Volume 1

Textbook of Perinatal Medicine

Dedication

This textbook is dedicated to the pioneers from throughout the world who created perinatal medicine

Volume 1

Textbook of Perinatal Medicine

Second Edition

Edited by

Asim Kurjak MD
Professor and Chairman
Department of Obstetrics and Gynecology
Medical School University of Zagreb
Croatia

and

Frank A. Chervenak MD
Given Foundation Professor and Chairman
Department of Obstetrics and Gynecology
Weill Medical College of Cornell University
New York Presbyterian Hospital
USA

informa
healthcare

First published in the United Kingdom in 1998
by The Parthenon Publishing Group Ltd

Second edition published in the United Kingdom in 2006 by Informa UK Ltd
4 Park Square, Milton Park, Abingdon, Oxon OX14 4RN. Informa Healthcare is a trading division of Informa UK Ltd. Registered Office: 37/41 Mortimer Street, London WIT 3JH. Registered in England and Wales Number 1072954.

Tel: +44 (0)20 7017 6000
Fax: +44 (0)20 7017 6699
E-mail: info.medicine@tandf.co.uk
Website: www.tandf.co.uk/medicine

A CIP record for this book is available from the British Library.

Library of Congress Cataloging-in-Publication Data
Data available on application

ISBN10 1 84214 333 6 (2-volume set)
ISBN13 978 1 84214 333 9

Distributed in North and South America by
Taylor & Francis
6000 Broken Sound Parkway, NW (Suite 300)
Boca Raton, FL 33487, USA

Within Continental USA
Tel: 1(800) 272 7737; Fax: 1(800) 374 3401
Outside Continental USA
Tel: (561) 994 0555; Fax: (561) 361 6018
E-mail: orders@crcpress.com

Distributed in the rest of the world by
Thomson Publishing Services
Cheriton House
North Way
Andover, Hampshire SP10 5BE, UK
Tel: +44 (0)1264 332424
E-mail: tps.tandfsalesorder@thomson.com

Composition by Keyword Group Ltd, Great Yarmouth, Norfolk, UK
Printed and bound in India by Replika Press Pvt. Ltd

Contents for Volume 1 and 2

List of principal contributors

A. Adra Department of Obstetrics & Gynecology, American University of Beirut Medical Center, Beirut, Lebanon

J. L. Alcázar Department Obstetrics & Gynecology, Clinica Universitaria de Navarra, Pamplona, Spain

Z. Alfirevic University Department of Obstetrics & Gynaecology, Liverpool Women's Hospital, Liverpool, UK

M. M. Anceschi Institute of Gynecology, Perinatology & Child Health, University of Rome "La Sapienza", Rome, Italy

A. Antsaklis Department of Fetal-Maternal Medicine, Alexandra Maternity Hospital, Athens, Greece

Z. Appelman Institute of Genetics, Kaplan Medical Center, Rehovot, Israel

B. Arabin Department of Perinatology, Isala Clinics, 8025 AB Zwolle, The Netherlands

J. Babnik Department of Obstetrics & Gynecology, University Medical Center, Ljubljana, Slovenia

J. M. Bajo Arenas Department of Obstetrics & Gynecology, Getafe University Hospital, Madrid, Spain

L. S. Bakketeig Department of Epidemiology, University of Southern Denmark, Odense, Denmark

R. Baraibar Department of Pediatrics, Institute Universitari Dexeus, Barcelona, Spain

Y. Baytur Celal Bayar University, Medical School, Department of Obstetrics and Gynecology, Manisa, Turkey

A. Beke First Department of Obstetrics & Gynecology, Semmelweis University Medical School, Budapest, Hungary

G. Benagiano Department of Gynecological Sciences, Perinatology & Child Care, University "la Sapienza", Rome, Italy

K. Benirschke University of California, San Diego, CA, USA

K. Biedermann Department of Obstetrics & Gynaecology, Kantonales Frauenspital Fontana Lürlibadstr. 118, CH-7000 Chur, Switzerland

D. J. Birnbach Department of Anesthesiology, University of Miami School of Medicine, Miami, Florida, USA

I. Blickstein Department of Obstetrics & Gynecology, Kaplan Medical Center, Rehovot, Israel

F. Bonilla-Musoles Department of Obstetrics & Gynecology, Valencia School of Medicine, Valencia, Spain

R. Bracci Institute of Preventive Pediatrics and Neonatology, University of Siena, Siena, Italy

B. Brambati Center of Prenatal Diagnosis, Milan, Italy

V. N. A. Breeveld-Dwarkasing Department of Pathobiology, Division of Veterinary Anatomy & Physiology, Faculty of Veterinary Medicine, Utrecht University, Utrecht, The Netherlands

B. Breyer University of Zagreb, Faculty of Electrical Engineering and Computing, Zagreb, Croatia

H. Budge Centre for Reproduction and Early Life, Institute of Clinical Research, University Hospital, Nottingham, UK

P. Buekens School of Public Health & Tropical Medicine, Tulane University, New Orleans, LA, USA

F. Carmona Institut Clinic de Ginecologis, Obstetricia i Neonatologia, Hospital Clinic-University of Barcelone, Catalonia, Spain

M. R. G. Carrapato Department of Paediatrics & Neonatology, Hospital de São Sebastiao, Santa Maria da Feira, Portugal

J. M. Carrera Fetal Medicine Service, Departamento de Obstetricia y Ginecologia, Instituto Universitario Dexeus, Barcelona, Spain

R. Chaoui Center for Prenatal Diagnosis & Human Genetics, Berlin, Germany

S. T. Chasen Weill College of Cornell University, New York, NY, USA

F. A. Chervenak The New York Presbyterian Hospital, Weill Medical College of Cornell University, NY, USA

S. Cicero Fetal Medicine Foundation, London, UK

W. R. Cohen Department Obstetrics & Gynecology, Weill Medical College of Cornell University, New York, NY, USA

C. Comas Prenatal Diagnosis Unit, Centro Gutenberg, Malaga, Spain

L. Cornette The Peter Congdon Neonatal Unit, Leeds General Infirmary, Leeds, UK

E. V. Cosmi Institute of Gynecology, Perinatology & Child Health, University of Rome "La Sapienza", Rome, Italy

L. de Crespigny Murdoch Children's Research Institute, Royal Children's Hospital, University of Melbourne, Victoria, Australia

A. Csaba First Department of Obstetrics & Gynecology, Semmelweis University Medical School, Baross, Budapest, Hungary

V. D'Addario Fetal Medicine Unit, Department Obstetrics & Gynecology, University of Bari, Italy

F. Daffos Département de Diagnostic Prénatal et de Foetologie, Institut de Puériculture de Paris, Paris, France

M. Dan Unit of Infectious Diseases, Wolfson Medical Center, Holon, Israel

J. E. Deaver Women's Health Research, Jamaica Hospital Medical Center, New York, NY, USA

R. Derom Association de Soutien a la Recherche Scientifique au Profit des Naissances Multiples, Destelbergen, Belgium

G. C. di Renzo Centre of Perinatal & Reproductive Medicine, University of Perugia, Perugia, Italy

E. Domenech Department Pediatrics, Faculty of Medicine of La Laguna, University Hospital of the Canary Islands, Tenerife, Spain

S. M. Donn Division of Neonatal-Perinatal Medicine, CS Mott Children's Hospital, University Michigan Health System, Ann Arbor, MI, USA

A. Drazancic Division of Neonatal-Perinatal Medicine, CS Mott Children's Hospital, University Michigan Health System, Ann Arbor, MI, USA

J. W. Dudenhausen Department Obstetrics, Charite Campus Virchow-Klinikum, Berlin, Germany

S. J. English The Peter Congdon Neonatal Unit, Clarendon Wing, Leeds General Infirmary, Leeds, UK

A. K. Ertan Department of Obstetrics & Gynecology, Saarland University Medical School, Homburg, Germany

J. Espinoza Perinatology Research Branch, National Institute of Child Health and Human Development, NIH, DHHS, Bethesda, Maryland and Department of Obstetrics and Gynecology, Wayne State University School of Medicine, Detroit, Michigan, USA

M. I. Evans Institute for Genetics, Mt Sinai School of Medicine, New York, NY, USA

E. Fabre Department of Obstetrics and Gynecology, Hospital Clinico Universitario, Avda. San Juan Bosco, 15, 50009 Zaragoza, Spain

S. J. Fasouliotis Department of Obstetrics & Gynecology, Hebrew University Ein-Kerem, Hadassah Medical Centre, Jerusalem, Israel

R. Floyd Department Obstetrics, Gynecology & Women's Health, University of Missouri-Columbia, School of Medicine, Columbia, Missouri, USA

M. Foley Department Obstetrics & Gynecology, National Maternity Hospital, Dublin, Ireland

J. A. Fortney Heilbrunn Department of Population and Family Health, Columbia University, New York 10032, USA

E. A. Friedman Obstetrics & Gynecology, Albert Einstein College of Medicine, New York, NY, USA

K. Fujimori Department of Obstetrics & Gynecology, School of Medicine, Fukushimas Medical University, Fukushima-City, Fukushima, Japan

K. Fukushima Department of Obstetrics & Gynecology, Graduate School of Medical Sciences, Kyushu University, Higashi-Ku, Fukuoka, Japan

K. Ghebremeskel Institute of Brain Chemistry and Human Nutrition, London Metropolitan University, London, UK

P. D. Gluckman National Research Centre for Growth and Development, Liggins Institute, University of Auckland, Auckland, New Zealand

F. Goffinet Research Epidemiology Unit for Perinatal & Women's Health, Port Royal Maternity Hospital, Paris, France

L. F. Goncalves Perinatology Research Branch, National Institute of Child Health and Human Development, NIH, DHHS, Bethesda, Maryland and Department of Obstetrics and Gynecology, Wayne State University School of Medicine, Detroit, Michigan, USA

C. Gordon Department of Rheumatology, City Hospital, Birmingham, UK

J. L. Graf Department of Pediatric Surgery, University of California, San Francisco, CA, USA

B. E. Grand Department of Fetal Medicine, Juan A. Fernández Hospital of Buenos Aires, Argentina

A. Grunebaum Weill Cornell Medical Center, New York, NY, USA

B. Hargitai First Department of Obstetrics & Gynecology, Semmelweis University Medical School, Baross, Budapest, Hungary

M. R. Harrison Department of Pediatric Surgery, University of California, CA, USA

L. Hellstrom-Westas Department of Pediatrics, University Hospital Lund, Lund, Sweden

J. Herczeg Teaching Hospital of the University of Szeged, Szeged, Hungary

P. Hilton Women's Services, Royal Victoria Infirmary, Newcastle upon Tyne, UK

W. Holzgreve Women's University Hospital Basel, Basel, Switzerland

H. Hopp Charity Clinic for Obstetics, Campus Benjamin Franklin, Berlin, Germany

T. Hosono Department of Medical Engineering, Osaka Electro-communication University, Shijo-nawate, Osaka, Japan

T. Ikeda Department of Obstetrics and Gynecology, Miyazaki Medical College, University of Miyazaki, Kihara, Kiyotake-Cho, Miyazaki, Japan

S. Iniesta Santa Cristina University Hospital, Universidad Autonoma de Madrid, Madrid, Spain

T. Kanzaki Kanzaki Lady's Clinic, Nishinomiya, Hyogo, Japan and Division Obstetrics & Gynecology, Osaka University, Osaka, Japan

I. Kassis Ichilov Hospital, University of Tel Aviv, Tel Aviv, Israel

T. Kawarabayashi Department of Obstetrics & Gynecology, School of Medicine, Fukuoka University, Fukuoka, Japan

A. Khurana The Ultrasound Laboratory, C 584 Defence Colony, New Delhi, India

T. Kimura Division of Obstetrics & Gynecology, Department of Specific Organ Regulation, Osaka University Graduate School of Medicine, Suita, Japan

D. A. Krantz NTD Laboratories Inc, East Meadow, NY, USA

I. Krause Department of Pediatrics, Schneider Children's Medical Center of Israel, Sackler School of Medicine, Tel Aviv University, Israel

S. Kupesic Department of Obstetrics & Gynecology, Zagreb University Medical School, Sveti Duh, Zagreb, Croatia

A. Kurjak Department of Obstetrics & Gynecology, University of Zagreb, Sveti Duh Hospital, Zagreb, Croatia

M. L. Kush University of Maryland School of Medicine, Department Obstetrics, Gynecology & Reproductive Sciences, Baltimore, MD, USA

H. J. Landy Division of Maternal-Fetal Medicine, Department Obstetrics & Gynecology, Georgetown University Hospital, Washington DC, USA

O. Lapaire Women's University Hospital Basel, Spitalstraae, Basel, Switzerland

M. Levene Department of Paediatrics, Leeds General Infirmary, Leeds, UK

L. Lewi Department Obstetrics & Gynecology, University Hospital Gasthuisberg, Leuven, Belgium

G. Lindmark Department of Women's and Children's Health, Uppsala University, Uppsala, Sweden

G. A. Little Dartmouth-Hitchcock Medical Center, Neonatology, Lebanon

J. A. Low Department of Obstetrics and Gynecology, Queen's University, Kingston, Ontario, Canada

R. Luzietti Centre of Perinatal & Reproductive Medicine, University of Perugia, Perugia, Italy

I. Z. MacKenzie Department of Obstetrics & Gynecolcogy, John Radcliffe Hospital, Oxford, UK

K. Maeda Department of Obstetrics and Gynecology, Tottori University, Nadamachi, Yonago, Japan

S. Maheshwari Department of Pediatric Cardiology, Narayana Hrudayalaya, Anekal Taluk, Bangalore, India

G. P. Mandruzzato Department Obstetrics & Gynecology, Istituto per l'Infanzia IRCCS "Burlo Garofolo", Trieste, Italy

T. Marton Department of Histopathology, Birmingham Women's Hospital, Edgbaston, Birmingham, UK

G. Maso Department Obstetrics & Gynecology, Istituto per l'Infanzia IRCCS "Burlo Garofolo", Trieste, Italy

A. Matias Department of Obstetrics & Gynecology, Faculty of Medicine, University Hospital of S Joao, Porto, Portugal

L. T. Mercé Assisted Reproduction Unit, International Ruber Hospital, Madrid, Spain

E. Merz Department of Obstetrics & Gynecology, Krankenhaus Nordwest, Frankfurt/Main, Germany

D. Miron Pediatric Department A, Ha'Emek Medical Center, Afula 18101, Israel

G. Monni Department of Obstetrics and Gynecology, Prenatal and Preimplantation Genetic Diagnosis, Fetal Therapy, Ospedale Microcitemico, Cagliari, Italy

N. Montenegro Department of Obstetrics & Gynecology, Faculty of Medicine, University Hospital of S Joao, Porto, Portugal

A. Morag Clinical Virology Unit, Hadassah University Hospitals, Jerusalem, Israel

C. Mortera Diagnostico Prenatal y Perinatal, Institut Dexeus, Cardio-Hemodinamica, Hospital Sant J de Deu, Barcelona, Spain

A. Mulic-Lutvica Department of Women's and Children's Health, Uppsala University, Uppsala, Sweden

Y. Murata Division of Obstetrics and Gynecology, Osaka University Graduate School of Medicine, Osaka, Japan

M. F. Murphy Department of Haematology, Oxford Radcliffe Hospitals NHS Trust, Oxford, UK

H. Nakano Department of Obstetrics & Gynecology, Graduate School of Medical Sciences, Kyushu University, Higashi-Ku, Fukuoka, Japan

L. J. Nelson Department of Philosophy, Santa Clara University, Santa Clara, CA, USA

C. Nelson-Piercy Department of Obstetrics, St Thomas's Hospital, London, UK

K. H. Nicolaides Fetal Medicine Foundation, London, UK

J. G. Nijhuis Department of Obstetrics, Academisch Ziekenhuis Maastricht, The Netherlands

J. Nizard Department of Obstetrics & Gynecology, Hôpital de Poissy-Saint-Germain en Laye, Poissy, France

Z. Novak-Antolic Department of Obstetrics & Gynecology, University Medical Center, Ljubljana, Slovenia

K. Olshtain-Pops Department of Clinical Microbiology & Infectious Diseases, Hadassah University Hospital, Jerusalem, Israel

K. Ozono Division of Obstetrics & Gynecology, Department of Specific Organ Regulation, Osaka University Graduate School of Medicine, Suita, Osaka, Japan

K. M. Paarlberg Department of Obstetrics & Gynecology, University Hospital Vrije Universiteit, Amsterdam, The Netherlands

M. Pajntar Department of Obstetrics & Gynecology, University Medical Center, Ljubljana, Slovenia

E. Papiernik University Rene Descartes, Maternite de Port Royal, Hopital Cochin, Paris, France

C. Paul Department of Obstetrics & Gynecology, King's College Hospital, Denmark Hill, London, UK

L. Pereira Maternal Fetal Medicine, Oregon Health & Science University, Portland, OR, USA

P. O. D. Pharoah FSID Unit of Perinatal and Paediatric Epidemiology, Department of Public Health, University of Liverpool, Liverpool, UK

T. Podymow Division of Nephrology & Hypertension, Weill Medical College of Cornell University, New York, NY, USA

R. K. Pooh Center for Maternal, Fetal & Neonatal Medicine, Kagawa National Children's Hospital, Zentsuji City, Kagawa, Japan

P. Prats Prenatal Diagnosis Unit, Department of Obstetrics and Gynaecology, Institut Universitari Dexeus, Barcelona, Spain

E. Quarello Department of Obstetrics and Gynecology, CHI Poissy St Germain, Universite Paris-Ouest, Poissy, France

E. J. Quilligan University California Irvine, Long Beach Memorial Hospital, Long Beach, CA, USA

R. Romero Perinatology Research Branch, National Institute of Child Health and Human Development, NIH, DHHS, Bethesda, MD, USA

G. Rosner Genetic Institute, Tel Aviv Sourasky Medical Center, Israel

P. Rozenberg Department of Obstetrics & Gynecology, Poissy-Saint Germain Hospital, Versailles-Saint Quentin University, Poissy Cedex, France

F. F. Rubaltelli Department of Neonatology, Ospedale Careggi Reparto, Florence, Italy

E. Rubinstein Section of Infectious Diseases, University of Manitoba, Winnipeg, MB, Canada

R. M. Sabatel López Department Obstetrics & Gynecology, University of Grenada, Spain

N. Sagawa Department of Obstetrics & Gynecology, Mie University Graduate School of Medicine, Tsu, Mie, Japan

S. Saito Department Obstetrics & Gynecology, Toyama Medical & Pharmaceutical University, Toyama-shi, Toyama, Japan

S. Sakamoto Toyko, Aiiku Maternal & Child Health Center, Boshi Aiiku-kai,, Minato-ku, Japan

E. Z. Saling Institut für Perinatale Medizin, Berlin, Germany

O. D. Saugstad Department of Pediatric Research, The National Hospital, Oslo, Norway

J. G. Schenker Department of Obstetrics & Gynecology, Hadassah University Hospital, Jerusalem, Israel

S. Scherjon Department of Obstetrics, LUMC, Leiden, The Netherlands

B. S. Schifrin Department of Obstetrics & Gynecology, Loma Linda University School of Medicine, Loma Linda, CA, USA

Y. Schlesinger Division of Infectious Diseases, Shaare Zedek Medical Center, Jerusalem 91031, Israel

J. J. Sciarra Department of Obstetrics and Gynecology, Northwestern University Medical School Chicago, IL, USA

N. J. Sebire Department of Histopathology, Camelia Botnar Laboratories, Great Ormond Street Hospital, London, UK

C. Sen Department of Obstetrics & Gynecology, Cerrahpasa Medical School, Istanbul, Turkey

M. Seoud Department of Obstetrics & Gynecology, American University of Beirut Medical Center, Beirut, Lebanon

B. Serra Departamento de Obstetricia y Ginecologia, Instituto Universitario Dexeus, Barcelona, Spain

F. Sethna Fetal Medicine Unit, Department Obstetrics & Gynecology, St George's Hospital NHS Trust, London, UK

M. Shapiro Department of Clinical Microbiology and Infectious Diseases, Hadassah University Hospital, Jerusalem 91120, Israel

N. Shinozuka Department of Obstetrics & Gynecology, Faculty of Medicine, Teikyo University, Japan

D. W. Skupski Division of Maternal-Fetal Medicine, New York Hospital Queens, Flushing, New York, NY, USA

D. T. Spira Department of Parasitology, Hebrew Univ, Hadassah Med School, Jerusalem, Israel

Z. Stembera WHO Collaborating Center for Perinatal Medicine and Human Reproduction, Institute for the Care of Mother and Child, Podolske Nabrezi 157m 147 10 Praha 4, Czech Republic

G. M. Stirrat Centre for Ethics in Medicine, University of Bristol, Bristol, UK

K. N. S. Subramanian Georgetown University Hospital, Washington DC, USA

G. Sylvestre The New York Presbyterian Hospital, Weill Medical College of Cornell University, New York, NY, USA

A. Tabor Copenhagen University Hospital, Department of Obstetrics & Gynaecology, Hvidovre Hospital, Hvidovre, Denmark

H. A. Tanriverdi Department Obstetrics & Gynecology, Karaelmas University Medical School, Kozlu / Zonguldak, Turkey

S. Tercanli University Women's Hospital, Basel, Switzerland

J. M. Thomas National Collaborating Centre for Women and Children's Health, London, UK

J. M. Troyano Division of US & Fetal Medicine, University Hospital of the Canary Islands, La Laguna, Tenerife, Spain

K. Tsukimori Department of Obstetrics & Gynecology, Graduate School of Medical Sciences, Kyushu University, Higashi-Ku, Fukuoka, Japan

F. A. van Assche Department of Gynecology, Catholic University of Leuven, Leuven, Belgium

P. P. van den Berg Department of Obstetrics and Gynecology, University Hospital Nijmegen, Nijmegen, The Netherlands

J. van Eyck Department of Perinatology, Isala Clinics, Zwolle, The Netherlands

H. P. van Geijn Department Obstetrics & Gynecology, University Hospital Vrije Universiteit, Amsterdam, The Netherlands

W. J. van Wijngaarden Department of Obstetrics and Gynaecology, Ziekenhuis Bronovo, Den Haag, The Netherlands

Y. Ville Department of Obstetrics & Gynecology, Poissy-Saint Germain Hospital, Versailles-Saint Quentin University, Poissy Cedex, France

L. S. Voto Fundacion Miguel Margulies, Buenos Aires, Argentina

N. Wake Department of Molecular Genetics, Medical Institute of Bioregulation, Kyushu University, Beppu, Oita, Japan

J. Walker Department of Obstetrics & Gynecology, St James University Hospital, Leeds, UK

C. P. Weiner Department Obstetrics, Gynecology & Reproductive Sciences, University of Maryland School of Medicine, Baltimore, MD, USA

S. Weiner Department of Obstetrics & Gynecology, Thomas Jefferson College of Medicine, Philadelphia, PA, USA

D. J. Williams Institute of Women's Health, University College London, Elizabeth Garrett Anderson Obstetric Hospital, London, UK

M. S. Wingate Department Maternal & Child Health, University of Alabama at Birmingham, Birmingham, Alabama, USA

D. C. Wood Jr Fetal Cardiology, Maternal Fetal Medicine, Department of Obstetrics and Gynecology Thomas Jefferson University, Philadelphia, Pennsylvania, USA

H. N. Winn Department of Obstetrics, Gynecology and Women's Health, University of Missouri-Columbia School of Medicine, Columbia, MI, USA

Y. Yaron Prenatal Genetic Diagnosis Division, Genetic Institute, Tel Aviv Sourasky Medical Center, Tel Aviv, Israel

L. Yeo Department of Obstetrics, Gynecology & Reproductive Sciences, Division of Maternal Fetal Medicine, UMDNJ – Robert Wood Johnson Medical School, New Brunswick, NJ, USA

K. A. Yunis Department of Pediatrics, American University of Beirut Medical Center, Beirut, Lebanon

P. Zalloua Department of Obstetrics & Gynecology, American University of Beirut Medical Center, Beirut, Lebanon

M. A. Zoppi Department of Obstetrics and Gynecology, Prenatal and Preimplantation Genetic Diagnosis, Fetal Therapy, Ospedale Microcitemico, Cagliari, Italy

Foreword

Perinatal medicine is among the most challenging and beautiful areas of study and practice. It deals with events before birth, when the fetus is a patient and during the immediate neonatal period. The World Association of Perinatal Medicine is dedicated to the study of all aspects of perinatal biology, physiology, screening, diagnosis, management and ethics, with the goal of continuous quality improvement in the care of maternal, fetal and neonatal patients.

This textbook is based on a previous work that was produced by the European Association of Perinatal Medicine in 1998. Because perinatal medicine is now a global area of study, it is appropriate that the current textbook is a product of the World Association of Perinatal Medicine. The bonds that link perinatologists together transcend geographic, political, religious and lingual differences, resulting in a globalization that optimizes clinical care.

This textbook consists of over 200 chapters divided into 20 sections, which span the depth and breadth of the field. Beginning with the history of perinatal medicine and ending with the challenges facing this specialty in developing countries, this book is a comprehensive text designed to provide insight and guidance to clinicians throughout the world with state of the art information, written by the world's leading perinatologists.

We are grateful to the authors of the 205 chapters and the editors of the 20 sections, who have worked so diligently with us to produce this textbook, which we believe bears testament to the importance and success of international collaboration in perinatal medicine.

Asim Kurjak
Frank A. Chervenak

Introduction

1 Birth and youth of prenatal and perinatal obstetrics*

E. Z. Saling

Introduction

Singular observations of the infant in the prenatal period, as well as the first elementary attempts at diagnostics and therapy, stretch back over generations, centuries and up to thousands of years. However, until the beginning of the 1960s, the only possible method of clinical 'assessment' of the intrauterine patient, apart from the fetal movements observed by the mother herself, was auscultation of the fetal heart beats with a simple stethoscope. The following statement made in 1966 by two English pediatricians Dobbs and Gairdner in an editorial in *Archives of Disease in Childhood* aptly sums up the situation:

> Up to now the formidable inaccessibility of the human foetus has meant that foetal medicine (apart perhaps from foetal electrocardiography [author's note: which was in a basic experimental state and should not be mistaken for cardiotocography.]) has virtually not existed. In an age when man has been able to measure most things from an atom to a galaxy, it is thus paradoxical that to measure his own size during the most critical and precarious period of his life, he still has to depend upon the extreme fallibility of the palpating hand.

Thus, today we can draw the following conclusion: systematic exploration of the intrauterine space during pregnancy and labor did not start until the 1960s. This, therefore, can be considered the beginning of prenatal medicine and the related clinical subspecialty 'prenatal and perinatal obstetrics'.

According to Dobbs and Gairdner, four innovative techniques brought about the real breakthrough. They stated:

> With the advent of the techniques of amnioscopy and foetal blood sampling and of amniocentesis and foetal transfusion, we witness the end of the long period of foetal inaccessibility, and we hopefully believe the start of the science of foetal medicine.[1]

Amniocentesis and fetal transfusion

As far as we have been able to ascertain, the first report about amniocentesis appeared in 1881 by Lambl, as a means of decompressing a hydramnion.[2] In 1930, Meness *et al.* performed the first amniography.[3] Not until 70 years after Lambl's first amniocentesis was this technique used by Bevis in 1952 for diagnosing Rh erythroblastosis.[4] This was an important prerequisite for both spectrophotometric analysis of amniotic fluid[5] and the first trials involving the treatment of the preterm fetus with severe Rh disease,[6] developed by Liley in Australia. Liley is especially renowned for the development of his 'Liley Scheme', which has been used as a nomogram for bilirubin limits. With this method, clinicians were provided with information enabling them to decide whether the fetus should be treated by intra-abdominal blood transfusion or if the pregnancy should be terminated when the fetus was sufficiently mature, in order to perform an exchange transfusion immediately postpartum. Today, amniocentesis is one of the standard techniques used in various fields of prenatal obstetrics.

Intrauterine transfusion, developed by Liley in 1963,[6] was used in cases of severe Rh erythroblastosis. This measure is one of the very first milestones of prenatal obstetrics in so far as it was the first real breakthrough in intrauterine, i.e. fetal, therapy. The effectiveness of intrauterine transfusion can be explained by the fact that the fetus resorbs through its peritoneum the compatible donor blood that is injected into the peritoneal cavity. Gradually, the donor erythrocytes reach the fetal blood circulation via the ductus thoracicus.

*This chapter covers a period of limited time and has therefore been taken over unchanged from the first edition

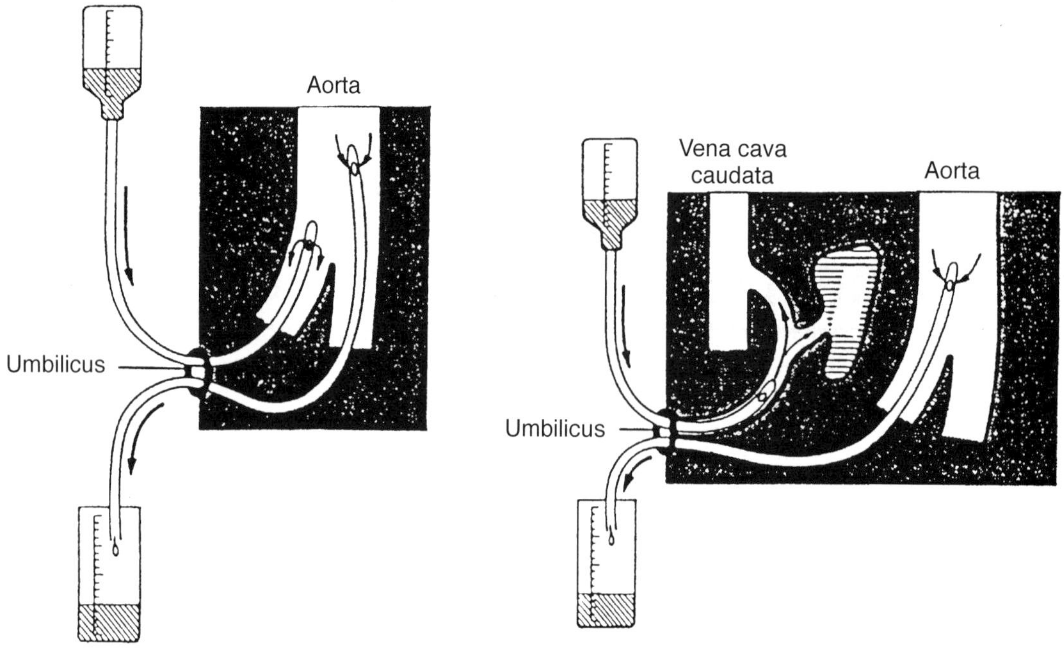

Figure I.1 Two options using the two-catheter technique for exchange transfusion in a newborn: infusion and simultaneous exfusion to and from the aorta (left) and infusion into the venous system and simultaneous exfusion from the aorta (right).

In the meantime intrauterine intraumbilical transfusions have been performed since 1986 mainly with the help of ultrasound[7] and even intracardial transfusions have been described.[8]

Fetal blood sampling

Of broader clinical importance, *fetal blood sampling during labor* – as a method of daily routine in the labor room – was the main step initiating the start of a completely new medicine, which up to that point was non-existent.

Before the introduction of fetal blood analysis (FBA), we were using other techniques, which, subsequently, brought us nearer this special new field. Several of the progressive steps described have been achieved by us as clinically engaged obstetricians. Today, these activities seem rather curious in so far as such efforts have belonged to the domain of neonatologists for some decades.

At the end of the 1950s we started examinations to determine the most effective method for resuscitation of an asphyxiated newborn immediately after delivery. At that time, the thorax compression methods, mouth-to-mouth respiration, intragastric O_2 insufflation and various other methods were still being used.[9] We came to the conclusion that most of these methods were not effective enough.[10] This motivated us to develop equipment for endotracheal O_2 respiration and we began to prove its efficiency. One component of the equipment was a laryngoscope for newborns, which, according to a recent recommendation in a textbook of anesthesiology,[11] is particularly suitable for the intubation of very small premature newborns.

An important development was that for the very first time we had been successful in catheterizing the aorta of the newborn immediately after delivery via the easily accessible umbilical arteries.[12] We used this method for a new two-catheter technique (Figure I.1) of exchange transfusion in erythroblastotic newborns[13] and, in addition, we withdrew samples for blood analysis from the central circulation of the asphyxiated newborn to prove the efficiency of the different techniques of resuscitation.[10] For these examinations, in cooperation with K. Damaschke, we developed a fast micromethod in order to determine the oxygen saturation in very small blood samples.[14]

A decisive step forward was the idea of *withdrawing fetal blood samples from the presenting part* of the fetus in cases of Rh erythroblastosis, thus enabling us to perform, before delivery, the most important serologic and hematologic examinations, such as the Coombs test, hemoglobin concentration, hematocrit and the blood group. This resulted in important progress in some cases of severe Rh erythroblastosis as it enabled us to begin exchange transfusions shortly – in six cases, 5–10 min – after delivery.[15]

The fast O_2 microanalysis, which had recently been developed, and the knowledge that blood samples could be taken so easily from the skin of the presenting part of the fetus provided us with the additional idea of performing fetal blood gas analyses. This was the birth of FBA. Almost at the same time, equipment for measuring pH in micro blood samples was developed and we were also able to examine fetal acid–base balance.

The first FBA *during labor with pH and O_2 saturation measurement* and *pCO_2 calculation* was performed on June 21, 1960. This was the first documented direct approach to the human fetus before birth.

Information on FBA was first published in the form of a report of a lecture presented at an official meeting of the Berlin Society of Obstetrics and Gynecology in 1961.[16] The first original article appeared in a journal in 1962.[17] In 1984, the latter publication became a so-called 'citation classic' of Current Contents after it had been identified by the Institute for Scientific Information in Philadelphia as one of the most cited items in its field.

Only a day later, on June 22, 1960, a blood sample for FBA was taken from the buttock of a fetus. In addition to the FBA during labor for the first time, for clinical purposes we performed an acidity measurement in blood from the umbilical artery and vein of this infant. Thus, the *complementary assessment of the newborn by also measuring the pH in umbilical vessels*, employed by many obstetricians today, was also created. The best routine assessment of the newborn immediately after delivery is achieved by the Apgar score for the basic clinical status, combined with our acidity values giving information about the biochemical status of the newly born baby. Historically, the two above-mentioned days were of special importance in the field of *combined examination of the acid–base balance in the fetus and neonate immediately after delivery*. The way in which we practiced the method can be seen in Figure I.2, in which the rubber stamp used in the labor room is described. The first publications describing the combined diagnosis of the newborns' condition, using the modified Apgar score as the clinical (physical) part and our acidity score as the biochemical part with the recommendation for routine clinical use, appeared in 1965[18] and 1966[19] in German as well as in 1968[20] and 1974[21] in English.

FBA received international attention through the activities of the Montevideo group. Joseph Bieniarz, a coworker of Roberto Caldeyro-Barcia for many years, with knowledge of the German language, undertook the task of reviewing German scientific literature. In this way, our first publication on FBA in 1962[17] and our studies published later in 1963[22] concerning normal fetal blood gas and acid–base values during labor, of which actual pH values (Figure I.3) were the most important, aroused particular interest in Montevideo. In 1964, Roberto Caldeyro-Barcia, who unfortunately passed away on November 2, 1996, organized a historic meeting. The invited guests were Stanley James, Edward Hon, Fred Kubli and myself. A photograph of the main participants and a short report on this international symposium can be found in the Editor's Preface in the first issue of the *Journal of Perinatal Medicine*.[23] After this meeting, FBA also attracted attention in North America and was introduced step by step in many places, its importance becoming accepted clinically and for research purposes.

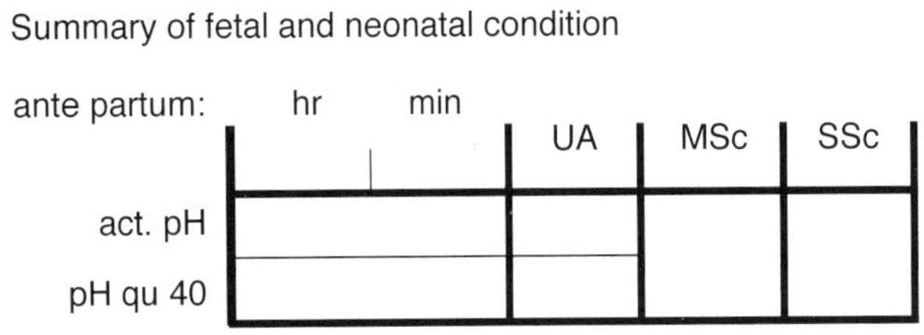

Figure I.2 Rubber stamp for summary of all results obtained concerning fetal and neonatal assessment.[19,20] In the first column the time in hours and minutes, actual pH and pH qu 40 (pH after equilibration of a blood sample with 40 mmHg pCO_2; this pH expresses the metabolic acidity and can directly be compared with actual pH values) of the lowest fetal blood pH measured during labor are recorded and in the second column (UA), the umbilical arterial actual pH and pH qu 40 immediately after delivery. The points achieved in our main score (MSc), a modified Apgar score, and in a subsidiary scoring system (SSc) are recorded in the left and right hand boxes, respectively. The subsidiary score contains the timed first breath, the first cry, the regular respiration and pink flash after delivery and is more objective and more reliable than the Apgar score.

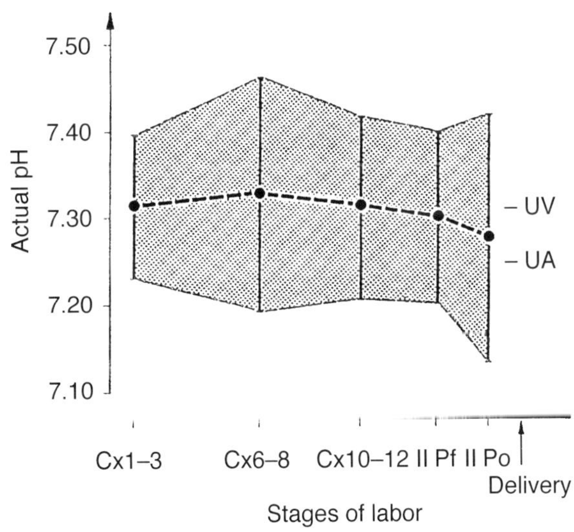

Figure I.3 Actual pH values of fetal scalp blood samples and of blood from umbilical vessels during different stages of normal labor ($x \pm 2$ s). Cx, cervix dilatation (cm); II, second stage; Pf, presenting part on pelvic floor; Po, on pelvic outlet.[18–20]

Amnioscopy

Another procedure that was developed at the beginning of the 1960s and which immediately became widespread is *amnioscopy*, a report on which was first published by us in 1962.[24] This procedure is based on the fact that hypoxic risks to the fetus in late pregnancy progress very slowly in most cases and that in more than 99% of these fetuses, passage of meconium actually occurs, which can then be detected amnioscopically (see below). A further advantage of amnioscopy is that amniotic fluid remains green for several days, and therefore it can safely be diagnosed by amnioscopic checks at intervals of 48 h. Amnioscopy continues to

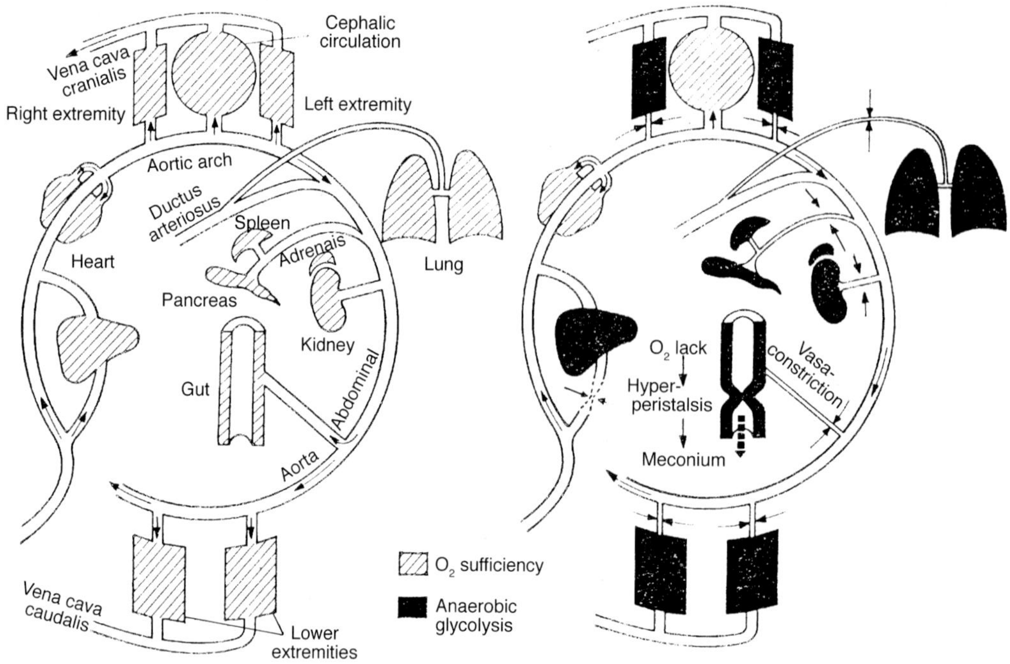

Figure I.4 Our first concept of the oxygen-conserving-adaptation of the fetal circulation.[26,27] Left: Normal arterial supply, with full oxygenation, to heart, brain and all other parts. Right: Reduction of oxygen supply leading to vasoconstriction in the extremities, abdominal viscera and lungs. Local hypoxemia leads to anaerobic glycolysis.

enjoy widespread popularity, particularly in countries with limited financial resources, because it is simple to use and does not require a great deal of equipment and takes only a short time. Furthermore, amnioscopy, as already mentioned, is very reliable in its early selection of fetuses at chronically advanced hypoxic risk. The method fails if a fetus with amnioscopically clear amniotic fluid, i.e. no passage of meconium, should die. This happened only eight times in more than 12,000 supervised high-risk pregnancies, i.e. only 0.6/1000.[25]

Some pathophysiological backgrounds that gave amnioscopy such a high diagnostic reliability are based on common circulatory reactions special to the fetus and can be explained by the concept we developed in 1966, namely, the *O_2-conserving adaptation of the fetal circulation*.[26,27]

This concept, now more than 30 years old, represents the basic principle for the Doppler diagnostics used today (Figure I.4). Our explanation in the 1960s was that the borderline oxygenated fetus reduces its O_2 consumption by restricted circulation of those organs that are not of vital importance and increases, relatively, the circulation in the vital organs such as brain and heart. Reduction of different areas of circulation has been found by Dawes in many animal experimental studies.[28,29] According to our concept, the intestinal organs are also affected, where the intestine reacts with hyperperistalsis. As a result, there will be a passage of meconium with high certainty during the last 4–6 weeks before the date of birth, which can be easily detected via amnioscopy.

The results of Doppler ultrasound investigations initially achieved by Arabin *et al.* in our Institute as early as 1987[30] provided an interesting new confirmation of our O_2-conserving adaptation concept, at this time already 20 years old. In severely growth-retarded fetuses even when a loss of enddiastolic blood flow velocities had already occurred in the umbilical artery and in the fetal aorta, there was an increase in the end-diastolic flow in the common carotid artery. Since then many further confirmations have been published in the same direction.

Many years after our publications the new term 'brain sparing effect' appeared in the Anglo-American literature. This was certainly regrettable as the colleagues who created this new term and 'rediscovered' the known principle overlooked two decisive facts:

(1) There was already a more appropriate term, which had been in existence for many years, without the necessity of formulating a new one.
(2) The new term, as far as it went, was incorrect since the pathophysiological situation concerned contains not only a 'brain sparing' but also a 'heart sparing' effect and possibly also sparing effects on other organs, for instance, the adrenals.

Some of the following comments about 'birth and youth of pre- and perinatal obstetrics' are mainly based on our previous report about 'historic landmarks of perinatal medicine in obstetrics'.[31]

Cardiotocography

In 1968, 8 years after FBA was introduced, *cardiotocography* also became available for clinical use. Cardiotocography is one of the important landmarks in prenatal obstetrics. Historic steps lead back to Pestalozzi, who in 1891 recorded the heartbeats of a twin in breech presentation with a sphygmograph[32] and also Hofbauer and Weiss, who recorded the first phonocardiogram in the year 1908.[33] Cremer was successful in designing the first electrocardiogram in 1906.[34] The first continuous cardiotachogram, conducted from an anencephalic fetus, was described by Caldeyro-Barcia and coworkers in 1958.[35] The electrode was inserted into the rump of the fetus through the abdominal wall of the mother, using the harpoon principle. The same principle was successfully used by Rech in 1931 in animal experiments.[36]

In 1966, with his 'one-poled' silver–silver chloride electrode (CLIP electrode), that could be inserted vaginally, Hon introduced direct fetal electrocardiotocography during labor.[37] An electrode is fixed on the fetal head; a second counter-electrode lies in the vagina where it is in contact with the mother. The spiral electrodes most widely used were developed by Junge in 1967.[38] All these recordings of the fetal heart rate, combined with the recording of the intrauterine contractions, pioneered by Caldeyro-Barcia and Hon, required the use of very complicated equipment and could, therefore, only serve experimental and scientific considerations. The real breakthrough leading to practical clinical usage came in the mid-1960s, when Hammacher, in cooperation with Hewlett and Packard, was successful in developing the cardiotocograph (CTG), which is still known by the same name today. The equipment was based on the phonocardiographic principle and enabled the elimination of all disturbing noises by electronically controlled comparisons of the time interval between two successive first heartbeats and two successive second heartbeats.[39] In this way it was possible to achieve reliable, specific registrations of the fetal heart rate. The first prototype of the equipment for routine use was tested by Hammacher in Düsseldorf in 1966. Widespread clinical usage started in 1968. The first systematic comparisons between pathological cardiotocograms and the acid–base balance of the fetus were published by us in 1968.[40] Doppler ultrasound cardiotocography found widespread popularity in the 1970s due to the simplicity of applying the wide-angled transducer operating on the abdominal wall of the mother. However, due to the considerable deviations from the real beat-to-beat variability that sometimes occurred, it was heavily criticized. It was not until the beginning of the 1980s that ultrasound cardiotocography was accepted in expert circles; this happened after the industry – namely the Toitu company in Japan – employed the so-called 'auto-correlation principle' in 1977, which made a recording available that was much more in accordance with the beat-to-beat variability.

From the very beginning we have warned against using cardiotocography as a single method and we introduced the combined fetal monitoring during labor for the first time by recommending the use of both methods – CTG routinely and, if indicated (abnormal CTG), additionally FBA. This was, already in 1968, the *start of combined electronic and biochemical monitoring* of the fetus.[40] This kind of monitoring remains the safest and most efficient way of supervision of the fetus during labor, provided it is used clinically according to our experience and to the recommended strategy. In the meantime a great number of papers have been published in which FBA formed either solely or partly the subject matter. We also contributed and tried to explain further basic aspects, additional clinical findings and recommendations as well as criticisms about misuse of modern fetal monitoring during labor.[41–46]

In connection with such a critical statement we once gave a humorous, less scientific but impressive and illustrative description of the advantages and disadvantages of cardiotocography in simple terms.[44] For this purpose we took an example from nature:

The cardiotocogram situation can be compared with the screaming of monkeys in the jungle: when danger is imminent they always scream. When there is a threat of hypoxia, the CTG is almost always suspicious or pathological. But monkeys have the typical attribute of screaming much too often; especially when there is no danger at all. The CTG often does this too, in the figurative sense. It is suspicious or pathological, but there are no real reasons to suspect dangerous fetal hypoxia – as measurements of the acid–base balance can clearly prove. This is unfortunately the reverse side of cardiotocography which many obstetricians either fail to recognize or push aside with naive credulity. If the newborn are vigorous after operative delivery – as regards their acidity and clinical state – then many colleagues excuse their management by saying that a hypoxia had just been avoided by well-timed intervention. Anyone who performs FBA, can give enough examples how often such excuses are self deception or a misguidance to the patient.

Unfortunately, too many clinicians and investigators did not follow the recommendations we had expressed from the very beginning, namely not to use cardiotocography as a single method to supervise the fetus but to combine it with FBA when an abnormal heart rate pattern appears. The adverse effects of the last 30 years are well known. They range from the polemic public discussions about fetal monitoring to recent debate about the rare intrapartum origin of cerebral palsy. We think most of such negative consequences could have been avoided with the use of combined electronic–biochemical supervision. So, for instance, the argument that false estimation of 'modern monitoring' was the main reason for the wrong conclusion, that cerebral palsy was so often caused by malpractice of obstetricians in the labor ward, is not correct from our point of view. This misleading assumption would never have been made if combined supervision of the fetus during labor (CTG plus FBA) – which has now been available for almost three decades – had always been correctly used everywhere as a standard method in routine practice, for the pathogenetic contradiction (cerebral palsy without proven hypoxia) would then have been obviously recognized at the very beginning and not now after almost 30 years.

Ultrasound scanning

Without doubt, one of the most important landmarks of prenatal obstetrics is *ultrasonic diagnostics.* It not only serves to supplement the typical attribute of the obstetrician's acknowledged palpatory skill, but in many respects competes with it as an instrument of equal or superior capability.

The 'father' of obstetrical and gynecological ultrasonic diagnostics is Ian Donald. Donald *et al.* in 1958 published the first scans of fetuses aged 14 gestational weeks.[47] Donald and Brown published pictures of a hydatid mole, a hydrocephalus and the first prenatal measurements of the biparietal diameter with the help of the A-mode procedure in 1961.[48] This was the beginning of fetal biometry and the diagnosis of gestational age later improved by measuring the crown–rump length. Sonographic placental diagnostics began when Gottesfeld demonstrated cross-sectional pictures of the placenta.[49,50] Important steps forward were made in the diagnosing of malformations through the progress achieved in ultrasonic techniques and by the detailed presentation of fetal organs, particularly with the gray-scale technique developed by Kossoff *et al.*[51]

Sonographic vitality diagnostics started with the first registration of fetal movements in the 7th week of gestation by Donald,[52] and also with the first registration of fetal heart movements with the help of the Doppler procedure performed by Callaghan *et al.* in 1964.[53] In 1967, Kratochwil and Eisenhut reported on evidence of fetal heart actions in the 6th week of gestation with the help of the A-mode procedure.[54] In 1973, Reinold reported on qualitatively different movement patterns of the fetus and their prognostic value.[55] In 1971, before real-time ultrasound had been developed, Boddy and Robinson gave proof of fetal thorax movements with the help of an A-scan.[56]

Stimulated by studies resulting from animal experiments by Dawes,[29] numerous systematic investigations of fetal breathing movements, among others by Gennser,[57] were undertaken with the help of real-time procedure. Studies on the complex behavioral pattern of the fetus in early pregnancy were published by De Vries *et al.*[58] and on behavioral states in advanced pregnancy by Nijhuis et al.[59]

Blood flow measurements using the ultrasound Doppler technique are a new landmark in prenatal supervision. With the help of this technique it was possible to make non-invasive measurements of the uterine and fetal blood flow, which allow conclusions to be drawn concerning the placental hemodynamics. The first report on the use of the Doppler technique for examining fetal blood flow in the umbilical artery was published in 1977 by Fitzgerald and Drumm.[60] Studies followed on the first measurements in the umbilical vein, by Gill,[61] and on measurements of blood flow in the fetal aorta, by Eik-Nes *et al.*[62] Campbell *et al.* presented a new important contribution in 1983 enabling us to measure the uteroplacental flow.[63]

Tocolysis

Another step forward during the 'youth era' was the application of betamimetics to inhibit contractions. The now classical term *tocolysis* was introduced by Mosler in 1964.[64] The use of tocolytics for prevention of prematurity is now obsolete as prematurity is caused mostly by ascending infection. At the present time, the real task of tocolytic substances applied antepartum is to postpone premature labor for a short period of a few days to perform lung maturity treatment of the highly endangered premature fetus.

There is no controversy as to the advantage of using betamimetics during labor for intrauterine resuscitation. The first clinical applications were undertaken in 1969 by the Galdeyro-Barcia group[65] and shortly afterward by Gamissans *et al.*[66] and Esteban-Altirriba *et al.*[67] It has been confirmed that acute hypoxic complications in the fetus can be relieved by the administration of a relatively high dose of bolus injection or an infusion to the mother. The use of tocolysis during labor has also proved to be of clinical value in cases with hypertonic or hyperactive uterine dysfunction. Tocolysis has also led to considerable improvements in the *external version* of the fetus from breech to vertex presentation. Unnecessary cesarean sections can be avoided using this method and a number of infants are spared the risk of vaginal breech delivery. We performed an external version near term under tocolysis for the first time in 1974, published in 1975.[68] The method, when properly applied, does not provide any serious risk to the fetus. Up to now, no infant has died as a result of the use of this method in over 2000 versions performed in our department.

Cervical ripening

Further progress in modern obstetrics was achieved by the introduction of *cervical ripening* by prostaglandin application into routine practice by Calder in 1975,[69] after Lippert had developed the prostaglandin gel principle in 1973 in this country for use in artificial abortion.[70] By means of general local administration (extra-amnially, intracervically, intravaginally) of prostaglandin E, numerous operative deliveries can be avoided in cases with an unripe cervix.

Lung maturation diagnostics

The clinical picture of 'respiratory distress syndrome' was first described by Hochheim in 1903.[71] In 1947, Gruenwald suggested that there was linkage with the surface tension in the lungs.[72] Clements called the postulated component reducing the surface tension 'pulmonary surfactant' and discussed its central importance as an antiatelectasis factor in 1956.[73] In 1959, for the first time, Avery and Mead suggested a relation between low surface activity and the occurrence of respiratory distress syndrome.[74] Graven reported in 1968 on the determination of phospholipids in human and monkey amniotic fluid and assumed an association between a low concentration of phospholipids and the probability of respiratory distress syndrome developing.[75] Gluck *et al.* were able to prove a close relation between the phospholipid content of the amniotic fluid and fetal lung maturity. They started their work in 1968 and in 1971, published the most often cited study on this particular subject.[76]

Lung maturation therapy

Neonatal morbidity and mortality have been decreasing during the past decades. The reasons for this are:

(1) There has been improvement in neonatal intensive care, particularly in artificial respiration techniques and application of surfactants.
(2) The widespread use of tocolytic substances has enabled us to delay premature delivery until lung maturation can be improved with the aid of various drugs. The glucocorticoids hold the leading position in this group.

In 1968, Buckingham *et al.* developed the hypothesis that glucocorticoids promote fetal lung maturation – on account of the stimulation of alkaline phosphatase proved in experiments on animals.[77] Liggins supported this hypothesis in 1969 with his observations during artificial induction of labor: the lungs of prematurely induced lambs that had been given glucocorticoids were clearly more mature than the lungs of lambs of the same gestational age that had not been treated in this way. He postulated, after this chance observation, that glucocorticoids bring about an acceleration in the formation of surface-active substances in the lung via enzyme induction.[78]

In 1972 Liggins and Howie, in their epochal prospective study, were able to transfer the experience achieved in animal experiments to human beings.[79] The occurrence of respiratory distress syndrome after antepartum administration of betamethasone to the mother could be reduced from 24% to 4.3% compared to the control group, who received no therapy. According to Liggins and Howie, the preventive effect of betamethasone is all the more efficient the lower the gestational age (26–32 weeks).

General discussion and conclusions

The last part of this contribution is directed to further historical facts, to some general views and to structural consequences. Basically, some points should be taken into consideration when describing the history of this new 'prenatal medicine' or 'prenatal obstetrics' as a whole. We believe that such a recapitulation is of importance as our mainly foreign colleagues, particularly the younger ones, no longer seem to be aware how, where and when this new medicine started.

The *foundation of scientific associations* concerned with this speciality developed accordingly. In 1967, the first national society, the German Society of Perinatal Medicine, was founded. One year later (1968), in Berlin, we started the first international society, the European Association of Perinatal Medicine.

The term 'perinatal' instead of 'prenatal' in the German and European societies has been chosen because, from the very beginning, we wanted to achieve close cooperation with neonatologists. In fact, it mainly concerned and represented the medical progress that prevailed in the prenatal area and was, for instance, reflected in 80–90% of topics of prenatal medicine at nearly all German congresses in this field, each of which attracted more than 2000 participants.

The Society of Perinatal Obstetricians in America was founded in 1977 and represents one of the most dynamic national societies in the world at the present time.

During our lifetime not only has outer space been opened up in such a spectacular fashion, but also on a biological level an equally important development has started rolling and has still by no means come to a halt; I mean the medical exploration of our own 'intrauterine space', our 'prenatal cradle'. Very few people are aware of this fact.

A disastrous conclusion drawn by many influential colleagues in our country and also in many other places was to think from the beginning that we were dealing with a special narrow and limited field – a field of medicine of particular interest to only a few colleagues and practiced mainly by the younger ones from time to time. And so it was thought, based on the conventional all-round structure of obstetrics and gynecology as a whole and according to the *status quo ante*, that all these revolutionary events could be taken into consideration and the rotation principle could still be maintained. The consequences of this grave error of judgment continue, even today, to give cause for concern to a wide extent in some parts of Europe.

Realization of structural consequences began at an appropriately early stage in the United States. The setting up of 'Units of Maternal–Fetal Medicine', begun in 1972, made successful the consequent use of the prenatal part of perinatal medicine within the framework of the complete field of obstetrics and gynecology.

The term 'fetal medicine', which is still used today in the form of 'maternal–fetal medicine', had probably not been considered enough when it was introduced at the very beginning for clinical purposes. Unfortunately, it does not include the embryonic period, which also belongs to our clinical competence. The consequence is that other subspecialties have been more aware of this and are using this term, for example, in the name of their society, namely, European Society of Human Reproduction and Embryology. We, therefore, prefer the general term 'prenatal medicine', which some colleagues use erroneously for only a special subordinated field, mainly for diagnostics of anomalies and some special therapeutic procedures in early pregnancy. As an alternative, the term 'pre- and perinatal obstetrics' would be appropriate, if preferred.

On the basis of the enormous progress already achieved in 1967, we recommended a structural reform of the discipline in our country and the setting up of units of modern obstetrics and prenatal medicine.[80] However, up to now many European university departments, particularly in our country, do not have such units. The consequences are depressing as regards highly qualified research activities and our international image. Due to the lack of the necessary requirements, not enough interested colleagues could remain working in this field for a longer period to become adequately specialized and to obtain appropriate career chances. Consequently, some of the European countries concerned have only a few internationally reputed 'perinatal obstetricians'.

The birth and youth of prenatal obstetrics and perinatal medicine were to a large extent a product of European clinicians and scientists, although many impulses in numerous fields of medicine since the Second World War have come from abroad, particularly from North America. It is therefore particularly commendable that the European Association of Perinatal Medicine again took up the initiative and, under the leadership of such a powerful and outstanding colleague as Asim Kurjak together with the participation of so many renowned experts, is publishing an extensive current review about our great field of perinatal medicine.

These great steps forward have by no means come to a halt, as many opposed to this direction of development have been artlessly suggesting for years. It would be most improbable if a practically newly opened extensive area – as represented by the intrauterine space up to the beginning of the 1960s – should be fully explored medically within only 38 years. The work will certainly go on and perhaps when the next generation period is over, several of the modern achievements, of which we are so proud today, may be regarded as obsolete. New pioneers will take over our role then, and the next generation will again continue this course of medical science and course of life.

REFERENCES

1. Dobbs RH, Gairdner D. Foetal medicine: Who is to practice it? *Arch Dis Child* 1966;41:453.
2. Lambl D. Ein seltener Fall von Hydramnion. *Zentralbl Gynäkol* 1881;14:14.
3. Meness TO, Miller JE, Holly LE. Amniography. *Am J Roentgenol* 1930;2:363.
4. Bevis DCA. Antenatal prediction of haemolytic disease of the newborn. *Lancet* 1952;I:395.
5. Liley AW. Liquor amnii analysis in the management of the pregnancy complicated by rhesus sensitization. *Am J Obstet Gynecol* 1961;82:1359.
6. Liley AW. Intrauterine transfusion of fetus in haemolytic disease. *Br Med J* 1963;ii:1107.
7. Berkowitz RL, Chitkara U, GoldbergJD, *et al.* Intravascular transfusion *in utero*: The percutaneous approach. *Am J Obstet Gynecol* 1986;154:622.
8. Hansmann M, Bald R, Gembruch U. Ultraschall-kontrollierte intrauterine Transfusion - intravasal-intrakardial, mit Austausch? *Ultraschall in Klinik und Praxis* 1986;Suppl 1:68.
9. Saling E. Zur Frage der optimalen Behandlung des scheintoten Neugeborenen. *Geburtshilfe Frauenheilkd* 1958;18:128.
10. Saling E. Über die Wirksamkeit von alteren und neuen Asphyxiebehandlungsmethoden. *Geburtshilfe Frauenheilkd* 1960;20:325.
11. Strauss H. Technische Hilfsmittel zur Intubation. In Biro P, Pasch Th, eds. *Die schwierige Intubation.* Göttingen: Hans Huber Bern, 1995:52.
12. Saling E. Austauschtransfusion beim Neugeborenen über die Aorta abdominalis. *Geburtshilfe Frauenheilkd* 1959;19:230.
13. Saling E. Die Zwei-Katheterverfahren fur den Blutaustausch beim Neugeborenen. *Dtsch Med Wochenschr* 1961;86:294.
14. Saling E, Damaschke K. Neue Mikro-Schnell-Methode zur Messung des Blutsauerstoffs auf elektrochemischem Wege. *Klin Wochenschr* 1961;39:805.
15. Saling E. The antenatal detection of haemolytic disease of the newborn. *Germ Med Mth* 1961;6:326.
16. Saling E. Neue Untersuchungsmoglichkeiten des Kindes unter der Geburt. *Zentralbl Gynäkol* 1961;83:1906.
17. Saling E. Neues. Vorgehen zur Untersuchung des Kindes unter der Geburt (Einfiihrung, Technik, Grundlagen). *Arch Gynäkol* 1962;197:108.
18. Saling E. Zustandsdiagnose beim Neugeborenen unmittelbar nach der Geburt. *Gynaecologia* 1965;160:133.
19. Saling E. *Das Kind im Bereich der Geburtshilfe.* Stuttgart: Thieme, 1966.
20. Saling E. *Foetal and Neonatal Hypoxia in Relation to Obstetric Practice.* London: Arnold (Publication), 1968.
21. Boenisch H, Saling E. A combined clinical – biochemical scoring of the newborn. Results of the past four years. *J Perinat Med* 1974;2:122.
22. Saling E. Die Blutgasverhaltnisse und der Säure-Basen-Haushalt des Feten bei ungestörtem Geburtsverlauf. *Z Geburtsh Gynäkol* 1963;161:262.
23. Caldeyro-Barcia R. Editorial. *J Perinat Med* 1973;1:5.

24. Saling E. Die Amnioskopie, ein neues Verfahren zum Erkennen von Gefahrenzuständen des Feten bei noch stehender Fruchtblase. *Geburtshilfe Frauenheilkd* 1962;22:830.
25. Dudenhausen JW, Saling E. Die Amnioskopie zur Uberwachung des Föten bei EPH-Gestose der Mutter. In Rippmann ET, Rippert C, eds. *EPH-Gestose*. Berlin: de Guyter, 1972:101–6.
26. Saling E. Die O_2-Sparschaltung des fetalen Kreislaufes. *Geburtshilfe Frauenheilkd* 1966;26:413.
27. Saling E. Oxygen-conserving adaptation of the foetal circulation. *Mod Trends Paediatr* 1970;3:51.
28. Dawes GS, Mott JC. Changes in O_2 distribution and consumption in foetal lambs with variations in umbilical blood flow. *J Physiol* 1964;170:524.
29. Dawes GS. Revolutions and clinical rhythm in prenatal life. Fetal respiratory movements rediscovered. *Pediatrics* 1973;51:965.
30. Arabin B, Bergmann PL, Saling E. Simultaneous assessment of blood flow velocity waveforms in uteroplacental vessels, the umbilical artery, the fetal aorta and the fetal common carotid artery. *Fetal Ther* 1987;2:17.
31. Saling E, Arabin B. Historic landmarks of perinatal medicine in obstetrics. *J Perinat Med* 1988;16:5.
32. Pestalozzi E. Graphische Darstellung des fötalen Herzimpulses. *Arch Gynäkol* 1891;39:137.
33. Hofbauer J, Weiss O. Photografische Registrierung der fötalen Herztöne. *Zentralbl Gynäkol* 1908;32:429.
34. Cremer M. Über die direkte Ableitung der Aktionsstrome des menschlichen Herzens vom Ösophagus und über das Elektrokardiogramm des Fötus. *Münch Med Wochenschr* 1906;53:811.
35. Caldeyro-Barcia R. Estudio de la anoxial fetal intrauterina mediante el EGG fetal y el registro continuo de la frecuencia cardiaca fetal. In *Proceedings of III Congr Latinoamer Obstet Ginec*, Mexico, 1958;2:383.
36. Rech W. Untersuchungen über die Herztätigkeit des Fetus. I. Teil. *Arch Gynäkol* 1931;145:714.
37. Hon EH. A foetal electrographic electrode. *Yale J Biol Med* 1966; 39:54.
38. Junge H. Über die kontinuierliche Kontrolle der fetalen Herztätigkeit durch Aufzeichnung des fetalen Herzfrequenzdiagramms. *Z Geburtshilfe Gynäkol* 1967;166:159.
39. Hammacher K. Neue Methoden zur selektiven Registrierung der fetalen Herzschlagfrequenz. *Geburtshilfe Frauenheilkd* 1962; 22:1512.
40. Saling E. Elektronische und biochemische Überwachung des Feten unter der Geburt. *Bull Soc Roy Belge Gynec Obstet* 1968; 38:289.
41. Brandt-Niebelschütz S, Saling E. Indications for operative termination of labor on cardiotocography and fetal blood analysis: The reliability of these methods. *J Perinat Med* 1994;22:19.
42. Saling E, Dudenhausen JW. The present situation of clinical monitoring of the fetus during labor. *J Perinat Med* 1973;1:75.
43. Saling E. Fetal scalp blood analysis. *J Perinat Med* 1981;9:165.
44. Saling E. Introduction and clinical aspects of biochemical monitoring of the fetus. *J Perinat Med* 1988;16(Suppl 1):23.
45. Saling E, Langner K. Fetal acid-base measurements in labor. In Spencer JAD, ed. *Fetal Monitoring*. Tunbridge Wells: Castle House Publications, 1989.
46. Saling E, Bartnicki. Clinical importance of biochemical monitoring of the fetus during labor with demonstration of typical cases. In Chatterjee MS, ed. *Biochemical Monitoring of the Fetus*. New York: Springer, 1993:1–12.
47. Donald I, MacVicar J, Brown TG. Investigation of abdominal mass by pulsed ultrasound. *Lancet* 1958;I:1188.
48. Donald I, Brown TG. Demonstration of tissue interfaces within the body by ultrasonic echo sounding. *Br J Radiol* 1961;34:539.
49. Gottesfeld KR. The practical application of ultrasound in obstetrics and gynecology. In *Diagostic Ultrasound*. New York: Plenum Press, 1966.
50. Gottesfeld KR, Thompson HE, Holmes JH, Taylor ES. Ultrasonic placentography – A new method for placental localization. *Am J Obstet Gynecol* 1966;96:538.
51. Kossoff G, Garrett WJ, Radovanovich G. Grey scale echography in obstetrics and gynecology. *Aust Radiol* 1974;18:62.
52. Donald I. Clinical application of ultrasonic techniques in obstetrical and gynaecological diagnosis. *Br J Obstet Gynaecol* 1962;69:1036.
53. Callaghan D, Rowland TC, Goldman DE. Ultrasonic observation of the fetal heart. *Obstet Gynecol* 1964;23:637.
54. Kratochwil A, Eisenhut L. Der früheste Nachweis der fetalen Herzaktion durch Ultraschall. *Geburtshilfe Frauenheilkd* 1967; 27:176.
55. Reinold E. Clinical value of fetal spontaneous movements in early pregnancy. *J Perinat Med* 1973;1:65.
56. Boddy K, Robinson JS. External method for detection of fetal breathing *in utero*. *Lancet* 1971;II:T231.
57. Gennser G. The dynamics of fetal respiratory movements in man. In Bennet MJ, Campbell S, eds. *Realtime Ultrasound in Obstetrics*. Oxford: S. Blackwells, 1980.
58. De Vries JIP, Visser GHA, Prechtl FIFR. The emergence of fetal behaviour. I quantitative aspects. *Early Hum Dev* 1982;7:301.
59. Nijhuis JG, Prechtl HFR, Martin CB Jr, Bots RSGM. Are there behavioural states in the human fetus? *Early Hum Dev* 1982;6:177.
60. Fitzgerald DE, Drumm JE. Non-invasive measurement of human fetal circulation using ultrasound. *Br Med J* 1977;2:1450.
61. Gill RW. Quantitative blood flow measurement in deep-lying vessel using pulsed Doppler with the Octoson. In White DN, Lyons EA. *Ultrasound in Medicine*. New York: Plenum Press, 1978;4:341.
62. Eik-Nes SH, Brubakk A, Ulstein M. Measurement of human fetal blood flow. *Br Med J* 1980;1:283.
63. Campbell S, Diaz-Recasens J, Griffin DR. New Doppler technique for assessing uteroplacental blood flow. *Lancet* 1983;I:675.
64. Mosler K-H. Bericht über das 3. Symposion über Physiologie und Pathologie der Wehentatigkeit. Würzburg 1964. *Zentralbl Gynäkol* 1965;87:197.
65. Caldeyro-Barcia R, MaganaJM, Castillo JB, *et al.* A new approach to the treatment of acute intrapartum fetal distress. In *Perinatal Factors Affecting Human Development*. Washington: Pan American Health Organization, 1969:248.
66. Gamissans O, Esteban-Altirriba J, Gomez S, *et al.* Estudio de la accion utero-inhibidora de un nuevo beta-adrenergico (derivado de la orciprenalina) en clinica obstetrica. *Ada Ginecol (Madrid)* 1968;19:445.
67. Esteban-Altirriba J, Gamissans O, Duran P, *et al.* Administration of beta-mimetic agents to the mother as a conservative therapy in cases of intrapartum fetal acidosis. In Saling E, Dudenhausen JW, eds. *Perinatale Medizin Band III*. Stuttgart: Thieme, 1972:198–208.
68. Saling E, Müller-Holve W. External cephalic version under tocolysis. *J Perinat Med* 1975;3:115.
69. Calder AA, Embrey MP, Tait T. Ripening of the cervix with extraamniotic prostaglandin E in viscous gel before induction of labour. *Br J Obstet Gynaecol* 1975;84:264.
70. Lippert Th, Moldy T. Induction of abortion by extraamniotic administration of prostaglandin gel. *J Obstet Gynaecol Br Commonw* 1973;80:1025.
71. Hochheim K. Über einige Befunde in den Lungen von Neugeborenen und die Beziehung derselben zur Aspiration von Fruchtwasser. *Zentralbl Pathol* 1903;14:537.
72. Gruenwald P. Surface tension as a factor in the resistance of neonatal lungs to aeration. *Am J Obstet Gynecol* 1947;53:966.
73. Clements JA. Surface tension of lung extracts. *Am J Physiol* 1956;187:592.
74. Avery ME, Mead J. Surface properties in relation to atelectasis and hyaline membrane disease. *Am J Dis Child* 1959;97:517.
75. Graven SN. Phospholipids in human and monkey amniotic fluid. *Pediatr Res* 1968;2:318.
76. Gluck L, Kulovich MV, Borer RC, *et al.* Diagnosis of respiratory distress syndrome by amniocentesis. *Am J Obstet Gynecol* 1971;109:440.
77. Buckingham S, McNary FF, Sommers SC, Rothschild J. Is lung an analogue of Moog's developing intestine? I. Phosphatases and pulmonary alveolar differentiation in fetal rabbits. *Fed Proc* 1968;27:328.
78. Liggins GC. Premature delivery of foetal lambs infused with glucocorticoids. *J Endocrinol* 1969;45:515.
79. Liggins GC, Howie RN. A controlled trial of antepartum glucocorticoid treatment for prevention of the respiratory distress syndrome in premature infants. *Pediatrics* 1972;50:515.
80. Saling E. Vorschläge zur Neuordnung der Geburtshilfe. *Geburtshilfe Frauenheilkd* 1967;27:572.

II Memories of the World Association of Perinatal Medicine

S. Sakamoto

The First International Congress of Perinatal Medicine, 1991, was the first global meeting of scientists, clinicians, midwives and persons who are concerned with perinatal medicine. Although academic exchange in this field had been active on the regional level, this congress was the first worldwide meeting of its kind following agreement at the Rio de Janeiro FIGO meeting in 1989.

How was the World Association of Perinatal Medicine (WAPM) born? Its history

On the occasion of the new publication on perinatology, we had better look back at the history of the international congress of perinatal medicine to know how the WAPM started its activity.

Since the 1960s, there has been a scientific breakthrough in perinatology, due to the remarkable development of medical science. As a result, many federations of perinatology were born: the European Congress of Perinatology, first started in 1968, the high-level scientific exchange system in the USA, the Asia Oceania Federation of Perinatology (1979) and the Latin–American Federation (1980s).

The idea of having an international-level body for perinatal medicine came to the mind of the pioneers. In Europe, Prof. E. Saling took up the initiative to set up the international congress of perinatology, which was unfortunately discontinued, and Prof. E. Cosmi proposed the foundation of the international-level federation on the occasion of the European Congress of Perinatology, Rome, in 1987, and preparatory work has just started. In 1989, on the occasion of the FIGO Congress, Rio de Janeiro, Prof. R. Caldeyro-Barcia, a famous perinatologist from Uruguay and former FIGO president, had a meeting with the invited participants from about 40 countries, around 70 doctors, for a discussion on how to set up the international body. The objectives were unanimously approved, but it was hard to decide on a method of setting up the proposed federation. Then I proposed 'Let's have one international congress under a suitable person in a suitable place, and at the end of the congress, Mr. Chairman, you should have a general assembly and ask the delegates again to vote whether the foundation of an international body is necessary or not?' Prof. Caldeyro-Barcia and all the participants agreed with this idea and finally nominated me as the president of the congress, requesting that the congress be held in the autumn of 1991 in Tokyo. Preparation for the congress was expected to be completed within 2 years.

The congress was held under the name of the First International Congress of Perinatal Medicine, in November 5–8, 1991, at the Keio Plaza Hotel in Tokyo, and was attended by 1580 participants from 45 countries, and a total of 516 invited and oral and poster papers were presented. It was a great success. Prof. R. Caldeyro-Barcia chaired the general assembly held immediately after the congress was over and about 60 delegates from 45 countries attended. They rated the first congress very highly and the foundation of an international body the, World Association of Perinatal Medicine, was unanimously accepted.

Thus, the WAPM was satisfactorily formed. All members signed as founders. Annual fees, etc. were carefully discussed, but as the discussion took time, the chairman proposed the election of officers and entrusted them with the preparatory work.

I was then elected as the first president of WAPM. Other officers were also elected.

I thought the second congress should be held in Europe and I proposed Prof. Cosmi as the president and Rome as the venue. As Cosmi and I worked for FIGO as members of the executive board, I knew he had a strong wish to be the president of the congress. Then, the chairman closed the session, with congratulatory remarks.

I believe that WAPM is really Prof. Robert Caldeyro-Barcia's legacy, just as FIGO, IFFS and IAMANEH are called Hubert de Watteville's legacy. And the First International Congress was nominated naturally as the first congress of WAPM.

His Imperial Majesty Akihito's opening address

His Imperial Majesty Akihito kindly attended the opening ceremony of the First International Congress of Perinatal Medicine and welcome party with Her Majesty Michiko.

The success of this congress, I believe, was due to his speech, which was full of deep thoughts and stimulating messages.

At the request of the sixth president of WAPM, Prof. Kurjak, I quote here our emperor's address:

> It is my heartfelt pleasure to convene the First International Congress of Perinatal Medicine in Tokyo, where the East meets the West. Perinatal cares, which address the safety and happiness of mother and child, have always been pursued in earnest by both obstetricians and pediatricians. At last, in 1968, the academic outline of perinatal medicine, called perinatology was established in Europe. Hence, perinatal medicine has become new and important area in academic fields. During the following two decades, with remarkable advancements in science, important discoveries were made, in succession, about the fetus, which previously had been kept in a black box. It is truly noteworthy that neonatology also has become a brilliant specialty, and academic findings are now vigorously exchanged in feedback between researchers. As a biologist, I fully understand that perinatology in a broad sense consists of maternal medicine, fetal medicine and neonatology.
>
> I am deeply impressed that scholars from many specialties reached beyond their own territories and exchange expertise to establish a new academic branch, the core of which is new life. I am convinced that deep reverence of life as well as love of mankind has made it possible. I would like to praise the pioneers and their followers who gather here today.
>
> When we reflect on the situation of mother and child at a global level, we realize that the achievements from advanced studies benefit only people in advanced nations. I am pained to think that young mothers, newborn babies and infants in many developing countries where people face problems associated with population explosion do not benefit from the fruits of advanced studies. All lives, great or small, have an equal right to enjoy happiness and maintain dignity. I pray that you take that initiative to extend helpful hands to these less fortunate people.
>
> In this International Congress, not only advancements from studies but also other efforts are joined to spread reality-based information. In that regard, the Congress will make great achievements. It is my sincere hope that the Congress will create a milestone.

The Emperor and Empress are extremely concerned with perinatal medicine. His Majesty spoke with infinite care to make sure no word was left unheard. Everyone at the opening ceremony could not help but be captivated by his Majesty's warm personality. It was the moment when people who have taken separate ways to reach the peak of perinatal medicine came together to achieve the ideas of the future.

Progress and development of fetal medicine up to the First Congress, 1991

Fetal care was initially developed to prevent fetal disorders by improving obstetrical care related to labor and delivery. It became clear that neonatal care, in collaboration with obstetrics and pediatrics, was essential in obtaining a better prognosis in newborn infants, which led to the establishment of perinatal medicine.

Since the 1960s, 20 years have passed. Perinatal medicine has achieved tremendous progress in safe care for mother and child. Furthermore, as neonatal care has developed to neonatology, fetal therapy is now becoming a new scientific field – fetal medicine. However, looking back, the scientific level at around 1980 was like this.

Development of perinatology

Experiments in perinatal medicine, such as pathophysiology of the fetus and neonatal hypoxia and metabolic analysis of thermogenesis of neonates, were carried out during the 1960s.

Progress in fetal medicine

Progress in fetal therapy can be divided into three phases according to therapeutic objectives. The first decade, 1960–1975, is defined as a period of fetal emergency care. Many trials were concentrated on diagnosis of fetal distress (this word has since been changed) and resuscitation of newborn infants.

The following decade, 1975–1985, was a period of long-term management of abnormal fetuses during pregnancy. The introduction of ultrasonographic observation brought about new diagnostic techniques in fetal inspection.

This decade, and the following 5 years (1985–1990), brought a new era of fetal therapy in which we can apply individualized diagnostic measures and therapeutic devices to different types of fetal disorders.

Establishment of fetal emergency care

Fetal emergency care was established by the progress in fetal monitoring. Cardiotocography and chemical diagnosis of fetal blood gave a very accurate diagnosis of fetal distress. Biochemical analysis of maternal hormone secretion and blood enzymatic distribution also provided criteria for placental dysfunction. These led to diagnosis of chronically affected fetuses.

Therapeutic effects, caused by oxygen inhalation and maternal infusion therapy, could be satisfactorily evaluated and gave more accurate timing of emergency care for the fetus. However, caution against unnecessary management due to overdiagnosis was advised elsewhere.

In this period, diagnostic criteria for fetal distress by different methods were proposed by distinguished researchers. Pathophysiological diagnosis for encephalopathy of the fetus and neonate, and fetal endocrinology have become subjects of extensive research.

Long-term management of fetus *in utero*

The second decade of progress in perinatology was defined between 1975 and 1985. Progress in ultrasonic diagnosis of the fetus resulted in the second advanced stage in fetal care. Abnormalities in fetal growth could be accurately diagnosed by fetometry. In addition, a cross-sectional view of the fetus gave us a new indication for therapeutic measures, such as fetal surgery, fetal biopsy, reproductive physiology, etc.

Blood flow determination by Doppler ultrasound enabled us to monitor circulatory conditions in the fetus. These contributed to long-term management of the fetus *in utero*.

Congenital hydrocephalus develops rapidly around the 28th week of gestation.

Close observation of cerebral thickness gives the exact timing of induction of labor. Radical neurosurgery to construct permanent drainage followed by delivery saves the baby from mental disorders.

Accurate diagnosis of placenta previa and precise determination of fetal growth could be easily obtained by ultrasonography.

Intrauterine blood transfusion, or even an exchange transfusion through the umbilical vein when blood incompatibility occurs, could be carried out by guided catheterization under ultrasonography.

Genetic diagnosis done by amniocentesis, chorionic villi sampling and neonatal blood sampling, developed during this period, was also one of the remarkable advances in fetal medicine. Some of the inborn errors of metabolism that affect the mental development of the newborn, such as methyl maronic acidemia or galactosemia, can be treated by maternal administration of cyanocobalamin or a low-galactose diet for the mother. Folic acid therapy has been recommended to prevent fetal spina bifida.

A typical medical intervention in the handicapped fetus with hydrocephalus is described as an example. Enlargement of BPD was clearly shown ultrasonographically. Progress of ventricular dilatation and thinning of the cerebral cortex by CT were carefully monitored along with fetal growth and maturation.

Our case was born at 36 weeks of gestation by cesarean section followed by neurosurgery of continuous drainage. Both the fetus' maturation tolerance to surgical stress and the prognostic limitation of the ventricular enlargement were carefully taken into consideration in determining the time of delivery.

By CT scanning, performed 1 week after surgery, a remarkable reduction in ventricular size was noted. The baby recovered smoothly and obtained normal mental development at the age of 1 year.

Individualization in fetal therapy

Advances in bioengineering and molecular biology in recent years contribute greatly to the scientific basis of perinatal medicine. Feto-maternal interaction of growth factors and endothelial functions of chorionic villi gave basic consideration of the pathogenesis of intrauterine growth retardation (IUGR).

Feto-maternal interaction was clearly demonstrated by IGF-1 regulation in relation to fetal growth. This is an example of research work picked up from many works.

Production of IGF-1 is switched over from the maternal liver to the placenta. Activity of IGF-1 in the placental environment is regulated by the autocrine function of the villi and paracrine function of villi and decidua. The hPL and placental GH stimulate IGF-1 and its binding protein production in the maternal liver. Binding protein is also regulated by protease from deciduas. These facts suggest that duplicate cycle for IGF-1 regulation functions during pregnancy. Fetal growth factors are independent of the maternal side; however, they show their activity substrate dependency on maternal transport of nutrients. IGFs mainly have three types of structure, IGF-1, -2 and -3, and they have different functions. Other growth factors concerning the fetal growth should be studied carefully.

Coagulation and fibrinolysis system – thrombomoduline

This system is another example of the new approach to analyze placental circulation in PIH. It became clear that trophoblast has an endothelial function maintaining smooth blood circulation in the intervillous space, where most slow and complicated blood streams exist, and easily forms infarction during abnormal conditions, in cases such as PIH. Our data clearly indicated decreased trophoblastic thrombomodulin activity in PIH, which referred to endothelial function. This is one of the explanations for the fact that remarkable IUGR takes place in severe PIH. Endothelial function in pregnancy is also an important field of study.

Fetal surgery

A direct therapeutic approach to the fetus, such as catheter replacement and experimental trial of gene manipulation, may lead to radical treatment *in utero*. Open fetal surgery may lead to complete correction of fetal anomalies. Direct catheter replacement in half-delivered fetuses with urethral obstruction at the 30th week through the incised uterine window was first performed in 1990. The window was closed and the amnion was supplied through a catheter. The baby was successfully managed for a considerable period *in utero* after surgery. Radical urethral reconstruction was performed in the neonatal period. This shows that fetal medicine is obtaining general consensus for clinical use.

Several years ago, the international symposium 'The Fetus as a Patient' was held with the high expectations by all perinatologists. Fetal medicine, which started from emergency care of fetal distress 25 years ago, is now able to apply total medical care to the fetus. Our hope symbolized in 'The Fetus as a Patient' is now being realized.

Finally, I would like to conclude by saying, 'Whenever, wherever, we have our hopes and dreams, they will certainly be realized and bring a brighter future in perinatal medicine'.

The above examples are samples of perinatal research and treatment performed around the 1980s. More developed research work had been performed by the pioneers, but member of which were quite limited.

In this book the most developed data will be described. You may find a dramatic development in perinatal medicine in the period from 1991 until 2005.

Closing remarks

While the 20th century was the era of advance in science and technology, with the emphasis on physics, the 21st century is the era of chemistry and the genome, and can be called the period of respect for life and establishment of human dignity. People who are sick or suffer from extreme poverty long for the normalization of the quality of life and the life worth living. It is our duty to deal with such evidence and respond to the wish of those countless people. Naturally, these actions require highly advanced science and appropriate as well as reasonable means of healing.

Medicine must not only be highly advanced but must also bring peace to lonely souls. Life-long education also is our own choice and duty, imposing on our experience. Physicians must be always disciplined to be humble. Medical care should not be ruled by temporal good intention or judgment, but should aim at the future of humankind, especially of the mother and child.

For the younger generation:

- What we should do, is taught by the mind and body of patients.
- What we should not do, we learn from the history of evidence, and valuable experience.

Last, I would like to close my remarks with my own view for medicine, which was first proposed in the 1991 Congress.

May our international festival of academia be a forum and an opportunity to turn human dreams to hopes, and hopes to reality, thus bringing to all humanity true peace and happiness. (1991)

III Perinatal medicine in the United States

E. J. Quilligan

It is always difficult to set a date as to when perinatal medicine began in the United States. During the 1940s, 1950s and 1960s there seemed to be a significant increase in research, both basic and clinical, regarding the pregnant mother and her fetus. This was fueled by the increase in federal grant funds, the increased numbers of full-time faculty in Obstetrics and Gynecology and the developing technology that would allow measurement of hitherto inaccessible fetal and maternal parameters. For example, the intrauterine catheter allowed the development of a new understanding of the work required by the uterus during labor and how abnormalities of the contraction pattern may lead to abnormal labor.[1] The development of more sophisticated electronics allowed the recording of the fetal heart rate throughout labor.[2]

Another factor important in the development of perinatal medicine was the growing awareness that a pregnant patient with medical complications, such as diabetes, needed completely different care from a non-pregnant diabetic. In the past it was usually the case that the obstetrician managed the pregnancy and an internist managed the diabetes. This occasionally led to difficulties as the two physicians were not working in concert. It was found that the well-prepared obstetrician could manage both with better outcomes for mother and fetus.

A more specific date can be set for the beginning of the subspecialty of maternal fetal medicine in the United States. The American Board of Obstetrics and Gynecology, under the leadership of Gordon W. Douglas, MD, organized a meeting in 1969 to determine the feasibility of subspecialty certification or boards in Obstetrics and Gynecology.[3] I was fortunate to chair the discussion on maternal fetal medicine. It was the consensus of our committee, and ultimately the Board, that there were adequate numbers of obstetricians and gynecologists who were primarily interested in maternal fetal medicine from a clinical and research standpoint to justify a subspecialty board or certification. A similar conclusion was reached with regard to oncology and reproductive endocrinology. The next 2 years were spent in developing the subspecialty divisions and getting the necessary approval from the American Board of Medical Specialties. It was decided that rather than being subspecialty boards, the parent board would offer certificates of special competence in the areas of maternal–fetal medicine, oncology and reproductive endocrinology. This was primarily due to the fact that the American Board of Medical Specialities had recently granted several subspecialty boards and had a temporary moratorium on new ones. We felt it was of no particular advantage to be a subspecialty board.

The American Board of Obstetrics and Gynecology did establish divisions of Maternal Fetal Medicine, Oncology and Reproductive Endocrinology in 1969. I was appointed the first head of the division of Maternal Fetal Medicine. There was one representative of the parent board in our division, Dr Harry Prystowsky. There were four additional members of the original division, Donald L. Hutchinson, MD, Edgar L. Makowski, MD, Joseph Seitchik, MD and Fredrick P. Zuspan, MD.

The purposes of our division were as follows: (1) to improve the health care of mother and fetus suffering from diseases peculiar to or related to gestation, by elevating the standard of education and training related to abnormal obstetrics, enhancing the recruitment of qualified physicians in this field, by improving the organization and distribution of patient care and increasing knowledge; (2) to evaluate the qualifications of educational programs offering training in maternal and fetal medicine for the purpose of providing improved patient care and adequate preparation and experience for the physician intending to become a specialist in this field; (3) to define periodically and to publish from time to time the details of formal training, which the division considers essential to attain eligibility for the examination; (4) to establish procedures whereby the knowledge and skills of a candidate for advanced certification may be evaluated, and examinations designed to determine the individual's competence as a specialist in maternal and fetal medicine and (5) to recommend to the Board for advanced certification of physicians who have demonstrated to the satisfaction of the Division their possession of special knowledge and a high degree of professional competence in the management of disorders of the mother and fetus.[4]

One of the first major decisions that had to be made was one that affected all the divisions, namely, how to treat those individuals who considered themselves subspecialists but had no formal training or had training that had not been Board approved: the grandfathers. Three choices were available: (1) have no grandfathers, make all candidates undergo board-approved training; (2) permit anyone who thinks they are qualified take the examinations, which would be for a specified period of time, and (3) allow all grandfathers to receive a certification. There was a lively discussion of this question with many feeling there should be no grandfathers. The threat of a protracted suit in one of the other divisions led us all to accept the second option: permit those who thought themselves qualified to take the examination. This option would be open only for a period of 2 years after the initial examination. The candidates choosing this option were required to submit an application, which described their residence training and any fellowship training they had taken. In addition, we required a case list of all complicated pregnancies they had managed during the previous 2 years as well as the total number of normal pregnancies they had managed during the same time period. A bibliography of all articles, book chapters and abstracts, including reprints of original articles, was a requirement. The type of application gave the Division the material needed to make a judgment as to whether an individual qualified as a grandfather.

The number and type of examinations were rather easily determined. The parent board had both written and oral examinations. All subspecialty divisions decided to follow that example. The scope of the written examination included (1) genetics, biochemistry of genes and chromosomes, gene transformation in man, cytogenetics and karyotyping, population genetics and genetic counseling; (2) teratology, knowledge of embryology, drugs that affect the fetus, viral effects on the fetus, bacterial effects on the fetus and radiation effects on the fetus; (3) maternal physiology; (4) fetal physiology; (5) effects of maternal disease on the fetus; (6) effects of pregnancy on maternal disease; (7) immunology; (8) evaluation of fetal welfare during pregnancy and labor; (9) newborn adjustments and adaptations to health and disease; (10) infection in mother and fetus, diagnosis and therapy; (11) immunologic disorders; (12) intrapartum disorders and (13) general knowledge of investigative concepts and techniques and the knowledge necessary to critically evaluate studies in maternal and fetal medicine. An individual passing the written examination was eligible to take the oral examination after 2 years of practice. The 2 years of practice was waived for grandfathers. Requirements for the oral examinations included a case list for the 2 years of practice and a thesis of original clinical or basic research. The oral examination was conducted by two examiners and a neonatologist questioning the candidate for 3 h on the thesis, case list and knowledge of maternal–fetal medicine including investigative concepts.[4]

The Division developed the required training program, which was of 2 years' duration with the following requirements: (1) training could be obtained in one or more institutions; (2) at all times there must be evidence of a patient population adequate to assure the candidate of a satisfactory experience; (3) comprehensive care of maternal and fetal disorders requires (a) a high-risk pregnancy unit with adequate numbers of pregnant patients presenting special problems defined as high risk, adequate supervision by individuals competent in the care of high-risk pregnant patients and adequate laboratory and monitoring equipment, (b) a genetics unit with a qualified geneticist and laboratory to perform genetic analysis including karyotyping and biochemical studies, (c) a newborn care unit with a noenatologist director and adequate numbers of newborns requiring intensive care and (d) a pathology service with a qualified fetal and newborn pathologist and (4) there should be a program director certified as a Diplomate of the American Board of Obstetrics and Gynecology who is judged to be qualified to direct such a program. The last requirement was soon changed to a person certified as a subspecialist in maternal–fetal medicine. Each new training program was inspected by one or more division members.

A significant number of changes have occurred since the initial candidates were examined in 1973. After the second oral examination the neonatologists were not used since this area was felt to be primarily in the realm of a new subspecialty within pediatrics, neonatology. In 1975 the case list for oral examination was reduced to 18 months before the application was submitted.[5] In 1977 obstetric anesthesia was added to the scope of the oral examinations and an obstetric anesthesiologist was a required part of the training program.[6] The 1978 bulletin did specify that 'The program must include two university-level courses, one in qualitative techniques which should include biostatistics and other areas such as epidemiology and research design and implementation. The second course must be relevant to the specific subspecialty. Both courses must be approved by the division. All courses must have an examination which the candidate must pass'. Also in 1978 the thesis requirement was changed to a paper in press or published within the past 3 years in a peer review journal.[7] In 1979 the ultrasound unit was required in the training program and ultrasound became a part of the written and oral examinations.[8] In 1986 a *Guide of Learning* was published by the Board, which gave a much more complete outline of the scope of knowledge required by a subspecialist.[9] Perhaps the most significant change occurred in 1998 when the division decided to lengthen the training to 3 years.[10] The Division, from its inception, felt that research was a very important part of the training program. This was evident in the first bulletin, which stated: 'The candidate must possess (a) an understanding and general knowledge of investigative concepts and techniques as they relate to maternal health and fetal development and (b) the knowledge necessary to evaluate studies relative to maternal and fetal medicine'. It was expected, though not specifically stated, that one of the 3 years be spent in research.

The type of practice for a maternal and fetal medicine subspecialist has changed significantly during the 30 years since the inception of the division. Initially, the subspecialist was primarily a consultant for pregnancy with complications. With the development of sophisticated ultrasound and the increasing understanding of genetic abnormalities, a significant portion of the subspecialist's time is spent doing ultrasound.

A reasonable question might be what is the result of the development of the subspecialty of maternal and fetal medicine? This can be answered both numerically and philosophically. Numerically, there are currently 62 approved programs in maternal and fetal medicine. There have been 1542 candidates certified. Philosophically, I believe it has resulted in significantly better care for the pregnant patient with complications. This is difficult to prove because there have been so many changes in practice during the same time period, such as the development of neonatal intensive care units, antepartum fetal monitoring and the development of ultrasound. All of these and more may have resulted in the significant decreases in perinatal mortality and stillbirth rate. The integration of care in a single individual who is focused on the pregnant patient with a complication such as diabetes or hypertension, in my opinion, must result in improved care.

REFERENCES

1. Caldeyro-Barcia R, Pose SV, Alverez H. Uterine contractility in polyhydramnios and the effects of withdrawal of the excess of amniotic fluid. *Am J Obstet Gynecol* 1957;73(6):1238–54.
2. Hon EH, Hess OW. The clinical value of fetal electrocardiography. *Am J Obstet Gynecol* 1960;79:1012–38.
3. Gerbie AB. *The American Board of Obstetrics and Gynecology: A Personalized History 1980–2000.* The American Board of Obstetrics and Gynecology.
4. The American Board of Obstetrics and Gynecology. *Bull Div Matern–Fetal Med* 1973.
5. The American Board of Obstetrics and Gynecology. *Bull Div Matern–Fetal Med* 1975.
6. The American Board of Obstetrics and Gynecology. *Bull Div Matern–Fetal Med* 1977.
7. The American Board of Obstetrics and Gynecology. *Bull Div Matern–Fetal Med* 1978.
8. The American Board of Obstetrics and Gynecology. *Bull Div Matern–Fetal Med* 1979.
9. The American Board of Obstetrics and Gynecology. *Bull Div Matern–Fetal Med* 1986.
10. The American Board of Obstetrics and Gynecology. *Bull Div Matern–Fetal Med* 1998.

IV A perspective on perinatal medicine

E. V. Cosmi

The process of fetal growth and development of the human fetus at birth has always attracted the attention of scientists. Hippocrates, 460–370 B.C., suggested that when the onset of labor is near 'the fetus becomes agitated and breaks the membranes'. Leonardo da Vinci said that 'the child grows daily more within the body of its mother that when it is outside of the body, and this teaches us ...'. In the 17th century Sir William Harvey suggested a direct role of the fetus in the initiation of parturition, a concept that was endorsed by Van Deventer in the same century and by Spielberg in 1882.

Subsequently many animal experimentations and human observations have attempted to discover the many mysteries of fetal and neonatal growth and development, the features of the cardiovascular and respiratory systems, some relevant aspects of energy metabolism, temperature control and their integration by hormonal and nervous mechanisms, the role of the placenta, the initiation of labor, the transition from the intrauterine to the extrauterine life of the fetus, etc.

Considering comparative physiology it has been recognized that general principles should hold in every species with peculiar adaptation to particular needs.

Some species lend themselves well to a particular type of study, e.g. the fetal lamb, because it is relatively large and comparable by weight to the human fetus and because the uterus of the ewe does not at once contract, has been used for various studies, including fetal breathing movements (FBMs) and lung maturity. The fetal rhesus monkey has been studied mainly because its brain is more closely related to that of the human fetus and of the newborn at birth; furthermore, since the lamb's brain is only 1.3% of body weight at birth, whereas that of the fetal rhesus monkey is 12%, the latter is a better model for studying the distribution of cardiac output (CO).[1]

Finally, the hemochorial placenta of the rhesus monkey and also that of the pig are more suitable for the study of placental transfer of gases, other supplies, and drugs than the cotyledonary placenta of the ewe.

The beginning of fetal physiology is rooted in the measurements of placental and fetal growth and in comparative studies of placental histology that were made long before physiologic data could be collected and properly understood. The pioneers of this approach are many; they include Sir Joseph Barcroft (1946)[2] and, around the 1960s, D. H. Barron, H. Prystowski, C. A. Villee, P. Grunewald, R. Margaria (Turin, Italy), R. E. Cooke, E. Ramsey, I. Leitsch, F. C. Hytten, E. G. Makowski, F. C. Battaglia, G. Meschia, A. N. Rudolph, G. S. Dawes and others.

Because perinatal biology encompasses marked differences among mammals in placentation, fetal and neonatal development, and in the adaptation made by the mother during pregnancy and lactation, the young of different species are often said to be at different maturity at birth. Nevertheless, most mammals and the human infants have one thing in common, i.e. they all must have developed, by the time they are born, the circulation and the lungs, which will permit maintenance of an independent existence outside the uterus. Initially, following acute experiments in animals, Barcroft[2] believed that the fetus was living *in utero* under conditions of anaerobiosis or semianaerobiosis, thereby introducing the concept of 'the Everest *in utero*', i.e. the fetus living under low oxygen tension. This concept was further supported by the low pO_2, pH and high pCO_2 found at birth in the umbilical arteries and vein of the human fetus. Chronic experiments performed in several pregnant animals and their fetuses have refuted this misconception and have shown instead that the oxygen supply and consumption, and the acid–base status of the fetus are similar to that of the mother.[3–8] These results have been substantiated in the human fetus by James *et al.*[9], Caldeyro-Barcia,[10] and Saling.[11] They have found that during labor and delivery fetal pO_2 and pH decrease whereas pCO_2 and buffer base increase.

The introduction of the micromethod of P. Astrup of blood sampling and acid–base status analysis has permitted the confirmation of these studies in animals and subsequent studies in the human fetus and neonate. Normally, although the PaO_2 of the fetus is around 30 Torr, hemoglobin-O_2 saturation is around 90%, also because of the double (maternal and fetal) Bohr effect on the O_2 transfer across the placenta.[12]

Another concept that was put forward was that although the fetus has a relatively high tolerance to noxious agents, many noxious factors can affect its normal intrauterine development, physiologic performance, and subsequent adaptation to the extrauterine life. These factors may originate in the mother, the placenta, or in the fetus itself. Other sources of trouble include environmental, nutritional, pharmacologic, and toxicologic factors; hematologic, hormonal, metabolic, immunologic, and genetic disorders; and infections diseases (for a review see Cosmi and Caldeyro-Barcia[12]).

Considerable efforts have been made to elucidate the morphology and the physiology of the placenta because the homeostasis of the mammalian fetus depends almost entirely on its function and on maternal homeostasis. Chorioallantoic placentas differ remarkably in shape and structure from one mammal to another and their classification on the basis of shape, morphometry, morphology, function, and the presence or absence of a maternal (decidual) component has resulted in considerable controversy.

In humans the implantation and subsequent development of the placenta depend on certain changes in the endometrium that culminate in the formation of the decidua. Basically, the human placenta has a chorioallantoic structure in which the precocious differentiated mesoderm of the allantois forms the umbilical cord.

Prof. P. M. Motta from the University 'La Sapienza' of Rome has contributed significantly with electron microscopy to clarify the process of implantation of the fertilized human ovum.[13]

In humans shortly after fertilization, the ovum is implanted and the trophoblast erodes the endometrial capillaries. At the end of the second week the endometrial veins have been eroded and communicate with the lacunar spaces. At about the 15th day, endometrial spiral arterioles are eroded and maternal inflow to the intervillous space is established. By the 16th day the entire surface of the ovum is covered with branching villi containing vascular primordia. Between days 20 and 21 after the beginning of nidation the chorionic villi show a well-defined ultrastructure with a relatively undifferentiated Langhans' layer and highly differentiated syncytiotrophoblast layer, located peripherally. By days 22 and 23 the embryonic vessels have formed an anastomotic network of channels within the villi. By 12 weeks, other villi are found, which fill the intervillous space. Each primary villus with his branching and rebranching villi constitutes a fetal cotyledon, which is the functional unit of the placenta. The villous core contains fetal capillaries, fibroblasts, the Hofbauer cells (which are morphologically similar to macrophages, originate from the mesemchyma, and possess pinocytotic and histiocytic activity), and other mesenchymal elements.[12]

One of the major advances in perinatal genetic diagnosis has been the introduction by Bruno Brambati (Milan, Italy) of chorionic villi sampling,[14] which can be performed at 9–10 weeks' gestation, thereby offering earlier diagnosis than amniocentesis and the analysis of the amniotic fluid (AF), which is performed between 14 and 18 weeks' gestation, or cordocentesis which is performed around 20 weeks' gestation for hematologic problems, infections, metabolic and enzymatic diseases. However, chorionic villi and cordocentesis are coupled with significantly higher complications than amniocentesis. The basement membrane contains immunoglobins IgG and IgA, which probably represent maternal blocking antibodies to trophoblastic antigens, thereby preventing the rejection of the placenta. Various proteins are produced by the placenta in increasing amounts during gestation. Some, such as pregnancy-specific β_1-glycoprotein (SP_1, $PS\beta_1G$), pregnancy-associated plasma protein C (PAPP-C) and α_2-glycoprotein (PAPP-α_2G), are probably trophoblast-specific antigens described by Bohn.[15] These are mainly released into the maternal circulation, where they can be measured and used as an index of placental function, whereas other proteins have enzymatic or hormonal activity. Recently, for prenatal genetic diagnosis the following tests have been introduced using maternal blood: (1) double test – determination of PAPP-A and human chorionic gonadotropin β (hCG-β) (free) performed between 9 and 13 weeks' gestation *vis à vis* fetal nuchal translucency; (2) triple test – determination of hCG-β or hCG-β (free), α-fetoprotein, and free estriol between 14 and 19 weeks; (3) quadruple test – as above plus determination of PS-β at the same gestational age; and (5) pentatest – as above plus inhibin. The reliability of these tests is much less than that of amniocentesis and fetal cell culture. However, they may be indicative of certain fetal chromosomal abnormalities.

Different types of fetal nucleated cells have been found in maternal blood by Adinolfi[16] and our group,[17] providing the possibility for non-invasive prenatal diagnosis of genetic abnormalities; however, the results of these and further studies have been inconclusive. The same holds for the study of fetal nucleated cells obtained by washing of the cervical fornix.

Lo *et al.*[18] and Farina *et al.*[19] have studied the DNA of fetal cells in maternal circulation for non-monogenic diseases such as abortion, pre-eclampsia, and IUGR. Although promising, this approach needs further studies.

The placenta, like the fetus and the mother, produces certain enzymes and hormones that influence not only its function but also those of the other two compartments – e.g. composition of the nutrients supply from the maternal circulation to the fetus, maternal and fetal metabolism, and eventually fetal growth. Conversely, placental function is influenced by fetal and maternal enzymes and hormones. The placenta possesses enzymes that are absent in the fetus, and enzymes lacking in the placenta are present in the fetus. The integrated placental and fetal functions act as a unit, and the *feto-placental unit* is indispensable for the production of most steroid hormones as suggested by Diczfalusy[20] (see below).

Several enzymes have been isolated and their activity varies during gestation, i.e. lysosomal hydrolase activity reflects the need for specialized functions (e.g. lysosomal hyaluronidase, which probably plays an important role in the regulation of placental permeability, increases with gestation).

The human placenta synthesizes and stores carbohydrates, lipids, proteins, nucleotides, and nucleic acids,[12] possesses mixed function oxidation systems and aryl hydrocarbon hydrolase involved in the transportation of xenobiotics and epoxides.[12] It is rich in 11β-ol-dehydrogenase, which *converts active steroids into inactive 11-ketosteroids*. Therefore, the question has been posed as to whether certain corticosteroids, e.g. betamethasone, administered to the mother reach the fetus in sufficient quantities to elicit their biological effect – i.e. acceleration of fetal lung maturity (FLM).[12] The placenta also contains monoamine oxidase and catechol-*O*-methyltransferase, which significantly effect the transfer of the catecholamines. Renin is also produced by the placenta. This enzyme is released into the AF. The placenta is unique in its capacity to form proteins and steroid hormones, i.e. hCG, hPL, hPRL, human chorionic thyrotropin, somatomedins C and A,[21] and adrenocorticotropic hormone (ACTH) related peptides, i.e. hCG, α-melanocyte-stimulating hormone, thyroid-stimulating hormone, and luteinizing hormone releasing factors, β-lipotropin, and β-endorphin, as demonstrated by Fraioli and Genazzani.[22]

The placenta produces large amounts of progestogens and estrogens in increasing concentrations during pregnancy. These hormones have important effects, such as the regulation of fetal growth, development, and sexual differentiation; uterine growth and contractility; the onset of labor; and uteroplacental blood flow. Estrogen production is not due solely to the placenta but to the interaction between the mother, placenta, and fetus, which *act as a unit*.[20] The production of E_3 involves the formation of precursors by fetal and maternal adrenals; 16α-hydroxylation of DHAS and E_1 or E_1 sulfate by the fetal and the maternal livers; and aromatization by the placenta. The concentration of E3 in body fluids increases steadily throughout a normal pregnancy.

Concerning the *fetal circulation* in the mature placenta, it is worth mentioning that in the definitive (tertiary) villi, arterioles and veins are given off from axially oriented trunks to supply and drain an extensive anastomosing capillary network, which lies superficially beneath the surface syncytium. Fetal blood is in close contact with maternal blood, being separated by a thin syncytiocapillary membrane.[23] Information on the fetal circulation has been derived principally from animal experiments, using a variety of methods, i.e. cineangiocardiography, blood gas analyses, blood flow measurements by electromagnetic flow meters, distribution of radioisotope-labeled microspheres, dye dilution, radioisotope methods, and Doppler ultrasound. Some of the findings from these experiments have been corroborated for the human in studies of the human fetus itself.

A variable portion of the blood returning from the fetal placenta via the umbilical vein is distributed to both right and left lobes of the liver and reaches the interior vena cava via the hepatic veins. The remainder of the blood returning from the placenta is shunted directly to the inferior vena cava via the ductus venosus in amounts varying between 20% and 90% of umbilical–portal blood flow. In the left atrium, blood from the inferior vena cava mixes with blood coming from the pulmonary veins in a ratio of about 4.5:1. Thus, the abdominal organs, the lower body, and the placenta are supplied with blood with a lower pO_2 than the coronary circulation, heart, neck, and brain.[24]

The right and the left ventricles work in parallel by virtue of the presence of the foramen ovale and the ductus arteriosus. Approximately 40% of the combined CO returns to the placenta, while only 7% flows through the lungs; the remainder perfuses body tissues. To define fetal CO, Assali *et al.* introduced the term 'effective CO' – i.e. the total volume of the blood that is distributed to the body and the placenta.[25] This represents the sum of the left ventricular output and the ductus arteriosus blood flow, and does not include coronary blood flow and the flow to the lungs. Rudolph had introduced the term 'combined ventricular output', which represents the total volume of blood ejected by both ventricles and includes pulmonary and coronary flows.[24]

It has been suggested that changes in differential CO that may occur in the fetus as a result of changes in the venous return or outflow impedance are adjusted homeometrically by the Frank–Starling relationship.[7,25,26] Rudolph[24] (from the Cardio-Vascular Institute of San Francisco, directed by Julius Comroe) has criticized this theory and indicated that the Frank–Starling mechanism is essentially inoperative in the fetal myocardium because of the large shunts between the left and the right sides of the heart, and because of the fact that the two ventricles work in parallel. Thus, in contrast to the adult, the fetus has only a limited ability to increase CO by increasing stroke volume. The increase in CO is accomplished primarily by increasing the heart rate (HR).

The cardiovascular system of the fetus is under the direct control of the autonomic nervous system through peripheral chemoreceptors and baroreceptors. In the human fetus the clearest evidence for autonomic activity is the transient bradycardia associated with uterine contraction and abolished by administration of atropine to the mother, as shown by Caldeyro-Barcia *et al.*[27] The fetal cardiovascular system is capable of responding to various humoral and pharmacological agents.

Moderate fetal hypoxemia and/or hypercapnia cause a rise in arterial pressure, vasoconstriction in the lungs, and little change in umbilical vascular resistance. At the same time, umbilical, coronary, carotid, and superior sagittal sinus blood flows increase, ensuring a better oxygen uptake and supply to vital organs. Fetal heart rate (FHR) increases initially in response to hypoxemia, but if hypoxemia persists and/or becomes more pronounced, bradycardia develops.

Fetal hypoxemia of a marked degree and/or acidemia also induce an increase in blood flow to vital organs (i.e. heart, brain, and adrenal glands), but cause a decrease in blood flow to non-vital organs (i.e. lungs, gut, spleen, kidneys, and the carcass). The selective vasoconstriction in the latter organs is accompanied by hypertension and bradycardia and later, if it persists, by anaerobic glycolysis and metabolic acidemia. Although hypertension tends to increase perfusion pressure and umbilical blood flow, with marked hypoxia and bradycardia umbilical blood flow will fall.[12]

The cardiovascular response of the fetus to hypoxia and acidosis with redistribution of the systemic circulation is a defense mechanism for conserving the oxygen supply to vital organs and for adjusting to the effects of accumulated metabolites, such as carbon dioxide and hydrogen ions. This defense mechanism is similar to that of diving mammals – e.g. the ability of the fetus of the seal and of other mammals to survive its mother's prolonged dives,[28,29] also called, less precisely, the brain sparing effect. However, it is limited, for although CO remains virtually constant, the blood redistributed to vital organs may be diverted away from the placenta, thereby further reducing the oxygen supply to the fetus.[12,24] A fall in CO will cause a marked reduction in umbilical blood flow. The survival time of the asphyxiated fetus depends on the concentration of glycogen in the myocardium before the asphyxial episodes.

FHR and ECG: FHR and ECG monitoring are the oldest and most frequently used methods of fetal surveillance.[30,31] The ultrasound technique, based on the Doppler principle,* is the method most widely used for recording FHR. Concern still exists as to its relative value, accuracy of interpretation, and prognostic significance. Caldeyro-Barcia *et al.*[30,31] combined the recording of uterine contractility with FHR monitoring. Subsequently, Hon *et al.*[32] applied a similar method and obtained analogous results.

Direct fetal ECG was obtained by placing a bipolar electrode directly on the fetus either transcervically or by maternal transabdominal puncture. With this method one detects changes in ECG pattern and FHR that may coincide with early alterations in fetal homeostasis and neonatal morbidity. The technique has been refined by the use of special nonpolarizable clips, suction, hooks, or other types of transcervical electrodes, monitoring devices and group averaging of a series of consecutive ECG complexes.[32,33] In Italy, fetal ECG has been studied extensively by Pardi *et al.*[34] Opinions pertaining to alterations in fetal ECG and their reliability and accuracy in predicting fetal distress vary considerably. Prolongation of the P–R and Q–T intervals, widening of the QRS complex, and isoelectric or inverted T-waves have been observed in conjunction with fetal hypoxia and acidosis. Shortening of the Q–T and P–R intervals with peaked, biphasic, and inverted P-waves, and inversion of the T-wave have been also recorded in the presence of severe fetal asphyxia. Forms of 'arrhythmias' have been observed – i.e. nodal extrasystoles, atrial flutter, atrial and ventricular premature beats in the form of persistent bigeminy, paroxysmal atrial tachycardia, and heart block. However, in both the human and the animal fetuses, no definite relationship was found between ECG abnormalities and the acid–base status of the fetus. Although ECG abnormalities could represent a possible early sign of fetal distress, their significance in relation to fetal homeostasis and neonatal outcome has not been settled.[4,12]

Doppler ultrasound has been recently introduced in the study of fetal circulation and several vessels including umbilical artery (UA), descending aorta, internal carotid artery, middle cerebral artery (MCA), ductus venosus and renal artery have been investigated. Preliminary statistical correlations between perinatal complications and abnormalities in indices of flow resistance have been reported, suggesting a potential role for Doppler ultrasound in the management of high-risk pregnancies. Several indices have been introduced to analyze flow velocity waveform, including pulsability index (PI) and resistance index, by several groups including Arduini and Rizzo,[35] Campbell and Bower,[36] Kurjak *et al.*,[37] and Chervenak and McCullough.[38] It has been found that absent or reversed diastolic blood flow of UA and low PI in MCA are often associated with alteration of FHR. However, no reference values on large population studies are available for flow velocity waveforms. Transcutaneous pO_2 and pulse oximetry and computerized FHR have also been introduced to improve the accuracy of the latter with variable results.

Fetal breathing activity in utero has been a matter of controversy for a long time. Rhythmic, periodic FBMs were observed and/or recorded in humans between 1888 and 1911 by Ahlfeld,[39] Weber,[40] Ferroni of Florence,[41] and Reifferscheid,[42] and in animals from 1781 until 1941.[12,43] These reports have been almost universally ignored or discounted as artifacts, and subsequent studies have in general denied that FBMs are normally present *in utero*, provided the fetus is not disturbed by physical stimuli or asphyxia. They have been rediscovered around 1970 in the fetal lamb by Dawes and coworkers,[44,45] Condorelli, Cosmi,

*This principle was theorized in 1794 by the Italian biologist Lazzaro Spallanzani, i.e. the bat's ability to 'see'. The bat gets bearing by sound rather than light.[12]

and Scarpelli.[29,46–48] Studies in human fetuses have demonstrated that FBMs are normal phenomena of intrauterine development.[12,43,48] Observation of both animal and human fetuses have indicated that FBMs might provide an index of fetal well-being.[42,44] In the human fetus, FBMs have been studied by injecting isotopes into AF, by means of force transducers placed on the maternal abdomen, and, more precisely, by ultrasound. Various systems have been used to quantify ultrasonic signals of FBMs, including A-mode, continuous Doppler systems, T-mode, time–distance recording systems, and real-time B-scan.[12,43]

Recently, we have measured nasal flow velocity waveforms (NFVW) with continuous or power Doppler, *vis à vis* the thoracic and abdominal movements, in more than 1800 human fetuses[49] and have observed that during gestation the fetal respiratory patterns are similar to those we had observed in preterm and term newborns,[50] i.e. they start at around 20 weeks' gestation as abdominal movements followed by thoracic movements and NFVW as gestational age advances. We have correlated FBMs during gestation with FLM and have found that the full development of FBMs indicates FLM.[49]

Amniotic fluid indices: *Amniocentesis* and the analysis of AF have been introduced successfully by Bevis,[51] Liley,[52] and Freda *et al.*[53] for the spectrophotometric analysis of AF at wavelengths between 300 and 700 nm in case of Rh alloimmunization and erythroblastosis fetalis. When AF contains bile pigments that absorb monochromatic light at wavelengths between 525 and 375 nm, there is an elevation above the expected slope of the curve, with a peak around 400 nm. The magnitude of this departure from the expected curve (between 525 and 375 nm) is proportional to the concentration of bilirubin and related pigments, while its width is constant and reflects the condition of the fetus.[12,52,53] Liley's method offers a more precise quantification of AF bilirubin concentration, but the upper limits of normality are too low, leading to an overestimation of the degree of fetal compromise. Freda's method takes into consideration the trend rather than the absolute concentration of bilirubin and related pigments. During the same year Freda introduced Rh gammaglobulins for the prevention of Rh alloimmunization;[54,55] since then, the disease has practically disappeared.

Amniocentesis has been widely used for *culturing and karyotyping* of AF cells by Valenti *et al.*[56] and Steele and Breg.[57] Recently, diagnosis of many genetic diseases has been performed particularly after the completion of the study of genome mapping and the introduction of fluorescence *in situ* hybridization and polymerase chain reaction techniques. It is possible to diagnose fetal sex and a variety of genetic disorders including Down's syndrome, Duchenne/Beker muscular dystrophy, deafness, cystic fibrosis, fragile X-syndrome, hemoglobinopathies, e.g. hemophilia, inborn errors of metabolism. Amniocentesis is performed between 14 and 18 weeks' gestation.

Fetal lung maturity: In recent years various laboratory tests for AF constituents to predict FLM have been developed. They can be divided into biochemical [determination of surfactant phospholipids (PLs)] and biophysical methods (e.g. surface tension, microviscosity).[12] Gluck *et al.*[58] were the first to demonstrate that the lecithin–sphiengomyelin ratio of AF provides an index of FLM. This ratio can be used to predict whether or not neonatal respiratory distress syndrome (NRDS) will develop in the infant if born within 24–48 h of amniocentesis. The same group measured other AF PLs, i.e. phosphatidylinositol and phosphatidylglycerol, and introduced the lung profile.[59] Clements *et al.* in 1972 introduced a simple and rapid screening method: the shake test.[60] Various tests have been introduced,[12] including lamellar body count and Doppler ultrasound.[61] These tests have good predictive values, high specificity, and sensitivity.

We have demonstrated that fetal urine contributes to AF PLs,[62] although in much lower concentrations than fetal pulmonary PLs.[63]

The pulmonary surfactants play a critical role in the survival of the fetus in the extrauterine life, especially in case of premature delivery and other forms of high-risk pregnancy, because a prompt and effective ventilation is required at birth. In turn, this depends on the alveolar stability (alveolar resistance to collapse) and thus on lung maturity. When FLM is not fully reached, delivery almost invariably results in NRDS. This disease is responsible for a major portion of perinatal mortality and morbidity (including neurologic and intellectual defects).

In recent years our understanding of perinatal lung development and of the pathophysiology of neonatal lung adaptation has increased considerably as a result of intensive studies by various investigators. Much experimental work has focused on the functional significance of the surfactant system of the lung during transition from fetal to neonatal life, on its role in the pathogenesis of NRDS, and on various methods that can facilitate the adaptation of the premature infant to extrauterine life.[64]

In 1903 Hochheim[65] first described the formation of hyaline membrane in the lungs of two infants dying from respiratory insufficiency in the neonatal period. Because of this finding, the term generally used to describe this disorder until 1959 was 'hyaline membrane disease' (HMD). Subsequently, it was realized that early pathologic hallmarks of HMD are atelectasis and intra-alveolar edema [in part perhaps representing unresorbed fetal pulmonary fluid (FPF)], whereas hyaline membranes, which develop at a later stage of the disease, may be absent in infants dying within a few hours of birth. The membranes are made up of degenerated epithelial cells, blood cells, fibrin, and components of the alveolar lining layer.

NRDS begins shortly after birth. The classical picture of tachypnea, expiratory grunting, sternal and intercostal inspiratory reactions, inability to maintain adequate oxygenation in room air, cyanosis, the diffuse hypolucency, and the air bronchogram at chest x-ray, all indicate alveolar instability, i.e. decreased functional residual capacity. Expiratory grunting represents an attempt by the newborn infant to overcome alveolar collapse. In fact, by prolonging the expiration and increasing the pressure within the alveoli, the neonate obtains a better diffusion of oxygen across the air–blood barrier. It is noteworthy that the method of therapy with mechanical ventilation of the lung under positive end-expiratory pressure is based on this premise. In fact, Gregory *et al.* noted that when cyanotic babies cried they turned pink as a result of Valsalva's maneuver.[66] The clinical picture of NRDS may be mimicked by 'transient tachypnea', or the so-called NRDS type II, due to slow resorption of FPF. However, this latter symptomatology usually disappears in less than 24 h, whereas that of NRDS lasts at least 24 h.[60]

The pathophysiology of NRDS was poorly understood until the discovery of pulmonary surfactants.[67,68] In 1959, Avery and Mead[69] were the first to demonstrate the deficiency of surfactants in saline extracts of lungs from infants who had died of NRDS. Several subsequent reports have confirmed that lungs of newborn infants with NRDS have a high surface tension[70,71] and therefore tend to collapse. This finding is in agreement with the abnormal characteristics observed in pressure–volume curves from lungs of infants with NRDS: high opening pressure required to inflate the alveoli; more important, poor ability to maintain a residual volume of air once all distending pressure is removed; and small hysteresis between inflation and deflation curves.[63,70,71]

Under normal conditions, the surface tension on expiration is extremely low because surfactants are present in the alveolar air–liquid interface. King and Clements[72] have suggested that the alveolar stability is determined by low surface compressibility. Colacicco and Scarpelli,[73,74] in their *in vitro* studies on surface properties of pulmonary dipalmitoyl lecithin, have indicated that surface tension is virtually zero and have thus substantiated the original 'zero surface tension, antiedema' theory of Pattle.[67] The implication of this is that surface tension is of primary importance in maintaining alveolar stability in the newborn infant as compared to older individuals, since the former have less rigid chest walls, and therefore the opposing force to alveolar collapse is low.[64,71] Many diverse theories have been proposed to define the etiology and pathogenesis of NRDS, most of which emphasize the prominent role of surfactant deficiency, secondary to prematurity. Liggins[75] showed in the 1960s that ablation of the anterior pituitary gland of the lamb fetus resulted in prolongation of pregnancy, whereas subsequent administration of ACTH or corticosteroids initiated labor. In the latter case, the preterm newborn seldom had serious lung problems such as RDS. This indicated, both to Liggins and Howie[76] and to Avery,[77] that administration of glucocorticoids to the mother might accelerate FLM. Liggins also demonstrated a primary role for progesterone in the maintenance of pregnancy in the sheep model, an observation that led to the estrogen–progesterone ratio hypothesis developed by Csapo.[78] Controlled clinical trials have been performed with i.m. injection of one, two, three doses of betamethasone (12 mg each, 24 h apart), dexamethasone (12 mg/day), or hydrocortisone (a single dose of 100 mg) to the mother. The results have been in general promising with few side effects. To avoid these it has been suggested by NIH consensus conferences and the European Study against Immature Lung that one course of betamethasone should be used, avoiding a second course of 1 week later.[79,80] Other drugs have been used both in animals and in humans to accelerate FLM, with less promising results than glucocorticoids.[79] Cosmi *et al.*[81,82] have injected supplementary surfactant (SS) obtained from pig lungs into the amniotic liquid close to the nostrils of the human fetus after the administration of aminophylline to the mother to induce FBMs, thereby favoring the entrance of SS into the fetal trachea and upper airways, in cases of severe fetal distress and/or preterm labor, and have obtained good results. These findings have been confirmed in humans by a Chinese group[83] and in animal experiments.[84] It should be noted that after the pioneering study of Fujiwara in 1980 supplementary surfactant has been used successfully for the treatment of rescue babies, i.e. with NRDS, and recently for early (prophylactic) treatment of NRDS (for a review see Cosmi *et al.*[80]).

Other important discoveries have been made in perinatal medicine, i.e. that prostaglandins have a definite role in parturition, followed by the observations that there is a surge of certain prostaglandins in maternal plasma and urine during parturition, that the administration of drugs such as aspirin and indomethacin suppresses uterine activity, and that administration of prostaglandin precursors (either exogenous, e.g. arachidonic acid, or endogenus, e.g. PLs from fetal urine into the AF[62]) is capable of inducing labor. It is now universally recognized that certain prostaglandins are clinically effective for induction of labor.

A link between infection and preterm delivery was proposed by Romero and Mazor[85] in 1988. The paradigm of infection-driven preterm labor has led to a better understanding of the cytokines produced by the placenta and the fetal membranes and by deciduas. It triggered the discovery of new uterotonins such as interleukin (IL) 1β, IL-6, tumor necrosis factor, endothelin-1, and transforming growth factor β-1, and of certain uterine relaxants, such as relaxin, prostaglandin inhibitors, thromboxane, and, more recently, nitric oxide. Cytokines and eicosanoids appear to interact on each other's production in a cascade.

At this point the complexities of the labor–delivery issue are abundantly clear as fetal–placental–maternal parameters search for a unifying mantle (placental insufficiency, fetal distress, and endorphins?) or new biologically active substances (peptides such as corticotrophin releasing hormone, placental activin, and oxytocin?).

The unique stresses, both positive and negative, that *Homo sapiens* brings to the 'evolutionary' picture are also quite considerable. For example, preterm labor is now linked to social, economic, and environmental factors, including low economic status, poor working conditions, environmental pollution, maternal malnutrition, and substance abuse with cocaine and other drugs, smoking and alcohol being particularly offensive.

Stress generically and related biologically active substances such as oxytocin, antidiuretic hormone, catecholamines, and certain placental hormones also involved in the perception of pain have been recognized as labor inducers. Indeed, humans and animals under stressful conditions tend to initiate labor. The best example is given by the siege of Leningrad during World War II, when half of the pregnant women either aborted or delivered preterm overnight.

Notable advances are being made by researchers and public health officials to ameliorate the social economic challenges and to find new therapeutic approaches, e.g. in the areas of pain relief, inhibition of preterm labor, and fetal therapy, including surgical approaches. The pioneering transabdominal intrauterine recording method induced five decades ago by Alvarez and Caldeyro-Barcia[10,12,30] has led to useful observations on the pharmacology of the human uterus and on the effects of uterine contractions on the fetus. Many utero-inhibitory drugs have been introduced and tested with different results.[86] A major advance of pain relief during labor and delivery has been the introduction of regional (epidural and spinal) blocks with the i.v. prophylactic hydration of the mother combined with 1000 NS or 500 dextrane solution 1 h before the block to avoid hypotension from sympathetic blockade.[86,87]

Many formidable challenges remain. For example, the mode of delivery, vaginal vs. cesarean section, is a matter of continuous debate; the biophysical approach to fetal monitoring during labor is moving into the era of computers and maybe of nanotechnology; the invasive technique of fetal scalp blood sampling and acid–base status determination have been replaced by pulse oximetry and other techniques. Ultrasound and Doppler technology, including three-dimensional imaging, have entered the labor world. New methods of pain relief are sought and used with increased frequency. New technologies are being introduced at such a pace that soon they will be extended to the home environment, where the use of telemedicine[88] can be applied, not only for monitoring uterine activity, blood pressure, and maternal glycemia, but also in the neonatal cardiorespiratory system for the diagnosis and treatment of apnea of prematurity and sudden infant death syndrome.[50] Assisted reproduction techniques also pose a particularly intriguing challenge to the perinatology team, i.e. the obstetrician, biologist, neonatologist, anesthesiologist, midwife, and nurse, because of the increased incidence of complications during pregnancy, labor, and delivery. Among the opportunities brought by the new technologies that address the fetus and its mother directly, are the questions of propriety and ethics,[38] which are among those covered in many symposia, workshops, congresses, and books on perinatal medicine.

It is noteworthy that in 1984 I founded in Erice (Sicily, Italy) a permanent School of Perinatal Medicine, which is very active. Furthermore, around the same year, I founded the Italian Society of Perinatal Medicine, which is composed of the above specialists. In 1988 I Founded the World Federation of Perinatal Medicine which in 1991 became the World Association of Perinatal Medicine.

It seems that we are now in a period of development of that art, which may be characterized as the period of assimilation into academic medicine and medical practice. To some degree or other, each one of us has known the aura of anxiety in which perinatal medicine is cast. To whom does it belong? Obviously, it belongs to the perinatologist. But then, who is the perinatologist? Of course he is each one of us. He is the obstetrician, the fetologist, the neonatologist, the pediatrician, the anesthesiologist, the basic scientist, ... He is in fact the amalgamation of all and in this amalgamation he loses the primordial title as he practices and becomes the perinatologist. At some centers he is so designated, and his discipline – perinatal medicine – is so recognized. But at too many other centers he continues to strive to dispel the anxiety and to complete the assimilation. There is no question that the fall of departmental barriers will result in even greater achievements in this new era of perinatal care. Eleanor Roosevelt once said that we are indeed one world and should strive to live our lives that way. Similarly, perinatal medicine is a unified body of knowledge, a science in its own right.

REFERENCES

1. Schutz AH. Fetal growth of man and other primates. *Quart Rev Biol* 1926;1:465.
2. Barcroft J. *Research on Pre-natal Life*. London: Blackwell, 1946.
3. Metcalfe J, Meschia G, Hellegers A, Prystowky H, Hukabee W, Barron DH. Observation on placental exchange of respiratory gases in pregnant ewes at high altitude. *Quart J Exp Physiol* 1962;47:74.
4. Adamsons K Jr, James LS, Towell ME, Lucey JF. Physiologic observation during induced anemia in utero in the rhesus monkey. *J Pediatr* 1965;67:1042.
5. Joelsson I, Cosmi EV. Effects of maternal anesthesia upon the cardiovascular system and acid–base state of the fetus. In Centaro A., Ragazzini F, eds. *Proceedings of a Symposium on Problems of Fetal Distress*. Padua, Italy: Piccin, 1967:771.

6. Condorelli S, Cosmi EV. L'impiego di elettrodi endocavitari sensibili alle modificazioni dei potenziali elettrici nello studio della velocità di circolo materno–fetale. *Acta Anaesthesiol Ital* 1970; 21:699.
7. Dawes GS. *Fetal and Neonatal Physiology*. Chicago: Year Book Medical Publishers Inc., 1968.
8. Metcalfe J. Placental gas transfer. *Anesthesiology* 1965;26:460.
9. James LS, Weisbrot JM, Prince CE, Holaday DA, Apgar V. Acid–base status of human infants in relation to birth asphyxia and onset of respiration. *J Pediatr* 1958;52:379.
10. Caldeyro-Barcia R. *The Physiology of Prematurity*. New York: Josia Macy Jr. Foundation, 1956.
11. Saling F. Mikroblutuntersuchungen am Feten: klinischer Einsatz and erste Ergebnisse. *Z Geburtshilfliche Gynakol* 1964;162:56.
12. Cosmi EV, Caldeyro-Barcia R. Fetal homeostasis. In Cosmi EV, ed. *Obstetric Anesthesia and Perinatology*. New York: Appleton–Century–Crofts, 1981:chap 7.
13. Motta PM, Nottola SA, Micara G, Familiari G. Ultrastructure of unfertilized oocytes and polispermic embryos in an IVF-ET programme. In Jones HW Jr, Schrader C, eds. *In Vitro Fertilisation and Other Assisted Reproduction*. New York: New York Academy of Sciences, 1988;541:367.
14. Brambati B, Simoni G. Diagnosis of fetal trisomy 21 in first trimester. *Lancet* 1983;1:586.
15. Bohn H. Die Antigen der menschlichen Placenta. *Klin Wochenschr* 1975;53:554.
16. Adinolfi A. On a non invasive approach to prenatal diagnosis based on the detection of fetal nucleated cells in maternal blood samples. *Prenat Diagn* 1991;11:799.
17. Ferranti G, Mezzanotte F, Cosmi EV. Fetal cells detection in maternal circulation. In Cosmi EV, ed. *New Technologies in Reproductive Medicine, Neonatology and Gynecology*. Lancaster, UK: Parthenon Publishing Group, 1999:39.
18. Lo YM, Corbetta N, Chamberlain PF, *et al*. Presence of fetal DNA in maternal plasma and serum. *Lancet* 1997;350:485.
19. Farina A, Rizzo N, Concu M, *et al*. Lower maternal PLAC1 mRNA in pregnancies complicated with vaginal bleeding (threatened abortion <20 weeks) and a surviving fetus. *Clin Chem* 2004;October 28.
20. Diczfalusy E. Endocrine functions of the human fetus and placenta. *Am J Obstet Gynecol* 1974;119:419.
21. Brinsmead MV, Liggins GC. Somatomedins and other growth factors in fetal growth. In Scarpelli EM, Cosmi EV, eds. *Reviews in Perinatal Medicine*. New York: Raven, 1979;3:207–42.
22. Fraioli F, Genazzani AR. Human placental β-endorphin. *Gynecol Obstet Invest* 1980;11:37.
23. Ramsey EM, Dodder NW. *Placental Vasculature and Circulation*. Stuttgart: Georg Thieme, 1980.
24. Rudolph AM. Cardiac output in the mammalian fetus. In Scarpelli EM, Cosmi EV, eds. *Reviews in Perinatal Medicine*. Baltimore: University Park Press, 1976;1:35.
25. Assali NS, Brinkman CR III, Nuwayhid B. Comparison of maternal and fetal cardiovascular functions in acute and chronic experiments in the sheep. *Am J Obstet Gynecol* 1974;120:411.
26. Kirkpatrik SE, Pitlick PT, Naliboff J, Friedman WF. Frank-Starling relationship as an important determinant of fetal cardiac output. *Am J Physiol* 1976;231:495.
27. Caldeyro-Barcia R, Mèndez-Bauer C, Pose S, Poseiro JJ. Fetal monitoring in labor. In Fallace HM, Gold EM, Lis EF, eds. *Maternal and Child Health Practices: Problems, Resources and Methods of Delivery*. Springfield, IL: C. Thomas, 1973:332.
28. Elsner R, Hammond DD, Parker HR. Circulatory responses to asphyxia on pregnant and fetal animals: A comparative study of Weddel seals and sheeps. *Yale J Biol Med* 1970;42:202.
29. Condorelli S, Cosmi EV. Cardio-vascular respiratory reflexes in the adult and fetal animal: Evidence for a reflex originating in skeletal muscle. In Nahas JJ, *et al*., eds. *Basis Fundamentales de l'anesthesie et de la reanimation obstetricales*. Paris: Libraire Arnette, 1972:275.
30. Caldeyro-Barcia R. Uterine contractility in obstetrics. Main lecture, *Second World Congress of the International Federation of Obstetricians and Gynecologists*. Montreal: Librairie Beauchemin Limitée, 1959;1:65.
31. Caldeyro-Barcia R, Mèndez-Bauer C, Poseiro JJ, *et al*. Control of human fetal heart rate during labor. In Cassels DE, ed. *The Heart and Circulation in the Newborn and Infant*. New York: Grune and Stratton, 1966:7.
32. Hon EH, *et al*. *An Atlas of Fetal Heart Rate Patterns*. New Haven: Harty, 1968.
33. Vasicka A, Hutchinson HT, Rylander WJ, Murray C. Simultaneous monitoring of uterine contractility and fetal heart rate using an intra-amniotic platinum electrode. *Obstet Gynecol* 1963;22:271.
34. Pardi G, Tucci E, Uderso A, Zanini D. Fetal electrocardiogram changes in relation to fetal heart rate patterns during labor. *Am J Obstet Gynecol* 1974;118:243.
35. Arduini D, Rizzo G. Normal values of pulsatility index from fetal vessels: A cross-sectional study on 1556 healthy fetuses. *J Perinat Med* 1990;18:165.
36. Campbell S, Bower SJ. Doppler velocimetry of the uterine artery as a screening test in pregnancy. In Chervenak FA, Isaacson GC, Campbell S, eds. *Ultrasound in Obstetrics and Gynecology*. London: Little, Brown and Company, 1993:579.
37. Kurjak A, alud I, Predanic M, Kupesic S. Transvaginal color and pulsed Doppler study of uterine blood flow in the first and early second trimester of pregnancy: Normal vs abnormal. *J Ultrasound Med* 1994;13:43.
38. Chervenak FA, McCullough LB. Ethical issues in obstetric ultrasound. In Chervenak FA, Isaacson GC, Campbell S, eds. *Ultrasound in Obstetrics and Gynecology*. London: Little, Brown and Company, 1993:277.
39. Ahlfeld F. Die intrauterine Tätigkeit der Thorax und Zwerchfellmuskulatur. Intrauterine Atmung. *Monatsschr Geburtshilfliche Gynakol* 1905;21:143.
40. Weber H. Über physiologische Atmungsbewegungen des Kindnes im Uterus. Inaugural dissertation, Universität Marbourg, 1888.
41. Ferroni E. Osservazioni e ricerche sui movimenti ritmici fetali intrauterini. *Ann Ostet Ginecol (Ital)* 1899;21:897.
42. Reifferscheid K. Über intrauterine Atembewegungen des Foetus. *Dtsch Med Wochenschr* 1911;37:887.
43. Duenhoelter JH, Pritchard JA. Fetal respiration: A review. *Am J Obstet Gynecol* 1977;129:326.
44. Dalton KJ, Dawes GS, Patrick JE. Fetal breathing and heart rate variability. In Rooth G, Bratteby LE, eds. *Perinatal Medicine*. Stockholm: Almqvist and Wiksell International, 1976:187.
45. Dawes GS. Effects of fetal hypoxemia on breathing movements and endocrine system. In Scarpelli EM, Cosmi EV, eds. *Reviews in Perinatal Medicine*. Baltimore: Baltimore University Park Press, 1976;1:333.
46. Cosmi EV, Condorelli S. Onset of breathing. In Mushin WW, *et al*., eds. *First International Seminar on Psycological Basis of Anesthesiology*. Padua, Italy: Piccin, 1975:239.
47. Cosmi EV. Drugs, anesthetics and the fetus. In Scarpelli EM, Cosmi EV, eds. *Reviews in Perinatal Medicine*. Baltimore: Baltimore University Park Press, 1976;1:191.
48. Scarpelli EM, Condorelli S, Cosmi EV. Cutaneous stimulation and generation of breathing in the fetus. *Pediatr Res* 1977;11:24.
49. Cosmi EV, Anceschi MM, Cosmi E, Piazze JJ, La Torre R. Ultrasonographic patterns of fetal breathing movements in normal pregnancy. *Int J Gynecol Obstet* 2003;80:285.
50. Cosmi EV, Sacco R, Anceschi MM, Bastianon V. Treatment of apnea of prematurity and SIDS with an electric stimulator including home care telemonitoring. In Cosmi EV, ed. *Proceedings of the Symposium "The Place for New Technologies in Gynecology, Obstetrics and Perinatology,"* CNR, Rome, June 26–29. Rome: Monduzzi, 1995:267–72.
51. Bevis DCA. Blood pigments in haemolytic diseases of the newborn. *J Obstet Gynaecol Br Emp* 1956;63:68.
52. Liley AW. Liquor amnii analysis in the management of the pregnancy complicated by rhesus sensitisation. *Am J Obstet Gynecol* 1961;82:1359.
53. Freda VJ, Gorman JG, Pollack W. Prevention of rhesus haemolytic disease (letter to the editor). *Lancet* 1965:690.
54. Freda VJ, Gorman JG, Pollack W. Rh factor: Prevention of isoimmunisation and clinical trial on mothers. *Science* 1966; 151:828.
55. Freda VJ. Recent obstetrical advance in the Rh problem. *Bull N Y Acad Med* 1966;42:474.
56. Valenti C, Shutta EJ, Keathy T. Prenatal diagnosis of Down's syndrome. *Lancet* 1968;27(2):220.
57. Steele M, Breg W Jr. Chromosome analysis of human amniotic fluid cell. *Lancet* 1966:383.
58. Gluck L, Kulovich MV, Borer RC, *et al*. Diagnosis of respiratory distress syndrome by amniocentesis. *Am J Obstet Gynecol* 1971;109:440.
59. Kulovich MV, Hallman M, Gluck L, *et al*. The lung profile. *Am J Obstet Gynecol* 1979;135:57.

60. Clements JA, Platzker ACG, Tierney DF, *et al.* Assessment of the risk of the respiratory distress syndrome by a rapid test for surfactant in amniotic fluid. *N Engl J Med* 1972;286:1077.
61. Piazze JJ, Anceschi MM, Picone G, Cerekja A, La Torre R, Cosmi EV. Association between maternal fetal Doppler velocimetry and fetal lung maturity. *J Perinat Med* 2003;31:484.
62. Condorelli S, Cosmi EV, Scarpelli EM. Extrapulmonary source of amniotic fluid phospholipids. *Am J Obstet Gynecol* 1974; 15:118.
63. Setnikar I, Agostoni E, Taglietti A. The fetal lung, a source of amniotic fluid. *Proc Soc Exp Biol Med* 1959;108:842.
64. Cosmi EV, Robertson B. Morphologic and functional aspects of neonatal adaptation. In Cosmi EV, ed. *Obstetric Anesthesia and Perinatology.* New York: Appleton–Century–Crofts, 1981: chap 16.
65. Hocheim K. Über einige Befunde in den Lungen von Neugeborenen und die Beziehung derselben zur Aspiration von Fruchtwasser. *Zentralbl Pathol* 1903;14:537.
66. Gregory GA, Kitterman JA, Phibbs PH, *et al.* Treatment of idiopathic respiratory-distress syndrome with continuous positive airway pressure. *N Engl J Med* 1971;17:1333.
67. Pattle RE. Properties function and origin of alveolar lining layer. *Nature* 1955;175:1125.
68. Clements JA. Surface tension of lung extract. *Proc Soc Exp Biol Med* 1957;95:170.
69. Avery MF, Mead J. Surface properties in relation to atelectasis and hyaline membrane disease. *Am J Dis Child* 1959;97:517.
70. Grunewald P, Johnson RP, Husteas RF, Clements JA. Correlation of mechanical properties of infant lungs with surface activity of extracts. *Proc Soc Exp Biol Med* 1962;109:369.
71. Scarpelli EM. *The Surfactant System of the Lung.* Lea & Fabiger, 1963.
72. King RJ, Clements JA. Surface active materials from dog lung II. Composition and physiological correlation. *Am J Physiol* 1972; 223:715.
73. Colacicco G, Cosmi EV, Ray AK, *et al.* Betamimetics, prostaglandins and lung maturity. Presented at the *8th World Congress on Gynaecology and Obstetrics,* Mexico. *Excerpta Med Cong Ser* 1976;396:144.
74. Cosmi EV, Condorelli S, Scarpelli EM. Pulmonary surfactant in anesthesia and resuscitation. *Acta Anaesthesiol* 1970; 31(Suppl):95.
75. Liggins GC. Premature parturition after infusion of corticotrophin or cortisol into foetal lambs. *J Endocrinol* 1968;42:323.
76. Liggins GC, Howie RN. A controlled trial of antepartum glucocorticoid treatment for prevention of the respiratory distress syndrome in premature infants. *Pediatrics* 1972;50:515.
77. Avery ME. Pharmacological approaches to the acceleration of fetal lung maturation. *Br Med Bull* 1975;31:13.
78. Csapo A. The diagnostic significance of the intrauterine pressure. *Obstet Gynaecol Surv* 1970;25:403.
79. Cosmi EV, Di Renzo GC, Anceschi MM. *The Surfactant System of the Lung: Prevention and Treatment of Neonatal and Adult Respiratory Distress Syndrome.* London: MacMillan Press, 1991.
80. Cosmi EV, Breart G, Halliday HL, Saugstad OD, Szabó I, Visser GHA. Antenatal and postnatal management of fetal lung immaturity in Europe. In *Prenatal and Neonatal Medicine.* London: Parthenon Publishing Group, 2001;6(Suppl 2):1–88.
81. Cosmi EV, La Torre R, Di Iorio R, Anceschi MM. Surfactant administration to the human fetus in utero: A new approach prevention of neonatal respiratory distress syndrome (NRDS). *J Perinat Med* 1996;24:191–3.
82. Cosmi EV, La Torre R, Piazze JJ, *et al.* Intraamniotic surfactant for prevention of neonatal respiratory distress syndrome (NRDS): Rationale and personal experience. *Eur J Obstet Gynecol Reprod Biol* 1997;71:135–9.
83. Zhang JP, Wang YL, Wang YH, Zhang R, Chen H, Su HB. Prophylaxis of neonatal respiratory distress syndrome by intramniotic administration of pulmonary surfactant. *Chin Med J* 2004;117:120.
84. Illia R, Solana C, Oliveti P, Toblli J, Imaz MU, Habich D. Evidence of fetal pulmonary aspiration of intraamniotic administered surfactant in animal experiment. *J Perinat Med* 2004; 32:354.
85. Romero R, Mazor M. Infection and preterm labor. *Clin Obstet Gynecol* 1988;31:553.
86. Cosmi EV. Drugs and anesthetics in the management of preterm labor and delivery. In Cosmi EV, ed. *Obstetric Anesthesia and Perinatology.* New York: Appleton–Century–Crofts, 1981:chap 15.
87. Marx GF, Cosmi EV, Wollman SB. Biochemical status and clinical condition of mother and infant at caesarean section. *Anesth Analg* 1969;48:986.
88. Di Renzo GC, Luzi G, Caserta G, Clerici G, Cosmi EV. The role of telemetry in perinatal monitoring. *J Perinat Med* 1994;22:517.

SECTION I

Neonatology

Section Editors: **M. Levene and M. R. G. Carrapato**

1 Transition at birth

O. D. Saugstad

Introduction

The transition from fetal to postnatal life is characterized by a number of dramatic changes in physiological, biochemical, immunological, and hormonal functions. The fetus is fully dependent on the maternal supply not only of oxygen and nutrients but also of a number of hormones and other important substances. The thermal control of the fetus is also taken care of by the mother. Intestinal and breathing movements as well as non-shivering thermogenesis are partially inhibited. Large organs such as the lungs and liver are not very active. The fetus is also asleep most of the time. These are some important reasons why the oxygen requirements and metabolism are low in fetal life. Cardiac output is low with a low systemic blood pressure. A relatively low blood glucose level and oxygen supply is therefore sufficient to ensure substrate for energy metabolism at this stage.

During the last trimester the fetus prepares itself to meet the extrauterine milieu; energy stores are established, minerals and trace elements are deposited, both white and brown fat accumulate, the lungs mature both structurally and biochemically. The last means that the surfactant system matures and the antioxidative defense develops in order for the fetus to breathe and to be able to withstand the sudden increased oxidative stress induced by the high oxygen concentration in ambient air. Many epithelial transport functions of different organs mature in late fetal and early neonatal life.

After birth, the newly born infant is responsible for its own oxygenation and ventilation. The partially inhibited status of the fetus is immediately reversed at birth. It is awake, aroused, breathing, and crying. Metabolism increases with a subsequent increased oxygen demand, and the newborn can initiate lipolysis and mobilize glucose. The higher oxygen consumption of the brain is one reason the newborn brain is more vulnerable to hypoxia than in fetal life. The sharp increase in oxygen exposure makes it necessary for the newborn infant to protect itself from oxygen toxicity. Transition to birth is therefore not only a matter of redistribution of the circulation, maturation of the lungs and the surfactant system with alveolar gas exchange, it is much more complex and probably only a small part of this is understood. In the following some of these aspects will be discussed.

Growth

General principles

The greatest growth rate in human life occurs in the fetal period. The increase from a fertilized egg to a term newborn infant is in weight 6×10^{12}, in length 5000-fold, and in surface area 61×10^{6}. After birth, growth slows down, still the greatest postnatal growth rate occurs immediately after birth.

Prenatal growth is dependent on maternal, placental, and fetal factors. In the first trimester growth occurs by increase in cell number, in the second trimester there is an increase both in number and in cellular size. In the third trimester growth is mainly by cellular growth since the rate of mitosis slows down. During the first two trimesters the fetus has reached approximately one-third of its term weight. In this period only 50 g of fat is accumulated in contrast to approximately 500 g deposited in the last trimester. Of the approximately 95 kcal/kg/day needed by the fetus 40 kcal are spent for growth. Prenatal growth is dependent on autocrine and paracrine growth factors such as insulin-like factors 1 and 2; however, insulin also plays a major role in prenatal growth. Macrosomia is a well-known effect of fetal hyperinsulinism, and these children have increased body fat at 1 year of age. Abnormal patterns in insulin-like growth factor (IGF) 2 gene expression may lead to the Bechwith Wiedemann syndrome. These infants are large with elevated insulin levels.

Postnatal growth is mainly regulated through pituitary growth hormones (GHs), thyroid hormone, and other hormones. GH is high in the fetus; however, the number of GH receptors is low. That GH plays some role in fetal growth is reflected in the poor growth of children with GH deficiency or GH receptor deficiency (Laron syndrome), and its action is mediated by IGFs. During the first weeks of extrauterine life GH falls, and already in the first day of life a pulsatile release of GH is detected with a pulse periodicity of

73 min, with higher peaks and more frequent pulses found in small for gestational age (SGA) than in appropriate for gestational age (AGA) infants. This pulsatility is controlled by the stimulatory GH-releasing hormone and the inhibitory somatostatin, both produced in the hypothalamus. Thyroid hormone is a major factor in postnatal growth and an acute elevation with a peak in thyroid stimulating hormone (TSH) is found immediately after birth, with a decline the first 5–6 days after birth. Leptin is produced in adipose tissue and also regulates growth. Its role in fetal life is unknown, but high concentrations are found in the umbilical cord with a gradual decrease over the next 3 months. Androgens decrease leptin values, so that girls have higher concentrations than boys from birth; the significance of this seem not to be understood.

The changes in body composition the fetus undergoes with the advancement of gestation is a progressive decrease in total water, extracellular water, sodium, and chloride and an increase in intracellular water, potassium, calcium, and magnesium. The postnatal body composition changes are characterized by an increase in adipose tissue with a peak around 4–6 months, a progressive decrease in body water with a relative increase of intracellular water.[1–6]

Fluid shift

In early fetal life approximately 95% of the fetus is water, which gradually decreases throughout gestation, being 80% at 8 months and 75% at term. Mode of delivery does not seem to influence this. Simultaneously with this decline in body water there is a drastic decrease in extracellular and a gradual increase in intracellular water. This tendency continues until 9 months of age, when body water constitutes 62%. However, the total body water related to surface area does not change very much in this period. Maximal intracellular water of 43% of body weight is reached at 2 months of age at the same time when extracellular water is 30%. The term newborn loses 5–10% of its body weight and the preterm more. This is mainly due to loss of water; however, it is not clear whether this loss is predominantly from the extra- or intracellular space or perhaps both.

In the newborn's first days of life the blood volume is to a large extent dependent on placental transfusion at the time of delivery, which can be up to 25–50 ml/kg within 3 min. Whether or not this increase in blood volume of 50% is harmful is not clear. A delayed cord clamping may lead to a gradual increase in hematocrit within a couple of hours. This is caused by plasma loss of 30 ml/kg the following 4 h due to a shift of fluid from the plasma into the interstitial space in addition to an increased urinary output.[7,8]

Recently, it has become clear that specific water channels, aquaporines, play an important role in water transport and water balance. Aquaporines 1 and 4 have been found in the brain, 9 in the skin, 2 in the kidney, etc. The newborn kidneys' reduced ability to concentrate the urine is probably due to the lack of aquaporines. Aquaporines are active also in the perinatal period and probably are important for removing fluid from the lung and in so-called transitoric tachypne of the newborn.

Carbohydrates

Glucose is the major source of energy in fetal life and the fetus is entirely dependent on glucose delivery from the mother. It seems that the human fetus does not produce glucose until the end of gestation, and the brain requires a continuous glucose supply that is received from the mother – at term at a rate of 4–7 mg/kg/min. This equals 6–10 g glucose/kg/day and represents approximately 60% of the calories needed by the fetus. Glucose is transported by facilitated carrier-mediated placental diffusion. Several facilitated glucose transporters have been identified and recently cloned. They comprise a family of structurally related families and are designated GLUT. The primary function of these is to mediate the exchange of glucose between blood and the cytoplasm of the cell. Several of these GLUT are present in early fetal life.

Blood glucose is lower in the fetus compared with the mother but there is a significant correlation between maternal and fetal levels at least if the maternal levels are not too low (< 4.4 mmol/l), below which fetal concentrations are independent of maternal levels. At birth, the transplacental supply of nutrients is abruptly interrupted. The newborn infant therefore has to produce glucose from its own endogenous stores until feeding is started. At birth blood glucose is 60–75% of maternal levels and then falls over the next 1–2 h stabilizing at 2.5–3.3 mmol/l (45–60 mg/dl) in healthy term infants within 24 h. Maternal glucose supplementation during labor and delivery seems to blunt this decrease. With the initiation of feeding it increases, and after 24 h is between 2.5–5.0 mmol/l (45–90 mg/dl).

Glucose can be metabolized to either lactate, which occurs in anaerobic conditions, or to acetyl coenzyme A (Ac-CoA) under aerobic conditions. Pyruvate can be metabolized to either lactate or Ac-CoA; this is partly regulated by the relative amounts of the isoenzymes of lactate dehydrogenase (LDH). In adult brain the LDH isoenzyme composition favors aerobic oxidation of glucose but in the fetal and newborn brain the LDH composition allows anaerobic glycolysis. The placenta is impermeable to both insulin and glucagon, which are produced by the fetus at least from the 10th week of gestation. Glucose stimulates insulin in the third trimester only.

In late gestation, approximately 50% of the glucose is converted to glycogen in the liver and muscle, and to fat in the liver and adipose tissue. Glucose storage is regulated primarily by insulin but also by glucocorticoids. Glycogen is low until approximately 36 weeks of gestation; however, it triples in the liver until term, when it reaches a maximum both in the liver and in the skeletal muscles. In other organs such as myocardium and lungs the peak is reached somewhat earlier, declining toward term. Postnatally, glycogen is the initial substrate for glucose, but only for a few hours. Within 24 h after birth the glycogen stores are more or less exhausted. Gluconeogenesis from fat and protein is therefore necessary to meet the metabolic demands, and this is in principle a postnatal event. Fat is therefore an important substrate for glucose production in the early newborn period. Although key enzymes for gluconeogenesis are present in the liver from early fetal life, gluconeogenetic activity is not expressed *in utero*, at least not until near term. In late gestation, fetal gluconeogenesis therefore occurs and may contribute to fetal glucose levels especially if the glucose supply from the mother is reduced, for instance, during maternal fasting or by intrauterine growth retardation. Initiation of lipolysis and gluconeogenesis is promoted by hormonal and enzymatic changes occurring in the first day of life. The insulin/glucagon ratio rapidly decreases after birth and the high postnatal concentrations of catecholamines, cortisone, and TSH contribute to this. In the newborn infant glycerol can be converted to glucose, contributing up to 20% of the hepatic glucose production. It has been shown that preterm infants of less than 28 weeks' gestation have the capability of gluconeogenesis from glycerol.[9–13]

Proteins

In the second and third trimester protein synthesis is especially high, however, with a reduced rate toward term. The term newborn infant has about 0.5 kg of protein after a many-fold linear increase in the last half of the gestation. Protein synthesis slows down toward term but is still high, approximately fivefold higher than adult levels. In fact, not only synthesis is high in fetal life, but breakdown of proteins is also increased, giving a high protein turnover in the fetus. There is a substantial difference between organs, with the highest rate of protein synthesis in the placenta, heart, and liver (half-life 1 day) compared with a half-life of 1 week in muscle. A number of growth factors may be responsible for this, such as IGF-1. For this reason the amino acid concentration in fetal plasma is higher than later in life, and the fetal/maternal amino acid ratio in plasma is high with a peak in the second trimester, when it is approximately 3:1, falling to 1.5:1 toward term. Intrauterine growth retardation is characterized by a falling fetal/maternal plasma amino acid ratio mainly due to an augmentation in the maternal levels.

Amino acids are transported across the placenta by both a direct active transfer of essential amino acids and placental cytosolic synthesis of non-essential amino acids. A number of amino acid transporters – at least 12 – have recently been identified. The rate of amino acid utilization is about 4 g/kg/day, similar to the estimated intake of very premature infants. A protein intake in the postnatal period of 2.8 g/kg/day is close to the minimal intake needed to ensure weight gain and nitrogen retention equal to intrauterine rates, and a protein intake of 3–4.3 g/kg/day is recommended. Some amino acids that are non-essential in postnatal life are essential in fetal life due to inadequate maturation of enzyme systems. One example of this is the absence of cysthionase, making the fetus completely dependent on the mother's cystine supply. During the first hours postnatally there is a rapid fall in plasma amino acid levels.[14,15]

Lipids

The fetus requires both essential and non-essential fatty acids from the mother, and fat represents one-sixth of the body weight at term.

Free fatty acid supply to the fetus may occur through a process of facilitated membrane translocation involving a plasma membrane protein, placental synthesis and release into the umbilical circulation, or lipolysis of triglycerides, lipoproteins, or phospholipids from either the maternal or the fetal side. The free fatty acid concentration and composition in the fetus reflect maternal values. It is well known that maternal manipulation with diet may change the growth and development of the fetus. For instance, mothers fed a diet high in docosahexenoic acid deliver babies with higher birth weight. These children seem to mature earlier and have a higher IQ at the age of 4 years. Triglycerides are hydrolyzed to fatty acids by lipoprotein lipases, which are secreted by capillary endothelium. Lipoprotein lipase is stimulated by insulin and is present in fetal life with low activities in muscle and heart but higher in the lungs. This may be of importance for surfactant synthesis and maturation. After birth, the activity of this enzyme increases both in preterm and term infants. However, in preterm infants the clearance of circulating triglycerides is reduced due to a lower enzyme activity than in the term infants, and this activity seems to be directly related to the degree of prematurity. In the human fetus, the enzymes for cholesterol and lipoprotein metabolism develop early in gestation. As low-density lipoprotein (LDL) receptor expression also increases in gestation serum cholesterol and LDL decrease to levels lower than that observed in early postnatal life. In breast-fed infants these metabolites increase rapidly and are doubled from day 1 to day 7 of life but are still only half of the adult levels.

In the last 8 weeks of gestation subcutaneous fat increases rapidly from approximately 20 to 350 g, and deep body fat from 10 to 80 g. The total fat content increases from 6 g at 22 weeks to 500 g at term.

Fatty acid catabolism is an important energy source in postnatal life. High concentrations of free fatty acids and glycerol soon after birth indicate the onset of lipolysis and lipid oxidation. Free fatty acids and glycerol increase sharply and peak around 120 min after birth. Beta-oxidation of fatty acids occurs in the mitochondria. Ac-CoA is transesterified to carnitine by carnitine acyltransferase located on the inner mitochondrial membrane. Fatty acid oxidation is limited in the fetal myocardium because of a low concentration of carnitine and a limited number of mitochondria. Liver, brain, placenta, and lung also have limited capacity to oxidize fatty acids. After birth, however, fatty acid oxidation increases substantially and remains high until the time of weaning.

Lipogenesis is found in fetal tissue from 12 weeks of gestation and is stimulated by insulin and inhibited by glucagon or cAMP. Fatty acid synthesis declines after birth when the diet is milk, which is rich in fat. Placental transfer of ketone bodies in contrast to glycerol has been described. The fetus uses ketone bodies as substrates for oxidation and lipogenesis.[10,16–19]

Mineral metabolism

The placenta actively transports calcium to the fetus to allow rapid fetal skeletal mineralization. From 20 to 26 weeks of gestation fetal levels are maintained about 0.25 mmol/l (1mg/dl) above the maternal level. In the last trimester calcium stores quadruples. In humans two-thirds of the mean 30 g calcium in a healthy term fetus are transported in the last trimester. At birth the constant calcium supply is interrupted and there is a normal fall in serum calcium in the first hours after birth, reaching a stable level after 24–48 h of age of about 2–2.25 mmol/l. During the next few days there is a subsequent gradual increase, resulting in serum calcium of about 2.5 mmol/l at 1 week of age. In one study serum ionized calcium concentrations decreased from a mean 1.45 mmol/l at birth to 1.33 mmol/l at 2 h and 1.23 mmol/l at 24 h of age.

At birth parathyroid hormone is low, increasing two- to fourfold during the first 2 days of life, giving an efficient response after 3–4 days. In contrast, calcitonin levels are high in the newborn, thereby inhibiting calcium mobilization from bone. Magnesium, zinc, and phosphorus are also transported actively across the placenta from the mother to the fetus. During the first week of life magnesium levels show small variations, correlating directly with serum calcium and inversely with phosphorus. Adequate zinc levels are needed for normal fetal growth and postnatally the requirements are approximately 2 mg/day. Zinc deficiency in infancy may lead to failure to thrive and reduced immunological function. Globally, zinc deficiency represents a major health problem in infancy.[20–23]

Hormones

The endocrine system is involved in growth, reproduction, cellular nutrition, as well as energy, thermal, cardiovascular and fluid homeostasis. Many hormones do not cross the placenta but are found in the fetus around 10–12 weeks of gestation. This is true for GH, insulin, prolactin, and thyroxin.

Prolactin may play an important role in regulating fluid balance in fetal life. At term its levels are 20-fold higher than adult levels and decline rapidly in the first weeks after birth. This reduction may be linked to the decline in total body water after birth. Prolactin may also have a maturational effect on the pulmonary surfactant system in combination with glucocorticoids and thyroidea hormones. Thyrotropin-releasing factor regulates TSH and prolactin secretion. As early as 12 weeks of gestation it is clear that the fetus produces thyroxin and around 13 weeks of gestation TSH-producing cells have been identified. TSH both stimulates growth and contributes to differentiation of the thyroid gland. TSH does not cross the placenta and tri-iodothyronine (T3) and thyroxine (T4) do not cross in sufficient quantity for the fetus. The fetus is therefore dependent on its own pituitary and thyroid hormones in addition to supply from the mother. In contrast, thyrotropin-releasing factor crosses the placenta and stimulates fetal TSH. Fetal total and free T4 as well as thyroxin-binding globulin values increase during the gestation and reach the level of the mean adult values around 36 weeks. In umbilical cord blood TSH is low and increases rapidly within the first 10–15 min after birth, and T4 reaches a peak after 48 h as a response to the high TSH concentration. TSH remains high the first days of life before it reaches its low normal adult levels. The half-time of T4 is much shorter in the neonatal period compared with adult life, making the thyroxin requirements many times higher than in the adult period.

From the eighth week of gestation the fetal adrenal converts prenenolone to dehydroepiandrosterone sulfate, which in the fetal liver and other tissues is hydroxylated to 16-hydroxy-dehydroepiandrosterone, which passes to the placenta and forms estriol. Since estrogen is important in maintaining pregnancy the fetus therefore contributes to this itself.

The fetal adrenal cortex promotes fetal organ enzyme maturation and in the last part of gestation adrenocortico-tropic hormone and cortisol levels increase in the fetus influencing maturation of enzyme systems in the lung, gastrointestinal tract, and possibly other organs. After birth, cortisol levels decrease, reaching adult levels by the age of 2–3 months.[2,22,24–27]

Stress at birth

There is a dramatic activation of the adrenal, the sympathetic, and the parasympathetic systems toward term. The sympathoadrenal system develops in fetal life and the newborn infant has large adrenals and extra chromaffin tissue in the paraganglia. The adrenal cortex matures toward term and releases substantial amounts of epinephrine and norepinephrine near

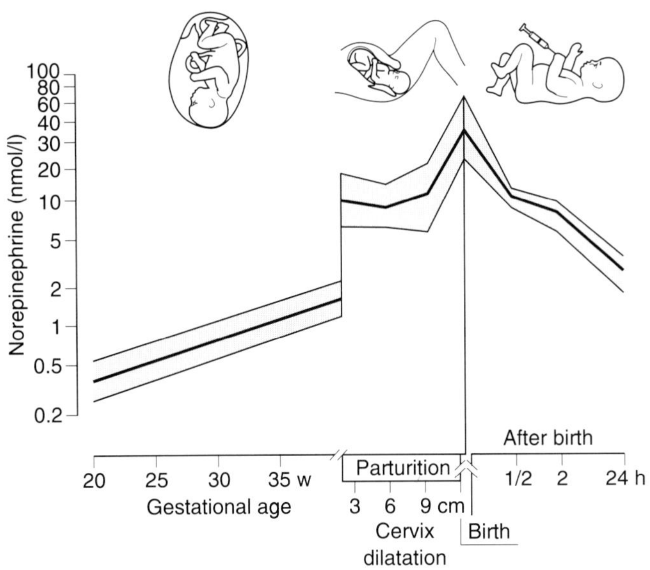

Figure 1.1 Norepinephrine concentration before, during, and after birth. From Lagercrantz.[28]

term. Corticosteroids around birth mature the surfactant system by inducing its synthesis, as well as antioxyenzymes in the lung, and further play a role in the labor process. Corticosteroids also induce the expression of phenylethanolamine-*N*-methyl-transferase, which converts norepinephrine to epinephrine. The transition at birth is characterized by high levels of catecholamines, angiotensin and vasopressin. The catecholamine levels are higher than in any other period of life under physiological circumstances. Norepinephrine constitutes approximately 85% of the total catecholamines and in plasma is normally increased 20-fold or more during the first stage of labor. Also, in the newborn infant the catecholamine levels are very high, continuing to rise immediately after birth then decreasing to the prelabor levels during the first 24 h or so (Figure 1.1). This is vital for successful postnatal adaptation.

The newly born infant is normally awake and alert. In these few hours, before it falls asleep, it is supersensitive to sensory stimulation. This arousal might be caused by the catecholamine surge at birth. An activation of catecholamines in the brain, especially in the locus ceruleus in the brainstem, takes place, and the turnover of norepinephrine increases several fold before birth. The high concentration of catecholamines also increases myocardial contractility, increases peripheral vascular resistance, promotes surfactant secretion, reduces production and increases absorption of lung water, mobilizes glucose and free fatty acids as energy substrates, and initiates non-shivering thermogenesis. The increase in circulating catecholamines at birth therefore probably is vital for cardiovascular adaptation at birth. Rhythmic lung inflation also increases plasma catecholamine levels as does cooling and umbilical cord clamping.

Sympathetic nervous activity, especially of the baroreceptors and chemoreceptors, increases during gestation and the influence of the parasympathetic system on the resting heart rate increases with maturation. In fetal life sympathetic tone is high and is important in maintaining fetal arterial blood pressure. The basal sympathetic tone fluctuates in the normal state and this is more important in fetal than in newborn life to generate blood pressure variability and is related to change in the behavioral state of the fetus. At birth the activity increases further, for instance, in renal sympathetic nerves, three- to fourfold; this is, however, observed only in full-term and not in preterm animals. This effect is also blunted by antenatal dexamethasone.[28,29]

Development of breathing

In the fetus spontaneous and rhythmic activity of the diaphragm and respiratory muscles occurs already from weeks 10–11 of gestation. The fetal breathing is, in contrast to postnatal breathing, not continuous, and with advancing gestational age fetal breathing movements become more sporadic and occur only during electrophysiological activity comparable to rapid eye movement (REM) states. From about 30 weeks of gestation the breathing seems to be more strongly influenced by the behavioral state and a powerful central inhibitory mechanism is functioning during non-REM activity. Near term the human fetus performs breathing movements approximately 25–30% of the time. In contrast to the adult in whom hypoxemia stimulates breathing, in the fetus it causes a rapid depression independently of the physiological state. This is also regulated centrally, possibly via some metabolites such as adenosine.

The first breath occurs normally at 10–30 s of life but is delayed in birth asphyxia and also in those given pure oxygen compared with room air. Immediately after birth breathing is irregular and deep but within minutes a regular breathing rhythm is established, and such a continuous breathing rhythm is activated by a number of stimulants. Separation of the placenta in itself stimulates respiration, perhaps by decrease of inhibitory substances such as adenosine and PGE_2, which are produced there. Since the concentration of, for instance, prostaglandin I_2 (PGI_2), decreases relatively slowly after birth, other factors must be responsible for the rapid initiation of respiration. Oxygenation of the lungs itself seems to stimulate respiration and may contribute to this establishment.

It is clear that respiratory control in the postnatal period is multifactorial. Airway mechanoreflexes, thermoregulation, chemoreflexes, and behavioral states are important. The influence of the behavioral states on breathing patterns in the newborn is important, especially since the newborn spends so much time asleep. During wakefulness and REM sleep, breathing is irregular; in quiet sleep, breathing is slower and more regular.

Immediately after birth thermal inputs play a major role in regulating the respiration. A cool environment stimulates breathing and it has been suggested that the increased metabolic drive this initiates in order to keep the infant in the thermo-neutral zone stimulates breathing. After a few weeks the thermo-neutral zone widens and this mechanism seems to be less influential. Instead vagal stimuli become more important and stretch receptors in the airways and lung parenchyma and chest wall determine both breathing depth and frequency. Lung inflation inhibits respiration, this phenomenon is known as the Hering–Breuer reflex and is more active in the newborn than in the adult and more active in the term than in the preterm infant. Further, it is more active during quiet sleep than in active sleep (REM sleep). The importance of mechanosensory receptors in the airways in regulating the respiration plays only a minor role immediately after birth and increases in the first weeks after birth.

The chemoreceptors in the carotid body respond both to pCO_2 and pO_2. In fetal life the set point for pO_2 is much lower than in postnatal life, which means they are silenced immediately after birth. The sensitivity of the chemoreceptors both in the carotid body and in the aorta then slowly shifts toward adult levels during the next few days. In fetal life the chemoreceptors increase their activity when paO_2 decreases below 2.7–3.3 kPa (20–25 mmHg). After birth, resetting of the chemoreceptors increases their activity if paO_2 decreases below 12–13.3 kPa (90–100 mmHg). The mechanism for this resetting is not fully understood and it has been suggested that the level of catecholamines, such as dopamine in the carotid body, may play a role. Four to seven weeks postnatally chemoregulation is established as the most important regulator of the respiration.

Hypercapnia affects the fetal breathing movements in REM-like sleep only, but much more weakly than after birth when resistance to hypercapnic respiratory stimulation disappears during the quiet sleep state. Sensitivity to CO_2 increases with increasing gestational age and is therefore less developed in the preterm than in the term infant. Hypoxia in the term newborn infant results in hyperventilation for some minutes followed by normalization or reduced ventilation due to a fall in respiratory frequency. This second phase of ventilatory depression is more marked in the preterm infant, who often will not go through the initial hyperventilation when exposed to hypoxia and thus has a response to hypoxia similar to the fetus.[30–33]

Perinatal transition of the lungs

The lung development goes through several stages: the embryonic (3–7 weeks postconception), pseudoglandular (5–17 weeks), canalicular (16–26 weeks), saccular (24–38 weeks), alveolar (36 weeks to 2 years postnatally). A detailed description of these is found in several textbooks. Suffice here to mention that in the canalicular stage the appearance of vascular canals multiplies to form the alveolar-capillary respiratory membrane, which is the air–blood barrier and the future gas exchange surface. The epithelium is thinner and gas exchange may take place at the end of this stage. The saccular stage is characterized by dilatation of terminal respiratory units into alveolar saccules and ducts, with a reduction in the interstitial tissue. The alveolar stage is characterized by the formation of secondary alveolar septa that partition the terminal ducts and saccules into mature alveoli. The alveolar septa become thinner during this stage, which also increases the surface area of the lungs significantly. Most alveoli (80%) are formed after birth.[31,34]

Inflation

In fetal life the lungs are fluid filled and a normal fluid volume is a major determinant of normal lung growth. Lung liquid is actively secreted by epithelial cells, but the formation and volume decrease toward term. At birth an abrupt stop is needed. It seems that labor itself more than mechanical squeezing of lung fluid clears the lung of its liquid. The secretory process in fetal life is abruptly switched to allow absorption from the lung lumen into the fetal circulation. Two hours after birth the lung liquid normally is cleared. Epinephrine, but not norepinephrine, seems to be important to induce Na^+ transport out of the lumen. Epithelial sodium (Natrium) channels (ENaC) are important regulators of lung liquid clearance and parallel the rise of cortisol in late gestation of guinea pigs. Recently, the role of water channels, so-called aquaporines, for clearing lung water after birth has been focused on (see the section 'Fluid Shift'). Transitory tachypnea of the newborn is considered by many as a condition in which an inadequate lung liquid clearance is found due to a low stress at birth (exemplified by C-section). At birth the infant must inflate its lungs to provide a large enough area for gas exchange in the course of a few minutes. The first respiratory effort must be large enough to overcome the great resistance caused by the surface tension of the lung liquid. Pulmonary surfactant lowers the surface tension and therefore facilitates the expansion of the lung. In the absence of surfactant a positive end expiratory pressure of about 28 cm H_2O to avoid lung collapse and maintain an adequate functional residual capacity is necessary.

Inflation of the lung of a normal infant at birth is probably nearly accomplished with the first cry if it is vigorous. Karlberg and coworkers recorded the first breath in a series of 11 normal term infants to occur at the age of 6–93 s. Opening of alveoli occurs serially, each unit going to full inflation before the next one opens. Lung inflation is extremely rapid and after only one-third of a second the lungs look inflated as assessed by chest x-ray. Pleural pressures vary from 10 to 70 cm H_2O subatmospheric during the first

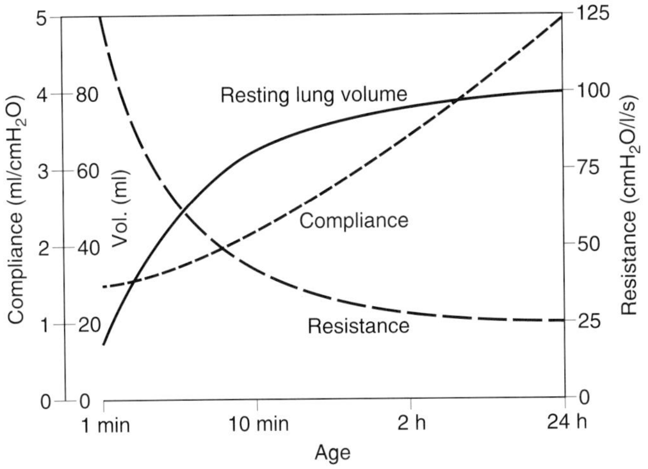

Figure 1.2 Change in lung mechanics in the first 24 h of life. From Godfrey.[36]

breath. Others have registered opening pressures around 30 cm H_2O. This large pressure is applied for only 0.5–1 s and during the first expiration there is a high positive pleural pressure of 20–30 cm H_2O. The pressure difference from inspiration to expiration in one single breath may therefore be formidable, up to 100 cm H_2O. Still, most children need an intrathoracic pressure of less than 10 cm H_2O to open their lungs vs. 4 cm H_2O in normal breathing. The tidal volumes of the first breaths in term infants were found by Karlberg and coworkers to vary between 12 and 67 ml.

Functional residual capacity increases quickly from about 17 ml/kg at 10 min of age to 25–35 ml/kg at 30 min, the same as 4 days of age. Lung compliance increases gradually during the first week of life and by 1–2 days of life the compliance is four- to fivefold greater than it was during the first few breaths. Simultaneously, resistance to airflow is decreased by one-half to one-fourth of the first registered values (Figure 1.2).

Following the initial inflation of the lung, the intra-alveolar lung fluid moves into the interstitium and is partially absorbed by the capillaries. Cold, light, noise, increased force of gravity, and falling pO_2 and pH all contribute to the initial gasping and subsequent breathing. The intrathoracic pressure an infant can generate is also dependent on the stability of the chest wall and the strength of the respiratory muscles. Following aeration of the lungs the pulmonary vascular resistance decreases and pulmonary blood flow increases, left atrial pressure increases, and the foramen ovale closes (see the section 'Transition of the Circulation').[35–38]

Gas exchange

In the umbilical vein blood pH has a mean of 7.33 in normal-term infants and in arterial umbilical blood reaches a minimum of about 7.20–7.25 a few minutes after birth and then is normally between 7.33 and 7.36 at 20 min of age. In some investigations pH already at 1 h reaches 7.40–7.42. pCO_2 in umbilical vein cord blood has a mean of 5.7 kPa (43 mmHg) and $paCO_2$ peaks around 8–9.3 kPa (60–70 mmHg) immediately after birth and then quickly normalizes to around 5.3 kPa (40 mmHg) or even a little lower than this by 20–60 min after birth. paO_2 in umbilical vein cord blood has a mean of 3.7 kPa (28 mmHg) and quickly rises to 6.7–8 kPa (50–60 mmHg) within the first 20–60 min after birth and then gradually increases toward adult levels over the next days, depending on how quickly the foramen ovale and the ductus arteriosus close.[39]

Surfactant

Pulmonary surfactant is synthesized, stored, secreted, and cleared in the type II cells in the alveoli. There are almost twice as many type II cells than the flat type I cells but they cover only 5–10% of the alveolar surface. In addition to surfactant, they synthesize and secrete many other bioactive components such as coagulation factors, cytokines, growth factors, and lysozyme and lysosomal enzymes. Active synthesis of surfactant begins in the second trimester and around 35–36 weeks adult pool size is obtained. At term only a fraction of the normal amount of surfactant is present in the alveoli. With lung inflation at birth a dramatic secretion of surfactant occurs and a normal pool of surfactant is established in the alveoli after a few hours.

Maturation of surfactant is delayed by 1–2 weeks in males compared with females and is not only dependent on the amount of surfactant produced but also on the surfactant composition. It has been shown in several mammalian species that considerable changes take place in the composition of surfactant as maturation of the fetus occurs. One of these is the increase of phosphatidyl choline and dipalmitoyl phosphatidyl choline with a concomitant decrease in phosphatidyl ethanolamine. This is reflected by an increasing lecithin/sphingomyelin ratio in amniotic fluid during the maturation process. The percentage of disaturated lecithin increases and reaches about 50 around 34 weeks of gestation. The acidic phospholipids of surfactant follow a different pattern. At around 34–35 weeks phosphatidyl glycerol becomes present and increases; simultaneously, phosphatidyl inositol peaks before it decreases toward term.[40]

Surfactant proteins

Experiments with several animal species have shown that the production of surfactant proteins in the fetal lung increases toward term. In humans mRNA for surfactant proteins A, B, and C were detected as early as 13 weeks of gestation and by 24 weeks their levels were 50% and 15% of the adult levels of mRNA for surfactant proteins B and C, respectively. In contrast, mRNA for surfactant protein A is very low before 24 weeks of gestation. In rat lung surfactant protein A increases substantially during the last 3–4 days of gestation, reaching a peak at the first day of life. In adult lungs its level doubles compared with the neonatal level. In humans surfactant protein A normally appears in amniotic fluid around 30–32 weeks of gestation and increases with surfactant lipids toward term. Surfactant protein B increases more gradually during gestation and continues to do so the first days after birth with a slight decrease in the adult. Glucocorticoids seem to increase the production of surfactant proteins A, B, C, and D. The hydrophilic surfactant proteins A and D are important for host defense and the hydrophobic proteins B and C for stabilization and rapid adsorption and spreading of the surfactant film. Surfactant protein B deficiency is a rare autosomal recessive disorder leading to lethal respiratory distress even in term infants. Recently, mutations in the transport of surfactant protein B from the lamellar bodies in type 2 cells to the surface have been detected giving a similar clinical picture as surfactant protein B deficiency. Surfactant protein C deficiency is an autosomal recessive disease and clinically not as dramatic as surfactant protein B deficiency, but it may lead to interstitial inflammation and pulmonary fibrosis.[41–43]

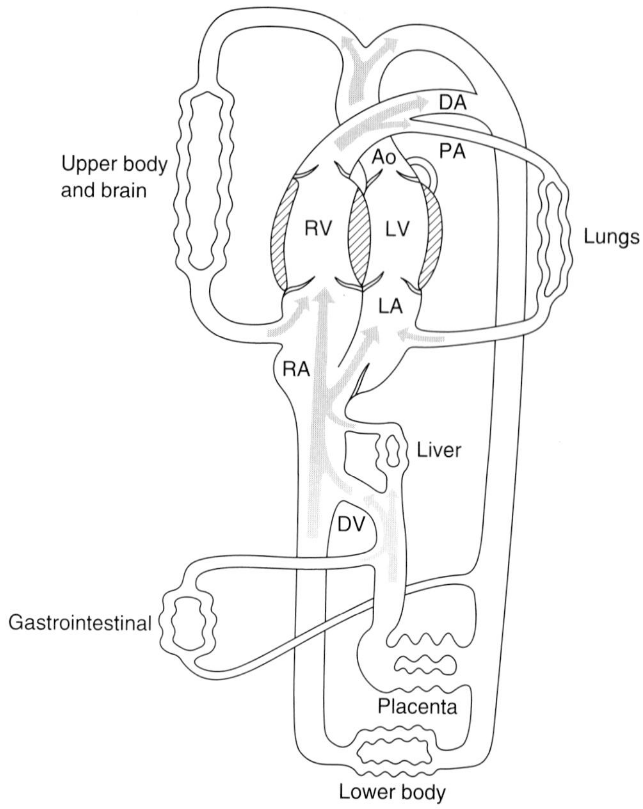

Figure 1.3 The fetal circulation. Ao: aorta, DA: ductus arteriosus, DV: ductus venosus, LA: left atrium, LV: left ventricle, PA: pulmonary artery, RA: right atrium, RV: right ventricle. From Rudolph.[44]

Transition of the circulation

Vascular changes

In fetal life the pulmonary and systemic vascular systems are coupled in parallel in contrast to the postnatal period when the blood circulation is coupled in series through the right side of the heart to the lungs and then through the left side of the heart to the systemic circulation to return to the right side of the heart through the systemic and the pulmonary vasculature (Figure 1.3). The fetal circulation is characterized by a low systemic and a high pulmonary vascular resistance, the opposite of the situation in postnatal life. The fetal circulation is designed to provide a large blood flow to the placenta and supply less to the lungs since the fetal lung has no gas exchange until birth. Due to the large surface of the placenta the fetal circulation has a low resistance, and the blood pressure therefore need not be high. The fetal circulation is further characterized by the presence of three shunts, which facilitate venous return from the placenta. These are the ductus venosus and the two right to left shunts reducing blood flow through the lungs (foramen ovale and ductus arteriosus). Through the foramen ovale (the opening between the right and left atrium) and the ductus arteriosus (the connection between the pulmonary trunk and the aorta), blood is bypassed away from lung tissue into the systemic circulation. The three shunts mentioned above therefore contribute to a separation between blood rich in oxygen and nutrients supplied from the placenta via the umbilical vein; this blood supplies the brain and myocardium.

During fetal life, blood is oxygenated in the placenta and returns to the fetal body via the umbilical vein, which joins the portal vein in the hepatic sinus. About 40% of the combined ventricular output goes through the placenta. This volume of blood, approximately 200 ml/kg fetal weight per minute, can be distributed through the ductus venosus directly into the inferior cava vein bypassing the hepatic micro-circulation, or it can pass via the portal veins through the hepatic circulation and then enter the inferior caval vein through the hepatic veins. In the fetal sheep about 70% of the venous return is derived from the lower portion of the body, and 20% from the superior vena cava. Of the remaining 10% approximately 7% comes from the pulmonary circulation – a fraction increasing toward term – and 3% from the myocardium. About 55% of the umbilical venous return passes through the ductus venosus and the rest mainly through to the right lobe of the liver.

The fetal liver is a highly compliant organ able to regulate the distribution of umbilical blood flow during fetal stress. Umbilical blood flow does not change significantly from normal values when fetal hypoxemia is induced by maternal hypoxia; however, the intrahepatic circulation is redistributed so that flow through the ductus venosus is increased. This increased flow is distributed to favor the brain, myocardium, and placenta in order to secure more oxygenated blood to these vital organs during hypoxemia. After traversal through the ductus venosus and entry into the inferior caval vein, oxygenated blood from the placenta does not mix with deoxygenated blood from the lower body. This blood when entering the inferior caval vein streams in parallel with blood from the lower body. When entering the right atrium the blood from the placenta and the blood from the lower body are split by *crista dividens* and blood originating from the ductus venosus preferentially crosses the foramen ovale into the left side of the heart and therefore the myocardium and the head are supplied with oxygen-enriched blood. Blood from the lower body and right liver lobe preferentially passes through the tricuspid valve into the right ventricle together with blood from the superior vena cava. Thus, blood with lower oxygen content is pumped out of the right ventricle and reaches the lower parts of the body.

Doppler studies in humans have demonstrated that the ductus venosus is a narrow vessel projecting a high-velocity jet posteriorly to reach the foramen ovale. The high peak velocity in the ductus venosus may give the blood sufficient momentum to reach the foramen ovale without extensive mixing with deoxygenated and nutrient poor blood. Blood streaming, therefore, not only occurs in parallel, but also side by side at different velocities when entering the right atrium.

Umbilical venous blood has a pO_2 of 4–4.7 kPa (30–35 mmHg). After mixing with portal venous and inferior caval blood the pO_2 is about 3.5–3.7 kPa (26–28 mmHg). Venous blood returning from the superior cava vein has a pO_2 of 1.6–1.9 kPa (12–14 mmHg) and this combines with the inferior caval vein stream passing through the tricuspid valve, giving a pO_2 in the right ventricle of 2.4–2.5 kPa (18–19 mmHg). The pO_2 of the blood entering the left ventricle and the ascending aorta is about 3.1–3.3 kPa (23–25 mmHg), slightly less than in the proximal part of the inferior caval vein due to mixing with blood from the pulmonary veins in the left atrium. The descending aortic blood, which is a mixture of blood passing through the ductus arteriosus and the aortic isthmus, has a pO_2 of 2.7–2.9 kPa (20–22 mmHg). Postnatally there is essentially no mixing of blood oxygenated in the lungs and systemic venous blood.

Fetal pulmonary vascular resistance falls with advancing gestational age primarily due to the great increase in the number of pulmonary vessels, expanding the total cross-sectional area of the vascular bed. Pulmonary blood flow and pulmonary artery pressure increase substantially in the fetal sheep from midgestation toward term.[44–49]

Establishment of the postnatal lung

The most dramatic changes in the circulation occur at birth when gas exchange through the lungs is established. Immediately after birth the umbilical placental blood flow is stopped and the pulmonary circulation is established adequately. Neither in the placenta nor in the umbilical cord vessels are adrenergic or cholinergic nerve fibers detected. So the regulation of cord flow is probably mainly due to vasoactive factors. Within a minute after birth umbilical blood flow is less than one-fifth of the fetal level. Simultaneously, a significant decrease in umbilical artery and vein diameters is observed within another minute. The mechanisms behind this are not fully understood but cooling, increased oxygen tension, and stretching of the cord may play a role. Locally produced mediators such as serotonin are powerful constrictors of umbilical vessels. The umbilical vessels also constrict by mechanical stimulation, particularly stretching, and the constriction is upheld by the immediate increase in systemic oxygen tension. Simultaneously, venous return through the inferior caval vein is reduced by removal of the placental circulation. Cessation of venous return reduces flow through the ductus venosus and this vessel therefore closes passively within 3–7 days after birth.

After birth, ventilation of the lungs with air results in a four- to tenfold increase in pulmonary blood flow, which is associated with a relatively rapid fall in pulmonary vascular resistance (Figure 1.4). These effects are mediated by mechanical lung changes, lowering of pCO_2, and increase in pO_2, each factor accounting for the pulmonary vasodilator effects seen after birth.

In addition to the structural adaptation of the pulmonary circulation after birth there are a number of vasoactive substances participating in the regulation of the pulmonary vascular tone in the perinatal period. The pulmonary vascular endothelium is central in the regulation of vascular tone. By stimulation the endothelial cells may release vasoactive substances into the circulation, or release lung tissue enzymes involved in the activation or inactivation of vasoactive mediators.

In recent years endothelium-derived relaxing factors such as nitric oxide (NO) have been identified and together with PGI_2 may be responsible for the rapid decrease in pulmonary vascular resistance that occurs at the onset of normal ventilation after birth. In fetal circulation there is an increased production of nitric oxide compared with adult levels. This nitric oxide contributes to the low vascular resistance and increased flow, for instance, in the gastrointestinal tract. Increased fetal oxygen tension increases the release of NO. The increase in pulmonary blood flow in response to the high oxygen concentration at birth as well as distention of the lung seems to be mediated, at least partly, by NO. This system seems to be especially potent near term, the reaction of the preterm is diminished. Endogenous NO production is augmented due to induction of especially endothelial nitric oxide synthase (eNOS). In the baboon both inducible NOS and eNOS activities increase during gestation, falling toward term. However, the total NOS activity seems to

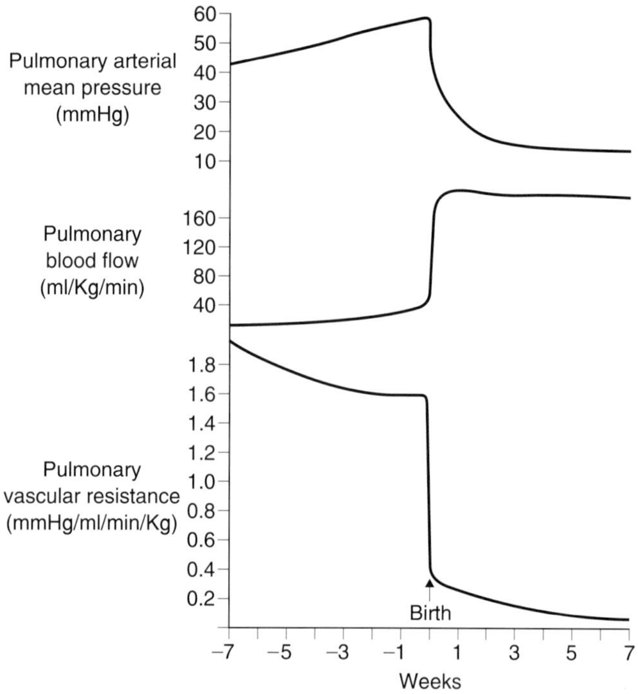

Figure 1.4 Changes in fetal pulmonary arterial pressure, pulmonary blood flow, and vascular resistance in the perinatal period. From Rudolph.[46]

be preserved. Both hypoxemia and diaphragmatic hernia decrease NOS expression. A lack of neuronal nitric oxide synthetase has been found in neonatal hypertrophic pyloric stenosis. Arachidonic acid metabolites are involved in the physiological regulation of the perinatal circulation. PGI_2 is a strong pulmonary vasodilatator. Mechanical stimulation of the lungs leads to PGI_2 production and ventilation of the fetal lung itself increases concentration of PGI_2 in pulmonary venous blood. The release of this metabolite is also stimulated by histamine, bradykinin, reactive oxygen species (ROS), and adenosine triphosphate (ATP), as well as angiotensin II, which is high immediately after birth.

Bradykinin is a potent vasoconstrictor in the umbilicoplacental circulation but otherwise is usually a vasodilatator. Bradykinin is released in fetal lungs during ventilation with air or during hyperbaric oxygenation. It is therefore possible that bradykinin could play a role in postnatal pulmonary circulatory changes. Endothelium-dependent vasoconstriction can also be stimulated by substances and factors such as acetylcholine, thrombin, serotonin, physical forces, and hypoxia. There are also endothelium-derived vascular constricting factors such as metabolites of arachidonic acid [thromboxane A_2 (TXA_2) and PGH_2], as well as endothelin and free radicals. In animal studies it has been shown that ROS are able to potently constrict the pulmonary vasculature and to dilate the ductus arteriosus. It has been shown both in the lungs and in the isolated ductus arteriosus that ROS stimulate the production of prostaglandins. In the lungs there seems to be a balance between dilating and constricting prostaglandins. The constrictor TXA_2 is elevated first, followed by the dilator PGI_2, when the pulmonary circulation is exposed to free oxygen radical generating systems. These substances therefore can have both constrictory and dilatory effects on the pulmonary circulation depending on the balance between TXA_2 and PGI_2. Superoxide radicals, for instance, can act by inactivating NO and also by activation of endothelial cyclooxygenase products. In addition, endothelin and angiotensin II have a prolonged effect on the tone and structure of blood vessels.

Remodeling of the pulmonary vasculature occurs immediately after birth, contributing to the decrease in pulmonary vascular resistance. In the precapillary arteries the endothelial cells shortly after birth become slimmer, the surface/volume ratio increases so the vessel wall becomes thinner, and the lumen diameter increases. Further, small, unopened muscular arteries are recruited to the pulmonary circulation during the first days after birth. Thus, a structural adaptation to extrauterine life consists of changes in cell shape and position. The structural remodeling during the first 2 weeks of life in the pig lungs contributes to the reduction in mean pulmonary artery pressure from 55 to 14 mmHg.

The baroreflex setting of heart rate mediated by baroreceptor fibers in the carotic body and aortic arch is active in both fetal and newborn life, but with different sensitivity and shifts toward higher pressures during development.[46,50,51]

Ductus arteriosus

The open ductus arteriosus in fetal life diverts blood away from the lungs toward the descending aorta. The patent ductus is regulated both by dilating and by contracting factors. Prostaglandins play an important role in maintaining the patency, and the ductus is especially sensitive to the dilating action of PGE_2. Oxygen is a potent constrictor of the ductus and becomes more effective the more mature the fetus is. This is due to the fact that in early fetal life the ductus has decreased muscular development, causing less contractile ability. In fetal lambs the ductus arteriosus is also more sensitive to the dilating effect of PGE_2 in the preterm than near term. This is due to a developmental alteration in the sensitivity of the vessels to prostaglandins. It is circulating PGE_2, probably produced in the placenta, which probably controls the ductus arteriosus *in utero*. After birth, when the oxygen tension increases, the ductal wall is itself capable of producing PGE_2. Reactive oxygen metabolites (ROS) may stimulate PGE_2 synthesis in the isolated ductal wall from fetal lambs. In the ductus arteriosus ROS can therefore contribute to dilatation by turning on prostaglandin synthesis in the ductal wall. The functional closure of the ductus, therefore, is promoted by an increase in oxygen tension, and a p450 hemoprotein located in the smooth muscle plasma membrane is a receptor of the oxygen-induced events. Further, a decrease in blood pressure within the ductus itself, a decrease in circulating PGE_2 (due to loss of placental prostaglandin synthesis and increase in prostaglandin removal by the lungs), and finally a decrease in PGE_2 receptors in the ductus wall also contribute to constriction of the ductus. In full-term infants closure of the ductus arteriosus occurs in two phases with a functional closure within the first hours after birth due to smooth muscle constriction, and the anatomic closure caused by closure of the lumen due to thickening of the intima and loss of smooth muscle cells. This is caused by progressive thickening of the intima, so it eventually occludes the constricted lumen. Smooth muscles migrate from media into the intima layer. Vascular endothelial growth factor plays an important role in this intimal 'cushion'.[52–54]

Myocardium

At the end of gestation, right and left ventricular systolic pressures are equal, 65–70 mmHg. The cardiac output of the right ventricle is, however, in fetal life 50% higher than the left ventricle mainly due to the fact that the left ventricle has a high afterload caused by the high vascular resistance of the head, neck, and forelimbs, while the right ventricle's afterload is lower because of the low umbilical–placental resistance. The removal of the low-resistance placental circulation results in an increase in systemic vascular resistance. The combined ventricular output in the fetal lamb is about 500 ml/kg/min; however, after birth there is an increase in total cardiac output and during the first few days each ventricle ejects approximately 350 ml/kg/min. During the next weeks in the newborn lamb there is a rapid decrease in cardiac output to a level of about 150 ml/kg/min and then it falls slowly to the adult level of 70–80 ml/kg/min. Cardiac output changes parallel changes in oxygen consumption.

O_2 consumption is almost identical in the adult and fetal hearts; however, the fuel used by them is different since the adult heart uses fatty acids and the fetal heart is an obligatory user of carbohydrates as a substrate for oxidative phosphorylation. In the fetal lamb 60% of these carbohydrates are lactate, 35% glucose and 5% pyruvate. This can explain why a fall in circulating glucose concentrations results in myocardial depression in fetal and neonatal life but not later in life. In fact, it has been shown that fatty acids are detrimental to fetal cardiac function. In order to use fatty acids as fuel they must be transformed to Ac-CoA, which is transesterified with carnitine and in this form is transported across the mitochondrial membrane by the transport enzyme carnitine-palmitoyl transferase (CPT). CPT is inhibited by malonyl-CoA, which is high in fetal life. Malonyl-CoA is regulated by glucagon and during the delivery glucagon concentration increases sharply, thereby reducing the concentration of malonyl-CoA and releasing CPT inhibition allowing fatty acid oxidation to proceed.

The contractile properties of the myocyte also differ in fetal and adult life. Only about 30% of fetal cardiac muscle consists of contractile elements compared with approximately 60% in the adult. The velocity of shortening of the myocyte is also lower in fetal life. Especially, preterm infants and to some degree also term infants have therefore a much reduced ability to tolerate an increase in afterload. The change from fetal to adult performance seems, however, to occur quickly after birth.

At birth, cardiac output increases considerably and the left ventricular level is doubled compared with fetal levels. This higher left ventricular inotropy and performance is due to sympathetico-adrenal stimulation after birth, and T3 seems to be important in maturation of the fetal myocardial response. After birth, myocardial contractility is greatly increased but because of the high demands on the circulation to provide the increased oxygen requirements for metabolism, there is also little reserve available, and thus volume loading results in only a small rise in cardiac output. In a fetus an increase in heart rate gives a fall in end diastolic volume and stroke volume unless ventricular diastolic filling is maintained. The rearrangement of the circulation after birth leads to an increased end diastolic left ventricular volume, which leads to an increased stroke volume. The days after birth a gradual decrease in cardiac output per kilogram is observed returning to the fetal levels.

Fetuses at midgestation have individualized heart rates that are stable. The control of heart rate variability seems to develop later and fetal heart rate variability is predictive of neonatal heart rate variability not until 30 weeks. With increasing gestation there is a reduced fetal heart rate variability and this demonstrates the development of the autonomic nerve system during gestation. Heart rate at birth is around 160–180 beats/min and decreases to 120 beats/min in sleeping newborn infants and to 140–160 beats/min in awake newborn infants. The postnatal situation compared with the fetal is characterized by a decrease in heart rate, postextrasystolic potentiation increases, and inotropic responses to catecholamine elevation, suggesting that the postnatal heart has greater potential reserves than in fetal life.[45,46,49]

Shift in oxygen transport

The newborn infant has a higher oxygen demand than the fetus and the oxygen consumption typically is increased between two- and threefold in the first days of life. O_2 consumption per kilogram of body weight is higher in the newborn than in the adult and the fetus. In adult life O_2 consumption is about half that in the immediate newborn period; however, when compared with body surface area this age difference seems to disappear. The delivery of oxygen to the tissues depends on (1) the oxygen content of the blood, (2) the cardiac output, (3) the distribution of the circulation, and (4) the affinity of oxygen to hemoglobin. In fetal blood there is a high affinity to oxygen. The postnatal decrease in hemoglobin O_2 affinity is caused by an increase in adult hemoglobin at the expense of fetal hemoglobin, and an increase from birth in the concentration of 2,3-diphosphoglycerate (DPG). During gestation until 34 weeks, fetal hemoglobin comprises about 90% of the total hemoglobin, falling to 80% at term, and from birth to 8 months of age there is a gradual decline in fetal hemoglobin to less than 2%. Fetal red cells have a higher oxygen affinity than adult cells, which is achieved by a reduced interaction between fetal hemoglobin and 2,3-DPG than in adult hemoglobin. The concentration of 2,3-DPG in fetal and adult cells is almost the same. 2,3-DPG present in the erythrocytes decreases the affinity to O_2 through an allosteric action with the hemoglobin molecule. DPG does not bind as strongly to fetal hemoglobin as the adult hemoglobin. In addition, it is low immediately after birth, making a high O_2 affinity immediately after birth with a p50 of approximately 2.7 kPa (20 mmHg) vs. 4 kPa (30 mmHg) at 8 months of age. Therefore, in the newborn period and early infancy when the fetal hemoglobin concentration is high, intraerythrocyte change in 2,3-DPG has little effect on p50; however, later in life the modulating effect of 2,3-DPG on oxygen affinity plays a more important role. In the fetal period the high oxygen-carrying capacity and greater oxygen affinity of fetal blood in fact compensate for the one-fifth to one-fourth oxygen tension of adult blood, ending with rather similar oxygen saturation at term and in adult life. Fetal blood also is slightly hypercarbic and acidotic, whereas the maternal blood is hypocarbic and alkalotic. The Bohr effect, that is, the shift in the oxygen equilibrium curve to the right by increased pCO_2 or decreased pH, giving a higher oxygen tension, is more pronounced with a lower pH and more efficient in the fetus. In addition, a higher temperature of the fetus contributes to a shift in the fetal dissociation curve to the right.[55–57]

Tissue injury

Energy metabolism

Most of the oxygen taken into the body is used in cell energy metabolism. The metabolic process is a redox process where energy is released in a stepwise fashion and stored as ATP. Energy metabolism can schematically be divided into three parts. In step 1 glucose, amino acids and fatty acids are broken down to Ac-CoA. In the second step Ac-CoA enters the tricarboxylic acid (Krebs) cycle, the final common pathway of all fuel substrates in aerobic cells. Here, acetyl groups are metabolized to form carbon dioxide and hydrogen ions. In step 3, the hydrogen ions enter the respiratory chain of the cell, a series of electron carriers linked to oxidative phosphorylation, with ATP formed in a stepwise manner. Oxygen is the final electron acceptor and is necessary for continuous oxidation of reduced coenzymes in the respiratory chain. Oxygen, therefore, can be considered as the 'garbage cleaner' of energy metabolism taking care of its waste products, the electrons, after having traversed through the respiratory chain.

The energy metabolism tends to keep the energy charge, EC $[EC=0.5([ATP]+[ADP]/[ATP]+[ADP]+[AMP])]$, of the cell at an optimal level, which is around 0.85. This can be achieved in two ways, either by increasing the ATP concentration or by increasing the catabolism of AMP. In hypoxia with lack of energy the cell might be forced to choose the latter alternative. An accelerated breakdown of AMP occurs. This is a hazardous compensation since the cell might lose its purine pool irreversibly. One of the intermediate breakdown products is, however, adenosine. This metabolite has important control feedback functions in brain hypoxia, partly because it is an active vasodilatator and thus contributes to a higher oxygen supply to hypoxic tissues and partly because adenosine in itself cuts down brain metabolism. When adenosine accumulates because of energy deficiency, this metabolite fights back by contributing to an increased oxygen supply and a decreased energy need. This is important also because a breakdown product from adenosine is hypoxanthine. This metabolite accumulates in tissues and body fluids during hypoxia and its extracellular concentration reflects the intracellular energy charge. However, hypoxanthine is also a potential oxygen radical generator during reoxygenation and it is therefore probably advantageous for the organism to try to keep the hypoxanthine concentration as low as possible.

Before the cell's energy charge falls markedly, several biochemical compensatory mechanisms are activated. First, glycolysis is accelerated many fold. Pyruvate is reduced to lactate, while nicotinamide adenine nucleotide (NADH) is oxidized to NAD^+. This is the basis for the use of lactate as a clinical marker of hypoxia. Lactate augmentation merely reflects the compensation mechanism. Although hypoxanthine and lactate parallel each other in many clinical settings, hypoxanthine nevertheless more correctly reflects the intracellular energy status of the cells.

As soon as oxygen delivery to the cells declines the mitochondria also change their metabolism to utilize available oxygen more efficiently. The compensation takes place 30–60 min after a reduction in oxygen supply. In the fetus or in the immediate newborn period mitochondrial adaptation already is maximal. A fetus has a respiratory capacity of about 300% of the adult, but by 10–14 days after birth the newborn and adult levels equate in this respect. What does this mean for the fetus and newborn? First, they are able to utilize the limited oxygen supply very efficiently. On the other hand, the fetus is unable to make cellular respiratory adaptations if hypoxia occurs. From this point of view, the fetus and newborn are more vulnerable to hypoxia than older patients.

Hypoxic injury to the perinatal brain

It has been known since Boyle's classical experiment in 1670 that newborn animals can resist hypoxia longer than adult ones. In the 1960s and 1970s it was shown that the preterm monkey can withstand hypoxia longer than the term one. In fact, in the fetal monkey there was an exponential relation between duration of hypoxia and gestational age when the outcome measure was neurologic brain injury (cerebral palsy). The younger the animal the longer it could resist hypoxia before brain injury occurred. Thus, mature fetal rats survive in pure nitrogen more than 25 times longer and 1-day-old rats about 10 times longer than adult rats. One part of the explanation for this seems to be that newborn animals can preserve cerebral circulation and thus ensure supply of substrates for energy metabolism better than in the adult. Further, it is known that oxygen demand of the brain is lower in fetal life and increases with gestation. The immature brain has smaller neurons, which are less branched with fewer synapses. The energy requirement is therefore lower and the cerebral metabolic rate of oxygen is lower in the immature brain compared with the adult. The fetal brain is also able to use alternative sources such as ketone bodies as fuel for energy metabolism. Further, the glycolytic capacity allows the immature brain to regenerate ATP at a higher rate than in the adult brain.

The perinatal period is also accompanied by dramatic neurochemical changes. The concentration of excitatory amino acids such as glutamate peaks around term and may contribute to a higher sensitivity to hypoxia in the term compared with the preterm infant.[58,59]

Apoptosis and necrosis

Apoptosis is an important part of development and homeostasis. For instance, in the developing brain perhaps up to half of the cells undergo apoptosis, in spite of the fact that the distinction between apoptotic and necrotic death is considered less clear than previously. These two modes of cell death are considered by many as a continuum running from apoptosis to necrosis more than two different entities. Infants who have undergone secondary energy failure after, for instance, birth asphyxia, have a tendency to lose their neurons by necrosis, while those dying *in utero* have experienced more apoptotic death. The same injury may induce apoptosis in the fetus or newborn and necrosis in the adult organism. To make it more complex the same cell may undergo apoptosis if the injury is mild and necrosis if it is severe. Oxidative stress plays an important role in initiating apoptosis, for instance, through opening up the mitochondrial permeability transition pore. This reduces the mitochondrial membrane potential and release of substances that are involved in apoptosis, for instance, cytochrome *c* and Apaf-1, both of which activate caspase-3, which is specifically involved in the apoptotic execution. As mentioned already, the fetus is more susceptible to oxidative stress than the term newborn and therefore also perhaps more susceptible to this mechanism.[60]

Development of antioxidants

In fetal life paO_2 is around 3.3 kPa (25 mmHg) and after birth rises quickly to 8 kPa (60 mmHg) over the next 30 min. In order to survive in an oxygen-rich atmosphere antioxidant systems must be well developed at birth. A number of defense systems have been described. In the lung and kidney, maturation of antioxyenzymes such as superoxide dismutases, glutathione peroxidase, and catalase seems to occur near term in animal fetuses. In fact, the maturation of these systems occurs in parallel with the maturation of the surfactant system. Furthermore, preterm infants with gestational age of 24–29 weeks have only 50% activity of Cu/Zn superoxide dismutase in cord erythrocytes compared with term infants. Glutathione is a major intracellular antioxidant and is found in high concentrations (mM) in eukaryotic cells. Glutathione is the substrate for glutathione peroxidase, which catalyzes oxidation of reduced to oxidized glutathione at the expense of hydrogen peroxide. The rate of glutathione synthesis from methionine is strongly reduced in preterm infants compared with term ones. These data therefore suggest that at least the intracellular defense against free radicals is low in many organs in fetal life and probably also in the human fetus. A preterm infant is therefore more vulnerable to increased oxidative stress and attacks of free radicals than a term one. In contrast to the intracellular defense, extracellular antioxidants seem to be adequately developed at term, and the concentration of several extracellular antioxidants such as ascorbate is very high in the umbilical cord (see Chapter 6).[61–64]

Thermal regulation

In fetal life the body temperature is efficiently regulated to be 0.5°C higher than the maternal. The tight linkage between fetal and maternal body temperature is called a 'heat clamp', which prevents the fetus from independent regulation of its temperature. At birth a dramatic change in the thermal environment occurs. During the first hours of life core body temperature can fall to less than 36°C if the newborn is not taken care of optimally. After 8 h, body temperature has usually returned to the normal adult range. Since the newborn infant has a relatively large body surface area and limited thermal insulation it is necessary to wrap the newborn infant adequately. The newborn infant in fact has the capability to regulate the temperature by sweating and can also respond to a cool environment by increasing the metabolic rate. This takes place without shivering, is activated by catecholamines, and the heat is generated mainly from brown fat, which is present in large amounts in the full-term infant. Although the fetus may mobilize brown fat the thermogenic responses still are very low. These require increased oxygen and substrate consumption. The combination of hypoxia and hypothermia therefore is dangerous.[25,65]

Skin

The transition from intra- to extrauterine life is dramatic for the skin, perhaps the largest organ of the body. It immediately must be a barrier to water loss; it takes part in thermoregulation, protects against infections, has an antioxidant function, and protects against UV light. The skin is a barrier to chemicals and is needed for tactile discrimination as well as being an important emotional and psychological link between the child and its caregivers. The skin of the term in contrast to the preterm infant also has a highly developed immunological system. *In utero* the skin is in a sterile environment but already in the birth canal it is colonized and specific cells in the epidermal layer take part in host defense.

Prenatally, lipid synthesis is necessary for production of vernix caseosa, forming a barrier that is needed for successful adaptation to postnatal life. The vernix also may function as an endogenous skin cleanser removing, for instance, carbon particles. Of interest is that both the stratum corneum of epidermis and the brain contain very high concentrations of ceramides. The close embryological relation between these two organs both derived ectodermally makes this an interesting observation. At birth the epidermis is pH neutral but rapidly over the first postnatal weeks, it develops an 'acid mantle' that is characteristic of human skin. This acidic surface can be destroyed by using alkaline soaps for infant bathing and is delayed in very low birth weight infants. The acid mantle is believed to be important in antimicrobial defense as well as in keeping the integrity of the epidermal barrier. Postnatally transepidermal water loss that increases after birth is an important regulator of DNA and lipid synthesis in the epidermis.[66]

Circadian rhythms

The clock for the circadian rhythms is set by the suprachiasmatic nucleus. It is fascinating that the neurons in this area of the brain *in vitro* oscillate within a period close to 24 h. This is regulated by light, which in a complex way affects gene expression of transcription factors. Efferent pathways from the suprachiasmatic nerve control the pineal function and regulate the rhythms of endocrine, cardiovascular, temperature, and even behavioral circadian variations.

From midgestation the suprachiasmatic nucleus is present in the fetus and diurnal rhythms are found in the human fetus after 20 weeks. Whether or not they are intrinsically regulated or are due to maternal control, for instance, via maternal melatonin rhythms, is unclear. However, in fetal life the maternal rhythms are mainly followed by the rhythm of the mother exemplified by cortisol fluctuations. In contrast, fetal autonomic activity that controls the heart rate follows a 12-h cycle and not the mother's 24-h rhythm. This 12-h rhythm disappears immediately after birth and around 2–4 weeks the 24-h rhythm is established. It takes 8–12 weeks before postnatal circadian rhythms in sleep and wakefulness as well as plasma cortisol and melatonin are established.[25,67]

Gene activation at birth

In the near future the transition at birth will be described by a shift in different gene activities and not only by physiological and biochemical changes. Labor affects the mRNA encoding for a number of enzymes such as tyrosine hydroxylase, dopamine-beta-hydroxylase. mRNA encoding for substance P increases many fold in the nucleus tractus solitarius the first days of life. Substance P probably plays a role in the central respiratory control by promoting the hypoxic drive from peripheral chemoreceptors. Depression of genes is also described at birth and in some circumstances there is a shift from one isoform to the other. One example is the expression of genes that encode the muscle-specific and non-muscle-specific isoforms of cytochrom oxidase subunit VIa during pre- and postnatal life of striated muscle in the mouse. The non-muscle form is the predominant isoform in fetal life and is gradually at the end of gestation and early neonatal life replaced by the muscle-specific isoform both in cardiac and in skeletal muscle.[68]

Conclusion

In order to understand both normal development as well as disease processes in the newborn infant it is necessary to have insight into the complex changes that occur in relation to birth. Previously, physiological processes have been emphasized giving us valuable knowledge on the perinatal transition of the cardiovascular and pulmonary systems. Recently, biochemical changes in relation to birth have been understood more fully as, for instance, the maturation of the surfactant system and antioxidative systems.

Presently, more and more data will accumulate, teaching us how the transition at birth is regulated at the gene level. In this way it could hopefully be possible to modulate the disease processes in relation to the birth processes in a much more efficient and powerful way than we understand today.

References

1. Ambler GR, Gluckman PD. Postnatal growth. In Gluckman PD, Heymann MA, eds. *Perinatal and Pediatric Pathophysiology*. London: Edward Arnold, 1993:170–90.
2. Girard J, Ferre P. Metabolic and hormonal changes around birth. In Jones CT, ed. *Biochemical Development of the Fetus and Neonate*. Amsterdam: Elsevier Biomedical Press, 1982:517–51.
3. Gospodarowicz D. The role of growth factors in organ growth and differentiation. In Jones CT, ed. *The Biochemical Development of the Fetus and Neonate*. Amsterdam: Elsevier Biomedical Press, 1982:101–25.
4. Milner RDG. Prenatal growth control. In Gluckman PD, Heymann MA, eds. *Perinatal and Pediatric Pathophysiology*. London: Edward Arnold, 1993:162–9.
5. Parkes MJ. The transition between growth-hormone independent and growth-hormone dependent growth. In Jones CT, Nathanielsz PW, eds. *The Physiological Development of the Fetus and the Newborn*. London: Academic Press, 1985:55–8.
6. Styne DM. Endocrine factors affecting neonatal growth. In Polin RA, Fox WW, Abman SH, eds. *Fetal and Neonatal Physiology*, 3rd ed. Philadelphia: Saunders, 2004:266–75.
7. Friis-Hansen B. Water and electrolyte balance before and after birth. In Rooth G, Saugstad OD, eds. *The Roots of Perinatal Medicine*. New York: Thieme-Stratton Inc., 1985:39–47.
8. Brace RA. Fluid distribution in the fetus and neonate. In Polin RA, Fox WW, Abman SH, eds. *Fetal and Neonatal Physiology*, 3rd edn. Philadelphia: Saunders, 2004:1341–50.
9. Khalan SC. Metabolism of glucose and methods of investigation in the fetus and newborn. In Polin RA, Fox WW, Abman SH, eds. *Fetal and Neonatal Physiology*, 3rd edn. Philadelphia: Saunders, 2004:449–64.
10. Milner RDG. Fat and carbohydrate metabolism. In Gluckman PD, Heymann MA, eds. *Perinatal and Pediatric Pathophysiology*. London: Edward Arnold, 1993:84–102.
11. Philips AF. Oxygen consumption and general carbohydrate metabolism of the fetus. In Polin RA, Fox WW, Abman SH, eds. *Fetal and Neonatal Physiology*, 3rd edn. Philadelphia: Saunders, 2004:465–78.
12. Simmons RA. Cell glucose transport and glucose handling during fetal and neonatal development. In Polin RA, Fox WW, Abman SH, eds. *Fetal and Neonatal Physiology*, 3rd edn. Philadelphia: Saunders, 2004:487–93.
13. Sunehag A, Ewald U, Gustafsson J. Extremely preterm infants (< 28 weeks) are capable of gluconeogenesis from glycerol on their first day of life. *Pediatr Res* 1996;40:553–7.
14. Hay WW, Regnault TRH. Fetal requirements and placental transfer of nitrogenous compounds. In Polin RA, Fox WW, Abman SH, eds. *Fetal and Neonatal Physiology*, 3rd edn. Philadelphia: Saunders, 2004:509–27.
15. Milner RDG. Protein and amino acid metabolism. In Gluckman PD, Heymann MA, eds. *Perinatal and Pediatric Pathophysiology*. London: Edward Arnold, 1993:71–8.
16. Herrera E, Lascuncion MA. Maternal-fetal transfer of lipid metabolites. In Polin RA, Fox WW, Abman SH, eds. *Fetal and Neonatal Physiology*, 3rd edn. Philadelphia: Saunders, 2004:375–88.
17. Van Arde JE, Wilke S, Feldman M, Clandinin MT. Accretion of lipid in fetus and newborn. In Polin RA, Fox WW, Abman SH, eds. *Fetal and Neonatal Physiology*, 3rd edn. Philadelphia: Saunders, 2004:388–404.
18. Persson B. Lipid metabolism. *Acta Obstet Gynecol Scand* 1969;48(Suppl 3):92–6.
19. Helland IB, Smith L, Saarem K, Saugstad OD, Drevon CA. Maternal supplementation with very-long-chain n-3 fatty acids during pregnancy and lactation augments children's IQ at 4 years of age. *Pediatrics* 2003;111:e39–44.
20. Husain SM, Mughal MZ, Tsang RC. Calcium, phosporous and magnesium transport across the placenta. In Polin RA, Fox WW, Abman SH, eds. *Fetal and Neonatal Physiology*, 3rd edn. Philadelphia: Saunders, 2004:314–22.
21. Loughead JL, Mimouni F, Tsang RC. Serum ionized calcium concentrations in normal neonates. *Am J Dis Child* 1988;142:516–8.
22. Prada JA. Calcium regulating hormones. In Polin RA, Fox WW, Abman SH, eds. *Fetal and Neonatal Physiology*, 3rd edn. Philadelphia: Saunders, 2004:303–14.
23. Hambridge KM, Krebs NF. Zink in the fetus and neonate. In Polin RA, Fox WW, Abman SH, eds. *Fetal and Neonatal Physiology*, 3rd edn. Philadelphia: Saunders, 2004:342–7.
24. Gluckman PD. The onset and organisation of hypothalamic control in the fetus. In Jones CT, Nathanielsz PW, eds. *The Physiological Development of the Fetus and the Newborn*. London: Academic Press, 1985:103–11.
25. Grimberg A, Kutikov JK. Hypothalamus: Neuroendometabolic center. In Polin RA, Fox WW, Abman SH, eds. *Fetal and Neonatal Physiology*, 3rd edn. Philadelphia: Saunders, 2004: 1871–80.
26. Sack J. The hypothalamic–pituitary–thyroidea axis. In Gluckman PD, Heymann MA, eds. *Perinatal and Pediatric Pathophysiology*. London: Edward Arnold, 1993:302–10.
27. Thorpe-Beeston JG, Nicolaides KH, Felton CV, Butler J, McGregor AM. Maturation of the secretion of the thyroid hormone and thyroid stimulating hormone in the fetus. *N Engl J Med* 1991;324:532–6.
28. Lagercrantz H. Stress, arousal, and gene activation at birth. *News Physiol Sci* 1996;11:214–8.
29. Segar JL. Neural regulation of blood pressure during fetal and newborn life. In Polin RA, Fox WW, Abman SH, eds. *Fetal and Neonatal Physiology*, 3rd edn. Philadelphia: Saunders, 2004: 715–26.
30. Johnson P. The development of breathing. In Jones CT, Nathanielsz PW, eds. *The Physiological Development of the Fetus and the Newborn*. London: Academic Press, 1985: 201–10.
31. Avery ME, Fletcher BD, Williams RG. *The Lung and Its Disorders in the Newborn Infant*. Philadelphia: WB Saunders Co, 1981.
32. Saugstad OD. Physiology of resuscitation. In Polin RA, Fox WW, Abman SH, eds. *Fetal and Neonatal Physiology*, 3rd edn. Philadelphia: Saunders, 2004:763–72.
33. Saugstad OD, Rootwelt T, Aalen O. Resuscitation of asphyxiated newborn infants with room air or oxygen: An international controlled trial: The Resair 2 study. *Pediatrics* 1998;102(1):e1.
34. Wert SE. Normal and abnormal structural development of the lung. In Polin RA, Fox WW, Abman SH, eds. *Fetal and Neonatal Physiology*, 3rd edn. Philadelphia: Saunders, 2004:783–801.
35. Barker PM, Southern KW. Regulation of liquid secretion and absorption by the fetal and neonatal lung. In Polin RA, Fox WW, Abman SH, eds. *Fetal and Neonatal Physiology*, 3rd edn. Philadelphia: Saunders, 2004:822–34.
36. Godfrey S. Growth and development of the respiratory system: Functional development. In Davis JA, Dopping J, eds. *Scientific Foundations of Paediatrics*, 2nd edn. London: Heineman, 1981:432–50.
37. Karlberg P, Cherry RB, Escardo FE, Koch G. Respiratory studies in newborn infants. II. Pulmonary ventilation and mechanics of breathing in the first minutes of life, including the onset of respiration. *Acta Paediatr* 1962;51:121–36.
38. Vyas H, Milner AD, Hopkins IE. Intrathoracic pressure and volume changes during the spontaneous onset of respiration in babies born by caesarean section and by vaginal delivery. *J Pediatr* 1981;99:787–91.
39. Sjostedt, S, Rooth G, Caligara F. The oxygen tension in the cord blood after normal delivery. *Acta Obstet Gynecol Scand* 1960;39:34–8.
40. Kulovich MV, Hallman MB, Gluck L. The lung profile. *Am J Obstet Gynecol* 1979;135:57–63.

41. Hamvas A, Nogee LM, White FV, *et al.* Progressive lung disease and surfactant dysfunction with a deletion in surfactant protein C gene. *Am J Respir Cell Mol Biol* 2004;30:771–6.
42. Nogee LM. Genetic mechanisms of surfactant deficiency. *Biol Neonate* 2004;85(4):314–8.
43. Whitsett JA. Composition of pulmonary surfactant lipids and proteins. In Polin RA, Fox WW, Abman SH, eds. *Fetal and Neonatal Physiology*, 3rd edn. Philadelphia: Saunders, 2004:1005–13.
44. Rudolph AM. *Congenital Diseases of the Heart.* Chicago: Year Book Medical Publishers, Inc., 1974.
45. Rudolph AM. Organisation and control of the fetal circulation. In Jones CT, Nathanielsz PW, eds. *The Physiological Development of the Fetus and the Newborn.* London: Academic Press, 1985:343–53.
46. Rudolph AM. Fetal circulation and cardiovascular adjustment at birth. In Rudolph AM, ed. *Pediatrics.* Appleton & Lange, 1987: 1219–23.
47. Soifer SJ, Fineman JR, Heyman MA. Cardiovascular system: The pulmonary circulation. In Gluckman PD, Heymann MA, eds. *Perinatal and Pediatric Pathophysiology.* London: Edward Arnold, 1993:519–25.
48. Kiserud T, Eik-Nes SH, Hellevik LR, Blaas HG. Ductus venosus – A longitudinal Doppler velocimeter study of the human fetus. *J Matern Fetal Investig* 1992;2:5–11.
49. Anderson PAW, Kleinman CS, Lister G, Talner N. Cardiovascular function during development and the response to hypoxia. In Polin RA, Fox WW, Abman SH, eds. *Fetal and Neonatal Physiology*, 3rd edn. Philadelphia: Saunders, 2004:635–69.
50. Kinsella JP, Shaul PW. Physiology of nitric oxide in the developing lung. In Polin RA, Fox WW, Abman SH, eds. *Fetal and Neonatal Physiology*, 3rd edn. Philadelphia: Saunders, 2004: 731–43.
51. Ignarro LJ, Buga GM. Cardiovascular system: Vascular smooth muscle and endothelial function. In Gluckman PD, Heymann MA, eds. *Perinatal and Pediatric Pathophysiology.* London: Edward Arnold, 1993:462–71.
52. Clyman RI. Cardiovascular system: Ductus arteriosus. In Gluckman PD, Heymann MA, eds. *Perinatal and Pediatric Pathophysiology.* London: Edward Arnold, 1993:525–9.
53. Clyman RI. Mechanisms regulating closure of the ductus arteriosus. In Polin RA, Fox WW, Abman SH, eds. *Fetal and Neonatal Physiology*, 3rd edn. Philadelphia: Saunders, 2004:743–8.
54. Clyman RI, Saugstad OD, Mauray F. Reactive oxygen metabolites relax the lamb ductus arteriosus by stimulating prostaglandin production. *Circ Res* 1989;64:1–8.
55. Lister G. Cardiovascular system: Oxygen transport. In Gluckman PD, Heymann MA, eds. *Perinatal and Pediatric Pathophysiology.* London: Edward Arnold, 1993:547–55.
56. Delivoria-Papadopolous M, McGowan JE. Oxygen transport and delivery. In Polin RA, Fox WW, Abman SH, eds. *Fetal and Neonatal Physiology*, 3rd edn. Philadelphia: Saunders, 2004:880–9.
57. Wood WG. Erythropoiesis and haemoglobin production during development. In Jones CT, ed. *Biochemical Development of the Fetus and Neonate.* Amsterdam: Elsevier Biomedical Press, 1982:127–62.
58. Myers RE. Experimental models of perinatal brain damage: Relevance to human pathology. In Gluck L, ed. *Intrauterine Asphyxia and the Developing Brain.* Chicago: Year Book Publishers, Inc., 1977:37–97.
59. Levene MI, Anthony MY. Perinatal asphyxia and neonatal seizures. In Gluckman PD, Heymann MA, eds. *Perinatal and Pediatric Pathophysiology.* London: Edward Arnold, 1993: 274–9.
60. Mehmet H, Bessley J, Edwards D. Apoptosis and necrosis. In Polin RA, Fox WW, Abman SH, eds. *Fetal and Neonatal Physiology*, 3rd edn. Philadelphia: Saunders, 2004:72–9.
61. Frank L, Sosenko IRS. Prenatal development of lung antioxidant in four species. *J Pediatr* 1987;110:106–10.
62. Frank L. Development of the antioxidant defences in fetal life. *Semin Neonatol* 1988;3:173–82.
63. Berger HM, Molicki JS, Moison RMW, Van Zoeren-Grobben D. Extracellular defence against oxidative stress in the newborn. *Semin Neonatol* 1998:183–90.
64. Pallardo FV, Sastre J, Asensi M, Rodrigo F, Estrela JM, Vina J. Physiological changes in glutathione metabolism in foetal and newborn rat liver. *Biochem J* 1991;274:891–3.
65. Power GG, Blood AB, Hunter CJ. Perinatal thermal physiology. In Polin RA, Fox WW, Abman SH, eds. *Fetal and Neonatal Physiology*, 3rd edn. Philadelphia: Saunders, 2004:541–8.
66. Hoath SB. Physiologic development of the skin. In Polin RA, Fox WW, Abman SH, eds. *Fetal and Neonatal Physiology*, 3rd edn. Philadelphia: Saunders, 2004:595–611.
67. McMillen C. Biological rhythms. In Gluckman PD, Heymann MA, eds. *Perinatal and Pediatric Pathophysiology.* London: Edward Arnold, 1993:254–6.
68. Parssons WJ, Williams RS, Shelton JM, Luo Y, Kessler DJ, Richards JA. Developmental regulation of cytochrome oxidase subunit VIa isoforms in cardiac and skeletal muscle. *Am J Physiol* 1996;270:H567–74.

2 Neonatal jaundice

F. Rubaltelli and C. Dani

Introduction

Neonatal jaundice is one of the most common conditions of the newborn. Neonatologists are concerned about this problem, not only for the risk of bilirubin encephalopathy in very low birth weight infants and in full-term infants with hemolysis due to different causes (rhesus and ABO hemolytic disease, glucose-6-phosphate dehydrogenase deficiency, etc.), but also because of the anxiety that jaundice in the full-term neonate gives to parents.

In neonates, jaundice becomes apparent at higher serum bilirubin concentrations in comparison to adults (5–7 mg/dl or 85–120 mmol/l in comparison to 2–3 mg/dl or 35–50 mmol/l). If we take into account clinically evident jaundice, we can say that almost 60–70% of term infants and almost all prematures present with jaundice. But, if we consider a cutoff of >12.9 mg/dl (220 mmol/l), which in full-term infants is the most accepted limit to consider jaundice as deserving attention, only 5% or less present with a serum bilirubin concentration higher than that.[1,2]

Neonatal jaundice is principally the result of transient deficiency of bilirubin conjugation, some deficiency of hepatic uptake and intracellular transport, and an increased enterohepatic circulation of the pigment. It is notable that bilirubin production in the newborn is two or more times greater than that in the adult per kilogram of body weight.[2] The serum bilirubin level at any point in time is dependent on the rate of bilirubin production minus the rate of bilirubin excretion.

The largest portion of bilirubin is derived from heme breakdown of hemoglobin, myoglobin, mitochondrial and microsomal cytochromes, catalase, and peroxidase. Heme degradation probably occurs by auto-oxidation after reduction of ferric (Fe^{3+}) heme to the ferrous state (Fe^{2+}) by the action of heme oxygenase and reduced form of nicotinamide adenine dinucleotide phosphate (NADPH) cytochrome *c* (P450) reductase.[3,4] The methene-bridge carbon of the heme is eliminated as carbon monoxide (CO). At the end of this process biliverdin is formed, and is subsequently reduced to bilirubin through the activity of biliverdin reductase. For each molecule of bilirubin formed, a molecule of CO is produced, which constitutes the basis for measuring bilirubin production by determination of the CO concentration in the expired air, or the carboxyhemoglobin content of the blood.[2]

Three isoforms of HO have been isolated: inducible heme oxygenase (HO-1), constitutive heme oxygenase (HO-2), and the more recently discovered and less active heme oxygenase isoform (HO-3).[5] HO-1 is a known stress response protein, whose transcription can be induced by a whole array of stresses, including endotoxin, transition metals, heme, hemoglobin, and other heme proteins.[6] Indeed, it has been suggested that HO-1 induction might represent a generalized response to oxidative stress[5,7,8] and that it could confer cellular protection against oxidant stress. However, recent studies suggest that HO-1 induction might not always be beneficial and that the release of redox-active iron from heme might induce an increase of oxidative stress.[9,10] Moreover, *in vitro* studies[11,12] suggested that the possible protective antioxidant action of HO-1 could occur within a narrow range, as when HO-1 is overexpressed, and free-iron release may obviate any cytoprotective effect against oxidative stress.[13]

Bilirubin solubility

Bilirubin is derived from heme by separation from methene-bridge. The configuration on the C-5 and C-14 bridges is very important, and bilirubin preferentially takes the *Z* form. Moreover, (*Z*,*Z*)-bilirubin IXa has a configuration that makes the formation of intramolecular hydrogen bridge linkages possible. For this reason it is almost insoluble in aqueous media (1–10 nmol/l at pH 7.4), but dissolves readily in a number of non-polar solvents. The degree to which bilirubin (B) ionizes with the propionic acid residue depends on the pH, and this is decisive both for the distribution of the molecule and for its toxicity:

$$B^{2-}+H \leftrightarrow BH^{-};\ BH^{-}+H+ \rightarrow BH_2$$

The dissociation constants cannot be determined with absolute precision owing to the problem of solubility, but they are found to be approximately $pK_1=4.4$ and $pK_2=6.5$.[14]

All modifications of the molecule that prevent the formation of hydrogen bridges cause an increase in water solubility. In the human, this takes the form of an esterification of the residue of propionic acid with glucuronic acid, which makes excretion in the bile possible. Obviously, monoconjugated bilirubin is less soluble than diconjugated bilirubin, and can thus precipitate in the biliary tract forming stones. Alkalinization (salt formation) or the addition of non-polar solvents, such as chloroform, methanol, ethanol, etc., also results in better solubility, and this is the key mechanism used in the laboratory to differentiate between direct-reacting (mostly the conjugated form) and indirect-reacting (unconjugated) bilirubin.

Distribution of bilirubin in the body

The distribution of bilirubin in the body is essentially determined by its firm binding to albumin. However, the presence of a visible jaundice seems to be due, at least in part, to the presence of bilirubin in the skin. Therefore, there is a dynamic competition between tissue-binding sites and albumin-binding sites. In fact, albumin binds bilirubin according to the law of mass action:

$$\text{Bilirubin} + \text{albumin} \leftrightarrow \text{albumin–bilirubin}$$

$$\frac{(\text{albumin–bilirubin})}{\text{albumin} \times \text{bilirubin}} = \text{KA}$$

Two classes of binding sites have been observed: a primary binding site with an extremely high affinity for bilirubin ($KA_1 = 7 \times 10^7$ l/mol at 37°C) and one or two other binding sites with a lesser affinity ($KA_2 = 5 \times 10^5$ l/mol). The concentration of free bilirubin is mostly determined by the molar relationship between bilirubin and albumin. However, bilirubin can be displaced from its binding site by certain drugs, such as sulfisoxazole, benzoate, salicylate, etc. Nowadays, every drug intended for use in newborns must be accompanied by the evidence that it has no effect on bilirubin–albumin binding.[15]

At the hepatic level, bilirubin is taken up at the sinusoidal membrane level, but about 40% is then regurgitated into the plasma again. The albumin–bilirubin complex seems to bind to specific receptors located on the basolateral surface of the sinusoidal plasmatic membrane of the hepatocyte much better than bilirubin alone.[16] In the hepatocyte, bilirubin reacts with binding proteins, the most important being glutathione *S*-transferase, thus preventing its regurgitation into the plasma. Bilirubin has a low solubility in water due to the fact that its hydrophilic groups are masked by hydrogen bonds; however, it is made hydrosoluble by esterification in the endoplasmic reticulum, with one or both propionic acid side chains reacting with a sugar residue to form mono- or diesters; in this way the formation of hydrogen bonds is prevented.[17]

The formation of bilirubin glycosides is catalyzed by uridine diphosphate (UDP) glycosyltransferase, an enzyme system that utilizes bilirubin as an acceptor substrate, and UDP sugars (especially glucuronic acid) that act as donor substrates. Transfer from binding proteins to the enzyme system does not necessarily require a higher affinity for the enzyme-binding site, because bilirubin is far more soluble in membranes than in the aqueous cytoplasm, and the reaction could therefore take place simply by means of a favorable partitioning. Furthermore, the bilirubin monoglucuronide could be converted to diglucuronide by the same enzyme system, following a 180° rotation of the monoglucuronide molecule, or it could even be excreted without modification in the bile.

Oxidative stress and neonatal hyperbilirubinemia

Several reports have emphasized the antioxidant role of bilirubin, which in human neonatal plasma seems to have a greater antioxidant potency than urates, α-tochoferol, or ascorbates.[18] In particular, unconjugated bilirubin is able to scavenge singlet oxygen with high efficiency to react with superoxide anions and peroxyl radicals, and to serve as a reducing substrate for peroxidases in the presence of hydrogen peroxide or organic hydroperoxides. Nevertheless, although the antioxidant effect of bilirubin as a scavenger of reactive oxygen species is well documented *in vitro*[19–22] as well as in animal studies,[23] its role *in vivo* has not been definitively cleared in preterm infants.[22–27]

Recently, two studies investigated the possible relationship between plasma bilirubin levels and oxidative stress in newborn infants[28,29] excluding the fact that bilirubin acts as an antioxidant agent *in vivo*. It was demonstrated that the decrease of plasma bilirubin level (probably induced by phototherapy) was associated with the concurrent increase of HO-1 activity in blood and the decrease of oxidative stress, suggesting an antioxidant effect of HO-1 exerted *in vivo* by mechanisms other than bilirubin formation. These protective mechanisms could involve the removal of the pro-oxidant heme, the removal of hydrogen superoxide during the degradation of heme, the induction of ferritin synthesis, which sequesters redox-active iron, and the regulation of superoxide anion production. Other possible mechanisms could involve the multiple ways by which CO modulates inflammatory processes, such as the reduction of neutrophil adhesion and extravasation,[30] the reduction of histamine release from mast cells and human basophils,[31,32] the inhibition of the expression of proinflammatory cytokines, such as TNFα and IL-1β, and an increase of anti-inflammatory cytokine IL-10.[33]

These studies confirmed the findings of Yigit *et al.*,[34] who found no correlation between oxidative stress and total bilirubin in preterm infants with non-hemolytic hyperbilirubinemia, and Gopinathan *et al.*,[35] who observed no correlation between plasma bilirubin level and total plasma antioxidant capacity in preterm infants. On the other hand, Belanger *et al.*[36] found an association between reduction of the antioxidant capacity of plasma after exchange transfusion, and the ensuing decrease of bilirubinemia. This result, however, as indicated by the authors, could be explained by factors other than bilirubin decrease, such as oxidative stress induced by a large amount of transfused blood and the consequent overload of iron through transfusion. Hammerman *et al.*[37] found a correlation between total bilirubin serum level and plasmatic antioxidant capacity, but the bilirubinemia of their patients was lower than that reported in other studies. To explain these conflicting results it may be considered that the correlation between plasma bilirubin level and the antioxidant capacity of the plasma could change at low and high values, and could be affected by phototherapy through its lowering effect on bilirubin, which, moreover, could also explain the lack of correlation between bilirubin and HO-activity.

Causes of neonatal jaundice

Physiological jaundice

The so-called physiological or developmental jaundice (which could be especially harmful for the small preterm infant) is due to an imbalance between increased pigment load and reduced hepatic handling. The latter seems mainly determined by the low activity of bilirubin UDP glucuronosyltransferase, the hepatic microsomal enzyme that conjugates bilirubin with one or two sugar moieties. It is now accepted that, even in the absence of impaired biliary secretion, a fraction of the esterified bilirubins formed in the liver normally refluxes from hepatocyte to the plasma. Measuring the esterified bilirubins in the plasma of newborn infants has made it possible to demonstrate definitively that neonatal jaundice is mainly due to an increased bilirubin production with subnormal conjugation.[38] On the other hand, infants with the lowest plasma concentration of total bilirubin exhibited the highest fraction of conjugates. The percentage of diconjugates relative to total conjugates is 15% on the first day of life. This value tends to increase slightly with age.[38] In premature infants, serum monoconjugates paralleled the course of total and unconjugated bilirubin, but the values were significantly lower than those found in full-term infants.[17,38]

From the practical point of view, we can rule out the diagnosis of physiological jaundice if plasma or serum bilirubin concentration exceeds at any time 12.9 mg/dl (220 mmol/l) in full-term infants or 5–8 mg/dl (85–138 mmol/l) in preterm infants,[39] if jaundice becomes evident in the first 24 h of life, if bilirubin concentration increases more than 5 mg/dl/day (85 mmol/ l/day), and if direct reacting plasma bilirubin exceeds 1.5–2 mg/dl (25–35 mmol/l) (it is important to determine conjugated bilirubin by a chromatographic method[17,38]).

Jaundice in breast-fed neonates

An increased incidence of early-onset jaundice has been reported in breast-fed infants, both full-term and preterm.[40,41] However, an increased bilirubin synthesis, demonstrated by an increased CO production, possibly secondary to caloric deprivation, has not been proven.[42] The process of bilirubin conjugation, investigated in breast-fed and formula-fed infants, by means of the determination of serum concentrations of unconjugated and esterified bilirubin, and the proportion of diesterified (as a percentage of esterified bilirubin) pigment, appeared not to be different between the two groups of infants, showing that bilirubin production and conjugation were not different.[43] In addition, a recent study comparing the incidence of neonatal jaundice in 605 infants exclusively breast-fed on demand, in 623 who received both breast- and formula feeding, and in 226 exclusively formula-fed demonstrates that the incidence of neonatal hyperbilirubinemia (>12.9 mg/dl or 220 mmol/l) in full-term infants is both insignificant (< 5%) and not correlated with demand breast-feeding.[1] These results were recently confirmed in a population of 2174 infants with gestational age ≥37 weeks where hyperbilirubinemia was not found to be correlated with breast-feeding, but rather with an increased weight loss, dehydration, and caloric deprivation, which could enhance the enterohepatic circulation of bilirubin.[44]

Hemolytic jaundice

Fetomaternal blood group incompatibility, particularly ABO and rhesus hemolytic disease, are the most common causes of severe jaundice. Nowadays, rhesus hemolytic disease is infrequently due to maternal prophylaxis with antirhesus immunoglobulins. However, ABO hemolytic disease still remains an important cause of indirect hyperbilirubinemia and anemia in full-term as well as preterm infants. Suspicion of ABO or rhesus hemolytic disease must be confirmed by a direct Coombs test carried out on the newborn blood.

Glucose-6-phosphate dehydrogenase (G-6-PD) deficiency

G-6-PD deficiency is frequently associated with neonatal jaundice and sometimes kernicterus. The pathogenesis of this jaundice remains in part unclear, because increased erythrocyte breakdown is not always the major factor in its development.[45] In some patients, overt hemolysis, due to different substances, is detected, and in others no signs of hemolysis are detectable (normal level of carboxyhemoglobin). In this group of patients it has been shown that a deficiency in bilirubin conjugation does exist.[45] It is possible that G-6-PD is also involved in some steps (possibly UDP glucuronic acid synthesis) of bilirubin conjugation.

Congenital non-obstructive, non-hemolytic jaundice

Crigler–Najjar disease is a rare disorder of bilirubin metabolism caused by a deficiency of hepatic UDP-glucuronyltransferase, and characterized by high serum levels of unconjugated bilirubin that appear in the first days after birth and continue through life. Based on the responsiveness of the serum bilirubin concentration to phenobarbital, this disease can be distinguished as either type 1, which does not respond to phenobarbital, or type 2, which responds to barbiturates and other drugs that induce enzyme synthesis. Type 2 is probably caused by a partial enzymatic deficiency. In type 1 and type 2 Crigler–Najjar disease, it is possible to detect traces of monoconjugated but not diconjugated bilirubin both in serum and in bile.[46]

Bilirubin entry into the brain

Some clinical observations suggest that several mechanisms may be involved with the entry of bilirubin pigment into the brain. In fact, bilirubin seems to enter into the brain both as free bilirubin acid and as bilirubin–albumin complex, by passage through a disrupted blood–brain barrier that is often caused by hyperosmolality and hypercarbia. It seems that even during physiological jaundice, there is a steady passage of unbound bilirubin across this barrier. Furthermore, these low levels of bilirubin do not seem to be harmful; in fact, it is also possible that cerebral stores of bilirubin oxidase are able to metabolize bilirubin *in loco*. Obviously, the entry of bilirubin into the brain can be significantly increased in the presence of high plasma bilirubin concentrations, particularly if the albumin-binding capacity is exceeded.[47] Ahlfors *et al.* reported that in term newborns unbound bilirubin levels between 0.9 and 2 μg/dl produce subtle and reversible changes in auditory brainstem response latency, and described the case of an infant who developed a kernicterus at a total bilirubin concentration of 31.7 mg/dl and unbound bilirubin concentration of 7.7 μg/dl.[48] However, in preterm infants bilirubin-induced changes in auditory brainstem response can begin at an unbound bilirubin level of 0.5 μg/dl and kernicterus becomes likely at 1–1.5 μg/dl.[49]

Effects of bilirubin on neurologic functions

It is well known that bilirubin acts to uncouple oxidative phosphorylation and, consequently, inhibits the respiratory chain by causing certain toxic effects.[50] However, a number of studies carried out on experimental animals show no difference either in bilirubin binding between different brain regions or in the rate of bilirubin disappearance from the cerebral tissues.[51] Moreover, it is still unclear as to why bilirubin has a preferential localization at the level of the basal ganglia. One proposed explanation relies on the possibility that bilirubin may be metabolized locally at different rates.[51] In fact, the typical findings of kernicterus are a yellow staining of the subthalamic, dentate, and inferior olivary nuclei and the globus pallidus. Cell culture models suggest that bilirubin initially interacts with cellular membranes, affects ion channels and neurotransmitters, and ultimately leads to deranged metabolism and cell death.[52] The clinical picture of kernicterus is also fairly uniform in these children, with convulsions and opisthotonus followed by hypotonia, high-pitched crying, and fever. The sequelae in the survivors consist of neurogenic hearing disorders, choreoathetosis with asymmetrical spasticity and paralysis of upward gaze, together with other neurologic manifestations. Ambulation, despite severe athetosis, is generally reached by the age of 5 years.[53]

Brain stem auditory-evoked potentials are altered by bilirubin in various ways.[54,55] In some studies, it has been observed to change the conduction latencies; in others, it lowered the conduction wave amplitude, both of which fit in with the follow-up observation of deafness in kernicteric babies. Some studies note reversibility of these altered potentials through lowering of high bilirubin levels.[4,56,57]

Bilirubin-induced membrane potential lowering may impair nerve conduction along the auditory pathway, which may be reversible if each cell endures only temporary malfunction or if a sufficient number of neurons in the nerve survive the toxicity to maintain function.

It is commonly accepted that (1) bilirubin may be toxic for cells, (2) kernicterus can occur when unconjugated bilirubin levels are high, and (3) the mechanism of bilirubin toxicity is mostly unknown.

Measurement of bilirubinemia

The majority of the published studies on bilirubin in infants were made measuring its level on capillary blood with spectrophotometric methods. Some studies compared capillary and venous measurement of bilirubinemia, but their results were conflicting.[58,59] Therefore, to confirm a high plasma bilirubin level in a venous sample is not recommended. Recently, new devices have permitted an easier and more reliable transcutaneous measurement of bilirubin. The Chromatics Colormate III™ (Chromatics Color Science International Inc., New York, NY, USA) is still based on the color of the skin, estimating serum bilirubin from skin reflectance (skin color), whereas the BiliCheck™ (Respironics, Murrysville, PA, USA) measures transcutaneous bilirubin by utilizing the entire spectrum of visible light (380–760 nm) reflected by the skin. Data obtained using BiliCheck™ suggest that this device provides measurements within 2–3 mg/dl (34–51 μmol/l) of the serum bilirubin concentration.[60] These devices could be used as screening tools but, in some circumstances, also as substitutes for serum bilirubin measurements, in particular, when its value is lower than 15 mg/dl (257 μmol/l).

Treatment of neonatal hyperbilirubinemia

Bilirubin is bound to albumin in the blood, and when its concentration exceeds the binding capacity of the carrier, unbound or free bilirubin concentration increases and results in its redistribution between the tissues (brain) and the vascular space (free bilirubin theory). Thus, not only is the serum bilirubin concentration important in judging whether an infant is at risk of bilirubin toxicity, but the albumin concentration and the bilirubin/albumin ratio are also of critical importance. In fact, Ahlfors suggests that when the bilirubin/albumin ratio is < 8 mg/g (136 mmol/g) and the neonate appears well, exchange transfusion is probably not necessary.[61]

Exchange transfusion, first performed in 1925 by Alfred Purvis Hart and then implemented by L. K. Diamond in 1947 using the umbilical vein to withdraw and to perfuse blood, was the only treatment available until 1958, when Cremer and colleagues[62] showed that both sunlight and blue light were able to reduce jaundice in newborns. In fact, phototherapy is now the most widely used method worldwide for the treatment of jaundiced babies.

The mechanisms by which light renders the insoluble bilirubin molecule (bilirubin IX-alpha *Z,Z*), at physiologic pH, soluble and rapidly excretable in the biliary tract are the transformation of the *Z,Z* configuration at the C4–C5 and C15–C16 double bonds to the *E* configuration in one or both double bonds, thus forming the configurational isomers *E,Z* or *Z,E* or *E,E*.[63–65] Of these isomers, the predominant one is the *Z,E* form. However, the *Z,E* change is reversible, and after phototherapy it reconverts in the bile or in the intestines to the *Z,Z* isomer. In addition, intramolecular cyclization of bilirubin can occur as a result of phototherapy, to form a structural isomer called lumirubin, which cannot be reconverted to native bilirubin. Moreover, lumirubin, which is formed at a lower rate in comparison to the configurational isomers, seems to be excreted more rapidly in the bile than the other isomers.

There is a striking regional selectivity that causes isomerization to take place at the double bond of the CH-bridges. Because of the specific preference evidenced by one-half of the bilirubin molecule in binding to human albumin, the *E* configuration in position 15 is the main isomer formed. This selectivity is lacking to a large extent in a number of the animals used in experimental studies. Finally, the available data suggest that bilirubin is bound to albumin at the site of the light effect, namely in the skin.

The extent to which isomerization, cyclization, or oxidation exerts the therapeutic effect of light is determined mainly by the quantum yield of the photochemical reactions and the speed of the transport processes up to the excretory phase.

The quantum yield of configurational isomerization is probably very high; isomers are formed very quickly, and they can be detected within a few minutes after light treatment. On the other hand, photocyclization proceeds more slowly, and depends on the wavelength employed. Moreover, the quantum yield of bilirubin oxidation is very low, and it is most probable that the excretion of catabolites formed in the process takes place rapidly. Since the excretion rate of lumirubin is very high, it is conceivable that, in phototherapy for neonatal jaundice, bilirubin photocyclization is the most effective mechanism of bilirubin photometabolism, followed by configurational isomerization, and, finally, photo-oxidation.

The bronze baby syndrome (BBS)

The BBS is a rare pathological condition that appears during phototherapy. The typical characteristic is a grayish-brown discoloration of the skin, serum, and urine. This condition was first described by Kopelman *et al.*,[66] who observed the typical discoloration in the skin of a newborn following phototherapy. They found that the onset of the syndrome was linked to an increase in conjugated bilirubin, implying a cholestatic disorder; moreover, they also related it to hemolytic anemia. Since then, various authors have attempted to explain the biochemical mechanism responsible for the onset of this syndrome.[67,68] In this connection, Kopelman *et al.* noted a reduced bilirubin-binding capacity in newborns suffering from BBS. They suspected that bilirubin photoproducts might be responsible both for the bronze discoloration and for the change in binding capacity ascertained by the salicylate method. Autopsy evidence later showed that this peculiar discoloration was also present in the kidneys, liver, and peritoneum. Clark *et al.*[67] and Rubaltelli *et al.*,[68] in particular, found anatomical signs of kernicterus in two newborns who died with this syndrome. They considered this observation to be the confirmation that the pigments responsible for BBS increase the risk of bilirubin neurotoxicity, as suggested by the reported decline in the albumin-binding capacity.[66,69]

In 1982, a notably higher concentration of porphyrins was found in the serum of patients with BBS.[70] Two cases of this syndrome, with very high serum porphyrins, probably due to some degree of cholestasis, were described.[71,72] The porphyrins were identified as Cu^{2+}-uro-, Cu^{2+}-copro-, and Cu^{2+}-protoporphyrin. In fact, the absorption spectrum of serum specimens from infants with BBS showed spectral features typical of bilirubin (peak absorption around 460 nm), as well as an intense band with a peak at about 400 nm and broad absorbance in the near-UV and the 600–700-nm region. The latter two features were not confirmed by the absorption spectra of control sera. The sera of bronze babies also exhibited a wide range of fluorescence emission spectra with peaks at 585, 619, and 670 nm. This finding indicates that absorption in the 400-nm band does not reflect the presence of residual hemoglobin in the serum because hemoproteins are known to be devoid of any appreciable fluorescence in the red region. Instead, the emission spectra observed are characteristic of porphyrin compounds.

Chromatographic separation led to the conclusion that the main component is Cu^{e+}-protoporphyrin IX, although small amounts of Cu^{e+}-coproporphyrin II and Cu^{e+}-uroporphyrin III are also present. These porphyrins do not seem to have an appreciable photosensitizing effect. Furthermore, there was no evidence of significant alterations in the UV spectrum of irradiated serum from infants with BBS or in cord blood serum with added synthetic Cu^{e+}-porphyrins. This is due to the well-known shortening of the half-life of excited porphyrin as a consequence of the binding of the Cu^{e+} ion on the tetrapyrrolic ring.[73]

These investigations show that the grayish-brown skin color is a result of the photolability of the Cu^{2+}-porphyrins. Indeed, Cu^{e+}-porphyrins in the serum of infants with BBS or in aqueous solutions are converted under irradiation with visible light into brown photoproducts with a higher absorption in near-UV and red spectral regions. Moreover, the presence of bilirubin increases the photodegradation rate of Cu^{e+}-porphyrins, suggesting that bilirubin acts as a photosensitizer in this process.

Guidelines for the treatment of unconjugated hyperbilirubinemia

Full-term newborn infants

Neonatal jaundice (total serum bilirubin concentration > 12.9 mg/dl (220 mmol/l) occurs in around 5% of normal neonates.[1] In the majority of cases it is a physiologic or developmental jaundice,[1,74] which does not need any treatment. However, it is important to exclude the presence of a rhesus or ABO hemolytic disease, and the possibility that the jaundice could be an early sign of an inborn error of metabolism, or sepsis, etc.

It is suggested that a direct Coombs test plus blood group and rhesus determination should be carried out on the cord blood of every neonate, and when jaundice is present, the neonatologist should evaluate the appropriateness of a serum bilirubin determination in relation to the day of appearance and intensity of the jaundice, etc. A serum bilirubin level of 20 mg/dl (340 mmol/l) in a normal full-term newborn infant is no longer considered an indication for exchange transfusion.[74] In the absence of a hemolytic disorder, and with a bilirubin level in the range 20–25 mg/dl (340–425 mmol/l), exchange transfusion might be considered, but this decision must be based on a careful evaluation of the risk/benefit ratio.

Following Wennberg's suggestions,[47] one should take into consideration not only the serum bilirubin level but also the albumin serum concentration: that is, by multiplying the albumin value in grams by 7, a value is obtained which corresponds to the level when an exchange transfusion is indicated.

It is recommended that phototherapy be started during the first 24 h of life if the serum bilirubin level exceeds 4–7 mg/dl (70–120 mmol/l), or during the second 24 h of life if it exceeds 11–15 mg/dl 190–260 mmol/l), and in all cases whenever it exceeds 15 mg/dl (260 mmol/l). Phototherapy should be carried out for at least 24 h, and should be interrupted when serum bilirubin concentration is decreased by ≥ 2 mg/dl (≥ 35 mmol/l).

However, the American Academy of Pediatrics has recently published guidelines for the management of hyperbilirubinemia in the newborn infant of 35 or more weeks' gestation, which report in depth on current recommendations for prevention, diagnosis, and treatment of neonatal jaundice.[75] The approach to jaundice in preterm infants appears more difficult because there are no specific evidence-based guidelines for the use of phototherapy and exchange transfusion in these infants. Different authors have reported a range of plasma bilirubin levels for intervention in various circumstances, but none of these indications has greater validity than another.[39] However, considering that in preterm infants kernicterus has almost disappeared probably because of aggressive phototherapy, it is probable that the current management of jaundice in these infants is correct.

Other possible therapeutic interventions are immunoglobulin therapy in immune hemolytic jaundice and administration of the heme oxygenase inhibitor Sn-mesoporphyrin. Alcock *et al.*, in a meta-analytical study on term and preterm infants with rhesus and ABO incompatibility, found that the rate of exchange transfusion decreased significantly in the immunoglobulin-treated group.[76] As for Sn-mesoporphyrin, its use is very promising both for the prevention and for the treatment of neonatal jaundice. However, this drug is as yet under research and is not commercially available (see Kappas[77]).

Premature newborn infants

In the past few years, a number of studies have shown that currently neither kernicterus nor clinical signs of bilirubin encephalopathy are found in premature babies (see the important review of Conolly and Volpe[78]). These findings were reported despite the fact that higher serum bilirubin concentrations were allowed compared with the studies reported in the 1960s and 1970s, when kernicterus was not a rare occurrence.[79,80] It is possible that the improved quality of health care has reduced the appearance of preterm kernicterus, the pathogenesis of which is still not completely understood.[80–85]

The definition of prematurity (< 37 weeks of gestational age) includes neonates of very different gestational ages. Moreover, a generous use of phototherapy has allowed a reduction of high serum bilirubin concentrations, and as a result exchange transfusion is no longer used very often. However, it seems rational to initiate light treatment independently of the age of the premature infant, whenever the serum bilirubin concentration is ≥ 8 mg/dl (135 mmol/l), provided that no hemolysis is present. In fact, exchange transfusion must be considered when bilirubin reaches the level of 18 mg/dl (305 mmol/l). Furthermore, for the premature newborn one can use Wennberg's formula[47] to identify infants needing exchange transfusion: multiplying by six the value of serum albumin concentration (in g) one obtains the threshold value for exchange transfusion.

REFERENCES

1. Rubaltelli FF. Unconjugated and conjugated bilirubin pigments during perinatal development. IV. The influence of breast-feeding on neonatal hyperbilirubinemia. *Biol Neonate* 1993; 64:104–9.
2. Maisels MJ, Pathak A, Nelson NM, Nathan DG, Smith CA. Endogenous production of carbon monoxide in normal and erythroblastotic newborn infants. *J Clin Invest* 1971;50:1–8.
3. Yoshinaga T, Sassa S, Kappas A. The occurrence of molecular interactions among NADPH-cytochrome-c reductase, heme oxygenase, and biliverdin reductase in heme degradation. *J Biol Chem* 1982;257:7786–93.
4. Yoshinaga T, Sassa S, Kappas A. A comparative study of heme degradation by NADPH-cytochrome-c reductase alone and by the complete heme oxygenase system. *J Biol Chem* 1982;257: 7794–802.
5. Keyse SM, Applegate LA, Tromvoukis Y, Tyrrell TM. Oxidant stress leads to transcriptional activation of the human heme oxygenase gene in cultured skin fibroblast. *Mol Cell Biol* 1990; 10:4967–9.
6. Lamb NJ, Quinlan GJ, Mumby S, Evans TW, Gutteridge JMC. Haem oxygenase shows pro-oxidant activity in microsomal and cellular systems: Implication for the release of low-molecular-mass iron. *J Biochem* 1999;344:153–8.
7. Vile GF, Basu-Modak S, Waltner C, Tyrrell RM. Heme oxygenase 1 mediates an adaptive response to oxidative stress in human skin fibroblasts. *Proc Natl Acad Sci USA* 1994;91:2607–10.
8. Lautier D, Luscher P, Tyrrell RM. Endogenous glutathione levels, modulate both constitutive and UVA radiation/hydrogen peroxide inducible expression of the human heme oxygenase gene. *Carcinogenesis* 1992;13:227–32.
9. Gutteridge JMC. Fate of oxygen free radicals in extracellular fluids. *Biochem Soc Trans* 1982;10:72–3.
10. Dennery PA, Spitz DR, Yang G, *et al.* Oxygen toxicity and iron accumulation in the lungs of mice lacking heme oxygenase-2. *J Clin Invest* 1998;101:1001–11.
11. Dennery Pa, Sridhar KJ, Lee CS, *et al.* Heme oxygenase-mediated resistance to oxygen toxicity in hamster fibroblasts. *J Biol Chem* 1997;272:14937–42.
12. Suttner DM, Sridhar K, Le CS, Tomura T. Hansen TN, Dennery PA. Protective effects of transient HO-1 overexpression on susceptibility to oxygen toxicity. *Am J Physiol* 1999;276: L443–51.
13. Dennery PA. Regulation and role of heme oxygenase in oxidative injury. *Curr Top Cell Regul* 2000;36:181–99.
14. Jāhrig K, Jāhrig D, Meisel P. *Phototherapy. Treating Neonatal Jaundice with Visible Light.* München: Quintessenz-Verlag s-GmbH, 1993.
15. Brodersen R. Binding of bilirubin to albumin. *CRC Crit Rev Clin Lab Sci* 1979;11:305–99.
16. Berk PD, Potter BJ, Stremmel W. Role of plasma ligand binding proteins in the hepatocellular uptake of albumin bound organic anion. *Hepatology* 1987;7:165–76.
17. Rubaltelli FF. Bilirubin metabolism in the newborn (editorial). *Biol Neonate* 1993;63:133–8.
18. Halliwell B, Gutteridge JM. Role of free radicals and catalytic metal ions in human disease: An overview. *Methods Enzymol* 1990;186:1–85.
19. Kentaro H, Satoshi Y, Akio F, Shun I, Teruyuki O, Yorihiro Y. Oxidative stress in newborn infants with and without asphyxia as measured by plasma antioxidants and free fatty acids. *Biochem Biophis Res Commun* 1999;257:244–8.
20. Hardy P, Peri KG, Lahaie I, Varma DR, Chemtob S. Increased nitric oxide synthase and action preclude choroidal vasoconstriction to hyperoxia in newborn pig. *Circ Res* 1996;79:504–11.
21. Abran D, Varma DR, Chemtob S. Increased thromboxane mediated contractions of retinal vessels of newborn pig to peroxides. *Am J Physiol* 1995;268:H628–32.
22. Chemtob S, Abran D, Hardy P. Peroxide-cyclooxygenase interactions in postasphyxial changes in retinal and choroidal hemodinamics. *J Appl Physiol* 1995;78:2039–46.
23. James L, Greenough A, Naik S. The effect of blood transfusion on oxygenation in premature ventilated neonates. *Eur J Pediatr* 1997;156:139–141.
24. Cooke RWI, Clark D, Nickel-Dwyer M, Weindling AM. The apparent role of blood transfusion in the development of retinopathy of prematurity. *Eur J Pediatr* 1993;152:833–6.
25. Shaw JCL. Iron absorption by the premature infants: The effect of transfusion and iron supplementation on the serum ferritin levels. *Acta Paediatr Scand* 1982;299:S83–9.
26. Lackman GM, Schnieder C, Bohner J. Gestational age-dependent reference values for iron and selected proteins of iron metabolism in serum premature human neonates. *Biol Neonate* 1998; 74:208–13.
27. Siimes MA, Addiego JE, Dallman PR. Ferritin in serum, diagnosis of iron deficiency and overload in infants and children. *Blood* 1974;43:581–90.
28. Dani C, Martelli E, Bertini G, *et al.* Bilirubin plasma level and oxidative stress in preterm infants. *Arch Dis Child Fetal Neonatal Ed* 2003;88:F119–23.
29. Dani C, Masini E, Bertini G, *et al. Pediatr Res*, in press.
30. Ndisang JF, Masini E, Mannaioni PF, Wang R. In Wong R, ed. *Carbon Monoxide and Cardiovascular Inflammation.* Boca Raton, FL: CRC Press, 2002:165–80.
31. Mirabella C, Baronti R, Berni LA, *et al.* Hemin and carbon monoxide modulate the immunological response of human basophils. *Int Arch Allergy Immunol* 1999;118:259–60.
32. Di Bello MG, Berni L, Gai P, *et al.* A regulatory role of carbon monoxide in mast cells function. *Inflamm Res* 1998;1:S7–8.
33. Otterberin LE, Bach FH, Alam J, *et al.* Carbon monoxide has anti-inflammatory effects involving the mitogen-activated protein kinase pathway. *Nat Med* 2000;6:422–8.
34. Yigit S, Yurdakok M, Kilinc K, Oran O, Erdem G, Tekinalp G. Serum malondialdehyde concentrations in babies with hyperbilirubinemia. *Arch Dis Child Fetal Neonatal Ed* 1999;80:F235–7.
35. Gopinathan V, Miller NJ, Milner AD, Rice Evans CA. Bilirubin and ascorbate antioxidant activity in neonatal plasma. *FEBS Lett* 1994;349:197–200.
36. Bellanger S, Lavole JC, Chessex P. Influence of bilirubin on the antioxidant capacity of plasma in newborn infants. *Biol Neonate* 1997;71:233–8.
37. Hammerman C, Goldstein R, Kaplan M, *et al.* Bilirubin in the premature: Toxic waste or natural defense? *Clin Chem* 1998;44:2551–3.

38. Muraca M, Blanckaert N, Rubaltelli FF, Fevery J. Unconjugated and conjugated bilirubin pigments during perinatal development. I. Studies on rat serum and intestine. *Biol Neonate* 1986;49:90–5.
39. Maisels MJ, Watchko JF. Treatment of jaundice in low birthweight infants. *Arch Dis Child Fetal Neonatal Ed* 2003;88: F459–63.
40. Maisels MJ, Gifford K, Antle CE, Leib GR. Jaundice in the healthy newborn infant: A new approach to an old problem. *Pediatrics* 1988;81:505–11.
41. Lucas A, Baker BA. Breast milk jaundice in premature infants. *Arch Dis Child* 1986;61:1063–7.
42. Stevenson DK, Bartoletti AL, Ostrander CR, *et al.* Pulmonary excretion of carbon monoxide in human infant as an index of bilirubin production. IV. Effects of breast-feeding and caloric intake in the first postnatal week. *Pediatrics* 1980;65:1170–2.
43. Rubaltelli FF, Muraca M, Vilei MT, Largajolli G. Unconjugated and conjugated bilirubin pigments during perinatal development. III. Studies on serum of breast-fed and formula-fed neonates. *Biol Neonate* 1991;60:144–7.
44. Bertini G, Dani C, Tronchin M, Rubaltelli FF. Is breastfeeding really favoring early neonatal jaundice? *Pediatrics* 2001;107:E41.
45. Kaplan M, Rubaltelli FF, Hammerman C, *et al.* Conjugated bilirubin in neonates with glucose-6-phosphate deficiency. *J Pediatr* 1996;128:695–7.
46. Rubaltelli FF, Novello A, Zancan L, Vilei MT, Muraca M. Serum and bile bilirubin pigments in the differential diagnosis of Crigler–Najjar disease. *Pediatrics* 1994;94:553–6.
47. Wennberg RP. Cellular basis of bilirubin toxicity. *NY State J Med* 1991;91:493–6.
48. Ahlfors CE. Unbound bilirubin in a term newborn with kernicterus. *Pediatrics* 2003;111:1110–2.
49. Amin Sb, Ahlfors C, Orlando MS, Daizell LE, Merle KS, Guillet R. Bilirubin and serial auditory brainstem response in premature infants. *Pediatrics* 2001;107:664–70.
50. Zetterstrom R, Ernster L. Bilirubin, an uncoupler of oxidative phosphorylation in isolated mitochondria. *Nature* 1956;178: 1335–7.
51. Hansen WR. Bilirubin in the brain. Distribution and effects on neurophysiological and neurochemical processes. *Clin Pediatr* 1994;33:452–9.
52. Ochoa EL, Wennberg RP, An Y, *et al.* Interaction of bilirubin with isolated presynaptic nerve terminals: Functional effects on the uptake and release of neurotransmitters. *Cell Mol Neurobiol* 1993;13:69–86.
53. Rubaltelli FF, Griffith PF. Management of neonatal hyperbilirubinemia and prevention of kernicterus. *Drugs* 1992;43:864–72.
54. Karplus N, Lee C, Cashore WJ, Oh W. The effect of brain bilirubin deposition on auditory brain stem evoked responses in rats. *Early Hum Dev* 1988;16:185–94.
55. Vohr BR, Lester B, Rapisardi G, *et al.* Abnormal brainstem function correlates with acoustic cry features in term infants with hyperbilirubinemia. *J Pediatr* 1989;115:303–8.
56. Nakamura H, Takada S, Shimabaku R, *et al.* Auditory nerve and brainstem responses in newborn infants with hyperbilirubinemia. Pediatrics 1985;75:703–8.
57. Wennberg RP, Ahlfors CE, Bickers R, *et al.* Abnormal auditory brainstem response in a newborn infant with hyperbilirubinemia: Improvement with exchange transfusion. *J Pediatr* 1982; 100:624–6.
58. Leslie GI, Philips JB, Cassady G. Capillary and venous bilirubin values: Are they really different? *Am J Dis Child* 1987;141: 1199–200.
59. Eidelman AI, Schimmel MS, Algur N, Eylath U. Capillary and venous bilirubin values: They are different-and how! *Am J Dis Child* 1989;143:642
60. Bertini G, Rubaltelli FF. Non-invasive bilirubinometry in neonatal jaundice. *Semin Neonatol* 2002;7:129–33.
61. Ahlfors CE. Criteria for exchange transfusion in jaundiced newborns. *Pediatrics* 1994;93:488–94.
62. Cremer RJ, Perryman PW, Richards DH. Influence of light on the hyperbilirubinemia of infants. *Lancet* 1958;1:1994–7.
63. Cohen A, Ostrow J. New concepts in phototherapy: Photoisomerization of bilirubin IX-alpha and the potential toxic effect of light. *Pediatrics* 1980;65:740–50.
64. Lightner D, Wooldridge T, McDonagh A. Configurational isomerization of bilirubin and the mechanisms of jaundice phototherapy. *Biochim Biophys Res Commun* 1979;86:235–43.
65. Lightner D, Woolridge T, McDonagh A. Photobilirubin: An early bilirubin photoproduct detected by absorbance difference spectroscopy. *Proc Natl Acad Sci USA* 1979;76:29–32.
66. Kopelman AE, Brown RS, Odel GB. The bronze baby syndrome: A complication of phototherapy. *J Pediatr* 1972;81:446–50.
67. Clark CF, Torii S, Hamamoto Y, Kaito H. The 'bronze baby' syndrome: Postmortem data. *J Pediatr* 1976;88:461–4.
68. Rubaltelli FF, Da Riol R, D'Amore ESG, Jori G. The bronze baby syndrome: Evidence of increased tissue concentration of copper porphyrins. *Acta Paediatr* 1996;85:381–4.
69. Ebbesen F. Low reserve albumin for binding of bilirubin in neonates with deficiency of bilirubin excretion and bronze baby syndrome. *Acta Paediatr Scand* 1982;71:415–20.
70. Jori G, Reddi E, Rubaltelli FF. Bronze baby syndrome: Evidence for an increased serum porphyrin concentration. *Lancet* 1982; 1:1073.
71. Jori G, Reddi E, Rubaltelli FF. Porphyrin metabolism in the bronze baby syndrome. In Stern L, Bard H, Friis HB, eds. *Intensive Care in the Newborn.* New York: Masson Publishing Co. 1993:41–5.
72. Rubaltelli FF, Jori G, Reddi E. Bronze baby syndrome: A new porphyrin-related disorder. *Pediatr Res* 1983;17:327–30.
73. Cauzzo G, Gennari G, Jori G, Spikes JD. The effect of the chemical structure on the photosensitizing efficiency of porphyrins. *Photochem Photobiol* 1977;25:389–95.
74. Newman TB, Maisels MJ. Evaluation and treatment of jaundice in the term newborn: A kinder, gentler approach. *Pediatrics* 1992;89:809–18.
75. American Academy of Pediatrics. Management of hyperbilirubinemia in the newborn infant 35 or more weeks of gestation. *Pediatrics* 2004;114:297–316.
76. Alcock GS. Immunoglobulin infusion for isoimmune haemolytic jaundice in neonates. *Cochrane Database Syst Rev* 2002;3: CD003313.
77. Kappas A. A method for interdicting the development of severe jaundice in newborns by inhibiting the production of bilirubin. *Pediatrics* 2004;113:119–23.
78. Connolly AM, Volpe JJ. Clinical features of bilirubin encephalopathy. *Clin Perinatol* 1988;17:371–9.
79. Harris RC, Lucey JF, MacLean RJ. Kernicterus in premature infants associated with low concentration of bilirubin in the plasma. *Pediatrics* 1958;21:875–83.
80. Gartner LM, Snyder RN, Chabon RS. Kernicterus: High incidence in premature infants with low serum bilirubin concentrations. *Pediatrics* 1970;45:906–17.
81. Jardine DS, Rogers K. Relationship of benzyl alcohol to kernicterus, intraventricular hemorrhage, and mortality in preterm infants. *Pediatrics* 1989;83:153–60.
82. Seidman DS, Paz I, Stevenson DK, *et al.* Neonatal hyperbilirubinemia and physical and cognitive performance at 17 years of age. *Pediatrics* 1991;88:828–33.
83. Van de Bor M, Ens D, Schreuder AM, *et al.* Hyperbilirubinemia in low-birthweight infants and outcome at 5 years of age. *Pediatrics* 1992;89:359–64.
84. O'Shea TM, Dillard RG, Klinepeter KL, *et al.* Serum bilirubin levels, intracranial hemorrhage, and the risk of developmental problems in very-low-birthweight neonates. *Pediatrics* 1992; 90:888–92.
85. Bergman I, Hirsch RP, Fria TJ, *et al.* Cause of hearing loss in the high-risk premature infant. *J Pediatr* 1985;106:95–101.

3 Management of hypotension in the neonatal period

S. J. English

Introduction

Hypotension is a commonly encountered problem on the neonatal intensive care unit. It occurs in up to 40% of very low-birth-weight (< 1500 g) infants, and is almost universally seen in the extreme preterm baby, most commonly in the first 48 h after birth. Its importance lies in its possible causal link with brain injury in these infants.[1–4]

There are numerous controversies surrounding the management of hypotension in the preterm infant. As more extremely preterm babies are surviving, our accepted definitions of hypotension are being challenged. The level of blood pressure required to maintain tissue perfusion in these babies is unknown, and the effects of standard therapy are relatively under-researched. As a result, the level of hypotension at which treatment is instigated, and the treatment chosen, largely remain subject to personal preference.

Definition

Normal blood pressure has proven difficult to define in preterm babies, partly because it varies with gestational and postnatal age,[5,6] but also because the range of blood pressure, which will ensure adequate organ perfusion, is not known. There have been a number of studies attempting to define the normal range of blood pressure in the neonate. These have resulted in two widely accepted definitions of hypotension:

(1) Mean arterial blood pressure less than the 10th centile for gestation/birth weight and postnatal age.[1]

(2) Mean arterial blood pressure less than gestational age in weeks. This is derived from the first definition, following the observation that the 10th centile for mean blood pressure is roughly equal to the gestational age.[5] It is worth remembering, however, that this is only valid in the first 48 h of life, and that blood pressure rises steeply over the first five postnatal days.

Most neonatal units use the gestational age as a guide when instituting treatment for hypotension. It is important, however, to assess other markers of tissue perfusion, such as capillary refill time, the presence of metabolic acidosis, and urine output when deciding whether to treat.

Pathogenesis

Hypovolemia

Hypovolemia causes hypotension by decreasing the preload, leading to reduced cardiac output. In neonates, hypovolemia may result from acute hemorrhage (antenatal or postnatal), or from fluid loss due to capillary leak, as seen in septicemia or acute abdominal pathology. It is generally accepted that hypovolemia is an uncommon primary cause of hypotension in the sick preterm infant.[7] It may, however, be implicated in a small number of babies, and should always be considered.

Myocardial dysfunction

There is good evidence that myocardial dysfunction plays an important role in the development of hypotension in preterm infants in the first few hours of life.[8] There are several factors that contribute to myocardial dysfunction, the foremost of which is immaturity of the myocardium. Hypoxic damage to the heart muscle, acidosis, sepsis, and the presence of a ductal shunt will all adversely affect myocardial function, leading to decreased cardiac output and hypotension. Congenital structural heart defects may also present with hypotension secondary to reduced cardiac output.

Downregulation of adrenergic receptors

There is growing evidence that a proportion of sick preterm infants have relative adrenal insufficiency, demonstrating a low cortisol response to human corticotrophin releasing hormone.[9–12] Because glucocorticoids have a role in regulating the expression of cardiovascular adrenergic receptors, these infants may be incapable of responding to endogenous or exogenous sympathomimetic agents.[13]

Measurement

Intra-arterial blood pressure monitoring through an umbilical or peripheral arterial catheter is widely accepted as the gold standard. Studies comparing oscillometric with invasive measurement demonstrate that, providing cuff size is standardized, oscillometric measurement seems to be accurate within the normal range.[14,15] However, concern has been expressed that at the lower levels it consistently overestimates the blood pressure, providing false reassurance to the clinician.[16] In situations where intra-arterial monitoring is not possible, it is important to also assess other markers of tissue perfusion.

Clinical relevance

Tissue perfusion

In neonatology, blood pressure is regularly used as a marker of systemic organ perfusion, and our efforts to maintain normal blood pressure are based on the belief that we are preserving tissue perfusion. Unfortunately, there are few data to support this. In preterm infants there is only a weak correlation between blood pressure and cardiac output.[17] Furthermore, since blood pressure is the function of blood flow and systemic vascular resistance, blood pressure may not reflect the blood flow in end organs, as the vascular resistance will vary. Several methods that may be useful for assessing systemic blood flow and tissue perfusion in neonates are being evaluated.

Left ventricular output is often used in adults to assess systemic blood flow. Measurements of ventricular outputs in neonates may be confounded by shunts through a patent ductus or foramen ovale. Systemic blood flow in the superior vena cava of newborn infants has been successfully measured, using Doppler echocardiography. Flow in the superior vena cava is thought to reflect blood flow in the upper body, particularly the brain, and appears to correlate well with left ventricular output in babies with a closed duct.[18]

Near-infrared spectroscopy (NIRS) has been used to measure hemoglobin flow and venous saturation in the forearm of hypotensive preterm babies.[19] Using this technique, it has been demonstrated that peripheral oxygen delivery and consumption are lower in hypotensive babies, but that oxygen extraction is similar to normotensive controls, with no rise in lactate concentration. This suggests that in hypotensive babies, peripheral oxygen delivery is still adequate for tissue demands, challenging the need to routinely correct hypotension. NIRS has also been used to monitor cerebral circulation in sick premature infants. Unfortunately, it has not been clearly demonstrated whether there is a direct relationship between mean arterial blood pressure and cerebral intravascular oxygenation.[20,21]

As NIRS and cardiac output measurements are not continuous, their role in the decision to treat a blood pressure level remains unclear. They do, however, question our present practice of using a single value below which treatment should be started. Further research in this area is obviously needed before techniques such as this have direct relevance to the management of hypotension.

Cerebral injury

Sick VLBW infants have reduced cerebral vascular autoregulation compared with term infants with the postulated effect that significant hypotension may lead to cerebral hypoperfusion.[22,23] Episodes of systemic hypotension have been linked to cerebral hemorrhage, ischemia, and an increased risk of long-term neurological sequelae.[1,3,4] Hypotension is thought to lead to intraventricular hemorrhage by causing ischemic damage to the germinal matrix, which bleeds on reperfusion. It is unlikely that overenthusiastic correction of hypotension is involved, as episodes of hypertension are not associated with the occurrence of intraventricular hemorrhage. There is no clear evidence that systemic hypotension, in itself, leads to periventricular leukomalacia,[3] although it may be a factor in babies who are also septic. Interestingly, there is little evidence to support the view that treating hypotension prevents any of these sequelae.

Management

The aim of treating hypotension is to preserve adequate organ perfusion and thus to prevent complications, such as cerebral injury. However, a cause for hypotension should always be sought before treatment is instituted. Important conditions to exclude include:

- Blood loss
- Pneumothorax
- Sepsis
- Patent ductus arteriosus
- High positive intrathoracic pressure (secondary to mechanical ventilation)
- Heart failure

If one of the above causes is identified, the primary treatment of the hypotension is to institute the specific treatment for the underlying condition. In most instances, a cause for hypotension in the neonatal period will not be determined, although myocardial dysfunction has been identified as a common factor, and treatment will be initiated on the basis of unit protocols. These normally follow a stepwise approach, beginning with volume support followed by inotropes and in some the use of steroids.

Volume support

As previously discussed, hypovolemia is an infrequent cause of hypotension in the sick preterm infant.[7] It is also difficult to diagnose in the immediate postnatal period, as indicators, such as urine output and capillary refill time, are unreliable. However, because it does occasionally occur, and it is relatively easy to treat, most units adopt a policy of moderate volume replacement prior to the institution of inotropes.

Fluids available for volume replacement may be either crystalloid or colloid. The main difference between the two is the oncotic pressure effect, according to Starling's law, and the theoretical difference in the length of time they remain in the intravascular space. However, the volume administered appears to be more important than the protein content in producing a sustained increase in blood pressure in preterm infants,[24] and isotonic saline has been shown to be as effective as 5% albumin for treating hypotension in this population.[25] Crystalloids are also significantly cheaper than colloids, and do not carry the same infection risk.

As colloid and crystalloid are equally effective in treating hypotension in the neonatal period, and considering the other advantages of using isotonic saline, it would seem that the safest approach to volume replacement would be to use 10–20 ml/kg 0.9% saline given over 30 min in the first instance. For babies who are likely to be hypovolemic secondary to protein losing conditions, such as babies who have undergone gastrointestinal surgery, 4.5% albumin should be reserved.

Dopamine and dobutamine

Since myocardial dysfunction plays an important role in the development of hypotension in preterm infants in the first few hours of life,[8] it is clear that inotropic agents should be of some benefit in the management of hypotension in these babies. The use of inotropes is, however, historically based rather than evidence based, and there are few data relating to associated mortality and morbidity.

Unsurprisingly, dopamine is more effective than volume expansion in restoring normal blood pressure in preterm infants.[26] Dopamine is an exogenous sympathomimetic amine that exerts its cardiovascular effects by the dose-dependent stimulation of dopaminergic and α- and β-adrenergic receptors. In the preterm population dopamine causes a dose-dependent increase in mean arterial blood pressure in doses of 5–20 μg/kg/min.[27–29]

The main hemodynamic effects of dopamine are to increase myocardial contractility and peripheral vascular tone. The increase in myocardial contractility is caused both by a direct stimulation of α- and β-adrenoceptors and indirectly through its action on β_2-adrenoceptors, stimulating the release of endogenous noradrenaline.[30] In adults, the vasotonic effects of dopamine are dose dependent. At doses $< 5\ \mu$g/kg/min dopamine stimulates peripheral dopaminergic receptors, resulting in the selective dilatation of renal, mesenteric, and coronary arteries. At higher doses $>10\ \mu$g/kg/min it causes vasoconstriction by stimulation of α-adrenergic receptors. The dose-dependent effects of dopamine on vascular tone in the preterm neonate are less clear,[29,30] although there are emerging concerns that it may have a potent vasoconstrictive effect on the pulmonary vasculature.[31]

Studies in adults suggest that, in sick hypotensive patients, there is a downregulation of adrenergic receptors, requiring much higher doses of dopamine to maintain blood pressure.[13] However, there have been no such studies in neonates. The fact that some preterm infants may also have relative adrenal insufficiency[9] may explain the occurrence of pressor resistance. Further research is clearly required in order to define a maximum dose for dopamine, as the use of high doses ($> 25\ \mu$g/kg/min) has not been studied.

Dobutamine is a relatively cardioselective sympathomimetic amine, which exerts its positive inotropic action by direct stimulation of cardiac α- and β-adrenoceptors. It has several theoretical advantages over dopamine: (1) it has limited chronotropic effect, (2) its use is not associated with an increase in systemic vascular resistance,[27] and (3) it does not rely on release of endogenous catecholamines for any part of its action.

There is relatively little research into the use of dobutamine in preterm neonates, and it is generally used as a second-line drug in patients unresponsive to dopamine. It is infused at rates of 5–20 μg/kg/min,[27,32–35] and has been shown to increase left ventricular performance in these doses.[36] The use of high doses ($> 25\ \mu$g/kg/min) has not been studied. Dobutamine can cause hypercontractile heart failure in the presence of left ventricular hypertrophy, resulting in paradoxical hypotension.[37] It should therefore be used with caution in babies with existing cardiac disease.

In the preterm infant, dopamine is significantly more effective than dobutamine in the treatment of systemic hypotension, with no differences in short-term complications, such as intraventricular hemorrhage and necrotizing enterocolitis.[38] No data are available on long-term outcome for either drug.

Other agents

Most neonatal units advocate the use of adrenaline or noradrenaline in cases where dopamine and dobutamine have failed to maintain 'normal' blood pressure.

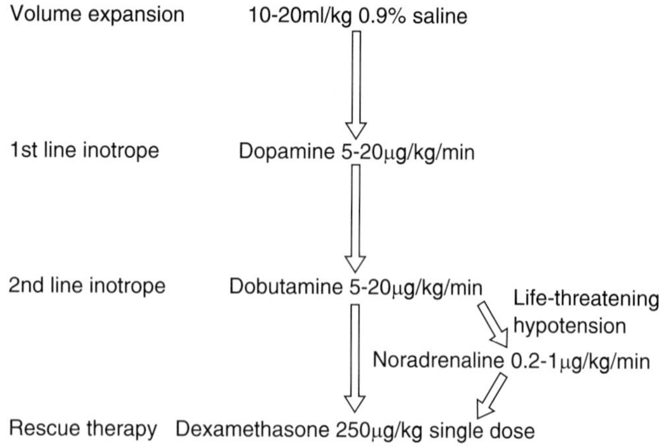

Figure 3.1 Flow chart for management of hypotension in neonates. From Dasgupta and Gill[49] with permission.

However, very few studies have looked at the use of these agents in preterm infants, most of the data originating from animal studies. Both adrenaline and noradrenaline, when used in addition to dopamine, do restore normal blood pressure in sick, hypotensive neonates without causing significant cerebral, myocardial, or renal vasoconstriction.[39,40] The use of these agents is, however, associated with a high mortality rate of over 50%.

Dopexamine, a relatively new synthetic catecholamine, with predominant β_2-adrenergic and dopaminergic activity, has been shown to be effective in raising blood pressure, and improving arterial pH and urine output.[41] In neonates who are hypotensive secondary to septic shock, methylene blue, an inhibitor of soluble guanylate cyclase, has been shown to be effective in increasing blood pressure.[42]

Further research is clearly needed in this area before the routine use of any of these agents can be recommended.

Steroids

Antenatal steroids are now commonly given to mothers in preterm labor. They have been shown to have an independent effect (from the effect on respiratory distress syndrome) on reducing the incidence of hypotension in the preterm infant.[43]

In neonates with hypotension, who are unresponsive to volume or pressor administration, there is growing evidence that steroids may be of some value. The theory is that infants with refractory hypotension may have relative adrenal insufficiency.[9–12] The resulting low levels of circulating cortisol in these babies may be insufficient to counteract any downregulation of cardiovascular adrenergic receptors, which occurs in critical illness,[13] rendering them resistant to treatment with sympathomimetic agents.

In infants with severe hypotension refractory to both volume expansion and inotropes, treatment with either single-dose dexamethasone or a 5-day course of hydrocortisone has been shown to be successful with discontinuation of inotropes within 54 h. This effect is sustained for many days following the administration of steroids.[12,44–46] Although the effect may not be evident for up to 6 h, in my experience it is usually seen within 2 h of treatment.

There are some groups who have advocated the use of hydrocortisone in smaller doses as prophylaxis against hypotension in at-risk VLBW infants.[47] Side effects from postnatal steroids, including the long-term risk of adverse neurological outcome, are well documented and probably prohibit prophylactic use.[48]

Based on the available evidence, the use of steroids in the treatment of severe, intractable hypotension, resistant to inotropes, is probably justified. This may be in the form of a single dose of 250 μg/kg dexamethasone or a 5-day tapering course of hydrocortisone starting at 2.5 mg/kg qds. Obviously, there is a balance of risks against benefits, but the short-term benefit of preventing death must outweigh the long-term risks, which are anyway unproven. Further research is obviously needed to determine the optimum dose and course.

Conclusion

The management of hypotension in preterm infants remains a controversial area in current neonatal practice. Research in this area is relatively limited, which in part is probably due to the difficulty in obtaining continuous measures of tissue perfusion. There is no consensus on either the definition of hypotension or the level at which treatment should be initiated. The effects of aggressive correction are relatively under-researched, and there are few data on morbidity and mortality in relation to the use of volume support and inotropes. The aim of management must be to attain adequate tissue perfusion and oxygenation, but there may be little or no relation between blood pressure and organ perfusion. Further research is required in methods of assessing tissue perfusion, which can be used alongside monitoring of blood pressure to guide the neonatologist in deciding when to intervene.

Continuous invasive arterial blood monitoring remains the preferred method of recording blood pressure. Decisions to treat hypotension should be based on the general condition of the infant, not on the mean arterial blood pressure alone. On the basis of the available evidence Figure 3.1 outlines a suggested guideline for the management of hypotension in the neonatal period.

REFERENCES

1. Watkins AMC, West CR, Cooke RWI. Blood pressure and cerebral haemorrhage and ischaemia in VLBW infants. *Early Hum Dev* 1989;19:103–10.
2. Miall-Allen VM, De Vries LS, Whitelaw AGL. Mean arterial BP and neonatal cerebral lesions. *Arch Dis Child* 1987;62:1068–9.
3. Dammann O, Allred EN, Kuban KC, *et al.* Systemic hypotension and white-matter damage in preterm infants. *Dev Med Child Neurol* 2002;44(2):82–90.
4. Low JA, Froese AB, Galbraith RS, *et al.* The association between newborn hypotension and hypoxemia and outcome during the first year. *Acta Paediatr* 1993;82(5):433–7.
5. Nuntnarumit P, Yang W, Bada-Ellzey HS. Blood pressure measurements in the newborn. *Clin Perinatol* 1999;26:981–96.
6. Lee J, Rajadurai VS, Tan KW. Blood pressure standards for very low birthweight infants during the first day of life. *Arch Dis Child Fetal Neonatal Ed* 1999;81:F168–70.
7. Dimitriou G, Greenough A, Mantagos J, Skinner S. Metabolic acidosis, core-peripheral temperature difference and blood pressure response to albumin infusion in hypotensive, very premature infants. *J Perinat Med* 2001;29(5):442–5.
8. Gill AB, Weindling AM. Cardiac function in the shocked very low birthweight infant. *Arch Dis Child* 1993;6817–21.
9. Scott SM, Watterberg KL. Effect of gestational age, postnatal age, and illness on plasma cortisol concentrations in premature infants. *Pediatr Res* 1995;37(1):112–6.
10. Tantivit P, Subramanian N, Garg M, *et al.* Low serum cortisol in term newborns with refractory hypotension. *J Perinatol* 1999;19(5):352–7.
11. Heckmann M, Wudy SA, Haack D, Pohlandt F. Serum cortisol concentrations in ill preterm infants less than 30 weeks gestational age. *Acta Paediatr* 2000;89(9):1098–103.
12. Ng PC, Lam CWK, Fok TF, *et al.* Refractory hypotension in preterm infants with adrenocortical insufficiency. *Arch Dis Child Fetal Neonatal Ed* 2001;84:F122–4.
13. Hausdorff WP, Caron MG, Lefkowitz RJ. Turning off the signal: Desensitization of β-adrenergic receptors. *FASEB J* 1990;4:33–40.
14. Kimble KJ, Darnall RA, Yelderman MD. An automated technique for estimating mean arterial pressure in critically ill newborns. *Anesthesiology* 1981;54:423–425.
15. Dellagramaticas HD, Wilson AJ. Clinical evaluation of the Dinamap non-invasive blood pressure monitor in pre-term neonates. *Clin Phys Physiol Meas* 1981;2:271–6.
16. Diprose GK, Evans DH, Archer LNJ, Levene MI. Dinamap fails to detect hypotension in very low birthweight infants. *Arch Dis Child* 1986;61:771–3.
17. Kluckow M, Evans N. Relationship between blood pressure and cardiac output in preterm infants requiring mechanical ventilation. *J Pediatr* 1996;129(4):506–12.
18. Kluckow M, Evans N. Superior vena cava flow in newborn infants: A novel marker of systemic blood flow. *Arch Dis Child Fetal Neonatal Ed* 2000;82:F182–7.
19. Wardle SP, Yoxall CW, Weindling AM. Peripheral oxygenation in hypotensive preterm babies. *Pediatr Res* 1999;45(3):343–9.
20. Tsuji M, Saul JP, du Plessis A, *et al.* Cerebral intravascular oxygenation correlates with mean arterial pressure in critically ill premature infants. *Pediatrics* 2000;106(4):625–32.
21. Wardle SP, Yoxall CW, Weindling AM. Determinants of cerebral fractional oxygen extraction using near infrared spectroscopy in preterm neonates. *J Cereb Blood Flow Metab* 2000;20(2):272–9.
22. Panerai RB, Kelsall AWR, Rennie JM, *et al.* Cerebral autoregulation dynamics in premature newborns. *Stroke* 1995;26:74–80.
23. Pryds O, Edwards AD. Cerebral blood flow in the newborn infant. *Arch Dis Child Fetal Neonatal Ed* 1996;74:F63–9.
24. Emery EF, Greenough A, Gamsu HR. Randomised controlled trial of colloid infusions in hypotensive preterm infants. *Arch Dis Child* 1992;67:1185–8.
25. So KW, Fok TF, Ng PC, *et al.* Randomised controlled trial of colloid or crystalloid in hypotensive preterm infants. *Arch Dis Child Fetal Neonatal Ed* 1997;76:F43–6.
26. Gill AB, Weindling AM. Randomised controlled trial of plasma protein fraction versus dopamine in hypotensive very low birth weight infants. *Arch Dis Child* 1993;69:284–7.
27. Roze JC, Tohier C, Maingueneau C, *et al.* Response to dobutamine and dopamine in the hypotensive very preterm infant. *Arch Dis Child* 1993;69:59–63.
28. Padbury JF, Agata Y, Baylen BG, *et al.* Dopamine pharmacokinetics in critically ill newborn infants. *J Pediatr* 1986;110:293–8.
29. Seri I, Abbasi S, Wood D, Gerdes JS. Regional hemodynamic effects of dopamine in the sick preterm neonate. *J Pediatr* 1998;133:728–34.
30. Seri I. Cardiovascular, renal, and endocrine actions of dopamine in neonates and children. *J Pediatr* 1995;126:333–44.
31. Liet J-M, Boscher C, Gras-Leguen C, *et al.* Dopamine effects on pulmonary artery pressure in hypotensive preterm infants with patent ductus arteriosus. *J Pediatr* 2002;140:373–5.
32. Klarr JM, Faix RG, Pryce CJE, Bhatt-Mehta V. Randomized, blind trial of dopamine versus dobutamine for treatment of hypotension in preterm infants with respiratory distress syndrome. *J Pediatr* 1994;125:117–22.
33. Greenough A, Emery EF. Randomized trial comparing dopamine and dobutamine in preterm infants. *Eur J Pediatr* 1993;152(2):164–5.
34. Hentschel R, Hensel D, Brune T, *et al.* Impact on blood pressure and intestinal perfusion of dobutamine or dopamine in hypotensive preterm infants. *Biol Neonate* 1995;68(5):318–24.
35. Miall-Allen VM, Whitelaw AGL. Response to dopamine and dobutamine in the preterm infant less than 30 weeks gestation. *Crit Care Med* 1989;17:1166–9.
36. Stopfkuchen H, Queisser-Luft A, Vogel K. Cardiovascular response to dobutamine determined by systolic time intervals in preterm infants. *Crit Care Med* 1990;18(7):722–4.
37. Germanakis I, Bender C, Hentscel R, *et al.* Hypercontractile heart failure caused by catecholamine therapy in premature neonates. *Acta Paediatr* 2003;92:836–8.
38. Subedhar NV, Shaw NJ. Dopamine versus dobutamine for hypotensive preterm neonates. *Cochrane Database System Rev* 2000;2:CD001242.
39. Seri I, Evans J. Addition of epinephrine to dopamine increases blood pressure and urine output in critically ill extremely low birthweight neonates with uncompensated shock. *Pediatr Res* 1998;43(4, Suppl 2):194.
40. Derleth DP. Clinical experience with norepinephrine infusions in critically ill newborns. *Pediatr Res* 1997;41(4, Pt 2):145.
41. Kawczynski P, Piotrowski A. Circulatory and diuretic effects of dopexamine infusion in low-birth-weight infants with respiratory failure. *Intensive Care Med* 1996;22(1):65–70.
42. Driscoll W, Thurin S, Carrion V, *et al.* Effect of methylene blue on refractory neonatal hypotension. *J Pediatr* 1996;129:904–8.
43. Moise AA, Wearden ME, Kozinetz CA, Gest AL. Antenatal steroids are associated with less need for blood pressure support in extremely preterm infants. *Paediatrics* 1995;95(6):845–50.
44. Bourchier D, Weston PJ. Randomised trial of dopamine compared with hydrocortisone for the treatment of hypotensive very low birth weight infants. *Arch Dis Child Fetal Neonatal Ed* 1997;76:F174–8.
45. Seri I, Tan R, Evans J. Cardiovascular effects of hydrocortisone in preterm infants with pressor-resistant hypotension. *Pediatrics* 2001;107(5):1070–4.
46. Gaissmaier RE, Pohlandt F. Single-dose dexamethasone treatment of hypotension in preterm infants. *J Pediatr* 1999;134:701–5.
47. Rajah V. Treatment of hypotension in very low birthweight infants (letter). *Arch Dis Child Fetal Neonatal Ed* 1998;78:F156.
48. Sweet DG, Halliday HL. A risk-benefit assessment of drugs used for neonatal chronic lung disease. *Drug Saf* 2000;22:389–404.
49. Dasgupta SJ, Gill AB. Hypotension in the very low birthweight infant: The old, the new, and the uncertain. *Arch Dis Child Fetal Neonatal Ed* 2003;88:F450–4.

4 Cytokines and neonatal disease

L. Cornette and H. Logghe

Fetal and neonatal inflammatory responses

This review is designed to guide the reader through the framework given in Figure 4.1, summarizing the concept of perinatal inflammation/infection and current factors that may influence the overall outcome under study. Several diseases in the newborn, such as sepsis, chronic lung disease and broncho-pulmonary dysplasia (CLD/BPD) and necrotizing enterocolitis (NEC) are characterized by the presence of inflammation. Given the mounting evidence suggesting a continuum between ante- and postnatal inflammation, and adverse neonatal outcome,[1,2] we will first study the fetal inflammatory response, prior to expanding on inflammatory responses emerging in the neonatal period.

By definition, an inflammatory response is a protective response to an infection or an injury, mediated by proinflammatory cytokines, i.e. low molecular weight glycoproteins, predominantly produced by the monocyte–macrophage cell line at the inflammatory site. Proinflammatory cytokines (e.g. IL-1β, IL-18, IFN-γ, TNF-α) are primarily responsible for initiating an effective defense (i.e. acute phase response) against exogenous pathogens, whereas anti-inflammatory cytokines (e.g. IL-4, IL-10) are involved in the downregulation of exacerbated inflammatory processes and the maintenance of homeostasis for proper functioning of the vital organs.[3]

Fetal inflammatory response syndrome

The majority of women delivering before 28 weeks, with or without preterm premature rupture of membranes (PrePROM), show evidence of intrauterine infection. A mechanism postulated is microbial invasion of the uterine cavity resulting in a fetal systemic cytokine or inflammatory response through aspiration, otitis, conjunctivitis or omphalitis.[4] However, only a small proportion of these women will have a positive amniotic fluid culture.[5] Intra-amniotic *inflammation* would therefore appear to be a better predictor for imminent preterm delivery rather than intra-amniotic *infection*.[6]

Such active participation of the fetus in a systemic antenatal inflammatory response is therefore commonly

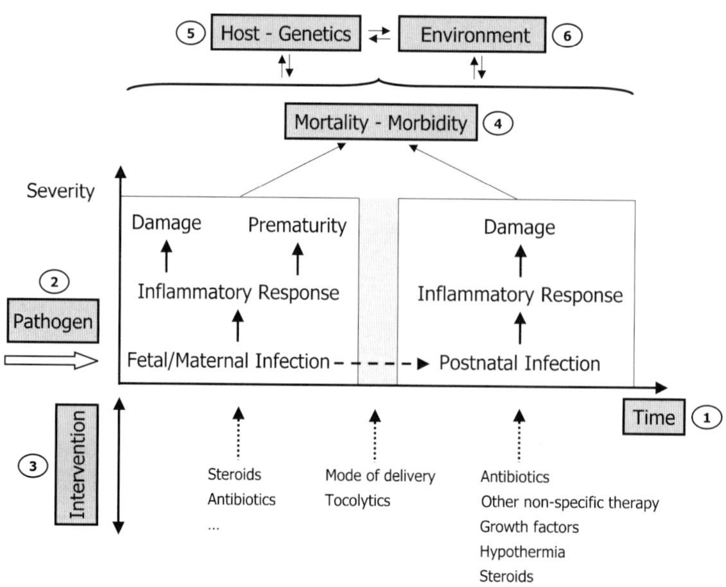

Figure 4.1 The fetal/neonatal inflammatory response. Illustration of antenatal and postnatal inflammatory responses and six factors that may influence the overall outcome.

studied using cordocentesis techniques. Indeed, the fetal inflammatory response syndrome (FIRS) was originally defined by relating increased fetal cord plasma IL-6 to the onset of spontaneous preterm labor (through increased fetal adrenal cortisol production and subsequent prostaglandine release).[7] More recent studies have revealed that the FIRS involves the synergistic action of different cytokines and several complex host defense mechanisms.[8] In addition, through the study of differential placental vs. fetal immune cytokine responses within animal models, we now know that an FIRS, rather than the maternal infection, causes fetal multiorgan injury.[9]

Fetal brain/fetal neurotoxicity

The fetal brain has been extensively studied within the context of intrauterine inflammation.[10,11] Funisitis, i.e. infection of the umbilical cord, and chronic chorio-amnionitis have been associated with an increased risk of intraventricular hemorrhage.[12,13] Fetal vasculitis has been linked with an 11-fold increased risk of development of periventricular echolucencies.[14] Histopathological examination of infant brain specimens shows overexpression of TNF-α in the microglia cells of periventricular leukomalacia (PVL) lesions, with cytokine production being highest in infected infants.[15]

However, a clear link between intrauterine infection/inflammation and neurological outcome in preterm babies is not confirmed in all studies, as much of the confusion arises from different timings of blood sampling across different studies. Cytokine levels in neonatal blood (day 2 or 3) are likely to be influenced by respiratory or infectious complications, as well as different levels of intensive care, and thus may be different from umbilical cord blood levels.[16] In order to establish a causal link between antenatal infection and neonatal brain disease in individual cases, one needs to provide evidence of placental infection, elevated inflammatory mediators in both umbilical cord and postnatal infant blood, presence of moderate to severe encephalopathy and/or neuroradiological confirmation of brain injury.

Proposed mechanisms for neurotoxicity associated with proinflammatory cytokines comprise (1) a direct cytolytic effect on neurones and oligodendrocyte precursors (either through *in situ* cytokine production or through systemic cytokines crossing the blood–brain barrier), (2) induction of excitatory amino acid release, (3) increased caspase activity resulting in amplified apoptosis, (4) abnormalities in the coagulation cascade or (5) fetal hypotension.[10,14,15,17] Further clarification of these and other mechanisms will increase the likelihood of successful therapeutic interventions.

Many studies focus on the interaction between cytokine and excitatory amino acid release (e.g. glutamate). It is now recognized that an antenatal inflammation-related insult to the central nervous system comprises both infection (proinflammatory cytokine release) and hypoxia-ischemia (excessive excitatory neurotransmitter release). The interaction between both entities is, however, complex. First, injury to the brain during antenatal infection may be secondary either to cytokinemia, i.e. cytokines crossing the blood–brain barrier, or to the interruption of placental blood flow resulting in asphyxia.[17] Second, animal work indicates that administration of a low dose of bacterial endotoxin (LPS) dramatically sensitizes the immature brain to injury and induces cerebral infarction in response to short episodes of hypoxia-ischemia that by themselves cause little or no injury.[18] Third, increased levels of IL-1 and TNF-α and neutrophil invasion into infarcted areas have been reported following hypoxia-ischemia in the absence of infection.[18–20] Fourth, complex interaction effects between both inflammation and excitotoxicity exist, as, for example, IL-1β perpetuates excitotoxic brain damage *in vivo*, whereas it ameliorates neuronal death *in vitro*.[20] Others have reported similar dual neurotrophic and detrimental effects exerted by cytokines following ischemia.[21] Finally, a complex interaction between hypoxia-ischemia and inflammation is also reflected in the neuropathology of white matter (WM) abnormalities observed in infants born to mothers with chorio-amnionitis.[22] Careful review of animal work suggests that cytokines can be neurotoxic through a process of 'sensitizing' the immature brain, i.e. lowering the threshold at which a hypoxic-ischemic insult triggers apoptosis.[23] Further clinical studies investigating the relationship between fetal infection/inflammation, feto-placental thrombosis and subsequent adverse neurological outcome will therefore be challenging.[24]

Other fetal morbidity

Fetal exposure to infection/inflammation, similar to antenatal administration of glucocorticoids can, on the one hand, result in maturation of the *lungs*. However, antenatal chorio-amnionitis can also prime the fetal lung to respond differently to postnatal events, increasing the risk of CLD/BPD (see below).[25]

Histological chorio-amnionitis has been associated with a noticeable reduction of volume and corticomedullary differentiation of the *thymus*, a reduced number of thymocytes and infiltration of macrophages into the parenchyma.[26]

Finally, a FIRS can result in preterm delivery (and, hence, possible neonatal morbidity), as increased fetal and not maternal serum IL-6 is one of several cytokines that precedes imminent preterm delivery.[8]

Neonatal inflammatory responses

Sepsis

The progression to septic shock in infants born to mothers with acute chorio-amnionitis is rarely seen in the immediate neonatal period. However, a significant association between funisitis and congenital sepsis has been described.[2]

Neonatal sepsis in the absence of chorio-amnionitis is predominantly mediated by IL-1, IL-6 and TNF-α. Sepsis-related mortality is well correlated with multiple-organ failure (MOF), caused by uncontrolled inflammation, immunodeficiency (prolonged neutropenia, lymphopenia, hypogammaglobulinemia) and endothelial injury with thrombotic microangiopathy. Septic newborns have low von Willebrand factor (vWF) cleaving metalloprotease activity (ADAMTS13), resulting in high amounts of circulating ultralarge vWF multimers that lead to microvascular platelet thrombosis and MOF.[27]

Little is known about the profile of pro- and anti-inflammatory cytokines in septic preterm infants, in whom the immune system may be considered as immature. An exaggerated proinflammatory response together with an inadequate anti-inflammatory compensation may result in an adverse clinical outcome, as a persistent high IL-6/IL-10 ratio implies a poor prognosis in very low-birth-weight patients.[1] Alternatively, a persistently high IL-10 concentration can be an early indicator of a poor prognosis in preterm neonates with sepsis.[28]

Necrotizing enterocolitis

NEC is a devastating intestinal disease that primarily occurs in low-birth-weight premature infants. Its etiology is not well known, and may consist of intestinal immaturity, intestinal ischemia, changes in microbiological environment related to enteral feeding practices, with an increased inflammatory response as the final common pathway. The evidence suggesting a causal association between chorio-amnionitis and subsequent NEC is very sparse, although some retrospective case–control studies suggest a significantly higher frequency of PrePROM and chorio-amnionitis in infants with NEC.[29]

Inflammatory mediators involved in NEC are tissue and circulating proinflammatory cytokines (IL-1, IL-6, IL-8, TNF-α), platelet-activating factor, leukotriene C4, iNOS, endothelin-1 and thromboxane. These mediators are believed to stimulate signal transduction and gene transcription, leading to apoptosis or programmed cell death, secondary inflammation, increased intestinal wall permeability and, ultimately, necrosis. Conversely, IL-10, IL-11, IL-12, erythropoietin and epidermal growth factor have been shown to play an important role in the prevention of intestinal injury. Using a neonatal rat model, the protective effect of maternal milk has been associated with increased ileal production of anti-inflammatory IL-10.[30] Also, enteric organisms such as non-virulent *Salmonella* strains are capable of attenuating intestinal inflammatory responses.[31]

Chronic lung disease/bronchopulmonary dysplasia

Many aspects of the inflammatory response in the context of CLD/BPD remain to be elucidated.

On the one hand, artificially induced lung inflammation through intra-amniotic injection of proinflammatory cytokines in rabbits results in increased lung volumes, increased surfactant production and improved gas exchange.[32] Likewise, fetal exposure to chorio-amnionitis can lead to enhanced lung maturation, similar to the effect yielded by antenatal glucocorticoids.[25] This is in line with the findings from the UK Epicure study, indicating that infants born below 26 weeks' gestation are more likely to die in the absence of chorio-amnionitis and antenatal administration of glucocorticoids.[33]

Alternatively, as previously mentioned, antenatal inflammation can disrupt the process of alveolarization, resulting in alveolar simplification and priming of the fetal lung, rendering it vulnerable for further injury postnatally.[25,34] Indeed, prolonged postnatal mechanical ventilation (> 7 days) of lungs that are primed in this way, together with postnatal infection (sepsis or pneumonia), may result in a secondary inflammatory response and the development of CLD/BPD.[35,36] Support for this hypothesis stems from the observation that predominantly memory cells from the immune system, i.e. lymphocytes and monocytes, are observed in broncheo-alveolar lavage fluids obtained from ventilated and antenatally inflamed animal lungs.[37]

Ongoing lung damage in the premature infant may also be caused by failure to downregulate inflammatory responses.[38] Data suggest that preterm newborns with lung inflammation may be unable to activate the anti-inflammatory cytokine IL-10. Comparing preterm infants with term infants in respiratory failure, the ability of lung macrophages to produce TNF-α is nearly identical, whereas a trend toward diminished levels of IL-10 expression exists in the preterm group.[39] Such data suggest an imbalance between pro- and anti-inflammatory responses, leading to CLD/BPD.

The role of transforming growth factor-β, i.e. a cytokine participating in adult chronic inflammatory diseases, is still to be elucidated in neonatal inflammatory processes.[40]

Retinopathy of prematurity (ROP)

ROP is an ischemia-induced proliferative retinopathy, affecting premature infants with low birth weight. The process of retinal neovascularization in ROP is complex, involving several angiogenic factors, such as vascular endothelial growth factor. Potential medical therapies for ROP include not only modulators of such angiogenic factors but also endogenous inhibitors and anti-inflammatory drugs. The latter drugs have proved to be efficacious against neovascularization in several animal models of oxygen-induced retinopathy, and are currently already trialled for adult diabetic retinopathy and age-related macular degeneration.[41]

Perinatal inflammatory responses, neonatal disease and neuro-morbidity

Both animal and clinical data suggest that intrauterine infection can be linked to adverse neurological outcome either via infection/inflammation-induced WM damage or via infection/inflammation-induced preterm birth.[42,43] A recent meta-analysis (23 studies) revealed a significant association between clinical chorio-amnionitis, cystic PVL (RR, 3.0; 95% CI, 2.2–4.0) and cerebral palsy (CP) (RR, 1.9; 95% CI, 1.4–2.5), whereas histologic chorio-amnionitis was associated with cystic PVL (RR, 1.6; 95% CI, 1.5–2.9) but less with CP (RR, 1.6; 95% CI, 0.9–2.7).[12] The same group recently described an increased risk for neurological sequelae in term infants with funisitis.[44]

It is also likely that postnatal infection/inflammation contributes to a long-term adverse neuro-development, as a recent UK trial indicated a four times higher risk of CP among infants with neonatal sepsis compared to those without.[45] A significant association between increased levels of inflammatory cytokines in the newborn and the development of spastic di-, quadri- and hemiplegia has been demonstrated,[24] with increased concentrations of cytokines (TNF-α, IL-1β, IL-6 and the anti-inflammatory IL-10) correlating with cerebral lesions detected by MRI.[46]

However, several variables account for the observation that not all studies suggest such an association between infection/inflammation and adverse outcome in newborn infants (see Figure 4.1), i.e. (1) timing issues, (2) nature of the infectious/inflammatory process, (3) established and new anti-insult strategies, (4) morbidity in organs other than the brain, (5) genetic influences and (6) environmental factors.

Timing issues

Clinical chorio-amnionitis is based on the acute presence of two or more of the following clinical signs: maternal temperature, maternal tachycardia, fetal tachycardia, maternal leucocytosis, uterine tenderness and foul-smelling amniotic fluid. However, intrauterine infection may also remain undetected for months as a *chronic* indolent inflammatory process. Also, bacterial vaginosis can result in intrauterine colonization present at conception; if the organisms are not cleared within 4–8 weeks after the expanding membranes seal the endometrial cavity, the infection may result in preterm delivery. Hence, in the absence of clear criteria to identify the severity and duration of *in utero* infection, it is not surprising that the clinical outcome is unpredictable, ranging from normal fetal development with histologic chorio-amnionitis as an incidental finding to severe chorio-amnionitis leading to *in* or *ex utero* death with long-term neurological sequelae.[25]

Type and presence of pathogen

Not only timing but also the nature of the infection may determine the outcome.[43] For example, administration of a low dose of *Escherichia coli* (O55:B5) endotoxin to rats, prior to short periods of hypoxia-ischemia, increases the overall brain injury.[18] However, the opposite effect is observed using a different bacterial toxin (lipoteichoic acid) in a similar rat model.[47] Amniotic fluid contaminated with *E. coli* but not with *Ureaplasma urealyticum* and *Mycoplasma* increases the risk of CLD/BPD,[48] although one could point out that the latter two species are more difficult to grow *in vitro*.

Evidence suggests that preterm delivery and neonatal morbidity may be better predicted by the degree and nature of the FIR to infection (i.e. the host response) than by the presence of (a combination of) pathogens (i.e. positive amniotic cultures).[8,49] It is within this context that functional polymorphisms of the different cytokines may play a role as they may determine each individual's genetic susceptibility and response to infection (see below).

Anti-insult strategies

As perinatal infection/inflammation seems to be an important risk factor for adverse neonatal outcome, the development of appropriately designed (brain) protective strategies will, to a great extent, become indispensable in neonatal care over the next decade.[50] However, the difficulties experienced hereto are at least threefold: (1) we are currently unable to prospectively identify those infants at greatest risk for developing (neuro)morbidity; (2) the presence of both beneficial and detrimental physiologic effects by cytokines complicates any targeted intervention; (3) the origin of perinatally acquired brain damage is currently thought to be multifactorial, possibly including hypoxia/perfusion failure, thyroid hormone deficiency, genetic factors, thrombotic processes, growth factor deficiency, excess free reactive oxygen production and antenatal infection.[51]

Antenatal strategies

Steroids. Endogenous glucocorticoids, released by the fetal adrenal cortex, downregulate the expression and action of cytokines both in the periphery and in the brain.[52] Likewise, antenatal administration of exogenous steroids can result in a reduced FIR.[53] Antenatal steroids administered to women at risk of preterm delivery decrease the risk of death, respiratory distress[54] and protect very low-birth-weight infants against the risk of neuro-morbidity.[55] However, antenatal steroids do not reduce the incidence of CLD/BPD, as the drug induces alveolar simplification and hence primes the lungs for postnatal ventilation-mediated injury.[25] In addition, whereas betametasone yields an initial suppressive effect on inflammation, it may ultimately result in 'late inflammation'.[56]

It thus seems that the exposure to infection/inflammation together with antenatal administration of glucocorticoids can both 'mature and injure' the fetus. The 'net effect' in terms of adverse neonatal outcome may depend on exposure to postnatal noxious interventions such as ventilation, high concentration of oxygen, etc. These time-dependent interactions between steroids and inflammation warrant further investigation.

Antibiotics. The administration of antibiotics following PrePROM results in a significant reduction in chorio-amnionitis, a delay in delivery and reduced neonatal morbidity (e.g. neonatal infection, use of surfactant, oxygen requirement, abnormal findings on cranial ultrasound).[57] Due to an increased risk of NEC, coamoxiclav should be avoided, while erythromycin seems a better choice, possibly because of a smaller endotoxin release by damaged bacteria.[58] The current treatment for clinical chorio-amnionitis is delivery of the fetus and subsequent treatment with antibiotics. Maternal treatment in such cases is ineffective because the amniotic cavity is largely a sequestered site, inaccessible to antibiotics.

Mode of delivery. Normal labor is always associated with some form of hypoxic stress, which may be detrimental if the fetal brain is more vulnerable to hypoxia in the presence of antenatal infection/inflammation. However, there is no clear evidence that suggests an elective cesarean section is more neuroprotective than normal labor in the case of (chronic or acute) chorio-amnionitis.

Postnatal strategies

Non-specific therapy for severe sepsis comprises antibiotics, aggressive fluid resuscitation, inotropes and ventilatory support. More specific strategies are aimed at tapering of sepsis-related immunodeficiency syndromes by using recombinant growth factors, such as granulocyte colony stimulating factor (CSF), granulocyte macrophage CSF and interferon. Recombinant activated protein C is an anti-inflammatory, antithrombotic and fibrinolytic agent that has been successfully used in severe sepsis in adults. However, its use is not approved in infants or children.[59]

Treatment of NEC currently consists of antibiotics and hemodynamic stabilization, with, in some cases, the need to proceed to surgery. However, a better understanding of the mechanisms underlying its pathogenesis is needed. For example, understanding the protective effects of maternal milk could be beneficial either in the prevention of NEC or in the development of future therapeutic strategies to cure NEC.[30]

Postnatal steroids are commonly administered in severe CLD/BPD, as data suggest that preterm newborns with lung inflammation may be unable to activate anti-inflammatory cytokine pathways.[39] Dose-related inhibition of cytokine synthesis is indeed observed when treating monocytes with dexamethasone *in vitro*.[60] Although early postnatal anti-inflammatory therapy could help in preventing CLD/BPD, prophylactic dexamethasone cannot be recommended, as there are a number of potential interactions between surfactant and cytokine effects on the preterm lung that have not been fully evaluated.[38] In addition, postnatal administration of steroids has been associated with neurodevelopmental impairment, warranting further randomized controlled evaluation of its risks vs. benefits.[61]

It is to be hoped that we will see multicenter clinical trials over the next decade, evaluating inflammatory protection and inflammatory response modification in the newborn infant. This requires further detailed animal work of immune modulatory drugs and their kinetics within the newborn age group.[62] Inflammatory protection can be achieved by exogenous administration of IL-10, although complex differential effects between its central and peripheral effects need further exploration.[63] The exogenous administration of response modifiers/receptor antagonists currently evaluated in animal models (e.g. IL-1β receptor antagonist or soluble TNF receptor) may not be without risk, as many of the proinflammatory cytokines exhibit fragile equilibria of biological activity.[64] As an example, the presence of TNF-α can have beneficial effects, whereas blocking TNF-α in adults with septic shock results in increased mortality.[65] Future strategies therefore must aim to 'redress the optimal cytokine balance' rather than 'prevent the inflammatory response'.

Morbidity in organs other than the brain

Is there evidence that a neonatal inflammatory response (e.g. sepsis, NEC) involves an increased risk of neuro-morbidity?

Sepsis/NEC

The role of proinflammatory cytokines during sepsis/NEC in the etiology of CP remains controversial. However, preliminary reports suggest a significant association between TNF-α, IL-8 and an abnormal cognitive and psychomotor outcome at the age of 24–28 months.[66]

Lung inflammation

A complex interaction exists between lung and brain inflammatory processes. Lung disease has been mimicked in transgenic mice that overexpress human IL-1β in the respiratory epithelium.[67] The expression of a number of genes participating in inflammation was also increased in their brains, although no major histological differences were detected compared to control animals. Ventilation of inflamed preterm lungs may also result in more lung inflammation, creating an excess of cytokines in the systemic circulation, which in turn may promote the development of CLD/BPD, and, in addition, may result in remote (brain) damage.[37]

Host-genetics

Single-nucleotide polymorphisms (SNPs) consist of single base substitutions in a DNA sequence. Almost all genes contain SNPs, but only a minority of SNPs result in amino acid variation in protein products. In addition, many of the functional SNPs occur in the promotor region rather than the gene itself and affect protein levels through altered transcription. Polymorphism-association studies compare the prevalence of a genetic marker in persons with a given condition to the prevalence in controls.[68] Gene polymorphisms that may influence perinatal outcome through alteration of the response to infection have been reported for the IL-1 receptor antagonist,[69] IL-6,[70] interferon-γ[71] and TNF-α.[72] Likewise, cytokine gene polymorphisms may modify the risk of brain injury and hence act as an endogenous inflammatory response modification mechanism.[22] As an example, the IL6-174(G|C) genotype has been associated with impaired neurological outcome in preterm children.[73]

Cytokines are able to mediate intravascular cell adhesion, coagulation and/or thrombosis, and vasoconstriction. In the presence of an existing thrombophilia or a cytokine polymorphism resulting in increased susceptibility to infection, the actions of these cytokines in the fetal brain may be enough to result in adverse neurological outcome.[74]

Such outcome-related research is complicated by the fact that one needs to examine the frequencies of several cytokine genotypes, in infants as well as in mothers, while taking into account demographics, newborn illness severity and several other risk factors. The ultimate goal is to use identified SNPs as a biologic guide to target new anti-inflammatory strategies toward the most genetically vulnerable premature infants (i.e. pharmaco-genomics).

Environment

Impaired neurodevelopment after a fetal/neonatal inflammatory response most likely occurs via a complex interaction between genetic and environmental processes, such as home environment, maternal education, socioeconomic and ethnic backgrounds.

Conclusion

We investigated the available evidence, suggesting a link between inflammatory responses and adverse neonatal outcome. Currently, there is no silver bullet to prevent an impaired neurodevelopmental outcome in the event of a fetal and/or neonatal inflammatory response. Future research needs to focus on (1) the relation between fetal, maternal and neonatal inflammatory processes, i.e. CLD/BPD and NEC; (2) the interaction between inflammatory responses and genetic or environmental factors; (3) the use of advanced techniques for laboratory research and neuro-imaging and (4) large and well-designed observational studies that use well-defined outcome variables for transparent logistic regression analyses in large samples of patients, with sufficiently long periods of follow-up.[64] Although such research will be complex, only then can we become successful in the identification of pre- and postnatal risk profiles that permit the introduction of new anti-inflammatory interventions in the newborn.

REFERENCES

1. Yoon BH, Romero R, Park JS, *et al.* The relationship among inflammatory lesions of the umbilical cord (funisitis), umbilical cord plasma interleukin 6 concentration, amniotic fluid infection, and neonatal sepsis. *Am J Obstet Gynecol* 2000;183:1124–9.
2. Watterberg KL, Demers LM, Scott SM, Murphy S. Chorioamnionitis and early lung inflammation in infants in whom bronchopulmonary dysplasia develops. *Pediatrics* 1996;97:210–5.
3. Ng PC, Li K, Wong RP, *et al.* Proinflammatory and anti-inflammatory cytokine responses in preterm infants with systemic infections. *Arch Dis Child Fetal Neonatal Ed* 2003; 88:F209–13.
4. Goldenberg RL, Hauth JC, Andrews WW. Intrauterine infection and preterm delivery. *N Engl J Med* 2000;342:1500–7.
5. Jacobsson B, Mattsby-Baltzer I, Andersch B, *et al.* Microbial invasion and cytokine response in amniotic fluid in a Swedish population of women with preterm prelabor rupture of membranes. *Acta Obstet Gynecol Scand* 2003;82:423–31.
6. Romero R, Yoon BH, Mazor M, *et al.* A comparative study of the diagnostic performance of amniotic fluid glucose, white blood cell count, interleukin-6 and gram stain in the detection of microbial invasion in patients with preterm premature rupture of membranes. *Am J Obstet Gynecol* 1993;169:839–51.
7. Gomez R, Romero R, Ghezzi F, Yoon BH, Mazor M, Berry SM. The fetal inflammatory response syndrome. *Am J Obstet Gynecol* 1998;179:194–202.
8. Romero R, Gomez R, Ghezzi F, *et al.* A fetal systemic inflammatory response is followed by the spontaneous onset of preterm parturition. *Am J Obstet Gynecol* 1998;179:186–93.
9. Bell MJ, Hallenbeck JM, Gallo V. Determining the fetal inflammatory response in an experimental model of intrauterine inflammation in rats. *Pediatr Res* 2004.
10. Yoon BH, Kim CJ, Romero R, *et al.* Experimentally induced intrauterine infection causes fetal brain white matter lesions in rabbits. *Am J Obstet Gynecol* 1997;177:797–802.
11. Yoon BH, Jun JK, Romero R, *et al.* Amniotic fluid inflammatory cytokines (interleukin-6, interleukin-1β, and tumor necrosis factor-α), neonatal brain white matter lesions, and cerebral palsy. *Am J Obstet Gynecol* 1997;177:19–26.
12. Wu YW, Colford JM. Chorio-amnionitis as a risk factor for cerebral palsy: A meta-analysis. *J Am Med Assoc* 2000;284: 1417–24.
13. Hitti J, Krohn MA, Patton DL, *et al.* Amniotic fluid tumor necrosis factor-alpha and the risk of respiratory distress syndrome among preterm infants. *Am J Obstet Gynecol* 1997;177:50–6.
14. Leviton A, Paneth N, Reuss ML, *et al.* Maternal infection, fetal inflammatory response, and brain damage in very low birth weight infants. Developmental Epidemiology Network Investigators. *Pediatr Res* 1999;46:566–75.
15. Kadhim H, Tabarki B, Verellen G, De Prez C, Rona AM, Sebire G. Inflammatory cytokines in the pathogenesis of periventricular leukomalacia. *Neurology* 2001;56:1278–84.
16. Hagberg H. No correlation between cerebral palsy and cytokines in postnatal blood of preterms: Commentary on the article by Nelson *et al.* on page 600. *Pediatr Res* 2003;53:544–5.
17. Shalak LF, Laptook AR, Jafri HS, Ramilo O, Perlman JM. Clinical chorio-amnionitis, elevated cytokines, and brain injury in term infants. *Pediatrics* 2002;110:673–80.
18. Eklind S, Mallard C, Leverin AL, *et al.* Bacterial endotoxin sensitizes the immature brain to hypoxic-ischaemic injury. *Eur J Neurosci* 2001;13:1101–6.
19. Bona E, Andersson AL, Blomgren K, *et al.* Chemokine and inflammatory cell response to hypoxia-ischemia in immature rats. *Pediatr Res* 1999;45:500–9.
20. Loddick SA, Rothwell NJ. Mechanisms of tumor necrosis factor alpha action on neurodegeneration: Interaction with insulin-like growth factor-1. *Proc Natl Acad Sci USA* 1999;96:9449–51.
21. Hagan P, Barks JD, Yabut M, Davidson BL, Roessler B, Silverstein FS. Adenovirus-mediated over-expression of interleukin-1 receptor antagonist reduces susceptibility to excitotoxic brain injury in perinatal rats. *Neuroscience* 1996;75:1033–45.
22. Dammann O, Durum SK, Leviton A. Modification of infection-associated risks of preterm birth and white matter damage in the preterm newborn by polymorphisms in the tumor necrosis factor locus? *Pathogenesis* 1999;1:171–7.
23. Hagberg H, Wennerholm UB, Sävman K. Sequelae of chorioamnionitis. *Curr Opin Infect Dis* 2002;15:301–6.

24. Nelson KB, Dambrosia JM, Grether JK, Phillips TM. Neonatal cytokines and coagulation factors in children with cerebral palsy. *Ann Neurol* 1998;44:665–75.
25. Jobe AH. Antenatal factors and the development of bronchopulmonary dysplasia. *Semin Neonatol* 2003;8:9–17.
26. Toti P, De Felice C, Stumpo M, *et al.* Acute thymic involution in fetuses and neonates with chorio-amnionitis. *Hum Pathol* 2000;31:1121–8.
27. Levy GG, Nichols WC, Lian EC, *et al.* Mutations in a member of the ADAMTS gene family cause thrombotic thrombocytopenic purpura. *Nature* 2001;413:488–94.
28. Romagnoli C, Frezza S, Cingolani A, *et al.* Plasma levels of interleukin-6 and interleukin-10 in preterm neonates evaluated for sepsis. *Eur J Pediatr* 2001;160:345–50.
29. Martinez-Tallo E, Claure N, Bancalari E. Necrotizing enterocolitis in full-term or near-term infants: Risk factors. *Biol Neonate* 1997;71:292–8.
30. Dvorak B, Halpern MD, Holubec H, *et al.* Maternal milk reduces severity of necrotizing enterocolitis and increases intestinal IL-10 in a neonatal rat model. *Pediatr Res* 2003;53:426–33.
31. Neish AS, Gewirtz AT, Zeng H, *et al.* Prokaryotic regulation of epithelial responses by inhibition of IkappaB-alpha ubiquitination. *Science* 2000;289:1560–3.
32. Bry K, Lappalainen U, Hallman M. Intra-amniotic interleukin-1 accelerates surfactant protein synthesis in fetal rabbits and improves lung stability after premature birth. *J Clin Invest* 1997;99:2992–9.
33. Costeloe K, Hennessy E, Gibson AT, Marlow N, Wilkinson AR. The EPICure study: Outcomes to discharge from hospital for infants born at the threshold of viability. *Pediatrics* 2000;106: 659–71.
34. Willet KE, Kramer BW, Kallapur SG, *et al.* Intra-amniotic injection of IL-1 induces inflammation and maturation in fetal sheep lung. *Am J Physiol Lung Cell Mol Physiol* 2002;282:411–20.
35. Speer CP. New insights into the pathogenesis of pulmonary inflammation in preterm infants. *Biol Neonate* 2001;79:205–9.
36. Van Marter LJ, Dammann O, Allred EN, *et al.* Chorioamnionitis, mechanical ventilation, and postnatal sepsis as modulators of chronic lung disease in preterm infants. *J Pediatr* 2002;140:171–6.
37. Kramer BW, Ikegami M, Jobe AH. Intratracheal endotoxin causes systemic inflammation in ventilated preterm lambs. *Am J Respir Crit Care Med* 2002;165:463–9.
38. De Dooy JJ, Mahieu LM, Van Bever HP. The role of inflammation in the development of chronic lung disease in neonates. *Eur J Pediatr* 2001;160:457–63.
39. Blahnik MJ, Ramanathan R, Riley CR, Minoo P. Lipopolysaccharide-induced tumor necrosis factor-alpha and IL-10 production by lung macrophages from preterm and term neonates. *Pediatr Res* 2001;50:726–31.
40. Marek A, Brodzicki J, Liberek A, Korzon M. TGF-β (transforming growth factor-β) in chronic inflammatory conditions – A new diagnostic prognostic marker? *Med Sci Monit* 2002;RA145–51.
41. Mechoulam H, Pierce EA. Retinopathy of prematurity: Molecular pathology and therapeutic strategies. *Am J Pharmacogenomics* 2003;3:261–77.
42. Dantzer R, Wollman EE, Vitkovic L, Yirmiya R. Cytokines, stress, and depression. Conclusions and perspectives. *Adv Exp Med Biol* 1999;461:317–29.
43. Dammann O, Kuban K, Leviton A. Perinatal infection, fetal inflammatory response, white matter damage, and cognitive limitations in children born preterm. Ment Retard Dev Disabil Res Rev 2002;8:46–50.
44. Wu YW, Malin BT, Johnson LL, Lin FY, Machin GA. Funisitis and neurologic abnormalities in term infants. *Pediatr Res* 2003;53:545A.
45. Wheater M, Rennie JM. Perinatal infection is an important risk factor for cerebral palsy in very-low-birth weight infants. Dev Med Child Neurol 2000;42:364–7.
46. Duggan PJ, Maalouf EF, Watts TL, *et al.* Intrauterine T-cell activation and increased proinflammatory cytokine concentrations in preterm infants with cerebral lesions. *Lancet* 2001;358: 1699–700.
47. Palmer C, Roberts RL, Towfighi J, Housman C. Endotoxin pretreatment protects neonatal rats from hypoxic ischemic brain injury. *Pediatr Res* 2001;49:122A.
48. Mittendorf R, Covert R, Montag A, *et al.* Association between fetal inflammatory response syndrome and bronchopulmonary dysplasia. *Pediatr Res* 2003;53:387A.
49. Yoon BH, Romero R, Moon JB, *et al.* Clinical significance of intra-amniotic inflammation in patients with preterm labor and intact membranes. *Am J Obstet Gynecol* 2001;185:1130–6.
50. Perlman JM. Markers of asphyxia and neonatal brain injury. *N Engl J Med* 1999;341:364–5.
51. Gressens P, Rogido M, Paindaveine B, Sola A. The impact of neonatal intensive care practices on the developing brain. *J Pediatr* 2002;140:646–53.
52. Goujon E, Parnet P, Aubert A, Goodall G, Dantzer R. Corticosterone regulates behavioral effects of lipopolysaccharide and interleukin-1 beta in mice. *Am J Physiol* 1995;269:154–9.
53. Crowley PA. Antenatal corticosteroid therapy: A meta-analysis of the randomized trials, 1972 to 1994. *Am J Obstet Gynecol* 1995;173:322 335.
54. Shimoya K, Taniguchi T, Matsuzaki N, *et al.* Chorio-amnionitis decreased incidence of respiratory distress syndrome by elevating fetal interleukin-6 serum concentration. *Hum Reprod* 2000;15:2234–40.
55. Leviton A, Dammann O, Allred EN, *et al.* Antenatal corticosteroids and cranial ultrasonographic abnormalities. *Am J Obstet Gynecol* 1999;181:1007–17.
56. Kallapur SG, Kramer BW, Moss TJ, *et al.* Maternal glucocorticoids increase endotoxin-induced lung inflammation in preterm lambs. *Am J Physiol Lung Cell Mol Physiol* 2003;284:633–42.
57. Kenyon SL, Taylor DJ, Tarnow-Mordi W, ORACLE Collaborative Group. Broad-spectrum antibiotics for preterm, prelabour rupture of fetal membranes: The ORACLE I randomised trial. ORACLE Collaborative Group. *Lancet* 2001;357:979–88.
58. Kenyon SL, Taylor DJ, Tarnow-Mordi W, ORACLE Collaborative Group. Broad-spectrum antibiotics for spontaneous preterm labour: The ORACLE II randomised trial. ORACLE Collaborative Group. *Lancet* 2001;357:989–94.
59. Matthay MA. Severe sepsis – A new treatment with both anticoagulant and anti-inflammatory properties. *N Engl J Med* 2001; 344:759–62.
60. Schultz C, Rott C, Temming P, Schlenke P, Moller JC, Bucsky P. Enhanced interleukin-6 and interleukin-8 synthesis in term and preterm infants. *Pediatr Res* 2002;51:317–22.
61. Barrington KJ. The adverse neuro-developmental effects of postnatal steroids in the preterm infant: A systematic review of RCTs. *BMC Pediatr* 2001;1:1.
62. Dembinski J, Behrendt D, Martini R, Heep A, Bartmann P. Modulation of pro- and anti-inflammatory cytokine production in very preterm infants. *Cytokine* 2003;21:200–6.
63. Mesples B, Plaisant F, Gressens P. Effects of interleukin-10 on neonatal excitotoxic brain lesions in mice. *Brain Res Dev Brain Res* 2003;141:25–32.
64. Dammann O, Leviton A. Brain damage in preterm newborns: Biological response modification as a strategy to reduce disabilities. *J Pediatr* 2000;136:433–8.
65. Fisher CJ, Agosti JM, Opal SM, *et al.* Treatment of septic shock with the tumor necrosis factor receptor: Fc fusion protein. The Soluble TNF Receptor Sepsis Study Group. *N Engl J Med* 1996;334:1697–702.
66. Lodha AK, Asztalos E, Moore AM. Elevated cytokines and poor neurodevelopmental outcome in prematurity and NEC. *Pediatr Res* 2003;53:386A.
67. Lappalainen U, Bry K. Lung disease in newborn mice overexpressing IL-1 in the lung. *Pediatr Res* 2003;53:461A.
68. Peters RG, Boekholdt SM. Gene polymorphisms and the risk of myocardial infarction – An emerging relation. *N Engl J Med* 2002;347:1963–5.
69. Witkin SS, Gerber S, Ledger WJ. Influence of interleukin-1 receptor antagonist gene polymorphism on disease. *Clin Infect Dis* 2002;34:204–9.
70. Terry CF, Loukaci V, Green FR. Cooperative influence of genetic polymorphisms on interleukin 6 transcriptional regulation. *J Biol Chem* 2000;275:18138–44.
71. Orsi N, Logghe H, Lynch K, *et al.* Carriage of the high secreting interferon gamma polymorphism is associated with an increased risk of preterm delivery and premature rupture of membranes. *Am J Obstet Gynecol* 2002;187:S120.
72. Hajeer AH, Hutchinson IV. Influence of TNF-α gene polymorphisms on TNF-α production and disease. *Hum Immunol* 2001;62:1191–9.
73. Harding D, Dhamrait S, Humphries SE, Montgomery H, Whitelaw A, Marlow N. Is interleukin-6 genotype associated with outcome after preterm birth? *Pediatr Res* 2003;53:540A.
74. Gibson C, MacLennan A, Goldwater P, Dekker G. Antenatal causes of cerebral palsy: Associations between inherited thrombophilias, viral and bacterial infection, and inherited susceptibility to infection. Obstet Gynecol Surv 2003;58:209–20.

5 Advances in neonatal ventilation

S. M. Donn and S. K. Sinha

Introduction

Ever since Hippocrates first described the use of intubation and positive pressure ventilation to support respiration approximately 2400 years ago, the goals of mechanical ventilation have remained essentially unchanged. We continue to attempt to achieve and maintain adequate pulmonary gas exchange, minimize the risk of lung injury, reduce the patient work of breathing, and optimize patient comfort. The introduction of surfactant replacement therapy, antenatal corticosteroid treatment, and the deployment of state-of-the-art mechanical ventilators have all changed the demographics of the 'old BPD' and presented new challenges in neonatal intensive care. Although we have made a start, the evidence as to how best to approach the problem is as yet insufficient on which to draw specific therapeutic conclusions or make clinical recommendations. Until we have created a sufficient evidence base, it seems prudent, therefore, to rely on the basic tenet of medicine, 'Primum Non Nocere: First, Do No Harm'. Therapy, in this case mechanical respiratory support, should be directed at avoiding the potentially damaging effects of oxygen therapy, the trauma from excessive pressure and/or volume, the adverse consequences of atelectasis; and the role of inflammation and infection in the pulmonary injury sequence, which is now well established. In addition, the new technology has given us the opportunity to observe the potentially deleterious effects of inappropriate airway flow, referred to as 'rheotrauma'.[1] The challenge is to identify the most appropriate device, technique, and strategies, especially as philosophies of respiratory management differ so widely among the individual clinicians and institutions.[2]

The past

The last three decades brought tremendous advances in the management of newborns with respiratory failure. The use of continuous distending pressure, first introduced by Gregory *et al.*,[3] was a remarkable step in maintaining the alveolar stability and improving survival in premature infants with respiratory distress syndrome (RDS). Mechanical ventilation of newborns resulted in the first report of a new disorder, bronchopulmonary dysplasia (BPD), also referred to as chronic lung disease (CLD), described by Northway *et al.* in 1967,[4] in which infants developed chronic parenchymal lung and airway injury characterized by inflammation and squamous metaplasia of the respiratory epithelium.

The 1970s brought the widespread practice of mechanical ventilation to neonatal intensive care, utilizing primarily continuous flow, time-cycled, pressure-limited ventilators. It dramatically extended the limits of viability, although the incidence of BPD continued to rise. In 1975, Philip attributed the pathogenesis of BPD to the combined effects of exposure to oxygen and positive pressure ventilation over time.[5]

The technological revolution accelerated in the 1980s with the advent of high-frequency ventilation (HFV). This new form of mechanical ventilation utilized delivered gas volumes that were smaller than the anatomical dead space at very high rates in an attempt to lower airway pressure and achieve more uniform gas distribution within the lung. Continuous 'non-invasive' monitoring was introduced, with transcutaneous gas monitoring and pulse oximetry becoming readily available. Toward the end of the decade, surfactant replacement therapy became a reality, overcoming the biochemical effects of the premature lung. Yet, CLD persisted.

The 1990s were characterized by the continued proliferation of technology. Real-time breath-to-breath pulmonary monitoring became feasible, and with it a host of new ventilator modes and modalities were introduced into clinical practice, such as synchronized intermittent mandatory ventilation (SIMV), assist-control (patient triggered), pressure-control, pressure-support, and volume-targeted ventilation. This decade also saw a dramatic change in the demographics and the nature of CLD. Infants surviving RDS were even smaller and more premature. Chronic lung changes (the 'new BPD')[6,7] were now characterized by a decrease in alveolarization of the lung, with less inflammation and scarring, but with diminished surface area and functional lung units. The incidence of CLD approached 30–40%, depending on how one chose to define it.

The present

Management strategies in the new millennium represent a broad spectrum with little consensus, ranging from non-invasive techniques to the highly invasive extracorporeal membrane oxygenation (ECMO). Almost all of the clinical trials conducted to date, which have utilized CLD as the primary outcome measure, have failed to demonstrate a benefit in lowering its incidence.

Continuous distending pressure

Continuous positive airway pressure (CPAP) is a form of distending pressure applied to the airways of a spontaneously breathing infant. It works by abolishing the upper airway occlusion and preventing atelectasis of the lungs, thus maintaining adequate functional residual capacity (FRC). CPAP as a primary strategy was popularized by the work of Wung and colleagues beginning in the early 1970s.[8] This approach was based on a dependence on spontaneous breathing, the avoidance of sedative and paralytic drugs, and the acceptance of 'abnormal' blood gases. The approach did result in a dramatic reduction in CLD, but it was never subjected to a randomized clinical trial. Moreover, only pulmonary and not long-term neurodevelopmental outcomes have been reported. In recent years, there has been a resurgence in the use of CPAP because it is a non-invasive technique and easy to apply. Several different devices and ways to administer CPAP are now available including the Infant Flow Driver® and Bubble CPAP®.[9,10]

The infant CPAP system™ (Electro Medical Equipment Ltd, Sussex, England) uses a dedicated flow driver and gas generator with fluid-flip, variable flow, CPAP. The Bernoulli effect directs gas flow toward each nostril, and the Coanda effect causes the inspiratory flow to flip and leave the generator chamber via the expiratory limb. This is supposed to assist spontaneous breathing and reduce the work of breathing by decreasing expiratory resistance and maintaining stable airway pressure throughout the respiratory cycle.

In the Bubble CPAP® system (Fisher and Paykel, Auckland, New Zealand), the blended gas is heated and humidified and then delivered to the infant through a secured nasal prong cannula. The distal end of the expiratory tubing is immersed under water, and at 4 l/min of gas flow the CPAP pressure generated is equal to the level of the CPAP probe. Varying the depth of the underwater link, the expiratory tube can vary the CPAP pressure. It has also been proposed that chest vibrations produced with Bubble CPAP® may contribute to gas exchange. Bubble CPAP® appears to

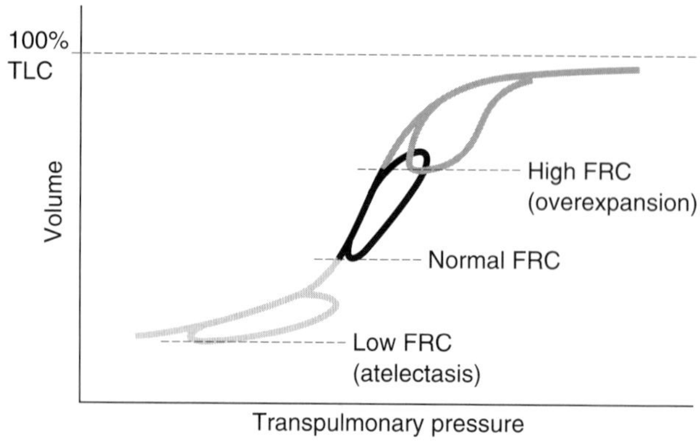

Figure 5.1 Static pressure–volume relationship. Optimal ventilation occurs at normal FRC, where compliance is best and incremental volume changes occur at the least pressure change. Ventilating above FRC results in overexpansion of the lung and increases the risks of baro- and volutrauma; ventilating below FRC may result in atelectasis and its attendant consequences.

be an effective and inexpensive option for providing respiratory support to premature infants.

There are as yet no controlled trials to compare the efficacy or superiority of one system over another. Many questions are as yet unanswered. Is there a 'best' way to provide CPAP? Does primary CPAP therapy delay or alter the benefit of surfactant replacement therapy in babies who ultimately require it? Is caloric expenditure higher than with mechanical ventilation? Does Bubble CPAP® confer any physiologic advantages?

Conventional mechanical ventilation (CMV)

CMV attempts to deliver physiologic tidal volumes to the patient with the lung at or near FRC. In doing so, we are utilizing the steepest portion of the pressure–volume relationship, where pulmonary compliance is the best and where the change in delivered volume occurs at the lowest increment in driving pressure. The concept is demonstrated nicely in Figure 5.1, a schematic pressure–volume graph. Ventilation at normal FRC, the middle loop, results in the best hysteresis and compliance axis, compared to either ventilating at high FRC, the upper loop, which leads to overexpansion and the risk of baro- and volutrauma, or ventilating at low FRC, the lower loop, which leads to atelectasis and the risk of atelectotrauma.[11–14]

The principles of mechanical ventilation are based on pulmonary physiology.[15] Oxygenation is a function of mean airway pressure. Mean airway pressure is usually adjusted by increasing the peak inspiratory pressure (PIP), the positive end-expiratory pressure (PEEP), and/or the inspiratory time. Ventilation refers to carbon dioxide removal and is the product of tidal volume and frequency (rate). The tidal volume is proportional to the difference between the PIP and the PEEP, a value referred to as the amplitude. It is crucial that clinicians understand that there are significant

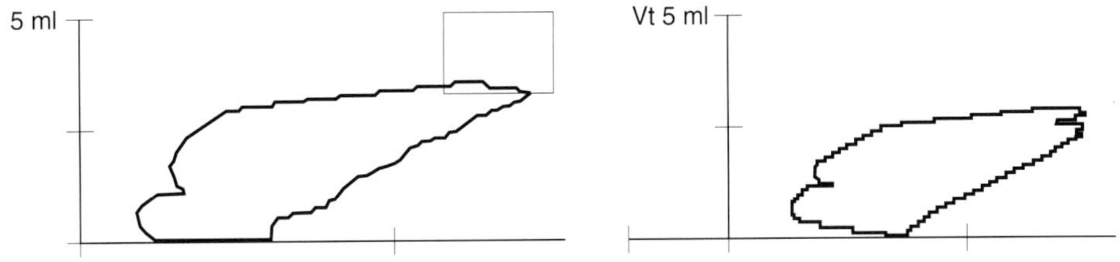

Figure 5.2 Left: Real-time pressure–volume loop demonstrating overinflation. Note the flattened portion at high pressure, where no additional volume is recruited. Right: A normal pressure–volume loop, showing satisfactory hysteresis.

differences among the various neonatal respiratory disorders and that differing pathophysiologic conditions call for different strategies. For instance, a preterm baby with RDS (low lung volume, homogenous disease) is very different from a term baby with meconium aspiration syndrome (high lung volume, heterogenous disease).

Mechanical ventilation is as much an art as a science. Great care must be taken to balance the life-saving benefit and the potentially injurious effects of positive pressure ventilation. Excessive inspiratory pressure can be detected by real-time pulmonary graphic monitoring.[16] This is shown in Figure 5.2. On the left, the pressure–volume relationship demonstrates hyperinflation, with exaggerated hysteresis and an upper inflection point on the inspiratory limb. A more normal pressure–volume relationship is shown on the graph on the right.

Until recently, the effects of airway flow on pulmonary mechanics have only been conceptual. Airway flow, which is the time rate of volume delivery, must be appropriately controlled. Rheotrauma refers to injury caused by inappropriate flow. If flow is excessive, it may result in turbulence, gas trapping, and inadvertent PEEP, leading to overdistension and the potential for thoracic air leaks. If flow is inadequate, it may create 'air hunger' or 'flow starvation' and increase the patient's work of breathing.

Turbulence, or non-laminar flow, can be created by excessive circuit flow. This can decrease the efficiency of gas exchange. If inspiratory airway flow exceeds expiratory airway flow, gas trapping and inadvertent PEEP may develop, increasing the risk of air leaks and contributing to elevated pulmonary vascular resistance. Paying close attention to respiratory time constants, the product of resistance and compliance, may help to avoid this.

Gas trapping can also be detected by real-time monitoring. Figure 5.3 demonstrates an abnormality in the expiratory flow waveform, which does not return to the zero flow baseline prior to the initiation of the next breath. This pattern calls for immediate adjustments in ventilator parameters, such as a reduction in flow, a decrease in the inspiratory time, or a slowing down of the ventilator rate if mandatory ventilation is being used.

For more than 30 years, neonatal ventilation has been accomplished using time-cycled, pressure-limited devices. This form of ventilation is easy to use and leaves all parameters to the discretion of the clinician. The baby may breathe spontaneously between the mechanical breaths from continuous flow in the ventilator circuit. These spontaneous breaths receive ventilatory support by PEEP only. Recent technological advances have introduced a variety of newer modes of ventilation, which were not available to neonatal populations before. They are also based on sound physiological principles, but often cause confusion. It is important that clinicians make themselves aware of the commonly used nomenclature. This can be best understood by using a hierarchical organization of ventilator modes:[17]

(1) Parent mode – determined by the control variable. This can be pressure, volume, or flow, and at any one time the mechanical breath can be controlled by only one of these.
(2) Daughter mode – determined by the breath type, which has four phases (phase variables):
    - Initiation of inspiration (trigger)
    - Inspiration (limit)
    - The change from inspiration to expiration (cycle)
    - Termination or expiration (baseline variable).

Pressure, volume, flow, and time are used as phase variables and determine the parameters of each ventilatory cycle. For example, in time-cycled, pressure-limited ventilation (TCPLV), the ventilator controls the airway pressure and the inspiratory phase lasts according to the time set by the clinician. On the other hand, in volume-controlled ventilation, the ventilator controls and measures the tidal volume generated by the machine irrespective of lung compliance. A ventilator is flow controlled if the gas delivery is limited by flow. This type of ventilator also controls the tidal volume even though it does not measure it directly.

Pressure-targeted ventilation

Modalities of ventilation that target pressure as the dependent or 'limit' variable include TCPLV; flow-cycled, pressure-limited ventilation (FCPLV); pressure-control ventilation (PCV); and pressure-support ventilation (PSV). What all of these have in common is a fixed pressure limit that the ventilator will not

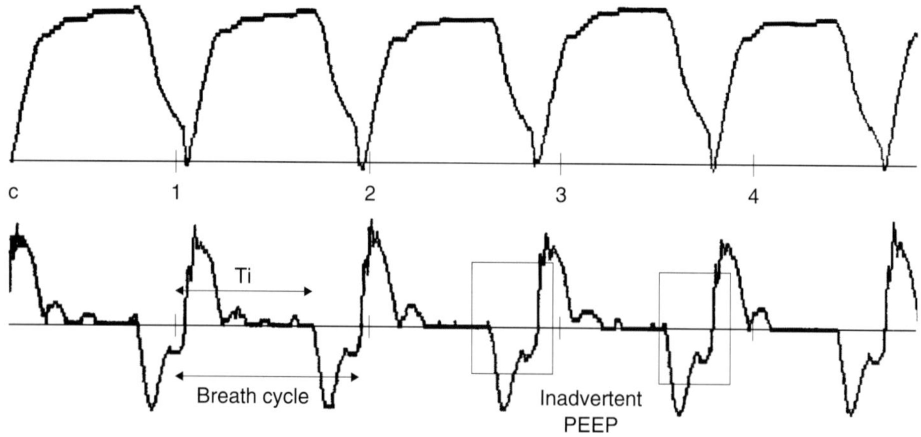

Figure 5.3 Real-time pressure (top) and flow (bottom) waveforms. The flow waveform demonstrates gas trapping. The expiratory portion (below baseline) does not return to a zero flow state (baseline) before the initiation of the subsequent breath, which prevents complete emptying of the lung.

exceed. Thus, delivery of tidal volume depends primarily on the patient's lung mechanics, of which compliance is the most contributory. TCPLV has a fixed inspiratory time and flow rate, FCPLV has a variable inspiratory time (set by the patient) and a fixed flow rate, and PCV has a fixed inspiratory time and variable inspiratory flow rate, which is proportional to patient effort. PSV is a spontaneous mode, used to support spontaneous breathing, generally during weaning. It can be used alone (if there is reliable respiratory drive) or in combination with synchronized intermittent mandatory ventilation (SIMV). Pressure-support breaths are flow cycled, so there is variable inspiratory time, and offer variable inspiratory flow proportional to the patient effort. Pressure-support breaths are pressure limited and may also be time limited.

Pressure-targeted modalities may be used in several modes. IMV involves the delivery of mechanical breaths at a fixed rate, selected by the clinician, with the patient able to breathe spontaneously between mechanical breaths. SIMV also involves a fixed mechanical rate, but the ventilator looks for spontaneous effort during a timing window in order to synchronize the start of a mechanical breath with the start of a spontaneous breath (see 'Triggered Ventilation', below). Assist-control ventilation provides a mechanical breath each time the patient breathes spontaneously, provided the trigger threshold is met, and also has a set control rate in case of patient apnea or inability to exceed the trigger threshold.

Volume-targeted ventilation

More recent technological advances have also enabled measurement of delivered tidal volumes and made possible the reintroduction of volume-targeted ventilation to newborn infants.[18] This form of CMV allows the clinician to select a specific tidal volume to be delivered to the patient. Pressure is permitted to fluctuate, creating a 'self-weaning' style of ventilation. Volume cannot truly be used as a cycling mechanism in the newborn, because of gas leaks around the uncuffed endotracheal tubes used in clinical practice, so it is better to refer to this form of CMV as volume-targeted, volume-limited, or volume-controlled ventilation. One of the advantages it offers over pressure-limited ventilation is that it responds to changes in pulmonary compliance. If compliance improves (e.g. following the administration of surfactant), pressure is decreased. Conversely, if compliance decreases (e.g. with pulmonary edema), pressure is increased to provide the desired tidal volume. Earlier, technological limitations of volume-targeted ventilation included high trigger sensitivity and asynchrony, slow response times (long trigger delays), highly compliant circuits (leading to increased compressible volume loss), and inability to both provide and measure the small tidal volumes required by premature infants. These have all been overcome (although not all of the devices providing volume-targeted ventilation can accurately measure tidal volume at the proximal airway).

Few studies to date have examined the effects of volume-targeted ventilation on neonatal outcomes. The investigation of Sinha *et al.*[19] randomized larger preterm infants to receive volume-targeted or pressure-targeted ventilation with tidal volume delivery tightly controlled. Infants assigned to the volume group had a shorter duration of ventilation, a strong trend to less CLD, and fewer severe neuroimaging abnormalities than the pressure group. Since this study, advances in the technology have enabled the delivery of even smaller tidal volumes and extended the capability to provide volume-targeted ventilation to the smallest premature infants. A large clinical trial is presently under way.

Hybrid forms of ventilation

Attempts have been made to combine the best features of both pressure-targeted and volume-targeted ventilation, resulting in a number of hybrid modalities.[18,20–22] Volume-guarantee® and pressure-regulated volume control® ventilation utilize a breath averaging technique to constantly adjust delivered tidal volume in response to changing patient lung mechanics. Volume-assured pressure support® adjusts the delivery of gas during a single breath to provide a minimum tidal volume by extending the inspiratory time and slightly ramping inspiratory pressure until the desired volume has been provided.[23] All three of these modalities appear promising but are in need of further investigation.

Proportional assist ventilation (PAV)[24] is an adaptive form of mechanical ventilation in which the inspiratory pressure is determined by the elastic and resistive properties of the patient. In the only published clinical trial, PAV was noted to be associated with lower mean airway and transpulmonary pressure at an equivalent fraction of inspired oxygen and similar carbon dioxide removal rate. Again, preliminary results are encouraging and ongoing evaluations may help to define the role of this modality.

Mandatory minute ventilation is a modality that combines SIMV and PSV. The desired minute ventilation (the product of tidal volume and frequency per minute) is set by the clinician, and as long as the patient is able to meet this target spontaneously, all of the breaths are pressure supported. If the minute ventilation falls below the desired level, the ventilator will provide additional 'catch-up' SIMV breaths using a breath-averaging technique. This form of ventilation is also being actively investigated.

Permissive hypercapnia

A recent lung-protective strategy that has been evaluated is permissive hypercapnia. This approach was based on an observation by Kraybill *et al.* in 1989,[25] in which infants displaying the highest carbon dioxide levels had the lowest incidence of BPD. The rationale behind permissive hypercapnia is that it decreases volutrauma, reduces the duration of ventilation, decreases the complications associated with hypocapnia, and increases oxygen unloading at the tissues by the Bohr effect. Two prospective controlled trials[26,27] did demonstrate a reduction in the duration of ventilation, but failed to show a decrease in the incidence of CLD. Although the strategy is attractive, further work is necessary to determine its place in the management of neonatal respiratory failure.

Triggered ventilation

Although IMV was the major ventilatory mode utilized for newborns for more than 25 years (Figure 5.4, left panel), it was not without hazard. One of its major drawbacks is the development of asynchrony, where the ventilator cycles at a programmed rate and the patient breathes independently, sometimes with and sometimes against the mechanical breath. Asynchrony has been shown to have adverse physiological consequences. 'Fighting the ventilator' may lead to inconsistent tidal volume delivery, increased work of breathing (and the need for higher mechanical support), inefficient gas exchange, and airleaks. Other organ systems may also be affected. Nearly 20 years ago, Perlman and Volpe[28] demonstrated the adverse effects of asynchrony on cerebral blood flow velocity and its high association with intraventricular hemorrhage.

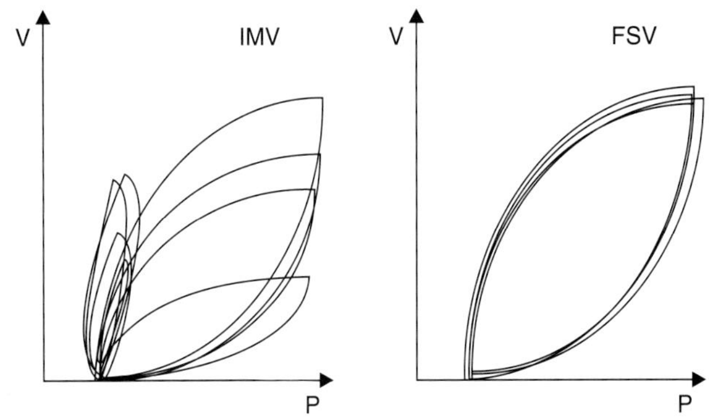

Figure 5.4 Graphic comparison of IMV (left) and flow synchronized ventilation (FSV; assist-control) (right). Note the wide variability of delivered tidal volumes in IMV, depending on whether the baby and ventilator are in or out of phase. In FSV, every breath is the same, since baby and ventilator are always 100% synchronous.

Figure 5.4 is a graphic comparison of IMV (left) and flow synchronized assist-control ventilation (right) and the difference is striking. In addition to the relatively feeble spontaneous breaths, supported only by PEEP, pressure-targeted IMV can result in widely variable tidal volumes, depending on whether the baby and the ventilator are in or out of phase with one another. Synchronization results in a consistently reproducible pattern of gas delivery with nearly identical pulmonary mechanics with each breath.

Synchronized or patient-triggered ventilation utilizes a patient-derived signal to initiate a mechanical breath. The signal is a surrogate of spontaneous breathing and may be a change in airway flow or pressure, abdominal movement, or thoracic impedance. One of the keys to successful triggered ventilation is a short response time or trigger delay. This is the interval between reaching the trigger threshold and the delivery of gas to the proximal airway. Long trigger delays mean that the baby may be considerably into the inspiratory cycle before receiving mechanical support, thus increasing the work of breathing and decreasing synchrony.[29]

Flow signals may also be used to terminate a breath, thus fully synchronizing the baby and the ventilator in both inspiration and expiration. This is referred to as flow-cycling. Flow-cycling is advantageous during assist-control ventilation as a safeguard against gas trapping and inversion of the inspiratory–expiratory ratio. If a baby becomes tachypneic during time-cycled assist-control, the fixed inspiratory time means that the expiratory time will become shorter and shorter as the baby breathes faster and faster. With flow-cycling, the inspiratory time will become shorter, since the breath terminates at a percentage of peak inspiratory flow rather than at a fixed time. Flow-cycling is also incorporated in PSV, where an inspiratory pressure 'boost' is applied to spontaneous breaths to help overcome the work of breathing imposed by the narrow lumen endotracheal tube, ventilator circuit, and demand valve. Pressure-support ventilation is primarily a weaning mode, but is also a form of synchronized ventilation[30] (Figures 5.5 and 5.6). Unfortunately, the evidence base for synchronized ventilation is also variable, and its role in the prevention of BPD still needs to be determined.[31–33]

High-frequency ventilation

HFV is generally divided into two subcategories. High-frequency jet ventilation (HFJV) uses a jet injector and pulsed or interrupted flow, usually in the range of 240–600 breaths/min. It involves passive exhalation and is thus dependent on the elastic recoil of the lungs for emptying. It is used in tandem with a conventional ventilator, which provides PEEP and conventional or sigh breaths. High-frequency oscillatory ventilation (HFOV) is different from HFJV and involves the use of distending pressure to inflate the lung to a static volume, and usually piston-driven displacement during inspiration and active exhalation. Typical rates for HFOV are 8–15 Hz. The gas volumes delivered are even smaller than those during HFJV. Management is relatively straightforward with oxygenation controlled by adjusting mean airway (distending) pressure and ventilation controlled by adjusting the amplitude of the oscillations.

HFJV was shown to be more effective than rapid rate CMV in the management of preterm infants with pulmonary interstitial emphysema, but few studies have examined its effect on CLD as a primary outcome measure. One study by Keszler *et al.*[34] did show a reduced incidence of CLD and a decreased need for home oxygen, but the comparison group was ventilated with IMV and the results of this study may not be applicable today.

HFOV has been more intensively studied, but the investigations have yielded conflicting results. In 1996, Gerstmann *et al.*[35] demonstrated increased survival without CLD, but Rettwitz-Volk *et al.*[36,37] found no differences in a 1998 report. Thome *et al.* showed a shorter time to extubation in an earlier trial, but a later study in 1999[38] found no differences in the incidence of death, CLD, or intraventricular hemorrhage. The two most recent studies, both published in 2002, also had discrepant results. The Neonatal Ventilation Study of Courtney *et al.*[38] found a small reduction in the incidence of CLD, whereas the UKOS study of Johnson *et al.* found no reduction.[39] The Courtney study utilized SIMV with inspiratory times of 0.25–0.4 s in the comparison group; the Johnson study utilized IMV with inspiratory times set at 0.4 s. Perhaps, the work of breathing was higher in the former study and may explain some of the differences in the results.

At present, the use of HFOV as a primary treatment strategy does not appear to be supported by the available evidence. The latest recommendation of the Cochrane Library[40] is consistent with this.

Extracorporeal membrane oxygenation

ECMO is a form of extracorporeal life support in which the circulation is diverted from the body to an artificial lung for gas exchange. ECMO was originally done through catheters placed in the right common carotid artery and right internal jugular vein (veno-arterial), but this necessitated permanent ligation of these vessels. Veno-arterial ECMO has now been largely replaced by veno-venous ECMO, using a double-lumen catheter in the right interval jugular vein. It has been shown to be efficacious in infants > 34 weeks of age or > 2000 g, who have reversible respiratory failure, unresponsive to 'conventional' treatment, and with a $> 80\%$ probability of death. Although ECMO is technically feasible in infants as small as 800 g, it requires systemic anticoagulation, and thus the risk of severe cerebral hemorrhage precludes its use in smaller newborns.

Neonatal ECMO utilization for respiratory failure has declined substantially as newer treatments, such as inhaled nitric oxide (iNO) and HFV, have evolved. However, it remains as the penultimate rescue technique in infants with suitable indications.[41]

iNO therapy

Nitric oxide in conjunction with appropriate ventilatory support is currently indicated in the management of newborns of term and near-term gestation with hypoxemic respiratory failure associated with evidence of pulmonary hypertension. Its use in the management of hypoxemic respiratory failure in the preterm infant, however, has not yet been established and any such use remains investigational.

The physiologic rationale for the clinical use of iNO in hypoxemic respiratory failure is based on its ability to achieve sustained and potent pulmonary vasodilation without causing systemic hypotension. Persistent pulmonary hypertension of the newborn (PPHN) is a disorder associated with diverse underlying pathologies, which is characterized by high pulmonary vascular resistance causing extrapulmonary right-to-left shunting of blood across the patent ductus arteriosus, foramen ovale, or both, leading to severe hypoxemia. iNO abolishes or decreases this shunt by lowering the pulmonary arterial pressure, often producing the immediate improvement in oxygenation seen in infants with PPHN.

The Neonatal Inhaled Nitric Oxide Study Group (NINOS)[42] and the Clinical Inhaled Nitric Oxide Research Group (CINRGI) are the pivotal multicenter-randomized trials that have demonstrated that iNO therapy improved oxygenation and reduced the need for ECMO treatment in term and near-term ($\geq$34 weeks' gestation) infants with hypoxemic respiratory failure and PPHN by 15–24%.

Finer recently reviewed the role of nitric oxide for respiratory failure in infants born at or near term.[43] Twelve eligible randomized-controlled trials were included in the analysis. iNO therapy was shown to reduce the incidence of combined outcome of death or the need for ECMO. The reduction was purely in the need for ECMO; mortality was not reduced. This finding primarily results from the efficacy of rescue ECMO for these infants.

The role of iNO in preterm infants with hypoxemic respiratory failure is controversial. Unblinded clinical studies and case reports have shown that iNO acutely improves oxygenation in preterm infants.[44] In a recent controlled trial, Schreiber *et al.*[45] showed a reduction in the combined outcome of survival without CLD in preterm infants given iNO early compared to those given placebo. The effect was only seen in infants who had less severe respiratory failure (oxygenation index <7) at entry and not in more sick babies. Another study, the INNOVO trial from the UK, failed to demonstrate any benefit,[46] but it recruited babies who had more severe respiratory failure. Additional trials are under way and until we know more, the role of iNO in preterm infants remains uncertain.

Monitoring

Continuous monitoring of the mechanically ventilated newborn has been a major technological advance. In the earlier era of mechanical ventilation, monitoring was intermittent and inferential. Assessments were made on the basis of a daily chest radiograph to crudely estimate lung volumes, and occasional blood gas measurements to evaluate gas exchange. Transcutaneous oxygen monitoring demonstrated the foibles of this approach. The development of pulse oximetry and continuous invasive therapy has enabled tighter control of oxygenation and ventilation, and the introduction of real-time pulmonary graphic monitoring[16] has finally given the clinician breath-to-breath feedback on the interaction between the ventilator and the patient. It allows for the customization or 'fine tuning' of ventilation for the individual baby and the evaluation of treatments that have a narrow therapeutic index. Monitoring is not a substitute for close clinical observation, but it can serve to augment the bedside care of ventilated newborns.

Weaning from mechanical ventilation

Weaning refers to the process in which the work of breathing is shifted from the mechanical ventilator to the patient. For the baby to be successfully weaned and extubated, there are a number of physiologic essentials. The baby must have reliable respiratory drive and be capable of sustaining alveolar ventilation once support is lessened, then removed. This requires neuromuscular competence. Adequate calories must be provided to fuel the work of breathing (but too many non-nitrogen calories can also increase carbon dioxide production). Factors known to impede the weaning process should be avoided or at least considered. They include electrolyte imbalance and metabolic alkalosis, anemia, infection, patent ductus arteriosus and/or congestive heart failure, neurologic dysfunction, and the effects of pharmacologic agents, such as analgesics and sedatives.

In general, the most harmful parameters should be decreased first. If the fraction of inspired oxygen is high, it should be weaned to less than 0.4 as oxygenation permits. If PIP or PEEP is high, it should likewise be decreased. The advent of triggered ventilation has altered weaning strategy, since reduction in the ventilator rate during assist-control does little if the patient is breathing above the control rate. Most studies to date have demonstrated that any form of triggered ventilation is superior to IMV in decreasing the time of ventilation.[47] Care should be taken to avoid fatiguing the baby by decreasing the ventilator rate during (S)IMV, since there is no support for spontaneous breathing other than PEEP. Perhaps, augmenting this with PSV will be the solution.

Controversies are still abound regarding adjunctive treatments during the weaning process. Although studies do support the use of methylxanthines, concerns exist regarding long-term safety. Similarly, diuretics and bronchodilators have been used with varying success, but some measure of efficacy should be assessed if treatment is to be continued. Corticosteroids have received a great deal of attention, primarily related to their use in the prevention and treatment of BPD. Neurodevelopmental concerns appear justified,[48,49] and the use of corticosteroids in the weaning/extubation process should be limited to short-term treatment of infants who have failed extubation because of upper airway edema.

Prior prospective indices to determine readiness for extubation have not been helpful. However, the ability to measure pulmonary mechanics, tidal volume, and minute ventilation has been shown to have a high positive predictive value in determining when to extubate a preterm infant recovering from RDS.[50] Alternatively, in the larger infant, one might consider extubation when the degree of support appears to equal the imposed work of breathing. This is another area ripe for investigation.

Optimizing mechanical ventilation

How can we optimize conventional ventilation? First, we need to ask good clinical questions. Second, we need to design the right tools to answer them. Third, we need to accurately and succinctly define our terminology and our outcome measures. A significant example of this is how we choose to define BPD.

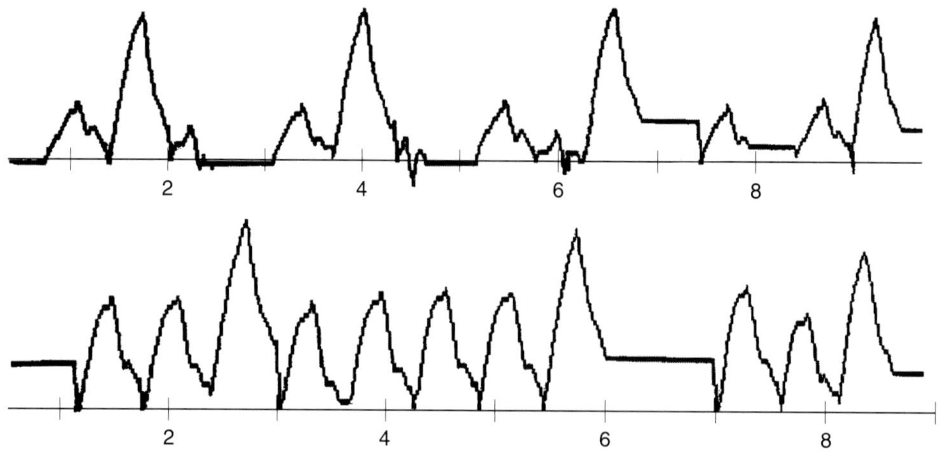

Figure 5.5 Top: Larger breaths are mechanical SIMV breaths, smaller breaths are spontaneous, supported only by PEEP. Bottom: Pressure support has been added to spontaneous breaths. These partially supported breaths are not quite as robust as the SIMV breaths (by choice), but are far better than the unsupported spontaneous breaths in the upper panel.

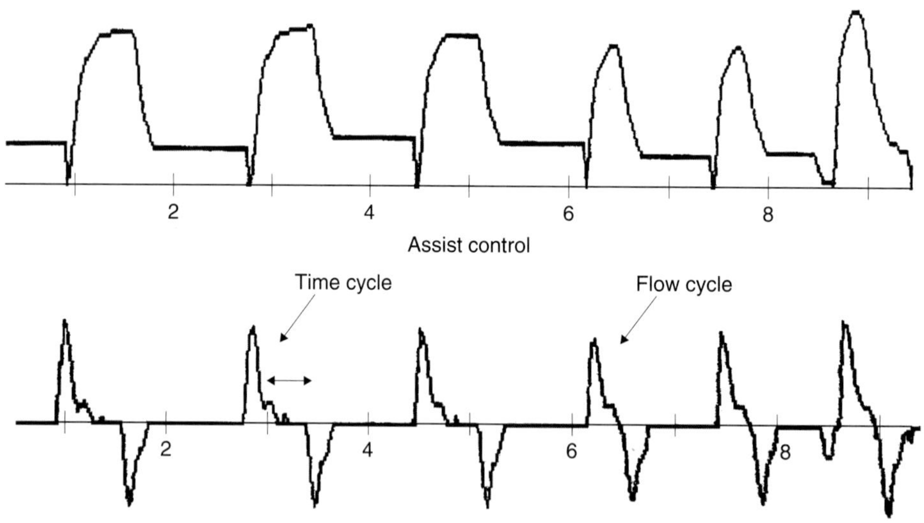

Figure 5.6 Pressure (top) and flow (bottom) waveforms demonstrating the differences between time-cycling and flow-cycling. In time-cycling, the inspiratory phase continues for a fixed period; expiration does not begin until the exhalation valve opens. This results in a plateau pressure. In flow-cycling, inspiration ends as a percentage of peak inspiratory flow. Thus, inspiration cycles directly into expiration and results in a more spiked pressure waveform.

There can be an enormous variation in the incidence of BPD within the same population, depending on how one chooses to define BPD. We need to find a better way to do this, and the work of Walsh *et al.* on determining a functional or physiological definition of CLD is an encouraging beginning.[51]

We clearly need to develop a better evidence base with respect to the multiple ways we can now ventilate babies. From this, we should be able to ask even better questions. It is possible that we have relied too heavily on meta-analysis, and we need to understand its limitations. Again, as an example, although the focus of most analyses has been on ventilation practices, which may very well be the most important variable affecting pulmonary outcomes, are the cited studies adequately controlled for other clinical parameters that can and do impact the pathogenesis of BPD, including nutritional practices, management of blood pressure and fluids, the approach to the PDA, the use of analgesics and sedatives, and respiratory drugs, antibiotic practices, ancillary care, and, very importantly, the variability in the host response?

The future

As we ask the important questions, other outcomes, besides just CLD, need to be considered. CLD is an intermediate outcome variable, but it may not be as important as looking at longer-range assessments, of which neurodevelopmental outcome is probably the most important. Similarly, short-term measures may also be significant. For instance, if there are no differences in either CLD or neurodevelopmental outcomes between two styles of ventilation, we should pay close attention to the short-term measures, such as patient comfort, cost-effectiveness, and acute complications, such as pneumothorax and days of ventilation.

What is the ideal mode of ventilation? It is one that delivers a breath that synchronizes with patient's own spontaneous respiratory effort. It maintains adequate and consistent tidal volume delivery and minute ventilation at low airway pressures. It is able to respond to sudden or unpredictable changes in pulmonary mechanics or patient demand. It provides the lowest possible work of breathing for the baby.

What is the ideal ventilator? It is one that achieves all of the important goals of mechanical ventilation. It provides a variety of modes and modalities that can ventilate even the most challenging pulmonary diseases. It has monitoring capabilities to adequately assess ventilator and patient performance. It has safety features and alarms that offer lung protective strategies. Most importantly, perhaps, it is used by a clinician willing to investigate its optimal uses and clinical applications.

Where do we go from here? The technology is only going to become more complex, the choices more numerous, and the decisions more perplexing. It will be imperative for us to harness the technology appropriately and, most importantly, safely.

Acknowledgment

We acknowledge the useful contribution from Dr Samir Gupta, Senior Clinical Fellow, and Mrs Victoria Hall, PA, in preparing this manuscript.

References

1. Attar MA, Donn SM. Mechanism of ventilator-induced lung injury in premature infants. *Semin Neonatol* 2002;7(5):353–60.
2. Donn SM, Sinha SK. Newer techniques of mechanical ventilation: An overview. *Semin Neonatol* 2002;7(5):401–8.
3. Gregory G, Kitterman J, Phibbs R. Treatment of the idiopathic respiratory distress syndrome with continuous positive airway pressure. *N Engl J Med* 1971;284:1333–40.
4. Northway WH Jr, Rosan RC, Porter DY. Pulmonary disease following respirator therapy of hyaline-membrane disease. Bronchopulmonary dysplasia. *N Engl J Med* 1967;276(7):357–68.
5. Philips AGS. Oxygen plus pressure plus time. The etiology of bronchopulmonary dysplasia. *Pediatrics* 1975;55:44–50.
6. Jobe AH, Bancalari E. Bronchopulmonary dysplasia. *Am J Respir Crit Care Med* 2001;163(7):1723–9.
7. Jobe A. The new BPD: An arrest of lung development. *Pediatr Res* 1999;46:641–3.
8. Wung JT, James LS, Kilchevsky E, *et al.* Management of infants with severe respiratory failure and persistence of fetal circulation without hyperventilation. *Pediatrics* 1985;76:488–92.
9. Morley, C. Continuous distending pressure. *Arch Dis Child Fetal Neonatal Ed* 1999;81:F152–6.
10. De PA, *et al.* Devices and pressure sources for administration of nasal continuous positive airway pressure (NCPAP) in preterm neonates. *Cochrane Database Syst Rev* 2002;4:CD002977.
11. McCulloch PR, Forkert PG, Froese AB. Lung volume maintenance prevents lung injury during high frequency oscillatory ventilation in surfactant-deficient rabbits. *Am Rev Respir Dis* 1988;137(5):1185–92.
12. Dos Santos CC, Slutsky AS. Invited review: Mechanisms of ventilator-induced lung injury: A perspective. *J Appl Physiol* 2000;89(4):1645–55.
13. Bond DM, Froese AB. Volume recruitment maneuvers are less deleterious than persistent low lung volumes in the atelectasis-prone rabbit lung during high-frequency oscillation. *Crit Care Med* 1993;21(3):402–12.
14. Froese AB. Role of lung volume in lung injury: HFO in the atelectasis-prone lung. *Acta Anaesthesiol Scand Suppl* 1989;90:126–30.
15. Harris T, Wood B. Physiologic principals. In Goldsmith J, Karotkin E, eds. *Assisted Ventilation of the Neonate.* Philadelphia, PA: WB Saunders Company, 1996:21–68.
16. Sinha SK, Nicks JJ, Donn SM. Graphic analysis of pulmonary mechanics in neonates receiving assisted ventilation. *Arch Dis Child Fetal Neonatal Ed* 1996;75(3):F213–8.
17. Carlo WA, Ambalavanan N, Chatburn RL. Classification of mechanical ventilation devices. In Sinha SK, Donn SM, eds. *Manual of Neonatal Respiratory Care.* Armonk, NY: Futura Publishing Company Inc., 2000:122–7.
18. Sinha S, Donn S. Volume-controlled ventilation: Variations on a theme. *Clin Perinatol* 2001;28(3):547–60.
19. Sinha SK, *et al.* Randomised trial of volume controlled versus time cycled, pressure limited ventilation in preterm infants with respiratory distress syndrome. *Arch Dis Child Fetal Neonatal Ed* 1997;77(3):F202–5.
20. Cheema IU, Ahluwalia JS. Feasibility of tidal volume-guided ventilation in newborn infants: A randomized, crossover trial using the volume guarantee modality. *Pediatrics* 2001;107(6): 1323–8.
21. Donn SM, Sinha SK. Newer modes of mechanical ventilation for the neonate. *Curr Opin Pediatr* 2001;13(2):99–103.
22. Dekeon M. Pressure control ventilation and pressure-regulated volume-controlled ventilation. In Sinha S, Donn S, eds. *Manual of Neonatal Respiratory Care.* Armonk, NY: Futura Publishing Company Inc., 2000:161–2.
23. Sinha SK, Donn SM. Volume controlled ventilation. In Goldsmith JP, Karotkin EH, eds. *Assisted Ventilation of the Neonate*, 4th edn. Philadelphia, PA: Elsevier, 2003.
24. Schulze A, Bancalari E. Proportional assist ventilation in infants. *Clin Perinatol* 2001;28(3):561–78.
25. Kraybill EN, Runyan DK, Bose CL, Khan JH. Risk factors for chronic lung disease in infants with birth weights of 750 to 1000 grams. *J Pediatr* 1989;115:115–20.
26. Amato MB, *et al.* Effect of a protective-ventilation strategy on mortality in the acute respiratory distress syndrome. *N Engl J Med* 1998;338(6):347–54.
27. Carlo WA, *et al.* Minimal ventilation to prevent bronchopulmonary dysplasia in extremely-low-birth-weight infants. *J Pediatr* 2002;141(3):370–4.
28. Perlman JM, Volpe JJ. Cerebral blood flow velocity in relation to intraventricular hemorrhage in the premature newborn infant. *J Pediatr* 1982;100(6):956–9.
29. Donn SM, Sinha SK. Controversies in patient-triggered ventilation. *Clin Perinatol* 1998;25(1):49–61.
30. Sinha SK, Donn SM. Pressure support ventilation. In Sinha SK, Donn SM, eds. *Manual of Neonatal Respiratory Care.* Armonk, NY: Futura Publishing Company Inc., 2000:157–60.
31. Greenough A. Update on patient triggered ventilation. *Clin Perinatol* 2001;28(3):533–46.
32. Baumer JH. International randomised controlled trial of patient-triggered ventilation in neonatal respiratory distress syndrome. *Arch Dis Child Fetal Neonatal Ed* 2000;82(1):F5–10.
33. Donn SM, Greenough A, Sinha SK. Patient triggered ventilation. *Arch Dis Child Fetal Neonatal Ed* 2000;83(3):F225–6.
34. Keszler M, *et al.* Multicenter controlled clinical trial of high-frequency jet ventilation in preterm infants with uncomplicated respiratory distress syndrome. *Pediatrics* 1997;100(4):593–9.

35. Gerstmann DR, *et al.* The Provo multicenter early high-frequency oscillatory ventilation trial: Improved pulmonary and clinical outcome in respiratory distress syndrome. *Pediatrics* 1996;98(6, Pt 1):1044–57.
36. Rettwitz-Volk W, *et al.* A prospective, randomized, multicenter trial of high-frequency oscillatory ventilation compared with conventional ventilation in preterm infants with respiratory distress syndrome receiving surfactant. *J Pediatr* 1998;132(2): 249–54.
37. Thome U, *et al.* Randomized comparison of high-frequency ventilation with high-rate intermittent positive pressure ventilation in preterm infants with respiratory failure. *J Pediatr* 1999;135(1): 39–46.
38. Courtney SE, *et al.* High-frequency oscillatory ventilation versus conventional mechanical ventilation for very-low-birth-weight infants. *N Engl J Med* 2002;347(9):643–52.
39. Johnson AH, *et al.* High-frequency oscillatory ventilation for the prevention of chronic lung disease of prematurity. *N Engl J Med* 2002;347(9):633–42.
40. Henderson-Smart DJ, *et al.* Elective high frequency oscillatory ventilation versus conventional ventilation for acute pulmonary dysfunction in preterm infants. *Cochrane Database Syst Rev* 2004;2:CD000104.
41. Schumacher RE, Baumgart S. Extracorporeal membrane oxygenation 2001: The odyssey continues. *Clin Perinatol* 2001; 28(3):629–53.
42. Anonymous. Inhaled nitric oxide in full-term and nearly full-term infants with hypoxic respiratory failure. The Neonatal Inhaled Nitric Oxide Study Group. *N Engl J Med* 1997;336(9):597–604 [erratum appears in *N Engl J Med* 1997;337(6):434].
43. Finer NN, Barrington KJ. Nitric oxide for respiratory failure in infants born at or near term. *Cochrane Database Syst Rev* 2001;2:CD000399 [update of *Cochrane Database Syst Rev* 2000;2:CD000399; PMID: 10796358].
44. Kinsella JP, *et al.* Inhaled nitric oxide in premature neonates with severe hypoxaemic respiratory failure: A randomised controlled trial (comment). *Lancet* 1999;354(9184):1061–5.
45. Schreiber M, *et al.* Inhaled nitric oxide in premature infants with the respiratory distress syndrome. *N Engl J Med* 2003;349: 2099–107.
46. Field D. The INNOVO trial: Preliminary results for NO use in preterm infants. *Arch Dis Child* 2003;88:A1.
47. Sinha SK, Donn SM. Weaning babies from mechanical ventilation. *Semin Neonatol* 2002;7:421–8.
48. Yeh T, *et al.* Outcomes at school age after postnatal dexamethasone therapy for lung disease of prematurity. *N Engl J Med* 2004;350:1304–13.
49. Finer N, *et al.* Postnatal steroids: Short term gain, long term pain? *J Pediatr* 2000;137:9–13.
50. Gillespie L, Whyte S, Sinha SK, Donn SM. Usefulness of the minute ventilation test in predicting successful extubation in newborn infants: A randomized controlled trial. *J Perinatol* 2003;23:205–7.
51. Walsh MC, Wilson-Costello D, Zadell A, Newman N, Fanaroff A. Safety, reliability, and validity of a physiologic definition of bronchopulmonary dysplasia. *J Perinatol* 2003;23:451–6.

6 Clinical care of the very preterm infant

L. Hellström-Westas, L. J. Björklund, M. Lindroth, S. Polberger and V. Fellman

Regionalization of care

The concept of regionalization of perinatal care was introduced in the late 1960s in Canada,[1] and during the 1970s, perinatal centers were established in developed countries. The goal was to identify the high-risk pregnancies and to transfer mothers to tertiary hospitals, which were organized, staffed, and equipped for the multidisciplinary task of providing optimal maternal and neonatal care. In Europe, the regionalization of preterm infants in the late 1990s was evaluated in a survey (EUROPET) showing that there were great variations in the regionalization programs between different countries.[2,3] In some countries, governmental policies exist; in others, national scientific societies issue guidelines, usually stressing intrauterine transfers and delivery in level III centers for very preterm infants. The size of the delivery units varies considerably, the average number of births per maternity unit being 500–3000. Large maternity units usually have adjacent level III neonatal intensive care units (NICU), although their organization varies.[4]

In USA, a trend toward deregionalization has occurred since the late 1980s, referring to a process of moving away from transfers to referral centers providing the highest quality of care to promoting competing hospitals with less expertise. The difference in functioning level is not clear to the public, and thus decisions on which caring centers to choose may be taken on non-medical grounds, such as convenient location.[5] Deregionalization may also be a result of too small tertiary neonatal units without the possibility of admitting all newborn patients requiring intensive care. As a result of the remarkable increase in survival of the very preterm infants during the past decades, the patient load in tertiary NICUs often exceeds their capacities. Thus, the criteria used for defining high-risk pregnancies tend to be stricter, i.e. only the most immature infants are transferred to level III units and less immature preterm infants with considerable morbidity risks are increasingly treated in level II units. This development is unfortunate, since the way that perinatal care is organized may have a substantial impact on clinical outcomes, such as mortality and disability rates. Birth at a hospital with a regional NICU is associated with a lower risk-adjusted mortality than birth at a hospital with no NICU, intermediate NICU of any size or small community hospitals.[6]

The size of the NICU has an impact on the outcome, as, for example, was reported in a Finnish national study where the lowest mortality and disability rates were reported in the largest academic NICU.[7] In a California study on preterm infants with birth weight less than 2000 g, risk-adjusted neonatal mortality was significantly lower for births that occurred in hospitals with level III NICUs with an average census of more than 15 patients/day.[8] No evidence-based recommendations are available on the optimal size of a NICU. However, a reasonable-sized NICU is mandatory for running a neonatal service with all the necessary functions: neonatologists available around the clock, experienced staff, full range of medical intensive care with cardiology and surgical services, including bedside operations, and capacities to expand the facilities during high-demand periods, e.g. due to preterm multiple births. Regional units should have an academic function, providing high-quality specialist training and performing research on their preterm cohorts as well as repeated quality assessments of treatment strategies. Further, tertiary academic units should participate in national and international networks, e.g. for collaborative use of quality improvement techniques, and translation of research into practice, which may result in accelerated and effective practice changes and implementation of evidence-based interventions.[9]

The rapid development of technology in newborn medicine, e.g. ventilators and incubators for preterm infants, leads to a continuous need for new investments in intensive care equipments. Centralization of neonatal care decreases the need for overlapping functions in level III and level II centers, especially investments in expensive technology. Regional resources for expensive front-line equipment should be allocated to the regional center, which should have responsibility for evaluating them scientifically and keeping them in continuous use, thus providing a high level of technical know-how to the staff. The performance of intensive care could be facilitated by a computerized clinical information system, which ensures precision in physician orders, improves medication management, facilitates reporting, and provides detailed documentation of care and continuous monitoring of parameters from technical equipment. Implementation of a computerized physician order entry has been shown to reduce medication turnaround times and medication errors.[10]

The limited health resources can be efficiently used with a well-organized tiered network with regionalization of highly specialized intensive care and several level II units for the intermediate care.[11] This organization model aims at a balance between efficiency and accessibility to services and requires transfer of the preterm infant after the intensive care period to the next level unit.

Transport

Regionalization of perinatal care requires a well-organized transfer service as well as presents an opportunity to establish a safe and efficient transfer network.[12] The goal should be that all high-risk pregnancies are identified antenatally and the transfer to the perinatal center with level III NICU should take place *in utero*. However, there will be a small group of preterm infants acutely delivered outside the tertiary perinatal center, as well as newborn infants with unexpected complications and postnatal disorders, who need to be transferred postnatally to the regional center.

Neonatal transport service requires an appropriate referral system, trained personnel, and management structures.[13] Depending on the population base and the geography different solutions can be applied. For emergency postnatal transports of very preterm infants to the level III units, it is crucial that the transport team is trained in neonatal intensive care of this patient group. Prior to the transfer, the infant should be stabilized and the intensive care should be continued and monitored during the transport. According to the EUROPET survey in 1996 on large NICUs in Europe, the average national inborn rate of preterm infants of less than 30–32 weeks' gestation exceeded 75% in the majority of countries.[14] Thus, the need for postnatal transports of very preterm infants is fortunately an uncommon situation, which, however, is a highly demanding task in order to avoid transport-related complications.

The neonatal intensive care unit

The goal should be to deliver all very preterm infants in a tertiary perinatal center with a neonatal unit well experienced in all aspects of intensive care. Active management has contributed to the improved prognosis for very preterm infants during the last decade[15,16] in addition to other factors, such as level of antenatal care and socioeconomic factors, and administration of antenatal steroids. Ideally, the NICU should be located close to the delivery unit and to the operating theatre, so that intrahospital transports can be avoided after delivery. It is necessary for neonatal units, which treat very preterm infants, to develop clinical routines for the care of these infants. Such routines should include guidelines for minimal handling and strategies for keeping the number of invasive procedures to a minimum. The noise level in the NICU is often high, and, consequently, measures should be taken to reduce noise and light and include environmental guidelines.

Immediate care at birth

The initial clinical care of the very preterm infants differs from the care of more mature infants in several aspects. In this context we will emphasize the initial care of extremely preterm infants born before 28 weeks' gestation. The very preterm infants have higher mortality and are more likely to develop intraventricular hemorrhages (IVH), symptomatic persistent ductus arteriosus, sepsis, necrotizing enterocolitis, and bronchopulmonary dysplasia (BPD) as compared to more mature infants.[7,17] They are also at higher risk of developing cerebral palsy and disturbances in attention and cognition. Close perinatal collaboration between obstetricians and neonatologists is essential for healthy survival of these infants.

Prior to delivery, the parents should be informed by the neonatal staff about expectations for survival and morbidity, based on recent statistics. The parents should always be allowed to express their own expectations, and if time allows also have the possibility of a visit to the NICU before the delivery. This goal can sometimes be difficult to achieve, not least with an expecting mother in active labor or with pre-eclampsia, nevertheless it should always be attempted. In vaginal deliveries, immediate postnatal stabilization of the very preterm infant can preferably take place in the delivery room, close to the parents.

The initial care of the very preterm infants should be very carefully planned.[18] Evaporative heat loss during the first minutes of life can cause severe cooling of these infants, and a low temperature on admission to the NICU is an independent risk factor of death.[17] Radiant heater open beds designed for resuscitation should be used. In addition, hypothermia can be prevented by wrapping the wet body of the infant in a plastic bag as soon as possible after birth.[19,20] After rapid stabilization, the infant can be placed directly in a preheated incubator. This transfer can be avoided by initial use of combination incubators with both radiant heater open-bed and double-wall incubator alternatives. The incubator is then moved to the NICU and used for the continuing care of the infant. In order to minimize the disturbance of the very preterm infant, all later procedures, e.g. insertion of umbilical lines, should be done without moving the infant from the incubator.

It is of vital importance that adequate equipment for resuscitation is available in the delivery room or operating theatre. For this purpose, mobile resuscitation beds are very useful. Modern pulse oximeters can give correct values for oxygen saturation and heart rate within a few minutes after birth,[21] and it is no longer acceptable to rely on intermittent heart rate auscultation and visual assessment of skin color. The pulse oximeter probe should preferably be placed on the right hand to assess preductal saturation.[22] The more common placement on one foot may result in lower readings early in life, with a risk of unnecessary oxygen treatment. Although current guidelines still recommend that 100% oxygen should be used for resuscitation,[23] there is increasing evidence suggesting that lower oxygen exposure is beneficial for newborn infants.[24,25] Healthy, full-term infants are not expected to reach preductal oxygen saturation above 90% until 10 min after birth,[25] and there is no reason to strive for higher levels in premature infants. The resuscitation bed must be equipped with an inspired gas blender for precise oxygen administration.[22] If oxygen saturation rises above 93%, oxygen supply should be rapidly reduced or discontinued.[26]

The initial ventilatory management of the very preterm infant is currently much debated.[27] In general, previous studies recommended that premature infants should be intubated and given prophylactic surfactant early after birth, but it has been questioned whether this is applicable to current babies.[28] These babies are often more immature, but may paradoxically both have an accelerated lung maturation at birth and have a highly vulnerable lung with a disposition to develop BPD.[29] Animal studies indicate that the immature lung may be particularly sensitive to ventilation-induced injury very early after birth,[30] and epidemiological studies imply that an aggressive initial respiratory management, including early intubation and surfactant, may be associated with an increased risk of BPD.[31] In many centers, there is now a trend against routine delivery room intubation in favor of early application of continuous positive airway pressure (CPAP).[32] A recent trial showed that delivery room intubation could be avoided in 53% of infants born at 24–25 weeks' gestation.[33] Another approach, aiming to avoid mechanical ventilation early in life, is to perform endotracheal intubation immediately after birth and give prophylactic surfactant, followed by rapid extubation to nasal CPAP. However, preliminary results from one study showed that in infants born at 27–29 weeks' gestation there was no added benefit from prophylactic surfactant when early CPAP was used.[34] It is not known if the same is true also for more immature infants. Ongoing multicenter trials on delivery room management of preterm infants may provide new evidence on treatment strategies.[27]

Although the preterm infant may appear severely depressed at birth, immediate intubation is usually not indicated. Even if a prophylactic surfactant strategy is chosen, there is no proven benefit from giving surfactant before the first breath.[35] Bag-and-mask ventilation of preterm infants may be difficult, and gas exchange will probably be very inefficient unless the baby contributes by making gasps.[36] Even so, the vast majority of small infants will respond to bag-and-mask ventilation with a rapid increase in heart rate. Once the baby starts breathing spontaneously, its efforts can be supported if adequate equipment is available. Unfortunately, the commonly used self-inflating resuscitation bags have severe limitations.[37] The oxygen supply is difficult to regulate, and the bags have a poorly working pressure limitation. Consequently, high pressures (> 40 cm H_2O) are easily generated, especially at high ventilatory rates. Tidal volumes are unknown and can potentially become very large. Moreover, there is usually no way of obtaining CPAP or positive end-expiratory pressure (PEEP), and therefore no way to effectively support the baby's spontaneous breathing.

The Neopuff® Infant Resuscitator (Fisher & Paykel, Auckland, New Zealand) is a commonly used T-piece system with adjustable PEEP and peak pressure that can be attached to a face mask or an endotracheal tube. It can easily be used to apply nasal or face mask CPAP immediately after birth (see Figure 6.1). It has been suggested that a relatively high distending pressure (up to 8 cm H_2O) should be used in this situation.[37] If the baby responds well, CPAP with the same device can be continued during transportation to the NICU. In an experimental setting, the Neopuff® device produced reliable and reproducible peak inspiratory pressures and PEEP.[38,39] However, there are at present no published clinical trials evaluating this method against other systems.

At all very preterm deliveries, surfactant should be immediately available. According to Scandinavian tradition, infants are not intubated for the sole purpose of giving surfactant. However, if the very preterm infant needs intubation for resuscitation, surfactant should be given as soon as the endotracheal tube is presumed to be in a correct position. Many infants respond rapidly and may soon be breathing room air on endotracheal tube CPAP, in which case early extubation can be considered.

Even if the infant is intubated and surfactant is administered in the delivery room, there is usually sufficient time to allow the parents to see their baby

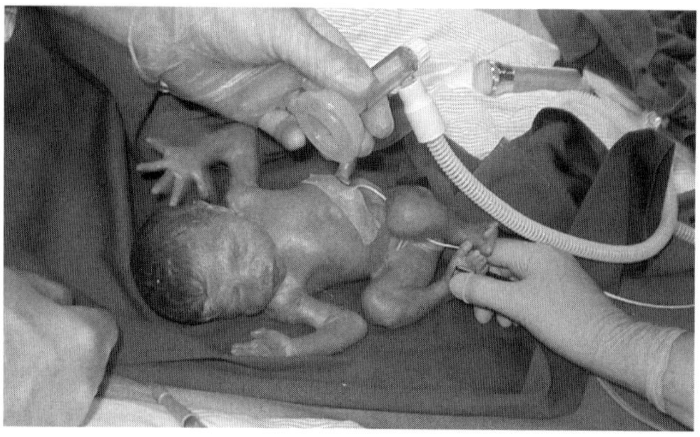

Figure 6.1 Immediate care after delivery. This vigorous and spontaneously breathing infant is just about to be assisted with face mask CPAP by the Neopuff®. An oxygen saturation probe is applied to the right foot. Photograph courtesy of Mats Blennow.

before transportation to the NICU. The father can usually take part in this transport, and photographs can be taken as a first memory. After arrival to the NICU and within the first hour of life, venous and arterial catheters are inserted for blood sampling, infusion of glucose and arterial blood pressure monitoring.

Nutrition

The beneficial effects of early enteral feeding on the development of the gut of the preterm infant are well recognized.[40,41] Recent data indicate improved short-term and long-term outcome in preterm infants fed human milk as compared to formula-fed infants.[42–44] Enteral feedings with small amounts of human milk (1–2 ml every 3 h) can usually be started within the first hours of life in very preterm infants.[45] The primary feed should be the infant's own mother's milk, but until it is available, heat-treated donor milk is used.

In order to reduce the number of invasive procedures, indwelling central venous catheters (CVCs) for fluid and drug administration can be used. Although the risks, e.g. thrombosis, with umbilical venous catheters are well known, this is for the very preterm infants an easy and rapid way of gaining venous access. Before use, the position should always be checked with x-ray and the catheter should always allow withdrawal of blood. An umbilical venous catheter, in correct position with the tip of the catheter in the inferior vena cava, is suitable for supplementary parenteral nutrition during the first days of life. Double-lumen catheters are useful, since they allow a steady infusion in one lumen, while intermittent injections can be given in the other lumen without the need for additional peripheral intravenous lines during the first days. After 3–4 days the umbilical venous catheter can be replaced by a peripherally inserted central venous catheter (PICC). When the tip of a PICC is optimally located in the upper vena cava (as checked by x-ray) it can often be used also for blood sampling.[46]

Initially, an infusion of glucose is given and replaced as soon as possible by a glucose–amino acid solution, providing glucose at a rate of 4–6 mg/kg/min.[47] Before the third day of life, there is usually no need to add electrolytes except calcium. To reduce the risk of hyperchloremic metabolic acidosis, sodium acetate should be used instead of sodium chloride in the intravenous solutions. Providing adequate nutrition and sufficient caloric intake is a problem during the first week of life in very preterm infants.[47] For this reason, intravenous lipids should be started in the first or second day of life, with close supervision of serum triglycerides. A multivitamin preparation is included in the lipid solution to reduce the risk of peroxidation. The initial daily dose of lipids is usually 0.5 g/kg, which, if tolerated without hyperlipidemia, is increased stepwise to 2 g/kg during the first week of life, and only rarely increased to 3 g/kg.[48]

The enteral milk feedings are gradually increased on a day-to-day basis. When the very preterm infant can tolerate 75–80% of the total volume intake by the enteral route, i.e. 130–160 ml/kg of a total daily volume intake of 170–200 ml/kg, the supplementary parenteral nutrition can be omitted. The infant's own mother's milk is the preferred source of the enteral nutrition. All mothers should be encouraged to express their milk during the preterm period and to breast-feed their infants after discharge from the neonatal unit. If the mother cannot supply her infant with milk, pasteurized banked donor milk is used, or a preterm formula. Administered human milk can be analyzed for macronutrient content (protein and energy)[49,50] and thus the fortification can be individually planned, aiming at a daily protein and energy intake of 3.5 (to 4.0) g/kg and 120 kcal/kg, respectively. Higher energy intakes are often required in infants with BPD. Weekly biochemical monitoring of protein status should be performed in the very preterm infants by, for example, measuring serum levels of urea and transthyretin (prealbumin).[51] Calcium and particularly phosphorus supplementation is needed for adequate bone mineralization in human milk-fed infants.[43]

Clinical monitoring

Respiratory and hemodynamic instability is common in very preterm infants. Close surveillance is essential, both during the early acute phase, characterized by postnatal adaptation and respiratory distress, and during the later stages when nosocomial infections and recurrent apneas are common. Initial clinical signs of infection may be subtle, but often precede deterioration in vital parameters. The clinical monitoring includes regular observations of vitality, color, heart rate, respiration, body temperature, bowel movements, and diuresis.

Fluid and electrolyte balance are closely related to evaporation and heat loss from the immature skin.[52] The insensible water loss from the immature skin is highest during the first 2 days of life, and then decreases during the first week.[53] The skin of the most immature infants sometimes becomes dry and cracked during the first week of life. Various methods for preventing this, e.g. by applying prophylactic ointment, have been evaluated, but have shown that this strategy may be associated with an increased risk of nosocomial sepsis.[54] Double-walled incubators with a high humidity, starting at 80%, should be used in these infants to diminish the inevitable water losses (see Figure 6.2). The daily fluid requirements average 85–100 ml/kg. However, the most immature infants may require more during the first days of life. Serum levels of electrolytes (sodium, potassium, and ionized calcium) should be measured and monitored daily during the initial course. Hypocalcemia can usually be corrected by i.v. administration of calcium, either as bolus or added to the intravenous infusion. Hypernatremia (serum sodium above 150 mmol/l) is usually caused by too low fluid intakes, or by too large insensible water loss, or by adding sodium too early to intravenous infusions. Non-oliguric hyperkalemia sometimes occurs during the first days of life in the most immature infants and does not seem to be related to kidney function.[55] Kidney function is difficult to evaluate in the very preterm infants during the first days of life. The serum creatinine levels are often affected by the maternal creatinine level, although very high serum creatinine and urea levels, and oliguria may be seen in infants with poor kidney function. Urinary output mainly reflects the fluid balance and is also a sign that the arterial blood pressure is sufficient. A diuresis of 1–2 ml/kg/h after 24 h of age is usually adequate. Blood transfusions are often needed in the initial care of very preterm infants. In many hospitals, diuretics are given routinely after blood transfusions. This strategy has no support by controlled studies, and the frequent use of diuretics may increase the risk of nephrocalcinosis.[56] Blood and urinary glucose levels should be checked regularly, particularly during the first weeks of life, in order to avoid both hypoglycemia and hyperglycemia. Almost all very preterm infants need phototherapy for hyperbilirubinemia, and initially serum bilirubin should be checked daily.[57] In computerized clinical information systems, algorithms for insensible water loss can be included providing continuous water balance monitoring. Thus, dehydration and hypernatremia can be avoided. Continuous glucose infusion, without interruption, is important for stable blood glucose values. The most immature infants may need insulin infusion for adequate glucose intake.

Continuous monitoring of vital parameters is necessary in the care of very preterm infants. These infants often need monitoring of electrocardiogram or heart rate, respiration, and oxygen saturation at least until they have reached 32–33 weeks' gestation. In the initial phase, blood pressure is preferably monitored through an indwelling umbilical or peripheral artery catheter, since non-invasive blood pressure monitoring is less reliable. Continuous transcutaneous measurement of blood gases, i.e. partial pressures of oxygen and carbon dioxide, is often very useful, although the fragile skin during the first days of life sometimes limits the time in which electrodes can be applied. Transcutaneous monitoring of PCO_2 levels can reduce the need for blood gas samples and give early indications of hypocarbia, which indicates that ventilator settings should be promptly reduced. Monitoring PCO_2 is important, since low $PaCO_2$ values are associated with decreased cerebral blood flow and development of periventricular leucomalacia, and also with the development of BPD.[58] Continuous monitoring of oxygen saturation is a standard procedure in all NICU's, and most units have guidelines for oxygen saturation limits in very preterm infants, often with a wide range between 85% and 95%. However, more research is needed in order to obtain evidence on whether the lower or the higher values of this range would be preferable.[59] High or unstable oxygen saturation is a risk factor for retinopathy of prematurity (ROP), and very preterm infants should be regularly examined by ophthalmologists from around 32 weeks' gestation until full term for early detection and treatment of ROP. Continuous monitoring of electrocortical activity with amplitude-integrated electroencephalography (aEEG), a simplified method utilizing one or two channels of filtered and time-compressed EEG, is increasingly being used in neonatal units. The

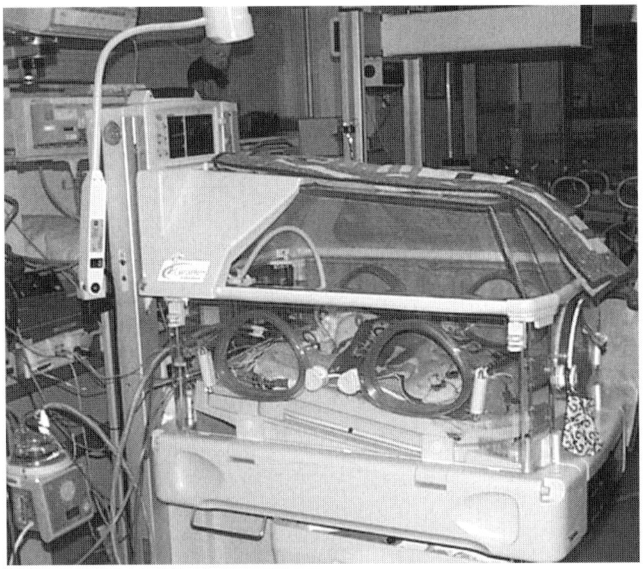

Figure 6.2 Double-walled incubators are used for optimal thermal management of very preterm infants. When the infants are stable an incubator cover can be used in order to reduce noise and light.

method shows changes over time in cerebroelectrical background activity and can be used also in preterm infants. Degree of electrocortical background depression in aEEG activity shows good correlation with grade of IVH and outcome.[60–62] The method also reveals subclinical seizure activity. Normal data for very preterm infants have been published recently.[63]

Infections

Perinatal infections (bacterial vaginosis, premature rupture of membranes, and chorioamnionitis) are important causes of very preterm birth. In contrast, early-onset bacterial infections (positive culture before 72 h age) in the offspring are uncommon, and blood cultures drawn at the time of arterial line insertion are usually negative. Increasing use of antibiotics before and during labor has led to a substantial decrease in early group B streptococcal infections, but simultaneously there has been an increase in prevalence of *Escherichia coli* sepsis.[64] These infections may have a rapidly progressive course with severe hypoxic respiratory failure and early demise.

Late-onset nosocomial bloodstream infections are much more common, occurring in between 10% and 30% of very low-birth-weight infants (VLBWI).[65] They are usually less severe than early infections, but are still associated with a significant morbidity. Coagulase-negative staphylococci (CoNS) are by far the most common pathogens, being implicated in around 50% of the cases.[66] CoNS infections often occur at around 10–14 days of age. The source of bacteremia is usually a CVC that has been colonized with CoNS, either by skin contamination during insertion or through the catheter hub during later manipulations.[67] Symptoms are unspecific and include apneas, increased oxygen requirement, respiratory insufficiency, and, sometimes, also arterial hypotension. Serum level of C-reactive protein is increased, but this may not be seen until after 12–24 h. Treatment with vancomycin is often started when an infection is first suspected, leading to a substantial overuse of this drug. It is not known how long one can safely wait before starting vancomycin treatment,[67] but in relatively stable infants it is usually possible to wait until there is an increase in serum levels of C-reactive protein. If an adequate amount of blood (1 ml) is taken for culture, vancomycin can be discontinued after 48 h if blood culture and ancillary tests are still negative.[67] Antibiotic treatment of CoNS bacteremia is often started without removal of the CVC, but if the baby has a delayed clinical response and if bacteremia persists, the line must be withdrawn.[68,69] CoNS bloodstream infections are not associated with an increased mortality,[70] but these infections often herald the start of a period of clinical deterioration with a need for mechanical ventilation, opening of the ductus arteriosus, development of BPD,[71,72] and an increased length-of-stay. There is also a concern that sepsis increases the likelihood of having an adverse neurodevelopmental outcome.

Candida infections occur particularly in extremely preterm infants. Colonization of mucoepithelial surfaces with *Candida* appears to be a prerequisite for systemic infection,[73] and invasive disease usually results from a colonizing *Candida* strain, rather than from some different isolate.[74] Colonization is most often vertical from the mother at birth, usually with *Candida albicans*, but horizontal colonization from care providers in the NICU also occurs, and is thought to be the primary mode of transmission for *Candida parapsilosis*.[74] Congenital cutaneous candidiasis is relatively uncommon, presenting with diffuse skin rash, in some cases burn-like desquamations, and sometimes pulmonary involvement in the first days of life.[69,75] There is usually no fungemia, but systemic treatment is definitely indicated in the very preterm infants. There is an association between the presence of intrauterine contraceptive devices or cerclage during pregnancy and congenital candidiasis.

Some very immature infants (mean gestational age 24 weeks) have invasive fungal dermatitis. Erosive skin lesions with crusting develop during the first 2 weeks of life. Blood culture is often positive, and the port of entry into the bloodstream is probably through dermal vessels.[75] One outbreak of systemic candidiasis was associated with the use of a petrolatum ointment emphasizing the risk that skin care products may damage the delicate dermal barrier in immature infants.[76] However, the intestinal epithelium is considered the primary portal of entry for most systemic *Candida* infections.[74] Such infections often occur in the second week of life or later, often in the aftermath of a CoNS infection treated with vancomycin, but sometimes as the first nosocomial infection in an extremely preterm infant. Other risk factors are mechanical ventilation, CVC, and treatment with broad-spectrum antibiotics, corticosteroids, or H_2 blockers. Symptoms are often unspecific. Abdominal distension and discoloration, and especially spontaneous intestinal perforation, should raise suspicion of invasive candidiasis.[75] Though *Candida* is known to cause end-organ invasion (meningitis, renal candidiasis, endocarditis, and endophthalmitis), this is rarely evident at the time of first symptoms. Serum level of C-reactive protein is usually moderately elevated. Thrombocytopenia is probably more pronounced in invasive candidiasis than in the other nosocomial infections.[66] The diagnosis of invasive candidiasis is difficult because blood cultures are often negative, but other diagnostic tests are currently under evaluation. Measurement of urinary D-arabinitol/L-arabinitol ratio may be used in neonates.[77,78]

CVCs are extremely important in the pathogenesis of neonatal candidiasis. These catheters are usually not the primary port of entry, but once in the bloodstream, *Candida* organisms can adhere to and even penetrate into the catheter wall,[78] which becomes the source of end-organ damage, at the same time making the organisms inaccessible to antimicrobial drugs. It has been stated that removal or replacement of the CVC should be completed within 24 h of notification of a positive blood culture for *Candida*.[78] A recent review stated that if a *Candida* infection is suspected and the patient is clinically stable and has not had previous antifungal therapy, fluconazole is a suitable empiric therapy.[79] Amphotericin B should be considered in severe or life-threatening infections pending results of cultures.

Infections with Gram-negative bacteria are relatively uncommon, but often present with a more rapid clinical deterioration and may be associated with shock, coagulation problems, and increased mortality.[66,70] In many neonatal units, there has recently been a substantial increase in infection with *Enterobacter*, usually resistant to cephalosporins[80]. An empiric antibiotic policy including ampicillin and cefotaxime was shown to be associated with an increased prevalence of resistant Gram-negative bacteria, especially *Enterobacter*, as compared with a policy including penicillin and an aminoglycoside.[81] Spread of *Enterobacter* among patients is well documented, and outbreaks have been contained by simple hygienic measures and restrictions in the use of cephalosporins.[82,83]

In view of the relative immune deficiency of premature infants and the necessary invasive care with multiple broken barriers, a high prevalence of nosocomial infections may seem inevitable. However, there is a great variation among centers in the incidence of such infections, which is not explained by different case mix.[65] It follows that these infections should to a large extent be seen as preventable complications of the treatment. A recent survey showed that the staff of units with a particularly low rate of nosocomial sepsis tended to see such infections as a breakdown in care that could have been prevented.[65]

Hand hygiene is of great importance in preventing the spread of bacteria and fungi between patients. The availability of waterless alcohol hand rubs in close proximity to the incubators makes compliance more likely. In adult wards, the education of patients about the importance of hand washing and asking that they remind their caregivers to wash has been very successful,[84] and perhaps we should teach the parents of premature babies to do the same. Good nutrition with an emphasis on enteral feeding with human milk probably diminishes the risk of infection. Indwelling venous catheters and intravenous lipids are important risk factors for CoNS bloodstream infection. Strategies for maximal barrier precautions and aseptic techniques during catheter placement are important, as well as strict guidelines for blood sampling through catheters and for hub manipulations. The use of 'antibiotic locks' to prevent catheter-related bloodstream infections seems to be a promising technique, but it remains to be evaluated in clinical trials.[85] The use of fluconazole prophylaxis to prevent neonatal candidiasis is probably safe and can be considered in high-risk patients, but larger studies are needed.[86]

Developmentally supportive care

Behavioral problems, including attention deficit and hyperactivity disorders, are common among surviving children who were born very preterm.[87,88] The reasons for this are not known, but it is believed that environmental influence from the extrauterine environment negatively affects the development of the immature central nervous system.[89,90]

One of the most important aspects of the care of preterm infants is promotion of emotional attachment between the infant and its parents. Family-focused neonatal care has been increasingly practiced during the last two decades. Systematic strategies for this include free visiting hours and early involvement of parents in care procedures, e.g. diaper changes and feeding, creation of good family memories with hand- and footprints, photographs and diaries, etc. Kangaroo care promotes attachment between the infant and its parents, and development of preterm infants.[91,92] Kangaroo care can often start during the first week of life (see Figure 6.3).[93]

It was previously shown that reduced light, and day-and-night light promoted sleep in preterm infants, and this effect persisted several months after discharge.[94] Incubator covers are increasingly being used to reduce light and noise. However, as a single procedure in neonatal care their effect has only been investigated in a few studies. In a small observational study there were only minor effects on quiet sleep from the incubator covers in stable preterm infants.[95] Neonatal Individualized Developmental Care and Assessment Program (NIDCAP) is based on formal observations of the preterm infants during a care procedure. The observations are made by medical personnel, often neonatal nurses, who have received special training in this

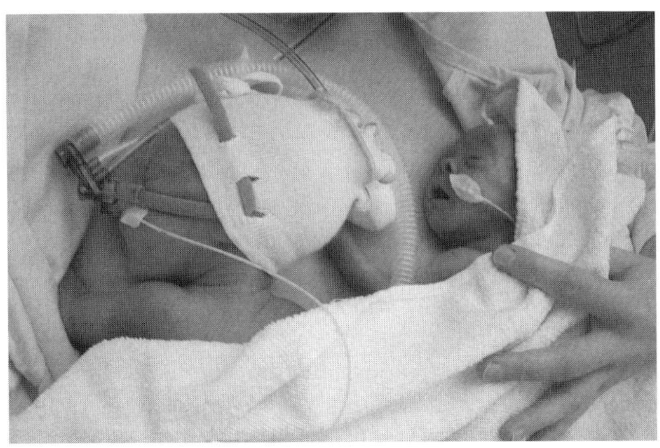

Figure 6.3 Kangaroo care of twins. The twin to the left is treated with nasal CPAP and fed mother's milk through a nasogastric tube. Photograph courtesy of Ann-Cathrine Berg.

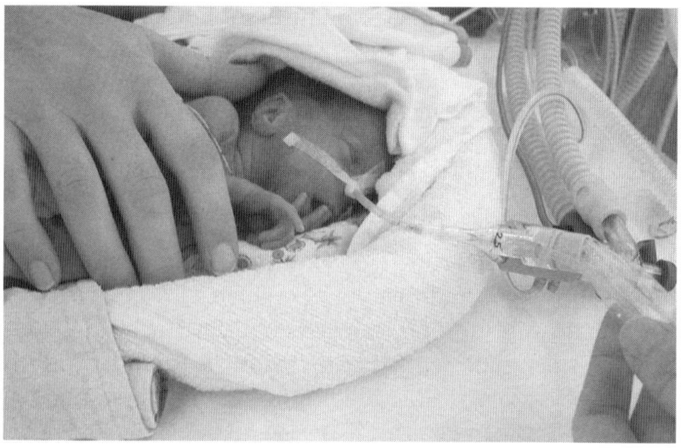

Figure 6.4 Giving support to an infant during care procedures is an important part of developmental care. This infant is supported by the hand of a parent during endotracheal suctioning. Photograph courtesy of Ann-Cathrine Berg.

method. Individual recommendations for the nursing care are made from the results of these observations (see Figure 6.4). Treatment with NIDCAP is associated with a shorter need for respiratory support and a shorter duration of stay in the NICU.[96,97] Recently, it was shown that NIDCAP is associated with structural changes of the brain, as shown by magnetic resonance imaging and diffusion tensor imaging techniques, and with increased neurophysiological maturation, as shown by EEG.[98]

Pain and treatment of pain

Pain is defined by the International Association for the Study of Pain as 'an unpleasant sensory and emotional experience associated with actual or potential tissue damage or described in terms of such damage'.[99] According to this definition, pain is always a subjective phenomenon with subjective reporting. Thus, individuals, such as preterm infants, not capable of reporting pain would not experience it. However, based on empirical evidence it has been proposed that physiological and behavioral responses are valid indicators of pain.[100]

Whether the fetus feels pain, and if so from which gestational age, has been a controversial issue. The thalamo-cortical fibers, which are considered crucial for nociception, are present between the 20th and 34th week of gestation. The afferent fibers grow into the cortical plate after the 26th week of gestation, but already between 20 and 26 weeks synaptic circuits occur between the subplate and the cortical plate indicating neuro-anatomical basis for the fetus to feel pain.[101] Evoked potentials suggest that thalamic inputs reach the cortex at 29 weeks.[102] Pain threshold is lower in preterm infants than in term infants and later in life.[103] Even in full-term infants the threshold remains low after injury.[104] This suggests that the exposure to multiple procedures in the neonatal period increases pain awareness. Newborn infants undergoing intensive care are subjected to repeated daily procedures. Very preterm infants are likely to experience a large number of invasive procedures during the neonatal care period.[105,106] The most immature infants may be exposed to several hundreds of potentially painful procedures, including, e.g. blood sampling and endotracheal intubation.[105] Neonatal pain experiences may alter later pain responses in children.[89] The gentle care of very preterm infants also includes some aspects of standard care procedures, e.g. painful stimuli from venous or arterial punctures for blood sampling. Painful stimuli can cause fluctuation in arterial blood pressure, which may affect cerebral blood flow. This could contribute to cerebral hemorrhages or ischemia.[107] However, it has also been shown that blood sampling from umbilical artery catheters can affect cerebral blood volume in preterm infants. This can be avoided by very slow withdrawal of blood from the catheter.[108] Other care procedures associated with changes in cerebral blood volume in very preterm infants include endotracheal suctioning and surfactant administration (Figure 6.4).[109,110] Because of the many procedures and long-lasting mechanical ventilation, routine opioid infusion or bolus injections were introduced during the early 1990s in many NICUs for pain relief during the first day(s) of life to preterm infants undergoing assisted ventilation and repeated procedures. Several behavioral pain scales have been developed for preterm infants, but are, however, not widely used in clinical routine.[111–113] In order to administer optimal analgesia, repeated assessments using pain scales are recommended.

Controversies still exist regarding the severity of pain and the need for pain relief for preterm infants undergoing intensive care. With the development of synchronized ventilation, preference of nasal CPAP, and indwelling lines to minimize procedures, the liberal use of opioids has recently been questioned. In the NEOPAIN study[113] infants were randomized to receive either morphine or placebo infusion. The results showed that opioid-treated infants did not have a more beneficial outcome than infants in the placebo group and in some cases they even had a worse outcome. Referring to this study, the goal would be *a priori* to reduce the amount of distress and pain by the use of non-pharmacological means, including individualized care. Only when obvious pain is present, such as procedural or postoperative pain, a routine administration would be advisable. Otherwise, the use of potentially hazardous analgesics should only be given if a pain scale assessment or behavioral observations indicate the presence of distress and pain despite non-pharmacological intervention to minimize it. This approach would produce a more focused pain treatment, probably with fewer side effects.

Ethical aspects

During the last 20 years there has been a growing concern about the ethical issues surrounding the most preterm infants who are at the limits of viability and intact survival. The majority of deaths, around 80%, in very premature infants occur in the first 3 days of life in spite of full intensive care.[114] Neonatologists caring for these infants need to address the question whether to continue care or to withdraw ongoing intensive care. Such discussion may arise when the patient suffers from severe brain or pulmonary injury and the chance of survival is low and the possibility of healthy survival is extremely low.[115] The first principle of treatment is always to act in the best interest of the patient and the family according to the Hippocratic rules, i.e. never to hurt or harm, if possible to relieve, sometimes to cure, and always to console.

When evaluating the question on withdrawal of intensive care, the situation should be analyzed using the traditional ethical principles of (1) benefit, (2) harm, (3) autonomy, and (4) justice. This analysis should be performed in a two-dimensional model taking into account the different interest groups, i.e. the infant, parents, caretakers, and even society.[116]

For the evaluation, a summary of all medical facts is needed, from which an estimated probable prognosis is derived. Sometimes, the decision is not difficult or controversial, such as in babies with Potter syndrome (absence of kidneys) or hydranencephaly. However, when outcome is not inevitably fatal or the interest of the parents and the infants diverge, the decision making needs a thorough discussion. In these instances, non-medical factors, such as social or economical factors, may influence the decision. A decision to withdraw treatment should always be taken by a senior consultant, and usually by a team of them, after careful discussions with all involved staff. The medical course and prognosis should be carefully and repeatedly explained to the parents, and their opinion should be taken into consideration. If parents cannot accept the recommendation to withdraw treatment, the discussions should be repeated. A special situation is prolonged delivery-room resuscitation of extremely premature infants at the limits of viability, where urgent decisions usually are needed in the interest of the infant. On such occasions, thorough discussion with the parents before delivery is of the greatest importance for the decision making.[117]

There is usually time to arrange for death to be filled with dignity also for the most immature infants. Good psychological care of the parents is essential, since they will continue to live with strong and sad memories of this time. A professional, warm, and empathic care by experienced staff will assist them in this difficult situation. The parents' wishes regarding social or cultural ceremonies, e.g. baptism, or for information to or presence of relatives or friends should be fulfilled. Rituals connected to death are important for coping with the loss and sorrow after the death. The terminal care of the dying baby should be carefully planned and performed, including sufficient sedation and analgesia, in order to prevent further suffering. A dying infant should be cared for in a single room together with the parents. One or two experienced staff members should participate and assist the parents in this situation.

The outcome of very preterm infants

The outcome of very preterm infants has significantly improved during the last two decades, and especially of those with a gestational age below 28 weeks.[118,119] Most follow-up studies of preterm cohorts are defined by birth weight, either including extremely low-birth-weight infants < 1000 g or VLBWI < 1500 g. The mortality rate is correlated to immaturity: the more preterm the infant, the higher the mortality.[7] The limit of viability seems to be about 23 weeks of gestation, since survival after 22 weeks of gestation is very rare, but after 23 weeks, about 10% according to regionalized long-term follow-up studies from the postsurfactant era, i.e. from the 1990s.[120–122] In a national cohort, the stillborn rate was 60% in infants delivered after 22 gestational weeks, 35% after 23 weeks, and 25% after 24 weeks,[7] suggesting that there may be a less active care during birth in the very immature infants resulting in intrapartal death or classification as dead if there is bradycardia at birth. In this cohort, the long-term survival of live-born infants born after 24 weeks of gestation was 40%, but less than one-half of them were classified as completely normally developed at 1.5 years of age.[120]

Despite increasing survival, the rate of neurodevelopmental impairment has remained similar, which results in an increased absolute number of infants with abnormalities.[122,123] Severe handicaps, such as cerebral palsy, deafness, blindness, and mental retardation, have in recent studies been reported to occur in 15–25%.[118,123] Even more common are cognitive dysfunction and learning disabilities. In a large VLBWI birth cohort study in The Netherlands, assessment at the age of 9 years showed that 56% of children in mainstream education needed special assistance at school or were below the age-appropriate level.[123] Similar results have been reported from other countries.[124] Most of the learning difficulties seem to be related to low overall IQ.[88]

Several perinatal risk factors have been associated with poor school performance, such as low-birth weight, need for assisted ventilation, and IVH.[125] Intrauterine growth restriction in preterm infants is associated with increased morbidity, and low postnatal growth, resulting in smaller size at school age and poorer school performance as compared to appropriately grown siblings.[126] The high incidence of sequelae in very preterm infants warrants long-term follow-up of regional cohorts for quality control of the demanding perinatal care and long-lasting neonatal intensive care.

REFERENCES

1. Swyer PR. The regional organization of special care for the neonate. *Pediatr Clin North Am* 1970;17:761–76.
2. Debauche C, Van Reempts P, Kollée L, *et al.* Maternal and neonatal transfer policies in Europe. *Prenat Neonatal Med* 1999;4(Suppl 1):5–14.
3. Kollée L, Chabernaud J, Van Reempts P, *et al.* Perinatal transport practices: A survey of inborn versus outborn very preterm infants admitted to European neonatal intensive care units. *Prenat Neonatal Med* 1999;4(Suppl 1):61–72.
4. Papiernik E, Zeitlin J, Milligan D, *et al.* Variations in the organization of obstetric and neonatal intensive care in Europe. *Prenat Neonatal Med* 1999;4(Suppl 1):73–87.
5. Hein HA. Regionalized perinatal care in North America. *Semin Neonatol* 2004;9:111–6.
6. Cifuentes J, Bronstein J, Phibbs CS, Phibbs RH, Schmitt SK, Carlo WA. Mortality in low birth weight infants according to level of neonatal care at hospital of birth. *Pediatrics* 2002;109:745–51.
7. Tommiska V, Heinonen K, Ikonen S, *et al.* A national short-term follow-up study of extremely low birth weight infants born in Finland in 1996–1997. *Pediatrics* 2001;107:e2.
8. Phibbs CS, Bronstein JM, Buxton E, Phibbs RH. The effects of patient volume and level of care at the hospital of birth on neonatal mortality. *J Am Med Assoc* 1996;276:1054–9.
9. Sharek PJ, Baker R, Litman F, *et al.* Evaluation and development of potentially better practices to prevent chronic lung disease and reduce lung injury in neonates. *Pediatrics* 2003;111:e426–31.
10. Cordero L, Kuehn L, Kumar RR, Mekhjian HS. Impact of computerized physician order entry on clinical practice in a newborn intensive care unit. *J Perinatol* 2004;24:88–95.
11. Tucker J, Parry G, Fowlie PW, McGuire W. ABC of preterm birth. Organisation and delivery of perinatal services. *Br Med J* 2004;329:730–2.
12. Cornette L. Contemporary neonatal transport: Problems and solutions. *Arch Dis Child Fetal Neonatal Ed* 2004;89:F212–4.
13. Lupton BA, Pendray MR. Regionalized neonatal emergency transport. *Semin Neonatol* 2004;9:125–31.
14. Zeitlin J, Papiernik E, Bréart G, the EUROPET group. Regionalization of perinatal care in Europe. *Semin Neonatol* 2004;9:99–110.
15. Shankaran S, Fanaroff A, Wright L, *et al.* Risk factors for early death among extremely low-birth-weight infants. *Am J Obstet Gynecol* 2002;186:796–802.
16. Håkansson S, Farooqi A, Holmgren PA, Serenius F, Högberg U. Proactive management promotes outcome in extremely preterm infants: A population-based comparison of two perinatal management strategies. *Pediatrics* 2004;114:58–64.
17. Costeloe K, Hennessy E, Gibson AT, Marlow N, Wilkinson AR, for the EPICure Study Group. The EPICure study: Outcomes to discharge from hospital for infants born at the threshold of viability. *Pediatrics* 2000;106:659–71.
18. Fowlie PW, McGuire WM. ABC of preterm birth. Immediate care of the preterm infant. *Br Med J* 2004;329:845–8.
19. Vohra S, Frent G, Campbell V, Abbott M, Whyte R. Effect of polyethylene occlusive skin wrapping on heat loss in very low birth weight infants at delivery: A randomized trial. *J Pediatr* 1999;134:547–51.
20. Björklund LJ, Hellström-Westas L. Reducing heat loss at birth in very preterm infants. *J Pediatr* 2000;137:739–40.
21. Kopotic RJ, Lindner W. Assessing high-risk infants in the delivery room with pulse oximetry. *Anesth Analg* 2002;94(Suppl 1): S31–6.
22. Finer NN, Rich WD. Neonatal resuscitation: Raising the bar. *Curr Opin Pediatr* 2004;16:157–62.
23. International guidelines for neonatal resuscitation: An excerpt from the guidelines 2000 for cardiopulmonary resuscitation and emergency cardiovascular care: International consensus on science. *Pediatrics* 2000;106:e29.
24. Lundstrom KE, Pryds O, Greisen G. Oxygen at birth and prolonged cerebral vasoconstriction in preterm infants. *Arch Dis Child Fetal Neonatal Ed* 1995;73:F81–6.
25. Saugstad OD. The role of oxygen in neonatal resuscitation. *Clin Perinatol* 2004;31:431–43.
26. Chow LC, Wright KW, Sola A, the CSMC Oxygen Administration Study Group. Can changes in clinical practice decrease the incidence of severe retinopathy of prematurity in very low birth weight infants? *Pediatrics* 2003;111:339–45.
27. Dunn MS, Reilly MC. Approaches to the initial respiratory management of preterm neonates. *Paediatr Respir Rev* 2003; 4:2–8.
28. Morley C, Davis P. Surfactant treatment for premature lung disorders: A review of best practices in 2002. *Paediatr Respir Rev* 2004;5(Suppl A):S299–304.
29. Van Marter LJ, Dammann O, Allred EN, *et al.*, for the Developmental Epidemiology Network Investigators. Chorioamnionitis, mechanical ventilation, and postnatal sepsis as modulators of chronic lung disease in preterm infants. *J Pediatr* 2002;140:171–6.
30. Ingimarsson J, Björklund LJ, Curstedt T, *et al.* Incomplete protection by prophylactic surfactant against the adverse effects of large lung inflations at birth in immature lambs. *Intensive Care Med* 2004;30:1446–53.
31. Van Marter LJ, Allred EN, Pagano M, *et al.*, the Neonatology Committee for the Developmental Epidemiology Network. Do clinical markers of barotrauma and oxygen toxicity explain interhospital variation in rates of chronic lung disease? *Pediatrics* 2000;105:1194–201.
32. Narendran V, Donovan EF, Hoath SB, Akinbi HT, Steichen JJ, Jobe AH. Early bubble CPAP and outcomes in ELBW preterm infants. *J Perinatol* 2003;23:195–9.
33. Finer NN, Carlo WA, Duara S, *et al.*, the National Institute of Child Health and Human Development Neonatal Research Network. Delivery room continuous positive airway pressure/positive end-expiratory pressure in extremely low birth weight infants: A feasibility trial. *Pediatrics* 2004;114:651–7.
34. Thomson MA. Continuous positive airway pressure and surfactant; combined data from animal experiments and clinical trials. *Biol Neonate* 2002;81(Suppl 1):16–9.
35. Kendig JW, Ryan RM, Sinkin RA, *et al.* Comparison of two strategies for surfactant prophylaxis in very premature infants: A multicenter randomized trial. *Pediatrics* 1998;101:1006–12.
36. Palme-Kilander C, Tunell R. Pulmonary gas exchange during facemask ventilation immediately after birth. *Arch Dis Child* 1993;68:11–6.
37. O'Donnell CPF, Davis PG, Morley CJ. Resuscitation of premature infants: What are we doing wrong and can we do better? *Biol Neonate* 2003;84:76–82.
38. Finer NN, Rich W, Craft A, Henderson C. Comparison of methods of bag and mask ventilation for neonatal resuscitation. *Resuscitation* 2001;49:299–305.
39. Hussey SG, Ryan CA, Murphy BP. Comparison of three manual ventilation devices using an intubated mannequin. *Arch Dis Child Fetal Neonatal Ed* 2004;89:F490–3.
40. Lucas A, Bloom SR, Aynsley-Green A. Gut hormones and "minimal enteral feeding." *Acta Paediatr Scand* 1986;75:719–23.
41. McClure RJ, Newell SJ. Randomised controlled study of clinical outcome following trophic feeding. *Arch Dis Child Fetal Neonatal Ed* 2002;82:F29–33.
42. Lucas A, Morley R, Cole TJ, Lister G, Leeson-Payne C. Breast milk and subsequent intelligence quotient in children born preterm. Lancet 1992;339:261–4.
43. Schanler RJ. The use of human milk for premature infants. *Pediatr Clin North Am* 2001;48:207–19.
44. Hylander MA, Strobino DM, Pezzullo JC, Dhanireddy R. Association of human milk feedings with a reduction in retinopathy among very low birthweight infants. *J Perinatol* 2001;21:356–62.
45. Bellander M, Ley D, Polberger S, Hellström-Westas L. Tolerance to early human milk feeding is not compromised by indomethacin in preterm infants with persistent ductus arteriosus. *Acta Paediatr* 2003;92:1074–8.
46. Polberger S, Jirwe M, Svenningsen NW. Silastic central venous catheters for blood sampling and infusions in newborn infants. *Prenat Neonatal Med* 1998;3:340–5.
47. Ziegler EE, Thureen PJ, Carlson SJ. Aggressive nutrition of the very low birthweight infant. *Clin Perinatol* 2002;29:225–44.
48. Putet G. Lipid metabolism of the micropremie. *Clin Perinatol* 2000;27:57–69.
49. Michaelsen KF, Skafte L, Badsberg JH, Jørgensen M. Variation in macronutrients in human bank milk: Influencing factors and implications for human milk banking. *J Pediatr Gastroenterol Nutr* 1990;11:229–39.

50. Polberger S, Räihä NCR, Juvonen P, Moro GE, Minoli I, Warm A. Individualized protein fortification of human milk for preterm infants: Comparison of ultrafiltrated human milk protein and a bovine whey fortifier. *J Pediatr Gastroenterol Nutr* 1999;29: 332–8.
51. Moro GE, Minoli I, Ostrom M, *et al.* Fortification of human milk: Evaluation of a novel fortification scheme and of a new fortifier. *J Pediatr Gastroenterol Nutr* 1995;20:162–72.
52. Modi N. Management of fluid balance in the very immature neonate. *Arch Dis Child Fetal Neonatal Ed* 2004;89:F108–11.
53. Ågren J, Sjörs G, Sedin G. Transepidermal water loss in infants born at 24 and 25 weeks gestation. *Acta Paediatr* 1998;87: 1185–90.
54. Edwards WH, Conner JM, Soll RF, Vermont Oxford Network Neonatal Skin Care Study Group. The effect of prophylactic ointment therapy on nosocomial sepsis rates and skin integrity in infants with birth weights of 501 to 1000 g. *Pediatrics* 2004;113:1195–203.
55. Gruskay J, Costarino AT, Polin RA, Baumgart S. Nonoliguric hyperkalemia in the premature infant weighing less than 1000 grams. *J Pediatr* 1988;113:381–6.
56. Betremieux P, Hartnoll G, Modi N. Should frusemide be prescribed after packed cell transfusions in the newborn? *Eur J Pediatr* 1997;156:88–9.
57. Maisels MJ, Watchko JF. Treatment of jaundice in low birthweight infants. *Arch Dis Child Fetal Neonatal Ed* 2003;88: F459–63.
58. Collins MP, Lorenz JM, Jetton JR, Paneth N. Hypocapnia and other ventilation-related risk factors for cerebral palsy in low birth weight infants. *Pediatr Res* 2001;50:712–9.
59. Cole CH, Wright KW, Tarnow-Mordi W, Phelps DL. Resolving our uncertainty about oxygen therapy. *Pediatrics* 2003;112: 1415–9.
60. Greisen G, Hellström-Westas L, Lou H, Rosen I, Svenningsen NW. EEG depression and germinal layer haemorrhage in the newborn. *Acta Paediatr Scand* 1987;76:519–25.
61. Hellström-Westas L, Rosén I, Svenningsen NW. Cerebral function monitoring during the first week of life in extremely small low birthweight infants. *Neuropediatrics* 1991;22:27–32.
62. Hellström-Westas L, Klette H, Thorngren-Jerneck K, Rosén I. Early prediction of outcome with aEEG in premature infants with large IVH. *Neuropediatrics* 2001;32:319–24.
63. Olischar M, Klebermass K, Kuhle S, *et al.* Reference values for amplitude-integrated electroencephalographic activity in preterm infants younger than 30 weeks' gestational age. *Pediatrics* 2004; 113:e61–6.
64. Stoll BJ, Hansen N, Fanaroff AA, *et al.* Changes in pathogens causing early-onset sepsis in very-low-birth-weight infants. *N Engl J Med* 2002;347:240–7.
65. Edwards WH. Preventing nosocomial bloodstream infection in very low birth weight infants. *Semin Neonatol* 2002;7:325–33.
66. Clark R, Powers R, White R, Bloom B, Sanchez P, Benjamin DK Jr. Nosocomial infection in the NICU: A medical complication or unavoidable problem? *J Perinatol* 2004;24(Pt 1):382–8.
67. Clark R, Powers R, White R, Bloom B, Sanchez P, Benjamin DK Jr. Prevention and treatment of nosocomial sepsis in the NICU. *J Perinatol* 2004;24(Pt 2):446–53.
68. Benjamin DK Jr, Miller W, Garges H, *et al.* Bacteremia, central catheters, and neonates: When to pull the line. *Pediatrics* 2001;107:1272–6.
69. Nistala K, Nicholl R. Should preterm neonates with a central venous catheter and coagulase negative staphylococcal bacteraemia be treated without removal of the catheter? *Arch Dis Child* 2003;88:458–9.
70. Benjamin DK Jr, DeLong E, Cotton CM, Garges CM, Steinbach WJ, Clark RH. Mortality following blood culture in premature infants: Increased with Gram-negative bacteremia and candidemia, but not Gram-positive bacteremia. *J Perinatol* 2004;24:175–80.
71. Gonzalez A, Sosenko IR, Chandar J, Hummler H, Claure N, Bancalari E. Influence of infection on patent ductus arteriosus and chronic lung disease in premature infants weighing 1000 grams or less. *J Pediatr* 1996;128:470–8.
72. Liljedahl M, Bodin L, Schollin J. Coagulase-negative staphylococcal sepsis as a predictor of bronchopulmonary dysplasia. Acta Paediatr 2004;93:211–5.
73. Chapman RL. Candida infections in the neonate. *Curr Opin Pediatr* 2003;15:97–102.
74. Bendel CM. Colonization and epithelial adhesion in the pathogenesis of neonatal candidiasis. *Semin Perinatol* 2003; 27:357–64.
75. Rowen JL. Mucocutaneous candidiasis. *Semin Perinatol* 2003;27:406–13.
76. Campbell JR, Zaccaria E, Baker CJ. Systemic candidiasis in extremely low birth weight infants receiving topical petrolatum ointment for skin care: A case–control study. *Pediatrics* 2000;105:1041–5.
77. Sigmundsdóttir G, Christensson B, Björklund LJ, Håkansson K, Pehrson C, Larsson L. Urine D-arabinitol/L-arabinitol ratio in the diagnosis of invasive candidiasis in newborn infants. *J Clin Microbiol* 2000;38:3039–42.
78. Benjamin DK Jr, Garges H, Steinbach WJ. Candida bloodstream infection in neonates. *Semin Perinatol* 2003;27:375–83.
79. Bliss JM, Wellington M, Gigliotti F. Antifungal pharmacotherapy for neonatal candidiasis. *Semin Perinatol* 2003;27:365–74.
80. Hervas JA, Ballesteros F, Alomar A, Gil J, Benedi VJ, Alberti S. Increase of Enterobacter in neonatal sepsis: A twenty-two year study. *Pediatr Infect Dis J* 2001;20:134–40.
81. de Man P, Verhoeven BAN, Verbrugh HA, Vos MC, van den Anker JN. An antibiotic policy to prevent emergence of resistant bacilli. Lancet 2000;355:973–8.
82. v Dijk Y, Bik EM, Hochstenbach-Vernooij S, *et al.* Management of an outbreak of Enterobacter cloacae in a neonatal unit using simple preventive measures. *J Hosp Infect* 2002;51:21–6.
83. Calil R, Marba STM, von Nowakonski A, Tresoldi AT. Reduction in colonization and nosocomial infection by multiresistant bacteria in a neonatal unit after institution of educational measures and restriction in the use of cephalosporins. *Am J Infect Control* 2001;29:133–8.
84. McGuckin M, Waterman R, Storr J, *et al.* Evaluation of a patient-empowering hand hygiene programme in the UK. *J Hosp Infect* 2001;48:222–7.
85. Garland J, Alex C, Henrickson K, Maki D. A randomised pilot trial of a vancomycin–heparin lock solution (VHLS) for prevention of catheter-related bloodstrem infection (CRBSI) in neonates. *Pediatr Res* 2002;51:298A.
86. Kaufman D. Strategies for prevention of neonatal invasive candidiasis. *Semin Perinatol* 2003;27:414–24.
87. Stjernqvist K, Svenningsen NW. Ten-year follow-up of children born before 29 gestational weeks: Health, cognitive development, behaviour, and school achievement. *Acta Paediatr* 1999;88:557–62.
88. Marlow N. Neurocognitive outcome after very preterm birth. *Arch Dis Child Fetal Neonatal Ed* 2004;89:F224–8.
89. Anand KJ, Scalzo FM. Can adverse neonatal experiences alter brain development and subsequent behavior? *Biol Neonate* 2000;77:69–82.
90. Nagy Z, Westerberg H, Skare S, *et al.* Preterm children have disturbances of white matter at 11 years of age as shown by diffusion tensor imaging. *Pediatr Res* 2003;54:672–9.
91. Charpak N, Ruiz-Pelaez JG, Figueroa de CZ, Charpak Y. A randomized, controlled trial of kangaroo mother care: Results of follow-up at 1 year of corrected age. *Pediatrics* 2001;108:1072–9.
92. Feldman R, Eidelman AI, Sirota L, Weller A. Comparison of skin-to-skin (kangaroo) and traditional care: Parenting outcomes and preterm infant development. *Pediatrics* 2002;110:16–26.
93. Törnhage CJ, Stuge E, Lindberg T, Serenius F. First week kangaroo care in sick very preterm infants. *Acta Paediatr* 1999;88:1402–4.
94. Mann NP, Haddow R, Stokes L, Goodley S, Rutter N. Effect of night and day on preterm infants in a newborn nursery: Randomised trial. *Br Med J* 1986;293:1265–7.
95. Hellström-Westas L, Inghammar M, Isaksson K, Rosén I, Stjernqvist K. Short term effects of incubator covers on quiet sleep in stable preterm infants. *Acta Paediatr* 2001;90: 1004–8.
96. Als H, Lawhorn G, Duffy FH, McAnulty GB, Gibes-Grossman R, Blickman JG. Individualized developmental care for the very low birth-weight preterm infant. *J Am Med Assoc* 1994;272:853–8.
97. Westrup B, Kleberg A, Stjernqvist K, Lagercrantz H. A randomized controlled trial to evaluate the effects of NIDCAP in a Swedish setting. *Pediatrics* 2000;105:66–72.
98. Als H, Duffy FH, McAnulty GB, *et al.* Early experience alters brain function and structure. *Pediatrics* 2004;113:846–57.
99. Merskey H, Albe-Fessard DG, Bonica JJ, *et al.* Pain terms: A list with definitions and notes on usage. Recommended by the IASP Subcommittee on Taxonomy. *Pain* 1997;6:249.

100. Anand KJ, Craig KD. New perspectives on the definition of pain. *Pain* 1996;67:209–11.
101. Mrzljak L, Uylings HB, Kostovic I, Van Eden CG. Prenatal development of neurons in the human prefrontal cortex: I a qualitative Golgi study. *J Comp Neurol* 1988;271:355–86.
102. Klimach VJ, Cooke RWI. Maturation of the neonatal somatosensory evoked response in preterm infants. *Dev Med Child Neurol* 1988;30:208–14.
103. Fitzgerald M, Anand KJ. Developmental neuroanatomy and neurophysiology of pain. In Schechter NL, Berde CB, Yaster M, eds. *Pain in Infants, Children, and Adolescents.* Baltimore: Williams & Wilkins, 1993:11–31.
104. Andrews K, Fitzgerald M. Cutaneous flexion reflex in human neonates: A quantitative study of the threshold and stimulus–response characteristics after single and repeated stimuli. *Dev Med Child Neurol* 1999;41:696–703.
105. Barker DP, Rutter N. Exposure to invasive procedures in neonatal intensive care unit admissions. *Arch Dis Child Fetal Neonatal Ed* 1995;72: F47–8.
106. Holsti L, Grunau RE, Oberlander TF, Whitfield MF. Specific Newborn Individualized Developmental Care and Assessment Program movements are associated with acute pain in preterm infants in the neonatal intensive care unit. *Pediatrics* 2004; 114:65–72.
107. Wells JT, Ment LR. Prevention of intraventricular hemorrhage in preterm infants. *Early Hum Dev* 1995;42:209–33.
108. Schulz G, Keller E, Haensse D, Arlettaz R, Bucher HU, Fauchere JC. Slow blood sampling from an umbilical artery catheter prevents a decrease in cerebral oxygenation in the preterm newborn. *Pediatrics* 2003;111:e73–6.
109. Skov L, Ryding J, Pryds O, Greisen G. Changes in cerebral oxygenation and cerebral blood volume during endotracheal suctioning in ventilated neonates. *Acta Paediatr* 1992;81:389–93.
110. Skov L, Hellström-Westas L, Jacobsen T, Greisen G, Svenningsen NW. Acute changes in cerebral oxygenation and cerebral blood volume in preterm infants during surfactant treatment. *Neuropediatrics* 1992;23:126–30.
111. Stevens B, Johnston C, Petryshen P, Taddio A. Premature infant pain profile: Development and initial validation. *Clin J Pain* 1996;12:13–22.
112. Debillon T, Zupan V, Ravault N, Magny JF, Dehan M. Development and initial validation of the EDIN scale, a new tool for assessing prolonged pain in preterm infants. *Arch Dis Child Fetal Neonatal Ed* 2001;85:F36–41.
113. Anand KJ, Hall RW, Desai N, *et al.*, NEOPAIN Trial Investigators Group. Effects of morphine analgesia in ventilated preterm neonates: Primary outcomes from the NEOPAIN randomised trial. *Lancet* 2004;363:1673–82.
114. Meadow W, Reimshisel T, Lantos J. Birthweight-specific mortality for extremely-low-birthweight infants vanishes by four days of life: Epidemiology and ethics in the neonatal intensive care unit. *Pediatrics* 1996;97:636–46.
115. Whitelaw A. Death as an option in neonatal intensive care. *Lancet* 1986;2:328–31.
116. Doyal L. The moral foundation of the clinical duties of care: Needs, duties, and human rights. *Bioethics* 2001;15:520–35.
117. Goldschmidt JP, Ginsburg HG, McGettigan MC. Ethical decisions in the delivery room. *Clin Perinatol* 1996;23:529–50.
118. Tin W, Wariyar U, Hey E. Changing prognosis for babies of less than 28 weeks' gestation in the north of England between 1983 and 1994. Northern Neonatal Network. *Br Med J* 1997;314: 107–11.
119. Darlow BA, Cust AE. Australian and New Zealand Neonatal Network improved outcomes for very low birth weight infants: Evidence from New Zealand national population based data. *Arch Dis Child Fetal Neonatal Ed* 2003;88:F23–8.
120. Tommiska V, Heinonen K, Kero P, *et al.* A national 2 year follow up study of extremely low birth weight infants born in 1996–1997. *Arch Dis Child Fetal Neonatal Ed* 2003;88:F29–35.
121. Doyle LW, Victorian Infant Collaborative Study Group. Outcome at 5 years of age of children 23 to 27 weeks gestation, refining the prognosis. *Pediatrics* 2001;108:134–41.
122. Yu VYH, Doyle LW. Regionalized long-term follow-up. *Semin Neonatol* 2004;9:135–44.
123. Hille ET, den Ouden AL, Bauer L, van den Oudenrijn C, Brand R, Verloove-Vanhorick SP. School performance at nine years of age in very premature and very low birth weight infants: Perinatal risk factors and predictors at five years of age. Collaborative Project on Preterm and Small for Gestational Age (POPS) Infants in The Netherlands. *J Pediatr* 1994;125:426–34.
124. Saigal S, Hoult LA, Streiner DL, Stoskopf BL, Rosenbaum PL. School difficulties at adolescence in a regional cohort of children who were extremely low birth weight. *Pediatrics* 2000;105: 325–31.
125. Bylund B, Cervin T, Finnström O, *et al.* Very low birth weight children at 9 years: School performance and behavior in relation to risk factors. *Perinat Neonatal Med* 2000;5:124–33.
126. Monset-Couchard M, de Bethmann O, Relier J-P. Long term outcome of small versus appropriate size for gestational age co-twins/triplets. *Arch Dis Child Fetal Neonatal Ed* 2004; 89:F310–4.

7 Can we establish a universal lower limit of viability? What are the medical and ethical implications?

M. R. G. Carrapato

Introduction

Over the last few decades, perinatal mortality has been greatly reduced and in most Western countries now stands in single figures, albeit with many geographical asymmetries. The overall good results achieved are primarily the consequence of National Health Policies toward rationalization of human and financial resources with modern technology playing a subsidiary role in the high-risk pregnancy and neonate. The development of neonatal intensive care has been shown to be effective in the survival of preterm infants without a significant increase in later morbidity, at least for the larger, more mature neonates.

The World Health Organization places 22 weeks of gestational age or 500 g birth weight as the lower limit, at least for the purpose of perinatal statistics, and the International Classification of Diseases describes the perinatal period as starting at 22 completed weeks. The European Association of Perinatal Medicine (EAPM) defines the perinatal period as that which starts 'from 22 completed weeks (154 days) gestation and ends 7 complete days after birth',[1] which implies that the lower limit of viability stands at 22 weeks of gestation. The question, with all its medical, legal, social and financial implications, is how close are we, as a whole, in this pursuit?

Lower limit of viability – fact or not quite?

Biological survival will depend on not just the presence of a given organ but on its functional maturation, a sequential evolution often referred to as the 'developmental windows'. Alveolarization, essential for survival, is a process that includes anatomical, physiological and biochemical differentiation starting from about 24 weeks' gestation, progressing until term and continuing throughout the postnatal period and childhood. 'Viability', therefore, would be around 24 weeks. To lower this limit, strategies ranging from antenatal steroids, postnatal surfactant and different ventilatory modes have been attempted with some success, but as an example, after 30 years of clinical practice, antenatal steroids show quite disappointing results at below 24 weeks' gestation[2,3] and they might also delay and alter postnatal alveolarization.[4–6] Nevertheless, in recent years increased survival of very immature infants has been reported ranging, from 2% to 35% at 23 weeks and in some perinatal centers in the USA these figures approach 50% among live-born infants, between 17% and 58% at 24 weeks and vary from 35% to 85% at 25 weeks.[7–21]

Survival and outcome data on extremely preterm infants, between 22 and 26 weeks, has been widely reported and reviewed.[7,10–12,15–18,22,23] Allen *et al.*, in a retrospective study of infants born between 22 and 25 weeks, showed that mortality at 6 months' corrected age was 75% for neonates born at less than 24 weeks' gestation, with no survivors at 22 weeks while at 25 completed weeks, survival was in the region of 80%.[23] Hack and Fanaroff and Kilpatrick *et al.* showed similar survival rates of around 40% and 80%, respectively for 24 and 26 weeks' gestational age, especially after the introduction of steroids and surfactant.[12,15] Cooke has reported an increasing survival rate of extremely preterm infants from the early 1980s to the 1990s: in the early period, from 1982 to 1985, there were no survivors at 23 weeks' gestational age while in the later part of the study, between 1990 and 1993, 35% of these infants survived to discharge.[7]

Tin *et al.*, in a prospective, population-based regional survey, also showed that the survival of very immature infants has improved progressively since the early 1980s, particularly after the introduction of surfactant in clinical practice, although the impact of surfactant was only evident in those babies of 25 or more gestational weeks.[9] A national population-based study carried out in the UK and Ireland in the mid-1990s, of all infants born between 22 and 25 weeks of gestation, revealed two survivors to discharge at 22 weeks, with increasing survival rates from 11% at 23 weeks to 44% at 25 weeks.[17] However, in the last decade, survival among live births even at 22 weeks has been reported as being from 14% to 19%.[24–26] In a survey of 21 European countries registered with the EAPM, representing a wide spectrum of different regions from Scandanavia to southern, central and eastern European countries, the mortality rate for infants weighing between 500 and 749 g at birth stood at 54.4% but showed very wide variations within countries, approaching a 90% mortality rate in the less affluent countries as opposed to 26% in the more developed regions.[27] It is quite obvious from the findings of this survey that obstetric and neonatal practices, as well as available resources and facilities, play a major role in the survival of these very immature infants, but, both human and financial resources apart, why should there be such a discrepancy in reported survival rates at the threshold of viability?

There can be several reasons and explanations. First of all, many of the earlier studies referred to birth weight rather than to gestational age and therefore included more mature babies who were growth retarded [although babies of the same gestational age with intrauterine growth retardation (IUGR) usually have a poor prognosis].[22,28–31] Then, again, with some of the earlier reports referring to gestational age, how accurate was dating based on menstrual estimates in the absence of scanning in early pregnancy? Even in recent data, gestational age is often inferred from the first day of the last menstrual period with scanning only prevailing if it differs more than 2 weeks from the menstrual dates.[32–36] At this 'threshold for viability', a few days or a couple of hundred grams will make all the difference when reporting survival rates. On the other hand, many studies are regional/population based,[7,9,14,17,35,36] while others refer either to individual perinatal tertiary centers with very few numbers as a whole or to multicenter collaborative studies[13,15,23,33,34,37–41] with quite different outcomes. Some studies refer to the outcome of pregnancy from the beginning of labor, including still and live births; others include only live births, while others only survival rates for infants admitted to the neonatal intensive care units. This selection bias may overestimate survival rates by as much as 100% at 23 weeks and even up to 50% at 24 weeks.[42]

From our own experience involving 20 perinatal units, 70% of all pregnancies of less then 25 weeks gestational age at the onset of labour ended in fetal death, with no live births at 22 weeks. Amongst live births, at 23 weeks we report only the anedoctal case, but at 24/25 weeks there was, on average, an overall survival of 46% at discharge, albeit with some interunit variation (MOSAIC Study, Portuguese Northern Region, 2003: prospective study of pregnancies between 22 and less then 32 weeks gestation). Over an eight year period from 1996–2003, similar results are reported in Portugal for live births from unselected populational studies, with 8% survival at 23 weeks, 34.6% at 24 weeks and 49.3% at 25 weeks (Portuguese National VLBW Register). At 26 weeks both Portuguese Mosaic and the VLBW Register show figures in the order of 64–67% survival to discharge.

Also, in some perinatal centers, both obstetricians and neonatologists may invest aggressively at these lower gestational ages while in others, no active management will be contemplated because both the fetuses and the babies are considered non-viable or because of the very poor overall outcome in the event of survival.[43–48] Whether the mode of delivery at this very low gestational age will make any appreciable difference to survival is very debatable and cesarean section has not been proved to be better.[24,27,49–53] Indeed, the increasing morbidity for the mother and the future consequences of a vertical incision at this stage of pregnancy should perhaps preclude a cesarean in favor of a vaginal delivery, at least for fetal reasons. Further to all the aforementioned explanations for such discrepancies in survival reporting, other confounding data related to pregnancy will also influence survival, and therefore the outcome, namely, IUGR, pre-eclampsia, PPRM/oligohydramnios, antepartum hemorrhage, infection chorioamnionitis, etc.[15,24,49,54,55] Gender and ethnicity, especially, meet with conflicting results at these very low gestational ages.[56–60]

What is the outcome for the survivors?

Survival is not (and should not be) the only goal in perinatal medicine when attempting to establish a 'lower limit of viability'. Outcome and quality of life should, at the beginning of a new century, be a major priority. Although several follow-up studies on these very immature babies have shown that increasing survival has not been mirrored by an increase in cerebral palsy (CP), the fact is that a proportionally higher number of infants are now survivors of very low gestational age and birth weight. Furthermore, the major neuromotor, psychomotor, neurosensory and cognitive disfunctions are found especially in the most immature infants, below 25 gestational weeks.[10–14,17] Over a period of 12 years, between 1983 and 1984, in the north of England, although the survival rate at gestational age greater than 24 weeks had improved (while at gestational age below 24 weeks the overall survivor rate remained unchanged at 4%), the proportion of survivors with severe disability remained unaltered at around 25%, with 10% being so profoundly disabled as to have to live a completely dependent life.[9] From the results of the European survey, based either on regional or on national data, it was also shown that chronic lung disease ranged from 16.7% to 60% at 36 weeks' corrected age, retinopathy of prematurity (ROP) from 5.5% to 40%, intraventricular hemorrhage Grade III from 15% to 35%, necrotizing enterocolitis from 3% to 23% and nosocomial infection from 23% to 50%. All these complications were common to all countries and were directly related to either the degree of prematurity or the survival rate, being especially prevalent at 26 weeks' gestation or less. As expected, the picture was somewhat reversed, the countries with the better survival rates showing a higher incidence of sequelae, especially in visual impairment and chronic lung disease. At the time of the survey in 1998, almost everyone in Europe was using antenatal steroids, particularly between 26 and 32 weeks' gestation, and postnatal surfactant, either prophylactically or as a rescue. In those days there were no criteria for the use of postnatal steroids. Seven countries out of 21 would never use them while, of the remaining 14, 6 would apply them early – mostly systemically, with the remainder only contemplating their use late in the course of respiratory distress syndrome (RDS), if ventilatory dependent.[27] [These figures might be somewhat distorted and not reflect usual medical practice in Europe since some neonatal units were, at the time, enrolled in a controlled trial of postnatal steroid studies – an open study of early corticosteroid treatment (OSECT).]

On this basis, it could be argued that as recently as the last decade, these very immature infants were receiving quite different treatment across the globe – even from center to center within the same area. However, Vohr *et al.*, reporting on the long-term outcome of a collaborative study of babies on the threshold of viability in the 1990s in the USA, and Wood *et al.*, from a population-based cohort in the UK and Ireland, reporting on behalf of the EPICure study group, both showed that of the surviving children with birth weights less than 750 g or gestational ages below 25 weeks, between 30% and 50% had moderate or severe neuromotor or neurosensorial disabilities and very often had multiple handicaps.[17,61] In a review of the world literature, Hack and Fanaroff estimated that of the survivors of 23 weeks' gestation, over a third had a severe disability from CP to blindness and/or deafness with subnormal cognitive function. At 24 weeks' gestation, the range of severe disability was from 22% to 45% and at 25 weeks, from 12% to 35% and, in general, these rates overlapped those of children born before the 1990s.[62]

It is quite plausible that some of the adverse outcomes in survivors at these low gestational ages may not be just the direct effect of prematurity and/or low-birth weight *per se* but also the result of the hostile intrauterine milieu leading to preterm delivery from inflammatory mediators, to IUGR, hypoxic-ischemic insults, metabolic imbalances, etc. These would perhaps explain the somewhat better, and paradoxical, reported outcome of multiple pregnancies at these very low gestational ages in contrast to the general outcome of multiples at the later stages of pregnancy, presumably because the reasons for preterm delivery would rest with multiplicity alone, in the absence of the adverse factors for singletons' preterm deliveries.[60]

Postnatal events, from nosocomial infection to anemia and hemodynamic instability, metabolic derangements of hyper/hypoglycemia and electrolytic disturbances, etc. may also play an adjuvant role in the overall picture of survival with multiple handicaps. But one area in particular should call for special caution: the possible role of iacterogenically induced disability. Many of these tiny babies are, from the very beginning, often subjected to a whole panoply of maneuvers and medications known to alter hemodynamics, blood flow and perfusion, from xantines to NSAIDs, namely, indometacin, diuretics, volume expanders, antimicrobials with known toxic side effects, paralyzing agents and sedatives, etc. In recent years, two 'old' tools in perinatal care have been submitted to re-evaluation and reappraisal, with growing concern as to their use and misuse.

Antenatal corticosteroids (ANC) have been shown to be associated with a significant reduction of RDS, neonatal death and intra/periventricular hemorrhage[63–65] with a possible synergistic effect with postnatal surfactant therapy.[66] A single course of ANC results in benefits without significant adverse effects, with long-term follow-up studies up to adulthood showing no adverse neurological or cognitive outcome.[67] Betamethasone has shown a reduced risk of cystic periventricular leukomalacia, and therefore has become the recommended steroid for enhanced lung maturation.[68] The available evidence of ANC in multiple pregnancies is somewhat conflicting regarding both use and outcome,[69] while its use in diabetic pregnancies is also controversial for the reduction of RDS, as the adverse steroid-induced hyperglycemia on fetal lung maturation may offset any beneficial effects.[70]

From animal data and observational human studies, there is increasing concern that repeated courses of ANC may lead to immediate and long-term harmful effects on growth, delay in lung and brain development,[71–76] and at present, only a single course is advocated with subsequent courses reserved for randomized control trials.[77] How much the widespread use of repeated courses of steroids in the 1990s may be playing a subsidiary role in the adverse outcome of some of these tiny survivors, in addition to prematurity and low-birth weight, remains an open question.

Postnatal steroids have been shown to promote early extubation in ventilatory-dependent extremely low-birth-weight infants but randomized control studies failed to demonstrate any significant reduction in death rates or in the development of chronic lung disease.[78,79] Furthermore, in addition to the immediate effects of hyperglycemia, hypertension, gastrointestinal tract bleeding and perfuration, there is growing concern that postnatal steroids may also be responsible for adverse outcome on growth, CP and neurosensory impairment.[79–86] For these reasons, at the present time, postnatal steroids should only be considered for the extubation of ventilatory-dependent babies and only upon informed consent of the parents.

More than 60 years after the initial report of retinal blindness in preterm babies subjected to excess O_2 supplementation, a high proportion of these tiny babies still survive these days with more or less severe ROP. The 'optimal' level (and 'correct' monitoring) for O_2 supplementation remains as yet unknown. A few years ago an observational study of the case notes of surviving infants delivered before 28 weeks' gestation showed a significant decrease of ROP (6% vs. 27.2%) if they were maintained at SaO_2 levels between 70% and 90%. Furthermore, it was also shown that there was much less time on ventilation, less oxygen dependency at 36 weeks' corrected age, a better weight gain and, especially, no increase in mortality or CP.[87] Not surprisingly, this publication caused considerable polemic[88–93] and ongoing debate.[94–98] Understandably, SaO_2 monitoring has become common practice in most neonatal intensive care units with considerable benefit, i.e. comfort, over repeated arterial punctures and complications from invasive procedures. However, there is very little correlation between PaO_2 and SaO_2 levels, both below 84% and above 94% for SaO_2 to keep an ideal PaO_2 level between 50 and 70 mmHg.[99] Also, SaO_2 monitoring is dependent on the methodology used[100,101] and other variables will have to be considered, namely, hemoglobin levels and associated medications that may interfere with cerebral and retinal blood flow and perfusion and not just SaO_2/PaO_2 levels. Nevertheless, ROP is a significant handicap, especially at the lower limit of viability, and caution should be used in reappraising the 'physiological' saturations inferred from the more mature infants and extrapolated to these extremely preterm babies, especially in the first few days of life.

Over and above the immediate and short-term sequelae, how do these tiny survivors perform at a later stage? The available long-term evidence – school age and above – generally shows that besides neuromotor and neurosensorial impairments, a high proportion of these children reveal significant learning difficulties and behavioral and educational problems, only adding further to the burden and placing an enormous responsibility on society as a whole, particularly for the allocation of financial and human resources to provide the necessary collateral help.[102–108] Furthermore, these children will grow to adulthood into a competitive world of 'perfection'. How sensitive are we to handle their multitude of needs and how prepared are we to integrate them into society with fairness and equity?

What are the ethical implications?

Ethics, the study of ideal conduct, classed as a branch of philosophy,[109] should be above cultural barriers, be universal and center upon respect for mankind: easily said, often not practiced. Deontology, the science of duty, the branch of knowledge that deals with moral obligations,[110] the science of professional duties and etiquette,[111] is often referred to as being synonymous with ethics. Laws vary from country to country and sometimes between states within the same country.

It would thus appear to be quite unrealistic to argue the attainability of a common denominator derived from such widespread philosophical, religious and moral views, to frame it within the various legal requirements, to dictate the codes of rules and to expect it to be internationally accepted, yet that is the essence of ethics.

In perinatal medicine, the overall ethical principles of autonomy, beneficence and non-maleficence are even more difficult to apply than in most branches of medicine due to the often conflicting interests of the mother (and partner) and the fetus. The fetus, regardless of its semantic definitions, its rights, its independent moral status and so forth[112,113] is an entity representing human life. The question is, of course, when does human life begin from the biological, moral, religious, legal and social perspectives? Perhaps the concept of 'a fetus as a patient, if not a person', might be the pragmatic answer, at least, for the immediate implications of medical and ethical decisions.[114,115] For similar reasons we approach the subject of neonatal ethics from a practicing angle, focusing on medical management and decisions at the threshold of viability. Far from guidelines, these thoughts, hopefully unbiased, express our concern and independent views on the complexities of universal medical ethics.

Reports in the past 10 years of survival at 22 weeks' gestation[24–26] and less than 400 g birth weight[116] have led to a change in legislation[117] and to a redefinition of the perinatal period,[1] and the aim for the survival of the most immature of babies became only natural and pressing. Accepting the (theoretical) concept of 22 weeks' gestation as the lower limit of viability, what then is the evidence to support this claim and what is the outcome? The answer to the first question is the proverbial case that confirms the exception, and as for the quality of survival, none of the reported survivors was free from neurological sequelae.[24–26,117,118]

And what about at 23 weeks (or 23 weeks and a couple of days)? From here on it is an open game and the stakes are high, with survival rates from 2% to 35% at 23 weeks to 35% to 85% at 25 weeks.[7,10–14] It is quite clear that there are enormous geographical asymmetries even within countries with similar demographies, and it is thus not surprising that some countries will place their lower limit of viability at 24–25 weeks' gestation.[27]

The ethical questions for practicing neonatologists are whether they should accept their own reality of survival and try to improve on quality rather than quantity, or whether they should try to compete with the more advanced countries and aim for the threshold of viability? Who should decide on that? Should it be an individual (local) decision or a matter of national (regional) policy? What are the ethics and moral implications of these decisions? Could it possibly be that in practice new technologies would change matters? What would be the financial resources needed, could they be afforded and, again, what would be the ethical implications of discrimination on financial grounds?

Of the general ethical principles of autonomy, beneficence and non-maleficence, the first does not apply to the neonate for obvious reasons. However, as a person with independent moral status, the newborn is entitled to the full demands and obligations of beneficence and of *primum non nocere*. In everyday practice the concept of 'in the best interest of the patient' has also gained access to neonatal medicine in order to surmount the subtleties of definition from 'sustained life' to 'quality of life'.[119–121] However, this begs the question, in the best interests of whom – the baby, the parents, or society, and who should decide? Handicap is a notion often defined by healthy, normal people, which may or may not be shared by the affected individuals themselves. Perhaps it is a question of degree: what is more acceptable, the survival of a severely physically handicapped but intellectually sound child or, on the contrary, an individual who is completely mentally dependent but who has no physical impairment? And who will be the judge? With the present low birth rate in most Western societies, 'perfection' is understandably always the goal. However, is it not also a sign of moral perfection when a society is prepared to accept the difference, showing compassion and solidarity with its less fortunate members? On one issue at least, everyone would agree that whatever the dilemmas and however difficult, decisions must never be taken upon account of sex, eugenics, religious or economic prejudice, and never based on a doctor's own cultural or religious beliefs.[122,123]

'Futile treatment' is currently used in medicine to mean that any treatment beyond a certain point would be unjustifiable. Neonatologists, often young, are frequently faced in the middle of the night with the crucial decision (based very often upon inaccurate information on gestational age) of whether or not to initiate active, aggressive management of the extremely immature infant at the threshold of viability.

When in doubt, active resuscitative measures should be started in the labor ward.[122] The decision to further continue intensive care can always be reversed after revaluation and counseling to the parents, but this does not imply that decisions to continue or withdraw treatment should rest upon them. Decisions to withdraw or withhold treatment should always be the responsibility of the most senior physician, after discussion with all the staff, including the nurses, and upon informing the parents. The 'phantom of the law' is often used as an argument for the continuation of futile intensive care. In fact, in most places what is unlawful is the preservation of life at all costs, against the dignity of the human being. As for the ethics of treatment withdrawal, once again, what is morally wrong is to prolong useless and hopeless treatments, contradicting the Hippocratic rules of 'not to harm, if possible to cure, but always to relieve and console'. Yet, the same European survey revealed that a considerable number of countries had no policies or consensus for DNR/withdrawal of life support therapies (67% and 48%, respectively).[27] Advancing technologies can often cause procrastination over medical decisions, which, when based on a particularly sophisticated tool, may be mistaken for good medical practice. Neuroimaging is often quoted in this context: but how reliable and infallible is neuroimaging in the prediction of function? It might assist but does not replace clinical judgment of when to withdraw or withhold life-supporting therapies – that would be quite unethical and unacceptable.

Most importantly, once the medical decision has been reached to withdraw advanced life-support treatment, the baby should be allowed to die in privacy, with dignity, surrounded by the warmth, care and love of his parents with the full support of the medical and nursing staff. Fortunately, in most cases, parents accept medical judgments based on sound clinical evidence, knowledge and good faith and are almost always relieved that the decision has been taken out of their hands. Occasionally, medical decisions to withdraw or withhold treatment do not meet with the parents' agreement or approval because of their particular philosophical, cultural or religious beliefs. Frustrating as this may be, professionals must understand and accept these feelings and must continue medical treatment until such time as further counseling may reverse the parents' decision. In the last resort, if consensual agreement cannot be reached in the best interest of human dignity for the baby, the question of treatment withdrawal may be addressed to the courts.[122]

Can a universal lower limit of viability be established?

It is quite obvious from the world literature and from individual realities that a threshold exists for each and everyone, whatever it might be. However commendable the pursuit and quest to emulate the best results, for the meantime, individual thresholds must be recognized. It is within this reality that decisions can be made when faced with the extremely preterm infant, and that an educated prognosis can be discussed with parents. Improvements can then be pursued based on continuous self-auditing, in strict adherence to the moral conduct of good medical practice toward the most vulnerable of all patients, the sick and extremely preterm infant.

Acknowledgments

Grateful thanks are due to the collaborators from the participating European countries for their invaluable assistance: Belgium, P. van Reempts; Croatia, J. Polak-Babic; Cyprus, Hadjidemetriou; Czech Republic, P. Zoban; England, N. Marlow; Estonia, H. Varrendi; Finland, A. L. Jarvenpaa; The Netherlands, W. E. Fetter, L. Kollee; Hungary, P. Temesvari; Iceland, A. Dagbjartsson; Italy, G. Bevilacqua; N. Ireland, H. Halliday; Norway, A. Meberg; Poland, J. Gadzinowski; Portugal, J. C. Peixoto; Serbia, K. Mulutina; Slovenia, M. Pajntar; Spain, E. Domenech; Sweden, G. Sedin; Switzerland, A. Moessinger; Turkey, G. Can, and also to my departmental colleagues Catarina Prior and Susana Tavares for their help with perusal of the literature.

REFERENCES

1. Dunn PM, McIlwaine G, eds. *Perinatal Audit.* A report produced for the European Association of Perinatal Medicine. London: The Parthenon Publishing Group, 1996:39.
2. Chapman SJ, Hauth JC, Bottoms SF, *et al.* Benefits of maternal corticosteroid therapy in infants weighing less or equal to 1000 gs at birth after preterm rupture of the amnion. *MJ Obstets Gynecol* 1999;180:677–82.
3. Elimian A, Verma U, Canterino J, Shah J, Visintainer P, Tejani N. Effectiveness of antenatal steroids in obstetric sub groups. *Obstet Gynecol* 1999;93:174–9.
4. Massaro D. Postnatal development of alveoli. Regulation and evidence for a critical period in rats. *J Clin Invest* 1985;76: 1294–9.
5. Stewart JD, Sienko AE, Gonzalez CL, Christensen HD, Rayburn WF. Placebo-controlled comparison between a single dose and a multidose of betamethasone in accelerating lung maturation of mice offspring. *Am J Obstet Gynecol* 1998;179:1241–7.
6. Ikegami M, Gobe AH, Newnham J, Polk DH, Willet KE, Sly P. Repetitive prenatal glucocorticoids improve lung function and increase growth in preterm lambs. *Am J Respir Crit Care Med* 1987;156:178–84.
7. Cooke RWI. Improved outcome for infants at the limits of viability. *Eur J Pediatr* 1996;155:665–7.
8. Synnes AR, Ling EW, Whitfield MF, *et al.* Perinatal outcomes of a large cohort of extremely low gestational age infants (twenty-three to twenty-eight completed weeks of gestation). *J Pediatr* 1994;125(6, Pt 1):952–960.
9. Tin W, Wariyar U, Hey E. Changing prognosis for babies of less than 28 weeks gestation in the north of England between 1983 and 1994. *Br Med J* 1997;314(7074):107–11.
10. Emsley HC, Wardle SP, Sims DG, Chiswick ML, D'Souza SW. Increased survival and deteriorating developmental outcome in 23–25 week-old gestation infants 1990–4 compared with 1984–9. *Arch Dis Child Fetal Neonatal* 1998;78(2):F99–104.
11. Hack M, Friedman H, Fanaroff AA. Outcomes of extremely low birthweight infants. *Pediatrics* 1996;98(5):931–7.
12. Hack M, Fanaroff AA. Outcome of children of extremely low birthweight and gestational age in the 1990s. *Early Hum Dev* 1999;53(3):193–218.
13. Lefebvre F, Glorieux J, St-Laurent-Gagnon T. Neonatal survival and disability rate at age 18 months for infants born between 23 and 28 weeks of gestation. *Am J Obstet Gynecol* 1996;174(3):833–8.
14. Finnström O, Otterblad OP, Sedin G, *et al.* Neurosensory outcome and growth at three years in extremely low birthweight infants: Follow up results from the Swedish national prospective study. *Acta Paediatr* 1998;87(10):1055–60.
15. Kilpatrick SJ, Schlueter MA, Piecuch R, Leonard CH, Rogido M, Sola A. Outcome of infants born at 24–26 weeks gestation: I survival and cost. *Obstet Gynecol* 1997;90(5):803–8.
16. Lorenz JM. Survival of extremely preterm infants in North America in the 1990s. *Clin Perinatol* 2000;27:255–62.
17. Wood NS, Marlow N, Costeloe K, Gibson AF, Wilkinson AR. Neurologic and developmental disability after extremely preterm birth. EPICure Study Group. *New Engl J Med* 2000;343:378–84.
18. Batton DJ, DeWitte DB, Espinosa R, *et al.* The impact of fetal compromise on outcome at the border of viability. *Am J Obstet Gynecol* 1998;178:909–15.
19. Bahado-Singh RO, Dash J, Deren O. Prenatal prediction of neonatal outcome in the extremely low birthweight infant. *Am J Obstet Gynecol* 1998;178:900–15.
20. El-Metwally D, Vohr B, Tucker R. Survival and neonatal morbidity at the limits of viability in 1990s; 22–25 weeks. *J Pediatr* 2000;137:616–22.
21. McElrath TF, Robinson JN, Ecker JF. Outcome of infants born at 23 weeks gestation. *Obstet Gynecol* 2001;97:49–52.
22. Stevenson DK, Wright LL, Lemons JA, *et al.* Very low birthweight outcomes of the National Institute of Child Health and Human Development Neonatal Research Network, January 1993 through December 1994. *Am J Obstet Gynecol* 1998;179: 1632–9.
23. Allen MC, Donohue PK, Dusman AE. The limit of viability – Neonatal outcome of infants born at 22–25 weeks' gestation. *N Engl J Med* 1993;329(22):1597–601.
24. Bottoms SF, Paul RH, Iams JD. Obstetric determinants of neonatal survival: Influence of willingness to perform cesarean delivery on survival of extremely low birthweight infants. *Am J Obstet Gynecol* 1997;176:960–6.
25. Lemons JA, Bauer CR, Oh W. Very low birthweight outcomes of the National Institute of Child Health and Human Development Neonatal Research Networks, January 1995 through December 1996. *Pediatrics* 2000;107:E1.
26. Chan K, Ohlsson A, Synnes A, Lee DS, Chien LY, Lee SK. Canadian Neonatal Network. Survival, morbidity and resource of infants of 25 weeks' gestational age or less. *Am J Obstet Gynecol* 2001;185:220–6.
27. Carrapato MRG, Costa R. The lower limit of viability in Europe. *Proceedings III International Conference on Perinatal Medicine of Romanian Association of Perinatal Medicine*, 1999:33–39.
28. Reiss I, Landmann E, Heckman M, Misselwitz B, Gortner L. Increased risk of bronchopulmonary displasia and increased mortality in very preterm infants being small for gestational age. *Arch Gynecol Obstet* 2003;269:40–4.
29. Bardin C, Zelkowitz P, Papageorgiou A. Outcome of small for gestational age and appropriate for gestational age infants born before 27 weeks gestation. *Pediatrics* 1997;100(2):E4.
30. Cooke RWI. Factors affecting survival and development in extremely tiny babies. *Semin Neonatol* 1996;1:267–76.
31. Spinillo A, Capuzzo E, Piazzi G, Baltaro F, Stronati M, Ometto A. Significance of low birthweight for gestational age among very preterm infants. *Br J Obstet Gynecol* 1997;104:668–73.
32. MacDonald H, Committee of Fetus and Newborn. American Academy of Pediatrics. Clinical report. *Pediatrics* 2002;110: 1024–7.
33. Horbar JD, for the investigators of the Vermont Oxford Trials Network Database Project. The Vermont Oxford Trials Network. Very low birthweight outcomes for 1990. *Pediatrics* 1993; 91:540–5.
34. O'Shea TM, Klinepeter KL, Goldstein DJ, Jackson BW, Dillard RG. Survival and development disability in infants with birthweight of 501–800 grams, born between 1979 and 1994. *Pediatrics* 1997;100:982–6.
35. Bohin S, Draper ES, Field DJ. Impact of extremely immature infants on neonatal services. *Arch Dis Child* 1996;74F: 110–3.

36. Cartlidge PHT, Stewart JH. Survival of very low birthweight and very preterm infants in a geographically defined population. *Acta Paediatr* 1997;86:105–10.
37. Robertson C, Sauve RS, Christianson HE. Province-based study of neurologic disability amongst survivors weighing 500 through 1249 grams at birth. *Pediatrics* 1994;93:636–40.
38. Casiro O, Bingham W, MacMurray B, Whitefield M, Saigal S, Vincer M, Long W. One-year follow-up of 89 infants with birthweights of 500–749 grams and respiratory distress syndrome randomised to two rescue doses of synthetic surfactant or air placebo. *J Pediatr* 1995;26:853–60.
39. Ferrara TB, Hoekstra RE, Couser RJ. Survival and follow-up of infants born at 23–26 weeks of gestational age: Effects of surfactant therapy. *J Pediatr* 1994;124:119–24.
40. Piecuch RE, Leonard CH, Cooper BA, Kilpatrick SJ, Schlueter MA, Sola A. Outcome of infants born at 24–26 weeks gestation. II Neurodevelopmental outcome. *Obstet Gynecol* 1997;90: 809–14.
41. Nishida H. Perinatal health care in Japan. *J Perinatol* 1997;17:70–4.
42. Evans DJ, Levene MI. Evidence of selection bias in preterm survival studies: A systematic review. *Arch Dis Child Fetal Neonatal Ed* 2001;84:F79–84.
43. Oei J, Askie LM, Tobienski R, Lui K. Attitudes of neonatal clinicians towards resuscitation of the extremely premature infant: An exploratory survey. *J Paediatr Child Health* 2000;36:357–62.
44. Munro M, Yu VY, Partridge JC, Martinez AM. Antenatal counselling, resuscitation practices and attitudes among Australian neonatologists towards life support in extreme prematurity. *Aust NZ Obstet Gynecol* 2001;41:275–80.
45. Campbell D, Fleischman AR. Limits of viability: Dilemmas, decisions and decision-makers. *Am J Perinatol* 2001;18:117–28.
46. Molholm HB, Greisen G. Preterm delivery and calculation of survival rate below 28 weeks of gestation. *Acta Paediatr* 2003;92:1335–8.
47. Rhoden NK. Treating baby Doe: The ethics of uncertainty. *Hastings Cent Rep* 1986;16:34–42.
48. Lorenz JM, Paneth N, Getton JR. Comparison of management strategies for extreme prematurity in the USA and Netherlands: Outcomes and resource expenditure. *Pediatrics* 2001;108: 1269–74.
49. Hagen R, Benninger H, Cliffings D, Evans S, French N. Very preterm birth – A regional study. Part I: Maternal and obstetric factors. *Brit J Obstet Gynecol* 1996;103:230–8.
50. Amon E, Steigerwald J, Winn H. Obstetric factors associated with survival of the borderline viable liveborn infant (500–750 gm) (abstract). *Am J Obstet Gynecol* 1995;418.
51. Jones HA, Lumley JM. The effects of the mode of delivery on neonatal mortality in very low birthweight infants born in Victoria, Australia: Cesarean section is associated with increased survival in breech-presenting, but not vertex-presenting infants. *Paediatr Perinat Epidemiol* 1997;1:181–99.
52. Grant A, Penn ZJ, Steer PJ. Elective or selective caesarean delivery of the small baby? A systematic review of the control trials. *Brit J Obstet Gynecol* 1996;103:1197–200.
53. Bauer J, Hentschel R, Zahradnik H, Karch U, Linderkamp O. Vaginal delivery and neonatal outcome in extremely-low-birth-weight-infants below 26 weeks of gestational age. *Am J Perinatol* 2003;20:181–8.
54. Gascon G, Skoll A, Lefevbre F, Glorieu G. The influence of maternal factors on the outcome at 18 months of babies born at 23 to 28 weeks gestation. *Am J Obstet Gynecol* 1995;172:418.
55. Iannuci TA, Tomich PG, Gianopoulos JG. Etiology and outcome of extremely low birthweight infants. *Am J Obstet Gynecol* 1996;174:1896–902.
56. Verloove-Vanhorick P, Veen S, Ens-dochum MH, Schrender AM, Brand R, Ruyz JH. Sex difference in disability and handicap at 5 years of age in children born at very short gestation. *Pediatrics* 1994;93:576–9.
57. Alexander GR, Kogan M, Bader G, Carlo W, Allen M, Mor J. US birthweight/gestational age – Specific neonatal mortality: 1995–1997 rates for whites, hispanics and blacks. *Pediatrics* 2003;111:61–6.
58. Allen MC, Alexander GR, Tompkins ME, Hulsey TC. Racial differences in temporal changes in newborn viability and survival by gestational age. *Paediatr Perinat Epidemiol* 2000;14:152.
59. Petrova A, Mehta R, Anwar M, Hiatt M, Hegyi T. Impact of race and ethnicity on the outcome of preterm infants below 32 weeks' gestation. *J Perinatol* 2003;23:404–8.
60. Draper ES, Manktelow B, Field DJ, James D. Prediction of survival for preterm births by weight and gestation age: Retrospective population based study. *Br Med J* 1999;319: 1093–7.
61. Vohr BR, Wright LL, Dusick AM. Neuro development and functional outcomes of extremly low birthweight infants in the National Institute of Health and Human Development Neonatal Research Network 1993–1994. *Pediatrics* 2000;105:1216–26.
62. Hack M, Fanaroff AA. Outcomes of children of extremely low birthweight and gestational age in the 1990s. *Semin Neonatal* 2000;5:89–106.
63. Wright LL, Harbar JD, Gunkel H, *et al.* Evidence from multicentre networks on the current use and effectiveness of antenatal corticosteroids in low birthweight infants. *Am J Obstet Gynecol* 1995;173:263–9.
64. National Institute of Health. Effect of corticosteroids for fetal maturation on perinatal outcomes. NIH Consensus Statement. *Natl Inst Health* 1994;12:1–24.
65. Crowley P. Prophylactic corticosteroids for preterm birth. *Cochrane Database Syst Ref* 2002;4:CD000065.
66. Jobe AH, Mitchell BR, Gunkel JH. Beneficial effects of the combined use of prenatal corticosteroids and postnatal surfactant in preterm infants. *Am J Obstet Gynecol* 1993;168:508–13.
67. Vermillion ST, Soper DE, Chasedunn-Roark J. Neonatal sepsis after betamethazone administration to patients with preterm premature rupture of membranes. *Am J Obstet Gynecol* 1999; 181:320–7.
68. Baud O, Foix-L'Hellas L, Kaminski M, Audibert F, Jarreau PH, Papiernik E. Antenatal glucocorticoid treatment and cystic periventricular leucomalacia in very premature infants. *N Engl J Med* 1999;34:1190–6.
69. Hashimoto LN, Hornung RW, Linsell CJ, Brewer DE, Donovan EF. Effects of antenatal glucocorticoid on outcome of very low birthweight multifetal gestations. *Am J Obstet Gynecol* 2002; 187:804–10.
70. Carlson KS, Smith BT, Post M. Insulin acts on the fibroblast to inhibit glucocorticoid stimulation of lung maturation. *J Appl Physiol* 1984;57:1577–9.
71. Walfisch A, Hallak M, Mazor M. Multiple courses of antenatal steroids: Risks and benefits. *Obstet Gynecol* 2001;98:491–7.
72. Kay HH, Bird IM, Coe CL, Dudley DJ. Antenatal steroids treatment and adverse fetal effects: What is the evidence? *J Soc Gynecol Investig* 2000;7:269–78.
73. Goldenberg RI, Wright LL. Repeated courses of antenatal corticosteroids. *Obstet Gynecol* 2001;97:316–7.
74. Newnham JP. Is prenatal glucocorticoid administration another origin of adult disease. *Clin Exp Pharmacol Physiol* 2001;28: 957–61.
75. Vermillion ST, Soper DE, Newman RB. Neonatal sepsis and death after multiple courses of antenatal betamethasone therapy *Am J Obstet Gynecol* 2000;183:810–4.
76. Aghajfari E, Murphy K, Matthews S, Ohlsson A, Amankwah K, Hannah M. Repeated doses of antenatal corticosteroids in animals: A systematic review *Am J Obstet Gynecol* 2002;186: 843–9.
77. National Institutes of Health Consensus Development Panel. Antenatal corticosteroids revisited: Repeat courses. National Institutes of Health Consensus Development Conference Statement, August 17–18, 2000. *Obstet Gynecol* 2001;98:144–50.
78. Halliday HL, Patterson CC, Halahakoon CW, on behalf of the European Multicentre Steroid Study Group. A multicentre, randomised, open study of early corticosteroid treatment (OSECT) in preterm infants with respiratory illness: Comparison of early and late treatment and of dexamethasone and inhaled budesonide. *Pediatrics* 2001;107:232–40.
79. Vermont Oxford Network Steroid Study Group. Early postnatal dexamethasone therapy for the prevention of chronic lung disease. *Pediatrics* 2001;108:741–8.
80. Nicholl RM, Greenough A, King M, Cheeseman P, Gamsu HR. Growth effects of systemic versus inhaled steroids in chronic lung disease. *Arch Dis Child Fetal Neonatal Ed* 2002;87: F59–61.
81. Stark AR, Carlo WA, Tyson JE, *et al.* National Institute of Child Health and Human Development Neonatal Research Network. Adverse effects of early dexamethasone in extremely-low-birth-weight infants. *N Engl J Med* 2001;344:95–101.
82. French NP, Hagan R, Evans SF, Godfrey M, Newham JP. Size at birth and subsequent developments. *Am J Obstet Gynecol* 1999;180:114–21.

83. Yeh TF, Lin YJ, Lin CH, *et al.* Early postnatal (> 12 hr) dexamethasone (D) therapy for prevention of BPD in preterm infants with RDS – A two-year follow-up study. *Pediatrics* 1998;101(5):http://www.pediatrics.org/cgi/content /full/105/5/e7.
84. Oshea TM, Kothadia JM, Klinepeter KL, *et al.* Randomised placebo-controlled trial in very low birthweight infants to reduce the duration of ventilation dependency: Outcome of study participants at one year adjusted age. *Pediatrics* 1999;104:15–21.
85. Shinwell ES, Karplus M, Reich D, *et al.* Early postnatal dexamethasone treatment and increased incidence of cerebral palsy. *Arch Dis Child Fetal Neonatal Ed* 2000;83:F177–81.
86. The Royal Women's Hospital, The Mercy Hospital for Women, Monash Medical Centre, The Royal Children's Hospital, The Newborn Emergency Transport Service, The Victorian Perinatal Data Collection Unit, Melbourne, Australia. Postnatal corticosteroids and sensorial neural outcome at 5 years of age. *J Paediatr Child Health* 2000;36:256–61.
87. Tin W, Milligan DWA, Pennfather P, Hey E. Pulse oximetry, severe retinopathy, and outcome at one year in babies of less than 28 weeks' gestation. *Arch Dis Child Fetal Neonatal Ed* 2001;F106–10.
88. Primhak R. Oxygen saturation and retinopathy of prematurity (letter to the editor). *Arch Dis Child Fetal Neonatal Ed* 2001;85:F75–8.
89. Tin W, Milligan DWA, Pennfather P. Oxygen saturation and retinopathy of prematurity (authors' response). *Arch Dis Child Fetal Neonatal Ed* 2001;85:F75–8.
90. Roberton NRC. Two sacred cows of neonatal intensive care (letter to the editor). *Arch Dis Child Fetal Neonatal Ed* 2001;85: F75–78.
91. Hey E. Two sacred cows of neonatal intensive care. (authors' response). *Arch Dis Child Fetal Neonatal Ed* 2001;85:F75–78.
92. McIntosh N. High or low oxygen saturation for the preterm baby. *Arch Dis Child Fetal Neonatal Ed* 2001;84:F149–50.
93. Marlow N. High or low oxygen saturation for the preterm baby. *Arch Dis Child Fetal Neonatal Ed* 2001;84:F149–50.
94. Tin W, Walker S, Lacamp C. Oxygen monitoring in preterm babies: Too high, too low? *Paediatr Respir Rev* 2003;4:9–14.
95. Sinha SK, Tin W. The controversies surrounding oxygen therapy in neonatal intensive care units. *Curr Opin Pediatr* 2003;15: 161–5.
96. Tin W, Wariyar U. Giving small babies oxygen: 50 years of uncertainty. *Semin Neonatol* 2002;7:361–7.
97. Tin W. Optimal oxygen saturation for preterm babies. Do we really know? *Biol Neonate* 2004;85:319–25.
98. Tin W. Oxygen therapy: 50 years of uncertainty. *Pediatrics* 2002;110:615.
99. Wasunna A, Whitelaw AGI. Pulse oximetry in preterm infants. *Arch Dis Child* 1987;62:957–61.
100. Gibson LY. Pulse oximeter in the neonate intensive care unit: A co-relational analysis. *Pediatr Nurs* 1996;21:511–5.
101. Grieve SH, McIntosh N, Laing IA. Comparison of two different pulse oximeters in monitoring preterm infants. *Crit Care Med* 1997;25:2051–4.
102. Nadeau L, Boivin M, Tessier R, Lefebvre F, Robey P. Mediators of behavioural problems in 7-year-old children born after 24–28 weeks of gestation. *J Dev Behav Pediatr* 2001;22:1–10.
103. Anderson P, Doyle LW. Victorian Infant Collaborative Study Group. Neural behavioural outcomes of school-age children born extremely low birthweight or very preterm in the 1990s. *J Am Med Assoc* 2003;289:3264–72.
104. Harding L, Walker LG, Lloyd D, Duffty P. A controlled study of children born at gestation 28 weeks or less: Psychological characteristics at seven to ten years of age. *Health Bull (Edinb)* 2001;59:81–90.
105. Darlow BA, Horwood LJ, Mogridge N, Clement RS. Survival and disability at 7–8 years of age in New Zealand infants less than 28 weeks' gestation. *NZ Med J* 1998;111:204–7.
106. Petrou S, Mehta Z, Hockley C, Cook-Mozaffari P, Henderson J, Goldacre M. The impact of preterm birth on hospital in-patient admissions and costs during the first five years of life. *Pediatrics* 2003;192:1290–7.
107. Bowen JR, Gibson FL, Hand PJ. Educational outcome at 8 years for children who were born extremely prematurely: A controlled study. *J Paediatr Child Health* 2002;38:438–44.
108. Taylor HG, Klein N, Hack M. School-age consequences of birthweight less than 750 g: A review and update. *Dev Neuropsychol* 2000;17:289–321.
109. Sebastian A. *Dictionary of the History of Medicine.* London: The Parthenon Publishing Group.
110. *Oxford English Dictionary.* Oxford: Oxford University Press.
111. Dorland, WAN. *Dorlands Illustrated Medical Dictionary.* Amsterdam: Elsevier.
112. McCullough LB, Chervenak FA. *Ethics in Obstetrics and Gynecology.* New York: Oxford University Press, 1994.
113. Elias S, Annas GJ. *Reproductive Genetics and the Law.* Chicago: Year Book Medical Publishers, 1987.
114. Chervenak FA, McCullough LB. The fetus as a patient: Implications for directive versus non-directive counselling for fetal benefits. *Fetal Diagn Ther* 1991;6:93–100.
115. Chervenak FA, McCullough LB. Ethics in perinatal medicine. In Kurjak A, ed. *Text Book of Perinatal Medicine.* London: The Parthenon Publishing Group, 2000.
116. Ginsberg HG, Goldsmith JP, Stedman CM. Hospital care techniques resulting in intact survival of a 380 g infant. *Acta Paediatr* 1992;Suppl 382:13–5.
117. Nishida H, Ishizuka Y. Survival rate of extremely low birthweight infants and its effect on the amendment of the Eugenic Protection Act in Japan. *Acta Paediatr Jpn* 1992;34(6):612–6.
118. Nishida H. Outcome of infants born preterm with special emphasis on extremely low birthweight infants. *Baillieres Clin Obstet Gynaecol* 1993;7(3):611–31.
119. Hull D. The viable child. *J R Coll Phys Lond* 1988;22:169–75.
120. Rennie JM. Perinatal management at the lower margin of viability. *Arch Dis Child* 1996;74:F214–8.
121. Dunn PM, Stirrat GM. Capable of being born alive? *Lancet* 1984;i:553–5.
122. FIGO. Recommendations on ethical issues in Obstetrics and Gynecology by the FIGO Committee for the study of ethical aspects of human reproduction: Ethical aspects in the management of severely malformed infants. London: FIGO, 1994.
123. Schenker JG. Codes of perinatal ethics. An international perspective. *Clin Perinatol* 2003;30:45–65.

8 The offspring of maternal diabetes: perinatal events and future outcome

M. R. G. Carrapato, S. Tavares, C. Prior and T. Caldeira

Introduction

The 1989 St Vincent's Declaration stated, as a 5-year goal, '... that the outcome of the diabetic pregnancy should approach that of non-diabetic pregnancies'[1] and indeed, over the last 25 years significant reductions in spontaneous abortions, stillbirths, congenital malformations and perinatal mortality have been achieved at least in centers with a special interest in diabetic pregnancy and in selected populations.[2–9] However, reports have shown even in Western countries, that spontaneous abortions may be as high as 17%, the stillbirth rate to be five times greater, congenital malformations to range from 4 to 10 times the usual rate, perinatal mortality to be fivefold, neonatal mortality to be 15 times greater and that infant mortality might be trebled as the result of diabetic pregnancies.[10–13] Although population-based studies from Norway have reported considerably better outcomes,[14] data from other countries have continued to show bad results. In a cross-sectional study conducted in 12 perinatal centers in France between 2000 and 2001 involving 435 diabetic pregnancies, both types 1 and 2, perinatal mortality was six times greater than the national rate, severe congenital malformations were double and preterm delivery eight times the national level. Cesarean rates at 59%, shoulder dystocia at 7.6% and macrosomia at 17.3% added to the burden. Preconceptional care was provided in only 48.5% and 24% of women with types 1 and 2 diabetes, respectively, even though women with type 1 diabetes were being followed at least biannually in diabetic centers.[15] Unplanned pregnancies, therefore, remained at levels similar to those observed in the 1990s[16] and close to the reported rates in a recent survey in the USA.[17] In a nationwide prospective study from The Netherlands between 1999 and 2000, although planned pregnancies were observed in 84% of women with type 1 diabetes and glycemic control was considered good ($HbA_1C < 7.0\%$), in about 75% of subjects the outcome was considerably worse than the general population, with pre-eclampsia 12 times greater, cesarean sections 43%, perinatal mortality 2.8%, congenital malformations 8.8%, macrosomia 45.1% with 27.4% of shoulder dystocia and neonatal hypoglycemia in approximately two-thirds of neonates.[18] These poor results have also been reported for type 2 diabetes: congenital malformations 11 times greater, a twofold risk of stillbirth, perinatal mortality 2.5 times higher, risk of neonatal deaths 3.5 times greater and a sixfold risk of death in the first year of life.[19,20]

It would therefore appear that over 15 years on from the St. Vincent's Declaration the goal of a similar outcome for diabetic and non-diabetic pregnancies has yet to be attained.

When addressing diabetic embryofetopathy several issues are necessarily raised: What are the problems? Why does it happen? What is the outcome? Can it be avoided?

Peri(neo)natal problems of the infant of the diabetic mother (IDM)

Pregestational diabetes mellitus (pre-GDM)

The potential complications affecting the conceptus of the diabetic women have been identified for centuries[21] and range from an increased incidence of fetal demise to congenital malformations and a multitude of immediate neonatal problems including macrosomia/intrauterine growth restriction, respiratory distress syndrome (RDS), hypoglycemia, polycythemia, hypocalcemia, hyperbilirubinemia, heart failure and cardiomyopathy, renal vein thrombosis and small left colon. Although these clinical manifestations are seen, especially in uncontrolled diabetic mothers, some of the morbidities, namely macrosomia, hypoglycemia, jaundice and RDS, are still more common in the IDM despite good metabolic control and, in general, these neonates still require a higher rate of neonatal intensive care unit admission than the control population.

Congenital malformations

Although a whole range of congenital malformations involving multiple organ systems, without specific syndromes, have been observed in pre-GDM, both types 1 and 2, some dysmorphies and malformations are more common, including the association of dysplastic external ears and oculo–auriculo–vertebral spectrum.[22] Caudal regression anomalies, in particular saccral agenesis (with a 200- to 600-fold risk ratio), neural tube and CNS defects (relative risk ranging from 3 for anencephaly to a 40- to 400-fold risk for holoprosencephaly), cardiac malformations, from ASD, VSD to TGV and truncus arteriosus (four to six times greater) to renal defects, from agenesis to ureter duplication with a risk ratio from 6 to 23 times, respectively, have all been repeatedly observed in diabetic pregnancies.[18,23–26] Most of these congenital malformations occur particularly in the offspring of uncontrolled diabetic women with very poor, or no, preconceptional care. They appear to be directly related to HbA_1C levels, ranging from levels similar to those of the general population, with 'excellent metabolic control' ($HbA_1C < 6.9\%$), to 5.1% (with 'good metabolic control', HbA_1C 7.0–8.5%) to 22.4% incidence with greater than 8.6% HbA_1C.[27] Reid and Ylinen have also shown similar results and correlation with HbA_1C, suggesting that a good metabolic control could greatly reduce the impact of congenital malformations in the outcome of diabetic pregnancies.[28,29] By enrolling diabetic women to intensive metabolic control before conception, Furhmann showed that major congenital malformations could be reduced to 1.1%, rising to high uncorrected rates for those presenting later in pregnancy.[30,31] Since then, many other authors have shown similar good results from preconceptional care aimed at good metabolic glycemic control.[4,5,7–9,32,33] From the available evidence, it would seem that tight metabolic control for at least 6–12 months prior to conception would greatly reduce the burden of congenital malformations to almost normal rates. Nevertheless, even in the best series, corrected rates for diabetes-related malformations are considerably higher than those for the rest of the population, despite good metabolic control, i.e. preconceptional care and HbA_1C levels.[4,5,7,18] This raises several points, from the evaluation of good metabolic control and the best parameters, to the question of compliance and whether hyperglycemia is the only teratogenic fuel *per se* or is additional to other predisposing or adjuvant factors, as outlined in the etiopathogeny of diabetic embryofetopathy.

Macrosomia

Ranging from 17% to 50% in the offspring of pre-GDM[15,18,34–36] macrosomia poses a major problem for both obstetricians and neonatologists. In an attempt to diagnose fetal macrosomia many different ultrasound parameters have been proposed with differing results, from estimated fetal weight to abdominal circumference, to the more sophisticated evaluation of fetal subcutaneous fat tissue thickness of various body segments (midarm and midthigh fat and lean mass, abdominal and subscapular fat mass and cheek fat), to fetal fat layer, intraventricular septal thickness, etc.[37–39] How reliably can it be diagnosed by the practising obstetrician, outside the major research institutes if, in effect, he is referring to a large for gestational age (LGA) fetus based on the estimated weight and abdominal circumference?[40,41] This is an important question. While both share common characteristics, the true macrosomic fetus will have other peculiarities due to its abnormal fat distribution, especially affecting the shoulder girdle, leading to dystocia and its complications. Should, therefore, all (true) macrosomic fetuses be delivered by cesarean section? Perhaps not, but in practice they are. As for the pediatrician, the term macrosomia is also often used to describe a large baby and, again, although sharing common problems of hypoglycemia, polycythemia, hypocalcemia and hyperbilirubinemia, the true macrosomic baby will also be a candidate for birth (intrapartum) asphyxia, brachial palsy and cardiomyopathy.

Moreover, rather than mentioning any given weight or babies' weight/gestational age, as is traditionally done for macrosomia, it would be more appropriate to refer to ponderal indices [PI = (fetal weight in grams/fetal length in cm^3) × 100] against the estimated centile for gestational age.[42–44] This approach, besides differentiating the normal LGA from the true macrosomic neonate, may also have other implications, particularly with regard to long-term outcome.

Hypoglycemia

Another issue relates to neonatal hypoglycemia and its never-ending controversies. What in fact is neonatal hypoglycemia and does it matter? Methodological problems of glucose measurements – capillary to venous blood, whole blood to plasma values, sample containers and transport, etc. – all account for the different definitions of hypoglycemia. Glucose concentration in whole blood is about 10–15% lower than in plasma and due to the usually high hematocrit of the IDM, plasma, rather than whole blood, should be used for the definition of hypoglycemia. Moreover, what low blood sugar level might be harmful? Will a (given) low blood sugar level in the absence of symptoms be less damaging than when coupled to clinical manifestations? And if, at the follow-up, these children are found to be performing below par, is it because of neonatal hypoglycemia or is it due to poor antenatal metabolic control? Conversely, could it possibly be that in order to overcome hypoglycemia, the neonate is able to utilize other substrates as an alternative to glucose for brain metabolism? The answer is a partial 'yes' for lactate in the immediate neonatal period, but quite unlikely for other, more important fuels, namely ketone bodies, given the sustained hyperinsulinism-inhibiting lypolysis. For these reasons, it would therefore be recommended to keep blood levels in the range of ≥2.6 mmol/l regardless of gestational and postnatal age, by promoting early enteral feeds. If oral feeds are not being tolerated or are contraindicated, i.v. glucose should be started at 5–6 mg/kg/min and may be subsequently increased according to the lack of response to 8–10 mg/kg/min. If the neonate has symptomatic hypoglycemia, especially related to neuroglycopenia, a bolus i.v. glucose administration of 0.25–0.5 g/kg should be given followed by glucose infusion at the required rate to maintain normal glycemia. As soon as possible, enteral feeds with either breast milk or formula should be promoted and gradually increased to avoid reactive hypoglycemia if glucose infusion is decreased too rapidly. Glucagon administration of 200–300 μg/kg may occasionally be required to enhance glucose release from glycogen storages and to increase hepatic acids oxidation.

Respiratory distress syndrome

Premature delivery remains a hazard due to either maternal or fetal well-being, mostly in poorly controlled women or with associated pregnancy complications or due to underlying disorders secondary to diabetes itself. Hyaline membrane disease (HMD) is more common in infants of diabetic mothers at any gestational age due to either inhibition or decreased surfactant synthesis, a consequence of fetal hyperinsulinism.[45–50] In general, both *in vivo* and *in vitro*, insulin opposes the glucocorticoid stimulating effect on lung maturation[51–53] by a complex cascade of impaired mechanisms, from blockade of fibroblast – pneumocyte – factor (FPF) release and directly inhibiting phospholipid synthesis by type 2 cells[54] to reducing surface protein synthesis[55] or both.

Antenatal corticosteroids have been shown to promote fetal lung maturation in normal pregnancies. Their use in diabetic pregnancy remains controversial as the adverse steroid-induced hyperglycemia on fetal lung maturation may offset any beneficial effects.[54] In addition, the acute rise of severe hyperglycemia in the mother needs to be taken into account and caution demands close monitoring during antenatal corticosteroid administration and several schemes have been proposed for supplementary insulin to counteract the unbalanced hyperglycemic status.[56,57]

Whether the routine assessment of fetal lung maturation by lamella body counts or lecithin/sphingomyelin ratios should be performed in reliably dated pregnancies, at term, is doubtful and lately is becoming less advocated.[58–62]

If HMD remains a common neonatal problem, RDS in the offspring of diabetic mothers is further aggravated not only by the concomitant polycythemia and hyperviscosity, hypoxia and pulmonary hypertension, occasionally heart failure, but also, especially by the high rate of cesarean sections, often without previous labor.

Hypocalcemia

Calcium homeostasis depends on the equilibrium between intestinal absorption and renal excretion under hormonal regulation. Parathormone mobilizes calcium from bone, promotes its renal tubular reabsorption and stimulates 1,25 hydroxy vitamin D production. Vitamin D increases calcium and phosphate intestinal absorption and regulates bone metabolism mediated by parathormone. Hypocalcemia, on the other hand, stimulates parathormone release. In pregnancy, calcium is actively transferred across the placenta from maternal circulation under the influence of the parathyroid hormone-related peptide (PTHrP) with maternal parathormone and vitamin D having very little influence due to their inability to cross the placenta. Fetal plasma calcium is higher than maternal levels, especially with advancing pregnancy (total and ionized calcium 10–11 mg/dl and 6 mg/dl, respectively), and consequently, the parathyroid glands show reduced activity.[63–65] At birth, following the suppression of maternal–fetal transferal of calcium, the plasma levels fall within the first 24 h of life, leading to parathormone release and the normalization of calcium levels by 2 weeks of life.[63,64] Total calcium concentrations in the neonate are dependent on gestational age, albumin levels and pH.

Hypocalcemia occurs in up to 50% of IDM, usually on the first 3 days of age, often associated to hyperphosphatemia and hypomagnesemia probably due to delayed parathyroid response and correlated to the duration and severity of maternal diabetes although the mechanisms remain elusive.[63–65] Pulmonary disease and/or asphyxia worsen the hypocalcemia.[63,65]

In the absence of clinical manifestations, it is debatable whether calcium determination should be performed routinely. On the contrary, with preterm delivery, respiratory compromise, asphyxia, sepsis, etc., calcium levels should be performed and corrected. Prolonged QTc (QT corrected for heart rate over 0.4 s) on the ECG requires special attention, but with the possibility of heart block, refractory bradycardia and hypotension, calcium administration should be carefully monitored.

Persistent hypocalcemia may be the result of the concomitant hypomagnesemia and is unlikely to be corrected if magnesium levels are not adjusted. With significant hyperphosphatemia ($Ca_2 \times PO_4 > 80$) calcium administration may lead to calcification of the soft tissues if the high phosphate levels are not lowered primarily.[63–66]

Polycythemia

The definition of polycythemia may include infants with or without symptoms having hematocrits greater than 65%. The reported incidence of polycythemia ranges from 0.4% to 12% in the newborns, but it affects up to 30% of infants of poorly controlled diabetic mothers.

Fetal red cells have a larger mean cell volume and are less deformable than more mature cells, leading to increased viscosity. Low fetal oxygenation and tissue hypoxia increase erythropoietin levels stimulating erythropoiesis and leading to high fetal hemoglobin. Some authors speculate that fetal plasma erythropoietin concentration is significantly correlated to maternal high-affinity HbA_1C[67–69] while others suggest that the increased erythropoiesis in fetus of diabetic pregnancies may be subsequent to fetal hypoxemia, the result of hyperglycemia, hyperinsulinemia and hyperketonemia, in line with Freinkel's concept of 'pregnancy as a tissue culture experience'.[70,71] The chronic hypoxemic state *in utero* may thus explain some cases of fetal death. In the neonate, symptomatic polycythemia may present with RDS, congestive heart failure and, occasionally, pulmonary hypertension. Neurological signs include jitteriness, irritability, seizures and apnea. Potential sequelae of polycythemia may be thrombosis, gangrene and stroke. The treatment of polycythemia, especially if symptomatic, is the standard partial exchange transfusion.

Jaundice

Physiological jaundice is a common neonatal problem due to transient glucoronyl transferase deficiency, immature hepatic intracellular uptake and transport, increased enterohepatic circulation and occurs in 60–70% of the newborns. However, clinically significant jaundice (total bilirubin greater than 12.9 mg/dl at term) affects only 5% of these babies.[72]

In the IDM, the risk of clinically important jaundice is up to 30% and is due to multifactorial causes from prematurity, to polycythemia and increased hemolysis, and macrosomia, with PI rather than weight/gestational age showing a better correlation with bilirubin levels.[69,73–75]

Gestational diabetes mellitus

GDM usually develops in the second half of pregnancy. With advancing pregnancy considerable demands are placed on insulin to meet increasing maternal metabolism. If the threshold is surpassed, maternal hyperglycemia may supervene. Although some studies also point to a higher incidence of congenital malformations in association with GDM, most cases are probably pre-GDM diagnosed in pregnancy, especially type 2, with prepregnancy body mass index (BMI) and advanced maternal age playing a very conspicuous role.[76–80] Congenital malformations aside, the whole spectrum of peri(neo)natal problems overlap those of pre-GDM and contribute to the high maternal–fetal and neonatal morbidities.

The incidence of GDM varies from 3% to 5% depending on whether screening is universal or only for women at risk.

In our Institution over the 2-year period from January 1, 2002 to December 31, 2003, from an unselected population of 5930 women, after a universal 1 h of 50-g glucose screening, followed by 3 h of 100-g OGTT, 211 women were confirmed as having GDM. Seven women diagnosed in the first weeks as having had possible pre-GDM detected only in pregnancy (mean BMI 32.5, mean age 32.4 years) were eliminated from the study.

Among the multigest and multipara, 7.2% had had previous GDM with 24% miscarriage and 4.3% late fetal death.

In the present pregnancy, the average gestational age at the time of diagnosis was 27 weeks and the mean HbA_1C was 4.3% (range 3.4–5.7%). Forty-one women (20.4%) required insulin treatment to maintain good metabolic control.

Complications of pregnancy included pregnancy-induced hypertension (8, 3.8%), pre-eclampsia (3, 1.4%), HELLP (3, 1.4%), placenta abruptio (3, 1.4%), thrombocytopenia (4, 1.9%), oligo/hydramnios (2, 0.9%), ACIU (2, 0.9%). There were no maternal or perinatal deaths.

Delivery was by cesarean section in 43.9% and by instrument delivery in 8.8% while for a control group of macrosomic babies of non-diabetic mothers these figures were 36.4% and 9.2%, respectively. The average birth weight at 38 weeks was 3121 g (SD 424 g) and length 48.55 cm (SD 1.77 cm).

Neonatal morbidities expressed in Table 8.1, compared to LGA neonates of non-diabetic mothers, were considerably better than in many series. Several points, though, need to be considered. The incidence of macrosomia [birth weight/gestational age (BW/GA) > 90th centile] was identified in only six (2.9%), a figure that is just above that of our unselected population (2.8%). However, if PI is applied instead of BW/GA, the incidence rises to 31 (16.1%) of babies with PI > 90th centile, especially with advancing gestational age (21.4% and 38.5% at 39 and 40 weeks, respectively), suggesting a population of short obese babies within our population of gestational diabetes in contrast to LGA neonates of non-diabetic mothers, which are large and long (Table 8.2). We would therefore consider PI to be a more accurate and true reflection of macrosomia than just BW/GA. Another area for concern is the high incidence of cesarean sections, which suggests labor-induced failure, because even correcting for PI, only 16.1% were macrosomic newborns, questioning the current practice of elective induction at 38 weeks' gestation. The proportion of small for gestational age within our diabetic population (10.3% vs. 13.64 % in our general population), suggests an adequate metabolic control.

Although there were very few cases of RDS in our neonates, mostly due to the paucity of very small, extremely preterm infants, we observed that of those with respiratory problems, more than one-half were pulmonary adaptation syndromes in neonates delivered by cesarean section at 37 weeks' gestation.

In summary, even within perinatal centers, although maternal and peri(neo)natal adverse results can be greatly improved, GDM remains a public health problem of considerable proportions.

Table 8.1 Comparative neonatal morbidities of IDM and LGA

Morbidity	IDM n	%	LGA N	%	χ^2 (P)
Fractured clavicles	4	2	9	5.4	0.79
Brachial plexus palsy	1	0.5	2	1.2	0.47
Congenital malformations	9*	4.3	9**	4.7	0.582
Prematurity	21	10.2	11	6.6	0.959
Hypoglycemia	6	3.1	4	2.4	0.663
RDS	8	4.1	4	2.4	0.342
Jaundice	63	32.6	28	16.8	< 0.001
Polycythemia	7	3.6	9	5.4	0.37
Hypocalcemia	9	4.7	2	1.2	0.054

*Hypospadias 2, hydronephrosis 2, hypoplasia of distal phalanx 1, CHD 4 (3 VSD, 1 ASD); **epispadias 1, hypospadias 1, hydronephrosis 1, CHD 5 (2 VSD, 3 ASD), craniofacial dysmorphy 1

Table 8.2 Body proportions of IDM and LGA per GA

	IDM (207/5930)						LGA (167/5930)				
GA (Weeks)	Weight (±SD)	>90th centile (%)	Length (±SD)	>90th centile (%)	PI (±SD)	>90th centile (%)	Weigh (±SD)	Length (±SD)	>90th centile (%)	PI(±SD) centile (%)	>90th centile (%)
41							4650 (±167.19)	54.8 (±1.85)	38.1	3.3 (±0.35)	61.9
40	3389 (±231.90)	0	49.0 (±1.79)	0	2.9 (±0.39)	38.5	4328 (±211.08)	52.1 (±1.27)	33.3	3.1 (±0.22)	54.2
39	3332 (±341.51)	0	49.1 (±1.73)	6.9	2.8 (±0.29)	21.4	4208 (±263.40)	51.87 (±1.63)	31.8	3.1 (±0.22)	43.3
38	3121 (±424.14)	5.2	48.5 (±1.77)	4.3	2.7 (±0.26)	15.3	3989 (±137.89)	50.9 (±1.57)	34.8	3.0 (±0.31)	60.9
37	2900 (±337.07)	0	47.8 (±1.80)	0	2.6 (±0.21)	5.0	3751 (±204.07)	51.0 (±1.24)	50	2.8 (±0.21)	38.9
36	2645 (±220.76)	0	46.5 (±1.62)	0	2.6 (±0.22)	0	3495 (±111.13)	49.8 (±2.68)	50	2.9 (±0.47)	50
35	2343 (±82.14)	0	44.0 (±2.74)	0	2.8 (±0.45)	5.0	3233 (±101.16)	47.0 (±2.60)	0	3.1 (±0.49)	100
TOTAL	3074.3 (±432.87)	2.9	48.4 (±1.94)		2.7 (±0.27)	16.1	4133.6 (±351.98)	51.55 (±1.81)		3.0 (±0.28)	

Why does it happen?

In a theoretical model, according to Freinkel's concept of pregnancy as a tissue culture experience, the whole pathogenesis and spectrum of fetal and neonatal mortality and morbidity could primarily be attributed to the excessive transferal of glucose from mother to fetus, inducing fetal hyperglycemia, leading to fetal pancreatic islet hypertrophy and β-cell hyperplasia with a consequent rise in insulin secretion.[81] Chronic fetal hyperinsulinism results in raised metabolic rates and oxygen consumption causing fetal hypoxemia, which, in turn, would be responsible for the increased rate of stillbirths and birth asphyxia as well as for the excessive erythropoietin production and polycythemia.[68–70,82,83] In addition, fetal hyperinsulinism would be responsible for increased fetal substrate intake, leading to fat synthesis, with the resulting adiposity, macrosomia and visceromegaly. Furthermore, fetal hyperinsulinism may also be responsible for the development of respiratory distress syndrome at birth by either inhibiting or decreasing lung surfactant synthesis.[45–50] Neonatal hypoglycemia may be a combination of several factors including sustained hyperinsulinism and lack of counter-regulatory hormonal responses impairing hepatic glucose production, deficient lipolysis and increasing peripheral glucose uptake.[84–86] It would seem, therefore, that uncontrolled maternal hyperglycemia could start the whole spectrum of diabetic embryofetopathy (Figure 8.1). It is quite possible, however, that other metabolic fuels, either besides or in association with glucose, from lipids to

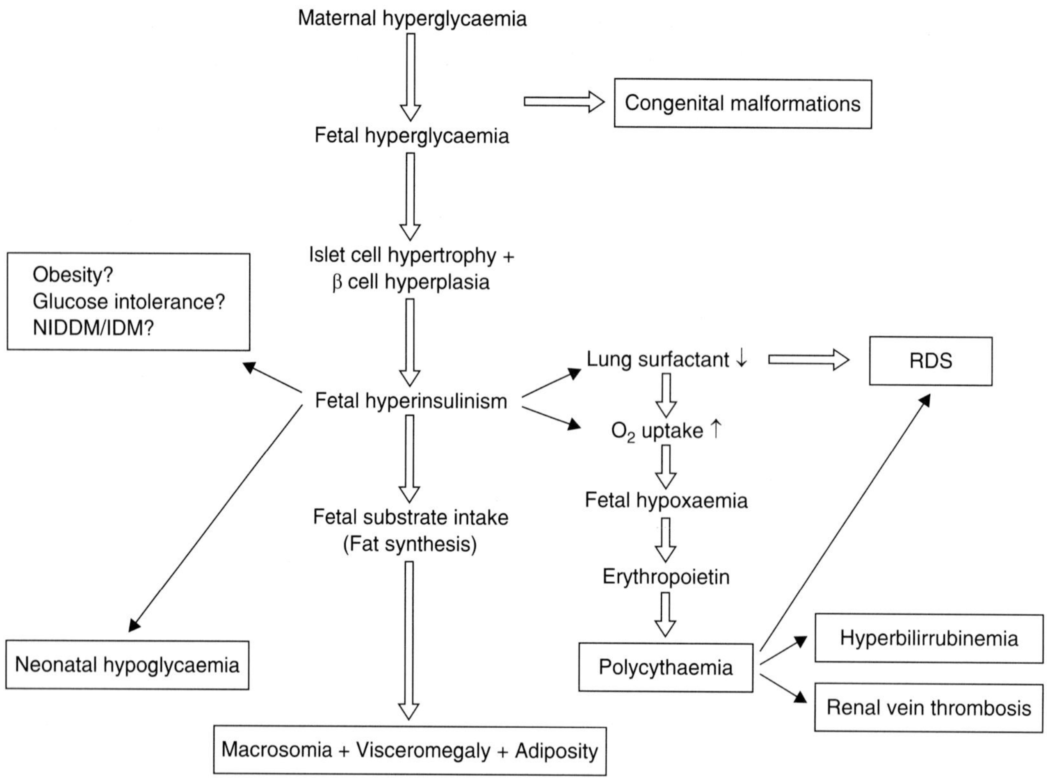

Figure 8.1 Diabetic embryofetopathy.

amino acids, may also cross the placenta in a concentration gradient inversely proportional to insulin availability, further contributing to the abnormal fetal milieu.[70,71,87] Depending on the timing of gestation, during critical developmental stages, the same metabolic fuels would have different effects on the fetus. Over the last 15 years there has been increasing evidence from animal and human studies to support the theory that in addition to sugars (glucose, galactose and mannose) other metabolic fuels, from ketones to deranged lipid peroxidation, may be responsible for the pathomechanisms of congenital malformations provided that they are present at certain (high) levels for a reasonable amount of time and especially at crucial 'developmental windows'.[88–91] Dietary supplementation of deficient substracts (arachidonic acid and myo-inositol), free oxygen radical scavenging enzymes and antioxidants have been shown *in vivo* and *in vitro* to reduce the rate of malformation in the offspring of diabetic animals.[92–95] Whether such strategies might be applicable to clinical practice remains a promising but open question.

Similarly, the same general principles of multifactorial pathomechanisms have been postulated for macrosomia, including and ranging from ketone bodies to free fatty acids, 'selected' amino acids and with a conspicuous role for IGF-1 and IGF-2 at the local level. Maternal insulin antibodies and insulin counter-regulatory hormones may, in addition, further contribute to the resulting macrosomia.[96–101]

Toward the end of the second trimester, at a time of increasing cerebral cortical differentiation and maturation, it is quite conceivable that a metabolic insult may result in altered neurological or intellectual behavior[102–106] and, during the third trimester, proliferation of fetal adipocytes, muscle cells and pancreatic β-cells may then be responsible for 'programming' the later development of several adult disorders.[107–111]

What is the outcome?

Neonatal complications of the IDM, in spite of the high morbidities involved, are now quite well managed with intensive neonatal care. It is questionable whether these babies are more prone to developing neurological, behavioral and learning disabilities and, if so, whether they are due to an unfavorable intrauterine metabolic environment or to other perinatal and early life events operating on different fetal determinants. Most of the early reports of severe brain damage are, reassuringly, now of historical interest.[112,113] Nevertheless, well-documented evidence points to mild to moderate psychomotor and psychosocial impairment in the offspring of these mothers. While it is quite possible that early neonatal events may play a role, available data also place a suspicious emphasis on intrauterine life.[102–105]

The long-term outcome, on the other hand, poses several questions. Some studies point to a higher incidence of childhood obesity in the offspring of these mothers while others fail to find such correlations. Conflicting results might be the result of the different methodologies involved, including different definitions and very often small numbers, without adequate control populations.[114–116]

Finally, a major issue is whether some adult diseases of metabolic and vascular disorders may have had a fetal origin. In recent years, there has been accumulating evidence, both from animal studies and from epidemiological data, to suggest that fetal β-cell hyperplasia and hyperinsulinism may induce irreversible changes leading to obesity, glucose intolerance and even overt non-insulin-dependent diabetes and, perhaps, a protective effect against type 1 diabetes later in life – a model very much in line with the 'Barker Hypothesis' of the fetal origins of adult disease.[107–111,117,118]. What might be the relative weight of genetics vs. intrauterine events remains to be confirmed[119,120] but it is quite interesting that at least in experimental models the prevention of hyperglycemia in pregnancy significantly reduces the prevalence of diabetes in the next generations.[111]

What can be done?

Based on the assumption that poor maternal homeostasis is at the core of the problem and that tight metabolic control might change the outcome of a diabetic pregnancy to normal, why then are such poor results being reported even in developed countries? Admittedly, most of these bad performances are for pre-GDM. But, even allowing for different data collection, lack of uniform criteria in definitions and case identification,[121–123] the fact remains that overall results are far from satisfactory. It can be argued that they are due to poor medical and social care – and they most probably are. It can also be argued that poor metabolic control has not been achieved or that 'good' is not necessarily 'optimal'. Alternatively, it can be put forward that there might be an abnormal genetic background contribution (evidence is pretty scanty) or that there might be other metabolic fuels besides glucose operating at different developmental stages of pregnancy, thus accounting for the etiopathogenesis of the whole syndrome. It is quite possible that some, or all, of these metabolic fuels may, *per se* or in synergie, play a significant role in the whole metabolic disturbance and it is quite conceivable that besides the classical approach to strict glucose control, other dietary manipulations with supplementation or replacement of deficient substracts might hold a promise for the near future. For the moment, however, priority should focus on intensive prenatal care for diabetic women and the identification of women for the development of GDM and, once diagnosed, placing them on a strict glycemic control throughout pregnancy. The cost-efficiency of screening all women for GDM is often discussed and, likewise, whether many of these women are overtreated unnecessarily. Argument, however, should concentrate not just on the immediate effects of GDM but on the long-term consequences for both the mother and her offspring.

Acknowledgment

The authors gratefully acknowledge the antenatal data on diabetic mothers supplied by Dr. Célia Araújo.

REFERENCES

1. Diabetes Care and Research in Europe. The St Vincent Declaration. WHO/IDF Europe. *Diabet Med* 1990;7:360.
2. Teramo K, Kuusisto AN, Raivio KO. Perinatal outcome of insulin-dependent diabetic pregnancies. *Ann Clin Res* 1979;11: 146–55.
3. Jervell J, Bjerkedal T, Moe N. Outcome of pregnancies in diabetic mothers in Norway 1967–76. *Diabetologia* 1980;8: 131–4.
4. Molsted-Pedersen L, Pedersen J. Congenital malformations in diabetic pregnancies. Clinical viewpoints. *Acta Paediatr Scand Suppl* 1985;320:79–84.
5. Hanson U, Persson B, Thunnel S. Relationship between haemoglobin A1c in early Type I (insulin-dependent) diabetic pregnancy and the occurrence of spontaneous abortion and fetal malformation in Sweden. *Diabetologia* 1990;33:100–4.
6. Roberts AB, Pattison NS. Pregnancy in women with diabetes mellitus, twenty years experience: 1968–1987. *N Z Med J* 1990; 103:211–3.
7. Kitzmiller JL, Gavin LA, Gin GD, Jovanovic-Peterson L, Main EK, Zigrang WD. Preconception care of diabetes. Glycemic control prevents congenital abnomalies. *J Am Med Assoc* 1991;265: 731–6.
8. McElvy SS, Miodovnik M, Rosenn B, Khoury JC, Siddiqi T, Dignan PS, Tsang RC. A focused preconceptional and early pregnancy program in women with type I diabetes reduces perinatal mortality and malformation rates to general population levels. *J Matern Fetal Med* 2000;9:14–20.
9. Diabetes Control and Complications Trial Research Group. The effects of intensive treatment of diabetes on the development and progression of long-term complications in insulin-dependent diabetes mellitus. *N Engl J Med* 1993;329:977–86.
10. Hawthorne G, Robson S, Ryall EA, Sen D, Roberts SH, Ward Platt MP. Prospective population-based survey of outcome of pregnancy in diabetic women: Results of the Northern Diabetic Pregnancy Audit, 1994. *Br Med J* 1997;315:279–81.
11. Casson IF, Clarke CA, Howard CV, *et al.* Outcomes of pregnancy in insulin-dependent diabetic women: Results of a five year population cohort study. *Br Med J* 1997;315:275–8.
12. Penney GC, Mair G, Pearson DW. Scottish Diabetes Pregnancy Group. Outcome of pregnancies in women with type 1 diabetes in Scotland: A national population-based study. *Br J Obstet Gyneacol* 2003;110:315–18.
13. Hadden DR, McCance D, Traub AI. Ten-year outcome of diabetic pregnancy in Northern Ireland: The case for centralization. *Diabet Med* 1998;15(Suppl 1):S16.
14. Hawthorne G, Irgens LM, Lie RT. Outcome of pregnancy in diabetic women in Northern England and Norway, 1994–7. *Br Med J* 2000;321:730–1.
15. Diabetic and Pregnancy Group, France. French multicentric survey of outcome of pregnancy in women with pregestational diabetes. *Diabetes Care* 2003;26:2990–93.
16. Gestation and Diabetes in France Study Group. Multicenter survey of diabetic pregnancy in France. *Diabetes Care* 1991;14: 994–1000.

17. American Diabetes Association. Preconceptional care of women with diabetes. *Diabetes Care* 2003;26 (Suppl 1):S91–93.
18. Evers IM, de Valk HW, Visser GH. Risk of complications of pregnancy in women with type I diabetes: Nationwide prospective study in the Netherlands. *Br Med J* 2004;328(7445):915–20.
19. Dunne F, Brydon P, Smith K, Gee H. Pregnancy in women with type 2 diabetes: Twelve-years outcome data 1990–2002. *Diabet Med* 2003;20:734–8.
20. Hadden DR, Cull CA, Croft DJ, Holman RR. Poor pregnancy outcome for women with type 2 diabetes. *Diabet Med* 2003;20: 506–7.
21. Le Corche E. Du diabetic dans ses rapports avec la vie intrauterine menstruation et la grossesse. *Ann Gynecol* 1885;24:257.
22. Wang R, Martinez-Frias ML, Graham JM Jr. Infants of diabetic mothers are at increased risk for the oculo-auriculo-vertebral sequence: A case-based and case-control approach. *J Pediatr* 2002;141:611–7.
23. Kucera J. Rate and type of congenital anomalies among offspring of diabetic women. *J Reprod Med* 1971;7:73–82.
24. Mills JL, Baker L, Goldman AS. Malformations in infants of diabetic mothers occur before the seventh gestational week. *Diabetes* 1979;28:292–3.
25. Barr M Jr, Hanson JW, Currey K, *et al.* Holoprosencephaly in infants of diabetic mothers. *J Pediatr* 1983;102:565–8.
26. Wren C, Birrel G, Hawthorne G. Cardiovascular malformations in infants of diabetic mothers. *Heart* 2003;89:1217–20.
27. Miller EM, Hare JW, Cloherty JP, *et al.* Major congenital anomalies and elevated hemoglobin A1c in early weeks of diabetic pregnancy. *N Engl J Med* 1981;304:1331–4.
28. Reid M, Hadden D, Harley JM, Halliday HL, McClure BG. Fetal malformations in diabetics with high haemoglobin A1c in early pregnancy (letter). *Br Med J (Clin Res Ed)* 1984;289:1001.
29. Ylinen K, Aula P, Stenman UH, Kesaniemi-Kuokkanen T, Teramo K. Risk of minor and major fetal malformations in diabetics with haemoglobin A1c values in early pregnancy. *Br Med J* 1984; 289:345–6.
30. Furhmann K, Reiher H, Semmler K, Fischer F, Fischer M, Glockner E. Prevention of congenital malformations in infants of insulin-dependent diabetic mothers. *Diabetes Care* 1983;6:219–23.
31. Furhmann K, Reiher H, Semmler K, Glockner E. The effect of intensified conventional insulin therapy before and durig pregnancy on the malformation rate in offspring of diabetic mothers. *Exp Clin Endocrinol* 1984;83:173–7.
32. Steel JM. Prepregnancy counseling and contraception in the insulin-dependent diabetic patient. *Clin Obstet Gynecol* 1985; 28:553–66.
33. DCCT 1996. The Diabetes Control and Complications Trial Research Group. Pregnancy outcomes in the diabetes control and complications trial. *Am J Obstet Gynaecol* 1996;174:1343–53.
34. Martin Carballo G, Fernandez Cano G, Grande Aragon C, Mendez Alavedra J, Hawkins Carranza F, Garcia Bouthelier R. Infants of diabetic mothers (IDM) I – Macrosomia and growth factors. *Ann Esp Pediatr* 1997;47:295–301.
35. Cordero L, Landon MB. Infant of diabetic mother. *Clin Perinatol* 1993;20:635–48.
36. Carvalheiro M. Diabetes in pregnancy: State of the art in Mediterranean countries, Portugal. *Ann 1st Super Sanita* 1997; 33:303–6.
37. Larciprete G, Valensise H, Vasapollo B, *et al.* Fetal subcutaneous tissue thickness (SCTT) in healthy and gestational diabetic pregnancies. *Ultrasound Obstet Gynecol* 2003;22:591–7.
38. Bethune M, Bell R. Evaluation of the measurement of the fetal fat layer, interventricular septum and abdominal circumference percentile in the prediction of macrosomia in pregnancies affected by gestational diabetes. *Ultrasound Obstet Gynecol* 2003;22: 586–90.
39. Greco P, Vimercati A, Hyett J, *et al.* The ultrasound assessment of adipose tissue deposition in fetuses of "well controlled" insulin-dependent diabetic pregnancies. *Diabet Med* 2003;20:858–62.
40. Buchanan TA, Kjos SL, Montoro MN, et al. Use of fetal ultrasound to select metabolic therapy for pregnancies complicated by mild gestational diabetes. Diabetes Care 1994;17:275–83.
41. Gilby JR, Williams MC, Spellacy WN. Fetal abdominal circumference measurements of 35 and 38 cm as predictors of macrosomia. A risk factor for shoulder dystocia. *J Reprod Med* 2000; 45:936–8.
42. Roje D, Ivo B, Ivica T, *et al.* Gestational age – The most important factor of Neonatal Ponderal Index. *Yonsei Med J* 2004;45: 273–80.
43. Patterson RM, Pouliot MR. Neonatal morphometrics and perinatal outcome: Who is growth retarded? *Am J Obstet Gynecol* 1987;157:691–3.
44. Dombrowski MB, Stanley MB, Johnson MP, Saleh AAS, Sokol RJ. Birth weight – Length ratios, ponderal indexes, placental weights, and birth weight – Placenta ratios in a large population. *Arch Pediatr Adolesc Med* 1994;148:508–12.
45. Bourbon JR, Farrell PM. Fetal lung development in the diabetic pregnancy. *Pediatr Res* 1985;19:253–67.
46. Tyden O, Berne C, Eriksson U. Lung maturation in fetuses of diabetic rats. *Pediatr Res* 1980;14:1192–5.
47. Warburton D. Chronic hyperglycaemia with secondary hyperinsulinemia inhibits the maturational response of fetal lamb lungs to cortisol. *J Clin Invest* 1983;72:433–440.
48. Warburton D, Parton L, Buckley S, Cosico L, Saluna T. Effects of glucose infusion on surfactant and glycogen regulation in fetal lamb lung. *J Appl Physiol* 1987;63:1750–6.
49. Levine DH. Hyperinsulinemia and decreased surfactant in fetal rabbits. *Dev Pharmacol Ther* 1985;8:284–91.
50. Rooney SA, Ingleson LD, Wilson CM, Gross I. Insulin antagonism of dexamethasone-induced stimulation of cholinephosphate cytidyltransferase in fetal rat lung in organ culture. *Lung* 1980;158:151–5.
51. Gross I, Smith GJ, Wilson CM, et al. The influence of hormones of the biochemical development in fetal rat lung in organ culture. II. Insulin. *Pediatr Res* 1980;14:834–8.
52. Smith BT, Girout CJ, Robert M, Avary ME. Insulin antagonism of cortisol action on lecithin synthesis by cultured fetal lung cells. *J Pediatr* 1975;87:953–5.
53. Pignol B, Bourbon J, Ktorza A, Marine L, Rieutort M, Tordet C. Lung maturation in the hyperinsulinemic rat fetus. *Pediatr Res* 1987;21:436–41.
54. Carlson KS, Smith BT, Post M. Insulin acts on the fibroblasts to inhibit glucocorticoid stimulation of lung maturation. *J Appl Physiol* 1984;57:1577–9.
55. Snyder JM, Kwun JE, O'Brien JA, Rosenfeld CR, Odom MJ. The concentration of 35-kDa surfactant apoprotein in amniotic fluids from normal and diabetic pregnancies. *Pediatr Res* 1988;24: 728–34.
56. Kaushal K, Gibson JM, Railton A, Hounsome B, New JP, Young RJ. A protocol for improved glycemic control following corticosteroid therapy in diabetic pregnancies. *Diabet Med* 2003; 20:73–5.
57. Mathiesen ER, Christensen AB, Hellmuth E, Hornnes P, Stage E, Damm P. Insulin dose during glucocorticoid treatment for fetal lung maturation in diabetic pregnancy: Test of an algorithm. *Acta Obstet Gynecol Scand* 2002;81:835–9.
58. Kjos SL, Berkowitz KM, Kung B. Prospective delivery of reliably dated term infants of diabetic mothers without determination of fetal lung maturity: Comparison to historical control. *J Matern Fetal Neonatal Med* 2002;12:433–7.
59. Langer O. The controversy surrounding fetal lung maturity in diabetes in pregnancy: A re-evaluation. *J Matern Fetal Neonatal Med* 2002;12:428–32.
60. DeRoche ME, Ingardia CJ, Guerette PJ, Wu AH, LaSala CA, Mandavilli SR. The use of lamellar body counts to predict fetal lung maturity in pregnancies complicated by diabetes mellitus. *Am J Obstet Gynecol* 2002;187:908–12.
61. Piper JM. Lung maturation in diabetes in pregnancy: If and when to test. *Semin Perinatol* 2002;26:206–9.
62. Moore TR. A comparison of amniotic fluid fetal pulmonary phospholipids in normal and diabetic pregnancy. *Am J Obstet Gynecol* 2002;186:641–50.
63. Abrams SA. Neonatal hypocalcemia. In: Rose BD, ed. Wellesley, MA: UpToDate, 2004.
64. Nold JL, Georgieff MK. Infants of diabetic mothers (review). *Pediatr Clin North Am* 2004;51:619–637.
65. Riskin A, Haney PM. Infant of a diabetic mother. In: Rose BD, ed. Wellesley, MA: UpToDate, 2004.
66. Choukair MK. *The Harriet Lane Handbook*. St Louis: Mosby-Year Book Inc., 2000.
67. Salvesen DR, Brudenell JM, Snijders RJ, Ireland RM, Nicolaides KH. Fetal plasma erythropoietin in pregnancies complicated by maternal diabetes mellitus. *Am J Obstet Gynecol* 1993;168: 88–94.
68. Salvesen DR, Brudenell MJ, Nicolaides KH. Fetal polycythemia and thrombocytopenia in pregnancies complicated by maternal diabetes mellitus. *Am J Obstet Gynecol* 1992;166: 1287–93.

69. Mimouni F, Miodovnik M, Siddiqi TA, Butler JB, Holroyde J, Tsang RC. Neonatal polycythemia in infants of insulin-dependent diabetic mothers. *Obstet Gynaecol* 1986;68:370–2.

70. Freinkel N, Metzger BE. Pregnancy as a tissue culture experience: The critical implications of maternal metabolism for fetal development. *Ciba Found Symp* 1978;63:3–28.

71. Freinkel N, Metzger BE. Emerging challenges in diabetes and pregnancy: Diabetic embryopathy and gestational diabetes. In Alberti KGMM, Krall LP, eds. *The Diabetes Annual*. Amsterdam: Elsevier Science Publishers, 1988;4:179–201.

72. Rubaltelli FF. Unconjugated and conjugated bilirubin pigments during perinatal development. IV. The influence of breastfeeding on neonatal hyperbilirubinemia. *Biol Neonate* 1993;64:104–9.

73. Peevy KJ, Landaw SA, Gross SJ. Hyperbilirubinemia in infants of diabetic mothers. *Pediatrics* 1980;66(3):417–19.

74. Jahrig D, Jahrig K, Stiete S, Beyersdorff E, Poser H, Hopp H. Neonatal jaundice in infants of diabetic mothers. *Acta Paediatr Scand Suppl* 1989;360:101–7.

75. Ballard JL, Rosenn B, Khoury JC, Miodovnik M. Diabetic fetal macrosomia: Significance of disproportionate growth. *J Pediatr* 1993;122:115–9.

76. Garcia-Patterson A, Erdozain L, Ginovart J, *et al.* In human gestational diabetes mellitus congenital malformations are related to pre-pregnancy body mass index and to severity of diabetes. *Diabetologia* 2004;47:509–14.

77. Cedergren MI, Kallen BA. Maternal obesity and infant heart defects. *Obes Res* 2003;11:1065–71.

78. Watkins ML, Rasmussnen SA, Honein MA, Botto LD, Moore CA. Maternal obesity and risk for birth defects. *Pediatrics* 2003;111:1152–8.

79. Sheffield JS, Butler-Koster EL, Casey BM, McIntire DD, Leveno KJ. Maternal diabetes mellitus and infant malformations. *Obstet Gynecol* 2002;100:925–30.

80. Mikhail LN, Walker CK, Mittendorf R. Association between maternal obesity and fetal cardiac malformations in African–Americans. *J Natl Med Assoc* 2002;94:695–700.

81. Pedersen J. Hyperglycaemia–hyperinsulinism theory and birthweight. In Pedersen J, ed. *The Pregnant Diabetic and Her Newborn*. Baltimore: Williams & Wilkins, 1977.

82. Carson BS, Phillipps AS, Simmons MA, Battaglia FC, Meschia G. Effects of a sustained insulin infusion upon glucose uptake and oxygenation of the ovine fetus. *Pediatr Res* 1980;14:147–52.

83. Widness JA, Susa JB, Garcia JF, *et al.* Increased erythropoiesis and elevated erythropoietin in infants born to diabetic mothers and in hyperinsulinic rhesus fetuses. *J Clin Invest* 1981;67:637–42.

84. Artal R, Platt LD, Kammula RK, Strassner HT, Gratacos J, Golde SH. Sympathoadrenal activity in infants of diabetic mothers. *Am J Obstet Gynecol* 1982;142:436–9.

85. Bloom SR, Johnston DI. Failure of glucagon release in infants of diabetic mothers. *Br Med J* 1972;4:453–4.

86. Stern L, Ramos A, Leduc J. Urinary catecholamine excretion in infants of diabetic mothers. *Pediatrics* 1968;42:598–605.

87. Milner RDG. Amino acids and beta cell growth in structure and function. In Merkatz IR, Adam PAJ, eds. *The Diabetic Pregnancy: A Perinatal Perspective*. New York: Grune & Stratton, 1979.

88. Reece EA, Homko C, Wiznitzer A. Metabolic changes in diabetic and nondiabetic subjects during pregnancy. *Obstet Gynecol Surv* 1994;49:64–71.

89. Hod M, Star S, Passonneau JV, Unterman TG, Freinkel N. Effect of hyperglycemia on sorbitol and myo-inositol content of cultured rat conceptus: Failure of aldose reductase inhibitors to modify myo-inositol depletion and dysmorphogenesis. *Biochem Biophys Res Commun* 1986;140:974–80.

90. Reece EA, Homko CJ, Wu YK. Multifactorial basis of the syndrome of diabetic embryopathy. *Teratology* 1996;54:171–82.

91. Eriksson UJ, Borg LA. Diabetes and embryonic malformations. Role of substrate-induced free-oxygen radical production for dysmorphogenesis in cultured rat embryos. *Diabetes* 1993;42: 411–9.

92. Hagay ZJ, Weiss Y, Zusman I, *et al.* Prevention of diabetes-associated embryopathy by overexpression of the free radical scavenger copper zinc superoxide dismutase in transgenic mouse embryos. *Am J Obstet Gynecol* 1995;173:1036–41.

93. Goldman AS, Baker L, Piddington R, Marx B, Herold R, Egler J. Hyperglycemia-induced teratogenesis is mediated by a functional deficiency of arachidonic acid. *Proc Natl Acad Sci USA* 1985;2:8227–31.

94. Khandelwal M, Wu YK, Borenstein M, Reece EA. Dietary phospholipid therapy, hyperglycaemia-induced membrane changes and associated diabetic embryopathy. *Am J Obstet Gynecol* 1995;172:265–71.

95. Khandelwal M, Reece EA, Wu YK, Borenstein M. Dietary myo-inositol in hyperglycemia-induced embryopathy. *Teratology* 1998;57:79–84.

96. Menon RK, Cohen RM, Sperling MA, Cutfield WS, Mimouni F, Khoury JC. Transplacental passage of insulin in pregnant women with insulin-dependent diabetes mellitus. Its role in fetal macrosomia. *N Engl J Med* 1990;323:309–15.

97. Reece EA, Homko C, Wiznitzer A. Metabolic changes in diabetic and nondiabetic subjects during pregnancy. *Obstet Gynecol Surv* 1994;49:64–71.

98. Rosenn BM, Miodovnik M, Khoury JC, Siddiqi TA. Deficient counterregulation: A possible risk factor for excessive fetal growth in IDDM pregnancies. *Diabetes Care* 1997;20:872–4.

99. Schwartz R, Gruppuso PA, Petzold K, Brambilla D, Hiilesmaa V, Teramo KA. Hyperinsulinemia and macrosomia in the fetus of the diabetic mother. *Diabetes Care* 1994;17:640–8.

100. Yan-Jun L, Tsushimo T, Minei S, et al. Insulin-like factors (IGFs) and IGF-binding proteins (IGFBP-1, -2, -3) in diabetic pregnancy: Relationship to macrosomia. *Endocr J* 1996;43: 221–31.

101. Roth S, Abernathy MP, Lee WH, et al. Insulin-like growth factors I and II peptide and messenger RNA levels in macrosomic infants of diabetic pregnancies. *J Soc Gynecol Invest* 1996;3:78–84.

102. Ornay A, Ratzon N, Greenbaum G, Peretz E, Soriano D, Dulitzky M. Neurobehaviour of school age children born to diabetic mothers. *Arch Dis Child Fetal Neonatal Ed* 1998;79(2):F94–9.

103. Ornay A, Wolf A, Ratzon N, Greenbaum G, Dulitzky M. Neurodevelopmental outcome at early school age of children born to mothers with gestational diabetes. *Arch Dis Child Fetal Neonatal Ed* 1999;81(1):F10–4.

104. Rizzo TA, Dooley SL, Metzger BE, Cho NH, Ogata ES, Silverman BL. Prenatal and perinatal influences on long-term psychomotor development in offspring of diabetic mothers. *Am J Obstet Gynecol* 1995;173:1753–8.

105. Rizzo TA, Metzger BE, Dooley SL, Cho NH. Early malnutrition and child neurobehavioural development: Insight from the study of children of diabetic mothers. *Child Dev* 1997;68:26–38.

106. Silverman BL, Rizzo TA, Cho NH, Metzger BE. Long-term effects of the intrauterine environment. The Northwestern University Diabetes in Pregnancy Centre. *Diabetes Care* 1998;21(Suppl 2): B142–9.

107. Dorner G, Plagemann A, Reinagel H. Familial diabetes aggregation in type I diabetics: Gestational diabetes an apparent risk factor for increased diabetes susceptibility in the offspring. *Exp Clin Endocrinol* 1987;89:84–90.

108. Dorner G, Steindel E, Thoelke H, Schliack V. Evidence for decreasing prevalence of diabetes mellitus in childhood apparently produced by prevention of hyperinsulinism in the foetus and newborn. *Exp Clin Endocrinol* 1984;84:134–42.

109. Martin AO, Simpson JL, Ober C, Freinkel N. Frequency of diabetes mellitus in mothers of probands with gestational diabetes: Possible maternal influence on the predisposition to gestational diabetes. *Am J Obstet Gynecol* 1985;151:471–5.

110. Pettitt DJ, Aleck KA, Baird HR, Carraher MJ, Bennett PH, Knowler WC. Congenital susceptibility to NIDDM. Role of intrauterine environments. *Diabetes* 1988;37:622–8.

111. Van Assche FA, Holemans K, Aerts L. Fetal growth and consequences for later life. *J Perinat Med* 1998;26:337–46.

112. Howarth JC, McRae KN, Dilling LA. Prognosis of infants of diabetic mothers in relation to neonatal hypoglycaemia. *Dev Med Child Neurol* 1976;18:471–9.

113. Persson B, Gentz J. Follow-up of children of insulin-dependent and gestational diabetic mothers: Neuropsychological outcome. *Acta Pediatr Scand* 1984;73:349–58.

114. Vohr BR, Lipsitt LP, Oh W. Somatic growth of children of diabetic mothers with reference to birth size. *J Pediatr* 1980;97: 196–9.

115. Vohr BR, McGarvey ST, Tucker R. Effects of maternal gestational diabetes on offspring obesity at 4–7 years of age. *Diabetes Care* 1999;22:1284–91.

116. Whitaker RC, Pepe MS, Seidel KD, Wright JA, Knopp RH. Gestational diabetes and the risk of offspring obesity. *Pediatrics* 1998;101:E9.

117. Van Assche FA, Aerts L, Holemans K, Danneels L. Fetal consequences of maternal diabetes. In Andreani D, Bompiani G, Di Mario U, Faulk WP, Galluzo A, eds. *Immunobiology of Normal and Diabetic Pregnancy*. New York: John Wiley, 1990.

118. Warram JH, Martin BC, Krolewski AJ. Possible mechanisms for the diminished risk of IDDM in the children of diabetic mothers. In Andreani D, Bompiani G, Di Mario U, Faulk WP, Galluzo A, eds. *Immunobiology of Normal and Diabetic Pregnancy.* New York: John Wiley, 1990.
119. Hales CN, Barker DJ. Type 2 (non insulin-dependent) diabetes mellitus: The thrifty phenotype hypothesis. *Diabetologia* 1992;35:595–601.
120. Phillips DI, Barker DJ, Hales CN, Hirst S, Osmond C. Thinness at birth and insulin resistance in adult life. *Diabetologia* 1994;37:150–4.
121. Johnston F. Outcome of pregnancy in diabetic women. Authors did not define criterion for case selection (author reply). *Br Med J* 2001;322:614.
122. Golding J. ALSPAC (Avon Longitudinal Study of Parents and Children) Study Team. Outcome of pregnancy in diabetic women. More investigation is needed into whether control of diabetes is really poorer in England than Norway. *Br Med J* 2001; 322(7286):614–5.
123. Hawthorne G, Irgens LM, Tie RT, Moe N, Jervell J. Retraction of paper on maternal diabetes (letter). *Br Med J* 2003;327:929.

9 Neonatal seizures

A. Beke and Z. Papp

Definition

Seizures have been defined as abnormal, paroxysmal, stereotypical clinical events that are initiated by the hypersynchronous activity of neurons in the brain.[1] They represent rapid alteration in the function of the nervous system by which the motor, behavioral or autonomic functions (or all of these) are clinically affected. Seizures are far commoner in the first month of life than at any other time. Neonatal seizures have been described in both clinical and electrical terms. Clinical seizures have been described as occurring in close association with electroencephalograph (EEG) seizure activity (epileptic in origin), and without accompanying EEG seizure activity (presumably non-epileptic in origin). All the clinical seizures described indicate the presence of significant central nervous system dysfunction. In this regard, the findings of EEG monitoring studies do not change a fundamental concept concerning seizures of the newborn: each newly diagnosed neonatal seizure represents a neurological emergency.[2]

Incidence

Conventionally, the neonatal period is limited to the first 4 weeks of life. However, some authors[3,4] define neonatal seizures as those that occur up to 44 weeks of postmenstrual age, to take into account premature birth. Although convulsive phenomena are the most frequent among the major neurological disorders in the neonatal period, their precise frequency is unknown because many of the subtle manifestations of neonatal convulsions may escape recognition. Conversely, jittery and tremulous movements, common at this period, are often mistaken for convulsive seizures, although their significance is completely different. The true incidence of neonatal seizures varies in different series from 0.15% to 1.4%.[5–10] Scher *et al.*[11] found that the incidence of seizures among all neonates admitted to the intensive care unit was 2.3%, and the group of preterm neonates of <30 weeks of gestational age had a seizure frequency of 3.9%, which was significantly higher than that of older preterm or full-term neonates. The very high incidence (up to 22.7%) reported in premature infants by Bergman *et al.*[6] is probably due to the frequency of non-epileptic events in this group.[1] Seay and Bray[12] reported seizures in 20% of infants admitted to the intensive care unit, weighing 2500 g or below. In general, an incidence of neonatal seizures of between 4 and 6 per 1000 infants seems to be a realistic figure. This figure is much higher among the most immature infants. Neonatal seizures appear to be associated with major morbidities and surgical interventions in very low-birth-weight infants. Continuous electroencephalographic monitoring could be warranted in infants following surgical treatment.[13]

Pathophysiology

The site of paroxysmal activity may arise from previously normal neurons. This fire due to a trigger and abnormal conduction occurs through neighboring neurons. Alternatively, the nouronal focus may be inherently abnormal and fires repetitively. Seizures in infants and children may be due to either or both mechanisms.[10] Seizures indicate the presence of a central nervous system dysfunction and may contribute to additional brain injury.[14–16]

Brain maturation progresses rapidly during the last weeks of gestation and in the postnatal period. Structural and functional development of the central nervous system is reflected in the rapidly changing bioelectrical activity and behavior of the brain. This has been extensively documented during the past decades in studies of various mammalian species[17,18] and human preterm and newborn infants.[19–21] In the term newborn, the archicortex (i.e. diencephalon and brain stem) is at a relatively more advanced stage of development than is the neocortex. A significant percentage of paroxysmal electrical discharges in the newborn brain, which arise from subcortical gray matter, might not be identified by EEG scalp recordings. Two possible explanations exist for clinical seizures without an electrographic signature:[22]

(1) Tonic posturing and motor automatism are epileptic but are generated in the brain stem, and the paroxysmal electrical epileptic activity is not manifested at the scalp and not recorded by surface EEG electrodes.
(2) Tonic posturing and motor automatisms are generated and elaborated at a brain-stem level by a non-epileptic mechanism.

It has been suggested that the latter explanation is more plausible.[23,24] Although the lack of a close association to EEG seizure activity would only suggest that tonic posturing and motor automatisms are not epileptic in origin, it is these clinical characteristics of the behaviors that provide the evidence for a non-epileptic mechanism. Tonic posturing and motor automatism may be evoked by tactile stimulation; a graded increase occurs in the magnitude of the response proportional to an increase in the intensity of the stimulus at a single site (temporal summation) or an increase in the number of sites of stimulation (spatial summation). The response may spread to muscle groups other than those originally stimulated (irradiation of the response). Both provoked and spontaneous tonic posturing and motor automatism may be suppressed by restraint or repositioning of the body or affected limbs. All of these features are typical of reflex behaviors[25–27] and are not characteristic of epileptic seizures. On this basis, it has been proposed that tonic posturing and motor automatisms result from depression of forebrain function and the consequent disinhibition of the brain-stem centers that facilitate primitive reflex behaviors.[23,24] This hypothesis is based not only on clinical observations but also on the correlation of these findings with experimental studies of reflex physiology in animals.[24,28] Primitive reflex behaviors are normally mediated by spinal mechanisms and facilitated by centers within the brain stem. These centers are tonically inhibited by the forebrain and may be stimulated by proprioceptive and entroceptive pathways activated by limb and truncal manipulation. When the forebrain is depressed, brain-stem centers are disinhibited, and primitive reflexes may occur spontaneously or be evoked by stimulation. It has been proposed that these behaviors, as a group, be designated 'brain-stem release phenomena' rather than epileptic seizures.[26,29] Although neurons are in place by the time of birth, their axonal and dentritic ramifications and synaptic connections are still incompletely developed in the neonatal human brain,[30,31] and myelination is limited to a few pathways not including the main hemispheric commissures.[32] The *hyperexcitability* of the immature cortex is explained by the underdevelopment of the myelinization and the characteristic phenomena;[33–35] the *modification* of the shapes of spikes depends on the developmental stage of dendrites; the *propagation* of discharges is determined by the state of maturity of the cortical and subcortical and interhemispherial connections.[36]

Kolmodin and Meyerson[37] found the age-related variations of the potential stable and others observed the role of the enzymatic reactions.[38,39] In addition, synaptic connection and transport across synaptic membranes is much less efficient in the immature brain.[40] Both inhibitory [γ-amino butyric acid (GABA)-ergic] and excitatory receptors are present in the human newborn but are not fully developed or are not completely functional because of the incomplete development of the appropriate circuitry.[41,42] There is evidence that the inhibitory dopamine transmitters have a predominant effect over excitatory transmitters in the developing brain.[43] The neonatal brain appears uniquely susceptible to seizure because neonatal GABA receptors are excitatory, and are functionally more active than *N*-methyl-D-aspartate (NMDA) receptors at this time of life.[44] The absence of generalized tonic–clonic seizures probably reflects both the lack of a sufficient degree of cortical organization (which is necessary to propagate and sustain the electrical discharge) and the failure of interhemispheric transmission, resulting from commissural immaturity. Experimental data suggest that neonatal seizures may have a deleterious effect on the developing brain, depleting cerebral glucose, which may interfere with DNA synthesis, glial proliferation and differentiation and myelinization.[45–47] Younkin *et al.*,[48] using nuclear resonance spectroscopy, showed a marked depletion of brain phosphocreatine and adenosine triphosphate during a subtle seizure, which was reversed following phenobarbital therapy and seizure cessation. Animal studies have shown that seizures impair neurogenesis and derange neuronal structure, function and connectivity ('cells that fire together'). The hippocampus has been well studied because it is particularly susceptible to seizure-induced injury. Seizures cause synaptic reorganization with aberrant growth (sprouting) of the dentate granule cell (DGC) axons (i.e. the mossy fibers).[49] There is also apoptosis in the inner granule cell layer of the dentate hilus, and bilateral hippocampal sclerosis has been found at autopsy in human babies who suffered prolonged seizures. Seizures lead to a mismatch between energy supply and demand, and although there is a rise in cerebral flow this may not be sufficient to meet the requirement.[50] Neonates have a low cerebral metabolic rate and a fragmentary neuronal network, making them less vulnerable to neuronal damage and cell loss than adults and more resistant to the toxic effects of glutamate. However, seizures undoubtedly can inhibit brain growth, modify neuronal circuits and increase neuronal excitability. Recurrent seizures during early development have been shown to result in impairment of visual-spatial learning and memory.[51,52] Status epilepticus and recurrent seizures have also been shown to predispose the brain to seizures in later life.[53] Magnetic resonance spectroscopy studies show areas of cerebral metabolic dysfunction in babies with seizures.[54] Status epilepticus can result in necrotic damage to the thalamus in immature rats.[55] The response of the developing brain to epileptic seizures and to status epilepticus is highly age specific. Neonates with their low cerebral metabolic rate and fragmentary neuronal networks can tolerate relatively prolonged seizures without suffering massive cell death, but severe seizures in experimental animals inhibit brain growth, modify neuronal circuits and can lead to behavioral deficits and to increases in neuronal excitability. Past infancy, the developing brain is characterized by a high metabolic rate, exuberant neuronal and synaptic networks and overexpression of receptors and enzymes involved in excitotoxic mechanisms. The outcome of seizures is highly model dependent. Status epilepticus may produce massive neuronal death, behavioral deficits, synaptic reorganization or chronic epilepsy in some models, and little damage in others. We now have some models that reliably lead to spontaneous seizures and chronic epilepsy in the vast majority of animals, demonstrating that seizure-induced epileptogenesis can occur in the developing brain. The mode of cell death from status epilepticus is largely (but not exclusively) necrotic in adult, while the incidence of apoptosis increases at younger ages. Seizure-induced necrosis has many of the biochemical features of apoptosis, with early cytochrome release from mitochondria and capsase activation. Wasterlain *et al.* speculate that this form of necrosis is associated with seizure-induced energy failure.[56] A recent finding is that neonatal seizures can permanently disrupt neuronal development, induce synaptic reorganization, alter plasticity and 'prime' the brain to increased damage from seizure later in life. This finding has led to a renewal of interest in the topic of neonatal seizures, particularly regarding treatment.[57]

Edwards *et al.* found that prenatal stress alters the seizure threshold and the development of kindled seizures in infant and adult rats. Their findings indicate that stress, particularly during the latter half of pregnancy, may play an important role in increasing vulnerability to seizures in the unborn offspring.[58] The idea that stem cells may play a role in the pathophysiology or potential treatment of specific epilepsy syndromes is relatively new.[59] Knowledge of the normal neurogenesis pathways in the mature brain has led to recent studies of neurogenesis in rodent models of acute seizures or epileptogenesis. Current evidence indicates that single brief or prolonged seizures, as well as repeated kindled seizures, increase DGC neurogenesis. Recent work also suggests that pilocarpine-induced status epilepticus increases rostral forebrain subventricular zone (SVZ) neurogenesis and caudal SVZ gliogenesis. These abnormalities include aberrant mossy fiber reorganization, persistence of immature DCG structure (e.g. basal dendrites) and abnormal migration of newborn neurons to ectopic sites in the dentate gyrus. Taken together, these findings suggest a proepileptogenic role of seizure- or injury-induced neurogenesis in the epileptic hippocampal formation. However, the induction of forebrain SVZ neurogenesis and directed migration to injury after seizures and other brain insults underscores the potential therapeutic use of neural stem cells as a source for neuronal replacement after injury.

Table 9.1 Electroclinical classification of neonatal seizures (from Younkin[2] with permission)

Clinical seizures with a consistent electrocortical signature
- A. Focal clonic
  - Unifocal
  - Multifocal
    - Alternating
    - Migrating
  - Hemiconvulsive
  - Axial
- B. Myoclonic
  - Generalized
  - Focal
- C. Focal tonic
  - Asymmetric truncal
  - Eye deviation

Clinical seizures with no electrocortical signature
- A. Motor automatisms
  - Oral–buccal–lingual movements
  - Ocular movements
  - Progression movements
    - Pedaling
    - Stepping
    - Rotary arm movements
  - Complex purposeless movements
- B. Generalized tonic
  - Extensor
  - Flexor
  - Mixed extensor/flexor
- C. Myoclonic
  - Generalized
  - Focal

The classification of neonatal seizures

Recently, neonatal seizures have been characterized and classified according to their presumed pathophysiology, with the suggestion that some neonatal seizures are epileptic in origin and others are not (Table 9.1).[2,60,61] Seizure recognition, characterization and classification create the foundation of care of the neonate who may be at risk for central nervous system dysfunction. For classification of neonatal seizures and for making a guide to clinical recognition a workshop was formed in the USA [participants: Subcommission on Classification and Terminology of Pediatric Epilepsy, Commission on Classification and Terminology, International League against Epilepsy (ILAE) and the Clinical Research

Centers for Neonatal Seizures, National Institute of Neurological Disorders and Stroke, National Institute of Health (NIH)]. The report of the newest classification was published by Mizrahi in 2004.[62] The classification system and the infants presented in the workshop are based on a prospective, clinical study of infants with seizures that have been documented by bedside, video-EEG monitoring. Each seizure was examined by all the investigators together, characterized and then classified by consensus.

Approximately 65% of neonatal seizures are not clearly associated with apparent cortical electrographic seizure activity on the basis of EEG recordings from surface electrodes.[24,63] Neonatal seizure types differ considerably from seizures observed commonly in older children, principally because the newborn infant is less able to sustain organized, generalized epileptiform discharges. The most widely accepted and most often clinically applied classification scheme is that proposed and recently updated by Mizrahi and Kellaway (Table 9.2). Some clinical seizures are characterized by just one type of movement. However, other seizures are more complex. They may begin with one type of movement, which is then followed by others in a sequence typical for that specific seizure. The most effective application of this classification is to use it as a basis to identify the individual components of a single seizure, rather than to classify an entire complex event.

Several seizure types frequently occur together in the same infant; subtle seizures are frequently associated with other types in the severely ill neonate.[5] In addition, various seizure types may be generated by different mechanisms – either epileptic or non-epileptic. The clinical characteristics of a specific seizure may designate its pathophysiology. Thus, the classification of a seizure may suggest a specific mechanism of generation, leading eventually to considerations of therapy and long-term prognosis.

Clonic seizures

Clonic seizures consist of rhythmic muscle jerking that can involve any part of the body and are often

Table 9.2 Classification of neonatal seizures (modified from Mizrahi[62])

I. Clonic
  A. Unifocal: (1) limb, (2) facial, (3) hemiconvulsive
  B. Multifocal: (1) alternating, (2) bilateral, asynchronous
  C. Axial: (1) abdominal, (2) diaphragmal

II. Tonic
  1. Focal: (1) ocular (sustained eye deviation), (2) limb posturing, (3) asymmetric
  2. Generalized: (1) symmetric – a. flexion, b. extension, c. mixed flexion–extension; (2) asymmetric

III. Myoclonic
  1. Generalized
  2. Focal
  3. Multifocal (fragmentary)

IV. Spasm (generalized)
  1. Flexion
  2. Extension
  3. Mixed extension–flexion

V. Motor automatisms
  A. Oral–buccal–lingual movements: (1) chewing, (2) sucking
  B. Ocular signs: (1) random eye movements, (2) blinking, rhythmic eye opening
  C. Limb (movements of progression): (1) pedaling, (2) swimming
  D. Complex purposeless movements

VI. Autonomic nervous system signs
  A. Respiratory: (1) tachypnea, (2) respiratory pause
  B. Cardiac: (1) tachycardia, (2) bradycardia
  C. Cardiovascular: (1) hypertension, (2) hypotension
  D. Vasomotor: (1) flushing, (2) pallor
  E. Pupillary dilatation
  F. Salivation
  G. Other

VII. No clinical signs – electrical seizure only

VIII. Unclassified

ILAE–NIH classification of neonatal seizures

associated with simultaneous epileptiform activity on EEG.[64] Two subtypes are recognized, focal clonic and multifocal.

Focal clonic seizures have limited, usually unilateral, involvement of the face, limbs or axial muscles and are often not associated with alterations of the level of consciousness. In many instances, there is an underlying focal lesion, e.g. focal cerebral infarction. However, it is important to realize that metabolic derangements, e.g. hypoglycemia, may present as focal seizures in the newborn.[16] Cockburn *et al.*[65] reported clonic seizures with late hypocalcemia.

Multifocal clonic seizures are observed more frequently in the term newborn, and are a relatively benign form. They involve non-synchronized clonic movements of the extremities, which differ from multifocal clonic seizures in older infants in that abnormal movements in newborns usually migrate in an unordered, non-Jacksonian fashion. For example, clonic movements of one hand may be followed by jerking of the opposite leg.[66] This particular seizure type may be explained by the immature stage of development of the cerebral cortex of the term infant. Thus, although there is sufficient interneuronal communication to permit sustained seizure activity, the immaturity of synaptic development and axonal myelination may prevent the organized spread of electrical impulses. Because of this, generalized tonic–clonic seizures, which are symmetric and synchronous, occur infrequently in the term newborn.[30]

Tonic seizures

Tonic seizures are most often generalized, featuring tonic extension of all limbs (which resembles 'decerebrate' posturing), or, occasionally, flexion of the upper limb with the extension of the legs (which resembles 'decorticate' posturing). Eye signs such as opening or closing movements of eyelids, staring, gaze deviation or the occurrence of a few clonic jerks may be a clue to their epileptic mechanism. Volpe[30] found tonic seizures to be particularly common among premature infants, and they accounted for 70% of fits seen in infants weighing 2500 g or less. This form of seizure occurs in infants with significant cerebral injury [e.g. massive intraventricular hemorrhage (IVH)] and is associated with a bad prognosis. In approximately 85% of cases, the abnormal posturing is accompanied by electrical seizure activity or autonomic phenomena and the response to anticonvulsant therapy is poor.[12,30] This observation gives rise to the possibility that such posturing represents abnormal brain-stem release phenomena as opposed to true epileptic seizures.[23,30,67] In these instances, although there is no corresponding electrical seizure activity, the interictal EEG is usually severely abnormal with marked voltage suppression.[29]

Myoclonic seizures

Myoclonic seizures, which may be focal, multifocal or generalized, are rare in the neonatal period. They may occur in infants of any gestational age and are associated with time-synchronized EEG discharges only in a minority of cases.[24] They are characterized by rapid, unilateral or bilateral, single or multiple flexion jerks of the upper extremities, but to a lesser extent. Myoclonic seizures often signify severe structural or metabolic cerebral disturbance. They often persist into infancy as more or less atypical infantile spasms.[68,69] A benign variety of neonatal myoclonus has been described, which occurs characteristically only during sleep. Focal and multifocal myoclonic activity may be observed, which is difficult to distinguish clinically from epileptic seizures. However, the correlation with the sleep state and the absence of associated EEG abnormalities may be helpful in this. It typically resolves spontaneously before 6 months of age.[70–72]

Spasms

Spasms may be flexor, extensor or mixed extensor and flexor, and may occur in clusters. Spasms cannot be provoked by stimulation or suppressed by restraint. Pathophysiology is epileptic.

Motor automatisms (subtle seizures)

Subtle seizures may be the most common type and are present to some degree in most term newborns with seizures. This category includes all paroxysmal steps of behavior in newborns that may be sustained, and that cannot be readily classified as myoclonic seizures. Subtle or minimal seizures are also termed 'motor automatisms' by some investigators.[73] The most common clinical manifestation is a variety of ocular movements, e.g. eye opening, tonic horizontal deviation of the eyes; orofacial movements, such as repetitive chewing, swallowing, drooling; rotatory limb movements or complex patterns, like pedaling, boxing, swimming or stepping, and autonomic disturbances, such as hyperpnea, vasomotor abnormalities, salivation or modification of the heart rate. Abnormal eye movements, especially in the horizontal plane are of special diagnostic value.[74,75] Unlike sustained eye deviation is typical of focal tonic seizure of epileptic origin; the ocular signs of motor automatisms are less well defined. They include random eye movements, eye opening and blinking.[62] Motor automatisms and generalized tonic posturing may coexist, since their pathophysiologic mechanisms are the same.

Autonomic nervous system signs are often combined with motor automatisms apneic seizures are common, sometimes in isolation,[76,77] but more often in association with ocular or other autonomic signs. Fenichel *et al.*[78] found that apneic seizures were not accompanied by bradycardia, as opposed to the much more frequent non-epileptic apneas of the premature infant, which last 20 s or more. Other studies involving simultaneous video-EEG investigations demonstrated that subtle clinical phenomena are frequently accompanied by simultaneous electrical discharges in premature infants.[79] The EEG signs that are associated with subtle seizures occur commonly in the temporal leads,[64] which is not surprising as similar clinical features are frequently observed in older children in complex partial seizures, which originate in the temporal lobes. Alterations in the autonomic function as a seizure manifestation raise particular diagnostic problems. Thus, although apneic episodes in the premature infant may rarely be a manifestation of seizure activity,[79] they are much more likely to be related to other mechanisms. In contrast, apnea in the term newborn appears to be associated more commonly with electrical seizure activity. Recently, the apneic episodes have been observed and differentiated in newborns and especially in prematures with a new polygraphic computerized method (SLEEP Labor). We can also determine the type of apnea exactly: central, obstructive or mixed. Figure 9.1 shows a polygraphic investigation demonstrating a central apnea (cenA-) following the electrical activity change on the FP1 channel. There is no significant change in ECG (examination of the author). Infantile spasms and episodic apnea (associated with electroencephalographic seizure activity) may also occur as neonatal seizures, but they are rare and currently do not warrant major classifications.[3]

Isolated seizures are relatively uncommon in the neonatal period. The occurrence of at least a few attacks is the rule. However, neonatal seizures tend to be self-limited and to last 24–96 h,[80–82] which complicates the assessment of therapy further.

Neonatal status epilepticus has been defined by Dreyfus-Brisac and Monod[83,84] as the repetition of clinical and/or purely electrical seizures with the interictal persistence of an abnormal neurological status. Cukier *et al.*[82] redefined the term with greater precision as the occurrence of electrical seizure discharges, each lasting at least 10 s and repeated for several hours, in association with an abnormal neurological state and unconsciousness. Clinical seizures may or may not be present. The latter definition does not include repeated clinical seizures without ictal EEG concomitants such as those that may occur in neonates who have been convulsing for many hours.[85] The term serial seizures is perhaps preferable to that of status epilepticus in the neonatal period because it does not refer to an abnormal interictal neurological state, which may be impossible to assess reliably on account of the interference of drug treatment.[3] With prolonged convulsive episodes, there is a tendency for individual seizures to change from well-marked to poorly organized attacks, clinically as well as electrically.

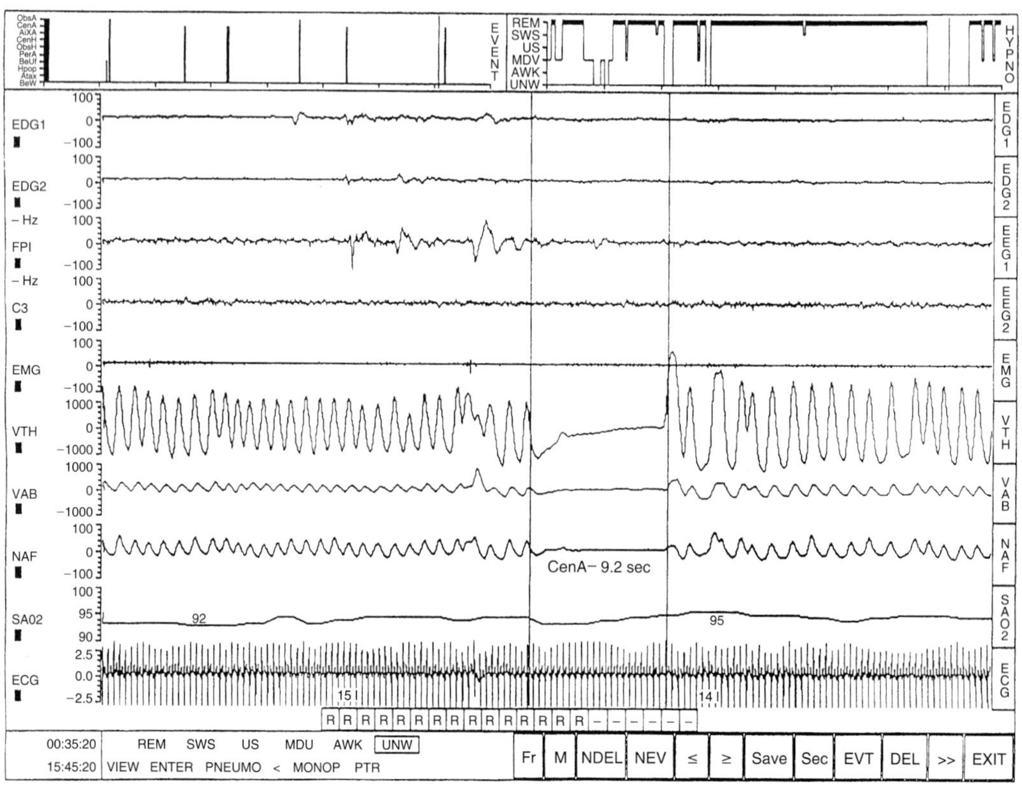

Figure 9.1 Central apnea demonstrated by polygraphy.

Etiology

Although the etiology of neonatal seizures is extremely diverse, most of them can be attributed to hypoxic-ischemic encephalopathy (about 65% of neonatal seizures), intracranial hemorrhage (about 15%), metabolic disturbances (hypoglycemia, hypocalcemia), intracranial infection and cerebral cortical dysgenesis. Table 9.3.

Hypoxic-ischemic encephalopathy is the most important cause of neonatal seizures in infants and in all gestational ages.[30] It has been estimated to account for approximately two-thirds of all cases. Seizures are a major manifestation of moderate or severe intrapartum hypoxic-ischemia encephalopathy in approximately 50% of affected term newborns and are associated with long-term neurological sequelae in at least 20–40% of cases.[30,86] Many cases are probably of prenatal origin, so a low weight for date and other signs of dysmaturity are common findings.[66] Postnatal respiratory insufficiency causes less than 10% of cases of hypoxic encephalopathy.[30] Ischemia is secondary to intrauterine asphyxia with cardiac insufficiency. Seizures begin most frequently during the first day of life,[87–89] and 60% of the patients with this condition have already had fits by 12 h.[30] The seizures are often isolated at the start. Of the cases of neonatal status epilepticus 75–85% have been attributed to hypoxic insult.[30] Seizures may be of any type and are often prolonged and refractory to anticonvulsant therapy. Brown[90] has pointed out that the seizures usually occur when infants show a transition in muscle tone. The interictal EEG is of the 'tracé paroxystique' or inactive tracing type in severe cases.[91] The convulsions may be extremely difficult to control by drugs. Levene *et al.*[92] have reported neonatal convulsions due to asphyxia to occur in 2 per 1000 full-term infants. Delivoria-Papadopoulos and Mishra studied the mechanism of cerebral hypoxia in the fetus and newborn that results in neonatal morbidity and mortality as well a long-term sequelae such as mental retardation, seizure disorders and cerebral palsy. Using electron spin resonance (ESR) spectroscopy they demonstrated that tissue hypoxia results in increased free-radical generation in the cortex of fetal guinea pigs and newborn piglets.[93] Normally, more than 80% of the oxygen consumed by the cell is completely reduced by cytochrome oxidase to reactions with the cytoplasm and mitochondria that produce a superoxide anion radical. To protect cells from the deleterious effects of free radicals, a number of enzymatic and non-enzymatic defenses such as catalase, superoxide dismutase, glutathione peroxidase, ascorbic acid and vitamin E are present in cells.

The hypoxia-induced increase in lipid peroxidation products was shown to be also associated with a decrease in cell membrane Na^+,K^+-ATPase activity. The direct demonstration of production of free radicals during hypoxia was documented by measuring the signal of spin adducts using ESR, which allows direct identification and characterization of free radicals.[94] The brain tissue hypoxia modified the NMDA receptor ion channel recognition and modulation sites. A higher increase in NMDA receptor agonist-dependent Ca^{2+} in synaptosomes was demonstrated. The increase in intracellular Ca^{2+} may activate several enzymatic pathways such as phospholipase A and metabolism of arachidonic acid by cyclooxygenase and lipoxygenase, conversion of xanthine dehydrogenase to xanthine oxidase by proteases and activation of nitric oxide synthase. In summary, studies demonstrated that cerebral tissue hypoxia results in increased free-radical generation that may lead to the oxidation of brain cell membrane lipids, membrane enzymes, receptor proteins as well as the nuclear DNA precipitating the hypoxic neuronal injury in the fetus and newborn.

Table 9.3 Correlation of time of onset of seizures and etiology (adapted from Hill and Volpe[73] with permission)

Most frequent time of onset	Etiology of seizures
< 48 h	Hypoxic-ischemic encephalopathy Intracranial hemorrhage Hypoglycemia Sepsis-meningitis Congenital viral infection Drug withdrawal Local anesthetic intoxication Pyridoxine dependency Non-ketotic hyperglycinemia Urea cycle disorders
48–72 h	Cerebral dysgenesis Cerebral infarction Ketotic hyperglycinemia Urea cycle disorders
> 7 days	Cerebral dysgenesis Organic acidopathies Amino acidopathies Urea cycle disorders Bacterial meningitis

Intracranial hemorrhage

This condition is often difficult to establish conclusively as a primary cause of seizure distinct from hypoxic-ischemic encephalopathy or traumatic injury, because of the frequent association of these conditions. There are three important types of hemorrhage according to localization:

Intraventricular hemorrhage is a very common lesion in extremely premature infants, but germinal matrix/IVH is associated relatively rarely with seizures. However, large IVHs, especially if there is associated intraparenchymal hemorrhagic infarction (which accounts for approximately 15% of all examples of IVH), may occur together with generalized tonic seizures, most often as part of a catastrophic deterioration evolving to coma and respiratory arrest. This clinical setting and type of seizure signify an ominous prognosis.[30]

Subdural hemorrhage is most commonly associated with traumatic delivery or non-accidental shaking injury. The associated cerebral contusion frequently results in focal clonic and subtle seizures. Such seizures most commonly begin during the first 48 h of life.[95] Subdural hemorrhage occurring as a result of tentorial tears is not necessarily fatal and may have a relatively good prognosis.

Primary *subarachnoid hemorrhage*, especially of a minor degree, is a very common occurrence in newborns and is usually not of major clinical significance. When seizures occur secondary to the subarachnoid hemorrhage in the full-term infant, they occur most commonly on the second day of life.[96] During the interictal period, affected infants often appear remarkably healthy, leading to the descriptive term 'well baby with seizures'. Spanish authors have reported neonatal convulsions and subarachnoid hemorrhage after paroxetine treatment in the third trimester of pregnancy.[97]

Neonatal stroke

Billard et al.[98] reported eight infants presenting focal seizures between the age of 8 and 72 h and all had evidence of cerebral infarction on the computed tomography (CT) scan. Only three of these infants showed evidences of subsequent handicap. Venkataraman *et al.* studied 11 full-term babies with neonatal stroke. Seizure was the most common presenting sign, with paucity of other focal neurological deficits.[99]

The few days before and after birth are a time of special risk for stroke in both mother and infant, probably related to activation of coagulation mechanisms in this critical period. Arterial ischemic stroke around the time of birth is recognized in about 1 in 4000 full-term infants, and may present with neurological and systemic signs in the newborn.[100] Neonatal seizures are most commonly the clinical finding that triggers assessment. In other children, prenatal stroke is recognized only retrospectively, with emerging hemiparesis or seizure after the early month of life. Risk factors for perinatal stroke include hereditary or acquired thrombophilias and environmental factors. Perinatal stroke underlies an important share of congenital hemiplegic cerebral palsy, and probably some spastic quadriplegic cerebral palsy and seizure disorders. There is much to be learned about the natural history of perinatal stroke, and there are as yet no evidence-based strategies for prevention or treatment.

Intracranial infection

Both the bacterial and the non-bacterial types of intracranial infection are common causes of neonatal seizures. Seizures secondary to bacterial meningitis are most likely to occur after the first week of life. Like the common metabolic disturbances, they are of particular concern because definitive therapy is of primary importance. Of the bacterial infections, meningitides secondary to group B streptococci, *Listeria monocytogenes* and *Escherichia coli* are the most common. In addition to bacterial meningitis, meningo-encephalitis may occur due to herpes simplex, Coxackie and toxoplasmosis. In the latter case, toxoplasmosis may be acquired in early pregnancy and extensive brain damage may have occurred by the time of delivery. Cytomegalovirus and rubella infections acquired in early pregnancy may also present with neonatal fits, without any signs of other infections. Septicemic infants, without meningitis, may also develop seizures. The cause of this can be the complication associated with infection and hypoglycemia or hypotension. Diarrhea due to infection may cause disturbances in the sodium balance, which may also cause seizures. Herpes simplex virus type 1 (HSV-1) encephalitis is the most common cause of acquired epilepsy in human. Chen *et al.* studied *in vitro* HSV-1-infected organotypic hippocampal slice culture to elucidate the underlying mechanisms of HSV-1-associated acute seizure activity. The results suggest that a direct change in excitability of the hippocampal CA3 neuronal network and HSV-1-induced neuron loss resulting in subsequent mossy fiber reorganization may play an important role in the generation of epileptiform activity.[101]

Metabolic disturbances

Although different kinds of metabolic derangement and certain intoxications are associated with convulsive phenomena in newborn infants, abnormalities of glucose and divalent cation homeostasis are the most frequent.

Hypoglycemia is most common in infants who are small for their gestational age and in infants of mothers with diabetes or gestational diabetes.[102] The brain can use few sources of energy, glucose being the most important. Hypoglycemia may cause devastating neurological damage when the brain's energy reserves are exhausted. The most important determinant of the occurrence of neurological signs in neonatal hypoglycemia appears to be the duration of this. Monod *et al.*[103] observed that among the prematures, hypoglycemia may be very low, without any seizures. Neurological symptoms consist most commonly of jitteriness, stupor, hypotonia and apnea, as well as seizures. The onset of the seizures is usually early, often on the second postnatal day. In many instances hypoglycemia occurs in the context of hypoxic-ischemic encephalopathy, IVH or infection. Secondary transient hypoglycemia may occur in association with meningitis or following exchange transfusion. Persistent hypoglycemia may be observed in certain inborn errors of metabolism, e.g. galactosemia, fructosemia, leucin sensitivity, glucos-6-phosphatase deficiency, etc. Other rare disorders that must be considered include the Beckwith–Wiedemann syndrome, pancreatic islet cell tumors and anterior pituitary hypoplasia. The importance of early diagnosis and treatment of hypoglycemia has become more critical. Recent data suggest that even moderate hypoglycemia in the premature newborn may be associated with poor outcome.[104]

Electrolyte disturbances

Divalent cations are regulators of the ion fluxes associated with membrane depolarization. Because of this, abnormalities in their homeostasis are more likely to result in electrical seizures than in the homeostasis in monovalent cations. However, both hyponatremia and hypernatremia have been associated with seizures because of derangements in cell volume. The most common cause of these disturbances is inappropriate fluid therapy. In infants with serious neurological or pulmonary disease, the syndrome of inappropriate secretion of antidiuretic hormone may result in severe hyponatremia and seizures.[30]

Hypocalcemia/hypomagnesemia

Infants with seizures due to hypocalcemia are usually alert between seizures and the seizures are often multifocal and migratory. Hypocalcemia occurs at two peak times in the newborn period. Early hypocalcemia, which occurs in the first 2–3 days of life, seems to be in association with other potential etiologic factors that appear to play a major role in the origin of the convulsions. The definition of hypocalcemia is taken to be serum calcium below 1.75 mmol/l (7 mg/dl). The ionized calcium is a more important predictor; unfortunately, this is a difficult measurement in clinical practice. Ionized calcium is responsible in part for axonal conduction as well as neuromuscular function. In addition, magnesium is an important comineral for the function of the neuromuscular junction.[10] Functional hypocalcemia can be diagnosed by assessing cardiac neuromuscular conduction on the electrocardiograph. Early-onset hypocalcemia is often observed in the context of hypoxic-ischemic encephalopathy, in newborns with low birth weight, in prematures with hyaline membrane disease and in infants of diabetic mothers. In rare cases, early severe hypocalcemia is due to parathyroid hypoplasia or aplasia. The commonest condition associated with absent parathyroid is Di George syndrome. An infusion of intravenous calcium may be useful for determining whether seizures are caused directly by the low calcium level. Late-onset hypocalcemia is relatively uncommon and presents as an isolated condition without other associated or underlying diseases. Classically, such hypocalcemic infants are large, term infants who have avidly consumed a milk preparation with a suboptimal ratio of phosphorus to calcium and phosphorus to magnesium, e.g. cow's milk. The neurological syndrome is consistent and distinctive, and it consists primarily of hyperactive tendon reflexes. Hypocalcemia fits are treated with intravenous 10% calcium gluconate and the seizures should stop soon after administration. Hypomagnesemia often coexists with hypocalcemia and convulsions are likely to occur at serum levels below 0.3 mmol/l. Giving magnesium alone to hypocalcemic infants caused both serum magnesium and calcium to rise.[65] Manzar mentioned a case of a newborn with late-onset seizure with hypocalcemia, hyperphosphatemia and raised parathyroid hormone. The infant did not have any stigmata of pseudohypoparathyroidism. The hypocalcemia was initially resistant to calcium therapy but responded to vitamin D analog therapy. Transient pseudohypoparathyroidism was entertained.[105]

Table 9.4 Inborn errors of metabolism that may cause neonatal seizures (adapted from Levene[10] with permission)

Maple syrup urine disease
Urea cycle defects
Tyrosinemia
Non-ketotic hyperglycinemia
Proprionic acidemia
Methyl malonic acidemia
Other organic acidemias

Table 9.5 Neonatal storage diseases that may cause neonatal fits (adapted from Levene[10] with permission)

Adrenoleukodystrophy
Alexander's disease
Alper's disease
Gaucher's disease
Krabbe's leukodystrophy
Niemann Pick disease
Tay Sachs disease
Zellweger's syndrome

Congenital abnormalities

Tables 9.4 and 9.5 list inborn errors of metabolism and neuronal storage diseases that may cause neonatal fits.[10]

Pyridoxine dependency is a rare, autosomal recessive disorder of the pyridoxine metabolism. Pyridoxine is a cofactor necessary for the synthesis of the inhibitory neurotransmitter GABA, a deficiency that may presumably produce severe neonatal seizures recalcitrant to all treatment except the administration of large doses of pyridoxine.[106] Fewer than 100 patients have been reported, and only four reports have included examples of brain imaging findings.

Gospe *et al.* found in their patient progressive magnetic resonance changes – dilatation of the ventricular system, cortical and white matter atrophy. The abnormalities may be due to chronic excitotoxicity caused by an imbalance of cerebral levels of GABA and glutamic acid.[107]

Kernicterus

Bilirubin is a neurotoxic substance that may cause a clinical syndrome in severely jaundiced infants, referred to as kernicterus. The most severe form of this condition includes opisthotonus, sunsetting and neonatal tonic seizures.

Any abnormality in the cerebral development may cause neonatal seizures but disorders of neuronal migration are particularly likely to be associated with abnormal neurological behavior and fits. Seizures in these infants are usually very difficult to control. Genetically determined disorders such as Sturge–Weber syndrome, tuberose sclerosis and incontinentia pigmenti may also rarely cause neonatal convulsion.[10] Hennel *et al.* found in their case with incontinentia pigmenti evolution of acute microvascular hemorrhagic infarcts in the periventricular white matter in the first week of life. The associated magnetic resonance angiogram findings consisted of decreased branching and poor filling of intracerebral vessels.[108] Table 9.6 lists some congenital cerebral abnormalities that may be associated with neonatal convulsion.[10] Wada *et al.* show a female patient who has enlargement of lateral ventricles and atrophy of the brain associated with infantile spasms. The ventriculomegaly was documented *in utero* at as early as the 28th week of gestation with lactic acidosis due to deficiency of the pyruvate dehydrogenase E1 (alpha) subunit, demonstrating that the changes characteristic of this disease can occur antenatally. The mechanism of infantile spasms in this disease may be linked to mosaicism of the brain cells involving the normal enzyme and the mutant enzyme.[109]

Table 9.6 Congenital cerebral abnormalities that may be associated with neonatal convulsions (adapted from Levene[10] with permission)

Pachygyria
Micropolygyria
Congenital porencephaly
Hydrocephalus
Holoprosencephaly
Neurofibromatosis
Sturge–Weber syndrome
Incontinentia pigmenti
Tuberose sclerosis
Hydranencephaly

Intoxications

Local anesthetics

Seizure may occur when local anesthetics are administered to the mother for episiotomy, or for other types of maternal analgesia. The major clinical features of toxicity include a very low Apgar score, apnea or severe hypoventilation, severe bradycardia and hypotonia and severe bradycardia. Seizures occur early and are commonly tonic in nature. These features are also seen in hypoxic-ischemic encephalopathy. There are two distinguishing features that aid in its differentiation from perinatal hypoxia: the absence of the pupillary response to light and the absence of eye movement with the oculocephalic (doll's eye) maneuver. The absence of these signs is unusual in hypoxic encephalopathy during the first 12 h of life. Management depends on prompt recognition. The half-life of the drug in the blood is approximately 8–10 h.

Methylxanthine

Both theophyllin and caffeine overdosage have resulted in seizures in the neonatal period.[8]

Drug withdrawal

Passive addiction of the newborn and drug withdrawal may be related to maternal ingestion of cocaine, narcotic-analgesics and sedative hypnotics. Many findings demonstrate that exposure to alcohol during brain development can permanently alter the physiology of the hippocampal formation, thus promoting epileptic activity, enhancing kindling and facilitating spreading depression.

Epileptic syndromes in the neonatal period

Subgroups can be recognized among the neonatal convulsions on the basis of the age at onset and/or characteristics of fits and associated neurological manifestations. Although there is some relationship between the age at the onset of seizures and the associated clinical manifestations on the one hand, and etiology and prognosis on the other, it is difficult to isolate well-defined 'epileptic syndromes' during the neonatal period. Most groupings are rather loose, and only familial seizures and a few rare syndromes such as neonatal myoclonic encephalopathy[110,111] stand out clearly.

Neonatal myoclonic encephalopathy[30] is a syndrome characterized clinically by the occurrence of erratic, fragmentary myoclonus of early onset, usually in association with other types of seizures and, from the EEG viewpoint, by a stable suppression–burst pattern persisting after 2 weeks of age.[110,112,113] Seizures associated with the myoclonus include partial motor seizures, massive myoclonias and tonic spasms that are not usually observed before 4–5 months of age. The onset is in the neonatal period and all affected infants have severe neurological impairment; half of them die before the age of 6 months.[112] Familial cases are frequent; a recessive inheritance is probable in some of the cases. The syndrome may result from undetermined metabolic defects or from brain malformations.[114] The relationship of neonatal myoclonic encephalopathy with early infantile epileptic encephalopathy (Ohtahara's disease) is not entirely clear. The two conditions have several clinical and EEG characteristics in common, including the occurrence of tonic spasms and a suppression–burst pattern. Lombroso[115] accepts that early myoclonic encephalopathy is distinct from the Ohtahara syndrome but considers the latter only as a variant of infantile spasms.

Benign familial epilepsy

An autosomal dominant syndrome of neonatal seizures unrelated to recognized etiologies has been described.[116] The gene for this transient, primary epilepsy of infancy has been recently assigned to chromosome 20q.[117] The onset of the seizures is usually on the second or third postnatal day, and in the interictal period the infants appear remarkably well. Seizures may occur at a frequency of 10–20 per day or even more. The disorder is usually self-limiting. Neurological development is normal. Because of the benign course yet striking clinical presentation, the history of affected family members might easily be missed unless specifically sought.[118]

The 'fifth-day fits' syndrome is characterized by repeated seizures that occur between the third and the seventh days of life in full-term neonates without any abnormal gestational and obstetric antecedent and without any neurological abnormality during the first days of life. According to Dehan *et al.*,[119] the attacks are of two main types: clonic focal or multifocal convulsions and apneic spells. They last on an average 20 h. The interictal EEG shows preserved rhythms and a normal organization of sleep. Bursts of alternating delta-rhythms or 'théta pointu alternant' are observed in three-quarters of the patients. Dehan *et al.* and other authors have underlined the benignity of fifth-day fits when all the criteria of the syndrome were present.[119–121]

Intrauterine seizures have been suspected in several reports.[122,123] Movements identified by mothers as probably convulsive in nature occur mainly in the last days or weeks of gestation. Pyridoxine dependency is a possible cause of intrauterine convulsions,[122,124] but other causes, especially brain dysplasia, can be suspected.

Mulley *et al.* in their review describe the significant number of new gene associations with epilepsy syndromes that have emerged during the past year, together with additional mutations and new electrophysiological data relating to previously known gene associations. Idiopathic epilepsies are predominantly a family of channelopathies. The corresponding ion channel mutations show measurable *in vitro* abnormalities that are likely to affect transmission between neurons. In their paper autosomal dominant juvenile myoclonic epilepsy was demonstrated to be a channelopathy associated with a GABAa receptor, (alpha) 1 subunit mutation. Benign familial neonatal infantile seizures were delineated as another channelopathy of infancy, by molecular characterization of sodium channel, (alpha) 2 subunit defects. A sodium channel, (alpha) 2 subunit defect was previously found to be associated with generalized epilepsy with febrile seizure plus (GEFS+). Similarly, the clinical spectrum associated with potassium channel, KQT-like mutations was extended to include the channelopathy, myokymia and neonatal epilepsy. Mutations in the non-ion channel genes, leucin-rich, glioma inactivated 1 gene and Aristaless related homebox gene (causative gene in X-linked infantile spasms) have emerged as important causes of their specific syndromes, with mutations in the last gene frequently underlying X-linked mental retardation with epilepsy.

There are now nine ion channel subunit genes implicated in 10 syndromes of idiopathic epilepsy.

The boundaries between clinically defined 'idiopathic' and 'cryptogenic' epilepsies are being blurred by the demonstration of sodium channel mutation in the infantile syndrome of severe myoclonic epilepsy in infancy. Genetic heterogeneity has been so far proven for three of the syndromes: autosomal dominant frontal lobe epilepsy, benign familial neonatal seizure and GEFS+. Considerable phenotypic heterogeneity occurs in association with mutations in four of the genes described in GEFS+: sodium channel, (beta) 1 subunit (SCN1B); sodium channel, (alpha) 1 subunit (SCN1A); sodium channel, (alpha) 2 subunit (SCN2A) and GABAa receptor, (gamma) 2 subunit (GABRG2).

Whether progress toward understanding the genetic basis for the rare epilepsies will relate to the development of therapies for the common epilepsies remains to be established, but progress to date has provided remarkable insights into the neurobiology of the epilepsies.[125]

Diagnosis

First- and second-line investigations in infants with seizures are listed in Table 9.7.[10]

Diagnostic evaluation must begin with a careful history and physical examination. From the maternal history it is important to determine the possibility of drug abuse, intrauterine infection and genetic or metabolic disorders. Laboratory investigations should focus initially on treatable causes, such as metabolic

Table 9.7 First- and second-line investigations in infants with seizures (adapted from Levene[10] with permission)

In all infants immediately
Clinical history
Blood sugar
Sodium
Calcium
Magnesium
Ultrasound brain scan
Lumbar puncture
Blood culture
If the above are negative and the infant is still fitting
Prenatal viral screen
Urine for amino acid chromatogram
Urine for organic acid profile
Sugar chromatography for galactose
Pyridoxine infusion
Computer tomography or magnetic resonance scan

disorders and infection. Lumbar puncture or treatment with meningitic doses of antibiotics and acyclovir may be indicated. Rapid diagnosis of the underlying etiology is of major importance to enable the institution of specific and definitive therapy as well as for accurate prediction of the outcome. However, in such instances the diagnosis of a specific underlying disease may have important genetic implications for the family. The time of the onset of seizures may assist in determining an underlying etiology. If the initial screening investigations fail to confirm the etiology, additional studies may be obtained, e.g. CT, cranial ultrasonography, magnetic resonance imaging, serum amino acids, blood pyruvate and lactate, urine amino acids and organic acids, maternal and fetal titer of TORCH [toxoplasma, others, rubella, cytomegalovirus, herpes (hepatitis)] group and syphilis, and urinary drug screen.[30,126]

Differential diagnosis

Jitteriness is a common movement disorder of the newborn, which may be misinterpreted as epileptic seizures. The major features that distinguish jitteriness from seizures are summarized in Table 9.8.[118] The distinction between jitteriness and seizures may be difficult at times because both may occur in a similar context, e.g. hypoxic-ischemic encephalopathy, hypoglycemia, hypocalcemia. Drug withdrawal is another common cause of jitteriness.[127]

EEG in diagnosis

Despite advances in neuroimaging techniques over the past decades that have helped identifying structural

Table 9.8 Clinical characteristics that distinguish jitteriness from seizures (adapted from Hill and Volpe[73] with permission)

Clinical features	Jitteriness	Seizures
Stimulus-sensitive movements	+	–
Movements cease with restraint	+	–
Associated abnormal eye movements	–	+
Quality of movement	Tremor	Clonic jerking

–, absent; +, present

lesions of the central nervous system, EEG continues to provide a valuable insight into brain function by demonstrating focal or diffuse background abnormalities and epileptiform abnormalities. It is an extremely valuable test in patients suspected of epilepsy and in patients with altered mental status and coma. Patterns in the EEG make it possible to clarify the seizure type; it is indispensable for the diagnosis of non-convulsive status epilepticus and for separating epileptic from other paroxysmal (non-epileptic) episodes. There are EEG patterns predictive of the cause of the encephalopathy (i.e. triphasic waves in metabolic encephalopathy) or the location of the lesion (i.e. focal polymorphic delta activity in lesions of the subcortical white matter). An EEG is most helpful in assessing normal or abnormal brain functioning in a newborn because of the serious limitation in performing an adequate neurological examination on the neonate who is intubated or paralyzed for ventilatory control. Under such circumstances, the EEG may be the only tool available to detect an encephalopathic process or the occurrence of epileptic seizures.[128] Neonatal EEG abnormalities may be transient and of benign significance, or may be persistent and severe, indicating neurological morbidity. The clinical usefulness of the EEG is enhanced by recording as soon as possible after the onset of symptoms of the suspected insult, although during the first day of life the stress of birth and the effect of anesthesia may complicate the interpretation of the tracing. If an EEG appears abnormal, recordings may be repeated in 48–72 h, and at weekly or biweekly intervals until discharge or normal patterns appear. Continuous EEG monitoring may be of value for the diagnosis of seizures in newborns that are treated with muscular paralysis to improve assisted ventilation.[129]

The major EEG correlates of neonatal seizures include focal or multifocal spikes or sharp waves and focal monorhythmic discharges. Care must be taken not to confuse epileptiform activity and normal sharp transients in recordings of premature newborns or 'tracé alternant' patterns of quiet sleep in term newborns with seizures. Abnormal motor activity is associated with EEG abnormalities on routine surface recordings in only approximately one-third of the recordings.[126] Several modifications of electroencephalographic techniques have been developed recently to improve the quantification of the frequency and the duration of the seizure activity. These include serial or continuous EEG recordings, and simultaneous video-EEG recordings. Cerebral function monitoring (CFM) is widely used to detect neonatal seizure but comparing with video recording, the observer usually detects generalized seizures but approximately half of all focal neonatal seizures may be missed using CFM only. The CFM may thus be useful for long-term monitoring alone. The digital EEG technology can improve the accuracy of EEG interpretation and lead to more accurate recognition of electroencephalographic features and thereby improve the diagnostic utility of EEG.[130] Clinical interpretation of the EEG during this age-period is difficult because of its rapidly changing morphology. The main characteristics of EEG maturation in preterm infants were a progressive spatiotemporal differentiation, with an increase of rhythmic activities and a decrease of discontinuity. A strong relationship was found between the postmenstrual age of the infants and EEG maturity, but there were exceptions to this rule. A longer duration of extrauterine life had a small accelerating influence on EEG maturation. The relationship between EEG pattern types and behavioral states becomes more stable with increasing age.[131]

Clinically significant and common EEG abnormalities noted in the neonatal period are the next:[132]

Isoelectric pattern in the absence of hypothermia or acute systemic disorders indicates severe and diffuse cerebral dysfunction and is associated with a high incidence of neurological sequelae in survivors.

The paroxysmal pattern, which is characterized by suppression–burst activity, must be distinguished from the discontinuous pattern of the normal preterm, and consists of irregular bursts of abnormal activity on an isoelectric or markedly attenuated ground. The paroxysmal pattern is usually associated with neurological sequelae.

Excessively slow background pattern occurs most commonly in abnormal term newborns, who lack the usual spectrum of beta, delta and transients, are poorly reactive and are not associated with normal wake–sleep cycles; the incidence of neurological sequelae is high.

Persistent asymmetry of the background (reduced by 50%) is sometimes associated with underlying structural lesions, including intracranial hemorrhage.

Excessive interhemispheric asynchrony is commonly noted in association with other EEG abnormalities.

Positive rolandic sharp waves may occur in association with IVH in the newborn, and the positive component is of high amplitude, may be broad in configuration and may be followed by a lower-amplitude negative wave, as well as with other separate focal abnormalities. Positive rolandic sharp waves have also been recorded in neonatal infants with nonhemorrhagic disorders and in apparently normal preterm infants.

Electroencephalographic seizures in preterm and term newborns are associated with a combined mortality and neurological morbidity of approximately 30%; they appear as ictal, repetitive focal or generalized spiking, rhythmic focal or generalized delta and occasionally rhythmic alpha or theta-like activities. There are few specific pathologic EEG patterns associated with specific illnesses (neonatal herpes encephalitis, congenital malformations or Aicardi syndrome).

Patrizi *et al.* observed the characteristics of EEG ictal activity in preterm and full-term infants.[133] They investigated the trend for a closer relationship between behavioral changes during the electroencephalographic seizure when the background activity was normal or moderately abnormal than when background activity was severely abnormal. In both, preterm and full-term infants, the most common site of seizure origin was the temporal lobe. Full-term infants commonly had sharp waves, spikes, sharp and slow waves and spike and slow waves at the onset of the ictus while rhythmic delta activity was most common in the preterm infants. Preterm infants typically had a regional onset to the ictus whereas full-term infants most frequently had a focal onset. There was no clear relationship between onset, morphology, frequency or propagation of the ictal discharge in both age groups. The results demonstrate that while the type of ictal discharge is related to gestational age, there is a rich variety in the onset, morphology and frequency of the ictal discharges in both groups. Generally, neonatal ictal patterns lack a close correlation with the underlying pathology.

Therapy

The newborn exhibiting seizure activity should be treated on an urgent basis with adequate support ventilation and perfusion, correction of any underlying metabolic derangements and the use of anticonvulsant medication.

Treatment of neonatal seizures is directed toward minimizing physiological and metabolic derangements that are associated with the epileptic process and to prevent recurrence of seizures. The choice of anticonvulsants in the treatment of neonatal seizures should consider the unique characteristics of neonatal seizures and the efficacy, toxicity and pharmacologic appropriateness of the drug. All aspects of toxicity are to be considered, but two factors of immediate concern in neonates are changes in heart rate and effects on brain growth.[132] The generally used order of antiepileptic drugs and their doses are indicated in Table 9.9.

Table 9.9 Treatment of neonatal seizures (adapted from Younkin[2] with permission)

Initial therapy

1. Phenobarbital 20 mg/kg i.v.; if seizures continue, phenobarbital 10 mg/kg i.v. every 15–30 min to a total of 40 mg/kg or to a serum level of 40 μg/ml
2. Phenytoin 20 mg/kg i.v.; if seizures continue, phenytoin 10 mg/kg intravenously to a serum level of 20 μg/ml. If seizures continue
3. Diazepam 0.1–0.3 mg/kg i.v. repeated as necessary, or 0.7–2.75 mg/h continuous intravenous infusion
   Lorazepam 0.05–0.10 mg/kg i.v. repeated as necessary
   Paraldehyde 200–400 mg/kg i.v. over first hour, then 16 mg/kg/h; adjust infusion rate based on EEG response

Since clinical detection of seizures is frequently inaccurate, it is helpful to have continuous and video-EEG monitoring during the initiation of therapy. The EEG is especially helpful in making decisions regarding additional diazepam or lorazepam, or in adjusting the rate of paraldehyde infusion

Maintenance therapy

1. Phenobarbital 3–4 mg/kg/day i.v., i.m. or orally, starting 12 h after the loading dose
2. Phenytoin 3–4 mg/kg/day i.v. starting after the loading dose
3. Primidone 12–20 mg/kg/day

Phenobarbital continues to be the first-line drug for the treatment of neonatal seizures. A loading dose of up to 40 mg/kg achieves therapeutic levels in the serum within a short time. Therapeutic levels are 20–40 mg/l (80–160 μmol/l). Babies who are not artificially ventilated can be rendered apneic by a single loading dose of 40 mg/kg, and it is usual to give two separate doses of 20 mg/kg in this situation. If clinical and EEG-revealed seizures persist despite a phenobarbital concentration greater than 40 μ/ml, phenytoin should be added; approximately one-third to half the babies with seizure respond to phenobarbital, about 90% respond to a combination of phenobarbital and phenytoin. The dose of phenytoin is 15 mg/kg given as an intravenous 'push' at a rate no greater than 1 mg/kg/min. Phenytoin is probably the best choice as second-line treatment in babies who fail to respond to phenobarbital, but problems with hypotension and arrhythmias have been reported when there is hidden myocardial damage accompanying hypoxic-ischemic encephalopathy.

Most of the benzodiazepines have been tried in the newborn. The use of diazepam is controversial. Diazepam has a very long half-life in babies, of approximately 30–75 h, and because of the respiratory depressant effects that occur when the levels accumulate this drug is not suitable for prolonged infusion. Lorazepam and clonazepam are also given; the latter is traditionally given intravenously or as an infusion. Hypersalivation and increased bronchial secretion are frequent side effects. Midazolam is a newer benzodiazepine that has proved effective in treating status epilepticus. Midazolam has been reported to cause myoclonic jerking and dystonic posturing in preterm babies when it was used for sedation. The neurodevelopment outcome was better in a group of preterms sedated with morphine, than it was when midazolam was used.

There is very little published experience with any other antiepileptic drug in the newborn. Paraldehyde was popular during the 1970s and 1980s, but it is now difficult to obtain. Sodium valproate has hepatotoxicity. Vigabatrin is not available in an intravenous form, and there is a risk of incurring visual field effects, which cannot be monitored precisely in babies. There is virtually no neonatal experience with lamotrigine or carbamazepine, or with other, new antiepileptic drugs, like oxcarbazepine, gabapentin, topiramate. In animal models the acute and chronic effects of hypoxia can be prevented by pretreatment with topiramate. Topiramate was administered before the hypoxic insult and prevented the expression of the hypoxia-induced seizure.[134] Anticonvulsant therapy must be tailored to the individual needs of the child. Most neonatal seizures are secondary to an acute cerebral insult and thus tend to resolve within 2–4 days. If there has been status epilepticus or if seizures have not been controlled with phenobarbital alone, we continue anticonvulsants for at least 3 months.[2]

Specifics of the pharmacology of antiepileptic drugs in neonates

Binding profile

Painter *et al.*[135] found that there is significant correlation between phenobarbital and phenytoin *in vitro* binding and the total protein and albumin concentration.

Phenobarbital is exclusively but weakly albumin bound. The finding that *in vivo* phenobarbital binding was not significantly correlated with total protein or albumin may be explained by the influence of other factors known to affect albumin binding, such as bilirubin concentration, pH changes, the elevations of free fatty acid concentration and drugs administered to critically ill neonates.

Half-life

Morselli *et al.*[136] studied the influence of age on the half-life of diazepam. The metabolic pathway of diazepam develops only some time after birth, so premature babies show a significantly longer half-life than full-term infants. Carbamazepine autoinduces its own biotransformation, usually during the first 4–6 weeks of treatment. Beginning at a relatively low dose and progressively increasing the dose can avoid the fall in drug concentration.

Toxicity

Phenytoin toxicity is known to cause cardiac arrhythmias and exacerbate seizures. Elevated free concentrations of phenobarbital are known to cause hypotension and respiratory depression. Phenytoin has less of a sedative effect than phenobarbital and clonazepam, thus allowing a more reliable clinical assessment of improvement.[137] Interpatient variability of the various antiepileptic drugs is extensive in newborns, and intraindividual variation occurs in all premature and full-term newborns during the neonatal period. The extensive variability means that the therapy should begin with a relatively small dose, which is increased stepwise until either seizures are controlled or side effects occur.[138]

The effect of antiepileptic drugs on the EEG

Bell *et al.*[139] show a marked depressant effect of phenobarbitone and diazepam on the EEG in newborn babies. The effect of sedation on the maximum interburst interval was greater than expected, particularly when compared to reports on adults.[140] The authors suppose that the drugs are acting on subcortical generators, such as the thalamus and reticular formation, which play a major role in maintaining the background EEG in newborns. Determination of effectiveness of therapy is important in the management of neonatal seizures. With the antiepileptic treatment the clinical control of the convulsions was obtained in more them 80% of the cases, while control of the electrical convulsions was obtained only in 62.5%. There was a highly significant association between favorable response to treatment and normal neurological examination at hospital discharge and at 1 year of age. It is necessary to confirm by means of EEG record the neonatal clinical convulsion before and after having established the anticonvulsive treatment, as the control of electrical convulsion improves the neurological outcome.[141]

Table 9.10 Prognosis of neonatal seizures – relation to neurological disease (adapted from Volpe[30] with permission)

Neurological disease	Normal development (%)*
Hypoxic-ischemic encephalopathy	50
Intraventricular hemorrhage**	10
Primer subarachnoid hemorrhage	90
Hypocalcemia	
Early onset	50†
Late onset	100
Hypoglycemia	50
Bacterial meningitis	50
Development defect	0

Prognosis is for those cases with the stated neurological disease when seizures are a manifestation (thus, value usually will differ from the overall prognosis for the disease)
*Values are rounded off to the nearest 5%; **usually, severe intraventricular hemorrhage associated with major periventricular hemorrhagic infarction; † represents primarily that prognosis approaches later-onset hypocalcemia if no or only minor neurological illness is present

Long-term treatment

There is little agreement on how long to continue anticonvulsant therapy in the neonate. We agree with the opinion of Levene, who stops all drugs when the infant has had no seizure for 7 days as long as they show no neurological abnormality.[10] In those in whom seizures recur or who are neurologically abnormal, medication is continued for 3 months, when they are reviewed. Drugs are stopped if the infant appears to be neurologically normal.

Prognosis

Several factors may influence the neurological outcome of neonates who have clinical seizures. These include the nature and degree of the underlying neuropathologic process, the possible adverse effects of epileptic activity on the developing brain, the secondary effects of the seizures (for example, hypoventilation or hypoperfusion) and the potential adverse effects of antiepileptic drugs. Several studies, however, suggest that seizures associated with certain etiologic factors have a worse prognosis than others (Table 9.10). Normal outcomes occur with increasing frequency in each of the following: hypoxic-ischemic encephalopathy, intracranial hemorrhage, hypoglycemia, unknown cause, hypocalcemia.[23] In monitored infants in whom outcome was assessed only at hospital discharge, the highest morbidity and mortality were associated with seizures due to hypoxic-ischemic encephalopathy and the lowest in infants with subarachnoid hemorrhage, hypoglycemia and hypocalcemia.[24,28] The outcome of neonatal seizures is mainly dependent on their cause. Newborns with seizure were three times more likely (16%) to develop cerebral palsy than were controls (6%). The adverse outcomes observed after neonatal encephalopathy included both cerebral palsy and global developmental delay without motor deficit. For years it has been held that intellectual difficulties can only accompany motor problems in the postasphyxia syndrome, and are not seen in isolation, but this view is now beginning to be challenged. Over the years the reported outcome of neonatal encephalopathy with seizures has been remarkably consistent, with about 25% adverse outcomes in babies with moderate encephalopathy and 66% adverse outcomes (33% dead, 33% disabled) in those with severe encephalopathy, usually defined as coma. The background electroencephalogram abnormality consistently performs best as an outcome predictor; babies with burst suppression or a markedly attenuated background pattern that persists for longer than 12 h after birth have an adverse outcome.[57]

The role of EEG and the clinical neurological status

The extreme ends of the spectrum of clinical neurological status during the newborn period are useful indicators of the outcome. Thus, infants with flaccid coma and seizures generally have an unfavorable outcome, whereas infants with consistently preserved consciousness, activity, reflexes and tone have a more favorable outcome.[96] Infants, who had non-epileptic seizures consisting of tonic posturing and motor automatisms most often had hypoxic-ischemic encephalopathy, interictal lethargy or obtundation, the nature of the abnormal EEG, and poor short-term outcome. In the infants who had epileptic seizures (focal-clonic or focal-tonic), an association was noted with focal structural lesions, subarachnoid hemorrhage and metabolic abnormalities; and with interictal alertness, normal background EEG activity and a relatively good short-term outcome. These clinical and electrographic features suggest a delimited process rather than diffuse injury, which is probably the important factor in the relatively good short-term outcome of these infants. Abnormal neurological examination on discharge was a good predictor of an unfavorable outcome and abnormal polysomnographic recording a moderate predictor.[142] Several investigators have demonstrated that the interictal EEG is a useful prognostic indicator in the term infants. In one large series, a normal interictal EEG was associated with an 86% chance of normal development at the age of 4 years.[96] In contrast, infants with flat, periodic or multifocal EEGs had only an 8% probability of a normal outcome. The burst–suppression pattern, which is included in this group of EEGs with a poor prognosis has a superficial resemblance to the tracé alternant pattern seen in quiet sleep in the normal term newborn. Moreover, 25–35% of term newborns with seizures will have EEGs that are borderline, or demonstrate less marked abnormalities associated with an uncertain prognosis. Bergman *et al.*[6] demonstrated that the outcome of neonates who had manifested seizures for more than 3 days was associated with moderate or severe neurological injury. Babies with normal clinical examination, cranial ultrasound, CT and EEG results at 7–14 days usually have a good prognosis. Estimates of the incidence of epilepsy in children with neonatal seizures vary from 15% to 20%.[96]

Maternal epilepsy

Risk of maternal seizure

Pregnancy in women with epilepsy is accompanied by increased maternal and fetal risk. During pregnancy, seizure can cause maternal and fetal hypoxia and acidosis. The increase in seizure has been reported to occur mostly during the first trimester[31] or evenly throughout pregnancy.[25,26] In animal studies, estrogen is generally proconvulsant; conversely, progesterone generally has an anticonvulsant effect.[46] Status epilepticus is an uncommon complication of pregnancy, but when it occurs it carries high maternal and fetal mortality rates (31% and 48%, respectively).[26] The effects of non-convulsive seizures on the developing fetus are not clear.

Antiepileptic drug pharmacokinetics during pregnancy and lactation

The ideal management of women with epilepsy during pregnancy and the postpartum period involves achieving an optimal balance between minimizing fetal and neonatal exposure to the deleterious influences both of antiepileptic drugs and of seizures.[143] During the past decade, consensus guidelines have emphasized minimizing the associated risk by optimizing a woman's antiepileptic drug regimen and initiating supplemental folic acid before conception, and high-dose folate supplementation prior to conception and during organogenesis. However, there are no current guidelines regarding the best management once a woman with epilepsy becomes pregnant. Because of large intraindividual and interindividual variability, some authors recommend at least monthly monitoring of antiepileptic drug concentration.[144] During mothers taking the most antiepileptic drugs indicate extensive transplacental transfer and low to moderate excretion into breast milk, the breast milk/maternal plasma concentration ratios less than 1.

In the newborn special care should be given to congenital malformations, vitamin K supplementation and symptoms of neonatal withdrawal. Breast-feeding should be allowed for the most anticonvulsive drugs unless the infant becomes symptomatic.[145]

Fetal anticonvulsant syndrome

The cause of this syndrome is probably multifactorial, but recent studies have indicated that antiepileptic drugs are a major offending factor.[15,20,21] If women with epilepsy are in need of antiepileptic drugs for seizure control, then monotherapy at the lowest effective dose should be employed. Offspring are at increased risk of major congenital malformation, a rate of 4–7% (2–3% in normal population), including congenital heart disease, cleft lip/palate, neural tube defects and urogenital defects. The risk of malformations increases with the number of antiepileptic drugs to which the fetus is exposed during pregnancy[10,11] and possibly with the daily amount or peak concentration of individual drugs. Data for valproic acid are suggestive of a dose–response effect for the risk of neural tube defects.[9,12,14,15]

Results of studies investigating cognitive outcome report an increased risk of mental deficiency in 1.4–6% of children of women with epilepsy (including both seizures[17] and *in utero* exposure to antiepileptic drugs[18]), compared with 1% of controls. Unlike major malformations, exposure to antiepileptic drugs during the last trimester may actually be the most detrimental for cognitive outcome.[19]

REFERENCES

1. Mizrahi EM. Consensus and controversy in the clinical management of neonatal seizures. In Volpe JJ, ed. *Clinics in Perinatology-Neonatal Neurology*. Philadelphia, PA: W.B. Saunders Company, 1989;16(2).
2. Younkin D. Neonatal seizures. In Nelson NM, ed. *Current Therapy in Neonatal–Perinatal Medicine – 2*. Philadelphia, PA: B.C. Decker Inc., 1990:321–7.
3. Aicardi J. *Epilepsy in Children*, 2nd edn. New York: Raven Press, 1994.
4. Giovanardi RP, Santucci M, Gobbi G, Parmeggiani A, Pini A, Ambrosetto G. Long-term follow-up of severe myoclonic epilepsy of infants. In Fukuyama Y, Kamoshita S, Ohtsuka C, Susuki Y, eds. *Modern Perspectives of Child Neurology*. Tokyo: Japanese Society of Child Neurology, 1991:205–13.
5. Aicardi J. Neonatal seizures. In Dam M, Gram L, eds. *Comprehensive Epileptology*. New York: Raven Press, 1991.
6. Bergman I, Painter MJ, Hirsch RP, Crumrine PK, David R. Outcome in neonates with convulsions treated in an intensive care unit. *Ann Neurol* 1983;14:642–7.
7. Goldberg HJ. Neonatal convulsions: A 10 year review. *Arch Dis Child* 1983;58:976–8.
8. Legido A, Clancy, RR, Berman HP. Neurologic outcome after electroencephalographically proven neonatal seizures. *Pediatrics* 1991;88(3):538–96.
9. Erikson M, Zetterstrom, R. Neonatal convulsions. Incidence and causes in the Stockholm area. *Acta Paediatr Scand* 1979;68:807–11.
10. Levene MI. Neonatal seizures. In Levene M, ed. *Neonatal Neurology*. New York: Churchill Livingstone, 1987:201–35.
11. Scher MS, Kosaburo A, Beggarly MM, Hamid MY, Steppe DA, Painter MJ. Electrographic seizures in preterm and full-term neonates; clinical correlates, associated brain lesions, and risk for neurologic sequalae. *Pediatrics* 1993;91(1):128–34.
12. Seay R, Bray PF. Significance of seizures in infants weighing less than 2500 grams. *Arch Neurol* 1977;34:381–2.
13. Kohelet D, Shochat R, Lusky A, Reichmann B. Risk factors for neonatal seizures in very low birthweight infants: Population-based survey. *J Child Neurol* 2004;19(2):123–8.
14. Fenichel GM. *Neonatal Neurology*. New York: Churchill Livingstone, 1980.
15. Freeman JM. Neonatal seizures. In Dreyfuss FE, ed. *Pediatric Epileptology*. Boston: John Wright, PSAG Inc., 1983:159–72.
16. Volpe JJ. Neonatal seizures; current concepts and classification. *Pediatrics* 1989;84:422–8.
17. Purpura DP. Synaptogenesis in mammalian cortex; problems and perspectives. In Sterman MB, McGinty D, Adinolfy M, eds. *Brain Development and Behaviour*. London: Academic Press, 1971: 23–40.
18. Shapiro S. Hormonal and environmental influences on rat brain development and behavior. In Sterman MB, McGinty D, Adinolfy M, eds. *Brain Development and Behaviour*. London: Academic Press, 1971:307–23.
19. Dreyfus-Brisac C. The electroencephalogram of fullterm newborns and premature infants. In Remond A, Lairy GC, eds. *Handbook of Electroencephalography and Clinical Neurophysiology*. Amsterdam: Elsevier, 1962;6(Pt B):6–23.
20. Nolte R, Schulte FJ, Michaelis R, Juergens U. Power spectral analysis of the EEG of newborn twins in active and quiet sleep. In Kellaway P, Petersen I, eds. *Clinical Electroencephalography in Children*. Stockholm: Almquist and Wiksell, 1968:89–96.
21. Watanabe K, Iwase K, Hara K. Development of slow-wave sleep in low birthweight infants. *Dev Med Child Neurol* 1974;16: 23–31.
22. Bergey GK, Swaiman KF, Schrier BK. Adverse effects of phenobarbital on morphological and biochemical development of fetal mouse spinal cord neurons in culture. *Ann Neurol* 1981;1:584–8.
23. Kellaway P, Mizrahi EM. Neonatal seizures. In Lüders H, Lesser RP, eds. *Epilepsy: Electroclinical Syndromes*. London: Springer Verlag, 1987:13–47.
24. Mizrahi EM, Kellaway P. Characterization and classification of neonatal seizures. *Neurology* 1987;37:1837–44.
25. Lindsley DB, Schreiner LH, Magoun HW. An electomyographic study of spasticity. *J Neurophysiol* 1949;12:197–203.
26. Mori S, Nishimura H, Aoki M. Brain stem activation of the spinal cord stepping generator. In Hobson JA, Brazier MAB, eds. *The Reticular Formation Revisited*. New York: Raven Press, 1980:241–65.
27. Sherrington CS, Creed RS, Denny-Brown DE. *Reflex Activity of the Spinal Cord*. London: Oxford University Press, 1932.
28. Kellaway P, Mizrahi EM. Electroencephalographic, therapeutic, and pathophysiologic studies of neonatal seizures. In Wasterlain CG, Vert P, eds. *Neonatal Seizures: Pathophysiology and Pharmacologic Management*. New York: Raven Press, 1990:1–13.
29. Kellawey P, Hrachovy RA. Status epilepticus in newborn. A perspective on neonatal seizures. In Deldago-Escueta AV, Wasterlain CG, Treiman, DM, eds. *Advances in Neurology. Status Epilepticus*. New York: Raven Press, 1983;34:93–9.
30. Volpe JJ. *Neurology of the Newborn*, 2nd edn. Philadelphia, PA: Saunders, 1987:129–58.
31. Yakovlev PI, Lecours AR. The myelogenetic cycles of regional maturation of the brain. In Minkowski A, ed. *Regional Development of the Brain in Early Life*. Philadelphia, PA: F. A. Davies, 1967:3–70.
32. Yamamoto N, Watanabe, Negoro T. Partial seizures evolving to infantile spasms. *Epilepsia* 1988;29:34–40.

33. Yakovlev PI. Maturation of cortical substrata of epileptic events. *World Neurol* 1962;3:299–304.
34. Purpura DP. Relationship of seizure susceptibility to morphologic and physiologic properties of normal and abnormal immature cortex. In Kellaway P, Petersen I, eds. *Neurologic and Electroencephalographic Studies in Infancy*. New York: Grune and Stratton, 1964.)
35. Purpura DP, Shoffer RJ, Scraff J. Intracellular study of spike potentials synaptic activities of neurons in immature neocortex. In Minkowski, ed. *Regional Development of the Brain in Early Life*. New York: Grune D. Stratton, 1967:117–121.
36. Wright FS, Bradley WE. Maturation of epileptiform activity. *Electroencephalogr Clin Neurophysiol* 1968;25:259–69.
37. Kolmodin GM, Meyerson BA. Ontogenesis of paroxysmal cortical activity in fetal sheep. *Electroencephalogr Clin Neurophysiol* 1952;21:589–600.
38. Bonasera N, Smorto M, Bonavita V. Izoniacid seizures in the developing rat and the content of pyridoxal-5-phosphat in the brain. *Brain Res* 1967;4:383–6.
39. Millichap JG. Development of seizure pattern in newborn animals. Significance of brain carbonic anhydrase. *Proc Soc Exp Biol Med* 1057;96:125–8.
40. Kato M, Malamut BL, Caveness WF, Hosokawa S, Wakisaka S, O'Neill RR. Local cerebral glucose utilization in newborn and pubescent monkeys during focal motor seizures. *Ann Neurol* 1980;7:204–12.
41. Ricci GF, Mecaelli O, De Feo MR. Ontogenesis of GABAergic and glutamergic receptors in the developing brain. In Wasterlain CG, Vert P, eds. *Neonatal Seizures*. New York: Raven Press, 1990:209–20.
42. Rondouin G. GABAergic inhibition and convulsive seizures. In Wasterlain CG, Vert P, eds. *Neonatal Seizures*. New York: Raven Press, 1990:221–30.
43. Johnston MV, Singer HS. Brain neurotransmitters and neuromodulators in pediatrics. *Pediatrics* 1982;70:57–68.
44. Holmes GL, Khazipov R, Ben-Ari Y. New concept in neonatal seizures. *NeuroReport* 2002;13:3–8.
45. Vannucci RC, Vasta F. Energy state of the brain in experimental neonatal status epilepticus. *Pediatr Res* 1985;19:396–9.
46. Wasterlain CG, Dwyer B. Brain metabolism during prolonged seizures in neonates. *Adv Neurol* 1983;34:241–60.
47. Wasterlain CG, Vert P, eds. *Neonatal Seizures*. New York: Raven Press, 1990.
48. Younkin DP, Delivoria-Papadopoulos M, Maris J, Donlon E, Clancy R, Chance B. Cerebral metabolic effects of neonatal seizures measured with in vivo 31P NMR spectroscopy. *Ann Neurol* 1986;20:513–9.
49. McCabe BK, Silvera DC, Cilio MR, *et al.* Reduced neurogenesis after neonatal seizures *J Neurosci* 2001;6:2094–103.
50. Boylan GB, Panerai RB, Rennie JM, *et al.* Cerebral blood flow velocity during neonatal seizures. *Arch Dis Child* 1999;80:105–10.
51. Sogawa Y, Monokoshi M, Silveira DC, *et al.* Timing of cognitive deficits following neonatal seizures: Relationship to histological changes in the hippocampus. *Dev Brain Res* 2001;131:73–83.
52. Rogalski Landrot I, Minokoshi M, Silveira DC, *et al.* Recurrent neonatal seizures: Relationship of pathology to the electroencephalogram and cognition. *Dev Brain Res* 2001;129:27–8.
53. Koh S, Storey TW, Santos TC, *et al.* Early-life seizures in rats increase susceptibility to seizure-induced brain injury in adulthood. *Neurology* 1999;53:912–21.
54. Miller SP, Weiss J, Barnwell, *et al.* Seizure-associated brain injury in term newborn in perinatal asphyxia. *Neurology* 2001;58: 542–8.
55. Kubova H, Druga R, Lukasiuk K, *et al.* Status epilepticus causes necrotic damage in the mediodorsal nucleus of the thalamus in immature rats. *J Neurosci* 2001;21:3593–9.
56. Wasterlain CG, Niquet J, Thompson KW, *et al.* Seizure-induced neuronal death in immature brain. *Prog Brain Res* 2002;135: 335–53.
57. Rennie JM, Boylan GB. Neonatal seizures and their treatment. *Curr Opin Neurol* 2003;16(2):177–81.
58. Edwards HE, Dortok D, Tam J, Won D, Burnham WM. Prenatal stress alters seizure thresholds and the development of kindled seizures in infant and adult rats. *Horm Behav* 2002;42(4):437–47.
59. Parent JM, Lowenstein DH. Seizure-induced neurogenesis: Are more new neurons good for an adult brain? *Prog Brain Res* 2002;135:121–31.
60. Aicardi J. Complex partial seizures in childhood. In Parsonage M, Grant RHE, Craig AG, Ward AA Jr, eds. *Advances in Epileptology: XIVth Epilepsy International Symposium*. New York: Raven Press, 1983:237–42.
61. Aicardi J. *Diseases of the Nervous System in Childhood*. London: Mac Keith Press, 1992.
62. Mizrahi EM. Classification on neonatal seizures. A guide to clinical recognition. *ILEA Workshop on Neonatal Seizures Classification-Script*, Houston, TX, 2004:July.
63. Roos RAC, Van Dijk JG. Reflex-epilepsy induced by immersion in hot water; case report and review of the literature. *Eur Neurol* 1988;28:6–10.
64. Mizrahi EM. Neonatal seizures: Problems in diagnosis and classification. *Epilepsia* 1987;28:546–55.
65. Cockburn F, Brown JK, Belton NR, Forfar JO. Neonatal convulsions associated with primary disturbance of calcium, phosphorus and magnesium metabolism. *Arch Dis Child* 1973;48:99–108.
66. Lombroso CT. Prognosis in neonatal seizures. In Deldago-Escueta AV, Wasterlain CG, Freiman DM, Orter RJ, eds. *Advances in Neurology. Status Epilepticus*. New York: Raven Press, 1983;42:101–13.
67. Sarnat HB. Pathogenesis of decerebrate seizures in the premature with intraventricular haemorrhage. *J Pediatr* 1975;87:154–5.
68. Lombroso CT. Seizures in the newborn period. In Vinken PJ, Bruyn GW, eds. *Handbook of Clinical Neurology. The Epilepsies*. Amsterdam: North-Holland, 1974;15:189–218.
69. Lombroso CT. Neonatal seizures. In Resor SR, Kutt H, eds. *The Medical Treatment of Epilepsy*. New York: Marcel Dekker, 1992: 115–25.
70. Coulter DL, Allen RJ. Benign neonatal sleep myoclonus. *Arch Neurol* 1982;39:191–2.
71. Resnik T, Mosh S, Perotta L, Chambers H. Benign neonatal sleep myoclonus. *Arch Neurol* 1986;43:266–8.
72. Daoust-Roy J, Seshia SS. Benign neonatal sleep myoclonus. *Am J Dis Child* 1992;146:1236–41.
73. Hill A, Volpe JJ. Neonatal seizures. In Roberton NRC, ed. *Textbook of Neonatology*, 2nd edn. New York: Churchill Livingstone, 1992:1043–55.
74. Blume WT. Clinical and electroencephalographic correlates of the multiple independent spike foci pattern in children. *Ann Neurol* 1978;4:541–7.
75. Watanwbe K, Hara K, Miyazaki S, Hakamada S, Kuroyanagi M. Apneic seizures in the newborn. *Am J Dis Child* 1982;15: 584–96.
76. Navelet Y, Wood RC, Robieux C, Tardieu M. Seizures presenting as apnea. *Arch Dis Child* 1989;64:357–9.
77. Fenichel GM. Seizure in newborns. In Fenichel GM, ed. *Neonatal Neurology*. Edinburgh: Churchill Livingstone, 1985: 25–52.
78. Fenichel GM, Olson BJ, Fitzpatrick JE. Heart rate changes in convulsive and nonconvulsive neonatal apnea. *Ann Neurol* 1980;7:577–82.
79 Radvanyi-Bouvet MF, Vallecalle MH, Morel-Kahn F, Relier JP, Dreyfus-Brisac C. Seizures and electrical discharges in premature infants. *Neuropediatrics* 1985;16:143–8.
80. Bour F, Plouin P, Jalin C, Frenkel A, Dulac O, Bonifas P. Les états de mal unilatéraux au cours de la période neonatale. *Rev EEG Neurophysiol Clin* 1983;13:162–7.
81. Camfield PR, Camfield CS. Neonatal seizures: A commentary on selected aspects. *J Child Neurol* 1987;2:244–51.
82. Cukier F, Sfaello Z, Dreyfus-Brisac C. Lés états de mal du nouveau-né terme et du prématuré dans un centre de réanimation néonatale. Aspects cliniques, électroencephalographiques et évolution. *Gaslini* 1976;8:100–6.
83. Dreyfus-Brisac C, Monod N. Neonatal status epilepticus. In Remond A, ed. *Handbook of Electroencephalography and Clinical Neurophysiology*. Amsterdam: Elsevier, 1977;15(Pt B): 39–52.
84. Monod N, Dreyfus-Brisac C, Sfaello Z. Presentation et prognostic de l'état de mal épileptique néonatal: Étude clinique et EEG de 150 cas. *Arch Fr Pédiatr* 1969;26:1085–102.
85. Dreyfus-Brisac C, Peschanski N, Radvanyi MF, Cukier-Hemeury F, Monod N. Convulsions du noveau-né. Aspects clinique, électroencéphalographique, étiopathogenique et prognostique. *Rev EEG Neurophysiol* 1981;11:367–78.
86. Sarnat HB, Sarnat MS. Neonatal encephalopathy following fetal distress. *Arch Neurol* 1976;33:696–705.
87. Fenichel GM. Hypoxic-ischemic encephalopathy in the newborn. *Arch Neurol* 1983;40:261–6.

88. Hill A, Volpe JJ. Seizures, hypoxic-ischaemic brain injury and intraventricular hemorrhage in the newborn. *Ann Neurol* 1981;10:109–21.
89. Minchon P, Niswandeer K, Chalmers I. Antecedents and outcome of very early neonatal seizures in infants born at or near term. *Br J Obstet Gynecol* 1987;94:431–5.
90. Brown JK. Convulsions in the newborn period. *Dev Med Child Neurol* 1974;15:823–46.
91. Dreyfus-Brisac C. Neonatal electroencephalography. In Scarpelli EM, Cosmi EV, eds. *Reviews of Perinatal Medicine.* New York: Raven Press, 1979;3.
92. Levene MI, Kornberg J, Williams THC. The incidence and severity of post-asphyxial encephalopathy in full-term infants. *Early Hum Dev* 1985;11:21–6.
93. Delivoria-Papadopoulos M, Mishra OP. Mechanisms of perinatal cerebral injury in fetus and newborn. *Ann N Y Acad Sci* 2000;900:159–68.
94. Maulik D, Zanelli SA, Numagami Y, Onishi T, Mishra OP, Delivoria-Papadopoulos M. Oxygen free radical generation during in utero hypoxia in the fetal guinea pig brain. *Brain Res* 1999;817:117–22.
95. Craig WS. Convulsive movements occurring in the first ten days of life. *Arch Dis Child* 1960;35:336–44.
96. Rose AL, Lombroso CT. Neonatal seizure states. *Pediatrics* 1970;45:404–25.
97. Salvia-Roiges MD, Garcia LI, Gonce-Mellgren A, Esque-Ruiz MT, Figueras-Aloy J, Carbonell-Estrany X. Neonatal convulsion and subarachnoid hemorrhage after in utero exposure to paroxetine. *Rev Neurol* 2003;36(8):724–6.
98. Billard C, Dulac O, Diebler C. Ramollissement cerebral ischemique du noveau-né. Une etiologie possible des états de mal convulsifs neonatals. *Arch Fr Pédiatr* 1982;39:677–83.
99. Venkataraman A, Kingsley PB, Kalina P, *et al.* Newborn brain infarction: Clinical aspects and magnetic resonance imaging. *CNS Spectr* 2004;9(6):436–44.
100. Nelson KB, Lynch JK. Stroke in newborn infants. *Lancet Neurol* 2004;3(3):150–8.
101. Chen SF, Huang CC, Wu HM, Chen SH, Liang YC, Hsu KS. Seizure, neuron loss, and mossy fiber sprounting in herpes simplex virus type 1-infected organotypic hippocampal cultures. *Epilepsia* 2004;45(4):322–32.
102. Pagliara AS, Karl IE, Haymond M. Hypoglycemia in infancy and childhood. Part 1. *J Pediatr* 1973;8:365–79.
103. Monod N, Dreyfus-Brisac C, Scafello Z, Pajot N, Morel-Kahn F, Guidasci S. Depistage et prognostic de l'état de mal néonatal. *Arch Fr Pédiatr* 1969;26:1085–102.
104. Lucas A, Morley R, Cole T. Adverse neurodevelopmental outcome of moderate hypoglycaemia. *Br Med J* 1988;297: 1304–8.
105. Manzar S. Transient pseudohypoparathyroidism and neonatal seizure. *J Trop Pediatr* 2001;47(2):113–4.
106. Johnson GM. Powdered goat's milk: Pyridoxyne deficiency and status epilepticus. *Clin Pediatr* 1982;21:494–5.
107. Gospe SM Jr, Hecht ST. Longitudinal MRI findings in pyridoxine-dependent seizures. *Neurology* 1998;51(81):74–8.
108. Hennel SJ, Ekert PG, Volpe JJ, Inder TE. Insight into the pathogenesis of cerebral lesions in incontinentia pigmenti. *Pediatr Neurol* 2003;29(2):148–50.
109. Wada N, Matsuishi T, Nonaka M, Naito E, Yoshino M. Pyruvate dehydrogenase E 1a subunit deficiency in a female patient. *Brain Dev* 2004;26(1):57–60.
110. Aicardi J, Goutieres F. Encéphalopathie myoclonique néonatale. *Rev EEG Neurophysiol Clin* 1978;8:99–101.
111. Schlumberger E, Dulac O, Plouin P. Early infantile epileptic syndrome(s) with suppression–burst; nosological considerations. In Roger J, Bureay M, Dravet C, Dreifuss FE, Perret A, Wolf P, eds. *Epileptic Syndromes in Infancy, Childhood and Adolescence,* 2nd edn. London: John Libbey, 1992:35–42.
112. Aicardi J. Epileptic syndromes in childhood. Overview and classification. In Ross E, Reynolds E, eds. *Paediatric Perspectives on Epilepsy.* Chichester: J. Wiley, 1985:65–71.
113. Dalla Bernardina B, Fontana E, Sgro V, *et al.* Generalised or partial atonic seizures – inhibitory seizures – in children with partial epilepsy. *Electroencephalogr Clin Neurophysiol* 1990;75: S31–2.
114. Aicardi J. Myoclonic epilepsies of infancy and childhood. In Fahn S, Marsden CD, Van Woert MH, eds. *Advances in Neurology. Myoclonus.* New York: Raven Press, 1986;43.
115. Lombroso CT. Early myoclonic encephalopathy, early infantile epileptic encephalopathy and benign and severe infantile myoclonic epilepsies: A critical review and personal contributions. *J Clin Neurophysiol* 1990;7:380–408.
116. Zonana J, Silvey K, Strimling B. Familial neonatal and infantile seizures: An autosomal dominant disorder. *Am J Med Gen* 1984;18:455–9.
117. Leppert M, Anderson VE, Quattlebaum T, *et al.* Benign familial neonatal convulsions linked to genetic markers on chromosome 20. *Nature* 1989;337:647–8.
118. Mellits ED, Holden KR, Freeman JM. Neonatal seizures. II. Multivariate analysis of factors associated with outcome. *Pediatrics* 1981;70:177–85.
119. Dehan M, Quilleron D, Navelet Y, *et al.* Les convulsions du cinquieme jour de la vie: Une nouveau syndrome. *Arch Fr Pédiatr* 1977;34:730–42.
120. Levy SR, Abroms IF, Marshall PC, Rosquette EE. Seizures and cerebral infarction in the full-term newborn. *Ann Neurol* 1985;17:366–70.
121. Pryor DS, Don N, Macourt DC. Fifth day fits: A syndrome of neonatal convulsions. *Arch Dis Child* 1981;56:753–8.
122. Bejsovec M, Kulenda Z, Ponca E. Familial intrauterine convulsions in pyridoxine dependency. *Arch Dis Child* 1967; 42:201–7.
123. Holmes GL. Neonatal seizures. In Pedley TA, Meldrum BS, eds. *Recent Advances in Epilepsy.* Edinburgh: Churchill Livingstone, 1985:207–37.
124. Miikati MA, Travathan E, Krishnamoorthy K, Lombroso CT. Pyridoxine-dependent epilepsy: EEG investigations and long-term follow-up. *Electroencephalogr Clin Neurophysiol* 1991; 78:215–21.
125. Mulley JC, Scheffer IE, Petrou S, Berkovic SF. Channelopathies as a genetic cause of epilepsy. *Curr Opin Neurol* 2003;16(2): 171–6.
126. Legido A, Clancy RR, Behrman PH. Recent advances in the diagnosis, treatment and prognosis of neonatal seizures. *Pediatr Neurol* 1988;4:79–86.
127. Hill A, Volpe JJ. Neonatal seizures. In Avery GB, Fletcher MA, Macdonald MG, eds. *Neonatology: Pathophysiology and Management for the Newborn,* 4th edn. Philadelphia, PA: J.B.Lippincott Company, 1994:1118–34.
128. Markand ON. Pearls, perils, and pitfalls in the use of the electroencephalogram. *Semin Neurol* 2003;23(1):7–46.
129. Eyre JA, Oozeer RC, Wilkingson, AR. Diagnosis of neonatal seizures by continuous recording and rapid analysis of the electroencephalogram. *Arch Dis Child* 1983;58:785–90.
130. Levy SR, Berg AT, Testa FM, Novotny EJ Jr, Chiappa KH. Comparison of digital and conventional EEG interpretation. *J Clin Neurophysiol* 1998;15(6):476–80.
131. Nolte R, Haas G. A polygraphic study of bioelectrical brain maturation in preterm infants. *Dev Med Child Neurol* 1978;20: 167–82.
132. Streletz LJ, Graziani LJ. Electroenchephalography and evoked potentials in neonates. In Nelson NM, ed. *Current Therapy in Neonatal–Perinatal Medicine.* Philadelphia, PA: B.C. Decker Inc.; London: The C.V. Mosby Company, 1986:329–32.
133. Patrizi S, Holmes GL, Orzalesi M. Allemand F. Neonatal seizures: Characteristics of EEG ictal activity in preterm and full-term infants. *Brain Dev* 2003;25(6):427–37.
134. Koh S, Jensen FE. Topiramate blocks perinatal hypoxia-induced seizures in rat pups. *Ann Neurol* 2001;50:366–72.
135. Painter MJ, Minnigh MB, Gaus L, Scher M, Brozanski B, Alvin J. Neonatal phenobarbital and phenytoin binding profiles. *J Clin Pharmacol* 1994;34:312–7.
136. Morselli PL, Pippenger CE, Penry JK. *Antiepileptic Drug Therapy in Pediatrics.* New York: Raven Press, 1983.
137. Albani M. Phenytoin in infancy and childhood. *Adv Neurol* 1983;34:457–64.
138. Dodson WE. Aspects of antiepileptic treatment in children. *Epilepsia* 1988;29(Suppl 3):S10–4.
139. Bell AH, Greisen G, Pryds O. Comparison of the effects of phenobarbitone and morphine administration on EEG activity in preterm babies. *Acta Paediatr* 1993;82:35–9.
140. Jorgensen EP. The EEG during severe barbiturate intoxication. *Acta Neurol Scand* 1970;46(Suppl 43):281.
141. Domenech Martinez E, Castro-Conde JR, Herraiz-Culebras T, Gonzales-Campo C, Mendez-Perez A. Neonatal convulsion: Influence of the electroencephalographic pattern and the

response to treatment on the outcome. *Rev Neurol* 2003;37(5): 413–20.
142. Garcias Da Silva LF, Nunes ML, Da Costa JC. Risk factors for developing epilepsy after neonatal seizures. *Pediatr Neurol* 2004;30(4):271–7.
143. Penell PB. Antiepileptic drug pharmacokinetics during pregnancy and lactation. *Neurology* 2003;61(69):35–42.
144. Yerby MS. Quality of life, epilepsy advances, and the evolving role of anticonvulsants in women with epilepsy. *Neurology* 2000;55:S21–31.
145. Baumeister FAM. Epilepsy and pregnancy from the neuropaediatric perspective. *Gynaekol Prax* 2003;27(3):425–31.
146. Gal P, Roop C, Robinson H, Erkan NV. Theophyllin induced seizures in accidentally overdosed neonates. *Pediatrics* 1980; 65:547–9.
147. Aicardi J. Epilepsy in brain-injured children. *Dev Med Child Neurol* 1990;32:191–202.

10 Oxygen toxicity

R. Bracci

Introduction

Although the toxic effects of oxygen have been known since the end of the 19th century,[1] the first evidence of a relationship between oxygen toxicity and neonatal diseases emerged in the early 1950s when retinopathy (ROP) was observed in premature infants breathing high concentrations of oxygen.[2] At about the same time, the red cells of the newborns were demonstrated to have increased susceptibility to oxygen damage.[3] This made it clear that oxygen species were particularly toxic to neonatal red cells, which were damaged by exposure to H_2O_2 and substances producing H_2O_2.

Great advances in our understanding of the toxic effects of oxygen were made in the years that followed, when oxygen toxicity was recognized to be due to the development of reactive oxygen species (ROS). The main ROS are the superoxide anion ($O_2^{\bullet-}$), hydrogen peroxide (H_2O_2), lipid peroxide (LOOH), peroxyl radicals $RO_2^{\bullet-}$ and the hydroxyl radical ($OH^\bullet$). Other important radicals are the highly reactive electron delocalized phenoxyl radical ($C_6H_5O^\bullet$) and nitric oxide ($NO^\bullet$).[4–8]

The term ROS includes free radicals, which are atoms or molecules with one or more unpaired electrons. Free radicals may react with other radicals, the unpaired electrons forming a covalent bond. The resulting molecule may decompose other molecules into toxic products. Free radicals may react with non-radical molecules in free-radical chain reactions, which are stopped by antioxidant enzymes or protein reactions. $O_2^{\bullet-}$ is the precursor of most ROS and a mediator in oxidative chain reactions. Dismutation of $O_2^{\bullet-}$ by superoxide dismutase (SOD) produces H_2O_2, which in turn may be fully reduced to water by glutathione peroxidase (GSH-Px) and catalase (Cat) or partially reduced to $OH^\cdot$. The latter reaction is called the Fentonl-Haber–Weiss reaction and is catalyzed by reduced transition metals.[4–9] ROS are involved in the following reactions:

$$O_2^{\bullet-} \xrightarrow{SOD} H_2O_2$$

$$H_2O_2 + GSH \xrightarrow{GSH\text{-}Px} H_2O + \text{Oxidized glutathione}$$

$$H_2O_2 \xrightarrow{Cat} H_2O + O_2$$

A deficiency of scavenging reduces the detoxification of H_2O_2 and $O_2^{\bullet-}$ and increases the formation of $OH^\bullet$ by metal activation following the Fenton reaction:[4–9]

$$Fe^{2+} + H_2O_2 \rightarrow Fe^{3+} + OH^\bullet + OH^-$$

There is no specific scavenger for this radical: once released, OH reacts with lipoproteins, cell membranes, lipids, proteins, DNA, amino acids and other molecules. $OH^\bullet$ is one of the strongest oxidants in nature and may damage tissues.

Oxidative tissue damage may be mediated by reactive nitroxide species.[9–11] The reaction product of $NO^\bullet$ and $O_2^{\bullet-}$ is the unstable molecule peroxynitrite ($ONOO^-$), which is regarded as highly reactive and hence destructive, although it seems to be trapped by cellular antioxidants and other factors at low concentration.[12–14]

It is important to remember that free-radical reactions are a normal occurrence in living organisms and ROS are not necessarily toxic. Vascular tone appears to be modulated by the contrasting effects of $NO^\bullet$ and $O_2^{\bullet-}$.[15] Production of $O_2^{\bullet-}$ by phagocytes is an important defense mechanism but extracellular release of free radicals by activated phagocytes is itself a mechanism of tissue damage during inflammation.[5,16] Oxidative balance, therefore, is an intriguing question, and much recent research has increased our knowledge of the relations between ROS and human diseases.

The oxidative stress

An excess of ROS, as well as reactive nitrogen species, in relation to detoxification capacity is called 'oxidative stress', a term used to describe imbalance between oxidants and antioxidants, which is a potential cause of damage. If oxidative stress is mild, cell defenses may increase by a complex mechanism, which generally involves enhanced gene expression of ROS scavenging activities.[6,17,18] Severe oxidative stress is generally followed by cell injury, which may proceed to necrosis or apoptosis.[4–6] The involvement of oxidative stress in the mechanism of apoptosis has been extensively studied.[19–22]

The pathological conditions leading to oxidative stress are extremely complex. It is therefore necessary to identify the biochemical basis of oxidative stress in order to prevent or treat oxygen toxicity.[4–7,9,23]

ROS production

Two main sites have been recognized as sources of ROS: the extracellular compartment with phagocyte activation and the endogenous source with mitochondrial function.[13] Both these sites are important in the pathogenesis of fetal and neonatal diseases.

Intracellular and extracellular production of ROS is provided by activated phagocytes.[24] ROS released inside phagocytes during infection and cytokine production can also alter the extracellular oxidative balance and harm tissues, since the cells undergo an efflux of $O_2^{\bullet-}$.[25] However, opsonization and activation of phagocytes is also known to occur during the hypoxanthine–xanthine oxidase reaction, and therefore during hypoxia–reoxygenation.[26]

Mitochondria are the primary sources of superoxide and it has been demonstrated that mitochondrial dysfunction is responsible for increased superoxide release. The mitochondrial electron transport chain contains redox centers, which may leak electrons to oxygen, constituting the primary source of $O_2^{\bullet-}$ in most tissues.[9] Research into myocardial physiology has demonstrated that under normal conditions, mitochondrial electron transport reduces 95% of oxygen to H_2O by tetravalent reduction without any free-radical intermediates and the remaining 5% is reduced by the univalent pathway in which free radicals are produced.[27,28]

During acidosis and hypoxia ischemia, mitochondrial dysfunction occurs and ROS production increases, while antioxidant defenses are depleted and metal ions may play a role in generating $OH^{\bullet}$.[29] ROS production by mitochondria may increase during hypoxia ischemia as a result of dramatic increases in cytosolic calcium concentrations. Since mitochondrial enzymes, such as pyruvate dehydrogenase and α-oxyglutarate dehydrogenase, are normally regulated by Ca cycling across the inner mitochondrial membrane, when intracellular Ca increases, cycling may become excessive and lead to increased ROS production, while structural alterations to the inner mitochondrial membrane may be followed by mitochondrial respiratory chain disorganization with further increases in ROS.[30–33] During asphyxia, $OH^{\bullet}$ production also increases as a result of the release of iron from safe sites.[27] Acidosis may therefore enhance $OH^{\bullet}$-mediated tissue injury.[34]

When oxygen is restored to ischemic tissue, free-radical reperfusion injury occurs by several mechanisms including the xanthine–xanthine oxidase reaction.[27,35] Reperfusion injury is considered the major source of oxidative stress and has been reported in heart, kidney, liver lung and intestine, particularly in necrotizing enterocolitis (NEC).[27,36]

Hyperoxia has been demonstrated to be associated with increased mitochondrial production of $O_2^{\bullet-}$.[9] The rate of mitochondrial $O_2^{\bullet-}$ production increases linearly with increasing oxygen concentration.[37] Under normobaric hyperoxic conditions, the only organs affected by ROS formation are the lungs, since they are the only ones in direct contact with atmospheric oxygen.[9] However, under hyperbaric conditions other tissues become exposed to a hyperoxic environment and increased ROS formation has been found in other organs.[9] Other sources of ROS include catecholamines, prostaglandins and xenobiotics, previously reduced by certain enzymes.[4–6]

Endothelial dysfunction caused by oxidative stress and leading to vascular disease has been extensively investigated.[38–41] The endothelium is normally protected against ROS; however, overproduction may occur via mitochondrial reactions, xanthine–xanthine oxidase reaction, vascular as well as phagocytic NAD(P)H oxidases and toxin-induced reactions. There is also a growing body of evidence linking blood cell and endothelial cell interactions in the enhanced production of ROS.[38–42] Oxidative stress to endothelium may be due to ROS or reactive NO-mediated peroxynitrite.[11] $O_2^{\bullet-}$ therefore promotes tissue damage by reacting with NO, reducing NO bioavailability and producing toxic $ONOO^-$.[38–41] The presence of non-protein bound iron during acidosis, hypoxia and infections causes $OH^{\bullet}$ release and may exacerbate ROS-mediated tissue injury.[10,19,41,43] The resulting vascular endothelial dysfunction elicits a number of maladaptive phenomena that impair normal healthy blood vessels. The normal vascular environment is lost, exposing the lumen to the possibility of thrombosis, while the decrease in NO production and enhanced endothelin 1 production leads to vasoconstriction,[38] which also seems to be enhanced by inhibition of PGI.[43] Endothelial injury due to oxidative stress has been demonstrated to play a key role in coagulation disorders by enhancing procoagulant activity.[44,45]

Antioxidants

The antioxidant system can be classified into two major groups: enzyme activities and low-molecular-weight antioxidants.[13] The enzyme group is represented in the reactions mentioned above. Other important antioxidant enzymes are thioredoxin reductase and glutathione transferase (GSH-T). It is important that $O_2^{\bullet-}$ dismutation be associated with balanced H_2O_2 detoxification. It has been suggested that overexpression of SOD may lead to deleterious effects if not balanced by GSH-Px.[46,47] This observation underlines the key role of GSH in protecting against oxidative stress.[48] The enzyme-based antioxidant system includes extracellular SOD, the only extracellular scavenger of $O_2^{\bullet-}$, which also plays a key role in scavenging $O_2^{\bullet-}$ produced in the extracellular compartment by phagocytes, endothelium and other mechanisms.[49]

The low-molecular-weight antioxidant group contains a large number of compounds that are capable of preventing oxidative damage by direct or indirect interactions with ROS. The effects of these molecules are complex, since the same molecule may have pro-oxidant or antioxidant effects depending on the bioavailability, metabolism and tissue properties as well as interactions between enzymic and non-enzymic antioxidants. Ascorbic acid may have pro-oxidant and antioxidant properties.[50] Coenzyme Q (CoQ) is a source of $O_2^{\bullet-}$ when partially reduced and an antioxidant when fully reduced.[51] One of the most studied antioxidants is α-tocopherol, but competition between different forms and their uptake and the synergistic or inhibitory role of other compounds are not yet understood. Furthermore, non-antioxidant effects of α-tocopherol have been demonstrated.[52] Iron-binding proteins have the major antioxidant activity, protecting against metal-induced $OH^{\bullet}$ production.[53]

ROS in fetus and neonate

Excessive oxidative stress and particularly $OH^{\bullet}$ can impair cell function and induce apoptosis in rapidly growing structures. An oxidized state can also be beneficial, since ROS may activate transcription factors and promote fetal development, but both of which are sensitive to uncontrolled oxidative stress.[54] The effects of ROS are secondary to its direct toxicity and indirect effects, such as vasoconstriction in the lung or systemic circulation.[55,56] Another important condition of oxidative stress produced by $O_2^{\bullet-}$ and NO-derived free radicals is impaired placental function, which may lead to fetal growth retardation.[57]

Oxidative stress in the fetus and the newborn may result from decreased antioxidants, increased ROS or both. The fetus has a lower antioxidant capacity than older babies and adults. Free-radical scavenger enzyme activities and many other components of the antioxidant system are low. Studies in various animals have shown that the main ROS-detoxifying enzymes, GSH-Px, Cat and SOD, increase during intrauterine life.[58,59] At least in the lungs and liver, detoxifying reactions ruled by SOD, GSH-Px and Cat are fully expressed only after birth.[58,59] Scavenger activities involving GSH-T have been studied in the fetus and newborn and seem to vary widely in different animal species.[60]

In the human newborn, the scavenger enzyme activities were first investigated in erythrocytes: Cat and GSH-Px were found deficient in most of the infants, and SOD only in some.[46,61,62] SOD activity is reported to increase in the lungs of the human fetus during intrauterine life.[63,64] Normal values of GSH-Px have been reported in leukocytes of full-term newborns.[65]

Non-enzyme antioxidant factors are reported to be lower in the fetus and newborn than in adults and older babies,[66–68] partly because of deficient placental transfer of some antioxidants.[54] However, antioxidant capacity of neonatal plasma is controversial since peroxy-radical trapping capacity and chain-breaking antioxidants, the same or higher than in adults, have been observed.[69,70] These differences can be ascribed to the study methods, the components of antioxidant capacity tested and the timing of blood sampling. Infant condition also plays a role since asphyxia and acidosis may reduce certain components of antioxidant power.[71] Plasma antioxidant capacity is not correlated with any neonatal pathology. On the contrary, other markers suggest ROS toxicity in neonates[70,72–74]. Irrespective of total antioxidant capacity, a deficiency in particular antioxidant factors, such as ceruloplasmin and transferrin, may play an important role in neonatal susceptibility to oxidative stress and particularly to metal-induced $OH^{\bullet}$ production.[75,76] Low concentrations of transferrin have been found in neonates, especially premature ones, and high plasma levels of ascorbic acid may create a condition of risk due to the pro-oxidant effect of iron. The finding of increased bleomycin-detectable iron in premature and some full-term infants is the evidence of the real risk of increased pro-oxidant effects of iron in neonates.[77] High saturation of transferrin is therefore probably a risk factor of oxidative stress. It is generally accepted that non-transferrin bound iron is a pathological manifestation and it is extremely rare in adults, in whom even the presence of non-protein-bound iron (NPBI) in iron overload is uncommon.[78] Levels of NPBI in the plasma of newborns are correlated with other markers of oxidative stress and high plasma NPBI has been found in hypoxic newborns with poor outcome.[79] Compensatory protection against oxidative stress in neonates is demonstrated by high activity of GSH reductase and high recycling of GSH in red cells.[80] However, several observations have shown that preterm infants have lower and age-related plasma concentrations of GSH and higher concentrations of GSSG than adults.[81] This is interesting since a low GSH/GSSG ratio is a reliable index of generalized oxidative stress.[82] Reliable markers, such as F2-isoprostanes, allantoin and the oxidized form of CoQ, provide further evidence of oxidative stress in neonates.[71,83,84] Oxidative stress in neonates has also been demonstrated by higher values of CoQ120 in those born by vaginal delivery than by elective cesarean section.[85]

Oxidative stress is involved in tissue damage induced by infection and sepsis. Although there is a general agreement that neonatal phagocytes, and, especially those of premature infants, have abnormalities of various functions,[86] active neonatal secretion of proinflammatory cytokines suggests a very complex situation in which oxidative stress following infection may be more dangerous in newborns, especially if premature, than in adults.[87]

The high levels of peroxides found in cord blood of fetuses with asphyxia are in line with the hypothesis of high ROS production in the placenta and umbilical structures during hypoxia.[88–90] However, it should be remembered that the oxidative balance of the fetus is not the same as that of the neonate because of the peroxidase content of the placenta.[91,92]

The first condition suspected to be responsible for increased oxygen toxicity, namely hyperoxia, has recently been demonstrated to cause the oxidative stress responsible for lung injury and possibly generalized tissue damage.[93] The definition of hyperoxia in newborns is closely related to oxygen requirements during the first hours of life, when the baby is suddenly exposed to higher oxygen tension than in the uterus. The oxidative stress recorded in animal experiments with hyperoxia could occur in neonates with oxygen tensions lower than previously considered.[93]

Endothelial injury by ROS following asphyxia or infection may lead to vasoconstriction and coagulation disorders that are particularly harmful to newborns due to the procoagulative state of the fetus and neonate.[44]

Links between ROS and endothelial cell injury seem to play a role in the development of pre-eclampsia, since increased oxidative stress has been demonstrated in pre-eclamptic women.[94,95] Although the pathogenesis of pre-eclampisa is poorly understood, it seems that oxidative stress plays an important role.[96]

ROS are involved in many diseases of newborns and adults, such as NEC, renal failure and septic shock. Neonatal conditions of particular interest concern red cells, lung, retina and brain.

Red cells

Several observations in animal and human erythrocytes have demonstrated that release of free radicals inside red cells may affect membrane structure during oxidation of hemoglobin.[97,98] Membrane structure may also be damaged by ROS uptake from the extracellular medium, where they may arise from ischemia–reperfusion, phagocyte activation, endothelial metabolism, hyperoxia, lipoprotein peroxidation and other sources.[99,100] Uptake of free radicals by red cells can be regarded as a mechanism protecting the tissues from oxidative injury, since the high-antioxidant enzyme activities of erythrocytes can scavenge extracellular ROS. However, excessive oxidative stress leads to hemolysis followed by free iron and free-radical release, and possible tissue damage.[101] In newborns, antioxidant activities are generally lower than in adults, and seem to be even lower in premature infants.[61,62,–102,103,105] Activities, such as GSH-Px, increase rapidly in the first days, presumably as a result of increased exposure to ROS.[106,107] Exposure of red cells to ROS after birth is also demonstrated by a decrease in GSH-T in the first days of life in response to ROS production.[108] Very active GSH recycling occurs in normal newborns, but asphyxia and acidosis have been reported to depress it, as well as ATP.[80] GSH recycling also seems deficient in infants with RDS and chronic lung disease (CLD).[109] Chemiluminescence assays have demonstrated higher ROS production in newborns than in adults.[110] This observation is in line with the demonstration of high lipid peroxidation and decreased CoQ10.[111] The red cells of newborns appear to be more susceptible to the toxic effects of oxidative stress than those of adults.[112] Besides low scavenger enzyme activities, newborn red cells have other characteristics, such as lipid content and composition, which predispose them to oxidative stress.[112] Vitamin E levels are not only much lower in the neonatal than in the adult red cell, but requirements of the vitamin are also higher, as shown by increased recycling.[113] ROS are generated in red cells not only under pathological but also under normal conditions.[114,115] Animal studies have demonstrated the key role of oxidative stress caused by intraerythrocyte iron release in a reactive form and hydroxyl radical production in the development of membrane protein damage.[102] Oxidative cross-linking of membrane proteins can produce clustering of the major erythrocyte membrane spanning protein band 3.[116,117] The clusters provide recognition sites for antibodies against senescent cells and trigger their removal from circulation. In the absence of efficient protection by antioxidant factors, oxidative stress therefore appears to be responsible for the release of iron in a reactive form, predisposing red cells to hemolysis through the formation of senescence antigen.[117] Paradoxically, recent observations show that auto-oxidation of Hb may occur *in vitro* at low oxygen tension.[118]

Studies in newborns have shown interesting analogies between experimental and clinical observations. The free iron content of red cells of newborns is higher than that of adults and is significantly correlated with pH and base deficit as well as with plasma lipid peroxide products, expressed by malondialdehyde (MDA) concentrations.[119] Incubation of newborn and adult red cells *in vitro* showed higher iron release in the former under aerobic and anaerobic conditions. It is interesting that during anaerobic incubation, increased $O_2^{\bullet -}$ production, free iron release and senescence antigen production showed the highest significant differences between adults and neonates.[110,120] *In vitro* studies show that incubated neonatal red cells release iron in reactive form. This iron is recovered in the incubation medium at the end of incubation, apparently irrespective of hemolysis, demonstrating that reactive iron may be released by stressed red cells and diffuse outside the cell.[121] This finding suggests that oxidative stress in erythrocytes may be involved in the increase in NPBI in plasma of asphyxiated neonates. In conclusion, several reports suggest that acidosis and hypoxia may generate red cell damage via ROS.

Pulmonary oxygen toxicity

Oxygen toxicity is particularly harmful for the lungs. The mechanism of damage is complex. Lung injury may be caused directly by ROS production in response to hyperoxia or indirectly by ROS due to phagocyte activation and inflammation. The two mechanisms seem to be integrated.

CLD, a severe complication of prematurity, was long thought to be due to high concentrations of oxygen in inspired air and barotrauma. ROS are now generally accepted to be largely responsible for lung injury in preterm infants since several studies using different methods have demonstrated products of ROS reactions in premature infants with CLD.[122–127] The particular toxicity of ROS in the immature lung is due to the low antioxidant capacity of premature infants, which does not increase rapidly as in the full-term lung, as well as to the possibly high toxicity of ROS in rapidly developing tissues.[128] Increased production of ROS under certain conditions may also play a role. The main sources of ROS production in the immature lung are ischemia–reperfusion, phagocytosis and increased mitochondrial activity, mainly due to hyperoxia. Mitochondrial oxidative stress following hyperoxia has been demonstrated by a decrease of intramitochondrial GSH/GSSG redox status.[129] High inspired oxygen fraction (FiO_2) may be responsible for lung injury and high lipid peroxidation, as demonstrated by high F2-isoprostane levels in the lungs of animals exposed to high oxygen concentrations.[130] Effects of hyperoxia in the lung and a close relationship between oxidative stress and inflammation have been demonstrated. Magnetic resonance studies have confirmed the previously reported experimental data on the consequences of hyperoxia in the lungs of premature newborn animals, namely, edema, congestion, immune cell infiltration and decreased number of alveoli per square meter.[131,132] Prolonged moderate hyperoxia induces airway hyper-responsiveness and histological changes similar to those of CLD.[133] Increased type IV collagenase in bronchoalveolar lavage suggests a role of this factor in lung damage and particularly in disruption of the extracelluar matrix. It is interesting that injury produced by oxidative stress involves matrix metalloproteinases (MMP) and tissue inhibitor of matrix metalloproteinase (TIMP), which are also involved in infections.[134] Increased MMP-8 and MMP-9 associated with decreased TIMP have been reported in amniotic fluid during infection and chorioamnionitis, a condition frequently associated with the development of CLD.[87] These findings are in line with reports of phagocyte activation and increased cytokine production. The finding of a large number of neutrophils and high concentrations of interleukin-8 and leukotrienes in bronchopulmonary lavage of infants with severe CLD demonstrates the role of inflammatory reactions and ROS production in the development of this disease.[135,136]

The toxic effects of ROS on the lungs appear to be due to iron-mediated $OH^\bullet$ release.[125] This radical alters surfactant composition and causes decreased surfactant production by injuring type II pneumocytes.[125,137] Peroxynitrate formation from $O_2^{\bullet -}$ and $NO^\bullet$ can also cause lung injury.[138] ROS can modify production of vasoactive substances by the endothelium, and this might be important in CLD since increased endothelin-1 has been demonstrated to be associated with inflammation and lung disease.[139] Oxidative stress has been studied in the lungs of premature rats and a complex orchestra of genes involved in inflammation, coagulation, fibrinolysis, extracellular matrix turnover, cell cycle, signal transduction and alveolar enlargement have been found to be affected by oxidative stress.[140] The combined effect of oxygen and inflammation on the origin of CLD also emerges from studies of bronchopulmonary lavage and tracheal aspirate in which increased levels of markers of oxidative stress, such as protein carbonyls and myeloperoxidase activity in neutrophils of premature infants who developed CLD, have been found.[141,142] Increased lipid peroxidation in plasma of premature infants with CLD and periventricular leukomalacia has been reported.[77] Conditions of oxidative stress possibly responsible for CLD and ROP have also been reported.[143] These observations suggest a combined effect of oxidative stress in the pathogenesis of CLD, brain damage and ROP.

Retinopathy

Although the origins of ROP are multifactorial (see Chapter 12), the role of oxygen toxicity, which was first detected half a century ago, has been confirmed by experimental and clinical studies. ROS have been recognized to play an important role, particularly in the first stage of eye injury when hyperoxia seems to affect the vascular endothelium arresting normal blood vessel development.[144] Hyperoxia also seems to inhibit vascular endothelium growth factor, and involvement of oxidative stress in vascular obliteration caused by apoptotic vascular endothelial cells has also been suggested.[144] The hypothesis of a complex mechanism of oxidative stress in the development of ROS is also suggested by observation of the role of iron intake,[145] decreased GSH/GSSG ratio[146] and NPBI[147] in patients with ROP. Morphological abnormalities of ROP, such as ‘gap junctions’, are an expression of lipoperoxidation, which has been demonstrated in the retina as a result of free-radical release.[148]

A relationship between free-radical release, induced retinal injury and cyclooxygenase pathway activity has been reported.[149] Abnormalities of retinal vasculature have demonstrated that reversal vasoconstriction by dilator prostaglandin during oxidative stress in newborns may facilitate neovascularization of the retina of premature animals.[150] The role of peroxides in inducing abnormal retinal vasculature has also been demonstrated by the marked vasoconstriction that these molecules produce in the retinal vasculature of premature animals.[151]

Brain injury

ROS may affect the brain by different interacting systems involving membrane damage, astrocyte dysfunction, abnormalities of *n*-methyl-D-aspartate receptors and, particularly, increased intracellular calcium and mitochondrial dysfunction.[152,153] ROS may also cause indirect injury by inducing cerebrovascular spasms.[154] Iron-induced $^\bullet OH$ production may occur during brain injury because the low transferrin content of cerebrospinal fluid (CSF) is saturated by iron released from cells with a high iron content, and free and unbound iron becomes available for the Fenton reaction.[152]

The brain is low in Cat and has moderate amounts of SOD and GSH-Px; its membrane lipids are rich in polyunsaturated fatty acids, which are sensitive to oxidative stress.[152] In the fetus and newborn, protection against ROS seems to be even poorer than in adults, especially in the glia, and sensitivity to oxidative stress seems particularly high in the first hours of life.[152–157] The first mechanism of brain damage due to ROS to be investigated was that of ischemia–reperfusion and hypoxanthine–xanthine oxidase reaction.[158] The importance of this mechanism emerged from the finding of high concentrations of hypoxanthine in blood and CSF during hypoxia, and from experimental data demonstrating inhibition of ROS release by allopurinol, an inhibitor of xanthine oxidase.[159] However, Delivoria *et al.*[160] demonstrated that hypoxia results in brain cell membrane damage, as shown by increased membrane lipid peroxidation and decreased Na^+,K^+-ATPase activity, irrespective of reoxygenation. High levels of isoprostane-8, another marker of oxidative stress, also suggest the responsibility of ROS in brain damage during asphyxia,[161] while electron spin resonance spectroscopy has shown that tissue hypoxia results in increased free-radical generation in the cerebral cortex.[162] Levels of conjugated dienes and fluorescent compounds, markers of lipid peroxidation, have also been detected in the brain of newborn animals with asphyxia, particularly during recovery from single or repeated episodes.[163] Histochemical studies of brains of neonatal rats after hypoxic ischemic injury demonstrated that iron increases rapidly in the first 24 h in regions of ischemic injury, suggesting oxidative stress induced by $OH^•$ produced via the Fenton reaction.[164] The effects of ROS are also due to brain hypoxia-induced generation of NO free radicals; peroxynitrite is formed when $O_2^{•-}$ predominates over the scavenger system and NO increases as an effect of increased NOS.[153]

However, during ischemia, a number of metabolic changes occur and prostaglandin metabolism and dopamine oxidation have been found to have a role in the release of ROS.[165] The recent availability of reliable markers of oxidative stress, such as isoprostanes and particularly F2-isoprostane and 8-isoprostane, has provided evidence of involvement of oxidative stress in the development of cerebral white matter injury, since these compounds were detected in the CSF of premature infants with white matter damage.[161] Further confirmation of this involvement was the finding of increased carbonyls, a marker of protein oxidation in the CSF of these neonates.[161] It is interesting that none of the observed infants had infections and their CSF, unlike in meningitis, did not contain chlorotyrosine, a marker of leukocyte oxidant activity.[166] Indirect evidence of the responsibility of ROS in brain damage of asphyxiated infants comes from the observation of NPBI in CSF.[167] Increased NPBI resulting from asphyxia or hemorrhage has an important role in the development of brain injury, one reason being that early differentiating oligodendroglia is poor in ROS detoxification systems and enables peroxide accumulation and $OH^•$ generation by the Fenton reaction.[152,168]

Several observations also suggest ROS involvement in brain injury during hyperoxia.[169,170] Decreases in cerebral blood flow in response to O_2 administration have been detected in human studies[170] and reduced blood flow was observed in premature newborns treated with high O_2 concentrations.[171] However, animals kept in hyperoxia showed a reduction in blood flow, which was not statistically significant.[172]

Considering the interaction between ROS and inflammatory mediators, oxidative stress to the endothelium may play an important role in the development of brain damage.[173]

Relationships between ROS and brain damage are suggested by the link between increased markers of oxidative stress and clinical observations.

Oxidative stress in premature and full-term newborns with asphyxia is demonstrated by high plasma levels of lipid hydroperoxides and evidence of the MDA reaction.[174,175] Markers of oxidative stress, such as HPLC determinations of MDA, 4-hydroxynonenal, total hydroperoxide and carbonyl groups, are significantly higher in asphyxiated babies.[174–177] It is interesting that markers of oxidative stress, such as total hydroperoxides, remain high for weeks in sick babies.[177] Isoprostanes, a reliable marker of oxidative stress, have been reported to be higher in cases of fetal distress.[178]

High levels of NPBI in plasma of the asphyxiated newborn are evidence of a role of ROS in the development of brain injury in hypoxia ischemia. The reports of Dorrepal *et al.*[179] indicated that this occurrence, which is peculiar to neonates, is associated with severe brain damage. Buonocore *et al.*[180] recently tested the predictivity of traditional indicators of brain damage in relation to neurodevelopmental outcome. They demonstrated that plasma NPBI is the most reliable marker of severe outcome in asphyxiated newborns.[180]

The markers of oxidative stress

If oxidative damage contributes significantly to neonatal pathology, it is essential to be able to accurately measure oxidative stress. Two basic approaches have been suggested: (1) attempting to trap ROS and measure levels of trapped molecules and (2) measuring the oxidative damage done by ROS.[181] Other frequently used approaches are inaccurate.[181] Erythrocyte enzyme activities, which were the first indication of the low antioxidant resistance of newborns, are not fully reliable since the enzyme activities of red cells are age dependent and values may be an expression of young or old red cell populations.[181] Measurement of total antioxidants usually involves major contributions from urate, ascorbate, bilirubin and albumin-SH groups, which are variable and may not accurately reflect antioxidant power.[181] However, plasma antioxidants, if measured in conjunction with other parameters, may be useful in the detection of imbalance between free radicals and antioxidants. Chromatographic profiles of antioxidants in human plasma can provide indications of single-component deficiencies, which may be useful to distinguish particular deficiencies or increased consumption of a factor involved in a particular disease.[182]

Lipid oxidation is a complex process and commonly used methods, such as thiobarbituric acid (TBA), are questionable. The TBA test should not be used because most TBA-reactive material in the human body is not related to lipid peroxidation.[181] Measurement of MDA by HPLC is more indicative of lipid peroxidation, although MDA is only one of the many aldehydes formed during this process.[181] It is more logical to measure 4-hydroxynonenal.[181] The best biomarker of lipid peroxidation is isoprostane, which is a specific end product of peroxidation of polyunsatured fatty acids.[181,183] Most work has been done with F2-isoprostane, which arises from arachidonic acid peroxidation. Neuroprostane or F4-isoprostane has also been measured.[183] They are best measured by mass spectrometry.[184] It is important to remember that isoprostanes are rapidly metabolized, so that increased values may indicate slower metabolism and not increased production.[181]

Measurement of ethane and pentane in expired air was among the first methods of detecting oxidative stress in asphyxiated neonates.[185] These assays have the advantage of being non-invasive and independent of the complex matrix of blood.[186] However, variations in the methods make it difficult to compare populations.[187] Simultaneous measurement of pentane and MDA has been carried out to assess oxidative stress. In studies on human hyperoxia, increased values of both the markers were found, but no correlation between pentane and MDA was observed, probably because they are metabolized differently.[188]

Profiles of aldehydes pentanal, hexanal, 2-hexanal, heptanal, 2-heptanal, 2-octenal, 2-nonenal and 4-hydroxy-nonenal formed during autoxidation of fatty acids, such as oleic, linoleic, α-linoleic, γ-linoleic and arachidonic, seem to improve the sensitivity of detection.[189]

Determination of protein carbonyl concentrations provides information regarding protein involvement in ROS reactions. The carbonyl assay as applied to tissues and body fluids measures the average extent of protein modification.[181] The use of proteomics to identify specifically oxidized proteins appears to be a promising method.[190] Research on plasma of newborns has shown interesting selectively oxidized proteins during asphyxia.[191]

Total hydroperoxides represent a measure of overall oxidative stress, given that they are the intermediate oxidative products of lipids, peptides and amino acids.[176]

Percentages of oxidized forms of CoQ10 have also been used to demonstrate oxidative stress in asphyxiated newborns.[71]

A major marker of oxidative stress is the GSH/GSSG ratio, which directly reflects alteration of intracellular redox status.[192] GSH is a cofactor of GSH-Px and also has the antioxidant effect of binding Cu^{2+}, contributing to delivery of copper to the apoprotein of copper enzymes and decreasing free metal available for the Fenton reaction. Filomeni *et al.*[192] showed a relationship between intracellular GSH levels and mitochondrial-dependent apoptotic pathways. Under oxidative stress, GSSG may be produced at a high rate and extruded from cells into the extracellular milieu.[192] Since blood glutathione may reflect GSH status in other less accessible tissues, measurement of GSH and GSSG in blood has been considered an essential index of overall oxidative status and a useful indicator of risk of disease.

The GSH/GSSG ratio has been used as a measure of oxidative stress in neonates. Decreased ratios were observed in premature infants with severe RDS and newborns resuscitated with 100% O_2.[193,194] Lower GSH/GSSG ratios were found in very low-birth weight (LBW) infants even when they were breathing room air.[195]

Levels of nitrotyrosine have been reported to be a marker of $ONOO^-$ production resulting from phagocyte activation in inflammatory processes.[196] Therefore, nitrotyrosine can also be used as a marker of oxidative stress, since total nitration is consistent with amplified cell levels of $O_2^{\bullet-}$ in the presence of NO and CO_2.[197]

Allantoin can be measured in body fluids and its plasma levels are high under conditions of oxidative stress.[198] Assays in urine give reliable results.[199]

8-Hydroxydeoxyguanosine has been reported to be a reliable marker of oxidative stress. This molecule can be assayed in urine and has been done in newborns. While no differences in relation to gestational age have been reported by some authors,[200] others[201] observed a negative correlation between 8-OHdG and gestational age, confirming that premature infants are more subject to oxidative stress.

Plasma levels of NPBI appear to be a reliable marker of oxidative stress and close relationships between these levels and plasma carbonyls have been reported.[197] At least in neonates, both assays can be regarded as markers of potential risk of pathology due to oxygen toxicity.

Isolevuglandins (structural isomers and stereoisomers of cyclooxygenase-generated levoglandins) may be formed via free-radical-mediated pathways and have been proposed as a sensor of lipid peroxidation initiated by myeloperoxidase.[202]

Prevention and therapy

Avoiding oxidative stress

ROS are normally produced in living organisms. Their properties and complex role in the development of diseases make prevention and antioxidant therapy very difficult in newborns as well as in adults. Obviously, avoidance of conditions, such as asphyxia, hyperoxia and retinal light exposure, under which excessive free-radical release occurs, are the best defense against development of imbalances in pro-oxidant and antioxidant factors in the neonate. It is also important to remember that infections and particularly sepsis may be a severe source of oxidative stress. Frequent reports of NPBI in plasma of neonates suggest that indiscriminate iron supplementation should be avoided.

The concept of optimal oxygenation of newborns has recently been revised in order to clarify whether the optimal oxygen saturation unanimously accepted for normal infants and adults is also the best for sick neonates, especially if premature. The relationship between Hb oxygen saturation, risk of oxidative stress and oxygen toxicity, is still a problem. Even a recent Cochrane review failed to define the target range for maintaining blood oxygen levels in preterm/LBW infants.[203] This is presumably due to the complex mechanism of oxygen toxicity, which may be expressed at different percentages of O_2 saturation under different conditions. Conventional indications suggest that optimal oxygen tension should be maintained between 50 and 70 mmHg.[204] High O_2 saturation seems to be necessary for infants with CLD and infants with prethreshold ROP.[205] However, in view of susceptibility of some neonates to oxidative stress, it has been suggested that oxygen saturation maintained within physiological limits could result in moderate hyperoxia that could generate an excess of ROS. Experimental studies in animals in the first 24 h of life demonstrated a threshold of oxygen-restricted metabolism at $PaO_2 = 40$ Torr.[206] Shulze *et al.*[207] did not observe signs of mismatch between systemic oxygen delivery and demand in LBW infants kept at O_2 93–96% and 89–92% saturation. A significant decrease in CLD and ROP without any differences in mortality were observed in extremely low-birth-weight (ELBW) infants kept at less than 95% O_2 saturation compared to those kept at more than 95%.[208] Important indications on the use of oxygen were recently reported by Cow *et al.*[209] in a 5-year study in a tertiary neonatal center, where oxygen therapy was adjusted to optimize neonatal care and decrease the incidence of ROP. They recommended avoidance of repeated increase and decrease in FiO_2 in response to the oxygen saturation monitor and maintenance of oxygen saturation within 'acceptable' limits. They also recommended an alarm setting for oxygen saturation below 85% and above 93% for the newborns under 32 weeks of age. More recently, comparison of two populations of high-risk newborns kept at O_2 saturations of 88–98% and 70–90% showed a significant reduction in ROP in the group at lower O_2 saturation, but no differences in mortality or poor outcome.[210,211]

Hyperoxia and oxidative stress may occur during neonatal resuscitation. In an attempt to avoid the risk of tissue damage caused by ROS in the first hours of life, when susceptibility to oxidative stress is particularly high, the effects of reduction of O_2 were investigated. Some animal studies demonstrated identical outcome variables, including blood pressure, lung hemodynamics, acid–base status, cerebral blood flow and brain oxygenation whether resuscitation was done with room air or 100% oxygen.[212] In other experiments with animals subjected to ischemia and hypoxia, reoxygenation with 100% oxygen was followed by better restoration of microcirculation, but no difference in biochemical markers of brain injury.[213] Comparison of short and long duration of oxygen treatment after cerebral asphyxia in newborn piglets confirmed the efficacy of reoxygenation with room air.[214] Potential risks associated with resuscitation with 100% oxygen are suggested by the observation of increased production of ROS with respect to room air.[215,216] Clinical studies have demonstrated that there were no differences in short-term outcome between newborns resuscitated with room air and 100% oxygen.[217,218] The same results were observed in a follow-up at 18 and 24 months.[219] Vento *et al.*[194] demonstrated that room air resuscitation was associated with significantly less oxidative stress. It is important to note that increased oxidative stress following resuscitation with 100% oxygen was demonstrated by the sensitive GSH/GSSG ratio, which is a marker of generalized oxidative stress.[192] The satisfactory results of room air resuscitation in terms of outcome and avoidance of oxidative stress were recently confirmed by the same authors.[220] A reduction in mortality and no evidence of harm were described in a Cochrane review.[221] However, the authors concluded that there is insufficient evidence on which to recommend a policy of using room air over 100% oxygen or vice versa for resuscitation of newborns.[221] Although the guidelines do not discourage high FiO_2, it seems reasonable to conclude that 100% oxygen should not be used routinely.

Antioxidants

Much research has recently been carried out to find substances with antioxidant activity.[222] These substances can be divided into those decompartmentalizing metal complexes, those limiting ROS production, those modifying antiradical defenses and enhancing intracellular or extracellular antioxidant levels, those incorporating lipophilic antioxidant into membranes and those scavenging superoxide.[222]

Substances inhibiting phagocyte activation or xanthine oxidase and arachidonic acid metabolism, or decompartmentalizing free iron and making it available for the Fenton reaction, have also been investigated, together with those scavenging ROS directly or repairing ROS-induced membrane injury, like calcium antagonists and β-blockers.

On the whole, the results obtained in newborns have been uncertain. Although substances such as ascorbate are considered to be antioxidants *in vitro* and *in vivo*, they may act as pro-oxidant factors by causing metal-induced release of ROS.[223] Several other antioxidant substances have been used in newborn animals and humans in an attempt to improve the worst prognosis of damage, presumed to be due to ROS. Many, such as SOD, showed the same disadvantages in newborns as in adults.[224] Other drugs, such as allopurinol, have shown good results in animals,[225] but no advantages in human newborns, especially those with hypoxic ischemic encephalopathy.[226] Indomethacin, which has been shown to have antioxidant effects in humans, reduces the incidence and severity of intraventricular hemorrhage, but it is not known whether this effect is due to antioxidant activity.[227] Involvement of metal-induced ROS in brain damage suggested treatment with chelating agents. Desferrioxamine seemed to have a protective effect in animals, which has not yet been demonstrated in humans.[228] No definite results have been obtained by retinol supplementation.[229] Among the antioxidants, melatonin has a special place since it has been reported to have several interesting effects, such as enhancement of antioxidant enzyme activities and neutralization of H_2O_2 singlet oxygen and peroxynitrite.[230] Melatonin also appears to scavenge $OH^{\bullet}$.[231] Administration of melatonin to neonates with RDS has been reported to lower concentrations of proinflammatory cytokines.[232] In septic newborns, melatonin also lowers levels of oxidative markers, such as MDA and 4-hydroxylalkonals, and improves prognosis.[233]

Some drugs commonly used in neonatology, such as aminophylline, are reported to have antioxidant properties.[234] Vitamin E is a powerful, widely tested antioxidant and although no definite agreement has been reached on its use, interesting results have been reported even in human newborns. Analysis of nine randomized controlled trials of prophylactic use of vitamin E supplementation in very LBW infants showed no statistically significant reduction in the incidence of ROP and hemorrhage confined to the germinal matrix, although a significant reduction in the incidence of intraventricular hemorrhage was found.[235] Some formulations of vitamin E are poorly absorbed[236] and the metabolism and membrane distribution of the vitamin is uncertain; apart from this, there is no doubt about the effectiveness of α-tocopherol in protecting membranes and plasma lipoproteins from lipoperoxidation. In view of the potential activity of α-tocopherol and its proven deficiency in newborns, administration of vitamin E at the commonly recommended doses should be considered in any high-risk neonates.[237,238] Doses from 10 to 25 mg/kg/day in the first 3 days of life should protect premature infants in the first weeks.[239] Serum levels should be monitored in order to avoid levels exceeding 3 mg/dl. Subsequently, human milk or formula should be sufficient to maintain adequate vitamin levels.[239] Conclusions of a recent Cochrane review are that vitamin E supplementation to preterm infants reduces the risk of intracranial hemorrhage, but increases the risk of sepsis; in very LBW infants it seems to reduce the risk of ROP and blindness.[240] There is no evidence to support the use of vitamin E at high doses or the aim of keeping serum tocopherol levels above 3.5 mg/dl.[240]

Peroxidation products in stored lipid emulsions have been shown to increase lipid peroxidation *in vivo* in newborns and adults.[241] Since parenteral nutrition has been associated with increased formation of ROS, it is necessary to protect intralipids from light and add vitamins.[242] However, adaptation to factors responsible for oxidative stress has been demonstrated by Pitkanen *et al.*,[242] who found attenuated lipid peroxidation in preterm infants after repeated doses of intravenous lipids.

Micronutrients also play a role in protection against oxidative stress. Selenium is a part of the GSH-Px molecule, and a close correlation exists between selenium and GSH-Px.[243] Very severe RDS has been reported in selenium-deficient human babies.[244] However, while the deficiency of GSH-Px has been demonstrated in premature infants deficient in selenium,[245] the quantity of selenium supplementation to premature infants has yet to be established.[246]

Finally, the protective effects of bilirubin against ROS have been conclusively proved.[247,248] Although hyperbilirubinemia can be regarded as a natural antioxidant factor, the risk of brain damage due to high plasma levels of this molecule, particularly in premature babies, should not be underestimated.

REFERENCES

1. Smith JL. The pathological effects due to increase of oxygen tension in the air breathed. *J Physiol (Lond)* 1899;24:19–35.
2. Patz A, Hoeck I, de la Cruz E. Studies on the effect of high oxygen administration in retrolental fibroplasia. *Am J Ophthalmol* 1952;35:1248–53.
3. Gordon HH, Nitowsky HM, Cornblath M. Studies of tocopherol deficiency in infants and children. Hemolysis of erythrocytes in hydrogen peroxide. *Am J Dis Child* 1955;90:669–81.
4. Halliwell B, Gutteridge JMC. *Free Radical Biology and Medicine*, 2nd edn. Oxford: Clarendon Press, 1989.
5. Halliwell B, Gutteridge JMC, Cross CE. Free radicals, antioxidants, and human disease: Where are we now? *J Lab Clin Med* 1992;119:598–620.
6. Halliwell B. Free radicals, antioxidants, and human disease: Curiosity, cause, or consequence? *Lancet* 1994;344:721–4.
7. Gutteridge JMC. Lipid peroxidation and antioxidants as biomarkers of tissue damage. *Clin Chem* 1995;41:1819–28.
8. Fridovich I. Superoxide dismutase: An adaptation to a paramagnetic gas. *J Biol Chem* 1989;264:7761–4.
9. Turrens JF. Mitochondrial formation of reactive oxygen species. *J Physiol* 2003;552:335–44.

10. Radi R, Cassina A, Hodara R, *et al.* Peroxynitrite reactions and formation in mitochondria. *Free Radic Biol Med* 2002;33: 1451–64.
11. Wink DA, Miranda KM, Effey MG. Effects of oxidative and nitrosatide stress in cytotoxicity. *Semin Perinatol* 2000;24:20–3.
12. Beckman JS, Viera L, Estevez A, *et al.* Nitric oxide and peroxynitrite in the perinatal period. *Semin Perinatol* 2000;24:37–41.
13. Granot E, Kohen R. Oxidative stress in childhood in health and disease states. *Clin Nutr* 2004;23:3–11.
14. Balavoine GG, Geletii YV. Peroxynitrite scavenging by different antioxidants. I. Convenient assay. *Nitric Oxide* 1999;3:40–54.
15. Halliwell B. Superoxide, iron, vascular endothelium and reperfusion injury. *Free Radic Res Commun* 1989;5:315–8.
16. Weiss SJ. Tissue destruction by neutrophils. *N Engl J Med* 1989; 320:365–76.
17. Wiese AG, Pacifici RE, Davies KJA. Transient adaptation to oxidative stress in mammalian cells. *Arch Biochem Biophys* 1995;318:231–40.
18. Jaiswal AK. Antioxidant response element. *Biochem Pharmacol* 1994;48:439–44.
19. Warren MC, Bump EA, Medeiros D, *et al.* Oxidative stress-induced apoptosis of endothelial cells. *Free Radic Biol Med* 2000;29:537–47.
20. Clutton S. The importance of oxidative stress in apoptosis. *Br Med Bull* 1997;53:662–8.
21. Takahashi A, Masuda A, Sun M, *et al.* Oxidative stress-induced apoptosis is associated with alterations in mitochondrial caspase activity and Bcl-2-dependent alterations in mitochondrial pH. *Brain Res Bull* 2004;62:497–504.
22. Salvayre R, Auge N, Benoisi H, *et al.* Oxidized low-density lipoprotein-induced apoptosis. *Biochim Biophys Acta* 2002; 1585:213–21.
23. Azzi A, Davies KJA, Kelly F. Free radical biology – Terminology and critical thinking. *FEBS Lett* 2004;558:3–6.
24. Grisham MB. Reactive oxygen species in immune responses. *Free Radic Biol Med* 2004;36:1479–80.
25. Ginsburg I, Kohen R. Cell damage in inflammatory and infectious sites might involve a coordinated "cross-talk" among oxidants, microbial haemolysis and ampiphiles, cationic proteins, phospholipases, fatty acids, proteinases and cytokines (an overview). *Free Radic Res* 1995;22:489–517.
26. Grisham MB, Hernandez LA, Granger DN. Xanthine oxidase and neutrophil infiltration in intestinal ischemia. *Am J Physiol* 1986;251:G567–74.
27. Becker LB. New concepts in reactive oxygen species and cardiovascular reperfusion physiology. *Cardiovasc Res* 2004;61: 461–70.
28. Ferrari R, Ceconi C, Curello S, *et al.* Role of oxygen free radicals in ischemic and reperfused myocardium. *Am J Clin Nutr* 1991;53:215S–22S.
29. Hess ML, Manson NH. Molecular oxygen: Friend and foe. The role of the oxygen free radical system in the calcium paradox, the oxygen paradox and ischemia/reperfusion iniury. *J Mol Cell Cardiol* 1984;16:969–85.
30. Buonocore G, Perrone S, Bracci R. Free radicals and brain damage in the newborn. *Biol Neonate* 2001;79:180–6.
31. Turrens JF. Superoxide production by the mitochondrial respiratory chain. *Biosci Rep* 1997;17:3–8.
32. Taylor DL, Edward D, Mehmet H. Oxidative metabolism, apoptosis and perinatal brain injury. *Brain Pathol* 1999;9:93–117.
33. Kroemer G, Dallaporta B, Reshe-Rigon M. The mitochondrial death/life regulator in apoptosis and necrosis. *Annu Rev Physiol* 1998;60:619–42.
34. Schafer FQ, Buettner GR. Acidic pH amplifies iron-mediated lipid peroxidation in cells. *Free Radic Biol Med* 2000;28: 1175–81.
35. Saugstad OD. Hypoxanthine as an indicator of hypoxia: Its role in health and disease through free radical production. *Pediatr Res* 1998;23:143–50.
36. Ikeda H, Suzuki Y, Suzuki M, *et al.* Apoptosis is a major mode of cell death caused by ischaemia and ischaemia/reperfusion injury to the rat intestinal epithelium. *Gut* 1998;42:530–7.
37. Turrens JF, Freeman BA, Levitt JG, Crapo JD. The effect of hyperoxia on superoxide production by lung submitochondrial particles. *Arch Biochem Biophys* 1982;217:401–10.
38. Fenster BE, Tsao PS, Rockson SG. Endothelial dysfunction: Clinical strategies for treating oxidant stress. *Am Heart J* 2003; 146:218–26.
39. Channon KM, Guzik TJ. Mechanisms of superoxide production in human blood vessels: Relationship to endothelial dysfunction, clinical and genetic risk factors. *J Physiol Pharmacol* 2002; 53(4):515–24.
40. Yokoyama M. Oxidant stress and atherosclerosis. *Curr Opin Pharmacol* 2004;4:110–5.
41. Ullrich V, Bachschmid M. Superoxide as a messenger of endothelial function. *Biochem Biophys Res Commun* 2000; 278:1–8.
42. Loscalzo J. Oxidant stress: A key determinant of atherothrombosis. *Biochem Soc Trans* 2003;31:1059–61.
43. Zou M, Jendral M, Ulrich V. Prostaglandin endoperoxide-dependent vasospasm in bovine coronary arteries after nitration of prostacyclin synthase. *Br J Pharmacol* 1999;126:1283–92.
44. Salvemini D, Cuzzocrea S. Oxidative stress in septic shock and disseminated intravascular coagulation. *Free Radic Biol Med* 2002;33:1173–85.
45. Kreuz WM, Veldmann AM, Fisher D, *et al.* Neonatal sepsis: A challenge in hemostaseology. *Semin Thromb Hemost* 1999; 25:531–35.
46. Rotilio G, Rigo A, Bracci R, *et al.* Determination of red blood cell superoxide dismutase and glutathione peroxidase in newborns in relation to neonatal hemolysis. *Clin Chim Acta* 1997;81:131–4.
47. Gardner R, Salvador A, Moradas-Ferreira P. Why does SOD overexpression sometimes enhance, sometimes decrease, hydrogen peroxide production? A minimalist explanation. *Free Radic Biol Med* 2002;32:1351–7.
48. Wu G, Fang YZ, Yang S, Lupton J, Turner ND. Glutathione metabolism and its implications for health. *J Nutr* 2004;134: 489–92.
49. Nozik-Grayck E, Dieterle CS, Piantadosi CA, *et al.* Secretion of extracellular superoxide dismutase in neonatal lungs. *Am J Physiol Lung Cell Mol Physiol* 2000;279:L977–84.
50. Abudu N, Miller JJ, Attaelmannan M, Levinson SS. Vitamins in human arteriosclerosis with emphasis on vitamin C and vitamin E. *Clin Chim Acta* 2004;339:11–25.
51. Beyer RE. The participation of coenzyme Q in free radical production and antioxidation. *Free Radic Biol Med* 1990;8:545–65.
52. Ricciarelli R, Zingg JM, Azzi A. The 80th anniversary of vitamin E: Beyond its antioxidant properties. *Biol Chem* 2002;383(3–4): 457–65.
53. Halliwell B, Gutteridge JMC. The antioxidants of human extracellular fluids. *Arch Biochem Biophys* 1990;280:1–8.
54. Dennery PA. Role of redox in fetal development and neonatal diseases. *Antioxid Redox Signal* 2004;6:147–53.
55. Weinberger D, Laskin DL, Heck DE, *et al.* Oxygen toxicity in premature infants. *Toxicol Appl Pharmacol* 2002;181:60–7.
56. Hooper SB, Coulter CL, Deayton JM, *et al.* Fetal endocrine responses to prolonged hypoxemia in sheep. *Am J Physiol* 1990; 259:R703–8.
57. Khullar S, Greenwood SL, McCord N, *et al.* Nitric oxide and superoxide impair human placental amino acid uptake and increase Na^+ permeability: Implications for fetal growth. *Free Radic Biol Med* 2004;36:271–7.
58. Frank L, Sosenko IRS. Prenatal development of' lung antioxidant enzymes in four species. *J Pediatr* 1987;110:106–10.
59. de Haan JB, Tymms MJ, Cristiano F, Kola I. Expression of copper/zinc superoxide dismutase and glutathione peroxidase in organs of developing mouse embryos, fetuses, and neonates. *Pediatr Res* 1994;35:188–96.
60. Jung K, Henke W. Developmental changes of antioxidant enzymes in kidney and liver from rats. *Free Radic Biol Med* 1996;20:613–7.
61. Jones PEH, McCance RA. Enzyme activities in the blood of infants and adults. *Biochem J* 1949;45:464.
62. Gross RT, Bracci R, Rudolph N, *et al.* Hydrogen peroxide toxicity and detoxification in the erythrocytes of newborn infants. *Blood* 1967;29:481–93.
63. Ochoa JJ, Ramirez-Tortosa MC, Quilez JL, *et al.* Oxidative stress in erythrocytes from premature and full term infants during the first 72 h of life. *Free Radic Res* 2003;37:317–22.
64. Dobashi K, Asayamat K, Hayashibe H, *et al.* Immunohistochemical study of copper–zinc and manganese superoxide dismutases in the lungs of human fetuses and newborn infants: Developmental profile and alterations in hyaline membrane disease and bronchopulmonary dysplasia. *Virchows Arch* 1993; 423:177–84.

65. Strange RC, Cotton W, Fryer AA, *et al.* Studies on the expression of Cu, Zn superoxide dismutase in human tissues during development. *Biochem Biophys Acta* 1988;964:260–5.

66. Bracci R, Calabri G, Bettini F, *et al.* Glutathione peroxidase in human leukocytes. *Clin Chim Acta* 1970;29:345–8.

67. Sullivan JL, Newton RB. Serum antioxidant activity in neonates. *Arch Dis Child* 1988;63:748–57.

68. Gopinathan V, Miller NJ, Milner AD, Rice-Evans CA. Bilirubin and ascorbate antioxidant activity in neonatal plasma. *FEBS Lett* 1994;349:197–200.

69. Rogers S, Witz G, Anwar M, *et al.* Antioxidant capacity and oxygen radical diseases in the preterm newborn. *Arch Pediatr Adolesc* 2000;154:544–8.

70. Luukkainen P, Aejmelaeus R, Alho H, *et al.* Plasma chain-breaking antioxidants in preterm infant with good and poor short-term outcome. *Free Radic Res* 1999;30:189–97.

71. Lindeman JH, van Zoeren-Grobben D, Schrijver J, *et al.* The total free radical trapping ability of cord blood plasma in preterm and term babies. *Pediatr Res* 1989;26:20–4.

72. Hara K, Yamashita S, Fujisawa A, *et al.* Oxidative stress in newborn infants with and without asphyxia as measured by plasma antioxidants and free fatty acids. *Biochem Biophys Res Commun* 1999;257:244–8.

73. Pitkanen OM, Hallman M, Andersson SM. Correlation of free radical-induced lipid peroxidation with outcome in very low birth weight infants. *J Pediatr* 1990;116:760–4.

74. Ahola T, Fellman V, Kjellmer I, *et al.* Plasma 8-isoprostane is increased in preterm infants who develop bronchopulmonary dysplasia or periventricular leukomalacia. *Pediatr Res* 2004;56:88–93.

75. Goil S, Truog W, Brnes C. Eight-epi-PGF$_{2\alpha}$: A possible marker of lipid peroxidation in term infants with severe pulmonary disease. *J Pediatr* 1998;132:349–51.

76. Lindeman JH, Houdkamp E, Lentjes EG, *et al.* Limited protection against iron-induced lipid peroxidation by cord blood plasma. *Free Radic Biol Med* 1992;16:285–94.

77. Lindeman JHN, Lentjes EG, van Zoeren-Grobben D, *et al.* Postnatal changes in plasma ceruloplasmin and transferrin antioxidant activities in preterm babies. *Biol Neonate* 2000;78:73–6.

78. Evans PJ, Evans P, Kovar IZ, *et al.* Bleomycin-detectable iron in the plasma of premature and full-term neonates. *FEBS Lett* 1992;303:210–2.

79. Breuer W, Hershko C, Cabantchik ZI. The importance of non-transferrin bound iron in disorders of iron metabolism. *Transfus Sci* 2000;23:185–92.

80. Berger HM, Mumby S, Gutteridge JMC. Ferrous ions detected in iron overloaded cord blood plasma from preterm and term babies: Implications for oxidative stress. *Free Radic Res* 1995;22:555–9.

81. Clahsen PC, Moison RMW, Holtzer CAJ, Berger HM. Recycling of glutathione during oxidative stress in erythrocytes of the newborn. *Pediatr Res* 1992;32:399–402.

82. Smith CV, Hansen TN, Martin NE, *et al.* Oxidant stress responses in premature infants during exposure to hyperoxia. *Pediatr Res* 1993;34:360–5.

83. O'Donovan DJ, Fernandes CJ. Mitochondrial glutathione and oxidative stress: Implications for pulmonary oxygen toxicity in premature infants. *Mol Genet Metab* 2000;71:352–8.

84. Berger MT, Polidori MC, Dabbag A, *et al.* Antioxidant activity of vitamin C in iron-overloaded human plasma. *J Biol Chem* 1997;272:15656–60.

85. Moison RM, de Beaufort A, Haasnoot AA. Uric acid and ascorbic acid redox ratio in plasma and tracheal aspirate of preterm babies with acute and chronic lung disease. *Free Radic Biol Med* 1997;23:226–34.

86. Compagnoni G, Lista G, Giuffrè B, *et al.* Coenzyme q(10) levels in maternal plasma: Correlation with mode of delivery. *Biol Neonate* 2004;86:104–7.

87. Johnston RB Jr. Function and cell biology of neutrophil and mononuclear phagocytes in the newborn infant. *Vaccine* 1998;16:1363–8.

88. Bracci R, Buonocore G. Chorioamnionitis: A risk factor for fetal and neonatal morbidity. *Biol Neonate* 2003;83:85–96.

89. Arnould T, Michiels C, Remacle J. Hypoxic human umbilical vein endothelial cells induce activation of adherent polymorphonuclear leukocytes. *Blood* 1994;83:3705–16.

90. Wang W, Pang CCP, Rogers MS, Chang AMZ. Lipid peroxidation in cord blood at birth. *Am J Obstet Gynecol* 1996;174:62–5.

91. Holcberg G, Kossenjans W, Miodovnik M, Myatt L. The interaction of nitric oxide and superoxide in the human fetal–placental vasculature. *Am J Obstet Gynecol* 1995;173:528–33.

92. Toh N, Inoue T, Kuraya M, *et al.* Antioxidative activities of a reductant in the ultrafiltrate of human placental homogenate. *Biol Res Pregnancy* 1987;8:47–52.

93. Murth KR, Joseph P, Kulkarni AP. 2-Aminofluorene bioactivation by human term placental peroxidase. *Teratogen Carcinogen Mutagen* 1995;15:115–26.

94. Saugstad OD. Is oxygen more toxic than currently believed? *Pediatrics* 2001;108:1203–5.

95. Wang Y, Walsh SW, Kay HH. Placental lipid peroxides and thromboxane are increased and prostacyclin is decreased in women with pre-eclampsia. *Am J Obstet Gynecol* 1992;167:946–9.

96. Walsh SW, Vaughan JE, Wang YP, *et al.* Placental isoprostane is significantly increased in preeclampsia. *FASEB J* 2001;15:79–81.

97. Moretti M, Phillips M, *et al.* Increased breath markers of oxidative stress in normal pregnancy and in preeclampsia. *Am J Obstet Gynecol* 2004;190:1184–90.

98. Goldberg B, Stern A, Peisach J. The mechanism of superoxide anion generation by its interaction of phenylhydrazine with hemoglobin. *J Biol Chem* 1976;251:3045–51.

99. Lync RE, Fridovich I. Permeation of the erythrocyte stroma by superoxide radical. *J Biol Chem* 1978;253:4697–9.

100. Winterbourn CC, Stern A. Human red cells scavenge extracellular hydrogen peroxide and inhibit formation of hypochlorous acid and hydroxyl radical. *J Clin Invest* 1987;80:1486–91.

101. Weiss SJ. Neutrophil-mediated methemoglobin formation in the erythrocyte. The role of superoxide and hydrogen peroxide. *J Biol Chem* 1982;257:2947–53.

102. Ferrali M, Signorini C, Ciccoli L. Iron release and membrane damage in erythrocytes exposed to oxidizing agents, phenylhydrazine, divicine and isuramil. *Biochem J* 1992;285:295–301.

103. Ripalda MJ, Rudolph N, Wong SL. Developmental patterns of antioxidant defense mechanisms in human erythrocytes. *Pediatr Res* 1989;26:366–9.

104. Phylactos AC, Leaf AA, Costeloe K, Crawford MA. Erythrocyte cupric/zinc superoxide dismutase exhibits reduced activity in preterm and low-birthweight infants at birth. *Acta Paediatr* 1995;84:1421–5.

105. Bracci R, Bagnoli F, De Donno ML, *et al.* Red cell superoxide dismutase and other erythrocyte enzyme activities in the newborn Infants with hyperbilirubinemia. *Ital J Biochem* 1979;28:73–5.

106. Bracci R, Buonocore G, Talluri B, Berni S. Neonatal hyperbilirubinemia. Evidence for a role of the erythrocyte enzyme activities involved in the detoxification of oxygen radicals. *Acta Paediatr Scand* 1988;77:349–56.

107. Vives Corrons JL, Pujades MA, Colomer D. Increase of enzyme activities following the in vitro peroxidation of normal human red blood cells. *Enzyme* 1988;39:1–7.

108. Neefjes VME, Evelo CTA, Daars LGM, *et al.* Erythrocyte glutathione S transferase as a marker of oxidative stress at birth. *Arch Dis Child Fetal Neonatal Ed* 1999;81:F130–3.

109. Moison RMW, Haasnoot AA, van Zoeren-Grobben D, *et al.* Red blood cell glutathione and plasma sulfhydryls in chronic lung disease of the newborn. *Acta Paediatr* 1997;86:1363–9.

110. Ciccoli L, Rossi V, Leoncini S, *et al.* Iron release, superoxide production and binding of autologous IgG to band 3 dimers in newborn and adult erythrocytes exposed to hypoxia and hypoxia–reoxygenation. *Biochim Biophys Acta* 2004;1672: 203–13.

111. Robles R, Palomino N, Robles A. Oxidative stress in the neonate. *Early Hum Dev* 2001;Suppl 65:S75–81.

112. Jain SK. The neonatal erythrocyte and its oxidative susceptibility. *Semin Hematol* 1989;26:286–300.

113. Jain SK, Wise R, Bocchini JJ. Vitamin E and vitamin E–quinone levels in red blood cells and plasma of newborn infants and their mothers. *J Am Coll Nutr* 1996;15:44–8.

114. Kondo M, Itoh S, Kusaka T, *et al.* The ability of neonatal and maternal erythrocytes to produce reactive oxygen species in response to oxidative stress. *Early Hum Dev* 2002;66:81–8.

115. Bracci R, Benedetti PA, Ciambellotti V. Hydrogen peroxide generation in the erythrocytes of newborn infants. *Biol Neonate* 1970;15:135–41.

116. Signorini C, Ferrali M, Ciccoli L. Iron release, membrane protein oxidation and erythrocyte aging. *FEBS Lett* 1995;362:165–70.

117. Kay MM. Mechanism of removal of senescent cell by human macrophages in situ. *Proc Natl Acad Sci USA* 1975;72:3521–5.
118. Rifkind JM, Zhang L, Levy A, *et al.* The hypoxic stress on erythrocytes associated with superoxide formation. *Free Radic Res Commun* 1991;12–13:645–52.
119. Buonocore G, Zani S, Perrone S, *et al.* Intraerythrocyte non protein bound iron and plasma malondialdehyde in the hypoxic newborn. *Free Radic Biol Med* 1998;25:766–70.
120. Ciccoli L, Rossi V, Leoncini S, *et al.* Iron release in erythrocytes and plasma non protein-bound iron in hypoxic and non hypoxic newborns. *Free Radic Res* 2003;37:51–8.
121. Bracci R, Perrone S, Buonocore G. Oxidant iniury in neonatal erythrocytes during the perinatal period. *Acta Paediatr Suppl* 2002;438:130–4.
122. Saugstad OD. Mechanisms of tissue injury by oxygen radicals: Implications for neonatal disease. *Acta Paediatr* 1996;85:1–4.
123. Bancalari E, Gerhardt T. Bronchopulmonary dysplasia. *Pediatr Clin North Am* 1986:33:1–23.
124. Mirro R, Armstead W, Leffler C. Increased airway leukotriene levels in infants with severe bronchopulmonary dysplasia. *Am J Dis Child* 1990;144:160–1.
125. Moison RMW, Palinckx JJS, Roest M, *et al.* Induction of lipid peroxidation of pulmonary surfactant by plasma of preterm babies. *Lancet* 1993;341:79–82.
126. Ogihara T, Okamoto R, Kim H-S, *et al.* New evidence for the involvement of oxygen radicals in triggering neonatal chronic lung disease. *Pediatr Res* 1996;39:117–9.
127. Varsila E, Pitkanen O, Hallman M, Andersson S. Immaturity-dependent free radical activity in premature infants. *Pediatr Res* 1994;36:55–9.
128. Frank L. Developmental aspects of experimental pulmonary oxygen toxicity. *Free Radic Biol Med* 1991;11:463–94.
129. O'Donovan DJ, Lynette K, Rogers DKK, *et al.* CoASH and CoASSG Levels in the lung of hyperoxic rats as potential biomarkers of intramitochondrial oxidant stresses. *Pediatr Res* 2002;51:346–53.
130. Vacchiano CA, Tempel GE. Role of nonenzymatically generated prostanoid, 8-iso-PGF(2-alpha), in pulmonary oxygen toxicity. *J Appl Physiol* 1994;77:2912–7.
131. Wilson WL, Mullen M, Olley PM, *et al.* Hyperoxia-induced pulmonary vascular and lung abnormalities in young rats and potential for recovery. *Pediatr Res* 1985;19:1059–67.
132. Appleby C, Towner RA. Magnetic resonance imaging of pulmonary damage in the term and premature rat neonate exposed to hyperoxia. *Pediatr Res* 2001;50:502–7.
133. Denis D, Fayon MJ, Berger P, *et al.* Prolonged moderate hyperoxia induced hyperresponsiveness and airway inflammation in newborn rats. *Pediatr Res* 2001;50:515–9.
134. Schock BC, Swett DG, Ennis M, *et al.* Oxidative stress and increased type-IV collagenase levels in bronchoalveolar lavage fluid from newborn babies. *Pediatr Res* 2001;50:29–33.
135. Grigg J, Arnon S, Chase A, Silverman M. Inflammatory cells in the lungs of premature infants on the first day of life: Perinatal risk factors and origin of cells. *Arch Dis Child* 1993;69:40–3.
136. Kotecha S, Chan B, Azam N, *et al.* Increase in interleukin-8 and soluble intercellular adhesion molecule-1 in bronchoalveolar lavage fluid from premature infants who develop chronic lung disease. *Arch Dis Child* 1995;72:F90–6.
137. Crim J, Longmore WJ. Sublethal hydrogen peroxide inhibits alveolar type II cell surfactant phospholipid biosynthetic enzymes. *Am Physiol* 1995;12:L129–35.
138. Ischiropoulos H, Almehdi AB, Fisher AB. Reactive species in ischemic rat lung injury: Contribution of peroxynitrite. *Am Physiol* 1995;13:L158–64.
139. Kojima T, Hattori K, Hirata Y, *et al.* Endothelin-1 has a priming effect on production of superoxide anion by alveolar macrophages: Its possible correlation with bronchopulmonary dysplasia. *Pediatr Res* 1996;39:112–6.
140. Wagenaar GT, Horst SA, van Gastelen MA, *et al.* Gene expression profile and histopathology of experimental bronchopulmonary dysplasia induced by prolonged oxidative stress. *Free Radic Biol Med* 2004;36(6):782–801.
141. Buss ICH, Darlow BH, Winterbourn CC. Elevated protein carbonyls and lipid peroxidation products correlating with myeloperoxidase in tracheal aspirates from premature infants. *Pediatr Res* 2000;47:640–5.
142. Schock BC, Sweet DG, Halliday HL, *et al.* Oxidative stress in lavage fluid of preterm infants at risk of chronic lung disease. *Am J Physiol Lung Cell Mol Physiol* 2001;281:L1386–91.
143. Winterbourn C, Chan T, Buss H, *et al.* Protein carbonyls and lipid peroxidation products as oxidation markers in preterm infant plasma: Association with chronic lung disease and retinopathy and effects of selenium supplementation. *Pediatr Res* 2000;48:84–90.
144. Smith LEH. Pathogenesis of retinopathy of prematurity. *Growth Horm IGF Res* 2004;14:S140–4.
145. Dani C, Reali MF, Bertini G, *et al.* The role of blood transfusions and iron intake on retinopathy of prematurity. *Early Hum Dev* 2001;62:57–63.
146. Papp A, Nemeth I, Karge E, *et al.* Glutathione status in retinopathy of prematurity. *Free Radic Biol Med* 1999;27:738–43.
147. Hairano K, Morinobu T, Kim H, *et al.* Blood transfusion increased radical promoting non-transferrin bound iron in preterm infants. *Arch Dis Child Fetal Neontal Ed* 2001;84:F188–93.
148. Armstrong D, Hiramitsu T, Gutteridge J, Nilsson SE. Studies on experimentally induced retinal degeneration. I. Effect of lipid peroxides on electroretinographic activity in the albino rabbit. *Exp Eye Res* 1982;35:157–71.
149. Chemtob S, Roy M-S, Abran D, *et al.* Prevention of postasphyxial increase in lipid peroxides and retinal function deterioration in the newborn pig by inhibition of cyclooxygenase activity and free radical generation. *Pediatr Res* 1993;33:336–40.
150. Abran D, Hardy P, Varma DR, Chemtob S. Mechanisms of the biphasic effects of peroxides on the retinal vasculature of' newborn and adult pigs. *Exp Eye Res* 1995;61:285–92.
151. Abran D, Varma DR, Chemtob S. Increased thromboxane-mediated contractions of retinal vessels of newborn pigs to peroxides. *Am J Physiol* 1995;37:H628–32.
152. Halliwell B. Reactive oxygen species and the central nervous system. *J Neurochem* 1992;59:1609–23.
153. Delivoria-Papadopoulos M, Mishra OP. Mechanism of perinatal cerebral injury in fetus and newborns. *Ann N Y Acad Sci* 2000; 900:159–68.
154. Cook DA, Vollrath B. Free radicals and intracellular events associated with cerebrovascular spasm. *Cardiovasc Res* 1995;30: 493–500.
155. Oka A, Belliveau MJ, Rosenberg PA, Volpe JJ. Vulnerability of oligodendroglia to glutamate: Pharmacology, mechanisms, and prevention. *J Neurosci* 1993;13:1441–53.
156. Abdelrahman A, Parks JK, Devereaux MW, *et al.* Developmental changes in newborn lamb brain mitochondrial activity and postasphxial lipid peroxidation. *Proc Soc Exp Biol Med* 1995; 209:170–7.
157. Volpe JJ. Neurobiology of periventricular leukomalacia in the premature infant. *Pediatr Res* 2001;50:553–6.
158. Poulsen JP, Oyasaeter S, Sanderud J, *et al.* Hypoxanthine, xanthine, and uric acid concentrations in the cerebrospinal fluid, plasma, and urine of hypoxemic pigs. *Pediatr Res* 1990;28:477–81.
159. Palmer C, Vannucci RC, Towfighi J. Reduction of perinatal hypoxic–ischemic brain damage with allopurinol. Pediatr Res 1990;27:332–6.
160. Goplerud JM, Mishra OP, Delivoria-Papadopoulos M. Brain cell membrane dysfunction following acute asphyxia in newborn piglets. *Biol Neonate* 1992;61:33–41.
161. Inder T, Mocatta T, Darlow B, *et al.* Elevated free radical products in the cerebrospinal fluid of VLBW infants with cerebral white matter injury. *Pediatr Res* 2002;52:213–8.
162. Maulik D, Numagami Y, Osnishi ST, *et al.* Direct measurement of oxygen free radicals during in utero hypoxia in the fetal guinea pig brain. *Brain Res* 1998;798:166–72.
163. DiGiacomo JE, Pane CR, Gwiazdowski S, *et al.* Effects of graded hypoxia on brain cell membrane injury in newborn piglets. *Biol Neonate* 1992;61:25–32.
164. Palmer C, Menzies SL, Roberts RL, *et al.* Changes in iron histochemistry after hypoxic–ischemic brain injury in the neonatal rat. *J Neurosci Res* 1999;56:60–71.
165. Olano M, Song DK, Murphy S, *et al.* Relationship of dopamine, cortical oxygen pressure, and hydroxyl radicals in brain of newborn piglets during hypoxia and post-hypoxic recovery. *J Neurochem* 1995;65:1205–12.
166. Inder T, Mocatta T, Darlow B, *et al.* Markers of oxidative injury in the cerebrospinal fluid of premature infant with meningitis and periventricular leukomalacia. *J Pediatr* 2002;140:617–21.
167. Savman K, Nilsson UA, Blennow M, *et al.* Non-protein-bound iron is elevated in cerebrospinal fluid from preterm infants with post hemorrhagic ventricular dilatation. *Pediatr Res* 2001;49: 208–12.

168. Back SA, Gan X, Li Y, *et al.* Maturation-dependent vulnerability of oligodentrocytes to oxidative stress-induced death caused by glutathione depletion. *J Neurosci* 1998;18:6241–53.
169. Jamieson, DD. Lipid peroxidation in brain and lungs from mice exposed to hyperoxia. *Biochem Pharmacol* 1991;41:749–56.
170. Watson NA, Beard SC, Ataf N, *et al.* The effect of hyperoxia on cerebral blood flow: A study in healthy volunteers using magnetic resonance phase-contrast angiography. *Eur J Anaesthesiol* 2000;17(3):152–9.
171. Niijima S, Shortland DB, Levene MI, *et al.* Transient hyperoxia and cerebral blood flow velocity in infants born prematurely and at full term. *Arch Dis Child* 1998;63(10):1126–30.
172. Fumagalli M, Mosca F, Knudsen GM, *et al.* Transient hyperoxia and residual cerebrovascular effects in the newborn rat. *Pediatr Res* 2004;55:380–4.
173. Leviton A, Dammann O. Coagulation, inflammation and risk of neonatal white matter damage. *Pediatr Res* 2004;55:541–45.
174. Supnet MC, David-Cu R, Walther FJ. Plasma xanthine oxidase activity and lipid hydroperoxide levels in preterm infants. *Pediatr Res* 1994;36:283–7.
175. Schmidt H, Grune T, Muller R, *et al.* Increased levels of lipid peroxidation products malondialdehyde and 4-hydroxynonenal after perinatal hypoxia. *Pediatr Res* 1996;40:15–20.
176. Buonocore G, Perrone S, Longini M, *et al.* Total hydroperoxide and advanced oxidation protein products in preterm hypoxic babies. *Pediatr Res* 2000;47:221–4.
177. Buonocore G, Perrone S, Longini M, *et al.* Oxidative stress in preterm neonates at birth and on the seventh day of life. *Pediatr Res* 2002;52:46–9.
178. Qin Y, Wang CC, Kuhn H, *et al.* Determinants of umbilical cord arterial 8-iso-prostaglandin F2alpha concentration. *Br J Obstet Gynaecol* 2000;107(8):973–81.
179. Dorrepal CA, Berger HM, Benders MJN, *et al.* Non protein-bound iron in postasphyxial reperfusion injury in the newborn. *Pediatrics* 1996;98:883–9.
180. Buonocore G, Perrone S, Longini M, *et al.* Non protein bound iron as early predictive marker of neonatal brain damage. *Brain* 2003;126:1224–30.
181. Halliwell B, Whiteman M. Measuring reactive species and oxidative damage in vivo and in cell culture: How should you do it and what do result mean? *Br J Pharmacol* 2004;142:231–55.
182. Polidori MC, Stahl W, Eichler O, *et al.* Profiles of antioxidants in human plasma. *Free Radic Biol Med* 2001;30:456–62.
183. Roberts LJ II, Morrow JD. Products of the isoprostane pathway: Unique bioactive compound and markers of lipid peroxidation. *Cell Mol Life Sci* 2002;59:808–20.
184. Lawson JA, Rokach J, Fitzgerald GA. Isoprostanes: Formation, analysis and use as indices of lipid peroxidation in vivo. *J Biol Chem* 1999;264:24441–4.
185. Varsila E, Hallman M, Andersson S. Free-radical-induced lipid peroxidation during the early neonatal period. *Acta Paediatr* 1994;83:692–95.
186. Nycyk JA, Drury JA, Cooke RWI. Breath pentane as a marker for lipid peroxidation and adverse outcome in preterm infants. *Arch Dis Child Fetal Neonatal Ed* 1998;79:67–9.
187. Springfield JR, Levitt MD. Pitfalls in the use of breath pentane measurements to assess lipid peroxidation. *J Lipid Res* 1994; 35:1497–504.
188. Loiseaux-Meunier MN, Bedu M, Gentou C, *et al.* Oxygen toxicity: Simultaneous measure of pentane and malondialdehyde in humans exposed to hyperoxia. *Biomed Pharmacother* 2001;55:163–9.
189. Ogihara T, Hirano K, Morinobu T, *et al.* Raised concentrations of aldehyde lipid peroxidation products in premature infants with chronic lung disease. *Arch Dis Child Fetal Neonatal Ed* 1999;80:F21–5.
190. Butterfield DA. Proteomics: A new approach to investigate oxidative stress in Alzheimer's disease brain. *Brain Res* 2004;1000(1–2):1–7.
191. Marzocchi B, Perrone S, Paffetti P, *et al.* Non protein bound and plasma protein oxidant stress at birth. *Pediatr Res* 2004;55:291A.
192. Filomeni G, Rotilio G, Ciriolo MR. Cell signaling and the glutathione redox system. *Biochem Pharmacol* 2002;64:1057–64.
193. Nemeth I, Boda D. Blood glutathione redox ratio as a parameter of oxidative stress in premature infants with RDS. *Free Radic Biol Med* 1994;16(3):347–53.
194. Vento M, Asensi M, Sastre J, *et al.* Resuscitation with room air instead of 100% oxygen prevents oxidative stress in moderately asphyxiated term neonates. *Pediatrics* 2001;107:642–7.
195. Smith CV, Hansen TN, Martin NE, *et al.* Oxidant stress responses in premature infants during exposure to hyperoxia. *Pediatr Res* 1993;34:360–5.
196. Eiserich JP, Hristova M, Cross CE, *et al.* Formation of nitric oxide-derived inflammatory oxidants by myeloperoxidase in neutrophils. *Nature* 1998;391:393–7.
197. Koeck T, Fu X, Hazen SL, *et al.* Rapid and selective oxygen regulated protein tyrosine "denitration" and nitration in mitochondria. *J Biol Chem* 2004;279:27257–62.
198. Grootveld M, Ehalliwell B. Measurement of allantoin and uric acid in human body fluids. A potential index of free radical reactions in vivo? 1987;243:803–8.
199. Mikami T, Kita K, Tomita S, *et al.* Is allantoin in serum and urine a useful indicator of exercise-induced oxidative stress in humans? *Free Radic Res* 2000;32:235–44.
200. Drury JA, Jeffers G, Cooke RW. Urinary 8-hydroxydeoxyguanosine in infants and children. *Free Radic Res* 1998;28:423–8.
201. Matsubasa T, Uchino T, Karashima S, *et al.* Oxidative stress in very low birth weight infants as measured by urinary 8-OHdG. *Free Radic Res* 2002;36(2):189–93.
202. Poliakov E, Brennan ML, Macpherson J, *et al.* Isolevuglandins, a novel class of isoprostenoid derivatives, function as integrated sensors of oxidant stress and are generated by myeloperoxidase in vivo. *FASEB J* 2003;17:2209–20.
203. Askie LM, Henderson-Smart DJ. Restricted versus liberal oxygen exposure for preventing morbidity and mortality in preterm or low birth weight infants (Cochrane review). *Cochrane Database Syst Rev* 2004;4:CD001077.
204. Wolkoff LI, Narula P. Issue in neonatal and pediatric oxygen therapy. *Respir Care Clin N Am* 2000;6:675–91.
205. Askie L. Appropriate levels of oxygen saturation for preterm infants. *Acta Pediatr Suppl* 2004;444:26–8.
206. Torrance SM, Wittnich C. Blood lactate and acid-base balance in graded neonatal hypoxia: Evidence for oxygen restricted metabolism. *J Appl Physiol* 1994;77(5):2318–24.
207. Schulze A, White K, Way RC, *et al.* Effect of the arterial oxygenation level on cardiac output, oxygen extraction, and oxygen comsumption in low birth weight infants receiving mechanical ventilation. *J Pediatr* 1995;126:777–84.
208. Sun SC. Relation of target SpO_2 levels and clinical outcome in ELBW infants on supplemental oxygen. *Pediatr Res* 2002; 51:350A.
209. Chow LC, Wright KW, Sola A, *et al.* Can changes in clinical practice decrease the incidence of severe retinopathy of prematurity in very low birth weight infants? *Pediatrics* 2003;111: 339–45.
210. Tin W, Milligan DWA, Pennefather P, *et al.* Pulse oximetry, severe retinopathy, and outcome at one year in babies of less than 28 weeks gestation. *Arch Dis Child Fetal Neonatal Ed* 2001;84:F106–10.
211. Tin W. Optimal oxygen saturation for preterm babies. *Biol Neonate* 2004;85:319–25.
212. Rootwelt T, Loberg M, Moen A, *et al.* Hypoxemia and reoxination with 21% or 100% oxygen in newborn pigs. Changes in blood pressure, base deficit, and hypoxanthine and brain morphology. *Pediatr Res* 1992;32:107–13.
213. Solas AB, Kalous P, Saugstad OD. Reoxygenation with 100 or 21% oxygen after cerebral hypoxia ischemia–hypercapnia in newborn piglets. *Biol Neonate* 2004;85:105–11.
214. Solas AB, Munkeby BH, Saugstad OD. Comparison of short-and long-duration oxygen treatment after cerebral asphyxia in newborn piglets. *Pediatr Res* 2004;54:125–31.
215. Kondo M, Itoh S, Isobe K, *et al.* Chemiluminescence because of the production of reactive oxygen species in the lungs of newborn piglets during resuscitation periods after asphyxiation load. *Pediatr Res* 2000;47:524–7.
216. Kutzsche S, Ilves P, Kirkeby OJ, *et al.* Hydrogen peroxide production in leukocytes during cerebral hypoxia and reoxygenation with 100% or 21% oxygen in newborn piglets. *Pediatr Res* 2001;49:834–42.
217. Ramij S, Abuja S, Thirupuram S, *et al.* Resuscitation of asphyxic newborn infants with room air or 100% oxygen. *Pediatr Res* 1993;34:809–12.
218. Saugstad OD, Rootwelt T, Aalen O. Resuscitation of asphyxiated newborn infants with room air or oxygen: An international controlled trial: The resair 2 study. *Pediatrics* 1998;102:e1.
219. Saugstad OD, Ramji S, Irani SF, *et al.* Resuscitation of newborn infants with 21% or 100% oxygen: Follow-up at 18 to 24 months. *Pediatrics* 2003;112:296–300.

220. Vento M, Asensi M, Sastre J, *et al.* Oxidative stress in asphyxiated term infants resuscitated with 100% oxygen. *J Pediatr* 2003;142: 240–6.
221. Tan A, Schulze A, O'Donnell CPF, Davis PG. Air versus oxygen for resuscitation of infants at birth (Cochrane review). *Cochrane Database Syst Rev* 2004;3:CD002273.
222. Rice-Evans CA, Diplock AT. Current status of antioxidant therapy. *Free Radic Biol Med* 1993;15:77–96.
223. Powers HJ, Loban A, Silvers K, Gibson AT. Vitamin C at concentrations observed in premature babies inhibits the ferroxidase activity of caeruloplasmin. *Free Radic Res* 1995;22(1):57–65.
224. Greenwald RA. Superoxide dismutase and catalase as therapeutic agents for human diseases. A critical review. *Free Radic Biol Med* 1990;8:201–9.
225. Palmer C, Vannucci RC, Towfighi J. Reduction of perinatal hypoxic–ischemic brain damage with allopurinol. *Pediatr Res* 1990;27:332–6.
226. Russell GAB, Cooke RWI. Randomised controlled trial of allopurinol prophylaxis in very preterm infants. *Arch Dis Child* 1995;73:F27–31.
227. Bada HS, Green RS, Pourcvrous M, *et al.* Indomethacin reduces the risk of severe intraventricular hemorrhage. *J Pediatr* 1989; 115:631–7.
228. Peeters Sholte C, Braun K, Koster J, *et al.* Effects of allopurinol and deferroxamine on reperfusion injury of the brain in newborn piglets after neonatal hypoxia-ischemia. *Pediatr Res* 2003; 54:516–22.
229. Mupanemunda RH, Lee DSC, Fraher IJ, *et al.* Postnatal changes in serum retinol status in very-low-birth-weight infants. *Early Hum Dev* 1994;38L:45–54.
230. Pieri C, Marra M, Moroni F, *et al.* Melatonin, a peroxyl radical scavenger more efficient than vitamin E. *Life Sci* 1994;55:PL271–6.
231. Tan DX, Chen LD, Poeggeler B, *et al.* Melatonin: A potent, endogenous hydroxyl radical scavenger. *Endocr J* 1993;1:57–66.
232. Gitto E, Reiter RJ, Cordaro SP, *et al.* Oxidative and inflammatory parameters in respiratory distress syndrome of preterm newborns: Beneficial effects of melatonin. *Am J Perinatol* 2004;21:209–16.
233. Gitto E, Karbownik M, Reiter RJ, *et al.* Effects of melatonin treatment in septic newborns. *Pediatr Res* 2001;50:756–60.
234. Lapenna D, Degioia S, Mezzetti A, *et al.* Aminophylline: Could it act as an antioxidant in vivo? *Eur J Clin Invest* 1995;25: 464–70.
235. Law MR, Wijewardene K, Wald NJ. Is routine vitamin E administration justified in very-low-birthweight infants? *Dev Med Child Neurol* 1990;32:442–50.
236. Italian Collaborative Group on Preterm Delivery. Absorption of intramuscular vitamin E in premature babies. *Dev Pharmacol Ther* 1991;16:13–21.
237. Marx MM, Cronin JH. Medications used in the newborn. In Clothery JP, Stark AR, eds. *Manual of Neonatal Care.* Boston: Little, Brown and Company, 1992;619–33.
238. Holland BM, Wardrop CAJ. Oxygen transport by the blood, haematinics and blood cell component therapy in the neonate. In Rylance G, Harvey D, Aranda JV, eds. *Neonatal Clinical Pharmacology and Therapeutics.* Oxford: Butterworth Heinemann, 1991:211–23.
239. Tanaka H, Mino M, Takeuchi T. A nutritional evaluation of vitamin E status in very-low-birthweight infants with respect to changes in plasma and red blood cell tocopherol levels. *J Nutr Sci Vitaminol* 1988;34:293–07.
240. Brion LP, Bell EF, Raghuveer TS. Vitamin E supplementation for prevention of morbidity and mortality in preterm infants. *Cochrane Database Syst Rev* 2003;3:CD003665.
241. Silvers KM, Sluis KB, Darlow BA, *et al.* Limiting light-induced lipid peroxidation and vitamin loss in infant parenteral nutrition by adding multivitamin preparations to Intralipid. *Acta Pediatr* 2001;90:242–9.
242. Pitkanen OM, Luukkainen P, Andersson S. Attenuated lipid peroxidation in preterm infants during subsequent doses of intravenous lipids. *Biol Neonate* 2004;85(3):184–7.
243. Van Callie-Bertrand M, Degenhart HJ, Fernandes J. Selenium status of infants on nutritional support. *Acta Paediatr Scand* 1984;73:816–9.
244. Darlow BA, Inder TE, Graham PJ. The relationship of selenium status to respiratory outcome in the very-low-birthweight infant. *Pediatrics* 1995;96:314–9.
245. Tubman TR, Halliday HL, McMaster D. Glutathione peroxidase and selenium levels in the preterm infant. *Biol Neonate* 1990;58:305–10.
246. Daniels L, Gibso R, Simmer K. Randomised clinical trial of parenteral selenium supplementation in preterm infants. *Arch Dis Child* 1996;74:F158–64.
247. Dennery PA, McDonagh AF, Spitz DR, *et al.* Hyperbilirubinemia results in reduced oxidative injury in neonatal Gunn rats exposed to hyperoxia. *Free Radic Biol Med* 1995;19:395–404.
248. Nakamura H, Uetani Y, Komura M, *et al.* Inhibitory action of bilirubin on superoxide production by polymorphonuclear leukocytes. *Biol Neonate* 1987;52:273–8.

11 Pathology of the neonate

B. Hargitai, T. Marton and Z. Papp

Introduction

Obstetrical care of high-standard and regular ultrasound scanning usually leads to prenatal diagnosis of developmental abnormalities and often prevents perinatal pathologists from encountering those in term, or near-term neonates. Therefore, dysmorphology and congenital abnormalities are more and more the subject of the fetopathology while growth abnormalities, hypoxic injuries, preterm birth and infection remain a major problem in neonatal medicine. Congenital tumor and genetic metabolic disease are rare in general, but may have a great impact on the life of the family, especially when they are part of a syndrome and have a high risk of recurrence. Stillbirth and early neonatal death rates, due to birth-related events, have significantly decreased in the last 40 years (from 7.9 to 0.5 per 1000 total births) in the UK[1] and a similar trend can be observed in many other European countries. The number of litigation cases following intrapartum neonatal death is increasing, and thus potentially the postmortem report has medico-legal importance. It is highly recommended for obstetricians to ask for a postmortem examination and to encourage the parents to give permission for a full autopsy. It is a good practice to have regular discussions with the perinatal pathologist and to provide the pathologist with detailed clinical information prior to postmortem examination.

Growth abnormalities and intrauterine growth restriction (IUGR). Assessment of IUGR during perinatal postmortem examination

Massive cell division and differentiation take place in the developing fetus and result in a linear growth until the 38th week of gestation. Any failure of the complicated biochemical routes and control system, shortfall in nutritional agents or oxygen supply, may lead to growth abnormalities. In obstetric practice, ultrasonographic assessment of biparietal diameter (BPD), femur length and other fetal measurements was found to be useful to date the pregnancy.[2] To estimate the duration of the pregnancy, the most frequently used method is to count the gestational weeks from the first day of the mother's menstrual period. Although many charts of fetal and neonatal measurements are available in textbooks, most of these were created decades ago.[3–5] Perinatal pathology centers have to update these data, especially to reflect characteristics of a given geographical and ethnical population.

During perinatal necropsy the appropriate measurements of the body (weight, crown–rump length, crown–heel length, foot length and head circumference) and organ weight always have to be taken and should be compared with the normal values, apt for the counted gestational age.

Neonates, born between the 37th and 41st gestational weeks are term neonates and those born before the 37th week are preterm neonates, expressing signs of prematurity. Both term and preterm babies can be of appropriate weight for the gestational age or may weigh less than the expected normal value. Babies who weigh 2500 g or less are called low-birth-weight neonates and those under 1500 g are designated as very low-birth-weight. Small-for-date or small-for-gestational-age infants measure less than the 3rd, 5th, or 10th centile or less than two standard deviations below the mean. Small-for-date infants are not necessarily growth restricted and babies suffering from IUGR are not always small-for-date.

IUGR is usually detected during the third trimester of pregnancy. In case of an early-onset growth restriction, the fetal organs are smaller but proportionally developed. The serial BPD measurements are lower and parallel with the normal values from the early pregnancy. This type of IUGR is usually associated with intrauterine infections, chromosome abnormalities – e.g. Down's syndrome – and many other malformation syndromes. Triploidy (Figure 11.4) is an example of early onset asymmetrical growth restriction. Late-onset IUGR is usually caused by environmental factors, such as malnutrition due to placental dysfunction or maternal undernutrition, reduced utero-placental perfusion related to maternal hypertension, pre-eclampsia, diabetes mellitus or maternal smoking. In late-onset IUGR the infant's body is disproportional, the head circumference is relatively large and the brain weight/liver weight ratio is elevated.

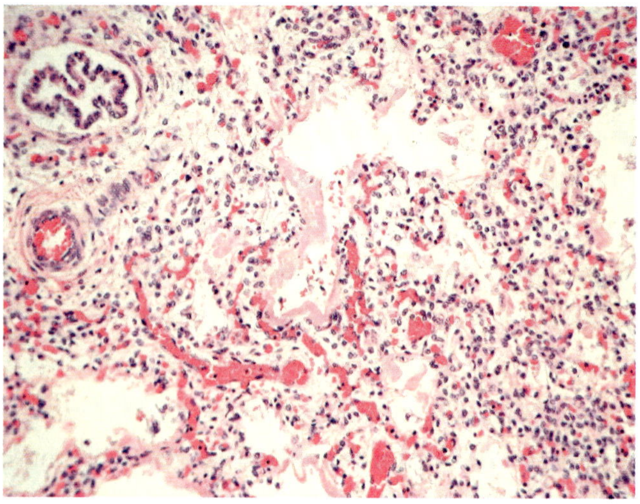

Figure 11.1 Eosinophilic membrane lines the inner surface of the airway.

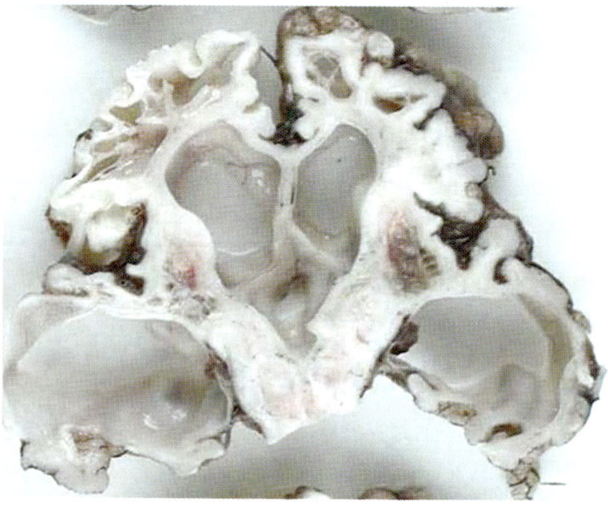

Figure 11.3 Postischemic change in the brain. The ventricles are dilated, and there are multiple cysts in the white matter (postnecrotic porencephaly).

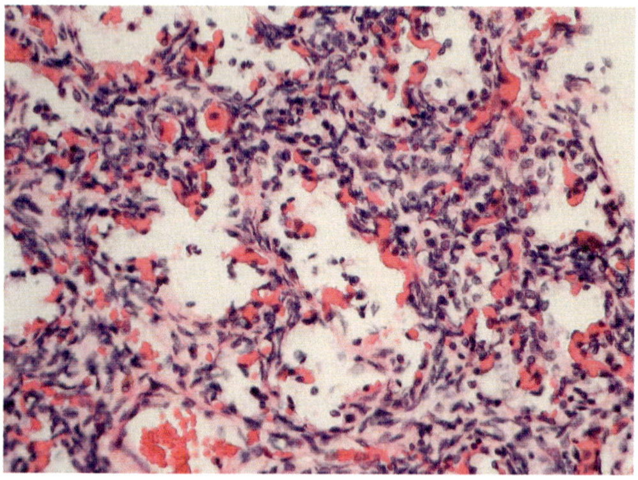

Figure 11.2 Simplified airways, widened interalveolar septa are present in chronic lung disease.

Pathological and histological assessment of IUGR requires accurate measurement of body weight, crown–heel length, crown–rump length, head circumference, foot length, organ weights, and microscopic examination of the parenchymal organs. Elevated brain weight/liver weight ratio [mean 2.8 (range 1.7–4.1)],[6,7] lower crown–rump length than head circumference, immature brain gyral pattern,[8] decreased nephron counts and presence of nephrogenic zone of the kidney after the 36th week of gestation,[9] bone growth plate abnormalities and specific placental findings are sensitive markers of IUGR.[10]

Infants who weigh more than the normal value for a particular gestational age are called heavy-for-date babies. This condition can be constitutional and usually is associated with high maternal body weight or higher parity. Maternal diabetes mellitus and gestational diabetes are often complicated with increased somatic size (macrosomia) when the diabetes of the mother is not sufficiently controlled. Macrosomia, unilateral hyperplasia or single organ overgrowth can be seen in so-called overgrowth syndromes. This group includes Beckwith–Wiedermann syndrome, characterized by hemihyperplasia, macroglossia, omphalocele and increased risk of pediatric neoplasms, most frequently Wilm's tumor. Simpson–Golabi–Bernel syndrome, an X-chromosome-linked disorder, is associated with macrosomia, congenital heart defects among other abnormalities.[11] Perlman syndrome, autosomal recessive, is characterized by macrosomia at birth, cardiac malformation, hypertrophy of the islets of Langerhans, bilateral renal hamartomas and sometimes nephroblastomatosis.[12] Weawer syndrome is characterized by accelerated growth and osseous maturation, bears considerable overlap with Soto's syndrome, both of them associated with congenital heart defects and higher risk of malignancy.[13]

Pathological sequels of intrauterine asphyxia

Intrauterine asphyxia is a common cause of fetal death and may lead to severe organ failure, such as long-term neurodevelopmental injuries, in the surviving infant. During the last two decades it has become evident that only a minority of cases of cerebral palsy and severe neurological damage begin at labor. In contrast, chronic or subacute intrauterine asphyxia is responsible for about 80% of cases.[14,15] In case of acute intrauterine asphyxia, pathological events lead to fetal demise or major damage within 24 h, while in chronic intrauterine asphyxia the estimated time course is 3 weeks or more. Specific causes of intrauterine asphyxia and associated pathological events can be identified in 50–80% of stillbirth cases.[16] Clinical data and pathological examination

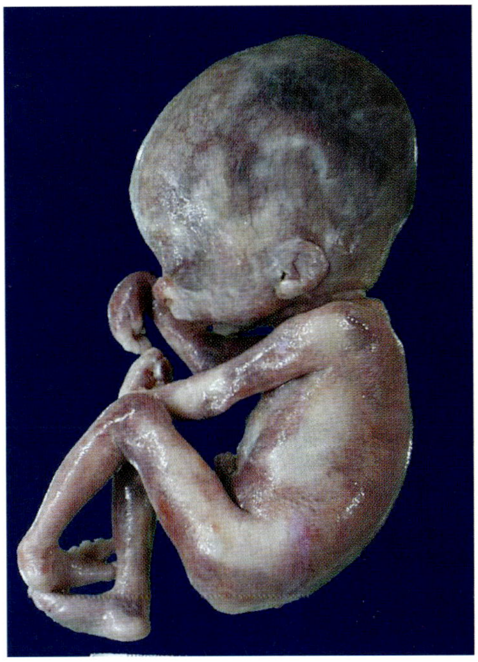

Figure 11.4 Triploidy: note the relatively large head and atrophic body, small jaw and low-set ear of this fetus.

may help to clarify the mechanism of damage and reveal maternal, placental or fetal causes, such as maternal disease, hemorrhage, placental malfunction, fetal malformation, second trimester loss of a twin in monochorionic pregnancy or infection.

During the course of the postmortem examination of a fetus or a neonate, which underwent intrauterine asphyxia, a combination of features associated with the predisposing causes as well as symptoms related to intrauterine hypoxic stress can be seen.

Acute intrauterine asphyxia is characterized by petechial hemorrhages on the epicardium along coronary arteries and at the base of the aorta and pulmonary trunk, visceral pleura, meconium in the airways, massive intrapulmonary hemorrhage, subcapsular hemorrhage of the liver, interstitial corticomedullary hemorrhage of the kidney and subcapsular hematoma of the adrenal glands. Microscopic examination reveals aspirated meconium, squames in the airways (Figure 11.5.), myocardial contraction band changes, cortical histiocytosis in the thymus and cystic degeneration of the adult cortical zone in the adrenals.

There are usually no petechial hemorrhages in subacute asphyxia/hypoxia. Microscopical shrinking of the cortex, prominent Hassal's corpuscles and histiocytosis can be observed in the thymus; with lymphocytolysis. The depletion of lymphocytes results in a typical 'starry sky' pattern. (Figure 11.6.) In the adrenals, lipid depletion and reaccumulation occur in the middle fetal cortex. (Figure 11.7.)

Chronic intrauterine hypoxia leads to fetal growth retardation with an asymmetric or disproportionate pattern, reduced muscle and subcutaneous fat. Microscopically, reaccumulation of lipid and fatty change

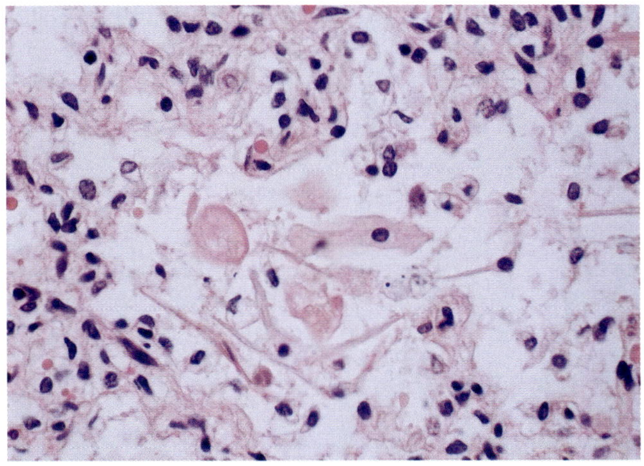

Figure 11.5 Squamous cells in the alveoli of a stillborn fetus.

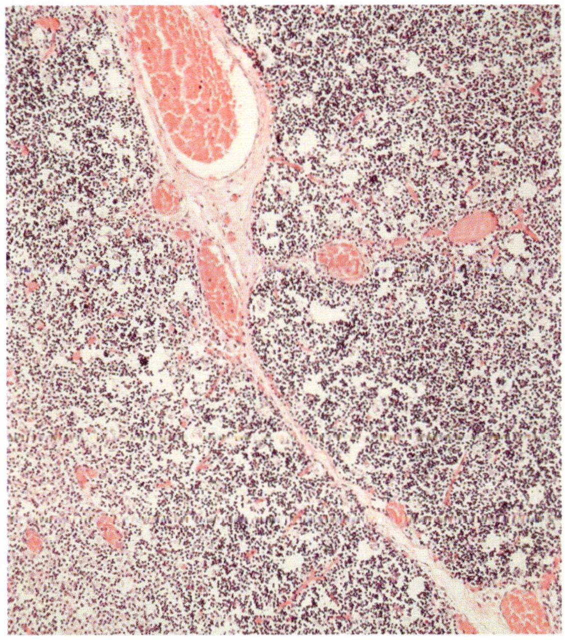

Figure 11.6 Starry sky reaction in the thymus of a neonate. The whitish small areas represent missing thymocytes as a result of subacute stress.

in the outer fetal cortex of the adrenal gland is characteristic. The thymus shows severe involutional changes with thin or diminished cortex and crowding of Hassal's corpuscles. (Figure 11.8.) In the enchondral growth plate of the bones irregular costo-chondral junction can be observed.

Intrauterine hypoxia leads to congestion in the central nervous system. Grossly, flattening of the gyri and compression of lateral ventricles can be seen. Microscopically, different stages of neuronal degeneration, necrosis and apoptosis are typical for hypoxic-ischemic changes in thalamus, midbrain, pons, hippocampus and basal ganglia. Angulation of the neurons, karyorrhexis and karyopicnosis are characteristic signs of neuronal apoptosis. (Figure 11.9.) Late consequences

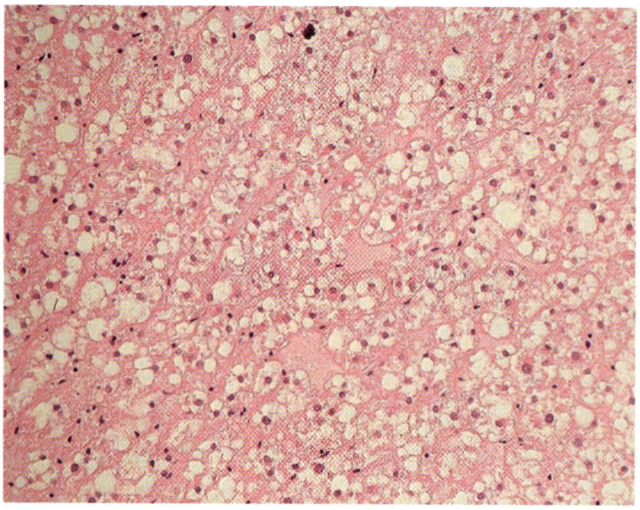

Figure 11.7 Severe lipid reaccumulation in the adrenal cortex.

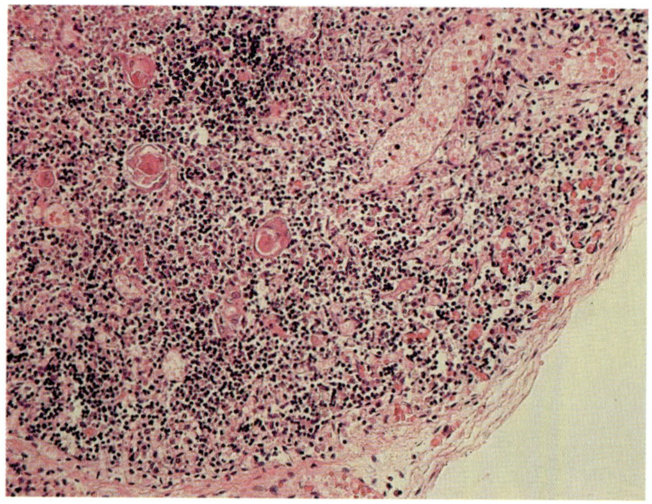

Figure 11.8 Atrophic cortex of the thymus, prominent Hassal's corpuscles.

of hypoxic-ischemic brain damage may include massive loss of brain tissue causing porencephaly, hydrocephaly, cystic changes and subsequent microcephaly.

Prematurity, immaturity

Neonates, delivering before 37 completed weeks of gestation are called preterm neonates. The direct causes of preterm labor are not entirely understood, although many associated pathological events have been studied, such as maternal diseases, socio-economic factors, previous reproductive events, effect of twinning and fetal factors. Structural and functional immaturity of preterm babies causes major problems in postnatal life during adaptation. Hypoglycemia, hypothermia, high blood potassium level and anemia are frequent complications. The pathological appearance of organ-specific alterations has been changed due to technical development of neonatal intensive care and new therapeutic methods.

Pathology of the respiratory system in premature infants

Infantile respiratory distress syndrome (IRDS) and hyaline membrane disease (HMD)

IRDS is a frequent condition in preterm infants and is characterized by a well-defined clinical picture: rapid increase in oxygen requirement and demand for ventilation, cyanosis, tachypnoe, intercostal and sternal recession, increasing expiratory pressure and a typical grunting noise at expiration. Radiological staging is possible but not always consistent with the degree of respiratory failure. In an advanced stage the picture of 'white lungs' appears on x-ray.

The underlying cause behind the acute respiratory failure of preterm neonates is the functional and structural immaturity of the lung. The reduced number and incomplete formation of airways, inefficient production of surfactant factor and lack of antioxidant defense lead to a number of immunopathological processes similar to diffuse alveolar damage syndromes. The exact mechanism of the initial epithelial injury is not known but ischemia, volu- and barotrauma and oxygen toxicity are likely to play a major role.[17] Most babies survive IRDS, and in about 50% of the cases there are no significant complications in the respiratory system. The outcome is less favorable with younger gestational age. The incidence is higher in males, and symptoms can be more severe in infants of diabetic mothers, in multiple pregnancies and after intrauterine asphyxia.[18]

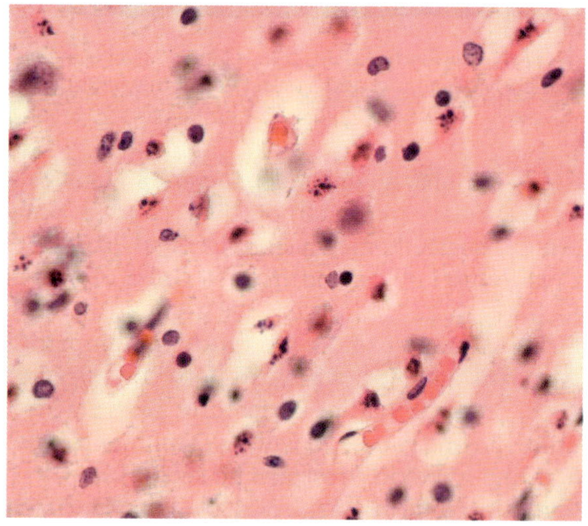

Figure 11.9 High number of apoptotic figures in the hippocampus of a neonate with hypoxic-ischemic encephalopathy.

In pretem babies who die in the first week of life with symptoms of IRDS, the lungs are heavy, purple colored and have a liver-like texture due to atelectasia. Microscopically, most airways are collapsed, but terminal airways are distended, the bronchial epithelial lining is necrotic. As soon as 1 h after birth, the hyaline membrane starts to develop lining the primitive airways, which consists of nuclear debris of epithelial cells as well as necrotic cell mass and exudates from inflammatory cells. A few hours later polymorphonuclears and macrophages migrate into the septae and after 2 days regenerative changes in the epithelium become visible. The hyaline membrane (Figure 11.1.) is strongly associated with IRDS, but can be present in acute asphyxia, in some infections (e.g. group B streptococcus infection) and in pulmonary hemorrhage.

The incidence of IRDS and HMD has been significantly reduced with surfactant administration and, especially the preventive use of natural surfactant has proved to be useful. Steroid administration before preterm labor is a common practice, the benefits and complications of which are still being investigated.[19,20]

Changing morphology of chronic lung disease (CLD)

Clinical definition of chronic lung disease requires a demand for assisted or supported ventilation after 28 days of life, radiological signs and previous acute respiratory failure of the infant, most frequently IRDS–HMD. The classical morphology of chronic lung injury has changed and is rarely seen today. Therefore, the term 'bronchopulmonary dysplasia' is not appropriate for the majority of the cases and 'CLD' is preferred currently.

Traditionally, three stages could be distinguished in BPD based on the histology of the lung.

- In the acute exudative early reparative stage (1–9 days) persisting hyaline membrane, lack of type II pneumocytes, bronchiolar epithelial necrosis, obliterative bronchiolitis, interstitial edema, congestion and initial septal fibrosis can be seen.
- In the subacute fibroproliferative stage (10–30 days) increasing interstitial and perialveolar fibrosis, necrotizing tracheobronchitis, smooth muscle proliferation, dilated bronchioli and terminal airways are present.
- In the late stage (after 1 month) prominent septal fibrosis, reduced number and anatomical distortion of terminal airways, metaplastic changes in bronchial epithelium, pulmonary hypertensive changes in pulmonary arterioles are typical findings.

The changing morphology of chronic lung disease might be a result of the longer survival time of the very immature, very low-birth-weight preterm infants and the technical improvement of intensive care, especially ventilation. Characteristic morphological changes include less exudative–fibroproliferative signs, but a dramatic fall in the number of airways and gas exchange surfaces. (Figure 11.2.) The proximal airways are collapsed and in contrast, the terminal structures are dilated. Patchy fibrosis may be present, but is not dominant. Inflammatory morphological changes are not common, although a significant inflammatory response is associated with CLD and there is an increased level of inflammatory cytokines. It is suggested that the current morphology of chronic lung disease might be the consequence of an alveolar developmental abnormality due to the lack of physiological signal during lung remodeling in the highly immature infants.[21,22]

Pulmonary air leak and pulmonary hemorrhage

Positive pressure ventilation may result in alveolar overdistension and rupture. The air can be pressed into the pleural cavities leading to pneumothorax. Air leakage into the pulmonary tissues results in pulmonary interstitial emphysema. Pneumopericardium is usually associated with other air leaks and is a severe complication with the risk of pericardial tamponade. Systemic air embolism is a very rare complication of ventilation and may lead to sudden death.

Intra-alveolar and interstitial hemorrhage is frequently associated with HMD. Massive hemorrhage is occasionally a terminal event, while alveolar and subpleural hemorrhage are rather associated with acute asphyxia.

Pathology of the central nervous system in premature infants (germinal matrix hemorrhage, intraventricular hemorrhage and periventricular leukomalacia)

A reasonable improved prognosis has been documented in the last decade; the incidence of intracerebral hemorrhage and ischemic white matter damage in preterm infants is still high and may be responsible for long-term neurodevelopmental sequels, such as hydrocephalus, spastic diplegia, hemiplegia, quadriplegia, learning difficulties and behavioral problems.[23,24]

The pattern of neuropathological changes in preterm brain differs from those that can be found in term neonates. Most frequent pathological findings in preterms are germinal matrix/intraventricular hemorrhage and periventricular leukomalacia, and in contrast with the term brain, the most vulnerable areas are the periventricular germinal matrix and white matter. Although basal ganglia are far more frequently affected in term babies, pontosubicular necrosis has been observed in a high ratio of preterm infants.[25] The fetal brain is characterized by an active neurogenesis, dense aggregation of precursor cells in the subependymal germinal layer and a paucity of myelin. Neuronal precursors migrate from the germinal layer into the cortex, where later glial cells are also produced, and by the 36th week of gestation only residual foci of the germinal matrix can be seen. The germinal matrix bears a delicate vascular pattern, consisting of vulnerable capillaries, having no muscular wall. Sudden changes in the blood pressure, disturbed autoregulation, higher fibrinolytic activity and increased permeability of vessel walls, caused by hypoxia, contribute to the pathogenesis of germinal matrix hemorrhage. Bleeding may occur in one focus but can be multiple, unilateral or bilateral. According to Papile's grading system, bleeding restricted to the germinal matrix represents grade 1; hemorrhage breaking into the lateral ventricle is regarded as grade 2; in more severe cases, dilatation of ventricles follows the hemorrhage, which is grade 3 and parenchymal damage (grade 4) can be observed in about 10% of the cases.[26] Germinal matrix and intraventricular hemorrhage usually develop in the first 3 days of life. High-grade intraventricular hemorrhage, associated with RDS, is a leading cause of death, and grades 1–4 hemorrhage is present in as many as 83% of very low-birth-weight preterm infants in our postmortem examinations. On histology, extravasation of red blood cells, tissue damage and a few days later many hemosiderin-laden macrophages and petrified neurons can be seen.

Periventricular leukomalacia is related to a sudden drop in the blood pressure and the most vulnerable sites are the vascular watershed areas, where the decreased perfusion leads to ischemia.[27] Recent studies have revealed a relationship between intrauterine infection, acute high-grade chorioamnionitis–funisitis and white matter injuries.[28,29] On macroscopical examination whitish–yellowish foci can be seen with a chalk-white rim, usually within the paraventricular white matter, in the temporal lobe and in the tapetum. The lesion tends to be multifocal and bilateral. Histologically, signs of coagulative necrosis, microglial and astrocytic reaction, groups of macrophages and mineralized neurons can be present. In the later stage, cystic changes develop in the injured sites leading to the typical picture of multicystic periventricular leukomalacia (Figure 11.3).

Necrotizing enterocolitis (NEC)

The onset of the NEC is usually during the first 2 weeks for preterm infants. Although the exact initial cause is not known, alimentary and iatrogenic aspects are investigated. Immaturity is strongly associated with this condition, but the etiological role of early enteral feeding is now challenged.[30,31] In contrast, perinatal asphyxia and RDS were not among the risk factors in the study of Kanto,[32] but umbilical cord catheterization increased the chance of NEC.[33] An infectious component has also been suspected by many investigators, but no pathogenic organism has been found yet.[34,35] Breast milk proved to have a protective role.[36]

The clinical picture of NEC is characterized by lethargy, pale skin tone, abdominal distension, bloody stools and vomitting. Radiology shows distended, gas-containing bowels and occasionally gas perforation into the abdominal cavity. The outcome is less favorable for very low-birth-weight infants, and for cases complicated by perforation, peritonitis, sepsis and intravascular coagulopathy.

Postmortem or postoperative examination of the bowels reveals a distended, thin or paper-like bowel wall, sites of perforation, greenish–brownish exudate on the visceral peritoneum. The number of villi of the small intestine is diminished and the wall shows different degrees of edema, hemorrhagic necrosis and gangrenous inflammation. The picture can be similar in the lower part of the intestinal tract.

Retinopathy of prematurity and other pathological conditions associated with prematurity

Retinopathy of preterm infants was described in the early 1940s, and was regarded as retrolental fibroplasia (Terry 1942). The frequency dropped when the adverse effect of concentrated oxygen was recognized, but rose again with the increasing survival time of very low-birth-weight infants. According to the current practice, high-risk babies (less than 1500 g and/or born before the 32nd week of gestation) are monitored in order to prevent retinal detachment and blindness, total retinal detachment being the most severe stage of this condition.[37] The site of the changes is the junction of the vascularized and avascular retina, where demarcation, fibrovascularization and neovascularization develop as a pathological reaction of the immature tissue for angiogenetic signals. The detailed pathway of this procedure is not yet fully understood.

There are other clinically important consequences of the altered metabolic functions, which do not have characteristic morphological appearance, such as hypothermia, hypoglycemia and higher blood potassium level. Anemia of preterm infants presents with extensive extramedullary hemopoiesis and occasionally fatty changes of the adrenal cortex.

The risk of sudden infant death syndrome is higher for preterm babies.

Preterm birth is very frequently complicated by perinatal infections, which are discussed in the next section.

Perinatal infections

Frequent pathological sequels of intrauterine infections

The incidence of the intrauterine infection reaches a peak in the second trimester. The two most frequent mechanisms are the ascending genital tract infections and the transplacental hematogenous spread. The pathogenesis of the intra-amniotic infections and the most common pathogenic agents are summarized in Table 11.1.

The consequences of intrauterine infection include early, spontaneous, preterm labor and premature rupture of membranes,[38] and occasionally generalized fetal infection. Developmental abnormalities and other clinical features related to particular intrauterine infections are well described in pediatric pathology.[4] Cytomegalovirus (CMV) infection is known to be

Table 11.1 Mechanism and common pathogens of intrauterine infections

	Virus	Bacteria	Fungi	Protozoa
Transcervical	Herpes simplex or genitalis, HIV-1 (infection during labor)	Group B streptococcus, *E. coli* and *H. influenzae*	*C. albicans*	
Transplacental	CMV, parvovirus, rubella and HIV-1	Group B streptococcus and *L. monocytogenes*		*Toxoplasma, Chlamydia psittaci, Treponema p.* and *Borrelia*

Table 11.2 Typical macroscopic and microscopic features of intrauterine infections in the fetus and in the placenta

	Macroscopic signs	Microscopic signs
Bacterial infection		
Placenta	Opaque or greenish–brownish membranes in transcervical infection Placental abscesses in case of transplacental spreading	Transcervical infection Acute, high-grade chorioamnionitis, fetal chorionic vessel vasculitis and funisitis Transplacental infection Acute villitis, deciduitis Microabscesses, microgranulomas, e.g. in listeriosis
Fetus	Macroscopic features of septic shock Leptomeningeal purulent exudate and congestion in meningitis Occasionally periventricular leukomalatia	Intrauterine pneumonia, infiltration with polymorphonuclear leukocytes in the airways, interstitial inflammatory reaction Microabscesses of the parenchymal organs
Viral infection		
Placenta		Subacute or chronic villitis, specific virus inclusions, e.g. parvovirus B19, CMV
Fetus	Hepatosplenomegaly Icterus, petechiae Hydrops IUGR Developmental malformation	Specific virus inclusions, e.g. parvovirus B19, CMV, HSV Hemolysis – hemosiderin deposition Focal necrosis, dystrophic calcification, e.g. HSV

associated with severe central nervous system damage, microcephaly with multifocal calcification, chorioretinitis, hearing loss and neonatal hepatitis, while rubella infection may lead to cardiac malformation, deafness and eye defects. The incidence of syphilis infection is very low and the vertical transmission rate for HIV showed a decreasing trend in the industrialized countries in recent years.[39,40] The statistics is less favorable in the developing countries.[41]

The patho-morphological signs of intrauterine infection have to be carefully looked for in case of stillbirth or neonatal death. Symmetric type of IUGR is a common association. Frequent macroscopic and microscopic features of viral and bacterial infections are summarized in Table 11.2.

Neonatal infection

Neonatal infection is frequent in preterm infants, with a higher risk and worse prognosis for low-birth-weight infants.

Sepsis occurring in the first 3 days of life, called early-onset neonatal sepsis, can be a devastating neonatal problem with a high mortality rate. Although neonatal sepsis is not very frequent (2–4 per 1000 live births) in developed countries, the rate increases for preterm infants and those born to mothers with infections or prolonged rupture of the fetal membranes. Group B streptococci and enterobacteriaceae are the main causes of early-onset sepsis in more developed countries.[42]

Late-onset neonatal sepsis (>72 h) is usually caused by Gram-positive agents, especially coagulase-negative staphylococci.[43,44]

Rarely, other streptococci, *Haemophilus influenzae, Serratia marcescens, Malassezia furfur, Salmonella, Pseudomonas aeruginosa, Campylobacter* and *Listeria monocytogenes* lead to neonatal infection. *Candida albicans* is the most common among fungal infections, which often colonizes the baby from birth, and sometimes causes pneumonia in infants treated with antibiotics.

The costs and benefits of intrapartum antibiotic prophylaxis therapy should be carefully evaluated and the therapeutic policies reconsidered in the light of the new data on increasing frequency of nosocomial infections.[45,46]

The most severe complications of early- and late-onset infections are pneumonia and meningitis, but enteral and urogenital infections, conjunctivitis and skin rashes may be also present. Pathological signs are frequently poor and non-specific. Macroscopically, skin rashes, congestion of the parenchymal organs, petechiae, adrenal hemorrhage, rarely leptomeningeal purulent exudates can be observed. Microscopically, inflammatory infiltrate of the airways is present in the congested, edematous lung tissue with interstitial reaction. Special stains may help to visualize the fungi. Samples for microbiological laboratory tests should be taken during postmortem examination.

Congenital tumors and tumor-like lesions

Epidemiology, biological behavior and etiology of congenital tumors

Neonatal tumors (including congenital tumors) occurring within the first 28 days of life represent an age-specific group of neoplastic lesions. The reported incidence (2003) ranged between 1 per 12,500 and 27,500 live births in the UK and the USA and varied from 17 to 121 per million births worldwide.[47]

Abnormal tissue swellings and masses present at birth are often regarded as congenital tumors, although many types of them do not fulfill the criteria of true neoplasias. These tumor-like lesions, traditionally called hamartomas and choristomas, are probably due to tissue developmental abnormalities, differentiation and migration defect of cells, resulting in a pathological architecture.

Benign and tumor-like lesions are reasonably frequent and usually harmless – such as infantile hemangioma, the smallest congenital nevi – but occasionally bear more clinical significance and complications, e.g. Kaposiform hemangioendothelioma associated with Kasabach–Merrit syndrome and fetal hydrops.[48] The biological behavior of neonatal tumors cannot always be predicted based on their morphological appearance. Benign congenital lesions may have a risk of malignant transformation, e.g. malignant melanoma can develop in giant congenital nevus.[49–51] Infantile hemangioma may show spontaneous regression; however, lesions of large size may cause cardiac failure or consumptional coagulopathy. The histologically benign cardiac fibroma or cardiac rhabdomyoma may represent a poor prognosis for its unfavorable location. In contrast, some tumors of malignant histological appearance tend to show a significantly better prognosis in early life, e.g. neuroblastoma, hereditary retinoblastoma and congenital fibrosarcoma.

A unique group of true congenital neoplasias are regarded as embryonal tumors. These are characterized by a uniformly primitive histological picture resembling the embryonal–fetal appearance of the organ in which they arise. This group includes neuroblastoma, nephroblastoma (Wilm's tumor), hepatoblastoma, retinoblastoma, embryonal rhabdomyosarcoma and medulloblastoma. Some embryonal tumors are familial, such as 40% of retinoblastomas and familial Wilm's tumors, while others associate with inherited syndromes, e.g. glycogenosis type I and hepatocellular carcinoma, or α-1 antitripsin deficiency and hepatoblastoma.

In a few sporadic malformation syndromes there is a higher risk of neonatal tumors, for example, in Beckwith–Wiedermann syndrome, where a higher risk of nephroblastoma, hepatoblastoma and adrenal cancer can be observed, or in Hirschsprung's disease, which is occasionally associated with neuroblastoma. There is a long list of many other inherited syndromes, including metabolic disorders, phacomatoses, DNA repair defects, immune deficiency syndromes, carrying a higher risk of different malignant tumors, but most of these develop only in later childhood.

Neonates with structural chromosomal anomalies may present with congenital tumors, trisomy 18 and 13 can be associated with teratomas, trisomy 18 with nephroblastoma and hepatoblastoma.[52] Acute megakaryocytic leukemia is a well-known complication of Down's syndrome in early neonatal age.[53]

On the other hand, the frequency of congenital abnormalities – spina bifida, abnormalities of ribs and eyes – was higher in children with solid tumors (Wilm's tumor, Ewing sarcoma, hepatoblastoma) than in population-based controls. This observation directs future studies in underlying gene disorders.[54]

Environmental factors including ionizing radiation, particular drugs taken during pregnancy and maternal CMV, varicella, influenza and HIV virus infections have been implicated in the etiology of neonatal (and pediatric) tumors.[55–57]

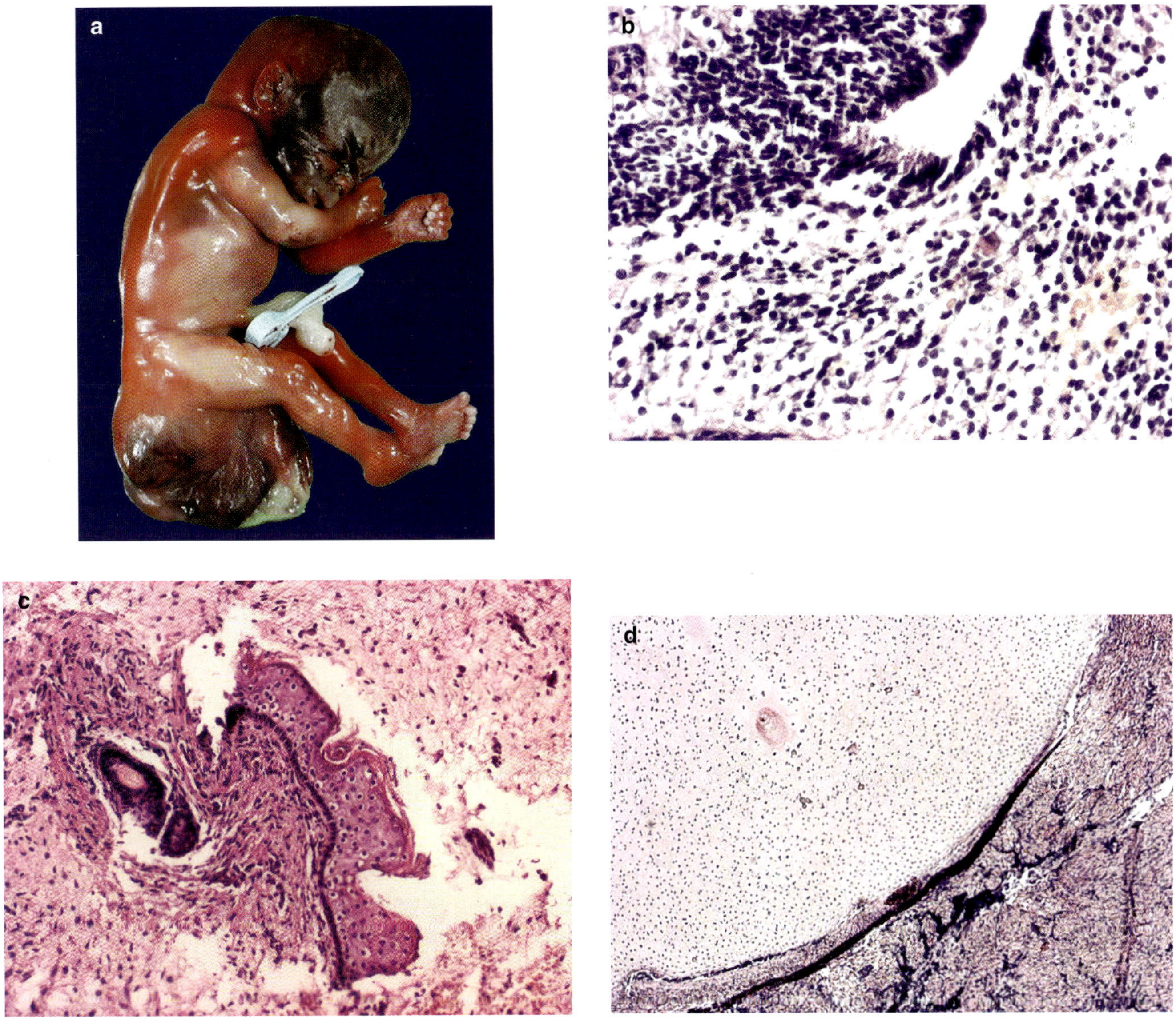

Figure 11.10 Sacrococcygeal teratoma in a fetus of 23 weeks of gestation. (a) Macroscopic picture of the large, mainly presacral tumor. (b, c and d) Microscopic examination reveals immature neural elements, squamous epithelium with a hair follicle, hyaline cartilage tissue.

Common types of solid neonatal tumors

The incidence of neonatal tumors is similar in different reports: teratoma and neuroblastoma, being the most common, followed by soft tissue tumors, renal and CNS tumors and leukemias.[47]

Congenital and neonatal teratoma

Fetal and neonatal germ cell tumors have a different clinical course and morphology from those occurring in older children or adults. Congenital teratoma has been described in numerous sites, most frequently in sacrococcygeal location, but ovarial, testicular, mediastinal, cervico-facial, retroperitoneal, abdominal and intracranial location have also been documented (Figure 11.10a–d). There are published cases of teratoma developing in the placenta or umbilical cord. Prenatal diagnosis, recognition of risk factors and intrauterine therapeutic interventions improved the outcome, although maternal complications, polyhydramnios, fetal cardiac failure, fetal hydrops and tumor rupture were not uncommon.[58–60]

Macroscopically, teratoma presents as a solid and cystic mass, potentially containing well-formed organoid structures. The traditional histological definition requires the presence of tissues from all three germ layers and most teratomas fulfill these criteria. Immature tissue is usually present in 20–50% of cases[4,61] and the histological grading is based on the amount of immature tissue;[62] however, immature neural elements do not indicate malignancy in this age group. True malignant tumors, most frequently yolk sac tumor, were present in 5.8% of teratomas, with

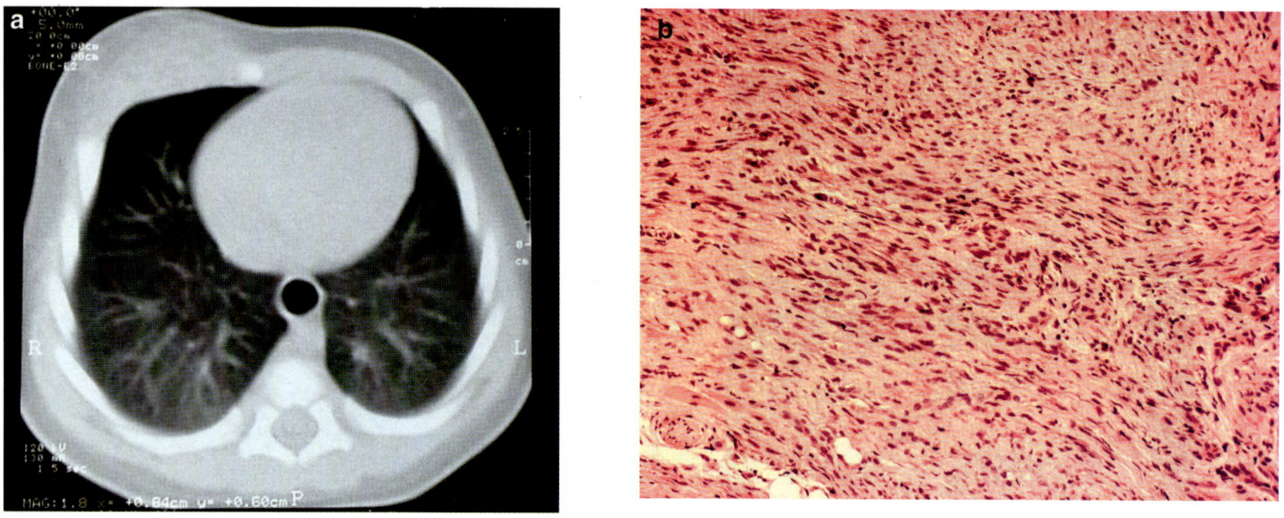

Figure 11.11 Soliter infantile myofibromatosis in a term baby. (a) CT scan shows soft tissue swelling around the second rib, on the right, suggesting infiltrative growth. (b) Characteristic microscopic appearance, with bindles of spindle cells, and small round primitive-looking cells. The soliter lesion bears an excellent prognosis.

the highest incidence (10%) in sacrococcygeal teratoma, and a tumor recurrence rate of 5% was reported in a recent review.[61]

Presacral sacrococcygeal teratoma has a worse prognosis than those in postsacral location, gastric teratoma has a good prognosis, while the outcome of the intracranial teratomas is poor with a few exceptions.[63–66] The main prognostic factors of fetal and neonatal teratoma are the size and the location, the completeness of surgical excision and the presence of malignant tumor (yolk sac tumor).

Congenital neuroblastoma

The incidence of congenital neuroblastoma is similar to that of teratoma; thus, it is the most frequent malignant tumor of the neonatal period. Ultrasonographic features of the tumor have been described and prenatal diagnosis gives an opportunity for appropriate planning and management.[67,68]

Congenital neuroblastoma usually presents with an abdominal or adrenal mass but extra-adrenal location, disseminated form, massive liver involvement and metastasis of the skin and placenta can occur.[69–72]

The morphological features are not different from those in older children, and the same histological criteria are used for classification.[73] Immunohistochemistry and electron microscopy confirm the histological diagnosis. Molecular genetics is a useful aid to detect prognostic factors. N-myc amplification, expression of bcl-2, an apoptosis suppressing protein, is associated with unfavorable histology and a bad prognosis.[74] The outcome of congenital neuroblastoma is generally favorable. A special pattern, characterized by a small primary tumor, disseminated spreading and low N-myc copy numbers, is termed as Stage IV-S neuroblastoma. Spontaneous regression is not an uncommon finding in this stage.[75–77] Only a small proportion of congenital neuroblastomas require aggressive therapy. Life-threatening respiratory complication might be related to massive hepatomegaly.

Soft tissue tumors

Fibromatosis This is a unique group of tumors with diverse clinicopathologic features.

The histological picture varies according to the specific types, but shares common features like the presence of intersecting bands of spindle cells in variably collagenized stroma. The lesions might be more cellular than the similar adult-type alterations and show an aggressive growth. In contrast with the occasionally formidable picture, the outlook is favorable. Spontaneous regression is not uncommon, although local recurrence may occur.[78]

Congenital myofibromatosis may present as a solitary lump and show spontaneous regression, while in its generalized form it carries a poor prognosis due to visceral involvement (Figure 11.11a and b). Fibromatosis colli is a palpable mass in the sternocleidomastoid muscle and occurs in young infants, while infantile digital fibromatosis may be present on the fingers and toes. Cranial fascitis and fibrous hamartoma of infancy are both rapidly growing lesions of the subcutaneous soft tissue, the former localized on the skull.

Sarcoma. Congenital infantile fibrosarcoma is a fibroblastic–myofibroblastic proliferation, a rapidly growing lesion resulting in a massive tumor. The histological appearance is sarcoma-like, but the prognosis is good, with a 5-year survival of more than 90%, and metastases are very rare.[78] Some cases have a characteristic chromosomal translocation with t(12;15)(p13;q25) and an *ETV6–NTRK3* gene fusion or *ETV6* gene rearrangement.[79] Embryonal rhabdomyosarcoma shares similar features in young infants and children, having a 5-year survival of 66%. Embryonal rhabdomyosarcoma displays loss of heterozygosity on chromosome 11p15.5, a tumor-related locus at 11q, numerical abnormalities, trisomy 8 and other abnormalities. However, these findings do not, as yet, have diagnostic or prognostic significance.[80,81]

Neural/neuroectodermal tumors

Neural tumors in young infants are usually associated with neurofibromatosis type 1 (NF1). Plexiform neurofibromas are histologically benign lesions with premalignant potential as in about 10% of the NF1 patients malignant peripheral nerve-sheath tumor develops from it. Congenital peripheral/primitive neuroectodermal tumor (PNET) has been reported in several sites.[82–84] PNET and Ewing sarcoma are now considered the same entity, based on their shared genetic abnormalities, being consistently associated with chromosomal translocation and functional fusion of the *EWS* gene to any of several structurally related transcription factor genes (*EWS-FLI-1*, *EWS-ERG*, *EWS-ETV1*, *EWS-E1AF*, etc.).[85]

Adipose tumors of the neonate

Lipoblastoma, a typical benign tumor of fat tissue in early childhood, occasionally may be present at birth. The circumscribed type is more common, with superficial location, while the diffuse type (lipoblastomatosis) originates from deep soft tissue, has an infiltrative growth pattern and recurs more frequently. Characteristic clonal karyotypic changes can be demonstrated and help to distinguish it from childhood and adult lipomas as well as from myxoid liposarcoma.[86]

Intracranial tumors

The most frequently diagnosed intracranial tumor is teratoma, PNET, medulloblastoma, astrocytoma, glioblastoma multiforme and ependymoma. Plexus choroideus papilloma, ganglioglioma and low-grade astrocytoma have the best prognosis, but the overall survival rate of perinatal brain tumors was only 28% in a recent review. Stillbirth is frequent and hydrocephalus-macrocephaly is often diagnosed prenatally.[87–90]

Congenital tumors of the kidney

Congenital mesoblastic nephroma is a benign tumor, and occasionally leads to fetal hydrops and polyhydramnios. Although the tumor mass can be huge and extends beyond the kidney, surgical treatment is usually curative. Histologically, the tumor consists of spindle cells of myofibroblastic origin. A more cellular variant is known that carries the same t(12;15)(p13;q25) and *ETV6–NTRK3* gene fusion as infantile fibrosarcoma.[91]

Rhabdoid tumor of the kidney is an aggressive tumor with bad prognosis and distinct morphological features. It is characterized by deletion of the *hSNF5/INI1* gene, which links it to other rhabdoid tumors of infancy that arise in the soft tissue and brain.[92]

Congenital and infantile Wilm's tumor is rare and shows a strong association with the presence of nephrogenic rests (persistent metanephric blastema) in the kidney.[93] Recent molecular genetic findings suggest a multistep model of the pathogenesis in Wilm's tumor and support the precursor role of nephrogenic rests.[94] Nephrogenic rest as well as nephroblastoma may be present in bilateral location. Nephroblastoma of early infancy has a good prognosis.[95,96]

REFERENCES

1. Members of the CESDI Organisation. *Confidential Enquiry into Stillbirths and Deaths in Infancy*. 8th Annual Report. London: Maternal and Child Health Research Consortium, 2001.
2. Degani S. Fetal biometry: Clinical, pathological, and technical considerations. *Obstet Gynecol Surv* 2001;56(3):159–67.
3. Gilbert-Barness E, ed. *Potter's Pathology of the Fetus and Infant*. Baltimore: Mosby, 1997.
4. Keeling JW, ed. *Fetal and Neonatal Pathology*, 2nd edn. Berlin: Springer-Verlag, 2001.
5. Wigglesworth JS, Singer DB, ed. *Textbook of Fetal and Perinatal Pathology*. Boston: Blackwell Scientific Publications, 1991.
6. Anderson JM. Increased brain weight–liver weight ratio as a necropsy sign of intrauterine undernutrition. *J Clin Pathol* 1972;25(10):867–71.
7. Mitchell ML. Fetal brain to liver weight ratio as a measure of intrauterine growth retardation: Analysis of 182 stillborn autopsies. *Mod Pathol* 2001;14(1):14–19.
8. Dorovini-Zis K, Dolman CL. Gestational development of brain. *Arch Pathol Lab Med* 1977;101(4):192–5.
9. Hinchliffe SA, Lynch MR, Sargent PH, Howard CV, Van Velzen D. The effect of intrauterine growth retardation on the development of renal nephrons. *Br J Obstet Gynaecol* 1992;99(4): 296–301.
10. Khong TY, Yee KT. Pathology of intrauterine growth retardation. *Am J Reprod Immunol* 1989;21(3–4):132–6.
11. Terespolsky D, Farrell SA, Siegel-Bartelt J, Weksberg R. Infantile lethal variant of Simpson–Golabi–Behmel syndrome associated with hydrops fetalis. *Am J Med Genet* 1995;59(3):329–33.
12. Perlman M, Levin M, Wittels B. Syndrome of fetal gigantism, renal hamartomas, and nephroblastomatosis with Wilms' tumor. *Cancer* 1975;35(4):1212–7.
13. Douglas J, Hanks S, Temple IK, *et al.* NSD1 mutations are the major cause of Sotos syndrome and occur in some cases of Weaver syndrome but are rare in other overgrowth phenotypes. *Am J Hum Genet* 2003;72(1):132–43.
14. Jacobsson B, Hagberg G. Antenatal risk factors for cerebral palsy. *Best Pract Res Clin Obstet Gynaecol* 2004;18(3): 425–36.
15. MacLennan A. A template for defining a causal relation between acute intrapartum events and cerebral palsy: International consensus statement. *Br Med J* 1999;319(7216):1054–9.
16. Magee JF. Investigation of stillbirth. *Pediatr Dev Pathol* 2001;4(1):1–22.
17. Krauss AN. New methods advance treatment for respiratory distress syndrome. *Pediatr Ann* 2003;32(9):585–91.
18. Weisman LE. Populations at risk for developing respiratory syncytial virus and risk factors for respiratory syncytial virus severity: Infants with predisposing conditions. *Pediatr Infect Dis J* 2003;22(Suppl 2):S33–7.
19. Garland JS, Alex CP, Pauly TH, *et al.* A three-day course of dexamethasone therapy to prevent chronic lung disease in ventilated neonates: A randomized trial. *Pediatrics* 1999;104(1, Pt 1): 91–9.
20. Shah PS. Current perspectives on the prevention and management of chronic lung disease in preterm infants. *Paediatr Drugs* 2003;5(7):463–80.

21. Bhandari A, Bhandari V. Pathogenesis, pathology and pathophysiology of pulmonary sequelae of bronchopulmonary dysplasia in premature infants. *Front Biosci* 2003;8:e370–80.
22. Coalson JJ. Pathology of new bronchopulmonary dysplasia. *Semin Neonatol* 2003;8(1):73–81.
23. Hoekstra RE, Ferrara TB, Couser RJ, Payne NR, Connett JE. Survival and long-term neurodevelopmental outcome of extremely premature infants born at 23–26 weeks' gestational age at a tertiary center. *Pediatrics* 2004;113(1, Pt 1):e1–6.
24. Vollmer B, Roth S, Baudin J, Stewart AL, Neville BG, Wyatt JS. Predictors of long-term outcome in very preterm infants: Gestational age versus neonatal cranial ultrasound. *Pediatrics* 2003;112(5):1108–14.
25. Skullerud K, Westre B. Frequency and prognostic significance of germinal matrix hemorrhage, periventricular leukomalacia, and pontosubicular necrosis in preterm neonates. *Acta Neuropathol (Berl)* 1986;70(3–4):257–61.
26. Papile LA, Burstein J, Burstein R, Koffler H. Incidence and evolution of subependymal and intraventricular hemorrhage: A study of infants with birth weights less than 1,500 gm. *J Pediatr* 1978;92(4):529–34.
27. Takashima S, Tanaka K. Development of cerebrovascular architecture and its relationship to periventricular leukomalacia. *Arch Neurol* 1978;35(1):11–6.
28. Wu YW, Colford JM Jr. Chorioamnionitis as a risk factor for cerebral palsy: A meta-analysis. *J Am Med Assoc* 2000;284(11):1417–24.
29. Yoon BH, Kim CJ, Romero R, *et al.* Experimentally induced intrauterine infection causes fetal brain white matter lesions in rabbits. *Am J Obstet Gynecol* 1997;177(4):797–802.
30. Flidel-Rimon O, Friedman S, Lev E, Juster-Reicher A, Amitay M, Shinwell ES. Early enteral feeding and nosocomial sepsis in very low birthweight infants. *Arch Dis Child Fetal Neonatal Ed* 2004;89(4):F289–92.
31. Stoll BJ. Epidemiology of necrotizing enterocolitis. *Clin Perinatol* 1994;21(2):205–18.
32. Kanto WP Jr, Wilson R, Breart GL, *et al.* Perinatal events and necrotizing enterocolitis in premature infants. *Am J Dis Child* 1987;141(2):167–9.
33. Rand T, Weninger M, Kohlhauser C, *et al.* Effects of umbilical arterial catheterization on mesenteric hemodynamics. *Pediatr Radiol* 1996;26(7):435–8.
34. Faustini A, Forastiere F, Giorgi Rossi P, Perucci CA. An epidemic of gastroenteritis and mild necrotizing enterocolitis in two neonatal units of a University Hospital in Rome, Italy. *Epidemiol Infect* 2004;132(3):455–65.
35. Sharma R, Garrison RD, Tepas JJ, *et al.* Rotavirus-associated necrotizing enterocolitis: An insight into a potentially preventable disease? *J Pediatr Surg* 2004;39(3):453–7.
36. McGuire W, Anthony MY. Donor human milk versus formula for preventing necrotising enterocolitis in preterm infants: Systematic review. *Arch Dis Child Fetal Neonatal Ed* 2003;88(1):F11–4.
37. Ells A, Hicks M, Fielden M, Ingram A. Severe retinopathy of prematurity: Longitudinal observation of disease and screening implications. *Eye* 2004;E-pub: June 25.
38. Goldenberg RL, Culhane JF. Infection as a cause of preterm birth. *Clin Perinatol* 2003;30(4):677–700.
39. Duong T, Ades AE, Gibb DM, Tookey PA, Masters J. Vertical transmission rates for HIV in the British Isles: Estimates based on surveillance data. *Br Med J* 1999;319(7219):1227–9.
40. Gibb DM. Reduction of mother-to-child transmission of HIV infection: Non-pharmaceutical interventions and their implementation. *Int J STD AIDS* 1998;9(Suppl 1):19–21.
41. Lepage P, Van de Perre P, Msellati P, *et al.* Mother-to-child transmission of human immunodeficiency virus type 1 (HIV-1) and its determinants: A cohort study in Kigali, Rwanda. *Am J Epidemiol* 1993;137(6):589–99.
42. Moore MR, Schrag SJ, Schuchat A. Effects of intrapartum antimicrobial prophylaxis for prevention of group-B-streptococcal disease on the incidence and ecology of early-onset neonatal sepsis. *Lancet Infect Dis* 2003;3(4):201–13.
43. Isaacs D, Barfield C, Clothier T, *et al.* Late-onset infections of infants in neonatal units. *J Paediatr Child Health* 1996;32(2):158–61.
44. Stoll BJ, Hansen N. Infections in VLBW infants: Studies from the NICHD Neonatal Research Network. *Semin Perinatol* 2003;27(4):293–301.
45. Baltimore RS. Neonatal sepsis: Epidemiology and management. *Paediatr Drugs* 2003;5(11):723–40.
46. Clark R, Powers R, White R, Bloom B, Sanchez P, Benjamin DK. Nosocomial Infection in the NICU: A medical complication or unavoidable problem? *J Perinatol* 2004;24(6):382–8.
47. Moore SW, Satge D, Sasco AJ, Zimmermann A, Plaschkes J. The epidemiology of neonatal tumours. Report of an international working group. *Pediatr Surg Int* 2003;19(7):509–19.
48. Martinez AE, Robinson MJ, Alexis JB. Kaposiform hemangioendothelioma associated with nonimmune fetal hydrops. *Arch Pathol Lab Med* 2004;128(6):678–81.
49. Hoss DM, Grant-Kels JM. Significant melanocytic lesions in infancy, childhood, and adolescence. *Dermatol Clin* 1986;4(1):29–44.
50. Leech SN, Bell H, Leonard N, *et al.* Neonatal giant congenital nevi with proliferative nodules: A clinicopathologic study and literature review of neonatal melanoma. *Arch Dermatol* 2004;140(1):83–8.
51. Richardson SK, Tannous ZS, Mihm MC Jr. Congenital and infantile melanoma: Review of the literature and report of an uncommon variant, pigment-synthesizing melanoma. *J Am Acad Dermatol* 2002;47(1):77–90.
52. Satge D, Van Den Berghe H. Aspects of the neoplasms observed in patients with constitutional autosomal trisomy. *Cancer Genet Cytogenet* 1996;87(1):63–70.
53. Al-Kasim F, Doyle JJ, Massey GV, Weinstein HJ, Zipursky A. Incidence and treatment of potentially lethal diseases in transient leukemia of Down syndrome: Pediatric Oncology Group Study. *J Pediatr Hematol Oncol* 2002;24(1):9–13.
54. Narod SA, Hawkins MM, Robertson CM, Stiller CA. Congenital anomalies and childhood cancer in Great Britain. *Am J Hum Genet* 1997;60(3):474–85.
55. Leotta N, Alvaro F, Dalla-Pozza L, Isaacs D. Concurrent HIV infection and neuroblastoma. *J Paediatr Child Health* 2003;39(3):236–8.
56. Marias BJ, Peinaar J, Gie RP. Kaposi sarcoma with upper airway obstruction and bilateral chylothoraces. *Pediatr Infect Dis J* 2003;22(10):926–8.
57. Reyes C, Abuzaitoun O, De Jong A, Hanson C, Langston C. Epstein-Barr virus-associated smooth muscle tumors in ataxia-telangiectasia: A case report and review. *Hum Pathol* 2002;33(1):133–6.
58. Chisholm CA, Heider AL, Kuller JA, von Allmen D, McMahon MJ, Chescheir NC. Prenatal diagnosis and perinatal management of fetal sacrococcygeal teratoma. *Am J Perinatol* 1999;16(2):89–2.
59. Chisholm CA, Heider AL, Kuller JA, von Allmen D, McMahon MJ, Chescheir NC. Prenatal diagnosis and perinatal management of fetal sacrococcygeal teratoma. *Am J Perinatol* 1999;16(1):47–50.
60. Hedrick HL, Flake AW, Crombleholme TM, *et al.* Sacrococcygeal teratoma: Prenatal assessment, fetal intervention, and outcome. *J Pediatr Surg* 2004;39(3):430–8.
61. Isaacs H Jr. Perinatal (fetal and neonatal) germ cell tumors. *J Pediatr Surg* 2004;39(7):1003–13.
62. Gonzalez-Crussi F, Winkler RF, Mirkin DL. Sacrococcygeal teratomas in infants and children: Relationship of histology and prognosis in 40 cases. *Arch Pathol Lab Med* 1978;102(8):420–5.
63. Canan A, Gulsevin T, Nejat A, *et al.* Neonatal intracranial teratoma. *Brain Dev* 2000;22(5):340–2.
64. Chien YH, Tsao PN, Lee WT, Peng SF, Yau KI. Congenital intracranial teratoma. *Pediatr Neurol* 2000;22(1):72–4.
65. Hunt SJ, Johnson PC, Coons SW, Pittman HW. Neonatal intracranial teratomas. *Surg Neurol* 1990;34(5):336–42.
66. Saleem SM, Hussain S, Nazir Z. Gastric teratoma – A rare benign tumour of neonates. *Ann Trop Paediatr* 2003;23(4):305–8.
67. Granata C, Fagnani AM, Gambini C, *et al.* Features and outcome of neuroblastoma detected before birth. *J Pediatr Surg* 2000;35(1):88–91.
68. Kurjak A, Zalud I, Jurkovic D, Alfirevic Z, Tomic K. Ultrasound diagnosis and evaluation of fetal tumors. *J Perinat Med* 1989;17(3):173–93.
69. Millman GC, Lodha AK, Moore AM, Cutz E. Disseminated congenital neuroblastoma presenting at birth. *Arch Dis Child* 2003;88(3):191.
70. Smith R, Chan HS, deSa DJ. Placental involvement in congenital neuroblastoma. *J Clin Pathol* 1981;34(7):785–9.
71. Nguyen TQ, Fisher GB Jr, Tabbarrah SO, Greer KE, Cooper PH. Tage IV-S metastatic neuroblastoma presenting as skin nodules at birth. *Int J Dermatol* 1988;27(10):712–3.

72. Yamashina M, Kayan H, Katayama I, Shibuya A. Congenital neuroblastoma presenting as a paratesticular tumor. *J Urol* 1988; 139(4):796–7.
73. Shimada H, Ambros IM, Dehner LP, *et al.* The International Neuroblastoma Pathology Classification (the Shimada system). *Cancer* 1999;86(2):364–72.
74. Goto S, Umehara S, Gerbing RB, *et al.* Histopathology (International Neuroblastoma Pathology Classification) and MYCN status in patients with peripheral neuroblastic tumors: A report from the Children's Cancer Group. *Cancer* 2001;92(10): 2699–708.
75. Haas D, Ablin AR, Miller C, Zoger S, Matthay KK. Complete pathologic maturation and regression of stage IVS neuroblastoma without treatment. *Cancer* 1988;62(4):818–25.
76. Hachitanda Y, Hata J. Stage IVS neuroblastoma: A clinical, histological, and biological analysis of 45 cases. *Hum Pathol* 1996; 27(11):1135–8.
77. Stokes SH, Thomas PR, Perez CA, Vietti TJ. Stage IV-S neuroblastoma. Results with definitive therapy. *Cancer* 1984;53(10): 2083–6.
78. Coffin CM, Dehner LP. Fibroblastic–myofibroblastic tumors in children and adolescents: A clinicopathologic study of 108 examples in 103 patients. *Pediatr Pathol* 1991;11(4):569–88.
79. Knezevich SR, McFadden DE, Tao W, Lim JF, Sorensen PH. A novel ETV6-NTRK3 gene fusion in congenital fibrosarcoma. *Nat Genet* 1998;18(2):184–7.
80. Coffin CM, Dehner LP. Soft tissue tumors in first year of life: A report of 190 cases. *Pediatr Pathol* 1990;10(4):509–26.
81. Chen Z, Coffin CM, Smith LM, *et al.* Cytogenetic–clinicopathologic correlations in rhabdomyosarcoma: A report of five cases. *Cancer Genet Cytogenet* 2001;131(1):31–6.
82. Daw JL, Wiedrich TA, Bauer BS. Congenital primitive neuroectodermal tumor of the hand: A case report. *J Hand Surg [Am]* 1997;22(4):743–6.
83. Smith LM, Adams RH, Brothman AR, Vanderhooft SL, Coffin CM. Peripheral primitive neuroectodermal tumor presenting with diffuse cutaneous involvement and 7;22 translocation. *Med Pediatr Oncol* 1998;30(6):357–63.
84. Yamada T, Takeuchi K, Masuda Y, Moriyama T, Kitazawa S, Maruo T. Prenatal imaging of congenital cerebral primitive neuroectodermal tumor. *Fetal Diagn Ther* 2003;18(3):137–9.
85. de Alava E, Gerald WL. Molecular biology of the Ewing's sarcoma/primitive neuroectodermal tumor family. *J Clin Oncol* 2000;18(1):204–13.
86. Chen Z, Coffin CM, Scott S, *et al.* Evidence by spectral karyotyping that 8q11.2 is nonrandomly involved in lipoblastoma. *J Mol Diagn* 2000;2(2):73–7.
87. Buetow PC, Smirniotopoulos JG, Done S. Congenital brain tumors: A review of 45 cases. *Am J Neuroradiol* 1990;11(4): 793–9.
88. Buetow PC, Smirniotopoulos JG, Done S. Congenital brain tumors: A review of 45 cases. *Am J Roentgenol* 1990;155(3): 587–93.
89. Isaacs H Jr. I. Perinatal brain tumors: A review of 250 cases. *Pediatr Neurol* 2002;27(4):249–61.
90. Isaacs H Jr. II. Perinatal brain tumors: A review of 250 cases. *Pediatr Neurol* 2002;27(5):333–42.
91. Argani P, Fritsch M, Kadkol SS, Schuster A, Beckwith JB, Perlman EJ. Detection of the ETV6-NTRK3 chimeric RNA of infantile fibrosarcoma/cellular congenital mesoblastic nephroma in paraffin-embedded tissue: Application to challenging pediatric renal stromal tumors. *Mod Pathol* 2000;13(1):29–36.
92. Argani P, Ladanyi M. Recent advances in pediatric renal neoplasia. *Adv Anat Pathol* 2003;10(5):243–60.
93. Beckwith JB, Kiviat NB, Bonadio JF. Nephrogenic rests, nephroblastomatosis, and the pathogenesis of Wilms' tumor. *Pediatr Pathol* 1990;10(1–2):1–36.
94. Charles AK, Brown KW, Berry PJ. Microdissecting the genetic events in nephrogenic rests and Wilms' tumor development. *Am J Pathol* 1998;153(3):991–1000.
95. Kullendorff CM, Wiebe T. Wilms' tumour in infancy. *Acta Paediatr* 1998;87(7):747–50.
96. Ritchey ML, Azizkhan RG, Beckwith JB, Hrabovsky EE, Haase GM. Neonatal Wilms tumor. *J Pediatr Surg* 1995;30(6):856–9.

SECTION II

Ethical and legal dimensions

Section Editors: **F. A. Chervenak and**
L. B. McCullough

12 Ethics: An essential dimension of perinatal medicine

F. A. Chervenak and L. B. McCullough

Introduction

Ethics is an essential dimension of perinatal medicine.[1–3] In this chapter, we develop a framework for clinical judgment and decision making about the ethical dimensions of perinatal medicine. We will emphasize a preventive ethics approach that anticipates the potential for ethical conflict and adopts ethically justified strategies to prevent those conflicts from occurring. Preventive ethics in perinatal medicine helps to build and sustain a strong physician–patient relationship.

This chapter has five parts. First, we define ethics, medical ethics, and the fundamental ethical principles of medical ethics: beneficence and respect for autonomy. Second, we show how these two principles should interact in perinatal medicine with emphasis on the clinical ethical concept of the fetus as a patient. Third, we describe different concepts of the ethical principles of justice. Fourth, we examine ethical issues in managed care with particular attention to the virtues of the physician as a professional. Fifth, we describe a new formal tool for critically appraising the literature of medical ethics, including perinatal ethics.

Ethics and medical ethics

Ethics is understood to be the disciplined study of morality. Medical ethics is therefore the disciplined study of morality in medicine, and concerns the obligations of physicians and health care organizations to patients, as well as the obligations of patients.[4] Medical ethics should be distinguished from the many sources of morality in pluralistic societies. These include law, our political heritage as free people, the world's religions, ethnic and cultural traditions, families, the traditions and practices of medicine (including medical education and training), and personal experience. Medical ethics since the 18th century European and American enlightenments has been secular.[5] It makes no reference to God or revealed tradition, but to what rational philosophical discourse produces. Therefore, ethical principles and virtues should be understood to apply to all physicians, regardless of their personal, religious, and spiritual beliefs.[6]

The traditions and practices of medicine constitute an important source of morality for physicians because they are based on the obligation to protect and promote the health-related interests of the patient. This obligation tells physicians what morality in medicine ought to be in very general and abstract terms. Providing a detailed and clinically applicable account of that obligation is the central task of medical ethics, using ethical principles.[4]

Ethical principles

The principle of beneficence

The ethical principle of beneficence requires one to act in a way that is expected reliably to produce the greater balance of benefits over harms in the lives of others.[6] Putting this principle into clinical practice requires a reliable account of the benefits and harms relevant to the care of the patient and how those benefits and harms should be reasonably balanced against each other, when not all of them can be achieved in a particular clinical situation. In medicine, the principle of beneficence requires the physician to act in a way that is reliably expected to produce a greater balance of clinical benefits, over clinical harms, for the patient.[4]

Beneficence-based clinical judgment has an ancient pedigree with its first expression found in the Hippocratic Oath and accompanying texts.[7] Beneficence-based clinical judgment aims to interpret reliably the health-related interests of the patient from a rigorous clinical perspective, which is provided by accumulated scientific research, clinical experience, and reasoned responses to uncertainty. Such a rigorous clinical perspective is thus not the function of the individual clinical perspective of any particular physician, and therefore should not be based merely on the clinical impression or intuition of an individual physician.

On the basis of this rigorous clinical perspective, which should be based on the best-available evidence, beneficence-based clinical judgment identifies the clinical benefits that can be achieved based on the competencies of medicine. The benefits that medicine is competent to seek for patients are the prevention and management of disease, injury, handicap, unnecessary pain, and suffering, and the prevention of premature or unnecessary death. Pain and suffering become unnecessary when they do not result in achieving the other benefits of medical care, e.g. allowing a woman to labor without effective analgesia.[4] Non-maleficence means that the physician should not, on balance, cause harm, and is best understood as expressing the limits of beneficence. This is also known as '*Primum non nocere*' or 'first do no harm'. This commonly invoked dogma is really a Latinized misinterpretation of the Hippocratic texts, which emphasized beneficence, while avoiding harm when approaching the limits of medicine.[4] There is an inherent risk of paternalism in beneficence-based clinical judgment. By this we mean that beneficence-based clinical judgment, if it is mistakenly taken by the physician to be the sole source of moral responsibility, and therefore moral authority in medical care, invites the unwary physician to conclude that beneficence-based judgments can be imposed on the patient irrespective of her autonomy. Paternalism is a dehumanizing response to the patient and therefore should be avoided in the practice of perinatal medicine.

The preventive ethics response to paternalism is for the physician to explain the diagnostic, therapeutic, and prognostic reasoning that leads to his or her clinical judgment about what is in the interest of the patient and her pregnancy, so that the patient can assess that clinical judgment for herself. The physician should first explain to the patient the major factors of this reasoning process, including matters of uncertainty. In neither medical law nor medical ethics does this require that the patient be provided with a complete medical education.[8] The physician should then explain how and why other clinicians might reasonably differ from his or her clinical judgment. The physician should then present a well-reasoned response to this critique. The outcome of this process should be that beneficence-based clinical judgments take on a rigor, which they sometimes lack, and the process of their formulation includes explaining them to the patient. In complex areas, such as perinatal medicine, beneficence-based clinical judgment will frequently result in the identification of a continuum of clinical strategies, which protect and promote health-related interests. Awareness of this feature of beneficence-based clinical judgment provides an important preventive ethics antidote to paternalism by increasing the likelihood that one or more of these medically reasonable, evidence-based alternatives will be acceptable to the patient. This feature of beneficence-based clinical judgment also provides a preventive ethics antidote to 'gag' rules that restrict physician's communications with the managed care patient.[9] All beneficence-based alternatives must be identified and explained to all patients, regardless of how the physician is paid, especially those who are well established in evidence-based perinatal medicine.

One advantage for the physician in carrying out this approach to communicating with the patient would be, we believe, to increase the likelihood of compliance.[10] This is an especially pertinent consideration in perinatal medicine, e.g. self-observation for unusual weight gain, bleeding, or signs of premature labor. Another advantage would be to provide the patient with a better-informed opportunity to make a decision about whether to seek a second opinion. The approach outlined above should make a decision less threatening to her physician, who has already shared with the patient the limitations of clinical judgment.

The principle of respect for autonomy

To complement the principle of beneficence, there is emphasis in the literature of medical ethics on the principle of respect for autonomy.[6] This principle requires one to always acknowledge and carry out the value-based preferences of the adult, competent patient, unless there is compelling ethical justification for not doing so, e.g. prescribing antibiotics for viral respiratory infections. The pregnant patient increasingly brings to her medical care her own perspective on what is in her and her pregnancy's interest. The principle of respect for autonomy translates this into autonomy-based clinical judgment. Because each patient's perspective on her interests is a function of her values and beliefs, it is impossible to specify in advance the benefits and harms of the patient's autonomy-based clinical judgment. Indeed, it would be inappropriate for the physician to do so, because the definition of her benefits and harms and their balancing are the prerogative of the patient. Autonomy-based clinical judgment is strongly antipaternalistic in nature.[4]

The responsible practice of perinatal medicine depends on an operationalized concept of autonomy to make it relevant to clinical practice. We therefore identify three sequential autonomy-based behaviors on the part of the patient: (1) absorbing and retaining information about her condition and alternative diagnostic and therapeutic responses to it, (2) understanding that information (i.e. evaluating and rank-ordering those responses and appreciating that she could experience the risks of treatment), and (3) expressing a value-based preference. The physician has a role to play in each of these. They are, respectively, (1) to recognize the capacity of each pregnant patient to deal with medical information (and not to underestimate that capacity), provide information (i.e. disclose and explain all medically reasonable alternatives, that is, supported in beneficence-based clinical judgment), and recognize the validity of the values and beliefs of the patient; (2) not to interfere with, but, when necessary, to assist the patient in her evaluation and ranking of diagnostic and therapeutic alternatives for managing her condition; and (3) to elicit and implement the patient's value-based preference.[4]

Beneficence and respect for autonomy in perinatal practice

The ethical principles of beneficence and respect for autonomy play a central role in perinatal practice. There are obviously beneficence-based and autonomy-based obligations to the pregnant patient: the physician's perspective on the pregnant woman's health-related interests provides the basis for the physician's beneficence-based obligations to her. Her own perspective on those interests provides the basis for the physician's autonomy-based obligations to her. Because of an insufficiently developed central nervous system, the fetus cannot meaningfully be said to possess values and beliefs. Thus, there is no basis for saying that a fetus has a perspective on its interests. Hence, there can be no autonomy-based obligations to any fetus. The language of fetal rights has no meaning and therefore no application to the fetus in perinatal clinical judgment and practice, despite its popularity in public and political discourse in the United States and other countries. The physician does have a perspective on the fetus's health-related interests, and the physician can have beneficence-based obligations to the fetus, 'but only when the fetus is a patient'.[4]

Clinical ethical concept of the fetus as a patient

The clinical ethical concept of the fetus as a patient is essential to perinatal clinical judgment and practice. Developments in fetal diagnosis and perinatal management strategies to optimize fetal outcome have become widely accepted, encouraging the development of this concept. This concept has considerable clinical significance, because when the fetus is a patient, directive counseling, that is, recommending clinical management for fetal benefit, is appropriate, and when the fetus is not a patient, non-directive counseling, that is, offering, but not recommending, a form of management for fetal benefit, is appropriate. However, these seemingly straightforward roles for directive and non-directive counseling are often difficult to apply in actual perinatal practice, because of uncertainty about when the fetus is a patient. This concerns moral status, i.e. whether others have an ethical obligation to the fetus to protect and promote its interests.

One prominent approach for establishing whether or not the fetus has the moral status of being a patient has involved attempts to show whether or not the fetus has independent moral status. Independent moral status for the fetus means that one or more characteristics that the fetus possesses in and of itself, and therefore independently of the pregnant woman or any other factor, generate and therefore ground clinical obligations to the fetus on the part of the pregnant woman and her physician.

Many fetal characteristics have been proposed as the basis for such independent moral status, including moment of conception, implantation, central nervous system development, quickening, and the moment of birth. It should come as no surprise that there is considerable variation among ethical arguments about when the fetus acquires independent moral status. Some take the view that the fetus has independent moral status from the moment of conception or implantation. Others believe that independent moral status is acquired in degrees, thus resulting in 'graded' moral status. Still others hold, at least by implication, that the fetus never has independent moral status so long as it is *in utero*.[11,12]

Despite an enormous amount of theological and philosophical literature on this subject, there has been no closure on a single authoritative account of the independent moral status of the fetus. This outcome should be expected because, given the absence of a single method that would be authoritative for all of the markedly diverse theological and philosophical schools of thought involved in this sometimes acrimonious debate, closure is impossible. For closure ever to be possible, debates about such a final authority within and between theological and philosophical traditions would have to be resolved in a way satisfactory to all, an inconceivable intellectual and cultural event. Claims about the independent moral status of the fetus, as the basis for claims about the fetus as a patient, have no stable or clinically applicable meaning. We therefore abandon these futile attempts to understand the fetus as a patient in terms of independent moral status of the fetus and turn to an alternative approach.

Our analysis of the clinical ethical concept of the fetus as a patient starts with the recognition that being a patient does not require that one possess independent moral status. Rather, being a patient means that one can benefit from the applications of the clinical skills of the physician. More precisely stated, a human being is properly regarded as a patient when two conditions are met: (1) the human being is presented to the physician and (2) there exist clinical interventions that are reliably expected to be efficacious, in that they are reliably expected to result in a greater balance of clinical benefits over harms for the human being in question.[13] We call this the dependent moral status of the fetus as a patient.

The authors have argued elsewhere that beneficence-based obligations to the fetus exist when the fetus is reliably expected later to achieve independent moral status as a child and a person. The fetus is a patient when the fetus is presented for medical interventions, whether diagnostic or therapeutic, that reasonably can be expected to result in a greater balance of benefits over harms for the child and person the fetus can *later* become during early childhood.[4] The clinical ethical significance of the concept of the fetus as a patient, therefore, depends on the links that can be established between the fetus and its later achieving independent moral status.

The viable fetus as a patient

One such link is viability. Viability is not an intrinsic property of the fetus because viability should be understood in terms of both biological and technological factors. It is only by virtue of both factors that a viable fetus can exist *ex utero* and thus achieve independent moral status. It is important to appreciate that these two factors do not exist as a function of the autonomy of the pregnant woman. When a fetus is viable, that is, when it is of sufficient maturity so that it can survive into the neonatal period and achieve independent moral status, given the availability of the requisite technological support, and when it is presented to the physician, the fetus is a patient.

Viability exists as a function of biomedical and technological capacities. These differ in different parts of the world. As a consequence, there is no worldwide, uniform gestational age to define viability. In the USA, we believe viability presently occurs at approximately 24 weeks of gestational age.[14]

When the fetus is a patient, directive counseling for fetal benefit is ethically justified. In perinatal practice, directive counseling for fetal benefit involves recommending against termination of pregnancy, recommending against non-aggressive management, or recommending aggressive management. Aggressive obstetric management includes interventions, such as fetal surveillance, tocolysis, cesarean delivery, or delivery in a tertiary care center when indicated. Non-aggressive obstetric management excludes such interventions. Directive counseling for fetal benefit, however, must always take account of the presence and severity of fetal anomalies, extreme prematurity, and obligations to the pregnant woman.

The strength of directive counseling for fetal benefit justifiably varies according to the presence and severity of anomalies. As a rule, the more severe the fetal anomaly, the less directive counseling should be for fetal benefit. In particular, when lethal anomalies, such as anencephaly, can be diagnosed with certainty, there are no beneficence-based obligations to provide aggressive management. Such fetuses are dying patients, and the counseling, therefore, should be non-directive in recommending between non-aggressive management and termination of pregnancy, but directive in recommending against aggressive management for the sake of maternal benefit.[15] By contrast, third-trimester abortion for Down's syndrome or achondroplasia is not ethically justifiable, because the future child with high probability will have the capacity to grow and develop as a human being.[16,17]

Directive counseling for fetal benefit in cases of extreme prematurity of viable fetuses is appropriate. In particular, this is the case for what we term just-viable fetuses, those with a gestational age of 24–26 weeks, for which there are significant rates of survival, but high rates of mortality and morbidity. These rates of morbidity and mortality can be increased by non-aggressive obstetric management, whereas aggressive obstetric management may favorably influence outcome. Thus, it appears that there are substantial beneficence-based obligations to just-viable fetuses to provide aggressive obstetric management. This is all the more the case in pregnancies beyond 26 weeks of gestational age. Directive counseling for fetal benefit is therefore justified in all cases of extreme prematurity of viable fetuses. Of course, such directive counseling is appropriate only when it is based on documented efficacy of aggressive obstetric management for each fetal indication. For example, such efficacy has not been demonstrated for routine cesarean delivery to manage extreme prematurity.

All directive counseling for fetal benefit must occur in the context of balancing beneficence-based obligations to the fetal patient against beneficence-based and autonomy-based obligations to the pregnant woman. Any such balancing must recognize that a pregnant woman is obligated only to take reasonable risks of perinatal interventions that are reliably expected to benefit the viable fetus or child later. A unique feature of perinatal ethics is that the pregnant woman's autonomy influences whether, in a particular case, the viable fetus ought to be regarded as presented to the physician.

Obviously, any strategy for directive counseling for fetal benefit that takes account of obligations to the pregnant woman must anticipate the possibility of conflict between the physician's recommendation and the pregnant woman's autonomous decision to the contrary. Such conflict should be managed preventively through the use of the informed consent process as an ongoing dialog throughout a woman's pregnancy, augmented as necessary by negotiation and respectful persuasion.[18]

The previable fetus as a patient

The only possible link between the previable fetus and the child it can become is the pregnant woman's autonomy, because technological factors cannot result in the previable fetus becoming a child. The link, therefore, between a previable fetus and the child it can become can be established only by the pregnant woman's decision to confer the status of being a patient on her previable fetus. The previable fetus has no claim to the status of being a patient independently of the pregnant woman's autonomy. The pregnant woman is therefore free to withhold, confer, or, having once conferred, withdraw the status of being a patient on or from her previable fetus, according to her own values and beliefs. The previable fetus is presented to the physician as a function of the pregnant woman's autonomy.[4]

Counseling the pregnant woman regarding the management of her pregnancy when the fetus is previable should be non-directive in terms of continuing the pregnancy or having an abortion if she refuses to confer the status of being a patient on her fetus. If she does confer such status in a settled way, at that point beneficence-based obligations to her fetus come into existence, and directive counseling for fetal benefit becomes appropriate for these previable fetuses. Just as for viable fetuses, such counseling must take account of the presence and severity of fetal anomalies, extreme prematurity, and beneficence-based and autonomy-based obligations to the pregnant woman.

For pregnancies in which the woman is uncertain about whether to confer such status, the authors propose that the fetus be 'provisionally' regarded as a patient. This justifies directive counseling against behavior that can harm a fetus in significant and irreversible ways, e.g. substance abuse, especially alcohol, until the woman settles on whether to confer the status of being a patient on the fetus.

In particular, non-directive counseling is appropriate in cases of what we term near-viable fetuses, that is, those that are 22–23 weeks of gestational age, for which there are anecdotal reports of survival. In our view, aggressive obstetric and neonatal management should be regarded as clinical investigation (i.e. a form of medical experimentation), not a standard of care.[14] There is no clinical obligation on the part of any pregnant woman to confer the status of being a patient on a near-viable fetus, because the efficacy of aggressive obstetric and neonatal management has yet to be proven.

The *in vitro* embryo as a patient

A subset of previable fetuses as patients concerns the *in vitro* embryo.[19] It might seem that the *in vitro* embryo is a patient, because such an embryo is presented to the physician. However, for beneficence-based obligations to a human being to exist, it must also be the case that medical interventions are reliably expected to be efficacious.

Whether the fetus is a patient depends on the links that can be established between the fetus and its eventual independent moral status. Therefore, whether medical interventions on the *in vitro* embryo should be reliably expected to be efficacious for the child later depends on whether that embryo later becomes viable. Otherwise, no benefit of such intervention can meaningfully be said to result. An *in vitro* embryo becomes viable only when it survives *in vitro* cell division, transfer, implantation, and subsequent gestation to such a time that it becomes viable. The process of achieving viability occurs only *in vivo* and is therefore entirely dependent on the woman's decision regarding the status of the fetus(es) as a patient, should assisted conception successfully result in the gestation of the previable fetus(es). Whether an *in vitro* embryo will become a viable fetus, and whether medical intervention on such an embryo will benefit the fetus and future child, are both functions of the pregnant woman's autonomous decision to withhold, confer, or, having once conferred, withdraw the moral status of being a patient on or from the previable fetus(es) that might result from assisted conception.

It therefore is appropriate to regard the *in vitro* embryo as a previable fetus rather than as a viable fetus. As a consequence, any *in vitro* embryo(s) should be regarded as a patient only when the woman into whose reproductive tract the embryo(s) will be transferred confers that status. Thus, counseling about preimplantation diagnosis should therefore be non-directive, just as it should be for previability counseling. One additional justification is that the woman may elect not to implant abnormal embryos. These embryos will not become patients, and so there is no basis for directive counseling regarding them. Information should be presented about prognosis for a successful pregnancy and the possibility of confronting a decision about selective reduction, depending on the number of embryos transferred. Counseling about how many *in vitro* embryos should be transferred should be rigorously evidence based.[20]

Justice and perinatal medicine

Ethical concerns about justice arise when economic, clinical, or other resources are scarce. Justice requires that in the distribution of resources, each should receive what is due to him or her. Different concepts of justice define 'due' in different ways. Each strives to result in a fair distribution of benefits, i.e. access to resources, and burdens, the risks that could follow from lack of such access.

Utilitarianism is a theory of justice that makes central the obligation to produce the greatest good for the greatest number in the management of scarce resources. To be successful in guiding practical, day-to-day decisions about the allocation of resources, utilitarianism requires an account of the greatest good. For society overall, it has been difficult, if not impossible, to define what the greatest good is. The value of utilitarianism is the balance it seeks to achieve among benefits and burdens of scarce resources, so that inequalities do not become inequities, i.e. unfair. Critics of utilitarians have pointed out that sometimes utilitarianism results in inequities, i.e. shared distributions of benefits and burdens.[21]

Two other concepts of justice have been developed to address this problem. The first of these is a libertarian concept of justice. This concept of justice was developed to correct for tyrannical burdens that pure utilitarianism could create. In particular, libertarianism was developed to give priority to individual freedom and property rights, as correctives to the potential excesses of utilitarianism and, in the political realm, of state power. Libertarians argue that in a market that places different values on different services and products, and in which there is an equal opportunity to develop one's talents, those who provide more highly valued services rightly earn more than those who provide less valued (though not necessarily less intrinsically valuable) services. Everyone should get to keep what he or she earns through these marketplace exchanges, reflecting the strong emphasis of the libertarian concept of justice on property rights. Libertarian theories emphasize fairness of process, rather than equality of outcomes.

The other concept of justice that has been developed is an egalitarian concept of justice. This concept was developed to protect vulnerable and disadvantaged members of society, who may lose out in a utilitarian distribution of scarce resources. This concept of justice corrects for unfair outcomes in the form of undue burdens on those least able to protect themselves.

These three and other concepts of justice remain in unresolved competition in ethics generally, in medical ethics,[22] and in perinatal ethics. It is fair to say that the medical ethics literature is strongly influenced by a concept of justice that calls for fair equality of opportunity (an element of libertarian justice) and protection of the least well-off (an element of egalitarian justice). However, it is also fair to say that no single concept of justice shapes health care policy in the United States. This lack of a conceptually coherent health care policy is a long-standing feature of American health care policy. In particular, unlike many other developed countries, the United States has yet to create a universal right to health care, though there are selective entitlements.

Managed care and the professional virtues

The practice of perinatal medicine is coming under managed care, which involves a set of strategies used by both private and public payers to control the cost of medical care. Two main business tools are used to achieve this goal: (1) creating conflicts of interests in how physicians are paid, diplomatically called 'sharing economic risk', and (2) increasingly strict control of clinical judgment and practice through such means as practice guidelines, critical pathways, physician report cards, and retrospective chart reviews. These business tools generate ethical challenges to perinatologists who seriously threaten the virtues that define the fiduciary character of medicine as a profession.[23]

In medicine, the physician is the patient's fiduciary. The physician should be competent and use clinical competence as a matter of routine and habit primarily to protect and promote patients' interests rather than pursue his or her own interests. Virtues are those traits and habits of character that routinely focus the concern and behavior of an individual on the interests of others and thereby habitually blunt the motivation to act on self-interest one's primary consideration. We believe that four virtues constitute the physician–patient relationship based on the physician as fiduciary.[4]

The first virtue is *self-effacement*. This professional virtue requires the physician not to act on the basis of potential differences between the patient and the physician, such as race, religion, national origin, gender, sexual orientation, manners, socioeconomic status, or proficiency in speaking English. Self-effacement prevents biases and prejudices from arising from these differences that could adversely impact on the plan of care for the patient.

The second professional virtue is *self-sacrifice*. This requires physicians to accept reasonable risks to themselves. As an example, perinatologists manifest this virtue in their willingness to perform a cesarean delivery for an HIV+ patient, following accepted standards. In both fee-for-service and managed care, the professional virtue of self-sacrifice obligates the physician to blunt economic self-interest and focus on the patient's need for relief, when the two are in conflict.

The third professional virtue, *compassion*, motivates the physician to recognize and seek to alleviate the stress, discomfort, pain, and suffering associated with the patient's disease and illness. Self-effacement, self-sacrifice, and compassion provide the basis for a powerful ethical response to the business tool of conflicts of interest by the physician.

This response is strengthened by the fourth professional virtue, *integrity*. This virtue imposes an intellectual discipline on the physician's clinical judgments about the patient's problems and how to address them. Integrity prescribes rigor in the formation of clinical judgment. Clinical judgment is rigorous when it is based on the best available scientific information or, when such information is lacking, on consensus clinical judgment and on careful thought processes of an individual physician that can withstand peer review. Integrity is thus an antidote to the pitfalls of bias, subjective clinical impressions, and unexamined clinical 'common sense' that can undermine evidence-based practice. Integrity provides the basis for the physician's ethical response to the business tool of control of clinical judgment and practice.

None of these four virtues is absolute in its ethical demands. The task of medical ethics is to identify both the application and the limits of these four virtues. The concept of legitimate self-interest provides the basis for these limits. Legitimate self-interest includes protecting the conditions for practicing medicine well, fulfilling obligations to persons in the physician's life other than the patient, and protecting activities outside the practice of medicine that the physician finds deeply fulfilling.

Managed care and the physician as fiduciary

The fee-for-service practice of medicine unconstrained by fiduciary obligations could and did in the past lead to harm to patients from non-indicated overutilization of resources. It is a violation of the standard of care to subject patients to unnecessary active intervention in order to achieve personal economic gain. Managed care unconstrained by fiduciary obligations puts patients at risk of harm by denying access to the standard of care. This will occur if patients are subjected to unnecessary risk from withholding appropriate care and intervention in order to achieve reduced cost.[23,24]

Financial incentives to the physician and supervision of clinician decision making with strict controls over utilization are the business tools managed care uses. Forms of payment by managed care plans, such as capitation and withhold, deliberately impose an economic conflict of interest on the physician.[25] Every time the physician uses a resource, e.g. consultation, diagnostic testing, or surgical procedures, the physician pays an economic penalty. The ethical challenge occurs when the patient's interests are subordinated to the pursuit of financial rewards and are thereby harmed by this underutilization.

The professional virtue of self-sacrifice prohibits the physician from making the avoidance of such financial risk, the *primary* consideration. Avoiding financial risk as one's primary consideration involves an ethically pathologic process that leads naturally and quickly to the abandonment of self-effacement (economically driven managed care for some patients, but not for others), compassion (patients' health-related concerns do not matter but are only a means to maximize revenues), and integrity (the standard of care is sacrificed to maximize revenues). Importantly, physicians are not sanctioned by society to engage in the destruction of medicine as a fiduciary profession, because it is a public trust, not a private fiefdom.

Physicians should not assume that managed care organizations (MCOs) are unwilling to negotiate contracts to reduce the severity of economic conflicts of interest. Physicians should therefore make a good faith effort to negotiate these matters. If the MCO refuses to negotiate and the economic risk of not signing the contract is very significant, then the physician should voluntarily accept the ethical responsibility to be alert to and manage these conflicts of interest well. First, integrity requires that the physician avoid the self-deception of underestimating any potential influence on clinical judgment and practice by the conflict of interest. Second, once these contracts are signed, the professional virtues add an important dimension to total quality management: diligent monitoring of conflicts of interest to prevent them from resulting in substandard care should be among the physician's 'accountabilities'. Third, the realities of managed care mean that, for the near term at least, increasing financial sacrifice may be required to protect the integrity of medicine as a fiduciary profession. Fourth, in group practice, there should be a fair sharing of economic self-sacrifice. In particular, individual efforts to tune the system to one's economic advantage in a group, for example, avoiding the care of high-risk pregnancies, and to the disadvantage of colleagues should be avoided.

The second business tool of managed care, increasingly strict control of clinical judgment and practice, is a heterogenous phenomenon. Some managed care plans are poorly capitalized and poorly managed. They compete by price, with little or no attention given to the quality of their services. A 'bottom line' mentality dominates with economic savings and net revenue maximization the overriding values. These poorly managed companies have little or no understanding of or interest in the fiduciary nature of medicine, and so their controls of clinical judgment and practice are driven almost entirely by economic considerations.

Physicians subject to management controls by such companies face the very difficult challenge of trying to get such companies to constrain their economic interests by their fiduciary obligations, a daunting task but not, we believe, impossible. The concerns of ethics, especially to protect the integrity of the fiduciary enterprise, may frequently be swept aside when they are not ignored altogether. However, as the fiduciaries of patients, physicians in such MCOs are the ultimate bulwark on which patients and society must be able to rely at the present time to protect patients from management's unbridled pursuit of economic self-interest. Physicians, therefore, should strenuously resist and seek to change management controls driven solely by economic considerations. Adhering to evidence-based medicine of perinatal practice becomes a powerful tool for achieving this goal. If physicians refused to cooperate with such poorly managed companies, systematic dissociation would result in a loss of market share or, more optimistically, better management.

Being physician controlled does not provide the MCO immunization against the ethical challenges of the business tools of managed care. These new physician-owned provider entities will not provide a solution in and of themselves to the ethical threats of conflict of interest and control of clinical judgment and practice. The virtue-based arguments we have made will apply to these new entities without exception.

There is no conclusive evidence that preserving medicine as a fiduciary profession is impossible, even given the enormous economic power of MCOs. Ethics teaches us that business and economic power are not absolute and should always be called to account for their consequences. Society has not given MCOs the moral authority or permission to destroy the fiduciary character of medicine as a consequence of the pursuit of economic interest and power. Nor has society given physicians the moral authority or permission to cooperate willfully in this destruction. Quite the

1. Does the article address a focused ethics question?
   a. Does the article address a clearly stated and focused ethical issue or problem?
   b. Is the issue important and why?
   c. Is justification for the importance presented?
   d. From whose perspective is importance claimed?

2. Are the arguments that support the results of the article valid?
   a. Is the literature search complete?
   b. Are the analysis and argument of cited papers reported clearly and accurately?
   c. What is the quality of the paper's ethical analysis and argument?

3. What are the results?
   a. What are the conclusions of the paper's ethical analysis and argument?

4. Will the results help me in clinical practice?
   a. Will the help be practical?
   b. Will the help be theoretical?
   c. How should the reader change his or her thinking, attitudes, practices or policies?

Figure 12.1 Critical appraisal tool.

opposite, society counts on physicians because ultimately society can count on no one else to preserve and advocate for the fiduciary character of the medical profession.

Argument-based ethics

Before turning to the presentation of a formal tool[26] for critically appraising the ethics literature, it is important to distinguish descriptive from normative medical ethics. The proposed formal tool is designed to be applied to the latter. Descriptive medical ethics uses empirical methods to obtain data that describe the actual ethical judgments, practices, and policies of physicians and health care organizations, of patients and their families, and of the larger society. These articles also report the results of ethically justified interventions for their clinical effects. Descriptive ethics articles use accepted methods of empirical research, such as interviews analyzed with qualitative methods and questionnaire research analyzed with quantitative methods.[27,28] Such empirical studies are common in the medical literature and should be critically appraised using appropriate methodology that has already been well described.[29–37]

The literature of normative medical ethics is argument based. It therefore uses the tools of ethical analysis and argument to explore the implications of ethical concepts for what clinical practice and organizational and health care policy ought to be, as we did above with respect to the clinical ethical concept of the fetus as a patient. Normative ethics scholarship offers reasoned conclusions about what clinical judgment, decision making, and behavior ought to be, rather than empirically based descriptions of what these are.

Formal assessment tool

The new critical appraisal tool presented here is adapted from recent work on critical appraisal of the medical literature reporting the results of qualitative research[26] (see Figure 12.1).

Does the article address a focused ethics question?

Normative ethics articles in perinatal medicine should have a clear, well-defined focus. This focus should be reflected in the title and made explicit in the introductory section of the paper. There are a number of possible domains for the focus of normative ethics literature, including theoretical issues (such as whether the fetus is a patient or a person), clinical issues for a specific patient population (the management of pregnancy in a diabetic patient), research issues for a specific population (surgical management of fetal spina bifida), organizational management issues (quality improvement and cost control of IVF services), and public policy issues (partial-birth abortion).

The importance of the issue should be explained, which can be theoretical or clinical. The issue may be important for research or for organizational and public policy. The importance of the issue should be justified. It is important that the article should identify the perspective from which importance of the issue is claimed, whether that of physicians, scientific investigators, patients, patient's families and other support networks, payers, health care organization leadership, and scholars and public officials concerned with health policy. The target audience for the article should be made clear.

Are the arguments that support the results of the article valid?

This question concerns whether the results of the article, i.e. the conclusions that it draws about what morality in medicine ought to be, are supported by high-quality ethical analysis and argument. The literature of normative ethics in perinatal medicine is now quite extensive, making it increasingly unlikely that there is no prior relevant literature that should be considered. Relevant literature should be cited and analysis and arguments from this literature should be presented clearly and accurately. In the basic and clinical science literature, investigators are increasingly expected to elucidate the search strategies, including keywords, databases, bibliographies, and other sources used. The same standard should begin to be met by the normative ethics literature. In assessing the search of an article, the critical reader should first ask, how adequate is the article's search strategy? In as much as all are major forms of scholarship in bioethics, are articles, book chapters, and books cited?

Is the literature carefully reviewed? By this we mean that the major positions on the issue should be presented in a clear and unbiased fashion. How these positions have developed and their critical interaction should be explained, so that the reader is provided with a reliable account of the best thinking on the subject. Major positions should be critically appraised for their strengths and weaknesses and how well they have responded to criticisms that advanced against them.

What is the quality of the paper's analysis and argument? Quality turns on both validity and soundness. Validity concerns the formal qualities of ethical analysis and argument. Are relevant clinical and other facts clearly identified and supported? Are key concepts and ethical appeals clearly stated and reasonably related to clinical information? Are these concepts and appeals used with consistent meaning throughout the argument? Do the reasons given for the position, the premises of the argument, fit together into a coherent whole? Is the conclusion that follows from those premises clearly stated? Normative ethics in perinatal medicine is not an 'ivory tower' enterprise; it concerns issues of vital importance in clinical practice and research and in organizational management and health policy. Physician readers are therefore entitled to expect authors of normative medical ethics scholarship to take a clinically relevant and applicable stand that is supported by the argument presented.[4,41]

Soundness concerns the substance of the ethical analysis and argument, including especially whether the conclusion should be regarded as reliable, i.e. one on which the physician can act with confidence that patient care will be improved as a result. Reliable arguments are those in which a clear warrant of defense is given for each premise or reason offered in support of the conclusion.

In preventing readers' bias,[42] it is helpful to identify the disciplines represented among the authors. The normative medical ethics literature is distinctive in that work of high quality by non-clinicians should influence the clinical judgment and decision making of physicians, just as a work on infectious diseases of the reproductive tract by microbiologists or on pharmacokinetics of gynecologic cancer chemotherapy by pharmacologists rightly influences clinical judgment and practice. Normative ethics work, therefore, should not be dismissed when only some, or even none, of the authors are physicians.

At the same time, the reader should beware of positive or negative bias toward an article, based on the reputation of the author(s) or of the journal. Just as in the basic and clinical sciences, the standing of authors in journals in obstetrics and gynecology or in the field of bioethics is no guarantee of quality in normative medical ethics.

What are the results?

The results of normative ethics are the conclusions of ethical analysis and argument. These conclusions should be clearly stated and easy to find in the article.

Will the results help me in clinical practice?

The results of normative ethics articles and books can be helpful in at least three ways. First, they may have important practical implications, especially if the paper incorporates evidence to support the clinical utility of acting on the conclusions of the paper. The quality of the empirical evidence cited should be assessed in the same way as evidence should be assessed in any medical or scientific article.[29–37] The results for clinical practice, research, organizational management, or policy should be assessed as well. Second, they may have important theoretical implications, which do not depend on whether an intervention was performed and evaluated. Identifying such theoretical implications results in critical assessment and revision of ethical frameworks and appeals based on them. Finally, readers of the normative ethics literature should ask themselves how they should change their thinking (clinical judgment and reasoning), attitudes (toward patients, their families, and legal institutions), clinical practice, or organizational policies. This is a crucial step in the literature on evidence-based medicine and is similarly crucial here.

Conclusion

In this chapter we have provided a general ethical framework for perinatal clinical judgment and practice. Implementing this framework on a daily basis is essential to creating and sustaining a professional physician–patient relationship in perinatal medicine. This framework emphasizes preventive ethics, i.e. the recognition that the potential for ethical conflict is built into clinical practice and the use of such clinical tools as informed consent and negotiation to prevent such conflict from occurring. This framework comprehensively appeals to the ethical principles of beneficence, respect for autonomy, and justice, and the professional virtues of self-effacement, self-sacrifice, compassion, and integrity. Finally, a formal tool can now be used to critically evaluate the literature of ethics in perinatal medicine.

REFERENCES

1. American College of Obstetricians and Gynecologists. *Ethics in Obstetrics and Gynecology*. Washington, DC: American College of Obstetricians and Gynecologists, 2002.
2. Association of Professors of Gynecology and Obstetrics. *Exploring Medical–Legal Issues in Obstetrics and Gynecology*. Washington, DC: APGO Medical Education Foundation, 1994.
3. FIGO Committee for the Study of Ethical Aspects of Human Reproduction. *Recommendations of Ethical Issues in Obstetrics and Gynecology*. London: International Federation of Gynecology and Obstetrics, 1997.
4. McCullough LB, Chervenak FA. *Ethics in Obstetrics and Gynecology*. New York: Oxford University Press, 1994.
5. Engelhardt HT Jr. *The Foundations of Bioethics*, 2nd edn. New York: Oxford University Press, 1995.
6. Beauchamp TL, Childress JF. *Principles of Biomedical Ethics*, 5th edn. New York: Oxford University Press, 2001.
7. Hippocrates. Oath of Hippocrates. In Temkin O, Temkin CL, eds. *Ancient Medicine: Selected Papers of Ludwig Edelstein*. Baltimore: Johns Hopkins University Press, 1976:6.
8. Faden RR, Beauchamp TL. *A History and Theory of Informed Consent*. New York: Oxford University Press, 1986.
9. Brody H, Bonham VL Jr. Gag rules and trade secrets in managed care contracts: Ethical and legal concerns. *Arch Intern Med* 1997;157:2037–43.
10. Wear S. *Informed Consent: Patient Autonomy and Clinician Beneficence within Health Care*, 2nd edn. Washington, DC: Georgetown University Press, 1998.
11. Callahan S, Callahan D, eds. *Abortion: Understanding Differences*. New York: Plenum Press, 1984.
12. Annas GJ. Protecting the liberty of pregnant patient. *N Engl J Med* 1988;316:1213–4.
13. Chervenak FA, McCullough LB. Ethics in obstetrics and gynecology: An overview. *Eur J Obstet Gynecol Reprod Med* 1997;75:91–4.
14. Chervenak FA, McCullough LB. The limits of viability. *J Perinat Med* 1997;25:418–20.
15. Chervenak FA, McCullough LB. An ethically justified, clinically comprehensive management strategy for third-trimester pregnancies complicated by fetal anomalies. *Obstet Gynecol* 1990;75: 311–6.
16. Chervenak FA, McCullough LB, Campbell S. Is third trimester abortion justified? *Br J Obstet Gynaecol* 1995;102:434–5.
17. Chervenak FA, McCullough LB, Campbell S. Third trimester abortion: Is compassion enough? *Br J Obstet Gynaecol* 1999; 106:293–6.
18. Chervenak FA, McCullough LB. Clinical guides to preventing ethical conflicts between pregnant women and their physicians. *Am J Obstet Gynecol* 1990;162:303–7.
19. Chervenak FA, McCullough LB, Rosenwaks Z. Ethical considerations in newer reproductive technologies. *Semin Perinatol* 2003;27:427–34.
20. Chervenak FA, McCullough LB, Rosenwaks Z. Ethical dimensions of the number of embryos to be transferred in in vitro fertilization. *J Assist Reprod Genet* 2001;18:583–7.
21. Sterba JF. Justice. In Reich WT, ed. *Encyclopedia of Bioethics*, 2nd edn. New York: Macmillan, 1995:1308–15.
22. Chervenak FA, McCullough LB. Professionalism and justice in the leadership of academic medical centers. *Acad Med* 2002;77: 45–7.
23. Chervenak FA, McCullough LB, Chez R. Responding to the ethical challenges posed by the business tools of managed care in the practice of obstetrics and gynecology. *Am J Obstet Gynecol* 1996;175:524–7.
24. Council on Ethical and Judicial Affairs of the American Medical Association. Ethical issues in managed care. *J Am Med Assoc* 1995;273:330–335.
25. Spece RG, Shimm DS, Buchanan AE, ed. *Conflicts of Interest in Clinical Practice and Research*. New York: Oxford University Press, 1996.
26. McCullough LB, Coverdale JH, Chervenak FA. Argument-based medical ethics: A formal tool for critically appraising the normative medical ethics literature. *Am J Obstet Gynecol* 2004;191: 1097–102.
27. Sulmasy DP, Sugarman J. The many methods of medical ethics (or thirteen ways of looking at a blackbird). In Sugarman J, Sulmasy DP, eds. *Methods in Medical Ethics*. Washington, DC: Georgetown University Press, 2001:3–18.
28. Sugarman J, Faden R, Weinstein J. A decade of empirical research in medical ethics. In Sugarman J, Sulmasy DP, eds. *Methods in Medical Ethics*. Washington, DC: Georgetown University Press, 2001:19–28.
29. Oxman AD, Cook DJ, Guyatt GH. Users' guides to the medical literature. VI. How to use an overview. *J Am Med Assoc* 1994; 272:1367–71.
30. Guyatt GH, Sackett DL, Cook DJ. Users' guides to the medical literature. II. How to use an article about therapy or prevention. A. Are the results of the study valid? *J Am Med Assoc* 1993; 270:2598–601.
31. Guyatt GH, Sackett DL, Cook DJ. Users' guides to the medical literature. II. How to use an article about therapy or prevention. B. What were the results and will they help me in caring for my patients? *J Am Med Assoc* 1994;271:59–63.
32. Wilson MC, Hayward RS, Tunis SR, Bass EB. Users' guides to the medical literature. VIII. How to use clinical practice guidelines. A. Are the recommendations valid? *J Am Med Assoc* 1995;274: 570–4.
33. Wilson MC, Hayward RS, Tunis SR, Bass EB. Users' guides to the medical literature. VIII. How to use clinical practice guidelines. A. What are the recommendations and will they help you in caring for your patients? *J Am Med Assoc* 1995;274:1630–2.
34. Giacomini MK, Cook DJ. Users' guides to the medical literature. XXIII. Qualitative research in health care. A. Are the results of the study valid? Evidence-Based Medicine Working Group. *J Am Med Assoc* 2000;284:357–62.
35. Giacomini MK, Cook DJ. Users' guides to the medical literature. XXIII. Qualitative research in health care. B. What are the results and how do they help me care for my patients? Evidence-Based Medicine Working Group. *J Am Med Assoc* 2000;284: 478–82.
36. Drummond MF, Richardson WS, O'Brien BJ, Levine M, Heyland D. Users' guides to the medical literature. XIII. How to use an article on economic analysis of clinical practice. A. Are the results of the study valid? Evidence-Based Medicine Working Group. *J Am Med Assoc* 1997;277:1552–7.
37. O'Brien BJ, Heyland D, Richardson WS, Levine M, Drummond MF. Users' guides to the medical literature. XIII. How to use an article on economic analysis of clinical practice. B. What are the results and how do they help me in caring for my patients? Evidence-Based Medicine Working Group. *J Am Med Assoc* 1997;277:1802–1806.
38. Brody BA. *Life and Death Decision Making*. New York: Oxford University Press, 1988.
39. Brody BA. *Taking Issue: Pluralism and Casuistry in Bioethics*. Washington, DC: Georgetown University Press, 2003.
40. DeGrazia D, Beauchamp TL. Philosophy. In Sugarman J, Sulmasy DP, eds. *Methods in Medical Ethics*. Washington, DC: Georgetown University Press, 2001:31–46.
41. Chervenak FA, McCullough LB. What is obstetric ethics? *J Perinat Med* 1995;23:331–41.
42. Owen R. Reader bias. *J Am Med Assoc* 1982;247:2533–4.

13 Ethical committees

J. G. Schenker

In the last two decades, ethical issues in medicine have come to the forefront of public consciousness, with concern focusing on several important areas. Advances in scientific and technological knowledge have created ethical dilemmas about what is right and wrong, about life and death issues, as well as issues of equality, justice, and personal preferences. Biomedical ethics also raised issues on patients' rights, which required steps to be taken to protect the patient's welfare and to promote the patients' autonomy.

Society's concern for ethical issues in medical practice has led to a growing need for the medical profession to become fully aware of the public view not only on individual patient–physician relationships, but also on how medical developments affect social structure and health policies. Health policy makers as well must examine the ethical basis of decision making, prioritization, and conflicts of interest as they influence health care locally, nationally, and internationally.

Biomedical ethical issues, guidelines, principles and regulations cut across national boundaries and often have universal implications. Although cultures differ, certain values are common to all. In this context, the most important is respect for human dignity, and this should not be negotiable. The establishment of international and interdisciplinary forums in which scientists and lay people can exchange views on topics of immediate concern, unhampered by administrative, political, or other considerations was needed. They are intended especially for the discussion of the scientific and technical bases of advances in biology and medicine and other related areas and their social, economic, ethical, administrative, and legal implications.

The range of ethical questions raised by new scientific achievements in the life science and methods of taking care of women's health, especially assisted reproduction, have been debated by international political and professional bodies. Within international committees, diverse geographic, ethnic, cultural, linguistic, and religious backgrounds are represented.

The Nuremberg Code

The first international code of ethics for research involving human subjects – the Nuremberg Code – was a response to the atrocities committed by Nazi research physicians that were revealed at the Nuremberg War Crimes Trials. Many of their experiments had entailed the deliberate killing of, or infliction of grievous injuries on, prisoners whose rights to consent or refuse were ignored. Thus, it was to prevent repetition by physicians of such attacks on the rights and welfare of human beings that human-research ethics came into being. The Nuremberg Code, issued in 1947,[1] laid down the standards for carrying out human experimentation, emphasizing the subject's voluntary consent:

(1) The voluntary consent of the human subject is essential. This means that the person involved should have legal capacity to give consent; should be so situated as to be able to exercise free power of choice without the intervention of any element of force, fraud, deceit, duress, overreaching, or other ulterior form of constraint or coercion; and should have sufficient knowledge and comprehension of the elements of the subject matter involved so as to enable him to make an understanding and enlightened decision. This latter element requires that before the acceptance of an affirmative decision by the experimental subject there should be made known to him the nature, duration, and purpose of the experiment; the method and means by which it is to be conducted; all inconveniences and hazards reasonably to be expected; and the effects upon his health or person that may possibly come from his participation in the experiment. The duty and responsibility for ascertaining the quality of the consent rests upon each individual who initiates, directs, or engages in the experiment. It is a personal duty and responsibility that may not be delegated to another with impunity.

(2) The experiment should be such as to yield fruitful results for the good of society, unprocurable by other methods or means of study, and not random and unnecessary in nature.

(3) The experiment should be so designed and based on the results of animal experimentation and knowledge of the natural history of the disease or other problem under study that the

anticipated results will justify the performance of the experiment.

(4) The experiment should be so conducted as to avoid all unnecessary physical and mental suffering and injury.

(5) No experiment should be conducted where there is an *a priori* reason to believe that death or disabling injury will occur, except, perhaps, in experiments where the experimental physicians also serve as subjects.

(6) The degree of risk to be taken should never exceed that determined by the humanitarian importance of the problem to be solved by the experiment.

(7) Proper preparations should be made and adequate facilities provided to protect the experimental subject against even remote possibilities of injury, disability, or death.

(8) The experiment should be conducted only by scientifically qualified persons. The highest degree of skill and care is required through all stages of the experiment of those who conduct or engage in the experiment.

(9) During the course of the experiment, the human subject should be at liberty to bring the experiment to an end if he has reached the physical or mental state where continuation of the experiment seems to him to be impossible.

(10) During the course of the experiment, the scientist in charge must be prepared to terminate the experiment at any stage if he has probable cause to believe, in the exercise of the good faith, superior skill, and careful judgment required of him, that a continuation of the experiment is likely to result in injury or death to the experimental subject. All research involving human subjects should be conducted in accordance with three basic ethical principles, namely, respect for persons, beneficence, and justice.

The Nuremberg Code document was criticized because it does not distinguish between different types of biomedical experimentation. The Nuremberg Code makes the subject's legal capacity to consent a prerequisite to experimentation, thus excluding from participating in research many people who might benefit from the results obtained, including children, the mentally ill, and others who are unable to give legal consent.

UNESCO – The United Nations Educational, Scientific and Cultural Organization

The United Nations Educational, Scientific and Cultural Organization (UNESCO) was established on November 16, 1945.[2] The main objective of UNESCO is to contribute to peace and security in the world by promoting collaboration among nations through education, science, culture, and communication to further universal respect for justice, for the rule of law, and for the human rights and fundamental freedoms that are affirmed for the peoples of the world without distinction of race, sex, language, or religion. At the international level, UNESCO has been one of the principal promoters of the reflection on ethics of living. In 1993, UNESCO created the International Bioethics Committee (IBC). The IBC[3] is a forum for debate and reflection and for the elaboration of UNESCO's normative actions, particularly with regard to the implementation of the Universal Declaration on the Human Genome and Human Rights. It is up to the IBC to keep up with progress in genetics while taking care to ensure respect for the values of human dignity and freedom in view of the potential risks of irresponsible attitudes in biomedical research. The IBC has drafted statutes and published reports on the ethical aspects of human embryonic stem cell research and its use in therapeutic research; ethical issues on genetic screening and the testing, treatment, storage, and use of genetic data on genetic screening; and human gene therapy.

WHO – World Health Organization

The Health Organization of the League of Nations was set up in Geneva in 1919. In 1945, the United Nations Conference on International Organization established a new, autonomous, international health organization – the World Health Organization (WHO). The objective of the WHO is the attainment by all peoples of the highest possible level of health.[4]

The WHO's constitution affirms fundamental ethical principles, such as the equality of rights and the unalienable dignity of all human beings. The WHO has set technical standards and proposed guidelines and codes of good practice in virtually all its fields of activity, including the widely publicized areas of organ transplantation, breast-milk substitutes, essential drugs, the marketing of pharmaceuticals, and, more recently, reproductive health, environmental health, and emerging diseases. The WHO also contributes to harmonizing legislation and terminology and fosters the dissemination and exchange of information on these subjects. Ethics continues to provide the basis for the WHO's activities and functions. Several WHO programs have their own ethical review committees; additional activities are carried by consultation on ethics and health at the global level.

The Declaration of Helsinki

The Declaration of Helsinki, promulgated in 1964 by the World Medical Association, is the fundamental document in the field of ethics in biomedical research and has had considerable influence on the formulation of international, regional, and national legislation and codes of conduct. The Declaration, revised in Tokyo in 1975, in Venice in 1983, and again in Hong Kong in 1989,[5] is a comprehensive international statement of the ethics of research involving human subjects. It is the mission of the physician to safeguard the health of the people. The physician's knowledge and conscience are dedicated to the fulfillment of this mission. Medical progress is based on research that ultimately must rest in part on experimentation involving human subjects. In current medical practice, most diagnostic, therapeutic, or prophylactic procedures involve hazards.

The purpose of biomedical research involving human subjects must be to improve diagnostic, therapeutic, and prophylactic procedures and the understanding of the etiology and pathogenesis of disease. In the field of biomedical research, a fundamental distinction must be recognized between medical research in which the aim is essentially diagnostic or therapeutic for a patient and medical research the essential object of which is purely scientific and without implying direct diagnostic or therapeutic value to the person subjected to the research.

In 1992, International Ethical Guidelines for Biomedical Research Involving Human Subjects were introduced by The Council for International Organizations of Medical Sciences and WHO based on ethical principles.[6] All research involving human subjects should be conducted in accordance with three basic ethical principles: respect for persons, beneficence, and justice. Respect for persons incorporates at least two fundamental ethical considerations: (1) respect for autonomy, which requires that those who are capable of deliberation about their personal choices should be treated with respect for their capacity for self-determination and (2) protection of persons with impaired or diminished autonomy, which requires that those who are dependent or vulnerable be afforded security against harm or abuse.

For all biomedical and clinical research involving human subjects, the investigator must obtain the informed consent of the prospective subject. Informed consent is based on the principle that competent individuals are entitled to choose freely whether to participate in research. Informed consent protects the individual's freedom of choice and respects the individual's autonomy. In the case of an individual who is not capable of giving informed consent (e.g. a fetus, a newborn, or a small child), the proxy consent of a properly authorized representative should be obtained. In all human research, ethical guidelines have differentiated between beneficial (therapeutic) and non-beneficial (non-therapeutic) research. The therapeutic research subject stands to gain as much from the research, whether it be a procedure or a drug, as to lose from it. In the non-therapeutic research, the subject cannot possibly benefit himself, and any benefits can therefore only add to others. The risks of a non-beneficial research fall solely on the research subject, whereas the benefits may extend beyond the research subject to the population as a whole.

The spirit of the Declaration of Helsinki is that, in medical research, the interests of science and society should never take precedence over considerations related to the well-being of the subject. Only a minimal level of risk may be allowed for volunteers to subject themselves for the benefit of others. However, it remains a problem to decide what sorts of levels of risk are acceptable in the case of pregnant women and where the subjects of non-therapeutic research are not autonomous (e.g. premature and newborn babies).

It is generally accepted that pregnant and nursing women are not suitable subjects of clinical trials other than those that are designed to respond to the health needs of such women or their fetuses or nursing infants. Clinical trials for conditions associated with or aggravated by pregnancy and to test the safety and efficacy of drugs, methods, and devices for detecting fetal abnormalities and well-being are of primary importance in the medical field of perinatology. The justification for the participation of pregnant women in clinical trials is that they should not be deprived arbitrarily of the opportunity to benefit from investigational drugs, vaccines, or other agents that promise therapeutic or preventive benefit. In all cases, risks to pregnant women, fetuses, and newborns should be minimized, as far as sound research design permits. As a general rule, pregnant or nursing women should not be the subjects of clinical trials except when such trials are designed to protect or advance the health of pregnant or nursing women or fetuses or nursing infants and for which women who are not pregnant or nursing would not be suitable subjects.

Some therapeutic research on fetuses *in utero* must be allowed. It contributes to the discovery of new methods for treating fetal health problems. There is a consensus that research on fetuses *in utero* should be treated as human subjects research, and governed by the policies for human subjects research. Because fetuses *in utero* and pregnant women are linked to each other, research on one may affect the other. Such research may have a differential impact on the pregnant woman and the fetus, with one benefiting while the other does not, and may be harmful to the other. At the extreme, the research that is beneficial to the one may actually be harmful to the other. The fundamental presupposition of all ethical policies is that the independent review process for human subjects research must consider the interests and rights of both parties in reviewing research protocols. Most guidelines have also imposed additional requirements on the acceptable level of risk to the fetuses involved in the research protocol. It is assumed that fetuses have some moral standing so that some concern must be devoted to their interests and rights.

Sir John Peel's report, published in 1972,[7] presented governmental guidelines concerning the ethics of fetal research. The recommendations were as follows:

- Viable fetuses should not be subjected to non-beneficial research.
- Research is permitted on the whole alive previable fetus, dead fetus, or its organs.
- Dead fetuses or tissues may be used in accordance with the provisions of the Human Tissue Act, which governs the postmortem use of human tissue.
- Parental informed consent should be obtained.
- The validity of the research should be assured.

The National Commission for the Protection of Human Subjects in Biomedical and Behavioral Research was established in July 1974[8] and issued its recommendations. The guidelines have certain things in common with the British guidelines but differ on some grounds. The common points are that dead fetuses and their tissues are to be afforded the respect of other dead human bodies and tissues. Fetuses with a chance of survival are to be treated like children. Willful damage to the fetus *in utero* may not be caused, presumably lest a mother change her mind about abortion. Significant differences are that in the United States, regulations fathers can veto the research, whereas in the British guidelines there is no such specific provision. In Britain it is proposed that non-beneficial research is to be done on the fetus *in utero* or on the viable fetus, whereas in the United States it may be done if there is minimal risk.

Council of Europe

In 1985, the Council of Europe created a multidisciplinary body with experts appointed by each member country. This committee has already produced documents on reproduction research on human subjects, prenatal diagnosis and screening, and genetic testing. Once the Committee of Ministers approves these documents, they become recommendations for the national parliaments, which may or may not decide to follow them. The European assembly and other committees have also issued reports related to bioethical problems. The Council of Europe, which represents all the democratic countries of Europe, has organized a European Convention on Bioethics. The Committee published protocols regarding human experiments and organ transplantation.[9]

FIGO Committee for the Study of Ethical Aspects of Human Reproduction

In 1985, the FIGO Committee for the Study of Ethical Aspects of Human Reproduction was established.[10] Its main objectives were the recording and study of general ethical problems emanating from the research and practice of human reproductive medicine, with the aim of providing guidelines for the attention of physicians and the public in developed and developing countries.

From its inception this committee was not intended to solve these ethical dilemmas, but rather to raise discussion by suggesting the perspectives that this group of health professionals, lawyers, and ethicists arrived at after carefully crafted analysis and debate over these issues. Given the rich field of ethical issues in women's health that derive from not only the reproductive life cycle, but also the economic and political status of women internationally – this committee will always confront new issues and even new aspects of old issues that challenge ethical perspectives and practice. There are continual variations on themes the committee has raised in the past through new medical developments. The social status of women, the constraints on health care dollars, and the health status of women have also increased the need for the committee to address the broader set of rights and economic issues that directly influence the health of women and the ethical setting of their care.

The committee was composed of a range of international members who represented developing and developed countries and had a significant interest and expertise in medical ethics. The members of the FIGO Committee are obstetricians, gynecologists, oncologists, lawyers, and public health workers, all of whom represent diverse geographic, ethnic, cultural, linguistic, and religious backgrounds. Among the 14 members, 13 were chairs of leading obstetric and gynecologic departments.

The initial task of the FIGO Committee for the Study of Ethical Aspects of Human Reproduction was to identify and study the important ethical problems confronting health care practitioners in human reproduction. The ethical problems identified were to be brought to the attention of physicians and the public in the developed and developing countries to provide ethical guidelines where appropriate. This task has assumed greater importance with the continuing challenge of ensuring that women are granted human and reproductive rights worldwide. Furthermore, the complexity of incorporating the many ethical aspects of reproductive issues in different societies, for issues such as cloning, or patenting of the human genome, argues for the need for such a consensus body.

There is no other body internationally that confronts these issues with a view toward the impact on the health care of women. Because of this, the opinions of the committee are used by women's health practitioners internationally to assist them in setting national or local standards, to expand the depth of discussion of these issues locally, and to support their advocacy for improvements in the health and status of women internationally. In the face of rapid cultural and scientific change, this is a critical role of ever-greater need. Women are clearly vulnerable in countries where their health care rights are either non-existent or threatened, and thus, these guidelines can be a powerful force to support the rights of women.

The work of the Committee: In its first Congress as a standing committee, the Ethics Committee presented three seminars: on medical ethics and medically assisted reproduction, on AIDS with emphasis on ethical aspects, and on refusal of obstetrical care (maternal health, fetal health, and neonatal health), which were published in the proceedings of the Rio Congress.

The early focus of the Committee, from 1985 to 1991, was clearly in areas central to obstetrics and gynecology practice, with a focus on such areas as sterilization, research on pre-embryo, and elective reduction of multiple pregnancies. In the same time period, however, the committee began to explore what the ethical responsibilities of societies of gynecology and obstetrics were for the broader issues of provision of reproductive health care and women's health in general. This led to a seminar during the FIGO Singapore Congress focusing on issues such as:

- How much are mothers worth?
- Distribution of resources between primary and tertiary reproductive care.
- Availability of resources for newborn care.
- Macroethical issues in obstetrics and gynecology.

This key seminar was chaired by Profs. Sureau and Schenker, and marked an important expansion of the thinking of the Committee beyond that of the common bioethical analysis of the time, which focused on principles such as benefit (beneficence), harm (maleficence), and patient autonomy in the area of human rights and justice. During this time, the Committee also began to align its meetings with regional meetings that paralleled the focus of the committee on ethical aspects of human reproduction. The first of these took place in Cairo in 1991 and focused on bioethics in human reproduction research in the Muslim World. The committee meeting foreshadowed an area of ongoing controversy in medicine – that of transplantation. At that time the group considered whether research on pre-embryos was required in order to broaden our knowledge of the developmental process, to improve the treatment of infertility and the control of reproduction, and to permit genetic screening with its potential for the prevention and treatment of birth defects. The Committee recognized and tried to incorporate the diverse spectrum of ethical, cultural, and religious values regarding the status of the pre-embryo. However, agreement was reached on some key areas even with these divergent views:

(1) First, research on pre-embryos is only ethically acceptable when its purpose is for the benefit of human health and only if animal models would not suffice.
(2) The Committee felt that no developing human pre-embryo might be kept alive beyond 14 days after fertilization (not including any time during which the embryo had been frozen).
(3) Research projects on pre-embryos should be authorized by ethical and/or other appropriate bodies in the country and, if allowed, appropriate informed consent must be obtained before undertaking research on pre-embryos, normally from both gamete donors. Furthermore, provision of gametes and pre-embryos should not be subject of commercial profit.
(4) The Committee was unable to reach a consensus as to whether research should be limited to surplus pre-embryos or should also include pre-embryos specifically generated for research, a debate that continues worldwide. The discussion over this issue established the precedent that committee statements required consensus, and where that was not possible, debates were either not included or included with the caveat that there was no consensus.

The deliberations are made public through committee statements published in scientific journals and in specific reports. The FIGO Committee has discussed and provided guidelines on general issues in women's health and advocacy, issues on genetics, embryo research, contraception, abortion, and reproductive endocrinology issues regarding pregnancy, maternal–fetal health, and neonates. The first bound publication of the collated Issues and Guidelines appeared in 1994, 1997, and 2000, and by 2003 had grown to a body of work that, with the translations into Spanish and French, covers 232 pages.[11]

The method of analysis adopted by the committee evolved early on and consisted of position papers on a topic identified by the committee that were circulated prior to committee meetings in the working language of the committee, English.

These research papers explicated the problem, the present status of knowledge, and the various ethical stances or issues that were identified in the literature. At times, the committee invited outside experts in areas where there was not felt to be adequate depth of expertise or where there were other FIGO committees working on the medical or rights aspects of the same issue. The papers were presented at the meeting and a consensus about the important background and ethical issues was identified.

Depending on the issues, further work on synthesizing these into a set of reflections or guidelines might take place at the meeting or over several meetings, until every word of each document was reviewed, read, and revised by all the members of the committee. Proposed statements were read line by line and edited by the entire committee to assure that not only the content was acceptable to the committee, but that the translations to French and Spanish would not contain errors because of the likely translation from English.

The committee statements and opinion are independent from FIGO member societies or the executive board. The documents represent the result of that carefully researched and considered discussion. This independence has been particularly helpful to FIGO in providing ethical guidance regarding the relationship of the federation to industry, initially formulated as internal 'Guidelines for Relations between Industry and FIGO' in 1991. The committee collaborates with international organizations – such as the WHO – on various aspects of women's health to ensure that the ethical aspects are fully covered.

The committee members represent a wide spectrum of religions and countries, and numerous members have co-coordinated with multiple international committees to encourage and ensure inclusion of these ethical aspects in regular and extraordinary meetings.

WAPM – World Association of Perinatal Medicine

In 1999, the World Association of Perinatal Medicine established an Ethical Committee. The main objectives of the committee are:[12]

- To study the ethical problems that emanate from practice and research in perinatal medicine.
- To provide guidelines for the practice of obstetrics and neonatology.
- To bring the ethical issues to the attention of physicians, nurses, paramedical staff, and the public.

National Ethics Committees

National ethics committees are set up by governments to advise on regulations or proposed legislation concerning moral bioethical programs that raise controversy among professionals and the public. National committees were originally created due to an increasing demand among doctors and researchers for some authoritative guidance as to what was permissible in issues where no law exists. The nature of the membership of such committees is of even greater importance. The chairman must be unrelated to the medical or research profession. The members of national ethics committees must represent a broad range of values and professional expertise in the fields of medicine, law, administration, media, economics, public policy, and moral philosophy. Within committees dealing with reproductive health, for example, at least 50% of the members must be women. Governmental or non-governmental bodies have issued reports on ethical and legal aspects, especially in the fields of perinatal care, assisted reproduction technologies, and human experimentation. Scientific progress is ahead of what society is willing to accept, and the reports of the bioethical committees protect the public by monitoring and, when necessary, regulating scientific practice. There is no single solution to a moral problem. A committee must incorporate a number of different moral ideals and reach a workable compromise. The law that these committees create must be in step with moral beliefs, or it will not be implemented. It is the task of the ethics committee to try to produce some consensus, based on all considerations, and to recommend it for practice. Several problems arise in the setup of the committees. Who should make moral decisions in controversial public issues? How is the committee's membership to be determined? In a pluralistic, mainly secular society there are no moral experts *per se*. Committees who serve public morality must conform to certain specifications of expertise. The committee members must be capable of understanding the scientific background of the subject matter of the issue. They must be acquainted with moral philosophy and understand the nature of ethics. The members must be intelligent and creative and not dogmatic. It is imperative that people who hold particular moral or religious views that make them impervious to the language of consensus are not included in the committee's team. They may be incapable of sympathy and flexibility and thus not be of use. The members must also be readily available to perform this extremely time-consuming task. One major disadvantage of these committees is that sometimes the advent of new technologies is ahead of committee deliberations. If a previous committee decision was opposed to specific new advances, their use may be delayed until the committee changes its original decision. In most Western countries, committees are set up ad hoc to address specific subjects of public bioethical concern. The Warnock Committee on Human Fertilization and Embryology (1984) had a great influence on subsequent legislation in the United Kingdom.[13] In the United States, legislation that seems to reinforce ethical conduct may actually replace the exercise of ethical judgment with unreflective obedience to law. The Belmont Report (1979) identified the basic ethical principles that should emphasize the conduct of biomedical and behavioral research involving human subjects and developed guidelines that should be followed to ensure that such research is conducted in accordance with those principles.[14] The guidelines provided by national committees are usually converted into laws by legislation that introduces criminal punishment for violation. The experience of Assisted Reproductive Technology (ART) practice demonstrated that countries with voluntary guidelines seem to enjoy public confidence, and public pressure for a change seems minimal. Countries with legislative surveillance seem to agree that it works well, although there are understandable complaints about the slowness of the legislative process and the difficulty of having regulations changed once they are in place, and thus, not be of use.

Summary

The range of ethical questions raised by new scientific achievements in the life science, and methods of taking care of women's health especially, has been debated by international political and professional bodies. Biomedical ethical issues, guidelines, principles, and regulations cut across national boundaries and often have universal implications. Although cultures differ, certain values are common to all. In this context, the most important value is respect for human dignity, and this should not be negotiable. The establishment of international and interdisciplinary forums in which scientists and lay people can exchange views on topics of immediate concern, unhampered by administrative, political, or other considerations, was needed. They are intended especially for the discussion of the scientific and technical bases of advances in biology and medicine and other related areas and their social, economic, ethical, administrative, and legal implications. Commissions appointed by institutions, governments, and international bodies serve to relieve the medical profession from making ethical decisions and to protect human subjects from any harm. The deliberations of these committees are usually followed by guidelines of operation, which in many cases have become abiding law. For these committees to be of full advantage, they must convene promptly as issues arise so as not to delay medical advances from being implemented.

REFERENCES

1. The Nuremberg Code. In Anna GJ, Grodin MA, eds. *The Nazi Doctors and the Nuremberg Code: Human Rights in Human Experimentation*. New York: Oxford University Press, 1992.
2. *Constitution*. London: UNESCO, 1945.
3. International Bioethics Committee. *Statutes of the International Bioethics Committee*. London: UNESCO, 1998.
4. WHO. From small beginnings. *World Health Forum* 1988; 9:29–34.
5. World Medical Association. Declaration of Helsinki. In Anna GJ, Grodin MA, eds. *The Nazi Doctors and the Nuremberg Code: Human Rights in Human Experimentation*. New York: Oxford University Press, 1992:311–343.
6. International ethical guidelines for biomedical research involving human subjects. In: Bankowski Z, Levine RJ, eds. *Proceedings of the 26th CIOMS Conference*, Geneva, Switzerland, February 5–7, 1992. Geneva: CIOMS, 1993:1–36.
7. Department of Health and Social Security, Scottish Home and Health Department, Welsh Office. *The Use of Fetuses and Fetal Material for Research: Report of the Advisory Group*. London: Her Majesty's Stationery Office, 1972.
8. US Department of Health, Education, and Welfare, Office of the Secretary. Protection of human subjects: proposed amendments concerning fetuses, pregnant women, and in vitro fertilization. *Fed Reg* 1977;42(9)2792–3.
9. The Council of Europe. Principles concerning medical research on human beings. *WHO Int Digest Health Legislation* 1990; 41:3–6.
10. Schenker JG, ed. *Recommendations on Ethical Issues in Obstetrics and Gynecology by the FIGO Committee for the Study of Ethical Aspects of Human Reproduction*. London: FIGO 1994:7–8,11.
11. *Recommendations on Ethical Issues in Obstetrics and Gynecology by the FIGO Committee for the Study of Ethical Aspects of Human Reproduction*. London: FIGO, 1994, 1997, 2000, 2003.
12. Schenker JG. Report from the Ethical Committee of the World Association of Perinatal Medicine. *J Perinat Med* 2000;28:3–6.
13. Warnock DM. *Report of the Committee of Inquiry into Human Fertilization and Embryology*. London: HMSO, 1984.
14. National Commission for the Protection of Human Subjects of Biomedical and Behavioral Research. *The Belmont Report: Ethical Principles and Guidelines for the Protection of Human Subjects of Research*. United States: Office for Protection from Research Risks, 1979:1–8.

14 Education in perinatal ethics

G. M. Stirrat

Introduction

Amazing advances, in genetics, reproductive technologies, and perinatal medicine occurred in the latter part of the 20th century. As Radcliffe-Richards[1] has said, 'Science keeps on throwing up new situations which, in some ways resemble familiar ones but in others are utterly unlike them; and we try to solve the resulting problems by stretching our old familiar categories to fit, but with ever increasing strains and cracks appearing everywhere'. Those of us who practice perinatal medicine are required to consider a wide range of ethical questions, sometimes on a daily basis. Some of them relate to our specialty while others are generic (e.g. consent, confidentiality and resource allocation). The problems can be complex and true dilemmas where the choices are between equally undesirable alternatives. Over 30 years ago, Campbell[2] wrote, 'moral dilemmas will continue to occur in medicine as long as choices have to be made which involve putting one set of values against another'. Unfortunately, ready-made answers cannot be found in textbooks (not even this one!), because the situations in which the problems arise and the stories of the people involved are all different from any other. The desired goals may also be different. For example, the prevention of disease and health promotion tends to raise different issues and require different solutions than the relief of symptoms, pain and suffering, or the cure of disease.

The 21st century will bring further advances in what can be done, but the prevailing ethical climate suggests that there will continue to be much less critical consideration of what 'ought' to be done. How then can we as individuals and as a community of physicians reduce the risk of Radcliffe-Richards's 'strains and cracks' causing the edifice of our professional practice to crumble around us? If you ask an architect, builder or constructional engineer that question, their answer will be 'Get the foundations right!'.[3] Would it not, therefore, seem prudent that those training to be perinatal physicians be properly grounded in the theories and principles behind the increasingly complex ethical decisions in which they will inevitably be closely involved in their subsequent career?

This chapter is based on several fundamental premises:

(1) Each one of us is required to think ethically and act morally (i.e., we are all 'moral agents'). This is not an optional extra.

(2) Ethics is about individuals living and working in community.[4] It is not just about 'me' and 'mine'. As Campbell[5] states, 'there can be no possibility of freedom for any one individual if that person acts without reference to all other moral agents'.

(3) Medical ethics is not solely a matter of moral theory, it is 'an ethics of relation and practice'.[4] Thus, ethics is *for* something and must be translatable into moral action. It has to work in real life.

(4) The dominant individualistic version of autonomous choice is fundamentally (and, in the long run, potentially fatally) flawed.[6,7] Stirrat and Gill,[7] among others, have suggested a principled version of patient autonomy that involves the provision of sufficient and understandable information and space for a patient, who has the capacity to make a settled choice about medical interventions on himself/herself and to do so responsibly in a manner considerate to others. A lifetime in clinical practice strongly suggests that this model best fits the optimal patient–doctor relationship in which there is a mutual, unspoken agreement between the parties that recognizes the duties and obligations each to the other with bilateral trust at the heart of this relationship. This is discussed further below.

(5) The discipline of medical ethics is *not* qualitatively different from ethics in general. The fundamental ethical principles underpinning medical practice should be shared by society in general. However, by virtue of being a profession, we clearly have special obligations to the patients we serve. In the United Kingdom the 'Duties of a Doctor' are clearly laid down by the General Medical Council (GMC)[8], whose primary roles are 'To protect the public by setting standards for professional practice, overseeing medical education, keeping a register of qualified doctors and

Table 14.1 Duties of a doctor (UK GMC)[8]

'Patients must be able to trust doctors with their lives and well-being. To justify that trust, we as a profession have a duty to maintain a good standard of practice and care and to show respect for human life'

As a doctor you must

- Make the care of your patient your first concern
- Treat every patient politely and considerately
- Respect patients' dignity and privacy
- Listen to patients and respect their views
- Give patients information in a way they can understand
- Respect the rights of patients to be fully informed in decisions about their care
- Keep your professional knowledge up-to-date
- Recognize the limits of your professional competence
- Be honest and trustworthy
- Respect and protect confidential information
- Make sure that your personal beliefs do not prejudice your patients' care.
- Act quickly to protect patients from risk if you have good reason to believe that you or a colleague may not be fit to practice
- Avoid abusing your position as a doctor
- Work with colleagues in the ways that best serve patients' interests

In all these matters you must never discriminate unfairly against your patients or colleagues. And you must always be prepared to justify your actions to them

Table 14.2 American Medical Association 'Principles of Medical Ethics'[9]

Preamble

The medical profession has long subscribed to a body of ethical statements developed primarily for the benefit of the patient. As a member of this profession, a physician must recognize responsibility not only to patients, but also to society, to other health professionals, and to self. The following Principles adopted by the American Medical Association are not laws, but standards of conduct which define the essentials of honorable behavior for the physician.

I. A physician shall be dedicated to providing competent medical service with compassion and respect for human dignity.

II. A physician shall deal honestly with patients and colleagues, and strive to expose those physicians deficient in character or competence, or who engage in fraud or deception.

III. A physician shall respect the law and also recognize a responsibility to seek changes in those requirements which are contrary to the best interests of the patient.

IV. A physician shall respect the rights of patients, of colleagues, and of other health professionals, and shall safeguard patient confidences within the constraints of the law.

V. A physician shall continue to study, apply and advance scientific knowledge, make relevant information available to patients, colleagues, and the public, obtain consultation, and use the talents of other health professionals when indicated.

VI. A physician shall, in the provision of appropriate patient care, except in emergencies, be free to choose whom to serve, with whom to associate, and the environment in which to provide medical services.

VII. A physician shall recognize a responsibility to participate in activities contributing to an improved community.

taking action when a doctor's fitness to practice is in doubt'. Table 14.1 outlines the duties of a doctor as set down by the GMC.[8] The Code of Medical Ethics of the American Medical Association (AMA)[9] states, 'a physician must recognize responsibility not only to patients, but also to society, to other health professionals, and to self'. The two main items on the agenda of the first meeting of the Association in 1847 were the establishment of a code of ethics and the creation of minimum requirements for medical education and training. Table 14.2 shows the principles adopted by the AMA as 'standards of conduct which define the essentials of honorable behavior for the physician'.

(6) Ethics is a necessary part of good clinical practice. Ethical judgments must take full account of all the circumstances of the case and be based on sound principles. Decisions must be consistent, free from contradiction and clinically relevant. Exercise by physicians of their clinical judgment is frequently attacked as paternalism. While, in some instances, this can be so, it may also be the doctor fulfilling his or her duty to the

patient by exercising his or her own autonomy, and as such, may be entirely justified. Indeed, there will be some occasions, particularly in perinatal medicine, when acquiescence to a requested intervention against one's clinical or ethical judgment will be abrogation of one's duty as a doctor!

(7) The patient–physician covenant relationship depends totally on the trust of the former that the latter will act at all times with the highest ethical standards. Indeed, not only is trust 'the fundamental virtue at the heart of being a good doctor', it also allows us all to function socially as individuals in a complex society,[10] and 'every genuine moral community is built on the trust that its members will look beyond personal interests and individual concerns towards a truly common good'.[11] The words 'trust' or 'trustworthy' can be found on several occasions in the GMC's 'Duties of a Doctor' (Table 14.1) and it is implicit in the AMA's 'Code of Ethics' (Table 14.2). (Among other authors, Draper and Sorell[12] argue that the patient has reciprocal duties, but it is not appropriate to discuss this further here.)

The Basis for Ethics

Since at least the time of Socrates (470–399 B.C.), people have asked questions like 'How do we know what is good?' 'How should I live?' 'How can we know which decision is right?' and 'What is justice?'. Ethics or moral philosophy addresses these fundamental questions in order to establish a basis for moral judgments. Morals are the specific judgments, codes or beliefs of particular groups or societies and the actions that follow from these.

The relationship between ethics and morals has been compared to that between DNA and cell proteins.[13] Within the DNA (ethics) lies the fundamental information for the cell to function. The proteins (morals) produced by the cell interpreting and following that information do two things – they express both the nature and character of the cell and also perform its specific function. In addition, cells must work together within and among bodily structures and organs. The cell that expresses its individuality at the expense of its neighbors is 'neoplastic' and may become malignant, ultimately causing the demise of the body. What this might suggest about the long-term consequences of the dominance of the primacy of the individual – 'I', 'me' and 'mine' – in today's society is among the factors that leads to my concern about the potentially fatal flaw in this view of autonomy.

Diversity of moral theory

In 1972, Campbell[2] wrote, 'The essence of morality is that there is uncertainty'. As a young obstetrician wrestling with a whole series of ethical dilemmas at that time, I found this very threatening. I was like Montaigne who said, 'Tell me of your certainties; I have doubts enough of my own'. Indeed, I venture to suggest that we all find uncertainty difficult to deal with. We would much prefer 'meanings that are completely clear' and 'truths that are completely certain'.[14] Campbell[2] stated:

> Many people seek to handle situations of uncertainty by elevating their personal convictions to the status of inherent and all-embracing rules, which must apply to every situation, whatever its complexities and ambiguities. Others try to reduce all moral dilemmas to questions of technical skill.

He considered that both of these reactions were commonly found among physicians and nurses, 'many of whom may feel that there is little to be argued about in medical ethics, either because they do not themselves see any moral ambiguities in their professional practice or because they consider all the decisions taken to be purely matters of clinical judgment'. Personal experience suggests that although such individuals still exist, the vast majority of health care professionals are anxious to learn how to make more reflective and consistent ethical judgments in the face of the problems that they face from day to day.

Of course, 'moral philosophy does not attempt to "solve" moral dilemmas'.[2] Rather, 'it attempts to provide a rational framework for understanding the complexities of moral judgment'.[2] It is entirely appropriate that we try to make sense out of uncertainty, and we do so by classification and codification of what we think we know. We need frameworks as reference points to allow us to progress through our lives as individuals in society, much as a ship traveling across the ocean. Indeed, Jonsen[15] suggests:

> ... moral principles are not unlike the sky-marks used in celestial navigation: a position is determined and a course marked by continual reference to fixed points – sun, stars, and planets. At the same time the navigator must look not only to the sky-marks but also to any visible landmarks and to the wind and waves. Thus while principles provide an indispensable general guiding direction, other features of the problem must be taken into consideration as the passage from moral question to moral answer is navigated.

It is, perhaps, not only inevitable, but also appropriate that a multiplicity of theoretical approaches to ethics should have arisen. Campbell has suggested, 'The diversity of ethical theories is about as wide as the diversity of ways of understanding the relationship between man and his environment'.[2]

The first of the two main theories is *deontology* or 'duties in action'. The best example is found in the writing of the philosopher Immanuel Kant in the 18th century. The essence of Kant's ethics is:

- Certain kinds of acts are intrinsically right and others intrinsically wrong determined by a set of rules.
- The rules must be universally applicable, coherent (i.e. not contradictory) within what Kant called 'a rational system of nature' and capable of being freely adopted by 'a community of rational beings'.
- Among the rules are 'do not kill, cause pain, disable, deprive of freedom or pleasure' and 'do not deceive, break promises, cheat, break laws, or neglect one's duty'.
- Each of us has a set of duties to our fellow men and women. One of the most important duties is to 'act so that you treat humanity, whether in your own person or in that of any other, always as an end, and never as a means only'. It is this maxim that has, for example, contributed to concerns about so-called 'savior sibling' procedures in which a child is conceived with the primary intention of being a source of compatible tissue for a seriously ill sibling.
- An action should not be judged to have been right or wrong by its consequences in individual situations.

No theory is without problems, and the main difficulties with this theory are defining the meaning of 'rational' and agreeing on universally applicable rules.

The second main theory, developed in the 19th century by Jeremy Bentham and John Stuart Mill, is *consequentialism*, in which the rightness or wrongness of an action is based solely on consequences.[16] They named their theory *utilitarianism*, and argued that the maximization of pleasure or happiness was what made acts right. This has been summarized as 'The greatest happiness of the greatest number'. Consequentialist theories can be further divided. *Act consequentialism* states that the right action is the one that produces the most good. In *rule consequentialism* the test is whether an action accords with a set of rules whose general acceptance would result in the most good. In each case, 'good' is determined solely by the beneficial consequences. The problem with consequentialism is that, although consequences are undoubtedly important in moral judgments and actions, happiness is highly subjective, and what is good (let alone the greatest good) is not always easy to determine. Moreover, benefiting the majority could result in ignoring vulnerable minorities. Where do the seriously disadvantaged in our society, such as the very preterm infant, the severely disabled child, the terminally ill or the elderly with dementia fit with this philosophy? A rule to protect the vulnerable could be set aside if it did not promote general happiness.

Clearly, these theories are not, of themselves, sufficient for the resolution of clinical problems in real life and several other views have been developed to try to deal with their inherent problems. The *Four Principle Approach*, otherwise known as 'principlism', shown in Table 14.3 (and see Beauchamp[17]), was formulated as a basis for working out practical solutions for problems in medical ethics.

Table 14.3 The Four Principles ('principlism')[17]

Principle	The obligation/duty
Beneficence	• To do what is in the patient's best interests • To provide benefits balanced against risks
Non-maleficence	• Not to cause harm and, indeed, seek to prevent it
Autonomy ('self-rule')	• To respect the right of the individual to make choices about her own life *in the context of equal respect for everyone else involved*
Justice	• To treat patients fairly and without unfair discrimination • Fairness in the distribution of benefits and risks

Critics say, with some justification, that these are merely a checklist without an underlying theory, are often in conflict with one another (with no internal resolution) and do not deal with emotional aspects or relationships. In particular, as has already been noted, the concept of autonomy is widely misunderstood. It does not necessarily mean doing what someone requests or demands at one point in time. It implies a settled view of the individual reached by deliberation as to what is in his or her own long-term best interests. It is also to be balanced with the autonomy of others, including, in this context, medical staff. Regrettably, the four principles are all too often used as a mantra to be applied by the lazy to every ethical issue without thought or discrimination. If, however, one recognizes their shortcomings and incorporates some other insights such as those discussed below, the four principles can provide a useful framework for analyzing ethical problems (see Table 14.4a).

Other useful perspectives can be found:

Narrative ethics:[18] This takes account of the patient's and the physician's context, emotions and relationships. Indeed, whatever one's approach, the patient's story must be part of the ethical relationship and one's own feelings are relevant to the moral choices. It is important that the latter be recognized, if only to ensure that one's feelings do not inappropriately influence the choice of the patient.

Virtue ethics: Instead of asking 'How should I act?' this asks 'How should I live?'.[19] This system tried to define excellence of character or behavior to which individuals or groups should aspire. One aspect is caring about someone, rather than just caring for him

Table 14.4 Making ethical judgments

(a) Analysis

Define the problem(s)

Analyze the problem(s)

- What are its elements? – e.g. medical, ethical, legal, etc.
- What parties are involved? – such as the patient, her family, one or more fetuses, statutory authorities (e.g. social workers, police), health care professionals, etc.
  - Who is the appropriate advocate for the fetus?
- How do their perspectives fit together or conflict with each other, and in the latter case, what are the appropriate mechanisms for resolution?
- What is its context? – e.g., social, ethnic, economic (within this may be issues about rationing)

Consider the underlying principles involved

- It may be useful to start with the four principles (beneficence, do no harm, autonomy and justice).[17]
  - What is in the patient's best interests?
  - How can I balance this with the avoidance of harm?
  - Is the patient competent? If so
    - Is she expressing her settled view on what she wants?
    - Am I respecting her right to make choices about her own life?
    - Does this conflict with the autonomy of others, and if so, how is this to be resolved?
  - If she is not competent (e.g. a minor or an unconscious adult), or if this is open to question (e.g. a child aged 12–13 years), how is this to be dealt with?
  - Are there any issues of justice? e.g.
    - Is the patient being unfairly discriminated against?
    - Is there any conflict between what I consider to be in the patient's best interest and what can be provided?
- What other perspectives could assist in resolution?
  - Have the patient's social context, emotions and relationships been adequately considered?
  - Am I sure that I am treating the patient as a person?
  - Are we both caring for and caring about the patient?

(b) Action

Move towards recommending actions that best meet the above criteria

- What are the proposed objectives? e.g. cure, relief of symptoms (e.g. pain and suffering) or prevention of disease?
  - Which objectives are essential and which desirable?
  - What alternatives are available (including doing nothing)?
  - What are the risks of acting (or failing to act) and what is their probability and severity?
  - Do the expected benefits outweigh the potential risks?
    - Has the patient been properly informed of the available options?
  - Is she competent to give consent?
    - If so, has the consent been obtained properly?
    - If yes, put chosen option into effect.
  - If she is not competent whom, if anyone, can legally give consent?

Dealing with potential or actual conflict

This difficult area cannot be dealt with comprehensively here, but examples include the following:

- The patient refuses to accept the recommended interventions.
  - If competent, she has the right to do so, even if it leads to harm of herself (or the unborn child). Do not coerce her. Among the things to do are:
    - If junior, inform more senior colleagues; if senior, seek advice through clinical governance channels.
    - Make sure that full contemporaneous notes are made.

(Continued)

Table 14.4 (Continued)

- She requests intervention that informed medical opinion suggests is not justified or in her best interests.
  - You are not bound to do as she asks, particularly if it is contrary to your principles.
  - Offer referral for another opinion or, if needs be, transfer care to another team. (In the United Kingdom, if the patient is requesting termination of pregnancy, you are obliged to refer to another practitioner.)
  - (Then as above.)
- Another party tries to intervene inappropriately, e.g.
  - The family or another third party asks for confidential information.
    - The presumption is that confidentiality must be kept.
    - Any breach can be justified only in exceptional circumstances.
      - It is preferable that this be with the knowledge of the patient.
      - However, if, for example, it is judged that the patient would be seriously harmed by knowing that her illness is terminal, but that it would be in her best interests that a close relative should know about it, information may be divulged without consent.
  - The family asks that the patient not be told the truth about her illness.
    - The assumption (possibly rebuttable with good grounds – see example above) must be to tell the truth at all times.
    - Not to do so can have regrettable consequences, e.g. who is she to trust when she discovers any deception?
    - *Remember that your primary duty of care is to your patient and not her family.*

Good communication skills in general, and knowing how to impart bad news in particular, are central to being a good doctor
Review the outcome

- Ethical issues do not lend themselves easily to audit, but it may be useful to record and review major cases from time to time.
- In individual cases, remember that a good or bad outcome does not necessarily mean that the intervention was right or wrong

or her, and it can provide a useful perspective in, for example, those faced with chronic and/or serious illness or disability.

Feminist approaches to ethics:[20] One form of feminist ethics attempts to balance the dominant masculine ethos of traditional ethics with a more feminine perspective. The ethics is one of caring for individuals and although caring resolutions may be different in their outcomes, they are linked by personal regard and respect given to individuals.

However, 'formal frameworks, for all their value, need to be supplemented with other ethical approaches, based more on interpretation and judgment than on formal deduction or algorithm'[18] and 'any particular theory, when applied deductively, is shown to be inadequate sooner or later'.[21]

Sherwin[22] suggests, 'No moral theory can do the work normally expected of it, because none provides reliable grounds for resolving all moral complexities through deductive application of its central principles' and 'Doing bioethics well requires appeal to the insights provided by multiple theories'. Ethical reflection depends on having a set of core ethical beliefs that describe clear cases of morally objectionable or praiseworthy behavior, which contribute the prototypes of ethical deliberation. Rather than trying to force us to choose a single, comprehensive theory to apply to all cases, she finds it preferable to view different theoretical perspectives as providing alternative 'frameworks' or 'templates' for different sorts of approaches to problems. She suggests that we use competing theories as a set of lenses through which we can get a clearer view of complex moral problems. Some lenses will provide a clearer understanding than others.

Dunstan's[4] criteria for the practice of ethics in medicine are good moral theories, the elucidation of principles to which implicit or explicit appeal can be made, the discipline of logic for the framing of good arguments and the exposure of bad ones, learning the 'art of moral reasoning', discipline in the use of words without clichés and 'wisdom above all'.

Making ethical judgments

There are two main ways in which ethical issues arise. The first is while dealing with patients and their clinical problems. The second is when faced with an issue in abstract (e.g. 'What do you think of cloning?'). Dealing with the former tends to inform one's approach to the latter and, incidentally, provides valuable insights not given to the non-clinician.

How then do we go about making ethical judgments in the clinical context? McCullough and Chervenak[21] advocate five individually necessary and jointly sufficient criteria for rigorous analysis:

- *Clarity*: terms and concepts must have precise meaning.
- *Consistency*: those terms must always be used with that precise meaning and reasoning must be free of contradiction.
- *Coherence*: ethical deliberations must be internally consistent and non-contradictory.
- *Applicability*: the results of ethical deliberations can be applied in the clinical and research settings.
- *Adequacy*: the judgments allow ethical conflicts to be identified, managed or, preferably, prevented.

It has to be emphasized that there is no magic formula and, indeed, Dan Callahan has suggested (personal communication, 2002) that 'ethical theory ultimately doesn't matter very much – 90 per cent is educated common sense'.

My own approach to making ethical judgments involves consideration of a series of questions under five task-oriented headings, as outlined in Table 14.4a and b, that move from ethical analysis to clinical action.

The purpose and process of education in ethics

If Callahan is correct that 90% of ethics is educated common sense, why should anyone need training in ethics? The key is in the qualifying adjective, 'educated'. I once bought a wooden plaque on Cape Cod that read, 'The one thing about common sense is that it is not so common!'. Josh Billings (the pen name of Henry Wheeler Shaw), the renowned 19th century humorist, said two wise things on the subject: 'Common sense is the knack of seeing things as they are, and doing things as they ought to be done' and 'Learning is the art of knowing how to use common sense to advantage'. Thomas Huxley's aphorism that 'Science is nothing but trained and organized common sense'[23] applies equally to ethics. He suggests that the former differs from common sense 'only as a veteran may differ from a raw recruit: and its methods differ from those of common sense only as far as the guardsman's cut and thrust differ from the manner in which a savage wields his club'. To change the metaphor, no one expects the child with an innate musical ability to sit down at the piano and immediately play Beethoven sonatas. The talent needs to be developed both by understanding the theory underpinning the music and also by practicing increasingly complex compositions. It must also be rewarding for the student! Thus it is with ethics.

I believe that far more is achieved if a teacher starts from where the students are and builds on their inherent abilities, rather than start from where the teacher is and expect the students to soak up facts and opinions that do not necessarily relate to their own experiences. In the United Kingdom the majority of students come to medical school from high school at about 18 years of age. Teaching of ethics in medicine in the University of Bristol begins shortly after the students commence their course and follows for several weeks, working with family practitioners meeting patients, learning about their problems and discerning the ethical issues involved. It subsequently runs as a vertical theme through all 5 years of the course. We never cease to be amazed at the maturity with which these talented young people address complex ethical issues often from their own experiences. This develops as the course progresses. They have the talent; it is our task to let it flourish.

Not long ago I had one of the most rewarding teaching experiences of my life at the other end of the age spectrum. I was asked to speak to an older women's group on a reproductive ethics topic. Instead of lecturing them on the subject (on which, if truth be told, I was not an expert), I had prepared four hypothetical cases of increasing ethical complexity. Members of the group presented each case, the facts of the matter were discussed and questions addressed. We then began to consider the ethics of each case. In a very short time, the key ethical issues had been raised and debated, and by the time the fourth case had been completed, we had discussed a range of issues that would not have disgraced a textbook of ethics. Of course we did not come up with many firm answers, but these women not only discovered that they could think (something their families had probably told them implicitly or explicitly that they could no longer do), but also that their opinions were meaningful. What is more, they were not only thinking ethics on that day, but had been doing so all their lives! They also learned that there were few absolute answers, but had derived the principles to address the dilemmas by their own efforts. It was gratifying to see their self-esteem rise as the session progressed, and they left rejoicing in the experience. Henry Brook Adams, the historian, wrote in 1907, 'a teacher affects eternity: he can never tell where his influence stops'. Our objective in education in ethics is no less!

Phases of Education in Ethics

The most effective way to achieve proper education in ethics is to begin early and build on it through school, college, medical school and continuing professional development:

(1) *Education in human relationships*: This should begin early in school and become a more formal study of ethics for all students in high school and college, where it should be part of the examined curriculum. The objective is for the student to learn how to think, not what to think.

(2) *Introduction to bioethics*: This should commence in medical school, concentrating on a patient-centered approach to medicine, and be part of the examined curriculum. This has been emphasized by the GMC

Table 14.5 Introduction to bioethics in medical school

Objective	Key issues
Increasing knowledge	• In ethics there are very few cut and dry solutions to problems. In part this is because the problems themselves are so varied • As a practical discipline, ethics involves fitting general principles to specific circumstances in a way that respects these variations, but this does not mean deciding arbitrarily or with prejudice • The course should cover the main principles of ethics in medicine (e.g. respect for autonomy, beneficence, justice) and ethical concepts to be used in making morally reasonable judgments (e.g. duty, rights, virtue, consequences) • The students should learn: o The relevant law and professional codes of conduct that determine specific obligations owed by doctors to patients, society and each other o How best to determine what is morally important and relevant in a given medical situation: without this moral understanding it is impossible to apply rules or concepts in a sensitive and constructive way o The centrality of the patient's narrative in determining what is important for her and her medical care
Developing skills	The course should aim to develop skills of analysis, judgment and rational argument about moral issues in medicine. The context should always be their relevance to the practice of medicine and good patient care
Improving attitudes	The student should be become aware of the wide variety of patients' attitudes to health, illness, doctors and society, the ways in which these impact on the medical relationship and the ways in which their own attitudes play a part in this relationship The ways in which ethical issues in medicine are not only about hard decisions for doctors, but about making decisions with patients in personal, social and institutional contexts should be explored This approach to patients' attitudes will inevitably involve the students confronting and rethinking their own, and this can be threatening for some Problematic attitudes should be identified, acknowledged by the student and, if possible, remedied

Based on the Ethics and Law in Medicine Vertical Theme Course in the University of Bristol Medical School, 2003–4

in 'Tomorrow's doctors – recommendations on undergraduate medical education'.[24] The focus should be not only on knowledge, but also on skills and attitudes, as shown in Table 14.5. Both clinical and research governance should be included. There is increasing emphasis on this course being interprofessional, involving students from a variety of health care professions. The confrontation of some issues will be traumatic for some students. Teachers must be sensitive to this. The earlier this is recognized and dealt with, the better. In addition, having been dean of a medical faculty, I realize that the problem of the failing student is more often a problem in attitude rather than ability. This too must be recognized early for remedial action to be instituted and, if necessary, the student encouraged to join an alternative course of study for which he or she is more suited. It is too late for this to be recognized for the first time after qualification, perhaps as a result of an event that resulted in harm to a patient.

(3) *A core generic course for health care professionals*: It is suggested that these practice-based modular courses be designed for doctors working in hospitals, family practice and public health, nurses, midwives, allied health professionals and health care managers. The courses would be an integral part of their continuous professional development. The design would have to recognize that not all participants are starting from the same point in their understanding of basic bioethics. A 'core and options' design would allow this to be the first part of a specialty-specific program (in our case perinatal medicine). Among the proposed objectives of these courses would be:

- To provide an introduction to (or revision of) basic theory in bioethics and to the relationship between ethics and the law.
- To develop consistent, critical and reflective attitudes to ethical decision making in the health care setting.

Table 14.6 Suggested basic bioethics modules for a core generic course for health care professionals, and indicative curriculum for a specific course in perinatal medicine

(a) Suggested basic bioethics modules

Module 1	Overview of bioethics – 'What ought I do?', dealing with uncertainty, etc.
Module 2	Competing theories, e.g. duties vs. consequences
Module 3	Other important concepts, e.g. principlism, virtue and narrative ethics, autonomy, paternalism
Module 4	Ethics and the law
Module 5	Ethics and the professions, e.g. confidentiality, informed consent and the vulnerable and failing doctor
Module 6	Making ethical judgments
Module 7	Methods of ethics support in practice

Among the suggested core topics might be

- Patients' rights, expectations and reality
- Consent, confidentiality, communication
- Legal framework in relevant countries
- Economics, to include resource allocation and prioritization
- Refusal of treatment
- Conflicts of interest, e.g.
  - Commercial enterprises in medical practice
- Clinical governance, e.g.
  - Managing and reducing risk, clinical error, poor performance, support structures
  - Clinical ethics committees
- Quality of life issues
- Decision making, to include:
  - Partnerships in decision making, e.g. interdisciplinary career perspectives, patient–parental perspectives
  - Dealing with uncertainty
  - 'Futile' treatment
  - Withdrawing or withholding treatment
  - Religious and secular influences on decision making
- Generic issues at the beginning and end of life
- Research governance, e.g.
  - Evidence based medicine
  - Properly informed consent
  - Innovative interventions
  - Fraud and misconduct
  - Research ethics committees

(b) Indicative curriculum for a specific course in perinatal medicine

- Human genetics
- Conception and birth
- New reproductive technologies; pre-embryo research; stem cells and cloning
- The law and perinatal medicine
- Screening, antenatal diagnosis and counseling
- Sex selection for medical and non-medical reasons
- Termination of pregnancy
- Feticide
- Non-selective embryo reduction
- The fetus as person and patient
- Patient choice and the maternal–fetal relationship
- Obstetric interventions 'on demand'
- Antepartum management of fetal anomalies
- Drug dependency in pregnancy
- Critical care obstetrics
- HIV infection in pregnancy
- Prematurity (particularly the very pre-term infant at or near the threshold of viability)
- Ethical aspects of the care of the newborn
- Ethical aspects of the care of the malformed or brain-damaged infant

Table 14.7 A guide to a bibliography for core ethical subjects and perinatal ethics

(a) Core ethical subjects

Medical Ethics Today
The BMA's handbook of ethics and law
BMJ Publishing Group, London, 2004
A comprehensive, concise and authoritative guide to medical ethics
Medical Ethics, 4th edn
Campbell A, Charlesworth M, Gillett G, Jones G
Oxford University Press, New York/Oxford, 1997
An invaluable primer for the subject accessible to the non-expert
Clinical Ethics, 5th edn
Jonsen AR, Siegler M, Winslade WJ
McGraw-Hill, New York, 2002
A 'must read' in this context. 'Facilitates solutions to everyday ethical problems'
Principles of Health Care Ethics
Edited by Gillon R
John Wiley, Chichester/New York, 1994
A detailed in-depth analysis of the field
Principles of Bio-medical Ethics, 5th edn
Beauchamp TL, Childress JF
Oxford University Press, New York/Oxford, 2001
Another excellent source book
Bioethics – An Introduction to the History, Methods and Practice
Jecker NS, Jonsen AR, Pearlman RA
Jones & Bartlett Publishers, Boston, 1997
It does as it says
Medical Ethics – A Case-Based Approach
Schwartz L, Preece PE, Hendry RA
Saunders, Edinburgh/New York, 2002
A useful guide
Medicine, Patients and the Law, 3rd edn
Brazier M
Penguin Books, London, 2003
A scholarly work by an eminent legal authority
Medical Ethics and the Law – The Core Curriculum
Hope T, Savulescu J, Hendrick J
Churchill Livingstone, Edinburgh/New York, 2003
A useful guide
Autonomy and Trust in Bioethics
O'Neill O
Cambridge University Press, Cambridge, England, 2002
A must for anyone who wishes to understand the true nature of autonomy
Three Methods of Ethics
Baron MW, Pettit P, Slote M
Blackwell Publishers, Oxford/Malden, MA, 1997
For those who wish to consider more deeply and contrast Kantian ethics, consequentialism and virtue ethics
The Health Care Professional as Friend and Healer
Edited by Thomasma DC, Kissell JL
Georgetown University Press, Washington, DC, 2000
This book builds on the work of Edmund Pellegrino. A 'must-read' in this context

(b) Perinatal ethics

Ethics and Perinatology
Edited by Goldworth A, Silverman W, Stevenson DK, Young EWD
Oxford University Press, New York/Oxford, 1995
A required text for this field
Ethics in Obstetrics and Gynecology
McCullough LB, Chervenak FA
Oxford University Press, New York/Oxford, 1994
Another valuable reference for this field
Ethics in Obstetrics and Gynecology
American College of Obstetricians and Gynecologists
ACOG, Washington, DC, 2002
A compilation of the subjects considered by the ACOG Ethics Committee and another invaluable source of material

(Continued)

Table 14.7 (Continued)

Recommendations on Ethical Issues in Obstetrics & Gynecology The FIGO Committee for the Ethical Aspects of Human Reproduction and Women's Health FIGO, 2000 A compilation of the subjects considered by the FIGO Ethics Committee and also an invaluable source of material
Ethical Issues in Maternal–Fetal Medicine Edited by Dickenson DL Cambridge University Press, Cambridge, England, 2002 Contains succinct but deep analyses of many relevant issues
Crucial Decisions at the Beginning of Life McHaffie H Radcliffe Medical Press, Oxford, 2001 A descriptive account of parents' experiences of treatment withdrawal from their infants
Should the Baby Live? The Problems of Handicapped Infants Kuhse H, Singer PO Oxford University Press, New York/Oxford, 1985 A controversial book that discusses issues that must be addressed in this context
Selective Non-treatment of Handicapped Newborns: Moral Dilemmas in Neonatal Medicine Weir RF Oxford University Press, New York/Oxford, 1988 A necessary source book in this context for understanding how better to deal with clinical and ethical dilemmas
The Worth of Child Murray TH University of California Press, Berkeley, CA, 1996 A deep and compassionate analysis of many of the relevant issues

- To increase awareness of ethical dilemmas faced in different health care settings.
- To understand better the ethical problems facing colleagues in different disciplines.
- To reinforce best practices in clinical and research governance.

The desired learning outcomes would include:

- A working knowledge of basic concepts and theories in clinical ethics.
- Greater confidence in confronting ethical issues encountered in clinical practice.
- A more consistent approach to dealing with similar ethical issues as they affect individual patients.
- A better understanding of the social and institutional context of decision making in health care.
- Improved interprofessional communication, learning and decision making.
- Improved communication of ethical issues with the patients and their families.

Table 14.6 outlines some suggested modules for such a course in basic bioethics. Formative and summary assessments would be incorporated and candidates could gain credits toward, for example, a master's degree in bioethics.

(4) *Specific course in perinatal medicine*: In this model, participants would have completed and gained credits in the generic course. This too could benefit from being interdisciplinary. Table 14.6b is a guide to the possible subjects to be included in the curriculum for such a course. Table 14.7a and b lists some suggested texts relevant to both the generic and the specific curriculum. It is for the users to adapt these suggestions to their requirements.

Does education in ethics make any difference?

It is not sufficient to assert that education in ethics is a good thing. Evaluation is required in support of the program to justify the commitment and expense, and to provide an evidence base for future work. But what outcomes can be used? Among those suggested are ethical sensitivity, attitudes, reasoning ability and decision making. There is some literature on promoting ethical sensitivity in modern medical practice,[25–30] but the main focus has been on medical students.[31,32] Although some attempts have been made to measure the general effectiveness of ethics training,[33–36] the work lacks substantial investigation and discussion of different methods of moral education. One study has attempted to evaluate the effects of an intensive ethics course on health care professionals, including physicians and nurses.[37] It was carried out during an open conference. Only about half of the participants provided direct patient care, and there were no data on the proportions of health care professionals taking part, so no real conclusions can be drawn from it. More rigorous work is required.

Summary

Ethics is the system of thought that analyzes and provides a rational framework for moral judgments. Among the key features of ethics are:

- It must be translatable into moral action.
- It is a public system rather than a private activity, and no one can act morally without reference to other individuals.
- The fundamental ethical principles underpinning medical ethics are those of society in general.
- Ethical analysis must be clear, internally consistent and free of contradiction.
- The judgments made must allow ethical conflicts to be identified, managed or, preferably, prevented.

The most effective way to achieve proper education in ethics is to begin early and build on it through school, college, medical school and continuing professional development. Among the purposes of education in ethics are the development of consistent, critical and reflective attitudes to ethical decision making, increasing awareness of ethical dilemmas in one's own practice and that of others and reinforcement of best practices in clinical and research governance.

REFERENCES

1. Radcliffe-Richards J. Maternal–fetal conflict. In Bewley S, Ward RH, eds. *Ethics in Obstetrics & Gynaecology*. London: RCOG Press, 1994:34–42.
2. Campbell AV. Moral dilemmas and ethical theories. In *Moral Dilemmas in Medicine*. Edinburgh: Churchill Livingstone, 1972:1–13.
3. Stirrat GM. Education in ethics. *Clin Perinatol* 2003;30:1–15.
4. Dunstan G. Should philosophy and medical ethics be left to the experts? In Bewley S, Ward RH, eds. *Ethics in Obstetrics & Gynaecology*. London: RCOG Press, 1994:3–8.
5. Campbell AV. The freedom that is health. In *Health as Liberation*. Cleveland, OH: The Pilgrim Press, 1995:1–24.
6. O'Neill O. Gaining autonomy and losing trust? In *Autonomy and Trust in Bioethics*. Cambridge: Cambridge University Press, 2002:1–27.
7. Stirrat GM, Gill R. Autonomy in medical ethics after O'Neill. *J Med Ethics* 2005;31:127–30.
8. General Medical Council. *Duties of a Doctor*. London: GMC, 1998.
9. American Medical Association. Council on Ethical and Judicial Affairs. Principles of medical ethics. In *Code of Medical Ethics*, 2000–2001 edn. American Medical Association: Chicago, 2001:xii.
10. O'Donovan LJ. A profession of trust: Reflections on a fundamental virtue. In Thomasma DC, Kissell JL, eds. *The Health Care Professional as Friend and Healer*. Washington, DC: Georgetown University Press, 2000:1–9.
11. Pellegrino ED. Being a physician: Does it make a moral difference? *Adv Otolaryngol Head Neck Surg* 1992;6:1–10.
12. Draper H, Sorell T. Patient's responsibilities in medical ethics. *Bioethics* 2003;16:335–52.
13. Stirrat GM. How to approach ethical issues. *Obstetrician Gynaecol (RCOG)* 2003;5:214–7.
14. Westphal M. Post-modern theology. In *Concise Routledge Encyclopaedia of Philosophy*. London: Routledge, 2000:699.
15. Jonsen A. Clinical ethics and the four principles. In Gillon R, ed. *Principles of Healthcare Ethics*. New York: John Wiley & Sons, 1994:13–21.
16. Baron MW, Pettit P, Slote M. The consequentialist perspective. In *Three Methods of Ethics*. Oxford: Blackwell, 1997:92–174.
17. Beauchamp TL. The 'four principles approach'. In Gillon R, ed. *Principles of Healthcare Ethics*. New York: John Wiley & Sons, 1994:3–12.
18. Brody H. The four principles and narrative ethics. In Gillon R, ed. *Principles of Healthcare Ethics*. New York: John Wiley & Sons, 1994:207–15.
19. MacIntyre A. *After Virtue: A Study in Moral Theology*, 2nd edn. London: Duckworth, 1985.
20. Tong R. Feminist ethics. In *Concise Routledge Encyclopaedia of Philosophy*. London: Routledge, 2000:278.
21. McCullough LB, Chervenak FA. A framework for ethics in a clinical setting. In *Ethics in Obstetrics and Gynecology*. Oxford: Oxford University Press, 1994:3–81.
22. Sherwin S. Foundations, frameworks and lenses. In *The Role of Theories in Bioethics*. Oxford: Blackwell, 1999:198–206.
23. Huxley TH. The method of Zadig. In *Collected Essays (1893–4)*. London: Macmillan, 1893.
24. General Medical Council. *Tomorrow's Doctors – Recommendations on Undergraduate Medical Education*. London: GMC, 1993.
25. Andre J. Learning to see: Moral growth during medical training. *J Med Ethics* 1992;18:148–52.
26. Herbert P, Mesline EM, Dunn EV, *et al.* Measuring ethical sensitivity in medical students: Using vignettes as an instrument. *J Med Ethics* 1990;16:141–5.
27. Herbert PC, Meslin EM, Dunn EV. Measuring the ethical sensitivity of medical students: A study at the University of Toronto. *J Med Ethics* 1992;18:142–7.
28. Savulescu J, Crisp R, Fulford KWM, Hope T. Evaluating ethics competence in medical education. *J Med Ethics* 1999;25:367–74.
29. Walker RM., Miles SH., Stocking CB, Siegler M. Physicians and nurses perceptions of ethics problems on general medical-services. *J Gen Int Med* 1991;6(5):424–9.
30. Zalewski Z. What philosophy should be taught to the future medical professionals? *Med Health Care Philos* 2000;3:161–7.
31. Goldie J, Schwartz L, McConnachie A, Morrison J. Impact of a new course on students' potential behaviour on encountering ethical dilemmas. *Med Educ* 2001;35:295–312.
32. Green B, Miller PD, Routh CP. Teaching ethics in psychiatry: A one-day workshop for clinical students. *J Med Ethics* 1995;21:234–8.
33. Bebeau MJ. Designing an outcome-based ethics curriculum for professional-education-strategies and evidence of effectiveness. *J Moral Educ* 1993;22(3):313–26.
34. Fischer GS, Arnold RM. Measuring the effectiveness of ethics education. *J Gen Int Med* 1994;9(11):655–6.
35. Holm S, Nielsen GH, Norup M, *et al.* Changes in moral reasoning and the teaching of medical ethics. *Med Educ* 1995; 29(6):420–3.
36. Self DJ, Davenport E. Measurement of moral development in medicine. *Camb Q Healthcare Ethics* 1996;5(2):269–77.
37. Malek JI, Geller G, Sugarman J. Talking about cases in bioethics: The effects of an intensive course on health care professionals. *J Med Ethics* 2000;26:131–6.

15 Words matter: nomenclature and communication in perinatal medicine

L. de Crespigny

Language

The general public now accepts the importance of using appropriate language. Their acceptance is in contrast with the attitude of many doctors who are quick to dismiss the importance of word choice in treating patients. The goal of this chapter is, first, to demonstrate that word choice by professionals involved in prenatal diagnosis is important and, second, to consider ethically appropriate word choices in our specialty.

Sexist and discriminatory language is now recognized as unacceptable. This is because we are aware that such language impacts negatively on others. As long ago as 1977, the United States Department of Labor revised 3000 of its approximately 30,000 titles for occupations. Advertisers are well aware of the importance of language and spend huge resources choosing names for products and developing phrases to describe them. Language is also the tool of trade of politicians. When there was an outcry over the government's harsh treatment of asylum seekers, the Australian Prime Minister, John Howard, recently declared that his party was endeavoring to govern in the interests of the mainstream of the Australian community. Shortly afterward, when the majority of Australians believed that he should dismiss the Governor General who had failed to act on child sexual abuse claims, he indicated that he would not be succumbing to the clamor of the mob. In other words, when the majority of Australians agreed with him, they represented the 'mainstream', but when most disagreed, it was 'the mob' talking.[1]

People now take care to avoid sexist and discriminatory language. Racist language, in particular, is acknowledged as being offensive and inappropriate. It is hurtful to, and places stress on, other people. Nobody working in prenatal diagnosis could fail to be aware of the unique stresses placed on a couple who are given bad news following a prenatal test. Despite this, however, there is remarkably little literature analyzing what word choice in prenatal diagnosis leaves couples feeling most comfortable. The importance of language has had very little focus in medicine generally – indeed, discussions on word choice may be perceived as trivial.

Language, reality, and moral judgment

Language makers and users of language are in a position to influence reality; language is a vehicle for them to construct, reinforce, and reproduce their particular bias or view of reality.[2] People's language can influence opinion: for example, a group might be called 'freedom fighters' if we support their cause, others may call the same group 'terrorists' if they wish to present them as evil.[3]

Doctors performing prenatal diagnosis are language makers in their specialist field. By their language they can subtly influence how their patients perceive a problem. We know that doctors have the potential to influence a patient's decision of what to do when a fetal anomaly is diagnosed. They can do this both by their choice of what information to impart and in the way they impart it. One group found that the proportion of women choosing pregnancy termination following the diagnosis of a facial cleft was 50%. It dropped to 5% following the introduction of 'emergency counseling by the cleft team'.[4] Women feel vulnerable and are susceptible to influence from their doctor following the diagnosis of fetal abnormality. There are few, if any, areas of medicine in which the language used by doctors is more important than in communicating with women having prenatal testing. Women feel stressed and may need to make one of the biggest decisions of their lives – to consider whether to have an abortion if a major abnormality is found.

Loftus and Palmer,[5] who summarized their results as follows, demonstrated the impact of language on memory:

> Two experiments are reported in which subjects viewed films of automobile accidents and then answered questions about events occurring in the films. The question, "About how fast were the cars going when they smashed into each other?" elicited higher estimates of speed than questions which used the verbs *collided*, *bumped*, *contacted*, or *hit* in place of *smashed*. On a retest one week later, those subjects who received the verb *smashed* were more likely to say "yes" to the question, "Did you see any broken glass?" even though broken glass was not present in the film. These results are consistent with the view that the questions asked subsequent to an event can cause a reconstruction in one's memory of that event.

The unique emotive experience suffered by women given a diagnosis of fetal abnormality far exceeds that of people watching a film. It is reasonable to assume that the doctor's language would have at least as much impact on patients as did the wording of questions to watchers of the crash film. In prenatal diagnosis there is the added factor that the doctor is seen as 'the expert'. Following the diagnosis of fetal abnormality, patients will often ask their doctor what is the best course of action. They will even attempt to read into a doctor's words or manner whether he or she thinks an abortion is warranted. It is not the role of the doctor to make a moral judgment about what is best for any particular patient. However, patients may be highly influenced not only by what the doctor says, but also by inferences from the doctor's word choice. The use of words such as 'baby' and 'mother' when the doctor means 'fetus' and 'pregnant woman' may result in the patient thinking that her doctor considers that her fetus has the status of a baby and she is already a mother. It might be expected that such a word choice may influence the patient's decision about abortion. In the crash film the questioner's language influenced the subjects' perception. Following detection of a fetal abnormality, the doctor's language at the time of diagnosis could affect the woman's decision on abortion. If her doctor, either directly or by word choice, infers that the fetus is a baby, this might also impact in the woman's ultimate ability to come to terms with her decision.

Medical language

In a field closely allied to prenatal testing, Bowker[2] explores the level of gender insensitivity in specialist language in the field of infertility. She cites examples demonstrating that the language used for similar problems leading to male and female infertility is often gender insensitive. For example, 'sperm antibodies' are described as being present in a male, while a woman whose cervical mucus develops such antibodies is described as having 'hostile mucus'. She claims that the choices of language are not always innocent and may be determined by belief systems that underlie them. Language may attempt to portray men in a more positive light and women in a negative one. She also notes that the term 'expected date of confinement' suggests punishment and imprisonment reflecting the male doctor's control over the place of birth and birthing practices. The terms 'expected date of delivery' or 'due date' are more gender sensitive. Bowker concludes that even when a doctor claims not to have a bias against women, the language that he uses to communicate to patients may be based on such a bias and may therefore have a harmful effect, even in the absence of a malicious intent.

A detailed analysis of the terms commonly used in obstetrical ultrasound practice would be valuable. Some language is clearly gender insensitive, such as cervical incompetence and the labeling of a woman as a 'recurrent aborter'. Some language is simply insensitive, such as intrauterine growth retardation (instead of restriction, to avoid a perceived association with intellectual retardation) or a fetal anomaly scan (instead of a fetal normality scan, to focus on the normal).

Doctors also use terms that could lead to misconceptions in the eyes of colleagues as well as the public. It has been suggested that 'myocardial infarction' should be replaced by 'coronary occlusion' since the goal of current treatment is to prevent the myocardial death that follows coronary occlusion.[6] The same author also proposed replacing the term 'hypertension', which falsely suggests that the condition is related to tension or stress, and replacing 'cardiac failure' with 'cardiac insufficiency'.

The medical profession has been slow to acknowledge the importance of language, dismissing it as being 'politically correct'. The term 'political correctness' is now used as a slogan of opprobrium, referring to someone who is an ideological monster.[7] Doctors dislike linguistic change and find it threatening, suggesting that there is something more acceptable about their own linguistic preference.[7] Why is it that the Right to Life movement long ago learned to use 'killing of babies' instead of 'abortion', while doctors often still speak as if language is mere political correctness and does not impact on peoples' opinions?

Language in obstetrics

Although doctors are often dismissive of politically correct language, our journals have over time reduced discriminatory language. The use of 'husbands and wives' when the author means 'men and women' would no longer be accepted, although these terms were used in a leading journal as recently as 1984.[8] Similarly, one would not now expect to find in a standard medical text a quote such as 'it has been said that bad girls get babies but good girls get myomata'.[9] While this may have been presented as a joke, it helps perpetuate sexism by suggesting 'good girls comply with the stereotypical portrayal of women as chaste and passive'.[10]

The RCOG Study Group on *Problems in Early Pregnancy: Advances in Diagnosis in Management*[11] has recommended that in early pregnancy loss, the term 'abortion' be replaced by 'miscarriage'. It is recommended that 'spontaneous miscarriage' replace 'spontaneous abortion', 'early embryonic demise' and 'fetal demise' replace 'blighted ovum' and 'missed abortion', respectively, and 'incomplete miscarriage' be used instead of 'incomplete abortion'.[12] The general community has long accepted that our language is important in influencing the way people see reality; this is also starting to be accepted in our specialty.

Language in prenatal diagnosis

Ethical dilemmas pervade the specialty of prenatal diagnosis. However, there has so far been little attempt to review the language we use and the impact it may have on other professionals, and even more importantly on our patients. It is time doctors were more considered and considerate in their word choice. The terms 'fetus' and 'pregnant woman' are grammatically more correct than 'baby' and 'mother'. The latter names are used by some (including antiabortionists) euphemistically with a more sinister motivation – namely, to blur reality. Antiabortionists use 'baby' and 'mother' as 'linguistic fig leaves' to suggest that abortion is wrong;[7] while the motivation of doctors using these terms is likely to differ from antiabortionists, it may be misinterpreted by patients.

How do we determine the most appropriate terminology for the language of our specialty? Should we survey our patients and let them decide terminology? One such survey showed pregnant women had a strong preference to be called 'patient' rather than 'mother', 'client', 'consumer', 'customer', 'lady', 'woman', or 'pregnant woman'.[13] Another study surveyed women in an antenatal clinic in an attempt to decide whether to use the term 'mother-to-be', 'pregnant woman', 'maternant', 'patient', 'client', or 'consumer'.[14] The authors concluded, 'Simple softer terms like mother-to-be please a vast majority'. While we do not know the gestation of these women, given that most women have healthy pregnancies, it must be assumed that most of these women believed they had, and in fact had, healthy pregnancies. How would their answers have changed if, immediately after filling out this questionnaire, their doctor had told them that their fetus had a major abnormality? The softer pleasing term of 'mother-to-be' suddenly seems inappropriate – the patient will probably choose not to be a mother this time. Would the doctor using the term 'mother-to-be' have an impact on their patient's decision whether or not to continue with the pregnancy? Would the patient think that the doctor is insinuating that since she is a mother-to-be and not a pregnant woman that the doctor therefore opposes an abortion? If the woman has an abortion, might her grief be prolonged because of her concern that the doctor had implied that she should have become a mother?

Mothers, and presumably mothers-to-be, do not kill their children/fetuses. Pregnant women, however, do have a right to abortion in some circumstances in most Western societies. We cannot expect patients in an outpatient survey to think through these issues. Sometimes word choice is better resolved by reflection and discussion, because the appropriate survey cannot be easily carried out. Word choice is not always best resolved by surveying patients – just as medical treatments are not. Doctors have a role in patient and community education.

Another study suggested that some patients preferred the term 'baby' to 'fetus'.[15] Researchers in Canada examined the results of a questionnaire sent to women who had been informed of ultrasound findings of 'serious anomalies', soft markers of aneuploidy, or obstetric complications. Approximately 900 patients were seen in the study year, the number who declined to participate was not recorded, but 117 agreed to participate in the survey. Surveys were returned by 65% of the 117. This shows the difficulty in both performing and analyzing the results of such a survey – questionnaires were analyzed from only 76 (8%) of the original approximately 900 eligible women.

More women felt strongly that they preferred to have their health care provider use the word 'baby' when giving them bad news. A smaller number felt it important to hear the word 'fetus'. There was a significant minority who considered the terms used to be unimportant. There was great diversity of opinion among the women.

It is not clear from this paper how many women had chosen pregnancy termination following diagnosis of a serious anomaly. It might be expected that many women who continue their pregnancy, who have made the decision that they are going to have a baby, would prefer the term baby to be used. This would apply particularly to the women in this study who completed the survey up to 9 months after their ultrasound visit, so would by then either have a baby or be very late in pregnancy.

In our use of language in the specialist field of prenatal testing we have a number of goals:

(1) *Maximize the information provided to pregnant women.* The words we use should be descriptive and easily understood by the majority of pregnant women.

(2) *Be respectful of women's choices.* While some have suggested that prenatal diagnosis is a 'select and destroy' mission, most support the concept of prenatal diagnosis enhancing autonomous choices of pregnant women. The enhancement of autonomy should apply not only to choice of tests, but also to what information they receive from these tests (does the woman wish to know 'everything' including all low-risk markers of aneuploidy?) and the decision whether to continue the pregnancy or have an abortion.[16]

(3) *Reduce risks of long-term psychological maladjustment.* Since we have few data on the impact of language on psychological adjustment to adverse pregnancy outcome, we must theorize on its impact. Surveying healthy women at an antenatal clinic does not answer this question.

(4) *Promote bonding in normal healthy pregnancies.* This is not only through our language, but also by the use of technology, for example, offering of three-dimensional (3D) and 4D ultrasound when available.

At times, points (3) and (4) may appear to be in conflict. In showing pregnant women ultrasound images, we may promote bonding only to discover later in the examination that there is a fetal abnormality. The bonding itself is not necessarily a problem if the patient later chooses pregnancy termination. Indeed, counselors go to great lengths to support bonding by offering photographs, footprints, etc. following termination for fetal abnormality, and such a policy is supported by patient groups. We should not shield women from the fact that the fetus they aborted looks human, but we can use language that indicates that even though it looks human, it does not have human characteristics such as a conscious life and an ability to plan. Careful use of language can support this message.

Rothman has coined the phrase 'tentative pregnancy'[17] to describe the state of limbo that women are in prior to completion of prenatal testing. Women cannot say with confidence that 'I am going to have a baby' until after the completion of prenatal testing. Those of us in prenatal diagnosis know that most women in whom a major fetal abnormality is diagnosed will choose pregnancy termination. Women who have had a previous pregnancy terminated because of fetal abnormality are uniquely aware of their 'tentative pregnancy'. Their relief and excitement at the completion of a normal midtrimester ultrasound examination are plainly visible. Women are increasingly aware that a midtrimester ultrasound examination is primarily for fetal anomaly detection and that a midtrimester scan is the final prenatal test. Although women anxiously await the results of any prenatal test, the defining moment for pregnant women has become the news of a normal midtrimester ultrasound examination. It is rare that subsequent events or testing cause a pregnant woman to rethink pregnancy termination.

Our language should support and enhance the autonomy of pregnant women.[18] It is a normal midtrimester ultrasound examination that indicates to most pregnant women that their fetuses will become babies. They will become mothers after the birth. They are now unlikely to request abortion – a fetal anomaly is now unlikely to be found. Our word choice should acknowledge that our language is focused on the woman, and not on the views of the doctor.

The *Oxford English Dictionary* defines 'mother' as a female parent, one who has borne a child. It is therefore grammatically incorrect to use the term 'mother' for a pregnant woman. Pregnant women and mothers have contrasting rights and responsibilities. Pregnant women have the right to abortion in certain circumstances in most Western countries, while it is illegal for a mother to kill or fail to care for her child.

The definitions of 'baby' are more variable. The *Oxford English Dictionary* includes both unborn and newly born human beings as a baby while the *Collins Dictionary* defines a baby as a child in the first year or two of life. It is proposed that 'fetal patient' (or the lay terms 'child' or 'baby') should be used when it is unlikely that termination of pregnancy would be requested.[18] For most women this is after normal results of prenatal testing. An exception is the woman who in early pregnancy clearly indicates that she would not consider termination of pregnancy for fetal abnormality; she has given the status of a fetal patient to her previable fetus. She is free to withdraw that status at any time.[18]

The goal should be to remain as neutral as possible in the choice of words prior to the completion of prenatal testing in an attempt to avoid inadvertent directive counseling. The term 'fetus' is neutral in that it does not imply the fetus has the status of a baby; it implies that pregnancy termination is still considered acceptable. Following completion of prenatal testing the term 'fetal patient' is advocated with 'child' or 'baby' as the analogous lay term.[18]

The term 'mother' is clearly defined, and should be used when grammatically correct. 'Mother' is appropriate when describing a woman who has borne a child and is inappropriate when describing a pregnant woman who has not borne a child.

What alternative proposals for word choice might be suggested?

(1) In an earlier paper the author argued that the terms 'pregnant woman' and 'fetus' should replace 'mother' and 'baby' throughout pregnancy.[19] Such language supports the claim that 'a pregnant woman ... should have the right to make decisions about her own body up until the time of birth .... In a difficult decision, the woman's present right to bodily integrity should prevail over the rights of the potential person'.[20]

The law puts great emphasis on the moment of birth. Late abortion is legal in many parts of the world, especially in the presence of a major fetal abnormality. In most Western countries late abortion is available for lethal abnormalities. Using the term 'fetus' throughout pregnancy supports the philosophy that women late in pregnancy may put their rights above those of the fetus in the unusual situation when these are in conflict.

There are good reasons for reserving the term 'baby' for after birth and 'fetus' for before birth. This word choice is consistent with the definition of baby in at least some dictionaries. It supports the autonomy of the pregnant woman throughout pregnancy.

On balance, however, the author suggests the use of 'baby' is preferred following completion of prenatal testing. A disadvantage of using the term 'fetus' late in pregnancy is that it might potentially prolong the 'tentative pregnancy' in the eyes of the pregnant woman. Women benefiting from modern obstetrical and neonatal care have good reason for being confident that 'they are going to have a baby' after completion of testing; it would be a pity if our language diminished that confidence. Very few women have reason to request abortion after standard tests are completed. There is little reason not to enhance such confidence by using the lay term 'baby' late in pregnancy.

(2) Those opposing abortion following potential fetal viability may argue that from viability the term 'baby' should be used. Given a normal midtrimester ultrasound examination, few women will have further prenatal tests in the few weeks prior to potential viability. Even fewer women suddenly change their mind at this late stage and decide that their apparently normal pregnancy is unwanted and they wish to have an abortion. To propose viability as being decisive in determining word choice would result in the doctor prolonging the tentative pregnancy to support his or her ethical position. For the patient, the completion of prenatal testing is the more critical time.

(3) Finally, even after reflection, some doctors may choose to call the fetus a 'baby' from conception. This is the position of the Right to Life movement, since it enhances their view that abortion is tantamount to killing babies. These doctors are using word choice to deliberately promote their personal views on the status of the fetus. Others may claim that they use the term 'baby' throughout pregnancy because it is more patient friendly – better understood by some women. However, the term 'fetus' is now widely used and understood in the lay context; few adults find this term confusing. Young children and some adults may be more comfortable with 'unborn baby' and 'mother-to-be' – these are acceptable alternatives to 'baby'.

Some might claim that the language proposed contradicts the language used by many pregnant women who prefer to think of their child as a baby. The doctor participating in such baby talk may please some pregnant women and may be preferred by many, or even most, women who will proceed to have a baby. However, the long-term interests of the patient may be better served by more neutral language, particularly if the outcome to the pregnancy is adverse. It would be unfortunate if patients interpreted the doctor's participation in baby talk as the euphemistic language of an antiabortionist.

It is important to consider the impact of our language on women continuing the pregnancies. But the life-long distress felt by many women following pregnancy loss means that this group deserves our special attention. These women are at greatest risk – and they will not have a baby. The critical issue is how language impacts on women who are considering pregnancy termination. The author's proposition is that by using neutral language, such as 'fetus' and 'pregnant woman', these terms are not only more accurate, but also assist in ensuring that the pregnant woman does not misinterpret the health care provider as having an antiabortion bias.

We need to be sensitive that women who give the status of a patient to the fetus, in other words women who have made a prior decision to continue the pregnancy, might prefer the use of 'baby' to 'fetus'. We should use whatever language is most supportive of our patients.

After a miscarriage or pregnancy termination, some couples like to think of and refer to their fetus as a baby. They may even name the fetus. Even women having a pregnancy termination may wish the fetus to be considered as a baby, and that preterm labor is being induced in the best interests of the baby. It is important that our language is supportive of our patients and flexible, so enhancing their best interests. No rigid framework is correct for all situations. This is not to say, however, that the doctor should support the 'baby talk' of a woman early in pregnancy, excited by the first images of her fetus on the ultrasound screen. Not all pregnant women appreciate that prenatal testing may mean that they withdraw the status of a baby from their fetus. We as professionals need to be aware that we should, in general, support neutral language, even when caring for excited couples early in pregnancy. Doctors would be less tempted to indulge in baby talk if they perceived there was any risk that this could result in more prolonged psychological sequelae for a woman who subsequently chose pregnancy termination in the presence of a fetal abnormality. The principle guiding the physician should be respect for the patient.

Our respect for the patient also extends to others in the family. The term 'father' should be avoided during pregnancy. A male partner or husband becomes an expectant father following normal prenatal test.[18] If the partner is a woman, she becomes the expectant parent at that time.

Conclusion

The best interests of our patients are served by using language that supports patient autonomy and is neutral. While it remains a 'tentative' pregnancy, i.e. prior to the completion of normal prenatal tests, the term 'fetus' should be used. Following normal prenatal testing, only in rare situations will the pregnant woman request an abortion. It is appropriate that the term 'fetal patient', or lay terms 'child' or 'baby', be then used. To be a mother, however, one must have borne a child.

Our language should support the autonomous views of the patient. The language proposed is not intended to be rigidly adhered to in all situations, but rather is an appropriate starting point, after which we as health providers need to be responsive to the position of the pregnant woman. It is important to individualize language to accommodate the views of individual patients. It is, however, time for doctors to acknowledge that their language can influence reality, particularly since they are frequently considered experts, not only in prenatal diagnosis, but also in morality. Doctors' language has a powerful influence not only on the way patients think, but potentially also on the decisions that they make.

REFERENCES

1. Henderson G. When the mainstream becomes a mob, blame the dingo pack. *The Age* 2002;March 12:11.
2. Bowker L. Terminology and gender sensitivity; a corpus-based study of the LSP of infertility. *Lang Soc* 2001;30:589–601.
3. Schulz MR. The semantic derogation of women. In Thorne B and Henley N, eds. *Language and Sex: Difference and Dominance*, 1975:64–75.
4. Moss A. Controversies in cleft lip and palate management. *Ultrasound Obstet Gynecol* 2001;18:420–1.
5. Loftus EF, Palmer JC. Reconstruction of automobile destruction: an example of the interaction between language and memory. *J Verb Learn Verb Behav* 1974;13:585–9.
6. O'Rourke MF. What's in a name? Would that which we call "cardiac failure," by any other name threaten less? *Med J Aust* 1997;166:372–3.
7. Burridge K. Polcor-Big Brother, Thomas Bowdler or June Dally-Watkins. In Peters PH, ed. *Style in Context: Language at Large.* Proceedings of Style Councils, 1996, 1997 and 1999.
8. Stray-Pedersen B, Stray-Pedersen S. Etiologic factors and subsequent reproductive performance in 195 couples with a prior history of habitual abortion. *Am J Obstet Gynecol* 1984;148:140–4.
9. Llewellyn-Jones D. *Fundamentals of Obstetrics and Gynaecology.* London: Faber & Faber, 1982;2.
10. Harres A. The representation of women in three medical texts *ARAL Ser* 1993;35(10)–53.
11. Grudzinskas JG, O'Brien PMS. *Problems in Early Pregnancy: Advances in Diagnosis and Management.* London: RCOG Press, 1997.
12. Hutchon DJR. Understanding miscarriage or insensitive abortion: Time for more defined terminology? *Am J Obstet Gynecol* 1998;179:397–8.
13. Denning AS, Tuttle LK, Bryant VJ, Walker SP, Higgins JR. Ascertaining women's choice of title during pregnancy and childbirth. *Aust N Z J Obstet Gynaecol* 2002;42:125–9.
14. Batra N, Lilford RJ. Not clients, not consumers and definitely not maternants. *Eur J Obstet Gynecol Reprod Biol* 1996;64:197–9.
15. Alkazaleh F, Thomas M, Grebenyuk J, *et al.* What women want: women's preferences of caregiver behavior when prenatal sonography findings are abnormal. *Ultrasound Obstet Gynecol* 2004;23:56–62.
16. de Crespigny L, Savulescu J. Is paternalism alive and well in obstetric ultrasound? Helping couples choose their children. *Ultrasound Obstet Gynecol* 2002;20:213–6.
17. Rothman BK. *A Tentative Pregnancy: Prenatal Diagnosis and the Future of Motherhood.* New York: Viking, 1986.
18. de Crespigny L, Chervenak F, McCullough L. Mothers and babies, pregnant women and fetuses. *Br J Obstet Gynaecol* 1999;106:1235–7.
19. de Crespigny L. What's in a name – is the pregnant woman a mother? Is the fetus a baby? *Aust N Z J Obstet Gynaecol* 1996; 36:435–6.
20. Special project: Legal rights and issues surrounding conception, pregnancy and birth "maternal rights v's fetal rights." Vanderbilt Law Review 819 at 849, 1986:39.

16 The beginning of human life – scientific and religious controversies

A. Kurjak and J. M. Carrera

One of the most controversial topics in modern bioethics, science, and philosophy is the beginning of individual human life. In the seemingly endless debate, strongly stimulated by recent technologic advances in human reproduction, a synthesis between scientific data and hypothesis, philosophical thought, and issues of humanities has become necessary to deal with ethical, juridical, and social problems.[1] Furthermore, in this field there is a temptation to ask science to choose between opinions and beliefs that tend to neutralize one another. Indeed, the question of when human life begins requires the essential aid of different forms of knowledge. Here, we become involved in the juncture between science and religion, which needs to be carefully explored.[2]

Obviously, the beginning of human life is seen differently by different individuals, groups, cultures, and religions. Fundamental to productive debate and reconciliation between minority and majority groups is an understanding of the ill-defined concept of 'the beginning of human life'.[3]

Entering this field, scientists have been remiss in failing to translate science into the terms that allow mankind to share their excitement of discovering life before birth. Regardless of the remarkable scientific development, curiosity, and speculations dating back to Hippocrates, life before birth still remains a big secret. Different kinds of intellectuals involved themselves in trying to contribute to the solution of the human life puzzle. They are led by the idea that each newborn child will only reach its full potential if its development *in utero* is free from any adverse influence, providing the best possible environment for the embryo/fetus. Considering the embryo/fetus, the amazing aspect of these parts of human life in which the pregnant woman and the embryo/fetus, although locked in the most intimate of relationships, are at all times two separate individuals should be always kept in mind. Accepting the embryo/fetus as a person opens a new set of questions about its personality and human rights.

The definition of life

Proper answers to the question of how to define human life are complicated. Nowadays, dilemmas consider the respect of human life from birth to death involving not just biology, but other sciences also. Philosophy, theology, psychology, sociology, law, and politics evaluate this topic from different points of view. Integration of all could result in a useful answer.

Some authors say that life as such does not exist – no one has ever seen it. Szent-Gyorgy says that the noun 'life' has no significance because there is no such thing as 'life'. Le Dantez holds that the expression 'to live' is too general, and that it is better to say a dog 'dogs' or a fish 'fishes' than 'a dog or a fish lives'.[4]

When defining life, it should be considered not just as it is today, but as it might have been in its primordial form and as it will be in the future. All present forms of life appear as something completely new. Life, then, is transferred and not conceived in each new generation. Furthermore, the phenomenon of life has existed on Earth for approximately 3.5 billion years. Consequently, although the genome of a new embryo is unique, the makeup of an embryo is not new. If life is observed through the cell, then every life (and human life also) is considered as a continuum. Human cells and mankind have existed on Earth continuously since the appearance of the first man. However, if the definition refers to a single human being or the present population, the statement that 'human life is a continuum' is not acceptable.[5]

'Life', in the true sense of the word, begins when the chemical matter gives rise, in a specific way, to an autonomous, self-regulating, and self-reproducing system. Life is connected with a living being, and it

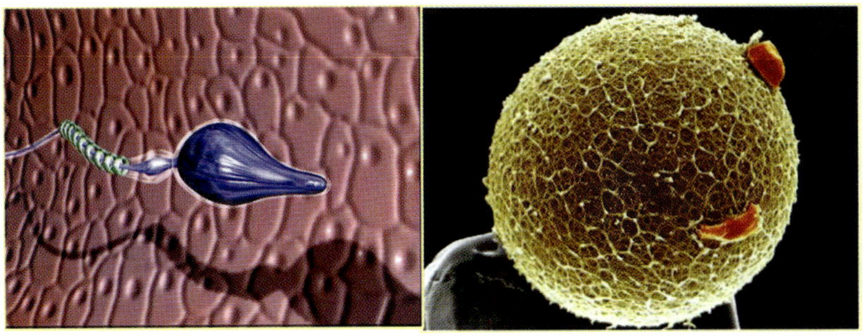

Figure 16.1 Schematic presentation of spermatozoa and oocyte.

creates its own system as an indivisible whole – it forms its individuality. One of the most important characteristics of living beings is reproduction.

Reproduction is a means of creating new life by transferring forms of an old one into a newly formed human being. Therefore, variability, individual development, and harmony characterize human beings. Individuality is the most essential characteristic of human beings consisting of new life. But also all human life forms through evolution, characterized by phenotype, behavior, and the capability to recognize and adapt. Human embryo and fetus gradually develop into these characteristics.

'Human life' poses a semantic problem. The placenta is 'human life', as is every individual cell or organ of the human body, but 'human life' is clearly not equivalent to 'human being'. It is therefore mandatory to differentiate between 'organic or vegetative human life' and 'potential personal human life'. The latter term allows various groups to identify a point of the continuum between abortion and birth to which they can ascribe appropriate values and rights.[3]

Although we should not forget that today's research is tomorrow's benefit,[6] concerning human life, conclusions should not be treated one-sidedly – from one perspective. This reality should be regarded in all its richness: the embryo gives the biologist and geneticist substance for consideration, but talking about the beginning of a human life requires philosophical/anthropological consideration, as well as theological and social sciences. In its protection, we have to include ethics and law. This approach leads to the conclusion that it is necessary to reject reductionism as well as integrism, and to find a 'golden middle' between these two methodologies.[1]

What does biology say?

Biology characterizes human beings by the dynamics of the system and its self-control (homeostasis), excitability (response to stimuli of different nature and origins), self-reproducibility, the heredity of the characters, and the evolutionary trend.[1] For biologists, it is important to specify which form of life phenomena we are referring to: cell, organism population, or species. The basic level of organization and the simplest form of life is the cell. Biologically speaking, human cellular life never stops – or if it did, the extinction of the human species would result – and is passed on from one generation to another. Human individual organismic life is defined within its life cycle, which is temporarily limited, i.e. it has a beginning and an end.[7] It is obvious that life is a highly dynamic phenomenon that could be described and explained through the careful study of life processes and interactions by the interdisciplinary approach. In human spermatozoa and oocyte, there are two essential cells involved in creating human life (Figures 16.1 and 16.2). It is clear that biologists are most qualified to render judgment on the structure and function of cells. To quote Scarpelli,[8] the very broad scope of biological science (from molecular to behavioral biology, and from unicellular to multisystem forms) brings with it the justifiable understanding that the biological scientist knows and is able to define the state of being 'alive' or 'life'. If not, the science fails.

The biological scientist, who may specialize within one or another domain of the broad scope, has particular and definitive knowledge and understanding of the living individual that is his specialty. If not, disorder will rise above failure.

Understanding of the beginning of human life and development of the embryo/fetus could provide definitive resolution. However, with the recent possibility of visualizing early human development virtually from conception, perinatologists should be those who by study, training, practice, and research are singularly qualified.[9]

While science provides us data about physical development of the human being, it does not provide information about its personality and personhood. These topics are philosophical rather than scientific.

Human embryogenesis

Only a proper understanding of the process of human embryogenesis enables answering scientifically the question of when the life cycle of a human individual

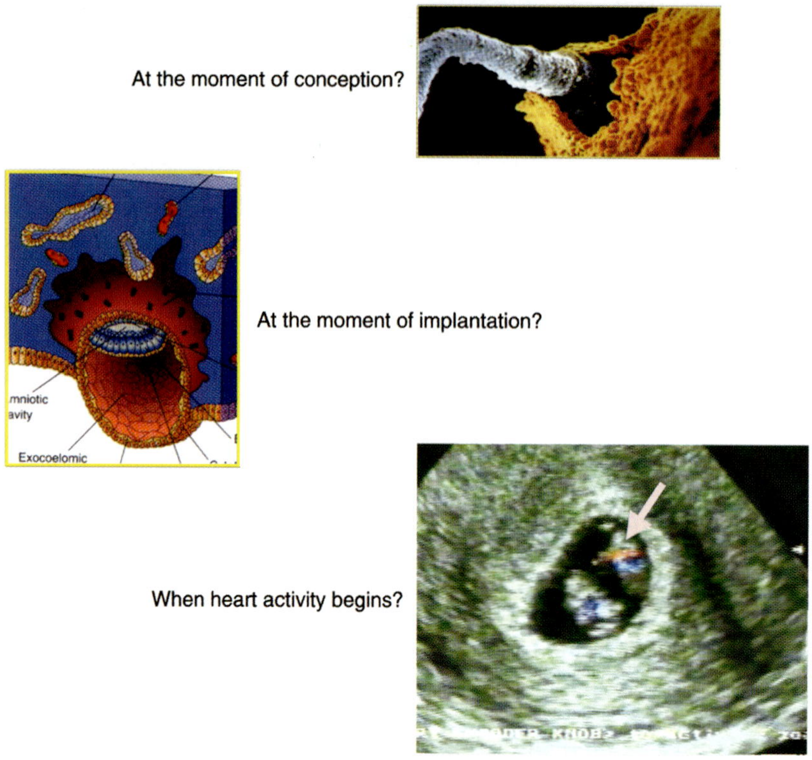

Figure 16.2 Some possible questions on the beginning of human life.

starts. Therefore, in the following text the main steps of the human developmental process are briefly described, primarily during the first 15 days following fertilization.

A human being originates from two living cells: the oocyte and the spermatozoon, transmitting the torch of life to the next generation. The oocyte is a cell approximately 120 μm in diameter with a thick membrane, known as the zona pellucida. The spermatozoon moves, using the flagellum or tail, and the total length of the spermatozoon including the tail is 60 μm.[10]

After syngamy, the zygote undergoes mitotic cell division as it moves down the fallopian tube toward the uterus. A series of mitotic divisions then leads to the development of the pre-embryo. The newly divided cells are called blastomeres. From 1 to 3 days after syngamy, there is a division into two cells, then four cells. Blastomeres form cellular aggregates of distinct, totipotent, undifferentiated cells that, during several early cell divisions, retain the capacity to develop independently into normal pre-embryos. As the blastocyst is in the process of attaching to the uterine wall, the cells increase in number and organize into two layers of cells. Implantation progresses as the outer cell layer of the blastocyst, the trophectoderm, invades the uterine wall and erodes blood vessels and glands. Having begun five or more days after fertilization with the attachment of the blastocyst to the endometrial lining of the uterus, implantation is completed when the blastocyst is fully embedded in the endometrium several days later. Even during these 5–6 days, modern medicine introduces the possibility of making preimplantation genetic diagnosis.

However, at this time, these cells are not yet totally differentiated in terms of their determination to specific cells or organs of the embryo. The term 'pre-embryo', then, includes the developmental stages from the first cell division of the zygote through the morula and the blastocyst. By approximately the 14th day after the end of the process of fertilization, all cells, depending on their position, will have become parts of the placenta and membranes or the embryo. The embryo stage, therefore, begins approximately 16 days after the beginning of the fertilization process and continues until the end of 8 weeks after fertilization, when organogenesis is complete.[11]

The pre-embryo is the structure that exists from the end of the process of fertilization until the appearance of a single primitive streak. Until the completion of implantation, the pre-embryo is capable of dividing into multiple entities, but does not contain enough genetic information to develop into an embryo; it lacks genetic material from maternal mitochondria and maternal and parental genetic messages in the form of messenger RNA or proteins. Therefore, during the pre-embryonic period it has not yet been determined with certainty that a biological individual will result, or would be one or more (forming of identical twins), so that the assignment of the full rights of an individual human person is inconsistent with biological reality.

One conclusion from this is that the pre-embryo requires the establishment of special rules in society: it cannot claim absolute protection based on claims of personhood; although meriting respect, it does not have the same moral value that a human person has. Today, one largely accepted opinion is that until the 14th day from fertilization, or at least until implantation, the human embryo may not be considered, from the ontological point of view, as an individual.

Genetic uniqueness and singleness coincide only after implantation and restriction have completed, which is about 3 weeks after fertilization. Until that period, the zygote and its sequelae are in a fluid process, are not a physical individual, and therefore cannot be a person.

It is well known that high percentages of oocytes that have been penetrated never proceed on to further development, and that many oocytes that do are thwarted so early in their development that their presence is not even recognized. It is suggested that 30% of conceptions detected by positive reactions to human chorionic gonadotropin (HCG) tests abort spontaneously before these pregnancies are clinically verified.

The newly conceived pre-embryo presents itself as a biologically defined reality. However, the status of the pre-embryo as an individual remains a great mystery. In the present scientific scene, especially with the progress of ultrasound technologies, prenatal psychology and therapeutics have opened a window into the prenatal life of embryo and fetus confirming the evidence that the embryo/fetus is a true subject in itself.[12]

Personality

Defining personality is very complex. There is still no clear definition of personality. One dictionary offers 'what constitutes an individual as distinct person', but does not define what the 'what' is. Another dictionary asserts 'the state of existing as a thinking intelligent being'. This definition might lead to the inference that personality increases *pro rata* with intelligence, or that some people may not have a personality at all if we followed Bertrand Russell's dictum that 'most people would rather die than think and many, in fact, do!'. Kenneth Stallworthy's *Manual of Psychiatry* is more helpful with the definition that 'personality is the individual as a whole with everything about him which makes him different from other people', because we can certainly distinguish fetuses from each other and from other people. With the next sentence – 'personality is determined by what is born in the individual in the first place and by everything which subsequently happens to him in the second' – we are really in the field.[1,3]

Viewpoints on the nature of 'personhood' and what it means ethically and legally vary widely. In his proposed Life Protection Act, Sass acknowledges that a fetus with formed synapses is not a 'person' in the usual sense of the word, connoting consciousness and self-consciousness.[13] Veatch sees the problem as defining the life that has full moral standing,[14] while Knutson[15] has noted that 'those who employ spiritual or religious definitions of when life begins tend to place the beginning of life earlier than those who employ psychological, sociological, or cultural definitions'.

Led by the truism, 'No insignificant person was ever born', human beings should be valued from birth to natural death. It is hard to establish proper values and exact definitions. This becomes especially problematic when prenatal life is considered. The above-stated truism opens an important question: 'Is the person-unborn a person in the first place and, if so, is the person-unborn a "significant" person?'.[1]

Let us evaluate further present controversies. There is no doubt that the embryo and fetus *in utero* are biologically human individuals prior to birth. The child who is born is the same developing human individual that was in the mother's womb. Birth alone cannot confer natural personhood or human individuality. This is confirmed by preterm deliveries of babies who are as truly human and almost as viable as those whose gestation goes to full term. All the known evidence supports the human fetus being a true ontological human individual and consequently a human person in fact, if not in law. *A human person cannot begin before the appropriate brain structures are developed that are capable of sustaining awareness.* The same applies to a grossly malformed fetus. It would still be a human individual even if its human nature was not perfect or its functions quite normal. Nobody questions the humanity of a Down's syndrome fetus or child. A fetus or child with severe open spina bifida is not less of a human being. The same should be said for the live anencephalic fetus or infant with only brain stem functions. It is a human individual even if it lacks a complete brain and usually survives birth by only a few hours or a day.

'Person' and 'personhood' are the legally operational terms in the USA and many other countries. Alternatively, 'person' and 'personhood' are replaced by terms such as 'viable outside the uterus', 'a woman's right to privacy', and 'a woman's right to choose'. In each case, viable, privacy, and choice, the life-support provider may legally order transfer of the dependent individual into a morbid environment. For this group, dilemma (which includes the stem cell, abortion, and cloning debates) is abated, but not resolved.[3]

Human society created several standards in defining 'person' or 'human being' based on what is familiar and easy recognizable.[1] For example, a human speaks, understands, and laughs. Absence of these characteristics (mutism, autism, and stoicism) is not a disqualification. On the contrary, the conclusion is that the characteristics we have come to associate with being a person may not be applicable to each individual person. Therefore, it is necessary to establish criteria for a definition of 'person' in society and in time (Figures 16.3 and 16.4). Some prominent Italian professors[12] committed themselves to caring

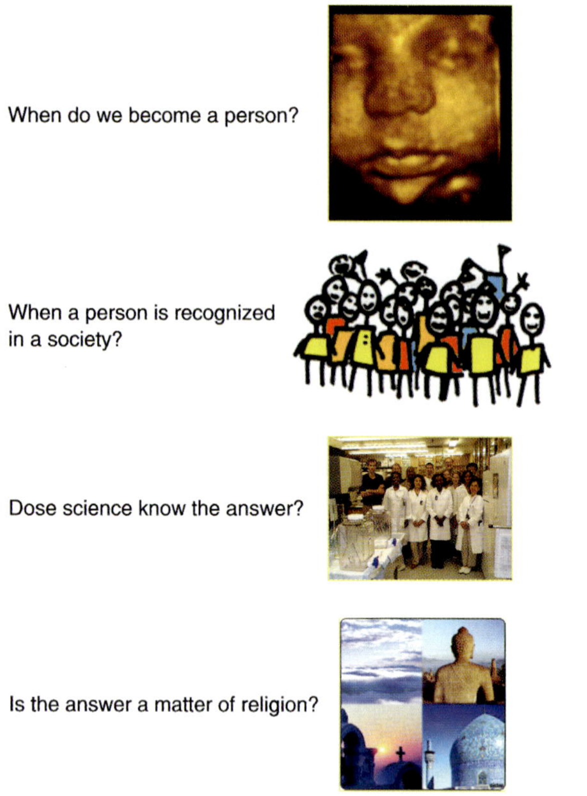

Figure 16.3 Some questions about the definition of a person.

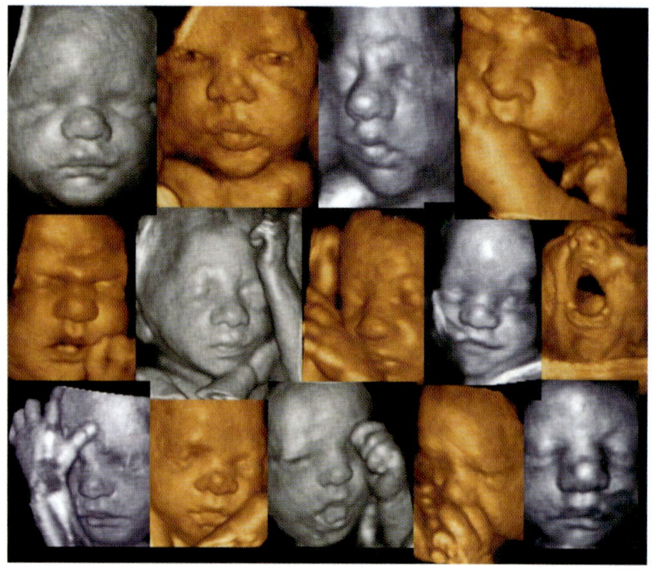

Figure 16.4 Different behavioral patterns of the fetuses in the second half of pregnancy. Are they different personalities?

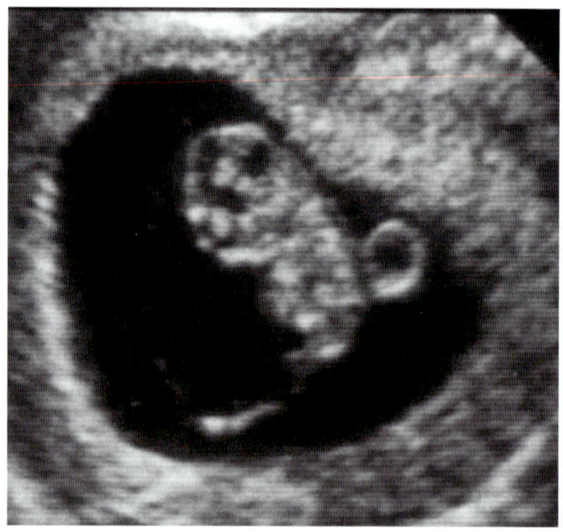

Figure 16.5 Transvaginal sonography of the 8-week embryo with yolk sac.

for the embryo in such a way, giving the same dignity to every patient, and the human conditions to grow and develop, to educate others inside and outside the specialty, and to carry out research involving all the components of society.

Embryo as a patient – bioethical aspects

The idea of the embryo/fetus as a miniaturized infant or adult is true to the extent that the embryonic/fetal physiologist must be able to apply knowledge of every system after birth, yet quite untrue in failing to recognize the many ways in which life before birth differs fundamentally from life after birth.[6] The newly conceived form presents itself as the biologically defined reality: it is an individual that is completely human in development, that autonomously, moment by moment without any discontinuity, actualizes its proper form in order to realize through intrinsic activity a design present in its own genome (Figures 16.5–16.10).[12] The embryo as a patient is best understood as the subset of the concept of the fetus as the patient. These two concepts opened a whole set of questions regarding ethical problems. The embryo as the patient is indivisible from its mother. However, balance is needed in protecting the interests of the embryo/fetus and the mother. One prominent approach to understanding the concept of the embryo/fetus as a patient has involved attempts to show whether or not the embryo/fetus has independent moral status, or personhood.[16–18] Independent moral status for the fetus would mean that one or more of the characteristics possessed either in or of the embryo/fetus itself, and therefore independently of the pregnant woman or any other factor, generate, and therefore ground, obligations to the embryo/fetus on the part of the pregnant woman and her physician.

A wide range of intrinsic characteristics have been considered for this role, e.g. moment of conception, implantation, central nervous system development, quickening, and moment of birth.[19] Given the variability of proposed characteristics, there are many

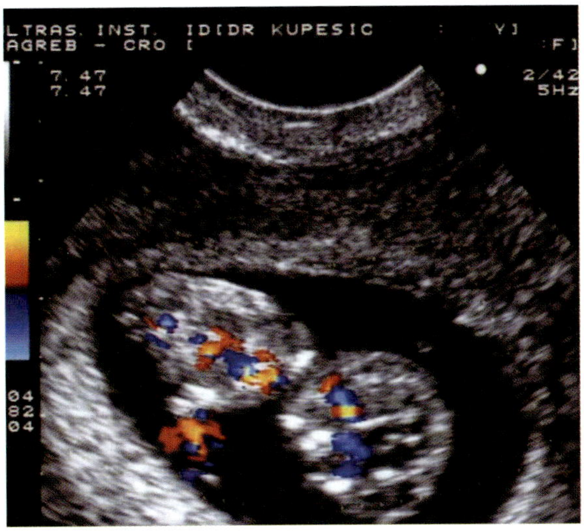

Figure 16.6 Color Doppler visualization of the entire embryonic circulation.

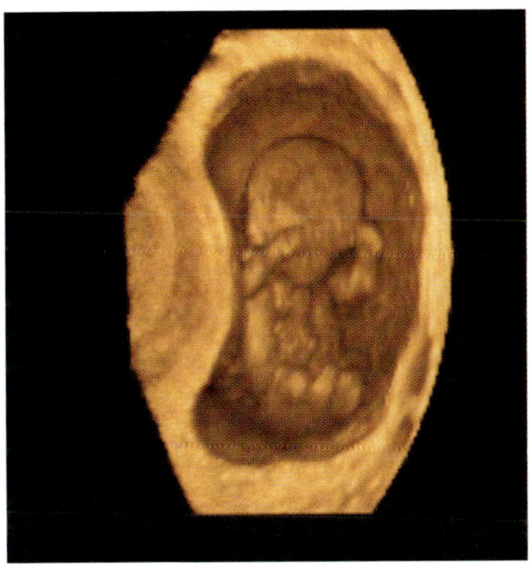

Figure 16.7 Ten weeks' gestation. Intrauterine content with early fetus. Many anatomical landmarks are visible.

views about when the embryo/fetus does or does not acquire independent moral status. Some take the view that the embryo/fetus possesses independent moral status from the moment of conception or implantation. Others believe that the embryo/fetus acquires independent moral status in degrees, thus resulting in 'graded' moral status. Still others hold, at least implicitly, that the embryo/fetus never has independent moral status so long as it is *in utero*.[18]

Being a patient does not require that one possesses independent moral status.[20] Being a patient means that one can benefit from the application of the clinical skills of the physician.[21] Put more precisely, a human being without independent moral status is properly regarded as a patient when the following conditions are met: that a human being is presented to the physician for the purpose of applying clinical interventions that are reliably expected to be efficacious,

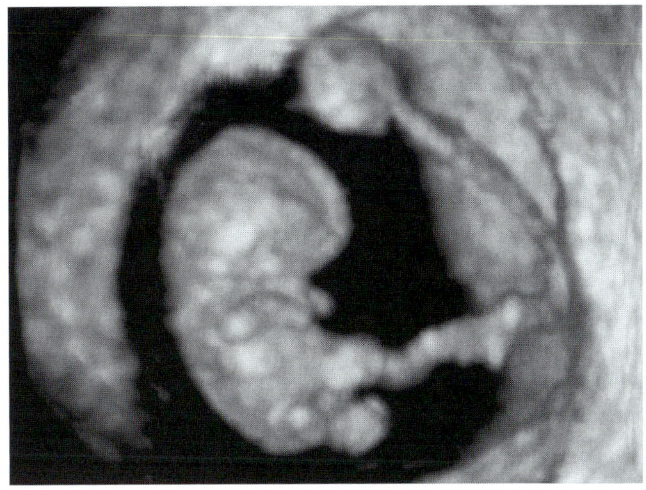

Figure 16.8 Nine-week embryo with vitelline duct and yolk sac seen in three dimensions.

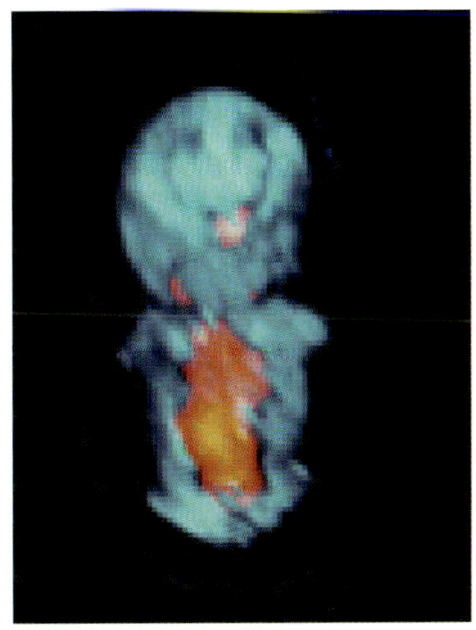

Figure 16.9 Eleven-week embryo with entire peripheral and central vascularization visualized by 3D power Doppler.

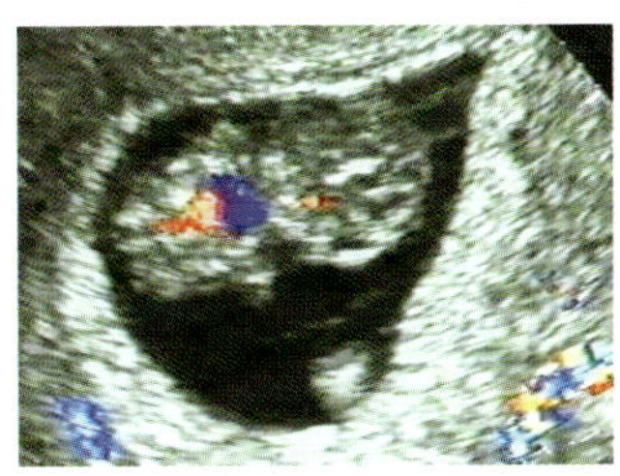

Figure 16.10 The earliest detection of brain circulation at 7 weeks and 4 days of gestation.

in that they are reliably expected to result in a greater balance of benefits over harms in the future of the human being in question.[19] In other words, an individual is considered a patient when a physician has beneficence-based ethical obligations to that individual.

To clarify the concept of the embryo/fetus as the patient, beneficence-based obligation is necessary to be provided. Beneficence-based obligations to the fetus and embryo exist when the fetus can later achieve independent moral status.[21] This leads to the conclusion that ethical significance of the unborn child is in direct link with the child to be born – the child it can become.

Legal status of the embryo

When discussing law, it should be always kept in mind that medicine is international, but law is not. Before the era of Aristotle, who taught that human life begins when the fetus is formed, human life was considered to begin at birth. Prior to birth, the fetus was not an independent human being but, like an organ, part of the mother.[22] Thus, the birth of a full-term infant has been used in the laws of various countries to signify the beginning of the human life that is to be protected.

Indeed, the status of the human embryo is not juridically defined and relies on the political, social, and religious influences in each country. Interestingly, nearly all countries of the Western world use the 12th week of pregnancy as the limit for legal abortion. It is not the end of the first trimester, which is 13.3 weeks, and there is no other particular biological event to justify this limit.

It is hard to answer the question when human life should be legally protected. At the time of conception? At the time of implantation? At the time of birth? (Figure 16.11). In all countries (except Ireland and Liechtenstein) juridical considerations are based on Roman law. Roman civil law says that the fetus has rights when it is born or if it is born-nasciterus.

Few countries agree with the definition of the beginning of human personality at the time of conception. The majority does not grant legal status to the human embryo *in vitro* (i.e. during the 14 days after fertilization). Thus, even in the absence of legal rights, there is no denying that the embryo constitutes the beginning of human life, a member of the human family. Therefore, whatever the attitude, every country has to examine which practices are compatible with the respect of that dignity and the security of human genetic material.[23]

Arguments for beginning of human life and human person at fertilization

The fundamental approaches of biomedical and social (secular) practice must begin with the understanding that the subject before birth is a person and that 'personhood' is conferred by successful fertilization of the egg. To hide from this in silence or ignorance should be unacceptable to all, as stressed by Scarpelli.[9]

The view that human life begins when sperm and eggs fuse to give rise to a single-cell human zygote, whose genetic individuality and uniqueness remain unchanged during normal development, is widely supported. Because the zygote has the capacity to become an adult human individual, it is thought it must be one already. The same zygote organizes itself into an embryo, a fetus, a child, and an adult. By this account, the zygote is an actual human individual and not simply a potential one, in much the same way as an infant is an actual human person with potential to develop to maturity and not just a potential person. As Scarpelli pointed out, outside the realm of religious dogma, there has been no one whose existence can be traced back to any entity other than the fertilized egg. The biological line of existence of each individual, without exception, begins precisely when fertilization of the egg is successful.[9]

The process of fertilization actually begins with conditioning of the spermatozoon in the male and female reproductive tracts. Thereafter, fertilization involves not only the egg itself, but also the various investments that surround the egg at the time it is released from the ovary follicle. Fertilization, therefore, is not an event, but a complex biochemical process requiring a minimum of 24 h to complete syngamy, that is, the formation of a diploid set of chromosomes. During this process, there is no commingling of maternal and paternal chromosomes within a single nuclear membrane (prezygote); after this process, the parental chromosomes material is commingled (zygote).

Among the many other activities of this new cell, most important is the recognition of the new genome, which represents the principal information center for the development of the new human being and for all its further activities. For the better understanding of the very nature of the zygote, two main features are to be at least mentioned here. The first feature is that the zygote exists and operates from syngamy on as a being, ontologically one, and with a precise identity. The second feature is that the zygote is intrinsically oriented and determined to a definite development. Both identity and orientation are due essentially to the genetic information with which it is endowed. That is why many do believe that this cell represents the exact point in time and space where a new human individual organism initiates its own life cycle.[1]

Arguments against the beginning of human life at fertilization

Today, one largely accepted opinion is that until the 14th day from fertilization – or at least, until implantation – the human embryo may not be considered, from the ontological point of view, as an individual. There are at least five main reasons in favor of this opinion:

(1) Before the formation of the embryonic disk, the embryo is 'a mass of cells, genetically human', 'a

cluster of distinct individual cells', which are each 'distinct ontological entities in simple contact with the others' (see Ref.[24], pp. 137–46). The genetically unique, newly developed DNA, a genome, is not established until 48 h after sperm penetration. The ovum and sperm lie side by side for more than 48 h before they finally merge. In biological terms, this renders conception as a process that occurs over time and not at a specific point in time.[3]

(2) Until approximately the 14th day after fertilization, all that happens is simply a preparation of the protective and nutritional systems required for the future needs of the embryo. Only when the entity called embryonic disk is formed can the embryo develop into a fetus.[25]

(3) The monozygotic twins phenomenon or chimeras can occur. In fact, this seems to be the strongest reason why the embryo is denied the quality of individuality, and proof that the zygote cannot be an ontologically human being. In approximately one-third of the cases the embryo divides at about the two-cell stage, and in the other two-thirds, the inner cell mass divides within the blastocyst from day 38. Occasionally, the division takes place from day 8 to day 12, but usually it is not complete, thereby forming conjoined identical twins or two-headed individuals.

The chimera, resulting from the recombination of two individua to become one individuum (and detectable through genetic testing) provides another argument against the equivalence of conception and the beginning of human life: no individuum has died, yet one has ceased to exist.

(4) Coexistence of the embryo with its mother is a necessary condition for an embryo belonging to the human species, and this condition can be obtained only at implantation.[18] However, there is evidence that development of a human embryo *in vitro* can continue well beyond the stage of implantation, and that mouse embryos implanted under the male renal capsule can reach the fetal stage. It is also argued, or at least implied, that so many human embryos die before or after implantation that it would be lacking in realism to accept that the human individual begins before implantation.

It is well known that high percentages of oocytes that have been penetrated never proceed on to further development, and that many oocytes that do are thwarted so early in their development that their presence is not even recognized. Up to 50% of ovulated eggs and zygotes recovered after operations were found so grossly abnormal that it would be very unlikely that they would result in viable pregnancies. It is also suggested that 30% of conceptions detected by positive reactions to HCG tests abort spontaneously before these pregnancies are clinically verified. The scientific literature is not unanimous on the incidence of natural wastage prior to, and during, implantation in humans, varying from 15% to as much as 50%. The vast majority of these losses are due to chromosomal defects caused during gametogenesis and fertilization.[26]

Genetic uniqueness and singleness coincide only after implantation and restriction have completed, which is about 3 weeks after fertilization. Until that period, the zygote and its sequelae are in a fluid process and are not a physical individual, and therefore cannot be a person.

Although in a set of twins one individuum can disappear, genetic and individual identities are now more or less equivalent. Many eminent Catholic writers, among them the Australian priest Norman Ford, author of *When Did I Begin?*, consider implantation to mark the beginning of human life; they maintain that the pre-embryo has only intrinsic potential and must be protected only from the time of implantation.[27]

(5) The product of fertilization may be a tumor, a hydatidiform mole, or chorioepithelioma. Though the mole is alive and of human origin, it is definitely not a human individual or human being. It lacks a true human nature from the start and has no natural potential to begin human development.

A teratoma is another clear instance of cells developing abnormally that results from the product of fertilization, but which could not be considered to be a true human individual with a human nature. It has no potential to develop into an entire fetus or infant. Clearly, the fetus with the teratoma would be a human individual, but not the attached teratoma itself. Obviously, not all the living cells that develop from the conceptus, the early embryo, or the fetus form an integral part of a developing human individual.[1]

Different religious teachings and historical aspects

The Catholic Church's teachings are clearly described in the Introduction of *Donum Vitae*: 'A human creature is to be respected and treated as a person from conception and therefore from that same time his (her) rights as a person must be recognized, among which in the first place is the invaluable right to life of each innocent human creature'.

In 1997 the Third Assembly of the Pontifical Academy for Life was held in Vatican City. It has been concluded that 'at the fusion of two gametes, a new real human individual initiates its own existence, or life cycle, during which – given all the necessary and sufficient conditions – it will autonomously realize all the potentialities with which he is intrinsically endowed'. The embryo, therefore, from the time the gametes fuse, is a real human individual, not a potential human individual. It was even added that recent findings of human biological science recognize that in zygotes resulting from fertilization, the biological identity of a new human individual is already constituted.[28,29]

In Western Europe and in North and South America these opinions are mostly based on Judeo-Christian theology; in Arabian countries, in Africa, and in Asia the influences of the Islamic and Buddhist religions prevail. Although their approach to the beginning of human life is impressively similar, each of these religions has different attitudes to the problem of embryo research, infertility and its therapy. In fact, while the Jewish attitude toward infertility is expressed in the Talmud sayings and in the Bible (synthesized in the first commandment of God to Adam: 'Be fruitful and multiply'), the Christian point of view establishes no absolute right to parenthood. According to the Islamic views, attempts to cure infertility are not only permissible, but also a duty.

Islamic teaching is based on Prophet Mohammed's description:

> The creation of each of you in his mother's abdomen assumes a "nufta" [male and female semen drops] for 40 days, then becomes "alaga" for the same [duration], then a "mudgha" [like a chewed peace of meat] for the same, then God sends an angel to it with instructions. The angel is ordered to write the Sustenance, life span, deeds and whether eventually his lot is happiness or misery, then to blow the Spirit into him. (Human developments as described in the Khur'an and Sunnah; Moore *et al.* In *Some Evidence for the Truth of Islam*, 1981)

The summary of this poetic and sacred description is: 'Soul breathing "ensoulment" occurs at 120 days of gestation from conception'.

To make this religious principle applicable to the practice, the Islamic Jurisprudence Council wrote a fatwa in 1990 that said: 'Abortion is allowed in the first 120 days of conception if it is proven beyond doubt that the fetus is affected with a severe malformation that is not amenable to therapy, and if his life, after being born, will be a means of misery to both him and his family, and his parents agree', so that there is no difficulty for either the prenatal diagnosis, or for the possible termination of pregnancy within the exposed limits.

Buddhism has imposed strict ethics on priests, but it has relatively lenient attitudes toward lay people, so if medical treatment for infertility is available, people should make use of it.

For about 2000 years the opinions of Aristotle, the great Greek philosopher and naturalist, on the beginning of the human being were commonly held. He argued that the male semen had a special power residing in it, pneuma, to transform the menstrual blood, first into a living being with a vegetative soul after 7 days, and subsequently into one with a sensitive soul 40 days after contact with the male semen.[30]

Aquinas adopted Aristotle's theory, but specified that rational ensoulment took place through the creative act of God to transform the living creature into a human being once it had acquired a sensitive soul. The first conception took place over 7 days, while the second conception, or complete formation of the living individual with a complete human nature, lasted 40 days.[24]

Hippocrates believed that entrance of the soul into the male embryo occurred on the 30th day of intrauterine life. It entered into the female embryo on the 40th day. Actually, this idea was a considerable improvement on the scheme found in the *Book of Leviticus*, where it is suggested that the soul does not enter the female until 40 days after the conception.[31]

In short, the rational soul enables the matter to become a human being, an animated body, an embodied soul, a human person.

Harvey's experiments with deer in 1633 proved Aristotle's theory of human reproduction wrong, without finding a satisfactory explanation of human conception. After modern scientists discovered the process of fertilization, most people took it for granted that human beings, complete with a rational soul, began once fertilization had taken place.

It is clear that the answer to the question 'When has the human being actually come to life?' could only be given by combining the cognition of different religions, philosophies, and various biological scientific disciplines. There is a very fine line between the competence of science and that of metaphysics, and it greatly depends on the individual's philosophical principles. These two, more or less autonomous intellectual disciplines have very often tried dominating one another, or ignoring each other. It is only recently that the majority of scientists and some theologians have come to realize that the separate meanings of scientific and religious 'truths' complement each other, thus representing methodologically independent entities. Current science is not interested in what Nature is, but in the facts that could be stated regarding it, thus trying to explain the term, rather then inventing it. The main difference between science and religion can be seen in the fact that scientific 'truths', unlike religious postulates, can and must be experimentally verified and the methods of scientific cognition can be easily explained and learnt. Whereas religion favors irrationality, science prefers an entirely rational approach to matters of importance. Intellectual cognition, when scientifically expressed, usually is in the form of mathematical formulas and presented quantitatively. Contrarily, religion tends to keep its truths in the form of metaphoric expressions, preferring qualitative presentation. Today, there is a tendency, on a higher level, to reopen the dialog between science and religion, which was present at the very beginning of our culture. Religion had existed long before science came to life, but science is not to be thought of as a continuation of religion. Each discipline should preserve its principles, its separate interpretations, and its own conclusions. In the end, both of them represent different components of the one and indivisible culture of mankind.

Clinical controversies

There are some clinical controversies pertinent in any discussion of when life begins. Spermatozoa are living cells. They present evidence that they are living by their motility. They are equipped with an effective mechanism for movement in the form of a tail that beats under the control of the cytoplasmic droplets within the head. These living cells, which have been manufactured in the testes, are released into the environment provided by the male reproductive tract. They are not yet capable of fertilization. The spermatozoon must first come under the influence of the male reproductive tract, where it acquires the ability to function in fertilization. Even after ejaculation, it is capable of penetrating the egg, and it is modified further by exposure to the female reproductive tract, taking on the ability or capacity to fertilize. The decision must be made as to whether the spermatozoon is a being (i.e. living and human with the potential for continued life once fertilization has occurred), albeit in another form, it is entitled to the right of protection as a person. Those who deny right for life to the spermatozoon might argue that it is not a complete human cell chromosomally – it contains only the haploid number of chromosomes. Paradoxically, those who take that point of view would insist that an individual born with fewer or more chromosomes than normal is human and entitled to all the rights of 'personhood'. As Mastroianni stressed, the decision to base the definition of 'human life' solely on the number of chromosomes in a given cell has far-reaching implications.[32]

Furthermore, life has been defined as being terminated when brain activity ends. If we were to say that life begins when brain activity starts, we would be admitting that the definition of the beginning of life is dependent on technology and not on ethics or morality.

Some suggested that the beginning of human life requires the neural fusion of the periphery with the center, as well as sufficient development of the brain itself.[33] Brody formulated the so-called symmetry concept: if the death of a human being requires the death of the brain, the beginning of human life shall correspond with the beginning of the life of the brain, considered to be at day 32 pc.[34] However, Sass has correctly pointed out that fusion is not established anatomically without neurons that form synapses, which would be expected from embryological development at 70 days (8 weeks) pc.[35]

In this light, let us take, for example, the accepted definition of birth, which some years ago was described as the complete expulsion of a fetus of 1000 g or 28 weeks of pregnancy. With advances in perinatal and neonatal intensive care, the line was drawn at 500 g, or approximately 22 weeks of gestation, some years later. This meant that a 20-week-old fetus was not born by definition, even if it was viable. This concept has changed. The same logic applies to a live fetus being accorded the term 'life', if we use such definitions as the beginning of brain activity or ultrasonic proof of heartbeat and movement. The establishment of each of these parameters is shifted to an earlier stage year by year by improving technological refinements in electronic and ultrasonic equipment. This leads us to the conclusion that to follow this line of reasoning means to give life, birth, and viability definitions determined by technology. The more advanced the technology, the earlier life begins.

In any consideration of the beginning of human life, it helps to think about when life ends. Let us consider the following. A 2-week-old newborn is hospitalized with massive brain injury suffered in an automobile accident. Despite all measures, no electrical or other brain activity can be detected during the next 2 days and the child is pronounced dead. Its body parts may survive after its death, as after the death of every person of whatever age. Hair and nails grow for days. Kidneys, heart, liver, and other organs may go on living for years if transplanted into another individual. Cells taken soon after death and cultured in a laboratory might live well beyond the 72 or more years this child might have lived, although the life of the infant has ended. The conclusion reached in this case – that death of the brain means the end of life – is generally accepted by physicians, courts, and the public.[4]

Returning to the question of when life begins, it is true that the DNA of the fertilized egg has the information necessary to form an individual, but so does virtually every other cell in the body. Nobody would claim full rights for the living cells of the infant killed in the accident, although each has a complete library of DNA. Nor would they for thousands of living skin cells we lose every time we wash our hands and face. Is there some stage in the development of the brain that is critical? Or is it the time at which the fetus can survive outside the womb, with or without the support of medical technology? Should we revert to a criterion used for many years, the time of quickening, when one can feel the fetus moving? These are questions still to be answered.

Visualization of early human development

Significant advances have been made in recent years in visualizing and analyzing the earliest human development. Most of them have been done by introduction of three-dimensional (3D) static and color Doppler and 4D sonography. Many new parameters about early human development are now studied directly by new ultrasound techniques.

A considerable number of biochemical, morphological, and vascular changes occur within the follicle during the process of ovulation and luteinization and most of them can be studied by transvaginal ultrasound with color Doppler and 3D facilities.[36] If the oocyte is fertilized, the embryo is transported into the uterus where, under favorable hormonal and environmental conditions, it will implant and develop into a new and unique individual. The introduction of transvaginal color Doppler improved the recognition of blood vessels enabling detailed examination of small vessels such as arteries supplying preovulatory follicle, corpus luteum, and endometrium.[25]

Perifollicular vascularization can help in identification of follicles containing high-quality oocytes, with a high probability of recuperating, fertilizing, cleaving, and implanting, while 3D ultrasound enables accurate morphological inspection and detection of cumulus oophorus. Follicles without visualization of the cumulus by multiplanar imaging are not likely to contain fertilizable oocytes. This information is especially useful in patients undergoing ovulation induction.

Following ovulation, the corpus luteum is formed as the result of many structural, functional, and vascular changes in the former follicular wall. Color Doppler studies of the luteal blood flow velocities enable evaluation of the corpus luteum function in the second phase of the menstrual cycle and in early pregnancy. When the placenta takes over the role of production of progesterone, the corpus luteum starts regressing.

After ovulation there is a short period during which the endometrial receptivity is maximal. During these few days a blastocyst can attach to the endometrium and provoke increased vascular permeability and vasodilatation at the implantation site. Trophoblast-produced proteolytic enzymes cause the penetration of the uterine mucosa and erode adjacent maternal capillaries. This results in the formation of the intercommunicating lacunar network – the intervillous space of the placenta. A small intradecidual gestational sac can be visualized by transvaginal sonography between 32 and 34 days.[37]

The secondary yolk sac is the earliest extraembryonic structure normally seen within the gestational sac in the beginning of the fifth gestational week (Figure 16.8). The yolk sac volume was found to increase from 5 to 10 weeks' gestation. When the yolk sac reaches its maximum volume at around 10 weeks, it has already started to degenerate, which can be indirectly proved by a significant reduction in visualization rates of the yolk sac vascularity.[24] Therefore, a combination of functional and volumetric studies by 3D power Doppler helps to identify some of the most important moments in early human development.

The embryonic heart begins beating on about days 22–23, accepting blood components from the yolk sac and pushing blood into the circulation. The embryonic blood begins circulating at the end of the fourth week of development.

The start of the embryo–chorionic circulation changes the source of nourishment to all intraembryonic tissues. The survival and further development of the embryo become dependent on the circulation of embryonic/fetal blood. If the embryo–chorionic circulation does not develop, or fails, the conceptus is aborted. The embryo cannot survive without the chorion (placenta) and the chorion will not survive without the embryo. Avascular degenerated chorionic villi constitute the hydatidiform mole.

Within the embryo, there are three distinct blood circulatory systems:[10]

(1) *Vitelline circulation* (from yolk sac to embryo)
(2) *Intraembryonic circulation*
(3) *Two umbilical arteries* (from embryo to placenta – fetoplacental circulation)

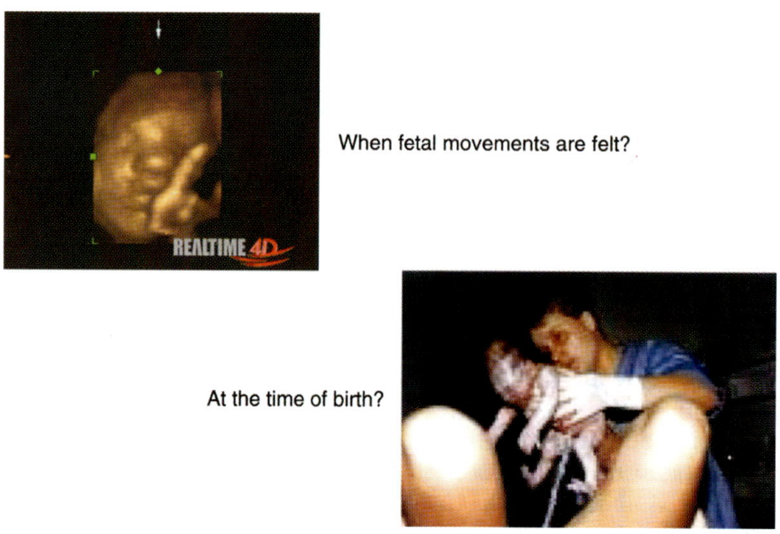

Figure 16.11 Another possible question about the beginning of human life.

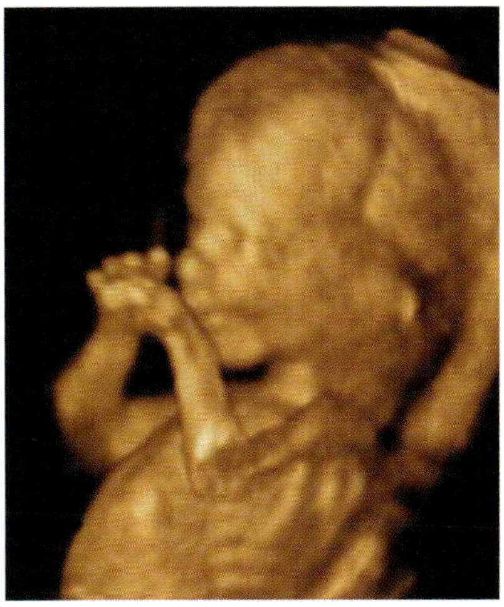

Figure 16.12 Hand near face movement of the fetus at 16 weeks of gestation, as seen by 3D ultrasound.

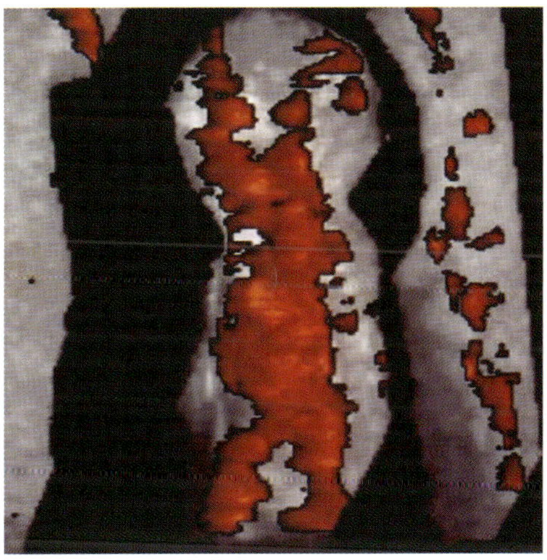

Figure 16.13 Early triplets clearly visualized by 3D sonography.

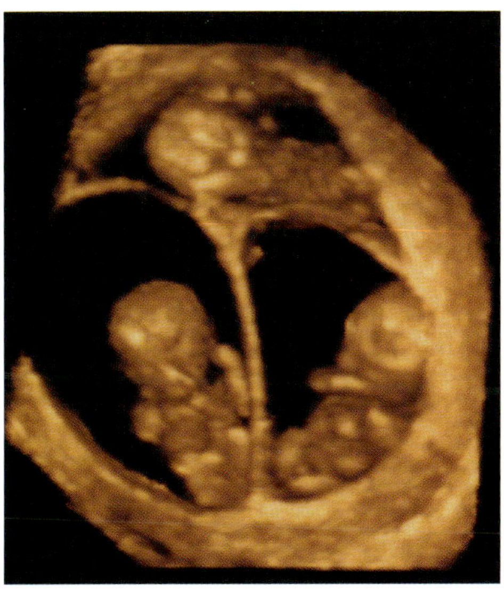

Figure 16.14 Illustrative example of the complex fetal movements recorded by 4D sonography at 12 weeks' gestation.

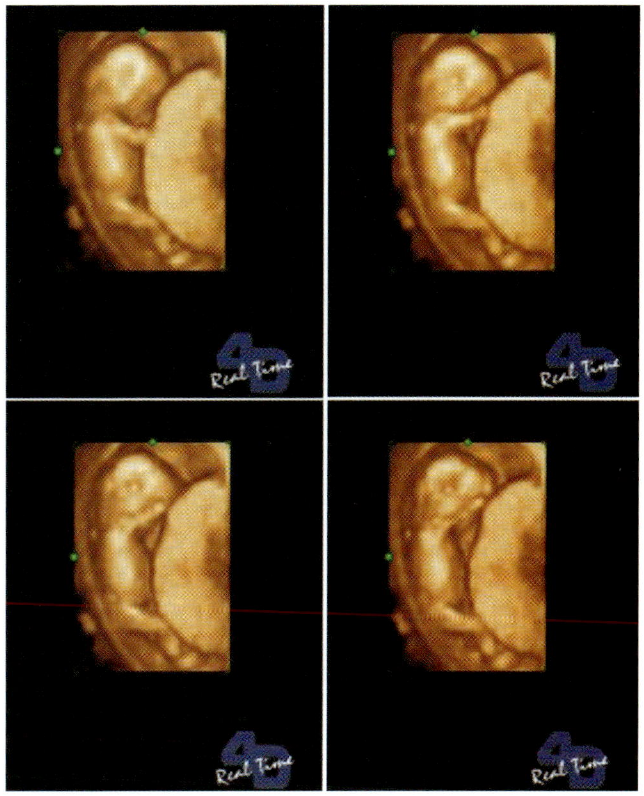

Figure 16.15 Fourteen-week fetus. Complete vascular anatomy of fetal and placental circulation shown by 3D power Doppler.

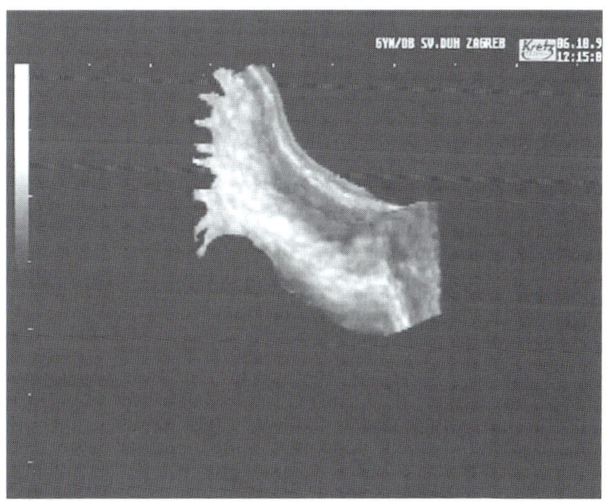

Figure 16.16 3D sonography visualization of the part of fallopian tube.

It is possible to visualize and assess them virtually from conception.[38–42]

At 5 weeks from the maternal side of the placenta, it is possible to obtain simultaneous 3D imaging of the developing intervillous circulation during the first trimester of pregnancy. 3D power Doppler reveals intensive vascular activity surrounding the chorionic shell starting from the first sonographic evidence of the developing pregnancy during the fifth week of gestation.

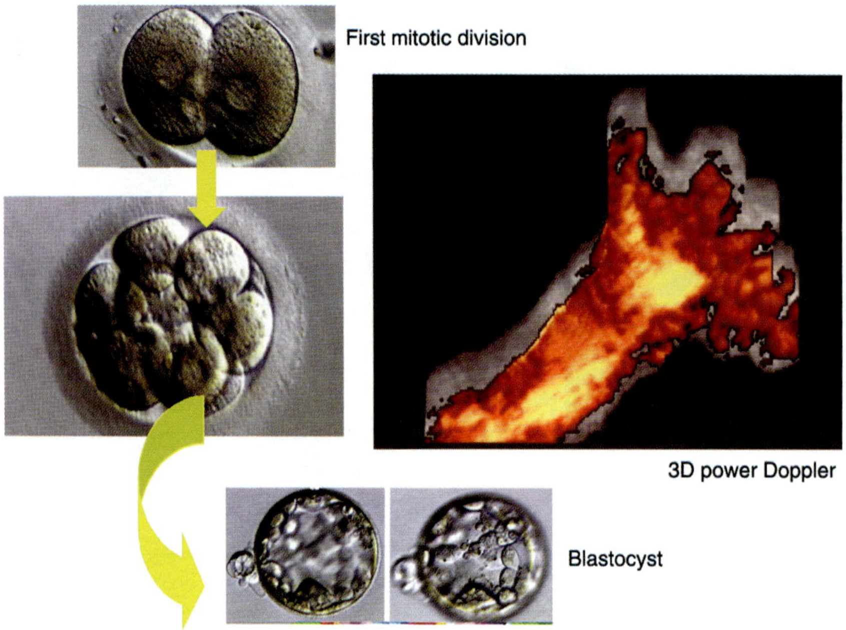

Figure 16.17 Visualization of the patency of fallopian tube by 3D power Doppler sonography, important for successful first mitotic division and transfer of early embryo to uterus.

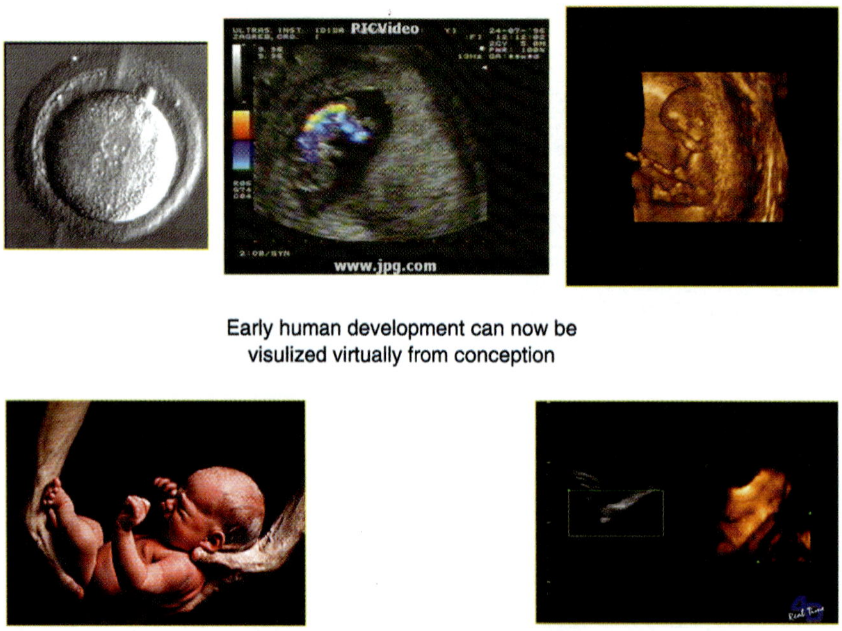

Figure 16.18 Illustrative example of the use of different medical methods to assess early human development.

At 7 weeks, 3D power Doppler images depict aortic and umbilical blood flow. Initial branches of umbilical vessels are visible at the placental umbilical insertion.

During the eighth and ninth weeks, the developing intestine is being herniated into the proximal umbilical cord.

At 9–10 weeks, herniation of the midgut is present. The arms with elbow and legs with knee are clearly visible, while feet can be seen approaching the midline.

At 11 weeks, 3D power Doppler imaging allows visualization of the entire fetal and placental circulation (Figures 16.6, 16.9, 16.10, and 16.12).

During the 11th and 12th week of pregnancy, development of the head and neck continues. Facial details such as nose, orbits, maxilla, and mandibles are often visible. Herniated midgut returns into the abdominal cavity.

New possibilities for studying embryonic movements and behavior

The latest development of 3D and 4D sonography enables the precise study of embryonic and fetal activity

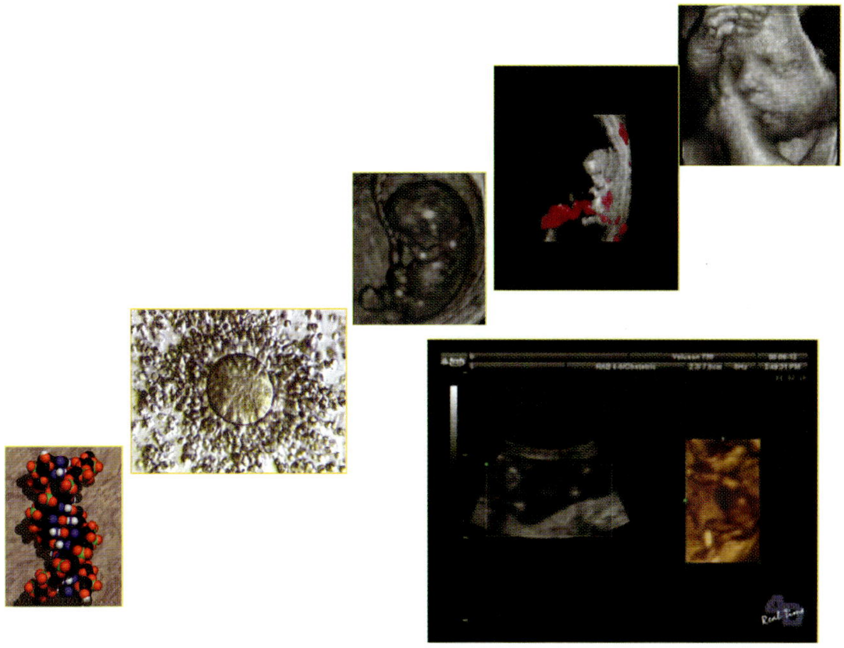

Figure 16.19 Integrated slide showing continuity of scientific visualization of the beginning of early human development from genetic material to oocyte, morphology of embryo, its vascularization, and fetal behavioral pattern assessed by 4D sonography.

and behavior (Figure 16.13).[43] With 4D ultrasound, movements of head, body, and all four limbs and extremities can be seen simultaneously in three dimensions.[44] Therefore, the earliest phases of the human anatomical and motor development can be visualized and studied simultaneously (Figures 16.11, 16.14, 16.18, and 16.19). It is clear that neurologic development – early fetal motor activity and behavior – needs to be re-evaluated by this new technique.[45–47] Our group studied the development of the complexity of spontaneous embryonic and fetal movements.[48] With the advancing of the gestational age, the movements become more and more complex. The increase in the number of axodendritic and axosomatic synapses between 8 and 10, and again between 12 and 15 weeks,[49] correlates with the periods of fetal movement differentiation and with the onset of general movements and complex activity patterns, such as swallowing, stretching, and yawning, seen easily by 4D technique. By 7–8 weeks of pregnancy, gross body movements appear. They consist of changing the position of the head toward the body. By 9–10 weeks of pregnancy, limb movements appear. They consist of changing the position of the extremities toward the body without the extension or flexion in elbow and knee. At 10–12 weeks of pregnancy, complex limb movements appear. They consist of changes in the position of limb segments toward each other, such as extension and flexion in elbow and knee (Figure 16.14).

Between 12 and 15 weeks of pregnancy, swallowing, stretching, and yawning activities appear. In addition to these activities, it is now feasible to study by 4D ultrasound a full range of facial expression including smiling, crying, and eyelid movement (Figure 16.15).

It is hoped that the new 4D technique will help us have a better understanding of both somatic and motoric development of the early embryo. It will also enable the reliable study of fetal and even parental behavior.[44]

Conclusion

The question of when a human life begins and how to define it could be answered only through the interconnecting pathways of history, philosophy, medical science, and religion (Figures 16.16–16.19). It has not been easy to determine where to draw the fine line between the competence of science and metaphysics in this delicate philosophical field. To a large extent the drawing of this line depends on one's fundamental philosophical outlook. To quote Beller:

> The point at which human life begins will always be seen differently by different individuals, groups, cultures, and religious faiths. In democracy there are always at least two sides, and the center holds only when the majority realizes that without a minority, democracy itself is lost. The minority in turn must realize its best chance lies in persuasion by reason and thoughtfulness rather than fanaticism.[3]

REFERENCES

1. Serra A, Colombo R. Identity and status of the human embryo: the contribution of biology. In de Dios Vial Correa, Sgreccia E, eds. *Identity and Statute of Human Embryo*. 1998;128.
2. Kurjak A. The beginning of human life and its modern scientific assessment. *Clin Perinatol* 2003;30:27–44.
3. Beller FK, Zlatnik GP. The beginning of human life. *J Assist Reprod Genet* 1995;12(8):477–83.
4. Kurjak A. When does human life begin? *Encyclopedia Moderna* 1992;383–90.
5. Godfrey J. The Pope and the ontogeny of persons (commentary). *Nature* 1995,273:100.
6. Liggins G (Mont). Foreword. In Nathanielsz PW, ed. *Life Before Birth and the Time to be Born*. Ithaca, New York: Promethean Press, 1992.
7. Gilbert SF. *Developmental Biology*. Sunderland, MA: Sinauer Associates, 1991;3.
8. Scarpelli EM. Postnatal through adult human life and the scientific deception. *Atti del I Congresso Nazionale della Societa Italiana di Medicina Materno Fetale*, Rome, March 17–21, 2003. Bologna, Italy: Medimond (International Proceedings), 2003:29–36.
9. Scarpelli EM. Personhood: a biological phenomenon. *J Perinat Med* 2001;29:417–26.
10. Jirasek JE. *An Atlas of the Human Embryo and Fetus*. New York: Parthenon Publishing, 2001.
11. ACOG Committee Opinion: Committee on Ethics. Preembryo research: history scientific background, and ethical considerations. *Int J Gynecol Obstet* 1994;45:291–301.
12. Declaration of Professors from Five Faculties of Medicine and Surgery of the Universities of Rome, Organizers of the Conference: *The Embryo as a Patient*. "La Sapienza" University Press, 2004.
13. Sass HM. Brain life and brain death: a proposal for normative agreement. *J Med Philos* 1989;14:45–59.
14. Veatch RM. The beginning of full moral standing. In Beller FK, Weir RF, eds. *The Beginning of Human Life*. Dordrecht: Kluwer, 1994:19.
15. Knutson AL. When does human life begin? Viewpoints of public health professionals. *Am J Public Health* 1967;57:2167.
16. Engelhardt HT Jr. *The Foundation of Bioethics*. New York: Oxford University Press, 1986.
17. Dunstan GR. The moral status of the human embryo. A tradition recalled. *J Med Ethics* 1984;10:38–44.
18. Chervenak FA, McCullough LB, Kurjak A. Ethical implications of the embryo as a patient. In Kurjak A, Chervenak FA, Carrera JM, eds. *The Embryo as a Patient*. New York: Parthenon Publishing Group, 2001:226–30.
19. Curran CE. Abortion: Contemporary debate in philosophical and religious ethics. In Reich WT, ed. *Encyclopedia of Bioethics*. New York: Macmillan, 1978:17–26.
20. Ruddick W, Wilcox W. Operating on the fetus. *Hastings Cent Rep* 1982;12:10–4.
21. McCullogh LB, Chervenak FA. *Ethics in Obstetrics and Gynecology*. New York: Oxford University Press, 1994.
22. Connery JR Jr. The ancients and medievals on abortion. In Horan DJ, Grant ER, Cunningham PC, eds. *Abortion and Constitution*. Washington, DC: Georgetown University Press, 1987:124.
23. Pierre F, Soutoul JH. Medical and legal complications (in French). *J Gynecol Obstet Biol Reprod (Paris)* 1994;23(5):516–9.
24. Ford NM. *When Did I Begin? Conception of the Human Individual in History, Philosophy and Science*. Cambridge: Cambridge University Press, 1991.
25. McLaren A. *Prelude to Embryogenesis, in the Ciba Foundation, Human Embryo Research, Yes or No?* London: Tavistock 1986; 5–23:12.
26. Abel F. Nascita e morte dell'uomo: prospettive della biologia e della medicina. In Biolo S, ed. *Nascita e morte dell'uomo. Problemi filosofici e scientifici della bioetica*. Genova: Marieti 1993:37–53.
27. McCormick KA. Who or what is the preembryo? *Kennedy Inst Ethics J* 1991;1:24.
28. Mahoney SJ. *Bioethics and Belief*. London: Sheed and Ward, 1984:80.
29. Johnson M. Delayed hominization. Reflections on some recent Catholic claims for delayed hominization. *Theol Stud* 1995;56:743–63.
30. Congregation for the Doctrine of the Faith. Instruction on respect for human life in its origin and on the dignity of procreation "Donum Vitae" (February 12, 1987). *Acta Apostolicae Sedis* 1988;80:70–102.
31. Beazley JM. Fetal assessment from conception to birth. In Kurjak A, ed. *Recent Advances in Ultrasound Diagnosis*. Amsterdam: Excerpta Medica 1980;2:128.
32. Kurjak A. Kada pocinje zivot. In Kurjak A, ed. *Ocekujuci novorodjence*. Zagreb: Naprijed, 1987:18–28.
33. Mastroianni L Jr. Ethical aspects of fetal therapy and experimentation. In Schenker JG, Weinstein D, eds. *The Intrauterine Life: Management and Therapy*. Amsterdam: Excerpta Medica, 1986:3–10.
34. Beller FK, Reeve J. Brain life and brain death: The anencephalic as an explanatory example. *J Med Philos* 1989;14:5–20.
35. Brody B. *Abortion and the Sanctity of Human Life: A Philosophical View*. Cambridge: MIT Press, 1975:109.
36. Sass HM. The moral significance of brain-life-criteria. In Beller FK, Weir RF, eds. *The Beginning of Human Life*. Dordrecht: Kluwer, 1994:57–70.
37. Kupesic S. The first three weeks assessed by transvaginal color Doppler. *J Perinat Med* 1996;24:310–7.
38. Kupesic S, Kurjak A, Ivancic-Kosuta M. Volume and vascularity of the yolk sac. *J Perinat Med* 1999;27:91–6.
39. Kurjak A, Predanic M, Kupesic S. Transvaginal color Doppler study of middle cerebral artery blood flow in early normal and abnormal pregnancy. *Ultrasound Obstet Gynecol* 1992;2: 424–8.
40. Kurjak A, Kupesic S. Doppler assessment of the intervillous blood flow in normal and abnormal early pregnancy. *Obstet Gynecol* 1997;89:252–6.
41. Kurjak A, Kupesic S, Hafner T. Intervillous blood flow in normal and abnormal early pregnancy. *Croat Med J* 1998;39(1):10.
42. Kurjak A, Kupesic S. Three-dimensional transvaginal ultrasound improves measurement of nuchal translucency. *J Perinat Med* 1999;27:97–102.
43. Kurjak A, Kupesic S, Banovic I, Hafner T, Kos M. The study of morphology and circulation of early embryo by three-dimensional ultrasound and power Doppler. *J Perinat Med* 1999;27:145–57.
44. Lee A. Four-dimensional ultrasound in prenatal diagnosis: Leading edge in imaging technology. *Ultrasound Rev Obstet Gynecol* 2001;1:144–8.
45. Campbell S. 4D, or not 4D: That is the question. *Ultrasound Obstet Gynecol* 2002;19:1–4.
46. de Vries JI, Visser GH, Prechtl HF. The emergence of fetal behaviour. I. Qualitative aspects. *Early Hum Dev* 1982;7: 301–22.
47. de Vries JI, Visser GH, Prechtl HF. The emergence of fetal behaviour. I. Qualitative aspects. *Early Hum Dev* 1985;12:99–120.
48. Kurjak A, Vecek N, Hafner T, Bozek T, Funduk-Kurjak B, Ujevic B. Prenatal diagnosis: What does four-dimensional ultrasound add? *J Perinat Med* 2002;30:57–62.
49. Kurjak A, Azumendi G, Vecek N, Kupesic S, Solak M, Varga D, Chervenak F. Fetal hand movements and facial expression in normal pregnancy studied by four-dimensional sonography. *J Perinat Med* 2003;31:496–508.
50. Okado N, Kojima T. Ontogenity of the central nervous system: Neurogenesis, fibre connection, synaptogenesis and myelinization in the spinal cord. In Prechtl HFR, ed. *Continuity of Neural Functions from Prenatal to Postnatal Life*. Oxford: Blackwell Scientific, 1984:46–64.

17 Preimplantation diagnosis

L. J. Nelson

Preimplantation genetic diagnosis (PGD) is a technique devised within the last 15 years used primarily to identify genetic disorders or defects in human embryos created by *in vitro* fertilization (IVF) prior to their implantation for gestation. The two dominant methods of PGD currently in use are polar body biopsy and blastomere biopsy on cleavage stage embryos, though fluorescence *in situ* hybridization has been used for PGD of common aneuploidies. PGD is an 'attractive means of preventing heritable genetic diseases', which, as an alternative to traditional prenatal genetic diagnosis following chorionic villus sampling (CVS) or amniocentesis, can avoid the need for selective abortion of the affected fetuses, even though it is strongly recommended that normality be confirmed by subsequent CVS or amniocentesis.[1] According to the National Society of Genetic Counselors, the primary reason for electing PGD over traditional prenatal diagnosis is the couple's objection to pregnancy termination.[2]

PGD is also used to detect aneuploidy (the major cause of inherited diseases) and to select chromosomally normal embryos for implantation, mostly in women of advanced maternal age undergoing IVF. The only known risk factor for aneuploidy is maternal age. While trisomies appear in 2% of recognized pregnancies of women 25 years old, this number increases up to 19% in women of 40 or more years of age.[3] One study found aneuploidy to be 52% in women aged 40–47 years.[4] PGD of aneuploidy has been shown to reduce the risk of children with trisomies, increase implantation rates, and decrease spontaneous abortions.[5]

Finally, in cases of parents who have children with bone marrow disorders, who are in need of human leukocyte antigen (HLA)-matched stem cell transplantation (e.g. acute lymphoid leukemia), and who wish to conceive another child to serve as a donor of stem cells, PGD can be employed to test embryos for causative gene mutations and simultaneously for HLA alleles with the goal of selecting and transferring only those unaffected embryos that are HLA matched to the sick child. A recent report documents this process as resulting in five singleton pregnancies and the birth of five HLA-matched healthy children.[6]

More than 1000 unaffected children have been born following PGD; this suggests that the procedure is both accurate and safe.[7] Even though PGD was described as experimental as recently as 1998,[8] it is now considered 'an established technique with specific and expanding applications for standard clinical practice', that is, 'a viable alternative to postconception diagnosis and pregnancy termination'.[1]

This chapter will review and comment on the central ethical issues raised by PGD. These fall into three major categories: (1) ethics and the provision of PGD, including the ethics of marketing PGD services, shared risk or refund programs, and disclosure and patient consent; (2) the moral status of the extracorporeal human embryo (those outside a woman's body) and its destruction following embryo selection; and (3) the ethically appropriate uses of PGD, including its use to prevent the birth of disabled persons and to select for sex and other traits for non-medical reasons. The last section examines the importance of each individual clinician making a personal decision, based on the exercise of an informed conscience, about the ethical propriety of his or her involvement in the provision of PGD services whether for the prevention of genetic disease and disability or for the selection of sex or some other trait unrelated to health.

Ethics and the provision of PGD

Marketing

Most of the utilization of IVF and, by implication, PGD, services is not covered by health insurance in the USA,[8] and this is likely true elsewhere in the world as well. Consequently, most individuals pay for these services directly out of their own private resources. With the average cost for an IVF cycle in the USA being $12,400,[9] the financial commitment for the individuals involved is substantial. Receiving direct payment from patients appeals to clinicians who are not required to wait weeks or months for insurer reimbursement, or to expend large amounts of time and effort in submitting reimbursement forms or obtaining pretreatment authorization. These factors make the provision of IVF and PGD an attractive and potentially profitable form of professional practice. The utilization of PGD adds several thousands of dollars in cost over and above those incurred for IVF.

Clinics providing IVF, PGD, and other reproductive health services often advertise in the mass media and make other efforts to attract patients (e.g. free informational seminars and internet sites). While advertising health care services is by no means inherently unethical, the traditional professional values of beneficence and loyalty to the patients' interests indicate that the provision of medical services ought not to resemble a common commercial transaction between strangers. Clinicians are in a fiduciary relationship with their patients and are obligated to act so as to deserve and maintain the patient's trust and confidence that their wishes and best interests are being faithfully served. Consequently, the marketing of infertility services ought to place the good of patients above other interests (especially a clinician's or clinic's own economic interests), should not induce patients to accept excessive, unneeded, or unproven services, and should adhere to high standards of honesty and accuracy in the information provided to the prospective patients.[10]

For example, one infertility clinic that used advertisements to entice persons to undergo IVF with language suggesting that 'the dream of having a child might still come true for you' can be criticized as selling profitable services at the expense of vulnerable people suffering from the anguish and disappointment of childlessness. Another IVF clinic used chemical rather than clinical pregnancies in calculating its 'success' rate, a misleading number as only a relatively small portion of chemical pregnancies result in live birth.[10] The success, that is, healthy live birth, rate of IVF and PGD varies by center, and the staff of each is ethically obligated to be scrupulously careful in calculating and disclosing its rates of success – and its rates of error as well. This is particularly important as many PGD centers have not reported their experience, and there currently is no systematic approach to presenting errors. Informal reports suggest an error rate in the range of 1–10%, depending on the disease and assay being evaluated.[1] The European Society for Human Reproduction and Embryology PGD consortium has reported clinical pregnancies in 17% of cases after testing for structural chromosomal abnormalities, 16% after sexing, and 21% after testing for monogenic diseases, while the International Working Group of Preimplantation Genetics has reported a pregnancy rate of about 24%.[11] The former also noted an error rate of 2–3%.

Shared risk programs

In addition to traditional fee-for-service pricing, some assisted reproduction programs offer IVF on a shared risk basis by refunding the patient(s) a portion of, or even all, specified fees (pretreatment screening and drug costs are typically excluded from refund) if the patient does not have a live birth or achieve an ongoing pregnancy. However, patients electing shared risk pay a significantly higher initial fee. These alternative payment plans have been criticized as being 'exploitative, misleading, and contrary to long-standing professional norms against charging contingent fees for medical services'.[12] There is also the objection that shared risk plans create a conflict of interest in which the clinician is induced to take steps to achieve pregnancy regardless of the impact on the patient in order to avoid paying the refund. Assuming fair and adequate disclosure of terms, defenders of the practice point out that it is a legitimate alternative payment plan given the usual absence of insurance coverage, which addresses patient concerns about the high cost of many cycles of IVF that fail to achieve pregnancy, a not uncommon outcome.

The claim that all such programs are misleading or exploiting those who are desperate to have a genetically related child by inducing them to purchase a more expensive set of services is not persuasive. While persons contemplating the utilization of expensive IVF services may well suffer greatly from their infertility and may feel some degree of desperation in their efforts to conceive a child, it is wrong to assume that they are inherently unable to determine their own best interests and make decisions with significant economic consequences. The clinicians involved are, of course, obligated to provide patients with sufficient information to make an informed choice of a shared risk plan rather than fee-for-service. The shared risk plans reviewed by the American Society for Reproductive Medicine (ASRM) Ethics Committee were found to meet this standard.[12]

The objection to shared risk plans as an unethical contingency fee is likewise misplaced. The American Medical Association Code of Medical Ethics states that 'a physician's fee should not be made contingent on the successful outcome of medical treatment'.[13] First, this prohibition is primarily aimed at physicians treating patients who are seeking compensation for their injuries through the legal system. A contingent fee arrangement would strongly tend to bias the physician's opinion in favor of more treatment and more expensive treatment than might be warranted. This concern is absent in assisted reproduction. Second, the prohibition is aimed at dispelling the implication that a good outcome is guaranteed and avoiding unrealistic patient expectations that follow from it. However, shared risks plans are offered precisely because the outcome of the procedure is in serious doubt and the provider is willing to accept some of the financial risk of failure with the patient at the latter's own election.

The final objection based on conflict of interest focuses on the likelihood of a clinician preferring (1) utilization of egg stimulation procedures that will not only produce more oocytes but also pose more risks to the woman's health and (2) transfer of a larger number of embryos in order to enhance the chances of pregnancy occurring but simultaneously increasing the chances of multiple gestation, which poses well-known risks to both offspring and parents. This objection has some merit. These dangers do exist, but they exist equally for IVF services provided on a fee-for-service basis. The solution is not to prohibit shared risk payment plans, but for clinicians both to carefully monitor their own behavior for strict conformance with the patient's best interests and to fully disclose to patients all of the risks and benefits, both to health and to wealth, of the different financing arrangements. Also, the ASRM Ethics Committee found no evidence that either danger mentioned here has actually materialized.[12]

Disclosure and informed consent

All clinicians should be scrupulous about the accuracy and the truthfulness of the methods they use to attract and secure patients who are dependent on professionals for knowledge about the health care services they receive. Likewise, all information provided by clinicians to patients wanting to utilize PGD should be complete, accurate, and devoid of ambiguity – in contrast with typical commercial information, which is often deliberately incomplete and ambiguous, and at least sometimes inaccurate. In particular, the risks, burdens, benefits, and probabilities of success, and the limits of PGD and IVF should be presented in a matter-of-fact manner and in terms easily accessible to persons unskilled in medical and scientific terminology. In particular, it is 'imperative that patients be aware of potential diagnostic errors and the possibility of currently unknown long-term consequences on the fetus [and subsequently born child] of the embryo biopsy procedure'.[1]

While the persons seeking PGD will almost certainly be competent adults with an above-average amount of education, they are also very likely to be struggling with the reproductive decisions they face and seriously worried about the outcomes. Clinicians providing PGD – and all other infertility and reproductive services – should be especially careful to avoid intentionally exploiting the anxiety and apprehension (or even desperation) of persons who know they are at risk of transmitting a genetic disease to their offspring.

Justice and ability to pay

Marked discrepancies in the use of prenatal genetic diagnosis already exist between affluent white women and other women in the USA.[8] As PGD becomes more available, this pattern will undoubtedly continue. It is certainly not inherently unethical for clinicians to offer health care services, such as cosmetic surgery, full body scans for detection of abnormalities, laser-assisted *in situ* keratomileusis (LASIK) vision correction, or PGD, which are available only to those who can afford to pay for them on their own. But the lack of broad availability of PGD for the less economically advantaged does becomes ethically problematic to the extent PGD satisfies fundamental human needs, but remains unavailable to them (like basic preventive and acute health care services) or produces additional social advantages for the well-to-do by enhancing their offspring, to which others cannot get access.[8] Insofar, as PGD can be legitimately considered as something owed as a matter of social justice to all persons in need, then it is the duty of the society in question to make PGD available to all. Finally, it is worth noting that it is seriously ethically questionable for public funds to be used in the development of PGD services when they are largely available only to persons of high socioeconomic status.

Moral status of the extracorporeal embryo

PGD is intended to result in the selective destruction (or the limbo of indefinite freezing) of extracorporeal human embryos following genetic analysis. Some consider PGD to be morally preferable to traditional prenatal genetic diagnosis because it precludes the need for an abortion to avoid the birth of a genetically abnormal child. This moral advantage to PGD can be understood in one of two ways. First, the woman who would have to undergo the abortion may find it morally preferable from her personal point of view to discard embryos prior to implantation rather than undergo a surgical or medical abortion with its attendant physical and psychological risks. Second, one could claim that discard is not morally wrong because extracorporeal embryos either lack moral status altogether or have less moral status than gestating embryos or fetuses, either of which makes destroying them *in utero* via abortion more morally problematic.

For many, the ethical acceptability of the destruction of human embryos turns much more on the inherent moral status or standing of the (gestating or extracorporeal) human embryo than on someone's moral preference for discard over abortion given that both end in the death of the human entity. If, as some contend, all human embryos have the same moral status as live-born persons,[14] then they are entitled to basic rights, including the right not to be killed arbitrarily or for the purpose of advancing the interests of other persons. In this view, PGD that resulted in the destruction of extracorporeal embryos, as well as abortion following traditional prenatal genetic diagnosis, would be seriously morally wrong. The opposing view would hold that embryos lack any moral status whatsoever as they lack any properties, such as sentience or other cognitive traits, that determine moral standing and hence can be destroyed at will.

Perhaps the more commonly held and the more ethically defensible position is that human embryos deserve some modest moral status because they are alive – embryos have some degree of potential to become human persons, and are in fact valued by moral agents whose views deserve at least some respect and deference from others, but they nevertheless do not possess the full and equal moral standing of persons because they lack interests and other moral claims to personhood. Having a modest level of moral status does not preclude the destruction of embryos for a morally serious reason or purpose, and the informed and conscientious choice of the persons who created the embryos to prevent the birth of a child with a serious genetic disease or abnormality is widely (though by no means universally) considered to be such a reason.

This ethical position roughly parallels that of current American constitutional law, which does not recognize embryos or fetuses as legal persons with rights (including the 14th Amendment rights not to be deprived of life, liberty, or property without due process of law and to have the equal protection of the laws), but recognizes considerable value in these entities through the State's substantial interest in preserving potential human life, an interest that becomes particularly compelling at viability.[15] This interpretation of constitutional personhood means that the State may ban postviability abortions (40 states have done so) unless an abortion is necessary to preserve the pregnant woman's life or health, but it may not totally ban previability abortions or otherwise place an undue burden on a woman's right to terminate her pregnancy.[16] In the absence of a state statute prohibiting the practice (and none exist at present), the discarding of embryos following PGD with the informed consent of the gamete sources cannot be considered a violation of the embryo's legal rights or be a form of criminal homicide in the USA. Whether the state could constitutionally ban PGD and IVF because they result in embryo discard is uncertain. Such a ban implicates not only the legal status of extracorporeal embryos, but also the constitutionally protected right of the persons whose gametes constitute the embryo to reproduce.[17]

However, the legal status of human embryos is not uniform around the world. Recently, the European Court of Human Rights ruled that the unborn are not human beings entitled to full human rights under applicable human rights conventions and that each national government must settle this legal issue for itself.[18] The legal status of embryos and the legal propriety of PGD vary in Europe. For example, PGD is currently illegal in Germany and Switzerland, although a recent study shows that a majority of Germans think the technique should be permitted for detecting genetic diseases.[19,20] The German Embryo Protection Law protects embryos from improper use and forbids genetic analysis of an embryo at the eight-cell stage or before.[21] One Austrian clinician has reported that the legal permissibility of PGD in Austria is unclear.[20] PGD has been authorized in France since 1994, but is strictly limited to cases in which there is a strong probability of the presence of a severe genetic disorder known to be incurable at the time of diagnosis.[22] The Human Fertilisation and Embryology Authority in the UK has licensed PGD for certain severe or life-threatening disorders at a limited number of clinics.[23] PGD is legally permitted in the Netherlands and Spain as well.[20]

Returning to the ethical analysis, the persons most humanly and ethically connected to human embryos are the individual men and women whose gametes wholly constitute the embryo. Almost all persons care deeply if their gametes or embryos are used for reproduction, and being a genetic parent is linked in profound ways to the individual's identity and the meaning he or she gives to life. Embryos ethically 'belong' to the people who created them, even if they are not property like inanimate objects.[24]

Consequently, even though embryos themselves have only a modest moral status, it is nonetheless seriously morally wrong to use the extracorporeal embryos of persons for any purpose without their informed consent. A corollary to this view is that the discarding of embryos secondary to PGD with the informed consent of the persons whose gametes created them is morally proper. In other words, the persons who created an embryo have the right of exclusive control over the disposition of those embryos, a right grounded in their interest in making the intimate, personal decision of when and how to reproduce. As no one else has a more significant moral connection to the embryos than the persons who created them, no one else has the moral authority to overrule their decision about the disposition of their embryos. Yet this right of disposition does not render embryos morally insignificant or allow them to be used for a morally trivial purpose; human embryos retain their modest moral status in any event.[24]

Ethics and the current uses of PGD

Before considering the ethics of the dominant use of PGD (the prevention of heritable genetic diseases), let us consider the other major uses mentioned previously: the identification (and discard) of chromosomally abnormal embryos in IVF and testing for HLA compatibility with an existing child. A moral objection to the former is actually an objection to the entire IVF process insofar as it results in the discard or indefinite cryopreservation of any human embryos, which have the moral status of persons with full and equal basic rights because this status would preclude their destruction or suspended animation. The objection to the intentional destruction of extracorporeal embryos for any purpose rests on the very controversial conclusion that such immature human entities are entitled to the very same moral respect owed to born persons. Moreover, the objection considers the benefits to the parents of a child born free of a serious, even devastating, genetic disease and to the child herself to be morally irrelevant, a conclusion that seems myopic and incomplete.

The use of PGD for HLA testing and selection of embryos who, when born, can serve as stem cell donors for their seriously ill siblings is certainly more controversial than the use of PGD for the detection of aneuploidy. The most commonly heard objection here is that the child to be conceived is being used as a means to benefit the already existing diseased child and her parents, and is not being brought into the world for her own sake, a violation of the Kantian principle of respect for persons. For this same reason the parents' motives for conception of a child are considered ethically improper. Some critics would also claim that the child would be harmed psychologically, once she finds out that she was brought into the world for the purpose of saving a sibling.

The moral objection to the child being conceived as a means to an end really has force only if the parents actually have this specific intent and treat the child in a manner consistent with it by, for example, putting the child up for adoption immediately after stem cell harvesting or abandoning her. No public report that documents such a state of affairs could be located; in fact, the children born in this manner appear to be loved and valuable members of the family just as their ill sibling is. People conceive children for a wide variety of reasons and motives – to have help in their old age, to fulfill cultural expectations, to make grandparents of their parents, to honor a command of God, to fulfill their own dreams of parenthood, and so on – not all of which are morally admirable or accepted as legitimate by most persons. The real moral test is not the purity of parental motives, but the quality of their behavior during pregnancy and after birth, which should show love, concern, and dedication to their child. Moreover, as existing children can properly serve as bone marrow donors for sick siblings, it follows by analogy that it is ethically acceptable for parents to make a child who will serve in the same role, assuming all children involved are loved and not subjected to procedures that are clearly contrary to their best interests.[11] Finally, it is implausible to assume that psychological harm will come to children who serve as donors when they are as likely to benefit from knowing they assisted in preserving their sibling's life.

The most common utilization of PGD is by a particular woman who wishes to avoid bearing a child with a genetic disease or abnormality that she (and commonly a spouse or partner) finds unacceptable. Actually, the risk of bearing such a child is reduced, but not eliminated, because PGD can only detect diseases or conditions with an identified genetic basis (such as certain single-gene defects and translocations), and it has an estimated error rate in the range of 1–10%, depending on the particular disease and assay being evaluated.[1] Errors are particularly bothersome when testing autosomal recessive or dominant conditions due to the phenomenon of allele-specific dropout.[25]

While the key purpose of traditional, non-directive prenatal diagnosis is to provide persons with information about the genetic constitution of the pregnancy and not to render any opinion on its termination, the same cannot be said of PGD.

> The purpose of PGD is not simply to inform couples about the genetic nature of their embryos. The explicit purpose is also to transfer healthy embryos and to discard those destined to be affected. Once a couple has chosen PGD, non-directiveness is no longer relevant.[8]

Therefore, the very purpose of PGD is to avoid the gestation and birth of a child who will have, or is likely to have, an identifiable genetic disease or disability of some sort. Nevertheless, clinicians remain ethically obligated not to impose on the prospective parents the values they bring to the assessment of a given embryo's genetic condition.

As a matter of general principle, prevention of the birth of a (genetically or otherwise) diseased or disabled child (such as one with profound mental retardation) is plainly a morally legitimate goal. If it were not, then it would make no sense to encourage pregnant (or prepregnant) women to avoid smoking tobacco or consuming large amounts of alcohol, to obtain competent prenatal care, or to take folic acid. But the prevention of such births is at least morally permissible, even if it is not morally obligatory.

There are two fundamental moral objections that can be levied at this particular goal: (1) the means taken to avoid the birth – the intentional discarding of embryos in the case of PGD – is morally wrong (this objection, based on the moral status of the embryo, was discussed above) and (2) the conception of 'disease or disability' being utilized by prospective parents and the clinicians assisting their reproduction is morally deficient. In addition, strong moral objections have been made to the use of PGD to determine conditions that cannot plausibly be called 'diseases', such as sex and the absence of desirable physical, mental, or social characteristics.

Disease and disability

Historically, medicine has offered prenatal diagnosis as a means of preventing the birth of children with the so-called serious inherited disorders, such as Tay Sachs, Trisomy 13, 18, and 21, cystic fibrosis, muscular dystrophy, Huntington's disease, Lesch–Nyhan, and neurofibromatosis. To one degree or another, each of these conditions may entail the imposition of pain, suffering, shortened life span, and/or significant inability to engage in typical activities of daily living on the individual with the condition. They also may place personal and economic burdens of one degree or another on the individual's parents, family, and even the society in which they live. These considerations lead some individuals to conclude that they would rather not give birth to a child with such a disorder; they then turn to medical professionals, such as those who provide PGD, to assist them in effectuating this decision. Embryo selection then prevents disability by avoiding the gestation of individuals who would (or likely) be significantly disabled or diseased if born.

Recently, disability activists have strongly challenged what they deem to be the basic assumption underlying PGD and traditional prenatal diagnosis: reducing the incidence of disease and disability is an obvious and unambiguous good. They rightly criticize certain views that can, and frequently do, support this assumption: that the disabled's enjoyment of life is necessarily less than for non-disabled people, that raising a child with a disability is a wholly undesirable thing, and that selective embryo discard or abortion necessarily saves mothers from the heavy burdens of raising disabled children.[26] Not all disabled persons are barred from having a satisfying life by their disability (although the social disadvantages and discrimination they encounter do decrease their quality of life), nor is it the case that raising a disabled child is always terribly burdensome or unrewarding.

However, the ethical critique of the disability activists goes much deeper than this quite proper debunking of broadly drawn and inaccurate assumptions about life with any disability. First, they contend that the medical system tends to exaggerate the 'burden' associated with having a disability and underestimates the functional abilities of the disabled:

> Conditions receiving priority attention for prenatal [genetic testing] are Down's syndrome, spina bifida, cystic fibrosis, and Fragile X, whose clinical outcomes are usually mildly to moderately disabling. Individuals with these conditions can live good lives.[26]

The activists also point out how medical language reinforces the negativity associated with disability by using such terms as 'deformity' or 'defective embryo or fetus'.

Second, and more importantly, the disability activists claim that the promotion and use of PGD and traditional prenatal diagnosis 'sends a message' to the public which negatively affects existing disabled people and fosters an increase in the oppression and prejudice from which they regularly suffer. The so-called 'message' of PGD – that the birth of disabled persons who are defective or deformed ought to be prevented – 'may have the effect of triggering additional oppression, reinforcing the general public's perception that disability is a tragic mistake (that could and should have been avoided) and that disabled people are therefore justifiably marginalized'.[26]

Some commentators within the disability community acknowledge that disability itself is not inherently a neutral condition; it may limit some options and impose real health problems and diminished human capacities. But they also emphasize that 'oppressive social conditions have so distorted the public's perceptions [of disability and disabled persons], as well as how disabled individuals themselves might internalize these perceptions, that it is difficult to assess the true impact of disability on the individual's life experiences'.[26] In other words, the real negative impact of disability in and of itself is exceedingly difficult to isolate because of deep and pervasive social discrimination against disabled individuals and widely shared, strongly negative social views on the meaning and personal impact of disability.

Insofar as individual clinicians do, in fact, exaggerate the problems and burdens of living as an individual with a disability or of living with a disabled person as a parent or family member, they are doing a moral disservice to the people they are duty bound to be helping. Adults who wish to reproduce are ethically obligated to do so in a responsible manner, and this means (insofar as it is possible in a world about which we have imperfect knowledge) gathering and assessing fair and accurate information about what the future might hold for them and the child they might produce. Clinicians (especially genetic counselors) should endeavor to provide this kind of information, supplemented – if at all possible – by the first-hand information that comes from those who have actually lived with disabilities of various kinds, as parents of the disabled, or from the disabled individuals themselves. For example, it is certainly true that not all individuals with Down's syndrome or their parents live painful, frustrated, or tragically diminished lives. The same is true for individuals with spina bifida, cystic fibrosis, Fragile X, and other genetic disorders.

On the other hand, these conditions are simply not utterly benign or neutral as each may, and often does, involve what can fairly be described as an 'undesirable event, such as pain, repeated hospitalizations and operations, paralysis, a shortened life span, limited educational and job opportunities, limited independence, and so forth'.[27] Even though not all instances of such disorders will involve the experience of such problems, a significant risk that an individual may encounter them always exists. A prospective parent who chooses to act on his or her conclusion that it is better for a child not to have, or to be at significant risk of having, such serious disorders is acting reasonably. 'We do no one – not disabled individuals, not women, not families – a service by minimizing the physical, mental, and emotional burdens that may result from parenting children with disabilities'.[27]

The claim of certain disability advocates that those who utilize PGD as patients or who offer it as clinicians are necessarily 'sending a message' to the public that it is ethically right to oppress or discriminate against the disabled, or that the birth of any disabled child is a tragic mistake which ought to have been avoided, is simply untenable. 'From the fact that a couple wants to avoid the birth of a child with a disability, it just does not follow that they value less the lives of existing people with disabilities, any more than taking folic acid to avoid spina bifida indicates a devaluing of the lives of people with spina bifida.'[27] The attempt on the part of a prospective parent to avoid the conception and birth of a child with a disability through PGD (and it is always just an attempt as there are no guarantees) does not mean that he or she would surely reject or fail to love a child born with a disability – or show disrespect to an existing disabled person.

While it is morally permissible for a prospective parent to discard an embryo with a genetic disease, it would be seriously wrong for him or her to 'discard' or reject a live-born child with the same disease. Adults who reproduce must take moral and legal responsibility for their reproductive decisions, and this necessarily includes accepting the risk that the child born to them may not be 'perfect' or not as healthy as they would like. Unlike an embryo that has only modest moral status whose very existence can properly be controlled by the persons who created it, a live-born child is an independent individual with full and equal moral status who has now joined the human community and who cannot be arbitrarily discarded or destroyed by its parents without a serious moral wrong being done. Rejecting or not loving a child solely because he or she has a disability is reasonably considered morally arbitrary and wrong because the child has full and equal moral status, while an extracorporeal embryo does not.

Society does not utilize PGD or traditional prenatal diagnosis, whatever 'society's' views on disability might be. Individual persons utilize such services with the assistance of individual clinicians, and they do so in order to make deliberate choices about their personal reproduction and about their particular lives rather than leave these entirely to chance. A choice that each individual makes about his or her own reproduction has no moral implication for how a similar choice ought to be made by another person: a choice not to implant an embryo with the gene for cystic fibrosis, while morally permissible, does not (indeed cannot) mean that the opposite choice by a different person is morally wrong. Nor does such a choice mean that the individual must therefore devalue persons living with cystic fibrosis. However, some commentators have argued that under certain circumstances persons have a positive ethical duty not to reproduce.[28]

Suppose PGD reveals the presence of a genetic abnormality, Down's syndrome, in an embryo. Someone could say that an individual woman who chooses not to have that embryo transferred into her uterus is rejecting persons with Down's syndrome, but there is another, more plausible interpretation as well.

> What I would say is 'I do not want my child to be born with Down's syndrome', meaning 'if I have a choice, I want the person who will be my child to be born into a body without such potentially significant limitations ...'. That is all [I am expressing]. For a person with a disability to take this as a personal rejection seems unreasonable to me.[29]

The claim of the disability activists that the meaning of PGD must be that 'people like us will never be born' is unfounded: of course, 'they will [be born], they just won't have the disability'. To me, this objection only really makes sense if people with disabilities are their disabilities, which they are not.[29]

In sum, discrimination against persons with disabilities is just as morally repugnant as discrimination against persons based on race, religion, or sex, but it is not at all clear that PGD reinforces or contributes to this in any manner. Regardless of how society might change (as it surely *ought* to change) its attitudes and practices to decrease or, better, eliminate the socially created disadvantages wrongly placed on the disabled – and regardless of how individual persons might change their views on the prospect of knowingly having a child with a serious disability – other persons

> will prefer not to have a child with a serious disability, no matter how wonderful the social services, no matter how inclusive the society. [T]his is a perfectly acceptable attitude, one that does not impugn their ability to be good parents. This attitude does not imply a devaluing of the lives of existing people with disabilities, any more than do programs to vaccinate children against polio or ensure that pregnant women get enough folic acid.[27]

It is this individual choice that PGD preserves, although the clinicians who offer PGD have a moral obligation to explore their own and their patients' attitudes about, and understanding of, disability so these individual decisions can be made fairly and responsibly with accurate information about the real world of life with and without disability.

PGD and selection for sex and other desirable characteristics

Three methods for prepregnancy or prebirth sex selection are available: (1) prefertilization separation of X-bearing from Y-bearing sperm with selection of the desired sex for artificial insemination or IVF (Microsort), (2) PGD with transfer of embryos of the desired sex, and (3) traditional prenatal diagnosis and selective abortion. However, given that IVF with PGD is expensive, technologically daunting, and imposes significant burdens on women, it has only limited usefulness as a method for sex selection, though it currently works much better than sperm sorting.[30] This may change as more reports of clinical experience with Microsort are made publicly available.

Interestingly, the Ethics Committee of the American Society for Reproductive Medicine has opined that 'policies to prohibit or condemn as unethical all uses of non-medically indicated preconception gender selection are not justified',[1] yet it has also held that

> ... initiation of IVF and PGD solely for sex selection holds even greater risk of unwarranted gender bias, social harm, and the diversion of medical resources from genuine medical need. It should therefore be discouraged.[31]

The National Society of Genetic Counselors has flatly stated that couples wanting 'sex selection for personal preference are not candidates for PGD'.[2] The primary ethical distinction between sperm sorting and PGD rests on the fact that the latter involves the creation and destruction of embryos, which have some moral status and are therefore entitled to some moral respect, while gametes have no moral status.

The selection of an embryo's sex via PGD is done for two basic reasons: (1) preventing the transmission of sex-linked genetic disorders, such as hemophilia A and B, Lesch–Nyhan syndrome, Duchenne–Becker muscular dystrophy, and Hunter syndrome and (2) choosing sex to achieve gender balance in a family with more than one child, to achieve a preferred order in the birth of children by sex, or to provide a parent with a child of the sex he or she prefers to raise.[31] While little extended ethical debate exists regarding the former, sex selection for the purpose of preventing the transmission of sex-linked genetic disease, the latter is the subject of heated ethical disagreement.

The ethical objections to sex selection for non-medical reasons can be grounded both in the very act of deliberately choosing one sex over the other and in the untoward consequences of sex selection, particularly if it is performed frequently. Sex selection can be considered inherently ethically objectionable because it makes sex a determinative reason to value one human being over another when it ought to be completely irrelevant: female and male children as such always ought to be valued equally and never differentially.

Sex selection can also be ethically criticized for the undesirable consequences it may generate. Choice by sex supports socially created assumptions about the relative value and meaning of 'male' and 'female' with the latter almost universally being considered seriously inferior to the former. By supporting assumptions that hold femaleness in lower social regard, sex selection enhances the likelihood that females will be the targets of infanticide, unfair discrimination, and damaging stereotypes. The experience in India and China indicates that sex selection is commonly used to ensure the birth of males over females.[32] At one point in China there were 153 boys for every 100 girls.[30] A more recent report indicates that in parts of China, there are 140 boys for every 100 girls (in contrast to the USA and world average of 105 boys for every 100 girls) and suggests that this will likely result in an increase in prostitution and the outright selling of women.[33] A preference for males as first-born could also disadvantage females, as research consistently shows that the first-born are more aggressive, more achieving, and of higher income and education than later-born children.[30]

Proponents of the ethical acceptability of sex selection would argue that the parents' desire for family balancing can be – and typically is – morally neutral. The defense of family balancing rests on the view that once a parent has a child of one sex, he or she can properly prefer to have a child of the other sex because the two genders are different and generate different parenting experiences.

To deny that the experience of parenting a boy is different from that of parenting a girl "seems breathtakingly simplistic, as if gender played no role either in a person's personality or relationships to others. Gender may be partly cultural (which does not make it less 'real'), but it probably is partly biological .... I see nothing wrong with wanting to have both the experiences".[30]

Thus, gender differences in fact exist and appear to be both cultural and biological in origin; actual physical and psychological differences exist between male and female children that affect parental child rearing experiences in important ways.[34] Even one noted feminist author has asserted that gender asimilarity and complementarity are morally acceptable reasons for wanting a child of a certain sex.[35]

The defender of sex selection for family balancing can also point out that parents who desire this different experience can do so without believing or acting as if one sex is better than the other and without imposing harmful gender roles (e.g. females are emotional, not rational) upon their children. As persons having such a preference may do so without believing that one sex is superior to another and with respect for the equal rights and status of females, proponents would argue that their preference should be respected incident to the exercise of their right to reproduce, especially in the absence of empirical evidence showing that the practice of sex selection actually harms females. Moreover, it can be argued that the modest moral respect due to embryos is not offended by a parental choice made on the basis of sex.

It also seems very unlikely that sex selection would significantly skew the male–female balance in the U.S. population or that of other developed Western nations. One U.S. study has shown that among the respondents who would use sex selection, 81% of the women and 94% of the men would want their first-born to be a boy, which would result in more males receiving the advantage of being first-born. But given that this same study found that only 25% of all respondents would use sex selection methods, it appears unlikely that this would dramatically add to the number of first-born males.

> Nevertheless, if sex selection became widely available, it might change the American family, making older sisters to younger brothers somewhat less common than they otherwise would be. Whether this change would be harmful enough to justify constraining choice [of sex], however, remains hard to say.[30]

Overall, the predictions of potential bad consequences due to sex selection seem too speculative to be determinative of its moral propriety.[31]

An opponent of sex selection for family balancing can argue that good parents, whether prospective or actual, ought never to prefer, favor, or give more love to a child of one sex over the other. For example, a morally good and admirable parent would never love a male child more than a female child, give the male more privileges than a female, or give a female more material things than a male simply because of sex or beliefs about the child's 'proper' gender. A virtuous and conscientious parent, then, ought not to think that, or behave as if, a child of one sex is better than one of the other sex, nor should a good parent believe or act as if, at bottom, girls are really different from boys in the ways that truly matter.

The argument in favor of sex selection for family balancing has to assume that gender and gender roles exist and matter in the lived world. For if they did not, then no reason would exist to differentiate the experience of parenting a male child from that of a female child. However, it is precisely the reliance on this assumption to which the opponent of sex selection objects: accepting – and perpetuating – gender roles inevitably both harms and wrongs both males and females, although females clearly suffer much more from them than males. While some gender roles or expectations are innocuous (e.g. men do not like asking for directions), the overwhelming majority (e.g. males are – and should be – aggressive, women are – and should be – self-sacrificing) are not. Consequently, given that sex selection is inevitably gendered and most gender roles and expectations restrict the freedom of persons to be who they wish to be regardless of gender, sex selection is at least strongly ethically suspect, if not outright wrong.

Some would claim that choosing the sex of our children is not the most morally worrisome application of PGD or other forms of medical intervention in reproduction; it is rather the prospect of our ability to choose the characteristics of our offspring. '[T]he real threat comes from the identification of an increasing number of genetic markers associated with conditions that are not life-threatening, but impairing or socially undesirable, such as hyperactivity, homosexuality, and obesity'.[36] Botkin notes that the moral reluctance to discard an embryo or abort a fetus for a less than serious medical condition already conflicts with the value of honoring parental autonomy 'in this most intimate of enterprises'.[8]

This conflict will be 'exacerbated by the rapid increase in genetic tests for a wide range of conditions, including late-onset conditions, conditions with a limited impact on health, and, possibly, behavioral or physical characteristics that fall within the normal range'.[8] Despite the apparent falsity of strict genetic determinism,

> ... we may only need a popular *perception* of genetic determinism, fueled by creative marketing and weak regulation, to move poorly predictive tests from the lab into the clinic ... [T]hese tests need not be very predictive to be adopted by some couples who want the very best that their sperm, eggs, and money can buy.[8]

In this regard, it is also worth recalling the ASRM's characterization of PGD as 'an established technique with specific and *expanding* applications for standard clinical practice'[34] (emphasis added).

Sex selection by PGD or traditional prenatal diagnosis is already available, although one recent study shows that a majority of physicians who offer PGD are not willing to do so for sex selection.[37] The existence of genetic tests linked (even tenuously) to certain desirable or undesirable social, psychological, or behavioral characteristics is highly likely to generate at least some demand from people who will pay the going rate for such tests up front in cash and who will be more than capable of giving informed consent to the procedure. The critical ethical question will be: should medical professionals provide any such tests (or sex selection for that matter) on request or, more likely, on demand?

The role of the individual clinician's conscience

It is quite common for bioethicists to call for a 'social' resolution of thorny questions like this that arise in medicine.[8,38] One type of social resolution comes from the law. However, an answer to the ethical and practical question of which genetic tests clinicians should offer will almost surely not come from the law, which is (at least in the USA) a typically politically charged, slow (it is consistently behind developments in science), expensive (for both lobbying and litigation), uncertain, and cumbersome method for regulating what physicians and other clinicians do, especially when it comes to human reproduction. A true social consensus about matters involving embryo destruction is even less likely, as witnessed by the current debate over therapeutic cloning and stem cell research, not to mention abortion. Some semblance of an answer may come from professional medical organizations in the form of 'recommendations' or 'guidelines', but they probably will be quite general and in need of interpretation and application to specific cases. Professional guidelines may also be intentionally ambiguously worded in order not to create a standard of care that could be legally enforced through civil lawsuits.

What then is a clinician involved in PGD to do? Should she perform PGD for sex selection for non-medical reasons or for roughly determining, say, IQ (which probably has some genetic basis)? There undoubtedly will be coherent and serious ethical arguments on both sides of the question, as the brief review of the debate over sex selection (above) indicates. Thoughtful and conscientious clinicians will undoubtedly disagree, but this is the same situation with other controversial areas in medicine, such as futility, the propriety of treatment in the absence of 'medical indications', physician-assisted suicide, and physician-performed euthanasia.[39]

Little true consensus exists regarding when physicians and other clinicians ought to refuse to do certain interventions because they do not benefit patients, harm patients or others, are inconsistent with the healing nature of medicine, disrespect the value of human life, or are outside the legitimate scope of medicine which should be devoted to promoting human health, not human happiness or simple human preference. As a result of this variability in ethical interpretation, each individual clinician has to make a personal decision, in light of his or her own conscience and understanding of the ethical requirements of responsible professional practice, about which genetic tests he will and will not perform incident to PGD.

Conscience is a form of self-reflection on, and a judgment about, whether a particular act (or omission) is morally right or wrong, good or bad, but it is never self-certifying from the moral point of view.[40] Conscience has to be properly informed by the pertinent moral principles and rules as well as relevant professional values. But conscience must, at some point or other, lead the individual to take a stand on pressing ethical issues – like which genetic tests of offer incident to PGD. And the stand must at least sometimes be '*this* I will *not* do'. The very meaning and integrity of an individual as a moral agent turns on this: the good things any person does can be made complete only by the things she refuses to do.[39]

When conscientiously refusing to do PGD for sex or a new marker associated with homosexuality or increased height, a clinician is not necessarily adopting the position that it is unethical for any other clinician to act in this manner, although she may believe this to be so and may attempt to persuade others to exercise their consciences in the same manner. An individual clinician who refuses to perform PGD for some specific purpose is primarily making a judgment about the ethical importance of acting in a way that preserves her *personal* moral integrity and expresses her need to assume personal moral responsibility for her actions. Clinicians cannot control the behavior of other professionals in their field, but they can and should choose to conform their own behavior to the ethical standards they personally embrace, even if the field as a whole has not taken a firm stand on the relevant issue.

Each and every clinician involved in assisted reproductive medicine (whether physician, nurse, genetic counselor, or technician) should practice as a responsible individual moral agent who has developed an informed conscience and not as a vending machine of professional services operated on patient demand. Every clinician should recognize that not all of her colleagues may come to the same conclusion as she and that her professional organizations may waffle on certain issues and issue only vague or ambiguous ethical exhortations. But the lack of agreement or consensus on ethical issues does not permit a morally conscientious individual to follow the path of least resistance and simply do whatever can technologically be done and whatever a willing patient will pay for.

Conclusion

PGD is a valuable addition to the repertoire of reproductive medicine as it gives individuals with a documented history of a genetic disorder the opportunity to begin a wanted pregnancy with little or even possibly no fear that they are transmitting this disorder to their offspring. An outstanding example of this is the recent report of PGD being successfully used to avoid the conception of a child that could have inherited a predisposition to early-onset Alzheimer disease.[41] But, if this service becomes embroiled in the detection of conditions having little or nothing to do with health and disease in order to satisfy patient demand or be a profitable business, its practitioners will get, and deserve, serious ethical criticism.

REFERENCES

1. Practice Committee Report of the American Society for Reproductive Medicine and Society for Assisted Reproductive Technology. Preimplantation genetic diagnosis 2001. www.asrm.org. Accessed June 2002.
2. National Society of Genetic Counselors. Preimplantation genetic diagnosis. www.nsgc.org/pr_diagnosis_10_01.asp. Accessed June 23, 2002.
3. Bahce M, Escudero T, Sandalinas M, Morrison L, Legator M, Munne S. Improvements of preimplantation diagnosis of aneuploidy by using microwave hybridization, cell recycling, and monocolour labeling of probes. *Mol Hum Reprod* 2000;6(9):849–54.
4. Marquez C, Sandalinas M, Bahce M, Alikani M, Munne S. Chromosome abnormalities in 1255 cleavage-stage human embryos. *Reprod BioMed Online* 2000;1:17–26.

5. Munne S. Preimplantation genetic diagnosis and human implantation – A review. *Placenta* 2003;24:S70–6.
6. Verlinsky Y, Rechitsky S, Sharapova T, Morris R, Taranissi M, Kuliev A. Preimplantation HLA testing. *J Am Med Assoc* 2004; 29(17):2079–85.
7. Kuliev A, Verlinsky Y. Thirteen years' experience of preimplantation diagnosis: Report of the Fifth International Symposium on Preimplantation Genetics. *Reprod BioMed Online* 2004;8(2): 229–235.
8. Botkin J. Ethical issues and practical problems in preimplantation genetic diagnosis. *J Law Med Ethics* 1998;26(1):17–28.
9. American Society for Reproductive Medicine. www.asrm.org/Patients/FactSheets/invitro.html. Accessed July 13, 2004.
10. Nelson LJ, Clark HW, Goldman RL, *et al.* Taking the train to a world of strangers: Health care marketing and ethics. *Hastings Cent Rep* 1989;19(5):36–43.
11. Sermon K, Van Steirteghem A, Liebaers I. Preimplantation genetic diagnosis. *Lancet* 2004;363:1633–41.
12. American Society for Reproductive Medicine Ethics Committee. Shared-risk or refund programs in assisted reproduction. www.asrm.org/Media/Ethics/shared.html. Accessed July 8, 2004.
13. American Medical Association, Council on Ethical and Judicial Affairs. *Code of Medical Ethics* 1997:94–5.
14. President's Council on Bioethics. *Human Cloning and Human Dignity: The Report of the President's Council on Bioethics*. New York: Public Affairs, 2003:174–5.
15. Nelson LJ, Marshall MF. *Ethical and Legal Analyses of Three Coercive Policies Aimed at Substance Abuse by Pregnant Women*. Report to the Substance Abuse Policy Research Program of the Robert Wood Johnson Foundation, award #030790, 1998.
16. Planned Parenthood of Southeastern Pennsylvania v. Casey, 505 U.S. 833, 1992.
17. Robertson J. *Children of Choice* Princeton: Princeton University Press, 1994:22–42.
18. European Court of Human Rights. Case of Vo v. France, 2004. Application no. 53925/00.
19. Preimplantation genetic diagnosis should be allowed in Germany, study reveals. www.medicalnewstoday.com/news.php?newsid=10048. Accessed July 8, 2004.
20. Feichtinger W. Preimplantation diagnosis (PGD) – A European clinician's point of view. *J Assist Reprod Genet* 2004;21(1):15–7.
21. Mueller S. Ethics and the regulation of preimplantation diagnosis in Germany. *Eubios J Asian Int Bioethics* 1997;7:5–6.
22. Comite Consultatif National d'Ethique. Reflections concerning an extension of preimplantation genetic diagnosis. www.ccne-thique.fr/english/pdf/aviso72.pdf. Accessed July 8, 2004.
23. Human Fertilisation and Embryology Authority and Advisory Committee on Genetic Testing. Consultation document on preimplantation genetic diagnosis. http://www.publications.doh.gov.uk/pub/docs/doh/preplant.pdf. Accessed July 8, 2004.
24. Meyer MJ, Nelson LJ. Respecting what we destroy: Reflections on human embryo research. *Hastings Cent Rep* 2001;31(1): 16–23.
25. Findlay I, *et al.* Allelic drop-out and preferential amplification in single cells and human blastomeres: Implications for preimplantation diagnosis of sex and cystic fibrosis. Hum Reprod 1995; 10(6):1609–18.
26. Saxton M. Why members of the disability community oppose prenatal diagnosis and selective abortion. In Parens E, Asch A, eds. *Prenatal Testing and Disability Rights*. Washington, DC: Georgetown University Press, 2000:147–64.
27. Steinbock B. Disability, prenatal testing, and selective abortion. In Parens E, Asch A, eds. *Prenatal Testing and Disability Rights*. Washington, DC: Georgetown University Press, 2000:108–23.
28. Purdy L. Genetics and reproductive risk: Can having children be immoral? In Mappes T, DeGrazia D, eds. *Biomedical Ethics*. Boston: McGraw Hill, 2001:52–7.
29. Baily MA. Why I had amniocentesis. In Parens E, Asch A, eds. *Prenatal Testing and Disability Rights*. Washington, DC: Georgetown University Press, 2000:64–71.
30. Steinbock B. Sex selection: Not obviously wrong. *Hastings Cent Rep* 2002;32(1):23–8.
31. Ethics Committee of the American Society for Reproductive Medicine. Sex selection and preimplantation genetic diagnosis. *Fertil Steril* 1999;72(4):595–8.
32. Allahbadia G. The 50 million missing women. *J Assist Reprod Genet* 2002;19(9):411–6.
33. Johnson T. Officials foresee prostitution, selling of women. *San Jose Mercury News* 2004;July 8:1A, 13A.
34. Ethics Committee of the American Society for Reproductive Medicine. Preconception gender selection for nonmedical reasons. *Fertil Steril* 2001;75(5):861–4.
35. Overall C. *Ethics and Human Reproduction*. Boston: Allen and Unwin, 1987:27.
36. Wachbroit R, Wasserman D. Patient autonomy and value-neutrality in nondirective genetic counseling. *Stanford Law Policy Rev* 1995;6(2):103–10.
37. Benson K, Udoff L, Escallon C. Physician attitude toward controversial applications of preimplantation genetic diagnosis. *J Genet Couns* 2003;12(6): 543–4.
38. Callahan D. Medical futility, medical necessity. *Hastings Cent Rep* 1991;21:30–5.
39. Nelson LJ. Medical futility and the clinician's conscience. In Mishin R, *et al.*, eds. *Health Care Crisis? The Search for Answers*. University Park: University Publishing Group, 1995:60–70.
40. Beauchamp TL, Childress JF. *Principles of Biomedical Ethics*. New York: Oxford University Press, 1994:475–83.
41. Verlinsky Y, Rechitsky S, *et al.* Preimplantation diagnosis for early-onset Alzheimer disease caused by V717L mutation. *J Am Med Assoc* 2002;287(8):1018–21.

18 Genetic counseling

Á. Csaba and Z. Papp

In the past decades, genetic counseling has assumed an increasingly significant role in medical science. Deep changes in societal expectations coupled with the transforming social structure have led a growing number of married couples to make use of services offered by genetic counseling. Whereas, at the time of Semmelweis, the saving of mothers' lives had constituted a breakthrough in obstetrical practice, the 20th century development of neonatology and perinatology leading to improved survival chances in fetuses and newborn babies, brought further significant progress. As birthrates decreased and families tended to be founded at older age, more and more pregnant women chose to take advantage of genetics. It became a more important, if not the most important, objective to enable families burdened with inheritable and accumulating problems to have healthy children. The natural selection process that works on a large scale was no longer acceptable for families desiring to have one or two children; therefore, the demand emerged in developed countries for the safest possible pregnancy care. As part of this development, genetic counseling developed and continues to assume an increasingly significant role. The recent, explosive progress in genetic research has made people believe that now every hereditary disease can be screened in time and prevented, that is, the birth of a sick baby can be avoided with absolute certainty. The requirement of living up to this expectation more comprehensively has led to establishing and launching genetic counseling centers, which have become an integral part of the maternity care system. It has become virtually the first priority for families to expect the health care system to prepare and inform them, and thus make it possible for them to accept pregnancy as a result of a well-informed and well-considered decision. Society has also recognized that for a number of reasons (healing, psychological, financial, societal, etc.) it is preferable to prevent diseases than treat them after their emergence.

The roots of genetic counseling go back a long time in history. The correction of the undesirable qualities of the human race and the curing of its diseases has preoccupied us since prehistoric times. In one of his works, *The State*, Plato (427–347 B.C.) described a way to improve people by 'selective breeding'. The English scientist Francis Galton was the first to be engaged more thoroughly and seriously in eugenics. (It was he who introduced the word eugenics in 1883.) In a book written in 1869 (*Hereditary Genius*), he proposed that outstanding men be married by a plan to well-to-do women for a talented race to emerge. In the first half of the 20th century, certain forces disgracefully used the science of genetics and its achievements as a distorted means of eugenics to underpin their racial theories (for the extinction of Jews, blacks, and homosexuals), and also in the early 20th century this culminated in political dictatorships ordering sterilization for individuals with high genetic risk. As a result, the application of genetic achievements was long stigmatized and it had a hard time regaining the appreciation it deserves.

Before discovering genetic rules, genetic counseling was based on empirical observations. In this process it was important to recognize that certain diagnoses were more frequent in certain couples' descendents.

The 20th century witnessed revolutionary progress in the science of genetics that coincided with increasing societal demands and therefore became an integral part of modern genetic counseling. In the beginning, in the age of 'classic genetic counseling', our means were quite limited. Genetic diseases were Mendelian disorders or diseases that were inheritable through one gene. Then, counseling extended merely to clarifying the genetic, i.e. hereditable nature of a certain disease and informing the patients about the risk of recurrence. This was the time when society's demand for the prevention of diseases emerged, but our scientific and technical possibilities were still rather restricted. Regrettably, we were in no position to offer a reassuring 'alternative' to the couples who approached us with their problems. Those asking for advice had to make do with mere information, the rigid percentage numbers of the risk of repetition, on the basis of which they could make their decision on whether to have a child. In many cases, however, the high risk of occurrence and/or recurrence communicated by the physician forever deterred the couple from having another child. To be sure, in other cases it was useful for the couple to know that with the knowledge about the heredity of the given problem, they could safely have another pregnancy without having to dread the recurrence of the disease that they had feared. In that period, there could occur such a situation (due to a lack of assisted reproduction techniques) when genetic counseling shed light on a disease inherited in a recessive manner, which might have led the couple to the conclusion that their descendents were exposed to a heightened risk. This could, unfortunately, result in the deterioration of the relationship, and even in their divorce, so that they both could increase their respective chances of having a healthy child. At last, the physician performing genetic counseling was also in a difficult position, since in many cases he was aware that he could not give the assistance that was needed, and he must have sensed the tension generated by the puzzlement of the couple seeking advice. (In certain cases, this feeling has, unfortunately, remained known to physicians providing genetic counseling.)

Theoretical and practical means of genetic counseling

Genetic counseling is centered on close interactive communication between those requesting and those giving advice. Genetic counseling centers operate in numerous countries of the world. Their task everywhere is to give information about hereditary diseases, to let patients know about the possible cures, and not the least to define the method of heredity. Knowing the type of heredity is indispensable for figuring out the risk of occurrence and/or recurrence, which is the most frequently asked and most important question for pregnant women or couples wanting babies, and therefore seeking counseling. Thus, genetic counseling can basically be divided into two major branches:

(a) Finding out if the disease of a newborn baby, older child, or adult is hereditary, making a diagnosis, and providing information about the possible treatment.
(b) Counseling during pregnancy concerning the occurrence and/or recurrence of hereditary (genetically determined) diseases in a family or those materializing in pregnancy, using prenatal diagnostic tools with the aim of ensuring the birth of healthy offspring.

Although the two branches obviously focus on the same diseases, they require different approaches. All over the world, genetic counseling is primarily done by biologists, geneticists, and various medical specialists, mainly pediatricians and obstetricians.[1–3] Pregnant women and their partners facing various genetic problems can base their decision on information and advice made available by these professionals' knowledge and expertise.[4] Counseling can follow two principles: the more widely used *non-directive* genetic counseling and the so-called *directive* genetic counseling.[5] Because the current era is dominated by legal claims against physicians, the non-directive method is more acceptable and more easily defendable, even though in many cases patients expect and demand a decision-shaping process closely guided by the physicians. When applying the non-directive method, the genetic counselor is ready to share information in a non-directive manner without committing to any potential alternative. It is very important that having thoroughly described the disease in question, the consultant should also inform the patient about the risk of occurrence and/or recurrence. After that, diagnostic alternatives should be described and offered – if there are any. This has to be done in a fashion so that the patients seeking counseling can understand the basic facts, and it may vary with the given circumstances. The patient's fear and anxiety must not be worsened by giving an opinion expressed in mystical, complicated sentences that are incomprehensible to ordinary people. By this point, the couples have already started the decision-making process. The physician leaves it to the patients to use the intensive interactive process to arrive at their final decision. Various prenatal screening and diagnostic methods have demonstrated revolutionary progress and have been made indispensable parts and means of modern genetic counseling.

Often screening tests could at least lower the excitement and nervousness, but it was prenatal diagnostics that made the real breakthrough in the practice of genetic counseling. At this point during counseling, one has to mention the inevitable necessity of explaining the differences between screening tests and diagnostic tests. Society mistakenly confuses the two examinations and attributes to them equal importance. In daily practice, this can result in erroneous decisions because many regard the reassuring results of the screening tests as a safe diagnosis. Too often, we can hear the following statement from a 40-year-old pregnant woman and her 50-year-old husband:

> As the biochemical markers (triple–quadro test) are normal, and the genetic ultrasound examination has not detected any visible abnormalities either, we can rest assured for we cannot have a child with chromosome abnormalities. We do not want amniocentesis.

Screening tests are performed to help us detect and 'take out' those who face a higher than average risk of certain pathological conditions of concern. Some procedures may serve a screening purpose in some cases, while they can have a diagnostic value in association with another disease. Sonography is one of these procedures, but it is only of a screening nature in the case of Down's syndrome, while it has a diagnostic value in the case of anencephaly, spina bifida, and hydrocephalus.

Among prenatal diagnostic tools we distinguish between *non-invasive* and *invasive* methods. Sonography, one of the most frequently and widely used, dynamically developing examination procedure belongs to the first group. In the non-invasive group, we also have the tests using maternal blood, of which tests with fetal cells obtained from maternal circulation deserve more attention. The arsenal of invasive prenatal diagnostics is also steadily broadening, but those applied first in the practice of genetic counseling remain its most frequent procedures. These are genetic amniocentesis and *chorionic villus sampling* (CVS). Invasive procedures, unfortunately, carry certain risks for the fetus and the pregnant woman. Their complications have a considerable influence on the patients' decision, since in many cases they perceive their situation as a choice between bad and worse. In this context, it is understandable that the essential factor on which they base their decision is the intention to opt for the less risky examination if they are given a choice. The pain and tension caused by the examination also appear as a problem in invasive examination, but this does not have a decisive influence when making the final choice. While these procedures are not painless, the pain is not extensive either.

This strong inter-relatedness between genetic counseling and prenatal diagnostics is largely determined and driven by ultrasound examinations that, as a result of rapid technological advancements, allow the physician to follow more closely the life of the embryo and the fetus.[6–8] Ultrasound is biologically harmless, so undergoing an ultrasound examination cannot pose a serious dilemma for pregnant women. However, despite the accumulation of an increasingly significant amount of expertise and knowledge, it is often difficult to evaluate and interpret the results of the examination. Modern medical examination equipment with largely improved detection capabilities makes even tiny 'suspicious signs' recognizable.[9] Nevertheless, these signs can lead to differing interpretations, thereby causing unwarranted concern among patients. The sonograph can record even tiny divergences from normal conditions that cannot be ignored, because written documents can later serve as legal evidence. Frequently, we are in no position to perform further non-invasive examinations to reassure the patients. This often renders invasive examinations advisable, potentially putting the patients in a difficult decision-making situation. Patients can become anxious or even fearful, because they are apt to treat machine-made images virtually as facts, and to interpret them as serious threats to the fetus. It is then a daunting task to dispel anxiety or fear because the patients tend to believe the 'objective' computer. Here too, the non-directive method is advisable, and it is important to point out not only the possible pathologic conditions, but also the possibility of a reassuring outcome. For this reason, it is essential to follow closely any abnormalities detected during ultrasound examinations in later stages of the pregnancy and after delivery. This approach can lead us to a stage when images currently interpreted as suspicious signs will not result in groundless tension and fears for the pregnant woman.

Practice standards regarding ultrasound examinations during pregnancy vary from country to country. In some countries, one or two examinations are deemed sufficient without providing much detail as to how these should be timed. Nearly a decade ago, we introduced in Hungary a carefully designed system that pays due consideration to the interests of pregnant women and to professional rationality. Our protocol advises four plus one examinations for the pregnant woman, with the first taking place during the first call (usually in the fifth to eighth weeks), the others later in the 10th to 12th, 18th to 20th, 28th to 30th, and 36th to 38th weeks. If necessary, we advise an intrauterine examination of the fetuses' heart (echocardiography).[10] The pregnant woman must understand that these examinations are part of a series of screening tests meant to check on the intrauterine development of the fetus. Countries advising or performing fewer examinations partly cite high costs and question the efficiency of the examinations. There are also skeptical opinions about whether ultrasound examinations can significantly improve morbidity and mortality indicators.[11] Some others, arguing against ultrasound examinations, also point to the misleading, wrongly reassuring effects of 'false-negative' diagnoses. Well-elaborated and organized sonographic training can, however, minimize such risks. It is imperative that examinations be carried out and interpreted by trained and experienced professionals.

Such invasive genetic examinations as amniocentesis, CVS, and fetal blood sampling have become indispensable means of prenatal diagnostics and genetic counseling. These examinations allow us to obtain genetic information, leading to major breakthroughs in the development of genetic counseling. Samples obtained during invasive procedures are helpful in performing several examinations, and the number of diseases that can be detected this way is steadily increasing. Beyond detecting chromosome irregularities, these are now important means of diagnosing monogenic inheritable diseases (Mendelian inheritance) as well. From the samples, we can also perform microbiological and serological examinations. The newest molecular genetic techniques are opening a previously unhoped-for dimension in prenatal diagnostics. Beyond the dangers arising from the invasive nature of such examinations (due to the higher risk of miscarriage), their more widespread use has raised numerous ethical questions as well. Even when we face increased risks of genetic, inheritable diseases, we must try our best to make sure that no sick children are born, while giving couples a realistic chance to have a healthy newborn. Here, we have a reverse situation: contrary to ultrasound examinations, in this case the interpretation of examination results leaves very few questions owing to diagnostic accuracy from the principle of methods applied. In these cases, however, the examination carries dangers that create significant tension, concern, and complicated decision situations. There can emerge a peculiar and difficult contradiction because the patients would like to have a healthy child, but the examination necessary to make this happen might endanger the further development of the fetus. When the woman makes this decision, the physician must stick with non-directive counseling, which allows him to inform patients about the benefits and drawbacks, but has him answer any further question about what decision to make in a non-directive fashion. The final decision has to come from the woman. The genetic counselor must not assume a 'divine role' and cannot be familiar with all relevant aspects of another person's life. Even in cases that seem identical, the final decisions can be different. A 37-year-old couple who already have three healthy children and where the woman can conceive without difficulty is likely to request karyotyping, whereas a couple having tried in vain to conceive a child for 15 years can be very concerned about the threat of miscarriage and may choose not to have such an invasive act performed.

During genetic counseling, certain 'semi-invasive' examinations can also be of assistance; these are widely used in screening because of their minimal level of invasiveness. Nevertheless, as a result of their being a screening test, they can produce false-positive results, generating serious concern in pregnant women. Biochemical marker tests done from samples of the mother's blood (AFP, BHCG, E2, PAPP-A, Inhibin) constitute one sort of genetic screening examination. Besides false-positive results, there are some false negative test results as well, which makes it essential to explain to patients that screening examinations do not provide the basis for establishing a diagnosis. In view of the existing risk factors of invasive examinations, one has to aim at putting together as reliable a screening examination protocol as possible. There are ongoing efforts to examine an increasing number of serum markers that can be combined with ultrasound examinations (e.g. nuchal translucency) to improve results. Because of fears of being held accountable and exposed to malpractice claims, the drawing of the point will regrettably increase the number of false-positive cases, which, in turn, will demand a larger capacity for intrauterine chromosome analysis.

Decision making: rights and responsibilities

Physicians who have provided genetic counseling for an anxious married couple have faced their distress and feelings of defenselessness. The very uncertainty shadowing the health of their desired offspring puts a considerable burden on the expectant woman and her spouse. Add to that the further risk of various other special circumstances, and the result can be an effectively unbearable load. Those couples seeking genetic counseling almost always carry the 'extra burden', that being the very reason why their physician sends them to consult a specialist.

Many decision-making situations crop up during genetic counseling. In certain cases, the first question to answer is whether or not the patient is ready for pregnancy, knowing the genetic risk. The individual seeking counseling must decide if she wants to have the proffered diagnostic test. Another decision may have to be made with regard to the patient's wish to carry on with or terminate the pregnancy in the case of a positive result (indicating disease).[2,12,13]

The diverse nature of genetic problems necessitates separating the following branches in order to better understand decision-making mechanisms:

(a) Those cases requiring invasive, high-risk intervention (chromosome defects).
(b) Monogenic diseases with a high risk of occurrence and/or recurrence.
(c) Low-risk genetic situations (taking medicine, diagnostic x-ray examinations).
(d) Uncertain conditions for which diagnostics are limited (certain infections and anatomical defects detectable by serology or ultrasound where the outcome cannot be predicted).

One important consideration is whether the available means can result in a rock-solid diagnosis, or the problem in hand cannot be diagnosed during pregnancy, although certain results may indicate pathological conditions. The decision-making mechanism seems to be affected by a couple of factors, including risk of recurrence, seriousness of the disease, risk of the procedure, maternal age, previous pathological pregnancies (malformations, miscarriages), number of healthy offspring, level of education, religious faith, and convictions of conscience.

The kind of genetic counseling we prefer lets the patients have the final word. Neither the right to make a decision nor the responsibility resulting from that decision can rest with the genetic counselor. This point is important because it makes many legal claims avoidable. The non-directive counseling process can be easily violated, because the patients can be manipulated by carefully determining the sequence of sentences. It must be our objective to be as neutral as possible, while providing comprehensive and honest information to patients. Our words ought not to give away which decision we might favor. Although it is true that we cannot exist without having certain ideals, values, and views, and that we are bound to form an opinion about what we say in a counseling situation, the patients should not sense that we might disagree with their decision or that we might judge them negatively as a result. For the pregnant woman and her partner to accurately feel the weight of their decision, it is necessary to stress that they can choose freely from the alternatives described to them. They have to see clearly the consequences of whatever decision they opt for.

It would be very difficult to conceive of any other counseling mechanism and decision-making process in democratic states where the wide-ranging rights of the individual are safeguarded. In democratic systems, however, one should not forget about obligations and responsibilities. Systems that exclusively emphasize rights, but not obligations, are moving toward anarchy. This anarchy would obviously apply to the field of genetic counseling as well. For free choice to be preserved, it is crucial that the decision made by the patients in no way influences further pregnancy care, and that the physicians continue to provide the broadest range of services possible.

The weight of the decision requires that pregnant women be given sufficient time to ponder the various dimensions of their choices. In most cases, the pregnant woman finds it reassuring to discuss her situation with her partner or physician and to seek the advice of her family before committing to one of the alternatives. It is highly possible that the patient and the counselor will have to see each other more than once.

During counseling, the physician should be understanding and patient – one cannot overemphasize the role empathy plays in the process. Dramatic statements, gestures, and other forms of non-verbal communication are equally impermissible during non-directive genetic counseling. A written report must be prepared about the counseling session and the patient's decision.

The complex nature of genetic counseling and its relatively short history are bound to raise several moral and ethical questions. Although there is an emerging consensus on the older problems, the new possibilities and achievements have caused significant rifts among physicians and scientists. These developments are increasingly prevalent in our everyday life, and their divisive effects can be felt in the society as well. When it comes to genetics and our endeavors to influence heredity, society tends to be sharply divided. In these situations, the individual's freedom and need to decide are at play simultaneously.

The counselor is not in an easy situation either. In these complicated and often very difficult decision-making situations the consultant's room for maneuver is rather limited due to the non-directive principle of counseling. One can feel every now and then that the advice seeker counts on the consultant's help when making her decision. Limited though the consultant's opportunities may be, he is still able to help by supplying clear and direct information relevant to the case. He is not to use either verbal or metacommunicative means, which might suggest that he is taking a firm stand on either side of the dilemma. At the same time, the verbal and metacommunicative behavior he does perform must not contradict each other, because that may confuse the other party. He must be patient and compassionate, but focused on the issues in hand, and should not let the advice seeker's attention wander. He must dissipate fears raised by 'rumors' and 'horror stories', but must never gloss over or retouch actual facts and dangers. The consultant must always be prepared and set forth possible alternatives along with their advantages, drawbacks, and consequences.[14] In many cases, the counselor is aware of the problem's serious and occasionally hopeless prognosis. The recurrence of this mental burden can pose a serious challenge for the physician. In cases of possible abortion, the genetic counselor's role goes beyond merely sharing information. From the moment that patients are confronted with the problem, we have to provide them with support. Besides the bare facts, we also need to point out the potential remedies. We must convey positive messages to the couple so that they can more easily deal with a tragedy. The description of the problem is never meant to deter; therefore, calm, a human voice, and compassion are the most important qualities of a genetic counselor. We stand a much better chance of achieving cooperation if, instead of telling the facts in a cold, matter-of-fact manner, we act kindly, and do not conceal the problem. The patients must never sense frustration and exhaustion on the part of the genetic counselor.

It is essential that the decision possibly reflects the common will of the couple, but at a minimum be preceded by a consultation between the partners. The couple frequently wishes to request the advice of the woman's gynecologist before making the final decision. This reinforces the strong bond of confidence that develops between the pregnant woman and her physician. This is especially true when genetic counseling is done by an obstetrician/gynecologist who may also be in charge of the patient's pregnancy.

The woman usually desires the most comprehensive information possible so that she can make an educated final decision. Questions like 'How would you decide in my place?' are often put to the genetic counselor. When responding, one has to follow the rules of non-directive counseling and accordingly give information about how the majority of other couples decide in similar situations. It needs to be pointed out to the patients that every individual's and every family's life is different, and therefore it is impossible to give a generalized answer. The decision is influenced, among other factors, by whether the family already has a healthy child, how many pregnancies the woman has had, how old the couple are, and how long they have been trying to conceive a child. Religion and beliefs certainly also play an important role. After the final decision is made, the couple must be given assistance to be able to deal with the consequences as smoothly as possible. A guilty conscience and the shadow of an irresponsible decision are difficult to dispel in a family, but proficiently executed counseling can prevent them from developing.

Ethical and moral aspects of genetic counseling

The diagnostics of monogenic diseases [heterozygote screening, Human Genome Project (HGP), eugenics]

The molecular genetic research brought to a high stage of development in the last years of the 20th century resulted in an even more detailed knowledge of the human genetic material. The HGP has established that the sequence of 3.1 billion letters of DNA shows that humans are made up of about 30,000–40,000 genes.[15,16] This may generate erroneous beliefs in society, because many think that any hereditary gene defect can be detected today, and therefore any given disease can be screened in the embryonic stage. True, more and more monogenic diseases may be diagnosed by polymerase chain reaction (PCR) or other molecular genetic techniques, but science has yet to enable us to detect every genetic defect. These examinations, combined with assisted reproduction techniques, in certain cases, make possible the detection of diseases in the pre-embryo conceived by *in vitro* fertilization (IVF). This doubtlessly important fact can be a strong propaganda factor for the unconditional supporters of this method and can contribute to solidifying it in practice and making its application more widespread by pushing its disadvantages into the background and making use of the media's help. Given that these are costly examinations, it is necessary to bring about a well-established international network of research. If the disease in question is serious, every effort is morally justifiable to organize prenatal diagnostics and make them available. However, HGP and our ever-deepening knowledge also mean that the genetic background of more and more 'conditions' can be examined, which conceals ethical dangers. Does humankind not try to implement positive eugenics when unearthing the genetic (hereditary) background of intelligence and physical features? Is there not a strange 'preordination', 'innate predestination', or 'special selection' for those who, because of their financial status, are able to take the opportunity provided by science however costly it may be in the beginning? Will it be possible to acquire or 'purchase' favored social status even before childbirth? Will these sayings come true: my child was born to be a banker, a doctor, a lawyer, a teacher or an athlete, an artist? Utopian as this assertion may seem, it is not unimaginable.

Let us play with the idea, and assume that the genetic code of every human disease and human quality, including physical and mental endowments as well as appearance, has become detectable through the HGP. In the present social environment, science and technology provide for the possibility of choosing and creating the socially most 'competitive', healthy descendants. If at the beginning it can be done through costly procedures, we have already reached the eugenics envisioned by Plato and Sir Francis Galton. Further, there could emerge in society castes firmly embedded for several generations, for with the help of genetic advantages, the descendants of the wealthier would become the leading stratum, while those with no access to these advantages would constitute the stratum of the subordinates and the employees. Would it be 'healthy', socially useful, or beneficial if everybody wished to be endowed with Einstein's IQ and Schwarzenegger's or Marylin Monroe's appearance? In our view, this vast acceleration of evolution's long and slow process could lead to unforeseeable tragic consequences.

A more delicate and much more topical aspect of this line of thinking is very much alive today: What are the pathological conditions that justify the induction of premature delivery as they exhaust its scope of indication? Who is to decide on these? If certain conditions (e.g. depression, rheumatoid arthritis, schizophrenia, arteriosclerosis, certain tumors, and autoimmune diseases) are proven to be inherited monogenically, is the pregnancy to be terminated if the fetus carries the faulty gene(s) and there is no known therapy? It is of paramount importance that the scope of therapy be extended so that more and more detected diseases can be treated. In order to prevent this, it is urgently necessary to create the proper legal framework of regulations and to introduce rational restrictions instead of outright prohibitions. Historical examples show that whatever can conceivably be done by man will be created sooner or later. We, therefore, cannot lull ourselves into illusions that mere prohibitions can prevent human cloning or that irrational restrictions can prevent the above vision from materializing.

Presymptomatic diagnostics (confidentiality of genetic data – relatives, insurance companies, employers, the family, and the individual)

Presymptomatic diagnostics and so-called 'susceptibility testing' are gaining increasing salience with reference to an increasing number of diseases.[17] *Presymptomatic testing* refers to identification of healthy individuals who may have inherited a gene for a late-onset disease, and if so will develop the disorder if they live long enough (e.g. Huntington disease). *Susceptibility (predictive) testing* identifies healthy individuals who may have inherited a genetic predisposition that puts them at increased risk of developing a multifactorial disease (e.g. heart disease, Alzheimer disease, or cancer), but who may never develop the disease in question. Do we have the right to inform the patient about the existence of untreatable diseases before symptoms appear? Is it necessary to do so? Are we obliged to do that? Is this individual ill at all? Can or need populations be screened for certain diseases? Indeed, the development of some diseases might be slowed down if changes in lifestyle were implemented. The knowledge, however, that the development of a serious disease is inevitable in a later stage of one's life could put a heavy burden on his everyday existence and might even change an individual's personality. Surviving in the knowledge that one is to expect to develop a malignant tumor by the age of 30–40 years is difficult. By the same token, possessing the relevant information might result in more careful diagnostic examinations, which should have a substantial effect on the life expectancy.

At the same time, this raises the question of who is entitled to know the information, i.e. *confidentiality*,[18,19] the individual affected and his relatives? One might think that only the individual affected should, but with the disease in question being a genetic one, are the relatives not affected, too? Do they not have the right to know their risk? Is the parent obliged to tell his or her child? Can the child request the performance of a predictive test? Can the parent make a decision on whether the examination should be performed for her minor child?[20] Presymptomatic and susceptibility testing in the absence of therapeutic options should be available if certain conditions are met. It is important that the individual be provided thorough information about the limits of testing, and the information contribute to enhancing the pathography and informing the family because, in many cases, it is impossible to predict the onset and seriousness of a particular disease and its symptoms. Awareness of susceptibility could induce a change in the lifestyle that could prevent or prolong the development of a disease. If a disease is inevitable, the individual will have the chance of planning for his or her short life, as in the case of Huntington disease. Such genetic information can influence plans for marriage and having children. Preimplantation genetics could possibly prevent the development of a particular disease in their children. But the basic question remains: Is it good or useful to know what for millennia mankind has had no way of knowing – the ultimate end of life, the number of years, the sequence of probable diseases? Is society prepared for this? Is the human soul strong enough to carry this burden? Do such examinations make sense as long as we lack adequate therapies? Do we have to do everything just because we can? The problem is further complicated by the shortcomings of available predictive genetic tests that still carry a factor of serious uncertainty about whether a disease will develop, and if it does, when exactly and to what extent. Given the onus of this information, if there is no medical advantage concerning prevention or treatment, these examinations can best be postponed until adulthood, when the individual is able to make decisions on crucial aspects of his own life.

Stigmatization, discrimination

Society tends to single out 'other-than-average' individuals, in many cases stigmatizing them. Given the sensitive nature of issues, such as reproduction, heredity, child-rearing skills, and the fact that society considers calculable and predictable health defects a serious drawback, exposing information about such issues is unethical. It is for the individual to decide whether or not his genetic profile ought to be made public. Employers, insurance companies, government administrations, and schools are prone to gather the widest possible spectrum of information about their associates.[21–23] The results of presymptomatic and susceptibility tests are beginning to become central issues for these institutions. These organizations would like to have unrestricted access to these data. The individual is essentially interested in the opposite, since the insurance company would surely demand a higher premium if it is ready to offer insurance at all.

Similarly, an employer would be disinclined to employ someone of whom it is known that in a few years he or she cannot do his or her job. At the same time, the fear of insurers and employers is also understandable, because the individual can also abuse such genetic information. Those declared 'healthy', who will not have to reckon with the development of a serious disease in the course of their lives, would not pay for insurance, and even the 'ill' would wait almost until the likely development of the disease before they would buy insurance. This could generate unmanageable burdens for insurance companies and could lead to the total collapse of the insurance system. Environmental or occupational (e.g. miners and chemical industry workers, pilots) hazards can play a significant role in the development of certain conditions (e.g. asthma, allergies, heart disease, or cancers); therefore, by applying for such jobs, people jeopardize their own health, which can become starting points of future lawsuits. (The employer could propose that the individual should work in a different department, since the desired job could accelerate the development of the disease. If the employee would still choose the job not recommended, which he should have a right to do, then he or she would lose his or her right to sue his company on these grounds.)

Considering the likely rapid dissemination of predictive tests, there is an urgent need to develop a well-thought-out, detailed legal framework. Prohibition cannot be allowed because it would deprive the individual of rather important information. The proper regulation would eliminate the situation of diametrically opposed interests among the parties and would make them interested in wide-ranging examinations. (For instance, at birth everyone should be genetically screened for 'susceptibility' and the resulting information should be made available to those concerned, but at the same time, discrimination and the possibility of abuse by the examined individual should be prohibited; emphasis should be placed on prevention, and adequate sets of incentives should be elaborated). Apparently, avoiding stigmatization and discrimination makes a very important goal, but the problem itself is highly complex. It is unacceptable to discriminate against anybody at school, work, or when taking out an insurance policy because of one's genetic background. It must not be allowed either that individuals misuse this information. Therefore, it is crucial to bring about well-considered, detailed regulation and legislative background. At present, the individual's and the family's personal rights must not suffer damage, and genetic information may be made public only with their consent.

Sex selection and sex determination

Both the prenatal and the preimplantation diagnostic procedures are suitable for the *determination of the sex* of the pre-embryo/embryo or the fetus. The majority of society does not prefer one sex to the other. In certain communities, however, the offsprings' sex is very important; therefore, sex determination presents itself as a problem in this controversial moral field. Many civilized societies do not allow carrying out invasive genetic examinations merely to select or determine sex, but loopholes exist in many countries. Where a pregnancy may be terminated at the married couple's request, the decision to do so is often made in the knowledge of the fetus' sex (as a result of karyotyping or an ultrasound examination). In these cases, we speak of sex determination done for non-medical reasons. Those in favor of this try to rely on demographic/statistical data arguing that in certain cases it would be favorable to permit it. There are certain research groups and countries where sex determination is permitted if a couple already has a child, and would like the next one to be of the other sex. Some claim that in countries with decreasing populations this could even become an instrument in stopping the declining numbers. In other countries (in Asia), this possibility is seen as one of the factors slowing down population growth.[24,25] They point out previous European experience when the selection of the descendant's sex was possible on the basis of the sperms, and practice showed that this did not change the proportion of the sexes in the population. In 2001, The American Society for Reproductive Medicine ruled that it is proper and ethical to help couples to choose the sex of their babies.[26]

By the same token, sex determination done for non-medical reasons also has several opponents. The most frequently heard argument against the use of preimplantation genetic diagnosis for non-medical sexing is that a medical method should not be used for non-medical reasons.[27] We are even more concerned that by legalizing this kind of sex determination, we will cross the Rubicon, for it would be classifying the sex of an individual as 'an abnormality'. This would be the first step toward the above-described, apparently utopian human interventions that on the surface would be 'done for genetic reasons', but in reality would serve a manipulated selection of human qualities. At a later point, this logic could have us argue that the decreasing population could be expanded if legal regulations allowed selection on the basis of intelligence or physique, or where the opposite is needed, the high-quality, efficient, and productive descendants could just as well slow down population growth.

In our view, to avoid abusing information about sex revealed by carrying out karyotyping for other reasons, careful regulation is needed, which effectively makes it impossible to terminate pregnancy just because the fetus belongs to one or the other sex.[28] Individual (personal) rights must be curtailed, and those uncritically embracing them should not ignore the rights of the fetus. Individualism is not identical to exemption from obeying rules and laws.

Today, sex determination may be justifiably indicated only if a family is affected by a hereditary disease connected to a sex chromosome, and when special molecular diagnostic tools making use of genetic engineering are not yet available. In such a case, if the test reveals that the fetus is male, the couple has the right to ask for the termination of pregnancy so that the disease will be avoided. In this case, we speak of sex determination done for medical reasons. If the preferred method of conception is IVF–ET and the disease in question is an X-determined, recessive one, the so-called preimplantation diagnostics is a possible option, which may ensure that only healthy female pre-embryos get implanted.[29]

The definition of illness and health

Differentiating between illness and health presents an increasingly complex problem. According to the World Health Organization's (WHO's) definition, health is a state of complete physical, mental, and social well-being, and is not merely the absence of disease or infirmity.[30] Holding the assertion that the absence of disease (an organic, physical decrease in or failure of function) does not in itself constitute health makes it difficult to define the conditions that ought to be regarded as healthy. Late-onset diseases, deviations from the statistical norm, and increased susceptibility to cancers are questionable states. These men and women are not ill for a long time, but they are handicapped from a certain point of view. Shall we or shall we not treat these states as diseases until we are able to cure already detected genetic predispositions? At the same time, millions of people live happy lives with certain diseases (blindness, absence of fingers, color blindness, deafness) presuming they are healthy. A number of geniuses would not have been born had they fallen victim to procured abortion because of conditions considered by society as illnesses.

There is another serious ethical challenge here. Do parents have the right to decide whether or not an obvious infirmity they carry is one that needs screening that might help avoid it in their children? And if they do not, who can decide? If it is left to the parents to make decisions, then strange situations should be expected. A good example is reported by Green.[31] A deaf–mute couple sought genetic counseling, their disease's nature being monogenically hereditary. Having been informed about their prospects, they asked for a molecular genetic diagnosis to be made on the 13-week-old fetus. To the pleasure of their consultant, the result was homozygote recessive, meaning they could expect a healthy offspring. Surprisingly, however, the couple was disappointed by the result, indicating:

We can't carry on with the pregnancy. How could we bring up a child totally alien to us, able to hear and communicate, while our friends and we live in a different way? We aren't capable of establishing the appropriate circumstances.

Terminating pregnancy because of genetic indications

The most challenging moments of genetic counseling arise when a decision has to be made on the disposition of a pregnancy. From the consultant's point of view, those situations are the most difficult when the problem is so severe and the prognosis is so bad that termination on a genetic basis may be proffered. Even in this case, the goal of non-directive counseling is to inform the patient about this option. The woman is about to resolve one of the most difficult situations of her life. The weight of the decision depends on the gestational age of the pregnancy and other factors. Decisions on serious conditions detected in the first trimester are made easier. Given that most diagnoses are made in the second trimester, when the fetus has already made its first movement, a very close relationship has sometimes developed between the fetus and the expectant mother by decision time. She may have seen its face during an ultrasound examination, and she may even know her offspring's sex. Realizing her widening waistline, the people around her may learn about the pregnancy, and this knowledge and having to wait, make it even more difficult for her to cope. The necessity to make a decision presents a major state of crisis, the extent of which depends, among other things, on the obstetrical anamnesis.

In such a case, the task is to give the relevant facts, help the patient to consider them thoughtfully and calmly, and encourage her to develop positive prospects for the future. It is important to outline the possible short-term and long-term consequences of the decisions, the risk of the defect being recurrent, and the details of its heredity. If the woman opts to continue her pregnancy, she needs to be briefed on what sort of aid she can rely on from the fields of medicine and social services, as well as family care. Those deciding to terminate the pregnancy must be informed about the procedure to relieve tension and distress. In any case, this should ease the anxiety regarding the operation itself. It must be stressed that if the couple opts to terminate the pregnancy, the procedure must be initiated as early as possible. The methods used for midterm abortions vary from country to country. Regardless of the method, the objective is to get the procedure over within the shortest possible time and in the least intrusive way. The patient ought to get back to her home as soon as possible to be able to deal with the tragedy with her loved ones. Access must be made available to post-termination counseling.

The woman's and partner's freedom of choice and representing the fetus' and the newborn's interest: considerations relating to faith and religion

One basic feature of modern genetic counseling is that the final decision is always made by those seeking assistance.[1] The justification for this appeals to individual rights of freedom and people's right to decide issues affecting their own lives. Obstetrics and genetics, however, are fields where a decision often has to do with another individual (i.e. the embryo, fetus, or newborn); therefore, it must not be practiced without limitations and relevant regulation. The problems of fetal life have often been put in the center of debates, not only in professional circles, but also as a political issue. The rigid attitude of the Roman Catholic Church is well known and stirs a lot of debates even within that faith community. The church turns a deaf ear to the issue of termination and does not accept contraception as a legitimate option (with a few exceptions). Thus, it is difficult to provide the opportunities offered by the achievements of prenatal diagnosis to Catholics. In some liberal circles' view, parents must be assured of having the widest possible sphere of authority. This cannot be readily accepted by a physician or an obstetrician-geneticist. In the USA, it is legally possible that termination be carried out until the 24th week of pregnancy at the request of the patient and without any medical indication. The test is whether an individual physician accepts the pregnant woman's decision to terminate her pregnancy.

The WHO's position is that after the 24th week, an end to pregnancy has to be considered as childbirth and as such, everything has to be done to save the life of the premature infant. Therefore, there are cases where several doctors and nurses make superhuman efforts for weeks to rescue a 490-g premature baby born after the 24th week, whereas the life of another baby, perhaps with a little better initial life expectancy, perhaps even weighing a little more, is taken in minutes because the parents changed their mind 'at the last minute'. Our era is burdened with lawsuits brought against thousands of doctors, and many tend to give in to patients' request as self-defense. There are cases of minor problems whose long-time prognosis is not known for certain. In such cases, the question is frequently asked, 'But surely our child will be healthy? You know we don't want a sick baby'. Well, this question is difficult to answer. One must not yield to pressure by irresponsibly allowing termination in such cases. The freedom of choice must be kept in focus, but between reasonable boundaries, too. Regulation established to protect fetal life enables us to do our job, living up to the principles of modern medicine, and actually protect life and health.

Preimplantation diagnostics: gene therapy

Assisted reproductive techniques are becoming more and more sophisticated, contributing to the expertise that makes it possible to subject the fertilized egg to ever more detailed genetic examinations still outside the mother's body. In the course of the procedure, blastomer, blastocyst, and polar-body biopsy take place, while the genetic analysis is performed with two major molecular genetic techniques, PCR and fluorescence *in situ* hybridization. The high cost of practice and the low pregnancy rate achieved are still considered the two major drawbacks of this new procedure. As our knowledge of the genetic background of diseases expands, the number of those for whom these examinations may be indicated is also increased. In the future, IVF may become more widespread, because it would prevent numerous terminations from occurring: pre-embryos carrying disease would not be implanted in the first place. Regulation must not be neglected in this field, because within a short time, society would be confronted with a deluge of unwarranted examinations. The financial and moral burden of this would surely prove unbearable. Positive eugenics must not be allowed to be realized this way.

Currently, the number of gene therapy procedures is negligible, but intensive research may make some treatments possible soon. This will herald a new age of genetics and, indeed, the whole of medicine. On the one hand, many couples as yet unable to rear children will have the opportunity to do so; on the other hand, one or another of these therapeutic methods might become a way of retrieving health, indeed, a new lease of life for many people.

Financial considerations

Science is capable of much more today in the fields of genetics and prenatal diagnostics than the health care system is able to offer to society. It is those costly interventions that make the difference. When setting priorities, their social usefulness must always be kept in mind. The needs of the wide social strata must never be sacrificed for the sake of a relatively narrow stratum. This principle will be there to be confronted in the field of genetics and prenatal diagnostics for a long time, because the procedures that have been introduced recently are highly costly. A breakthrough in this field may also be expected, but only if efficient screening/diagnostic methods and treatments are available, which are advantageous to the masses of society and for which financial consequences (insurance, work, pensions) are beneficial. The cost–benefit principle may not be accepted without reservation, but it defines what sort of examinations can be routinely carried out in a health care system with a finite budget.

Summary

The basic and clinical science of genetics has made vast progress in a few decades. In accordance with this, genetic counseling has reached the limelight of public attention. Given the fact that the subject of counseling is of momentous consequences and has important effects for both the short and the long term, its ethical aspect is paramount. What was inconceivable just half a century ago has become a routine procedure, and for the majority of previously hopeless couples it is now possible to have healthy descendants. Visions articulated by Plato millennia ago have come close to being realized. While ancient Sparta used exposure of infants on Mount Taigetos as a means of creating a healthy society, today we try to prevent the birth of ill children by examining and improving tiny DNA spirals and base pairs. The question is indeed whether mankind is mature enough to use this knowledge for choosing the right way ahead and utilizing the achievements for society's benefit. It is crucial that the relevant regulation be designed. The center of the ethical questions is occupied by the treatment of important personal information and the method of its being made public. The way the problems are dealt with is always changing, just as society is in a constant process of change. It is important, however, that we always be ready to offer proper help to those in need when they need it.

REFERENCES

1. Papp Z. Change in public demand for genetic counselling in the past 25 years. In Chervenak FA, Kurjak A, Papp Z, eds. *The Fetus as a Patient: The Evolving Challenge*. Boca Raton: Parthenon Publishing Group, 2002;11:130–45.
2. Sjogren B, Uddenberg N. Decision making during the prenatal diagnostic procedure. A questionnaire and interview study of 211 women participating in prenatal diagnosis. *Prenat Diagn* 1988;8(4):263–73.
3. Marteau T, Drake H, Bobrow M. Counselling following diagnosis of a fetal abnormality: The differing approaches of obstetricians, clinical geneticists, and genetic nurses. *J Med Genet* 1994;31:864–7.
4. Johnson KA, Brensinger JD. Genetic counseling and testing: Implications for clinical practice. *Nurs Clin North Am* 2000;35:615–26.
5. Seller MJ. Ethical aspects of genetic counseling. *J Med Ethics* 1982;8:185–8.
6. Berkowitz RA. Should every pregnant woman undergo ultrasonography? *N Engl J Med* 1993;329:874–5.
7. Chervenak FA, McCullough LB. Ethics and emerging subdiscipline of obstetric ultrasound, and its relevance to the routine obstetric scan. *Ultrasound Obstet Gynecol* 1991;1:18–20.
8. Romero R. Routine obstetric ultrasound. *Ultrasound Obstet Gynecol* 1993;3:303–7.

9. Egan JF, Malakh L, Turner GW, *et al*. Role of ultrasound for Down syndrome screening in advanced maternal age. *Am J Obstet Gynecol* 2001;185:1028–31.
10. Caughey AB, Lyell DJ, Filly RA, *et al*. The impact of the use of the isolated echogenic intracardiac focus as a screen for Down syndrome in women under the age of 35 years. *Am J Obstet Gynecol* 2001;185:1021–7.
11. Chervenak FA, McCullough LB. Ethical dimensions of ultrasound screening for fetal anomalies. *Ann NY Acad Sci* 1998;847:185–90.
12. Hunfield JAM, Wladimiroff JW, Passchier J, *et al*. Emotional reactions in women in late pregnancy (24 weeks or longer) following the ultrasound diagnosis of a severe or lethal fetal malformation. *Prenat Diagn* 1993;13:603–12.
13. Chitty LS, Barnes CA, Berry C. For debate: Continuing with pregnancy after a diagnosis of lethal abnormality: Experience of five couples and recommendations for management. *Br Med J* 1996;313:478–80.
14. Donnai D. The management of the patient having fetal diagnosis. *Baillieres Clin Obstet Gynaecol* 1987;1:737–45.
15. Macer D. Whose genome project? *Bioethics* 1991;5:183–211.
16. Murray TH, Livny E. The Human Genome Project: Ethical and social implications. *Bull Med Libr Assoc* 1995;83:14–21.
17. Macer DRJ. Ethics and prenatal diagnosis. In Milunsky A, ed. *Genetic Disorders and the Fetus: Diagnosis, Prevention and Treatment*. Baltimore: John Hopkins University Press, 1998: 999–1024.
18. Grady C. Ethics and genetic testing. *Adv Intern Med* 1999;44: 389–411.
19. Rawbone RG. Future impact of genetic screening in occupational and environmental medicine. *Occup Environ Med* 1999;56:721–4.
20. Savulescu J. Predictive genetic testing in children. *Med J Aust* 2001;175:379–81.
21. Billings PR, Kohn MA, de Cuevas M, *et al*. Discrimination as a consequence of genetic testing. *Am J Hum Genet* 1992;50: 476–82.
22. Rothenberg K, Fuller B, Rothstein M, *et al*. Genetic information and the workplace: Legislative approaches and policy challenges. *Science* 1997; 275:1755–7.
23. Lapham EV, Kozma C, Weiss JO. Genetic discrimination: Perspectives of consumers. *Science* 1996;274:621–4.
24. Williamson NE. Sex preference and its effect on family size and child welfare. *Draper Fund Rep* 1982;(11):22–5.
25. Malpani A, Malpani A, Modi D. The use of preimplantation genetic diagnosis in sex selection for family balancing in India. *Reprod Biomed Online* 2002;4(1):16–20.
26. Gottlieb S. US doctors say sex selection acceptable for non-medical reasons. *Br Med J* 2001;323:828.
27. Pennings G. Personal desires of patients and social obligations of geneticists: Applying preimplantation genetic diagnosis for non-medical sex selection. *Prenat Diagn* 2002;22:1123–29.
28. Sachs BP, Korf B. The Human Genome Project: Implications for the practicing obstetrician. *Obstet Gynecol* 1993;81:458–62.
29. Botkin JR. Ethical issues and practical problems in preimplantation genetic diagnosis. *J Law Med Ethics* 1998;26:17–28.
30. Preamble to the Constitution of the World Health Organization as adopted by the International Health Conference, New York, June 19–22, 1946. Signed July 22, 1946. Official Records of the World Health Organization, 1948;2:100.
31. Green RM. Prenatal autonomy and the obligation not to harm one's child genetically. *J Law Med Ethics* 1997;25:5–15.

19 Selective reduction

M. I. Evans, D. W. Britt, D. Ciorica and J. C. Fletcher†

Introduction

Millions of babies have been born benefiting from infertility therapies including more than 1 million *in vitro* fertilization (IVF) babies over the past 25 years. These fulfilling outcomes, however, have been accompanied by serious side effects. The twin pregnancy rate has doubled to more than 1 in 45. Multiple pregnancies have continually risen. Prematurity and related sequelae closely correlate with fetal number (Figure 19.1, Table 19.1).[1] Infertility treatments have become so pervasive that more than 70% of all twins and 99% of higher-order multiples are initiated by them (Table 19.2). With increasing public and professional attention, some of the very high-order multiples have diminished, particularly secondary to lower transfer numbers of embryos in IVF. There are some suggestions that the incidence of triplets and higher is slowly diminishing, but the incidence is still very high.

Perceived pregnancy losses in multiple pregnancies are mostly correlated to how early in pregnancy one establishes the denominator.[2,3] Some perinatal reports are overly optimistic because these physicians do not start counting until they begin to see patients at nearly 20 weeks, at which time most losses have already occurred.[3,4] Many other articles have addressed these issues, which will not be repeated here.[4–6]

In the 1980s, about 75% of multifetal pregnancy patients seeking reduction had pregnancies initiated with ovulation induction agents such as Pergonal.[7] However, even with the first month of the lowest dose of Clomid, quintuplets have occurred. Over the years, cases induced by assisted reproductive technologies (ARTs), such as IVF, have become increasingly common. Currently, about 70% of patients we see seeking reduction have pregnancies generated by ARTs.[8]

Despite the increased utilization of ARTs,[8] the proportion of cases significantly hyperstimulated, and resulting in quintuplets or more, has dramatically decreased to less than 10% of all cases seen by us. Regardless, the 2000 report of the Society of Assisted Reproductive Technologies (SART) suggested that, of all pregnancies achieved by ARTs, in the USA 58.5% are singletons, 28% twins, 7.5% triplets or higher, and 5.9% were unknown.[9,10] In our experience with referred cases of ovulation stimulation, the proportion of cases that are quintuplets or more has likewise fallen but not as remarkably.[11]

The vast majority of multifetal cases occur to physicians with the best of equipment and with the best of intentions who have an unfortunate and reasonably unpredictable or unpreventable mal-occurrence. Despite this, clearly some cases might have been prevented if increased vigilance had been used.[11–13]

Patient issues

The demographics of patients considering multifetal pregnancy reduction (MFPR) have evolved considerably over the past 10–15 years.[11,12] The most dramatic change has been the introduction of donor eggs, which has opened the door to 'older women'. Over

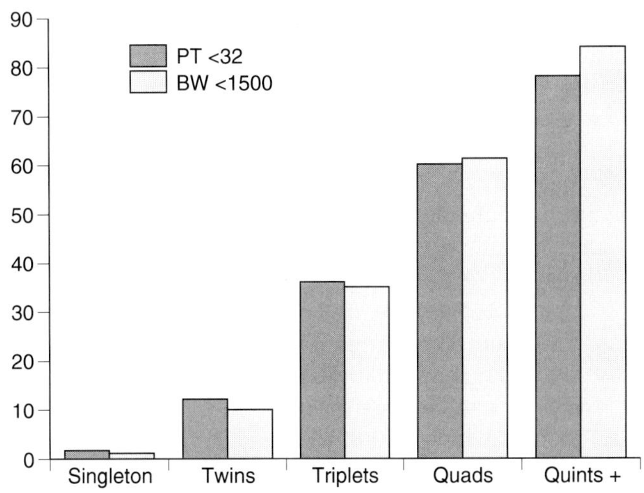

Figure 19.1 Risks of prematurity as a function of fetal number. 2002 United States Centers for Disease Control Data. Dark shaded area represent preterm birth < 32 weeks. Light shaded area represents birth weight < 1500 g.

†Deceased

Table 19.1 Multiple births in the USA (data taken from *National Vital Statitics Report,* 2003;52(10):22)

Year	Twins	Triplets	Quadruplets	Quintuplets and higher multiples
2002	125,134	6898	434	69
2001	121,246	6885	501	85
2000	118,916	6742	506	77
1999	114,307	6742	512	67
1998	110,670	6,919	627	79
1997	104,137	6,148	510	79
1996	100,750	5,298	560	81
1995	96,736	4,551	365	57
1994	97,064	4,233	315	46
1993	96,445	3,834	277	57
1992	95,372	3,547	310	26
1991	94,779	3,121	203	22
1990	93,865	2,830	185	13
1989	90,118	2,529	229	40
% Change from 1989–2002	38.9%	172.8%	89.6%	72.5%

Table 19.2 Ratio of observed to expected multiples

Births	Observed	Expected	Ratio
Twins	125,134	44,686	2.80:1
Triplets	6,898	496	13.9:1
Quadruplets	434	6	72.3:1
Quintuplets and higher multiples	69	0.07	985.7:1

Total births in 2002 – 4,021,726

Table 19.3 Maternal age and ART (SART data, 2001) (from Evans *et al.*[11])

All cases	81,915
Fresh non -donor	60,780
< 35	28,778
35–37	14,416
38–40	11,301
41–42	4,365
42+	2,190

10% of all patients seeking MFPR that we see are over 40 years of age; nearly half of them are using donor eggs. As a consequence of the shift to older patients, many of who already had previous relationships and children, there is an increased desire by these patients to have only one further child. The number of experienced centers willing to do two to one reductions is still very limited, but we believe it can be justified in the appropriate circumstances.[11,13] We expect the proportion of all patients with multiples reducing to a singleton to continually rise.

For patients who are 'older', particularly using their own eggs, the issue of genetic diagnosis comes into play. By 2001, more than 50% of patients in the USA having ART cycles were over 35 (Table 19.3).[1,9,10,14] In the 1980s and early 1990s, the most common approach was to offer amniocentesis at 16–17 weeks on the remaining twins. A 1995 paper suggested a 11% loss rate in these cases, which caused considerable concern.[15] However, the issue was settled by a much larger collaborative series in 1998 that showed that loss rates were no higher than comparable controls of MFPR patients who did not have amniocentesis.[16] The collaborative data demonstrate a loss rate of 5%, which was certainly no higher than the group of patients post-MFPR who did not have genetic studies.

As the centers with the most MFPR experience also happened to be the ones that also had the same accomplishments with chorionic villus sampling (CVS), combinations of the procedures were very logical. There are two main schools of thought as to the best approach to first trimester genetic diagnosis, i.e. should it be before or after the performance of MFPR? Published data in the early 1990s on doing the CVS first followed by reductions suggested a 1–2% error rate as to which fetus was which, particularly if the entire karyotype is obtained before going on to reduction.[17] Therefore, for the first 10–15 years, the approach we used was to generally do the reduction first at approximately 10.5 weeks in patients reducing down to twins or triplets, followed by CVS approximately 1 week later.[11,14] However, in patients going to a singleton pregnancy, essentially putting 'all of their eggs in one basket', we believed the best approach was to know what was in the basket before reducing the other embryos.[11,12] In these cases we performed a CVS on usually all the fetuses or one more than the intended stopping number, and performed a fluorescent *in situ*

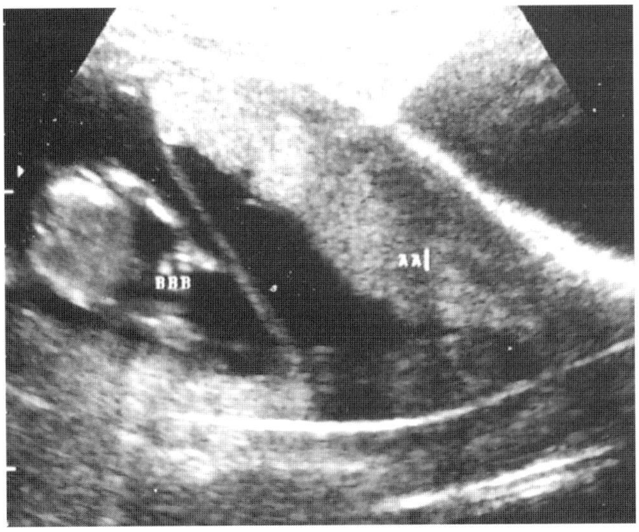

Figure 19.2 Transcervical CVS being performed on posterior placenta. For this patient, anterior placenta can be reached either transcervically or transabdominally

hybridization (FISH) analysis with probes for chromosomes 13, 18, 21, X, and Y (Figure 19.2). Whereas about 30% of overall anomalies seen on karyotype would not be detectable by FISH with these probes,[18] there is always residual risk.[19] The absolute risk given both a normal FISH and a normal ultrasound including nuchal translucency[20] is only about 1/500. We believe that risk is lower than the increased risk from the 2-week wait necessary to get the full karyotype. We have now commonly extended this approach to all patients who are appropriate candidates for prenatal diagnosis regardless of the fetal number. Over the past few years, more than half our patients have combined CVS and MFPR procedures. With data now suggesting increased risks of chromosomal and other anomalies in patients conceiving by IVF and especially with intracytoplasmic sperm injection (ICSI), the utilization of prenatal diagnosis will likely increase even further.[21–26]

The other approach used by another group was to perform the CVS and complete karyotype first and have the patient come back for the reduction. Although 'mistakes' were common 10 years ago, the chance of error has been considerably reduced, and they believed the benefits of the full karyotype justified the wait. The issue as to the better of these two approaches is currently unsettled and would require a very large series to differentiate among small risks.

Procedures

MFPR is a clinical procedure developed in the 1980s when a small number of centers in both the USA and Europe attempted to reduce the usual and tremendously adverse sequelae of multifetal pregnancies by selectively terminating or reducing the number of fetuses to a more manageable number. The first European reports by Dumez,[27] and the first American report by Evans *et al.*,[28] followed by a further report by Berkowitz *et al.*,[29] and later Wapner *et al.*[30] described a surgical approach to improve the outcome in such cases.

Even these early reports appreciated the ethical dilemma faced by couples and physicians under such difficult circumstances.[13] In the mid-1980s, needles were inserted transabdominally and maneuvered into the thorax for the injection of KCl or mechanical disruption of the fetus by mechanical destruction, air embolization, or potassium chloride injections despite relatively mediocre ultrasound visualization. Transcervical aspirations were also initially tried, but with little success. Some centers also used transvaginal mechanical disruption, but data suggested a significantly higher loss rate than with the transabdominal route.[31] Today, virtually all experienced operators perform the procedure inserting needles transabdominally under ultrasound guidance.

Outcome

Several centers with the world's largest experience have, for more than a decade, collaborated to leverage the power of their data. In 1993, the first collaborative report showed a 16% pregnancy loss rate through 24 completed weeks.[17] While by today's standards, that was not a very satisfactory number, it did represent a major improvement for higher-order multiple pregnancies. Further collaborative papers have shown continued dramatic improvements in the overall outcomes of such pregnancies (Table 19.4).[11] The 2001 collaborative data demonstrated that the triplets reduced to twins and quadruplets reduced to twins now perform essentially as if they had started as twins.[11] Even with the tremendous advances in neonatal care for premature babies, the 95% take-home baby rate for triplets and the 92% take-home baby rate for quadruplets clearly represent dramatic improvements over natural statistics. Not only has the pregnancy loss rate been substantially lowered, but so has the rate of very dangerous early prematurity. Both continue to be correlated with the starting number. Data from the past few years show that the improvements are, not surprisingly, greatest from the higher starting numbers (Figure 19.3).

The lowest pregnancy loss rates are for those cases reduced to twins with increasing losses for singletons followed by triplets. However, the rate of early premature delivery has been, not surprisingly, highest with triplets followed by twins and lowest with singletons. Mean gestational age at delivery was also lower for higher-order cases. Birth weights following MFPR decreased with starting and finishing numbers reflecting increasing prematurity.[32]

While data in the literature are conflicting, our experiences suggest that triplets reduced to twins do

Table 19.4 Multifetal pregnancy reduction – percentage of losses and deliveries by years (from Evans *et al.*[11])

	Total	Losses (weeks) % < 24	Losses (weeks) % > 24	Deliveries (weeks) % 25–28	Deliveries (weeks) % 29–32	Deliveries (weeks) % 33–36	Deliveries (weeks) % 37+
1986–1990	508	13.2	4.5	10.0	21.1	15.7	35.4
1991–1994	724	9.4	0.3	2.8	5.4	21.1	61.0
1995–1998	1356	6.4	0.2	4.3	10.2	31.5	47.4

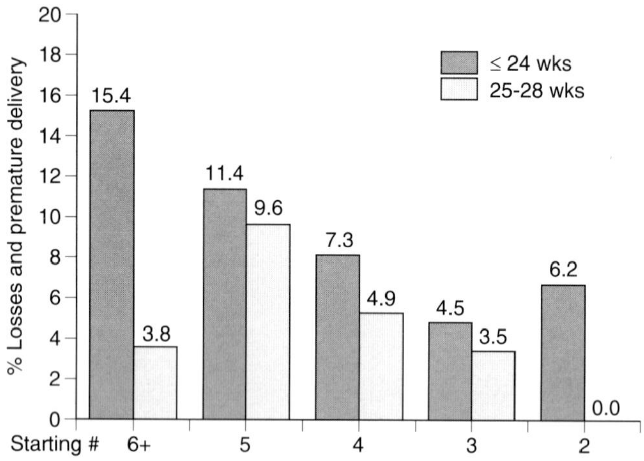

Figure 19.3 Multifetal pregnancy reduction: losses and very prematures by starting number. Adapted from Evans *et al.*[11] with permission.

much better in terms of loss and prematurity than do unreduced triplets. We believe that if a patient's primary goal is to maximize the chances of surviving children, then reduction of triplets to twins achieves the best live born results. More recent analyses suggest that while mortality is lowest with twins, morbidity is lowest with remaining singletons.

There has continued to be a debate in some circles over whether to reduce triplets or not. Yaron *et al.*[33] compared triplets to twins data to unreduced triplets with two large cohorts of twins. The data show substantial improvement of reduced twins as compared to triplets. The data from the most recent collaborative series suggest that pregnancy outcomes for cases starting at triplets or even quadruplets reduced to twins do fundamentally as well as starting as twins. These data therefore support some cautious aggressiveness in infertility treatments to achieve pregnancy in difficult clinical situations. However, when higher numbers occur, good outcomes clearly diminish. A paper published in 2001 suggested that reduced triplets did worse than continuing ones.[34] However, analysis of that series showed a loss rate following MFPR twice that seen in our collaborative series[11] and poorer outcomes in every other category for remaining triplets. Several other recent papers have likewise shown higher risks for 'unreduced' triplets than for reduced cases.[35–38] It is clear that one must use extreme caution in choosing comparison groups (Table 19.5). An ever-increasing situation involves the inclusion of a monozygotic pair of twins in a higher-order multiple.[39] Our experience suggests that provided the 'singleton' seems healthy, the best outcomes are achieved by reduction of the monozygotic twins. Obviously, if the singleton is not healthy, then keeping the twins is the next choice.

Pregnancy loss is only one of the deleterious outcomes. Very early preterm delivery correlates with the starting number. However, it has not been well appreciated that about 20% of babies born at less than 750 g develop cerebral palsy.[40] In Western Australia, Peterson *et al.* showed that the rate of cerebral palsy was 4.6 times higher for twins than singletons per live births, but 8.3 times higher when calculated per pregnancy.[41] Pharoah and Cooke calculated cerebral palsy rates per 1000 first-year survivors as 2.3 for singletons, 12.6 for twins, and 44.8 for triplets.[42]

In the 2001 collaborative report, the subset of patients who reduced from two to one (not for fetal anomalies) included 154 patients. These data suggested a loss rate comparable to three to two, but, in about one-third of the two to one cases, there was a medical indication for the procedure – e.g. maternal cardiac disease or prior twin pregnancy with severe prematurity, or uterine abnormality.[11] In recent years, however, the demographics are changing, and the vast majority of such cases are from women in their forties, or even fifties, some of whom are using donor eggs and who, more for social than medical reasons, only want a singleton pregnancy.[42,43] New data suggest that twins reduced to a singleton do better than remaining as twins.[13] Consistent with the above, more women are desiring to reduce to a singleton. In a recent series of triplets, we found the average age of outpatients reducing to twins to be 37 years and to a singleton 41 years.[44] While the reduction in pregnancy loss risk for three to one is not as much as for three to two, (15–7% and 15–5%, respectively), the gestational age at delivery for the resulting singleton is higher, and the incidence of births < 1500 g is 10 higher for twins than for singletons.[1] These data have made counseling of such patients far more complex than previously (Figures 19.4 and 19.5). Not surprisingly, there are often differences between members of the couple as to

Table 19.5 Comparison of reduced vs. unreduced triplets (from Evans *et al.* The optimal management of first trimester triplets: Reduce. *The Central Association of Obstetricians and Gynecologists Annual Meeting,* Las Vegas, NV, October 27–30, 2002)

	MFPR cases (%) Deliveries (weeks)				
Years	**< 24**	**24–28**	**29–32**	**33–36**	**37+**
Reduced triplets					
1980s	6.7	6.1	9.1	36.9	47.9
1990–1994	5.7	5.2	9.9	39.2	45.2
1995–1998	4.5	3.2	6.9	28.3	55.1
1998–2002	5.1	4.6	10.8	41.8	37.6
	Mean GA	PMR			
	35.5	10.0/1000			
1998–2002 (3→1)	8.0	4.0	12.0	4.0	72.0
	Mean GA	PMR			
	39.5	0/1000			
Unreduced triplets					
1998 (Leondires)	9.9				
	Mean GA	PMR			
	33.3	55/1000			
1999 (Angel)	8.0				
	Mean GA	PMR			
	32.3	29/1000			
1999 (Lipitz)	25.0				
	Mean GA	PMR			
	33.5	109/1000			
2002 (Francois)	8.3				
	Mean GA	PMR			
	31.0	57.6/1000			

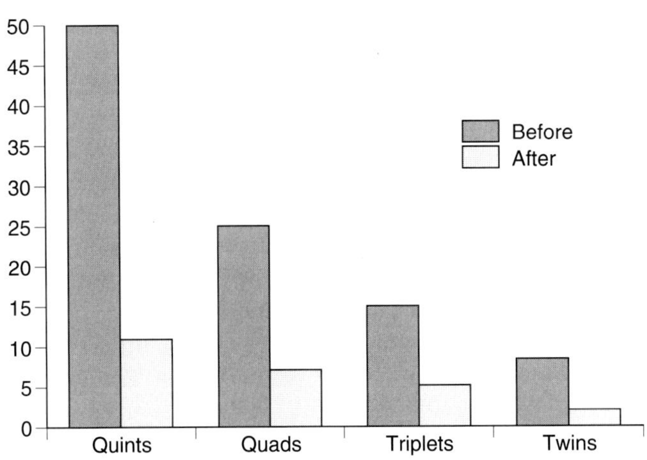

Figure 19.4 Risk reduction as a function of starting number.

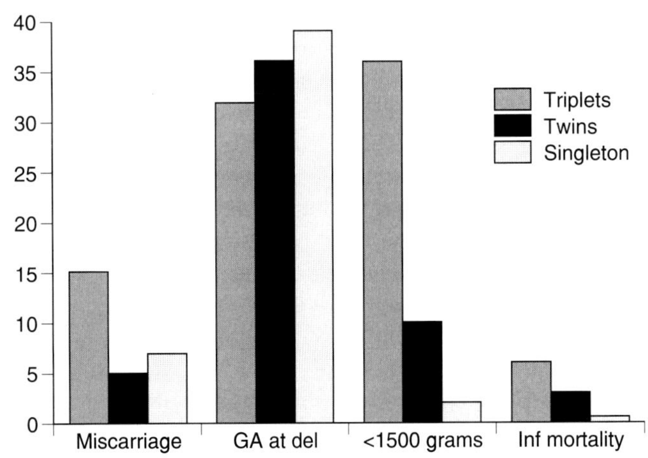

Figure 19.5 Risks starting with triplets. Reduction of triplets to twins has lower loss rates but higher incidence of prematurity, low birth weight, and infant mortality than reducing to a singleton.

Table 19.6 Frame comparison

	Medical frame	Conceptionalist frame	Lifestyle frame
Intensity of commitment to having children	High	High	High
Intensity of training in medicine, dentistry, hard sciences, and the law	High	Low	Modest
Intensity of commitment to belief that life begins at conception	Modest	High	Modest
Intensity of commitment to career	High	Low	High
Source of moral authority for resolution	Relative survivability of fetuses	Minimization of beliefs damage to moral though a 'barely sufficient' reduction	Having a 'normal' life in a culture that values both careers and family for women

the desirability of twins or singleton.[45] There are also profound public health and financial implications to these decisions, as 2000 United States Data show that of $10.2 billion spent per year on initial newborn care, 57% of the money is spent on the 9% of babies born at < 37 weeks.[46] This progress is much more likely to rise than fall.

Societal issues

There will never be a complete societal consensus on MFPR. Opinions have never followed the classic 'pro-choice/pro-life' dichotomy.[2,7,11,14] We believe that the real debate over the next 5–10 years will not be whether or not MFPR should be performed with triplets or more. A serious argument will be put forth over whether or not it will be appropriate to offer MFPR routinely for twins, even natural ones for whom the outcome has commonly been considered 'good enough'.[44] Our data suggest that reduction of twins to a singleton actually improves the outcome of the remaining fetus.[44] No consensus on the appropriateness of routine two to one reductions, however, is ever likely to emerge. We do, however, expect the proportion of patients reducing to a singleton to steadily increase over the next several years.

The ethical issues surrounding MFPR will also always be controversial. Over the years, much has been written on the subject. Opinions will always vary substantially from outraged condemnation to complete acceptance. No short paragraph could do justice to the subject other than to state that most proponents do not believe this is a frivolous procedure, but see it in terms of the principle of proportionality, i.e. therapy to achieve the most good for the least harm.[13,47–49]

How patients 'hear' and internalize data and make decisions with respect to reduction has been a subject of our investigation for several years. Much of the literature on medical decision making has emphasized a rational choice model in which emotions, feelings, and values are treated as complications that must be considered as the second stage of an analysis that puts hard data regarding relative risks into center stage.[50,51] Even in the literature that talks about genuine alternative models of decision making (systematic vs. heuristic, for example), a central assumption is that these are individual differences in style that can be identified through what people say.[52,53]

We have investigated this problem from a different direction, arguing that where controversial, high-anxiety decisions are concerned, patients treat these decisions as an ongoing part of the social reality that they are creating to live in and raise a family.[54] These realities, composed of supportive people and institutions together with complexes of supportive values, norms, and attitudes, are the source of frames that the patients use to view the data.[47–49] The decisions they make and how they justify those decisions may help resolve incompatible elements in the realities in which they find themselves enmeshed.

The one thing in common for all such patients is a very strong desire to have a family (Table 19.6). But there does not appear to be a single set of supportive institutions, people, and norms that is conducive to going through the pain, stress, and resource expenditure of IVF and then consider partial reduction as a pregnancy-management strategy. Rather, we think there are three viable alternative resolutions. The first of these, a rational *medical frame*, looks superficially like what one would expect from the rational analysis model. But the commitment to factual analysis comes from the patients having selected themselves into the hard sciences, medicine, dentistry, engineering, or law – disciplines in which 'facts' are crucial. Such women will want to see the numbers regarding the relative risk associated with different reduction choices and will want to engage in a rigorous discussion of the data and their implications. And they will be likely to choose a final number for reduction that maximizes the chances of a 'take-home' baby.

The lens of scientific objectivity is not the only frame through which women who have gone through IVF in order to have a child will examine these data. For those who have immersed themselves in a social reality that has a strong emphasis on norms against abortion and/or reduction – such that they themselves have such normative beliefs and are heavily involved in churches that reinforce similar beliefs – a detached examination of the 'facts' is simply not possible. These 'facts' hold no special moral authority. Their beliefs and those of the individuals and social institutions in which they have selected themselves have a moral authority as well. The balance that such women will likely seek is one that reduces their relative risk to acceptable limits. So, unless the consequences are dire, they will not reduce or choose to reduce only to three. We labeled such a resolution a *conceptionalist frame*.

Finally, there are those for whom the demands of career and/or existing children constitute powerful elements in their constructed realities. For such women – and this includes many of the older patients we encountered – the essential balance that they seek is a more secular one, a *lifestyle frame*, one that emphasizes creating a family situation in which having a family can be balanced with having a career. Such women will more than likely choose reduction to two or even one embryo, depending on the number of other children they have and the level of resources the family has.

Where women have selected themselves into and/or been trained to accept the legitimacy of rigorously determined statistics regarding relative risk (a *medical frame*), reduction choices *can* be straightforward – or at least, they can appear to be relatively straightforward. This is usually not the case, however, for women who must forge a resolution among potentially incompatible elements, as for women who are struggling to reconcile the potentially oppositional elements of religious beliefs and involvement with risks associated with higher-level pregnancies (*conceptionalist frame*) or those who are struggling to reconcile the potentially conflicting identities of home and career (*lifestyle frame*). We have been able to examine some of these issues in a few studies to date. In one we were able to trace the extreme fluctuations in anxiety and stress as women progress through IVF and then must confront the painful choice of reduction.[48] In a second, we were able to show that the meaning of detecting a fetal anomaly changes depending on the needs of the patient and her spouse for some confirmation regarding their choice.[47]

Summary

MFPR has become a well-established and integral part of infertility therapy and the attempts to deal with sequelae of aggressive infertility management. In the mid-1980s, the risks and benefits of the procedure could only be guessed.[10–14] Now we have very clear and precise data on the risks and benefits as well as an understanding that the risks increase substantially with the starting and finishing number of fetuses in multifetal pregnancies. The collaborative loss rate numbers, i.e. 4.5% for triplets, 8% for quadruplets, 11% for quintuplets, and 15% for sextuplets or more, seem reasonable ones to present to patients for the procedure performed by an experienced operator. Our own experience and anecdotal reports from other groups suggest that less-experienced operators have worse outcomes.

Pregnancy loss is not the only poor outcome. The other main issue of concern is very early preterm delivery and the profound consequences for such infants. Here again, there is an increasing rate of poor outcomes correlated with the starting number. The finishing numbers are also critical, with twins having the best viable pregnancy outcomes for cases starting with three or more. Triplets and singletons do not do as well. However, an emerging appreciation that singletons have prematurity rates less than twins is making the counseling far more complex. We continue to hope, however, that MFPR will become obsolete as better control of ovulation agents and ARTs make multifetal pregnancies uncommon.

REFERENCES

1. Martin JA, Hamilton BE, Ventura SJ, *et al. Births: Final Data for 2001*. National Vital Statistics Reports. Hyattville, MD: National Center for Health Statistics, 2002;51(2).
2. Evans MI, Rodeck CH, Stewart KS, Yaron Y, Johnson MP. Multiple gestation: Genetic issues, selective termination, and fetal reduction. In Gleisher N, Buttino L Jr, Elkayam U, Evans MI, Galbraith RM, Gall SA, Sibai BM, eds. *Principles and Practices of Medical Therapy in Pregnancy*, 3rd edn. Norwalk, CT: Appleton and Lange Publishing Co., 1998:235–42.
3. Evans MI, Ayoub MA, Shalhoub AG, Feldman B, Yaron Y. Spontaneous abortions in couples declining multifetal pregnancy reduction. *Fetal Diagn Ther* 2002;17:343–6.
4. Keith LG, Blickstein I, eds. *Triplet Pregnancies*. London: Parthenon Press, 2002.
5. Luke B, Brown MB, Nugent C, Gonzalez-Quintero VH, Witter FR, Newman RB. Risks factors for adverse outcomes in spontaneous versus assisted conception twin pregnancies. *Fertil Steril* 2004; 81(2):315–9.
6. Anwar HN, Ihab MU, Johnny BR, Tarek SH, Abdallah MA, Antoine AA. Pregnancy outcomes in spontaneous twins versus twins who were conceived through *in vitro* fertilization. *Am J Obstet Gynecol* 2003;189(2):513–8.
7. Evans MI, Dommergues M, Wapner RJ, *et al.* Efficacy of transabdominal multifetal pregnancy reduction: Collaborative experience among the world's largest centers. *Obstet Gynecol* 1993;82:61–7.
8. Evans MI, Ciorica D, Britt DW, Fletcher JW. Do reduced multiple pregnancies do better than higher numbers. In Penna L, Keith L, Guest, eds. *Multiple Pregnancy.* London: Parthenon Publishers, in press.
9. Toner JP. Progress we can be proud of: US trends in assisted reproduction over the first 20 years. *Fertil Steril* 2002;78(5):943 50.

10. Wright VC, Schieve LA, Reynolds MA, Jeng G, Kissin D. Assisted reproductive technology surveillance – United States, 2001. *MMWR Surveill Summ* 2004;53(1):1–20.
11. Evans MI, Berkowitz R, Wapner R, *et al.* Multifetal pregnancy reduction (MFPR): Improved outcomes with increased experience. *Am J Obstet Gynecol* 2001;184:97–103.
12. Adashi EY, Barri PN, Berkowitz R, *et al.* Infertility therapy-assisted multiple pregnancies (births): An on-going epidemic. *Reprod Med Online* 2003;7:515–42.
13. Evans MI, Fletcher JC. Multifetal pregnancy reduction. In Reece EA, Hobbins JC, Mahoney MJ, Petrie R, eds. *Medicine of the Fetus and Its Mother.* Philadelphia: Lippincott Harper Publishing Co., 1992;1345–62.
14. Evans MI, Littman L, St Louis L, *et al.* Evolving patterns of iatrogenic multifetal pregnancy generation: Implications for aggressiveness of infertility treatments. *Am J Obstet Gynecol* 1995; 172:1750–3.
15. Tabsh KM, Theroux NL. Genetic amniocentesis following multifetal pregnancy reduction twins: Assessing the risk. *Prenat Diagn* 1995;15:221–3.
16. McLean LK, Evans MI, Carpenter RJ, Johnson MP, Goldberg JD. Genetic amniocentesis (AMN) following multifetal pregnancy reduction (MFPR) does not increase the risk of pregnancy loss. *Prenat Diagn* 1998;18:186–8.
17. Brambati B, Tului L, Baldi M, Guercilena S. Genetic analysis prior to selective termination in multiple pregnancy: Technical aspects and clinical outcome. *Hum Reprod* 1995;10:818–25.
18. Evans MI, Henry GP, Miller WA, *et al.* International, collaborative assessment of 146,000 prenatal karyotypes: Expected limitations if only chromosome-specific probes and fluorescent in situ hybridization were used. *Hum Reprod* 1999;14:1213–6.
19. Homer J, Bhatt S, Huang B, Thangavelu M. Residual risk for cytogenetic abnormalities after prenatal diagnosis by interphase fluorescence in situ hybridization (FISH). *Prenat Diagn* 2003; 23:556–71.
20. Greene RA, Wapner J, Evans MI. Amniocentesis and chorionic villus sampling in triplet pregnancy. In Keith LG, Blickstein I, Oleszcuk JJ, eds. *Triplet Pregnancy.* London: Parthenon Publishing Group, 73–84.
21. Zadori J, Kozinszky Z, Orvos H, Katona M, Kaali SG, Pal A. The incidence of major birth defects following *in vitro* fertilization. *J Assist Reprod Genet* 2003;20(3):131–2.
22. Pinborg A, Loft A, Schmidt L, Andersen AN. Morbidity in a Danish national cohort of 472 IVF/ICSI twins, 1132 non-IVF/ICSI twins and 634 IVF/ICSI singletons: Health-related and social implications for the children and their families. *Hum Reprod* 2003;18(6):1234–43.
23. Place I, Englert Y. A prospective longitudinal study of the physical, psychomotor, and intellectual development of singleton children up to 5 years who were conceived by intracytoplasmic sperm injection compared with children conceived spontaneously and by *in vitro* fertilization. *Fertil Steril* 2003;80(6): 1388–97.
24. Retzloff MG, Hornstein MD. Is intracytoplasmic sperm injection safe? *Fertil Steril* 2003;80(4):851–9.
25. Kurinczuk JJ. Safety issues in assisted reproduction technology. From theory to reality – just what are the data telling us about ICSI offspring health and future fertility and should we be concerned? *Hum Reprod* 2003;18(5):925–31.
26. Tournaye H. ICSI: A technique too far? *Int J Androl* 2003;26(2): 63–9.
27. Dumez Y, Oury JF. Method for first trimester selective abortion in multiple pregnancy. *Contrib Gynecol Obstet* 1986;15:50.
28. Evans MI, Fletcher JC, Zador IE, Newton BW, Struyk CK, Quigg MH. Selective first trimester termination in octuplet and quadruplet pregnancies: Clinical and ethical issues. *Obstet Gynecol* 1988;71:289–96.
29. Berkowitz RL, Lynch L, Chitkara U, *et al.* Selective reduction of multiple pregnancies in the first trimester. *N Engl J Med* 1988; 318:1043.
30. Wapner RJ, Davis GH, Johnson A. Selective reduction of multifetal pregnancies. *Lancet* 1990;335:90–3.
31. Timor-Tritsch IE, Peisner DB, Monteagudo A, Lerner JP, Sharma S. Multifetal pregnancy reduction by transvaginal puncture: Evaluation of the technique used in 134 cases. *Am J Obstet Gynecol* 1993;168:799–804.
32. Torok O, Lapinski R, Salafia CM, Bernasko J, Berkowitz RL. Multifetal pregnancy reduction is not associated with an increased risk of intrauterine growth restriction, except for very high order multiples. *Am J Obstet Gynecol* 1998;179:221–5.
33. Yaron Y, Bryant-Greenwood PK, Dave N, *et al.* Multifetal pregnancy reduction (MFPR) of triplets to twins: Comparison with non-reduced triplets and twins. *Am J Obstet Gynecol* 1999; 180:1268–71.
34. Leondires MP, Ernst SD, Miller BT, *et al.* Triplets: Outcomes of expectant management versus multifetal reduction for 127 pregnancies. *Am J Obstet Gynecol* 1999;72:257–60.
35. Lipitz S, Shulman A, Achiron R, *et al.* A comparative study of multifetal pregnancy reduction from triplets to twins in the first versus early second trimesters after detailed fetal screening. *Ultrasound Obstet Gynecol* 2001;18:35–8.
36. Angel JL, Kalter CS, Morales WJ, *et al.* Aggressive prerinatal care for high-order multiple gestations: Does good perinatal outcome justify aggressive assisted reproductive techniques? *Am J Obstet Gynecol* 1999;181:253–9.
37. Sepulveda W, Munoz H, Alcalde JL. Conjoined twins in a triplet pregnancy: Early prenatal diagnosis with three-dimensional ultrasound and review of the literature. *Ultrasound Obstet Gynecol* 2003;22(2):199–204.
38. Francois K, Sears C, Wilson R, Elliot J. Twelve year experience of triplet pregnancies at a single institution. *Am J Obstet Gynecol* 2001;185:S112.
39. Yakin K, Kahraman S, Comert S. Three blastocyst stage embryo transfer resulting in a quintuplet pregnancy. *Hum Reprod* 2001; 16(4):782–4.
40. Task Force of American College of Obstetricians and Gynecologists. *Neonatal Encephalopathy and Cerebral Palsy: Defining the Pathogenesis and Pathophysiology*. Washington, DC: ACOG, 2003.
41. Petterson B, Nelson K, Watson L, *et al.* Twins, triplets, and cerebral palsy in births in Western Australia in the 1980s. *Br Med J* 1993;307:1239–43.
42. Pharoah PO, Cooke T. Cerebral palsy and multiple births. *Arch Dis Child Fetal Neonatal Ed* 1996;75:F174–7.
43. Templeton A. The multiple gestation epidemic: The role of the assisted reproductive technologies.
44. Evans MI, Kaufman MI, Urban AJ, Krivchenia EL, Britt DW, Wapner RJ. Fetal reduction from twins to a singleton: A reasonable consideration. *Obstet Gynecol,* 2004;104:102–9.
45. Kalra SK, Milad MP, Klock SC, Crobman WA. Infertility patients and their partners: Differences in the desire for twin gestations. *Obstet Gynecol* 2003;102:152–5.
46. St John EB, Nelson KG, Oliver SP, Bishno RR, Goldenberg RL. Cost of neonatal care according to gestational age at birth and survival status. *Am J Obstet Gynecol* 2000;182:170–5.
47. Britt DW, Risinger ST, Mans M, Evans MI. Devastation and relief: Conflicting meanings in discovering fetal anomalies. *Ultrasound Obstet Gynecol* 2002;20:1–5.
48. Britt DW, Risinger ST, Mans M, Evans MI. Anxiety among women who have undergone fertility therapy and who are considering MFPR: Trends and scenarios. *J Matern Fetal Neonatal Med,* 2003;13:1–8.
49. Britt DW, Evans WJ, Mehta SS, Evans MI. Framing the decision: Determinants of how women considering MFPR as a pregnancy-management strategy frame their moral dilemma. *Fetal Diagn Ther* 2004;19:232–40.
50. Redelmeier DA, Rozin P, Kahneman D. Understanding patients' decisions: Cognitive and emotional perspectives. *J Am Med Assoc* 1993;270:72–6.
51. Chapman GB, Elstein AS. Cognitive processes and biases in medical decision making. In Chapman GB, Sonnenberg FA, eds. *Decision Making in Health Care: Theory, Psychology and Applications*. New York: Cambridge University Press, 2000: 183–210.
52. Steginga SK, Occhipinti S. The application of the heuristic-systematic processing model to treatment decision making about prostate cancer. *Med Decis Making* 2004;24.
53. Hamm RM. Theory about heuristic strategies based on verbal protocol analysis: The emperor needs a shave. *Med Decis Making* 2004;24:681–6.
54. Britt DW, Campbell EQ. Assessing the linkage of norms, environments and deviance. *Soc Forces* 1977:532–49.

20 Neonatal ethics

K. N. S. Subramanian

Background

Neonatal medicine has undergone significant changes over the last four decades. The increasing survival of smaller and younger infants is possible because of medical and technological innovations, such as antenatal steroid administration to a pregnant mother in preterm labor, the availability of surfactant to the premature infants, ventilators of different kinds (conventional, high frequency, etc.), inhaled nitric oxide (iNO), and extra corporeal membrane oxygenation (ECMO) to name a few. The mortality rate has improved over time in the USA[1,2] and the rest of the world,[3,4] and it has significantly declined in all weight categories. But there also is a need to have uniformity in the denominators we use for defining mortality and morbidity of these infants. Currently, the mortality rates are expressed as deaths per 1000 live born babies, deaths per all premature infants, by specific weight categories, by admissions to neonatal intensive care units (NICUs), or by deliveries in one hospital, geographic region, or country. The rates vary significantly depending on which terminology is used. Although rates of significant morbidities or serious handicaps have reduced or have remained steady across many gestational ages or weight groups over the years,[5] there is still a high rate of handicaps in lower birth weight or early gestational age groups.[6–8]

With increased survival and an increase in the total number of handicapped infants, society is confronted with the need for special assistance for these children. Decisions regarding resuscitation at the lower ends of gestational age (< 24 weeks) and birth weight (<400 g) become increasingly difficult. Decisions regarding the congenitally malformed or infants with chromosomal problems (like Trisomy 13 and 18), identified during pregnancy, pose an ethical and moral challenge for the various participants. The pregnant woman and the father of the fetus, along with the family and physicians and other health care providers, struggle with these decisions at times of extreme vulnerability and uncertainty. Numerous publications and guidelines by professional and legal organizations attempt to clarify the issues and guide the parents, health care providers, and hospitals. Management of these issues compels the clinicians to make decisions 'in the moment of clinical truth'.[9]

Significant medical and technological innovations have invaded the NICU. Thoughtful use of such advances might help to save more lives but attention should be paid to whether these advances decrease morbidity over time. Surfactant use from 1990 has significantly increased survival and reduced morbidity. Administration of antenatal steroids to pregnant mothers with preterm labor has increased both pulmonary maturity and survival. Short-term outcomes of these infants appear to be favorable but long-term outcomes are being evaluated. On the other hand, the introduction of ECMO and ventilators occurred without any controlled studies in NICUs. Later studies suggested limited benefit for some of these therapies. It is critical to evaluate any new medical or surgical therapies before implementing them on a widespread basis in NICUs.

In this chapter some of these issues, such as the lower limit of viability (periviable or how small is too small?), withdrawal and/or withholding life support including nutrition and fluids, economics, role of parents and health care providers, global perspectives, and a common framework for neonatal ethical issues, will be reviewed.

Threshold of viability or how small is too small?

The current published statistics about survival and morbidity rates of extremely low birth weight (ELBW) and very low birth weight (VLBW) babies will be presented to assist in addressing the issue of viability. Survivability of infants correlates with gestational age and birth weight. African-American infants comprise 36.8% of the ELBW (<1000 g) babies born in the USA but account for only 15.5% of all live births. Biomedical and biopsychosocial factors may be contributing to this disproportionate increase in ELBW in African-American births, and these dynamics need further investigation.

It is important to know the outcomes of these ELBW and VLBW infants, especially below 25 weeks of gestation, to assist in decision making regarding withholding or withdrawing support. Infants born and admitted to the NICU at or < 23 weeks have a less than 10% chance of survival. Less than 1% survival was reported in ELBW infants with birth weights < 400 g. In a large multicenter review in the USA, the survival rate from birth until discharge for infants born between 1996 and 2000 and with birth weights of 401–500 g was 17%.[10] Earlier reports by other investigators were more dismal in terms of survival of infants <500 g.[11,12]

In a prospective study from England and Ireland,[12] the survival rates expressed as a percentage of live births in 1995 for infants at 23, 24, and 25 weeks of gestation were 11%, 26%, and 44%, respectively. Expressed as a percentage of the admission to NICUs, the survival rates improved to 20%, 34%, and 52%, respectively. For the same cohort of infants, the survival rates expressed by birth weight for infants weighing < 500, 500–749, and 750–999 g were 6%, 32%, and 55%, respectively.

Birth-weight-specific statistics of admissions to NICUs in the USA have shown higher survival rates. The National Institute of Child Health and Human Development (NICHD) network[2] reported that survival rates for infants at 23, 24, and 25 weeks of gestation were < 20%, 47%, and 68%, respectively. In the same report, survival rates from birth until discharge for infants born between January 1993 and December 1994 with birth weights of 501–750, 751–1000, 1001–1250, and 1251–1500 g were 49%, 85%, 93%, and 96%, respectively. Among these survivors, chronic lung disease developed in 19%, intraventricular hemorrhage in 32% (with 11% having severe grades), and periventricular leukomalacia in 6%. The incidence of necrotizing enterocolitis ranged from 3% to 9% and that of late-onset sepsis varied from 9% to 34%, inversely related to birth weights. Infants in these weight groups stayed in the hospital for an average of 2–4 months. The report also notes that the mortality rate declined by 42% from 1988 to 1994 in all weight groups but with no significant drop in the morbidity rates of infants < 750 g (38% in 1988 and 37% in 1994).

In 1997, a report compared the survival and morbidity rates of infants weighing 501–800 g born in North Carolina, USA,[5] during three time periods from 1979 to 1984, 1984 to 1989, and 1989 to 1994. Survival rates increased from 20% to 36% to 59%, respectively. On the other hand, the major neurosensory impairments at 1 year of age remained relatively the same, at 25%, 28%, and 21%, during the same three periods. Hussain and Rosenkrantz[13] reported in a 2003 composite of many studies from developed nations a survival rate of < 3.5% at 22 weeks, 21% at 23 weeks, 46% at 24 weeks, and 66% at 25 weeks of gestation.

The cohort of infants born in 1995 in England and Ireland at < 25 completed weeks were prospectively followed for > 6 years. The report in 2005 suggested that the cognitive and neurological deficits were common at school age (21%).[14] A comparison with their classroom peers showed even more impairment (41%). The rates of mild, moderate, and severe disabilities were 34%, 24%, and 22%, respectively, in these survivors. Twelve percent had cerebral palsy. Even more sobering were the rates of survival with no disability among this group at 6 years of age: 1%, 3%, and 8% for those born at 23, 24, and 25 weeks of gestation, respectively.

While this information will keep changing in the future as mortality and morbidity rates change, one can attempt to address the issue of how small is too small. Biologically, at < 22 weeks of gestational age, the physiological and anatomical maturity of the lung will unlikely support extrauterine function and hence survival.[15–17] Over the last 10 years there seems to be a leveling of improvement in survival in these gestational age groups. This leveling suggests that we may have reached the threshold of viability with the current technology and support. Sharing this information and institutional, regional, national, and global mortality and morbidity reports with parents will be the first step in addressing the issue of viability.

Parents' role

In the USA, parents are generally considered appropriate surrogate decision makers for their children. They are also considered to have the required authority and best interests of the infant in their minds when making decisions about medical care for their children.

Attitudes of parents and health care providers regarding outcomes of ELBW infants, including quality of life, have been evaluated in many reports.[18–20] Saigal reported that when presented with hypothetical clinical vignettes, health care providers in NICU were significantly more negative than the parents of the teenaged ELBW children.[18] The parents rated the quality of life as good for their children even though they acknowledged that their children have a greater burden than other normal birth weight children. These studies suggest that parents are appropriate decision makers in most cases.

It is evident from the available data that the mortality and morbidity rates are high for infants born at < 24 weeks and/or weighing < 500 g. At 23 and 24 weeks, even though survival has improved, reported handicaps of survivors should give a pause to those in NICU in pursuing a course of aggressive action in the delivery room and subsequently in the unit. It is important to have the global, national, regional, and institutional data on not only survival but also outcomes of these ELBW infants so the information can be shared with the parents to assist in decision making. Because the statistics differ depending on which denominators are used, one should be clear and consistent in the communication.

The issue of sanctity of life vs. quality of life is a running debate in neonatal and obstetric specialties, as well as with the prospective parents. Those who believe in sanctity of life may suggest that it is worth intervening with aggressive support for any live product of conception. Many have difficulty in accepting this notion as necessarily directing anyone to initiate or sustain treatments regardless of the mortality and morbidity. They suggest that it may be preferable to assess intervention after birth so that the decision can be made with more information at hand. On the other hand, the slippery slope argument about the quality of life judgment is well known. This issue remains a continuing debate in society and adds to the uncertainty in decision making.

Economics

As a result of advancing technology hospital bills have increased dramatically, and the total lifetime costs may go up even higher if the infant needs any type of rehabilitation or follow-up care. The cost of care in NICUs in the USA is now reported as exceeding four billion dollars. A 2003 California study[21] reported an average hospital cost of $224,000 for an infant with birth weight between 500 and 700 g compared to $4300 for infants between 2250 and 2500 g and $1000 for those with birth weights greater than 3000 g. In the same study, hospital costs averaged $202,400 for an infant born at 25 weeks compared to $2600 for an infant born at 36 weeks and $1100 for a 38-week infant. Similarly, another study[22] reported a median cost of $103,600 for infants born between 501 and 750 g, going down to $31,200 for those between 1251 and 1500 g. The hospital costs were highest for infants born at 25–26 weeks of gestation with a median of $101,600, dropping to $18,700 for infants born at > 32 weeks. Another 1987 California study[23] calculated that the average cost per first-year survivor in infants in NICUs with birth weights less than 750 g was $273,900; for those who weighed 750–999 g, the average cost was $138,800. In a May 16, 1988, article, *Newsweek* quoted the total cost for a surviving fetal infant as $366,480 with additional costs during rehabilitation. However, the aggregate cost of NICU is still far less than the cost of adult intensive care units providing care for those at the end of life.

This brief discussion of the economics of caring for critically ill infants in the NICU is necessary to understand the full impact on families, society, and the surviving infant with special needs. The infant's family undergoes severe emotional and financial stress with the birth of an extremely premature infant, and they are often confused, angry, and frustrated by the resulting issues. This concern needs to be understood by the medical team, and the public and society need to address it in an open forum.

Withholding/withdrawal of nutrition and fluids

The benefits and burdens of any medical intervention should be assessed so that a determination can be made regarding the withholding/withdrawal (WH/WD) of nutrition and fluids. Most will agree that if the burdens outweigh the benefits, the withholding or withdrawal of support to adults, children, or neonates is acceptable. Currently, most reports suggest that for adults with terminal conditions it is appropriate for the patient to request WH/WD of nutrition and fluids as well (*JAMA* 1990).[24,25] Most agree that appropriate family members, especially if authorized to make medical decisions, can request WH/WD of nutrition and fluids for a terminally ill adult patient. Increasingly, pediatric patients are also reported as appropriate candidates for requests for WH/WD in terminal conditions.[26–28] The premise behind such requests is that tube feeding or intravenous alimentation should be considered a medical intervention just like intubation or other treatments. Others would argue that withdrawal of nutrition and fluids, especially from neonates, should not be recommended.

In an excellent review by Carter and Leuthner,[29] the authors hold that WH/WD of nutrition and fluids in newborn infants is also appropriate. They state that the 'medical facts such as underlying diagnosis, response to previously given treatments, likely response to appropriate treatments or interventions not yet offered and ultimate prognosis for the infant's condition' should be considered and discussed in detail with the team, parents, and extended family. In addition, parents' expectations, culture, religion, traditions, and other social values should be brought to bear on this decision for their infant. The health care team should not usurp the authority of the parents without documentation (from independent experts) that they are not capable of making such decisions. The institution's policies and state legal statues should be reviewed and taken into account. Offering oral feeding in infants should be acceptable as well as pain medications as part of palliative care. Hospice care, if available, for such infants when the WH/WD of care including nutrition and fluids is indicated as a good alternative. More discussion by physicians, the health care community, parental groups, and society is necessary to guide the decision making about WH/WD of nutrition and fluids in the newborn in the future.

Global perspectives

It is clear that ethical decision making does not take place in the abstract. Societies, nations, cultures and traditions, and religions play an intricate part in such decision making. In developing nations, and now in developed nations as well, the economy also plays a

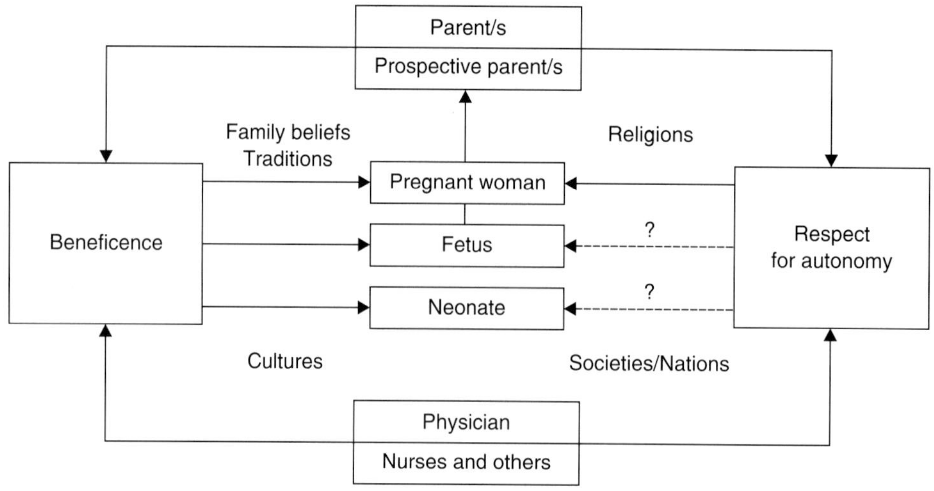

Figure 20.1 Common framework for perinatal/neonatal ethics. Modified from Subramanian and McCullough.[41]

role in such decisions at the macro level of national health care policy and at the micro level in the decision making of a patient (the principle of justice). In many countries, such as India, Nepal, and Sri Lanka[30] quality of life and economy clearly play a crucial role in parental and societal decisions regarding WH/WD of support. In Singapore[31] using an individualized prognostic strategy, 'a consensual decision that respects parental authority and promotes physician beneficence with the best interest of the infant placed in the center of analysis' is being reached. In Israel[32] the maternal birth place and level of religious observance were associated with aggressive intervention in hypothetical cases. In neonatal care, specific guidelines, such as those in The Netherlands and Japan,[33,34] led to infants at 22 or <25 weeks of gestation being resuscitated, but resulted in significant mortality and morbidity. Similarly, a study in California, USA, requiring resuscitation of all infants >22 weeks of gestation or >450 g, resulted in significant mortality and morbidity, leading to a recommendation of providing other than comfort care as exceptional for infants <23 weeks or <500 g. A report from Scotland[35] outlined that eight European countries compared the 'legal, ethical and professional settings within which decision making for neonates took place'. Overly aggressive treatment was discouraged and comfort care recommended. Most of the countries prohibited 'active intentional ending of life', except Dutch pediatricians. Reports from the USA,[36,37] Australia,[38,39] and Austria[40] suggest that infants born at tertiary centers with neonatal and perinatal specialties had a better survival rate at these gestational ages. Those transferred *in utero* to tertiary centers at 23, 24, and 25 or 26 weeks of gestation showed lower morbidity and had a better prognosis. Globally, the viability limit seems to be slowly but steadily converging around 22–24 weeks based on biological and experiential data.

Common framework for perinatal and neonatal ethics

Attempting to create a common framework for neonatal and perinatal ethics is a daunting task. We proposed in 1987, a model[41] based on the ethical principles of beneficence and respect for autonomy, incorporating the families, religion, culture and traditions, societies, and nations as part of the fabric of decision making (Figure 20.1). With minor modifications it probably still holds as an anatomical framework for clinicians to work through difficult ethical dilemmas.

The principles of beneficence and respect for autonomy are clearly addressed in the model. The fetus and future neonate along with the pregnant woman are at the center of this schema generating both beneficence- and autonomy-related obligations. Even though there are ethical obligations generated toward the parent/s, the neonatologist's primary patient is the neonate. The future parent/s is included at the top of the model to reflect the relationship in the neonatal period. The physician is at the base of the model generating ethical obligations to prospective parents, the pregnant woman, and the fetus during the perinatal period and to the neonate and the parents in the postnatal period and beyond. It is recognized that these ethical dilemmas are affected by the context in which they occur and hence the schema recognize the need to add religious beliefs, traditions, family beliefs and values, cultures, societies, and nations as the very fabric on which this model is built. There are primarily beneficence-based ethical obligations to the fetus and neonate, but the model included autonomy-based obligations as secondary in the model because some may believe they exist. This structural guidance could be applied to ELBW infants, infants with congenital anomalies such

Table 20.1 Guidelines for care of extremely preterm infants [from Boyle RJ, c472. *NeoReviews* 2004;5(11): November]

Canadian Pediatric Society (1994)
- 22 weeks' gestation: treatment should be started only at the request of fully informed parents or if it appears that the gestational age was underestimated
- 23–24 weeks' gestation: there is a role for parental wishes, the option of resuscitation, and a need for flexibility in deciding to start or withhold resuscitation, depending on the infant's condition at birth
- 25 weeks' gestation: resuscitation should be attempted for all infants who do not have fatal anomalies

Colorado Collective for Medical Decisions (2000)
- 22 weeks' gestation: comfort care is the only appropriate choice
- 23 weeks' gestation: most participants would advise comfort care, but if parents understood the high risks, they would be willing to initiate a course of intensive care.
- 24 weeks' gestation: participants are able to support either decision, as long as a collaborative process with good sharing of information occurred
- 25 weeks' gestation: most participants were uncomfortable with withholding care, but some were willing to support a parental request for comfort care if there had been good education and an effort at collaboration

American Academy of Pediatrics/American Heart Association Neonatal Resuscitation Program (2000)
- Non-initiation of resuscitation in the delivery room is appropriate for newborns who had confirmed gestation of less than 23 weeks or birth weights of less than 400 g

Thames Regional Perinatal Group (2000)
- Less than or equal to 22 weeks' gestation: compassionate care only
- 23–24 weeks' gestation: resuscitation depends on infant's condition at birth
- 25–27 weeks' gestation: full resuscitation and supportive care

as Trisomy 13, Trisomy 18, anencephalic and other terminally ill infants.

This model extends Pellegrino's proposed framework[9] for clinical ethical dilemmas to the complex perinatal and neonatal areas. This model recommends a collaborative approach to decision making between the parent/s, physician, and other health care providers acting in the best interest of the baby. Parents should be able to make these decisions for their infant unless they are shown to be incompetent or incapable as assessed by independent specialists such as psychiatrists or, of course, the courts. Obtaining the opinion of ethics consultant or ethics committee will help the clinician and family in guiding the decision making. Many families have found the objective view of another expert or group of people helpful in facilitating the discussion and clarification of the facts of the ethical dilemma being faced and the options available.

The four 'C's of clinical ethical decision making include: (1) communication, (2) clarification, (3) consistency, and (4) caring. Maintaining a high level of communication between parents and health care providers is necessary in the NICU where issues are extremely complex and highly charged with emotions. Clarification of issues that arise among health care givers and between parents and medical and nursing staff is crucial for problem solving even before a dilemma arises. Providing consistent information available to date by all care givers (provided good communication exists between providers) will allow for a trusting environment in which decision making is encouraged. An attitude of caring from the very beginning provides the necessary environment in which parents feel comfortable in discussing any and all issues about their infants. All four of these facilitate decision making by the parents and health care providers during difficult times.

Guidelines

Currently, there exist guidelines from various organizations including the American Academy of Pediatrics (AAP), AAP Committee on Fetus and Newborn,[42,43] AAP Committee on Bioethics,[44] NICHD concensus conference,[45] American College of Obstetricians and Gynecologists (ACOG), ACOG Committee on Obstetric Practice,[46] Canadian Pediatric Society,[47] Thames Regional Perinatal Group,[48] Colorado Collective for Medical Decisions,[49] International Guidelines for Neonatal Resuscitation,[50] New York State Task Force on Life and Law,[51] and from other countries (Table 20.1). At 22 weeks or < 23 weeks or < 400 g, most guidelines recommend giving only comfort or compassionate care, which is consistent with available data on mortality, morbidity, and biological information. Most guidelines will also suggest comfort care at 23 weeks unless parents, after understanding the high risks, want to initiate aggressive attempts. At 24 weeks, resuscitation will depend on the assessment of the baby's condition at birth and the parents' understanding of the mortality, morbidity, and prognosis; choosing to intervene to give a trial of life is an appropriate alternative. In some of the recommendations (Italy 2004, New York 1988), $\geq$24 weeks or > 500 g are used as cutoff points for resuscitation. At 25 weeks and beyond, most guidelines recommend full resuscitation. However, some maintain that a parental request not to resuscitate should be followed even at 25 weeks. Most guidelines base the recommendations on gestational age. Because growth-restricted mature infants are included in the statistics presented by birth weight, a hard birth weight cutoff is more difficult to use in deciding viability.

All guidelines consistently recommend the need for clear communication among physicians, nurses, and parents both before delivery and afterward. Collaborative decision making between parents and physicians, along with other health care providers, is the best way to chart a course that is appropriate for the individual baby and parents, especially in infants expected to be < 24 weeks of gestation or < 500 g in birth weight. Any strict cutoff by gestational age or birth weight at this edge of viability should be avoided because the prognosis for the individual infant remains uncertain in terms of both mortality and morbidity. Parents who understand the high risks involved in aggressive interventions at the borderline gestational ages should be given the option of assessment at birth and resuscitation. Further action will depend on the infant's condition and the NICU course. Even prior to delivery, one should discuss with parents that, if assessment after birth indicates a significantly poor prognosis, withdrawal of support should be an option. There should always be room for individual decision making based on the specifics of the situation, such as a parent with infertility, advanced age, multiple pregnancy losses, etc. Even though ethically there is no difference between withholding and withdrawing care, emotionally the latter may be harder for parents or some health care providers. For some, withholding may be preferable to withdrawing, but clear communication before and throughout the hospital course will help in making the right decision.

Collaborative or consensus decision making between the parents, physician, and team with careful, clear communication and discussion is the best way to resolve any ethical dilemmas. In situations where disagreement exists between the health care team and parent(s), additional consultations with a colleague and other specialists and/or ethics consultants and committee meetings should help clarify the issues and resolve the differences. In those difficult situations where differences remain, one or the other party can seek legal action. Usually, courts are not in the best position to resolve these difficult moral and ethical issues except on narrow legal grounds. In many situations Law and Ethics may not see eye-to-eye in resolving the dilemma.

Summary

In summary, the tremendous advances made in the last four decades in neonatal medicine have also brought difficult ethical dilemmas for health care providers and parents. Over these years the lower limit of viability dropped from 28–32 weeks to 22–23 weeks of gestation. As we reach the physiological and anatomical limits of lung development and extrauterine survival we also reach a natural barrier of lower limit of viability. Of course, this can change if there are some additional advances in existing treatments such as liquid ventilation or providing nutrition in a novel way, or new interventions such as artificial placenta or uterus. But this 'medical miracles around the corner' argument or outliers in terms of survival of < 23 weeks gestation infants cannot be used for decision making occurring now. Advances in technology and the ability to prolong life should be tempered with the benefits and burdens to the patient. Principles of beneficence and respect for autonomy obligations weigh heavily in neonatal ethical dilemmas in the milieu of principle of justice and cultures, traditions, religions, and nations. Weighing the benefits/burden to the patient should guide everyone in the decision making. Both obstetrician and neonatalogist have beneficence-generated obligations toward the fetus and neonate. The neonatologist has both beneficence- and autonomy-generated obligations toward the pregnant mother and father during antenatal consultations and subsequently to the parent/s when the neonate comes into the NICUs. Collaborative/consensus/shared decision making with parents, physicians, and others, applying the ethical principles outlined in the model, will result in the best practice in NICU for these infants. Judicial uses of the ethics consultant or committee and other experts may facilitate better communication and clarification in difficult circumstances. Providing communication in a clear, consistent, and caring way (four Cs) and sharing all the information about mortality, morbidity, and prognosis before and after delivery of a high-risk infant facilitates decision making.

Acknowledgments

My thanks to Ms Ninian Kring for preparing the tables and figures and Ramya Sivasubramanian, JD for reviewing the manuscript and providing valuable suggestions. I also thank all the infants that I had the privilege of taking care of over the years and their parents for the opportunity to serve and learn from and all the staff, residents, fellows, and colleagues at Georgetown University Hospital NICU.

REFERENCES

1. Lemons JA, Bauer CR, Oh W, *et al.* Very low birth weight outcomes of the National Institute of Child Health and Human Development Neonatal Research Network, January 1995 through December 1996. NICHD Neonatal Research Network. *Pediatrics* 2001;107(1):E1.
2. Stevenson DK, Wright LL, Lemons JA, *et al.* Very low birth weight outcomes of the National Institute of Child Health and Human Development Neonatal Research Network, January 1993 through December 1994. *Am J Obstet Gynecol* 1998;179(6, Pt 1): 1632–9.
3. Horbar JD, Badger GJ, Lewit EM, Rogowski J, Shiono PH. Hospital and patient characteristics associated with variation in 28-day mortality rates for very low birth weight infants. Vermont Oxford Network. *Pediatrics* 1997;99(2):149–56.
4. Wood B, Katz V, Bose C, Goolsby R, Kraybill E. Survival and morbidity of extremely premature infants based on obstetric assessment of gestational age. *Obstet Gynecol* 1989;74(6): 889–92.
5. O'Shea TM, Klinepeter KL, Goldstein DJ, Jackson BW, Dillard RG. Survival and developmental disability in infants with birth weights of 501 to 800 grams, born between 1979 and 1994. *Pediatrics* 1997;100(6):982–86.
6. Vohr BR, Wright LL, Dusick AM, *et al.* Neurodevelopmental and functional outcomes of extremely low birth weight infants in the National Institute of Child Health and Human Development Neonatal Research Network, 1993–1994. *Pediatrics* 2000; 105(6):1216–26.
7. Botting N, Powls A, Cooke RW, Marlow N. Cognitive and educational outcome of very-low-birthweight children in early adolescence. *Dev Med Child Neurol* 1998;40(10):652–60.
8. Ment LR, Vohr B, Allan W, *et al.* Change in cognitive function over time in very low-birth-weight infants. *J Am Med Assoc* 2003;289(6):705–11.
9. Pellegrino ED. The anatomy of clinical–ethical judgments in perinatology and neonatology: A substantive and procedural framework. *Semin Perinatol* 1987;11(3):202–9.
10. Lucey JF, Rowan CA, Shiono P, *et al.* Fetal infants: The fate of 4172 infants with birth weights of 401 to 500 grams – the Vermont Oxford Network experience (1996–2000). *Pediatrics* 2004;113(6):1559–66.
11. Allen MC, Donohue P K, Dusman AE. The limit of viability – neonatal outcome of infants born at 22 to 25 weeks' gestation. *N Engl J Med* 1993;329(22):1597–601.
12. Costeloe K, Hennessy E, Gibson AT, Marlow N, Wilkinson AR. The EPICure study: Outcomes to discharge from hospital for infants born at the threshold of viability. *Pediatrics* 2000; 106(4):659–71.
13. Hussain N, Rosenkrantz TS. Ethical considerations in the management of infants born at extremely low gestational age. *Semin Perinatol* 2003;27(6):458–70.
14. Marlow N, Wolke D, Bracewell MA, Samara M. Neurologic and developmental disability at six years of age after extremely preterm birth. *N Engl J Med* 2005;352(1):9–19.
15. Barbet JP, Houette A, Barres D, Durigon M. Histological assessment of gestational age in human embryos and fetuses. *Am J Forensic Med Pathol* 1988;9(1):40–4.
16. DiMaio M, Gil J, Ciurea D, Kattan M. Structural maturation of the human fetal lung: A morphometric study of the development of air–blood barriers. *Pediatr Res* 1989;26(2):88–93.
17. deMello DE, Reid LM. Embryonic and early fetal development of human lung vasculature and its functional implications. *Pediatr Dev Pathol* 2000;3(5):439–49.
18. Streiner DL, Saigal S, Burrows E, Stoskopf B, Rosenbaum P. Attitudes of parents and health care professionals toward active treatment of extremely premature infants. *Pediatrics* 2001;108(1):152–7.
19. McHaffie HE, Laing IA, Parker M, McMillan J. Deciding for imperilled newborns: Medical authority or parental autonomy? *J Med Ethics* 2001;27(2):104–9.
20. Hansen MM, Durbin J, Sinkowitz-Cochran R, Vaughn A, Langowski M, Gleason S. Do no harm: Provider perceptions of patient safety. *J Nurs Adm* 2003;33(10):507–8.
21. Gilbert WM, Nesbitt TS, Danielsen B. The cost of prematurity: Quantification by gestational age and birth weight. *Obstet Gynecol* 2003;102(3):488–92.
22. Rogowski J. Using economic information in a quality improvement collaborative. *Pediatrics* 2003;111(4, Pt 2):e411–8.
23. Fischer AF, Stevenson DK. The consequences of uncertainty. An empirical approach to medical decision making in neonatal intensive care. *JAMA* 1987;258(14):1929–31.
24. Winter SM. Terminal nutrition: Framing the debate for the withdrawal of nutritional support in terminally ill patients. *Am J Med* 2000;109(9):723–6.
25. Hastings Center. *Guidelines on the Termination of Life-Sustaining Treatment and Care of the Dying.* Briarcliff Manor, NY: The Hastings Center, 1987.
26. Burns JP, Mitchell C, Griffith JL, Truog RD. End-of-life care in the pediatric intensive care unit: Attitudes and practices of pediatric critical care physicians and nurses. *Crit Care Med* 2001;29(3): 658–64.
27. Cranford RE. Withdrawing artificial feeding from children with brain damage. *Br Med J* 1995;311(7003):464–5.
28. Johnson J, Mitchell C. Responding to parental requests to forego pediatric nutrition and hydration. *J Clin Ethics* 2000;11(2): 128–35.
29. Carter BS, Leuthner SR. Decision making in the NICU – strategies, statistics, and "satisficing". *Bioethics Forum* 2002;18(3–4):7–15.
30. Subramanian KN, Paul VK. Care of critically ill newborns in India. Legal and ethical issues. *J Leg Med* 1995;16(2):263–75.
31. Ho NK. Ethical issues in neonatal paediatrics – the Singapore perspective. *Ann Acad Med Singapore* 1995;24(6):910–14.
32. Hammerman C, Kornbluth E, Lavie O, Zadka P, Aboulafia Y, Eidelman AI. Decision-making in the critically ill neonate: Cultural background v individual life experiences. *J Med Ethics* 1997;23(3):164–9.
33. Oishi M, Nishida H, Sasaki T. Japanese experience with micropremies weighing less than 600 grams born between 1984 to 1993. *Pediatrics* 1997;99(6):E7.
34. Nishida H, Sakamoto S. Ethical problems in neonatal intensive care unit – medical decision making on the neonate with poor prognosis. *Early Hum Dev* 1992;29(1–3):403–6.
35. McHaffie HE, Cuttini M, Brolz-Voit G, *et al.* Withholding/withdrawing treatment from neonates: Legislation and official guidelines across Europe. *J Med Ethics* 1999;25(6):440–6.
36. Yeast JD, Poskin M, Stockbauer JW, Shaffer S. Changing patterns in regionalization of perinatal care and the impact on neonatal mortality. *Am J Obstet Gynecol* 1998;178(1, Pt 1):131–5.
37. Bode MM, O'Shea TM, Metzguer KR, Stiles AD. Perinatal regionalization and neonatal mortality in North Carolina, 1968–1994. *Am J Obstet Gynecol* 2001;184(6):1302–7.
38. Doyle LW, Casalaz D. Outcome at 14 years of extremely low birthweight infants: A regional study. *Arch Dis Child Fetal Neonatal Ed* 2001;85(3):F159–64.
39. Doyle LW, Cheung MM, Ford GW, Olinsky A, Davis NM, Callanan C. Birth weight <1501 g and respiratory health at age 14. *Arch Dis Child* 2001;84(1):40–4.
40. Hohlagschwandtner M, Husslein P, Klebermass K, Weninger M, Nardi A, Langer M. Perinatal mortality and morbidity. Comparison between maternal transport, neonatal transport and inpatient antenatal treatment. *Arch Gynecol Obstet* 2001;265(3): 113–8.
41. Subramanian KN, McCullough LB. A common framework for perinatal and neonatal medical ethics. *Semin Perinatol* 1987;11(3):288–90.
42. American Academy of Pediatrics Committee on Fetus and Newborn. The initiation or withdrawal of treatment for high-risk newborns. *Pediatrics* 1995;96(2, Pt 1):362–3.
43. MacDonald H, & the Committee on Fetus and Newborn: Perinatal care at the threshold of viability. *Pediatrics* 2002;110:1024–7.
44. American Academy of Pediatrics Committee on Bioethics. Ethics and the care of critically ill infants and children. *Pediatrics* 1996;98(1):149–52.
45. Higgins RD, Delivoria-Papdopoulos M, Raju N.K.T. *et al.* Executive summary of the workshop on the border of viability. 2005;1392–6.
46. American Academy of Pediatrics Committee on Fetus and Newborn. Perinatal care at the threshold of viability. American College of Obstetricians and Gynecologists Committee on Obstetric Practice. *Pediatrics* 1995;96(5, Pt 1):974–6.

47. Canadian Pediatric Society, Fetus and Newborn Committee. Management of the woman with threatened birth of an infant of extremely low gestational age. Maternal–Fetal Medicine Committee, Society of Obstetricians and Gynaecologists of Canada. *Can Med Assoc J* 1994;151(5):547–53.
48. Thames Regional Perinatal Group. Guidelines relating to the birth of extremely immature babies (22–26 weeks gestation). http://www.gapm.org/publication.php. Accessed March 2000.
49. Colorado Collective for Medical Decisions. *Neonatal Guidelines and Video.* Denver, CO: Colorado Collective for Medical Decisions.
50. Niermeyer S, Kattwinkel J, Van Reempts P, *et al.* International guidelines for neonatal resuscitation: An excerpt from the Guidelines 2000 for Cardiopulmonary Resuscitation and Emergency Cardiovascular Care: International Consensus on Science. Contributors and Reviewers for the Neonatal Resuscitation Guidelines. *Pediatrics* 2000;106(3):E29.
51. Anonymous. *Fetal Extrauterine Survivability.* Report of the Committee on Fetal and Extrauterine Survivability to the New York State Task Force on Life and the Law. New York: New York State Task Force on Life and the Law, 1988.

21 Medicolegal aspects of perinatal medicine: European perspective

J. Walker

Introduction

A pregnant woman has similar rights to any other patient and these are protected by the normal human rights assigned to her by society. Therefore, her informed consent is required before intervention and her right to refuse treatment is accepted. However, there is a complication – she carries another potential individual; therefore, her rights and control over her pregnancy are influenced by the rights assigned to the fetus and how much of these rights are allocated to the mother to hold.

Irrespective of the rights the child has *in utero*, after birth, its rights are paramount, and although the parents may control these rights to a degree, this is not absolute and their control can be taken away in the best interests of the baby. Also, in some situations, the rights of the newborn baby can be considered to be present in retrospect; in other words, damage done prior to delivery that results in problems after birth can give rights of complaint to the baby that were not there at the time of the event. Therefore, potentially, the rights of this one individual, the child, and the rights of others over it, can change at the moment of birth and, in some instances, this change of rights can then be applied retrospectively.

This has caused increasing ethical dilemmas over the years because of the increasing knowledge of pregnancy physiology and, more importantly, the increasing ability to assess and visualize the fetus. This means that the fetus is increasingly seen as an individual that has access to medical care and is a factor in medical decision making. This has led to the concept of the 'fetus as a patient' and, by definition, medical rights.[1] Generally, what is good for the baby is good for the mother, so there is no conflict. It is when the mother disagrees with her carers about what is best for the baby that conflict appears.[2,3]

With advances in medical technology and the ability to salvage pregnancies that failed previously, society has begun to believe that medicine can achieve anything. This means that if damage occurs, there has to have been error and negligence. Since the fetus is usually the one that is damaged, it is the baby, or its guardian, who will have to proceed with litigation, even though the fetus may not have had rights at the time of the event. If a neonatal death occurs, this may increasingly lead to potential criminal proceedings,[4,5] but this can depend on the legal rights of the fetus and whether it is born alive or not. It is in these areas of litigation and fetal rights that there is so much difference between countries.

The rights of the fetus

There is no universal truth and this is never truer than for ethical and legal issues. Perinatal doctors in different countries work in different environments. What is acceptable in one country may not be acceptable in another, not because it is right or wrong, but because of differences in ethical, legal or social mores.[5] In medicine, we are taught to 'first do no harm', but in the case of perinatal medicine, we also need to consider 'to whom?'. The problem is that there can be conflict between the concept of the 'fetus as a patient' and the rights of the mother.

This situation is covered by the term beneficence.[1] Beneficence is the moral principle that one should aim to help and failure to do this when one is in the position to do so is morally wrong. However, one is obligated to act to benefit others when one can do so with minimal risk, inconvenience or expense. In perinatal medicine there is potentially two patients to consider. How much of a conflict this is depends on both legal and moral belief. In general, the life of the mother takes precedence because the health of the mother is important for the health not only of that baby but also of any siblings. However, the main governor of the decision-making process is the legal rights of the fetus.

If the fetus has the same rights as a newborn baby, decisions can be made on behalf of the baby against the wishes of the mother, so-called court-ordered care. There is also the chance of the newborn suing for any damage sustained *in utero* from maternal or other's actions, so-called Wrongful Life decisions.[6]

However, where the fetus has no legal rights, the mother's wishes are paramount. It is only variations in law or ethical constraints that will restrict her and her carers' actions. However, this maternal control exists only up to the moment of birth, when full neonatal rights exist and the control transfers to the baby or its guardians. This change in legal status occurs in a matter of minutes and can be confusing to the mother, attendant staff and society as a whole.

Generally, in European law, the starting point is that a child *en ventre sa mere* is a part of its mother and therefore its rights are held by the mother.[7] However, in English common law an unborn child has rights to inherit property as follows:

> There is nothing in law to prevent a man from owning property before he is born. His ownership is contingent, for he may never be born at all; but it is nonetheless real and present ownership. A man may settle property on his wife and the children to be born of her. Or he may die intestate and his unborn child will inherit his estate.

This is traditionally called 'present ownership', that is, a right possessed by the unborn child at that time, but conditional on being born alive. If the child is stillborn, the inheritance (or rights) will revert to someone else. This is referred to as the 'born alive rule'.[7]

Therefore, any right the fetus has in English common law is dependant on being born alive. This means that actions leading to death of the baby before birth do not come under the normal crimes against the person, but if the baby is born alive and then dies then the baby's existence, and therefore rights, exists and action can be taken. Overall, the legal situation in Europe is somewhat confused and is constantly evolving, as will be described. Within the European Community, there is a further complication since the countries are governed by similar European laws on human rights, although there are still differences with the application due to the local law in each country.

The right to life

When the European Human Rights Act came into force in 2000, it was felt by many that the 'Right to Life' stated in Article 2 could be extended to the unborn fetus. This would protect it from termination of pregnancy and give it equal rights to those of the mother when considering medical decisions. However, a case based on this belief has recently been heard in the European Court of Human Rights, and it was decided that the rights of the fetus are not covered by Article 2. This is an important landmark decision not based on law but more on lack of consensus of what is right.

The case involved Mrs Vo, one of two women of the same name admitted to the same hospital at the same time, one for a medical examination when 6 months pregnant, the other to have a coil removed. The wrong Mrs Vo went for coil removal. In an attempt to remove the non-existent coil, Mrs Vo's amniotic sac was pierced and the pregnancy had to be terminated. The doctor was charged with unintentional homicide, the French equivalent of involuntary homicide. He was initially acquitted, but was then convicted on appeal and sentenced to 6 months in prison and fined 10,000 francs. He then appealed to the Court of Cassation – France's highest court – which overturned the ruling on the grounds that the fetus was not a human being and not entitled to the protection of criminal law.

Mrs Vo then took the case before the Grand Chamber of the European Court (application no. 53924/00). She alleged that France's failure to extend the law on unintentional homicide to the unborn violated the State's Article 2-based obligation to respect life. However, the court found 14 votes to 3 in favor of France.

The Court felt that the decision of when the right to life begins was a question to be decided at the national level. They noted that there was no European consensus on the scientific and legal definition of the beginning of life, particularly in France, where the issue had been the subject of public debate. At best, it could be said that the consensus was that the embryo/fetus belonged to the human race. Its potential and capacity to become a person required some protection in the name of human dignity, without making it a person with the right to life for the purposes of Article 2 or legal status in conflict with the mother. Therefore, the Court was convinced that it was neither desirable, nor even possible as matters stood, to answer the question whether the unborn child was a person for the purposes of Article 2 of the Convention. The main judgment of the Court was to accord each State a degree of autonomy, or a 'margin of appreciation' as it is called, to work out the right legal position for itself. So on this view, Article 2 did not apply. A minority of the judges felt that there was no issue since 'even if one accepts that life begins before birth, that does not automatically and unconditionally confer on this form of human life a right to life equivalent to the corresponding right of a child after its birth'.

Therefore, by a majority of 13 votes to 4, the court was in favor of the inapplicability of Article 2, implying a lack of rights for the unborn child and setting a precedent on the legal status of unborn babies that will be applied across European countries.

Wrongful Life and Wrongful Birth

After the baby is born, it has equal rights to the mother and the rest of society. To some extent these rights can be applied retrospectively and the events that occurred or did not occur prior to birth can, in theory, be litigated against if they adversely affect the baby after birth. There are two particular situations, Wrongful Life and Wrongful Birth, where the plaintiff claims that the baby would rather not have been born, i.e. be terminated. Since this usually involves failure of prenatal diagnosis and termination of pregnancy, it can produce conflict with the various legal and moral arguments.

Definitions

Wrongful Life is when the child takes the action against another party for allowing it to be born in a deformed or harmed way caused by actions or inaction prior to birth. In other words, it would rather have been terminated and litigates for damages to help it live as comfortably as possible.

Wrongful Birth is when the mother sues other people for being burdened with a disabled child, something she could have avoided.

In essence, these suits are genetic or prenatal diagnosis litigation cases where termination could have been offered. Again, much of the debate has occurred in France but affects all countries.

The Nicholas Perruche case

In 1982, when Josette Perruche was in her early pregnancy, her 4-year-old daughter developed rubella. She told her doctor that if she had been infected, she wanted a termination rather than risk giving birth to a handicapped child. She had two blood tests, 2 weeks apart, which gave contradictory results. Mrs Perruche was reassured that all was well. However, Nicholas was born with the rubella syndrome and, after investigation, it was discovered that the laboratory had made an error. A case was brought on behalf of Nicholas against the doctors alleging that failure by the doctors to diagnose the condition in the womb had prevented a termination of pregnancy and led to Nicholas being born with deformity. The French Court found in his favor, stating in its ruling: [8]

> ... since mistakes committed by the doctors and the laboratory while carrying out their contract with Mrs Perruche prevented her from exercising her choice to end the pregnancy to avoid the birth of a handicapped child, the latter can ask for compensation for damages resulting from this handicap.

There was great discontent over the court ruling. Cathrine Fabre, of the Federation of French Families, said at the time, 'we cannot approve the idea of claiming for compensation for being alive'.

Further cases were brought where families argued that if doctors had detected the disabilities prior to birth, they would have had the pregnancies terminated.[9] This case went on appeal to the highest court in France, the Cour de Cassation. The court ruled that disabled children were entitled to compensation if their mothers were not given the chance of an abortion. The court stated that the Perruche precedent remained 'as long as a causal link can be established with an error committed by a doctor'.

Following this, doctors and campaigners for the disabled reacted furiously, describing the decision by the court as an incitement to eugenics. The case was widely described as establishing in French law a disabled child's 'right not to be born'. The Collective to Stop Discrimination against the Disabled (CCH), which was set up after the Perruche case, feared that parents would be attacked for giving birth to a handicapped child as a result of the decision. 'This is a real act of phobia. Now parents are going to be attacked and seen as irresponsible because they gave birth to a handicapped child', it said. 'The ruling means that the handicapped have no place in our society', said Yves Richard, a lawyer representing the medical profession. 'There is a real risk of this starting a process that ends with the search for the perfect child'.

Doctors expressed increasing concern that the verdict would push doctors to terminate pregnancies when they were unsure about the normality of the fetus. Some started to refuse to carry out routine antenatal scans as they were worried that they would be sued if a disabled baby was born that they had failed to diagnose. The doctors threatened strike action.

Ethicists and legal specialists also attacked the rulings. 'To allow a child to be born cannot be considered as a mistake – that must be written into law', said Laurent Aynes, a professor in civil law at Paris' Sorbonne University. Many called on the government to change the law on the subject. Initially, they held out against legislation, but were forced to act by public pressure and by the decision of some medical staff to stop carrying out prenatal scans. The bill was passed, and it states that nobody can claim to have been harmed simply by being born. By doing this, the government's ruling brought to an end a year's legal and moral debate.[8]

However, the new parliament bill prohibited Wrongful Life cases only, not Wrongful Birth suits. This means that the obstetrician or technician can still be sued, and the parents – not the affected child – will be able to seek damages, but only on the grounds of a 'blatant error' by doctors, the argument being that the birth of the disabled child is damaging the life of the mother.

The Dutch experience

After a court awarded damages to a severely disabled girl for the fact that she was born, Members of Parliament (MPs) called for The Netherlands to follow

France and ban damage claims for Wrongful Life. Doctors fear the judgment could lead to a sharp increase in defensive prenatal testing.

The case was of 9-year-old Kelly Molenaar whose parents had informed a midwife at the Leiden University Medical Centre that a relative of the father was disabled because of a chromosomal abnormality. The midwife reassured them and did not carry out further prenatal diagnostic tests or refer the case to a clinical geneticist. The abnormality was not detected early enough for intervention and Kelly was born with multiple mental and physical disabilities. She cannot walk, talk or properly recognize her parents; has deformed feet; is believed to be in constant pain and has had several heart operations. By the age of 21 months, she had been admitted to hospital nine times due to 'inconsolable crying'.[10]

The court accepted that damage to Kelly resulted from the midwife's error. The appropriate referral would have resulted in a termination and Kelly would not have been born. Damages against the hospital amounting to the cost of Kelly's care and upbringing until her 21st birthday were awarded to her parents. But the court went further, ruling that Kelly herself was liable to damages. The court judged that the damage experienced by Kelly was in a legal sense a predictable consequence of the midwife's mistake. Therefore, the court accepted the possibility of a claim for Wrongful Life. The amount of the damages is still to be decided.

The hospital's lawyers are considering an appeal to the Supreme Court to quash the judgment and MPs are urging the ministries of health and justice to respond to the decision. Boris Dittrich (MP) has called for Dutch law to be changed to prohibit Wrongful Life claims as has happened in France.

Joseph Hubben, Professor of Health Law at the Free University of Amsterdam, said:

> To recognize a disabled life as a source of financial damages gives the wrong signal to society. Disabled people should be fellow citizens not someone who should have been aborted.

He also argued that the decision would increase pressure for more prenatal diagnostic testing not just from parents but also from doctors.

The UK experience

In 2004, a UK mother was successful in suing her hospital after giving birth to a child with genetic abnormalities. She claimed damages, saying that if she had been informed of the child's disability, she would have had him killed before birth. The baby had had extensive scanning but no abnormality was detected. The baby boy was born in 1999 with a genetic abnormality that causes bladder, bowel and genitalia defects. The Hospital, Leeds Teaching Hospitals NHS Trust, had to pay an undisclosed amount of damages to assist the woman in the raising of the child. A spokesman for the Leeds Teaching Hospitals NHS Trust said, 'This was an extremely complex case and one which was defended by the trust because it raised important clinical questions'.

Summary of the European situation

As can be seen, the European situation is confusing, but it would seem that Wrongful Life cases are not being allowed, not only because of the litigation fears it brings, but also because of the moral aspects deciding that a disabled child is better off not being born. However, Wrongful Birth cases are increasing. These cases, unlike the usual litigation case, which relates to damage sustained, center around the doctor or technician's failure to diagnose a pre-existing abnormality and therefore prevent the mother from having the opportunity to terminate the pregnancy. This produces major problems and concern for obstetric units because any scan may sometimes 'miss' an abnormality. Also, which abnormalities 'merit' consideration for termination? This is accentuated by a case currently under consideration in the UK where a member of the public has asked for a judicial review of a case of a late termination of pregnancy for a cleft lip and palate.

The upper gestational limit of termination varies from country to country. In France, the law allows termination of pregnancy with no upper gestational age limit. In Italy, termination of pregnancy after the time of viability may be legally carried out only when continuation of pregnancy represents, either for physical or psychological reasons, a danger to the mother's life. In the UK, the most recent abortion act states that a termination of pregnancy can be carried out for a serious handicap right up to term as long as the baby is born dead.

What, however, is a serious handicap? A paper, in 2001, demonstrated that of the 270 children born with cleft lip and/or palate, 23 were positively diagnosed by ultrasound prior to birth.[11] Out of these 23 cases, two ended in termination of pregnancy, which is just less than 10%. The assumption from this and other studies is that if the diagnosis were available to more couples, then more terminations for cleft lip and palate would be requested. It also implies that there are many causes of fetal abnormality that parents may wish to terminate and that are not currently universally diagnosed or termination offered. In a European survey, only 2% of doctors would offer a termination for cleft lip/palate.[12] Do we need to extend the screening of babies to cover a wider range of abnormalities and offer all termination of pregnancy? If we do not offer them termination and/or the abnormalities are missed, will litigation follow to cover any surgical and other care costs? Who is to decide what a serious handicap is and whether a termination is justified?

Litigation – the European perspective

This problem relating to Wrong Birth cases is adding to the already increasing litigation culture in Europe. There are significant differences between Europe and the USA. In Europe:

(1) The litigation is usually brought by claimants paying for the legal costs. However, this is often supported by government grant (Legal Aid in the UK) although some *No Win, No Fee* cases are beginning to appear.
(2) The cases are heard in front of judges, not juries, which means that the cases are usually less emotive but lead to law of precedent.
(3) The awards are largely for cost of care required, not suffering. This means that the cost of an award for a child with cerebral palsy may be in the region of 4 million UK pounds but if the child dies, the award may only be £20,000.

The cost of litigation is mounting and, at present, the total *potential* payouts for litigation in the UK is more than the total cost of running three London teaching hospitals or providing all maternity care for England for a year. However, this is a misleading statistic, as the total amount *paid out* in *settling* claims each year is only about 1% of the total National Health Service (NHS) budget, not a huge sum.[13] In 1998, the rate of litigation was 0.81 closed claims per 1000 finished consultant episodes. The problem is that 65% of the cost, but not the numbers, are obstetric cases. Because of the rising litigation cost, medical malpractice insurance for obstetricians has escalated. This has led to the UK government bringing in 'Crown Indemnity', meaning that the NHS (the Crown) will cover the cost of litigation.[14] Therefore, it is the health authority that is sued and not the individual doctor. Also, all cases brought against hospitals are defended in England by lawyers working for the National Health Service Litigation Authority (NHSLA), a centralized body. Any costs up to £100,000 are paid by the individual hospitals but above that, the costs are met by the Clinical Negligence Scheme for Trusts (CNST), which was set up in 1995 to indemnify acute NHS Trusts against litigation. The CNST grades hospitals according to risk, and when a Trust undergoes this assessment it can earn a rebate of up to 30% of its indemnity payments if it can demonstrate significantly good performance in terms of certain risk management processes.[15] This can be a six-figure sum.

Therefore, litigation in Europe is becoming an increasing drain on health care resources and governments are stepping in to provide the financial cover in various ways. However, this does not come without strings; although individuals are no longer targeted for litigation, the government agencies are wielding increasing power to insist on risk management procedures and the appropriate training and supervision of staff. So although individuals are no longer responsible to reduce the litigation threat, the hospitals themselves have financial gains to be made if their staff follows the necessary guidelines and practices. This can be an important driver of improved care.[15]

Obstetric decision making

Decision making by doctors is a complex business influenced by training, culture and knowledge of outcome. A good example of this is the decision to deliver the premature fetus by cesarean section. Obstetricians in the different European countries were asked about what would be the earliest gestation at which they would intervene by cesarean section in the fetal interest in three different scenarios:

(1) when parents wanted everything possible done to save this baby,
(2) when parents were against aggressive management or
(3) when it was your child.

In the first situation, the median lowest gestational age at which obstetricians would be willing to perform an emergency cesarean section for fetal indication varied from 24 completed weeks in Sweden and Germany to 26 in The Netherlands, the UK, Italy and Spain. Knowledge that parents were against aggressive management would increase this figure by 1 week in Spain, France, The Netherlands, Luxembourg and Sweden. Interestingly, the most conservative approach, i.e. the latest gestation, was found in scenario 3, where it was your own child.[12] These results imply that if you want to achieve a live birth, then going early can be justified; but it is not if the best interests of the parents and the baby are taken into account. The recent Growth Restriction Intervention Trial (GRIT) study would tend to confirm the rightness of this view since delayed delivery reduced long-term disability.[16]

Neonatal decision making

As previously stated, at birth, the baby takes on individual rights, which may initially rest with the parents but ultimately can be practiced independently through an appointed guardian. This can cause confusion before birth, sometimes just minutes before; the maternal rights were paramount, now the baby's rights can be in conflict.

Here again, retrospective rights pertain. In English law, termination of pregnancy is allowed right up to term for significant fetal abnormality; however, the baby must be born dead. If the baby is born alive and then dies due to the result of prematurity or of the procedure itself, the doctor who carried out the procedure that led to the baby's death can be charged with manslaughter. This means that late termination usually requires feticide. This adds to the stress and unpleasantness of the procedure for the parents and the staff carrying out the procedure, although others might feel that it is more humane.[17] The fact that the killing of a handicapped fetus is allowed but is not minutes later after birth adds to the confusion.

However, Dr Eduard Verhagen, of the Groningen Academic Hospital and Dr Louis Kollée of Radboud University Medical Centre in The Netherlands have asserted that euthanasia of infants is occurring worldwide. They called on the Dutch government to regularize the killing of handicapped newborn babies by providing guidelines that will protect physicians from murder charges. They felt that there should be a panel to consider guidelines for euthanasia for people with 'no free will', i.e. severely handicapped infants. The practice varies throughout Europe, most commonly in The Netherlands and France, but doctors are divided on whether it should be controlled by law.[18] Interestingly, nurses are more in favor than doctors.

An associated problem is when to initiate and/or withdraw care from an infant with a severe abnormality or gross prematurity. This problem was highlighted by the 'Baby Messenger' case in the US, where a severely ill preterm infant was resuscitated against his parents' wishes and was removed by his parents from ventilator support and allowed to die in their arms. The father was initially charged with manslaughter, although subsequently acquitted.[19]

The approach to the resuscitation of premature babies varies among countries with many producing clear guidelines of when small or abnormal babies should be treated or when treatment should be withdrawn.[20] The different approaches are based on various methodologies, including

- the 'statistical' approach, whereby treatment is withheld from infants defined as underweight and/or immature,
- the 'initiate and re-evaluate' approach, whereby aggressive treatment is begun and then re-evaluated relative to the infant's progress and parents' wishes and
- a 'treat until certainty' approach, whereby each infant is treated until death or discharge.

Each of these approaches has advantages and disadvantages. The Danish Council of Ethics produced a protocol that combines a minimum gestational age, maturity and parental wishes. Generally, infants younger than 24 or 25 weeks are not treated aggressively but this can be modified if the infant looks mature and can be resuscitated using 'low-technology modalities' and minimal handling.[19] Also, the approach can be modified by considerations of parental wishes. The long-term outcome for the baby is greatly influenced by the ability of his parents to provide the care it requires. Therefore, the threshold can be moved down by parents wishing to care for a child that fails to meet the criterion or can be moved up by parents requesting to withhold treatment from a newborn that meets the threshold requirement. Under these guidelines, Baby Messenger would not have been resuscitated. Even had the neonatologist decided that the gestational threshold had been met, the baby's immediate condition following birth did not meet the maturity criterion. This, together with the parent's refusal of ventilator support, should have meant that he should not have been resuscitated. The council's recommendations are based on two main factors, the infant's best interests and economic justice:

> The basis for the [modified threshold] recommendation is that the panel considers the 35% occurrence of severe handicaps in children born after a pregnancy term of 24–25 full weeks to be high in relation to the number of surviving infants; the panel also takes into account the comparison of the expenditure incurred with the possible alternative applications for that amount.[9]

Therefore, the infant's best interests and the cost to society are considered and not just survival. A 35% risk of severe impairment may be too high for a parent, physician or policy maker to accept. However, there is also a chance that the child may lead a relatively normal life. While this may seem a reasonable decision for parents to make, it does result in large numbers of healthy infants being allowed to die to avoid a smaller number of handicapped infants. One benefit of targeting care is to benefit those who would gain most.

> It seems reasonable to exercise reticence in the treatment of extremely preterm infants in order to benefit the slightly less premature, since the prospects of better results increase with age and fewer resources are consumed, allowing more to be helped.[10]

In a survey in different European countries, doctors were asked how they would care for a case of extreme prematurity (24 weeks' gestational age, birth weight of 560 g, Apgar score of 1 at 1 min). Most physicians in every country but The Netherlands would resuscitate this baby and start intensive care.[20] On subsequent deterioration of clinical conditions caused by a severe intraventricular hemorrhage, attitudes diverge: most neonatologists in Germany, Italy, Estonia and Hungary would favor continuation of intensive care, whereas in other countries some form of limitation of treatment would be the preferred choice. Parental wishes appear to play a role, especially in Great Britain and The Netherlands. Interestingly, again nurses are more likely than doctors to want to withhold resuscitation in the delivery room and to ask parental opinion regarding subsequent treatment choices. Among doctors who would resuscitate, only in Great Britain and The Netherlands would a substantial percentage change the decision, knowing that parents were against resuscitation. In Estonia, Hungary, Italy, Germany and Spain, most doctors would withhold treatment in case of emergencies, such as cardiac arrest, whereas doctors in Great Britain, The Netherlands and Sweden would withdraw mechanical ventilation. Only in France and The Netherlands would definitive actions be taken to end life. Therefore, the range of care throughout Europe, in the same clinical situation, varied from active care until there was no hope to positively ending life.

Interestingly, the parents' responses to these decisions are varied, partly depending on the outcome, with 22% of the parents expressing reservations about the length of the dying process. Some reported that this had taken from 3 to 36 h. Deaths that medical teams had predicted would be quick had, according to the parents' recollections, taken from 1.5 to 31 h. When a baby died swiftly, it seemed to confirm the decision to stop, but when babies lingered, doubts were raised.[20]

Conclusions

So there is no pan-European perspective; each country has its own approach. The Danes have a varied statistical approach to what should and should not be done; the Dutch similarly have a definite cut-off point, with a pragmatic approach toward withdrawal of treatment and even active ending of life; the British wait and see, discuss the case with their colleagues and the parents and largely let nature take its course but will withdraw treatment when clear possibilities of a successful outcome have gone and the Germans will work to save the baby until it dies. This does not appear to be influenced by religious factors but by the social norms of the society in which the doctors work.

Similarly, the approach toward termination is extremely liberal and uninfluenced by religious prejudice. This is helped by the largely pan-European legal position that the fetus has no rights before birth, as this is the main pillar of the right to life battle. The recent findings in the European courts have ended this fight for the foreseeable future.

However, there is an increasing European problem of litigation with the number and cost of cases increasing. The UK leads the way in this situation and has tried to solve the insurance costs by the government footing the bill. This has just led to spiraling costs. The newer Wrongful Birth cases has opened up what appears to be an endless source of new cases, which can be of significant cost. Again, Governments have had to intervene to legislate in these situations, not because of the rights or wrongs but for the social good.

REFERENCES

1. Chervenak FA, McCullough LB. The fetus as a patient: an essential concept for the ethics of perinatal medicine. *Am J Perinatol* 2003;20(8):399–404.
2. Draper H. Women, forced caesareans and antenatal responsibilities. *J Med Ethics* 1996;22(6):327–33.
3. Harris LH. Rethinking maternal–fetal conflict: Gender and equality in perinatal ethics. *Obstet Gynecol* 2000;96(5, Pt 1):786–91.
4. Molenaar JC. The legal investigation of a decision not to operate on an infant with Down's syndrome and a duodenal atresia: A report from The Netherlands. *Bioethics* 1992;6(1):35–40.
5. McHaffie HE, Cuttini M, Brolz-Voit G, *et al.* Withholding/withdrawing treatment from neonates: Legislation and official guidelines across Europe. *J Med Ethics* 1999;25(6):440–6.
6. Bottis MC. Wrongful birth and wrongful life actions. *Eur J Health Law* 2004;11(1):55–9.
7. Wellman C. The concept of fetal rights. *Law Philos* 2002;21(1): 65–93.
8. Spriggs M, Savulescu J. The Perruche judgment and the "right not to be born". *J Med Ethics* 2002;28(2):63–4.
9. Dorozynski A. Highest French court awards compensation for "being born". *Br Med J* 2001;323(7326):1384.
10. Sheldon T. Court awards damages to disabled child for having been born. *Br Med J* 2003;326(7393):784.
11. Shaikh D, Mercer NS, Sohan K, Kyle P, Soothill P. Prenatal diagnosis of cleft lip and palate. *Br J Plast Surg* 2001;54(4):288–9.
12. Cuttini M. The European Union Collaborative Project on Ethical Decision Making in Neonatal Intensive Care (EURONIC): Findings from 11 countries. *J Clin Ethics* 2001;12(3):290–6.
13. Walsh P. Editorial. *AVMA Med Legal J* 2003;9:108.
14. Palmer RN. United Kingdom 'Crown' indemnity for medical negligence – an overview of the first 18 months of the new scheme. *Med Law* 1992;11(7–8):623–7.
15. Wood J. Clinical negligence scheme for trusts and maternity care: Let's redesign services, not patch up outdated systems. *Clin Risk* 2003;9:86–8.
16. Thornton JG, Hornbuckle J, Vail A, Spiegelhalter DJ, Levene M. Infant wellbeing at 2 years of age in the Growth Restriction Intervention Trial (GRIT): Multicentred randomised controlled trial. *Lancet* 2004;364(9433):513–20.
17. Dommergues M, Cahen F, Garel M, Mahieu-Caputo D, Dumez Y. Feticide during second- and third-trimester termination of pregnancy: Opinions of health care professionals. *Fetal Diagn Ther* 2003;18(2):91–7.
18. Cuttini M, Casotto V, Kaminski M, *et al.* Should euthanasia be legal? An international survey of neonatal intensive care units staff. *Arch Dis Child Fetal Neonatal Ed* 2004;89(1):F19–24.
19. Gross ML. Avoiding anomalous newborns: Preemptive abortion, treatment thresholds and the case of Baby Messenger. *J Med Ethics* 2000;26(4):242–8.
20. De Leeuw R, Cuttini M, Nadai M, *et al.* Treatment choices for extremely preterm infants: An international perspective. *J Pediatr* 2000;137(5):608–16.

22 Malpractice issues in perinatal medicine: The United States perspective

B. S. Schifrin, M. R. Lebed and J. McCauley

Introduction

It was probably inevitable that the law and medicine would come into conflict irrespective of the fact that despite some obviously different approaches, these learned professions share more than they conflict. While medicine is fundamentally inductive and law deductive, both fields are centered in advocacy for the client. When it comes to medicine, the law tries to reconcile a body of science with the art of clinical practice. When it comes to the law, medicine tries to reconcile a body of laws with notions of fault and accountability. The relationship is abetted when the goals of better, more efficient care and prompt and effective methods of dealing with error and adverse outcome are agreed upon. On the other hand, when each profession deems the other side to hold some unscrupulous advantage, when the 'playing field is perceived to be not level', and when myth and misdirection are rampant and malpractice premiums have become excessive or insurance coverage unavailable, then the worst of the relationship comes to the fore and political and legislative resources are recruited to help control the dialog and the invective and define or create new rules of engagement. In the end, care is compromised as are notions of justice and access to the law.

Historic perspective of malpractice in the United States

Malpractice suits were unheard of until 1848. Prior to that there was no control over the practice of medicine or its numerous schools of practice. There was no need: patients generally were fatalists, believing that any adverse medical outcome was the will of God. It became an issue after 1848 only because allopathic physicians, to eliminate other 'schools of medicine', created objective standards of practice, created national medical societies and national standards, elected to support litigation under tort law rather than contract law, and established the 'deep pockets' of malpractice insurance – a profitable industry for attorneys.

But it was only with the beginning of the 1960s that more educated, informed, and assertive patients began to question their physicians in the same manner that they evaluated their other goods and services. In general, this was poorly accepted by physicians, who for the most part maintained a traditional authoritarian stance in the care of their patients. The legislative crises of the 1970s, and the subsequent 'crises' of the 1980s, 1990s, and today brought with them tort reform, health maintenance organizations (HMOs), increasing regulation, decreasing autonomy, strained relations between physicians, hospital administrations, and allied health care providers, and decreased physician and patient satisfaction. Although much has changed from the mid-1800 s there is one historic consistency: the major litogen (a promoter of lawsuits) is not outcome but physician behavior.

Malpractice law

Malpractice law is part of tort, or personal injury, law that affects large segments of society, including product liability, automobile accidents, airplane crashes, and other examples of unintended harm. As mentioned above, it was the physicians, themselves, who determined that due to their superior status, they were not subject to contract law with patients, who were not their equal, and set the higher civil law standard of Tort law. The objectives of malpractice litigation are straight forward: (1) to resolve disputes fairly with equal opportunity for 'justice' on both sides, (2) to compensate persons injured through negligence, and (3) to prevent unsafe practices – i.e. raise the standard of care[1] – all without resorting to armaments or fisticuffs.

A plaintiff prevails in a lawsuit by proving the four Ds: that the defendant (1) owed a Duty of care to the plaintiff, (2) that there was a Deviation from an acceptable standard of care, and (3) that there was a non-trivial injury to the plaintiff (Damages) that was Directly caused by the deviation from the standard of care.[1] A failure to demonstrate any one of the four means that the requirements, under the law, are not met. To begin the process, a patient approaches a lawyer. The reasons patients sue are many.[2–5]

For patients and family members, the physical and emotional devastation of medical error cannot be easily overcome. As a rule, however, this circumstance has been made even more difficult because there was no satisfactory explanation to the patient of the reason for the adverse outcome, no admission of negligence, no opportunity for questions, and no consolation for loss.[6,7] In reality, the patients want a forthright explanation of what happened, and want to understand if they had played a role in it. And if, just if, a mistake had been made, they expect an apology and an offer to compensate for the expense and aggravation. They are real people and whether the injury was the result of negligence or not, they, not the physicians burdened with a lawsuit, are the real victims. When asked, 'What was wrong with the care you or your child received?' or 'What complaints do you have about physicians?', patients respond rather specifically (Table 22.1).[4] As underscored by these data, the attorney is often the last person who is contacted, not the first. Indeed, most often patients are directed to an attorney by a member of the medical community.

Table 22.1 Why patients sue (Hickson *et al.*[4])

Cited deficiencies of care	
Recognizing fetal distress	53%
Managing fetal distress	57%
Timely cesarean section	35%
Physician unavailable	29%
Birth injury (forceps)	28%
Consultation or transfer	10%
What prompted the lawsuit?	
Person outside family	33%
Medical personnel	23/41 (56%)
Lawyer	8/41 (20%)
Money for long-term care	24%
Physician deception	24%
Child would have no future	20%
Find out what happened	20%
Prevent malpractice/revenge	19%
Complaints about physicians	
Not informed about injury potential	70%
Misled patient	48%
Would not talk or answer questions	32%
Would not listen	13%

Indeed, many are amazed, when looking at medical malpractice cases, by the cold-blooded attitude so many defendants have taken toward patients who have been seriously, and sometimes grotesquely, harmed. Inhumanity and indifference to the suffering of others is in itself another form of injury. When patients file suit, they are often made to feel as though they had done something wrong, as if seeking legal redress and compensation was in some sense an affront to the system, a personal assault on the physician. Many plaintiffs feel pressured by all the parties involved to agree to a settlement. In some instances, such advice may come from the plaintiff attorney or even the sitting judge. Indeed, on occasion extraordinary amounts of offered settlement are turned down, not because of the size of the award, but because all the details of their case would then come out publicly – they would have their day in court.

Physicians believe themselves to be operating in an environment of zero tolerance for error. It is embedded in their oath and dedication to 'do no harm', in their professed desires to help others, and magnified by a historic paternalistic tendency to extend unrealistic expectations to their patients. [8] The physician who has erred is wounded, and suffers the consequences of guilt, fear of reprisal (from the patient, hospital, regulatory agencies), embarrassment (peer), and sorrow for having harmed someone (Levinson).[5,9] Because medicine, for centuries, has been loathe to identify negligent care (even in closed, protected settings), this system of justice has enfranchised the plaintiff's attorney, not especially trained for the purpose, to determine the medical and the legal merits of the case (they are not the same!) Under the contingency-fee relationship prevalent in the United States, the attorney takes a percentage of the award as a fee (often around 35%) to compensate for the costs, expenses, and time absorbed in pursuing the case irrespective of the outcome; they take nothing if the defendant prevails. These expenses are not trivial; bringing a 'damaged child' case to court, for example, may easily cost $100,000 of up front expenses. It is not undertaken lightly.[10]

But before the attorney can proceed, one of his first expenses will involve consultation with a medical expert (a physician) to determine whether the potential case satisfies the two most critical criteria of the four Ds: was there a Deviation from a reasonable standard of care and was there a Direct causal relationship between that failure and the adverse outcome? Damages and Duty, generally, are self-evident. Traditionally, the 'standard of care' is defined as the quality of care (customs and behavior) that would be expected of a reasonable practitioner in similar circumstances. These standards are drawn from members of the profession itself as well as documents that reflect a consensus on appropriate standards (plural) of care.

It should be emphasized that there is no single standard of care. Satisfying the need to do something *reasonable under the circumstances*, indeed, may permit mutually exclusive choices to be within the standard of care. Because the law holds the arcane nature of medicine, 'a learned profession', to be beyond the grasp of common citizens, it requires the testimony of experts in the same field as the defendant.[11,12] Neither the courts nor the legislatures can reasonably establish detailed conduct for professional practice without 'practicing medicine'.[13]

Ideally, medical witnesses will be readily available and forthright and medical standards will be determinable from readily available medical records that are well documented, readable, and responsive to questions of whether or not the medical conduct met a reasonable standard of care. The medical consultant/potential expert witness will possess both current knowledge and experience with the issues at hand, but, at any time in the review process, is honor bound to use all available relevant information and to apply broadly understood, minimal, standards of care – not their own personal standards. An expert witness must elaborate the standard for medical care at the time of the plaintiff's injury and give an opinion on whether the defendant's conduct met this standard. The standard is not unique to the expert, but rather must reflect general principles applicable to all practitioners, but at the same time, specific to the individual patient's circumstances. Ideally, it should be supported by scholarly literature. While it need not prescribe a single course of action, it must either (for the plaintiff) proscribe the defendant's conduct or (for the defense) endorse the defendant's conduct as an acceptable alternative. Therein lies the conflict.

While the courts expect that medicine, as a learned, science-based discipline, will have articulated standards for practice in most circumstances, they also recognize that not all standards are formalized or even well defined, not all clinical circumstances can be circumscribed in some obvious standard of care, and there is 'art' to the practice of medicine. To overcome these hurdles the courts, using their own legal (not medical) standards of witness acceptability, allow appropriately qualified expert witnesses to express expert opinions. Indeed, the expert witness is the only party in the lawsuit who may express opinions; everyone else is only entitled to the 'facts' of the case. Ideally, the expert will not be an advocate, except perhaps of his own opinion, and will honestly present his or her understanding of the applicable standards without tailoring his responses to serve the single-minded ends of the lawyer engaging the expert.

Obtaining expert testimony has always been the most difficult part of medical malpractice litigation. Historically, experts were readily available to testify against competing medical disciplines, including homeopathic physicians and chiropractors, although they were expected to remain silent about the misconduct of members of their own profession (*omerta*). To abolish these vituperative, economic rivalries, the courts established the doctrines of 'school of practice' and 'locality rule' as the bases for qualifying expert witnesses.

The school of practice rule permits the differentiation of physicians into self-designated specialties depending on whether the case concerns procedures and expertise that are intrinsic to the specialty or general medical knowledge and techniques that are common to all physicians. Thus, obstetrical cases may involve family practitioners, midwives, obstetrician-gynecologists, as well as members in training; the potentially significant differences in their individual standards may indeed require expert witnesses from each of these specialties.

Before the standardization of medical training and certification that prevails today, there was a tremendous gulf between the skills and abilities of university-trained physicians and the graduates of 'less reputable' schools issuing diplomas. Thus, in many parts of the country, a physician's ability to serve as an expert would be determined by comparison with the other physicians in the community, or at least in similar neighboring communities. For obvious reasons, this rule essentially precluded injured patients from finding supportive expert testimony – effectively preventing most medical malpractice litigation. Reasonably, there is no longer a justification for any rule that impedes evaluation of what have become national standards of care on the sole basis that it is the norm for a given community. While most states have explicitly abolished the locality rule, it is being reinvigorated in some states as a tort reform measure (and *omerta*) to deal with the problems of access to care and facilities in rural areas.

A national standard of care implies that the rural and urban physicians will have the same training and exercise the same level of judgment and diligence. The rule does not require that the rural physician have the same medical facilities, consultants, or other resources available. If the community does not have facilities for an emergency cesarean section, for example, the physician cannot be found negligent for failing to do this surgery within the 15 min that might be the standard in a well-equipped urban hospital. The physician, however, to comply with the standard of care, must inform the patient of the limitations of the available facilities and recommend prompt transfer if indicated. He must also make reasonable efforts to deal with the inevitability of requiring an emergency section – even in a rural community. Proper informed consent allows patients to balance the convenience of local care against the risks of inadequate facilities.

At trial, judges and jurors (the triers of fact) have no alternative but to judge the testimony of witnesses whether expert or percipient (fact) on the personal credibility of the witness. For the experts and the defendants, positive factors such as academic degrees, specialty board certification, and publications enhance credibility. So do such factors as physical appearance, race, gender, command of English, and personality. Irrespective of these personal traits, the objective is to be believed. The defendant also has to be believed but his/her role is much more focused; he/she has but one chore: to convince *anyone* who will listen (judge, juror, attorney, stenographer, bailiff, passerby) that he/she is a thoughtful, caring, concerned human being who did what was professionally reasonable under the circumstances. The defendant has no other job. Performing research, providing expert opinion, or combating the opinions of the opposing expert are all, we believe, someone else's function. As mentioned above, the defendant's demeanor in deposition or trial (as well as with patients) has a great deal to do both with the likelihood of lawsuit and its resolution. For the expert witness, the foremost requirements are effective presentation and teaching ability. The expert must educate the judge and jury on the technical matters at hand.

Until 1993, federal courts had used the 'general acceptance' test, set forth in Frye v. United States, to assess the admissibility of expert scientific testimony.[14] In 1993, the United States Supreme Court modified the standard for determining the admissibility of expert scientific testimony in federal trials. In Daubert, the court stated that the Frye test did not comport with the Federal Rules of Evidence and that 'a rigid "general acceptance" requirement would be at odds with the "liberal thrust" of the Federal Rules and their "general approach to relaxing the traditional barriers to opinion testimony"'.[14] Accordingly, the court emphasized that a trial judge must screen the proposed scientific testimony to ensure that the testimony is relevant and reliable before allowing it to be presented at trial.[14–16]

If scientific, technical, or other specialized knowledge will assist the trier of fact to understand the evidence or to determine a fact in issue, a witness qualified as an expert by knowledge, skill, experience, training, or education may testify thereto in the form of an opinion or otherwise. It is a judicial decision not a medical one.[16,17]

The court set forth four factors that may be used to assist the trial judge in determining 'whether the expert is proposing to testify to scientific knowledge that will assist the trier of fact to understand or determine a fact in issue'. The factors that may be considered when determining the validity of a scientific theory or technique are: (1) whether the theory or technique can be tested, (2) whether the theory has been subject to peer review and publication, (3) the rate of error, and (4) the acceptance of the theory or technique within the community. The court cautioned that '[t]he focus must be solely on principles and methodology, not on the conclusions that they generate'. The court emphasized that these factors are not exclusive.

Thus, under Daubert, a defendant doctor may be considered negligent for treatment and diagnosis even though he presents evidence from a number of medical experts genuinely of the opinion that the defendant's care followed customary medical practice. The court must determine for itself the appropriateness and the logic of the professional opinion and find reassurance that the body of opinion relied upon was not created for defensive purposes (see below). It is a curiosity that an expert's position may fail a Daubert challenge in one case but may continue to be offered in other cases! It seems counterintuitive that a lay judge is qualified to be asked to determine the qualifications and credibility of an expert. Some believe that the selection of medical experts be the purview of medically trained peers. Indeed, there is an argument to be made that the specialty societies develop a list of 'true' experts that are available to either side or the judge himself.

At least in Federal Court the expert's legal activities over the last 5 years must be listed with the court prior to his appearance. Federal rules also give a judge the authority to (1) limit cumulative evidence, i.e. more than one expert testifying to the same issues unrelated to qualifications, (2) retain experts to assist the court, or (3) with mutual consent appoint a single expert witness. Despite these available options, especially in 'damaged child' cases, there is an increasing tendency to line up a broad array of qualified experts on both sides, including an obstetrician, perinatologist, placental pathologist, neonatologist, neurologist, nurse, economist, neuroradiologist, etc. There is at least some evidence that this proliferation of experts (and costs), more likely driven by the defense, is counterproductive. Bors-Koefoed *et al.* found that the use of multiple defense expert witnesses decreased the chances of a successful defense.[18]

Many jurisdictions have attempted to insinuate the expert witness into the proceedings prior to the case being filed. In several states a report or affidavit of merit from the expert is required to launch the suit, in others only the testimony by the lawyer that he has contacted an expert is required. By and large there is no standard format for expert reports. While they are often quite minimal and non-specific there is an increasing trend to make them more substantive and even to limit in some states the allegations to those specifically identified in the report. There is also no requirement that the 'expert' who gave an affirmative opinion to the attorney, whether he signed the letter of merit or not, will subsequently be involved in the case, a deplorable circumstance as will be discussed below. Even if he/she were later involved, there are no mechanisms short of deposition or interrogatory to amplify on the experts' allegations. In some states, the expert cannot be deposed before trial and indeed his identity is unknown to the opposing side until he is called to the stand – widely referred to as 'trial by ambush'.

While the expert's opinion is normally protected by the doctrine of witness immunity, this does not protect the witness from fraud or from professional malpractice liability[19] or from other forms of harassment. 'The goal to insuring that the path to truth is unobstructed and the judicial process is protected, by fostering an atmosphere where the expert witness will be forthright and candid in stating his or her opinion, is not advanced by immunizing the expert witness from ... negligence in forming the opinion'.[19] In one instance, a consulting expert was sued for failing to testify on behalf of the plaintiff in trial. The expert believed that causation could not be satisfactorily proven.

It is perhaps instructive here to deal with the terms, 'meritorious' and 'frivolous' as applied to malpractice cases. In brief, whether the case is meritorious or not is a function not of the result, but of whether there is a substantive question about the standard of care and its relationship to the outcome. In a frivolous case, there is no substantive question, the four Ds cannot be shown or linked, or any question of negligence is readily answered in the negative simply with the most cursory examination of the evidence. Often, the complaints that prompt the visit to the attorney derive from actual or perceived slights by the physician related to a poor 'bedside manner', a disputed bill, a lack of timely response, etc. In this respect, it is important to understand how, given the unrequited emotional needs associated with adverse outcomes, malpractice litigation serves the purpose of emotional vindication.[20,21] Such complaints are usually dismissed out of hand by the attorney in the first interview with the patient or secondarily on the basis of the review by the consulting expert. It is not widely appreciated but the vast majority of patients who approach lawyers with complaints about their physicians are turned down (probably greater than 90%). Some patients are actually grateful to know that they did not receive substandard care, and equally important, that they themselves did not contribute to the adverse outcome. Despite any anger or frustration they may have with the conduct or deportment of the physician they often harbor notions of their own complicity in an adverse outcome, especially when there has been a brain-damaged baby. If they had only not skipped an appointment, not used the hot tub, not gained so much weight, etc Being turned down in a request to sue a physician may have positive benefits of closure. It may indeed help them to forgive themselves. While it is quite uncommon to pursue a lawsuit based solely on an emotional misdemeanor by the physician, it becomes a powerful incentive to bring a lawsuit if the care has also been negligent. As will be seen in the statistics below, many negligent physicians are exculpated or avoid lawsuits entirely not because of the facts of the case, but by a becoming demeanor to the patient or to the jury. Other physicians have been found negligent, not because of their care, but by their indifference toward the patient. It is this author's experience that the minute the jury perceives that the physician does not care vindication of his medical conduct is not possible.

Thus, to label as 'frivolous', as many physicians have, all cases that plaintiffs lose, or are settled 'for economic reasons' or are dismissed trivializes the tort system, the lawyers, the patients, the opposing expert witness and, in its way, impedes the solution of the malpractice problem and foments more error. This posture reveals an inadequate understanding of the dynamics of expert allegations, settlements, jury verdicts, and even the process of peer review.

Given the affirmative report by his expert, the attorney is legally *obligated* to pursue discovery – the accession of all the relevant clinical data from the medical records or other sources. To flesh out the records and to understand something of the personality of the defendants, depositions are taken of the relevant treating or factual witness – sometimes including the custodian of records, etc. and the various medical experts.

The defense against the allegation of failing to meet the standard of care of a malpractice case centers around issues of customary practice, clinical practice guidelines, informed consent, and differentiating error from complication. In judging the conduct of the physician in a court of law, the court is guided by a notion called 'reasonable conduct'. Indeed, it is sufficiently vague as to require the participation of an expert witness to state what is and what is not 'reasonable' conduct. At least theoretically, the creation of clinical practice guidelines would simplify and implement broadly understood practices subscribing to a quality of care that could be objectively measured. At the same time, the quality of care would be improved and iatrogenic injury diminished.

There has been a broad implementation of 'clinical practice guidelines' from various hospitals, professional organizations, and the government itself. A clinical practice guideline is any guide to the clinical management of a patient. These guidelines vary widely according to the purpose for which they are written and who has been selected to write them. They may be driven by medicolegal issues, by the cost of care, or by the quality of care. While great emphasis has now been placed on the process of writing guidelines, many providers have become concerned with the basic precepts of guidelines, including the possible emergence of 'cookbook' medicine, the effect of patient variability, and the need to keep guidelines flexible, current, and credible.[22,23]

Clearly, one impetus for the creation of clinical practice guidelines for specific medical conditions and their treatment was the notion that they would help avoid or defend malpractice claims. Indeed, someday they might replace the 'reasonable conduct' standards and their dependence on expert testimony in medical cases and thereby discourage both defensive medical practices and spurious claims – after all, it is the medical profession and not the juries that establish the standard of care; the jury just attempts to find out what were the standards that the medical profession had set for itself in any given situation and then to determine whether those guidelines were appropriately and reasonably followed. There are several problems with the use of 'guidelines'. First, they may not be usable (admissible in evidence) at all. Because of the wide range of reasons for creating guidelines (care, costs, medicolegal protection) in many states, such guidelines constitute 'hearsay' in great measure because their author is not in court to be cross-examined. Finally, having followed the guidelines may not mean malpractice was not committed. Scrupulous adherence to the relevant guidelines for an amputation, for example, avails nothing if the wrong leg has been amputated. Thus, it is that the notion that compliance with guidelines renders the clinician immune from lawsuit has not been upheld. Consensus, after all, is not necessarily wisdom, or applicable in all cases!

When the opinions of the opposing experts conflict irreconcilably over this issue, the jury comes face to face with the logical conundrum. Is the disagreement related to lack of awareness of the standards or is one of the experts lying? The jury assesses the credentials and the credibility and various other sources of information, to help them decide which expert is more credible in relating the individual patient's care to the prevailing standards.

One of the most widely quoted and misunderstood guidelines requires that institutions be capable of instituting an emergency cesarean section within 30 min of decision.[24] Some institutions cannot meet these guidelines reliably while others maintain a standard that can result in an emergency cesarean section in 10 min or less. While several studies have attempted to determine the reasonableness of 'the 30-min rule', neither the studies nor the guidelines take into account certain realities or certain remedies.[24] The 30-min rule is shorthand designation for a more encompassing principle that, under certain conditions, performance of a cesarean section should be carried out as quickly as possible consistent with concern for the health and well-being of the mother and fetus, preferably within 30 min. But what is the standard if there is already one cesarean section in progress, or two? Under these circumstances, a delay becomes 'reasonable under the circumstances', notwithstanding the fact that the standard of care required an earlier cesarean section. However, if a physician is late in realizing the need for cesarean section or is ready to operate within 20 min but fritters away 10 min beforehand, his conduct cannot possibly comport with a reasonable standard of care, even if the patient is delivered within 30 min. Further, it stands to reason, that institutions normally unable to consistently meet the 30-min rule must modify their practices and exhibit a willingness to prepare for cesarean section early (even if it proves unnecessary) in anticipation of problems and make special arrangements for unique situations such as vaginal birth after cesarean (VBAC). Thus, the failure to meet the 30-min rule is rarely by itself a telling plaintiff's allegation. Much more frequently, the plaintiff's allegation is that the failure to properly interpret the fetal monitoring tracing or to properly estimate the feasibility of safe vaginal delivery hopelessly delayed the decision in the first place, irrespective of the 'decision to incision' interval.

There is frequent debate over whether 'official' pronouncements such as the 30-min rule are to be construed as monolithic 'standards of care'. More reasonably, it seems, that irrespective of whether these writings are entitled practice parameters, guidelines, standards, apocrypha, hints, clues, etc., the imprimatur of an official body, gives any statement about care the force of a 'standard'. Indeed, during litigation, both sides are apt to offer these professional publications as standards to support their case irrespective of the disclaimer that these recommendations are guidelines rather than standards of care. Thus, guidelines, whatever their provenance, are never 'medicolegally binding' and can be directly and reasonably contravened by a thoughtful, alternative choice of care – that is annotated!

Informed consent

Similarly, the patient has rights, no matter how appropriately they may be exercised, to influence decisions about her care. In dealing with matters of informed consent, most courts in the United States look to what a reasonable patient would want to know, not what a 'reasonable physician' would have said. The courts have on several occasions been asked to intervene in circumstances involving the refusal of treatment by a pregnant woman, refusal that nominally threatens the life and well-being of her fetus and herself. While the courts' responses have been varied, there is general consensus among the specialties that these ethical (not legal) issues should *not* be resolved in court and that considerable ethical weight should be given to the mother's decision as long as the consent has been proper and there has been no coercion. Lawsuits based entirely on informed consent are quite uncommon, but most such cases in obstetrics seem to involve VBAC, the use of operative delivery, and the decision to induce labor with a previous history of shoulder dystocia. If the consent document signed by the potential VBAC patient, for example, is to truly represent that her consent is truly 'informed', it must reveal the patient's understanding that she may either undergo an elective repeat cesarean section or, if she is a suitable candidate, attempt a VBAC. She must understand that not all patients are candidates for VBAC and that not all VBAC attempts will result in successful vaginal delivery. She must be aware that some of the determinable clinical factors that affect the success of VBAC become apparent only in labor. The patient must also understand that all pregnancies carry a small risk to both mother and fetus, whether or not the mother has had a previous cesarean section. In patients with a previous cesarean section, the risk of uterine rupture during a VBAC is approximately 1% and this occasionally may result in serious, potentially life-threatening complications for the mother or the baby. If the patient initially agrees to attempt VBAC, she needs to understand that she is entitled to an updating of the likelihood of success and to change her mind at any reasonable time and to obtain a cesarean section even during labor. Finally, the patient should understand that no decision, however thoughtfully made, or however reasonably pursued, guarantees a normal outcome for the mother or the infant.

The reader may now compare this approach with the deliberations in an informed consent case that was decided by the Wisconsin Supreme Court and that stretched the limits to which some physicians would go to reduce their cesarean delivery rate. In this case a patient presented with a history of two previous cesarean sections, the first undertaken for arrest of labor after 17 h (the second was elective); she had agreed prior to labor to attempt VBAC.[25] During labor, in the face of slow progress and severe abdominal pain, she changed her mind and repeatedly requested a cesarean section. Just as often the obstetrician maintained that it was unnecessary. The obstetrician commented, '... if I performed cesarean section on every woman who wanted one then all deliveries would be by cesarean section'. Intimidated, the patient no longer requested cesarean section. Ultimately, the uterus ruptured and the child was hopelessly injured despite delivery within 30 min. The physician defended his conduct on the ground that the original informed consent should prevail throughout the labor and that the standard of care had been met by the 'timely' delivery within 30 min. He noted that the patient had reaffirmed upon admission her earlier willingness to undergo a trial of labor and he maintained that labor continued 'without objection'.

The court (inviting the implication that the patient had been coerced) rejected the defense position that the patient's resignation implied acceptance of a continued trial of labor.[25] The court did not comment on the change in the *medical situation* (dysfunctional labor, unexplained abdominal pain) that required medical reconsideration of the case and updating of the informed consent. The court did, however, conclude that the *legal situation* had changed:

> Where two or more medically acceptable options for treatment are present, the competent patient has the absolute right to select from among those treatment options after being informed of the relative risks and benefits of each approach. But consent, once given, is not categorically immutable and the patient was entitled to withdraw her consent to VBAC. That indisputable withdrawal, placed the patient and her physician in their original position – a blank slate on which the parties must again diagram their plan which in this case would have resulted in cesarean section.

It was foreseeable that as a backlash to the alarm generated by this verdict along with other reports and settlements, many hospitals no longer permit VBAC deliveries and an increasing number of malpractice insurers are limiting their indemnification of physicians performing VBAC deliveries![26]

Complication or error?

The 'recognized risk defense', asserts that the undesirable outcome or injury in question is nothing more than an unavoidable complication – an understandable and acceptable risk of a properly considered and provided treatment. Accordingly, so long as the patient is reasonably apprised of the more serious and the commonplace risks and participates in the decision, in theory there can be no issue of negligence. A typical example is subgaleal or intracranial hemorrhage in the newborn following vacuum-assisted delivery. Indeed, every obstetrical text devotes significant space to such complications but only rarely do they include a full discussion about preventability or even the distinction between complication and negligence. Is intracranial/subgaleal hemorrhage following vacuum extraction, for example, an *unavoidable* risk or, in some instances, the result of negligence and how would that be determined?[27] Similarly, is brachial plexus injury after shoulder dystocia a foreseeable event related to excessive lateral traction on the fetal neck, anticipated by multiple risk factors, or is it a totally unpredictable, unpreventable injury *always* unrelated to the care of the physician during delivery. In the courtroom, the plaintiff's attorney will use the statistics on complications as follows. A 'recognized complication' does *not* preclude that the complication was caused by negligence. Indeed, none, all, or only some of these complications may represent negligence. For example, if 2% of all drivers run red lights, running red lights is a known complication of driving, but it is also a case of negligence. The most likely situation is that some of the injury is potentially avoidable. Thus, that a given adverse outcome is a known complication of a procedure tells an attorney nothing. The attorney wants to know why the complication occurs and, more importantly, why it occurred in this particular case.

Pursuing the case

If the case is pursued, it may be settled by an agreement of the parties or may go to trial. While the physician believes himself disadvantaged in this system of finding fault, in reality the law gives health care providers considerable advantage. They are advantaged by the presumption of non-negligence.

They do not have to be right in their care, just reasonable. The law denies the jury the right to decide medical issues and even requires expert witnesses from the profession itself. After an agreement to settle the case or after an adjudication that finds the defendant negligent, his insurance company bears the costs of both economic losses (lost earnings and medical bills) and non-economic losses, so-called 'pain and suffering'. The system is maintained in balance by the provision of insurance for both hospitals and physicians based on a pooling of risk, historically through separate lines of insurance.[13,28] This minimizes the risk of bankruptcy by a single large payout and because resources are available to compensate patients. The cost of insurance coverage for hospitals is typically linked to the history of claims from year to year, an arrangement known as 'experience rating'. Physicians, on the other hand, unless their experience is extreme, are generally not risk rated, a potentially contrived actuarial practice.[29]

In practice, this theoretically balanced system falls short of its objectives, as illustrated in the 'ire and angst' of contemporary malpractice litigation.[13] This chapter, written at the end of 2004, will therefore attempt to review some of the competing, nay dueling, agendas that are being brought to bear in the medical, legal, and political arenas. The enterprise redounds with myth and divisive and often contradictory data – sometimes of dubious provenance. The dust of the latest in these, increasingly disagreeable, epochal skirmishes for the malpractice 'high road' has not yet settled and is unlikely to be settled to everyone's satisfaction in the near future. In the authors' view, this situation prevails because each side, for its particular reasons, is unwilling to make the tort system work as it was designed to. Indeed some of the issues raised are ethical in nature, beyond the purview of the courts and the legislature.

Malpractice mythology – the failure of medicolegal education

An enduring feature of the malpractice upheaval in the United States (and almost nowhere else) is the ignorance of malpractice doctrine in the medical community and beyond. Not only is there widespread fear of being sued, but there is also a great misperception about the requirements for proof of malpractice, the outcomes of lawsuits, and the reasons patients sue. There is little appetite to deal with the major litogen (a factor promoting lawsuit) – physician behavior.

Some current mythology: 'Malpractice relates to the incompetence of a few bad physicians'; 'Anyone can sue, everyone wins'; 'Every case resulting in CP will come to lawsuit'; 'The system is unfair and favors the plaintiff'; 'Patients who sue are greedy, ingrates'; 'Judges and juries cannot understand medicine'; 'Losing a lawsuit raises premiums and besmirches the physician's name in the community'; 'The plaintiff's attorney and the expert are the enemy, along with the judge, jury, insurance company'; 'Malpractice doesn't make care better'; 'The majority of suits in medicine are frivolous whether they are settled, dropped, go to jury trial, or lose'; 'We're living in a time when people have a higher expectation from physicians – that until proven otherwise, it's the doctor's fault'; 'The system is overrun with runaway juries and jackpot justice, with sinister lawyers and opportunistic plaintiffs preying on virtuous corporations, hospitals, and doctors in search of that big payout from the lawsuit lottery'.[30]

There is almost a universal belief that the injured child's appearance in the courtroom elicits sufficient sympathy from the jury for the plaintiff to win the case. Physicians, however, win about 80% of lawsuits that do go to court. It is naive to believe that these were the cases in which the plaintiff's attorney forgot to bring the affected child into the courtroom. More reasonably, it is the thoughtful, compassionate physician, who manifests his sympathy and compassion, who most easily obtains the jury's favor and a favorable verdict.

The defendant is often unaware of the statistics that about 40% of cases are dropped and about 50% settle, sometimes as befitting the merits of the case and sometimes as a calculated strategy that limits exposure of assets. The physician who is terrified by an *ad damnum* clause (demand for damages) that greatly exceeds his insurance policy limits is rarely in our experience reassured by his own attorney that the risk to his/her assets is essentially nil. The authors are unaware of any malpractice suit involving an obstetrician who was covered by a reasonable policy and who, despite a verdict that exceeded the policy limits, had to pay any money out of his own pocket. Despite counseling, the frightened obstetrician does 'not want to be the first one'. To some extent the defense attorney may be excused for failing to understand how impoverished the physician's medicolegal education is. As one American physician put it:

> I fought in the battle of the bulge in World War II. We were trained, we were fighting a good cause and we were armed. I felt safer then than I do in a malpractice suit.

Education is the antidote to disabling myth. Medical and legal organizations have long recognized the importance of legal medicine and have repeatedly recommended its study by physicians in training – with minimal success. In 1952, the American Medical Association (AMA) advised that 'No medical student should be permitted to receive his medical degree without instruction in legal duties'. Four decades later, less than 50% of medical schools had medicolegal courses, considering the subject too unimportant to teach. Even fewer schools have any formal instruction on communication and dispute management skills. Many medical schools feel that the intense curriculum leaves no room for such instruction, and that the ability to communicate and deal with conflict is part of the student selection process, which is to be refined following their didactic medical school training, during their apprentice/mentor training of internship and residency.

Kollas, in 1997, studied the medicolegal knowledge base of senior residents in internal medicine. Only 28% felt they had been adequately trained in the subject. Only 26% could list the requirements for proof of malpractice, i.e. the four Ds.[31,32]

A national survey of physicians in 1999 revealed that 58% had faced malpractice charges and that more than 20% had been sued at least three times. Almost 70% expected to be sued during their career. Despite the fact that physicians win the vast majority of cases that go to court, more than 75% of physicians polled felt that lay juries were not capable of deciding malpractice cases! While ready to admit that everyone makes mistakes and that they had made mistakes in other cases, virtually all physicians believe that the cases filed against them had no merit.[33] Something (read tort reform) must be done, physicians cry, to stem the tide, to eliminate the reign of terror by the plaintiff's attorneys. Plaintiff's attorneys and some consumer groups also want to stem the tide as they see it – the tide of medical error, the tide of unsympathetic, unapologetic, and ill-informed physicians.[34]

When all of these myths are wiped away, the most devastating myth or fiction about malpractice, the one that resides deepest beneath the surface, is that the allegation of malpractice represents the allegation of incompetence, or misanthropy, or malice. In fact, it simply represents an allegation of fallibility – being human and being capable of error. Imagine the response of the physician who believes that he or she is being accused of malice – the intention to do harm. The allegation of malice is precluded by the precepts of tort law and is rendered improper by the Hippocratic Oath by which the physician swears to 'First, do no harm' and, by implication, to 'intend no harm', i.e. malice. Judges and jurors understand that the physician, like the speeding driver, did not intend harm. But the physician's good intentions are not the test of reasonable performance and the profession will be unlikely to regulate itself without fundamental understanding that the legal rules of evidence in negligence cases, including malpractice, exclude the accusation of the intent to harm. When misunderstanding about the law is combined with an appreciable incidence of medical error and a high resistance among physicians to report errors,[35] then it seems that the 'culture of secrecy' derives in part from a 'culture of fear'.[36] Thus, despite the attention to the subject of medical error and the formation of organizations devoted to patient safety, there has been little demonstrable evidence of a reduction in medical error. The solution will involve changes not only in the conduct of care but also in the educational, ethical, and emotional components associated with medical errors.[37]

We will attempt, in passing, to deal with these notions, but perhaps the following experiences will assist the reader to focus on the issue of patients' expectations of a perfect outcome. The senior author delivered his first baby as a medical student about 1963. After the delivery, the first words out of the mother's mouth were, 'Is my baby alright?' He would deliver his last baby about 40 years later and the first question this mother asked was exactly the same as the question asked by the mother 40 years earlier. In the intervening 40 years, the ultrasounds, computers, and monitors of every description have allowed us to visualize the fetus, characterize its genetic composition, and determine its behavior, its growth, and its tolerance to hypoxia. As a result, there has been a dramatic reduction in the risk of fetal anomaly or death, especially during labor. Labor rooms have become intensive care suites with remote surveillance capabilities. Indeed, it has never in history been safer to deliver a baby, or perversely, to be sued for negligent care. Everyone, patients and physicians included, understands that there are no guarantees with pregnancy and under the best of circumstances, considering the stakes, not all outcomes are perfect. As with all medical care, there is always an element of uncertainty – about care and about outcome. Are lawsuits generated by those patients who fail to understand this principle or by physicians who, confronted with a bad outcome, fail to educate their patients or respond compassionately?

With regard to the notion that the presentation of the handicapped child in the courtroom dooms the defense case because of sympathy for the child, the author has witnessed the following situation in the courtroom in the case of a neurologically handicapped infant. After their deliberations, the jury returned to the courtroom to announce their verdict before the judge and the various parties. When the judge asked for the decision of the jury, the foreman arose and asked the judge if he could first make a preliminary statement on behalf of each of the jury. With tears in his eyes, the foreman acknowledged that over the course of the trial the members of the jury felt that they had come to know and care for the parents and the afflicted child. He further stated that he wanted to extend from each member of the jury both their best wishes for the future and their considerable concern about the future support of the child. They did not find the physician negligent.

In medicine today there is considerable enthusiasm for 'evidence-based medicine', epidemiologically driven decisions, and structured reimbursement. There seems much less appetite for 'evidence-based law'. The initiatives derived from evidence-based medicine seem driven as much by motives of cost control as by the hope for better health care services. Similarly, the avoidance of error, such as the use of automated medication ordering and dispensing, and the efforts of risk management (safeguarding assets) while contributory may not directly enhance the quality of care. The extraordinary response to the Institute of Medicine study has led to a nationwide movement to find ways to reduce error and increase patient safety. The foundation of these efforts is based on increasing the ease and confidentiality of error reporting, as well as the facilitation of root cause analysis systems, team approach techniques, and improved communication and dispute management techniques, all with the goal of improving patient care.

In this way, the avoidance of error and the efforts of risk management (safeguarding assets) have become as important as, if not more important than, ensuring the quality of care. The breadth of malpractice mythology and the detestation and fear of the malpractice system by the physicians and organized medicine have distracted our attention from the public's concern about the ineffectual efforts to improve outcome whether by the adoption of higher standards, improved educational processes, or the meaningful activities of peer review committees and professional societies.

Peer review

In 1973, the U.S. Congress enacted legislation requiring physicians to initiate Peer Review Organizations to monitor the utilization and the quality of hospital and physician services in the federally funded Medicare program. Now more than 30 years later we must acknowledge the lack of a gold standard, medical or legal, for reviewing allegations of negligence and dealing meaningfully with medical error. Peer reviews produce inconsistent agreement and operate without formal rules or guidelines for review.[38] They are left to the local hospital,[39] and although the American College of Obstetricians and Gynecologists (ACOG) has attempted to provide outside review to individual hospitals, there is no analysis of such efforts.[10] The majority of 'true' peer review exercises are driven by adverse outcomes and do not represent systemic reviews of the numerous latent processes promoting adverse outcome. These are left to the occasional review of a 'sentinel event'. With peer review the rules for reviewing records and for obtaining agreement about either the severity of any departure or the impact on the offending physician are inconstantly applied and haphazardly administered. Peer review requires the presence of the physician – an overt acknowledgment of the fact that medical records are often silent about important questions whose understanding is necessary to determine the standard of care. Despite the physician's presence, the deliberations of the peer review committee are not backed up by systemic reviews of the physician's conduct in similar cases. The system is not designed to promote either patient education or an apology.

Peer review in obstetrics is especially problematic. The medical records of the infant may not be present, and there may not be anyone (neonatologists/pediatrician) present to discuss the infant's course and the impact of the obstetrical care on that course. The patient, moreover, is rarely, if ever, questioned about her perceptions of the care! Invariably, there is no long-term follow-up, especially if the infant is transferred to another hospital. Imagine, therefore, a discussion at a Peer Review Meeting of the medical conduct in a case of shoulder dystocia and brachial plexus injury. The medical record is silent about the use of fundal pressure – as it should be: fundal pressure should not be used to relieve shoulder dystocia. As a result, the physician who had carefully documented a normal sequence of maneuvers was exonerated. During the malpractice case, however, incontrovertible evidence was produced that the 263-lb anesthesiologist was exerting sufficient force on top of the patient's abdomen to produce considerable pain and broad ecchymoses. The case was settled on behalf of the plaintiff!

Other complaints of lack of due process, poor reproducibility, and motivation by non-medical/non-scientific considerations plague discussions of the peer review process whether involving the practicing physician by a hospital department, the review of a manuscript submitted for publication, the funding of grants submitted for research, or the evaluation of expert testimony by professional societies (Judson, Cohen, Pegalis, American College of Physicians).[41,42]

Peer reviews are conducted by people from the same department of the hospital and in many states are safeguarded from legal scrutiny under the common law privilege of self-critical analysis, a privilege that protects and encourages quality assessment, but that secrecy, in the final analysis, may be counterproductive for the ultimate objective of improved patient care and better transparency of medicines self-governance.[34,43] At its most collegial, colleagues of the physician being reviewed are likely to minimize error on the notion that when their turn comes, similar cordiality and extenuation will prevail. After all, the objective of the process of review is not to find fault or apportion blame, but to improve outcomes for the future.[44] The greatest failure of error is the failure to learn from it.

Gawande in an article in *The New Yorker* describes a surgical peer review exercise and the limitations of this process. He admits that he had made a serious medical error, but he was not obligated to face the peer review committee directly and the committee did not deal directly with the error itself in any remedial way.[45] Under the heading of 'the banality of injury', Gawande acknowledges that medial error is ubiquitous and makes the point that medical error is *not* the province of a select few culprits as common wisdom suggests. He avers, 'There are no "incompetent, unethical, negligent few", no basket of "bad apples" that conspire to taint all of medicine'.

Sometimes, however, peer review meetings may not be cordial and the meeting may become the venue for limitation of privileges or dismissal. Here, the purpose is not educational or remedial but political or economic, described under such appellations as 'economic credentialing' or 'sham peer review'. At these times, generally, hostility may prevail, the physician will have a lawyer present, and the battle will be joined. It is the law, not medicine, that must safeguard due process in these cases. If it can be shown that the peer review process was being used for purposes other than those related to medical care, the deliberations of the committee may no longer be protected. In either circumstance, it is an expensive, unsatisfying experience for which physicians have little appetite – whatever the outcome.

There is evidence that the knowledge of an adverse outcome (hindsight bias) may cause the peer review committee, like the expert in a malpractice case, to criticize retrospectively the decisions of the treating doctor.[46–48] While it might be better to withhold outcome information in both circumstances, it seems neither practical nor enforceable. While a 1988 study of anesthetic mishaps from a national database found strong agreement among anesthesiologist reviewers,[49] a later study about on agreement among anesthesiologists assessing 12 actual malpractice cases whose verdict was known has implications both for malpractice and peer review.[50] Here, the intraobserver agreement among observers was high (> 80%). Of the eight cases with complete or virtually complete agreement between respondent anesthesiologists, three (37.5%) disagreed with the verdict rendered by the actual juries. In addition, anesthesiologists showed significant disagreement (> 30%) among themselves in four of the case scenarios, indicating there may not be agreement regarding the standard of care in these clinical circumstances. Finally, anesthesiologists predicted jury verdicts poorly, with success rates of 50% or less in 7 of the 12 case scenarios. It should be pointed out that these reviews are usually parochial matters for only rarely does the peer review evaluation benefit from information obtained from the patient or in the hospital review, from bona fide experts in the field. These potential sources of enlightenment are available in the courtroom.

While there are correlations between the risk of lawsuit and such features of character as medical school prestige, physician intuition, gender, and even the apparently perverse inverse relationship between current medical knowledge and the likelihood of being sued, the fact is that most obstetricians are sued at least once in their professional life.[51] Repeat offenders may sometimes occur, but are not a common problem. As Gawande poignantly asks, 'How do we keep good physicians from harming patients?' He and others invite the inference that it is not the peer review process that can accomplish this, in part because of the dynamics mentioned above, but also because the contributing causes to adverse events are often not detected by current medical review processes.[38] We may also ask, what is the value of either peer review or even malpractice suits in improving care?[38,45]

A study (generally known as the Harvard study) commissioned by New York State in 1986, and released in 1990, showed that although actual malpractice is relatively rare, it is nevertheless underreported. If anything, the study group believed that there were too few lawsuits.[52–54] Further, they wrote, 'Physicians tended to equate a finding of negligence with a judgment of incompetence. Thus, although willing to admit that 'all doctors make mistakes', physicians were often unwilling to label substandard care as negligent and were opposed to compensation for iatrogenic injury. Given medicine's delayed response to the problem of medical error, including the limitations of peer review, the public's only alternative therefore was for individual patients to try to hold individual practitioners, one at a time, to whatever medical standards could be upheld by lawyers and expert witnesses.[55] It may be true that to 'address the problem of iatrogenic injuries seriously, we must reform the system of malpractice litigation'. What seems equally true is that the problems of iatrogenic injury and physician conduct cannot be contingent on changing the tort system alone.

The role of the physician

These complaints about the system also serve to camouflage the physician's role in the genesis of malpractice suits. 'It has been estimated that, the risk of lawsuit "seems not to be predicted by patient characteristics, illness complexity, or even physicians' technical skills". Instead, risk appears related to patients' dissatisfaction with their physicians' ability to establish *rapport*, develop trust, provide access, administer care and treatment consistent with reasonable *expectations*, deal effectively with conflict, and *communicate* effectively'.[4] In an article by Hickson *et al.*, patients who saw physicians with the highest number of lawsuits were more likely to complain that their physicians 'would not listen or return telephone calls', were 'rude', and 'did not show respect'.[2] Such complaints, furthermore, were similar to those documented in interviews with families who sued their physicians. Patients are less likely to sue (about 50% less) even for moderate and severe mistakes if the physician informs them of the mistake (basically, apologizes).

For the reasons mentioned above, physicians are untrained in the art of apology. It may seem counterintuitive for many physicians that one can accept responsibility for an outcome without admitting blameworthiness.[56,57]

In an analysis of 500 claims in obstetrics and gynecology, B-Lynch *et al.* show that 46% were misguided allegations and about half were due to incompetent care, an error of judgment, lack of expertise, poor supervision, or inadequate staffing. The other half were due to poor communication and 'misguided allegations', for which they recommend an alternative course of dispute resolution combined with improved communication.[58] Parenthetically, the more time the physician spends with a patient the greater is the satisfaction of *both* patient and physician.[59] In a survey reported by the ACOG,

Table 22.2 Malpractice-induced activities (from ACOG, 1990)

Modality	Percentage
Testing	76.2
Monitoring	73.3
Documenting	72.2
Informed consent	61.6
Consulting MDs	58.0
Patient information	51.2
Referrals	47.2
Staff presence	21.8

physicians reported wholesale changes in their practices (Table 22.2) and their fees as a result of malpractice suits – including greater consultation with the patient.[60]

In 1997, a highly publicized article recommended that when doctors make a mistake that harms a patient, they should tell the patient what happened, apologize, and do whatever it takes to repair the damage.[61] Basic professional ethics aver that patients have a right to know what happened to them. It seems like the right thing to do as part of the physician's responsibility to his patient and it may be therapeutic for the physician who may feel guilt and distress. Telling the truth may also strengthen the patient's faith in the doctor while a cover-up that fails, as many do, may anger the patient and make him/her more inclined to sue. Cover-ups also antagonize juries. Medicine is a human enterprise and error (i.e. fallibility) is part of being human. 'We are programmed for error'.

Understandably, the notion of admitting error has drawn skeptical review from the medical community, the insurance companies, and the defense bar.[62] They fear that admitting mistakes will 'open the floodgates' to lawsuits and hurt their reputations and careers. They fear also that without tort reform to decrease the number of malpractice suits and large settlements, and to reduce the punitive implications of existing reporting, few doctors could risk owning up to errors. The notion that telling the truth, apologizing, and reaching out to a family in grief can defuse some of the anger and polarization that characterize a typical lawsuit becomes hostage to the notion that every word you utter in consolation or contrition is an admission that can be used against you in a court of law. On top of that, defense lawyers then order doctors to say nothing until all the facts are in, and then to say nothing. It seems obvious to state that until legislative protections maintaining such admissions are enacted, it is very likely that lawyers will continue to order doctors to say nothing until all the facts have been ascertained through discovery, and then to say nothing. But is this a medicolegal problem, or is it an ethical problem?[61,63,64] Baldwin suggests that increased levels of moral reasoning may diminish the risk of malpractice suit,[65] making legislative protection unnecessary.

The Joint Commission on Hospital Accreditation (JACHO) standards require the disclosure of sentinel events and other unanticipated outcomes of care to patients and to their family members when appropriate. Hospital administrators, fearing medical liability suits, are reluctant to comply with this standard.[66] If disclosure is taken a step further to the offer of an apology, hospitals and physicians are even more likely to gravitate to traditional 'defend and deny' behaviors. Apology as it turns out is yet one more control that physicians exert over the risk of lawsuit. Thus, a prompt explanation of what is understood about what happened and its probable effects; assurance that an analysis will take place to understand what went wrong; follow-up based on the analysis to make it unlikely that such an event will happen again; and an apology will likely reduce the risk of lawsuit and heal, rather than harm, the physician-patient relationship.[67] In fact, a growing number of hospitals, doctors, and insurers have come to accept that genuine disclosure and apology may reduce error-related payouts and the frequency of litigation.[9,59,68,69] Further, a growing number of states are passing ('I'm sorry') laws that protect an apology from being used against a doctor in court.[68] Despite the ethical imperatives underlying such disclosure, it seems likely that more such fundamental protections will be needed before these practices become commonplace.

Common areas of litigation during labor

General problems relating to litigation in medicine include documentation, communication, institution of a chain of command, or internal systems conflicts, when there are unresolved disagreements between individuals, departments, and all levels of health care providers, such as between physicians and nurses or physicians and administrators. Of most concern are the attitudinal problems involving the interaction of nurses and physicians, which receive too little emphasis and are particularly difficult to change. Their potential serious impact on the ability of an obstetrical unit to provide 'high-reliability care' has been discussed at length by Simpson and Knox.[70] Of the many specific types of cases, only some will be briefly discussed here: (1) the failure to properly interpret fetal monitoring tracings, (2) the poor conduct of operative vaginal delivery, (3) the management of the large infant and shoulder dystocia resulting in either in brain damage with death or subsequent CP, or (4) the infant with brachial plexus injury (sometimes both).

Along with the measures taken by physicians in response to the threat of malpractice (Table 22.2), the profession, especially obstetrics, has embarked upon a series of defensive 'scientific' initiatives to *modify* its vocabulary and its accountability. Defensive medicine is a practice designed not for the purpose of answering clinical questions or directing therapy, but for the purpose of preventing lawsuits or counteracting plaintiff testimony in court. The ACOG, for example, has recommended the elimination of such universally applied terms of art as 'fetal distress', 'perinatal asphyxia', and 'stat cesarean section' and have modified the definitions of 'low-' and 'mid-forceps'.[71–73] Further articles have created definitive, unyielding requirements for the diagnosis of birth-related injury and suggest that labor related injury is rare and perhaps irreducible.[74]

Irrespective of motivation, these publications have not been accompanied by any decrease in lawsuits, any improvement in outcome, or any less defensive posture on the part of the obstetrical community. These efforts to make our specialty 'fair of speech' and litigation-proof discount important mechanisms of injury, diminish notions of medical judgment, inhibit scientific inquiry into the timing and mechanism of fetal injury, and delay the testing of new paradigms for dealing with adverse outcome. These articles attempt to influence the defense in these cases in several ways. An inexperienced lawyer may turn down a meritorious case because, as the guideline states, 'It is not possible to ascertain retrospectively whether earlier obstetric intervention could have prevented injury or cerebral damage in any individual case where no detectable sentinel hypoxic event occurred', or because the umbilical artery pH was > 7.0 despite obvious injury during labor or delivery. In addition, by insisting that extreme derangements in pH values are required to begin to make the correlation between labor events and subsequent neonatal injury, these criteria modify the level of proof normally required in malpractice suits. The burden of proof in these suits requires that the level of confidence in the relationship between the events and the outcome be more probable than not. It is well to compare these pronouncements with a widely respected authority of neonatal brain injury.

> Brain injury in the intrapartum [period] does occur, [it] affects a large absolute number of infants worldwide ... and represents a large source of potentially preventable neurological morbidity. Among the many adverse consequences of the explosion in obstetrical litigation has been a tendency in the medical profession to deny the importance or even existence of intrapartum brain injury. (Volpe, *Neurology of the Newborn*, 3rd ed., 1995)

These issues have also been discussed at some length for the brain-damaged infant[75,76] and for brachial plexus injury.[77]

Fetal cardiotocography (CTG)

In part, because of the pivotal role it plays in malpractice cases, there have been attacks on fetal monitoring that have come both from within the profession and from without. In an article in the Stanford University Law Review, Margaret Lent, a young defense lawyer, argues that the widespread use of electronic fetal monitoring (EFM) is both medically and legally unsound.[78] Ms Lent points to selected clinical trials to demonstrate that EFM does not reduce fetal mortality, morbidity, or CP rates. She argues that because EFM has a very high false-positive rate and its usage correlates strongly with a rise in cesarean section rates so that it offers no medical advantage over auscultation. Similarly, she argues, EFM provides no protection in the courtroom. Though obstetricians believe that they should use EFM because its status as the standard of care will protect them from liability, Ms Lent argues that given its failings it may in fact expose them to liability. She further argues that auscultation, at least as safe and effective as EFM, is also more likely to protect physicians from liability. Ms Lent concludes that obstetricians have an obligation to their patients and to themselves to adopt auscultation as the new standard of care. She finds 'no excuses left to defend the continued use of EFM'. The medical literature can be used to justify any position on monitoring, including those of Ms Lent. Thus, it may be shown that CTG increases the risk of CP and that 'substandard care' protects against subsequent CP.

While failure on the part of the health care provider to recognize clear fetal heart rate abnormalities is frequently alleged in malpractice cases, to isolate the CTG tracing under these circumstances frequently oversteps its permissive role in obstetrical care. A normal CTG pattern permits ongoing labor *only* as long as safe vaginal delivery is a reasonable option. If the pattern turns abnormal (rising baseline, decreasing variability along with variable/late decelerations), especially in the second stage, then the questions are several. Can the pattern be ameliorated (by reducing the oxytocin, moderating the pushing efforts)? If the pattern cannot be ameliorated what is the feasibility of safe vaginal delivery given the estimated fetal weight, previous obstetrical history, position, presentation of the fetal head, and progress in labor to this point? Experience suggests that the vast majority of cases hinge far more on the reasonableness of the conduct of obstetrical care (especially the second stage) than on the interpretation of the fetal monitor. Regardless, reviewers of malpractice cases consistently find that the CTG tracing has been frequently misinterpreted in allegations of negligence.[79]

The legal climate

Most changes in both the medical and the legal professions are evolutionary and it is often difficult to define any sea change. The last three decades, however, have witnessed a number of remarkable and epochal changes in the medicolegal climate in the United States, with doubtless more to come. Many of the changes derive from periodic surges in malpractice premiums, reduced availability of insurance coverage, and the exodus of major insurers from the market first in the early 1970s, again in the mid-1980s, a lesser event in the 1990s, and more recently in the new millennium. In each epoch, affected providers clamored for policy changes to inhibit litigation.[80] In the 1970s, legislatures established joint underwriting associations to serve as insurers of last resort,[81] special state patient compensation funds were introduced to absolve commercial insurers of responsibility for specified dollar portions of malpractice payments, and public reinsurance mechanisms were established to fill gaps in the underwriting market. By the late 1970s, the malpractice crisis had abated – only to recur less than a decade later. In Washington State between 1984 and 1986, for example, malpractice premiums for obstetrics jumped approximately 100%. As a consequence, obstetricians marched on legislatures or joined many family physicians and midwives in an exodus from obstetric practice. Those remaining in practice became more reluctant to care for high-risk obstetric patients and less willing to accept indigent patients and reduced fees, irrespective of the fact that indigent patients, in fact, appear less likely to sue.[82] In many rural areas across the United States obstetric care became virtually unobtainable. Periodically, these circumstances galvanized legislative activity in virtually every state and led to further far-reaching reforms of existing tort and insurance law[83,84] with some stabilization of premiums – at least initially. After almost a decade of essentially flat premiums, premiums are rising exponentially, which is said to be due to the increasing size of awards and insurers leaving the medical malpractice business because of diminishing returns on investment. This has been aggravated by rising health care costs ($1.6 trillion in 2002 and increasing yearly), and efforts to control physician income. The average annual increase in health care costs from 2000 to 2004 was 12–16% with predictions that, whether or not the result of negligent care, they will rise by a further 8% in 2005, with likely little containment beyond that.[85]

It is important to emphasize that premium levels are responsive to a variety of factors besides litigation dynamics, including previous losses, past and expected investment returns, business strategies, and the degree of state regulation of rate changes.[86] A January 2004 study found that nationwide, average premiums for all physicians between 2000 and 2002 rose by 15% – a rate of rise almost twice as fast as per capita total health care spending. Certain specialties had even greater increases, including obstetricians/gynecologists (22%) and internists and general surgeons (33%).[87] Neurosurgeons, obstetricians, orthopedists, and emergency room physicians are particularly likely to have premium rate increases. The rates for obstetricians/gynecologists vary nationally, but according to ACOG, between 2002 and 2003 about half of obstetricians/gynecologists were experiencing increases of 10–49% in their insurance premiums.

Premiums may influence physicians' decisions to join and leave the labor force, their choice of a medical specialty, and their decision of where to locate, creating the potential for undeserved patient populations in certain specialties or geographic areas. Rising malpractice premiums may also encourage physicians to practice 'defensive medicine', performing more tests and procedures than necessary in order to reduce exposure to lawsuits. Parenthetically, however, defensive medicine (ordering a test not for the purpose of furthering patient care, but for the legal protection of the physician) is indefensible in court. Imagine the physician-defendant responding to a question about the indication for a certain test with the answer: 'I didn't want to get sued'. Both rising malpractice premiums and defensive medicine practices may contribute to the rising health care costs and thus to an increase in health insurance premiums.

The choices for the obstetricians – short of some windfall protection scheme – are leave practice, move to a 'more compliant' state, give up obstetrics, obtain employment where malpractice insurance is provided, raise fees, discontinue seeing patients with restrictive payment structures, or go bare, i.e. do not obtain any malpractice insurance. For many, there is no good option and their future will hinge on the least inimical choice. Beyond physicians, these rapidly rising medical malpractice premiums have again become an issue of increasing concern about the health care system for policy makers and the general public.

Underwriter data claims payments

The insurance industry also has its problems. In 2003, insurers were paying out in claims and expenses $1.38 for every medical malpractice premium dollar collected. (National Underwriter Data Services). Results have deteriorated steadily from 1998, when the rate of return was −7.6. Medical malpractice insurers' return on net worth was −7.4% in 2002, down from −4.7% in 2001.[88] Results in 2002 were the worst in the following states: Arkansas, Nevada, Montana, Mississippi, Illinois, and Missouri, with a return on net worth ranging from −33.7% in Arkansas −24.4% in Missouri. In reality, even in the good years, premiums rarely cover payouts. The system works in part because premiums are invested and with at least a modest return permit the insurance company to make a profit. This is abetted by the fact that malpractice suits, especially, take a long time to resolve – about 4 years on average.

The average claim payment rose almost 8% per annum from $95,000 in 1986 to $320,000 in 2002 despite the fact that the frequency of claims per 100 doctors has remained more or less constant. Only about 30% of claims result in insurance payouts, but expenses for cases, especially obstetrical (brain-injured baby cases), where there is no payout are considerable[18]. Concurrently, insurance companies, along with the population at large, faced reduced income from investments to help offset underwriting losses.

Another study in 2004 found that hospital professional liability and physician liability claims costs have increased at a steady 9.7% since 2000 and are likely to rise at the same rate in 2004. Frequency, or the number of claims, is growing at 3% a year; claim severity (the dollar amount) is increasing by 6.5% annually. Hospital liability claim costs for 2004 are expected to reach almost $150,000 per claim, compared with $79,000 per claim in 1996. The average claim against a physician is expected to reach $178,000, compared with $120,000 in 1996.[89]

Jury awards and settlements

In early 2005, a Towers Perrin study found that over the 28 years since 1975, when they were first identified separately, medical malpractice cost increases have outpaced those in other tort areas, rising at an average of 11.8% a year, compared with 9.2% for all other tort costs. In 2003, medical malpractice, at almost $27 billion, cost each American an average of $91 a year. This compares with $5 a year in 1975.[85] Recent data suggest that while jury awards are stabilizing and the frequency of claims may be decreasing, the severity of malpractice claims is increasing and the range of awards is moving upward.[89] Median medical malpractice jury awards have held steady at about $1 million over the 3 years 2000–2002.[90] Awards ranged from a low of $11,000, almost double the amount of the previous year, to a high of $95 million. The average award in 2002 hit $6.25 million, up from $3.91 million in 2001. However, only a small fraction of cases go to trial and very large awards are frequently reduced after the fact and after the publicity.

The costs of perinatal injury are quite high, relative not only to the costs of settlement and defense but also to personal and professional upheaval for all concerned. As Simpson and Knox have pointed out,[70] the perspective of human and system factors reveals themes, context, and conditions common to accidental injury in other high-risk domains. According to the Jury Verdict Research, in 2000 the median jury award for neonatal neurological injury had increased to $5 million compared to $725,000 in 1994, with 76% of the jury awards valued at greater than $1 million (compared to 40% in 1994).[90] Higher awards were more likely to occur when the hospital was the sole defendant than when both were defendants.

Conventional wisdom holds several contributing factors to account for the increased incidence of malpractice claims. (1) People are more litigious; it is part of our culture and extends everywhere from lawyers themselves to city governments. (2) Given the media coverage and watchdog groups, there has been an increasing understanding by the public of the fallibility of physicians. The Public Citizen Health Research Group, and the more recently formed groups emphasizing both medical error and the need to improve care as part of tort reform, have also helped fuel the public's demand for change.[34] (3) Another factor is the diminishing intimacy of the patient-doctor relationship fomented in part by larger changes in the way health care is distributed (HMOs), by increasing overhead and by deteriorating reimbursement schedules. (4) Then, there is the increasing availability of medical experts to testify in malpractice cases (the breakdown of *omerta*). (5) Also, there is the increasing assertiveness of the courts and the increasing sophistication of the plaintiff's bar with more careful selection of meritorious suits. (6) Last, there is the need for assistance with financing medical bills. Indeed, there is a seeming increase in the frequency of lawsuits for the 'damaged child', in part due to the large verdicts sometimes realized but also due to the increasing incidence of CP related to the increasing survival of low birth weight infants and the costs thereof.

Several clinical practices and media attention would seem also to be impacting on the frequency and type of lawsuit. As an example, the United States Food and Drug Administration (FDA) issued a national advisory on the risks of vacuum extractors.[91] This was rapidly followed by a nationwide television program emphasizing some of the disastrous results with vacuums. In turn, there has been a dramatic increase both in the reporting of adverse events associated with vacuum deliveries to the FDA and in the number of lawsuits alleging negligent care in the use of vacuums. Similarly, the methods undertaken to lower the cesarean section rate in the United States have perhaps been accomplished at the expense of an increased risk of ruptured uterus, shoulder dystocia, and lawsuit.[92] While all authorities would agree that any woman with one previous cesarean section and no other adverse features may be eligible for an attempt at VBAC – if she chooses to do so after being carefully explained the options, some HMOs have refused to accede to the mother's choice and have required that *every* patient with a previous cesarean be given a trial of labor – a horrific, medically indefensible recommendation. One institution in California that adopted this policy was assessed almost $25 million as a result of 48 women who suffered adverse outcome as a result of this policy.

Prevalence of medical malpractice

When hospital medical records from New York State were examined as part of the Harvard study, the incidence of adverse events or injuries resulting from medical 'interventions' or treatment was 3.7%. The percentage of adverse events due to what the physician team characterized as 'negligence' (not necessarily a legal definition) was 1%. However, only one in eight who suffered from an adverse event due to negligence filed a medical malpractice claim, and only 1 in 15 received compensation. Most adverse events resulted in only minimal and transient disability and most of the patients' medical care expenses were paid for by health insurance. This helps to explain why only a small percentage of patients who are injured as a result of negligence file medical malpractice claims. However, a significant proportion (22%) of patients who did not file medical malpractice claims suffered moderate or greater incapacity. In the second phase of the study, researchers confirmed that some of the tort claims filed provided little or no evidence of medical malpractice or even an adverse event, suggesting that the tort system is 'very error-prone', at least in its initial stages (related to the expert). This inefficiency in both the medical and the legal systems, notwithstanding, the study noted that 'if anything, there are too few lawsuits'. The inference here is that more patients with adverse outcomes related to negligence should be suing.[52,53,93,94]

There are several studies of closed claims in obstetrics and their relationship to negligence or their adherence to guidelines. Julian *et al.* reviewed the files of 220 obstetric closed-claim cases to identify common factors predisposing to claims and to suggest preventative measures.[95] Identification of common obstetric risks and correct management of these risks was poor in these cases. Only 54% of the risks were recognized; of these, only 32% were correctly managed. A high percentage of risks were thought to be directly related to the obstetric outcome leading to the claim (66%). The authors feel obstetric closed claims can be studied and suggestions made to aid obstetricians in providing care. They concluded that obstetric malpractice closed claims are amenable to study; physicians and their patients would benefit from better data collection systems to identify risks in individual pregnancies, along with available resources to aid their management of patients. They felt that suits can be avoided through modification of physician behavior.[95]

In 1989, Rosenblatt and Hurst reviewed all closed obstetric claims in the records of a major physician-sponsored malpractice insurer from 1982 to 1989.[96] Of the 54 files closed during the 6.5-year period covered by this study, 21 (39%) involved physician reports of bad outcomes that did not lead to a formal claim. Of the 33 formal claims, 14 (42%) were dismissed, either by the plaintiff's attorney or by the courts. Eighteen of the remaining 19 claims were settled before trial, with an average payment to the plaintiff of $185,000. The one suit that went to trial resulted in a defense verdict. A review of the case histories demonstrated that in the majority of cases when a payment was made, probable medical negligence had taken place. Non-meritorious claims were not compensated. For those cases in which a payment was made, the size of the settlement was commensurate with the seriousness of the injury, which almost always involved damage to the infant. Poor physician judgment was the most common source of error.[96]

The surviving, handicapped infant continues to represent the highest payout/case. There are numerous representative reviews of closed cases (Table 22.3). An analysis of 353 closed claims involving obstetrician-gynecologists revealed that the 40 highest-paid claims (11.3%) accounted for 88.7% of the total dollars spent. The majority of these 23 (57.5%) were obstetrical, including the five highest claims and 17 of the first 20 highest-paid awards. Obstetrical negligence represented over $5 million (76.5%) of the total expense. Of the 40 cases, 23 (60%) were resolved with a compromise settlement, 9 claims (22.5%) were resolved with indemnity payment on the basis of verdict or pretrial compromise; 7 (17.5%) had no indemnity payment because of a jury verdict or voluntary dismissal. These seven were in the highest-paid claims group only because of expenses.[91,96]

Of the 40 cases, none were considered frivolous, 28 (70%) were judged to be meritorious, and 12 (30%) were judged to be non-meritorious. Seven of the latter settled without indemnity costs, including four that went to trial with a defense verdict and three that were dismissed, leaving five others in this group with proper treatment and indemnity costs. Expenses to defend all 12 cases of proper treatment totaled over $500,000. Irrespective of the absence of strict negligence, each of these 'non-meritorious claims' illustrated substantial deficits with the medical record or system failures – inviting the allegation of negligence and lawsuit (making the case appear meritorious). These analyses clearly reveal that bad outcomes may not be the fault of the physician, but that physician behavior in the conduct of the case and the conduct of the medical record contribute heavily to successful allegations of malpractice.

Ogburn *et al.* reviewed 153 closed claims involving perinatal injury or death filed from 1980 through 1982 with the St. Paul Fire and Marine Insurance Company.[97] The claims included were those in which an indemnity was paid or $1,000 or more was expended on the legal defense. Cases were classified according to the presence or absence of medical negligence. Most of the complications leading to claims arose during labor and delivery. Many claims resulted from the failure to evaluate or treat in a manner consistent with accepted standards of care. Many lacked documentation of the physician's recognition of the risk factors involved. In the opinion of the reviewers, medical negligence occurred in 47% of the cases. Indemnity payment occurred with most (but not

Table 22.3 Operative delivery notes

Operative delivery note (A)

Op del note:

MF, OP≫OA, mid epis, no lac

Apgar 8, 9 P and M intact

EBL 400, M and B left DR in good cond.

Signature

Translation:

Operative delivery note:

Midforceps, occiput posterior (OP) to occiput anterior (OA), midline episiotomy, no lacerations

Apgar scores 8, 9 at 1, 5 min. Placenta and membranes expressed intact

Estimated blood loss 400 ml. Mother and infant left the delivery room in good condition

Operative delivery note (B)

Procedures: *Trial of forceps, midforceps rotation, episiotomy repaired*

Findings: *Gyneocoid pelvis, normal active phase, +3 station, minimal molding, direct OP, epidural anesthesia, second stage=2.5 h, pushing inadequate, patient tired*

EFW=3000. Prev. baby=2800

Indications: *Persistent occiput posterior, prolonged second stage, secondary arrest of descent, tired patient*

Informed consent: *Discussed options with patient and husband, who agree and understand that if any difficulty is encountered, the forceps will be abandoned and cesarean section undertaken*

The operating room has been alerted

Methods: *Midline episiotomy Kielland forceps. Direct application to OP without difficulty*

Gentle rotation: ROT to OA. Kiellands removed, Simpson forceps applied. Gentle traction – delivered as OA

Fetal outcome: *3200-g male infant, APGAR 8, 9 (see individual features in chart)*

Resuscitation: Oxygen only, no evidence of trauma to skull forceps, marks reveal appropriate placement

Maternal outcome: *Perineum intact, episiotomy repaired, no lacerations. Placenta and membranes intact. Estimated blood loss: 300 cc*

Mother left delivery room in good condition

all!) of the claims judged to be associated with medical negligence. Payment to the claimant was also made in a number of cases in which the reviewer thought no malpractice had occurred. The authors concluded that these results suggest that improvements are needed in prenatal and perinatal health care as well as in the legal system used to address the problem of perinatal medical negligence.[97]

In a study published in 2003, Ransom et al, tried to estimate whether guideline compliance affected medicolegal risk in obstetrics and whether malpractice claims data can provide useful information about compliance.[98] From the claims experience of a large health system delivering approximately 12,000 infants annually, they retrospectively identified 290 delivery-related (diagnosis-related groups 370–374) malpractice claims and 262 control deliveries between 1988 and 1998. Clinical pathways for vaginal delivery and cesarean section, implemented in 1998, were used as a standard of care. They compared rates of non-compliance with the pathways in the claims and control groups. They found that non-compliance with the clinical pathways was significantly more common among claims than controls (43.2% vs. 11.7%, $P<0.001$; odds ratio=5.76, 95% CI 3.59, 9.2). In 81 (79.4%) of the claims involving non-compliance with the pathway, the main allegation in the claim related directly to the departure from the pathway. The excess malpractice risk attributable to noncompliance explained approximately one-third (104 of 290) of the claims filed (attributable risk=82.6%). They concluded that malpractice data are a useful resource in understanding breakdowns in processes of care and that adherence to clinical pathways might (1) reduce clinical variation, (2) improve the quality of care, and (3) protect clinicians and institutions against malpractice litigation.

A study by Greenwood *et al.* from the National Perinatal Epidemiology Unit, Oxford, United Kingdom compared the prevalence of criteria suggesting acute intrapartum hypoxia in children with CP according to whether a lawsuit was brought alleging obstetrical negligence.[99] The subjects were singleton children with CP born between 1984 and 1993, excluding cases with a recognized postnatal cause for CP. Only one-fifth (27/138) of all singleton CP children were the subject of a lawsuit. The greater the number of criteria suggesting intrapartum insult the more likely was a legal claim ($P<0.01$), but 36% (4/11) of those satisfying all required criteria did not make a claim. Of the 27 claims, 12 were discontinued, 8 were settled, and in 7 the legal process was still pending at the time of writing the article. Furthermore, the presence of the three essential criteria for acute intrapartum hypoxia did not increase the likelihood of a legal claim being settled.[99]

Other studies have focused on the costs and outcomes of litigation but not on culpability.[18] Closed claims provide valuable data, but because, on average, a medical liability case takes 3–5 years to come to closure,[86] opportunities for timely intervention in unsafe practices are lost. The research value is further compromised when the details of cases that reach settlement are suffocated by 'gag clauses' that mandate silence not only on the amount of award, but also on the allegations and the admission or even acknowledgment of wrong-doing, thereby removing an obvious incentive to make care better. Hatlie and Sheridan have suggested that gag orders are counterproductive.[34]

Medical records

Unfortunately, the opinions that serve to launch medical or medicolegal proceedings are most often based on a review of medical records that are frequently silent on the intentions of the provider or their exercise of 'medical judgment'. They may be silent, as well, on fundamental details of the obstetrical care. As a result, medical records, which represent both a medical document and a legal document, often promote or perpetuate cases and confound their defense. A cost analysis of 3205 multispecialty claims showed an average cost per claim of $22,584.[100] Deficits in the medical record, e.g. inadequate instructions, delayed entries, inadequate notes, and consent-form issues, more than double the average cost. System failures nearly triple the average cost. Thus, while an erroneous decision may be defensible if the reasons leading to it are recorded in the chart, the changed record and the contradictory record are almost impossible to defend. Until medical records objectively communicate the findings, the attention paid, the comprehension that was achieved and offer a reasonable plan followed by appropriate and consistent action, their appearance in court will continue to be an uphill battle for the physician and he/she will get little credit for the thought process or use to his/her advantage the testimony of 'a witness whose memory never dies'.

As an aside, the reader is invited to compare the two enclosed notes regarding a midforceps procedure (Table 22.3). In the first example, the note invites lawsuit if there is an adverse outcome. The note provides no indication for, or details about, the procedure. It is more a personal memorandum than a responsible medical description relevant for decisions about care in future pregnancies, for example. The second note, on the other hand, would seem to protect against lawsuit in several ways. The note (1) clearly bespeaks thoughtfulness, (2) bespeaks understanding of the medical issues and alternatives, and (3) underscores the physician's efforts to provide a forthright explanation to the patient and her husband – all powerful disincentives to lawsuit. Naked may be the best disguise!

One can readily blame the plaintiff's attorney for bringing to suit an apparently frivolous case, but who is to blame (i.e. what has been learned?) for the negligent care and adverse outcome in situations where no suit is brought despite negligent care or where no award is made despite a suit, and the physician's care is vindicated? Should the plaintiff's attorney be blamed for pursuing a case that his expert has told him, based on a review of the medical records only, is negligent care? Each of the articles that evaluated closed cases found appreciable amounts of agreed upon negligent care. Each emphasizes (1) the need for better data, 2) the inculpating role of physician behavior, and 3) the importance of the review of malpractice claims to identify problem-prone clinical processes and suggest interventions that may improve outcome and reduce negligence.[101]

It must be readily apparent from even these limited studies that not all meritorious suits succeed and not all non-meritorious suits (not the same as frivolous) lose. These articles leave it open to speculation why patients victimized by obvious medical negligence do not sue or why they are not compensated by the system in the face of agreed upon negligence. Clearly, patients without demonstrable evidence of negligence bring suit and sometimes they are rewarded in the system. The system does not work perfectly, but these studies from various specialties and perspectives strongly suggest that it is not a lottery. Given the non-medical issues that incite or color a case, physicians squander much of the advantage they have in the system! Thus, it is with some justification that critics of malpractice litigation point out that it is unrealistic to expect that increased levels of litigation will make compensation for injuries more 'just' or health care better. A *reductio ad absurdum* argument suggests that immunity from lawsuit, perhaps the true goal behind physicians' notion of tort reform, will, by eliminating lawsuits, achieve these goals. Some conventional tort reforms appear to be effective in reducing litigation costs and stabilizing insurance markets; they are not, however, designed to remedy the fundamental failings of the malpractice system – making care better and making the physician–patient relationship better. Fulfillment of these objectives may not require more sweeping tort reform; perhaps more sweeping 'thought reform' may be required or, alternatively, trying to make the system work as it was supposed to. These reforms can only come from the medical community.

Legal vulnerability

The last several decades have also witnessed the development of new bases for lawsuit in reproductive matters, including wrongful birth and wrongful life. In the former, the parents with an injured child may bring suit alleging that negligent treatment or advice deprived them of the opportunity to avoid conception or terminate a pregnancy. The latter, brought on behalf of the child born with birth defects, alleges that the child would not have been born but for negligent advice to, or negligent treatment of, the parents. It should be emphasized that such allegations are actionable in some states but not in others. While not strictly related to malpractice, a mother who pleaded with her hopelessly premature infant's caretakers to discontinue resuscitation was not heeded, resulting in the survival of a severely handicapped child and a provisional $42 million verdict for the plaintiff.

Tort reform measures

Most liability reform acts have four major components: (1) reforms directly addressing the size of awards – under the heading of caps on damages; (2) reforms intended to modify liability rules, to control the number of claims and size of payouts by eliminating joint and several liability for cases in which a plaintiff found to be partially at fault becomes responsible for a disproportionate share of the damages; 3) reforms limiting access to the cồurts, through shortening statutes of limitation – a reduction in the length of time during which lawsuit can be brought; and 4) periodic payments – the latitude to pay future economic damages over time. Some initiatives have legislated review panels to pass on the merit of a case prior to the institution of suit, while others have attempted to remove the infant who is brain damaged during birth from the medicolegal arena by the institution of no-fault insurance. Still other initiatives have attempted to increase the percentage of any award that goes to the patient by limiting the attorney's fees.

The most popular of these, caps on premiums, have had the benefit of moderating the increases in insurance payments. A publication from the Rand Corporation has emphasized that in cases with modest claims there is indeed a reduction in indemnity payouts, but they cast doubt on the likely benefit of caps on the high-award cases where economic damages are large and 'pain and suffering' may be much smaller. It seems axiomatic that caps should not apply to frivolous suits where the cap should be zero.[102]

In the 1970's 22 states legislated some form of prelitigation processes, including screening panels and mandatory binding and non-binding arbitration: only two remain active and neither has been effective. The costs of constitutional battles over due process rights for binding processes and the failed reduction of litigated cases in non-binding processes, led to further soaring legal costs, rather than reductions. The only lasting 'tort reform', although, as discussed later, with questionable material impact on malpractice frequency and awards, has been caps on non-economic damages, with the gold standard being that of California's Medical Injury Compensation Reform Act of 1975 (MICRA).[102]

Tort reform, the mantra of both the ACOG and the Bush administration to deal with high medical malpractice costs, makes sense only from the political aspect.[30] Capping awards on malpractice suits may offend trial lawyers, but it helps or holds harmless special interests in the insurance, drug, and health care industries. It provides no assistance to patients who suffer grievous harm as a result of negligent care nor does it improve the delivery of medical care. To many, a $250,000 cap (the cap placed on non-economic damages in California) is poor acknowledgment indeed for the physical and emotional damage done to people who have suffered total paralysis, permanent blindness, or severe brain injury because of medical errors. Indeed, many states burdened with high premiums have already set their own caps, but generally at more reasonable levels. It would seem more useful to consider making it harder for insurance companies to gain rate increases.

Guidelines for judges and juries might be enacted to help determine what compensation is reasonable in a given circumstance. Similar guidelines could help ensure that punitive damages, sometimes masquerading as non-economic damages, are high enough to deter bad conduct; $250,000 would hardly amount to a slap on the wrist.

The problem with frivolous lawsuits is best addressed by raising the hurdles for filing a malpractice suit, for example, requiring an expert judgment on the merits of a case before it can proceed through the courts. As mentioned above, there seems to be no place for the expert witness to certify a case as meritorious if that same expert will not appear on the record for (public) report, deposition, and trial if necessary.

The notion that the crisis of escalating malpractice insurance premiums is forcing doctors out of business remains murky. Insurance companies have substantially raised premiums for malpractice coverage for doctors in high-risk specialties like obstetrics and neurosurgery in some states, leading at least some doctors to curtail their services, retire, or move. But when the Government Accountability Office visited five of the hardest hit states in 2003, it found only scattered problems and was unable to document wide-scale lack of access to medical care.[86]

None of the tort reform proposals deal with the underlying need to diminish malpractice and to identify harmed patients and provide them with fair, prompt compensation, or provide tools for health care providers to properly prepare patients and deal effectively with unanticipated outcomes. Although, they do resolve the desire of the health care industry and the insurance companies for fewer big court awards, they do not materially impact the frequency of suit. But they do act as a rollback of the legal rights of patients who are injured.

The Center for Justice and Democracy, a consumer advocacy group, recently commented:

> It may be hard to understand why 'tort reform' is even on the national agenda at a time when insurance industry profits are booming, tort filings are declining, only 2% of injured people sue for compensation, punitive damages are rarely awarded, liability insurance costs for businesses are minuscule, medical malpractice insurance and claims are both less than 1% of all health care costs in America, and premium-gouging underwriting practices of the insurance industry have been widely exposed.

Despite claims by the insurance industry, there is no evidence that soaring malpractice premiums are the result of sharp increases in the amounts of money paid out for malpractice claims. And, tellingly, industry executives have carefully acknowledged that tort reforms will not result in substantial premium reductions – only an improvement in care can do that.[30,103]

Caps do not limit lawsuits. More reasonably, caps are intended to increase the hurdles to a lawsuit by diminishing the economic value of a suit. In cases where there is little economic loss (irrespective of negligence), victims may not be able to find lawyers to take their cases (www.saynotocaps.org/newsarticles/WSJEffectof Caps.html) because malpractice cases can cost plaintiff's lawyers hundreds of thousands of dollars out of pocket to prosecute, with no guarantee of recouping those expenses. As pointed out by the Rand Corporation study, caps have little impact on lawsuits where there are substantial economic losses, e.g. brain-damaged infant, maternal death. A one-size-fits-all cap cannot encompass the unique facts in any case and, in fact, more reasonably creates a system of 'one-size-fits-none'.[102] It unfairly discriminates against victims with no economic losses, such as children, stay-at-home moms, the elderly, the poor, and the mentally handicapped. The media unflinchingly promulgates numerous cases of tragic, ineffable medical error where such arbitrary limits (originally set in 1979) seem inadequate and, if not inadequate, arbitrary.

Caps will not lower doctors' malpractice insurance premiums.(www.saynotocaps.org/reports/Premium Deceit.pdf: The Failure of Tort 'Reform' to Cut Insurance Rates) Average premiums are actually 16% higher in states with caps. In states that have recently adopted caps, most notably Texas and Florida, insurance rates are continuing to increase. Indeed the only thing keeping rates down in California – a state often cited as a model for caps is insurance industry regulation provided by Proposition 103.

The amount of money awarded on pain and suffering is not known. In the majority of awards, those reached by settlement out of court, there is no distinction between economic and non-economic damages. In jury trials economic and non-economic damages are awarded separately, but there appears to be no calculation of either the amount or the propriety. Nor has there been any compilation of those extreme awards that are reduced, sometimes drastically, by judicial review. In three cases where the jury awarded over $220 million, the total cumulative amount received was $14 million (6 cents on the dollar!). There was no publication of the reduction! (Public Citizen.pdf.)[104] When adjusted for the sky-rocketing rate of health care inflation, total payouts in malpractice cases remained flat until 2001. In the 3 years since, total payouts have declined each year (newsarticle/LowerPayouts.htm).

Many states have enacted legal reforms that have effectively eliminated any lawsuits that could be construed as 'frivolous' by requiring a 'certificate of merit' from a physician certified in the same medical specialty as the doctor being sued. There have also been laws enacted to prevent 'venue shopping' for a more favorable jury. Indeed, a Republican state senator from Pennsylvania declared that 'There is no such thing as a frivolous lawsuit any more' in Pennsylvania. In addition, again in Pennsylvania, one of the 'red alert states', there has been a significant increase in the number of physicians over the past several years, prompting one state legislator to call such claims of a doctor exodus as 'scare tactics'.

It is far from clear that malpractice costs are driving up the costs of health care. Malpractice costs account for less than 2% of the U.S. health care budget. The Congressional Budget Office, in a report released in January 2004, found that legislation to cap damages in medical malpractice lawsuits would 'do little to hold down health care spending' or eliminate the practice of 'defensive medicine'. There is little evidence that the threat of malpractice lawsuits contributes to the practice of defensive medicine. Rather, it has been suggested that doctors order additional tests because it is good medical practice; doctors make money from additional testing; and managed care discourages unnecessary testing, or 'bad' defensive medicine.[86]

Faulty underwriting and misfeasance by malpractice underwriters are additional factors contributing to the rise in premiums. In Pennsylvania in the late 1990s, six major malpractice insurers became insolvent because of risky premium underpricing, poor investment strategies, and Enron-style malfeasance, leaving doctors to pay for their mismanagement (InsolvencySummary.pdf.).

There is no basis for the notion that insurance companies routinely settle lawsuits just to make them go away. This seems more like a strategy for self-destruction and is contradicted by the closed-claims data presented above (factsandfigures/fibsysfacts.html).

There can be little doubt that there is an immediate question of affordability that must be dealt with acutely. Indeed, several states have contributed significant amounts of public money to subsidize insurance premiums. Physicians remain the highest-paid professionals in the state, according to U.S. Census data. Indeed, the incomes of obstetricians – the physicians most affected by higher premiums – are rising. For many, on average, doctors spend 1–5% of their gross revenues on medical malpractice insurance. It seems obvious also that many doctors supplement their incomes with fees from attorneys for providing 'independent medical evaluations' in malpractice cases.

Alternative system reforms

Experts have suggested a number of approaches, including special health courts with judges trained to deal with malpractice issues, required mediation, mandatory reporting of errors by doctors, and prompt offers of compensation. Some of these will be reviewed briefly here. Not strictly a part of tort reform, alternative dispute resolution has much to recommend it.[58]

The *strict liability (no-fault) administrative system* supports creation of a just patient safety culture and encourages reporting (and prevention) of adverse events. It has the advantages of dispensing with trial and supports open disclosure to the patient (not the public) as the deliberations are administrative. In this system the provider is accountable for all avoidable medically related losses and the matter can be resolved promptly. It eliminates the requirement of proving negligence, but the patient must establish that their injury was actually caused by the treatment. As a generalization, eligibility is based on avoidability rather than providers being strictly responsible for medically related losses. There is, unfortunately, the common perception that 'no-fault' means 'no accountability'. Examples include the Neurological Injury Compensation Association (NICA) in Florida and Virginia.[104–108]

Although, the system of No-Fault is modeled after that of Workers Compensation and Automobile No-Fault claims, the complexity of determining causal and avoidable injury medical injury claims is very different. And although it removes negligence as a basis for the claim, it does not replace the regulatory system of reporting and the resultant physician fear, nor does it address the inbred philosophy of 'do no harm', 'zero tolerance'. Since premiums in any no-fault system are based on injury rates, this creates an incentive to conceal injuries and reduce the admission of high-risk specialists to medical staffs. It may also discriminate against patients at high risk for injury. It is uncertain how the establishment of a no-fault system will impact cost. Some test programs have demonstrated that costs of a general no-fault system would exceed those of the present tort system. Finally, the introduction and administration of a no-fault medical injury system, whether public or private, will be complicated and likely politically encumbered.

Preventable events (ACEs) represents consensus on what constitutes an avoidable event.[106] These are predetermined events that should not occur in quality health care delivery. They encourage prevention of avoidable events that can trigger eligibility for an early compensation offer. ACEs make 'avoidability', and therefore eligibility for compensation, transparent to providers and patients alike. They standardize eligibility for compensation and provide quicker identification of eligible cases. There is, however, no comprehensive ACE list currently available, and there is concern as to who is to develop the categories of avoidable events. Brain-damaged infants, for example, would not be covered. Development of the list will, of course, require an array of expert consensus (selected by whom?). The use of ACEs provides a basis to determine eligibility for alternative and conventional compensation systems. It can also be paired with a standardized compensation fee schedule.

Mediation

Mediation represents a highly efficient option for non-adversarial resolution of health care conflicts. It is a process in which the parties to the conflict themselves, not lawyers, craft their own unique resolution to a conflict. Mediation is essentially facilitated communication and negotiation using a neutral third party. The process itself is non-binding and does not prevent the patient from moving forward to litigation. However, if a resolution is reached, it becomes binding under contract law and may even be brought as an order of the court. Mediation is highly cost-efficient and time sparing, in that it makes response to adverse events and their resolution more timely, and boasts a greater than 90% resolution rate. It is widely accepted and highly successful in many 'industries' such as real estate and education, but has met with much resistance in the health care industry, especially in medical malpractice. It intensifies the pressure on patients to settle, thus reducing or avoiding litigation. Because confidentiality has been stripped from the mediation process in medical malpractice disputes by medical regulatory boards and reporting agencies, the successful application of the mediation process in physician–patient conflicts has therefore been crippled. Although confidentiality in error reporting is the foundation of most of the proposed legislation, it has not been extended to the resolution of conflicts arising from alleged medical errors. The statutory obligation physicians have to report settlements of disputes involving quality of care issues creates a perverse incentive for physicians to move forward in litigation, especially when one considers the high attrition rate of malpractice claims and the likelihood of a physician prevailing in those cases that persist. It is likely that even in the face of tort reform mediation will remain an infrequently used medium for the resolution of physician–patient disputes.

Arbitration

As with mediation, arbitration provides economical and prompt adjudication of adverse events. Like mediation, it provides prompt, private settlement and compensation, yet is also subject to reporting requirements and regulatory oversight. The processes differ, however, in a few major factors. With arbitration the decision maker is a third party, the arbitrator(s), and the process is highly formalistic and adversarial. There are two forms of arbitration, binding and non-binding. The latter is similar to mediation in that if either party disagrees with the arbitrator's decision, they may move on to litigation. The former, however, is a binding decision that cannot be appealed. Binding arbitration for malpractice claims has met with considerable legal opposition and non-binding arbitration has met with low utilization and increased litigation costs. Such systems intensify the pressure on patients to settle, thus reducing or avoiding litigation. They may be used with the current tort system – as well as with no-fault and ACEs. Kaiser Permanente, for example, requires enrollees to sign a 'willingness to arbitrate' agreement. With this approach, the health plan undertakes to resolve disputes through arbitration rather than go through the courts. This of course is not the same as a waiver of liability.

Specialized medical malpractice courts

There are three types of specialized courts under consideration: the Health Court, the Medical Board Administrative Adjudication System, and the Tripartite Panel.

Health Court: This involves the creation of an alternative court system within the federal court system. This proposal will, as touted by the consumer advocate group Common Good, presumably make judgments more reliable and provide clearer lessons for deterrence of adverse outcome. In theory, it can provide more timely access, faster resolution of claims, along with more reliable and standardized compensation. It requires appointment of special expert courts to hear medical cases or administer compensation based on avoidable events. Health courts also make the system more transparent by providing public access to settlement and adjudication findings. It will require judges who have special knowledge or training in medicine. Although proponents believe that this form of adjudication will offer more consistent and informed decisions than the traditional trier of fact, a lay jury, many studies find that in comparison with expert's reviews, the present jury system is quite consistent.

Health courts may be paired with ACEs and a standardized compensation schedule – and may even add a trial option to an administrative system. There are precedents for these types of courts in certain tax and patent infringement and workers' compensation laws.

Medical Board Administrative Adjudication System: In 1988, the AMA, 31 medical specialty associations, the Physician Insurer's Association of America (PIAA), and the Counsel of Medical Specialty Societies created the Medical Liability Project to develop an equitable and efficient method to handle malpractice claims.[109,110] They proposed a claims adjudication process based on fault and suggested that the states' medical boards act as the trier of fact in addition to their regulatory and disciplinary roles. This system would initially screen cases, offer free legal counsel for cases passing review, and offer limited judicial review. In a parallel development, the AMA considers that the provision of expert testimony constitutes 'the practice of medicine' and that it should be subject to peer review by state medical boards. The AMA encourages the state medical associations to work with the licensing boards to develop effective disciplinary measures for fraudulent testimony.

Tripartite Panel: Also in 1988, the PIAA proposed an administrative system similar to that used for workers' compensation in the hope that patients would elect this more speedy system through the offer of incentives. The panel would consist of a judge, a physician, and a lay person and function much like the few state screening panels that remain active. In cases where malpractice was found, all medical expenses would be paid under a specific method of computation, all non-economic awards would be based on a fixed schedule of benefits, and there would be a limit on attorney's fees.

Pretrial screening panels

This is a system that is modeled after state programs that are presently functioning, with those of Maine and Vermont the most recognized. To enlist the Panel, the patient provides written notice to the physician and with the superior court to be acted upon within 90 days. The superior court selects a Panel Chair from a pool of retired judges and/or mediators with judicial or legal experience. The Chair selects from a court issued list one attorney and one physician panelist, of the same or relevant specialty. The parties may challenge the selection for cause. There is a Prehearing Discovery, then a Pretrial Screening Hearing that follows the format of an arbitration. Depositions are admissible, but expert testimony is unusual. The panel has prior access to written briefs, complete medical records, deposition transcripts. The panel then acts as the trier of both fact and law, under the standard used by lay juries, 'preponderance of the evidence'. It evaluates the case on the basis of the four Ds of negligence. Unanimous decisions by the panel on negligence and causation are admissible in court, in favor of either the patient or the provider. The decision of the panel, like in non-binding arbitration, does not bind either party from pursuing litigation and trial. Some systems allow recovery of costs by the losing party, but as stated previously, if it is the plaintiff, actual recovery is unlikely.

Enterprise liability

Enterprise liability provides an incentive for prioritization of enterprise-wide safety. It shifts liability from the individual provider to a provider organization such as an integrated medical staff, IPO, large group practice, or hospital capable of influencing care across the systems. Enterprise liability essentially makes these organizations 'strictly liable' in both a legal and an economic sense by their responsibility for liability premiums for all staff involved in the organization, which could potentially impact the present punitive reporting system and allow for a freer flow of error reporting. Such a system would promote institutional safety, and potentially stabilize liability insurance fees. Legal provisions (Stark laws) may prohibit liability insurance coverage of non-employee physicians. It works equally well with alternatives as well as the current tort system. The Department of Health and Human Services Office of Inspector General (OIG) historically has been concerned that a hospital's subsidy of malpractice insurance premiums for potential referral sources, including hospital medical staff, may implicate the antikickback statute, because the payments may be used to influence referrals. 'There is a particular concern where subsidies are offered in a conditional or selective manner that reflects current or anticipated referrals from the subsidized practitioners'. Hospitals may be able to subsidize the malpractice insurance of local obstetricians without triggering antikickback sanctions, according to an advisory opinion issued by the OIG. In this opinion, OIG outlines a specific case in which it would not impose antikickback sanctions against a medical center that provides subsidies to four community-based obstetricians who hold staff privileges at the medical center but are not employees of the facility.[111]

Tort reform in many of its guises, however, has historically not been universally 'friendly' to the physician. In 1988, the U.S. Congress established a National Practitioner Data Bank authorizing the collection of data about physicians and dentists from malpractice settlements, awards, and disciplinary actions; these data were to be supplied by insurers, hospitals, and HMOs.[112] Queries of the Data Bank might be made by hospitals and physicians, but there is to be no access by the public or actual or prospective litigants including patients and attorneys although expanded access to this information is the subject of much debate. This tracking by the Data Bank has probably decreased the willingness of physicians to settle cases, but has probably not decreased the frequency of malpractice. The non-departmental public body (NPDB) reporting system is primarily based on the reporting of any formal written claim of malpractice that results in even one penny changing hands, regardless of admission of blame or severity of injury. Such reports carry great weight in considerations for staff privileges, provider contracts, and malpractice premium rates. Hatlie and Sheridan have argued that the NPDB should be abandoned.[34]

Even more recently, there has been increasing attention on the amount of medical error that has heretofore gone unnoticed and undocumented. The AMA has created a Patient Safety Initiative and the Federal Government is considering legislation that will likely reorient the approach to error. Indeed, since the publication of the prestigious IOM's 'To Err is Human', which claims that between 44,000 and 98,000 hospitalized patients die per year as a result of medical error, and subsequent studies such as that of Chaudhry and coworkers, patient safety has become the mantra of the Joint Commission on Accreditation, which has now embellished the requirements for disclosure of error.[36,66,113] Programs for the evaluation of root cause analyses of reported errors and the resulting error reducing actions have become, as they should, a national priority.

Also potentially threatening to the physician are those tort reforms that are linked (politically) to the establishment of enhanced physician review panels, the creation of 'three strikes and you are out' rules, etc. In Texas, for example, along with a stringent tort reform bill passed in 2003, the Texas legislature gave the Texas State Board of Medical Examiners new authority to regulate medical practice through the passage of S.B. 104. This bill gave the board increased funding for expert consultants and staff. These resources were used to assess the approximately 6000 complaints the board receives each year. As a result, Board enforcements have increased dramatically. Before the augmentation, cases were filed against physicians immediately, which immediately affected their records. The new system provides more due process, but is more far wide-ranging. Opponents of this feature of Texas Health litigation argue that standard of care issues should be left to local community medical societies or hospital peer review and credentialing societies. But when the boot is on the other foot and these organizations engage in sham peer review or economic credentialing, physicians complain about their unfair practices (see below). Physician groups complaining about S.B. 104 want the presumption of innocence, the right to access details of the complaints against them, the right of discovery, the right to present witnesses and cross-examine witnesses, and the right to appeal. How seductive is the illusion of a new idea – all of these features are present in current malpractice law, the beneficiary of 200 years of accumulated jurisprudence. Public Citizens's Health Research Group ranked Texas 23 out of the 50 states.

Reviews of the impact of tort reform on premiums suggest that while premiums do respond to increases in payments, they do not increase dollar for dollar (http://www.nber.org/papers/w10709). This suggests that other factors may also be important in explaining the recent jump in malpractice premiums, such as a less competitive insurance industry or a decline in insurers' investment income. There is little evidence that changes in malpractice premiums are linked to changes in either the total number of physicians or the number of physicians working in obstetrics/ gynecology, surgery, or internal medicine. There is weak evidence to suggest that the entry decisions of young physicians and the exit decisions of older physicians may be affected by malpractice premiums. There is stronger evidence to suggest that rural physicians are more sensitive to a change in premiums – a 10% increase in premiums results in a 1% decrease in rural physicians per capita and a 2% decrease in older rural MDs (http://www.nber.org/papers/w10709).

Although there is no change in the frequency of most treatments, some data suggest that physicians may increase the use of screening procedures in response to higher premiums. Such practices however have had little effect on total Medicare expenditures, suggesting that the costs associated with defensive medicine practices may be small, at least for this age group. Thus, it is far from clear that state tort reforms will avert local physician shortages or lead to greater efficiencies in care. The stabilization of premiums, the initial response to most rounds of tort reform, may not indeed be the result of the tort reform legislation. Normally, it takes years before legislative tort reform has a direct impact on malpractice premiums and several, but not all, state courts have invalidated the cap on damages, the component of the law with the greatest potential to reduce premiums.[114,115] Malpractice premiums are affected by a constellation of additional factors, including the general investment climate, interest rate cycles, and insurance regulations.

Whether driven by legislation or not, it seems reasonable that stable malpractice insurance premiums offered by experienced, reputable companies are important reasons for maintaining physician availability and equilibrium.

There is no evidence that tort reform has resulted in better care or more realistic confrontation of error. Tort reform simply 'tinkers with certain aspects of the system in a piecemeal fashion without having to grapple with fundamental reform of either the health care delivery system, the reimbursement system or physician behavior'.

Tort reform and finances – litigation and risk management

There is universal agreement that the medical needs of those with adverse outcome require more attention, whether they are related to negligence or not. There is also universal agreement that the present functioning of the medicolegal system is an anachronism – neither is it efficient or error-free in reaching a settlement nor is the distribution of money equitable. In the United States, only about 28 cents of every premium dollar goes to injured patients after an average delay of 4.9 years to dispose of a case.

Is no-fault insurance better? To determine whether Florida's implementation of a no fault system for birth-related neurological injuries reduced lawsuits and the total spending associated with such injuries, and whether no-fault was more efficient than customary tort procedures in distributing compensation, Sloan *et al.* compared claims and payments before and after implementation of a no-fault system in 1989.[6] They found that the number of tort claims for permanent labor-delivery injury and death indeed fell by about 16–32%. However, when no-fault claims were added to tort claims, the total frequency of claims rose by 11–38%. Further, of the estimated 479 children who suffered birth-related injuries annually, only 13 were compensated under no-fault. The total combined payments to patients and all lawyers did not decrease, but under no-fault, a much larger portion of the total went to patients. Thus, less than 3% of the total payments went to lawyers under no-fault versus 39% under tort – a new equilibrium. Some claimants with birth-related injuries were winners, taking home a larger percentage of their awards than their tort counterparts. Lawyers clearly lost under no-fault, but so did many children with birth-related neurologic injuries who did not qualify for coverage because of the narrow statutory definition.

Solving the malpractice problem

While the focus of clinical risk management intuitively rests on the analysis of adverse events, it seems clear that this is the most inefficient way of reducing or eliminating harm to the patient. In the current climate, risk management tends to deal more with avoidance of blame and litigation than with the avoidance of harm to patients.

One of health care's principal patient safety success stories is anesthesiology. In the 1980s, in the midst of a separate medical liability crisis, the rate of anesthesia-related deaths was one in 10,000; 6000 people per year who had undergone anesthesia died or suffered brain damage, and anesthesiologists' liability insurance premiums had sharply escalated.[68] Following a national news magazine broadcast that pilloried the field for these outcomes, the American Society of Anesthesiologists (ASA) decided to seize the opportunity presented by the crisis to improve anesthesiology safety.

It started with the hiring of a systems engineer. Through close scientific examination of 359 anesthesia errors, every aspect of anesthesia care – equipment, practices, and caregivers – was analyzed. Eventually, with the commitment of leadership and resources toward the task, the many system failures revealed by the study were re-engineered, and anesthesia-related death rates fell dramatically.

The ASA uses case analysis to identify liability risk areas, monitor trends in patient injury, and design strategies for prevention. Today, the ASA Closed Claims Project – created in 1985 – contains 6448 closed insurance claims. Analyses of these claims have, for example, revealed patterns in patient injury in the use of regional anesthesia, in the placement of central venous catheters, and in chronic pain management. Results of these analyses are published in the professional literature to aid practitioner learning and promote changes in practices that improve safety and reduce liability exposure.

Closed claims data analysis is the one way in which the current medical liability system helps to inform improvements in care delivery. However, reliance on closed claims for information related to error and injury is cumbersome at best. It may take years for an insurance or malpractice claim to close. These are years in which potentially vital information on substandard practices remains unknown. Providing patient safety researchers with access to open claims, now protected from external examination, could vastly improve efforts aimed at identifying worrisome patterns in care and designing appropriate safety interventions.

In addition to anesthesiology's early work in identifying the human factors and system failures that cause error, anesthesiology has also promoted reliance on standards and guidelines to support optimal anesthesiology care. Anesthesiology has also been at the forefront in the use of patient simulation for research, training, and performance assessment. With simulation, no patients are at risk of exposure to novice caregivers or unproven technologies.[116] Anesthesiology is still far from perfect. But, its 'institutionalization of safety' continues to serve the field well as it tackles the continuing threats to patient safety that are endemic to modern medicine.

Medicine is different from industry in that the medical system has not adjusted to the realities of human fallibility. The circumstances of the contemporary malpractice situation continue to compromise both the provision and the safety of health care as well as our notions of justice, of access to the law and to health care. This state of affairs benefits neither the patient nor, in the long run, the physician. While in some instances the fear of lawsuit has increased the amount of surveillance and may have even had a salutary effect on outcome, there is little argument that the present format for dealing with allegations of negligence provides any incentive to the profession to practice better medicine, provide better peer review, or, in the occasional instance, restrict the future practice of the physician whatever his conduct. True reform will require a systemic approach to error in medicine as elsewhere and some refinement of our ethics and an appreciation of the paradoxes of contemporary malpractice. To lower the risk of malpractice we must continue to attempt to raise the standards of care. We need this more than we need the identification of the 'bad apples' of our specialty. We must increase communication with the patient and remain their advocate. We must address the formal teaching of communication skills, conflict management, and team development techniques throughout medical school and residency. We must construct effective error reporting and systems analysis programs that promote error reduction, while protecting physicians from being punished by arbitrary and ineffective reporting systems. We must not squander our greatest asset – the medical record – and we must stop playing the role of victim. Often the ultimate failure is often not the individual provider but the latent, systemic errors, errors for which our systems are programmed, but which are functionally immune from lawsuit. A lawsuit cannot make 'the system' a defendant. Finally, we must be willing to participate in the process of uncovering error and make the patients our allies in these efforts.

REFERENCES

1. Keeton WP DD, Keeton RE, Owens DG. *Prosser and Keeton on the Law of Torts*, 5th edn. St. Paul, MN: West Publishing, 1984.
2. Hickson GB, Clayton EW, Entman SS, *et al.* Obstetricians' prior malpractice experience and patients' satisfaction with care. *J Am Med Assoc* 1994;272(20):1583–7.
3. Hickson GB, Federspiel CF, Pichert JW, Miller CS, Gauld-Jaeger J, Bost P. Patient complaints and malpractice risk. *J Am Med Assoc* 2002;287(22):2951–7.
4. Hickson GB, Clayton EW, Githens PB, Sloan FA. Factors that prompted families to file medical malpractice claims following perinatal injuries. *J Am Med Assoc* 1992;267(10):1359–63.
5. Ambady N, Laplante D, Nguyen T, Rosenthal R, Chaumeton N, Levinson W. Surgeons' tone of voice: A clue to malpractice history. *Surgery* 2002;132(1):5–9.
6. Sloan FA, Whetten-Goldstein K, Hickson GB. The influence of obstetric no-fault compensation on obstetricians' practice patterns. *Am J Obstet Gynecol* 1998;179(3, Pt 1):671–6.
7. Gibson S. *Wall of Silence: The Untold Stories of the Medical Mistakes That Kill and Injure Millions of Americans*. Washington, D.C.: Lifeline Press; 2003.
8. Moore J, Berry D, Knox GE. Dispelling urban myths in healthcare risk management. *J Healthc Risk Manag* 1999;19(2):2–10.
9. Gallagher TH, Waterman AD, Ebers AG, Fraser VJ, Levinson W. Patients' and physicians' attitudes regarding the disclosure of medical errors. *J Am Med Assoc* 2003;289(8):1001–7.
10. Kritzer H. *The Justice Broker: Lawyers and Ordinary Litigation*. New York: Oxford University Press, 1990.
11. Hyams AL, Shapiro DW, Brennan TA. Medical practice guidelines in malpractice litigation: An early retrospective. *J Health Polit Policy Law* 1996;21(2):289–313.
12. Peters K. The role of the jury in modern malpractice law. *Iowa Law Rev* 2002:909-69.
13. Studdert DM, Mello MM, Brennan TA. Medical malpractice. *N Engl J Med* 2004;350(3):283–92.
14. Fry v. United States F, 1013 (1923).
15. Shea vs. Esensten F, 3d 625m 629 (8th Cir.), 1997.
16. Daubert v. Merrell Dow Pharmaceuticals I, 509 U.S. 579, 1993.
17. Kumho Tire Co. LVC, 119 S. Ct. 1167, 1999.
18. Bors-Koefoed R, Zylstra S, Resseguie LJ, Ricci BA, Kelly EE, Mondor MC. Statistical models of outcome in malpractice lawsuits involving death or neurologically impaired infants. *J Matern Fetal Med* 1998;7(3):124–31.
19. LLMD of Michigan IvJ-C, Co., 1999.
20. Ross BK. ASA closed claims in obstetrics: Lessons learned. *Anesthesiol Clin North Am* 2003;21(1):183–97.

21. Meyers AR. 'Lumping it': The hidden denominator of the medical malpractice crisis. *Am J Public Health* 1987;77(12):1544–8.
22. Meeker CI. A consensus-based approach to practice parameters. *Obstet Gynecol* 1992;79(5, Pt 1):790–3.
23. Meeker WC. The future impact of clinical practice guidelines. *J Manipulative Physiol Ther* 1995;18(9):606–10.
24. Lavery JP, Janssen J, Hutchinson L. Is the obstetric guideline of 30 minutes from decision to incision for cesarean delivery clinically significant? *J Healthc Risk Manag* 1999;19(1):11–20.
25. Schreiber v. Physicians Insurance Company, Wisconsin, 223 Wis. 2d 417, 1996.26.
26. *Ob-Gyn News* 2003;February 1.
27. Plauche WC. Subgaleal hematoma. A complication of instrumental delivery. *J Am Med Assoc* 1980;244(14):1597–8.
28. Calbresi G. *The Cost of Accidents: A Legal and Economic Analysis*. New Haven, CT: Yale University Press, 1970.
29. Schwartz W, Mendelson D. Physicians who have lost their malpractice insurance: Their demographic characteristics and the surplus-lines companies that insure them. *J Am Med Assoc* 1989; 262:1335–41.
30. Brooks R. Malpractice mythology (editorial). *New York Times* Jan 9, 2005.
31. Kollas CD. Medicolegal program for resident physicians. *Pa Med* 1997;100(9):28–9.
32. Kollas CD, Frey CM. A medicolegal curriculum for internal medicine residents. *J Gen Intern Med* 1999;14(7):441–3.
33. Malpractice. *Med Econ* 1999;August.
34. Hatlie MJ, Sheridan SE. The medical liability crisis of 2003: Must we squander the chance to put patients first? *Health Aff (Millwood)* 2003;22(4):37–40.
35. Chaudhry SI, Olofinboba KA, Krumholz HM. Detection of errors by attending physicians on a general medicine service. *J Gen Intern Med* 2003;18(8):595–600.
36. Institute of Medicine. *To Err Is Human: Building a Safer Health System*. Washington, DC: National Academies Press Publications, 2000.
37. Kalra J. Medical errors: Overcoming the challenges. *Clin Biochem* 2004;37(12):1063–71.
38. Morris JA Jr, Carrillo Y, Jenkins JM, *et al.* Surgical adverse events, risk management, and malpractice outcome: Morbidity and mortality review is not enough. *Ann Surg* 2003;237(6):844–51; discussion 51–2.
39. Spaeth RG, Pickering KC, Webb SM. Quality assurance and hospital structure: How the physician–hospital relationship affects quality measures. *Ann Health Law* 2003;12(2):235–47, Table of Contents.
40. Gluck PA, Scarrow PK. Peer review in obstetrics and gynecology by a national medical specialty society. *Jt Comm J Qual Saf* 2003;29(2):77–84.
41. Posner KL, Caplan RA, Cheney FW. Variation in expert opinion in medical malpractice review. *Anesthesiology* 1996;85(5):1049–54.
42. Gunn IP. Evidence-based practice, research, peer review, and publication. *CRNA* 1998;9(4):177–82.
43. Donohue SK. Health care quality information liability & privilege. *Ann Health Law* 2002;11:147–58, Table of Contents.
44. Posner KL, Kendall-Gallagher D, Wright IH, Glosten B, Gild WM, Cheney FW Jr. Linking process and outcome of care in a continuous quality improvement program for anesthesia services. *Am J Med Qual* 1994;9(3):129–37.
45. Gawande AA. Ubiqity of error. *New Yorker* 2003.
46. Caplan RA, Posner KL, Cheney FW. Effect of outcome on physician judgments of appropriateness of care. *J Am Med Assoc* 1991;265(15):1957–60.
47. Hugh TB, Tracy GD. Hindsight bias in medicolegal expert reports. *Med J Aust* 2002;176(6):277–8.
48. Meadow W, Lantos JD. Expert testimony, legal reasoning, and justice. The case for adopting a data-based standard of care in allegations of medical negligence in the NICU. *Clin Perinatol* 1996;23(3):583–95.
49. Caplan RA, Posner K, Ward RJ, Cheney FW. Peer reviewer agreement for major anesthetic mishaps. *Qual Rev Bull* 1988; 14(12):363–8.
50. Cheney FW, Posner K, Caplan RA, Ward RJ. Standard of care and anesthesia liability. *J Am Med Assoc* 1989;261(11):1599–603.
51. Reding R. The role of intuition in medical malpractice. *Zentralbl Chir* 1999;124(Suppl 3):50–2.
52. Brennan TA, Hebert LE, Laird NM, *et al.* Hospital characteristics associated with adverse events and substandard care. *J Am Med Assoc* 1991;265(24):3265–9.
53. Brennan TA, Leape LL. Adverse events, negligence in hospitalized patients: Results from the Harvard Medical Practice Study. *Perspect Healthc Risk Manag* 1991;11(2):2–8.
54. Localio AR, Lawthers AG, Brennan TA, *et al.* Relation between malpractice claims and adverse events due to negligence. Results of the Harvard Medical Practice Study III. *N Engl J Med* 1991;325(4):245–51.
55. Mohr JC. American medical malpractice litigation in historical perspective. *J Am Med Assoc* 2000;283(13):1731–7.
56. Hobgood C, Peck CR, Gilbert B, Chappell K, Zou B. Medical errors – what and when: What do patients want to know? *Acad Emerg Med* 2002;9(11):1156–61.
57. Witman AB, Park DM, Hardin SB. How do patients want physicians to handle mistakes? A survey of internal medicine patients in an academic setting. *Arch Intern Med* 1996;156(22): 2565–9.
58. B-Lynch C, Coker A, Dua JA. A clinical analysis of 500 medico-legal claims evaluating the causes and assessing the potential benefit of alternative dispute resolution. *Br J Obstet Gynaecol* 1996;103(12):1236–42.
59. Michael S, Woods MD. Healing words: The power of apology in medicine. info@doctorsintouch.com, 2004.
60. American College of Obstetricians and Gynecologists (ACOG). *Professional Liability and Its Effect: Report of 1990 Survey of ACOG Membership*. Washington, DC: American College of Obstetricians and Gynecologists, 1990.
61. Finkelstein D, Wu AW, Holtzman NA, Smith MK. When a physician harms a patient by a medical error: Ethical, legal, and risk-management considerations. *J Clin Ethics* 1997;8(4):330–5.
62. Grady D. Doctors urged to admit mistakes. *New York Times* 1997;December 9.
63. Hebert PC, Levin AV, Robertson G. Bioethics for clinicians: 23. Disclosure of medical error. *Can Med Assoc J* 2001;164(4):509–13.
64. Nowicki M, Chaku M. Do healthcare managers have an ethical duty to admit mistakes? *Healthc Financ Manage* 1998;52(10): 62–4.
65. Baldwin DC Jr, Adamson TE, Self DJ, Sheehan TJ, Oppenberg AA. Moral reasoning and malpractice. A pilot study of orthopedic surgeons. *Am J Orthop* 1996;25(7):481–4.
66. Lamb RM, Studdert DM, Bohmer RM, Berwick DM, Brennan TA. Hospital disclosure practices: Results of a national survey. *Health Aff (Millwood)* 2003;22(2):73–83.
67. Physician apology. *Wall Street Journal* 2004;May 18.
68. Zimmerman R. Doctors' new tool to fight lawsuits: Saying 'I'm sorry.' Malpractice insurers find owning up to errors soothes patient anger. 'The risks are extraordinary'. *J Okla State Med Assoc* 2004;97(6):245–7.
69. Mazor KM, Simon SR, Yood RA, *et al.* Health plan members' views about disclosure of medical errors. *Ann Intern Med* 2004;140(6): 409–18.
70. Simpson KR, Knox GE. Common areas of litigation related to care during labor and birth: Recommendations to promote patient safety and decrease risk exposure. *J Perinat Neonatal Nurs* 2003;17(2):110–25; quiz 26–7.
71. ACOG. Operative vaginal delivery. *Tech Bull* 1994;196.
72. ACOG. Inappropriate use of the terms fetal distress and birth asphyxia. *Committee Opin* 1998;197.
73. Schifrin BS. Polemics in perinatology: Disengaging forceps. *J Perinatol* 1988;8(3):242–5.
74. ACOG. Fetal and neonatal neurologic injury. *Tech Bull* 1992;163.
75. Schifrin BS. The CTG and the timing and mechanism of fetal neurological injuries. *Best Pract Res Clin Obstet Gynaecol* 2004; 18(3):437–56.
76. Dear P, Newell S. Establishing probable cause in cerebral palsy. How much certainty is enough? *Br Med J* 2000;320(7241):1075–6.
77. O'Leary JA. *Shoulder Dystocia and Birth Injury: Prevention and Treatment*. New York: Mcgraw-Hill, 1992.
78. Lent M. The medical and legal risks of the electronic fetal monitor. 51 Stan L Rev 807, April 1999.
79. Ennis M, Vincent CA. Obstetric accidents: A review of 64 cases. *Br Med J* 1990;300(6736):1365–7.
80. Rosenblatt RA, Bovbjerg RR, Whelan A, Baldwin LM, Hart LG, Long C. Tort reform and the obstetric access crisis. The case of the WAMI states. *West J Med* 1991;154(6):693–9.
81. Weiler P. *Medical Malpractice on Trial*. Cambridge, MA: Harvard University Press, 1991.
82. Burstin HR, Johnson WG, Lipsitz SR, Brennan TA. Do the poor sue more? A case-control study of malpractice claims and socio-economic status. *J Am Med Assoc* 1993;270(14):1697–701.

83. Sloan FA, Whetten-Goldstein K, Githens PB, Entman SS. Effects of the threat of medical malpractice litigation and other factors on birth outcomes. *Med Care* 1995;33(7):700–14.
84. *The Effects of Medical Professional Liability on the Delivery of Obstetrical Care.* Washington, DC: Institute of Medicine, National Academy Press, 1989.
85. Towers-Perrin. *2006 Health Care Cost Survey*, 2005.
86. *Medical Malpractice Insurance: Multiple Factors Have Contributed to Increased Premium Rates.* Washington, DC: General Accounting Office, 2003.
87. *Limiting Tort Liability for Medical Malpractice.* Washington, DC: Office CB, 2004.
88. Nordman E, Cermak D, McDaniel K. *Medical Malpractice Insurance Report: A Study of Market Conditions and Potential Solutions to the Recent Crisis.* National Association of Insurance Commissioners, 2004. www.naic.org. Accessed August 15, 2005.
89. AON Risk Services. *2005 Hospital Profession Liability and Physician Ability Benchmark Analysis.* AON Risk Services, 2004.
90. Jury Verdict Research. *Medical Malpractice: Verdicts, Settlements and Statistical Analysis*, updated edition. LRP Publications, 2005.
91. FDA. Advisory. Food and Drug Administration, 1998.
92. Sachs BP, Kobelin C, Castro MA, Frigoletto F. The risks of lowering the cesarean-delivery rate. *N Engl J Med* 1999;340(1):54–7.
93. Brennan TA, Leape LL, Laird NM, *et al.* Incidence of adverse events and negligence in hospitalized patients: Results of the Harvard Medical Practice Study I. 1991. *Qual Saf Health Care* 2004;13(2):145–51; discussion 51–2.
94. Brennan TA, Localio AR, Leape LL, *et al.* Identification of adverse events occurring during hospitalization. A cross-sectional study of litigation, quality assurance, and medical records at two teaching hospitals. *Ann Intern Med* 1990;112(3):221–6.
95. Julian TM, Brooker DC, Butler JC Jr, *et al.* Investigation of obstetric malpractice closed claims: Profile of event. *Am J Perinatol* 1985; 2(4):320–4.
96. Rosenblatt RA, Hurst A. An analysis of closed obstetric malpractice claims. *Obstet Gynecol* 1989;74(5):710–4.
97. Ogburn PL Jr, Julian TM, Brooker DC, *et al.* Perinatal medical negligence closed claims from the St. Paul Company, 1980–1982. *J Reprod Med* 1988;33(7):608–11.
98. Ransom SB, Studdert DM, Dombrowski MP, Mello MM, Brennan TA. Reduced medicolegal risk by compliance with obstetric clinical pathways: A case–control study. *Obstet Gynecol* 2003;101(4):751–5.
99. Greenwood C, Newman S, Impey L, Johnson A. Cerebral palsy and clinical negligence litigation: A cohort study. *BJOG* 2003; 110(1):6–11.
100. Richards BC, Thomasson G. Closed liability claims analysis and the medical record. *Obstet Gynecol* 1992;80(2):313–6.
101. Kravitz RL, Rolph JE, McGuigan K. Malpractice claims data as a quality improvement tool. I. Epidemiology of error in four specialties. *J Am Med Assoc* 1991;266(15):2087–92.
102. Pace NZ, Golinelli D. *Capping Non-Economic Awards in Medical Malpractice Trials – California Jury Verdicts under MICRA.* Santa Monica: Rand Corporation, 2004.
103. Malpractice mythology (editorial). *New York Times* 2005; January 9.
104. Sloan FA, Whetten-Goldstein K, Stout EM, Entman SS, Hickson GB. No-fault system of compensation for obstetric injury: Winners and losers. *Obstet Gynecol* 1998;91(3):437–43.
105. Whetten-Goldstein K, Kulas E, Sloan F, Hickson G, Entman S. Compensation for birth-related injury: No-fault programs compared with tort system. *Arch Pediatr Adolesc Med* 1999; 153(1):41–8.
106. Bovbjerg RR, Tancredi LR, Gaylin DS. Obstetrics and malpractice. Evidence on the performance of a selective no-fault system. *J Am Med Assoc* 1991;265(21):2836–43.
107. Saphier CJ, Thomas EJ, Studdert D, Brennan TA, Acker D. Applying no-fault compensation criteria to obstetric malpractice claims. *Prim Care Update Ob Gyns* 1998;5(4):208–9.
108. Skolbekken JA. Shoulder dystocia – malpractice or acceptable risk? *Acta Obstet Gynecol Scand* 2000;79(9):750–6.
109. Meredith V, Cook CB, Penman A. Use of the physician insurers association of America database as a surveillance tool for diabetes-related malpractice claims in the U.S. *Diabetes Care* 1998;21(7): 1096–100.
110. PIAA releases results of latest malpractice claims study. *J Okla State Med Assoc* 1994;87(6):283–4.
111. News O-G. Medical Malpractice. *Ob-Gyn News* 2004;October 15:Sect. 25.
112. Waters TM, Studdert DM, Brennan TA, *et al.* Impact of the National Practitioner Data Bank on resolution of malpractice claims. *Inquiry* 2003;40(3):283–94.
113. Chaudhry S. Fighting for justice. *Br Med J* 2005;330(7483):114.
114. Zuckerman S, Bovbjerg RR, Sloan F. Effects of tort reforms and other factors on medical malpractice insurance premiums. *Inquiry* 1990;27(2):167–82.
115. Zuckerman S, Koller CR, Bovbjerg RR. Information on malpractice: A review of empirical research on major policy issues. *Law Contemp Probl* 1986;49(2):85–111.
116. Gaba DM. The future vision of simulation in health care. *Qual Saf Health Care* 2004;13(Suppl 1):i2–10.

SECTION III

Evidence-based medicine and epidemiology

Section Editors: **Z. Alfirevic and L. Cabero-Roura**

23 Epidemiology in perinatal medicine

L. S. Bakketeig

Definitions

For a long time, it has been recognized that events during pregnancy and childbirth influence the health and development of the newborn. This recognition has led to the establishment of perinatology as a medical specialty that bridges the gap between the obstetrician's concern for the pregnant woman and the pediatrician's care of the newborn.

Population-based studies of these phenomena are labeled 'perinatal epidemiology', which has evolved into a major subspecialty of epidemiology, representing an important contribution to perinatal medicine. Traditionally, perinatal epidemiologists have focused on exposures and outcomes occurring in the perinatal period, which most commonly covers the time from conception through to birth and the first part of life (1 week, 1 month or the first year of life). In recent years, though, it has been realized that events or exposures that take place *in utero*, or shortly after birth, can also affect development and health even into adult life. We also have come to realize that even events occurring long before pregnancy, sometimes intergenerationally, can affect our reproduction.

An Austrian pediatrician suggested nearly 75 years ago that stillbirths and deaths during the first week of life should be treated as one statistical entity in the analysis of causes of death.[1] The term 'perinatal mortality' was increasingly used from the 1940s onward.[2–4] The increasing attention being paid to perinatal mortality was caused by the observation that the fall in infant mortality (death during the first year of life) in the first half of the 20th century derived mainly from the reduction in mortality of infants surviving beyond the first week of life.[5] It appeared that the progress made was mostly a result of the success in combating deaths due to infectious diseases in early infancy. Mortality among infants shortly after birth, as well as fetal mortality, had decreased far less.[5]

Perinatal mortality is the most commonly used death rate as an indicator of perinatal health. The other death rates used in perinatal epidemiology are stillbirth, neonatal, postneonatal and infant death rates, as illustrated in Figure 23.1. The death rates are defined as the number of deaths per 1000 births, or per 1000 live births for the last three rates.

Perinatal surveillance

Perinatal surveillance can be based on the perinatal and infant death rates, but also on other health indicators such as the frequency of different congenital anomalies or the frequency of preterm births or low-birth-weight (LBW) births. Some countries, for example, the Scandinavian countries, have established medical birth registries where all births in the country are monitored. Thus, the occurrence of different adverse outcomes can be monitored and changes in frequencies can be detected and further investigated. The thalidomide disaster in the early 1960s was the main reason why such a medical registration system was established in Norway in 1967. This was the first national population-based registration of births ever established.[6] Later, similar registration systems were established in Denmark, Sweden and Finland.

The medical registration of births contains information on the parents (a few items on civic and medical information), the course of pregnancy and delivery and, finally, some information about the newborn baby. Therefore, the medical birth registration information can be used for perinatal audit purposes beyond the surveillance of congenital anomalies. Perinatal audit represents a current assessment of the quality of perinatal care, based on the structure of care, the process of care and the outcome of care. The information collected through the medical birth registration represents a valuable basis for assessing at least the process and the outcome of care, while data on the structure of care will have to be collected separately.

The medical birth registration forms the basis of the Medical Birth Registries in the Nordic countries. The child and its parents are identified by unique identification numbers. This facilitates the linkage of the information with other data sources, like the death registry, the census data and the education registry. Also,

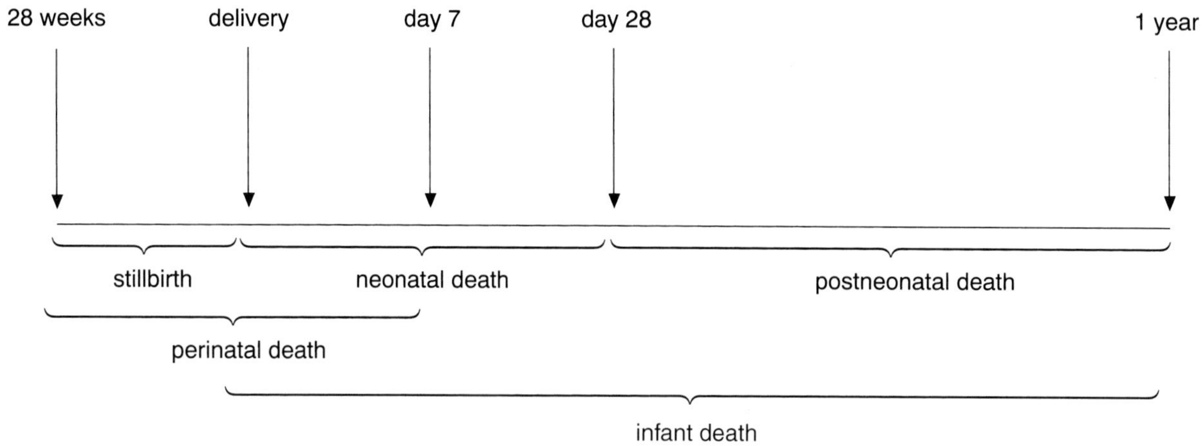

Figure 23.1 Time of death surrounding birth and during the first year of life.

the identification number makes it possible to link the medical birth registries with other morbidity registries, such as the cancer registries, which represent high-quality data sources in the Nordic countries.

Risk factors

Perinatal epidemiology focuses on different risk factors associated with pregnancy and childbirth. Births with an adverse outcome are compared with controls and whether one group has more often been exposed to the risk factor under study than the controls (case–control study). An outstanding example of such a study is the discovery of the strong association between the use of diethylstilbestrol in pregnancy to prevent miscarriages and the risk of cancer vaginalis in the female offspring of these women when they reach their early reproductive years.[7]

The other approach in studying associations between exposures and adverse outcomes is the use of cohort studies, where two groups of women are selected, one exposed and the other not exposed to the suspected risk factor, and then comparing the outcomes in the groups. In Table 23.1, an example is shown of such a cohort study, which focuses on the risk of small-for-gestational-age (SGA) births in groups of women with established risk factors at the start of their pregnancies, and evaluates the additional risk associated with cigarette smoking. The data shown in the table are based on a longitudinal study of fetal growth.[8] For women with no known risk factors at the beginning of the pregnancy, 6.5% will have an SGA birth. If the women smoke cigarettes, the risk increases to 11.8% [relative risk (RR) = 1.8]. If the women have had a previous LBW birth (birth weight below 2500 g), then the risk of an SGA birth is more than doubled (RR = 2.4), and if they smoke cigarettes, there is a further doubling of the risk (RR = 5.4).

Case–control and cohort studies are both observational studies. Furthermore, within perinatal epidemiology as well as other areas of epidemiology, observational studies are the dominant tools in addition to more descriptive and even hypotheses-generating studies. The more powerful experimental approaches are obviously less suitable. However, in evaluating perinatal care, one can use randomized controlled trials, applying either individual or cluster randomization. This approach can also be applied in the evaluation of preventive programs. Here, the cluster randomization approach ought to be used more often. For example, in evaluating a new program for antenatal care, instead of randomizing individuals, one could randomize areas, counties, municipalities or clinics to alternative programs and then compare the results.[9]

Recurrence risks

The feasibility of linking parents and child in the medical birth registries makes it possible to study the recurrence of pregnancy and childbirth events within sibships. This has been done extensively, based on the Norwegian Medical Birth Registry data over the last 25 years, starting with a paper in 1977, which demonstrated the strong tendency to repeat preterm, LBW and SGA births in successive pregnancies in the same woman.[10]

As it turned out, as shown in Table 23.2, LBW was the best predictor of subsequent LBW birth, preterm birth was the best predictor of later preterm birth and SGA birth was the best predictor of subsequent SGA births. These and later analyses have indicated that women are 'programmed' to have births of a similar size in subsequent pregnancies.

The first babies included in the Norwegian Medical Birth Registry from 1967 onward have now long since started to reproduce themselves, which facilitates the study of intergenerational effects. As it turns out, birth weight correlates across generations, but gestational

Table 23.1 The frequency of SGA births in cohorts of women with different risk factors, including cigarette smoking, at start of pregnancy (derived from Bakketeig et al.[8])

Risk factor		SGA births			
	Women (*n*)	*N*	Percentage	Relative risk	95% Confidence interval
None*					
Non-smoker	3190	208	6.5	1.0	
Smoker	1515	179	11.8	1.8	(1.5, 2.2)
Previous LBW birth					
Non-smoker	286	44	15.4	2.4	(1.7, 3.3)
Smoker	238	84	35.3	5.4	(4.2, 7.0)
Low prepregnancy weight (< 50 kg)					
Non-smoker	164	20	12.2	1.9	(1.2, 3.0)
Smoker	175	45	25.7	3.9	(2.9, 5.4)

*Defined as the absence of the following risk factors: previous LBW birth, low prepregnancy weight, previous perinatal death or chronic maternal diseases (essential hypertension, heart disease or renal disease)

Table 23.2 Prediction of LBW, preterm and SGA second births based on birth weight and gestational age of first birth (76,398 mothers with first two births in 1967–73) (from Bakketeig[10])

First birth	Risk of second birth					
	LBW		Preterm		SGA	
	%	Relative risk	%	Relative risk	%	Relative risk
LBW	15.2	5.6	15.4	3.7	20.5	4.1
Preterm	11.8	4.1	16.4	4.0	11.5	1.5
SGA	7.7	2.8	6.6	1.4	22.1	3.9

Table 23.3 Recurrence risks across generations

	Relative risk
Preterm birth (< 37 weeks)	1.18
LBW birth (< 2500 g)	2.25
SGA birth (sex and parity specific)	2.57

age correlates to a lesser extent.[11] A recent analysis is based on 105,104 mother/child pairs recruited from females in the Norwegian Medical Birth Registry born since 1967 and reproducing through 1995. Based on 101,579 single mother/child units, the recurrence risks across generations are shown in Table 23.3. The recurrence risk or LBW is of the same magnitude as the recurrence within sibships.[10] However, for gestational age, the recurrence risk across generations is much weaker compared to the recurrence within sibships. This could indicate that genetic factors affect fetal growth more than the duration of pregnancy and that gestational age might be more affected by environmental factors. Further studies of paternal effects and the association among paternal and maternal half-siblings might help to clarify these relationships.

Future perspectives of perinatal epidcmiology

The idea that health in adult life may reflect circumstances in childhood, or even earlier in life, dates back many years.[12] The notion that at least some adult diseases may originate *in utero* has recently captured attention across a wide range of biomedical sciences. Editorial comments have ranged from being enthusiastic, claiming a 'paradigm shift',[13] to being more critical and skeptical.[14]

Barker has introduced a series of hypotheses of relationships between perinatal events and later health.[15] For example, Barker *et al.* have examined the association between blood pressure and measures of size and shape at birth, indicating that the ratio of birth weight to placental weight is an important predictor of subsequent blood pressure, where men who were light at birth, but with a relatively heavy placenta, had the highest blood pressure.[16]

Most of these associations will require more sophisticated studies before the issues can be resolved. In the Nordic countries we have some advantages in approaching some of these challenges, particularly since we have relatively homogenous populations where the individuals can be traced over time due to our identification number system, which thus facilitates longitudinal studies with follow-up over a long time.[17]

Epidemiology certainly has an extremely important role to play in perinatal medicine, and genetic epidemiology and molecular epidemiology are likely to introduce new and more effective analytical methods, which will provide the basis for improved prevention of adverse outcomes of perinatal events, regardless of when these outcomes occur.

Acknowledgment

I wish to thank Liv Knurvik for skillful technical assistance in preparing this manuscript.

REFERENCES

1. Peller S. Proper delineation of the neonatal period in perinatal mortality. *Am J Public Health* 1965;55:1005–11.
2. Wallgren A. The neonatal mortality in Sweden, from a pediatric point. *Acta Paediatr Scand* 1942;29:372–86.
3. Baird D, Thomson AM, Duncan EHL. The causes and prevention of stillbirths and first week deaths. *J Obstet Gynaecol Br Emp* 1953;60:17–30.
4. World Health Organization. *Epidemiological and Vital Statistics*. Report 57. Geneva: WHO, 1957:506–11.
5. Taylor W. The changing pattern of mortality in England and Wales. I. Infant mortality. *Br J Prev Soc Med* 1954;8:1–9.
6. Bjerkedal T, Bakketeig LS. Surveillance of congenital malformations and other conditions of the newborn. *Int J Epidemiol* 1975;4:31–6.
7. Schlesselman JI. *Case–Control Studies*. New York: Oxford University Press, 1982.
8. Bakketeig LS, Jacobsen G, Hoffman HJ, *et al*. Pre-pregnancy risk factors of small-for-gestational age births among parous women in Scandinavia. *Acta Obstet Gynaecol Scand* 1993;72:273–9.
9. Bakketeig LS. Methodological problems and possible endpoints in the evaluation of antenatal care. *Int J Technol Assess Health Care* 1992;8(Suppl 1):33–9.
10. Bakketeig LS. The risk of repeated preterm or low birth weight delivery. In Reed DM, Stantey FJ, eds. *The Epidemiology of Prematurity*. Munich: Urban and Schwarzenberg, 1977.
11. Magnus P, Bakketeig LS, Skjærven R. Correlations of birth weight and gestational age across generations. *Ann Hum Biol* 1993; 20:231–8.
12. Kuh D, Davey Smith G. When is mortality risk determined? Historical insights into a current debate. *Soc Hist Med* 1993; 6:101–23.
13. Robinson RJ. Is the child father of the man? (editorial) *Br Med J* 1992;304:789–90.
14. Paneth N, Susser M. Early origin of coronary heart disease ("the Barker hypothesis") (editorial). *Br Med J* 1995;310:411–2.
15. Barker DJP, ed. Fetal and infant origins of adult disease. *Br Med J* 1992.
16. Barker DJP, Bull AR, Osmond C, *et al*. Fetal and placental size and risk of hypertension in adult life. *Br Med J* 1990;301:259–62.
17. Bakketeig LS. Perinatal epidemiology – a Nordic challenge. *Scand J Soc Med* 1991;19:145–7.

24 Structure of perinatal care systems

G. A. Little

Pregnancy outcomes are clearly dependent on the availability and effective delivery of reproductive care. Advances in knowledge and technology have resulted in improvement in national perinatal statistics such as survival of low-birth-weight infants, but the degree of improvement is dependent on the care environment. Structure, the systematic organization of perinatal care, is a primary determinant of the degree of success in meeting the needs of a population.

Constant improvement of pregnancy outcomes is a logical objective. The optimal state of health involves functioning at full individual potential, without disease or abnormality. The ultimate positive expression of reproductive health would be pregnancies without adverse medical outcomes occurring as intended events within a healthy emotional and social environment. A zero adverse outcome rate may not seem attainable at this time, but there is no reason to believe that there is an irreducible minimum of poor outcome that cannot eventually be overcome.

This chapter discusses the organization of perinatal care in the effort to improve outcomes of pregnancy. While each geopolitical entity – population, region or country – must be analyzed and subjected to individualized planning and intervention, there are common concepts that apply.

The problem

Throughout the world, disease associated with reproduction represents a dominant part of medical need and is a major contributor to mortality and long-term morbidity. Even if that part of reproductive system pathology not necessarily associated with pregnancy, such as infertility and sexually transmitted diseases, is removed, the human and economic costs of pregnancy-related disease remain very high in both developed and less fortunate countries.

The disparity between developed and developing regions is especially dramatic in the area of reproductive health. Thirty-nine of the 50 million yearly deaths worldwide (approximately four-fifths) occur in the developing countries, where maternal, perinatal, and communicable causes are said to be responsible for 40% of deaths as compared to 5% in developed countries. Pregnancy-related conditions are estimated to be responsible for 18% of the burden of disease in women between 15 and 44 years of age, and in children under 5 years of age about 19% of loss of healthy life is said to be due to perinatal complications.[1] Of five essential groups of clinical interventions for developing countries identified in a world development report – prenatal and delivery care, family planning services, management of the sick child, treatment of tuberculosis, and case management of sexually transmitted diseases – three involve perinatal and reproductive health.[2,3]

Within developed countries there have been remarkable advances in outcomes in recent decades, but there are persistent differences between countries. Furthermore, expenditure of greater resources per capita and availability of proportionately more providers does not necessarily result in better outcomes. The United States, despite greater application of resources to neonatal intensive care, does not appear to have better birth-weight-specific mortality than some other countries.[4]

Indicators

Perinatal systems of care have traditionally used vital statistics indicators to quantify relative magnitude of outcomes. The following are illustrative of indicators that are based on events that are relatively easy to define and record, such as death, birth weight, and gestational age.

Maternal mortality, usually defined as death of a woman during or within 42 days of pregnancy of any cause other than accidental or incidental, remains a problem in the industrialized world, where deaths approximate 10–20 per 100,000 live births. This indicator is said to document the widest disparity of human reproductive outcomes yet reported, with some sections of the world, notably sub-Saharan Africa and South Asia, apparently experiencing an incidence as much as 200 times higher than the safest areas.[5]

Fetal mortality, neonatal mortality, and infant mortality serve as valuable indicators by themselves or when included in various rates and ratios. Perinatal mortality, including all newborns, live and stillborn, of 1000-g weight and greater and up to 168 h or 7 days of age (early neonatal), is used frequently. Neonatal mortality (deaths up to 28 days) is part of infant mortality (deaths in the first year), and the two, independently or when analyzed together, give valuable insights into the health of a population and availability of care. For example, it has become evident that improvement in infant mortality in some countries such as Egypt has exceeded the rate of improvement in neonatal mortality, suggesting that advances in perinatal care of the fetus and neonate may lag behind advances in care of conditions of infancy, as programs such as oral rehydration for diarrheal diseases make an impact.[6]

Low-birth-weight rate and *birth-weight-specific mortality* provide information about the general health of a population and the relative success of intervention, especially for the population of prematurely born babies (< 37 weeks' gestation). Within the United States, for example, the low-birth-weight rate varies by a factor of 3 or 4 for various subpopulations and has not responded favorably to interventions, while birth-weight-specific mortality has improved considerably, probably due to neonatal intensive care and regional programs. The result is a situation where individual low-birth-weight babies do relatively well and birth-weight-specific mortality is perhaps the best in the world, but the number of low-birth-weight babies per thousand births remains higher than in many other countries.

Figure 24.1 serves to illustrate the breadth of possible perinatal outcome indicators. Identified values can be used to derive indicators. Traditional outcomes based on vital statistics address a small portion of the value and outcome spectrum. The clinical value compass model can be applied to all aspects of a care delivery process including the parent perspective of the neonatal intensive care experience.[7] Perinatal care systems in all stages of development will rely on vital statistics based indicators. Those in complex environments that are market driven with a strong interest in consumer- or family-centered care may also employ a variety of indicators.

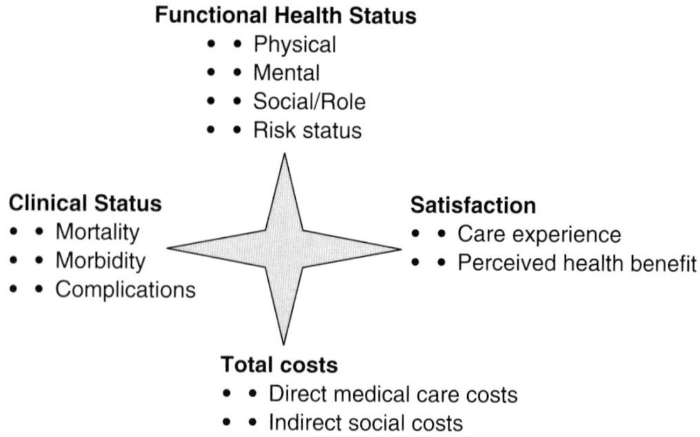

Figure 24.1 The clinical value compass model has been used to derive the four parental neonatal intensive care outcome groupings. A wide range of outcome indicators can be developed for each of these groupings. Derived from Conner and Nelson[7].

Risk assessment, need identification, and resource allocation

Risk assessment is a key concept in perinatal care systems. The process of evaluating the possibility that a patient has or will have a specific problem is an integral part of all medical practice including perinatal medicine. *Needs* are identified and quantified for both individual patients and populations. *Resources* can then be allocated to meet identified or anticipated needs.

Risk assessment has furthered care and improved outcomes through identification of populations and individuals at increased risk for specific conditions. It also can result in false positives and negatives. Furthermore, there is legitimate concern that the concept of risk has meant to some that pregnancy is never normal except retrospectively. These shortcomings must be managed.

A method entitled the *risk approach* has been developed to improve availability and use of existing health-care resources and systems, especially in resource-poor areas. Health problems, including their associated risk factors and populations, are identified, the status of function of the existing health-delivery system is assessed, interventions to deal with risk and performance are put in place, and these are followed by monitoring and evaluation.[8] This process has been applied to construct programmatic approaches to population-based maternal and child health care. Shortcomings have been discussed, including the inability in some situations to recognize or evaluate all forms of risk, inadequate preparation or training of personnel, lack of complete understanding of the determinants of risk including cultural factors, and inability to achieve a balance between preventive and curative services.[9,10]

Patient care and the need for structure

The individual perinatal patient has benefited greatly from advances in care. For example, if access to preventive and acute care is available and timely, all of the five main causes of maternal mortality – hemorrhage, unsafe abortions, hypertensive disorders, sepsis, and obstructed labor – can be managed successfully. Most of the common causes of fetal and neonatal mortality and morbidity, such as peripartum asphyxia, prematurity, and infections, respond to assessment of fetal well-being, obstetric intervention, neonatal resuscitation, and intensive care. Although there are many diagnostic and therapeutic challenges that remain, such as prevention of permaturity, the simple fact is that most of the world's perinatal pathology can be detected and

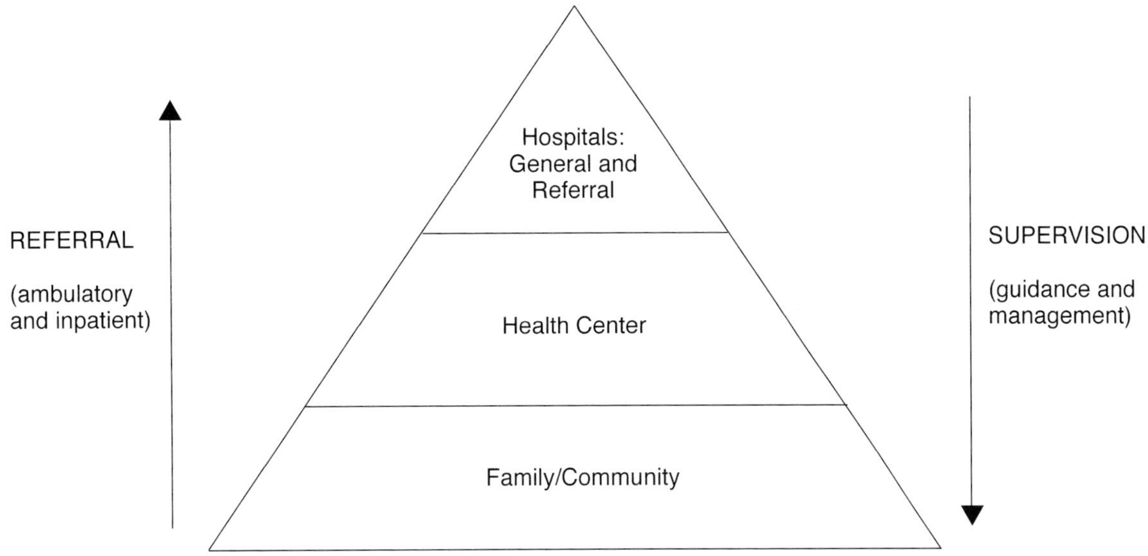

Figure 24.2 The World Health Organization health-care pyramid. Modified from World Health Organization[3].

treated successfully with available knowledge and structured care.

Because it is not possible to meet all needs in all places, a structured system that allows for efficient use of resources and maximizes outcomes is a logical objective.

The health-care pyramid

The World Health Organization (WHO) has presented an ideal health-care pyramid with three levels: family/community, health center, and district hospital.[3] With slight modification (see Figure 24.2), this model can serve as a conceptual framework for the structure of perinatal health care in countries and societies at all stages of development. The basic importance of the family/community sector is emphasized; it is here that the need for clinical intervention arises and moves to health center and hospital when necessary (see referral arrow, Figure 24.2). The arrow on the right pointing down suggests a family/community objective for supervision in the WHO model; the guidance and management terms were added to this illustration to suggest proactive clinical and educational interventions that originate in health-care institutions.

A problem associated with improving pregnancy outcomes is the need for both comprehensive preventive and acute care for an entire population. One without the other will not be successful. As the health-care pyramid suggests, an effective and efficient framework or structure of component activities is necessary.

Perinatal systems

Systems consist of components functioning together for common goals and objectives. Understanding of the complexity and breadth of activities associated with perinatal care is essential if systems are to be effective.

Perinatal system activities

Table 24.1 provides an overview of the basic activities associated with systematic efforts to improve pregnancy outcomes of a population. Patient care is essential and must be facilitated by administration and management. If standards of care and outcomes are to be maintained and improved, ongoing data collection, evaluation, and research must take place to provide the substrate for quality improvement. Training and education of personnel must be available either from within the system itself or from a cooperating resource.

System development

Much of the effort of system development in technically-advanced nations has focused on hospital inpatient services. The hospital is usually the community institution where knowledge and technology are concentrated, with individual members of the community coming to that location. In developing and less fortunate environments, a single regional institution such as a district hospital receives designated governmental support, while in more affluent areas there may be multiple hospital alternatives that, in fact, may compete.

Perinatal systems and their patients originate from communities and families. The focus on hospitals as an identified community resource and site of many if not most births leads to a challenge for systems to adaquately address needs in the ambulatory and education sectors. Preconception and prenatal care tends to be less well addressed in many systems as inpatient services.

Table 24.1 Perinatal system activities

Patient care	Date acquisition, evaluation, and research	Administration	Education
Primary (basic)	Vital statistics	Clinical services	Public
Pregnancy planning	Pregnancy outcomes	System development and maintenance	Patient
Preconception	Maternal	Institutions	Prevention
Prenatal	Neonatal/infant	Clinics	Preparation
Peripartum	Technology assessment	Hospitals	Training
Postpartum	Professional/provider	Quality assessment and improvement	Continuing
Maternal	Medical and social science	Fiscal	System (outreach)
Infant			
Specialty (consultative, referral)			
Genetics			
High-risk obstetrics			
(Maternal–fetal)			
Neonatal (medical and surgical)			
Psychological and social			
Ancillary services			
Radiology/imaging			
Anesthesia			
Laboratory			
Transportation			
(Interhospital care)			
Maternal–fetal			
Neonatal			

In an ideal situation, need assessment followed by resource allocation to guide initial development of a basic perinatal system for a defined population is a relatively uncomplicated exercise. As previously discussed, vital statistics and perinatal indicators can help to quantify the magnitude of the need and support solutions that direct resources toward systems and comprehensive program activities. The reality of perinatal systems development is complex, with each situation involving different medical, economic, social, and political determinants.

Perinatal regionalization in the United States: evolution of a systems approach

During the 1960s and early 1970s, significant advances in perinatal care, especially in hospital-based services, were occurring in the United States, Canada, and many countries in Europe and elsewhere. Neonatal intensive care in particular was emerging, as was the concept of interhospital transfer, including care instituted prior to and during movement to established centers. Perinatal providers and their organizations, including the American Academy of Pediatrics (AAP) and the American College of Obstetricians and Gynecologists (ACOG), became convinced that a systems or programmatic approach to perinatal care could improve outcomes. With the assistance of a private foundation, The National Foundation – March of Dimes, the AAP, and the ACOG, joined by the American Medical Association and the American Academy of Family Physicians, formed an *ad hoc* Committee on Perinatal Health.

Toward Improving the Outcome of Pregnancy: Recommendations for the Regional Development of Maternal and Perinatal Health Services was formally released in 1976.[11] The first sentence states that to make optimal care available for each person, 'a systems approach is essential'.

The publication, now known as TIOP I, while directed broadly at maternal and perinatal services, focused heavily on the third trimester and neonatal period and on the hospital or inpatient sectors primarily. Central to the recommendations and subsequent influence of TIOP I was a three-level categorization of perinatal services. The level framework was promoted to introduce cooperative interaction and organization into a system having as its only objective the improvement of pregnancy outcome (see Figure 24.3).[11,12]

By the mid-1980s, perinatal regionalization, including the level concept of organization, had been

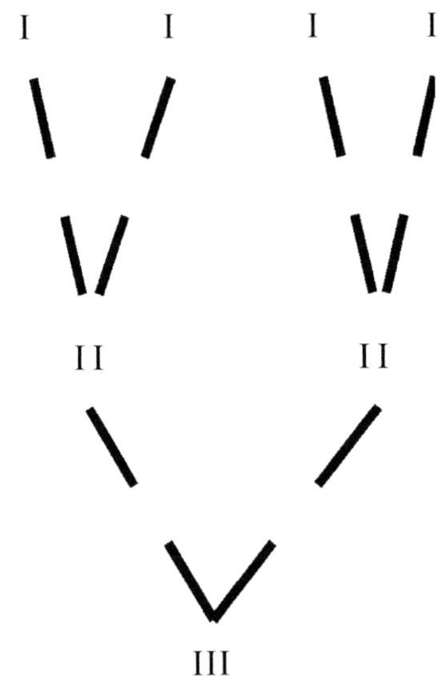

ACTIVITY	LOCATION
Usual level of patient entry Risk assessment Uncomplicated care Stabilization of unexpected problems Data collection Sponsor of local education	Community or district clinics and hospitals
Level I activities plus: diagnosis and treatment of selected high-risk pregnancies and neonatal problems education for part of network	Large community hospitals with many support services
Level I and II activities plus: diagnosis and treatment of most perinatal problems regional transport research and outcome surveillance regional education regional administration	Large medical centers with comprehensive, often academic, programs

Figure 24.3 Levels of hospital perinatal services originally recommended in the United States in 1976. Derived from Frigoletto and Little[12].

implemented throughout the United States, with most authorities agreeing that it had been responsible for improvement in outcomes.[13] The degree of governmental involvement in the form of leadership and regulation varied widely across the 50 states. The three-level categorization was broadly accepted, although some argued for a four-level system with a few perinatal centers, usually academic, to provide the most technologically demanding care as another level. Others argued for a two-level system involving primary, routine, or specialty care and a referral level for subspecialty care. Some felt that the level system inappropriately centralized care, although the TIOP documents clearly state that that is not intended.

Recently, the AAP released, after considerable collection of practice data and debate, a new categorization of levels of newborn care that maintained a basic three-level framework with subcategorization based on functional capabilities.[14] The rationale utilized, while applied to neonatal care, is seemingly also applicable to obstetric units. As perinatal services in hospitals and within systems are interrelated, assigning the level of perinatal service is an important aspect of structure.

By the late 1980s, a great deal of concern was being expressed by US professionals and health planners that so-called 'deregionalization' was occurring and that outcomes might be worsening or at best the rate of improvement was inadequate. Some argued that the levels categorization had outlived its usefulness. It is important to place this concern into a context of a nationwide deliberation about the entire system of care and health-care reform. A movement to review and revise TIOP I emerged.

TIOP II, *Toward Improving the Outcome of Pregnancy, The 90s and Beyond* was released in 1993 by a reconstituted and expanded Committee on Perinatal Health.[15] In it are included a review of past development of US prenatal services, consideration of indicators of outcome, and recommendations for improvement that are broad and strongly state that successful interventions such as intensive obstetrical and neonatal hospital-based interventions must be maintained, while a newly energized focus on ambulatory care, especially in the preconception, prenatal, and postpartum intervals, should be instituted. The levels categorization is supported but with a recommendation that review and revision on a local or state basis should be undertaken as part of an emphasis on the need for regional systems to be community focused. Also stressed are health awareness and promotion, universal access to care, and a recognition that social and fiscal, as well as medical, factors must be addressed. TIOP II is also not a *laissez-faire* document; it recommends that community resources as well as professionals should play a role in a system that includes a forum, usually government led, for addressing accountability, access, and progress.[16]

Thus, in the United States, the need for structure in the delivery of perinatal care, which includes risk identification, patient referral and possible transport to a site of available service, and categorization of levels of care has been debated and largely accepted. Agreement on the specifics of system implementation and management is not as universal. In some states, structure has evolved informally, while in others, considerable structure has been mandated. The care-related activities presented in Table 24.1 are largely in place, while some, such as continuous quality improvement involving an entire geopolitical unit such as a state, are not. The current movement toward managed care and competition on the one hand supports the development of systems of care that are internally structured and largely self-contained, while on the other hand urging the freedom to compete and limited external structure and review. In many areas, there are regionalized perinatal networks that function in parallel, with limited interaction including assessment.

In this millineum the US perinatal system continues to evolve while there is ongoing questioning of resource allocation. The dominence of hospital-based services including obstetric high-risk and neonatal intensive care is being debated from the perspective of whether it improves outcomes.[17] Availability of neonatal intensive care capacity is thought to be responsible for a significant portion of improvement in outcomes such as low-birth-weight survival, with obstetric care contributing a smaller but definite portion.[18] There is research that supports a concern that neonatal intensive care capacity may be excessive and not able to contribute further to improved pregancy outcomes.[19]

A cross-national study of reproductive care involving the United States, Australia, Canada, and the United Kingdom determined that the United States has more neonatal intensive care capacity with 6.1 neonatologists per 10,000 live births compared with 3.7, 3.3, and 2.7 for the other countries, respectively. Neonatal bed capacity was also greater in the United States. Birth-weight-specific mortality outcomes were not the best in the United States where proportionately less resources are allocated to such efforts as preconception, prenatal, and other maternal and child health services.[4] This study questions the effectiveness of the current distribution of reproductive care resources, as did TIOP II,[15] and should serve as a resource for other perinatal systems in development and evolution.

Present and future challenges

Access to clinical care

The implementation and improvement of perinatal systems remains challenging across the spectrum of economic development and political structure. In the less developed situations, certain key system components, such as the first referral level for emergency obstetric care and the ability to perform operative interventions like cesarean sections, are yet to be made universally available. In others, access may be less than optimal due to organizational or economic factors. System structure may have to be modified or individualized to meet prioritized acute care needs. In situations where care is readily available and perhaps even oversubscribed, such as neonatal care, there are challenges related to the relative priority of technologies and services. Dissemination of evidence-based innovations has been pointed out as a challenge in all industries including health care.[20]

Data acquisition and analysis

The ability to use existing computer technology to provide data about events and outcomes in a practical and real-time fashion is now available to perinatal system management. Individual providers, centers or hospitals, and systems can record data economically, and through analysis derive information to effect improvement and change. Efforts such as the Oxford Database for Perinatal Trials, the emergence of measures of acuity,[21,22] and the growing worldwide presence of collaborative networks, such as the Vermont–Oxford Neonatal Network[23] with its international cumulative database of 400- to 1500-g-birth-weight babies from over 400 units, provide opportunity for evidence-based collaborative research.[24] These tools need to be supported, developed further, and used by perinatal systems.

Quality improvement

The concept of continuous quality improvement employed with success in business and in health care is not foreign to perinatal care. In fact, an emphasis on measurement and improvement of outcomes has always been a fundamental part of perinatal care, as evidenced by the Apgar score and neonatal follow-up efforts. Perinatal systems can benefit from advances in quality management being championed in other sectors, including competitive business. Data acquisition and analysis are essential in this effort and the productive linkage of data with quality improvement is a systems function.[25]

Expectations and accountability

Perinatal systems, their institutions, and their personnel are formally and informally considered to be accountable for their actions and outcomes. Accountability is well defined in some areas such as procedures on patients in hospitals and less evident in other concerns such as who is responsible for patients who receive inadaquate prenatal care. Problems such as maternal mortality in developing countries and infant mortality in subpopulations of some advanced countries may become part of a political process that asks for identification of the responsible party and improvement. In such situations the media may become involved by publicizing issues and demanding accountability and change.

Families and communities in this era of patient or consumer involvement in health care have expectations. They can profoundly influence care. For example, perinatal parents have successfully advocated for change leading to the presence of fathers at operative delivery and increased involvement in decision making in the neonatal intensive care unit.[26]

A basic principle of public health is to involve the entire population in analysis and efforts for improvement. Many perinatal systems across the economic and political spectrum of countries study parts of the total population. Accountability or responsibility for less than the total cohort is inadequate. If more than one perinatal network, program, or system exists within a population, then responsibility must rest somewhere, often with the government, for total cohort accountability.

REFERENCES

1. Murray CJL, Lopez AD. *Global Comparative Assessments in the Health Sector: Disease Burden, Health Expenditures and Intervention Packages*. Geneva: World Health Organization, 1994.
2. The World Bank. *World Development Report 1993: Investing in Health*. New York: Oxford University Press, 1993.
3. World Health Organization. *Care of Mother and Baby at the Health Centre: A Practical Guide*. Report of a Technical Working Group, WH0/FHE/MSM/94.2. Geneva: World Health Organization, 1994.
4. Thompson LA, Goodman DC, Little GA. Is More Neonatal Intensive Care Always Better? Insights from a Cross-National Comparison of Reproductive Care. *Pediatrics* 2002;109(6): 1036–43.
5. Tinker A, Koblinsky MA. *Making Motherhood Safe*. Washington, DC: The World Bank, 1992.
6. Little GA, El Kassas M, Eissa AN. The Egyptian National Neonatal Care Program: A practical strategy to improve neonatal outcomes. *Int Child Health* 1996;VII:31–8.
7. Conner JM, Nelson EC. Neonatal intensive care: Satisfaction measured from a parent's perspective. *Pediatrics* 1999; 103(Suppl 1):336–49.
8. World Health Organization. *The Risk Approach in Maternal and Child Health*. WHO Offset Publication No. 39. Geneva: World Health Organization, 1978.
9. McCarthy BJ, Kowal D. The risk approach in maternal and child health. In Wallace HM, Giri K, Serrano CV, eds. *Health Care of Women and Children in Developing Countries*, 2nd edn. Oakland: Third World Publishing, 1995.
10. Backett EM, Davies AM, Petros-Barvazian A. *The Risk Approach in Health Care*. Public Health Papers, No. 76. Geneva: World Health Organization, 1983.
11. Committee on Perinatal Health. *Toward Improving the Outcome of Pregnancy (TIOP #1): Recommendations for the Regional Development of Maternal and Perinatal Health Services*. White Plains, NY: National Foundation-March of Dimes, 1976.
12. Frigoletto FD, Little GA, eds. *Guidelines for Perinatal Care*, 2nd edn. Elk Grove, Washington: American Academy of Pediatrics, American College of Obstetrians and Gynecologists, 1988.
13. Phibbs CS, Bronstein JM, Boxton E, *et al.* The effects of patient volume and level of care at the hospital of birth on neonatal mortality. *J Am Med Assoc* 1996;276:1054–9.
14. American Academy of Pediatrics, Committee on Fetus and Newborn. Policy statement, levels of neonatal care. *Pediatrics* 2004;114(5):1341–7.
15. Committee on Perinatal Health. *Toward Improving the Outcome of Pregnancy, The 90's and Beyond (TIOP #2)*. White Plains, NY: National Foundation – March of Dimes, 1993.
16. Little GA, Merenstein GB. Toward improving the outcome of pregnancy, 1993: Perinatal regionalization revisited (commentary). *Pediatrics* 1993;92(4):611–2.
17. Grumbach K. Specialists, technology, and newborns – Too much of a good thing. *New Engl J Med* 2002;346:1574–5.
18. Richardson DK, Gray JE, Gortmaker SL, *et al.* Declining severity adjusted mortality: Evidence of improving neonatal intensive care. *Pediatrics* 1998;102(4):893–9.
19. Goodman DC, Fisher ES, Little GA, *et al.* The relation between the availability of neonatal intensive care and neonatal mortality. *New Engl J Med* 2002;346:1538–44.
20. Berwick DM. Disseminating innovations in health care. *J Am Med Assoc* 2003;15:1069–975.
21. International Neonatal Network. The CRIB (clinical risk index for babies) score: A tool for assessing initial neonatal risk and comparing information of neonatal intensive care units. *Lancet* 1993; 342:193–8.
22. Richardson DK, Gray JE, McCormick MC, *et al.* Score for neonatal acute physiology: A physiology severity index for neonatal intensive care. *Pediatrics* 1993;91(3):617–23.
23. Horbar JD. The Vermont Oxford Neonatal Network: Integrating research and clinical practice to improve the quality of medical care. *Semin Perinatol* 1995;19:124–31.
24. Lucey JF, Rowan CA, Shiono P, *et al.* Fetal infants: The Fate of 4172 infants with birth weights of 401–500 grams – The Vermont–Oxford Network Experience (1996–2000). *Pediatrics* 2004;113(6):1559–66.
25. Horbar JD, Rogowski JD, Plsek P, *et al.* Collaborative quality improvement in neonatal intensive care. *Pediatrics* 2001;107(1): 14–22.
26. Harrison H. The principles for family-centered neonatal care. *Pediatrics* 1993;92(5):643–50.

25 Perinatal quality indicators and perinatal audit

G. Lindmark and J. Langhoff-Roos

Health-care services should be evaluated not only in quantitative terms, which is still often the case, but also with respect to the quality. The qualitative dimensions of health care are fundamental for its impact on health. Clients, not least in maternal health care, increasingly demand to be considered as individuals and not only as objectives of the health-care activities. Resources are restricted even in the most affluent parts of the world and do not allow unlimited use of health-care interventions. Critical scrutiny and assessment of the quality of health care are therefore mandatory.[1]

In maternal and perinatal health care, the survival of mother and baby without short- or long-term morbidity is the first and fundamental need. However, in childbearing there are other needs related to social, cultural and existential dimensions, which also have to be considered in the care of mothers and infants. One obvious reason to acknowledge these dimensions is their importance for acceptance of and compliance with care.

To maintain and improve quality in health care, it is necessary to clearly define the goals and objectives related to patient's needs, and assess the resources available.[2] For such a process to be possible, good communication and collaboration must be present. It is also essential that health workers at all levels feel themselves as subjects and a part of the process and not as objects of scrutiny or criticism.

To define quality as the extent to which the care is meeting the expectations and needs of the patient is attractive, and implies that also other outcomes than the strict medical ones must be considered. However, the expectations of health care do not come only from the patient but also from society and from the agencies that cover the cost of the care. Therefore, not only individual but also public health outcomes must be considered, and the effective use of available resources will therefore be a quality aspect of great interest. When comparisons of the quality of perinatal care are performed, it is common to relate only to indicators of outcome or process and not mention indicators of structural input. Also, single-process or -outcome indicators – like rates of cesarean section and perinatal mortality – have been used to measure quality without considering the relation with other important aspects of care.

It will be increasingly important to define quality also as cost-effectiveness, in any case if the aim is to offer universal high-quality care to all mothers and newborns.

Indicators of quality

A weighted sum of all essential indicators, including fetal and maternal, short-term and long-term outcomes as well as maternal satisfaction and the impact on future pregnancies and deliveries, would be the ideal measure of quality. This will imply that an unrealistically high amount of resources are spent to collect quantitative as well as qualitative data – at least in the same population. The most important source for quality improvement activities is the routinely collected indicators at the local and regional levels. However, we still need to supplement this with results from other and larger regions. Published descriptive–analytical clinical research will also in the future constitute one of the backbones of regional quality assessment activities.

Decisions on the best indicators must consider not only their relevance for assessment of the objectives of care, but also their feasibility. For an indicator to be useful it must be constructed from data that are possible to collect within the available resources, and both these variables and the indicator itself must be clearly defined. The usefulness of quality indicators for comparisons over time or between regions depends on agreement on these definitions and continuous data collection by all the participating health facilities.

Quality assessment of the *structure* of care includes organization, resources, qualifications of staff and availability of structured and adequate programs of care. The *process* or utilization of resources in the provision of health care can be assessed so that each activity for screening, prevention, diagnosis or therapy is correctly applied and used for the intended or appropriate purpose. Assessment of process quality should ascertain that the care is carried out according to evidence-based guidelines or recommendations.

In perinatal care the *result* of the health-care process in terms of mortality and morbidity traditionally has been discussed most often. Nowadays, patient satisfaction and provision of relevant and reliable information are products of care generally appreciated as important not just in cases with perinatal complications but also in the majority of cases in which everything is normal from a strictly medical perspective.

These quality indicators are useful for constructive discussions about the content and quality of perinatal health care. The variations in outcome are not related to physical resources in a simplified way, but must be discussed in the wider context of attitudes, practices and training of health staff at all levels. Assessment of results of care should not be limited to intermediate variables such as the results of tests or examinations, but should focus on essential patient-related indicators. In perinatal care, it is common that a screening procedure or an intervention during pregnancy is validated by parameters that are indirectly related to the actual health outcome of mother or infant or even to the result of another test or examination. Variables that are indirectly related to health outcome, such as low birth weight and preterm birth and to some extent low Apgar score, may be useful, however, if there is a direct relationship with short- and long-term morbidity.

Data collection

Since quality assessment includes both the general level of care in all cases as well as serious adverse events, variables and indicators must include both information about all mothers and newborns and special information in selected cases of special interest. The data collection system must therefore include both routine registration of basic information and more detailed information on complicated events – usually to be retrieved from the medical record.

Existing routinely collected data, for example, from medical birth registers, should be used whenever possible, in order to limit the resources needed.[3] Studies show that the quality of routine data in maternity services can be adequate for quality control.[4]

In some countries, routine data may be retrieved from clinical information systems in hospitals or primary care, or civil registers of births and deaths. In the Scandinavian countries, national medical birth registers provide important information. In some countries, routine surveys of reproductive health outcomes are performed at regular intervals and data from routine child health care may be used for quality assessment purposes. However, register data and standard data collected without a specific purpose or unrelated to specific quality improvement activities may be of questionable validity. Registers may also be unreliable regarding causes of death, diagnoses of complications or autopsy data. Terms such as hypoxia, placental dysfunction or pre-eclampsia are frequently used without clear and uniform definitions of the variables.

For comparisons – not only of trends over time in one specific region, but also between regions or using the data compiled for international comparisons – it is essential that all variables are defined according to international standards.

Definitions of basic concepts such as perinatal mortality, gestational age and diagnoses describing maternal and infant condition must be uniform. It is particularly important that all extremely preterm deliveries and infants with the lowest birth weight are included, because of their high risk of mortality and morbidity.

The patient record is an important quality instrument if it is standardized and contains specified and well-defined data. It is nowadays often in a computer format and can be used directly to produce data for special purposes. However, there must be specified definitions for registration to make a variable useful for quality assessment. All data that are the result of a subjective interpretation are also less reliable than absolute values of test results.

Specific surveys and interviews, as well as observations of the process of care, are valuable instruments for assessment of quality, but cannot usually be routinely used since they are more resource demanding and also require training and skills of the data collectors. Thus, these methods will be limited to specific, short-period projects.

Validity of data

The most common problem in the initial discussions about choice of indicators is that people underestimate the difficulties of performing continuous data collection in routine care over long periods of time. The validity of the data registration must therefore be given attention before the data registration begins, as well as regularly over time. Also it is important that definitions and indications are not changed too often. A change should not be considered unless a significant improvement is foreseen to follow, considering both the initial rather poor validity of data during the first phase and the loss of longitudinal aspects of data collection.

In order to secure valid registration of indicators it is important that health personnel are provided with regular and immediate feedback based on registered data and that regular proper validation based on internal registry analyses and external studies based on case notes are performed.

Validation of reported indicators depends on whether the data are aggregated, anonymous case based or case based linked to a personal ID. At an aggregated level, validation may be achieved by logic checks for outliers, at a case-based anonymous level by logic checks for relations between indicators (such

Table 25.1 Obstetric clinical indicators developed by the American College of Obstetricians and Gynecologists

Maternal indicators
Maternal mortality
Unplanned readmission within 14 days
Cardiopulmonary arrest
In-hospital initiation of antibiotics 24 h or more after term vaginal delivery
Unplanned removal, injury or repair of organ during operative procedure
In-hospital maternal red blood cell transfusion or hematocrit < 22 vol% or hemoglobin of < 7.0 g or decrease in hematocrit of 11 vol% or hemoglobin of 3.5 g or more
Maternal length-of-stay more than 5 days after vaginal delivery or more than 7 days after cesarean delivery
Eclampsia
Delivery unattended by the 'responsible' physician*
Postpartum return to delivery room or operating room for management
Induction of labor for an indication other than diabetes, premature rupture of membranes, pregnancy-induced hypertension, postterm gestation, IUGR, cardiac disease, isoimmunization, fetal demise or chorioamnionitis
Cesarean delivery required
Primary cesarean delivery for fetal distress.
Primary cesarean delivery for failure to progress
Delivery of an infant with a birth weight < 2500 g or respiratory distress syndrome following induction of labor
Neonatal indicators
Perinatal mortality of a fetus or infant surviving less than 28 days and weighing 500 g or more at delivery
Intrapartum death, in hospital, of a fetus or infant weighing 500 g or more
Neonatal mortality of an inborn infant with a birth weight of 750–999 g in an institution with a neonatal intensive care unit**
Delivery of an infant weighing < 1800 g in an institution without a neonatal intensive care unit**
Transfer of a neonate to a neonatal intensive care unit in another institution
Term infant admitted to a neonatal intensive care unit
Apgar score of 4 or less at 5 min
Birth trauma (#767 in ICD-9 directory), such as shoulder dystocia, cephalohematoma, Erb palsy and clavicular fracture but not caput
Diagnosis of fetal 'massive aspiration syndrome' (#770.1 in ICD-9-CM)
Inborn term infant with clinically apparent seizures recorded before discharge

*To be defined by each institution; **an inborn infant is one born in this hospital rather than transferred from another institution

as compatibility – cesarean section vs. sphincter rupture), whereas at a case-based level where case notes are traceable a proper external validation may be carried out.

Sets of indicators for quality assessment

Many quality assurance projects have used process indicators in health care, often recorded as proportions of cases subject to various interventions. Several national and international agencies and scientific societies have developed lists of essential quality indicators for maternal and perinatal care.[5] An example of a set of clinical quality indicators for monitoring results is the one developed by the American College of Obstetrics and Gynecology (Table 25.1).[2] Other sets reflect a more public-health-oriented perspective. Usually, they are a mix of imput from clinicians (obstetricians or midwives) and public health professionals. Clinicians usually focus more on indicators of specific areas to be improved by clinical interventions (process–outcome indicators), indicators such as cesarean section, sphincter rupture and asphyxia at delivery. Public health professionals focus more on areas that are public health issues (structure–outcome indicators), such as maternal age, marital status, congenital malformations, length of hospital stay for childbirth, etc.

By comparison these sets of indicators are quite heterogenous and show a considerable amount of diversity, reflecting differences in interest, but also characterized by a number of common indicators that were found to be essential, such as maternal, perinatal and infant death.

A recent European collaborative effort, PERISTAT – a part of the European Commission's Health Monitoring Programme – has developed indicators of perinatal health for health professionals, policy makers, researchers and health service users who wish to monitor and evaluate perinatal health. The aim of this project, which included 13 countries, was to facilitate monitoring and comparison by harmonizing indicator definitions and encouraging the collection of comparable data based on the following priorities:

- Assess maternal and infant mortality and morbidity associated with events in the perinatal period.
- Describe the evolution of risk factors for perinatal health outcomes in the population of childbearing women, including demographic, socioeconomic and behavioral characteristics.

Table 25.2 PERISTAT[6] working list of indicators

Category	Core	Recommended	Future development
Neonatal health	Fetal mortality rate Neonatal mortality rate Infant mortality rate Distribution of birth weight Distribution of gestational age	Prevalence of congenital anomalies Distribution of Apgar score at 5 min	Causes of perinatal death Prevalence of cerebral palsy Prevalence of hypoxic-ischemic encephalopathy
Maternal health	Maternal mortality ratio	Maternal mortality by cause of death Severe maternal morbidity Prevalence of trauma to the perineum	Prevalence of fecal incontinence
Population characteristics or risk factors	Multiple birth rate by number of fetuses Distribution of maternal age Distribution of parity	Percentage of women who smoke during pregnancy Distribution of mothers' education	Distribution of mother's country of origin
Heath-care services	Distribution of births by mode of delivery	Percentage of all pregnancies following fertility treatment Distribution of timing of the first prenatal visit Distribution of births by mode of onset of labor Distribution of place of birth Percentage of infants breast-feeding at birth Percentage of very preterm births delivered in units without a neonatal intensive care unit	Indicator of support to women Indicator of maternal satisfaction

- Monitor the use and consequences of medical technology in the care of women and infants during pregnancy, delivery and the postpartum period.

In 2003 a list of recommended indicators (Table 25.2) was published on the Internet together with the figures for the year 2000 from most of the participating countries.[6]

Analysis of indicators

Differences in quality indicators are usually interpreted as mainly related to the care itself, but it is important to consider also differences in the population. Even when comparing area-based populations, differences in maternal characteristics such as parity, multiple pregnancy, preterm birth rate, etc. influence the rates of interventions and outcome. Differences in social and economic conditions may be important for outcomes, but are difficult to assess in a reliable way.

Analyses also depend on the level at which data are reported. Aggregated data merely provide a basis for frequencies and predefined tables, whereas case-based data allow *ad hoc* analyses involving all the variables or indicators recorded. When cases have an ID-number with a link to the newborn's personal ID, longitudinal follow-up of maternal and infant morbidity and mortality and even intergenerational studies are possible.

When data are reported at a case-based level, regional differences may be adjusted by multivariate analyses. This is often used in epidemiological analyses for a scientific purpose. Multivariate analyses have the advantage that adjustment may be made in a model that considers several variables/risk factors and ends up in a single odds ratio with confidence intervals. The disadvantages are that the analysis considers only very simple mathematical relations, that the procedure is not easy to explain and that the analysis often is perceived as something happening in a black box.

Standard populations or risk stratification

Another way to adjust for differences in maternal characteristics is to apply 'standard populations'. One of the first standard populations used in perinatal quality assessment is the 'standard primipara'.[7] The standard primipara is a 20- to 35-year-old parturient without pregnancy complications, admitted in spontaneous labor at term with vertex presentation. This standard primipara is only one of several possible standard populations that adjust for clinically relevant preconditions, and – not least – reflect a risk of interventions and complications that occur in a specific group of mothers. Thus, the results from these analyses are relevant for that specific group of women when informed to choose mode of delivery.

It is possible to construct a structure of mutually exclusive standard populations that constitute the whole population.[8] In this way the variables primi/multiparity, preterm/term, vertex/breech–transverse, singleton/multiple pregnancy and elective delivery (induction of labor/cesarean section) have been used to define standard populations.

National birth statistics stratified by place of birth and standard population may be useful for clients choosing place of birth and midwives and obstetricians as a basis for discussions on quality improvement issues.[9]

To compare regional differences in cesarean section rates in a population with an average rate of 23%, a specific low-risk standard population was defined and used.[10] The low-risk standard population, which constituted 49% of the population, consisted of women of all parities without previous cesarean section, spontaneous labor at term, vertex presentation and without specific pregnancy complications or fetal malformations. The average rate in this standard population was 5.8%. Places of birth were categorized by a higher, lower or average rate of cesarean section in the low-risk group. With this method it could be demonstrated that neonatal morbidity was increased in centers where the cesarean section rates were either higher or lower than average.

Audit of perinatal deaths

Perinatal audit can be performed at different levels: local, regional and national. The levels are of importance when discussing the methodology and outcome of an audit.

Audit at the *local level* is often performed on materials that cannot be compared in a quantitative way because of the small sample sizes. However, it is very useful for improvement in structure and process. Depending on whether the audit is performed by a selected group (leaders) or by all involved in the care (all midwives, all obstetricians, a keen pathologist, all neonatologists), the audit process will be perceived as a superior control or as constructive discussion on how to improve within the team. It is very important that audit meetings of the latter type are supervised in a permissive way to underline the fact that by discussing our mishaps openly we share with each other experience that probably will reduce the risk of repetition. This can also reduce the guilt that many carry subsequent to a more or less preventable adverse outcome.

For practical reasons audit at a *regional level* will not take place very close to the obstetrical or neonatal department where the event took place. Regional audits, however, can work as a forum for discussion of guidelines and attitudes. Also, since the distance between the auditors and the local department where implementation should take place is not very far, often at least one participant in the activity will represent the local department or hospital. Quantitative analyses of common events will sometimes be possible at a regional level, and comparisons between regions are often valuable for initiating quality improvement activities. The results of qualitative activities, such as auditing in different regions, however, may be difficult to compare unless audit procedures are identical and the auditors are well matched. In addition, historical comparisons in the same region imply that criteria are explicit and identical and that auditors do not change their sense of judgment over time.

At the *national level* epidemiological analyses of clinical indicators and well-defined categories can be used for surveillance and provision of subgroups for audit, in order to identify health-care structures or processes that should be changed to improve perinatal health care on a national level.

The premise for a valuable international audit is that indicators and categories are similarly defined. The major advantage of the higher level is the larger sample sizes, which in many cases reach a magnitude suitable for statistical analyses with confidence intervals that allow differences to be detected and addressed.

Classification of perinatal deaths

One of the main objects of perinatal care is to avoid serious adverse outcomes. Most perinatal audit activities have focused on perinatal deaths, which is the most important fetal adverse outcome to be avoided. However, perinatal deaths are heterogenous, and chains of events and causes of death differ widely. Clearly, some deaths are potentially more avoidable than others. A perinatal death classification, which stratifies the perinatal deaths in appropriate groups aiming for quality improvement, including qualitative analyses by audit, and comparison between regions may be helpful as a basic tool. It should rely on simple, routinely recorded variables for allocation into mutually exclusive groups, which should be associated with specific areas for health-care interventions.

In an investigation that analyzed the differences in perinatal mortality rate between Denmark and Sweden, a new perinatal death classification was proposed in order to categorize the perinatal deaths in relevant groups for further qualitative audit. This classification was discussed and evaluated at a Nordic Baltic collaborative workshop with obstetricians, pediatricians and perinatal epidemiologists. The final classification system was named the Nordic–Baltic Perinatal Death Classification[11] (Table 25.3). Perinatal deaths with fetal malformations were placed in a separate category, and subsequently the rest were categorized by time of death (before, during or after delivery), gestational age, Apgar score, plurality and birth weight [considering intrauterine growth retardation (IUGR)] into mutually exclusive groups.

This classification can be applied both to medical records data and, because of the simple structure, to register data.

Table 25.3 The Nordic–Baltic Perinatal Death Classification[11]

I	Fetal malformation
II	Antenatal death. Single growth-restricted fetus ≥28 weeks of gestation
III	Antenatal death. Single fetus ≥28 weeks of gestation
IV	Antenatal death. Before 28 weeks of gestation
V	Antenatal death. Multiple pregnancy
VI	Intrapartum death. After admission. ≥28 weeks of gestation
VII	Intrapartum death. After admission. Before 28 weeks of gestation
VIII	Neonatal death. 28–33 weeks of gestation. Apgar score > 6 after 5 min
IX	Neonatal death. 28–33 weeks of gestation. Apgar score < 7 after 5 min
X	Neonatal death. > 33 weeks of gestation. Apgar score > 6 after 5 min
XI	Neonatal death. > 33 weeks of gestation. Apgar score < 7 after 5 min
XII	Neonatal death. Before 28 weeks of gestation
XIII	Unclassified

Thirteen mutually exclusive groups

Qualitative audit

It is possible to continue the analysis of cases in subgroups in a qualitative way. Applying the Nordic–Baltic perinatal death classification, a panel from Denmark and Sweden found that there were significantly more intrapartum deaths of non-malformed infants in Denmark than in Sweden. By subsequent qualitative audit on case notes blinded by nationality, a panel of Nordic obstetricians concluded that there was more insufficient care and a higher rate of potentially avoidable deaths among the Danish cases. It was proposed that a cardiotocographic recording should be done on admission, and that swifter intervention during delivery should be implemented in Denmark.[12]

Register-based subanalysis

When comparing Lithuania with the Nordic countries, the higher perinatal mortality in Lithuania was mainly explained by a doubled rate of malformed infants, a three-fold increase in intrapartum and two- to five-fold increase in neonatal deaths of non-malformed infants.[13] Since qualitative audit by case notes was not feasible, a register-based subanalysis of the type of malformation was performed. The higher rate of malformed perinatal deaths was explained by a four times higher mortality from neural tube defects.

Perinatal deaths in Europe

In the Euronatal Study, a research project contracted by the European Union for the period 1996–2000, factors related to differences in populations and health care were studied to explain the differences in perinatal death rates. To determine whether suboptimal factors were present in the cases of perinatal deaths, a regional case-based audit was performed in 10 European regions.[14] Using the Nordic–Baltic perinatal death classification, the groups in which care and treatment were most likely to have a significant impact on the outcome were audited: singleton fetal deaths and intrapartum deaths of 28 weeks of gestation or more, and neonatal deaths in children born after 34 weeks of gestation or more.

Suboptimal factors were mostly identified in the antenatal care period, often related to professional care delivery, with failure to detect severe IUGR as the most prominent factor. Maternal smoking was also a significant suboptimal factor among potentially avoidable deaths.

Perinatal quality assessment and audit in low-income countries

In low-income countries, regions are not always clearly defined and referral systems are often not working even if there is a structure proposed. The most common situation is that the regional center with its better resources is overloaded with fairly normal deliveries whereas the complicated cases may not even reach the first level of care. The denominator for any area-based assessment of outcome is therefore very uncertain and also the process-related indicators will reflect only what happens to a minor part of the obstetric population. Still, there is an agreement that especially in settings with limited resources and large health problems, quality assessment of care is even more important than in affluent regions. It is essential that quality assessment activities in low-income countries are focused and their results implemented to improve quality of care.

The baseline registration of data in low-income countries is usually limited to a delivery book in which all mothers who are coming for delivery are noted. This registration is done on admission, and the information about complications and interventions that occur later is usually not complete. Usually, the outcome of the baby is not registered beyond a notation of stillbirth. In uncomplicated cases the neonatal observation time is very short and can be a few hours. If the newborn baby needs special care, it is separated from the mother and the information is not available in her file.

Therefore, routine registration needs to be improved at several levels before it is valid for regional quality assessment activities. Until then local and focused quality improvement activities are needed to motivate staff for relevant routine registrations.

Perinatal audit is such an activity, which is suitable for all levels irrespective of the standard of care and has been found to increase motivation in staff and quality of care. This process, however, needs good leadership and careful introduction to overcome initial suspicion and cultural barriers.

REFERENCES

1. Meeker CI. Quality improvement: then and now. *Clin Obstet Gynecol* 1994;37:115–21.
2. Loegering L, Reiter RC, Gambone JC. Measuring the quality of health care. *Clin Obstet Gynecol* 1994;37:122–36.
3. Hall M. Audit of antenatal care. *Fetal Matern Med Rev* 1993;5:19–27.
4. Cleary R, Beard RW, Coles J, *et al.* The quality of routinely collected maternity data. *Br J Obstet Gynaecol* 1994;101:1042–7.
5. Zeitlin J, Wildman K, Breart G, *et al.* Selecting an indicator set for monitoring and evaluating perinatal health in Europe: Criteria, methods and results from the PERISTAT project. *Eur J Obstet Gynecol Reprod Biol* 2003;111(Suppl 1):S5–14.
6. PERISTAT. Monitoring and evaluating perinatal health in Europe. http://europeristat.aphp.fr.
7. Cleary R, Beard RW, Chapple J, *et al.* The standard primipara as a basis for inter-unit comparisons of maternity care. *Br J Obstet Gynaecol* 1996;103:223–9.
8. Robson MS. Can we reduce the caesarean section rate? *Best Pract Res Clin Obstet Gynaecol* 2001;15:179–94.
9. Danish Medical Birth Statistics. http://www.dsog.dk.
10. Gould JB, Danielsen B, Korst LM, *et al.*, California Perinatal Quality Care Collaborative. Cesarean delivery rates and neonatal morbidity in a low-risk population. *Obstet Gynecol* 2004; 104:11–9.
11. Langhoff-Roos J, Borch-Christensen H, Larsen S, Lindberg B, Wennergren M. Potentially avoidable perinatal deaths in Denmark and Sweden 1991. *Acta Obstet Gynecol Scand* 1996;75:820–5.
12. Westergaard HB, Langhoff-Roos J, Larsen S, Borch-Christensen H, Lindmark G. Intrapartum death of nonmalformed fetuses in Denmark and Sweden in 1991. A perinatal audit. *Acta Obstet Gynecol Scand* 1997;76:959–63.
13. Langhoff-Roos J, Larsen S, Basys V, Lindmark G, Badokynote M. Potentially avoidable perinatal deaths in Denmark, Sweden and Lithuania as classified by the Nordic–Baltic classification. *Br J Obstet Gynaecol* 1998;105:1189–94.
14. Richardus JH, Graafmans WC, Verloove-Vanhorick SP, Mackenbach JP, The EuroNatal Audit Panel, The EuroNatal Working Group. Differences in perinatal mortality and suboptimal care between 10 European regions: Results of an international audit. *Brit J Obstet Gynecol* 2003;110:97–105.

26 Audit in perinatal medicine

J. M. Thomas and S. Paranjothy

Definition

Research is concerned with discovering the right thing to do, audit is concerned with ensuring that the right thing is done.[1] Clinical audit aims to improve patient care and outcome by reviewing the care provided to patients against explicit quality criteria and implementing change to improve the quality of care as a result. The structure, processes and outcomes of care can be selected and systematically evaluated against explicit criteria. Where indicated, changes are implemented at an individual, team or service level and further monitoring is used to confirm improvement in health-care delivery.[2]

Is audit effective at improving the quality of care?

A review of the evidence by the National Institute for Clinical Excellence (NICE) concluded that audit is an effective method for improving the quality of care. The same review also described the audit methods associated with successful audit projects.[2] These findings are drawn upon in this document to give practical advice for undertaking audit.

What can be audited?

Audit may evaluate the structure (organization or provision) of services, the process of care or the outcome of care against an agreed standard.

Measure of structure or service provision

Audit can provide an overview of service provision. For example, research evidence shows that the outcome for patients with ovarian cancer is better if they are operated on by an appropriately trained gynecologist and managed within the framework of a multidisciplinary team.[3–9] An audit of the referral and management of patients with ovarian cancer can provide an overview of service provision in this area. Good-quality health-care services need to be patient centered and acceptable to those who use them. Measuring the views of those who use services enables health care providers to assess the service delivered from the patient's perspective.

Process measure

Process measures are clinical practices that have been evaluated in research and shown to have an influence on outcome. For example, research evidence shows that the use of antenatal steroids has improved perinatal outcome. Evaluation of this process of care would entail measuring the proportion of appropriate women who received antenatal steroids. Process measures may be used to assess the quality of care and have some advantages over outcome measures:

- They provide a more direct measure of the quality of care provided.
- They occur more frequently, so smaller samples are needed.
- The findings are easier to interpret.
- As smaller audits are needed, they cost less to achieve.

Outcome measure

Outcome measure is the physical or behavioral response to an intervention, for example, the health status (dead or alive), cure following surgery for stress incontinence, level of knowledge or satisfaction (e.g. users' views on the care they have received). Outcomes can be desirable, for example, improvement in the patient's condition or quality of life, or undesirable, e.g. adverse effects of a treatment. The assessment of outcomes such as cancer survival rates is fundamental to measuring quality of care but the use of outcomes alone in assessing quality of care has the following limitations. Outcomes are not a direct measure of the care provided; ascribing causal factors to variation in care may be problematic, e.g. social and health inequalities may contribute to variation in mortality rates. Not all patients who experience substandard care will have a poor outcome. Many factors contribute to the eventual outcome (e.g. disease severity, health status and social and health inequalities);

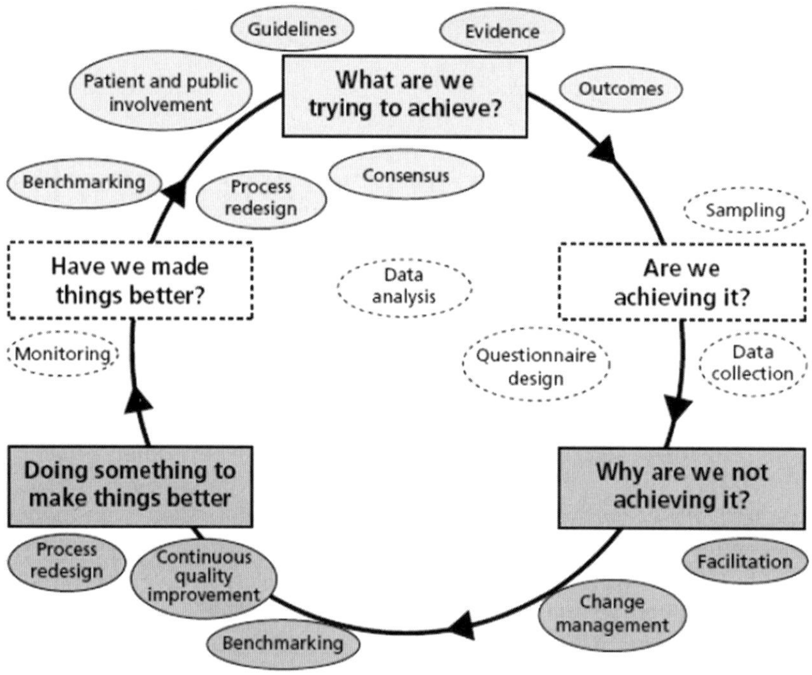

Figure 26.1 The clinical audit cycle.

therefore, mechanisms to account for these differences are required (e.g. case-mix adjustment for comorbidity). Outcomes may be delayed. Research evidence about the impact of some care processes on outcome is limited. Adverse outcomes occur less frequently, so larger samples will be needed.

Despite all the difficulties associated with the interpretation of outcome measures, mortality and morbidity measures are important and this is a major justification for regular monitoring. 'Critical incident' or 'adverse event' reporting involves the identification of patients where an adverse event has occurred, such as the Confidential Enquiries into Maternal Deaths (CEMD), the Confidential Enquiry into Stillbirths and Deaths in Infancy (CESDI) and the National Confidential Enquiry into Perioperative Deaths (NCEPOD). These are examples[6] of outcome reporting. However, only adverse events are reported and usually only adverse events are considered.

The audit cycle

Audit can be considered to have five principal steps, commonly referred to as the audit cycle (Figure 26.1):

1. selection of a topic
2. identification of an appropriate standard
3. data collection to assess performance against the prespecified standard
4. implementation of changes to improve care if necessary
5. data collection for a second, or subsequent, time to determine whether care has improved.

Audit projects require a multidisciplinary approach with the involvement of stakeholders (including consumers or users of the service provided) and the local audit department at the planning stage. Good planning and resources are also necessary to ensure their success.

Selecting a topic for audit

It is essential to establish clear aims and objectives at this stage so that the audit is focused and addresses specific issues within the selected topic. A key consideration is how will the results of this audit be used to change or improve practice.

In selecting a topic for audit, priority should be given to common health concerns, areas associated with high rates of mortality, morbidity or disability and those where good research evidence is available to inform practice or aspects of care that use considerable resources. If successful change is to occur it is important to involve those who will be implementing change at this stage of the audit process.

Identifiying an appropriate audit standard

Review criteria

These are defined as 'systematically developed statements that can be used to assess specific health-care decisions, services and outcomes'. In audit, review criteria are generally used for assessing care; this approach is sometimes referred to as criterion-based audit (Table 26.1). The criterion is the reference point against which current practice is measured.

Table 26.1 Examples of audit and review criteria

Audit topic	Review criteria
Induced abortion	Screening for lower genital tract organisms and treatment of positive cases among women undergoing induced abortion should be carried out to reduce postabortion infective morbidity
Cesarean section	A thromboprophylaxis strategy should be part of the management of women delivered by cesarean section
Hysterectomy	Transcervical resection of the endometrium or endometrial ablation should be available and offered to women with dysfunctional uterine bleeding as an alternative to hysterectomy

High-quality evidence-based guidelines can be used as the starting point for developing criteria. Where this is not possible, criteria should be agreed by a multidisciplinary group including those involved in providing care and those who use the service. Where criteria are based on the views of professionals or other groups, formal consensus methods are preferable. Review criteria should be explicit rather than implicit and need to[2]

- lead to valid judgments about the quality of care, and therefore should be based on research evidence about the importance of those aspects of care,
- relate to aspects of care that are important either to patients or in terms of clinical outcome and
- be measurable.

Standard and target level of performance

This is defined as 'the percentage of events that should comply with the criterion' (e.g. the proportion of women undergoing induced abortion who were screened for lower genital tract organisms, the proportion of women delivered by cesarean section who received thromboprophylaxis, the proportion of women with dysfunctional uterine bleeding who were offered transcervical resection of the endometrium or endometrial ablation). Information about the levels of performance that can be achieved may be helpful when making plans for improvement. Target levels of performance should be examined periodically. The most common approach for setting target levels of performance is informal agreement among the group leading the audit or among health professionals. In some settings, external standards can be useful. However, in many audits no explicit targets are set and the aim is to improve upon current performance.

Target levels of performance have been used most in screening programs. For example, in screening for cervical cancer there are quality criteria to be met, such as the proportion of cervical smears that have endocervical cells.

The term 'standard' has been used to refer to different concepts, sometimes as an alternative word for 'clinical guidelines' and 'review criteria', either with or without a stated target level of performance and, somewhat confusingly, also to refer to the observed or desired level of performance. However, it has been defined as 'the percentage of events that should comply with the criterion' in the interests of clarity.

Benchmarking

This is the 'process of defining a level of care set as a goal to be attained'. There is insufficient evidence to determine whether it is necessary to set target levels of performance in audit. However, in some audits, benchmarking techniques could help participants in audit to avoid setting unnecessarily low or unrealistically high target levels of performance. Reference to the levels achieved in audits undertaken by other professionals is useful. National audits may provide data for benchmarking. For example, the National Sentinel Caesarean Section Audit Report[7] gives regional and national data for comparison on topics such as the use of regional anesthesia in women having cesarean section.

Data collection to assess performance against the prespecified standard

Data collection in criterion-based audit is generally undertaken to determine the proportion of cases where care is in accordance with the criteria. In practice, the following points need to be considered.

What data items to collect

Consideration needs to be given to which data items are needed in order to answer the audit question. For example, if undertaking an audit on cesarean section rates, collecting information on the number of cesarean sections alone will not give sufficient information to measure the cesarean section rate. Data on the number of other births that took place are also required. In general, for audit projects with clear aims, objectives and well-defined review criteria, it is easier to identify those data items that require collection. Definitions need to be clear so that there is no confusion about what is being collected. The definitions will depend on the review criterion that is being assessed. For example, if collecting data on rupture of membranes, it may need to be specified whether this is spontaneous or artificial. Data collectors should always be aware of their legal responsibilities regarding confidentiality and having electronic patient data such as those under the Data Protection Act in the UK and the Caldicott Principles.[8] Under the Data Protection Act 1998, it is an offence to collect personal details of patients such as name, address or other items that are potentially identifiable for the individual without consent. It is rarely necessary or acceptable to use patient identifiers, such as names and addresses, but some form of pseudoanonymized identifiers may be used. Clinical audit may be considered part of direct patient care and therefore consent to the use of data for audit can be implied through consent to treatment, provided that information is given to patients that their data may be used in this way. Audit project protocols should be submitted to the local research and development committee and ethics committees to seek approval if necessary. Guidance on how to do this can be obtained from the respective bodies.

Data collection

Sources of data include:

- Routinely collected data if available (e.g. birth registers); this enables repeated data collections with a minimum of extra effort.
- Clinical records.
- Data collection through direct observation or from questionnaire surveys of staff or patients.

Routinely collected data can be used if all the data items required are available. It will be necessary to check the definitions for data items that are used within the routine database to ensure their usefulness for the aims of the audit. Also, the completeness and coverage of the routine source needs to be known.

Where the data source is clinical records, training of data abstractors and use of a standard *pro forma* can improve the accuracy and reliability of data collection. The use of multiple sources of data may also be helpful. However, this can be problematic, as it will require linking of data from different sources with common unique identifiers.

Questionnaire surveys of staff or patients are often used for data collection. There are several validated questionnaires on a wide range of topics that may be adapted to a specific audit project. There is also literature on developing these (see Appendix).

Developing a questionnaire

There is a large amount of literature on how to develop questionnaires.[10,11] Some of the general principles involved are presented here. Questionnaires are often used as a tool for data collection. Questions may be open or closed. Generally, questionnaire design using open questions, e.g. 'What was the indication for cesarean section?', followed by space for free-text response, is easier. However, analysis of these data is difficult, as there will be a range of responses and interpretation can be problematic. Open questions may be more difficult and time-consuming to answer and can lead to non-response, which results in loss of data.

Questionnaires can be composed entirely of closed questions (i.e. with all possible answers predetermined). More time is needed to develop this type of questionnaire but the analysis is generally easier. An example of this type of questionnaire is given below:

Which of the following statements most accurately describes the urgency of this cesarean section?

A. Immediate threat to the life of the fetus and the mother.
B. Maternal or fetal compromise that is not immediately life threatening.
C. No maternal or fetal compromise but needs early delivery.
D. Delivery timed to suit the woman and staff.

Closed questions assume that all possible answers to the question are known but not the distribution of responses. Time and consideration needs to be given to the options available for response as, if a desired response is not available, the question may just be missed out and it may put people off completing the rest of the questionnaire. For some questions, the 'other' category can be used with the option 'please specify', which gives an opportunity for the respondent to write in a response. However, if this is used, thought must be given *a priori* as to how these free-text responses will be coded and analyzed. In some situations, not having a category of 'other' may lead to the question not being answered at all, which means that data will be lost.

If questionnaires are developed for a specific project, they need to be piloted and refined to ensure their validity and reliability before use as a tool for data collection. While those who developed the questionnaire understand the questions being asked, the aim of piloting is to check that those who have to fill in the questionnaire are able to understand and respond with ease. Questionnaires that are not user friendly are associated with lower response rates, the quality of data collected will be poor and hence results will be of little value.

Data management

Thought needs to be given to who will collect the data, as well as the time and resources that will be involved. In small audit projects it may be feasible for the principal investigators to go through clinical notes for data abstraction. However, for larger projects, e.g. a prospective audit on induction of labor practices within a maternity unit, it may be more appropriate for those involved in the care of the woman giving birth (e.g. midwives or obstetricians) to fill in standard data collection sheets. Where available, audit support staff should be involved.

Data that are collected on paper forms are usually entered onto electronic databases or spreadsheets such as Microsoft Access®, Epi Info® or Microsoft

Excel® for cleaning and analysis. Data entry may be done by optical character recognition (OCR) software, optical mark readers (OMR) or manually. OCR is the most accurate for questionnaire data using tick boxes but less accurate for free-text responses. The method of data entry needs to be taken into account when designing the questionnaire or data collection sheet. For manual data entry, accuracy is improved if double data entry is used. However, this can be a time-consuming exercise. If the facilities and resources are available, electronic collection of data can be considered. In this case, data are entered immediately, at source, into a computer. While this is quick and requires minimal storage space, it can be difficult to handle unexpected responses and as information is entered directly into a computer it cannot be verified or double entered.[9]

Consideration also needs to be given to the coding of responses on the database. For ease of analysis of closed questions it is generally better to have numeric codes for responses. For example, yes/no responses can be coded to take the value 0 for no and 1 for yes. Missing data will also need to be coded, for example, with the number 9. Missing data should be distinguished from those where the response is 'not known' (if this was an option on the questionnaire).

It is advisable to incorporate consistency checks as data are being entered, in order to minimize errors. For example, if there are two questions:

(1) How many previous pregnancies of at least 24 weeks of gestation has this woman had?
(2) How many previous cesarean sections has she had?

A consistency check will highlight entries with responses other than 0 to question (2) if the response to question (1) is 0.

Data analysis

Simple statistics are often all that is required. Statistical methods are used to summarize data for presentation in the form of summary statistics (means, medians or percentages) and graphs.[12]

Statistical tests are used to find out the likelihood that the data obtained have arisen by chance and how likely it is that a real difference exists between two groups. Before data collection has started it is essential to know what data items will be collected, whether comparisons will be made and the statistical methods that will be used to make these comparisons.

Data items that have categorical responses (e.g. yes/no or A/B/C/D) can be expressed as percentages. Some data items are collected as continuous variables, for example, the mother's age, height and weight. These can either be categorized into relevant categories and then expressed as percentages or, if they are normally distributed, the mean and standard deviations can be reported. These summary statistics (percentages and means) are useful for describing the process, outcome or service provision that was measured.

Comparisons of percentages between different groups can be made using a chi-square test; *t* tests can be used to compare means between two groups, assuming that these are normally distributed. Non-parametric statistical methods can be used for data that are not normally distributed. These comparisons are useful in order to determine whether there are any real differences in the observed findings, for example, when comparing audit results obtained at different time points or in different settings. In some situations a sample-size calculation may be necessary to ensure that the audit is large enough to detect a clinically significant difference between groups, if one exists. In this situation, it is important to consult a statistician during the planning stages of the audit project.

These simple statistics can be easily done using Microsoft Excel spreadsheets and Microsoft Access databases. Other useful statistical software packages include Epi Info, SAS, SPSS, STATA and Minitab.

Implementation of changes to improve care if necessary

Data analysis and interpretation will lead to the identification of clinical areas that should be addressed. There are many methods by which this can be done. The feedback of audit findings is most commonly used; for example, presentation at regular audit meetings will stimulate discussions and solutions may be agreed. The NICE review[2] identified several audits in which change in care had occurred. Simple methods were occasionally effective, for example:

- feedback of data collected
- provision of clear data, perhaps using modern information systems, supported by active teamwork
- support from the organization for teamwork
- use of several methods together within the context of an implementation plan.

Change does not always occur in audit and consideration of the reasons for failure may take place after the second data collection. Resistance to change among local professionals or in the organizational environment or team should be considered. Patients themselves may have preferences for care that make change difficult.

The significance of teamwork, culture and resistance to change has led several authors to propose frameworks for planning implementation. These usually include analysis of the barriers to change and use of theories of individual, team or organizational behavior to select strategies to address the barriers. For some topics, such as adverse incidents, systems for continuous data collection may be justified.

Organization of audit

The NICE review[2] found that some methods of organizing audit programs were better than others. The following features are associated with successful audit:

- structured programs with realistic aims and objectives
- leadership and attitude of senior management
- a non-directive, hands-on approach
- support of staff, strategy groups and regular discussions
- emphasis on teamwork and support
- an environment conducive to conducting audit.

Common reasons why audits fail

- *Failure to participate and attitudes to audit*: Involving all stakeholders (including service users) in the project can encourage participation. It is important to recognize the attitudes of those whose behavior is being audited, and to modify the audit process to accommodate these views.
- *Failure to continue and complete the audit cycle*: This makes it impossible to determine whether the audit has led to any improvements in care.
- *Failure to provide a supportive environment for audit*: Perceived lack of support at all stages, together with a range of structural and organizational problems, is associated with poor progress in conducting audit. Research has pointed to a theory–practice gap for clinicians carrying out audit, one solution being to change the organizational culture to one in which clinical audit is supported and actively encouraged.
- *Lack of resources, especially time*: This includes lack of protected time to investigate the audit topic, collect and analyze data, and the time to complete an audit cycle. It follows that audit should be recognized as an important part of clinical practice and those directly involved in audit need to be allocated protected time.
- *Lack of training in audit methodology and evidence-based skills*: Health professionals and audit support staff require adequate knowledge and skills for undertaking audit, and they should be keen to learn. Barriers identified in the literature include a lack of training in evidence-based audit skills and the failure to apply what has already been established.
- *Cost*: It must be recognized that audit requires appropriate funding and that improvements in care resulting from clinical audit can increase costs.

REFERENCES

1. Smith R. Audit and research. *Br Med J* 1992;305:905 (see comments).
2. NHS, National Institute for Clinical Excellence, Commission for Health Improvement, Royal College of Nursing, University of Leicester. *Principles for Best Practice in Clinical Audit.* Oxford: Radcliffe Medical Press, 2002. www.nelh.nhs.uk/BestPractice ClinicalAudit.pdf. Accessed September 11, 2003.
3. Junor EJ, Hole DJ, Gillis CR. Management of ovarian cancer: Referral to a multidisciplinary team matters. *Br J Cancer* 1994;70:363–70.
4. Woodman C, Baghdady A, Collins S, Clyma JA. What changes in the organisation of cancer services will improve the outcome for women with ovarian cancer? *Br J Obstet Gynaecol* 1997;104: 135–9.
5. Department of Health. *The NHS Cancer Plan.* London: Department of Health, 2000.
6. Penney GC. Audit. In O'Brien PMS, Broughton Pipkin F, eds. *Introduction to Research Methodology for Specialists and Trainees.* London: RCOG Press, 1999:95–106.
7. Royal College of Obstetricians and Gynaecologists, Clinical Effectiveness Support Unit. *The National Sentinel Caesarean Section Audit Report.* London: RCOG Press, 2001.
8. Department of Health. *Data Protection Act 1998. Protection and Use of Patient Information.* London: Department of Health, 1998.
9. McKenzie-McHarg K, Ayres S. Data management. In O'Brien PMS, Broughton Pipkin F, eds. *Introduction to Research Methodology for Specialists and Trainees.* London: RCOG Press, 1999:140–6.
10. Gillham B. *Developing a Questionnaire.* London: Continuum, 2000.
11. McColl E, Jacoby A, Thomas L, *et al.* Design and use of questionnaires: A review of best practice applicable to surveys of health service staff and patients. *Health Techn Assess* 2001; 5(31):1–256.
12. Brocklehurst P, Gates S. Statistics. In O'Brien PMS, Broughton Pipkin F, eds. *Introduction to Research Methodology for Specialists and Trainees.* London: RCOG Press, 1999:147–60.

27 Systematic reviews in perinatal medicine

Z. Alfirevic

The principles of evidence-based medicine are not disputed. What constitutes the evidence, however, is hotly debated. Traditionally, medical textbooks and review articles written by experts and opinion leaders have been the main sources of evidence. Recommendation on diagnostic and therapeutic interventions in such material was predominantly based on personal clinical experience and easily accessible literature. Although there has always been some concern about the possible biases inherent in this traditional approach to teaching and information sharing, a more formal criticism gathered momentum in the early 1990s. For example, Antman *et al.* published in *JAMA* a comparison between treatment recommendations for myocardial infarction extracted from review articles and textbook chapters on the one hand and randomized clinical trials on the other.[1] The evidence that thrombolytic therapy saves lives had been available in the early 1970s, when a combined reduction in deaths from 10 clinical trails with around 2500 enrolled patients reached statistical significance. Unfortunately, there were no attempts to analyze the results from the different studies together and further clinical trials continued well into the 1990s with tens of thousands of patients exposed unnecessarily to placebo and many given no treatment at all. Even more worryingly, it took more than 15 years for this evidence to start appearing in medical textbooks and authoritative review articles. In perinatal medicine, the evidence that antenatal corticosteroids can reduce not only neonatal respiratory distress syndrome, but also the risk of neonatal intracranial hemorrhage and perinatal death was available from the early 1970s. Even if early studies could have been seen as hypothesis generating, the reluctance to consider the totality of evidence on this topic in the late 1980s was inexcusable.

Systematic reviews have emerged as one of the most effective ways of bridging the gap between already available evidence and clinical recommendations. The main differences between traditional and systematic reviews are summarized in Table 27.1. The numbers of published systematic reviews have risen quite considerably in the last decade (Figure 27.1) and such reviews are now considered not only an integral part of clinical guidelines, but also a prerequisite for any planned research on diagnostic and therapeutic interventions. The term meta-analysis is often used as a synonym for a systematic review in this context because of the misconception that systematic review must always include a quantitative synthesis of the data to yield a summary statistics (meta-analysis). This is clearly not the case, as systematic reviews may fail to identify studies suitable for statistical pooling.

Table 27.1 The main differences between traditional and systematic reviews

	Narrative reviews	Systematic reviews
Defined clinical questions	Rarely	Common
Reproducible, clearly defined literature search	No	Mandatory
Defined exclusion criteria for potentially eligible studies	Rarely	Common
Prespecified comparisons and outcomes of interest	No	Common
Statistical pooling of the results (meta-analysis)	No	Common
Peer review before publication	Rarely	Common

Cochrane Reviews

Major advances in the scientific rigor and availability of systematic reviews in perinatal medicine have come from the Cochrane Collaboration – an international, not-for-profit organization established in 1993.[2] The aim of the Cochrane Collaboration is to facilitate the preparation, maintenance and dissemination of up-to-date systematic reviews of the effects of health-care interventions. The Cochrane Collaboration Pregnancy and Childbirth Group (CCPC) was the first registered review group within the Cochrane Collaboration and

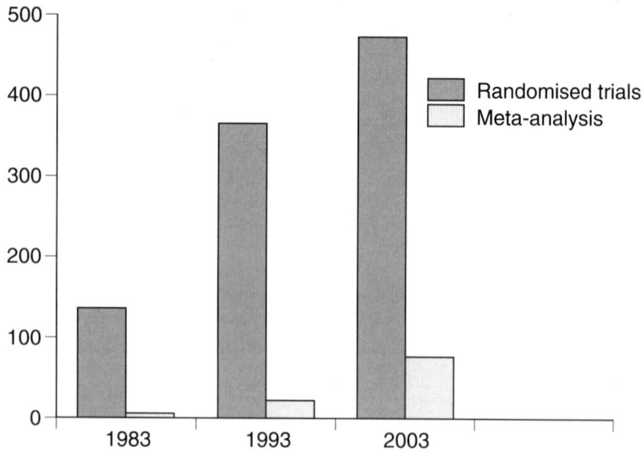

Figure 27.1 Progressive increase in the number of randomized trials and meta-analyses related to pregnancy included in the PubMed *(number of hits for three separate 12-month periods using keywords: pregnan* or labor or labour).*

was subsequently joined by around 50 other topic-based groups, each of them working under the guidance of an international editorial team. The CCPC remains the largest and most productive Cochrane review group with more than 400 registered reviewers from 27 countries.

The distinguishing features of the Cochrane Reviews published quarterly in the electronic publication *The Cochrane Library* are transparent peer-reviewed protocols published in anticipation of each new review, significant input from consumers and consumer advocates throughout the reviewing process[3] and a commitment to keep Cochrane Reviews regularly updated. The main criticism of Cochrane Reviews is a limitation of any evidence based solely on randomized trials.

The criticism that systematic reviews of randomized trials ignore the wealth of knowledge generated by observational studies and basic science is valid. However, the restriction of Cochrane Reviews to randomized trials is primarily pragmatic. The methodology for systematic searches of observational studies is nowhere near as sophisticated as searches restricted to randomized trials. The current register of randomized trials compiled by the Cochrane Pregnancy and Childbirth Group contains more than 10,000 trial reports the majority of which are yet to be included in the Cochrane Reviews. It is anticipated that any similar register of all literature relevant to the evaluation of health interventions related to pregnancy could contain more than a million records.

Other types of systematic reviews

Two other types of systematic reviews have gathered momentum recently as a welcome addition to the already established analyses of aggregate data from randomized trials – systematic reviews of diagnostic and screening tests and individual patient data analysis.

Systematic reviews of diagnostic tests differ from standard reviews in the assessment of study quality and the statistical methods used to combine results (pooled sensitivities, specificities, likelihood ratios and summary receiver operating curves).[4] Most published systematic reviews of diagnostic tests are hindered by the poor quality of the included studies. It is also important to note that the evaluation of diagnostic accuracy of a test is only one aspect of clinical usefulness; the most accurate test can still be clinically useless or, even worse, harmful.

Methods of undertaking a meta-analysis of several studies may involve collecting either aggregate data or data on each patient individually. The advantages of the latter approach, described as the 'yardstick',[5] include a more complete analysis of 'time of event' outcomes and a more powerful analysis of whether treatment is more or less effective in particular subgroups. The drawbacks can include the increased use of time, staff and financial resources and the lack of availability of the original data for some trials.

Summary

Systematic reviews have made an important contribution to perinatal medicine by reinforcing the evidence on effective therapies like antenatal corticosteroids in threatened preterm labor and highlighting ineffective interventions like thyreotropin-releasing hormone in the same clinical scenario. Equally important has been the role of systematic reviews in identifying gaps in our knowledge. The challenge for the future is to provide regularly updated unbiased summaries of observational, randomized and qualitative data in a format that is understandable to both patients and health professionals. We have nothing to fear. The time currently spent on information gathering and the haphazard critical appraisal of incomplete evidence will be much better spent communicating with our patients and helping them to achieve perinatal care and outcomes that truly suit their needs.

REFERENCES

1. Antman EM, Lau J, Kupelnick B, Mosteller F, Chalmers TC. A comparison of results of meta-analyses of randomized control trials and recommendations of clinical experts. Treatments for myocardial infarctions. *J Am Med Assoc* 1992;268:240–8.
2. Sakala C, Gyte G, Henderson S, Neilson JP Horey D. Consumer–professional partnership to improve research: The experience of the Cochrane Collaboration's Pregnancy and Childbirth Group. *Birth* 2001;133–7.
3. Chalmers I. The Cochrane Collaboration: preparing, maintaining and disseminating systematic reviews of the effects of health care. *Ann N Y Acad Sci* 1993;703:156–65.
4. Deeks JJ. Systematic reviews of evaluations of diagnostic and screening tests. *Br Med J* 2001;323:157–62.
5. Stewart LA, Parmar MKB. Meta-analysis of the literature or of individual patient data: Is there a difference? *Lancet* 1993; 341:418–22.

28 Cost benefit in perinatal medicine

Z. Stembera

Greatly increased advances in medicine lead on the one hand to a high quality of care expected and demanded by both health-care professionals and patients, but on the other hand the resources available for responding to the expectations and demands are becoming increasingly stretched. Even in high-income countries, the available resources are scarce in relation to these demands.

Because of this, more and more studies have been reported in the expert medical literature of these countries in the last two decades trying to solve the disproportion between the increasing investments in health care and the principal factors that have led to basic improvements in health by means of methods of economic evaluation.

The key question on how best to choose between the different and competing ways of using the resources that are available has considerable importance in perinatal medicine, whose share in the costs of health care is quite high. There are three reasons for this. First, the number of users – pregnant and childbearing women and their infants – is quite high. Second, the number of preventive screening examinations and preventive hospitalizations during the course of pregnancy has increased. Third, the number of special, sometimes very expensive, examinations using technological advances in medicine has increased.

The approach to preparation of these studies and to their exploitation shows considerable variations. It is different in the professionals within the perinatal field, who wish to make optimal use of the budgets and resources that are available to them, than in the planners, who must decide on the appropriate level of funding for maternity care. There are also differences between the views of the patient, of the hospital, as well as of the government or the community at large.

Methods of economic evaluation

When discussing the already classical studies of Drummond *et al.*[1] and Mugford and Drummond,[2] it is necessary first to state some basic considerations related to the role of economics in the evaluation of care:

(1) The first consideration must be that the care for which the resources are used is likely to do more good than harm. Only afterward comes the consideration of both the most cost-effective or efficient use of the resources available for perinatal care and the extent to which society's resources should be allocated to perinatal care.
(2) Economic evaluation requires a contrast between alternative courses of action, in term of both costs and consequences.
(3) There are three main stages of economic evaluation. First, the likely costs and benefits must be enumerated; second, they must be measured; third, they must be expressed in comparable units.
(4) Among the most important methods of economic evaluation of perinatal care programs are cost-minimization, marginal, cost-effectiveness, cost–utility and cost–benefit analyses.

The nature and scale of any economic evaluation will vary according to the question that is being asked. While all approaches involve to some extent deriving a balance sheet of the costs and benefits of the different strategies compared, some approaches are more complex than others.

Cost-minimization analysis

This, probably the simplest, analysis comes from the presumption that benefits of treatments that are compared are equal, which makes it possible to compare the resource costs without any need to measure benefits. A different length of hospitalization of a woman subsequent to a spontaneous delivery and physiological pregnancy, who delivered a healthy, term newborn, whose adaptation to extrauterine life was normal in the first hours of life, could serve as an example. This is the problem that is being solved at present in the

Czech Republic. Before the transformation of health care to the conditions of market mechanism, that is, before 1990, hospitalization after delivery in the given case lasted for 5–6 days, whereas in the majority of high-income countries with advanced perinatal care, such hospitalization lasts for half that time on average without adversely affecting the health condition of the woman or her child.

From the given example concerning the calculation of decreased costs with the same benefit, it explicitly emerges that it is possible to save the costs of hospitalization for 2–3 days. On the other hand, however, new costs arise for the home visits for the mother and infant when women are discharged earlier from hospital after delivery. This has to last at least until the time of separation of the umbilical stump in the child, and healing of the perineal wound in the woman. Even if, in comparison with the more expensive hospital care, the cheaper home care clearly decreases the costs of postnatal care, this change opens new concerns:

(1) A decrease in satisfaction of Czech women (predominantly primiparae) in consequence of the shorter spell of rest after delivery and the early care of the newborn at home.[3]
(2) A choice of the optimal method for cord care associated with a reduction of the number of home visits by midwives.[4] However, these types of studies fall within other methods of economic evaluation.

Marginal analysis

This analysis would be particularly useful in the case of routine and repeated testing, which is so common in the care of women during pregnancy and childbirth. But the key question is: How many of them should we use? There may be a general agreement that certain screening tests should be applied to high-risk pregnancies. But should they be applied routinely to all pregnant women and possibly also repeatedly? When analyzing the majority of screening tests performed in the course of pregnancy, it should be first taken into account that there exist complex factors affecting the mother's health. It is consequently extremely difficult to evaluate the effectiveness of the analyzed test, because many other variables that influence maternal and fetal health are interacting at the same time and confound the findings. These variables are considerably different in developing and industrial countries, where the most important ones influencing the outcome of pregnancy include socioeconomic factors, level of education, desire for pregnancy and maternal age. Taking into account the above background information and limitations, we shall try to ascertain the effectiveness of these screening tests and subsequent measures from the following two aspects:

(1) *Biological*: Each intervention is considered in terms of what it intended to achieve.
(2) *Programmatic*: Do the maternal health programs successfully deliver the biologically effective intervention to the intended target population?

The widely used practice of ultrasound imaging of the fetus during pregnancy can be employed as a typical example. From the biological point of view this method is routinely performed up to the 20th week of pregnancy since it

(1) defines more precisely the expected date of confinement, hence reducing the induction rate in pregnancies mistakenly diagnosed as post-term;
(2) allows an earlier diagnosis of twin pregnancies, leading to reduced premature labor connected with an increased mortality and morbidity of these newborns and
(3) improves the detection of malformed fetuses, which is followed by termination of pregnancy if the pregnant woman agrees, thereby reducing the number of impaired babies.

Repeated routine ultrasound examinations at the beginning of the third trimester improve a timely diagnosis of fetal growth retardation and placenta previa, leading to reduced mortality and morbidity in newborns.

In a series of studies, the routine and repeated performance of ultrasound examinations during the course of pregnancy was compared with only selective examinations for predicting the expected date of delivery and for assessing subsequent measures upon the occurrence of adverse outcomes. From the programmatic point of view, the health resource implications of such screening programs between the two strategies of care can be considered on the basis of costs, which include equipment, trained staff and clinic accommodation. These then vary with the number of cases treated and differ between the two types of care offered. Of the studies mentioned concerning the effectivness of ultrasound screening programs, only a few refer explicitly to health resource implications.[5] However, since several of the above-mentioned pregnancy complications are studied at the same time in the course of one ultrasound examination, it is very difficult, if not impossible, to earmark out of the total cost of this examination, the partial cost of diagnosing only one of these conditions. For instance, in the Czech Republic, it was possible to successively eliminate anencephaly out of the population of newborns by means of routine ultrasound screening, which is performed in 94% of all pregnant women before the 20th week of pregnancy.[6]

In an effort to limit some relatively expensive and, in the majority of cases, invasive tests connected with a certain, albeit very small, physical risk, while enabling a reliable and timely diagnosis of a serious pathological condition, the procedure was divided from the programmatic point of view into two levels. The timely diagnosis of some chromosomal or genetic disorders in the fetus can be taken as an example. By means of a routine screening program using relatively cheap and non-invasive tests, a high-risk group is selected from the total population of women on the first level. Only in the small group of women selected in this way are reliable diagnostic methods allowing a timely identification of the disease used, for example, chorionic villus sampling or examination of fetal cells after obtaining a sample of amniotic fluid by amniocentesis. Over the past few years in the Czech Republic, such a programmed procedure has decreased the incidence of neural tube defects and Down's syndrome by 50%, as in the majority of high-income countries.[7]

Cost-effectiveness analysis

Cost-effectiveness analysis of any intervention requires calculation of the change in costs divided by the change in outcome of the intervention; the outcomes are measured in units of health (for example, survival rates, or life-years saved).

Change in cost

The best economic analysis will consider all costs, regardless of who has to pay: the health insurance company, the hospital, the patient, the family or the community at large. A distinction has to be made between charges and costs. Only in some cases will the charge for a service equal the cost, and only under such circumstances can charge be substituted for costs.

Change in survival rates

A differentiated approach to the change in survival rate can be demonstrated with the example of care for newborns of very low birth weight. When evaluating the effectivness of the care for these newborns in the sense of their survival, the following considerations are taken into account:

(1) Birth weight of the newborn: The lower the birth weight, the longer the period of hospitalization in the neonatal intensive care unit (NICU) and the higher the costs of the treatment, because the two factors are combined.
(2) Whether the evaluation concerns a country-wide or regional program, all live births or only neonatal intensive care in the hospital.
(3) Whether the newborn was delivered in a perinatologic center where there is an NICU, or whether the newborn was transported to the NICU only after delivery, because out-born newborns have a different prognosis.
(4) Whether all liveborns are evaluated, or whether certain newborns are excluded, for example, those with lethal malformations, whose death is not influenced by the quality of intensive perinatal care.

The results of this deliberation determine which newborns must be accounted for in the denominator of any calculation of survival rate.

An internationally recommended objective criterion for the intensive care of newborns of a very low birth weight differentiated in this way is the birth-weight-specific neonatal death rate (potentially after exclusion of lethal malformations), which can be further differentiated into death during the first 7 days after delivery (early neonatal death) or during the subsequent 3 weeks (late neonatal death).[8,9]

Cost–utility analysis

In cost–utility analysis, the social value of the outcome is determined. The analysis requires calculation of the change of costs, which is the same as for cost-effectiveness analysis, divided by the change in outcome adjusted for the quality-adjusted life saved, or quality-adjusted life-years saved. From the point of view of utility, the outcome is also the satisfaction gained from consumption of a service.

Change in quality-adjusted life-years or survival rate

The major difficulty is the inability to define what constitutes a normal quality of life, and what is the possibility of measuring the health status and health-related quality of life. The broad definition of health as formulated by the World Health Organization (WHO) is 'a state of complete physical, mental and social well-being and not merely the absence of disease or infirmity'. WHO has also developed a classification of impairment, disability and handicap.[10] Conventionally, an outcome with normal health and quality of life is allotted a utility of 1, and death is allotted a utility of 0.[11] Any outcome of less than normal health or quality of life has a value of less than 1. But many handicapped children lead productive lives, and their health-related quality of life might be fairly good. In this respect, measurement of health-related quality of life adds a different, additional and important dimension to the standard description of cognitive and motor functioning in outcome studies. It is therefore clear that the available adult measures cannot be applied directly to children, whose life experiences and daily activities differ substantially from those of adults. Therefore, the six-component multi-attributable system known as the Health Utilities Index was worked out to describe the quality of life of children, and this includes sensory and communication ability, happiness, self-ability, freedom from moderate to severe pain, learning and school difficulty and physical ability.[12] In spite of this, there still remain a series of factors that may influence the measurement of the health-related quality of life of these children, for example:

(1) Children of different ages have varying capabilities, and with increasing age they develop new and more advanced skills and challenges. Therefore, the dimensions of any measure of health-related quality of life have to take these changes into consideration.[13]
(2) Health status measured by health professionals, self-assessment and parental score might not be consistent.[14]
(3) Children with the same disability might view their quality of life very differently.

A particular problem represents the justification of estimating the health status at the time of a striking decline in neonatal monitoring of very immature newborns, although improvements in morbidity of these children have not been significant. Offering intensive care to all newborns of borderline viability without having the possibility of predicting reliably the quality of life gained in every individual case is being questioned by both parents and health-care providers. It is well recognized that parents, health professionals and members of society may have different views on both the dimensions of importance and the values placed on different health states.[15] The fundamental question, however, is whose values are important for consideration of allocation of health-care resources and for decision making.

Another criterion for analogous decision making, for example, between neonatal intensive care and other programs, is the probability of the length of life gained by means of intensive care. Most surviving adults admitted to intensive care will be dead within a shorter time than the neonates admitted to the NICU, of whom the surviving ones may well live for 70 years or more.

However, cost–utility is also used from the point of view of utility to women. For example, pregnant women may be anxious about their genetic history, or because of their age that they may be carrying a fetus with one or more abnormalities. It is precisely the above-mentioned two-level screening performed in these women that will affect an unnecessary prolongation of their anxiety up to the time of assessment of the correct diagnosis on the second level, since there exists a certain percentage of false-positive results on the first level. The anxiety of the women will be also prolonged if the correct final diagnosis is made by amniocentesis, which can only be performed in the second trimester. On the other hand, the examination by means of chorionic villus sampling can be performed earlier, in the first trimester.

However, routine ultrasound screening also has a psychosocial benefit in some cases. A mother's attitude to her pregnancy can be positively affected by the observation of the first fetal movements on the screen of the ultrasound apparatus, even more than by their perception.[16] It is, in this way, possible to create a relationship with the child before it is born.

Another example of utility to women represents the lower satisfaction of women in connection with the shortened time of hospitalization after delivery that is mentioned in the section Cost-Minimization Analysis.

Cost–benefit analysis

This method of economic analysis in perinatal care, the last one to be mentioned, similarly allows the outcome to be converted into monetary terms. The cost–benefit analysis of perinatal intensive care requires the subtraction of additional costs per live birth from additional earnings per live birth; the results can be expressed in units of currency and would be termed the net economic benefit, or net economic loss if negative.

The data used for the change in cost are the same ones as mentioned in the section Cost-Effectiveness Analysis. The major difficulty is to estimate the lifetime earnings of a survivor, when such imponderables as life expectancy, career choice (including the possibility of unemployment) and inflation have to be predicted so far into the future. Affected children may have different skills and capacities than unaffected children, different health care, education and other needs throughout their lives.

Another important point of view when taking into account the timing of costs and benefits is a generational view, when, for example, the favorable result of treatment of a pregnant woman 40 years ago may have an adverse effect on the fertility of her offspring, as happened in the case of diethylstilbestrol.[17]

The already classical randomized trial of MacDonald *et al.*[18] concerning the economic evaluation of electronic fetal heart monitoring vs. intermittent auscultation achieved the same outcome of care. Since, however, the whole course of labor in every individual woman was always followed by one midwife, and if, rather than her salary bill, the time necessary for such a follow-up should be measured, we would find that hardly any workplace would have a sufficient number of staff for such a procedure.

Costs and benefits arise from changes in the uses not only of a community's, but also of a family's, resources. Returning back to the example of early postnatal discharge from hospital, it is likely that more family resources will be needed for informal home care and support for a mother who comes back home very soon after delivery.

International comparative studies

The cost-effective analysis for better health outcome is also solved in the form of international comparative studies. In some of the above-mentioned problems, for example, because the costs have to be standardized if different areas are compared, further sources of confusion arise when comparing different countries due

Table 28.1 Increase of costs for hospitalization of pregnant women. The data are based on a comparison of two groups of pregnant women: Czech Republic (*n*=106,680) and Hessen (58,430) in 1994. The costs are calculated in accordance with the rate table of the Czech Health Insurance Company in Czech crowns

Length of hospitalization (days)	Hospitalization of pregnant women in population (%)		Cost increase, difference (%)	(Czech crowns, millions)
	Czech Republic	Hessen		
1–7	10.9	10.1	0.7	0.8
8–21	9.8	7.6	2.2	10.4
> 21	6.6	3.1	3.5	47.8
Total	27.3	20.8	6.4	59.0

Table 28.2 Decrease of costs for the care of low-birth-weight newborns in consequence of their decreased incidence in the population. The data are based on a comparison of two groups of newborns: Czech Republic (*n*=107,721) and Hessen (*n*=59,198) in 1994. The costs are calculated in accordance with the rate table of the Czech Health Insurance Company in Czech crowns

Birth weight (g)	Incidence of low-birth-weight newborns in population (%)		Cost decrease, difference (%)	(Czech crowns, millions)
	Czech Republic	Hessen		
<1000	0.30	0.37	0.07	69.9
1000–1499	0.55	0.62	0.07	34.1
1500–1999	1.07	1.23	0.16	18.6
2000–2499	3.55	3.82	0.27	7.3
Total	5.47	6.04	0.57	129.9

to the fluctuations in the respective currency rates over time.

Of these studies, the World Bank data[19] on infant mortality and life expectancy in 21 high-income and 27 low-income countries are meaningful. For each country, the differences between actual and predicted values were calculated for health expenditure per capita on the basis of per capita gross national product and health. From the results of this comparison, it emerged that for high-income countries, the marginal return of health expenditure per capita as measured by mortality is negligible. This means that improvement in health and reduction in mortality can be expected to arise not from further increases in costs, but from greater efficiency in the use of resources, more reliance on preventive measures, advances in lifestyle, behavior and medical technology.[20]

It was the preventive measures to which a comparative epidemiological study was devoted, concerning the effect of bed rest during pregnancy upon two internationally accepted indicators of maternal morbidity: rate of eclampsia and neonatal rate of low birth weight.[21] The incidence of these indicators in the Czech Republic was compared with the incidence in Hessen (one of the federal states of the Federal Republic of Germany), where there is a lower rate of prenatal hospital admissions, while the system of perinatal care and the perinatal mortality rate are similar. From the economic point of view, it was calculated under the conditions of the Czech Republic that:

(1) The increase of expenses for hospitalization of women is higher by 7% in the Czech Republic (predominantly because of hospitalization for different lengths of time for preventive reasons) (Table 28.1).
(2) There is a decrease of expenses for specialized care in the NICU due to a 0.5% lower incidence of low-birth-weight infants in the population (further differentiated into four groups according to birth weight) (Table 28.2).

The two-fold lower sum spared from the NICU costs against the sum paid for the higher percentage of preventively hospitalized women does not include the benefit attained in the second analyzed indicator, that is, the decreased incidence of eclampsia (one case per 2556 deliveries per year in the Czech Republic compared with a greater than two-fold incidence in

Hessen, that is, one case per 1328 deliveries per year). However, it is not possible to express this benefit in monetary terms.

Conclusions

In the economy at large, the costs and benefits of activities are made visible through the market system. However, the market mechanism in general either does not apply, or works imperfectly in the health-care field. This is also true of the use of the terms 'cost' and 'benefit' during economic evaluation of perinatal care. Economists thus have to use other approaches in estimating the benefits of health-care programs. The most promising approach appears to be the evaluation of health improvements not in monetary terms. Also, the monetary cost is often an inadequate measure of the true economic cost. From this point of view, the main methods that economists consider in the evaluation of health-care alternatives and in the comparison of health-care programs were described. These methods of economic evaluation should also ensure wise spending during allocation of resources.

The application of the methods of economic evaluation in perinatal care cannot overcome the moral dilemmas that arise in the choice of different screening or therapeutic methods or allocation of resources. It does, however, provide a framework within which such factors become less easily avoided and more readily discussed from the point of view of both the care givers and the care receivers.

REFERENCES

1. Drummond MF, Stoddart GL, Torrance GW. *Methods for the Economic Evaluation of Health Care Programmes.* Oxford: Oxford University Press, 1986.
2. Mugford M, Drummond MF. The role of economics in the evaluation of care. In Chalmers I, Enkin M, Keirse MJ, eds. *Effective Care in Pregnancy and Childbirth.* Oxford: Oxford University Press, 1991:86–96.
3. Goldberg H, Velebil P, Stembera Z, *et al.*, eds. *Czech Republic Reproductive Health Survey 1993.* Atlanta, GA: Centers for Disease Control and Prevention, 1995.
4. Mugford M, Somchaiwong M, Waterhouse I. Treatment of umbilical cords. Report of a randomised controlled trial. *Midwifery* 1986;2:177–86.
5. Bakketeig LS, Eik-Nes SH, Jacobsen G, *et al.* Randomised controlled trial of ultrasonographic screening in pregnancy. *Lancet* 1984;2:207–9.
6. Sípek A, Gregor V, Chudobová M. Incidence of birth defects and effectivity of prenatal diagnosis in the Czech republic 1993 (in Czech). *Cs Pediatrie* 1996;2:114–23.
7. International Clearinghouse for Birth Defects Monitoring System. *ICBDMS, Annual Report 1994.* Rome: ISSN 0743-5703, 1996: 52–123.
8. Dunn PM, McIlwaine G. Perinatal audit. *Prenat Neonat Med* 1996;1:160–94.
9. World Health Organization. *International Statistical Classification of Diseases,* 10th revision. (Statistical presentation.) Geneva: World Health Organization, 1993;2:124–38.
10. World Health Organization. *International Classification of Impairments. Disabilities and Handicaps.* Geneva: World Health Organization, 1980.
11. Bennett KJ, Torrance GW. Measuring health state preference and utilities rating scale time trade-off, and standard gamble techniques. In Spilker B, ed. *Quality of Life and Pharmacoeconomics in Clinical Trials.* Philadelphia: Lippincott-Raven, 1996:253–65.
12. Torrance GW, Furlong W, Feeny D, *et al.* Multiattribute preference functions: Health Utilities Index. *Pharmacoeconomics* 1995;7:503–20.
13. Saigal S, Szatmari P, Rosenbaum P, *et al.* Cognitive abilities and school performance of extremely low birthweight children and matched term control children at age 8 years: A regional study. *J Pediatr* 1991;118:751–60.
14. Saigal S, Feeny D, Rosenbaum P, *et al.* Self-perceived health status and health-related quality of life of extremely low birthweight teenagers: Comparison with term controls. *J Am Med Assoc* 1996;276:453–9.
15. Saigal S, Rosenbaum PL, Feeny DH, *et al.* Comparison of preferences of health professionals and parents for health outcomes of neonatal intensive care (abstract). *Pediatr Res* 1996;39:1654.
16. Reading AD, Campbell S, Cox DN, *et al.* Health beliefs and health care behaviour in pregnancy. *Psychosom Med* 1982;12: 379–83.
17. Herbst AL, Ulfelder H, Postkanzer DC. Adenocarcinoma of the vagina: Association of maternal stilbestrol therapy with tumor appearance in young women. *N Engl J Med* 1971;284:878–81.
18. MacDonald D, Grant A, Sheridan-Pereira M, *et al.* The Dublin randomised trial of intrapartum fetal heart monitoring. *Am J Obstet Gynecol* 1985;152:524–39.
19. The World Bank. *World Development Report 1993: Investing in Health.* New York: Oxford University Press, 1993.
20. Shmueli A. Cost-effective outlays for better health outcomes. *World Health Forum* 1995;16:287–92.
21. Stembera Z, Holub J. Hospitalization during pregnancy: Professional versus economic aspect (in Czech). *Ces Gynek* 1996;61: 332–7.

SECTION IV

Ultrasound

Section Editors: **A. Kurjak and Y. Ville**

29 3D–4D ultrasound evaluation of the embryo and the early fetus

F. Bonilla-Musoles, L. E. Machado, F. Raga, F. Bonilla Jr and F. Machado

Introduction

Following the USA Food and Drug Administration (FDA) approval of 3D in November 1997, interest in the technique has soared to the extent that reports on 3D in obstetrics and gynecology are now in the thousands. Moreover, any international or national ultrasound congress or meeting of our specialty has main lectures, courses or workshops dedicated to this issue.

Today, 3D is an integrated part of ultrasound (US), not only in obstetrics and gynecology but also in other medical streams.

Most important, the FDA with its strict guidelines has highlighted the importance of this technology for the future of medicine.

Because of the most recent advances in informatics, several important innovations have appeared recently.

The first 3D instruments that appeared in 1991 took 25 s to store an image and minutes to hours to reconstruct the 3D rendering. Then, the defocused instruments[1,2] formed 3D images in real-time. Current software has improved to the extent that images are stored in tenths of a second, and spatial images can be reconstructed immediately, in 1 s. In this way, images are obtained in quasi-real-time showing embryonic or fetal movements, the so-called 4D.

The newest instruments limit the field of vision (a disadvantage similar to 2D) and eliminate distorted echoes. They also store transparency systems allowing immediate visualization and avoiding loss of time. The smaller and easier-to-handle transducers and the better proportionate image quality are also definitive improvements.

But not only has 3D changed and improved in only 2 years, in our opinion two amazing improvements have been introduced:

- The combination in quasi-real-time at the same time and in the same frame of the 2D and 3D images. This advantage allows a rapid and better orientation and, for those with scarce experience, easier identification of structures and planes.
- The integration of successive images in only 1 s, allowing the visualization of embryonic or fetal movements.

But these are not the final effects of the new computer technology. Recently, we used new Japanese prototypes of 3D machines, which were able to produce six images per second, with a store capacity of minutes (the existing machines store only 10 s) and an incredible image quality.

Today, more than 11 commercial establishments make use of 3D, but not all are good. Many use ill-equipped 'work stations' that necessitate spending time (and money) after the exam. These are not real 3D machines, and one should not forget that what the patient, and the sonographer, wants is to visualize the baby in the frame.

In our opinion, and until very recently, none of the workstations are good enough. Recently, a new one with important advantages has been approved by the FDA (although it is not yet approved in the European Community):

- The software program is cheap (€15,000).
- Adaptable to all US machines (also the small ones) and transducer images.
- Excellent image quality.
- Immediate free-hand 3D rendering image of excellent quality.
- No limitation of storing space, as with all existing 3D transducers.
- Very rapid 3D rendering, allowing the study of the heart motion.
- Adaptable to old stored clinical cases, and not only in US machines but in videos, PCs, DVDs, etc.

Some problems remain to be solved:

- There is a shortage of learning centers where interested professionals can learn about new techniques, learn how to use the new instruments and become acquainted with the variety of equipment that is constantly appearing on the market.
- Health-care professionals must not only be aware that all commercial instruments have the latest technological advantages, they must also know that every month new machines are being offered with new and better technology.
- The three first and most important statistics on fetal malformations (reported by Merz, Pretorius, and Bonilla-Musoles) need to be reproduced by other investigators. All the articles that have recently appeared show isolated cases, superficial malformations, or use with few cases.

In summary, we would recommend starting to work with 3D, *it is the future.*

History of 3D

3D reports started 10 years ago. The first descriptions were devoted to emphasis on the diagnostic possibilities in obstetrics or gynecology.[2–67]

Sporadic reports of normal[2,4–8,10,11,13,15,16,26,68–84] and malformed fetuses[2,18–20,38,49,54,70–72,80–82,85–110] followed.

Soon after, descriptive images of specific organs and areas were available:

- craneum and fontanelles[111,112]
- central nervous system[113–118]
- head[21,119,120]
- face[12,22,39,91,105,119,121–124]
- lips[108,125]
- forehead[126]
- eyes[127]
- thorax and vertebral column[14,27,34,37,111,122,128–132]
- heart[60,110,126,133–143]
- fingers[28,75,80,131,144–147]
- genitalia, normal or ambiguous.[148–153]

Comparative 2D/3D biometric studies of fetal weight[154–162] and organ volumes[12,156,157,163–165] showed that 3D provides more accurate results.

Specific organ studies allowed for nomograms regarding:

- anatomic structures (e.g. long bones)
- volumetry of organs (e.g. the gestational sac and lung)[83,156,157,166–169]
- functions (e.g. the heart)[60,86,126,133–138,170]
- vascularization[160,171–179]
- estimation of the fetal weight or fat content through calculation of the muscle circumference.[180]

Extensive casuistics have shown that 3D improves the diagnostic accuracy of 2D in more than 70% of malformations.[18–20,70,71,73,96–105,181,182] Also, the more recent specific reports on selected malformations, such as facial,[91,55] lips,[125] head, neck and spine,[70,111] abdominal wall[59,183] and limbs[90,147] have confirmed these findings.

With regard to the first-trimester fetus, many abdominal or transvaginal (TV) descriptions have been published.[6,7,10,52,69–73,107,112,184–200] The most outstanding are those related to studies of the cerebral cavities.[5,8,69–73,115,116,118,184,185,201–203] Also, uterine-introduced 10-MHz transducers have been used[191] without success.

Gestational sac and secundines have been volumetrically studied.[32,35,204,205]

A new field of publications concerning the early diagnosis of malformations has appeared. These publications show the ability to study important markers of chromosomal anomalies, such as the nucal translucency,[70,73,195] ectopia cordis,[196] trisomy 18-affected fetuses[199] or conjoined twins.[71,88,186,197]

Outside the prenatal diagnosis some important articles have been published related to assisted reproduction,[56,199,206–215] the cervix in pregnancy,[216] urogynecology,[138,217,218] gynecological and breast cancer.[120,219–225]

This chapter deals with the appearance chronology of embryonic and fetal structures up to week 16 based on our own previous published investigations.[5–8,69–73,185]

Abdominal US

As when using 2D, the TV approach is superior to the transabdominal for 3D in the first trimester. Abdominal 3D should not be recommended.

Nevertheless, in this chapter we show the 3D schedule images of the abdominal US, because all machines are equipped with abdominal transducers, but not all make use of TV transducers, which are optional additions.

In our book *Atlas de ecografia obstetrica* of 1988, the schedule of appearance of embryonic and fetal structures according to the gestational week was established.

This embryologic–echographic schedule is still completely adaptable today to the first-trimester abdominal 3D (Graphics 29.1 and 29.2).

Because of the lack of interest and the difficulty in obtaining good 3D first-trimester abdominal images, there is a scarcity of publications. However, with care, 3D images of exceptional quality can be obtained.

Fifth week

The gestational sac can be observed with the following characteristics:

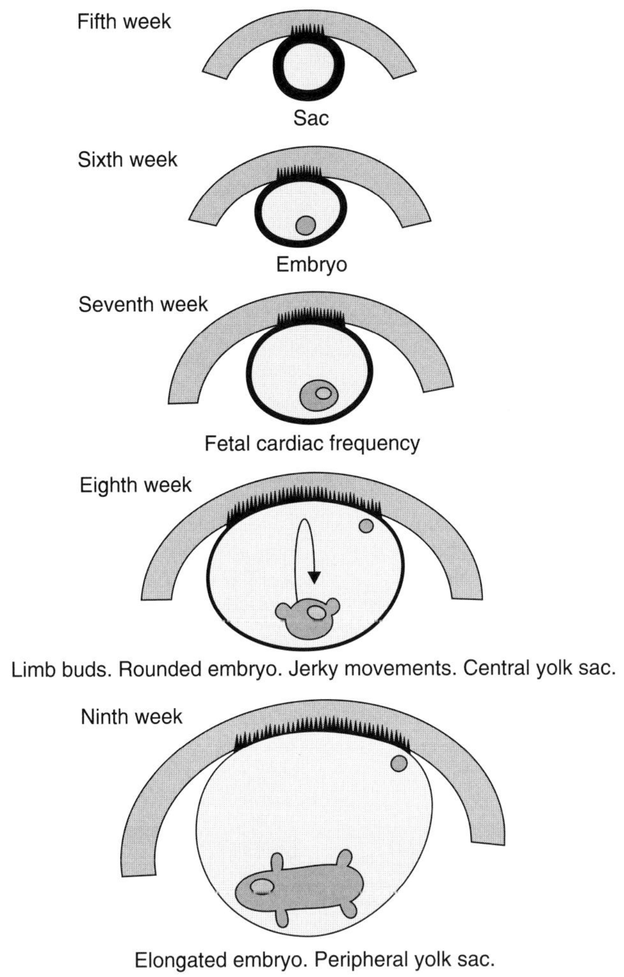

Graphic 29.1

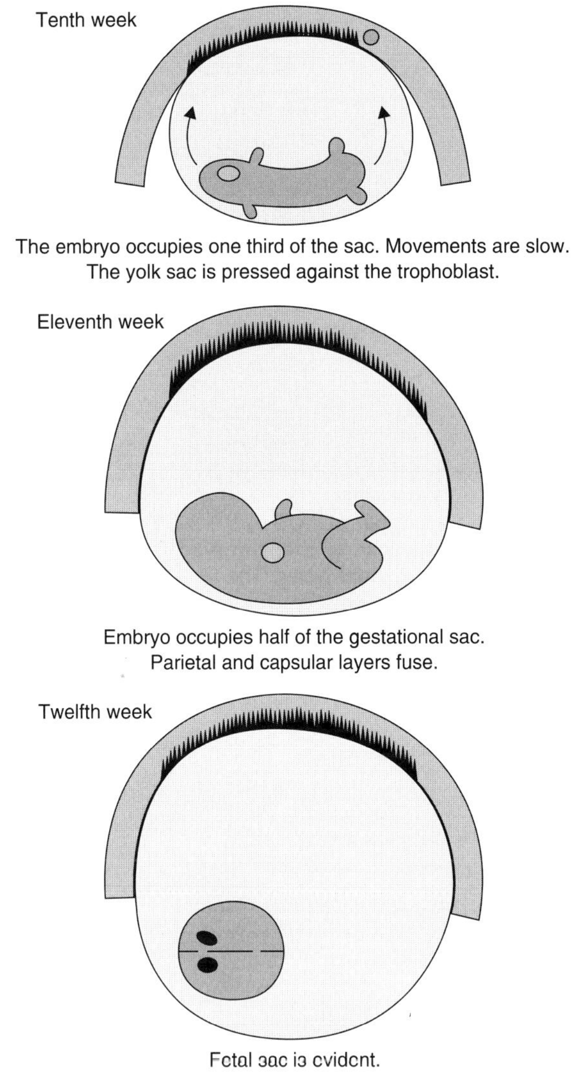

Graphic 29.2

- oval or round with limpid boundaries
- homogenous trophoblastic rim greater than 5 mm
- no internal contour irregularities
- progressive growth (1 mm/day)

Viewing the abdominal 3D gestational sac at this age is not easy, and there is no improvement when compared with 2D. At present, only the TV route is useful.

The sac's shape is round between the fifth and sixth weeks and becomes oval later on. Irregular forms, such as enlarged, comma shaped, should not be considered abnormal if not accompanied by other anomaly/ies, such as:

- irregular growth: no growth, too slow, too rapid
- decidual refringency changes
- contour irregularities
- embryo not visible (vanishing), etc.

Abnormal sac forms in normal evolution pregnancies are common in cases of myomas, ovarian cysts, distended bladder or sigmoid, etc.

The gestational sac wall thickness decreases as the gestation progresses due to the progressive atrophy of the deciduas capsularis and parietalis.

Following the visualization of the embryo, the crown–rump length should be measured. This measurement should be made from the cephalic pole to the rump taking care to measure the embryonic curvature. The crown–rump length should be measured across the dorsal curvature.

Sixth week

The most important finding is the embryonic visualization. It appears as an echorefringent round structure located in the inferior pole because of its specific gravity, which is greater than that of the amniotic fluid. Its length is of approximately 10 mm.

The gestational sac grows approximately 1.15 mm/day, so that at the end of the sixth week it measures 20 mm, up from 10 mm at the beginning of this week.

The embryonic growth is 1 mm/day, reaching 15–17 mm at the end of the sixth week.

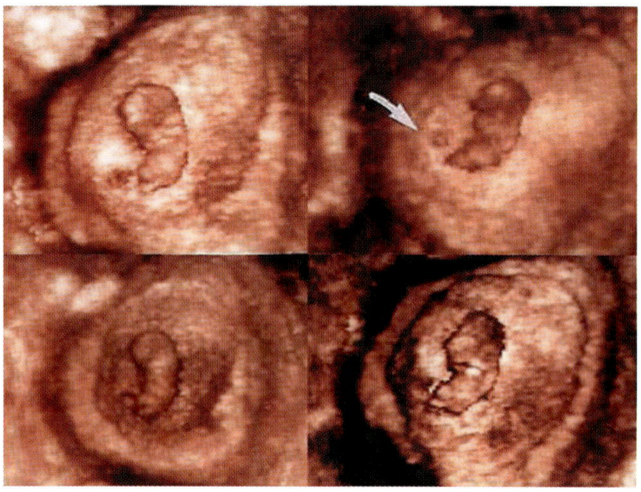

Figure 29.1 Abdominal 3D US in 9+6 weeks. Observe the profile of the embryo lying over the placenta, showing well-defined cranial and caudal poles. The yolk sac can be seen in the upper pictures (arrow). The remaining pictures show the lower limbs.

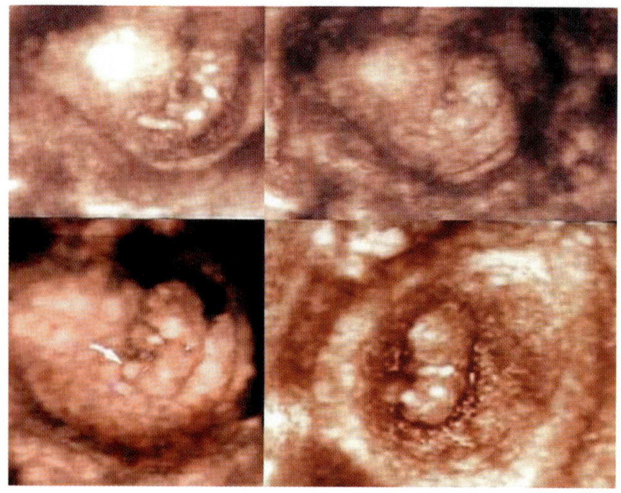

Figure 29.2 Abdominal 3D US first trimester, 10+1 weeks. The fetal head, abdomen and extremities are clearly defined. The ossification nuclei of the jaw and the face profile along with the four limbs are visible. The physiological herniation is depicted in the two lower pictures.

Seventh week

Along with the increasing size of the embryo and sac, the most important feature is the visualization of the cardiac activity. The embryo remains round.

Eighth week

The limb buds appear in an embryo, which is still round. So-called jerky embryonic movements are detectable. We say 'so-called' because the embryo in fact moves up and down repeatedly within the sac.

The yolk sac can be observed in a location near the gestational sac.

Ninth week

For the first time, the embryo appears elongated with definite cranial and caudal poles. The limbs are fully developed, although the fingers are not yet visible. The yolk sac is in a more peripheral location.

From this week on, 3D visualization is superior to 2D due to the amount of amniotic fluid (Figure 29.1).

Tenth week

So-called slow and lazy movements appear. They are characterized by fetal rotations around its longitudinal axis, balancing and movement of the extremities.

The fetus occupies more than a third of the space in the gestational sac; it can be viewed well with 3D along with the yolk sac (Figures 29.2–29.4).

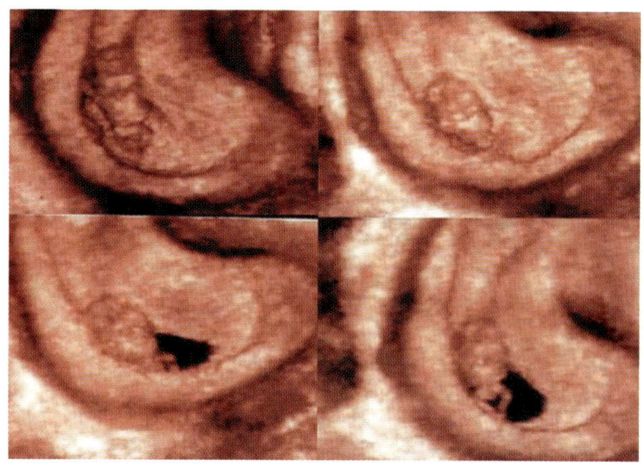

Figure 29.3 3D abdominal US. 10+3 weeks. Frontal view of the fetus showing semiextended legs. The fetus is resting on the placenta (left upper and lower pictures), seen in a frontal view where the face can be observed (bottom right) and the feet already formed (bottom pictures).

Eleventh week

There is fusion of the parietal and capsular decidual layers, eliminating in this way what is considered a gestational sac.

The fetus now occupies one-half of the amniotic cavity. Structures in the head, abdomen and limbs are clearly visible.

Twelfth to sixteenth week

In week 12, the skull is fully formed (Figures 29.5 and 29.6). Facial and abdominal structures can be

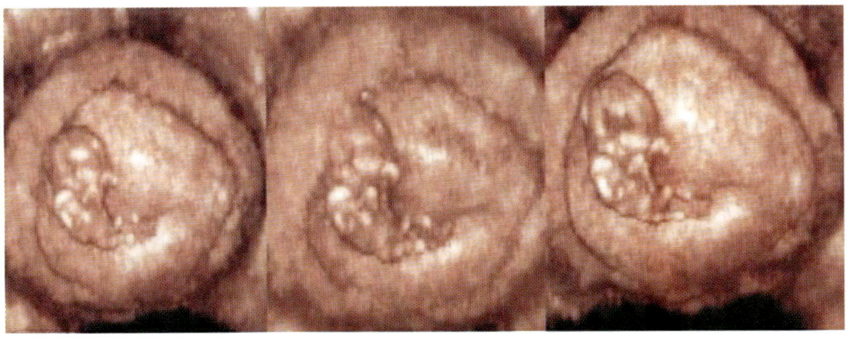

Figure 29.4 Abdominal 3D US. 10+4 weeks. The extremities are complete. The fetus lies over the placenta. Fully developed fetus with well-formed arms and legs lying over the placenta.

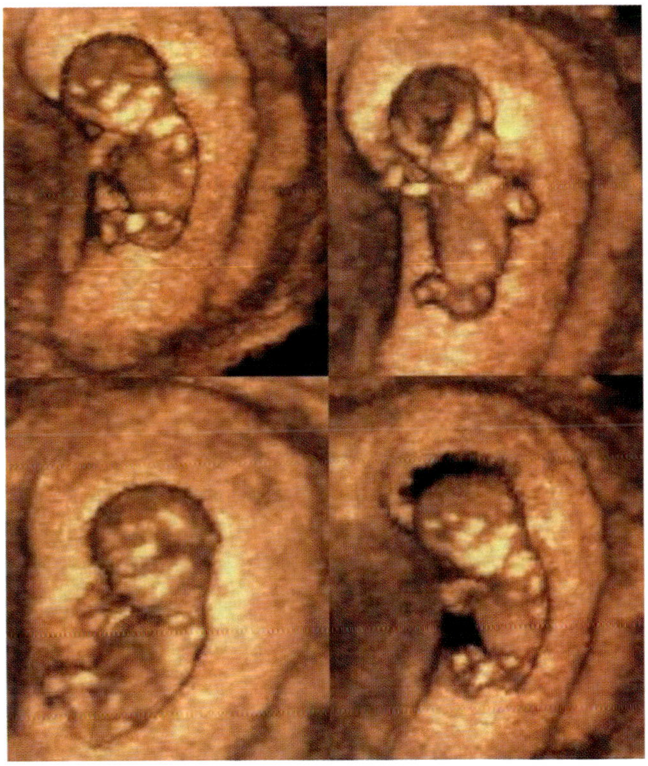

Figure 29.5 Abdominal 3D US in first trimester. 13 weeks. In this fully developed fetus the physiological herniation has disappeared. The orbits, nose, mouth and limbs with hands and feet can be seen.

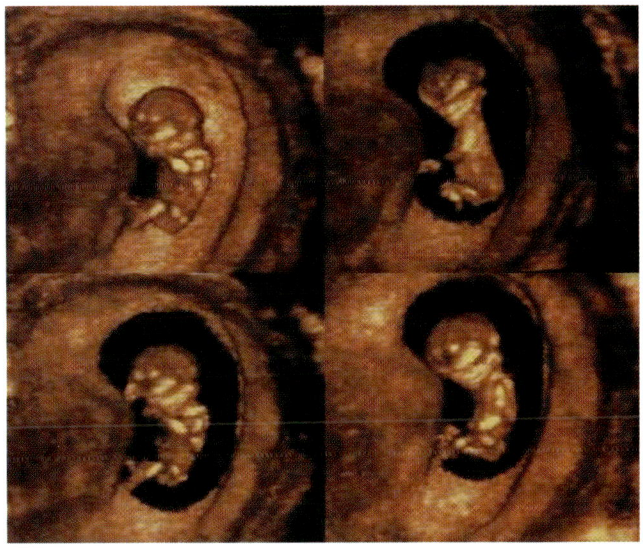

Figure 29.6 Thirteen weeks days. This image shows hands and feet with fingers and toes.

observed. Hands and feet are fully developed. Fingers and toes are identified.

From week 13 on the normal fetal development can be followed (Figures 29.7–29.12).

Twin pregnancy

Twin pregnancy can be diagnosed after week 6, when two gestational sacs are clearly visible, each with its own embryo.

It is not acceptable to miss a diagnosis of twins by transabdominal US examination after the eighth week of pregnancy (Figure 29.11).

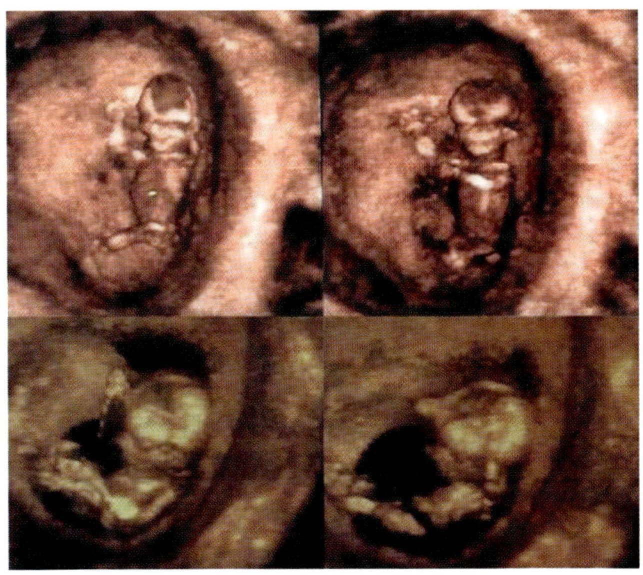

Figure 29.7 Top: Fourteen weeks and 1 day of gestation. Observe the frontal view of the fetus with uplifted arms, the superciliary arches, the nose, ears and hands. Bottom: Fourteen weeks and 4 days of gestation. Fetal profile, superfiliary arches, eyes, sutures and fontanelles.

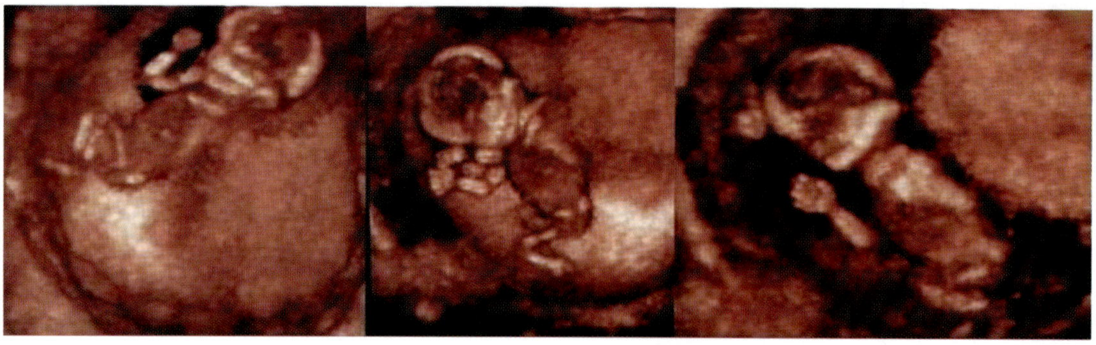

Figure 29.8 Fourteen weeks and 5 days of pregnancy. This lying fetus reveals arms and hands with clearly defined fingers. The mouth can be seen on the profile view of the face (left).

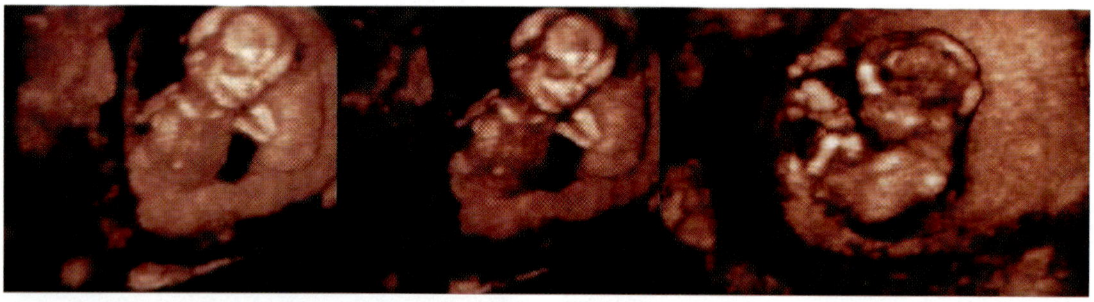

Figure 29.9 Fifteen weeks plus 1 day of pregnancy. Frontal view of a fetus. Skull bones along with sutures, fontanelles, orbital sockets, mouth and lower limb bones. The right figure shows the profile, forehead, eyes, nose and mouth.

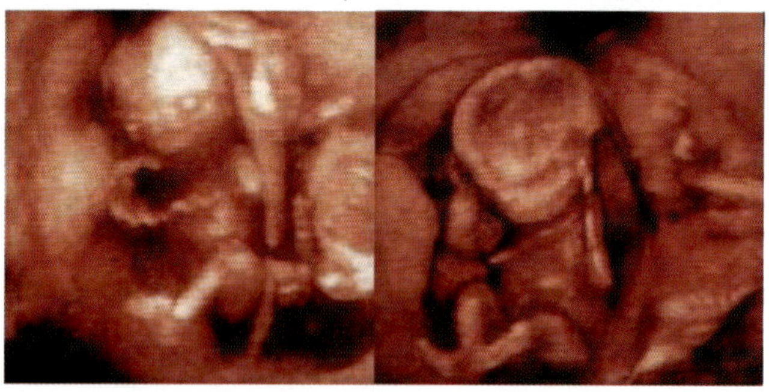

Figure 29.10 Gestations of 14 weeks plus four and five days. Left: The fetus shows open eyes. Right: The eyes are closed.

Transvaginal 3D US

Fourth week (from 4+0 to 4+6 days)

The first structures observed with 3D as with TV 2D are obtainable between weeks 4 and 5.

The first image that indicates the possibility of pregnancy is the persistence proximal to the menstrual days of a decidual transformed endometrium accompanied by a vascular active corpus luteum (Figure 29.13).

What is first observed is the gestational sac (day 31±1), and the visualization threshold is now established when the β-human chorionic gonadotropin (β-hCG) values have surpassed 1000 mUI.

Being able to observe in the three orthogonal planes and with 3D rendering allows observation of the exact site of implantation in the endometrium (Figures 29.14–29.21).

The gestational sac appears round or oval, perfectly delimited by an echogenic zone greater than 3 mm: the trophoblastis rim. At this time, the size of the gestational sac is 2–3 mm (Graphic 29.3).

One day later, the yolk sac appears. It is round, central, well delimited and measures 3–4 mm in diameter (day 32±1 day). It is linked through the omphalomesenteric duct to the embryo.

On day 33 (±1 day) the embryo can be seen laminar, small, wide, refringent and 2 mm in length. The yolk sac is always visible facing the ventral surface of the embryo.

In cases of multiple pregnancies, monochorial or bichorial, sacs and embryos can be observed (Figures 29.22–29.26): two sacs and two embryos in bichorionic or two embryos in one sac in cases of monoamnionic twin gestation.

Fifth week

By the end of week 5, all these structures are evident, the embryo enlarges and is connected to the yolk sac by a long and slender duct (Figures 29.27–29.29).

From the fifth week on, different organs and structures appear and will be visible according to the schedule showed in Graphics 29.4 and 29.5.

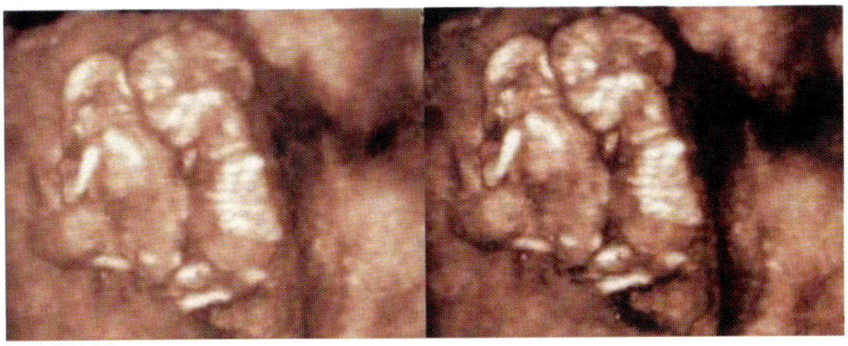

Figure 29.11 Monochorionic twin gestation at 13 weeks and 3 days. Discordant fetuses are already evident. The fetus on the left is already evident. The fetus on the left is already smaller.

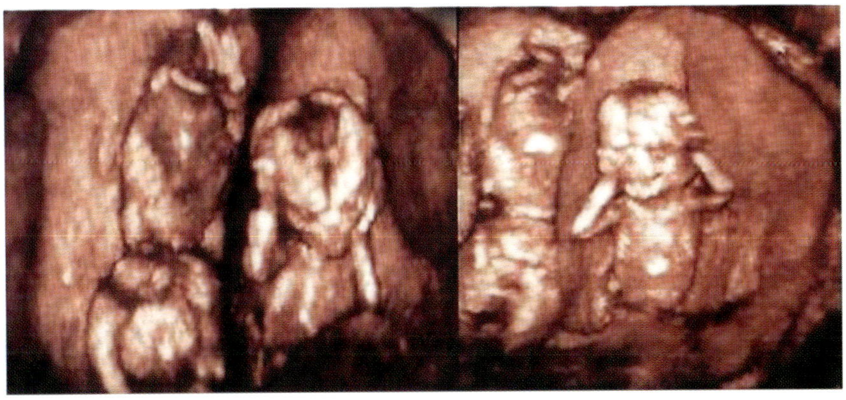

Figure 29.12 Dichorionic diamnionic twin pregnancy at 14 weeks and 5 days. Both fetuses are aligned longitudinally, one in cephalic and the other in breech position. The face, sutures and fontanelles of one of them can be observed.

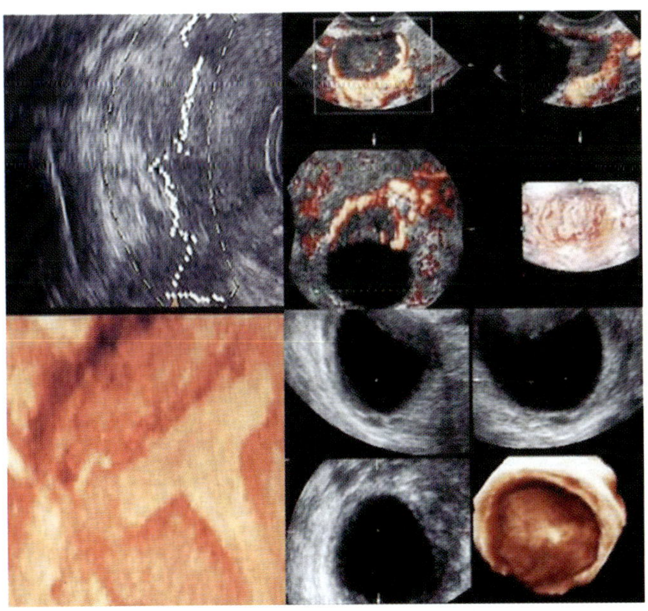

Figure 29.13 Left: 2D and 3D images of the decidua. Right: The corpus luteum with its vascularization. The gestation is not yet defined.

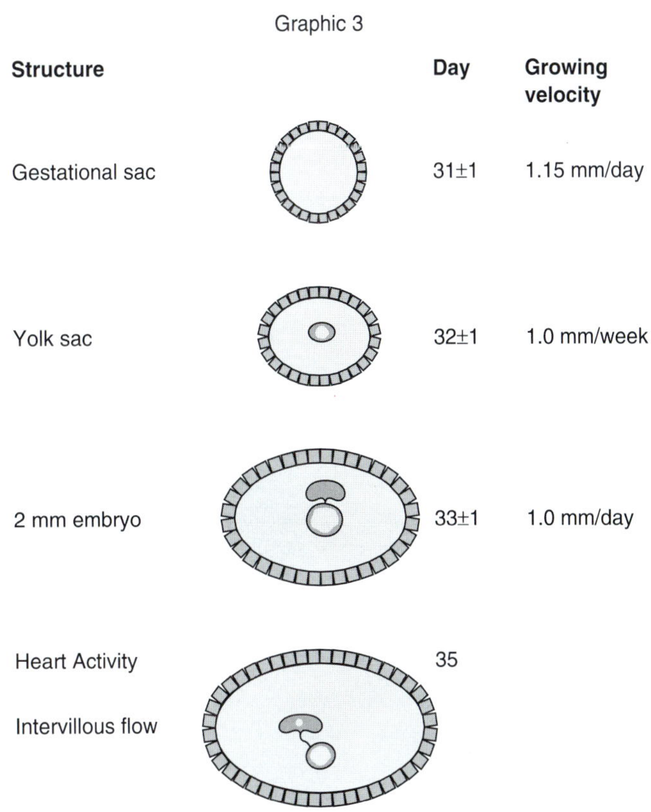

Graphic 29.3

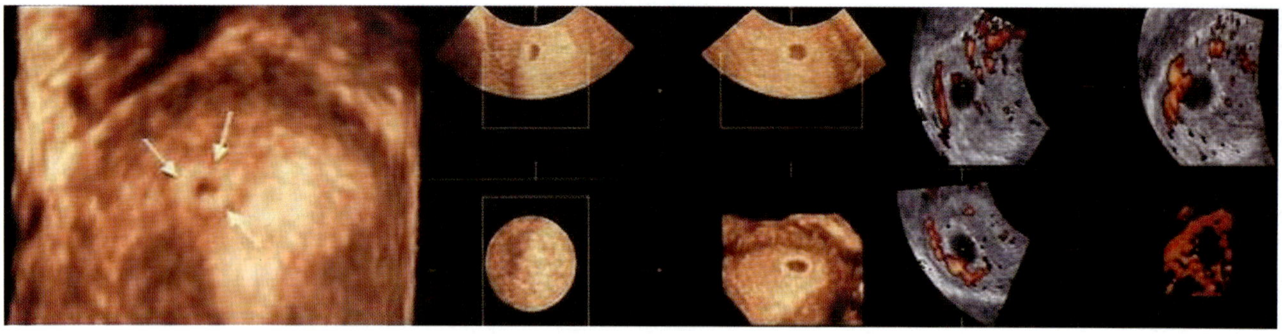

Figure 29.14 Beginning of pregnancy. Weeks 4–5. Round or oval implanted gestational sac and its vascularization.

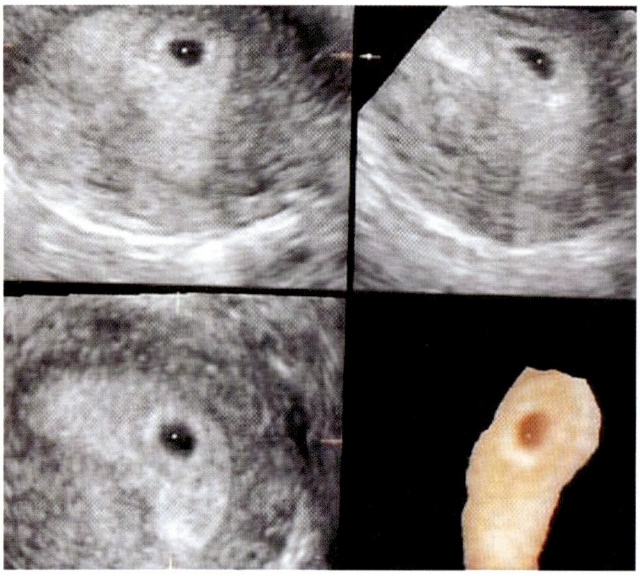

Figure 29.15 Four weeks and 3 days of pregnancy. The decidua and the gestational sac are showed. Observe the rim.

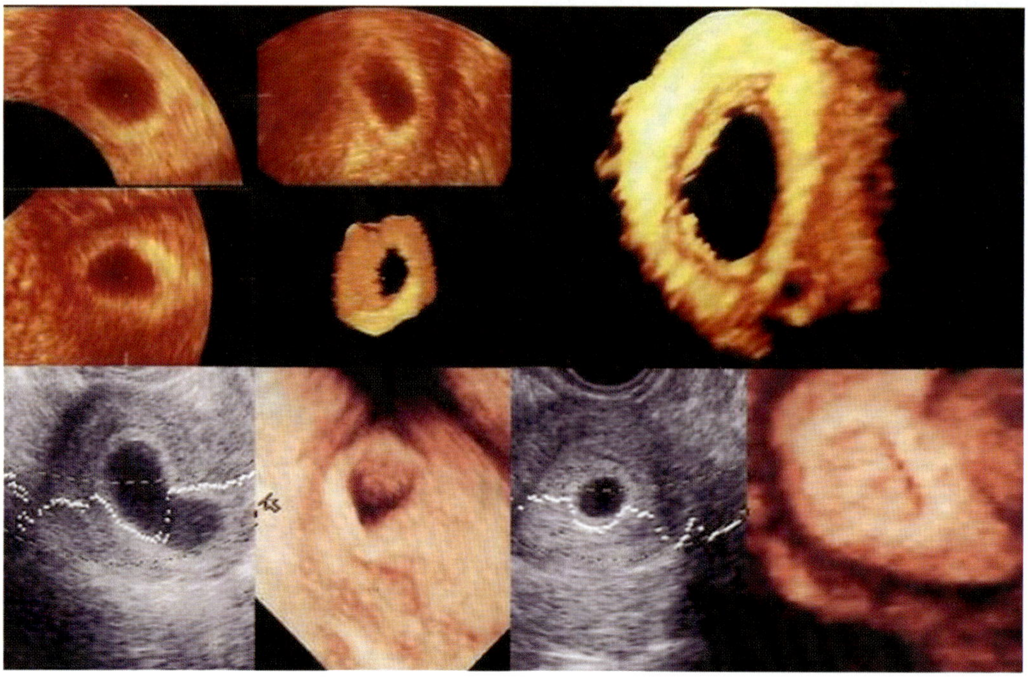

Figure 29.16 3D normal gestational sacs. The trophoblastic rim is clearly depicted and can be measured. Its thickness has to be bigger than 5 mm.

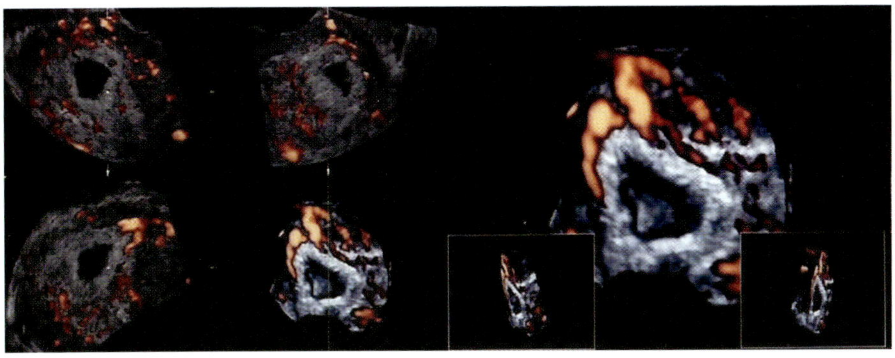

Figure 29.17 4D color Doppler of a normal gestational sac vascularization. Observe the trophoblastic rim.

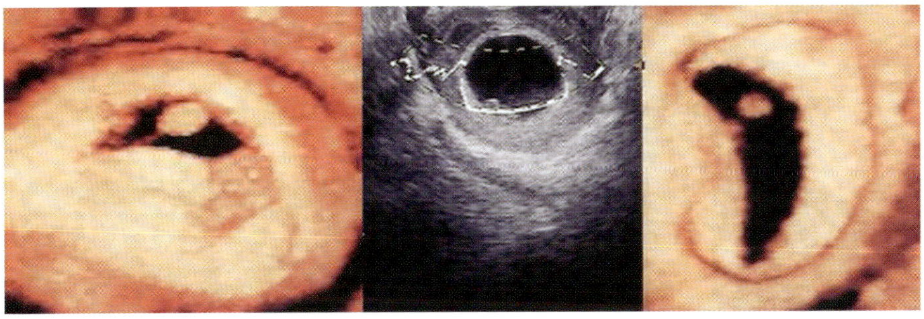

Figure 29.18 Day 32. The yolk sac appears. A small segment of the omphalomesenteric duct can be observed in the left image.

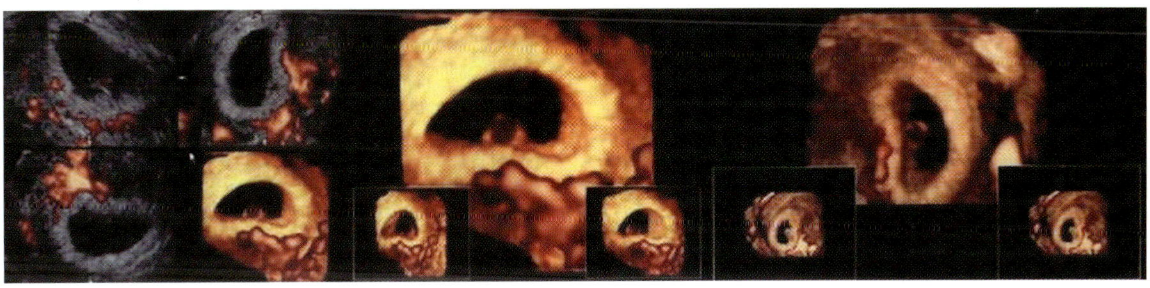

Figure 29.19 4D pictures of normal yolk sacs, gestational sacs trophoblast and vascularization.

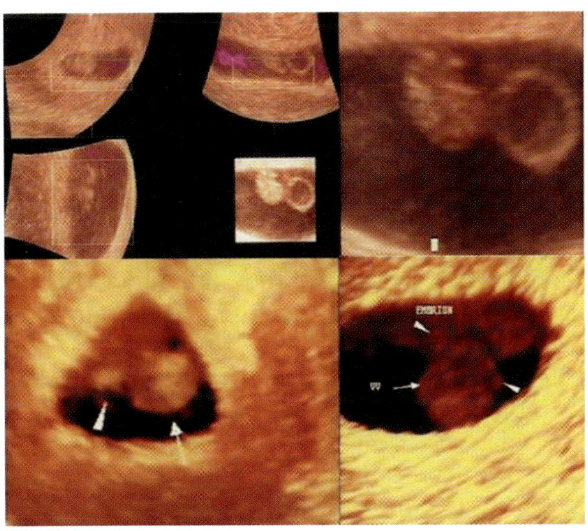

Figure 29.20 Day 33 the embryo is visible measuring 2–3 mm. The yolk sac faces the abdominal embryonic wall. The embryo's growth is very rapid, and only days after it is bigger than the yolk sac.

Sixth week

In only 1 week, the embryo enlarges, allowing the observation of two well-differentiated poles: the cranial and the caudal. Also, the limb buds can be visualized, especially the superior, which appear earlier. This finding occurs earlier than what we have seen in TV 2D US.

Another interesting finding is that at this age, in the distal portion of the caudal pole the cauda is visible. This structure is not observable with other US techniques.

In this week, it is especially remarkable to study the secundines.

The amnios appears as a very thin membrane on the surface of the dorsum of the embryo, just on the opposite side from where the yolk sac is visible. The amnion will soon surround the entire embryo, leaving out the extraembryonic mesenchyme and the yolk sac (Figures 29.30–29.33).

The yolk sac remains visible until weeks 13 to 14. It is always round and grows very slowly, 1 mm a week.

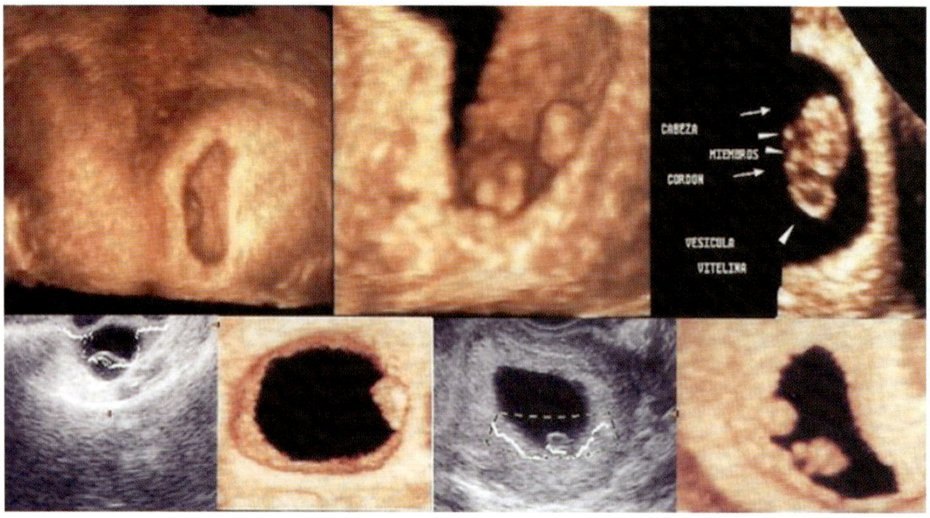

Figure 29.21 Visualization of the embryo. Days 33–35. The embryo takes a laminar form. Two poles are depicted.

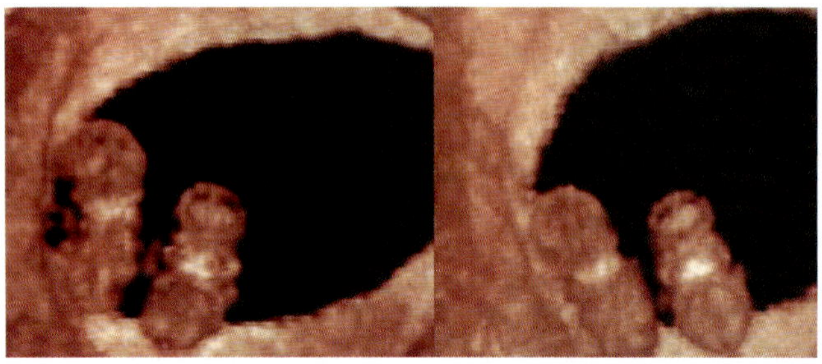

Figure 29.22 Seventh week monochorionic monoamniotic twin pregnancy.

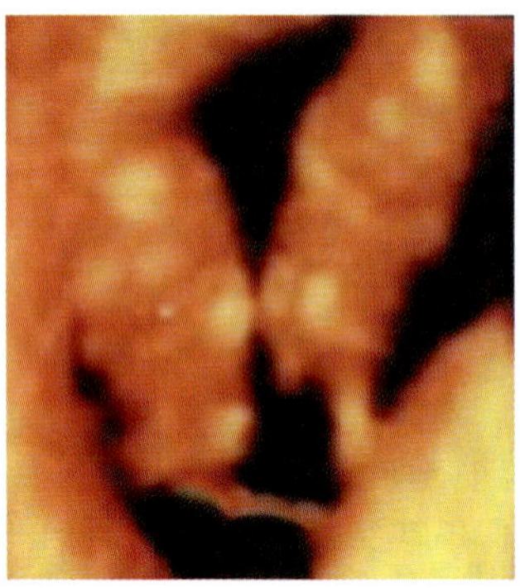

Figure 29.23 Eight-week monochorionic twin.

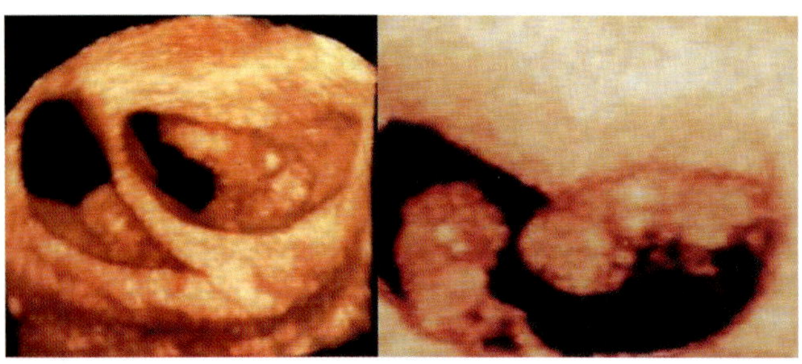

Figure 29.24 Comparison between bichorial biamniotic with lambda sign twin (left) with a monochorial monoamniotic one (right).

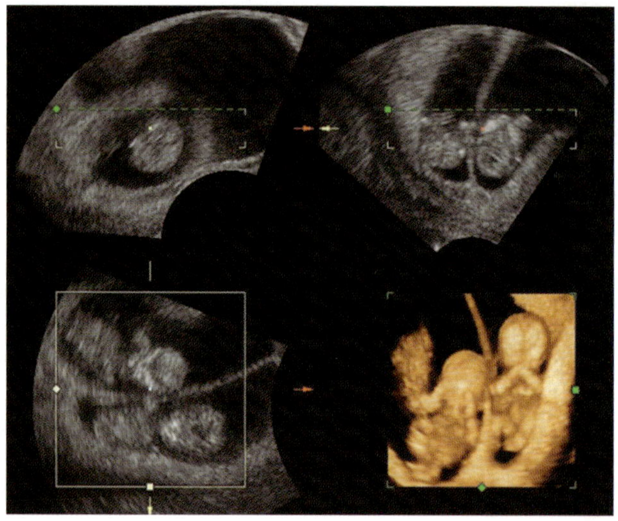

Figure 29.25 Orthogonal planes and 3D rendering of a 12th-week twin pregnancy.

As the cord forms, its anchoring site narrows and thins out.

Seventh week

The embryo clearly shows the limb buds. This detail is used to establish the gestational age (Figures 29.34 and 29.35).

The cephalic pole is flexed. It is very interesting that in the back of the embryo two parallel layers are observable, which represent the first vision of what will be the fetal spine. This finding is only visible with 2D TV US in the eighth week.

Eighth week

The configuration of the embryo is completed. The cranial pole is large and voluminous. The profile, face, orbits, mouth, jaw and maxilla can be identified.

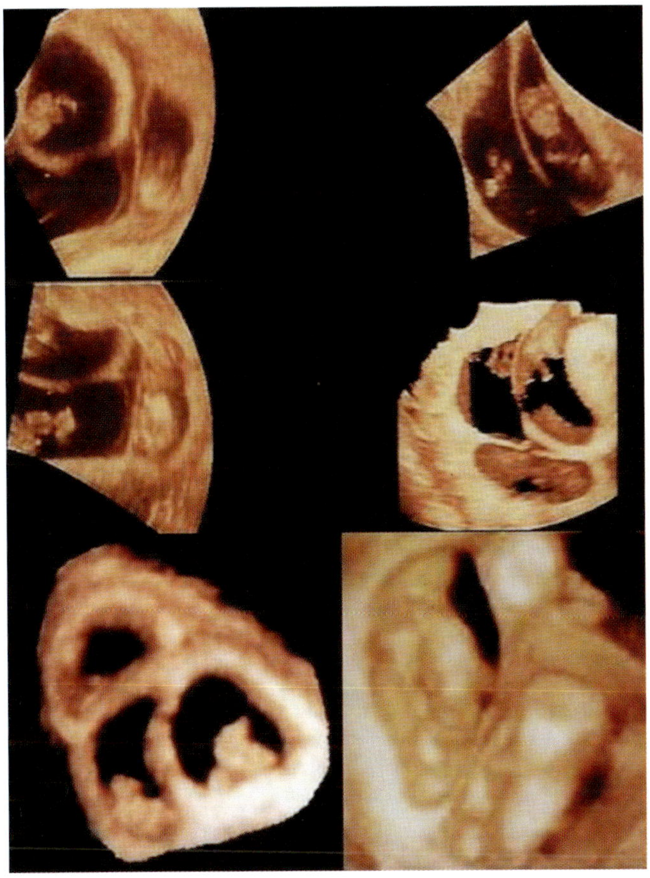

Figure 29.26 Different cases of triplets. Top: Week 10. Bottom: Weeks 6 (left) and 13 (right).

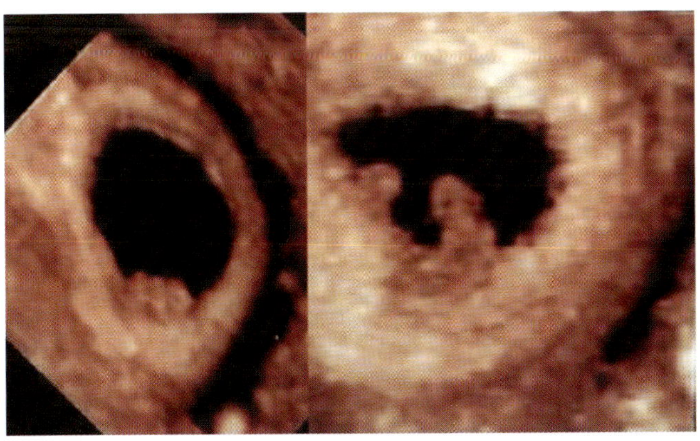

Figure 29.27 Five weeks' pregnancy. Elongated embryo with two poles. The yolk sac is visible on the left of the right image.

The caudal pole shows large limb buds with stubby ends that resemble hands and feet. Joints and articulations are visible.

The spine is completely formed, and appears as a white line in the dorsum. The superior portion (axis and atlas) still remains separate.

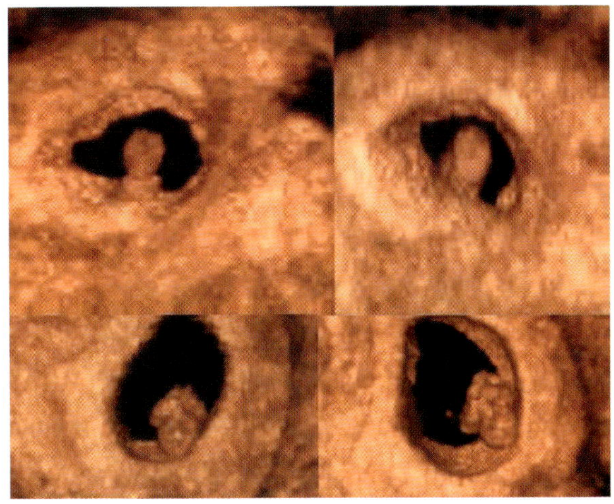

Figure 29.28 Five weeks' pregnancy. These four images show the embryo, still smaller and elongated, and the yolk sac round and facing the embryo.

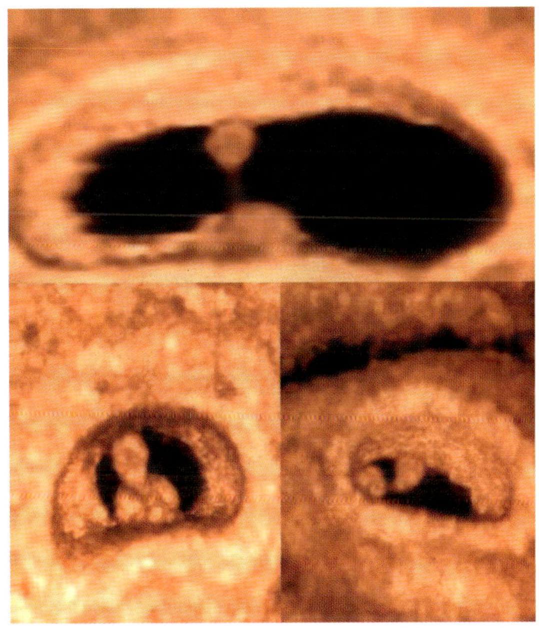

Figure 29.29 The same case as Figure 29.10. Five weeks' pregnancy showing the embryo with a thin omphalomesenteric duct linking the yolk sac.

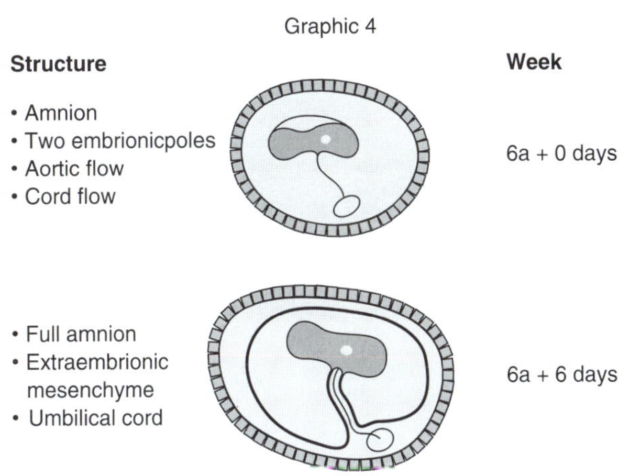

Graphic 29.4

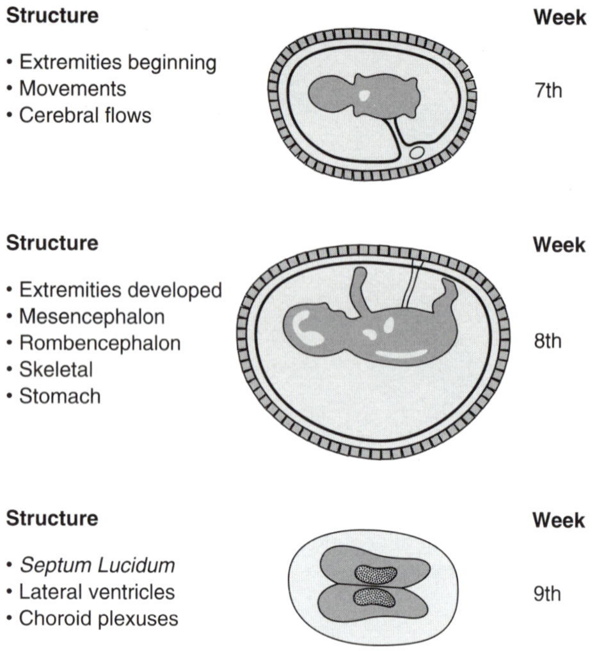

Graphic 29.5

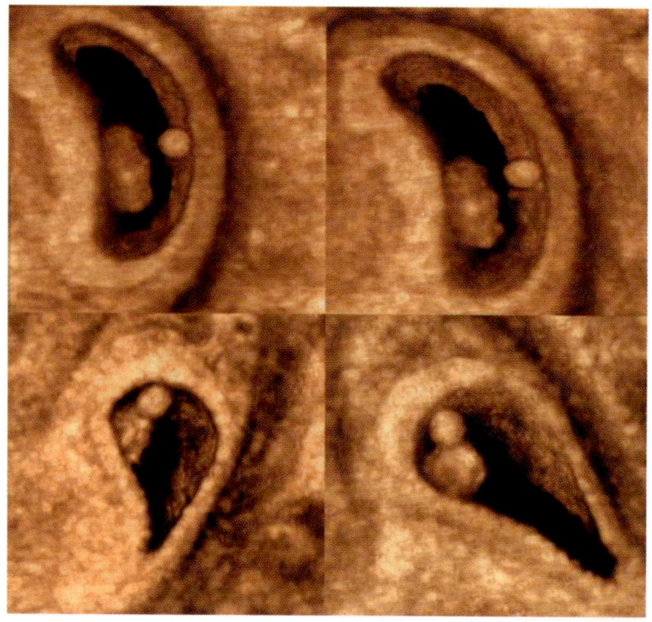

Figure 29.30 Beginning of week 6. The embryo is much bigger than in week 5, shows clearly two poles, the craneal and the caudal, and the upper and lower buds of the extremities are depicted. The cauda appears between the lower buds of the extremities.

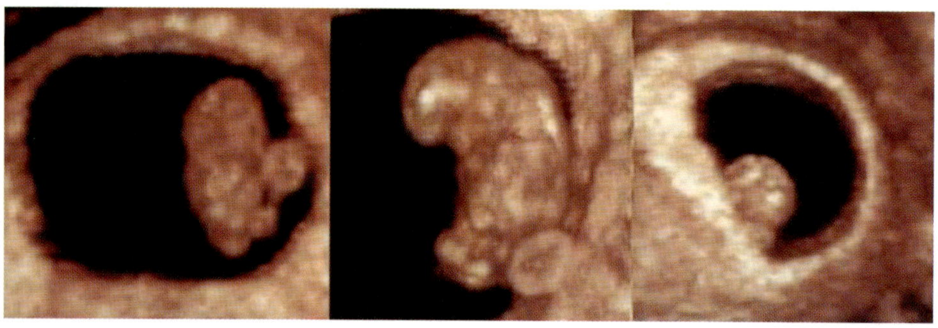

Figure 29.31 End of week 6. The embryo shows a bigger size, the cephalic pole is slightly angulated and the extremities buds are longer.

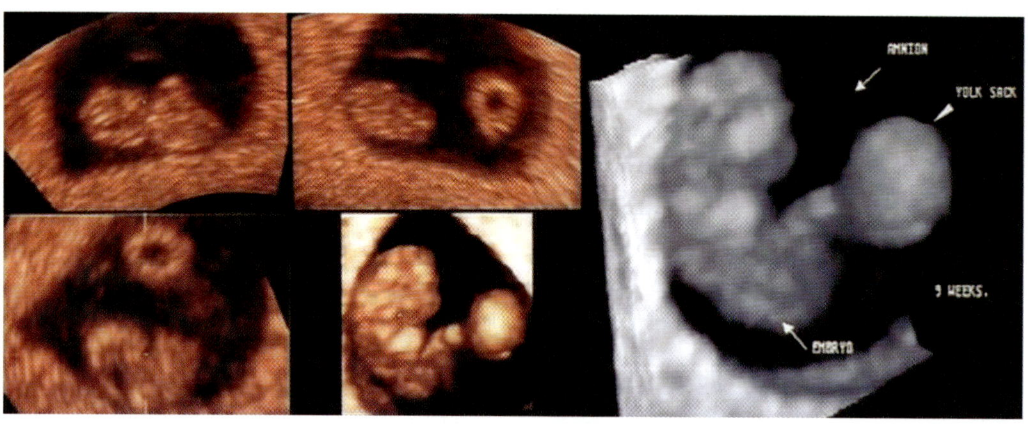

Figure 29.32 These two figures show the 3D image of the whole omphalomesenteric duct and the yolk sac in week 6.

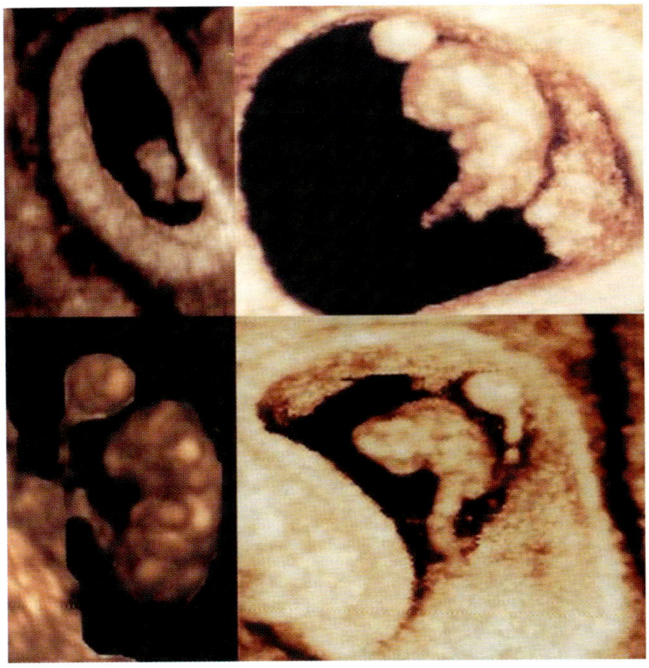

Figure 29.33 End of week 6. The embryo shows in detail the curved cephalic pole and an elongated, sometimes thick, sometimes thin but very long omphalomensenteric duct.

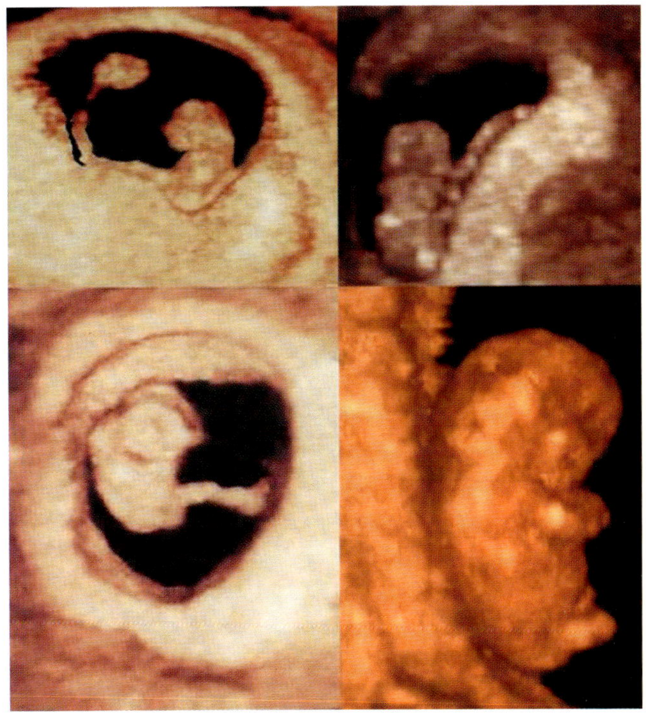

Figure 29.35 Seventh week of pregancy, fetuses showing the cauda, the buds and a very long omphalomesenteric duct.

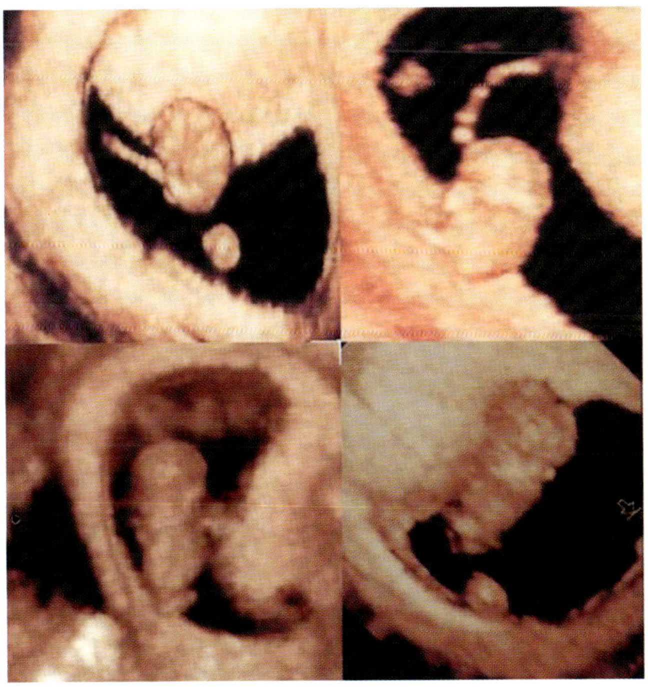

Figure 29.34 Seventh week of pregnancy. Observe the cephalic pole, the extremity buds and a long coiled umbilical cord. The yolk sac lies away from the embryo.

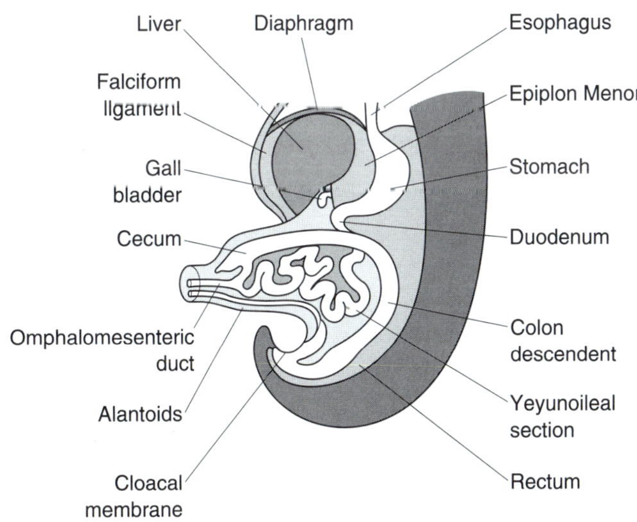

Graphic 29.6

It is important to note that during this week the physiologic herniation can be seen. It is a round and well-defined structure, refringent and linked to the abdominal wall at the site of the umbilical cord insertion (Graphic 29.6).

Its refringency is that of the abdominal wall, its size is small, less than 7 mm, and it always disappears between the 11th and the 12th weeks.

Although at this week the profile, forehead, nose and mouth are visible, they will be clearly defined by the 10th week (Figures 29.36–29.39).

Ninth week

During this week the head appears always flexed anteriorly and the finger and toe buds appear (Figures 29.40–29.42).

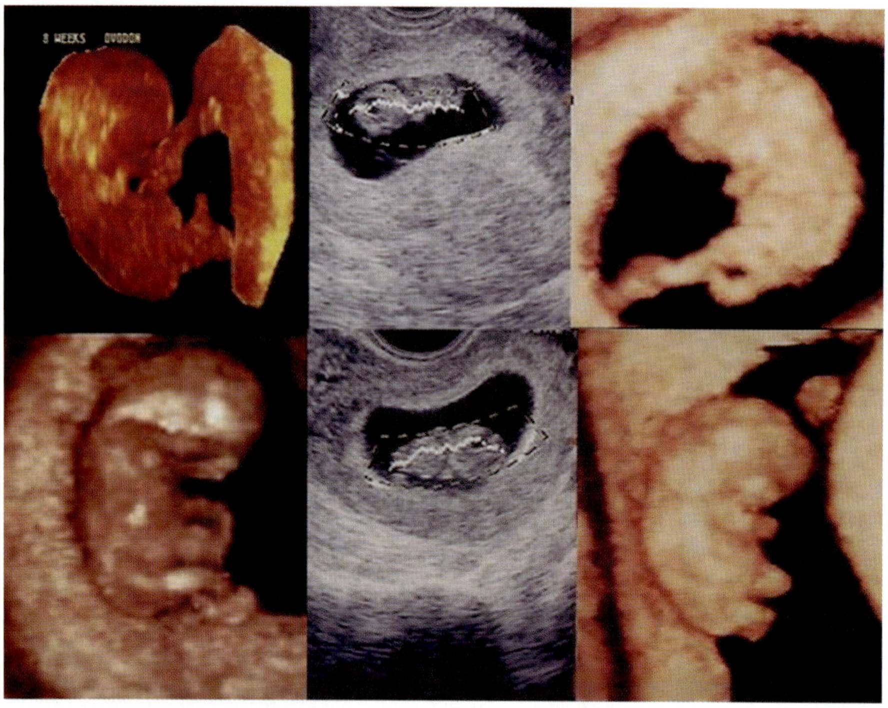

Figure 29.36 Eight weeks' pregnancy. The embryo shows full extremities. The profile can be identified. The umbilical cord is fully formed.

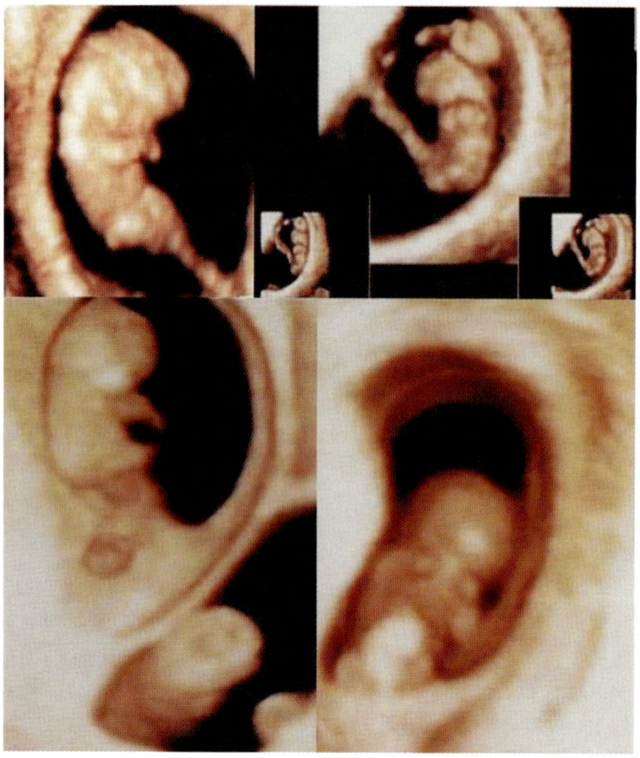

Figure 29.37 Frontal and sagittal 4D view of an eighth week embryo.

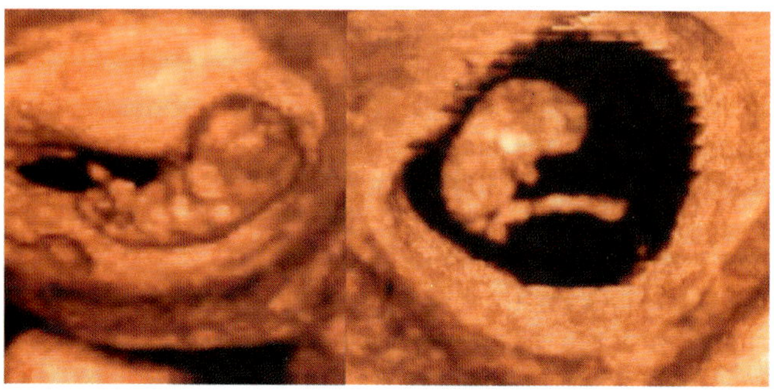

Figure 29.38 This picture shows the ossification nuclei of jaw and maxilla. The mouth is visible as well as the complete extremities.

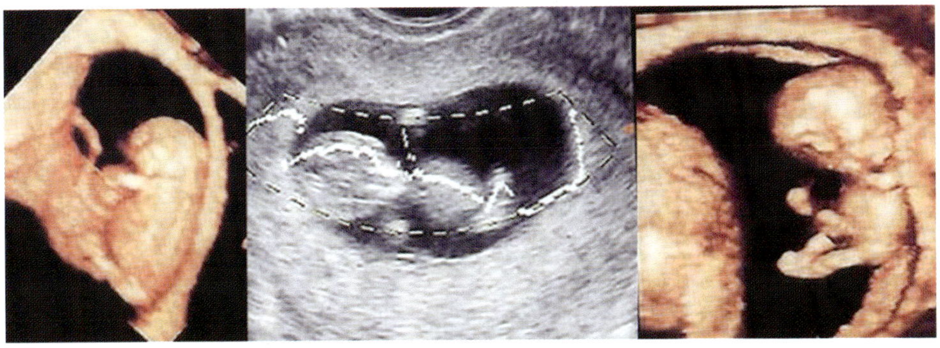

Figure 29.39 Eighth week twin pregnancy showing in both fetuses the hands and the feet.

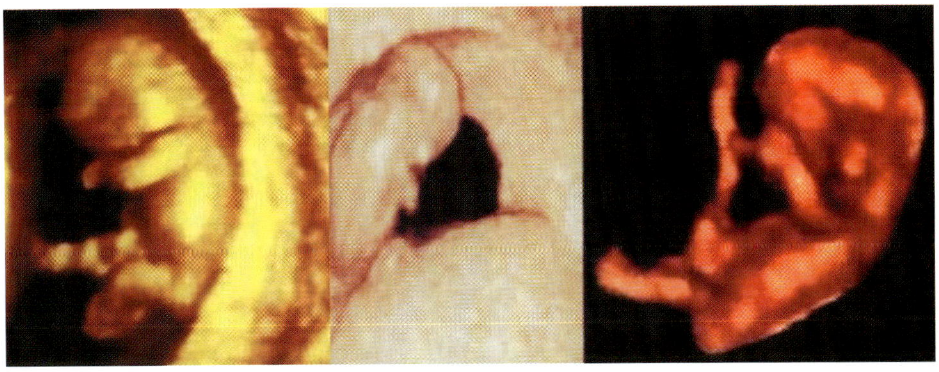

Figure 29.40 Ninth week pregnancy showing the back with the medullary canal (center), a coiled (left) and an uncoiled (right) cord and the physiological herniation (right).

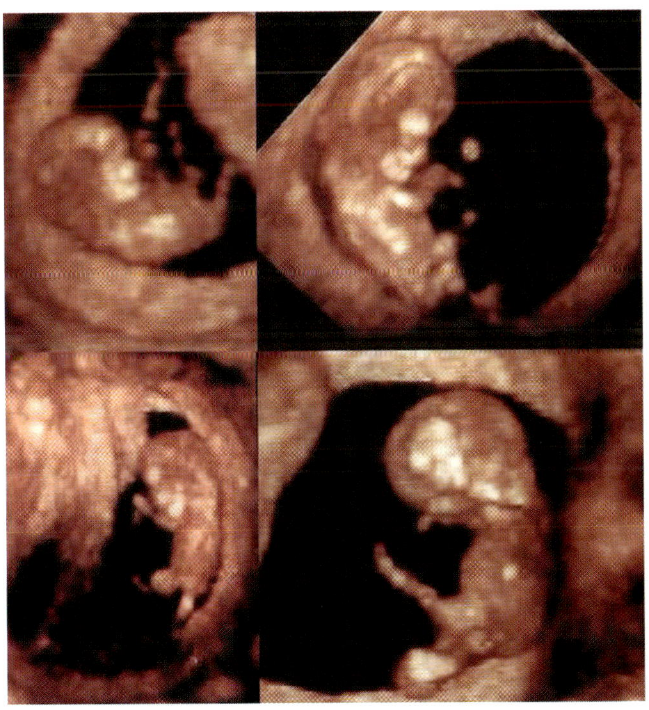

Figure 29.41 These pictures showed different varieties of normal physiological herniations. Also, the fetal profile is clearly depicted, showing the mouth, Jaw and maxilla. See the feet.

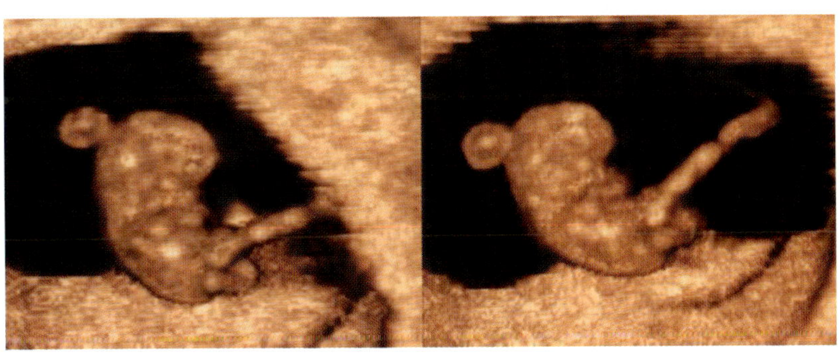

Figure 29.42 Ninth week pregnancy. The fetus shows the yolk sac near the occipital bone. The profile, eyes, abdominal wall with the physiologic herniation, extremities and umbilical cord are clearly depicted.

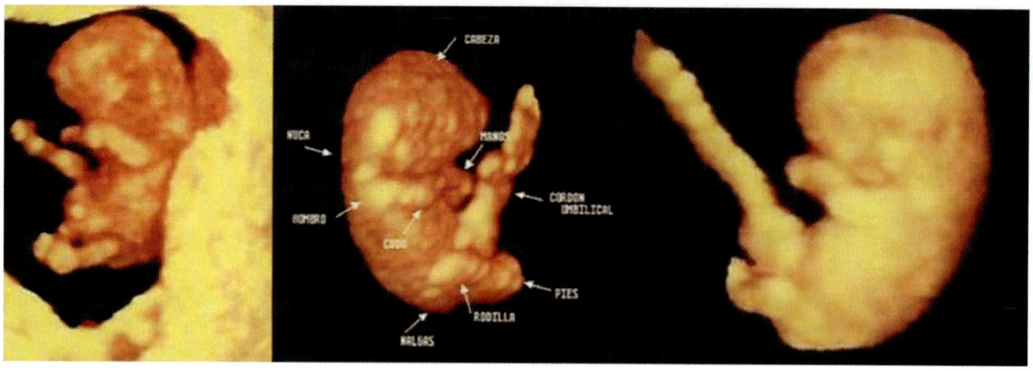

Figure 29.43 Ten-week fetuses showing a long umbilical cord with physiologic herniation. Hands and feet are visible.

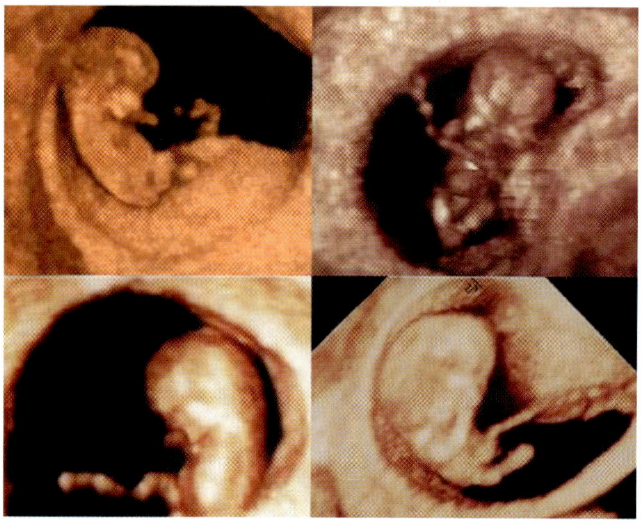

Figure 29.44 Ten weeks. Frontal and sagittal view showing the mouth, nose, supercilliary arch, hands and feet. The umbilical cord is very long and coiled.

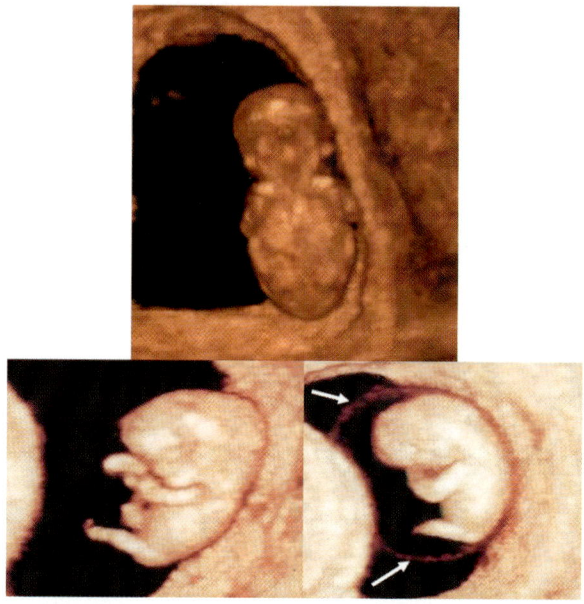

Figure 29.46 Top: Shoulder of a 10-week fetus looking at the sky. Observe the ears and the claviculae. Bottom: Ten-week normal fetus surrounded by the amnion (arrows).

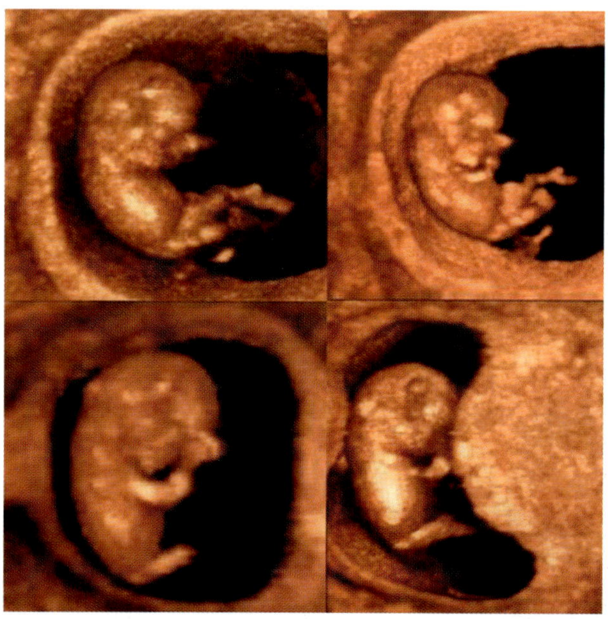

Figure 29.45 Ten weeks. The hands show the finger bones. Eyes are also visible.

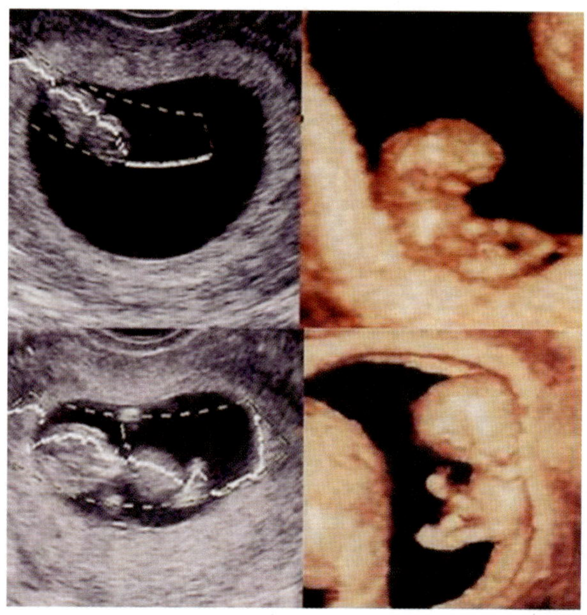

Figure 29.47 Ten weeks' pregnancy. The fetus shows the profile and the eyes and it is surrounded by the amnion (arrows). Extremities, hands and feet are clearly depicted.

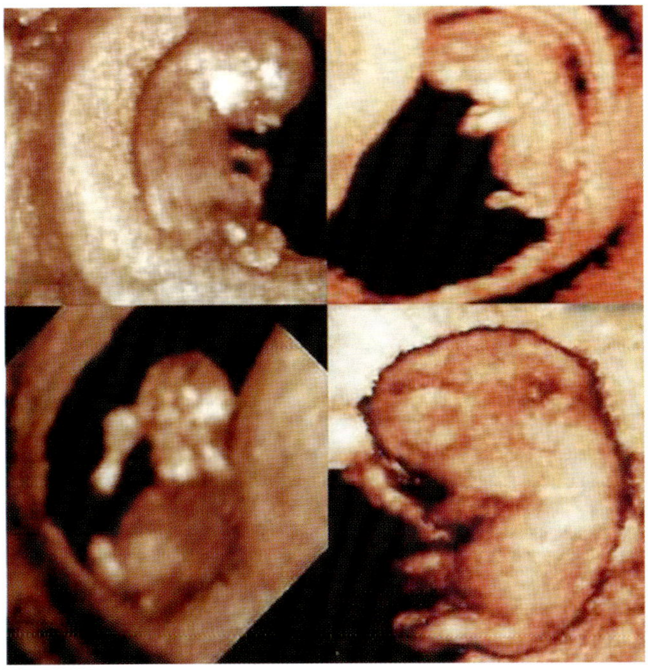

Figure 29.48 Eleventh-week fetuses. The herniation is getting smaller.

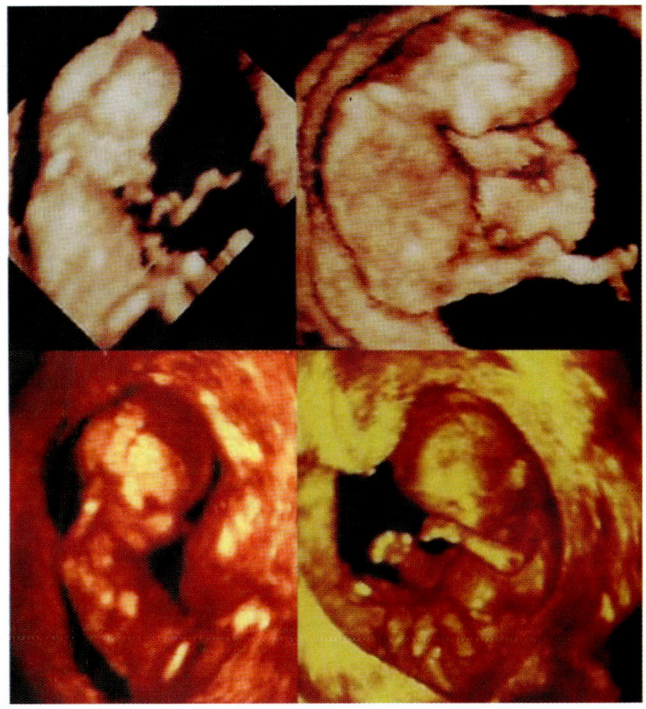

Figure 29.50 Visualization of fetuses of 13 weeks, showing intense arm and leg movements.

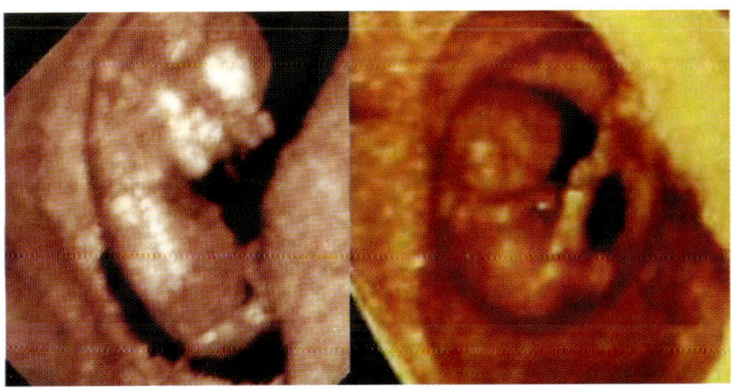

Figure 29.49 Twelve weeks. Visualization of the whole fetus, umbilical cord and placenta.

Tenth week

The fetus is completely formed. Generally, the head is flexed over the thorax, but even so, we are able to see the face with big orbits, lips, mouth, etc. We can visualize prominent fontanelles and sutures on the forehead.

On the remainder of the fetal body the arms are well developed with elbow and knee flexions as well as hands and feet visible (Figures 29.43–29.46).

The umbilical cord is very long and thick, proportionally larger and thicker than at the end of the pregnancy. By using the transparency system, we can observe for the first time, and identify, the femur, tibia, fibula, humors, radius and ulna. At the beginning of the 11th week the superciliar arch, the orbits, eyes, forehead, nose, ears and jaw can be observed (Figures 29.44, 29.45 and 29.47).

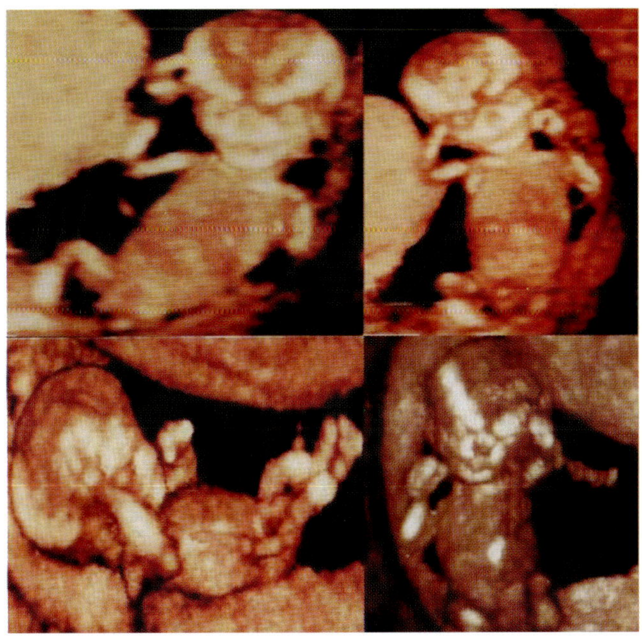

Figure 29.51 Frontal view of 13th-week fetuses showing the development of the face. Special details can be observed from the development of the nose, eyes and mouth.

Other organs and structures

The fingers and toes are clearly observed in the 11th and 12th weeks, and are better defined than what is seen with 2D TV US (Figures 29.48 and 29.49).

It is of interest to note how these structures move independently. It is possible to notice that the thumb

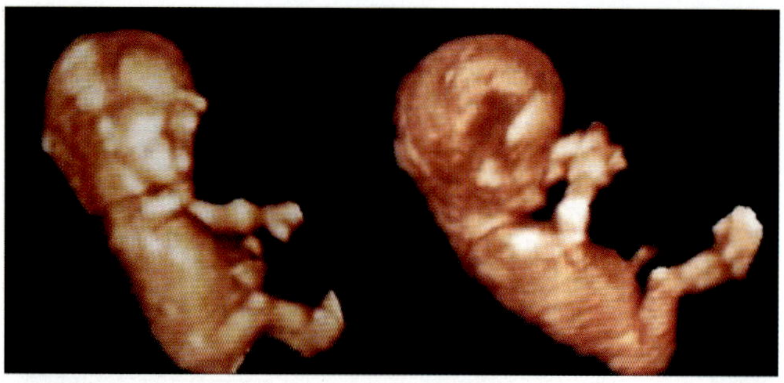

Figure 29.52 4D 13th-week fetus showing completely developed arms and legs.

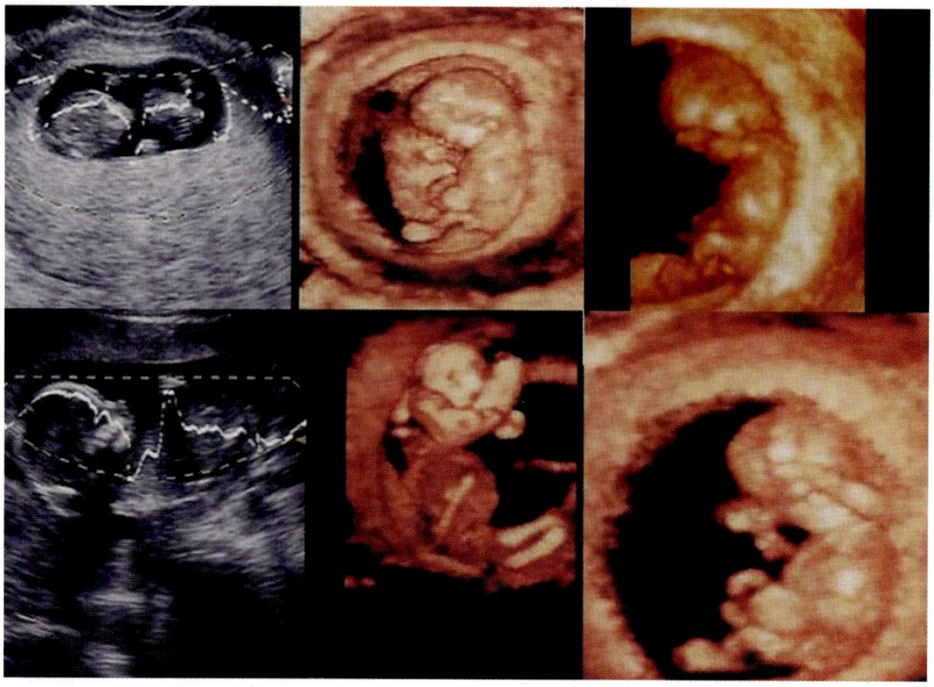

Figure 29.53 3D and 4D visualization of 13th-week fetuses. The herniation has disappeared. The femur, tibia and ulna are visible.

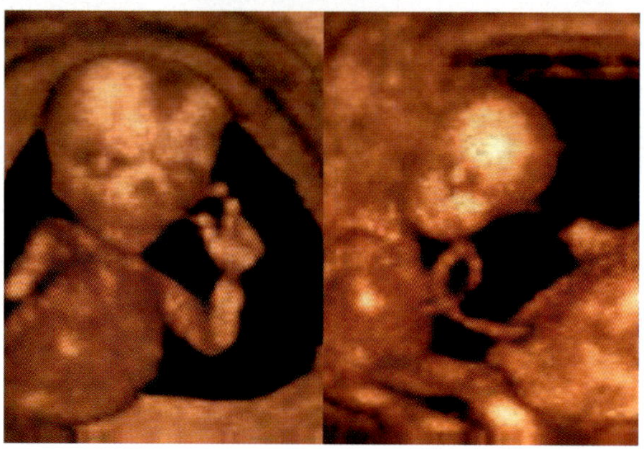

Figure 29.54 Fourteenth-week fetuses showing the face, the fingers and the palm, as well as the arm bones.

apposes the other fingers. The phalanges can be observed in the fingers and toes (Figure 29.54).

Although we have observed movement since the seventh week, by the eighth week we can observe the fetus flexing its arms and legs across the abdomen. These movements, as well as others like opening and closing the mouth, etc., are better observed by using the 4D system available today (Figure 29.50).

We consider the use of the transparency and x-ray systems essential for the study of the spine and pelvic bones after week 12. In this way, the medullary canal, the vertebrae and the ossification nuclei in the ribs can be visualized. It is important to remember that the high portion of the spine is not completely closed until the end of week 12 (axis and atlas). This is of great importance for cases of hygroma colli (see the corresponding chapter), and we think that this will also serve in the future for early diagnosis of neural tube defects (Figure 29.56).

At the same time, the ribs can be seen, the principal pelvic bones (ischium and ilium) and their ossification. All of this will be useful to measure the intervertebral spaces.

Normally, fetuses are flexed, and cover their faces with their hands. But after the 10th week, they can deflex, showing in this manner their faces. The orbits and eyes are more visible and the lids are evident (Figures 29.51–29.58).

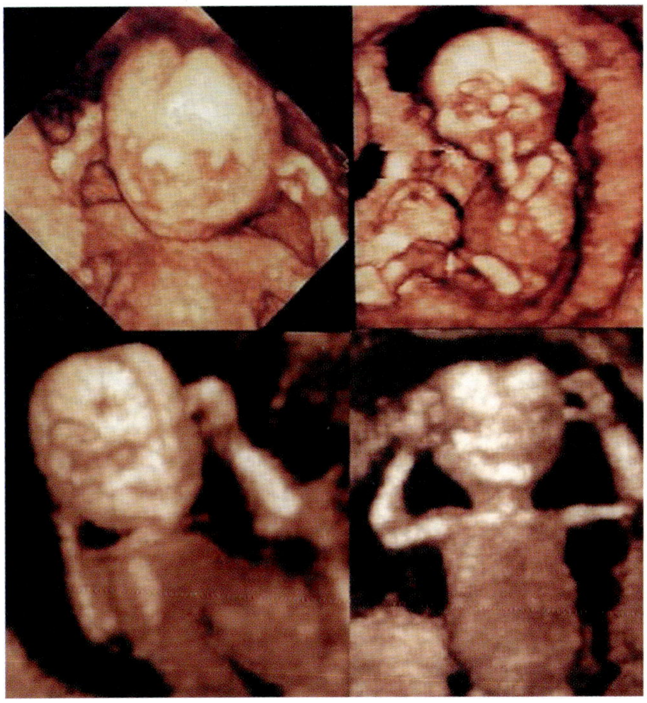

Figure 29.55 Fourteenth-week fetuses showing the whole face.

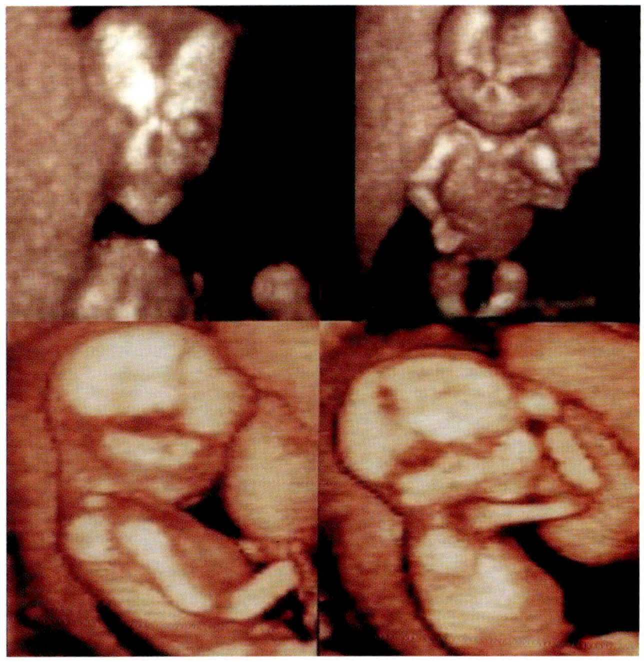

Figure 29.57 Frontal and sagittal view of fetuses between weeks 14 and 16 showing the development of the whole skull. See the clear view of all bones and sutures.

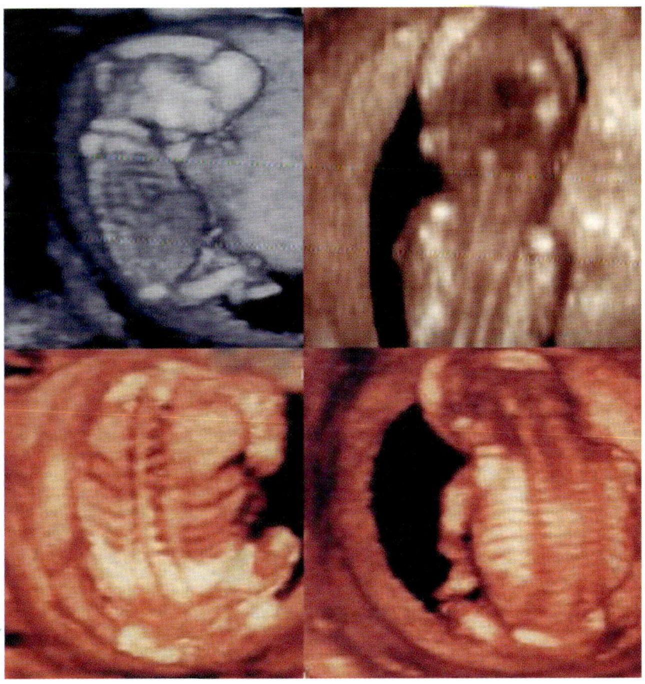

Figure 29.56 Either the use of the transparence system or introducing the ROI into the thorax allows study of the thoracic cage, ribs, vertebrae and medullary channel.

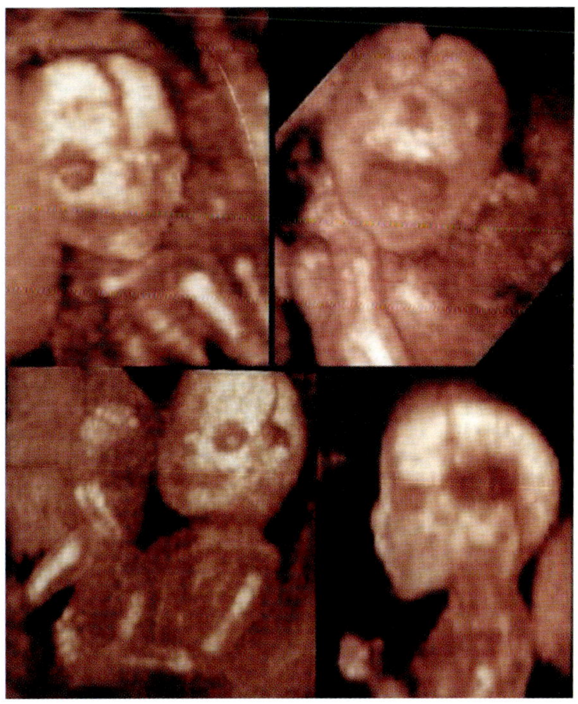

Figure 29.58 Eighteen weeks' pregnancy. The upper images show a fetus with the mouth open. The bottom images show the skull bones, fontanelles and sutures.

The nose is more protuberant and is completely formed between weeks 10 and 13. The mouth, lips and jaw are perfectly defined. The sutures and fontanelles will approximate progressively (Figures 29.51, 29.53 and 29.57).

Finally, in some cases we have observed the fetal sex clearly as early as the 13th week only in male fetuses. The labia of female fetuses can occasionally be distinguished clearly during the 16th week.

REFERENCES

1. Laudy JAM, Janssen MMM, Struyk PC, Stijmen T, Wallenburg H, Wladimiroff JW. Fetal liver volume measurements by three-dimensional ultrasonography: A preliminary study. *Ultrasound Obstet Gynecol* 1998;12:93–6.
2. Lee A, Deutinger J, Bernaschek G. Voluvision: Three-dimensional ultrasonography of the fetal malformations. *Am J Obstet Gynecol* 1994;170:1312–4.
3. Achiron R. The art of ultrasound in obstetrics: From abstraction to hyper-realism (editorial). *Ultrasound Obstet Gynecol* 1995;6:1–3.
4. Baba K, Okai T, Kozuma S. Real-time processable three-dimensional fetal ultrasound. *Lancet* 1996;348:1307.
5. Bonilla-Musoles F, Raga F, Blanes J, Osborne N, Siles CH. Three-dimensional ultrasound in reproductive medicine: Preliminary report. *Hum Reprod Update* 1995;1:4 (item 21 CD ROM).
6. Bonilla-Musoles F, Raga F, Osborne N, Blanes J. Control of inserted devices (IUD's) by using three-dimensional ultrasound (3D). It is the future? *J Clin Ultrasound* 1996;24:263–7.
7. Bonilla-Musoles F, Raga F, Osborne N, Blanes J. The use of three-dimensional (3D) ultrasound for the study of normal and pathologic morphology of the human embryo and fetus: Preliminary report. *J Ultrasound Med* 1995;14:757–65.
8. Bonilla-Musoles F. Three-dimensional visualization of the human embryo: A potential revolution in prenatal diagnosis. *Ultrasound Obstet Gynecol* 1996;7:393–7.
9. Dolz N, Osborne NG, Blanes J, *et al.* Polycystic ovarian syndrome: Assessment with colour Doppler angiography and three-dimensional ultrasound. *J Ultrasound Med* 1999;18: 303–13.
10. Gregg A, Steiner H, Staudach A, Weiner CP. Accuracy of 3-D sonographic volume measurements. *Am J Obstet Gynecol* 1993; 168:348.
11. Gregg A, Steiner H, Bogner G, Staudach A, Weiner CP. The gestational sac and 3-D volumetry. *Am J Obstet Gynecol* 1993;168:348.
12. Hamper UM, Trapanatto V, Sheth S, Dejo NG, Caskey C. Three-dimensional US: Preliminary clinical experience. *Radiology* 1994;191:397–401.
13. Hata T, Aoki S, Manabe A, Hata K, Miyazaki K. Visualization of fetal genitalia by three-dimensional ultrasonography in the second and third trimesters. *J Ultrasound Med* 1998;17:137–9.
14. King DL, King DL Jr, Shao MY. Three-dimensional spatial registration and interactive display of position and orientation of real-time ultrasound images. *J Ultrasound Med* 1990;9:625–32.
15. Kirbach D, Whittingham TA. 3-D Ultrasound – The Kretztechik Voluson approach. *Eur J Ultrasound* 1994;1:85–9.
16. Lee A, Kratochwil A, Deutinger J, Bernaschek G. Three-dimensional ultrasound in diagnosing phocomelia. *Ultrasound Obstet Gynecol* 1995;5:238–40.
17. Merz E, Bahlmann F, Weber G, Macchiella O. Volume 3D-scanning. A new dimension in the evaluation of fetal malformations. *Ultrasound Obstet Gynecol* 1993;3:131–6.
18. Müller GM, Weiner CP, Yankowitz J. Three-dimensional ultrasound in the evaluation of fetal head and spine anomalies. *Obstet Gynecol* 1996;88:372–8.
19. Nelson TR, Pretorius DH. Three-dimensional ultrasound of fetal surface features. *Ultrasound Obstet Gynecol* 1992;2:166–74.
20. Nelson TR, Downey DB, Pretorius DH, Fenster A. *Three-Dimensional Ultrasound.* Philadelphia: Lippincott Williams and Wilkins, 1999.
21. Pretorius DH, Nelson TR. Prenatal visualization of cranial sutures and fontanelles with three-dimensional ultrasonography. *J Ultrasound Med* 1994;13:871–6.
22. Pretorius DH, Nelson TR. Three-dimensional ultrasound. *Ultrasound Obstet Gynecol* 1995;5:219–21.
23. Raga F, Bonilla-Musoles F, Blanes J, Bailao LA, Osborne N. Uterine anomalies with three-dimensional ultrasound (Müllerian duct malformations). *Assoc Reprod Rev* 1996;6:126–41.
24. Rempen A. The shape of the endometrium evaluated with three-dimensional ultrasound: An additional predictor of extrauterine pregnancy. *Hum Reprod* 1998;13:450–4.
25. Riccabona M, Johnson D, Pretorius DH, Nelson TR. Three-dimensional ultrasound: Display modalities in the fetal spine and thorax. *Eur J Radiol* 1995;22:141–5.
26. Rotten D, Billon C, Rua P. Three-dimensional ultrasound imaging of the female breast and human fetus in utero. Preliminary results. *Ultrasound Imaging* 1989;11:149–50.
27. Steiner H, Gregg AR, Bogner G, Weiner CP, Staudach A. First trimester 3-D ultrasound volumetry of the gestational sac. *Ultrasound Obstet Gynecol* 1993;3(s):168.
28. Steiner H, Staudach A, Spitzer D, Schaffer HI. Three-dimensional ultrasound in obstetrics and gynecology; technique, possibilities and limitations. *Hum Reprod* 1994;9:1773–8.
29. Sohn CH, Rudofsky G. Die dreidimensionale Ultraschall-diagnostik. Ein neues Verfahren für die klinische Rourine? *Ultraschall Klin Prax* 1989;4:219–24.
30. Sohn CH, Grotepass J. Die 3 dimensionale Organdatstellung mittels Ultraschall. *Ultraschall Med* 1990;11:295–301.
31. Sohn C;Stolz W, Nuber B, Hesse A, Hornung B. Die dreidimensionale Ultraschalldiagnostik in Gynäkologie und Geburtshilfe. *Geburtsh Frauenheilk* 1991;51:335–40.
32. Sohn C, Bastert G. Dreidimensionale Ultraschalldatstellung. *Deutsch Med Wschr* 1992;117:467–72.
33. Sohn CH, Stolz W, Kaufmann M, Bastert G. Die dreidimensionale Ultraschalldarstellung benigner und maligner Brusttumoren. Erste klinische Erfahrungen. *Geburtsh Frauenheilk* 1992;52:520–5.
34. Sohn C, Bastert G. Die 3D-Sonographie in der pränatalen Diagnostik. *Z Geburtsh Perinatol* 1993;197:11–9.
35. Sohn C, Bastert G. *Dreidimensionale Ultraschalldiagnostik.* Heidelber: Springer Publishers, 1994.
36. Sohn C, Bastert G. The technical requirements of stereoscopic three-dimensional ultrasound imaging. *Sonoace Int* 1996;3:16–25.
37. Suren A, Osmers R, Kuhn W. 3D color power angio imaging: A new method to assess intracervical vascularization in benign and pathological conditions. *Ultrasound Obstet Gynecol* 1998;11:133–7.
38. Tan SL. Clinical applications of Doppler and three-dimensional ultrasound in assisted reproductive technology. *Ultrasound Obstet Gynecol* 1999;13:153–6.
39. Tulandi T, Watkin K, Tan SL. Reproductive performance and three-dimensional ultrasound volume determination of polycystic ovaries following laparoscopic ovarian drilling. *Int J Fertil Womens Med* 1997;42:436–40.
40. Ulm MR, Kratochwil A, Ulm B, Solar P, Aro G, Bernaschek G. Three-dimensional ultrasound evaluation of fetal tooth germs. *Ultrasound Obstet Gynecol* 1998;12:240–3.
41. Van Wymersch, Favre R. Interét de l'échographie tridimensionnelle en Obstétrique et Gynécologie. *Ref Gynecol Obstet* 1995;3:82–7.
42. Watkin KL, Khalife S, Nuwayhid B, *et al.* Three-dimensional reconstruction of freehand abdominal and vaginal ultrasonic images. *Ultrasound Obstet Gynecol* 1993;3(s):185.
43. Weber G, Merz E, Bahlmann F, Macchiella D. Sonographische Beurteilung von Ovarialtumoren- Vergleich zwischen trans-vaginaler 3D-Technik und konventioneller 2dimensionaler Vaginosonographie. *Ultraschall Med* 1997;18:26–30.
44. Weinraub Z, Maymon R, Shulman A, *et al.* Three-dimensional saline contrast hysterosonography and surface rendering of uterine cavity pathology. *Ultrasound Obstet Gynecol* 1996;8:277–82.
45. Wisser J, Schar J, Kurmanavicius J, Huch R, Huch A. Anwendung von 3D-Ultraschall als neuer Weg zur Bestimmung von Geburtstraumen am Beckenboden. *Ultraschall Med* 1999;19:15–8.
46. Wu MH, Hsu CC, Huang KE. Detection of congenital Müllerian duct anomalies using three-dimensional ultrasound. *J Clin Ultrasound* 1997;25:487–92.
47. Zarca D, Bady J, Levaillant JM, Rotten D. Des images et des nombres. *Gynecol Int* 1996;5:6–10.
48. Zosmer N, Jurkovic K, Gruboeck K, Geipel A, Jauniaux E, Campbell S. Three-dimensional fetal echocardiography: The identification of arterial connections on planar reformatted sections. *Ultrasound Obstet Gynecol* 1994;4(s):359.
49. Zosmer N, Jurkovic D, Jauniaux E, Gruoeck K, Lees C, Campbell S. Selection and identification of standard cardiac views from three-dimensional volume scans of the fetal thorax. *J Ultrasound Med* 1996;15:25–32.
50. Bonllla-Musoles F, Machado L. *Ultrasonidos y Reproducción.* Madrid: Panamericana Ed., 2000.
51. Bonilla-Musoles F. *Ecografia Vaginal, Doppler y Tridimensional.* Madrid: Panamericana Ed., 2000.
52. Andrist LA, Katz VI, Elijah R. Developing a plan for routine 3D surface rendering in Obstetrics. *J Def Model Simul* 2001;17:16–21.
53. Andrist LA, Katz VI, Elijah R. Visualization of fetal anomalies with surface 3-dimensional ultrasound: A case study. *J Def Model Simul* 2001;17:88–93.

54. Axt-Flietner R, Hendrick HJ, Ertan K, Remberguer R, Smith W. Course and outcome of a pregnancy with a giant fetal cervical teratoma diagnosed prenatally. *Ultrasound Obstet Gynecol* 2001;18:543–6.
55. Baba K, Ishihara O, Hayashi N, Saito M, Taya J, Kinoshita K. Three-dimensional ultrasound in embryo transfer. *Ultrasound Obstet Gynecol* 2000;16:372–3.
56. Bahlmann F. Three-dimensional color power angiography of an aneurysm of the vein of Galen. *Ultrasound Obstet Gynecol* 2000;15:341.
57. Bega G, Kuhlman K, Lev-Toaff A, Kurtz A, Wapner R. Application of three-dimensional ultrasonography in the evaluation of the fetal heart. *J Ultrasound Med* 2001;20:307–13.
58. Bonilla-Musoles F, Raga F, Blanes J, Navarro J, Machado L, Osborne N. Current status of three dimensional ultrasound in reproductive medicine. *Middle East Fertil Soc J* 2000;5:169–77.
59. Bonilla-Musoles F, Raga F, Blanes J, Osborne N, Machado L. Ecografía tridimensional en uroginecología. *Progresos Obstet Ginecol* 2001;44:237–44.
60. Bordes A, Bory AM, Benchaid M, Rudigoz RC, Salle B. Reproducibility of transvaginal three-dimensional endometrial volume measurements with virtual organ computer-aided analysis (VOCAL) during ovarian stimulation. *Ultrasound Obstet Gynecol* 2002;19:76–80.
61. Chaoui R, Kalache KD, Hartung J. Application of three-dimensional power Doppler ultrasound in prenatal diagnosis. *Ultrasound Obstet Gynecol* 2001;17:22–9.
62. Kiyokawa K, Masuda H, Fuyuki T, *et al.* Three-dimensional hysterosalpingo-contrast sonography (3D-HyCoSy) as an outpatient procedure to assess infertile women: A pilot study. *Ultrasound Obstet Gynecol* 2000;16:648–54.
63. Lee W, Deter R, Ebersole J, Huang R, Blanckaert K, Romero R. Birth weight prediction by three-dimensional ultrasonography: Fractional limb volume. *J Ultrasound Med* 2001;20:1283–92.
64. Merz E, Miric-Tesanic D, Welter C. Value of the electronic scalpel (cut mode) in the evaluation of the fetal face. *Ultrasound Obstet Gynecol* 2000;16:564–8.
65. Platt LD. Three-dimensional ultrasound, 2000. *Ultrasound Obstet Gynecol* 2000;16:295–8.
66. Poehl M, Hohlagschwandtner R, Doerner V, Dillinger B, Feischtinger W. Cumulus assessment by three-dimensional ultrasound for in-vitro fertilization. *Ultrasound Obstet Gynecol* 2000;16:251–3.
67. Raine-Fenning N, Campbell B, Collier J, Brincat M, Johson I. The reproducibility of endometrial volume acquisition and measurements with the VOCAL imaging program. *Ultrasound Obstet Gynecol* 2002;19:69–75.
68. Bernaschek G, Deutinger J. Voluvision fetaler Fehlbindungen. *Ultraschall Klin Prax* 1993;8:154–7.
69 Bonilla-Musoles F, Raga F, Blanes J, *et al.* A tridimensao ecografica em obstetricia e ginecologia: Futuro da nosa especialidade? *Ginecol Obstet Attual (Brazil)* 1995;7:29–45.
70. Bonilla-Musoles F, Raga F, Osborne N, Blanes J. La triple dimensión ecográfica en el estudio del embrión y del feto normales durante el primer trimestre del embarazo e inicio del segundo. In Carrera JM, Kurjak A, eds. *Medicina del embrión.* Barcelona: Masson, 1997:163–88.
71. Bonilla-Musoles F, Raga F, Osborne N, Blanes J, Coelho F. Three-dimensional hysterosonography (3D-HSSG), for the study of endometrial tumors; comparison with conventional transvaginal sonography, hysterosalpingosonography and hysteroscopy. *Gynecol Oncol* 1997;65:245–52.
72. Bonilla-Musoles F, Raga F, Villalobos A, Osborne N, Blanes J. First-trimester neck abnormalities: Three-dimensional evaluation. *J Ultrasound Med* 1998;17:419–26.
73. Bonilla-Musoles F, Raga F, Bonilla F Jr, Blanes J, Osborne NG. Early diagnosis of conjoined twins using two-dimensional color Doppler and three-dimensional ultrasound. 1998;90:552–6.
74. Devonald KJ, Ellwood D, Griffiths K, *et al.* Volume imaging: Three-dimensional appreciation of the fetal head and face. *J Ultrasound Med* 1995;14:919–26.
75. Jurkovic D, Jauniaux E, Campbell S. Three-dimensional ultrasound in obstetrics and gynecology. In Kurjak A, Chervenak FA, eds. *The Fetus as a Patient.* Carnforth, UK: Parthenon Publishing Group, 1995:135–40.
76. Kuo HC, Chang FM, Wu CH, Yao BL, Uu CH. The primary application of three-dimensional ultrasonography in obstetrics. *Am J Obstet Gynecol* 1992;166:880–6.
77. Kupesic S, Kurjak A. Septate uterus: Detection and prediction of obstetrical complications by different forms of ultrasonography. *J Ultrasound Med* 1998;17:631–6.
78. Kyei-Mensah A, Maconochie N, Zaidi J, Pittrof R, Campbells UN, Tan S. Transvaginal three-dimensional ultrasound: Reproducibility of ovarian and endometrial volume measurements. *Fertil Steril* 1996;66:718–22.
79. Machado LE, Bonilla-Musoles F, Chamusca L, *et al.* Diagnóstico de toracópagos mediante el empleo de ecografía tridimensional. *Obstet Ginecol Esp* 1999;8:19–27.
80. Maymon R, Halperin R, Weinraub Z, Herman A, Schneider O. Three-dimensional transvaginal sonography of conjoined twins at 10 weeks: A case report. *Ultrasound Obstet Gynecol* 1998; 11:292–4.
81. Matsumi H, Kozuma S, Baba K, *et al.* Three-dimensional ultrasound is useful in diagnosing the fetus with abdominal wall defects. *Ultrasound Obstet Gynecol* 1996;8:356–8.
82. Pretorius DH, Nelson TR, Baergen R. 3-Dimensional ultrasound and power Doppler imaging of placental vasculature (abstract). *Acad Radiol* 1995;2:1154.
83. Pretorius DH, Nelson TR. Three-dimensional ultrasound in gynecology and obstetrics. A review. *Ultrasound Q* 1998;14: 218–33.
84. Meyer-Wittkopf M, Rappe N, Sierra F, Barth H, Schmidt S. Three-dimensional (3-D) ultrasonography for obtaining the four and five chamber view: Comparison with cross-sectional (2-D) fetal sonographic screening. *Ultrasound Obstet Gynecol* 2000; 15:397–402.
85. Blaas H-G, Eik-Nes SH, Kiserud T, Berg S, Angelsen B, Olstad B. Three-dimensional imaging of the brain cavities in human embryos. *Ultrasound Obstet Gynecol* 1995;5:228–32.
86. Chevernak A, Kurjak A, Comstock CH. *Ultrasound and the Fetal Brain.* Progress in Obstetric and Gynecological Sonography Series. Lancashire, UK: The Parthenon Publishing Group, 1995: 221–36.
87. Fujiwaki R, Hata T, Hata K, Kitao M. Intrauterine sonographic assessments of embryonic development. *Am J Obstet Gynecol* 1995;173:1770–4.
88. Kelly IMG, Gardener JE, Brett AD, Richards RR, Lees WR. Three-dimensional US of the fetus. Work in progress. *Radiology* 1994;192:253–9.
89. Liang RI, Huang SE, Chang FM. Prenatal diagnosis of ectopia cordis at 10 weeks of gestation using two-dimensional and three-dimensional ultrasonography. *Ultrasound Obstet Gynecol* 1997; 10:137–9.
90. Lin MT, Chen GD, Lin LY, Lee MS. Measurements of follicle size and the volume of follicular fluid by 3-dimensional ultrasound scanning compared with aspirated findings in IVF programs. *J Obstet Gynecol Rep China* 1991;30:47–50.
91. Ludomirski A, Khandelwal M, Uerpairojkit B, Reece EA, Chan L. Three-dimensional ultrasound evaluation of fetal facial and spinal anatomy. *Am J Obstet Gynecol* 1996;Suppl 174:318.
92. Merz E, Weber G, Macchiella O, Bahlmann F. 3D-Volumensonographie in der transvaginalen Diagnostik. *Ultraschall Klin Prax* 1993;8:154–62.
93. Merz E, Bahlmann AF, Weber G. 3D-Volumensonographie in der transvaginalen Diagnostik. *Med Bild* 1994;8:43–51.
94. Merz E, Weber G, Bahlmann AF, Macchiella O. Transvaginale 3D-Sonographie in der Gynakologie. *Der Gynäkol* 1995;28: 270–5.
95. Merz E, Balhmann F, Weber G. Three dimensional ultrasonography in prenatal diagnosis. *J Perinat Med* 1995;23:213–22.
96. Merz E, Weber G, Bahlmann AF, Miric-Tesanic D. Application of transvaginal and abdominal three-dimensional ultrasound for the detection or exclusion of malformations of the fetal face. *Ultrasound Obstet Gynecol* 1997;9:237–43.
97. Merz E. Aktuelle technische Möglichkeiten der 3D-Sonographie in der Gynakologie und Geburtshilfe. *Ulltraschall Med* 1997;18: 190–5.
98. Merz E. Three-dimensional ultrasound – A requirement for prenatal diagnosis? *Ultrasound Obstet Gynecol* 1998;12:225–7.
99. Merz E, Bahlmann F, Welter C, Miric-Tesanic D. Transvaginale 3D-Sonographie in der Frühgraviditat. *Gynäkologe* 1999;32:213–9.
100. Merz E, Miric-Tesanic D, Bahlmann F, Sedlaczek H. Prenatal diagnosis of fetal ambiguous gender using three-dimensional sonographic. *Ultrasound Obstet Gynecol* 1999;13:217–8.
101. Merz E. *3-D Ultrasound in Obstetrics and Gynecology.* Philadelphia: Lippincott Williams and Wilkins, 1998.

102. Meyer-Wittkopf M, Cook A, Mclennan A, Summers P, Shar-Land GK, Maxwell DJ. Evaluation of three-dimensional ultrasonography and magnetic resonance imaging in assessment of congenital heart anomalies in fetal cardiac specimens. *Ultrasound Obstet Gynecol* 1996;8:303–8.
103. Nelson TR, Pretorius, DH. 3D-ultrasound volume measurements (abstract). *Med Phys* 1993;201:927.
104. Nelson TR, Pretorius DH, Skansky M, Hagen-Ansert S. Three-dimensional echocardiographic evaluation of fetal heart anatomy and function: Acquisition, analysis and display. *J Ultrasound Med* 1996;15:1–12.
105. Nelson TR, Pretorius DH. Visualization of the fetal thoracic skeleton with three-dimensional sonography: A preliminary report. *Am J Roentgenol* 1995;164:1485–8.
106. Pellicer A, Villalobos A, Raga F, Simon C, Ardiles J, Bonilla-Musoles F. Three-dimensional ultrasound in low responders. *Fertil Steril* 1998;70:671–5.
107. Pretorius DH, Nelson TR, Jaffe JS. Three-dimensional US of the fetus. *Radiology* 1990;177:194.
108. Schwartz G. Three-dimensional volume measurement. *Ultrasound Obstet Gynecol* 1998;11:4–5.
109. Endres LK, Cohen L. Reliability and validity of three dimensional fetal brain volumes. *J Ultrasound Med* 2001;20:1265–70.
110. Michailidis GD, Simpson JM, Tulloh R, Economides D. Retrospective prenatal diagnosis of scitimar syndrome aided by three-dimensional power Doppler imaging. *Ultrasound Obstet Gynecol* 2001;17:449–52.
111. Pretorius TH, Nelson TR, Jaffe JS. Three-dimensional sonographic analysis based on colour flow Doppler and grey scale image data. A preliminary report. *J Ultrasound Med* 1992;11: 225–32.
112. Riccabona M, Nelson TR, Pretorius DH, Davidson TE. Distance and volume measurements using three-dimensional ultrasound. *J Ultrasound Med* 1995;14:881–6.
113. Guerra FA, Isla AI, Aguilar RC, Fritz EG. Use of free-hand three-dimensional ultrasound software in the study of the fetal heart. *Ultrasound Obstet Gynecol* 2000;16:329–4.
114. Hull AD, James G, Salerno CC, Nelson T, Pretorius DH. Three-dimensional ultrasonography and assessment of the first-trimester fetus. *J Ultrasound Med* 2001;20:287–93.
115. Naylor C, Carlson D, Santulli T, Platt L. Use of three-dimensional ultrasonography for prenatal diagnosis of ambiguous genitalia. *J Ultrasound Med* 2001;20:1365–9.
116. Pretorius DH, Nelson TR. Fetal three-dimensional ultrasonography. Today or tomorrow? *J Ultrasound Med* 2001;20:283–6.
117. Schild RL, Fimmers R, Hansmman M. Fetal weight estimation by three-dimensional ultrasound. *Ultrasound Obstet Gynecol* 2000; 16:445–52.
118. Toots-Hobson P, Kuhllar V, Cardozo L. Three-dimensional ultrasound: A novel technique for investigating the urethral sphincter in the third trimester of pregnancy. *Ultrasound Obstet Gynecol* 2001;17:421–4.
119. Favre R, Nisand K, Bettahar K, Grange G, Nisand I. Measurement of limb circumference with three-dimensional ultrasound for fetal weight estimation. *Ultrasound Obstet Gynecol* 1993;3: 176–9.
120. Welsh AW, Taylor MJO, Cosgrove D, Fisk NM. Free hand three-dimensional Doppler demonstration of monochorionic vascular anastomoses in vivo: A preliminary report. *Ultrasound Obstet Gynecol* 2001;18:317–24.
121. Gruboeck K, Jurkovic D, Lawton F, Savras M, Tailor A, Campbell S. The diagnostic value of endometrial thickness and volume measurements by three-dimensional ultrasound in patients with menopausal bleeding. *Ultrasound Obstet Gynecol* 1996;8:272–6.
122. Merz E, Macchiella, D, Bahlmann F, Weber G. Three-dimensional ultrasound for the diagnosis of fetal malformations. *Ultrasound Obstet Gynecol* 1992;2:137–44.
123. Merz E. Volume (3D) scanning in the evaluation of fetal malformation. *Ultrasound Obstet Gynecol* 1994;4(ls): 339.
124. Riccabona M, Nelson TR, Pretorius DH, Davidson TE. In vivo three-dimensional sonographic measurement of organ volume: Validation in the urinary bladder. *J Ultrasound Med* 1996;15: 637–42.
125. Riccabona M, Pretorius DH, Nelson TR, Johson D, Budorick NE. Three-dimensional ultrasound: Display modalities in obstetrics. *J Clin Ultrasound* 1997;25:157–67.
126. Sohn CH, Grotepa SJ, Schneider W, *et al.* Erste Untersuchungen zur Dreidimensionalen Darstellung mittels Ultraschall. *Z Geburtsh Perinatol* 1988;192:241–8.
127. Sohn CH, Grotepa SJ, Schneider W, *et al.* Dreidimensionale Darstellung in der Ultraschalldiagnostik. Erste Ergebenisse. *Dtsch Med Wschr* 1988;113:1743–7.
128. Pretorius DH, Nelson TR. Three-dimensional US in obstetrics. In Fleischer AC, Manning FA, Jeanty P, Romero R, eds. *Principles and Practice of Ultrasonography in Obstetrics and Gynecology*, 5th edn. Norwalk: Appleton and Lange, 1995:119–26.
129. Sklansky MS, Nelson TR, Pretorius TH. Usefulness of gated three-dimensional fetal echocardiography to reconstruction and display structures not visualized with two-dimensional imaging. *Am J Cardiol* 1997;80:665–8.
130. Sklansky MS, Nelson TR, Pretorius DH. Three-dimensional fetal echocardiography: Gated versus nongated techniques. *J Ultrasound Med* 1998;17:451–7.
131. Steiner H, Merz E, Staudach A. Three-dimensional fetal facing. *Hum Reprod Update* 1995;1:item 6.
132. Schild RL, Holdhaus S, D'Alquen J. Quantitative assessment of subendometrial blood flow by three-dimensional ultrasound is an important predictive factor of implantation in an in-vitro fertilization programme. *Hum Reprod* 2000;15:89–94.
133. Chiba Y, Hayashi K, Yamazaki S, Takamizawa K, Sasaki H. New technique of ultrasound, thick slicing 3D imaging and the clinical aspects in the perinatal field. *Ultrasound Obstet Gynecol* 1994;4:337.
134. Meinel K, Guntermann E. Transparente 3D-Sonographie bei fetalen Fehlbildungen. *Ultraschall Med* 1998;19:120–5.
135. Pretorius DH, Nelson TR. Three-dimensional ultrasound imaging in patient diagnosis and management: The future (opinion). *Ultrasound Obstet Gynecol* 1991;1:381–3.
136. Pretorius DH, House M, Nelson TR, Hollenbach KA. Evaluation of normal and abnormal lips in fetuses: Comparison between three and two dimensional sonography. *Am J Roentgenol* 1995;165:1233–7.
137. Sohn CH, Grotepa SJ, Menge KH, Ameling W. Klinische Anwendung der dreidimensionalen Ultraschall Dartellung. *Dtsch Med Wsch* 1989;114:534–7.
138. Bonilla-Musoles F, Serra V, Machado LE, *et al.* Tridimension y diagnóstico prenatal. *Cuadernos Med Reprod* 2001;7:123–38.
139. Blaas HG, Eik-Nes SH, Berg S. Three-dimensional fetal ultrasound. *Baillieres Best Pract Res Clin Obstet Gynaecol* 2000;14: 611–27.
140. Hafner E, Schuchter K, Van Leeuwen M, *et al.* Three-dimensional sonographic volumetry of the placenta and the fetus between weeks 15 and 17 of gestation. *Ultrasound Obstet Gynecol* 2001; 18:116–20.
141. Meyer-Wittkopf M, Cole A, Cooper SG, Schmidt S, Sholler GF. Three-dimensional quantitative echocardiographic assessment of the ventricular volume in healthy human fetuses and in fetuses with congenital heart disease. *J Ultrasound Med* 2001;20:317–27.
142. Meyer-Wittkopf M, Cooper SG, Vaughan J, Sholler GF. Three-dimensional echocardiographic (3D) analysis of congenital heart disease in the fetus: Comparison with cross-sectional (2D) fetal echocardiography. *Ultrasound Obstet Gynecol* 2001;6:485–92.
143. Monteagudo A, Timor-Tritsch IE, Mayberry P. Three-dimensional transvaginal neurosonography of the fetal brain: "Navigating" in the volume scan. *Ultrasound Obstet Gynecol* 2000;16:307–13.
144. Budorik NE, Pretorius OH, Johnson DO, Nelson TR, Tartar MK, Lou KW. Three-dimensional ultrasonography of the fetal distal lower extremity: Normal and abnormal. *J Ultrasound Med* 1998;17:649–60.
145. Carson PL, Moskalika P, Govil A, *et al.* The 3D and 2D colour flow display of breast masses. *Ultrasound Med Biol* 1997;23:837–49.
146. Carson PL, Adler DO, Fowlkes LB, Harnist K, Rubin J. Enhanced colour flow imaging of breast cancer vasculature: Continuous wave Doppler and three-dimensional ultrasound display. *J Ultrasound Med* 1992;11:377–85.
147. Pretorius DH, Richards RD, Budorick NE. Three-dimensional ultrasound in the evaluation of fetal anomalies. *Radiology* 1997; 205(s):245.
148. Berardi JC, Mouilis M, Dlanete A, Godart J, Ecole-Pick MJ. Echographie en 3-dimensions (3D) en Obstetrique. Avantages et limites. *J Gynecol Obstet Biol Rep* 1997;26:520–4.
149. Johnson DD, Pretorius DH, Budorick N. Three-dimensional ultrasound of conjoined twins. *Obstet Gynecol* 1997;90:701–2.
150. Johnson DD, Pretorius DH, Riccabona M, Budorick NE, Nelson TR. Three-dimensional ultrasound of the fetal spine. *Obstet Gynecol* 1997;89:434–8.
151. Pohls UG, Rempen A. Fetal lung volumetry by three-dimensional ultrasound. *Ultrasound Obstet Gynecol* 1998;11: 6–12.

152. Lever AS, Pinheiro LW, Bega G, Kurtz AB, Goldberg BB. Three-dimensional multiplanar sonohysterography: Comparison with conventional two-dimensional sonohysterography and x-ray hysterosalpynography. *J Ultrasound Med* 2001;20:295–306.
153. Nelson TR, Pretorius DH, Hull A, Riccabona M, Skansky M, James G. Sources and impact of artefacts on clinical three-dimensional ultrasound imaging. *Ultrasound Obstet Gynecol* 2000;16:374–83.
154. Brunner M, Obruca A, Bauer P, Feichtinger W. Clinical application of volume estimation based on three-dimensional ultrasonography. *Ultrasound Obstet Gynecol* 1995;6:358–61.
155. Budorick NE, Pretorius DH, Tartar MK, Johnson DO, Nelson TR, Lou KV. Three-dimensional US of the fetal hands: Normal and abnormal findings. *Radiology* 1996;201(P):160.
156. Bega G, Lev-Toaff A, Kuhlman K, *et al.* Three-dimensional multiplanar transvaginal ultrasound of the cervix in pregnancy. *Ultrasound Obstet Gynecol* 2000;16:351–8.
157. Hata T, Yanagihara T, Matsumoto M, *et al.* Three-dimensional sonographic features of fetal central nervous system anomaly. *Acta Obstet Gynecol Scand* 2000;79:635–9.
158. Kupesic S, Kurjak A. Contrast-enhanced, three-dimensional power Doppler sonography for differenciation of adnexal of masses. *Obstet Gynecol* 2000;96:452–8.
159. Kurjak A, Kupesic S. The use of echo-enhancing contrasts in gynecology. *Ultrasound Rev Obstet Gynecol* 2001;1:85–95.
160. Lev-Toaff AS, Ozhan S, Pretorius D, Bega G, Kurtz AB, Kuhlman K. Three-dimensional multiplanar ultrasound for fetal gender assignment: Value of the mid-sagittal plane. *Ultrasound Obstet Gynecol* 2000;16:345–50.
161. Schild RL, Wallny T, Fimmers R, Hansmman M. The size of the fetal thoracolumbar spine: A three-dimensional ultrasound study. *Ultrasound Obstet Gynecol* 2000;16:468–72.
162. Timor-Tritsch IE, Monteagudo A, Mayberry P. Three-dimensional ultrasound evaluation of the fetal brain: The three horn view. *Ultrasound Obstet Gynecol* 2000;16:302–6.
163. Budorick NE, Pretorius DH, Johnson DO, Tartar MK, Lou KW, Nelson TR. Three-dimensional ultrasound examination of the fetal hands: Normal and abnormal. *Ultrasound Obstet Gynecol* 1998;12:227–34.
164. Pretorius DH, Nelson TR. Fetal face visualization using three-dimensional ultrasonography. *J Ultrasound Med* 1995;4: 349–56.
165 Steiner H, Spitzer D, Weiss-Wichert PH, Graf AH, Staudach A. Three-dimensional ultrasound in prenatal diagnosis of skeletal dysplasia. *Prenat Diagn* 1995;15:373–7.
166. Duncan KR, Baker PN, Johnson IR. Estimation of fetal lung volume using enhanced 3 dimensional ultrasound: A new method and first results. *Br J Obstet Gynecol* 1997;86:971–2.
167. Feichtinger W. Transvaginal three-dimensional imaging. *Ultrasound Obstet Gynecol* 1993;3:375–8.
168. Leventhal M, Pretorius DH, Sklansky MS, Budorick NE, Nelson TR. Three-dimensional ultrasound of the normal fetal heart. A comparison with two-dimensional imaging. *J Ultrasound Med* 1998;17:341–8.
169. Ludomirski A, Uerpairojkit B, Whiteman VE, Reece EA, Chu GP, Chan L. New technology in three dimensional obstetrical ultrasonography: Technique, advantages and limitations. *Am J Obstet Gynecol* 1996;Suppl 174:328.
170. Chou C-Y, Hsun K-F, Wang S-T, Huang S-C, Tzeng C-C. Accuracy of three-dimensional ultrasonography in volume estimation of cervical carcinoma. *Gynecol Oncol* 1997;65: 89–93.
171. Bahmaei A, Hughes SW, Clark T, *et al.* Serial fetal lung volume measurement using three-dimensional ultrasound. *Ultrasound Obstet Gynecol* 2000;16:154–8.
172. Chaoui R, Kalache KD. Three-dimensional power Doppler ultrasound of the fetal great vessels. *Ultrasound Obstet Gynecol* 2001;17:455–6.
173. Dyson RL, Pretorius DH, Budorick NE, *et al.* Three-dimensional ultrasound in the evaluation of fetal anomalies. *Ultrasound Obstet Gynecol* 2000;16:321–8.
174. Kupesic S. Clinical implications of sonographic detection of uterine anomalies for reproductive outcome. *Ultrasound Obstet Gynecol* 2001;18:387–400.
175. Kupesic S. The present and future role of three-dimensional ultrasound in assisted reproduction. *Ultrasound Obstet Gynecol* 2001;18:191–4.
176. Lee W, Kirk JS, Comstock CH, Romero R. Vasa previa: Prenatal detection by three-dimensional ultrasonography. *Ultrasound Obstet Gynecol* 2000;16:384–7.
177. Lee SL, Tan A. Lymphangiectasis with iniencephaly. *Ultrasound Obstet Gynecol* 2001;18:552–3.
178. Sladkevicius P, Ojha K, Campbell S, Nargund G. Three-dimensional power Doppler imaging in the assessment of fallopian tube patency. *Ultrasound Obstet Gynecol* 2000;16: 644–7.
179. Woelfer B, Salim R, Banerjee S, Elson J, Regan L, Jurkovic D. Reproductive outcomes in women with congenital uterine anomalies detected by three-dimensional ultrasound screening. *Obstet Gynecol* 2001;98:1099–103.
180. Feichtinger W. Follicle aspiration with interactive three-dimensional digital imaging (Voluson*): A step toward real-time puncturing under three-dimensional ultrasound control. *Fertil Steril* 1998;70:374–7.
181. Jackson DN, Braun I, Keel-Thompson K. Volume mode planar imaging in patients with non-surface fetal abnormalities: Techniques and efficacy. *J Med Ultrason* 2000;27:14–9.
182. Jackson DN, Aptekar LH, Keel-Thompson K. Technique of 3D volume mode sectional planar imaging. *Ultrasound Obstet Gynecol* 2000;16(s):26.
183. Merz E. Einsatz der 3D-Ulltrschalltechnik in der pranatalen Diagnostik. *Ulltraschall Med* 1995;16:154–61.
184. Blaas HG, Eik-Nes SH, Berg S, Torp H. In-vivo three-dimensional ultrasound reconstructions of embryos and early fetuses. *Lancet* 1998;ii:1182–6.
185. Bonilla-Musoles F, Raga F, Blanes J, Coelho F. La tridimensión ecográfica en tumores ováricos. *Obstet Ginecol Esp* 1995; 4:193–210.
186. Bonilla-Musoles F, Machado L, Raga F, *et al.* Ecografia tridimensional interactiva Doppler color en el primer trimestre del embarazo. In Kurjak A, Carreras JM, eds. *Medicina Perinatal.* Barcelona: Masson, 2000:213–30.
187. Bonilla-Musoles F, Martinez Molina V, Blanes J, Raga F, Villalobos A. Three-dimensional ultrasound investigation for identification and control of intrauterine devices. In Merz E, ed. *3-D Ultrasound in Obstetrics and Gynecology.* Philadelphia: Lippincott Williams and Wilkins, 1999:31–6.
188. Brinkley JF, McCallum WD, Muramatsu SK. Fetal weight estimation from length and volumes found by three dimensional ultrasonic measurements. *J Ultrasound Med* 1984;3:162–9.
189. Brinkley LF, McCallum WD, Muramatsu SK. Fetal weight estimation from ultrasonic three-dimensional head and trunk reconstructions: Evaluation in vitro. *Am J Obstet Gynecol* 1982;144:715–20.
190. Hafner E, Philipp T, Schuchter K, Dillinger-Paller B, Philipp K, Bauer P. Second-trimester measurements of placental volume by three-dimensional ultrasound to predict small-for gestational-age infants. *Ultrasound Obstet Gynecol* 1998;12:97–102.
191. Hata T, Aoki S, Akiyama M, Yanaglhara T, Miyazaki K. Three-dimensional ultrasonographic assessment of fetal hands and feet. *Ultrasound Obstet Gynecol* 1998;12:235–9.
192. Hata T, Yanagihara T, Hayashi K, *et al.* Three-dimensional ultrasonographic evaluation of ovarian tumours preliminary study. *Hum Reprod* 1999;14:858–61.
193. Hosli JM, Tercanli S, Herman A, Kretschmann M, Holzgreve W. In-vitro volume measurement by three-dimensional ultrasound: Comparison of two different systems. *Ultrasound Obstet Gynecol* 1998;11:17–22.
194. Kossoff G. Three-dimensional ultrasound. Technology push or market pull. *Ultrasound Obstet Gynecol* 1995;5:217–8.
195. Lees WR, Gardener JE, Gilliams A. Three-dimensional US of the fetus. *Radiology* 1991;181:131–2.
196. Mo MH, Chao-Chin H, Ko-En H. Detection of congenital müllerian duct anomalies using three-dimensional ultrasound. *J Clin Ultrasound* 1997;25:487–92.
197. Merz E, Bahlmann AF, Weber G. Volume scanning in the evaluation of fetal malformations: A new dimension in prenatal diagnosis. *Ultrasound Obstet Gynecol* 1995;5:222–7.
198. Ploeckinger-Ulm B, Ulm MR, Lee A, Kratochwil A, Bernaschek G. Antenatal depiction of fetal digits with three-dimensional ultrasonography. *Am J Obstet Gynecol* 1996;175:571–4.
199. Bonilla-Musoles F, Machado L, Bailao LA, Osborne N, Raga F. Abdominal wall defects. Two-versus three-dimensional ultrasonographic diagnosis. *J Ultrasound Med* 2001;20:379–89.
200. Jackson DN, Aptekar I, Thompson KK, Aptekar M. Counselling impact of three-dimensional imaging in perinatal consultation. *Ultrasound Rev Obstet Gynecol* 2001;1:216–47.
201. Bonilla-Musoles F, Raga F, Blanes J, Osborne N, Coelho F. Three dimensional hysterosonographic evaluation of the normal endometrium: Comparison with transvaginal sonography and three-dimensional ultrasound. *J Gynecol Surg* 1997;13:101–7.

202. Bonilla-Musoles F, Raga F, Osborne N, Blanes J. Three-dimensional evaluation of embryonic and fetal malformations: Comparison with two-dimensional ultrasound. In Kurjak A, ed. *Perinatology.* Lancaster, UK: Parthenon Publishing Group, 1998:228–35.
203. Bonilla-Musoles F, Raga F, Blanes J, *et al.* Avances en el diagnóstico prenatal: Empleo de la angiografía digital Doppler y la tridimensión ecográfica. *Rev Iberoam Fertil* 1997;14: 295–318.
204. Harita G, Gabriel R, Carre-Pigeon F. Primary application of three-dimensional ultrasonography to early diagnosis of ectopic pregnancy. *Eur J Obstet Gynecol* 1995;60:110–20.
205. Lee A, Kratochwil A, Stümpflen L, Deutinger J, Bernaschek G. Fetal lung volume determination by three-dimensional ultrasonography. *Am J Obstet Gynecol* 1996;175:588–92.
206. Campbell S. 4D or not 4D: That is the question. *Ultrasound Obstet Gynecol* 2002;19:1–5.
207. Kratochwil A, Lee A, Schoisswohl A. Networking of three-dimensional sonography volume data. *Ultrasound Obstet Gynecol* 2000;16:335–40.
208. Kurjak A, Kupesic S, Anic T, Kosuta D. Three-dimensional ultrasound and power Doppler improve the diagnosis of ovarian lesions. *Gynecol Oncol* 2000;76:28–32.
209. Maymon R, Herman A, Ariely S, *et al.* Three-dimensional vaginal ultrasonography in obstetrics and gynecology. *Hum Reprod Update* 2000;5:475–84.
210. Pedersen MH, Larsen T. Three-dimensional ultrasonography in obstetrics and gynecology. *Ugeskr Laeger* 2001;163:594–9.
211. Pooh RK, Pooh K. Transvaginal 3D and Doppler ultrasonography of the fetal brain. *Semin Perinatol* 2001;25:38–43.
212. Sabbagha R. The endometrium and the role of three-dimensional sonohysterography. *Ultrasound Rev Obstet Gynecol* 2001;1: 72–84.
213. Salerno CC, Pretorius H, Hilton SW, *et al.* Three-dimensional ultrasonographic imaging of the neonatal brain in high-risk neonates; preliminary study. *J Ultrasound Med* 2000;19:549–56.
214. Song TB, Moore TR, Lee JY, Kim EK. Fetal weight prediction by high volume measurement with three-dimensional ultrasonography. *Obstet Gynecol* 2000;96:157–61.
215. Bonilla-Musoles F, Machado LE, Raga A. Three- and four-dimensional images of fetal malformations. In Kurjak A, Jackson D, eds. *An Atlas of Three- and Four-Dimensional Sonography in Obstetrics and Gynecology.* London: Taylor & Francis, 2004: chap 5, 67–127.
216. Bega G, Lev-Toaff A, Kuhlman K, Kurtz A, Goldberg B, Wapner R. Three-dimensional ultrasonographic imaging in obstetrics. *J Ultrasound Med* 2001;20:391–408.
217. Umek WH, Obermair A, Stutterecker D, Häusler G, Leodolter S, Hanzal E. Three-dimensional ultrasound of the female urethra: Comparing transvaginal and transrectal scanning. *Ultrasound Obstet Gynecol* 2001;17:425–30.
218. Wang P. Obstetrical three-dimensional ultrasound in the visualization of the intracranial midline and corpus callosum of fetuses with cephalic position (letter). *Prenat Diagn* 2000;20:518–20.
219. Kupesic S, Kurjak A, Ujevic B. B-mode, color Doppler and three-dimensional ultrasound in the assessment of endometrial lesions. *Ultrasound Rev Obstet Gynecol* 2001;1:50–71.
220. Kupesic S, Bekavac I, Bejelos D, Kurjak A. Assessment of endometrial receptivity by transvaginal color Doppler and three-dimensional power Doppler ultrasonography in patients undergoing in-vitro fertilization procedures. *J Ultrasound Med* 2001; 20:125–34.
221. Kurjak A, Kupesic S, Jacobs Y. Preoperative diagnosis of the primary fallopian tube carcinoma by three-dimensional static and power Doppler sonography. *Ultrasound Obstet Gynecol* 2000; 15:246–50.
222. Kurjak A, Kupesic S, Sparac V, Kosuta D. Three-dimensional ultrasonographic and power Doppler characterization of ovarian lesions. *Ultrasound Obstet Gynecol* 2000;16:365–71.
223. Kurjak A, Hafner T, Kos M. Three-dimensional sonography in prenatal diagnosis: A luxury or a necessity? *J Perinat Med* 2000; 28:194–209.
224. Lee T-H, Shih J-C, Peng SS-F, Lee C-N, Shyu M-K, Hsieth F-J. Prenatal depiction of the angioarchitecture of an aneurysm of the vein of Galen with three-dimensional color power angiography. *Ultrasound Obstet Gynecol* 2000;15:345.
225. Pal A, Babinski A, Vajda G, Kovacs L. Diagnosis of Asherman's syndrome with three-dimensional ultrasound. *Ultrasound Obstet Gynecol* 2000;15:341.
226. Ayida G, Kennedy S, Barlow D, Chamberlain P. Contrast sonography for uterine cavity assessment: A comparison of conventional two-dimensional with three-dimensional transvaginal ultrasound. *Fertil Steril* 1996;66:848–50.
227. Baba K, Satoh K, Sakamoto S, Okai T, Ishi IS. Development of an ultrasonic system for three-dimensional reconstruction of the foetus. *J Perinat Med* 1989;17:19–24.
228. Balen FG, Allen CM, Gardener JE, Siddle NC, Lees WR. 3-Dimensional reconstruction of ultrasound images of the uterine cavity. *Br J Radiol* 1993;66:588–91.
229. Benoit B. Early fetal gender determination. *Ultrasound Obstet Gynecol* 1999;13:299–300.
230. Blohmerju, Bollmann R, Heinrich G, Paepke S, Lichtenegger W. Die dreidimensionale Ultraschalluntersuchung (3D-Sonographie) der weiblichen Brustdrüse. *Geburtsh Frauenh* 1996;56:161–5.
231. Bonilla-Musoles F, Raga F, Osborne N, Blanes J. Ecografia tridimensional en Obstetricia y Ginecologia. *Obstet Gynecol Españ* 1994;3:233–50.
232. Bonilla-Musoles F, Raga F, Osborne N. Three-dimensional ultrasound evaluation of ovarian masses. *Gynecol Oncol* 1995;59: 129–35.
233. Bonilla-Musoles F, Pellicer A, Raga F, Osborne N, Blanes J. Review: Three-dimensional (3D) ultrasound in reproduction, obstetrics and gynecology. *Assoc Reprod Rev* 1995;5:170–88.
234. Bonilla-Musoles F, Raga F, Villalobos A, Blanes J, Branco J, Martinez Molina V. Demonstration of early pregnancy with three-dimensional ultrasound. In Merz E, ed. *3-D Ultrasound in Obstetrics and Gynecology.* Philadelphia: Lippincott Williams and Wilkins, 1999:81–94.
235. Casanas-Roux F, Nissole M, Marbaix E, Smets M, Bassil S, Gonnez J. Morphometric, inmunohistological and three-dimensional evaluation of the endometrium of menopausal woman treated by oestrogen and Crinone, a new slow-release vaginal progesterone. *Hum Reprod* 1996;11:357–63.
236. Chan L, Lin M, Uerpairojkit B, Hartman D, Reece EA, Helm W. Evaluation of adnexal masses using three-dimensional ultrasonographic technology: Preliminary report. *J Ultrasound Med* 1997; 16:349–54.
237. Chang FM, Hsu KF, Ko HC, *et al.* Fetal heart volume assessment by three-dimensional ultrasound. *Ultrasound Obstet Gynecol* 1997;9:42–8.
238. D'Arcy TJ, Hughes SW, Chiu WSC. Estimation of fetal lung volume using enhanced 3-dimensional ultrasound: A new method and first results. *Br J Obstet Gynecol* 1996;103:1015–20.
239. Favre R. Echographie tridimensionelle dans le despistage des malformations. *J Med Foetale* 1994;19:22–9.
240. Hata T, Manabe A, Makihara K, Kohkichi H, Koh-Ji M, Daisaku S. Assessment of embryonic anatomy at 6–8 weeks of gestation by intrauterine and transvaginal sonography. *Hum Reprod* 1997;12:1873–6.
241. Hata T, Aoki S, Manabe A, Hata K, Miyazaki K. Three-dimensional ultrasonography in the first trimester of human pregnancy. *Hum Reprod* 1997;12:1800–4.
242. Hata T, Manabe A, Aoki S, Miyazaki K, Yoshino K, Yamamoto K. Three-dimensional intrauterine sonography in the early first trimester of human pregnancy: Preliminary study. *Hum Reprod* 1998;13:740–3.
243. Hata T, Aoki S, Hata K, Miyazaki K, Akahane M, Mochizuki T. Three-dimensional ultrasonographic assessment of fetal development. *Obstet Gynecol* 1998;91:218–23.
244. Jurkovic D, Geipel A, Gruboeck K, Jauniaux E, Natucci M, Campbell S. Three-dimensional ultrasound for the assessment of uterine anatomy and detection of congenital anomalies: A comparison with hysterosalpingography and two-dimensional sonography. *Ultrasound Obstet Gynecol* 1995;5:233–7.
245. Jurkovic D, Jauniau E. *Ultrasound and Early Pregnancy.* Progress in Obstetric and Gynecological Sonography Series. Lancaster, UK: The Parthenon Publishing Group, 1996.
246. Kelly IMG, Gardener JE, Lees WR. Three-dimensional fetal ultrasound. *Lancet* 1991;i(339):1062–4.
247. King DL, King DL Jr, Shao MY. Evaluation of in vitro measurements accuracy of a three-dimensional ultrasound scanner. *J Ultrasound Med* 1991;10:77–82.
248. Kossoff G, Griffiths A, Warren PS. Real-time quasi three-dimensional viewing in sonography, with conventional grey-scale volume imaging. *Ultrasound Obstet Gynecol* 1994;4:211–6.
249. Kratochwil A. Versuch der 3-dimensionalen Darstellung in der Geburtshilfe. *Ultraschall Med* 1992;13:183–6.
250. Kurjak A, Kupesic S, Breyer B, Sparac V, Jukic S. The assessment of ovarian tumour angiogenesis: What does three-dimensional power Doppler add? *Ultrasound Obstet Gynecol* 1998;12:136–46.

251. Kyei-Mensah A, Zaidi J, Pittrof R, Shaker A, Campbell S, Tan SL. Transvaginal three-dimensional ultrasound; accuracy of follicular volume measurements. *Fertil Steril* 1996;65:371–6.

252. Laudy JAM, Janssen MMM, Struyk PC, Stijmen T, Wladimiroff JW. Three-dimensional ultrasonography of normal fetal lung volume: A preliminary study. *Ultrasound Obstet Gynecol* 1998; 11:13–6.

253. Lee A, Deutinger J, Bernaschek G. Three-dimensional ultrasound: Abnormalities of the fetal face in surface and volume rendering mode. *Br J Obstet Gynecol* 1995;102:302–6.

254. Lee A, Eppel W, Sam C, Kratochwil A, Deutinger J, Bernaschek G. Intrauterine device localization by three-dimensional transvaginal sonography. *Ultrasound Obstet Gynecol* 1997;10:289–93.

255. Levaillant JM, Rotten D, Billon C, Leguerinel Y, Rua P. Three-dimensional ultrasound imaging of the female breast and human fetus in utero. Preliminary results. *Ultrasound Imaging* 1989;11: 149–50.

256. Levaillant JM, Benoit B, Bady J, Rotten D. Echographie tridimensionelle apport technique et clinique en echographie osbtetricale. *Reprod Hum Horm* 1995;3:341–7.

257. Lev-Toaff AS, Rawool NM, Kurtz AB, Forssberg F, Gold-Berg BB. Three-dimensional sonography and 3D-transvaginal US: A problem solving tool in complex gynecologic cases. *Radiology* 1996; 20(P):384.

258. Machado LE, Chamusca L, Chagas K, *et al.* Ecografia tridimensional (3D) en tiempo "quasi real" en la segunda mitad del embarazo. *Obstet Ginecol Esp* 1999;8:7–18.

259. Mo M-H, Chao-Chin H, Yue-Shan L. Three-dimensional ultrasound and hysteroscopy in the evaluation of intrauterine retained fetal bones. *J Clin Ultrasound* 1997;25:93–5.

260. Merz E, Macchiela O, Bahlmann F, Weber G. Fetale Fehlbildungsdiagnostik mit Hilfe der 3D-Sonographie. *Ultraschall Klin Prax* 1991;6:147–52.

261. Merz E. Three-dimensional ultrasound in the evaluation of fetal anatomy and malformations. In Chervenak FA, Kurjak A, eds. *Current Perspectives on the Fetus as a Patient.* London: Parthenon Publishing Group, 1996:75–87.

262. Pretorius DH, Johnson DD, Budorick NE, Jones MC, Lou KV, Nelson TR. Three-dimensional ultrasound of the fetal lip and palate. *Radiology* 1997;205(s):245.

263. Raga F, Bonilla-Musoles F, Blanes J, Osborne N. Accuracy of three-dimensional ultrasound diagnosis in congenital müllerian anomalies. *Fertil Steril* 1996;65:523–8.

264. Rotten D, Levaillant JM, Constancis E, Collet Billon A, Le Guerinel Y, Rua P. Three-dimensional imaging of solid breast tumours with ultrasound: Preliminary data and analysis of its possible contribution to the understanding of the standard two-dimensional sonographic images. *Ultrasound Obstet Gynecol* 1991;1:384–90.

265. Schild RL, Fimmers R, Hansmann M. Kann die 3 D-Volumetrie von fetalem Oberarm und Oberschenkel konventionelle 2D-Gewichtsschätzungen verbessern? *Ultraschall Med* 1999;19: 31–7.

266. Schild RL, Wallny T, Fimmer R, Hansmann M. Fetal lumbar spine volumetry by three-dimensional ultrasound. *Ultrasound Obstet Gynecol* 1999;13:335–9.

267. Shih JC, Shyu M-K, Lee C-N, Wu C-H, Un C-J, Hsieh F-J. Antenatal depiction of the fetal ear with three-dimensional ultrasonography. *Obstet Gynecol* 1998;91:500–5.

268. Sivan E, Chan L, Uerpairojkit B, Chu G-P, Reeze EA. Growth of the fetal forehead and normative dimensions developed by three-dimensional ultrasonographic technology. *J Ultrasound Med* 1997;16:401–6.

269. Steiner H, Staudach A, Spitzer D, Graf AH, Wiennerroither H. Bietet die 3D-Sonographie neue perspektive in der Gynakologie und Geburtshilfe? *Geburtsh Frauenheilk* 1993;53:779–82.

270. Steiner H, Spitzer D, Diem A, Batka M, Staudach A. Outcome nach artifizielle Fruchtwasser-Instillation (AFI) bei früher Oligohydramnie. *Geburtsh Frauenheilk* 1993;53:559–63.

271. Steiner H, Staudach A, Schaffer H. Drei dimensionale Ultraschalldiagnostik in der Gebursthilfe und Gynakologie. *Med Bild* 1994;1:19–23.

272. Steiner H, Staudach A, Zajc M, Wienerroither H. Verbesserte Diagnostik am fetalen Skelett mittels 3D-Sonographie. *Ultraschall Klin Prax* 1994;8:154–7.

273. Steiner H, Gregg AR, Bogner G, Graf AH, Weiner CP, Staudach A. First trimester three-dimensional ultrasound volumetry of the gestational sac. *Arch Gynecol Obstet* 1994;255:165–70.

274. Steiner H. Potential der dreidimensionalen (3D) Sonographie in del Fehlbildungs diagnosrik. *Gynäkologe* 1995;28:315–20.

275. Sohn C, Grotepass J, Swobodnik W. Moglichkeiten der 3-dimensionalen Ultraschalluntersuchung. *Ultraschall Med* 1989;10:307–13.

276. Jackson DN, Braun I, Keel-Thompson K. Comparison of rapid MRI (HASTE) procedure to volume mode planar imaging in the management of fetal abnormalities. *J Med Ultrason* 2000;27: 1–13.

277. Jones D, Reyes M, Gallagher P, Fricks P, Touloukian R, Copel J. Three-dimensional sonographic imaging of a highly developed fetus in fetu with spontaneous movement of the extremities. *J Ultrasound Med* 2001;20:1357–64.

278. Kuno A, Akiyama M, Yamashiro C, Tanaka H, Yanagihara T, Hata T. Three-dimensional sonographic assessment of fetal behavior in the early second trimester of pregnancy. *J Ultrasound Med* 2001;20:1271–7.

279. Michailidis GD, Simpson JM, Karidas C, Economides DL. Detailed three-dimensional fetal echocardiography facilitated by an internet link. *Ultrasound Obstet Gynecol* 2001;18:325–8.

280. Orden MR, Gudmundsson S, Kirkinrn P. Contrast-enhanced sonography in the examination of benign and malignant adnexal masses. *J Ultrasound Med* 2000;19:783–9.

281. Weisman CF, Forstner R, Prokop E, Rettenbacher T. Three-dimensional targeting: A new three-dimensional ultrasound technique to evaluate needle position during breast biopsy. *Ultrasound Obstet Gynecol* 2000;16:359–64.

282. Bonilla-Musoles F, Machado LE. *3D–4D in Obstetrics.* Madrid: Panamericana Ed., 2004.

30 Malformations of the gastrointestinal system

V. D'Addario and L. Di Cagno

A correct ultrasonic examination of the fetal gastrointestinal tract includes the visualization of the following structures:

- the stomach (Figure 30.1)
- the small and large bowels (Figure 30.2)
- the liver with its main vessels and the gallbladder (Figure 30.1)
- the abdominal wall and the insertion of the umbilical cord (Figure 30.3)
- the diaphragm (Figure 30.4).

The systematic evaluation of the above-mentioned structures allows the recognition of several congenital anomalies of the gastrointestinal system. The reported sensitivity of ultrasound in diagnosing gastrointestinal malformations varies from 24% to 86%, according to different authors' results. This wide variation is due to the different study designs (mainly the number of scans performed during pregnancy), inclusion criteria and levels of examination. Since many gastrointestinal malformations appear late in pregnancy, the best results are obtained when the screening design includes a scan also in the third trimester.

The malformations of gastrointestinal tract and abdominal wall can be divided into four groups:

(1) anterior abdominal wall defects
(2) diaphragmatic defects
(3) bowel disorders
(4) non-bowel cystic masses.

Anterior abdominal wall defects

The congenital abdominal wall defects include gastroschisis, omphalocele and body stalk anomaly.[1] The ultrasonic prenatal diagnosis of these defects is relatively simple and possible in the first half of pregnancy. However, it must be remembered that there is a physiological herniation of the small intestine outside the abdominal cavity between the 5th and the 11th weeks of gestation (Figure 30.5) and therefore a prenatal diagnosis of abdominal wall defect cannot be made in the earliest stage of pregnancy.[2]

Gastroschisis

This malformation consists of a paraumbilical full-thickness defect of the anterior abdominal wall, which is usually located to the right side of the umbilical cord insertion, associated with evisceration of abdominal organs.

The incidence ranges from 1:10,000 to 1:15,000 live births.

Gastroschisis is considered a sporadic event with a multifactorial etiology, but cases of familial occurrence have been reported. Young maternal age, maternal cigarette use and vasoactive drugs consumption during the first trimester are considered as possible etiological factors.

The malformation results from vascular compromise of either the umbilical vein or the omphalomesenteric artery. The abdominal wall defect is generally small but the amount of bowel protruding from the defect and floating freely in the amniotic fluid may be disproportionately large. The herniated organs include mainly bowel loops that are not protected by a membrane but are usually covered by an inflammatory exudate, possibly resulting from chemical irritation by exposure to amniotic fluid.

The ultrasonographic diagnosis of gastroschisis is suggested by the finding of a partly solid, partly cystic mass adjacent to the anterior abdominal wall and freely mobile in the amniotic fluid (Figure 30.6), which has a cauliflower-like appearance. The differential diagnosis from omphalocele is based on the presence of a normal insertion of the umbilical cord, the lateral location of the mass and the absence of a membrane covering the herniated mass.

In contrast to omphalocele, gastroschisis is rarely associated with other malformations and chromosomal anomalies, but additional gastrointestinal abnormalities (malrotation, atresia, volvulus and infarction) may occur in 20–40% of the cases.[3,4] A high percentage of fetuses with gastroschisis (77%) present intrauterine growth retardation and preterm labor occurs in one-third of cases. The extent of bowel damage is variable and strictly affects the prognosis. Most of the bowel damage is caused by constriction at the site of the abdominal wall defect: the sonographic

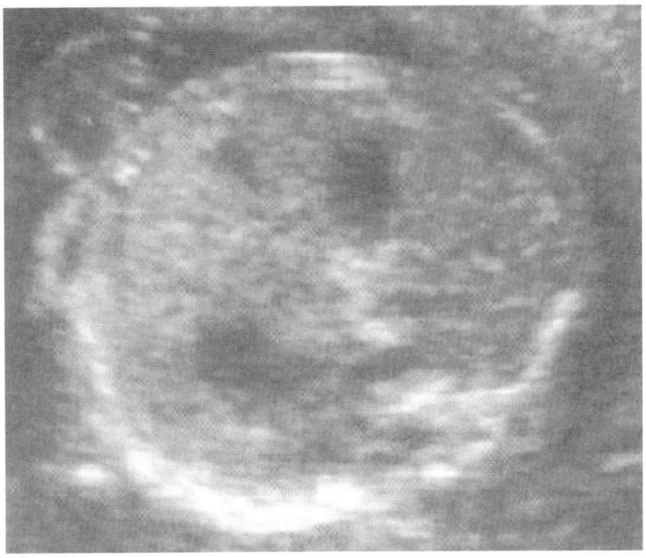

Figure 30.1 Transverse scan of the fetal abdomen showing the stomach, the liver, the intraepatic tract of the umbilical vein and the gallbladder.

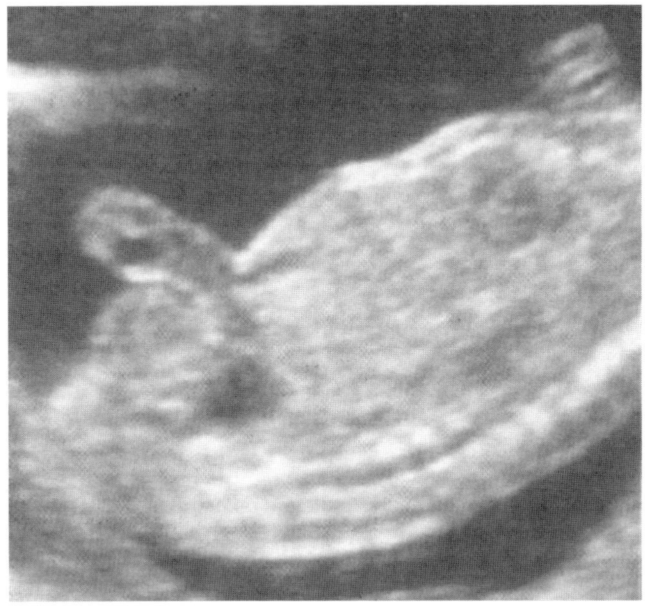

Figure 30.3 Insertion of the umbilical cord into the abdominal wall.

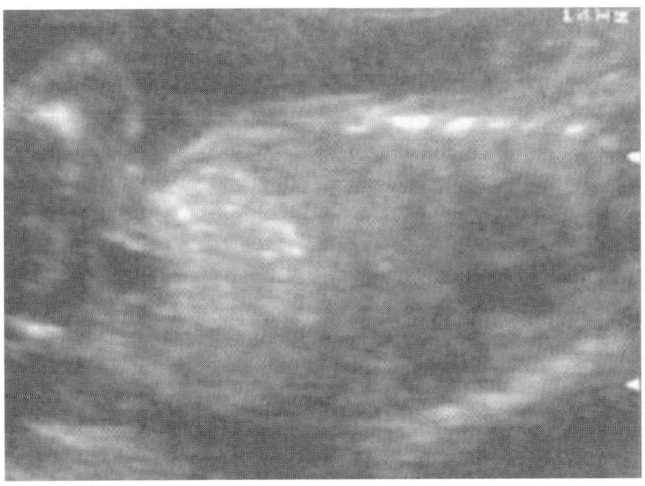

Figure 30.2 The echogenic bowel is seen below the liver.

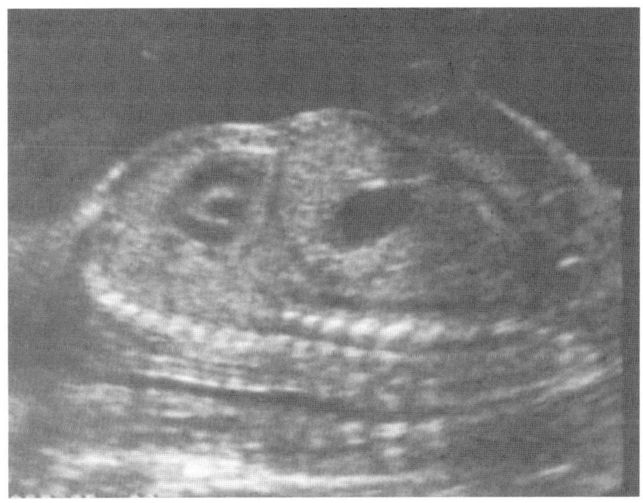

Figure 30.4 Longitudinal scan of the fetal chest and abdomen showing the diaphragm between the lung and the liver.

evidence of small bowel dilatation and mural thickening correlates with severe intestinal damage and poor clinical outcome.

The mode of delivery of fetuses affected by gastroschisis is still controversial although there is no striking evidence for cesarean section over vaginal delivery. Maternal transfer before delivery to a tertiary care center is recommended. The mortality rate ranges from about 8 to 28%.

Omphalocele

Omphalocele is a ventral wall defect characterized by an incomplete development of abdominal muscles, fascia and skin and the herniation of intra-abdominal organs (bowel loops, stomach and liver) into the base of the umbilical cord, with a covering by amnioperitoneal membrane. The defect is thought to be caused by an abnormality in the process of body infolding. The classic omphalocele is a midabdominal defect, although there is also a high or epigastric omphalocele (typical of the pentalogy of Cantrell) and a low or hypogastric omphalocele (as seen in bladder or cloacal extrophy), due to cephalic and caudal folding defects, respectively. The incidence of omphalocele ranges from 1:4000 to 1:7000 live births. It is more frequent in older women; most cases are sporadic, although a familial occurrence with a sex-linked or autosomal pattern of inheritance has been reported.

The ultrasonographic appearance of omphalocele varies according to the type of defect, the presence of ascites and the organs herniated. The principal diagnostic features are the umbilical cord insertion into the membrane covering the abdominal wall defect,

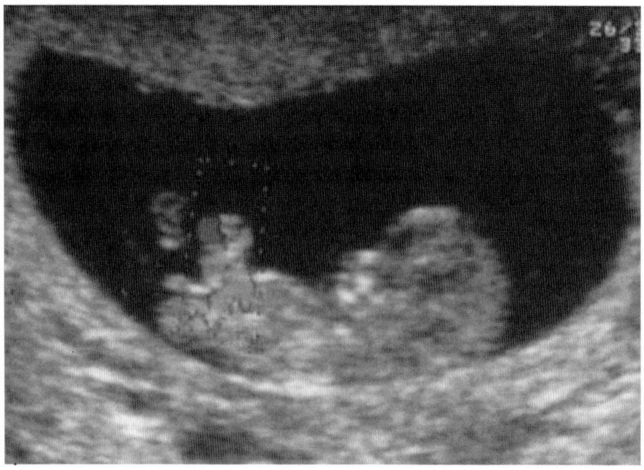

Figure 30.5 Physiological herniation of the midgut at 10 weeks of gestation.

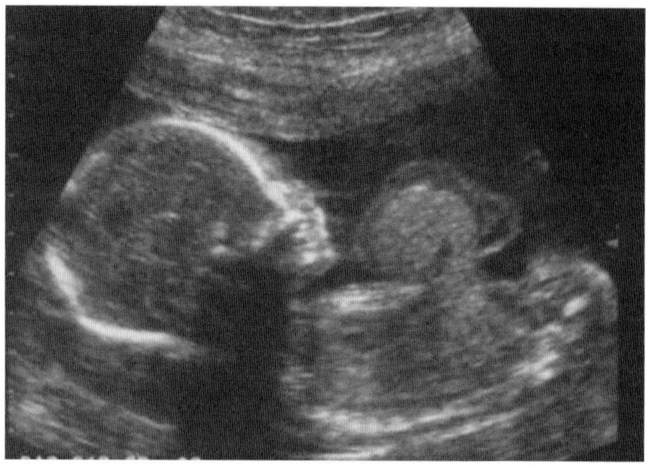

Figure 30.7 Omphalocele: a round solid mass, covered by a thin membrane, protrudes from the anterior abdominal wall.

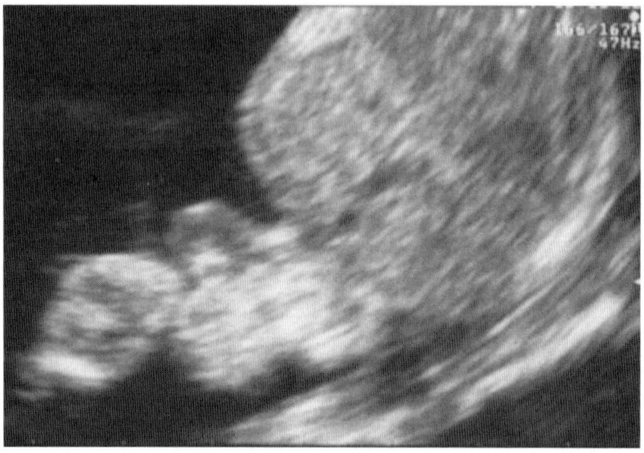

Figure 30.6 Gastroschisis: a cauliflower-like mass protrudes from the abdominal cavity into the amniotic fluid.

the presence of the intrahepatic portion of the umbilical vein coursing through the central portion of the defect and the presence of a limiting membrane that can occasionally rupture (Figure 30.7).

There are different syndromes that include omphalocele, such as pentalogy of Cantrell (midline supraumbilical abdominal defect, lower sternum defect, deficiency of diaphragmatic pericardium, anterior diaphragm defect and cardiac abnormality) and Beckwith–Wiedemann syndrome (macroglossia, visceromegaly and omphalocele). Although most cases of omphalocele are sporadic, a familial occurrence of this anomaly with a sex-linked or autosomal pattern of inheritance has been reported.

The most important prognostic variable is the presence of associated malformations (50–70% of cases) or chromosomal abnormalities (30% of cases).[5] Some authors have demonstrated that small defects involving only the bowel are associated with an increased risk of chromosomal abnormalities, as opposed to large defects that have an exposed liver. The main associated malformations are cardiac anomalies (up to 47% of cases), genitourinary abnormalities (40% of cases) and neural tube defects (39% of cases). Fetal mortality is highly dependent on associated malformations but respiratory complications also account for a significant percentage of morbidity and mortality.

The mode of delivery of fetuses with omphalocele has been debated in the literature. The goal of management is to deliver the fetus as close to term as possible in tertiary care centers. Cesarean section may be necessary to avoid dystocia or sac rupture in large omphaloceles. In the case of small defects vaginal delivery is recommended.

Body stalk anomaly

The body stalk anomaly is a severe abdominal wall defect caused by the failure of formation of the body stalk; it is characterized by the absence of umbilical cord and umbilicus and the fusion of the placenta to the herniated viscera. The incidence is 1:14,000 births. This malformation is caused by a developmental failure of the cephalic, caudal and lateral embryonic folds.

The ultrasonographic diagnosis is suggested by the finding of a large anterior wall defect attaching the fetus to the placenta or uterine wall, the absence of umbilical cord and the visualization of abdominal organs in a sac outside the abdominal cavity (Figure 30.8).[6,7] The position of the fetus may lead to scoliosis and kyphosis. Multiple malformations such as neural tube defects, and gastrointestinal and genitourinary anomalies may be associated. The body stalk anomaly is a uniformly fatal condition.

Diaphragmatic defects

The classification of these malformations is based on the location of the diaphragmatic defect:

(1) diaphragmatic hernia (Bochdaleck and Morgagni types)
(2) septum transversum defects (defect of the central tendon)
(3) hiatal hernia (congenital large esophageal orifice)
(4) eventration of the diaphragm
(5) agenesis of the diaphragm.

A diaphragmatic hernia is a defect in the diaphragm, due to failure of the pleuroperitoneal canal to close between 9 and 10 weeks of gestation, thus determining the protrusion of the abdominal organs into the thoracic cavity.

The incidence of congenital diaphragmatic hernia is 1:3000–1:5000 live births. This entity can be either sporadic or a familiar disorder but its etiology is quite unknown. The most common type of diaphragmatic hernia is the Bochdalek type, which is a posterolateral defect mostly located on the left side (80% of cases), less frequently on the right side (15%) or bilateral (5%). Stomach, spleen and colon are the most frequently herniated organs. When the hernia is on the right side, the main organs involved are the liver and the gallbladder.

The Morgagni type is usually a very small hernia that occurs in 1–2% of cases. It is a parasternal defect located in the anterior portion of the diaphragm; it involves the liver, which may limit the degree of herniation. In the case of eventration of the diaphragm, this structure appears to be weak so that the abdominal contents are displaced in the thoracic cavity.

Eventration of the diaphragm consists of an upward displacement of abdominal organs into the thoracic cavity secondary to a congenitally weak diaphragm, which has the aspect of an aponeurotic sheet. It occurs in 5% of diaphragmatic defects and is more common on the right side.

Diaphragmatic hernia can be either a sporadic or a familiar disorder and although the etiology is unknown, this abnormality has been described in association with maternal ingestion of drugs such as thalidomide, quinine and anticonvulsants. There are two hypotheses to explain the mechanism responsible for the origin of a diaphragmatic defect: (1) delayed fusion of the diaphragm and (2) a primary diaphragmatic defect. In addition to this classification, another one has been proposed concerning a late onset of this anomaly:

(1) Herniation occurring early during bronchial branching causing a severe bilateral pulmonary hypoplasia and lately death.
(2) Herniation at the stage of distal bronchial branching leading to unilateral hypoplasia, with survival depending on the balance between pulmonary vascular and ductal resistances.
(3) Late herniation in pregnancy, which causes a compression of otherwise normal lung and a good prognosis.
(4) Postnatal herniation without pulmonary pathology and with good chances of viability.

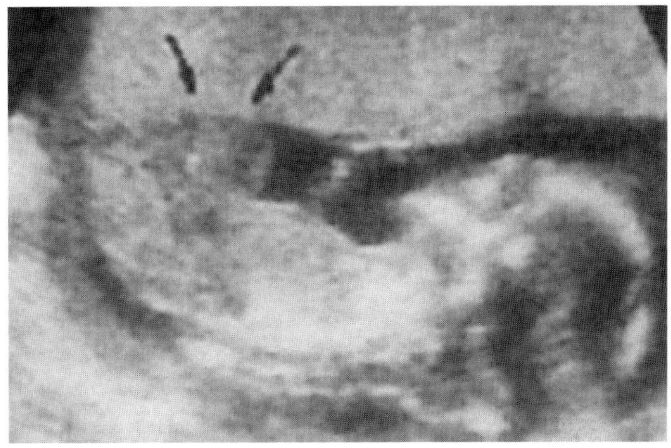

Figure 30.8 Body stalk anomaly: a large anterior abdominal wall defect attaches the fetus directly to the placenta.

The prenatal sonographic diagnosis of diaphragmatic hernia is mainly based on the visualization of abdominal organs at the same level of the four-chamber view of the heart in the transverse section of the fetal chest. The heart is usually shifted on the right side of the chest (Figure 30.9).

The visualization of the fluid-filled bowel or the stomach bubble in the thoracic cavity is highly diagnostic. The presence of peristalsis of bowel loops may help make the differential diagnosis with other conditions such as cystic adenomatoid malformation of the lung, bronchogenic cysts and mediastinal cysts. Polyhydramnios is common and is secondary to the bowel obstruction.

The rate of associated anomalies is 25–75%, increasing to 95% in stillborns. Such anomalies include central nervous system, cardiac and chromosomal abnormalities, omphalocolo and oral cleft.

The prognosis for this malformation is still very poor and becomes poorer if other malformations are associated. The poor prognosis mainly depends on the severity of pulmonary hypoplasia induced by the prolonged compression of the lungs by the herniated viscera. For this reason experimental prenatal surgery has been suggested to prevent the lung damage. The different outcome is related to variation in the timing of entry of abdominal organs into the chest (the earlier is the entrance, the worse is the prognosis). Due to the complexity of this malformation and the different diagnosis and treatment, the ultrasound examination is very essential. Management relies on protecting the controlateral lung hoping that it is normally formed, which depends on the gestational age at diagnosis. If the fetus is less than 24 weeks' gestation, parents may choose to terminate the pregnancy, to continue the pregnancy with postnatal care or even to consider repair of the defect *in utero*. Between 24 and 32 weeks, parents may choose between conventional postnatal therapy and fetal surgery. Anytime a diaphragmatic defect is diagnosed, prenatal karyotyping and detailed ultrasound examination to detect associated anomalies

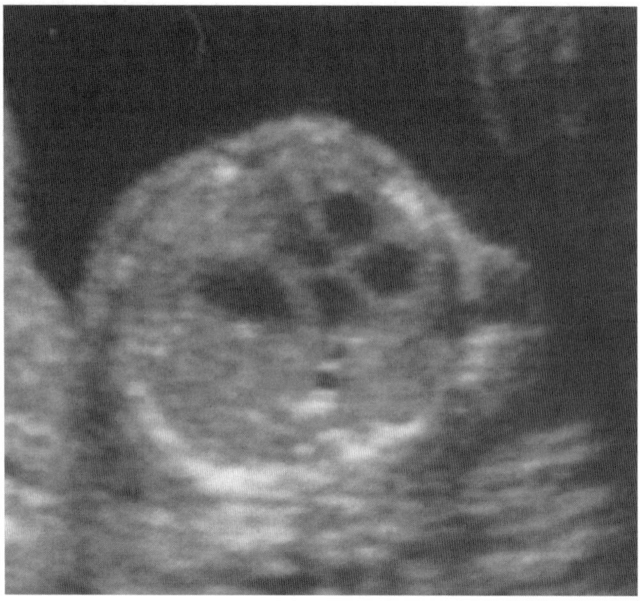

Figure 30.9 Transverse section of the fetal chest in a case of diaphragmatic hernia: the heart is displaced to the right side by the presence of the stomach and bowel loops in the thoracic cavity.

are recommended. There are no indications for preterm delivery or for cesarean section. The delivery should be planned in a tertiary care center.

Bowel disorders

Prenatal ultrasound examination allows the detection of the majority of gastrointestinal malformations because they are often associated with a dilated bowel, cystic masses or intra-abdominal calcifications, although the prenatal diagnosis generally does not influence the mode or the timing of delivery (except in the cases with polyhydramnios, which can cause premature labor or delivery). Moreover, it allows maternal referral to a center with appropriate perinatal, neonatal and surgical expertise, which, in some cases, may improve the outcome.

Esophageal atresia

This anomaly consists of the absence of a segment of the esophagus and is often associated with a tracheo-esophageal fistula (86–90% of cases). Five types of esophageal atresia may be distinguished:

(1) Isolated (type I)
(2) Associated with a fistula connecting only the proximal part of the esophagus and the trachea (type II)
(3) Associated with a fistula connecting the lower part of the esophagus and the trachea (type III)
(4) Associated with proximal and distal fistulas (type IV)
(5) Tracheo-esophageal fistula without esophageal atresia (type V).

Among different types the most common is the esophageal atresia associated with a fistula connecting the proximal part of the esophagus and the trachea (80% of the cases). The incidence varies between 1:800 and 1:5000 live births and the etiology is unknown.

The prenatal diagnosis is possible in only 10% of the cases and should be suspected in the presence of polyhydramnios with absent stomach bubble in several and repeated ultrasound examinations or visualizing a dilated proximal tract of the esophagus with absent stomach (Figure 30.10); however, this malformation can occur even in the presence of a normal or small stomach, due to the frequently associated tracheo-esophageal fistula.[8]

Associated anomalies are present in 50–70% of the cases, including cardiac, genitourinary, chromosomal (trisomy 21), additional gastrointestinal and musculoskeletal anomalies. A characteristic association is the 'VACTERL' (Vertebral, Anorectal anomalies, Cardiac anomalies, Tracheo-esophageal fistula, Esophageal atresia, Renal anomalies and Limb anomalies). Fetal karyotyping is suggested. The prognosis depends on the associated malformations and on the severity of polyhydramnios, which can facilitate preterm delivery.

Duodenal atresia or stenosis

The incidence of this malformation is 1:10,000 live births and its genesis goes back to the 11th week of gestation due to the failure of canalization of the primitive bowel. In most cases the etiology is unknown. Atresia is more common than stenosis (70% of cases) and could be associated with chromosomal abnormalities (trisomy 21), skeletal defects and other anomalies.[9]

The most typical sonographic finding is the characteristic 'double bubble' sign caused by the simultaneous dilatation of the stomach and the proximal duodenum (Figure 30.11). The diagnosis is usually made in the late second trimester.[10] Up to half the duodenal atresia cases are complicated by polyhydramnios and this can contribute to preterm labor, but the main cause of death are the associated anomalies. This malformation can present late complications (motility disorders, megaduodenum, gastro-esophageal and duodenal-gastric reflux, gastritis and blind loop syndrome) and late death even months or years after management.

Bowel obstruction

The incidence of bowel stenosis and atresia is 2–3:10,000 births and the most common locations are distal ileum (36%) and proximal jejunum (31%). There are four types of intestinal atresias:

(1) Type I: presence of a transverse diaphragm of mucosa or submucosa (20%).
(2) Type II: presence of blind ends of bowel loops connected by a fibrous band (32%).

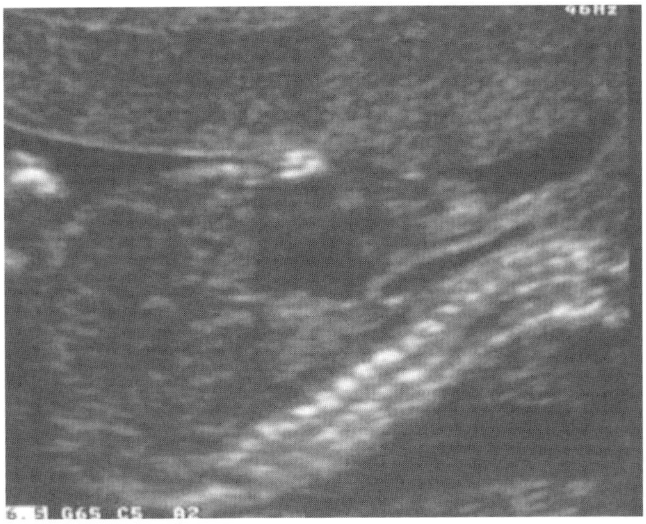

Figure 30.10 Esophageal atresia: the diagnosis is suspected by the association of absent stomach and dilatation of the proximal tract of the esophagus.

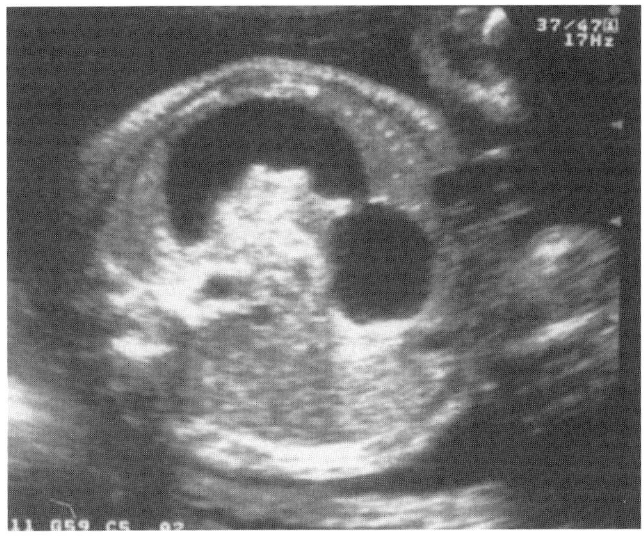

Figure 30.11 Duodenal atresia: the dilated stomach and proximal duodenum are clearly recognized.

(3) Type III: complete separation of blind ends with a corresponding mesenteric defect (48%).
(4) Type IV: absence of a large tract of small bowel with the typical 'apple peel' deformity, resulting from loss of the superior mesenteric artery.

These defects are usually sporadic, although familial cases have been described.

According to the site of the obstruction the defects are divided into (1) jejuno-ileal atresia and stenosis, (2) colonic atresia and (3) imperforate anus.

The sonographic prenatal appearance varies according to the level of the defect. In the case of jejuno-ileal atresia multiple dilated bowel loops in the fetal abdomen may be seen in association with polyhydramnios (Figure 30.12).[11,12] In colon atresia (which usually occurs proximal to the splenic flexure with a significant segment of absent colon with distal microcolon) the sonographic finding is similar to distal ileal occlusion and the differential diagnosis may not be possible. In the imperforate anus dilated intestinal loops with increased peristalsis may be seen as well as intraluminal hyperechogenic small areas referring to meconium (Figure 30.13).[13]

The diagnosis of bowel obstruction is usually made in the third trimester: the lower the obstruction the later is the appearance of the sonographic signs.

The prognosis of these malformations mainly depends on the level of obstruction (the lower the obstruction, the better the outcome), the length of remaining intestine and birth weight. Other important prognostic factors are the presence of associated malformations (especially gastrointestinal anomalies including bowel malrotation, esophageal atresia, microcolon and intestinal duplication), meconium peronitis and intrauterine growth restriction.

Meconium peritonitis

This condition is the consequence of *in utero* perforation of the bowel with spread of meconium into the peritoneal cavity leading to a local sterile chemical peritonitis. The peritonitis may be localized, with the development of a dense calcified mass or fibrous tissue, or diffuse, with a fibrous reaction leading to bowel adhesions and pseudocyst formation. Inflammatory reaction leads to an exudative process and ascites. Its incidence is 1:35,000 live births. Bowel perforation involves the proximal tract, with some form of obstruction such as intestinal atresia (65% of cases), meconium ileus, volvulus, gastroschisis or Meckel's diverticulum.

The prenatal sonographic appearance of meconium peritonitis varies according to the underlying anatomical finding: the main signs are intrabdominal calcifications (85% of cases), polyhydramnios, fetal ascites caused by exudate and bowel dilatation.

Postnatal management depends on the etiology of meconium peritonitis; up to one-third of all cases have cystic fibrosis.

Echogenic bowel

Sonographically, 'echogenic bowel' is defined as echogenicity of the bowel loops equal to or greater than the density of the iliac wing (Figure 30.14). A total of 1:200 midtrimester fetuses present this feature, which might depend on a slow or delayed transit of the meconium along the bowel. This finding has been considered as a 'soft marker' of chromosomal abnormalities but actually the increased risk of chromosomopathy in the presence of such an isolated marker is extremely low.[14] The risk increases when further sonographic markers are present. The echogenic bowel may also be the first sign of cystic fibrosis or can be

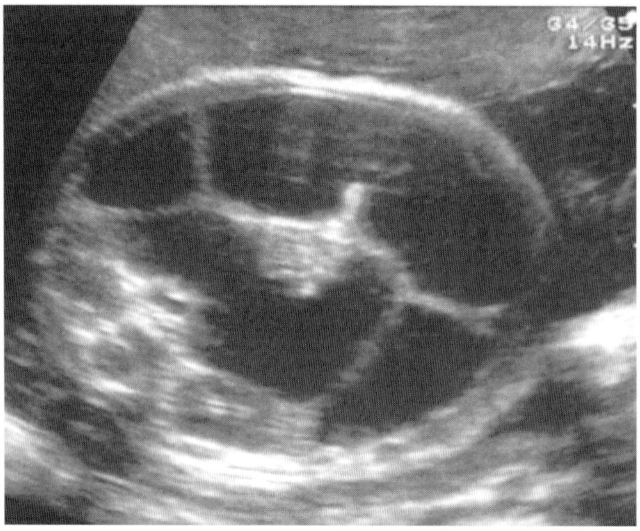

Figure 30.12 Jejunal atresia: multiple dilated bowel loops are present in the fetal abdomen.

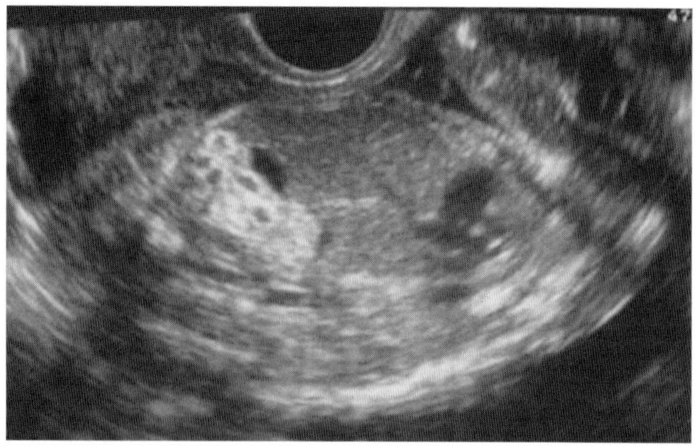

Figure 30.14 Echogenic bowel.

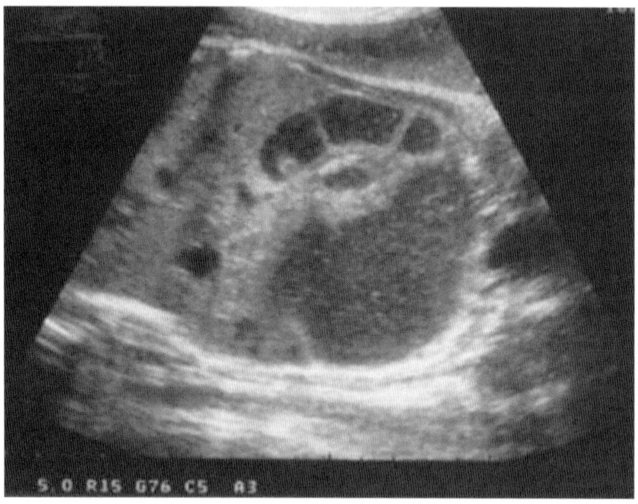

Figure 30.13 Imperforate anus in a third-trimester fetus: a dilated distal colon is seen containing multiple small echogenic foci due to meconium.

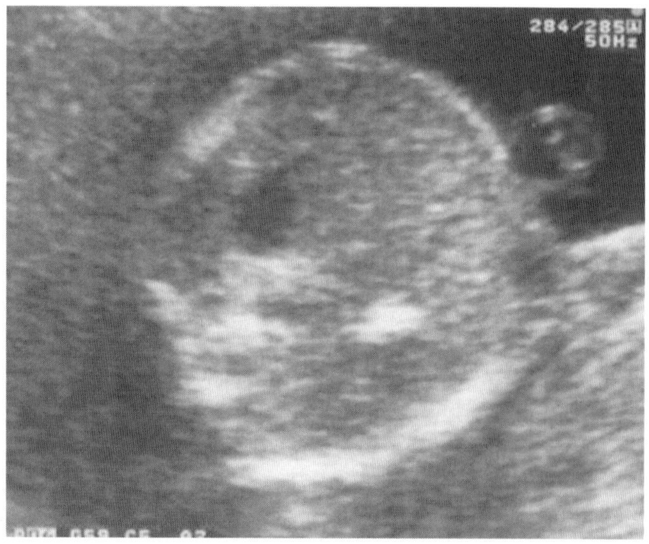

Figure 30.15 Hepatic hamartoma appearing as an isolated intraepathic area.

seen in cases of intraamniotic bleeding.[15] However, it is important to stress that the recognition of hyperechogenic meconium does not always represent a pathological condition but might be a normal variant and an isolated finding.[16]

Non-bowel cystic masses

Choledocal cysts

Choledocal cyst is a rare congenital cystic dilatation of the common bile duct. The incidence is about 1:2000. The cysts can be single or, in rare cases, multiple involving the intrahepatic or extrahepatic portion of the biliary tree. Choledocal cysts are classified into four types: (1) fusiform dilatation of the common bile duct, (2) diverticular dilatation of the common bile duct, (3) intramural dilatation of the common bile duct and (4) intrahepatic biliary duct dilatation. Its sonographic appearance is that of a cystic structure located in the upper right abdomen with dilated proximal ducts. Differential diagnosis includes duodenal atresia, hepatic cyst, dilated gallbladder, ovarian cyst and biliary atresia. The cystic size and the association with biliary obstruction affect the prognosis.[17]

Mesenteric and omental cyst

This benign malformation consists of cystic structures located in the small or large bowel mesentery or in the omentum filled with serous or chilous fluid. Its sonographic appearance is that of a thin-walled, unilocular or multilocular cystic mass. It is difficult to make a differential diagnosis with other intraabdominal cystic conditions such as choledocal, ovarian and hepatic cysts.

Hepatic masses

Hepatic masses might originate from an obstruction of the hepatic biliary system or might have a tumoral origin (hemangioma, hamartoma, etc.).

Their sonographic appearance changes depending on the origin: mesenchymal hamartomas usually appear as irregular hyperechoic areas (Figure 30.15), while hemangioma appears hypoechoic, hyperechoic or mixed depending on the degree of fibrosis and the stage of involution.[18] Hepatoblastomas and adenomas have a solid appearance. Polyhydramnios may be associated; many cases of reduction in volume or even disappearance *in utero* have been described.

The management is expectant in terms of monitoring the size and evolution of the tumor; for large tumors cesarean section is indicated.[19]

REFERENCES

1. Martin RW. Screening for fetal abdominal wall defects. *Obstet Gynecol Clin North Am* 1998;25(3):517–26.
2. Kurkchubasche AG. The fetus with an abdominal wall defect. *Med Health R I* 2001;84(5):159–61.
3. Oguniemy D. Gastroschisis complicated by midgut atresia, absorption of bowel, and closure of the abdominal wall defect. *Fetal Diagn Ther* 2001;16(4):227–30.
4. Morris-Stiff G, al-Wafi A, Lari J. Gastroschisis and total intestinal atresia. *Eur J Pediatr Surg* 1998;8(2):105–6.
5. Boyd PA, Bhattacharjee A, Gould S, Manning N, Chamberlain P. Outcome of prenatally diagnosed anterior abdominal wall defects. *Arch Dis Child Fetal Neonatal Ed* 1998;78(3).
6. Cadkin A, Strom C. Prenatal diagnosis of body stalk anomaly in the first trimester of pregnancy. *Ultrasound Obstet Gynecol* 1997;10(6):419–21.
7. Takeuchi K, Fujita I, Nakajima K, Kitagaki S, Koketsu I. Body stalk anomaly: Prenatal diagnosis. *Int J Gynaecol Obstet* 1995; 51(1):49–52.
8. Shulman A, Mazkereth R, Zalel Y, Kuint J, Lipitz S, Avigad I, Achiron R. Prenatal identification of esophageal atresia: The role of ultrasonography for evaluation of functional anatomy. *Prenat Diagn* 2002;22(8):669–74.
9. Sugimoto T, Yamagiwa I, Obata K, *et al.* Choledochal cyst and duodenal atresia: A rare combination. *Pediatr Surg Int* 2002; 18(4):281–3.
10. Lawrence MJ, Ford WD, Furness ME, Hayward T, Wilson T. Congenital duodenal obstruction: Early antenatal ultrasound diagnosis. *Pediatr Surg Int* 2000;16(5–6):342–45.
11. Uerpairojkit B, Charoenvidhya D, Tanawattanacharoen S, Manotaya S, Wacharaprechanont T, Tannirandorn Y. Fetal intestinal volvulus: A clinico-sonographic finding. *Ultrasound Obstet Gynecol* 2001;18(2):186–7.
12. Ogunyemi D. Prenatal ultrasonographic diagnosis of ileal atresia and volvulus in a twin pregnancy. *J Ultrasound Med* 2000; 19(10):723–6.
13. Has R, Gunay S. "Whirlpool" sign in the prenatal diagnosis of intestinal volvulus. *Ultrasound Obstet Gynecol* 2002;20(3): 307–8.
14. Al-Kouatly HB, Chasen ST, Streltzoff J, Chervenak FA. The clinical significance of fetal echogenic bowel. *Am J Obstet Gynecol* 2001;185(5):1035–8.
15. Berlin BM, Norton ME, Sugarman EA, Tsipis JE, Allitto BA. Cystic fibrosis and chromosome abnormalities associated with echogenic fetal bowel. *Obstet Gynecol* 1999;94(1):135–8.
16. Slotnik RN, Abuhamad AZ. Study of fetal echogenic bowel (FEB) and its implications. *J Ultrasound Med* 1999;18(1):88.
17. Chen CP, Cheng SJ, Chang TY. Prenatal diagnosis of choledochal cyst using ultrasound and magnetic resonance imaging *Ultrasound Obstet Gynecol* 2004;23(1):93–4.
18. Macken MB, Wright JR Jr, Lau H, *et al.* Prenatal sonographic detection of congenital hepatic cyst in third trimester after normal second-trimester sonographic examination. *J Clin Ultrasound* 2000;28(6):307–10.
19. Tsao K, Hirose S, Sydorak R, *et al.* Fetal therapy for giant hepatic cysts. *J Pediatr Surg* 2002;37(10).

31 Ultrasound diagnosis of urinary tract anomalies

P. Prats, N. Maiz, A. Rodriguez, C. Pedrero, M. Torrents,
F. Astudillo and J. M. Carrera

Embryology and anatomy of the nephrourologic system

The nephrourologic system has the functions of production and conduction of the urine toward the exterior by means of two independent nephrourologic tracts, but with the same functions that converge toward a reservoir that is the bladder, where the urine produced by the kidneys is stored, and it is excreted to the exterior through the urethra.

Embryology

The nephrourologic system has its embryonic origin in the intermediate mesoderm, located on both sides of the dorsal wall of the body. As the embryonic development advances it suffers transformations and specifications that will be translated into different anatomical parts of the urinary tract.

It would be possible to say that the embryonic development of the nephrourologic system occurs in two areas but in a synchronous way.

The superior nephrourologic system consists of kidneys (nephrons), collecting tubules, papillary ducts, calyces, renal pelvis and ureters.

Toward the fifth week of gestation, the paraspinal mesoderm differentiates into pronephros and mesonephros, which present some structural changes to become the metanephric blastema (that would be undifferentiated mesenchyma from the nephrogenic crest, which will give place to the future kidneys).

At the sacral level, there are also some paraspinal structures of mesodermic origin named ureteral gemmae from where some canals arise in caudocephalad direction address denominated mesonephric ducts or wolffia ducts that in their ascent penetrate inside the metanephric blastemas and ramify in their interior until a total of 15 generations.

In the seventh week of gestation, the functional units of the kidney, the nephrones, begin to differ due to the inductive influence of the ureteral gemma.

In the 20th week of gestation, the collecting system has already been formed: collecting tubules, papillary ducts, calyces, renal pelvis and ureters and 30% of the total population of nephrones.

Starting from this week and until the 36th week of gestation, an exponential increment in the total number of nephrones will take place.

The lower nephrourologic system consists of bladder and urethra. Both structures are unique and they take charge of transporting the urine produced in the superior nephrourologic system toward the exterior.

They arise from the mesoderm and the paramesonephric ducts (that also participate in the formation of the genital system) that will give place at the pelvic level to an embryonic structure called cloaca.

The cloaca, among the fourth and sixth weeks of gestation, presents a tabication by means of the urorectal septum that divides the cloaca into two parts: a posterior one that will be the rectum and another anterior one that will be the primitive urogenital sinus whose superior portion together with the allantois will give place to the bladder that will receive posterolaterally the ureters from the ureteral gemmae.

The inferior portion of the primitive urogenital sinus will give place to the membranous urethra and vaginal introitus in females and to the membranous and prostatic urethra in males.

Normal anatomy and variants

With the transvaginal ultrasonography, the kidneys and the bladder can be detected in the fetus from the ninth week of gestation. From the 12th week, the kidneys look like bilateral echogenic structures in the paraspinal region (Figure 31.1). The renal pelvis can be identified central to the medial hipoecogénicas. The bladder is in the pelvis and looks like a round anechoic structure that is well defined. Its position can be confirmed with the Doppler technique to identify the two umbilical arteries that surround it.

From 18–20 weeks of gestation, the kidneys can be defined clearly as oval masses lateral to the psoas

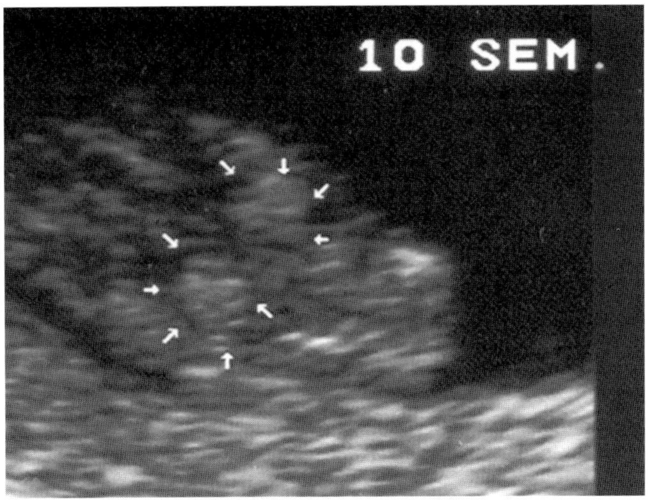

Figure 31.1 Kidneys at 10 weeks of gestation. Bilateral echogenic structures in the paraspinal region.

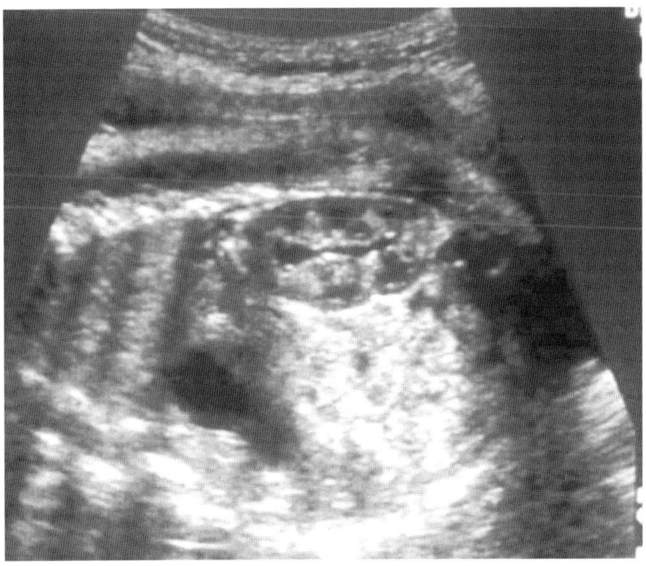

Figure 31.2 Sagittal scan of the kidney.

muscles and below the suprarenal glands using coronal or sagittal sections. These look like hypoechoic triangular that delimit the superior pole of the kidneys. In the traverse plane, the kidneys look like round paravertebral structures and the renal pelvis looks like anechoic areas medial to the kidneys (Figures 31.2 and 31.3). The renal pelvis is measured better in the anteroposterior projection, whether the fetus' column is up or down. The normal limit is 4 mm until 33 weeks of gestation and 7 mm from this date until the term. The normal values of the renal dimensions have been published, including the renal longitude, the anteroposterior diameter and the renal circumference.

With high-resolution devices, the renal pyramids can be seen as hypoechoic areas in the renal cortex, which should not be confused with renal cysts.

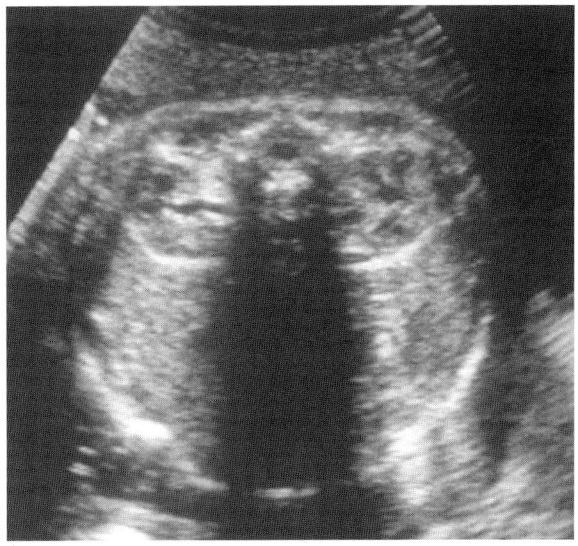

Figure 31.3 Coronal scan of the kidney.

The ureters are not usually seen, and if they are identified they are suspected for a renal obstruction or vesicoureteral reflux.

In the first trimester, the bladder looks like a round anechoic structure with the rectum behind. It is often possible to differentiate it from the intestine that surrounds it. However, it is better to measure the wall thickness at the umbilical artery level when this surrounds the bladder. The normal limit for the bladder wall thickness is 2 mm.

Ultrasonographic study

The ultrasonographic study of the fetal urinary system involves the evaluation of the kidneys, the bladder and the volume of amniotic fluid. It is also necessary to eliminate the associated anomalies.

Fetal kidneys

First, it is imperative to confirm if two kidneys are present. If a kidney is not present, it is necessary to look for it in ectopic positions like the pelvis. If it is not found, it is necessary to consider the possibility of unilateral renal agenesis. The bilateral renal agenesis usually associates to a severe oligoamnios, mainly starting from 17 weeks of gestation. When a renal anomaly is detected, it is fundamental to explore the contralateral kidney to confirm or to exclude a bilateral renal illness.

The size and echogenicity of both the kidneys should be valued. The hyperechoic kidneys can be normal, but it is also necessary to think about the possibility of a cystic renal disease, particularly when they are big.

The presence of macroscopic cysts usually indicates a multicystic kidney, but it is necessary to make sure that the cysts do not spread, because there are cases of multicystic kidneys with a great central cyst and smaller outlying cysts that can be mistaken for

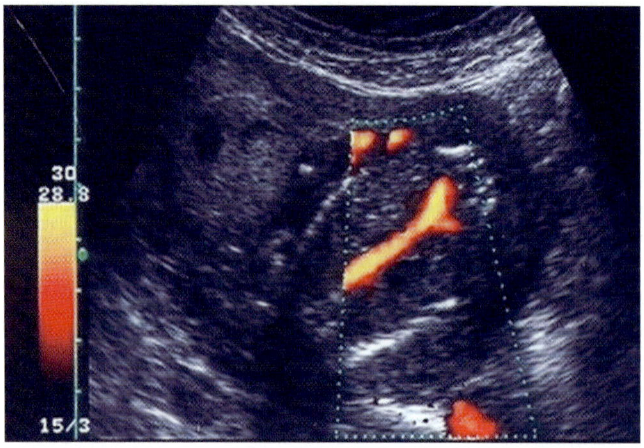

Figure 31.4 Bilateral renal agenesis. Absence of the renal arteries.

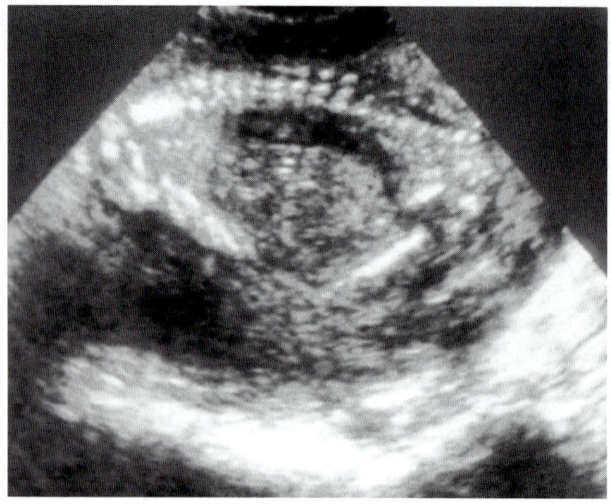

Figure 31.5 Bilateral renal agenesis. Note the enlarged adrenal gland.

hydronephrosis. If there is only one cyst, it can be considered a simple cyst.

The collector system of both kidneys should be evaluated not only with respect to the size but also the number. If two collector systems are seen it is necessary to discard a double kidney and to explore the bladder to rule out an ureterocele.

The dilatation of the collector system forces us to consider the possibility of a renal obstruction. The grade of dilatation of renal pelvis, ureter and bladder usually suggests the level of obstruction. When there is a dilatation of the collector system it is necessary to value the renal cortex echogenicity and the presence or absence of renal cysts to rule out secondary renal dysplasia.

Bladder

Bladder exploration includes size evaluation and – when it is large – the visualization of the posterior urethra, because if this is dilated it is necessary to think of an obstruction of the vesical exit. The thickness of the vesical wall can be measured at the level of the umbilical artery. It is necessary to rule out the existence of the ureterocele, particularly when there is a renal duplicity. In a period of 30–40 min, it is usually possible to demonstrate vesical filling and drainage.

Volume of amniotic fluid

This volume can be evaluated in different ways. Most echographers carry out a subjective evaluation first and then they adopt more objective approaches if they find that there is too much or too little. It seems that the best technique is the calculation of the index of amniotic fluid from the measures in the four uterine quadrants and its half-value. Severe oligoamnios of the second trimester usually has a bad prognosis and if it excludes premature rupture of membranes and a severe intrauterine growth restriction (IUGR), it usually indicates the presence of a severe bilateral renal illness.

Urinary tract malformations

Renal agenesis

Renal agenesis is the absence of one or two of the kidneys. The incidence of unilateral renal agenesis is 1 per 1000 births, and bilateral is 1 per 4000 births.[5] The etiology is ignored. Some cases of unilateral agenesis could be secondary to an intrauterine regression of a dysplastic multicystic kidney.[6] The embryological origin of the renal agenesis is the lack of union or penetration of the ureteral sprouting in the metanephric blastema, so that the primitive collecting tubules do not induce nephrone formation starting from metanephric mesoderm.[7]

Diagnosis

Bilateral agenesis: Echographic diagnosis is carried out for:

- The absence of kidneys in renal fossae that is difficult to evaluate because of the oligohydramnios in many cases
- Severe oligoamnios
- No bladder visualization[8]
- The absence of renal arteries by means of the color Doppler study[9,10] (Figure 31.4)
- The 'lying down adrenal sign' where the renal fossae is not occupied by the suprarenal glands[11] (Figure 31.5)
- Fetuses in podalic presentation where transvaginal ultrasound will help to improve the image[12,13]
- The infusion of intraamniotic and intraperitoneal physiologic salt solution to improve the image quality[14,15]

Unilateral agenesis: For diagnosis a meticulous evaluation of both renal fossae must be carried out. Ultrasound findings will be:

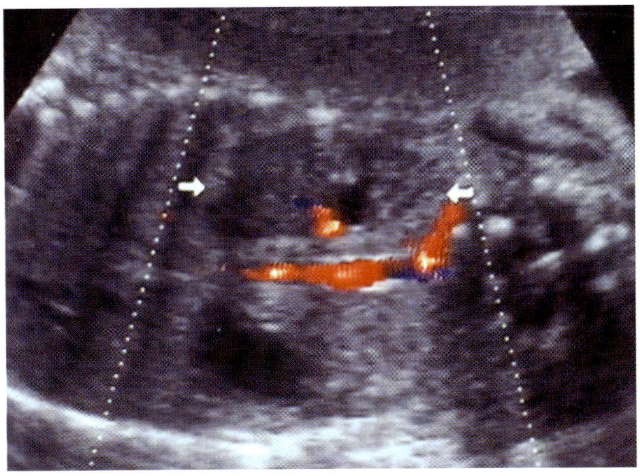

Figure 31.6 Unilateral renal agenesis. Renal artery in Doppler color. Notice the absence of the renal artery.

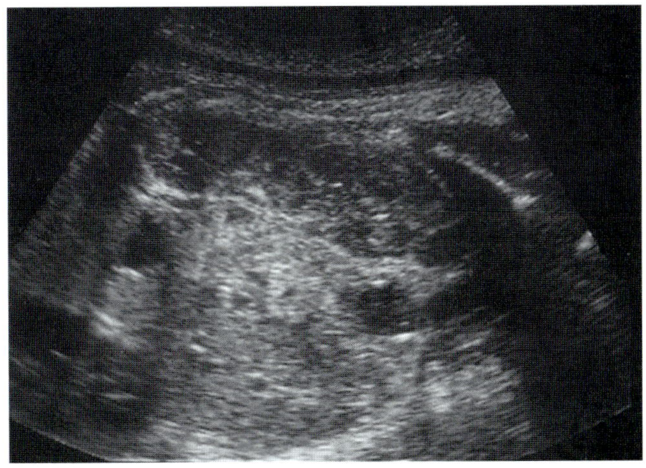

Figure 31.7 Unilateral renal agenesis. Note the large kidney.

- Absence of kidney in the renal fossa
- Absence of ipsilateral renal artery by means of color Doppler (Figure 31.6)
- Absence of pelvic kidney or renal ectopy, for this the renal pelvis and contralateral kidney needs to be evaluated.

The contralateral kidney can be increased in size because of compensatory hypertrophy[16] (Figure 31.7).

Differential diagnosis

Differential diagnosis will be mainly carried out for other causes of severe oligoamnios:

- Renal pathology
- Bilateral multicystic kidneys. The kidneys are usually evident for their cysts
- Infantile polycystic kidney disease. The kidneys are usually big and echogenic
- Uretral obstruction. The bladder is usually much evident
- IUGR. The kidneys and the bladder are present. It is usually accompanied by an alteration in the flow wave speed (FWS) of the umbilical artery
- Premature rupture of membranes (PRM). It usually has an antecedent of loss of vaginal liquid. The kidneys and the bladder are present.

Associated anomalies

Bilateral agenesis

- The Potter sequence (wide and plane nose, ears of low implantation, hypertelorism, receding chin, deformities of extremities) appears as a consequence of the severe oligoamnios
- Fifty percent present other associated anomalies
    - Cardiovascular
    - VATER (vertebral defects, anal atresia, tracheoesophageal, radial and renal anomalies)
    - Gastrointestinal (anal and duodenal atresia, omphalocele)
    - Phrenic hernia
    - Musculoskeletal: sirenomelus, digital anomalies
    - Central nervous system (CNS): neural tube defects
- Associated syndromes
    - Fraser syndrome
    - Brain-occulo-facial skeletal syndrome
    - Acrorenal–mandibular syndrome
    - Branchiootorenal syndrome.

Unilateral agenesis

- Anomalies of the contralateral kidney in 48% of the cases
    - Vesicoureteral reflux
    - Obstruction of vesicoureteral junction
    - Obstruction of pelviureteral junction.

Prognosis

- Bilateral agenesis: The prognosis is very poor. All newborns die in the first few hours or days similar to the consequence of lung hypoplasia
- Unilateral agenesis: In general, the prognosis of these newborns is very good, although it will much depend on any anomalies associated with the contralateral kidney.

Management

- Bilateral agenesis: A pregnancy interruption may be offered due to the lethal prognosis. If the mother decides to continue with the pregnancy it will be opted by a conservative behavior, a vaginal delivery will always be attempted, and reanimation maneuvers will not be made in the neonate
- Unilateral agenesis: During the pregnancy normal controls are followed. As much as during the pregnancy as in the newborn the appearance of anomalies will be watched over in the contralateral kidney.

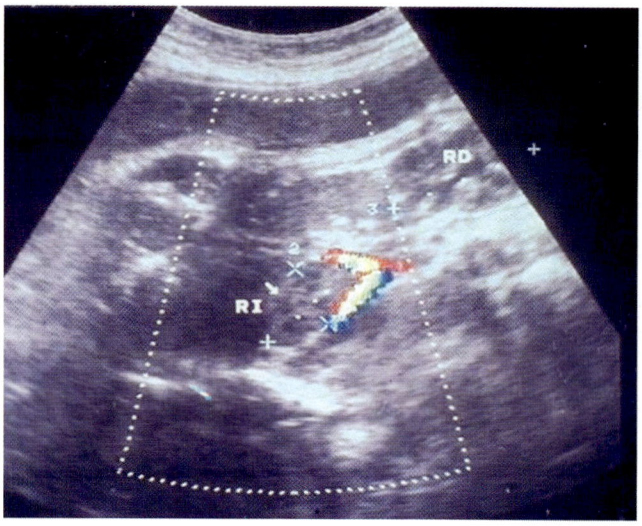

Figure 31.8 Ectopic pelvic kidney. Between iliac arteries.

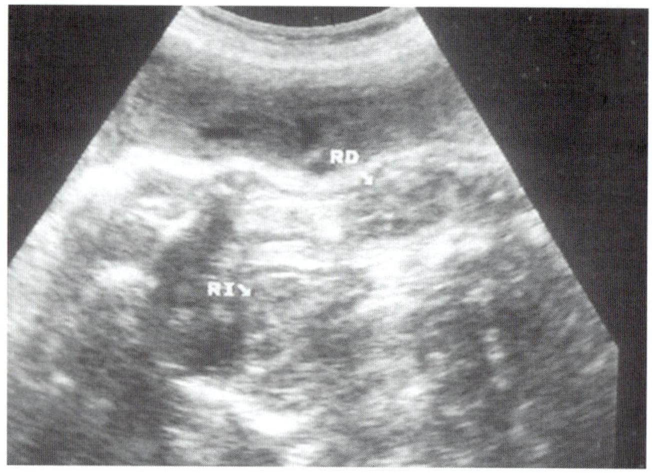

Figure 31.9 Ectopic pelvic kidney. Between iliac arteries.

The recurrence risk of the bilateral renal agenesis is approximately 4%.[17] About 9% of first grade relatives of the fetuses or newborns with renal impotence will have asymptomatic renal malformations. If the renal agenesis is part of a syndrome, the recurrence risk will depend on the inheritance type.

Renal ectopy

Ectopic kidney is that which is located outside the renal fossa. The most frequent locations are the pelvis (pelvic kidney) and the crusader of the other side (ectopia renal crusade); other less frequent ones are lumbar or thoracic. The incidence is approximately 1/1200 and 1/1900, respectively.[18,19]

Pelvic kidney

The lack of ascent of the kidneys originates the pelvic kidneys and other ectopic forms.

Diagnosis The echographic signs that will be found are:

- *Absence of the kidney in the renal fossa.* In these cases it is very important to make an exploration of the fetal pelvis and the contralateral side in search of a possible ectopic kidney
- *Localization of the kidney adjacent to the bladder or the wing of the ileum.*[18] In some cases, it may be difficult for its echogenicity to be similar to the adjacent intestine (Figures 31.8 and 31.9).

Differential diagnosis

- Unilateral renal agenesis.

Associated anomalies. Other anomalies have been described as:

- Gynecological anomalies
- Gastrointestinal, cardiovascular anomalies and skeletal defects [18]
- Unique umbilical artery
- Contralateral kidney anomalies, as vesicoureteral reflux.

Prognosis The prognosis is very good, although it will depend on the associated anomalies of the contralateral kidney.

Crossed ectopic kidney

During the renal ascent, a kidney crosses to the other side, resulting in crossed renal ectopy.

Diagnosis

- Absence of kidney in the renal fossa
- Big contralateral kidney and bilobate.[20]

Differential diagnosis

- Unilateral renal agenesis with compensatory hypertrophy. In these cases, the kidney is not bilobed and it does not present a second collector system
- Renal tumor. The contraleteral kidney is present. A collector system is not identified in the tumor.

Associated anomalies

- Vertebral anomalies (myelomeningocele, sacral agenesis)
- Anal atresia
- Urinary anomalies like ureterovesical reflux, hydronephrosis, urinary infections etc.

Prognosis If it is presented in an isolated way the prognosis is good.

Horseshoe kidney

Horseshoe kidney is the union of the lower, or occasionally, the upper extremities of the two kidneys by a band of tissue extending across the vertebral column. The incidence is 1 per 400–600 births.[21,22] Because of their proximity, the kidneys fuse before completing their ascent, so that the root of the inferior mesenteric artery will avoid completing their ascent.

Diagnosis

Because of subtle findings, it is underdiagnosed. The echographic diagnosis is based on the demonstration of the presence of a renal tissue bridge that connects both the kidneys. Generally, in the inferior poles, it can be identified both in the transverse and coronal sections.

Associated anomalies

- *Urogenital anomalies*: Hydronephrosis, vesicoureteral reflux, hypospadias, and cryptorchidism
- *Extraurological anomalies*: Anomalies of CNS (neural tube defects[23]), cardiovascular, gastrointestinal anomalies, and musculoskeletal defects[24]
- *Chromosomal anomalies*: Turner's syndrome,[25] Trisomy 18[26,27]
- *Renal tumors*. In children it has been associated to the Wilms' tumor,[28] and in adults it has been associated to a higher incidence of adenocarcinoma[29] and transitional cells tumor.[30]

Prognosis

The prognosis is excellent. A higher incidence of vesicoureteral reflux, renal stone, infection and hydronephrosis must be kept in mind.

Obstructive uropathies

The fetal kidney responds in different ways to an obstruction depending on the gestational age in which it occurs. Very precocious obstructions, in the first trimester or beginning of the second, will give place to polycystic dysplastic kidneys. Later obstructions (after the 22nd week) can produce hydronephrosis.

A particular difficulty in the diagnosis of renal obstruction is the high proportion of false-positive estimates in 36–81%. This is due to the mild hydronephrosis that is solved at the end of the pregnancy or in the neonatal stage. In order to avoid these false positives, limiting values of the anteroposterior diameter of the renal pelvis have been defined, for which the obstruction should be suspected. Unfortunately, these cut-off points vary: from 4 to 10 mm in the second trimester and from 7 to 10 mm in the third trimester.

For some authors, the best echographic approach to predict postnatal uropathies is an anteroposterior diameter of the renal pelvis greater than or equal to 7 mm in the third trimester with a 69% positive predictive value.[31,32] Other authors have calculated echographic false negatives below 10%[33] and negative predictive values of 98%.[34]

Diameters of the renal pelvis above 15 mm have a high predictive value of renal pathology that needs postnatal surgery.[35]

The group that has more problems is those that have pelvic diameters from 4 to 10 mm from the 20th week because 10–30% of children will present a vesicoureteral reflux that could damage the renal function without follow-up.[31]

These cases should be re-evaluated toward the 28th week of gestation and in the neonatal period to rule out a possible progression of the pyelectasis.

A sign of serious concern of the hydronephrosis is the presence of caliectasis, because it bends the necessity of surgery with regard to when the hydronephrosis is only present.[36]

Another aspect is the association between the dilatation of the urinary tract and chromosomal anomalies. In most of the cases, they are part of a multisystemic alteration secondary to a genetic alteration.[37] In the case of isolated mild hydronephrosis, the association with chromosomopathies is less clear; according to Nicolaides it would be a 3% in isolated hydronephrosis.[38]

Obstruction at the pyeloureteral junction level

Obstruction at the pyeloureteral junction level is the most common cause of obstruction at renal level, with an unknown real incidence; some authors have calculated it in 1/2000 born alive.[39] It is more common in males, and in 30% it is bilateral; when it is unilateral it is more frequently on the left side.

It is produced by a stenosis at the pyeloutereral junction level.

The obstruction is in most of the cases functional, so it would result in a urine propulsion failure.

Histologically, the ureter frequently shows signs of chronic inflammation with disruption and disorganization of the collagen and muscular fibers in its wall. In 69% of the cases a muscular anomaly exists so that there is an absence of the longitudinal fibers.[40]

With less frequency there are anatomical causes of obstruction like fibrous adhesions, bands, anomalous ureteral insertion and obstruction for double kidneys.

Diagnosis In the sonographic scan a dilated renal pelvis will be seen with or without dilation of the renal calyces and without ureteral or vesical dilation (Figures 31.10–31.13).

In cases of severe obstructions dilation of the renal chalices takes place with weight loss of the renal cortex (Figure 31.14). In rare cases, an abdominal cyst will be present or it will rupture with consequent perirenal urinoma (Figure 31.15).

The volume of the amniotic fluid is usually normal; however, it can cause polyhydramnios for increase of urine production. The appearance of oligoamnios is not normal.

Differential diagnosis It is necessary to consider other causes of lower renal obstruction where the ureters appear usually dilated like those of the vesicoureteral junction, vesical exit and the bilateral vesicoureteral reflux. It will also be necessary to consider polycystic kidneys, simple renal cysts or urinomas.

Associated anomalies In the cases of pyeloureteral obstruction we should study both kidneys in detail in search of possible associated anomalies (25–27%) as agenesis, multicystic dysplasia, vesicoureteral reflux, as well as possible extrarenal anomalies (12–19%) like cardiovascular anomalies, neural tube or digestive anomalies and chromosomal anomalies.[41]

Prognosis The postnatal prognosis is usually good and the hydronephrosis grade is usually correlated with the renal function.[35]

Prenatal management is usually conservative with the echographic follow-up in the third trimester. In the newborn, antibiotic profilaxis is prescribed and a complete evaluation is carried out with echography, isotopic renogram and cystourethrography. The examinations are delayed for about 10 days except in the cases that present severe bilateral affectation.[42]

In most cases postnatal management is conservative except when an increment of the hydronephrosis or decrease of the differential renal function exists, where pyeloplasty is the surgery of choice.[43]

Though most of the cases are sporadic family forms of dominant inheritance have been described.[44]

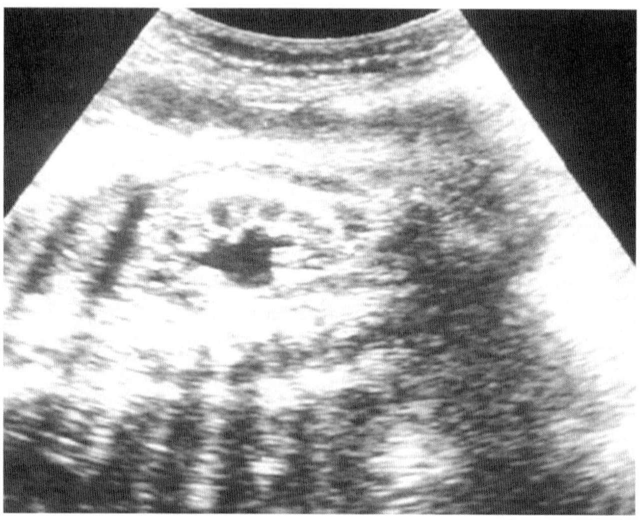

Figure 31.10 Mild dilatation of the renal pelvis.

Obstruction of the ureterovesical junction

This is the second cause of hydronephrosis, affecting 1/6500 newborns.[39] It is more common in males (ratio 2:1). It can be bilateral in 25% of the cases.

The obstruction is generally due to a regional malfunction or an estenosis at the ureteral end, without evidence of vesicoureteral reflux or obstruction of the vesical exit. This is also called primary megaureter or megaureter without reflux.

Diagnosis The affected kidney is shown with pyelectasis and a tortuous ureteral course (Figures 31.16 and 31.17).

The intravesical urine volume and amniotic fluid volume are usually normal, although they can be diminished in some cases of severe bilateral obstructions.

Differential diagnosis The dilated ureter can be easily differentiated from intestine because the urine is anechoic while the intestinal content transmits low echogenicity.

A differential diagnosis with the vesicouereteral reflux should be carried out, which can have the same prenatal echographic appearance and not to be able to exclude until the realization of a cystouretography in the neonatal period. It will also be necessary to carry out the differential diagnosis with strange cases of obstructions in the exit of the bladder that produce a massive uretral reflux and in the cases of double kidneys where the ureteral dilatation is produced by an ureterocele, in this situation it is usual that the superior pole is hydronephrotic and that the ureterocele is visualized inside the bladder.

Associated anomalies The contralateral kidney will present anomalies in 16% of the cases, including

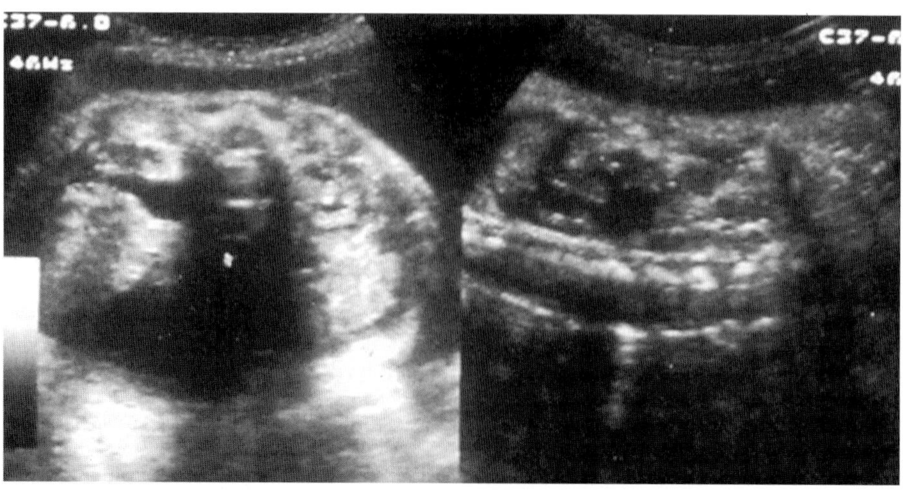

Figure 31.11 Mild dilatation of the renal pelvis.

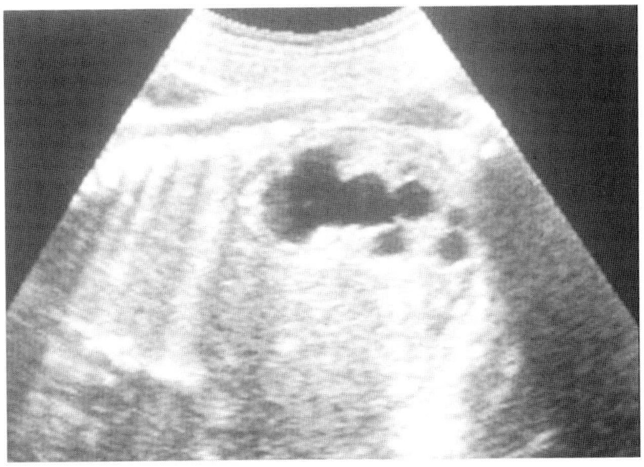

Figure 31.12 Moderate dilatation of the collecting system and the renal pelvis.

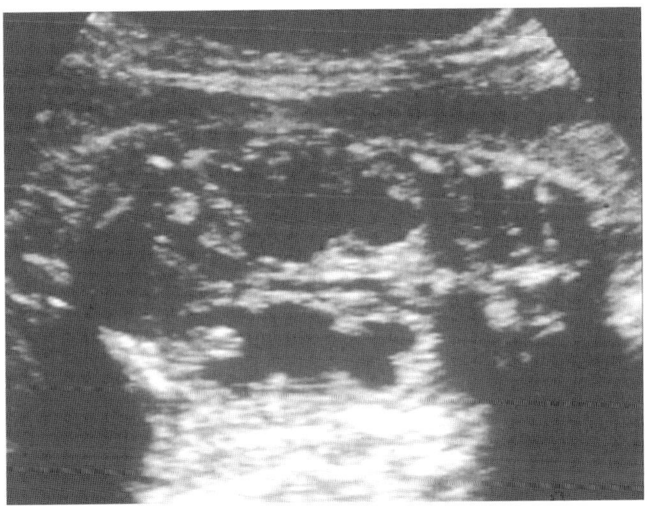

Figure 31.13 Moderate dilatation of the collecting system and the renal pelvis.

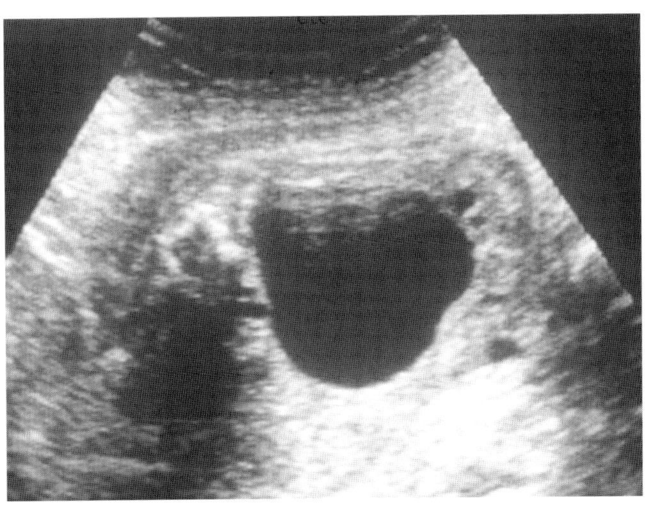

Figure 31.14 Hydronephrosis. Severe dilatation of the renal pelvis and calyces. Enlarged kidney.

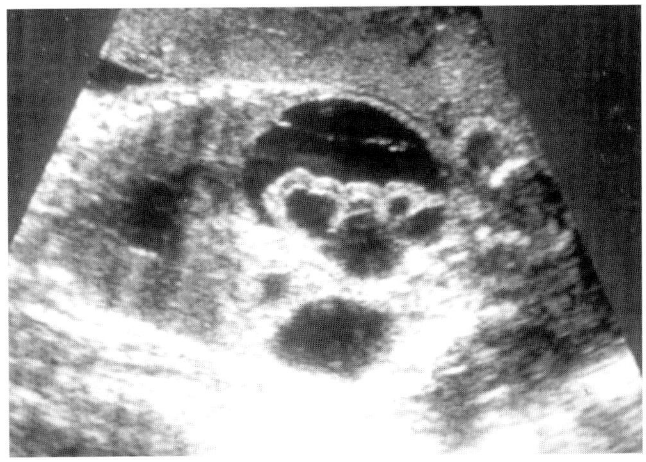

Figure 31.15 Urinoma. Note the thinning of the cortex.

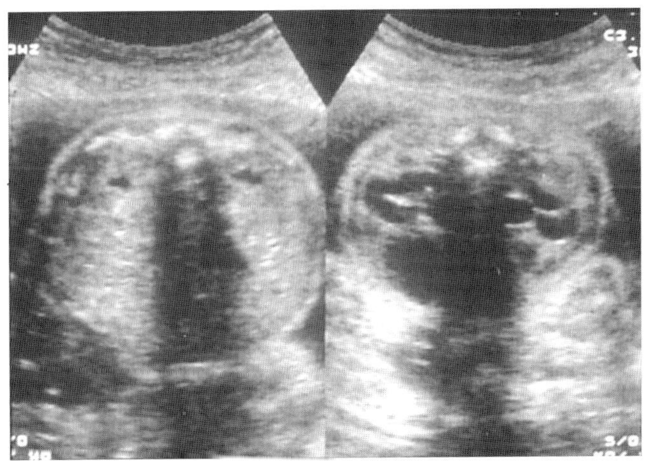

Figure 31.16 Dilatation of the ureters.

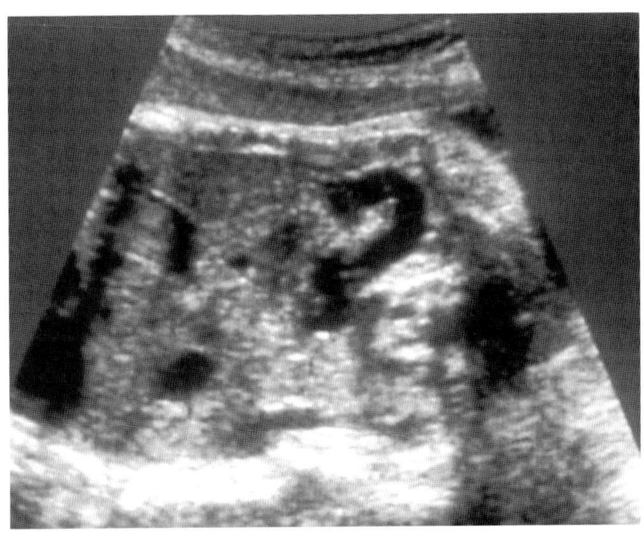

Figure 31.17 Dilatation of the ureters.

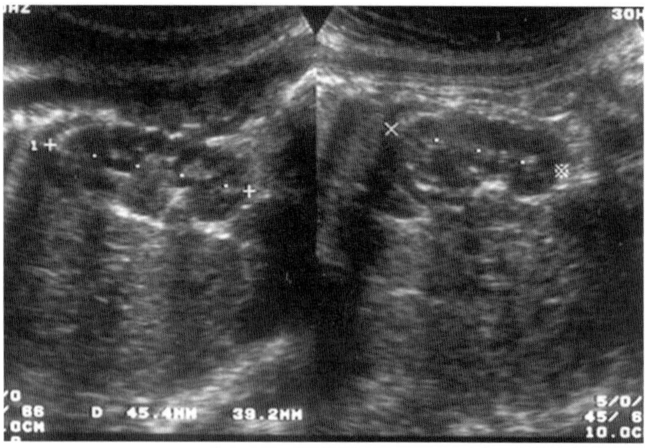

Figure 31.18 Duplex kidney. A sagittal scan through a duplex kidney shows two collecting systems.

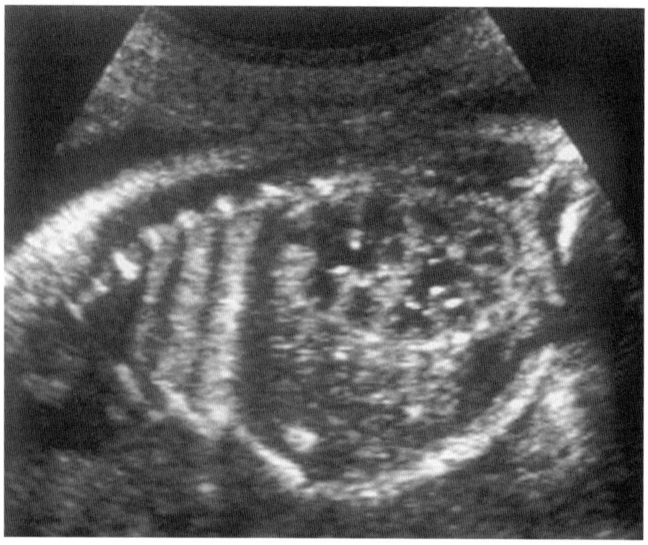

Figure 31.19 Duplex kidney. A sagittal scan through a duplex kidney shows two collecting systems.

pyeloureteral obstruction, multicystic renal dysplasia, pelvic kidney, renal agenesis and vesicoureteral reflux.[45]

Prognosis It is generally good so that up to 40% resolves postnatally in a spontaneous way. Ureters with diameters of less than 6 mm are associated with low surgery incidence, while those that have a diameter above 10 mm have a higher incidence of surgical corrections.[46,47]

A neonatal follow-up should be carried out with cystourethrography and a renogram to evaluate the renal function. Those that present a poor renal function will be candidates for surgery with ureteral reimplantation.

It is sporadic with a low recurrence risk.

Secondary obstruction to ureterocele and ectopic ureter

The ureterocele is a cystic dilation of the distal ureter in its intravesical portion.

An ectopic ureter is that which is not inserted near the posterolateral angle of the trigone.

An ectopic ureter can end in the urethra, in the neck of the urinary bladder or in the trigone, in an inferomedial localization regarding the normality. In girls, it can also be inserted in the vestibule of the vagina, vagina or uterus and in males in the seminal vesicle, ductus deferens or ejaculatory ducts.

The incidence is difficult to determine. There are studies that estimate it in 1/9000 newborns.[39]

The ureteroceles frequently associates in girls (up to 80%) with double renal systems being located in these cases the ureterocele in the superior system.[48]

However, in 40% of children the ureteroceles drain to a unique collector system. The ureteroceles and the ectopic ureteres are bilateral in 10–15% of the cases.

The double systems occur for the development of two ureteral gemmae starting from the mesonephric duct. In the double systems, the place where it drains is reversed, so the ureter of the superior pole drains into a more inferior and more medial place and the inferior pole drains into a superior and lateral place. The presence of ureterocele will produce hydronephrosis in the superior pole, which can produce dysplasia and deterioration of the renal function. In the inferior pole, it can also have hydronephrosis but it is usually due to vesicoureteral reflux.

Diagnosis In the absence of hydronephrosis, it may be difficult to diagnose prenatally a double system. In these cases, a meticulous echographic study would demonstrate a kidney of increased size with two collector systems. The prenatal diagnosis of the double system is usually carried out during the second half of the pregnancy with the presence of two or more of the following signs: limited hydronephrosis to a kidney pole, double renal pelvis not communicated, ipsilateral megaureter and ureterocele[49] (Figures 31.18 and 31.19).

When hydronephrosis exists, the superior pole is usually affected and the ureterocele can be demonstrated if the bladder is full. The ureterocele cannot be seen for different reasons: dysplasia of the superior pole that makes little urine excretion, empty bladder, large ureterocele that confuses with the own bladder. An ectopic ureter will be suspected when hydronephrosis exists in the superior system of a double system, and this dilated ureter seems to end below the base of the bladder without ureterocele. The utility of the magnetic resonance has been described in doubtful cases[50] (Figures 31.20 and 31.21).

The ureteroceles can be large enough to produce obstruction of the exit of the urine from the bladder. They can be bilateral in 15% of the cases[51] (Figures 31.22–31.24).

The amniotic fluid is usually normal in unilateral cases.

Differential diagnosis With the reflux and the vesicoureteral obstruction. Also with posterior urethral

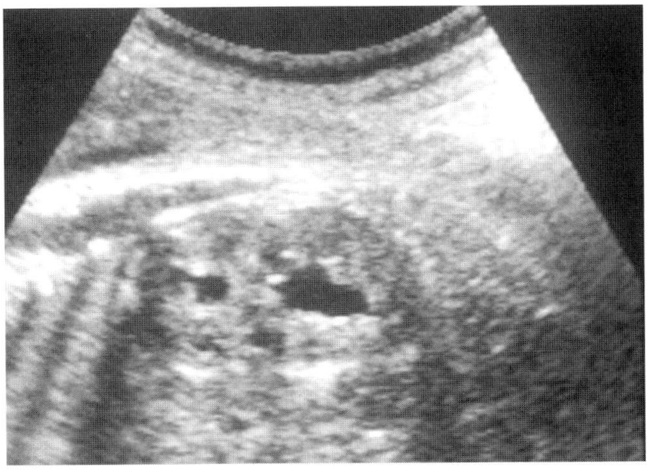

Figure 31.20 Duplex kidney. A sagittal scan through a duplex kidney shows two collecting systems.

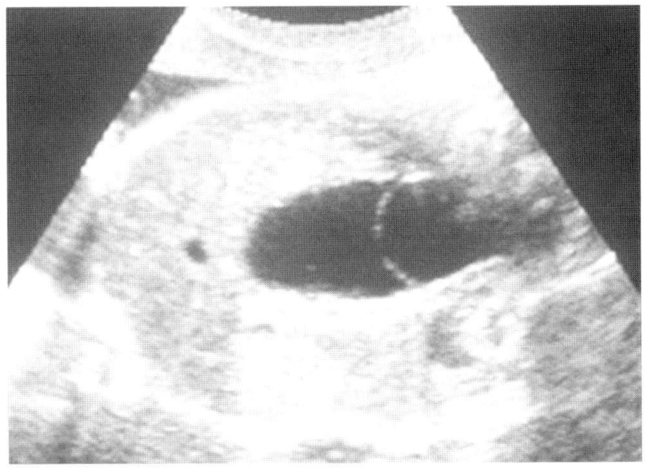

Figure 31.22 Ectopic ureterocele in the bladder.

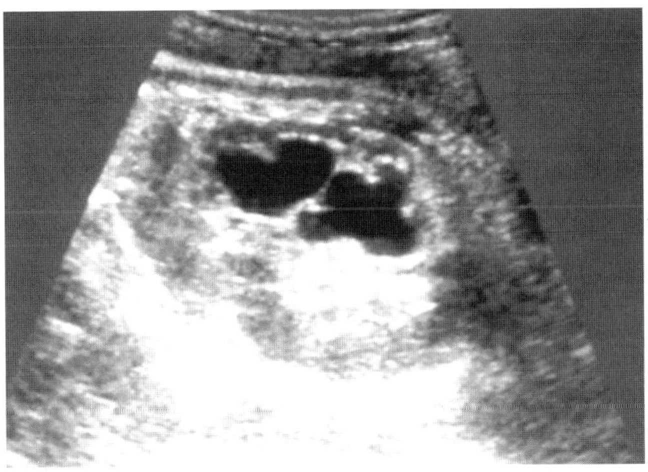

Figure 31.21 Duplex kidney. A sagittal scan through a duplex kidney shows two collecting systems.

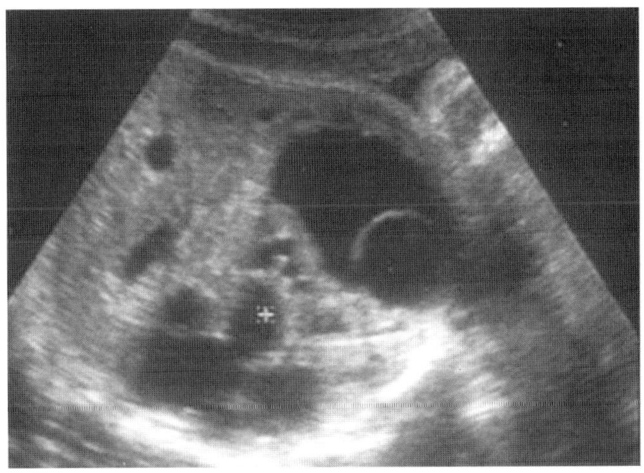

Figure 31.23 Ectopic ureterocele in the bladder.

valves in cases of ureteroceles that occlude the urethra, the posterior urethral valves occur only in males.

Associated anomalies The vesicoureteral reflux is presented in the inferior pole in 50% of the fetuses with ureterocele in the superior pole.[52] Higher association with other anomalies does not exist.

Prognosis It is better when a prenatal diagnosis is carried out. The necessity to carry out second surgery is reduced when it has been diagnosed prenatally.[53] The renal function will depend on the grade of dysplasia of the superior pole that is usually higher in ectopic ureters than in ureteroceles. In cases of severe reflux in the inferior pole, dysplasia and worsening of the renal function can also exist.

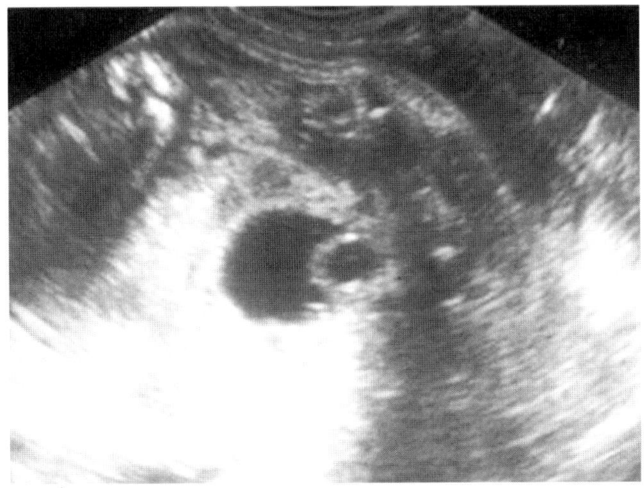

Figure 31.24 Ectopic ureterocele in the bladder.

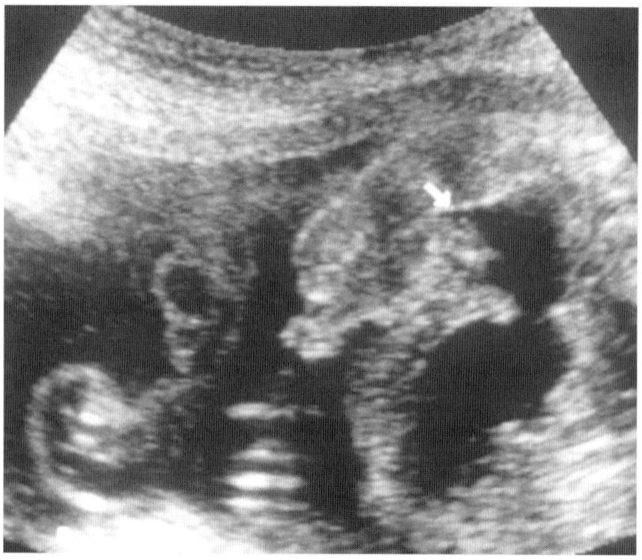

Figure 31.25 Dilated bladder and a 'keyhole' deformity of the posterior urethra.

Prenatal follow-up ultrasound will be carried out to evaluate the progression of the hydronephrosis.

In the postnatal period, it will be re-evaluated with echography, renogram and cystourethrography. In cases with good renal function the ureterocele can be punctured through the urethra by cystoscopy, which although has a risk of increasing the reflux in 30% does not seem to increase the necessity of second surgeries.[54] The non-functional superior poles are usually resected.[55–57]

It is sporadic with a low risk of recurrence.

Posterior urethral valves

This is the most frequent cause of severe obstructive uropathy in children, constituting 9% of the cases of fetal urinary obstruction.[55] The approximate incidence is 1 in each 5000–8000 children. It only affects males.

It is produced by folds of membranous tissue with a fibrous estruma that go from the prostatic urethra to the external urinary sphincter producing a more or less severe difficulty of the urine exit from the bladder.[59] The etiology is unknown; one of the theories is an anomalous insert of the mesonephric conduit into the cloaca.[60]

Diagnosis It is usually diagnosed in the second and third trimester. The characteristic echographic findings will be bladder dilatation with wall thickening (due to a detrusor thickening) and dilatation of the posterior urethra. It can exist in renal dysplasia recognized echographically for echogenic kidneys whether or not accompanied by cortical cysts[61] (Figure 31.25).

It is usually associated with a variable grade of bilateral ureterohydronephrosis[60] (Figure 31.26). The vesical distension can give place to its rupture causing urinary ascites, this ascites is considered a sign of good prognosis, since it liberates the kidneys of the

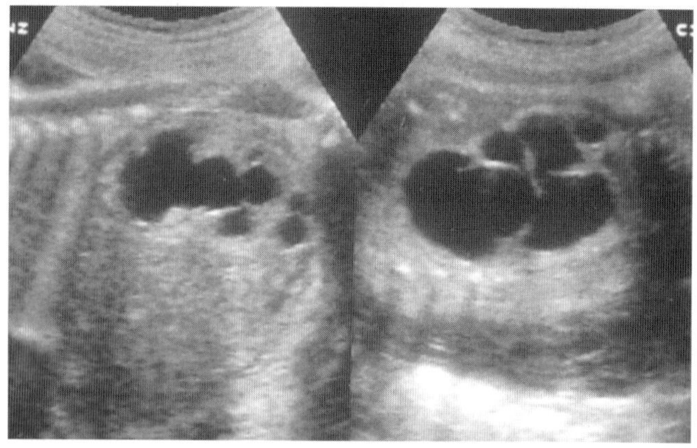

Figure 31.26 Kidney showing moderate dilatation.

pressure due to obstruction and therefore diminishes the risk of dysplasia.[55–62,63]

They can also break the renal chalices giving place to perirenal urinomas, which is a sign of bad prognosis since it is associated with renal dysplasia.[64]

It can exist as an asymmetric hydronephrosis by a massive reflux to a kidney that is practically destroyed; this can be a protection mechanism for the contralateral kidney.[65]

The amniotic fluid can be diminished, which is a sign of poor prognosis.

Differential diagnosis It is mainly with severe bilateral vesicoureteral reflux. Sometimes diagnosis is not easy. It may be useful to observe that in the reflux the bladder wall is usually thin, the dilatation of the posterior urethra also will not be seen.

We will also carry out the differential diagnosis with the ureteral atresia in which a marked vesical distension usually exists, of precocious detection in the first trimester or second initial trimester usually accompanied by oligoamnios.

We will also consider other rare causes of obstruction of the exit of the bladder like the congenital megalourethra, where a distal obstruction in the penile urethra exists and cystic images among the fetal legs can be observed in the ultrasound,[66] the cloacal persistence and hydrometrocolpos associated with a urogenital sinus that only takes place in girls,[67] and the microcolon-megalocysts syndrome where bilateral hydronephrosis and vesical dilatation can exist but it can be polyhydramnios and stomach distention. It affects the females more and it is of recessive autosomal inheritance.[68,69]

Associated anomalies They will be associated with a sequence of anomalies in variable grade secondary to the obstruction: megalocysts, megaloureter, hydronephrosis, paraurethral diverticula and dilatation of the proximal urethra. Other associated urinary anomalies are: megalourethra,[70] cryptorchidism, hypospadias and urethral duplications. Anomalies in other organs are also very frequently found (up to 43% of the fetuses)[71] like: tracheal hypoplasia, persistent ductus arteriosus, skeletal anomalies, imperforate anus, VACTERL syndrome[72] and frequent association of chromosomal anomalies.

When a precocious oligoamnios exists, lung hypoplasia will occur and the typical findings of the Potter's syndrome (low ear implantation, micrognathia, hypertelorism, limbs contracture) will be observed.

It can be the cause of the prune belly syndrome (thickening of the abdominal wall muscles, urinary tract alterations and undescended testes) due to the abdominal distension secondary to the vesical distension.

Prognosis The prognosis is variable depending on the graveness of the obstruction that in turn will be translated in the ultrasound findings, so that the most serious cases, diagnosed before the 24th week, will have a perinatal mortality or chronicle renal failure in 53%, while those diagnosed later will have a bad evolution risk of 7%.

The precocious oligoamnios, signs of renal dysplasia as the echogenic kidneys, cortical cysts, the perirenal urinoma and the association with other anomalies are the signs of a poor prognosis.

A determination of urine electrolytes is used to evaluate the renal function, with serial determinations to avoid the stagnated urine (Table 31.1). According to the result it will also be able to classify as good or bad prognosis.

It will also be convenient to carry out a fetal karyotype.

In the fetuses diagnosed before 32 weeks without signs of renal dysplasia but with oligoamnios the decompression of the urinary tract should be evaluated by means of the realization of a vesico-amniotic bypass.[74] After the 32nd week, it will be necessary to evaluate the finalization of the gestation for the decompression of the urinary tract in the proximate neonatal period. Nowadays, an option of intrauterine fetal therapy exists, which can be carried out by means of valvular resection with endoscopy. The criteria for this intrauterine surgery will be the absence of echographic dysplasia findings, normal karyotype and some appropriate values of electrolytes in the vesicocentesis.[75,76]

It is sporadic with a low recurrence risk.

Atresia urethral

The real incidence is ignored. It affects males more.

Etiology is ignored. It is characterized by the complete obstruction from the urethra secondary to the obliteration of the membranous urethra.

Diagnosis It can be seen as a very dilated bladder with oligoamnios in the ecograph. Detection can be carried out very early, on occasion starting from the 10th week. Frequently, an anhydramnios exists with such a loosened bladder that it is difficult to explore the fetal anatomy (Figures 31.27–31.29).

In some occasions, a vesicocutaneous fistula is developed being able to be the amniotic liquid normal.[77]

Table 31.1 Poor prognostic values in fetal urine

Sodium	100 mEq/l
Chlorine	90 mEq/l
Osmolarity	280 mOsm/l
Calcium	2 mmol/l
Phosphate	2 mmol/l
B_2 microglobulin	2 mmol/l

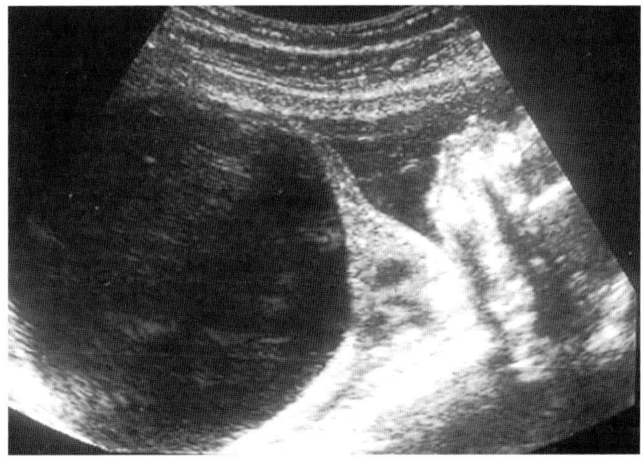

Figure 31.27 Axial plane through the fetal abdomen demonstrating fetal megacystis.

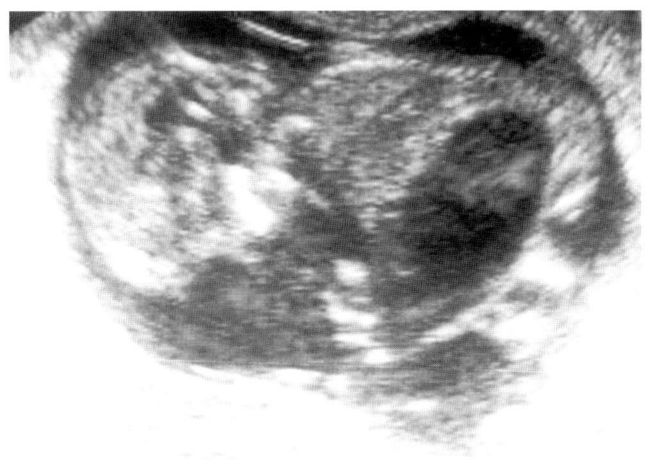

Figure 31.28 Axial plane through the fetal abdomen demonstrating fetal megacystis.

Differential diagnosis With other causes of vesical exit obstruction: posterior urethral valves, megalourethra, megacystis-microcolon syndrome, persistent cloaca and severe vesicoureteral reflux.

Associated anomalies They are very frequent (more than 50%) but difficult to diagnose because of the oligoamnios. Among them are: heart anomalies, diaphragmatic hernia, polydactily, VACTERL syndrome and chromosomal anomalies.

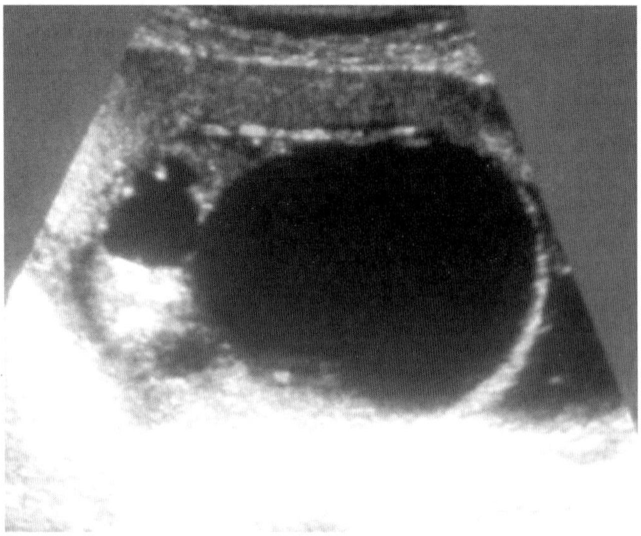

Figure 31.29 Kidney showing moderate dilatation.

It is one of the causes of the prune belly syndrome.[79]

Prognosis It is always poor and almost always lethal. Due to the oligoamnios or anhydramnios they develop a lung hypoplasia. The development of a vesicocutaneous fistula can improve the neonatal survival; however, they usually develop a renal failure that makes them need a renal transplantation with a bigger surgical reconstruction or hemodialysis.[77]

Due to the possibility of an early diagnosis an appropriate option is the interruption of the pregnancy. If the gestation is continued the possibility of the realization of a vesicoamniotic shunt will be evaluated.[80]

It is sporadic with a low recurrence risk.

Vesicoureteral reflux

This is the backward flow of urine from bladder into ureter and the pyeloureteral system.

This reflux occurs in around 1% of all the children. Fetal vesicoureteral reflux presents a masculine prevalence, of up to 80% and a high frequency (20%) of high grade reflux (III–IV).[81,82] Around 60% is bilateral. It represents 11% of the prenatal hydronephrosis cases.[83]

The etiology seems to be multifactorial. The neonatal reflux seems to have its origin in a distortion of the vesicoureteral junction *in utero*, secondary to the high casting pressures that some fetuses present.[81]

Pathology

- Urinary tract infection, which is more frequent in this group, is typically associated to parenchymatous affectation
- Up to 50% of the infants with sterile vesicoureteral reflux can present parenchymatous renal anomalies, which suggests a congenital etiopathology of renal lesion independent of the urinary infection.[84,85]

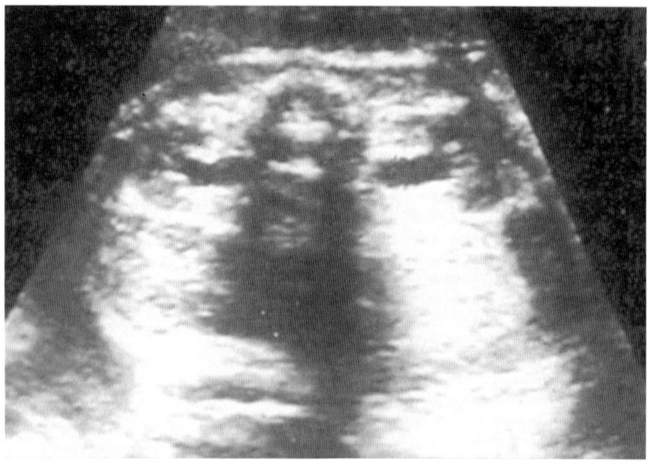

Figure 31.30 Moderate pyelectasis with vesicoureteral reflux.

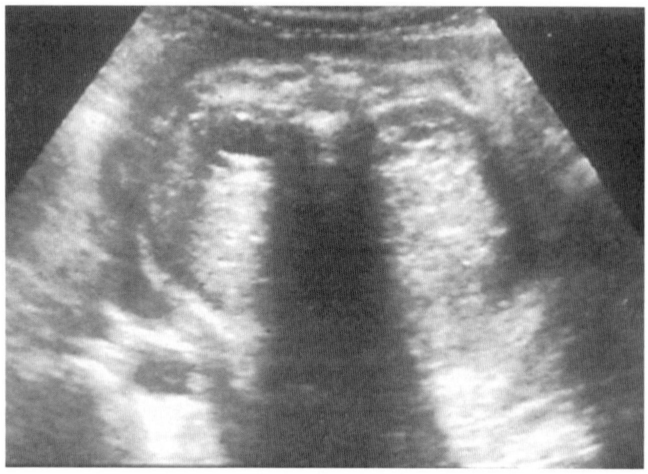

Figure 31.31 Moderate pyelectasis with vesicoureteral reflux.

Diagnosis

- *Hydronephrosis*. It is the main echographic finding. It can be unilateral or bilateral (Figures 31.30 and 31.31)
- *Hydroureter* and a dilated bladder with a thinner wall. These are findings that we could find in the most severe cases. It may be confused with some posterior ureteral valves
- The amniotic fluid volume is normal
- The moderate *pyelectasis* (4–10 mm) can also be associated to vesicoureteral reflux.

Differential diagnosis

Other hydronephrosis causes should be considered

- Unilateral: obstruction of pyeloureteral or vesicoureteral junction
- Bilateral: posterior urethral valves.

Associated anomalies

These are mainly anomalies of the contralateral kidney

- Obstruction of the pyeloureteral junction
- Multicystic kidney

- Renal agenesis
- Renal or ureteral duplicity.

Prognosis

- Many resolve completely spontaneously. A total of 60% grade III, 50% grade IV and 28% grade V were resolved in 14 months[83]
- 30% of these fetuses present renal scars, and two-thirds of them present widespread renal lesions
- The reflux is the cause of 25% of the renal failure in children and 15% in adults.

Management

- If there is a hydronephrosis:
  - *Prenatal control*: *In utero*, we must make an echographic follow-up of the hydronephrosis and of the volume of amniotic fluid.
  - *Postnatal control*:
    - Echography starting from 48 h of life
    - Antibiotic prophylaxis
    - Serial cystourethrography
- If there is a moderate pyelectasis
    - Postnatal echography
    - Echography up to 3 months
    - Urologic follow-up.

Treatment will be surgical in those cases that present new renal scars, a high reflux grade, a progressive reflux, or persistent urinary infections.

The recurrence risk in brothers of the affected cases is 34%[86] and in children of the affected cases is 66%.[87]

Renal cystic diseases

Renal cystic disease compromises a mixed group of heritable, developmental and acquired disorders. Because of their diverse etiology, histology and clinical presentation, no single scheme of classification has gained acceptance.[88]

The Potter classification (Potter 1972),[89] does cover the most important conditions seen prenatally (Table 31.2).

Many of the terms used to describe kidney malformations, such as the Potter classification, are confusing since they are based on histology and do not take account of recent advances in molecular biology and genetics. A more straightforward approach is to divide the abnormalities into groups based on the underlying cell biology, such as aberrant early development or defects in 'terminal' maturation.[90]

The aberrant early development group includes dysplastic kidney[90]:

1. Large multicystic dysplastic (Potter type IIa).
2. Small organs with a combination of hypoplasia/dysplasia (Potter type IIb).
3. Severely obstructed kidneys (Potter type IV).

Table 31.2 Potter classification of cystic renal disease

Type I	Autosomal recessive (infantile) polycystic renal disease
Type II	Multicystic renal dysplasia
Type III	Autosomal dominant (adult) polycystic renal disease
Type IV	Obstructive cystic dysplasia

Kidney malformations associated with syndromes are also included within this category.[90]

Defects in terminal maturation are observed in polycystic kidney disease (PKD). Initial nephron and collecting duct formation is unremarkable in these kidneys, but there is a later cystic dilatation of these structures causing secondary loss of adjacent normal structures. The most common types are autosomal dominant and autosomal recessive PKD. Both may present prenatally.[90]

Polycystic kidney diseases

Two forms of PKD will be discussed in this chapter:

1. Autosomal recessive polycystic kidney disease (infantile) (ARPKD).
2. Autosomal dominant polycystic kidney disease (adult) (ADPKD).

Both diseases may present prenatally or during infancy.

Cysts only arise from collecting ducts in ARPKD, whereas they arise from all areas of the nephron or collecting duct in ADPKD. In addition, there are usually numerous small cysts in ARPKD whereas there are fewer, larger cysts in the dominant disease. Associated abnormalities in other organ systems are quite different in both conditions.[90]

Autosomal recessive polycystic kidney disease (Potter I)

This condition is characterized by symmetric enlargement of both kidneys secondary to renal collecting tube dilatation. This is associated with varying degrees of hepatic fibrosis and biliary ectasia.[91]

It is an autosomal recessive condition with an incidence of 1/40,000–50,000 live births.[92]

There is likely to be a defect in the collecting ducts resulting in the formation of cystic dilatations of the collecting tubules.[93] The hepatic fibrosis could be due to overgrowth of the biliary epithelium. The gene for ARPKD is located on chromosome 6p.[103]

Pathology The kidneys are symmetrically enlarged, and this is produced by cystic dilatations of the collecting tubules, which are arranged radially throughout the renal parenchyma.[93] The earlier-forming distal collecting tubules are more severely affected than the proximal collecting tubules. There is no proliferation of the connective tissue.

Table 31.3 Manifesations of ARPKD according to the subclassification of Blyth and Ockenden

Type	Proportion of dilated renal tubules (%)	Extent of portal fibrosis	Lifespan
Perinatal	90	Minimal	Hours
Neonatal	60	Mild	Months
Infantile	20	Moderate	10 years
Juvenile	<10	Gross	50 years

Clinically the disease has been classified into four subtypes[94] (Table 31.3).

Diagnosis The typical appearance is of enlarged kidneys showing increased echogenicity associated with small or absent bladder and oligohydramnios[95,96] (Figure 31.32).

These sonographic features may not be present until the third trimester, however, and it is well documented that fetuses with their condition may look absolutely normal at the 20-week scan. Thus, this condition cannot be excluded until well into the third trimester.[97–99]

A few cases diagnosed by transvaginal scanning at 12–14 weeks' gestation have been reported.[100]

Careful measurements of both kidneys are important to the diagnosis because affected kidneys have a faster growth profile than normal kidneys.[101]

Molecular genetics studies provide a useful adjunct to ultrasound for diagnosing ARPKD and these should be discussed with high-risk families. It is possible to make a prenatal diagnosis at 11–12 weeks gestation from chorionic villus sampling.

Magnetic resonance imaging (MRI) has also been used to diagnose ARPKD *in utero*, but this technique is not in regular use in most centers.[102]

Associated anomalies The main association is hepatic fibrosis.

Differential diagnosis The differential diagnosis for ARPKD is quite large. However, one important consideration is autosomal dominant polycystic kidney disease (adult), which can look identical except that liquor volume is usually normal. The other main diagnoses are outlined in Table 31.4.

Prognosis The outcome is predicted from the severity of the renal disease, with the poorest outlook for the perinatal type. Infants usually die from respiratory failure rather than renal problems, although aggressive ventilatory support and emergency nephrectomy may improve the outcome.

The outcome is progressively better with later presentation and decreasing severity of renal involvement.

Long-term complications include severe systemic hypertension, urinary tract infection and hepatic fibrosis with portal hypertension leading to hypersplenism and gastroesophageal varices.[104]

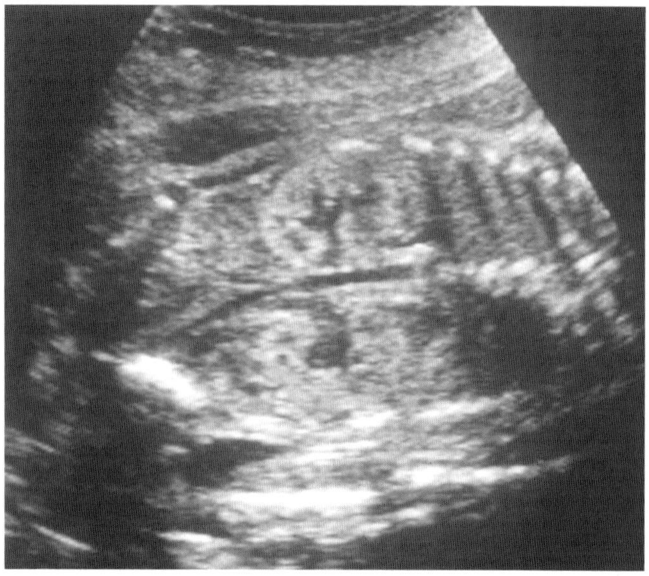

Figure 31.32 Autosomal recessive polycystic kidney disease. The images show enlarged kidneys with echogenic parenchyma and oligohydramnios. The bladder is not visible.

Management When scanning demonstrates bilaterally enlarged echogenic kidneys with oligohydramnios and there is family history of autosomal recessive polycystic renal disease, the outlook is likely to be very poor. In such a setting a termination of the pregnancy could be offered to the mother before viability.

When there is no family history and the amniotic fluid is normal, other conditions that have better prognosis should be considered. In such cases, conservative management is more appropriate.

The presence of associated abnormalities recommends karyotype. Follow-up scans are of value to assess liquor volume in pregnancy.

There is a 25% risk of recurrence.

Autosomal dominant polycystic renal disease (Potter III)

This condition is much more common than ARPKD. However, it is much less common or ADPKD to present prenatally or in early childhood. The ADPKD classically of both kidneys present cystic dilatation of the nephrons. It is the most common of the hereditary renal cystic disease, with an incidence of 1/1000 live births.[105]

The condition is caused by a mutation near the telomere of chromosome 16 in 90% cases.[106] Five percent of cases are caused by abnormality of chromosome 4.[107] Ninety percent of cases are linked to the *PKD1* gene on the short arm of chromosome 16[106] and 5% are linked to the *PKD2* gene on chromosome 4.[107]

Prenatal diagnosis is possible by gene probes from chorion sampling.[104]

Pathology It is a systemic disorder characterized by cysts formation in ductal organs, particularly the kidneys and liver. Cysts may also be present within the pancreas, spleen and CNS.[88] In the kidneys only 5% of nephrons are cystic in the early part of the disease.

Diagnosis In adults, almost all patients present one cyst, at least, at age of 30 years.[108,109] The sonographic appearance is well known: enlarged hyperechogenic kidneys, with a mixture of small and large cysts[110] (Figure 31.33).

Some cases diagnosed prenatally have been reported. The most common sonographic finding is large kidneys.[111–113] The sonographic appearance is similar to the ARPKD: symmetrically enlarged and hyperechogenic kidneys. The bladder is generally present and the amniotic fluid is normal. The corticomedullary junction may appear accentuated or may be indistinct.[114] Some reports have described the presence of macroscopic cysts within the echogenic kidneys.[90]

Brun *et al.*[27] determined a new specific echographic pattern: moderately enlarged kidneys (1–2 SD > mean) with, in the majority of cases, a hyperechogenic cortex and relatively hypoechogenic medulla that occurs in the third trimester. This hyperechogenic cortex is probably related to the presence of multiple microcysts within renal cortex.

Sonographic diagnosis is usually made in the third trimester with a mean of 28 weeks.[114] Some cases of earlier sonographic diagnosis have been reported but mostly in cases with known family history.[115,116]

Follow-up scans are essential because in the second trimester the kidneys can look normal.

Very rarely, the condition can be unilateral.[117,118]

Differential diagnosis Several conditions may exhibit enlarged hyperechogenic kidneys. This echographic feature may correspond to different renal diseases with different outlooks and perinatal outcomes: obstructive dysplasia, multicystic renal dysplasia, autosomal recessive polycystic renal disease, genetical syndromes (Perlman sd., Beckwith–Wiedemann sd., Bardet–Biedl sd., Meckel sd.), nefroblastomatosi, renal vein thrombosis, toxic injured, infections (cytomegalovirus), isquemia, aneuploydy, and sometimes, normality.

In autosomal dominant polycystic kidney disease few cases are diagnosed prenatally. The diagnosis is based on family history, amniotic fluid, associated abnormalities and genetic analysis.

Associated anomalies The most important associated anomalies are cysts in the liver, spleen and pancreas. Noncystic anomalies include cardiac disease, skeletal anomalies, pyloric stenosis and intracranial aneurysms.[88] Tract urinary malformations associated with this condition have also been described.[114]

Prognosis The condition is often asymptomatic and usually presents in the fifth decade with hypertension and end-stage renal failure.[105]

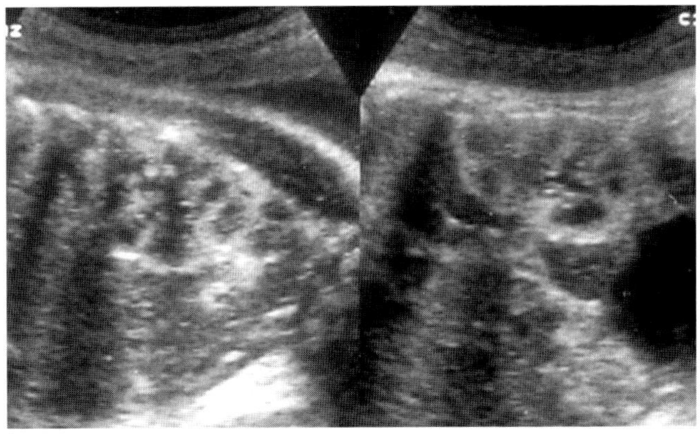

Figure 31.33 Adult polycystic kidney disease. Brightly echogenic kidneys with accentuation of the cortico-medullary junction and a small bladder with decreased fluid.

The outlook for those cases diagnosed *in utero* is difficult to determine because to date only 83 cases of adult-type polycystic renal disease presenting prenatally or in the first few months of life have been reported. MacDermott *et al.*[104] reported that in prenatal cases, 43% of babies die within the first year of life and 67% of survivors develop hypertension. The best indicators for outcome are the presence of oligohydramnios and the perinatal outcome from a previously affected sibling.

Management Management of the pregnancy depends in large part on the parents' knowledge of the condition.

The diagnosis of this condition requires very careful counseling with regards to both the short-term and long-term outlooks.

Follow-up scans in the third trimester are of value to assess liquor volume.

There is a 50% risk of recurrence.

Dysplastic kidneys — multicystic renal dysplasia (Potter II)

The diagnosis is inferred from the 'bright' echogenic appearance caused by the lack of normal renal parenchyma and structurally abnormal kidneys.

Dysplastic kidneys can be of any size, ranging from massive distended with multiple large cysts up to 9 cm in diameter, which are commonly termed 'multicystic dysplastic kidneys' (MCDK), to normal or small kidneys, with or without cysts. Dysplasia can be unilateral or bilateral. MCKD is one of the most common causes of abdominal masses in the newborn.[90]

It is the most common form of renal cystic disease in childhood. It has an incidence of 1/3000 live births and is more common in boys.[119,120] The majority is unilateral, but it can be bilateral up to 23% of cases.[119]

MCDK are attached to atresia of the ureter and renal pelvis. This may be related to incomplete but severe obstruction to the kidney early in nephrogenesis.[121]

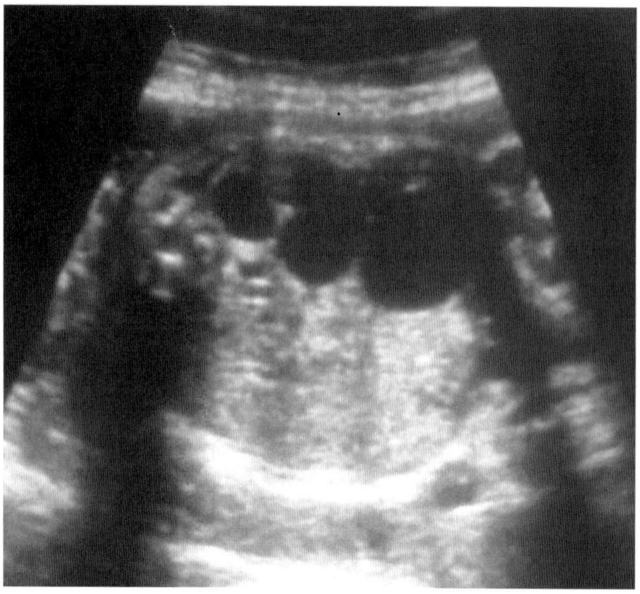

Figure 31.34 Multicystic dysplastic kidney disease. The kidney appears enlarged with multiple cysts. The contralateral kidney is normal.

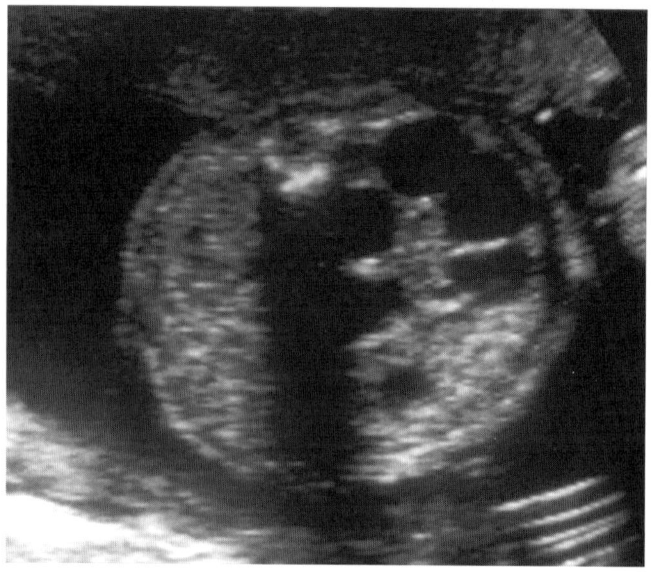

Figure 31.35 Multicystic dysplastic kidney disease. The kidney appears enlarged with multiple cysts. The contralateral kidney is normal.

Pathology The kidney is replaced by multiple smooth-walled cysts of varying size.[88] Between the cysts is a dense stroma but usually no normal renal tissue.[122,123] Typically, the renal artery is either absent or very small.

Diagnosis The prenatal diagnosis for the unilateral condition is variable and depends on its severity. It is usually straightforward in the mid-trimester scan.

The classical presentation of MCDK is a multiloculated abdominal mass consisting of multiple thin-walled cysts, which do not appear to be connected. The kidneys are usually enlarged with an irregular outline and no renal pelvis can be demonstrated (Figures 31.34 and 31.35). Circumferential cysts may occasionally be detected in kidneys of more normal size, particularly in association with lower tract obstruction. Parenchymal tissue between the cysts is often hyperechogenic[90] (Figures 31.36 and 31.37). Bladder and amniotic fluid are usually normal in the unilateral condition.[120,121]

The bilateral form is usually diagnosed earlier because oligohydramnios is present and bladder is not seen. MCDK usually affects the whole kidney; however, occasionally, only part of the kidney is involved, usually the upper pole of a duplex kidney.[124]

Careful attention should be paid to assessment of the contralateral kidney because the incidence of contralateral renal anomalies is high (39%). A search should be made for nonrenal anomalies.[110]

There is a high association between dysplasia and obstruction: dysplastic kidneys are classically attached to atresic ureter; renal dysplasia is associated with lower urinary tract malformations.[90]

Color Doppler assessment may be useful in determining the diagnosis since the renal artery is always small or absent in MCKD and the Doppler waveform, when present, is markedly abnormal with reduced systolic peak and absent diastolic flow (Figure 31.38).

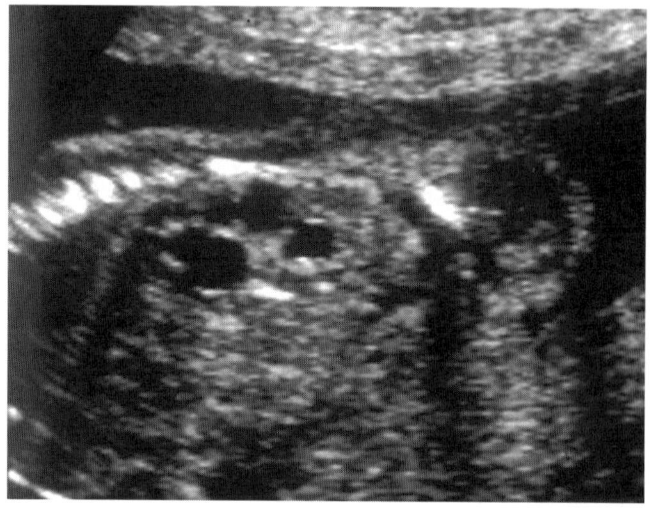

Figure 31.36 Multicystic dysplastic kidney disease. Parenchymal tissue between the cysts is often hyperechogenic.

Differential diagnosis includes upper urinary tract dilatations and other cystic abdominal masses.

Associated anomalies Associated anomalies are seen in the contralateral kidney in 30–50% of cases: vesicoureteric reflux is the most common, followed by renal agenesis, renal hypoplasia and pelviureteric junction obstruction.[125,126]

Detection of dysplastic kidneys should stimulate a detailed examination of the fetus for other structural abnormalities, including heart, spine, gastrointestinal, CNS, cleft palate, limb anomalies and umbilical cord

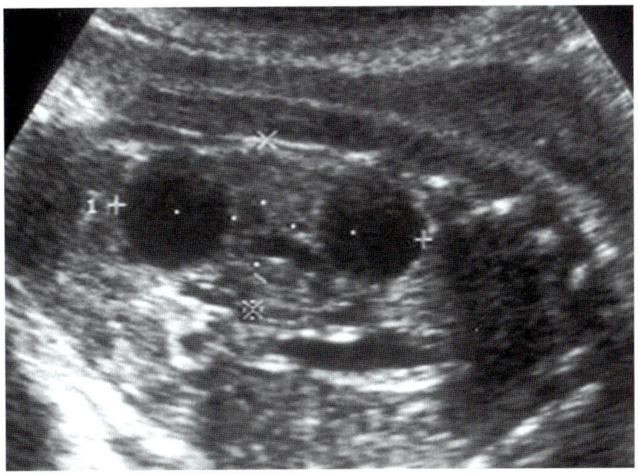

Figure 31.37 Multicystic dysplastic kidney disease. Parenchymal tissue between the cysts is often hyperechogenic.

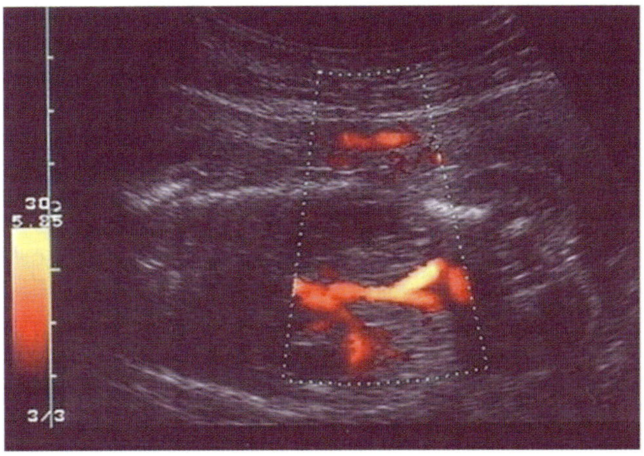

Figure 31.38 Multicystic dysplastic kidney disease. Color Doppler shows that the renal artery is always small or absent.

as up to 35% may have extra-renal anomalies. These are more likely to occur in fetuses with bilateral than unilateral MCDKD.[127] Chromosome analysis should also be discussed with the parents, particularly when structural abnormalities are detected or dysplasia is bilateral. Risks of chromosomal defects are low if there is isolated renal dysplasia.

Kazebnik *et al.*[127] reported 102 prenatally detected cases. In their experience the condition is unilateral in 76% of cases, 10% have normal karyotype, but in all cases they found associated nonrenal anomalies.

Prognosis Unilateral multicystic dysplastic kidney has a good outcome provided the contralateral kidney is normal. If an associated renal anomaly is present, the prognosis depends on the severity of the associated abnormality. The presence of multiple anomalies confers a poorer prognosis.

Bilateral multicystic kidneys have a very poor prognosis, and all babies succumb, in the early neonatal period, to pulmonary hypoplasia.

Management Unilateral multicystic kidney can be managed conservatively with follow-up scans in the third trimester to assess both the multicystic and contralateral kidney.

Bilateral multicystic kidney has a very poor prognosis, and a termination of pregnancy is an appropriate management strategy.

The risk of recurrence is small, about 2–3%, but it can be higher if it is associated with a genetic syndrome.

Obstructive cystic dysplasia (Potter IV)

It occurs secondary to obstruction in the first or early second trimester of pregnancy.[128]

The incidence of this condition is difficult to determine because only a small proportion of obstructed kidneys progress to renal dysplasia. There is an approximate incidence of 1 in 8000 live births, with 40% being bilateral dysplasia.[92,129]

This condition is caused by early renal obstruction.

Unilateral disease can be caused by a pelviureteral or vesicoureteric junction obstruction.

Bilateral obstructive dysplasia is caused by severe bladder outlet obstruction (urethral atresia or posterior urethral valves).

Pathology The kidney is usually small with disorganized epithelial structures surrounded by fibrous tissue. Cortical cysts are often present.[129]

Diagnosis The sonographic appearance is small echogenic kidneys with peripheral cysts. In the bilateral condition, bilateral hydronephrosis may be present, bladder with thick walls and usually collapsed and severe oligohydramnios may be seen.

The renal cortex assessment is very important. The presence of cortical cysts and hydronephrosis is suggestive of dysplasia.[129] Although increased echogenicity is a good sign of renal dysplasia, normal renal echogenicity does not exclude this condition[128] (Figures 31.39 and 31.40).

Occasionally, the obstructive dysplasia can affect part of a kidney.[130]

Differential diagnosis The differential diagnosis is established between multiple conditions, as shown in Tables 31.4 and 31.5.

Associated anomalies The main anomalies seen are cardiac and the VACTERL association (*v*ertebral anomalies, *a*norectal atresia, *c*ardiac anomalies, *t*racheo-*e*sophageal fistula, *r*enal anomalies and *l*imb abnormalities). Other less common associations are hydrocephalus, cloacal malformation, malrotation and ambiguous genitalia.[131]

Prognosis The prognosis depends on whether the condition is bilateral or unilateral. Bilateral disease

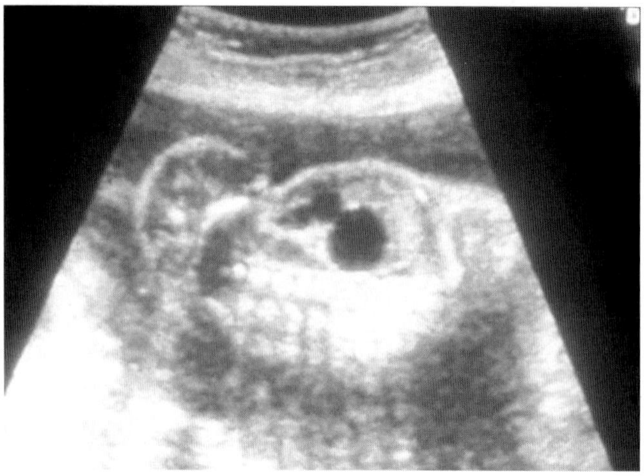

Figure 31.39 Obstructive cystic dysplasia. Peripheral cortical cysts and echogenic parenchyma.

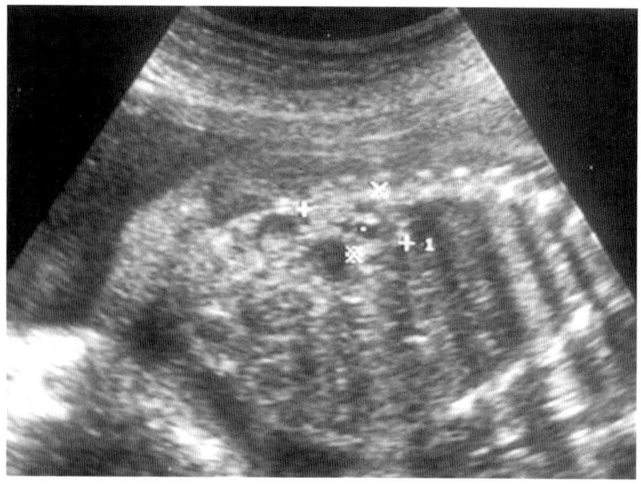

Figure 31.40 Obstructive cystic dysplasia. Peripheral cortical cysts and echogenic parenchyma.

has a poor prognosis, and most of newborn succumb in neonatal period to pulmonary hypoplasia. In unilateral disease, the outcome depends on the presence of renal anomalies affecting the contralateral kidney and the presence or absence of associated abnormalities.

Management. Due to the very poor outcome of the bilateral condition, interruption of pregnancy can be offered to the parents.

Unilateral condition can be managed conservatively in the absence of contralateral kidney disease and associated abnormalities.

The condition is sporadic.

Echogenic large kidneys or 'bright' kidneys

Large 'bright', or hyperechogenic kidneys are occasionally seen at the time of a routine ultrasound scan or indeed later in pregnancy when a woman is scanned for another clinical indication.[132]

They represent a difficult diagnostic dilemma, particularly in the presence of a normal liquor volume, since their underlying etiologies are relatively diverse. A list of the more common underlying pathologies is shown in Table 31.6.[90] Only a few of these conditions can be identified prenatally, usually on the basis of associated abnormalities, liquor volume and targeted invasive test. In many instances, however, definitive diagnosis is dependent upon postnatal investigations.

Sonographic detection of large, 'bright' kidneys should stimulate a detailed examination of the rest of the fetus paying particular attention to the rest of the renal tract and other measurements. If the bladder is enlarged, with or without dilated ureters, then the findings reflect an obstructive uropathy. If the kidneys and all measurements lie above the 95th percentile, then an overgrowth syndrome (Beckwith–Wiedemann, Perlman, Simpson–Golabi–Behmel syndrome, etc.) could be considered (Figures 31.41 and 31.42). Karyotyping should be discussed, particularly when other malformations are detected.

If the fetus has isolated hyperechogenic kidneys and a normal karyotype with no evidence of renal tract obstruction, then the etiology lies between renal dysplasia, autosomal recessive polycystic kidney dysplasia, autosomal recessive polycystic dysplasia, nephrocalcinosis or a variant of normal.

Accurate prediction of the prognosis can be difficult, although liquor volume is a key indicator since reduced volume or its absence indicates that the outcome is likely to be poor and the pregnancy will frequently end in a neonatal death subsequent to pulmonary hypoplasia, as well as renal failure. In these circumstances, termination of pregnancy is a reasonable option.

In the presence of normal amniotic fluid, serial scanning should be undertaken to monitor the size of the kidneys and renal function as indicated by liquor volume.

Simple renal cysts

The incidence of simple renal cysts varies with gestational age. Scanning at 14–16 weeks' gestation is 1/1100[132] and at 20 weeks is 1/2400.[133]

The etiology is unclear, but there are two main theories[134]:

(1) They are retention cysts resulting from the obstruction of renal tubules secondary to local vascular damage or inflammation.
(2) The second to fourth generations of uriniferous tubules fail to degenerate or unite with later generations of collecting tubules, persisting as cystic collections.

The cysts are usually solitary and unilocular with no communication with the renal pelvis. The rest of the kidney is normal.[133]

Table 31.4 Echogenic kidneys: antenatal ultrasound appearances and clinical findings

Condition	Renal size	Cysts present?	Hydronephrosis	AF	Cysts in parents' kidneys	Family history	Associated findings
ARPKD	Large	No	No	↓	No	Yes, in sibling	Hepatic fibrosis
ADPKD	Large	Sometimes	No	Normal	Yes > 20 yr	Yes, in parent	Occasionally cysts in parents' liver, spleen
Obstructive cystic dysplasia	Small	Often	Yes	Depends on degree of renal obstruction	No	No	Hydronephrosis usually urethral obstruction
Finnish type nephrotic syndrome	Large	No	No	Normal	No	Yes, in sibling	Raised serum AFP
Beckwith–Wiedemann syndrome	Large	No	No	Normal ↑	No	Occasionally	Macrosomia, large liver, macroglossia, omphalocele
Perlman syndrome	Large	No	Sometimes	Normal ↑	No	Yes, in sibling	Macrosomia, hepatoesplenomegaly ascites, micrognathia, depressed nasal bridge
Meckel Grubel syndrome	Large	Sometimes	No	↓	No	Yes, in sibling	Polydactyly encephalocele
Trisomy 13	Large	Sometimes	No	Normal	No	No	Facial clefting, holoprosencephaly, cardiac defects, polydactyly
CMV infection	Large	No	No	Normal	No	No	Microcephaly, hydrocephaly, intracranea calcification, large liver and spleen, hydrops
Renal vein thrombosis	Large, usually unilateral	No	No	Normal	No	No	Maternal diabetes, maternal pyelonephritis
Normal	Normal	No	No	Normal	No	No	

Table 31.5 Syndromes associated with renal cystic disease

Syndrome	Clinical features
Meckel Gruber	Large echogenic kidneys, polydactyly, encephalocele
Patau	Hyperechogenic large kidneys, polydactyly, holoprosencephaly, facial clefting
Jeune	Echogenic kidneys, dwarfism, small thorax
Beckwith–Wiedemann	Large echogenic kidneys, macrosomia, hepatosplenomegaly, macroglossia, omphalocele
Short rib polydactyly (Majewski type)	Large echogenic kidneys, dwarfism, polydactyly, small thorax
Laurence–Moon (Bardet–Biedl)	Renal cysts, retinal dystrophy, polydactyly, mental deficiency, hypogonadism
Zellweger	Cystic kidneys, hypotonicity, limb contractures, congenital cataracts, hypoplastic corpus callosum, heterotopia
Perlman	Macrosomia, hepatosplenomegaly, ascitis, micrognathia, depressed nasal bridge
Tuberosa esclerosis	Epilepsy, mental retardation, cutaneous lesions, cardiac rhabdomyomas (*in utero*)

Table 31.6 Conditions associated with large, 'bright' kidneys

	AF	Renal cysts	Renal pelvis dilatation	Macrosomy	Other abnormalities	Heart abnormalities	Inheritance	Alternative prenatal diagnosis
Dysplasia	N/Oligo	+/–	+/–	–	+/–	–	10%(AD)	–
Obstruction	N/Oligo	+/–	+	–	+/–	–	Sporadic	
ARPKD	N/Oligo	–	–	–	–	–	AR	DNA
ADPKD	N/Oligo	+	–	–	–	–	AD	DNA
Beckwith–Wiedemann	N/Poly	–	+/–	+	+	–	AD or Disomy	Cyto/DNA
Perlman	N/Oligo	–	+/–	+	+	–	AR	–
Simpson–Golabi–Behmel	?	?	?	+	+	+/–	X-linked	DNA
Trisomy 13	Oligo	–	+/–	–	+	+/–	Sporadic	Cyto
Meckel Gruber	Oligo	–	–	–	+	+/–	AR	DNA
Nephrocalcinosis	N	–	–	–	–	–	Sporadic	–

Diagnosis The cysts appear as a unilocular round or oval anechoic structure with well-defined borders, usually near the periphery of the kidney. Cysts vary in size (2–4 mm).[133]

The differential diagnosis is established between:

(1) Hydronephrosis of the upper pole moiety of a duplex kidney.
(2) Perinephric urinoma.
(3) Cysts arising from structures close to the kidneys (duplication or mesenteric cysts).

Associated anomalies Most simple cysts are asymptomatic and rarely associated with structural or other abnormalities. Occasionally they are associated with[133,136,137]:

(1) Pelviureteric junction obstruction
(2) Posterior urethral valves
(3) Turner syndrome
(4) Trisomy 13
(5) Trisomy 18
(6) Trisomy 21(5% are associated with simple renal cysts)

Prognosis The outcome is good for fetuses with simple cysts.[133]

When cysts do become symptomatic, simple aspiration under ultrasound control is the treatment of choice.[138]

Management Simple cysts seen in the first half of pregnancy can be followed up with scans during the third trimester. The majority resolve and those that persist do not need any postnatal investigations.

Renal tumors

Congenital renal tumors are rare. The incidence is 1 per 125,000 newborns.[139] The most frequent tumor

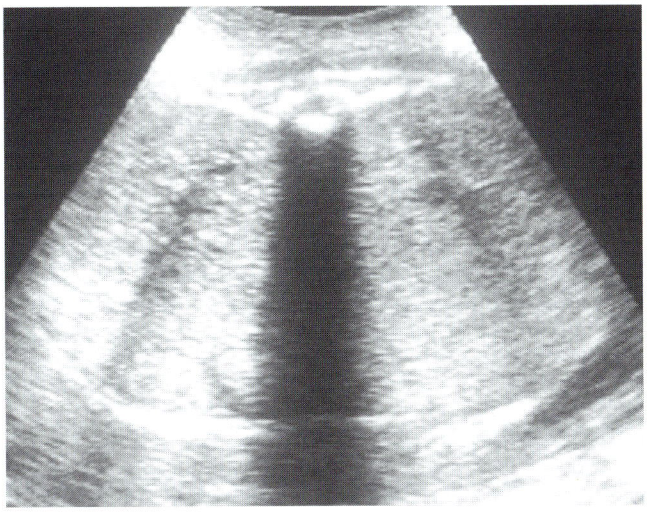

Figure 31.41 Meckel–Gruber syndrome. Distended abdomen due to the cystic renal dysplasia.

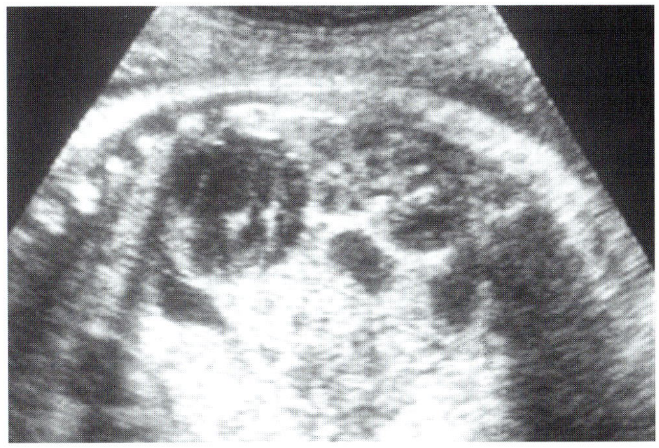

Figure 31.43 Neuroblastoma. Solid tumor and heterogenous.

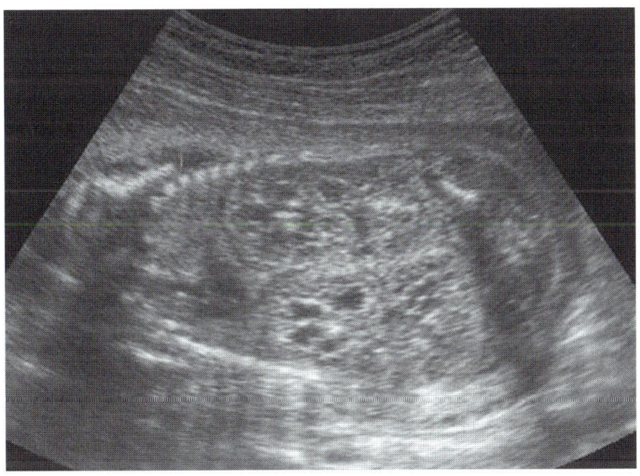

Figure 31.42 Large and bright kidneys with oligohydramnios.

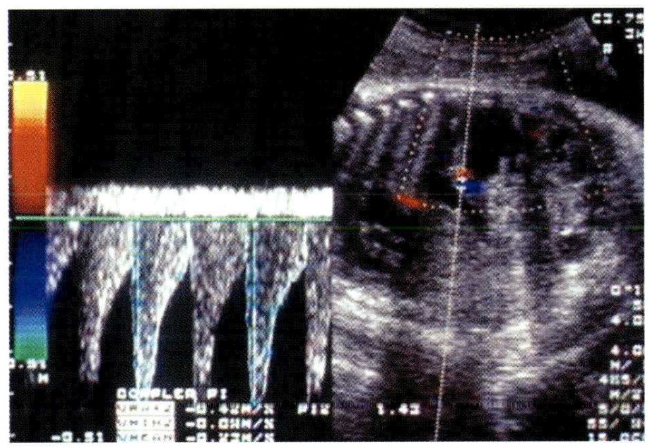

Figure 31.44 Neuroblastoma. Solid tumor and heterogenous. Color Doppler shows artery blood flow.

is the mesoblastic nephroma. It is a benign tumor that presents continuity with the normal nephrons. Wilms' tumor is rare in the fetus.

The etiology is unknown.

Diagnosis

The diagnosis will generally be made before the presence of a polyhydramnios and an abdominal mass at level of renal fossa in third trimester[140] (Figures 31.43 and 31.44).

- The mesoblastic nephroma is unilateral and on ultrasonography appears as a solid mass. Occasionally, cysts can be identified, many of them are located near the renal hilus, and almost all affect the renal parenchyma. On occasions, the tumor can be adjacent to the kidney and compress it. The mesoblastic nephromas is usually well defined
- It can have polyhydramnios in 70% of the cases, resulting from the polyuria secondary to the hypercalcemia[141]
- The hydrops is uncommon, and it has a poor prognosis[142]
- Wilms' tumor presents very similar echographic characteristics and an anatomopathological study should be carried out for its diagnosis.[143]

Differential diagnosis

- Neuroblastoma. It usually displaces inferior to the kidney
- Suprarenal hemorrhage
- Retroperitoneal teratoma
- Extralobar subphrenic sequestrum.

Associated anomalies

- The mesoblastic nephroma unusually associates to anomalies
- Wilms' tumor associates to anomalies in 15% of the cases: aniridia, genitourinary abnomalies and hemihypertrophy.[144]

Genetic markers

The genes WT1 and WT2 located in chromosome 11 have been implicated in the development of the Wilms' tumor, as well as the gene WT3 of chromosome 16 in Beckwith–Wiedemann syndrome and Denys–Drash syndrome.[144]

Prognosis

Treatment is surgical and it is usually curative. The presence of hydrops involves a very bad prognosis.[142]

Management

- During the pregnancy it is necessary to control the polyhydramnios to avoid premature childbirth and the premature rupture of membranes (PROM)
- Childbirth should take place in a tertiary level hospital, where there are neonatology unit, pediatric surgery and pediatric oncology.

This tumor appears sporadically.

REFERENCES

1. Twining P. Anomalías fetales. *Diagnóstico ecográfico* 2002;13: 270–8.
2. Larsen WJ. *Human Embryology.* London: Churchill Livingstone, 1993.
3. Wendell Smith CP, Williams PL, Treadgold S. *Basic Human Embryology.* London: Pitman Publishing, 1984.
4. Elder JS. *Tratado de Pediatría Nelson,* 16ª edición. Transtornos urológicos Embriología 2;1767–96.
5. Bronshtein M, Amil A, Achiron R, Noy I, Blumenfeld Z. The early prenatal diagnosis of renal agenesis: Techniques and possible pitfalls. *Prenat Diagn* 1994;14:291–7.
6. Mesrobian HG, Rushton HG, Bulas D. Unilateral renal agenesis may result from *in utero* regression of multicystic renal dysplasia. *J Urol* 1993;150:793–4.
7. Moore KL, Persaud TVN. *The Developing Human: Clinically Oriented Embryology.* Philadelphia: WB Saunders, 1998.
8. Romero R, Cullen M, Grannum P, *et al.* Antenatal diagnosis of renal anomalies with ultrasound, III: Bilateral renal agenesis. *Am J Obstet Gynecol* 1985;151:38–43.
9. Mackenzie FM, Kingston GO, Oppenheimer L. The early prenatal diagnosis of bilateral renal agenesis using transvaginal sonography and color Doppler ultrasonography. *J Ultrasound Med* 1994;13:49–51
10. Sepulveda W, Stagiannis KD, Flack NJ, Fisk NM. Accuracy of prenatal diagnosis of renal agenesis with color flow imaging in severe second-trimester oligohydramnios. *Am J Obstet Gynecol* 1995;173:1788–92.
11. Hoffman CK, Filly RA, Callen PW. The "lying down" adrenal sign: A sonographic indicator of renal agenesis or ectopia in fetuses and neonates. *J Ultrasound Med* 1992;11:533–6.
12. Benacerraf BR. Examination of the second trimester fetus with severe oligohydramnios using transvaginal scanning. *Obstet Gynecol* 1990;175:491–3.
13. Hill LM, Rivello D. Role of transvaginal sonography in the diagnosis of bilateral renal agenesis. *Am J Perinatol* 1991;8: 395–7.
14. Gembruch U, Hansmann M. Artificial instillation of amniotic fluid as a new technique for the diagnostic evaluation of cases of oligohydramnios. *Prenat Diagn* 1988;8:33–45.
15. Nicolini U, Santolaya J, Hubinont C, Fisk N, Maxwell D, Rodeck C. Visualization of fetal intra-abdominal organs in second-trimester severe oligohydramnios by intraperitoneal infusion. *Prenat Diagn* 1989;9:191–4.
16. Glazebrook KN, McGrath FP, Steele BT. Prenatal compensatory renal growth: Documentation with US. *Radiology* 1993;189: 733–5.
17. Roodhooft AM, Birnholz JC, Holmes LB. Familiar nature of congenital absence and severe dysgenesis of both kidneys. *N Engl J Med* 1984;310:1341–5.
18. Hill L, Peterson CS. Antenatal diagnosis of fetal pelvic kidneys. *J Ultrasound Med* 1987;6:393–6.
19. Hill LM, Grzybek P, Mills A, Hogge WA. Antenatal diagnosis of fetal pelvic kidneys. *Obstet Gynecol* 1994;83:333–6.
20. Greenblatt AM, Beretsky I, Lankin DH, *et al. In utero* diagnosis of crossed renal ectopia using high resolution real-time ultrasound. *J Ultrasound Med* 1985:4:105–7.
21. Moore KL, Pesrsaud TVN. The urogenital system. In: *The Developing Human: Clinically Oriented Embryology,* 6th edn. Philadelphia: WB Saunders, 1998;II:330.
22. Weizer AZ, Silverstein AD, Auge BK, Delvecchio FC, Raj G, Albala DM, Leder R, Preminger GM. Determining the incidence of horseshoe kidney from radiographic data at a single institution. *J Urol* 2003;170:1722–6.
23. Hunt GM, Whitaker RH. The pattern of congenital renal anomalies associated with neural-tube defects. *Dev Med Child Neurol* 1987;29:91–5.
24. Boatman DL, Kolln CP, Flocks RH. Congenital anomalies associated with horseshoe kidney. *J Urol* 1972;107:205–7.
25. Canki N, Warburton D, Byrne J. Morphological characteristics of monosomy X in spontaneous abortions. *Ann Genet* 1988;31: 4–13.
26. Kravtzova GI, Lazjuk GI, Lurie IW. The malformations of the urinary system in autosomal disorders. *Virchows Arch A Pathol Anat Histol* 1975;368(2):167–78.
27. Scott JE, Renwick M. Screening for fetal urological abnormalities: How effective? *Br J Urol Int* 1999;84:693–700.
28. Huang EY, Mascarenhas L, Mahour GH. Wilms' tumor and horseshoe kidneys: A case report and review of the literature. *J Pediatr Surg* 2004;39:207–12.
29. Rubio Briones J, Regalado Pareja R, Sanchez Martin F, Chechile Toniolo G, Huguet Perez J, Villavicencio Mavrich H. Incidence of tumoural pathology in horseshoe kidneys. *Eur Urol* 1998;33: 175–9.
30. Smith-Behn J, Memo R. Malignancy in horseshoe kidney. *South Med J* 1988;81:1451–2.
31. Ismaili K, Hall M, Donner C, Thomas D, Vermeylen, Avni FE. Results of systematic screening for minor degrees of fetal renal pelvis dilatation in an unselected population. *Am J Obstet Gynecol* 2003;188:242–6.
32. Ismaili K, Hall M, Avni FE. Management of isolated fetal dilatations of the kidney pelvis. *Rev Med Brux* 2003;24:29–34.
33. Eckoldt F, Heinick C, Wolke S, Stover B, Heling KS. Prenatal diagnosis of obstructive uropathies-positive predictive value and effect on postnatal therapy. *Z Geburtshilfe Neonatol* 2003;207: 220–4.
34. Moorthy I, Joshi N, Cook JV, Warren M. Antenatal hydronephrosis: Negative predictive value of normal postnatal ultrasound a 5 year study. *Clin Radiol* 2003;58:964–70.
35. Barrer AF, Cave MM, Thomas DFM, Lilford RJ, Irvine HC, Arthur RJ, Smith SEW. Fetal pelvi-ureteric junction obstruction: Predictions of outcome. *Br J Urol* 1995;76:649–52.
36. Lepercq J, Beaudoin S, Bargy F. Outcome of 116 moderate renal pelvis dilatations at prenatal ultrasonography. *Fetal Diagn Ther* 1998;13:79–81.
37. Benacerraf Br, Mandell J, Estroff JA, *et al.* Fetal pyelectasis: A possible association with Down syndrome. *Obstet Gynecol* 1992; 76:58–60.
38. Nicolaides KH, Cheng HH, Abbas A, Snijders RJM, Gosden C. Fetal renal defects: Associated malformations and chromosomal defets. *Fetal Diagn Ther* 1992;7:1–11.
39. James CA, Watson AR, Twining P, Rance CH. Antenatally detected urinary tract abnormalities: Changing incidence and management. *Eur J Pediatr* 1998;157:508–11.
40. Antonakoupoulus GN, Fuggle WJ, Newman J, *et al.* Idiopathic hydronephrosis. *Arch Pathol Lab Med* 1985;109:1097.
41. Bosman G, Reuss A, Nijman JM, Wladimiroff JW. Prenatal diagnosis, management and outcome of fetal uretero-pelvic junction obstruction. *Ultrasound Med Biol* 1991;17:117–20.

42. Grapin C, Auber F, de Vries P, Audry G, Heladort P. Postnatal management of urinary tract anomalies after antenatal diagnosis. *J Gynecol Obstet Biol Reprod (Paris)* 2003;32:300–13.
43. McAleer IM, Kaplan GW. Renal function before and after pyeloplasty: Does it improve? *J Urol* 1999;162:1041–4.
44. Buscemi M, Shanke A, Mallet E. Dominantly inherited ureteropelvic junction obstruction. *Urology* 1985;24:568–71.
45. Rickwood AMK, Jee LD, Williams MPL, Anderson PAM. Natural history of obstructed and pseudo-obstructed megaureters detected by prenatal ultrasonography. *Br J Urol* 1992;70:322–5.
46. Manzoni C. Megaureter. *Rays* 2002;27:83–5.
47. McLellan DL, Retik AB, Bauer SB, Diamond DA, Atala A, Mandell J, Lebowitz RL, Borer JG, Peters CA. Rate and predictors of spontaneous resolution of prenatally diagnosed primary nonrefluxing megaureter. *J Urol* 2002;168:2177–80.
48. Sherer DM, Hulbert WC. Prenatal sonographic diagnosis and subsequent conservative surgical management of bilateral ureteroceles. *Am J Perinatol* 1995;12:174–7.
49. Vergani P, Ceruti P, Locatelli A, Mariani E, Paterlini G, Zorloni C, Ghidini A. Accuracy of prenatal ultrasonographic diagnosis of duplex renal system. *J Ultrasound Med* 1999;18:463–7.
50. Sozubir S, Lorenzo AJ, Twickler DM, Baker LA, Ewalt DH. Prenatal diagnosis of a prolapsed ureterocele with magnetic resonance imaging. *Urology* 2003;62:144.
51. Kang AH, Bruner JP. Antenatal ultrasonographic development of ureteroceles. Implications for management. *Fetal Diagn Ther* 1998;13:157–9.
52. Winters WD, Lebowitz RL. Importance of prenatal detection of hydronephrosis of the upper pole. *Am J Radiol* 1990;155:125–9.
53. Upadhyay J, Bolduc S, Braga L, Farhat W, Bagli DJ, McLorie GA, Khoury AE, El-Ghoneimi A. Impact of prenatal diagnosis on the morbidity associated with ureterocele management. *J Urol* 2002;167:2560–5.
54. Castagnetti M, Cimador M, Sergio M, de Grazia E. Transurethral incision of duplex system ureteroceles in neonates: Does it increase the need for secondary surgery intravesical and ectopic cases? *Br J Urol Int* 2004;93:1313–7.
55. Elder JS. Antenatal hydronephrosis fetal and neonatal management. *Pediatr Clin North Am* 1997;44:1299–321.
56. Edkoldt F, Heling KS, Stover B, Woderich R, Wolke S. Retrospective analysis of differential therapeutic measures in children with double kidney and ureter and hydronephrosis. *Urologe A* 2003; 42:1087–91.
57. Arena F, Nicotina A, Cruccetti A, Centonze A, Arena S, Romeo G. Can histologic changes of the upper pole justify a conservative approach in neonatal duplex ectopic ureterocele? *Pediatr Surg Int* 2002;18:681–4.
58. Cendron M, D'Alton ME, Crombleholme TM. Prenatal diagnosis and management of the fetus with hydronephrosis. *Semin Perinatol* 1994;18:163–81.
59. Dinnen MD, Duffy PG. Posterior urethral valves. *Br J Urol* 1996; 78:275–81.
60. Manzoni C, Valentini AL. Posterior urethral valves. *Rays* 2002; 27:131–4.
61. McHugo J, Whittle M. Enlarged fetal bladders: Aetiology, management and outcome. *Prenat Diagn* 2001;21:958–63.
62. Silveri M, Adorisio O, Pane A, Zaccara A, Bilancioni E, Giorlandino C, De Gennaro M. Fetal monolateral urinoma and neonatal renal function outcome in posterior urethral valves obstruction: The pop-off mechanism. *Pediatr Med Chir* 2002;24: 394–6.
63. De Vries SH, Klijn AJ, Lilien MR, De Jong TP. Development of renal function after neonatal urinary ascitis due to obstructive uropathy. *J Urol* 2002;168:675–8.
64. Lee E, Thonell S. Posterior urethral valves causing urinomas: Two case reports. *Australas Radiol* 2002;46:101–5.
65. Peters CA. Lower urinary tract obstruction: Clinical and experimental aspects. *Br J Urol* 1998;81(Suppl 2):22–32.
66. Perrotin F, Ayeva-Derman M, Lardy H, Cloarec S, Lansac J, Body G. Prenatal diagnosis and postnatal outcome of congenital megalourethra. Report of two cases. *Fetal Diagn Ther* 2001;16: 123–8.
67. Geifman-Hotzman O, Crane SS, Winderl L, Holmes M. Persistent urogenital sinus: Prenatal diagnosis and pregnancy complications. *Am J Obstet Gynecol* 1997;176:709-11.
68. McNarama HM, Onwude JL, Thornton JG. Megacystis-microcolon-intestinal hypoperistalsis syndrome: A case report supporting autosomal recessive inheritance. *Prenat Diagn* 1994; 14:153–4.
69. Hsu CD, Craig C, Pavlik J, Ninios A. Prenatal diagnosis of megacystis-microcolon-intestinal hypoperistalsis syndrome in one fetus of a twin pregnancy. *Am J Perinatol* 2003;20:215–8.
70. Sharma AK, Kothari SK, Goel D, Agarwal LD, Tamani RN. Megalourethra with posterior urethral valves. *Pediatr Surg Int* 1999;15:591–2.
71. Hayden SA, Russ PD, Pretorius DH, Manco-Johnson ML, Chilwell WH. Posterior urethral obstruction. Prenatal sonographic findings and clinical outcome in fourteen cases. *J Ultrasound Med* 1988;7:371–5.
72. Krapp M, Geipel A, Germer U, Krokowski M, Gembruch U. First-trimester sonographic diagnosis of distal urethral atresia with megalourethra in VACTERL association. *Prenat Diagn* 2002; 22:422–4.
73. Hutton KAR, Thomas PFM, Arthur RJ, Irving HC, Smith SEW. Prenatally detected posterior urethra valves: Is gestational age at detection a predictor of outcome? *J Urol* 1994;152:698–701.
74. Holmes N, Harrison MR, Baskin LS. Fetal surgery for posterior urethral valves: Long-term postnatal outcomes. *Pediatrics* 2001; 108:E7.
75. Quintero RA, Johnson M, Muñoz H. *In utero* endoscopic treatment of posterior urethral valves. *Prenat Neonat Med* 1998;3: 208–16.
76. Quintero RA, Morales WJ, Allen MA, Bornick PW, Johnson P. Fetal hydrolaparoscopy and endoscopic cystotomy in complicated cases of lower urinary tract obstruction. *Am J Obstet Gynecol* 2000;183:324–33.
77. González R, De Filippo R, Jednak R, Barthold JS. Urethral atresia: Long-term outcome in 6 children who survived the neonatal period. *J Urol* 2001;165:2241–4.
78. Reinberg Y, Chelimsky G, González R. Urethral atresia and the prune-belly syndrome. Report of 6 cases. *Br J Urol* 1993;72: 112–4.
79. Jennings RW. Prune belly syndrome. *Semin Pediatr Surg* 2000;9: 115–20.
80. Leeners B, Sauer I, Schefels J, Cotarelo CL, Funk A. Prune belly syndrome: Therapeutic options including *in utero* placement of a vesicoamniotic shunt. *J Clin Ultrasound* 2000;28:500–7.
81. Elder JS. Commentary: Importance of antenatal diagnosis of vesicoureteral reflux. *J Urol* 1992;148:1750–4.
82. Scott JE, Renwick M. Screening for fetal urological abnormalities: How effective? *Br J Urol Int* 1999;84:693–700.
83. Farhat W, McLorie G, Geary D, Capolicchio G, Bagli D, Merguerian P, Khoury A. The natural history of neonatal vesicoureteral reflux associated with antenatal hydronephrosis. *J Urol* 2000;164(3, Pt 2):1057–60.
84. Orsola A, Fraga Rodriguez GM, Parra Roca J, Estorch Cabrera M, Monserrat Esplugas E, Garat Barredo JM, Ginovart Galiana G, Cubells Riero J. Congenital renal abnormalities in neonates with fetal vesicoureteral reflux. Detection by 99m-technetium(m)-dimercaptosuccinic acid renal scintigraphy (in Spanish). *An Pediatr (Barc)* 2003;59(4):345–51.
85. Nguyen HT, Bauer SB, Peters CA, Connolly LP, Gobet R, Borere JG, *et al.* 99m Technetium dimercapto-succinic acid renal scintigraphy abnormalities in infants with sterile high grade vesicoureteral reflux. *J Urol* 2000;164:1674–8.
86. Noe HN. The long-term results of prospective sibling reflux screening. *J Urol* 1992;148:1739–42.
87. Noe HN, Wyatt RJ, Peeden JN Jr, Rivas ML. The transmission of vesicoureteral reflux from parent to child. *J Urol* 1992;148(6): 1869–71.
88. Thomsen MS, Levine E, Meilstrup JW, Van Slyke Ma, Edgar KA, *et al.* Renal cystic diseases. *Eur Radiol* 1997;7:1267–75.
89. Potter EL. *Normal and Abnormal Development of the Kidney.* Chicago, IL: Year Book Medical Publishers Inc, 1972.
90. Winyard P, Chitty L. Dysplastic and polycystic kidneys: Diagnosis, associations and management. *Prenat Diagn* 2001;21:924–35.
91. Zerres K. Autosomal recessive polycystic disease. *Clin Invest* 1992;70:794–801.
92. Tsuda H, Matsumota M, Imanaka M, Ogita S. Measurement of fetal urine production in mild infantile polycystic kidney disease – a case report. *Prenat diagn* 1994;14:1083–5.
93. Osathanondh V, Potter EL. Pathogenesis of polycystic kidneys. Type I due to hypoplasia of intersticial portions of collecting tubules. *Arch Pathol* 1964;77:466–73.
94. Blyth H, Ockenden BG. Polycystic disease of kidneys and liver presenting in childhood. *J Med Genet* 1971;8:257–84.
95. Romero R, Cullen R, Janty P, Grannunm P, Reece EA, *et al.* The diagnosis of congenital renal anomalies with ultrasound II.

Infantile polycysytic kidney disease. *Am J Obstet Gynecol* 1984;150:259–62.

96. Wissser J, Hebisch G, Froster U, Zerres K, Stallmach T, *et al.* Prenatal sonographic diagnosis of autosomal recessive polycystic kidney disease during the early second trimester. *Prenat Diagn* 1995;15:868–71.
97. Mahony B, Cullen PW, Filly R, Golbus M. Progression of infantile polycystic kidney disease in early pregnancy. *J Ultrasound Med* 1984;3:277–9.
98. Barth R, Gillot A, Capeless E, Clemmons J. Prenatal diagnosis of autosomal recessive polycystic kidney disease: Variable outcome in one family. *Am J Obstet Gynecol* 1992;166:560–7.
99. Zerres K, Hansmann M, Mallmann R, Gembruch U. Autosomal recessive polycystic kidney disease. Problems of prenatal diagnosis. *Prenat Diagn* 1988;8:215–29.
100. Bronshtein M, Bar-Hava I, Blumenfeld Z. Clues and pitfalls in the early prenatal diagnosis of "late onset" infantile polycystic kidney. *Prenat Diagn* 1992;12:293–8.
101. Kogutt MS, Robichaux W, Boineau F, Drake G, Simonton S. Asymmetric renal size in autosomal recessive polycystic kidney disease: a unique presentation. *Am J Radiol* 1993;160:835–6.
102. Cassart M, Massez A, Metens T, Rypens F, Lambot MA, Hall M, Avni F. Complementary role of MRI after sonography in assessing bilateral urinary tract anomalies in the fetus. *AJR Am J Roentgenol* 2004;182:689–95.
103. Guay-Woodford LM, Meucher G, Hopkins SD, Avner ED, Germino GG, Guillot AP. The severe form of autosomal recessive polycystic kidney disease maps to chromosome 6p21.1-p12: Implications for genetic counseling. *Am J Hum Genet* 1995;56:1101–7.
104. MacDermot KD, Saggar-Malik AK, Economides SJ. Prenatal diagnosis of autosomal dominant polycystic kidney disease (PKD1) presenting *in utero* and prognosis for very early onset disease. *J Med Genet* 1998;35:13–6.
105. Parfrey PS, Bear JC, Morgan J, Cramer BC, MaManamon PJ, *et al.* The diagnosis and prognosis of autosomal dominant polycystic kidney disease. *N Engl J Med* 1990;323:1085–90.
106. Reeders ST, Breuning MH, Davies KE, *et al.* A highly polymorphic DNA marker linked to adult type polycystic kidney disease on chromosome 16. *Nature* 1985;317:542–4.
107. Kimberling WJ, Kimar S, Gabow P. Autosomal dominant polycystic kidney disease: Localization of the second gene to chromosome 4p13-q23. *Genomics* 1995;18:467–72.
108. Demetriou K, Tziakouri C, Anninou K, Eleftheriou A, Koptides M, Nicolau A, Deltas CC, Pierides A. Autosomal dominant polycystic kidney disease-type 2. Ultrasound, genetic and clinical correlations. *Nephrol Dial Transplant* 2000;15:205–11.
109. Nicolau C, Torra R, Bianchi L, Vilana R, Gilabert R, Darnell A, Bru C. Autosomal dominant polycystic kidney disease types 1 and 2: Assessment of US sensitivity for diagnosis. *Radiology* 1999;213:273–6.
110. Aubertin G, Cripps S, Coleman G, McGillivray B, Yong SL, Van Allen M, Shaw D, Arbour L. Prenatal diagnosis of apparently isolated unilateral multicystic kidney: Implications for counseling and management. *Prenat Diagn* 2002;22:388–94.
111. Journel H, Guyor C, Barc RM, Belbeoch P, Quemener A, Jouan H. Unexpected ultrasonographic prenatal diagnosis of autosomal dominant polycystic kidney disease. *Prenat Diagn* 1989;9: 663–71.
112. Michaud J, Russo P, Girgnon A, Dallaire L, Bicht D, Rosenblatt D, Lamathe E, Lambert M. Autosomal dominant polycystic kidney disease in the fetus. *Am J Med Genet* 1994;51:240–6.
113. Friedmann W, Vogel M, Dimer JS, Luttkus A, Buscher U, Dudenhausen JW. Perinatal differential diagnosis of cystic kidney disease and urinary tract obstruction: anatomic pathologic, ultrasonographic and genetic findings. *Eur J Obstet Gynecol Reprod Biol* 2000;89:127–33.
114. Brun M, Maugey-Laulomk B, Eurin D, Didier F, Avnis EF. Prenatal sonographic patterns in autosomal dominant polycystic kidney disease: a multicenter study. *Ultrasound Obstet Gynecol* 2004; 24:55–61.
115. Tsatsaris V, Gagnadoux MF, Aubry MC, Gubler MC, Dumez Y, Dommergues M. Prenatal diagnosis of bilateral isolated fetal hyperechogenic kidneys. Is it possible to predict long term outcome? *BJOG Br J Obstet Gynaecol* 2002;109:1388–1393.
116. Ceccherini I., Lituania M., Cordone MS., Perfumo F., Gusmano R., Callea F., Archidiacono N., Romeo G. *Autosomal dominant polycystic kidney disease: prenatal diagnosis by DNA análisis and sonographic at 14 weeks.* Prenat Diagn 1989;9:751–758.
117. Hartmann SS. *Unilateral adult polycystic kidney.* J Ultrasound Med 1982;1:371–374.
118. Middlebrook PF., Nizalik E., Schillinger JF. *Unilateral renal cystic disease: a case presentation.* J Urol 1992;148:1221–1223.
119. Gough DCS., Postlethwaite RJ., Lewis MA., Bruce J. *Multicystic renal dysplasia diagnosed in the antenatal period: a note of caution.* Br J urol 1995;76:244–248.
120. Rickwood AMK., Anderson PAM., Williams MPL. Multicystic renal dysplasia detected by prenatal ultrasonography. Natural history and results of conservative management. Br J Urol 1992; 69:538–540.
121. Van Eijk L., Cohen-Overbeek TE., Den Hollander NS., Nijman JM., Wladimiroff JW. *Unilateral multicystic dysplasia kidney: a combined pre-and postnatal assessment.* Ultrasound Obstet Gynecol 2002;19:180–183.
122. D´Alton M., Romero R., Grannum P., Jeanty P. Antenatal diagnosis of renal anomalies with ultrasound IV: bilateral multicystic kidney disease. Am J Obstet Gynecol 1986;54:532–537.
123. Hashimoto B., Filly R., Callen P. Multicystic dysplastic kidney in utero: changing appearance in ultrasound. Radiology 1986;159: 107–109.
124. Diard F., le Dosseur P., Cadier L., Calabet A., Bondionny JM. *Multicystic dysplasia in the upper component of the complete duplex kidney.* Pediatr Radiol 1984;14:310-313.
125. De Klerk DF., Marshall FF., Jeffs RD. *Multicystic dysplastic kidney.* J Urol 1977;118:306–308.
126. Karmazyn B., Zerin J. Lower urinary tract abnormalities in children with multicystic dysplastic kidney. Radiology 1997;203: 223–226.
127. Lazebkik N., Bellinger MF., Fergurson JE., Hogge JS., Hogge Wa. Insights into the pathogeniss and antural history of nfetuses with multicystic dysplastic kidney disease. Prenat Diagn 1999;19: 418–423.
128. Saunders RC., Nassbaum AR., Solez. *Renal dysplasia: sonographic findings.* Radiology 1988;167:623–626.
129. Mahony BS., Filly R., Callen PW., Hricak H., Golbus M., Harrison MR. *Fetal renal dysplasia: sonographic evaluation.* Radiology 1984;152:143–146.
130. Newman LB., McAlister WH., Kissane J. Segemental renal dysplasia associated with ectopic ureteroceles in childhood. Urology 1974;3:23–26.
131. Blane CE., Barr M., Dipietro MA., Sedman AB., Bloom DA. *Renal obstructive dysplasia: ultrasound diagnosis and therapeutic implications.* Pediatr Radiol 1991;21:274–277.
132. Braithwaite JM, Armstrong MA, Economides DL. Assessment of fetal anatomy at 12 to 13 weeks of gestation by transabdominal and transvaginal sonography. *Br J Obstet Gynaecol* 1996;103:82–5.
133. Blazer S, Zimmer E, Bumenfeld Z, Zelikovic I, Bronshtein M. Natural history of fetal simple renal cysts detected in early pregnancy. *J Urol* 1999;162:812–4.
134. Paduano L, Giglio L, Bembi B, Peratoner L, D'Ottavio G, Benussi G. Clinical outcome of fetal uropathy. I. Predictive value of prenatal echography positive for obstructive uropathy. *J Urol* 1992;146:1094–6.
135. Siegel MJ, McAlister WH. Simple cysts of the kidney in children. *J Urol* 1980;123:75–8.
136. Herman TE, Siegel MJ. Renal cysts associated with Turner' syndrome. *Pediatr Radiol* 1994;24:139–40.
137. Ariel I, Wells TR, Landing BH, Singer DB. The urinary system in Down syndrome: a study of 124 autopsy cases. *Pediatr Pathol* 1991;11:879–88.
138. Steinhardt GF, Slovis TL, Perlmutter AD. Simple renal cysts in infants. *Radiology* 1985;155:349–50.
139. Apuzzio JJ, Unwin W, Adhate A, Nichols R. Prenatal diagnosis of fetal renal mesoblastic nephroma. *Am J Obstet Gynecol* 1986;154:636–7.
140. Goldstein I, Shoshani G, Ben-Harus E, Sujov P. Prenatal diagnosis of congenital mesoblastic nephroma. *Ultrasound Obstet Gynecol* 2002;19:209–11.
141. Fung TY, Fung YM, Ng PC, Yeung CK, Chang MZ. Polyhydramnios and hypercalcemia associated with congenital mesoblastic nephroma: Case report and a new appraisal. *Obstet Gynecol* 1995;85(5, Pt 2):815–7.
142. Liu YC, Mai YL, Chang CC, Chen KW, Chow SN. The presence of hydrops fetalis in a fetus with congenital mesoblastic nephroma. *Prenat Diagn* 1996;16:363–5.
143. Applegate KE, Ghei M, Perez-Atayde AR. Prenatal detection of a Wilms' tumor. *Pediatr Radiol* 1999;29(1):65–7.
144. Vadeyar S, Ramsay M, James D, O'Neill D. Prenatal diagnosis of congenital Wilms' tumor (nephroblastoma) presenting as fetal hydrops. *Ultrasound Obstet Gynecol* 2000;16:80–3.

32 Fetal echocardiography

C. Mortera and J. M. Carrera

Introduction

Prenatal diagnosis of fetal cardiovascular malformations is generally based on the use of ultrasound and echocardiography techniques during pregnancy.[1,2]

Anatomical cardiac anomalies[3,4] are identifiable throughout the use of two-dimensional (2D) echocardiography, providing fetal anatomical cardiac structures.[2,4] Current use of 3D echocardiography provides images that may improve the anatomical structural relationship.[5,6] However, Doppler echocardiography studies allow for additional dynamic information to the cardiologist[7] and interested obstetrician[8,9] in prenatal diagnosis. Consequently, the application of such methods in normal and abnormal fetal cardiac structures and function leads to an accurate congenital heart disease diagnosis inside the uterus.[10,11]

In order to successfully diagnose cardiac malformations throughout the use of fetal echocardiography, a number of integrated conceptual areas need to be thoroughly understood to achieve a complete cardiovascular diagnosis. First, a profound knowledge of cardiovascular fetal physiology[12] and anatomy as well as fetal cardiovascular pathology and cardiac rhythm disturbances is required. Second, it is required to understand the causes and concepts of heart failure to identify the signs and causes of fetal heart failure.[13]

However, the goal of prenatal echocardiography is to make a prediction of the pregnancy outcome, offering medical[14] and surgical cardiac prognosis about the short- and long-term surgical management.[15]

Fetal cardiovascular anatomy

The fetal cardiovascular system is developed during the first 9 weeks of gestation. Interestingly, the heart is the only organ in the fetus capable of functioning while it is being developed. The 'foramen ovale' and 'ductus arteriosus' are the only features that are different in a developed fetal heart[16] when compared to an adult heart. The right atrium is presented as a slightly larger cavity than the left atrium. The superior and inferior vena cava are identifiable as they meet with the right atrium. Pulmonary veins tend to be smaller in size due to the reduced pulmonary blood flow; however, they become apparent in mature fetuses.

The tricuspid and mitral valves present similar features under echocardiographic analysis (Figure 32.1). Two papillary muscles constitute the subvalvular apparatus of the mitral valve, while only one is observed in the tricuspid valve. The tricuspid septal leaflet is distinctly apparent because it attaches to the septum at a closer location than the mitral valve from the apex of the heart. This separation in valve positioning allows for effective visual recognition if the ventricles are pathologically inverted.

To ensure normal ventriculoarterial connections,[8,17] a 'crossing' by the pulmonary and aortic outflow tracts and arteries must be identified when examined with echo (Figure 32.2). A parallel position of both great vessels at their origin from the heart would mean a 'transposition of the great arteries'.[8]

In order to differentiate the aortic arch from the ductal arch (Figure 32.3), three supra-aortic vessels must be attached to the curve of the aortic arch before it extends into the descending aorta. The position beneath the ductal arch is recognizable by its continuity from the pulmonary artery into the ductus arteriosus and the descending thoracic aorta.

Fetal cardiovascular physiology

The normal fetal heart structure and blood circulation differ physiologically[12] from those of the adult. The placenta and the feto-placenta circulation become the major source of oxygen in the uterus during fetal life as opposed to the adult lung autonomous respiratory system.

Two major fetal intracardiac shunts appear, one at the foramen ovale level and the other at the ductus arteriosus. These allow for a *right to left* direction of the almost total fetal cardiac output. Approximately half of this circulatory blood volume will be sent to the placenta to be oxygenated, returning subsequently to the fetus, resulting in two major circulations: the fetal circulation and the feto-placental circulation.[16]

Feto-placenta venous circulation is characterized by the entry of the umbilical vein through the fetal

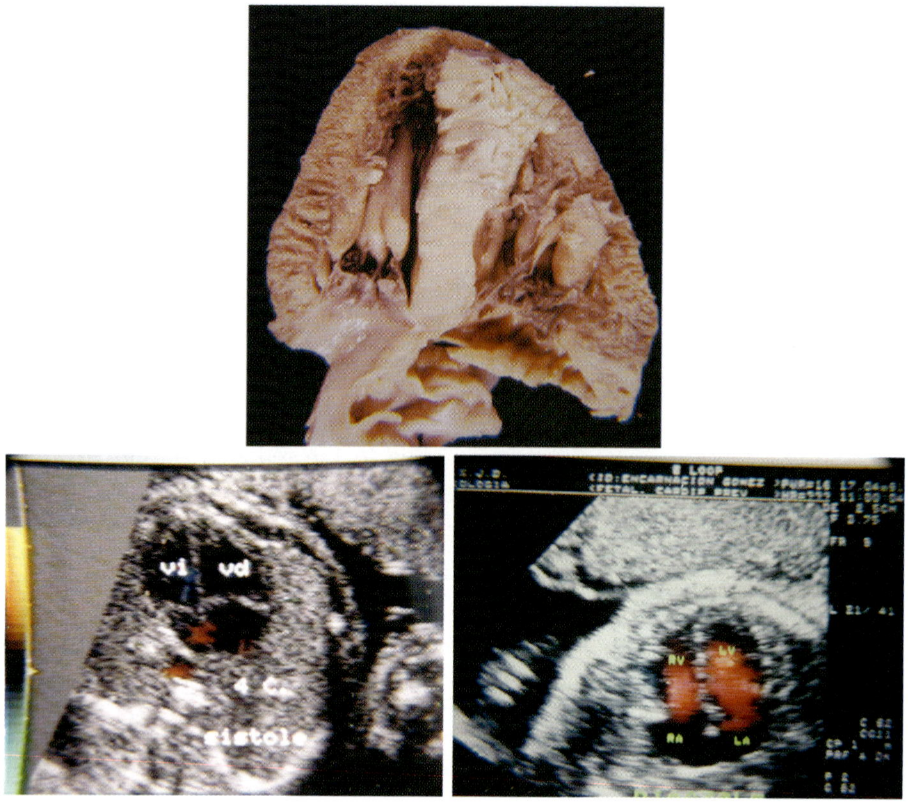

Figure 32.1 Normal four-chamber view. Systolic and diastolic color flow Doppler phases at the A–V valves. Anatomic correlation with the heart specimen.

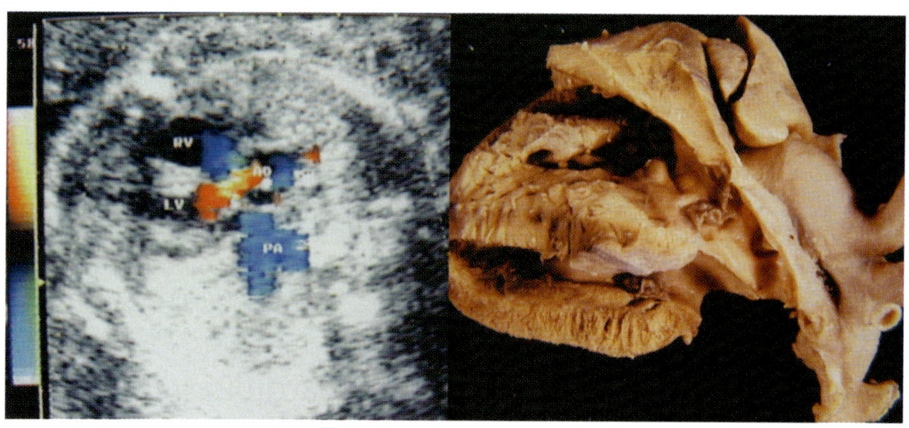

Figure 32.2 Normal longitudinal color flow Doppler cut at lateral dorsum. Crossing of the outflow tracts and arteries and anatomic correlation.

liver. Oxygenated blood travels from the placenta entering the fetus through the 'ductus venosus', which is an extension of intrahepatic umbilical vein. It has been found that the flow dynamics of the circulatory system in this specific area are crucial for the fetal oxygenation process. The diameter of the ductus venosus is reduced as it meets the inferior vena cava. This reduction in diameter accelerates the oxygenated blood, creating a directional jet toward the foramen ovale and left atrium. The entry of this oxygenated bloodstream is cyclically regulated by the fetal heart rate. The change in volume in the right atrial cavity imposes the cardiac filling pattern. This allows the oxygenated blood to be propelled through the left atrium and left ventricle toward the coronary arteries and fetal brain. Less oxygenated blood returning from the peripheral fetal body, coming from the superior vena cava and inferior vena cava, enters the right atrium, right ventricle and the pulmonary artery. At this last point most of the blood is diverted through the ductus arteriosus toward the descending aorta, leaving the pulmonary circulation at minimum flow.

The lower part of the fetal body has low oxygen requirements. This area is supplied by a part of the

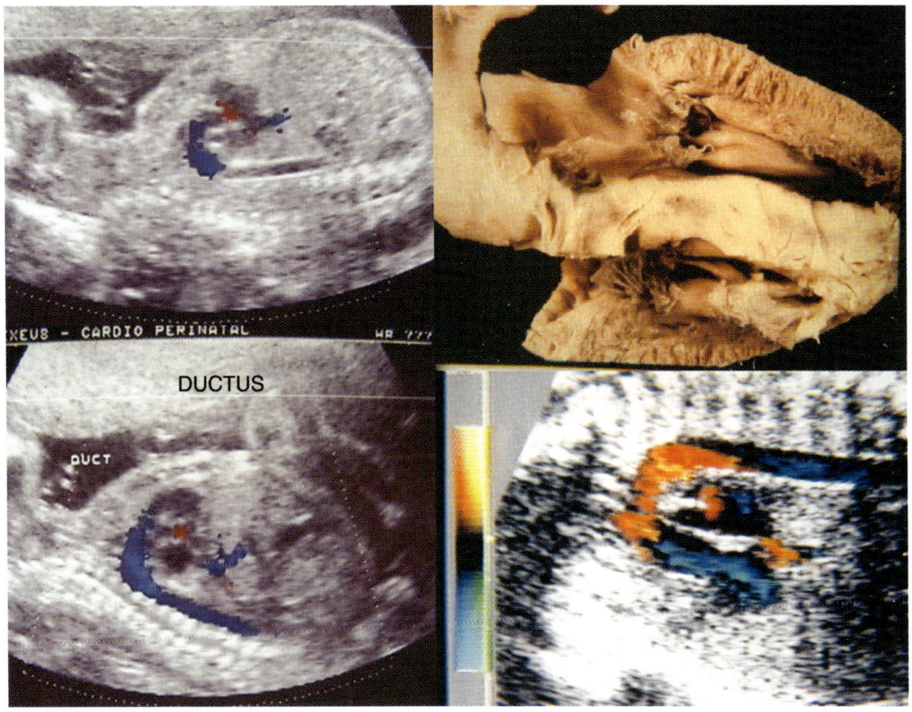

Figure 32.3 Normal aortic arch at posterior/anterior dorsum. Normal ductus arteriosus arch at posterior dorsum.

less oxygenated blood coming from the descending aorta. The rest of the blood at this level is directed toward the placenta through the umbilical arteries and umbilical cord. The blood oxygenation process takes place at the placenta, which is then returned to the fetus, closing the feto-placenta circulation.

Thus, two main circulatory systems are developed during the fetal life: fetal and feto-placenta circulation. Both the circulatory systems are maintained by the fetal heart. Consequently, high fetal cardiac output is required to keep both the circulations functioning. This translates into elevated heart rates (130–160 beats per minute, (bpm)), which are also partially imposed by the limited ventricular compliance of the fetal heart.

Another representative feature only present in the fetal circulatory system is the similar systolic pressure levels between the right ventricle/pulmonary artery and the left ventricle/aorta at a systemic level. Therefore, *right to left intracardiac shunts* are dependable on systemic vascular resistance as well as changes in cardiac and vascular blood volume adjustment.

Assessing the fetal heart

Instrumentation and technique

The study of the fetal heart requires the combination of several dynamic ultrasound techniques and sequential cardiac analysis.[18]

The intracardiac fetal echocardiographic studies require a range-gated 2D and pulsed Doppler to perform selective interrogation of blood flow across the A–V valves, ventricles and great arteries, ductus arteriosus, descending aorta as well as the aortic arch. The scanning should also include the hepatic duct and veins, the inferior vena cava, atrial flows, foramen ovale and when possible the pulmonary veins. The equipment should also include CW Doppler for sampling high-velocity jets.

Color flow mapping increases the diagnostic accuracy and understanding of fetal cardiovascular circulation.[8,9] Color flow display must be performed with the instrumentation settings at a high pulse repetition frequency in order to avoid aliasing. Intracardiac blood velocities are higher than in the periphery, therefore color Doppler settings must be set up at high frame rates, reduced angle and high filter to obtain good color resolution. However, diagnostic misinterpretation of color intracardiac Doppler may occur in complex congenital heart disease if previous analysis of 2D cardiac malformed anatomy has not been properly done.

(1) 2D echocardiography identifies anatomical structures, spatial relationship, position of the heart, myocardial thickness and myocardial function. The superimposition of color Doppler technique allows performing of selective cardiovascular flow dynamics in each heart structure.
(2) 'Pulsed Doppler' is used for selective flow studies in each cavity or vessel and the instrument setting has to be adjusted according to the sampling site. 'Continuous Doppler' is necessary to identify high-velocity blood signals as well as to quantify intracardiac and intravascular pressure gradients. 'Color Doppler' opacification of the

blood flow in cardiac cavities and vessels allows detection of abnormal turbulent accelerated flows produced by valve regurgitation and stenosis or other cardiac defects.

(3) 'M-mode color Doppler flow' is used to measure accurately the cavity size and vessels as well as to evaluate cardiac rhythm disturbances and cardiac function.

(4) Fetal position within the uterus must be understood to evaluate the spatial orientation of the different heart structures in order to trace the best Doppler signal and map the color flow Doppler displayed in anatomical position.

'Anterior dorsum' and 'posterior dorsum' are usually the best fetal positions to study the color flow displayed in the aortic arch and the aorta as well as the ductus arteriosus arch.

'Posterior dorsum' is the most favorable position to obtain the four-chamber view to evaluate the ventricular filling pattern across the A–V valves, obtaining information about atrial and ventricular size and anatomy, integrity of the atrioventricular septum and inlet septum, the A–V valves and atrioventricular connections.

'Lateral dorsum' identifies best the opacification of the right and left outflow tracts and outlet septum, as well as ventriculoarterial connections.

Transabdominal cardiac Doppler studies can be performed with adequate level of cardiac definition from 17 weeks of gestation onward, using a 3.5-MHz transducer. Cardiac scanning should include at least three anatomical and functional cuts to demonstrate structural and functional normal assessment.

Normal anatomic and functional fetal echocardiographic features

A number of normal features should be identified in the echocardiographic evaluation of the fetus:

(1) The normal position of the heart within the thorax is of levocardia (the heart is usually to the left, opposite to the liver and superior to the stomach). In the four-chamber view, the thoracic aorta should be in the left, in close proximity with the left atrium. The fetal heart lies in a more horizontal position due to the large liver.

(2) Septal integrity should be present, although weakening of the inlet/outlet septum may give the impression of a ventricular septal defect (VSD) in the early stages of pregnancy; no posterior confirmation has been possible, probably due to a transitional echo view, which cuts part of the left outflow tract and the interventricular septum.

(3) The patent foramen ovale should be a visible atrial communication of approximately the same size as the ascending aorta but no larger than 6 mm along pregnancy and with a detectable moving membrane.

(4) Normal separation between the septal leaflet implantation of the mitral and tricuspid valves should identify the right and left A–V valves (Figure 32.4).

(5) Myocardial contractility presents an out of systolic phase, paradoxical septal movement; however, movement of the anterior and posterior heart walls should be identified for evaluating ventricular myocardial movement and function.

(6) A pericardial space translucency may be visualized in the absence of a pericardial effusion.

(7) The heart rate should be between 120 and 180 bpm.

(8) Normal ventriculoarterial connections should be established when normal crossing of both ventricular outflow tracts and arteries is seen (Figure 32.2).[8]

(9) Normal vessel relationship is seen by the transverse three-vessel view from left to right – the pulmonary artery, the Ao and the SCV are seen in the same transverse plane.[19]

(10) The aortic arch should give rise to the three supra-aortic arteries.

(11) The ductus arteriosus arch should be identified as a vascular structure in continuity with the descending aorta, in a right-angle curvature when it meets the aorta.

(12) The superior vena cava and inferior vena cava should be visualized in continuity entering the right atrium.

(13) The pulmonary veins should be seen entering the left atrium.

Normal Doppler fetal hemodynamics

Peripheral venous return of the umbilical vein and ductus venosus

Doppler sample at the umbilical vein level shows that a low-velocity non-pulsatile wave form is slightly influenced by diaphragmatic respiratory movements. The intrahepatic umbilical vein continues with the ductus venosus as it meets the inferior vena cava. The diameter of the ductus venosus is reduced as it meets the inferior vena cava. This reduction in diameter accelerates the blood flow converting the non-pulsatile Doppler venous wave of the umbilical vein into a high-velocity triphasic wave form directly influenced by the cycling cardiac filling pattern. The first peak (S) represents the systolic cardiac phase; the second peak (D) represents the diastolic phase, which is followed by the atrial contraction inflection (A).

Right/left atrium and foramen ovale

Doppler interrogation of the foramen ovale demonstrates a right–left shunting. Premature closure of the foramen ovale has been described.[20] Doppler tracing in the pulmonary veins is also triphasic as in the systemic veins; the lowest-velocity deflection occurs

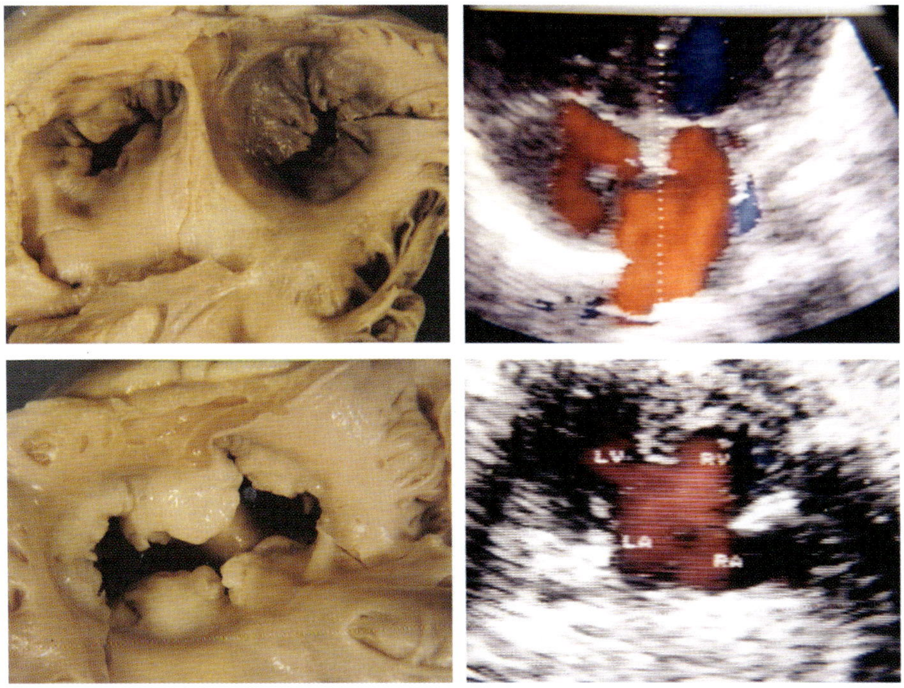

Figure 32.4 Inflow of the heart with two normal A–V valves. Color Doppler also identifies the PFO. Inflow of a heart specimen with one common A–V valve in atrioventricular septal defect. Echo/anatomy correlation.

during atrial contraction. Timing of the phases in the venous flow of the pulmonary veins may be useful in diagnosing premature atrial contractions.

Increase in right atrial or ventricular filling pressure may lead to right heart failure. This increase in resistance to umbilical venous flow accentuates the atrial contraction and the corresponding Doppler inflection wave at the 'ductus venosus', creating a negative deflection wave that may exceed the zero line at the venous return; this Doppler form should be recognized as a sign of heart failure.

The less oxygenated blood returning from the peripheral fetal body, coming from the superior vena cava and inferior vena cava as the blood enters the right atrium, presents a Doppler venous flow with the triphasic waveform related to the same cardiac filling cycle; this waveform exhibits more pronounced atrial inflection but less flow velocity than the waves obtained in ductus venosus.

Inflow heart and atrioventricular valves

Doppler interrogation of the inlet heart examines the diastolic filling function. Doppler waveforms through the tricuspid and mitral valves are similar, representing the ventricular filling pattern: the first peak E is followed by the A wave. Due to atrial contraction an increase in A occurs in the early phases of pregnancy and may represent a transient restricted compliance of the ventricles; normal velocity across the A–V valves increases along pregnancy. High heart rate may produce single wave changes in morphology. A–V valve stenosis or volume overload alters the morphology and increases velocity across the valves.

Regurgitation of an A–V valve is detected within the atrial cavity. Although quantification of a regurgitant flow by Doppler is difficult, detection of a significant regurgitant jet in fetal life represents a considerable hemodynamic dysfunction.[13]

The integrity of the atrioventricular septum in continuity with the inlet septum should be seen as color Doppler fills the ventricles. Weakening of the inlet septum may give the impression of a VSD in the early stages of pregnancy; but no posterior confirmation has been possible, probably due to a transitional echo cut; however, an A–V septal defect has to be excluded (Figure 32.4).

Outflow heart, semilunar valves and arteries

Color Doppler has become an extremely effective tool in identifying crossing flow patterns vs. parallel flows at the arterial level. The different color opacification of each artery indicates opposing flow directions that represent normal crossing of the pulmonary and the aortic outflow tracts and arteries[8] and normal ventriculoarterial connection (Figure 32.2). A single color representation in both arteries identifies the parallel relationship of the great arteries, being the most frequent anatomical arterial relationship seen in transposition of the great arteries (Figure 32.5). However, careful attention should be paid to fetal spatial orientation in the uterus in lateral dorsum to evaluate arterial crossing relationship by color Doppler.[21]

Color Doppler also gives information about the integrity of the outlet septum when both the outflow tracts are identified. Subarterial and infundibular VSD will be seen during this examination.

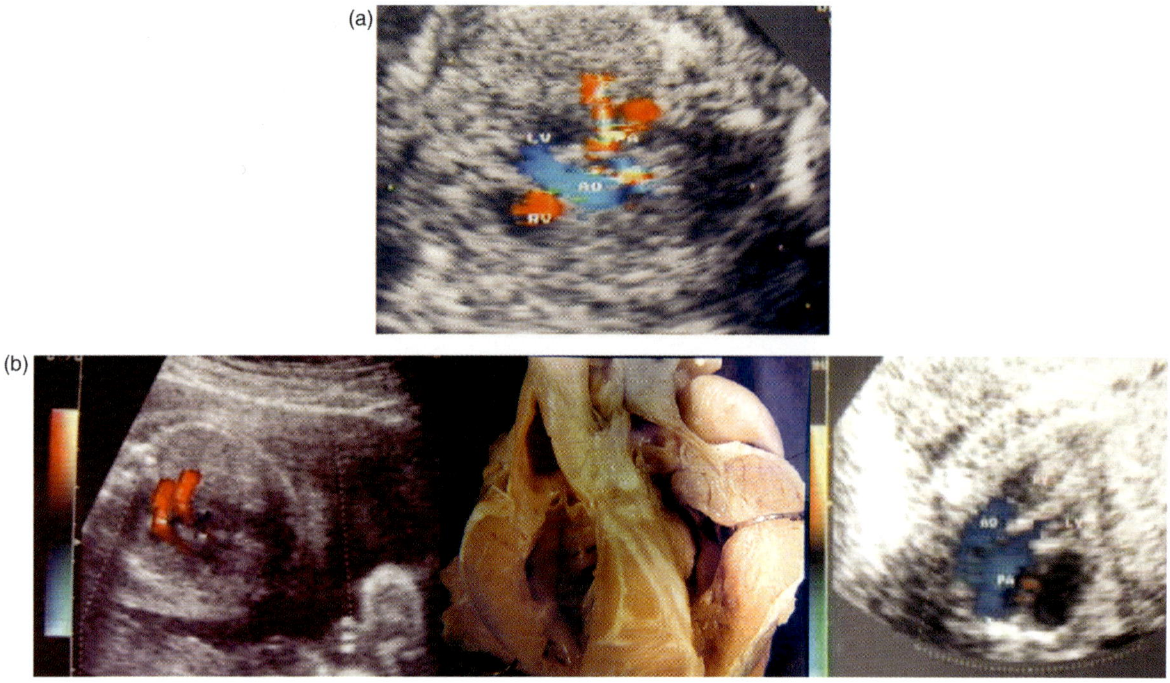

Figure 32.5 (a) Normal outflow right and left ventricular tracts and arteries. The opposite code opacification shows the normal crossing relationship. (b) Heart specimen from a transposition of the great arteries. Color flow Doppler shows parallel opacification of both arteries.

Semilunar valve systolic flow examination by Doppler not only allows measuring of time intervals to assess systolic function, but may also give information about the presence of valve stenosis or regurgitation. Blood velocity across a semilunar valve should not exceed 130 cm/s; an increase above this velocity could be due to valvular stenosis or increased blood volume. A turbulent high Doppler flow is usually produced by valve stenosis; the degree of obstruction is the key for measuring the severity of this lesion. In fetal life, each semilunar valve allows the passage of approximately half of the blood volume that will transverse the valve after birth; this reduced blood volume will cause an underestimation of the obstruction and of the valve pressure gradient, making the fetal assessment difficult. Valvular regurgitation produces a backward flow into the left or right ventricular outflow tract, which in the fetus with normal heart rate (>130 bpm) represents structural valvular dysfunction.

Ductus arteriosus and the descending aorta

The pulmonary artery receives approximately half of the total blood flow ejected by the right fetal heart. At this point most of the blood is diverted through the 'ductus arteriosus' toward the descending aorta, leaving the pulmonary circulation at minimum flow. The ductus arteriosus is a vascular structure in continuity with the descending aorta, forming almost a right-angle curvature when it meets the aorta; the ductus at this level may impose a degree of flow restriction; however; this is compensated by the active systolic contraction of the right ventricle. Doppler waveform shows a slight increase in systolic velocity as the ductus meets the aorta. However, an abnormal increase in systolic and diastolic velocity above 130 cm/seg. is produced during ductal constriction with marked elevation of systolic and diastolic velocity. Patients under indometacin treatment should be Doppler controlled to detect signs of ductal constriction (Figure 32.6) and medication should be stopped. A sudden increase in ductal constriction leads to increase in afterload with tricuspid regurgitation.[22,23]

Systolic arterial Doppler wave in the abdominal aorta is followed by continuous diastolic flow as blood entering the intra-abdominal umbilical arteries goes into the umbilical cord toward the placenta.

Abnormal anatomical and functional echocardiographic fetal features

Abnormal features of echocardiography include the following:

(1) Malposition of the heart is established when atrial and visceral organs (liver/stomach) are seen in the wrong position: the usual place for these structures is termed as 'situs solitus'. 'Situs inversus' involves reversal of the normal atrial and ventricular positions. 'Situs ambiguous' describes an undefined medial visceral position. Dextrocardia, mesocardia, levocardia are terms that define the location of the cardiac apex.

(2) Comparative disproportion between atrial and ventricular cavities, as well as arterial size, may lead to demonstration of pathological dilatation

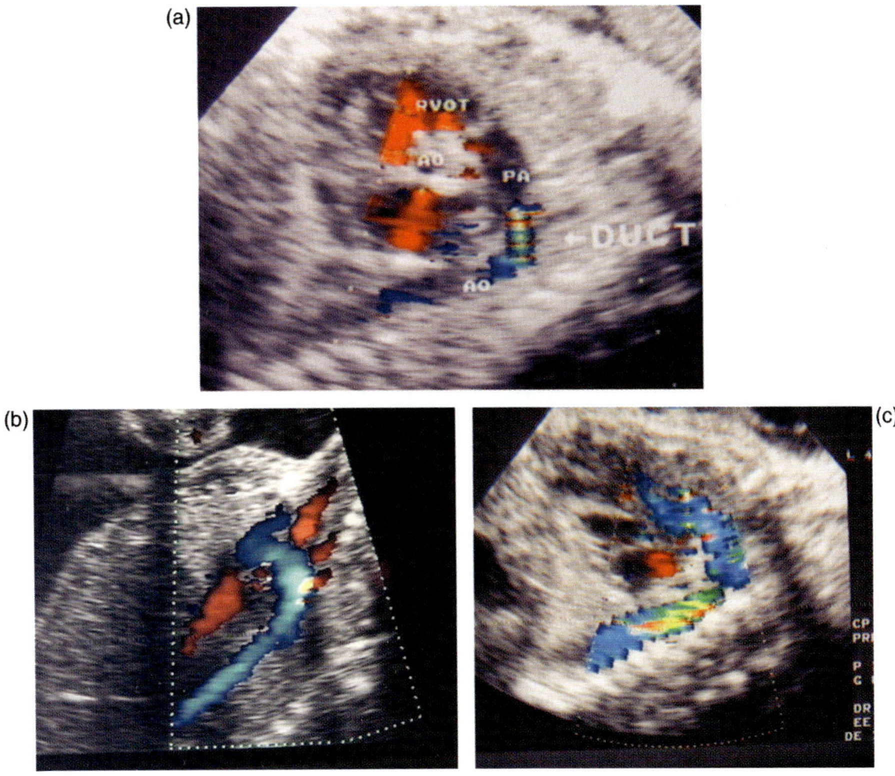

Figure 32.6 (a) Ductus arteriosus constriction under indometacin therapy. Color flow Doppler shows a turbulent ductal flow. (b) Normal aortic arch. (c) Coarctation of the Ao. Color flow detects a turbulent flow at the descending aorta.

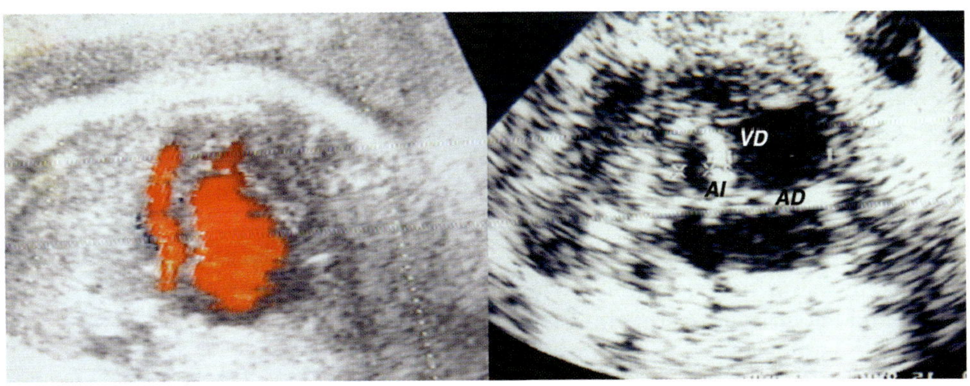

Figure 32.7 Four-chamber cut in left heart asymmetry due to hypoplastic left heart.

or reduced diameter of these heart structures (Figures 32.7 and 32.8).

(3) A single ventricular cavity.
(4) A single atrium.
(5) A single atrioventricular valve (Figure 32.4).
(6) Specific valvular anomalies. Ebstein's anomaly.
(7) Parallel ventricular outflow tracts and arteries (Figure 32.5).
(8) A single arterial trunk (truncus).
(9) A septal defect.
(10) Ventricular inversion.
(11) Regurgitant valvular jets (by Doppler).
(12) Cardiomegaly.
(13) Signs of heart failure: pericardial effusion, ascitis and hydrops.
(14) Arteriovenous fistula.
(15) Arrhythmias; taquyarrhythmia, bradycardia.

Fetal cardiovascular pathology. Identification by 2D echocardiography and color Doppler

Congenital heart disease appears as a result of 'structural malformations' developed during the early phases of fetal life.[2,3] The severity of each malformation marks the future prognosis of the newborn, with perinatal death as high as 50%,[4] when congenital heart

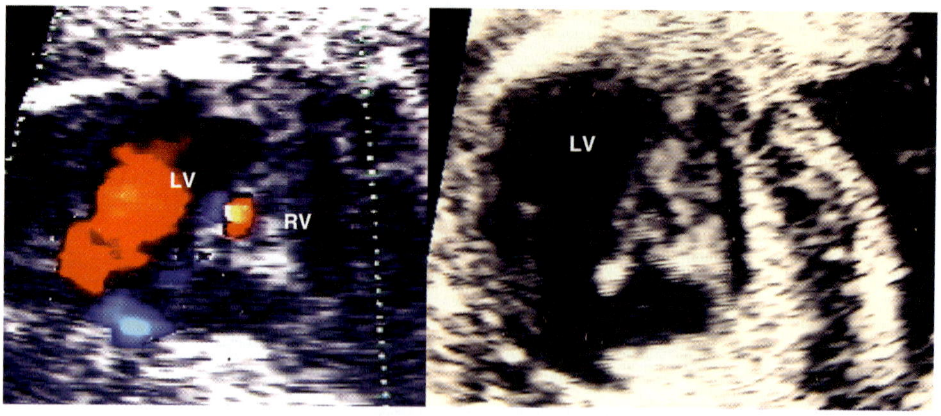

Figure 32.8 Tricuspid atresia and hypoplastic right heart. The Color Doppler helps to identify a small right ventricular cavity.

disease has been diagnosed in fetal life.[24] Chromosomal abnormalities may be found in as high as 42% of the fetal cases referred because of congenital heart disease.[25] However, 'functional cardiac anomalies' may occur as a transitory disturbance during fetal intrauterine growth and usually present a good prognostic outlook at term.

In an attempt to simplify congenital heart disease complexity, cardiac malformations may occur at two basic levels following a segmental approach:[7]

(1) The inflow level, including malformations at systemic and pulmonary veins, atriums, atrial septum, inlet valves, inlet/trabecular septum and ventricular cavities.
(2) The outflow level, which includes ventricles, outlet septum, outflow tracts, semilunar valves and arteries.

Inflow level

The veins are identified by using the four-chamber view as they meet the right and left atriums. Anomalous connections of the systemic veins as well as pulmonary veins may be visually identified.[26] The relative sizes of the right and left atriums should be compared. Usually, the right atrium is larger than the left atrium. Early closure or reduction of the foramen ovale[20] (atrial septal aneurysm) may be identified as well as a distended foramen. The ventricles should be of similar size although right ventricular dominance may be normally present.

Congenital cardiac malformations and conditions at inflow level include:

(1) Anomalous venous connections of the systemic venous return or the pulmonary veins.
(2) Atrial septal defects: ostium primun, ostium secundum and sinus venosus defects and patent foramen ovale with septal aneurismatic membranous septum.
(3) Atrioventricular valve anomalies: mitral/tricuspide atresia, mitral/tricuspid stenosis/hypoplasia (Figures 32.8 and 32.9). Atrioventricular valve regurgitation. Single common valve, Ebstein's anomaly.
(4) Ventricular development: hypoplastic left heart, hypoplastic right heart, single ventricle (univentricular heart), single inlet, double inlet, atrioventricular canal complete and partial, and ventricular inversion (atrioventricular discordance) corrected transposition.
(5) Ventricular septal defect: inlet portion (perimembranous), trabecular (muscular) and apical.
(6) Pericardium (effusion).
(7) Myocardium: ventricular anatomy (right ventricle heavily trabeculated containing the tricuspid valve with a confluent papillary muscle/left ventricle smooth endocardial walls with the mitral valve and two well-defined papillary muscles. Left ventricular myocardial contractility, function and hypertrophy.
(8) Cardiomyopathies: hypertrophic (diabetes, etc.), dilated (endocardial fibroelastosis, etc.).
(9) Cardiac tumors.

Outflow level

Color Doppler has become an extremely effective tool in identifying 'crossing flow patterns' vs. 'parallel flows'.[8] The different color code opacification of each artery indicates opposing blood flow directions that represent normal ventriculoarterial connections (Figure 32.5).[4] The key to the diagnosis is to demonstrate the origin of the pulmonary artery arising from the left ventricle and the aorta arising from the right ventricle.

Single color code opacification in both arteries identifies parallel arterial relationship, which represents a discordant ventricular–arterial connection, so-called transposition of the great arteries (Figure 32.5). Single opacification of one single arterial trunk, truncus.

Congenital cardiac malformation and conditions at the outflow level include:

(1) Aortic valve/pulmonary valve: atresia, stenosis and regurgitation.
(2) Hypoplastic aortic arch/pulmonary trunk.

(a)

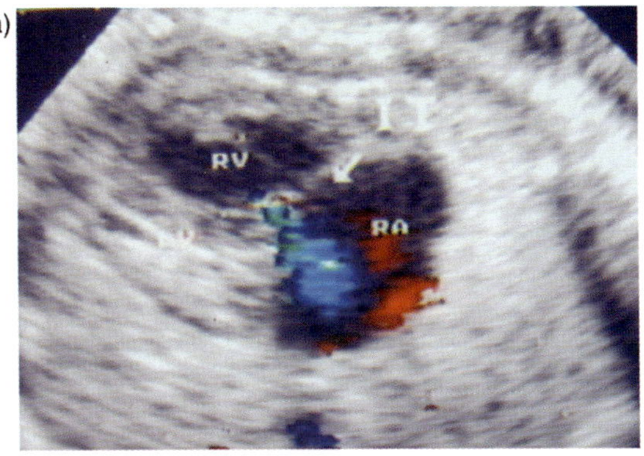

(b)

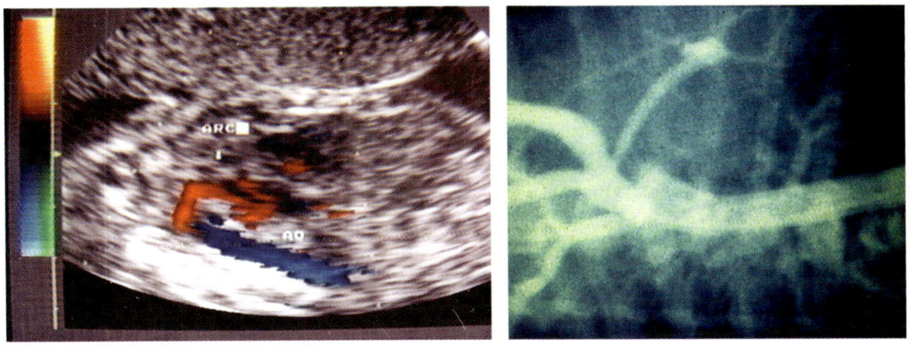

Figure 32.9 Hypoplastic left heart syndrome with mitral atresia and aortic atresia. (a) Single ventricular cavity corresponding to the right ventricle. Tricuspid regurgitation is seen. (b) Echocardiograph/angiogram to show the retrograde aortic arch opacification as no blood is ejected through the aortic valve.

(3) Coarctation of the aorta (Figure 32.6)/aortic arch interruption.
(4) Coronary artery anomalies.
(5) Absent pulmonary valve syndrome.
(6) Single arterial trunk (truncus arteriosus).
(7) Tetralogy of Fallot (Figure 32.10)/pulmonary atresia + VSD.
(8) Double-outlet right ventricle (Figure 32.11).
(9) Double-outlet right ventricle and transposition of the great arteries (Figure 32.11).
(10) Ventricular septal defect: infundibular, perimembranous, subarterial and trabecular.
(11) Aorto/pulmonary window.
(12) Anomalies of the aortic arch.
(13) Hypoplastic aortic arch and coarctation of the aorta (Figure 32.6) vs. interrupted aortic arch.

The diagnosis of structural and functional heart disease is possible during fetal life, although, not always with the amount of precision required. There are a number of congenital heart malformations that are extremely difficult to establish before birth as the fetal heart is not yet fully adapted to the future adult circulation that will take place after birth.

In the newborn with congenital heart disease, as the pulmonary circulation and lung oxygenation process begin, cardiac malformations will develop further. The intracardiac fetal shunts will close down as pulmonary artery pressure is reduced to one-quarter of the systemic pressure.

During pregnancy some fetal heart defects such as ostium secundum atrial defect, anomalous pulmonary venous return and some small ventricular septal defects will be impossible to evaluate. Also, in some cases of Fallot's tetralogy in which fetal pulmonary blood obstruction is not yet well established during the prenatal period, it may be difficult to identify the obstruction as the main functional/anatomical feature of this malformation. During fetal life, malformations and vascular anomalies such as persistent ductus arteriosus, aortopulmonary window, coarctation of the aorta and interruption of the aortic arch are extremely difficult to diagnose because no dysfunctional changes take place before birth, although indirect cardiac signs such as enlargement of the right heart cavities have been described.

Coronary artery anomalies are also difficult to suspect. The diagnosis of atrioventricular or semilunar valve stenosis is similarly difficult; the degree of obstruction to blood flow is the key to measuring severity in these lesions. In fetal life, each cardiac valve allows the passage of only half of the blood volume that will transverse the valve after birth because of the fetal intracardiac circulation pattern; this reduced blood volume will cause an underestimate of the obstruction and valve pressure gradient making the diagnosis by Doppler difficult.

Diagnosis and prognosis of fetal heart failure

The echocardiographic examination of the cardiovascular system provides much information about the

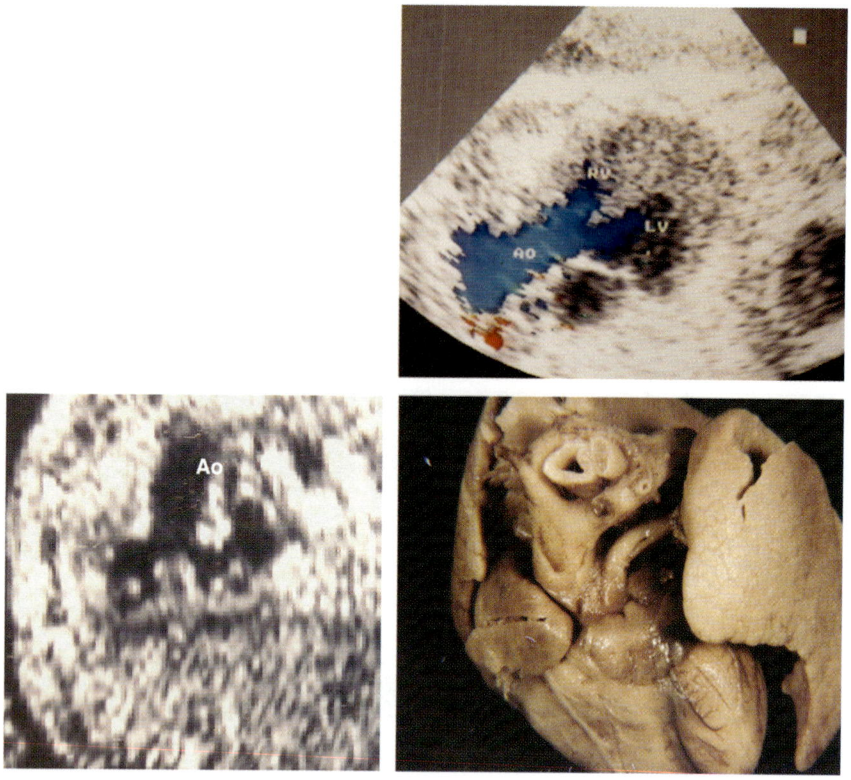

Figure 32.10 Tetralogy of Fallot. The heart specimen shows reduced pulmonary artery compared to the ascending aorta. A double aortic arch was present as well. Aortic–septal overriding can be seen by echocardiography, demonstrating the subarterial VSD.

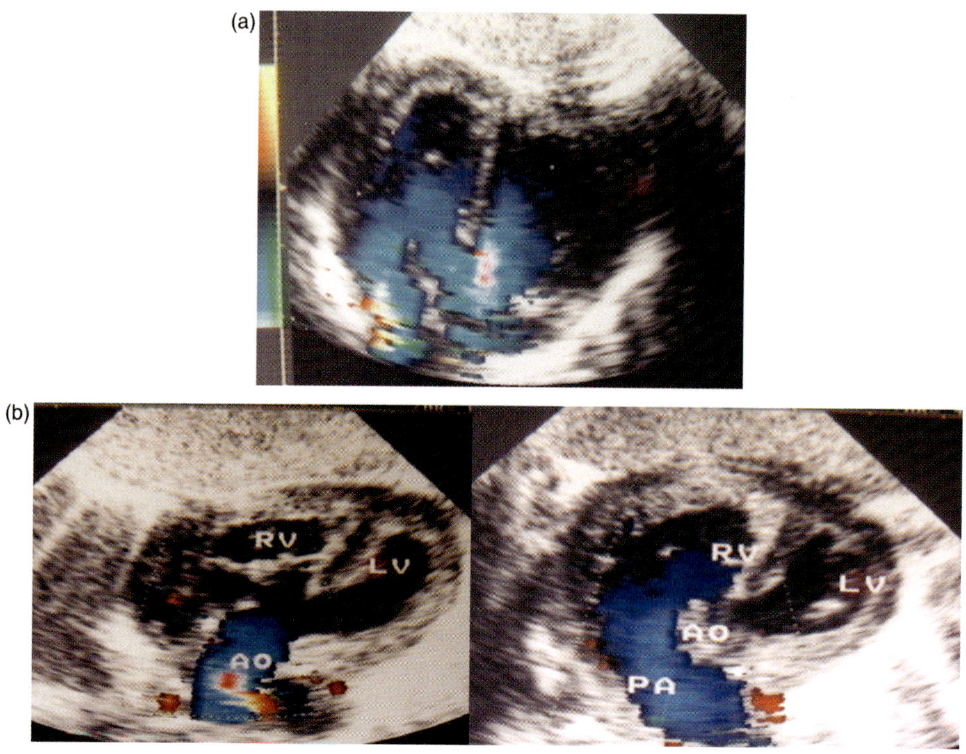

Figure 32.11 Double-outlet right ventricle. (a) Two parallel outflow tracts and arteries are seen coming from the right ventricle with subpulmonary VSD in double-outlet right ventricle with TGA. (b) Double-outlet right ventricle with normally related arteries with subaortic VSD.

well-being of the fetus. Heart failure is established when low cardiac output produces inadequate tissue perfusion. This results in a series of complex hormonal reflexes and vascular adaptations to improve direct flow to the vital organs. Peripheral vasoconstriction increases the fetal systemic resistances in response to cardiovascular stress with excess production of catecholamines and naturetic factor together with other complex humeral agents to maintain arterial redistribution of fetal cardiac output for the survival of the fetus.

The diagnosis of fetal heart failure is established through the analysis of a number of cardiovascular features:

(1) The cardio-thoracic size. Cardiomegaly is the universal sign of heart failure. This is measured using the CT cardiac/chest circumference ratio. Normal, < 0.5.
(2) Myocardial function. Assessment of cardiac function by global myocardium fiber shortening fraction is calculated by using the difference between the diastolic and systolic dimensions divided by the diastolic diameter. Normal, > 0.30.
(3) Increased atrial reversal contraction at the venous Doppler triphasic pattern in the hepatic duct and inferior vena cava. This may be a sign of increased end diastolic ventricular pressure. Increased A:S ratio peak atrial reversal divided by peak ventricular systole (Figure 32.12). Normal values should be less than 7%. In the fetus with congenital heart disease the venous filling patterns should be normal with the exception of tricuspid/pulmonary atresia with intact septum of restrictive filling compliance lesions.
(4) Analysis of Doppler detection of valve leak at the heart.

Fetal cardiac arrhythmias

Fetal cardiac disrrythmias[27,28] are rhythm disturbances caused by irregular cardiac beats, 'extrasystoles', or by regular accelerated tachycardias produced by ectopic heartbeats greater than 180 bpm. On the contrary, bradycardia are slow regular heart rhythms, below 80 bpm.

Cardiac disrrythmias account for 1–2% of rhythm alterations during pregnancy. Fetal arrythmias are also associated with a higher incidence of congenital heart disease. However, irregular cardiac rhythms caused by extrasystoles account for 80–85% of benign rhythm disturbances in normal fetus with no need for specific treatment. Management of these disrrythmias during pregnancy only requires maternal rest and withdrawal of stimulants.

Taquy-bradycardias[29] are frequently a cause of heart failure and hydrops. They usually require *in utero* treatment via maternal administration of antiarrhythmic agents, premature delivery and cardiac pacing of the newborn as in the case of congenital heart block.

Classification of cardiac arrhythmias

Irregular heartbeats (Figure 32.13)

Extrasystoles

Extrasystoles constitute the most frequent arrhythmia in the fetus and in the newborn; no treatment is required, only observation.

They have been associated with high fetal catecholamines, maternal hyperthyroidism and stimulants.

Sinus arrhythmia

In this disorder, there is variability between the sinus atrial contractions. It is recognized by the variable space between Doppler pulsed waves.

Premature atrial contraction

Premature atrial contraction is the most frequent ectopic arrhythmia often causing extrasystoles. It may be the origin of supraventricular tachycardia.

Premature ventricular contraction

Premature ventricular contractions are ventricular ectopic beats; they are rare in the fetus.

Regular fast heart rate

Sinus tachycardia

This is a persistent cardiac rhythm above 160 bpm but below 200 bpm, that may be related to the fetal response to catecholamines, anemia, etc.

Pathological tachycardias

They are regular fast heart rhythms above 200 bpm, divided into two main groups: supraventricular and ventricular tachycardia.

(1) Supraventricular tachycardia (Figure 32.14) includes:

- *Atrial tachycardia*, produced by an ectopic atrial beat.
- *Atrial flutter*, a rapid atrial contraction of 300–400 bpm. The atrial activity is blocked at the atrioventricular (A–V) node with ventricular response of 220 bpm. The p wave can be identified at the movement of the atrial wall by m-mode echo.
- *Intranodal tachycardia*, the most common fetal and newborn tachycardia, it presents with a ventricular response between 220 and 280 bpm and a 2/1 atrioventricular block.
- *Atrioventricular tachycardia with accessory pathway*, with conduction via the Kent or Mahian intranodal and extranodal pathway conduction. In the Wolf–Parkinson–White syndrome, tachycardias are produced by a

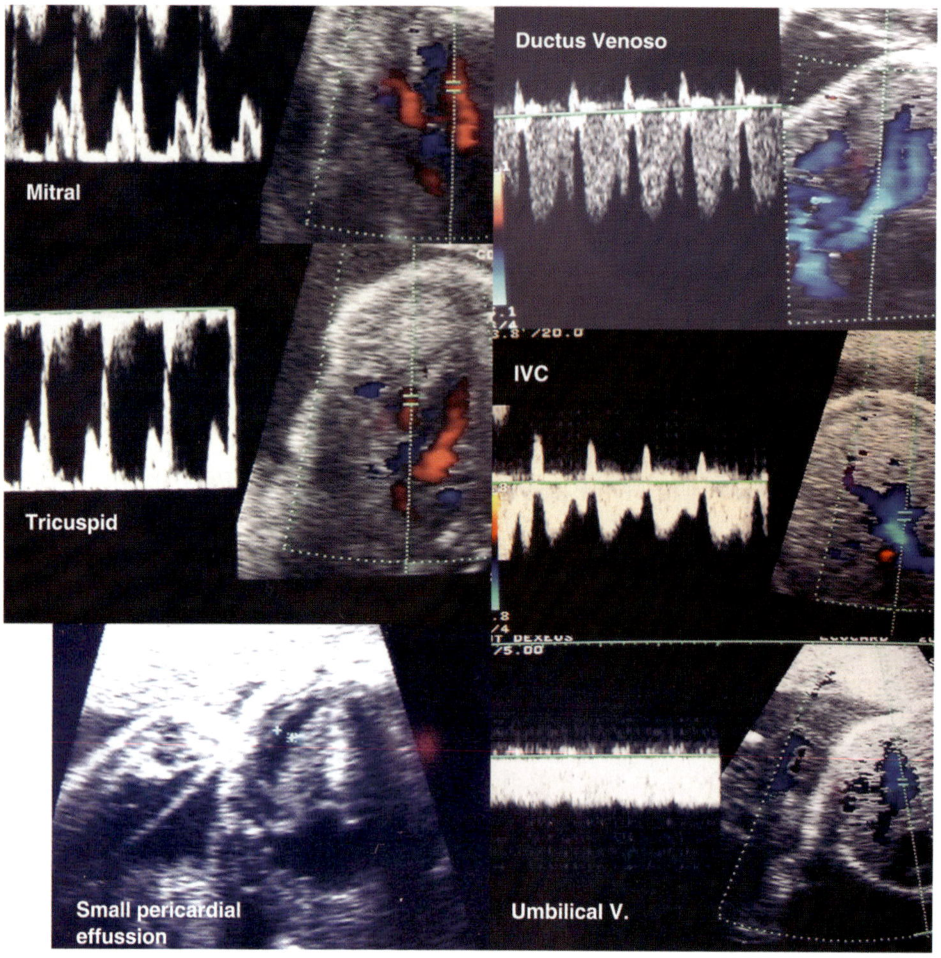

Figure 32.12 A number of Doppler signs can predict fetal heart failure: increased 'a' in A–V flow; deep diastolic phase at ductus venosus flow; prominent and negative 'a' wave at the inferior vena cava; small pericardial effusion; pulsatile deflection at the umbilical flow.

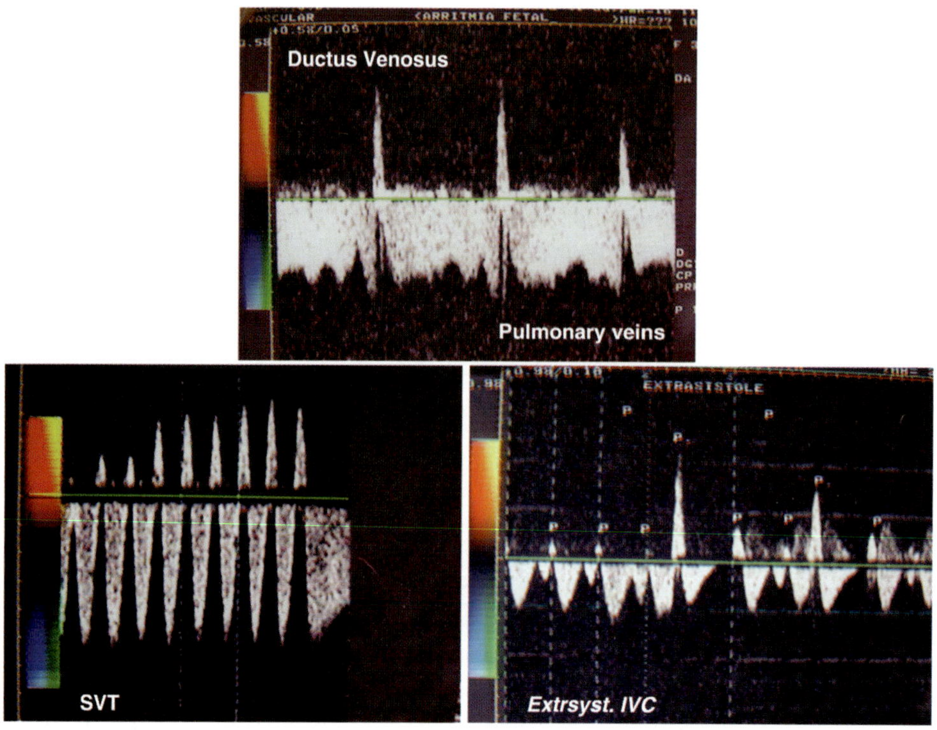

Figure 32.13 Supraventricular ectopic beats seen at ductus venosus flow and inferior vena cava (negative deflections) and run of supraventricular tachycardia.

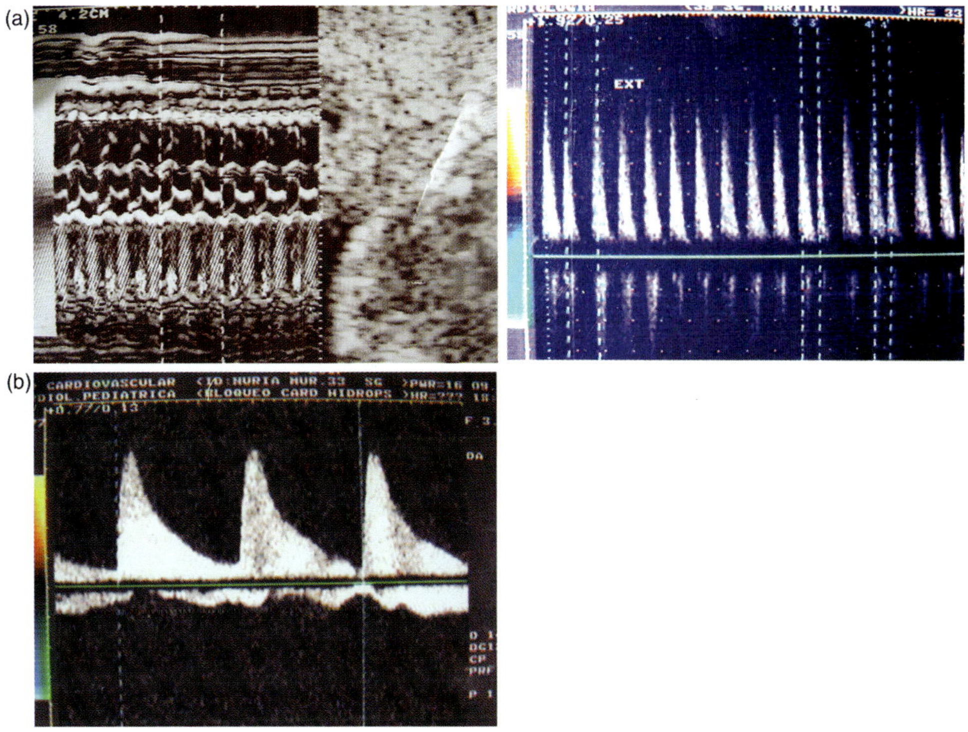

Figure 32.14 (a) Supraventricular tachycardia using M-mode echocardiography to establish a 2/1 atrioventricular rate comparing the atrial wall movements and the aortic valve opening. (b) Ventricular bradycardia in a congenital complete A–V block.

circular re-entry mechanism; atrial activity is not visualized by echo; therefore, no specific diagnosis of this syndrome can be reliably made *in utero*.

(2) Ventricular tachycardia are rare in the fetus and newborn and are usually associated with myocardial dysfunction or intramyocardial tumor. The ventricular heart rate is not as fast as in the supraventricular tachycardia and is in the range of 180 bpm. This disrrhythmia may present runs of tachycardia with irregular heartbeats and no relationship can be established between atrial and ventricular contractions.

Regular slow heart rate

Bradycardias

Bradycardia is a slow cardiac rhythm with heart rates below 80 bpm. The bradycardia includes the following:

(1) *Transient sinus bradycardia* can occur during ultrasound examination. In this situation vagal stimulation over the head of the fetus may produce transient bradycardia with spontaneous recovery. Persistent bradycardia may be the consequence of fetal hypoxia or congenital heart block with or without structural congenital heart disease.

(2) *Congenital heart block* is the result of a delay or a block in the transmission of atrial electrical impulse along the atrioventricular conduction system. Three degrees may be present.

- 'First-degree block' is produced by a delay in the A–V conduction system; it is not recognized by echo.
- 'Second-degree heart block' occurs when an incomplete A–V conduction delay results in an isolated atrial impulse, which is not conducted through the A–V node, resulting in a missed ventricular contraction.
- 'Third-degree heart block' produces an atrioventricular dissociation. The atrial contraction is independent of the ventricles; it follows the sinus beats at atrial rate of 150 bpm. Atrioventricular conduction is blocked and ventricular contraction is established at an autonomous ventricular rate of 50–60 bpm (Figure 32.14). Atrioventricular dissociation is the usual presentation of congenital heart block.

Congenital heart block and persistent fetal bradycardia are associated either with congenital heart disease or with a structurally normal heart. However, a normal fetal heart and congenital heart block can be related to autoimmune maternal disease as lupus erythematosus,[30] Sjogren's syndrome and rheumatoid arthritis, not always diagnosed before pregnancy. Anti-Ro and anti-LA antibodies are most likely to be detectable in maternal blood.[31]

Congenital heart block with heart rates above 60 bpm seems to have a reasonable outcome. A pacemaker should be implanted in the newborn when ventricular heart rate is below 70 bpm. Fetal hydrops and heart failure are related to slow ventricular heart rate below 50 bpm. Fetal management should include maternal administration of terbutaline or sympathomimetics agents, as well as premature delivery and pacemaker implantation in the newborn.[32]

REFERENCES

1. Allan LD, Tynan MJ, Campbell S, Wilkinson J, Anderson RH. Doppler echocardiography and anatomical correlates in the fetus. *Br Heart J* 1987;57:528–33.
2. Allan LD. A practical approach to fetal heart scanning. *Semin Perinatol* 2000;24:324–30.
3. Cohen MS. Fetal diagnosis and management of congenital heart disease. *Clin Perinatol* 2001;28:11–29.
4. Mortera C, Salvador JM, Torrens M, Carrera JM. Diagnostico prenatal de las Cardiopatias Congenitas mediante Ecocardiografia Doppler. In *Doppler en Obstetricia Hemodinamica Perinatal.* Masson-Salvat, 1992:chap 21.
5. Chaoui R, Hoffmann J, Heling KS. Three-dimensional (3D) and (4D) color Doppler fetal echocardiography using spatio-temporal image correlation. *Ultrasound Obstet Gynecol* 2004;23(6):535–45.
6. Maulik D, Nanada NC, Singh V, *et al.* Live three-dimensional echocardiography of human fetus. *Echocardiography* 2003; 20(8):715–21.
7. Mortera C. Diagnostico Prenatal de las Cardiopatias Congenitas: Valor de la Ecocardiografia. Doctoral thesis, Universidad de Barcelona, 1989.
8. Mortera C, Carrera JM, Torrents M. Doppler pulsado codificado en color: Mapa Doppler color de la circulacion fetal. In *Doppler en Obstetricia Hemodinamica Perinatal.* Masson-Salvat, 1992: chap 20.
9. Copel JA, Morotti R, Hobbins JC, Keinman CS. The antenatal diagnosis of congenital heart disease using fetal echocardiography: Is color flow mapping necessary? *Obstet Gynecol* 1991; 78(1):1–8.
10. Chiba Y, Kanzaki T, Kobayashi H, *et al.* Evaluation of fetal structural heart disease using color flow mapping. *Ultrasound Med Biol* 1990;16(2):221–9.
11. Kovalchin JP, Silverman NH. The impact of fetal echocardiography. *Pediatr Cardiol* 2004;25:299–306.
12. Rychick J. Fetal cardiovascular physiology. *Pediatr Cardiol* 2004;25:201–9.
13. Huhta JC. Guidelines for the evaluation of heart failure in the fetus with or without hydrops. 2004;25:274–86.
14. Small M, Copel JA. Indications for fetal echocardiography. *Pediatr Cardiol* 2004;25:250–22.
15. Mortera C. Fetal ultrasound in the preliminary diagnosis of cardiac anomalies for management of the newborn with interventional cardiac catheterization. The perinatal medicine of the new millennium. *The Fifth World Congress of Perinatal Medicine,* 2001:177–80.
16. Rudolph AM. *Congetinal Heart Disease.* Chicago: Year Book Medical, 1974:chap 2, 17–28.
17. DeVore GR. The aortic and the pulmonary outflow tract screening examination in the human fetus. *J Ultrasound Med* 1992; 11: 345–8.
18. Allan. Technique of fetal echocardiography. *Pediatr Cardiol* 2004;25:223–33.
19. Yoo SJ, Lee YH, Kim ES, *et al.* Three-vessel view of the fetal upper mediastinum: An easy means of detecting abnormalities of the ventricular outflow tracts and great arteries during obstetric screening. *Ultrasound Obstet Gynecol* 1997;9:173–82.
20. Eyck J, Stewart PA, Wladimiroff JW. Human fetal foramen ovale flow velocity waveforms relative to fetal breathing movements in normal term pregnancies. *Ultrasound Obstet Gynecol* 1991;1: 5–7.
21. Cohen MS. Fetal diagnosis and management of congenital heart disease. *Clin Perinatol* 2001;28:11–29.
22. Allan LD, Sharland GK, Chita SK, *et al.* Chromosomal anomalies in fetal congenital heart disease. *Ultrasound Obstet Gynecol* 1991:8–11.
23. Wessels MW, Frohn-Mulder IM, Cromme-Dijkhuis AH, Wladimiroff W. In utero-diagnosis of infradiaphragmatic total anomalous pulmonary venous return. *Ultrasound Obstet Gynecol* 1996;8:206–9.
24. Mortera C, Maroto C, Maroto I. Echocardiografia Doppler de la circulacion fetal. In *Principios y practica del Doppler Cardiaco.* New York: McGraw-Hill, 1995:365–89.
25. Achiron R, Lipitz S, Kidrons D, Berant M, Hegesh J, Rotstein Z. In utero congestive heart failure due to maternal indomethacin treatment for polyhydramnios and premature labour in a fetus with antenatal closure of the foramen ovale. *Prenatal Diagn* 1996;16:652–6.
26. Kim HS, Sohn S, Park MY, Choi JY. Coexistence of ductal constriction and closure of the foramen in utero. *Pedatr Cardiol* 2003;24(6):588–90.
27. McCurdy CM, Reed KL. Fetal arrhythmias. In *Doppler en Obstetrics and Gynecology.* New York: Raven Press, 1995:chap 26, 253–270.
28. Kleiman CS, Copel JA. Electrophysiological principles and fetal antiarrhythmic therapy. *Ultrasound Obstet Gynecol* 1991;1: 284–97.
29. Lynn LS, Marx G. Diagnosis and treatment of structural fetal cardiac abnormality and dysrhthmia. *Semin Perinatol* 1994;18.3: 215–27.
30. Silverman E, Mamula M, Hardin JA, *et al.* Importance of the immune response to Ro/La particle in the development of congenital heart block and neonatal lupus erythematosus. *J Rheumatol* 1991;18:120–124.
31. Schmidt KG, Ulmer HE, Silverman NH, *et al.* Perinatal outcome of fetal complete atrioventricular block. A multicenter experience. *J Am Coll Cardiol* 1991;91:1360–6.
32. Comas C, Mortera C, Figueras J, *et al.* Bloqueo Auriculoventricular Completo Congénito Diagnóstico Prenatal y Manejo Perinatal. *Rev Española de Cardiol* 1997;50(7):498–506.

33 Three-dimensional ultrasound in prenatal medicine

E. Merz

Introduction

During the past two decades three-dimensional (3D) ultrasound has evolved from a relatively tedious laboratory technique to a highly sophisticated technique for daily routine examinations, particularly in prenatal diagnosis.

In 1989 the first commercially available ultrasound scanner (Combison 330) with special 3D probes for transabdominal and transrectal scanning was launched by Kretztechnik AG, Austria.[1] This system allowed fully automated volume acquisition and multiplanar reconstruction of the 3D data set in three orthogonal planes. Due to rapid developments in computer and transducer technology, image quality and processing speed improved tremendously in the following years. With the latest 4D technology of Voluson® 730 Expert (GE Medical Systems Kretz Ultrasound), volume acquisition and volume display can be accelerated in such a way that the fetus can be visualized three-dimensionally in real-time. This gives the examiner a direct impression of the fetal surface and movements.

Additional 3D/4D techniques have been developed within the past 2–3 years: glass body rendering, volume contrast imaging in the A and C planes (VCI-A and VCI-C, respectively) and spatio-temporal image correlation (STIC).

Table 33.1 Steps required in transvaginal and transabdominal 3D ultrasound (after Merz[3])

Data acquisition
• Orientation in the 2D image
• Definition of the region of interest (ROI)
• Volume acquisition
3D visualization
• Multiplanar display
• Surface-rendered image (surface mode, light mode)
• Transparent image (maximum mode, x-ray mode)
• Vascular image (combination of surface or transparent rendering and color Doppler)
• Animated image (rendering of image sequences)
Volume/image processing
• Electronic scalpel
• Filtering
• Contrast and brightness control
• Color image
Storage of volumes, rendered images and image sequences

Technical aspects

All 3D/4D ultrasound examinations consist of four main steps:[2,3] (1) data acquisition, (2) 3D/4D visualization, (3) volume analysis/image processing and (4) storage of volumes, rendered images or image sequences (cine clips) (Table 33.1).

3D data acquisition

For volume acquisition, the ultrasound beam has to be moved over the object of interest. This procedure can be performed manually with external acquisition systems or automatically with internal acquisition systems.

External acquisition systems

These freehand systems do not require a specially designed transducer. The scans are performed using a freehand technique with a conventional 2D probe, whose position and movement in space are tracked by an add-on system.[4–6] However, the freehand systems are not able to achieve 4D ultrasound.[3]

Internal acquisition systems

These systems use specific probes with a fully automated scanning technique.[1,3,7] The automated scanning movement can be achieved by using mechanical gears and/or electronic scanning techniques such as steered phased arrays and/or curved/linear arrays in which different groups of elements are excited.[1] These probes can be used for 3D and 4D ultrasound as well.

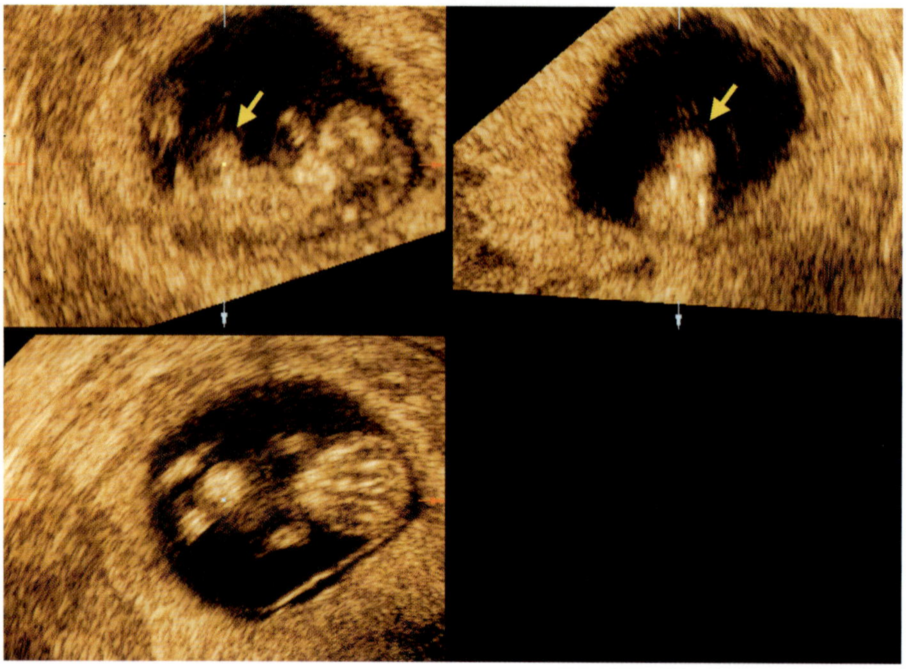

Figure 33.1 Fetus with physiologic umbilical hernia (←) (9 weeks) in the multiplanar display. Upper left, midsagittal scan; upper right, transverse scan; lower left, coronal scan.

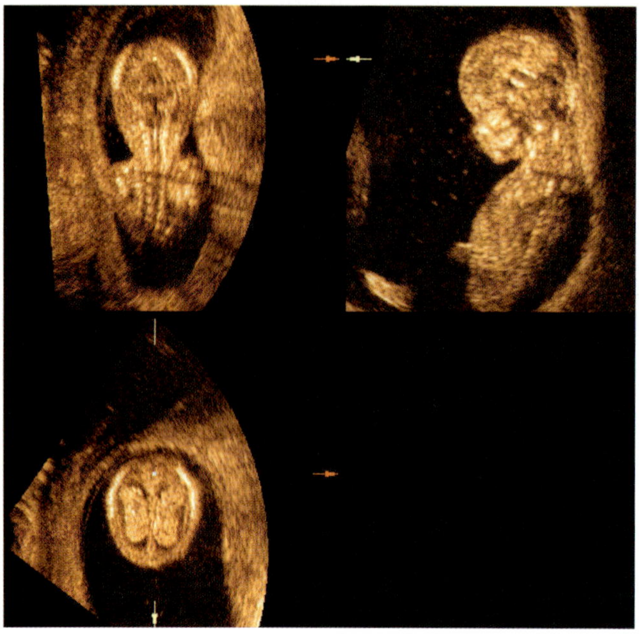

Figure 33.2 Multiplanar display of a fetus at 13 weeks of gestation. Upper left, coronal scan; upper right, midsagittal scan; lower left, transverse scan of the head.

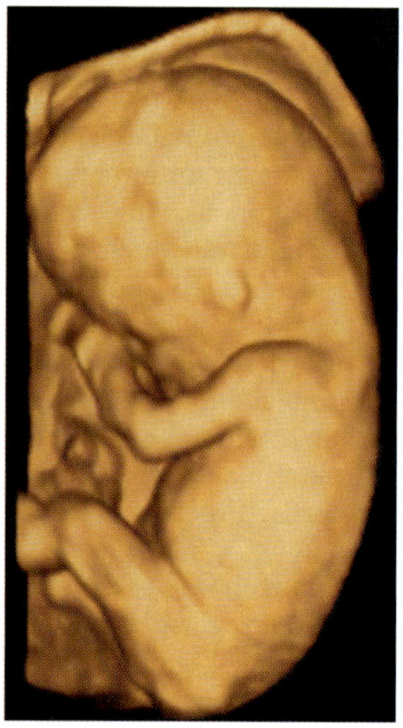

Figure 33.3 Surface view of a fetus at 12 weeks of gestation.

3D display

In contrast to conventional 2D ultrasound, which provides only one gray scale imaging mode to demonstrate the fetus, present 3D technology offers the ability to review the fetus in several different display modes:

Triplanar (= multiplanar) mode

The triplanar mode allows reslicing of acquired volumes in any direction.[3,8,9] Thus, any arbitrary plane can be shown, even image planes that are not accessible with conventional 2D ultrasound. The simultaneous display of all three perpendicular sectional planes provides an ideal basis for a detailed tomographic survey of the fetus and allows the demonstration of a specific plane to be precisely controlled (Figures 33.1 and 33.2).

Surface mode

The surface mode can provide 3D images of the outer and inner fetal surfaces (Figures 33.3–33.5, 33.15).[2,3,10,11]

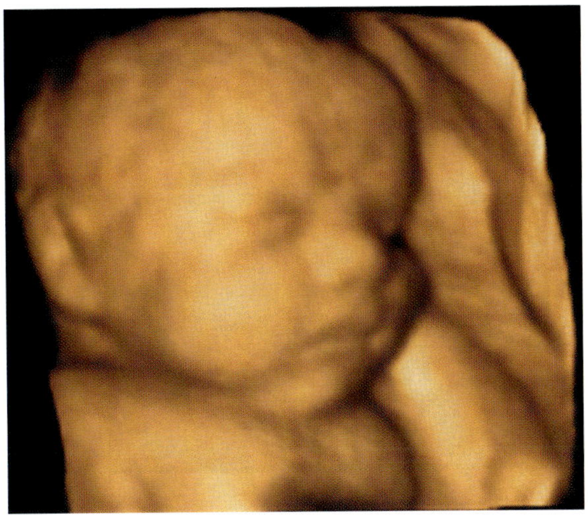

Figure 33.4 Surface view of a fetal face at 32 weeks of gestation.

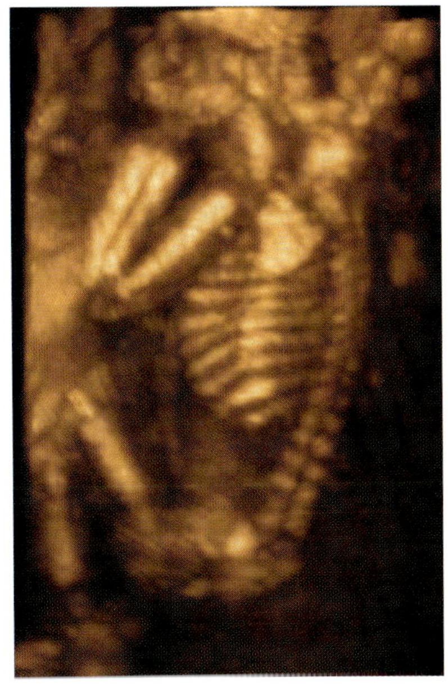

Figure 33.6 Transparent view (maximum mode) of a normal fetal skeleton at 20 weeks of gestation.

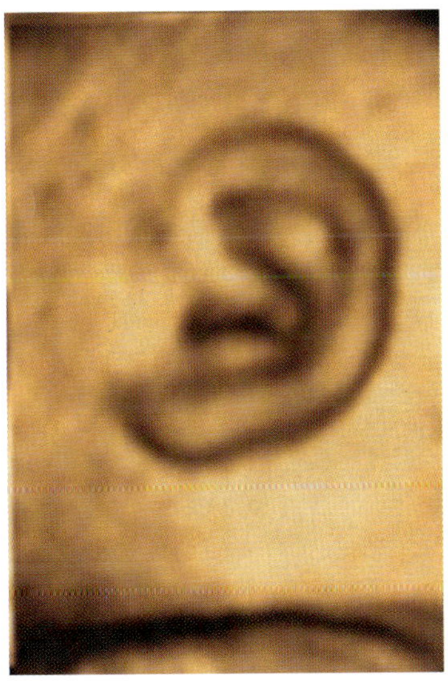

Figure 33.5 Surface view of a fetal ear at 38 weeks of gestation.

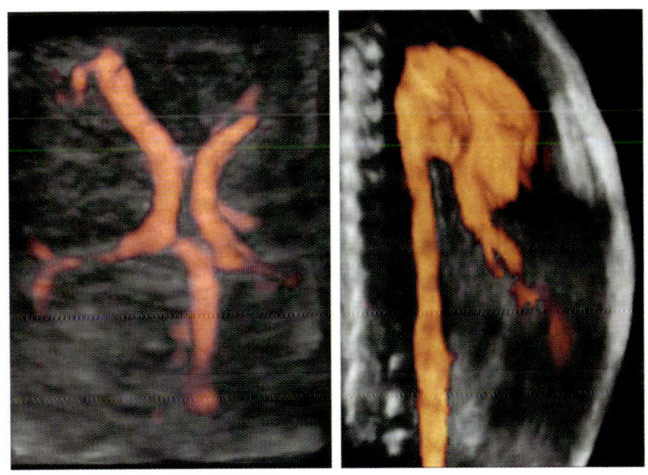

Figure 33.7 Glass body rendering: the combination of transparent mode and power Doppler displays the vascular system of the fetus. Left, circle of Willis (35 weeks); right, fetal heart and aorta (30 weeks).

For this purpose the region of interest has to be framed with a volume box. For many years this volume box was only variable in size but nowadays it is variable in size and shape. Various rendering algorithms (surface mode, soft surface mode, light mode and soft light mode) can be used in surface rendering, either individually or in different combinations.[3]

A basic requirement for all 3D surface rendering is the presence of an adequate fluid pocket in front of the structure being imaged. Overlying or adjacent structures such as the placenta, fetal limbs and loops of the umbilical cord tend to obscure the structure of interest and must be removed with the electronic scalpel.[12]

Transparent mode

The transparent mode provides a complete survey of the fetal skeleton (Figure 33.6).[13,14] Two different rendering algorithms (maximum mode and x-ray mode) can be used, either individually or in combination with the smooth surface mode or the gradient light mode.

Glass body rendering

The combination of 3D color Doppler or power Doppler and gray-scale 3D images enables the physician to analyze the fetal vascular system (Figure 33.7).

3D cine mode

In order to obtain an overall 3D impression of the object of interest, a certain number of rendered views are displayed in a fast sequence. In this way the observer can see the object of interest rotating on the screen. The 3D cine mode can be used with the surface mode, the transparent mode and the glass body rendering.

4D display

4D ultrasound

With the acquisition of up to 35 volumes/s, both the surface and the movements of the fetus can be demonstrated on the screen. This enables the parents to observe the movements of the fetus and allows the examiner to study the behavior of the fetus. The 4D cine loop allows the examiner to scroll back through volumes to achieve the best surface demonstration of the region of interest (Figure 33.8). For 4D volume rendering, two rendering modes are always applied simultaneously.

4D cine sequence

A 4D image cine sequence can be created with a Voluson® 730 series machine in the real-time 4D mode. After storage as an AVI file, such a sequence can be shown with a movie program in any personal computer.

DiagnoSTIC™

STIC is a new technique for assessment of the fetal heart, based on the automatic acquisition technology. It allows off-line multiplanar analysis of the fetal heart. For DiagnoSTIC™, a slow-motion (7.5, 10 or 12.5 s) volume scan of the fetal heart is performed. The data are then rearranged and stuck together by correlation of its temporal and spatial domains. An EGC trigger is not necessary. The result is a 4D real-time data set presenting one heart cycle in motion. This data set can also be rotated and analyzed in the triplanar view while the heart is beating at any stage of the cycle.

STIC-color (spatio-temporal image correlation with color Doppler)

In this technique the STIC technique is combined with color Doppler information. This facilitates the recognition and confirmation or exclusion of congenital heart defects (septal defects, transposition of the great vessels, etc.) (Figure 33.9).[3,15–18]

Volume contrast imaging

In VCI the probe is applied in the same way as in conventional 2D ultrasound and so is an easy approach to 4D, even for the novice. This volume rendering process is based on thick slice tissue data[3] and it is possible to select a slice thickness between 3 and 20 mm. Displayed as a thick slice, the VCI technique allows a 4D volumetric data acquisition.

The development of this tool has facilitated a marked improvement in tissue contrast resolution in real-time and therefore enables inhomogeneous areas or subtle lesions to be detected. It provides additional information simultaneously with conventional 2D imaging, without the processing time of off-line 3D reconstruction. In VCI technology a mixture of surface mode and transparent maximum mode rendering is employed.

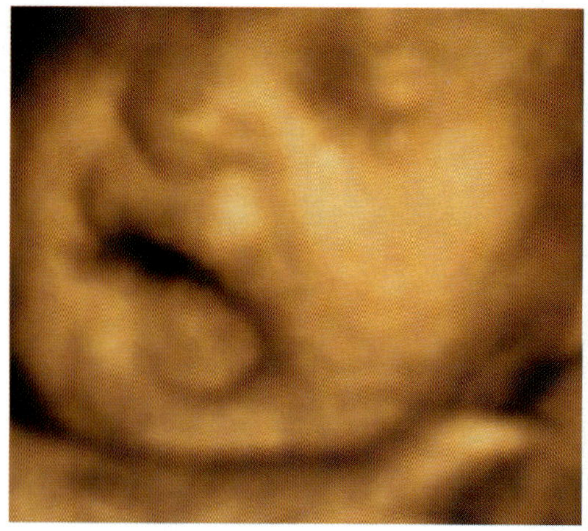

Figure 33.8 Surface-rendered view of fetal yawning at 32 weeks. The 4D cine loop allows scrolling back to the most interesting movement.

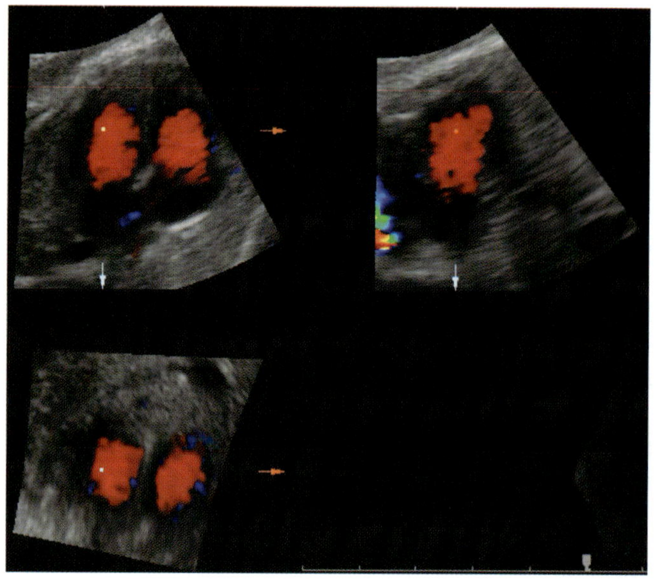

Figure 33.9 Fetal heart at 36 weeks. The STIC technique combined with color Doppler displays blood flow in all three orthogonal planes at the same time.

Volume contrast imaging in the A plane

VCI-A provides the examiner with an easy 4D approach. It reveals the same anatomical region as in the 2D ultrasound image, but the tissue contrast is better with VCI-A (Figure 33.10).

Volume contrast imaging in the C plane

VCI-C allows an easy 4D real-time approach in the coronal plane of the region of interest (Figure 33.11). VCI-C offers great potential in prenatal diagnosis because it scans planes that are not accessible with conventional B-mode scanning. This is particularly important when the fetus is in an unfavorable position.

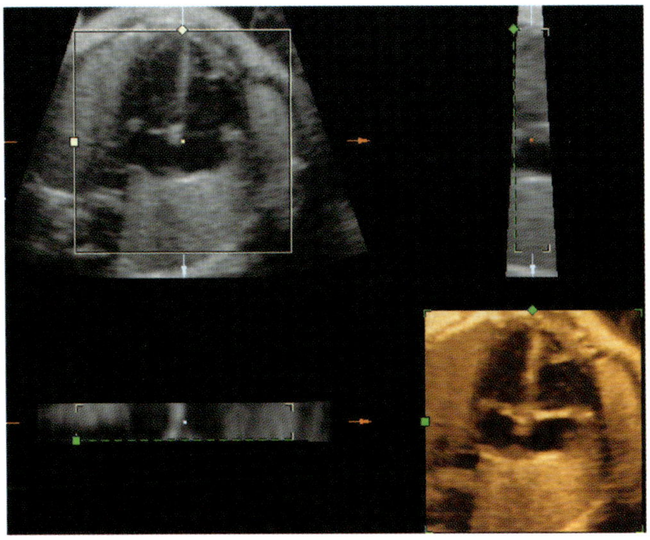

Figure 33.10 VCI-A of the fetal heart (29 weeks). This technique shows the same anatomical region as in the 2D ultrasound (upper left), but the contrast is better in VCI-A (lower right).

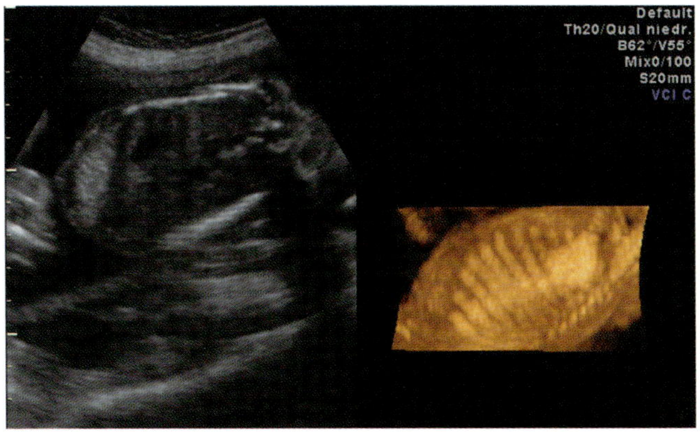

Figure 33.11 VCI-C. This simple technique yields detailed morphologic information of the plane perpendicular to the marked green line in the conventional 2D plane. Here: 3D information of the fetal chest in the tangenti view (20 weeks).

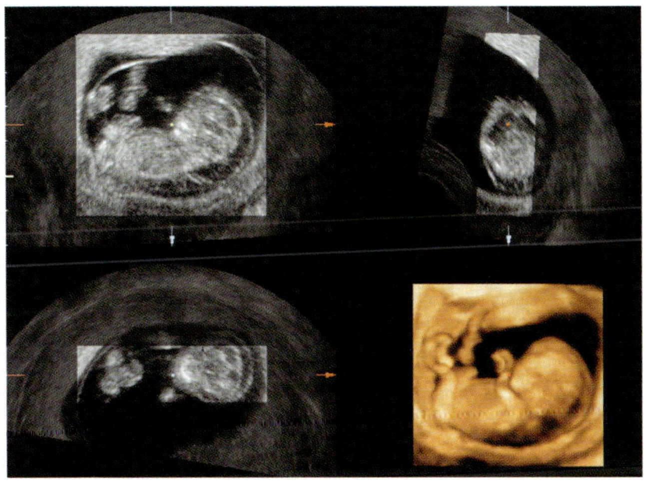

Figure 33.12 Multiplanar demonstration of a fetus with increased nuchal translucency thickness of 6.2 mm (→) (11 + 4 weeks). Karyotype: trisomy 18. Upper left, precise midsagittal scan; upper right, transverse scan at neck level; lower left, coronal scan; lower right: surface view.

Volume/image processing

In many cases the acquired data sets require post-processing. In order to obtain a high-quality surface image, adjacent or overlapping structures that are obscuring the fetus have to be removed with an electronic scalpel. Low-level echoes in the amniotic fluid may be filtered out by increasing the threshold value. In color Doppler the angio threshold removes small motion artifacts and color noise.

Image brightness and contrast can be set to any desired value in all 3D/4D display modes just as in 2D ultrasound. In glass body rendering, the color and gray-scale areas can be adjusted independently of one another. All changes are immediately visible on the monitor. These interactive control features make it easy to display any object with optimal brightness and contrast.[3,19]

Storage of volumes, rendered images and image sequences

Long-term storage

3D/4D ultrasound gives us the capability to store volumes, rendered images, 3D and 4D cine sequences digitally. Today, various media are available for the long-term storage of these volumes, such as removable hard disks, magneto-optical disks and DVD.

When findings of interest are stored digitally on non-degrading media, the examiner can retrieve the volumes at any time and navigate through them in the absence of the patient.[7] This is of particular value in the diagnosis of fetal anomalies, as it enables the examiner to take the time to fully scrutinize equivocal findings without upsetting the patient by lingering at a particular site with the probe, which is often a problem in conventional 2D examinations.[3]

Clinical applications

For the examination in the first trimester the transvaginal 3D/4D probe is usually applied, and for the second and third trimester examinations, the abdominal 3D/4D probe is used. If the fetus is in a cephalic presentation the transvaginal 3D/4D probe can also be used in the second or third trimester to assess the fetal brain in a higher resolution.[9,20]

The advantage of all the different 3D/4D rendering modes is that it is possible to visualize the normal embryonic and fetal development at all stages.[21–23] The first view of the fetal face has an important psychological effect on the parents to whom the detailed

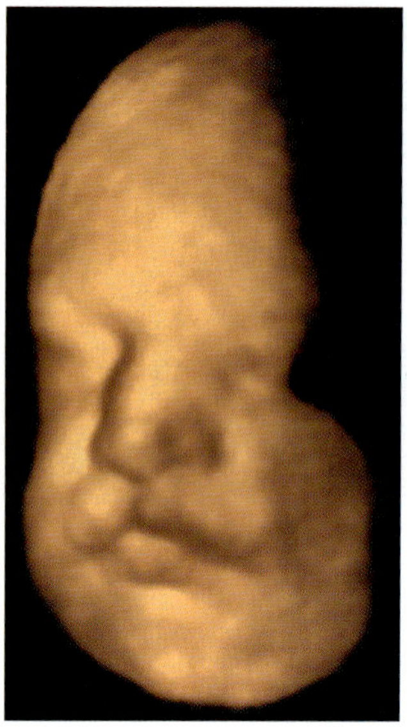

Figure 33.13 Surface-rendered view of a small cleft lip at the right side (38 weeks).

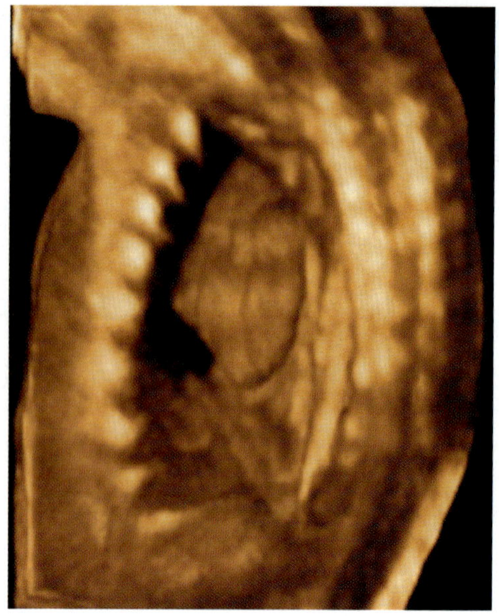

Figure 33.15 Surface-rendered view of a fetus with left-sided hydrothorax at 30 weeks of gestation. The fetal chest has been partly 'removed' with the electronic scalpel, displaying the surface of the small left lung.

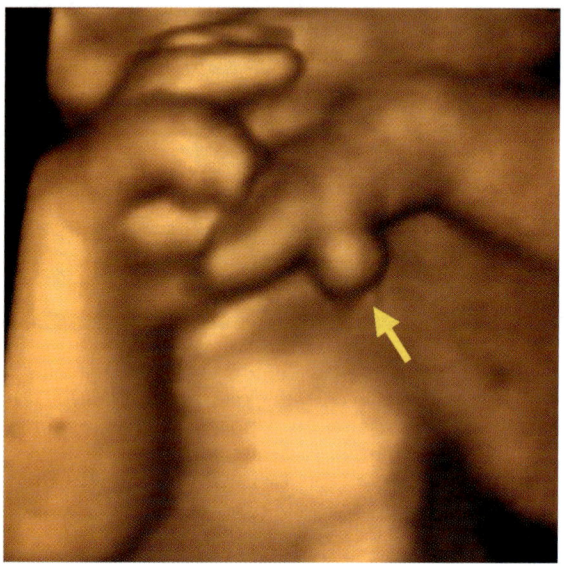

Figure 33.14 Surface-rendered view of the left hand with postaxial hexadactyly (←) (31 weeks).

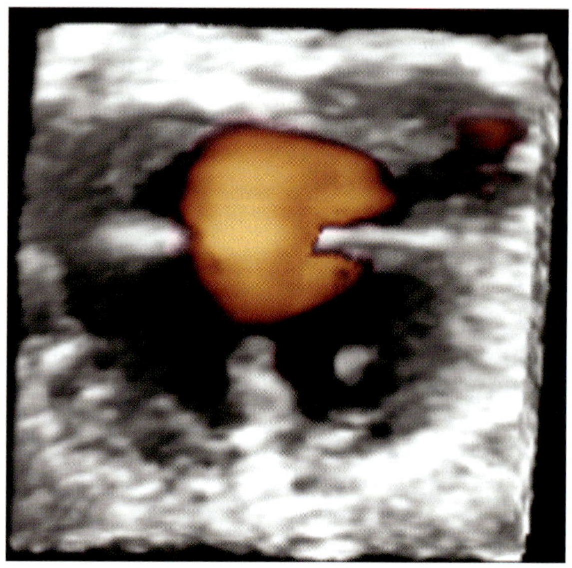

Figure 33.16 Glass body rendering (surface-rendered image) of an AV canal (23 weeks). The combination of transparent mode and power Doppler displays the defect in the valvular plane.

images are much better recognizable than the 2D pictures. With the use of glass body rendering (3D and power Doppler) even the vascular system can be observed by the parents.

For the sonographer, however, the detection of a fetal malformation is of more importance.[24–33] Despite the fact that with conventional 2D ultrasound examinations most of the fetal abnormalities can be detected by the experienced examiner, 3D/4D ultrasound provides additional information, particularly for the experienced examiner.[7] 3D ultrasonography can depict many image planes that are inaccessible with conventional 2D ultrasound. In the first trimester the triplanar demonstration is particularly helpful in the verification of a true midsagittal section, which is necessary for an exact nuchal translucency (NT) measurement (Figure 33.12).[34–36] In NT demonstration and measurement, the examination time can be dramatically reduced, especially in case of an unfavorable fetal position, and the quality of the requested image can be improved.[36]

In the second and third trimesters the photo-realistic surface view of the fetus offers interesting opportunities for the detection of abnormalities, especially in subtle defects (Figures 33.13 and 33.14).[24–33] In some cases it is also possible to find defects that were not revealed with conventional 2D ultrasound.[7] In other cases the surface mode can also provide impressive 3D images of the inner fetal surfaces (Figure 33.15).

4D ultrasound provides an excellent real-time 3D view of the fetus. With the STIC technique, even 4D fetal echocardiography has become a reality. The triplanar demonstration of the beating heart enables a comprehensive assessment of the fetal heart morphology including the great vessels. Due to the fact that the volume can be rotated and resliced in all dimensions even complex anomalies of the fetal heart can be demonstrated precisely. The combination of STIC and color Doppler allows an exact control of the cardiac blood flow while the heart is in motion (Figure 33.16).

The interactive display in 3D/4D ultrasound is particularly useful for the detection of specific abnormalities, making it possible to identify fetal surface abnormalities and define the extent of a defect in all dimensions. The same applies to the targeted exclusion of fetal anomalies. Particularly in cases with an increased recurrence risk, the various display options of 3D/4D ultrasound provide a selective exclusion of a fetal defect and parents can see for themselves that the 3D surface image demonstrates a normal fetus.

REFERENCES

1. Wiesauer F. Methodology of three-dimensional ultrasound. In Kurjak A, Kupesic S, eds. *Clinical Application of 3D Sonography*. London: Parthenon Publishing Group, 2000;1–6.
2. Merz E. 3-D ultrasound in prenatal diagnosis. *Curr Obstet Gynaecol* 1999;9:93–100.
3. Merz E. 3D Ultrasound in prenatal diagnosis. In: Merz E, ed. *Ultrasound in Obstetrics*. Stuttgart: Thieme, 2004.
4. Sakas G, Schreyer L, Grimm M. Preprocessing, segmenting and volume rendering 3D ultrasonic data. *IEEE Comput Graphics Appl* 1995;15:47–54.
5. Guerra FA, Isla AI, Aguilar RC, Fritz EG. Use of free-hand three-dimensional ultrasound software in the study of the fetal heart. *Ultrasound Obstet Gynecol* 2000;16:329–34.
6. Prager R, Gee A, Treece G, Berman L. Freehand 3D ultrasound without voxels: Volume measurement and visualisation using the Stradx system. *Ultrasonics* 2002;40(1–8):109–15.
7. Merz E, Bahlmann F, Weber G, Macchiella D. Three-dimensional ultrasonography in prenatal diagnosis. *J Perinatal Med* 1995;23:213–22.
8. Kratochwil A. Importance and possibilities of multiplanar examination in three-dimensional sonography. In Merz E, ed. *3-D Ultrasound in Obstetrics and Gynecology*. Philadelphia: Lippincott, Williams and Wilkins, 1998;105–8.
9. Timor-Tritsch IE, Monteagudo A, Mayberry P. Three-dimensional ultrasound evaluation of the fetal brain: The three horn view. *Ultrasound Obstet Gynecol* 2000;16:302–6.
10. Benoit B. Three-dimensional surface mode for demonstration of normal fetal anatomy in the second and third trimesters. In Merz E, ed. *3-D Ultrasound in Obstetrics and Gynecology*. Philadelphia: Lippincott, Williams and Wilkins, 1998:95–100.
11. Pretorius DH, House M, Nelson TR. Fetal face visualization using three-dimensional ultrasonography. *J Ultrasound Med* 1995;14:349–56.
12. Merz E, Miric-Tesanic D, Welter C. Value of the electronic scalpel (cut mode) in the evaluation of the fetal face. *Ultrasound Obstet Gynecol* 2000;16:364–8.
13. Yanagihara T, Hata T. Three-dimensional sonographic visualization of fetal skeleton in the second trimester of pregnancy. *Gynecol Obstet Invest* 2000;49:12–6.
14. Benoit B. The value of three-dimensional ultrasonography in the screening of the fetal skeleton. *Childs Nerv Syst* 2003;19:403–9.
15. DeVore GR, Falkensammer P, Sklansky MS, Platt LD. Spatio-temporal image correlation (STIC): New technology for evaluation of the fetal heart. *Ultrasound Obstet Gynecol* 2003;22:380–7.
16. Goncalves LF, Lee W, Chaiworapongsa T, *et al.* Four-dimensional ultrasonography of the fetal heart with spatiotemporal image correlation. *Am J Obstet Gynecol* 2003;189:1792–802.
17. Chaoui R, Hoffmann J, Heling KS. Three-dimensional (3D) and 4D color Doppler fetal echocardiography using spatio-temporal image correlation (STIC). *Ultrasound Obstet Gynecol* 2004;23:535–45.
18. Vinals F, Poblete P, Giuliano A. Spatio-temporal image correlation (STIC): A new tool for the prenatal screening of congenital heart defects. *Ultrasound Obstet Gynecol* 2003;22:388–94.
19. Nelson TR, Pretorius DH. Interactive acquisition, analysis and visualization of sonographic volume data. *Int J Imaging Syst Technol* 1997;8:26–37.
20. Pooh RK, Pooh KH. The assessment of fetal brain morphology and circulation by transvaginal 3D sonography and power Doppler. *J Perinat Med* 2002;30:48–56.
21. Bonilla-Musoles F. Three-dimensional visualization of the human embryo: A potential revolution in prenatal diagnosis. *Ultrasound Obstet Gynecol* 1996;7:393–7.
22. Benoit B, Hafner T, Kurjak A, Kupesic S, Bekavac I, Bozek T. Three-dimensional sonoembryology. *J Perinat Med* 2002;30: 63–73.
23. Rotten D, Levaillant JM. Two- and three-dimensional sonographic assessment of the fetal face. 1. A systematic analysis of the normal face. *Ultrasound Obstet Gynecol* 2004;23:224–31.
24. Merz E, Bahlmann F, Weber G. Volume (3D) scanning in the evaluation of fetal malformations – a new dimension in prenatal diagnosis. *Ultrasound Obstet Gynecol* 1995;5:222–7.
25. Pretorius DH, House M, Nelson TR, Hollenbach KA. Evaluation of normal and abnormal lips in fetuses: Comparison between three- and two-dimensional sonography. *AJR Am J Roentgenol* 1995;165:1233–7.
26. Lee A, Deutinger J, Bernaschek G. Three-dimensional ultrasound: abnormalities of the fetal face in surface and volume rendering mode. *Br J Obstet Gynaecol* 1995;102:302–6.
27. Mueller GM, Weiner CP, Yankowitz J. Three-dimensional ultrasound in the evaluation of fetal head and spine anomalies. *Obstet Gynecol* 1996;88:372–8.
28. Merz E, Weber G, Bahlmann, Miric-Tesanic D. Application of transvaginal and abdominal three-dimensional ultrasound for the detection or exclusion of malformations of the fetal face. Ultrasound *Obstet Gynecol* 1997;9:237–43.
29. Lee W, Kirk JS, Shaheen KW, Romero R, Hodges AN, Comstock CH. Fetal cleft lip and palate detection by three-dimensional ultrasonography. *Ultrasound Obstet Gynecol* 2000;16:314–20.
30. Dyson RL, Pretorius DH, Budorick NE, *et al.* Three-dimensional ultrasound in the evaluation of fetal anomalies. *Ultrasound Obstet Gynecol* 2000;16:321–8.
31. Kos M, Hafner T, Funduk-Kurjak B, Bozek T, Kurjak A. Limb deformities and three-dimensional ultrasound. *J Perinat Med* 2002;30:40–7.
32. Xu HX, Zhang QP, Lu MD, Xiao XT. Comparison of two-dimensional and three-dimensional sonography in evaluating fetal malformations. *J Clin Ultrasound* 2002;30:515–25.
33. Krakow D, Williams J III, Poehl M, Rimoin DL, Platt LD. Use of three-dimensional ultrasound imaging in the diagnosis of prenatal-onset skeletal dysplasias. *Ultrasound Obstet Gynecol* 2003; 21:467–72.
34. Chung, BL, Kim HJ, Lee KH. The application of three-dimensional ultrasound to nuchal translucency measurement in early pregnancy (10–14 weeks): A preliminary study. *Ultrasound Obstet Gynecol* 2000;15:122–5.
35. Eppel W, Worda C, Frigo P, Lee A. Three- versus two-dimensional ultrasound for nuchal translucency thickness measurements: Comparison of feasibility and levels of agreement. *Prenat Diagn* 2001;21:596–601.
36. Welter C, Merz E. Nuchal translucency-screening using 2D and 3D ultrasound. *Ultrasound Obstet Gynecol* 2003;22(Suppl 1):13.

34 Ultrasound-guided fetal invasive procedures: current status

J. M. Troyano, M. Alvarez de la Rosa and I. Martinez-Wallin

Since the early 1980s various forms of fetal puncture (fine needle aspiration) have been used for diagnostic purposes.[1–5] In the beginning, the only possible way of entering the fetal environment was with the help of a fetoscope, but the spectacular development of ultrasonography has permitted the invasion of the intrauterine environment using tools that are increasingly safe, especially in the tighter sections. Needles with improved characteristics have been developed that are now being used in new biopsy techniques.[3,6,7]

Fetal puncture for diagnosis is technically possible, provided it is done by adequately trained hands, but the essential problem lies in establishing the correct procedure, which is not quite defined yet.[8]

Technique generalization

Whatever the location of the fetal puncture, a certain number of requirements are imperative.

(1) The operator must have sufficient working experience in invasive echography.
(2) The room should be fit to be used for surgery: it is necessary to have an aseptic room for echographic intervention. A sterile wrap is recommended for the ultrasound probe. We use a surgical glove for an airtight seal.
(3) The characteristics of the surgical equipment used for obtaining samples are described in the following.

As the tendency is to obtain samples with maximum diagnostic utility and minimal risk to the integrity of the pregnancy, it is of utmost importance, with few exceptions, to use needles no smaller than 18 g.

It is clear that the tools used will not always be harmless. A simple example is the device still used for skin biopsies for diagnosing some types of *genodermatosis*, which consists of a pair of clipper forceps measuring 2.5 mm in size.

These methods often require the use of an anesthetic, and in some cases general anesthesia, before incision of the maternal abdomen using a scalpel and introduction of a guiding trocar sheath of the thickness of a Verre's needle.

The complications arising from the use of 2.5-mm-thick needles and the transabdomen forceps method are similar to those of the fetoscope. Further, the method itself is highly variable: a great variety of needles of relatively small size (18-g standard) are available, giving very good biopsies, including samples of skin and samples of visceral solid areas (Figure 34.1).[2,7]

Among the organs that are intrauterinally reachable, the most difficult to sample, after the skin, is the kidney, essentially due to the histological constitution of the parenchymal stratum.[9]

Only those samples that include the corticomedular stratum are considered satisfactory. Getting such samples is affected by the fetal availability in respect of its intrauterine position, the distance and the interposed tissue to the kidney (skin, muscle) and perirenal fat and the very capsule.

The use of a 14–16-g catheter with isometric aspiration techniques with constant vacuum in these cases allows us to obtain acceptable samples in 69–80% of all instances, while the use of a 18–20-g catheter gives acceptable specimens only in 25–30% of cases. This means that isometric (fine needle) puncture–aspiration techniques do not always offer the results hoped for with solid organs, mainly the kidney; wider catheters need to be used, which is far from the 'harmless philosophy' that should prevail in these processes.

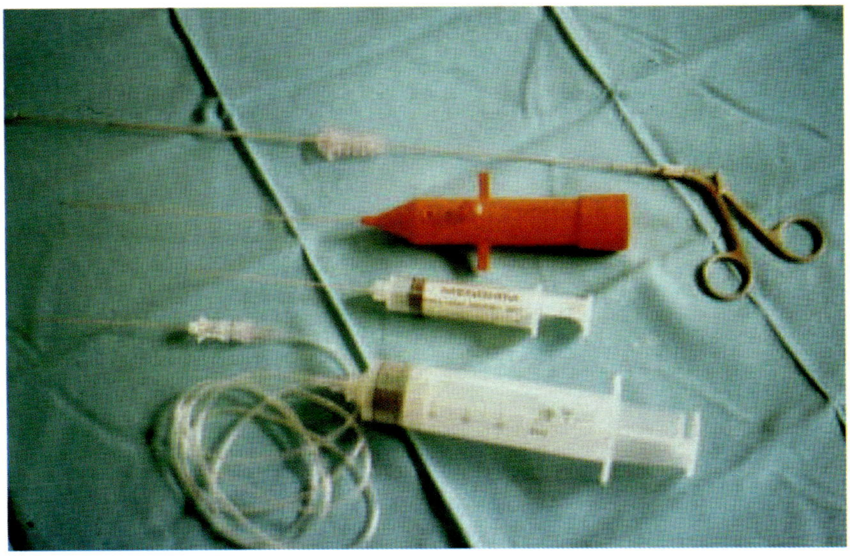

Figure 34.1 Different types of needles and system for fetal biopsy.

For these cases and others that could occur, depending on the tissue characteristics, the use of equipment such as an *aspiration biopsy set* yields cylindrical specimens of a maximum length of 2–5 mm. The set includes an 18-g bisided trocar syringe in all its circumference, acting as a circular blade, and a conical sheath with vacuum suction embolous contriving through its interior. It allows optimal safety conditions and histological quality comparable with those of the *Tru-Cut* method.

Of all the viscous solid organs within reach, the one that offers the least problems is the liver. Its spongy tissue constitution and its great size and volume in the fetal abdomen allows optimal accessibility and consequently offers samples in practically 100% of cases, using a conventional fine needle of 18–20 g.

The obtaining of muscle tissue samples presents one of the greatest difficulties due to the topographic and anatomical characteristics of the skeleton and the important motor innervation. For this reason it is necessary to correctly select the spot and the muscular area least susceptible to the formation of indelible functional lesions.

The most accessible topographic areas are the external faces of the thighs, but the vastus externus muscle is technically more accessible (Figure 34.2); it is a zone covered by the subtrochanteric fascia-lata descending in an oblique direction toward the fetal femur, The use of the *sure cut* system's 18-g needle with vacuum aspiration allows a success rate of over 75%. Conventional spinal needles with complementary aspiration with a 50-cc syringe vacuum allow us to obtain samples only with great difficulties.

When the puncture area has liquid characteristics, the echographic view is wide ranged, allowing a large field of action.

(4) In general, technically it is preferable to choose the most direct route, avoiding any obstacles, avoiding the placenta entirely if possible.
(5) Once the crucial point to puncture has been determined, the needle should be introduced within the field of view of the probe, frame by frame, until the fetus is reached.
(6) It is recommended to locate the puncture point approximately without making direct contact with it in the first instance, and to determine the angle of the needle at the chosen spot. It is of the greatest importance to enter with a single *sudden jab* to avoid sudden fetal jolts or movements.
(7) It is advisable in all *free-hand* fetal punctures for the operator to take into account the dynamic variations of the fetal position.
(8) For better manipulation, an assistant should be in charge of carrying out the isometric aspiration process at a prudent distance, approximately 1 m away from the surgical table, placing a serum of the same length between the needle and the syringe.
(9) Except in circumstances such as pericardic and pleural overflow that need an operating time of about 15–30 min, the procedure should be carried out without any anesthesia.

Aspiration in cystic disorders will fundamentally orientate the diagnosis. Aspiration on ovarian cysts is only indicated in cases that are complex due to the dynamic volume or due to rare structural types, with the aim of therapy rather than diagnosis.

We take suspicious chylous collections only where the presence of high lymphocyte concentrations gives

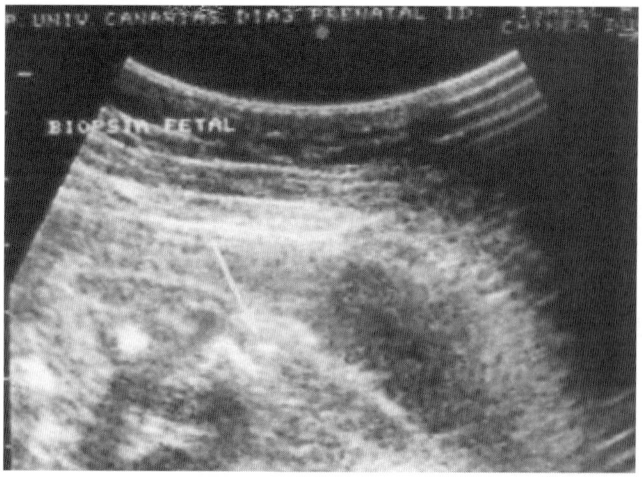

Figure 34.2 Subtrochanteric muscle biopsy: echographic monitoring. The arrow indicates the puncture position oblique to the fetal femur.

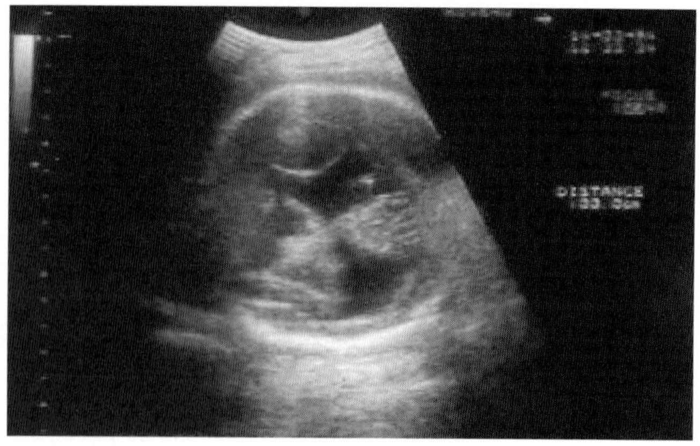

Figure 34.4 Ventriculocentesis: obtaining cephaloraquideus liquid determines the presence of viral bodies through polymerase chain reaction.

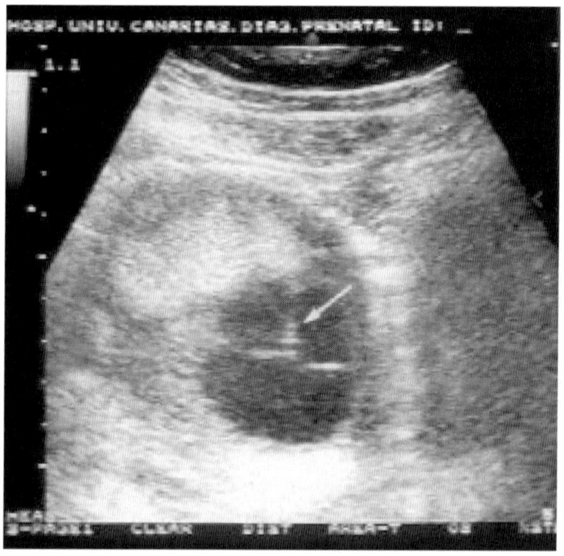

Figure 34.3 Cystic lynphangioma: percutaneous puncture determines qualitative and genetic characteristics (lymphocytes).

a practically certain diagnosis and a genetic study is possible in very few days, justifying this type of procedure (Figure 34.3).

Puncturing pericardic discharges has diagnostic as well as therapeutic aims.

Among brain punctures, the most representative, *ventriculocentesis*, allows us to carry out serological marker studies in RCL, independent of any derived therapeutic attitude, although the efficiency of the derivative procedures in hydrocefalia is uncertain (Figure 34.4).

Of all the structurally cystic processes, the obtaining of fetal urine in dilated urological pathology has the greatest diagnostic value. The biochemical analysis of fetal urine allows us to distinguish irreversible tubular lesions and normal renal function.

There is no doubt that the incorporation of biological molecular techniques and DNA studies allows us to establish in many of cases, alterations of any determined genetic locus[10–13].

Occasionally, we may find that we do not have enough material to base a prenatal diagnosis upon due to a lack of family records of deceased relations. In such cases the absence of this information constitutes a serious obstacle to the diagnosis, as it must then be based on only on a small corionic-villi, funicular or amniotic sample.[11,14]

In such a situation sampling directly from the fetal tissue is of special relevance for the diagnosis or for ruling out any suspicion of family inheritance.

> The taking of fetal samples by biopsy techniques is justified only in cases when the prenatal diagnosis of any specific pathological illness is not possible, or is frankly difficult, using any of the existing conventional techniques.

Liver biopsy

Technique

Fetal transabdominal aspiration-puncture using 18-g needles with a conic catheter or spinal needles of the same thickness with isometric vacuum aspiration using a 50-cc syringe and serum system. Once introduced into the fetal kidney, soft, brief *inward–outward* movements should be made in the same direction as the puncture.

The aspiration system should be extracted first and the needle last to avoid contaminating any other tissue. The spot to be punctured should be situated between the belly button and the edge of the ribcage. This fate is helped by the physiological hepatomegaly, introducing the needle approximately 1 cm under strict echographic monitoring. Preferably the external third of the right lobe should be chosen as it offers a minor principal vascularization; if not, the suprahepatic vessels should be avoided (Figure 34.5).

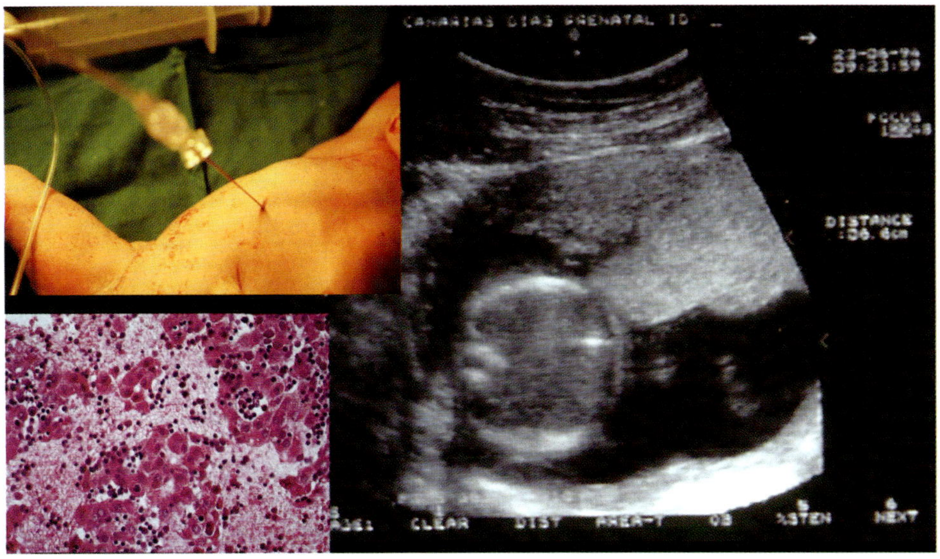

Figure 34.5 Liver biopsy: echographic monitoring and histological samples of fetal liver (19 weeks). Extramedullar hematopoietic foci can be detected.

If the diagnosis being sought is histological, the sample should be preserved in formaldehyde; if it is enzymatic, the sample should then be sealed airtight in carbonic snow.

The gestational age recommended is around 20 weeks, provided that the hepatic metabolism and main enzymatic processes are well or are practically established.

Indications

The indications are prenatal diagnosis, mainly of enzymatic alterations and of lethal metabolic character istics.[15,16]

Deficiencies of ornitil transcarbamylase (OTC): This mitochondrial enzyme of the urea cycle is synthesized in the liver or the intestines. Sex-linked disorders tied to the sex are revealed in the screening data of mothers who have urine excretion of orotic acid.

Primary hyperoxaluria (PH): This is severe, charted renal insuffiency of rapid evolution that is characterized by the presence of calcic oxalate deposits in the renal tubule, microlithiasis and interstitial fibrosis. The hepatic level is accompanied by a total absence of alanine and inactivity of the catalytic gliosilate aminotransferase and immunoreactive proteins. This leads to death.

For diagnosis it is very important to have the previous family clinical history.

Carbamoyl phosphate synthetase deficiency: This is an enzymatic defect of the urea cycle with recessive autosomic inheritance.

Other autosomic recessive disorders may be detected by means of hepatic biopsy, including the following:

(1) Non-ketotic hyperglycinemia
(2) Prenatal diagnosis of infantile neuronal ceroid-
(3) lipofuscinosis
(4) Biliary atresia (type I cysts)
(5) Long-chain 3-hydroxyacyl-CoA dehydrogenase.[17–20]

Table 34.1 Experience with seven prenatal punctures for liver biopsy

	Number of cases
Reasons for biopsy	
OTC diseases in the same family	4
Previously affected brother	1
Mitochondrial respiratory deficit	1
Non-ketotic hyperglycinemia	1
Results	
Prenatally confirmed diagnosis of OTC deficiency	2
Prenatally non-confirmed diagnosis with neonatal exitus by hyperammonemia	1
Prenatally confirmed as non-affected fetuses	4

Complications

Prenatal liver biopsy has a few risks at the tissue level, due to its visceral characteristics. These risks are derived from major vascular tears, which involve great bleeding, resulting in fetal death. In our experience (seven prenatal punctures), we have observed no complications (Table 34.1).

Fetal puncture in the evaluation of renal status

The correction of a theoretic renal obstruction problem is possible, in spite of the difficulties and risks that it holds, even if in the majority of cases it is not necessary. We should start by stating that an ultrasound

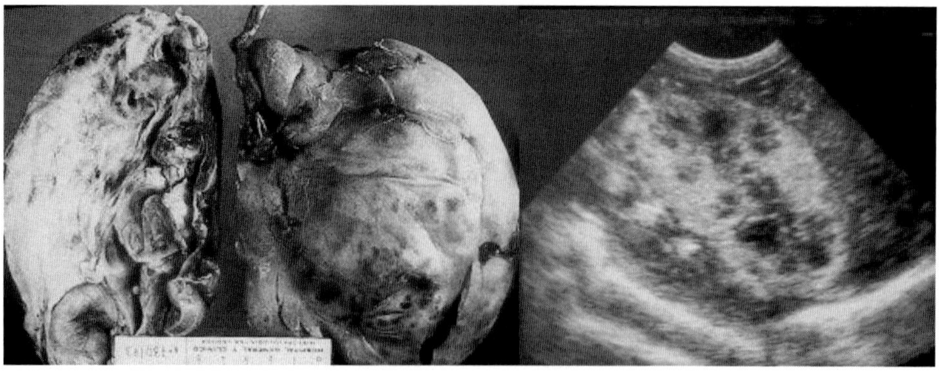

Figure 34.6 Fibrocortical dysplasia associated with corticomedullar cyst and renomegaly.

Table 34.2 Fetal nephrouropathy. Echographic prediction

Tissue marker	Sensibility (%)	Specificity (%)
Corticomedular cysts	70	100
Hyperecongenity	60	90
Hydronephrosis	75	70
Hydronephrosis + cysts	90	100

echography diagnosis of the obstructed renal pathology does not necessarily imply an irreversible function alteration. In this sense the amniotic volume can be used as an indirect marker of the actual renal function, but this does have the inconvenience that it includes the possible measuring of the intrinsic clearance function.

When taking into account the possibility of practicing an intrauterine derived therapy, it must be noted that this can only be justified in a fetus in whose kidneys there has been no irreversible damage. However, this makes it essential to establish a precise evaluation of the renal function in order to adequately select those fetuses that will benefit from prenatal therapy.

The most conflictive situation is renal dysplasia. Fibrosis, dysplasia and cartilaginosis are found simultaneously in this condition, frequently associated with corticomedular cysts, although not always so (Figure 34.6).

Approximately 90% of all kidney dysplasias are associated with dilated or obstructive disorders. It can be remarked that in these cases any derived therapeutic action is unnecessary.

High-resolution echography has become the leading kidney evaluation process; however, it does have a few diagnostic limitations (Table 34.2).

In our experience the obstruction of a kidney without visible cysts or hyperechos does not, however, exclude dysplasia. This quite alarming fact occurs approximately in 25–30% of all cases.[8–21]

From this we can deduce that echography on its own cannot be used to diagnose all renal dysplasias, and for this reason fetuses with pelvic dilation are subsidiary of derived drainage.

A biochemical study of fetal urine is important data for management of these fetuses. The composition of the fetal urine stays constant, practically throughout the pregnancy and with hypotonic characteristics. This fact automatically demonstrates an optimal and reliable renal function and in contrast iso- or hypertonic urine indicates a deficiency in renal function with an infastous prediction.

The biochemical markers that are closely related to the renal function are defined by Na^+, Cl^- and osmotic urine.

Another determining factor in the normal renal clearance function derived from the near high reabsorbing tubular activity is establishing specific proximal tubular lesion selective markers.

These markers correspond to lysosomal proteins exclusive of the proximate tubular structure and become expressed by *N*-acetyl-D-glucosaminidase (NAG). Low molecular weight proteins filtered by the glomerular system and reabsorbed practically in their totality by the proximal tube, if present in fetal urine and in the amniotic fluid in large quantities (higher than 8 U/l), are indicative of tubular tissue destruction.

The detection of β-2 microglobuline would be interpreted in the same manner (Figures 34.7 and 34.8).

We found that the levels of biochemical markers are significantly low in physiological urine in comparison with cases affected with irreversible renal disorder. The same outcome is found with the tissue markers NAG and β-2 microglobuline (Table 34.3).

When we compare the relationship between the ionic concentrations and the osmolarity (Na^+ and Cl^-) of the fetal urine and those of the amniotic liquid, we do not find significant differences between fetuses with conserving and fetuses with pathological functionalities. But comparing the levels of NAG and β-2 microglobuline, a significantly greater concentration of the two markers has been observed in the amniotic liquid of the affected fetuses (Tables 34.4 and 34.5).

The increase in concentration of NAG and β-2 microglobuline is possibly due to the cumulative effect of the amniotic clearance mechanism.

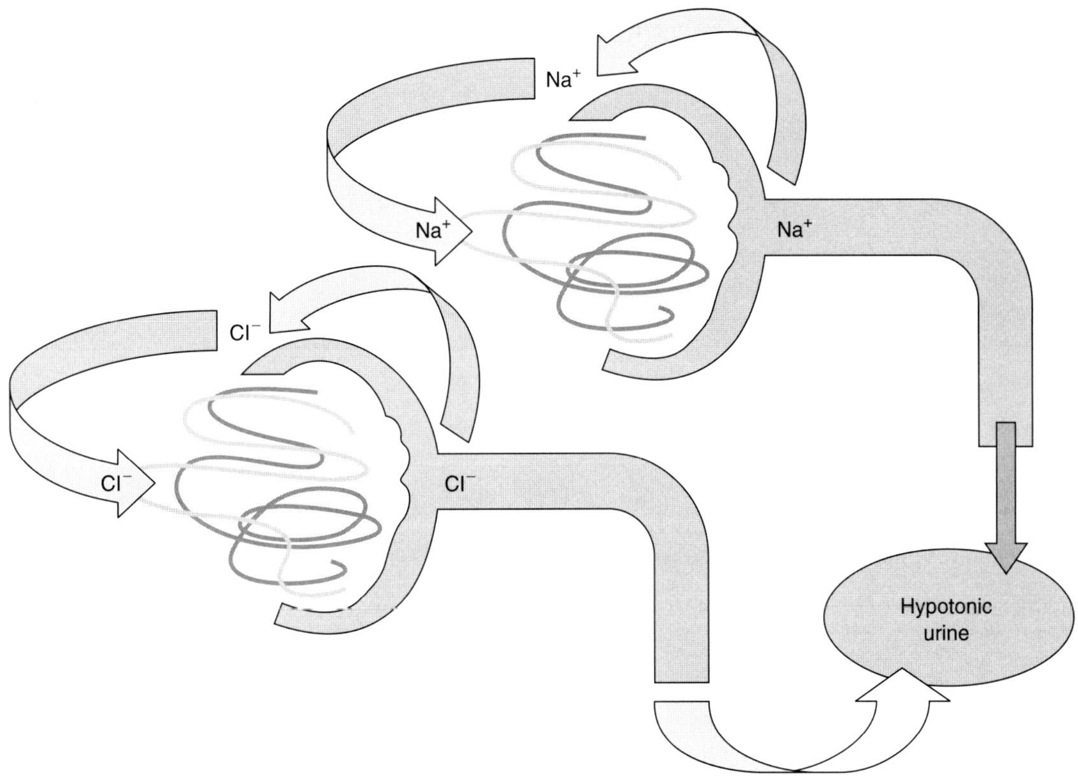

Figure 34.7 Biochemical markers that have a close relation with a renal function are defined by the NA+, Cl– and osmotic urine derived from the near high reabsorbing tubular activity. Fetal urine characteristics remain constant, practically throughout the pregnancy, with hypotonic features.

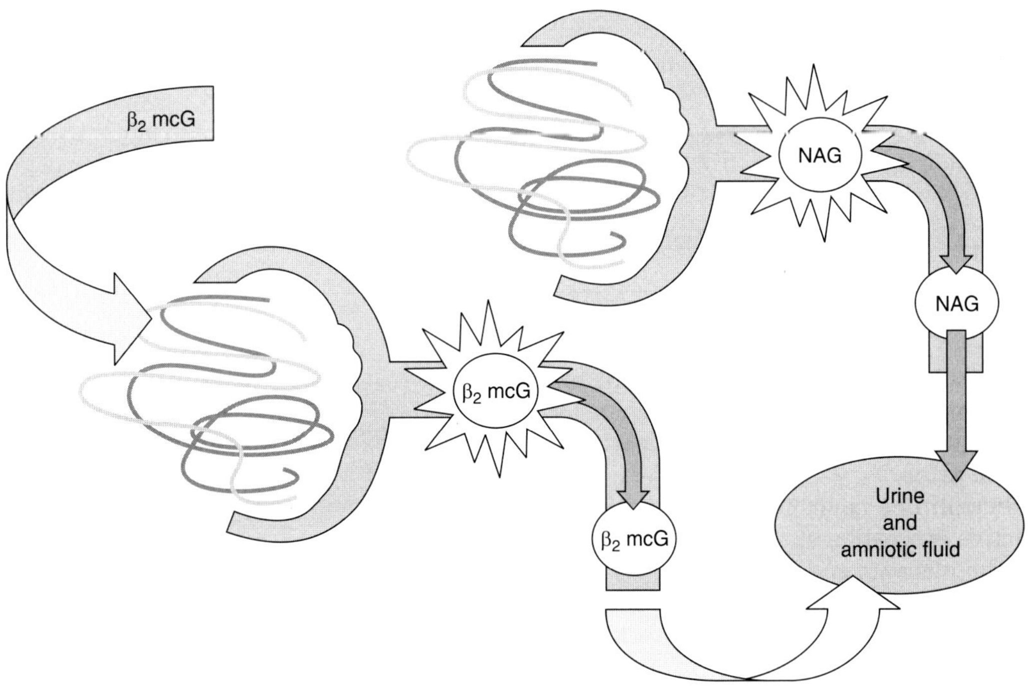

Figure 34.8 A determining factor of a normal renal clearance function corresponds to lysosomal proteins exclusive of the proximate tubular structure (NAG); if it is present in fetal urine and in the amniotic fluid in large quantities, it is indicative of tubular tissue destruction. β-2 Microglobuline would be viewed similarly.

Table 34.3 Fetal urinary aspiration: pathological biochemical markers and their values

	18–20 weeks	20–30 weeks	> 32 weeks
Na^+ (mEq/ml)	120.0	126.44 ± 11.50	139.60
Cl^- (mEq/ml)	119.0	132.50 ± 7.18	141.00
OsM (mOsm)	240	261.50 ± 24.20	281.00
NAG (U/l)	18.0	25.83 ± 0.85	25.73
β–2 Microglobuline (ml/l)	26.0	38.97 ± 1.30	38.72
K^+ (mEq/ml)	3.1	3.41 ± 0.66	3.90
Creatinine (ml/l)	1.2	2.54 ± 0.83	3.70

Table 34.4 Physiological values: urine vs. amniotic liquid

Urine/amniotic liquid	18–20 weeks	20–30 weeks	> 32 weeks
Na^+ (mEq/ml)	42/137	42/140	47/140
Cl^- (mEq/ml)	23/109	47/109	41/108
OsM (mOsm)	98/267	102/273	102/271
NAG (U/l)	2.0/3.6	2.7/3.62	2.0/4.69
β-2 Microglobuline (ml/l)	4.7/4.5	5.1/5.0	5.3/5.8
K^+ (mEq/ml)		41/140	
Creatinine (ml/l)		1.9/.6	

Table 34.5 Pathological values: urine vs. amniotic liquid

Urine/amniotic liquid	18–20 weeks	20–30 weeks	> 32 weeks
Na^+ (mEq/ml)	120/132	126.4/140	139.6/140
Cl^- (mEq/ml)	119/107	132.5/149	141/158
OsM (mOsm)	240/267	261.5/273	281/296
NAG (U/l)	18/16.9	25.83/20.34	25.73/20.8
β-2 Microglobuline (ml/l)	26/22.3	38.9/28.74	38.72/30.0
K^+ (mEq/ml)	3.1/138	3.4/140.6	3.9/148
Creatinine (ml/l)	1.2/0.7	2.54/0.82	3.7/0.9

This opens the field of study of nephrouropathies through the determination of these and other parameters in the amniotic liquid, without the need for an invasive study of the fetal urine.[21]

The K^+ and creatinine concentrations are different in their predictive evaluation as there is a large clearance effect in the placenta and great variability in its ionic charge, which makes the potassium filtration very dispersed; on the other hand, 90% of the K^+ concentration is intracellular.[8,21]

In summary, we can venture in Table 34.6 a prediction of renal viability in relation to the parameters described, taking into account the fact that these values are applicable to any gestational age.

Intrauterine determination of the characteristics of fetal urine offers the possibility of absolute diagnosis of normal renal clearance function.

Table 34.6 Fetal urine: biochemical markers applicable to any gestational age, echographic image indications and amniotic liquid volume to determine the renal function status

Prediction	Bad	Good
Echographic image	Hyperecongenity + cyst	Normal echography
Amniotic liquid	Oligoamnios	Normal
Fetal urine		
Na^+	> 100 mEq/ml	< 100 mEq/ml
Cl^-	> 90 mEq/ml	< 90 mEq/ml
Osmolarity	> 210	< 210
NAG	> 8 U/l	< 8 U/l
β-2 Microglobuline	> 4 mg/l	< 4 mg/l
K^+	Indifferent	Indifferent

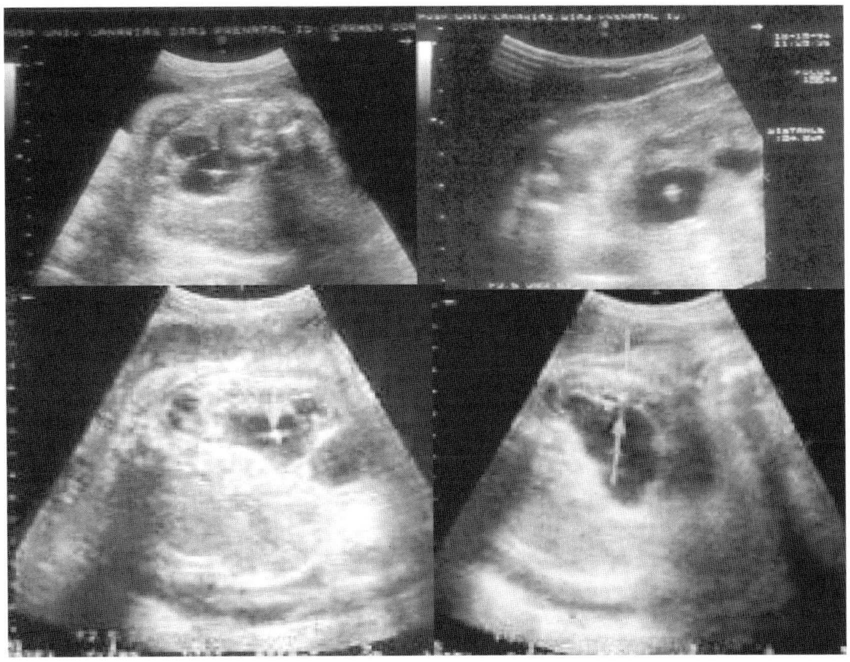

Figure 34.9 Aspirative nephrostomy: echographic monitoring.

Urine aspiration puncture for diagnosis is technically feasible, using conventional 18-g spinal needles having an aspiration system connected to a 20-cc syringe. The way to approach this depends on the fetal position available.

With the posterior back position we will not find any great inconvenience in puncturing the bladder, whilst for a lateral or anterior back position a nephrostomic aspiration is chosen (Figure 34.9).

In neither are there any noticeable complications, at least in our experience.[8,21]

Nephrostomic aspiration allows us firstly to reevaluate the echostructural characteristics of the expanded kidney parenchyma and, secondly, as long as we use the 16-g sure cut aspiration system, to carry out at the same time a renal biopsy without any technical difficulties.

For this, once the nephrostomic urine aspiration has been carried out, without taking the needle out move it toward the renal parenchyma and carry out the aspiration with a *swinging* movement over the corticomedular area.

Obtaining samples of 2-mm length is enough for detection of the histological characteristics that define a kidney dysplasia.[8,9,21–23]

However, once the technical problems involving tissues have been solved, the use of 16-g catheters from the aspiration biopsy set (Figure 34.3) allows us to obtain samples in 65% of cases. If conventional 18-g catheters are used, samples are obtained in only 30% of the cases though they are safe (J. Troyano and I. Donald, unpublished observations).

Skin biopsy

As already stated in the general section about fetal biopsies, skin biopsy entails the most serious difficulties in obtaining adequate or sufficient samples that will allow correct histopathological diagnosis or prediction.

The most important aspect is the obtaining of valid samples; for this we need at least 1-mm strips of skin and no smaller in surface area and that also include a layer of the epithelial stratum, comprising conjunctive areas and basal membrane. Only in this way can an acceptable reading be obtained.[24]

The second aspect to be taken into account is the surgical biopsy material. We have already indicated previously that the use of 2.5-mm clipping tongs (forceps/clippers), introduced into the amniotic environment using a trocar, will allow the obtaining of skin samples in 100% of all cases, and it is true that the residual skin lesions, and any pregnancy complications there may be, will not provide any noticeable benefits in relation to the diagnostic data.

The use of conventional needles and isometric aspiration, using the *slice* technique, which consists in inserting the needle sideways over the skin and making *scratching* or *scraping* movements, this will allow us to obtain skin strips of optimum quality with minimum damage to the integrity of the pregnancy (Figure 34.10).[25–28]

The third aspect to consider is the place selected for taking the sample, as depending on the disorder that we aim to diagnose prenatally, the biopsy area

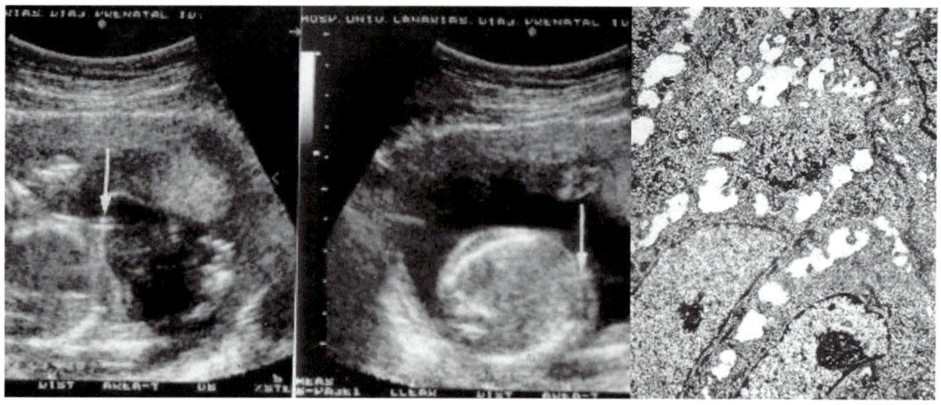

Figure 34.10 Left: Skin biopsy in fetal abdomen, scratched sideways. Right: Mature histological cutaneous samples in which keratohyalin and hemidesmosomes are detected.

will be different. The same area of fetal skin wrap will not always be valid or suit the purpose of the biopsy.

Technique

Skin samples should, if possible, be taken from different areas of the fetus.

The pregnancy stage recommended for this is around 20 weeks, as after this time, the pilose follicles begin to develop and keratinization mechanisms set it. A study of the elements involved in the keratinization (keratohyalin and tonofibers), gives preliminary indications of the disorder.

On the other hand, at this stage in the pregnancy the dermoepidermal junction has definitively been established, and the gradual rise of intercellular desmosomes is a great help for the diagnosis of different forms of epidermolysis.

The sequence should follow the following steps:

- Echographic monitoring
- If possible, the placenta must be avoided
- Take into consideration the fetal position as on some occasions it will be necessary to obtain samples from different skin areas
- Rigorous sterilization
- Optional local anesthesia, depending on the surgical timing
- Oblique needle incidence in the thickness and surface of the skin, making a scraping or scratching movement without pulling back
- Try to obtain at least 1-mm strips. The use of vacuum needles allows the collection of various fragments from the interior without the need for withdrawing the needle
- Immediately, proceed to wash the samples in saline serum for the histological staining and fixing process or for electron microscopy analysis.

Indications

Indications are most frequently based on diagnosis of some type of genodermatosis or congenital dermoepidermic disorders, of dominant autosomic transmission

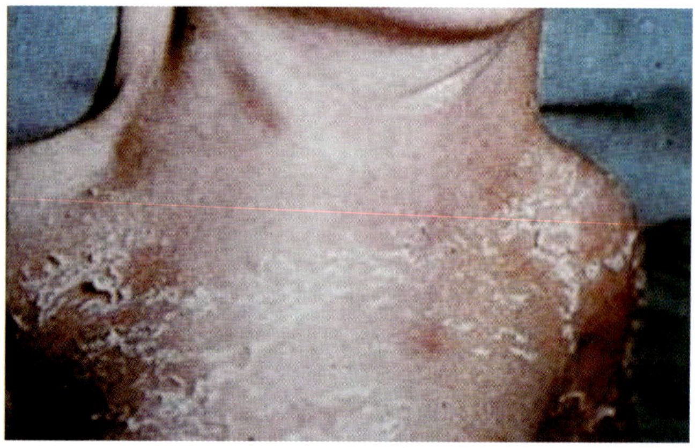

Figure 34.11 Keratinization disorder.

and recessive types, the majority being lethal in the short or medium term.

These disorders can be classified as follows:

- *Bullous epidermolysis*: Fetuses with large blistered areas that, once the blisters break, set off intensive erosive zones with a fast loss of electrolytes are affected[6,10,29,30]
- *Anhidrotic ectodermic dysplasias*: Recessive disorder linked to the sex. The fetuses are born without pilose follicles, without any hair or sudoriparous glands. They develop hyperthermic through disregulation and general dryness syndromes[31]
- *Keratinization disorders*: Also called *collodion baby syndrome*, characterized by the appearance of *reptilian skin* due to epidermic membranes that are *shed quickly*. Severe and lethal dehydrating disorders[32,33]
- *Pigmentary atopies*: Ocular syndromes with severe intolerance to light and early or premature development of skin cancers.[31,34,35]

The diagnostic problems faced with these dermatoses are due to the development of a lesion which has different topographic origins, and so the need to select

Table 34.7 Diagnoses possible from fetal skin biopsies

Keratinization disorders: The puncture spot is in the trunk and buttocks (Figure 34.11)
Harlequin fetus
Collodion baby
Sjögren–Larsson syndrome
Congenital icthyosis
Ampollous diseases: The puncture spot is in the waist, skin folds, abdomen and buttocks (Figure 34.12)
Herlitz ampollous junctional disease
Hallopeau–Siemens ampollous dermolytic disease
Inverse dystrophic ampollous disease
Cockayne–Touraine dystrophic ampollous disease
Pigmentary disorders: The puncture spot in the skin of the head (scalp) (Figure 34.13)
Negative tirosinase oculocutaneous albinism
Chediak-Higashi disease
Anhidrotic ectodermic disease

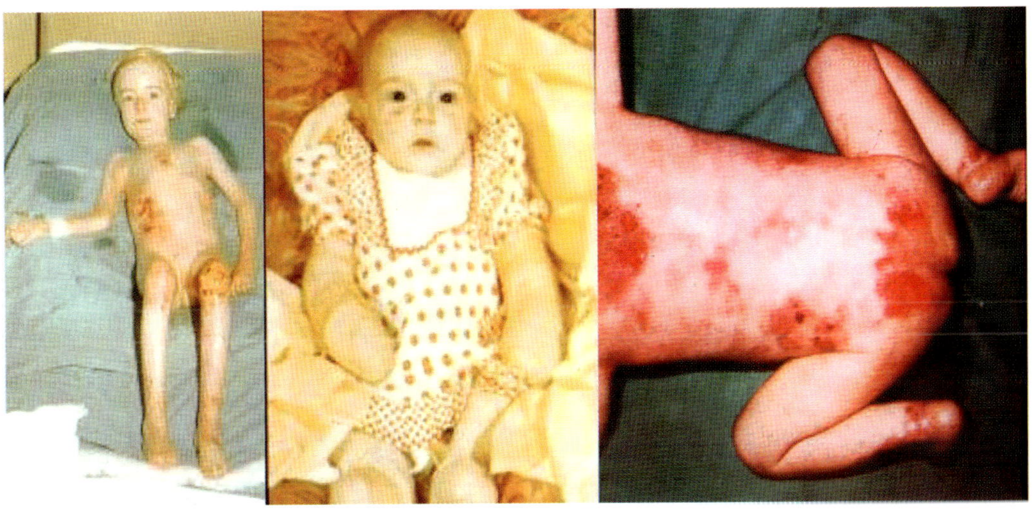

Figure 34.12 Ampollous disease.

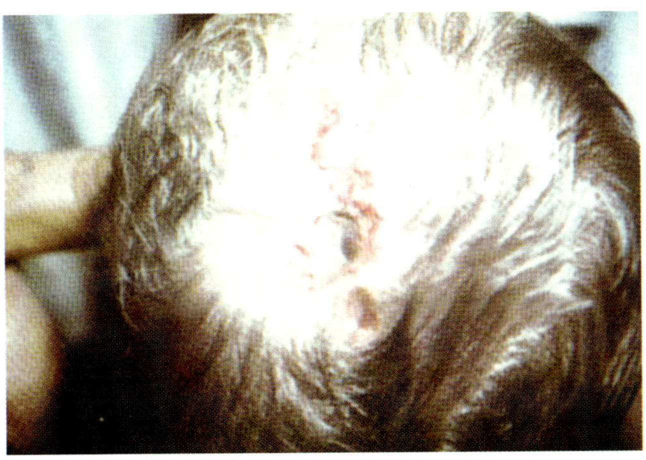

Figure 34.13 Pigmentary disorder (scalp lesions).

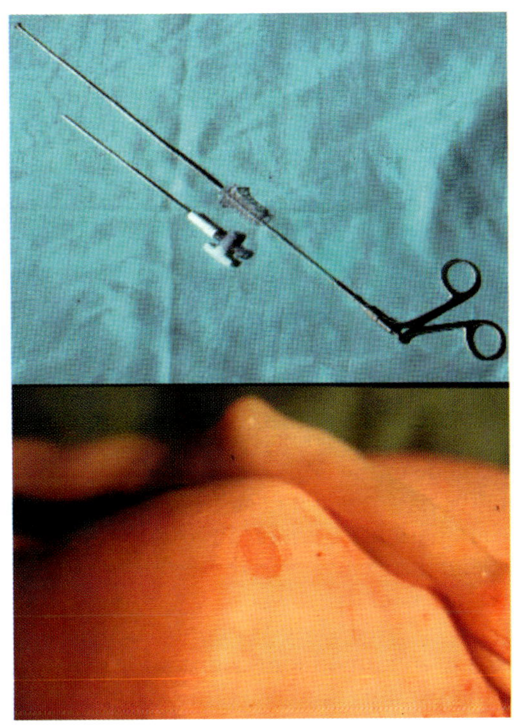

Figure 34.14 Residual cutaneous lesion after biopsy with clipper system.

the puncture spot has to be in accordance with the illness that one is trying to detect.

The diagnostic possibilities of skin biopsies are summarized in Table 34.7.

It is essential to have an objective family history in order to determine the biopsy spot.[34,36,37]

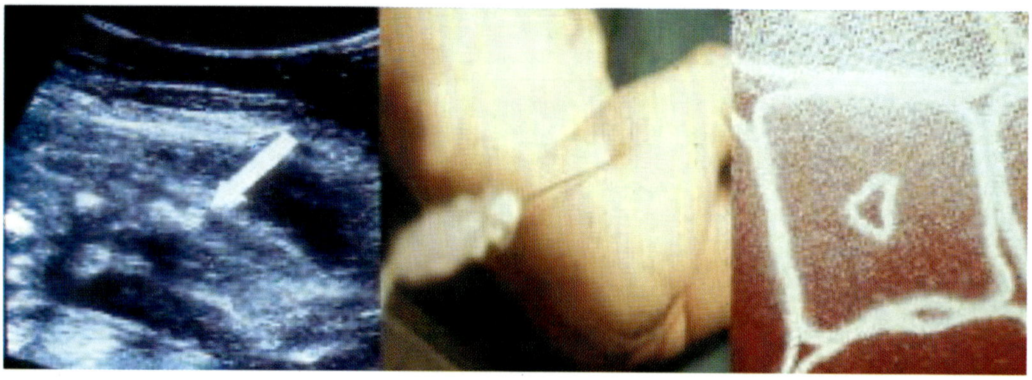

Figure 34.15 Subtrochanteric muscle biopsy: detection of dystrophine by immunofluorescence indicates healthy muscle.

Complementary requirements

The study of the samples will be based on the ultrastructural features stated previously. A great deal of experience in fetal dermatology using electron microscopy is required to make the diagnosis.

It is essential to have an objective family history knowledge in order to determine the prenatal dermoepidermic structural markers.

It is recommended that previous samples be maintained for use as a *study bank*.

Complications

Presently the tendency is to propose minimally invasive techniques using conventional needles **7** (38).

The use of conventional needles does not pose more risks than amniocentesis. On the other hand, trocar techniques and 2.5-mm biopsy provoke around 5% of miscarriages due to iatrogenic amniorexis, although some indelible fetal skin lesions have been described similarly (Figure 34.14). This does not occur in cases where the *scalp* technique is carried out with the use of conventional needles.

Muscle biopsy

This is carried out preferably for prenatal diagnosis of Duchenne's muscular dystrophy (DMD), although it is also possible to detect other hereditary myopathies as long as there is some clinical family history of these disorders.[11,38,39]

For the diagnosis of DMD, it is usual for DNA analysis to be used. When the recombinations within the DMD gene or the DNA analysis are not sufficiently informative or if it is not clear from the family history if there are possible carriers, direct examination of the muscle and its analysis is the only way to give an objective prenatal diagnosis.

The marker used is dystrophine; its determination by means of immunofluorescence allows us to differentiate the features of affected muscles from those of the healthy ones. The absence of this protein from the skeletal muscles is practically pathognomonic of DMD[11,14,39,40] (Figure 34.15).

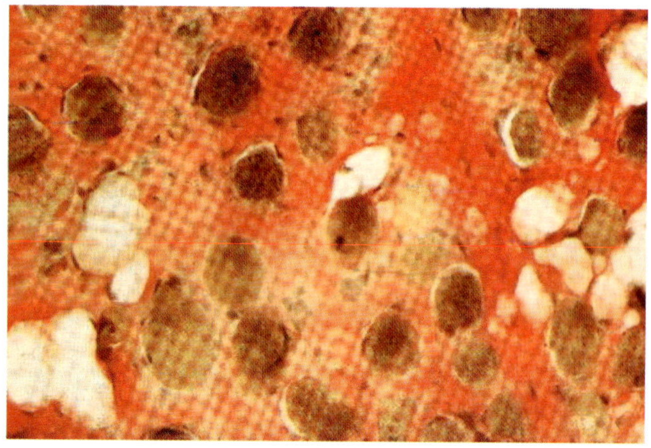

Figure 34.16 DMD with degenerated muscle as an associated sign: fat and connective infiltration, morphological cellular alterations and leucocyte infiltration.

At other times prenatal diagnosis of DMD may be impossible when there is only one previously affected male in the family, and there is no identifiable deletion.

The absence of dystrophine in a skeleton muscle, is in itself sufficient for determination of screening of the DMD. Nevertheless this diagnosis can be reinforced by detecting a rise in phosphocreatinkinase of more than 10 times its normal value in fetal blood.

Among the possibilities that can reinforce a prenatal DMD diagnosis or prediction we have:

- Sex linked
- High values of phosphocreatinkinase
- Absence of dystrophine
- Degenerated muscle
- Fat infiltration
- Connective infiltration
- Nuclear and cellular morphological alterations (Figure 34.16).

Technique

Any skeletal muscle is suitable, preferably the external face of one of the thighs or knuckles, avoiding topographic places with innervation or vital vascularization; indelible functional lesions will thus be avoided. The use of conventional 18-g needles or, even better, the sure cut method that has been described previously is preferred[8,38,41–43] (Figure 34.2).

Subtrochanteric punctures are carried out in a descending manner, as oblique as possible, orientated toward the fetal femur (Figure 34.2).

The puncture success rate is 75%.

It is essential to determine muscle dystrophy by immunoflourescence, being advisable but not determining the detection of phosphocreatinkinase and the study of the muscular structure at a morphological muscular level, fat and connective infiltration.

No complications are described.

The fetus may be studied using invasive techniques. These techniques are only justified when there are serious situations such as the possibility of an inherited illness or there is any other disorder detected during pregnancy; the need for diagnosis through biopsy is particularly important in the latter. Thoracocentesis, pericardiocentesis and other thoracoabdominal punctures are primarily carried out for therapy, and extracted material is studied for its components.

Other punctures on fetal tumor formations (sacrococcygeal teratomas, solid cervical teratomas, etc.) or liquid collections, such as pericariocentesis, do not have an acceptable justification from a therapeutic or diagnostic point of view, as echographic evaluation and currently used biophysical methods (color Doppler among these) give an acceptable identification of their vascularization and origin, including suspicious neoplasms[44,45] (A. Kurjak, unpublished data).

In agreement with our philosophy, we would like to express this thought:

> *The fetus has been endowed by nature to confront several inconveniences provided by its 40 weeks of development. It is a real 'Titan' that can face any adversity, and its adaptability is exceptional.*
>
> *Let us not disturb it!*
> *Let us not invade its privacy aggressively!*
> *Let us observe it minutely. When it needs us, which generally happens in few occasions, it will advise us; then let us help it.*
>
> J. M. Troyano-Luque (1993)

REFERENCES

1. Bahado-Singh RO, Morotti R, PirhorenJ, Lopez JA, Mahoney MJ. Invasive techniques for prenatal diagnosis: current concepts. *J Assoc Acad Minor Phys* 1995;6:28–33.
2. Cadrin C, Golbus MS. Fetal tissue sampling indications, techniques, complications and experience with sampling of fetal skin, liver and muscle. *West J Med* 1993;159:269–72.
3. Golbus MS, Sagebield RW, Filly RA, *et al.* Prenatal diagnosis of congenital icthyosiform erythroderma (epidermolytic hyperkeratosis) by fetal skin biopsy. *N Engl J Med* 1980;302:93.
4. KouseffBG, Matsouca LY, Stenn RS, *et al.* Prenatal diagnosis of Sjögren–Larsson syndrome. *J Pediatr* 1082;101:998.
5. Robjn AJ, David B, Gardner A, Rodeck CH. Prenatal diagnosis of oculocutaneous albinism by electron microscopy of fetal skin. *J Invest Dermatol* 1983;80:210–2.
6. Dolan CR, Smith LT, Syber UP. Prenatal detection of epidermolysis bullosa fetalis with pyloric atresia in a fetus by abnormal ultrasound and elevated alphafetoprotein. *Am J Genet* 1993; 47:395–400.
7. Rodeck CH. Fetoscopy guided by real time ultrasound for pure fetal samples, fetal skin samples and examination of the fetus *in utero. Br J Obstet Gynaecol* 1980;87:449–56.
8. Troyano JM, Padron E, Clavijo M. Fetal biopsy and puncture. Actual status. In *Balkan Ohrid's School of Ultrasound. Advanced Ultrasound II.* Ohrid, Macedonia: Dobri S. Filipche, 1996;9: 51–61.
9. Campbell WA, Yamase HT, Salafia CA, Vintilizeos AM, Rodis JF. Fetal renal biopsy: Technique development. *Fetal Diagn Ther* 1993; 8:135–43.
10. Dunnill MG, Rodeck CH, Richards AJ, *et al.* Use of type VII collagen gene (COL7A1) markers in prenatal diagnosis of recessive dystrophic epidermolysis bullosa. *J Med Genet* 1995;32:749–50.
11. Evans MI, Farrell SA, Greb A, Ray P, Johnson MP, Hoffman EP. *In utero* fetal muscle biopsy for the diagnosis of Duchenne musçular dystrophy in a female fetus 'suddenly at risk'. *Am J Med Genet* 1993;46:309–12.
12. Fox J, Hack AM, Fenton WA, *et al.* Prenatal diagnosis of ornithine transcarbamylase deficiency with the use of DNA polymorphisms. *N Engl J Med* 1986;315:1205.
13. Matilla I, Corral J, Miranda M, *et al.* Prenatal diagnosis of Werdnig–Woffmann disease: DNA analysis of a mummified umbilical cord using closely linked microsatellite markers. *Prenat Diagn* 1994;14:219–22.
14. Kuller JA, Hoffman EP, Fries MH, Golbus MS. Prenatal diagnosis of Duchenne muscular dystrophy by fetal muscle biopsy. *Hum Genet* 1992;90:34–40.
15. Illum N, Lavard L, Danpure ZJ, Aerenlund Jensen H, Skovby F. Primary hyperoxaluria type 1: Clinical manifestation in infancy and prenatal diagnosis. *Child Nephrol Urol* 1992;12:225–7.
16. Rodeck CH, Patrick AD, Pembrey ME, Tzannatos C, Whitfield AE. Fetal liver biopsy for prenatal diagnosis of ornithine carbamyl transferase deficiency. *Lancet* 1982;1:297–9.
17. Goebel HH, Vesa J, Reiter B, *et al.* Prenatal diagnosis of infantile neuronal ceroid lipofuscinosis: A combined electron microscopic and molecular genetic approach. *Brain Dev* 1995;17:83–8.
18. Murotsuki J, Vehara S, Okamura K, Yajima A, Oura I, Miyabayashi S. Fetal liver biopsy for prenatal diagnosis of carbamoyl phosphate synthetase deficiency. *Am J Perinatol* 1994;11:160–2.
19. Tsushida Y, Kawarasaki H, Iwanaka T, Uchida H, Nakanishi H, Uno K. Antenatal diagnosis of biliary atresia (type 1 cyst) at 19 weeks gestation: Differential diagnosis and etiologic implications. *J Pediatr Surg* 1995;30:607–9.
20. Von Dobeln V, Venizelos N, Westgren M, Hagenfeldt L. Long chain 3-hydroxylacyl-CoA dehydrogenase in chorionic villi, fetal liver, and fibroblasts and prenatal diagnosis of 3-hydroxylacyl-CoA dehydrogenase. *J Inherit Metab Dis* 1994;17:185–8.
21. Troyano JM, de la Fuente P, eds. *Prenatal Features of Fetal Kidney Physiopathology and Their Intra and Extrauterine Treatment. A Multi-disciplinary Problem.* Santa Cruz de Tenerife: University Hospital of the Canary Islands, 1993:35–9.
22. Greco P, Loverro G, Carusso G, Clement R, Selvaggi L. Diagnostic potential of fetal renal biopsy. *Prenat Diagn* 1994;14:415.
23. Gubler MC, Levy M. Prenatal diagnosis of nail–patella syndrome by intrauterine kidney biopsy. *Am J Med Genet* 1993;47:122–4.
24. Elias S, Emerson DS, Simpson JL, Shulrnan LP, Holbrook KA. Ultrasound-guided fetal skin sampling for prenatal diagnosis of genodermatoses. *Obstet Gynecol* 1994;83:337–41.

25. Bakharev VA, Aivazyan AA, Karetnikova NA, Mordovtsev VN, Yantousky Y. Fetal skin biopsy in prenatal diagnosis of some genodermatoses. *Prenat Diagn* 1990;10:1–12.
26. Buckshee K, Parveen S, Mittal S, Verma K, Singh M. Percutaneous ultrasound-guided fetal skin biopsy: A new approach. *Int J Gynaecol Obstet* 1991;34:267–70.
27. Holbrook KA, Wapner R, Jackson L, Zaeri N. Diagnosis and prenatal diagnosis of epidermolysis bullosa herpetiformis (Dowling–Meara) in a mother, two affected children and an affected fetus. *Prenat Diagn* 1992;12:725–39.
28. Suzumori K, Kanzak I. Prenatal diagnosis of harlequin ichthyosis by fetal skin biopsy: Report of two cases. *Prenat Diagn* 1991;11: 451–7.
29. McGrath JA, McMillan JR, Dunnill MG, *et al.* Genetic bases of lethal junctional epidermolysis bullosa in an affected fetus: Implications for prenatal diagnosis in one family. *Prenat Diagn* 1995;15:647–54.
30. Shirnizu H, Onodera Y, Ikeda S, Ogawa H, Suzumori K, Nishikawa T. Prenatal diagnosis of epidermolysis bullosa: First successful trial in Asia. *Dermatology* 1994;188:46–9.
31. Shimizu H, Ishko A, Kikushi A, Akiyarna M, Susumori K, Nishikawa T Prenatal diagnosis of tyrosinase negative oculocutaneous albinism by an electron microscopic dopa-reaction test of fetal skin. *Prenat Diagn* 1994;14:442–50.
32. Akiyama M, Kim DK, Main DM, Otto CE, Holbrook KA. Characteristic morphologic abnormality of harlequin ichthyosis detected in amniotic fluid cells. *J Invest Dermatol* 1994;102: 210–3.
33. Rizzo WB. Sjögren–Larsson syndrome. *Semin Dermatol* 1993; 12:210–8.
34. Akeo K, Shirai S, Okisaka S, *et al.* Histology of fetal ages with oculocutaneous albinism. *Arch Ophthalmol* 1996;114:613–6.
35. Shimizu H, Niizeki H, Suzurnori K, *et al.* Prenatal diagnosis of oculocutaneous albinism by analysis of the fetal tyrosinase gene. *J Invest Dermatol* 1994;103:104–6.
36. Holbrook KA, Smith LI, Elias S. Prenatal diagnosis of genetic skin disease using fetal skin biopsy samples. *Arch Dermatol* 1993;129:1437–54.
37. Normand J, Karasek MA. A method for the isolation and serial propagation of keratinocytes, endothelial cells and fibroblasts from a single punch biopsy of human skin. *In Vitro Cell Dev Biol Anim* 1995;31:447–55.
38. Evans MI, Krivchenia EL, Johnson MP, *et al. In utero* fetal muscle biopsy alters diagnosis and carrier risks in Duchenne and Becket muscular dystrophy. *Fetal Diagn Ther* 1995;10:71–5.
39. Fanin M, Pegoraro E, Angelini C. Absence of dystrophin and spectrin in regenerating muscle fibers from Becket dystrophy patients. *J Neurol Sci* 1994;123:88–94.
40. Lindahl M, Backman E, Henriksson KG, Gorospe JR, Hoffman EP. Phospholipase A2 activity in dystrophinopathies. *Neuromusc Disord* 1995;5:193–9.
41. Benzie RJ, Ray P, Thompson D, Hunter AG, Ivey B, Salvador L. Prenatal exclusion of Duchenne muscular dystrophy and fetal muscle biopsy. *Prenat Diagn* 1994;14:235–8.
42. Evans MI, Hoffman EP, Cadrin C, Johnson MP, Quintero RA, Golbus MS. Fetal muscle biopsy: Collaborative experience with varied indications. *Obstet Gynecol* 1994;84:913–7.
43. Evans MI, Quintero RA, King M, Kureshi F, Hoffman EP, Johnson MP. Endoscopically assisted, ultrasound-guided fetal muscle biopsy. *Fetal Diagn Ther* 1995;10:167–72.
44. Troyano JM, Clavijo MT, Clemente I, Marco OY, Rayward J, Mahtani VG. Kidney and urinary tract diseases: Ultrasound and biochemical markers. *Ultrasound Rev Obstet Gynecol* 2002; 2(2):92–109.
45. Bebatar A, Vaughan J, Nicolini U, Trotter S, Corrin B, Lincoln C. Prenatal pericariocentesis: Its role in the management of intrapericardial teratoma. *Obstet Gynecol* 1992;79(5, Pt 2):859.

35 The role of ultrasound examination of the cervix in pregnancy

P. Rozenberg and Y. Ville

Introduction

Preterm delivery is the main cause of perinatal mortality and morbidity.[1] Its prevalence has been stable for the last 20 years accounting for 5.9% and 11% of all deliveries in France and in the USA, respectively.[2–4] This is mainly due to poor therapeutic results and the inadequacy of the diagnostic criteria for preterm labor. Risk scoring for preterm birth has both low sensitivity and positive predictive value.[5–8] Only 15% of women with a previous history of preterm delivery will do so in a subsequent pregnancy.[8] Routine digital cervical examinations during pregnancy increase the risk for admission in hospital without decreasing the incidence of prematurity.[9] In threatened preterm labor as defined by painful contractions, cervical changes on digital examination and frequency of contractions both remain poor predictors of preterm delivery.[10–13]

Different strategies have been developed to refine the risk of preterm delivery, including the use of transvaginal sonography (TVS) to measure and examine the length and shape of the cervix. TVS has been studied in three different populations: (1) symptomatic women with threatened preterm labor, i.e. regular and painful contractions together with changes on digital examination of the cervix; (2) asymptomatic women at high risk of delivering prematurely, as defined by a history of preterm delivery, late miscarriage, conization, maternal exposure to diethylstilbestrol (DES) during fetal life, uterine malformation or a current multiple pregnancy; and (3) asymptomatic women without any relevant history.

Threatened preterm labor

The risk of preterm delivery is significantly associated with two ultrasound features: shortening of the cervical length and cervical wedging

Cervical length (CL) measured by TVS, < 20, < 25, or < 30 mm, on admission had positive and negative predictive values (PPV and NPV, respectively) of 100% and 72%, 70% and 82%, and 65% and 100%, on preterm delivery, respectively. These patients delivered preterm despite tocolytic therapy during hospitalization.[14] Thus, the risk of preterm delivery is especially high in women whose CL on admission is < 20 mm, whereas a CL ≥ 30 mm is reassuring. Preterm delivery is also significantly associated with the presence of cervical wedging together with a short CL. This led to sensitivity, specificity, PPV, and NPV of 100%, 74.5%, 59.4%, and 100%, respectively.[15]

Ultrasound examination is more accurate than digital examination of the cervix in preterm labor

In preterm labor with intact membranes, Gomez *et al.*[10] showed that despite cervical dilatation of < 3 cm, CL and cervical wedging ($P < 0.005$) were highly predictive of preterm delivery, but digital examination of the cervix (dilatation and effacement) failed to do so. Survival analysis demonstrated a shorter admission-to-delivery interval for patients with an abnormal CL ($P < 0.005$). In preterm labor following completion of a course of IV tocolysis, cervical sonography performed better than digital examination to predict delivery before 36 and even 34 weeks, with a best cut-off of 30 mm on receiver operating characteristic (ROC) curve analyses.[11,16] The PPV and NPV were of 15% and 36%, and 97% and 100% in singleton and twin pregnancies, respectively, when assessed at between 23 and 33 weeks. When analyzed for delivery before 37 weeks, this held true for singletons but not for twins.

The comparison of cervical fetal fibronectin (fFN) assay and TVS of the cervix to predict preterm delivery remains a controversial issue

We found that prediction performances of vaginal fFN assay ≥ 50 ng/ml and of a CL of ≤ 26 mm in threatened preterm labor at between 24 and 34 weeks were similar

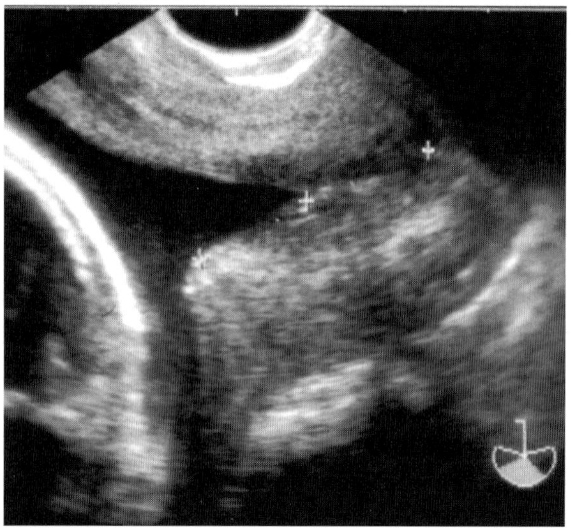

Figure 35.1 Dilatation of the IO.

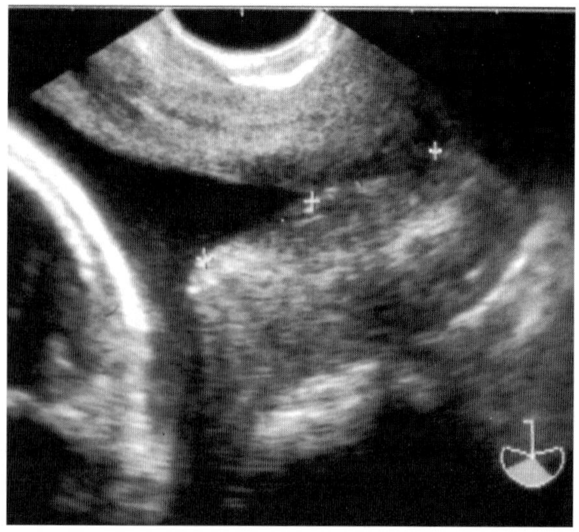

Figure 35.2 Sacculation of the membranes into the cervix.

with a high NPV of 86.6% and 89.1%, respectively.[17] The combination of both tests performed better with an NPV of 94.4% but the positive predictive value remained at around 50% although the odds ratio (OR) for delivering before 34 weeks was high (13.9; 95% CI, 3.7–52.2).

Rizzo *et al.*[18] reported that cervical fFN ≥60 ng/ml performed better than the association of CL and the presence of funneling on ultrasound. Furthermore, in patients with cervical fFN ≥60 ng/ml a shorter admission-to-delivery interval was found in the presence of an abnormal cervical index.

More recently, multiple logistic regression analysis found that only positive fFN testing (OR 11.25, P= 0.005) and functional CL ≤20 mm (OR 8.18, P=0.027) were independently associated with preterm delivery.[19] In the group with CL of 20–31 mm positive fetal fFN was found in 71.4% of patients delivered within 28 days and in 7.4% delivered after 28 days (P=0.001). fFN testing could therefore be performed only in patients with a short cervix to discriminate further those at true high risk of prematurity, with sensitivity, specificity, PPV, and NPV of 86%, 90%, 63%, and 97%, respectively, in predicting delivery within 28 days.

Asymptomatic women at high risk of preterm delivery

There are four types of clinical studies addressing this issue: (1) observational studies examining the natural course, (2) observational studies examining the course of those treated with cervical cerclage, (3) nonrandomized interventional studies, and (4) randomized interventional trials.

Observational studies of ultrasound features suggestive of cervical incompetence

Three ultrasound features are suggestive of cervical incompetence.

Dilatation of the internal os (IO) (Figure 35.1) was the first ultrasound feature suggesting cervical incompetence and thus increased risk of preterm delivery. Dilatation of the IO > 5 mm before 30 weeks' gestation is associated with preterm delivery in 33.3% vs. 3.5% when the IO remained closed (P < 0.01). Digital cervical examination noted dilatation of the IO in only 10 of the 26 (38.5%) patients in whom ultrasound showed cervical dilatation.[20]

Sacculation or prolapse of the membranes into a shortening cervix (Figure 35.2), either spontaneous or induced by transfundal pressure, can be seen even when digital cervical examination shows a long and closed cervix.[21]

Another study, in which ultrasound examinations were performed at between 15 and 24 weeks, compared three methods to detect cervical incompetence: transfundal pressure, coughing, and standing.[22] The transfundal pressure was the most predictive (sensitivity, specificity, PPV, and NPV of 83.3%; 97.2%; 88.2%; and 95.8%, respectively).

Shortening of the cervix in the absence of uterine contractions is also suggestive of cervical incompetence. A CL < 10th percentile (22 mm) and funneling at the IO (Figure 35.3) at between 16 and 30 weeks were associated with delivery within 2–4 weeks and before 35 weeks [33% vs. 0 (P=0.01); 67% vs. 0%, (P < 0.001); and 100% vs. 19%, P < 0.001, respectively].[23] Within this high-risk group, women with medical or obstetrical complications (including multiple gestation and ruptured membranes), symptoms of preterm labor, and history of incompetent cervix

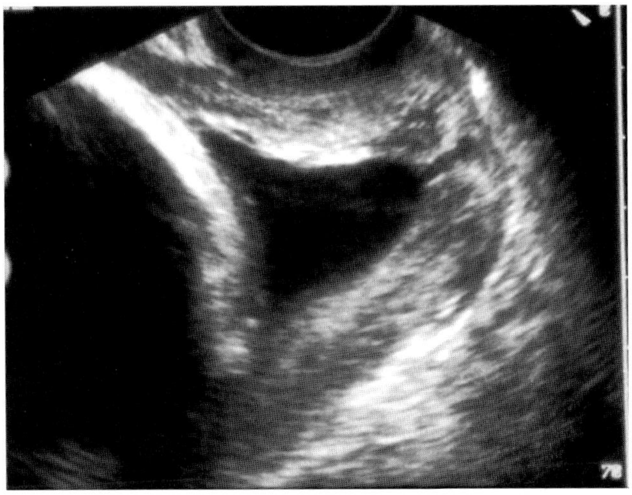

Figure 35.3 Funneling with shortening of the functional cervical length.

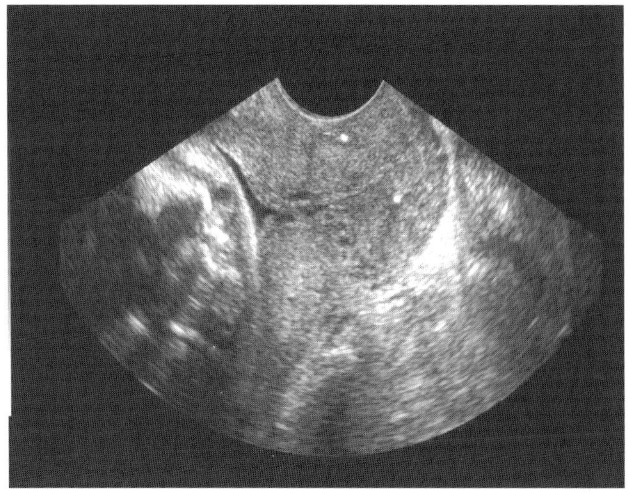

Figure 35.4 Increase in cervicle length after cerclage is often a temporary result.

that required cerclage were excluded. A short cervix or funneling beyond 20 weeks of gestation was also associated with an increased risk of preterm delivery before 35 weeks but not with an increased risk of delivering within 2–4 weeks following TVS.

Prospective longitudinal evaluation of a large cohort of 469 high-risk pregnancies by TVS and transfundal pressure on 1265 occasions at between 15 and 24 weeks[24] compared various sonographic cervical parameters to predict spontaneous preterm birth. ROC curve analysis showed that CL $\leq$25 mm alone performed as well as a combination of risk factors, CL, funneling, and transfundal pressure. The sensitivity for delivery at $<$28, $<$30, $<$32, and $<$34 weeks' gestation was 94%, 91%, 83%, and 76%, respectively, while the NPV was 99%, 99%, 98%, and 96%, respectively. Shortening of CL at weekly assessment helps in differentiating cervical competence from cervical incompetence in high-risk women ($-$0.3 vs. $-$4.1 mm/week; $P<0.001$).[25] Ultrasound diagnosis of cervical incompetence was defined as progressive shortening of the endocervical canal to 20 mm or less before 24 weeks' gestation.

In this high-risk group, CL $<$25 mm by TVS of the cervix performs better than CL $<$16 mm by digital cervical examination in assessing the risk of delivery before 35 weeks with relative risks of 4.8 and 2.0, respectively.[26]

In multiple pregnancies at between 24 and 28 weeks, a CL $\leq$25 mm by TVS was the best predictor of preterm delivery before 32 weeks, before 35 weeks, and before 37 weeks.[27] There is a continuous increase of 5–17% and 80% for this risk with CL shortening down to 40 and 20, and 8 mm, respectively.[28] CL of $\leq$20 mm seems to perform as well as any combination of clinical and ultrasound features at predicting preterm birth,[29] whereas CL $>$35 mm before 26 weeks seems to accurately identify a subgroup of twin pregnancies at low risk for premature delivery (3–4%).[30,31]

Although series are smaller, the predictive value of TVS of the cervix seems to hold true in triplets.[32,33] CL of $\leq$25 mm between 21 and 24 weeks' gestation was the best cutoff for the prediction of spontaneous preterm birth $<$28 weeks' gestation (86%, 79%, 40%, and 97% for sensitivity, specificity, PPV, and NPV, respectively).[34]

Follow-up studies in cervical incompetence diagnosed by TVS and treated by cerclage

It has been established that cervical cerclage is followed by a measurable increase in CL (Figure 35.4). This applies to both rescue cerclage[35,36] and elective procedures.[35,37,38] However, the relation of this increase with outcome is controversial and the longer the precerclage CL the more likely a delivery near term.[39] The value of CL shortening following cerclage is also controversial. A decrease of at least 10 mm is significant to predict delivery before 36 weeks.[36,37,40] However, this may not be significant when 34 weeks is considered as a cutoff.[38]

The value of non-randomized interventional studies based on ultrasound diagnosis of cervical incompetence is controversial

TVS together with transfundal pressure can be used in high-risk women to define cervical incompetence at between 16 and 24 weeks whenever this causes dilatation of the IO or protrusion of the membranes.[41]

Serial TVS suggests that evidence for cervical incompetence can be established by 24 weeks.[42] In a retrospective analysis, Kurup and Goldkrand[43] compared the outcome in three categories of cerclage: elective cerclage indicated by the patient's history, ultrasound-indicated cerclage performed in asymptomatic patients with cervical changes by ultrasound, and rescue procedure performed in symptomatic patients. This shows that the performance of ultrasound-indicated cerclage in terms of preterm delivery rate and gestational age at delivery was better than emergency procedures. The benefit of cerclage in this group is, however, uncertain when compared to elective cerclage on the basis of a relevant history.[44,45] This, therefore, suggests that a new indication for cerclage can be defined as cervical changes on serial TVS in a high-risk group.

Randomized trials assessing ultrasound-based indications for cerclage in high-risk women

There are two such randomized trials published and their results are apparently contradictory. Althuisius *et al.* studied patients with a history of delivery before 34 weeks with suspected cervical incompetence or preterm rupture of membranes at < 32 weeks without preceding contractions.[46] In subsequent singleton pregnancies, they were randomized into two groups, with a 1/2 ratio, for either prophylactic cerclage ($n=23$) or a follow-up cervical TVS ($n=44$). In the follow-up group, a CL < 25 mm before 27 weeks led to a second randomization for either therapeutic cerclage or expectant management. The obstetrical characteristics of the prophylactic cerclage and observational groups were similar. There was no significant difference in the rate of delivery before 34 weeks (13.0% vs. 13.6%) in these two groups. A CL < 25 mm before 27 weeks was found in 18 (41%) patients in the observational group with a mean CL of 18.2 ± 5.9 mm at a mean gestation of 19.1 ± 2.9 weeks. The incidence of deliveries < 34 weeks was significantly lower in the therapeutic cerclage group when compared (1/10 vs. 5/8) with the bed rest group ($P=0.04$).

There might therefore be a double benefit in performing cerclage for ultrasound indication only among asymptomatic patients at high risk:

- First, this would allow a significant reduction in the amount of prophylactic cerclage. Indeed, in this study, cerclage was performed in only 40% of the cases.
- Second, therapeutic cerclage before 27 weeks may reduce the incidence of premature delivery before 34 weeks among patients with a CL < 25 mm.

More recently, Althuisius *et al.*[47] published the final results of their trial on 35 women with definite risk factors of cervical incompetence and shortening of the cervix down to < 25 mm at before 27 weeks; 19 were allocated randomly to the cerclage group and 16 to the bed rest group. Both groups were comparable for mean CL and mean gestational age at the time of randomization. Preterm delivery before 34 weeks was significantly more frequent in the bed rest group than in the cerclage group (7 of 16 vs. none, respectively; $P=0.002$). The compound neonatal morbidity, defined as admission to the neonatal intensive care unit or neonatal death, was significantly higher in the bed rest group than in the cerclage group (8 of 16 vs. 1 of 19, respectively; $P=0.005$).

The other randomized trial by Rust *et al.*[48] led to different conclusions but addressed a different population. Screening in the general population and detecting 25% cervical funneling or CL < 25 mm at between 16 and 24 weeks were randomized into cerclage group or expectant management by Rust *et al.* Except for the cerclage, all patients were treated identically before and after randomization. Cerclage did not affect the perinatal outcome in any of the two trials.

Several differences between these studies[47,48] may explain these contradictory results. Low-risk patients were screened for a short CL to be included in the Rust trial. In Althuisius', all but one patient had risk factors for cervical incompetence.

The main difference is therefore the initial selection of potential candidates. In the Rust trial, measurement of the CL was performed in patients who had risk factors for preterm birth. In Althuisius' trial, it was performed in patients who had risk factors for cervical incompetence.

All three trials included patients with short CL, which implies a high risk of preterm delivery but not necessarily a high risk of cervical incompetence. Rust *et al.* hypothesized that these ultrasonographic findings of the cervix during the second trimester demonstrate a potential final common pathway of multiple pathophysiological processes, such as infection, immunologically mediated inflammatory stimuli, and subclinical abruptio placentae. This hypothesis is supported by a 14.8% incidence of abruptio placentae in their study. Abruptio placentae were not found in any of the women in Althuisius' study. This difference in the prevalence of abruptio placentae confirms that the study populations in both trials are basically different.

TVS of the cervix in clinical trials in the general population

There is a relation between the risk of preterm delivery and the functional length of the cervix in the general population. In a prospective multicenter observational study, Iams *et al.*[49] performed TVS of the cervix in women with a singleton pregnancy at 24 weeks ($n=2915$) and 28 weeks ($n=2531$) of gestation. Delivery before 35 weeks occurred in 126 (4.3%) of the 2915 patients examined at 24 weeks. CL was normally distributed at 24 weeks (35.2 ± 8.3 mm) and at 28 weeks (33.7 ± 8.5 mm). The risk of preterm delivery was inversely correlated with the length of the cervix.

Heath *et al.*[50] measured CL by TVS at 23 weeks in 2567 singleton pregnancies in women attending routine antenatal care. The risk for delivery at 32 weeks decreased from 78% at a CL of 5 mm to 4% at 15 mm and 0.5% at 50 mm.

To *et al.*[51] measured the CL in 6819 singleton pregnancies at 22–24 weeks and looked for the presence of funneling to evaluate possible additional risk. Funneling of the IO was present in about 4% of pregnancies and the prevalence decreased from 98% when the CL was 15 mm to less than 1% at lengths > 30 mm. The rate of preterm delivery was 6.9% in those with funneling compared to 0.7% in those without funneling ($P < 0.0001$). However, logistic regression analysis demonstrated that funneling did not provide a significant additional contribution to CL in the prediction of spontaneous delivery before 33 weeks.

Taipale *et al.* and Hassan *et al.*[52,53] confirmed the relation between the risk of preterm delivery and the functional length of the cervix but showed the limitations of this screening method in the general population. Indeed routine TVS of the cervix performed between 18 and 22 weeks helped to identify patients at risk of preterm delivery; nonetheless, the low prevalence of preterm births in these populations (2–3%) at low obstetrical risk is a limitation to the development of such a method of screening, which would bring either a high false-positive rate if the cutoff is 29 mm (3.6%) or a low sensitivity if the cutoff is 15 mm (8.2%).[52,53]

Non-randomized interventional studies among patients in whom ultrasound images are suggestive of a shortened cervix reported encouraging results.[54] CL was ≤15 mm in 1.6% of the cases at 23 weeks in an unselected population of singleton pregnancies.[54] The attending physician decided upon performing a cerclage or expectant management. The two groups did not differ in ethnic or obstetrical characteristics. The median CL was 10 mm in both groups. In the cerclage group, the prevalence of preterm delivery before 32 weeks was 5%, whereas it was 52% in the expectant management group.

There is one randomized trial among patients with ultrasound images suggestive of cervical incompetence that was initiated following the results of Heath's study. To *et al.*[50] chose a cutoff CL of < 15 mm at 23 weeks in the general population, with an overall low incidence of preterm deliveries. In their study, CL was the measured indicator. Randomization into cerclage or expectant management did not lead to any difference in the mean maternal age or in neonatal morbidity.

Conclusion

TVS of the cervix is an objective evaluation of cervical biometry as well as an anatomical survey looking for funneling and protrusion of the membranes through the cervix. Dynamic functional examination of the cervix evaluates the changes in the IO in response to uterine contractions or transfundal pressure. It has the advantage of screening for dilatation of the IO even when the external os is unchanged. Similarly, it enables early detection of shortening of the supravaginal portion of the cervix, which is not amenable to clinical examination. We can hope that this early diagnosis will improve the efficacy of tocolytics.

TVS is a more discriminant approach than digital examination of the cervix in terms of both PPV and NPV. Among high-risk symptomatic patients (threatened preterm delivery), the data in the literature are sufficient to justify the systematic use of TVS for a more accurate evaluation of the risk of preterm delivery before any decision of hospital admission.

Cervical ultrasound may also be useful in selecting patients with complete or partial cervical incompetence among asymptomatic women at high risk (history of preterm delivery, late miscarriage, conization, maternal DES treatment, uterine malformation, or a current multiple pregnancy). Among asymptomatic patients at high risk, progressive cervical incompetence may be a primary uterine condition that could trigger premature labor. Looking for funneling or protrusion of the membranes into the cervix is therefore extremely useful. In their absence, cervical incompetence should be sought by transfundal pressure. Compared with a single cervical measurement at 16–18 weeks and 6 days' gestation, serial measurements up to 23 weeks 6 days significantly improved the prediction of spontaneous preterm birth.[21,25,66] A shortened cervix, although non-specific and rarely observed in the absence of uterine contractions, could also be the only warning of cervical incompetence. On the basis of Guzman's studies, ultrasound surveillance of such patients should begin by the 15th week.

In the general population, TVS of the cervix should be a useful complement to ultrasound examination performed at 22–24 weeks of gestation and help clinicians to better identify patients at low risk of preterm delivery (NPV =96.7% and PPV =47.6%).[53] High-risk patients as defined by short CL or the presence of cervical funneling could benefit from weekly cervical ultrasound assessment in order to define further intervention including cerclage, tocolytics, and steroids injection for lung maturation.

REFERENCES

1. Hall MH, Danielian P, Lamont RF. The importance of preterm birth. In Elder MG, Lamont RF, Romero R, eds. *Preterm Labor.* New York: Churchill Livingstone, 1997:1–28.
2. Blondel B, Du Mauzaubrun C, Bréart G. *Enquête nationale périnatale 1995. Rapport de fin d'étude.* Paris: INSERM, February 1996.
3. Ventura SJ, Martin JA, Curtin SC, Mathews MS. *Final Data for 1997: National Vital Statistics Reports.* Hyattsville, MD: National Center for Health Statistics, 1998;47(18).
4. Ventura SJ, Martin JA, Curtin SC, Mathews MS. *Report of Final Natality Statistics, 1996; Monthly Vital Statistics Report.* Hyattsville, MD: National Center for Health Statistics; 1998;46 (11, Suppl).
5. McLean M, Walters WA, Smith R. Prediction and early diagnosis of preterm labor: A critical review. *Obstet Gynecol Surv* 1993; 48:209–25.
6. Keirse MJ. An evaluation of formal risk scoring for preterm birth. *Am J Perinatol* 1989;6:226–33.

7. Shiono PH, Klebanoff MA. A review of risk scoring for preterm birth. *Clin Perinatol* 1993;20:107–25.
8. Creasy RK, Merkatz IR. Prevention of preterm birth: Clinical opinion. *Obstet Gynecol* 1990;76(Suppl 1):2S–4S.
9. Buekens P, Alexander S, Boutsen M, Blondel B, Kaminski M, Reid M. Randomised controlled trial of routine cervical examinations in pregnancy. European Community Collaborative Study Group on Prenatal Screening. *Lancet* 1994;344:841–4.
10. Gomez R, Galasso M, Romero R, *et al.* Ultrasonographic examination of the uterine cervix is better than cervical digital examination as a predictor of the likelihood of premature delivery in patients with preterm labor and intact membranes. *Am J Obstet Gynecol* 1994;171:956–64.
11. Iams JD, Paraskos J, Landon MB, Teteris JN, Johnson FF. Cervical sonography in preterm labor. *Obstet Gynecol* 1994;84:40–6.
12. Berghella V, Tolosa JE, Kuhlman K, Weiner S, Bolognese RJ, Wapner RJ. Cervical ultrasonography compared with manual examination as a predictor of preterm delivery. *Am J Obstet Gynecol* 1997;177:723–30.
13. Iams JD, Newman RB, Thom EA, *et al.* The National Institute of Child Health and Human Development Network of Maternal–Fetal Medicine Units. Frequency of uterine contractions and the risk of spontaneous preterm delivery. *N Engl J Med* 2002;346: 250–5.
14. Murakawa H, Utumi T, Hasegawa I, Tanaka K, Fuzimori R. Evaluation of threatened preterm delivery by transvaginal ultrasonographic measurement of cervical length. *Obstet Gynecol* 1993;82:829–32.
15. Timor-Tritsch IE, Boozarjomehri F, Masakowski Y, Monteagudo A, Chao CR. Can a "snapshot" sagittal view of the cervix by transvaginal ultrasonography predict active preterm labor? *Am J Obstet Gynecol* 1996;174:990–5.
16. Crane JM, Van den Hof M, Armson BA, Liston R. Transvaginal ultrasound in the prediction of preterm delivery: Singleton and twin gestations. *Obstet Gynecol* 1997;90:357–63.
17. Rozenberg P, Goffinet F, Malagrida L, *et al.* Evaluating the risk of preterm delivery: A comparison of fetal fibronectin and transvaginal ultrasonographic measurement of cervical length. *Am J Obstet Gynecol* 1997;176:196–9.
18. Rizzo G, Capponi A, Arduini D, Lorido C, Romanini C. The value of fetal fibronectin in cervical and vaginal secretions and of ultrasonographic examination of the uterine cervix in predicting premature delivery for patients with preterm labor and intact membranes. *Am J Obstet Gynecol* 1996;175:1146–51.
19. Hincz P, Wilczynski J, Kozarzewski M, Szaflik K. Two-step test: The combined use of fetal fibronectin and sonographic examination of the uterine cervix for prediction of preterm delivery in symptomatic patients. *Acta Obstet Gynecol Scand* 2002; 81:58–63.
20. Okitsu O, Mimura T, Nakayama T, Aono T. Early prediction of preterm delivery by transvaginal ultrasonography. *Ultrasond Obstet Gynecol* 1992;2:402–9.
21. Guzman ER, Vintzileos AM, McLean DA, Martins ME, Benito CW, Hanley ML. The natural history of a positive response to transfundal pressure in women at risk for cervical incompetence. *Am J Obstet Gynecol* 1997;176:634–8.
22. Guzman ER, Pisatowski DM, Vintzileos AM, Benito CW, Hanley ML, Ananth CV. A comparison of ultrasonographically detected cervical changes in response to transfundal pressure, coughing, and standing in predicting cervical incompetence. *Am J Obstet Gynecol* 1997;177:660–5.
23. Andrews WW, Copper R, Hauth JC, Goldenberg RL, Neely C, Dubard M. Second trimester cervical ultrasound: Association with increased risk for recurrent early spontaneous delivery. *Obstet Gynecol* 2000;95:222–6.
24. Guzman ER, Walters C, Ananth CV, *et al.* A comparison of sonographic cervical parameters in predicting spontaneous preterm birth in high-risk singleton gestations. *Ultrasound Obstet Gynecol* 2001;18:204–10.
25. Guzman ER, Mellon C, Vintzileos AM, Ananth CV, Walter C, Gibson K. Longitudinal assessment of endocervical canal length between 15 and 24 weeks' gestation in women at risk for pregnancy loss or preterm birth. Transfundal pressure, coughing, and standing in predicting cervical incompetence. *Obstet Gynecol* 1998;92:31–7.
26. Berghella V, Tolosa JE, Kuhlman K, Weiner S, Bolognese RJ, Wapner RJ. Cervical ultrasonography compared with manual examination as a predictor of preterm delivery. *Am J Obstet Gynecol* 1997;177:723–30.
27. Goldenberg RL, Iams JD, Miodovnik M, *et al.* The preterm prediction study: Risk factors in twin gestations. *Am J Obstet Gynecol* 1996;175:1047–53.
28. Skentou C, Souka AP, To MS, Liao AW, Nicolaides KH. Prediction of preterm delivery in twins by cervical assessment at 23 weeks. *Ultrasound Obstet Gynecol* 2001;17:7–10.
29. Guzman ER, Walters C, O'Reilly-Green C, *et al.* Use of cervical ultrasonography in prediction of spontaneous preterm birth in twin gestations. *Am J Obstet Gynecol* 2000;183:1103–7.
30. Imseis HM, Albert TA, Iams JD. Identifying twin gestations at low risk for preterm birth with a transvaginal ultrasonic cervical measurement at 24 to 26 weeks' gestation. *Am J Obstet Gynecol* 1997;177:1149–55.
31. Yang JH; Kuhlman K; Daly S; Berghella V. Prediction of preterm birth by second trimester cervical sonography in twin pregnancies. *Ultrasound Obstet Gynecol* 2000;15:288–91.
32. Ramin KD, Ogburn PL, Mulholland TA, Breckle RJ, Ramsey PS. Ultrasonographic assessment of cervical length in triplet pregnancies. *Am J Obstet Gynecol* 1999;180:1442–5.
33. To MS, Skentou C, Cicero S, Liao AW, Nicolaides KH. Cervical length at 23 weeks in triplets: Prediction of spontaneous preterm delivery. *Ultrasound Obstet Gynecol* 2000;16:515–8.
34. Guzman ER, Walters C, O'Reilly-Green C, *et al.* Use of cervical ultrasonography in prediction of spontaneous preterm birth in triplet gestations. *Am J Obstet Gynecol* 2000;183:1108–13.
35. Funai EF, Paidas MJ, Rebarber A, O'Neill L, Rosen TJ, Young BK. Change in cervical length after prophylactic cerclage. *Obstet Gynecol* 1999;94:117–9.
36. Guzman ER, Houlihan C, Vintzileos A, Ivan J, Benito C, Kappy K. The significance of transvaginal ultrasonographic evaluation of the cervix in women treated with emergency cerclage. *Am J Obstet Gynecol* 1996;175:471–6.
37. Althuisius SM, Dekker GA, van Geijn HP, Hummel P. The effect of therapeutic McDonald cerclage on cervical length as assessed by transvaginal ultrasonography. *Am J Obstet Gynecol* 1999;180:366–9.
38. El-Azeem SA, Samuels P, Fullana M, Walker H, Iams JD. Perioperative transvaginal sonography as an adjunct to cervical cerclage. *Am J Obstet Gynecol* 2000;182(1):Abstract 117 (Society for Maternal–Fetal Medicine 2000 20th Annual Meeting).
39. Dijkstra K, Funai EF, O'Neill L, Rebarber A, Paidas MJ, Young BK. Change in cervical length after cerclage as a predictor of preterm delivery. *Obstet Gynecol* 2000;96:346–50.
40. Andersen HF, Karimi A, Sakala EP, Kalugdan R. Prediction of cervical cerclage outcome by endovaginal ultrasonography. *Am J Obstet Gynecol* 1994;171:1102–6.
41. Guzman ER, Rosenberg JC, Houlihan C, Ivan J, Waldron R, Knuppel R. A new method using vaginal ultrasound and transfundal pressure to evaluate the asymptomatic incompetent cervix. *Obstet Gynecol* 1994;83:248–52.
42. Macdonald R, Smith P, Vyas S. Cervical incompetence: The use of transvaginal sonography to provide an objective diagnosis. *Ultrasound Obstet Gynecol* 2001;18:211–6.
43. Kurup M, Goldkrand JW. Cervical incompetence: elective, emergent, or urgent cerclage. *Am J Obstet Gynecol* 1999;181:240–6.
44. Guzman ER, Forster JK, Vintzileos AM, Ananth CV, Walters C, Gipson K. Pregnancy outcomes in women treated with elective versus ultrasound-indicated cervical cerclage. *Ultrasound Obstet Gynecol* 1998;12:323–7.
45. Berghella V, Daly SF, Tolosa JE, *et al.* Prediction of preterm delivery with transvaginal ultrasonography of the cervix in patients with high-risk pregnancies: Does cerclage prevent prematurity ? *Am J Obstet Gynecol* 1999;181:809–15.
46. Althuisius SM, Dekker GA, van Geijn HP, Bekedam DJ, Hummel P. Cervical incompetence prevention randomized cerclage trial (CIPRACT): Study design and preliminary results. *Am J Obstet Gynaecol* 2000;183:823–9.
47. Althuisius SM, Dekker GA, Hummel P, Bekedam DJ, van Geijn HP. Final results of the cervical incompetence prevention randomized cerclage trial (CIPRACT): Therapeutic cerclage with bed rest versus bed rest alone. *Am J Obstet Gynecol* 2001;185: 1106–12.
48. Rust OA, Atlas RO, Reed J, van Gaalen J, Balducci J. Revisiting the short cervix detected by transvaginal ultrasound in the second trimester: Why cerclage therapy may not help. *Am J Obstet Gynecol* 2001;185:1098–1105.
49. Iams JD, Goldenberg RL, Meis PJ, *et al.*, the National Institute of Child Health and Human Development Maternal Fetal Medicine

Unit Network. The length of the cervix and the risk of spontaneous premature delivery. *N Engl J Med* 1996;334:567–72.

50. Heath VC, Southall TR, Souka AP, Elisseou A, Nicolaides KH. Cervical length at 23 weeks of gestation: Prediction of spontaneous preterm delivery. *Ultrasound Obstet Gynecol* 1998;12:312–7.
51. To MS, Skentou C, Liao AW, Cacho A, Nicolaides KH. Cervical length and funneling at 23 weeks of gestation in the prediction of spontaneous early preterm delivery. *Ultrasound Obstet Gynecol* 2001;18:200–3.
52. Taipale P, Hiilesmaa V. Sonographic measurement of uterine cervix at 18–22 weeks' gestation and the risk of preterm delivery. *Obstet Gynecol* 1998;92:902–7.
53. Hassan SS, Romero R, Berry SM, *et al.* Patients with an ultrasonographic cervical length 15 mm have nearly a 50% risk of early spontaneous preterm delivery. *Am J Obstet Gynecol* 2000;182:1458–67.
54. Heath VCF, Souka AP, Erasmus I, Gibb DMF, Nicolaides KH. Cervical length at 23 weeks of gestation: The value of Shirodkar suture for the short cervix. *Ultrasound Obstet Gynecol* 1998;12:318–22.
55. To MS, Skentou C, Liao AW, Cacho A, Nicolaides KH. Lancet 2004.

36 Labor and puerperium

A. Mulic-Lutvica and O. Axelsson

Labor

There is no doubt that labor is a dangerous period of our life and may result in birth-related disorders. Preterm and postdate deliveries, multiple gestations, preterm rupture of the membranes, intrauterine growth disturbances, breech presentations and intrapartum bleeding are associated with considerable perinatal morbidity and mortality. Healthy newborns with expected good quality of life are the main goal of modern obstetrics. Numerous different methods have been developed to achieve this goal. One of the most widely used is without doubt ultrasound. Although the value of ultrasound in antenatal care is well established, it is surprising that the clinical knowledge of its advantages during the intrapartum or postpartum period is sparse. Nowadays, however, it is becoming increasingly common for obstetricians to use bedside ultrasound and to have ultrasound equipment permanently available in labor and delivery suites. By means of an ultrasound admission test, a selection of high-risk patients should be made. The uterus with its contents, including the fetus, placenta, umbilical cord and amniotic fluid, as well as the cervix, can be assessed in detail by ultrasound (Figure 36.1). Even the maternal pelvis has become the subject of growing interest among sonographers. Ultrasound can also be useful during the performance of some obstetrical procedures including external version of a breech fetus, intrapartum twin management, or manual or instrumental placental evacuation as well as for confirmation of an empty uterus after the completed procedure. Intrapartum ultrasound imaging is difficult due to discomfort in women caused by pain, supine hypotension and loss of the 'acoustic window' after rupture of the membranes, low station of the presenting part and lack of appropriate ultrasound equipment in the labor and delivery suite as well as inadequately trained examiners.[1–3]

Ultrasound admission test

Laboring women with inadequate or no prenatal care should be carefully examined with ultrasound when arriving at the labor and delivery unit.

Diagnosis of fetal life or death

Ultrasound diagnosis of fetal life or death is simple, prompt and accurate. The fetal heart should be identified and the absence of fetal heart motion by real-time ultrasound and/or color Doppler implies fetal death. A completely quiescent fetus without body or breathing movements is an additional sign of fetal death. If the fetus has been dead for several days, the ultrasound signs of fetal death are oligohydramnios, overlapping skull bones, hyperflexion of the spine and the presence of hydrops.

Fetal number

The presence of two separate heads, two spines and two heart motions is enough to identify a twin pregnancy. However, it is rare but not impossible to miss a multiple gestation even by ultrasound in a busy labor and delivery room, and especially if one of the fetuses is dead. Moreover, as the number of fetuses increases, the accuracy of intrapartum ultrasound diagnosis decreases. One of the possible explanations may be crowding and shadowing of one fetus by another, which creates a very confusing ultrasound image. Therefore, a thorough systematic approach should be adopted. All quadrants of the uterus must be explored in order to avoid missing a multiple gestation. Furthermore, ultrasound can be used to estimate the amount of amniotic fluid, and to give information on fetal presentation, growth discordance, signs of hydrops and fetal malformations. A correct intrapartum diagnosis and painstaking management of delivery with the assistance of ultrasound are essential for an optimal outcome in cases with multiple gestations.

Fetal presentation

The presenting part of the fetus, be it head, breech, shoulder or compound presentation, can be simply and accurately diagnosed by ultrasound. It should always be done before labor induction, cesarean sections, preterm deliveries, deliveries of multiple gestations and in cases of planned vaginal deliveries after previous cesarean sections.

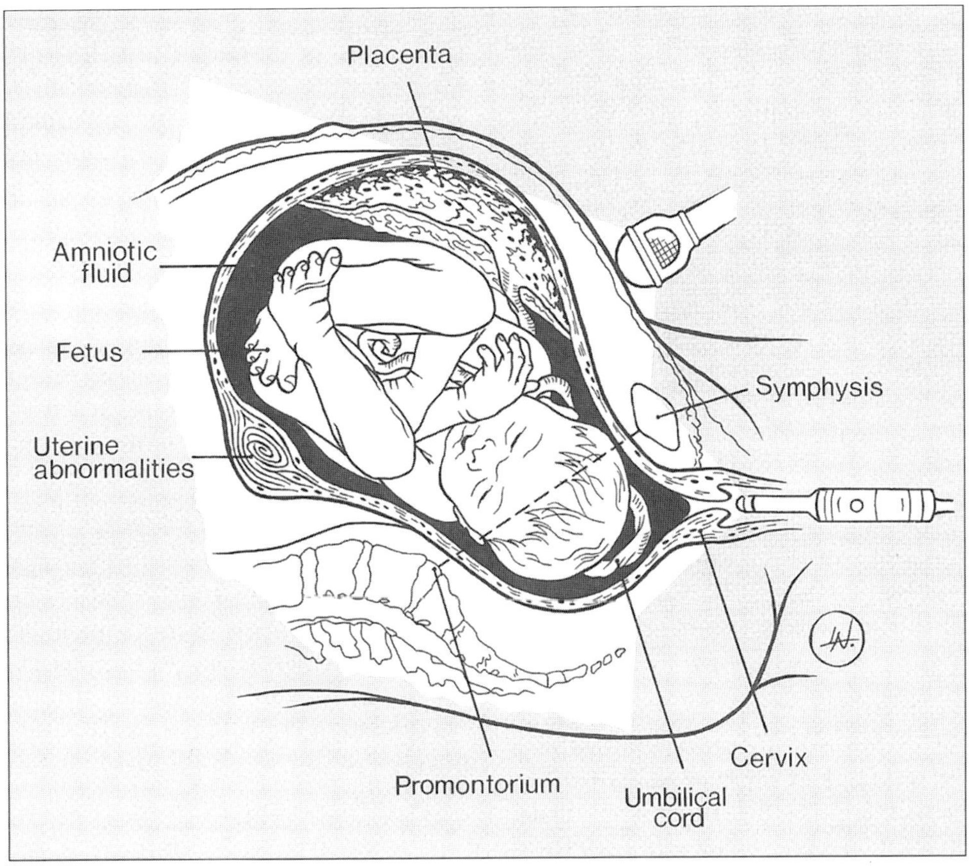

Figure 36.1 Potential use of intrapartum ultrasound.

Placenta location

Intrapartum vaginal bleeding and transverse lie are diagnoses in which ultrasound can be of assistance to confirm or rule out placenta previa or low-lying placenta. Prior to cesarean delivery, ultrasound can be an aid to locate the placenta and help to decide the type of uterine incision.

Intrapartum assessment of amniotic fluid

Ultrasound has made it possible to assess the amount of amniotic fluid. Several semiquantitative methods for evaluation of amniotic fluid volume, such as the largest vertical pocket and amniotic fluid index (AFI), have been published. A single largest vertical pocket of < 2 cm was labeled as oligohydramnios and a pocket of > 8 cm as hydramnios. Phelan and coworkers[4] described a four-quadrant method to measure the amount of amniotic fluid. A value of AFI < 5 cm was designated as oligohydramnios and a value of AFI > 24 cm as polyhydramnios. The umbilical cord and fetal limbs should be excluded from the measurement.[4–6] Since its introduction in clinical praxis, AFI has been widely accepted as an accurate method to estimate amniotic fluid volume. In antepartum surveillance, an AFI < 5 cm was considered to be associated with an increased risk of adverse pregnancy outcome and cesarean section for fetal distress.[7–9] Likewise, an intrapartum AFI < 5 cm was considered to be associated with neonatal metabolic acidosis.[5,10] Premature rupture of membranes, growth deficiency, postdate pregnancy and fetal renal anomalies are related to a reduced amount of amniotic fluid. A marked reduction in amniotic fluid increases the risk of cord compression and fetal death during labor, especially in postdate pregnancies.[6] Oligohydramnios in early labor should alert the obstetrician, and it is recommended that careful intrapartum surveillance be used. However, in the past several years AFI has been questioned as the appropriate method of defining oligohydramnios. Results from randomized trials showed that the use of AFI compared with the largest vertical pocket was associated with a significantly higher rate of suspected oligohydramnios.[11] The use of the test may increase interventions without improving neonatal outcome.[11,12] A meta-analysis of 42 reports found only one study that correlated intrapartum AFI with the rate of umbilical arterial pH < 7.00.[13]

Moreover, Moses[14] showed in a randomized study of 499 pregnancies that neither the AFI nor the single-pocket technique that was undertaken as a fetal admission test intrapartum identified a pregnancy that was at risk of an adverse outcome. As regards amnioinfusion for umbilical cord compression, in a systematic review of 12 studies it appears to reduce the occurrence of variable decelerations, lower the use of cesarean section for suspected fetal distress and is associated with a reduction in puerperal infection.[15–17] Amnioinfusion can also reduce the incidence of meconium aspiration.[17,18] Hofmeyr[18] performed a systematic review of two studies of 285 women related to prophylactic vs. therapeutic amnioinfusion for oligohydramnios in labor. There is no advantage of prophylactic amnioinfusion over therapeutic amnioinfusion carried out only when fetal heart rate (FHR) decelerations or thick meconium staining of the liquor occurred.[18] Likewise, in one study of 66 women serial amnioinfusion for preterm rupture of membranes did not detect significant differences concerning cesarean section rate, low Apgar score or neonatal death rate. The author does not recommend the use of serial amnioinfusion for preterm rupture of membranes.[19] Ultrasound may be useful to monitor this procedure.

Fetal malformations

Preterm labor, breech presentations and multiple gestations imply an increased risk of fetal malformations. Ultrasound can be used to look for fetal malformations in these clinical situations. The detection of an unsuspected fetal malformation may change the obstetrical management.[20] Anencephaly or infantile polycystic kidneys have a dismal prognosis, and cesarean section should be avoided on fetal indications. The vaginal probe and a diagnostic amnioinfusion may permit a definitive diagnosis of bilateral renal agenesis or Potter syndrome with severe oligohydramnios. That diagnosis is not possible with the poorer resolution of the transabdominal (TA) approach.[21] In addition, color Doppler ultrasonography is useful to demonstrate the presence or absence of renal arteries. Diaphragmatic hernia as well as some structural or functional abnormalities of the fetal heart may require prompt surgical or medical treatment after delivery, so an accurate diagnosis before delivery is a prerequisite for appropriate neonatal management. Conjoined twins or sacrococcygeal teratoma may cause soft tissue dystocia, and cesarean section should be advised. In addition, ultrasound detection of a severe fetal malformation in preterm labor can exclude the need for tocolytic therapy.

Estimation of fetal weight

Accurate knowledge of fetal weight in early labor is important. Many clinical situations in an acute care setting require quick decision making, often based on estimated birth weight. Intrauterine growth retardation, preterm labor, post-term gestations, suspicion of macrosomia and twin and breech presentations are some of the clinical situations in which prediction of fetal weight may influence the management decision. Clinical estimation of fetal weight by abdominal palpation may be highly inaccurate, especially in the extremes of fetal size.[22,23] Since the introduction of ultrasound in obstetrics, a variety of equations using biparietal diameter (BPD), head circumference (HC), abdominal diameter (AD), abdominal circumference (AC) and femur length (FL) have been evaluated to find the most accurate way to predict fetal weight. It is now generally accepted that ultrasound estimation of fetal weight is more reliable than clinical estimation. Ultrasound has contributed to an improvement in estimation of birth weight,[22–26,29–31] although a few reports have questioned its accuracy.[27,28] The accuracy of ultrasound estimation of fetal weight is $\pm$10–15%. To avoid errors caused by a low station of the fetal head and molding or dolichocephaly in breech presentations, formulas based on FL and AC or adjusting BPD using cephalic index or HC should be used intrapartum.[24,25,29–32] In spite of inherent difficulties, the accuracy of intrapartum estimations of fetal weights performed by the house staff in a busy labor and delivery unit is comparable to that reported by more experienced examiners.[24,25] Furthermore, Pattersson[24] found that amniotic fluid volume, cervical dilatation or station of the fetal head did not influence the accuracy of intrapartum estimation of fetal weight.

Fetal well-being during labor

The biophysical profile (BPP)

Several methods for assessing the fetal well-being and identifying a fetus at risk of intrauterine death or injury have been evaluated. Manning[33,34] originally described the BPP. The ability to see the fetus, its activities and environment yielded the concept of the 'fetus as a patient'. The four components included in the BPP based on ultrasound parameters are fetal breathing movements, fetal body movements, fetal tone and AFI. A reassuring BPP score of > 8 confers a high probability of perinatal survival, and it accurately predicts antepartum umbilical venous pH.[34,35] FHR and fetal body movements are the most sensitive indicators of impending asphyxia antepartum. Oligohydramnios is associated with chronic fetal stress, and the absence of fetal body movements is predictive of impending fetal demise.[34] As labor progresses, a decrease in the fetal motor activity is a normal finding.[36,37] Fetal apnea is also a normal phenomenon during labor and has no adverse prognostic significance.[37] Sasson *et al.*[38] did not find a correlation between the intrapartum BPP and umbilical pH. Chua and coworkers[39] tried to select the best screening test to identify fetal compromise during labor. They concluded that women in early labor with an equivocal admission test should be assessed by an additional test like AFI, umbilical artery Doppler or vibroacustic stimulation, which might be of some help to detect a fetus with an increased risk of adverse outcome. Although observational studies[33–35,40] found that BPP score gives the best prediction of both acute and chronic fetal compromise, a systematic review of RCTs (four studies of 2849 patients) do not support the use of the BPP as a test of fetal well-being in high-risk pregnancies.[41] However, the power of these studies is not strong enough to prove that the BPP score is without value.[42] Kim *et al.*[40] has recently found that cessation of any ultrasound component of BPP intrapartum significantly increased the risk of cesarean delivery and admission to the neonatal intensive care unit.

Intrapartum Doppler

Antepartum Doppler studies have shown an association between Doppler velocimetry and fetal well-being,[43] and the use of Doppler for antepartum surveillance in high-risk pregnancies can significantly reduce perinatal mortality in these cases.[43–46] The first intrapartum Doppler studies were performed with continuous and pulsed wave Doppler. Later, color Doppler and the transvaginal (TV) approach came into use. The most commonly examined vessels are the umbilical artery, uterine artery, fetal middle cerebral artery and aorta. There are three semiquantitative parameters that evaluate velocity waveform: pulsatility index (PI), resistance index (RI) and systolic/diastolic ratio (S/D). Uterine contractions, fetal breathing movements and frequent alterations in maternal position during painful contractions, as well as engagement of the fetal head in the bony pelvis, may make it difficult to get intrapartum Doppler signals.[47] Fairlie and colleagues[48] have, however, shown that the reproducibility of umbilical artery Doppler recordings during labor was comparable to the corresponding reproducibility from antepartum recordings. There is no significant change in the umbilical artery resistance during normal labor.[47–50] Neither amniotomy nor oxytocin infusion changes the umbilical artery resistence.[48] Likewise, epidural block with enough replacement has no negative effect on the S/D ratio.[51] Although Feinkind and coworkers[52] found that intrapartum screening with Doppler was sensitive enough to identify the fetus at risk of poor perinatal outcome, its use as a labor admission test is uncertain. At least two studies observed that intrapartum umbilical artery Doppler velocimetry is not a good predictor of fetal distress among unselected patients.[53,54]

Only in a high-risk population has a correlation been observed between the umbilical S/D ratio and umbilical cord pH.[48,52] The intrapartum umbilical artery S/D ratio might be of help in differentiating between variable decelerations caused by hypoxia or by mechanical occlusion.[55] It can also distinguish between true- and false-positive intrapartum late decelerations.[56] In the uterine arteries and their branches, a markedly reduced blood flow during normal labor has been noticed by several investigators.[47,49,51] Apart from intrauterine growth retardation and pre-eclampsia, preterm labor is also associated with a significantly higher uterine artery S/D ratio, probably due to decidual vascular abnormalities.[51] The few studies on fetal aortal blood flow have shown decreased flow during labor if intrapartum analgesia with pethidine and with a paracervical block were used.[47,57] In cases with no analgesia or with epidural blocks, an increased intrapartum fetal aortic blood flow was noted.[57] Doppler studies of fetal cerebral blood flow in labor may help to explain the pathophysiology of intrapartum asphyxia. Published data are, however, considerably controversial.[58–62] The aims of future investigations should be to elucidate the possible factors influencing the waveform pattern and the possible reasons for discrepancy in current reports.

Term and preterm premature rupture of the membranes (PROM, PPROM)

In cases of PROM, ultrasound assessment may be of diagnostic help in the labor and delivery unit. The amniotic fluid volume assessment, BPP and cervix status are ultrasound parameters of importance for evaluation of fetal well-being as well as for estimation of the conditions for induction of labor. To look for evidence of subclinical infection, a diagnostic amniocentesis may be performed. In patients with PROM, it has been shown that the overall BPP of the healthy fetus is not altered.[63,64] The most important parameters to evaluate fetal well-being are the amount of amniotic fluid and fetal breathing movements. Thus, PROM with severe oligohydramnios is accompanied by variable decelerations due to cord compression, an increased risk of metabolic acidosis, chorioamnionitis and a higher rate of cesarean section.[9,63–65] It seems that FHR alone and BPP are poor predictors of intrautorino infection. In a prospective study of 225 pregnancies complicated by PPROM with delivery between 24 and 32 weeks' gestation, AFI < 5 cm was the only significant risk factor independently associated with early-onset neonatal sepsis and chorioamnionitis.[66] Nowak also concluded that oligohydramnios might be associated with increased risk of chorioamnionitis.[67] While Vintzileos[68] recommended frequent estimation of the BPP as a simple test to predict the fetus at risk of developing sepsis, and questioned amniocentesis as a method to detect the fetus at risk of infection, Yoon[69] found amniotic fluid white blood cell count to be the best predictor of positive amniotic fluid culture, histological and clinical chorioamnionitis and neonatal morbidity. In a review of 12 studies, Hofmeyr found that amnioinfusion to prevent infection in women with membranes ruptured for more than 6 h was associated with a reduction in puerperal infection.[19] Amnioinfusion for umbilical cord compression in labor reduced FHR decelerations, cesarean section for suspected fetal distress, neonatal hospital stay > 3 days and maternal hospital stay > 3 days.[15] The assessment of fetal age, weight and presentation is important when determining optimal management. Tsoi *et al.*[70] studied 101 women presented with preterm prelabor amniorrhexis. He measured cervix length by TV ultrasound and concluded that prediction of delivery within 7 days is provided by cervical length, gestation and presence of contractions at presentations.

Threatened preterm labor

More than 70% of the women presenting with threatened preterm labor do not progress to active labor and delivery. When confronted with a potential of preterm labor, ultrasound evaluation can provide important information, such as gestational age, fetal weight, presentation, BPP and the status of the cervix. Doppler velocimetry can detect cases associated with uteroplacental impairment. Severe fetal malformations and placental abruption should be excluded prior to the institution of tocolytic therapy. Gestational age and birth weight are the most important predictors of neonatal survival. None of the various formulas for estimation of fetal weight seems to have superiority when applied to preterm labor.[71] In very-low-birth weight fetuses, ultrasound estimation of fetal weight is very accurate and correlates with neonatal survival.[72] Fetal presentation can drastically change the delivery management. The value of the BPP to predict impending preterm delivery has been studied.[73] The individual biophysical parameters, especially fetal tone rather than the total score, demonstrate a strong relationship with the time interval to delivery.[74] It has been shown that the presence or absence of fetal breathing movements might be helpful in differentiating between true and false preterm labor.[73] Rising fetal prostaglandin levels during either term or preterm labor affect the fetal respiratory center, and provide a possible explanation for the cessation of fetal breathing movements during labor.[75,76] A recently published systematic review regarding the accuracy of absence of fetal breathing movements in predicting preterm birth confirmed that the absence of fetal breathing has the potential to be a useful test in predicting preterm birth both within 7 days and within 48 h of testing.[77] Future research is needed.

Cervical sonography allows determination of cervical length, funneling, the cervical index (funnel length + 1/endocervical length), originally described by Andersen and colleagues,[78] and dynamic changes in cervical anatomy.[79] With the TV approach, errors due to a low presenting part, maternal obesity or an overdistended bladder can be avoided.[80] The transperineal or translabial approach is a good alternative for departments where vaginal probes are not available in the labor and delivery suite. Prolapse of the amniotic sac through a dilated internal cervical os can also be observed and has been described as the 'hourglass membranes'.[81]

Although ultrasound assessment of the cervix seemed to be better than digital examination to predict preterm delivery,[78–83] qualitative analysis of nine studies using a cervical length cutoff of 18–30 mm showed that TV ultrasound assessment of cervical dilatation or length has poor predictive value.[84] The sensitivity for predicting preterm birth varied from 68% to 100% and the specificity ranged from 54% to 90%. In the most recently published studies of women with threatened preterm labor, cervical length cutoff of <15 mm seemed to have a higher probability to predict preterm delivery within 7 days.[85,86] Thus, sonographic measurement of cervical length helps to distinguish between true and false labor and to avoid overdiagnosis of preterm labor.[85,86]

Intrapartum vaginal bleeding

Two major clinical causes of vaginal intrapartum bleeding, which may require ultrasound expertise, are placenta previa and placental abruption. The TA approach may result in high false-positive (2–7%) and false-negative (2–8%) rates for placenta previa, depending on the time of scanning.[87,88] An overdistended bladder, maternal obesity, the posterior location of the placenta, the presence of fresh blood clots and an acoustic shadowing from the fetal head are the factors that make the diagnosis of placenta previa difficult. Considerable improvement has been achieved by TV ultrasound, where a false-positive rate of 1% and a false-negative rate of 2% have been observed.[87] The focal zone of the vaginal probe is 2–8 cm, which provides optimal imaging of the internal os. It is enough to insert the probe at a distance of 2 cm remote from the external os to avoid severe bleeding.

Tan *et al.*[89] studied the role of TV sonography in the diagnosis of placenta previa and performed TV sonography in 70 women diagnosed to have placenta previa by TA sonography. The diagnostic accuracy of the TV approach was 92.8%, compared with 75.7% for the TA route. They concluded that TV sonographic localization of the placenta is superior to the TA approach for types 1 and 2 placenta previa, but no better for types 3 and 4. TV color Doppler seems promising in the diagnosis of placenta previa accreta.[90,91] The ultrasound appearance of placental abruption can vary. A high false-negative rate is a problem. The normal anechoic retroplacental area with signs of venous flow identified by pulsed Doppler should not be interpreted as a placental abruption.[92] Nyberg *et al.*[93] reported results of 57 cases of placental abruption, retrospectively reviewed. The location of the hemorrhage was subchorionic in 81%, retroplacental in 16% and preplacental in 4% of the cases. The fetal mortality rate was 20% with a placental abruption including 20% of the placenta. The ultrasound findings varied with the size and location of the hematoma, as well as with the time of the sonogram. Furthermore, the risk of fetal demise was greater in retroplacental and preplacental cases than in cases with subchorionic hematoma. In most of the cases with clinically suspected abruption, ultrasound findings are negative.[94] It is likely that the free passage of blood through the cervical os prevented the formation of a hematoma large enough to be visualized.[95] An acute hemorrhage is usually hyperechoic to isoechoic, and then gradually becomes anechoic during the following 1–2 weeks.[95,96] Rivera *et al.*[97] suggest that the use of ultrasound and non-stress testing in the expectant management of placental abruption could result in a decrease in maternal and perinatal mortality and morbidity. It must, however, be remembered that a negative ultrasound finding should not postpone essential treatment when there is a clinical suspicion of placental abruption.

Dystocia in early and late labor

Dystocia – poor progress of labor – is one of the leading indications for operative delivery, and it has previously been shown that mechanical problems in labor are responsible for a great number of all cesarean sections.[98] Cephalopelvic disproportion should be suspected in cases with an unengaged fetal head during labor, or in women with previous cesarean section due to dystocia. Efforts have been made to establish ultrasound diagnostic criteria to estimate cephalopelvic disproportion during early labor, based on results from ultrasound determination of the true conjugate and the transverse diameter of the pelvic inlet before labor.[99,100] This requires, however, special equipment and considerable expertise. Dystocia in late labor can be caused by persistent occiput position. Clinical evaluation of the position of the fetal head by digital palpation is sometimes uncertain and inaccurate due to scalp edema, which causes difficulties in recognition of the sutures and the fontanelles. Akmal *et al.*[101] studied the accuracy of intrapartum routine digital examination in defining the position of the fetal head and found that digital examination during labor failed to identify the correct fetal position in the majority of 496 cases. Likewise, he found among 64 women that digital examination during instrumental delivery failed to identify the correct fetal head position in 26.6% of cases.[102] Ultrasound diagnosis of persistent occiput posterior position is simple, by visualization of the facial bones and orbits anteriorly and the spine posteriorly. In contrast, persistent occiput anterior position is confirmed when the facial bones and orbits are placed posteriorly and the spine anteriorly. The risk of cesarean section can be estimated during the early stage of active labor by the sonographically determined occiput position.[103] Rayburn *et al.*[104] studied 86 patients with arrested labor and showed that intrapartum ultrasound significantly improved the diagnosis of persistent occiput position, and could be of help in the management of delivery. Chou[105] confirmed this recently. If midpelvic forceps or vacuum extraction is to be performed, precise knowledge of the position of the fetal head is mandatory; a more proper forceps application and proper axis of traction may then be applied. Persistent occiput anterior position associated with labor dystocia is indicative of fetal macrosomia, and shoulder dystocia can be expected.[104] A new method to assess the descent of the fetal head in labor with transperineal ultrasound has been presented.[106] Head deflection may cause either a brow or a face presentation and then an abnormally broad diameter makes the passage through the maternal pelvis difficult. Such head deflection can be detected by ultrasound. Clinically, face presentation can be mistaken for breech presentation, especially if there is facial edema. Ultrasound examination can accurately exclude such an unpleasant surprise in the delivery unit. Knowledge of the position of the mentum anterior and occiput posterior is mandatory for allowing vaginal delivery in cases with face presentation, and this can be confirmed by ultrasound. With a brow presentation, engagement of the fetal head and delivery usually cannot take place if it persists. The brow presentation can, however, be converted to either a vertex or face presentation to allow vaginal delivery.[107] With a transverse lie during early labor, the position of the head and back as well as the location of the placenta should be identified before an external version or a cesarean section is undertaken. When the back is anterior, the risk of cord prolapse is greater. Information obtained from ultrasound can facilitate the performance of the cesarean section.

Breech presentation

A recently published review of RCTs concerning the preferred method of delivery for breech at term, showed that cesarean delivery occurred in 550/1227 (45%) of those women allocated to a vaginal delivery protocol.[108] Perinatal mortality and morbidity was greatly reduced in the planned cesarean section group (RR=0.31, 95% CI 0.19–0.52). Reviewers concluded that planned cesarean section for breech at term should be the preferred method of delivery. Result of this review has considerably influenced obstetrical praxis regarding the delivery mode for breech at term.

Nowadays, there is enough evidence that external cephalic version reduces not only breech presentation at delivery, but also cesarean section rate.[109] Ultrasound may be of help during an external version of a breech fetus at term. Ferguson *et al.*[110] performed successful external version in 11 of 15 women at term who presented in active labor. In contrast, a review of three RCTs of 889 women shows that external cephalic version (ECV) is not useful in preterm breech presentations.[111] However, if ECV fails and vaginal breech delivery is the patient's preference or if a breech presentation is diagnosed during early labor, a thorough and targeted ultrasound evaluation should be performed. Valuable information that can be obtained by ultrasound includes:

(1) type of breech (frank, complete or footling)
(2) estimated birth weight
(3) amniotic fluid volume assessment
(4) placental location (rule out placenta previa)
(5) rule out malformations (anencephaly, infantile polycystic kidneys).

Additional information that substantially influences the decision making can also be obtained by ultrasound, i.e.:

(1) fetal head position (hyperextension)
(2) nuchal or extended arm
(3) nuchal cord
(4) cord presentation
(5) cephalopelvic disproportion.

The gold standard for evaluation of the maternal pelvis has long been x-ray pelvimetry. This technique can expose both fetus and mother to possible long-term radiation hazards.[107] Rojansky *et al.*[99] proposed a simple ultrasound method for diagnosis of hyperextension of the fetal head by measurement of the cranio-spinal angle, and a method to measure the obstetrical conjugate by TA ultrasound. He studied 72 laboring women with breech presentations and performed both traditional x-ray and ultrasound evaluation of the head position, type of breech and pelvic adequacy. A highly significant correlation between the two methods was demonstrated. He suggests that the ultrasound approach is reliable and may replace the x-ray method in management of breech presentation in labor. Although similar suggestions have been proposed previously,[100,112,113] sonographic pelvimetry has not yet become a routine praxis.

Ultrasound indications for cesarean sections, according to Rojansky, are: a cranio-spinal angle of 150°, an obstetrical conjugate of <10 cm and certain non-frank breech presentations. Ballas *et al.*[114] suggest that hyperextension of the fetal head (angle > 90°) that was present on radiographic assessment should be a contraindication to labor. Among 20 babies reported to have an angle > 90°, 8 of 11 delivered vaginally sustained cervical cord lesions. The nine babies delivered by cesarean section had no cervical damage. Sherer[115] suggests an additional indication for abdominal delivery, namely 'nuchal arm' (extension of an arm behind the fetal head). This condition can be diagnosed by ultrasound. He pointed out that nuchal arm is a cause of severe birth trauma, and can result in persistent Erb's palsy, torticollis and convulsions. Ultrasound can identify a nuchal cord with single or multiple coils, although its clinical value is still controversial.[116] Lange *et al.*[117] defined cord presentation as the finding on ultrasound of loops of the umbilical cord below the fetal body and occupying the lower segment. Estimation of birth weight should be performed in patients with breech presentations, who prefer vaginal delivery; weights between 2000 and 4000 g are reasonable limits within which a trial of labor can be permitted.[118,119] When fetal weight is estimated in breech presentations, dolichocephaly should be identified by the cephalic index, and corrections made for this. For the purpose of avoiding errors due to dolichocephaly, formulas based on FL, AD or AC should be used.[31,32]

Intrapartum management of multiple gestations

Ultrasound is an indispensable diagnostic tool for intrapartum management of multiple gestations. Presentations and estimated weights are most important when deciding on the mode and route of delivery. Estimation of fetal weight in twin gestations during labor seems to be reliable regardless of presentation, gestational age or the presence of discordant twins.[120,121] The general goal is vaginal delivery unless the presenting twin is lying non-longitudinally. A retrospective study comparing neonatal morbidity in term twins delivered by cesarean section with vaginal delivery found that neonatal respiratory disorders were significantly more common in the first group.[122] In vertex/vertex twins, vaginal deliveries are most often planned. It has to be remembered, however, that in about 20% of the cases, the second twin will change position once the first is delivered.[123] Therefore, ultrasound assessment should always be performed after delivery of the presenting twin, so that a transverse lie can be turned into a longitudinal lie.[123–126] Moreover, ultrasound should be used to assess the FHR of the second twin, and may be of help if a suddenly compromised second twin needs a swift delivery by internal version and extraction. The same maneuver should be done if external version of the second twin to longitudinal lie fails. If there is a vertex/non-vertex presentation, the ultrasonic estimated birth weight will be of vital importance when deciding on the route of delivery. Estimated birth weights between 2000 and 4000 g can be allowed for breech deliveries,[124] provided there is a pelvic adequacy, no substantial growth discordance, no cord presentations, nuchal cord, extended arm or head deflection. A retrospective study of 408 twin deliveries showed that external cephalic version of the second twin and subsequent vaginal delivery in vertex/non-vertex was successful in 75% of the cases. Internal podalic version and assisted breech delivery was performed in 20 cases and the remaining two were delivered by cesarean section. Apgar scores were not significantly different among the various groups and no complications arouse from external cephalic version performed on the second non-vertex twin.[127]

Induction of labor

Pre-eclampsia, intrauterine growth retardation, postdate pregnancies and diabetic pregnancies are common causes of labor induction. In postdate pregnancies, the presence of severe oligohydramnios, fetal macrosomia and unfavorable cervix can be revealed by ultrasound. Bishop[128] originally described evaluation of the cervix before induction of labor by digital vaginal examination. The results of numerous studies concerning the evaluation of the cervix by ultrasound are contradicting.[129–136] An unfavorable cervix results in failed induction in 3–5% of the cases. A careful evaluation of the cervix before induction of labor may help to avoid complications, such as failed inductions, leading to cesarean section. Since the introduction of TV ultrasound cervicometry, it has been possible to assess the cervical status more objectively, and our ability to predict the course of labor seemed to be improved.[129] A sagittal section of the cervix can be seen between the anterior anechogenic bladder and echogenic rectum. Although the cervical length and dilatation can be objectively measured by ultrasound, the consistency of the cervix can be assessed only by digital vaginal examination. Therefore, a combination of digital examination and vaginal ultrasound assessment was recommended. The Bishop score would seem to be the best and most cost-effective method to assess the cervix and predict the likelihood of success of labor induction and the duration of such an induction. It seems that TV ultrasound does not predict successful labor induction in post-term pregnancy as well as digital cervical examination.[130] Reis *et al.*[131] obtained similar results concerning induction at term. They found ultrasound measurement of the cervix and fibronectin test failed to predict accurately the outcome of induced labor. Digital examination and obstetric history were the only variables independently associated with labor duration and predicted accurately vaginal delivery within 24 h. Roman *et al.*[137] showed that neither the Bishop score nor the cervical length by ultrasound was a good predictor for the outcome of labor induction in an unfavorable cervix. In contrast, recently published studies as regards the value of ultrasound in the prediction of successful induction of labor found sonographic parameters (cervical length, occipital position posterior, cervical angle) superior to the Bishop score.[132,133] The same authors studied induction of labor for prolonged pregnancy and found cervical length and parity to be significant independent prediction of the likelihood of cesarean section, prediction of induction to delivery interval and the likelihood of vaginal delivery within 24 h of induction.[134,135] In postdate pregnancies or diabetic pregnancies, fetal macrosomia should be ruled out since large-for-date infants have an increased risk of traumatic birth injury.[136–138] Formulas based on FL and AC has the best correlation with actual birth weight in macrosomia.[139] Great efforts have been made to diminish the number of cases of shoulder dystocia, which is a nightmare for the obstetrician.[140–143] A cut-off value of 1.4 cm for the difference between the chest diameter and BPD[143] or 2.6 cm for the difference between AD and BPD[144] can be helpful in estimating the risk of shoulder dystocia, and can thus be helpful in deciding the appropriate route of delivery. The fetal subcutaneous tissue/FL ratio is an additional gestational age-independent parameter for the intrapartum identification of a macrosomic fetus.[145] Vaginal birth after cesarean section has been advocated as a safe method to reduce the increasing cesarean section rate.[146] Prior to a trial of labor, the myometrial thickness in the area of the prior cesarean scar can be examined by ultrasound. It has been shown that defects in the lower uterine segment or abnormal uterine thickness can be visualized by ultrasound.[148]

Third stage of labor

Herman *et al.*[149] investigated the third stage of labor by dynamic ultrasound. They showed that, immediately after delivery of the fetus, the placenta-free uterine wall became thick and the uterine wall at the site of the placenta remained thin. As soon as the contraction phase began, the wall behind the placenta contracted gradually and only when it attained its final thickness did the placenta detach. No hematoma was observed between the placenta and the uterine wall. Ultrasound during the third stage of labor can help clarify whether the placenta has already detached or still is adherent to the uterine wall. Directly after the delivery of the placenta, the uterine cavity is visualized as a thin bright central line. Krapp *et al.*[91] have shown that the disappearance of blood flow between the basal part of the placenta and the myometrium is the hallmark of normal placental separation: persistent blood flow due to abnormal vascular connections is suggestive of placenta accreta. Although this method can be helpful in making an early diagnosis and thus preventing heavy postpartum hemorrhage by early manual removal of the placenta, the clinical application is of limiting value due to the lack of appropriate ultrasound equipment at delivery suites.

Intrapartum uterine rupture

The actual site of uterine rupture is usually difficult to visualize by ultrasound.[150] Indirect ultrasound signs of uterine rupture are retroperitoneal hematoma and free peritoneal blood, most often localized in the cul-de-sac, the paracolic gutters or the subdiaphragmatic areas.[151,152] Sometimes, an extruded fetus or placenta can be seen. Although the clinical signs and symptoms of uterine rupture are most important, the use of ultrasound may be of additional aid in diagnosing this dangerous complication.

Puerperium

Normal ultrasound appearance of the postpartum uterus

The puerperium is defined as the period of 6–8 weeks after birth during which the reproductive tract anatomically and physiologically returns to the non-pregnant state. When faced with puerperal abnormalities, it is useful to know the normal ultrasound appearance, and the dynamic changes of the uterus during the puerperium, to better distinguish pathological from normal conditions. The involution changes concerning the size, shape and position of the uterus, as well as the appearance of the uterine cavity, can be evaluated by ultrasound.[153–160] In the early puerperium, TA ultrasound examinations are to be recommended. The woman should have a moderately filled urinary bladder. Gentle compression with the probe should be used and measurements should be made between uterine contractions to avoid uterine distortion. During the middle or late puerperal period, the TV approach is preferable. Color Doppler[161–163] and TV duplex Doppler[164] with high resolution have made it possible to study the vascular changes of the uterine involution non-invasively, and these methods have improved our ability to recognize puerperal abnormalities. The puerperal uterus should be assessed in sagittal, coronal and transverse sections (Figures 36.2 and 36.3). The coronal section is preferable for investigation of uterine malformations. Some ultrasound pictures are typical for the puerperium (Figures 36.4 and 36.6).[165] The involution of the uterus is a dynamic process that has no parallel in normal adult life. The uterine dimensions and the uterine cavity diminish progressively and substantially during the puerperium. There are two physiological lifesaving processes occurring soon after placenta delivery: thrombotamponade (enhanced blood clotting activity) and myotamponade (compression of the vessels by myometrial contraction). The appearance of ultrasound finding during early puerperium reflects these physiological changes. The normal shape of the uterus in the sagittal plane during the first postpartum days has been described as a 'hockey stick',[166] or a 'crescent'[156] (Figures 36.4a and 36.6a). This form of the uterus is typical only in the early puerperium and it is artificial. An extremely high degree of uterine deformability is caused by a heavy uterine corpus, a hypotonic lower uterine segment and supine position of the examined woman. In the second postpartum week, the shape changes and becomes more globular. The position of the uterus also changes. In the early period the uterus arches over the sacral promontory in a retroverted position. Wachsberg *et al.*[166] pointed out the importance of this uterine angulation and its effect on the measurements of uterine length. The uterus rotates (Figure 36.5) along its internal cervical os and in the majority of women it achieves an anteverted position in the beginning of the second postpartum week. This position is then retained. In only a few women does the uterus return to a retroverted position at the end of puerperium.[165] Concomitantly with the changes in dimension, shape and position of the uterus, the uterine cavity goes through a marked process of involution. During the first three postpartum days,

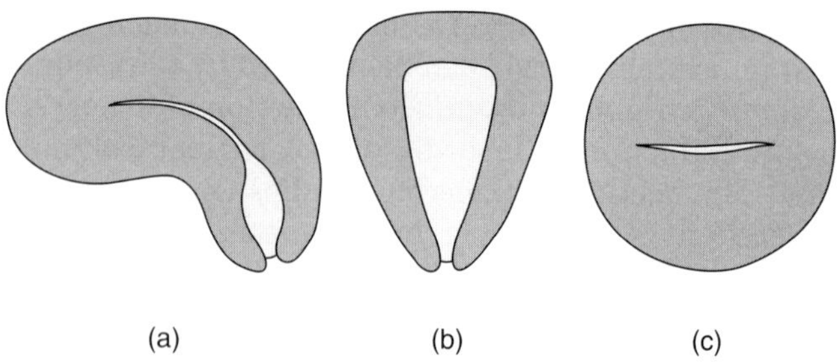

Figure 36.2 Three standard sections of the puerperal uterus: a longitudinal (a), a coronal (b) and a transverse (c).

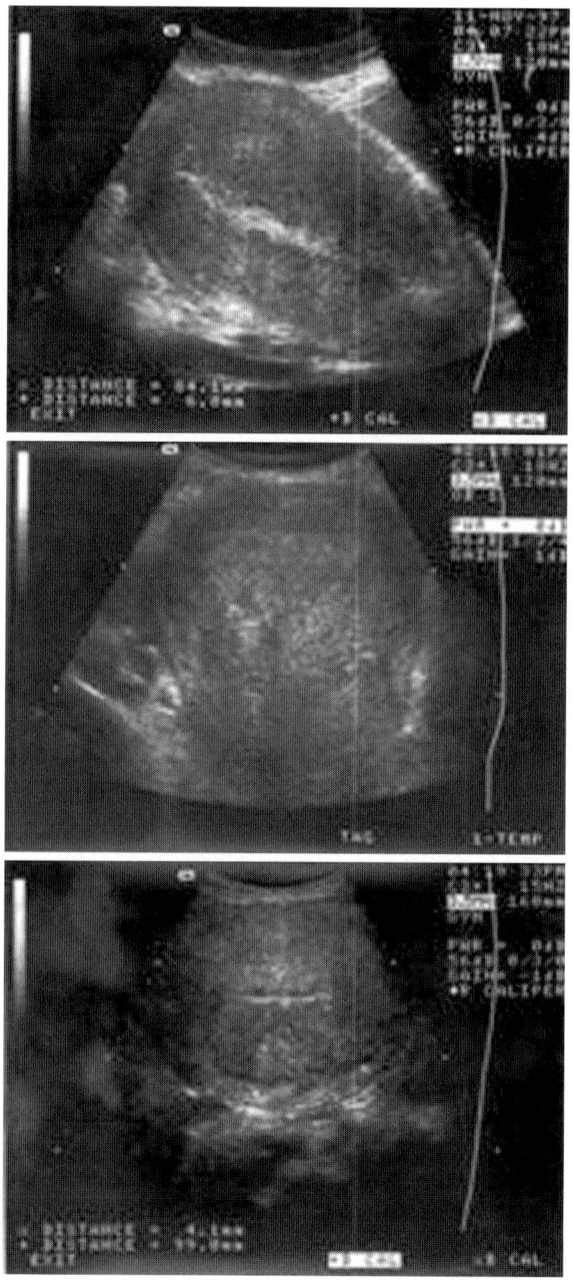

Figure 36.3 TA ultrasound scans of a normal puerperal uterus on day 1: a longitudinal scan (a), a coronal scan (b) and a transverse scan (c).

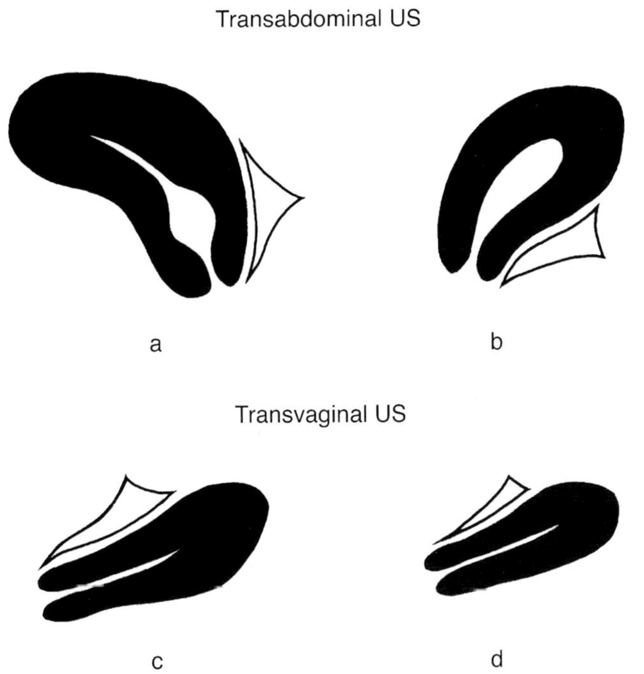

Figure 36.4 The normal ultrasound appearance of the uterus and uterine cavity during the puerperium. TA approach: (a) during the first 3 days postpartum, a 'hockey stick'-shaped retroverted uterus with an empty cavity in the upper part and fluid collection with mixed echo pattern in the lower uterine segment; (b) on days 7–14 postpartum, the uterus is oval-shaped and anteverted with fluid/mixed echo in the whole uterine cavity. TV approach: (c) 4 weeks postpartum, the size of the uterus is considerably diminished; the cavity is empty and is seen as a thin central line; (d) 8 weeks postpartum, the involution process is complete and the uterus has achieved non-pregnant dimensions and appearance.

lifesaving uterine contraction approaches the anterior and posterior uterine walls and just virtual cavity appears. It is empty and decidua appears as a thin white line from the fundus to the level of the internal cervical os (Figure 36.6a). Sometimes this line can be irregular and thicker, which probably depends on the amount of retained decidua. The separation of the placenta and membranes generally occurs in the spongy layer; however, the level varies. Already in 1931, Williams wrote concerning the line of separation of the placenta and membranes: 'While separation generally occurs in the spongy layer, the line is very irregular so that in places a thick layer of decidua is retained, in others only a few layers of cells remain, while in still others the muscularis is practically bare'.[167] The variation in the sonographic appearance of the cavity could be seen as a demonstration of these physiological variations in the retained decidua. The thin white line seen on ultrasound might possibly represent cases in which only the basal decidual layer is retained or if the muscularis is practically bare (Figure 36.6a), whereas the thicker and more irregular lines might represent cases with retention of the more spongy decidual layer and perhaps fragments of membranes. It is unusual to find a collection of fluid or any echogenic masses in the upper part of the cavity at that time. In the lower uterine segment, however, a collection of fluid with mixed echo patterns is almost always present. It comprises blood clots and probably small fragments of retained membranes.[165,166,168,169] This finding has no clinical significance and the mass is usually expelled spontaneously. Small echogenic or

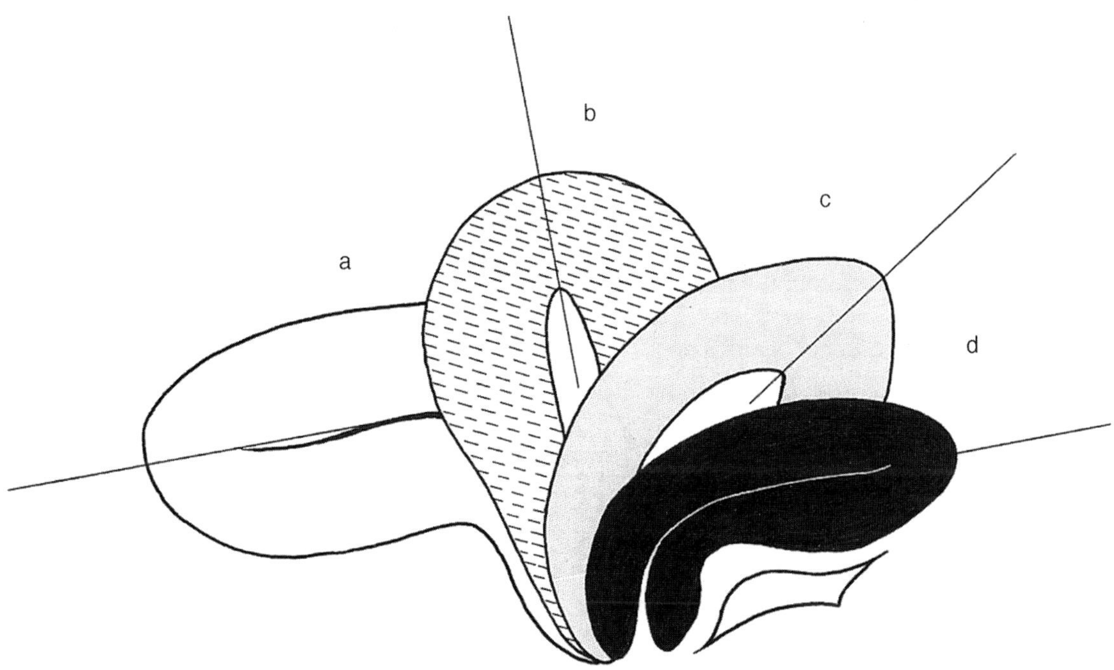

Figure 36.5 The normal rotation process of the uterus during the puerperium. The uterus usually rotates about 100–180° and changes its position from retroverted to an anteverted position during the involution period.

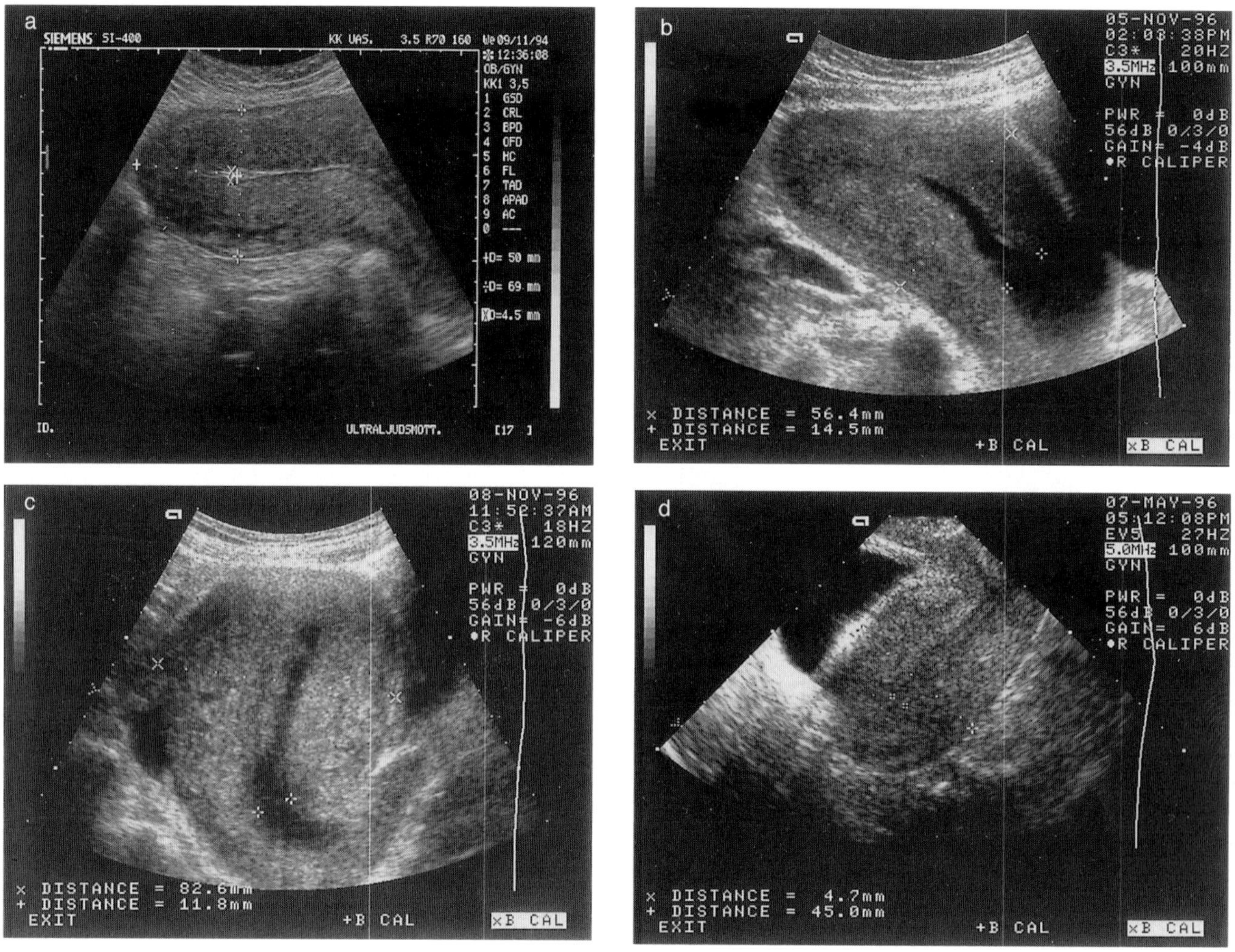

Figure 36.6 The normal ultrasound appearance of the postpartum uterus, TA approach (a, b, c) and TV approach (d). (a) On the first postpartum day the uterus has a hockey stick shape, a retroverted position and a thin endometrium. Prominent vascular channels are seen in the posterior myometrial wall. (b) One week postpartum, pure fluid is seen in the uterine cavity. (c) Two weeks' postpartum, the uterus has an oval shape, an anteverted position and a heterogenous pattern is seen in the whole uterine cavity. (d) Four weeks postpartum, the uterus is considerably diminished in size. It is empty and the uterine cavity is seen as a thin line.

echolucent dots in the cavity are harmless physiological findings.[168] In contrast, Sokol *et al.*[170] found in 16 of 40 women echogenic material in the uterine cavity within 48 h after normal vaginal delivery. On the posterior wall of the uterus, the prominent uterine vascular channels are regularly seen.[160] From days 7–14, endometrial fluid can be seen in the whole cavity, not only in the lower segment (Figure 36.6b and c). Moreover, echogenic and non-echogenic areas are seen in the whole uterine cavity, probably comprising a mixture of blood, blood clots and offcasts of necrotic decidua (Figure 36.6c). The diameter of the cavity in the upper part of the uterus may then be quite wide, which reflects a normal healing process of the placental site inside the uterine cavity, necrotic changes of retained decidua and an abundant shedding of lochia. In contrast, Edwards *et al.*[171] found an echogenic mass in a great proportion of normal puerperal women. At 4 weeks postpartum, the uterus is again empty and the uterine cavity is seen as a thin central line (Figure 36.6d). Sometimes, a small amount of fluid can be seen. By 8 weeks' postpartum, the involution process is complete, and the uterus has non-pregnant dimensions. It lies in an anteverted position in 88% of the cases.[165] In 12% of cases, the uterus has a retroverted position corresponding well to the normal prevalence of retroversion of the uterus in the general population. Decidua and necrotic vessel ends are exfoliated, the placental site is recovered and a new endometrium is regenerated from the basal layer of the decidua adjacent to the myometrium. In 1953, Sharman performed endometrium biopsies and identified fully restored endometrium from the 16th postpartum day.[172] Ultrasonically, the cavity appears as a thin white line. This corresponds to an inactive endometrium and reflects the hypoestrogenic state of the puerperium (the physiologic menopause). It is not common to find fluid or echogenic masses in the uterine cavity at that time. There are conflicting data about the presence of gas in the uterine cavity during the normal puerperium. Previous studies have suggested a correlation between gas and endometritis caused by *Escherichia coli* or

Clostridium perfringens.[159,173] These conditions are, however, nowadays very rare. Wachsberg and Kurtz[174] detected gas in the uterine cavity in 21% of the normal population, and suggested that gas in the uterine cavity did not necessarily indicate endometritis, but could be considered as a normal finding. Other investigators have not been able to confirm this.[165,168,169] Whether or not a small amount of gas is seen in the uterine cavity has, however, no clinical significance. Lavery and Shaw[160] described the prominent uterine vascular channels in the normal early postpartum period. With color Doppler, a venous blood flow could be demonstrated, which usually disappears during the second and third postpartum weeks. Besides conventional ultrasound, Doppler technology is used to study hemodynamic events occurring during the puerperium.[161–164,175,176] Normal pregnancy requires the growth of many new vessels. Consequently, during puerperium dramatically regressive changes occur. The physiological destruction of the uterus involves not only muscle cells and decidua but also arteries. Tekay[161] and Kirkiinen[162] assessed the peripheral vascular resistance of the uterine arteries in the postpartum period and found that the PI value started to increase in the early puerperium, remained unchanged during the next 6 weeks and finally increased to reach the non-pregnant values about 3 months after delivery. The prediastolic notch is also detected in the early puerperium and these hemodynamic changes can be partly explained by the immediate contraction of the uterus.[161,162] Fluid collections in the fossa of Douglas are not a common finding during the puerperium.[165,169]

Retained placental tissue

Retained placental tissue in the uterine cavity postpartum is associated with a high risk of excessive bleeding, either immediate or delayed. Immediate postpartum bleeding requires urgent management; manual evacuation of the uterine cavity is warranted. Ultrasound can be a valuable aid to confirm an empty uterine cavity after the evacuation by demonstrating the easily visible bright echogenic linear echo in the middle part of the uterus. Delayed postpartum hemorrhage occurs in about 1–2% of cases. It is most often the result of abnormal involution of the placenta site in the uterine cavity and endometritis, but it may be caused by retention of placental tissue. In developed countries, one-half of the postpartum women who are admitted to hospital with this condition undergo uterine surgical evacuation. In developing countries, it is the major contributor to maternal death.[177] Two etiological factors were identified as risk factors, namely primary postpartum hemorrhage and a history of manual removal of a retained placenta. Uterus curettage was performed in 63% of cases. Histological confirmation of the residual placental tissue was obtained in 37% following ultrasound diagnosis and in 33% without previous ultrasound examination. The decision whether to perform uterine evacuation for retained placental tissue depends on both the clinical finding and the ability to visualize retained placenta by ultrasound. Although prompt curettage seems to be necessary in many cases, it usually does not remove identifiable placental tissue.[178] Moreover, it is more likely to traumatize the implantation site and induce more bleeding. Consequently, the rate of complications is high. Hoveyda *et al.*[179] reported in his review regarding secondary postpartum hemorrhage that the frequency of perforation of the uterus was 3% and hysterectomy about 1%. Alexander *et al.*[177] identified 45 papers on the management of women with secondary postpartum hemorrhage and they concluded that no information was available from randomized trials to inform the management of women with this condition. Since curettage in the postpartum period can be dangerous, it is of great value to have a tool that can diagnose retained placental tissue. Many conflicting data exist about the ultrasound appearance of retained placenta tissue. The first studies were performed with old static ultrasound equipment.[154,173,180] They described various ultrasound images of retained placental tissue, and the rate of false-positive diagnosis was high. Despite the markedly improved imaging possibilities in the 1990s, confirmation or exclusion of retained placental tissue is still difficult.[163,164,168,169,173,179,180–182] We cannot expect the same ultrasound picture during the early (Figure 36.8a) and late periods (Figure 36.7b) of the puerperium. The ultrasound appearance of retained placental tissue may vary depending on the presence of different kinds of intrauterine contents. Necrotic decidua, blood, blood clots and inflammatory necrotic changes may essentially influence the ultrasound image. Nevertheless, the most common finding associated with retained placental tissue is an echogenic mass[164,168,169,180–181] (Figures 36.7a and 36.8a). In contrast, Edwards *et al.*[171] found in his study an echogenic mass on day 7 in 51% of normal cases, in 21% on day 14 and in 6% on day 21. He questioned the ultrasound finding of an echogenic mass in the uterine cavity as a sign of retained placental tissue. The definition of an echogenic mass was not specified. Even Sokol *et al.*[170] found 'echogenic material' in 40% of cases during 48 h after normal delivery. However, echogenic material was localized in the lower uterine segment in 14 of 16 women. On the other hand, ultrasound appears as a valuable tool to confirm an empty cavity. Lee and Mandrazzo[173] found an empty cavity in 20 of 27 patients with late puerperal bleeding. In only one case was retained placental tissue confirmed. The same authors reported that histological confirmation was obtained in eight of nine patients with ultrasound-suspected retained placental tissue. If the ultrasound finding shows an empty uterus with a thin white decidua/endometrium, pure endometrial fluid or only small

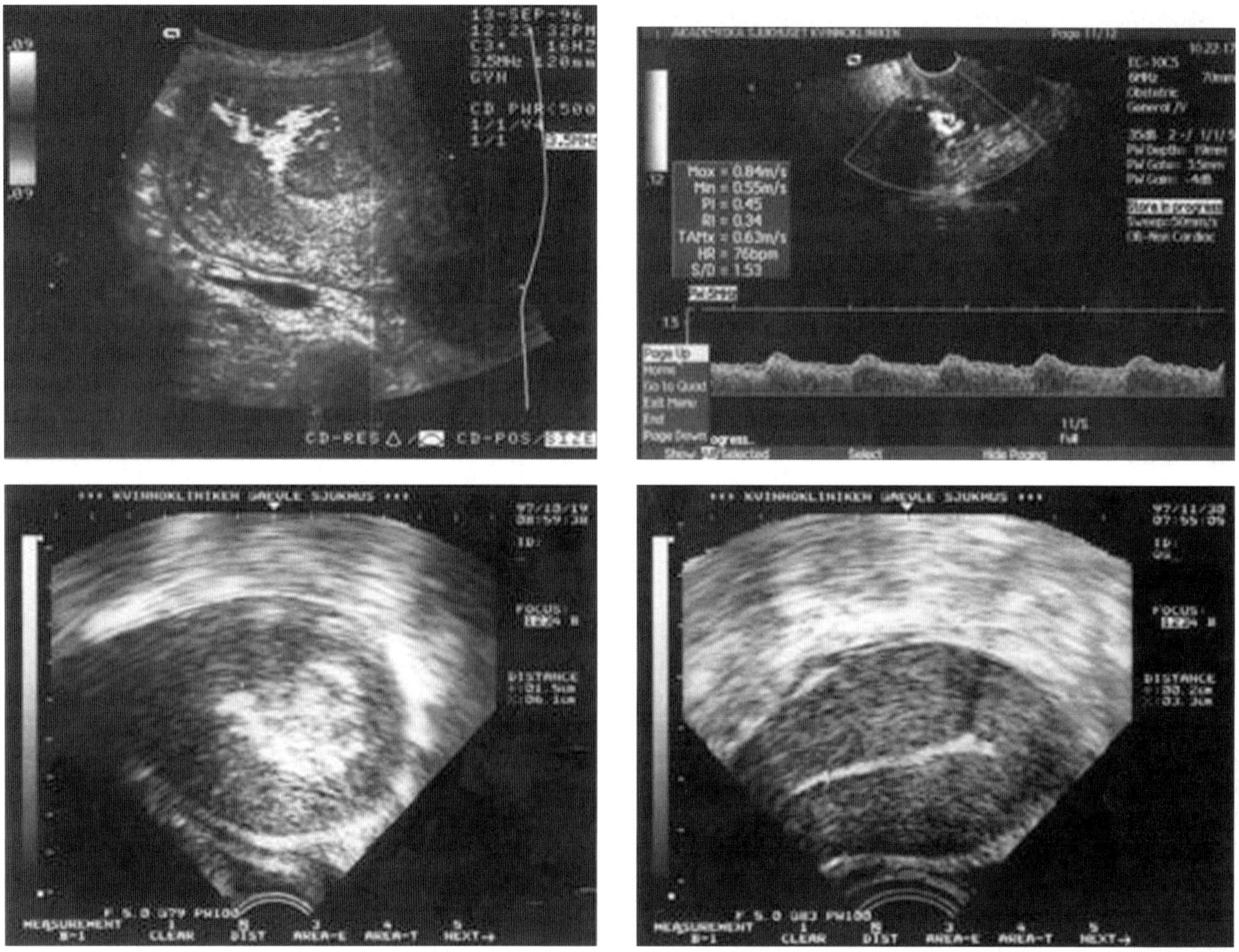

Figure 36.7 Puerperal abnormalities as seen by the TV (a,b) or TA (c,d) approach. (a) Retained placental tissue is seen as an echogenic mass surrounded by a distinct halo and easy detectable flow on the side of the mass. (b) Retained placental tissue that has persisted for a long time postpartum and is seen as 'a stippled pattern'. (c) After cesarean section, gas is observed in the uterine cavity with clean and dirty shadowing well visualized. (d) A necrotic myoma that caused dysfunctional puerperal bleeding is seen in the uterine cavity.

echolucent or hyperechogenic dots, a clinically significant amount of retained placental tissue is unlikely.[164,165,168,169] Patients with persistent dysfunctional postpartum bleeding are highly suspected of having retained placental tissue, and they often show a typical ultrasound image with a 'stippled pattern' of scattered hyperechogenic foci[168] (Figure 36.7b). Later on, the retained placental tissue becomes increasingly echogenic and the scattered appearance disappears[168] (Figure 36.8c). A heterogenous pattern may cause confusion since retained placental tissue and necrotic decidua with organized blood clots can give similar images during the first or second postpartum week. Neil *et al.*[182] compared ultrasound with clinical assessment for the diagnosis of retained placental tissue related to secondary postpartum hemorrhage. They concluded that both clinical assessment and ultrasound scan have limited diagnostic accuracy. TA two-dimensional imaging alone is not specific enough. TV ultrasound has been advocated[164] with the use of a high-frequency (6.5 MHz) TV probe to better differentiate between retained placental tissue and blood clots mixed with necrotic decidua. TV pulsed and color Doppler are promising noninvasive methods to improve the diagnostic accuracy of ultrasound concerning retained placental tissue.[161–163] Achiron *et al.*[164] looked at the myometrial arterial blood flow around intracavitary contents and found that patients with an RI below 0.35 had residual tissue (Figure 36.8b). These patients are suitable for invasive treatment. An RI above 0.45 should exclude diagnosis. Values between 0.35 and 0.45 were designated as a 'gray zone'. These patients could be treated conservatively with repeated ultrasound examinations, and curettage should be performed only if conservative treatment failed. Alcazar *et al.*[175] found an RI value < 0.45 to be suggestive of retained placental tissue. We observed easily detectable flow, always on the side of the circumscript echogenic mass, which was histologically proven to be retained placental tissue (Figures 36.7a and 36.8a). It may be speculated that this highly vascularized area is

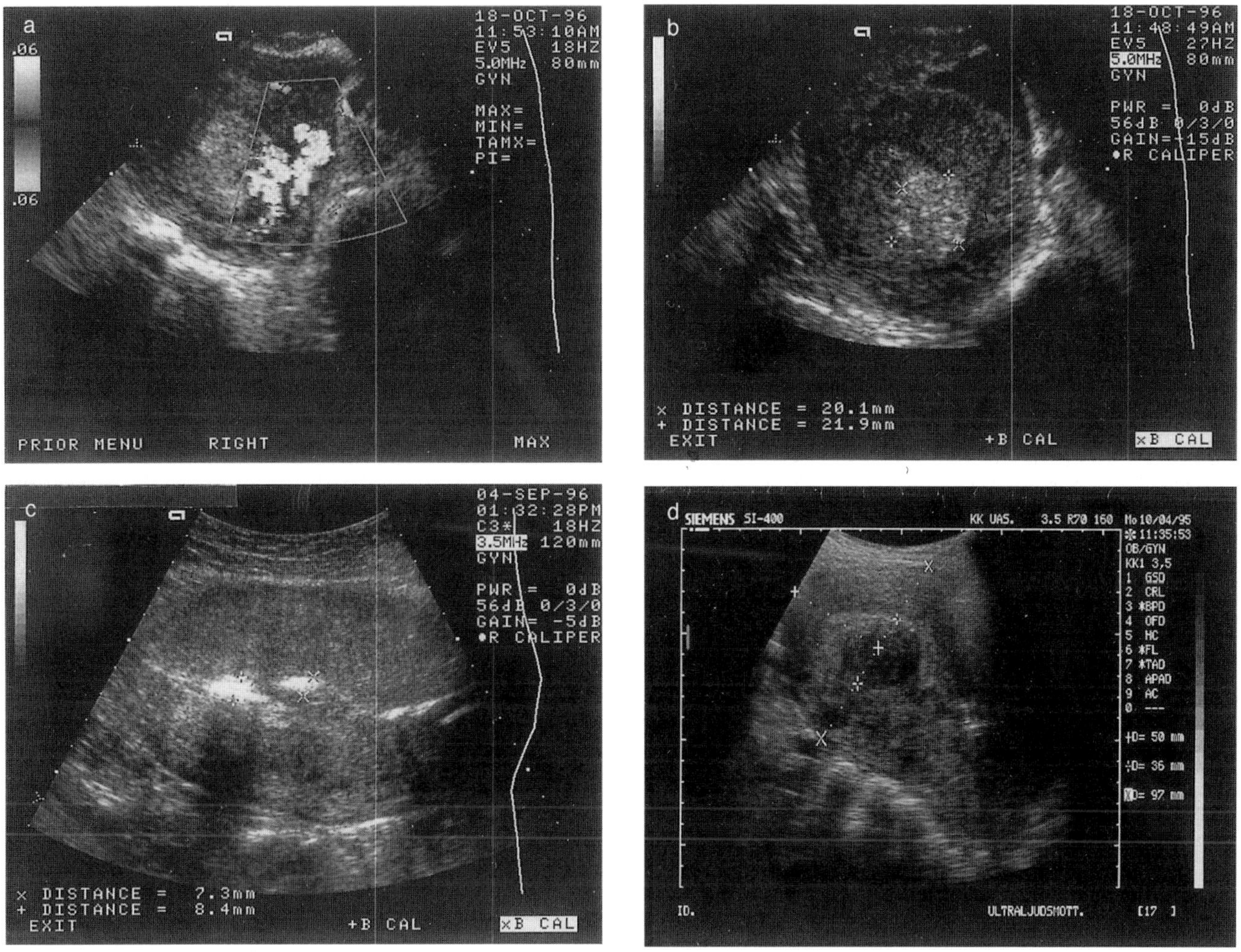

Figure 36.8 Puerperal abnormalities revealed by ultrasound: (a) retained placental tissue 2 days postpartum; (b) low-resistance blood flow on the side of the mass; (c) retained placental tissue 6 weeks postpartum; (d) a thin, echogenic endometrium soon after curettage.

responsible for the blood supply to retained placental tissue. Kelly *et al.*[183] described a rare case of severe secondary postpartum hemorrhage – arteriovenous malformation of the uterus. By color Doppler ultrasound, a localized area of increased vascularity within the myometrium may be detected. Pulsed Doppler usually reveals a low-resistance turbulent flow. Thus, uterine artery embolization may be performed and unnecessary curettage should be avoided. In contrast, Van Schobroeck[176] found enhanced myometrial vascularity (EMV) to be a common transient ultrasound finding if asymptomatic and it does not require treatment. On the other side, if in symptomatic patients residual placental tissue is suspected on ultrasound, EMV is an additional ultrasonic finding, which can help in guiding the appropriate management. The accuracy of TV sonohysterography has recently been evaluated and compared with TV ultrasound.[163,184] This new method seems to be more effective for evaluation of residual trophoblastic tissue. Power Doppler and three-dimensional ultrasound seem to be new unexplored modalities that could improve our abilities to diagnose clinically significant retained placental tissue. All of these new modalities need further evaluation before their usefulness can be recommended.

Postpartum endometritis

Whenever the obstetrician is faced with postpartum bleeding accompanied by signs of endometritis, the most important question is whether there is retained placental tissue in the cavity or not. Previously, it has been considered that ultrasound finding of retained placental tissue and endometritis overlap. Recent studies have, however, contradicted this view.[169] Only if endometritis is the result of retained placental tissue can a similar ultrasound appearance be observed. An isolated endometritis without retained placental tissue has no pathognomonic ultrasound finding. Confusion can sometimes arise in the presence of large retained and organized blood clots in the uterine cavity, which may mimic retained placental tissue. Clinical improvement following conservative treatment with antibiotics and uterotonic medications speaks against the presence of retained placental tissue. Uterine involution could be delayed in cases of endometritis, particularly if endomyometritis is present.[185] The detection of gas in the uterine cavity has been considered as a sign of endometritis. Madrazo[159] found endometrial gas in 15% of the patients with proven puerperal endometritis. Wachsberg and Kurtz,[166] however, observed gas in 21% of women postpartum; none of these women developed endometritis. Whenever gas is present in the uterine cavity a follow-up ultrasound should be performed to confirm its disappearance. It usually resolves during the first two postpartum weeks. If ultrasound is performed after intrauterine manipulations or cesarean sections, it should be kept in mind that highly echogenic foci caused by air are normal findings that must not be misinterpreted as retained placental tissue or endometritis. Kirkiinen found that blood flow to the infected uterus could be different from normal.[162] Deutchman and Hartman[185] have described an uncommon result of endometritis – postpartum pyometra. A lucent area within the uterus with no echogenic components is suggestive of pus. Ultrasound can assist in the proper diagnosis and be of help in guiding a drainage procedure.

Septic pelvic thrombophlebitis, well known as an 'enigmatic puerperal fever', is another uncommon complication of the puerperium. It most commonly presents in the early postpartum period and antibiotic treatment is usually unsuccessful. Rudoff *et al.*[186] suggest ultrasound examination in case of clinical suspicion of pelvic thrombophlebitis. Although ultrasound diagnosis of ovarian vein thrombophlebitis is well described,[187–189] the diagnosis is still difficult and ultrasound expertise is needed. Asymmetric dilatation of the ovarian or other pelvic vein may sometimes be observed.[187] Furthermore, a complex or hypoechoic mass near the lower pole of the kidney, particularly in a clinical setting of an enigmatic puerperal fever should suggest thrombophlebitis. An echogenic intracaval mass is considered diagnostic and anticoagulation treatment should be added.[189]

Cesarean section

Nowadays, when cesarean section rates are continuously rising, a higher incidence of all puerperal complications should be expected. The ultrasound appearance of the uterus after cesarean section usually shows three distinctive patterns: (1) gas in the cavity, (2) a small rounded area at the incision site that reflects tissue reaction due to localized edema[190–192] and (3) some echogenic dots at the incision site, which are related to the type of closure and the suture material used.[192] All these characteristics are normal findings and no correlation with pathological conditions is found. The ultrasound appearance of endometrial gas is an intensively hyperechogenic focus equivalent in echogenic to bowel gas with clean or dirty shadowing or reverberation artifacts[174,193] (Figure 36.7c). Fat and calcium have a similar ultrasound appearance. The gas usually disappears during the first two weeks after surgery. The involution rate of the uterus following cesarean section is not different from the involution rate after vaginal delivery. Nakai *et al.*[194] studied uterine blood flow resistance after cesarean section and concluded that the RI for the uterine artery did not show any change during the early postpartum period. The significant infectious morbidity is associated with cesarean section. Ultrasound may be useful in postpartum women with clinical suspicion of a postoperative complication like phlegmona,[191] abscess, pyometra, hematometra, wound infection and subfascial hematoma. If surgical drainage is chosen as therapy, ultrasound guidance can be helpful. Ultrasound can also confirm the suspicion of an intra-abdominal postoperative hemorrhage by visualization of free fluid in the abdomen. Baker *et al.*[190] described bladder flap hematoma after a low uterine transverse cesarean section. A solid or complex mass between the posterior bladder wall and the anterior uterine wall may be observed by ultrasound. An abscess appears as a cystic structure with internal debris surrounded by thicker irregular walls. An infected hematoma initially has a similar ultrasound appearance. During the resolution process, it may change and appears more solid. However, the physician must be aware that ultrasound diagnosis is just a complement and the clinical condition of the patient should guide the therapeutic approach.

Uterine myoma

Myoma may obstruct the birth canal, and thus be a cause for cesarean section. Intracavitary myoma may cause problems, such as placental detachment, with subsequent postpartum bleeding. Ultrasound is the best tool to make a correct diagnosis (Figure 36.7d). A myoma is characterized by hypoechogenicity. Due to degenerative processes, a myoma may appear as a bizarre heterogenous pattern of solid and fluid areas, and thus be misinterpreted as retained placental tissue. Pinpoint tenderness on palpation may direct the ultrasound examination and reveal the presence of a necrotic myoma.

Developmental abnormalities of the uterus

The prevalence of the congenital uterine malformations in the general population is unknown. Failed fusion of the two Mullerian ducts to form the genital organs may cause reproductive, fetal and maternal hazards. In addition to an increased risk of premature labor and abnormal fetal presentations, retained placental tissue with postpartum hemorrhage may be a consequence of this uterine abnormality. It is well known that uterine anomalies may remain undiscovered except when they are associated with reproductive or obstetric problems.

Already in 1976, Bennett suggested puerperal ultrasonic hysterography as a screening procedure prior to radiological examination in women whose reproductive performance suggests a diagnosis of congenital malformation of the uterus.[195] Since then a few studies concerning the issue have been published.[196,197] Szoke and Kiss[196] examined in 1977 patients in whom manual examination revealed a uterus differing in shape from the normal, the patient had a breech presentation in her previous or present pregnancy and the involution of the uterus was slow. The ultrasound echo technique was applied and uterine anomalies were found in five cases postpartum. In 1984, Land *et al.*[197] performed ultrasonic hysterography in 104 patients between the second and fifth postpartum days. An unexpectedly high number of women (16%) showed an abnormal uterine configuration. The coronal section seems to be the most appropriate section to reveal uterine cavity anatomy. It is difficult to obtain the coronal section by abdominal examination in non-pregnant patients. However, the puerperium when the uterus is extremely large is an exception. The ultrasound examination should be performed in the early puerperium because a large uterus lies in near proximity to the ultrasound probe and the highly echogenic decidua outlines well the shape of the cavity. Puerperal ultrasound can detect such an abnormality, providing an explanation for complications in labor and the puerperium.

Postpartum urinary retention

Postpartum urinary retention is a relatively common condition and the incidence ranges between 1% and 18%.[198] According to the International Continence Society, 100 ml is considered as the upper limit of residual urine. Ultrasound is the method of choice when assessing urinary bladder and residual urine postpartum. Invasive catheterization with the discomfort and the risk of infection can be avoided. Conventional bladder scanner is not to be recommended during the puerperium. A large uterus may contain fluid and thus a misinterpretation may be done. Many different techniques for bladder volume measurement are used and the accuracy of the method varies widely.

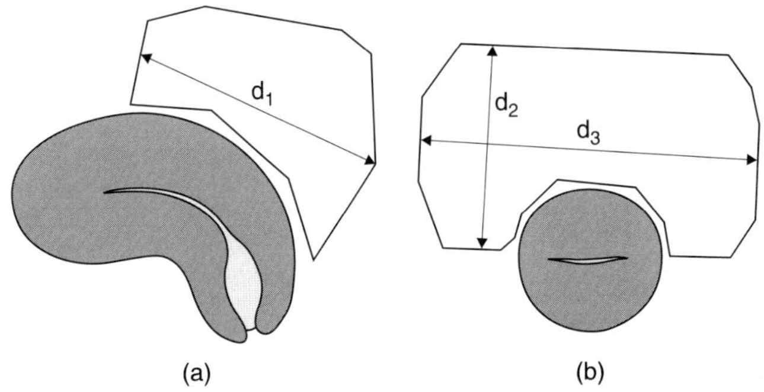

Figure 36.9 Residual urine volume measurement.

We prefer a method where the longest distance of the maternal bladder (d_1) is measured in a longitudinal section, and then two perpendicular diameters (d_2 and d_3) are measured in the transverse section (Figure 36.9). The estimated amount of residual urine can be calculated using the formula for approximation of the ellipsoid:

Volume (ml) $= (d_1 \times d_2 \times d_3)/2$ (Figure 36.9).

REFERENCES

1. Treacy B, Smith C, Rayburn W. Ultrasound in labor and delivery. *Obstet Gynecol Surv* 1990;45:213–19.
2. Deutchman ME, Sakornbut EL. Diagnostic ultrasound in labor and delivery. *Am Fam Physicians* 1995;51:145–54.
3. Benito CW, Guzman ER, Vintzileos AM. The use of ultrasonography in the labor and delivery suite. *Clin Perinatol* 1996;23:117–39.
4. Phelan JP, Ahn MO, Smith CV. Amniotic fluid index measurements during pregnancy. *J Reprod Med* 1987;32:601.
5. Chauhan SP, Rutherford SE, Sharp TW, *et al.* Intrapartum amniotic fluid index and neonatal acidosis, a pilot study to determine the correlation. *J Reprod Med* 1992;37:868–70.
6. Phelan JP. The role of ultrasound assessment of amniotic fluid volume in the management of the post-date pregnancy. *Am J Obstet Gynecol* 1985;151:304.
7. Robson SC, Crawford RA, Spencer JA. Intrapartum amniotic fluid index and its relationship to fetal distress. *Am J Obstet Gynecol* 1992;166:78.
8. Gonik B, Bottoms SF, Cotton DB. Amniotic fluid volume as a risk factor in preterm premature rupture of the membranes. *Obstet Gynecol* 1985;65:456.
9. Romero R, Gomez R, Galasso M. Is oligohydramnios a risk factor in term premature rupture of the membranes? *Ultrasound Obstet Gynecol* 1994;4:95.
10. Sarno AP, Ahn MO, Harbinder SB. Intrapartum Doppler velocimetry, amniotic fluid volume, and fetal heart rate as predictors of subsequent fetal distress. *Am J Obstet Gynecol* 1989;161:1508.
11. Chauhan SP, Doherty DA, Magann EF. Amniotic fluid index versus single deepest pocket technique during modified biophysical profile: A randomised clinical trial. *Am J Obstet Gynecol* 2004;19(2):661–7.
12. Alfirevic Z, Luckas M, Walkinshow SA, McFarlane M, Curran R. A randomised comparison between amniotic fluid index and maximum pool depth in the monitoring of post-term pregnancy. *Br J Obstet Gynecol* 1997;104:207–11.
13. Chauhan SP, Sanderson M, Hendrix NW, Magann EF, Devor LD. Perinatal outcome and amniotic fluid index in the antepartum and intrapartum periods: A meta analysis. *Am J Obstet Gynecol* 1999;181:1473–8.
14. Moses J, Doherty DA, Magann EF, Chauhan SP, Morrison JC. A randomised clinical trial of the intrapartum assessment of amniotic fluid volume: Amniotic fluid index versus the single deepest pocket technique. *Am J Obstet Gynecol* 2004;190(6):1564–9.
15. Hofmeyr GJ. Amnioinfusion for umbilical cord compression in labour. *Cochrane Database Syst Rev* 2001;3. Oxford: Update Software.
16. Moen MD, Besinger RE, Tomich PG, Fisher SG. Effect of amnioinfusion on the incidence of postpartum endometritis in patients undergoing caesarean delivery. *J Reprod Med* 1995;40:383–6.
17. Sadovsky Y, Amon E, Bade ME. Prophylactic amnioinfusion during labor complicated by meconium: A preliminary report. *Am J Obstet Gynecol* 1989;161:613.

18. Hofmeyr GJ. Prophylactic versus therapeutic amnioinfusion for oligohydramnios in labour. *Cochrane Database Syst Rev* 2000;2:CD000176.
19. Hofmeyr GJ. Amnioinfusion for preterm rupture of membranes. *Cochrane Database Syst Rev* 2000;2:CD000942.
20. Vintzileos AM, Campbell WA, Nochimson DJ. Antenatal evaluation and management of ultrasonically detected fetal anomalies. *Obstet Gynecol* 1987;69:640.
21. Benacerraf BR. Examination of the second-trimester fetus with severe oligohydramnios using transvaginal scanning. *Obstet Gynecol* 1990;75:491–3.
22. Hadlock FP, Harrist DB, Carpenter RJ. Sonographic estimation of fetal weight. *Radiology* 1984;150:535.
23. Hadlock FP, Harrist RB, Sharman RS, *et al.* Estimation of fetal weight with the use of head, body and femur measurements – A prospective study. *Am J Obstet Gynecol* 1984;151:333–7.
24. Pattersson RM. Estimation of fetal weight during labor. *Obstet Gynecol* 1985;65:330–2.
25. Platek DN, Divon MY, Anyaegbunam A, Merkattz I. Intrapartum ultrasonographic estimates of fetal weight by the house staff. *Am J Obstet Gynecol* 1991;165:842–5.
26. Yarkoni S, Reace EA, Wan M. Intrapartum fetal weight estimation: A comparison of three formulae. *J Ultrasound Med* 1986; 5:707–10.
27. Chauhan SP, Lutton TC, Bailey KJ, Morrison JC. Intrapartum prediction of birth weight: Clinical versus sonographic estimation based on femur length alone. *Obstet Gynecol* 1993;81:695–7.
28. Chauhan SP, Lutton PN, Bailey KJ, *et al.* Intrapartum clinical sonographic and parous patients' estimates of newborn birth weight. *Obstet Gynecol* 1992;79:956–8.
29. Shanley KT, Landon MB. Accuracy and modifying factors for ultrasonic determination of fetal weight at term. *Obstet Gynecol* 1994;84:926.
30. Shepard MJ, Richard VA, Berkowitz RL, *et al.* An evaluation of two equations for predicting fetal weight by ultrasound. *Am J Obstet Gynecol* 1982;142:47–54.
31. Doubilet PM, Greenes RA. Improved prediction of gestational age from fetal head measurements. *Am J Roentgenol* 1982;142:47.
32. Kasby CB, Poll V. The breech head and its ultrasound significance. *Br J Obstet Gynaecol* 1982;89:106.
33. Manning FA, Morrison I, Lange IR. Fetal assessment based on fetal biophysical profile scoring. *Am J Obstet Gynecol* 1985;151: 343.
34. Manning FA. Dynamic ultrasound based fetal assessment: The fetal biophysical profile score. *Clin Obstet Gynecol* 1995;38: 26–44.
35. Manning FA, Morrison I, Harman CR, *et al.* Fetal assessment based on fetal biophysical profile scoring in the management of the growth restricted fetus. *Ultrasound Obstet Gynecol* 1987;16:399–401.
36. Whitman BK, Davison BM, Lyons E. Real-time ultrasound observation of fetal activity in labor. *Br J Obstet Gynaecol* 1979;86:278.
37. Boylan P, Lewis PJ. Fetal breathing in labor. *Obstet Gynecol* 1980;56:35.
38. Sasson DA, Castro LC, Davis JL. The biophysical profile in labor. *Obstet Gynecol* 1990;76:360.
39. Chua S, Arulkumaran S, Kurup A, *et al.* Search for the most predictive test of fetal well being in early labor. *J Perinat Med* 1996;24:199–206.
40. Kim SY, Khandelwal M, Gaughan JP, Agar MH, Reece EA. Is the intrapartum biophysical profile useful? *Obstet Gynecol* 2003;102(3):471–6.
41. Alfirevic Z, Neilson JP. Biophysical profile for fetal assessment in high-risk pregnancies. *Cochrane Database Syst Rev* 2000;4. Oxford: Update Software.
42. David KJ, Mahomed K, Stone P, Wijngaarden W, Hill LM. *Evidence Based Obstetrics.* Amsterdam: Elsevier Science, 2003.
43. Jouppila P, Kiirkiinen P. Umbilical vein blood flow as an indicator of fetal hypoxia. *Br J Obstet Gynaecol* 1984;91:107.
44. Farmakides G, Weiner Z, Mammapolos M, Nikolaides P. Doppler velocimetry. *Clin Perinatol* 1994;21:849–61.
45. Almström H, Axelsson O, Gnattingius S. Comparison of umbilical artery velocimetry and cardiotocography for surveillance of small for gestational age fetuses. A multicenter randomised controlled trial (abstract). *J Matern Fetal Invest* 1991;1:127.
46. Alfirevic Z, Neilson JP. Doppler ultrasonography in high-risk pregnancies: Systematic review with metaanalysis. *Am J Obstet Gynecol* 1995;172:1379–87.
47. Kurjak A, Dudenhausen J, Kos M, *et al.* Doppler information pertaining to the intrapartum period. *J Perinat Med* 1996;24:271–6.
48. Fairlie FM, Lang GD, Sheldon CD. Umbilical artery flow velocity waveforms in labour. *Br J Obstet Gynaecol* 1989;96:151.
49. Fleischer A, Anyaegbunam A, Shulman H, *et al.* Uterine and umbilical artery velocimetry during normal labor. *Am J Obstet Gynecol* 1987;157:40.
50. Brar HS, Platt LD, De Vore GR, *et al.* Qualitative assessment of maternal uterine and fetal umbilical artery blood flow and resistance in labouring patients by Doppler velocimetry. *Am J Obstet Gynecol* 1988;158:952.
51. Strigini FA, Lencioni G, De Luca G, *et al.* Uterine artery velocimetry and spontaneous preterm delivery. *Obstet Gynecol* 1995;85: 374–7.
52. Feinkind L, Abulafia O, Delke I, *et al.* Screening with Doppler velocimetry in labor. *Am J Obstet Gynecol* 1989;161:765–70.
53. Malcus P, Gudmundsson S, Marsal K, Kwok HH, Vengadasalam D, Ratnam SS. Umbilical artery Doppler velocimetry as a labor admission test. *Obstet Gynecol* 1991;77:10–6.
54. Sarno AP, Ahn MO, Brar HS, Phelan JP, Platt LD. Intrapartum Doppler velocimetry, amniotic fluid volume, and fetal heart rate as predictors of subsequent fetal distress an initial report. *Am J Obstet Gynecol* 1989;161:1508–4.
55. Weis E, Hitschold T, Berle P. Umbilical artery blood flow velocity waveforms during variable decelerations of the fetal heart rate. *Am J Obstet Gynecol* 1991;164:534–9.
56. Brar HS, Platt LD, Paul RH. Fetal umbilical blood flow velocity waveforms using Doppler ultrasonography in patients with late decelerations. *Obstet Gynecol* 1989;73:363–6.
57. Lindblad A, Bernow J, Marshal K. Obstetric analgesia and fetal aortic blood flow during labor. *Br J Obstet Gynaecol* 1987; 94–306.
58. Ueno N. Studies on fetal middle cerebral artery blood flow velocity waveform in the intrapartum period. *Nippon Sanka Fujinka Gakkai Zasshi* 1992;44:97.
59. Vyas S, Campbell S, Bower S, Nicolaides K. Maternal abdominal pressure alters fetal cerebral blood flow. *Br J Obstet Gynaecol* 1990;97:140.
60. Mirrro R, Gonzales A. Perinatal anterior cerebral artery Doppler flow indexes: Methods and preliminary results. *Am J Obstet Gynecol* 1987;156:1227.
61. Maesel A, Lingman G, Marsal K. Cerebral blood flow during labor in human fetus. *Acta Obstet Gynecol Scand* 1990;69:493.
62. Yagel S, Anteby E, Lavy Y, *et al.* Fetal middle cerebral artery blood flow during normal active labour and in labour with variable decelerations. *Br J Obstet Gynaecol* 1992;99:483.
63. Vintzileos AM, Campbell WA, Nochimson DJ. The use of fetal biophysical profile improves pregnancy outcome in premature rupture of the membranes. *Am J Obstet Gynecol* 1987;157:236.
64. Vintzileos AM. Antepartum surveillance on preterm rupture of membranes. *J Perinat Med* 1996;24:319.
65. Goldstein I, Romero R, Merill S. Fetal body and breathing movements as predictors of intra-amniotic infection in preterm premature rupture of membranes. *Am J Obstet Gynecol* 1988;159:363.
66. Vermillion ST, Kooba AM, Soper DE, *et al.* Amniotic fluid index values after preterm premature rupture of the membranes and subsequent perinatal infection. *Am J Obstet Gynecol* 2000;183:271–6.
67. Nowak M, Oszukowski P, Szpakowski M, *et al.* Intrauterine infections. I. The role of C-reactive protein, white blood cell count and erythrocyte sedimentation rate in pregnant women in the detection of intrauterine infection after preliminary rupture of the membranes. *Ginekol Pol* 1998;69:615–22.
68. Vintzileos AM, Campbell WA, Nochimson DJ. Fetal biophysical profile versus amniocentesis in predicting infection in premature rupture of the membranes. *Obstet Gynecol* 1986;68:488.
69. Yoon BH, Jun JK, Park KH, *et al.* Serum C-reactive protein, white blood cell count, and amniotic fluid blood cell count in women with preterm premature rupture of membranes. *Obstet Gynecol* 1996;88:1034–40.
70. Tsoi E, Fuchs I, Henrich W, Dudenhausen JW, Nicolaides KH. Sonographic measurement of cervical length in preterm prelabor amniorrhexis. *Ultrasound Obstet Gynecol* 2004;24(5):550–3.
71. Main DM, Hadley CB. The role of ultrasound in the management of preterm labor. *Clin Obstet Gynecol* 1988;31:53.
72. Weinberger E, Cyr DR, Hirsh JH. Estimating fetal weights less than 2000g. An accurate and simple method. *Am J Roentgenol* 1984;141:973.

73. Besinger RE, Compton AA, Hayashi RH. The presence or absence of fetal breathing movements as a predictor of outcome in preterm labor. *Am J Obstet Gynecol* 1987;157:753–7.
74. McFarlin BL, Baumann P, Sampson MB, *et al.* The biophysical profile as a tool for prediction of preterm delivery. *Obstet Gynecol* 1995;50:413–14.
75. Weitz CM, Ghodaonkar RB, Dubin NH. Prostaglandin F metabolite concentration as a prognostic factor in preterm labor. *Obstet Gynecol* 1986;67:496.
76. MacKenzie IZ. Induction of labor – A review of the use of prostaglandins. *J Obstet Gynecol* 1988;Suppl 8:s7.
77. Honest H, Bachmann LM Sengupta R, Gupta JK, Kleijnen J, Khan KS. Accuracy of absence of fetal breathing movements in predicting preterm birth a systematic review *Ultrasound Obstet Gynecol* 2004;24:94–100.
78. Andersen HF, Nugent CE, Wanty SD, Hayashi RTH. Prediction of risk for preterm delivery by ultrasonographic measurement of cervical length. *Am J Obstet Gynecol* 1990;163:859.
79. Dessel HJHM, Friijns JHM, Kok FT, Wallenburgh HCS. Ultrasound assessment of cervical dynamics during the first stage of labour. *Eur J Obstet Gynecol Reprod Biol* 1994;53:123–7.
80. Gomez R, Galasso M, Romero R, *et al.* Ultrasonographic examination of the uterine cervix is better than cervical digital examination as a predictor of the likelihood of premature delivery in patients with preterm labor and intact membranes. *Am J Obstet Gynecol* 1994;171:956–64.
81. McGahan JP, Phillips HE, Bowen MS. Prolapse of the amniotic sac "hourglass membranes": Ultrasound appearance. *Radiology* 1981;140:463–6.
82. Romero R. The uterine cervix and preterm delivery (abstr. 0518). Presented at the *VI World Congress of Ultrasound in Obstetrics and Gynecology*, Rotterdam, October 1996:257.
83. Iams JD, Paraskos J, Landon MB, *et al.* Cervical sonography in preterm delivery. *Obstet Gynecol* 1994;84:40–6.
84. Vendittelli F, Volumenie J. Transvaginal ultrasonography examination of the uterine cervix in hospitalized women undergoing preterm labour. *Eur J Obstet Gynecol Reprod Biol* 2000;90:3–11.
85. Tsoi E, Akmal S, Rane S, Otigbaah C, Nicolaides KH. Ultrasound assessment of cervical length in threatened preterm labor. *Ultrasound Obstet Gynecol* 2003;(6):552–5.
86. Fuchs IB, Henrich W, Osthues K, Dudenhausen JW. Sonographic cervical length in singleton pregnancies with intact membranes presenting with threatened preterm labor. *Ultrasound Obstet Gynecol* 2004;(5):554–7.
87. Laing FC. Placenta previa: Avoiding false-negative diagnosis. *J Clin Ultrasound* 1981;9:109.
88. Timor-Trish IE, Rottem S. *Transvaginal Sonography*. New York: Elsevier, 1987:1–13.
89. Tan NH, Abuy M, Woo JL. The role of transvaginal sonography in the diagnosis of placenta praevia. *Aust N Z J Obstet Gynaecol* 1995;35:42–5.
90. Patel F, Bornet C, Moodley J. The use of transvaginal color-Doppler ultrasound in the diagnosis of placenta previa accreta. *Ultrasound Obstet Gynecol* 1996;8(Suppl 1):78.
91. Krapp M, Baschat AA, Hankeln M, Gembruch U. Gray scale and color-Doppler sonography in the third stage of labor for early detection of failed placental separation. *Ultrasound Obstet Gynecol* 2000;15:138–42.
92. McGahan JP, Phillips HE, Reid MH. The anechoic retroplacental area. *Radiology* 1980;134:47.
93. Nyberg DA, Cyr DR, Mack LA, *et al.* Sonographic spectrum of placental abruption. *Am J Roentgenol* 1987;148:161–4.
94. Hurd WW, Miodovnik M, Hertzberg V. Selective management of abruptio placentae: A prospective study. *Obstet Gynecol* 1983;61:467–72.
95. McGahan JP, Phillips HE, Reid MH. Sonographic spectrum of retroplacental hemorrhage. *Radiology* 1982;142:481.
96. Spirt BA, Kagan EH, Rozanski RM. Abruptio placenta: Sonographic and pathologic correlation. *Am J Roentgenol* 1979;133:877–81.
97. Rivera Alsima ME, Saldana LR, Maklad N. The use of ultrasound in the expectant management of abruptio placentae. *Am J Obstet Gynecol* 1983;146:924–7.
98. Macara LM, Murphy KW. The contribution of dystoci to the caesarean section rate. *Am J Obstet Gynecol* 1994;171:71–7.
99. Rojansky N, Tanos V, Lewin A, Weinstein D. Sonographic evaluation of fetal head extension and maternal pelvis in cases of breech presentation. *Acta Obstet Gynecol Scand* 1994;73:607–10.
100. Deutinger J, Bernaschek G. Vaginosonographical determination of the true conjugate and the transverse diameter of the pelvic inlet. *Arch Gynecol* 1987;240:241–6.
101. Akmal S, Tsoi E, Kametas N, Howard R, Nicolaides KH. Intrapartum sonography to determine fetal head position. *J Matern Fetal Neonatal Med* 2002;12(3):172–7.
102. Akmal S, Tsoi E, Kametas N, Hargreaves C, Nicolaides KH. Comparison of transvaginal digital examination with intrapartum sonography to determine fetal head position before instrumental delivery. *Ultrasound Obstet Gynecol* 2003;21(5):437–40.
103. Akmal S, Tsoi E, Nicolaides KH. Intrapartum sonography to determine fetal occipital position: Interobserver agreement. *Ultrasound Obstet Gynecol* 2004;24(4):421–4.
104. Rayburn WR, Siemers KH, Legino LJ. Dystoci in late labor: Determining fetal position by clinical and ultrasonic techniques. *Am J Perinatol* 1989;6:161–89.
105. Chou MR, Kreiser D, Taslimi MM, Druzin ML, El-Sayed YY. Vaginal versus ultrasound examination of fetal occiput position during the second stage of labor. *Am J Obstet Gynecol* 2004;191(2):521–4.
106. Barbera A, Pombar X, Perugino G, *et al.* A new method to assess fetal head descent in labor with transperineal, ultrasound. *Ultrasound Obstet Gynecol* 1996;8(Suppl 1):95.
107. Pritchard JA, MacDonald PC, Gant NF. *Williams Obstetrics*, 17th edn. Norwalk: Appleton-Century-Crofts, 1985:660.
108. Hofmeyr GJ, Hannah ME. Planned caesarean section for term breech delivery. *Cochrane Database Syst Rev* 2001;3. Oxford: Update Software.
109. Hofmeyr GJ, Kulier R. External cephalic version for breech presentation at term. *Cochrane Database Syst Rev* 2000;4. Oxford: Update Software.
110. Ferguson JE, Dyson DC. Intrapartum external cephalic version. *Am J Obstet Gynecol* 1985;152:297.
111. Hofmeyr GJ. External cephalic version for breech presentation before term. *Cochrane Database Syst Rev* 2000;4. Oxford: Update Software.
112. Kratochwil A, Zeibekis N. Ultrasonic pelvimetry. *Acta Obstet Gynecol Scand* 1972;240:241–6.
113. Schlensker KH. Ultrasonographic examinations of the true conjugate. *Geburshilfe Frauenheilkd* 1979;37:333–7.
114. Ballas S, Toaff R. Hyperextension of the fetal head in breech presentation radiological evaluation and significance. *Br J Obstet Gynaecol* 1976;83:201–4.
115. Sherer DM. Sonographic detection of a nuchal arm in the intrapartum assessment of the breech-presenting fetus (letter). *J Ultrasound Med* 1993;12:524.
116. Giacomello F. Ultrasound determination of nuchal cord in breech presentation (letter). *Am J Obstet Gynecol* 1988;159:531.
117. Lange IR, Masning FA, Morrison I. Cord prolapse: Is antenatal diagnosis possible? *Am J Obstet Gynecol* 1985;151:1083.
118. Gimovsky ML, Paul R. Singleton breech presentation in labor. Experiences in 1980. *Am J Obstet Gynecol* 1982;143:733.
119. Scorza WE. Intrapartum management of breech presentation. *Clin Perinatol* 1996;23:31–49.
120. Chauhan S, Washburne J, Martin J. Intrapartum assessment by house staff of birth weight among twins. *Obstet Gynecol* 1993;82:523.
121. Lukacs HA, MacLennan AH, Verco PW. Ultrasonic fetal weight estimation in multiple and singleton pregnancy. *Aust Paediatr J* 1984;20:59–61.
122. Chasen ST, Madden A, Chervenak FA. Caesarean delivery of twins and neonatal respiratory disorders. *Am J Obstet Gynecol* 1999;181:1052–6.
123. Houlihan C, Knuppel RA. Intrapartum management of multiple gestations. *Clin Perinatol* 1996;23:91.
124. Chervenak F, Johnson R, Youcha S. Intrapartum management of twin gestation. *Obstet Gynecol* 1985;65:119.
125. Chervenak F, Johnson RE, Berkowitz RL, Hobbins JC. Intrapartum external version of the second twin. *Obstet Gynecol* 1983;62:160.
126. Hays PM, Smeltzer JS. Multiple gestations. *Clin Obstet Gynecol* 1986;29:264.
127. Kaplan B, Peled Y, Rabinerson D, *et al.* Successful external version of B twin after the birth of A twin for vertex non vertex twins. *Eur J Obstet Gynecol Reprod Biol* 1995;58:157–60.
128. Bishop EH. Pelvic scoring for elective induction. *Obstet Gynecol* 1964;24:266.
129. Boozarjomehri F, Timor-Trisch I, Chao C. Transvaginal sonography – An objective evaluation of the cervix in labor: Presence of cervical

wedging is associated with shorter duration of labor for induction. *Am J Obstet Gynecol* 1994;170:374.
130. Sujata C, Crane JMG, Hutchens DRN, Young DC. Transvaginal ultrasound and digital examination in predicting successful labor induction.
131. Reis FM, Gervasi MT, Florio P, *et al.* Prediction of successful induction of labor at term, role of clinical history, digital examination, ultrasound assessment of the cervix and the fetal fibronectin assay. *Am J Obstet Gynecol* 2003;189:1361–7.
132. Rane SM, Guirgis RR, Higgins B, Nicolaides KH. The value of ultrasound in the prediction of successful induction of labor. *Ultrasound Obstet Gynecol* 2004;24(5):538–49.
133. Yang SH, Roh CR, Kim JH. Transvaginal ultrasonography for cervical assessment before induction of labor. *J Ultrasound Med* 2004;3:375–82.
134. Rane SM, Guirgis RR, Higgins B, Nicolaides KH. Pre induction sonographic measurement of cervical length in prolonged pregnancy the effect of parity in the prediction of the need for Caesarean section. *Ultrasound Obstet Gynecol* 2003;(1):45–8.
135. Rane SM, Pandis GK, Guirgis RR, Higgins B, Nicolaides KH. Pre induction sonographic measurement of cervical length in prolonged pregnancy the effect of parity in the prediction of induction to delivery interval. *Ultrasound Obstet Gynecol* 2003;22:40–4.
136. Mastrogiannis DS, Knuppel RA. Critical management of the very low birth weight infant and macrosomic fetus. *Clin Perinatol* 1996;23:51–89.
137. Roman H, Verspyck E, Vercoustre L, *et al.* Does ultrasound examination when the cervix is unfavourable improve the prediction of failed labor induction? *Ultrasound Obstet Gynecol* 2004;(4):357–62.
138. Wikström I, Bergström AR, Meirik O. Traumatic injury in large for dates infants. *Obstet Gynecol Surv* 1989;44:616–17.
139. Hirata GI, Medearis AI, Horenstein J. Ultrasonographic estimation of fetal weight in the clinically macrosomic fetus. *Am J Obstet Gynecol* 1990;162:238.
140. Wiznitzer A. Obstructed labor and shoulder delivery. *Curr Opin Obstet Gynecol* 1995;7:486–914.
141. Pearson JF. Shoulder dystocia. *Curr Obstet Gynecol* 1996;6:30–4.
142. Smith RB, Lane C, Pearson JF. Shoulder dystocia: What happens at the next delivery? *Br J Obstet Gynaecol* 1994;101:713–5.
143. Eliot JP, Garite TJ, Freeman RK, *et al.* Ultrasonic prediction of fetal macrosomia in diabetic patients. *Obstet Gynecol* 1982;60: 159–62.
144. Cohen B, Penning S, Major C, *et al.* Sonographic prediction of shoulder dystocia in infants of diabetic mothers. *Obstet Gynecol* 1996;88:10–3.
145. Santolaya-Forgas TJ, Meyer WJ, Gauthier DW, Kahn D. Intrapartum fetal subcutaneous tissue /femur length ratio: An ultrasonographic clue to fetal macrosomia. *Am J Obstet Gynecol* 1994;171:1072–5.
146. Martins ME. Vaginal birth after caesarean section. *Clin Perinatol* 1996;23:141–53.
147. Rayburn W, Haraman M, Legino L, *et al.* Routine preoperative ultrasonography and caesarean section. *Am J Perinatol* 1988; 5:297–9.
148. Michaels WH, Thompson HO, Boutt A, *et al.* Ultrasound diagnosis of defects in the scarred lower uterine segment during pregnancy. *Obstet Gynecol* 1988;71:112.
149. Herman A, Weinraub Z, Bukovsky I, *et al.* Dynamic ultrasonographic imaging of the third stage of labor: New perspectives into third-stage mechanisms. *Am J Obstet Gynecol* 1993; 168:1496–9.
150. Bedi DG, Salmon A, Wisett MZ, *et al.* Ruptured uterus: Sonographic diagnosis. *J Clin Ultrasound* 1986;14:529–33.
151. Schiotz HA. Rupture of the uterus in labour. An unusual case followed with sonography. *Arch Gynecol Obstet* 1991;249:43–5.
152. Suonio S, Saarikoski S, Kääriäinen J, Virtanen R. Intrapartum rupture of uterus diagnosed by ultrasound: A case report. *Int J Gynecol Obstet* 1984;22:411–3.
153. Robinson HP. Sonar in the puerperium. *Scott Med J* 1972;17: 364–6.
154. Szoke B, Kiss D. The use of the ultrasonic echo technique in examining the normal and pathological involution in the puerperium. *Int J Gynecol Obstet* 1976;14:513–6.
155. Rodeck CH, Newton JR. Study of the uterine cavity by ultrasound in the early puerperium. *Br J Obstet Gynaecol* 1976;83:795–801.
156. Defoort P, Benijts G, Martens G, Thiery M. Ultrasound assessment of puerperal uterine involution. *Eur J Obstet Gynecol Reprod Biol* 1978;8:95–7.
157. Van Rees D, Bernstine R, Crawford W. Involution of the postpartum uterus: An ultrasonic study. *J Clin Ultrasound* 1981;9:55–7.
158. Seeds JW, Chescheir NC, Wade RV. Postpartum ultrasound. In *Practical Sonography in Obstetrics and Gynecology*, 2nd edn. New York: Lippincott-Raven, 1986:347–8.
159. Madrazo BL. Postpartum sonography. In *The Principle and Practice of Ultrasonography in Obstetrics and Gynecology*, 3rd edn. East Norwalk: Appleton-Century-Crofts, 1985:449–56.
160. Lavery JP, Shaw LA. Sonography of the puerperal uterus. *J Ultrasound Med* 1989;8:481–6.
161. Tekay A, Jouppila P. A longitudinal Doppler ultrasonographic assessment of the alterations in peripheral vascular resistance of uterine arteries and ultrasonographic findings of the involuting uterus during the puerperium. *Am J Obstet Gynecol* 1993; 168:190–8.
162. Kirkinen P, Dudenhausen J, Baumann H, *et al.* Postpartum blood flow velocity waveforms of the uterine arteries. *J Reprod Med* 1988;33:745–4.
163. Zalel Y, Gamzu R, Lidor A, Goldenberg M, Achiron R. Color Doppler imaging in the sonohysterographic diagnosis of residual trophoblastic tissue. *J Clin Ultrasound* 2002;30:222–5.
164. Achiron R, Goldenberg M, Lipitz S, Mashiach S. Transvaginal duplex Doppler ultrasonography in bleeding patients suspected of having residual trophoblastic tissue. *Obstet Gynecol* 1993; 81:507–11.
165. Mulic-Lutvica A, Bekuretzion M, Axelsson O, *et al.* Ultrasonic evaluation of the uterus and uterine cavity after normal, vaginal delivery. *Ultrasound Obstet Gynecol* 2001;18:491–8.
166. Wachsberg RH, Kurtz AB, Levine CD, *et al.* Real-time ultrasonographic analysis of the normal postpartum uterus: Technique, variability and measurements. *J Ultrasound Med* 1994;13:215–21.
167. Williams JW. Regeneration of the uterine mucosa after delivery with special reference to the placental site. *Am J Obstet Gynecol* 1931;22:664.
168. Hertzberg BS, Bowie JD. Ultrasound of the postpartum uterus, prediction of retained placental tissue. *J Ultrasound Med* 1991; 10:451–6.
169. Sakki A, Kirkiinen P. Ultrasonography of the uterus at early puerperium. *Eur J Ultrasound* 1996;4:99–105.
170. Sokol ER, Casele H, Haney EI. Ultrasound examination of the postpartum uterus what is normal? *J Maternal Fetal Neonat Med* 2004;15:95–9.
171. Edwards A, Ellwood DA. Ultrasonographic evaluation of the postpartum uterus. *Ultrasound Obstet Gynecol* 2000;16:640–3.
172. Sharman A. *Reproductive Physiology of the Post-Partum Period.* Edinburgh: Livingston, 1966.
173. Lee CY, Madrazo B, Drukker BH. Ultrasonic evaluation of the postpartum uterus in the management of postpartum bleeding. *Obstet Gynaecol* 1981;58:227–32.
174. Wachsberg RH, Kurtz AB. Gas within the endometrial cavity at postpartum US. A normal finding after spontaneous vaginal delivery. *Radiology* 1992;183:431–3.
175. Alcazar JL, Lopez-Garcia G, Zornoza A. A role of color velocity imaging and pulsed Doppler sonography to detect retained trophoblastic tissue. *Ultrasound Obstet Gynecol* 1996;8(Suppl 1):41.
176. Van Schoubroeck D, Van den Bosch T, Scharpe K, Lu C, Van Huffel S, Timmerman D. Prospective evaluation of blood flow in the myometrium and uterine arteries in the puerperium. *Ultrasound Obstet Gynecol* 2004;23:378–81.
177. Alexander J, Thomas P, Sanhghera J. Treatments for secondary postpartum haemorrhage. *The Cochrane Library* 2002;4.
178. Dewhurst C. Secondary postpartum hemorrhage. *J Obstet Gynaecol Br Commonw* 1966;73:53–8.
179. Hoveyda F, MacKenzie IZ. Secondary postpartum haemorrhage: Incidence, morbidity and current management. *Br J Obstet Gynaecol* 2001;108:927–30.
180. Malvern J, Campbell S, May P. Ultrasonic scanning of the puerperal uterus following secondary postpartum hemorrhage. *J Obstet Gynaecol Br Commonw* 1973;80:320–4.
181. Carlan SJ, Scott WT, Pollack R, *et al.* Appearance of the uterus by ultrasound immediately after placental delivery with pathologic correlation. *J Clin Ultrasound* 1997;25(6):301–8.
182. Neill AMC, Nixon RM, Thornton S. A comparison of clinical assessment with ultrasound in the management of secondary postpartum haemorrhage. *Eur J Obstet Gynecol Reprod Biol* 2002;104:113–5.
183. Kelly SM, Belli AM, Campbell S. Arteriovenous malformation of the uterus associated with secondary postpartum hemorrhage. *Ultrasound Obstet Gynecol* 2003;21:602–5.

184. Wolman I, Hartoov J, Amster R, *et al.* Transvaginal sonohysterography for the early detection of residual trophoblastic tissue. *Ultrasound Obstet Gynecol* 1996;8(Suppl 1):37.

185. Deutchman ME, Hartmann KJ. Postpartum pyometra: A case report. *J Fam Pract* 1993;36:449–52.

186. Rudoff JM, Astranskas LJ, Rudoff JC, *et al.* Ultrasonographic diagnosis of septic pelvic thrombophlebitis. *J Ultrasound Med* 1988; 7:287–91.

187. Warhit JM, Fagelman D, Goldman MA, *et al.* Ovarian vein thrombophlebitis: Diagnosis by ultrasound and CT. *J Clin Ultrasound* 1984;12:301.

188. Wilson PC, Lerner RM. Diagnosis of ovarian vein thrombophlebitis by ultrasonography. *J Ultrasound Med* 1983;2:187.

189. Sherer DM, Fern S, Mester J, *et al.* Postpartum ultrasonographic diagnosis of inferior vena cava thrombus associated with ovarian vein thrombosis. *Am J Obstet Gynecol* 1997;177(2):474–5.

190. Baker ME, Bowie JD, Killam AP. Sonography of post cesarean-section bladder-flap haematoma. *Am J Roentgenol* 1984;144: 757–9.

191. Lavery JP, Howell RS, Shaw L. Ultrasonic demonstration of a phlegmona following caesarean section – Case report. *J Clin Ultrasound* 1985;13:134–6.

192. Burger NF, Dararas B, Boes EGM. An echogenic evaluation during the early puerperium of the uterine wound after caesarean section. *J Ultrasound Med* 1983;2:18.

193. Carson PL. Clean and dirty shadowing at US a reappraisal. *Radiology* 1991;181:231–6.

194. Nakai Y, Imanaka M, Nishio J, *et al.* Uterine blood flow velocity waveforms during early postpartum course following caesarean section. *Eur J Obstet Gynecol Reprod Biol* 1997;74(2):121–4.

195. Bennett MJ. Puerperal ultrasonic hysterography in the diagnosis of congenital uterine malformations. *Br J Obstet Gynaecol* 1976; 83(5):389–92.

196. Szoke B, Kiss D. The use of ultrasonic echo technique in the diagnosis of developmental anomalies of the uterus. 1977.

197. Land JA, Stoot JE, Evers JL. Puerperal ultrasonic hysterography. *Gynecol Obstet Invest* 1984;18(3):165–8.

198. Weissman A, Grisarn D, Shenhav M, *et al.* Postpartum surveillance of urinary retention by ultrasonography: The effect of epidural analgesia. *Ultrasound Obstet Gynecol* 1995;6:130–4.

37 Safety of diagnostic ultrasound in obstetrics

B. Breyer, A. Kurjak and K. Maeda

Introduction

Diagnostic ultrasound has become an integral component of perinatal care. Even after widespread use for almost four decades there has not been a single known instance of identifiable adverse effects caused by the diagnostic intensity of ultrasound. Nevertheless, the need for continuing vigilance for biosafety is well recognized. It has long been recognized that, given certain circumstances, ultrasound exposure can influence biological systems. Diagnostic medical insonation, however, is generally assumed to be safe.

This chapter addresses some complex issues about safety, and presents a review of available data from the literature as well as from the personal experience of the authors.

Physical background

Ultrasound waves

Ultrasound waves convey mechanical energy through matter by passing energy from particle to particle. Longitudinal waves induce pressure variations along their way. In soft tissues, these waves are the most common type. Other modes, like transverse or shear waves, can spread an appreciable distance, only in solids. When transmitted into bodily liquids, such waves are absorbed within a very small distance. Waves that spread only very short distances are not really of interest from a diagnostic point of view, but when considering safety, such absorption within a short distance is exactly the type of phenomenon that may be of concern. All waves attenuate very strongly in bone.

Describing ultrasound waves

Ultrasound waves and pulses can be described using the following parameters:

(1) *Propagation speed.* The average speed for longitudinal waves in human soft tissue is 1540 m/s. In calcified bones, the speed is about twice that in soft tissues. In gases, it is about 330 m/s. Shear waves travel more slowly.
(2) *Wavelength* (λ) is inversely proportional to frequency. It greatly influences the resolution of diagnostic machines. The higher the frequency, the shorter the wavelength. For example, the wavelength in the body at 3 MHz is approximately 0.5 mm.
(3) The *pulse length* for Doppler measurements is often longer than for B-mode imaging. These pulses are transmitted at a repetition frequency typically of the order of a few kilohertz.
(4) The *attenuation* of ultrasound is proportional to frequency. Absorption causes heating of tissues.
(5) *Ultrasound pressure amplitude* is the maximum pressure induced by the compressional wave at a point in the tissue. If we operate with continuous wave (CW) [as in fetal cardiotocographic (CTG) monitoring] the wave is continuous. If, however, we use pulses (such as in imaging), ultrasound is transmitted in the form of short pulses and the maximum positive (compressional), maximum negative (rarefaction) and average pressure during the pulse or during the total time must be taken into account.

Energy is measured in watt seconds or joules; *power* is measured in watts; *intensity* is measured in watts per square meter or centimeter. The *attenuation* property is measured in decibels per centimeter per megahertz.

In diagnostic applications, ultrasound waves are mainly used in the form of beams and are usually transmitted in the form of pulses. In pulse applications, the energy flow exists in time only during the pulse. Considering an example when the pulse duration is one-thousandth of the repetition period, the intensity during the pulse is about 1000 times higher than the overall time average intensity.

Ultrasound beams can be focused in various ways, but the important feature from the safety standpoint is that focusing concentrates ultrasound energy and thus, potentially, increases the hazard. For safety consideration, only transmission focusing is relevant. In scanning applications the beam moves, while in Doppler spectrometry and M-mode imaging one tends to keep the beam in one position for a prolonged time.

The ultrasound pulse consists of a few pressure oscillations around the static atmospheric pressure. When considering safety, the positive peak pressure p_c and the negative peak pressure p_r play a role. At high intensities, the positive peak pressure may become a few times higher than the negative peak pressure. These effects are much more expressed in liquids in which there is little attenuation compared to human tissues in which attenuation is much greater.

Acoustic parameters used to describe ultrasound exposure

In order to concisely and exactly describe ultrasound waves with regard to their potential hazard a multitude of parameters are used. Intensity is the first such parameter. Later, it was recognized that this was not enough and therefore additional parameters were introduced:

(1) *Acoustic power* output is the total acoustic power that exits from a transmitting transducer. In commercial B-mode instruments, the power ranges between 0.3 and 280 mW; in color Doppler mapping, between 15 and 400 mW; in pulsed Doppler spectrometry, between 10 and 450 mW.[1–3]

(2) *Spatial peak temporal average intensity* (I_{SPTA}) is the intensity averaged over time, but measured in the position of the spatial peak (focus). When considering the potential hazard of heating, we take this I_{SPTA} into account. In commercial B-mode instruments, this ranges between 0.3 and 990 mW/cm^2; in color Doppler mapping, between 20 and 2000 mW/cm^2; and in pulsed Doppler spectrometers, between 170 and 9000 mW/cm^2.

(3) The intensity at the point of maximum pressure in a pulse is the *pulse peak intensity*. This is the temporal peak intensity.

(4) When considering the potential hazard of cavitation, *spatial peak pulse average* (I_{SPPA}) is among the significant parameters. In commercial pulsed Doppler instruments, this ranges between 1 and 770 W/cm^2.

(5) *Peak negative pressure* is also among the parameters for evaluation of the cavitation probability. It is easier to measure than the peak positive pressure, which may be greatly distorted in shape. The peak pressure varies in all types of modern equipment between 0.4 and 5 MPa.[1–3]

The above parameters play a role in the body, but are far easier to measure in water. In addition, it is much easier to standardize them in water. Two approaches are used: the measurement of all parameters in water or the immediate calculation of the *in situ* values taking into account conventional standard attenuation values, e.g. 0.3 dB/cm MHz. Bone is considered to be very attenuating so that nearly all the energy is absorbed within a short path. Various organ or situation models have been conceived to represent specific situations, e.g. full bladder and uterus with an embryo.

Instrument properties and acoustic output

In purely practical terms, it is necessary to know what properties of the scanners are important for their safe use, both when acquiring a new machine and when using existing ones. Some properties are inherent to the instrument while others depend on the application and the way in which the instrument is used.

Heating of tissues is proportional to I_{SPTA} *in situ*. The general trend is an increase in the output of diagnostic ultrasound instruments.[1] Since the 1980s, there have been instruments in the market with I_{SPTA} above 1 W/cm^2 in pulsed Doppler operation regimens.[2] The actual intensity greatly depends on the mode of operation and settings (ALARA principle[4,5] should be followed). The lowest intensity is used in fetal heart monitors (CW Doppler systems with the intensity below 100 W/cm^2), and then, in order of increasing intensities: B-mode imaging scanners, two-dimensional (2D) Doppler machines and pulsed Doppler instruments. In many instruments, it is possible to operate in various regimens. High-end scanners normally have the possibility of quasi-parallel operation in various regimens, e.g. gray scale, 2D flow mapping and Doppler spectrometry, at the same time. In fact, the scanner switches quickly between the various modes.

The actual acoustic power and pressure in the pulses greatly depend on the mode of operation; depth and length of examination also influence the exposure. The frequency influences the penetration ability and thus may influence the acoustic power used. For example, the use of higher-frequency intracavitary probes implies two opposite effects; that is, the scanning distance (range) is reduced but the frequency is increased and, therefore, the attenuation per centimeter is reduced. Thus, the acoustic energy traversing the region of interest is about the same.

In the current commercially available instrumentation, I_{SPTA} varies with the mode: in B-mode imaging the median is 35 mW/cm^2; in M-mode the median is about 100 mW/cm^2; in 2D velocity mapping (color Doppler) the median is about 290 mW/cm^2 and in pulsed Doppler the median is 1200 mW/cm^2. The factor of increase of intensity between the various modes is about three from mode to mode.[1–3]

Another source of heat may be heating of the transducer because of internal dissipation. When intracavitary probes are used, this may be a factor for serious consideration. The extent of heating depends on the probe design and materials used.

Cavitation is less likely with short pulses. In B-mode imaging, the pulse length is usually less than 0.5 μs, but in pulsed Doppler applications it can be up to 20 μs. It is possible to control this length by varying the 'sample volume'. Shorter 'sample volumes' generally yield smaller I_{SPTA}.

Ultrasound therapy

In order to have an idea of what these intensities may mean it is worth mentioning that the ultrasound machines used in physical therapy operate at intensities between 0.5 and 3 mW/cm^2. Therapy using these machines is based on tissue heating, particularly heating of boundaries between soft and connective tissue and bones. There exists an extensive body of data[1–3] on ultrasound machine outputs.

There is the ever-developing ultrasound-treatment field that includes lithotripsy, physiotherapy and 'ultrasound knives' of various types, particularly of brain and liver surgery. Therefore, it is sensible to consider how these applications, where the biological effect is the essence of the application, compare to diagnostic applications where, in ideal cases, information is gathered without causing any biological effect.

Physiotherapy devices use continuous waves or very long pulses of intensity between 0.5 and 3 W/cm^2. The mechanism used is heating. The therapist must continuously move the probe in order not to overheat some structure in the patient.

Lithotripsy is done with short pulses that 'bang' on the stones. Their average intensity is fairly low compared to the effects on the stones. However, their acoustic pressures are very high, reaching nearly 10 MPa. The range of pressures overlaps with the diagnostic equipment.

The important difference between these therapy applications and the diagnostic applications is the frequency, normally 10–50 times lower in therapy.

The application of ultrasound for treatment of disease in the mother may inadvertently lead to damage to the fetus if serious precautions are not taken.

Safety of diagnostic ultrasound in obstetrics

Obstetrics is a particularly sensitive field. A general rule is that fast growing and developing tissues are more sensitive to outside influences. This applies to embryonic and fetal tissues in particular. The potential hazard varies in extent and nature during the intrauterine development.

Before implantation, physical stress can cause abortion. After implantation, various tissues and organs become susceptible to damage at different times. Between 5 and 10 weeks of gestation, the neural tube is prone to damage; the forebrain development is particularly important until the 20th week of gestation. The development of the right and left side of the brain is not symmetrical in time, nor is the end result. Thus, it is important to be aware of possible neurological effects and that such effects may show as some sort of sidedness.

Heating and its effects

The human body is a thermodynamic system. Chemical reactions depend on the temperature. The sensitivity of the reactions dictates the very narrow temperature span in which the human body operates well.

A very long temperature increase of 1.5°C above 37°C does not present a health hazard for humans.[6–10] It has been shown that exposure of mouse embryos for 5 min to a temperature increase of 4°C is hazardous for their development. The temperature range between the two extremes both in temperature and duration is the present 'gray zone' of knowledge. The consensus is that exposure of adult proliferative tissue to heat at 42°C for up to 2 h[11] can cause only reparable damage. The effects are proportional to I_{SPTA} and the absorption coefficient. The absorption coefficient is proportional to frequency. Absorption also depends on the tissue type. In the case of longitudinal waves, absorption is at least an order of magnitude greater in bone than in soft tissues. Bodily fluids absorb very little so that they are unlikely to heat up due to the traversing of ultrasound. Tissues with high connective tissue content absorb more. However, they allow little attenuated ultrasound to reach structures positioned beyond them. On the other hand, the absorption of shear waves is very high in soft tissues and, thus, if any shear wave is induced in a bone it will be absorbed within a millimeter in the adjacent soft tissue. This may then significantly increase the temperature on such a boundary. Blood vessels and perfusion in the target area act as a cooling system and take the heat away. If the perfusion is poor, the heat may accumulate. Fatty tissue and bones are structures with relatively poor perfusion and little consequent cooling. The heating may have multiple maxima, i.e. near the transducer at the focus and at specific media interfaces. The main problem may be the heating of nervous tissue caused by absorption within itself, by heating at the adjacent bone/soft tissue boundaries (skull vertebrae). The same applies to bone marrow.[12] While it is known that hyperthermia can be teratogenic in animals, there is no study in large mammals confirming that diagnostic ultrasound-induced hyperthermia causes such effects. It should be borne in mind that a higher body temperature, e.g. due to fever, may increase the damaging ultrasound energy.

Non-thermal effects

Effects other than thermal are conceivable. In 1972, Hill considered the possibility of mechanical effects.[13]

Either cavitation or other forces induced by altering compression and rarefaction forces may damage the molecules of which the body is composed. Transient cavitation is known to have damaging potential, as collapsing bubbles generate shock waves that disrupt nearby structures. The temperature at the point of implosion is extremely high (a few thousand degrees). In addition, relatively stable, oscillating bubbles induce microstreaming of liquids around them, possibly causing changes in metabolism or mechanical damage to cell membranes. If cavitation is a possible cause of hazard then the mechanical index (MI)[14,15] accepted by the Food and Drug Administration (FDA)[16] might yield some means of comparing various scanners and modes of operation.

In order to measure the pressure *in situ,* it is necessary to take into account the attenuation in the intervening tissue. Using this convention, the attenuation is taken to be 0.3 dB/cm MHz. It is a good idea to have this index displayed on the screen in order to choose the operation regimen that yields the required data while maintaining the MI as low as possible.

Streaming[17,18] of absorbing and attenuating liquids due to ultrasound passage is due to the variation of energy concentration along the path (actually it is the change of the impulse). It depends on the attenuation coefficient of the liquid and its viscosity. Particles in the liquid can contribute to streaming. A particular type of streaming is microstreaming around an oscillating gas bubble.

The basic biological effect that would cause concern in the case of collapsing bubbles is the generation of free radicals. This could lead to alteration of chromosomes. If the free radicals are formed outside the membrane, the time needed for transport of such radicals to the nucleus is longer than their half-life. However, there is no confirmed evidence of chromosomal effects, particularly in living mammals.

Another possible non-thermal mechanism may be due to direct mechanical vibration of cell membranes. This might cause changes in ion (calcium in particular) permeability.[4]

The soft tissue to gas boundary may present a particularly favorable situation for mechanical effects because the gas side presents very low resistance. Rarefaction pressures may present a potential hazard when using high-energy Doppler with the beam hitting the lung.[19] However, the fetal lung is not at such risk as it is not filled with air. The reports of change in neurological development such as speech and handedness[20–22] have not been confirmed by independent studies.

Clinical aspects

The whole body of knowledge concerning the biological effects of ultrasound is relevant only if it helps in the estimation of whether diagnostic ultrasound as used today is hazardous for the patients and, if so, to what extent. It should be noted that even a significant change in rare conditions (for example, those that appear once in 10,000) may not be detectable, because the statistics require too great a number of controlled cases. In such investigations, we must concentrate on the type of damage that is most likely to occur, based on the understanding of the underlying mechanisms. Because of the bone/soft tissue interface the central nervous system is the most likely candidate for thermal damage. Damage of a small area in the brain may not yield easily detectable consequences unless it affects a sensory mechanism (vision, hearing, etc.). Other organs, once they consist of a large number of cells, can repair partial mechanical damage. If the damage happens early, destruction of a small number of cells may have very serious late consequences in the form of defective development.

While there is no independently confirmed experimental proof of such damage, the indications are that any effects are obtained only when the temperature rises by more than 2°C for a few minutes. With scanned beams and modern equipment, it is very improbable that such a long time would be spent at one spot.

The application of echo/contrasts ought to be restricted to adult scanning for the time being, because the existence of microbubbles may increase the probability of non-thermal effects.

In vitro experiments yield a variety of demonstrated effects.[13,23,24] Such experiments can help indicate the direction of investigation in whole organisms, but they lack the important property of living tissues, namely, that the individual cells are interconnected in a tissue unlike cells suspended in a culture. Under such conditions, the probability of non-thermal mechanisms occurring is much higher than in whole tissues.

All the experimental indications of damage caused by diagnostic ultrasound, although independently confirmed, indicate that the probability is low. This means that in practice caution is advised, but no absolute recommendation against the use of diagnostic ultrasound measurements is advised.

Standards and labeling recommendations

There are no easy methods for measuring the temperature increase in a patient *in vivo*. Thus, it is necessary to resort to estimates based on experimental work. Present solutions to this problem are certainly approximate and partial, but the pressure of the reality warrants such approaches. The National Council on Radiation Protection and Measurements (NCRP) and The American Institute of Ultrasound in Medicine/ National Electrical Manufacturers Association (AIUM/ NEMA)[14] have developed models. The latter body has devised an index for estimating the heating likelihood, which is not expected to exceed under normal circumstances. This so-called thermal index (TI) may be displayed on the screen to give the operator real-time relative guidance on the potential heating of the tissues scanned. The value applies to the situation *in situ*. There exists no internationally accepted standard for any of the proposed indicators of thermal hazard. The AIUM/NEMA TI provides an estimate of temperature increase. By convention, TI is the ratio of total acoustic power to the acoustic power required to raise tissue temperature by 1°C. Although its basis is an approximate calculation of the actual temperature increase for a 'standard' tissue at a distance, it may not be interpreted literally. It is a relative indication of the possible temperature increase. The subvariants of the TI are meant for specific situations, i.e. TIS for homogenous soft tissue, TIC for temperature increase of bone near the surface (e.g. skull) and TIB for temperature increase at the bone boundary in the beam focus area. Using this labeling standard, if the scanner is not capable of producing a TI >1, it does not have to be displayed. Other national and international bodies have conceived other means of estimation. The capability of an ultrasound system to cause heating may be described by the ratio of acoustic power to the maximum temperature rise. The idea is to perform an actual worst-case calculation and to define the conditions (and instrument settings) that yield the maximum temperature increase so that all else is less hazardous. This is still under development, as a consensus about the tissue and beam properties has not been achieved.[11] Various sources give differing data[9,25–28] on ultrasound absorption in tissues and its action upon them. Nevertheless, the ultimate aim should be a consensus in recommendations given by various bodies and organizations. This should be based on realistic estimates of the possibility of ultrasound-induced heating. This is, among other things, an important guideline for the industry to discontinue the increase in ultrasound energy outputs in new apparatus models.

This leads to guideline conclusions by expert groups, e.g. European Federation of Societies of Ultrasound in Medicine and Biology (EFSUMB) Watchdogs or the AIUM bioeffects committee, which came to the consensus that when using the I_{SPTA} of 720 mW/cm^2, the maximum temperature rise *in situ* would not exceed 2°C, and thus will be safe to use. The present FDA regulation gives I_{SPTA} values of 720, 430, 94, 17 mW/cm^2 for peripheral vessel, cardiac, fetal and ophthalmic (i.e. eye lens) applications, respectively. The regulation is not limited to I_{SPTA} but includes an MI. Measurements in humans would be difficult or unduly aggressive and thus are impossible. Experiments on excised tissue or experimental animals cannot be directly extrapolated to humans but give important guidelines as to where to look for danger. The time-limited soft tissue experiments with ultrasound pulses equivalent to pulsed Doppler mode have shown heating below 2.5°C in various experiments. However, higher temperature increases have been measured in animals at skull bone/brain boundaries.[11]

The safety of Doppler ultrasound

In general, it is emphasized that ultrasonic examination should be performed only for medical indications, and diagnostic ultrasound users should recognize the sensitivity of young biological tissues of developing embryos and fetuses exposed to intense ultrasound.[10] The users also should know the ultrasonic intensity of their devices, the mechanisms of ultrasound bioeffect, and the prudent use of the devices, because they are responsible for the ultrasound safety. An important ultrasound bioeffect is thermal effect due to temperature rise induced by ultrasound absorption, because malformations were reported in the exposure of animal embryos and fetuses to high temperature in biological experiments. No hazardous thermal effect is expected when the temperature rise of exposed tissue is less than 1.5°C, and local temperature is lower than 38.5°C.[29] Five minutes' exposure to 41°C temperature can be hazardous to the tissue. Inertial cavitation and other mechanical effects are concerned in the non-thermal bioeffects of ultrasound.

The intensity of Doppler ultrasound

No hazardous thermal effect is expected in common B-mode imaging device because of minimum heat production due to low ultrasound intensity, i.e. the World Federation of Ultrasound in Medicine and Biology (WFUMB)[29] concluded that the use of simple imaging equipment is not contraindicated on thermal grounds. The real-time B-mode, simple 3D and 4D imaging devices, ultrasonic fetal heartbeat detector and fetal monitor are included in the category. Diagnostic ultrasound safety was established in Japan, after the Japanese Industrial Standard regulated the output power of diagnostic ultrasound devices below 10 mW/cm^2 in 1980, which was 1/100 of hazardous CW ultrasound[30–32] intensity at 1 W/cm^2. However, ultrasound safety has been discussed again after the introduction of Doppler flow velocity measurement, because pulsed Doppler method required definitely higher power than B-mode ultrasound.

Maximum intensity of commercial Doppler ultrasound is 1–3 W/cm^2. It is definitely higher than that of B-mode imaging, and it is the level of ultrasound physiotherapy for the tissue heating. Ultrasound safety is important even in physiotherapy, e.g. the therapeutic transducer should be always moved on the bone, so young bone and pregnant women are contraindicated for physiotherapy. The difference between therapeutic ultrasound and pulsed Doppler is exposure duration, i.e. it is short in Doppler flow measurement and long in therapeutic ultrasound. Therefore, thermal effect is a big concern in Doppler ultrasound bioeffect. Temperature rises not only at the sample volume, but also in all tissues passed by the ultrasound beam. The International

Table 37.1 Relation of non-hazardous exposure time (*t* min) to the temperature rise above 37°C and absolute temperature is calculated by Eq. (2), which is obtained from the results of experimental heating of animal fetuses[34]

Temperature rise (°C)	Absolute temperature (°C)	Non-hazardous exposure time; *t* (min)	log *t*
1	38	1000.0	3.00
2	39	251.8	2.40
3	40	63.10	1.80
4	41	15.85	1.20
5	42	3.98	0.60
6	43	1.0	0

Society of Ultrasound in Obstetrics and Gynecology (ISUOG) has also discussed the safe use of Doppler ultrasound.[33] Ultrasound intensity is less in color/power Doppler flow mapping due to the scanning procedure than in pulsed Doppler because of stable irradiation. Temporal averaging intensity of common color Doppler ultrasound is also less than 720 mW/cm^2, which is lower than in pulsed Doppler devices, and lower than the FDA regulation.[16] Thermal effect is discussed in the first place, due to possible teratogenicity of heating. Exposure duration is important for the safety of Doppler velocimetry.

The effect of heating on mammal fetuses

A teratogenic effect was reported by the biologists after the exposure of animal embryos and fetuses to high temperature, that is, malformations were found in various species by experimental heating. The temperature was 39–50°C. Teratogenic effect on mammals are summarized in the report of the National Council for Radiation Protection and Measurement (NCRP).[34] A discrimination line is found between the hazardous and non-hazardous areas in the NCRP report. There is no malformation if the fetus is heated in the area under the discrimination line, which is determined by connecting the points of high temperature/short exposure and low temperature/long exposure. Non-hazardous exposure is as short as 1 min in 43°C, and infinite in physiological body temperature. In case of ultrasound irradiation, TI indicates the temperature rise, therefore absolute temperature is obtained by summing 37°C and the temperature rise derived from TI.

Non-hazardous exposure time of the fetus to the heating

The guideline on the safety of mammals against heat can be found in the revised safety statement of AIUM[35] published in 1998, which is based on the NCRP report in 1992, where an inverse relation was found between hazardous temperature level and exposure time. AIUM[35] stated that the fetus tolerates 50 h at 2°C rise (absolute temperature is 39°C), and 1 min at 6°C rise (43°C). They also showed the relation of the temperature rise (T) above 37°C and non-hazardous exposure time (t min) by Eq. (1), and non-hazardous time (t min) is shown by Eq. (2), which is revised from Eq. (1):

$$T\ (^\circ\mathrm{C}) = 6-[(\log_{10} t)/0.6] \quad (1)$$

$$t = 10^{(3.6-0.6T)} \quad (2)$$

The relation of non-hazardous exposure time and the temperature rise as well as absolute temperature is shown by Eq. (2) (Table 37.1, Figure 37.1). The safety regarding the thermal effect of ultrasound can be discussed by the relation of exposure time and temperature, when the heat production of Doppler ultrasound is estimated from TI, which indicates the temperature rise above 37°C in the worst case of temperature rise in ultrasound exposure to standardized tissue model, i.e. maximum temperature rise is known by TI.

Maintaining the safety of Doppler sonography

General safety of diagnostic ultrasound device

Electrical and mechanical safety is assured in ultrasound devices by the manufacturer under international and domestic guidelines. In a Doppler scanner, TI, MI, transducer temperature and other related indices are displayed on the monitor screen,[36] enabling the users to maintain the safety of ultrasound diagnosis by themselves. Obstetric setting should be confirmed before Doppler flow velocity measurements during pregnancy. Ultrasonic examinations should be done under medical indications. Although the ISUOG safety statement[33] reported that there is no reason to withhold the use of scanners that have received current FDA clearance in the absence of gas bodies, AIUM[35] stated that for the current FDA[16] regulatory limit of 720 mW/cm^2, the best available estimate of the maximum temperature increase can exceed 2°C. Pulsed ultrasound intensity threshold to

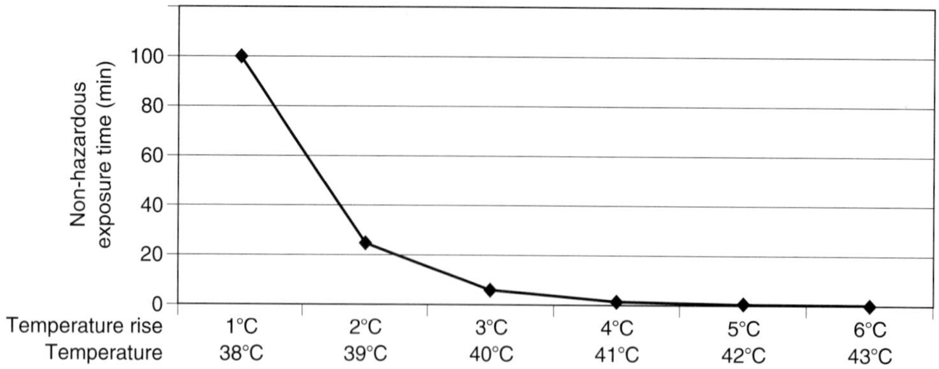

Figure 37.1 Relation of non-hazardous exposure time to the temperature rise between 1°C and 6°C above 37°C (38–43°C of absolute temperature) in experimental heating of animal fetuses[34] [graphed by Eq. (2)].

suppress cultured cell-growth curve was 240 mW/cm^2 in our studies.[32] The FDA regulation may be still controversial from the opinions and reports.

Thermal effect of Doppler scanner

The TI is a useful index of temperature rise induced by ultrasound exposure. Standard tissue models are exposed to ultrasound and TI is determined in the worst case, i.e. the highest temperature rise is the base of TI.[36] One TI stands for 1°C temperature elevation, and in the same manner, temperature rises for 3°C above 37°C, and absolute temperature is 40°C, if TI is 3. Local temperature rise is estimated only by TI at present, therefore TI is the index to estimate tissue temperature in ultrasound examination, to study the ultrasonic thermal effect, and to avoid the possible thermal hazard of intense ultrasound. TI and temperature rise are low in the soft tissue exposure, and high in the bone exposure. Soft tissue TI (TIS) is, therefore, used in the case of embryo that has no bone before 10 weeks of pregnancy, and bone TI (TIB) is applied for the fetus with bone after 10 weeks. Cranial TI (TIC) is the index for the intracranial flow examination.

No hazardous thermal effect is expected when the temperature rise of exposed tissue is less than 1.5°C, and local temperature is lower than 38.5°C, while a 5-min duration of 41°C can be hazardous to the tissue. Its temperature rise is 4°C above 37°C, and TI can be 4. Ultrasound examination is totally safe in the exposure with TI <1. In daily practice, therefore, TI should be <1, particularly in the long fetal examination, the screening of pregnancy or the research study of no limit. The output power is reduced if TI >1 on the monitor, then TI decreases to the level <1.[36] Clear flow velocity waveform is recorded and even output power is reduced to 60% in the experiment on the small hand artery.

The revised safety statement of AIUM[35] stated that an equal or less than 2°C temperature rise above 37°C showed no adverse effects with exposure duration up to 50 h, and that the upper limit of safe exposure duration was 16 min at 4°C rise and 1 min at 6°C rise above normal, respectively. The AIUM opinion on the effect of high temperature is similar to the report of NCRP,[34] and the safety statement is acceptable if the temperature rise is accurately determined by the TI, because TI indicates the worst tissue temperature elevation due to ultrasound exposure in clinical study.

Although the revised safety statement is useful in a retrospective safety confirmation after ultrasound exposure of known exposure time and TI, fetal exposure to the temperature rise for 4–6°C may be controversial, where absolute temperature is 41–43°C. Non-hazardous exposure time at temperatures higher than 40°C is critically short in the NCRP report[34] and AIUM statement,[35] where the safety margin remains very narrow,[2] excess heating may not be completely avoided and it may be imperfect to precisely keep strict exposure time at the highest temperature. The aim of this report is, therefore, to propose a practically applicable safe exposure time in the prospective situation before a Doppler ultrasound diagnosis.

Two modes in the time of exposure to diagnostic ultrasound

Two modes can be classified in the use of Doppler ultrasound. The TI <1 (AIUM) or the temperature rise below 1.5°C (WFUMB) after temperature equilibrium can be adopted for the infinite exposure. Therefore, this mode is suitable for research work, where exposure duration is rarely determined before the study. TI may also be <1 in the screening of the fetus during pregnancy and in fetal heart rate monitoring.

A pulsed Doppler study is another situation where the user requires improved Doppler flow wave by using TI >1. In some ultrasound lectures, the speakers stated that in the Doppler studies safety was proved by shortened exposure when TI >1. The technique is the same as in the NCRP report,[34] which proved non-hazardous by the short exposure to high temperature. Therefore, the Doppler examination with TI >1 can be also non-hazardous by the short exposure.

The relation of non-hazardous exposure to high temperature, high temperature rise and large TI is

Table 37.2 Thermal index (TI), tissue temperature, non-hazardous exposure time in the NCRP report,[34] the safety factors and exposure time to ultrasound are listed. Although the user can voluntarily set the safety factor and exposure time, we recommend choosing the safety factor at 50 and exposure time at 5 min when TI is 2

TI	Absolute temperature (°C)	Non-hazardous exposure time of NCRP report (min)	Exposure time (min) obtained by dividing non-hazardous exposure time of NCRP report by various safety factors			
			Safety factor			
			3	10	50	100
6	43	1	0.3	0.1	0.02	0.01 (no use)
4	41	16	5	0.2	0.03	0.02 (no use)
3	40	64	21	6	*1*	0.6
2	39	256	85	25	*5*	2.5

achieved by using Eq. (2) (Table 37.1 and Figure 37.1). Exposure time is as long as 250 min, about 4 h, when TI is 2 and temperature is 39°C, 1 h if TI is 3 and temperature 40°C, and 15 min even if TI is 4, where the temperature is 41°C according to the reports of NCRP[34] and AIUM.[35] These criteria are extremely useful in the retrospective confirmation of Doppler ultrasound safety of past examination. However, the prospective exposure time setting before examination should be further discussed.

Prospective exposure time setting before Doppler examination

Exposure time is preset before the Doppler examination, where the TI is voluntarily increased to >1 with the intention of improving Doppler flow. The NCRP report is the base of decision, where non-hazardous exposure time is determined by the temperature rise estimated by TI (Tables 37.1 and 37.2, Figure 37.1). It is unique in the present proposal that the non-hazardous exposure time obtained is divided by the 'safety factor' of 3–100, and actual exposure time is obtained. The procedure was the same as the past regulation of simple ultrasound devices in Japan, where hazardous threshold intensity of CW ultrasound in our experimental study was divided by the safety factor of 100 and output intensity was regulated to be lower than 10 mW/cm^2. There was no problem in the safety of dagnostic ultrasound before the introduction of Doppler flow studies. Though the factor is voluntarily changed by the user, appropriate values will be discussed in this paper. As ultrasound intensity may increase by about three times in the case of standing wave, 3 is the lowest safety factor. The intensity increases due to the distortion of ultrasound wave, and the possible estimation error of TI[11] or others are further added to the safety factor.

For example, non-hazardous exposure time is 252 min at 39°C (Table 37.1), where the temperature rises for 2°C and corresponding TI is 2. If the safety factor is 50, 252 min is divided by 50, and the exposure time is 5 min. By the same procedure, 1 min of exposure time is preset when TI is 3 (Table 37.2). The safety factor of 100 may be too conservative, though the factor can be selected by the user. Mildly longer exposure than the preset value may be included in the safety factor in most cases. Possibly 50 is the appropriate safety factor in the actual Doppler examination. The exposure time setting is coincidentally close to the safety statement of the British Medical Ultrasound Society (BMUS),[37] where the exposure time is 4 min when TI is 2 and 1 min if TI is 2.5.

The users can voluntarily change the safety factor and prolong the exposure time, because they are responsible for the ultrasound safety. However, they may also be responsible at the same time for the increased risk factor caused by the reduction of the safety factor.

Other thermal issues

Ultrasound thermal effect has been discussed mainly in relation to teratogenicity in the first trimester, whereas animal fetal skull or the brain surface was heated and the temperature elevation was more than 4°C by the exposure to intense ultrasound.[38] Thermal damage of the brain cannot be denied in this case. Therefore, the use of maximum intensity level of Doppler ultrasound is inadvisable in the flow study even in late pregnancy.

Caution should be used regarding the temperature of the tissue exposed to Doppler ultrasound in febrile patients, where the basic temperature is higher than 37°C. For example, if TI is 2 in a 38°C febrile patient, the temperature rise above the physiologic condition is 3°C, the situation is the same as TI 3 in non-febrile normal temperature cases, and therefore, 1 min of exposure time is allowed if the safety factor is 50.

Exposure duration should be recorded by the user in every study of voluntarily increased exposure time, while TI which appeared on the monitor screen is recorded on the photograph or computer memory. The safety indices including TI and MI are recommended to be described in the 'Methods' section of the reports of Doppler ultrasound study on human subjects.

Transducer temperature in transvaginal scan

The transvaginal scan user should be careful about the direct heating of the attached tissue due to high surface temperature of the transducer, which directly attaches to the vaginal wall, and because the subjects are closer to the transducer than to the abdominal ultrasound. The transducer temperature, which is displayed on the monitor screen, should be lower than 41°C. Every intracavitary scan user should also be careful of the transducer temperature.

Mechanical effects of diagnostic ultrasound

MI is used for the estimation of mechanical bioeffect. It is rarefactional sound pressure expressed in megapascals, divided by the square root of ultrasound frequency (MHz). The MI indicates the non-thermal bioeffect of ultrasound, particularly in the collapse of gas bubbles in various liquids. Although gynecologic examination by contrast medium is still infrequent, its common use in adult circulation should be carefully studied in the mechanical bioeffect. Although common B-mode imaging devices are low in the thermal effect, its mechanical effect is similar to the Doppler devices because instantaneous intensity of its ultrasound pulse is not much different from Doppler machines, and therefore, even simple imaging devices should be carefully handled in relation to mechanical effect. It is rare to use contrast medium in obstetrical tissue; free radicals formed in the liquid due to inertial cavitation hardly reach the floating cells because of their short life, and no cavitation may occur within the cell due to the high viscosity of cell plasma. However, the biological effects of acoustic streaming, capillary blood cell stasis by the standing wave, or direct ultrasonic pressure require further basic studies. As hemorrhage is found in the lung of neonatal animals after the exposure to intense ultrasound, MI <1 is recommended particularly in neonatal lung examination. The International Electrotechnical Commission (IEC) is working on the classification of diagnostic ultrasound devices by the MI.

Conclusion

Diagnostic ultrasound safety has been mainly discussed on the thermal effect. Simple real-time B-mode, 3D and 4D imaging devices, fetal heart detector and fetal monitor are not contraindicated due to thermal effect, because of their very low ultrasound intensity. Doppler flow machines are mainly discussed with thermal effect, because of their definitely high ultrasound intensity. Safe fetal exposure time to ultrasound determined by the NCRP criteria on the exposure to high temperature estimated by TI is useful in the retrospective evaluation of past ultrasound examination. In prospective estimation of ultrasound safety in daily practice, the principle of safe diagnostic ultrasound is the reduction of ultrasonic intensity and exposure time when displayed TI is >1. The research work and pregnancy screening follow the principle. Moderately higher TI is allowed in clinical study when the users require more improved Doppler flow wave by increased intensity, where a limited short exposure time is prescribed and the users adhere to the preset time by their own responsibility. We recommend using the non-hazardous exposure time of the NCRP report after dividing it by the safety factor of 50, where exposure time is 5 min if TI is 2, and 1 min if TI is 3. Higher TI or longer exposure may be applied by reducing the safety factor under the users' responsibility. Attention should be paid to the decreased safety in the febrile patient. Transvaginal transducer should be used under 41°C. The mechanical effect may be similar in simple B-mode Doppler devices. MI is recommended to be <1 in ultrasound examination, particularly in the studies on air in neonatal lung.

REFERENCES

1. Starrit HC, Duck FA. A comparison of ultrasound exposure in therapy and pulsed Doppler fields. *Br J Radiol* 1992;65: 557–63.
2. American Institute of Ultrasound in Medicine (AIUM). *Acoustical Data for Diagnostic Ultrasound Equipment.* AIUM, 1993.
3. Henderson J, Willson K, Jago JR, Whittingham TA. A survey of acoustic outputs of diagnostic ultrasound equipment in current clinical use. *Ultrasound Med Biol* 1995;21:699–705.
4. International Commission on Radiation Protection. *Recommendation for Radiation Protection,* ICRP Publication 26. New York: Pergamon Press, 1977.
5. International Commission on Radiation Protection. *Recommendation for Radiation Protection,* ICRP Publication 60. New York: Pergamon Press, 1991.
6. MacDonald W, Newham J, Gurrin L, Ewans S. Effect of frequent prenatal ultrasound on birthweight: Follow up at one year of age. *Lancet* 1996;348:482.
7. Lyons EA, Dyke C, Toms M, Cheang M. *In utero* exposure to diagnostic ultrasound: A 6 year follow-up. *Radiology* 1988; 166:687–90.
8. Smith CB. Birthweights of fetuses exposed to diagnostic ultrasound. *J Ultrasound Med* 1984;3:395–6.
9. Saari Kemppainen A, Karjalainen O, Ylostalo P, Heinonen OP. Ultrasound screening and perinatal mortality: Controlled trial of systemic one-stage screening in pregnancy. The Helsinki Ultrasound Trial. *Lancet* 1990;336:387–91.
10. Barnett SB, ter Haar G, Ziskin MC, Nyborg WL, Maeda K, Bang J. Current status of research on biophysical effects of ultrasound. *Ultrasound Med Biol* 1994;20:205–18.

11. Barnett SB, Kossoff G, eds. Results of the WFUMB Symposium on Safety and Standardization in Medical Ultrasound. *Ultrasound Med Biol* 1992;18 (special issue).
12. Barnett SB, Edwards MJ, Martin P. Pulsed ultrasound induces temperature elevation and nuclear abnormalities in bone marrow cells of guinea pig femurs (abstract). Presented at the *6th World Congress of Ultrasound in Medicine*, Copenhagen, Denmark, 1991:3405.
13. Hill CR. Ultrasonic exposure thresholds for changes in cells and tissues. *J Acoust Soc Am* 1972;52:667–72.
14. American Institute of Ultrasound in Medicine. *AIUM/NEMA Standard for Real-time Display of Thermal and Mechanical Acousitc Output Indices on Diagnostic Ultrasound Equipment.* AIUM Publications, 1992.
15. Food and Drug Administration. *Guide for Measuring and Reporting Acoustic Output of Diagnostic Ultrasound.* Rockville, MD: Food and Drug Administration, Devices and Radiological Health, 1992.
16. Food and Drug Administration. *Revised 510(K) Diagnostic Ultrasound Guidance for 1993.* Rockville, MD: Food and Drug Administration, 1993.
17. Nyborg WL. Acoustic streaming due to attenuated plan waves. *J Acoust Soc Am* 1953;25:68–75.
18. Starrit HC, Duck FA, Humphrey VF. An experimental investigation of streaming in pulsed diagnostic ultrasound beams. *Ultrasound Med Biol* 1989;15:363–73.
19. Tarantal AF, Canfield DR. Ultrasound induced lung hemorrhage in the monkey. *Ultrasound Med Biol* 1994;20:65–72.
20. Salvesen KA, Vatten LJ, Eik-Nes S, Hugdahl K, Bakketig LS. Routine ultrasonography *in utero* and subsequent handedness and neurological development. *Br Med J* 1993;307:159–64.
21. Campbell JD, Elford RW, Brant RF. Case control study of prenatal ultrasonography exposure in children with delayed speech. *Can Med Assoc J* 1993;149:1435–40.
22. Salvesen KA, Vatten LJ, Bakketig LS, Eik-Nes S. Routine ultrasonography *in utero* and speech development. *Ultrasound Obstet Gynecol* 1994;4:101–3.
23. Holland CK, Zheng X, Apfel RE, Alderman JL, Fernandez L, Taylor KJW. Direct evidence of cavitation *in vivo* from diagnostic ultrasound. *Ultrasound Med Biol* 1996;22:917–25.
24. Hefer-Lauc M, Latin V, Breyer B, Floegel M, Mueler WEG, Lauc G. Glycoprotein and ganglioside changes in human trophoblasts after exposure to pulsed Doppler ultrasound. *Ultrasound Med Biol* 1995;21:579–84.
25. Barnett SB, Kossoff G, eds. *Safety of Diagnostic Ultrasound.* Carnforth, UK: Parthenon Publishing, 1997.
26. American Institute of Ultrasound in Medicine. *Medical Ultrasound Safety.* AIUM Publications, 1994.
27. International Electrotechnical Commission. *IEC International Standard,* IEC/CEI 1157. Geneva: Bureau Central de la Commission Electrotechnique Internationale, 1992.
28. Dyson M. The susceptibility of tissues to ultrasound. In Docker FM, Duck FA, eds. *The Safe Use of Diagnostic Ultrasound.* BIR, 1991:24.
29. Barnett SB, Kossoff G. WFUMB symposium on safety and standardisation in medical ultrasound: Issues and recommendations regarding thermal mechanisms for biological effects of ultrasound, Hornbick, 1991. *Ultrasound Med Biol* 1992;18:v–xix, 731–814.
30. Ide M. Japanese policy and status of standardisation. *Ultrasound Med Biol* 1986;12:705–8.
31. Maeda K, Ide M. The limitation of the ultrasound intensity for diagnostic devices in the Japanese industrial standards. *IEEE Trans Ultrason Ferroelectr Freq Control* 1986;UFFC-33:241–4.
32. Maeda K, Murao F, Yoshiga T, Yamauchi C, Tsuzaki T. Experimental studies on the suppression of cultured cell growth curves after irradiation with CW and pulsed ultrasound. *IEEE Trans Ultrason Ferroelectr Freq Control* 1986;UFFC-33:186–193.
33. ISUOG Bioeffects and Safety Committee. Safety statement, 2000 (reconfirmed 2002). *Ultrasound Obstet Gynecol* 2002;19:105.
34. National Council on Radiation Protection and Measurements. *Exposure Criteria for Medical Diagnostic Ultrasound: I. Criteria Based on Thermal Mechanisms.* NCRP Report No. 113, 1992.
35. American Institute of Ultrasound in Medicine. AIUM official statement changes; revised statements; clinical safety. *AIUM Reporter* 1998;154(1):6–7.
36. American Institute of Ultrasound in Medicine/National Electrical Manufacturers Association. *Standard for Real Time Display of Thermal and Mechanical Acoustic Output Indices on Diagnostic Ultrasound Equipment.* AIUM, 1992.
37. The Safety Group of the British Medical Ultrasound Society. Guidelines for the safe use of diagnostic ultrasound equipment. *Br Med Ultrasound Soc Bull* 2000;3:29–33.
38. Barnett SB, Rott HD, Ter Haar GR, Ziskin MC, Maeda K. The sensitivity of biological tissue to ultrasound. *Ultrasound Med Biol* 1997;23:805–12.
39. European Committee for Ultrasound Radiation Safety. *Eur J Ultrasound* 1996;4:145.
40. ter Haar G. Commentary: Safety of diagnostic ultrasound. *Br J Radiol* 1996;69:1083–5.
41. EFSUMB. European Committee for Ultrasound Radiation Safety – the Watchdogs, clinical safety statement. *Eur J Ultrasound* 1996;3:283.

38 Behavioral perinatology assessed by four-dimensional sonography

A. Kurjak, J. M. Carrera, W. Andonotopo,
G. Azumendi, M. Medic and A. Salihagic-Kadic

Three-dimensional (3D) ultrasound has been available for more than 10 years. However, the 3D image freezes the object and therefore does not provide information on movements or any information about the dynamic changes in the object of interest. A technique was needed that would enable 3D imaging to be performed in a real-time mode. This technique has been recently introduced and has been called 4D sonography, because time becomes a parameter within the 3D imaging sequence. This new diagnostic tool enables the continuous monitoring of the fetal face and other surface features of the fetus such as fetal extremities. This permits exciting new possibilities for the study of fetal behavior.

Four-dimensional ultrasound provides a new tool for observation of the fetal face. Simultaneous imaging of complex facial movements was not possible using real-time 2D ultrasound. Four-dimensional ultrasound integrates the advantage of the spatial imaging of the fetal face with the addition of time. This new technology therefore allows the appearance and duration of each facial movement and expression to be determined and measured.

In a relatively short period of time 4D sonography has stimulated many multicentric studies on fetal behavior and even fetal awareness with more convincing imaging and data than those obtained by conventional ultrasonic and non-ultrasonic methods. The purpose of this article is to review and illustrate presently available data on 4D ultrasound fetal behavior imaging in all three trimesters of pregnancy.

Neurophysiology of fetal behavior

For centuries, maternal registration of fetal movements and obstetrician auscultation of fetal heartbeats were the only methods of follow-up of fetal well-being *in utero*. However, during the past few decades, the development of ultrasonic techniques has enabled the direct visualization of the fetus *in utero*, as well as the real-time assessment of fetal activity. Ultrasonic studies have revealed the fascinating diversity of fetal intrauterine activities. It has been shown that fetal activity occurs as early as the late embryonic period, which is far earlier than a mother can sense. Furthermore, qualitative and quantitative aspects of behavioral patterns expand rapidly as the pregnancy progresses, and the random movements of the fetal body, which are the earliest sign of fetal activity, change into the well-organized behavioral patterns observed late in gestation. Analysis of the dynamics of fetal behavior has led to the conclusion that fetal behavioral patterns directly reflect the developmental and maturational processes of the fetal central nervous system (CNS). Nevertheless, the ultrasound findings and their relevance in the assessment of the development of the CNS can be interpreted only in comparison with the structural developmental events in the particular period of gestation. Therefore, understanding the relation between fetal behavior and developmental processes in different periods of gestation may make possible the distinction between normal and abnormal brain development, as well as the early diagnosis of various structural or functional abnormalities.

Structural development of human CNS

All the neurons and glial cells originate from the embryonic ectoderm, precisely a structure called the neural plate. During the fourth postconceptional week, the neural plate bends into a neural tube, whose further growth reshaping and histological characteristics directly reflect complicated histogenetic processes. The results of those processes are specific transitional embryonic zones, which cannot be observed in an

Table 38.1 Dynamics of the most important progressive processes in the development of the human brain

	Beginning	The most intensive period	Ending
Proliferation	3–4 weeks of gestation	8–12 weeks of gestation	Approximately 20 weeks of gestation
Migration	Simultaneously with proliferation	18–24 weeks of gestation	38 weeks of gestation
Synaptogenesis	8 weeks of gestation	13–16 weeks of gestation, after 24 weeks of gestation, eighth month to second year of postnatal life	Puberty

adult brain. Three embryonic zones, ventricular, intermediary and marginal (seen from ventricular to pial surface), are present in all parts of the neural tube, whereas the telencephalon contains two additional zones, subventricular and subplate.[1]

Histogenetic processes are proliferation, migration and differentiation of neurons and glial cells, as well as the synaptogenesis and development of chemical specificity of neurons. The dynamics of the main hystogenetic processes is shown in Table 38.1.

It is important to point out that proliferation of neurons and glial cells occurs only in the ventricular zone and in the subventricular zone of the telencephalon. All the future neurons and glia originate from these zones, form other transitional zones during their migration toward the pial surface and finally reach their permanent position and form the permanent synapses. The early appearance of interneuronal connections, shown in Table 38.1, implicates a possibility of an early functional development. However, these first synapses exist only temporarily and disappear due to the normal developmental processes. That is, simultaneously with these progressive processes, so-called reorganization processes occur. Some embryonic zones, types of neurons and glia and synapses that play a crucial role in certain periods of fetal brain development eventually disappear, significantly changing the structure and function of the brain. Reorganization processes include apoptosis, disappearance of redundant synapses, axonal retreat and transposition, and transformation of the neurotransmitters' phenotype. The temporal overlapping of the major histogenetic processes during the fetal brain development can be seen only in primates.

Obviously, the development of the human brain is not completed at the time of delivery. In an infant born at term, characteristic cellular layers can be observed in motor, somatosensor, visual and auditory cortical areas. Although proliferation and migration are completed in a term infant, synaptogenesis and neuronal differentiation continue very intensively.[2] The brain stem demonstrates a high level of maturity, whereas all histogenetic processes actively persist in the cerebellum.[3] Therefore, only subcortical formations and the primary cortical areas are developed completely in a newborn. Associative cortex, barely visible in a newborn, is scantily developed in a 6-month-old infant. Postnatal formation of synapses in associative cortical areas, which intensifies between the eighth month and the second year of life, precedes the onset of the first cognitive functions, such as speech. Following the second year of age, many redundant synapses are eliminated. The elimination of synapses begins very rapidly, and continues slowly until puberty, when the same number of synapses as seen in adults is reached.[3]

Functional development of the fetal nervous system

The functional development of the human fetus cannot be studied directly, but ultrasonic studies have made possible the visualization of the fetal motor activity *in utero*. The ultrasonic studies of fetal spontaneous motor activity and the motor responses to stimulation, in comparison with the morphological studies and experiments on animal models, have given us an insight into the complex dynamic of fetal development. An overview of the functional development of the fetal nervous system, which will be discussed further in the text, is given in Table 38.2.

Fetal motor development

The first synapses in the human nervous system appear approximately simultaneously with the formation of the cortical plate, i.e. around the eighth postconceptional week.[4,5] It is the period when the earliest electrical activity and transmission of information[6] occurs. The first spontaneous fetal movements were observed at 7.5 postconceptional weeks. These movements, consisting of slow flexion and extension of the fetal trunk accompanied by the passive displacement of the arms and legs[7] and appearing in irregular sequences, were described as 'vermicular'.[8] In a little while, they are replaced by various general movements, which include the head, trunk and limb, such

Table 38.2 Chronology of the functional development of fetal nervous system. Detailed description is given in the text

Weeks of gestation	Motor system	Sensor system	Circadian rhythm
6	Earliest spontaneous movements, gross body movements	Development of taste buds; development of nociceptors	
7		Generalized movements after cutaneous stimulation	
8	Movements of extremities, head and trunk; isolated limb movements	Localized movements after cutaneous stimulation	
9			
10	Sporadic breathing movements; spontaneous movements observed over 15% of 24-h time	Peripheral afferents from nociceptors to spinal cord begin to form – reflexive reactions to pain; cutaneous reflexes seen in hands	
11			
12			
13			Spontaneous movements and breathing movements associated with heart rate acceleration
14	Facial movements – swallowing, yawning, grimacing; very intensive motor activity, 15 different types of body movements can be observed; sporadic eye movements	Legs sensitive to cuntaneous stimulation – reflexes	
15		Secretion of leptin and VIP-possible regulators of appetite	
16			
17			
18		Alterations in cerebral blood flow in response to painful stimuli	
19			
20		Nociceptors present all over the body	
21			
22			
23		Elevation of cortisol and beta endorphin levels in response to painful stimuli	
24	Breathing movements eye observed over 14% of 24-h period		Consolidation of movements – alternation of EM and NEM periods
25		Cochlear function established (22–25 weeks); response to vibroacoustic stimulation without lag time	
26			
27			
28			
29			

Table 38.2 (Continued)

Weeks of gestation	Motor system	Sensor system	Circadian rhythm
30	Number of breathing movements change in response to alteration in CO_2 concentration in maternal blood	Fetus responds to purely acoustic stimulation	
31			
32	The number of spontaneous movements begins to decrease		
33			REM and SEM periods can be distinguished
34	Breathing movements sensitive to the maternal plasmatic glucose concentration		
35			
36			
37			
38			Constant duration of EM and NEM periods; integration of eye movements with other parameters of fetal activity (heart rate, movements)
39			
40			

as 'rippling' seen at 8 weeks, 'twitching' and 'strong twitching' at 9 and 9.5 weeks, respectively, and 'floating', 'swimming' and 'jumping' at 10 weeks.[9] Isolated limb movements appear almost simultaneously with the generalized movements.

Simultaneously with the onset of spontaneous movements, the earliest cutaneous reflex activity can be observed, allowing the assumption of the existence of the first afferent–efferent circuits (Table 38.2). The first reflex movements are massive and indicate a very limited number of synapses in a cutaneous reflex pathway.[10] At that time, head tilting after perioral stimulation is noted. During the eighth week of gestation these massive reflex movements are replaced with local movements, probably due to an increase in the number of axodendritic synapses. Hands become sensitive at 10.5 weeks and lower limbs begin to participate in these reflexes approximately at 14 weeks.[10–14] From the 10th week onward, the number and frequency of movements increase. By 14–19 weeks, the fetus is very active, with the longest period of inactivity lasting only 5–6 min. In the 15th week, 15 different movements can be observed. Besides the general body movements and isolated limb movements, retroflection, anteflection and rotation of the head can easily be seen. Moreover, face movements such as mouthing, yawning, hiccups, suckling and swallowing can be added to a wide repertoire of fetal motor activity in this period (see Table 38.2).[15] However, in such an early gestational period, the dynamic pattern of neuronal production and migration, as well as the immature cerebral circuits, are considered too immature for the cerebral involvement in the motor behavior (for a review see Kostovic *et al.*[16]). Only at the end of this period do a quantifiable number of synapses appear in the structures preceding the cerebral cortex, probably forming a substrate for the first cortical electric activity, noted at the 19th week.[16] Studies of anencephalic fetuses have also provided apparent evidences that around 17–20 gestational weeks, motor behavior becomes influenced by the supraspinal structures. That is, in these fetuses the incidence of movements was normal or even increased, but the complexity of movement patterns changed dramatically and movements were stereotyped and simplified.[17,18]

The number of spontaneous movements tends to increase until the 32nd week of pregnancy, when their frequency begins to decrease.[19–21] By term, the average number of generalized movements per hour was found to be approximately 31, with the longest period between movements ranging from 50 to 75 per min.[22] This decrease is considered a result of cerebral maturation processes, rather than a consequence of the decrease in the amniotic fluid volume. Simultaneously with the decrease in the number of generalized movements, an increase in the facial movements, including opening/closing of the jaw, swallowing and chewing, can be observed. These movements can be seen mostly in the periods of absence of generalized movements and that pattern is considered to be the reflection of the normal neurological development of the fetus.[19] However, the changes in not only the number of movements but also their complexity are shown to be the result of maturational processes. Our recent 4D ultrasound study, which will be described later in the text, has shown an even wider repertoire of fetal face and hand movements in the third trimester of gestation than has been previously described.[23] Obviously, the story of fetal intrauterine activity is far from being completed and the development of new recording techniques could enrich our perspective of the intrauterine life. It has been demonstrated that the fetal movement patterns in the second half of pregnancy are almost identical to those observed after birth,[24,25] although the repertoire of movements in newborns includes some patterns that cannot be observed in the fetus, such as the Moro reflex.[26] The detailed description of fetal movement patterns at different gestational ages, studied by conventional as well as 4D ultrasound, will be given later in the text.

Many factors, such as cigarette smoking[27] or injection of corticosteroids for fetal lung maturation,[28] were proved to decrease the number of spontaneous fetal movements. Furthermore, fetal activity is increased in mothers suffering some kind of emotional stress.[29] The quality of fetal movement patterns is altered in fetuses suffering intrauterine growth restriction. The movements become slower, monotonous, resembling cramps, and their variability in strength and amplitude is reduced. These changes could indicate the existence of brain lesions in growth-restricted and possibly hypoxic fetuses. That is, despite the earlier assumptions, the alterations in the amplitude and complexity of movements in these fetuses do not appear due to oligohydramnios. In cases of premature rupture of fetal membranes and a subsequently reduced volume of amniotic fluid, movements occur less frequently, but their complexity resembles that of movements performed in the normal volume of amniotic fluid (for a review see Prechtl and Einspieler[30]). Obviously, the qualitative as well as quantitative analysis of fetal movements reveals the integrity of the fetal nervous system, and can be used for the detection of various cerebral dysfunctions, and probably neuromuscular diseases.[29,30]

Development of specialized movements

Studies on animals, especially various species of mammals, as well as their comparisons with the ultrasonic recordings of human fetuses, have revealed that some specialized movement patterns, crucial for the survival of newborns, such as swallowing or rhythmic respiratory movements, develop and mature during gestation. Although these patterns differ somewhat from adult patterns, in the near-term fetuses they are developed sufficiently to enable the survival of the fetus.

In the human fetus, breathing movements occur around the 10th week of gestation.[31] Early in gestation, they are present almost continually and are associated with the activity in the postural muscles of the neck and limbs. However, the frequency and complexity of the breathing pattern change as pregnancy progresses. The total breathing time in a 24-h interval extends, as well as the duration of individual breathing and non-breathing intervals.[32,33] Changes in breathing patterns are considered to be a result of the maturation of the fetal lungs and respiratory and sleep centers in the fetal CNS. In the 38th and 39th weeks of gestation, frequency of movement decreases to 41 respirations per minute and the movements become as regular as in the postnatal period.[34] Approximately at the 30th week of gestation, the regulation of fetal breathing movements by the plasmatic level of carbon dioxide is established and the number of respirations increases following an excess of carbon dioxide in maternal blood.[35,36] This sensitivity to the alterations in the plasmatic carbon dioxide level is connected to the maturation of fetal respiratory neural centers, which is thought to occur during the last 10 weeks of pregnancy (see Table 38.2).[37] The process of maturation of fetal breathing movements is accelerated in some conditions such as premature rupture of membranes. For instance, decrease in fetal breathing has been observed following premature rupture of membranes[38,39] and during the three days prior to the initiation of labor.[37,40] Kisilevsky *et al.* compared the body movements and breathing patterns in normal fetuses at 24–33 weeks of gestation and fetuses threatening to deliver prematurely. High-risk fetuses had a reduced level of body movements and an earlier onset of extended periods of breathing, which occurred at 30 weeks in contrast to 33 weeks in the control group.[41] However, in this study, accelerated maturation of breathing was not observed in the presence of ruptured membranes. Fetuses delivered prematurely had less breathing than those delivered at term. Maternal consumption of alcohol or methadone and, according to some authors, even cigarette smoking, is known to decrease the incidence of breathing movements.[42–44] On the other hand, aminophiline, used for the treatment of bronchial asthma, as well as conjugated estrogens and betamethasone increase the frequency of breathing.[45,46] An increased number of fetal movements following the elevation of the glucose concentration in maternal blood has been noted at the 34th week of gestation.[47,48]

Another indispensable prerequisite for the survival of the newborn is the ability to feed, i.e. to ingest food. In the human fetus, swallowing has been noted as early as 11 weeks of gestation,[49] with daily swallowing rates near term of 200–500 ml.[50,51] Swallowing of amniotic fluid proteins and growth factors contributes to the growth and maturation of the fetal gastrointestinal tract, and possibly to the fetal somatic growth.[52] That is, the amniotic fluid provides 10–14% of the nitrogen requirements of the normal fetus, and esophageal atresia is often associated with lower birth weight.[53] Many authors agree that swallowing patterns develop *in utero* in all species in which there is significant fetal fluid excretion (urine and lung liquid) into the amniotic cavity. Thus, fetal swallowing contributes to the regulation of amniotic fluid volume.[52] In some, although not all cases with fetal esophageal atresia, the volume of amniotic fluid is increased. The normal volume of amniotic fluid in some of these cases could be explained by the coexistence of tracheoesophageal fistula, which could allow the intake of liquid during respiratory movements (for a review see Ross and Nijland[54]). Furthermore, polyhydramnios sometimes, though not always, develops in anencephalic fetuses. However, some of these fetuses have an intact swallowing reflex, whereas cases with normal amniotic fluid volume and decreased fetal swallowing have been described (for a review see Ross and Nijland[54]). Spontaneous fetal swallowing is, like most motor patterns, correlated with neurobehavior. The development of dypsogenic mechanisms and their influence on fetal swallowing will be described later in the text. Here, we have to emphasize that fetal swallowing patterns differ significantly from those seen in the adult and that the fetus daily swallows 5–10 times more fluid per body mass unit.[55]

Development of the fetal sensor system

The combination of ultrasonic studies, pathoanatomical examinations and studies of premature infants has provided a wide spectrum of evidence that the ability to register vibrations, acoustic stimuli and even light is acquired during intrauterine life. It is well known that the fetus can sense pain and respond to painful stimulus with a variety of responses, such as movements, circulatory and hormonal responses, although the question of the emotional response to pain or memorization of the unpleasant events *in utero* still remains unresolved. The fetus can also sense the taste of amniotic fluid and even functions such as appetite, satiety and thirst seem to be developed during intrauterine life (see Table 38.2).

Fetal vestibular and auditory system

It is generally accepted that reflexes of the brain stem, which include vestibulary, olfactory and auditory reflexes, develop early in gestation.[56] Vestibular ganglionic cells mature earlier than the neurons of lateral and inferior vestibule nuclei, which are functional from 9 gestational weeks onward.[57] Vestibule stimulation is thought to contribute to the development of fetal movements. That is, the gravity-free environment in the uterus appears to promote the development of vestibulary reflexes.[58] According to electrophysiological examinations of the evoked potentials in prematurely delivered healthy infants, cochlear function develops between 22 and 25 weeks of gestation, whereas its maturation continues during the first 6 months after delivery.[59–61] Maternal heartbeats and motility of the gastrointestinal tract during digestion appear to generate 90 dB of noise[62] *in utero*. However, fluid in the fetal ear as well as the immaturity of the cochlea complicate the transmission of sound, so that only strong acoustic stimuli can produce fetal reflex movements, such as startle motion of the trunk and/or flexion of the extremities, accompanied by changes in the heart rate. These are seen during or soon after vibroacoustic stimulation.[61] Applying acoustic stimulation with a wide spectrum of frequencies directly on the maternal abdomen, Shahidullah and Hepper have registered reflex movements with a short lag time in 20-week-old fetuses, and movements without the lag time in 25-week-old fetuses.[63] However, these movements were explained as a reflex response to vibroacoustic stimulation or proprioceptor stimulation. Kisilevsky *et al.* reported an increased number of fetal movements and heart rate during acoustic stimulation performed with the sound transmitter placed 10 cm above the maternal abdomen, in 30-week-old fetuses.[64]

Fetal vision

The intrauterine environment is not completely deprived of light. Moreover, some experimental results indicate that the development of visual and auditory organs could not be possible without any light or acoustic stimulation.[62] Although the structural development of sensor pathways is a prerequisite for functional development, the final organization of the brain circuitries relies predominantly on guidance from external output.[16] In the cortical area,[17] synaptogenesis persists between 24 weeks and 8 months after delivery,[65] whereas myelination of the optical tract begins at 32 weeks of gestation[66] and cones of the central foveola reach adult proportions late in childhood.[67]

Fetal pain

During the past decade, fetal perception of pain has been not only an object of interest for scientists, but also an important issue in public debates, in relation to late abortion and an increasing number of intrauterine operations. The pain consists of two components: perception of the stimulus and an emotional reaction or unpleasant feeling with regard to the noxious stimulus. These occur in two anatomically and physiologically distinct systems in the brain. The response to painful stimulation can be regarded at three different levels:

somatosensory response, pain-induced autonomic and endocrinological reflexes and pain-related behavior (for a review see Vanhatalo and van Nieuvenhuizen[68]). In the human fetus, the first nociceptors appear at the seventh week of gestation and by the 20th week, these are present all over the body. Peripheral afferents begin to make synapses to the spinal cord, approximately during weeks 10–30.[69] The myelination of these pathways[70] and the development of functional spinal reflex circuitry occur almost simultaneously.[70,71] Higher parts of the pain pathways include the spinothalamic tract, established at 20 weeks and myelinated by 29 weeks of gestation,[72] and thalamo-cortical connections, which begin to grow into the cortex at 24–26 weeks.[66] Finally, at 29 weeks, evoked potentials can be registered from the cortex, indicating that the functional connection between periphery and cortex operates from that time onward.[12,71]

The earliest reactions to painful stimuli are motor reflexes, resembling withdrawal reflexes. These reactions are completely reflexive and are guided by the spinal cord. Higher perception or processing of painful sensation does not exist at this stage.[10] However, some investigators indicate that facial reflexes in response to somatic stimulation, which could indicate the emotional reaction to pain, develop rather early in gestation.[13] These reflexes are thought to be coordinated by subcortical systems and probably reflect development of these lower brain circuitries.[73] As for the autonomic responses to pain, an elevation of cortisol and beta-endorphin levels in plasma in response to needle pricking of the innervated hepatic vein was registered in a 23-week-old fetus, whereas the stimulation of the uninnervated umbilical cord had no effect.[74,75] Alterations in cerebral blood flow, i.e. blood flow redistribution during invasive procedures, were noted in an 18-week-old fetus.[76] These results indicate that painful stimuli trigger a wide spectra of reactions in the CNS, such as activation of the hypothalamic pituitary axis or autonomic reflexes, even without reaching the cortex. Furthermore, we have to emphasize that these hormonal, autonomic and metabolic responses can be neutralized by analgesics such as fentanyl.[76,77] The reduction of fetal responses to pain is extremely important because many studies have shown the influence of the early pain experiences on the later behavioral variables or on the later developmental outcomes.[78] One of the most important effects of painful experience is a prolonged stress response.[79] It includes fluctuations in blood pressure and cerebral blood flow, and hypoxemia, which may predispose to intracranial hemorrhage.[76] Experiments on animals have revealed that elevated cortisol levels, equivalent to those secreted during the stress response in humans, were associated with degenerative changes in the fetal hypothalamus.[80] Finally, long-term follow-up studies of fetuses treated in the intensive care units (ICU) and exposed to pain and/or stress have demonstrated the correlations between the stay in ICU and altered pain thresholds and abnormal pain-related behavior later in life.[79,81] All these findings underline the importance of a stress-free environment for normal physiological and psychological development.

Fetal taste, appetite and satiety

It is generally believed that appetite and satiety functions develop during the intrauterine period in all precocial species. In the human fetus, taste buds are developed from the seventh week of gestation onward.[82] Sucrose increases swallowing in the human fetus, whereas the incidence of swallowing movements decreases following the injection of Lipiodol, a bitter extract of poppy seeds, into the amniotic fluid.[82] The main endocrine regulators of appetite, leptin and neuropeptide Y (NPY) are secreted as early as 15 and 18 weeks, respectively, in the human fetus, but the ontogeny and functions of their regulatory pathways have not been delineated in the human fetal brain.[83–85] However, experiments on animals have shown the increase of swallowing upon ingestion of NPY.[86] Swallowing was increased following the injection of leptin, which is in contradiction with leptin function in adults.[87] Therefore, some authors postulated that the presence of NPY pathways and the immaturity of leptin pathways may potentiate feeding and facilitate weight gain in newborns, despite high body fat levels.[52]

Development of dipsogenic mechanisms

Experiments on animal models, especially fetal lambs, have shown that dipsogenic mechanisms begin to modulate fetal swallowing during intrauterine life. For instance, in fetal lambs, swallowing and arginine vasopressin secretion increase following the central administration of hypertonic saline and angiotensin II.[88,89] Ross *et al.* have identifed the hypertonicity-activated neurons in dipsogenic hypothalami nuclei, such as the parvocellular and magnocellular division of periventricular nucleus and supraoptic nucleus in near-term ovine fetus.[90–92] These authors also suggested that exaggerated fetal swallowing under physiologic conditions (5–10 times more liquid in proportion to the adult) might be the result of tonic activation of angiotensin II receptors and production of nitric oxide.[93,94] Nevertheless, the fetus appears to have a reduced sensitivity to osmotic stimuli[95–97] when compared to the adult, despite the intact dipsogenic nuclei. Reduced swallowing during systemic hypotension despite the elevated renin plasma levels, together with the increased amount of liquid swallowed under normal conditions, indicates that fetal dipsogenic response might differ from that of the adult.[98]

Cyclic behavior and development of circadian rhythms

Fetal life *in utero* is organized in cyclical patterns. Periods of activity alternate with periods of rest.

The observation of human infants resulted in the hypothesis that the alternations of activity and inactivity periods reflect the elementary ultradian rhythm of the fetal CNS, uninfluenced by external input.

For instance, eye movements, which become observable at 16–18 weeks of gestation, begin to consolidate at 24–26 weeks of gestation, and the periods of eye movements (EM) begin to alternate with non-eye movement (NEM) periods. During the last 10 weeks of gestation, both switching and maintaining mechanisms responsible for this ultradian rhythms mature, and constant mean values of duration of EM and NEM periods are achieved by 37–38 weeks. At that time, EM and NEM last 27–29 min and 23–24 min, respectively, which is similar to the values in the neonate.[99] In the adult human, rapid eye movements (REM) are present during active sleep, alternate with the slow eye movements (SEM) or deep sleep and are accompanied by changes in electrocortical activity.[100] In the fetus, REM and SEM can be registered at 33 weeks of gestation. At 36–38 weeks of gestation, they become integrated with other parameters of fetal activity, such as heart rate and fetal movements, into organized and coherent behavioral states.[101]

In fetal animals, simultaneous measurements of fetal electrocortical activity, eye and body movements have shown that deep sleep, characterized by high-voltage waves and decreased fetal activity, occurred during 54% of the total time each day. The total length of REM sleep period, characterized by low-voltage waves and rapid eye movements, lasted 40% of the total time each day. Wakeful state (6% of the day) is characterized by low-voltage waves.[102] In human premature newborns, born 4 weeks prior to term, 60–65% of the total sleeping period is REM sleeping, whereas in a term newborn, the REM sleeping period is 50% of the total 16 h of sleep.[103] The intensive activity of neuronal circuits during REM sleep is thought to contribute to the development of the CNS.[103]

The circadian system is a kind of biological clock that receives information from the environment and sends efferent outputs that orchestrate circadian rhythms.[104] In mammals, the major role in orchestration of these rhythms is played by the suprachiasmatic nucleus (SCN) of the hypothalamus, which oscillates with a period of close to 24 h. Biological oscillations of SCN are entrained by the light/darkness cycle, which is registered by retinal receptors and transmitted by the retino-hypothalamical tract. Efferent pathways from SCN include projections into the various nuclei of the hypothalamus, and possibly, endocrine SCN secretion. In the human fetus, as well as other mammal species, SCN is developed by midgestation, but its maturation continues after birth, as shown by an increase in the number of neurons containing adrenalin vasoperssine and vasoactive intestinal polipeptide (VIP) during the first year of postnatal life (for a review see Kelly[104]). Circadian rhythms in behavior, cardiovascular function and hormones are present in human fetuses, as well as in fetal sheep and monkey, and are entrained to the light/darkness cycle. However, the question whether that rhythm is generated by the fetus itself or influenced by maternal rhythms remains to be resolved, although some animal experiments indicate the importance of the maternal SCN. In this case, the transmission of the signal to the fetus would necessarily require an endocrine mediator, but no such molecule has been identified yet. The latest results suggest the role of the maternal pineal hormone melatonin. This hormone is present in humans, as well as in other mammals, and its plasma concentrations exhibit daily variations, with the peak during the night. Therefore, its role in sleep induction has been suggested (for a review see Kelly[104]). Seasonal alterations in melatonin concentrations have also been reported. Daily oscillations of melatonin concentrations in plasma are present throughout gestation,[104] and various human tissues including the CNS express some types of melatonin receptors.[105,106] However, its role in the orchestration of fetal circadian rhythms remains to be confirmed.

Basic technology of 4D sonography

The rapid development of digital ultrasound systems allows 3D image reconstructions and, lately, 4D real-time inspection of anatomical regions and pathological changes. However, 3D images are static and do not provide information on movements and dynamic changes of the object of interest.[23] Moreover, fetal movements are the source of significant artifacts and volume scanning should be performed during the fetal inactive phase, i.e. whenever the fetus is active, qualitative 3D image is unobtainable. This fact limits the usage of classic 3D ultrasound. Four-dimensional ultrasound overcomes this disadvantage, making it possible to obtain qualitative 3D images regardless of fetal movements. The only limiting factor for 4D sonography is the quantity of adjacent amniotic fluid.

The acquisition of volume data sets is performed by 2D scans with special transducers (linear, convex, transvaginal) designed for 2D scans, 3D and real-time 4D volumes.[107] The real-time 4D mode is obtained from simultaneous volume acquisition and computing of 3D images, which is in fact multidimensional ultrasound.[108] The movement of the ultrasound beam over the region of interest (ROI) is automatic. Such a design enables simplified 3D and 4D acquisition. Ultrasound probes include a scanning mechanism moved by a built-in electromotor. The processing speed allows continuous acquisition and processing of 4D volumes.

The volume acquisition begins with a 2D image and superimposed volume box. The initial 2D image is the central 2D image of the volume. According to the dimensions of the volume box, the volume scan sweeps between the margins of the volume box. The

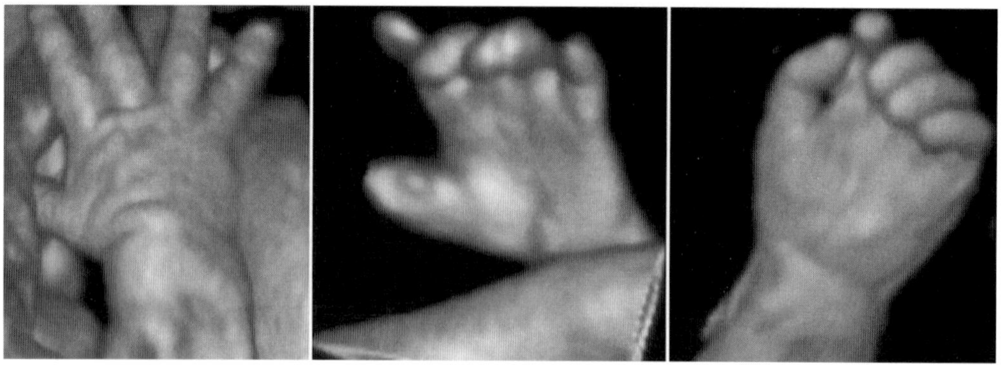

Figure 38.1 3D surface rendering of the normal hand movement. Note the alteration of the palm position.

volume box is set to frame the ROI. The following steps are important for producing reliable 4D images:

(1) Orientation in real-time 2D mode.
(2) Selection of ROI.
(3) Starting the volume scan. Volume data are shown in a multiplane display on the monitor (transverse, sagittal and coronal).

During the 3D and 4D acquisition, sweep time depends on the volume box size, scan quality and adjusted scan parameters such as depth, number of focuses and other parameters that affect the B-mode image frame rate.

Four-dimensional rendering

The pixel is the smallest element of 2D images, while the voxel is the smallest information unit in 3D and 4D imaging. Volume rendering provides visualization of animated voxel-based images on a 2D screen. Because of the development of instant computer technology and fast data transmission, volume acquisition and data processing are accelerated to enable 3D rendering in real time (4D). Fast volume data processing enables calculation of 5–30 volumes per second depending on the system hardware and size of the render box. As 4D imaging is almost a real time, there is always some delay as a result of the time needed to reconstruct 3D images from 2D scans. It is always desirable to achieve as many volumes per second (volume rate) as possible. The number of volumes per second is some kind of trade-off between image quality and frame rate. The quality of 3D and 4D images mostly depends on 2D image quality. Prior to volume acquisition it is important to achieve the best 2D image quality, adjusting depth, focus position and number of focuses, frequency and gain. All 2D image artifacts will be also present on 3D and 4D image reconstruction. Good 4D image acquisition depends on ROI size and volume box size, ROI position or direction of view and accessibility to the object. The render box determines the contents that will be rendered. Structures that are not selected by volume box will be cut from 3D reconstruction.

ROI can be sized, moved and rotated in all directions arbitrarily by the operator. Volume data can be acquired from different 2D modes: gray-scale imaging, CFI and power Doppler imaging. There are different rendering modes available: surface, transparent (maximum, minimum, x-ray) and light, some of them can be active simultaneously in real time.

Volume rendering is a process of visualization of 3D structures on an animated 2D screen and rendering modes determine how the 3D image will be presented on screen.

Surface rendering or gray-scale rendering

In the surface rendering mode, only signals from the surface of ROI are extracted and displayed in the plastic appearance. Surface rendering examination of the fetus focuses the sonographer's attention exclusively on the fetal external anatomy (Figure 38.1).

This mode is capable of clear visualization of fetal normal surface anatomy or surface anomalies such as myelomeningocoele, omphalocele, cleft lip/palate, macroglossia and limb defects (Figures 38.2–38.6). Furthermore, visualization of the spatial relationship between surface structures enables accurate diagnosis of subtle malformations and anomalies such as micrognathia, overlapping fingers, hexadactilia and auricular malposition or malformation.

Surface rendering gives the best result when ROI structures are surrounded by fluid or hypoechoic tissue. By selecting the threshold level, voxels with gray values below the threshold value selected are not shown on the reconstructed image. Selecting the threshold parameter influences the quality of the surface rendered image.

The surface image can be displayed in 'textural' mode. The gray values can be colored by different color maps, but the most successful map for 4D image is the 'body heat' map. The texture mode can also be 'smoothed', showing smooth surfaces on 4D

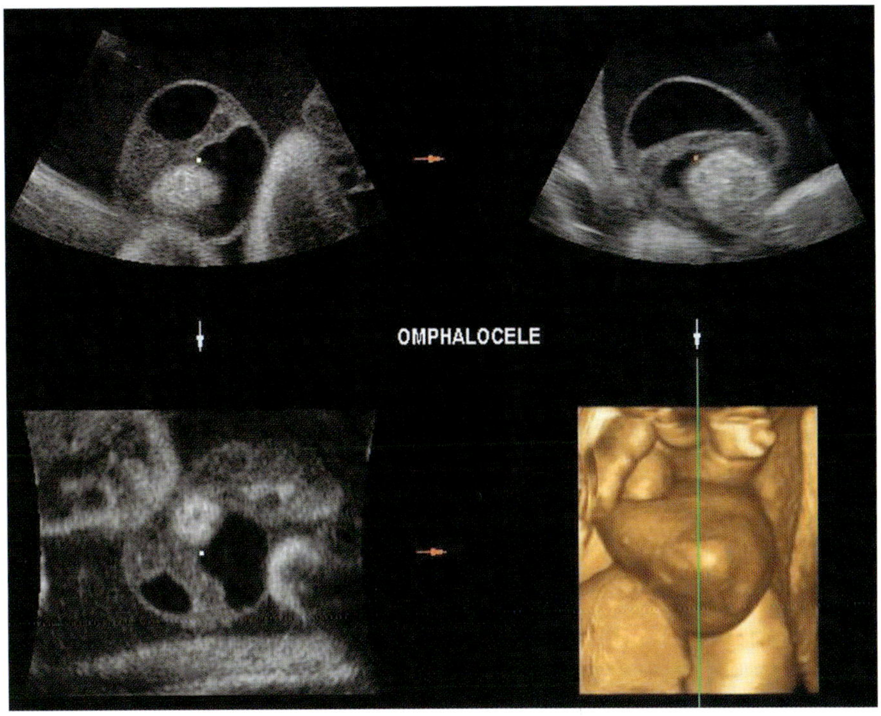

Figure 38.2 3D surface rendering of omphalocele.

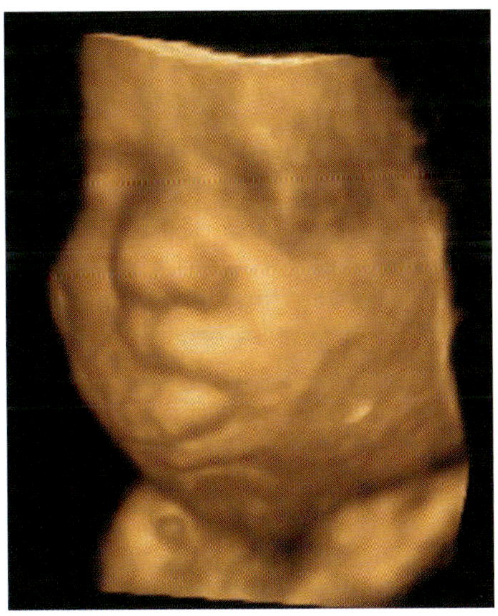

Figure 38.3 3D surface rendering of macroglossia.

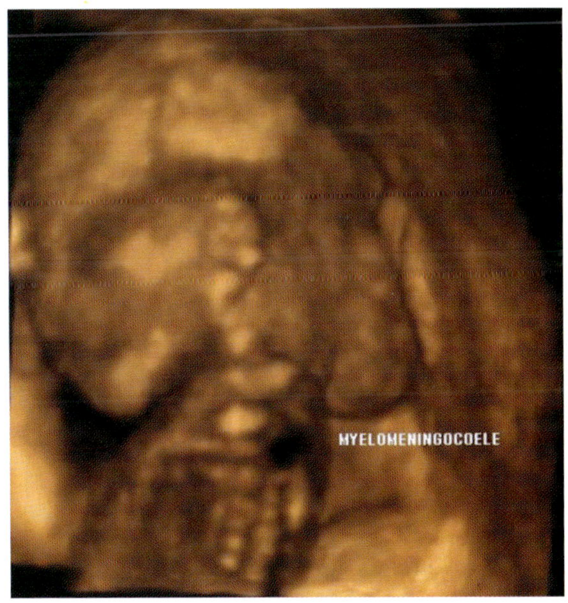

Figure 38.4 3D surface rendering of myelomeningocoele.

reconstructions. Texture and smooth surface displays are suitable for use in applications such as fetal face, abdominal wall, genitals, umbilical cord (Figure 38.7) and the surfaces of the urinary bladder.[109–111]

The surface can be displayed in 'light' mode. Closer structures are brighter, while distant structures are displayed darker. A variation of the light mode is 'gradient light mode', showing virtual illumination from a spot light sourco.[112]

Transparent mode

In the transparent mode, contrary to the surface mode, only the signals from the inner layers of the ROI are extracted, providing spatial reconstruction of the internal structure of the ROI. According to the echogenicity of extracted signals there are two submodalities: maximum and minimum modes. In the maximum mode there are only the signals of the highest echogenicity, whereas in the minimum mode only the signals of the

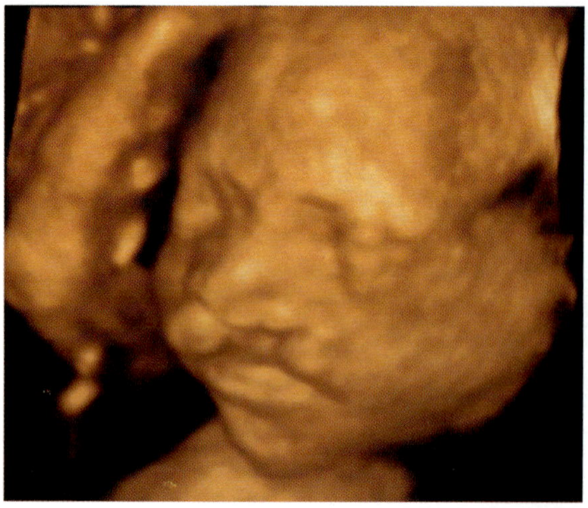

Figure 38.5 3D surface rendering of bilateral cleft lips.

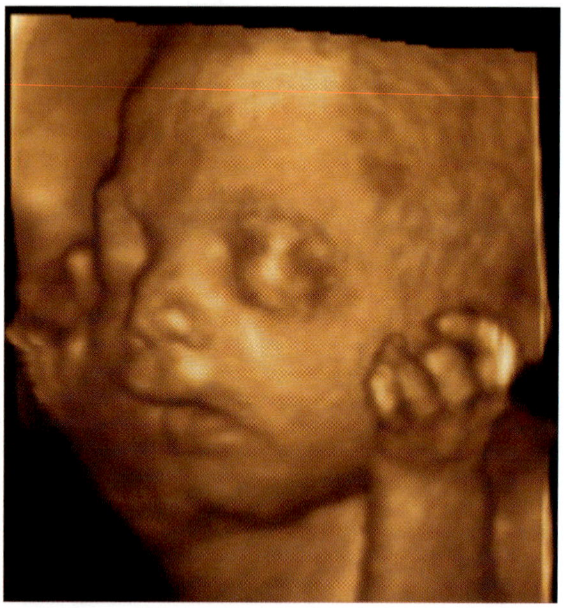

Figure 38.6 3D surface rendering of arthrogryposis of the fingers showing rigid and fixed posture.

lowest echogenicity are extracted from the entire volume. In the transparent mode only maximum gray values are displayed. This mode is suitable for visualization of fetal bones, endometrium and breast.

Minimum mode

Minimum gray values are displayed for visualization of vessels, cystic structures and parenchyma of different organs.[113]

Maximum mode

Maximum gray values are displayed. It is suitable for visualization of fetal bone structures and is the method of choice for imaging of the spatial relationships between bones.[114] Moreover, this modality offers an option of complete visualization of curved bones such as ribs or clavicle on a single image.

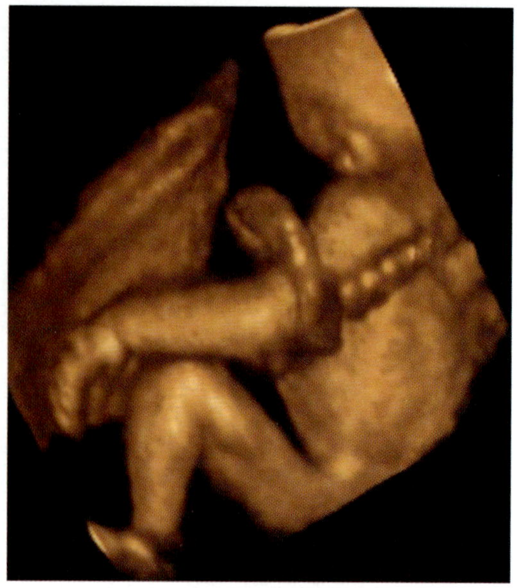

Figure 38.7 3D surface rendering of umbilical cord around the arm.

Evaluation of the complete skeleton, particularly the thoracic skeleton in the developing fetuses, often is difficult with 2D ultrasound because of curvature of the bones. Ribs can be completely observed using the 3D ultrasound transparency mode. This modality reduces the echogenicity of soft tissues, leaving behind echogenic structures, namely, the bones. The curvature and relationship of the rib ends to the vertebral bodies and the anterior chest wall can be demonstrated as well as the entire length.

The vertebral column is originally curved anteroposteriorly. If it is pathologically curved laterally, it is impossible to display the whole vertebral column in a single sectional image by 2D ultrasound. The advantage of 3D ultrasound (Figure 38.8) is the ability to visualize both curvatures at the same time. Anomalies such as scoliosis, kyphosis, lordosis and spina bifida may be overlooked by 2D ultrasound, but are easy to recognize by using the 3D maximum mode. Congenital malformations of the fetal spine can be identified more easily using 3D surface and transparent mode reconstruction together. Specific vertebral body levels may be accurately identified by simultaneous evaluation of axial planes of the spine within the volume rendered image. It is difficult to acquire the entire spine in a single volume and thus multiple volumes are often necessary to evaluate the spine completely.

Volume contrast imaging (VCI)

Using 4D it is possible to make high-contrast 2D images. The rendered algorithm is a combination of surface texture mode and minimum transparency 4D

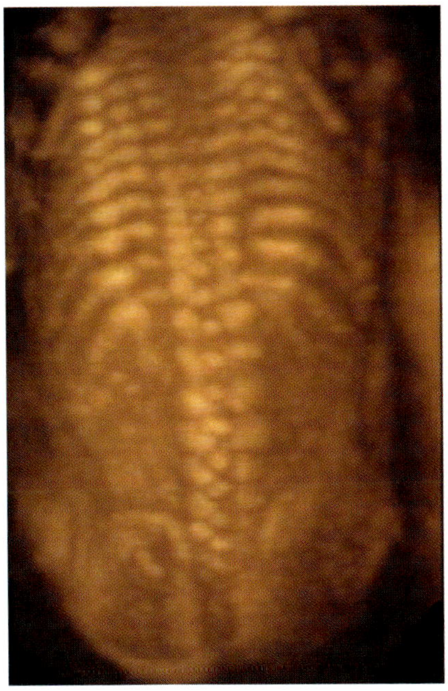

Figure 38.8 3D maximum mode showing the vertebral column.

mode. It is possible to display a couple of millimeters thin volume slice showing very good contrast between different tissues. The user can define the thickness of the slice that is scanned using 4D image rendering. The reconstructed image shows improved tissue contrast. VCI is used for better visualization of nodular or diffuse lesions in parenchyma of organs such as liver and spleen.

Spatio-temporal image correlation (STIC) in fetal echocardiography

STIC is a new method for clinical investigation of the fetal heart. The reconstructed volume scan offers a user-friendly technique to acquire data from the fetal heart and its visualization in a 4D sequence. The volume acquisition occurs in two ways. First, data are obtained by a single, automatic volume sweep. In the second step, the system examines the data in proportion to their spatial and temporal domain and processes a 4D sequence. This sequence presents the heart beating in real time in a multiplanar display. After the volume acquisition, the heart can be assessed off-line, without depending on the patient.[115,116]

Removing overlaying structures

This option is called Magic-Cut or the electronic scalpel. During 3D and 4D scanning in most cases there are structures that interfere or are superimposed on the reconstructed image. The Magic-Cut tool enables successful removal of overlaying structures using 3D imaging. Unwanted structures can be cut off from the image in all three directions along the *x*, *y* and *z* axes. There is also a possibility of using this tool to remove some structures from real-time 4D volumes. The cutting tool enables the operator to have improved visualization of the object from all directions.[117]

Data review and networking

Volume data sequences can be stored on the hard disk of the ultrasound unit or in different media (CD-R, MO-Disc) in various formats: 2D image, 2D cine (selected sequence of 2D images), 3D volume (sequence of 3D rotating images) and 4D volume. Since the complete volume data set is saved, it is possible to review saved examinations without any loss of image quality. Stored data can be interactively processed with the possibility of additional 3D reconstruction.

Three-dimensional and 4D imaging provides additional dimensions to conventional 2D sonography. The main advantage of ultrasound in general is dynamic imaging of the human body. Four-dimensional imaging is following this tradition, permitting visualization of dynamic changes inside the body and its organs. Using 4D ultrasound in obstetrics, it is possible for the first time to monitor the quality and quantity of fetal movements on 3D real-time reconstructed images.

Assessment of fetal behavior

Prenatal motility is considered to reflect the developing nervous system but it also involves the functional and maturational properties of fetal hemodynamics and the muscular system. Despite medical reports from 100 years ago and 25 years of systematic research initiated by Prechtl and associates, the study of prenatal behavior is in its infancy.

Fetal behavior can be defined as fetal activities observed or recorded with ultrasonographic equipment. As it is not yet possible to assess the functional development of the CNS directly, investigators have started to analyze fetal behavior as a measure of neurological maturation.[118]

A turning point in the assessment of fetal behavior was the introduction of real-time ultrasound. This technique allowed the investigation of spontaneous fetal motor activity *in utero*.[117,119] For the first time, studies of spontaneous prenatal movements and behavior *in utero* were carried out and published. Since fetal body movements give important information about the condition of the fetus, their quantitative as well as qualitative aspects were analyzed. de Vries *et al.* described the developmental pathway of fetal movements in a longitudinal study of 12 healthy nulliparous women.[15] They reported not only how to describe a particular movement, but also how these movements were performed in terms of speed and amplitude.[15]

Assessment of fetal movements

Using ultrasound imaging, de Vries *et al.* focused on the first half of pregnancy, while Roodenburg *et al.*

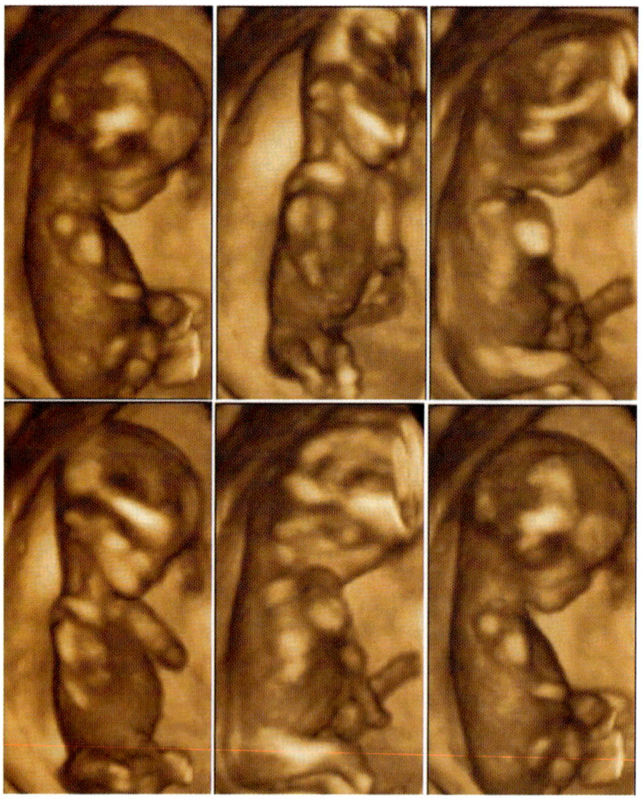

Figure 38.9 4D ultrasound sequence of the fetus at 12 weeks of gestation showing general movements. The complex movements of the limb, trunk and head are clearly visible and cause a shift in fetal position. In the first sequence, the right limb is bent in the elbow joint. In the next sequence, the fetus has dropped the hand and has begun to deflect the elbow joint. In the last sequence, further elevation of the hand is seen.

investigated the second half of pregnancy.[24,120] In a classic paper, de Vries and her team classified at least 13 different movement patterns.[24]

Classification of movement patterns[121]

(1) Just discernible movements (between 7 and 8.5 weeks)
(2) Startle
(3) General movements (Figure 38.9)
(4) Hiccup
(5) Breathing
(6) Isolated arm or leg movement
(7) Isolated retroflexion of the head
(8) Isolated rotation of the head
(9) Isolated anteflexion of the head
(10) Jaw movements
(11) Hand–face contact – in this pattern of movement, the hand slowly touches the face, the fingers frequently extend and flex (Figures 38.12–38.15)
(12) Stretch
(13) Rotation of the fetus.

Relying on the observations of apparently typical spontaneous human fetal movements, de Vries *et al.* recorded variations in general movements that they believed suggested abnormalities of the CNS.[122] Following their lead, other researchers have selected, as a dependent variable, general movements or 'gross movements' involving the whole body.[123] Fetal motor behavior has been described.[124–127] The descriptor of general movements has been applied to the movements of preterm newborns.[128,129] Unfortunately, the lack of definition specificity, long-term follow-ups and the reliability of descriptions have limited the usefulness of some of these studies. Nevertheless, careful observation and analysis of fetal movements could be useful in the assessment of the integrity of the fetal CNS, as will be described later in the text.

The Zagreb group has evaluated the advantages of 4D over 2D real-time sonography in the assessment of early fetal behavior.[117] With 4D transvaginal sonography these authors found body movements at 7 weeks of pregnancy (Table 38.3).[117] The observed body movements consisted of the changing position of the head toward the body. Therefore, this technology enables the visualization of the moving phenomenon 1 week earlier than 2D ultrasound. At 7 weeks of gestation, the dominant embryonic feature is the head, which is strongly flexed anteriorly. Upper and lower limb buds are visible on the lateral aspects of the embryo. However, embryonic movements are not frequent and consist mainly of moving of the head toward the rest of the body. At 8–9 weeks, the head is less flexed and the changes in the position of the head toward the body are clearly visible.

General movements are the first complex fetal movement patterns observable by 2D ultrasound.[15] They can be recognized from 8–9 weeks of pregnancy and continue to be present until 16–20 weeks after birth.[130] According to Prechtl these are gross movements, involving the whole body.[121] Movements of the limbs, trunk and head are of variable speed but smooth in appearance. They wax and wane in intensity, force and speed, and they have a gradual beginning and end.[121] The qualitative characteristics of general movements can be altered by some pathological conditions, such as in fetuses of women with type 1 diabetes mellitus or fetuses with anencephaly.[17,131] The range of movements varies from forceful and jerky in character and of large amplitude in anencephalic fetuses (Figure 38.10) to monotonous and rigid or chaotic in diabetic pregnancies. Qualitative alterations of general movements (Figure 38.11) seem to be useful in the assessment of the severity of associated neurological disability. The complex sequences of extension and flexion of the legs and arms (Figure 38.9) may be assessed better with 4D ultrasound. Furthermore, 4D sonography seems to be the method of choice for detecting subtle changes such as superimposed rotations and changes in the direction of the movements. The application of this new technique could improve the analysis of fetal movements and could allow the definition of precise criteria for the assessment of the integrity of the fetal nervous system.

Table 38.3 The incidence of spontaneous embryonic/fetal movement according to gestational age (adapted from Kurjak *et al.*[117])

Gestational age (weeks)	CRL (mm)	No movements	Gross body movements	Limb movements	Complex limb movements
7–8	0–15	31	12	0	0
9–10	16–30	26	11	7	0
11–12	31–50	19	16	12	8

CRL, crown–rump length

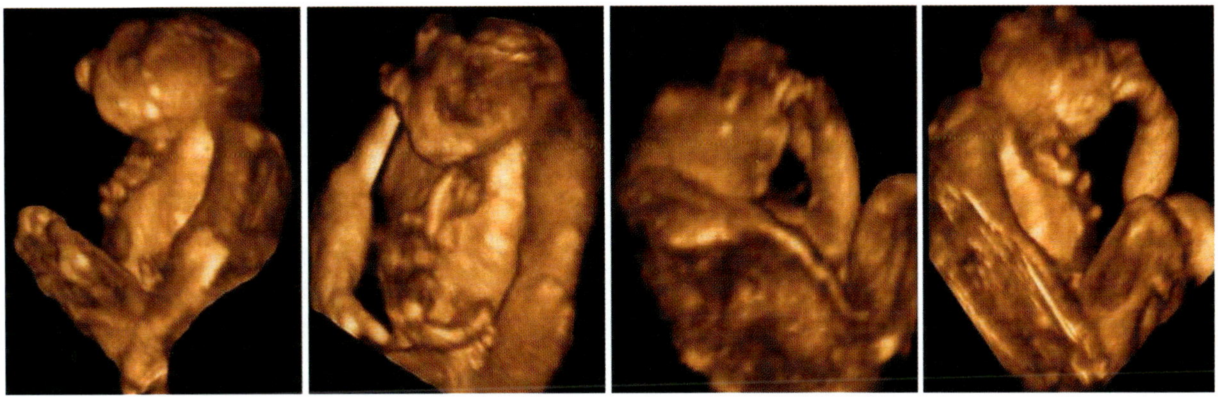

Figure 38.10 4D sequence of anencephalic fetus at 19 weeks of pregnancy. Only hand to head movements in one direction of the left arm could be seen; their onset was abrupt and jerky. Body movements in anencephalic fetus showed a lack of positional changes, with a waxing and waning in intensity. Using this technique, the function of lower-level CNS responsible for these forceful, monotonous changes is evaluated.

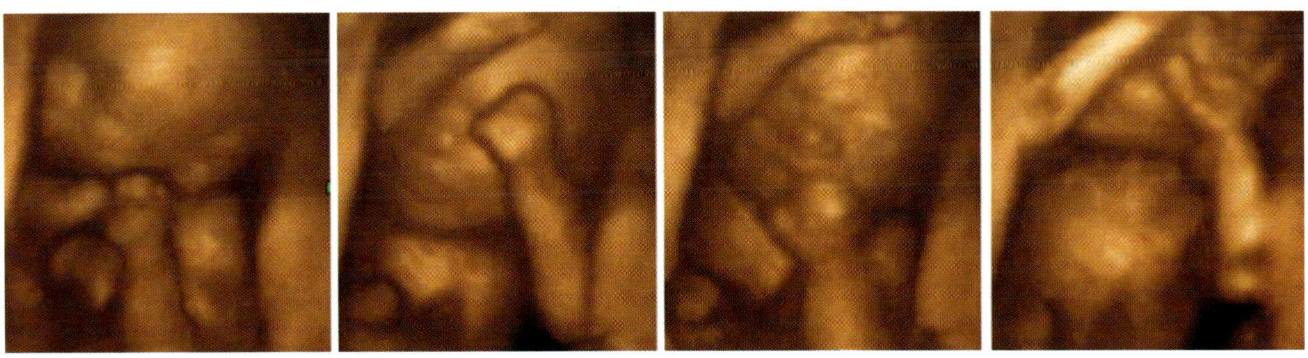

Figure 38.11 4D sequence of normal fetus at the same age as in Figure 38.10. Hand movement could be observed in any direction. We could see head movement (retroflexion and rotation) followed by palm opening position simultaneously. Qualitative alteration of movements can be used as a marker of the severity of associated neurological disability.

According to the literature, there is a period between 8 and 12 weeks concerning the first appearance of limb movements.[15,131] de Vries *et al.* found isolated arm and leg movements at 8 weeks of pregnancy.[15] With 4D ultrasound, the limb movements were detected at 8–9 weeks of gestation (Table 38.3).[117] In this period, limbs are elongated and their segments are discernible. Isolated arm and leg movements were clearly visible and consisted of changes in position of the extremities toward the body without observable flexion or extension in the joints.

Limb movements become more complex with advancing gestational age. Specific movements can be recognized at 14 weeks by 2D ultrasound. The organization of the movement pattern occurs as their frequency increases.[126] It seems that the fetal arms explore the surrounding environment and cross the midline, while the palmar surface is oriented toward

Table 38.4 Developmental motor characteristics of low-risk fetuses (adapted from Geerdink and Hopkins[128])

Gestational age (weeks)	Description
8	Trunk flexion and extension
12	Isolated random-appearing movement of extremities
14	All movement patterns present; an increased frequency of movement that is more 'organized' in appearance compared with movement at 12 weeks; arms appear to 'explore' while legs extend against uterine wall; arm crosses midline, extending palmar surface to opposite uterine wall
16	Decreased frequency of movements from 14 weeks, with pincer grasp, thumb in mouth
20	More bilateral movement (e.g. legs extend together against uterine wall, arms flex and hands are often held together near the face)
26–32	Independent movement of extremities to all parts of the uterus and specific body parts; no cephalocaudal development, but apparent distal–proximal development in extremities
37–38	Decreased frequency of movements; hand often molded to occiput or dorsum of hand rests against uterine wall

the uterine wall. The fetal legs are extended to the uterine wall. This phenomenon can be seen 2 weeks earlier using 4D ultrasound.[117] However, these movement patterns are less organized in comparison with those observed at 14 weeks by 2D ultrasound. Complex limb movement consists of changes in the position of the limb segments toward each other, seen by 4D ultrasound. More limb joints are active and move simultaneously, for example, as extension or flexion in arm and elbow or hip and knee. The elevation of the hand, extension of the elbow joint, with a slight change in direction and rotation, can be seen simultaneously.

Sparling and Wilhelm also described spontaneous movements in fetuses from 12 to 35 weeks of gestation (Table 38.4) and recorded the characteristics of hand movement.[126] Many movements appeared to be directed to a body part or the uterine wall. The hands of the fetuses moved with a variety of frequencies and apparent force. Joint ranges of motion changed throughout the movements rather than remaining the same, as in floating. These movements suggested primary and secondary circular reactions in which a movement is repeated, presumably because it has functional importance to the organism.[127,129] During later gestational periods, the fetuses' hands are directed to and manipulate body parts and features of the environment, such as the umbilical cord.

Our recent study, using 4D sonography, shows that the number of isolated arm movements decreases gradually from 13 through 16 weeks (Table 38.5a). All recordings were made during 15-min periods. The incidence varied between 50 and 120 with a median value of 60 at 13 weeks, between 17 and 27 with a median value of 23 at 14 weeks, between 0 and 6 with a median value of 2 at 15 weeks and between 18 and 28 with a median value of 25 at 16 weeks. The highest range was registered at 13 weeks of gestation. Data from Table 38.5(b) demonstrate the incidence of hand to head movements (Figure 38.15). There is a notable decrease in their incidence, followed by a plateau at 14 weeks of gestation. The incidence varied from 4 to 29 at 13 weeks and from 0 to 7 at 16 weeks of gestation. Table 38.5(c) shows the incidence of hand at mouth movements (Figure 38.13). The incidence varied between 0 and 4 with a median value of 2 at 13 weeks and between 0 and 2 with a median value of 2 at 16 weeks. The highest range was found at 15 weeks of gestation. At 13 weeks, a plateau was observed and was present until 16 weeks. Although this plateau was evident, mild fluctuations occurred. In contrast to most other movement patterns, hand near mouth movements (Table 38.5d) decreased gradually from 13 weeks onward, with a single fluctuation in the 14th week (it varied between 0 and 3 with a median value of 1). The incidence of hand to face movement (Figures 38.12 and 38.15) is characterized by a decrease

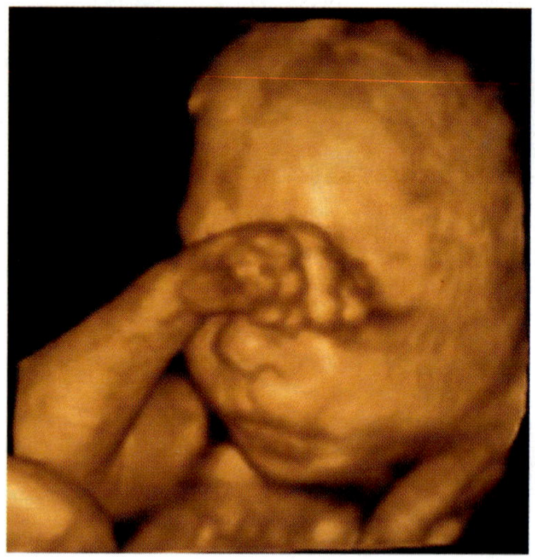

Figure 38.12 This picture shows the hand to face contact.

Table 38.5 The incidence of several characteristics of hand movements from 13 to 16 gestational weeks shown by 4D sonography: (a) isolated hand movement, (b) hand to head movements, (c) hand to mouth movements, (d) hand near mouth movements, (e) hand to face movements, (f) hand near face movements, (g) hand to ear movements and (h) hand to eye movements (adapted from Kurjak *et al.*[23])

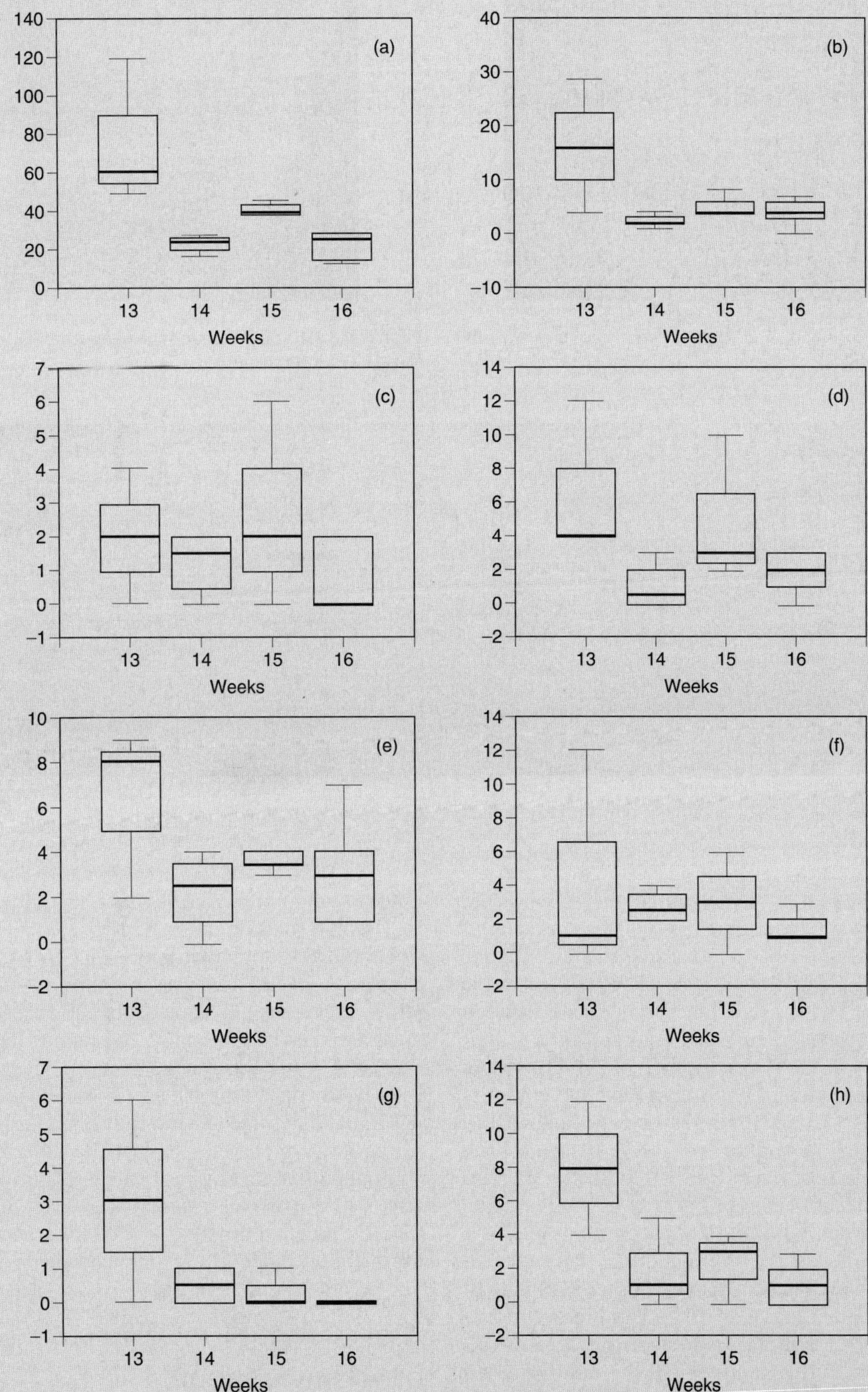

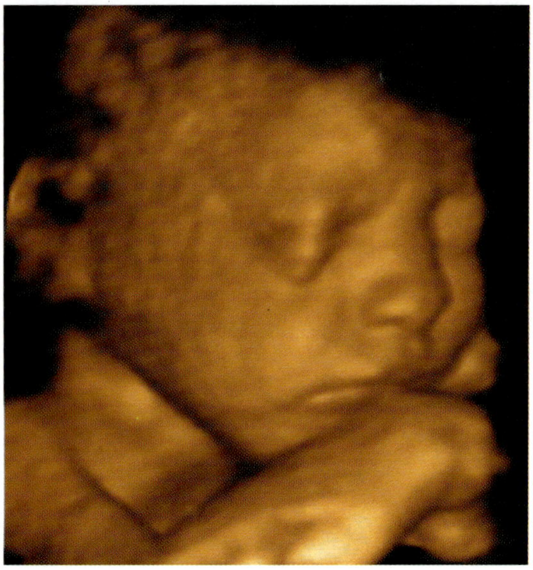

Figure 38.13 The hand movement in direct contact with the mouth.

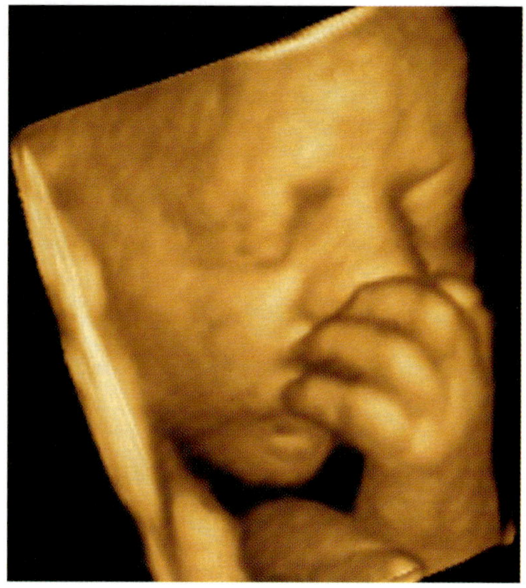

Figure 38.14 3D image showing the direction of hand movement to the nose.

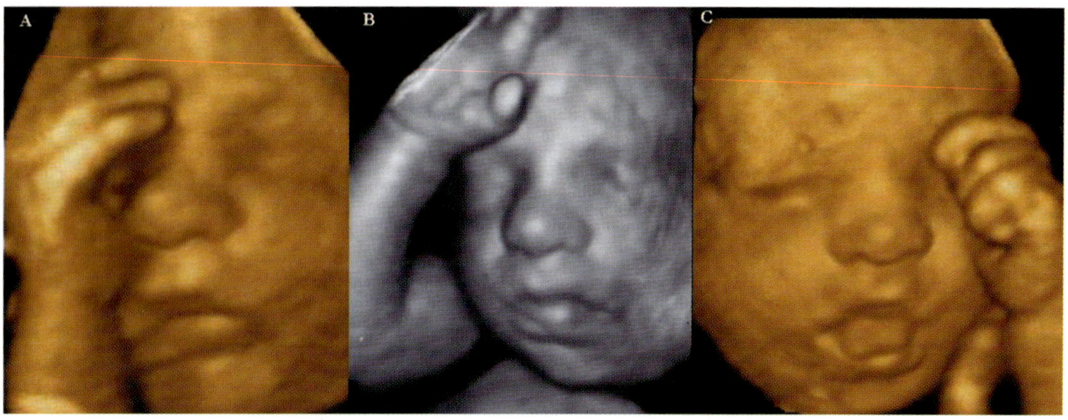

Figure 38.15 Several 3D images of hand direction to the face (a), to the head (b) and to the eye (c).

at 14 weeks followed by a plateau (Table 38.5e). From 13 weeks onward, the hand near face movement pattern was visible in all 15 fetuses, with an incidence of 2–9 and a median value of 8. At 16 weeks, the range was from 1 to 7 with a median value of 3. Although the plateau was observed, mild fluctuation was evident, especially at 15 weeks. From Table 38.5f, we can see that the incidence of hand near face movement is stable between 13 and 16 weeks of gestation with a slight increase at 14 and 15 weeks. At 13 weeks, the range was the widest (from 0 to 12), with the median value of 3. The incidence of hand to ear movements decreased between 13 and 16 weeks (Table 38.5g). It varied between 4 and 12 with a median value of 8 at 13 weeks and between 0 and 3 with a median value of 0 at 16 weeks. The incidence of the hand to eye movement (Figure 38.15) pattern showed the same developmental trend as the incidence of the hand to head and hand to face movement patterns (Table 38.5h). At 13 weeks, the incidence was between 4 and 12 occurrences per 15 minutes' observation time with a median value of 8. At 16 weeks, the range was from 0 to 3 with a median value of 1.[23]

Other developmental tendencies in hand movement have been noted.[132] Movements such as thumb in mouth and bilateral leg extension against the uterine wall were considered as functionally important. The frequently observed leg extension against the uterine wall was believed by the authors to be a possible precursor to later participation in the birthing process. Early movements of the arms appeared to assist the fetus in identifying components of its environment. Attributing function to any of these early movements, however, does not imply that the assigned function is preliminary to or necessary for the appearance of a spontaneous behavior.[25,132]

Assessment of fetal facial expressions by 4D ultrasound

Recent studies have demonstrated that during the second and third trimesters it is possible to study the

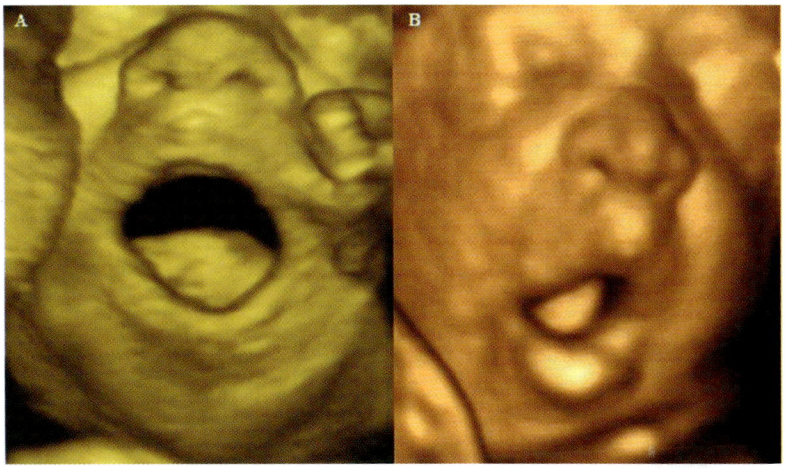

Figure 38.16 Yawning expression of the fetus. An involuntary wide opening of the mouth, with maximal widening of the jaw, followed by quick closure, often with retroflexion of the head and sometimes elevation of the arms.

full range of fetal facial activities. In addition to yawning, sucking and swallowing described by 2D real-time imaging, it is now possible to study the full range of facial expressions including smiling, crying and eyelid movements.[23,133]

The fetal behavioral patterns have been evaluated in 10 gravidas in the third trimester, between 30 and 33 weeks of gestation.[23] The incidence of eyelid movements ranged between 4 and 20 with a median value of 17, mouthing movements ranged between 2 and 19 with a median value of 12 and mouth and eyelid movements ranged between 0 and 13 with a median value of 5. The incidence of pure mouth movements such as opening of the mouth ranged between 4 and 13 with a median of 5, tongue expulsion ranged between 0 and 2 with a median of 2, yawning ranged between 0 and 2 with a median of 1 and pouting ranged between 0 and 9 with a median of 3. The incidence of facial expressions such as smiling ranged between 2 and 7 with a median of 2 and scowling between 2 and 4 with a median of 2. It is evident that eyelid and mouthing movements are predominant at this gestational age. The continuity between fetal and neonatal behavior has also been suggested.[132] These findings may stimulate multicentric studies of fetal behavior and responsiveness as a sign of neurological maturation. In the long term, fetal behavioral studies may become a means of assessing fetal well-being.[23]

Classification of facial movement patterns

The Zagreb group has attempted to evaluate 4D sonography in the assessment of fetal facial expression. They have classified eight different facial expressions:

(1) *Yawning*: This movement is similar to the yawn observed after birth: an involuntary wide opening of the mouth, with maximal widening of the jaws followed by quick closure, often with retroflexion of the head and sometimes elevation of the arms. This movement pattern is non-repetitive (Figure 38.16).
(2) *Swallowing*: This indicates that the fetus is drinking amniotic fluid. Swallowing consists of displacements of the tongue and/or larynx. Swallowing activity develops earlier than sucking in the course of fetal development.
(3) *Sucking*: This consists of rhythmical bursts of regular jaw opening and closing at a rate of about one per second, placing the finger or thumb on the roof of the mouth behind the teeth and sucking with lips closed. Thumb sucking is a very frequent fetal behavioral pattern (Figure 38.17).
(4) *Smiling*: A facial expression characterized by turning up the corners of the mouth (Figure 38.21).
(5) *Tongue expulsion*: A facial expression characterized by expulsion of the tongue (Figure 38.18).
(6) *Grimacing*: The wrinkling of the brows or face in frowning to express displeasure (Figure 38.22).
(7) *Mouthing*: A facial expression characterized by mouth manipulation to investigate an object. Mouthing is most common in the fetus and it may develop into a persistent, stereotyped behavior pattern (Figure 38.19).
(8) *Isolated eye blinking*: A reflex that closes and opens the eyes rapidly. Brief closing of the eyelids by involuntary normal periodic closing, as a protective measure, or by voluntary action (Figures 38.20 and 38.21).

They have also tried to identify emotional expressions as a combination of several of the facial expressions mentioned above (Figures 38.20–38.22).

The early results, presented above, indicate that fetal facial grimaces, resembling the emotional expressions in humans, are present during the third trimester of gestation. However, the precise criteria for distinction of these expressions in the fetus remain to

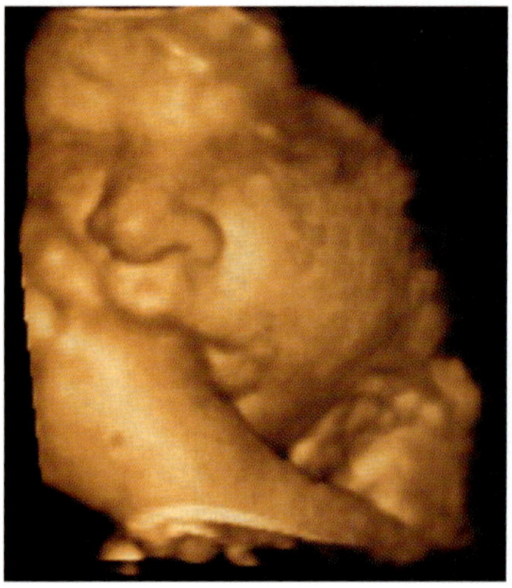

Figure 38.17 This picture shows sucking expression. The fetus is placing the thumb into the mouth, probably on the roof of the mouth and sucking with lips closed.

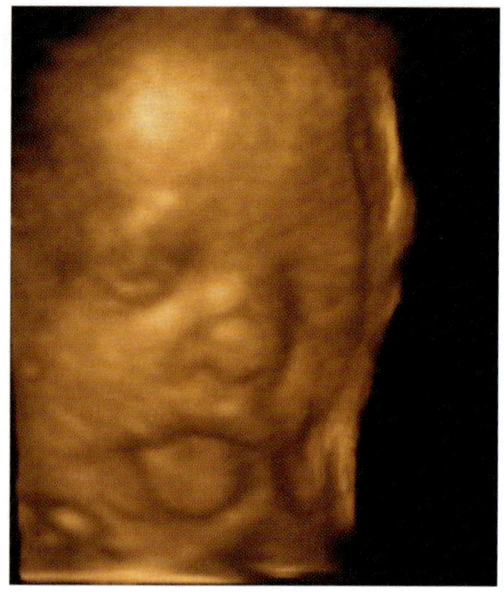

Figure 38.18 Facial expression characterized by tongue expulsion.

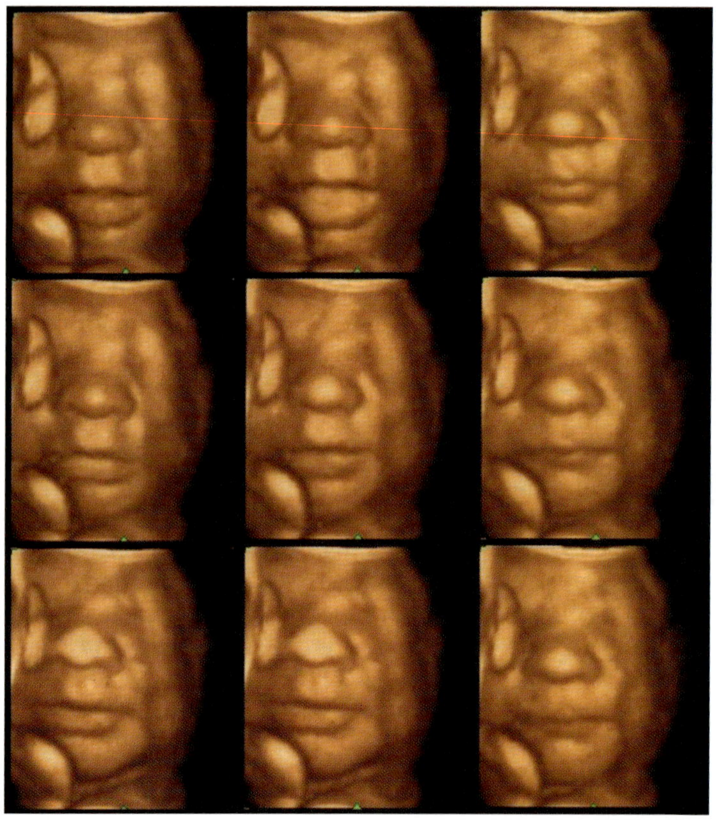

Figure 38.19 In this image sequence, mouthing can be observed as a facial expression pattern. We can see a series of rhythmic movements involving the mandible and tongue, characterized by constant frequency and duration until disappearance.

be established. A possibility of study of fetal facial expressions allows new research questions to be dealt with and indicates a great potential for 4D sonographic studies in the psychological and fetal behavioral sciences. Facial expressions are an important channel of non-verbal communication. The characteristics of facial expressions can provide the expert a different means of understanding the hidden side of the fetus *in utero*, a side that may not be accessible in the form of any verbalizations. However, clear evidences that fetal emotional processing exists in the third trimester of gestation or that it is related to facial expressions are still lacking and extensive multicentric studies should be conducted in order to clarify this idea. We believe that the fetal facial expressions and fetal behaviors related to emotions could reveal a part of the emotional aspect of intrauterine life. If this assumption becomes confirmed, it is possible to

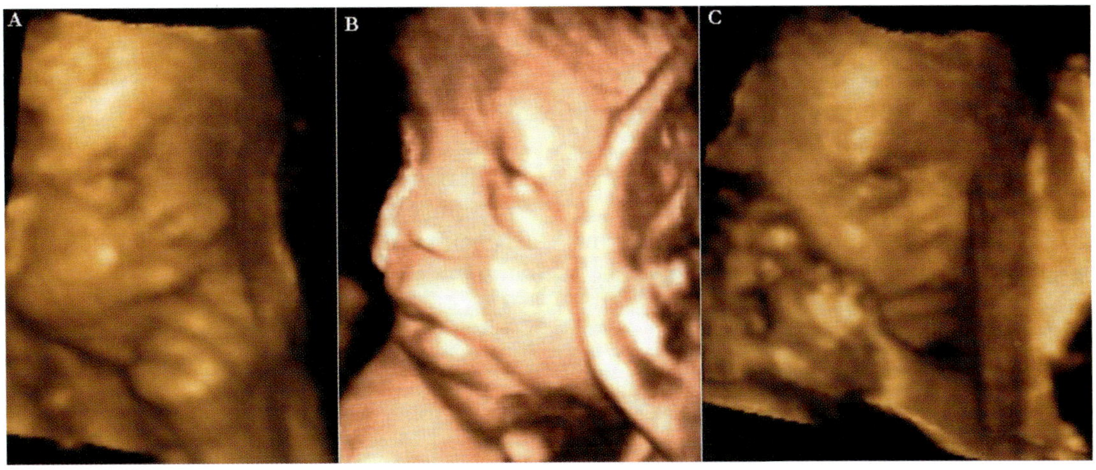

Figure 38.20 The picture shows fear expressions of the fetus. We can see the hand to the mouth movement together with opening of the eyelid. We assumed that this complex expression could be related to the imminent possibility of fetal danger, a nearby threat, a displeasure position or bodily harm. http://face-and-emotion.com/dataface/emotion/x_fear.html

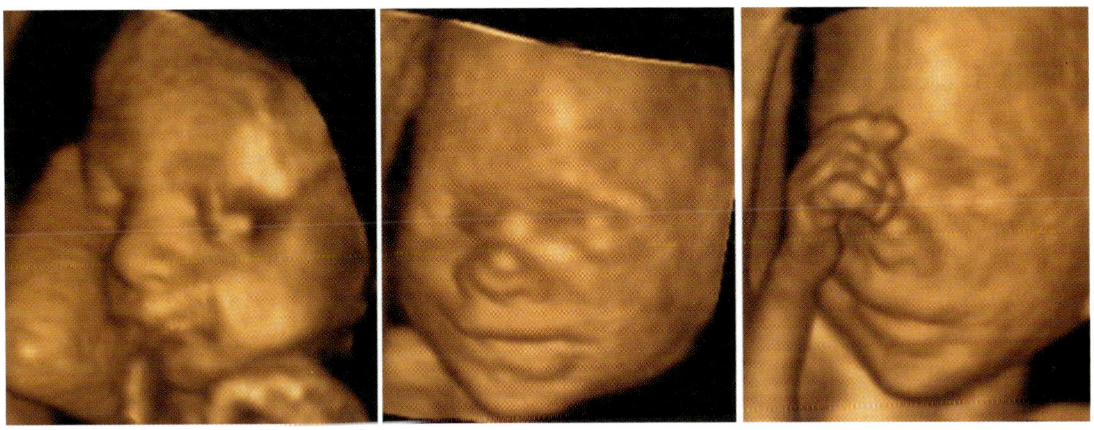

Figure 38.21 Several facial expressions characterized by turning up of the corners of the mouth shows the smiling fetus.

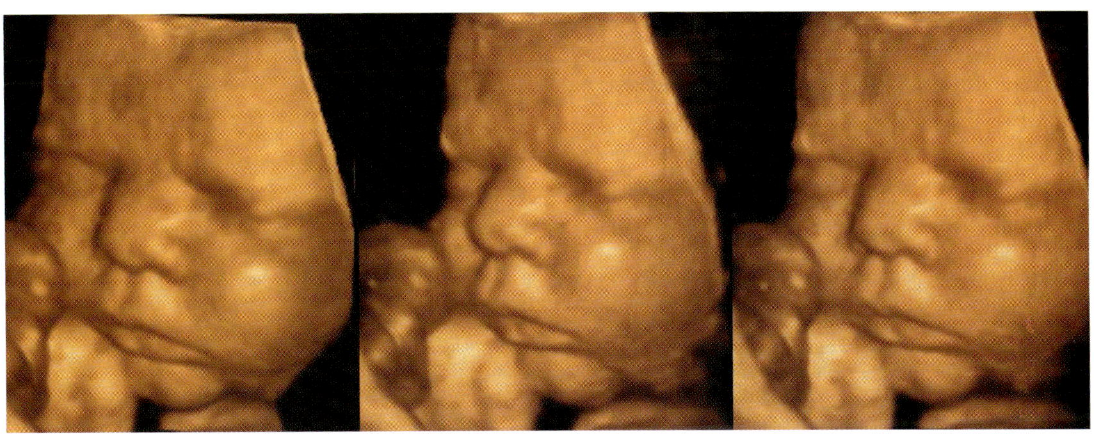

Figure 38.22 In this picture the fetus shows wrinkling of the brows or frowning face, may be to express displeasure or anger. The frontalis muscle can also be responsible for the appearance of grimacing. However, the main agent responsible for the appearance of scowling is the corrugator muscle.

imagine that we could construct a system that relates discrete emotions, like happiness, anger, sadness, etc., and various intensities of fetal facial expressions *in utero* to external events. A system might be able to be constructed where componential and general internal states like pleasure control each parameter unit and establish a pleasure score of the fetus that can be used to drive facial expressions.

Conclusions

Behavioral perinatology assessed by 4D sonography should be an interdisciplinary area of research involving concepts and conducting studies of the dynamic interplay between behavioral processes in fetal, neonatal and infant life.[134–136] Understanding the technical aspects of 4D ultrasound is important for utilizing its full potential. Furthermore, image postprocessing should be considered as a part of examination. Sometimes, additional information about the range of interest can be provided with post-processing.

The study of fetal behavior has provided us with an important contribution to understanding the hidden function of the developmental pathways of the fetal CNS and the potential to investigate neurologic deficits *in utero*.

REFERENCES

1. Judaš M, Kostoviæ I. *Temelji neuroznanosti*, 1st edn. Zagreb: Mladost, 1997:24–31, 353–60, 622–42.
2. Schacher S. Determination and differentiation in the development of the nervous system. In Kandel ER, Schwartz JH. *Principles of Neural Science*, 2nd edn. Amsterdam: Elsevier Science Publishing 1985:730–2.
3. Kostović I. Prenatal development of nucleus basalis complex and related fibre system in man: A histochemical study. *Neuroscience* 1986;17:1047–77.
4. Molliver ME, Kostovic I, Van der Loos H. The development of synapses in cerebral cortex of the human fetus. *Brain Res* 1973;50:403–7.
5. Kostovic I. Zentralnervensystem. In Hinrichsen KV, ed. *Humanembryologie*. Berlin: Springer-Verlag, 1990:381–448.
6. Kurjak A, ed. *Očekujući novorođenče*. Zagreb: Mladost, 1984:18, 30.
7. Ultrasound studies of human fetal behaviour. *Early Hum Dev* 1985;12(2):91–8.
8. Ianniruberto A, Tajani E. Ultrasonographic study of fetal movements. *Semin Perinatol* 1981;4:175–81.
9. Goto S, Kato TK. Early movements are useful for estimating the gestational weeks in the first trimester of pregnancy. In Levski RA, Morley P, eds. *Ultrasound '82*. New York: Pergamon Press, 1983:577–82.
10. Okado N. Onset of synapse formation in the human spinal cord. *J Comp Neurol* 1981;201(2):211–9.
11. Okado N. Development of the human cervical spinal cord with reference to synapse formation in the motor nucleus. *J Comp Neurol* 1980;191(3):495–513.
12. Fitzgerald M. *An Update on Current Scientific Knowledge*. London: Department of Health, 1995.
13. Humphrey T. Some correlations between the appearance of human fetal reflexes and the development of the nervous system. *Prog Brain Res* 1964;4:93–135.
14. de Vries JIP, Visser GHA, Prechtl HFR. Fetal motility in the first half of the pregnancy. In Prechtl HFR, ed. *Continuity of Neural Functions from Prenatal to Postnatal Life*. Philadelphia, PA: Lippincott, 1984:44–64.
15. de Vries JIP, Visser GHA, Prechtl HFR. The emergence of fetal behavior I. Qualitative aspects. *Early Human Dev* 1982;7: 301–22.
16. Kostovic I, Judas M, Petanjek Z, Simic G. Ontogenesis of goal-directed behavior: Anatomo-functional considerations. *Int J Psychophysiol* 1995;19(2):85–102.
17. Visser GHA, Laurini RN, Vries JIP, *et al.* Abnormal motor behaviour in anencephalic fetuses. *Early Human Dev* 1985;12:173–83.
18. Visser GHA, Prechtl HFR. Perinatal neurological development. *Proceedings of the Third International Conference on Fetal and Neonatal Physiological Measurements*, 1989:335–46.
19. D'Elia A, Pighetti M, Moccia G, Santangelo N. Spontaneous motor activity in normal fetus. *Early Human Dev* 2001;65(2): 139–44.
20. Natale R, Nasello-Paterson C, Turlink R. Longitudinal measurements of fetal breathing, body movements, and heart rate accelerations, and decelerations at 24 and 32 weeks of gestation. *Am J Obstet Gynecol* 1985;151:256–63.
21. Eller DP, Stramm SL, Newman RB. The effect of maternal intravenous glucose administration on fetal activity. *Am J Obstet Gynecol* 1992;167:1071–4.
22. Patrick J, Campbell K, Carmichael L, Natale R, Richardson B. Patterns of gross fetal body movements over 24-hour observation intervals during the last 10 weeks of pregnancy. *Am J Obstet Gynecol* 1982;142:363–71.
23. Kurjak A, Azumendi G, Vecek N, *et al.* Fetal hand movements and facial expression in normal pregnancy studied by four-dimensional sonography. *J Perinat Med* 2003;31(6):496–508.
24. de Vries JIP, Visser GHA, Prechtl HFR. The emergence of fetal behavior. II Quantitative aspects. *Early Hum Dev* 1985;12:99–120.
25. de Vries JIP, Visser GHA, Prechtl HFR. The emergence of fetal behavior. III. Individual differences and consistencies. *Early Hum Dev* 1988;16:85–103.
26. Prechtl HF. Fetal behaviour. *Eur J Obstet Gynecol Reprod Biol* 1989;32(1):32.
27. Graca LM, Cardoso CG, Clode N, *et al.* Acute effects of maternal cigarette smoking on fetal heart rate and fetal movements felt the mother. *J Perinat Med* 1991;19:385–90.
28. Katz M, Meizner I, Holcberg G, Mazor M, *et al.* Reduction or cessation of fetal movements after administration of steroids for enhancement of lung maturation. *Isr J Med Sci* 1988;24:5–9.
29. Kurjak A. Kada ivot počinje. *OKO* 1981;232:14.
30. Prechtl HFR, Einspieler C. Is neurological assessment of the fetus possible? *Eur J Obstet Gynecol Reprod Biol* 1997;75:81–4.
31. Patrick J, Gagnon R. Fetal breathing and body movement. In Creasy RK, Resnik R, eds. Maternal–fetal medicine: Principles and practice, 2nd edn. Philadelphia, PA: W. B. Saunders Company, 1989:268–84.
32. Natale R, Nasello-Paterson C, Connors G. Patterns of fetal breathing activity in the human fetus at 24 to 28 weeks of gestation. *Am J Obstet Gynecol* 1988;158:317–21.
33. Patrick J, Campbell K, Carmichael L, *et al.* Patterns of human fetal breathing during the last 10 weeks of pregnancy. *Obstet Gynecol* 1980;56:24–30.
34. Patrick J, Campbell K, Carmichael L, *et al.* A definition of human fetal apnea and the distribution of fetal apneic intervals during the last 10 weeks of pregnancy. *Am J Obstet Gynecol* 1978;136:371–7.
35. Ritchie K. The response to changes in the composition of maternal inspired air in human pregnancy. *Semin Perinatol* 1980;4:295–9.
36. Richardson B, Campbell K, Campbell L, *et al.* Effects of external physical stimulation on fetuses near term. *Am J Obstet Gynecol* 1981;139:344–52.
37. Richardson B, Natale R, Patrick J. Human fetal breathing activity during induced labour at term. *Am J Obstet Gynecol* 1979; 133:247–55.
38. Roberts AB, Goldstein I, Romero R, *et al.* Fetal breathing movements after preterm rupture of membranes. *Am J Obstet Gynecol* 1991;164:821–5.
39. Kivikoski A, Amon E, Vaalamo PO, *et al.* Effect of third-trimester premature rupture of membranes on fetal breathing movements: A prospective case–control study. *Am J Obstet Gynecol* 1988; 159:1474–7.
40. Besinger RE, Compton AA, Hayashi RH. The presence or absence of fetal breathing movements as a predictor of outcome in preterm labor. *Am J Obstet Gynecol* 1987;157:753–7.
41. Kisilevsky BS, Hains SMJ, Low JA. Maturation of body and breathing movements in 24–33 week old fetuses threatening to deliver prematurely. *Early Hum Dev* 1999;55(1):25–38.
42. Fox HE, Steinbrecher M, Pessel D, *et al.* Maternal ethanol ingestion and occurrence of human breathing movements. *Am J Obstet Gynecol* 1978;132:354–61.
43. Richardson B, O'Grady JP, Olsen GD. Fetal breathing movements in response to carbon dioxide in patients on methadone maintenance. *Am J Obstet Gynecol* 1984;150:400–4.
44. Manning FA, Wym Pugh E, Boddy K. Effect of cigarette smoking on fetal breathing movements in normal pregnancy. *Br Med J* 1975;1:552–8.

45. Ishigava M, Yoneyama Y, Power GG, *et al.* Maternal teophylline administration and breathing movements in late gestation human fetus. *Obstet Gynecol* 1996;88(6):973–8.
46. Cosmi EV, Cosmi E, La Torre R. The effect of fetal breathing movements on the utero-placental circulation. *Early Pregnancy* 2001;5(1):51–2.
47. Natale R, Patrick J, Richardson B. Effects of maternal venous plasma glucose concentrations on fetal breathing movements. *Am J Obstet Gynecol* 1978;132–41.
48. Patrick J, Natale R, Richardson B. Patterns of human fetal breathing activity at 34 to 35 weeks gestational age. *Am J Obstet Gynecol* 1978;507–13.
49. Diamant NE. Development of esophageal function. *Am Rev Respir Dis* 1985;131:S29–32.
50. Pritchard JA. Fetal swallowing and amniotic fluid volume. *Obstet Gynecol* 1966;28:606–16.
51. Abramovich DR, Garden A, Jandial L, *et al.* Fetal swallowing and voiding in relation to hydramnios. *Obstet Gynecol* 1979;54:15–20.
52. Abramovich DR. Fetal factor influencing the volume and composition of liquor amnii. *J Obstet Gynaaecol Br Commonw* 1970;77:865–77.
53. Pitkin RM, Reynolds WA. Fetal ingestion and metabolism of amniotic fluid protein. *Am J Obstet Gynecol* 1975;123:356–63.
54. Ross MG, Nijland JM. Development of ingestive behavior. *Am J Physiol* 1998;274(4, Pt 2):R879–93.
55. Ross MG, El Haddad M, DeSai M. Unopposed orexic pathways in the developing fetus. *Physiol Behav* 2003;79(1):79–88.
56. Humphrey T. The embryologic differentiation of the vestibular nuclei in man correlated with functional development. *International Symposium on Vestibular and Occular Problems.* Tokyo: Society of Vestibular Research, University of Tokyo, 1965: 51–6.
57. Hooker D. Fetal reflexes and instinctual processes. *Psychosom Med* 1942;4:199–220.
58. Starr A, Amlie RN, Martin WH, Saunders S. Development of auditory function in newborn infants revealed by auditory brainstem potentials. *Pediatrics* 1991;60:831–8.
59. Morlet T, Collet L, Solle B, *et al.* Functional maturation of cochlear active mechanisms and of the medial olivocochlear system in humans. *Acta Otolaringol (Stockh)* 1993;113:271–7.
60. Morlet T, Collet L, Duclaux R, *et al.* Spontaneous and evoked otoacoustical emissions in preterm and full term neonates. Is there a clinical application? *Int J Ped Otorhinolaryngol* 1995;33:207–11.
61. Leader LR, Baille P, Martin B, *et al.* The assessment and significance of habituation to a repeated stimulus by human fetus. *Early Human Dev* 1982;7:211–8.
62. Liley AW. Fetus as a person. Speech held at the 8th meeting of the psychiatric societies of Australia and New Zealand. *Fetal Ther* 1986;1:8–17.
63. Shahidullah S, Hepper P. The developmental origins of fetal responsiveness to an acoustic stimulus. *J Reprod Infant Psychol* 1994;12:143–54.
64. Kisilevsky BS, Pang LH, Hains SMJ. Maturation of human fetal responses to airborne sound in low- and high-risk fetuses. *Early Human Dev* 2000;58:179–95.
65. Huttenlocher PR, deCourten CH. The development of synapses in striate cortex of man. *Hum Neurobiol* 1987;6:1–9.
66. Magoon EH, Robb RM. Development of myelin in human optic nerve tract. A light and electron microscopic study. *Arch Ophthalmol* 1981;99:655–9.
67. Hendrickson AE, Youdelis C. The morphological development of the human foveola. *Ophthalmology* 1981;91:603–12.
68. Vanhatalo S, van Nieuvenhuizen O. Fetal pain? *Brain Dev* 2000;22(3):145–50.
69. Fitzgerald M. Development of pain mechanisms. *Br Med Bull* 1991;47:667–75.
70. Okado N, Kojim T. Ontogeny of central nervous system: Neurogenesis, fibre connections, synaptogenesis and myelination in the spinal cord. In Prechtl HFR, ed. *Continuity of Neural Functions from Prenatal to Postnatal Life.* Philadelphia, PA: Lippincott, 1984:31–45.
71. Anand KJS, Hickey PR. Pain and its effects in the human neonate and fetus. *N Engl J Med* 1987;317:1321–9.
72. Anand KJS, Phil D, Carr DB. The neuroanatomy, neurophysiology, and neurochemistry of pain, stress and analgesia in the newborns and children. *Ped Clin North Am* 1989;36;795–882.
73. Holstege G. Descending motor pathways and the spinal motor system: Limbic and non-limbic components. *Prog Brain Res* 1991;87:307–421.
74. Giannakoulopoulos X, Sepulveda W, Kourtis P, *et al.* Fetal plasma cortisol and beta endorphin response to intrauterine needling. *Lancet* 1994;344:77–81.
75. Giannakoulopolous X, Teixeira J, Fisk N, *et al.* Human fetal and maternal noradrenaline responses to invasive procedures. *Pediatr Res* 1999;45:494–9.
76. Smith RP, Gitau R, Glover V, *et al.* Pain and stress in the human fetus. *Eur J Obstet Gynecol Reprod Biol* 2000;92:161–5.
77. Anand KJS, Sippell WG, Aynsley-Green A. Randomized trial of fentaniyl anaesthesia in preterm babies undergoing surgery: Effects of the stress response. *Lancet* 1987;1:62–6.
78. Guinsburg R, Kopelman BI, Anand KJS, *et al.* Physiological, hormonal and behavioural responses to a single fentanyl dose in intubated and ventilated preterm neonates. *J Pediatr* 1998;132:954–9.
79. Anand KJS. Clinical importance of pain and stress in preterm neonates. *Biol Neonate* 1998;73:319–24.
80. Uno H, Lohmiller L, Thieme C, *et al.* Brain damage induced by prenatal exposure to dexamethasone in fetal rhesus macaques. I. Hippocampus. *Brain Res Dev Brain Res* 1990;53:157–67.
81. Grunau RVE, Whitfield MF, Petrie JH, *et al.* Early pain experience, child and family factors, as precursors of somatization: A prospective study of extremely premature infants and fullterm children. *Pain* 1994;56:353–9.
82. Bradley RM, Mistretta CM. The developing sense of taste. In Denton VDA, Coghlan JP, eds. *Olfaction and Taste.* New York: Academic Press, 1975:91–8.
83. Kawamura K, Takebayashi S. The development of noradrenaline-, acetylcholinesterase-, neuropeptide Y- and vasoactive intestinal polypeptide-containing nerves in human cerebral arteries. *Neurosci Lett* 1994;175:1–4.
84. Cetin I, Morpurgo PS, Radaelli T, *et al.* Fetal plasma leptin concentrations: Relationship with different intrauterine growth patterns from 19 weeks to term. *Pediatr Res* 2000;48:646–51.
85. Jaquet D, Leger J, Levy-Marchal C, *et al.* Ontogeny of leptin in human fetuses and newborns: Effect of intrauterine growth retardation on serum leptin concentrations. *J Clin Endocrinol Metab* 1998;83:1243–6.
86. Roberts TJ, Caston-Balderrama A, Nijland MJ, *et al.* Central neuropeptide Y stimulates ingestive behavior and increases urine output in the ovine fetus. *Am J Physiol Endocrinol Metab* 2000;279:E494–500.
87. Roberts TJ, Nijland MJ, Caston-Balderrama A, *et al.* Central leptin stimulates ingestive behavior and urine flow in the near term ovine fetus. *Horm Metab Res* 2001,33.144–50.
88. Ross MG, Kullama LK, Ogundipe OA, *et al.* Ovine fetal swallowing response to intracerebroventricular hypertonic saline. *J Appl Physiol* 1995;78:2267–71.
89. Ross MG, Kullama LK, Ogundipe OA, *et al.* Central angiotensin II stimulation of ovine fetal swallowing. *J Appl Physiol* 1994;76(3):1340–5.
90. McDonald TJ, Li C, Nijland MJM, *et al.* Fos response of the fetal sheep anterior circumventricular organs to an osmotic challenge in late gestation. *Am J Physiol* 1997.
91. Xu Z, Nijland MJ, Ross MG. Plasma osmolality dypsogenic thresholds and c-fos expression in the near-term ovine fetus. *Pediatr Res* 2001;49:678–85.
92. Caston Balderrama A, Nijland MJM, McDonald TJ, *et al.* Central fos expression in fetal and adult sheep following intraperitoneal hypertonic saline. *Am J Physiol* 1999;276:H725–35.
93. El Haddad MA, Chao CR, MA SX, *et al.* Neuronal NO modulates spontaneous ANG II-stimulated fetal swallowing behavior in the near-term ovine fetus. *Am J Physiol Regul Integr Comp Physiol* 2002;282:R1521–7.
94. El Haddad MA, Chao CR, Sayed AA, *et al.* Effects of central angiotensin II receptor antagonism on fetal swallowing and cardiovascular activity. *Am J Obstet Gynecol* 2001;185:828–33.
95. Davison JM, Gilmore EA, Durr J. Altered osmotic thresholds for vasopressin secretion and thirst in human pregnancy. *Am J Physiol* 1984;246:F105–9.
96. Ross MG, Sherman DJ, Schreyer P, *et al.* Fetal rehydration via amniotic fluid: Contribution of fetal swallowing. *Pediatr Res* 1991;29:214–7.
97. Nijland MJM, Kullama LK, Ross MG. Maternal plasma hypoosmolality: Effects on spontaneous and stimulated ovine fetal swallowing. *J Matern Fetal Med* 1998;7:165–71.
98. Ross MG, Sherman DJ, Ervin MG, *et al.* Fetal swallowing: Response to systemic hypotension. *Am J Physiol* 1990;257:R130–4.
99. Inoue M, Koyanagi T, NakaharaH. Functional development of human eye-movement in utero assessed quantitatively with real-time ultrasound. *Am J Obstet Gynecol* 1986;155:170–4.

100. Aserinski E, Kleitman N. Two types of occular motility occurring in sleep. *J Appl Physiol* 1955;8:1–10.
101. Parmelee AH, Stern E. Development of states in infants. In Clemente CD, Purpura DP, Mayer FE, eds. *Sleep and the Maturing Central Nervous System*. New York: Academic Press, 1972:100–215.
102. Ruckenbush Y, Gaujoux M, Eghbali B. Sleep cycles and kinesis in the fetal lamb. *Electroencephalogr Clin Neurophysiol* 1977;42:226–33.
103. Kelly DD. Sleep and dreaming. In Kandell ER, Schwartz JH, eds. *Principles of Neural Science*, 2nd edn. Amsterdam: Elsevier Science Publishing, 1985:651.
104. Seron Ferre M, Torres C, Parraguez VH, *et al.* Perinatal neuroendocrine regulation. Development of the circadian time-keeping system. *Mol Cell Endocrinol* 2002;186:169–73.
105. Vanececk J. Cellular mechanisms of melatonin action. *Physiol Rev* 1998;78:687–721.
106. Yie SM, Niles LP, Younglavi EV. Melatonin receptors on human granulosa cell membranes. *J Clin Endocrinol Metab* 1995;80: 1747–9.
107. Hu W, Wu MT, Liu CP, *et al.* Left ventricular 4D echocardiogram motion and shape analysis. *Ultrasonics* 2002;40:949–54.
108. Kossoff G. Basic physics and imaging characteristics of ultrasound. *World J Surg* 2000;24:134–42.
109. Timor-Tritsch IE, Platt LD. Three-dimensional ultrasound experience in obstetrics. *Curr Opin Obstet Gynecol* 2002;14:569–75.
110. Lee W. 3D fetal ultrasonography. *Clin Obstet Gynecol* 2003;46:850–67.
111. Arzt W, Tulzer G, Aigner M. Real time 3D sonography of the normal fetal heart – clinical evaluation. *Ultraschall Med* 2002;23:388–91.
112. Yanagihara T, Hata T Three-dimensional sonographic visualization of fetal skeleton in the second trimester of pregnancy. *Gynecol Obstet Invest* 2000;49:12–6.
113. Mangione R, Lacombe D, Carles D, *et al.* Craniofacial dysmorphology and three-dimensional ultrasound: A prospective study on practicability for prenatal diagnosis. *Prenat Diagn* 2003;23:810–8.
114. Kurjak A, Hafner T, Kos M, *et al.* Three-dimensional sonography in prenatal diagnosis: A luxury or a necessity? *J Perinat Med* 2000;28:194–209.
115. De Vore GR, Falkensammer P, Sklansky MS, *et al.* Spatio-temporal image correlation (STIC): New technology for evaluation of the fetal heart. *Ultrasound Obstet Gynecol* 2003;22:380–7.
116. Vinals F, Poblete P, Giuliano A. Spatio-temporal image correlation (STIC): A new tool for the prenatal screening of congenital heart defects. *Ultrasound Obstet Gynecol* 2003;22:388–94.
117. Kurjak A, Vecek N, Hafner T, *et al.* Prenatal diagnosis: What does four-dimensional ultrasound add? *J Perinat Med* 2002;30:57–62.
118. Nijhuis JG, ed. *Fetal Behaviour: Developmental and Perinatal Aspects*. Oxford: Oxford University Press, 1992.
119. Azumendi G, Kurjak A. Three-dimensional and four-dimensional sonography in the study of the fetal face. *Ultrasound Rev Obstet Gynecol* 2003;3:1–10.
120. Roodenburg PJ, Wladimiroff JW, van Es A, *et al.* Classification and quantitative aspects of fetal movements during the second half of normal pregnancy. *Early Hum Dev* 1991;25:19–35.
121. Prechtl HFR. Qualitative changes of spontaneous movements in fetus and preterm infant are a marker of neurological dysfunction. *Early Hum Dev* 1990;23:151–8.
122. de Vries JIP, Laurini RN, Visser CHA. Abnormal motor behaviour and developmental postmortem findings in a fetus with Fanconi anaemia. *Early Hum Dev* 1994;36:137–142.
123. Prechtl HFR. Qualitative changes of spontaneous movements in fetus and preterm infant are a marker of neurological dysfunction. *Early Hum Dev* 1990;23:151–8.
124. Ververs IAP, de Vries JIP, van Geijn HP, *et al.* Prenatal head position from 12–38 weeks, I: Developmental aspects. *Early Hum Dev* 1994;39:83–91.
125. Hepper PG, Shahidullah S, White R. Handedness in the human fetus. *Neuropsychologia* 1991;29:1107–11.
126. Sparling JW, Wilhelm IJ. Quantitative measurement of fetal movement: Fetal-posture and movement assessment (F-PAM). *Phys Occup Ther Pediatr* 1993;12:97–114.
127. Piaget J. *The Origins of Intelligence in Children*. New York: International Universities Press, 1952.
128. Geerdink JJ, Hopkins B. Effects of birthweight status and gestational age on the quality of general movements in preterm newborns. *Neonate* 1993;63:215–24.
129. Butterworth G, Hopkins B. Hand–mouth coordination in the new-born baby. *Br J Dev Psychol* 1988;6:303–14.
130. Hopkins B, Prechtl HFR. A qualitative approach to the development of movements during early infancy. In Prechtl HFR, ed. *Continuity of Neural Functions from Perinatal to Postnatal Life*. Oxford: Blackwell Scientific Publications, 1984:179–97.
131. Kainer F, Prechtl HF, Engele H, *et al.* Assessment of the quality of general rnovements in fetuses and infants of women with type-I diabetes mellitus. *Early Hum Dev* 1997;50:13–25.
132. Kurjak A, Stanojevic M, Andonotopo W, Salihagic-Kadic A, Carrera JM, Azumendi G. Behavioral pattern continuity from prenatal to postnatal life – a study by four-dimensional (4D) ultrasonography. *J Perinat Med* 2004;32:346–53.
133. Kozuma S, Baba K, Okai T, *et al.* Dynamic observation of the fetal face by three-dimensional ultrasound. *Ultrasound Obstet Gynecol* 1999;13:283–4.
134. Arabin B. Two-dimensional real-time ultrasound in the assessment of fetal activity in single and multiple pregnancy. *Ultrasound Rev Obstet Gynecol* 2004;4(2).
135. Arabin B, Van Straaten I, Van Eyck J. Fetal hearing. In Kurjak A, ed. *Textbook of Perinatal Medicine*. London: Parthenon Publishing, 1998:756–75.
136. Arabin B, Bos R, Rijlaarsdam R, Mohnhaupt A, van Eyck J. The onset of inter-human contacts: Longitudinal ultrasound observations in early twin pregnancies. *Ultrasound Obstet Gynecol* 1996;8(3):166–73.

39 Fetal central nervous system

R. K. Pooh and K. Pooh

Introduction

Recent advances in prenatal imaging technologies such as transvaginal ultrasound, three-dimensional (3D) ultrasound, and magnetic resonance imaging have been remarkable and have contributed to prenatal evaluation of fetal abnormalities *in utero*. Owing to these technologies, fetal malformations have been reliably diagnosed with increasing accuracy and at earlier gestation. As regards to fetal central nervous system (CNS) assessment, a new field of *neurosonography*[1] has been established. Many of the congenital CNS anomalies, which were disclosed in the late pregnancy or after birth, have been recently demonstrated by use of high frequency transvaginal sonography before viability. More advances of technological development will clarify unknown neuropathological facts during fetal period.

Diagnostics of the fetal CNS is one of the most difficult fields in perinatology. There are several reasons why the prenatal CNS evaluation is difficult: (1) lack of essential knowledge of CNS anatomy and pathology; (2) rapid changes of normal CNS development during pregnancy; and (3) inexperience in the use of CNS neuroimaging techniques.

When beginners start prenatal CNS imaging, the above three may be the most frequent reasons for difficulties encountered in prenatal assessment. However, after overcoming those problems, there still exist difficulties in assessment of fetal CNS diseases, because of difficulty in prediction of neurological prognosis and existence of gray zone between normality and abnormality.

CNS development

The brain is a 3D structure and should be comprehended in the three orthogonal views of sagittal, coronal, and axial sections. During fetal period, the embryonal premature CNS structure develops to mature structure (Figure 39.1). Within this rapid change of development, various developmental disorders and/or insults result in various phenotypes of fetal CNS abnormalities. For understanding fetal CNS diseases, basic knowledge of the development of the nervous system is essential. The developmental stages and their major disorders are described in Table 39.1.

It is believed that the brain anatomy must be complicated and there must be lots of terms to remember. In this chapter, essential anatomical structures are selected for neuroimaging and comprehension of fetal CNS diseases. Figures 39.2 and 39.3 show the basic anatomy in the axial, sagittal, and anterior coronal sections of the brain. For understanding hydrocephalus, ventriculomegaly, and/or other intracranial lesions, the ventricular system (Figure 39.4) and cerebrospinal fluid (CSF) circulation (Figure 39.5) should be understood.

Technology

Transabdominal sonographic technique, by which it is possible to observe the fetal internal organs through the maternal abdominal wall and uterine wall, is the most widely used method for fetal imaging diagnosis. Using the transabdominal approach, fetal brain structure mostly in the axial section and fetal back structure including the vertebrae and spinal cord in the sagittal section can be well demonstrated. However, in the transabdominal approach to the fetal CNS, there are several obstacles such as maternal abdominal wall, placenta, and fetal cranial bones.

Introduction of high-frequency transvaginal transducer has contributed to establishing 'sonoembryology'[2] and recent general use of transvaginal sonography in early pregnancy has enabled early diagnoses of major fetal anomalies.[3] During middle and late pregnancy, fetal CNS is generally evaluated through the maternal abdominal wall. The brain, however, is a 3D structure, and should be assessed in the basic three planes of sagittal, coronal, and axial sections. Sonographic assessment of the fetal brain in the sagittal and coronal sections requires an approach from fetal parietal direction (Figure 39.6). Transvaginal sonography of the fetal brain has opened up a new field in medicine, 'neurosonography'.[1] The transvaginal approach to the normal fetal brain during the second and third trimester was introduced in the beginning of the 1990s. It was the

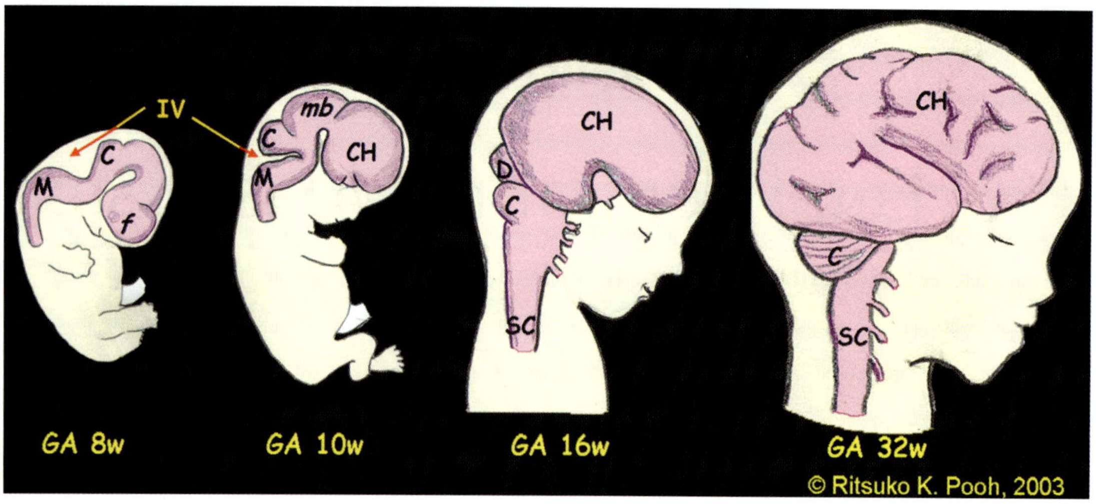

Figure 39.1 Developing brain and spinal cord during pregnancy. Fetal central nervous system changes in size and appearance from early premature structure into late mature structure with gyral formation. CH, cerebral hemisphere; C, cerebellum; D, diencephalons; M, medulla; SC, spinal cord; f, forebrain; mb, midbrain; IV, fourth ventricle.

Table 39.1 Developmental stages and major disorders

Development stage	Disorders
Primary neurulation (3–4 weeks' gestation)	Spina bifida aperta, cranium bifidum
Caudal neural tube formation (secondary neurulation, from 4 weeks' gestation)	Occult dysraphic states
Procencephalic development (2–3 months' gestation)	Holoprosencephaly
	Agenesis of the corpus callosum, agenesis of the septum pellucidum, septo-optic dysplasia
Neuronal proliferation (3–4 months' gestation)	Micrencephaly, macrencephaly
Neuronal migration (3–5 months' gestation)	Schizencephaly
	Lissencephaly, pachygyria polymicrogyria
Organization (5 months' gestation–years postnatal)	Idiopathic mental retardation
Myelination (birth–years postnatal)	Cerebral white matter hypoplasia

first practical application of 3D CNS assessment by 2D ultrasound.[4] Transvaginal observation of the fetal brain offers sagittal and coronal views of the brain from fetal parietal direction[5–8] through the fontanelles and/or the sagittal suture as ultrasound windows. Serial oblique sections[3] via the same ultrasound window reveal the intracranial morphology in detail. This method has contributed to the prenatal assessment of congenital CNS anomalies and acquired brain damage *in utero*.

Three-dimensional ultrasound is one of the most attractive modalities in the field of fetal ultrasound imaging. There are two scanning methods, namely free-hand scan and automatic scan. Automatic scan by dedicated 3D transducer produces motor-driven automatic sweeping and is called fan scan. With this method, a shift and/or angle-change of the transducer is not required during scanning and scan duration needs only several seconds. After acquisition of the target organ, multiplanar imaging analysis is possible. Combination of both transvaginal sonography and 3D ultrasound[9–12] may be a great diagnostic tool for evaluation of the 3D structure of fetal CNS. There are several useful functions in 3D ultrasound as follows:

- Surface imaging of the fetal head
- Bony structural imaging of the calvaria and vertabrae
- Multiplanar imaging of the intracranial structure
- Three-dimensional sono-angiography of the brain circulation

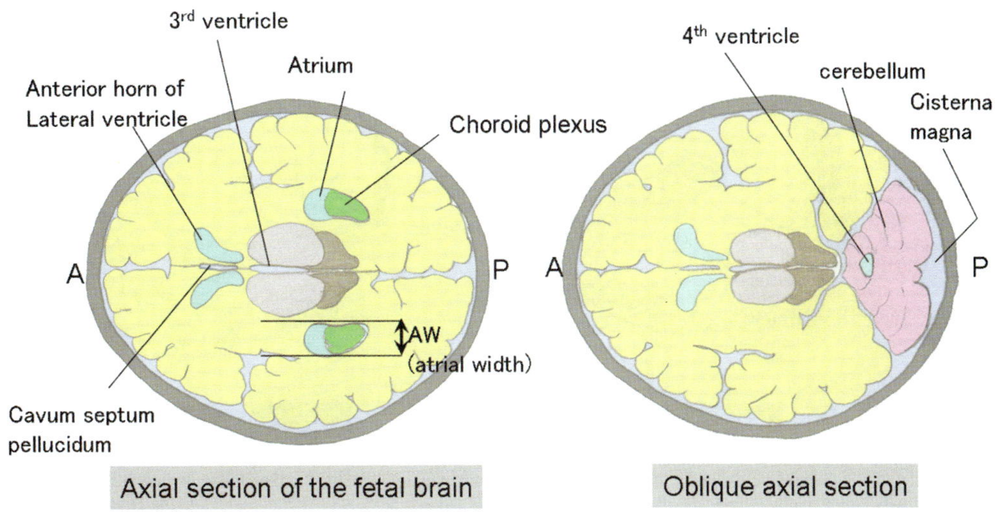

Figure 39.2 Basic anatomical knowledge for neuroimaging in the axial and oblique axial sections.

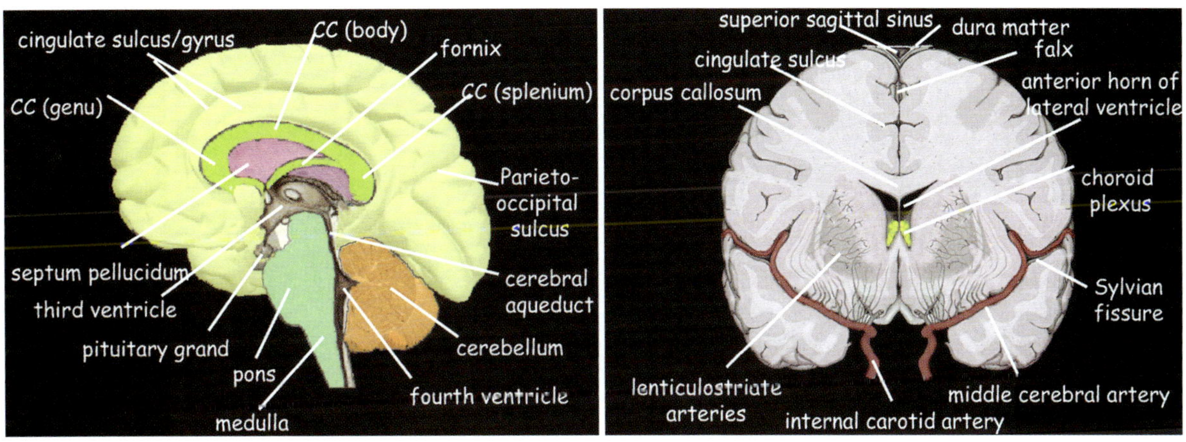

Figure 39.3 Basic anatomical knowledge of sagittal (left) and anterior coronal cutting sections of the brain. CC, corpus callosum.

- Volume calculation of target organs such as intracranial cavity, ventricle, choroid plexus, and intracranial lesions
- Simultaneous volume contrast imaging by 4D ultrasound.

In multiplanar imaging of the brain structure, it is possible to demonstrate not only the sagittal and coronal sections but also the axial section of the brain, which cannot be demonstrated from parietal direction by a conventional 2D transvaginal sonography. Parallel slicing provides a tomographic visualization of internal morphology similar to magnetic resonance imaging (MRI). Volume extracted image and volume calculation of the fetal brain in early pregnancy was reported in the 1990s.[13,14] We used VOLUSON 730 Expert (GE Medical Systems, Milwaukee, USA) with transvaginal 3D transducer and 3D View version 3.2 software (Kretztechnik AG, Zipf, Austria) for volume extraction and volume estimation of the brain structure. Furthermore, with application of 4D ultrasound, real-time images with increased contrast resolution can be obtained in not only the same plane as 2D cutting section but also vertical plane to 2D image.[15] Fetal neuroimaging with advanced 3D/4D technology

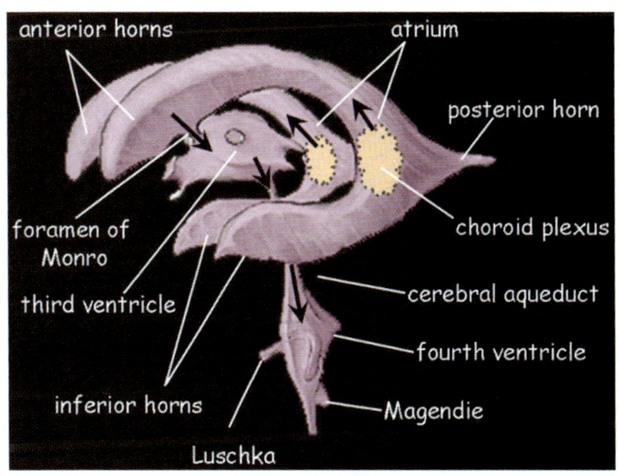

Figure 39.4 Basic anatomical knowledge of ventricular system and cerebrospinal fluid (CSF) flow.

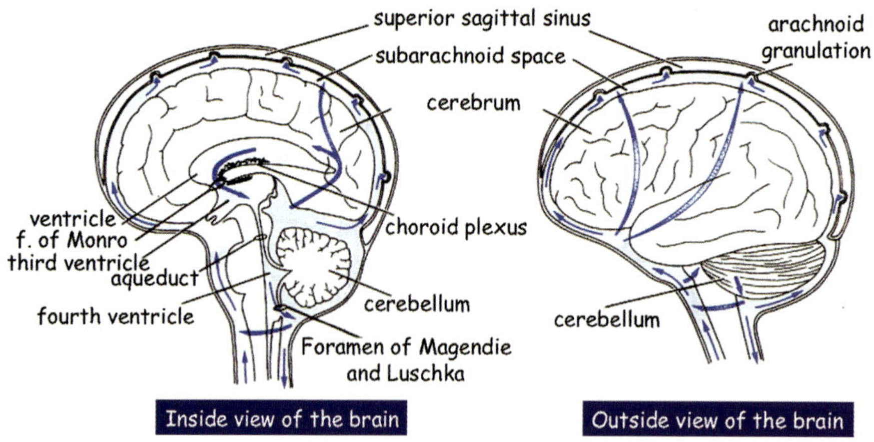

Figure 39.5 Cerebrospinal fluid (CSF) circulation. Inside and outside views of the brain. CSF is produced from choroid plexus of ventricles. CSF runs through the third ventricle, aqueduct and fourth ventricle, goes to the surface of the brain and spinal cord, and is then absorbed by arachnoid granulation. From *Handbook on hydrocephalus for patients*, Research Committee of 'Intractable Hydrocephalus', Japanese Ministry of Health and Welfare, © 1993, with permission. (Schema by courtesy of chairman of the Committee, Prof. K. Mori.)

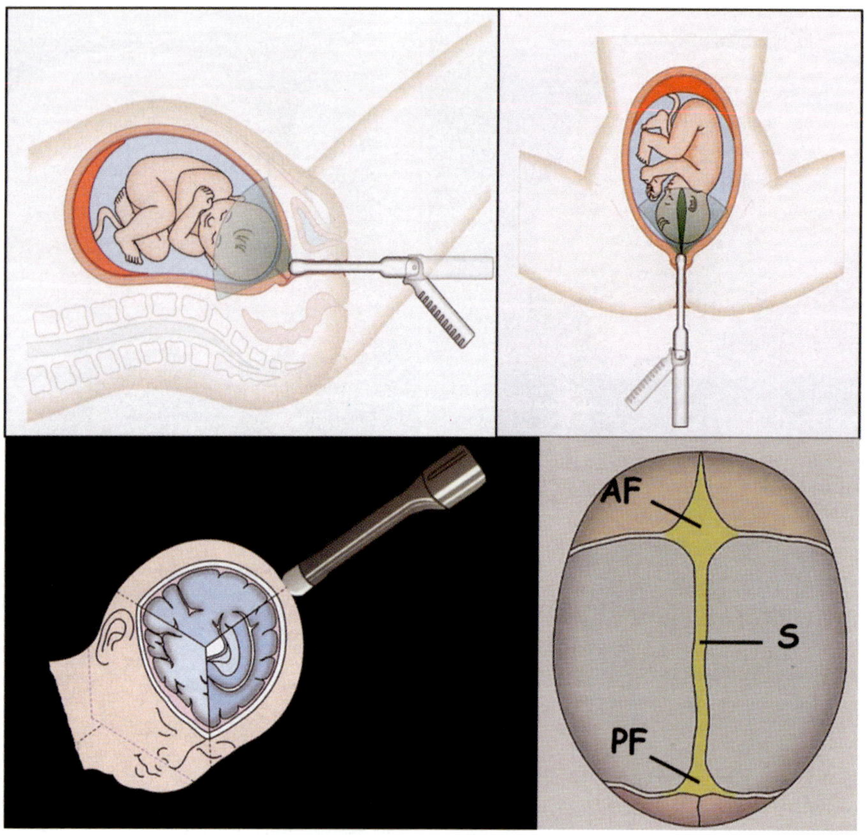

Figure 39.6 Schema of transvaginal sonography. (Upper left) Lateral view of vertex presenting fetus and transvaginal transducer. (Upper right) Frontal view of transvaginal approach. Clear imaging is possible by rotating and angle-changing of the transducer. (Lower left) Scheme of transfontanelle/trans-sutural approach of the fetal brain. (Lower right) Cranial bony structure from parietal direction. AF, anterior fontanelle; S, sagittal suture; PF, posterior fontanelle. These spaces are used as ultrasound windows.

is easy, noninvasive, and reproducible. It produces not only comprehensible images but also objective imaging data which can be graphed in volume calculation. Easy storage/extraction of raw volume data set enables off-line analysis and consultation with neurologists and neurosurgeons.[16,17]

Recent fast MRI is being used increasingly as a correlative imaging modality because it uses no ionizing radiation, provides excellent soft tissue contrast, has multiple planes for reconstruction, and a large field of view.[18] Recent advances in fast MRI technology, such as half-Fourier and the 0.5-signal-acquired single-shot

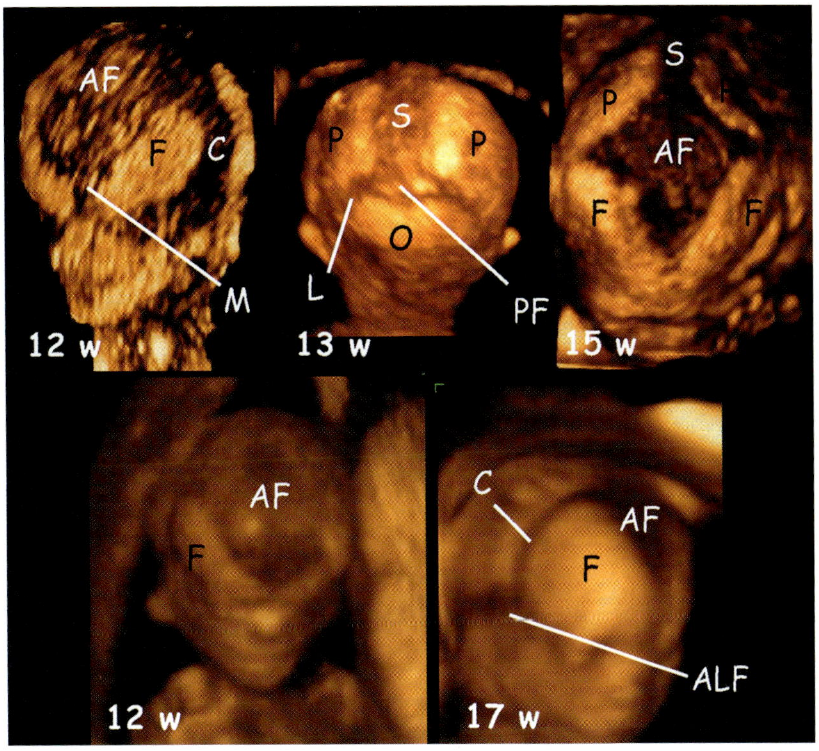

Figure 39.7 Fetal cranial structure in early gestation (3D ultrasound images). (Upper left) 12 weeks, from the oblique front. (Upper middle) 13 weeks, from the back. (Upper right) 15 weeks, from the top of head. (Lower left) 12 weeks, from the front. (Lower right) 17 weeks. Oblique position. Premature shape of cranial bones, sutures, and fontanelles at 12–13 weeks changes its appearance to the neonatal shape. AF, anterior fontanelle; PF, posterior fontanelle; ALF, anterolateral fontanelle; F, frontal bone; P, parietal bone; O, occipital bone; C, coronal suture; M, metopic suture; S, sagittal suture; L, lambdoid suture.

fast spin-echo (SE), half-Fourier rapid acquisition with relaxation enhancement (RARE) sequences, has remarkably improved the T2-weighted image resolution despite a short acquisition time, and minimized fetal and/or maternal respiratory motion artifacts without the need for fetal sedation.[19] MRI has a great potential especially in the evaluation of CNS and several reports have been published on normal and abnormal CNS anatomy by using fast MRI techniques.[20–23]

Normal fetal CNS imaging

The calvaria and its major sutures develop between 12 and 18 weeks of fetal life, with dura as guiding tissue in the morphogenesis of the skull.[24] The cranial bones are detectable by sonography from 10 weeks of gestation on. At 12 weeks, premature cranial bones and sutures in between are detectable (Figure 39.7). The sagittal suture, lambdoid sutures, and posterior fontanelle are recognizable from 13 weeks. As the fetal parietal portion has the anterior/posterior fontanelles and sagittal suture, which is the widest suture among the fetal cranial sutures,[25] transvaginal approach to the fetal brain using these spaces as ultrasound windows demonstrates the detailed brain structure without obstacles of the cranial bone, and is the most reasonable way for brain assessment. Recent advanced 3D ultrasound has been able to depict vertebral body, intervertebral disk space, and vertebral lamina (Figures 39.8 and 39.9).

From 8 weeks of gestation, the premature sonolucent ventricular system is detectable (Figure 39.10). Before 16 weeks of gestation, lateral ventricles are occupied by the choroid plexus (Figure 39.11). Basic knowledge of images in several cutting sections obtained by transvaginal scanning is shown in Figure 39.12. Three orthogonal views by 3D ultrasound are useful for obtaining easy orientation. Multiplanar image analysis is possible (Figure 39.13). Using new technology of 3D tomographic ultrosound imaging (TUI), the brain structure can be observed in parallel cutting slices of any section (Figure 39.14). TUI demonstrates the brain just like magnetic resonance imaging (MRI). Furthermore, off-line analysis allows us to change slice width and to rotate all images in any angle. Three-dimensional transvaginal power Doppler demonstrates clear anatomical vascular formation (Figure 39.15). Vertebrae and spine should be observed carefully for detection of back abnormalities such as spina bifida or scoliosis. Fetal sagittal sectional screening is preferable (Figure 39.16).

Volume analysis by 3D ultrasound provides exceedingly informative imaging data.[15] Volume analysis of the structure of interest provides an intelligible evaluation of the brain structure in total, and longitudinal and objective assessment of enlarged ventricles and intracranial occupying lesions. Any intracranial organ can be chosen as a target for volumetry no matter how distorted its shape and appearance may be (Figure 39.17).

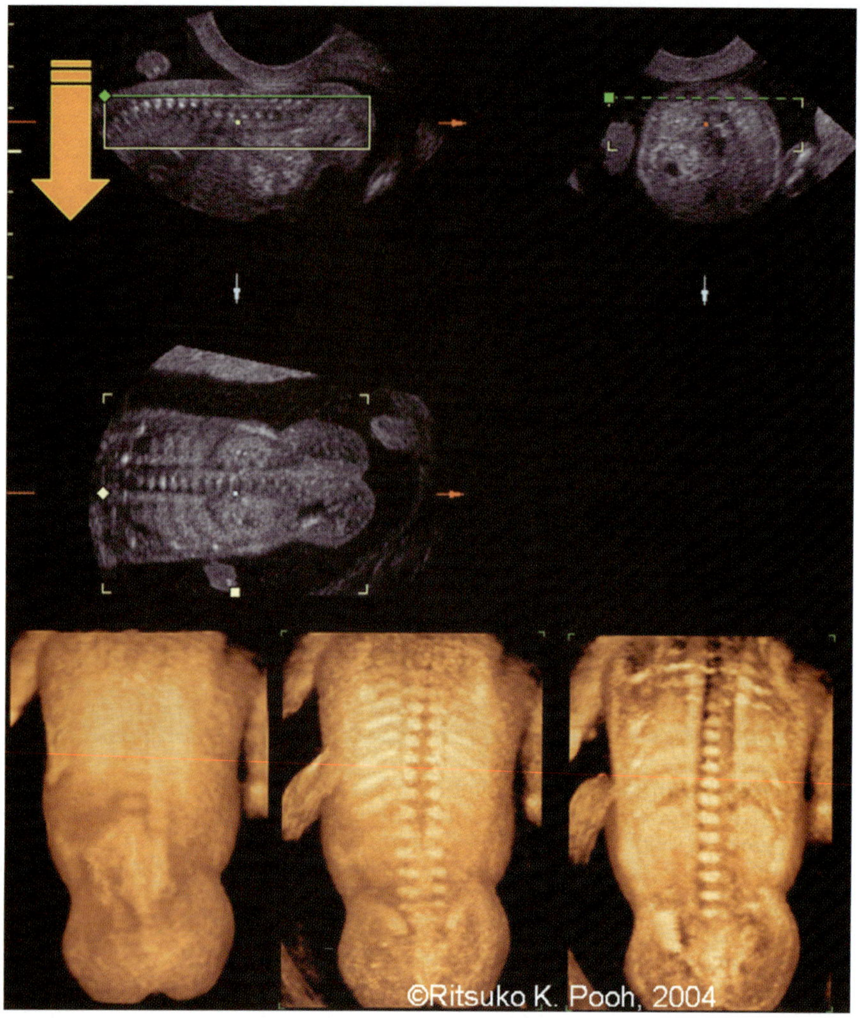

Figure 39.8 Three orthogonal views and 3D reconstructed image of normal fetus at 16 weeks of gestation. Movement of region of interest (arrow) provides 3D reconstruction image of the surface level (lower left), neural arch level (lower middle), and vertebral body level (lower right).

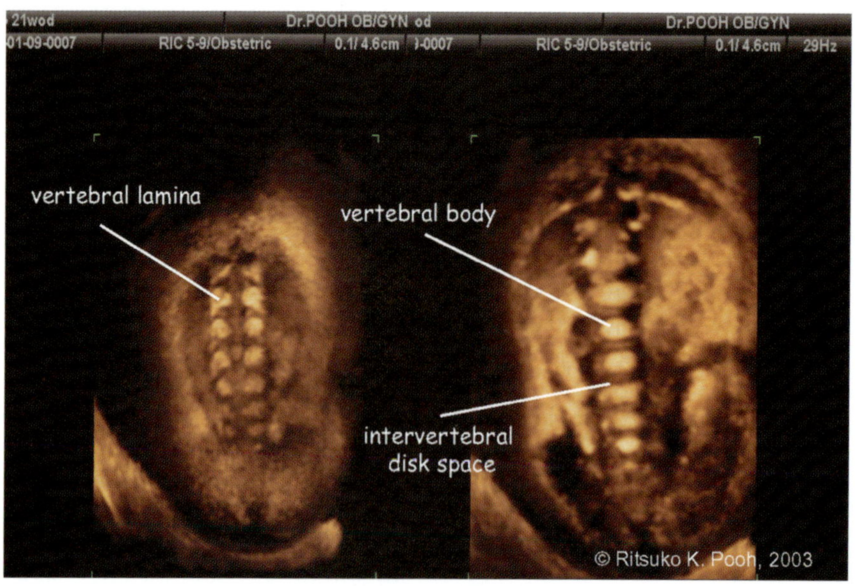

Figure 39.9 Fetal vertebral structure by 3D ultrasound at 21 weeks of gestation.

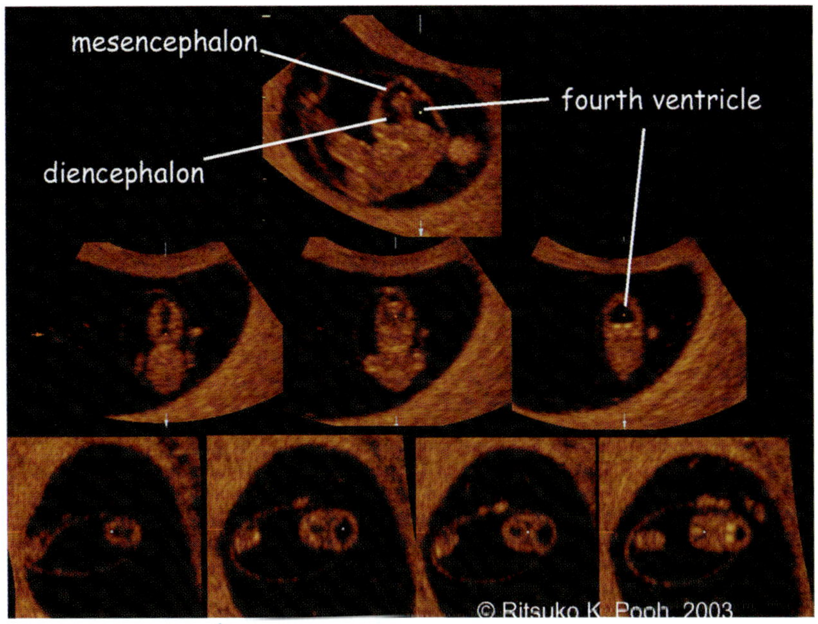

Figure 39.10 Normal intracranial structure at 8 weeks of gestation in parallel cutting slices of three orthogonal views. Sagittal, coronal, and axial sections from above. Premature sonolucent ventricular system is visible.

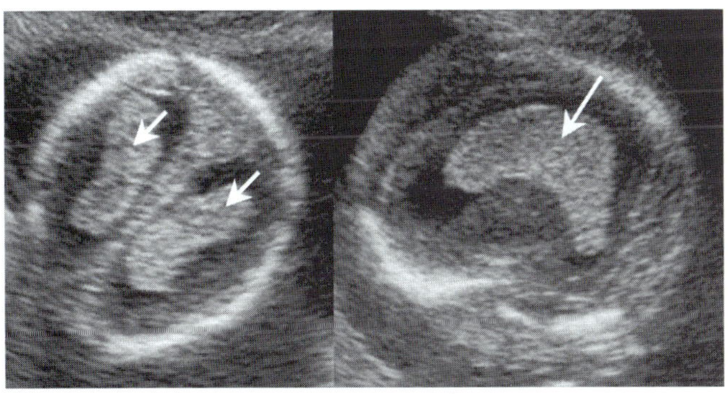

Figure 39.11 Normal intracranial structure at 14 weeks of gestation. Axial view (left) and parasagittal view (right). Choroid plexus (arrows) occupies most of the lateral ventricle.

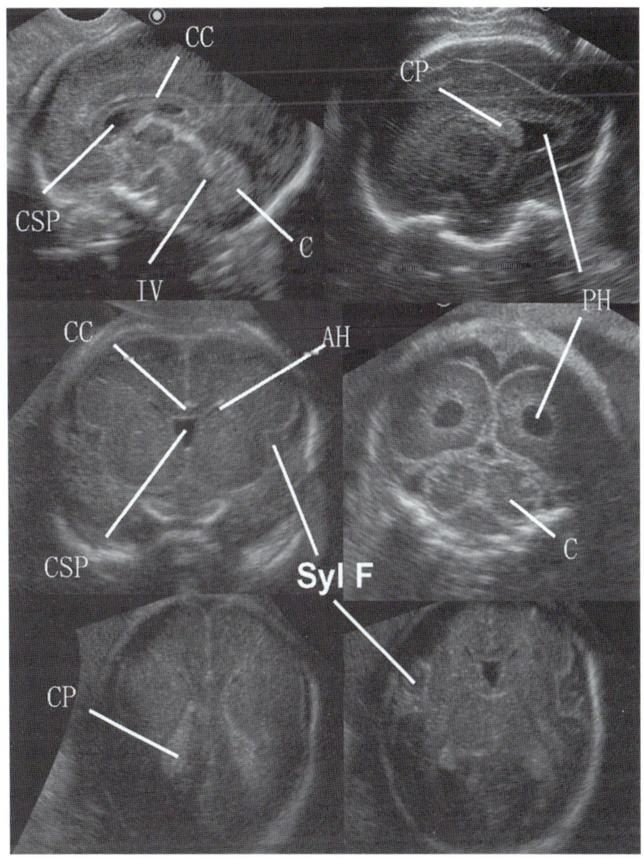

Figure 39.12 Normal views of fetal brain at 26 weeks of gestation. Sagittal (upper), coronal (middle) and axial (lower) sections. CC, corpus callosum; CSP, cavum septum pellucidum; C, cerebellum; IV; fourth ventricle; AH, anterior horn of the lateral ventricle; PH, posterior horn of the lateral ventricle; CP, choroid plexus; Syl F, sylvian fissure.

Hydrocephalus and ventriculomegaly *in utero*

Both 'hydrocephalus' and 'ventriculomegaly' are terms used to describe dilatation of the lateral ventricles. However, these two should be distinguished from each other. Hydrocephalus signifies dilated lateral ventricles resulted from increased amount of cerebrospinal fluid and intracranial pressure, while ventriculomegaly is a dilatation of lateral ventricles without increased intracranial pressure due to hypoplastic cerebrum or other intracerebral abnormalities such as agenesis of corpus callosum. Of course, ventriculomegaly can sometimes change into the hydrocephalic state. In sonographic imaging, those two

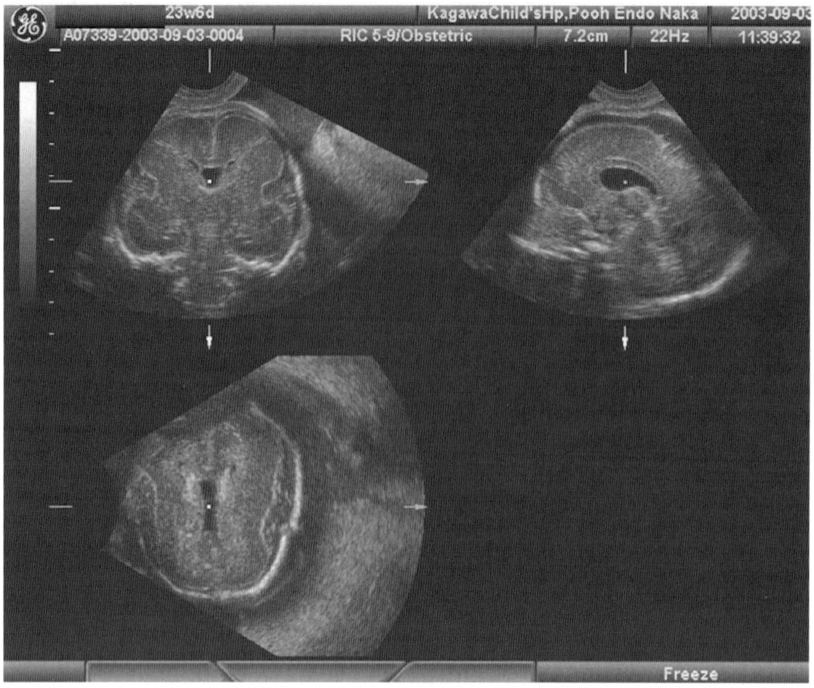

Figure 39.13 Three-dimensional multiplanar image analysis (normal brain at 23 weeks of gestation). Three orthogonal views are useful for obtaining orientation of the brain structure. Coronal (left upper), sagittal (right upper), and axial (left lower) images can be visualized on a single screen. Any rotation of the brain image around any (*x*,*y*,*z*) axis is possible.

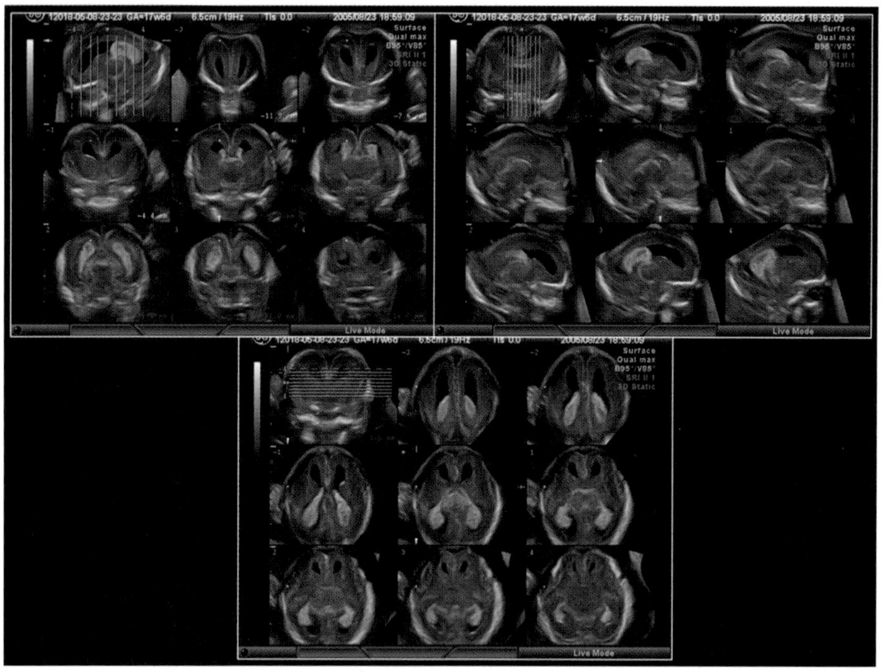

Figure 39.14 Normal intracranial structure at 19 weeks of gestation in parallel cutting slices of three orthogonal views. Sagittal, coronal, and axial sections from above.

intracranial conditions can be differentiated by visualization of subarachnoid space and appearance of choroids plexus. In normal condition, subarachnoid space, visualized around both cerebral hemispheres is preserved during pregnancy (Figure 39.18). Choroid plexus, which secretes CSF within the ventricles, is a soft tissue and easily affected by pressure. Obliterated subarachnoid space and dangling choroid plexus in the case of hydrocephalus (Figures 39.19 and 39.20). In contrast, the subarachnoid space and choroid plexus are well preserved in cases of ventriculomegaly (Figure 39.21). It is difficult to evaluate obliterated subarachnoid space in the trans-abdominal axial section and this method may not differentiate

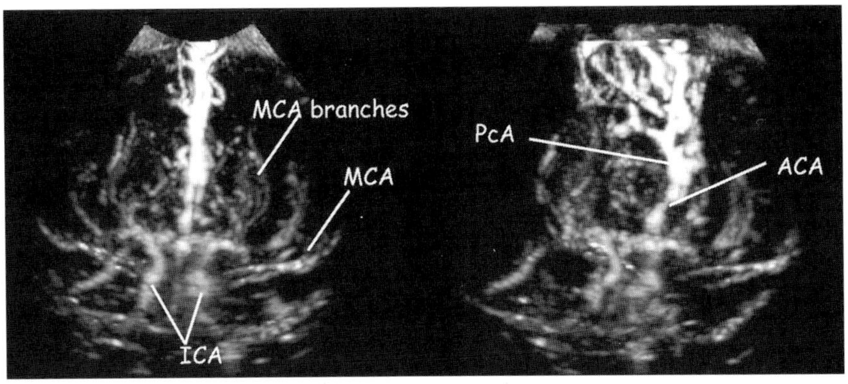

Figure 39.15 Three-dimensional power Doppler image of fetal brain circulation. (Left) View from the front. Bilateral internal carotid arteries (ICA) and middle cerebral arteries (MCA) and branches of MCA are demonstrated. (Right) Oblique view. Anterior cerebral artery (ACA) and pericallosal artery (PcA) are demonstrated.

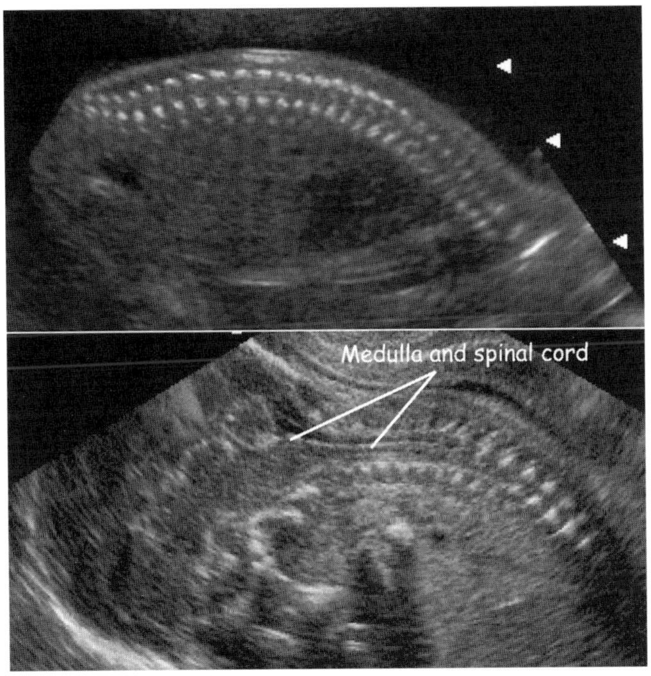

Figure 39.16 Normal vertebral structure in the sagittal section at 19 weeks of gestation. Lower figure shows the medulla and spinal cord in the craniospinal region.

accurately hydrocephalus with increased intracranial pressure from ventriculomegaly without pressure. Therefore, it is suggested that the evaluation of fetuses with enlarged ventricles should be performed in the parasagittal and coronal views by transvaginal way or 3D multidimensional analysis. In some cases with hydrocephalus, the septum pellucidum is destroyed and both ventricles are fused to each other (Figure 39.19). This condition should be differentiated from lober type of holoprosencephaly. Furthermore, intracranial venous blood flow may be related to increased intracranial pressure. In normal fetuses, blood flow waveforms of dural sinuses, such as superior sagittal sinus, vein of Galen, and straight sinus have pulsatile pattern (Figure 39.22).[26] However, in cases with progressive hydrocephalus, normal pulsation disappears and blood flow waveforms display a flat pattern (Figure 39.23).[26] In cases with progressive hydrocephalus, there may be seven stages of progression (Figure 39.24): (1) increased fluid collection of lateral ventricles; (2) increased intracranial pressure; (3) dangling choroids plexus; (4) disappearance of subarachnoid space; (5) excessive extension of the dura and superior sagittal sinus; (6) disappearance of venous pulsation; and finally (7) enlarged skull. In general, both hydrocephalus and ventriculomegaly are still evaluated by the measurement of biparietal diameter (BPD) and atrial width (AW) in transabdominal axial section. As a screening examination, the measurement of AW is useful with a cut-off value of 10 mm.[27,28] As described above, however, hydrocephalus and ventriculomegaly should be differentiated from each other and hydrocephalic state should be assessed by changing appearance of the intracranial structure. To evaluate enlarged ventricles, examiners should carefully observe the structures mentioned below and specify causes of hydrocephalus:

- choroids plexus, dangling or not
- subarachnoid space, obliterated or not
- ventricles, symmetry or asymmetry
- visibility of third ventricle
- pulsation of dural sinuses
- ventricular size (3D volume calculation if possible)
- other abnormalities.

Genetic hydrocephalus is rare but important in counseling couples on subsequent pregnancy. X-linked hydrocephalus (HSAS, hydrocephalus due to stenosis of the aqueduct of Sylvius), MASA (mental retardation-aphasia-shuffling gait-adducted thumbs) syndrome, X-linked complicated spastic paraparesis (SP1), and X-linked corpus callosum agenesis (ACC) are all due to mutations in the L1 gene.[29] The gene encoding L1 is located near the telomere of the long arm of the X chromosome in Xq28. Therefore, it was suggested to refer to this clinical syndrome with the

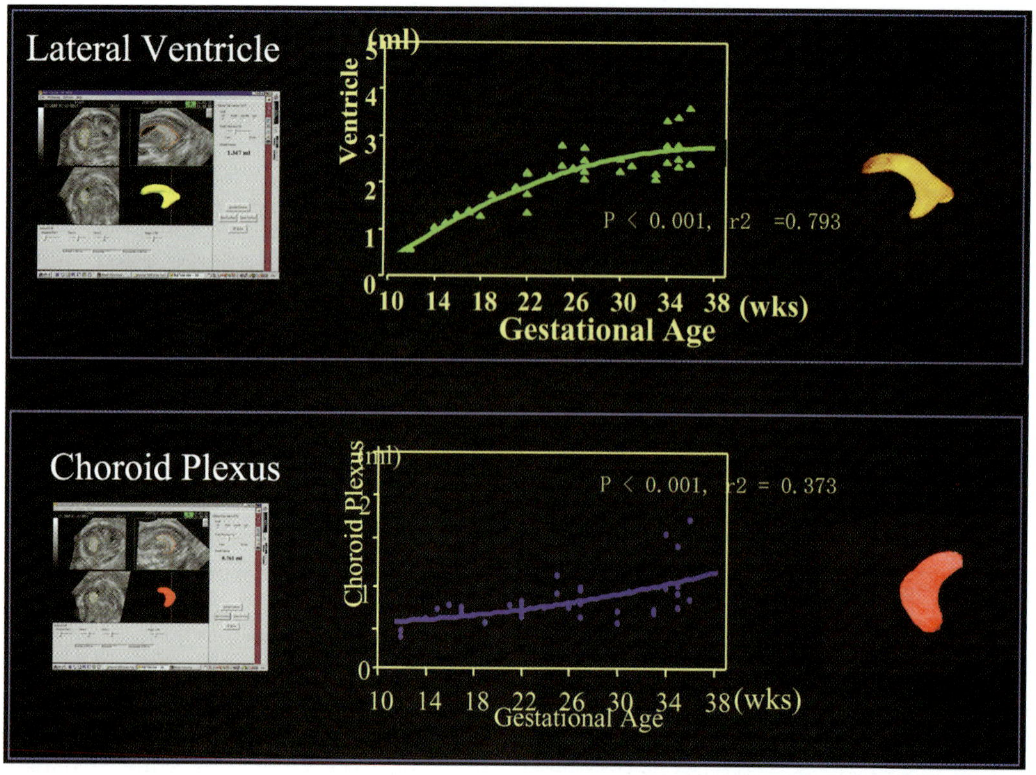

Figure 39.17 Three-dimensional volume extraction and volumetric analysis of lateral ventricle and choroid plexus. On three orthogonal sections, the target organ can be traced automatically or manually with rotation of volume imaging data. After tracing, volume extracted image (right) is demonstrated and volume calculation data is shown. Middle graphs show normograms of ventricular size (upper) and choroid plexus size (lower) during pregnancy.

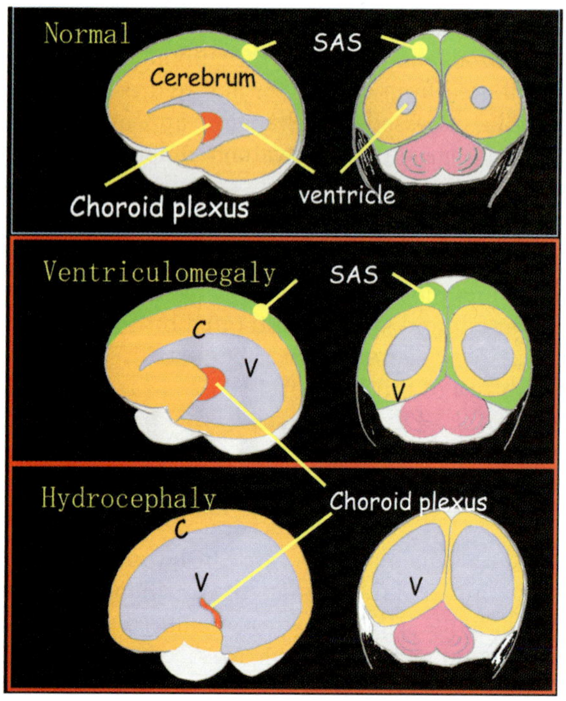

Figure 39.18 Schema of ventriculomegaly and hydrocephaly. In cases of ventriculomegaly without increased intracranial pressure, subarachnoid space (SAS) and choroid plexus appearances are well preserved, while in cases of hydrocephaly with increased intracranial pressure, dangling choroid plexus and gradual disappearance of SAS are seen.

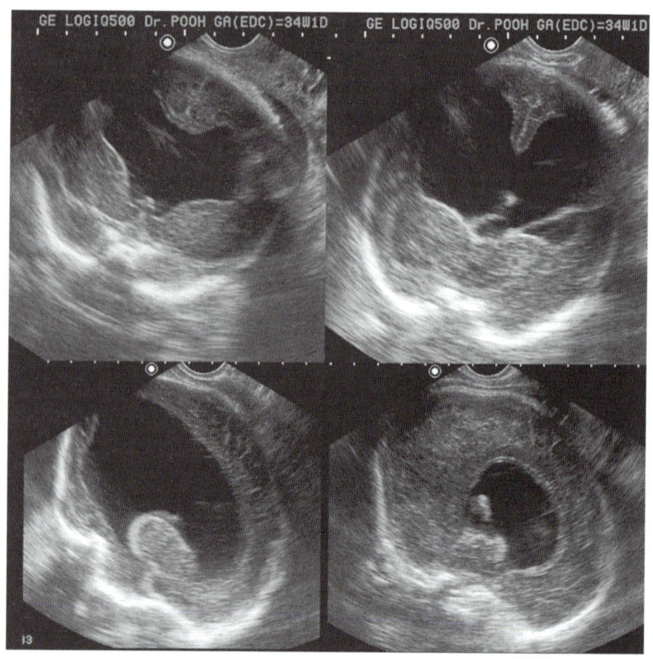

Figure 39.19 Ultrasound images of hydrocephalus at 34 weeks of gestation. (Upper) Coronal images. Septum pellucidum was destroyed maybe due to enlargement of bilateral ventricles and both ventricles were fused. Dangling choroid plexus is seen. (Lower) Parasagittal and sagittal images. Dangling choroid plexus and obliterated subarachnoid space are seen.

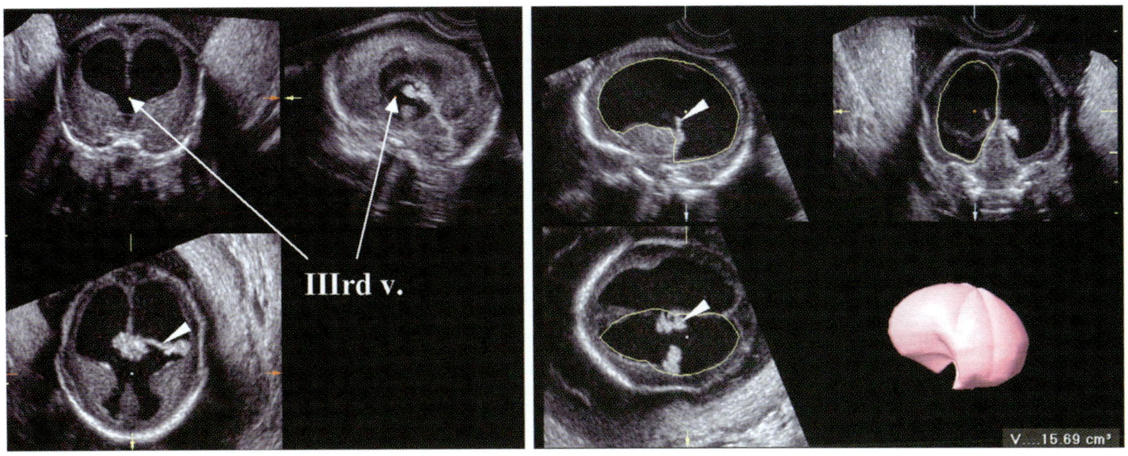

Figure 39.20 Hydrocephalus due to aqueductal obstruction at 19 weeks of gestation. (Left) Three orthogonal views with anterior coronal (upper left) and median sagittal (upper right) and axial (lower left) slices. Bilateral ventriculomegaly and third ventriculomegaly (IIIrd v.) are seen. No enlargement of fourth ventricle indicates obstruction of the aqueduct. (Right) Three orthogonal views with parasagittal (upper left), posterior coronal (upper right), and axial (lower left) slices. Subarachnoid space is already obliterated and dangling choroid plexus (arrowheads) is seen. Lower right pink figure shows extracted 3D ventricular image by VOCAL mode. Ventricle in this case was 10 fold size of normal 19-week-ventricle.

acronym CRASH, for corpus callosum hypoplasia, retardation, adducted thumbs, spastic paraplegia, and hydrocephalus.[29] It has been reported that mutations which produce truncations in the extracellular domain of the L1 protein are more likely to produce severe hydrocephalus, grave mental retardation or early death than point mutations in the extracellular domain or mutations affecting only the cytoplasmic domain of the protein.[30] For the families, prenatal CNS diagnosis of male infants is important. Morphology-based approach becomes feasible between postmenstrual weeks 15 and 20. Prior to this gestational age, the diagnosis should rely on molecular biology tests.[31]

Borderline ventriculomegaly is defined as a width of the atrium of the lateral cerebral ventricles of 10–15 mm. The majority with prenatally detected isolated mild ventriculomegaly are developmentally normal.[32] Pilu and his colleagues[33] reviewed 234 cases of borderline ventriculomegaly including an abnormal outcome in 22.8% and concluded that borderline ventriculomegaly carries an increased risk of cerebral maldevelopment, delayed neurological development, and possibly, chromosomal aberrations.

The treatment of hydrocephalus includes a miniature reserver,[34,35] shunt procedure, and neuroendoscopy. Ventriculoperitoneal shunt is the most popular procedure. Effectiveness of shunt procedure for congenital hydrocephalus has been proven from earlier. However, it has been known that there are various complications of shunting, such as shunt infection obstruction of the shunt tube, over drainage, under drainage, and slit ventricle syndrome. To reduce these complications, various types of shunt devices, such as antisiphon device or pressure programmable valve shunt device have been developed. Third ventriculostomy by neuroendoscopy has recently been performed in children with obstructive hydrocephalus, and the number of shunt-independent cases has been increased. It has been controversial, however, whether infants less than the age of 1 year have a higher risk of treatment failure after neuroendoscopic procedures than older children. Some conclude that neuroendoscopy presents an effective alternative for the treatment of hydrocephalus in cases under the age of 1 year.[36] However, third ventriculostomy still does not seem to be effective in neonates because of their prematurity of absorption ability in neonates and small infants.

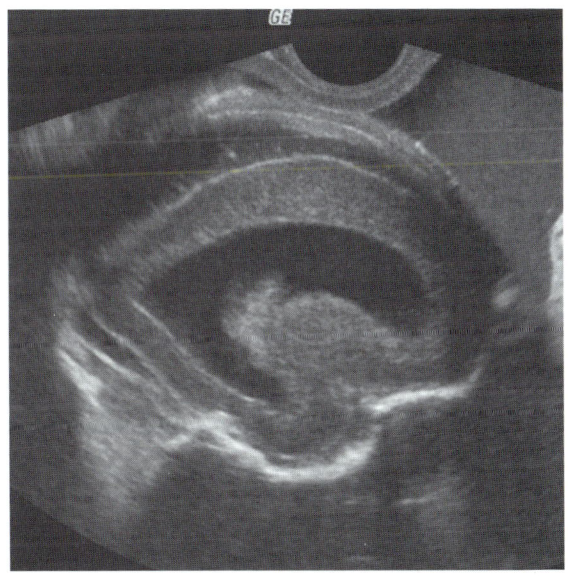

Figure 39.21 Ultrasound image of ventriculomegaly at 29 weeks of gestation. Enlarged ventricle exists but subarachnoid space is well preserved and no dangling choroid plexus is seen. From these findings, nonincreased intercranial pressure (ICP) is estimated. This condition should be differentiated from hydrocephalus with increased ICP.

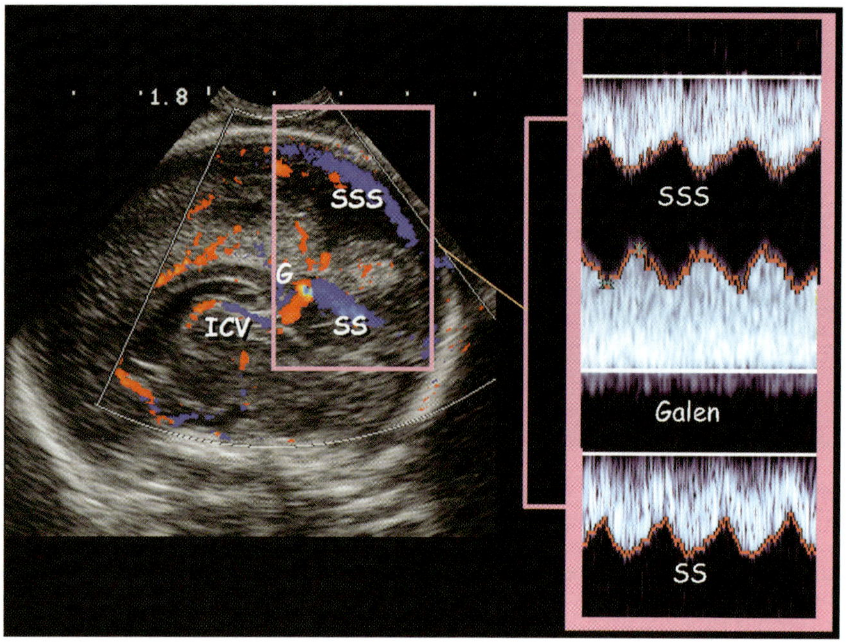

Figure 39.22 Normal cerebral venous circulation. (Left) Sagittal image of color Doppler. SSS, superior sagittal sinus; ICV, internal cerebral vein; G, vein of Galen; SS, straight sinus. (Right) Normal blood flow waveforms of dural sinuses. In normal fetuses, venous flow always has pulsations.

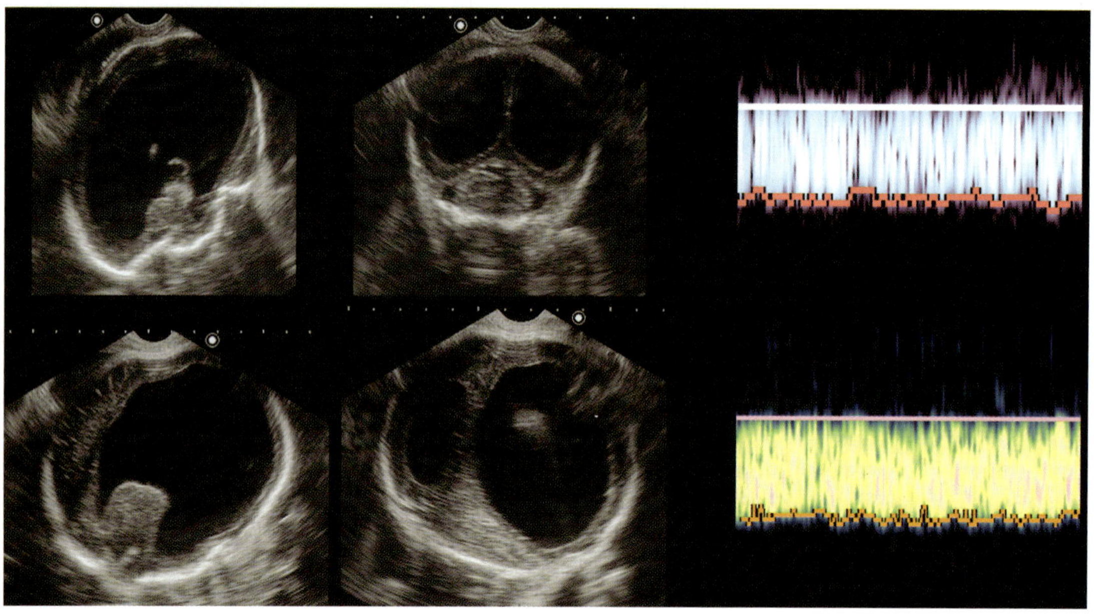

Figure 39.23 Disappearance of venous pulsation in cases with hydrocephalus. Normal dural sinuses have pulsatile patterns of flow waveform (Figure 39.22). In cases with progressive hydrocephalus, venous pulsation disappeared (right figures) maybe because of excessive extension of the dura and dural sinuses.

Congenital CNS anomalies

Cranium bifidum

Prevalence: Anencephaly; 0.29/1000 births,[37] overall neural tube defect (NTD); 0.58–1.17/1000 births.[38–40] Many reported remarkable reduction of prevalence of NTDs after using folic acid supplementation and fortification,[37–40] although some reported no decline of anencephaly rate.[41]

Definition: As in spina bifida, cranium bifidum is classified into four types of encephaloschisis (including anencephaly and exencephaly), meningocele, encephalomeningocele, encephalocystocele, and cranium bifidum occulutum. Encephalocele occurs in the occipital region in 70–80%. Acrania, exencephaly, and anencephaly are not independent anomalies. It is considered that dysraphia (absent cranial vault, acrania) occurs in very early stage and disintegration of the exposed brain (exencephaly) during the fetal period results in anencephaly.[42]

Etiology: Multifactorial inheritance, single mutant genes, specific teratogens (valproic acid), maternal

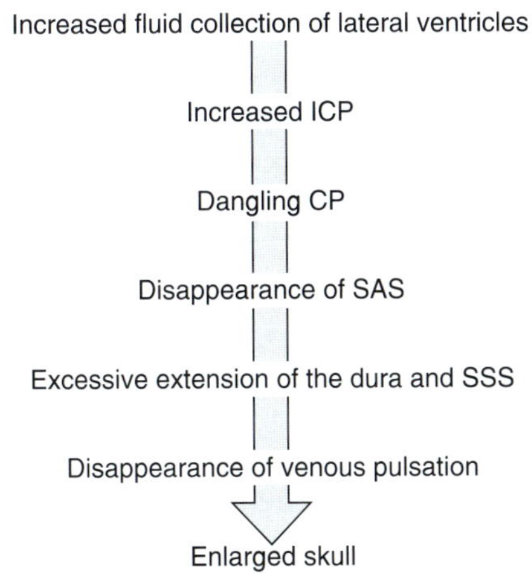

Figure 39.24 Progressive stages of hydrocephalus. ICP, intracranial pressure; CP, choroid plexus; SAS, subarachnoid space.

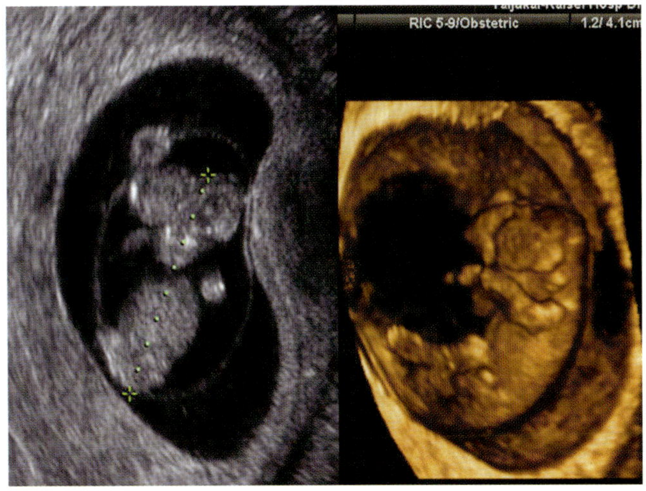

Figure 39.25 Acrania at 10 weeks of gestation. (Left) Ultrasound coronal image at 10 weeks. Note the normal appearance of amniotic membrane, which indicates that this condition is not amniotic band syndrome. (Right) Three-dimensional ultrasound image of the same fetus as in the left image.

diabetes, environmental factors, predominant in females.

Pathogenesis: Failure of anterior neural tube closure or a restricted disorder of neurulation.

Associated anomalies: Open spina bifida (iniencephaly), Chiari type III malformation, bilateral renal cystic dysplasia, and postaxial polydactyly with occipital cephalocele (Meckel–Gruber syndrome), hydrocephalus, polyhydramnios.

Prenatal diagnosis: Acrania in Figure 39.25, anencephaly in Figure 39.26, and early detection of iniencephaly in Figure 39.27.

Differential diagnosis: Amniotic band syndrome (ABS). In cases of ABS, cranial destruction occurs secondarily to an amniotic band, similar appearance is observed. However, ABS has completely different pathogenesis from acrania/excencephaly.

Prognosis: Anencephaly is a uniformly lethal anomaly. Other types of cranium bifidum, various neurological deficits may occur, depending on types and degrees.

Recurrence risk: Used to be high recurrence risk of 5–13%; however, the risk has recently declined by use of folic acid supplementation and fortification.

Obstetrical management: Termination of pregnancy can be offered in cases with anencephaly.

Neurosurgical management: For other cranium bifidum, surgical operation aims at transposition of cerebral tissue into the intracranial cavity. Ventriculoperitoneal shunt for hydrocephalus.

Spina bifida

Prevalence: 0.22/1000 births,[37] overall NTD; 0.58–1.17/1000 births.[38–40] Many reported remarkable reduction of prevalence of NTDs after using folic acid supplementation and fortification.[37–41]

Definition: Spina bifida aperta, manifest form of spina bifida is classified into four types: meningocele, myelomeningocele, myelocystocele, and myeloschisis. Spina bifida occuluta is a generic term of spinal diseases covered with normal skin tissue, and does not indicate spinal diseases which cannot be diagnosed by external appearance. Cutaneous abnormalities near the spinal lesion are found; skin bulge (subcutaneous lipoma), dimple, hair tuft, pigmentation, skin appendage and hemangioma. In cases with thickened film terminale, dermal sinus, or diastematomyelia (split cord malformation), abnormal tethering and fixation of the spinal cord occur.

Etiology: Multifactorial inheritance, single mutant genes, autosomal recessive, chromosomal abnormalities (trisomy 18, 13), specific teratogens (valproic acid), maternal diabetes, environmental factors, predominant in females.

Pathogenesis: Spina bifida aperta: an impairment of neural tube closure. Spina bifida occuluta: caudal neural tube malformation by the processes of canalization and retrogressive differentiation.

Associated anomalies: Chiari type II malformation, hydrocephalus, scoliosis (above L2), polyhydramnios, additional non-CNS anomalies.

Prenatal diagnosis: Figures 39.28–39.31.

Differential diagnosis: Sacrococcygeal teratoma.

Prognosis: Disturbance of motor, sensory, and sphincter function. Depends on lesion levels. Below S1, unable to walk unaided; above L2, wheelchair dependent; variable at intermediate level.

Recurrence risk: Decreased, almost no recurrence rate[43] by use of folic acid supplementation and fortification.

Obstetrical management: In cases with spina bifida aperta, especially with defect of skin, cesarean section is preferable to protect the spinal cord and nerves and prevent infection.

Neurosurgical management: Spina bifida aperta: in cases with defect of normal skin tissue, immediate closure of spina bifida after birth reduces spinal infection. Spinal cord reconstruction is the most important

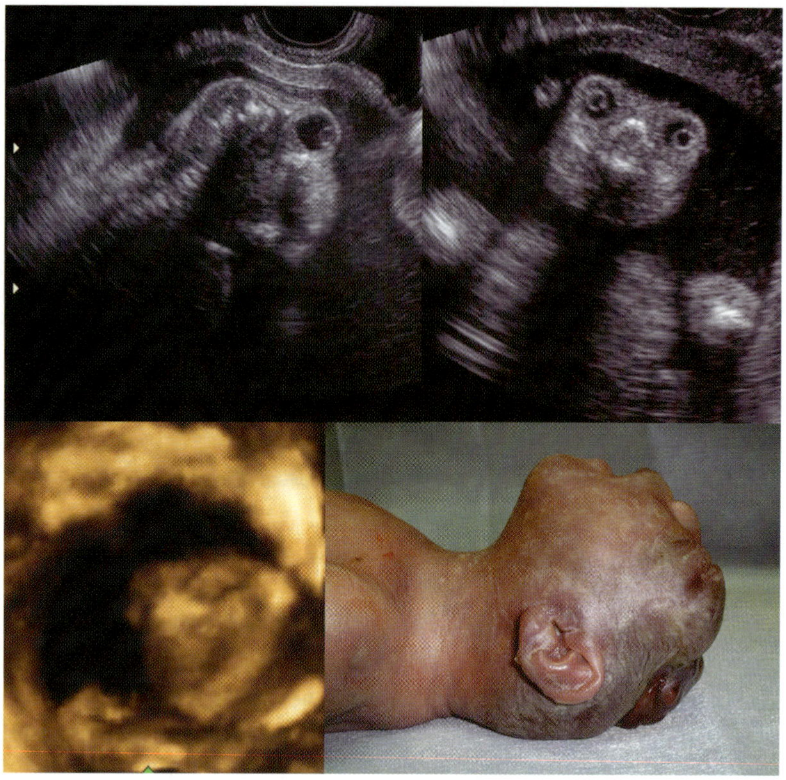

Figure 39.26 Anencephaly in middle gestation. (same case as in Figure 39.25). (Upper left) Ultrasound sagittal image at 23 weeks of gestation. (Upper right) Ultrasound coronal image. (Lower left) Three-dimensional ultrasound image. (Lower right) External appearances of stillborn fetus at 25 weeks of gestation. It is clear that excencephalic brain tissue scattered in the amniotic space compared with this case at 10 weeks.

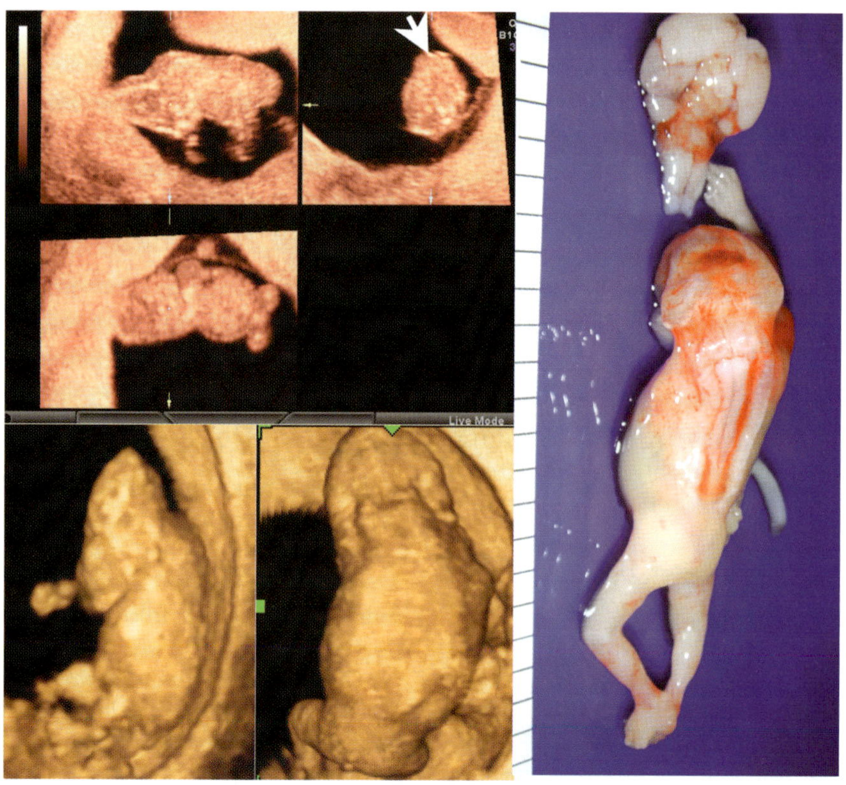

Figure 39.27 3D detection of a fetus with iniencephaly and acrania at 10 weeks of gestation. (Upper left) Three orthogonal views of the fetus. Spina bifida (arrow) was demonstrated in the coronal section. (Lower left) Three-dimensional images show the fetal lateral and dorsal views. (Right) External appearance of aborted fetus at the end of 11 weeks of gestation. The brain and a part of spinal cord were detached at delivery.

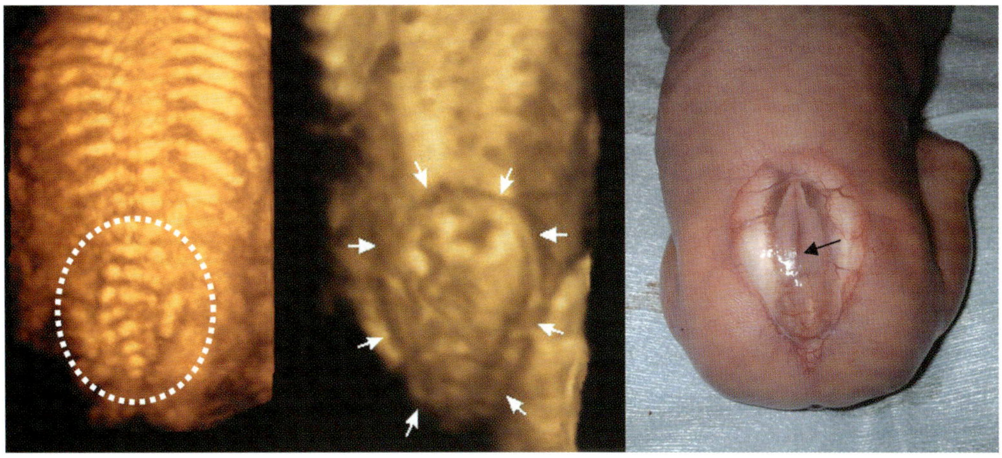

Figure 39.28 Prenatal ultrasound image of myelomeningocele, spina bifida at 20 weeks of gestation. (Left) Three-dimensional bony demonstration of lumber spina bifida. Three-dimensional ultrasound shows the exact level of spina bifida. (Middle) Three-dimensional surface reconstruction of large myelomeningocele (white arrows). (Right) External appearance of aborted fetus at 21 weeks of gestation. Note the central canal of the spinal cord (black arrow) in large myelomeningocele.

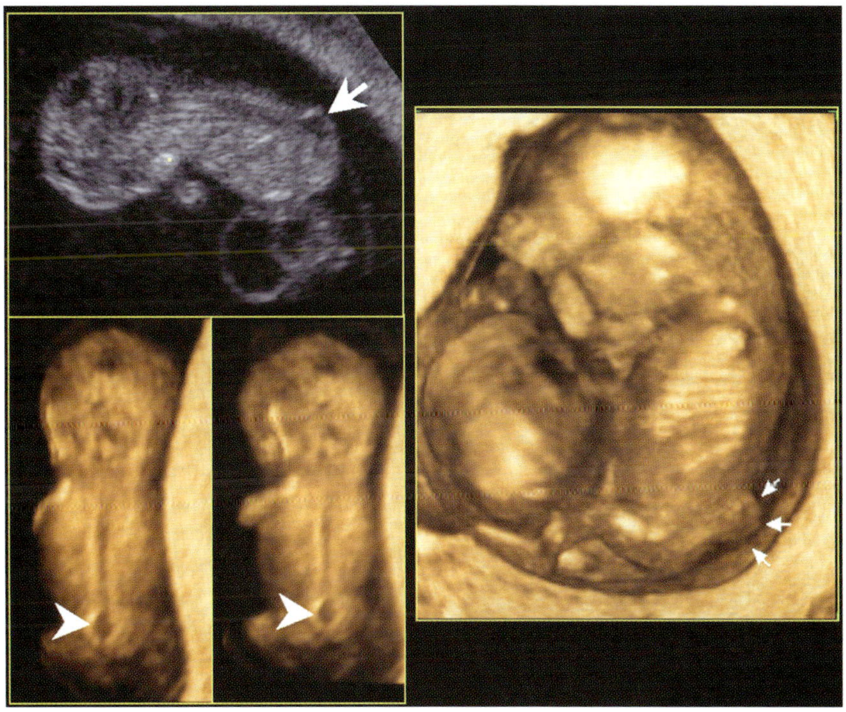

Figure 39.29 Myelomeningocele in early pregnancy. Two-dimensional sagittal view at 9 weeks of gestation (upper left) shows the cystic lesion (arrow). Three-dimensional dorsal views at 9 weeks (lower left) clearly demonstrate a neural tube defect at the lower lumber and sacral level (arrowheads). Right figure shows the same fetus at 12 weeks of gestation. Arrows indicate the lumbosacral myelomeningocele.

role of operation. Miniature Ommaya reservoir placement and subsequent ventriculoperitoneal shunt are required for hydrocephalus (see Chapter 5). For symptomatic Chiari malformation, posterior fossa decompressive craniectomy and/or tonsillectomy is performed. Spina bifida occuluta: the aim of surgical treatment is decompression of the spinal cord and cutting off tethering to the spinal cord (Figures 39.32 and 39.33).

Chiari malformation

Prevalence: Depends on prevalence of spina bifida (Chiari type II malformation). According to recent remarkable reduction of prevalence of NTDs after using folic acid supplementation and fortification, prevalence has declined. Other types are rare.

Definition: Chiari classified anomalies with cerebellar herniation in the spinal canal into three types by contents of herniated tissue: contents of type I is a

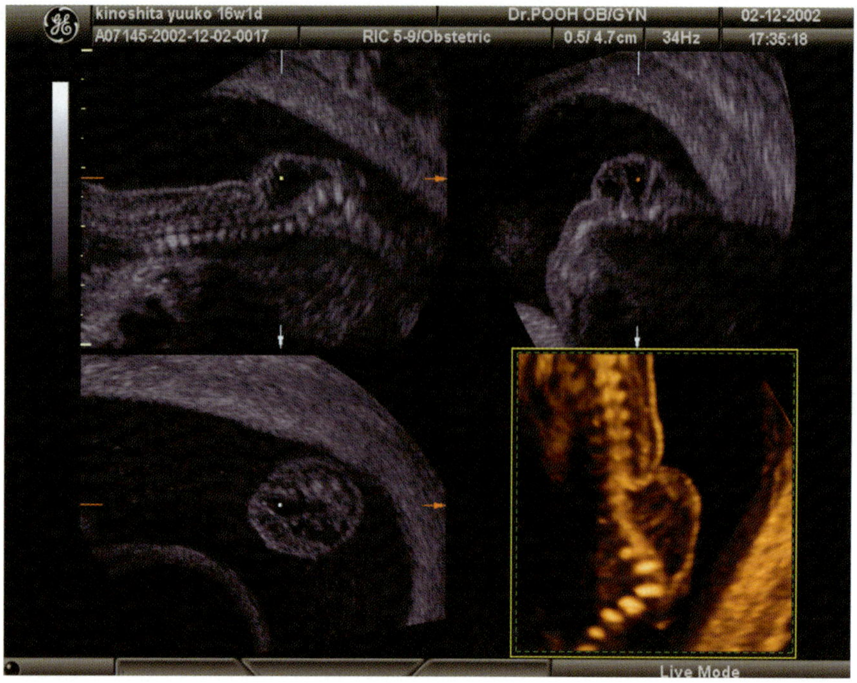

Figure 39.30 Three-dimensional ultrasound image of myelomeningocele with kyphosis at 16 weeks of gestation. Three orthogonal views and surface reconstruction image. (Upper left) Sagittal ultrasound image. Spinal cord completely protrudes into the sac surface from spinal canal and severe kyphosis is seen (upper right). Axial ultrasound view. (Lower left) Coronal ultrasound view of myelomeningocele. Lower right figure demonstrates the sagittal vertebral bony structure by 3D thick slice.

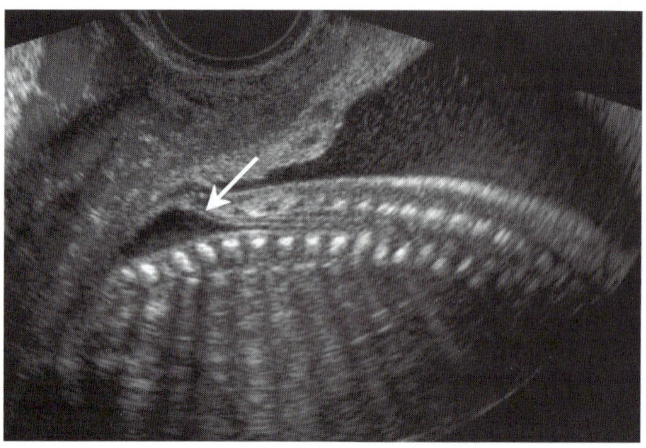

Figure 39.31 Two-dimensional sagittal section of myelomeningocele at 19 weeks of gestation. The spinal cord (arrow) protrudes from spinal canal toward the sac surface of myelomeningocele.

lip of cerebellum, type II part of cerebellum, fourth ventricle and medulla oblongata, pons, and type III large herniation of the posterior fossa. Thereafter, type IV with just cerebellar hypogenesis was added. However, this classification occasionally leads to confusion in neuroimaging diagnosis. Therefore, at present, the classification as given below is advocated:

Type I: Herniation of only cerebellar tonsil, not associated with myelomeningocele.

Type II: Herniation of cerebellar tonsil and brain stem. Medullary kink, tentorial dysplasia, associated with myelomeningocele.

Type III: Associated with cephalocele or craniocervical meningocele, in which cerebellum and brainstem are herniated.

Type IV: Associated with marked cerebellar hypogenesis and posterior fossa shrinking.

Synonyms: Arnold–Chiari malformation.

Etiology: Depends on the types.

Pathogenesis: Schematic picture and macroscopic findings, MRI images are in Figures 39.32 and 39.33. Chiari malformation occurs according to: (1) inferior displacement of the medulla and the fourth ventricle into the upper cervical canal; (2) elongation and thinning of the upper medulla and lower pons and persistence of the embryonic flexure of these structures; (3) inferior displacement of the lower cerebellum through the foramen magnum into the upper cervical region; and (4) a variety of bony defects of the foramen magnum, occiput, and upper cervical vertebrae.[44]

Associated anomalies: Hydrocephalus caused by obstruction of fourth ventricular outflow or associated aqueductal stenosis. Myelomeningocele or myeloschisis (type II), cephalocele or craniocervical meningocele (type III), cerebellar hypogenesis (type IV), and syringomyelia (type I).

Prenatal diagnosis: Prenatal ultrasound diagnosis by features; lemon sign which indicates deformity of the frontal bone, banana sign which indicates abnormal shape of cerebellum without cisterna magna space (Figure 39.34), medullary, kink small clivus-supraocciput angle.[45] Figure 39.35 shows the sagittal ultrasound imaging of Chiari type II malformation compared to normal structure.

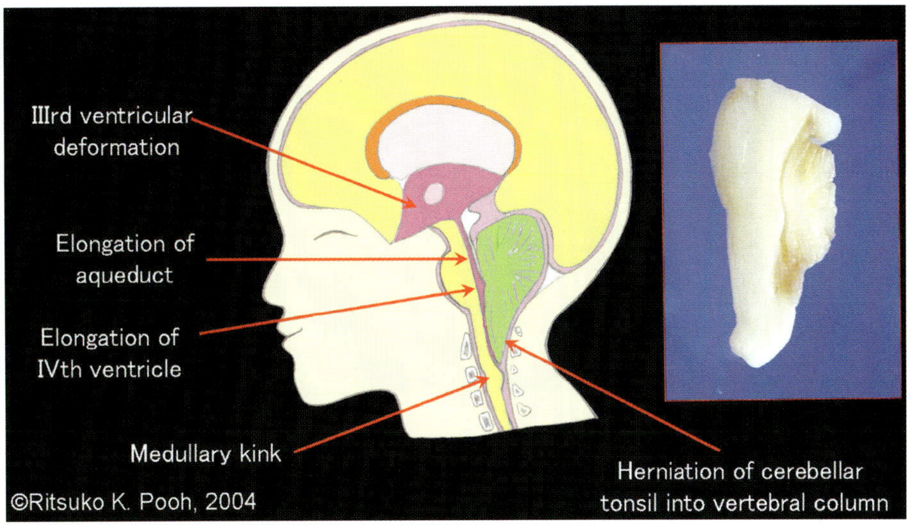

Figure 39.32 Schema and macroscopic finding of Chiari type II malformation. Chiari type II malformation is characterized by inferior displacement of the lower cerebellum through the foramen magnum with obliteration of the cisterna magna, inferior displacement of the medulla into the spinal canal, and elongation of the fourth ventricle and aqueduct. Right picture shows the macroscopic view of the elongated aqueduct, fourth ventricle, and cerebellum from the specimen of an aborted fetus at 21 weeks of gestation.

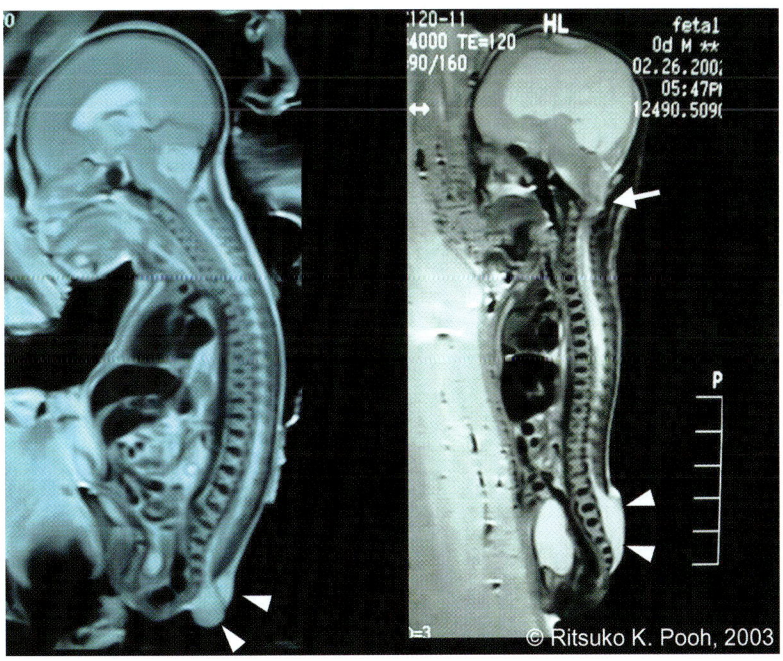

Figure 39.33 Magnetic resonance (MR) images of aborted fetuses at 20–21 weeks of gestation. (Left) At 20 weeks of gestation. Sacral myelomeningocele (arrowhead) and Chiari type II malformation are demonstrated. (Right) At 21 weeks of gestation. Lumbosacral myelomeningocele with Chiari type II malformation is seen. In this case, myelomeningocele is complicated with holoprosencephaly. Normal karyotype. Severe medullary kink (arrow) is seen.

Differential diagnosis: Craniosynostosis.

Prognosis: Nearly every case of myelomeningocele is accompanied by morphological Chiari II malformation. Many cases with Chiari II are asymptomatic. However, clinical features due to Chiari malformation, such as feeding disturbances, laryngeal stridor, or apneic episode, are found in approximately 9–30% of cases. In cases with these clinical features, vital prognosis is often poor.

Recurrence risk: Depends on types of Chiari malformation. Decreased according to decline of NTD recurrence rate by use of folic acid supplementation and fortification.

Neurosurgical management: Neurosurgical decompression of foramen magnum (FMD) for any type of Chiari malformation. Syringo-subarachnoid shunt for Chiari type I.

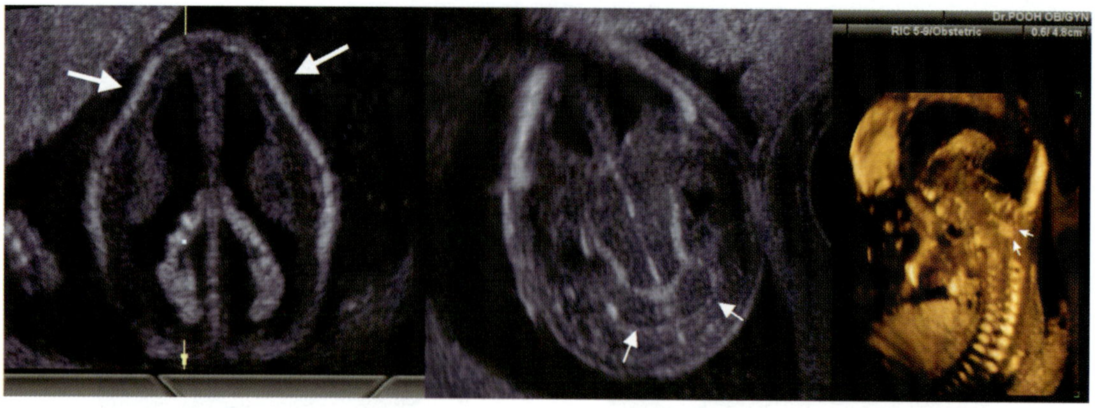

Figure 39.34 Chiari type II malformation at 16 weeks of gestation. Chiari type II malformation is observed in most cases with myelomeningocele and myeloschisis. (Left) Typical lemon sign (arrows). (Middle) Typical banana sign (arrows). (Right) Three-dimensional reconstruction internal image of Chiari type II malformation (arrows).

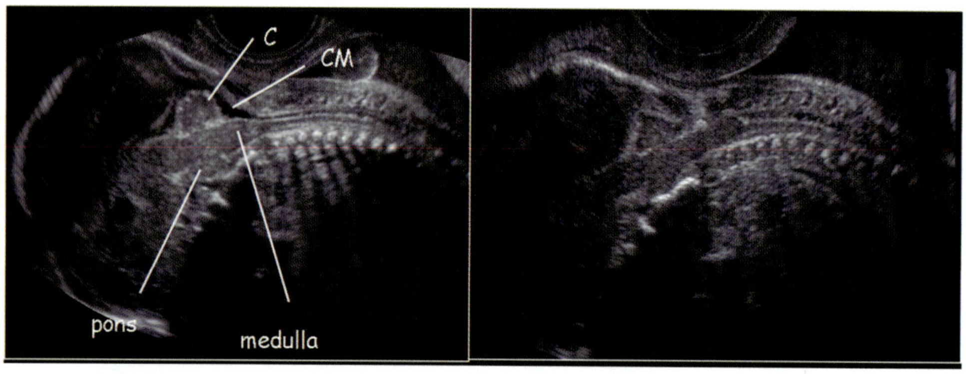

Figure 39.35 Medullary kink in a case of Chiari II malformation at 19 weeks of gestation. (Left) Medullary kink (arrowhead) associated obliterated cisterna magna is demonstrated. (Right) Comparative normal image in the same cutting section at the same gestation. The cisterna magna, cerebellum, and medullospinal portions are clearly demonstrated.

Holoprosencephaly

Incidence: 1 in 15,000–20,000 live births, however, initial incidence may be more than 60-fold in aborted human embryos.[45,46]

Classification:[44] Holoprosencephalies are classified into three varieties:

- Alobar type: a single-sphered cerebral structure with a single common ventricle, posterior large cyst of third ventricle (dorsal sac), absence of olfactory bulbs and tracts and a single optic nerve.
- Semilobar type: with formation of a posterior portion of the interhemispheric fissure.
- Lobar type: with formation of the interhemispheric fissure anteriorly and posterorly, but not in the midhemispheric region. The fusion of the fornices is seen.[47]

Etiology: 75% of holoprosencephaly has normal karyotype, but chromosomes 2, 3, 7, 13, 18, and 21 have been implicated in holoprosencephaly.[44] Particularly, trisomy 13 has most commonly been observed. Autosomal dominant transmission is rare.

Pathogenesis: Failure of cleavage of the prosencephalon and diencephalon during early first trimester (5–6 weeks) results in holoprosencephaly.

Associated anomalies: Facial abnormalities such as cyclopia, ethmocephaly, cebocephaly, flat nose, cleft lip and palate are invariably associated with horoprosencephaly. Extracerebral abnormalities are also invariably associated, such as renal cysts/dysplasia, omphalocele, cardiac disease and/or myelomeningocele.

Prenatal diagnosis: Alobar type in Figure 39.36 and semilobar type in Figure 39.37. Figure 39.38 shows facial appearance in cases of holoprosencephaly.

Differential diagnosis: Hydrocephalus, hydranencephaly.

Prognosis: Extremely poor in alobar holoprosencephaly. Uncertain in lobar type. Various but poor in semilobar type.

Recurrence risk: 6%,[48] but much lower in sporadic or trisomy cases, much higher in genetic cases.

Management: Chromosomal evaluation is offered.

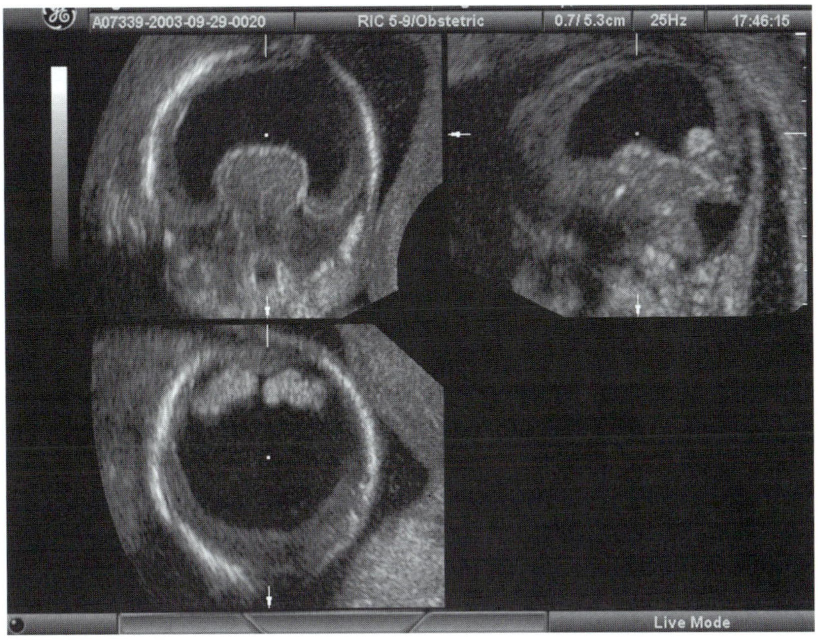

Figure 39.36 Alobar holoprosencephaly at 15 weeks of gestation. Three orthogonal images of intracranial structure show a complete single ventricle within a single-sphered cerebral structure.

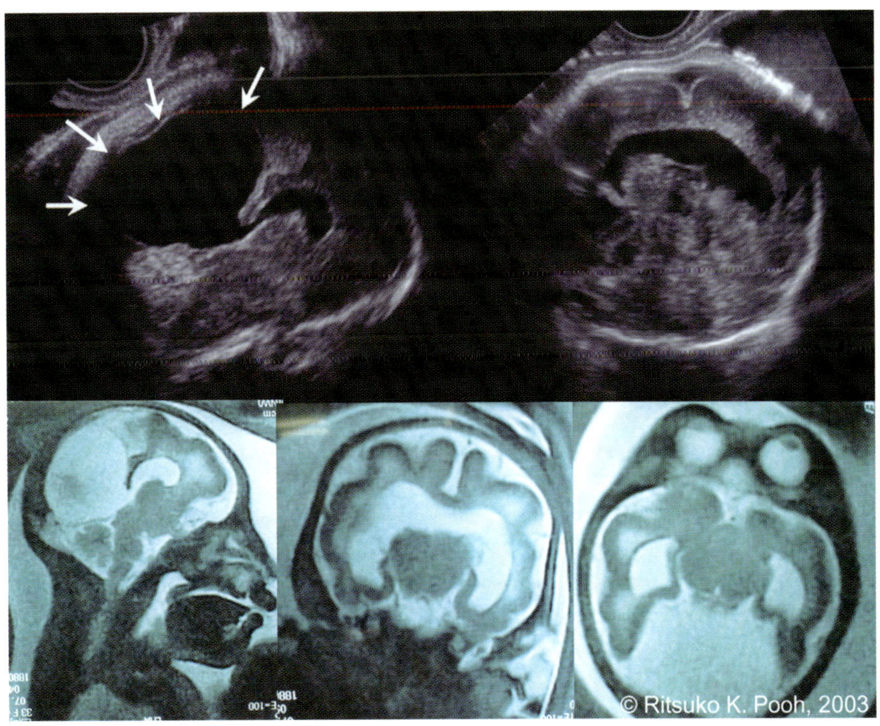

Figure 39.37 Semilobar holoprosencephaly at 33 weeks of gestation. Upper left shows dorsal sac (arrows) in the median section. Upper right demonstrates the fused ventricle. Lower figures are fetal MR images. Sagittal (left), coronal(middle), and axial (right) sections. A blind end of nasal cavity and hypotelorism are seen in the sagittal and axial MR images, respectively.

Agenesis of the corpus callosum

Prevalence: Uncertain, but 3–7/1000 in the general population is estimated.

Definition: Absence of the corpus callosum, which may be divided into (complete) agenesis, partial agenesis, or hypogenesis of the corpus callosum (Figure 39.39).

Complete agenesis: complete absence of the corpus callosum.

Partial agenesis (hypogenesis): absence of splenium or posterior portion in various degrees.

Etiology: Chromosomal aberration in 20% of affected cases, such as trisomy 18, 8, and 13. Autosomal dominant, autosomal recessive, X-linked recessive, part of

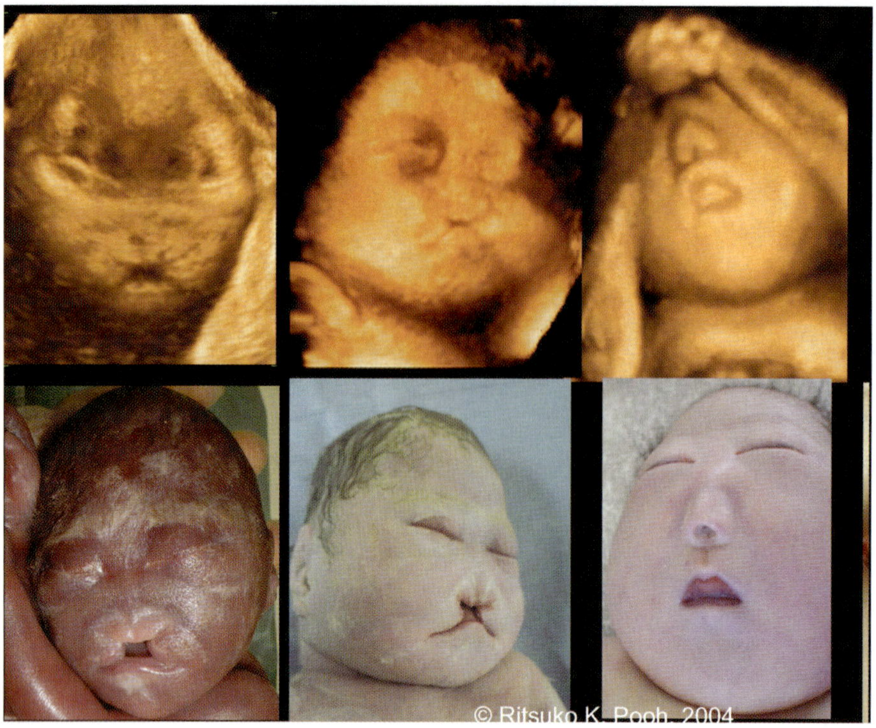

Figure 39.38 Facial abnormality in cases of holoprosencephaly. Upper figures are prenatal 3D facial images and lower figures show postpartum face appearance of each baby. (Left) Alobar holoprosencephaly at 20 weeks. (Middle and right) Semilobar type in late pregnancy. Hypotelorism and exophthalmos are common. Left and middle cases had cleft lip and palate and obstruction of the nasal cavity. Right case had a single and obstructed nasal cavity.

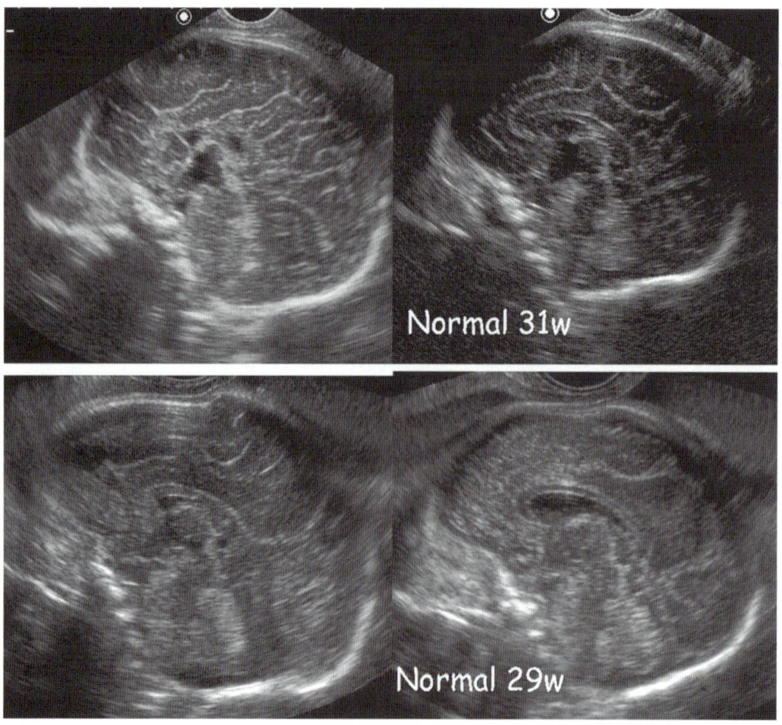

Figure 39.39 Complete agenesis (upper) and hypogenesis (lower) of the corpus callosum. All images are transvaginal median (mid-sagittal) images. Right images are normal images of the corpus callosum at the same gestational age as each left image.

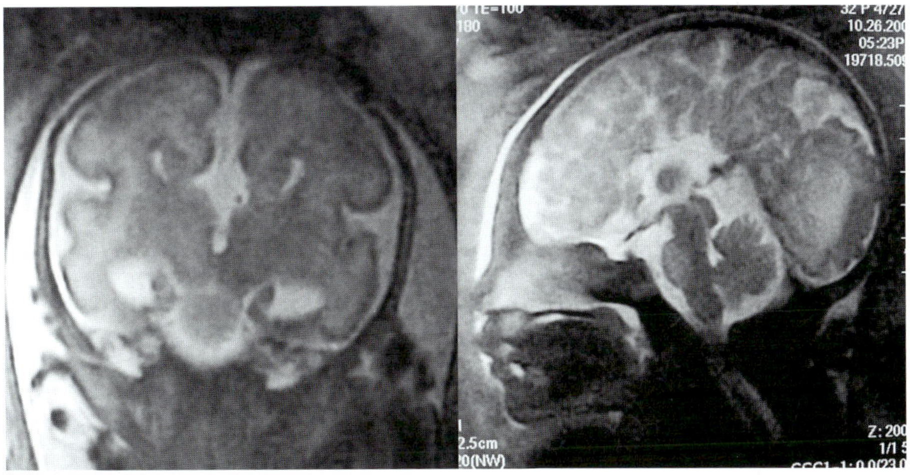

Figure 39.40 Fetal MR images of complete agenesis of the corpus callosum at 33 weeks of gestation. Anterior coronal section (left) and median section (right). No communicated bridge is seen. Note the bull's horn like appearance of the anterior horns of lateral ventricle in the coronal image.

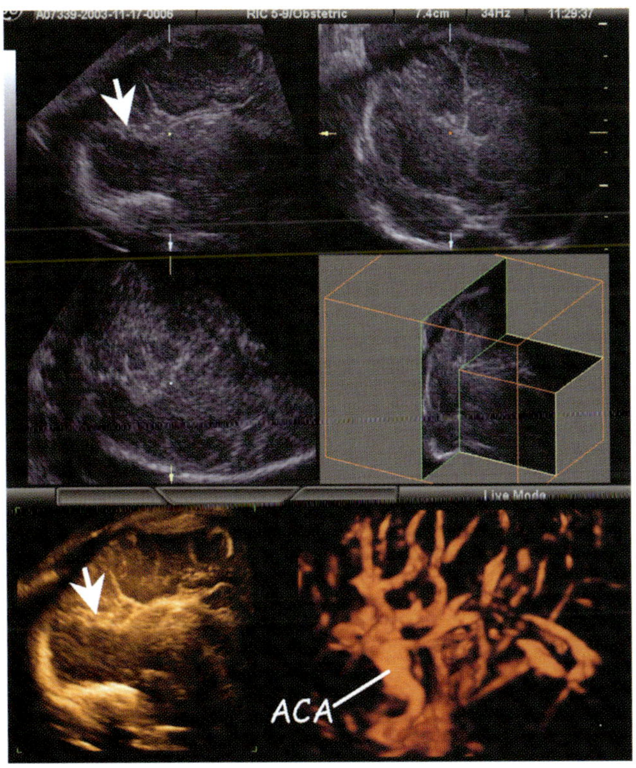

Figure 39.41 Agenesis of the corpus callosum with abnormal gyration at 36 weeks of gestation. Upper figure shows the three orthogonal view of the brain with agenesis of the corpus callosum with an abnormal gyrus (arrow). Lower left figure is a thick slice of the sagittal section. Abnormal gyration (arrow) is more clearly demonstrated. Lower right shows the intracranial angiostructure by 3D power Doppler. Normal pericallosal artery does not exist and radial formation of the branches of anterior cerebral arteries (ACA) is seen.

mendelian syndrome such as Walker–Warburg syndrome, and X-linked dominant such as Aicardi syndrome.

Pathogenesis: Uncertain, but callosal formation may be associated with migration disorder.

Associated anomalies: Colpocephaly (ventriculomegaly with disproportionate enlargement of trigones, occital horns, and temporal horns, not hydrocephaly), superior elongation of the third ventricle, interhemnispheric cyst, lipoma of the corpus callosum.

Prenatal diagnosis: Fetal MRI in Figure 39.40 and median sonographic images in Figure 39.41. Colpocephaly is shown in Figure 39.42.

Diagnosis: As the corpus callosum is depicted after 17 or 18 weeks of gestation by ultrasound, it is impossible to diagnose agenesis of the corpus callosum prior to this age.[49]

Prognosis: Various, depends on associated anomalies. Most cases with isolated agenesis of the corpus callosum without other abnormalities are asymptomatic and prognosis is good. Complete agenesis has a worse prognosis than partial agenesis.[50] Epilepsy, intellectual impairment, or psychiatric disorder[51] may occur later on.

Recurrence risk: Depends on etiology. Chromosomal, 1%; autosomal recessive, 25%; X-linked recessive male, 50%.

Management: Standard obstetrical care. Chromosomal evaluation is offered. In cases with interhemispheric cyst, postnatal fenestration or shunt procedure may be performed.

Absent septum pellucidum: septo-optic dysplasia

Incidence: Unknown, rare.

Definition: Absent septum pellucidum: absence of the septum pellucidum with or without associated anomalies. The septum pellucidum can be destroyed by concomitant hydrocephalus or by contiguous ischemic lesions such as porencephaly. An isolated absent septum pellucidum[52] exists but is rare. Septo-optic dysplasia: absence of the septum pellucidum and unilateral or bilateral hypoplasia of the optic nerve.

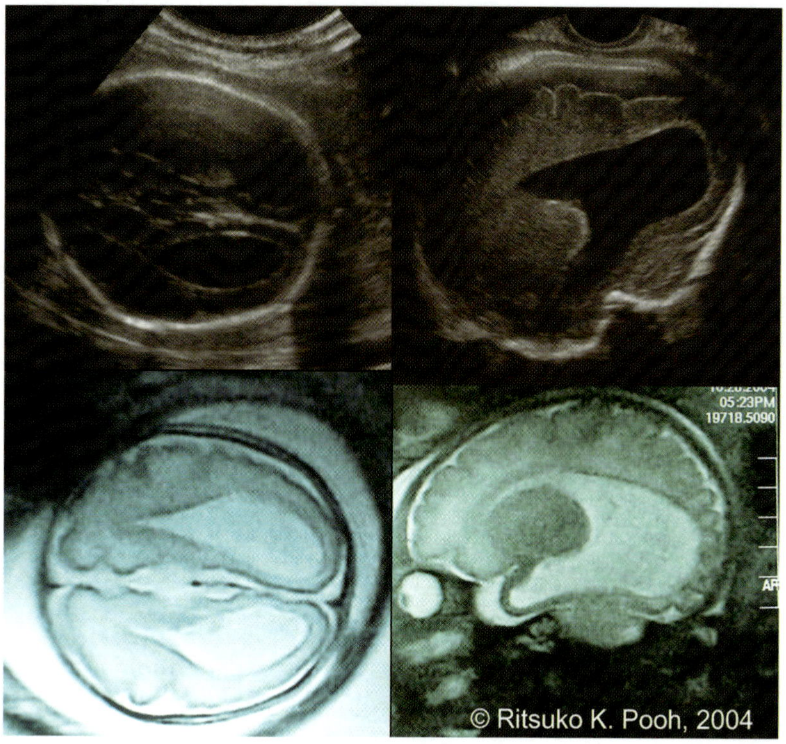

Figure 39.42 Fetal ultrasound and MR images of characteristic ventricular shape in a case with agenesis of the corpus callosum. (Upper left) Ultrasound axial image. (Upper right) Ultrasound parasagittal image. (Lower left) MR axial image. (Lower right) MR parasagittal image. Note the tear-drop appearance of the lateral ventricles in the axial section. Ventricular appearance in the parasagittal section is called 'colpocephaly'.

Synonyms: de Morsier syndrome (septo-optic dysplasia).

Etiology: maternal drug (multidrug, valproic acid,[53] cocaine[54]), autosomal recessive, HESX1 homeodomain gene mutation.[55]

Pathogenesis: May occur as a vascular disruption sequence, with other prosencephalic or neuronal migration disorders.

Associated anomalies: Schizencephaly, gyral abnormalities, heterotopias, hypotelorism, ventriculomegaly, communicating lateral ventricles, bilateral cleft lip and palate, hypopituitarism.

Differential diagnosis: Dysgenesis of the corpus callosum, lobar holoprosencephaly.

Prognosis: Depends on associated anomalies. Variable degree of mental deficit, multiple endocrine dysfunction. In cases with isolated absent of septum pellucidum, prognosis may be good.

Recurrence risk: Unknown.

Management: Confirmation of diagnosis after birth is important for genetic counseling. Endocrine dysfunction should be searched and corrected. Shunt procedure in cases with progressive ventriculomegaly.

Lissencephaly

Incidence: Unknown, rare.

Definition: Characterized by a lack of gyral development and divided into two types:

Lissencephaly type I: a smooth surface of the brain. Cerebral wall is similar to that of an approximately 12-week-old fetus.[56] Isolated lissencephaly. Miller–Dieker syndrome with additional craniofacial abnormalities, cardiac anomalies, genital anomalies, sacral dimple, creases, and/or clinodactyly.

Lissencephaly type II: cobblestone appearance. Walker–Warburg syndrome with macrocephaly, congenital muscular dystrophy, cerebellar malformation, retinal malformation. Fukuyama congenital muscular dystrophy with microcephaly and congenital muscular dystrophy.

Synonyms: Agyria, pachygyria, Walker–Warburg syndrome was known as HARD±E syndrome (*h*ydrocephalus, *a*gyria, *r*etinal *d*ysplasia, with or without *e*ncephalocele).

Etiology: Isolated lissencephaly is link to chromosome 17p13.3 and chromosome Xq24-q24. Miller–Dieker syndrome is also linked to chromosome 17p13.3. Walker–Warburg syndrome is autosomal recessive inheritance. Fukuyama congenital muscular dystrophy is linked to chromosome 9q31, fukutin.[57]

Pathogenesis: Defective neuronal migration with four, rather than six, layers in the cortex.

Associated anomalies: Polyhydramnios, less fetal movement, colpocephaly, agenesis of the corpus callosum, Dandy–Walker malformation are observed in Miller–Dieker syndrome. Micrognathia, flat nose,

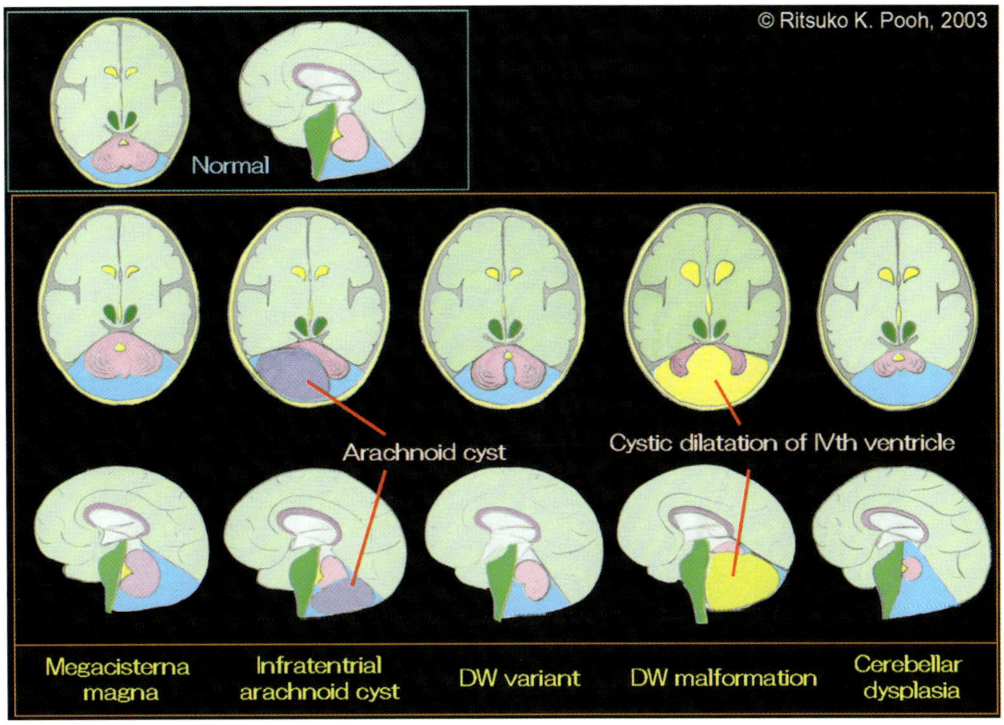

Figure 39.43 Differential diagnosis of 'hypoechoic lesion' of the posterior fossa.

high forehead, low-set ears, cardiac anomalies, genital anomalies in male are often observed in Walker–Warburg syndrome.

Prenatal diagnosis: Prenatal diagnosis[58–60] of lissencephaly without previous history of an affected child probably cannot be reliably made until 26–28 weeks' gestation.[42]

Prognosis: Type I: hypotonia, paucity of movements, feeding disturbance, seizures. The prognosis is poor, and death occurs. Type II: severe seizures, mental disorders, severe muscle disease with hypotonia. Death in the first year is common.

Recurrence risk: Depends on etiology.

Management: Karyotyping is recommended to detect the chromosomal defect. Standard obstetrical care.

Schizencephaly

Incidence: Rare.

Definition: A disorder characterized by congenital clefts in the cerebral mantle, lined by pia-ependyma, with communication between the subarachnoid space laterally and the ventricular system medially (Figure 6-52); 63% is unilateral and 37% bilateral. Frontal region in 44% and frontoparietal 30%.[56]

Etiology: Uncertain. In certain familial cases, a point mutation in the homeobox gene, EMX2 was found.[61,62] Cytomegalovirus infection was also related in some cases.[63]

Pathogenesis: Neuronal migration disorder.

Associated anomalies: Ventriculomegaly, microcephaly, polymicrogyria, gray matter heterotopias, dysgenesis of the corpus callosum, absence of the septum pellucidum, and optic nerve hypoplasia.

Differential diagnosis: Porencephaly, arachnoid cyst, or other intracranial cystic masses. MRI is useful in diagnosis of schizencephaly.[64]

Prognosis: Variable. Generally suffer from mental retardation, seizures, developmental delay and motor disturbances.

Recurrence risk: Unknown.

Management: Ventriculoperitoneal shunt for progressive hydrocephalus.

Dandy–Walker malformation, Dandy–Walker variant, megacisterna magna

Incidence: Dandy–Walker malformation has an estimated prevalence of about 1/30,000 births, and is found in 4–12% of all cases of infantile hydrocephalus.[65] Incidence of Dandy–Walker variant and megacisterna magna is unknown.

Definition: At present, the term Dandy–Walker complex[66] is used to indicate a spectrum of anomalies of the posterior fossa that are classified by axial computed tomography (CT) scans as it follows. Dandy–Walker malformation, Dandy–Walker variant, and megacisterna magna seem to represent a continuum of developmental anomalies of the posterior fossa.[66] Figure 39.43 shows the differential diagnosis of hypoechoic lesion of the posterior fossa.

- (Classic) Dandy–Walker malformation: cystic dilatation of fourth ventricle, enlarged posterior fossa, elevated tentorium, and complete or partial agenesis of the cerebellar vermis.

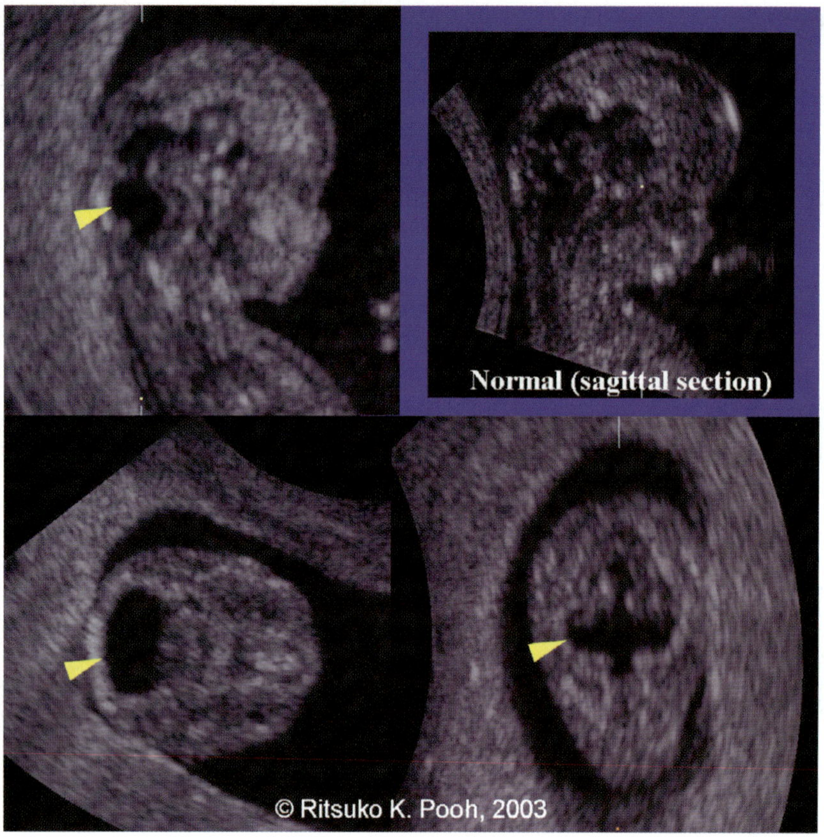

Figure 39.44 Early stage of Dandy–Walker malformation at 11 weeks of gestation. Abnormal dilatation of the posterior fossa (arrowheads). Upper right figure is a sagittal image at the same gestational age in a normal case. Amniocentesis revealed trisomy 9 mosaicism and the fetus died *in utero* at 19 weeks.

- Dandy–Walker variant: variable hypoplasia of the cerebellar vermis with or without enlargement of the posterior fossa.
- Megacisterna magna: enlarged cisterna magna with integrity of both cerebellar vermis and fourth ventricle.

Etiology: Mendelian disorders such as Warburg, chromosomal aberration such as 45,X, partial monosomy/trisomy, viral infections, and diabetes.

Pathogenesis: During development of the fourth ventricular roof, a delay or total failure of the foramen of Magendie to open occurs, allowing a buildup of CSF and development of the cystic dilation of the fourth ventricle. Despite the subsequent opening of the foramina of Luschka (usually patent in Dandy–Walker malformation), cystic dilatation of the fourth ventricle persists and CSF flow is impaired.

Associated anomalies of Dandy–Walker malformation: Hydrocephalus. Other midline anomalies, such as agenesis of the corpus callosum and holoprosencephaly and occipital encephalocele. Extracranial abnormalities such as congenital heart disease, NTDs, and cleft lip/palate. A frequency of additional anomalies ranging between 50% and 70%.

Prenatal diagnosis: Dandy–Walker malformation is shown in Figures 39.44 and 39.46; Dandy–Walker variant is shown in Figure 39.45. To observe the agenesis of the cerebellar vermis, axial cutting section is preferable. To observe the elevated tentorium, sagittal section is preferable.

Differential diagnosis: infratentorial arachnoid cyst, other intracranial cystic tumor, hydrocephalus, and cerebellar dysplasia (Figure 39.47).

Prognosis: Progressive hydrocephalus, not observed in neonates but often progressive during the first month. In cases diagnosed *in utero* or during the neonatal period, outcome is generally unfavorable. Nearly 40% die, and 75% of survivors exhibit cognitive deficits. Prognosis of Dandy–Walker variant is good. Clinical significance of megacisterna magna is uncertain.

Recurrence risk: Depends on etiology. Generally 1–5% (Dandy–Walker malformation).

Management: Cyst–peritoneal shunt, cyst–ventriculoperitoneal shunt.

Arachnoid cyst

Prevalence: 1% of intracranial masses in newborns.

Definition: Congenital or acquired cyst, lined by arachnoid membranes, and filled with fluid collection which is of the same character as the CSF. The number of cysts is mostly single, but two or more cysts can be occasionally observed. Location of arachnoid cyst is

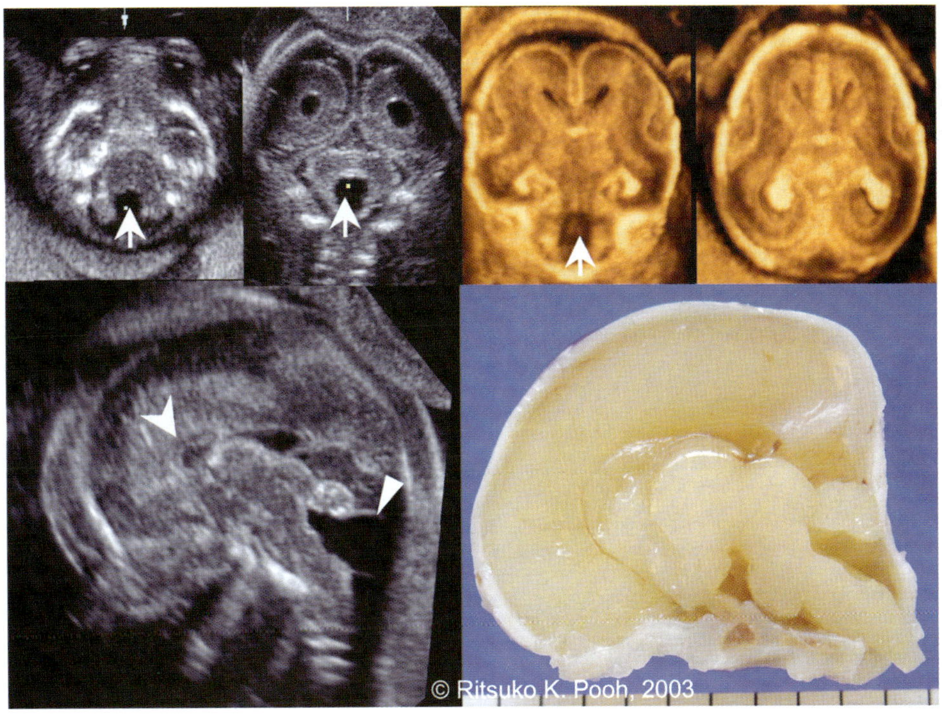

Figure 39.45 Dandy–Walker variant at 20 weeks of gestation. Upper figures show the 2D axial, 2D posterior coronal, and 3D thick slices of oblique coronal and axial sections from the left. Hypoplasia of the vermis (arrows) is demonstrated and no marked ventriculomegaly was seen. Lower left figure shows the median section. Partial agenesis of the corpus callosum (arrowhead), floated celebellum (triangle arrowhead), and cystic formation of the posterior fossa are seen. Lower right figure shows the median cutting section of the specimen of an aborted fetus at 21 weeks of gestation. This case had other complicated anomalies and the karyotype was partial trisomy of chromosome 10.

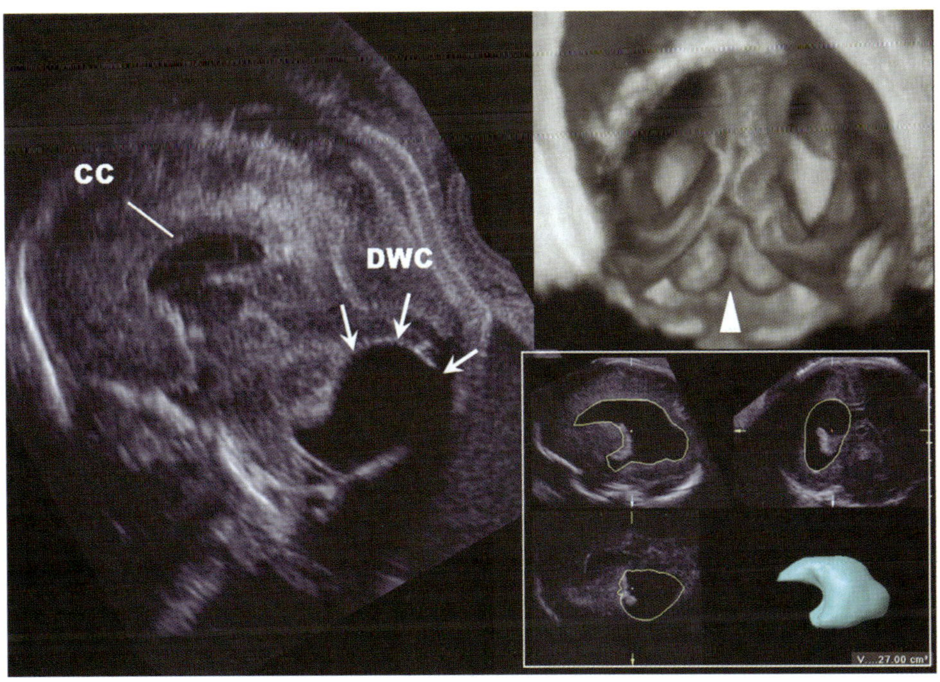

Figure 39.46 Dandy–Walker malformation at 28 weeks of gestation. Left figure shows the median section of the brain. Corpus callosum (CC) is normally demonstrated and Dandy–Walker cyst (DWC, arrows) is seen in the posterior fossa. Right upper figure is a 3D view of the posterior coronal section. Hypoplastic vermis of the cerebellum (arrowhead) is seen. Right lower figures, three orghogonal views and an extracted ventricular appearance, demonstrate moderate ventriculomegaly in this case.

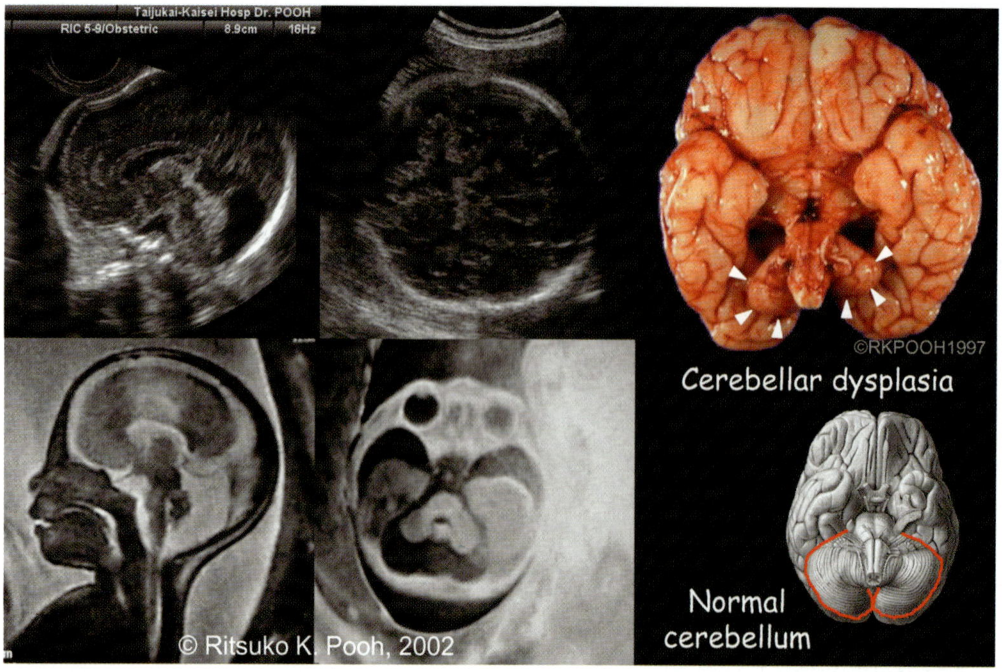

Figure 39.47 Cerebellar dysplasia in a case of trisomy 18. (Upper left) Transvaginal median image. Small cerebellum within a normal size of posterior fossa. (Upper middle) Transabdominal axial image. (Lower left) Fetal MR sagittal image. (Lower middle) MR axial image. (Upper right) Macroscopic photograph of cerebellar dysplasia in another case of trisomy 18. Compared with normal cerebellum shown in the right lower figure, hypoplastic cerebellum is easily identified.

various; approximately 50% of cysts occur from the Sylvian fissure (middle fossa), 20% from the posterior fossa, and 10–20% each from the convexity, suprasellar, interhemisphere, and quadrigeminal cistern. Interhemisperic cysts are often associated with agenesis or hypogenesis of the corpus callosum.

Etiology: Unknown.

Pathogenesis: Congenital arachnoid cyst is formed by maldevelopment of the arachnoid membrane. CSF accumulation in the subarachnoid space or intra-arachnoid layers from a choroid plexus-like tissue within the cyst wall, leads to a progressive distension of the lesion.

Associated anomalies: Unilateral or bilateral hydrocephalus, macrocrania.

Prenatal diagnosis: Figures 39.48–39.50. Detection in the first trimester was reported.[67]

Differential diagnosis: Porencephaly, schizencephaly, third ventriculomegaly, intracranial cystic type tumor, vein of Galen aneurysm, Dandy–Walker malformation, large cisterna magna, external hydrocephalus.

Prognosis: Generally good. Postnatally, many are asymptomatic and remain quiescent for years, although others expand and cause neurological symptoms by compressing adjacent brain, ventriculomegaly, and/or expanding the overlying skull.

Recurrence risk: Unknown.

Obstetrical management: Arachnoid cysts may increase or decrease its size. Therefore, expectant management of antenatally diagnosed cases is suggested.[68] In cases with accompanying hydrocephalus, mode and timing of delivery may be modified.

Postnatal management: In cases with these symptoms or with prospects of neurological symptoms, treatment should be considered. Operation methods include:

- Cyst fenestration by craniotomy
- Cyst fenestration by neuroendoscopy
- Cyst-peritoneal shunt.

Craniotomy, shunting, or neuroendoscopic method is still controversial.[69,70]

Craniosynostosis

Incidence: Unknown.

Definition: Premature closure of cranial suture, which may affect one or more cranial sutures. Simple sagittal synostosis is most common. Various cranial shapes depend on affected suture(s).

Sagittal suture	Scaphocephaly or dolichocephaly
Bilateral coronal suture	Brachycephaly
Unilateral coronal suture	Anterior plagiocephaly
Metopic suture	Trigonocephaly
Lambdoid suture	Acrocephaly
Unilateral lambdoid suture	Posterior plagiocephaly
Coronal/lambdoid/metopic or squamous/sagittal suture	Cloverleaf skull
Total cranial sutures	Oxycephaly

Syndromes

Crouzon syndrome: acrocephaly, synostosis of coronal, sagittal and lambdoid sutures. With ocular proptosis, maxillary hypoplasia.

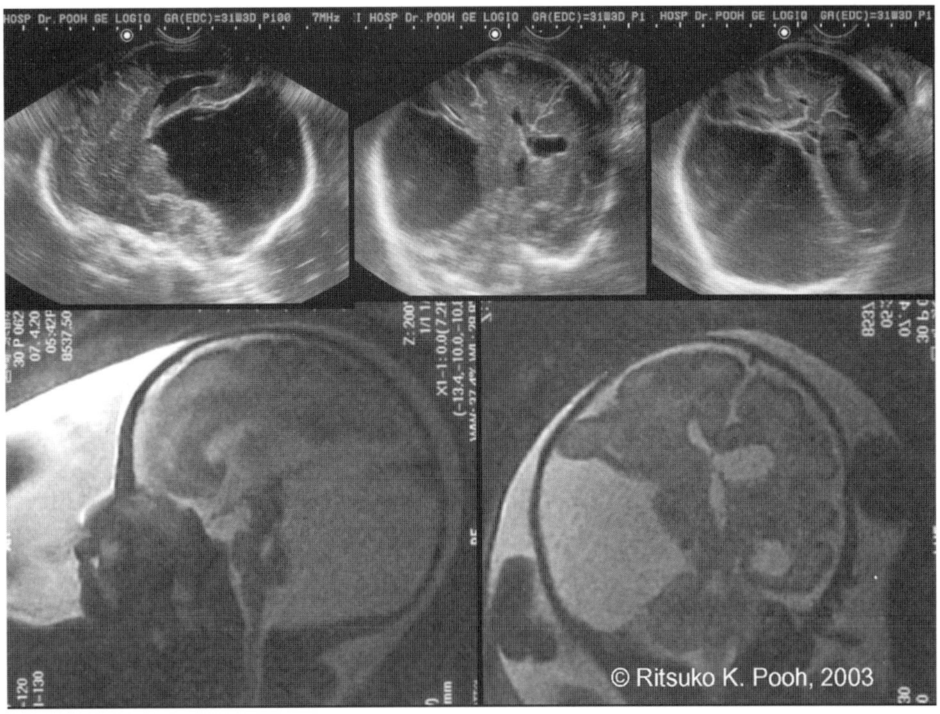

Figure 39.48 Fetal arachnoid cyst at 31 weeks of gestation. (Upper) Transvaginal ultrasound image. Sagittal (left) and coronal (middle, right) sections. (Lower left) Fetal MR sagittal image. The cyst occupies supra- to infratentorial space. Not only cerebrum but also the cerebellum is compressed by the cyst. (Lower right) Fetal MR coronal image. Midline is conspicuously arcuated. Unilateral scalp and skull bone are extended due to the existence of the huge cyst. Note the difference between right and left head size.

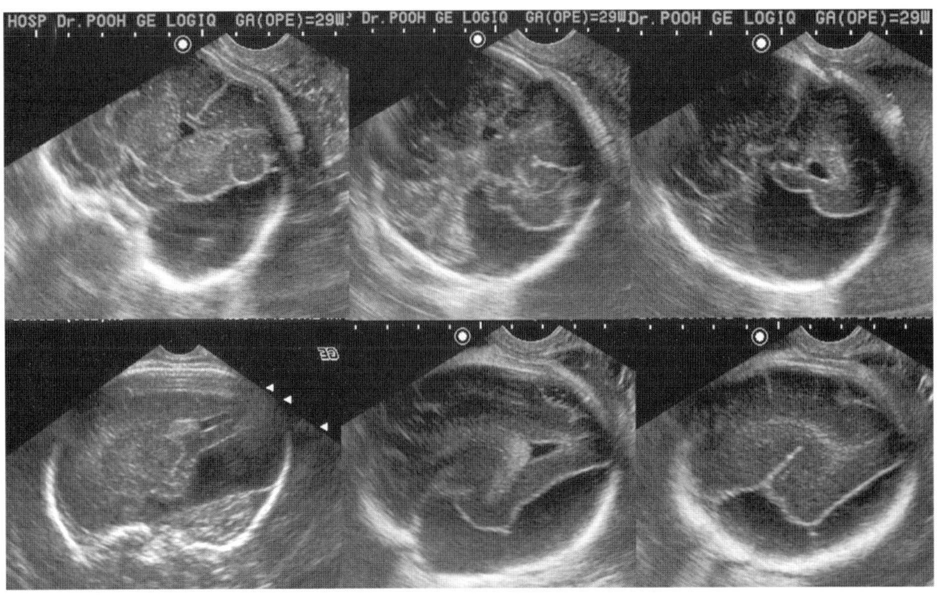

Figure 39.49 Transvaginal ultrasound images of middle fossa arachnoid cyst at 29 weeks of gestation. (Upper) Serial coronal sections. (Lower) Serial sagittal sections. Compressed adjacent cerebrum is demonstrated.

Apert syndrome: brachycephaly, irregular synostosis, especially coronal suture. With midfacial hypoplasia, syndactyly, broad distal phalanx of thumb and big toe.

Pfeiffer syndrome: brachycephaly, synostosis of coronal and/or sagittal sutures. With hypertelorism, broad thumbs and toes, partial syndactyly.

Antley–Bixler syndrome: brachycephaly, multiple synostosis, especially of coronal suture. With maxillary hypoplasia, radiohymeral synostosis, choanal atresia, arthrogryposis.

Etiology: Crouzon (AD, variable), Apert (AD, usually new mutation), Pfeiffer (AD), Antley–Bixler (AR). In five autosomal dominant craniosynostosis syndromes

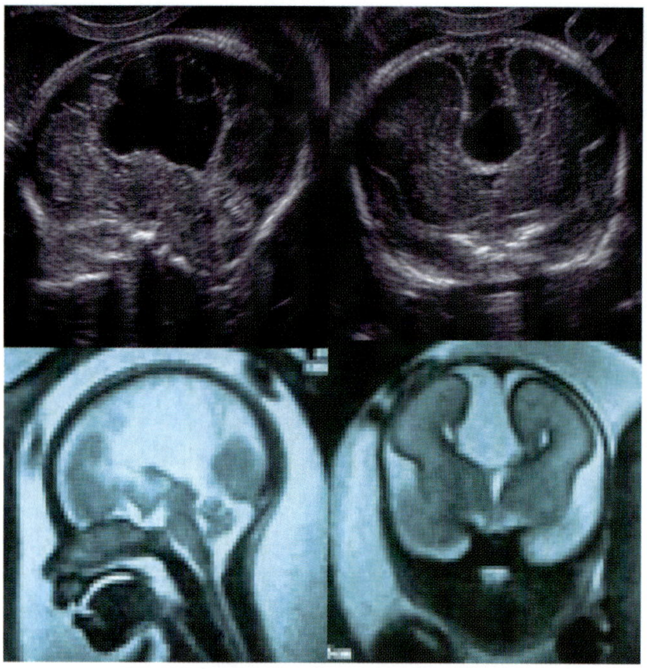

Figure 39.50 Ultrasound and MR images of interhemispheric cyst at 24 weeks of gestation. (Upper left) Ultrasound median section. (Upper right) Ultrasound anterior coronal section. (Lower left) MR median section. (Lower right) MR anterior coronal secrion. Cystic lesion exists between hemispheres. Intracystic cyst is visible in the ultrasound images.

(Apert, Crouzon, Pfeiffer, Jackson–Weiss, and Crouzon syndromes with acanthosis nigricans) result from mutations in FGFR genes.[71]

Pathogenesis:[72] (1) Cranial vault bones with decreased growth potential; (2) asymmetrical bone deposition at perimeter sutures; (3) sutures adjacent to the prematurely fused suture compensate in growth more than those sutures not contiguous with the closed suture; (4) enhanced symmetrical bone deposition occurs along both sides of a nonperimeter suture continuing prematurely closed suture.

Associated anomalies: Hypertelorism, syndactyly, polydactyly, exophthalmos.

Prenatal diagnosis: Figure 39.51 shows prenatal appearance in Apert syndrome and Figure 39.52 shows the postnatal findings. Abnormal craniofacial appearance can be detected by 2D/3D ultrasound.[73,74]

Prognosis: Various. In some of trigonocephaly and syndromic types, prognosis is poor.

Recurrence risk: Depends on etiology.

Management: Operative aim of cranioplasty is improvement of intracranial pressure and cosmetic change.

Vein of Galen aneurysm

Incidence: Rare.

Definition: Direct arteriovenous fistulas between choroidal and/or quadrigeminal arteries and an overlying single median venous sac.

Synonyms: Vein of Galen malformation.

Etiology: Unknown.

Pathogenesis: Venous sac most probably represents persistence of the embryonic median prosencephalic vein of Markowski, not the vein of Galen, per se.[75]

Associated anomalies: cardiomegaly, high cardiac output, secondary hydrocephalus, macrocrania, cerebral ischemia (intracranial steal phenomenon), subarachnoid/cerebral/intraventricular hemorrhages.

Prenatal diagnosis: 2D and 3D color/power Doppler detection is possible.

Differential diagnosis: Arachnoid cyst, porencephalic cyst, intracranial teratoma. Color/power Doppler is helpful for differential diagnosis.

Prognosis: According to earlier review, outcome did not differ between treated and nontreated group and over 80% of cases resulted in death.[76] However, recent advances in treatment have improved outcome, such that 60–100% survive and over 60% have a good neurological outcome.[77,78]

Recurrence risk: Unknown.

Management: Evaluation of the fetal high-output cardiac state for the proper obstetrical management. Percutaneous embolization by microcoils is recent main postnatal treatment and remarkably improved outcome.

Choroid plexus cysts

Incidence: 0.95–2.8% of all fetuses scanned.[79–81]

Definition: Cysts with fluid collection within the choroids plexus, which may exist unilaterally or bilaterally. They are depicted in the second trimester and usually resolve by the 24th week.

Etiology: Normal variant, chromosomal aberration such as trisomy 18 and others.

Pathogenesis: Choroid plexus is located within the ventricular system and produces CSF. Within the choroidal villi, choroid plexus cysts exist, surrounded by the loose stroma of the choroid plexus.[82]

Associated anomalies: In cases of trisomy 18, associated anomalies include growth retardation, congenital heart diseases such as ventricular septum defect and double outlet right ventricle, overlapping finger, facial anomaly, cerebellar dysplasia, and others.

Prenatal diagnosis: Figure 39.53. Macroscopic photo is shown in Figure 39.54. It is impossible to distinguish normal from abnormal karyotypes only by location and appearance of choroid plexus cyst. Detection of additional anomalies is important for differential diagnosis.

Differential diagnosis: Intraventricular hemorrhage.

Prognosis: Choroid plexus cysts, per se, are usually asymptomatic and benign, but rarely, symptomatic and disturbs CSF flow.[83,84] Isolated choroids plexus cysts may be normal variation.

Recurrence risk: Unknown.

Management: Fetal karyotyping examination should be offered if additional abnormalities are found.

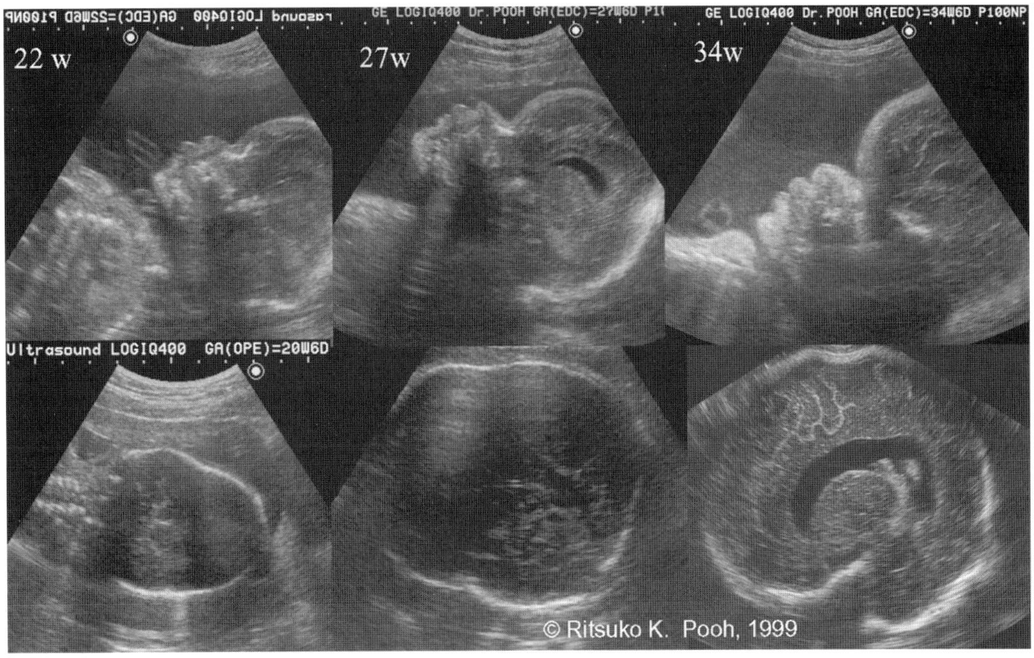

Figure 39.51 Prenatal craniofacial appearance of Apert syndrome. (Upper) Longitudinal changing appearance of frontal bossing and low nasal bridge at 22, 27, and 34 weeks of gestation in a case of Apert syndrome. (Lower left) Irregular cranial shape at 20 weeks. (Lower middle) Cranial shape at 34 weeks. Note the bilateral indentation. (Lower right) Intracranial sagittal ultrasound image at 34 weeks. Mild ventriculomegaly is seen.

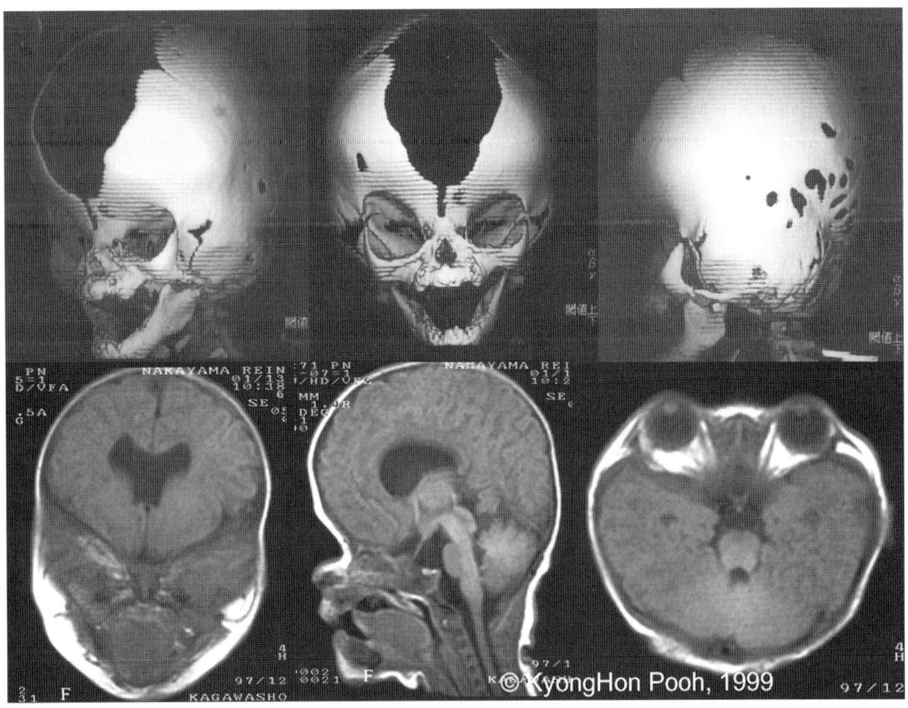

Figure 39.52 Three-dimensional reconstruction CT and MR images of Apert syndrome (the same case as in Figure 39.51). (Upper) Three-dimensional reconstruction CT. Fusion of bilateral coronal suture and squamous suture, defect of frontoparietal cranial structure, and craniofacial bony dysplasia are recognizable. (Lower) Postnatal MR images. Marked shortening of anterior cranial fossa is seen. Mild ventriculomegaly and absent septum pellucidum are seen.

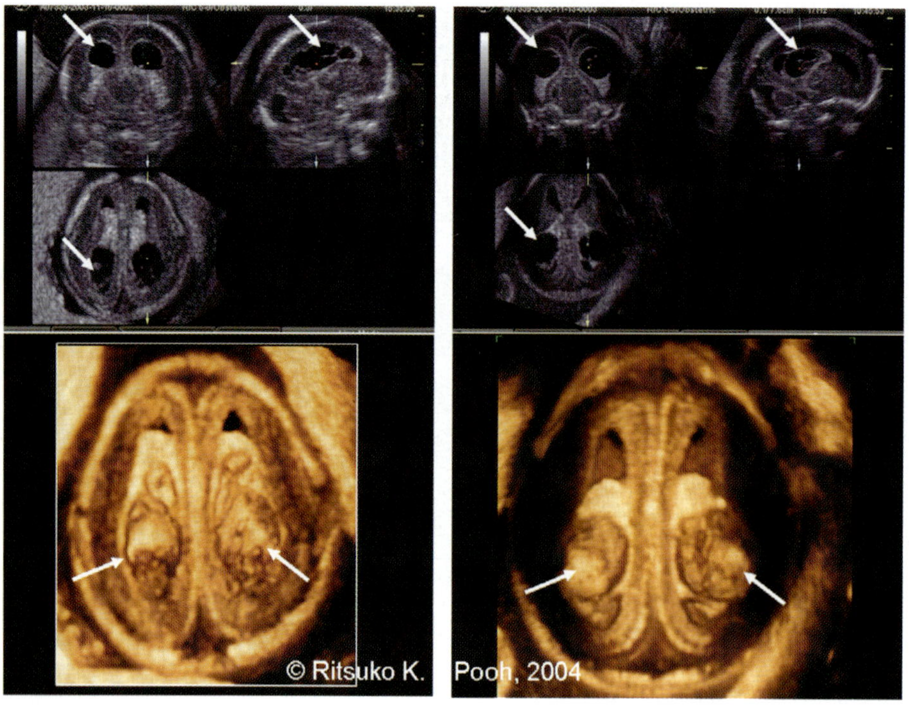

Figure 39.53 Choroid plexus cysts (CPC) in cases of trisomy 18 (left) and normal karyotype (right). (Left figures) Three orthogonal views and inside 3D view of CPC in a case of trisomy 18 at 17 weeks of gestation. Various additional anomalies were detected. (Right figures) Three orthogonal views and inside 3D view of CPC in a case with normal karyotype at 16 weeks. No additional abnormalities. Normal postnatal course. It is impossible to distinguish normal from abnormal karyotypes only by location and appearance of choroid plexus cyst. Detection of additional anomalies is important for differential diagnosis.

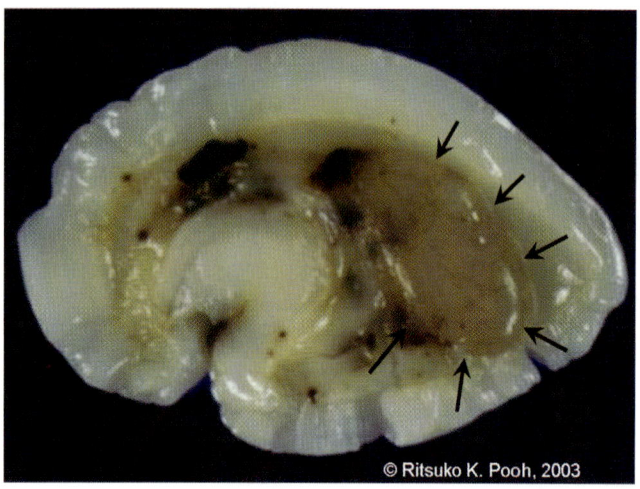

Figure 39.54 Macroscopic appearance of choroid plexus cyst. Arrows indicate the choroid plexus cyst. The specimen was from an aborted fetus of trisomy 18 at 20 weeks of gestation.

Acquired brain abnormalities *in utero*

In terms of encephalopathy or cerebral palsy, *timing of brain insult, antepartum, intrapartum, or postpartum?* is one of the serious controversial issues including medico-socio-legal-ethical problems.[85] Although brain insults may relate to antepartum events in a substantial number of term infants with hypoxic–ischemic encephalopathy, the timing of insult cannot always be clarified. It is a hard task to give antepartum evidences of brain injury predictive of cerebral palsy. Fetal heart rate monitoring cannot reveal the presence of encephalopathy, and neuroimaging by ultrasound and MRI is the most reliable modality for disclosure of silent encephalopathy. Many cases with cerebral palsy with acquired brain insults, especially, term-delivered infants with reactive fetal heart rate tracing and good Apgar score at delivery, are not suspected of having encephalopathy and are often overlooked for months or years. Recent imaging technology has revealed brain insult *in utero*.

Brain tumors

Incidence: Extremely rare.

Definition: Tumors located in the intracranial cavity.

Histological types: Brain tumors are divided into *teratoma*, most commonly reported and nonteratomatous tumor. Nonteratomatous tumors include *neuroepithelial tumor*, such as medulloblastoma, astrocytoma, choroids plexus papilloma, choroids plexus carcinoma, ependymoma, ependymoblastoma, and *mesenchymal tumor* such as craniopharyngioma, sarcoma, fibroma, hemangioblastoma, hemangioma and miningoma, and others of lipoma of the corpus callosum, subependymal giant-cell astrocytoma associated with tuberous sclerosis (often accompanied by cardiac rhabdomyoma).[86,87]

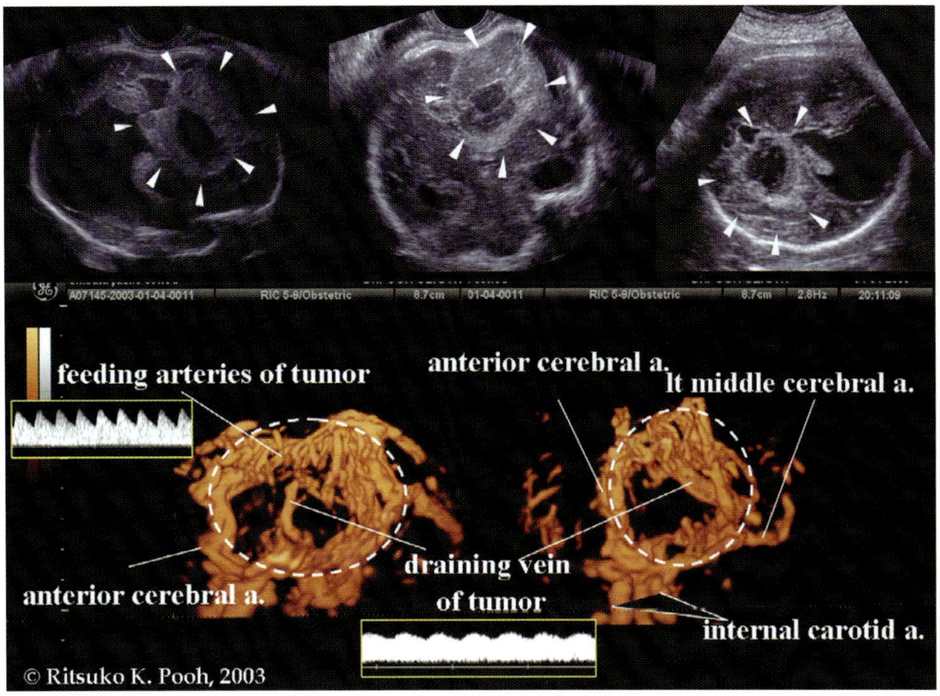

Figure 39.55 Ultrasound images and tumoral vascular visualization by 3D power Doppler in a fetus of intracranial tumor with interventricular hemorrhage (35 weeks and 5 days of gestation). (Upper) Sagittal, coronal, and axial ultrasound images. Huge tumor (arrowheads) with hemorrhage within the tumor in the fronto-parietal lobe, complicated with unilateral hydrocephalus with intraventricular hemorrhage (arrow). (Left lower) Oblique sagittal view from fetal left side. (Right lower) Oblique coronal view from fetal frontal side. Tumor is fed by numerous feeding arteries from anterior cerebral artery. Feeder arteries have low resistant flow waveform. One large vein which drains blood from tumor is visible. The draining vein has pulsatile flow.

Location of tumor: Supratentorial predominance in neonatal tumor. Infratentorial predominance in medulloblastoma. Choroid plexus papilloma is located within the lateral ventricles.

Associated abnormalities: Macrocrania or local skull swelling, epignathus, secondary hydrocephalus, Intracranial hemorrhage, intraventricular hemorrhage, polyhydroamnios, heart failure by high-cardiac output,[88] hydrops.

Diagnosis: Intracranial masses with solid, cystic or mixture pattern with or without visualization of hypervascularity by ultrasound and fetal MRI. Brain tumor should be considered in cases with unexplained intracranial hemorrhage.

Prenatal diagnosis: Prenatal diagnosis of intracranial tumor and its vascularization by 3D power Doppler is shown in Figure 39.55.

Differential diagnosis: Arachnoid cyst, vein of Galen aneurysm, porencephaly, schizencephaly, periventricular leukomalacia, subdural hemorrhage.

Prognosis: Fetal demise, stillborn may occur. Prognosis in neonates is generally poor, but depends on timing of diagnosis and the histological type of tumor. Choroid plexus papilloma has minimal mortality rate and high likelihood of neonatal outcome. Mortality rate of teratomas is over 90%, medulloblastoma over 80%. Other tumors have various prognoses.

Recurrence risk: Unknown.

Management: Cesarean section may be considered. Neurosurgical tumor resection including subtotal hemispherectomy by craniotomy and chemotherapy are possible treatments for neonatal tumors. Radiation therapy is usually not indicated in neonates.

Subependymal pseudocysts

Prevalence: 2.6–5% of all neonates, 1% of premature newborns, unknown in fetuses.

Definition: Cystic formation, which is located in the caudothalamic groove or in the caudate nucleus, lateral to the wall of the anterior horns of lateral ventricles.

Synonyms: Periventricular pseudocysts.[89,90]

Etiology: Infection (cytomegalovirus, rubella), subependymal hemorrhage, metabolic diseases, chromosomal deletions (del q6, delp4) cocaine exposure and others.

Pathogenesis: Cystic cavity is lined by a pseudocapsule, consisting of aggregates of germinal cells and glial tissue, but no epithelium can be found. Origin of pseudocysts is uncertain. Maybe cystic matrix regression or germinolysis.

Associated anomalies: Congenital infection such as cytomegalovirus, congenital heart diseases, associated CNS abnormalities.

Prenatal diagnosis: Figure 39.56.

Differential diagnosis: Periventricular leukomalacia.

Prognosis: Good in cases with isolated subependymal pseudocysts. In cases with accompanied abnormalities, such as cardiac disease, cytomegalovirus

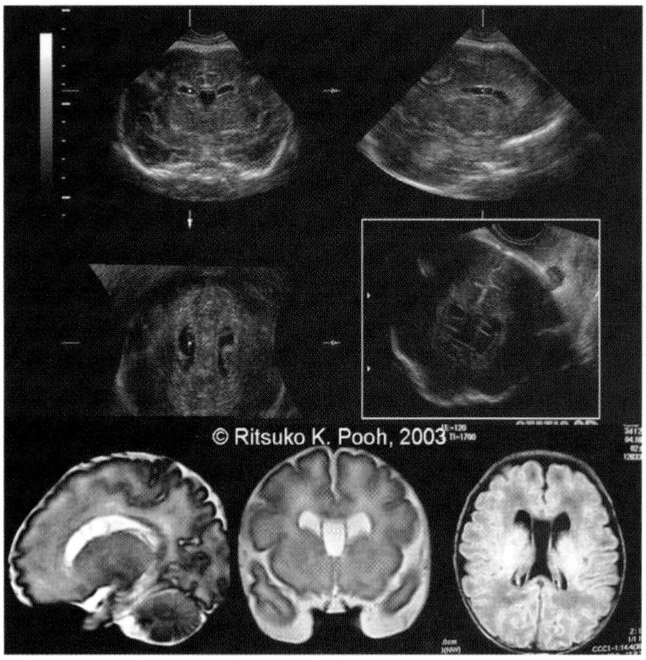

Figure 39.56 Subependymal cysts (fetal ultrasound images and neonatal MR images). (Upper) Coronal and sagittal images. (Middle left) Axial image. (Middle right) Anterior coronal section. Note bilateral bead-like cystic formation. (Lower) MR sagittal, coronal, and axial images at 3 days after birth. No neurological symptoms at the age of 1 year.

infection, other intracranial abnormalities, or cases with atypical pseudocysts, prognosis may be poor.[89–91]

Recurrence risk: Unknown.

Management: In many cases, cysts regress in several months after birth. Normal obstetrical/neonatal care.

Porencephaly

Incidence: Unknown.

Definition: Fluid-filled spaces replacing normal brain parenchyma; may or may not communicate with the lateral ventricles or subarachnoid space.

Synonyms: Porencephalic cyst.

Etiology: Ischemic episode, trauma[92] demise of one twin, intercerebral hemorrhage, infection.

Pathogenesis: Easy to occur when immature cerebrum has some factors with propensity of dissolution and cavitation, (high content of water, myelinated fiber bundles, deficient astroglial response). Timing of ischemic injury (maybe as early as second trimester) is strongly related to porencephaly, hydranencephaly.[93]

Associated anomalies: Intercerebral hemorrhage, interventricular hemorrhage, hydrocephalus.

Prenatal diagnosis: Figure 39.57. Some cases *in utero* have been reported.[94,95]

Differential diagnosis: Schizencephaly, arachnoid cyst, intracranial cystic tumor, other cysts. Porencephalic cyst never causes a mass effect, which is observed in cases with arachnoid cyst or other cystic mass lesions. This condition is acquired brain insult and differentiated from schizencephaly of migration disorder.

Prognosis: Various, depends on timing and size of lesion. Seizures, neurological deficits, and cerebral palsy often occur.[96]

Recurrence risk: Unknown.

Management: Ventriculoperitoneal shunt if hydrocephalus progresses.

Hydranencephaly

Incidence: 1–2.5/10,000 births.

Definition: Absence of the cerebral hemispheres and a sac-like structure containing CSF surrounding the brainstem and basal ganglia.

Etiology: Ischemic episode, trauma, demise of one twin, intercerebral hemorrhage, infection. There are several theories but bilateral occlusion of the supraclinoid segment of the internal carotid arteries[97] or of the middle cerebral arteries is one of the causes of subtotal defects of cerebral hemisphere.

Pathogenesis: Easy to occur when immature cerebrum has some factors with propensity of dissolution and cavitation, (high content of water, myelinated fiber bundles, deficient astroglial response). Timing of ischemic injury (maybe as early as second trimester) is strongly related to porencephaly and hydranencephaly.

Prenatal diagnosis: Recently, hydranencephaly from 11 weeks of gestation has been reported.[98]

Associated anomalies: Large head (Figure 39.58).

Differential diagnosis: Massive hydrocephalus, alobar holoprosencephaly, porencephaly.

Prognosis: Extremely poor.

Recurrence risk: Unknown.

Management: No active treatment. Shunt procedure for progressive increase of infant's head.

Intracranial hemorrhage

Incidence: Unknown, rare *in utero*.

Definition: Hemorrhage, bleeding inside of the cranium. Intracranial hemorrhage includes subdural hemorrhage, primary subarachnoid hemorrhage, intracerebellar hemorrhage, intraventricular hemorrhage, and intraparenchymal hemorrhage other than cerebellar.[99]

Etiology: Trauma, alloimmune and idiopathic thrombocytopenia, von Willebrand's disease, specific medications (warfarin) or illicit drug (cocaine) abuse, seizure, fetal conditions including congenital factor-X and factor-V deficiencies, intracranial tumor, twin–twin transfusion, demise of a co-twin, vascular diseases, or fetomaternal hemorrhage, extracorporeal membrane oxygenation (ECMO).[100]

Associated anomalies: Hydrocephalus, hydranencephaly, porencephaly, or microcephaly.

Prenatal diagnosis: Figure 39.59.

Differential diagnosis: Intracranial tumor.

Prognosis: Poor in premature infants. Apnea, seizures, and other neurological symptoms.

Recurrence risk: Depends on etiology.

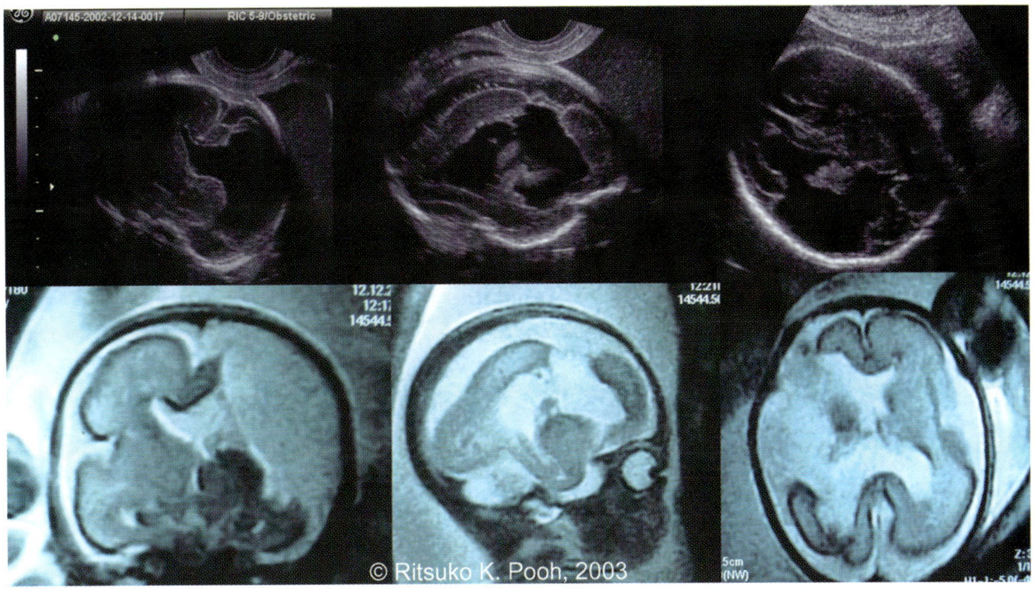

Figure 39.57 Fetal ultrasound and MR images of porencephaly at 25 weeks of gestation. (Upper left) Transvaginal ultrasound coronal image. Defect of parietolateral part of the unilateral cerebrum. This case has also absent septum pellucidum. (Upper middle) Parasagittal ultrasound image. Porencephalic part is fused with the unilateral ventricle. Echogenesity of inside ventricular wall indicates intraventricular hemorrhage. (Upper right) Transabdominal ultrasound axial image. (Lower) Fetal MR images on the same day. Coronal, parasagittal, and axial sections from the left side.

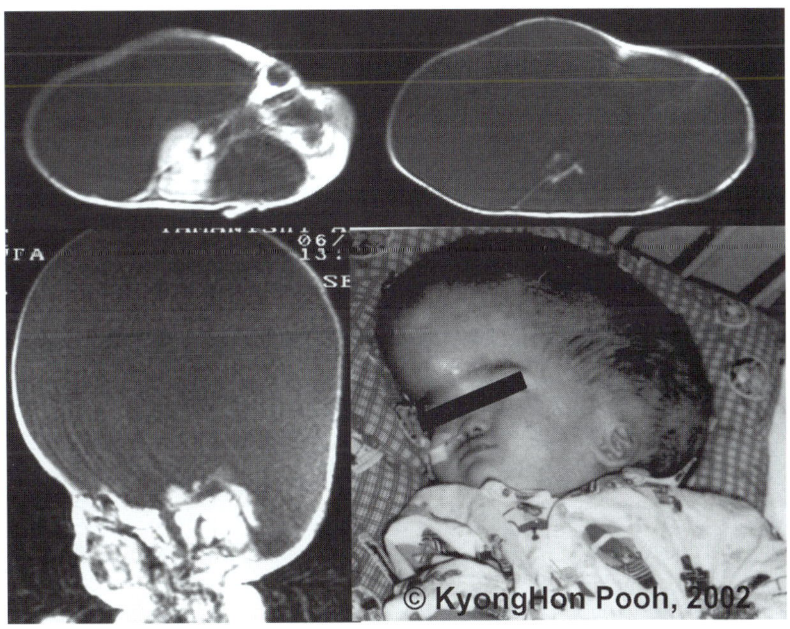

Figure 39.58 Hydranencephaly. Hydranencephaly is characterized by absence of the cerebral hemispheres with an incomplete or absent falx and a sac-like structure containing cerebral spinal fluid surrounding the brainstem and basal ganglia. In this case, tentorium and falx cerebri are recognized. Cerebral cortex is depicted in only a small part of occipital lobe. Brain stem and cerebellum are preserved to be normal. Cause of hydranencephaly may be obstruction of the bilateral internal carotid arteries. Note the remarkable increase of head circumference.

Management: Ventriculoperitoneal shunt if hydrocephalus progresses.

Fetal periventricular leukomalacia (PVL)

Incidence: 25–75% of premature infants at autopsy are complicated with periventricular white matter injury. However, clinically, incidence may be much lower; 5–10% of infants less than 1500 g birth weight. In term infants, PVL is very rare.

Definition: Multifocal areas of necrosis found deep in the cortical white matter, which are often symmetrical and occur adjacent to the lateral ventricles. PVL represents a major precursor for neurological and intellectual impairment, and cerebral palsy in later life.

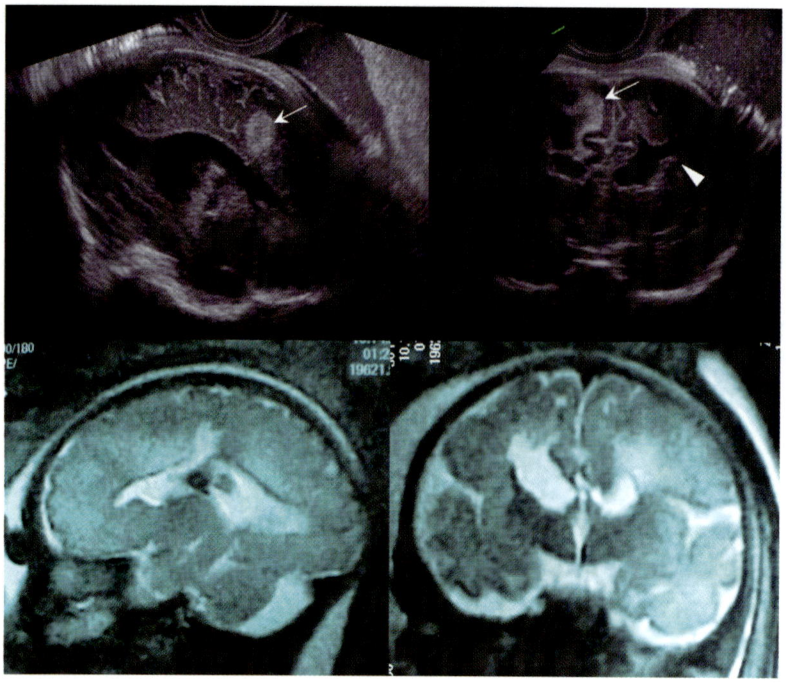

Figure 39.59 Ultrasound and MR images in a fetus with cerebral hemorrhage and mild ventriculomegaly at 35 weeks of gestation. Ultrasound parasagittal (upper left) and anterior coronal (upper right) images of the brain. Arrows indicate intracerebral hemorrhage. Arrowhead shows a porencephalic part fused with the lateral ventricle. Lower figures are MR images showing the same cutting sections as upper ultrasound images.

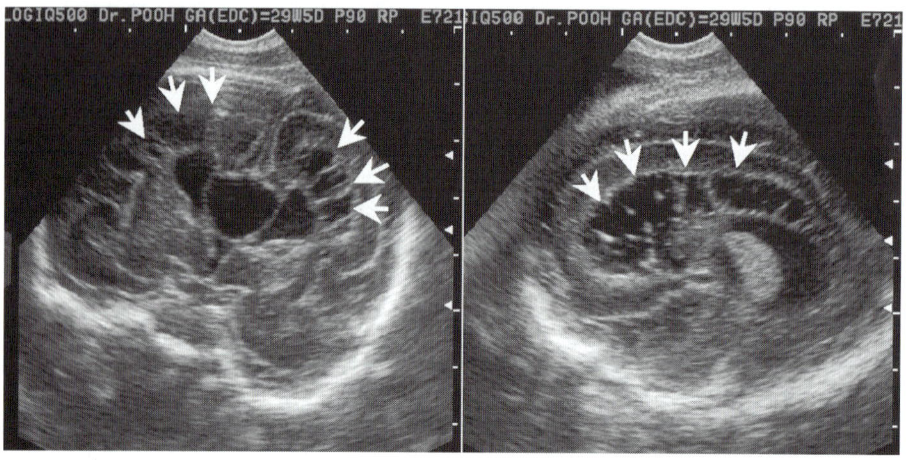

Figure 39.60 Fetal periventricular leukomalacia (PVL) at 29 weeks of gestation. Bilateral widespread type PVL (arrows) was seen. No particular maternal episode existed before and during pregnancy.

Etiology: Birth trauma, asphyxia and respiratory failure, cardiopulmonary defects, premature birth/low birth weight, associated immature cerebrovascular development and lack of appropriate autoregulation of cerebral blood flow in response to hypoxic-ischemic insults.[101]

Pathogenesis: Distinctive and consists primarily of both focal periventricular necrosis and more diffuse cerebral white matter injury. Two most common sites are at the level of the cerebral white matter near the trigone of the lateral ventricles and around the foramen of Monro. Volpe[93] describes three factors, namely (1) periventricular vascular anatomical and physiological factors, (2) cerebral ischemia, and (3) intrinsic vulnerability of cerebral white matter of premature newborn, are strongly related to PVL.

Prenatal diagnosis: Figure 39.60.

Differential diagnosis: Subarachnoid (periventricular) pseudocysts, porencephaly, other intracranial cystic formation.

Prognosis: Neurological features of PVL in neonatal period are probable lower limb weakness and as features of long-term sequelae, spastic diplegia, intellectual deficits and visual deficits are observed.[93]

Recurrence risk: Unknown.

Management: Early rehabilitation.

REFERENCES

1. Timor-Tritsch IE, Monteagudo A. Transvaginal fetal neurosonography: Standardization of the planes and sections by anatomic landmarks. *Ultrasound Obstet Gynecol* 1996;8:42–7.
2. Timor-Tritsch IE, Peisner DB, Raju S. Sonoembryology: An organ-oriented approach using a high-frequency vaginal probe. *J Clin Ultrasound* 1990;18:286–98.
3. Pooh RK. B-mode and Doppler studies of the abnormal fetus in the first trimester. In Chervenak FA, Kurjak A, eds. *Fetal Medicine*. Carnforth, UK: Parthenon Publishing, 1999;46–51.
4. Monteagudo A, Reuss ML, Timor-Tritsch IE. Imaging the fetal brain in the second and third trimesters using transvaginal sonography. *Obstet Gynecol* 1991;77:27–32.
5. Monteagudo A, Timor-Tritsch IE, Moomjy M. In utero detection of ventriculomegaly during the second and third trimesters by transvaginal sonography. *Ultrasound Obstet Gynecol* 1994;4: 193–8.
6. Monteagudo A, Timor-Tritsch IE. Development of fetal gyri, sulci and fissures: A transvaginal sonographic study. *Ultrasound Obstet Gynecol* 1997;9:222–8.
7. Pooh RK, Nakagawa Y, Nagamachi N, *et al.* Transvaginal sonography of the fetal brain: Detection of abnormal morphology and circulation. *Croat Med J* 1998;39:147–57.
8. Pooh RK, Maeda K, Pooh KH, Kurjak A. Sonographic assessment of the fetal brain morphology. *Prenat Neonat Med* 1999;4:18–38.
9. Pooh RK. Three-dimensional ultrasound of the fetal brain. In Kurjak A, ed. *Clinical Application of 3D Ultrasonography*. Carnforth, UK: Parthenon Publishing, 2000;176–80.
10. Pooh RK, Pooh KH, Nakagawa Y, Nishida S, Ohno Y. Clinical application of three-dimensional ultrasound in fetal brain assessment. *Croat Med J* 2000;41:245–51.
11. Timor-Tritsch IE, Monteagudo A, Mayberry P. Three-dimensional ultrasound evaluation of the fetal brain: the three horn view. *Ultrasound Obstet Gynecol* 2000;16:302–6.
12. Monteagudo A, Timor-Tritsch IE, Mayberry P. Three-dimensional transvaginal neurosonography of the fetal brain: 'Navigating' in the volume scan. *Ultrasound Obstet Gynecol* 2000;16:307–13.
13. Blaas HG, Eik-Nes SH, Kiserud T, Berg S, Angelsen B, Olstad B. Three-dimensional imaging of the brain cavities in human embryos. *Ultrasound Obstet Gynecol* 1995;5:228–32.
14. Blaas HG, Eik-Nes SH, Berg S, Torp H. *In-vivo* three-dimensional ultrasound reconstructions of embryos and early fetuses. *Lancet* 1998;352:1182–6.
15. Pooh RK, Pooh KH. Fetal neuroimaging with new technology. *Ultrasound Rev Obstet Gynecol* 2002;2:178–81.
16. Pooh RK, Pooh KH. Transvaginal 3D and Doppler ultrasonography of the fetal brain. *Semin Perinatol* 2001;25:38–43.
17. Pooh RK, Pooh KH. The assessment of fetal brain morphology and circulation by transvaginal 3D sonography and power Doppler. *J Perinat Med* 2002;30:48–56.
18. Levine D. Magnetic resonance imaging in prenatal diagnosis. *Curr Opin Pediatr* 2001;13:572–8.
19. Huisman TA, Wisser J, Martin E, Kubik-Huch R, Marincek B. Fetal magnetic resonance imaging of the central nervous system: A pictorial essay. *Eur Radiol* 2002;12:1952–61.
20. Ertl-Wagner B, Lienemann A, Strauss A, Reiser MF. Fetal magnetic resonance imaging: indications, technique, anatomical considerations and a review of fetal abnormalities. *Eur Radiol* 2002;12:1931–40.
21. Kubik-Huch RA, Huisman TA, Wisser J *et al.* Ultrafast MR imaging of the fetus. *AJR Am J Roentgenol* 2000;174:1599–606.
22. Levine D, Barnes PD. Cortical maturation in normal and abnormal fetuses as assessed with prenatal MR imaging. *Radiology* 1999;210:751–8.
23. Huppert BJ, Brandt KR, Ramin KD, King BF. Single-shot fast spin-echo MR imaging of the fetus: a pictorial essay. *Radiographics* 1999;19:S215–27.
24. Smith DW, Tondury G. Origin of the calvaria and its sutures. *Am J Dis Child* 1978;132:662–6.
25. Pooh RK. Fetal cranial bone formation: Sonographic assessment. In Margulies M, Voto LS, Eik-Nes S, eds. *9th World Congress of Ultrasound in Obstetrics and Gynecology*. Bologna, Italy: Monduzzi Editore, 1999;407–10.
26. Pooh RK, Pooh KH, Nakagawa Y, Maeda K, Fukui R, Aono T. Transvaginal Doppler assessment of fetal intracranial venous flow. *Obstet Gynecol* 1999;93:697–701.
27. Alagappan R, Browning PD, Laorr A, McGahan JP. Distal lateral ventricular atrium: reevaluation of normal range. *Radiology* 1994;193:405–8.
28. Almog B, Gamzu R, Achiron R *et al.* Fetal lateral ventricular width: What should be its upper limit? A prospective cohort study and reanalysis of the current and previous data. *J Ultrasound Med* 2003;22:39–43.
29. Fransen E, Lemmon V, Van Camp G, Vits L, Coucke P, Willems PJ. CRASH syndrome: Clinical spectrum of corpus callosum hypoplasia, retardation, adducted thumbs, spastic paraparesis and hydrocephalus due to mutations in one single gene, L1. *Eur J Hum Genet* 1995;3:273–84.
30. Yamasaki M, Thompson P, Lemmon V. CRASH syndrome: Mutations in L1CAM correlate with severity of the disease. *Neuropediatrics* 1997;28:175–8.
31. Timor-Tritsch IE, Monteagudo A, Haratz-Rubinstein N, Levine RU. Transvaginal sonographic detection of adducted thumbs, hydrocephalus, and agenesis of the corpus callosum at 22 post-menstrual weeks: The mass spectrum or L1 spectrum. A case report and review of the literature. *Prenat Diagn* 1996;16:543–8.
32. Patel MD, Filly AL, Hersh DR, Goldstein RB. Isolated mild fetal cerebral ventriculomegaly: Clinical course and outcome. *Radiology* 1994;192:759–64.
33. Pilu G, Falco P, Gabrielli S, Perolo A, Sandri F, Bovicelli L. The clinical significance of fetal isolated cerebral borderline ventriculomegaly: Report of 31 cases and review of the literature. *Ultrasound Obstet Gynecol* 1999;14:320–6.
34. Wakayama A, Morimoto K, Kitajima H *et al.* Extremely low birth-weight infant with hydrocephalus; management of hydrocephalus using a miniature Ommaya's reservoir. *No Shinkei Geka* 1991;19:795–800.
35. Morimoto K, Hayakawa T, Yoshimine T, Wakayama A, Kuroda R. Two-step procedure for early neonatal surgery of fetal hydrocephalus. *Neurol Med Chir* 1993;33:158–65.
36. Fritsch MJ, Mehdorn M. Endoscopic intraventricular surgery for treatment of hydrocephalus and loculated CSF space in children less than one year of age. *Pediatr Neurosurg* 2002;36: 183–8.
37. Martinez de Villarreal L, Perez JZ, Vazquez PA, *et al.* Decline of neural tube defects cases after a folic acid campaign in Nuevo Leon, Mexico. *Teratology* 2002;66:249–56.
38. Ray JG, Meier C, Vermeulen MJ, Boss S, Wyatt PR, Cole DE. Association of neural tube defects and folic acid food fortification in Canada. *Lancet* 2002;360:2047–8.
39. Persad VL, Van den Hof MC, Dube JM, Zimmer P. Incidence of open neural tube defects in Nova Scotia after folic acid fortification. *Can Med Assoc J* 2002;167:241–5.
40. Mathews TJ, Honein MA, Erickson JD. Spina bifida and anencephaly prevalence – United States, 1991–2001. *MMWR Recomm Rep* 2002;51:9–11.
41. Green NS. Folic acid supplementation and prevention of birth defects. *J Nutr* 2002;132:2356S–2360S.
42. Monteagudo A, Timor-Tritsch IE. Fetal neurosonography of congenital brain anomalies. In Timor-Tritsch IE, Monteagudo A, Cohen HL, eds. *Ultrasonography of the Prenatal and Neonatal Brain*, 2nd edn. New York: McGraw-Hill, 2001;151–258.
43. Stevenson RE, Allen WP, Pai GS *et al.* Decline in prevalence of neural tube defects in a high-risk region of the United States. *Pediatrics* 2000;106:677–83.
44. Volpe JJ. Neural tube formation and prosencephalic development. *Neurology of the Newborn*, 4th edn. Philadelphia, PA: WB Saunders, 2001;3–44.
45. D'Addario V, Pinto V, Del Bianco A *et al.* The clivus-supraocciput angle: A useful measurement to evaluate the shape and size of the fetal posterior fossa and to diagnose Chiari II malformation. *Ultrasound Obstet Gynecol* 2001;18:146–9.
46. Cohen MM Jr. Perspectives on holoprosencephaly. I. Epidemiology, genetics and symdromology. *Teratology* 1989;40:211–35.
47. Pilu G, Ambrosetto P, Sandri F *et al.* Intraentricular fused fornices: A specific sign of fetal lobar holoprosencephaly. *Ultrasound Obstet Gynecol* 1994;34:259–62.
48. Cohen MM. An update on the holoprosencephalic disorders. *J Pediatr* 1982;101:865–9.
49. Pilu G, Porelo A, Falco P, Visentin A. Median anomalies of the brain. In Timor-Tritsch IE, Monteagudo A, Cohen HL, eds.

Ultrasonography of the Prenatal and Neonatal Brain, 2nd edn. New York: McGraw-Hill, 2001;259–76.
50. Goodyear PW, Bannister CM, Russell S, Rimmer S. Outcome in prenatally diagnosed fetal agenesis of the corpus callosum. *Fetal Diagn Ther* 2001;16:139–45.
51. Taylor M, David AS. Agenesis of the corpus callosum: A United Kingdom series of 56 cases. *J Neurol Neurosurg Psychiatry* 1998; 64:131–4.
52. Schmidt-Riese U, Zieger M. Ultrasound diagnosis of isolated aplasia of the septum pellucidum. *Ultraschall Med* 1994;15:286–92.
53. McMahon CL, Braddock SR. Septo-optic dysplasia as a manifestation of valproic acid embryopathy. *Teratology* 2001;64:83–6.
54. Dominguez R, Aguirre Vila-Coro A, Slopis JM, Bohan TP. Brain and ocular abnormalities in infants with in utero exposure to cocaine and other street drugs. *Am J Dis Child* 1991;145: 688–95.
55. Dattani MT, Martinez-Barbera JP, Thomas PQ *et al*. Mutations in the homeobox gene HESX1/Hesx1 associated with septo-optic dysplasia in human and mouse. *Nat Genet* 1998;19:125–33.
56. Volpe JJ. Neuronal proliferation, migration, organization and myelination. *Neurology of the Newborn*, 4th edn. Philadelphia, PA: WB Saunders, 2001;45–99.
57. Kobayashi K, Nakahori Y, Miyake M *et al*. An ancient retrotransposal insertion causes Fukuyama-type congenital muscular dystrophy. *Nature* 1998;394(6691):388–92.
58. McGahan JP, Grix A, Gerscovich EO. Prenatal diagnosis of lissencephaly: Miller–Dieker syndrome. *J Clin Ultrasound* 1994; 22:560–3.
59. Greco P, Resta M, Vimercati A *et al*. Antenatal diagnosis of isolated lissencephaly by ultrasound and magnetic resonance imaging. *Ultrasound Obstet Gynecol* 1998;12:276–9.
60. Kojima K, Suzuki Y, Seki K *et al*. Prenatal diagnosis of lissencephaly (type II) by ultrasound and fast magnetic resonance imaging. *Fetal Diagn Ther* 2002;17:34–6.
61. Granata T, Farina L, Faiella A *et al*. Familial schizencephaly associated with EMX2 mutation. *Neurology* 1997;48:1403–6.
62. Brunelli S, Faiella A, Capra V *et al*. Germline mutations in the homeobox gene EMX2 in patients with severe schizencephaly. *Nat Genet* 1996;12:94–6.
63. Iannetti P, Nigro G, Spalice A, Faiella A, Boncinelli E. Cytomegalovirus infection and schizencephaly: Case reports. *Ann Neurol* 1998;43:123–7.
64. Denis D, Maugey-Laulom B, Carles D, Pedespan JM, Brun M, Chateil JF. Prenatal diagnosis of schizencephaly by fetal magnetic resonance imaging. *Fetal Diagn Ther* 2001;16:354–9.
65. Osenbach RK, Menezes AH. Diagnosis and management of the Dandy–Walker malformation: 30 years of experience. *Pediatr Neurosurg* 1991;18:179–85.
66. Barkovich AJ, Kjos BO, Normal D *et al*. Revised classification of the posterior fossa cysts and cyst-like malformations based on the results of multiplanar MR imaging. *AJNR Am J Neuroradiol* 1989;10:977–88.
67. Bretelle F, Senat MV, Bernard JP, Hillion Y, Ville Y. First-trimester diagnosis of fetal arachnoid cyst: prenatal implication. *Ultrasound Obstet Gynecol* 2002;20:400–2.
68. Elbers SE, Furness ME. Resolution of presumed arachnoid cyst in utero. *Ultrasound Obstet Gynecol* 1999;14:353–5.
69. Ciricillo SF, Cogen PH, Harsh GR *et al*. Intracranial arachnoid cysts in children. A comparison of the effects of fenestration and shunting. *J Neurosurg* 1991;74:230–5.
70. Nakamura Y, Mizukawa K, Yamamoto K, Nagashima T. Endoscopic treatment for a huge neonatal prepontine-suprasellar arachnoid cyst: A case report. *Pediatr Neurosurg* 2001;35:220–4.
71. Hollway GE, Suthers GK, Haan EA *et al*. Mutation detection in FGFR2 craniosynostosis syndromes. *Hum Genet* 1997;99: 251–5.
72. Delashaw JB, Persing JA, Broaddus WC, Jane JA. Cranial vault growth in craniosynostosis. *J Neurosurg* 1989;70:159–65.
73. Benacerraf BR, Spiro R, Mitchell AG. Using three-dimensional ultrasound to detect craniosynostosis in a fetus with Pfeiffer syndrome. *Ultrasound Obstet Gynecol* 2000;16:391–4.
74. Pooh RK, Nakagawa Y, Pooh KH, Nakagawa Y, Nagamachi N. Fetal craniofacial structure and intracranial morphology in a case of Apert syndrome. *Ultrasound Obstet Gynecol* 1999;13:274–80.
75. Raybaud CA, Strother CM, Hald JK. Aneurysms of the vein of Galen: Embryonic considerations and anatomical features relating to the pathogenesis of the malformation. *Neuroradiology* 1989;31:109–28.
76. Hoffman HJ, Chuang S, Hendrick EB, Humphreys RP. Aneurysms of the vein of Galen. Experience at The Hospital for Sick Children, Toronto. *J Neurosurg* 1982;57(3):316–22.
77. Campi A, Rodesch G, Scotti G, Lasjaunias P. Aneurysmal malformation of the vein of Galen in three patients: clinical and radiological follow-up. *Neuroradiology* 1998;40(12):816–21.
78. Friedman DM, Verma R, Madrid M, Wisoff JH, Berenstein A. Recent improvement in outcome using transcatheter embolization techniques for neonatal aneurysmal malformations of the vein of Galen. *Pediatrics* 1993;91(3):583–6.
79. Sullivan A, Giudice T, Vavelidis F, Thiagarajah S. Choroid plexus cysts: Is biochemical testing a valuable adjunct to targeted ultrasonography? *Am J Obstet Gynecol* 1999;181:260–5.
80. Reinsch RC. Choroid plexus cysts – association with trisomy: Prospective review of 16,059 patients. *Am J Obstet Gynecol* 1997;176:1381–3.
81. Morcos CL, Platt LD, Carlson DE, Gregory KD, Greene NH, Korst LM. The isolated choroid plexus cyst. *Obstet Gynecol* 1998;92: 232–6.
82. Farhood AI, Morris JH, Bieber FR. Transient cysts of the fetal choroid plexus: Morphology and histogenesis. *Am J Med Genet* 1987;27:977–82.
83. Lam AH, Villanueva AC. Symptomatic third ventricular choroid plexus cysts. *Pediatr Radiol* 1992;22:413–16.
84. Parizek J, Jakubec J, Hobza V *et al*. Choroid plexus cyst of the left lateral ventricle with intermittent blockage of the foramen of Monro, and initial invagination into the III ventricle in a child. *Childs Nerv Syst* 1998;14:700–8.
85. Pooh RK, Maeda K, Pooh KH. *An Atlas of Fetal Central Nervous System Disease. Diagnosis and Management.* London: Parthenon CRC Press, 2003.
86. Wakai S, Arai T, Nagai M. Congenital brain tumors. *Surg Neurol* 1984;21:597–609.
87. Volpe JJ. Brain tumors and vein of Galen malformation. *Neurology of the Newborn*, 4th edn. Philadelphia, PA: WB Saunders, 2001;841–56.
88. Sherer DM, Abramowicz JS, Eggers PC, Metlay LA, Sinkin RA, Woods JR Jr. Prenatal ultrasonographic diagnosis of intracranial teratoma and massive craniomegaly with associated high-output cardiac failure. *Am J Obstet Gynecol* 1993;168:97–9.
89. Lu JH, Emons D, Kowalewski S. Connatal periventricular pseudocysts in the neonate. *Pediatr Radiol* 1992;22(1):55–8.
90. Malinger G, Lev D, Ben Sira L, Kidron D, Tamarkin M, Lerman-Sagie T. Congenital periventricular pseudocysts: prenatal sonographic appearance and clinical implications. *Ultrasound Obstet Gynecol* 2002;20(5):447–51.
91. Bats AS, Molho M, Senat MV, Paupe A, Bernard JP, Ville Y. Subependymal pseudocysts in the fetal brain: Prenatal diagnosis of two cases and review of the literature. *Ultrasound Obstet Gynecol* 2002;20(5):502–5.
92. Eller KM, Kuller JA. Porencephaly secondary to fetal trauma during amniocentesis. *Obstet Gynecol* 1995;85:865–7.
93. Volpe JJ. Hypoxic–ischemic encephalopathy: Neuropathology and pathogenesis. *Neurology of the Newborn*, 4th edn. Philadelphia, PA: WB Saunders, 2001;296–330.
94. Meizner I, Elchalal U. Prenatal sonographic diagnosis of anterior fossa porencephaly. *J Clin Ultrasound* 1996;24:96–9.
95. de Laveaucoupet J, Audibert F, Guis F *et al*. Magnetic resonance imaging (MRI) of ischemic brain injury. *Prenat Diagn* 2001;21: 729–36.
96. Scher MS, Belfar H, Martin J, Painter MJ. Destructive brain lesions of presumed fetal onset: Antepartum causes of cerebral palsy. *Pediatrics* 1991;88:898–906.
97. Stevenson DA, Hart BL, Clericuzio CL. Hydranencephaly in an infant with vascular malformations. *Am J Med Genet* 2001;104: 295–8.
98. Lam YH, Tang MH. Serial sonographic features of a fetus with hydranencephaly from 11 weeks to term. *Ultrasound Obstet Gynecol* 2000;16:77–9.
99. Sherer DM, Anyaegbunam A, Onyeije C. Antepartum fetal intracranial hemorrhage, predisposing factors and prenatal sonography: A review. *Am J Perinatol* 1998;15:431–41.
100. Hardart GE, Fackler JC. Predictors of intracranial hemorrhage during neonatal extracorporeal membrane oxygenation. *J Pediatr* 1999;134:156–9.
101. Rezaie P, Dean A. Periventricular leukomalacia, inflammation and white matter lesions within the developing nervous system. *Neuropathology* 2002;22:106–32.

40 Ultrasound of the fetal thorax

A. Khurana

Technological advances in transducer and software technology have in recent years remarkably improved visualization of structures in the fetal thorax (Figures 40.1–40.4) way beyond the minimum requirement recommended by the American Institute of Ultrasound in Medicine[1] over the last few decades. Additionally, novel methods of *in utero* treatment, the evolution of neonatal surgical techniques and anesthesia, the newer understanding of the natural course of several malformations and the pressing social and legal need for informed parental counseling have placed a new responsibility on the shoulders of the practicing ultrasonologist.

There is now a pressing demand for an accurate diagnosis, the formulation of a prognosis and the institution of appropriate management whether it be expectant observation, *in utero* therapy or a referral to a tertiary care center.

This presentation reviews current concepts in the evaluation of the fetal thorax (excluding cardiac conditions).

Embryology

Knowledge of the embryology of the thoracic viscera is imperative to understand the outcome of congenital thoracic malformations and their direct bearing on fetal lung developments and ultimate fetal and neonatal outcomes.

Development of the lung begins at 5 weeks.[2] The epithelium of the respiratory system develops from the endoderm. The connective tissue, cartilage and muscle develop from splanchnic mesoderm and neural crest cells.

At 26 days the foregut evaginates to form a laryngotracheal diverticulum. This then gets separated from the foregut by longitudinal folds, which progress to form the tracheoesophageal septum. The lungs develop in four stages. From 5 to 17 weeks all elements are developed except those involved in gas exchange. This is also called the pseudoglandular period. From 16 to 25 weeks (canalicular period) the lumen of bronchi and

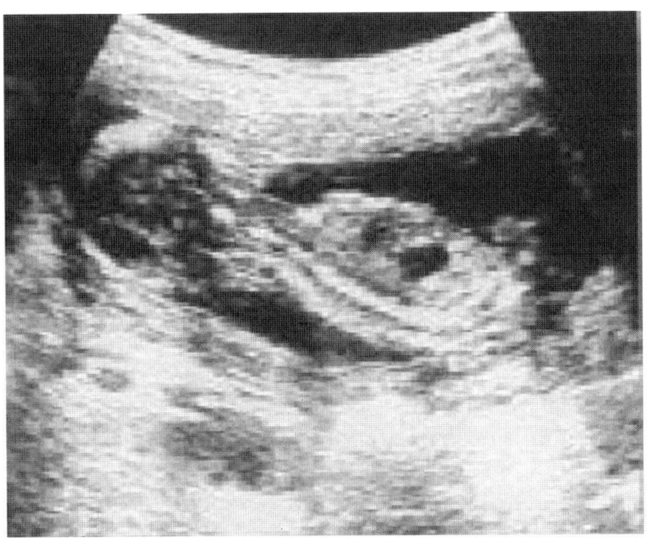

Figure 40.1

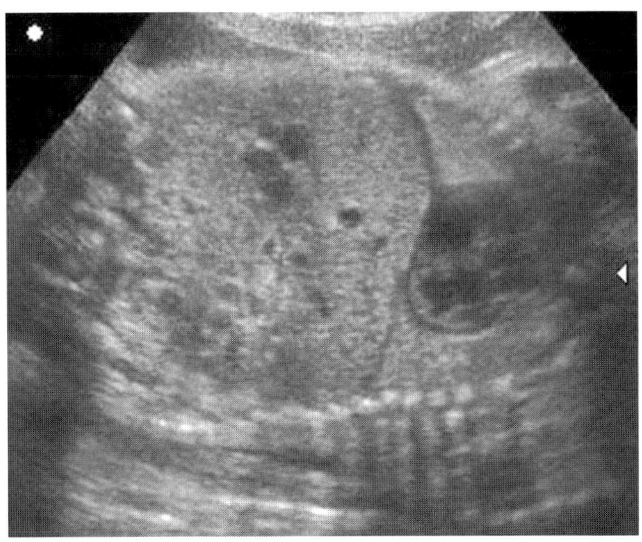

Figure 40.2

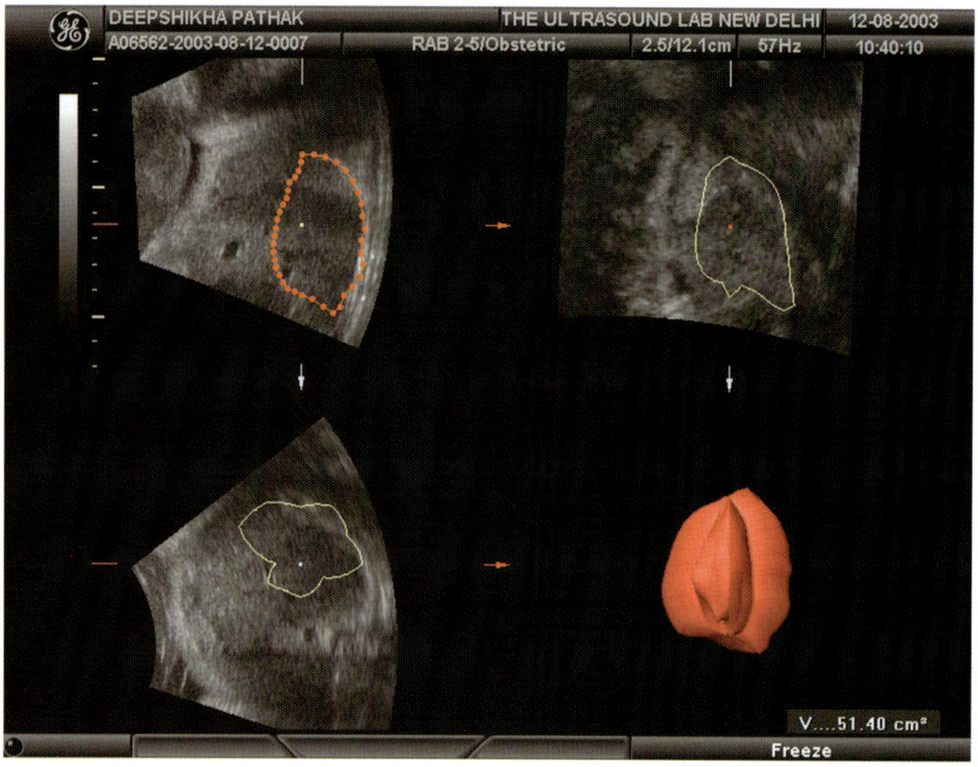

Figure 40.3

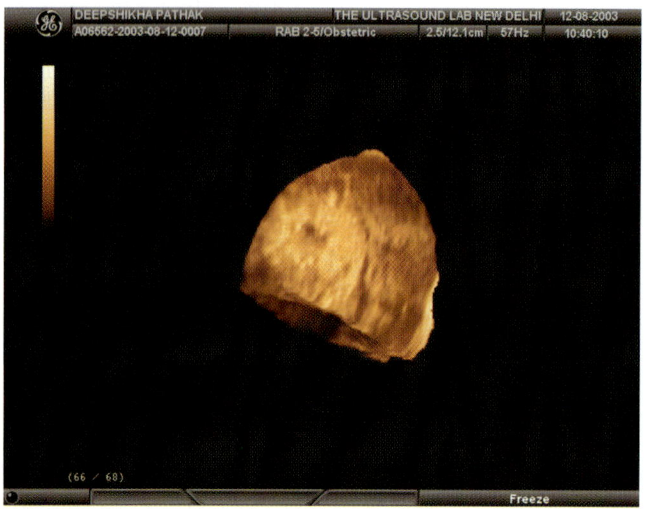

Figure 40.4

bronchioles become larger, and respiratory bronchioles and alveolar ducts develop. Some terminal sacs develop and the tissue becomes more vascular. From 25 weeks to birth, many more terminal sacs develop, the epithelium becomes very thick, capillaries bunch into alveoli, Type I alveolar cells develop and Type II alveolar cells begin producing surfactant. From late fetushood and up to childhood, squamous epithelium forms and alveoli continue to form after birth.[3]

Sonoanatomy of the fetal thorax

The fetal thorax extends from the clavicles to the fetal diaphragm. The diaphragm is continuous, thin and hypoechoic (Figure 40.5) and moves with respiratory movements in the third trimester of pregnancy. The thorax is bounded by the sternum anteriorly, the spine posteriorly and the ribs circumferentially. The heart is the most prominent structure in the thorax. The lungs are seen surrounding it. The left lung is limited in its extent by the heart (Figure 40.6). The lungs are homogenously echogenic and largely isoechoic with other mediastinal structures. The heart occupies one-third to half of the thorax and its location and axis are important to identify and evaluate non-cardiac conditions as well. Cardiac and mediastinal shifts have a tremendous bearing on the prognosis of a chest lesion. No fluid is seen in normal pleural spaces. The pleural and pericardial space should be evaluated to assess for hydrops, which again is a prognostic factor in the assessment of a chest mass. With some effort and resort to color flow mapping (Figure 40.7) and power Doppler studies, the aortic arch, pulmonary artery, ductus arteriosus, pulmonary veins, trachea, esophagus and thymus can be adequately evaluated.[4–6]

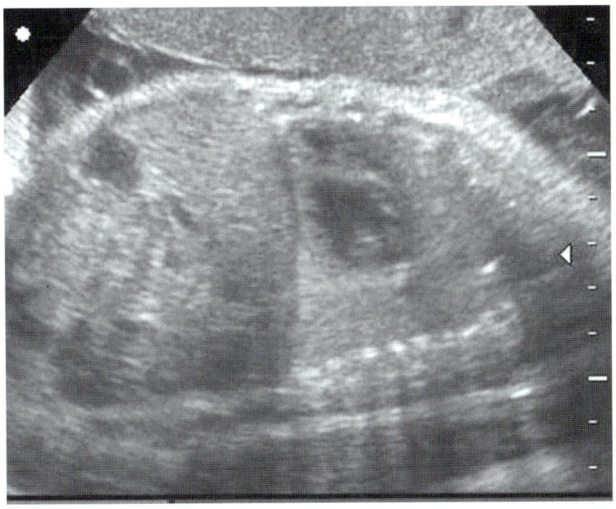

Figure 40.5

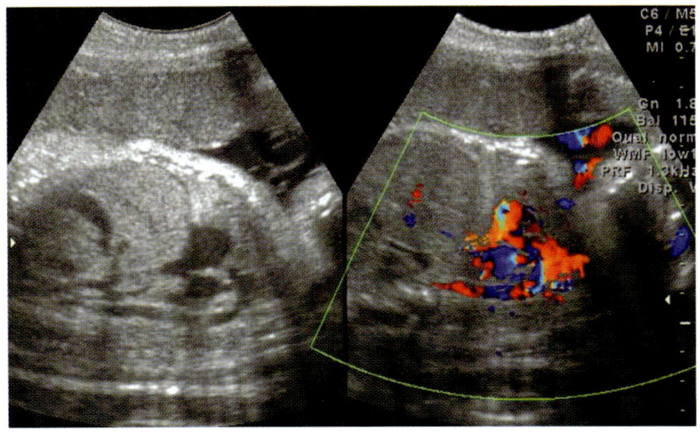

Figure 40.7

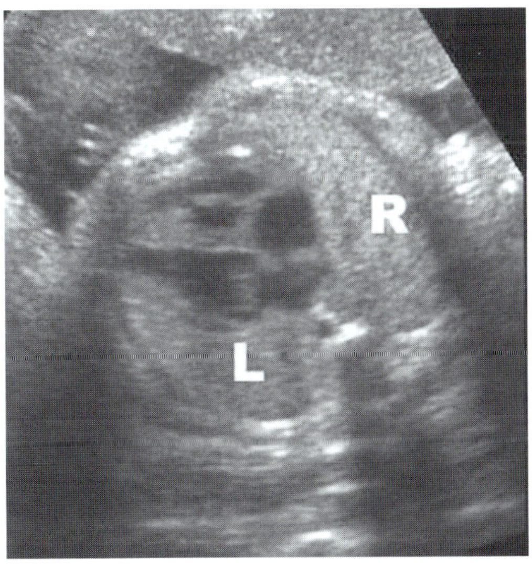

Figure 40.6

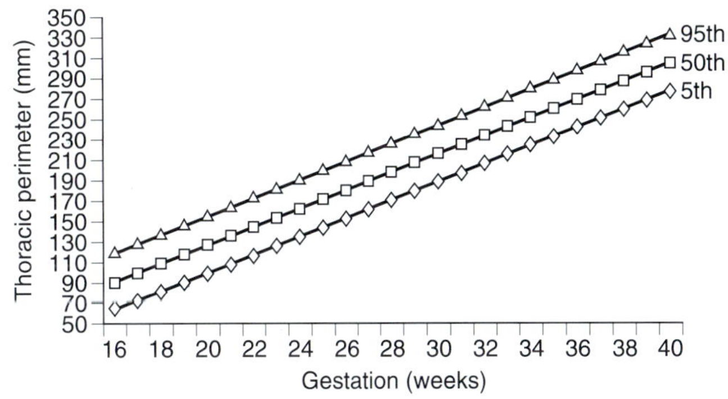

Figure 40.8

Pulmonary hypoplasia

Adequate lung development is central to fetal viability.[7,8] Hypoplastic lungs show a low lung to body weight ratio and histologically demonstrate a reduced number of alveoli.[9] Pulmonary hypoplasia is rarely primary and rarely unilateral.[10,11] It is usually secondary and consequent to any prolonged severe oligoamnios,[12–15] in skeletal dysplasias with a small bony thorax, in sizable intrathoracic masses,[16,17] consequent to neuromuscular dysfunction as in the Pena–Shokeir syndrome,[18] in trisomy 12, 18 and 21 and in conditions with decreased pulmonary artery perfusion.[19]

Thoracic perimeter measurements[20–23] (Figure 40.8) are made at the level of the four-chamber view and should exclude the soft tissue areas beyond the ribs. The thoracic perimeter/abdominal perimeter ratio[24–26] is steady through the late second trimester and in the third trimester: >0.80. Lung lengths[27] although well studied (Figure 40.9) are not easily reproducible. Fetal lung volumes by three-dimensional reconstruction techniques (Figure 40.10) are reliable and reproducible.[28,29]

The pathogenesis of pulmonary hypoplasia commences with inadequate thoracic space for growth, inadequate breathing movements of whatever cause, inadequate fluid within the lung and suboptimal quantities of amniotic fluid.[30] Lung echogenicity does not correlate with lung maturity.

General features of chest masses

Not all lung masses can be delineated in the 18–20 weeks anomalies scan although embryologically they do

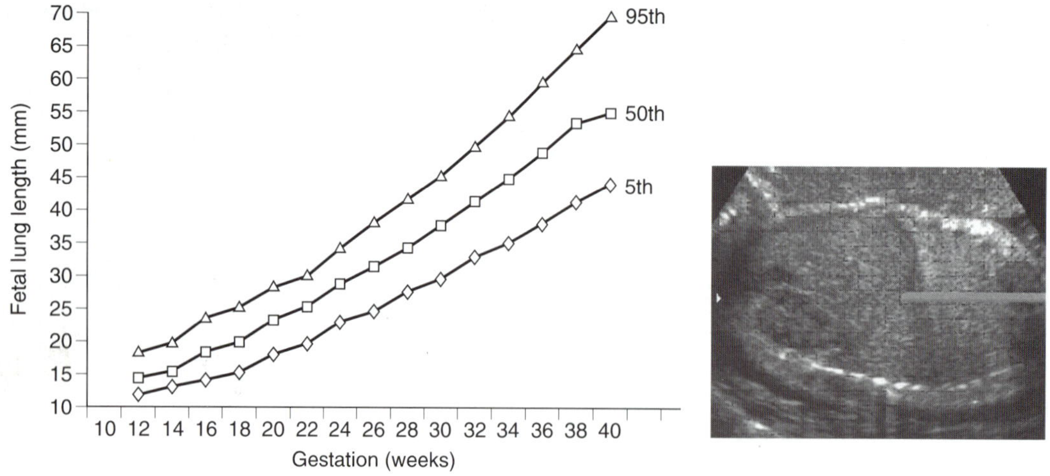

Figure 40.9

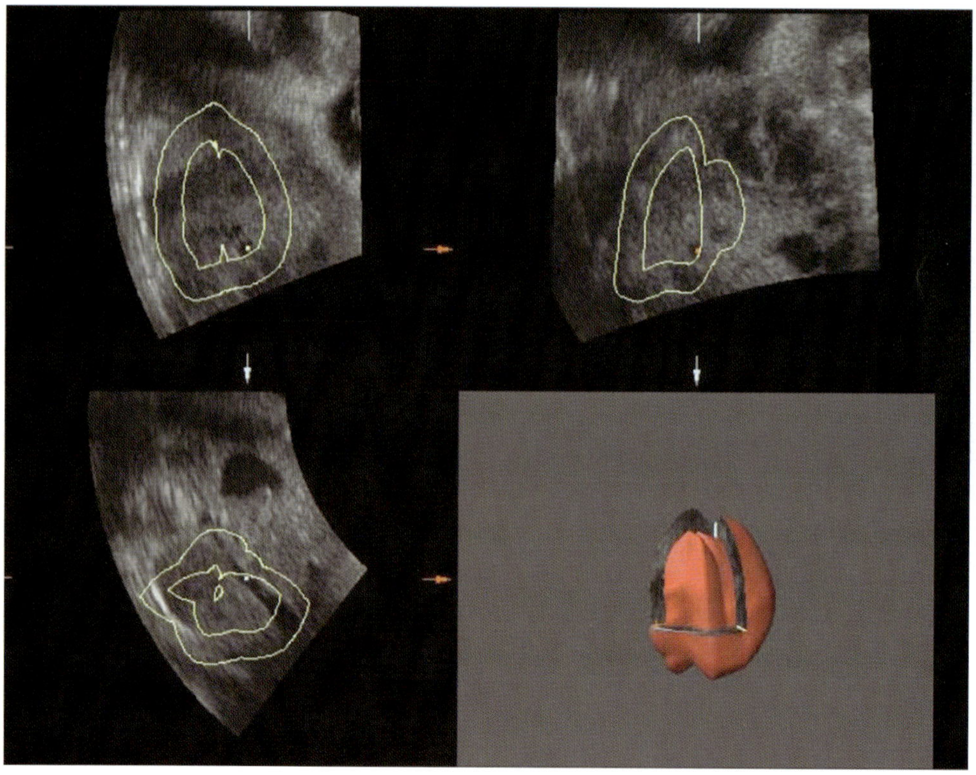

Figure 40.10

exist.[31,32] Depending on their size and growth they result in unilateral or bilateral hypoplasia of the lungs. Prognosis depends on the size of the lesion, heart and mediastinal displacements, the resence of hydrops, associated structural anomalies, underlying chromosomal abnormalities and the bearing of associated polyhydramnios on preterm premature rupture of membranes and prematurity.[33–35]

Common chest masses include congenital diaphragmatic hernia (CDH) and congenital cystic adenomatoid malformations (CCAM). Other lung masses include bronchogenic cysts, neurenteric cysts, congenital lobar emphysema (CLE), bronchial atresia, pulmonary gigantism, bronchopulmonary sequestration (BPS) and mediastinal masses. The mediastinal lesions include teratomas,[36] thymomas,[37] goiter, cardiac lesions such as rhabdomyoma, myxoma and fibroma,[38–40] esophageal duplication cysts,[41] enteric cysts,[41] neurenteric cysts[42–44] and thoracic neuroblastoma. Mediastinal lesions are rare but important in the perspective of a differential diagnosis of a mass adjacent to the mediastinum but arising from the adjacent lung or from the abdomen.

Congenital diaphragmatic hernia

CDH has an incidence of 1–4.5/10,000 live births.[45] The incidence is higher in the fetus and a fair number are lost *in utero* or in the neonatal period prior to clinical identification. CDH is more common on the left side but not infrequently right sided or bilateral. The diaphragm forms between the 6th and 14th weeks of pregnancy by fusion of the septum transversum, pleuroperitoneal membranes, mesentery of the esophagus and the body wall. Failure of fusion especially of the pleuroperitoneal membranes results in a herniation of abdominal contents into the thorax when the gut returns to the abdomen. The disorder is progressive and the organs that herniate include the stomach, liver, spleen, small bowel and colon. Left-sided CDH usually involves the stomach. Right-sided CDH usually involves herniation of the liver. The herniation may be small, isoechoic and intermittent[46] and may therefore go unrecognized except when the problem is specifically looked for. Over four of five fetuses die in the neonatal period usually because of pulmonary hypoplasia and pulmonary hypertension. Pulmonary hypertension is consequent to the poorly understood but well documented medial wall muscular hypertrophy of the small pulmonary arteries extending up to the preacinar vessels. Newborns have a high incidence of feeding problems, gastroesophageal reflux, chronic lung disease and neurodevelopmental delays.[45,47] Sonographic signs[48] include a low abdominal perimeter, failure to visualize the fetal stomach in the fetal abdomen (Figure 40.11), visualization of the herniated viscera in the thorax (Figures 40.12 and 40.13), cardiomediastinal shift, pleural effusions and hydrops. There may also be failure to delineate the diaphragm in its entire extent. Right-sided hernias are difficult to identify because of isoechoic lung and these should be evaluated by color Doppler to confirm the location of the portal vein in the thorax (Figures 40.14 and 40.15). Although identification of the liver is not critical for a diagnosis of CDH, it has a major bearing on the prognosis.[49,50] This is so because after surgical repair the ductus venosus and umbilical vein often get kinked or compromised, thereby contributing to morbidity and often mortality. When bowel segments are not fluid-filled, as is common in the second trimester, they may appear as a non-specific chest mass (Figure 40.16). Careful

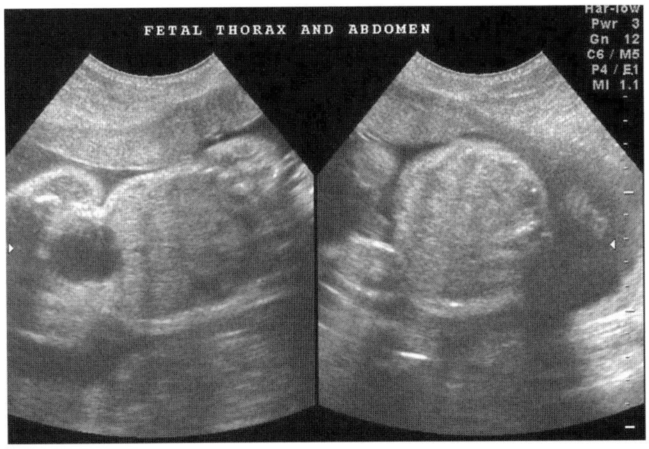

Figure 40.11

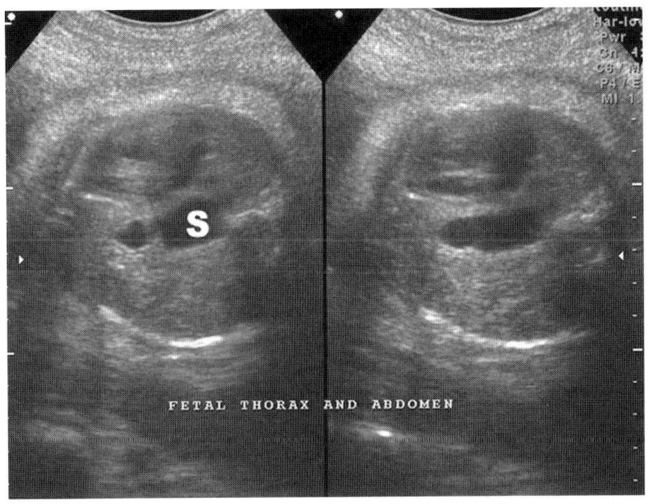

Figure 40.12

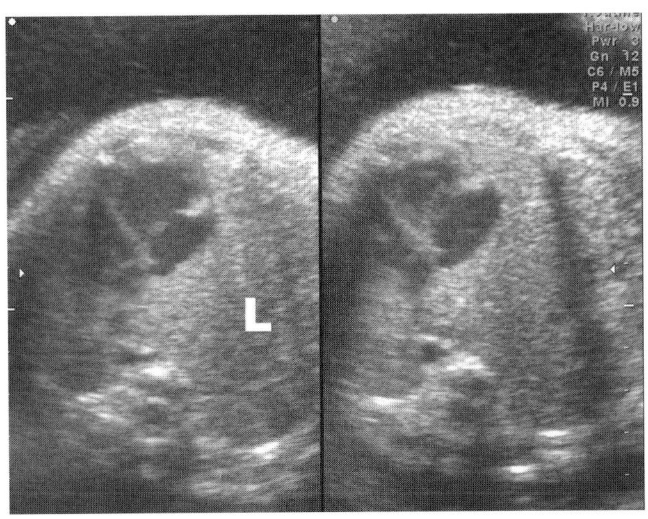

Figure 40.13

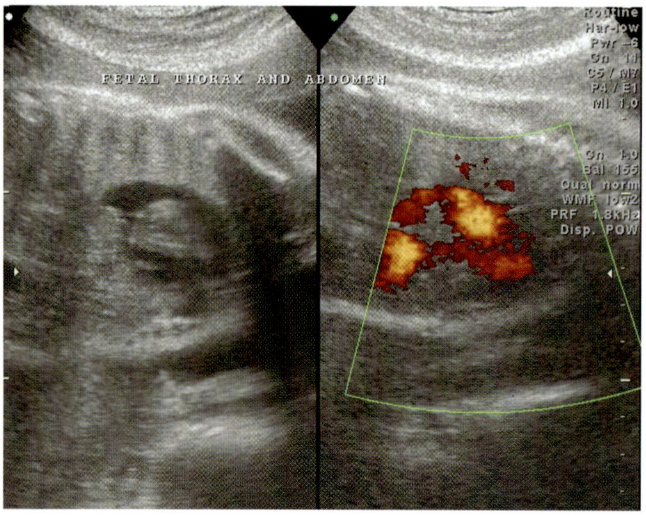

Figure 40.14

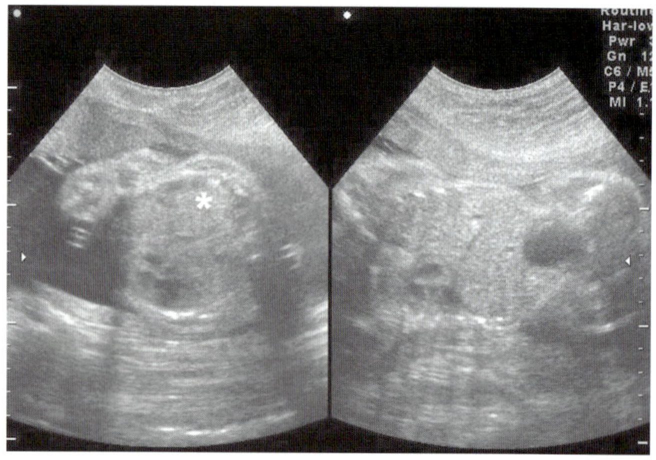

Figure 40.16

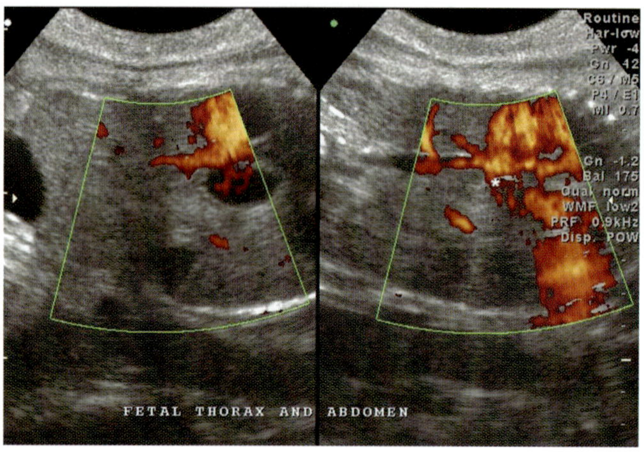

Figure 40.15

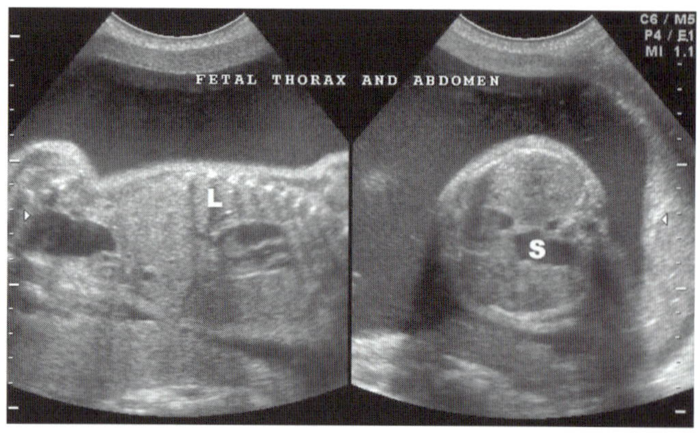

Figure 40.17

real-time scanning would reveal peristalsis in the third trimester. Occasionally, a gallbladder may be seen in the CDH. Bilateral hernias may be difficult to detect because of no cardiomediastinal shift. Ascites within a herniation may be mistaken for a pleural effusion.

Not all fetuses with a CDH have a poor prognosis.[51–54] Prognosis depends on gestational age at diagnosis, particularly if 24 weeks or earlier, large size, dilated stomach, the presence of the liver, even its left lobe in left-sided lesions, small contralateral lung, bilateral herniation (Figure 40.17) and the presence of associated anomalies (Figure 40.18). Because of the higher incidence of CDH in certain syndromes, facial and cardiac surveys merit special attention. These syndromes include trisomy 18, Fryn's, lethal pterygium, Beckwith–Wiedemann, Cornelia De Lange, Apert's and Goldenhahr.[55,56]

Fetal therapy has found a reasonable place in the treatment of CDH.[57] The aim of surgery is to prevent lung hypoplasia. Although fetal therapy initially involved reduction of the hernia by open repair *in utero*, current practice involves clipping of the trachea. Currently, videofetoscopic techniques are under evaluation. Tracheal occlusion results in increased lung volume and accelerated lung maturity similar to the pathophysiology seen in laryngeal and tracheal atresia.[58]

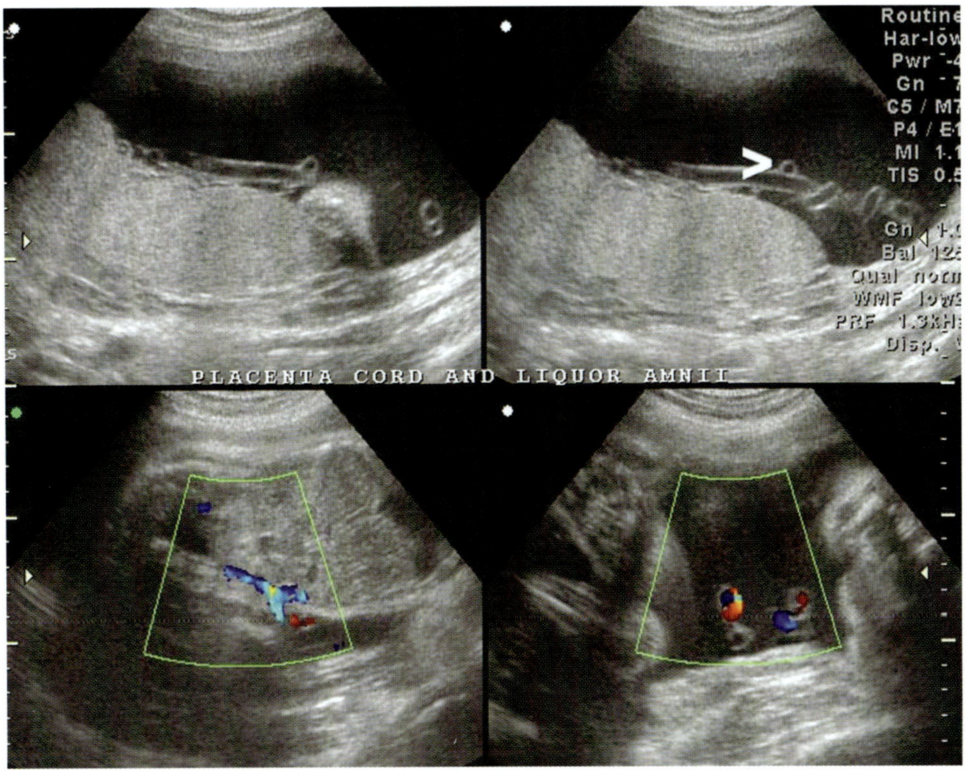

Figure 40.18

Congenital cystic adenomatoid malformations

CCAMs occur consequent to failure of induction of mesenchyme by bronchiolar epithelium. Lack of normal cellular development is considered to be consequent to focal bronchial atresia. The lesion is hamartomatous and characterized by focal abnormal proliferation of bronchiolar-like air spaces and absence of alveoli.[59] It is usually unilateral. Some may be associated with sequestration in the same lung. Diagnosis depends on the demonstration of a mass in the thorax.[60] This may be macrocystic (cysts 2–10 mm) (Figure 40.19), microcystic (cysts 0.3–0.5 mm) (Figure 40.20) or mixed[31,32] (Figure 40.21). These may cause a cardiomediastinal shift, ipsilateral and contralateral lung compression, pulmonary hypoplasia and hydrops. The lesion may regress spontaneously[61] (Figure 40.22). Prognosis depends on associated pulmonary hypoplasia, pulmonary hypertension, hydrops, associated anomalies, polyhydramnios and prematurity. Microcystic lesions are more likely to cause pulmonary hypoplasia and hydrops. The arterial supply is via a pulmonary artery and drainage into a pulmonary vein. Treatment of the lesion consists of expectant management, monitoring for hydrops or premature/term delivery followed by lobectomy if necessary.[33] Referral to a tertiary care center is important because emergency thoracic surgery is often needed. Recurrence is rare in later pregnancies. Since Klinefelter's syndrome and trisomy 18 are known for an association with CCAMs, it is appropriate to obtain a karyotype when the condition is diagnosed.

In utero aspiration of a larger cyst, thoracoamniotic shunting of a larger cyst and *in utero* resections have been attempted and are methods of gaining time to achieve viability. *In utero* resection has been tried only in fetuses with the poorest prognosis since the procedure itself carries a high morbidity and mortality.

Bronchopulmonary sequestration

Also known as pulmonary sequestration and accessory lung, BPS is a congenital malformation consisting of lung parenchyma, which is separated from normal lung. It receives arterial supply of systemic origin and does not communicate with the normal tracheobronchial tree. Sequestrations arise from a supernumerary anomalous outpouching of the foregut. If these arise prior to closure of the pleura they have no separate pleural envelope and are called intralobar

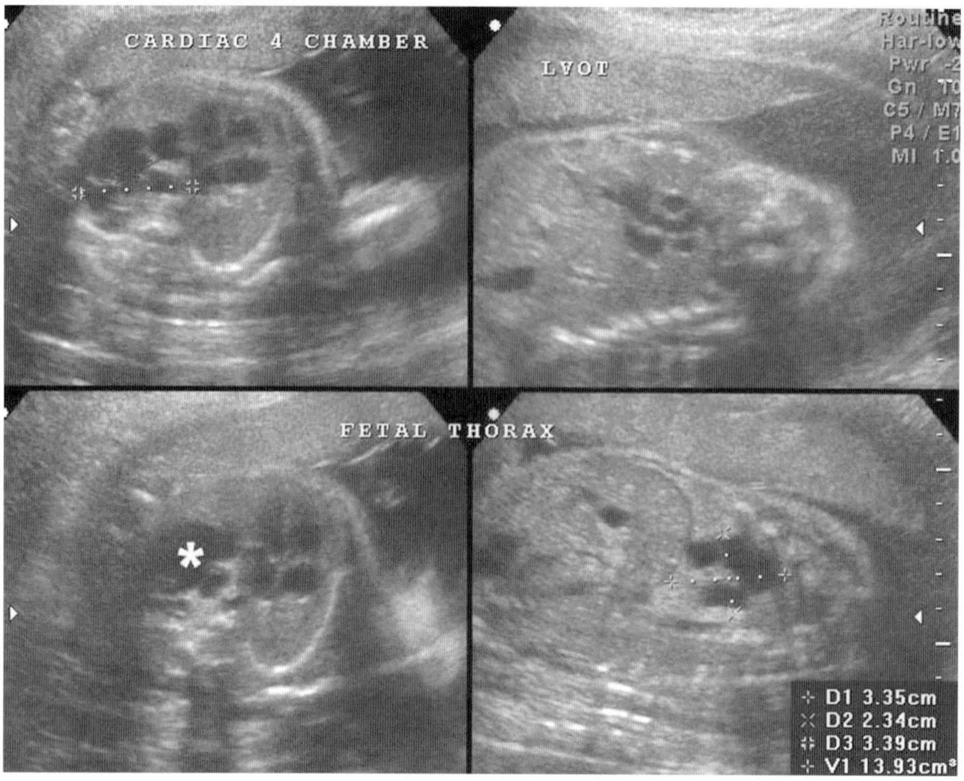

Figure 40.19

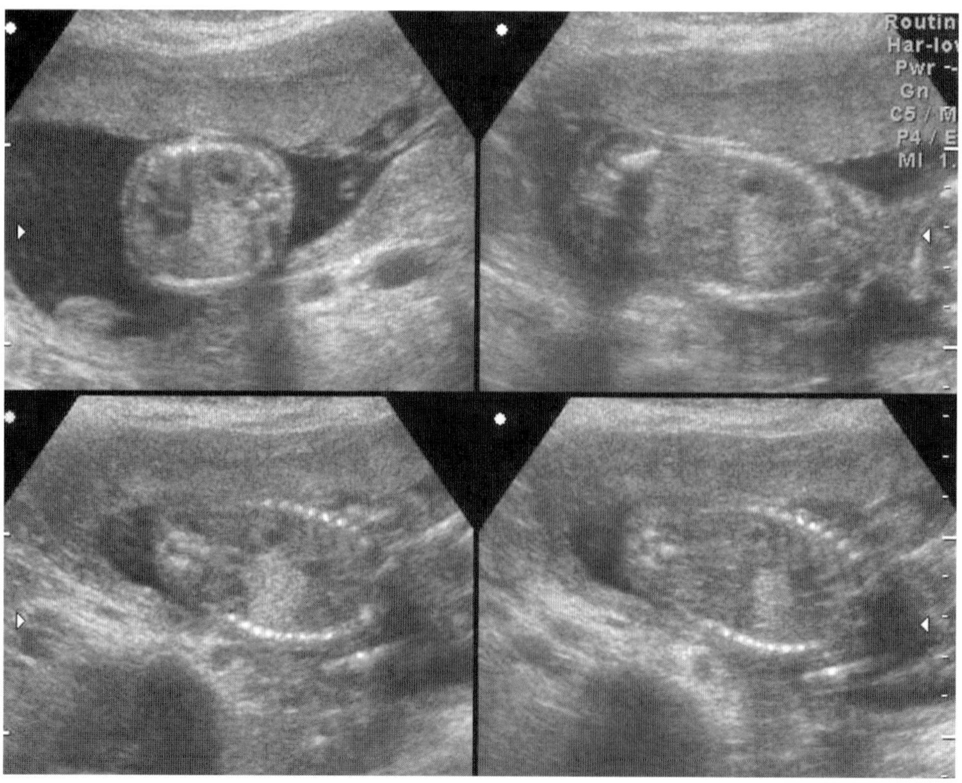

Figure 40.20

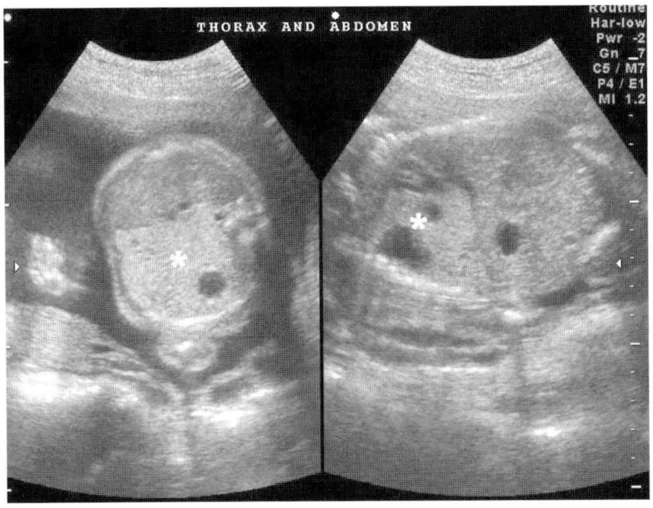

Figure 40.21

sequestrations. If these originate after closure of the pleura they are called extralobar sequestrations and have their own pleura. Intralobar sequestrations drain into pulmonary veins and extralobar sequestrations usually drain into a systemic vein, usually the azygos, hemiazygos or inferior vena cava. Extralobar sequestrations may be thoracic or extrathoracic and may even communicate with the esophagus.[62] They are occasionally associated with other thoracic and foregut anomalies such as CDH, CCAMs, bronchogenic cysts and neurenteric cysts. A wide variety of extrapulmonary anomalies including congenital heart disease, renal anomalies and hydrocephalus have been reported to coexist with sequestrations. Many sequestrations show extensive subpleural lymphatics, which account for ipsilateral pleural effusions. Typical sonographic appearances[63] include a lobar or triangular echogenic lesion in the lung base, usually left basal (Figure 40.23). Color Doppler studies reveal a systemic arterial supply[64] (Figure 40.24). There is a variable mediastinal shift and hydrops.

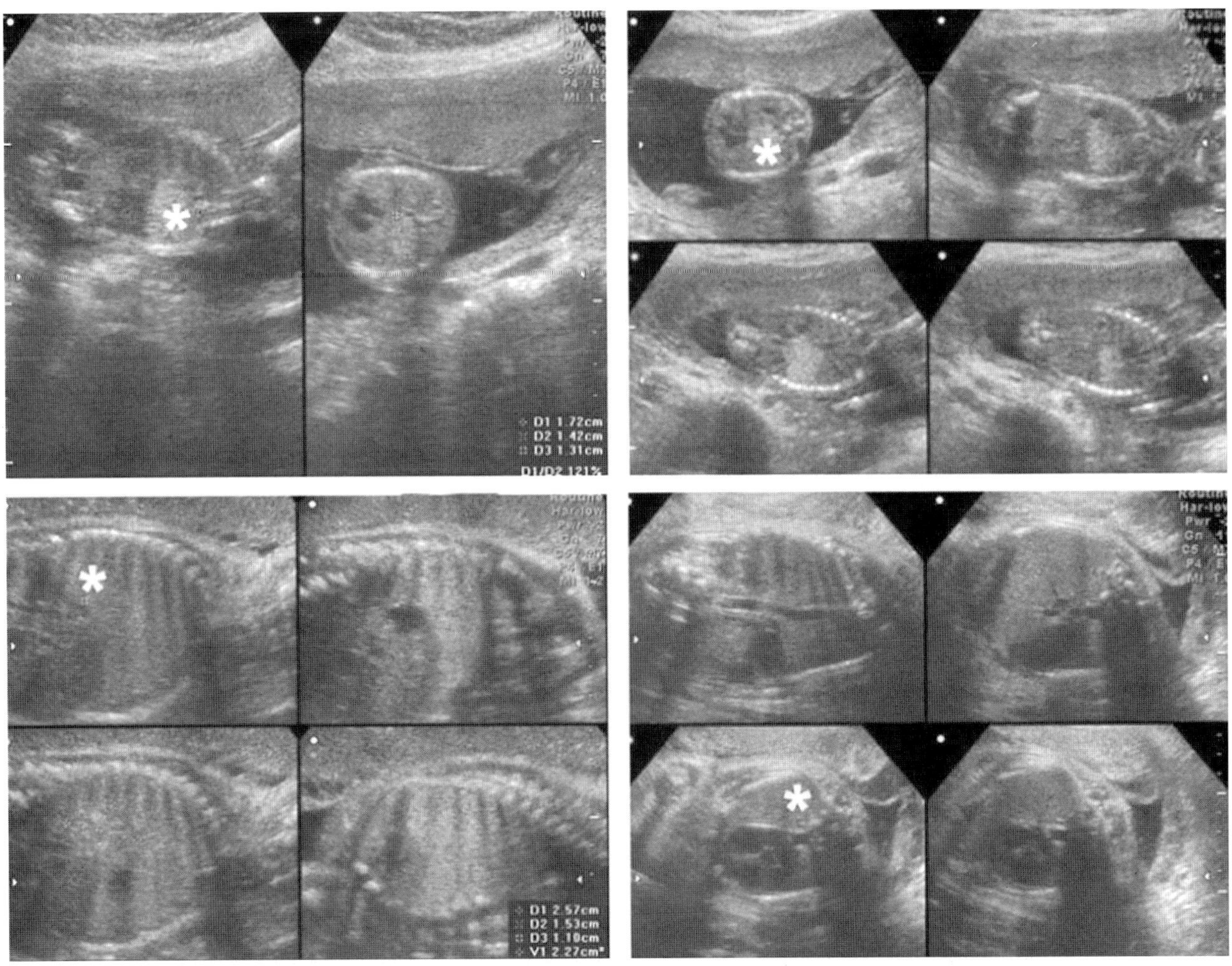

Figure 40.22

Several sequestrations regress spontaneously.[65] No specific features indicate which sequestrations are likely to resolve. Persistent sequestrations may stabilize or may need surgical resection (postnatal).

Bronchogenic cysts

These arise as a consequence of abnormal foregut budding and show variable echogenicity and variable progress. They may be mediastinal or peripheral and often show associated foregut malformations and hemivertebrae. The usual manifestation is an echogenic lesion representing fluid-filled lung beyond the stenosis. The left upper lobe is the most frequent site. Occasionally, these are multiple. These are usually innocuous and do not require specific obstetric management. Their importance lies in being one of the differential diagnoses of a fetal lung mass.[60]

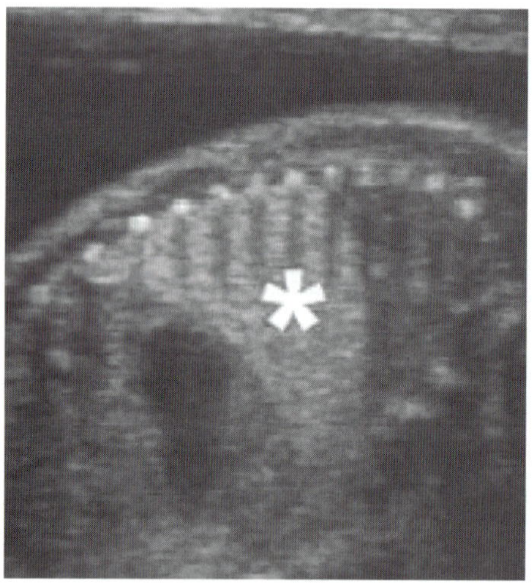

Figure 40.23

Laryngeal and tracheal atresia

These are rare congenital anomalies, which are associated with demise soon after birth, unless treated antenatally. These arise consequent to subglottic laryngeal atresia, tracheal stenosis or atresia, or tracheal webs or cysts and are also known as congenital high airways obstruction (CHAOS). Embryologically, persistent fusion of the sixth bronchial arches is apparently involved. Pathologically, failure of efflux of fluid from the fetal lung results in exaggerated lung development. Ultrasound features[66,67] include symmetric enlargement of both lungs (Figure 40.25) with anterior displacement of the heart. The lungs are homogenously echogenic, often similar to autosomal recessive infantile polycystic kidneys, since the underlying lesion consists of numerous fluid-filled spaces. The diaphragm is flat or inverted and cutaneous edema is common as is hydrops. Polyhydramnios is seen consequent to esophageal compression. The distal trachea and bronchii may be identified as tubular bulging fluid-laden structures in the mediastinum. Over half the fetuses with this abnormality have renal agenesis, facial anomalies and central nervous system malformations. To salvage a fetus with this anomaly it is necessary to establish a functional airway before the fetus is removed from placental support.[68]

Congenital lobar emphysema

Although this condition has clinical manifestations in the pediatric age group, it can be seen in the fetus as a solid lung mass akin to a microcystic CCAM or an ELS. It is usually located in the upper lobe unlike ELS. There is one case report of a spontaneous regression after indometacin treatment.[69]

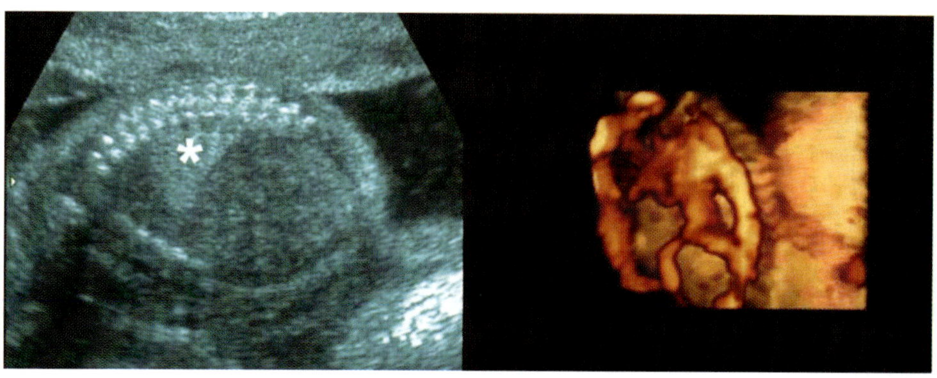

Figure 40.24

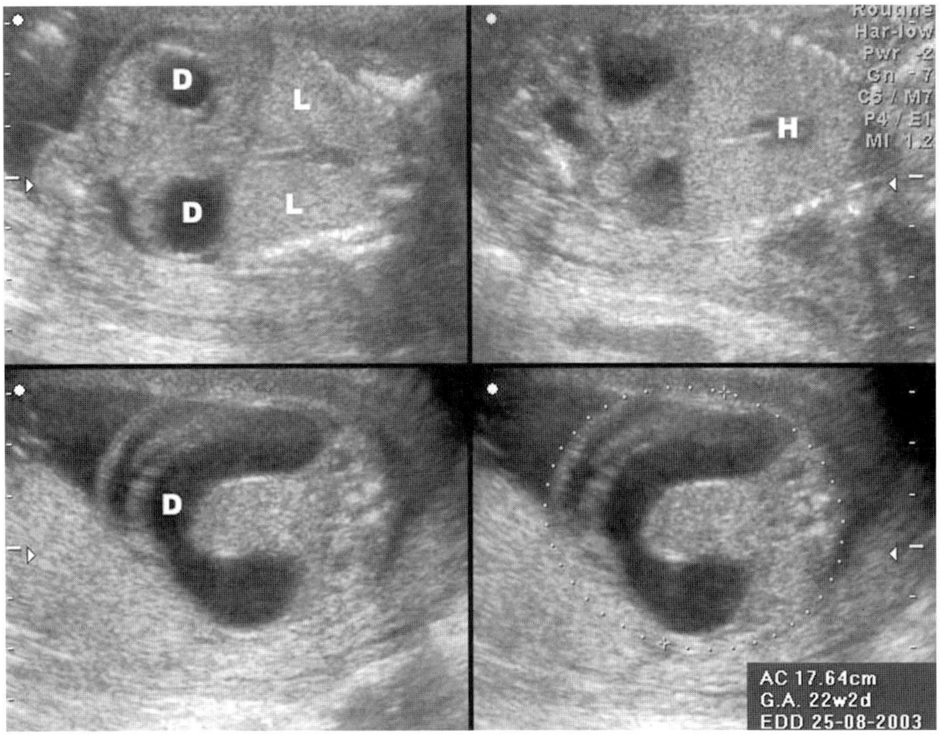

Figure 40.25

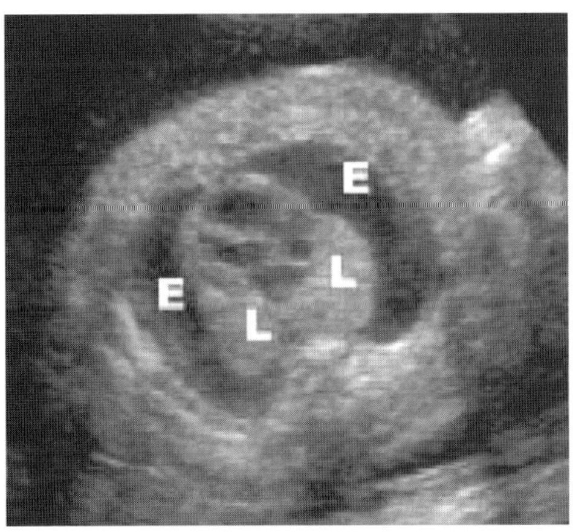

Figure 40.26

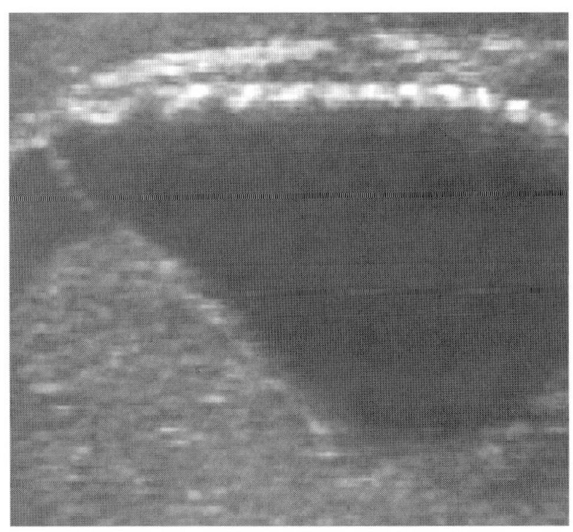

Figure 40.27

Pleural effusion

Unlike a small amount of pericardial fluid, which may be physiological, a fetal pleural fluid collection is always abnormal.

Primary pleural effusions are accumulations of pleural fluid, which may be idiopathic (Figures 40.26 and 40.27) or consequent to thoracic duct malformations[70]. They are unilateral or, if bilateral, markedly asymmetric. Mediastinal shifts are common and there are no associated findings except hydrops, which is an ominous finding. Pulmonary hypoplasia is common in large chronic effusions. The condition may resolve spontaneously and does very well after thoracentesis or thoraco-amniotic shunting.[71,72]

Secondary pleural effusions are consequent to other fetal anomalies and are often the earliest sign of immune or non-immune hydrops fetalis (NIHF).[73] The causes, therefore, include anemia, infection, cardiac anomalies, anomalies with large arteriovenous shunts, chromosomal abnormalities, skeletal dysplasias and thoracic malformations. Secondary effusions are usually bilateral and often associated with early onset of other signs of hydrops (Figure 40.28).

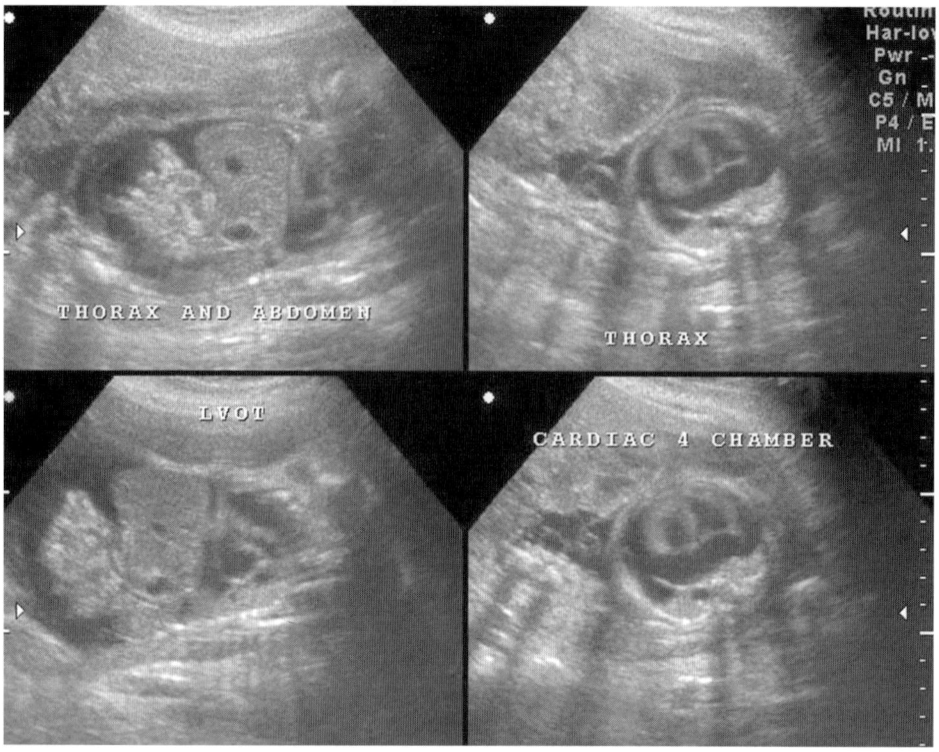

Figure 40.28

Prior to instituting any treatment procedure it is wise to exclude an abnormal fetal karyotype and assess fetal anemia.

Conclusion

The current approach to a thoracic lesion involves knowledge of sonographic features in order to make an accurate diagnosis. This should be followed by a careful evaluation for associated dysmorphic anomalies and identification of hydrops. An appropriate workup for fetal anemia and fetal karyotype should be considered next. The prognosis then needs to be formulated in the perspective of prevention of pulmonary hypoplasia, the possibility of spontaneous regression and referral to a tertiary care center. Ultrasound-guided interventions in such a fetus would include amniocentesis or cordocentesis for a complete diagnosis, and, from a therapeutic viewpoint, cyst aspiration, thoracentesis or a thoraco-amniotic shunt.

REFERENCES

1. American Institute of Ultrasound in Medicine. Guidelines for the performance of the antepartum obstetrical ultrasound examination. *J Ultrasound Med* 1996;15:185.
2. Moore KL, Persaud TVN. The respiratory system: Development of bronchi and lungs. In: *Before We Are Born: Essentials of Embryology and Birth Defects,* 5th edn. Philadelphia: WB Saunders, 1998:246.
3. Hislop AA, Wigglesworth JS, Desai R. Alveolar development in the human fetus and infant. *Early Hum Dev* 1986;13:1.
4. Felker RE, Cartier MS, Emerson DS, *et al.* Ultrasound of the fetal thymus. *J Ultrasound Med* 1989;8:669.
5. Jeanty P, Romero R, Hobbins JC. Fetal pericardial fluid: A normal finding of the second half of gestation. *Am J Obstet Gynecol* 1984;149:529.
6. Cooper C, Mahony BS, Bowie JD, *et al.* Ultrasound evaluation of the normal fetal upper airway and esophagus. *J Ultrasound Med* 1985;4:343.
7. Kilbride HW, Yeast J, Thibeault DW. Defining limits of survival: Lethal pulmonary hypoplasia after midtrimester premature rupture of membranes. *Am J Obstet Gynecol* 1996;175:675.
8. Vergani P, Ghidini A, Locatelli A, *et al.* Risk factors for pulmonary hypoplasia in second trimester premature rupture of membranes. *Am J Obstet Gynecol* 1994;170:1359.
9. Askenazi SS, Perlman M. Pulmonary hypoplasia: Lung weight and radial alveolar count as criteria of diagnosis. *Arch Dis Child* 1979;54:614.
10. Bromley B, Benacerraf BR. Unilateral lung hypoplasia: Report of three cases. *J Ultrasound Med* 1997;16:599.
11. Yancey MK, Richards DS. Antenatal sonographic findings associated with unilateral pulmonary agenesis. *Obstet Gynecol* 1993;81:847.
12. McNamara MF, McCurdy CM, Reed KL, *et al.* The relation between pulmonary hypoplasia and amniotic fluid volume: Lessons learned from discordant urinary tract anomalies in monoamniotic twins. *Obstet Gynecol* 1995;85:867.

13. Nicolini U, Fisk NM, Rodeck CH, *et al.* Low amniotic pressure in oligohydramnios – Is this the cause of pulmonary hypoplasia? *Am J Obstet Gynecol* 1989;161:1098.
14. Alcorn D, Adamson TM, Lambert TF, *et al.* Morphological effects of chronic tracheal ligation and drainage in the fetal lamb lung. *J Anat* 1977;123:649.
15. Hislop A, Hey E, Reid L. The lungs in congenital bilateral renal agenesis and dysplasia. *Arch Dis Child* 1979;54:32.
16. Fewell JE, Lee CC, Kitterman JA. Effects of phrenic nerve section on the respiratory system of fetal lambs. *J Appl Physiol* 1981; 51:293.
17. Harrison MR, Bressack MA, Churg AM, *et al.* Correction of congenital diaphragmatic hernia in utero: II. Simulated correction permits fetal lung growth with survival at birth. *Surgery* 1980; 88:260.
18. Ohlsson A, Fong KW, Rose TH, *et al.* Prenatal sonographic diagnosis of Pena–Shokeir syndrome type I, or fetal akinesia deformation sequence. *Am J Med Genet* 1988;29:59.
19. Mitchell JM, Roberts AM, Lee A. Doppler waveforms from the pulmonary arterial system in normal fetuses and those with pulmonary hypoplasia. *Ultrasound Obstet Gynecol* 1998; 11:167.
20. Nimrod C, Davies D, Iwanicki S, *et al.* Ultrasound prediction of pulmonary hypoplasia. *Obstet Gynecol* 1986;68:495.
21. DeVore GR, Horenstein J, Platt LD. Fetal echocardiography: VI. Assessment of cardiothoracic disproportion – A new technique for the diagnosis of thoracic hypoplasia. *Am J Obstet Gynecol* 1986; 155:1066.
22. Songster GS, Gray DL, Crane JP. Prenatal prediction of lethal pulmonary hypoplasia using ultrasonic fetal chest circumference. *Obstet Gynecol* 1989;73:261.
23. Chitkara U, Rosenberg J, Chervenak FA, *et al.* Prenatal sonographic assessment of the fetal thorax: Normal values. *Am J Obstet Gynecol* 1987;156:1069.
24. Vintzileos AM, Campbell WA, Rodis JF, *et al.* Comparison of six different ultrasonographic methods for predicting lethal fetal pulmonary hypoplasia. *Am J Obstet Gynecol* 1989;161:606.
25. D'Alton M, Mercer B, Riddick E, *et al.* Serial thoracic versus abdominal circumference ratios for the prediction of pulmonary hypoplasia in premature rupture of the membranes remote from term. *Am J Obstet Gynecol* 1992;166:658.
26. Yoshimura S, Masuzaki H, Gotoh H, *et al.* Ultrasonographic prediction of lethal pulmonary hypoplasia: Comparison of eight different ultrasonographic parameters. *Am J Obstet Gynecol* 1996;175:477.
27. Roberts AB, Mitchell JM. Direct ultrasonographic measurement of fetal lung length in normal pregnancies and pregnancies complicated by prolonged rupture of membranes. *Am J Obstet Gynecol* 1990;163:1560.
28. D'Arcy TJ, Hughes SW, Chiu WS, *et al.* Estimation of fetal lung volume using enhanced 3-dimensional ultrasound: A new method and first result. *Br J Obstet Gynecol* 1996;103:1015.
29. Lee A, Kratochwil A, Stumpflen I, *et al.* Fetal lung volume determination by three-dimensional ultrasonography. *Am J Obstet Gynecol* 1996;175:588.
30. Rizzo G. Use ultrasound to predict preterm delivery: Do not lose the opportunity (editorial). *Ultrasound Obstet Gynecol* 1996; 8:289.
31. Adzick NS, Harrison MR, Crombleholme TM, *et al.* Fetal lung lesions: Management and outcome. *Am J Obstet Gynecol* 1998; 179:884.
32. Bromley B, Parad R, Estroff JA, *et al.* Fetal lung masses: Prenatal course and outcome. *J Ultrasound Med* 1995;14:927 (quiz, 1378).
33. Thorpe-Beeston JG, Nicolaides KH. Cystic adenomatoid malformation of the lung: Prenatal diagnosis and outcome. *Prenat Diagn* 1994;14:677.
34. Rice HE, Estes JM, Hedrick MH, *et al.* Congenital cystic adenomatoid malformation. A sheep model of fetal hydrops. *J Pediatr Surg* 1994;29:692.
35. Dommergues M, Louis-Sylvestre C, Mandelbrot L, *et al.* Congenital adenomatoid malformation of the lung: When is active fetal therapy indicated? *Am J Obstet Gynecol* 1997;177:953.
36. Todros T, Gaglioti P, Presbitero P. Management of a fetus with intrapericardial teratoma diagnosed in utero. *J Ultrasound Med* 1991;10:287.
37. de Miguel Campos E, Casanova A, Urbano J, *et al.* Congenital thymic cyst: Prenatal sonographic and postnatal magnetic resonance findings. *J Ultrasound Med* 1997;16:365.
38. Gushiken BJ, Callen PW, Silverman NH. Prenatal diagnosis of tuberous sclerosis in monozygotic twins with cardiac masses. *J Ultrasound Med* 1999;18:165.
39. Green KW, Bors-Koefoed R, Pollack P, *et al.* Antepartum diagnosis and management of multiple fetal cardiac tumors. *J Ultrasound Med* 1991;10:697.
40. Schmaltz AA, Apitz J. Primary heart tumors in infancy and childhood. Report of four cases and review of literature. *Cardiology* 1981;67:12
41. Reed JC, Sobonya RE. Morphologic analysis of foregut cysts in the thorax. *AJR Am J Roentgenol* 1974;120:851
42. Fernandes ET, Custer MD, Burton EM, *et al.* Neurenteric cyst: Surgery and diagnostic imaging. *J Pediatr Surg* 1991;26:108.
43. Macualay KE, Winter TC III, Shields LE. Neurenteric cyst shown by prenatal sonography. *AJR Am J Roentgenol* 1997;169:563.
44. Wilkinson CC, Albanese CT, Jennings RW, *et al.* Fetal neurenteric cyst causing hydrops: Case report and review of the literature. *Prenat Diagn* 1999;19:118.
45. Katz AI, Wiswell TE, Baumgart S. Contemporaries controversies in the management of congenital diaphragmatic hernia. *Clin Perinatol* 1998;25:219.
46. Lewis DA, Reickert C, Bowerman R, *et al.* Prenatal ultrasonography frequently fails to diagnose congenital diaphragmatic hernia. *J Pediatr Surg* 1997;32:352.
47. Bernbaum J, Schwartz IP, Gerdes M, *et al.* Survivors of extracorporeal membrane oxygenation at 1 year of age. The relationship of primary diagnosis with health and neurodevelopmental sequelae. *Pediatrics* 1995;96:907.
48. Guibaud L, Filiatrault D, Garel L, *et al.* Fetal congenital diaphragmatic hernia: Accuracy of sonography in the diagnosis and prediction of the outcome after birth. *AJR Am J Roentgenol* 1996; 166:1195.
49. Albanese CT, Lopoo J, Goldstein RB, *et al.* Fetal liver position and perinatal outcome for congenital diaphragmatic hernia. *Prenat Diagn* 1998;18:1138.
50. Bootstaylor BS, Filly RA, Harrison MR, *et al.* Prenatal sonographic predictors of liver herniation in congenital diaphragmatic hernia. *J Ultrasound Med* 1995;14:515.
51. Dommergues M, Louis-Sylvestre C, Mandelbrot L, *et al.* Congenital diaphragmatic hernia: Can prenatal ultrasonography predict outcome? *Am J Obstet Gynecol* 1996;174:1377.
52. Geary MP, Chitty LS, Morrison JJ, *et al.* Prenatal outcome and prognostic factors in prenatally diagnosed congenital diaphragmatic hernia. *Ultrasound Obstet Gynecol* 1998;12:107.
53. Sharland GK, Lockhart SM, Heward AJ, *et al.* Prognosis in fetal diaphragmatic hernia. *Am J Obstet Gynecol* 1992;166:9.
54. Losty PD, Vanamo K, Rintala RJ, *et al.* Congenital diaphragmatic hernia – Does the size of the defect influence the incidence of associated malformations? *J Pediatr Surg* 1998;33:507.
55. Sheffield JS, Twickler DM, Timmons C, *et al.* Fryns syndrome: Prenatal diagnosis and pathologic correlation. *J Ultrasound Med* 1998;17:585.
56. Harrison MR, Adzick NS, Estes JM, *et al.* A prospective study of the outcome for fetuses with diaphragmatic hernia. *J Am Med Assoc* 1994;271:382.
57. Geary M. Management of congenital diaphragmatic hernia diagnosed prenatally: An update. *Prenat Diagn* 1998;18:1155.
58. Silver MM, Thurston WA, Patrick JE. Perinatal pulmonary hyperplasia due to laryngeal atresia. *Hum Pathol* 1988;19:110.
59. Moerman P, Fryns JP, Vandenbergthe K, *et al.* Pathogenesis of congenital cystic adenomatoid malformation of the lung. *Histopathology* 1992;21:315.
60. Mayden KL, Tortora M, Chervenak FA, *et al.* The antenatal sonographic detection of lung masses. *Am J Obstet Gynecol* 1984; 148:349.
61. Budorick NE, Pretorius DH, Leopold GR, *et al.* Spontaneous improvement of intrathoracic masses diagnosed in utero. *J Ultrasound Med* 1992;11:653.
62. Gerle RD, Jaretzki AD, Ashley CA, *et al.* Congenital bronchopulmonary-foregut malformation. Pulmonary sequestration communicating with the gastrointestinal tract. *N Engl J Med* 1968; 278:1413.
63. Lopoo JB, Albanese CT, Goldstein RB, *et al.* Fetal pulmonary sequestration: A favorable cystic lung lesion. *Obstet Gynecol* 1999;94:567.
64. Hernanz-Schulman M, Stein SM, Neblett WW, *et al.* Pulmonary sequestration: Diagnosis with color Doppler sonography and a new theory of associated hydrothorax. *Radiology* 1991;180:817.

65. Langer B, Donato L, Riethmuller C, *et al.* Spontaneous regression of fetal pulmonary sequestration. *Ultrasound Obstet Gynecol* 1995;6:33.
66. Scott JN, Trevenen CL, Wiseman DA, *et al.* Tracheal atresia: Ultrasonographic and pathologic correlation. *J Ultrasound Med* 1999;18:375.
67. Choong KKL, Trudinger B, Chow C, *et al.* Fetal laryngeal obstruction: Sonographic detection. *Ultrasound Obstet Gynecol* 1992; 2:357.
68. DeCou JM, Jones DC, Jacobs HD, *et al.* Successful ex utero intrapartum treatment (EXIT) procedure for congenital high airway obstruction syndrome (CHAOS) owing to laryngeal atresia. *J Pediatric Surg* 1998;33:1563.
69. Richards DS, Langham MR Jr, Mahaffey SM. The prenatal ultrasonograhic diagnosis of cloacal exstrophy. *J Ultrasound Med* 1992; 11:507.
70. Longaker MT, Laberge JM, Dansereau J, *et al.* Primary fetal hydrothorax: Natural history and management. *J Pediatr Surg* 1989;24:573.
71. Benaceraff BR, Frigoletto FD Jr. Mid-trimester fetal thoracentesis. *J Clin Ultrasound* 1985;13:202.
72. Wilkins Haug LE, Doubilet P. Successful thoracoamniotic shunting and review of the literature in unilateral pleural effusion with hydrops. *J Ultrasound Med* 1997;16:153.
73. Weber AM, Philipson EH. Fetal pleural effusion: A review and meta-analysis for prognostic indicators. *Obstet Gynecol* 1992;79:281.

41 Three-dimensional ultrasound of blood flow in the fetal cardiovascular system

R. Chaoui

Introduction

In the past 5 years three-dimensional (3D) ultrasound moved from an advertising toy with the highlight of baby facing to a new powerful diagnostic tool in prenatal medicine. This was mainly achieved by the development of fast processors enabling rapid 3D image acquisition and the advent of new software allowing new 3D image display.

The use of color and power Doppler ultrasound in the 1990s improved the prenatal diagnosis of malformations involving the cardiac and vascular systems.[1–3] Malformations of the cardiovascular system are often complex and difficult to understand when only gray-scale imaging is used. Two-dimensional color or power Doppler ultrasound can help in a better assessment of fetal abnormalities, but they generally enable the visualization of only those vessels with a straight course or lying in a 2D plane.[4–6] In most cases the examiner is reconstructing mentally a spatial image of the vessels examined.[5]

In recent years, a few case reports and studies demonstrated that the 3D power Doppler ultrasound (3D-PDU) helps in the reconstruction of the vessels of interest and thus improves the understanding of the spatial appearance of the vascular tree.[4,7,8] Images produced were very similar to results known from radiology acquired either by x-ray[9–11] or by MR-angiography. This chapter aims to present the actual possibilities of 3D ultrasound of the cardiovascular system in normal and abnormal pregnancies, looking for possible future applications of this method in prenatal diagnosis.

Technical background

The main aspects that have to be considered when evaluating a 3D imaging system are (1) the volume data acquisition and (2) the image rendering display.

Volume data acquisition

The acquisition of a volume with information on the fetal heart or the fetal vessels can be achieved either in 3D static mode, which means a volume consisting of a series of still images, or in 4D mode, which reflects the beating character of the heart. The latter can be acquired either in live real-time 3D or as off-line 4D, which was recently made possible by the advent of the new software of spatial and temporal image correlation (STIC).[12,13] In these acquisitions heart and vessels can be visualized either on gray-scale mode, or in combination with color Doppler,[14] power Doppler or B-flow. The acquisition of a volume with gray-scale information is reduced to the demonstration of the lumen of the heart or the vessels, whereas in Doppler or B-flow techniques blood flow is visualized. To acquire a volume with a potentially good 3D/4D image, the examiner should spend time in optimizing the presetting of the color and power Doppler or B-flow or increasing the contrast on the gray scale.

Image rendering

Image rendering is the process of creating a 3D visual representation of the parameters of interest. Generally the principle used is the 'planar geometric projection' of the 3D image, i.e. a 2D image representing the 3D data. For the 4D image it will be a 2D projection with cine-loop. The impression of the third dimension is generally given by the on-line rotation of the image on the screen and by different shadowing of anterior and posterior structures. Color maps can be used as well as different postprocessing means of increasing the brightness and transparency of color. The examiner can decide whether to visualize the vessels of interest alone or in combination with gray-scale information in the so-called 'glass body' rendering (Figure 41.1). Interestingly, the system also allows a gradual increase of the transparency, allowing at the beginning the visualization of the surface in gray scale

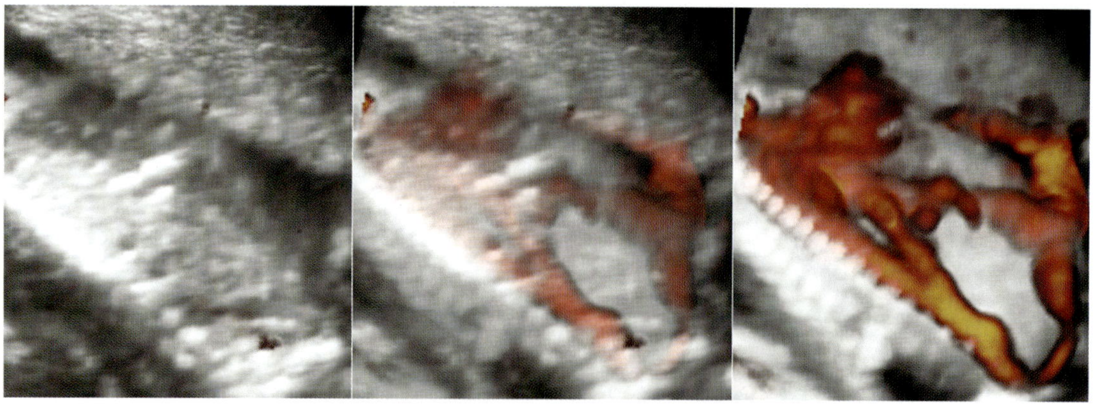

Figure 41.1 A longitudinal view of the abdomen seen from the right side in glass body mode. From left to right the transparency is gradually increased allowing a progressive visualization of power Doppler information.

but with progression of transparency, the visualization of the vessels inside the structure of interest (Figure 41.1).[7] For information using no Doppler assistance but only the gray-scale information, there are two volume rendering features permitting a 3D/4D appearance: the transparent minimum mode and the transparent inversion mode.

Most of the experience shared in this chapter was acquired with a Voluson 730 Expert system (GE Kretztechnik, Zipf, Austria) using mechanical transducers for acquisition and the 4D view software for 3D/4D volume reconstruction. The 4D of the fetal heart was achieved either with live 3D or by using the integrated STIC software as described elsewhere. Only the latter permitted a 4D of color or power Doppler information of the heart. It is expected that in the near future other companies will provide new software with new possibilities of 3D/4D acquisition and rendering, but the fields of interest will probably remain unchanged.

Clinical application

The clinical application of 3D/4D in prenatal visualization of the fetal cardiovascular system is closely related to the regions of interest known from the application of color and power Doppler ultrasound. We refer to reviews on the benefit of using color Doppler in fetal diseases.[2,3] Some years ago[4] we examined in a study the application of 3D-PDU in prenatal diagnosis on 45 normal and 87 abnormal pregnancies including mainly vascular abnormalities. In this study we used a prototype system and satisfactory image information was collected in only 56 out of the 87 abnormal cases examined (64%). The following eight regions were found to be of interest: vessels of the placenta, umbilical cord, abdomen, kidneys, lung, brain and fetal tumors as well as the heart and great vessels. In the following findings, the main regions of interest with the possible anomalies involving the vascular system were demonstrable on 3D ultrasound. The fetal heart will be discussed separately in the second part of this section.

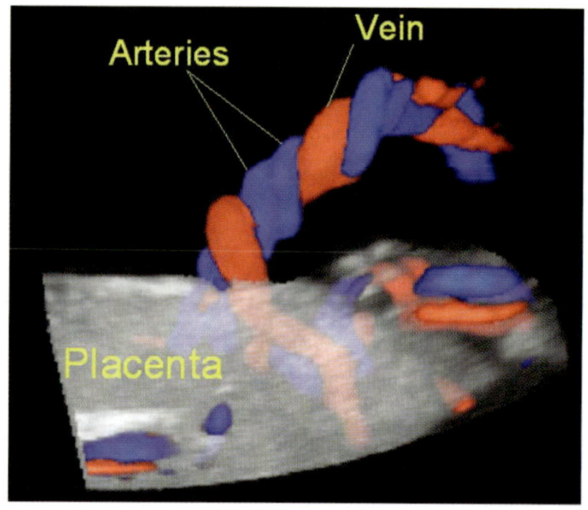

Figure 41.2 3D color Doppler ultrasound showing a posterior placenta with central insertion of the umbilical cord.

Peripheral vascular system in 3D

Umbilical cord and placenta

From our experience it seems to be the structure most easily accessible to 3D throughout pregnancy. Intraplacental vessel network architecture can be visualized with this method.[15] The umbilical cord can be rendered at different places from its insertion on the placental side (Figures 41.2 and 41.3) to its attachment on the fetal abdominal wall.[4] Abnormalities like placenta previa, vasa previa[16] or velamentous insertion (Figure 41.3) can be demonstrated, as well as the single umbilical artery or less important conditions such as the connecting vessels in twin pregnancies, nuchal cord or true and false knot (Figure 41.4) or the free course of the umbilical cord (Figure 41.5).

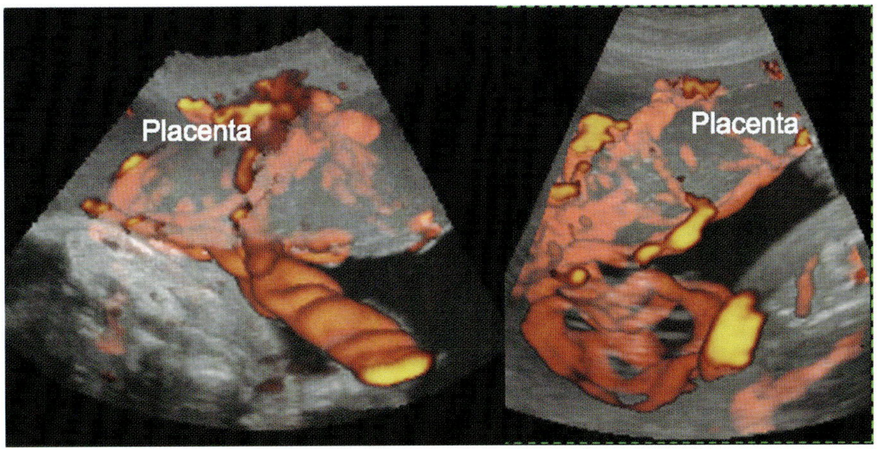

Figure 41.3 3D power Doppler ultrasound showing a central insertion of the umbilical cord (left) and a velamentous insertion (right).

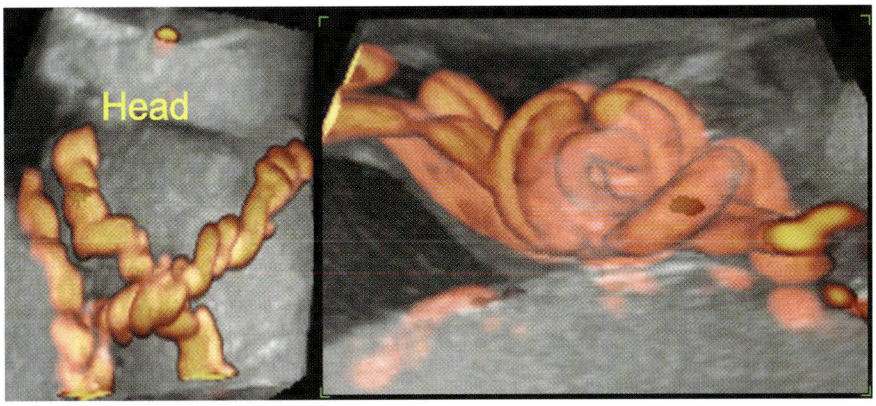

Figure 41.4 Fetus seen from behind with the umbilical cord around the neck (left). False knot of the umbilical cord.

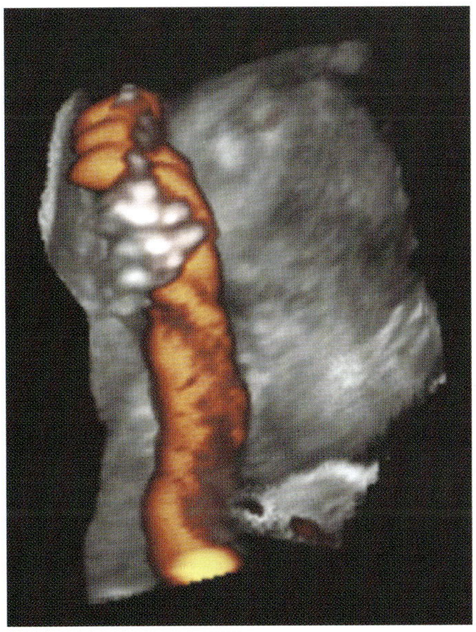

Figure 41.5 Fetus holding the umbilical cord with the hand in front of its face.

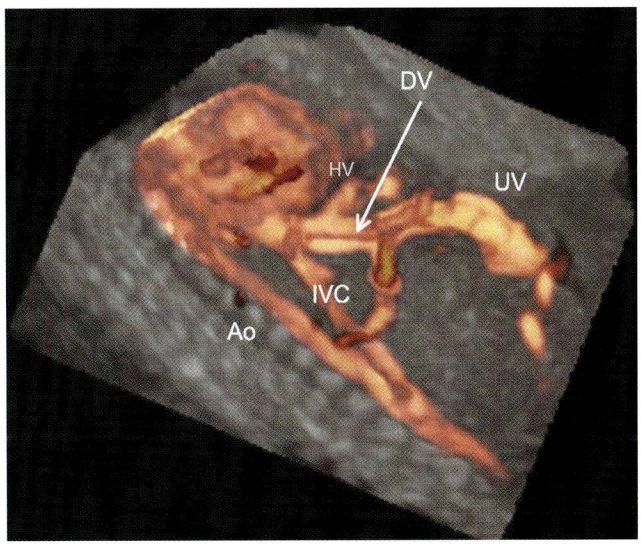

Figure 41.6 Longitudinal view of the abdomen view from the right side showing the descending aorta (Ao), the inferior vena cava (IVC), the umbilical vein (UV) with ductus venosus (DV) as well as hepatic veins.

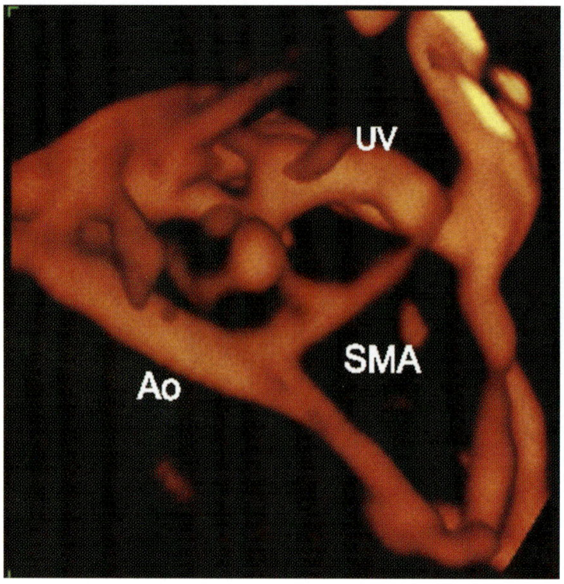

Figure 41.7 Longitudinal view from the right side in a fetus with gastroschisis, showing in comparison to Figure 41.6 the distortion in the course of the umbilical vein (UV), and the descending aorta (Ao). The superior mesenteric artery is stretched and arises in the direction of the abdominal wall.

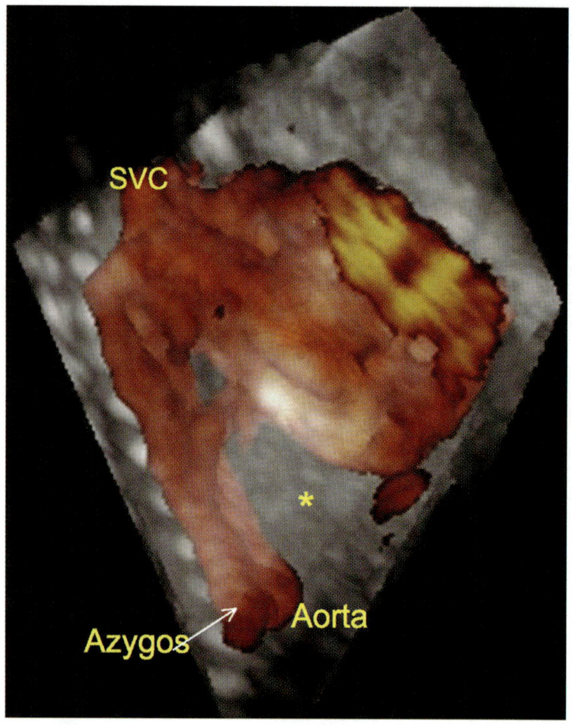

Figure 41.9 Fetus with left isomerism (polysplenia): with an interruption of the inferior vena cava (*), which is absent on 3D-PDU. Venous blood from the inferior part of the body returns via the azygos vein, which is dilated and seen side by side near the aorta.

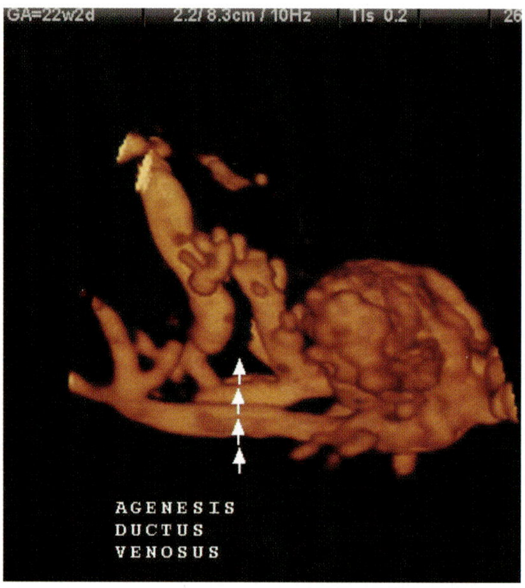

Figure 41.8 Longitudinal view of the intra-abdominal vascular tree in a 22-week fetus with agenesis of ductus venosus and connection of the umbilical vein into the hepatic vein system.

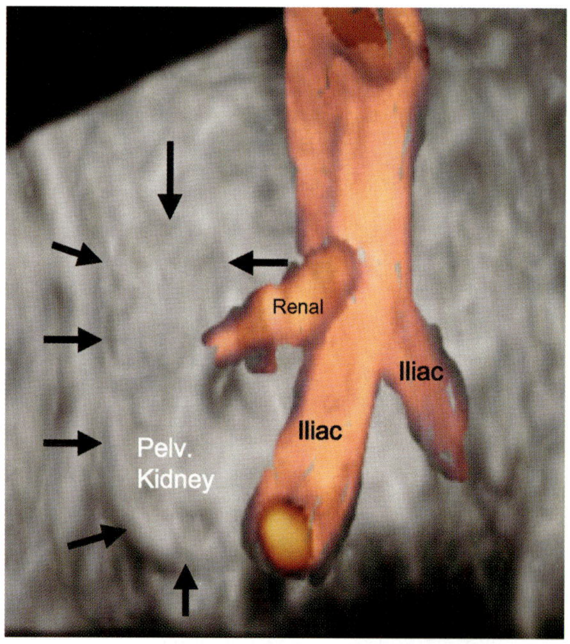

Figure 41.10 Pelvic kidney showing the abnormal renal artery arising in the region of the bifurcation of the iliac arteries.

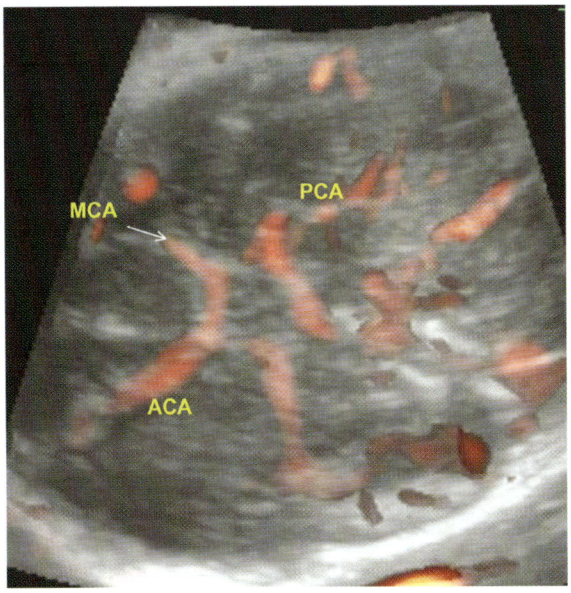

Figure 41.11 Circulus of Willis as demonstrated with 3D PDU, with the anterior (ACA), middle (MCA) and posterior (PCA) cerebral arteries.

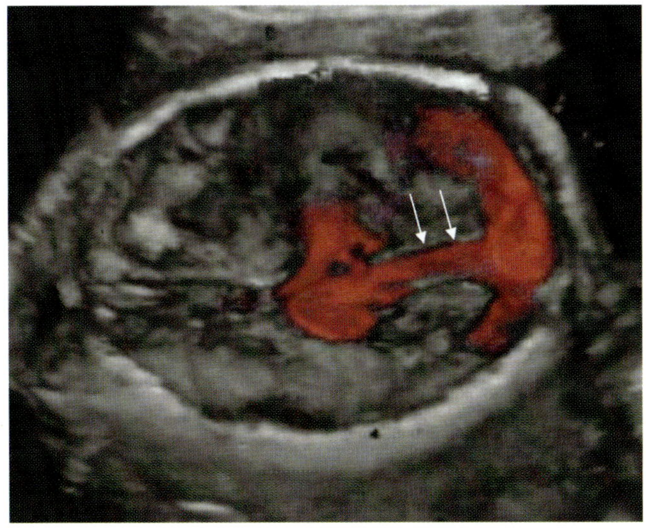

Figure 41.12 3D PDU of a vein of Galen aneurysm at 22 weeks' gestation with the dilated vessel between the hemispheres and in the posterior fossa.

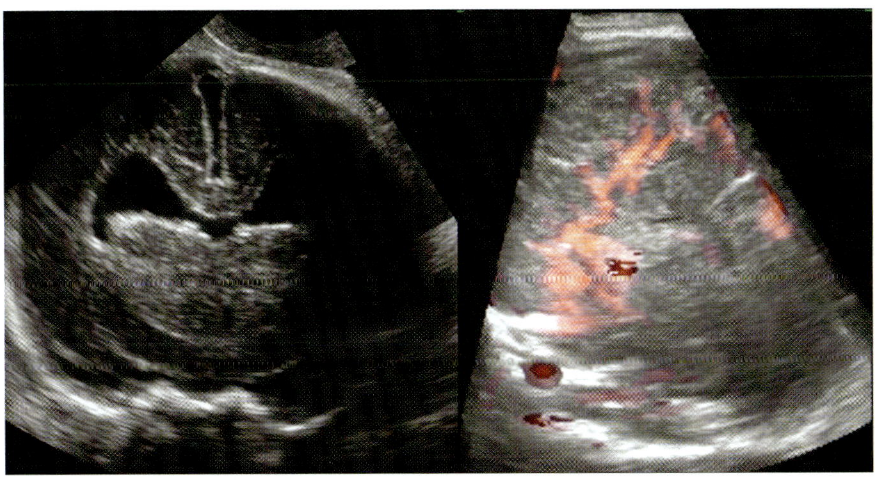

Figure 41.13 Fetus with trisomy 13 and lobar holoprosencephaly as seen by transvaginal ultrasound (left). 3D power Doppler shows the aberrant bizarre course of the anterior cerebral artery.

Intra-abdominal vessels

The vessels of interest are the umbilical vein, the ductus venosus, the portal vein system, the hepatic veins, the splenic vessels, the inferior vena cava and the abdominal aorta (Figure 41.6). The visualization of the lower abdomen gives a good orientation in visualizing the umbilical arteries around the urinary bladder in normal conditions. Since the application of color Doppler and the intensive study of the ductus venosus, abnormalities of the intrahepatic venous system were detected to be more common than expected. Conditions to study by 3D power Doppler could involve the abnormal cord insertion on the abdomen (omphalocele, gastroschisis) (Figure 41.7), abnormal umbilical vein size (varix or ectasia), but the main field of interest seems to be the absence of ductus venosus (Figure 41.8) with the different possibilities of connection of the umbilical vein. In these conditions 3D power Doppler demonstrates the spatial course of the aberrant vessel. Another interesting condition is the abnormal course of vessels in isomerism, i.e. interruption of the inferior vena cava with azygous continuity (Figure 41.9).

Renal vessels

The visualization of renal vessels is known to increase the accuracy of diagnosis of kidney malformations in the fetus. The renal vascular tree is well visualized

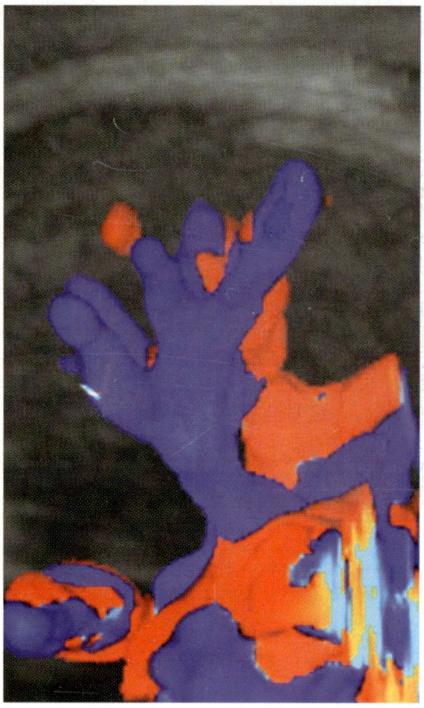

Figure 41.14 Pulmonary veins and arteries are demonstrated with 3D color Doppler ultrasound.

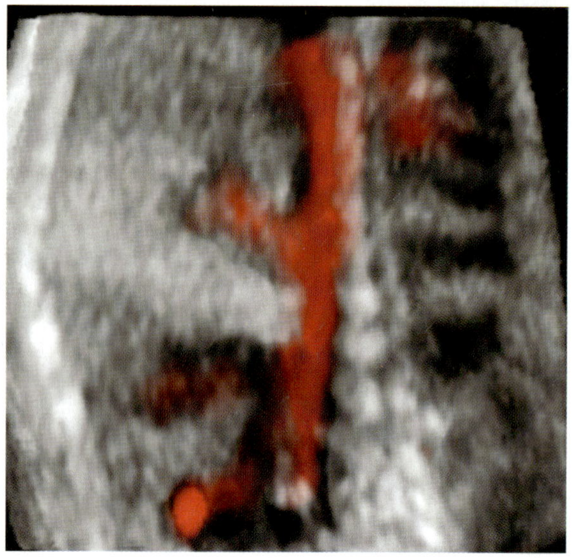

Figure 41.15 In this fetus with an echogenic lung segment the diagnosis of bronchopulmonary sequestration is supported by the demonstration of an aberrant vessel arising from the descending aorta (arrow).

(a)

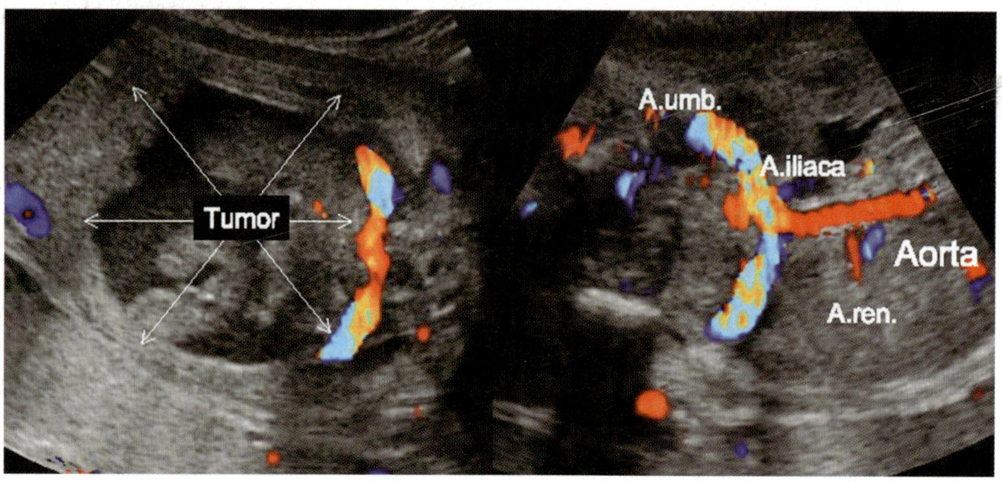

(b)

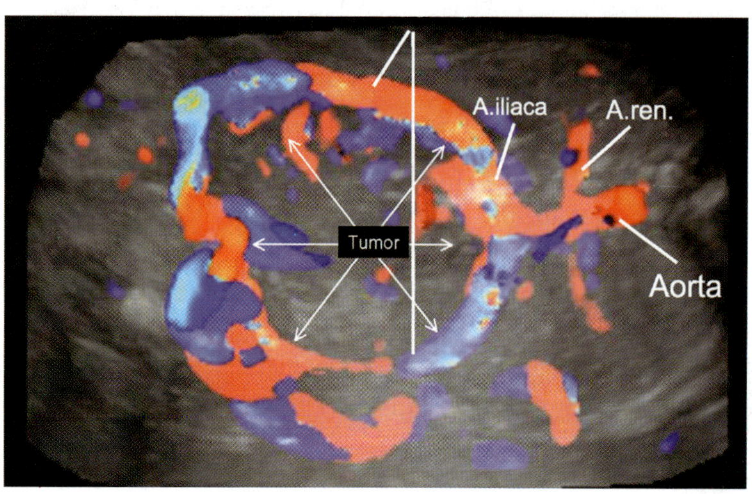

Figure 41.16 (a) In this fetus at 27 weeks with sacrococcygeal teratoma there was an intra-abdominal mass as well (arrows). In different planes one recognizes the descending aorta, one renal artery and the bifurcation of iliac arteries with the arising of umbilical arteries (A.umb). (b) The 3D rendering gives the complete aspect of the tumor and the surrounding vessels.

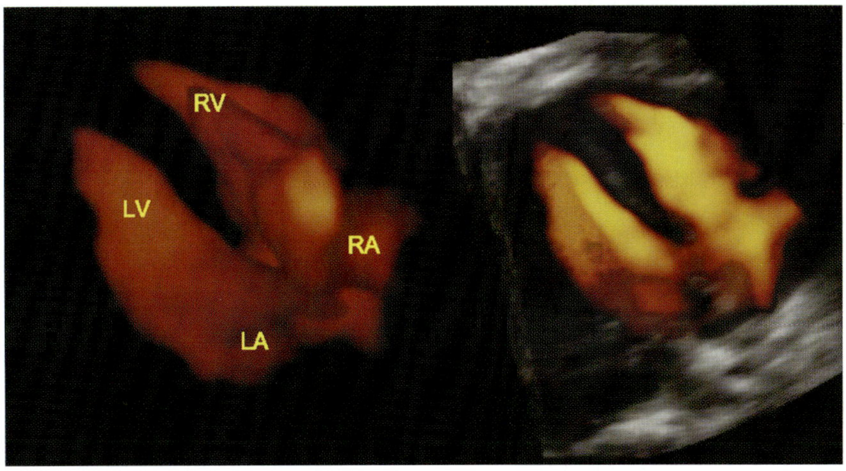

Figure 41.17 3D-PDU of a normal four-chamber view (left) with right and left atria (RA, LA), right and left ventricles (RV, LV) in 3D power mode (left) and glass body mode.

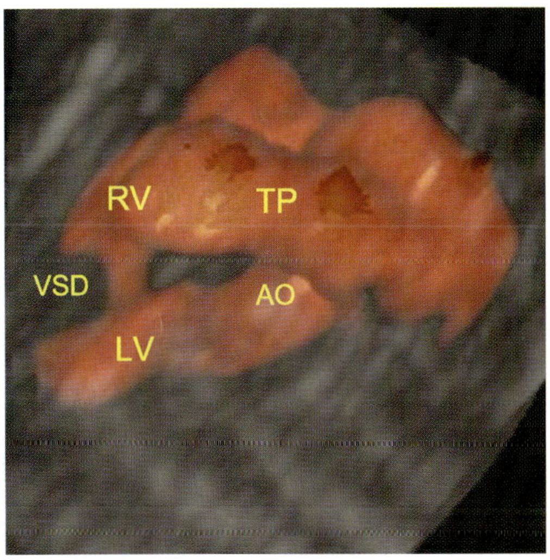

Figure 41.18 A muscular ventricular septal defect (VSD) connecting both right and left ventricles, whereas the vessels show a regular crossing.

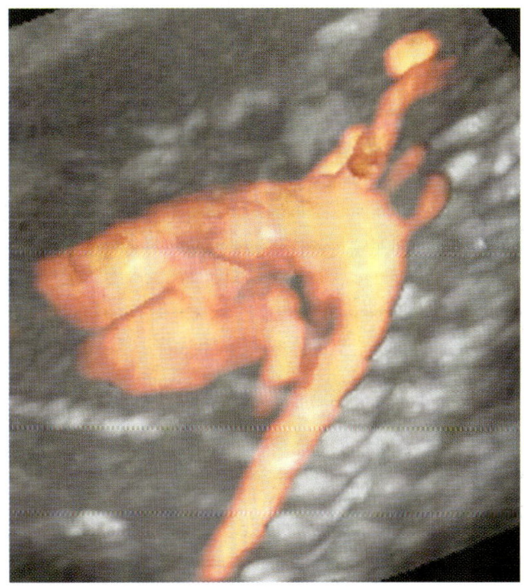

Figure 41.19 Aortic arch with the origin of the cephalic vessels. Behind the brachiocephalic artery the superior vena cava is seen.

in a coronal plane with the descending aorta showing a horizontal course. Conditions with possible benefit of 3D-PDU application are agenesis of one or both kidneys, arteries in duplex kidney, horseshoe or pelvic kidney (Figure 41.10), but the 3D rendering adds only a little information to 2D color and was probably overestimated in our few investigations.

Intracerebral vessels

The anatomy of intracranial vessel architecture became more important in recent years and is closely related to the structural anatomy of the brain. A transversal insonation allows easy reconstruction of the circulus of Willis (Figure 41.11), whereas a more sagittal approach enables the visualization of the pericallosal artery with its ramifications.[17] Choosing a lower velocity, scale flow in the cerebral veins and sagittal sinus can be imaged as well. The main fields of interest are the abnormal anterior cerebral artery in agenesis of corpus callosum, the aneurysm of the vein of Galen (Figure 41.12) and the disturbed vascular anatomy in cerebral malformations [holoprosencephaly (Figure 41.13), hydrocephaly, encephalocele, etc.]. Improved image information can be achieved by using transvaginal ultrasound of the fetal brain in fetuses with vertex position (Figure 41.13).

Lung vessels

Proximal and peripheral lung arteries and veins can be seen from their origin in peripheral pulmonary segments (Figure 41.14). Fields of interest are the analysis of the 3D vessel architecture in cystic lung malformation, congenital diaphragmatic hernia and bronchopulmonary sequestration (Figure 41.15). The

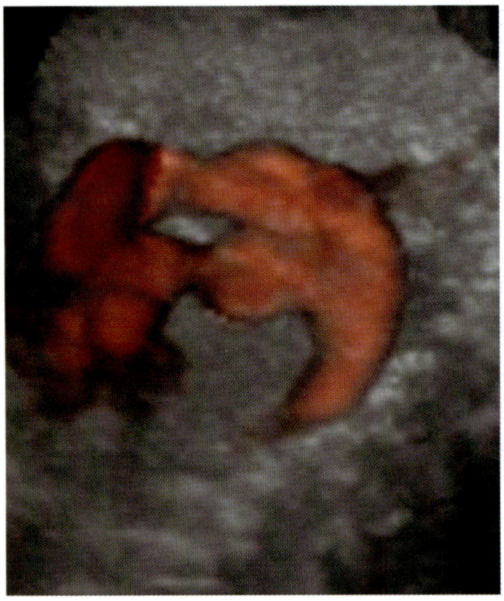

Figure 41.20 Parallel course of the great vessels in transposition of the great vessels.

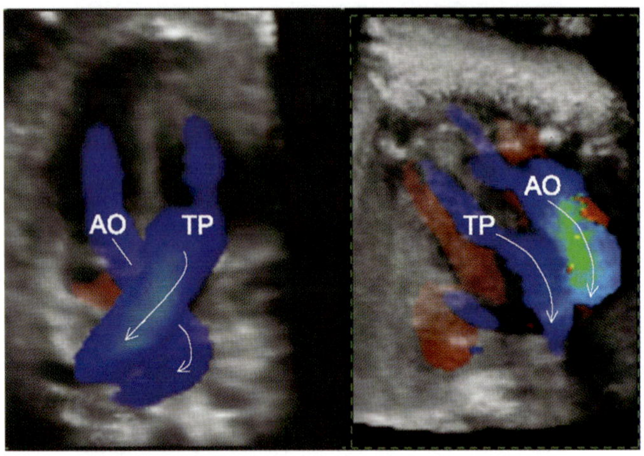

Figure 41.21 3D and 4D volume rendering with transparent gray scale and surface color Doppler of two fetuses: on the left a normal finding with the regular crossing of the great vessels, on the right a fetus with transposition of the great arteries with parallel course of both vessels.

role of color or power Doppler in predicting pulmonary hypoplasia failed and it is not expected that the 3D demonstration of the vessels could be in this field of great interest in the near future.

Fetal tumors or aberrant vessels

Aberrant vessels can be visualized in the presence of several malformations like lung sequestration, chorioangioma, lymphangioma or in (sacrococcygeal) teratoma, acardiac twin, etc. Visualization of fetal tumors is of interest not only for the risk of cardiac failure due to the presence of arterio-venous fistulae, but also to assess compression of shifting of neighboring organs (Figure 41.16a and b). Some fields of

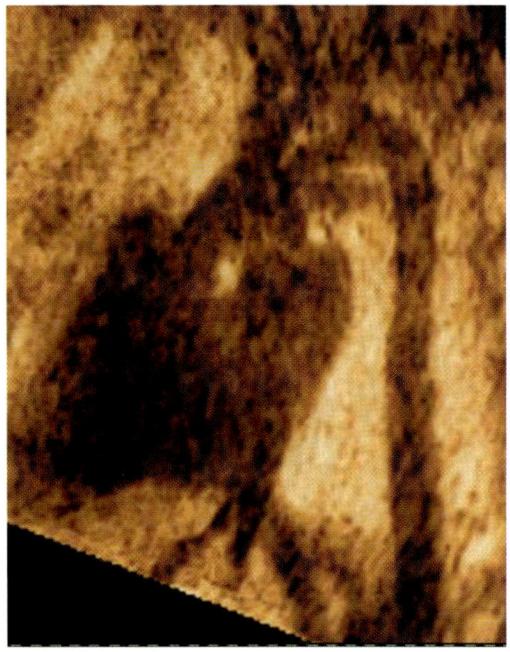

Figure 41.22 Longitudinal view of the heart, the aortic arch and the hepatic vessels in transparent minimum mode.

interest are chorangioma, teratoma, lung sequestration, acrania (TRAP), hemangioma, renal tumors, cardiac rhabdomyomas, etc.

The fetal heart in 3D and 4D

An extended fetal echocardiographic examination is achieved by acquiring and documenting different cross-sectional planes.[1,18] An examiner acquiring these cardiac cross-sectional planes during different cycles is automatically reconstructing mentally the heart in the third and fourth dimensions (3D + time). In the last decade 3D and 4D fetal echocardiography was investigated intensively in laboratories using external workstations, static volume sweep, matrix transducers and recently, a new ultrasound equipment with integrated software (STIC^{TM}) was introduced, allowing reliable 3D and 4D fetal echocardiography.[12,14]

Surface rendering can be applied to the fetal heart by using the interface between the cavities and the cardiac walls. The views are, however, either the known views from 2D ultrasound (four and five chambers) or could be new views as well, which are still to be defined.[19] Such views could focus on demonstrating the AV-valves or the interventricular or interatrial septum. The future will show which views are appropriate for clinical application. This part will not be covered in this chapter, which mainly focuses on the 3D appearance of blood flow. The first steps were acquired by combining power Doppler mode with 3D to get the image of the four cavities (Figure 41.17)[4] or the spatial arrangement of the great vessels.[11] These views could help in the demonstration

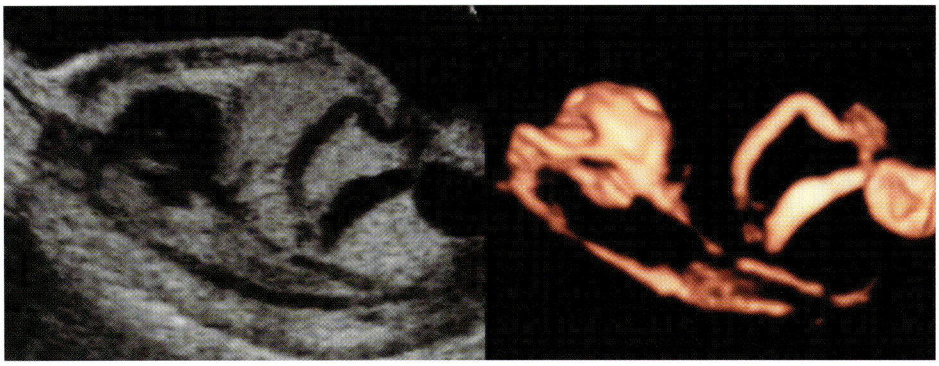

Figure 41.23 A longitudinal view of a fetal abdomen in minimum mode (left) and inversion mode (right). No blood flow is visualized but hypoechoic structures such as gallbladder and urinary bladder in addition to the usual vessels.

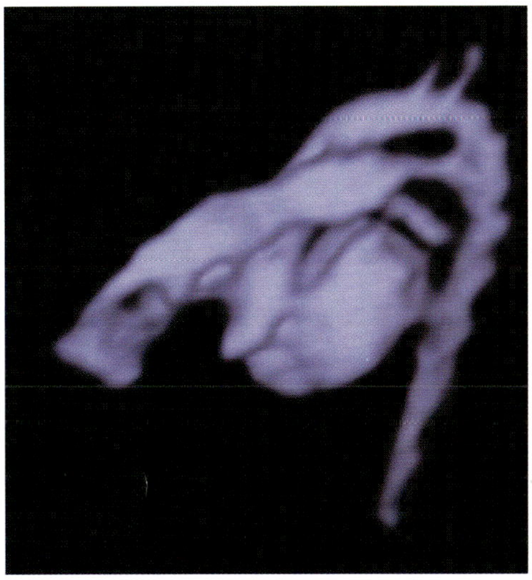

Figure 41.24 Crossing of the great vessels as demonstrated with the inversion mode.

of interventricular communications as a ventricular septal defect (Figure 41.18). Their main potential could be the demonstration of the crossing of the great vessels and the aortic arch under normal conditions (Figure 41.19) vs. transposition of the great arteries (Figure 41.20).[4] The application of STIC with color Doppler and 'glass body mode' allows a more precise and dynamic appearance of the relationship of the vessels to each other (Figure 41.21).[14]

An interesting rendering mode is the 'transparent minimal mode' rendering (Figures 41.22 and 41.23, left), in which blood vessels can be seen as hypoechoic structures in a projection. Especially in a longitudinal view, the aortic and ductus arch can be seen properly. The use of the new software of 'inversion mode' permits the demonstration of a negative image of the projection in minimum mode, but the image gets more plasticity and appears more 3D than the minimal mode (Figures 41.23, right and 41.24).

The breakthrough 2 years ago was achieved by the software allowing the acquisition of a STIC volume combined with color Doppler or power Doppler information. We presented extensively this technique elsewhere.[14] Using this technique the examiner is able to assess the hemodynamic spatial changes throughout the cardiac cycle. The 3D/4D volume rendering of color or power Doppler STIC provides images similar to an angiography when the feature glass body is chosen.

The potential of 3D is that it not only facilitates the understanding of the spatial arrangement of the chambers showing their size and shape, but the course of the great vessels can also be better understood. Crossing of vessels vs. parallel course, abnormal course as seen in double aortic arch, right arch with a sling[20] or simply tortuous hypoplastic aorta or pulmonary artery in different anomalies may be fields for future research.[21]

REFERENCES

1. Chaoui R, McEwing R. Three cross-sectional planes for fetal color Doppler echocardiography. *Ultrasound Obstet Gynecol* 2003; 21(1):81–93.
2. Chaoui R. Color Doppler sonography in the assessment of the fetal heart. In Nicolaides KH, Rizzo G, Hecher K, eds. *Placental and Fetal Doppler*. London: Parthenon Publishing, 2003:171–86.
3. Chaoui R. Color Doppler sonography in the diagnosis of fetal abnormalitites. In Nicolaides KH, Rizzo G, Hecher K, eds. *Placental and Fetal Doppler*. London: Parthenon Publishing, 2000:187–203.
4. Chaoui R, Kalache KD, Hartung J. Application of three-dimensional power Doppler ultrasound in prenatal diagnosis. *Ultrasound Obstet Gynecol* 2001;17(1):22–9.
5. Chaoui R, Kalache KD. Three-dimensional color power imaging: Principles and first experience in prenatal diagnosis. In Merz E, ed. *3D Ultrasonography in Obstetrics and Gynecology*. Philadelphia: Lippincot Williams & Wilkins, 1998:135–42.
6. Chaoui R, Kalache KD, Bollmann R. Three-dimensional color power Doppler in the assessment of fetal vascular anatomy under normal and abnormal conditions. In Kurjak A, ed. *Three-Dimensional Power Doppler in Obstetrics and Gynecology*. New York: Parthenon Publishing Group, 2000:113–9.
7. Lee W, Kalache KD, Chaiworapongsa T, *et al*. Three-dimensional power Doppler ultrasonography during pregnancy. *J Ultrasound Med* 2003;22(1):91–7.

8. Hartung J, Kalache KD, Chaoui R. Three-dimensional power Doppler ultrasonography (3D-PDU) in fetal diagnosis. *Ultraschall Med* 2004;25(3):200–5.
9. Heling KS, Chaoui R, Bollmann R. Prenatal diagnosis of an aneurysm of the vein of Galen with three-dimensional color power angiography. *Ultrasound Obstet Gynecol* 2000;15(4): 333–6.
10. Gagel K, Heling KS, Kalache KD, Chaoui R. Prenatal diagnosis of an intracranial arteriovenous fistula in the posterior fossa on the basis of color and three-dimensional power Doppler ultrasonography. *J Ultrasound Med* 2003;22(12):1399–403.
11. Chaoui R, Kalache KD. Three-dimensional power Doppler ultrasound of the fetal great vessels. *Ultrasound Obstet Gynecol* 2001;17(5):455–6.
12. DeVore GR, Falkensammer P, Sklansky MS, Platt LD. Spatio-temporal image correlation (STIC): New technology for evaluation of the fetal heart. *Ultrasound Obstet Gynecol* 2003;22(4):380–7.
13. Vinals F, Poblete P, Giuliano A. Spatio-temporal image correlation (STIC): A new tool for the prenatal screening of congenital heart defects. *Ultrasound Obstet Gynecol* 2003;22(4):388–94.
14. Chaoui R, Hoffmann J, Heling KS. Three-dimensional (3D) and 4D color Doppler fetal echocardiography using spatio-temporal image correlation (STIC). *Ultrasound Obstet Gynecol* 2004;23(6): 535–45.
15. Pretorius DH, Nelson TR, Baergen RN, Pai E, Cantrell C. Imaging of placental vasculature using three-dimensional ultrasound and color power Doppler: A preliminary study. *Ultrasound Obstet Gynecol* 1998;12(1):45–9.
16. Lee W, Kirk JS, Comstock CH, Romero R. Vasa previa: prenatal detection by three-dimensional ultrasonography. *Ultrasound Obstet Gynecol* 2000;16(4):384–7.
17. Pooh RK, Pooh KH. The assessment of fetal brain morphology and circulation by transvaginal 3D sonography and power Doppler. *J Perinat Med* 2002;30(1):48–56.
18. Chaoui R. The examination of the normal fetal heart using two-dimensional echocardiography. In Yagel S, Silvermann N, Gembruch U, eds. London: Martin Dunitz, 2003:141–9.
19. Chaoui R, Hoffmann J, Heling KS. Basal cardiac view on 3D/4D fetal echocardiographiy for the assessment of AV-valves and great vessels arrangement (abstract). *Ultrasound Obstet Gynecol* 2004; 22:228.
20. Chaoui R, Schneider MBE, Kalache KD. Right aortic arch with vascular ring and aberrant left subclavian artery: Prenatal diagnosis assisted by three-dimensional power Doppler ultrasound. *Ultrasound Obstet Gynecol* 2003; 22(6):661–3.
21. Chaoui R, Kalache KD, Heling KS, Schneider M. 3D-power doppler echocardiography: Usefulness in spatial visualization of fetal cardiac vessels (abstract). *Ultrasound Obstet Gynecol* 2003;22.

42 Specific aspects of ultrasound examination in twin pregnancies

E. Quarello and Y. Ville

Introduction

Although twins account for only 2% of all pregnancies, they are responsible for 20% of perinatal morbidity and the incidence of twinning has increased by 50% over the last 20 years. Embryologically, two-thirds of the twins are dizygotic, resulting from fertilization of two oocytes by two spermatozoids. One-third of the twins are therefore monozygotic, resulting from the splitting of one fertilized egg. Depending on the time of splitting after fecundation, one-third of monochorionic twins will be dichorionic, which occurs within the first 4 days. The majority, however, will therefore be monochorionic. It is only when splitting occurs after 8 days in 5% of these that the twins are monoamniotic. When splitting occurs after 12 days, the Siamese twins will share some organs. Among twin pregnancies, the incidence of perinatal mortality and morbidity is two to six times higher in monochorionic pregnancies. Both specific and non-specific complications justify closer surveillance by ultrasound. Indeed, ultrasound examination in twins is subjected to technical difficulties related to the presence of two fetuses in the uterine cavity and this has an impact both on biometry and on morphological and functional assessment. Specific features should also be surveyed during ultrasound examination of all twin pregnancies.

Determination of chorionicity and amnionicity (Figure 42.1)

Gestational sacs count should not be performed before 6 weeks. Indeed before that, one sac could be left unnoticed. Embryos can be counted from 7 weeks onward and yolk sacs can be identified between 8 and 12 weeks. Amnionicity should not be confirmed before 9 weeks. Prior to 9 weeks of gestation, amnionicity cannot be assessed reliably, even with the use of high-frequency vaginal ultrasound probes.[1] Chorionicity is the main determinant of both specific and non-specific complications in twin pregnancies. This is therefore the main aim of ultrasound examination in twins. Eighty percent of twin pregnancies are dichorionic. Diagnosis of chorionicity should be made in the first trimester of pregnancy, ideally between 9 and 12 weeks; however, this is still reliable until 14 weeks but it becomes uncertain thereafter when the twins are of the same sex.

Chorionicity can be established based on:

- Gestational sacs count
- Presence of the lambda sign before 14 weeks, as opposed to the T-sign in monochorionic pregnancies
- Presence of the twin peak thereafter
- Identification of two distinct placental masses
- Determination of different fetal genders
- Examination of the intertwin fetal membranes

The 'lambda' sign[2] and the 'twin peak'[3] are specific features of dichorionic pregnancies but have been described at two different gestational periods. They both appear as a thick hyper- or isoechoic triangular base of the intertwin membranes on a single placental mass. These feature the triangular projection of villous tissue at the union of two fused chorionic plates. In monochorionic placentae, a single chorionic layer cannot therefore project on the placenta; this features an abrupt junction on the placenta described as the T-sign. A lambda sign is the guarantee for a dichorionic pregnancy with a sensitivity close to 100%.[4] It can be found throughout pregnancy but the significance of its absence is reliable only before 14 weeks. Non-visualization of the lambda sign with the presence of the T-sign has a positive predictive value for monochorionicity close to 100%.

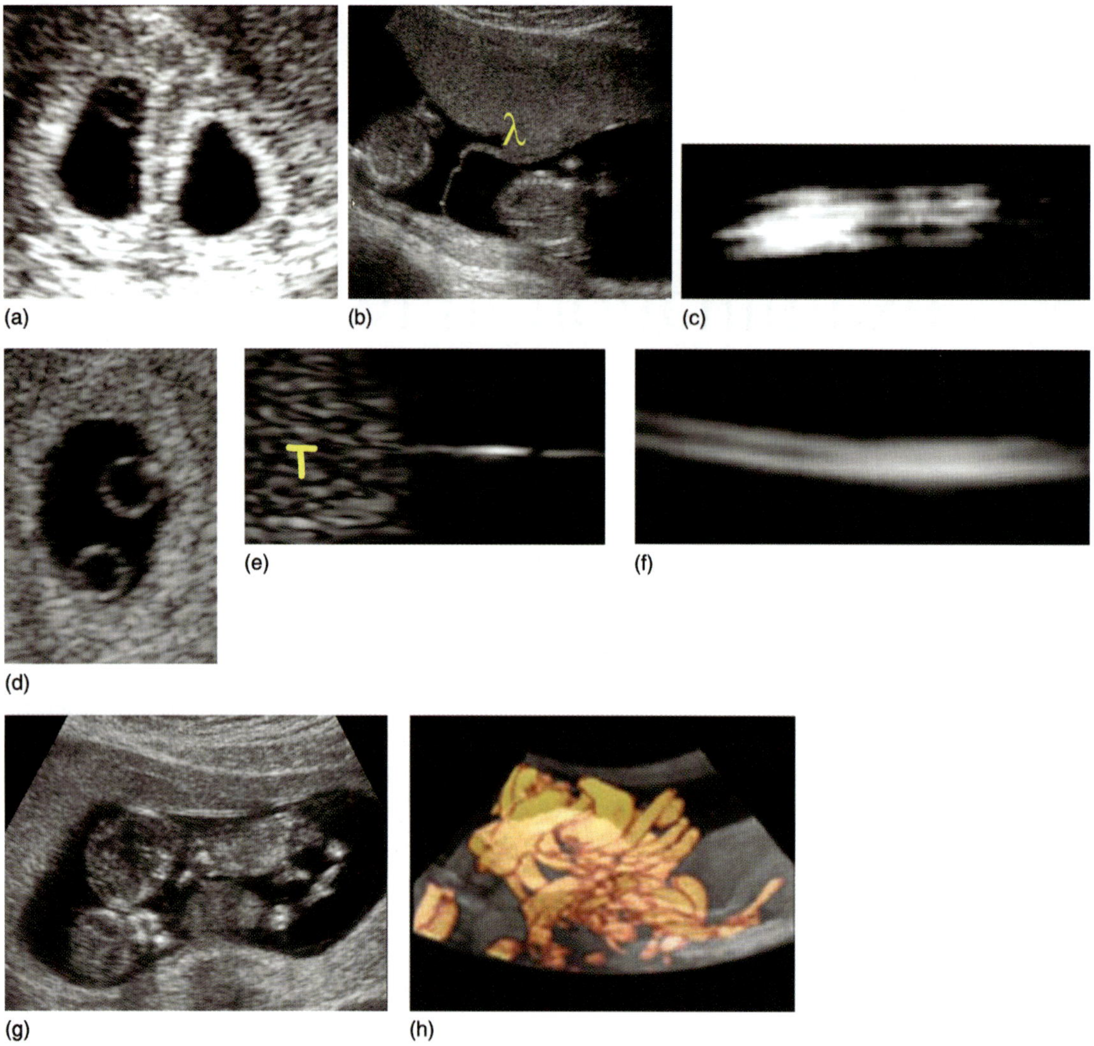

Figure 42.1 Assessment of chorionicity and amnionicity. (a) Dichorionic pregnancy (DCP) before 9 weeks showing two gestational sacs. (b) DCP showing the lambda sign of the fused chorions. (c) Interamniotic membrane in a DCP at 22 weeks counting more than two layers. (d) Monochorionic pregnancy (MCP) before 9 weeks showing one gestational sac and two yolk sacs. (e) MCP at 12 weeks showing the T-sign at the membrane attachment on the placenta without chorion interposition. (f) Interamniotic membrane in an MCP at 22 weeks counting only two layers. (g) Monoamniotic twins at 12 weeks. (h) Cord entanglement in a monoamniotic twin pregnancy at 17 weeks.

The presence of two placental masses is predictive of a dichorionic pregnancy; however, this may feature a placenta bipartita in up to 15% of these cases. Monochorionicity cannot be confirmed by the presence of a single placental mass since two separate placentae are frequently fused after 15 weeks. The presence of vascular anastomoses on the chorionic plate joining the two funicular circulations is a specific feature of monochorionicity but its detection is time-consuming and its reproducibility remains to be established.

Different fetal genders are specific of dichorionicity because they would confirm a dizygotic pregnancy. The reverse is not true.

Intertwin membrane is the result of the fusion of two amniotic and two chorionic layers in dichorionic pregnancies. This is made of only two amniotic layers in monochorionic diamniotic pregnancies. In the late second and third trimesters, ultrasound examination can assess the thickness of the intertwin membranes using cutoff measurements of 1.5 or 2 mm or, better, counting two or four layers in monochorionic and dichorionic pregnancies, respectively. Technically, this requires the use of magnification and the lowest gain possible and an angle of insonation to the membranes close to 45°. A right angle, although theoretically more suitable, is subjected to more artifactual images.

Amnionicity can be determined upon:

- Visualization of the interamniotic membrane. However, non-visualization of the membrane in a diamniotic pregnancy can arise due to technical difficulties, mainly before 8 weeks of pregnancy or in obese patients.
- Visualization of the yolk sacs and extra-amniotic spaces. The number of yolk sacs and extra-amniotic

spaces matches the number of amniotic sacs. Two yolk sacs are seen in monochorionic diamniotic pregnancies and only one in monoamniotic pregnancies.[5] These can be seen as non-contiguous in dichorionic pregnancies.
- Cords entanglement in monoamniotic twins can be best visualized using color Doppler. Doppler flow within the cord mass should also show a biphasic arterial flow.
- Conjoined twins can only be seen in monoamniotic pregnancies and can be suspected when visualizing close proximity of both twins, which also show concomitant movements.

Examination before 15 weeks is critical and a well-documented picture should be kept in the notes in order to confirm chorionicity whenever clinically relevant later on in pregnancy.

Nuchal translucency measurement in twin pregnancies

Nuchal translucency measurement can be used in twins to reliably screen for fetal aneuploidy. The false-positive rate for each dichorionic twin is 5% and is therefore similar to that in singletons. However, in monochorionic twins, nuchal translucency is measured above the 95th percentile for crown–rump length (CRL) in either twin inasmuch as 8.5% of the cases. Sebire *et al.* reported an 88% detection rate for a false-positive rate per pregnancy of around 10% and 15% in dichorionic and monochorionic pregnancies, respectively.[6] Discordance of nuchal translucency measurements between monochorionic twins is also predictive of the development of twin-to-twin transfusion syndrome (TTTS) with a sensitivity of 33% and a positive predictive value of 28%. The likelihood ratio of developing TTTS at 10–14 weeks of gestation is 4.2 (95% CI, 3.0–6.0).[6]

Specific complications of monochorionic twins

Twin-to-twin transfusion syndrome (Figure 42.2)

In all monochorionic pregnancies, a single placental mass implies that the two fetuses share some placental units with a shared vascularization of these cotyledons. An imbalance in placental sharing will arise in around 15% of monochorionic pregnancies.[6] Indeed, the natural history of monochorionic twins as observed by serial ultrasound examination suggests that up to 28% of all monochorionic twins scanned at 12 weeks will show some discrepancy either in abdominal circumference or in amniotic fluid volume, with membrane folding at 16–18 weeks, but only up to half of these (14% of the starting number) will develop TTTS in the second or early third trimester.[6,7] TTTS results from an acute hemodynamic imbalance through the vascular placental anastomoses. The donor twin becomes hypovolemic, oliguric and around two-thirds of these will also show some degree of growth restriction. Oligohydramnios develops in this sac. There is hypervolemia in the recipient twin, which is therefore polyuric leading to polyhydramnios in its sac and is exposed to high-output cardiac failure. Although a net transfer of blood is likely to initiate it, this is not the only mechanism involved in the syndrome. In order to maintain volemia, the fetal renin–angiotensin system is activated in the donor twin and suppressed in the recipient with preferential maternal–fetal transfer of fluid to the recipient.[8] A paradoxical effect of a transfer of renin toward the recipient twin through the placental anastomoses could also contribute to the development of hypertension and cardiomyopathy in this fetus. A velamentous insertion of the cord of either twin on the placenta is found in up to 30–50% of all monochorionic pregnancies and this is likely to play a significant role in creating hemodynamic imbalance between the two feto-placental circulations.

The diagnosis of TTTS requires that the pregnancy is monochorionic and relies on the association of polyuria-related polyhydramnios in the recipient twin together with oliguria-related oligohydramnios in the donor twin. Polyhydramnios is defined as a vertical deepest pool of amniotic fluid of at least 8 cm before 20 weeks and 10 cm thereafter and oligohydramnios is present when the deepest fluid is at most 2 cm. Up to 28% of all monochorionic twins seen at 12 weeks on ultrasound will develop some discrepancy in the volume of amniotic fluid and/or a discrepancy in size[6] by 16–18 weeks. This does not meet the criteria for TTTS and has led to a long-standing misunderstanding on the diagnosis and the prognosis of TTTS. It is only half of these, that is, 14% of the starting number, that will develop the polyoligohydramnios sequence. The fetal size, although the recipient is usually appropriately grown and the donor is usually smaller, is not an important criterion for the diagnosis of TTTS.

When oligohydramnios is confined to anhydramnios, the intertwin membranes are difficult to visualize and the donor twin is 'stuck' on the placenta or the uterine wall. This can lead to a false diagnosis of monoamniotic pregnancy or the suspicion of various malformations in the compressed donor twin. Pushing the abdominal wall with regard to the donor twin will demonstrate that this twin cannot move due to anhydramnios. Hypervolemia in the recipient often shows a cardiothoracic index of more than 0.55 with a thick myocardium and the presence of tricuspid regurgitation, which has no prognostic value when the recipient is not hydropic. The best first-line treatment consists of fetoscopic surgery to coagulate the anastomotic chorionic plate vessels.[9]

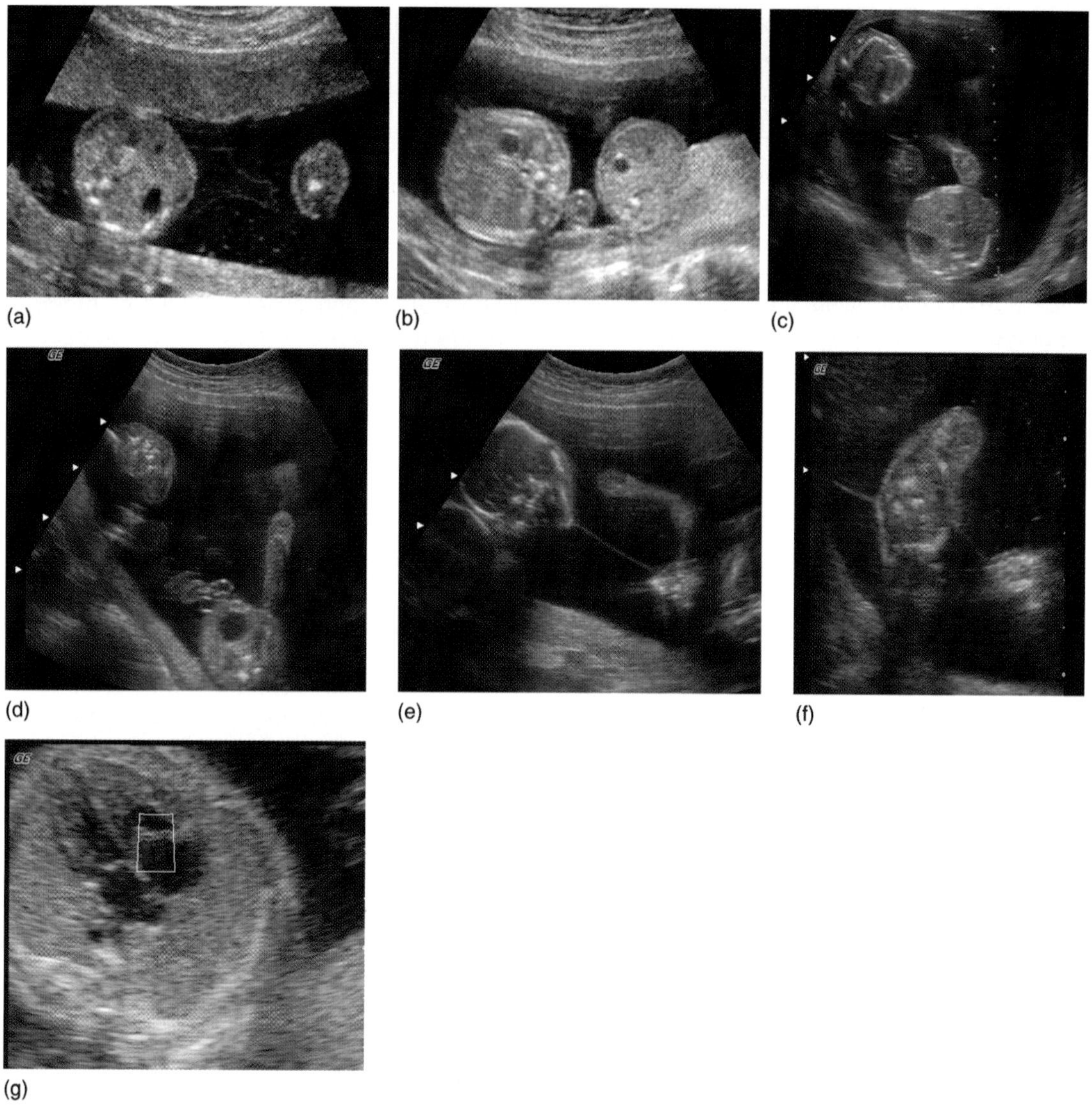

Figure 42.2 (a) Folding of the membranes (arrow) in a monochorionic twin pregnancy at 17 weeks. (b) Cross-section through the fetal abdomen of two monochorionic twins discordant for growth at 20 weeks. (c) Cross-section through the fetal abdomen of the stuck donor twin in anhydramnios against the uterine wall (d) and the recipient twin in polyhydramnios (r) in twin-to-twin transfusion syndrome. (d) Cross-section through the fetal pelvis of the stuck donor and the recipient showing absent and distended bladder, respectively. (e) The donor in anhydramnios is wrapped in its membranes as shown in a sagittal plane (f) and in a cross-section through the pelvis showing an empty bladder. This 'sling-sign' could lead to the false impression that the amniotic fluid volume is normal on both sides of a floating intertwin membrane. (g) Examination of the recipient's four-chamber view of the heart with color Doppler showing tricuspid regurgitation.

Arterial and venous fetal Doppler can be normal or show absent or reverse end diastolic flow in the umbilical arteries. Absent or reverse flow in the a-wave of the ductus venosus usually corresponds to severe hypoxemia or cardiac overload in the donor or the recipient twin, respectively. Peak systolic velocities in the middle cerebral artery are sensitive to anemia and to polycythemia showing values above 1.5 MoM or below 0.7 MoM, respectively.[10] However, a difference in hemoglobin is unusual *in utero* in most cases of TTTS.[11]

Quintero[12] has proposed a classification of TTTS in four stages, which has the advantage of homogenizing the diagnostic criteria. Stage 1 corresponds to the association of polyhydramnios in the recipient and oligohydramnios in the donor, where the bladder is visible. Stage 2 is similar but the bladder cannot be visualized in the donor. In Stage 3, Doppler examination shows marked abnormalities with absent or reversed end diastolic flow or absent or reversed a-wave in the umbilical arteries or in the ductus venosus, respectively. Stage 4 is characterized by the presence of hydrops in either twin. Stage 5 is when one or both twins have died *in utero*.

TTTS can also develop into monoamniotic pregnancies. Polyuric polyhydramnios is then seen together with a small or unseen bladder in its co-twin.

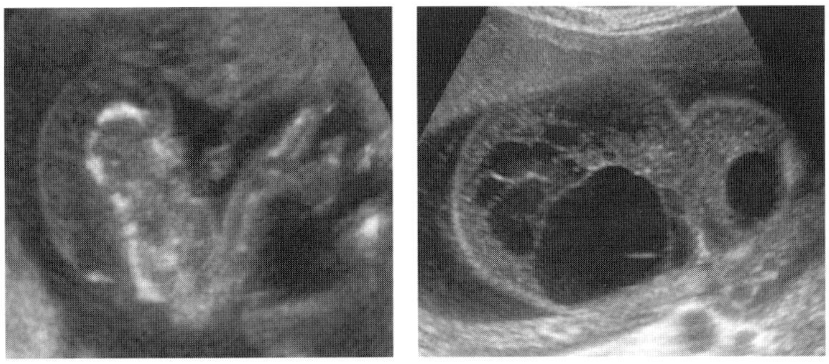

(a) (b)

Figure 42.3 (a) Monochorionic twin pregnancy showing an acardiac twin at 13 weeks showing rudimentary head, spine and lower extremities. (b) Edematous acardiac mass at 25 weeks.

Acardiac twin

An acardiac twin is defined by the presence of one monochorionic twin without a clearly anatomically defined heart; the co-twin is usually normal. Vascularization of the monochorionic placenta almost invariably shows the presence of two superficial anastomoses between the two cord insertions: one artery-to-artery and one vein-to-vein anastomose flowing in opposite directions. There is usually a single umbilical artery in the cord of the acardiac twin and this sets the basis for an increased cardiac workload in the normal twin, also named the pump twin. The acardiac mass can grow and develop to various degrees, increasing the mass of tissue that the normal twin heart has to bear (Figure 42.3). This can therefore lead to the development of high-cardiac output hydrops in up to 50% of pump twins. The bigger the acardiac mass, the higher the likelihood of hemodynamic decompensation of the pump twin.[13] The acardiac twin usually bears several major malformations, allowing for embryological classification,[13] the most frequent being the acardiac acephalus; however, rudimentary organs, especially limbs and spine, are often present. Early in the pregnancy, this is often mistaken for either an early embryonic demise or a placental tumor. The key to the diagnosis is the use of color Doppler showing retrograde perfusion of the acardiac mass, and eventually demonstrating the placental anastomoses.

Monoamniotic pregnancies

The fetuses will be seen in close proximity and both crossing of their limbs and cord entanglement as seen by color Doppler will establish the diagnosis.

Conjoined twins

These are 4–5% of all monochorionic monoamniotic twins. The embryological classification refers to the part of their body through which they are attached, the most frequent type being thoracopagus.[14] Organ sharing can be symmetrical or asymmetrical. The extreme form of the latter constitutes the fetus-in-fetu, where a rudimentary fetal mass can be found as a hyperechogenic tumoral mass into an otherwise usually normal fetus, child or even adult.

There is a clear benefit for an early diagnosis of a unique embryonic mass often characterized by the presence of two beating hearts. Embryonic/fetal movements are always simultaneous and a single umbilical cord with more than three vessels can be identified.

Amniotic fluid volume in twin pregnancies

Oligohydramnios, anhydramnios and the 'stuck-twin phenomenon'

All causes of oligohydramnios in the singleton can affect one or both twins and should be investigated in the same way. The stuck-twin phenomenon can therefore affect both monochorionic and dichorionic pregnancies to the same extent. However, when oligohydramnios affects only one twin, the twin with a normal amount of fluid is often unduly credited for having polyhydramnios and a wrong diagnosis of TTTS is often suspected. It is therefore critical to use an objective measurement of the amniotic volume, mainly using the deepest pool measurement.[15] Another important pitfall is to consider that the two layers of membranes tightly wrapped around the stuck-twin, featuring the 'sling-sign'[16] could be mistaken as free-floating membranes separating two cavities with a normal amount of fluid in each sac. Etiologies that are more prone to affect twins include low urinary tract obstruction, severe intrauterine growth retardation and preterm prelabor rupture of the membranes.

Polyhydramnios in twins

All malformations seen in singletons, such as anencephaly, bowel atresia, are more frequent in twins. Monochorionic twins, however, are the only ones to see acute polyhydramnios developing polyhydramnios due to TTTS.

Cervical changes in twin pregnancies

Although twin pregnancies are 1% of all pregnancies and 2% of all deliveries, twins account for 15% of all maternal morbidity and mortality. This is mainly due to preterm delivery with 12% of all preterm neonates being twins.

The advantage of cervical ultrasound over digital examination has also been clearly shown in twins. Relative risk of preterm delivery within a week of cervical ultrasound examination has been reviewed by Ong *et al.*[17] as 4.1 (95% CI, 1.10–15.47) and 11.7 (95% CI, 4.23–32.17), respectively, for values lower than the thresholds of 25 and 20 mm.

Growth discordance in twins

This is the second most frequent complication in twins and the second contributor to neonatal mortality and morbidity. Conflict of interest may arise between twins so as to define the optimal timing for delivery. In the second and third trimesters of pregnancy, the cutoff value for EBW estimate is at least 20%.

Malformations in twins

The presence of two embryos/fetuses increases the risk as compared to singletons. A recent series[18] has gathered data on 260,000 twin pregnancies among 12 million births. Five thousand and five hundred twin pregnancies carry at least one malformed twin outside specific risks associated with monochorionicity representing 2.14% vs. 1.72% for singletons. A total of 101 malformation sequences have been reported, 37 of which are more prevalent in twins. The prevalence of fetal malformations in twins is therefore around 25% with relative risks of 8–60%. Dizygotic twins only carry non-specific malformations. Monochorionic twins will bear malformations both non-specific and specific to monochorionicity. Specific malformations include those arising from a delay in zygotic splitting or midline abnormalities as well as those resulting from a sequence of events following severe hemodynamic imbalance through placental anastomoses. Furthermore, only 5–20% of monozygotic pregnancies are concordant for fetal malformations.[19] These differences can also arise from postzygotic genetic abnormalities, different susceptibility to their exposure to environmental factors.

Intrauterine fetal death of one twin

Perinatal mortality in twins is up to sevenfold higher than in singletons.[20] Intrauterine death of one twin can result from non-specific fetal complications such as those seen in singletons, including cord compression and severe growth restriction, as well as from specific complications related to hemodynamic imbalance, including TTTS and collapse. In monochorionic twins, the death of one fetus will threaten its co-twin by causing an abrupt and profound drop in systemic blood pressure subsequent to the exsanguinations of the survivor in its dead co-twin and its placenta through the intertwin anastomoses. Peak systolic velocities in the midcerebral arteries of the survivor measured above 1.5 MoM within 24 h of the co-twin's death will predict anemia/hypovolemia in this twin (sensitivity 90% for a 10% false-positive rate).[10] Exsanguination will lead to fetal death or severe ischemic sequelae in the survivor in 25% and 25% of the cases, respectively. Ischemia-related malformations include cerebral lesions such as periventricular leukomalacia, porencephaly, hydrocephalus and migrational anomalies, renal ischemia and mesenteric ischemia leading to bowel atresia. These lesions will only be amenable to prenatal diagnosis from 2 to 3 weeks following the acute event.

In dichorionic pregnancies, the co-twin will only be exposed to a persistent cause of death and prematurity.[21,22]

REFERENCES

1. Monteagudo A, Timor-Tritsch IE, Sharma S. Early and simple determination of chorionic and amniotic type in multifetal gestations in the first fourteen weeks by high-frequency transvaginal ultrasonography. *Am J Obstet Gynecol* 1994;170:824–9.
2. Bessis R, Papiernick E. Echographic imagery of amniotic membranes in twin pregnancies. *Prog Clin Biol Res* 1981;69A: 183–7.
3. Finberg HJ. The 'twin peak' sign: A reliable evidence of dichorionic twinning. *J Ultrasound Med* 1992;11:571–7.
4. Sepulveda W, Sebire NJ, Hughes K, Odibo A, Nicolaides KH. The lambda sign at 10–14 weeks of gestation as a predictor of chorionicity in twin pregnancies. *Ultrasound Obstet Gynecol* 1996;7: 421–3.
5. Bromley B, Benacerraf B. Using the number of yolk sac to determine amnionicity in early first trimester monochorionic twins. *J Ultrasound Med* 1995;14:415–9.
6. Sebire NJ, Souka A, Skentou H, Geerts L, Nicolaides KH. Early prediction of severe twin-to-twin transfusion syndrome. *Hum Reprod* 2000;15:2008–10.
7. Sebire NJ, d'Ercole C, Carvelho M, Sepulveda W, Nicolaides KH. Inter-twin membrane folding in monochorionic pregancies. *Ultrasound Obset Gynecol* 1998;11:324–7.
8. Mahieu-Caputo D, Dommergues M, Delezoide AL, *et al.* Twin–twin transfusion syndrome. Role of the fetal renin–angiotensin system. *Am J Pathol* 2000;156:629–36.
9. Senat MV, Deprest J, Boulvain M, Paupe A, Winer N, Ville Y. Endoscopic laser surgery versus serial amnioreduction for severe twin-to-twin transfusion syndrome. *N Engl J Med* 2004;351(2): 136–44.
10. Senat MV, Loizeau S, Couderc S, Bernard JP, Ville Y. The value of middle cerebral artery peak systolic velocity in the diagnosis of

fetal anemia after intrauterine death of one monochorionic twin. *Am J Obstet Gynecol* 2003;189:1320–4.

11. Denbow M, Fogliani R, Kyle P, Letsky E, Nicolini U, Fisk NM. Haematological indices at fetal blood sampling in monochorionic pregnancies complicated by feto-fetal transfusion syndrome. *Prenat Diagn* 1998;18:941–6.
12. Quintero R, Morales WJ, Allen MH. Staging of twin-to-twin transfusion syndrome. *J Perinat* 1999;19:550–5.
13. Moore TR, Gale S, Benirschke K. Perinatal outcome of 49 pregnancies complicated by acardiac twining. *Am J Obstet Gynecol* 1990;163:907–12.
14. Spencer R. Parasitic conjoined twins: External, internal, detached. *Clin Anat* 2001;14:428–44.
15. Hill LM, Krohn M, Lazebnik N, Tush B, Boyles D, Ursiny JJ. The amniotic fluid index in normal twin pregnancies. *Am J Obstet Gynecol* 2000;182:950–4.
16. al-Kouatly HB, Skupski DW. Intrauterine sling: A complication of the stuck twin syndrome. *Ultrasound Obstet Gynecol* 1999;14: 419–21.
17. Ong S, Smith A, Smith N, Campbell D, Wilson A. Cervical length assessment in twin pregnancies using transvaginal ultrasound. *Acta Obstet Gynecol Scand* 2000;79:851–3.
18. Mastroiacovo P, Castilla EE, Arpino C, *et al.* Congenital malformations in twins: An international study. *Am J Med Genet* 1999;83: 117–24.
19. Schinzel AAGL, Smith DW, Miller JR. Monozygotic twinning and structural defects. *J Pediatr* 1979;95:921–30.
20. Benirschke K, Kim CK. Multiple pregnancy. *N Engl J Med* 1973; 14:1276–83.
21. Bajoria R, Wee LY, Anwar S, Ward S. Outcome of twin pregnancies complicated by single intrauterine death in relation to vascular anatomy of the monochorionic placenta. *Hum Reprod* 1999;14:2124–30.
22. Fusi L, Gordon H. Twin pregnancy complicated by single intrauterine death. Problems and outcome with conservative management. *Br J Obstet Gynaecol* 1990;97:511–6.

43 Echocardiography in early pregnancy: a new challenge in prenatal diagnosis

C. Comas, J. M. Martínez, A. Galindo, O. Gómez, C. Millán and G. Azumendi

Summary

Within the last decade, two significant events have contributed to the increasing interest in early fetal echocardiography: first, the introduction of high-frequency vaginal ultrasound probes that allow detailed visualization of cardiac structures at an early stage of gestation, making early detection of fetal malformations possible, and second, the close relationship observed between some first-trimester sonographic and Doppler markers and congenital heart defects, which allows early identification of a high-risk group at 11–14 weeks of gestation. In this context, from the early 1990s, many authors have examined the potential role of the transvaginal (TV) approach to obtain earlier diagnosis of fetal cardiac malformations. Further studies have appeared in the literature showing that early TV echocardiography in experienced hands is a fairly sensitive investigative tool. Although some malformations are detected as early as 11 weeks' gestation, the optimal gestational age to perform the early scan is at least 13 weeks' gestation. TV ultrasound is the preferred approach, although most of the authors agree that results can be improved if transabdominal ultrasound is also incorporated. The further application of color Doppler enhances visualization. The sensitivity and specificity of early fetal echocardiography for the detection of heart anomalies are acceptable compared to those obtained by midgestational echocardiography, showing a slight reduction in detection rates and an increase in false-positive and -negative rates. The cardiac anomalies detected at this early stage of pregnancy are mainly defects involving the four-chamber view, indicating that defects solely affecting the outflow tracts are difficult to diagnose in the first trimester of pregnancy. Heart defects diagnosed early in pregnancy tend to be more complex than those detected later with a higher incidence of associated structural malformations, chromosomal abnormalities and spontaneous abortions. The neonate follow-up or postmortem examination in case of termination of pregnancy is essential to assess the actual role of early fetal echocardiography. At present, early fetal echocardiography is a promising technique, which can be of considerable value for patients at high-risk. This technique is, however, currently limited to a few specialized centers.

The aim of this review is to explore the possibilities of examining the fetal heart at this early stage of pregnancy. This article also presents our experience in the first multicenter trial in early fetal echocardiography performed in Spain. In accordance with other studies, this experience stresses the usefulness of early echocardiography when performed by expert operators on the fetus, specifically at risk for cardiac defects. Our review of these 48 additional cases contributes to the expanding literature on the ability of TV ultrasonography to detect fetal heart defects in early pregnancy.

Introduction

Prenatal detection of fetal congenital heart defects (CHD) remains the most problematic issue of prenatal diagnosis.[1] Major CHD are the most common severe congenital malformations with an incidence of about 5 in 1000 live births, whenever complete ascertainment is done and minor lesions are excluded.[1,2] Congenital heart anomalies have a significant effect on the affected children's life with up to 25–35% mortality rate during pregnancy and the postnatal period, and it is during the first year of life that 60% of this mortality occurs. Moreover, major CHD are responsible for nearly 50% of all neonatal and infant deaths due to congenital anomalies, and it is likely to be significantly higher if spontaneous abortions are considered. Although CHD used to appear isolated, they are frequently associated with other defects, chromosomal anomalies and genetic syndromes. Their incidence is six times greater than chromosomal abnormalities and four times greater than neural tube defects.[1–3]

Most major CHD can be diagnosed prenatally by detailed transabdominal second-trimester echocardiography at 20–22 weeks' gestation.[1,3–6] The identification of pregnancies at high risk for CHD needing referral to specialist centers is of paramount importance in order to reduce the rate of overlooked defects.[6,7] However, the main problem in prenatal diagnosis of CHD is that the majority of cases take place in pregnancies with no identifiable risk factors. Therefore, there is wide agreement that cardiac ultrasound screening should be introduced as an integral part of the routine scan at 20–22 weeks. When applied to the low-risk population, scrutiny of the four-chamber view allows only the detection of 40% of the anomalies, while additional visualization of the outflow tracts and the great arteries increases the rate up to 60–70%.[3–5]

Recently, the finding of an increased nuchal translucency (NT)[8,9] or an altered ductus venosus (DV) blood flow[10,11] at 10–14 weeks' gestation has been associated with a high risk for CHD and their prevalence increases exponentially with the thickness of NT[8] regardless of the fetal karyotype. Since earlier diagnosis of congenital malformations is increasingly demanded, the option of an early fetal echocardiography must be taken into account.[12–14] The use of high-frequency vaginal ultrasound probes along with substantial improvements in magnification and processing of the imaging, together with the introduction of color Doppler, has extensively contributed to the development of the technique, allowing better visualization of cardiac structures earlier in pregnancy.[12,15,16] Although most of the groups perform early fetal echocardiography between 13 and 16 weeks' gestation, we can name it as so when performed before the 18th week of gestation. Despite several studies that stated that fetal heart examination could be incorporated in first- or early second-trimester examinations, its use is currently still limited to a few specialized centers.

Technical issues

Regarding early fetal echocardiography, some institutions use predominantly the transvaginal (TV) approach,[14,17–22] while others prefer the transabdominal one.[23–26] Most of the authors reporting early fetal echocardiography prefer the TV approach because of its increased resolution associated with higher-frequency transducers and also because given that equivalent transducers frequencies, the TV probes provide better-quality images.[27] However, most importantly, authors with background training as pediatric cardiologists are more likely to use the transabdominal approach in contrast with most of the obstetricians, who are well used to the TV route. The superiority of TV sonography is usually well accepted before the 14th week. Between the 15th and the 18th weeks both transabdominal and TV routes seem to offer similar advantages and disadvantages, and beyond the 18th week the transabdominal echocardiography seems to achieve better results.[1,5,16,27,28]

The combination of two-dimensional echocardiography with color Doppler flow imaging proved generally helpful, in particular by visualization of blood flow on both great arteries and of two divided ventricular inflows. The addition of color Doppler flow studies provides substantial improvement in the diagnostic accuracy of early echocardiography, as was also shown by DeVore for transabdominal sonography in the second half of pregnancy.[29]

When performing early fetal echocardiography, we first recommend scanning by the TV route, following the examination by the transabdominal probe when a complete study is not possible. The highest frequency must always be used, whatever the route chosen. Obviously, a high-resolution real-time ultrasound has to be used. For color Doppler evaluation, the energy output levels have to be lower than 50 mW/cm^2 spatial peak-temporal average. Since color Doppler is dissipated over a wide area of interest, thermal effects resulting from Doppler insonation should not be a matter of concern, unlike pulsed Doppler in which the whole energy of the beam is focused at a specific location. Besides, the embryonic development of the heart has been completed by the time the scan is performed.

Ultrasound anatomy of the normal heart

Embryonic heartbeat can be detected as early as the 5th week of gestation, and normal development of its function shows an increasing heart rate from 80–90 beats/min at 5 weeks' gestation to 170–180 beats/min at the end of the 9th to 10th week. As pregnancy progresses, the control of the heart rate matures with increasing vagal dominance, and the baseline rate declines to 145–155 beats/min with the appearance of beat-to-beat variation, most likely resulting from the functional adaptation to the development of the heart and autonomic nervous system maturation, and remains more or less constant during the rest of intrauterine life.[30,31]

The structural development of the heart begins on day 16 and is completed by the 10th week. Early fetal echocardiography has the same goals as the standard one, and we advocate performing it in a segmental approach. The first objective of the examination is to assess the normality of the four-chamber view through a transverse section of the fetal chest: normal situs solitus; normal size and axis of the heart in relation to the chest; both atria equal in size, with the foramen ovale flapping within the left atrium; both ventricles equal in size and contractility; atrial and ventricular septa of normal appearance; tricuspid and

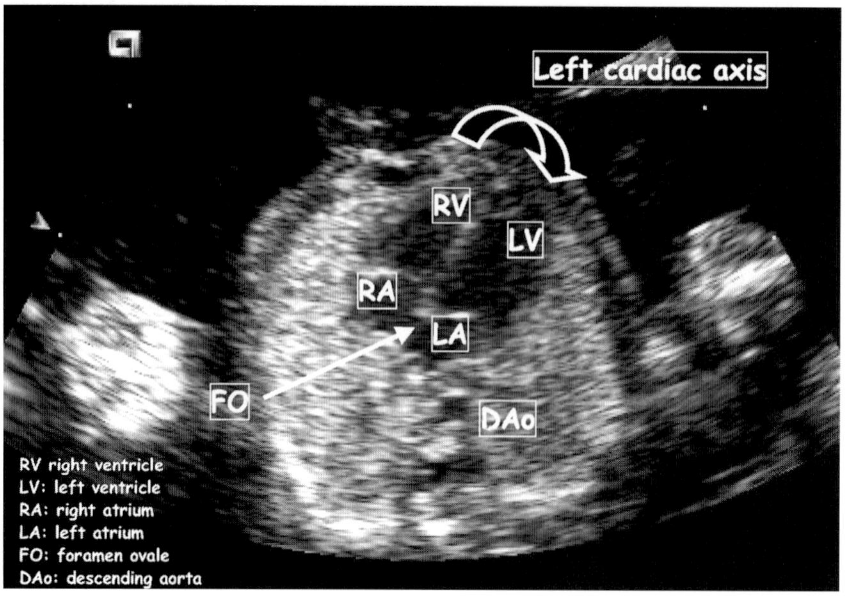

Figure 43.1 Early fetal echocardiography by 2D in a structurally normal heart. The four-chamber view: normal situs solitus; normal size and axis of the heart in relation to the chest; both atria equal in size, with the foramen ovale flapping within the left atrium; both ventricles equal in size and contractility; atrial and ventricular septa of normal appearance; tricuspid and mitral valves normally inserted.

mitral valves normally inserted, opening and closing together. Color and pulsed Doppler are particularly useful to confirm normal inflow to the ventricles and to detect turbulent flow or jets suggesting valve regurgitation. It is useful to assess the four chambers in different views, apical, basal and long axis, with the interventricular septum perpendicular to the ultrasound beam in order to visualize better the integrity of the septum. Then, the origin and double crossing of the great arteries must be correctly identified: the left ventricle outflow tract, with the continuity between the interventricular septum and the anterior wall of the ascending aorta; the right ventricle outflow tract, more superior, anterior, almost perpendicular to the axis of the ascending aorta and connecting to the descending aorta in the three vessels view. Color Doppler is also of help to better visualize the outflow tracts to confirm anterograde flow through the semilunar valves and great arteries, and makes easier the examination of both aortic and ductal arches and their confluence. Pulsed Doppler may be used to assess blood flow through the aortic and pulmonic valves in order to confirm the normal anterograde flow and to detect very high velocities suggesting valve stenosis. Finally, color and pulsed Doppler are also very useful to identify normal systemic and pulmonary venous return. Figures 43.1–43.10 illustrate images obtained at early fetal scan by two-dimensional echocardiography and color Doppler in a structurally normal heart. In our experience, the average duration of the complete fetal cardiac scan is over 15 min. It essentially depends on the gestational age at the examination, and can be even shorter if there is a favorable fetal lie. In our setting, a subsequent transabdominal echocardiography is scheduled for all our patients at 20–22 weeks' gestation.

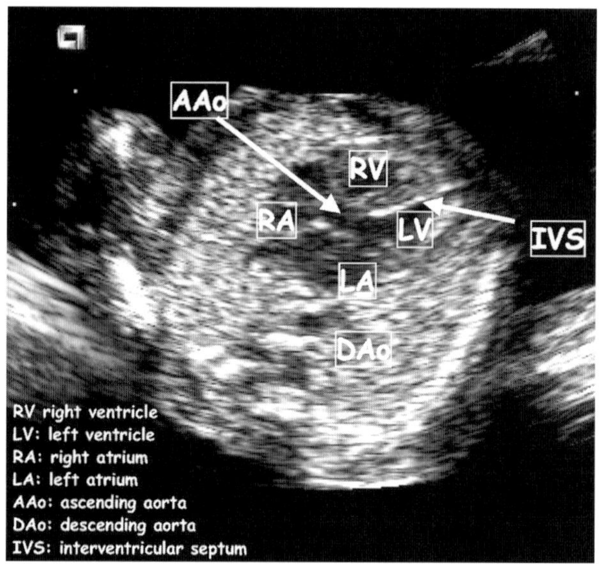

Figure 43.2 Early fetal echocardiography by 2D in a structurally normal heart. The five-chamber view: left ventricle outflow tract in the long axis view showing the continuity between the interventricular septum and the anterior wall of the ascending aorta.

Most of the authors agree that the best window of time to perform the early echocardiography is between 13 and 16 weeks of gestation, since a complete cardiac examination is rarely achieved before the 13th week of gestation.[14,17,18,20–22,26] Articles on early fetal echocardiography demonstrate an increase

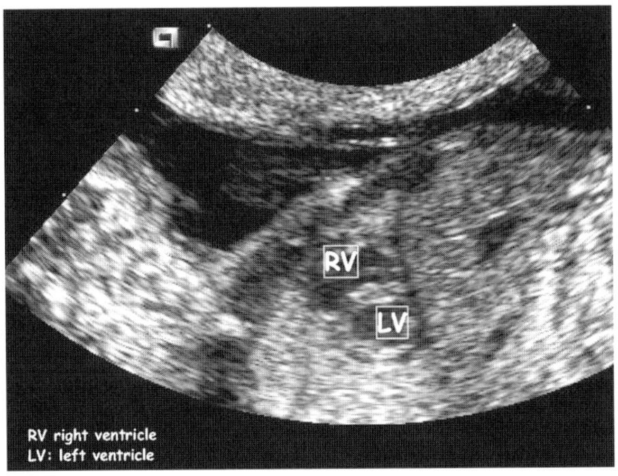

Figure 43.3 Early fetal echocardiography by 2D in a structurally normal heart. The short axis view showing an anterior right ventricle and a posterior left ventricle.

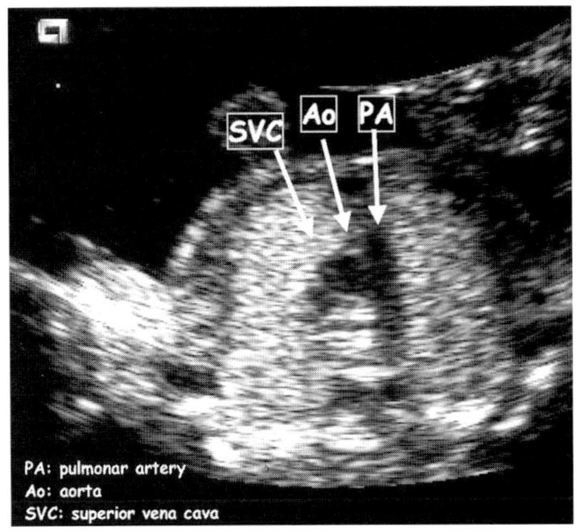

Figure 43.4 Early fetal echocardiography by 2D in a structurally normal heart. The three-vessel view: cross sections of the pulmonary artery, ascending aorta and superior vena cava in a transverse view of upper mediastinum. In normal conditions, the structures in the three-vessel view are in descending order of size from the left to the right.

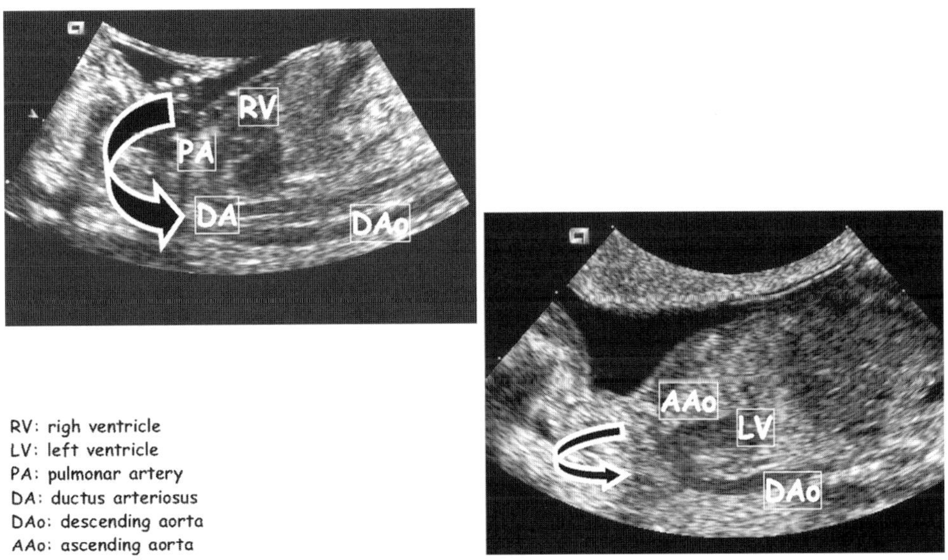

Figure 43.5 Early fetal echocardiography by 2D in a structurally normal heart. The left sagital view of ductal and aortic arches.

in visualization rates of the four-chamber view and the outflow tracts in the last decade, with visualization rates greater than 90% at 13 weeks' gestation.[28] To maximize the reduction of uninterpretable examinations, early fetal echocardiography should be preferably performed at 13 completed weeks' gestation. Using current technology, the four-chamber view and the outflow tracts are often demonstrated by two-dimensional echocardiography only, but color Doppler imaging enhances and makes the identification of the structures faster, increasing the success rate of the examination, and allows even earlier identification of the structures.

Diagnosis of CHD

The first diagnosis of CHD by early echocardiography was reported by Gembruch *et al.*[32] in 1990. A complete atrioventricular canal defect, with complete heart block and atrioventricular valve regurgitation, was diagnosed at 11 weeks + 4 days' gestation using a 5-MHz TV probe. The same year, Bronshtein *et al.*[33] reported the diagnosis of a ventricular septal defect (VSD) with overriding aorta and a further case of an isolated VSD with pericardial effusion, both cases at 14 weeks' gestation. Since then, an increasing number of case reports and series on the early diagnosis of CHD have been reported,

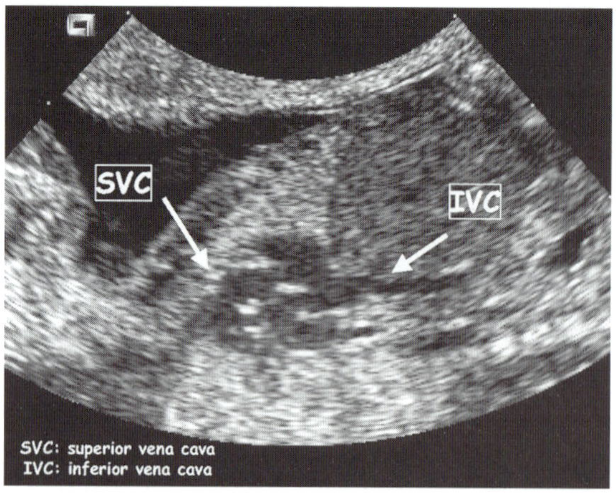

Figure 43.6 Early fetal echocardiography by 2D in a structurally normal heart. Systemic venous return to the right atrium through the superior and inferior venae cavae.

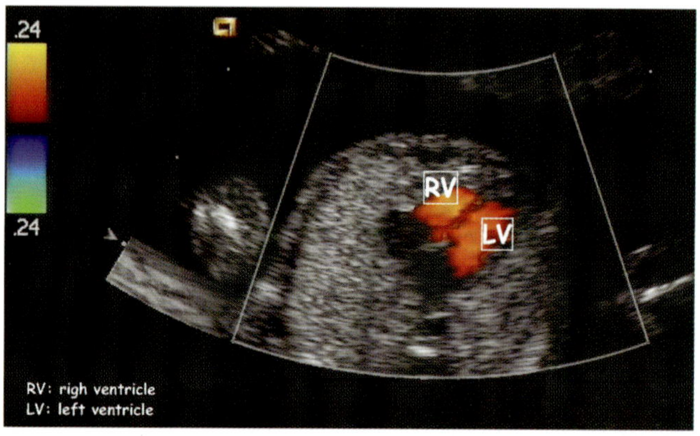

Figure 43.7 Early fetal echocardiography by 2D and color Doppler in a structurally normal heart. Color Doppler in the four-chamber view is particularly useful to confirm normal inflow to the ventricles and to detect turbulent flow or jets suggesting valve regurgitation.

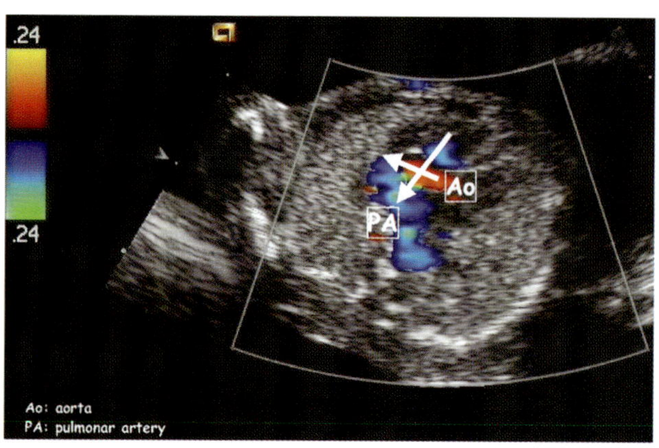

Figure 43.8 Early fetal echocardiography by 2D and color Doppler in a structurally normal heart. Color Doppler is particularly useful to demonstrate the crossing of the great arteries.

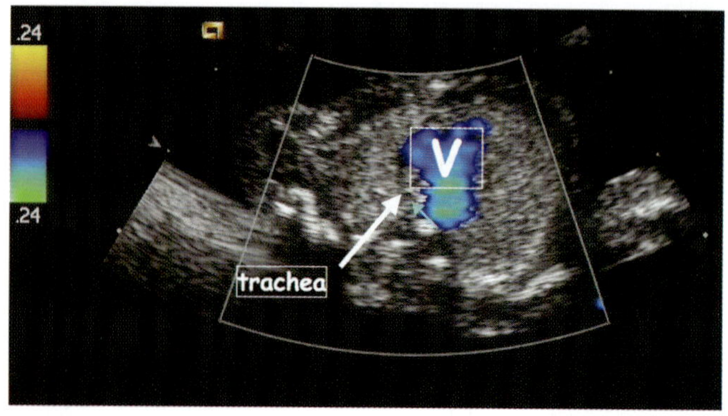

Figure 43.9 Early fetal echocardiography by 2D and color Doppler in a structurally normal heart. Color Doppler is particularly useful to demonstrate the normal V confluence of the ductal and aortic arches (V sign). Note that normally the trachea is located behind the aortic arch.

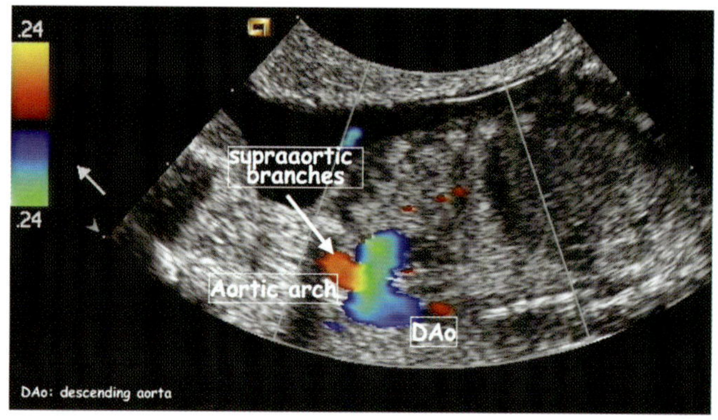

Figure 43.10 Early fetal echocardiography by 2D and color Doppler in a structurally normal heart. Color Doppler is particularly useful to demonstrate the aortic arch.

in both high-risk and low-risk populations. Tables 43.1 and 43.2 summarize some of the largest and the most significant studies on the detection of CHD using early fetal echocardiography in high-risk and low-risk pregnancies.[14,17–22,24–26,34–39] Obviously, studies in unselected population report less encouraging results with lower visualization rates and detection rates. The largest series so far is the one published by Bronshtein *et al.*[20] They report the diagnosis of 173 cases of CHD over 36,323 fetuses evaluated by TV ultrasound at 11–17 weeks' gestation over a 14-year period of time, with 99% of the scans performed at 14–16 weeks' gestation and 86% of them in low-risk population. Recently, two institutions went further and reported their experience performing the echocardiography as early as between 10 and 13 weeks' gestation.[22,26]

Table 43.1 Results of early fetal echocardiography to diagnose cardiac defects in a high-risk population (only series with at least 10 cardiac defects diagnosed)

Reference	Route	GA	Success (%)	Risk	*N*	Cases	11–16 weeks	20–22 weeks
Gembruch[14]	TV	11–16	90.3	High	114	13	92%	100%
Zosmer[24]	TA	13–17		High	323	27	89%	96.3%
Simpson[25]	TA	12–15	98.7	High	229	17	76%	94%
Huggon[26]	TA	10–14	86.8	High	478	68	94%	
Haak[22]	TV	10–13	95.5	High	45	13	54%	
Bronshtein[20]	TV	11–17	> 99	High	6175	46	> 90%	
Comas[21]	TV	12–17	94.6	High	337	48	79%	96%
Lopes[39]	TV	12–16	94.9	High	275	37	89%	

TV, transvaginal; TA, transabdominal; Route, main approach; GA, range of gestational age at scan (weeks); Success, visualization success rate for the complete early fetal echocardiography; *N*, total number of pregnancies scanned; Cases, total number of cardiac defects (pre- and postnatally); 11–16 weeks, percentage of cardiac defects identified at early echocardiography; 20–22 weeks, percentage of cardiac defects identified at midtrimester echocardiography

Table 43.2 Detection rate of cardiac defects at early ultrasound to screen for congenital malformations in a low-risk population

Reference	GA	Success (%)	Risk	Normal	Cases	11–16 weeks	20–22 weeks
Achiron[18]	13–15	98	Low	660	6	50%	50%
Hernadi[34]	12		Low	3991	3	33%	100%
D'Ottavio[35]	13–15		Low	3490	8	25%	80%
Yagel[17]	13–16	99	Low	6924	66	64%	81%
Economides[36]	12–13		Low	1632	3	0%	33%
Whitlow[37]	11–14		Low	6443	10	40%	60%
Guariglia[38]	10–16		Low	3592	11	18%	56%
Rustico[19]	13–15	< 50	Low	4785	41	10%	32%
Bronshtein[20]	11–17	99	Low	30148	127	97%	99%

GA, range of gestational age at scan (weeks); Success, visualization success rate for the extended cardiac examination (four chambers outflow tracts); Normal, total number of pregnancies screened; Cases, total number of cardiac defects (pre- and postnatally); 11–16 weeks, percentage of cardiac defects identified at early scan; 20–22 weeks, percentage of cardiac defects identified at midtrimester scan

The most frequent fetal heart anomalies diagnosed at early echocardiography are summarized in Table 43.3 (true-positive cases).[14,18–21,24–26,34,35,37,39] Note that only the main anomaly for each fetus is presented in the table, even though some fetuses had several cardiac anomalies. It should be noted that defects such as small, isolated VSD or valvular stenosis are not reported in these studies. Table 43.4 summarizes the published cases of cardiac anomaly not detected in early pregnancy (false-negative cases).[14,19–21,24–26,34–37,39]

The results of these studies support the use of early fetal echocardiography to detect the majority of major CHD in both low-risk and high-risk populations during the first and the early second trimesters of pregnancy. The cardiac anomalies detected at this early stage of pregnancy are mainly the defects involving the four-chamber view, such as large VSDs, atrioventricular septal defects (AVSDs) and malformations resulting in asymmetry of the ventricles, indicating that defects solely affecting the outflow tracts are

Table 43.3 Fetal heart anomalies diagnosed at early echocardiography (true-positive cases at early fetal echocardiography)

True +	A	B	C	D	E	F	G	H	I	J	K	L	M	N	O	P	Q	R	Overall
Gembruch[14]				6		1	1				2		2						12
Zosmer[24]			3	3	2	1	4	2	3	1			4				1		24
Rustico[19]				2		1	1	1											5
Simpson[25]			3	2				3	2				2	1					13
Huggon[26]			5	29		12	9	1			1			1	1	1			60
Bronshtein[20]	4	1	4	13	2	9	25		31*	22	5		18		17	3	2	13	169
Comas[21]			4	8		10	4	1	3		2	2	1			3			38
Achiron[18]				2					2		1				1	1	1		8
Hernadi[34]						1													1
D'Ottavio[35]							2										2		4
Whitlow[37]					1		1									1			3
Rustico[19]		1					2		1										4
Lopes[39]			2	6		11	5	1	1	1	1	3	2						33
Overall	4	2	21	71	5	46	54	9	43	24	12	5	29	2	19	9	6	13	374

A, abnormal veno-atrial connections; B, atrial septal defects; C, tricuspid atresia or dysplasia; D, atrioventricular septal defect; E, single ventricle; F, VSDs; G, aortic atresia, aortic stenosis and HLH; H, pulmonary atresia or stenosis; I, tetralogy of Fallot; J, transposition of great arteries; K, truncus; L, double-outlet right ventricle; M, aortic arch anomalies; N, isomerism; O, myocardiopathy; P, ectopia cordis; Q, complex cardiac defect, others; R, vascular ring

*This series include cases with tetralogy of Fallot and double-outlet right ventricle

Table 43.4 Fetal heart anomalies not detected at early echocardiography (false-negative cases at early fetal echocardiography)

False –	A	B	C	D	E	F	G	H	I	J	Overall
Gembruch[14]					1						1
Hernadi[34]	1			1							2
D'Ottavio[35]	1				3	2			1		7
Economides[36]	1					1	1				3
Whitlow[37]	2	1				2	1	1			7
Zosmer[24]					1	1			1		3
Rustico[19]	1				4	1	2		1		9
Simpson[25]	3									1	4
Comas[21]	4	1			3	1	1				10
Huggon[26]	2		2			1			2		7
Bronshtein[20]					1	1		1	1		4
Lopes[39]	3							1			4
Overall	18	2	2	1	13	10	5	3	6	1	61

A, VSDs; B, atrial septal defects; C, abnormal veno-atrial connections; D, tricuspid atresia or dysplasia; E, atrioventricular septal defect; F, aortic atresia, aortic stenosis and HLH; G, tetralogy of Fallot; H, transposition of great arteries; I, aortic arch anomalies; J, myocardiopathy

Table 43.5 Our experience: epidemiological data (from Comas *et al.*[21])

	Group I	Group II	Group III	Overall (Groups I+II+III)
Study period: September 1999 to May 2001				
n (Pregnancies)	68 (4 twins)	130	132	330 (334 fetuses)
GA (mean, range)	14.9 (12–17)	13.7 (12–16)	14.3 (13–16)	14.2 (12–17)
MA (mean, range)	33 (26–46) 30% > 34 years	33 (17–45) 37% > 34 years	32 (19–42) 38% > 34 years	33(17–46) 36% > 34 years
Ultrasound system	Toshiba SSH-140 5.0–7.5 MHz TV 3.0–6.5 MHz TA	Acuson 128 XP 5.0–7.0 MHz TV 3.5–5.0 MHz TA	Acuson 128 XP Aspen 5.0–7.0 MHz TV 3.5–5.0 MHz TA	
Optimal visualization	65/72 (90.3%)	119/130 (91.5%)	132/132 (100%)	316/334 (94.6%)
Overall follow-up	44/72 (61.1%)	108/130 (83.1%)	129/132 (97.8%)	281/334 (84.1%)

GA, gestational age (weeks); MA, maternal age (years); TV, transvaginal; TA, transabdominal

difficult to diagnose in the first trimester of pregnancy. Heart defects diagnosed early in pregnancy tend to be more complex than those detected later, with a higher incidence of associated structural malformations, chromosomal abnormalities and spontaneous abortions. It is widely accepted that the spectrum of CHD diagnosed during prenatal life is different from that observed in postnatal series, with a higher incidence of associated extracardiac lesions and a significant relationship with chromosomal abnormalities in comparison with postnatal life.[3–5,17] Furthermore, when the cardiac defects are detected during early pregnancy, they are even more complex, probably corresponding to the most severe spectrum of the disease,[21,25,26] and cause more severe hemodynamic compromise in the developing fetus. A common finding is the presence of a hygroma or hydrops associated with CHD, whereas this is not so when the diagnosis is done later in pregnancy.[1,5,21] As a result, many of these fetuses are not going to survive long into the second trimester, but this does not argue against early diagnosis. Indeed, when the intrauterine demise of the fetus occurs days or weeks before the delivery, the pathological examination is certainly more difficult to perform. All these considerations should be taken into account when counseling the parents about complex CHD.

This review presents our experience in the first multicenter trial in early fetal echocardiography performed in Spain.[21] In accordance with other studies, this experience stresses the usefulness of early echocardiography when performed by expert operators on the fetus specifically at risk of cardiac defects. Our review of these additional 48 cases contributes to the expanding literature on the ability of TV ultrasonography to detect fetal heart defects in early pregnancy.

Our experience in early prenatal diagnosis of congenital heart anomalies

Methods

A multicenter study was made of 334 fetuses from 330 selected high-risk pregnant women, including four twin pregnancies. The women were attending the prenatal diagnosis units of Institut Universitari Dexeus in Barcelona (Group I), Hospital 12 de Octubre in Madrid (Group II) or Institut Clínic d' Obstetrícia, Ginecologia i Neonatologia del Hospital Clínic in Barcelona (Group III) for ultrasound examination because of an increased *a priori* risk of heart anomalies. These are referral centers for prenatal diagnosis of CHD. Fetal echocardiography was performed combining TV and transabdominal probes between 12 and 17 weeks' gestation. When possible, we selected the 14th week of gestation as the optimal time for TV scan because the visualization of heart structures is better at this time. This is a prospective design study, performed from September 1999 to May 2001, where the overall group was reviewed focusing on the feasibility of diagnosing fetal CHD by early echocardiography. Informed consent was obtained from each patient and the study was approved by our ethics committees.

Epidemiological data are summarized in Table 43.5, for the overall group and according to the reference unit. Maternal age ranged from 17 to 46 years (mean 33 years with 36% of women over 34 years). The median gestational age at scan was 14.2 weeks (range 12–17 weeks). The distribution of gestational ages was as follows: 23 cases at 12 weeks, 76 cases at 13 weeks, 101 cases at 14 weeks, 72 cases at 15 weeks, 54 cases at 16 weeks and 8 cases at 17 weeks.

Fetal echocardiography was performed in a population with an increased *a priori* risk of CHD. Criteria for inclusion were a family history of CHD (n=37), ultrasound markers for chromosomal abnormalities (n=186), such as increased NT (>99th centile) or abnormal DV flow (pulsatility index for veins in the DV 95th centile), suspected cardiac or extracardiac anomalies at the early second-trimester scan (n=43), maternal pregestational diabetes (n=33), pregnancy affected by a chromosomal abnormality (n=8), exposition to teratogens (n=3), genetic sonography (n=22) and a screening test (n=2). The last two cases refer to two twin pregnancies in which the main indication for the echocardiography was an ultrasound marker for chromosomal abnormality in one fetus, but the echocardiographic examination was performed to both the fetuses for practical reasons. For NT and DV assessment, measurements were made between 10 and 16 weeks' gestation. NT was systematically assessed in all cases, while DV blood flow was only measured in Groups I and II. We have used our own published nomograms to define increased NT or abnormal DV.[40] Genetic sonography was offered to a high-risk population refusing invasive karyotyping test.

For each fetus, visualization of the four-chamber view (with both atria, atrioventricular valves and ventricles), the origin and double crossing of the great arteries, aortic and ductal arches and systemic venous return, was attempted in a segmental approach. Two-dimensional mode and color/pulsed Doppler flow imaging were used in all cases, while M-mode was occasionally performed. The operators kept a record of optimal visualization (complete visualization of heart structures) or partial visualization (incomplete visualization of heart structures). In cases of partial visualization, only when an anomaly was suspected was a second scan arranged 2 weeks later. Ultrasound examinations were performed using a multifrequency real-time vaginal probe (5.0–7.5 MHz) and convex abdominal probe (3.0–6.5 MHz) on a Toshiba ultrasound system (Toshiba SSH-140A, Toshiba Co., Tokyo, Japan), Acuson 128 XP or Aspen (Acuson Inc., Mountain View, CA) and General Electric Logic 400 or Logic 500 (GE Medical Systems, Milwaukee, WI). The ultrasound examination was mainly performed transvaginally, completed nearly always by the transabdominal route. For color Doppler evaluation, the energy output levels were lower than 50 mW/cm^2 spatial peak-temporal average. The duration of complete heart examination was less than 30 min. All the examinations were made by three experienced operators (CC, JMM and AG).

When indicated, fetal karyotyping by chorionic villus sampling or amniocentesis was offered. According to the policy of our institutions, invasive testing was recommended as a result of advanced maternal age (>35 years), family history of aneuploidy, biochemical screening for Down's syndrome higher than 1/270 or ultrasound anomalies (including malformations or NT >95th centile). Fluorescence *in situ* hybridization (FISH) studies to test for 22q11 deletion were also offered when a heart malformation affecting the great arteries was suspected. When possible, in those who continue their pregnancies, a follow-up detailed ultrasound scan was carried out at 20–22 weeks' gestation. When karyotyping was not performed, chromosomal abnormalities were excluded at neonatal examination.

Reliability was assessed by conventional transabdominal echocardiography at 20–22 weeks, by postnatal follow-up in the first 3 months of life and/or by autopsy in cases of termination of pregnancy (TOP). Minor cardiac anomalies described in the literature as difficult or impossible to diagnose early (atrial septal defects or patent ductus arteriosus) were not considered when calculating the validity of the early echocardiography.

Results

The rate of optimal visualization of the fetal heart was 94.6% (316/334). In 48 out of 334 (14.4%) fetuses the final diagnosis was abnormal, including 48 cases of structural heart abnormalities (Table 43.6). In 38 out of 48 cases with heart defects the diagnosis was suspected at early echocardiography. These true-positive cases were as follows: 13 cases of abnormal outflow tracts, 8 cases of atrioventricular defect, 4 cases of hypoplastic left heart (HLH), 5 cases of tricuspid atresia or dyspasia, 3 cases of isolated VSD, 3 cases of ectopia cordis, 1 case of aortic coartation and 1 severe complex heart defect. True positive diagnoses are summarized in Table 43.7. Figures 43.11–43.15 illustrate some examples of detected CHD early in pregnancy.

There were 10 false-negative cases (2 cases of HLH, 3 cases of atrioventricular defect, four cases of VSD and 1 case of tetralogy of Fallot) (Table 43.8). There were no false-positive diagnoses. When considering the validity of the early echocardiography, we have excluded one case of isolated pericardial effusion, two cases of significant tricuspid regurgitation within a structurally normal heart, a child affected by an ostium secundum atrial septal defect, a structural normal heart in a Down's syndrome affected by a patent ductus arteriosus who had neonatal surgery.

Karyotyping was performed in 290 cases of our series (86.8%), including all cases with cardiac abnormalities. In the whole series, 51 cases had an abnormal karyotype. These chromosomal abnormalities included trisomy 21 (n = 28), 45XO (n = 7), trisomy 18 (n = 6), trisomy 13 (n = 2), 22q11 microdeletion (n = 1), triploidy (n = 1), trisomy 7 (n = 1), partial trisomy 15 (n = 1), rearrangement (n = 1) and others (n = 3). Among the heart defects, 27 cases (56.3%) had an abnormal karyotype (13 trisomy 21, 5 trisomy 18, 3 Turner' syndrome, 2 trisomy 13, 1 trisomy 7, 1 partial trisomy 15, 1 rearrangement and 1 with a 22q11 microdeletion detected by FISH), and 31 cases (64.6%) showed additional sonographic extracardiac anomalies, including mainly cystic hygroma, congenital diaphragmatic hernia (CDH),

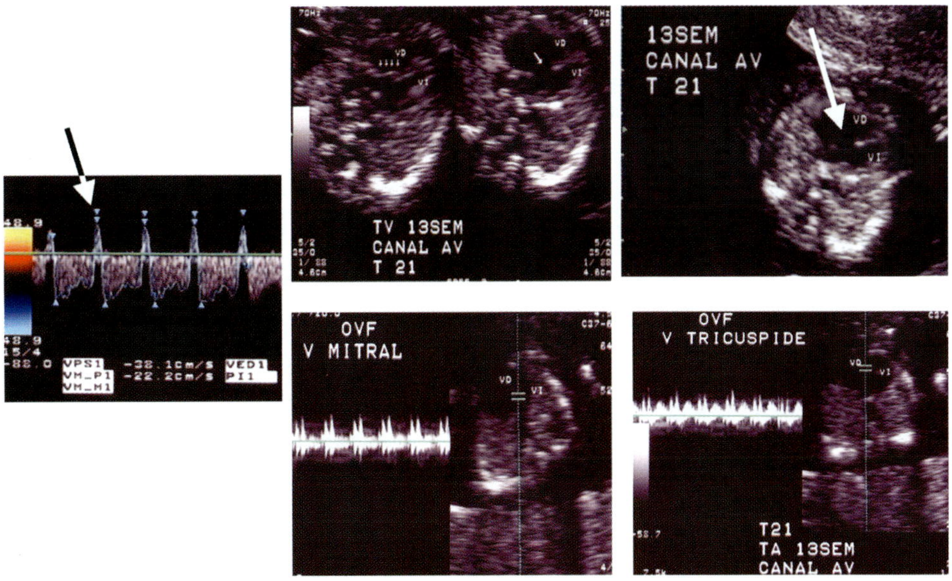

Figure 43.11 AVSD detected at 13 weeks' gestation in a fetus affected by cystic hygroma and trisomy 21. Note the abnormal reversed A wave in the DV.

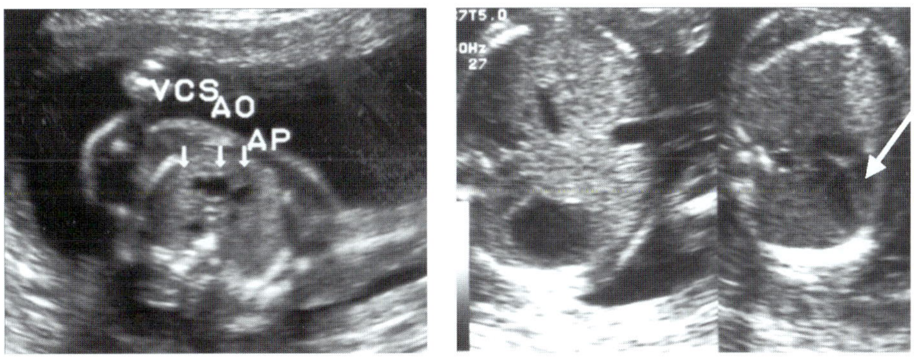

Figure 43.12 Tetralogy of Fallot detected at 16 weeks' gestation in a fetus affected by cystic hygroma and normal karyotype. Note the left cardiac deviation and the dominance of the aorta compared with the small pulmonary artery at the three-vessel view in the upper mediastinum.

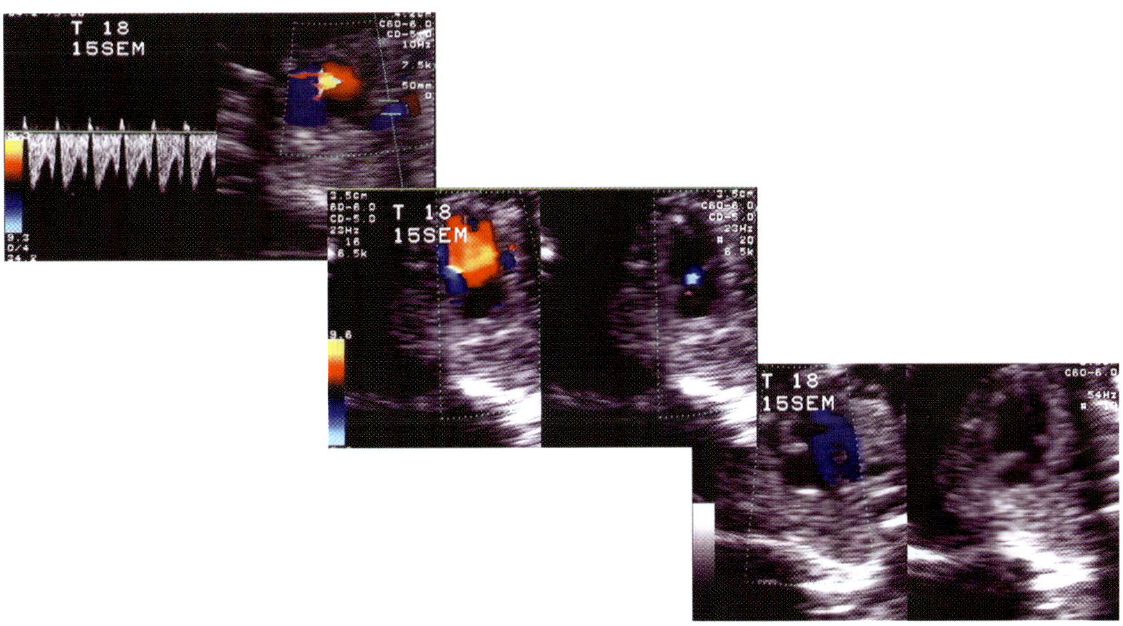

Figure 43.13 AVSD with unbalanced right ventricle dominance and double-outlet right ventricle at 15 weeks' gestation. Note the abnormal reversed A wave in the DV.

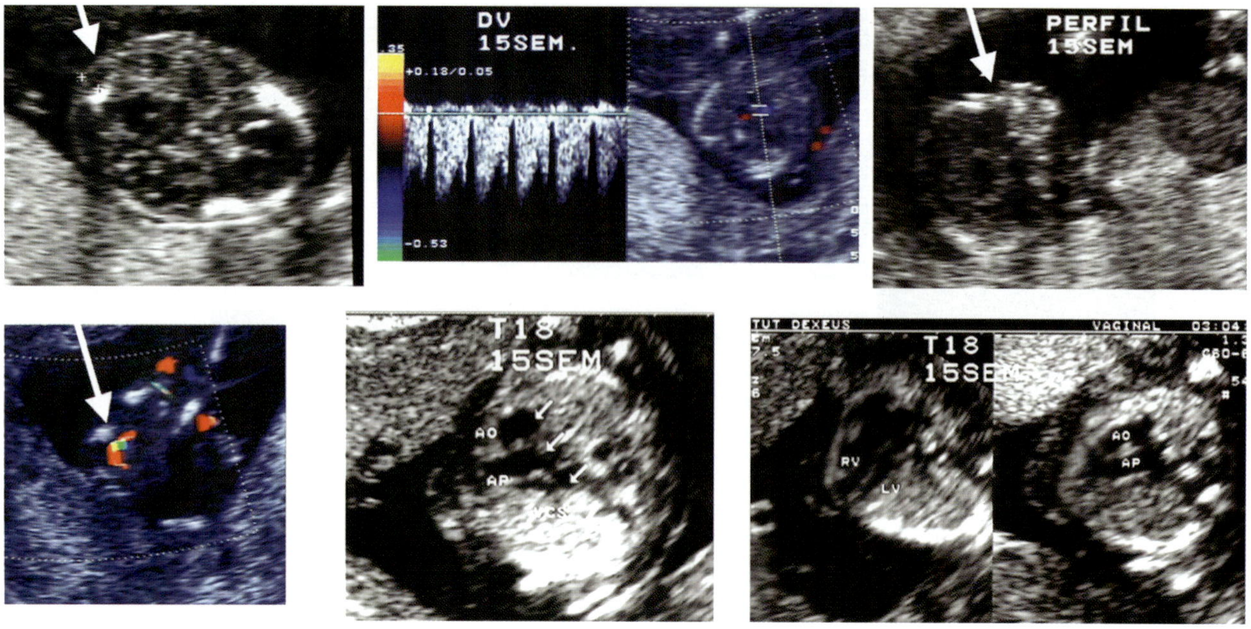

Figure 43.14 HLH and double-outlet right ventricle at 15 weeks' gestation in a trisomy 18. Note the identification of multiples markers of chromosomal abnormality (increased NT, abnormal DV flow, absent nasal bone, single umbilical artery).

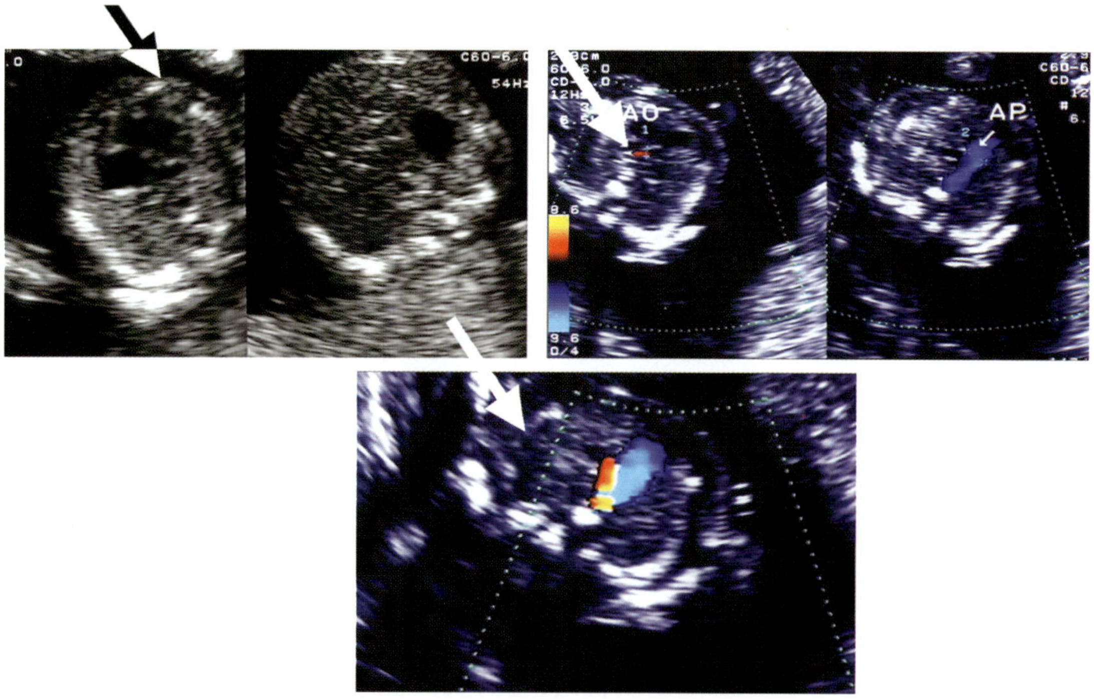

Figure 43.15 HLH and aortic stenosis at 17 weeks' gestation in a Turner syndrome. Note the left cardiac axis deviation, the opposite color flow in the V sign at the upper mediastinum level and the severe reduction of the aortic outflow tract compared to the main pulmonary artery.

abnormal situs visceralis, single umbilical artery, bilateral dysplastic kidneys, hydrops, limb–body wall complex, omphalocele, exencephaly, holoprosencephaly, pyelectasis, choroid plexus cysts, hemivertebra and pleural effusion.

In the CHD group, increased NT at 10–16 weeks' gestation was noted in 21 fetuses (43.8%), while abnormal DV blood flow was found in 18 out of 37 fetuses with DV assessment (48.6%).

The outcome of fetuses with a CHD was poor. In 37 cases a TOP was performed at the parents' request before 20 weeks' gestation and in one case a selective feticide was offered in a twin pregnancy discordant for a CHD. The outcome of the surviving fetuses was

Table 43.6 Our experience: CHD (from Comas *et al.*[21])

	Overall (Groups I+II+III)
Prevalence	48/334 (14.4%)
True positive	38/48 (79.2%)
False negative	10
False positive	0
Chromosomal abnormalities	27/48 (56.3%)
Extracardiac abnormalities	31/48 (64.6%)
Increased NT	21/48 (43.8%)
Abnormal DV	18/37 (48.6%)
Outcome	37 TOP
	One selective feticide
	Two postnatal death
	Eight surviving
Follow-up	33/48 (68.8%)
Autopsy available	25/41 (61.0%)

NT, nuchal translucency; DV, ductus venosus; TOP, termination of pregnancy

poor, with two cases of neonatal death (one VSD and one HLH) and eight surviving children [one VSD, three atrioventricular defects, one pulmonary stenosis, one VSD diagnosed of Noonan's syndrome, one case of tetralogy of Fallot and one single ventricle with transposition of great arteries (but the child died 3 months after palliative surgery)]. Pathological examination was performed in 25 cases. In 16 cases, the autopsy was not available, because of the selective feticide in a twin pregnancy or because the termination was performed in another hospital without fetal necropsy, or due to the unavailability of an adequate material for pathological exam (fragmentation) or because the parents declined the examination.

In our series of early echocardiography, a complete follow-up was possible in 281 cases (84.1%), 61.1% in Group I, 83.1% in Group II and 97.8% in Group III. When a heart defect was detected, a complete follow-up was possible in 33 out of 48 cases (68.8%).

Fetal heart rate

The diagnosis of fetal arrhythmia early in pregnancy may give rise to the suspicion of a fetal chromosomal abnormality,[34–36] an increased risk of a later miscarriage[35,37,38,41] or the presence of CHD.[42] The factors that control fetal heart rate in the first trimester are

Table 43.7 Our experience: fetal heart anomalies diagnosed at early echocardiography (true-positive cases at early fetal echocardiography) (from Comas *et al.*[21])

Case	CHD	GA	Associated findings	Karyotype	Follow-up
1	AVSD	17	Increased NT	Trisomy 21	TOP, no autopsy
2*	Hypoplastic RV Tricuspid atresia Abnormal great arteries	16	Single UA	Normal	TA-echo confirmative Selective feticide
3	AVSD	14	Increased NT	Trisomy 21	TOP, no autopsy
4	AVSD	13	Cystic hygroma	Trisomy 21	TOP, no autopsy
5	VSD	17	Cystic hygroma	Normal	Surviving Follow-up confirmative Noonan syndrome
6	VSD Abnormal great arteries	15	Abnormal situs Single UA	22q11 deletion	TOP, autopsy: abnormal situs visceralis, VSD, hypoplastic RV, truncus
7	AVSD	12	Increased NT	Trisomy 21	TOP, no autopsy
8	Abnormal great arteries	14	Cystic hygroma	Normal	Surviving, postnatal echo: tetralogy of Fallot
9	HLH, DORV, pulmonary atresia	16	Bilateral renal dysplasia	Normal	TOP, autopsy confirmative
10	VSD, DORV	16	Increased NT trisomy 15	Partial	TOP, autopsy confirmative
11	Truncus	15	Polimalformative fetus	Trisomy 13	TOP, autopsy confirmative
12	VSD, DORV, pulmonary atresia	12	Exencephaly	Normal	TOP, no autopsy

Table 43.7 Continued

Case	CHD	GA	Associated findings	Karyotype	Follow-up
13	VSD, DORV	16	Ventriculomegaly, single UA	Normal	TOP, no autopsy
14	Tetralogy of Fallot	16	Increased NT, bilateral renal dysplasia, omphalocele	Normal	TOP, no autopsy
15	Tetralogy of Fallot	13	Increased NT, bilateral renal	Trisomy 7	TOP, no autopsy dysplasia
16	AVSD	16		Normal	Surviving Follow-up confirmative
17	AVSD	13	Increased NT Hydrops	Trisomy 21	TOP, autopsy confirmative
18	AVSD	13	Increased NT Omphalocele	Trisomy 21	TOP, autopsy confirmative
19	VSD	16	Holoprosencephaly	Trisomy 13	TOP, autopsy confirmative
20	VSD	13	Increased NT	Trisomy 21	TOP, autopsy confirmative
21	HLH	13	Exencephaly	Normal	TOP, no autopsy
22	HLH	12	Increased NT	45XO	TOP, no autopsy
23	HLH	12	Increased NT, hydrops	45XO	TOP, autopsy confirmative
24	Aortic coartation	16	Cystic hygroma, hydrops	45XO	TOP, no autopsy
25	Tricuspid atresia	16	Increased NT	Normal	TOP, autopsy confirmative
26	Tricuspid atresia	16	Increased NT	Normal	TOP, autopsy confirmative
27	Ectopia cordis	12	Limb–body wall complex	Normal	TOP, no autopsy
28	Ectopia cordis	14	Limb–body wall complex	Normal	TOP, autopsy confirmative
29	Ectopia cordis, tricuspid atresia	14	Increased NT Limb–body wall complex	Trisomy 18	TOP, autopsy confirmative
30	Tricuspid dysplasia	13	Increased NT	Trisomy 21	TOP, no autopsy
31	VSD, overriding aorta	13	Increased NT Omphalocele	Trisomy 18	TOP, no autopsy
32	DORV + mitral atresia	13	Increased NT	Trisomy 18	TOP, no autopsy
33	VSD, tricuspid atresia	14	Increased NT	Normal	TOP, autopsy confirmative
34	Pulmonary stenosis	15		Normal	Surviving Follow-up confirmative
35	Single ventricle, TGA	15		Normal	Surviving Follow-up confirmative**
36	VSD, pulmonary atresia	16	Increased NT	Rearrangement	TOP, autopsy confirmative
37	AVSD	16	Increased NT Abnormal situs	Trisomy 21	TOP, autopsy confirmative
38	HLH + abnormal situs	16	Increased NT	Normal	TOP, autopsy confirmative

Fetal data of true-positives cases (CHD, gestational age at diagnosis, associated findings, karyotyping studies and follow-up)
CHD, congenital heart defect; GA, gestational age (weeks); TOP, termination of pregnancy; TA-echo, transabdominal conventional second-trimester echocardiography; AVSD: atrioventricular septal defect; VSD: ventricular septal defect; LV: left ventricle; RV: right ventricle; ASD: atrial septal defect; DO: double outlet; HLH: hypoplastic left heart; TGA: transposition of great arteries; UA: umbilical artery; CDH: congenital diaphragmatic hernia; NT: nuchal translucency

*Twin pregnancy; **death at 3 months of life after palliative surgery

Table 43.8 Our experience: fetal heart anomalies not detected at early echocardiography (false-negative cases at early fetal echocardiography)

Case	CHD	GA¹	GA²	Method Diagnosis	Associated findings	Karyotype	Outcome
1*	HLH	14	20	TA-echo	Congenital Diaphragmatic hernia	Normal	Neonatal death after surgery
2	Ostium primum, ASD, HLH	14	20	Autopsy	Hydrops Cystic higroma	Normal	TOP
3	AVSD	14	20	TA-echo	Single umbilical artery Short femur	Trisomy 21	TOP
4	AVSD	16	33	TA-echo		Normal	Surviving
5	AVSD	15	23	TA-echo	Echogenic foci Pleural effusion	Trisomy 21	Surviving
6	VSD	12	14	Autopsy	Pyelectasis	Trisomy 21	TOP
7	VSD	15	28	TA-echo	Choroid plexus cysts Hemivertebra	Trisomy 18	Neonatal death
8	VSD	13	15	Autopsy	NTD	48,XXY+18	TOP
9	Tetralogy of Fallot	13	20	TA-echo	Pyelectasis	Trisomy 21	TOP
10	VSD	13	21	TA-echo		Normal	Surviving

Fetal data of false-negative cases (CHD, gestational age at diagnosis, associated findings, karyotyping studies and outcome)
CHD, congenital heart defect; GA¹, gestational age of the echocardiographic examination in early pregnancy (weeks); GA², gestational age at diagnosis (weeks); TOP, termination of pregnancy; HLH, hypoplastic left heart; TA-echo, transabdominal echocardiography; ASD, atrial septal defect; AVSD, atrioventricular septal defect; VSD, ventricular septal defect; NTD, neural tube defects
*Twin pregnancy

uncertain, so the underlying cause of the abnormal pattern in chromosomally abnormal fetuses remains obscure. A delay in maturation of sympathetic and parasympathetic systems as well as an abnormally developed and responsive myocardium have been proposed.[30,43] An alternative explanation could be that fetal arrhythmias are a reflection of an underlying structural heart disease, and are a common feature in trisomic fetuses.[35,42,44,45] Baschat *et al.*[46] reported four cases of severe CHD associated with bradycardia (likely to be atrioventricular block) during early echocardiography at 11–14 weeks' gestation. All cases had either increased NT or generalized edema and complex CHD. Most authors find a high correlation between abnormal heart rate and increased NT in chromosomally abnormal fetuses, thus supporting the hypothesis that cardiac defects may be involved in the physiologic basis of NT.[35,36,47]

NT and DV

NT measurement at 10–14 weeks' gestation is a widely accepted method to screen for chromosomal abnormalities. Recent studies have suggested the potential role of an increased NT thickness [8,9,11,48–51] or an abnormal DV flow pattern [10,11,52,53] at early pregnancy as a screening tool for CHD, in addition to its role in screening for chromosomal defects. The risk of CHD after the finding of an increased NT seems to vary between 4% and 9%.[24,54] Recently, Galindo *et al.* have examined the prevalence, distribution and spectrum of cardiac defects in 353 chromosomally normal fetuses with increased NT, with a complete follow-up in 97% of the cases.[55] This multicenter Spanish study presents an overall prevalence of heart defects of 9.1%, increasing significantly from 5.3% in those with NT >95th centile to 24% when thickness >6 mm. Interestingly, most of the cardiac defects can be prenatally detected. A wide range of cardiac anomalies were observed in this series, with the most common being AVSDs and tricuspid atresia. Hyett *et al.* reported that about 55% of the major CHD were associated with a fetal NT thickness above 95th centile at 10–14 weeks of gestation.[8] However, others have failed to demonstrate such a strong association,[49,50,53,54,56–58] suggesting that the routine assessment of the four chambers and great vessels at mid-second trimester remains the most important screening tool for the detection of major CHD.[56,59] Theoretically, both types of screening used in combination should improve the overall sensitivity of prenatal diagnosis of the major cardiac defects.

The physiopathogenic mechanism of this relationship is not easy to explain.[11,44,45,53,59,60–63] Pathological examination of fetuses with increased NT thickness at 10–14 weeks have demonstrated a high prevalence of cardiac defects and abnormalities of the great arteries and of subtle defects, such as widening of the aortic valve and ascending aorta, narrowing of the aortic isthmus and persistence of the left superior vena cava. Another proposed mechanism to explain the increased NT is an early cardiac function impairment suggested by an abnormal DV flow pattern. However, Matias *et al.*[10] reported that most of the chromosomally normal fetuses with increased NT but normal DV flow did not have CHD. This finding might contradict a cardiac involvement in the pathogenesis of the increased NT in most of the fetuses, and suggest that only fetuses with abnormal DV blood flow are those at high risk of CHD. On the other hand, in cases with CHD and both enlarged NT and abnormal DV, because the type of cardiac defects cannot always explain the hemodynamic changes found in these fetuses, some other mechanisms seem to be involved.[53]

Based on ultrasonographic and postmortem morphological studies, the findings in increased NT fetuses can be classified into three categories.[64] First, an association between increased NT and cardiac anomalies, combined with an abnormal DV flow pattern, has been described in some cases, leading to the theory that cardiac failure causes NT enlargement. Second, various types of abnormalities have been found in the extracellular matrix of the nuchal skin of fetuses with increased NT. Third, abnormal lymphatic development has been demonstrated in fetuses with increased NT. Many hypotheses on NT enlargement are based on associations and speculations. Therefore, within this context, it is not clear whether all these cardiovascular anomalies are the cause of the increased NT or both events are the result of another pathophysiologic mechanism.

Chromosomal abnormalities

The detection of CHD may be the first clue to the diagnosis of a chromosomal abnormality or a genetic syndrome. The incidence of chromosomal defects in CHD diagnosed prenatally may be as high as 30–40%, and 15% when the CHD is presented isolated. These figures increase up to 40–60% when the CDH is diagnosed during the first trimester.[20-22,26] This is much higher than the incidence in live borns. Also, the high rate of spontaneous abortion loss in early pregnancy suggests a higher rate of chromosomal abnormalities in first-trimester fetuses with CHD. Therefore, whenever CHD are diagnosed, karyotype evaluation is mandatory, including FISH test to rule out 22q11 deletion.[65–68]

Recently, the early finding of isolated tricuspid regurgitation or disproportion of the cardiac chambers and/or outflow tracts, has been regarded to be highly associated with fetal chromosomal abnormalities, even in the absence of structural heart disease, as it had been previously described during the second trimester.[26,69,70] The chromosome defect most frequently found to be associated with tricuspid regurgitation was trisomy 21, but all types of karyotype anomalies were seen in association.[69] In view of these results, the authors propose to assess the four-chambers view and the outflow tracts for disproportion and to use color Doppler to rule out tricuspid regurgitation in each first- or early second-trimester ultrasound to screen for chromosomal anomalies.[26,27] Since these unexpectedly good results were obtained in particularly high-risk fetuses, they remain to be confirmed in an unselected population.

Advantages and limitations

The first benefit of performing early fetal echocardiography would be an early reassurance of normality in order to relieve anxiety and reduce emotional trauma to the parents at high risk of CHD. Early prenatal diagnosis of CHD will allow us to optimize the genetic counseling to the parents by permitting further testing, such as fetal karyotyping, and in those cases with severe defects it may provide the parents with the option of an earlier and safer TOP.[13,14,17] In selected cases, there is the possibility of pharmacologic therapy. Furthermore, the correct timing and place for delivery may be planned and arranged well in advance.

However, there are certain disadvantages of the early scanning, which reduce its diagnostic accuracy compared with the conventional examination at 20–22 weeks' gestation.[1,5,13,14,17] The TV technique requires a substantial amount of operator experience, yet it cannot be learned from the second-trimester examination as the early transabdominal scan. Unfavorable fetal position or limited angles of insonation due to the less mobile capacity of the TV probe may not be overcome. Also, spatial orientation can be challenging by the TV scan. In such cases, we recommend a transabdominal scan that will help us to quickly assess the situs and obtain a good spatial orientation. The small size of the fetal heart is an important limiting factor to obtain an optimal sonographic visualization, and also to obtain a successful pathological examination, particularly before the 13th week of gestation. At 13–14 weeks of gestation the transverse diameter of the heart at the four-chambers view ranges between 5 and 8 mm, and the great artery diameter at the level of the semilunar valves ranges between 0.8 and 1.8 mm[5]. Moreover, this exploration is more time-consuming and requires a high level of training of the examiner. Finally, the biggest disadvantage of first-trimester echocardiography is the later manifestation of structural and functional changes in some CHD. Some cardiac lesions are progressive in nature, such as mild pulmonary and aortic stenosis or coarctation and even HLH syndrome. Some obstructive lesions, as a result of a reduced blood flow, may increase the severity of the lesions, resulting in restricted growth in the chambers or arteries. This may be the biggest disadvantage of performing the early scan. Progression usually is toward a more severe form of lesion that may be sometimes discernible only in the second or even in the third trimester, although in some rare cases a regression to a less severe form may be observed. In this sense, the false-negative cases published in the literature are particularly instructive demonstrating these limitations (Table 43.4). Another disadvantage of early fetal echocardiography is the possible detection of defects that could resolve spontaneously in later pregnancy, such as muscular ventricular septal defects, resulting in unnecessary anxiety in the parents.

Therefore, a normal early examination does not preclude a subsequent abnormal heart development at the second-trimester ultrasound, or even in the third trimester or the postnatal period. After a normal early fetal echocardiography, a conventional transabdominal echocardiography at 20–22 weeks of gestation is strongly recommended.

Pathological confirmation

Pathological confirmation in the case of an early TOP or perinatal death is particularly important in those areas where ultrasound diagnosis is the most challenging. Only a complete diagnosis will make an individual genetic counseling possible and will validate the accuracy of early fetal echocardiography as a diagnostic technique. Therefore, we recommend that a precise pathological report has to be compulsory for an adequate assessment of the reliability of early fetal echocardiography. This is still a major drawback in most of the studies.[1,5,21,26]

TOP is an option only before 22 weeks of gestation in our country. Whenever a termination takes place, it is of vital importance to obtain permission for autopsy in order to confirm the diagnosis and to search for any other associated malformations. Ideally, this should be performed by a pathologist who is familiar with the small size of the specimen and with special examination techniques, such as dissection microscopy.[5,21,22,45] Current methods of terminating early pregnancies other than using prostaglandins are less recommended because they do not usually allow the retrieval of suitable specimens for appropriate examination to correlate ultrasound and pathological findings.[45] This method allows a more gentle extraction of the embryo or fetus so that a pathological examination for verification of the prenatally diagnosed malformation can be performed. A pathological investigation after TOP following the diagnosis of a CHD should be always recommended, preferably in referral laboratories, being of paramount importance to validate early echocardiography. In particular, semilunar valve and aortic arch defects are usually underdiagnosed. We are aware of some cases in which Doppler findings, such as turbulent flow and very high velocities, are more reliable to diagnose valve stenosis than pathological examination, even during the second trimester. Indeed, this is a problem and a major challenge not only for ultrasonographers but also for pathologists.

Indications of early fetal echocardiography

Since most CHD are detected in low-risk pregnancies, and knowing the high prevalence of heart defects in a non-selected population (incidence of CHD in low-risk population 1/238),[20] some authors suggest that an early detailed cardiac examination should be performed in all pregnant women.[17,20] Indeed, very few cardiac defects have been identified in the pregnancies in which a family history was the main indication for the early fetal echocardiography, which is consistent with the recurrence rate of 2–3% for siblings. The main value of the early scan in such family-risk cases lies in the reassurance that it gives to the parents. As we have previously stated, in most of the studies the early echocardiography is somewhat less reliable and may result in higher false-negative and false-positive results in comparison with the 20–22 weeks' transabdominal echocardiography. Besides, early echocardiography is the most time-consuming and requires a high level of expertise of the examiner. Therefore, it is difficult to offer this scan as a screening test to the general population. In this context, the identification of a high-risk collective is of paramount importance.

Currently, the importance of the aforementioned limitations of early fetal cardiac examination justifies restriction of its use to fetuses at high risk of having cardiac anomalies.[5,10,14,18,21,22,26] The indications proposed for early fetal echocardiography are:

- Increased NT (greater than 95th or 99th centile) is the main indication of referral in all recently reported studies.
- Abnormal DV blood flow, regardless of the measurement of the NT.
- Fetuses affected by other structural malformations: hygroma, hydrops, omphalocele, situs inversus and arrhythmia.
- Suspected cardiac anomalies at screening ultrasound.
- Pregestational diabetes of the mother.
- High-risk family, with a previously affected child, a first-degree relative affected by a congenital heart

disease or a genetic disease in which CHD are common.
- Women at high risk of chromosomal abnormality declining invasive test for karyotyping.
- Pregnancies affected by a chromosomal abnormality.

Currently, as long as the sensitivity, specificity and predictive value of early echocardiography is still unclear, this examination should be generally reserved for patients at high risk of CHD. However, only the accumulation of results from carefully collaborative studies such as the present series will clearly define the role of early TV echocardiography.

Conclusions

Fetal echocardiography performed by expert operators is reliable for an early reassurance of normal cardiac anatomy

(1) Transvaginal sonography enables good visualization of fetal heart earlier in gestation. The four-chamber view and the extended examination to the great vessels can be imaged in almost 100% at 13–14 weeks of gestation. Less than 5% of patients will need a repeated scan because of inadequate visualization.
(2) The combination of TV and transabdominal routes and the application of color Doppler enhances visualization.
(3) Most CHD are detected in a low-risk population. As we cannot perform a targeted fetal echocardiography as a screening test, we need to improve the identification of high-risk group pregnancies. Increased NT at 10–14 weeks' scan and, maybe, DV blood flow assessment seem to be the newest and the most promising risk factors for fetal CHD, and may be particularly useful during the first trimester.
(4) Currently, early fetal echocardiography should be offered to high-risk pregnancies. Some authors advocate routine early-extended cardiac examination in low-risk pregnancies. At present, as long as the sensitivity, specificity and predictive value of early echocardiography are still unclear, this examination should be generally reserved for patients at high risk of CHD.
(5) Whenever a normal heart is diagnosed in the early scan, it has to be supplemented with the conventional transabdominal examination at 20–22 weeks' gestation.

Fetal echocardiography performed by expert operators is reliable to diagnose most major structural heart defects in the first and early second trimesters of pregnancy

(1) Cardiac defects diagnosed early in pregnancy tend to be more complex than those detected later on and cause more severe hemodynamic compromise in the developing fetus.
(2) Many CHD can be detected at the beginning of the second trimester.
(3) The incidence of associated structural malformations, chromosomal abnormalities and spontaneous abortions is significantly high.
(4) A complete workup including pathological and karyotype evaluation should be warranted in order to provide the parents with proper genetic counseling, which is extremely difficult to obtain if spontaneous loss of pregnancy occurs.
(5) The small size of specimens at this time of gestation renders pathological examination difficult and requires high expertise and careful inspection, irrespective of the technique used for termination.
(6) Clinical follow-up in the neonate and post-mortem examination if TOP is undertaken are essential to assess the actual role of early fetal echocardiography.

REFERENCES

1. Campbell S. Isolated major congenital heart disease (opinion.). *Ultrasound Obstet Gynecol* 2001;17:370–9.
2. Mitchell SC, Korones SB, Berendes HW. Congenital heart disease in 56,109 births. Incidence and natural history. *Circulation* 1971;43:323–32.
3. Allan L, Sharland G, Milburn A, *et al.* Prospective diagnosis of 1006 consecutive cases of congenital heart disease in the fetus. *J Am Coll Cardiol* 1994;23:1452–8.
4. Allan LD. Fetal cardiology. *Curr Opin Obstet Gynecol* 1996;8:142–7.
5. Gembruch U. Prenatal diagnosis of congenital heart disease. *Prenat Diagn* 1997;17:1283–98.
6. Todros T. Prenatal diagnosis and management of fetal cardiovascular malformations. *Curr Opin Obstet Gynecol* 2000;12: 105–9.
7. Levi S, Schaaps JP, De Havay P, *et al.* End result of routine ultrasound screening for congenital anomalies. The Belgian Multicentric study 1984–92. *Ultrasound Obstet Gynecol* 1995;5: 366–371.
8. Hyett J, Perdu M, Sharland G, Snijders R, Nicolaides KH. Using nuchal translucency to screen for major cardiac defects at 10–14 weeks of gestation: Population based cohort study. *Br Med J* 1999;318:81–5.
9. Devine PC, Simpson LL. Nuchal translucency and its relationship to congenital heart disease. *Semin Perinatol* 2000;24:343–51.
10. Matias A, Huggon I, Areias JC, Montenegro N, Nicolaides KH. Cardiac defects in chromosomally normal fetuses with abnormal ductus venosus blood flow at 10–14 weeks. *Ultrasound Obstet Gynecol* 1999;14:307–10.
11. Bilardo CM, Müller MA, Zikulnig L, Schipper M, Hecher K. Ductus venosus studies in fetuses at high risk for chromosomal or heart abnormalities: Relationship with nuchal translucency measurement and fetal outcome. *Ultrasound Obstet Gynecol* 2001;17:288–94.
12. Johnson P, Sharland G, Maxwell D, Allan L. The role of transvaginal sonography in the early detection of congenital heart disease. *Ultrasound Obstet Gynecol* 1992;2:248–51.

13. Bronshtein M, Zimmer EZ, Gerlis LM, Lorber A, Drugen A. Early ultrasound diagnosis of congenital heart defects in high-risk and low-risk pregnancies. *Obstet Gynecol* 1993;82:225–9.
14. Gembruch U, Knopfle G, Bald R, Hansmann M. Early diagnosis of fetal congenital heart disease by transvaginal echocardiography. *Ultrasound Obstet Gynecol* 1993;3:310–17.
15. Achiron R, Tadmor O. Screening for fetal anomalies during the first trimester of pregnancy: Transvaginal versus transabdominal sonography. *Ultrasound Obstet Gynecol* 1991;1:186–91.
16. D'Amelio R, Giorlandino C, Masala L, *et al.* Fetal echocardiography using transvaginal and transabdominal probes during the first period of pregnancy: A comparative study. *Prenat Diagn* 1991; 11:69–75.
17. Yagel S, Weissman A, Rotstein Z, *et al.* Congenital heart defects: Natural course and in utero development. *Circulation* 1997;96: 550–5.
18. Achiron R, Rotstein Z, Lipitz S, Mashiach S, Hegesh J. First trimester diagnosis of congenital heart disease by transvaginal ultrasonography. *Obstet Gynecol* 1994;84:69–72.
19. Rustico MA, Benettoni A, D' Ottavio G, *et al.* Early screening for fetal cardiac anomalies by transvaginal echocardiography in an unselected population: The role of operator experience. *Ultrasound Obstet Gynecol* 2000;16:614–9.
20. Bronshtein M, Zimmer Z. The sonographic approach to the detection of fetal cardiac anomalies in early pregnancy. *Ultrasound Obstet Gynecol* 2002;19:360–5.
21. Comas C, Galindo A, Martínez JM, *et al.* Early prenatal diagnosis of major cardiac anomalies in a high-risk population. *Prenat Diagn* 2002;22:586–93.
22. Haak MC, Twisk JWR, Van Vigt JMG. How successful is fetal echocardiographic examination in the first trimester of pregnancy? *Ultrasound Obstet Gynecol* 2002;20:9–13.
23. Carvalho JS, Moscoso G, Ville Y. First trimester transabdominal fetal echocardiography. *Lancet* 1998;351:1023–7.
24. Zosmer N, Souter VL, Chan CS, Huggon JC, Nicolaides KH. Early diagnosis of major cardiac defects in chromosomally normal fetuses with increased nuchal translucency. *Br J Obstet Gynecol* 1999;106:829–33.
25. Simpson JM, Jones A, Callaghan N, Sharland GK. Accuracy and limitations of transabdominal fetal echocardiography at 12–15 weeks of gestation in a population at high risk for congenital heart disease. *Br J Obstet Gynecol* 2000;107:1492–7.
26. Huggon IC, Ghi T, Cook AC, Zosmer N, Allan LD, Nicolaides KH. Fetal cardiac abnormalities identified prior to 14 weeks' gestation. *Ultrasound Obstet Gynecol* 2002;20:22–9.
27. De Vore GR. First trimester fetal echocardiographic: Is the future now? *Ultrasound Obstet Gynecol* 2002;20:6–8.
28. Haak MC, van Vugt JM. Echocardiography in early pregnancy: A review of the literature. *J Ultrasound Med* 2003;22:271–80.
29. DeVore GR. Color Doppler examination of the outflow tracts of the fetal heart: A technique for identification of cardiovascular malformations. *Ultrasound Obstet Gynecol* 1994;4:463–71.
30. Wladimiroff JW, Seelen JC. Doppler tachometry in early pregnancy. Development of fetal vagal function. *Eur J Obstet Gynecol Reprod Biol* 1972;2:55–63.
31. Schats R, Jansen CAM, Wladimiroff JW. Embryonic heart activity: Appearance and development in early human pregnancy. *Br J Obstet Gynaecol* 1990;97:989–94.
32. Gembruch U, Knopfle G, Chatterjee M, Bald R, Hansmannn M. First-trimester diagnosis of fetal congenital heart disease by transvaginal two-dimensional and Doppler echocardiography. *Obstet Gynecol* 1990;75:496–8.
33. Bronshtein M, Siegler E, Yoffe N, Zimmer EZ. Prenatal diagnosis of ventricular septal defect and overriding aorta at 14 weeks' gestation using transvaginal sonography. *Prenat Diagn* 1990;10:697–705.
34. Hernadi L, Torocsik M. Screening for fetal anomalies in the 12th week of pregnancy by transvaginal sonography in an unselected population. *Prenat Diagn* 1997;17:753–9.
35. D'Ottavio G, Meir YJ, Rustico MA, *et al.* Screening for fetal anomalies by ultrasound at 14 and 21 weeks. *Ultrasound Obstet Gynecol* 1997;10:375–80.
36. Economides DL, Braithwaite JM. First trimester ultrasonographic diagnosis of fetal structural abnormalities in a low risk population. *Br J Obstet Gynaecol* 1998;105:53–7.
37. Whitlow BJ, Chatzipapas IK, Lazanakis ML, Kadir RA, Economides DL The value of sonography in early pregnancy for the detection of fetal abnormalities in an unselected population. *Br J Obstet Gynaecol* 1999;106:929–36.
38. Guariglia L, Rosati P. Transvaginal sonographic detection of embryonic-fetal abnormalities in early pregnancy. *Obstet Gynecol* 2000;96:328–32.
39. Lopes LM, Brizot ML, Lopes MAB, Ayello VD, Schultz R, Zugaib M. Structural and functional cardiac abnormalities identified prior to 16 weeks' gestation in fetuses with increased nuchal translucency. *Ultrasound Obstet Gynecol* 2003;22:470–8.
40. Comas C, Antolín E, Torrents M, *et al.* Early screening for chromosomal abnormalities: New strategies combining biochemical, sonographic and Doppler parameters. *Prenat Neonat Med* 2001; 6:95–102.
41. Van Lith JMM, Visser GHA, Mantingh A, Beekhuis JR. Fetal heart rate in early pregnancy and chromosomal disorders. *Br J Obstet Gynaecol* 1992;99:741–4.
42. Martinez JM, Comas C, Ojuel J, Borrell A, Puerto B, Fortuny A. Fetal heart rate patterns in pregnancies with chromosomal disorders or subsequent fetal loss. *Obstet Gynecol* 1996;87:118–21.
43. Hyett JA, Noble PL, Snijders RJM, Montenegro N, Nicolaides KH. Fetal heart rate in trisomy 21 and other chromosomal abnormalities at 10–14 weeks of gestation. *Ultrasound Obstet Gynecol* 1996;7:239–44.
44. Achiron R, Tadmor O, Mahiach S. Heart rate as a predictor of first-trimester spontaneous abortion after ultrasound-proven viability. *Obstet Gynecol* 1991;78:330–3.
45. Laboda LA, Estroff JA, Benacerraf BR. First trimester bradycardia: A sign of impending fetal loss. *J Ultrasound Med* 1989;8:561–3.
46. Baschat AA, Gembruch U, Knopfle G, Hansmann M. First-trimester fetal heart block: A marker for cardiac anomaly. *Ultrasound Obstet Gynecol* 1999;14:311–4.
47. Yagel S, Anteby E, Ron M, Hochner-Celnikier D. The role of abnormal fetal heart rate in scheduling chorionic villus sampling. *Br J Obstet Gynaecol* 1992;99:739–40.
48. Hyett JA, Moscoso G, Papapanagiotou G, Perdu M, Nicolaides KH. Abnormalities of the heart and great arteries in chromosomally normal fetuses with increased nuchal translucency thickness at 11–13 weeks of gestation. *Ultrasound Obstet Gynecol* 1996;7:245–50.
49. Moscoso G. Fetal nuchal translucency: A need to understand the physiological basis. *Ultrasound Obstet Gynecol* 1995;5:6–8.
50. Mavrides E, Cobian-Sanchez F, Tekay A, *et al.* Limitations of using first-trimester nuchal translucency measurement in routine screening for major congenital heart defects. *Ultrasound Obstet Gynecol* 2001;17:106–10.
51. Hyett JA, Perdu M, Sharland GK, *et al.* Increased nuchal translucency at 10–14 weeks of gestation as a marker for major cardiac defects. *Ultrasound Obstet Gynecol* 1997;10:242–6.
52. Huisman TWA, Bilardo CM. Transient increase in nuchal translucency thickness and reversed end-diastolic ductus venosus flow in a fetus with trisomy 18. *Ultrasound Obstet Gynecol* 1997;10:397–9.
53. Haak MC, Twisk JW, Bartelings MM, Gittenberger-de Groot AC, van Vugt JM. Ductus venosus flow velocities in relation to the cardiac defects in first-trimester fetuses with enlarged nuchal translucency. *Am J Obstet Gynecol* 2003;188:727–33.
54. Martinez JM, Echevarría M, Borrell A, Puerto B, Ojuel J, Fortuny A. Fetal heart rate and nuchal translucency in detecting chromosomal abnormalities other than Down syndrome. *Obstet Gynecol* 1998;92:68–71.
55. Galindo A, Comas C, Martínez JM, *et al.* Cardiac defects in chromosomally normal fetuses with increased nuchal translucency at 10–14 weeks of gestation. *J Matern Fetal Neonatal Med* 2003;13: 163–70.
56. Bilardo CM, Pajkrt E, De Graaf IM, *et al.* Outcome of fetuses with enlarged nuchal translucency and normal karyotype. *Ultrasound Obstet Gynecol* 1998;11:401–6.
57. Maymon R, Jauniaux E, Cohen O, *et al.* Pregnancy outcome and infant follow-up of fetuses with abnormally increased first trimester nuchal translucency. *Hum Reprod* 2000;15:2023–7.
58. Carvalho JS. Nuchal translucency, ductus venosus and congenital heart disease: An important association – A cautious analysis. *Ultrasound Obstet Gynecol* 1999;14:302–6.
59. Snijders RJM, Noble P, Sebire N, Souka A, Nicolaides KH. UK multicentre project on assessment of risk of trisomy 21 by maternal age and fetal nuchal translucency thickness at 10–14 weeks of gestation. *Lancet* 1998;351:343–6.
60. Brady AF, Pandya PP, Yuksel B, *et al.* Outcome of chromosomally normal livebirths with increased fetal nuchal translucency at 10–14 weeks' gestation. *J Med Genet* 1998;35:222–4.
61. Schwärzler P, Carvalho JS, Senat MV, Masroor T, Campbell S, Ville Y. Screening for fetal aneuploidies and fetal cardiac abnormalities

by nuchal translucency thickness measurement at 10–14 weeks of gestation as part of routine antenatal care in an unselected population. *Br J Obstet Gynaecol* 1999;106:1029–34.
62. Michailidis GD, Economides DL. Nuchal translucency measurement and pregnancy outcome in karyotypically normal fetuses. *Ultrasound Obstet Gynecol* 2001;17:102–5.
63. Hyett J, Moscoso G, Nicolaides K. Abnormalities of the heart and great arteries in first trimester chromosomally abnormal fetuses. *Am J Med Genet* 1997;69:207–16.
64. Haak MC, van Vugt JM. Pathophysiology of increased nuchal translucency: A review of the literature. *Hum Reprod Update* 2003;9:175–84.
65. Berg KA, Clark EB, Astemborski JA, *et al.* Prenatal detection of cardiovascular malformations by echocardiography: An indication for cytogenetic evaluation. *Am J Obstet Gynecol* 1998;69:494–7.
66. Schwanitz G, Zerres K, Gembruch U, *et al.* Prenatal detection of heart defects as an indication for chromosome analysis. *Ann Genet* 1990;33:79–83.
67. Gembruch U, Baschat AA, Knopfle G, *et al.* Results of chromosomal analysis in fetuses with cardiac anomalies as diagnosed by first- and early second-trimester echocardiography. *Ultrasound Obstet Gynecol* 1997;10:391–6.
68. Lazanakis MS, Rodgers K, Economides DL. Increased nuchal translucency and CATCH 22. *Prenat Diagn* 1998;18:507–10.
69. Huggon IC, DeFigueiredo DB, Allan LD. Tricuspid regurgitation in the diagnosis of chromosomal anomalies in the fetus at 11–14 weeks of gestation. *Heart* 2003;89:1071–3.
70. Simpson JM, Sharland GK. Nuchal translucency and congenital heart defects: Heart failure or not? *Ultrasound Obstet Gynecol* 2000;16:30–6.

44 Prenatal diagnosis of fetal cytomegalovirus infection

Y. Ville, O. Picone, G. Makridemas and M. Leruez-Ville

Congenital cytomegalovirus (CMV) infection is likely to have become the most prevalent infection-related cause of congenital neurological handicap as rubella vaccination has become universal in developed countries.[1] However, prenatal diagnosis and screening policies have been rather incoherent for the last 25 years and obstetricians have shown great reluctance to tackle this issue.[2] Indeed, although the infection is frequent in 1–2% of all neonates excreting CMV in their urine, 90% of these will remain asymptomatic.[3] However, among symptomatic neonates, half will be severely infected and one-third of these will die, while 60% will develop significant neurological and developmental sequelae. Among the moderately symptomatic neonates, 65–75% will develop normally, whereas 25–35% will have some degree of handicap at long-term follow-up. Furthermore, between 5% and 15% of the asymptomatic cases will also develop long-term developmental abnormalities, mainly sensorineuro hearing loss, which can be bilateral in up to 50% of the cases.[1,3,4] Epidemiological risk factors have been extensively reviewed elsewhere.[5] Maternal age below 25 years, low socioeconomic status and presence of children of age 1–3 years in the home are the most constantly quoted factors.[5] Preconceptional maternal immunity [relative risk (RR) 0.31; 95% CI 0.17–0.58] and maternal age of 25 years or older [RR 0.19; 95% CI 0.07–0.49] are highly protective against congenital infection.[6]

The possibilities for prenatal diagnosis have emerged more rapidly than those for establishing the prognosis of an infected fetus[2] and the possibilities of treatment are still experimental. In this chapter, we will address the possibilities and limits of prenatal imaging and biology in assessing both the diagnosis and the prognosis of fetal CMV infection.

Prenatal ultrasound examination

Overall, less than half of fetal infections are diagnosed by ultrasound[7–16] and multiple organ system involvement is present in more than 50% of the cases[17] at the time of prenatal diagnosis, ranging from 15% to 100% (Table 44.1), and is very likely subjected to reporting bias.

Indeed, a review of the pediatric literature suggests that most symptomatic congenitally infected neonates obviously escaped ultrasound screening and one should be aware that ultrasound alone is not a sensitive test for fetal infection or affection. Longitudinal observational surveys of intrauterine infection cases are lacking because the other half of prenatally diagnosed cases were recognized as a result of maternal screening. The majority of these cases reported to date were terminated on the basis of proven fetal infection without ultrasound findings or before they could eventually develop.[10,18] However, three small prospective series reported a 15–25% sensitivity for antenatal ultrasound.[14–18]

The predictive value of ultrasound, like that of any other diagnostic test, increases with the prevalence of the disease and therefore works better in a population preselected by screening for maternal seroconversion. However, even in such a high-risk population, at least 90% of infected fetuses are expected to be asymptomatic.[17] The ultrasound features of this progressive disease will also vary significantly with time and serial ultrasound follow-up is likely to perform better than routine cross-sectional examination at any fixed gestation.[2]

The pathophysiology of fetal CMV infection allows one to expect progressive and sometimes only subtle or transient findings on ultrasound in cases of fetal infection (Figure 44.1). Indeed, irrespective of the mode of transmission to the mother, CMV is a viremic herpes virus with a prolonged latency within maternal monocytes, which will eventually reach the fetus via the umbilical circulation.

The placenta, where the virus replicates, will act not only as a barrier against CMV but also as a reservoir, which may release the virus into the fetal circulation at any stage of the pregnancy, irrespective of the time of seroconversion.[55,56] Within 4–8 weeks

Table 44.1 Fetal abnormalities diagnosed *in utero* in cases of congenital cytomegalovirus infection, except cerebral abnormalities (Table 44. 2)

Series	Congenital CMV (*n*)	Fetuses with US findings (*n*)	IUGR	Hydrops	Ascites	Pericardial effusion	Pleural effusion	Skin edema	Hyperechogenic bowel	Hepatomegaly	Splenomegaly	Liver calcifications	Cardiomegaly	Placentomegaly	Oligohydramnios	Polyhydramnios
Enders *et al.*[9]	189	41	12	4	15	3	—	2	2	3	1	—	2	2	4	1
Liesnard *et al.*[10]	68	4	—	—	—	—	–	—	2	—	—	—	—	—	—	—
Lipitz *et al.*[8]	51	11	6	2	1	—	1*	—	2 (1*)	—	—	—	—	—	—	—
Azam *et al.*[11]	26	5	—	—	1*	—	—	—	1	1	—	—	—	1*	—	—
Lazzarotto *et al.*[18]	25	3	1	—	—	—	—	—	—	2	1	—	—	—	—	—
Drose *et al.*[13]	19	18	4 (1*)	—	4	1	3	1	—	—	—	3 (1*)	3 (1*)	5	6	7
Revello *et al.*[14/15]	19	4	1*	—	2 (1*)	—	—	—	—	—	—	—	—	—	—	—
Preece *et al.*[19]	9	—	—	—	—	—	—	—	—	—	—	—	—	—	—	—
Hohlfeld *et al.*[20]	8	2	—	1*	1*	—	—	—	—	—	—	—	—	—	—	—
Malinger *et al.*[21]	8	8	—	—	—	—	—	—	—	—	—	2	—	—	—	—
Lamy *et al.*[22]	7	2	—	—	—	—	—	—	—	—	—	—	—	—	—	—
Steinlin *et al.*[23]	7	—	—	—	—	—	—	—	—	—	—	—	—	—	—	—
Lynch *et al.*[24]	6	6	2 (1*)	1	1	—	—	—	1	—	—	—	—	—	3	—
Schneeberger *et al.*[25]	4	1	1*	—	—	—	—	—	—	—	—	—	—	—	—	—
Grose *et al.*[26]	3	2	1	—	—	1	—	—	—	—	—	—	—	—	1	—
Hogge *et al.*[27]	3	2	—	—	1*	—	—	—	—	—	—	—	—	—	—	—
Tassin *et al.*[28]	3	3	2	—	1	1	—	—	—	1	—	—	—	1	2	—
Agius *et al.*[29]	2	—	—	—	—	—	—	—	—	—	—	—	—	—	—	—
Ahlfors *et al.*[30]	2	—	—	—	—	—	—	—	—	—	—	—	—	—	—	—
Duvekot *et al.*[31]	2	1	1*	—	—	—	—	—	—	—	—	—	—	—	—	—
Forouzan *et al.*[32]	2	2	—	—	—	—	—	—	2	—	—	—	—	—	—	—
Gabrielli *et al.*[33]	2	—	—	—	—	—	—	—	—	—	—	—	—	—	—	—
Inoue *et al.*[34]	2	—	—	—	2	—	—	2	—	—	—	—	—	—	2	—
Morris *et al.*[35]	2	—	—	—	—	—	—	—	—	—	—	—	—	—	—	—
Nigro *et al.*[36]	2	—	—	—	—	—	—	—	—	—	—	—	—	—	—	—
Saigal *et al.*[37]	2	—	—	—	—	—	—	—	—	—	—	—	—	—	—	—
Fillioux *et al.*[38]	1	1	—	1 with tachycardia	1	—	1	—	—	—	—	—	—	—	—	—
Price *et al.*[39]	1	1	—	—	1	—	—	—	—	—	—	—	—	1	—	1
Achiron *et al.*[40]	1	1	—	—	—	—	—	—	—	—	—	—	—	—	—	—
Chaoui *et al.*[41]	1	1	1	—	—	—	—	—	—	—	1	—	—	—	—	—

Table 44.1 (*Continued*)

Series	Congenital CMV (*n*)	Fetuses with US findings (*n*)	IUGR	Hydrops	Ascites	Pericardial effusion	Pleural effusion	Skin edema	Hyperechogenic bowel	Hepatomegaly	Splenomegaly	Liver calcifications	Cardiomegaly	Placentomegaly	Oligohydramnios	Polyhydramnios
Heinrich *et al.*[42]	1	1	—	—	1	1	—	—	—	—	—	—	—	—	—	—
Nigro *et al.*[43]	1	1	1	—	—	—	—	—	—	—	—	—	—	1	—	—
Nigro *et al.*[44]	1	1	1	—	—	—	—	1	—	—	—	—	—	—	—	—
Nigro *et al.*[45]	1	1	—	—	1	—	—	—	—	—	—	1	—	—	—	—
Nigro *et al.*[46]	1	1	—	—	—	—	—	—	1	—	—	—	—	—	1	—
Peters *et al.*[47]	1	1	1	—	1	—	—	—	—	—	—	1	1	1	1	—
Pletcher *et al.*[48]	1	1	—	—	—	—	—	—	1	—	—	—	—	—	—	—
Rousseau *et al.*[49]	1	1	1	—	—	—	—	—	1	—	—	—	—	—	1	—
Seguin *et al.*[50]	1	1	1	—	—	—	—	—	—	—	—	—	—	—	—	—
Soussotte *et al.*[51]	1	—	1	—	—	—	—	—	—	—	—	—	—	—	—	—
Vogler *et al.*[52]	1	—	—	—	—	—	—	—	—	—	—	—	—	—	—	—
Yamashita *et al.*[53]	1	1	—	—	1	—	—	—	—	—	—	1	—	—	—	—
Watt-Morse *et al.*[54]	1	1	—	—	1	—	—	—	—	—	—	—	1	—	—	—
Total	490	130	37 (4*)	9 (1*)	32 (4*)	7	5 (1*)	6	13 (2*)	7	3	7 (1*)	5 (1*)	9 (1*)	17	8

IUGR, *in utero* growth restriction; US, ultrasound

*Isolated abnormality

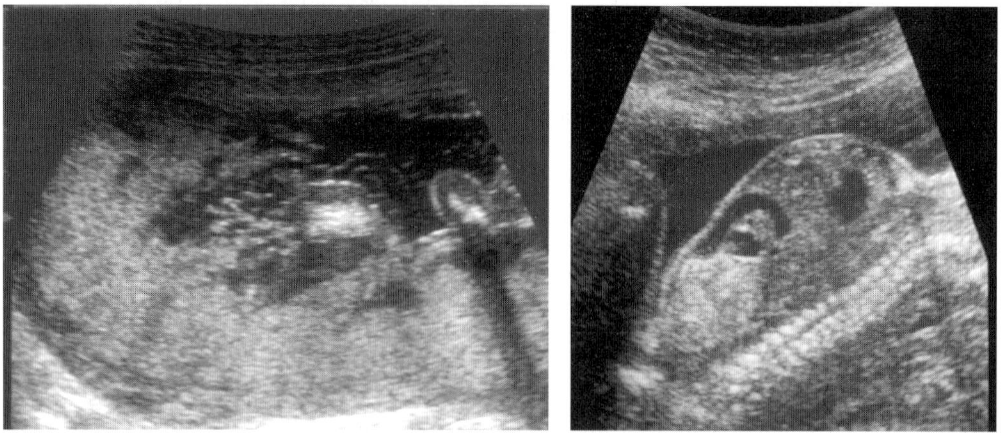

(a) (b)

Figure 44.1 Placentitis showing a thick and heterogenous placenta (a). Hyperechogenic bowel and hepatomegaly (b) are not specific features of systemic fetal infection.

following maternal viremia, an early but inconstant sign of vertical infection is therefore likely to be placentitis, as defined by a thickness of 4 cm or more and a heterogenous appearance typically with calcifications coexisting with hypoechoic areas[13].

Once the virus reaches the fetal circulation, the fetal kidney is hit early and preferentially, which may cause transient oligohydramnios and, less often, renal hyperechogenicity. This appears to be more frequent than polyhydramnios.[13] Viral enterocolitis often shows with the transient or persistent appearance of at least grade-2 hyperechogenic bowel as an early ultrasound finding, which may be accompanied by high human chorionic gonadotropin and alpha-fetoprotein levels in maternal blood.[32,47,48,57] This usually represents meconial ileus or bowel perforation and meconial peritonitis.[58,59] Several weeks can elapse until other features of fetal infection, if any, show up on antenatal ultrasound, and some of the former may have disappeared by then.

Overt systemic disease will appear as hepatosplenomegaly and possibly ascites in the fetus as a result of cholestatic hepatitis and liver insufficiency.[41] Less often, generalized edema and ascites will suggest anemia-related hydrops due to the combined effect of liver failure and marrow infection. This spectacular presentation has also proven to be eventually transient with both ultrasound and biological normalization at follow-up.[54] Cardiomyopathy, expressed as cardiomegaly with a thick myocardium, which may contain punctuate calcifications, is a rare finding that could also participate in the development of fetal hydrops, eventually associated with tachyarythmia.[13,41] Calcifications of the fetal liver, spleen and even lungs could appear and remain as a result of a systemic disease.[60]

Intrauterine growth restriction (IUGR) may develop as a result of fetal infection or placental infection or both. It can therefore be advisable to screen for CMV as a part of the assessment of any IUGR fetus below the fifth percentile. Indeed, this could be a completely isolated finding irrespective of placental or fetal Doppler values.[61,62]

Affection of the fetal brain shows mainly late and multiple suggestive and heterogenous ultrasound features of fetal infection and fetal affection[21] (Table 44.2). These can be present when the previously described features have resumed, therefore, weeks or months after the onset of maternal and even fetal infection.

Microcephaly is a major form of the disease; however, this may prove to be a very difficult diagnosis to establish, especially in a growth-retarded fetus.[72,73]

Ventriculomegaly, unilateral or bilateral, is a common entry to the diagnosis as around 5% of all ventriculomegaly diagnosed *in utero* is of infectious origin.[74] It can be of two types. Destructive ventriculomegaly is often moderate and will often precede microcephaly, showing even subtle enlargement of pericerebral spaces (Figure 44.2) as an early sign of microencephaly. Obstructive ventriculomegaly can occur as a result of obstruction of the foramen of Monroe and/or of Magendie and Lushka by ventriculitis-related edema or intraventricular hemorrhage.[46] The same mechanisms can lead to less common presentations such as mega cisterna magna, cerebellar hypoplasia or hemorrhage, pseudo-Dandy Walker malformations and schizencephaly.[21,66]

More subtle anomalies can be identified as associated findings with any of the features described above or as isolated findings, making the diagnosis more difficult. Non-specific vasculitis in the fetal thalami and basal ganglia,[67] described as candle-stick images, punctuate echogenicity within the brain parenchyma or underlying the rim of the lateral ventricles together with strands across the lateral ventricles.[40,75] Germinolysis-related subependymal cysts can also be overlooked by routine fetal ultrasound examination when fetal infection is not known).[21,40,64] Rare cases of corpus callosum abnormalities have also been described *in utero* and postnatally.[21,69]

Abnormal myelinization and gyration of the fetal brain is another pitfall for fetal brain ultrasound examination and the development of fetal MRI is a recent and definite asset in the complete assessment of high-risk fetuses.[21,51,63] Lissencephaly could reflect injury before 16 or 18 weeks whereas polymicrogyria could reflect injury at 18–24 weeks. Cases with normal gyral patterns have probably been injured during the third trimester showing diffuse heterogeneity in the white matter.[63] Both T1 and T2 sequences are therefore useful.

It is noteworthy that although the relationship between the ultrasound features described above and fetal CMV infection is well established, CMV is rarely reported in series of cases bearing these anomalies. This further emphasizes the poor performance of ultrasound in diagnosing fetal CMV infection in the general population.

Maternal and fetal biology

When the presence of CMV infection is suspected on the basis of any of the ultrasound findings described above, it can be excluded only if maternal serology shows negative immunoglobulin G (IgG) and negative IgM. Indeed, IgM, which can be present both in primary and non-primary infections, is often negative at the time of a positive fetal ultrasound examination several weeks or months following maternal infection. At that time, both maternal viruria and viremia are also likely to be negative although they have been found positive for 3–12 months following maternal infection.[76]

The diagnosis of fetal infection is made by recovery of the virus or by amplification of its genome in the amniotic fluid (AF) retrieved by amniocentesis.[5,77] Indeed, the AF is colonized once the virus has infected the fetal kidneys and replicates in the tubular epithelium to be passed in the urine. Viral DNA therefore accumulates in the AF as it does in the urine of infected individuals postnatally. This provides with clear guidelines for performing amniocentesis in CMV infection during pregnancy. Following seroconversion or reactivation, the process leading to CMV excretion in the fetal urine will take an average of 6–8 weeks and this interval should be recognized in order to avoid false-negative prenatal diagnosis.[77] This should also be performed when fetal urination is well established, and therefore not before 22 weeks.

Detection of infectious CMV in AF may be performed by the use of rapid virus isolation in cell cultures ('shell vial culture')[77,78] as well as CMV DNA detection by polymerase chain reaction (PCR) amplification. Sensitivity varies between 45% and 100% for both PCR and culture, the lowest figures being obtained when amniocentesis was performed before 21 weeks, and less than 6–8 weeks from maternal seroconversion.[7,19,21,42–44,79–81] However, the free interval can be even longer depending on the placental ability to contain infection.[55] The overall false-negative rate of amniocentesis is around 12% (52/365) [0–25%][8–10,14,15,18,24,43–45,77,80–84] and has been reported to be much lower and even down to 0% when the conditions of sampling were ideal.[14,15,20]

The variation in sensitivity may also account for the differences in PCR methods used. Each PCR method reported in the literature has its own protocol (e.g. single-round PCR, nested PCR or commercial tests) and tests different volumes of fetal specimen, leading to variable sensitivities. Moreover, the CMV genome sequences amplified in these PCR tests varied with various fragments of the immediate early protein gene or of the glycoprotein B gene being most frequently used. Genetic diversity in those two genes is well recognized,[85] but the design of primers and probes did not always account for this.

False-positive PCR results have also been reported when the neonate was not infected in 9/179 (5%) (0–30%), questioning the quality of the technique.[9,11,14,15,18,43–45,80,83,84] False-positive diagnosis may be explained by contamination of the AF with the maternal blood during amniocentesis, if the mother had a positive CMV DNAemia at the time of sampling. Indeed, Revello *et al.* showed that CMV DNA may be recovered in the blood of nearly 50% of immunocompetent patients up to 3 months after CMV primary infection.[76] Another explanation could be laboratory contamination occurring during PCR testing. Indeed, in some of these studies a nested CMV PCR was used, which is known to be a very sensitive technique but at high risk of contamination. Generalization of semiautomated real time PCR might help to overcome the risk of contamination and achieve absolute specificity for prenatal diagnosis of CMV infection. These results, however, establish PCR as a reliable technique in reference laboratories. The question of performing a second amniocentesis when the result of the first examination is negative remains unanswered. However, to date, information available on 13 cases with a false-negative result[9,24] did not show any symptom at the age of up to 36 months, although one neonate was growth restricted.

Another question without an answer today is that of the risk of fetal iatrogenic infection when maternal viremia is positive at the time of amniocentesis. However, the commonly understood pathophysiology of vertical transmission of CMV to the fetus makes this possibility unlikely.

Prenatal diagnosis in fetal blood

There are few data available on the prenatal diagnosis of CMV infection in fetal blood.

The sensitivity of IgM detection in fetal blood is around 50%.[10,77] The sensitivity of CMV rapid or classic culture is even lower, ranging from 0% to 40%.[10,11,77,80] This is probably due to the small volume

Table 44.2 Fetal brain abnormalities diagnosed *in utero* in cases of congenital cytomegalovirus infection

Series	Congenital CMV (*n*)	Ventriculomegaly	Hydrocephaly	Microcephaly	Brain and periventricular calcifications	Agenesis or abnormal corpus callosum	Reduced gyration	Choroid plexus cyst	Cystic structure in cerebellum	Lissencephaly	Hypoplastic or small cerebellum	Subependymal cysts
Enders *et al.*[9]	189	7	7	12	3	2	—	—	2	2	2	—
Guerra *et al.*[16]	68	4 (2*)	—	—	—	—	—	—	—	—	—	—
Boppana** *et al.*[61]	56	4	—	—	3—	—	3	—	—	—	—	—
Liesnard *et al.*[10]	55	1	2 (1*)	2	—	—	1	—	—	—	—	—
Lipitz *et al.*[8]	51	3	—	—	1	—	—	1	—	—	—	—
Azam *et al.*[11]	26	1	—	2 (1*)	—	—	—	—	—	—	—	—
Lazzarotto *et al.*[18]	25	2 (1*)	—	—	1	1	—	—	—	—	—	—
Drose *et al.*[13]	19	—	6 (1*)	2 (1*)	3	—	—	—	—	—	—	—
Barkovich** *et al.*[63]	11	9	—	6	7	1	2	—	1	—	7	6
Malinger *et al.*[21]	8	5	—	—	6	1	4	—	—	—	2 (1*)	3
Lamy *et al.*[20]	7	—	—	—	2*	—	—	—	—	—	—	—
Lynch *et al.*[24]	6	3	—	—	1	—	—	—	—	—	—	—
Butt** *et al.*[64]	4	4	—	—	4	—	—	—	—	—	—	2
Revello *et al.*[14/15]	4	2	—	—	—	—	—	—	—	—	—	—
Hogge *et al.*[27]	3	—	—	1	1	—	—	—	—	—	—	—
Tassin *et al.*[28]	3	1	2	1	2	—	—	—	—	—	—	—
Inoue *et al.*[34]	2	2	—	—	—	—	—	—	—	—	—	—
Nigro *et al.*[43/44/45]	2	—	—	1	—	—	—	—	—	—	—	—
Ries** *et al.*[65]	2	2	—	—	2	—	—	—	—	—	—	—
Seguin *et al.*[50]	2	—	—	1	—	—	—	—	—	—	—	—
Twickler *et al.*[66]	2	2	—	2	—	—	—	—	—	—	—	—
Achiron *et al.*[40]	1	1	—	—	1	—	—	—	—	—	—	1
Chaoui *et al.*[41]	1	1	—	—	—	—	1	—	—	—	—	—
Estroff *et al.*[67]	1	1	—	—	1	—	—	—	—	—	—	—

Table 44.2 (*Continued*)

Series	Congenital CMV (*n*)	Ventriculomegaly	Hydrocephaly	Microcephaly	Brain and periventricular calcifications	Agenesis or abnormal corpus callosum	Reduced gyration	Choroid plexus cyst	Cystic structure in cerebellum	Lissencephaly	Hypoplastic or small cerebellum	Subependymal cysts
Graham *et al.*[68]	1	1	—	—	1	—	—	—	—	—	—	—
Mehta** *et al.*[69]	1	1	—	—	1	1 (with lipoma)	—	—	—	—	—	—
Mittelman-Handwerker *et al.*[70]	1	1	—	—	—	—	—	—	1	—	1	1
Nigro *et al.*[43/44/45]	1	—	—	—	—	—	—	1	—	—	—	—
Nigro *et al.*[46]	1	1	—	—	—	—	—	—	—	—	—	—
Peters *et al.*[47]	1	1	—	1	1	—	—	—	—	—	—	—
Pletcher *et al.*[48]	1	1	—	—	—	—	—	—	—	—	—	—
Rousseau *et al.*[49]	1	—	—	1	—	—	—	—	—	—	—	—
Soussotte *et al.*[51]	1	—	—	1	1	—	1	—	—	—	—	1
Toma** *et al.*[71]	1	—	—	1	1	—	—	—	—	—	—	—
Watt-Morse *et al.*[54]	1	1	—	—	—	—	—	—	—	—	—	—
Total	304	32 (3*)	13 (2*)	21 (2*)	21 (2*)	6	12	2	2	—	4 (1*)	14

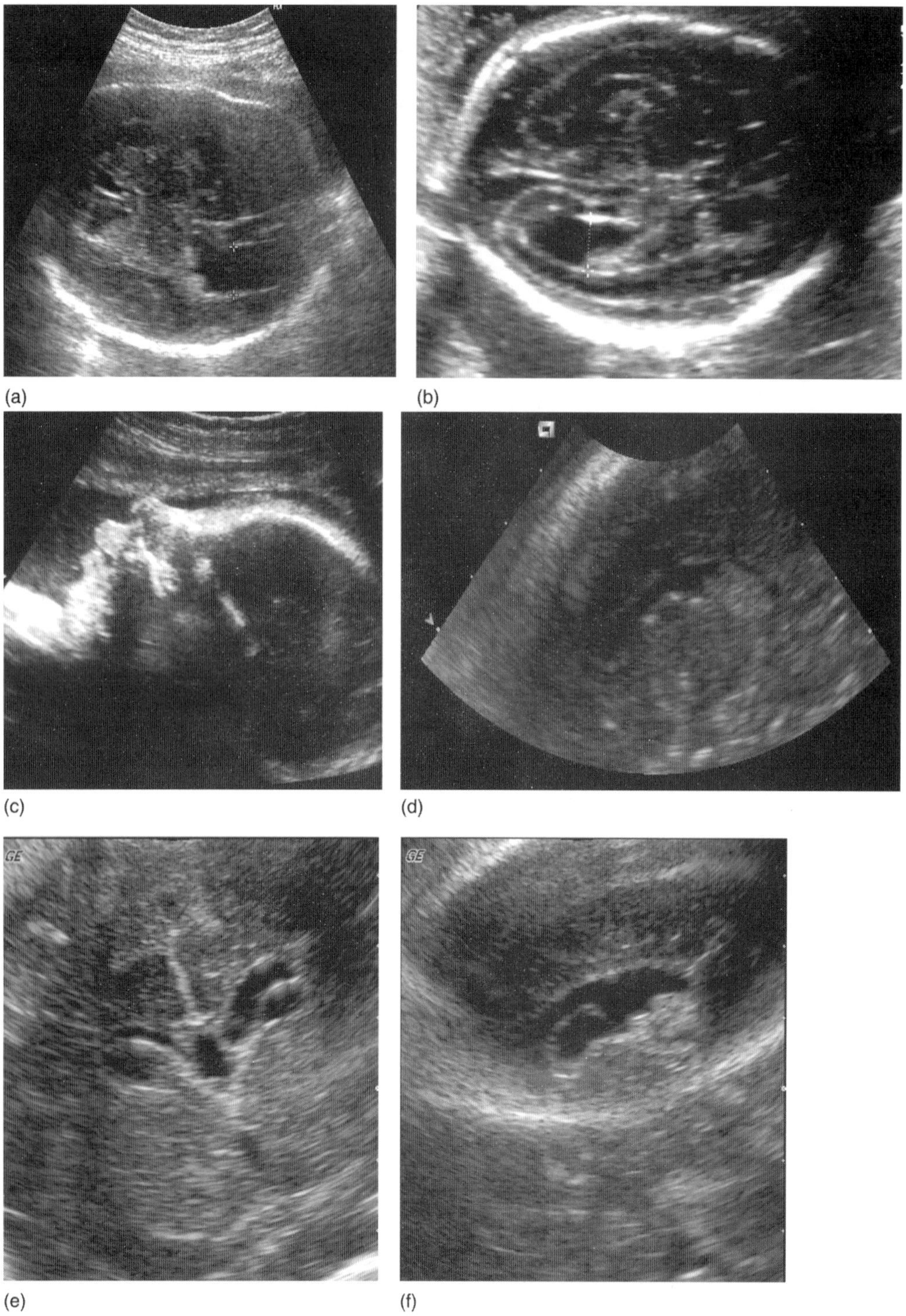

Figure 44.2 Cerebral features include ventriculomegaly (a) often preceding microencephaly (b), which in turn can precede microcephaly as illustrated by a sloping forehead on the profile view of the face (c). More subtle features include parenchymal punctiform calcifications (d), subependymal cyst (e) and hyperechogenicity of the germinal matrix (f).

retrieved by cordocentesis, and PCR methods should be preferred. However, the sensitivity achieved by PCR in fetal blood varied greatly in three studies published, ranging from 40% to 92%.[9,10,77] Enders *et al.*[9] reported a 100% sensitivity when combining amplification of CMV DNA in AF and in fetal blood.

To date, CMV detection in fetal blood is, therefore, generally considered to be unsuitable for prenatal diagnosis. However, the value of viral quantification (DNA and IgM) in fetal blood to identify fetuses at risk of developing severe congenital infection is emerging and this issue will be discussed in a later chapter.[9,14,15,77]

Conclusion

CMV infection in pregnancy is not only diagnosed from suggestive ultrasound features but also often suspected as a result of an individual or population-based screening. Interpretation of maternal serology and indication for invasive and non-invasive testing require some knowledge of the natural history of CMV transplacental infection.

Amniocentesis remains the gold standard invasive test to diagnose fetal infection, and in the absence of ultrasound features this should be performed after 22 weeks and at least 6 weeks following maternal seroconversion.

REFERENCES

1. Stagno S, Pass RF, Gretchen Cloud MS, *et al.* Primary cytomegalovirus infection in pregnancy. *J Am Med Assoc* 1986; 256:1904–8.
2. Ville Y. The megalovirus. *Ultrasound Obstet Gynecol* 1998;12: 151–3.
3. Fowler KB, Stagno S, Pass RF, Britt TJ, Boll TJ, Alford CA. The outcome of congenital cytomegalovirus infection in relation to maternal antibody status. *N Engl J Med* 1992;326:663–7.
4. Peckham C, Stark O, Dudgeon JA, Martin JAM, Hawkins G. Congenital cytomegalovirus infection: A cause of sensorineural hearing loss. *Arch Dis Child* 1987;62:1233–7.
5. Gaytant MA, Steegers E, Sommekrot BA, Merkus H, Galama JM. Congenital cytomegalovirus infection: Review of the epidemiology and outcome. *Obstet Gynecol Surv* 2002;57:245–56.
6. Fowler KB, Stagno S, Pass RF. Maternal immunity and prevention of congenital cytomegalovirus infection. *J Am Med Assoc* 2003; 26:1008–11.
7. Hagay ZJ, Biran GB, Ornoy A, Reece EA. Congenital cytomegalovirus infection: A long-standing problem still seeking a solution. *Am J Obstet Gynecol* 1996;174:241–5.
8. Lipitz S, Yagel S, Shalev E, Achiron R, Mashiach S, Schiff E. Prenatal diagnosis of fetal primary cytomegalovirus infection. *Obstet Gynecol* 1997;89:763–67.
9. Enders G, Bader U, Lindermann L, Schalsta G, Daiminger A. Prenatal diagnosis of congenital cytomegalovirus infection in 189 pregnancies with known outcome. *Prenat Diagn* 2001;21: 362–77.
10. Liesnard C, Donner C, Brancart F, Gosselin F, Delforge ML, Rodesch F. Prenatal diagnosis of cytomegalovirus infection: Prospective study of 237 pregnancies at risk. *Obstet Gynecol* 2000;95:881–8.
11. Azam AZ, Vial Y, Fawer CL, Zufferey J, Hohlfeld P. Prenatal diagnosis of congenital cytomegalovirus infection. *Obstet Gynecol* 2001;97:443–8.
12. Lazzarotto T, Guerra B, Spezzacatena P, *et al.* Prenatal diagnosis of congenital cytomegalovirus infection. *J Clin Microbiol* 1998;36:3540–4.
13. Drose JA, Dennis MA, Thickman D. Infection *in utero*: US findings in 19 cases. *Radiology* 1991;178:369–74.
14. Revello MG, Zavattoni M, Furione M, Baldanti F, Gerna G. Quantification of human cytomegalovirus DNA in amniotic fluid of mothers of congenitally infected fetuses. *J Clin Microbiol* 1999;37:3350–2.
15. Revello MG, Zavattoni M, Sarasini A, *et al.* Prenatal diagnostic and prognostic value of human cytomegalovirus load and IgM antibody response in blood of congenitally infected fetuses. *J Infect Dis* 1999;180:1320–3.
16. Guerra B, Lazzarotto T, Quarta S, *et al.* Prenatal diagnosis of symptomatic congenital cytomegalovirus infection. *Obstet Gynecol* 2000;183:476–82.
17. Crino JP. Ultrasound and fetal diagnosis of perinatal infection. *Clin Obstet Gynecol* 1999;42:71–80.
18. Lazzarotto T, Varani S, Guerra B, Nicolosi A, Lanari M, Landini MP. Prenatal indicators of congenital cytomegalovirus infection. *J Pediatrics* 2000;137:90–5.
19. Preece PM, Blount JM, Glover J, Fletcher GM, Peckham CS, Griffiths PD. The consequence of primary cytomegalovirus infection in pregnancy. *Arch Dis Child* 1983;58:970–5.
20. Hohlfeld P, Vial Y, Maillard-Brignon C, Vaudaux B, Fawer CL. Cytomegalovirus fetal infection: Prenatal diagnosis. *Obstet Gynecol* 1991;78:615–18.
21. Malinger G, Lev D, Zahalka N, *et al.* Fetal cytomegalovirus infection of the brain: The spectrum of sonographic findings. *Am J Neuroradiol* 2003;24:28–32.
22. Lamy H, Mulongo K, Gadissieux JF, Lyon G, Gaudy V, Van Lierde M. Prenatal diagnosis of fetal cytomegalovirus infection. *Am J Obstet Gynecol* 1992;166:91–4.
23. Steinlin MI, Nadal D, Eich GF, Martin E, Boltshauser EJ. Late intrauterine cytomegalovirus infection: Clinical and neuroimaging findings. *Pediatr Neurol* 1996;15:249–53.
24. Lynch L, Daffos F, Emanuel D, *et al.* Prenatal diagnosis of fetal cytomegalovirus infection. *Obstet Gynecol* 1991;165:714–8.
25. Schneeberger PM, Groendaal F, de Vries LS, van Loon AM, Vroom TM. Variable outcome of a congenital cytomegalovirus infection in a quadruplet pregnancy after primary infection of the mother during pregnancy. *Acta Paediatr* 1994;83:986–9.
26. Grose C, Meehan T, Weiner CP. Prenatal diagnosis of congenital cytomegalovirus infection by virus isolation after amniocentesis. *Pediatr Infect Dis* 1992;11:605–7.
27. Hogge WA, Buffone GJ, Hogge JS. Prenatal diagnosis of cytomegalovirus (CMV) infection: A preliminary report. *Prenat Diagn* 1993;13:131–6.
28. Tassin GB, Maklad NF, Stewart RR, Bell ME. Cytomegalic inclusion disease: Intrauterine sonographic diagnosis using findings involving the brain. *Am J Neuroradiol* 1991;12:117–22.
29. Agius G, Baillargeau E, Ranger S, Castets M. Infection congénitale à Cytomégalovirus chez des jumeaux dizygotes. *Arch Fr Pediatr* 1985;42:63–4.
30. Ahlfors K, Ivarsson SA, Nilsson H. On the unpredictable development of congenital cytomegalovirus infection. A study in twins. *Early Hum Dev* 1988;18:125–35.
31. Duvekot JJ, Theewes BA, Wesdrop JM, Roumen FJ, Bouckaert PX. Congenital cytomegalovirus infection in a twin pregnancy: A case report. *Eur J Pediatr* 1990;149:261–2.
32. Forouzan I. Fetal abdominal echogenic mass: An early sign of intrauterine cytomegalovirus infection. *Obstet Gynecol* 1992;80: 535–7.
33. Gabrielli L, Lazzarotto T, Foschini MP, *et al.* Horizontal *in utero* acquisition of cytomegalovirus infection in a twin pregnancy. *J Clin Microbiol* 2003;41:1329–31.
34. Inoue T, Matsumura N, Fukuoka M, Sagawa N, Fujii S. Severe congenital infection with fetal hydrops in a cytomegalovirus seropositive healthy women. *Eur J Obstet Gynecol* 2001;95:184–6.
35. Morris DJ, Sims D, Chiswick M, Das VK, Newton VE. Symptomatic congenital CMV infection after maternal recurrent infection. *Pediatr Infect Dis* 1994;13:61–4.
36. Nigro G, Clerico A, Mondaini C. Symptomatic congenital cytomegalovirus infection in two consecutive sisters. *Arch Dis Child* 1993;69: 527–8.
37. Saigal S, Lunyk O, Larke B, Chernesky MA. The outcome of children with congenital cytomegalovirus infection. *Am J Dis Child* 1982;136:986–01.
38. Fillioux F, Kelsey DK, Bose CL, Veasy LG, Gooch CL. Hydrops fetalis with supraventricular tachycardia and cytomegalovirus infection. *Clin Peadiatr* 1985;534–6.
39. Price JM, Fisch AE, Jacobson J. Ultrasonic findings in fetal cytomegalovirus infection. *J Clin Ultrasound* 1978;6:215–94.
40. Achiron R, Pinhas-Hamiel O, Lipitz S, Heiman Z, Reichman B, Maschiach S. Prenatal ultrasonographic diagnosis of fetal cerebral ventriculitis associated with asymptomatic maternal cytomegalovirus infection. *Prenat Diagn* 1994;14:523–6.
41. Chaoui R, Zodan Marin T, Wisser J. Marked splenomegaly in fetal cytomegalovirus infection: Detection supported by 3-dimensional power Doppler ultrasound. *Ultrasound Obstet Gynecol* 2002;20: 299–302.
42. Heinrich W, Meckies J, Dudenhausen JW, Vogel M, Enders G. Recurrent CMV infection during pregnancy: Ultrasound diagnosis and fetal outcome. *Ultrasound Obstet Gynecol* 2002;19:608–11.

43. Nigro G, La Torre R, Anceschi MM, Mazzocco M, Cosmi E. Hyperimmunoglobulin therapy for a twin fetus with cytomegalovirus infection and growth restriction. *Am J Obstet Gynecol* 1999;180:1222–6.
44. Nigro G, La Torre R, Mazzocco M, *et al.* Multi system cytomegalovirus fetopathy by recurrent infection in a pregnant women with hepatitis B. *Prenat Diagn* 1999;19:1070–2.
45. Nigro G, Mazzocco M, Anceschi M, La Torre R, Antonelli G, Cosmi E. Prenatal diagnosis of fetal cytomegalovirus infection after primary or recurrent maternal infection. *Obstet Gynecol* 1999;94:909–14.
46. Nigro G, La Torre R, Sali E, *et al.* Intraventricular hemorrhage in a fetus with cerebral cytomegalovirus infection. *Prenat Diagn* 2002;22:558–61.
47. Peters MT, Lowe TW, Carpenter A, Kole S. Prenatal diagnosis of congenital cytomegalovirus infection with abnormal triple-screen results and hyperechoic fetal bowel. *Am J Obstet Gynecol* 1995;173:953–4.
48. Pletcher BA, Williams MK, Mulivor RA, Barth D, Linder C, Rawlinson K. Intrauterine cytomegalovirus infection presenting as fetal meconium peritonitis. *Obstet Gynecol* 1991;78:903–5.
49. Rousseau T, Douvier S, Reynaud I, *et al.* Severe fetal cytomegalic inclusion disease after documented maternal reactivation of CMV during pregnancy. *Prenat Diagn* 2000;20:333–6.
50. Seguin J, Cho CT. Congenital cytomegalovirus infection in one monozygotic twin. *J Am Med Assoc* 1988;260:22.
51. Soussotte C, Maugey-Laulom B, Carles D. Contribution of transvaginal ultrasonography and fetal cerebral MRI in a case of congenital cytomegalovirus infection. *Fetal Diagn Ther* 2000; 15:219–33.
52. Vogler C, Kohl S, Rosenberg HS. Cytomegalovirus infection and fetal death in a twin. *J Reprod Med* 1986;31:207–10.
53. Yamashita Y, Iwanaga R, Goto A, *et al.* Congenital cytomegalovirus infection associated with fetal ascites and intrahepatic calcifications. *Acta Paediatr Scand* 1989;78:965–7.
54. Watt-Morse ML, Laifer SA, Hill LM. The natural history of fetal cytomegalovirus infection as assessed by serial ultrasound and fetal blood sampling: A case report. *Prenat Diagn* 1995;15: 567–70.
55. Goff E, Griffith BP, Booss J. Delayed amplification of cytomegalovirus infection in the placenta and maternal tissues during late gestation. *Am J Obstet Gynecol* 1987;156:1265–70.
56. Kumazaki K, Ozono K, Yahara T, *et al.* Detection of cytomegalovirus DNA in human placenta. *J Med Virol* 2002;68:363–9.
57. McGregor SN, Tamura R, Sabbagha R, Brenhofer JK, Kambich MP, Pergament E. Isolated hyperechoic fetal bowel: Significance and implications for management. *Am J Obstet Gynecol* 1995;173: 1254–8.
58. Dechelotte PJ, Mulliez NM, Bouvier RJ, Vanlieferinghen PC, Lmemery D. Pseudo-meconium ileus due to cytomegalovirus infection: A report of three cases. *Pediatr Pathol* 1992;12:73–82.
59. Huang YC, Lin TY, Huang CS, Hseun C. Ileal perforation caused by congenital or perinatal cytomegalovirus infection. *J Pediatr* 1997;129:931–4.
60. Stein B, Bromley B, Michlewitz H, Miller WA, Benacerraf BR. Fetal liver calcifications: Sonographic appearance and post-natal outcome. *Radiology* 1995;197:489–92.
61. Boppana SB, Fowler KB, Vaid Y, *et al.* Neuroradiographic findings in the newborn period and long term outcome in children with symptomatic congenital CMV infection. *Pediatrics* 1997;99:409–14.
62. Conboy TJ, Pass RF, Stagno S, *et al.* Early clinical manifestations and intellectual outcome in children with symptomatic congenital cytomegalovirus infection. *J Pediatr* 1987;111:343–8.
63. Barkovich AJ, Lindan CE. Congenital cytomegalovirus infection of the brain: Imaging analysis and embryologic considerations. *Am J Neuroradiol* 1994;15:703–15.
64. Butt W, Mackay RJ, De Crespigny L, Murton LJ, Roy RND. Intracranial lesions of congenital cytomegalovirus infection detected by ultrasound scanning. *Pediatrics* 1984;73:611–4.
65. Ries M, Deeg KH, Heininger U. Demonstration of perivascular echogenicities in congenital cytomegalovirus infection by colour Doppler imaging. *Eur J Pediatr* 1990;150:34–6.
66. Twickler DM, Perlman J, Maberry MC. Congenital cytomegalovirus infection presenting as cerebral ventriculomegaly on antenatal sonography. *Am J Perinatol* 1993;10:404–6.
67. Estroff JA, Richard BP, Teele RL, Benacerraf BR. Echogenic vessels in the fetal thalami and basal ganglia associated with cytomegalovirus infection. *J Ultrasound Med* 1992;11:686–8.
68. Graham D, Guidi SM, Sanders RC. Sonographic features of *in utero* periventricular calcification due to cytomegalovirus infection. *J Ultrasound Med* 1982;1:171–2.
69. Mehta N, Hartnoll G. Congenital CMV with callosal lipoma and agenesis. *Pediatr Neurol* 2001;24:222–4.
70. Mittelman-Handwerker S, Pardes JG, Post RC, Sumala M, Rosenberg JC, Chervenak FA. Fetal ventriculomegaly and brain atrophy in a woman with intrauterine cytomegalovirus infection. *J Reprod Med* 1986;31:1061–4.
71. Toma P, Magnano GM, Mezzano, P, Lazzini F, Bonacci W, Serra G. Cerebral ultrasound images in prenatal cytomegalovirus infection. *Neuroradiology* 1989;31:278–89.
72. Noyola DE, Demmler GJ, Williamson WD, *et al.* Cytomegalovirus urinary excretion and long term outcome in children with congenital cytomegalovirus excretion. *Pediatr Infect Dis* 2000;19: 505–10.
73. Ahlfors K, Ivarsson SA, Bjerre I. Microcephaly and congenital cytomegalovirus infection: A combined prospective and retrospective study of a Swedish infant population. *Pediatrics* 1986; 78:1058–63.
74. Holzgreve W, Feil R, Louwen F, Miny P. Prenatal diagnosis and management of fetal hydrocephaly and lissencephaly. *Child's Nerv Syst* 1993;9:51–4.
75. Fakhry J, Khoury A. Fetal intracranial calcifications; the importance of periventricular hyperechoic foci without shadowing. *J Ultrasound Med* 1991;10:51–4.
76. Revello MG, Zavattoni M, Sarasini A, Percivalle E, Simoncini L, Gerna G. Human cytomegalovirus in blood of immunocompetent persons during primary infection: Prognostic implications for pregnancy. *J Infect Dis* 1998;177:1170–5.
77. Revello MG, Gerna G. Diagnosis and management of human cytomegalovirus infection in the mother, fetus and new born infant. *Clin Microbiol Rev* 2002;15:680–713.
78. Gleaves CA, Smith TF, Shucter EA, Pearson GR. Rapid detection of cytomegalovirus in MRC-5 cells inoculated with urine specimens by using low-speed centrifugation and monoclonal antibody to an early antigen. *J Clin Microbiol* 1984;19: 917–9.
79. Baldanti F, Sarasini FM, Zavattoni PE, Gerna G. Polymerase chain reaction for prenatal diagnosis of congenital cytomegalovirus infection. *J Med Virol* 1995;47:462–6.
80. Donner C, Liesnard C, Content J, Busine A, Aderca J, Rodesch F. Prenatal diagnosis of 52 pregnancies at risk for congenital cytomegalovirus infection. *Obstet Gynecol* 1993;82:481–6.
81. Antsaklis A, Daskalakis G, Mesogitis S, Koutra P, Michalas S. Prenatal diagnosis of fetal primary cytomegalovirus infection. *Br J Obstet Gynaecol* 2000;107:84–8.
82. Ruellan-Eugene G, Barjot P, Campet M, *et al.* Evaluation of virological procedures to detect fetal human cytomegalovirus infection: Avidity of IgG antibodies, virus detection in amniotic fluid and maternal serum. *J Med Virol* 1996;50:9–15.
83. Bodeus M, Hubinont C, Bernard P, Bouckaert A, Thomas K, Goubau P. Prenatal diagnosis of human cytomegalovirus by culture and polymerase chain reaction: 98 pregnancies leading to congenital infection. *Prenat Diagn* 1999;19:314–7.
84. Gouarin S, Palmer P, Cointe D, *et al.* Congenital HCMV infection: A collaborative and comparative study of virus detection in amniotic fluid by culture and PCR. *J Clin Virol* 2001;21:47–55.
85. Chou S. Comparative analysis of sequence variation in gp116 and gp55 components of glycoprotein B of human cytomegalovirus. *Virology* 1992;88:388–90.
86. Kiriazopoulou V, Bondis J, Frantzidou F, *et al.* Prenatal diagnosis of fetal cytomegalovirus infection in seropositive pregnant women. *Eur J Obstet Gynecol* 1996;69:91–5.
87. Nicolini U, Kustermann A, Tassis B, *et al.* Prenatal diagnosis of congenital cytomegalovirus infection. *Prenat Diagn* 1994;14:903–6.

45 Fetal hydrops

T. Marton and P. M. Cox

Fetal hydrops

Fetal hydrops is a combination of generalized soft tissue edema and fluid (effusion) in one or more body cavity.

Hydrops still has a high mortality causing fetal demise in more than 50% of the detected cases and postnatal mortality following live birth is also around 50%.[1] There may be many causes. According to the traditional classification, the hydrops can be divided into immune and non-immune types. A more clinically (fetal medicine) oriented approach could be to divide cases into those due to fetal anemia- and non-anemia-related hydrops. The practical reason for this categorization is that fetal anemia is still the most common cause of hydrops and in most cases fetal anemia is easily detectable *in utero*. It can often be treated with intrauterine transfusion and thus anemia-related hydrops has a better prognosis than other forms.

In different parts of the world, there are different causes of hydrops. For example, in underdeveloped countries, rhesus (Rh) isoimmunization still remains a major cause; whereas in southern China, fetal α-thalassemia is the main causative factor. In contrast, in the developed world structural and chromosomal anomalies and parvovirus B19 infection are the most frequent causes of hydrops.

This chapter aims to be a comprehensive library of the various fetal conditions that play a role in fetal hydrops and presents a few characteristic features.

Anemia-related hydrops

It is well known that fetal anemia can be readily detected with the help of ultrasound/Doppler, measuring the middle cerebral artery velocity. For details see the relevant chapter of this book. The causes of fetal anemia should be subdivided, as they affect the prognosis for the pregnancy and fetus.

Immune hydrops

Historically, immune hydrops (due to maternal anti-D isoimmunization) was the commonest cause of fetal anemia and hydrops. Fortunately, these severe cases of anti-D isoimmunization are now very rarely seen, as a result of anti-D immunoglobulin (Ig) prophylaxis for rhesus-negative mothers. In the absence of prophylaxis, the disease still occurs. Immune hydrops is the result of a maternal IgG-mediated hemolytic disease of the fetus, the severest form of which is erythroblastosis fetalis.

There are further antigens that can cause immune-mediated fetal hemolytic disease including Rh anti-C, -c, -E, -e, anti-Kell, anti-MNS, anti-Duffy and anti-A or anti-B.

Isoimmunization due to the non-Rh groups such as Kell, MNS and Kidd have assumed increasing importance as the incidence of Rh-D sensitization has decreased.

Anti-Kell disease has a particularly poor prognosis, probably because the anemia is partly hemolytic and partly the result of suppressed erythropoiesis.[2] A significantly higher incidence of polyhydramnios was found among fetuses with Kell isoimmunization and the maternal serum titer is much lower than in the Rh-D group.[3]

Genetically determined hemolytic disease of the fetus

There are a number of genetically determined hemolytic diseases of the fetus, which can rarely lead to fetal hydrops (see Box 45.1).

Box 45.1 Genetically determined hemolytic anemias causing fetal hydrops

Glucose phosphate isomerase deficiency [autosomal dominant (AD) in adult cases, neonatal and fetal form most likely autosomal recessive (AR)][4] causes hemolytic crisis, very rarely fetal anemia and hydrops

Glucose-6-phosphate dehydrogenase (G6PD) deficiency (X-linked dominant) hemolytic episodes

Pyruvate kinase deficiency of erythrocyte (AR)[5]

Non-infectious disorders of erythrocyte production

α-Thalassemia (AD) is a common cause of fetal hydrops in the Chinese population.[6] Thalassemias are a group of inherited abnormalities of the hemoglobin synthesis. Hemoglobin has an α and a β chain. Homozygous α-thalassemia (deletion of both α-chain alleles of the corresponding region of chromosome 16) is responsible for the fetal hydrops (Bart syndrome). Clinical classification, such as thalassemia major, intermedia and minor refers only to the clinical severity of the disease. It is also apparent that, at least in some cases, compound heterozygosity is responsible for the hydropic change of the fetus. Anemia in thalassemia is the result of short turnover time of erythrocytes with a reduced hemoglobin content.

Other inherited forms of dyserythropoiesis are listed in Box 45.2. These represent rarities.

Box 45.2 Inherited dyserythropoietic conditions associated with fetal hydrops

Congenital dyserythropoietic anemia (AD)[7] is characterized by ineffective erythropoiesis and multinuclear erythroblasts

Congenital erythropoietic porphyria (AR)[8]

Diamond–Blackfan syndrome (AD)[9] causes congenital hypoplastic anemia

Leukemia (associated with Down's syndrome)[10]

Fetal anemia as a consequence of fetal blood loss

Internal fetal hemorrhage may lead to severe anemia due to blood loss. The commonest site of hemorrhage is the brain, but intrathoracic and intra-abdominal hemorrhages may also occur. Spontaneous fetal hemorrhage should always prompt a search for maternal antiplatelet antibodies to exclude alloimmune thrombocytopenia.[11,12]

Placental subchorial/intervillous hemorrhage can also originate from the fetus.

Fetomaternal hemorrhage (i.e. hemorrhage from the fetal into the maternal circulation) is common. Tiny hemorrhages are probably universal. Massive hemorrhage may be acutely fatal but smaller or recurrent bleeds may lead to an anemic, hydropic fetus. A maternal Kleihauer–Betke test is an essential part of the investigation of hydrops.[13]

Hemorrhage can also occur into a necrotic congenital tumor.

Human parvovirus B19 infection

Parvovirus is one of the most important factors causing anemia and hydrops.

In pregnant women, it can cause miscarriage (6.5%),[14] hydrops and intrauterine death, although most infected women give birth to healthy neonates without any intervention.[15] In a meta-analysis of 165 reported cases of antenatal human parvovirus B19 (HPVB19) cases, there was a 10.2% excess risk of fetal death. Transplacental transmission was confirmed in 69 (24.1%) of 286 reported maternal infections. According to a separate meta-analysis HPVB19 infection was present in 57 out of 299 (19.1%) non-malformed cases of non-immune hydrops fetalis.[16] Parvovirus not only affects the erythroid cell lines, inhibiting erythrocyte production, but also infects the cardiac myocytes. In most cases, the hydrops is a consequence of severe anemia, though at least in some chronic cases it appears that a direct effect on the heart cannot be excluded.

Infections in which anemia plays a role in the hydrops are seen below.

Non-anemia-related hydrops

Infection-induced fetal hydrops[17]

The most common infections causing fetal hydrops are parvovirus B19 (see earlier section), cytomegalovirus,[18] Herpes simplex virus, *Toxoplasma gondii*, *Treponema pallidum*, Coxsackievirus type B and adenovirus. Congenital Chagas' disease is also reported to be associated with hydrops.[19]

The mechanism by which the different infections cause hydrops varies. For example, Herpes simplex virus causes liver damage, whilst Coxsackie- and adenoviruses lead to myocarditis and fetal tachyarrhythmia.[20,21]

Congenital syphilis results in generalized chronic infection,[22] with anemia, thrombocytopenia and, later, ascites. In congenital syphilis, the mother can be seronegative with an infected fetus,[23] and this may also be true for parvovirus (personal observation).

Structural anomalies

(1) Tumors or tumor-like/hamartomatous lesions within the body cavities may cause hydrops with compression or obstruction of the major vessels of the systemic venous return. The lesions that belong to this group are shown in Box 45.3. Fetal lung lesions associated with hydrops are almost always lethal.[24]

Occlusions of the superior or inferior venae cavae and ductus venosus are also reported to result in hydrops.

Box 45.3 Obstruction of systemic venous return

Thorax

Congenital cystic adenomatoid malformation of the lung[25,26]

Pulmonary extralobar sequestration[27]

Large diaphragmatic hernia

Intrathoracic teratoma

Intrathoracic lymphangioma[28]

Cardiac or pericardial tumor[29]

Laryngeal atresia

Abdominal tumor or tumor-like lesion

Abdominal teratoma

Cystic kidneys

Obstructive uropathy

Hepatoblastoma

Ovarian cyst

Other tumor

(2) Cardiac disease, including developmental abnormalities, tachyarrhythmia and bradycardia may cause fetal hydrops. A list of these conditions is given in Box 45.4.

Box 45.4 Congenital heart conditions in fetal hydrops

Congenital heart disease[30]

Atresia of the aortic or pulmonary trunk

Various malformations of the great arteries

Atrioventricular septal defect

Right or left ventricular hypoplasia, divided right ventricle[31]

Cardiomyopathy[32]

Fetal bradycardia

Congenital heart block[33]

Maternal systemic lupus erythematosus

Lupus anticoagulant

Fetal tachycardia with myocarditis

Adenovirus

Coxsackievirus

Parvovirus

Chagas' disease

Wolff–Parkinson–White syndrome[34,35]

(3) Vascular shunts result in high-output cardiac failure and subsequent hydrops.

This occurs in fetal sacrococcygeal teratoma[36–38] and in arteriovenosus malformations at various locations in the body. In the head, vein of Galen aneurysm, intracranial arteriovenosus malformation and intracranial teratoma have been described.[39] Cervical, abdominal,[40] or cutaneous hemangiomas, arteriovenuous malformations of the liver and lung, large placental chorangioma and angiomatosis of the fetus are also rare causes of hydrops.

Hydrops can occur as a complication of monochorionic twinning, often because of high-output cardiac failure of one twin.[41] In twin-to-twin transfusion syndrome, volume overload in the recipient leads to failure and hydrops, while in TRAP sequence reversed perfusion of a large acardiac co-twin by the pump-twin is the cause. There are also reported cases with myocardial infarct of the recipient in twin-to-twin transfusion syndrome[42] and transient hydrops of the donor after amniocentesis.[43]

(4) Other circulatory problems.

It has been suggested that long and/or overcoiled umbilical cord with increased vascular resistance may, in some instances, cause circulatory failure and consequent hydrops.[44]

Chromosome abnormality (including Turner syndrome)

X monosomy (45,XO – Turner syndrome) is the most common chromosome aneuploidy related to hydrops. It appears that failure of the lymph vessel development causes the hydropic change.[45] It is also apparent that in 90% of the hydropic Turner syndrome fetuses the heart weight is under the 2.5th percentile and it has been suggested that this is a major cause of fetal demise in Turner syndrome fetuses.[46]

Trisomy 21 hydrops or nuchal swelling was diagnosed in approximately 40% [cystic hygroma and increased nuchal fold thickness (30.5%), hydrops (9.6%)] according to a large series.[47]

Other karyotypic abnormalities associated with hydrops include trisomy 18, trisomy 13, trisomy 15 and trisomy 10 mosaicism.

Metabolic and storage disease

Metabolic and storage disease represents less than 1% of all hydrops cases. These are individually rare, but important because of autosomal recessive inheritance, and thus have 25% recurrence risk. The relevant enzyme defects are listed in Box 45.5.

Box 45.5 Lysosomal and glycogen storage diseases that cause hydrops

Lysosomal storage disease[48]

Mucopolysaccharidosis type VII[49]
Mucolipidoses I (sialidosis III)[50]
Mucolipidosis II (I-cell disease)
Gaucher disease[51]
Farber disease[52]
GM1-gangliosidosis[53]
Niemann–Pick disease[54]
Moroquio disease[55]

Glycogen storage disease

Type IIb (glycogen storage disease limited to the heart)[56]
Type IV[57]

Further genetic causes

Box 45.6 contains the most frequent genetic syndromes that cause hydrops. Osteochondrodysplasias are important because of the inheritance, and the number of recognized syndromes is growing.

Box 45.6 Osteochondrodysplasias and other genetic syndromes causing hydrops

Osteochondrodysplasias

- Blomstrand-type chondrodysplasia [(AR) short limbs, polyhydramnios, hydrops fetalis, facial anomalies, increased bone density and a remarkable advanced skeletal maturation]
- Greenberg dysplasia [(AR) radiological features: 'moth-eaten' appearance of the markedly short long bones, bizarre ectopic ossification centers and marked platyspondyly with unusual ossification centers][58]
- Conradi–Hunermann, chondrodysplasia punctata [(X linked – D) disorganization of the spine, premature echogenity of femoral epipheses and frontal bossing with depressed nasal bridge, polyhydramnios][59]
- Osteogenesis imperfecta congenita (AD)
- Achondrogenesis type IA [(AR) polyhydramnios, subgaleal edema, microcephaly, a narrow thorax, pericardial effusion and a severe short-limbed dwarfism with unossified tubular bones and vertebral bodies][60]
- Achondrogenesis type IB [(AR) sulfate transporter gene mutation, severe rhisomelia, narrow chest, flat face, polyhydramnios, possible umbilical hernia]
- Achondrogenesis type II [(AD) Marked micromelic dwarfism, barrel shaped, small chest, polyhydramnios]
- Short rib polydactyly syndrome type II [(AR) short ribs, polydactyly (pre- or postaxial), possible polycystic kidneys, median cleft lip][61]
- Short rib polydactyly syndrome type IV [(AR) markedly narrow ribs, micromelia, shortened limbs with postaxial heptasyndactyly polycystic renal dysplasia]
- Fibrochondrogenesis (AR)
- Kniest-like dysplasia (AR)
- Campomelic dysplasia (AR)

Other genetic syndromes associated with hydrops

- Arthrogryposis multiplex
- Lethal multiple pterygium syndrome
- Fetal akinesia
- Beckwith–Wiedemann syndrome
- Simpson–Golabi–Behmel syndrome[62]
- Smith–Lemli–Opitz syndrome
- Tuberous sclerosis
- Congenital arteral calcification

Miscellaneous

According to recent studies, fetal hemochromatosis appears to be the result of fetal liver disease and in the late second trimester of pregnancy results in severe panhypoproteinemia with non-immune hydrops.[63,64]

Maternal indometacin therapy mainly in the third trimester has been reported causing early closure of ductus arteriosus and consequent fetal hydrops.[65]

One case of iatrogenic intrauterine hypothyroidism and subsequent fetal hydrops has also been published, which was caused by maternal propylthiouracil medication for maternal Grave's disease.[66] In another case report, fetal hyperthyreosis and hydrops were caused by a hyperthyroid mother with Grave's disease by antithyroid antibodies.[67] Mother also had a history of three prior perinatal deaths between 26 and 28 weeks' gestation, all associated with fetal hydrops. After maternal therapy with propylthiouracil, resolution of non-immune hydrops was documented and a healthy neonate subsequently delivered to term.

Investigations in hydrops[68,69]

Pathologic examination of fetuses with non-immune hydrops requires a multidisciplinary approach. The first and most important is the macroscopic description and identification of structural abnormalities. Developmental abnormalities may draw attention to the possibility of a chromosome abnormality; thus, cytogenetic studies are essential. (If cytogenetic culture fails, fluorescence *in situ* hybridization studies should be performed to exclude common trisomies.) The pathologist has to be careful to save living cells for further biochemical studies in case of suspicion of a metabolic disease. Osteochondrodysplasias cannot be diagnosed without proper x-ray documentation and, if necessary, involvement of an experienced radiographer. Molecular biology and DNA investigation are also important. Microbiology with bacterial, viral cultures and, if necessary, PCR investigation may also be useful. Light microscopic examination is essential, and in a significant proportion of the cases is enough to make a diagnosis. Fortunately, CMV, parvovirus and adenovirus antibodies are available to prove infection in paraffin-embedded blocks of the fetal tissues. According to published figures, a meticulous examination, including clinical studies, such as Kleihauer–Betke test and maternal autoantibodies, leaves approximately 10–20% of cases unexplained.[68,69]

The proverb that a *good clinical history is half the diagnosis* is very true with regard to the pathologist's work while undertaking an autopsy of a hydropic fetus. Nowadays, fetal hydrops is generally investigated prenatally. Clinical data can draw attention to subtle signs (which would otherwise be missed, especially in autolytic fetuses) and make the pathologist widen the investigation in the relevant direction. Samples are taken that cannot be taken later, such as frozen tissue for metabolic studies or DNA, frozen sections for immunohistochemistry, specially fixed tissue for electron microscopy, instruction to the cytogenetic or histochemistry laboratory to save cells for biochemical studies, etc.

It is essential to seek and document any prenatal finding, as it is an important feedback to the clinician and provides the parents with information.

In summary, because of the wide spectrum of causes of hydrops, a multidisciplinary approach to diagnosis is recommended based on proper communication and exchange of information between the clinician and the pathologist.

REFERENCES

1. Wy CA, Sajous CH, Loberiza F, Weiss MG. Outcome of infants with a diagnosis of hydrops fetalis in the 1990s. *Am J Perinatol* 1999;16(10):561–7.
2. McKenna DS, Nagaraja HN, O'Shaughnessy R. Management of pregnancies complicated by anti-Kell isoimmunization. *Obstet Gynecol* 1999;93(Pt 5):667–73.
3. Babinszki A, Lapinski RH, Berkowitz RL. Prognostic factors and management in pregnancies complicated with severe Kell alloimmunization: Experiences of the last 13 years. *Am J Perinatol* 1998;15(12):695–701.
4. Ravindranath Y, Paglia DE, Warrier I, Valentine W, Nakatani M, Brockway RA. Glucose phosphate isomerase deficiency as a cause of hydrops fetalis. *N Engl J Med* 1987;316(5):258–61.
5. Gilsanz F, Vega MA, Gomez-Castillo E, Ruiz-Balda JA, Omenaca F. Fetal anaemia due to pyruvate kinase deficiency. *Arch Dis Child* 1993;69(5):523–4.
6. Chui DH, Waye JS. Hydrops fetalis caused by alpha-thalassemia: An emerging health care problem. *Blood* 1998;91(7):2213–22.
7. Williams G, Lorimer S, Merry CC, Greenberg CR, Bishop AJ. A variant congenital dyserythropoietic anaemia presenting as a fatal hydrops foetalis. *Br J Haematol* 1989;72(2):289–90.
8. Pannier E, Viot G, Aubry MC, *et al.* Congenital erythropoietic porphyria (Gunther's disease): Two cases with very early prenatal manifestation and cystic hygroma. *Prenat Diagn* 2003;23(1):25–30.
9. McLennan AC, Chitty LS, Rissik J, Maxwell DJ. Prenatal diagnosis of Blackfan–Diamond syndrome: Case report and review of the literature. *Prenat Diagn* 1996;16(4):349–53.
10. Robertson M, De Jong G, Mansvelt E. Prenatal diagnosis of congenital leukemia in a fetus at 25 weeks' gestation with Down syndrome: Case report and review of the literature. *Ultrasound Obstet Gynecol* 2003;21(5):486–9.
11. Birchall JE, Murphy MF, Kaplan C, Kroll H. European collaborative study of the antenatal management of feto-maternal alloimmune thrombocytopenia. *Br J Haematol* 2003;122(2):275–88.
12. Khouzami AN, Kickler TS, Callan NA, Shumway JB, Perlman EJ, Blakemore KJ. Devastating sequelae of alloimmune thrombocytopenia: An entity that deserves more attention. *J Matern Fetal Med* 1996;5(3):137–41.
13. Biankin SA, Arbuckle SM, Graf NS. Autopsy findings in a series of five cases of fetomaternal haemorrhages. *Pathology* 2004;35(4):319–24.
14. Levy R, Weissman A, Blomberg G, Hagay ZJ. Infection by parvovirus B 19 during pregnancy: A review. *Obstet Gynecol Surv* 1997;52(4):254–9.
15. Odibo AO, Campbell WA, Feldman D, *et al.* Resolution of human parvovirus B19-induced nonimmune hydrops after intrauterine transfusion. *J Ultrasound Med* 1998;17(9):547–50.
16. Yaegashi N, Niinuma T, Chisaka H, *et al.* The incidence of, and factors leading to, parvovirus B19-related hydrops fetalis following maternal infection; report of 10 cases and meta-analysis. *J Infect* 1998;37(1):28–35.
17. Barron SD, Pass RF. Infectious causes of hydrops fetalis. *Semin Perinatol* 1995;19(6):493–501.
18. Beksac MS, Saygan-Karamursel B, Ustacelebi S, *et al.* Prenatal diagnosis of intrauterine cytomegalovirus infection in a fetus with non-immune hydrops fetalis. *Acta Obstet Gynecol Scand* 2001;80(8):762–5.
19. Okumura M, Aparecida dos Santos V, Camargo ME, Schultz R, Zugaib M. Prenatal diagnosis of congenital Chagas' disease (American trypanosomiasis). *Prenat Diagn* 2004;24(3):179–81.
20. Benirschke K, Swartz WH, Leopold G, Sahn D. Hydrops due to myocarditis in a fetus. *Am J Cardiovasc Pathol* 1987;1(1):131–3.
21. Oyer CE, Ongcapin EH, Ni J, Bowles NE, Towbin JA. Fatal intrauterine adenoviral endomyocarditis with aortic and pulmonary valve stenosis: Diagnosis by polymerase chain reaction. *Hum Pathol* 2000;31(11):1433–5.
22. Hollier LM, Harstad TW, Sanchez PJ, Twickler DM, Wendel GD Jr. Fetal syphilis: Clinical and laboratory characteristics. *Obstet Gynecol* 2001;97(6):947–53.
23. Levine Z, Sherer DM, Jacobs A, Rotenberg O. Nonimmune hydrops fetalis due to congenital syphilis associated with negative intrapartum maternal serology screening. *Am J Perinatol* 1998;15(4):233–6.
24. Adzick NS, Kitano Y. Fetal surgery for lung lesions, congenital diaphragmatic hernia, and sacrococcygeal teratoma. *Semin Pediatr Surg* 2003;12(3):154–67.
25. Laberge JM, Flageole H, Pugash D, *et al.* Outcome of the prenatally diagnosed congenital cystic adenomatoid lung malformation: A Canadian experience. *Fetal Diagn Ther* 2001;16(3):178–86.
26. Diamond IR, Wales PW, Smith SD, Fecteau A. Survival after CCAM associated with ascites: A report of a case and review of the literature. *J Pediatr Surg* 2003;38(9):E1–3.

27. Brus F, Nikkels PG, van Loon AJ, Okken A. Non-immune hydrops fetalis and bilateral pulmonary hypoplasia in a newborn infant with extralobar pulmonary sequestration. *Acta Paediatr* 1993; 82(4):416–8.
28. Jung E, Won HS, Lee PR, Lee IS, Kim A, Nam JH. The progression of mediastinal lymphangioma *in utero*. *Ultrasound Obstet Gynecol* 2000;16(7):663–6.
29. Grebille AG, Mitanchez D, Benachi A, *et al*. Pericardial teratoma complicated by hydrops: Successful fetal therapy by thoracoamniotic shunting. *Prenat Diagn* 2003;23(9):735–9.
30. Knilans TK. Cardiac abnormalities associated with hydrops fetalis. *Semin Perinatol* 1995;19(6):483–92.
31. Marton T, Hajdu J, Papp Z. A rare case of non-immune hydrops fetalis: double-chambered right ventricle. A case report. *Fetal Diagn Ther* 2001;16(4):251–3.
32. Pedra SR, Smallhorn JF, Ryan G, *et al*. Fetal cardiomyopathies: Pathogenic mechanisms, hemodynamic findings, and clinical outcome. *Circulation* 2002;106(5):585–91.
33. Eronen M, Heikkila P, Teramo K. Congenital complete heart block in the fetus: Hemodynamic features, antenatal treatment, and outcome in six cases. *Pediatr Cardiol* 2001;22(5):385–92.
34. Khositseth A, Ramin KD, O'Leary PW, Porter CJ. Role of amiodarone in the treatment of fetal supraventricular tachyarrhythmias and hydrops fetalis. *Pediatr Cardiol* 2003;24(5):454–6.
35. Krapp M, Kohl T, Simpson JM, Sharland GK, Katalinic A, Gembruch U. Review of diagnosis, treatment, and outcome of fetal atrial flutter compared with supraventricular tachycardia. *Heart* 2004;89(9):913–7.
36. Brace V, Grant SR, Brackley KJ, Kilby MD, Whittle MJ. Prenatal diagnosis and outcome in sacrococcygeal teratomas: A review of cases between 1992 and 1998. *Prenat Diagn* 2000;20(1):51–5.
37. Neubert S, Trautmann K, Tanner B, Steiner E, Linke F, Bahlmann F. Sonographic prognostic factors in prenatal diagnosis of SCT. *Fetal Diagn Ther* 2004;19(4):319–26.
38. Westerburg B, Feldstein VA, Sandberg PL, Lopoo JB, Harrison MR, Albanese CT. Sonographic prognostic factors in fetuses with sacrococcygeal teratoma. *J Pediatr Surg* 2000;35(2):322–5.
39. Bhattacharya B, Cochran E, Loew J. Pathologic quiz case: A 27-week female fetus with massive macrocephaly and generalized anasarca. Congenital immature intracranial teratoma with skull rupture and high output cardiac failure. *Arch Pathol Lab Med* 2004;128(1):102–4.
40. Albano G, Pugliese A, Stabile M, Sirimarco F, Arsieri R. Hydrops foetalis caused by hepatic haemangioma. *Acta Paediatr* 1998;87(12):1307–9.
41. Hayakawa M, Oshiro M, Mimura S, *et al*. Twin-to-twin transfusion syndrome with hydrops: A retrospective analysis of ten cases. *Am J Perinatol* 1999;16(6):263–7.
42. Marton T, Hajdú J, Hruby E, Papp Z. Intrauterine left chamber myocardial infarction of the heart and hydrops fetalis in the recipient fetus due to twin to twin transfusion syndrome. *Prenat Diagn* 2004;22(3):241–3.
43. Morine M, Maeda K, Higashino K, *et al*. Transient hydrops fetalis of the donor fetus in twin–twin transfusion syndrome after therapeutic amnioreduction. *Ultrasound Obstet Gynecol* 2003;22(2): 182–5.
44. Machin GA, Ackerman J, Gilbert-Barness E. Abnormal umbilical cord coiling is associated with adverse perinatal outcomes. *Pediatr Dev Pathol* 2000;3(5):462–71.
45. Chitayat D, Kalousek DK, Bamforth JS. Lymphatic abnormalities in fetuses with posterior cervical cystic hygroma. *Am J Med Genet* 1989;33(3):352–6.
46. Barr MJ, Oman-Ganes L. Turner syndrome morphology and morphometrics: Cardiac hypoplasia as a cause of midgestation death. *Teratology* 2002;66(2):65–72.
47. Rotmensch S, Liberati M, Bronshtein M, *et al*. Prenatal sonographic findings in 187 fetuses with Down syndrome. *Prenat Diagn* 1997;17(11):1001–9.
48. Stone DL, Sidransky E. Hydrops fetalis: Lysosomal storage disorders in extremis. *Adv Pediatr* 1999;46:409–40.
49. Cheng Y, Verp MS, Knutel T, Hibbard JU. Mucopolysaccharidosis type VII as a cause of recurrent non-immune hydrops fetalis. *J Perinat Med* 2003;31(6):535–7.
50. Godra A, Kim DU, D'Cruz C. Pathologic quiz case: A 5-day-old boy with hydrops fetalis. Mucolipidoses I (Sialidosis III). *Arch Pathol Lab Med* 2003;127(8):1051–2.
51. Mignot C, Gelot A, Bessieres B, *et al*. Perinatal–lethal Gaucher disease. *Am J Med Genet* 2003;120A(3):338–44.
52. van Lijnschoten G, Groener JE, Maas SM, Ben-Yoseph Y, Dingemans KP, Offerhaus GJ. Intrauterine fetal death due to Farber disease: Case report. *Pediatr Dev Pathol* 2000;3(6):597–602.
53. Tasso MJ, Martinez-Gutierrez A, Carrascosa C, Vazquez S, Tebar R. GM1-gangliosidosis presenting as nonimmune hydrops fetalis: A case report. *J Perinat Med* 1996;24(5):445–9.
54. Meizner I, Levy A, Carmi R, Robinsin C. Niemann–Pick disease associated with nonimmune hydrops fetalis. *Am J Obstet Gynecol* 1990;193(1, Pt 1):128–9.
55. Applegarth DA, Toone JR, Wilson RD, Yong SL, Baldwin VJ. Morquio disease presenting as hydrops fetalis and enzyme analysis of chorionic villus tissue in a subsequent pregnancy. *Pediatr Pathol* 1987;7(5–6):593–9.
56. Atkin J, Snow JW Jr, Zellweger H, Rhead WJ. Fatal infantile cardiac glycogenosis without acid maltase deficiency presenting as congenital hydrops. *Eur J Pediatr* 1984;142(2):150.
57. Cox PM, Brueton LA, Murphy KW, *et al*. Early-onset fetal hydrops and muscle degeneration in siblings due to a novel variant of type IV glycogenosis. *Am J Med Genet* 1999;86(2):187–93.
58. Greenberg CR, Rimoin DL, Gruber HE, DeSa DJ, Reed M, Lachman RS. A new autosomal recessive lethal chondrodystrophy with congenital hydrops. *Am J Med Genet* 1988;29(3):623–32.
59. Pryde PG, Bawle E, Brandt F, Romero R, Treadwell MC, Evans MI. Prenatal diagnosis of nonrhizomelic chondrodysplasia punctata (Conradi–Hunermann syndrome). *Am J Med Genet* 1993;47(3): 426–31.
60. Chen CP, Liu FF, Jan SW, Lin YN, Lan CC. A case of achondrogenesis type IA with an occipital encephalocele. *Genet Couns* 1996;7(3):193–9.
61. Montemarano H, Bulas DI, Chandra R, Tifft C. Prenatal diagnosis of glomerulocystic kidney disease in short-rib polydactyly syndrome type II, Majewski type. *Pediatr Radiol* 1995;25(6):469–71.
62. Terespolsky D, Farrell SA, Siegel-Bartelt J, Weksberg R. Infantile lethal variant of Simpson–Golabi–Behmel syndrome associated with hydrops fetalis. *Am J Med Genet* 1995;59(3):329–33.
63. Moerman P, Pauwels P, Vandenberghe K, *et al*. Neonatal haemochromatosis. *Histopathology* 1990;17(4):345–51.
64. Wisser J, Schreiner M, Diem H, Roithmeier A. Neonatal hemochromatosis: A rare cause of nonimmune hydrops fetalis and fetal anemia. *Fetal Diagn Ther* 1993;8(4):273–8.
65. Pratt L, Digiosia J, Swenson JN, Trampe B, Martin CB Jr. Reversible fetal hydrops associated with indomethacin use. *Obstet Gynecol* 1997;90(4):676–8.
66. Yanai N, Shveiky D. Fetal hydrops, associated with maternal propylthiouracil exposure, reversed by intrauterine therapy. *Ultrasound Obstet Gynecol* 2004;23(2):198–201.
67. Treadwell MC, Sherer DM, Sacks AJ, Ghezzi F, Romero R. Successful treatment of recurrent non-immune hydrops secondary to fetal hyperthyroidism. *Obstet Gynecol* 1996;87(5, Pt 2):838–40.
68. Lallemand AV, Doco-Fenzy M, Gaillard DA. Investigation of nonimmune hydrops fetalis: Multidisciplinary studies are necessary for diagnosis – review of 94 cases. *Pediatr Dev Pathol* 1999; 2(5):432–9.
69. Rodriguez MM, Chaves F, Romaguera RL, Ferrer PL, de la Guardia C, Bruce JH. Value of autopsy in nonimmune hydrops fetalis: Series of 51 stillborn fetuses. *Pediatr Dev Pathol* 2002;5(4):365–74.

SECTION V

Doppler ultrasound

Section Editors: **S. Weiner and A. K. Ertan**

46 3D/4D color and power Doppler ultrasound in obstetrics

G. Bega and S. Weiner

Introduction

Two-dimensional ultrasound (2DUS)-derived color and power Doppler imaging is commonly used in fetal imaging. The information derived from 2DUS color and power Doppler images is displayed in a cross-sectional image plane. It is from these cross-sectional ultrasound planes that we develop a 3D perception of the vascular anatomy. Nevertheless, the ability to visualize, fully understand and differentiate between normal and abnormal vascular anatomy with 2DUS is often limited. These limitations become especially important in complex anatomical abnormalities. Recent developments in digital signal processing and transducer design have made possible the acquisition of volume ultrasound data with color and power Doppler, which can also be interactively manipulated through the volume. In three-dimensional ultrasound (3DUS) or volume ultrasound, a volume (rather than a slice) of ultrasonographic data is acquired and stored. The stored data can be analyzed and displayed in numerous ways and new and more sophisticated tools are being introduced at a very fast rate. Although these new and relatively complex applications are not widely known or understood in the field of ultrasound, there seems to be little doubt that these tools will become a routine part of our diagnostic imaging toolset. One of the most significant advantages of acquiring a volume ultrasound data is the ability to navigate through the saved volume and demonstrate any arbitrary plane and, most importantly, even planes that are otherwise impossible to be obtained by the conventional 2DUS. In the multiplanar display, three perpendicular planes are displayed simultaneously. Correlation between these three planes is used to confirm the given desired plane, such as the midsagittal or midcoronal plane. This process generally involves placing the planar center point at the point of interest in one of the planes and observing the location of the corresponding center points in the other two planes.[1,2]

In this chapter, we intend to review the current and potential future applications of 3DUS and four-dimensional ultrasound (4DUS) color and power Doppler ultrasound in obstetrics. In the section Technical Considerations, the reader will be introduced to the basics of 3DUS volume acquisition, display, analysis, volume calculation and perfusion studies. The main clinical applications will be presented with a special section on techniques of 3D color and power Doppler in fetal echocardiography. The somewhat limited literature as related to 3D color and power ultrasound will be reviewed as well. Last but not least, networking capabilities will be discussed.

Technical aspects of acquisition and display

3DUS acquires 2D planar ultrasound data in a volume and as such represents an extension of the conventional 2DUS imaging. Considering this, 3DUS does not necessarily replace 2DUS but rather extends its capabilities in time and space. Being a 2DUS-based technique makes 3DUS vulnerable to all drawbacks and limitations of 2DUS. As such, problems related to image resolution, penetration, depth, artifacts and body habitus are also present in 3DUS and are even made worse and compounded across a volume of data. Consequently, image and color and power Doppler setting optimization plays a huge role in acquiring adequate information that could be used clinically. Using 3DUS, color and power Doppler techniques generally require an additional investment of time, which in experienced hands typically goes anywhere from 5 to 20 min and at times, depending on the complexity of the case and the experience of the examiner, significantly more. This additional time is not so much related only to scanning and acquiring the data, which is only a portion of the learning curve, but also to exploring the saved volume data afterward in a meaningful way. The fact that this information can be digitally saved, either temporarily in the hard disk of the equipment or permanently in a removable

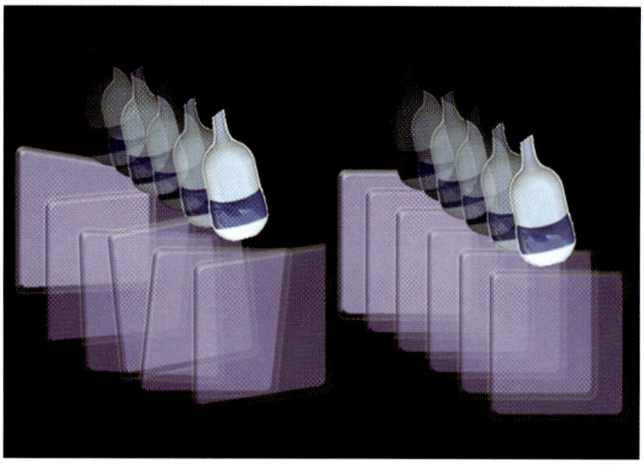

Figure 46.1 This image illustrates the principle of image registration and the effect of a dedicated 3D volume transducer with a built-in position-sensing device in it. The images on the right represent a volume acquired with a free-hand transducer and the images on the left represent a volume acquired with a dedicated volume transducer and appear well registered. The controlled acquisition and reliable registration are prerequisites for obtaining clinically useful ultrasound volumes with color or power Doppler.

disk, such as CD-ROMs or DVD-ROMs, makes the exploration of the saved volume data after the patient is discharged a real possibility.

It is important to understand the concept of volume data and how they are acquired. The acquisition of one single volume of ultrasound data is called a 3DUS acquisition and the volume is commonly called a 3D volume. The introduction of dedicated transducers in the mid-1990s made possible the continuous acquisition of 3D volumes and on the fly display of either multiplanar or rendered views. This continuous acquisition displaying motion views of moving targets, such as the fetus or the fetal heart, was called the fourth dimension and the imaging technique 4D. There are basically three methods of acquiring volumes of ultrasound data for 3DUS imaging. The first and the oldest one is the free-hand method, which utilizes a normal 2DUS transducer with a position-sensing device mounted that can acquire multiple 2DUS images as the probe is manually swept through the region of interest. This method typically acquires one 3DUS volume and in principle cannot acquire 4D data, as that would require the operator to continuously move his/her hand at fast acquisition speeds, which is impossible in reality. The second method is the acquisition of volumes with a dedicated 3DUS transducer (Figure 46.1). A mechanical device moves the transducer elements at a preselected speed and a preselected angle automatically in a fan shape through the region of interest.[3,4] While color and power Doppler ultrasound volumes can be reliably obtained with mechanically swept dedicated transducers, their acquisition time is typically slow as there simply is more information to acquire and process. There is a special fetal heart package that displays heart volumes with either color or power Doppler data in 4D, called spatiotemporal image correlation (STIC). This technique, which will be discussed in more detail at the fetal echocardiography section, is an exception to the fact that currently mechanically swept transducers cannot display 4D color and power data. The third method is the volume acquisition through matrix array transducers. These newly introduced dedicated volume transducers have a very high number of transducer elements (typically, as of this writing from 3000 to 4000 elements) and produce a thick ultrasound beam in all directions. All elements of the matrix array transducer transmit and receive. Interestingly, the first imaging and data processing take place in the transducer itself as it contains a built-in data processor. These transducers are electronically steered and have no need for mechanical sweeping. As such, they can produce very high acquisition speeds even with color or power Doppler.[5,6] These transducers are the future in volume imaging and will make a revolution in our capabilities of investigating fetal and/or placental vasculature with 3D/4D color and power Doppler. For the time being, matrix array technologies are mainly being investigated in adult echocardiography, but slowly studies are being conducted in obstetrics as well.[7] All of these methods rely on specialized 3D software, which allows processing of the acquired volumes either on-line through a built-in computer or off-line on a workstation.

In this chapter, we will present work with the dedicated mechanical volume transducers (the second method) as for the moment this is the best and the most commonly used technique of acquiring clinically useful data in obstetrics.

Image optimization

One of the most common problems practitioners encounter in their learning curve of acquiring 3D color and power Doppler is optimization of the settings. While there is no fixed recipe for every occasion, there is a set of principles and techniques that if understood well should be helpful in obtaining adequate information. First, we start with the 2D color or power Doppler information. Normal 2DUS principles of visualizing vessels with color and power Doppler should be followed (and the following work better in a 3D volume acquisition as well), such as:

(a) Be as parallel to the vessel or vessels of interest as possible.
(b) Adjust the gain to avoid 'bleeding' in the vessel wall by decreasing the gain at the minimally acceptable level, typically no more than 50–70%.
(c) Adjust the wall filter – usually the medium settings work better.
(d) Set the dynamic motion differentiation to avoid background noise signals.
(e) Sensitivity works better in medium scale.

(f) Priority set on high generally brings a better signal.
(g) Pulse repetition frequency (PRF) should be adjusted according to the particular vessel size and blood flow, typically a higher PRF is needed for higher-velocity vessels (i.e. intracardiac flow) and a lower PRF is needed for small and/or branching vessels (i.e. brain), especially placental or retroplacental (venous) vessels.
(h) Start in 2D gray-scale image with the highest frame rate possible. This translates into a volume with the highest quality, as there will be more frames in a volume. Factors that affect the frame rate are the angle opening in the 2D beam (use the narrowest angle you can), the number of focal zones and the amount of depth (the less the better). Harmonic imaging helps significantly in imaging in the near field but not much in the far field, but it is important to know that it does slow down the frame rate.

The 2D power and color Doppler ultrasound principles above should be incorporated to adequate 3D volume acquisition principles such as:

(a) Start with the slowest acquisition speed that is practically possible in order to leave time for the transducer to acquire the maximum amount of information. Typically, the slower the speed of acquisition the higher the quality of the volume obtained.
(b) Ask the mother to hold still for the expected time frame that the acquisition takes place, that is, anywhere between 5 and 15 s depending on the size of the volume box and the angle of acquisition.
(c) Try to acquire volumes at quiet fetal states to avoid motion artifacts.

Analyze the volume right after acquisition for possible acquisition-related artifacts due to fetal breathing, respiration or movement. Explore the B or the C window as those are the computer-generated views where the hidden artifacts can be depicted. Window A is the acquisition plane and as such may or may not show artifacts.

Flow volume and perfusion studies

For the first time 3DUS allows very accurate volume measurements. Multiple studies have shown that volume measurements are feasible and nomograms of several different organ systems in the fetus have been generated.[8–12] A very interesting aspect of obtaining power and color Doppler volumes is that this information can give an overall estimation of the blood supply of a given anatomical area. Many efforts have been made by the industry to further postprocess this information with the purpose of quantifying the amount of blood supply. One of the most useful programs is the so-called 3D-shell imaging method. In this method, a 3D volume is acquired with power Doppler, then a volume of interest (VOI) inside the initial acquired volume can be traced. Inside the VOI the gray scale and color histograms can be evaluated together or separately and expressed as a mean value. The expected clinical value of these power and color Doppler volume quantification methods is better estimation of blood flow within the area of interest (i.e. tumor). For this purpose, four indices have been proposed: (1) average gray value of non-color voxels (MG); (2) vascularization index (VI): ratio of number of color voxels to total number of voxels inside VOI; (3) flow index (FI): ratio of sum of color intensities to number of color voxels inside VOI and (4) ratio of sum of color intensities to total number of voxels outside VOI (VFI). Importantly, while these measurements provide a useful method in quantifying blood flow and vascularity in the acquired volumes, their information is based on digitized color voxel information. The accuracy of this information may change (i.e. improve) as software updates or better probes emerge that improve color or power Doppler sensitivity. Published nomograms for vascularity cannot be used for imaging with other types of machines or with different generations of the same probe because of variable color sensitivity. Nevertheless, the information obtained can provide important qualitative assessment of vascularization and blood flow changes in different normal and abnormal physiologic states. While a few studies have been conducted in gynecology, no studies have been reported in obstetrics yet.

Clinical applications

Color and power Doppler information in a volume have shown to be very useful in visualizing the fetal anatomy (Figures 46.2–46.10). Several authors have reported their positive experiences with the use of 3D Doppler.[13,14] Studies have shown that 3D color and power Doppler, as used with a free-hand 3D ultrasound system, was useful in imaging tumors (chorioangioma, teratoma, hygroma, lung sequestration), the fetal brain (vein of Galen aneurism, corpus callosus agenesis, vascular malformations), kidneys (agenesis of the kidneys, renal arteries), fetal abdominal vessels, umbilical cord anomalies and placental disorders.[14] Lee *et al.* demonstrated that 3D color and power Doppler, as acquired with an automated 3D probe, could visualize placental angiogenesis as early as 7.1 weeks of gestation, cerebral and neck vessels as early as 12.9 weeks of gestation, brain vessels, cord insertion, placenta and vasa previa.[15] In an interesting study, Kalache described the use of 3D power Doppler ultrasound to identify vascular congenital anomalies of the fetal portosystemic and umbilical venous system. He found 8 out of 310 fetuses with portosystemic venous malformations. When an umbilical vein or ductus venosus anomaly is suspected, the operator has to construct the 3D orientation of the vessels from cross-sectional 2D images. Power Doppler in 3D allows visualization of low-velocity

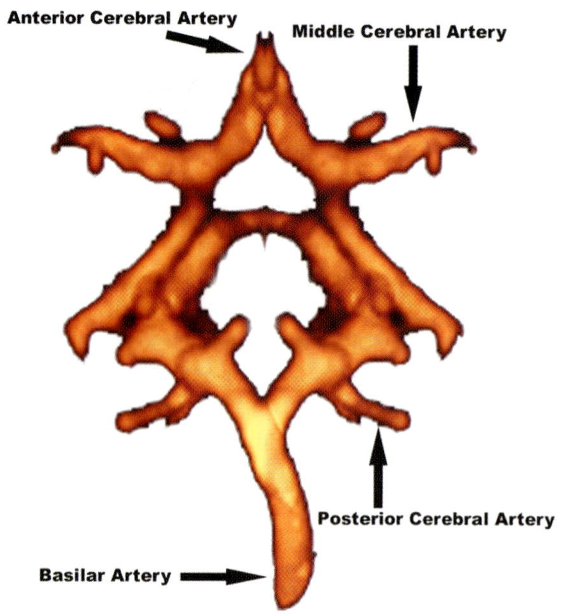

Figure 46.2 This is a 3D power Doppler (without the gray scale) display of the Circulus of Willis at 26 weeks' gestation. Note the anterior, middle and posterior cerebral arteries as well as the basilar artery.

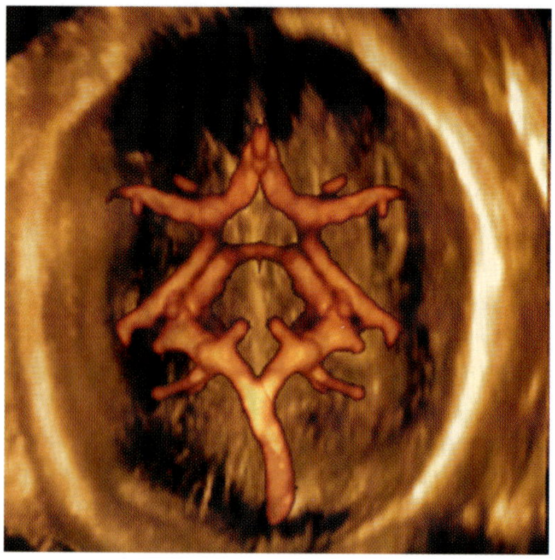

Figure 46.3 The same case as Figure 46.2. A volume rendered in transparent mode in gray scale and 3D power Doppler information in the same display. This display is generally used to display the brain vasculature in power Doppler as well as the brain gray-scale information simultaneously for better orientation and correlation. Typically, the color Doppler rendering can be combined with the gray scale at different percentages to the liking of the operator.

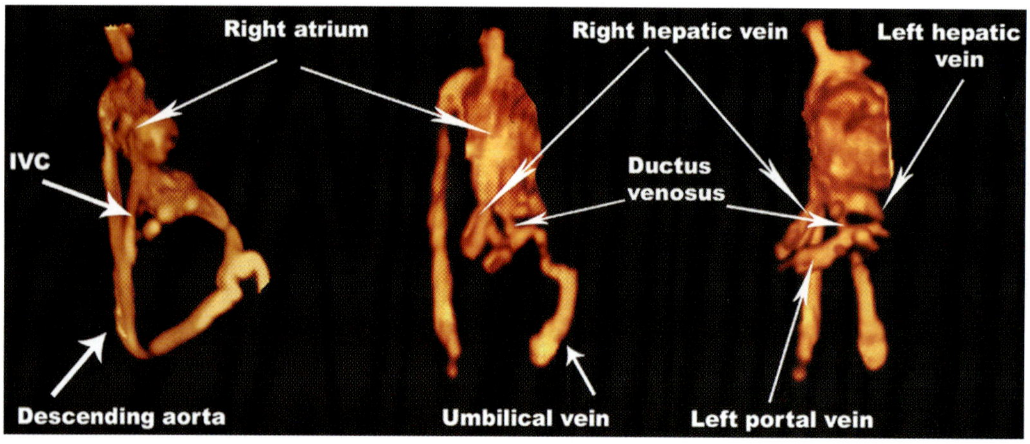

Figure 46.4 This is a 3D power Doppler rendered volume of the fetal cardiovascular system of a normal 23-week-gestation fetus. This volume has been rendered only with the 3D power Doppler without the presence of any gray-scale information. As this is the volume data, it can be rotated to depict different views of the anatomy. Note the detailed visualization of the descending aorta, inferior vena cava (IVC), right atrium, umbilical vein, right hepatic and left veins, left portal vein and ductus venosus.

flow; blood flow is displayed independent of its velocity and the vessels are visualized throughout the volume, ensuring spatial orientation.[16] Figures 46.5–46.7 demonstrate how 3D color and power Doppler can have an important role in visualizing the complex anatomical arrangements otherwise quite difficult with 2D ultrasound.

Hull *et al.* reported their experience in using 3D color and power Doppler in imaging the placenta.[17] They found that 3D ultrasound with color Doppler imaging allowed a more accurate diagnosis of placenta percreta. They had seen several patients in whom the use of 3D ultrasound with color flow and power Doppler imaging allowed refinement of the diagnosis of placental invasion, correctly predicting placenta percreta with bladder invasion. They feel that the multiplanar capability is the key to 3D ultrasound utility. Other useful applications of 3D color and power Doppler reported by this group are placental cord insertion and vasa previa visualization.[17]

Fetal echocardiography

3D volume acquisition speed has been improved significantly over the last 5 years. In the past, it was generally believed that increases in acquisition speeds

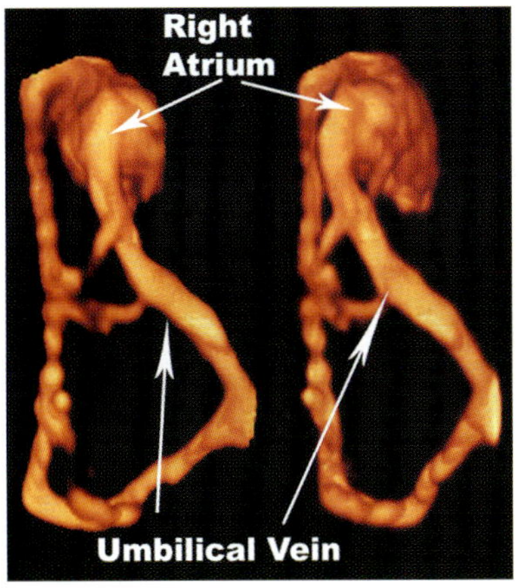

Figure 46.5 Power Doppler rendered volume of a fetus at 20 weeks' gestation with Noonan syndrome. Note the absence of ductus venosus and the umbilical vein draining directly to the right atrium. Note the distorted angio-architecture as compared to the normal fetus in Figure 46.4.

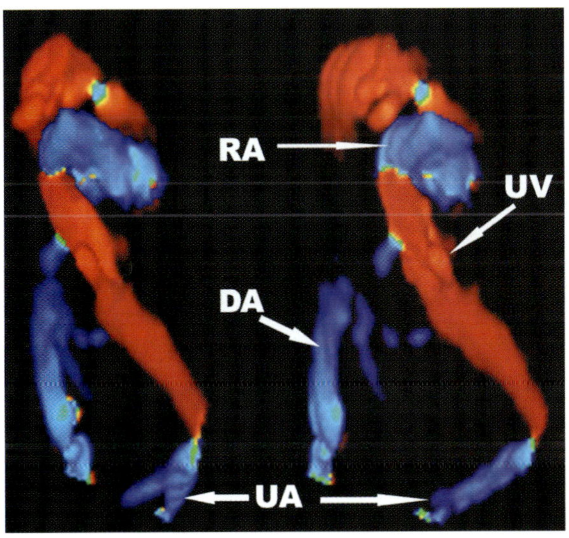

Figure 46.6 The same patient as in Figure 46.5, but the volume has been rendered in a 3D color Doppler again without the gray-scale information. The information provided from 3D color Doppler is similar to the one provided by 3D power Doppler, but in color Doppler we have additional information regarding the direction of flow. RA, right atrium; DA, ductus venosus; UV, umbilical vein; UA, umbilical arteries.

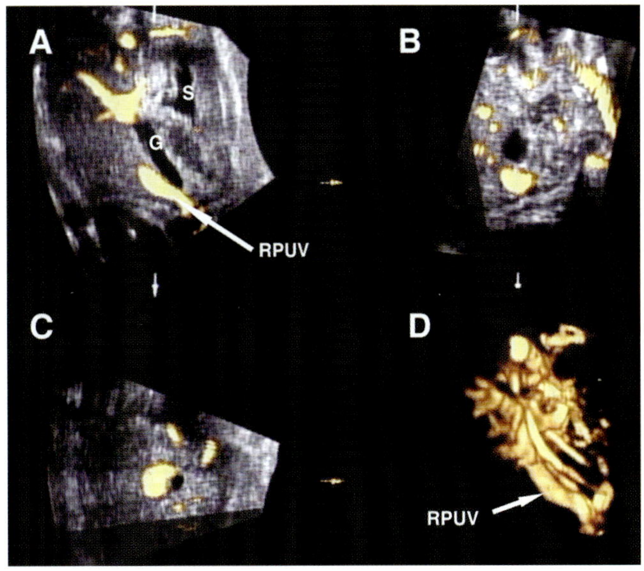

Figure 46.7 Multiplanar display and a rendered display of a fetus at 25 weeks' gestation with persistent right umbilical vein. (A) Transverse plane through the fetal abdomen at the level obtained to measure the abdominal circumference: S, stomach; G, gallbladder; RPUV, right persistent umbilical vein. The right umbilical vein passes lateral and to the right side of the gallbladder connecting the left portal vein. This is the intrahepatic form of the right umbilical vein. (B) A perpendicular view to plane A. (C) A coronal view to plane A. (D) The rendered 3D power Doppler view with the arrow pointing at the persistent right umbilical vein. Note that all these four windows are interactive with each other. Windows A and D can be correlated to identify the right umbilical vein both in cross-sectional and in rendered view.

will have a great impact in 3D fetal echocardiography. While the Voluson 730 Expert (GE MEDICAL, Milwaukee, WI, USA) can achieve speeds of acquisition up to 32 frames/s, in acquiring fetal heart volumes these high speeds do not necessarily translate into higher-quality volumes. Indeed, the opposite is true. Slower volumes yield higher-quality information as there are more 2D frames incorporated in the volume. To overcome this obstacle, a new volume acquisition technology was introduced. This technology is called STIC. With STIC, an extra slow (by 3DUS standards) acquisition from 7.5 to 15 s is performed over a preselected area of the fetal heart, typically at the level of the four-chamber view. The acquisition angle varies from 15° to 40° and again is user selectable. The same image optimization criteria apply just as the ones mentioned above. After the acquisition, postprocessing of spatial and temporal data is performed so that the 2D acquired images are correlated in time and space. This information is displayed in a classic multiplanar view and/or in a cine sequence depicting heart motion with total control on interactive reslicing and/or rendering the same as you would in a static 3D volume. Typically, in gray scale, this acquisition has a very high b-mode frame rate (approximately 150 frames/s) due to the relatively small region of interest.

STIC technique was initially introduced only in gray scale but later the acquisition of fetal heart volumes with STIC could be achieved with color and/or power Doppler information. This development opened up a whole new area in evaluating the fetal heart with 3DUS. STIC represents the first significant development in 3D fetal heart scanning that has the potential to perform a full fetal echo exam out of a single fetal heart volume at the level of the four-chamber view. Studies done before and after the introduction of STIC were able to demonstrate that a volume of the fetal heart can provide all the standard imaging views for a fetal echo[4,18] (Figures 46.13–46.15).

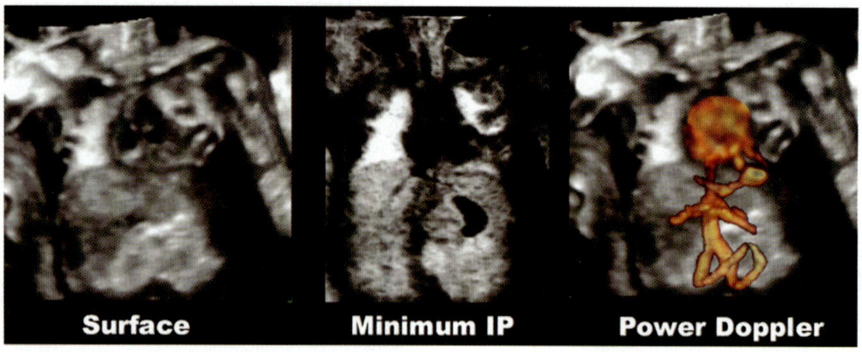

Figure 46.8 A composite image of a frontal view through the fetal body of a normal fetus at 20 weeks' gestation. The volume was acquired with and without power Doppler. The volumes are displayed in 3D surface rendering to visualize tissue interfaces of heart, lung, liver and bowel (first to the right), minimum intensity projection to visualize fluid-filled structures, such as heart and stomach, and surface and 3D power Doppler to visualize the relationships between vascular orientation and fetal body.

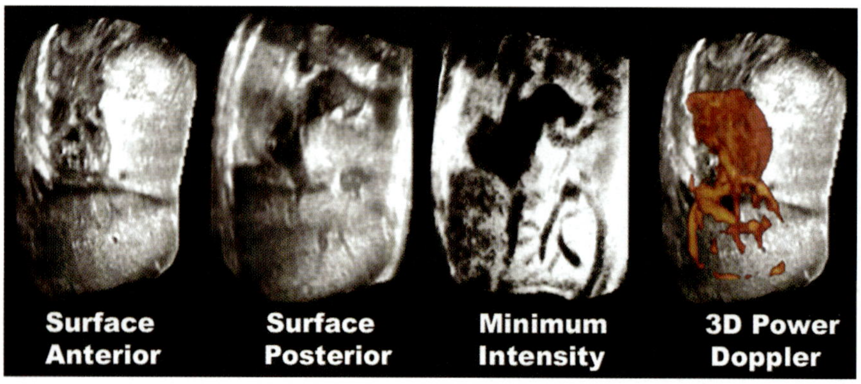

Figure 46.9 A composite image of several different volumes of a frontal view through the fetal body of a fetus at 22 weeks' gestation with congenital diaphragmatic hernia. In surface anterior view, the volume has been rendered with surface rendering settings at a very anterior level right behind the sternum to show the fetal liver, the diaphragm and the heart displaced in the right. In surface posterior view the volume has been rendered again with surface rendering settings, but at a posterior level to show the fetal stomach up in the chest, the disappearance of the diaphragm posteriorly and to the left as well as the left lobe of the liver going up in the chest. In minimum intensity view, the volume has been rendered with minimum intensity settings (good for fluid-filled structures) at a posterior level to better display the fetal stomach up in the chest as well as the left lobe of the liver vessels up in the chest. In 3D power view, the volume has been rendered with both surface and 3D power Doppler to better visualize the fetal heart and liver vessels in relationship to the chest wall and the diaphragm. Note the distorted angio-architecture as compared to the normal fetus in Figure 46.8.

Several reports have been demonstrating the value of STIC to the evaluation of the fetal heart with 3DUS.[20–24] Recently, Chaoui published a comprehensive prospective study in which he examined the potential of color Doppler STIC in the evaluation of normal and abnormal fetal hearts. He included 35 normal fetuses and 27 fetuses with congenital heart defects (CHD) examined between 18 and 35 weeks of gestation. Volume acquisition was achieved by initiating the image capture sequence from the transverse four-chamber view. Volumes were stored for later off-line evaluation using a personal computer-based workstation in a multiplanar mode and as spatial volume rendering. Successful acquisition was possible in all 62 cases. Spatial volume rendering was attempted in 18 fetuses with CHD. Four normal fetuses had inadequate visualization using color Doppler STIC, as the region of interest was perpendicular to the ultrasound beam. In two fetuses with CHD, inadequate visualization was related to an enlarged heart in late gestation, in which the entire cardiac volume could not be acquired. The third case was an 18-week fetus with complex CHD and transposed great vessels in which artifacts were related to confluent color signals as a result of low resolution in the reconstructed plane. He concluded that STIC in combination with color Doppler ultrasound is a promising new tool for multiplanar rendering of the fetal heart.[24]

While the potential of this technique is clear, there are a number of potential pitfalls that are worth mentioning. The acquisition is still relatively slow, from 7.5 to 15 s and as such fetal breathing and gross body

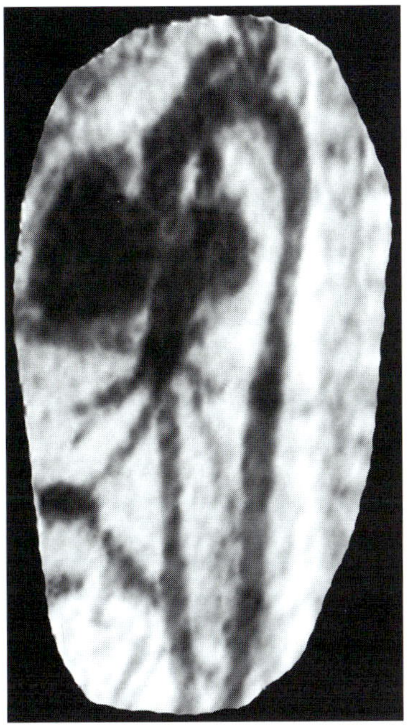

Figure 46.10 A 3D volume of the fetal heart and vessels of a normal fetus at 22 weeks rendered with minimum intensity projection. This is a unique and very helpful view that visualizes the vessels in gray scale without any color or power Doppler information. This rendering parameter can be employed in all acquisition modes (3D, 4D and STIC) and can be a useful addition to the information provided by the 3D color or power Doppler.

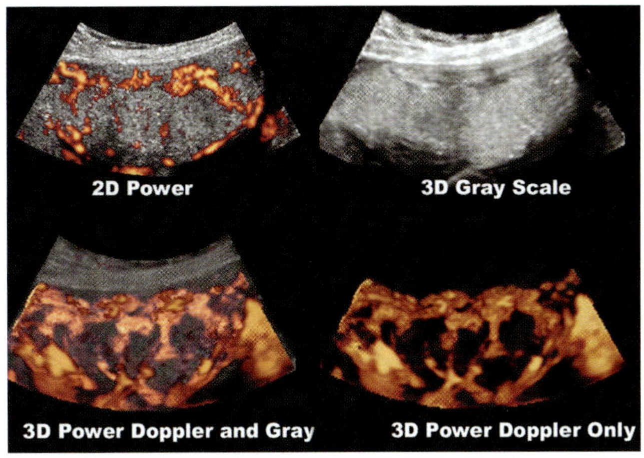

Figure 46.12 A composite image of four different image displays of the placenta. In 2D power Doppler view in the upper right we see scattered power Doppler signal in a thin 2D ultrasound slice. In 3D gray scale we see a rendered view through the placenta in gray scale. In 3D power Doppler and gray scale we see the great depth perception and detail of placental vasculature provided by 3D power Doppler in a 3D volume. In 3D power Doppler only we can see more clearly the vascular anatomy of the placenta without the gray scale superimposed on it.

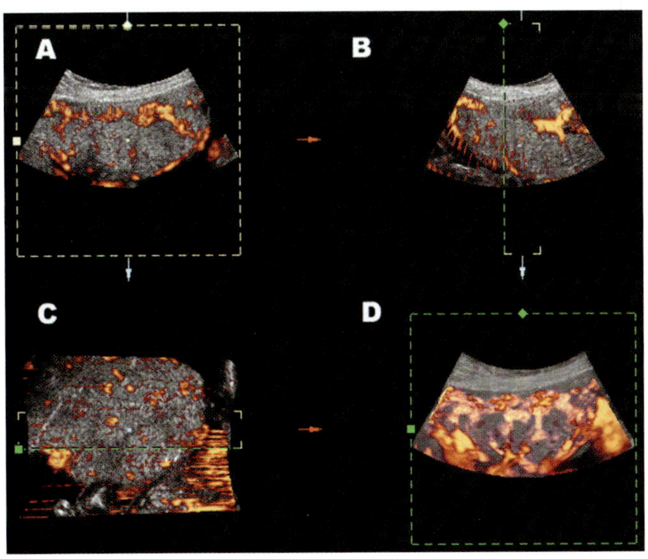

Figure 46.11 Multiplanar and rendered display of a placental volume acquired with 3D color Doppler at 20 weeks' gestation: (A) the acquisition plane, in this case along the long axis of the placenta; (B) the short axis; (C) the coronal view and (D) the 3D color Doppler and gray-scale rendered view of the placenta. Note that the rendered view represents a rather thin slice through the placenta and not the whole placental volume. The thickness of this particular volume can be judged and appreciated at (B), where you can see the green interrupted lines.

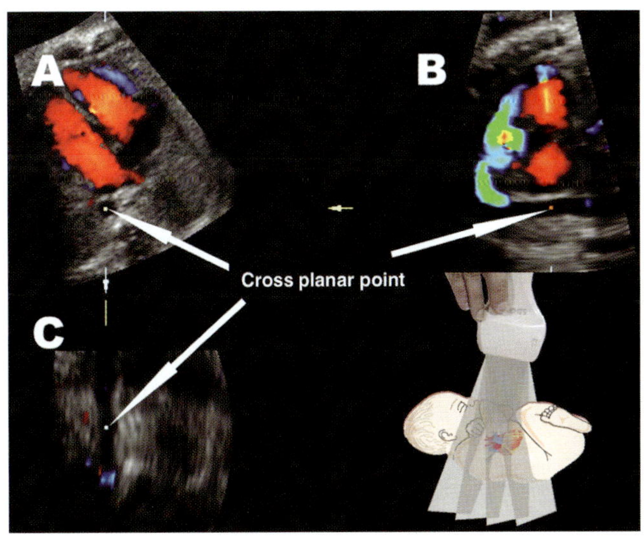

Figure 46.13 A composite image of a multiplanar view of the fetal heart acquired with 3D STIC color Doppler at the four-chamber view level. In the lower left, there is a diagram illustrating the acquisition of a fetal heart volume with a dedicated volume transducer where the transducer is kept stationary and the mechanically steered transducer elements sweep through the volume of the heart at a predetermined angle and speed. After the acquisition of the volume, the cross-planar center point is placed at the descending aorta in plane (A) and oriented at the 6 o'clock position. This rotation will ensure that we can obtain the ductal arch at (B) and the descending aorta in (C). A STIC volume with color Doppler depicts in red the atrioventricular flow (A) and in blue the outflow tracts (B).

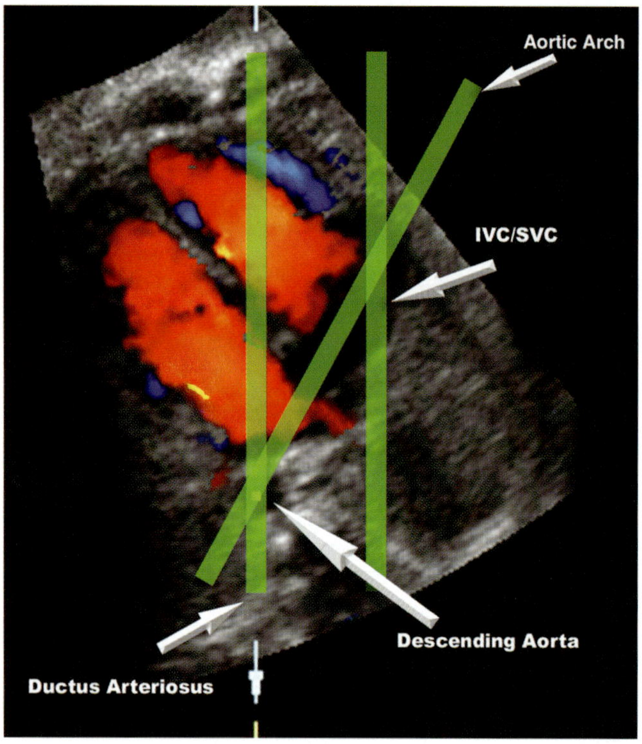

Figure 46.14 This image shows the four-chamber view image with color Doppler extracted from a STIC 3D color Doppler volume. The green lines represent the scan planes where the additional views of the heart, such as IVC/superior vena cava (SVC) or aortic arch, can be obtained. The vertical axis of the display can be aligned with these scan planes by rotating the image plane and simultaneously maintaining the descending aorta as the pivot point by placing the cross-planar point in it. Typically, the ductus arteriosus plane is the plane that goes through the descending aorta (placed at 6 o'clock) upward, intersecting the left atrium, right ventricle and sternum. The IVC/SVC plane is a plane parallel to the plane of the ductus arteriosus and to the right of it close to the level of the right atrium. The aortic arch is a plane that can be found by rotating the four-chamber view plane around 35–40° from the ductus arteriosus plane and maintaining the descending aorta as the pivot point by keeping the cross-planar point there.

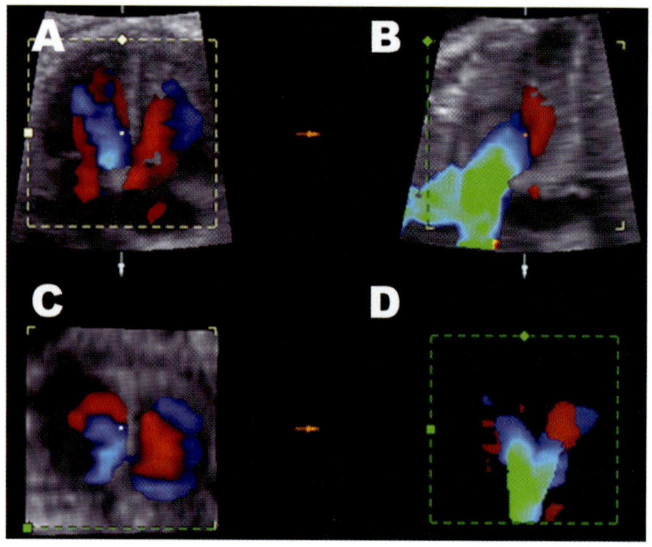

Figure 46.15 This image is a multiplanar and rendered view of a fetal heart volume obtained with STIC and color Doppler at the level of the four-chamber view in a patient with transposition of the great arteries. In (A) the heart is seen at the level of the four-chamber view and the atrio-ventricular flow is seen in red. In (B) we see a plane through the fetal heart that is perpendicular to (A) that shows a cross section of the outflow tracts in blue. In (C) we see a cross-sectional view of the heart right under the atrio-ventricular valves. In (D) there is a rendered view of the outflow tracts (in blue color). Note the fact that the outflow tracts do not crisscross as normally expected to, but they exit the ventricle in a parallel fashion indicative of a d-transposition of the great vessels.

movement do commonly occur. Careful evaluation of the windows B and C in the multiplanar display after the acquisition is crucial to ensure that no artifacts are present. Adjusting the volume box tightly around the region of interest helps, as it generally increases the frame rate. The best frame rates recommended are the ones above 15 Hz, typically with higher rates in smaller hearts and slower rates in bigger hearts. An important adjustment is the acquisition angle, as the default settings tend to be very narrow. Optimal angles vary from 15° to 30° and are related to the gestational age. The earlier the gestational age the narrower the angle.

Networking

A potential benefit of 3DUS lies in ultrasound documentation, storage and networking. Digitally saved volumes of patient data can be readily transferred to a remote site for interpretation or second opinion consultation. Further research is needed to define the indications, the potential advantages and limitations of volume data transfer across networks, but it is clear that this is a better method for sharing ultrasound information as one does not have to rely only on still 2D images or videotapes, but has the whole anatomy, which can be manipulated at any plane. Using this technology, one would expect that in the future, primary clinical sites in remote areas would have access to expert consultation and off-line interpretation, enabling high-quality and cost-effective medical care. The digitally stored patient volumes can be accessed and analyzed by physicians and sonographers in facilitating training in ultrasound. As this information is digital, it can be encrypted for patient data safety considerations, and efficiently compressed with loss-less algorithms to be shared across hospital networks.

Summary

It is important to emphasize that 3DUS color and power Doppler information is based on acquisition and reformatting of conventional 2DUS data. Therefore, it is not surprising that 3DUS is prone to the same problems that affect 2DUS, such as unfavorable body habitus, motion and shadowing artifacts and poor scanning technique. Although 3DUS with color and power Doppler may improve the overall comprehension of the vascular anatomy, it does not make up for poor scanning technique. Poor resolution in 2DUS will very likely result in suboptimal image quality in the volume data as well. Imaging the vessels in perpendicular planes with the beam will also result in poor imaging as the best results are achieved with parallel vessel orientation to the ultrasound beam. The resolution of the three perpendicular planes in the multiplanar display varies according to their deviation from the plane during acquisition. Typically, the coronal reconstructed plane, which is unique to 3DUS, has the lowest resolution of the three planes in the multiplanar display. There definitely is a learning curve associated with the adequate use of this technology. Professionals contemplating the introduction of this modality into their practices should consider dedicating time and effort for additional training in its principles. As this technology improves and becomes more widely available, clinical indications for its use will continue to emerge. There is a great need for comprehensive and rigorous research studies that would hopefully standardize optimal acquisition and analysis of 3D color and power Doppler studies for specific fetal indications.

REFERENCES

1. Nelson T, Downey D, Pretorius D, Fenster A. *Three Dimensional Ultrasound.* Philadelphia, PA: Lippincott Williams and Willkins, 1999.
2. Riccabona M, Pretorius DH, Nelson TR, Johnson D, Budorick NE. Three-dimensional ultrasound: Display modalities in obstetrics. *J Clin Ultrasound* 1997;25(4):157–67.
3. Kavic MS. Three-dimensional ultrasound. *Surg Endosc* 1996; 10(1):74–6.
4. Bega G, Kuhlman K, Lev-Toaff A, Kurtz A, Wapner R. Application of three-dimensional ultrasonography in the evaluation of the fetal heart. *J Ultrasound Med* 2001;20:307–13.
5. Ota T, Kisslo J, Von Ramm OT, Yoshikawa J. Real-time, volumetric echocardiography: Usefulness of volumetric scanning for the assessment of cardiac volume and function. *J Cardiol* 2001;37 (Suppl 1):93–101.
6. Kisslo J, Firek B, Ota T, *et al.* Real-time volumetric echocardiography: The technology and the possibilities. *Echocardiography* 2000;17:773–9.
7. Sklansky MS, DeVore GR, Wong PC. Real-time 3-dimensional fetal echocardiography with an instantaneous volume-rendered display: Early description and pictorial essay. *J Ultrasound Med* 2004;23(2):283–9.
8. Liang RI, Chang FM, Yao BL, Chang CH, Yu Ch, Ko HC. Predicting birth weight by upper-arm volume with use of three-dimensional ultrasonography. *Obstet Gynecol* 1997;177(3):632–8.
9. Lee W, Comstock CH, Kirk J, *et al.* Birthweight prediction by three-dimensional ultrasonographic volumes of the fetal thigh and abdomen. *J Ultrasound Med* 1997;16:799–805.
10. Pohls UG, Rempen A. Fetal lung volumetry by three-dimensional ultrasound. *Ultrasound Obstet Gynecol* 1998;11(1):6–12.
11. Laudy J, Janssen M, Struyk P, Stijnen T, Wladimirof J. Three dimensional ultrasonography of normal fetal lung volume: A preliminary study. *Ultrasound Obstet Gynecol* 1998;11:13–6.
12. Lee A, Kratochwil A, Stumpflen I, Deutinger J, Bernaschek G. Fetal lung determination by three dimensional ultrasonography. *Am J Obstet Gynecol* 1996;175(3):588–92.
13. Matijevic R, Kurjak A. Three dimensional color and power imaging: Experience in prenatal diagnosis. In Kurjak A, ed. *Clinical Application of 3D Sonography.* New York: Parthenon Publishing, 2000:155–60.
14. Chaoui R, Kalache K. Three dimensional color power imaging: Principles and first experience in prenatal diagnosis. In Merz E, ed. *3D Ultrasound in Obstetrics and Gynecology.* Philadelphia: Lippincot Williams&Wilkins, 1998:135–41.
15. Lee W, McNie B, Chaiworapongsa T, *et al.* Three-dimensional power Doppler ultrasonography during pregnancy. *J Ultrasound Med* 2003;22:91–7.
16. Kalache K, Romero R, Goncalves L, *et al.* Three-dimensional color power imaging of the fetal hepatic circulation. *Am J Obstet Gynecol* 2003;189(5):1401–6.
17. Hull AD, Pretorius DH. Three-dimensional power Doppler in the study of placental and umbilical cord abnormalities. In Kurjak A, ed. *Clinical Application of 3D Sonography.* New York: Parthenon Publishing, 2000:167–70.
18. DeVore GR, Polanco B, Sklansky MS, Platt LD. The 'spin' technique: A new method for examination of the fetal outflow tracts using three-dimensional ultrasound. *Ultrasound Obstet Gynecol* 2004;24(1):72–82.
19. Devore GR, Falkensammer P, Sklansky MS, Platt LD. Spatio-temporal image correlation (STIC): New technology for evaluation of the fetal heart. *Ultrasound Obstet Gynecol* 2003;22:380–7.
20. Vinals F, Poblete P, Giuliano A. Spatio-temporal image correlation (STIC). A new tool for the prenatal screening of congenital heart defects. *Ultrasound Obstet Gynecol* 2003;22:388–94.
21. Goncalves LF, Lee W, Espinoza J, *et al.* Four dimensional fetal echocardiography with spatio-temporal image correlation (STIC): A systematic study of standard cardiac views assessed by different observers (abstract). *Ultrasound Obstet Gynecol* 2003; 22:50.
22. Chaoui R, Kalache K, Heling KS. Potential of off-line 4D fetal echocardiography using new acquisition and rendering technique (STIC) (abstract). *Ultrasound Obstet Gynecol* 2003;22:50.
23. Chaoui R, Schneider MBE, Kalache KD. Right aortic arch with vascular ring and aberrant left subclavian artery: Prenatal diagnosis assisted by three-dimensional power Doppler ultrasound. *Ultrasound Obstet Gynecol* 2003;22:661–3.
24. Chaoui R, Hoffmann J, Heling KS. Three-dimensional (3D) and 4D color Doppler fetal echocardiography using spatio temporal image correlation (STIC). *Ultrasound Obstet Gynecol* 2004;23: 535–45.

47 Non-invasive detection of fetal anemia by Doppler ultrasonography

L. Pereira

Introduction

Cases of hemolytic disease of the newborn were described as early as 1609 in France;[1] however, it was not until 1932, over 300 years later, that the association of erythroblastosis with fetal hydrops, jaundice and hemolytic anemia was characterized by Diamond *et al.*[2] Shortly thereafter, the discovery of the Rhesus (Rh) blood group by Landsteiner and Weiner in 1940, and their demonstration of agglutination when rhesus monkey red blood cell antiserum was mixed with Rh-positive, but not Rh-negative blood, stands as one of the most important hematologic discoveries of the 20th century.[3] From this landmark achievement, treatment of hemolytic disease of the newborn with transfusion therapy and ultimately prevention of Rh sensitization with anti-D immune globulin became possible. However, despite the availability of postnatal transfusion therapy, the medical practice of this era was limited by an inability to screen for hemolytic disease antenatally.

The discovery that Rh sensitization could be quantified by assessing the spectral absorption curve of amniotic fluid at 450 nm (ΔOD_{450}) was first described by Bevis and Walker and then further characterized by Liley in 1961.[4–6] From this important observation, successful antenatal management strategies were developed for Rh alloimmunized patients and for those alloimmunized with non-Rh antigens as well.

Years of experience have taught us that amniocentesis ΔOD_{450} assessment is a reliable predictor of fetal anemia in most cases of alloimmunization. However, because amniocentesis ΔOD_{450} assessment is limited to hemolytic causes of fetal anemia and because it has the potential to cause fetal–maternal hemorrhage and worsen sensitization, active research for nearly 30 years has focused on attempts to detect fetal anemia non-invasively.

Ultrasonographic evaluation of fetal anemia

Serial ultrasound evaluations for fetal hydrops in cases of suspected anemia have become a routine component of perinatal medicine. The observation of hydrops on ultrasound is highly specific for severe anemia, with most hydropic fetuses having hemoglobin levels that are less than 5 g dl^{-1}. The finding of fetal hydrops in cases of suspected anemia should lead directly to therapeutic interventions aimed at restoring blood volume. However, basing treatment on the presence of hydrops alone may miss over 50% of fetuses with hemoglobin concentrations below 6.0 g dl^{-1}.[7]

Partly because of this shortcoming, many investigators have attempted to detect fetal anemia prior to the onset of hydrops. Rightmire *et al.* published one of the first successful endeavors at non-invasive diagnosis of fetal anemia in non-hydropic fetuses in 1986. The authors developed a model of combined Doppler measurements of the fetal aorta, inferior vena cava, and umbilical vein, which was able to predict fetal anemia with a mean error of only 3.8 hematocrit units in a retrospective study.[8] Nicolaides *et al.* prospectively measured six different ultrasonographic parameters, including umbilical vein diameter and placental thickness, but concluded that in the absence of hydrops, none of these successfully distinguished mild from severe fetal anemia.[9] This observation was confirmed by Whitecar *et al.* who reported on a variety of parameters including amniotic fluid volume, intrahepatic and extrahepatic umbilical vein diameters, hepatic length, and splenic perimeter.[10] Most of these parameters have proven unreliable clinically. Attempts to accurately predict fetal anemia by measurement of the mean blood velocity in the fetal aorta have likewise not been clinically applicable.[11]

Measurement of peak systolic velocity as opposed to mean blood velocity seems to have improved the clinical utility of Doppler velocimetry. One author has reported on the utility of measuring peak systolic velocity in the splenic artery for the detection of fetal anemia in cases of Rh factor alloimmunization[12] and no fewer than seven prospective studies have reported on the reliability of peak systolic velocity measurements in the middle cerebral artery for detection of fetal anemia in pregnancies complicated by red cell alloimmunization (including Kell sensitization) and parvovirus B19 infection.[13–19]

Evidence supporting middle cerebral artery peak systolic velocity measurements for fetal anemia

In 1995, Mari *et al.* reported that middle cerebral artery peak systolic velocity Doppler measurements could accurately predict fetal anemia in a prospective series of 16 pregnancies complicated by maternal red cell alloimmunization.[13] This report was followed in 2000 by a larger multicentered study in which 111 fetuses at risk for anemia were followed prospectively.[15] In this cohort, 23 fetuses had moderate to severe anemia without hydrops and in all 23, middle cerebral artery peak systolic velocities were above 1.5 multiples of the median (MoM). In this study, 83 women were RhD alloimmunized, 18 were Kell sensitized, and another 9 were alloimmunized to non-RhD antigens. The authors also published reference tables for fetal hemoglobin levels and middle cerebral artery peak systolic velocities, which have served as the basis for further research studies and are useful reference guides for current clinical management (Tables 47.1 and 47.2).

In 2000, Teixeira *et al.* published results from a prospective cohort study of 26 fetuses (24 cases of RhD and 2 cases of RhC alloimmunization), and using a peak systolic velocity above 1 standard deviation (SD), reported a sensitivity of 73% and specificity of 93% for fetal hematocrit values below 3 SD.[14] A large prospective, intent to treat trial of 125 cases of red cell alloimmunization was published by Zimmermann *et al.* in 2002 and confirmed the findings of previous authors.[17] This trial reported that for the detection of moderate to severe fetal anemia, middle cerebral artery peak systolic velocities over 1.5 MoM had a sensitivity of 88% and specificity of 87%.

Further studies have provided evidence that middle cerebral artery peak systolic velocity Doppler can be used to estimate actual hemoglobin concentrations[18] and to predict the timing of a second *in utero* blood transfusion.[20]

In addition to cases of red cell alloimmunization, two studies have found that, in a total of 42 cases of parvovirus B19 infection, middle cerebral artery peak systolic velocity assessment could detect fetal anemia with sensitivity between 94% and 100% and specificity between 93% and 100%.[16,19]

Table 47.1 Middle cerebral artery peak systolic velocity (MCA-PSV) as a function of gestational age (from Mari *et al.*[15])

Weeks of gestation	MCA-PSV ($cm\ s^{-1}$) (multiples of the median)			
	1.00	1.29	1.50	1.55
18	23.2	29.9	34.8	36.6
20	25.5	32.8	38.2	39.5
22	27.9	36.0	41.9	43.3
24	30.7	39.5	46.0	47.5
26	33.6	43.3	50.4	52.1
28	36.9	47.6	55.4	57.2
30	40.5	52.2	60.7	62.8
32	44.4	57.3	66.6	68.9
34	48.7	62.9	73.1	75.6
36	53.5	69.0	80.2	82.9
38	58.7	75.7	88.0	91.0
40	64.4	83.0	96.6	99.8

Table 47.2 Fetal hemoglobin (Hgb) as a function of gestational age(from Mari *et al.*[15])

Weeks of gestation	Fetal Hgb ($g\ dl^{-1}$) (multiples of the median)				
	1.16	1.00	0.84	0.65	0.55
18	12.3	10.6	8.9	6.9	5.8
20	12.9	11.1	9.3	7.2	6.1
22	13.4	11.6	9.7	7.5	6.4
24	13.9	12.0	10.1	7.8	6.6
26	14.3	12.3	10.3	8.0	6.8
28	14.6	12.6	10.6	8.2	6.9
30	14.8	12.8	10.8	8.3	7.1
32	15.2	13.1	10.9	8.5	7.2
34	15.4	13.3	11.2	8.6	7.3
36	15.6	13.5	11.3	8.7	7.4
38	15.8	13.6	11.4	8.9	7.5
40	16.0	13.8	11.6	9.0	7.6

Technique for measuring the middle cerebral artery peak systolic velocity

Measurement of peak systolic velocity in the middle cerebral artery should be technically straightforward in most cases. Obtain an axial view of the fetal

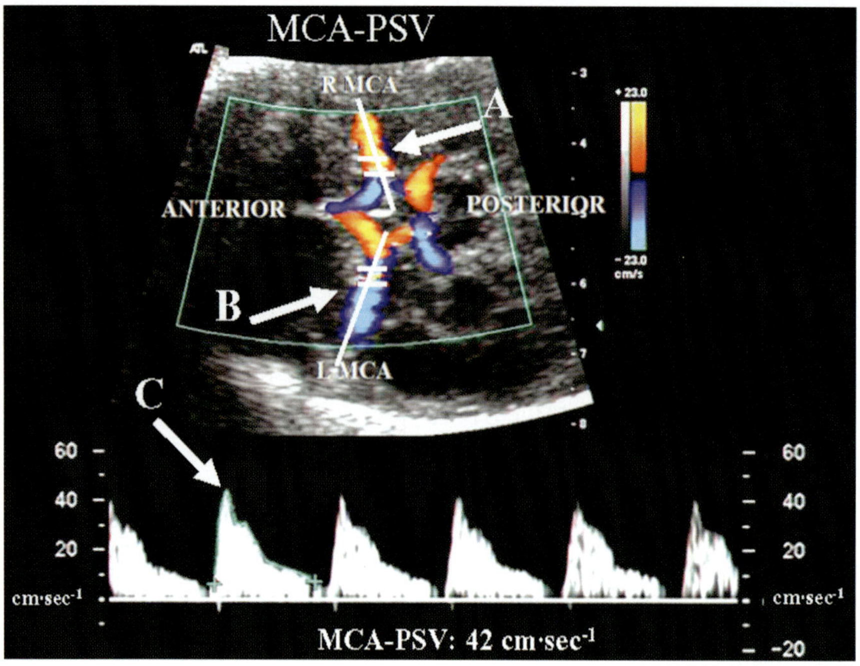

Figure 47.1 Doppler assessment of the fetal MCA. (A) Correct position of Doppler cursor over anterior MCA. (B) Correct position of Doppler cursor over posterior MCA. (C) Correct measurement of the PSV. MCA, middle cerebral artery; PSV, peak systolic velocity.

calvarium, as if one were measuring the biparietal diameter. Center and magnify the image until the fetal calvarium fills the image window. Following identification of midbrain structures, including the thalami and cavum septum pellucidum, move the transducer in a slight caudal direction and identify the circle of Willis using color Doppler. The bilateral middle cerebral arteries should then be visualized flowing anteriorly and outward just behind the orbits. The sample volume line should be parallel to the walls of the vessel, as close to a 0 angle of insonation as possible (Figure 47.1). Either the ipsilateral or the contralateral middle cerebral artery can be measured, but angle correction should not be used. The peak systolic velocity should be measured in the proximal middle cerebral artery, 2 mm after its origin from the internal carotid artery. Placement of the sample volume line in the proximal MCA is crucial since systolic velocity decreases with distance from the point of origin of the MCA.[15,21]

The sample volume should be made relatively small so that the Doppler signal does not incorporate the internal carotid artery. The peak systolic velocity should be measured at the highest point of the Doppler waveform. The measurement should be repeated several times during periods of fetal apnea, while the fetus is relatively stationary. The highest Doppler measurement obtained should be recorded. With this procedure, multiple sources have previously reported low intraobserver and interobserver variability rates between 2.3% and 4.0%.[13,21,22]

Management with middle cerebral artery peak systolic velocity compared to conventional management with amniocentesis ΔOD_{450}

Based on the results of the previously mentioned studies,[13–19] clinical reliance upon serial middle cerebral artery peak systolic velocity Dopplers is becoming more common. However, few studies have compared Doppler velocimetry to conventional management with amniocentesis. At the time of publication of this chapter, only two published trials had compared the two management strategies.

The first study, published by Nishie *et al.* followed 28 non-hydropic fetuses and found that conventional management and middle cerebral artery peak systolic velocity Doppler were both accurate predictors of fetal anemia in cases of red cell alloimmunization.[23] The authors suggested in their conclusion that management with middle cerebral artery peak systolic velocity Doppler could decrease the number of invasive procedures performed in their population.

A second study, by Pereira *et al.*, also reported outcomes on 28 cases of red cell alloimmunization followed by both middle cerebral artery peak systolic velocity Doppler and conventional management with amniocentesis.[24] In this study, management by middle cerebral artery peak systolic velocity Doppler compared favorably to conventional management, with a sensitivity of 91% and a specificity of 100% for moderate to severe fetal anemia. The authors concluded that compared to conventional management, management by middle cerebral artery peak systolic velocity Doppler may have a better predictive value for moderate to severe anemia in red cell alloimmunization, eliminate the need for amniocentesis, and reduce the number of percutaneous umbilical cord blood samplings (PUBS) performed on non-anemic fetuses.

The main benefit of management with middle cerebral artery peak systolic velocity Doppler is a reduction in invasive procedures and avoidance of potential complications. Transplacental fetal hemorrhage, which may worsen sensitization, occurs following 2–11% of amniocenteses.[25–27] Another 1–2% of amniocenteses are complicated by rupture of amniotic membranes, premature labor, vaginal bleeding, or infection, while fetal loss occurs in approximately 0.5% of cases.[28] Complications associated with PUBS are even more common, with at least 50% of procedures complicated by umbilical cord vessel bleeding and a procedure-related loss rate of 2–3%.[29]

In the USA, there are approximately 14,000 cases of alloimmunization annually.

Extrapolating from published trends, management with middle cerebral artery peak systolic velocity Doppler could avoid 24,500 amniocenteses and over 1500 PUBS per year in the US population.[24] With a complication rate of 0.5% for amniocentesis and a conservative estimate of 2% for PUBS, one pregnancy loss or preterm delivery per 100 patients (over 140 annually) could be avoided by using middle cerebral artery peak systolic velocity Doppler over conventional management – and these would likely occur in mildly anemic or non-anemic fetuses. Furthermore, an additional benefit would occur from avoiding procedure-related bleeding complications that increase sensitization and worsen disease.

Limitations of middle cerebral artery peak systolic velocity

Management of suspected fetal anemia by middle cerebral artery peak systolic velocity Doppler has limitations. The accuracy of middle cerebral artery peak systolic velocity Doppler appears to diminish after 35 weeks' gestation, leading to higher false-positive rates for prediction of anemia.[17,30] Furthermore, multiple intrauterine transfusions increase fetal blood viscosity, which may alter the predictive accuracy of middle cerebral artery peak systolic velocity Doppler.[20,31] The reliability of middle cerebral artery peak systolic velocity Doppler in predicting fetal anemia after three or more transfusions has not been tested prospectively, and false-negative cases have been reported.[17,20] At present, serial amniocenteses for ΔOD_{450} assessment should be considered in fetuses greater than 35 weeks' gestation and in those who have received three or more *in utero* transfusions. The use of amniocentesis after 35 weeks' gestation also allows for concomittant fetal lung maturity testing, which can impact the timing of delivery.

The predictive accuracy of middle cerebral artery peak systolic velocity Doppler in fetuses with compromised left-sided cardiac output from structural heart disease has not yet been established. Anomalies such as mitral stenosis or hypoplastic left heart syndrome that compromise left ventricular cardiac output may result in decreased middle cerebral artery peak systolic velocities. Amniocentesis ΔOD_{450} measurements should not be affected by the presence of congenital heart disease and may be superior to Doppler in this setting.

Another limitation of middle cerebral artery peak systolic velocity Doppler occurs in the setting of fetal hydrops. The middle cerebral artery peak systolic velocity in hydropic fetuses may be diminished by compromised cardiac output. In these cases, the fetus may not be able to maintain adequate cardiac output, resulting in a lower middle cerebral artery peak systolic velocity than would be expected for the degree of anemia. False-negative middle cerebral artery Dopplers have been previously reported in hydropic fetuses with severe anemia.[17,32]

Potential pitfalls in measuring middle cerebral artery peak systolic velocity

Serial middle cerebral artery peak systolic velocity Doppler measurements must be conducted in strict adherence with proper technique as previously discussed to maintain diagnostic accuracy. Measurements taken in the distal middle cerebral artery or with an angle of insonation above 20° may underestimate the peak systolic velocity and decrease sensitivity.

Intermittent vascular constriction of the middle cerebral artery can occur and may explain several reported cases where an elevated middle cerebral artery peak systolic velocity measurement has not been reproducible.[17,19]

Multiple factors influence fetal cerebral hemodynamics and can influence middle cerebral artery Doppler studies. Variations in fetal heart rate, both bradycardia[33,34] and tachycardia,[35] alter flow through the middle cerebral artery. Fetal behavioral state and activity level also result in dynamic changes in middle cerebral artery perfusion.[36] For these reasons, the middle cerebral artery peak systolic velocity should be measured during periods of fetal apnea and when fetal activity is minimal.

Alterations in middle cerebral artery Doppler waveforms should be anticipated during active labor and in fetuses with severe intrauterine growth restriction (IUGR). The reliability of middle cerebral artery peak systolic velocity in detecting anemia during active labor has not been established, and Yagel *et al.* reported a 40% reduction in middle cerebral artery

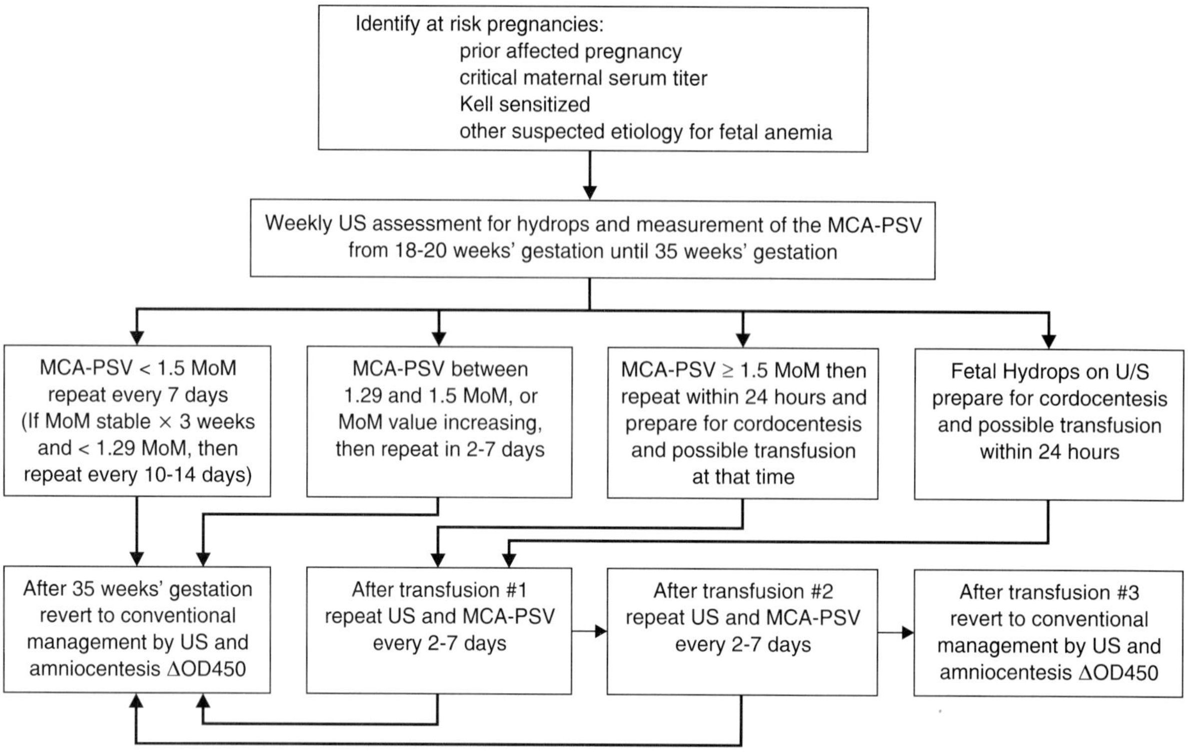

Figure 47.2 Antenatal surveillance for fetal anemia using MCA-PSV. MCA, middle cerebral artery; PSV, peak systolic velocity; US, ultrasound; MoM, multiples of the median.

blood flow impedence during labor.[37] Fetuses with severe IUGR display similar reductions in cerebral blood flow impedence independent of hematocrit.[38,39] This is likely due to 'brain-sparing', which has been characterized by a decrease in the middle cerebral artery pulsatility index as a cephalization of blood flow in response to fetal hypoxemia.[39–41]

Algorithm for fetal surveillance using middle cerebral artery peak systolic velocity

For clinical purposes, a sample algorithm for management of suspected fetal anemia using middle cerebral artery Doppler velocimetry is shown in Figure 47.2 and can be summarized as follows:

Identify pregnancies at risk for fetal anemia such as patients with prior affected pregnancies, antibody titers that have reached a critical threshold level, anti-Kell antibodies, congenital parvovirus, suspected fetomaternal hemorrhage (e.g. strongly positive Kleihauer–Betke test or unexplained elevated maternal serum alphafetoprotein level). Beginning at 18–20 weeks of gestation, perform weekly sonograms to measure the middle cerebral artery peak systolic velocity and evaluate for evidence of fetal hydrops. If the middle cerebral artery peak systolic velocity is less than 1.5 MoM, then repeat it weekly for the next 3 weeks. If over that time, the middle cerebral artery peak systolic velocity remains stable and is under 1.29 MoM, then it is probably safe to follow the middle cerebral artery peak systolic velocities every 10–14 days.

If serial middle cerebral artery peak systolic velocities remain between 1.29 and 1.5 MoM or are increasing in MoM values, then repeat the middle cerebral artery peak systolic velocity measurement in 7 days or less. If at any time the middle cerebral artery peak systolic velocity is $\geq$1.5 MoM, then plan to repeat the measurement in 12–18 h and plan for a cordocentesis with preparations for a possible *in utero* transfusion at that time.

If there is a sonographic evidence of fetal hydrops, then plan for a cordocentesis and transfusion even if the middle cerebral artery peak systolic velocity is $<$ 1.5 MoM.

Continue to follow at-risk fetuses as outlined above until the fetus reaches 35 weeks of gestation or has received three or more *in utero* transfusions, then revert back to conventional management by amniocentesis ΔOD_{450} measurements.

Areas for future research with middle cerebral artery peak systolic velocity

Areas for future research include studies to determine how well middle cerebral artery Dopplers predict anemia in fetuses with genetic syndromes (thrombocytopenia-absent radius, Fanconi syndrome), hemoglobinopathies (alpha-thalassemia), or viral infections that can cause a myocarditis as well as an anemia. There have been case reports of fetuses with hydrops due to parvovirus B19 that were not anemic at the time of umbilical cord sampling and recovered without transfusion.[42,43] In these cases, hydrops may be due to myocarditis caused by the tropism of parvovirus B19 for myocardial cells. Perhaps in these cases, middle cerebral artery peak systolic velocity will prove a valuable modality for avoiding an unnecessary cordocentesis.

The possibility of measuring middle cerebral artery peak systolic velocity Dopplers in fetuses with platelet or neutrophil disorders, such as neonatal alloimmune thrombocytopenia, should be explored remembering that the basis for elevated middle cerebral artery peak systolic velocities is not actual hematocrit but decreased blood viscosity.

Suspected fetal hemorrhage

Acute or chronic fetomaternal hemorrhage may lead to anemia, hydrops, and intrauterine death. In suspected cases, the diagnosis of fetomaternal hemorrhage is typically made by demonstration of fetal erythrocytes in maternal circulation by Kleihauer–Betke acid-elution stain. Measurement of the maternal serum alpha-fetoprotein level may also be useful in cases of suspected fetomaternal hemorrhage.

As in cases of red blood cell alloimmunization, the appearance of hydrops in the setting of fetomaternal hemorrhage remote from term should generally be treated with intrauterine transfusion as these fetuses are at risk for *in utero* demise.[44–46] Based on limited data, it appears that middle cerebral artery peak systolic velocities may be useful for detection of fetal anemia in these cases. Baschat *et al.*, in 1998, reported a case of acute fetomaternal hemorrhage in which the middle cerebral peak systolic velocity was elevated at presentation (hematocrit < 11%) and then normalized after *in utero* transfusion (hematocrit 27%).[47]

Some authors have reported that intraplacental Dopplers may be useful in predicting adverse pregnancy outcomes (IUGR, pre-eclampsia) in cases of fetomaternal hemorrhage. In 1996, Jaffe and Woods reported results from 32 patients followed due to abnormal first-trimester Doppler studies. In these patients, an abnormal ratio of intraplacental resistive index (RI) to umbilical artery RI (defined as > 1) between 22 and 25 weeks' gestation was associated with adverse pregnancy outcomes in 17/21 women compared to 2/11 controls.[48] A second study in 1997 by Haberman and Friedman compared intraplacental pulsatility index (PI) to umbilical artery PI and reported a higher rate of IUGR and pre-eclampsia when the intraplacental PI to umbilical artery PI ratio was over 1.[49]

In rare cases, fetal anemia may be due to fetal intracranial hemorrhage, usually subdural hematomas.[50,51] Coagulation deficiencies such as neonatal alloimmune thrombocytopenia should be suspected when a fetal intracranial hemorrhage is identified in the absence of antecedent trauma.[52] The reliability of middle cerebral artery Doppler assessment in the setting of intracranial hemorrhage has not been established at this time.

Summary

The clinical management of fetuses at risk for anemia is currently evolving. Based on the results of several prospective trials, the accuracy of middle cerebral artery peak systolic velocity Doppler has been established for the prediction of fetal anemia in cases of red cell alloimmunization. Limited evidence seems to support its accuracy in cases of parvovirus B19 infection as well. When conducted in strict adherence with proper technique, the reliability and accuracy of middle cerebral artery peak systolic velocity Doppler is high, and intraobserver variability uniformly low. In the near future, evidence may support the application of middle cerebral artery peak systolic velocity Doppler to a broad spectrum of conditions that may cause fetal anemia. At the present time, however, reliance solely on middle cerebral artery peak systolic velocity Doppler should be limited to cases where its accuracy has been established and normal left ventricular cardiac output preserved. In cases where the accuracy of middle cerebral artery peak systolic velocity Doppler has not been established, and in centers in which middle cerebral artery peak systolic velocity Dopplers are not performed regularly, simultaneous management by conventional amniocentesis ΔOD_{450} measurements should probably be continued. Exciting research in the field of Doppler velocimetry is ongoing, and in the near future further advances in our ability to detect fetal anemia non-invasively are certain to emerge.

REFERENCES

1. Bowman J. Hemolytic disease (erythroblastosis fetalis). In Creasy RK, Resnik R, eds. *Maternal–Fetal Medicine*. Philadelphia: WB Saunders, 1999:736–67.
2. Diamond LK, Blackfan KD, Baty JM. Erythroblastosis fetalis and its association with universal edema of the fetus, icterus gravis neonatorum and anemia of the newborn. *J Pediatr* 1932;1:269.
3. Landsteiner K, Weiner AS. An agglutinable factor in human blood recognized by immune sera for rhesus blood. *Proc Soc Exp Biol Med* 1940;43:223.
4. Bevis DCA. Blood pigments in hemolytic disease of the newborn. *J Obstet Gynaecol Br Emp* 1956;63:68–75.
5. Walker AHC. Liquor amnii studies in the prediction of haemolytic disease of the newborn. *Br Med J* 1957;2:376–8.

6. Liley AW. Liquor amnii analysis in the management of the pregnancy complicated by rhesus sensitization. *Am J Obstet Gynecol* 1961;82:1359–70.
7. Nicolaides KH, Rodeck CH, Mibashan RS, Kemp JR. Have Liley charts outlived their usefulness? *Am J Obstet Gynecol* 1986; 155:90–4.
8. Rightmire DA, Nicolaides KH, Rodeck CH, Campbell S. Fetal blood velocities in Rh isoimmunization: Relationship to gestational age and to fetal hematocrit. *Obstet Gynecol* 1986;68:233–6.
9. Nicolaides KH, Fontanarosa M, Gabbe SG, Rodeck CH. Failure of ultrasonographic parameters to predict the severity of fetal anemia in rhesus isoimmunization. *Am J Obstet Gynecol* 1988;158:920–6.
10. Whitecar PW, Moise KJ Jr. Sonographic methods to detect fetal anemia in red blood cell alloimmunization. *Obstet Gynecol Surv* 2000;55:240–50.
11. Nicolaides KH, Bilardo CM, Campbell S. Prediction of fetal anemia by measurement of the mean blood velocity in the fetal aorta. *Am J Obstet Gynecol* 1990;162:209–12.
12. Bahado-Singh R, Oz U, Deren O, *et al.* Splenic artery Doppler peak systolic velocity predicts severe fetal anemia in rhesus disease. *Am J Obstet Gynecol* 2000;182:1222–6.
13. Mari G, Adrignolo A, Abuhamad AZ, *et al.* Diagnosis of fetal anemia with Doppler ultrasound in the pregnancy complicated by maternal blood group immunization. *Ultrasound Obstet Gynecol* 1995;5:400–5.
14. Teixeira JMA, Duncan K, Letsky E, Fisk NM. Middle cerebral artery peak systolic velocity in the prediction of fetal anemia. *Ultrasound Obstet Gynecol* 2000;15:205–8.
15. Mari G, Deter RL, Carpenter RL, *et al.* Noninvasive diagnosis by Doppler ultrasonography of fetal anemia due to maternal red-cell alloimmunization. *N Engl J Med* 2000;342:9–14.
16. Delle Chiaie L, Buck G, Grab D, Terinde R. Prediction of fetal anemia with Doppler measurements of the middle cerebral artery peak systolic velocity in pregnancies complicated by maternal blood group alloimmunization or parvovirus B19 infection. *Ultrasound Obstet Gynecol* 2001;18:232–6.
17. Zimmermann R, Durig P, Carpenter RJ Jr, Mari G. Longitudinal measurement of peak systolic velocity in the fetal middle cerebral artery for monitoring pregnancies complicated by red cell alloimmunisation: A prospective multicentre trial with intention-to-treat. *Br J Obstet Gynecol* 2002;109:746–52.
18. Mari G, Detti L, Oz U, Zimmermann R, Durig P, Stefos T. Accurate prediction of fetal hemoglobin by Doppler ultrasonography. *Obstet Gynecol* 2002;99:589–93.
19. Cosmi E, Mari G, Delle Chiaie L, *et al.* Noninvasive diagnosis by Doppler ultrasonography of fetal anemia resulting from parvovirus infection. *Am J Obstet Gynecol* 2002;187:1290–3.
20. Detti L, Oz U, Guney I, Ferguson JE, Bahado-Singh RO, Mari G. Doppler ultrasound velocimetry for timing the second intrauterine transfusion in fetuses with anemia from red cell alloimmunization. *Am J Obstet Gynecol* 2001;185:1048–51.
21. Akiyama M, Detti L, Abuhamad A, Bahado-Singh R, Mari G. Is the middle cerebral artery peak systolic velocity measurement affected by the site of vessel sampling? Presented at the *Twenty-third Annual Meeting of the Society for Maternal–Fetal Medicine*, San Francisco, CA, February 7, 2003:381.
22. Mari G, Abuhamad A, Brumfield J, Ferguson JE II. Doppler ultrasonography of the middle cerebral artery peak systolic velocity in the fetus: Reproducibility of measurement. Presented at the *Twenty-second Annual Meeting of the Society for Maternal–Fetal Medicine*, New Orleans, LA, January 14, 2002:669.
23. Nishie EN, Brizot ML, Liao AW, Carvalho MHB, Toma O, Zugaib M. A comparison between middle cerebral artery peak systolic velocity and amniotic fluid optical density at 450 nm in the prediction of fetal anemia. *Am J Obstet Gynecol* 2003;188:214–9.
24. Pereira L, Jenkins T, Berghella V. Conventional management of fetal alloimmunization compared to management by middle cerebral artery peak systolic velocity. *Am J Obstet Gynecol* 2003;189(4):1002–6.
25. Bowman JM, Pollock JM. Transplacental fetal hemorrhage after amniocentesis. *Obstet Gynecol* 1985;66:749–54.
26. Woo Wang MYF, McCutcheon E, Desforges JF. Fetomaternal hemorrhage from diagnostic transabdominal amniocentesis. *Am J Obstet Gynecol* 1967;97(8):1123–8.
27. Peddle LJ. Increase of antibody titer following amniocentesis. *Am J Obstet Gynecol* 1968;100(4):567–9.
28. Simpson JL. Incidence and timing of pregnancy losses: Relevance to evaluating safety of early prenatal diagnosis. *Am J Med Genet* 1990;35:165–73.
29. Ghidini A, Sepulveda W, Lockwood CJ, Romero R. Complications of fetal blood sampling. *Am J Obstet Gynecol* 1993;168: 1339.
30. Moise KJ Jr. Management of rhesus alloimmunization in pregnancy. *Obstet Gynecol* 2002;100:600–11.
31. Stefos T, Cosmi E, Detti L, Mari G. Correction of fetal anemia on the middle cerebral artery peak systolic velocity. *Obstet Gynecol* 2002;99:211–5.
32. Abdel-Fattah SA, Soothill PW, Carroll SG, Kyle PM. Noninvasive diagnosis of anemia in hydrops fetalis with the use of middle cerebral artery Doppler velocity. *Am J Obstet Gynecol* 2001;185:1411–5.
33. Gembruch U, Baschat AA. Circulatory effects of acute bradycardia in the human fetus as studied by Doppler ultrasound. *Ultrasound Obstet Gynecol* 2000;15:424–7.
34. Mari G, Moise KJ Jr, Deter RL, Carpenter RJ Jr, Wasserstrum N. Fetal heart rate influence on the pulsatility index in the middle cerebral artery. *J Clin Ultrasound* 1991;19:149–53.
35. Gokay Z, Ozcan T, Copel JA. Changes in fetal hemodynamics with ritodrine tocolysis. *Ultrasound Obstet Gynecol* 2001;18:44–6.
36. Shono M, Shono H, Sugimori H. Dynamic changes in the middle cerebral artery perfusion in normal full-term human fetuses in relation to the timing of behavioral state. *Early Hum Dev* 2000;58:57–67.
37. Yagel S, Anteby E, Lavy Y, et al. Fetal middle cerebral artery blood flow during normal active labour and in labour with variable decelerations. *Br J Obstet Gynecol* 1992;99:483–5.
38. Wladimiroff J, Tonge H, Stewart P, *et al.* Severe intrauterine growth retardation: Assessment of its origin from fetal arterial flow velocity waveforms. *Eur J Obstet Gynecol Reprod Biol* 1986;22:23–8.
39. Vyas S, Nicolaides KH, Bower S, Campbell S. Middle cerebral artery flow velocity waveforms in fetal hypoxaemia. *Br J Obstet Gynaecol* 1990;97:797–803.
40. Mari G, Deter R. Middle cerebral artery flow velocity waveforms in normal and small-for-gestational age fetuses. *Am J Obstet Gynecol* 1992;166:1262–70.
41. Johnson P, Stojilkovic T, Sarkar P. Middle cerebral artery Doppler in severe intrauterine growth restriction. *Ultrasound Obstet Gynecol* 2001;17:416–20.
42. Humprey W, Magoon M, O'Shaughnessy R. Severe nonimmune hydrops secondary to parvovirus B19 infection: Spontaneous reversal *in utero* and survival of a term infant. *Obstet Gynecol* 1991;78:900–2.
43. Pryde PG, Nugent CE, Pridjian G, Barr M Jr, Faix RG. Spontaneous resolution of nonimmune hydrops fetalis secondary to human parvovirus B 19 infection. *Obstet Gynecol* 1992;79: 859–61.
44. Cardwell MS. Successful treatment of hydrops fetalis caused by fetomaternal hemorrhage: A case report. *Am J Obstet Gynecol* 1988;158:131–2.
45. Thorp JA, Cohen GR, Yeast JD, *et al.* Nonimmune hydrops caused by massive fetomaternal hemorrhage and treated by intravascular transfusion. *Am J Perinatol* 1992;9:22–4.
46. Montgomery LD, Belfort MA, Karolina A. Massive fetomaternal hemorrhage treated with combined intravascular and intraperitoneal fetal transfusions. *Am J Obstet Gynecol* 1995;173: 234–4.
47. Baschat AA, Harman CR, Alger LS, Weiner CP. Fetal coronary and cerebral blood flow in acute fetomaternal hemorrhage. *Ultrasound Obstet Gynecol* 1998;12:128–31.
48. Jaffe R, Woods JR. Doppler velocimetry of intraplacental fetal vessels in the second trimester: Improving the prediction of pregnancy complications in high-risk patients. *Ultrasound Obstet Gynecol* 1996;8:262–6.
49. Haberman S, Friedman ZM. Intraplacental spectral Doppler scanning: Fetal growth classification based on Doppler velocimetry. *Gynecol Obstet Invest* 1997;43:11–9.
50. Bose C. Hydrops fetalis and *in utero* intracranial hemorrhage. *J Pediatr* 1978;93:1023–4.
51. Hanigan WC, Ali MB, Cusack TJ, Miller TC, Shah JJ. Diagnosis of subdural hemorrhage *in utero*. *J Neurosurg* 1985;63:977–9.
52. Daffos F, Forestier F, Muller JY, *et al.* Prenatal treatment of alloimmune thrombocytopenia. *Lancet* 1984;2(8403):632.

48 Doppler ultrasound studies of the fetal pulmonary circulation

D. C. Wood Jr. and J. P. Räsänen

The fetal lungs may be quickly evaluated for size and function by observation using real-time ultrasound: there should be adequate amniotic fluid but there should be no thoracic fluid spaces, cysts or echo dense areas. The size of the lungs should occupy about 2/3 the area of the thoracic cavity in a transverse plane at the level of the four-chamber view of the heart. The heart should have a normal 45° axis from the sternal/spine axis in the levocardia position and occupy the other third of the chest cavity. The pulmonary outflow tract should emerge from the heart aiming toward the left shoulder and cross anteriorly over the aortic outflow tract that aims toward the right shoulder. While these observations of normality in the first half of the second trimester will typically rule out most forms of congenital heart disease, pulmonary obstructions and anomalous venous connections will typically be missed at anatomic fetal ultrasound. In the second half of pregnancy, diaphragmatic fetal breathing movements may reassure the observer of normal physiologic growth of the lungs, but this does not rule out lethal pulmonary hypoplasia. However, changes in lung size and heart position may be signs of potential neonatal pulmonary hypoplasia and hypertension problems (Figure 48.1).

The fetal pulmonary circulation consists of the pulmonary arteries, ductus arteriosus and pulmonary veins, all of which may be identified with ultrasound by 16 weeks' gestation. However, subtle differences in the circulation of the fetal lungs and the vascular connections to the heart require interrogations of the venous and arterial Doppler color and spectral flow patterns. These investigations may be both difficult and time consuming because of fetal lie and movement, maternal habitus and the presence of fetal breathing and may require an advanced ultrasound system. It is important to remember that normal appearing fetal lungs and normal cardiac situs can be seen with any major structural cardiac abnormality including pulmonary atresia and totally anomalous pulmonary venous connection.

Pulmonary angiogenesis

The cardiovascular system is the first organ developed in the embryonic period: primitive blood vessels are in place to accommodate the output of the heart, which begins to beat in the human fetus as early as 19 gestational days. Endothelial cells are the earliest specialized cells. They form endothelial tubes and recruit precursors to smooth muscle cells that form the arteries, arterioles, veins and venules. Proliferation, migration, matrix production and contractile protein

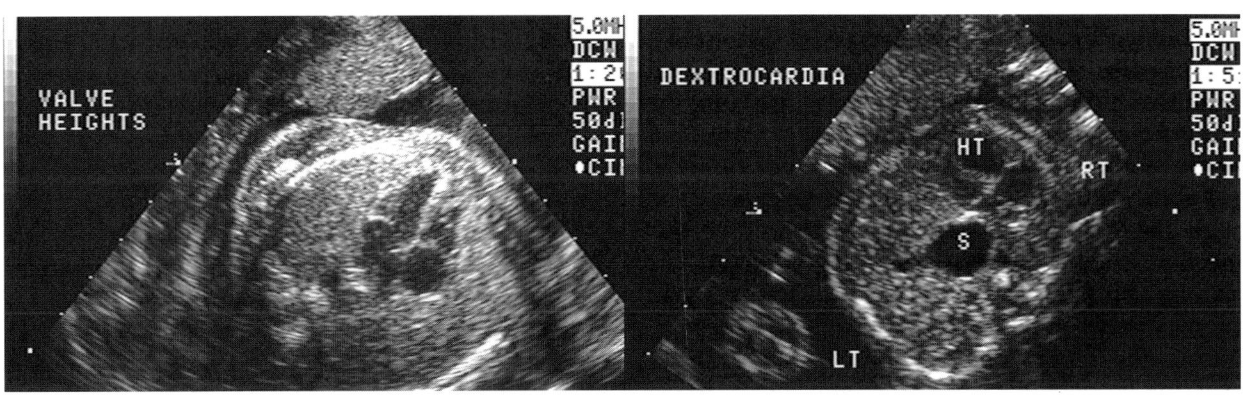

Figure 48.1 Four-chamber heart in the transverse thorax view with normal size lungs and diaphragmatic hernia with small lungs.

expression characterize early circulatory development.[1] Vasculogenesis within the primitive lungs may be considered to be of constant capillary production, fusion and regression. During the embryonic period, the lung appears as a ventral diverticulum of the foregut that becomes separated in a caudo-cranial direction from the future esophagus by the laryngyotracheal grooves. By day 26, that developing bud divides and grows into the surrounding mesenchyme into right and left lungs.[2] Blood is pumped from the heart into the common truncus arteriosus which divides into paired right and left branches which connect to the dorsal aorta via various arches, most of which will regress and disappear. The sixth or most proximal arch connection to the distal aorta is maintained throughout fetal life, typically on the left side, as the ductus arteriosus. The sixth arch vessel gives rise to the main branches of the pulmonary arteries, and, with the helical division of the truncus and muscular division of the conotruncus, becomes the main pulmonary artery, the anterior vessel originating from the right ventricular outflow tract. At the same time, a bud develops from the dorsal surface of the sinoatrial part of the heart, which divides and connects with the pulmonary plexus. As the atria expand, this single pulmonary vein is carried into the right atrium but eventually becomes absorbed into the left atrium as four separate ostia. Therefore, the pulmonary veins actually drain into the systemic venous system until about day 30, when they become the proximal pulmonary veins of the left atrium. In anomalous migratory patterns, the pulmonary veins can continue with their connection as a common venous sack, draining to the ascending vein of Marshall to the innominate vein to the superior vena cava, to a connection below the diaphragm to the hepatic veins, or continue in part or completely attached to the right atrium or the vena caval connections to the right atrium.

Pulmonary development in the postembryonic fetus has been studied extensively in various animal models and has generally divided into three overlapping morphological stages: the pseudoglandular lung, the canalicular lung and the sacular stage of the viable lung.[3] Development of the human pulmonary vasculature is closely timed to cardiac development. In the human embryo at 5 weeks, it has been shown that the upper poles of the right and left lungs are supplied by primitive pulmonary arteries, which arise from the sixth aortic arch between the pulmonary trunk and the dorsal aorta. The lower poles are supplied from the dorsal aorta via intersegmental arteries that penetrate through the diaphragm. Anomalous growth at this connection leads to pulmonary sequestration. As the branching bronchi develop, so do the aligned pulmonary veins and arteries.

During the early pseudoglandular period (5–17 weeks), the bronchial system has formed such that at each airway generation, there is an accompanying artery, in addition to supernumerary bronchial arteries which supply the major airways and pulmonary arteries.[4] The lung therefore possesses two vascular systems: a low pressure pulmonary system and a high pressure bronchial system. By the end of the pseudoglandular period, Kitaoka *et al.* counted 20 generations of airways with their accompanying arteries; the adult human lung averages 24 generations.[5] During this period, the growth in veins and arteries is enormous, not in total length or volume, but in the number of generations.

The canalicular stage (16–26 weeks) represents the development of the gas exchange tissues. During this period, pulmonary capillary expansion corresponds to epithelial cell differentiation that permits the formation of thin air–blood barriers and surfactant production. The tremendous growth of the capillary system into the lung parenchyma gives rise to the concept of 'canals' and gives the lungs a spongy appearance. Arteries and veins develop both in length and diameter as they follow the growth of the preacinar airways.

The saccular stage of lung development (24 weeks to birth) is demarcated by the expansion of the alveolar spaces. The interstitium between the airspaces contain the capillary system and the development of a network of elastic fibers where the postnatal interalveolar wall will be located. The arterial pathways increase in length and diameter. It has been shown that the diameter of the artery is a function of the distance from the previous branching such that the diameters are constant at a given distance from the end of the alveolar tree.[6] Arterial growth is faster centrally than in the periphery. Distally, the number of additional branches grows exponentially. The intrapulmonary veins begin to grow the circular muscular layer of mature vessels during the saccular period. The function of the lung tissue changes dramatically with birth but the structure is not radically altered (Figure 48.2).

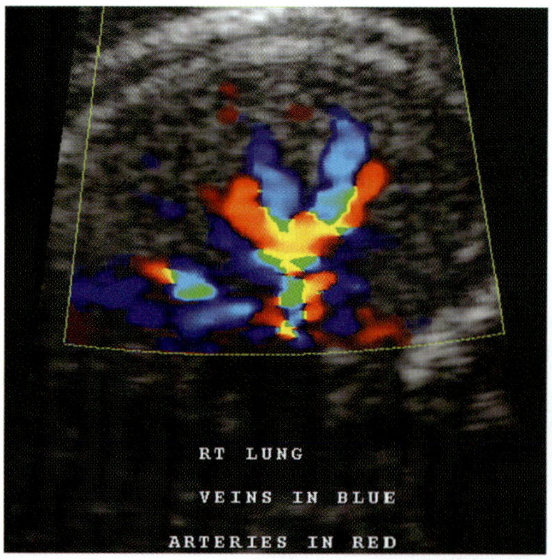

Figure 48.2 Color Doppler image of pulmonary vascularity.

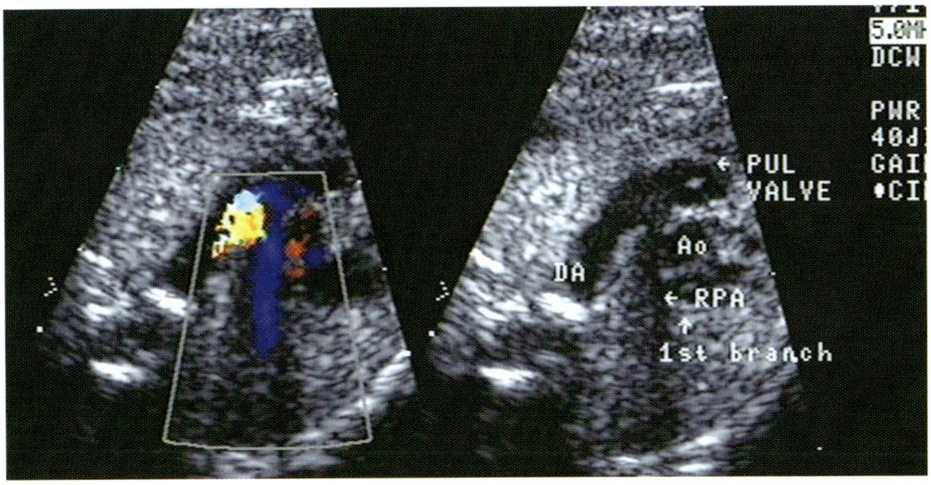

Figure 48.3 Site of pulmonary Doppler imaging.

Pulmonary vascular resistance (impedance)

Fetal pulmonary arterial vascular impedance decreases significantly during the second half of pregnancy. The linear decrease in the vascular impedance during the second trimester and in the beginning of the third trimester may be related to the growth of the lung and to the increase in the number of resistance vessels. During the latter part of the third trimester pulmonary vascular impedance does not decrease further. In a cross-sectional study of 100 uncomplicated singleton pregnancies we evaluated human fetal pulmonary blood flow by Doppler techniques to analyze the relationships between proximal and distal pulmonary arterial blood velocity waveforms and to determine normal pulmonary arterial vascular impedance and physiologic parameters in proximal and distal branch pulmonary arteries. We found that high resistance, high pressure and low blood flow characterize the fetal pulmonary circulation throughout pregnancy.[7]

Using color Doppler to identify and align the vessel in a position parallel to the pulsed Doppler beam, a narrow sample volume was placed into the proximal part of the branch pulmonary artery immediately after the bifurcation of the main pulmonary artery. Using color Doppler guidance in a high resolution magnification imaging mode, distal pulmonary arteries beyond the first bifurcation of the branch pulmonary artery were identified and waveforms were obtained during fetal apnea and in the absence of fetal body movements (Figure 48.3). Waveforms were also measured at the aortic and pulmonary valve levels and at the ductus arteriosus. Proximal left and right pulmonary artery diameters were measured from captured real-time images. In each fetus, a sagittal section right lung length was measured from the tip of the apex to the base of the lung on the dome of the diaphragm during fetal apnea, as described by Roberts and Mitchell.[8] Proximal right pulmonary artery Doppler measurements were obtained successfully in 98% of cases and proximal left pulmonary artery Doppler measurements in 96% of cases, respectively. In the distal pulmonary artery, success rate on the right side was 88% and on the left side 94%.

During the second half of pregnancy the pulsatility index (PI) values in both proximal and distal left and right pulmonary arteries decreased and the systolic peak velocities and time to peak velocity (TTP) intervals increased significantly. In the proximal branch pulmonary arteries, a near linear decrease in the PI values was detected until 34–35 weeks of gestation, while in the distal pulmonary arteries, after 31 weeks of gestation there was no significant decrease in the PI-value. Respectively, peak systolic velocities in the proximal branch pulmonary arteries increased in a linear fashion until 30 weeks of gestation and remained unchanged until term. Proximal and distal pulmonary arterial TTP-intervals were significantly shorter at 18–22 weeks of gestation and at term (36–40 weeks) than at the pulmonary valve. The TTP-interval at the ductus arteriosus was shown to be significantly longer than at the pulmonary or aortic valves. TTP-intervals at the aortic valve were significantly longer than at the pulmonary valve. In this study population, the fetal heart rate did not change significantly during the second half of pregnancy. There were no significant differences in PI values, peak systolic velocities, TTP-intervals or pulmonary artery diameters between right and left proximal and distal pulmonary arteries. Both proximal right and left pulmonary arterial diameters, as well as the right lung length, increased significantly during the second half of pregnancy, demonstrating a 2.5-fold increase in their respective measurements.

In the proximal pulmonary arteries the PI-values and peak systolic velocities were significantly higher

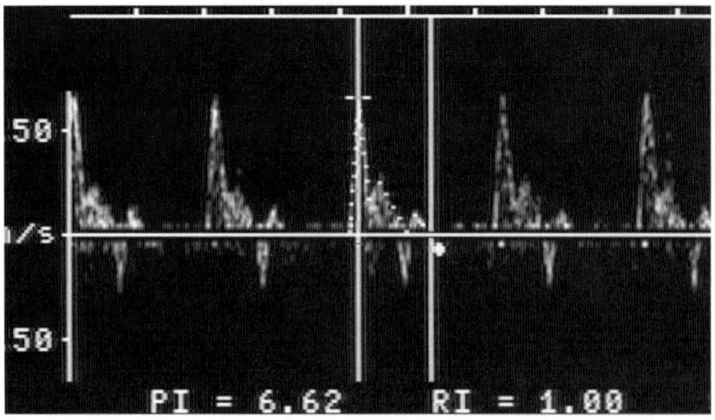

Figure 48.4 Distal pulmonary artery waveforms.

and TTP-intervals were significantly longer when compared with the distal pulmonary arteries. The ratio between the peak systolic velocities in proximal and distal pulmonary arteries decreased significantly with advancing gestational age. However, the ratio between the proximal and distal branch pulmonary artery PI values did not vary significantly during the study period. This study demonstrated that ultrasound techniques may be used to evaluate human fetal pulmonary circulation as early as 18 weeks of gestation.

The shape of the proximal branch pulmonary arterial Doppler velocity waveform profile is unique in the fetal circulation (Figure 48.4). It is characterized by rapid initial flow acceleration followed by a very early and rapid deceleration phase, producing a needle-like systolic peak followed by a short, but relatively stable systolic flow segment culminating in a gradual decay in systolic flow. At the beginning of diastole, proximal branch pulmonary artery blood flow patterns demonstrate a short reverse flow interval following either no or a small amount of diastolic flow. The fetal branch pulmonary artery Doppler tracing is similar to that obtained by direct invasive blood flow recordings in fetal lambs.[9] Fetal growth during the second half of pregnancy is characterized by a 2.5-fold increase in the lung length, as well as in the diameters of proximal pulmonary arteries. The significant decrease in the PI values in both proximal and distal pulmonary arteries during the study period suggests a significant decrease in the pulmonary vascular impedance. There is no difference in changes in the pulmonary vascular impedance between the right and left lungs during the second half of pregnancy.

The PI patterns in the distal and proximal pulmonary arteries during the second half of pregnancy are different. In the distal pulmonary arteries the decrease in the PI values reaches the plateau stage around 31 weeks of gestation, while in the proximal pulmonary arteries the PI values decrease in a linear fashion until 34–35 weeks of gestation. In fetal lambs, a 40-fold increase in the total number of the fifth and sixth generation vessels and a fourfold increase in the lung weight characterize the latter part of gestation.[10] The medial width of these vessels remains unchanged throughout the gestation. In our study, distal pulmonary arteries represent at least the third generation vessels, and in these segments, the linearly decreasing vascular impedance during the latter part of the second trimester represents the increase in the number of resistance vessels. The vascular impedance does not decrease markedly during the third trimester of pregnancy.

It is assumed that the phenomenon of wave reflection in a vascular bed is closely related to impedance. From the heart to the periphery, the pulsatility of pressure waves progressively increases while the flow velocity waves decline. This explains the difference between the proximal and distal branch pulmonary artery PI values. The forward propagating waves of pressure and flow demonstrate the same configuration, but after wave reflection, the retrograde flow waves are inverted, while the retrograde pressure waves are not. Wave reflections occur mainly in arterial system at the level of arterial–arteriolar junctions.[11]

Vasodilatation decreases the wave reflection and impedance while increasing flow.[12] The changes in the branch pulmonary arterial vascular impedance are similar to changes in the fetoplacental vascular impedance during the same pregnancy period. The continuing angiogenesis in both the fetoplacental unit and fetal lung causes diminished wave reflections associated with progressively declining vascular impedance. If the angiogenesis or angiomorphology is abnormal in the fetoplacental unit this vascular pathology results in increased vascular impedance associated with enhanced wave reflections (increased systolic to diastolic ratio).[13] We speculate that the failure of angiogenesis in fetal lungs could cause similar changes in vascular impedance, increasing the pulsatility of the Doppler waveform. The plateau stage, especially in the distal pulmonary artery vascular impedance during the third trimester, could be explained by acquired vasoconstriction in the pulmonary circulation, even though the number of resistance vessels is increasing in a linear fashion during this period according to animal studies.[14] However, other factors affect the regulation of the pulmonary circulation. For example, prostaglandin I_2 production is increased after lung distention, distortion or spontaneous ventilation of fetal lungs without changes in O_2 environment producing pulmonary vasodilatation.[15]

The changes in the peak systolic velocities support the concept that during the last trimester, the decrease in pulmonary vascular impedance reaches the plateau stage. Fetal lamb studies have revealed that an increase in the pulmonary vascular resistance due to hypoxia reduces the magnitude and duration of the forward flow in pulmonary arteries, while acetylcholine, which is a potent pulmonary vasodilator, produces a marked increase in the magnitude

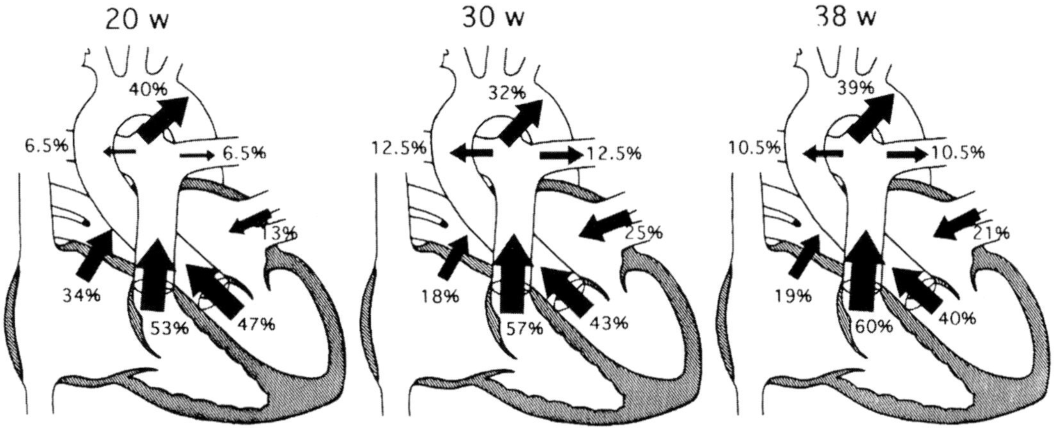

Figure 48.5 Distribution of fetal cardiac output.

and duration of systolic flow and reduces or eliminates backflow.[16] However, peak systolic velocities are not only affected by changes in afterload or vascular impedance, but also by fetal cardiac contractility, compliance, size of the vessels, and the distance between the point of measurement and the fetal heart will affect peak systolic velocities.

TTP-intervals increased significantly from 18 to 22 weeks of gestation to term in all the vessels examined, while the fetal heart rate was unchanged. At the pulmonary valve level the TTP-interval was significantly longer than in the proximal and distal pulmonary arteries and significantly shorter than in the aortic valve level and ductus arteriosus. These findings are partially in agreement with Machado *et al.*, concerning difference between aortic and pulmonary TTP-intervals[17] and with Choi *et al.* and Hata *et al.* demonstrating significant increases in aortic, pulmonary and ductal TTP-intervals with increasing gestation.[18,19] Invasive animal studies have shown significant increase in both mean systemic and pulmonary arterial pressures with advancing gestation. Mean pulmonary arterial pressure is higher than mean systemic pressure throughout gestation.[20] These findings parallel significant increases in cardiac output, peak systolic velocities, vessel size and by significant decrease in the placental vascular impedance. The difference in the mean arterial pressures and TTP-intervals may therefore be explained by the differences in end organ impedance: the placenta for the systemic circulation and the lung parenchyma for the pulmonary circulation. There is a structural obstruction in the ductus arteriosus that accelerates outflow into the descending aorta and increase the PI above that of the main pulmonary artery.[21] We speculate that during the latter part of the second trimester and in the beginning of the third trimester, the decrease in the vascular impedance may be related to the growth of the lung and especially to the increase in the number of resistance vessels. During the latter part of the third trimester, the pulmonary vascular impedance does not decrease further.

Pulmonary blood flow effects on fetal combined cardiac output

The human fetal pulmonary circulation has an important role in the distribution of the cardiac output.[22] The latter part of the second and the beginning of the third trimester is characterized by a decrease in the pulmonary vascular resistance and an increase in the proportion of pulmonary blood flow of the fetal combined cardiac output. This proportion is higher in human fetuses than suggested by previous animal studies. The proportion of blood flow across the foramen ovale decreases. Later during the last trimester, the pulmonary vascular resistance increases again. The proportion of pulmonary blood flow of the fetal combined cardiac output remains about 20% during this period, and is proportionate to that of the foramen ovale blood flow. Right ventricular dominance persists and even increases towards the end of pregnancy (Figure 48.5).

We studied 63 normal singleton fetuses in uncomplicated pregnancies referred for fetal echocardiography in a cross-sectional manner between 19 and 39 weeks of gestation (median 28 weeks) to establish the relative outputs of the left and right ventricles. The normal distribution of human fetal combined cardiac output from the left and right ventricles was determined and the weight-indexed pulmonary (*R*pi) and systemic (*R*si) vascular resistances and the changes during the second half of pregnancy were established.

Volumetric blood flow was calculated by using the formula: Q=fetal heart rate × valve area × time velocity integral. Left ventricular cardiac output

(LVCO) equals the blood flow through the aortic valve. Right ventricular cardiac output (RVCO) equals the blood flow through the pulmonary valve. Combined cardiac output (CCO) is the sum of LVCO and RVCO. Total pulmonary artery blood flow (Q_P) was calculated by combining right and left pulmonary artery blood flows. We calculated blood flows across the aortic and pulmonary valve annuli, right and left pulmonary arteries and ductus arteriosus. Foramen ovale blood flow was estimated by the formula $Q_{FO}=\text{LVCO}-Q_P$.

Biometric weight-indexed pulmonary and systemic vascular resistances were calculated by using the formula: $R_i=P/Q_i$, where P is the blood pressure (mmHg) and Q_i is the weight indexed volume blood flow (ml/min/kg). These indexes were analyzed at 20, 30 and 38 weeks of gestation. Systemic blood flow (Q_{Si}) was calculated by pulmonary volume blood flow from CCO. The mean transpulmonary pressure gradient was assumed to be equal to mean systemic blood pressure. At 20 weeks of gestation human fetal blood pressure is about 30–35 mmHg.[23] At 30 and 38 weeks of gestation fetal blood pressure values were assumed from values in newborns at the same gestational age.[24]

From 20 to 30 weeks of gestation the proportion of pulmonary blood flow (Q_P) of the CCO doubled (from 13 to 25%), while the proportion of flow across the foramen ovale (Q_{FO}) decreased by half (from 34 to 18%). After 30 weeks of gestation the proportions of Q_P and Q_{FO} remained unchanged. At 38 weeks of gestation, the proportion of RVCO (60%) was higher than that of LVCO (40%). The proportion of flow across the ductus arteriosus (Q_{DA}) did not change significantly. The correlation between RVCO calculated from blood flow across the pulmonary valve to the combined Q_{DA} and Q_P was excellent. R_Pi decreased from 20 to 30 weeks of gestation but increased from 30 to 38 weeks of gestation. However, R_Si continuously increased from 20 to 38 weeks of gestation. Thus, the R_{Pi}/R_{Si} decreased from 20 to 30 weeks of gestation and later remained unchanged.

The area and TVI of aortic and pulmonary valves, ductus arteriosus and branch pulmonary arteries increased significantly with advancing gestational age as did right and left ventricular stroke volumes. RVSV/LVSV ratio was greater at term of pregnancy than at 20 weeks of gestation. Fetal CCO, RVCO and LVCO increased more than 10-fold from 20 weeks to term, and Q_{DA}, Q_{FO} and Q_P also increased significantly with advancing gestation. The PV area, RVSV and RVCO were greater than AV area, LVSV and LVCO. The ratio between diameters of the pulmonary valve and the ductus arteriosus increased significantly from 20 weeks of gestation toward the term of pregnancy. The DA area was always greater than LPA or RPA area, but the ratio of LPA or RPA to DA area increased significantly with advancing gestation. There were no significant differences in the area, TVI or volume blood flow between right and left pulmonary arteries. The proportions of Q_P and Q_{FO} of the CCO remained unchanged from 30 to 38 weeks of gestation.

During the third trimester, the proportion of Q_P of the LVCO is about 50% suggesting that the Q_P contribution to the LVCO increases with advancing gestation. These measurements concur with previously published estimates.[25] Our results show that the proportion of Q_P of the human fetal CCO is clearly higher than suggested in previously published animal studies, where the proportion of Q_P of the CCO was estimated at less than 10%.[26,27]

Volume blood flow across the FO is very difficult to assess directly. The cross-sectional area of the FO is difficult to calculate accurately because of the shape and relative size and position of the flap tissue of the septum primum and the fact that the blood velocity waveform is multiphasic during the cardiac cycle.[28] However, our measurements correlated with published diameters of the FO and showed linear increase with advancing gestation.[29] In our study, the Q_{FO} increased fourfold, but its proportion of the CCO decreased by half from 20 weeks to term. At 20 weeks of gestation it represents about 73% of the LVCO, but after 30 weeks of gestation its proportion has decreased to about 50% of the LVCO. In the human fetus, the Q_{FO} has an important role, because highly oxygenated blood returning from the placenta is directed via the ductus venosus across the FO to the left atrium.[30] Thus the most oxygenated blood from the placenta is supplied to the fetal coronary and cerebral circulations. Our findings suggest that during the third trimester, the FO becomes relatively restrictive and therefore unable to increase its proportion of the CCO. This supports proportional right ventricular dominance in the human fetus during the last trimester of pregnancy. After 20 weeks of gestation, the right ventricular output becomes dominant. At 38 weeks of gestation RVCO (60%) significantly exceeds LVCO (40%) as a proportion of the CCO, which may explain the appearance of relative RV > LV disproportion seen in late third-trimester fetuses.

Effects of indomethacin treatment on pulmonary circulation

Maternally administered indomethacin used as tocolysis is transferred across the placenta to the fetus.[31] Maternal and fetal serum levels of indomethacin are identical after few hours of maternal oral administration of indomethacin.[32] Indomethacin is known to reduce fetal urine output leading to decreased amniotic fluid volume.[33] Another well-known effect of indomethacin on the fetus is the constriction or even occlusion of the ductus arteriosus.[34] It is evident that the prevalence of indomethacin-induced fetal ductal constriction increases with advancing gestational age.[35,36] These

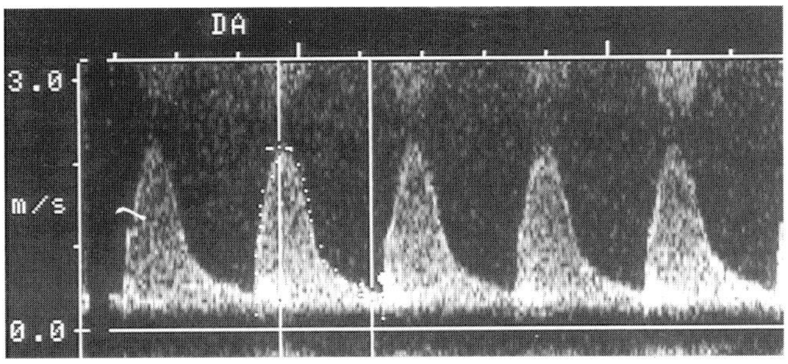

Figure 48.6 Ductal constriction with high velocity and increased diastolic flow.

fetal side effects of indomethacin are usually reversible after either reducing the indomethacin dose or stopping the indomethacin therapy.[37] Maternal indomethacin therapy affects human fetal pulmonary arterial vascular impedance.[38]

In a cross-sectional study, we compared Doppler echocardiographic findings in three groups of fetuses between 24 and 34 weeks of gestation. Fifty-two normal fetuses were without maternal medication, while 33 fetuses without constriction of the ductus arteriosus, 15 fetuses with mild to moderate and 8 fetuses with severe ductal constriction occlusion during maternal indomethacin therapy. The indication for maternal indomethacin therapy was preterm labor; the daily indomethacin dose varied between 50 and 200 mg. Blood velocity waveforms across the ductus, aortic and pulmonary valves, and proximal right or left pulmonary artery were obtained. The constriction of the ductus arteriosus was defined as mild to moderate when the pulsatility index of the ductus arteriosus varied between 1.0 and 1.9. The ductal constriction was defined as severe if the PI value was less than 1.0. During the second half of pregnancy normal values for the PI of the ductus arteriosus are between 1.9 and 3.0.[39] Occlusion of the fetal ductus arteriosus was diagnosed when no blood flow across the ductus arteriosus could be identified by color, continuous or pulsed Doppler techniques but tricuspid regurgitation was identified (Figure 48.6).

Pulsatility indices were measured in the peripheral pulmonary arteries and left and right ventricular outflows. Combined cardiac outputs were calculated. The pulsatility of the peripheral pulmonary arteries was constantly greater in the indomethacin fetuses than in the control group. After 26 weeks gestation, the values in the mild to moderate group were significantly higher than in the control group. In the study groups I and II, LVCO, RVCO and CCO were similar to the control group. In the study group III, RVCO and CCO were lower than in the control group. Only LVCO did not differ from the control group. Human fetal pulmonary arterial vascular impedance is increased by maternal indomethacin therapy even without ductal constriction. In the presence of mild to moderate DC the magnitude of the increase in the vascular impedance is related to the gestational age. In the group with severe ductal constriction or occlusion of DA pulmonary vascular impedance is similar to the control group. In this group, decreased RVCO and CCO without significantly increased LVCO show that these fetuses were unable to redistribute the cardiac output from the right to the left ventricle. Interestingly, the newborns with ductal occlusion in utero did not show any signs of pulmonary hypertension during the neonatal period.

Prostaglandins are potent vasoactive substances, which have a role in the pulmonary vascular changes occurring after birth. Prostaglandins D2, E1 and I2 have been shown to be fetal pulmonary vasodilators in near term animal models.[40] Indomethacin, which is a prostaglandin synthetase inhibitor, may affect fetal pulmonary function by decreasing lung liquid production and altering pulmonary hemodynamics. During rhythmic distention of the lungs in the fetal lambs, prostaglandin synthetase inhibitors have been demonstrated to abolish the fourfold decrease in pulmonary vascular resistance seen without prostaglandin inhibitors.[41,42] However, indomethacin has not been shown to change the pulmonary vascular response to increased oxygen tension in fetal lambs.[43] In the presence of indomethacin-induced ductal constriction in fetal lambs, the smooth muscle has been found to be significantly increased and the external diameter decreased in the fifth generation resistance vessels in the lung tissue compared to control fetuses.[44] Also, in fetal lambs the acute mechanically induced occlusion of the ductus arteriosus decreases the total fetal cardiac output by about 34%.[45] We have earlier demonstrated that pulmonary vascular impedance decreases significantly during the second half of pregnancy until 34–35 weeks of gestation and thereafter it remains unchanged. Likewise, weight-indexed pulmonary vascular resistance decreases significantly from 20 to 30 weeks of gestation and increases again from 30 to 38 weeks of gestation.[22]

Maternal indomethacin therapy without constriction of the fetal ductus arteriosus is associated with higher PI values in the branch pulmonary arteries than in the control fetuses. This finding suggests that prostaglandins have a role in the regulation of the human fetal pulmonary circulation. In fetuses with mild to moderate ductal constriction, the PI values were higher and the average weekly change in the PI values was significantly different from the control group. This suggests that after 27–28 weeks of gestation the human fetus is able to regulate branch pulmonary arterial vascular tone in response to increased pulmonary arterial pressure. In the group with severe constriction or occlusion of the ductus arteriosus the PI values of the branch pulmonary arteries were not different from the control group showing that further increase in the pulmonary arterial pressure overcomes the regulatory capacity of the pulmonary circulation. In these fetuses right ventricular and combined cardiac outputs were less than in the control group, while the left ventricular cardiac output remained similar to the control group demonstrating that these fetuses were not able to redistribute the cardiac output from the right to the left ventricle.

The effects of right ventricular loading conditions on pulmonary circulation

The equation for ventricular ejection force estimates the energy transferred from the ventricular myocardial shortening to work done by accelerating blood into the circulation. This information can be used for the assessment of the ventricular systolic function. Ventricular ejection force does not require estimation of ventricular volumes and is independent of ventricular configuration. Newton's second law of motion defines force as the product of mass and acceleration: force = mass × acceleration. The mass of blood accelerated across the aortic and pulmonary valves over a time interval is calculated by multiplying the density of blood, which is 1.055, with the cross-sectional area (CSA) and the TVI at the valve. The acceleration component is calculated by dividing peak systolic velocity by the time to peak velocity interval.[46] Ventricular ejection force (EFo) is calculated by using the formula: $EFo = (1.055 \times CSA \times TVI_{ac}) \times (PSV/TTP)$. In adults, a close correlation has been found between the mean left ventricular ejection force and ejection fraction suggesting that Doppler echocardiography can be used for the noninvasive assessment of right and left ventricular performance. The mean left ventricular ejection force has been shown to be more sensitive for the diagnosis of mild to moderate left ventricular systolic dysfunction than the peak aortic blood velocity or mean acceleration.[47]

Human fetal right and left ventricular ejection forces both increase 10-fold during the second half of gestation.[48,49] There is no significant difference between the right and left ventricular ejection forces *in utero*. Right ventricular performance is modified by abnormal loading conditions: it is increased by a chronic volume overload and decreased by an acute pressure overload. These findings demonstrate that the human fetal right ventricle is able to adapt its systolic function when it is facing chronically increased volume load. Pressure overload against the right ventricle must be dramatically increased as in severe ductal constriction or occlusion before the right ventricular ejection force (RVEF) decreases demonstrating the capability of the right ventricle to maintain its systolic performance.[50] In growth-retarded fetuses both ventricular ejection forces are reduced compared to normal fetuses as related to the severity of fetal compromise. Animal studies have suggested that early systolic flow is less affected by changes in afterload and preload than flow during late systole.[51,52]

To determine whether abnormal loading conditions can modify human fetal right ventricular ejection force, we studied 73 normal fetuses, 27 fetuses with hypoplastic left heart syndrome, 14 fetuses with mild to moderate constriction of the ductus arteriosus and 7 fetuses with severe constriction or occlusion of the ductus arteriosus. In the normal and ductal constriction/occlusion groups, blood velocity waveforms were recorded at the level of the aortic and pulmonary valves, and in the group with hypoplastic left heart syndrome (HLHS) at the level of the pulmonary valve. The ventricular ejection forces were calculated. In the HLHS group, seven patients terminated the pregnancy after diagnosis and there was one stillborn fetus. Except for one newborn, who had a heart transplant operation, others underwent three-stage palliative cardiac surgery. All the fetuses in the HLHS group had a normal karyotype. In the ductal occlusion or constriction groups there were no perinatal or neonatal deaths.

In the normal group, right and left ventricular ejection forces increased and were equal during the second half of gestation. The average weekly increases were greater in the hypoplastic left heart syndrome group than in the normal group. In the group with mild to moderate ductal constriction, both ventricular ejection forces were similar to those of the normal group. The average weekly increase was lower in the group with severe ductal constriction or occlusion than in the normal group, but the LVEF did not differ from that of the normal group. This study showed that chronic volume overload increases and relatively acute pressure overload decreases human fetal RVEF.

Increased chronic volume load (HLHS group) was associated with increased ejection force developed by the right ventricle. This demonstrates the capacity of the right ventricle to adapt its systolic performance and to maintain adequate cardiac output. This also shows that chronic volume overload the right ventricular ejection force rises with other parameters of ventricular size, i.e. mass, end-diastolic volume and stroke volume. In fetuses with anemia due to red cell alloimmunization, intravascular transfusion, which represents acute volume overload transiently, decreases fetal cardiac output with a recovery to baseline levels by the day following the correction of the anemia.[53,54] It has been proposed that relative hyperviscosity secondary to the acute correction of anemia during the transfusion increases the afterload. The transient decrease in the cardiac output could also represent the time period needed for the adaptation of the ventricles to the acute volume overload.

Severe ductal constriction or occlusion significantly decreased right ventricular ejection force, possibly because of tricuspid regurgitation in this group. However, right ventricular ejection force was similar in fetuses with holosystolic tricuspid regurgitation to those without tricuspid regurgitation. Rizzo *et al.*[55] showed that in fetal intrauterine growth restriction secondary to uteroplacental insufficiency, both ventricular ejection forces were symmetrically decreased. A direct relationship was present between ejection force and umbilical vein pH values, suggesting that decreased ejection force was primarily caused by myocardial dysfunction. In ductal constriction or occlusion groups, there were no signs of placental insufficiency and the growth of the fetuses was appropriate for gestational age in all cases. Also during fetal ductal constriction the umbilical artery PI is similar to or even significantly less than without constriction suggesting that fetal ductal constriction and indomethacin therapy itself are not detrimentally affecting placental impedance.[56,57] It seems that the human fetus with normal placental function is able to maintain right ventricular ejection force development until there is a dramatic increase in the right ventricular afterload. This demonstrates the capability of the right ventricle to maintain its systolic function, which seems to be disturbed only after the pulmonary artery diastolic pressure is significantly increased. We believe that in cases of severe ductal constriction or occlusion, which develops in a short time interval, the right ventricular systolic pressure is increased without myocardial hypertrophy leading to increased systolic wall tension and myocardial oxygen consumption. During that period, the FO becomes relatively restrictive because its fixed dimension and ability to increase blood flow is limited, which results in a decreased combined cardiac output.

Effects of maternally administered oxygen on fetal pulmonary circulation

Maternal hyperoxygenation decreases human fetal pulmonary arterial vascular impedance and increases pulmonary blood flow between 31 and 36 weeks of gestation. Earlier in pregnancy, between 20 and 26 weeks of gestation, maternal hyperoxygenation does not alter human fetal pulmonary circulation. These findings show that the reactivity of the human fetal pulmonary circulation to oxygen develops between these two study periods and oxygen tension in the fetus has a role in the regulation of the fetal pulmonary circulation. Fetal oxygen tension has a role in the regulation of the pulmonary circulation and in the distribution of fetal cardiac output during the latter part of the third trimester when the human fetal pulmonary arterial bed is under acquired vasoconstriction, directing right ventricular cardiac output from the pulmonary circulation to the systemic circulation. Maternal hyperoxygenation, at least after 31–36 weeks of gestation, mimics the changes in the fetal central hemodynamics, which occur after birth.[58]

To determine the role of oxygen tension on the human fetal pulmonary arterial circulation during the second half of gestation we studied 20 women between 20 and 26 weeks of gestation and 20 women between 31 and 36 weeks of gestation with normal singleton pregnancies. They were randomized to receive either 60% humidified oxygen or medical compressed air (room air) by face mask. Fetal aortic and pulmonary valve, ductus arteriosus, and right, left and distal pulmonary artery blood velocity waveforms were obtained by Doppler ultrasound before, during and after maternal administration of either 60% oxygen or room air. Left and right ventricular cardiac outputs, and DA (Q_{DA}), RPA and LPA (Q_P) volume blood flows were calculated. Foramen ovale blood flow was estimated. PI values of DA, RPA, LPA and DPA were calculated. Maternal hyperoxygenation did not change any of the measured fetal parameters between 20 and 26 weeks, while between 31 and 36 weeks the PI values of RPA, LPA and DPA decreased and the PI of DA increased. Q_P increased, and Q_{DA} and Q_{FO} decreased. LVCO and RVCO were unchanged. All changes returned to baseline after maternal hyperoxygenation were discontinued. Reactivity of the human fetal pulmonary circulation to maternal hyperoxygenation increases with advancing gestation.

The mean increase in the Q_P was 24.5% and the mean decrease in the Q_{DA} was 17.1% from the baseline values. One fetus at 36 weeks of gestation developed a reversal of diastolic blood flow in the DA during maternal hyperoxygenation (from the aorta to the pulmonary artery). The estimated Q_{FO} remained stable in groups 1, 2 and 4 during the study period whereas maternal hyperoxygenation after 30 weeks gestation decreased foramen ovale blood flow significantly. The FO blood flow decreases because the pulmonary volume blood flow increases significantly without any change in the LVCO. In fetal lambs, the FO blood flow decreases by an average of 50% during maternal hyperbaric oxygenation at near term gestation.[59] Both distal and proximal pulmonary arteries showed a similar decrease in the PI values during maternal hyperoxygenation suggesting that both sampling sites gave the same information about the pulmonary vascular reactivity.

This study supports the concept that in the human fetus the reactivity of the pulmonary arterial bed to changes in the fetal oxygen tension develops after 21–26 weeks of gestation and is detectable by noninvasive Doppler ultrasound techniques between 31 and 36 weeks of gestation. This suggest that human fetal pulmonary circulation is under acquired vasoconstriction at least after 31–36 weeks of gestation with blood flow directed from the pulmonary circulation to the systemic circulation. The reactivity of the pulmonary arterial circulation to oxygen with advancing gestation has been explained by an increasing amount of smooth muscle in small pulmonary arteries.[14] The decrease in the pulmonary vascular resistance is mainly caused by the release of endothelium derived nitric oxide, which leads to vasodilatation of the pulmonary arterial bed.[60,61]

The decrease in the pulmonary vascular impedance and the increase in the pulmonary blood flow by maternal hyperoxygenation between 31 and 36 weeks of gestation were accompanied by opposite changes in the fetal ductus arteriosus. The decrease in the DA PI has been associated with the constriction of the DA and the increase in the DA PI has been found in the cases with increased right ventricular cardiac output.[39] This study shows that the changes in the DA PI may also reflect fetal pulmonary vascular impedance. The decrease in the pulmonary vascular impedance directs blood flow from the systemic circulation to the pulmonary circulation. This mainly affects the diastolic flow component in the DA by decreasing it or even reversing the direction of the blood flow during diastole. This leads to increased PI in the DA, because the end-diastolic velocity and the mean velocity during the cardiac cycle decrease. In normal circumstances, the direction of the blood flow in the human fetal DA during the diastole is from the pulmonary artery to the aorta. This study supports previous animal data that the increase in the pulmonary blood flow and the decrease in the pulmonary vascular impedance during maternal hyperoxygenation are not caused by the constriction of the ductus arteriosus.[7,27,62] In the presence of the ductal constriction peak systolic, end-diastolic and mean velocities across the ductus arteriosus are increased in the human fetus leading to decreased PI value. These findings agree with those of Burchell *et al.* where children and adults with patent ductus arteriosus and pulmonary hypertension when breathing of a low oxygen mixture either initiated or increased the blood flow from the pulmonary artery to the aorta whereas the breathing of 100% oxygen caused opposite changes.[63]

Pulmonary hypoplasia

Pulmonary hypoplasia is a term that describes lungs that are sufficiently small enough to impede the exchange of respiratory gases leading to severe neonatal pulmonary disease or death.[64] It occurs secondarily to other fetal anomalies that restrict volumetric lung expansion. It can be associated with mediastinal shift or cardiac malposition. However, pulmonary hypoplasia is different from pulmonary agenesis where there is complete absence of a lung and from pulmonary aplasia where there is absence of a broncus or bronchiolar pathway as survival is likely with either of those two malformations. As gas exchange does not occur in the fetal lung, it is difficult to prove that fetal lungs may be functionally hypoplastic. Pulmonary hypoplasia is defined as incomplete or underdevelopment of lung tissue present at autopsy as determined by the wet lung to body weight ratio, reduced alveoli count or by reduced lung DNA content.[65] Fetal detection of pulmonary hypoplasia is based on ultrasound imaging techniques based on a reduced chest size for gestational age. The thoracic to abdominal ratio of 0.89 is relatively constant throughout gestation and a ratio of less than 0.77 is consistent with pulmonary hypoplasia.[66]

The association between pulmonary hypoplasia and reduced amniotic fluid volume was first observed in infants with bilateral renal agenesis.[67] Abnormalities that result in olighydramnios include renal agenesis, renal dysplasia and those that restrict urinary flow into the amniotic sac. Urethral atresia or stenosis, urethral valve and bladder outlet obstructions also restrict urinary flow. In pregnancies with prolonged leakage of amniotic fluid or premature rupture of the membranes may also be subject to pulmonary hypoplasia. With these conditions, it has been proposed that compression or forced flexion of the fetal trunk secondary to restricted movement.[68] It has been shown that fetal lung expansion becomes restricted within 48h of diminution of amniotic fluid but that process may be reversed by amnioinfusion.[69] A reduction in fetal breathing patterns in patients with reduced amniotic fluid may also contribute to pulmonary hypoplasia, although there are conflicting reports.[70–72]

Fluid in the fetal thorax either as primary hydrothorax or from hydrops fetalis is one of the most common causes of pulmonary hypoplasia with overall mortality reported at over 50%.[73] If fluid is drained from the chest in fetal hydrothorax by catheter or needle aspiration, lung growth may be restored.[74] Other 'space occupying lesions' of the fetal thorax include cardiomegaly (mitral valve insufficiency associated with giant left atrium and aortic stenosis, Ebstein's anomaly of the tricuspid valve and tricuspid valve dysplasia), pericardial effusion and neuroblastoma.

The incidence of congenital diaphragmatic hernia is estimated at 1 in 3000–5000 births. As a result of incomplete closure of the pleuroperitaneal membranes, the abdominal contents may enter the thorax and result in a mediastinal shift. This may effect the growth of the effected side and the contralateral lung, and may cause esophageal obstruction resulting in polyhydramnios. Postnatal survival is approximately 50% depending upon the degree of pulmonary hypoplasia.[75] In the absence of a congenital closure defect, the diaphragm may be affected by abnormal development of function as in phrenic nerve agenesis and Pena–Shokeir syndrome leading to an elevation or eventration of the dome of the diaphragm.[76] Central neural defects that as associated with absent fetal breathing movements may also lead to pulmonary hypoplasia including anencephaly, microcephaly and encephalocele.[77]

Congenital cystic adenomatoid malformation (CCAM) of the lung is a failure of maturation of certain bronchial structures during the pseudoglandular stage of development. The lesion is typically unilobar and consists of cystic areas that may be identified on ultrasound. Type I lesions have a single or multiple large cysts and represent 50% of CCAMs. Type II has multiple smaller cysts and may be associated with gastrointestinal or renal anomalies. Type III lesions are large with cysts often too small to measure and carry a poor prognosis. When associated with developing hydrops fetalis, preterm surgical intervention has been offered.[78]

Pulmonary hypoplasia is also associated with skeletal dysplasias because of a narrowed or constricted fetal thorax.[79,80] These anomalies may include Jeunes syndrome (asphyxiating thoracic dystrophy), achondrogenesis, achondroplasia, osteogenesis imperfecta, thanatophoric dwarfism and hypophosphasia. Ultrasound measurements of fetal lung or chest size as a ratio to normal gestational biometric measurements have been advanced as predictors of pulmonary hypoplasia.[81–84] Yoshimura *et al.* analyzed several methods of prediction for fetal lung hypoplasia, concluding that the lung area against gestational age and the ratio of the thoracic circumference to the abdominal circumference were the most clinically useful.[85] Recently, estimates of lung volumes from three-dimensional ultrasound have been used in an attempt to estimate lung maturity and predict hypoplasia.[86–89] We and others believe that a method that evaluates function as well as relative size may prove to be a more reliable predictor of post natal pulmonary dysfunction from pulmonary hypoplasia. Pulmonary blood flow parameters may be measured by the methods previously mentioned. We have seen in the fetus later found to have lethal pulmonary hypoplasia that the proximal and distal pulmonary artery flow patterns are reduced in peak velocity while pulsatility indices are increased. Those patients with space occupying lesions such as diaphragmatic hernias may have a blunted or no response to a maternal hyperoxia test after 32 weeks gestation.[90] One of the more easily obtained waveform patterns recorded during these studies has been the proximal pulmonary venous flow, which normally increases significantly with maternal hyperoxia. Mitchell *et al.* showed a high resistance pattern quite different from that of normal fetuses in the peripheral pulmonary arteries in 10 fetuses with bilateral multicystic dysplastic kidney disease all of whom died from associated pulmonary hypoplasia.[91] Yoshimura *et al.* made similar observations in the proximal pulmonary artery flow patterns with lethal pulmonary hyperplasia in hydrops fetalis, thanatophoric dwarfs and Potter syndrome.[92] Roth *et al.* have found an association with lethal pulmonary hypoplasia with the lack of pulmonary artery flow patterns with power color Doppler techniques.[93] Chaoui *et al.* have shown that abnormal pulmonary artery flow patterns may be seen as early as 19–23 weeks gestation in fetuses with lung hypoplasia.[94]

A test for the prediction of lethal pulmonary hypoplasia

To determine the predictive accuracy of our test for neonatal death from pulmonary hypoplasia, we measured the Doppler changes in fetal pulmonary artery blood flow in room air and during maternal hyperoxygenation. Women carrying fetuses with those congenital anomalies as illustrated above or with prolonged olighydramnios often associated with pulmonary hypoplasia were offered participation in the study as part of a comprehensive fetal echocardiogram. Each fetus at $\leq$30 weeks gestation had the Doppler blood flow pattern in the first branch of either the right or the left pulmonary artery measured before and again during at least 10 min exposure to maternal breathing of 60% oxygen by mask. An increase in the relative fetal pulmonary blood flow with oxygen (a decrease of at least 25% of the PI) was considered a reactive test. A change of less than 20% in the flow pattern during maternal hyperoxygenation was a nonreactive test and suggested pulmonary hypoplasia. The primary outcome for this study was neonatal outcome of death from pulmonary hypoplasia. In the 29 pregnancies that met criteria for our study, 14 fetuses who had a nonreactive hyperoxygenation test, 11 (79%) died of pulmonary hypoplasia. Of the 15 that had a reactive hyperoxygenation test, only 1 (7%) died in the neonatal period. Sensitivity, specificity, positive, and negative predictive values were 92%, 82%, 79% and 93%, respectively, with an odds ratio of 51 (95% CI 4.6–560).[95] We have now performed over 100 of these oxygen challenge tests with excellent results in sensitivity and specificity.

The oxygen challenge method evaluates fetal pulmonary function and therefore may prove to be a more reliable predictor of postnatal pulmonary dysfunction from pulmonary hypoplasia as compared to those that evaluate relative anatomic size. Maternal hyperoxygenation increases fetal pulmonary blood flow by decreasing pulmonary arterial vascular impedance. The changes we have observed between 31 and 36 weeks of gestation mimics the changes in the fetal hemodynamics after birth.[15] During normoxia, when the human fetal pulmonary arterial bed is under acquired vasoconstriction, right ventricular cardiac output is directed away from the lungs and into the systemic circulation via the ductus arteriosus. Increased blood oxygen content decreases pulmonary vascular resistance and thus increases pulmonary blood flow in the normal fetus. The reactivity of the pulmonary arterial circulation to oxygen with advancing gestation has been explained by an increasing amount of smooth muscle in small pulmonary arteries.[14] The decrease in the pulmonary vascular resistance is mainly caused by the release of endothelium-derived nitric oxide, which leads to vasodilatation of the pulmonary arterial bed.[60,61]

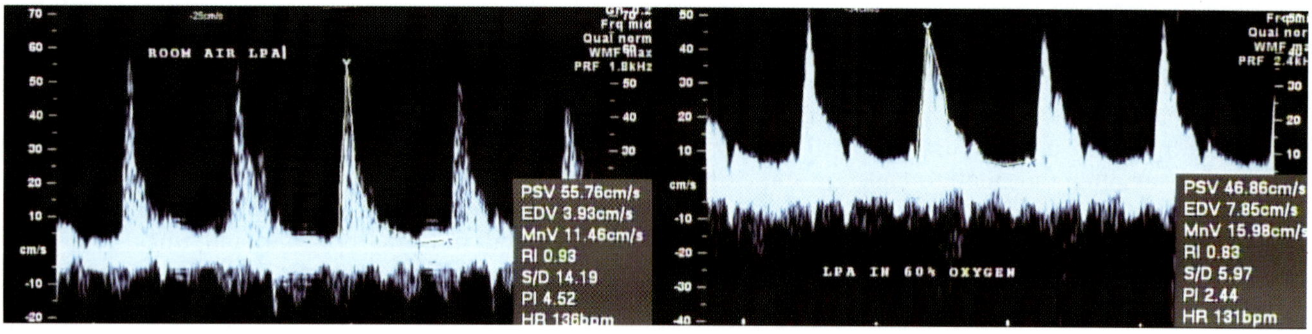

Figure 48.7 Positive change in Doppler flow patterns of pulmonary vascular reactivity with oxygen.

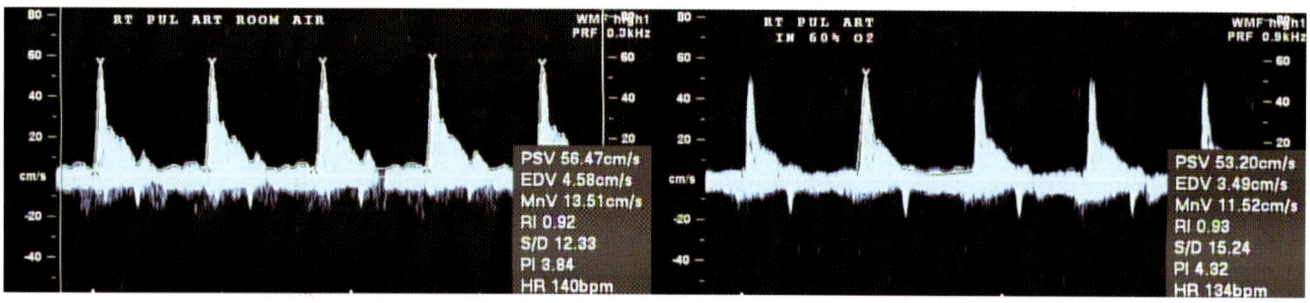

Figure 48.8 Negative change in Doppler flow patterns of pulmonary vascular reactivity with oxygen.

The method to accurately predict those fetuses who will die from pulmonary hypoplasia is important for parental counseling and subsequent decision-making regarding obstetric and neonatal management. As the oxygen challenge is an extension of our comprehensive fetal echocardiogram, we also measure the cardiac circumference to thoracic circumference ratio (CC/TC) and the thoracic circumference to the biometric abdominal circumference ratio (TC/AC) as well as M-mode measurements of the ventricles in systole and diastole. These measurements typically show normal size heart for gestational age, but the CC/TC and TC/AC are widely divergent relative to the cause of the small lungs. For example, oligohydramnios may show a relative cardiomegaly whereas a diaphragmatic hernia will have a relatively small heart to thoracic size. Likewise, we have seen exaggerated fetal breathing movements in fetuses that have lethal pulmonary hypoplasia and an absence of such movements in fetuses with long standing oligohydramnios who have a normal physiologic response to maternal oxygen and go on to a normal neonatal course. Difficulty in performing the examination occurs, especially in the fetus with diaphragmatic hernia, who has hard to image lungs and who typically increases both its gross body movements and breathing movements when exposed to an increased oxygen environment.

Intrauterine growth restricted (IUGR) fetuses with oligohydramnios can have a negative response to maternal hyperoxygenation. Those fetuses may present in extremis with abnormal Doppler measurements in the MCA, FLUA and DV, suggesting redistribution of cardiac output by cephalization, placental insufficiency and congestive heart failure with increased central venous pressure. The blunted or absent response to oxygen appears to be an extension of redistribution of cardiac output as these fetuses, who were delivered within hours of their oxygen tests, did reasonably well in the newborn period and were eventually discharged home (Figures 48.7 and 48.8).

Cystic adenomatoid malformation

Probably the most common lung lesion detected *in utero* by ultrasound is cystic adenomatoid malformation. This appears as an echo bright portion within a lobe of the lung and maybe associated with large, small mixed or micro cysts, appearing as a solid mass. It is characterized by dysplastic or hamartomatous tissue often mixed with normal tissue and typically confined to a single lobe. Regression is common, but when large and/or associated with hydrops it may be lethal because of pulmonary hypoplasia. As it is likely to be the result of early maldevelopment of terminal brochiolar structures, color or power Doppler in the area of the lesion may show pulmonary arterial flow around but not into the lesion (Figure 48.9).

Pulmonary sequestration

Pulmonary sequestration is a rare anomaly identified *in utero* by a difference in echo density of a particular

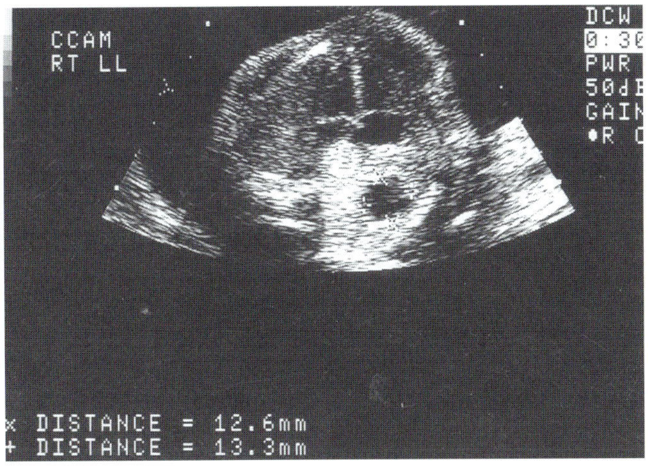

Figure 48.9 Cystic adenomatoid malformation.

lobe of the lung. It is seen as either above or below the diaphragm and is defined as either intrapulmonary or extrapulmonary depending on its position relative to the visceral pleura. It may present with mediastinal shift or cardiac malposition and occasionally with hydrops from impingement or torsion of the inferior vena cava. The sequestered lobe receives its blood supply from the aorta rather than the pulmonary artery with venous return usually to the right atrium via the inferior vena cava. The majority of sequestrations are extrapulmonary and occupy the lower portion of either hemi-thorax. Color directed pulsed Doppler may be used to identify the arterial origin from the descending aorta and thereby differentiate sequestration from cystic adenomatoid malformation. Most subdiaphragmatic sequestationas identified *in utero* regress and may not require neonatal surgical resection (Figure 48.10).

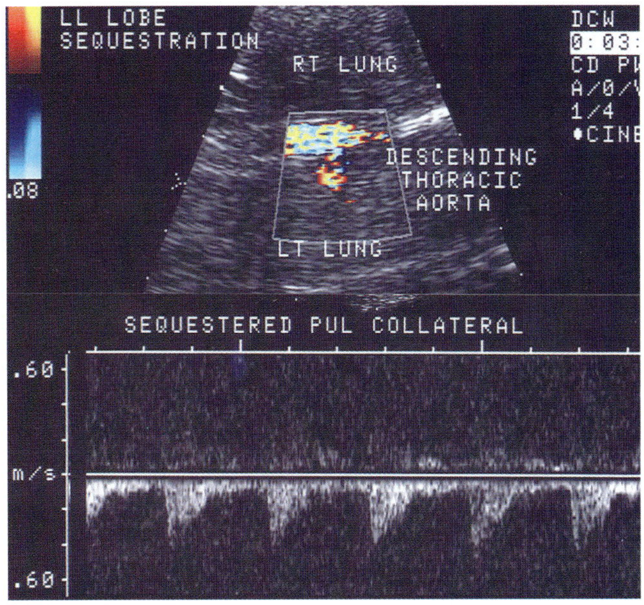

Figure 48.10 Color Doppler of sequestration flow pattern.

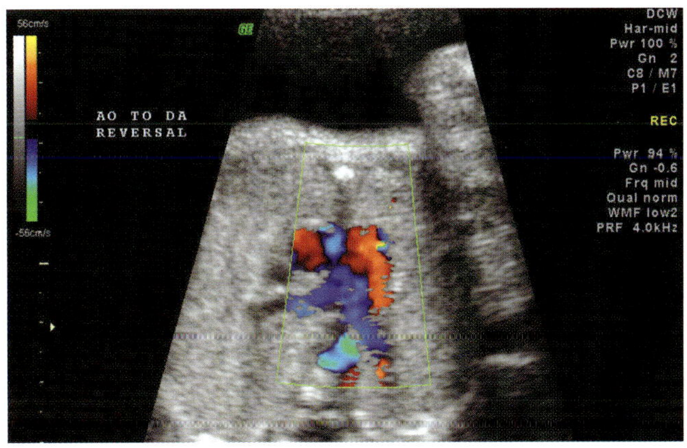

Figure 48.11 Color Doppler of normal pulmonary artery bifurcation with pulmonary valve atresia and reversed ductus arteriosus flow pattern.

Congenital pulmonary blood flow abnormalities

Observable abnormalities of fetal pulmonary circulation may be related to structural congenital heart disease or to thoracic space occupying lesions. The pulmonary artery should be superior and anterior to and slightly larger than the aorta in the four-chamber view of the fetal heart. The pulmonary artery blood flow is directed toward the fetal left shoulder and ductus arteriosus. Likewise, the normal connections of the pulmonary veins are easily identified from the four-chamber image just as the LVOT comes into view. Anomalous connection of the pulmonary veins should be ruled out when major structural congenital heart defects are identified. By combining high-resolution ultrasound magnification with the color flow and narrow sample size pulsed Doppler techniques we have described, blood flow connection abnormalities of the veins and arteries including sequestered lobes of the fetal lung may be identified. However, hydrothorax, cystic masses and diaphragmatic hernias may impede pulmonary blood flow to the extent that the flow may be difficult or impossible to observe or measure in one or both of the fetal lungs. Congenital malformations of pulmonary circulation should be considered in the presence of other forms of congenital heart disease. Direction of the fetal ductus arteriosus should be evaluated with both color and pulsed Doppler when arterial connection or obstruction is suggested in order to identify a ductal dependent lesion (Figure 48.11).

Major pulmonary venous abnormalities can generally be ruled out by imaging the right and left venous ostia as they connect into the left atrium on either side of the descending aorta when seen in the four-chamber view of the heart in a transverse image of the thorax (Figure 48.12). Exceptions to expect are when there is visceral heterotaxy when the stomach

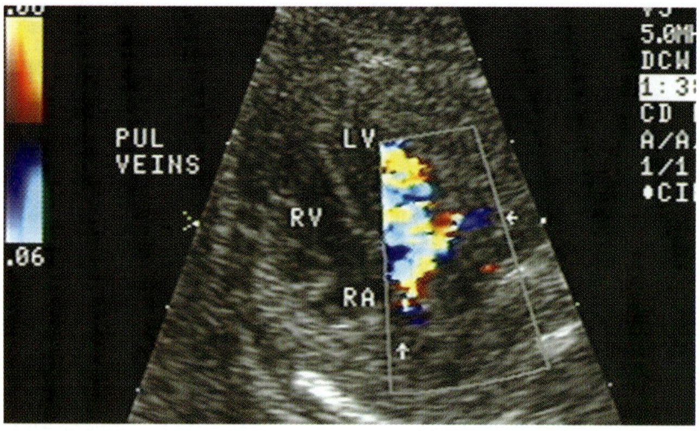

Figure 48.12 Color Doppler of normal pulmonary venous connections.

and heart may be on opposite sides of the fetus and/or when there is a common atrium or large atrial septal defect. Ipsilateral venous connections may be seen in these diagnoses but may be difficult to identify by fetal echocardiography. Both partially anomalous and totally anomalous pulmonary venous connections are typically associated with a disproportion of right-sided chambers larger than the left-sided structures. More obvious is total anomalous pulmonary venous connection (TAPVC) to the coronary sinus where a dilated coronary sinus can be identified as an eccentric line parallel to the mitral valve annulus in the four-chamber view. However, a dilated coronary sinus may also be seen with normally connected pulmonary veins when the left superior vena cava drains into the coronary sinus behind the lower left corner of the left atrium. The extra line in the left atrium may also signify the membrane in cortriatriatum (triatrial heart) where the common pulmonary venous sack is attached to the posterior left atrial wall but may drain anomalously into the right atrium or via restricted fenestrations into the left atrium. The most common type of TAPVC is when the common pulmonary venous sac is not attached to the left atrium but to a vein that ascends to join the innominate vein which then flows into the right superior vena cava and right atrium. The form of TAPVC most likely to become obstructed in the early newborn period is when the common pulmonary venous sack is attached to a vein that descends below the diaphragm and connects to a hepatic venous structure. Partially anomalous pulmonary venous veins are difficult to identify as they may enter the right atrium, coronary sinus, the right or left superior vena cava, the inferior vena cava or into the azygous venous system as single attachments with otherwise normally connecting pulmonary veins. In cases of hypoplastic left heart syndrome, the pulmonary veins may appear dilated for gestational age, but may be anomalously connected and associated with pulmonary venous stenoses. Stenosis of pulmonary veins may be difficult to identify in fetal life from ultrasound because of the relative paucity of pulmonary blood flow. Pulmonary venous dimensions can usually be measured successfully after 22 weeks' gestation. Pulmonary venous blood flow is best measured with color directed pulsed Doppler techniques in a lateral approach to the four-chamber view.

We believe that all fetal ultrasound anatomic survey examinations should include identification and relative quantification of the outflow tracts of the heart. The pulmonary artery should arise above the anterior right ventricle aiming toward the left shoulder at the ductus arteriosus, while the aorta arises centrally from the left ventricle aiming toward the right shoulder in a 90° crossing fashion relative to the main pulmonary artery. The ascending aorta and the main pulmonary artery should be about the same size. Pulmonary outflow obstructions may not become obvious on fetal ultrasound until the third trimester. A form of hypoplastic right heart where there is pulmonary atresia with intact ventricular septum may have a normal four-chamber view in the second trimester and normal sized pulmonary arteries at birth. In these cases, the pulmonary valve may acquire more severe obstruction with fetal growth resulting in a reversal of flow through the ductus arteriosus. We have seen this in the recipient twin in twin-to-twin transfusion syndrome as well as in singleton pregnancies. In these situations, the left ventricle begins to become disproportionately larger than the right ventricle during the second trimester as blood flow patterns change. Color Doppler is useful in proving a normal pulsed Doppler flow pattern into the main pulmonary artery. Normally, the forward flow pattern from the right ventricle into the pulmonary artery is a hollow envelope rarely exceeding 0.7 m/s. Pulmonary stenosis can be recognized by a course spectral flow pattern measuring greater than 1.0 m/min and often associated with tricuspid valve regurgitation. Pulmonary outflow obstruction should be considered with presumptive fetal diagnoses of Ebstein's malformation of the tricuspid valve, double outlet right ventricle (DORV), transposition of the great arteries (d or l-TGA), ventricular septal defect, tetralogy of Fallot and in cases of early diagnosis of transient cystic hygroma associated with Noonan's syndrome. In those cases with the physiology of tetralogy of Fallot with pulmonary atresia, color Doppler is useful in identifying collateral arterial vessels feeding the lungs from the aorta. It is important to differentiate this disease from truncus arteriosus. Collateral vessels can also be seen using color Doppler in cases of pulmonary sequestration.

We use a team approach of prenatal counseling by the perinatologist, neonatologist, pediatric cardiologist and cardiothoracic surgeon for the family of any fetus with congenital heart disease that may require prenatal or early neonatal intervention. Any suggestion of a fetal anomaly of venous or arterial connection or obstruction must be confirmed after delivery by newborn echocardiography or at cardiac catheterization.

REFERENCES

1. Morrell NW, Weiser MCM, Stenmark KR. Development of the pulmonary vasculature. In Gaultier C, Bourbon JR, Post M, eds. *Lung Development*. New York: Oxford University Press, 1999.
2. Burri PH. Lung development and angiogenesis. In Gaultier C, Bourbon JR, Post M, eds. *Lung Development*. New York: Oxford University Press, 1999.
3. Kikkawa Y. Morphology and morphologic development of the lung. In Scarpelli EM, ed. *Pulmonary Physiology of the Fetus, Newborn and Child*. Philadelphia, PA: Lea and Febiger, 1975.
4. Rabinovitch M. Developmental biology of the pulmonary vasculature. In Polin RA, Fox WW, eds. *Fetal and Neonatal Physiology*, 2nd edn. Philadelphia, PA: WB Saunders, 1998.
5. Kitaoka Y, Burri PH, Weibel ER. Development of the human fetal airway tree: analysis of the numerical density of airway endtips. *Anat Rec* 1996;244:207–13.
6. Hislop A, Reed L. Growth and development of the respiratory system-anatomic development. In Davis JA, Dobbing J, eds. *Scientific Foundations of Pediatrics*. London: Heinemann, 1972.
7. Rasanen J, Huhta JC, Weiner S, Wood DC, Ludomirski A. Fetal branch pulmonary artery vascular impedance during the second half of pregnancy. *Am J Obstet Gynecol* 1996;174:1441–9.
8. Roberts AB, Mitchell JM. Direct ultrasonographic measurement of fetal lung length in normal pregnancies and pregnancies complicated by prolonged rupture of membranes. *Am J Obstet Gynecol* 1990;163:1560–6.
9. Lewis AB, Heymann MA, Rudolph AM. Gestational changes in pulmonary vascular responses in fetal lambs in utero. *Circ Res* 1976;39:536–41.
10. Tessler FN, Kimme-Smith C, Sutherland ML, Schiller VL, Perrella RR, Grant EG. Inter- and intra-observer variability of Doppler peak velocity measurements: An in-vitro study. *Ultrasound Med Biol* 1990;16:653–7.
11. O'Rourke MF. Vascular impedance in studies of arterial and cardiac function. *Physiol Rev* 1982;62:571–621.
12. Downing GJ, Maulik D, Phillips C, Kadado TR. In vivo correlation of Doppler waveform analysis with arterial input impedance parameters. *Ultrasound Med Biol* 1993;19:549–59.
13. Giles WB, Trudinger BJ, Paird PJ. Fetal umbilical artery flow velocity waveforms and placental resistance: Pathological correlation. *Br J Obstet Gynaecol* 1985;92:31–8.
14. Levin DL, Rudolph AM, Heymann MA, Phibbs RH. Morphological development of the pulmonary vascular bed in fetal lambs. *Circulation* 1976;53:144–51.
15. Heymann MA. Regulation of the pulmonary circulation in the perinatal period and in children. *Intensive Care Med* 1989;15:S9–12.
16. Eik-Nes SH, Brubakk AO, Ulstein M. Measurement of human fetal blood flow. *Br Med J* 1980;1:283–4.
17. Machado MVL, Chita SC, Allan LD. Acceleration time in the aorta and pulmonary artery measured by Doppler echocardiography in the midtrimester normal human fetus. *Br Heart J* 1987;58:15–18.
18. Choi JY, Noh CI, Yun YS. Study on Doppler waveforms from the fetal cardiovascular system. *Fetal Diagn Ther* 1991;6:74–83.
19. Hata T, Senoh D, Makihara K, Aoki S, Hata K, Takamiya O, Kitao M. Fetal cardiac time intervals determined by Doppler echocardiography. *J Perinat Med* 1989;17:85–92.
20. Morin FC III, Egan EA. Pulmonary hemodynamics in fetal lambs during development at normal and increased oxygen tension. *J Appl Physiol* 1992;73:213–18.
21. Huhta JC, Moise KJ, Fisher DJ, Sharif DS, Wasserstrum N, Martin C. Detection and quantitation of constriction of the fetal ductus arteriosus by Doppler echocardiography. *Circulation* 1987;75:406–12.
22. Rasanen J, Wood DC, Weiner S, Ludomirski A, Huhta JC, The role of the pulmonary circulation on the distribution of human fetal cardiac output during the second half of pregnancy. *Circulation* 1996;94:1068–73.
23. Schmidt KG, Di Tommaso M, Silverman NH, Rudolph AM. Doppler echocardiographic assessment of fetal descending aortic and umbilical blood flows. Validation study in fetal lambs. *Circulation* 1991;83:1731–7.
24. Versmold HT, Kitterman JA, Phibbs RH, Gregory GA, Tooley WH. Aortic blood pressure during the first 12 hours of life in infants with birth weight 610 to 4220 grams. *Pediatrics* 1981;67:607–13.
25. St John Sutton M, Groves A, MacNeill A, Sharland G, Allan L. Assessment of changes in blood flow through the lungs and foramen ovale in the normal human fetus with gestational age: A prospective Doppler echocardiographic study. *Br Heart J* 1994;71:232–7.
26. Rudolph AM, Heymann MA. Circulatory changes during growth in the fetal lamb. *Circ Res* 1970;26:289–99.
27. Morin FC III, Egan EA, Ferguson W, Lundgren CEG. Development of pulmonary vascular response to oxygen. *Am J Physiol* 1988; 254:H542–6.
28. Soyeur D, Schaaps JP, Kulbertus H. Pulsed Doppler assessment of fetal blood flow across the foramen ovale and pulmonary vascular bed. *Eur Heart J* 1990;11:90.
29. Phillipos EZ, Robertson MA, Still KD. The echocardiographic assessment of the human fetal foramen ovale. *J Am Soc Echocardiogr* 1994;7:257–63.
30. Kiserud T, Eik-Nes SH, Blaas HG, Hellevik LR. Foramen ovale: An ultrasonographic study of its relation to the inferior vena cava, ductus venosus and hepatic veins. *Ultrasound Obstet Gynecol* 1992;2:389–96.
31. Traeger A, Noschel H, Zaumseil J. The pharmacokinetics of indomethacin in pregnant and parturient women and their newborn infants. *Zentralbl Gynakol* 1973;95:635–41.
32. Moise KJ, Ou CN, Kirshon B, Cano LE, Rognerud C, Carpenter RJ. Placental transfer of indomethacin in the human pregnancy. *Am J Obstet Gynecol* 1990;162:549–54.
33. Kirshon B, Moise KJ, Wasserstrum N, Ou CN, Huhta JC. Influence of short-term indomethacin therapy on fetal urine output. *Obstet Gynecol* 1988;72:51–3.
34. Moise KJ, Huhta JC, Sharif DS *et al.* Indomethacin in the treatment of premature labor. Effects on the fetal ductus arteriosus. *N Engl J Med* 1988;319:327–31.
35. Tulzer G, Gudmundsson S, Tews G, Wood DC, Huhta JC. Incidence of indomethacin-induced human fetal ductal constriction. *J Matern Fetal Invest* 1992;1:267–9.
36. Moise KJ. Effect of advancing gestational age on the frequency of fetal ductal constriction in association with maternal indomethacin use. *Am J Obstet Gynecol* 1993;168:1350–3.
37. Huhta JC, Cohen AW, Wood DC. Premature constriction of the ductus arteriosus. *J Am Soc Echocardiogr* 1990;3(1):30–4.
38. Rasanen J, Debbs RH, Wood DC, Weiner S, Huhta JC. The effects of indomethacin on pulmonary arterial vascular impedance and cardiac output. *Ultrasound Obstet Gynecol* 1999;13(2):112–16.
39. Tulzer G, Gudmundsson S, Sharkey AM, Wood DC, Cohen AW, Huhta JC. Doppler echocardiography of fetal ductus arteriosus constriction versus increased right ventricular output. *J Am Coll Cardiol* 1991;18:532–6.
40. Cassin S. Role of prostaglandins and thromboxanes in the control of the pulmonary circulation in the fetus and newborn. *Semin Perinatol* 1980;4:101–7.
41. Wlodek ME, Harding R, Thorburn GD. Effects of inhibition of prostaglandin synthesis on flow and composition of fetal urine, lung liquid, and swallowed fluid in sheep. *Am J Obstet Gynecol* 1994;170:186–95.
42. Velvis H, Moore P, Heymann MA. Prostaglandin inhibition prevents the fall in pulmonary vascular resistance as a result of rhythmic distension of the lungs in fetal lambs. *Pediatr Res* 1991;30:62–8.
43. Morin FC, Egan EA, Norfleet WT. Indomethacin does not diminish the pulmonary vascular response of the fetus to increased oxygen tension. *Pediatr Res* 1988;24:696–700.
44. Levin DL, Mills LJ, Weinberg AG. Hemodynamic, pulmonary vascular, and myocardial abnormalities secondary to pharmacologic constriction of the fetal ductus arteriosus. A possible mechanism for persistent pulmonary hypertension and transient tricuspid insufficiency in the newborn infant. *Circulation* 1979; 60:360–4.
45. Tulzer G, Gudmundsson S, Rotondo KM, Wood DC, Yoon GY, Huhta JC. Acute fetal ductal occlusion in lambs. *Am J Obstet Gynecol* 1991;165:775–8.
46. Kenny JF, Plappert T, Doubilet P *et al.* Changes in intracardiac blood flow velocities and right and left ventricular stroke volumes with gestational age in the normal human fetus: A prospective Doppler echocardiographic study. *Circulation* 1986;74:1208–16.
47. Isaaz K, Ethevenot G, Admant P, Brembilla B, Pernot C. A new Doppler method of assessing left ventricular ejection force in chronic congestive heart failure. *Am J Cardiol* 1989;64:81–7.
48. St John Sutton M, Gill T, Plappert T, Saltzman DH, Doubilet P. Assessment of right and left ventricular function in terms of

force development with gestational age in the normal human fetus. *Br Heart J* 1991;61:285–9.
49. Rizzo G, Capponi A, Rinaldo D, Arduini D, Romanini C. Ventricular ejection force in growth-retarded fetuses. *Ultrasound Obstet Gynecol* 1995;5:247–55.
50. Rasanen J, Debbs RH, Wood DC, Weiner S, Weil SR, Huhta JC. Human fetal right ventricular ejection force under abnormal loading conditions during the second half of pregnancy. *Ultrasound Obstet Gynecol* 1997;10(5):325–32.
51. Noble MIM, Trenchard D, Guz A. Left ventricular ejection in conscious dogs: II. Determinants of stroke volume. *Circ Res* 1966;19:148–52.
52. Noble MIM. The contribution of blood momentum to left ventricular ejection in the dog. *Circ Res* 1968;23:663–70.
53. Copel JA, Grannum PA, Green JJ *et al.* Fetal cardiac output in the isoimmunized pregnancy: A pulsed Doppler-echocardiographic study of patients undergoing intravascular intrauterine transfusion. *Am J Obstet Gynecol* 1989;161:361–5.
54. Moise KJ, Mari G, Fisher DJ, Huhta JC, Cano LE, Carpenter RJ. Acute fetal hemodynamic alterations after intrauterine transfusion for treatment of severe red blood cell alloimmunization. *Am J Obstet Gynecol* 1990;163:776–84.
55. Rizzo G, Nicolaides KH, Arduini D, Campbell S. Effects of intravascular fetal blood transfusion on fetal intracardiac Doppler velocity waveforms. *Am J Obstet Gynecol* 1990;163:1231–8.
56. Moise KJ, Mari G, Kirshon B, Huhta JC, Walsh SW, Cano L. The effect of indomethacin on the pulsatility index of the umbilical artery in human fetuses. *Am J Obstet Gynecol* 1990;162:199–202.
57. Khowsathit P, Tian ZY, Wood DC, Cohen AW, Huhta JC. Indomethacin-induced placental vasodilation: Association with fetal ductal constriction. *J Matern Fetal Invest* 1995;5:30–2.
58. Rasanen J, Wood DC, Debbs R, Cohen J, Weiner S, Huhta JC. Reactivity of the human fetal circulation to maternal hyperoxygenation increases in the second half of pregnancy, a randomized study. *Circulation* 1998;97:257–62.
59. Assali NS, Kirschbaum TH, Dilts PV. Effects of hyperbaric oxygen on uteroplacental and fetal circulation. *Circ Res* 1968;22:573–88.
60. Mital S, Konduri GG. Vascular K^+ ATP channels mediate O_2 induced pulmonary vasodilation in fetal lambs (abstract). *Pediatrics* 1996;98:527.
61. Mital S, Konduri GG. Oxygen causes pulmonary vasodilation by stimulating synthesis and release of ATP in fetal lambs (abstract). *Pediatrics* 1996;98:533.
62. Heymann MA, Rudolph AM, Nies AS, Melmon KL. Bradykinin production associated with oxygenation of the fetal lamb. *Circ Res* 1969;25:521–34.
63. Burchell HB, Swan HJC, Wood EH. Demonstration of differential effects on pulmonary and systemic arterial pressure by variation in oxygen content of inspired air in patients with patent ductus arteriosus and pulmonary hypertension. *Circulation* 1953;8:681–94.
64. Harding R, Hooper SB. Regulation of lung expansion and lung growth before birth. *J Appl Physiol* 1996;81:209–24.
65. Askenazi SS, Perlman M. Pulmonary hypoplasia: lung weight and radial alveolar count as critical diagnosis. *Arch Dis Child* 1979; 54:631–9.
66. Chitkara U, Rosenberg J, Chervenak FA *et al.* Prenatal sonographic assessment of the fetal thorax: normal values. *Am J Obstet Gynecol* 1989;156:1069–74.
67. Potter EL. Bilateral renal agenesis. *J Pediatr* 1946;29:68–76.
68. Rotschild A, Ling EW, Puterman ML, Farquharson D. Neonatal outcome after prolonged preterm rupture of the membranes. *Am J Obstet Gynecol* 1990;162(1):46–52.
69. Savich RD, Guerra FA, Lee CC, Padbury JF, Kitterman JA. Effects of acute oligohydramnios on respiratory system of fetal sheep. *J Appl Physiol* 1992;73(2):610–17.
70. Roberts AB, Mitchell J. Pulmonary hypoplasia and fetal breathing in preterm premature rupture of membranes. *Early Hum Dev* 1995;41(1):27–37.
71. Fisk NM, Talbert DG, Nicolini U, Vaughan J, Rodeck CH. Fetal breathing movements in oligohydramnios are not increased by aminoinfusion. *Br J Obstet Gynaecol* 1992;99(6):464–8.
72. Ohlsson A, Fong K, Hannah M *et al.* Prediction of lethal pulmonary hypoplasia and chorioamnionitis by assessment of fetal breathing. *Br J Obstet Gynaecol* 1991;98(7):692–7.
73. Longaker MT, Laberge JM, Dansereau J *et al.* Primary fetal hydrothorax: natural history and management. *J Pediatr Surg* 1989;24(6):573–6.
74. Blott M, Nicolaides KH, Greenough A. Pleuroamniotic shunting for decompression of fetal pleural effusions. *Obstet Gynecol* 1988;71(5):798–800.
75. Harrison MR, Adzick NS, Estes JM, Howell LJ. A prospective study of the outcome for fetuses with diaphragmatic hernia [see comments]. *J Am Med Assoc* 1994;271(5):382–4.
76. Persutte WH, Lenke RR, Kurczynski TW, Brinker RA. Antenatal diagnosis of Pena–Shokeir syndrome (type I) with ultrasonography and magnetic resonance imaging. *Obstet Gynecol* 1988;72(3 Pt 2): 72–5.
77. Dornan JC, Ritchie JW, Meban C. Fetal breathing movements and lung maturation in the congenitally abnormal human fetus. *J Dev Physiol* 1984;6(4):367–75.
78. Adzick NS, Harrison MR, Crombleholme TM, Flake AW, Howell LJ. Fetal lung lesions: Management and outcome. *Am J Obstet Gynecol* 1998;179(4):884–9.
79. Merz E, Miric-Tesanic D, Bahlmann F, Weber G, Hallermann C. Prenatal sonographic chest and lung measurements for predicting severe pulmonary hypoplasia. *Prenat Diagn* 1999; 19(7):614–19.
80. Lachman RS, Rappaport V. Fetal imaging in the skeletal dysplasias. *Clin Perinatol* 1990;17(3):703–22.
81. Ohlsson A, Fong K, Rose T *et al.* Prenatal ultrasonic prediction of autopsy-proven pulmonary hypoplasia. *Am J Perinatol* 1992; 9(5–6):334–7.
82. Nimrod C, Davies D, Iwanicki S, Harder J, Persaud D, Nicholson S. Ultrasound prediction of pulmonary hypoplasia. *Obstet Gynecol* 1986;68(4):495–8.
83. D'Alton M, Mercer B, Riddick E, Dudley D. Serial thoracic versus abdominal circumference ratios for the prediction of pulmonary hypoplasia in premature rupture of the membranes remote from term. *Am J Obstet Gynecol* 1992;166(2):658–63.
84. Songster GS, Gray DL, Crane JP. Prenatal prediction of lethal pulmonary hypoplasia using ultrasonic fetal chest circumference. *Obstet Gynecol* 1989;73(2):261–6.
85. Yoshimura S, Masuzaki H, Gotoh H, Fukuda H, Ishimaru T. Ultrasonographic prediction of lethal pulmonary hypoplasia: Comparison of eight different ultrasonographic parameters. *Am J Obstet Gynecol* 1996;175(2):477–83.
86. Laudy JA, Janssen MM, Struyk PC, Stijnen T, Wladimiroff JW. Three-dimensional ultrasonography of normal fetal lung volume: A preliminary study. *Ultrasound Obstet Gynecol* 1998;11(1):13–16.
87. Pohls UG, Rempen A. Fetal lung volumetry by three-dimensional ultrasound. *Ultrasound Obstet Gynecol* 1998;11(1):6–12.
88. D'Arcy TJ, Hughes SW, Chiu WS *et al.* Estimation of fetal lung volume using enhanced 3-dimensional ultrasound: a new method and first result. *Br J Obstet Gynaecol* 1996;103(10):1015–20.
89. Lee A, Kratochwil A, Stumpflen I, Deutinger J, Bernaschek G. Fetal lung volume determination by three-dimensional ultrasonography. *Am J Obstet Gynecol* 1996;175(3 Pt 1):588–92.
90. Rasanen J, Wood DC, Debbs RH, Tolosa J, Huhta JC. Diagnosis of lung hypoplasia by Doppler ultrasound in human fetuses (abstract). *Society of Perinatal Obstetricians*, Miami, 1998.
91. Mitchell JM, Roberts AB, Lee A. Doppler waveforms from the pulmonary arterial system in normal fetuses and those with pulmonary hypoplasia. *Ultrasound Obstet Gynecol* 1998;11(3):167–72.
92. Yoshimura S, Masuzaki H, Miura K, Muta K, Gotoh H, Ishimaru T. Diagnosis of fetal pulmonary hypoplasia by measurement of blood flow velocity waveforms of pulmonary arteries with Doppler ultrasonography. *Am J Obstet Gynecol* 1999;180 (2 Pt 1):441–6.
93. Roth P, Agnani G, Arbez-Gindre F *et al.* Use of energy color Doppler in visualizing fetal pulmonary vascularization to predict the absence of severe pulmonary hypoplasia. *Gynecol Obstet Invest* 1998;46(3):153–7.
94. Chaoui R, Kalache K, Tennstedt C, Lenz F, Vogel M. Pulmonary arterial Doppler velocimetry in fetuses with lung hypoplasia. *Eur J Obstet Gynecol Reprod Biol* 1999;84(2):179–85.
95. Broth RE, Wood DC, Rasanen J *et al.* Prediction of lethal pulmonary hypoplasia: The hyperoxygenation test for pulmonary artery reactivity. *Am J Obstet Gynecol* 2002;187(4):940–5.

49 Uteroplacental and umbilical circulation: physiologic changes in pregnancy

A. K. Ertan, H. A. Tanriverdi and W. Schmidt

Doppler sonography in obstetrics is a widely accepted functional method of examining the uteroplacental and fetal unit. It is a noninvasive method and became almost a standard technique in antenatal care. This method became an important tool for qualifying high-risk pregnancies. Color Doppler ultrasound represents blood flow changes as a color image, superimposed on the real-time ultrasound image being examined. In this way different vessels of the uteroplacental circulation can be accurately identified. Also, by identifying the vessel at a fixed point, e.g. where the uterine artery crosses the external iliac artery, it is possible to examine the same point in the circulation. Endovaginal color Doppler transducers allow easy and quick visualization of even the smallest vessels in the uteroplacental and fetal circulation. This, in turn, has enabled us to build a picture of the physiological changes in uteroplacental and fetal blood flow before and during the early stages of pregnancy.[1]

One of the first steps toward realizing the potential of Doppler ultrasound is to gain a clear understanding of the physiological changes that occur in the uteroplacental circulation during normal pregnancy. With this knowledge, we can obtain a clearer understanding of the pathophysiological changes that occur in the presence of disease.

Indices

Although measurement of volume flow changes in an organ would be ideal, *in vivo* the current methods for determining true flow are too inaccurate for deriving meaningful conclusions that can be of clinical value. Consequently, we rely on indices of resistance and velocity derived from the flow velocity waveforms (FVW) of a vessel.

Blood flow velocity in the fetal circulating system depends on the type of vessel. The arteries always have a pulsatile pattern (Figure 49.1), whereas veins have either a pulsatile or a continuous pattern (Figure 49.2).

Analyzing Doppler sonographic FVWs quantitatively is more difficult than analyzing them qualitatively. Qualitative analysis also overcomes erroneous measurements in small vessels. There are plenty of indices for qualitative analysis. The following are the most frequently used indices:

- systolic/diastolic ratio (S/D ratio, Stuart 1980)
- resistance index (RI, Pourcelot 1974)
- pulsatility index (PI, Gosling and King 1977).

In analyzing sonographic results and calculating indices, the following characters are used:

S = temporal peak of maximum frequency
D = end-diastolic maximum frequency
C = temporal average of maximum frequency, F_{mean}
I = instantaneous spatial average frequency
E = temporal average of spatial average frequency.

Calculations of formulas are as follows (Figure 49.3):

$$\text{S/D ratio} = S/D$$
$$\text{RI} = (S-D)/S$$
$$\text{PI} = (S-D)/C$$

The indices presented above also overcome a very serious problem involved with the angle between the ultrasound beam and the direction of blood flow (insonation angle). These indices are relatively angle independent and are therefore easily applied in clinical practice.

In practice, none of the indices is superior to the other[2–4] and any index may be used. Although S/D ratio is easily calculated, RI is the easiest to interpret. RI values approach 0 if resistance decreases and 1 if resistance increases. If end diastolic flow is absent,

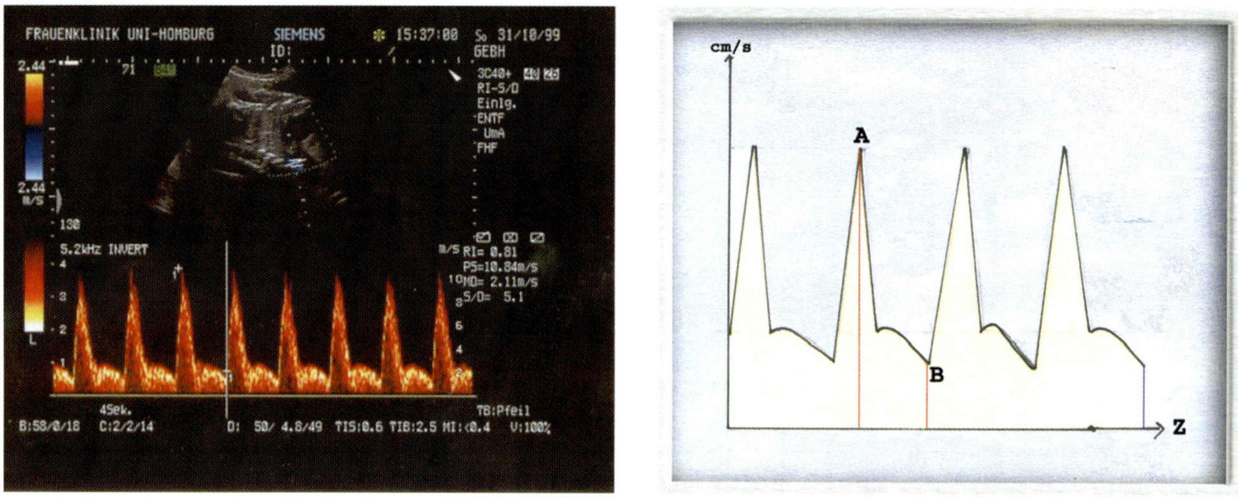

Figure 49.1 Doppler sonography of fetal aorta with a pulsatile pattern.

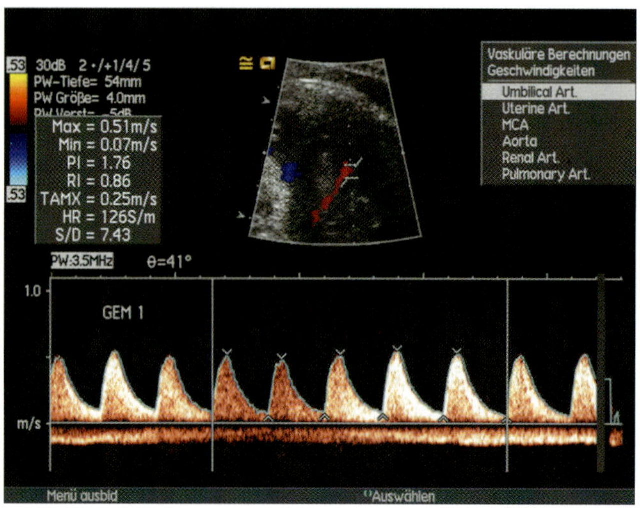

Figure 49.2 Umbilical artery with a pulsatile (upper line) and umbilical vein with a continuous pattern (lower line).

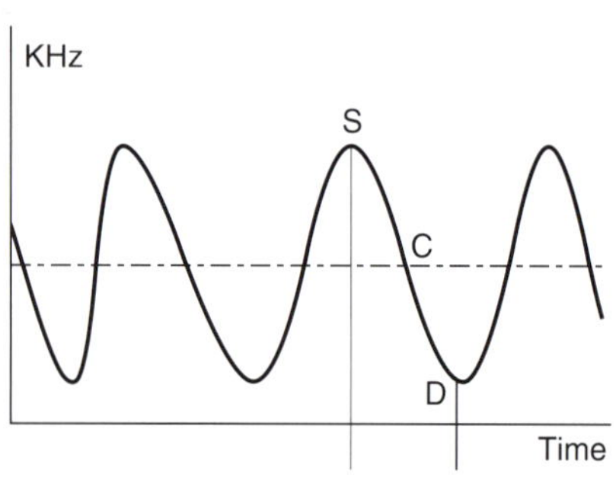

(I.)

S/D ratio : $\frac{S}{D}$

Resistance index (RI): $\frac{S-D}{S}$

Pulsatility index (PI): $\frac{S-D}{C}$

(II.)

Figure 49.3 Scheme of the Doppler curve (a). *S*=systolic, *D*=diastolic, *C*=temporal average of maximum frequency. Calculation of formulas of the main Doppler sonographic indices (b.)

PI is the only index making evaluation of blood flow possible, because in this situation S/D will equal to infinity and RI to 1. The PI is more complex because it requires the calculation of the mean velocity, but modern Doppler sonographic devices provide those values in real time.

Physiologic color Doppler sonographic changes of the embryonic and uteroplacental vessels in early pregnancy

The results of a recent study performed by Ertan *et al.*,[5] evaluating the uteroplacental and fetal circulation during early pregnancy in non-complicated pregnancies, showed that vascular impedance to blood flow in all the examined vessels decreased significantly throughout the first gestational trimester. Resistance to flow was highest in the main uterine artery and decreased toward the spiral artery. When the FVW patterns of the arteries under investigation were analyzed, specific changes were observed. In all of the cases during early gestational development, an early diastolic notching was determined in the uterine arteries. The FVWs of the fetal aorta and umbilical arteries were similar: until week 10 the arteries were typically without a diastolic flow. From week 16 onward, diastolic velocities were present in all signals at the fetal aorta and umbilical arteries.

Changes in uterine artery circulation in early pregnancy

The uterine artery FVW was characterized by an early diastolic notch and a gradually increasing flow velocity during early pregnancy. The peak systolic velocities (PSV) increase, whereas the S/D ratio and RI decrease progressively during early pregnancy. The end-diastolic velocity increases progressively. In all of the cases during early gestational development, an early diastolic notching was determined, but there was a gradually flattening in the depth of the notch (Figure 49.4). At the third trimester of pregnancy this notch disappeared. The RI of the uterine arteries decreased gradually, which means that the resistance of the arteries lessens during pregnancy progression.

Changes in umbilical circulation in early pregnancy

The color signal of the umbilical artery was recorded for the first time at 7 weeks' gestation.

From week 10 onward it was possible to show the end-diastolic velocity and from week 16 onward diastolic signals were present in all cases (Figures 49.5 and 49.6). The PSV between weeks 7 and 9 remained constant and from week 9 onward it increased, while the S/D ratio and RI decreased progressively during the first 16 weeks of gestation.

Changes in fetal aorta circulation in early pregnancy

It was possible to record the color signal of the fetal aorta for the first time at 7 weeks' gestation. The main problems in achieving Doppler signals of the aorta were fetal body movements and trying to make measurements with a correct angle, less than 60°.

The FVW was similar to the umbilical artery. Until week 10 of gestation the FVW was typically without a diastolic flow (end-diastolic zero flow). From week 16 onward, diastolic velocities were present in all aortic signals (Figure 49.7). The PSV increased and the S/D ratio and RI decreased progressively during the first 16 weeks of gestation.

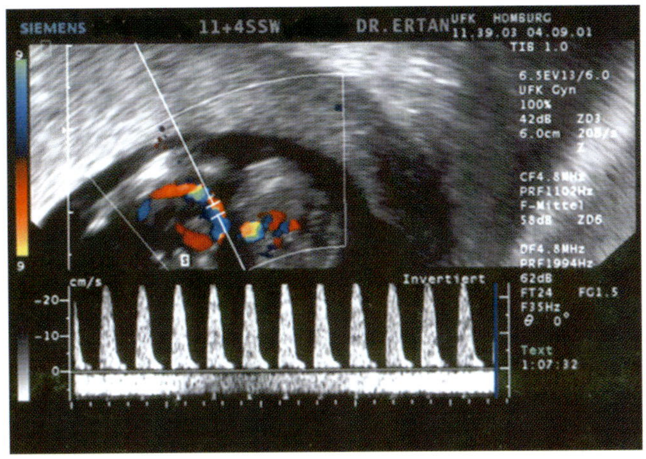

Figure 49.5 Doppler velocity waveforms of umbilical artery (end-diastolic zero flow) and continuous venous blood flow of umbilical vein in 11+4 weeks of pregnancy.

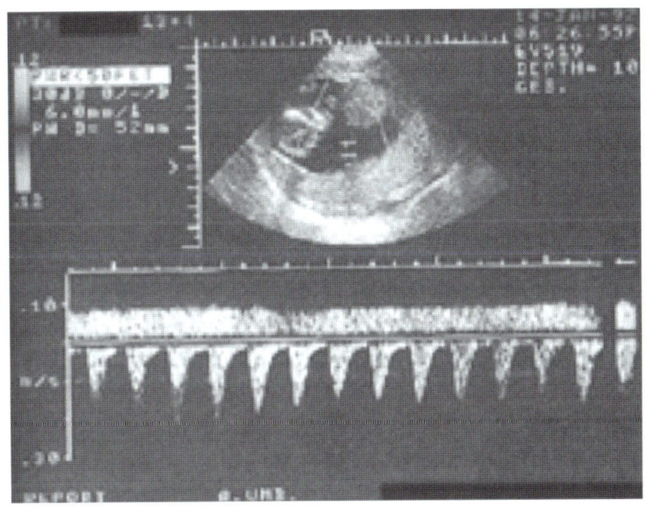

Figure 49.6 Doppler velocity waveforms of umbilical artery with an end-diastolic flow (lower line) in 13+4 weeks of pregnancy.

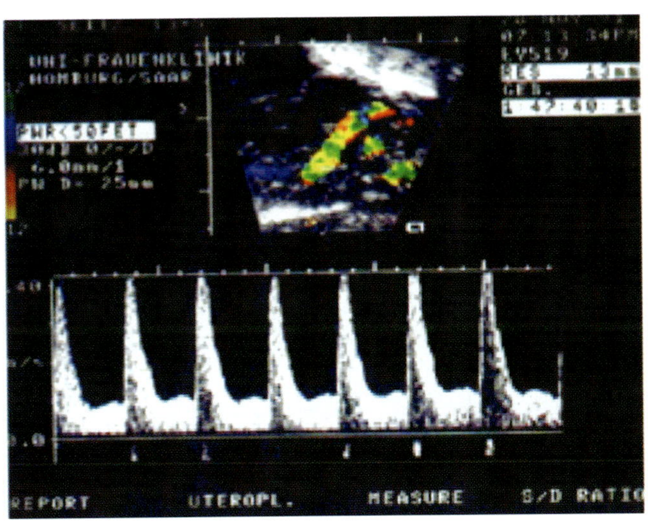

Figure 49.4 Doppler sonography of uterine artery in the first trimester of pregnancy (7+6 weeks) with early notch.

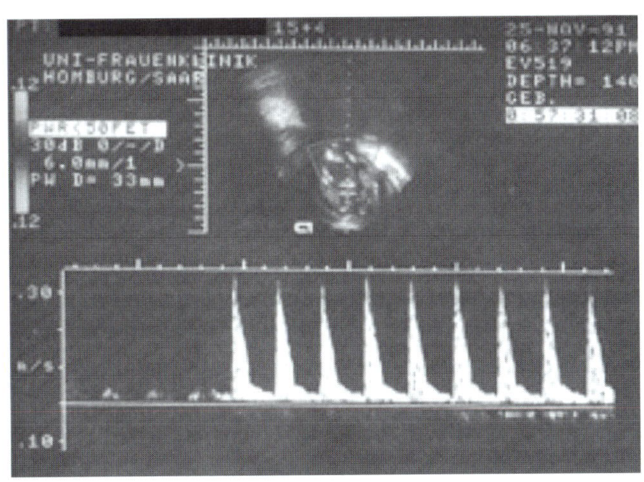

Figure 49.7 Doppler velocity waveforms of fetal aorta with an end-diastolic flow in 15+4 weeks of pregnancy.

Uteroplacental and fetal circulation after midpregnancy

The maternal side: uterine circulation

The uterine artery is a branch of the internal iliac artery. It courses along the lateral wall of the pelvis before crossing the external iliac artery and reaching the uterus at the level of the cervix. After giving off a cervical branch, it ascends along the lateral wall of the body of the uterus in a tortuous manner, before anastomosing with the Fallopian branch of the ovarian artery. As it passes along the body of the uterus it gives off the arcuate arteries, which encompass the uterine body. These in turn give off radial arteries that penetrate into the inner third of the myometrium, where they become the basal arteries. The spiral arteries, a continuation of the basal arteries, supply the endometrium, their coiled form allowing contraction during menstruation[1] (Figure 49.8).

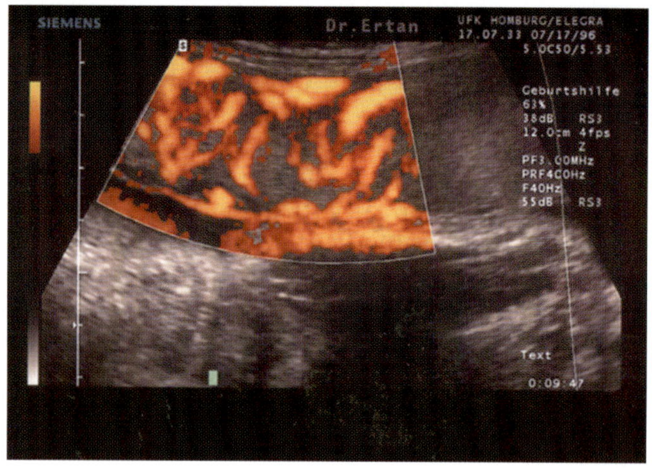

Figure 49.8 Power Doppler of arcuate and intraplacental arteries.

Using transvaginal color Doppler sonography, it is possible to identify the uterine artery in early pregnancy at the level of the cervical os, as it enters the uterus, and as it ascends into the uterine body (Figure 49.9). It is possible to examine the uterine artery by the transabdominal approach after 12 weeks' gestation, when the uterus becomes an abdominal organ. The FVWs obtained from the uterine artery do not significantly change from when it enters the cervix up to the point that it reaches the body of the uterus. It is important to measure at this level, before the uterine artery enters the uterus and branches into the arcuate arteries. An arcuate artery can exhibit a relatively low resistance pattern even when the uterine artery has high resistance with persistent notching present (Figure 49.10). It is therefore necessary to ensure that the uterine artery is examined as it reaches the uterus at the level of the cervix, if the changes in the uterine circulation are to be interpreted as a whole. Similarly, if the sample site is too low on the cervix, the cervical branch of the uterine artery will be examined; this can show high resistance when the main uterine artery waveform is normal.[1]

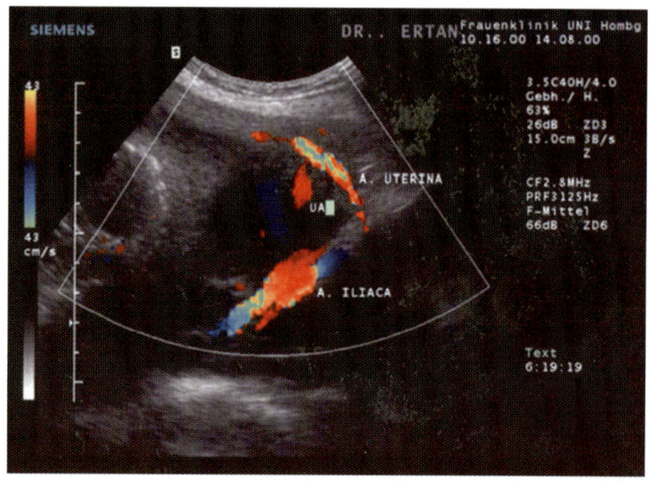

Figure 49.9 Color Doppler sonographic view of the main uterine artery crossing the iliac artery.

Blood flow velocities in the uterine artery depend on the localization of the placenta and the gestational age.[6] If the placenta is laterally located, blood flow velocities in the ipsilateral uterine artery are more important than the flow velocities of the contralateral vessel. Differences between flow velocities of the right and left uterine arteries are evident in the early stages of pregnancy. But in the third trimester, the difference between the S/D ratio of the vessels decreases to 0.3–0.4.[2] If an abnormal flow pattern is observed in the uterine arteries in midpregnancy, it most probably indicates the defective perfusion of the fetoplacental unit, which predicts a high probability of developing pre-eclampsia and/or intrauterine growth retardation (IUGR).[7]

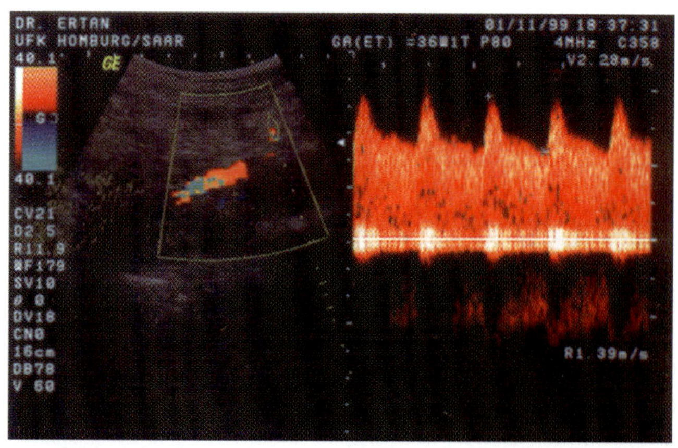

Figure 49.10 Flow in different parts of the uteroplacental circulation can be measured with color Doppler technology, here the relatively low resistance pattern of the uteroplacental arteries.

In the early stages of pregnancy end-diastolic flow velocities in placental arteries are low, but systolic flow is evident.[2] With trophoblastic invasion and maturation of the uteroplacental vessels, beyond the second trimester the high-pressure system is converted to a low-pressure system, and vascular resistance declines.[8] The biologic variability after the middle of the second trimester becomes almost stable.

Before 24 weeks' gestation early diastolic notching, due to the immature uteroplacental vascular system, is normally observed. Beyond this gestational age, persistent early diastolic notching is associated with pre-eclampsia[9–11] (Figures 49.11 and 49.12).

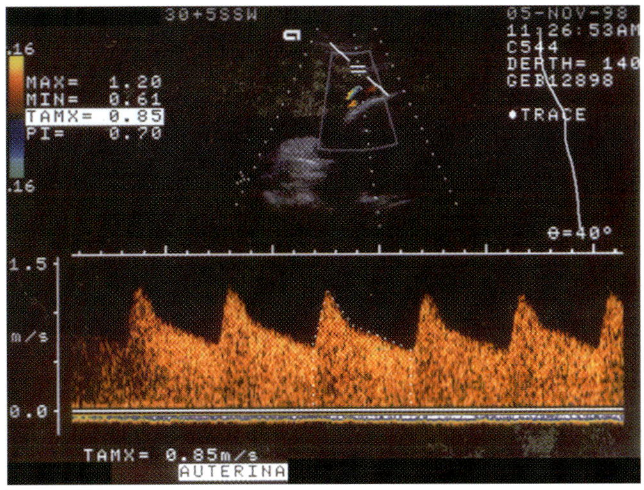

Figure 49.11 Normal Doppler FVW of uterine artery in the third trimester.

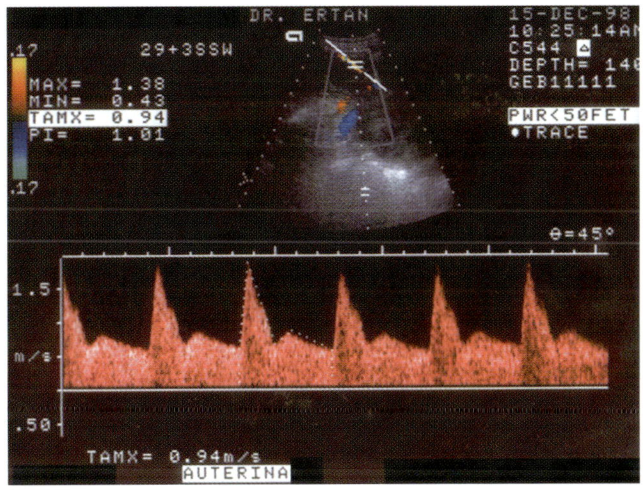

Figure 49.12 Pathological waveforms of uterine artery in 29 + 3 weeks of pregnancy with IUGR and pre-eclampsia.

The fetal side: umbilical arteries, fetal aorta and middle cerebral artery (MCA)

Umbilical arteries

Blood flow velocity in the umbilical arteries increases with progressive gestational age (Figure 49.13). As a result, the S/D ratio continuously decreases due to increasing arterial blood flow. With progressive gestational age, end-diastolic flow becomes evident during the whole heart cycle, matching with the previous longitudinal studies of Fogarty *et al.*[2] and Huneke *et al.*,[12] as with many cross-sectional studies.[13–16]

Trudinger *et al.*[17] put forth the following mechanisms to explain this development:

- continuous maturation in placental villi
- continuous widening of placental vessels causing a continuous decrease in vascular resistance
- continuous increase in fetal cardiac output
- continuous changes in the vessel compliance
- continuous increase in fetal blood pressure.

Especially in the third trimester of pregnancy, depending on the above factors, normal values become scattered on nomograms. This scattering is more prominent in the S/D ratio than the PI. RI is not affected by the above factors after 28 weeks' gestation.

Descending fetal aorta

Beside the umbilical arteries, routine Doppler sonographic measurements on the descending fetal aorta are possible. As the gestational age increases, the S/D ratio of fetal aorta decreases insignificantly, paralleling the results of Hecher *et al.*[18] The FVW of the fetal aorta shows a continuous forward stream during the whole heart cycle, but when compared to the FVW of the umbilical arteries, the end-diastolic flow is less than the systolic component. Because of this, the S/D ratio in the fetal aorta is greater than the S/D ratio in the umbilical arteries. As pregnancy progresses, the diameter of the vessel gets wider and as a result peripheral resistance decreases, and diastolic flow increases. Nevertheless, this does not cause a significant decrease in the S/D ratio in the fetal aorta. RI and PI are not affected significantly, and show a similar course as in the umbilical arteries.

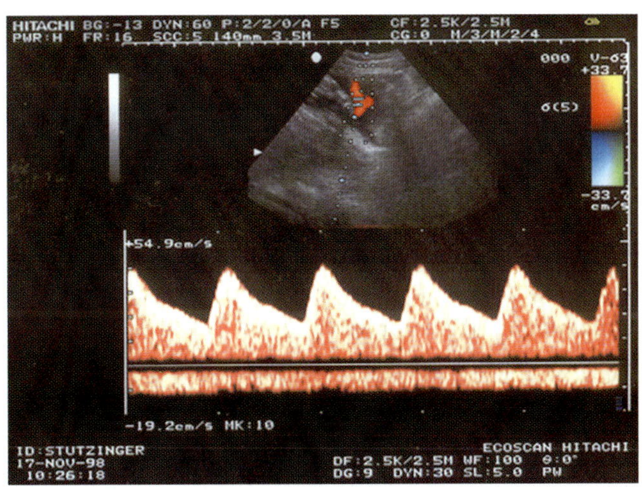

Figure 49.13 Blood velocity waveform in umbilical artery in late pregnancy.

Middle cerebral artery

The most favorably positioned vessel for Doppler sonographic examination of the fetal brain perfusion is the MCA. Biologic variability of vessels perfusing the fetal brain is excessive due to the fetal activity status. As pregnancy progresses, the vascular resistance decreases.[19] During the early stages of pregnancy, end-diastolic flow velocities in cerebral vessels are weak, but velocities increase toward the end of gestation. Hyperactivity of the fetus, increase of intrauterine pressure (e.g. polyhydramnios) and external pressure to the fetal head (e.g. by the probe) might erroneously increase end-diastolic flow velocities.[20] Different investigators have undertaken studies utilizing data obtained from the umbilical arteries and MCA to develop indices for evaluation of intrauterine risk.

Dependency of Doppler FVWs on gestational age

The amount of perfusion in trophoblastic tissue is related to gestational age. For this reason, in interpreting the Doppler sonographic findings, gestational age should be taken into account as well. In general, the accepted time for starting Doppler sonographic examinations is the beginning of the second trimester. This is the right time to allow for modifications in antenatal care in a high-risk pregnancy. For specific conditions, earlier timing of measurements may be considered.[21]

The main objective in using fetomaternal Doppler sonographic nomograms is to improve perinatal outcome in high-risk pregnancies. The curves presented below depict normal fetal and maternal Doppler sonographic values standardized according to gestational age, and can be used in routine practice (Figures 49.14–49.25).

Doppler sonographic nomograms are used for differentiation of normal and abnormal blood FVWs, which helps to determine high-risk pregnancies. By taking threshold values of pathologic pregnancies into consideration, nomograms are capable of differentiating between the normal and the abnormal.[22] While using these nomograms, it must always be kept in mind that the values on these nomograms should not be taken as mathematical equations, and that limitations of sensitivity and specificity exist.

Using nomograms in practice

Just like the defense mechanism of peripheral vasoconstriction in an adult in the face of hemorrhagic shock, the 'brain sparing' mechanism (brain sparing effect) becomes active in a fetus with hypoxia or chronic placental insufficiency. As a result of the brain sparing effect, resistance either in the umbilical artery or in the fetal descending aorta increases. As a consequence, Doppler indices related to these vessels

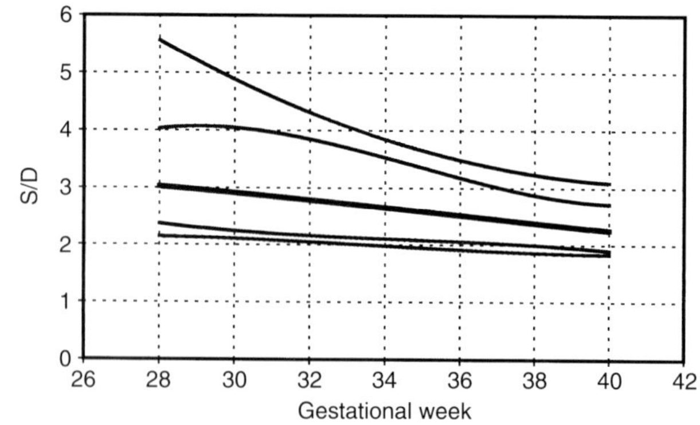

Figure 49.14 Umbilical artery S/D ratio nomogram.

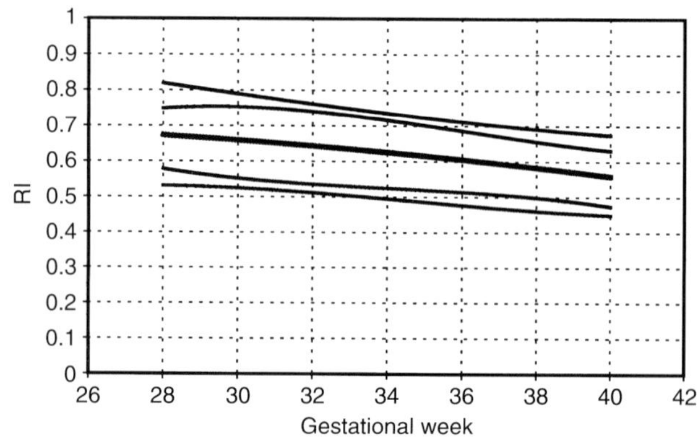

Figure 49.15 Umbilical artery RI nomogram.

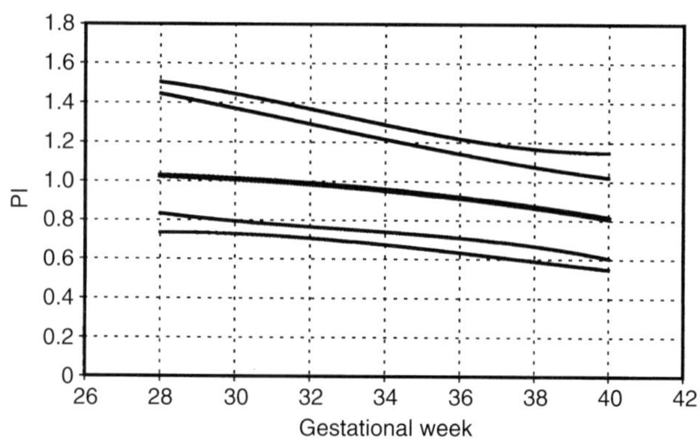

Figure 49.16 Umbilical artery PI nomogram.

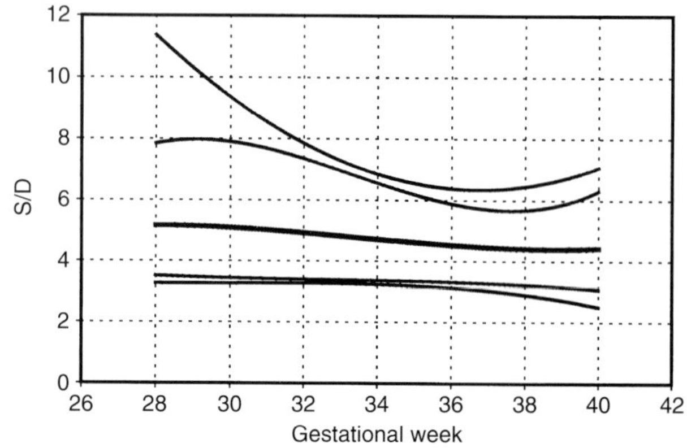

Figure 49.17 Descending fetal aorta S/D ratio nomogram.

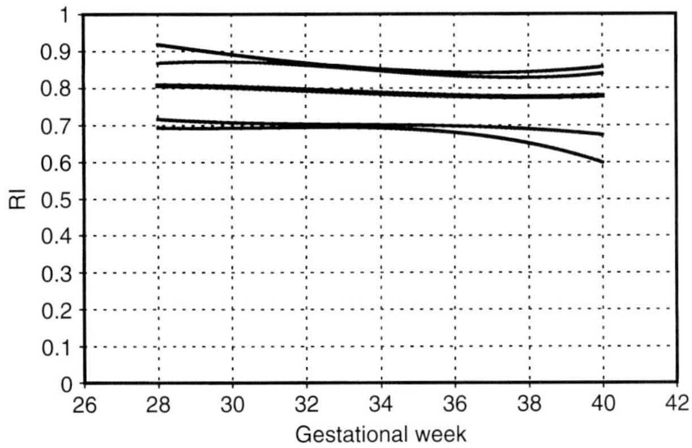

Figure 49.18 Descending fetal aorta RI nomogram.

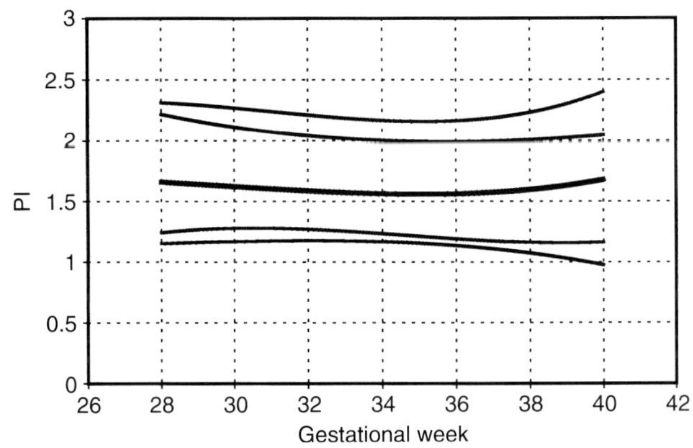

Figure 49.19 Descending fetal aorta PI nomogram.

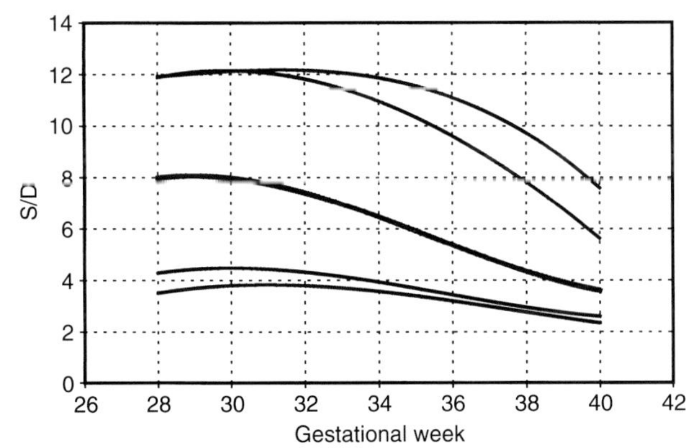

Figure 49.20 Middle cerebral artery S/D ratio nomogram.

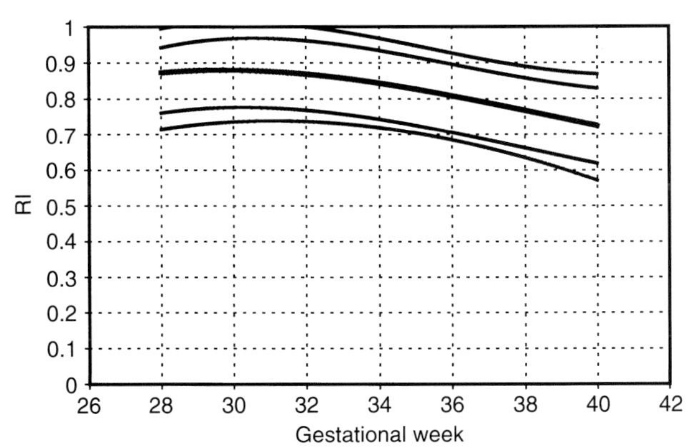

Figure 49.21 Middle cerebral artery RI nomogram.

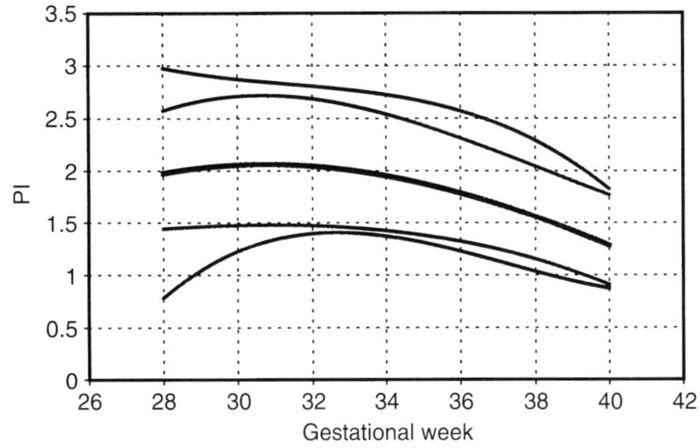

Figure 49.22 Middle cerebral artery PI nomogram.

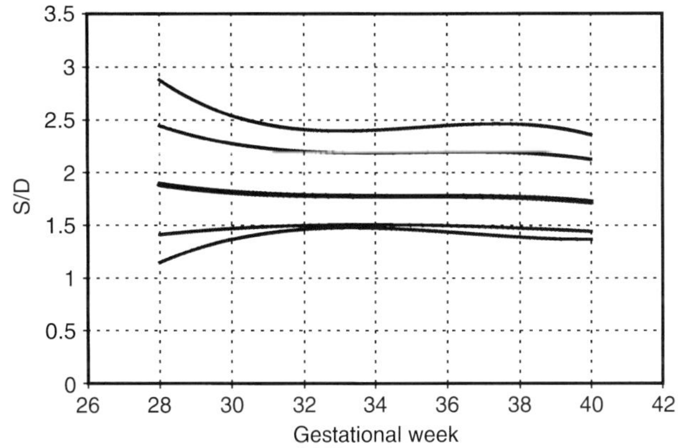

Figure 49.23 Uterine artery S/D ratio nomogram.

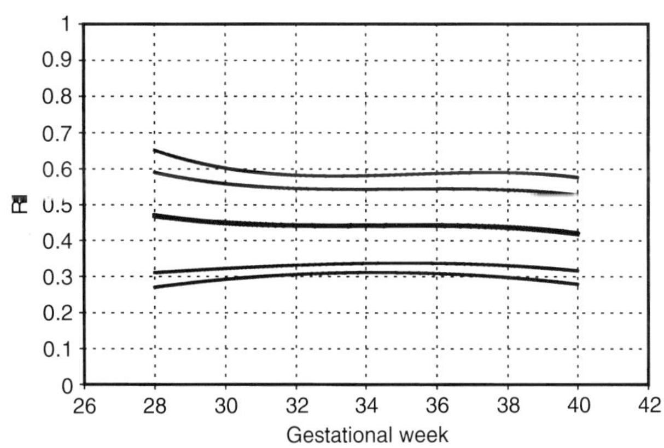

Figure 49.24 Uterine artery RI nomogram.

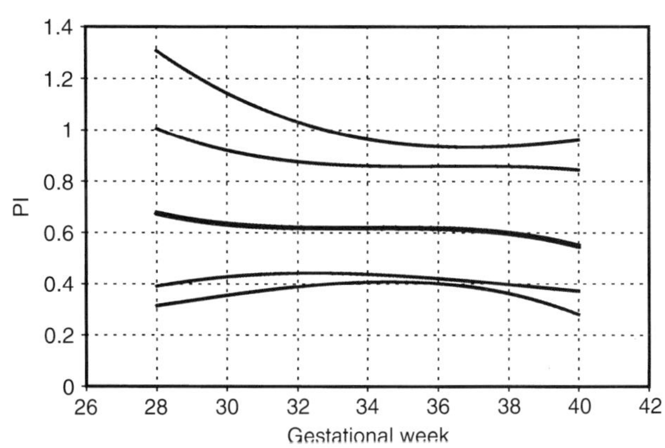

Figure 49.25 Uterine artery PI nomogram.

increase. The end-diastolic blood flow increases in the MCAs by the same effect. Doppler indices for this vessel decrease consequently.

Some points should be considered while using Doppler sonographic nomograms:

(1) Among the measurements performed on the umbilical artery and the fetal descending aorta, values between the 90th and 95th percentiles should be considered as borderline and repeat follow-ups should be planned. Values exceeding the 95th percentile are considered abnormal.
(2) Doppler values between the 5th and 10th percentiles in the MCA should be considered as borderline and repeat follow-ups should be planned. Values below the fifth percentile are considered abnormal.
(3) Measurements taken after 24 weeks' gestation from the uterine arteries are more valuable. The early diastolic notching and values exceeding the 95th percentile are considered as abnormal. One point to remember is that notching by itself predicts an elevated risk of pre-eclampsia.

Conclusion

In normal pregnancies, uteroplacental flow velocities become almost stable after the middle second trimester; meanwhile, fetal blood flow velocities also alter. With advancing gestational age, the S/D ratio in the umbilical artery and MCA decreases. Although the S/D ratio in the descending aorta is almost stable during pregnancy, advancing gestational age narrows the biologic variability of the flow spectrum. Accordingly, it is recommended to use gestational age-matched nomograms to define threshold values, and to differentiate and predict pathologic pregnancies.

The key points relating to physiological changes in the uteroplacental and fetal circulation can be summarized as follows:

(1) The technique of Doppler ultrasound is a non-invasive method of examining the uteroplacental and fetal circulation. Color Doppler sonography allows the uteroplacental and fetal circulation to be investigated throughout pregnancy.
(2) The main changes in FVW in the fetal and uteroplacental vessels occur in the first trimester of pregnancy and go on slowly in the remaining periods. Fetal and uteroplacental velocities increase gradually during early pregnancy and velocimetric indices show a progressive decrease of the uteroplacental resistances. In early pregnancy the umbilical artery and fetal aorta FVWs are initially of high resistance, with absent end-diastolic flow. Resistance falls rapidly toward the end of the first trimester; and end-diastolic flow is usually present by the 16th week of gestation. Resistance continues to fall throughout the remainder of the pregnancy.
(3) In normal pregnancy there is a gradual fall in resistance, an increase in diastolic flow and a disappearance of the diastolic notch in the uterine artery FVW.
(4) Pre-eclampsia, IUGR and placental abruption are associated with inadequate placentation/ function, and a relationship exists between these complications and the failure of physiological change in the uteroplacental circulation.

Acknowledgments

The authors thank Aykut Barut, MD (Zonguldak, Turkey), Hakan Sade, MD (Zonguldak, Turkey), and Mehmet Vural, MD (Zonguldak, Turkey) for their technical and editorial assistance in the preparation of this manuscript.

REFERENCES

1. Harrington K, Thompson O, Aquilina J. Uteroplacental and umbilical circulation: Physiological changes in pregnancy. In Kurjak A, ed. *Textbook of Perinatal Medicine*. New York: Parthenon Publishing, 1998:422–6.
2. Fogarty P, Beattie B, Harper A, Dornan J. Continuous wave Doppler flow velocity waveforms from the umbilical artery in normal pregnancy. *J Perinat Med* 1990;18:51–7.
3. Deutinger J. Physiology of Doppler blood flow in maternal blood vessels in pregnancy. *Gynakologe* 1992;25:284–91.
4. Fendel H, Fendel M, Pauen A, Liedtke B, Schonlau H, Warnking R. Doppler studies of arterial blood flow in the uterus during labor. *Z Geburtshilfe Perinatol* 1984;188:64–7.
5. Ertan AK, Wagner A, Tanriverdi HA, Schmidt W. Physiologic color Doppler sonographic changes of the embryonic and uteroplacental vessels in early pregnancy. *Ultrasound Rev Obstet Gynecol* 2003;3:219–22.
6. Schneider KT. Standards in der Perinatalmedizin – Dopplersonographie in der Schwangerschaft. *Frauenarzt* 1997;38:452–8.
7. Bower S, Schuchter K, Campbell S. Doppler ultrasound screening as part of routine antenatal scanning: Prediction of pre-eclampsia and intrauterine growth retardation. *Br J Obstet Gynaecol* 1993;100:989–4.
8. Brosens I, Dixon HG, Robertson W. Fetal growth retardation and the arteries of the placental bed. *Br J Obstet Gynaecol* 1977;84: 656–64.
9. Campbell S, Pearce JM, Hackett G, Cohen-Overbeek T, Hernandez C. Qualitative assessment of uteroplacental blood flow: Early screening test for high-risk pregnancies. *Obstet Gynecol* 1986;68:649–53.
10. Hoffmann H, Chaoui R, Bollmann R, Bayer H. Potential clinical application of Doppler ultrasound in obstetrics. *Zentralbl Gynakol* 1989;111:1277–84.

11. Trudinger BJ, Giles WB, Cook CM. Uteroplacental blood flow velocity-time waveforms in normal and complicated pregnancy. *Br J Obstet Gynaecol* 1985;92:39–45.
12. Huneke B, Holst A, Schroder HJ, Carstensen MH. Normal values for relative Doppler indices. A/B ratio, resistance index and pulsatility index of the uterine artery and umbilical artery in normal pregnancy. A longitudinal study. *Geburtshilfe Frauenheilkd* 1995; 55:616–22.
13. Arabin B, Bergmann PL, Saling E. Simultaneous assessment of blood flow velocity waveforms in uteroplacental vessels, the umbilical artery, the fetal aorta and the fetal common carotid artery. *Fetal Ther* 1987;2:17–26.
14. Arduini D, Rizzo G. Normal values of pulsatility index from fetal vessels: A cross-sectional study on 1556 healthy fetuses. *J Perinat Med* 1990;18:165–72.
15. Schulman H, Fleischer A, Stern W, Farmakides G, Jagani N, Blattner P. Umbilical velocity wave ratios in human pregnancy. *Am J Obstet Gynecol* 1984;148:985–90.
16. Thompson RS, Trudinger BJ, Cook CM. Doppler ultrasound waveform indices: A/B ratio, pulsatility index and Pourcelot ratio. *Br J Obstet Gynaecol* 1988;95:581–8.
17. Trudinger BJ, Ishikawa K. Use of Doppler ultrasound in the high-risk pregnancy. *Clin Diagn Ultrasound* 1990;26:119–37.
18. Hecher K, Spernol R, Szalay S, Stettner H, Ertl U. Reference values for the pulsatility index and the resistance index of blood flow curves of the umbilical artery and fetal aorta in the 3d trimester. *Ultraschall Med* 1989;10:226–9.
19. Vetter K. The significance of Doppler blood flow measurement in recognizing placental insufficiency. *Arch Gynecol Obstet* 1988; 244(Suppl):S12–8.
20. Vyas S, Nicolaides KH, Bower S, Campbell S. Middle cerebral artery flow velocity waveforms in fetal hypoxaemia. *Br J Obstet Gynaecol* 1990;97:797–803.
21. Mires GJ, Christie AD, Leslie J, Lowe E, Patel NB, Howie PW. Are 'notched' uterine arterial waveforms of prognostic value for hypertensive and growth disorders of pregnancy? *Fetal Diagn Ther* 1995;10:111–8.
22. Ertan AK, Hendrik HJ, Tanriverdi HA, Bechtold M, Schmidt W. Fetomaternal Doppler sonography nomograms. *Clin Exp Obstet Gynecol* 2003;30:211–6.

50 Doppler sonography in high-risk pregnancy

A. K. Ertan, H. A. Tanriverdi and W. Schmidt

One of the main aims of routine antenatal care is to identify the 'at risk' fetus in order to apply clinical interventions which could result in reduced perinatal morbidity and mortality.[1] Doppler sonography in obstetrics is a widely accepted functional method of examining the utero-fetoplacental unit.

Doppler ultrasound is a noninvasive technique whereby the movement of blood (usually in a vessel) is studied by detecting the change in frequency of reflected sound. Doppler ultrasound has been used in obstetrics since 1977 to study the feto-placental (umbilical) circulation,[2] and since the 1980s to study the utero-placental (uterine) circulation[3] and fetal circulation.[4] Recently, this method has become an important tool for qualifying high-risk pregnancies.

Information obtained with Doppler sonography helps obstetricians in managing patients in situations like pregnancies complicated by intrauterine growth restriction (IUGR), Rhesus alloimmunization, multiple pregnancies, and anamnestic risk factors. Examination of the uteroplacental and feto-maternal circulation by Doppler sonography in the early second trimester helps predicting pregnancy complications like preeclampsia, IUGR and perinatal death.[5–13]

This chapter aims to introduce Doppler sonographic examinations in high-risk pregnancies. Doppler blood flow velocity waveforms (FVWs) of the fetal side (umbilical artery, descending aorta, and middle cerebral artery) are discussed.

The safety of Doppler ultrasound in obstetrics

The safety of Doppler ultrasound in obstetrics remains a concern. The data available to date suggest that diagnostic ultrasound has no adverse effects on embryogenesis or fetal growth. In addition, ultrasonographic scanning has no long-term effects on cognitive function or noted changes of visual or hearing functions. However, although B and M mode scans are safe during pregnancy, color, power and pulsed Doppler procedures should be performed with caution due to possible thermal effects. Lastly, a new method, the three-dimensional technique, was introduced. While there are no studies regarding the safety of this new technique, the short acquisition time and the postprocessing analysis may decrease exposure and thus reduce the risk of possible effects of the ultrasound waves on fetal development.[14]

In particular, the use of pulsed Doppler involves the use of higher intensities compared to diagnostic ultrasound, and hence may cause significant tissue heating and thermal effects. However, these thermal effects depend on the presence of a tissue/air interface and may therefore not be clinically significant in obstetric ultrasound examinations.[15] Clearly, while there is continuing concern regarding the safety of Doppler ultrasound, it should only be used in cases of proven value or controlled investigational circumstances.

Indications of Doppler sonography in obstetrics

Prospective randomized studies of fetal vessels and their collective evaluation have shown no benefit of Doppler sonography in screening the nonselected population.[16] In high-risk pregnancies, however, there is definitive evidence that the use of Doppler studies can significantly reduce the number of antenatal examinations and the number of necessary inductions of labor and cesarean deliveries for fetal distress. Doppler sonography reduces the perinatal mortality, the number of elective deliveries, the incidence of intrapartum distress, and the occurrence of hypoxic encephalopathy.[17] A definite benefit has been established for Doppler sonography in selected cases (Table 50.1).

Table 50.1 Indications for Doppler sonography in obstetrics

Suspicion of intrauterine growth restriction (IUGR)
Pregnancy-induced hypertension (PIH)/preeclampsia/eclampsia
Suspicion for a fetal malformation or disease
Multiple pregnancy with discordant growth
Investigation of fetal cardiac anomaly or heart disease
Fetal heat rate abnormalities/arrhythmia
Preexisting maternal diseases with vascular relevance
Prior history of IUGR or intrauterine fetal death
Prior history of PIH/pre-eclampsia/eclampsia

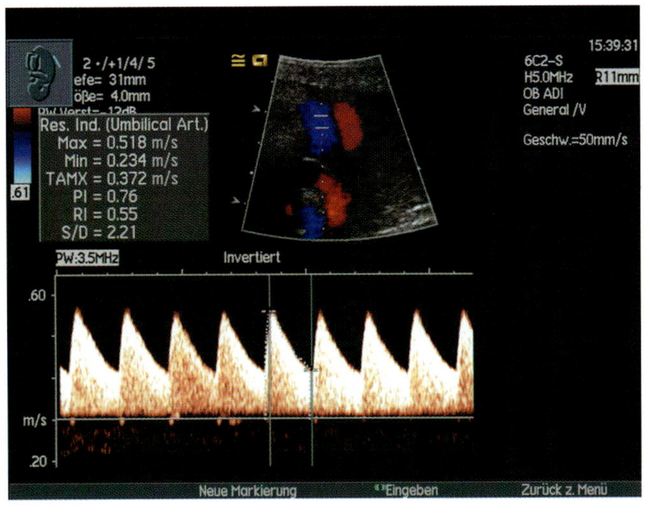

Figure 50.1 Normal flow velocity waveforms of the umbilical artery in the third trimester.

Changes in Doppler sonographic results during the course of pregnancy and complicated pregnancies

During the course of pregnancy and in some specific pregnancy complications, Doppler sonographic results of fetomaternal vessels display changing values. Chronic placental insufficiency is a major research application for Doppler sonography in high-risk pregnancies. Various fetal vessels are examined to determine/diagnose perinatal problems.

Umbilical artery

It has been shown in a longitudinal, observational study that Doppler ultrasound of the umbilical artery (UA) is more helpful than other tests of fetal well-being (e.g., heart rate variability and biophysical profile score) in distinguishing between the normal small fetus and the 'sick' small fetus.[18] However, its exact role in optimizing management, particularly timing of delivery, remains unclear, and is currently being investigated by many study groups. The optimal timing of delivery in pregnancies complicated by highly pathological Doppler flow findings is still an issue to be resolved. The established approach to resolve this question and to improve the perinatal morbidity and mortality by the use of Doppler examination is being investigated in multicenter clinical trials,[19] e.g., the trial of umbilical and fetal flow in Europe Group (TRUFFLE-Protocol, unpublished data).

Blood flow velocity in the UA increases with the advancing gestation. As a result impedance to blood flow continuously decreases due to increasing arterial blood flow in the systole and diastole. End-diastolic velocity is often absent in the first trimester[2,20] and the diastolic component increases with advancing gestation[21] (Figure 50.1). With advancing gestational age end-diastolic flow becomes evident during the whole heart cycle (Figure 50.1). This has been proven by previous longitudinal studies of Fogarty *et al.*[22] and Hünecke *et al.*,[23] as with many cross-sectional studies.[21,24]

Trudinger *et al.*[25] explained this phenomenon with the following mechanisms:

- Continuous maturation in placental villi
- Continuous widening of placental vessels cause a continuous decrease in vascular resistance
- Continuous increase in fetal cardiac output
- Continuous changes in the vessel compliance
- Continuous increase in fetal blood pressure.

Especially in the third trimester of pregnancy, depending on the above factors normal values become scattered on nomograms. This scattering is more prominent in the S/D ratio than the pulsatility index (PI). Resistance index is not affected by the above factors after 28 weeks' gestation.

FVWs of the UA are slightly different at the abdominal wall and the placental site, with indices higher at the fetal abdominal wall than the placental insertion.[26] The difference, however, is minimal, and therefore in clinical practice it is not important to obtain the FVWs always at the same level. FVWs must always be obtained during fetal apnea periods because fetal breathing affects the waveforms.

In case of an abnormal test, clinical experience and randomized controlled trials showed significant association with an adverse perinatal outcome.

Intrauterine growth restriction

The IUGR fetus is a fetus that does not reach its potential growth. Environmental factors responsible may be

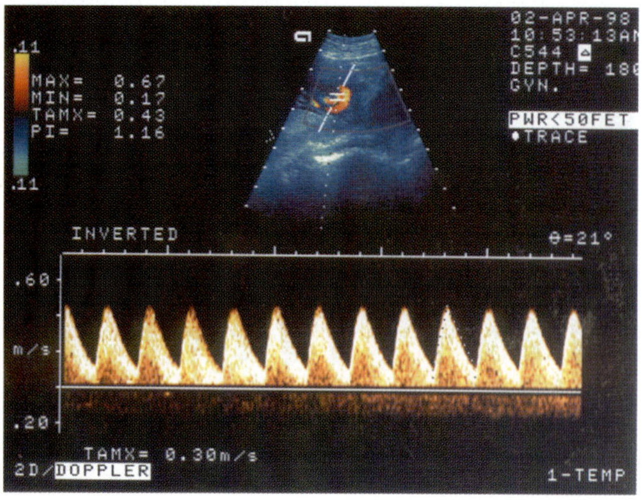

Figure 50.2 Abnormal flow velocity waveforms of the umbilical artery in the third trimester (high resistance index).

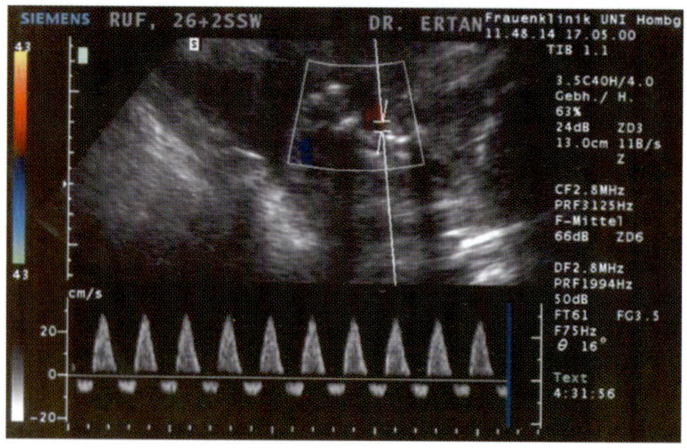

Figure 50.4 Reverse flow (RF) of the umbilical artery.

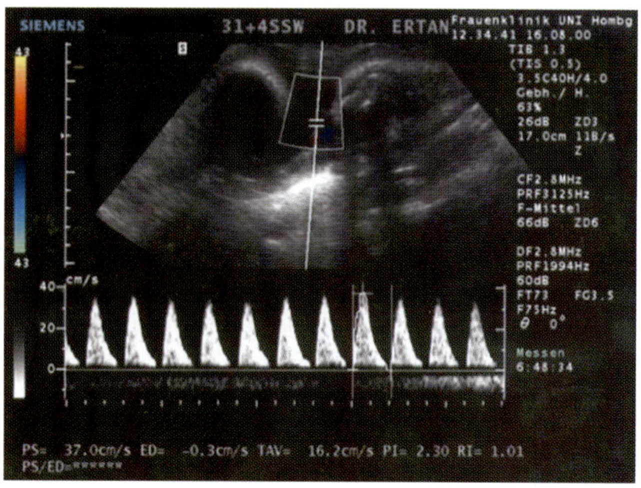

Figure 50.3 Absent end-diastolic flow (AEDF) of the umbilical artery in the third trimester.

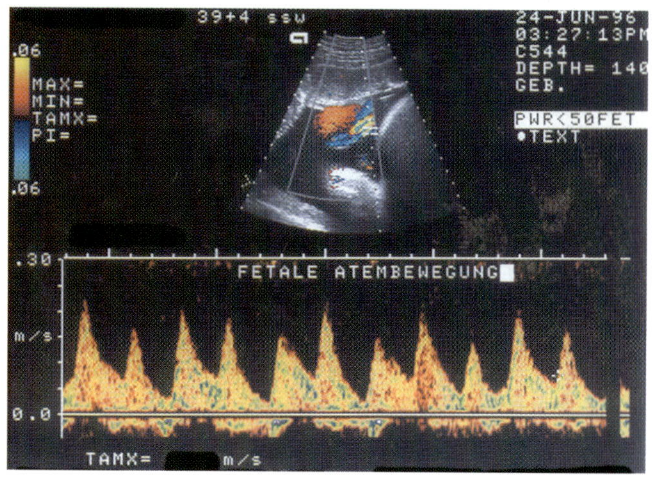

Figure 50.5 Pitfalls in umbilical artery Doppler velocimetry (fetal breathing).

due to maternal, uteroplacental and fetal factors. Many authors have reported on the association between an abnormal UA Doppler FVW and IUGR.

Differentiating the fetus with pathologic growth restriction that is at risk for perinatal complications from the constitutionally small but healthy fetus has been an ongoing challenge in obstetrics. Not all infants whose birth weight is below the 10th percentile have been exposed to a pathologic process *in utero*; in fact, most small newborns are constitutionally small and healthy. Doppler sonography has become the most important investigation method to differentiate between these fetuses.

It should be noted that Doppler sonography is not suitable for the primary diagnosis of fetal growth restriction, but it provides an excellent adjunctive method for risk differentiation in suspicious cases.

Pathophysiology of abnormal FVWs in placental insufficiency[27]

In the presence of placental insufficiency, there is greater placental resistance, which is reflected in a decreased end-diastolic component of the UA FVWs.[28–32] An abnormal UA FVW has an S/D ratio above the normal range. As their placental insufficiency worsens, the end-diastolic velocity decreases (Figure 50.2), then become absent (Figure 50.3), and finally it is reversed (Figure 50.4). Some fetuses have decreased end-diastolic velocity that remains constant with advancing gestation and never become absent or reversed, which may be due to a milder form of placental insufficiency (Figure 50.2). Pitfalls can be caused because of, e.g., fetal breathing (Figure 50.5).

Abnormal UA Doppler studies, but not normal results were found to be associated with lower arterial and venous pH values, an increased likelihood of intrapartum fetal distress, more admissions to the neonatal intensive care unit (NICU), and a higher incidence of respiratory distress in IUGR fetuses.[33] Therefore, intensive antenatal surveillance in fetuses with suspected IUGR if the UA Doppler FVWs are normal was not recommended by the authors. Conflicting data were presented by McCowan *et al.*[34] They confirmed that abnormal UA Doppler studies are associated with a poor perinatal outcome in IUGR fetuses but also concluded that the perinatal outcome in small for gestational age fetuses with normal UA Doppler studies is not always benign (i.e., low ponderal index, postnatal hypoglycemia, admission to the NICU). Recently, Ertan *et al.*[35] suggested that reversed flow should be seen as a particular clinical entity with higher incidences of perinatal and overall mortality, and severe intrauterine growth restriction compared to absent end-diastolic flow (Figures 50.3 and 50.4).

In our clinical experience, when an IUGR fetus is suspected, the UA, fetal descending aorta (FDA), and middle cerebral artery (MCA) are the first fetal vessels to be assessed. The ductus venosus (DV), umbilical vein, inferior vena cava Doppler examinations are secondary vessels to be examined, only when an abnormal FVW is detected on the arterial vessels. Adding serial Doppler evaluation of the UA, MCA, and DV to IUGR surveillance will enhance the performance of the biophysical score in the detection of fetal compromise and therefore optimizing the timing of intervention.[36]

Table 50.2 Antenatal complications of the reversed (*n*=30) and absent end-diastolic flow cases (*n*=30)

Type of complication	Reverse flow, *n* (%)	Absent flow, *n* (%)
Pregnancy-induced hypertension	19 (63.3)	19 (63.3)
HELLP syndrome	1 (3.3)	6 (20)
Gestational diabetes	1 (3.3)	2 (6.7)
Fetal Infection	1 (3.3)	0
Abruptio placenta	0	4 (13.3)
Birth weight in g (M±SD)	1071±112	1214±82
Intrauterine growth retardation* (< 5 percentile)	25 (83.3)	19 (63.3)
Oligohydramnios*	21 (70)	13 (43.3)

HELLP: hemolysis, elevated liver enzymes, low platelets.
* $p < 0.05$.

Comparison of perinatal outcome in fetuses with reverse or absent end-diastolic flow in the umbilical artery/fetal descending aorta[35]

An abnormal FVW is a good predictor for poor perinatal outcome in high-risk pregnancies.[37–41] The absence or reversal of end-diastolic flow in the umbilical artery (UA) and fetal aorta is widely accepted as an ominous sign of fetal compromise, with a very high perinatal mortality (35–100%) and morbidity.[27,39,42,43]

The incidence of absent end-diastolic flow is low, and of reversed flow it is even lower (reverse flow/absent end-diastolic flow ratio=1:10).[27,42,43] Studies so far analyzed the fetal outcome in reversed and absent end-diastolic flow cases together as one clinical entity. The difference between the prognosis of fetuses with reversed flow and absent end-diastolic flow is still unknown.

We undertook a study, in which the highly pathologic flow profiles, consisting of absent end-diastolic flow and reverse flow at the UA and fetal aorta were compared for perinatal outcome. The aim of this study was to clarify whether reverse flow at the UA and fetal aorta worsens perinatal outcome more than absent end-diastolic flow at the same vessels and to assess the possibility of making predictions about the further course of pregnancy.

Materials and methods

During a 10-year period 30 cases with reverse flow in the umbilical artery and/or fetal aorta (group I) were detected. We selected matched pairs of 30 cases with absent end-diastolic velocities (group II). The selection criterion into the groups was an absent or reverse flow at the time of delivery. Fetal malformations and chromosomal anomalies were excluded from both groups. For matching of the absent end-diastolic flow group fetuses to the reversed flow group same gestational ages, estimated fetal weights and gestational ages at delivery were stipulated.

Results

Maternal complications were similar in bothgroups. Intrauterine growth retardation and oligohydramnios incidences were significantly more common ($p < 0.05$, Table 50.2) in the reverse flow group (83% and 70% versus 73% and 43%).

The median time interval between the registration of reverse flow and death of fetuses was 2.5 days. After diagnosis of reverse flow, 11 fetuses (91.7%) died within a week (three on the same day, two on the next day, three on the second day, and the remaining four cases on days 3–8).

Table 50.3 Perinatal and neonatal parameters of the reverse ($n=18$) and absent end-diastolic ($n=29$) flow cases (live-born)

	Reverse flow, *n* (%)	Absent end-diastolic flow, *n* (%)
5 Apgar ≤7	7 (39)	13 (45)
pH ≤7.2	6 (33)	9 (31)
Cerebral hemorrhage	5 (27.8)	5 (17.2)
Infections	8 (44.4)	8 (27.6)
Anemia	8 (44.4)	9 (31.0)
Hypocalcemia*	3 (16.7)	0
Hyaline membrane syndrome	12 (67)	19 (66)
Icterus	8 (44.4)	12 (41.4)
Shock lung	3 (16.7)	2 (6.9)
Lung emphysema	2 (11.1)	0
Retinopathy	1 (5.6)	3 (10.4)
Muscle hypotony	1 (5.6)	3 (10.4)

* $p<0.05$.

The mean gestational age at live birth was 31 weeks in both groups. Of the 18 survivors in group I, 17 (94.4%) were delivered by cesarean section. This was not significantly different from group II. The main indication for the cesarean section was fetal distress. The mean birth weight, 1071 (112 g) vs. 1214 (82 g) was not statistically different between the groups.

The mean values and the frequency of pathological Apgar scores (7) at 1, 5, and 10 min, the arterial cord blood pH values, and the mean values of umbilical arterial PO_2, PCO_2 and HCO_3 were not different among the groups.

All the fetuses with absent and reversed end-diastolic flow were admitted to the NICU, and there was no difference in the duration of NICU treatment required. The rates (83% vs. 86%, respectively, for groups I and II) and duration of mechanical ventilation were not different among the groups.

Neonatal cerebral hemorrhage occurred more often in group I, but without statistical significance (27.8% vs. 17.2%). Neonatal morbidity (Table 50.3) included infections, hyaline membrane syndrome, icterus, and anemia and shock lung, without statistical difference between the groups. Only hypocalcemia was found more often in group I ($p<0.05$).

There was a significantly higher overall and perinatal mortality in the reversed end-diastolic flow group (53% and 27%) as compared to the absent end-diastolic flow group (10% and 7%) ($p<0.05$).

Discussion

Reverse flow in umbilical velocimetry is associated with dismal perinatal outcome. Perinatal mortality ranges from 35% to 100%, and postnatal morbidity is significant.[37,43–45] The above presented study[35] confirmed the adverse fetal outcome in fetuses with reversed end-diastolic flow in the UA and/or fetal aorta with a high overall mortality (53.3%) and perinatal mortality (26.8%).

Because of the low incidences of reverse flow cases, most authors have studied the effect of both reverse flow and absent end-diastolic flow velocity, often referred to an 'ARED-flow', on the fetal outcome together as one entity.[46] Reverse flow was considered to be the last phenomenon preceding fetal death.[37,47,48]

Absent or reversed end-diastolic flow in the UA or fetal aorta, is closely associated with intrauterine growth retardation due to uteroplacental insufficiency and higher rates of pre-eclampsia.[39,40,43] On the other hand, fetuses with intrauterine growth retardation have a high risk of developing absent or reversed end-diastolic flow.[44]

These fetuses with reverse flow had a very high incidence of oligohydramnios, intrauterine growth retardation and maternal pregnancy induced hypertension. Therefore, pregnant women with these complications should be evaluated with Doppler sonography to detect the compromised fetuses.

Several authors found an increasing association between reversed flow of the umbilical artery and the rate of fetal malformations, especially congenital heart anomalies, ranging from 12% to 50%.[43,49] These malformations of fetuses were associated with a low growth potential, not only for the fetus (intrauterine growth retardation) but also for the placenta, regardless of whether the placenta/neonatal weight was normal or below normal.[39] For a better understanding of this correlation, an additional study of subgroups with fetal malformations including more cases would be required.[49]

A close association between the reversed flow and neonatal cerebral hemorrhage has been reported.[44] The inappropriate autoregulation of the cerebral blood flow which is induced by extreme prematurity is the major risk factor for intracerebral hemorrhage.[50]

Normal fetal blood velocity values are considered reassuring and are generally believed to characterize a normal fetal oxygenation.[51] Absent or reversed end-diastolic flow velocity in the UA is associated with fetal hypoxia.[47,52,53] Although normal results of blood-gas analysis from umbilical vessels were observed in some cases with reversed or absent end-diastolic flow velocities, infants with this severe Doppler flow pathologies are at a high risk for neonatal asphyxia.[51] It was further suggested that fetuses with reverse flow should immediately be delivered after diagnosis.[48] 'Once the diastolic component of umbilical artery flow velocity waveforms becomes absent or reversed, the fetus is in a state of hypoxia and acidosis, and fetal death is impending'.[49] Our results showed almost the same frequency of neonatal acidosis in 33% (pH ≤ 7.2) in the reverse flow group, compared to 31% in cases with absent end-diastolic flow velocities. As significant reduction in the proportion of villous tissue occupied by the peripheral villi in pregnancies with absent or reversed end-diastolic flow was well documented previously,[54,55] in our presented cases the higher intrauterine death rates in the reverse flow group denotes an extreme placental insufficiency.

The incidence of infection, hyaline membrane syndrome and icterus was not influenced by reverse or absent end-diastolic flow. The incidence of anemia and shock lung was especially high, and hypocalcemia occurred statistically more frequent in the neonates with reversed end-diastolic flow. There was no difference in NICU admission and mechanical ventilation rates and duration of NICU stay. The overall neonatal morbidity was not significantly different between the groups. This suggests that both highly pathological Doppler findings are affecting the surviving neonates adversely. However, the higher rates of intrauterine and neonatal deaths in the reversed flow cases should be noticed.

The highly pathological Doppler findings (absent and reverse end-diastolic flow) of the umbilical artery and fetal aorta, which are attributable to severe impairment of placental circulation, and represent compromised fetal condition with high incidence of perinatal and neonatal mortality. In our opinion, the finding of a reverse flow spectrum of the umbilical arteries or fetal aorta should be accepted as a more abnormal Doppler finding, compared to absent end-diastolic flow. If absent or reversed end-diastolic flow is detected, a very close antenatal follow-up is advised and delivery should be considered if biophysical parameters and venous Doppler indices become abnormal.

Chromosomal abnormalities

It was shown that absent end-diastolic flow in the UA is associated with chromosomal abnormalities like trisomies, triploidies, or chromosomal deletions.[56] Setting out from the point that structural anomalies are more frequent in fetuses with chromosomal aberrations, the authors recommended a rapid acquisition of a karyotype in fetuses with congenital anomalies and an absent end-diastolic flow in the UA.[35]

Impact on perinatal consequences

Abnormal UA FVWs are associated in IUGR fetuses with one of the following outcomes: early delivery, reduced birth weight, oligohydramnios, NICU admission, and prolonged hospital stay.[27,57] In a meta-analysis it was shown that the use of UA Doppler sonography in pregnancies complicated by IUGR reduces perinatal mortality up to 38% and improves perinatal outcome.[17] A review consisting of 7000 high-risk pregnancies[58] found that Doppler ultrasound was associated with a trend toward reduction in perinatal death especially in pregnancies complicated with pre-eclampsia or IUGR. The Doppler ultrasound use was also associated with fewer inductions of labor and fewer hospital admissions, without reports of adverse perinatal effects. The reviewers concluded that the use of Doppler ultrasound in high-risk pregnancies is likely to reduce perinatal mortality.

Neonatal intraventricular hemorrhage

Fetal status as well as neonatal complications of prematurity in IUGR both contribute to adverse perinatal outcome and increase the risk for the development of intraventricular hemorrhage (IVH). Data suggest that absent and reversed end-diastolic flow in the UA early in gestation carries a high risk of subsequent neonatal IVH.[59] However, this observation is not independent of other perinatal variables: prematurity and difficult births remain the most important determinants of this complication.

Neuromotor outcome

Valcomonico *et al.*[57] evaluated the association of UA Doppler velocimetry with long-term neuromotor outcome in IUGR fetuses with normal ($n=17$), reduced ($n=23$), and absent or reversed ($n=31$) UA end-diastolic flow. The infants who survived the neonatal period were observed for a mean of 18 months. Their postural, sensorial, and cognitive functions were evaluated at 3, 6, 9, 12, and 18 months of age. Although, due to a small number of cases the results did not reach statistical significance, the incidence of permanent neurological sequelae increased as the UA end-diastolic flow decreased (35% with absent or reversed flow, 12% with reduced flow, and 0% with normal flow). Recently, in another study[60] 23 IUGR fetuses with absent or reversed UA end-diastolic flow were matched with fetuses with appropriate growth. All children were followed for 6 years, and intellectual development, neuromotoric development was significantly diminished in fetuses with abnormal FVWs. Only social development was not impaired in fetuses with abnormal UA FVWs. Similar results were previously published by our working group too.[38,61]

Intrapartum studies

A review of intrapartum UA Doppler velocimetry for adverse perinatal outcome gave disappointing results.[62] Out of 2700 pregnancies, which were evaluated for the intrapartum use of Doppler velocimetry, the technique proved to be a poor predictor for outcome measures like low Apgar scores, intrapartum fetal heart rate abnormalities, umbilical arterial acidosis, and cesarean section for fetal distress.

Umbilical artery Doppler ultrasound in unselected patients

Theoretically, the use of routine UA Doppler ultrasound in unselected or low-risk pregnancies would be to detect those pregnancies in which there has been failure to establish or maintain the normal low-resistance umbilical and uterine circulations (a pathological process leading to placental dysfunction and associated with intrauterine growth retardation and pre-eclampsia), before there is clinical evidence of fetal compromise. In practice, observational and longitudinal studies of Doppler ultrasound in unselected or low-risk pregnancies have raised doubts about its application as a routine screening test, and authors have cautioned against its introduction into obstetric practice without supportive evidence from randomized trials.[63–65] The relatively low incidence of significant, poor perinatal outcomes in low-risk and unselected populations presents a challenge in evaluating the clinical effectiveness of routine UA Doppler ultrasound, as large numbers are required to test the hypothesis.

Multiple gestation

The S/D ratio of twins at the UA is in agreement with singleton pregnancies in the third trimester.[66] Twins with an abnormal UA FVW tend to be born earlier, have a higher perinatal mortality and morbidity, and have more frequent structural anomalies than fetuses without abnormal Doppler results.[67]

In cases of twin–twin transfusion syndrome, a poor placental implantation site, or chromosomal anomalies discordant growth between the twins may occur. This is a very high-risk situation, with high perinatal mortality and morbidity. The diagnosis is made mainly by ultrasound biometry. The best predictor for diagnosis of discordant twins appears to be the presence of either a difference in the UA S/D ratio greater than 15% or a different estimated fetal weight greater than 15%.[68] Recently, it has been reported that abnormal UA velocimetry can be observed in small twins more often in monochorionic than dichorionic twins.[69] Doppler ultrasound abnormalities of the UA in either twin are associated with poor perinatal outcome in twin–twin transfusion syndrome.

The biophysical profile and multivessel Doppler ultrasound in IUGR

Biophysical profile scoring (BPS) and Doppler surveillance are the primary methods for fetal assessment in IUGR. As placental insufficiency worsens, the fetus adapts by progressive compensation. Previously it has been suggested that the sequential changes in arterial and venous flow occur before some biophysical parameters (fetal tonus, movement, breathing, amniotic fluid volume, and nonstress test) decline.[70,71] Baschat *et al.*[36] evaluated whether multivessel Doppler parameters (UA, UV, MCA, DV, and inferior vena cava) precede biophysical fetal parameters in fetuses with severe IUGR. They found that combining multivessel Doppler and composite BPS will provide significant early warning and a definitive indication for action in the management of severe IUGR, and suggested that delivery timing may be based on this new gold standard.

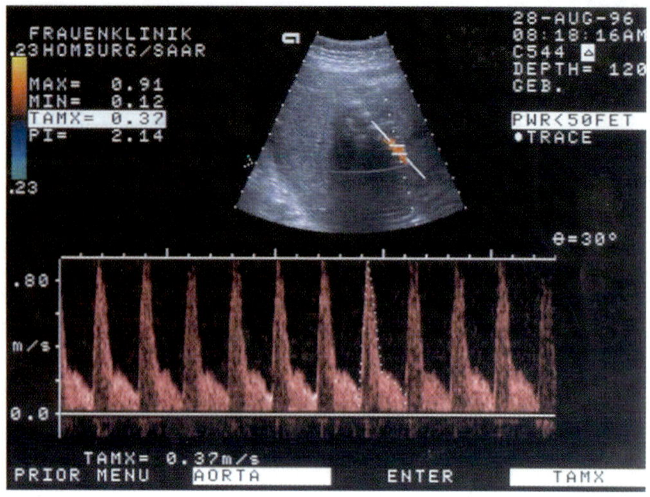

Figure 50.6 Normal flow velocity waveforms of the fetal descending aorta in the third trimester.

Fetal descending aorta

Besides the UA, routine Doppler sonographic examination at the descending fetal aorta is possible. FVWs of the FDA are usually recorded at the level of the diaphragm. In fact, FVWs at the level of the diaphragm and distally to the origin of the renal arteries are different.[72] Normal blood FVWs in the FDA is highly pulsatile, with a minimal diastolic component (Figure 50.6). The descending part of the aorta provides perfusion to the fetal abdominal organs, umbilical–placental circulation, and lower extremities. The flow velocity waveform of the FDA shows a continuous forward stream during the whole heart cycle, but when compared to the FVW of the UA, the end-diastolic flow is less than the systolic component. Due to this reason the S/D ratio in the fetal aorta goes further than the S/D ratio in the UA. As pregnancy advances, the fetal aortic diameter gets wider, which decreases peripheral resistance and increases diastolic flow component. Nevertheless, this does not cause a significant S/D ratio decrease in the FDA.[73] Resistance and pulsatility indices (RI and PI, respectively) in the last trimester are also not affected significantly, and show a similar course as in the UA.

Increased placental impedance combined with redistribution of blood flow from nonvital to vital organs may result in changes in the aortic FVWs. An elevated S/D ratio, RI and PI (Figure 50.7) is associated with both IUGR and adverse perinatal outcomes, such as severe growth restriction, necrotizing enterocolitis, fetal distress, and perinatal mortality.[74–81] Absent end-diastolic flow at the FDA is also a predictor of fetal heart rate abnormalities (Figure 50.8). It was shown that absent flow in the FDA was detected 8 days prior to the onset of decelerations at fetal heart rate monitoring.[78] The sensitivity and specificity of absent end-diastolic flow in the FDA for prediction of IUGR with fetal heart rate abnormalities are 85% and 80%, respectively.[80,81]

Abnormal FVWs of the FDA were also evaluated for intellectual function and minor neurological dysfunction.[38,61,82,83] At 7 years of age, verbal and global performances as well as neurological examination were significantly better in the fetuses with normal aortic FVWs.

Albeit most of the studies showed Doppler velocimetry abnormalities of the FDA is a predictive test for the onset of decompensation due to placental insufficiency in the IUGR fetuses (Figures 50.8 and 50.9), it cannot be recommended as a screening or diagnostic test for IUGR in an unselected obstetric population.[84]

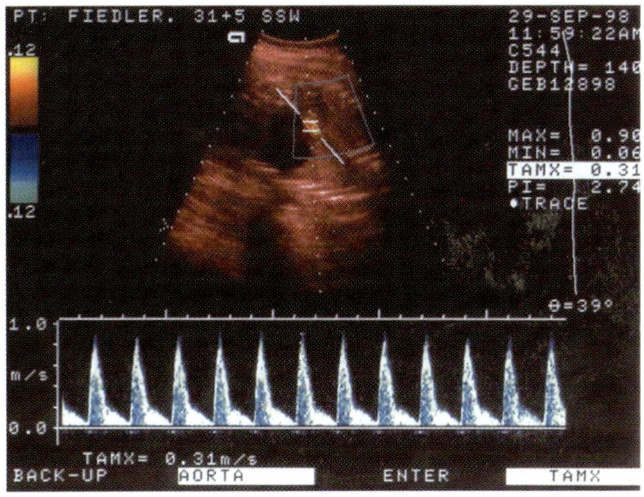

Figure 50.7 Abnormal flow velocity waveforms of the fetal descending aorta in the third trimester (high resistance index).

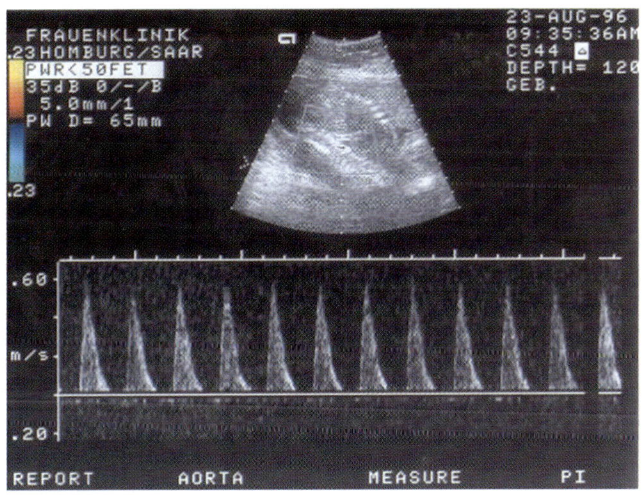

Figure 50.8 Absent end-diastolic flow (AEDF) of the fetal descending aorta (FDA) in the third trimester.

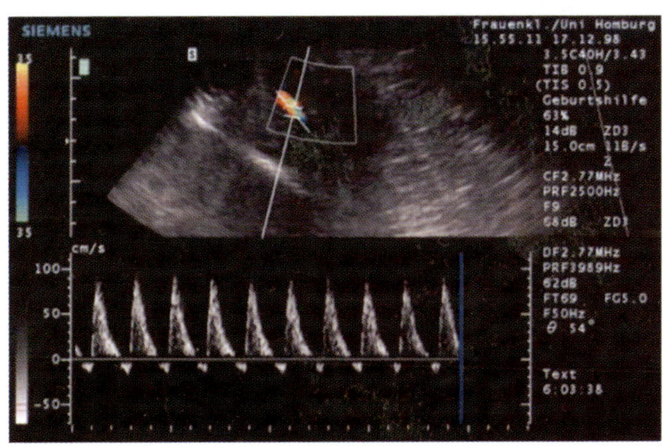

Figure 50.9 Reverse flow (RF) in the fetal descending aorta.

Middle cerebral artery

The circle of Willis is composed anteriorly of the anterior cerebral arteries (branches of the internal carotid artery that are interconnected by the anterior communicating artery) and posteriorly of the two posterior cerebral arteries (branches of the basilar artery that are interconnected on either side with internal carotid artery by the posterior communicating artery).[85] These two trunks and the MCA, another branch of the internal carotid artery, supply the hemispheres on each side (Figure 50.10). All of the defined arteries have different FVWs, therefore, it is important to know which artery is being examined during clinical practice.[86]

The most favorably positioned vessel for Doppler sonographic examination of fetal brain perfusion is the MCA. As the pregnancy advances, the vascular resistance in the MCA decreases (Figure 50.11),[87] and the Doppler indices change. During the early stages of pregnancy, end-diastolic flow velocities in cerebral vessels are small or absent, but velocities increase towards the end of gestation. In the normal developing fetus, the brain is an area of low vascular impedance and receives continuous forward flow throughout the cardiac cycle. IUGR due to placental insufficiency is likely to be caused by redistribution of fetal blood flow in favor of the fetal brain and 'stress organs', at the expense of less essential organs such as subcutaneous tissue, kidneys, and liver. Finally, the already

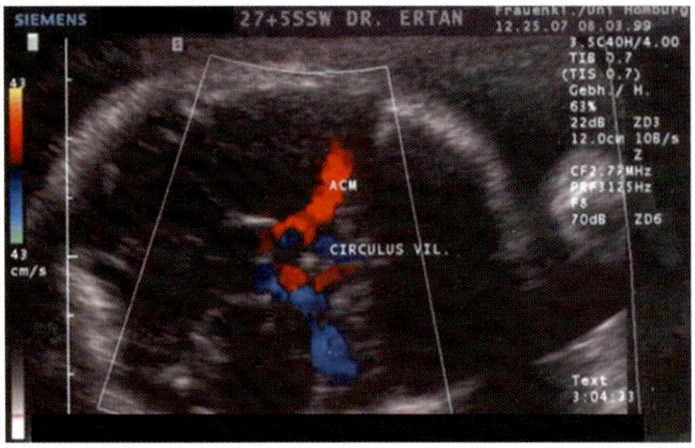

Figure 50.10 Circle of Willis and middle cerebral artery visualized with color Doppler.

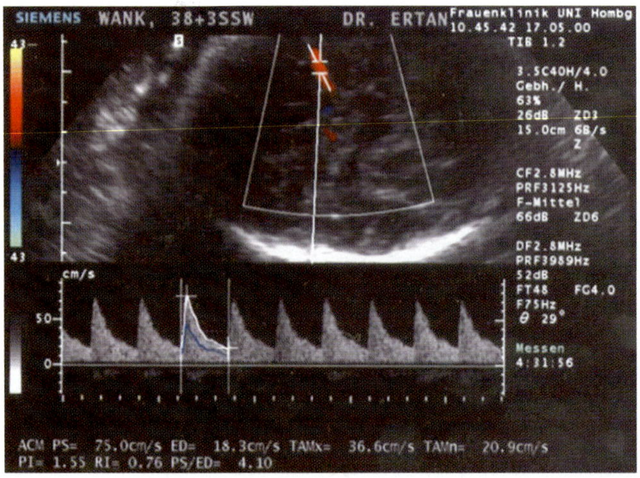

Figure 50.11 Normal flow velocity waveforms of the middle cerebral artery in the third trimester.

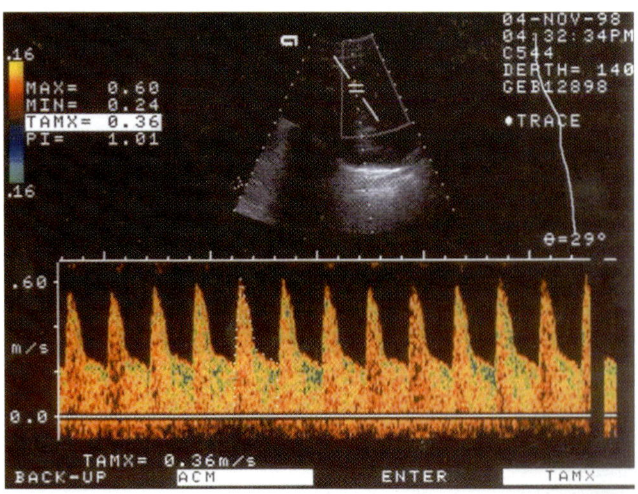

Figure 50.12 Abnormal flow velocity waveforms of the middle cerebral artery in the third trimester ('brain sparing effect').

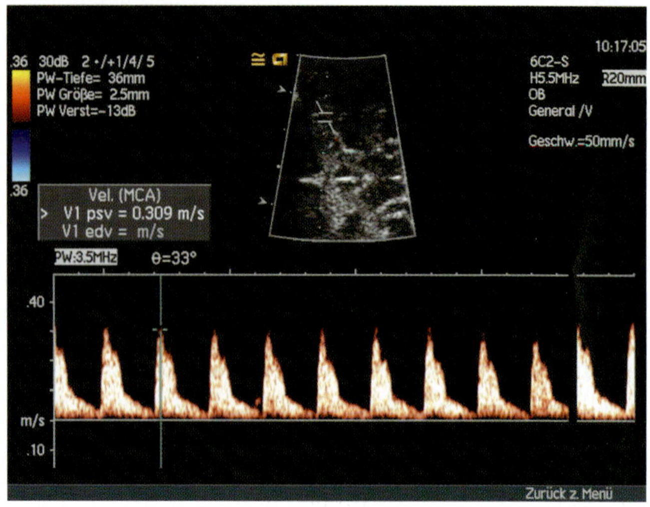

Figure 50.13 Low end-diastolic flow ('normal PI') after the brain sparing effect ('decentralization') this presumably reflects the preterminal stage due to development of brain edema.

low resistance to blood flow in the brain drops further to enhance brain circulation (Figure 50.12). This results in increased end-diastolic velocities, and a decrease in the S/D ratio of the MCA ('brain sparing effect').[88]

Abnormalities of the UA flow correlated with fetal compromise better than intracerebral artery blood flow impairment. This suggests that high placental impedance precedes the onset of the 'brain sparing effect'. In a study, in which 576 high-risk pregnancies were evaluated for the UA and MCA velocimetry, neither test was able to predict adverse perinatal outcome in the normal growing fetus.[89] Results showed that simultaneous assessment of UA and MCA velocimetry in IUGR fetuses did not improve the perinatal outcome. When the UA velocimetry was normal, the MCA velocimetry did not improve the prediction of IUGR or adverse perinatal outcome. However, when the velocimetric values of both arteries were abnormal, the risk of being growth restricted and having an adverse perinatal outcome was doubled.

It has been reported that the MCA PI is below the normal range when pO_2 is reduced.[90] Maximum reduction in PI is reached when the fetal pO_2 is 2–4 standard deviations below normal for gestation. When the oxygen deficit becomes greater, there is a tendency for the MCA PI to rise; this presumably reflects the prefinal stage due to development of brain edema (Figure 50.13).

Hyperactivity of the fetus, increase of intrauterine pressure (e.g., polyhydramnios), and external pressure to the fetal head (e.g., by the probe) might erroneously increase end-diastolic flow velocities in the MCA.[91] Different investigators have undertaken studies – utilizing data obtained from the UA and MCA – to develop indices for evaluation of intrauterine risk.[85]

Prediction of fetal hemoglobin in red cell alloimmunization

Fetal anemia caused by red cell alloimmunization can be detected noninvasively by Doppler ultrasound on the basis of an increase in the peak systolic velocity in the MCA.[92,93] Although there is no strong correlation between these two parameters when the fetus is nonanemic, the correlation becomes stronger as the hemoglobin levels decrease.[93] Prospective evaluation of the MCA peak systolic velocity to detect fetuses at risk for anemia in red cell alloimmunization showed that 90 of the 125 anticipated invasive procedures could be avoided.[94]

In anemic fetuses, change in hematocrit leads to a corresponding alteration in blood viscosity and to an impaired release of oxygen to the tissues. Increased cardiac output and vasodilatation are the main mechanisms by which the fetus attempts to maintain the oxygen and metabolic equilibrium in various organs. It is likely that when the fetus is nonanemic or mildly anemic, there are only minor or insignificant hemodynamic changes. Therefore, the blood velocity does not change. When the fetus becomes more anemic, various mechanisms compensate to maintain the oxygen and metabolic equilibrium in the various organs. The MCA peak systolic velocity changes proportionally to the hemoglobin deficiency.

Doppler measurements appear to be valuable for estimating hemoglobin concentration in fetuses at risk for anemia. Doppler sonography of the MCA has the potential to decrease the need for invasive testing (amniocentesis, cordocentesis) and its potential risks.[95]

Fetal venous circulation

In recent years research on the fetomaternal circulation has focused more on the venous side of the fetal circulation. Physiologically, blood flow velocities in the umbilical vein (UV) and the portal circulation are steady and nonpulsatile. However, it has been shown that both fetal body and breathing movements can interrupt the FVWs. In a recent review, it was concluded that several pathologic conditions such as non-immune hydrops, severe IUGR, and cardiac arrhythmias also result in an abnormal, pulsatile venous blood flow.[96] However, the relationship between fetal venous blood flow patterns and imminent fetal asphyxia or fetal death is still unknown. Recently, studies on venous circulation in the fetal brain[97] and pulmonary venous circulation in the diagnosis of pulmonary hypoplasia were performed.[98] Venous Doppler also has applications in several other disorders (Table 50.4).

Table 50.4 Indications for fetal venous Doppler sonography

Fetal arrhythmias
Suspected twin-twin transfusion syndrome
Nonimmune hydrops fetalis (NIHF)
Suspected stenosis in the cardiac outflow tract
Congenital heart disease
Severe centralization of the fetal circulation (brain sparing)
Suspicious fetal heart rate tracings

An understanding of the fetal venous circulation provides a platform for the clinical management of perinatal problems, especially timing of delivery in high-risk pregnancies, a subject that is dealt with later in this section.

Summary

Doppler ultrasound is a noninvasive technique that is commonly used in high-risk pregnancies. Examination of fetomaternal vessels using Doppler sonography has been subject of intensive investigation in recent years. However, to date, randomized controlled trials were able to establish only limited clinical value of Doppler velocimetry to improve perinatal outcome in high-risk situations. Umbilical artery, fetal descending aorta and middle cerebral artery Doppler velocimetric studies are acceptable tools in the diagnosis and management of intrauterine growth restricted fetuses, and in the reduction of perinatal mortality in high-risk pregnancies. The majority of severely compromised fetuses also show pathological venous velocimetry, which might give valuable clinical information for surveillance in high-risk pregnancies and their optimal perinatal management. In addition, Doppler sonography might have a role in predicting long-term neuromotor outcome. Large-scale randomized controlled trials are needed to establish the clinical utility of Doppler ultrasound in obstetrics.

Acknowledgments

The authors thank Mr. Aykut Barut, MD (Zonguldak/Turkey), Hakan Sade, MD (Zonguldak/Turkey), and Mehmet Vural, MD (Zonguldak/Turkey) for their technical and editorial assistance in the preparation of this manuscript.

REFERENCES

1. Ertan AK, Tanriverdi HA, Schmidt W. Doppler sonography in obstetrics. In Kurjak A, Chervenak FA, eds. *Donald School Textbook of Ultrasound in Obstetrics and Gynecology.* New Delhi, India: Jaypee Brothers, 2003;395–421.
2. FitzGerald DE, Drumm JE. Non-invasive measurement of human fetal circulation using ultrasound: A new method. *Br Med J* 1977;2:1450–1.
3. Campbell S, Diaz-Recasens J, Griffin DR *et al.* New Doppler technique for assessing uteroplacental blood flow. *Lancet* 1983;1: 675–7.
4. Eik-Nes SH, Marsal K, Brubakk AO, Kristofferson K, Ulstein M. Ultrasonic measurement of human fetal blood flow. *J Biomed Eng* 1982;4:28–36.
5. Bower S, Schuchter K, Campbell S. Doppler ultrasound screening as part of routine antenatal scanning: prediction of pre-eclampsia and intrauterine growth retardation. *Br J Obstet Gynaecol* 1993; 100:989–94.
6. Caforio L, Testa AC, Mastromarino C *et al.* Predictive value of uterine artery velocimetry at midgestation in low- and high-risk populations: A new perspective. *Fetal Diagn.Ther* 1999;14: 201–5.
7. Campbell S, Pearce JM, Hackett G, Cohen-Overbeek T, Hernandez C. Qualitative assessment of uteroplacental blood flow: Early screening test for high-risk pregnancies. *Obstet Gynecol* 1986;68:649–53.
8. Harrington K, Cooper D, Lees C, Hecher K, Campbell S. Doppler ultrasound of the uterine arteries: the importance of bilateral notching in the prediction of pre-eclampsia, placental abruption or delivery of a small-for-gestational-age baby. *Ultrasound Obstet Gynecol* 1996;7:182–8.
9. Harrington K, Goldfrad C, Carpenter RG, Campbell S. Transvaginal uterine and umbilical artery Doppler examination of 12–16 weeks and the subsequent development of pre-eclampsia and intrauterine growth retardation. *Ultrasound Obstet Gynecol* 1997;9:94–100.
10. Irion O, Masse J, Forest JC, Moutquin JM. Prediction of pre-eclampsia, low birthweight for gestation and prematurity by uterine artery blood flow velocity waveforms analysis in low risk nulliparous women. *Br J Obstet Gynaecol* 1998;105:422–9.
11. Hoffmann H, Chaoui R, Bollmann R, Bayer H. Potential clinical application of Doppler ultrasound in obstetrics. *Zentralbl Gynakol* 1989;111:1277–84.
12. Trudinger BJ, Giles WB, Cook CM. Uteroplacental blood flow velocity–time waveforms in normal and complicated pregnancy. *Br J Obstet Gynaecol* 1985;92:39–45.
13. Zimmermann P, Eirio V, Koskinen J, Kujansuu E, Ranta T. Doppler assessment of the uterine and uteroplacental circulation in the second trimester in pregnancies at high risk for pre-eclampsia and/or intrauterine growth retardation: Comparison and correlation between different Doppler parameters. *Ultrasound Obstet Gynecol* 1997;9:330–8.
14. Hershkovitz R, Sheiner E, Mazor M. Ultrasound in obstetrics: a review of safety. *Eur J Obstet Gynecol Reprod Biol* 2002; 101:15–18.
15. Barnett S, Kossoff G, Edwards M. Is diagnostic ultrasound safe? Current international consensus on the thermal mechanism. *Med J Aust* 1994;160:33–7.
16. Schneider KT. [Doppler ultrasound: patient safety and incorporation of the method into clinical management]. *Gynakol Geburtshilfliche Rundsch* 1993;33(Suppl 1):113–15.
17. Alfirevic Z, Neilson JP. Doppler ultrasonography in high-risk pregnancies: Systematic review with meta-analysis. *Am J Obstet Gynecol* 1995;172:1379–87.
18. Soothill PW, Ajayi RA, Campbell S, Nicolaides KH. Prediction of morbidity in small and normally grown fetuses by fetal heart rate variability, biophysical profile score and umbilical artery Doppler studies. *Br J Obstet Gynaecol* 1993;100:742–5.
19. Romero R, Kalache K, Kadar N. Timing the delivery of the preterm severely growth-restricted fetus: venous Doppler, cardiotocography or the biophysical profile? *Ultrasound Obstet Gynecol* 2002; 19:118–21.
20. Stuart B, Drumm J, FitzGerald DE, Duignan NM. Fetal blood velocity waveforms in normal pregnancy. *Br J Obstet Gynaecol* 1980;87:780–5.
21. Thompson RS, Trudinger BJ, Cook CM. Doppler ultrasound waveform indices: A/B ratio, pulsatility index and Pourcelot ratio. *Br J Obstet Gynaecol* 1988;95:581–8.
22. Fogarty P, Beattie B, Harper A, Dornan J. Continuous wave Doppler flow velocity waveforms from the umbilical artery in normal pregnancy. *J Perinat Med* 1990;18:51–7.
23. Huneke B, Holst A, Schroder HJ, Carstensen MH. Normal values for relative Doppler indices. A/B ratio, resistance index and pulsatility index of the uterine artery and umbilical artery in normal pregnancy. A longitudinal study. *Geburtshilfe Frauenheilkd* 1995; 55:616–22.
24. Schulman H, Fleischer A, Stern W, Farmakides G, Jagani N, Blattner P. Umbilical velocity wave ratios in human pregnancy. *Am J Obstet Gynecol* 1984;148:985–90.
25. Trudinger BJ, Giles WB, Cook CM, Bombardieri J, Collins L. Fetal umbilical artery flow velocity waveforms and placental resistance: Clinical significance. *Br J Obstet Gynaecol* 1985;92:23–30.
26. Maulik D, Yarlagadda AP, Youngblood JP, Willoughby L. Components of variability of umbilical arterial Doppler velocimetry – A prospective analysis. *Am J Obstet Gynecol* 1989;160:1406–9.
27. Ertan A, Hendrik H, Schmidt W. Hochpathologische Doppler-Flow-Befunde und perinatale Auffälligkeiten. In Schmidt W, Kurjak A, eds. *Farbdopplersonographie in Gynäkologie und Geburtshilfe.* Stuttgart: Thieme Verlag, 2000;177–87.
28. Fleischer A, Schulman H, Farmakides G, Bracero L, Blattner P, Randolph G. Umbilical artery velocity waveforms and intrauterine growth retardation. *Am J Obstet Gynecol* 1985;151:502–5.
29. Devoe LD, Gardner P, Dear C, Faircloth D. The significance of increasing umbilical artery systolic–diastolic ratios in third-trimester pregnancy. *Obstet Gynecol* 1992;80:684–7.
30. Rochelson B, Schulman H, Farmakides G *et al.* The significance of absent end-diastolic velocity in umbilical artery velocity waveforms. *Am J Obstet Gynecol* 1987;156:1213–18.
31. Trudinger BJ, Cook CM, Giles WB *et al.* Fetal umbilical artery velocity waveforms and subsequent neonatal outcome. *Br J Obstet Gynaecol* 1991;98:378–84.
32. Gudmundsson S, Marsal K. Umbilical and uteroplacental blood flow velocity waveforms in pregnancies with fetal growth retardation. *Eur J Obstet Gynecol Reprod Biol* 1988;27:187–96.
33. Baschat AA, Weiner CP. Umbilical artery Doppler screening for detection of the small fetus in need of antepartum surveillance. *Am J Obstet Gynecol* 2000;182:154–8.
34. McCowan LM, Harding JE, Stewart AW. Umbilical artery Doppler studies in small for gestational age babies reflect disease severity. *Br J Obstet Gynaecol* 2000;107:916–25.
35. Ertan AK, He JP, Tanriverdi HA, Hendrik HJ, Limbach H, Schmidt W. Comparison of perinatal outcome in fetuses with reverse or absent enddiastolic flow in the umbilical artery/fetal descending aorta. *J Perinat Med* 2003;31:307–12.
36. Baschat AA, Gembruch U, Harman CR. The sequence of changes in Doppler and biophysical parameters as severe fetal growth restriction worsens. *Ultrasound Obstet Gynecol* 2001;18: 571–7.
37. Brar H, Platt L. Reverse enddiastolic flow velocity on umbilical artery velocimetry in high-risk pregnancy: An ominous finding with adverse pregnancy outcome. *Am J Obstet Gynecol* 1988; 159:559–61.
38. Ertan A, Jost W, Hendrik H, Lauer S, Uhrmacher S, Schmidt W. Perinatal events and neuromotoric development of children with zero flow in the fetal vessels during the last trimester. In Cosmi EVDRG, ed. *2nd World Congress of Perinatal Medicine.* Bologna: Monduzzi Editore Spa, 1993;1049–52.
39. Jacobson S, Imhof R, Manning N *et al.* The value of Doppler assessment of the uteroplacental circulation in predicting preeclampsia or intrauterine growth retardation. *Am J Obstet Gynecol* 1990;162:110–14.
40. Trudinger B, Cook C, Giles W, Connelly A, Thompson R. Umbilical artery flow velocity waveforms in high-risk pregnancy. Randomized controlled trial. *Lancet* 1987;8526:188–90.
41. Marsal K. Rational use of Doppler ultrasound in perinatal medicine. *J Perinat Med* 1994;22:463–74.
42. Rühle W, Ertan A, Gnirs J, Schmidt W. Dopplersonographie in der Geburtshilfe-Beitrag zum Verständnis des "Reverse Flow" in der Arteria umbilicalis. *Ultraschall Med* 1991;12:134–8.

43. Schmidt W, Rühle W, Ertan A, Boos R, Gnirs J. Dopplersonographische-Perinatologische Daten bei Fällen mit enddiastolischem Block bzw. Reverse Flow. *Geburts Frauenheilkd* 1991;51: 288–92.
44. Karsdorp V, Vugt J, Van Geijin H *et al.* Clinical significance of absent or reversed enddiastolic velocity waveforms in umbilical artery. *Lancet* 1994;344:1664–8.
45. Zelop C, Richardson D, Heffner L. Abnormal umbilical artery Doppler velocimetry in structurally normal singleton fetuses. *Obstet Gynecol* 1996;87:434–8.
46. Montenegro N, Santos F, Tavares E, Matias A, Barros H, Leite L. Outcome of 88 pregnancies with absent or reversed enddiastolic blood flow (ARED flow) in the umbilical arteries. *Eur J Obstet Gynecol Reprod Biol* 1998;79:43–6.
47. Illyes M, Gati I. Reversed flow in the human fetal descending aorta as a sign of severe fetal asphyxia preceding intrauterine deaths. *J Clin Ultrasound* 1988;16:403–7.
48. Woo J, Liang S, Lo R. Significance of an absent or reversed enddiastolic flow in Doppler umbilical artery waveforms. *J Ultrasound Med* 1987;6:291–7.
49. Hsieh F, Chang F, Ko T, Chen H, Chen Y. Umbilical artery flow velocity waveforms in fetuses dying with congenital anomalies. *Br J Obstet Gynecol* 1988;95:478–82.
50. Weindling A, Wilkinson A, Cook J, Calvert S, Fox T, Rochefort M. Perinatal events which precede periventricular hemorrhage and leukomalacia in the newborn. *Br J Obstet Gynecol* 1985;92: 1218–23.
51. Bilardo C, Nicolaides K, Campbell S. Doppler measurements of fetal and uteroplacental circulations: relationship with umbilical venous blood gas measured at cordocentesis. *Am J Obstet Gynecol* 1990;162:115–20.
52. Gudmundsson S, Dubiel M. Doppler velocimetry in the evaluation of fetal hypoxia. *J Perinat Med* 2001;29:399–407.
53. Campbell S, Vyas S, Nicolaides K. Doppler investigation of the fetal circulation. *J Perinat Med* 1991;19:21–6.
54. Biagiotti R, Sgambati E, Brizzi E. Placental morphometry in pregnancies complicated by intrauterine growth retardation with absent or reversed end diastolic flow in the umbilical artery. *Ital J Anat Embryol* 1999;104:201–7.
55. Kingdom J, Huppertz B, Seaward G, Kaufmann P. Development of the placental villous tree and its consequences for fetal growth. *Eur J Obstet Gynecol Reprod Biol* 2000;92:35–43.
56. Rizzo G, Pietropolli A, Capponi A, Arduini D, Romanini C. Chromosomal abnormalities in fetuses with absent end-diastolic velocity in umbilical artery: Analysis of risk factors for an abnormal karyotype. *Am J Obstet Gynecol* 1994;171:827–31.
57. Valcamonico A, Danti L, Frusca T *et al.* Absent end-diastolic velocity in umbilical artery: Risk of neonatal morbidity and brain damage. *Am J Obstet Gynecol* 1994;170:796–801.
58. Neilson JP, Alfirevic Z. Doppler ultrasound for fetal assessment in high risk pregnancies. *Cochrane Database Syst Rev* 2000, CD000073.
59. Baschat AA, Gembruch U, Viscardi RM, Gortner L, Harman CR. Antenatal prediction of intraventricular hemorrhage in fetal growth restriction: What is the role of Doppler? *Ultrasound Obstet Gynecol* 2002;19:334–9.
60. Wienerroither H, Steiner H, Tomaselli J, Lobendanz M, Thun-Hohenstein L. Intrauterine blood flow and long-term intellectual, neurologic, and social development. *Obstet Gynecol* 2001;97:449–53.
61. Ertan AK, Jost W, Mink D, Schmidt W. Neuromotoric development of children after AED-flow during pregnancy. In Kurjak A, Latin V, Rippmann E, eds. *Advances in the Pathophysiology of Pregnancy*. Milan: CIC Edizioni Internazionali, 1995;55–62.
62. Farrell T, Chien PF, Gordon A. Intrapartum umbilical artery Doppler velocimetry as a predictor of adverse perinatal outcome: A systematic review. *Br J Obstet Gynaecol* 1999;106:783–92.
63. Sijmons EA, Reuwer PJ, van Beek E, Bruinse HW. The validity of screening for small-for-gestational-age and low-weight-for-length infants by Doppler ultrasound. *Br J Obstet Gynaecol* 1989;96: 557–61.
64. Beattie RB, Dornan JC. Antenatal screening for intrauterine growth retardation with umbilical artery Doppler ultrasonography. *Br Med J* 1989;298:631–5.
65. Goffinet F, Paris-Llado J, Nisand I, Breart G. Umbilical artery Doppler velocimetry in unselected and low risk pregnancies: A review of randomised controlled trials. *Br J Obstet Gynaecol* 1997;104:425–30.
66. Giles WB, Trudinger BJ, Cook CM, Connelly A. Umbilical artery flow velocity waveforms and twin pregnancy outcome. *Obstet Gynecol* 1988;72:894–7.
67. Gaziano EP, Knox H, Ferrera B, Brandt DG, Calvin SE, Knox GE. Is it time to reassess the risk for the growth-retarded fetus with normal Doppler velocimetry of the umbilical artery? *Am J Obstet Gynecol* 1994;170:1734–41.
68. Divon MY, Girz BA, Sklar A, Guidetti DA, Langer O. Discordant twins – A prospective study of the diagnostic value of real-time ultrasonography combined with umbilical artery velocimetry. *Am J Obstet Gynecol* 1989;161:757–60.
69. Gaziano E, Gaziano C, Brandt D. Doppler velocimetry determined redistribution of fetal blood flow: correlation with growth restriction in diamniotic monochorionic and dizygotic twins. *Am J Obstet Gynecol* 1998;178:1359–67.
70. Hecher K, Campbell S, Doyle P, Harrington K, Nicolaides K. Assessment of fetal compromise by Doppler ultrasound investigation of the fetal circulation. Arterial, intracardiac, and venous blood flow velocity studies. *Circulation* 1995;91:129–38.
71. Senat MV, Schwarzler P, Alcais A, Ville Y. Longitudinal changes in the ductus venosus, cerebral transverse sinus and cardiotocogram in fetal growth restriction. *Ultrasound Obstet Gynecol* 2000; 16:19–24.
72. Lingman G, Marsal K. Fetal central blood circulation in the third trimester of normal pregnancy – A longitudinal study. I. Aortic and umbilical blood flow. *Early Hum Dev* 1986;13:137–50.
73. Hecher K, Spernol R, Szalay S, Stettner H, Ertl U. Reference values for the pulsatility index and the resistance index of blood flow curves of the umbilical artery and fetal aorta in the 3rd trimester. *Ultraschall Med* 1989;10:226–9.
74. Soothill PW, Nicolaides KH, Bilardo K, Hackett GA, Campbell S. Utero-placental blood velocity resistance index and umbilical venous pO_2, pCO_2, pH, lactate and erythroblast count in growth-retarded fetuses. *Fetal Ther* 1986;1:176–9.
75. Jouppila P, Kirkinen P. Blood velocity waveforms of the fetal aorta in normal and hypertensive pregnancies. *Obstet Gynecol* 1986; 67:856–60.
76. Laurin J, Lingman G, Marsal K, Persson PH. Fetal blood flow in pregnancies complicated by intrauterine growth retardation. *Obstet Gynecol* 1987;69:895–902.
77. Hackett GA, Campbell S, Gamsu H, Cohen-Overbeek T, Pearce JM. Doppler studies in the growth retarded fetus and prediction of neonatal necrotising enterocolitis, haemorrhage, and neonatal morbidity. *Br Med J (Clin Res Ed)* 1987;294:13–16.
78. Arabin B, Siebert M, Jimenez E, Saling E. Obstetrical characteristics of a loss of end-diastolic velocities in the fetal aorta and/or umbilical artery using Doppler ultrasound. *Gynecol Obstet Invest* 1988;25:173–80.
79. Tonge HM, Wladimiroff JW, Noordam MJ, van Kooten C. Blood flow velocity waveforms in the descending fetal aorta: comparison between normal and growth-retarded pregnancies. *Obstet Gynecol* 1986;67:851–5.
80. Bonatz G, Schulz V, Weisner D, Jonat W. Fetal heart rate (FHR) pathology in labor related to preceding Doppler sonographic results of the umbilical artery and fetal aorta in appropriate and small for gestational age babies. A longitudinal analysis. *J Perinat Med* 1997;25:440–6.
81. Marsal K, Laurin J, Lindblad A, Lingman G. Blood flow in the fetal descending aorta. *Semin Perinatol* 1987;11:322–34.
82. Ley D, Tideman E, Laurin J. Abnormal fetal aortic velocity waveform and intellectual function at 7 years of age. *Ultrasound Obstet Gynecol* 1996;8:160–5.
83. Ley D, Laurin J, Bjerre M, Marsal K. Abnormal fetal aortic velocity waveform and minor neurological dysfunction at 7 years of age. *Ultrasound Obstet Gynecol* 1996;8:152–9.
84. Divon MY, Ferber A. Doppler evaluation of the fetus. *Clin Obstet Gynecol* 2002;45:1015–25.
85. Mari G, Detti L. Doppler ultrasound application to fetal medicine. In: Fleischer A, Manning F, Jeanty P, Romero R, eds. *Sonography in Obstetrics and Gynecology (Principles and Practice)*. New York: McGraw Hill, 2001;247–83.
86. Mari G, Moise KJ Jr, Deter RL, Kirshon B, Carpenter RJ Jr, Huhta JC. Doppler assessment of the pulsatility index in the cerebral circulation of the human fetus. *Am J Obstet Gynecol* 1989;160:698–703.
87. Vetter K. The significance of Doppler blood flow measurement in recognizing placental insufficiency. *Arch Gynecol Obstet* 1988; 244(Suppl):S12–18.

88. Arabin B, Bergmann PL, Saling E. Simultaneous assessment of blood flow velocity waveforms in uteroplacental vessels, the umbilical artery, the fetal aorta and the fetal common carotid artery. *Fetal Ther* 1987;2:17–26.
89. Strigini FA, De Luca G, Lencioni G, Scida P, Giusti G, Genazzani AR. Middle cerebral artery velocimetry: Different clinical relevance depending on umbilical velocimetry. *Obstet Gynecol* 1997;90:953–7.
90. Sepulveda W, Shennan AH, Peek MJ. Reverse end-diastolic flow in the middle cerebral artery: an agonal pattern in the human fetus. *Am J Obstet Gynecol* 1996;174:1645–7.
91. Vyas S, Nicolaides KH, Bower S, Campbell S. Middle cerebral artery flow velocity waveforms in fetal hypoxaemia. *Br J Obstet Gynaecol* 1990;97:797–803.
92. Mari G, Adrignolo A, Abuhamad AZ *et al.* Diagnosis of fetal anemia with Doppler ultrasound in the pregnancy complicated by maternal blood group immunization. *Ultrasound Obstet Gynecol* 1995;5:400–5.
93. Mari G, Deter RL, Carpenter RL *et al.* Noninvasive diagnosis by Doppler ultrasonography of fetal anemia due to maternal red-cell alloimmunization. Collaborative Group for Doppler Assessment of the Blood Velocity in Anemic Fetuses. *N Engl.J Med* 2000;342:9–14.
94. Zimmerman R, Carpenter RJ Jr., Durig P, Mari G. Longitudinal measurement of peak systolic velocity in the fetal middle cerebral artery for monitoring pregnancies complicated by red cell alloimmunisation: a prospective multicentre trial with intention-to-treat. *Br J Obstet Gynaecol* 2002;109:746–52.
95. Mari G, Detti L, Oz U, Zimmerman R, Duerig P, Stefos T. Accurate prediction of fetal hemoglobin by Doppler ultrasonography. *Obstet Gynecol* 2002;99:589–93.
96. Huisman TW. Doppler assessment of the fetal venous system. *Semin Perinatol* 2001;25:21–31.
97. Laurichesse-Delmas H, Grimaud O, Moscoso G, Ville Y. Color Doppler study of the venous circulation in the fetal brain and hemodynamic study of the cerebral transverse sinus. *Ultrasound Obstet Gynecol* 1999;13:34–42.
98. Yoshimura S, Masuzaki H, Miura K, Muta K, Gotoh H, Ishimaru T. Diagnosis of fetal pulmonary hypoplasia by measurement of blood flow velocity waveforms of pulmonary arteries with Doppler ultrasonography. *Am J Obstet Gynecol* 1999;180:441–6.

51 Effect of exercise on fetoplacental Doppler flow

H. A. Tanriverdi, A. K. Ertan and W. Schmidt

The effects of maternal exercise on placental bed blood flow

Sustained bouts of maternal exercise have both acute and chronic effects on placental bed blood flow. During exercise, blood flow is diverted away from the viscera to the exercising muscle and skin.[1] The magnitude of the reduction in flow is directly proportional to the exercise intensity and the muscle mass used (which varies with the type of exercise), and with common types of exercise performed at usual exercise intensities, the reduction usually exceeds 50%. This exercise-induced decrease in visceral flow persists throughout pregnancy but, in late pregnancy, the magnitude of the decrease is blunted in women who continue to exercise regularly.[2–4] Once the exercise ceases, flow rapidly returns to normal. Thus, during a routine exercise session both glucose and oxygen delivery to the placental site are acutely reduced and the magnitude of the decrease varies with exercise type and intensity, maternal fitness and the time point in pregnancy when the exercise is carried out.[4,5]

However, women who perform weight-bearing exercise regularly during pregnancy augment the pregnancy-associated increases in plasma volume, intervillous space blood volume, placental volume and cardiac output.[5,6] The fact that regular weight-bearing exercise augments the changes in these parameters by between 10% and 50% also suggests that it increases the rate of placental bed blood flow at rest. If this inference is correct, then exercise training during pregnancy should actually increase the glucose and oxygen delivery to the placental site throughout mid- and late pregnancy.

The main concern about exercise in pregnancy is that reduced uterine blood flow may cause hypoxia in the fetus.[7] Recent studies using Doppler ultrasonography found an increase in the systolic/diastolic (S/D) ratio of uterine circulation, indicating an increase in resistance of the main vessels that supply the uterus.[8,9]

Although uteroplacental blood flow may decrease with exercise, compensatory mechanisms may exist to ensure adequate fetal oxygenation. In studying ewes, Chandler reported an increase in uterine extraction of oxygen that occurred with the decreased uterine blood flow after maternal exercise.[10] Curet *et al.* reported altered distribution of uterine blood flow in favor of the placenta in ewes.[11]

Complicated pregnancies and exercise

Two worrisome antenatal complications of pregnancy are intrauterine growth restriction (IUGR) and preterm labor. Strenuous exercise in pregnancy has been assessed and is not harmful to the mother or the fetus in healthy women if it is of limited duration. Heavy work or exercise also does not appear to increase the risk of a preterm delivery or IUGR in women at low risk for an adverse pregnancy outcome.[12]

The influence of exercise during pregnancy and its effect on birth weight and pregnancy outcome remains uncertain. The most recent technical bulletin from the American College of Obstetricians and Gynecologists (ACOG)[13] suggests that lower birth weights are observed among vigorously exercising women, but there is no information linking exercise with an adverse outcome of the fetus. The effect of maternal exercise on prenatal complications is also unknown. A recent review from the Cochrane database was unable to demonstrate important benefits or risks to the mother or fetus with exercise in pregnancy.[12]

Small patient numbers or failure to take into consideration the confounding variables in larger samples hampers the studies assessing exercise with birth weight and pregnancy outcome. Because the labor force is composed of more working women, many who exercise at conception and continue during pregnancy, the impact of exercise on pregnancy outcome in working women is very important. Influences of exercise, stress and occupation on pregnancy outcome are difficult to examine because of confounding variables not taken into account in large investigations and the lack of an adequate sample size in smaller studies.

As physical stress is relatively easy to standardize, several groups have studied changes in pregnant women as a result of sporting exertion, particularly the measurable physiological changes in the organisms of the mother and child. Although using different types of exercise – produced by ergometer, treadmill and running tests – all authors came to the conclusion that light and medium physical exercise has no significant adverse effect on the mother or the fetus.[14–16]

Doppler flow measurements of the fetoplacental unit after physical exercise of the mother have been performed with varying results by several investigators.[16–30] Only one study compared Doppler flow in uncomplicated and complicated pregnancies after physical exercise of the mother.[31] In this study Hackett *et al.* studied 34 women (12 uncomplicated and the other 22 complicated by hypertension, IUGR fetus or both) in the third trimester of singleton pregnancies. The patients underwent a bicycle exercise test during which pulsed Doppler sonographic assessment of the uteroplacental circulation was performed. Exercise appeared to increase the pulsatility of the uteroplacental Doppler waveform in all cases. The changes in the waveforms were more exaggerated in the complicated pregnancies, particularly when the resting waveform had been abnormal. These changes indicate an increase in uteroplacental vascular resistance with exercise, suggesting a deleterious effect of physical exertion in the third trimester, particularly in the presence of hypertension or IUGR fetus.

The effect of physical exertion on the fetoplacental unit in pregnancies complicated by IUGR or hypertensive disorders is of special clinical interest, because these fetuses are known to be at risk for long-term neurological morbidity.

Doppler sonographic examination during exercise in complicated pregnancies: Own results

We conducted a study including measurements of the fetal aorta, fetal middle cerebral artery, umbilical artery and uteroplacental vessels in appropriate-for-gestational-age (AGA) and IUGR fetuses to investigate changes of the fetoplacental unit after defined maternal exercise in the third trimester of pregnancy.

Materials and methods: A total of 33 pregnant women with AGA fetuses and 10 patients with IUGR fetuses in the third trimester were examined. Multiple pregnancies, cases with maternal renal disease, maternal diabetes, maternal cardiovascular pathology other than hypertension and fetuses with chromosomal or structural anomalies were excluded from the evaluation. IUGR was defined as a fetal abdominal circumference < 5th percentile for the gestational age of our reference ranges.[33]

The exercise period began with an acclimatization period of 3 min (30 W), followed by 10 min of moderate exertion (1.25 W/kg body weight for each woman). A bicycle ergometer from Mijnhardt (Mijnhardt-Jäger b.v., Bunnik, The Netherlands) was used.

Immediately after the exercise period, Doppler flow measurements were performed. The test period was 35 min. In the IUGR group fetal heart rate (FHR) monitoring was performed for an additional 15 min before and after the exercise.

Doppler flow recordings of the umbilical arteries, fetal aorta, middle cerebral and uterine arteries were performed. During all Doppler examinations the patients were positioned semirecumbent to avoid 'vena cava syndrome'.

Doppler flow velocity waveforms were obtained from a free-floating central part of the umbilical artery in the absence of body movements, fetal breathing or cardiac arrhythmia with the sample volume covering the whole vessel. Care was taken to keep the insonation angle in the umbilical artery at a minimum. The fetal aorta was localized in its abdominal part at the origin of the renal arteries. The angle between ultrasound beam and fetal aorta was kept below 55°. The middle cerebral artery was visualized at about 1 cm of its origin in the circle of Willis in an axial view. The insonation angle in the middle cerebral artery was always below 15°. Care was taken to minimize fetal head compression, because this is known to influence the flow velocity waveforms of the middle cerebral arteries.

For uterine artery Doppler, the transducer was placed in the right or left lower part of the abdomen. Color Doppler imaging was used to localize the main uterine artery cranial to the crossing of the external iliac artery. The examination was repeated on the opposite side. The insonation angle was kept below 55° at the uterine arteries.

Abnormal umbilical, uterine and fetal aorta Doppler results were those > 2 standard deviations (SD) above the mean for gestational age of our local reference ranges.[34] Fetal brain sparing was supposed when the RI was < 2 SD below the mean of our local reference ranges for the middle cerebral artery.[34]

Glucose and lactate levels were measured in capillary blood samples taken from the finger pad before and after exercise ('Monotest-Lactat in Halbmicro-Technik', Boehringer Mannheim). The pulse and blood pressure of the mother were automatically registered at 3-min intervals during the test (Dinamap, Critikon, Tampa, FL, USA).

Results

Normal pregnancies

The mean performance on the bicycle ergometer was 79 W (±11 W). Gestational age at delivery was 40.0 weeks (±8 days). The mean birth weight was 3270 g (0383 g).

Mode of delivery: Twenty-four (73%) women delivered vaginal spontaneously, one (3%) vaginal operative and eight (24%) by cesarean section.

Table 51.1 Changes of RI during exercise in AGA pregnancies ($n=33$)

	RI (mean ± SD)			
		After exertion		
	Before exertion (baseline)	1–6 min	7–12 min	13–18 min
Fetal aorta	0.8 ± 0.21	0.82 ± 0.29	0.81 ± 0.22	0.82 ± 0.26
P value		< 0.01	ns	< 0.05
Middle cerebral artery	0.82 ± 0.48	0.77 ± 0.32	0.84 ± 0.54	0.83 ± 0.41
P value		< 0.01	ns	ns
Umbilical artery	0.62 ± 0.12	0.6 ± 0.12	0.62 ± 0.12	0.62 ± 0.1
P value		ns	ns	ns
Uterine artery	0.44 ± 0.15	0.41 ± 0.1	0.44 ± 0.12	0.44 ± 0.1
P value		ns	ns	ns

RI, resistance index; ns, difference not significant; SD, standard deviation

Doppler flow results of normal pregnancies ($n=33$) (Table 51.1)

Umbilical artery: The observed RI was within the normal range before and after exertion. However, in four (12%) fetuses the measurements reached the threshold range after exercise.

Fetal aorta: The mean RI before exercise was 4.9 (±1.3). In eight (24%) fetuses the RI was at the threshold range (between 0.83 and 0.86) and in one (3%) fetus at the pathological range (> 0.86). A significant increase in the RI was determined following exertion ($P < 0.01$). However, the mean value did not reach the pathological level. An increase in the RI of the aorta shortly after exertion was observed in 21 (63%) fetuses [in 5 (24%) within the threshold range, in 16 (76%) in the pathological range].

Middle cerebral artery: Before exercise, RI was in the normal range in all cases. A significant reduction in the RI was determined shortly after the exertion phase ($P < 0.01$). Twenty minutes after exertion, the results were almost the same as the baseline records.

Uterine artery: The observed RI was within the normal range before and after exertion.

Fetal heart rate: The FHR remained nearly unchanged before and after exertion (Figure 51.1). In one case fetal bradycardia (lasting approximately 2 min at the end of the exertion phase) was observed. This patient developed pre-eclampsia in the last 2 weeks of pregnancy.

Maternal parameters: The maternal blood pressure and the maternal heart rate increased during the exertion phase but returned to the initial values at the end of the test.

The maternal glucose levels decreased by 21% ($P < 0.001$) after exercise, while the lactate values increased almost twofold from 14.6 to 27.6 mg% ($P < 0.001$).

IUGR pregnancies

The mean performance on the bicycle ergometer was 68 W (±10 W). Gestational age at delivery was 37.6 weeks (±19 days). The mean birth weight was 2065 g (±526 g).

Mode of delivery: Five (50%) women delivered vaginal spontaneously and five (50%) by cesarean section.

Doppler flow results of IUGR pregnancies ($n=10$) (Table 51.2)

Umbilical artery: In three (30%) fetuses the baseline value was in the threshold and in another three (30%) fetuses it was pathological. After exercise the RI was in the threshold range in one (10%) fetus and pathological in four (40%) fetuses.

The RI in the umbilical artery was pathologic in three fetuses already before exercise. This had a marked influence on the mean RI value, because of the very small sample size. Thus, the calculated mean values of all measurements were in the pathological range from the beginning. After exclusion of these three cases, the RI became normal and no significant changes in the RI of umbilical arteries occurred during the test.

Fetal aorta: RI before exercise was within the pathological range in three (30%) fetuses and in two (20%) fetuses within the threshold range. The RI following exertion increased significantly ($P < 0.05$).

Doppler values of four (40%), five (50%) and six (60%) fetuses were within the pathological range, respectively, for measurements after exertion between 1 and 6 min, 7 and 12 min and 13 and 18 min.

The mean values of fetal aortic RI values in IUGR fetuses were higher than in AGA fetuses ($P < 0.05$). In contrast to the AGA group, in the IUGR group all

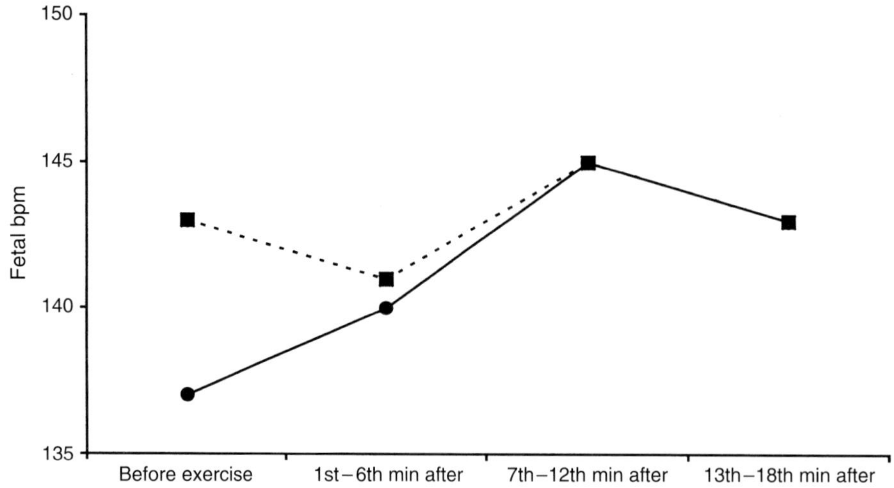

Figure 51.1 Fetal heart rate during the test period (mean ±SD) in AGA (squares) and in IUGR (circles) pregnancies.

Table 51.2 Changes of RI during exercise in IUGR pregnancies (*n*=10)

	RI (mean ±SD)			
		After exertion		
	Before exertion (baseline)	1–6 min	7–12 min	13–18 min
Fetal aorta	0.85±0.37	0.87±0.42	0.89±0.51	0.89±0.51
P value		<0.05	<0.05	<0.05
Middle cerebral artery	0.8±0.38	0.77±0.29	0.74±0.11	0.76±0.33
P value		<0.05	<0.05	<0.05
Umbilical artery	0.82±0.82	0.83±0.81	0.84±0.72	0.77±0.39
P value		ns	ns	ns
Umbilical artery (without extremes)	0.64±0.11	0.66±0.18	0.64±0.09	0.69±0.17
P value		ns	ns	ns
Uterine artery	0.41±0.19	0.52±0.2	0.47±0.12	0.47±0.07
P value		ns	ns	ns

RI, Resistance index; ns, difference not significant; SD, standard deviation

RI values after exercise were within the threshold or the pathologic range and did not return to normal values after exercise.

Middle cerebral artery: The RI revealed a stepwise reduction until 7–12 min after exertion ($P < 0.05$) and made a 'plateau' until 13–18 min after exertion. In six (60%) fetuses, the RI following exertion was lower than the baseline values.

In growth-retarded fetuses, the RI returned to normal levels more slowly than in AGA fetuses. In contrast to AGA fetuses, at the end, RI in IUGR fetuses remained well below the values registered at baseline ($P < 0.05$).

Uterine artery: There were no significant changes in RI of the uterine vessels during the test.

Fetal heart rate: The FHRs before and after exercise remained unchanged (Figure 51.1).

Maternal parameters: Maternal blood pressure and heart rate increased during exercise but regained normal values rapidly after exercise. The maternal glucose levels decreased about 24% ($P < 0.001$), while the lactate concentrations doubled from 11.6 to 24.2 mg% ($P < 0.001$).

Discussion

This study reports Doppler flow measurements of the placental vascular bed, the fetal aorta, umbilical artery together with the fetal cerebral arteries in the human AGA and IUGR fetus after physical exercise of the mother.

There are conflicting data regarding the question of uteroplacental supply during and after physical exercise by the mother in uneventful pregnancies and pregnancies at risk. The main hypothesis for guiding this study was that maternal exercise has both acute and chronic effects on placental bed blood flow. During the exercise, maternal blood flow is diverted away from the viscera to the exercising muscle and skin (fetoplacental blood steal effect). The magnitude of the reduction in flow is directly proportional to the exercise intensity and the muscle mass used (which varies with the type of exercise), and with common types of exercise performed at the usual exercise intensities, the reduction usually exceeds 50%. This exercise-induced decrease in visceral flow persists throughout pregnancy.[35]

The present Doppler flow results of the fetal aorta and fetal middle cerebral arteries in normal pregnancies showed significant differences before and after exertion. The RI in the aorta increased following exertion and remained higher for a considerable time (approximately 20 min), although the findings did not become pathological. In IUGR fetuses, the increase of the RI in the fetal aorta was more important with resistance indices being in the pathological range during the time period of the test.

The RI in the cerebral artery reduced significantly following exercise and returned very quickly approximately to its initial value in AGA fetuses. In IUGR cases, reduction of the RI could be observed until the end of the test without return to pretest values, thus indicating an initially decreased fetal cerebral circulation in IUGR cases after maternal exercise. RI of the placental vascular bed and the umbilical arteries remained unchanged throughout the test period. In three cases of IUGR, we found elevated RI values in the umbilical artery prior to maternal exercise. After exclusion of those cases, RI values in the umbilical artery were in the physiological range during the test in AGA and IUGR fetuses. These findings are in good accordance with the results reported in the literature.[30,36–41] Furthermore, FHR remained unchanged after maternal exercise in AGA and IUGR fetuses. This is partly in accordance with previous studies.[30,42–47] Differences in study protocols might account for these differences.

The presented results support evidence of fetal cerebral vasodilatation leading to redistribution of fetal blood volume to the cerebrum as a physiologic answer after moderate maternal exercise during the third trimester of pregnancy. In IUGR fetuses, cerebral vasodilatation (brain sparing phenomenon) lasted longer than in AGA fetuses and did not return to initial levels during the test period, pointing toward an altered fetal oxygenation under these circumstances. Furthermore, our results suggest that maternal exercise does not significantly alter uterine and umbilical perfusion in AGA and IUGR pregnancies suggesting absence of change in the uterine vascular bed resistance.

Other studies concerned with Doppler sonography during exercise in pregnant women

In 1956, Morris *et al.*[48] already studied changes in uterine circulation following physical exertion by the mothers. The authors found a statistically significant lengthening of the uterine clearance half-time of NaCl and hence a reduction in circulation during exertion.[48] At rest, in contrast, the clearance half-time was shorter and uterine circulation improved. The main point critical to the results of this study was that during the examination procedure the patient rested in a supine position, thus inducing possible vena cava occlusion syndrome.

Several investigators reported unchanged uteroplacental blood flow and umbilical perfusion after bicycle stress test in the third trimester.[30,49–52] Morrow *et al.* found higher resistance indices in the uterine arteries and elevated fetal heart rates after exercise by the mother in the third trimester. The RI in the umbilical artery, however, was unaltered.[53] Erkkola *et al.* demonstrated in a series of uncomplicated pregnancies an increase in RI of the uterine arteries and the maternal blood pressure after exercise, whereas no change in the RI occurred in the umbilical artery. Of note, the FHR increased significantly after exercise.[54]

The predictive value of maternal aerobic exercise for pregnancy-induced hypertension was studied by Hume *et al.* in a small series.[55] Pre-eclampsia developed in four patients with RI values being elevated in the umbilical artery after recovery in these four patients. It was concluded that aerobic exercise of the mother might be a valuable tool in predicting hypertensive pregnancy complications.[55] On the other hand, decreased umbilical artery RI values were reported after maternal exercise in the third trimester, thus indicating an improved placental circulation following exercise in healthy women.[28]

Hackett *et al.*[56] performed a bicycle exercise test in 34 women in the third trimester. Twelve pregnancies were uncomplicated, whereas 22 of the cases were complicated by small-for-gestational-age fetuses or maternal hypertension. Increase in pulsatility indices was more prominent in complicated pregnancies than in uncomplicated gestations, thus indicating an important reduction of uteroplacental blood flow by maternal exercise in complicated pregnancies.[56] In a more recent study, a fetal cerebral vasodilatation with decrease in umbilical resistance induced by submaximal maternal dynamic exercise was reported. FHR remained unchanged in this study.[18]

Conclusions

(1) *In healthy pregnant women* without obstetric or medical complications, the benefits of exercise seem to outweigh the risks. Therefore, pregnant women should continue to exercise, provided careful guidelines are followed. However, pregnant women may have to modify their exercise regimens because of the physiologic changes associated with pregnancy. Although lower birth weights are noted among offspring of women who exercise during pregnancy, these birth weights are still within normal ranges. Currently, there are no data to confirm that exercise during pregnancy has deleterious effects on the fetus.

(2) Maternal exercise does not significantly alter uterine and umbilical perfusion in AGA and IUGR pregnancies suggesting absence of change in the uterine vascular bed resistance. However, submaximal maternal exercise was followed by a fetal cerebral vasodilatation and an increase of resistance in the fetal aorta, which was more evident in IUGR fetuses. This might be due to a slight fetal hemoglobin desaturation in those cases. These findings underline the need of close antenatal surveillance of IUGR fetuses by Doppler flow measurements in order to detect circulatory deterioration in those fetuses and to reduce long-term morbidity. This is an important and relevant task of modern perinatal medicine.

Appendix

Guidelines for exercise during pregnancy

The ACOG has published a set of guidelines for exercise during pregnancy and the postpartum period. The most recent ACOG guidelines are listed in Table 51.3. These recommendations are made for women who do not have any additional risk factors for adverse maternal or perinatal outcome.[13]

Contraindications to exercise

According to ACOG[13] conditions that should be considered, contraindications to exercise during pregnancy include the following:

Absolute contraindications to aerobic exercise during pregnancy

- Hemodynamically significant heart disease
- Restrictive lung disease
- Incompetent cervix/cerclage
- Multiple gestation at risk for premature labor
- Persistent second- or third-trimester bleeding
- Placenta previa after 26 weeks of gestation
- Premature labor during the current pregnancy
- Ruptured membranes
- Pre-eclampsia/pregnancy-induced hypertension

Relative contraindications to aerobic exercise during pregnancy

- Severe anemia
- Unevaluated maternal cardiac arrhythmia
- Chronic bronchitis
- Poorly controlled type 1 diabetes
- Extreme morbid obesity
- Extreme underweight (body mass index < 12)
- History of extremely sedentary lifestyle
- IUGR in current pregnancy
- Poorly controlled hypertension
- Orthopedic limitations
- Poorly controlled seizure disorder
- Poorly controlled hyperthyroidism
- Heavy smoker

Warning signs to terminate exercise while pregnant

- Vaginal bleeding
- Dyspnea prior to exertion
- Dizziness
- Headache
- Chest pain
- Muscle weakness
- Calf pain or swelling (need to rule out thrombophlebitis)

Table 51.3 American College of Obstetricians and Gynecologists' guidelines for exercise during pregnancy and postpartum

1. Regular exercise (at least three times per week) is preferable to intermittent activity
2. Avoid exercise in the supine position after the first trimester. This position is associated with decreased cardiac output in most pregnant women, causing a decreased distribution of blood to splanchnic beds including the uterus
3. Pregnant women should stop exercising when fatigued and not exercise to exhaustion
4. Non-weight-bearing exercises such as cycling or swimming will minimize the risk of injury and facilitate the continuation of exercise during pregnancy
5. Adequate diet should be ensured
6. Avoid types of exercise in which loss of balance could be detrimental to maternal or fetal well-being, especially in the third trimester. Further, any type of exercise involving the potential for even mild abdominal trauma should be avoided
7. Adequate hydration, appropriate clothing and optimal environmental surroundings during exercise should be ensured
8. The physiologic and morphologic changes of pregnancy persist 4–6 weeks postpartum. Thus, prepregnancy exercise routines should be resumed gradually based on a woman's physical capability

- Preterm labor
- Decreased fetal movement
- Amniotic fluid leakage

Conclusions and recommendations of ACOG for exercise during pregnancy[13]

- Recreational and competitive athletes with uncomplicated pregnancies can remain active during pregnancy and should modify their usual exercise routines as medically indicated. The information on strenuous exercise is scarce; however, women who engage in such activities require close medical supervision.
- Previously inactive women and those with medical or obstetric complications should be evaluated before recommendations for physical activity during pregnancy are made. Exercise during pregnancy may provide additional health benefits to women with gestational diabetes.
- A physically active woman with a history of or risk for preterm labor or fetal growth restriction should be advised to reduce her activity in the second and third trimesters.

Acknowledgments

The authors thank A. Barut (Zonguldak, Turkey), H. Sade (Zonguldak, Turkey) and M. Vural (Zonguldak, Turkey) for their technical and editorial assistance in the preparation of this manuscript.

REFERENCES

1. Rowell LB. Human cardiovascular adjustments to exercise and thermal stress. *Physiol Rev* 1974;54:75–159.
2. Clapp JF III, Capeless EL. The changing glycemic response to exercise during pregnancy. *Am J Obstet Gynecol* 1991;165: 1678–83.
3. Clapp JF III, Little KD, Capeless EL. Fetal heart rate response to sustained recreational exercise. *Am J Obstet Gynecol* 1993;168: 198–206.
4. Clapp JF III, Stepanchak W, Tomaselli J, Kortan M, Faneslow S. Portal vein blood flow-effects of pregnancy, gravity, and exercise. *Am J Obstet Gynecol* 2000;183:167–72.
5. Clapp JF III. Exercise during pregnancy. A clinical update. *Clin Sports Med* 2000;19:273–86.
6. Clapp JF III. The effects of maternal exercise on fetal oxygenation and feto-placental growth. *Eur J Obstet Gynecol Reprod Biol* 2003;110(Suppl 1):S80–5.
7. Ezmerli NM. Exercise in pregnancy. *Prim Care Update Ob Gyns* 2000;7:260–5.
8. Hackett GA, Cohen-Overbeek T, Campbell S. The effect of exercise on uteroplacental Doppler waveforms in normal and complicated pregnancies. *Obstet Gynecol* 1992;79:919–23.
9. Morrow RJ, Ritchie JW, Bull SB. Fetal and maternal hemodynamic responses to exercise in pregnancy assessed by Doppler ultrasonography. *Am J Obstet Gynecol* 1989;160:138–40.
10. Chandler KD, Bell AW. Effects of maternal exercise on fetal and maternal respiration and nutrient metabolism in the pregnant ewe. *J Dev Physiol* 1981;3:161–76.
11. Curet LB, Orr JA, Rankin HG, Ungerer T. Effect of exercise on cardiac output and distribution of uterine blood flow in pregnant ewes. *J Appl Physiol* 1976;40:725–8.
12. Magann EF, Evans SF, Weitz B, Newnham J. Antepartum, intrapartum, and neonatal significance of exercise on healthy low-risk pregnant working women. *Obstet Gynecol* 2002;99:466–72.
13. ACOG Committee opinion. Number 267, January 2002: Exercise during pregnancy and the postpartum period. *Obstet Gynecol* 2002;99:171–3.
14. Van Hook JW, Gill P, Easterling TR, Schmucker B, Carlson K, Benedetti TJ. The hemodynamic effects of isometric exercise during late normal pregnancy. *Am J Obstet Gynecol* 1993;169: 870–3.
15. Pijpers L, Wladimiroff JW, McGhie J. Effect of short-term maternal exercise on maternal and fetal cardiovascular dynamics. *Br J Obstet Gynaecol* 1984;91:1081–6.
16. Revelli A, Durando A, Massobrio M. Exercise in pregnancy: A review of maternal and fetal effects. *Obstet Gynecol Surv* 1992;47:355–63.
17. Manders MA, Sonder GJ, Mulder EJ, Visser GH. The effects of maternal exercise on fetal heart rate and movement patterns. *Early Hum Dev* 1997;48:237–47.
18. Bonnin P, Bazzi-Grossin C, Ciraru-Vigneron N, *et al.* Evidence of fetal cerebral vasodilatation induced by submaximal maternal dynamic exercise in human pregnancy. *J Perinat Med* 1997;25: 63–70.
19. Veille JC. Maternal and fetal cardiovascular response to exercise during pregnancy. *Semin Perinatol* 1996;20:250–62.
20. Erkkola RU, Pirhonen JP, Kivijarvi AK. Flow velocity waveforms in uterine and umbilical arteries during submaximal bicycle exercise in normal pregnancy. *Obstet Gynecol* 1992;79:611–5.
21. Ruissen C, Jager W, von Drongelen M, Hoogland H. The influence of maternal exercise on the pulsatility index of the umbilical artery blood velocity waveform. *Eur J Obstet Gynecol Reprod Biol* 1990;37:1–6.
22. Hume RF Jr, Bowie JD, McCoy C, *et al.* Fetal umbilical artery Doppler response to graded maternal aerobic exercise and subsequent maternal mean arterial blood pressure: Predictive value for pregnancy-induced hypertension. *Am J Obstet Gynecol* 1990; 163:826–9.
23. Veille JC, Bacevice AE, Wilson B, Janos J, Hellerstein HK. Umbilical artery waveform during bicycle exercise in normal pregnancy. *Obstet Gynecol* 1989;73:957–60.
24. Morrow RJ, Ritchie JW, Bull SB. Fetal and maternal hemodynamic responses to exercise in pregnancy assessed by Doppler ultrasonography. *Am J Obstet Gynecol* 1989;160:138–40.
25. Baumann H, Huch A, Huch R. Doppler sonographic evaluation of exercise-induced blood flow velocity and waveform changes in fetal, uteroplacental and large maternal vessels in pregnant women. *J Perinat Med* 1989;17:279–87.
26. Moore DH, Jarrett JC, Bendick PJ. Exercise-induced changes in uterine artery blood flow, as measured by Doppler ultrasound, in pregnant subjects. *Am J Perinatol* 1988;5:94–7.
27. Steegers EA, Buunk G, Binkhorst RA, Jongsma HW, Wijn PF, Hein PR. The influence of maternal exercise on the uteroplacental vscular bed resistance and the fetal heart rate during normal pregnancy. *Eur J Obstet Gynecol Reprod Biol* 1988;27:21–6.
28. Rafla N, Beazely J. The effects of maternal exercise on fetal umbilical artery waveforms. *Eur J Obstet Gynecol Reprod Biol* 1991;1: 119–23.
29. Durak E, Jovanovic-Peterson L, Peterson C. Comparative evaluation of uterine response to exercise on five aerobic machines. *Am J Obstet Gynecol* 1990;162:279–84.
30. Drack G, Kirkinen P, Baumann H, Müller R, Huch R. Doppler ultrasound studies before and following short-term maternal stress in late pregnancy. *Z Geburtshilfe Perinatol* 1988;192:173–7.
31. Hackett GA, Cohen-Overbeek T, Campbell S. The effect of exercise on uteroplacental Doppler waveforms in normal and complicated pregnancies. *Obstet Gynecol* 1992;79:919–23.
32. Ertan AK, Schanz S, Tanriverdi HA, Meyberg R, Schmidt W. Doppler examinations of fetal and uteroplacental blood flow in AGA and IUGR fetuses before and after maternal physical exercise with the bicycle ergometer. *J Perinat Med* 2004;32:260–5.
33. Schmidt W, Hendrik H, Gauwerky J, Junkermann H, Leucht W, Kubli F. Diagnosis of intrauterine growth retardation by intensive ultrasound biometry. *Geburtshilfe Frauenheilkd* 1987;42:543–8.
34. Ertan A, Hendrik H, Tanriverdi H, Bechtold M, Schmidt W. Fetomaternal Doppler sonography nomograms. *Perinatoloji* 2001; 9:174–80.

35. Clapp J. The effects of maternal exercise on fetal oxygenation and feto-placental growth. *Eur J Obstet Gynecol Reprod Biol* 2003; 110:80–5.
36. Erkkola RU, Pirhonen JP, Kivijarvi AK. Flow velocity waveforms in uterine and umbilical arteries during submaximal bicycle exercise in normal pregnancy. *Obstet Gynecol* 1992;79: 611–5.
37. Ruissen C, Jager W, von Drongelen M, Hoogland H. The influence of maternal exercise on the pulsatility index of the umbilical artery blood velocity waveform. *Eur J Obstet Gynecol Reprod Biol* 1990;37:1–6.
38. Veille JC, Bacevice AE, Wilson B, Janos J, Hellerstein HK. Umbilical artery waveform during bicycle exercise in normal pregnancy. *Obstet Gynecol* 1989;73:957–60.
39. Morrow RJ, Ritchie JW, Bull SB. Fetal and maternal hemodynamic responses to exercise in pregnancy assessed by Doppler ultrasonography. *Am J Obstet Gynecol* 1989;160:138–40.
40. Moore DH, Jarrett JC, Bendick PJ. Exercise-induced changes in uterine artery blood flow, as measured by Doppler ultrasound, in pregnant subjects. *Am J Perinatol* 1988;5:94–7.
41. Steegers EA, Buunk G, Binkhorst RA, Jongsma HW, Wijn PF, Hein PR. The influence of maternal exercise on the uteroplacental vascular bed resistance and the fetal heart rate during normal pregnancy. *Eur J Obstet Gynecol Reprod Biol* 1988;27:21–6.
42. Erkkola RU, Pirhonen JP, Kivijarvi AK. Flow velocity waveforms in uterine and umbilical arteries during submaximal bicycle exercise in normal pregnancy. *Obstet Gynecol* 1992;79:611–5.
43. Ruissen C, Jager W, von Drongelen M, Hoogland H. The influence of maternal exercise on the pulsatility index of the umbilical artery blood velocity waveform. *Eur J Obstet Gynecol Reprod Biol* 1990;37:1–6.
44. Veille JC, Bacevice AE, Wilson B, Janos J, Hellerstein HK. Umbilical artery waveform during bicycle exercise in normal pregnancy. *Obstet Gynecol* 1989;73:957–60.
45. Morrow RJ, Ritchie JW, Bull SB. Fetal and maternal hemodynamic responses to exercise in pregnancy assessed by Doppler ultrasonography. *Am J Obstet Gynecol* 1989;160:138–40.
46. Moore DH, Jarrett JC, Bendick PJ. Exercise-induced changes in uterine artery blood flow, as measured by Doppler ultrasound, in pregnant subjects. *Am J Perinatol* 1988;5:94–7.
47. Steegers EA, Buunk G, Binkhorst RA, Jongsma HW, Wijn PF, Hein PR. The influence of maternal exercise on the uteroplacental vascular bed resistance and the fetal heart rate during normal pregnancy. *Eur J Obstet Gynecol Reprod Biol* 1988;27:21–6.
48. Morris N, Osborn S, Wright H, Hart A. Effective uterine blood flow during exercise in normal and preeclamptic pregnancies. *Lancet* 1956;361:481–3.
49. Veille JC. Maternal and fetal cardiovascular response to exercise during pregnancy. *Semin Perinatol* 1996;20:250–62.
50. Ruissen C, Jager W, von Drongelen M, Hoogland H. The influence of maternal exercise on the pulsatility index of the umbilical artery blood velocity waveform. *Eur J Obstet Gynecol Reprod Biol* 1990;37:1–6.
51. Moore DH, Jarrett JC, Bendick PJ. Exercise-induced changes in uterine artery blood flow, as measured by Doppler ultrasound, in pregnant subjects. *Am J Perinatol* 1988;5:94–7.
52. Steegers EA, Buunk G, Binkhorst RA, Jongsma HW, Wijn PF, Hein PR. The influence of maternal exercise on the uteroplacental vascular bed resistance and the fetal heart rate during normal pregnancy. *Eur J Obstet Gynecol Reprod Biol* 1988;27:21–6.
53. Morrow RJ, Ritchie JW, Bull SB. Fetal and maternal hemodynamic responses to exercise in pregnancy assessed by Doppler ultrasonography. *Am J Obstet Gynecol* 1989;160:138–40.
54. Erkkola RU, Pirhonen JP, Kivijarvi AK. Flow velocity waveforms in uterine and umbilical arteries during submaximal bicycle exercise in normal pregnancy. *Obstet Gynecol* 1992;79:611–5.
55. Hume RF Jr, Bowie JD, McCoy C, *et al.* Fetal umbilical artery Doppler response to graded maternal aerobic exercise and subsequent maternal mean arterial blood pressure: Predictive value for pregnancy-induced hypertension. *Am J Obstet Gynecol* 1990; 163:826–9.
56. Hackett GA, Cohen-Overbeek T, Campbell S. The effect of exercise on uteroplacental Doppler waveforms in normal and complicated pregnancies. *Obstet Gynecol* 1992;79:919–23.

52 Doppler velocimetry in intrauterine growth restriction: a practical clinical approach

G. P. Mandruzzato, Y. J. Meir and G. Maso

Introduction

Intrauterine growth restriction (IUGR) according to the current definition is that of a fetus that fails to reach its potential growth. The term IUGR should only be used with regard to the fetus, while small for gestational age (SGA) should be used only with regard to the newborn.[1] This distinction must be kept in mind very clearly. It is true that perinatal mortality and morbidity are significantly increased in cases presenting a birth weight less than the 10th percentile for gestational age (therefore defined as SGA) and also less than the 15th percentile.[2] However, it has been shown that symptoms of hypoxemia are observable in cases presenting a birth weight greater than the 50th percentile, but showing a restriction of growth by ultrasound biometry during fetal life, with the same frequency as in SGA newborns.[3] IUGR can be associated to many conditions (malformations, karyotype aberrations, infections, maternal diseases), but the most frequent and most dangerous complications are represented by chronic fetal hypoxemia. This is the consequence of obliterative placental vasculopathy, which reduces the maternal–fetal supply first of nutrients and later on of oxygen. This ominous condition is encountered in about 30% of IUGR fetuses and is the cause of poor perinatal outcome (intrauterine death or damage, acute hypoxemia in labor, neonatal death and morbidity early and late as well). Moreover, it has been postulated that IUGR can also be responsible for diseases occurring in adult life.

Chronic fetal hypoxemia induces changes in many fetal vital functions (hemodynamics, heart activity, fetal movements and behavior, amniotic fluid turnover) and one of the first to be observed is blood flow redistribution. As Doppler technology enables us to study these changes in a non-invasive way, it has become a fundamental tool for assessing the fetal oxygenation and the fetal response to hypoxemia, thus becoming a useful guide in the clinical management of IUGR fetuses.

Characteristics of Doppler velocity waveform

The Doppler velocity waveform (DVWF) reflects the velocities of blood during a cardiac cycle. The so-called 'angle-independent parameters' are commonly used for studying the characteristics of the DVWF. The velocities of the systolic phase are compared to that of the diastolic one according to different formulas. The simplest is the systolic/diastolic (S/D) ratio obtained by dividing the two. The resistance index (RI) is obtained by dividing the systolic velocity for the systolic minus the diastolic. Probably, the most comprehensive parameter is the pulsatility index (PI) because it takes into consideration not only systolic and diastolic velocities but also the mean of the velocities. However, the characteristics of the DVWF, and hence the different parameters, are mainly influenced by the diastolic phase, reflecting the peripheral resistance downstream the explored segment of the vessels, especially in the case of investigations performed on arteries. When the peripheral resistance is markedly increased, the forward blood flow may be absent or also reverted. These particular patterns of the DVWF are called absent/reverse end diastolic (ARED) flow. After the introduction of the color flow mapping (CFM) technique, it is possible to identify very tiny vessels and vascular structures also, which can be sampled by the Doppler technique. Hence, it is possible to build a map of fetal hemodynamic patterns in normally evolving pregnancies and in those affected by hypoxemia as well.

Fetal and umbilical hemodynamics in normal pregnancies

In case of normally evolving pregnancy, Doppler investigation on somatic and cerebral fetal arteries (FA) shows a fairly constant pattern of the DVWF, indicating an almost stable peripheral resistance or a small progressive reduction. Using the same technology on the umbilical arteries (UA), a significant progressive reduction of peripheral resistance can be observed possibly related to the increasing need of nutrients and oxygen by the growing fetus.

The main objects of investigation are UA and fetal thoracic descending aorta. With the progress of ultrasound imaging technology and the use of CFM, allowing identification and sampling of even tiny vessels, many other arteries like cerebral (internal carotid and middle and anterior cerebral), renal, mesenteric, adrenal, splenic, iliac aortic arch and coronary have been studied.

As a consequence, a very comprehensive overview of the fetal physiologic hemodynamics has been obtained, which is the fundamental basis for studying and understanding the possible changes occurring in pathologic pregnancies.

Arterial Doppler changes in hypoxemic IUGR

As already mentioned, the most frequent and severe complication of IUGR is represented by the chronic fetal hypoxemia, which is a consequence of the placental obliterative vasculopathy. With Doppler technology, it is possible to study the hemodynamic changes occurring in this condition in UA and those occurring in FA.

The first step of the fetal adaptation to hypoxemia is represented by blood flow redistribution inducing vasoconstriction in the somatic arteries and vasodilatation in the cerebral arteries. This phenomenon is called 'brain sparing effect' and is finalized to preserve sufficient oxygenation to the central nervous system. It has been postulated that such a 'sparing effect' occurs also at the level of the adrenal and coronary arteries. Therefore, peripheral resistance is increased in the somatic and splanchnic arteries and reduced in the cerebral arteries.

When placental obliterative vasculopathy occurs, the peripheral resistance is also increased in UA. It has been shown that PI elevation is proportional to the obliteration of the placental vascular bed.[4]

From the clinical point of view, it is possible to assess both the cause (UA) and the effect (FA) of hypoxemia using Doppler investigation.

Doppler patterns of IUGR

Doppler study on UA and fetal thoracic descending aorta has been performed in 653 IUGR fetuses. In all the cases, gestational age has been established on the basis of ultrasonic biometry carried out in early pregnancy [by measuring the crown–rump length (CRL)] and not later than 20 weeks of gestation (by measuring the biparietal diameter). IUGR has been diagnosed if the fetal biometry (abdominal circumference) showed a deviation of more than 2 weeks in the expected curve of growth that has been established in our institute. Cases presenting fetal abnormalities (anatomical and/or chromosomal) have been excluded from this study. After IUGR recognition, Doppler investigation is done at weekly or minor intervals, depending on the severity of the growth restriction and the maternal clinical conditions by measuring the PI values. Cases presenting PI values greater than the second standard deviation are considered abnormal. Fetal biometry has been performed weekly if severe restriction was observed and/or abnormal PI was present, and at 14-day intervals in cases presenting normal Doppler values. Computer-assisted cardiotochography (CTG) according to the Oxford System 8002 has been performed for monitoring fetal conditions.

The IUGR cases have been divided into four groups according to the characteristics of the Doppler patterns. In the first group, 71 cases presenting ARED flow have been included (10.8%). In the second group, the cases ($n=64$, 9.8%) presenting abnormal PI (over the second SD) in both vascular districts are collected. In the third group are the cases ($n=85$, 13%) presenting abnormal PI only in the aorta while still depicting normal values in the UA. The fourth group is represented by cases showing normal PI values in both aorta and UA ($n=433$, 66.3%).

The prevalence of fetal distress (FD) has been calculated for each group. FD has been diagnosed on the basis of short-term variation (ST) below 3 ms in pregnancy and on the basis of the presence of late decelerations or bradycardia and/or fetal acidemia on the fetal blood sample during labor, requiring cesarean delivery. Overall, the prevalence of FD was 31% but with a statistically significant difference in the four groups.

FD has been observed in 100% of the cases in the first group. This prevalence is reduced to 74% in the second group and even more, 33%, in the third. In the fourth group this figure is 12%.

Sensitivity and specificity of Doppler for predicting FD has been calculated separately for FA and UA. The sensitivity is 62.69 for FA and 35.18 for UA. The specificity is 81.56 for FA and 96.71 for UA. The reason for the difference depends on the pathophysiological background of the hemodynamic changes of the two vascular districts. Fetal vessel changes, as in the aorta, represent the adaptation to hypoxemia while UA changes are the consequence of increased peripheral resistance provoked by placental obliterative vasculopathy.

Practically, by studying hemodynamics in UA we can assess the cause of chronic fetal hypoxemia, whereas by studying the fetal vessels we can assess the phenomenon of fetal adaptation to the reduced oxygen supply.

As already discussed, it has been shown that PI values are proportional to the obliteration of the placental vascular bed, but evidence has also shown that DVWF becomes altered only when at least 60% of the placental vascular bed is obliterated[5] and oxygen supply to the fetus is strongly reduced. Hence, the specificity of PI in UA is much higher than that observed in FA.

Therefore, according to the Doppler patterns, the first group (ARED) represents a condition of restriction of oxygen supply to the fetus inducing a severe hypoxemia. Unfavorable perinatal outcome (death or handicaps in survivors) has been observed only in this group. The second and third groups represent a condition of reduced oxygen supply and fetal adaptation and possible FD. The fourth group represents IUGR fetuses not affected by chronic hypoxemia.

The clinical consequences can be indicated as follows:

Group 1: Timing of prompt delivery should be taken into consideration.

Groups 2 and 3: Close surveillance and timing of the delivery according to fetal monitoring and maternal corticosteroids administration if gestational age is lower than 34 weeks. Vaginal delivery after spontaneous onset of labor is possible in about 50% of the cases.

Group 4: Clinical and instrumental control at weekly or 14-day intervals. In the majority of cases, vaginal delivery after spontaneous onset of labor occurs.

Particular attention should be paid to IUGR cases when ARED flow is observed. This hemodynamic condition is encountered in about 10% of IUGR fetuses, and is usually associated with a low gestational age, with a mean of 30 weeks.

As the outcome is largely different in the case of end-diastolic flow absent (EDFA) as compared to reverse flow (RF), being better in the first condition, the characteristics of the management should be different. In fact, it has been shown that perinatal mortality and handicap rates are significantly higher in the case of RF.[6]

Conclusions

IUGR can be associated with many fetal adverse conditions (malformations, chromosomal aberrations, infections) but the most important cause of both restriction of growth and poor perinatal outcome is represented by chronic fetal hypoxemia (CFH). This condition is the consequence of placental obliterative vasculopathy, which affects the maternal–fetal supply of nutrients first and later on of oxygen. As a consequence, hemodynamic changes occur in UA and FA as well. These modifications are easily observable with Doppler technology by analyzing the characteristics of the DVWF.

As CFH occurs in about 30% of IUGR, therefore requiring close control and possibly active management, the crucial point, after IUGR recognition, is represented by the identification or the exclusion of CFH. By studying DVWF on UA and FA, it is possible to assess the characteristics of the blood flow from the mother to the fetus and to monitor the aspects of the fetal adaptation if CFH is present. Fetal thoracic descending aorta is easy to identify and sample by using pulsed Doppler.

According to the DVWF patterns and PI values, it is possible to distinguish the IUGR fetuses affected by CFH from those that are not. As a consequence, the characteristics of the control can be differentiated.

Moreover, if CFH is present, it is possible to monitor its evolution by obtaining information about clinical practical validity, in order to optimize the management and the timing of the delivery if necessary.

REFERENCES

1. Committee on Practice Bulletins – Gynaecology. American College of Obstetricians and Gynecologists. Intrauterine growth restriction. Clinical management guidelines for obstetrician-gynecologists. *Int J Gynaecol Obstet* 2001;72(1):85.
2. Seeds JW, Peng T. Impaired growth and the risk of fetal death: Is the tenth percentile the appropriate standard? *Am J Obstet Gynecol* 1998;178:658.
3. De Jong CLD, Francis A, Van Geijn HP, Gardosi J. Fetal growth rate and adverse perinatal events. *Ultrasound Obstet Gynecol* 1999;13:86.
4. Giles W, Trudinger B, Baird PF, *et al.* Umbilical artery flow velocity waveforms and placental resistance: Pathological correlation. *Br J Obstet Gynaecol* 1985;92:31.
5. Trudinger B, Cook CM. Doppler umbilical and uterine flow waveforms in severe pregnancy hypertension. *Br J Obstet Gynaecol* 1990;97:142.
6. Mandruzzato GP, Bogatti P, Fisher-Tamaro L, Gigli C. The clinical significance of absent or reverse end diastolic flow in the fetal aorta and umbilical arteries. *Ultrasound Obstet Gynecol* 1991;1:192.

53 Doppler evaluation of the fetal venous system

G. Maso, G. Conoscenti and G. P. Mandruzzato

Introduction

Fetal blood flow measurements have become an important tool in the surveillance of high-risk pregnancies. There is a vast amount of literature on umbilical arteries and the fetal arterial system, but fetal venous circulation has only recently been evaluated.

The introduction of high-resolution ultrasonography, combined with color Doppler imaging (CDI), offered a breakthrough in the study of the fetal venous system, considerably enhancing our understanding in normal physiologic conditions, as well as in abnormal circumstances.

This review will focus on the embryologic, anatomic and physiologic characteristics of fetal venous circulation. The knowledge of the development and physiology represents the basis to understand the structural anomalies and the hemodynamic changes that occur in the venous district in pathological conditions.

Embryology of the fetal venous system

In a 4-week embryo, three pairs of veins are found. The vitelline veins run from the yolk sac to the sinus venosus via liver sinusoid, and are connected to each other via anastomoses around the duodenum. The umbilical veins (UVs) transport oxygenated blood from the chorion to the sinus venous, bypassing the liver. They merge with the cardinal veins, the third pair of embryonic veins, which originate from the body of the embryo and open into the right and left horns of the sinus venosus of the primitive heart.

The fetal liver and its development in the septum transversus play an important role in modifying the primitive vitelline and UVs into their final morphology. With the rapid growth of the liver, the UVs connect with the liver sinusoids. The asymmetric development of the heart and the rotation of the intestinal tract cause a major change in the venosus circulation by forming a single venous blood stream from the left to the right.

In the 6-mm embryo, the complete right UV, the cranial part of the left UV, the left vitelline vein and part of the anastomoses obliterate and a new vessel, the ductus venosus (DV), develops. This is a shunt vessel between the left UV and the right hepatocardinal channel, which will become the upper inferior vena cava (IVC). At this stage, all the placental blood enters the right atrium through the left distal UV, the DV and the proximal right vitelline vein, which bypass the liver sinusoids. The upper two anastomoses of the distal vitelline veins fuse to form the portal vein, whereas the distal anastomoses form the superior mesenteric and splenic veins and the proximal parts become the hepatic veins (Figure 53.1).

IVC and superior vena cava (SVC) originate from the cardinal veins, which form the main drainage system of the embryo's body (Figure 53.2). The anterior and posterior cardinal veins drain the cranial and caudal parts of the body of the embryo, respectively. The left brachiocephalic vein is formed during the eighth week from the right anterior and the right common cardinal veins, through left to right anastomoses, whereas the left anterior cardinal vein disappears. Azygos and hemiazygos veins originate from the upper portion of the division of the supracardinal veins, whereas the caudal part becomes the caudal part of the IVC.[1–4]

Anatomy of the fetal venous system

Two venous systems can be identified within the fetal liver: an afferent system, or umbilical–portal system, taking blood from the placenta and the gut to the liver, and an efferent system, provided by the hepatic veins, taking blood from the liver to the heart (Figure 53.3). The DV shunts oxygenated blood from the umbilical–portal system directly to the heart.

In the afferent venous system, the UV enters the abdomen within the falciform ligament, ascending steeply toward the liver and runs along its surface in

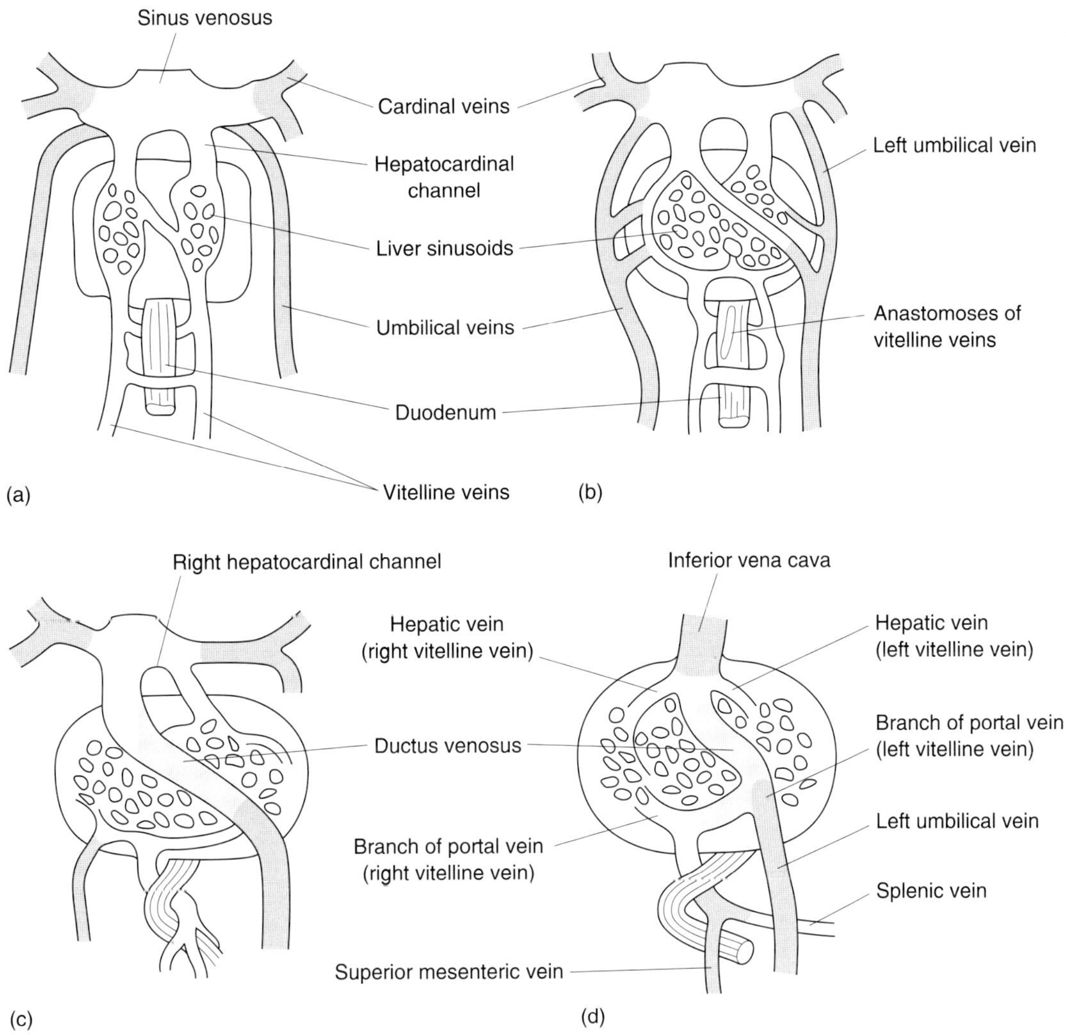

Figure 53.1 Embryology of umbilical, portal and hepatic venous systems. Reprinted from Hoffstetter *et al.*[2] with permission.

the cephalad direction. It then joins a confluence of vessels termed the portal sinus. This is a wide L-shaped vessel at the distal part of the UV, connecting the right and left intrahepatic portal veins. These perfuse the right and left hepatic lobes, respectively. There are two main left intrahepatic portal veins (superior and inferior). The right intrahepatic portal vein shows a more abundant branching pattern. The vein originating from the confluence of the splenic and superior mesenteric veins outside the liver represents the extrahepatic portal vein.

The DV originates from the portal sinus as the latter turns at an almost right angle into the right lobe of the liver. The diameter of the DV is approximately one-third that of the UV. This is a branchless, hourglass-shaped vessel ascending in the direction of the diaphragm, which joins distally with the hepatic left vein and the IVC, just proximal to the entrance into the right atrium (Figure 53.4). The existence of a 'sphincter' that regulates the blood flow through the DV to the heart has been postulated, and it has been assumed that the control of this anatomic structure is dependent on the concentration of oxygen.

The efferent system is represented by a number of vessels arising from the right and left hepatic lobes (right, middle and left hepatic veins), which drains into the subdiaphragmatic vestibulum. The hepatic veins, DV and IVC open into the subdiaphragmatic vestibulum, an inverted funnel-shaped vascular space just below the diaphragm, ending at the right atrium.[3–5]

Physiology of the fetal venous system

The anatomical relationship in the hepatic afferent venous system supports the well-established concept that oxygenated blood flow from the placenta is distributed through the UV to the portal sinus, which supplies the left and right intrahepatic portal veins and the DV. Deoxygenated blood from the extrahepatic portal veins is diverted almost exclusively to the right hepatic lobe. The alignment of UV and DV,

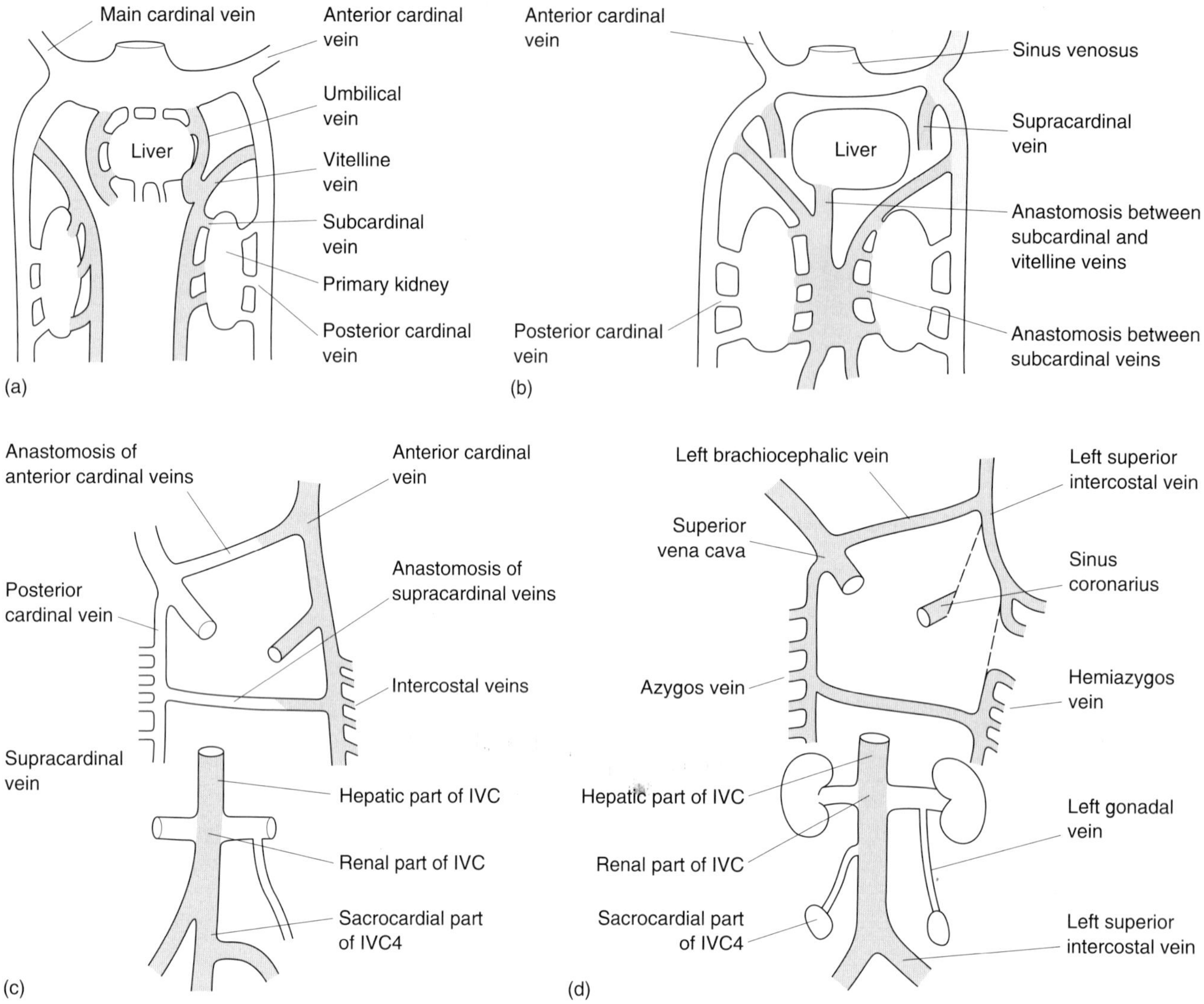

Figure 53.2 Embryology of inferior and superior vena cavae. Reprinted from Hoffstetter *et al.*[2] with permission.

although not in anatomical continuity for the interposed portal sinus, favors the preferential streaming of oxygenated blood to the DV and consequently to the heart (Figures 53.3 and 53.4). Approximately 50% of the UV blood flow enters the DV and accounts for 98% of the blood flow through the DV. The portal blood is mainly directed to the right lobe of the liver.

As far as the vessels of the efferent venous system are concerned, it is possible to observe that the right hepatic vein runs parallel to the IVC, whereas the left and middle hepatic veins run parallel to the DV. It has been postulated that this spatial rearrangement is the consequence of distribution of more oxygenated blood flow. The left hepatic lobe, in fact, is primarily supplied with the blood flow from the UV via the left portal vein.

Moreover, it has been shown that there is streamlining of blood flow within the thoracic IVC: blood from the DV and the left hepatic vein flows in the dorsal and leftward part, whereas blood from the right lobe, the distal IVC and the right hepatic lobe flows in the ventral and rightward stream part of IVC. The ventral and rightward stream, together with blood from SVC, is directed to the right atrium and through the tricuspid valve into the right ventricle, ejected into the main pulmonary artery and shunted, via ductus arteriosus, into the descending aorta. The dorsal and leftward stream is directed toward the foramen ovale, thereby delivering well-oxygenated blood flow directly to the left heart and, via ascending aorta, to the myocardium and the brain.[3,6,7]

Normal Doppler findings

The application of high-resolution and color Doppler ultrasonography has allowed the structural and functional evaluation of the fetal venous system.

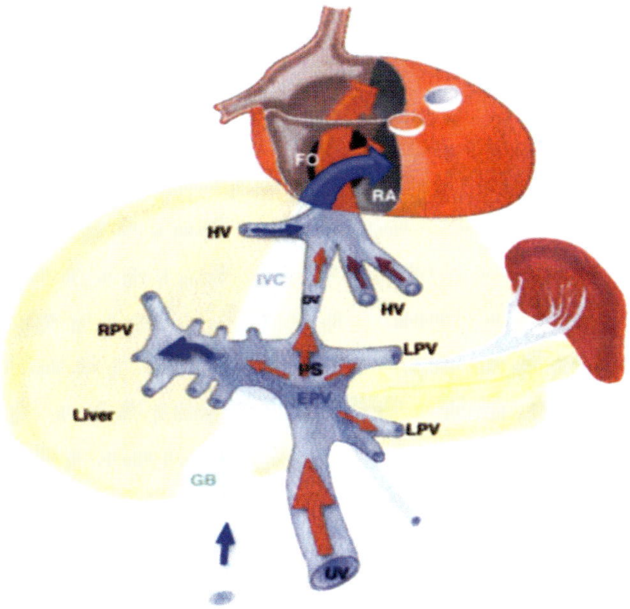

Figure 53.3 Representation of fetal umbilical and hepatic venous system. The arrows indicate the direction of flow. The colors show the degree of oxygenation (red, high; purple, medium; blue, low). FO, foramen ovale; RA, right atrium; DV, ductus venous; UV, umbilical vein; HV, hepatic veins; IVC, inferior vena cava; PS, portal sinus; LPV, left portal vein; RPV, right portal vein; EPV, extrahepatic portal vein; GB, gallbladder. Reprinted from Mavrides *et al.*[5] with permission.

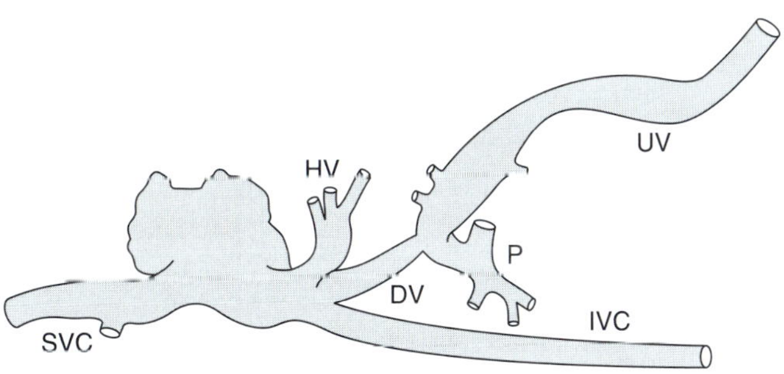

Figure 53.4 Sagittal view of the fetal venous system. RA, right atrium; DV, ductus venous; UV, umbilical vein; HV, hepatic veins; IVC, inferior vena cava; P, portal system; SVC, superior vena cava.

During sonography, the UV can be detected in a sagittal or transverse section of the abdomen. In the transverse section, it curves toward the right-hand side of the upper abdomen (Figure 53.5).

The DV can be visualized in its full length in a midsagittal longitudinal section of the trunk or in an oblique transverse section through the upper abdomen. Its origin from the UV can be found where CDI indicates higher velocities compared with the flow in UV, and sometimes this produces an aliasing effect. The blood flow velocities accelerate due to the narrow lumen of the DV, the maximum inner width of the narrowest portion being 2 mm (Figures 53.6 and 53.7).

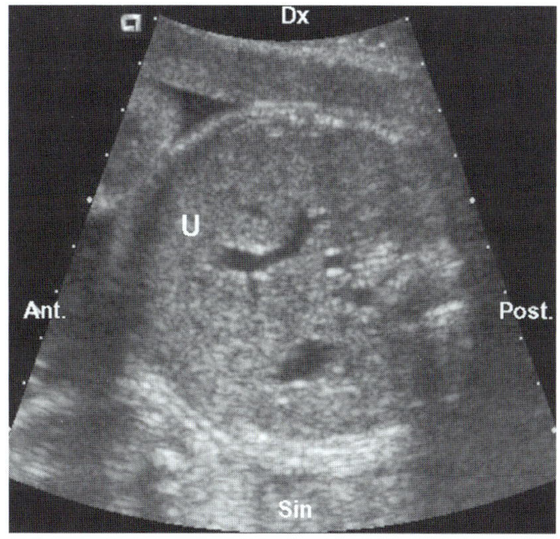

Figure 53.5 Transverse view of the fetal abdomen. The UV curves toward the right-hand side.

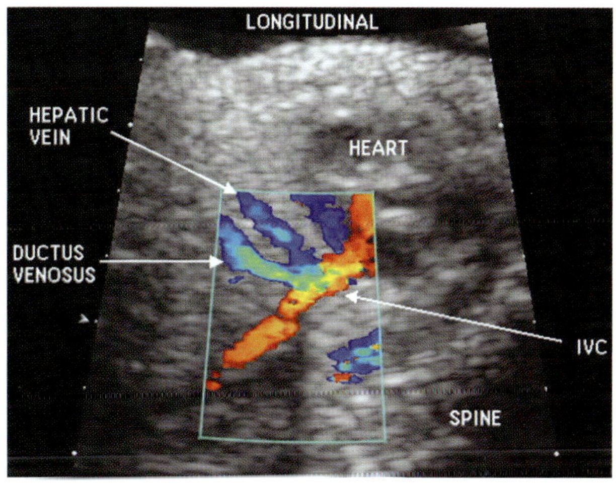

Figure 53.6 Midsagittal view of the fetal upper abdomen. DV and hepatic vein merge into the IVC forming the subdiaphragamatic infundibulum, a funnel-shaped vascular space just below the diaphragm, ending into the right atrium.

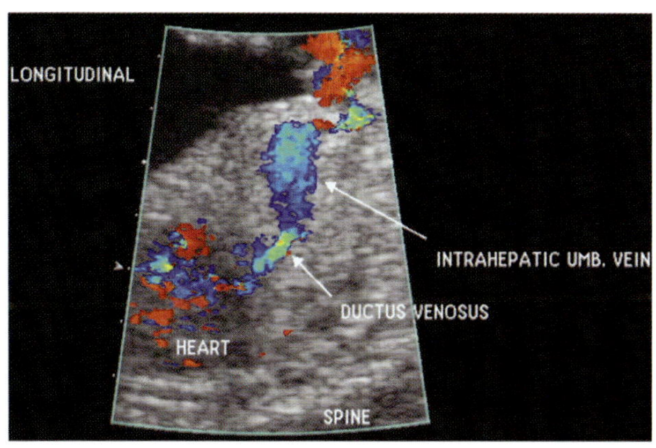

Figure 53.7 Midsagittal section of the fetal trunk: DV is visualized in its full length arising from the UV. The CDI indicates higher velocities compared with the flow in the UV: aliasing effect is present.

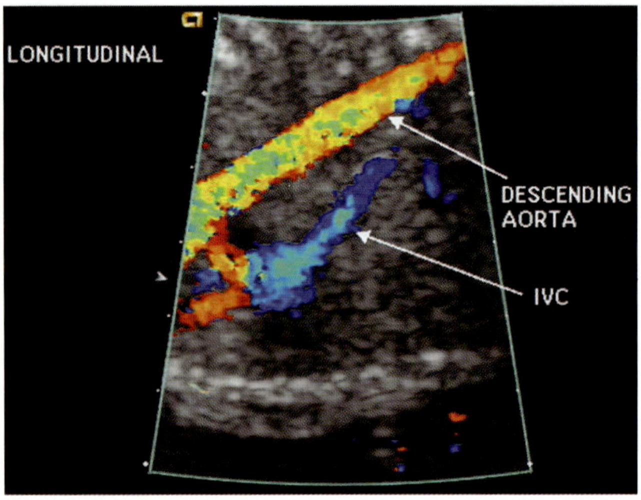

Figure 53.8 Coronal plane of the upper abdomen: the IVC runs anterior, to the right of and nearly parallel to the descending aorta.

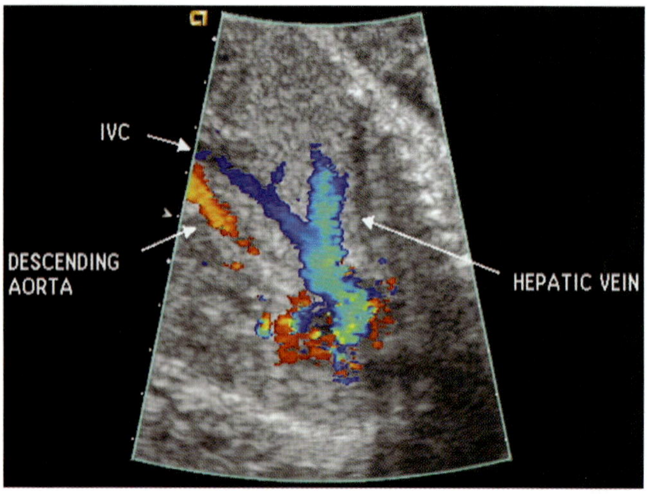

Figure 53.9 Coronal section through the right hepatic lobe. The right hepatic vein and IVC merge into the subdiaphragmatic infundibulum.

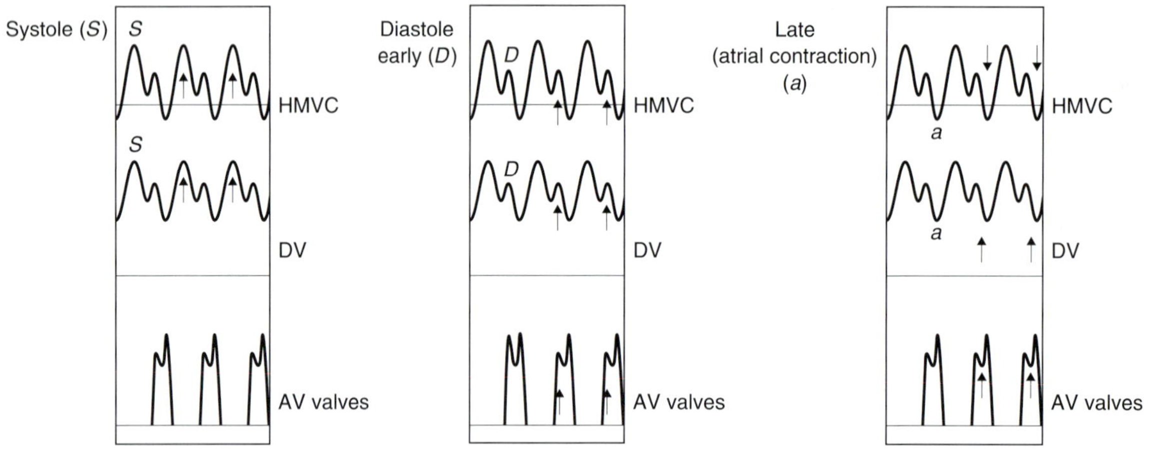

Figure 53.10 Doppler waveform patterns in the DV, HV and IVC, and their relationship with the cardiac cycle (AV, atrioventricular valves; S, systole; D, early diastole). A physiologic reverse flow is evident in IVC/HV during atrial contraction (a). With permission from Hecher K. The fetal venous circulation. In Harrington K, Campbell S, eds. *A Colour Atlas of Doppler Ultrasonography in Obstetrics*, 71–9.

The IVC could be well evaluated either in the longitudinal or coronal section; it runs anterior, to the right of and nearly parallel to the descending aorta (Figure 53.8).

The hepatic veins can be visualized either in a transverse scan section through the upper abdomen or in a sagittal–coronal section through the hepatic lobes (Figure 53.9).

The typical waveform for blood flow in the venous vessels, excluding the UV and portal veins, consists of three phases related to the cardiac cycle (Figure 53.10). The highest pressure gradient between the venous vessel and the right atrium occurs during ventricular systole (S), resulting in the fastest blood flow velocities forward from the fetal heart. Early diastole (peak D) with opening of the atrio-ventricular valves and passive early filling of the ventricles (peak E of the biphasic atrio-ventricular flow waveform) is associated with a second forward peak flow. The lowest velocities (a) in fetal venous vessels can be observed during the atrial contraction of the late diastole (peak A of the biphasic atrio-ventricular flow waveform).

The DV flow pattern is characterized by a triphasic forward flow (Figure 53.11): it is directed toward the heart through the whole cardiac cycle. Even in early pregnancy, there is no retrograde flow during atrial contraction.

In the IVC and hepatic veins (Figures 53.12 and 53.13), a physiological reverse flow during atrial contraction is observed. The percentage of reverse flow in the IVC decreases with advancing gestational age.

As for the site of sampling, it is of vital importance in the evaluation of the fetal venous system.

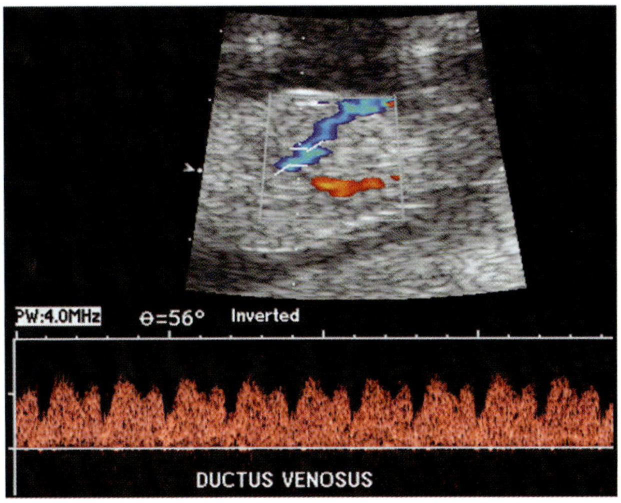

Figure 53.11 Triphasic forward Doppler flow waveform in the DV. It is directed toward the heart through the whole cardiac cycle. A nadir of forward flow is observed during atrial contraction.

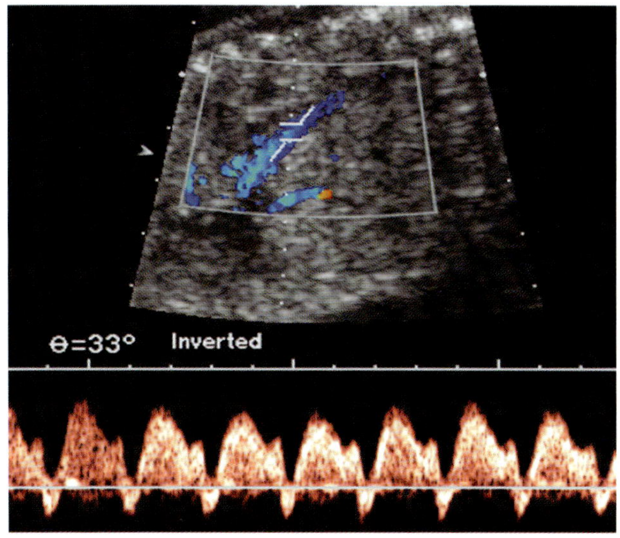

Figure 53.13 Doppler flow waveforms in the IVC: a physiological slight reversal flow is recorded during atrial contraction (a).

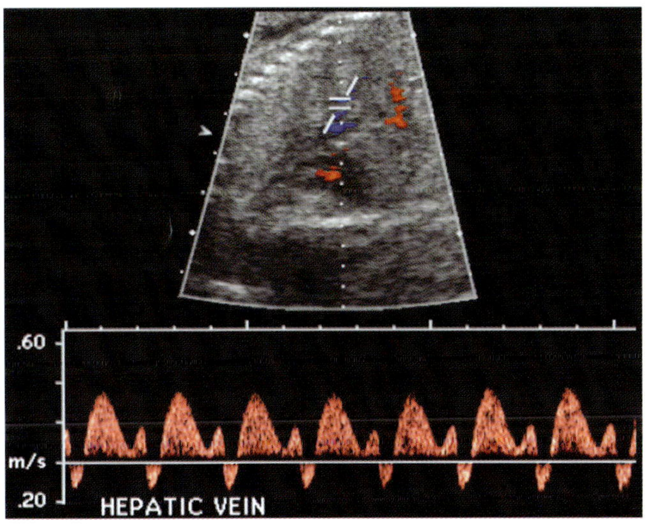

Figure 53.12 Doppler flow waveforms in the HV: a physiological slight reversal flow is recorded during atrial contraction (a).

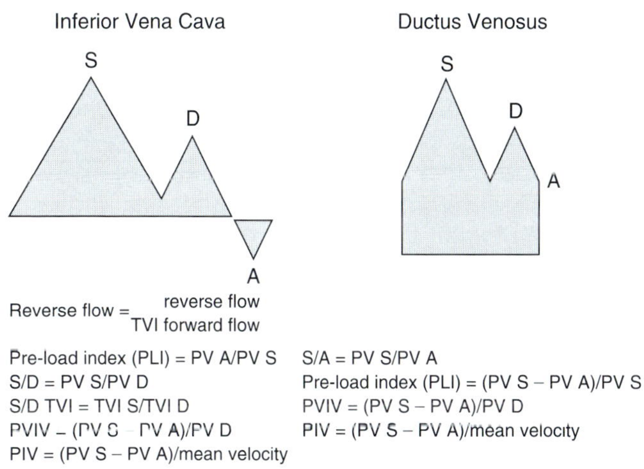

Figure 53.14 Angle-independent indices reported in the literature for the IVC and the DV. S, systole; D, diastole; A, atrial contraction; TVI, time velocity integral; PV, peak velocity; PLI, preload index; PVIV, peak velocity index for vein; PIV, pulsatility index for vein.

It has been shown that the highest velocities of the DV are at the inlet, immediately above the UV, relative to the outlet into the IVC. It has been established that the inlet part of the DV should be evaluated for Doppler waveform analysis.

As for the IVC, large standard deviations for various Doppler waveform variables and a mixture of overlapping signals from different bloodstreams have been shown at the subdiaphragmatic venous infundibulum. It has been established that the site of sampling is between the renal vein and the DV: this is the place of the highest reproducibility.[6–9]

More than 10 different angle-independent indices of the IVC and the DV have been proposed and reference ranges have been compiled (Figure 53.14). 'Pulsatility index for veins' and 'Peak velocity index for vein' are now commonly used for the highest correlation with adverse outcome variables, such as fetal acidemia and perinatal mortality.[9–11] Even if flow volume and absolute velocity measurements can be evaluated, it has been demonstrated to have higher inaccuracy and intraobserver variation compared to qualitative ratios. This is mainly due to vulnerable errors of the evaluation of vessel diameter measurements and unreliable or high angle of insonation.

The mean and peak velocities increase significantly in venous vessels with advancing gestational age. The highest and lowest velocities are found in the DV and the right hepatic vein, respectively. Conversely, the angle-independent indices decrease during gestation and this is consistent with a reduction in cardiac afterload because of the decrease in placental resistance. It may also reflect increased ventricular compliance. The reduction in cardiac afterload causes a decrease in end-diastolic ventricular pressure and therefore an increase in venous blood flow velocity toward the heart during atrial contraction.[10,11]

As shown for arterial Doppler evaluation, from a methodological point of view, it is essential to avoid measurements during fetal breathing movements. Changes in intrathoracic pressure during breathing movements have significant effects on Doppler waveforms. Inward movement of the abdominal wall during inspiration is accompanied by an increase of blood flow velocities, whereas a decrease in velocities is evident during expiration. As the shape of Doppler waveforms shows changes during the breathing movements, indices or velocity ratios should be evaluated during fetal apnea (Figures 53.15 and 53.16).[6,7,12]

The easiest vessel to investigate is the UV. Reference ranges for quantitative UV blood flow has been also compiled, according to the following formulae: UV volume flow (ml/min) = time averaged velocity (mm/s) × cross-sectional vessel area (mm^2); UV absolute flow (ml/min) = vessel cross-sectional area (mm^2) × mean velocity × 60. However, methodological differences in blood flow study have limited the quantitative evaluation of the UV in clinical practice. Qualitative analysis of the UV waveform in normal conditions shows a continuous forward flow without pulsations after the first trimester (Figure 53.17). Mild sinusoidal pulsations synchronous with the fetal heart rate (FHR) have been described in some normal fetuses between 34 and 38 weeks and during fetal breathing movements (20% of the cases in the free-loop portion). These have to be distinguished from the pathological pulsations in cases of severe fetal compromise and nonimmune hydrops[6,13–15] (Figure 53.18).

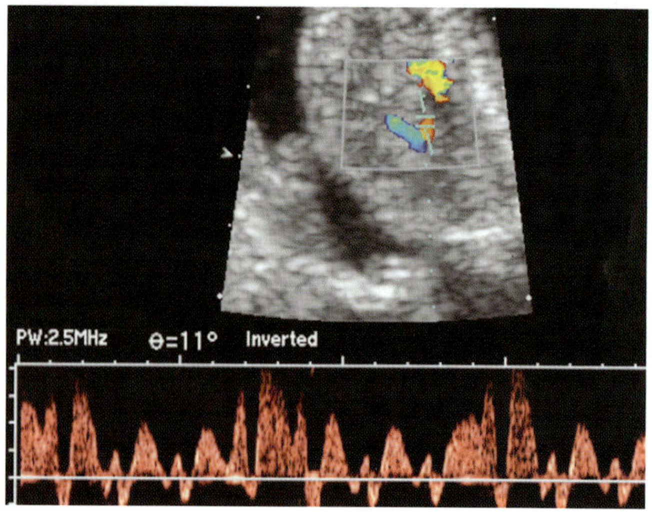

Figure 53.16 Doppler flow waveforms during breathing movements in the IVC.

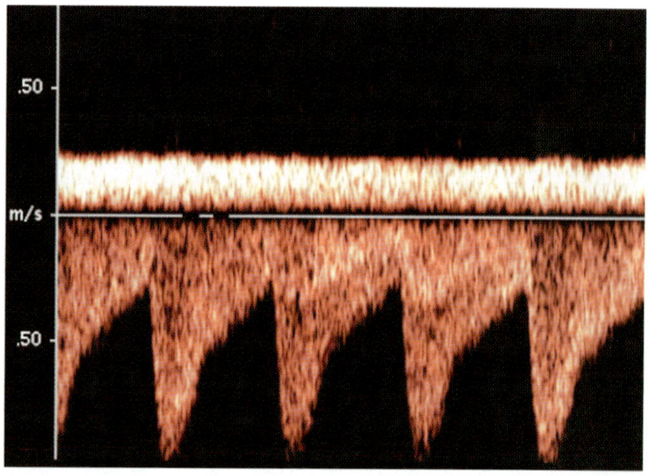

Figure 53.17 Qualitative analysis of the UV waveform: a physiologic continuous forward flow without pulsations is observed after the first trimester.

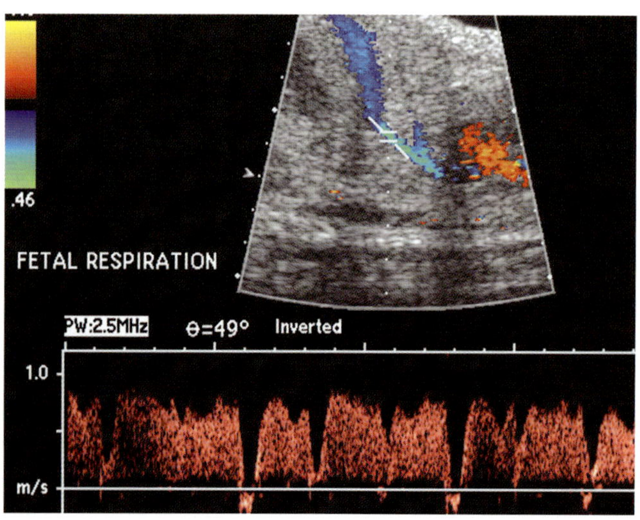

Figure 53.15 Doppler flow waveforms during breathing movements in the DV.

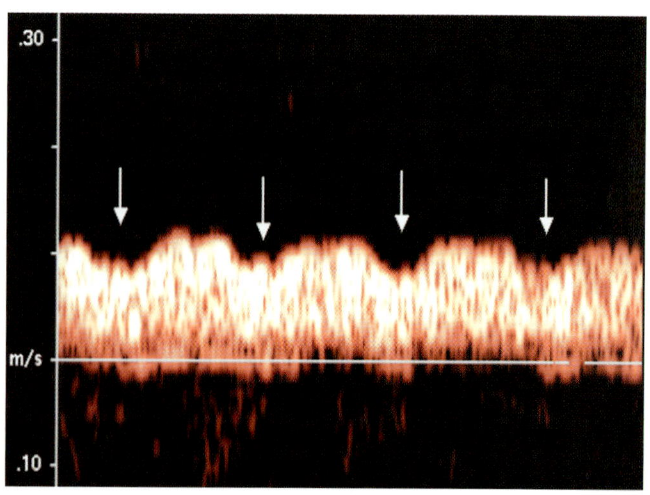

Figure 53.18 Umbilical vein pulsations with notches synchronous with atrial contractions. Diphasic pulsations due to the increased central venous pressure and/or opening of the DV may be secondary to congestive heart failure or imminent fetal hypoxemia/acidemia.

Table 53.1 Classification of the fetal venous system anomalies (from Fasouliotis *et al.*[3])

A. Cardinal veins
   a. Complex malformations, heterotaxic syndrome
   b. Isolated malformation

B. Umbilical veins
   a. Primary failure to create critical anastomoses
      – Complete: abnormal connection of UV (venosus shunts) into iliac vein, IVC, SVC and right atrium
      – Partial: persistence of right umbilical vein (PRUV) with or without DV
   b. Secondary occlusion

C. Vitelline veins
   a. Primary failure to create critical anastomoses
      – Complete agenesis of portal system
      – Partial agenesis of right or left portal branch (portosystemic shunt)

D. Anomalous pulmonary venous connection (total or partial)

Structural anomalies of the fetal venous system

A brief review of the embryologic landmarks was given in order to understand the fetal venous system structural anomalies (see section 'Embryology of the fetal venous system'.

The abnormal development of fetal venous vessels may be related to either of two different pathogenesis: the primary failure to transform or to form the critical anastomoses and the secondary occlusion of an already transformed system.

Four major groups of anomalies can be identified on the basis of the etiology (primary or secondary), the vessel involved and the embryologic precursor (Table 53.1): (A) abnormal connection of the cardinal veins; (B) abnormalities of the UV; (C) abnormalities of the vitelline veins; and (D) anomalous pulmonary venous connection (not discussed in this chapter).

Anomalies of the fetal venous system may be also classified simply considering either (1) the abnormalities of the caval venous system or (2) the anomalies of umbilical, portal and hepatic veins. The abnormal connections of the cardinal veins are part of the heterotaxy syndromes.

An interrupted or absent IVC with azygos vein continuation or the persistence of the left SVC are the result of primary failure to create the anastomoses in embryologic period and may be a sign of cardiosplenic syndromes.

The anatomical correlations of aorta to the IVC and the spine, and the venous connections to the atria are very helpful to diagnose left and right atrial isomerisms. In situs solitus, the aorta is located to the left of the spine, whereas in situs inversus the location is reversed. In right isomerism, the aorta and the IVC are on the same side of the spine, either right or left. Aplasia of the spleen should be a sign of right isomerism. In left isomerism, the aorta runs medial to the spine, the IVC is not identified and the azygos vein runs dorsal and lateral to the aorta, either on the right-hand side or on the left-hand side. In this subtype of heterotaxy syndrome, multiple spleens are usually present. A situs ambiguus is a common finding in both types of isomerism: the stomach can be in a left, right or medial position. Also, the position of the liver can be variable.[2–4,6,16,17]

Abnormalities of the IVC and the SVC are often associated with major impairments of the development of the heart, intestinal tract and body symmetry, influencing significantly the prognosis.[2–4,6] The anomalies of the umbilical veins represent the major and most common group of structural anomalies of the fetal venous system.

Primary failure to form the critical anastomoses results in an aberrant vessel that shunts the blood flow from the placenta to the systemic veins. This spectrum of anomalies may involve the iliac vein, the IVC or the SVC, or the direct connection with the right atrium. Agenesis of the DV is a common feature of these groups of anomalies. Two forms may be identified. The first one is represented by the direct connection of the UV with the systemic venous circulation, bypassing the liver. This is often associated with Noonan syndrome, pleural effusion and hydrops. The second form includes cases in which the UV is adequately connected with the portal vein, but fails to establish a communication with the persistent proximal part of the right vitelline vein. The result is a prolonged hypoperfusion of the liver that may lead to portal hypertension.[2–4,17–19]

Partial failure to form critical anastomoses in left and right veins is quite common. Persistence of the right umbilical vein (PRUV) is the most common anomaly observed. Three types may be identified: (1) the intrahepatic form (the UV is connected with the right portal vein instead of the left portal vein); (2) the RUV is connected directly to the iliac vein, the IVC or the right atrium; (3) both the UVs persist.[16,17]

The first type is commonly identified as an isolated finding, and is considered a benign variant, whereas the other two are often associated with complex structural anomalies, especially cardiac malformations, or signs of congestive heart failure.

The pathophysiologic mechanisms of PRUV, primary or secondary, seem to be related to occlusion by thromboembolic events arising from the placenta. Teratogenic agents have been advocated as inducing primary failure of the critical anastomoses.

The anomalies of the vitelline veins are extremely rare and only a few cases have been reported in prenatal literature. Primary failure to form the critical anastomoses may lead to complete agenesis of the portal system or to partial agenesis of the right or left portal vein. In the complete form, enterohepatic circulation is shunted systemically.

Partial forms of absence of the portal system might represent a more benign form of vitelline veins' abnormalities.[2–4]

Venous system Doppler and fetal diseases

UV pulsations with moderate to severe notches synchronous with atrial contraction have been described as an ominous sign. They are associated with various fetal pathological conditions such as nonimmune hydrops (NIH), fetal arrhythmia, fetal congestive heart failure, placental anomalies, fetal growth restriction (FGR), absent/reverse end-diastolic flow (ARED) in the umbilical artery (UA) and abnormal FHR patterns.

Different pathophysiological mechanisms may lead to UV pulsations. Single pulsation, caused by changes in forward flow from the placenta, might be related to ARED flow in the UA during diastole or bradicardia, umbilical cord occlusion and true knot on the cord during systole. Diphasic pulsations, because of increased central venous pressure and/or opening of the DV, can be secondary to congestive heart failure or imminent fetal hypoxemia/acidemia (Figure 53.18).[20]

NIHF is a severe clinical condition of varying etiologies with poor prognosis. Differentiating between NIHF caused by congestive heart failure and other noncardiac causes is essential to formulate a prognosis.

In the presence of NIHF and umbilical pulsations, the right ventricular shortening fraction is significantly decreased, and abnormal venous return to the heart is consistent with decreased cardiac output, leading to congestive heart failure and poor fetal outcome.

Structural heart diseases involving ventricular outflow, with or without hydrops, are frequently associated with abnormal venous blood flow. Altered pump function with increased workload causes a decrease or even reversal of blood flow during atrial contraction. In cases with tricuspid regurgitation, increased reversed phase in the IVC is frequently associated to fetal hydrops. Increased central venous pressure due to regurgitant flow into the atrium can cause hydrops, which implies poor prognosis.

The diagnosis of the different types of fetal arrhythmias is possible by simultaneous waveform recordings from abdominal aorta and IVC. High-velocity reverse flow due to increased right pressure is found either in atrial contraction against a closed tricuspid valve, or in tricuspid regurgitation. The first occurs during premature atrial contraction with complete atrioventricular block, and the second during premature ventricular contraction.

Premature beats of supraventricular or ventricular origin can be differentiated depending on the characteristic differences in blood flow velocity waveforms of the venous vessels (IVC) during atrial contraction. During premature beats of atrial origin an exaggerated reverse flow is recorded earlier than expected during the heart cycle. In cases of premature beats of ventricular origin, the reverse flow is evident at the moment of end diastole, with a typical lag pattern in blood flow velocity after ventricular premature beat.[6–20]

Venous Doppler analysis is also essential to manage supraventricular tachycardia. From the observation of venous flow patterns (IVC, DV), it is possible to delay antiarrhythmic treatment if the heart rate is below 210 beats/min. Above this critical heart rate frequency, an abnormal monophasic forward flow is observed in the DV and the IVC. This pattern is related to direct impediment of diastolic filling, causing elevation of atrial and venous pressures. Due to the presence of a parallel fetal flow circuitry, the increase of the left atrial pressure leads to right side congestive heart failure and ventricular dysfunction.[6,21,22]

Fetuses with intrauterine growth restriction (IUGR) are usually delivered on the basis of abnormal results of nonstress tests such as FHR monitoring, biophysical profile or the presence of maternal pathological conditions. Although the introduction of arterial Doppler ultrasound evaluation has resulted in a significant decrease in perinatal mortality and morbidity, the transition between adaptation and decompensation because of fetal hypoxemia/acidemia is difficult to identify accurately.

The decision regarding the optimal timing of delivery, to avoid iatrogenic delivery of a mild affected premature neonate before irreversible asphyxia-related damage, is still a dilemma. The arterial multivessel evaluation (umbilical artery, descending aorta, middle cerebral artery) is commonly used in clinical practice to assess fetal well-being in high-risk pregnancy. However, this assessment has a limited value in determining the time of delivery.[6,23–28]

Although maximal decrease in vascular cerebral resistance has been found to precede the onset of late decelerations by an average of 2 weeks, it has been unsuitable to monitor IUGR fetuses closely during the last 2 weeks preceding the occurrence of acute distress or intrauterine death.

The Doppler study of the fetal venous blood flow in the IVC and the DV and other venous vessels (sinus trasversus, right hepatic vein) have raised new

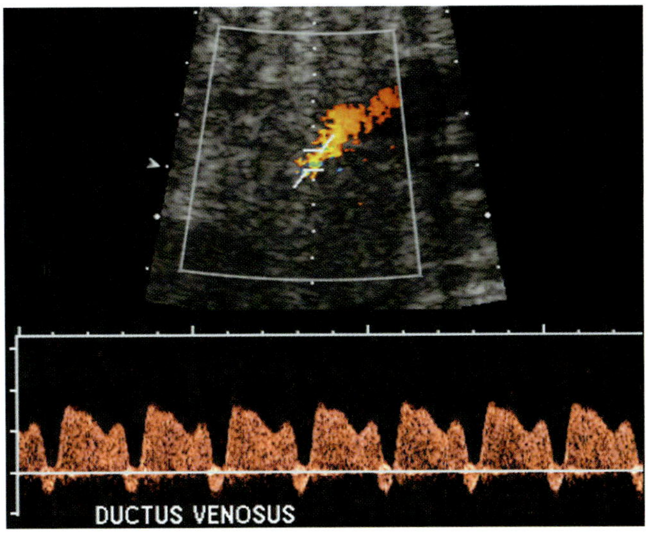

Figure 53.19 Abnormal DV waveform: reversal flow during atrial contraction is the consequence of increased end-diastolic pressure.

expectations by investigating fetal hemodynamic changes more accurately.

Two mechanisms can be considered for the onset of abnormal venous Doppler waveform: the increase of right ventricular afterload and myocardial failure. As long as the fetus is able to compensate for reduced placental supply by redistribution, preferential myocardial oxygenation delays the development of right heart failure, despite an increasing afterload. Progressive changes in fetal venous circulation may indicate failure of the compensatory mechanism and herald the development of right heart failure due to myocardial hypoxemia.[6,9,10]

It has been shown that the evaluation of Doppler venous waveforms are correlated to computerized analysis of FHR monitoring: reverse flow in DV is significantly correlated with values of short-term variation below 3.5 ms, ominous sign of hypoxemia/acidemia[29,30] (Figure 53.19).

Recent studies are focusing on the role of fetal venous Doppler evaluation, combined or integrated with other methods of fetal surveillance, such as biophysical profile and computerized cardiotocography, in the timing of delivery and the physiopathological sequence of the deterioration. Besides promising results, it has not been yet assessed as to what is the best method for timing the delivery of preterm severe IUGR fetuses.[30–32]

The widely held view that, in any case, venous Doppler abnormalities would precede deterioration of biophysical parameters has not been observed.

Ferrazzi *et al.*[30] reported that more than 50% of the fetuses delivered because of an abnormal FHR pattern did not have venous Doppler abnormalities.

Hecher *et al.*[31] observed that among fetuses born before 32 weeks of gestation, persistent abnormalities in FHR tracings preceded the occurrence of an abnormal DV pulsatility index in about 53% of the cases; simultaneous anomalies were detected in 5% of the cases.

Muller *et al.*[27] found that absent/reverse flow in the DV in a group of cases with umbilical artery ARED flow was significantly predictive of poor outcome. Delivery was indicated by non-reassuring status defined as either cardiotocographic (CTG) pathological pattern or when suspicious FHR traces were associated with absence or reversal in DV flow during atrial contraction. However, it is not indicated as to how many cases of normal DV Doppler flow waveforms were delivered for an abnormal CTG pattern.

Baschat *et al.*[32] reported that the deterioration of arterial/venous parameters occurred before an abnormal biophysical profile within 24 h in the majority of the cases.

These data show that hemodynamic changes of blood flow and decompensation, as detected by an abnormal FHR trace, biophysical profile or venous Doppler, are widely variable among fetuses and do not follow a predictable physiopathological cascade. It has been postulated that many variables have to be considered in the clinical practice. It has been shown that gestational age has a significant impact on the predictive value of venous Doppler for the timing of delivery. Moreover, in managing cases of severe preterm IUGR, the high risks involved in the sequelae of prematurity have to be considered.[33]

Probably, the combination of Doppler evaluation of the fetal circulation, to assess cardiac function, and biophysical parameters/computerized CTG, to assess central nervous system involvement, should allow more precise information about the pathophysiology and assessment of fetal growth restriction. A multicenter randomized clinical trial should be addressed to assess what is the best method of monitoring and timing the delivery of severe premature growth restricted fetuses; two ongoing trials, GRIT (Growth Restriction Intervention Trial) and TRUFFLE (Trial of Umbilical and Fetal Flow in Europe) studies, might clarify this issue.[33–35]

Conclusions

In recent years, high-resolution sonography, combined with CDI, has advanced our ability to investigate the fetal venous system. These noninvasive techniques have enhanced our understanding of the fetal venous circulation in physiologic conditions and provide us the possibility to evaluate circulatory changes in abnormal circumstances.

From the literature, it can be speculated that fetal venous Doppler may be a helpful diagnostic tool and may influence the management of fetal diseases such as cardiovascular pathologies, hydrops and fetal growth restriction.

As for the latter condition, the longitudinal Doppler analysis of fetal arterial and venous districts provides us essential information about the progressive deterioration that occurs in chronic hypoxemia. Even though abnormal venous Doppler has a high likelihood of perinatal mortality/morbidity, further studies are needed to clarify the role of fetal venous Doppler in the timing of delivery. The understanding of the variables that affect the physiopathological changes in severely compromised fetuses should provide us this crucial information.

REFERENCES

1. Hamilton WJ, Mossman HW. *Human Embriology*, 4th edn. Cambridge: Heffer, 1972:272–82.
2. Hoffstetter C, Plath H, Hansmann M. Prenatal diagnosis of abnormalities of the fetal venous system. *Ultrasound Obstet Gynecol* 2000;15(3):231–41.
3. Fasouliotis SJ, Achiron R, *et al.* The human fetal venous system: Normal embryologic, anatomic, and physiologic characteristics and developmental abnormalities. *J Ultrasound Med* 2002; 21(10):1145–58.
4. Achiron R, Hegesh J, Yagel M, *et al.* Abnormalities of the central veins and umbilico-portal system: Prenatal ultrasonographic diagnosis and proposed classification. *Ultrasound Obstet Gynecol* 2000;16:539–48.
5. Mavrides E, Moscoso G, Caravalho JS, *et al.* The anatomy of the umbilical, portal and hepatic venous systems in the human fetus at 14–19 weeks of gestation. *Ultrasound Obstet Gynecol* 2001; 18(6):598–604.
6. Hecher K, Campbell S. Characteristics of fetal venous blood flow under normal and during fetal disease. *Ultrasound Obstet Gynecol* 1996;7:68–83.
7. Moll W. Venous return in the fetal–placental cardiovascular system. *Eur J Obstet Gynaecol* 1999.
8. Hecher K, Campbell S, Snijders R, *et al.* Reference ranges for fetal venous and atrioventricular blood flow parameters. *Ultrasound Obstet Gynecol* 1994;4:381–90.
9. Hecher K, Snijders R, Campbell S, *et al.* Fetal venous, intracardiac, and arterial blood flow velocities in intrauterine growth restriction: Relationship with fetal blood gases. *Am J Obstet Gynecol* 1995; 173:10–15.
10. Rizzo G, Capponi A, Arduini D, *et al.* The value of fetal arterial, cardiac and venous flows in predicting pH and blood gases measured in umbilical blood at cordocentesis in growth retarded fetuses. *Br J Obstet Gynecol* 1995;102(12):963–9.
11. DeVore GR, Horenstein J. Ductus venosus index: A method for evaluation of right ventricular preload in the second trimester. *Ultrasound Obstet Gynecol* 1993;3:338–42.
12. Gardiner H, Brodszki J, Marsal K. Ventriculovascular physiology of the growth-restricted fetus. *Ultrasound Obstet Gynecol* 2001; 18(1):47–53.
13. Ferrazzi E, Rigano S, Bozzo M, *et al.* Umbilical vein blood flow in growth-restricted fetuses. *Ultrasound Obstet Gynecol* 2000; 16(5):432–8.
14. Reed KL, Anderson CF. Changes in umbilical venous velocities with physiologic perturbation. *Am J Obstet Gynecol* 2000;182(4): 738–40.
15. Boito S, Struijk PC, Ursen NT, *et al.* Umbilical venous volume flow in the normally developing and growth-restricted human fetus. *Ultrasound Obstet Gynecol* 2002;19(3):229–34.
16. Volpe P, Marasini M, Caruso G, *et al.* Prenatal diagnosis of ductus venosus agenesis and its association with cytogenetic/congenital anomalies. *Prenatal Diagn* 2002;22(11):995–1000.
17. Jaeggi ET, Fouron JC, Hornberger LK, *et al.* Agenesis of the ductus venosus that is associated with extrahepatic vein drainage: Prenatal features and clinical outcome. *Am J Obstet Gynecol* 2002;187(4):1031–7.
18. Cohen SB, Lipitz S, Mashiach S, *et al.* In utero ultrasonographic diagnosis of an aberrant umbilical vein associate with hepatic hyperechogenicity. *Prenatal Diagn* 1997;17(10):978–82.
19. Baz E, Zikulnig L, Hackeloer BJ, *et al.* Abnormal ductus venosus blood flow: A clue to umbilical cord complication. *Ultrasound Obstet Gynecol* 1999;13(3):204–6.
20. Gudmunsson S. Importance of venous flow assessment for clinical decision-making. *Eur J Obstet Gynecol Reprod Biol* 1999;84(2): 173–8.
21. Gembruch U, Krapp M, Germer U, *et al.* Venous Doppler in the sonographic surveillance of fetuses with supraventricular tachycardia. *Eur J Obstet Gynecol Reprod Biol* 1999;84(2):187–92.
22. Gembruch U, Krapp M, Baumann P. Changes of venous blood flow velocity waveforms in fetuses with supraventricular tachycardia. *Ultrasound Obstet Gynecol* 1995;5(6):394–9.
23. Ozcan T, Sbracia M, d'Ancona RL, *et al.* Arterial and venous Doppler velocimetry in the severely growth-restricted fetus and associations with adverse perinatal outcome. *Ultrasound Obstet Gynecol* 1998;12(1):39–44.
24. Baschat AA, Gembruch U, Reiss I, *et al.* Demonstration of fetal coronary blood flow by Doppler ultrasound in relation to arterial venous and flow velocity waveforms and perinatal outcome 'the heart sparing effect.' *Ultrasound Obstet Gynecol* 1997;9(3): 162–72.
25. Tchirikov M, Rybakowski C, Huneke B, *et al.* Umbilical vein blood volume flow rate and umbilical arterial pulsatility as 'venous-arterial index' in the prediction of neonatal compromise. *Ultrasound Obstet Gynecol* 2002;20(6):580–5.
26. Hofstaetter C, Gudmundsson S, Hansmann M. Venous Doppler velocimetry in the surveillance of severely compromised fetuses. *Ultrasound Obstet Gynecol* 2002;20(3):233–9.
27. Muller T, Nanan R, Rehen M, *et al.* Arterial and ductus venosus Doppler in fetuses with absent or reverse end-diastolic flow in the umbilical artery: Correlation with short-term perinatal outcome. *Acta Obstet Gynecol Scand* 2002;22(9):786–91.
28. Baschat AA, Gembruch U, Reiss I, *et al.* Relationship between arterial and venous Doppler and perinatal outcome in fetal growth restriction. *Ultrasound Obstet Gynecol* 2000;16(5):407–13.
29. Senat MV, Schwarzler P, Alcais A, *et al.* Longitudinal changes in the ductus venosus, cerebral transverse sinus and cardiotocogram in fetal growth restriction. *Ultrasound Obstet Gynecol* 2000; 16(1):19–24.
30. Ferrazzi E, Bozzo M, Rigano S, *et al.* Temporal sequence of abnormal Doppler changes in the peripheral and central circulatory systems of the severely growth-restricted fetus. *Ultrasound Obstet Gynecol* 2002;19:140–6.
31. Hecher K, Bilardo CM, Stigler RH, *et al.* Monitoring of fetuses with intrauterine growth restriction: A longitudinal study. *Ultrasound Obstet Gynecol* 2001;18(6):564–70.
32. Baschat AA, Gembruch U, Harman CR, *et al.* The sequence of changes in Doppler and biophysical parameters as severe growth restriction worsens. *Ultrasound Obstet Gynecol* 2001;18(6): 598–604.
33. Bilardo CM, Wolf H, Stigter RH, *et al.* Relationship between monitoring parameters and perinatal outcome in severe, early intrauterine growth restriction. *Ultrasound Obstet Gynecol* 2004; 23:119–25.
34. Romero R, Kalache KD, Kadar N Timing the delivery of the preterm severely growth-restricted fetus: Venous Doppler, cardiotocography or the biophysical profile? *Ultrasound Obstet Gynecol* 2002;19(2):118–21.
35. Baschat AA. Integrated fetal testing in growth restriction: Combining multivessel Doppler and biophysical parameters. *Ultrasound Obstet Gynecol* 2003;21:1–8.

SECTION VI

Basic science

Section Editors: **H. Nakano and Y. Murata**

54 Molecular background of parturition: lessons from knockout models

T. Kimura, K. Ogita, T. Tsutsui, K. Shimoya,
M. Koyama and Y. Murata

Introduction

Parturition, which is the last step of new life inside the mother's body, is considered to be the result of multiple biochemical and physiological steps. For example, during the first 9 months of human gestation, the uterus is in a quiescent state, and unresponsive to contractile stimuli (phase 0). After this prelude to parturition, the uterus should prepare for labor (phase 1). During labor, the uterus contracts to dilate the cervix and to force the fetus through the birth canal (phase 2). After the final process of labor, the uterus involutes to normal size (phase 3).[1] The beginning of parturition can be considered as a transition from phase 0 and phase 1, which is undetectable clinically. The initiation of labor is the transition from phase 1 to phase 2, which is determined clinically by the onset of regular and painful uterine contractions leading to cervical dilatation and descent of the fetal presenting part.

During phase 0 and phase 1, various endocrine and immunological factors should control uterine function for it to maintain quiescence and to prepare for labor. During phases 2 and 3, stimulating molecules for uterine smooth muscle contraction and molecules related to uterine contractile systems must play a crucial role (Figure 54.1). Several papers have appeared that describe up- and down-regulation of these molecules, although few of them told us how critical these functions were for maintenance of pregnancy, as well as initiation and progress of parturition *in vivo*. The biggest advantage in using the knockout mouse model is to elucidate the actual function of these molecules *in vivo* by disrupting the specific gene responsible for the phenotype. In some cases, natural human disease caused by the gene deletion/mutation would also give us a clue for elucidating the function of the genes and substrates in parturition. This chapter will focus on the reproductive phenotypes of gene-targeted mice or human genetic diseases in which genes that were deleted are suspected of having functions for reproduction.

Endocrine system

A drastic change in the endocrine milieu occurs during pregnancy. For example, plasma estrogen concentrations at term of pregnancy are over 1000-fold of those in the non-pregnant period. Steroid hormones play a crucial role in the development of reproductive organs. Most of the knockout mouse models related to steroidgenesis showed underdeveloped sexual organs and infertility, which were inadequate for analysis of parturition. Some peptide hormones are mainly secreted from the brain, and they modulate the functions of the peripheral organs. The peptide hormone oxytocin, which directly activates uterine contractilities, will be discussed later.

Steroid hormones

Estrogen and its receptors

In the endocrine system, steroid hormones (estrogens, progestagens, glucocorticoids and androgens) and their receptors have been considered to be involved in the regulation of parturition. Near term of pregnancy, the concentrations of circulating estrogens are drastically elevated. In humans at near term of pregnancy, there is more than a 100-fold increase of plasma estrogen concentrations. High concentrations of estrogens are believed to enhance uterine sensitivity and to induce labor-stimulating molecules. As most of the estrogens are synthesized by aromatase (P450arom, *cyp19*) in the placenta of near term in human and

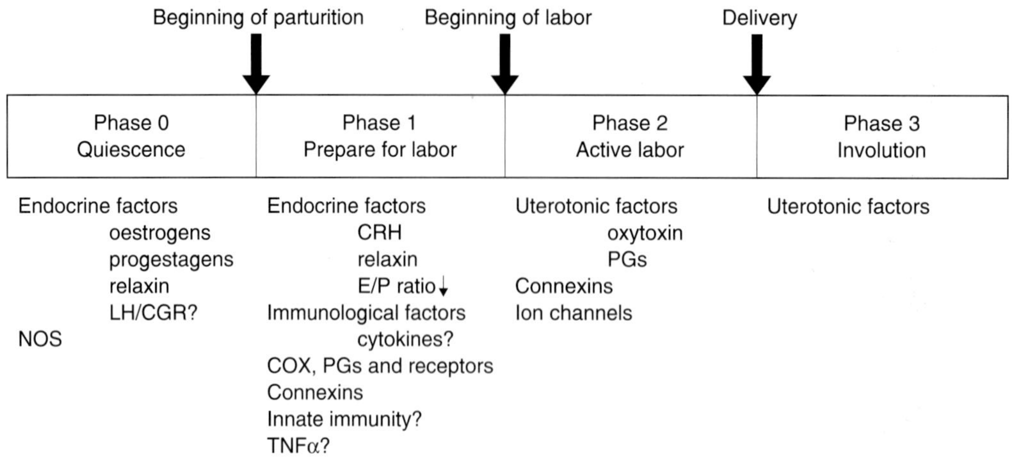

Figure 54.1 Various molecules have been reported to regulate four phases during pregnancy and postpartum. In phase 0, uterine smooth muscle should maintain quiescence even under severe distention and stretching by the conceptus. Transition from phase 0 to phase 1 is clinically undetectable, albeit this is the true initiation of parturition. Once phase 1 begins, the process to delivery is irreversible. Transition from phase 1 to phase 2 can be recognized as the onset of labor; however the attempt to stop labor at this point could already be impossible, as discussed in a lot of papers on tocolysis. Modified from Cunningham *et al.*[1]

higher primates, the antenatal histories of the aromatase-deficient patients are of great interest. Among the 16 cases reported, all appeared to be born at term with labor.[2–7] The gestational courses of two cases were precisely described. In one case, the mother suffered from progressive virilization during pregnancy[7] and in the other case the mother was administered tocolytic reagent for several weeks.[2] In both cases, labor occurred spontaneously at term and the mothers delivered their babies vaginally. Maternal estradiol and estriol concentrations near term were $< 3\%$ and $< 1\%$, respectively. These results from a natural 'knockout' human model indicated that extremely high amounts of estrogens during the third trimester are not necessary for the process of human parturition. Aromatase knockout (ArKO) female mice were completely infertile because of a hypoplastic uterus and ovary.[8] Adult male and female ArKO mice had higher concentrations of testosterone and androstendione, the precursors of estrogens. Concentrations of these androgens during the fetal and neonatal periods were not evaluated.

The estrogen effect is mediated by two distinct nuclear receptors, namely estrogen receptor (ER) α and ERβ. Female ERα knockout mice showed a hypoplastic uterus and were completely infertile.[9] Although they were infertile and implantation did not occur, decidualization could be induced with mechanical stimulation by progesterone dependent manner.[10] On the other hand, female ERβ knockout mice possessed a hormonally responsive uterus and grossly normal ovaries, and they were subfertile in terms of the frequency and size of the litters. Their parturition was not disturbed. The nature of this subfertility was caused by ovarian dysfunction.[11] ERα is necessary for the development and function of the uterus and ovary; however, ERβ appears to play a role that is more limiting on the ovary.

Progesterone and its receptors

In rodents, progesterone withdrawal is the most important trigger for parturition. As progesterone is the fundamental precursor of all other steroidgenesis, it is impossible to down-regulate progesterone synthesis without disturbing other steroidgenesis by specific gene disruption. There are two progesterone receptor (PR) isoforms, PR-A and PR-B. It is hypothesized that PR-B acts in a competitive manner to PR-A function. PR-A knockout female mice revealed extensive abnormalities, including anovulation, defective sexual behavior, a hypertrophic uterus and underdeveloped mammary glands, which led to infertility.[12] PR-B knockout female mice were fertile and sustained normal parturition at term.[13]

Glucocorticoid and its receptor

In sheep, up-regulation of fetal glucocorticoid triggers their parturition.[14] In mice, glucocorticoid receptor (GR) knockout caused severe respiratory failure after birth, and more than 80% of GR −/− pups died. The impaired feedback loop of the hypothalamo–pituitary–adrenal axis led to higher plasma corticosterone concentrations (approximately 2.5-fold) in GR−/−and GR+/−neonates. After mating GR+/− male and GR+/−female, 75% of pups are expected to have higher glucocorticoid concentrations *in utero*. However, there were no observations of preterm birth or other parturition failure in these cases, as well as in GR+/−or GR−/−pregnant females.[15] These observations reveal that knockout mouse models involving estrogen, progestagen and glucocorticoid systems are unsuitable for the study of parturition. The natural human model (fetuses suffering from aromatase deficiency) suggests that extremely high concentrations of estrogens in the third trimester are not necessary for maintenance of pregnancy and initiation of labor. To elucidate the function of estrogens, progesterone and glucocorticoid in parturition using the gene-targeting mice model, development of a novel tissue- and phase-specific gene-targeting strategy such as the Cre-loxP plus Tet-Off system should be mandatory.

Androgens

Androgens may also play an important role in parturition. Infusion of androstendione into pregnant rhesus monkeys increased uterine contractility, maternal plasma estradiol and oxytocin concentrations, as well as fibronectin in the amniotic fluid, and then induced preterm birth.[16] In humans, there were two reports of mothers with P450 aromatase deficiency and a mother with congenital adrenal hyperplasia caused by mutant P450 oxidoreductase. In both studies, the mothers suffered from virilization with hyperandrogenism in their antenatal periods.[7,17] However, these mothers did not experience preterm birth. Therefore, excess of circulating androgens, the high levels of which caused virilization in adult women, might have no effect on human parturition. The most potent form of androgens is dehydrotestosterone, which is converted from testosterone by steroid 5α-reductases. There are two isoforms of the enzyme, type 1 and type 2. Steroid 5α-reductase type 2 mutation in humans and mice causes male pseudohermaphroditism, characterized by normal internal genitalia but with external genitalia resembling those of the female. Steroid 5α-reductase type 1 knockout (5αR1-null) mice showed normal reproductive behavior in both male and female, and the female became pregnant normally. However, approximately 70% of pregnant 5αR1-null mice failed to undergo delivery at term.[18] These mutant mice showed normal luteal regression, withdrawal of circulating progesterone and normal uterine contractility to oxytocin and prostaglandin (PG) $F_{2\alpha}$. Administration of antiprogestin RU 486 or ovariectomy recovered parturition in 5αR1-null mice. Steroid 5α-reductase type 1 localized in the endometrial epithelium and cervical epithelium. Progesterone and 20α-hydoxyprogesterone concentrations in uterine tissue were higher in 5αR1-null mice at term of pregnancy. The cervix of 5αR1-null mice failed to ripen at term and relaxin administration prevented their parturition defect by enhancing cervical ripening.[19] These observations suggest that parturition defect in 5αR1-null mice was caused by local aberrant progesterone metabolism, rather than systemic androgen metabolism.

Peptide hormones

Corticotrpin-releasing hormone (CRH)

In primate and human pregnancy, the placenta produces a large amount of CRH. McLean *et al.*[20] reported that CRH may act as a 'placental clock', i.e. serum concentration of CRH could predict preterm birth or timing of labor in humans. CRH was shown to potentiate both oxytocin- and $PGF_{2\alpha}$-induced myometrial activity;[21,22] however, the actual function of CRH in the pregnant uterus is still unclear. In rodents, the placenta does not produce CRH. The CRH-deficient mouse might not be a good model for testing placental CRH function; however, it could still help to understand the function of the fetal hypothalamo–pituitary–adrenal axis at parturition, as Liggins suggested.[14] CRH −/− mice born from CRH +/− female mated with CRH +/− male grew normally and were fertile without glucocorticoid replacement. CRH −/− female mated with CRH −/− male delivered their pups between 19 and 20 days of gestation, although the authors did not compare the date with that of wild-type mothers. The CRH −/− pups born from CRH −/− dams died because of severe lung dysplasia, and maternal glucocorticoid substitution rescued the pups.[23] These observations indicated that both fetal and maternal hypothalamo–pituitary–adrenal axes do not play a crucial role in mouse parturition. However, maternal glucocorticoid administration helps fetal lung maturation similar to humans' clinical settings for the preterm baby.

Relaxin and its receptor

Relaxin is a polypeptide hormone composed of two amino-acid chains as a member of the insulin family. Relaxin has been believed to promote maturation of the uterine cervix at parturition. Recent meta-analysis of recombinant or porcine relaxin administration to pregnant women indicated that there was a reduction in the risk of the cervix remaining unfavorable or unchanged with induction, with relaxin administration. However, the cesarean rate was similar.[24] Relaxin-null mutant mice have been developed, and they were fully fertile. Some of the relaxin-null pregnant females had protracted labor, although the mean gestational period was similar to that of the wild type. Relaxin-null dams exhibited normal nursing behavior, and the pups could not suckle milk from the breast because of underdevelopment of the nipples.[25] In pregnant relaxin-null mice, decrease of collagen content was not observed in the nipples and vagina. Increase of water content in pubic symphysis was smaller than that observed in wild-type mice, suggesting that the female reproductive tract and nipples were harder than in the wild-type mice.[26] In relaxin-null mice, myometrial oxytocin receptor and ERa expressions in late pregnancy (day 18.5) were attenuated.[27] LGR7, which was at first cloned as an orphan receptor with structural homology to gonadotrophin and thyrotrophin receptors, was proved as a receptor for relaxin.[28] LGR7 knockout female mice exhibited normal fertility, but some of the pups (approximately 15%) died at parturition. Protracted delivery was also observed in LGR7-null mice. Length of the gestation period was similar to that of wild-type mice. Underdevelopment of the nipple was also observed.[29] On the whole, relaxin plays a role in the preparation for parturition, although it is not a critical factor for completion of birth.

Growth hormone receptor (GHR)

The GH/insulin-like growth factor 1 system exerts direct and indirect effects on gonadal function and the reproductive system. However, the phenotypes on parturition for GH-deficient patients are not well documented. In mice, female reproduction of GHR/GH binding protein-deficient (GHR-KO) mice was precisely investigated. GHR-KO mice had fewer numbers of ovulatory follicles and corpola lutea. When they became pregnant, GHR-KO mice conceived fewer pups, and the pups were smaller. On the other hand, their placentas were larger than those of wild-type mice. The date of parturition was delayed by 1 day; however, the mechanism of this delay was not characterized.[30,31]

Gonadotrophin receptors

There are two dominant gonadotrophin receptors, namely follicle-stimulating hormone receptor (FSHR) and luteinizing hormone/chorionic gonadotrophin receptor (LH/CGR). FSHR-null mice showed infertility due to hypoestrogenism. FSHR +/− mice revealed age-dependent reproductive deficits and developed unilateral uterine masses.[32] LH/CGR-null female mice showed a hypoplastic uterus and ovary. Follicular growth beyond the antral stage was arrested. Replacement therapy with estradiol and progesterone rescued the hypoplastic uterus completely, although female mice were infertile.[33] In humans, activation and inactivation mutants of FSHR and LHR were reported. Similar phenotypes to knockout mice were reported in both patients having inactivating FSHR and LH/CGR mutations.[34] It has been shown that LH/CGR is expressed in the human uterus. A very preliminary experiment suggests that administration of human CG to the patients of preterm labor might decrease the incidence of birth.[35] If the patients with LH/CGR inactivation mutation are conceived by oocyte donation–*in vitro* fertilization–embryo transfer program, the clinical course of their pregnancy could reveal the importance of uterine LH/CGR functions on maintenance of pregnancy and parturition.

Immunological system

There is an idea that parturition resembles 'rejection of conceptus as a semiallograft' from the mother. However, if maternal immune recognition were crucial for parturition, neither strained mice nor severe combined immunodeficiency mice would deliver their pups. Classical T-cell-mediated adapted immunity does not seem to play a significant role in preterm labor and term parturition in humans and mice, because the duration of gestation does not decrease in proportion to the number of previous deliveries. There are various reports suggesting the relation between physiological or pathological parturition and cytokines, chemokines, growth factors and their receptors. We suspect these phenomena reflect that the reproductive system may employ inflammation reaction for maternal adaptation or modulation to maintain pregnancy and/or parturition.

Interleukins (ILs)

IL-1 and its receptor

IL-1 is one of the central modulators of immune reaction/inflammation. Systemic administration of IL-1 can induce preterm birth in mice,[36] and pretreatment of IL-1 receptor antagonist prevents this IL-1-induced preterm labor.[37] Knockout model mice disrupting the IL-1 system (IL-1β-null mice,[38] IL-1β converting enzyme-null mice,[39] IL-1 type 1 receptor-null mice[40]) were fully fertile. In IL-1β type 1 receptor-null mice, litter size was significantly smaller than in wild-type mice.[41] Intracervical or intrauterine challenge of lipopolysaccharides or heat-killed *Ecshericia coli* is considered as a model for intrauterine infection. Preterm delivery could be induced in both IL-1β-null[42] and IL-1 type 1 receptor-null pregnant mice[43] by the intrauterine infection model. The challenge to delivery periods was similar to that observed in wild-type mice. Up-regulation of IL-1-induced cytokine/growth factors [IL-6, tumor necrosis factor (TNF) a, interferon (IFN) γ] and constitutive nuclear factor κB p65 protein expression were attenuated in IL-1β-null mice.[44] These data suggest that the intrauterine infection-induced preterm birth in the murine model does not require the maternal IL-1 signaling system.

Interleukin 6

IL-6 has numerous biologic activities, including induction of acute-phase proteins, regulation of hematopoiesis and terminal differentiation of B-cells. Various reports indicated the induction of IL-6 in chorioamnionitis/intrauterine infection, which causes preterm labor.[45,46] IL-6-null mice were fully fertile and there was no disturbance in parturition.[47] Signal transduction of IL-6 is mediated by the gp130 protein, a subunit signal transducer molecule of the dimeric IL-6 receptor and also a subunit of the receptors for leukemia inhibitory factor, oncostatin M, IL-11, ciliary neurotrophic factor and cardiotrophin 1. gp-130-null mice were lethal *in utero*, due to hypoplastic myocardium and impaired hematopoiesis.[48] Administration of exogenous IL-6 to wild-type pregnant mice did not lead to preterm birth. Intrauterine bacterial inoculation into IL-6-null pregnant mice induced preterm birth, at a rate similar to that in wild-type mice.[49] These observations revealed that IL-6 is neither necessary nor sufficient for the murine intrauterine infection preterm birth model.

Other interleukins and their receptors

IL-8 is considered to play an important role in cervical ripening before and during labor in the human uterus (reviewed by Kelly[50]). However, mice lacking IL-8 receptor homolog revealed a normal phenotype on their reproduction.[51] IL-2 receptor γ chain is shared for multiple cytokine receptors for IL-2, IL-4, IL-7, IL-9 and IL-15. Mice lacking the IL-2 receptor γ chain gene had an irregular estrous cycle; however, they were fertile. Interestingly, IL-2 receptor γ chain-null mice lacked uterine natural killer cells (uNK cells) on day 13 of gestation, but their parturition, litter size and body weight of offspring were similar to those of wild-type mice.[52] IL-15-null mice, which lack natural killer differentiation in lymphoid tissue, also had no uNK cells.[53] Their course of pregnancy and parturition was not disturbed. uNK cells are a major cellular component of decidua, and have been considered to play an important role in limiting normal trophoblast invasion and in immunological modulation of the fetal–maternal interface (e.g. reviewed by Croy *et al.*[54]). The course of pregnancy observed in uNK cells-deficient mice raised a big question about the functional significance of these cells.

IL-10 inhibits proliferation and cytokine synthesis in type 1 T-cells and can induce immunological non-responsiveness or anergy, acting preferably for Th1/Th2 balance hypothesis during pregnancy. However, IL-10-null mice conceived with larger numbers of implantation sites, heavier weight of pups and similar duration of gestation. There was no tendency to increase resorption of the fetus during pregnancy and preterm birth.[55]

TNF-α was implicated in the etiology of preterm birth. Amniotic fluid levels of TNF-α were elevated in patients with preterm labor or intrauterine infection. Recently, a relation between polymorphism in the promoter region of the TNF-α gene and preterm rupture of membrane[56] or bacterial vaginosis[57] has been reported. TNF-α-null mice were fully fertile.[58] There are two types of TNF receptors, and TNF receptor type 1-null mice showed early senescence and poor fertility, due to ovarian dysfunction.[59] However, these experimental models showed normal parturition process, although the number of pups was apparently smaller in TNF receptor type 1-null mice.[59]

Innate immune system

The innate immune system, which recognizes non-specific pathogen-derived molecules by toll-like receptors (TLRs), causes an inflammatory response including production of various cytokines and metalloproteinases. A unique target molecule for each TLR has been determined. For example, TLR-2 recognizes di- and tripalmitoylated peptides, TLR-3 recognizes double-strand RNAs, and TLR-4 recognizes the lipid-A component of lipopolysaccharides. Myeloid differentiation factor 88 (MyD88), the downstream adapter molecule, plays a crucial role in signal transduction from TLRs to inflammation reaction. These molecules are expressed in the placenta,[60] and one genetic polymorphism for TLR-4 (Asp 299 Gly) resulting in decreased receptor function may associate with a predisposition to preterm birth in humans.[61] Various knockout mice had already established for TLRs and MyD88, and all of them were healthy and fertile (reviewed by Kaisho and Akira[62]). Knockout mice of the molecules related to the innate immune system might provide useful models with which to analyze susceptibility to preterm birth resulting from infection.

Molecules stimulate/modulate uterine contractility

Oxytocin and its receptor

Oxytocin is one of the most potent uterotonic agents identified and is widely used in routine clinical settings for augmentation and induction of labor. Oxytocin has also been considered essential for milk let-down during lactation. Oxytocin is synthesized not only in the hypothalamic paraventricular and supraoptic nuclei, but also in the pregnant uterine endometrium[63] and fetal membrane.[64] As the oxytocin receptor up-regulation is observed in term myometrium[65] as well as in term deciduas,[66] oxytocin may act by both endocrine and paracrine manner to promote labor. Oxytocin-null mice were produced[67,68] and they were fully fertile and able to deliver litters at term. Their milk ejection reflex was severely disturbed, leading to the death of the pups by starvation. If the pups had been nursing, they would have survived. It was speculated that endogenous Arg^8-vasopressin compensated the oxytocin action, because the dissociation constants of Arg^8-vasopressin and oxytocin to oxytocin receptor are similar. However, the physiological responsiveness of oxytocin receptor to Arg^8-vasopressin was 1/10–1/100 of the oxytocin responses,[69,70] meaning that a pharmacological dose of vasopressin is required to induce physiological uterine contraction. Therefore, this hypothesis is unlikely. Oxytocin-null male mice showed social amnesia (less developed social memory) and aggression,[71,72] although their sexual behavior appeared to be normal.

In mice, initiation of labor is primarily determined by luteolysis, and corpus luteum expresses the oxytocin receptor. Continuous infusion of oxytocin to wild-type or oxytocin-null mice revealed that oxytocin can either delay labor at low doses or initiate preterm labor at high doses. A low dose of oxytocin prevented luteolysis and retarded progesterone withdrawal. The dose required to prevent luteolysis was lower in oxytocin-null mice than in wild-type mice, probably due to up-regulation of the oxytocin receptor in corpus luteum of oxytocin-null mice.[73] In wild-type and oxytocin-null mice, contrary to the up-regulation of the oxytocin receptor in term myometriun, the receptor in corpus luteum was down-regulated at term of pregnancy, which led to luteolysis and initiation of labor. The substances that compensate contractile activity of oxytocin should be further elucidated.

There was a report that the oxytocin receptor knockout mice were lethal (personal communication).[74] However, Nishimori's group successfully developed oxytocin receptor-null mice, and their phenotype on parturition appeared to be similar to that of oxytocin-null mice (Takayanagi *et al.*,[74a] in preparation). Further investigations of their phenotype with regard to reproduction, parturition and behavior are ongoing.

PGs and their receptors

PGs are synthesized from arachidonic acid, which is mainly released from cell membrane phospholipids by the activity of cytosolic phosholipase A_2. The arachidonic acid is then converted to PGH_2, which is the precursor for other PGs, prostacyclin (PGI_2) and thromboxane (TX) A_2, via the action of cyclooxygenase (COX) 1 or COX-2. Then, specific PG isomerases/synthetases convert PGH_2 to the specific forms. PGs are widely synthesized and distributed in the body. Particularly around parturition, they are synthesized and secreted from the placenta, fetal membrane and uterine myometrium. Numerous reports have indicated an up-regulation of PGE_2 and $PGF_{2\alpha}$ (or other PGs) and modulation of their receptors around parturition (reviewed by Olson *et al.*[74]).

Cytosolic phospholipase A_2-α ($cPLA_2$-α)

$cPLA_2$-α preferentially hydrolyses fatty acids and lysophosholipids to provide precursors for PGs and platelet activating factor. $cPLA_2$-α-null females could not deliver between day 18.5 and day 20.5; instead, they delivered a smaller number of live pups at days 21.5–22.5, and the offspring did not survive.[75,76] Cesarian section at term was able to yield viable neonates. Administration of a progesterone antagonist RU486 was able to rescue parturition defect of $cPLA_2$-α-null mice and restore the pups' viability. These observations suggest that the parturition defect of $cPLA_2$-α-null mice was caused mainly by the defect of luteal regression, rather than by the shortage of PGs as uterine-stimulating substrates.

Cyclooxygenases

COX-1 carries out 'house keeping' functions such as cytoprotection of stomach mucosa, platelet aggregation and regulation of blood flow. COX-1 is expressed in many cell types and, in general, it shows constitutive activity. COX-1-null female mice showed normal fertility, but their parturition was delayed, leading to neonatal death. Bolus administration of $PGF_{2\alpha}$ at day 19.5 resulted in labor within 24 h and restored the pups' viability.[77] In wild-type mice, they showed up-regulation of COX-1 and oxytocin receptor in the uterus near term of pregnancy, and induction of both molecules was diminished in COX-1-null mice. Double knockout of COX-1 and oxytocin restored their parturition at term.[77] This observation supported the idea that oxytocin acts as a luteosupportive factor to corpus luteum in pregnant mice.[73] Uterine $PGF_{2\alpha}$ production at term was impaired in both COX-1-null and COX-1/oxytocin-null mice, and uterine $PGF_{2\alpha}$ concentrations were very low in both types of mice. It is very interesting to know which molecule compensates the uterotonic function after luteolysis, with a smaller amount of $PGF_{2\alpha}$ and without oxytocin in COX-1/oxytocin-null mice.

COX-2-null mice showed severe renal pathology (dysplasia) and female infertility.[78,79] The uterus of COX-2-null mice could not decidualize after typical pseudopregnant stimuli, and showed implantation failure when wild-type fertilized eggs were transferred.[80] Pharmacological inhibition of COX-2 by selective COX-2 inhibitor (celecoxib) in COX-1-null mice induced complete implantation failure, suggesting that COX-2 is necessary for preparation of uterine receptivity.[81] The actual function of COX-2 in murine parturition cannot be analyzed by gene-targeting models. Administration of lipopolysaccharides induced preterm birth in COX-1-null mice, with induction of COX-2 messenger RNA (mRNA) and $PGF_{2\alpha}$ in the uterus. Selective COX-2 inhibitor was more potent to inhibit lipopolysaccharide-induced preterm birth than selective COX-1 inhibitor. These pharmacological studies using COX-1-null mice suggested that COX-2 plays a pivotal role when preterm birth is induced by infection.[82]

Membrane prostaglandin receptors

After the first molecular cloning of the receptor for TXA_2, the receptors for prostaglandin prostanoids have been cloned by homology screening. They are classified as the G-protein-linked rhodopsin receptor family with seven transmembrane domains (reviewed by Nasumiya *et al.*[83]). Specific receptors for PGD_2, TXA_2, PGI_2, PGE_2 and $PGF_{2\alpha}$ have been cloned and are referred to as DP, TP, IP, EP and FP, respectively. There are four subtypes for EP (EP1–EP4). Several isoforms of EP1, EP3, FP and TP have also been reported. $PGF_{2\alpha}$ action is mediated by FP, which is coupled with G-protein, leading to the increase of intracellular calcium $[Ca^{2+}]_i$ concentration and stimulation of myometrial contraction. The action of PGE_2 is more complex. Activation of EP1, EP3A and EP3D leads to elevation of $[Ca^{2+}]_I$, whereas EP2 and EP4 activate adenylate cyclase, which leads to myometrial relaxation. In the myometrium, it has been reported that there is up-regulation of EP2 and suppression of FP during pregnancy[84] and increase of FP, EP3 and suppression of EP2[85] at the onset of labor. As cyclic adenosine monophosphate induces uterine muscle relaxation and elevation of $[Ca^{2+}]_i$ activates the uterus, these observations are reasonable for maintenance of uterine quiescence and stimulation of parturition during the course of pregnancy.

Mice lacking EP1, EP2 and EP3 genes are healthy and fertile. In EP3-null mice, febrile response induced by IL-1β was attenuated.[86] Most of the EP4-null mice died due to a persistent ductus arteriosus. Less than 5% of the EP4-null mice survived and they were fertile.[87,88] No authors have mentioned precisely the course of parturition of EP-deficient mice.

In contrast, mice lacking FP gene were fertile, but females could not deliver pups at term. This prolonged pregnancy caused degeneration of the placenta and intrauterine fetal death. By cesarian section, the fetus could be rescued; however, administration of $PGF_{2\alpha}$ or oxytocin at term was not effective to induce labor. Up-regulation of the oxytocin receptor in the uterus at term was abolished. Oophorectomy on day 19 recovered the parturition process of FP-null mice, and they delivered pups normally. Oophorectomy also restored the oxytocin receptor up-regulation in the pregnant uterus at term.[89] In FP-null nice, induction of COX-2 in the uterus on day 20 was totally abolished. On the other hand, COX-1 in the uterus was up-regulated on day 17 and decreased at the time of parturition in wild-type mice; however, this decline of COX-1 level was also disturbed in FP-null mice. Induction of uterine connexin (Cx) 43 mRNA was abolished in FP-null mice. After oophorectomy on day 19, COX-2 up-regulation, COX-1 down-regulation and Cx43 up-regulation at the time of spontaneous labor normalized to the wild-type level. Administration of exogenous progesterone after oophrectomy in FP-null mice inhibited parturition. Treatment of FP-null mice with COX-non-selective or COX-2 selective inhibitors after oophrectomy also prolonged the time from oophrectomy to delivery.[90,91] These findings suggest that progesterone withdrawal is the critical factor to determine the onset of mouse parturition, and COX-2-derived prostaglandins compensate the uterine stimulative activity, although there is no FP in the myometrium.

Nuclear prostaglandin receptors

Recently, the existence of specific prostaglandin transporters, which mediate influx of PGs into the cells, has been demonstrated. Moreover, trafficking of COX-2 to nuclear envelope was also determined. These data suggest the existence of specific nuclear receptors for PGs (reviewed by Helliwell *et al.*[92]). Peroxisome proliferator activated receptors (PPARs) are putative targets for the nuclear action of PGs and other eicosanoids.

It has been shown that PPARγ preferentially binds to 15d-PGJ_2, the final metabolites of PGD2. As human gestational tissues contain PGD synthases and PGD_2 in amniotic fluid,[93] the function of PPARγ in the pregnant uterus is of great interest. PPARγ is also considered as a target molecule of thiazolidinedione drugs, which are widely used as insulin sensitizers. PPARγ-null mice were lethal *in utero*, due to defects in placental vascularization.[94] Using Cre-loxP recombination system, conditional PPARγ knockout mice were obtained. Female mice, in which the PPARγ gene was conditionally deleted in epithelial cells, T- and B-cells and ovary cells, showed impaired fertility with smaller litter size. In this mouse strain, uterine PPARγ was intact and parturition was not disturbed.[95]

PPARδ-null mice also showed high (approximately 90%) embryonic lethality. The connections between placenta and decidua were abnormally loose. The labyrinth was smaller; however, the vascular structure was fully developed, different from the placentas observed in PPARγ-null mice.[96] PGI_2 was considered as a mediator for embryo implantation,[97] and PGI_2 is revealed as one of the natural ligands for PPARδ.[98] In contrast to these observations, surviving PPARδ-null mice were generally healthy and fertile, albeit they displayed more than a 60% reduction in adipose mass. PPARα-null mice showed normal fertility.[99] Taken together, PPARs (especially PPARγ and PPARδ) play an important role during placentation. Their function in parturition has not been determined from knockout mice models, although several of their natural ligands (various eicosanoids and unsaturated fatty acids) were detected in gestational tissues during pregnancy.

Connexins

Cxs are the protein subunits of intracellular gap junction channels. In mammals, there are at least 15 Cx family genes. Among them, Cx43 is up-regulated in pregnant myometrium at term and this induction is considered to ensure the coordinate contraction of uterine smooth muscle during labor to produce expulsive force effectively. Mice lacking Cx43 died postnatally because of congenital obstruction of the right ventricular outflow.[100] Another subtype of Cxs, Cx32 or Cx40 genes, were 'knocked in' into the Cx43-null mice to elucidate the functional specificity of Cxs. Both Cx43-null heterozygous Cx32 and heterozygous Cx40 knock-in mice (−/Cx32 and −/Cx40, respectively) could deliver their pups, suggesting that these molecules are possibly compatible in uterine function at parturition. Cx43-null heterozygous Cx32 knock-in dams failed to nurse their pups, due to impairment of milk ejection.[101] These model mice could not indicate the necessity of gap junction in term myometrium for regulation of uterine contraction.

Ion channels

Ion channels are necessary for proper electrophysiological responses of the excitatory organs (nerves, muscles, etc.); however, few reports are available about their gene-targeting model and reproduction. SK channels are potassium selective, voltage independent and activated by increases of $[Ca^{2+}]_i$, which occur during an action potential and induce repolarization of membrane potential. There are three subtypes of SK channels. A tetracyclin-based genetic switch sequence was introduced into the 5′-flanking of mouse SK3 gene. Administration of doxycyclin to the mouse abolished the SK3 gene transcription effectively. On the other hand, homozygous mutant shows over-expression of SK3 gene and protein (approximately threefold). The phenotype after down-regulation by doxycyclin was almost negligible. On the other hand, the homozygous female showed protracted labor and the majority (7/10) of the pups died during parturition *in utero*. In adult mice, the respiratory response during hypoxic attack was abnormal; they could not increase their respiratory rate and apnea occurred. Doxycyclin administration, which abolished the SK3 expression, rescued these phenotypes.[102] Overexpression of Ca^{2+}-activated K^+ channel affected the uterine contractility most severely at parturition.

Nitric oxide synthases (NOS)

Nitric oxide may play an important role in the regulation of myometrial relaxation and cervical ripening. Three major isoforms of NOS, viz. neuronal NOS (nNOS), endothelial NOS (eNOS) and inducible NOS (iNOS), are expressed in the non-pregnant and the pregnant uterus. Knockout mice of these three NOSs were reported to be fertile and there were no abnormalities on their parturition.[103–105] Calcitonin gene-related peptide (CGRP) inhibits the contractile activities of smooth muscles. CGRP-induced vascular smooth muscle relaxation was mediated by nitric oxide. CGRP also inhibited KCl-induced contraction in uterine myometrium. However, this inhibition was observed in all nNOS-null, eNOS-null and iNOS-null mice models equivalently to the wild-type mouse.[106] These observations suggest that the nitric oxide–NOS system may not be necessary to ensure myometrial relaxation during pregnancy, although there is a possibility that the another type of NOS could compensate the function of the targeted NOS.

Conclusion

Since our first review of the knockout mouse model and parturition,[107] various gene-targeting model mice have been produced. Especially after finishing the human genome project in 2002 and the near completion of the mouse genome project, knockout mice are the ultimate strategy to investigate genes of unknown functions. All of the observations listed here and in other reviews[108,109] indicate that a few deficient genes, which are conventionally considered as a very important factor to regulate parturition, successfully disturbed their parturition. Moreover, in most of the knockout mice whose parturition was intruded, the process of luteolysis rather than the uterotrophic or uterotonic action was actually impaired (Figure 54.2). Gene targeting of the endocrine system often resulted in infertility, because of the hypoplastic reproductive system. Most of the gene-targeting mice related to the immune system and the substrates related to uterine contraction could successfully deliver their pups. Conventional uterotonic pathways such as oxytocin and the prostaglandin system could be preserved by redundant manner except for the function of the targeted molecule concerned with luteolysis. Some interesting knowledge could be obtained from human diseases from gene mutations, such as fetal aromatase deficiency. We clinicians should observe precisely the course of pregnancy and parturition in patients who are suffering from genetic disorders, even when they showed normal sequence.

For the future, an unexpected phenotype can be obtained from double- or triple-gene knockout mice. A good example was reported by Embree-Ku and Boekelheide,[110] indicating that absence both of p53 and FasL genes in female mice led to dystocia. Further analysis should be done to determine the unexpected pathway from these apoptosis-related genes to uterine contraction at parturition. Using the available resources of knockout model mice, we could further analyze the mechanism of parturition with some physiological and/or pharmacological manipulation. We also expect to find novel strategies against preterm birth through these experimental models, which is still a leading cause of mortality and morbidity of the infant.

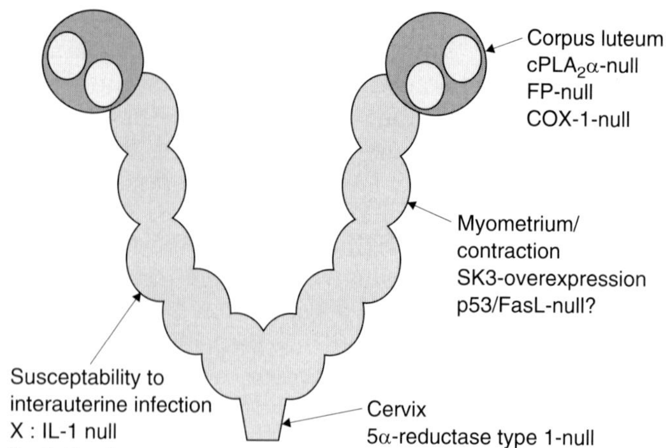

Figure 54.2 Summary of gene-targeted mice whose phenotype is affected on parturition. Note that most of the target points of knockout mice were corpus luteum: the failure of luteolysis. The relationship between deficiency of the immunological system and susceptibility to infection-induced preterm birth is of great interest; however, only negative data are available.

Acknowledgments

We thank Ms. Naoko Hagino for excellent secretarial help. This work was supported in part by grants-in-aid for scientific research (Nos. 14571557, 15390505, 15591746 and 16390476) from the Ministry of Education, Science and Culture of Japan (Tokyo, Japan).

REFERENCES

1. Cunningham FG, Gant NF, Leveno KJ, Gilstrap LC III, Hauth JC, Wenstrom KD, eds. *Williams Obstetrics*, 21st edn. New York: McGraw-Hill, 2001:251–307.
2. Shozu M, Akasofu K, Harada T, Kobota Y. A new cause of female psudohermaphroditism: Placental aromatase deficiency. *J Clin Endocrinol Metab* 1991;72:560–6.
3. Ito Y, Fisher CR, Conte FA, Grumbach MM, Simpson ER. Molecular bases of aromatase deficiency in adult female with sexual infantism and polycystic ovaries. *Proc Natl Acad Sci USA* 1993;90:11673–7.
4. Conte FA, Grumbach MM, Ito Y, Fisher CR, Simpson ER. A syndrome of female pseudohermaphrodism, hypergonadotropic hypogonadism, and a multycystic ovaries associated with missence mutations in the gene encoding aromatase (P450arom). *J Clin Endocrinol Metab* 1994;78:1287–92.
5. Morishima A, Grumbach MM, Simpson ER, Fisher C, Qin K. Aromatase deficiency in male and female siblings caused by a novel mutation and the physiological role of estrogens. *J Clin Endocrinol Metab* 1995;80:3689–98.
6. Carani C, Qin K, Simoni M, *et al.* Effect of testosterone and estradiol in a man with aromatase deficiency. *N Engl J Med* 1997;337:91–5.
7. Deladoey J, Fluck C, Bex M, Yoshimura N, Harada N, Mullis PE. Aromatase deficiency caused by a novel P450arom mutation: Impact of absent estrogen production on serum gonadotropin concentration in a boy. *J Clin Endocrinol Metab* 1999;84:4050–4.
8. Fisher CR, Graves KH, Parlow AF, Simpson ER. Characterization of mice deficient in aromatase (ArKO) because of targeted disruption of the *cyp 19* gene. *Proc Natl Acad Sci USA* 1998;95:6965–70.
9. Lubahn DB, Moyer JS, Golding TS, Course JF, Korach KS, Smithies O. Alteration of reproductive functions but not prenatal sexual development after insertional disruption of mouse estrogen receptor gene. *Proc Natl Acad Sci USA* 1993;90:11162–6.
10. Curtis SW, Hewitt S, Goulding EH, Eddy EM, Korach KS. Studies using the estrogen receptor alpha knockout uterus demonstrate that implantation but not decidualization-associated signaling is estrogen dependent. *Biol Reprod* 2002;67:1268–77.
11. Krege JH, Hodgin JB, Couse JF, *et al.* Generation and reproductive phenotypes of mice lacking estrogen receptor-β. *Proc Natl Acad Sci USA* 1998;95:15677–82.
12. Lydon JP, MeMayo FJ, Funk CR, *et al.* Mice lacking progesterone receptor exhibit pleiotropic reproductive abnormalities. *Genes Dev* 1995;9:2266–78.
13. Mulac-Jericevic B, Lydon JP, DeMayo FJ, Conneely OM. Defective mammary gland morphogenesis in mice lacking the progesterone receptor B isoform. *Proc Natl Acad Sci USA* 2003;100:9744–9.
14. Liggins GC. Premature parturition after infusion of corticotrophin or cortisol into fetal lambs. *J Endocrinol* 1968;42:323–9.
15. Cole TJ, Blendy JA, Monaghan P, *et al.* Targeted disruption of the glucocorticoid receptor gene blocks adrenergic chromaffin cell development and severely retards lung maturation. *Genes Dev* 1995;9:1608–21.
16. Mecenas CA, Giussani DA, Owiny JR, *et al.* Production of premature delivery in pregnant rhesus monkeys by androstendione infusion. *Nat Med* 1996;2:443–8.
17. Arlt W, Walker EA, Draper N, *et al.* Congenital adrenal hyperplasia caused by mutant P450 oxidoreductase and human androgen synthesis: Analytical study. *Lancet* 2004;363:2128–35.
18. Mahendroo MS, Cala KM, Russell DW. 5a-reduced androgens play a key role in murine parturition. *Mol Endocrinol* 1996; 10:380–92.
19. Mahendroo MS, Porter A, Russell DW, Word RA. The parturition defect in steroid 5a-reductase type 1 knockout mice is due to impaired cervical ripening. *Mol Endocrinol* 1999;13:981–92.
20. McLean M, Bistis A, Davies J, Woods R, Lowry P, Smith R. A placental clock controlling the length of human pregnancy. *Nat Med* 1995;1:460–3.
21. Quartero HW, Noort WA, Fry CH, Keirse MJ. Role of prostaglandins and leukotriens in the synergistic effect of oxytocin and corticotropin-releasing hormone (CRH) on contraction force in human gestational myometrium. *Prostaglandins* 1991;42:137–50.
22. Benedetto C, Petraglia F, Maroziol L, *et al.* Corticotropin releasing hormone increases prostaglandin F2 alpha activity on human myometrium in vitro. *Am J Obstet Gynecol* 1994;171:126–31.
23. Muglia L, Jacobson L, Dikkes P, Majzoub JA. Corticotropin-releasing hormone deficiency reveals major fetal but not adult glucocorticoid need. *Nature* 1995;373:427–32.
24. Kelly AJ, Kavanagh J, Thomas J. Relaxin for cervical ripening and induction of labour. *Cochrane Database Syst Rev* 2001: CD003103.
25. Zhao L, Roche PJ, Gunnersen JM, *et al.* Mice without a functional relaxin gene are unable to deliver milk to their pups. *Endocrinology* 1999;140:445–53.
26. Zhao L, Samuel CS, Tregear GW, B1ck F, Wintour EM. Collagen studies in late pregnant relaxin null mice. *Biol Reprod* 2000;63: 697–703.
27. Siebel AL, Gehring HM, Reytomas IGT, Parry LJ. Inhibition of oxytocin receptor and estrogen receptor-a expression, but not relaxin receptors (LGR7), in the myometrium of late pregnant relaxin gene knockout mice. *Endocrinology* 2003;144:4272–5.
28. Hsu SY, Nakabayashi K, Nishi S, *et al.* Activation of orphan receptors by the hormone relaxin. *Science* 2002;295:671–4.
29. Krajnc-Franken MAM, van Disseldorp AdJM, Koenders JE, Mosselman S, van Duin M, Gossen JA. Impaired nipple development and parturition in LGR7 knockout mice. *Mol Cell Biol* 2004;24:687–96.
30. Danilovich N, Wernsing D, Coschigano KT, Kopchick II, Bartke A. Deficiencies in female reproductive function in GH-R-KO mice; role of IGF-I. *Endocrinology* 1999;140:2637–40.
31. Zaczek D, Hammond J, Suen L, *et al.* Impact of growth hormone resistance on female reproductive function: New insights from growth hormone receptor knockout mice. *Biol Reprod* 2002;67: 1115–24.
32. Danilovich N, Roy I, Sairam MR. Emergence of uterine pathology during accelerated biological aging in FSH receptor-haploinsufficient mice. *Endocrinology* 2002;143:3618–27.
33. Lei ZM, Mishra S, Zou W, *et al.* Targeted disruption of luteinizing hormone/human chorionic gonadotropin receptor gene. *Mol Endocrinol* 2001;15:184–200.
34. Arnhold IJP, Latronico AC, Batista MC, Mendonca BB. Menstrual disorders and infertility caused by inactivating mutations of the luteinizing hormone receptor gene. *Fertil Steril* 1999;71: 597–601.
35. Toth P, Lukacs H, Gimes G, *et al.* Clinical importance of vascular LH/hCG receptors – A review. *Reprod Biol* 2001;1:5–11.
36. Romero R, Mazor M, Tartakovsky B. Systemic administration of interleukin-1 induces preterm parturition in mice. *Am J Obstet Gynecol* 1991;165:969–71.
37. Romero R, Tarakovsky B. The natural interleukin 1 receptor antagonist prevents interleukin-1-induced preterm delivery in mice. *Am J Obstet Gynecol* 1992;167:1041–5.
38. Zheng H, Fletcher D, Kozak W, *et al.* Resistance to fever induction and impaired acute-phase response in interleukin-1β deficient mice. *Immunity* 1995;3:9–19.
39. Li P, Allen H, Banerjee S, *et al.* Mice deficient in IL-1β-converting enzyme are defective in production of mature IL-1β and resistant to endotoxin shock. *Cell* 1995;80:401–11.
40. Leon LR, Conn CA, Glaccum M, Kluger MJ. IL-1 type 1 receptor mediates acute phase response to turpentine, but not lipopolysaccharide, in mice. *Am J Physiol* 1996;271:R1668–75.
41. Abbondanzo SJ, Cullinan EB, McIntyre K, Labow MA, Stewart CL. Reproduction in mice lacking a functional type 1 IL-1 receptor. *Endocrinology* 1996;137:3598–601.
42. Reznikov LL, Fantuzzi G, Selzman CH, *et al.* Utilization of endoscopic inoculation in a mouse model of intrauterine infection-induced preterm birth: Role of interleukin 1 beta. *Biol Reprod* 1999;60:1231–8.
43. Hirsch E, Muhle RA, Mussalli GM, Blanchard R. Bacterially induced preterm labor in the mouse does not require maternal interleukin-1 signaling. *Am J Obstet Gynecol* 2002;186:523–30.
44. Reznikov LL, Shames BD, Barton HA, *et al.* Interleukin-1beta deficiency results in reduced NF-kappaB levels in pregnant mice. *Am J Physiol Regul Integr Comp Physiol* 2000;278:R263–70.
45. Matsuzaki N, Taniguchi T, Shimoya K, *et al.* Placental interleukin-6 production is enhanced in intrauterine infection but not in labor. *Am J Obstet Gynecol* 1993;168:94–7.
46. Hillier SL, Witkin SS, Krohn MA, Watts DH, Kiviat NB, Eschenbach DA. The relationship of amniotic fluid cytokines and

preterm delivery, amniotic fluid infection, histologic chorioamnionitis, and chorioamnion infection. *Obstet Gynecol* 1993;81:941–8.

47. Poli V, Balena R, Fattori E, *et al.* Interleukin-6 deficient mice are protected from bone loss caused by estrogen depletion. *EMBO J* 1994;13:1189–96.
48. Yoshida K, Taga T, Saito M, *et al.* Targeted disruption of gp 130, a common signal transducer for the interleukin 6 family of cytokines, leads to myocardial and hematological disorders. *Proc Natl Acad Sci USA* 1996;93:407–11.
49. Yoshimura K, Hirsch E. Interleukin-6 is neither necessary nor sufficient for preterm labor in a murine infection model. *J Soc Gynecol Investig* 2003;10:423–7.
50. Kelly RW. Inflammatory mediators and cervical ripening. *J Reprod Immunol* 2002;57:217–24.
51. Cacalano G, Lee J, Kikly K, *et al.* Neutrophil and B cell expansion in mice that lack the murine IL-8 receptor homolog. *Science* 1994;265:682–4.
52. Miyazaki S, Tanebe K, Sakai M, *et al.* Interleukin 2 receptor gamma chain (γc) knockout mice show less regularity in estrous cycle but achieve normal pregnancy without fetal compromise. *Am J Reprod Immunol* 2002;47:222–30.
53. Ashkar AA, Black GP, Wei Q, *et al.* Assessment of requirements for IL-15 and IFN regulatory factors in uterine NK cell differentiation and function during pregnancy. *J Immunol* 2003;171:2937–44.
54. Croy BA, He H, Esadeg S, *et al.* Uterine natural killer cells: Insights into their cellular and molecular biology from mouse modeling. *Reproduction* 2003;126:149–60.
55. White CA, Johansson M, Roberts CT, Ramsay AJ, Robertson SA. Effect of interleukin-10 null mutation on maternal immune response and reproductive outcome in mice. *Biol Reprod* 2004;70:123–31.
56. Roberts AK, Monzon-Bordonaba F, van Deerlin PG, *et al.* Association of polymorphism within the promoter of the tumor necrosis factor alpha gene with increased risk of preterm rupture of the fetal membranes. *Am J Obstet Gynecol* 1999;180:1297–302.
57. Macones GA, Parry S, Elkousy M, Clothier B, Ural SH, Strauss JF III. A polymorphism in the promoter region of TNF and bacterial vaginosis: Preliminary evidence of gene–environment interaction in the etiology of spontaneous preterm birth. *Am J Obstet Gynecol* 2004;190:1504–8.
58. Pasparkis M, Alexopoulou L, Episkopou V, Kollias G. Immune and inflammatory responses in TNFa-deficient mice: A critical requirement for TNFa in the formation of primary B cell follicles, follicular dendritic cell networks and germinal centers, and in the maturation of the humoral immune response. *J Exp Med* 1996;184:1397–411.
59. Roby KF, Son D-S, Terranova PF. Alterations of events related to ovarian function in tumor necrosis factor receptor type I knockout mice. *Biol Reprod* 1999;61:1616–21.
60. Homlund U, Cebers G, Dahlfors AR, *et al.* Expression and regulation of the pattern recognition receptors toll-like receptor-2 and toll-like receptor-4 in the human placenta. *Immunology* 2002;107:145–51.
61. Lorenz E, Hallman M, Marttila R, Haataja R, Schwartz D. Association between the Asp299Gly polymorphisms in the toll-like receptor 4 and premature births in the Finnish population. *Pediatr Res* 2002;52:373–6.
62. Kaisho T, Akira S. Dendritic-cell function in toll-like receptor- and MyD88-knockout mice. *Trends Immunol* 2001;22:78–83.
63. Lefebvre DL, Giaid A, Bennett H, Lariviere R, Zing HH. Oxytocin gene expression in rat uterus. *Science* 1992;256:1553–5.
64. Chibbar R, Miller FD, Mitchell BF. Synthesis of oxytocin in amnion, chorion, and decidua may influence the timing of human parturition. *J Clin Invest* 1993;91:185–92.
65. Kimura T, Takemura M, Nomura S, *et al.* Expression of oxytocin receptor in human pregnant myometrium. *Endocrinology* 1996;137:780–5.
66. Takemura M, Kimura T, Nomura S, *et al.* Expression and localization of human oxytocin receptor mRNA and its protein in chorion and decidua during parturition. *J Clin Invest* 1994;93:2319–23.
67. Nishimori K, Young LJ, Guo Q, Wang Z, Insel TR, Matzul MM. Oxytocin is required for nursing but is not essential for parturition or reproductive behavior. *Proc Natl Acad Sci USA* 1996;93:11699–704.
68. Young WS III, Shepard E, Amico J, *et al.* Deficiency in mouse oxytocin prevents milk ejection, but not fertility or parturition. *J Neuroendocrinol* 1996;8:847–53.
69. Kimura T, Makino Y, Saji F, et al. Molecular characterization of a cloned human oxytocin receptor. *Eur J Endocrinol* 1994;131:385–90.
70. Kawamata M, Mitsui-Saito M, Kimura T, Takayanagi Y, Yanagisawa T, Nishimori K. Vasopressin-induced contraction of uterus is mediated solely by the oxytocin receptor in mouse, but not in human. *Eur J Pharmacol* 2003;472:229–34.
71. Ferguson JN, Young LJ, Hearn EF, Matzuk MM, Insel TR, Winslow JT. Social amnesia in mice lacking the oxytocin gene. *Nat Genet* 2000;25:284–8.
72. Winslow JT, Hearn EF, Gerguson J, Young LJ, Matzuk MM, Insel TR. Infant vocalization, adult aggression, and fear behavior of an oxytocin null mutant mice. *Horm Behav* 2000;37:145–55.
73. Imamura T, Luedke CE, Vogt SK, Muglia LJ. Oxytocin modulates the onset of murine parturition by competing ovarian and uterine effects. *Am J Physiol Regul Integr Comp Physiol* 2000;279:R1061–7.
74. Olson DM, Zaragoza DB, Shallow MC, *et al.* Myometrial activation and preterm labour: Evidence supporting a role for the prostaglandin F receptor – A review. *Placenta* 2003;24:S47–54.
74a. Takayanagi Y, Yoshida M, Bielsky IF, et al. Pervasive social deficits, but normal parturition, in oxytocin receptor–deficient mice. *Proc Natl Acad Sci USA* 2005;102:16096–101.
75. Bonventre JV, Huang Z, Reza Taheri M, *et al.* Reduced fertility and postischaemic brain injury in mice deficient in cytosolic phospholipase A2. *Nature* 1997;390:622–5.
76. Uozumi N, Kume K, Nagase T, *et al.* Role of cytosolic phspholipase A2 in allergic response and parturition. *Nature* 1997;390:618–21.
77. Gross GA, Imamura T, Luedke C, *et al.* Opposing action of prostaglandins and oxytocin determine the onset of murine labor. *Proc Natl Acad Sci USA* 1998;95:11875–9.
78. Dinchuk JE, Car BD, Focht RJ, *et al.* Renal abnormalities and an altered inflammatory response in mice lacking cyclooxygenase II. *Nature* 1995;378:406–9.
79. Morham SG, Langenbach R, Loftin CD, *et al.* Prostaglandin synthetase 2 gene disruption causes severe renal pathology in the mouse. *Cell* 1995;83:473–82.
80. Lim H, Paria BC, Das SK, *et al.* Multiple female reproductive failures in cyclooxygenase 2-deficient mice. *Cell* 1997;91:197–208.
81. Reese J, Zhao X, Ma WG, Brown N, Maziasz TJ, Dey SK. Comparative analysis of pharmacologic and/or genetic disruption of cyclooxygenase-1 and cyclooxygenase-2 function in female reproduction in mice. *Endocrinology* 2001;142:3198–206.
82. Gross G, Imamura T, Vogt SK, *et al.* Inhibition of cyclooxygenase-2 prevents inflammation-mediated preterm labor in the mice. *Am J Physiol Regul Integr Comp Physiol* 2000;278:R1415–23.
83. Nasumiya S, Sugimoto Y, Ushikubi F. Prostanoid receptors: Structures, properties, and functions. *Physiol Rev* 1999;79:1193–226.
84. Matsumoto T, Sagawa N, Yoshida M, *et al.* The prostaglandin E2 and F2 alpha receptor genes are expressed in human myometrium and are down-regulated during pregnancy. *Biochem Biophys Res Commun* 1997;238:838–41.
85. Brodt-Eppley J, Myatt L. Changes in expression of contractile FP and relaxatory EP2 receptors in pregnant rat myometrium during late gestation, at labor, and postpartum. *Biol Reprod* 1998;59:878–83.
86. Ushikubi F, Segi E, Sugimoto Y, *et al.* Impaired febrile response in mice lacking the prostaglandin receptor subtype EP3. *Nature* 1998;395:281–4.
87. Nguyen MT, Camenisch T, Snouwaert JN, *et al.* The prostaglandin receptor EF4 triggers remodeling of the cardiovascular system at birth. *Nature* 1997;390:78–81.
88. Segi E, Sugimoto Y, Yamasaki A, *et al.* Patient ductus arteriosus and neonatal death in prostaglandin receptor EP4-deficient mice. *Biochem Biophys Res Commun* 1998;246:7–12.
89. Sugimoto Y, Yamasaki A, Segi E, *et al.* Failure of parturition in mice lacking the prostaglandin F receptor. *Science* 1997;277:681–3.
90. Tsuboi K, Sugimoto Y, Iwane A, Yamamoto K, Yamamoto S, Ichikawa A. Uterine expression of prostaglandin H2 synthase in late pregnancy and during parturition in prostaglandin F receptor-deficient mice. *Endocrinology* 2000;141:315–24.
91. Tsuboi K, Iwane A, Nakazawa S, Sugimoto Y, Ichikawa A. Role of prostaglandin H2 synthase 2 in murine parturition: Study on ovariectomy-induced parturition in prostaglandin F receptor-deficient mice. *Biol Reprod* 2003;69:195–201.
92. Helliwell RJA, Berry EBE, O'Carroll SJ, Mitchell MD. Nuclear prostaglandin receptors: Role in pregnancy and parturition? *Prostaglandins Leukot Essent Fatty Acids* 2004;70:149–65.

93. Shiki Y, Shimoya K, Tokugawa Y, *et al.* Changes of lopocalin-type prostaglandin D synthase level during pregnancy. *J Obstet Gynecol Res* 2004;30:65–70.
94. Barak Y, Nelson MC, Ong ES, *et al.* PPAR gamma is required for placental, cardiac and adipose tissue development. *Mol Cell* 1999;4:585–95.
95. Cui Y, Miyoshi K, Claudio E, *et al.* Loss of the peroxisome proliferation-activated receptor gamma (PPARγ) does not affect mammary development and propensity for tumor formation but leads to reduced fertility. *J Biol Chem* 2002;277:17830–5.
96. Barak Y, Liao D, He W, *et al.* Effects of peroxisome proliferator-activated receptor d on placentation, adiposity, and colorectal cancer. *Proc Natl Acad Sci USA* 2002;99:303–8.
97. Lim H, Gupta RA, Ma WG, *et al.* Cyclo-oxygenase-2-derived prostacyclin mediates embryo implantation in the mouse via PPARdelta. *Genes Dev* 1999;13:1561–74.
98. Forman BM, Chen J, Evans RM. Hypolipidemic drugs, polyunsaturated fatty acids, and eicosanoids are ligands for peroxisome proliferator-activated receptors alpha and delta. *Proc Natl Acad Sci USA* 1997;94:4312–7.
99. Lee SS, Pineau T, Drago J, *et al.* Targeted disruption of the alpha isoform of the peroxisome proliferator-activated receptor gene in mice results in abolishment of the pleiotropic effects of peroxisome proliferators. *Mol Cell Biol* 1995;15:3012–22.
100. Reaume AG, de Sousa PA, Kulkarni S, *et al.* Cardiac malformation in neonatal mice lacking connexin 43. *Science* 1995;267:1831–4.
101. Plum A, Hallas G, Magin T, *et al.* Unique and shared functions of different connexins in mice. *Curr Biol* 2000;10:1083–91.
102. Bond CT, Sprengel R, Bissonnette JM, *et al.* Respiration and parturition affected by conditional overexpression of the Ca2+-activated K+ channel subunit, SK3. *Science* 2000;289:1942–6.
103. Huang PL, Dawson TM, Bredt DS, Snyder SH, Fishman MC. Targeted disruption of the neuronal nitric oxide synthase gene. *Cell* 1993;75:1273–86.
104. Laubach VE, Shesely EG, Smithies O, Sherman PA. Mice lacking inducible nitric oxide synthase are not resistant to lipopolysaccharide-induced death. *Proc Natl Acad Sci USA* 1995;92:10688–92.
105. Shesely EG, Maeda N, Kim H-S, *et al.* Elevated blood pressures in mice lacking endothelial nitric oxide synthase. *Proc Natl Acad Sci USA* 1996;93:13176–81.
106. Naghashpour M, Dahl G. Relaxation of myometrium by calcitonin gene-related peptide is independent of nitric oxide synthase activity in mouse uterus. *Biol Reprod* 2000;63:1421–7.
107. Kimura T, Ogita K, Kusui C, Ohashi K, Azuma C, Murata Y. What knockout mice can tell us about parturition. *Rev Reprod* 1999;4:73–80.
108. Gross G, Imamura R, Muglia LJ. Gene knockout mice in the study of parturition. *J Soc Gynecol Investig* 2000;7:88–95.
109. Muglia LJ. Genetic analysis of fetal development and parturition control in the mouse. *Pediatr Res* 2000;47:437–43.
110. Embree-Ku M, Boekelheide K. Absence of p53 and FasL has sexually dimorphic effects on both development and reproduction. *Exp Biol Med* 2002;27:545–53.

55 Mechanism of human uterine contraction

T. Kawarabayashi and Y. Inoue

Introduction

The uterus is one of the smooth muscle organs that carry out their physiological roles through contractile activities that are tonic and/or phasic contractions, which vary according to the function of each organ. The contractile activities are characterized by three elements (amplitude, duration and frequency), and their combinations determine the type of motility. On the other hand, the arrangement of the smooth muscle bundles, which are composed of smooth muscle cells, determines the direction of the force. The contractile properties of smooth muscle organs are generally correlated with the electrical activity of the plasma membrane; however, the influence of electrical activity varies from organ to organ. Some muscles do not generate action potentials, while others produce active responses. As for the relationship between action potential and contraction, it can be said that the pattern, duration and frequency of action potentials determine the pattern of contractions including each duration and frequency. Moreover, differences in electrical properties might be expected to correlate with the different mechanisms by which bioactive substances and drugs affect the activity of each smooth muscle organ. Therefore, various types of smooth muscles can be classified according to their excitability. For example, stomach and trachea are classified as poorly excitable muscles, and vas deferens and ureter as quiescent, but highly excitable muscles. As for the myometrium, it is placed in the group of spontaneously active and readily excitable muscles like the tenia of cecum, intestine and portal vein. The contractility of this muscle group is greatly influenced by changes in electrical activity. However, one of the most important roles of the uterus is to retain a fetus by suppressing contractility until such time as adequate fetal growth can be achieved, and then to expel the fetus by rhythmic contraction. Long-term and short-term control mechanisms are essential to achieve this dual role. The activity of the myometrium is highly influenced by hormonal conditions to keep the fetus *in utero*, and a variety of stimulants (oxytocin, prostaglandins, catecholamines, etc.) that promote expulsion of the fetus. The course of pregnancy and parturition vary between different species, and myometrial functions would be expected to show similar variation. In the human, a periodicity consisting of 1 min of contraction and a few minutes of relaxation is essential for both mother and fetus. The mother can perform pushing efforts during the contraction phase, and the fetus can recover from the hypoxic state during the relaxation phase. This periodicity probably determines the fundamental characteristics of human uterine contractility.

Electrical activity in the human myometrium

Few studies have recorded the intracellular electrical activity of the human myometrium, though there have been many studies on the electrophysiological properties of animal myometrium. In 1971, Nakajima reported intracellular action potential of human isthmic myometrium using a microelectrode. His description was limited to the mean resting potential (−46.4 mV), and the configuration of the action potential (plateau type). In 1982, therefore, we initiated electrophysiological experiments in human myometrium using the single sucrose-gap method. The specimens consisted of small strips of pregnant human isthmic myometrium dissected from the lower uterine segment at the time of term cesarean section with patients under epidural anesthesia under informed consent, prior to the administration of oxytosis. This material can be easily and consistently obtained from the human uterus without complications. We used the single sucrose-gap method to make a simultaneous record of spontaneous electrical and mechanical activity; this is the most stable method for recording long-term activities.

Passive electrical properties

Resting membrane potential

The resting membrane potential of a spontaneously active smooth muscle, such as intestine and myometrium, is lower than that of a non-spontaneously active smooth muscle. In these muscles, the resting potential is defined as the maximum polarization between action potentials recorded by the microelectrode method. If the tissue shows bursts of spontaneous activity, the value obtained during the quiescent period is taken as the membrane potential. In pregnant human myometrium, it is easier to measure the resting membrane potential because of the long-lasting quiescent period, since the frequency of the action potential is very low in comparison with that of the rat. However, it is obvious that many factors, such as faulty impalement, deficiencies in the microelectrodes, tip potentials of the microelectrodes, stretching of the tissue, bathing temperature and so on affect the membrane potential. Therefore, it is difficult to compare the date reported by different investigators even for the same tissue. The actual value of the resting membrane potential in term-pregnant human myometrium is about −46 to −50 mV,[1,2] and this is compatible with the values in term-pregnant rat myometrium.[3,4] Even in isolated pregnant human myometrial cells dissected from the incisional edge of the lower uterine segment at the time of cesarean delivery, the mean resting membrane potential is −49.4 mV, the same as in intact tissue.[5]

The resting membrane potential of the myometrium is highly influenced by external potassium and sodium in animals. In the rat, when potassium is increased from the normal concentration (5.9 mM in Krebs solution), the membrane gradually depolarizes.[6] On the other hand, when sodium is decreased, the membrane depolarizes and contracture develops in pregnant mouse[7] and rat[6] myometrium. It is considered that the contracture produced by sodium removal is largely calcium dependent, and that an increase in calcium conductance, secondary to membrane depolarization and sodium–calcium exchange, is involved in the calcium-dependent contracture.[8] In myometrium of pregnant woman, the resting membrane potential is primarily influenced by the permeability for potassium ion, but sodium permeability also has an important role.[2]

Length constant

We can obtain the electrical response of pregnant human myometrium evoked by various intensities of stimulation recorded at three different distances from the stimulating partition. The amplitudes of the electrotonic potentials show outward rectification. Linear relations between the applied inward current intensities and the amplitudes of the electrotonic potential were seen at more than three places. There was a long–linear relationship between spatial decay of the electrotonic potential produced at a given current intensity and the distances from the partition. This indicates an exponential decay of the electrotonic potential along the tissue. The length constant describes the efficiency with which a current will spread through the tissue. This content is significant in determining the propagation of action potentials through the tissue. The mean value of the length constant was 1.0 ± 0.1 mm, which was the distance at which the electronic potential decayed to $1/e$. This value is shorter than that measured in the longitudinal muscle of term-pregnant rat myometrium (2.9 mm),[3] but is similar to that observed in the circular muscle of midpregnant rat myometrium (1.02 mm).[9]

Membrane time constant

The membrane time constant is calculated from the relationship between the time to reach the half amplitude of the electrotonic potential at a steady sate and the distance between the recording electrode and the stimulating electrode. The slope of the line represents the relationship of $\tau m/2\lambda$, where τm and λ are the time constant of the membrane and the length constant of the tissue, respectively. The time constant is used as an indicator of membrane resistance. An increase in membrane permeability can therefore be measured as a decrease in τm. The time constant of pregnant human myometrium is 396 ± 46 ms[2]; this value is larger than that of the pregnant rats (180–228 ms).[3,10]

Effect of the reproductive state on passive electrical properties

The cells of the myometrium are spindle-shaped, ranging in size from 2 to 10 µm in diameter, and from 200 to 600 µm in length, depending on the species and hormonal state of the individual. The muscle cells are largest during the later stages of pregnancy, primarily because of the stimulatory influence of the sex steroids and the muscle distention caused by fetal growth.[11] Measurements of longitudinal muscle cells isolated from the uteri of 21-day pregnant rats (delivering day), showed an average size of $232 \pm 74 \times 16.2 \pm 7.0\,\mu$m.[12] Hormones, especially estrogen, and muscle distention also affect the electrical properties of the myometrium.[13] In rat, the resting membrane potential gradually depolarizes (from −43 to −36 mV in circular, −45 to −41 mV in longitudinal muscle), and there is a progressive increase in the length constant (from 2.5 to 2.9 mm in longitudinal muscle) and time constant (from 180 to 228 ms in longitudinal muscle) throughout pregnancy and delivery.[3,4] Thus, a spontaneous action potential is more easily generated and propagated through the myometrium as pregnancy progresses. The overall excitability of the myometrium in late pregnancy culminates in the initiation and progress of labor. The same may occur in human myometrium, though this has not been verified because of the difficulty in obtaining early and midpregnancy myometrium.

Active electrical properties

Action potentials

In a small animal with a bicornuate uterus, such as the rat or mouse, the myometrium consists of a well-defined outer longitudinal layer and an inner circular layer separated by an extensive vascular plexus; the electrophysiological characteristics of each muscle are different. The predominant types of action potentials in rat uteri at midpregnancy are spike in the longitudinal muscle and plateau in the circular muscle.[14] In human myometrium, it is difficult to dissect the longitudinal and circular muscle and therefore difficult to distinguish the action potentials characteristic of these two layers. However, spike- and plateau-type action potentials can be distinguished from the pattern of traces using the microelectrode method[2] and single sucrose-gap method.[15] Plateau potentials are more frequently observed, but these do not allow the prediction of whether the pattern of action potentials will be spike or plateau type before the onset of spontaneous activity. However, all contractions are well synchronized with the action potential, and even a single spike effectively triggers a small contraction; the tension does not revert to the resting level but is summated to a fused tetanus if the intervals between spikes are short enough. The amplitude of the contraction depends on the frequency of the spike potentials. In the plateau-type, the initial spike triggers the contraction, and the duration of the contraction is considerably prolonged in proportion to the plateau duration, though the amplitude is not greatly increased.[15]

The configuration of spontaneous action potentials in human myometrium is very similar to the pattern observed in rats; however, the time courses are remarkably different (about 10 s in rat vs. 60 s in human). The duration of both plateau-type and spike-type action potentials gradually decreases and finally disappears in excess calcium (7 mM) and calcium-free solutions, as well as with application of the calcium antagonist, diltiazem.[16] Moreover, superfusion with sodium-deficient (15.5 mM) and calcium-free solution increases the amplitude of the electrotonic potential and inhibits any active response, in comparison with the responses in the calcium-free solution.[2] Calcium ions can therefore be considered to play an essential role in constituting the action potential, and sodium ions influence the generation of the action potential.[9]

Pacemaker potentials

Myometrium is a spontaneously active and highly excitable muscle. Most of the uterine muscles show spontaneous rhythmic action potentials, which arise in pacemaker cells, and are transmitted over the organ as a whole. As in other visceral smooth muscles and the heart, uterine pacemaker activity is characterized by a slow depolarization of the muscle cell membrane culminating in generation of the action potential. As the pacemaker cells are not localized to a specific area of the myometrium, these cells can only be recognized by the pattern of electrical activity. It is said that all uterine muscle cells are capable of becoming pacemakers.[17] The frequency of pacemaker activity determines the rate of contraction. In pregnant rat myometrium, the slow depolarization is associated with a gradual increase in membrane resistance, presumably due to a reduction in potassium conductance, as judged from the increase in amplitude of the electrotonic potential recorded from a single cell.[3] It is also possible that the slow depolarization results from an increase in sodium permeability, since the pacemaker potential is dependent on the presence of sodium in the external environment and is unaffected by the removal of calcium.[18] Recently, we found hyperpolarization (below -60 mV) -activated inward currents (I_h) in circular but not in longitudinal muscle in pregnant rat uterus under voltage–clamp conditions. Since I_h is activated at the resting membrane potential, it is likely that this current contributes spontaneous activity in circular muscle cells of rats in late pregnancy.[19]

The pacemaker potential is also observed in pregnant human myometrium. The membrane potential gradually depolarizes and the action potential is ultimately evoked. Though steady current pulses are applied, evoked potentials are not regular and the pattern gradually changes in accordance with the periodicity of the membrane. The pacemaker potential is greatly influenced by temperature; the frequency of spontaneous contractions increased markedly, but their duration decreased when temperature of the bathing fluid was increased from 26°C to 39°C. External magnesium ion suppresses the gradient of the pacemaker potential and the duration of each action potential.[20–22]

Ion channels in the human myometrium

Calcium channels. It is well known that contractions of the myometrium are related to an increase in the concentration of intracellular free calcium ion, and it is also known that a large difference in calcium concentrations exists between the extracellular fluid ($\sim 10^{-3}$ M) and intracellular cytosol ($\sim 10^{-7}$ M). Therefore, calcium influx from the extracellular space into the cytosol is very important in regulating myometrial contractility. Two types of channels for calcium influx have been suggested.[23] One is a potential-sensitive calcium channel that opens when the membrane depolarizes and is normally responsible for the action potential. The other type is a receptor-operated channel, which is controlled or operated by a receptor for a stimulant substance. Nowadays, it is well known that voltage-dependent calcium channels (VDCC) represent the major machinery for intracellular calcium mobilization and two types of VDCC, L (long-lasting)-type (dihydropyridine-sensitive) and T (transient)-type, are identified. Therefore, we evaluated the difference in the expression of mRNA of two types of calcium channels between the longitudinal and circular muscle layers of rat myometrium during pregnancy. Changes in the expression of mRNA encoding L-type (α1C) and T-type (α1G, α1H and α1I) calcium channels in longitudinal and circular muscle cells of the rat myometrium were examined using a comparative kinetic RT/PCR method. During the course of pregnancy, α1C mRNA expression showed an N-shaped change in longitudinal muscle, but simply increased after midpregnancy in circular muscles. The mRNAs for α1G and α1H, but not that for α1I, were expressed in both longitudinal and circular muscles. In longitudinal muscle, the change in α1H mRNA was similar to that in α1C mRNA during gestation, but the expression of α1G mRNA changed significantly only at term (day 22). In circular muscle, a1H mRNA expression was stable at any stage during pregnancy, but α1G mRNA significantly increased on day 15 and at term. No relationship was observed between VDCC mRNA expressions and either proliferation or hypertrophy of circular muscle during pregnancy. These results suggest that the expression levels of L-type channels change dynamically and may contribute directly to the regulation of cell excitability and that the T-subtype that increases during pregnancy differs between longitudinal and circular muscle cells.[24]

In pregnant human myometrium, two different types of VDCC have been observed at the single-channel level using the patch clamp technique,[2] and the inward calcium current was characterized by activation and inactivation properties.[25] One of these had a single-channel conductance of 12 pS, and was only activated by depolarizing pulses from a holding potential of −100 mV; this channel was inactivated at a holding potential of 60 mV. The second type had a single-channel conductance of 29 pS activated by depolarizing pulses from a holding potential of −60 mV. Summate currents also showed different time courses for current relaxation, i.e. the 12 pS calcium channel (transient type: T-type) was rapidly inactivated, whereas the 29 pS calcium channel (long-lasting type: L-type) was slowly inactivated. The majority of the 12 pS calcium channels are likely to be inactivated at a normal resting potential of about −50 mV, as indicated by the experiments that used the whole-cell voltage–clamp technique.[2] The physiological importance of the L-type current must be related to the formation of plateau potential, judging from its higher threshold potential and slower inactivation. Activation of the T-type calcium channel may be responsible for the spike component, and it may trigger activation of the long-lasting-type calcium channel. Recently, three types of T-type channel a1 subunits, α1G (Ca_v3.1), α1H (Ca_v3.2) and α1I (Ca_v3.3), have been cloned and we examined the electrophysiological characteristics of three cloned human α1H isoforms of the T-type calcium channel Ca_v3.2 expressed in pregnant human uterus. Then, our results suggested that molecular-structure variation within the III-IV linker influenced the voltage dependence of activation and inactivation, and kinetics. Although the role of T-type calcium channels in uterus remains unknown, changes in the uterine expression of these α1H isoforms may influence the physiological function during pregnancy.[24]

Sodium channels. Sodium ions may play an important role in generating the pacemaker potential and the action potential in uterine muscle. In the longitudinal muscle layer of pregnant rat myometrium, a fast sodium channel current (tetrodotoxin sensitive) was recorded from freshly isolated single cells using whole-cell voltage–clamp technique, and it was suggested that the fast sodium channel current might play a role in cell-to-cell conduction and possibly in regulation of spontaneous electrical activity.[26]

In cultured cells obtained from pregnant human myometrium, a large voltage-activated inward current was identified as sodium channel conductance by the following criteria: (1) removal of sodium from the bath eliminated the current; (2) the current was blocked by the sodium-channel-blocking agent, tetrodotoxin and (3) the current was observed in the absence of calcium.[27] The sodium current was large (maximal inward current 7.2 $\mu A/cm^2$) and of short duration (decayed within 10 ms); the onset of activation was −40 mV, with a peak inward current at −10 mV. Steady-state voltage inactivation of this channel showed half-maximal inactivation at −67 mV, indicating that this channel is largely inactivated at normal resting potentials. The sodium currents do not appear to contribute to the rising phase of the action potential in human myocytes.[27] Further study is required to clarify the physiological role of sodium channels.

Potassium channels. The potassium channels are involved in terminating action potentials and in returning the membrane potential to its resting level. Furthermore, the resting potential is primarily set by the permeability to potassium ion, and changes in the membrane potential can affect the initiation of the action potential and, hence, contraction. In the myometrium of pregnant women, it is believed that the changes in potassium permeability primarily affect the resting potential,[2] and that this might be involved in the action of catecholamine β_2-agonist and the effect of high calcium on the duration of action potentials.[16,20] Though a single-channel potassium current has not yet been recorded from the human myometrium, several studies of potassium current obtained from the myometrial cells of experimental animals by the patch–clamp technique have been reported.[28–30] It has been suggested that calcium-activated potassium channels, which are controlled by intracellular calcium, are not activated by calmodulin, but rather that calcium binds directly to the gating site for channel activation.[29] Furthermore, three potassium currents (fast, intermediate and slow) are found in rat myometrium; the fast current is predominant in cells from estrus rats, whereas intermediate current is more frequent in cells from diestrus rats. In addition, norepinephrine potentiates the fast current and reduces the intermediate current.[30] Using rat or pig myometrial potassium channels incorporated into lipid bilayers, it has been shown that myometrial β–adrenergic receptors may be coupled to a guanosine tri phosphate (GTP)-dependent protein that can directly gate calcium-activated potassium channels.[31] Current research is directed at understanding the mechanisms of potassium channels through the molecular biological technique. One of the most conspicuous channels is the high (big)-conductance potassium channel, BK channel. It has a large single-channel conductance of around 250 pS and is a calcium-activated channel (K_{Ca}). A major role for BK_{Ca} channels is likely to be the restoration of resting conditions following an action potential. Thus, the calcium influx and depolarization occurring during the action potential in smooth muscle would both contribute to an increase in the probability of opening of BK_{Ca} channels resulting in repolarization of the membrane. This would decrease the probability of opening of the VDCC and in this way reduce excitability and facilitate relaxation.[32] As for human myometrium, it is reported that the mRNA for BK_{Ca} channels is abundant in human myometrium.[33] As the other potassium channels, delayed rectifier potassium channel,[34,35] transient A-type potassium channel[2] and ATP-sensitive potassium channel (K_{ATP})[36] are reported.

Effect of the reproductive state on active electrical properties

Near the end of pregnancy the circular muscle activities of the rat uterus exhibit characteristic changes that are a prerequisite for normal delivery. These changes consist of a progressive alteration in the configuration of action potentials from a single, plateau type in early and midpregnancy to a repetitive train discharge at term.[4,37] The action potentials cause brief, irregular contractions during early and midpregnancy and regular contractions of longer duration at term. Furthermore, uterine volume (muscle stretching) and circulating estrogens may be more important than the fetoplacental unit in the evolution of circular muscle activity in the pregnant rat.[13] The protein synthesis inhibitor, cycloheximide, can suppress the evolution of activity and delay parturition.[38] The action potential of longitudinal muscle exhibits a burst discharge of spikes and the pattern does not change throughout pregnancy. However, estradiol hyperpolarizes the membrane and a burst of spikes is generated from sustained depolarization. Progesterone, by contrast, slightly hyperpolarizes the membrane and typical burst discharges occur without sustained depolarization. Simultaneous treatment with progesterone and estradiol produces a plateau potential.[3] Although sex steroids affect membrane properties, the changes that occur during pregnancy cannot be explained by the action of such hormones. There is only one report that describes the electrical activity of human myometrium in early pregnancy.[15] The action potential is composed of long plateau potential or abortive spikes superimposed on the long plateau. The duration tends to be longer than in-term pregnancy.

Relationship between electrical activity and contraction

Contraction of the myometrium is related to the concentration of intracellular free calcium ion; the increase in intracellular calcium might arise from an influx of calcium from the extracellular space, the translocation of calcium ions in or near the cell membrane and/or the release of calcium from internal stores. Myometrium of pregnant women usually generates spontaneous action potentials and extracellular calcium might enter the cell through the calcium channels during these action potentials. In our sucrose-gap experiments, contractions were always synchronized with the corresponding action potentials. Therefore, the amount of calcium that enters during the action potential is sufficient to activate the contractile mechanism and to release additional calcium from internal stores, thereby amplifying the transmembrane signals.[39] On the other hand, the periodicity of 1-min contraction and a few minutes of relaxation is essential for the mother and fetus during the stress of parturition. A long and hypertonic contraction decreases uteroplacental blood flow, causes fetal hypoxia, and small contractions cannot expel the fetus further. The myometrium has a spontaneous periodicity and thereby generates action potentials and contractions of appropriate duration. Under physiological conditions, the contractility of the uterus is regulated by changing the electrical activity. It might be very easy to regulate the frequency, duration and probably amplitude of spontaneous contractions evoked by each action potential by changing the resting membrane potential.

In obstetric practice both periodic contractions and sufficient periods of relaxation are the most important factors for the well-being of the fetus and the progress of delivery. Considering these fundamental characteristics of the human uterine contraction, relaxation mechanisms are essential for the fetus and the mother, and should be better understood along with the stimulation of the contractions. A reduction in intracellular calcium is essential for relaxation. Currently, two pathways are speculated for the myometrium to lower the intracellular calcium ions to produce relaxation. One is a calcium pump in the plasma membrane or the membrane of the sarcoplasmic reticulum, and the other is a sodium–calcium exchange mechanism that is an antiporter present in the plasma membrane carrying sodium in one direction and calcium in the other. In the myometrium of pregnant women, we suggested the presence of the sodium–calcium exchange mechanism and the specific inhibitory effect of magnesium ion. This mechanism might prevent the long tonic contractions, to protect the fetus from hypoxia during pregnancy and parturition.[40]

Propagation of excitation

In the human uterus, the resting tonus maintains uterine shape and fetal position. Resting tonus is maintained by random activation of the myometrium by action potentials. However, well-coordinated contraction is essential for the successful expulsion of the fetus after the onset of labor. In order to achieve this coordination, many myometrial cells have to contract at the same time, and local contractions obtained by the coordination of the cells have to be synchronized over the whole of the uterus as parturition progresses. Since small muscle strips of myometrium of pregnant women exhibit spontaneous periodicity with 1-min contraction and a few minutes relaxation, this periodicity may facilitate coordinated contraction. In our clinical study, the qualitative characteristics of uterine contractions in labor were evaluated by a double-guard-ring tocodynamometer attached to the fundus and the caudal part of the uterus. The synchronizing ratio of two contraction waves was significantly higher in the active phase than in the latent phase of labor, and nearly regular upward or downward observed in each case.[41] Furthermore, the percentages of both concurrent and synchronous contractions were higher than those of Braxton Hichs contractions, and both values increased significantly between 5 and 6 cm of cervical dilation.[42] On the other hand, small contraction waves (30 s or less duration of each wave) recorded by a guard-ring tocodynamometer were observed in 7.5% of the cardiotocographs examined, and the rate of small-wave appearance in each gestational week tended to decrease gradually as the pregnancy progressed. This was not observed after 41 weeks of gestation and was frequently observed in cases of effective β_2-stimulant intravenous infusion for the treatment of preterm labor.[43] The synchronizing ratio of peaks of small contraction waves was almost the same as the ratio in the active phase of labor.[41] Thus, synchronization of local contractions results in the effective contractions of human parturition. However, the uterus does not have any specific conduction pathways for excitation. Instead, the action potential spreads into the surrounding cells in three dimensions in accordance with their cable-like properties. The length constant of the membrane gradually increases throughout pregnancy in the rat, as described earlier, and the conduction velocity of the action potential in longitudinal preparations of pregnant rat myometrium increases from 9.2 cm/s at late pregnancy to 10.5 cm/s during delivery.[44] Gap junctions, which are assumed to be the structure involved in electrical and chemical communication between cells, increase during parturition and disappear after delivery in experimental animals.[45] This structure is observed in human myometrium from women in preterm labor.[46] These changes may contribute to the propagation of excitation during parturition.

Effects of ions and drugs on electrical activity and contraction

Calcium

Extracellular calcium has been shown to play an important role in the activation of smooth muscle and the amplitude of the tension can be related to the external calcium concentration and, consequently, to the calcium influx in pregnant rat myometrium.[47,48] Moreover, the inward calcium current may affect potassium conductance during the plateau potential in the circular muscle of pregnant rat myometrium, and the potassium conductance provides the plateau duration, and consequently the duration of the contraction.[49] In myometrium of pregnant women, spontaneous contraction is strongly affected by external calcium; 2.5 mM calcium in Krebs solution is the most efficient concentration in terms of frequency, amplitude and duration of whole contractions. Both excess calcium and low calcium suppresses the generation of spontaneous contraction; however, the mechanism of these two types of suppression may differ. Calcium ions may play dual roles in the electrical activity of the myometrium: an excitatory role in action potential and an inhibitory role accomplished by membrane stabilization and calcium-mediated potassium activation. Therefore, the effects of excess calcium on spontaneous contractions may depend on the balance of excitatory and inhibitory effects. If the increase of calcium influx during the action potential is predominant, the amplitude of the contraction will increase; however, the contraction will be diminished if the generation of action potentials is suppressed by membrane stabilization and activation of the outward potassium current. In contrast, low calcium may decrease the influx of calcium and consequently suppress the contraction, since both the amplitude and the duration of contraction are generally decreased in low-calcium solution.[16,22]

Magnesium

Magnesium sulfate has been used as a tocolytic agent to prevent preterm labor. The effect of magnesium on the spontaneous electrical and mechanical activities of the circular muscle of term pregnant rat uterus suggests that the effect is largely due to suppression of the plateau potential.[50] According to the whole-cell voltage–clamp method on freshly isolated single pregnant rat myometrial cells, magnesium inhibits the calcium current, affecting mainly the transient component.[51] In myometrium of pregnant women, frequency, amplitude and duration of spontaneous contractions all decrease with increases in external magnesium; the frequency change is the most significant.[22] Magnesium ion suppresses the gradient of pacemaker potential, and consequently the frequency of contraction.[20]

Oxytocin

The initiation of either term or preterm labor is considered to be a final common phenomenon induced by augmented uterine contractions, regardless of the incipient cause. And it is well known that oxytocin plays an important role in the initiation of labor in both term and preterm parturients. However, a satisfactory direct comparison of the functional roles of oxytocin in term and preterm labor had not been elucidated. We had demonstrated that the inhibitory effects of both peptidyl and non-peptidyl oxytocin antagonists on spontaneous uterine contractions of pregnant rats became greater as the pregnancy progressed. This change was accompanied by a significant increase in myometrial oxytocin receptor density.[52] Then, we made a direct comparison of the functional roles of oxytocin in term and preterm labor in rats. First, we determined the myometrial oxytocin receptor density and maternal plasma concentrations of oxytocin and progesterone on gestational days 18, 20 and 22 (morning) and at the onset of delivery (day 22 afternoon) in rats with labor at term and at the onset of delivery (day 20 afternoon) in rats in preterm labor induced by the combined use of bilateral ovariectomy and estradiol injection. We also evaluated the effects of a non-peptidyl oxytocin antagonist on the initiation of both term and preterm labor. Consequently, the number of tritiated oxytocin-binding sites in myometrial membranes rapidly increased on gestational day 22 (morning). Plasma progesterone level decreased in an inverse fashion. A rapid increase in circulating oxytocin concentration was observed at the onset of delivery, and both the plasma oxytocin concentration and the receptor density had the same values in rats with preterm labor as in rats with term labor. The oxytocin antagonist delayed the initiation of labor in rats with term and preterm labor in a dose-dependent manner.[53]

On the other hand, the direct effect of oxytocin on spontaneous electrical and mechanical activities in myometrium of pregnant women has been investigated using the single sucrose-gap method.[54] Oxytocin potentiates spontaneous contractions by enhancing the plateau part of action potentials; the spike-type configuration becomes plateau. This potentiation depends on the external calcium concentration, and the effects on frequency and amplitude of contractions may vary. In our microelectrode experiments, two types of spontaneous action potentials were seen in the myometrium of pregnant women; a long plateau and a spike-like action potential. With no change in the resting membrane potential, low concentrations of oxytocin evoked an action potential with plateau phase, increased the amplitude and duration of the plateau potential or increased the frequency of generation of action potentials. Oxytocin also lowered the threshold for evoking an action potential. Higher concentrations depolarized the membrane with an associated reduction in membrane resistance.[55] Oxytocin evokes action potentials and contractions in high frequency; the duration of the action potential is short and the contraction is small in the presence of diltiazem (calcium antagonist). The results of the potassium contracture experiment also suggest that oxytocin evokes a contracture in the absence of an action potential by releasing calcium from intracellular storage sites.

This possibility is supported by another study measuring intracellular calcium using Fura-2 in isolated cells of pregnant rat myometrium.[12] Then, we examined the changes in responsiveness of freshly isolated longitudinal muscle cells from rat uterus to oxytocin during gestation by measuring contractility as well as intracellular free calcium concentration. We have demonstrated the pregnant stage-dependent contraction of freshly isolated myometrial cells in response to an extracellular hormone, oxytocin, in Ca^{2+}-containing medium. The oxytocin effect appeared to be through oxytocin receptor since the effect could be blocked by a specific oxytocin antagonist. The magnitude of the contraction of the isolated cells in response to extracellular oxytocin was in the order of 21-day $\gg$ 18-day > 15-day pregnant rat longitudinal muscle cells. In a concentration-dependent manner, oxytocin elicited a rapid increase in intracellular calcium ion of longitudinal muscle cells isolated from different stages of the pregnant rat uterus, especially at the term of pregnancy. The time (4–5 s) required to reach a maximum increase in intracellular calcium ion of the isolated longitudinal muscle cells in response to oxytocin was the shortest among all previously reported studies. The results also indicated that the freshly prepared longitudinal muscle cells maintained their functional calcium signaling system. The order of the responsiveness of the isolated longitudinal muscle cells to oxytocin was 21-day $\gg$ 18-day > 15-day pregnant rats in terms of rate, affinity and magnitude. Oxytocin appears to transmit its signal mainly through stimulating a voltage-dependent and/or receptor-operated non-selective calcium channel. However, the possibility that a part of the oxytocin action occurs through stimulating the release of calcium from intracellular store sites of longitudinal muscle still remains.[56]

The excitatory effect of oxytocin is modified by external magnesium ion in the myometrium of pregnant women. Relatively high magnesium (2.4 mM) suppresses the spontaneous activities; however, oxytocin enhances the contractions and the plateau part of action potentials to a greater extent than does the magnesium-free solution. In the potassium contracture experiment, the oxytocin-induced contracture during the tonic phase is potentiated by magnesium. Magnesium may potentiate the excitatory effect of oxytocin at superficial sites of the plasma membrane, allowing the possibility of intracellular action.[57] The interaction between calcium and magnesium is probably very significant in the regulation of the action of oxytocin on uterine contractility.

It is obvious that oxytocin is involved in the initiation and progress of labor in many species and also plays an important role in lactation. From another point of view about the initiation of labor and lactation, we clarified the possibility that oxytocin might modulate oxytocin neurons in the paraventricular nuclei of female rats throughout pregnancy and parturition. Our results show that the firing rates of paraventricular neurons in virgin and pregnant rats decreased in activity; however, the neurons of delivering and lactating rats exhibited excitatory responses. This excitation reversed to inhibition again after the lactating period ended. It is suggested that negative feedback by oxytocin in virgin and pregnant rats might reverse to positive feedback in delivering and lactating animals as a result of changes in hormonal conditions. This reverse might be closely related to the initiation of delivery.[58]

Catecholamines

The effects of catecholamines on the myometrium differ among animal species, and even in the same animal, depending on the hormonal status of the individual and each muscle layer. For example, in a rat at midpregnancy longitudinal muscle possesses mainly β-adrenoceptors, while circular muscle has a-adrenoceptors.[14] However, in late gestation, activation of the a-adrenoceptors occurs in the longitudinal muscle, while the circular muscle switches from α- to β-adrenoceptor dominance.[59]

In the myometrium of pregnant women, noradrenaline always exhibits α-excitatory action at 10^{12}–10^{6} g/ml; however, β-inhibition of β_2-stimulant is also observed.[20] It is suggested on the basis of animal studies that activation of a-receptors in the longitudinal muscle is mainly mediated by slow depolarization of the membrane (due to an increase in chloride conductance), which leads to an increase in spike frequency; in the circular muscle, it is mediated by prolongation of the plateau of action potentials (due to an increase in calcium conductance). β-Action of the myometrium also includes membrane hyperpolarization due to an increase in potassium conductance and an increase in cyclic adenosine monophosphate (cAMP) production underlies the suppression of spontaneous contraction.[60] Catecholamine action may fundamentally affect uterine contractility during pregnancy and parturition.

In obstetric practice, adrenergic β_2-stimulants have been widely used as tocolytic agents to prevent preterm delivery. However, commercially available tocolytic agents often have severe adverse effects (such as tachycardia, tremor of the hands and lung edema) because they simultaneously exert weak a and β_1 effects on the cardiovascular system. Another concern about β_2-stimulants as tocolytic agents is that their tocolytic effect is inconsistent among patients and the so-called myometrial desensitization phenomenon in which the recurrence of contractions might be related to a decrease in cAMP production.[61] Recently, we produced a new β_2-stimulant (KUR-1246) with a higher selectivity for uterine β_2-receptors (and thus weaker side effects).[62] Then, we performed the experiment to evaluate the usefulness of this new β_2-adrenergic stimulant as a tocolytic agent and to clarify the mechanisms that underlay the diverse inhibitory effects of β_2-stimulants that were seen in human myometria *in vitro*. Consequently, KUR-1246 was approximately 80 times and 7 times more selective for β_2-receptors than isoproterenol and ritodrine, respectively. The inhibitory effect of KUR-1246 was as strong as the inhibitory effect of the conventional β_2-adrenergic stimulants. A wide range of inhibitory effects was observed, even when high concentrations of isoproterenol or KUR-1246 were applied. There was a correlation between the degree to which isoproterenol suppressed contractions and the number of [^{3}H]dihydroalоprenolol-binding sites on the membrane in each muscle strip. These results suggest that KUR-1246 should be a very useful β_2-adrenergic stimulant for use as a tocolytic agent because of its high selectivity for the β_2-receptor and its potent inhibitory effect. The diversity of the inhibitory effects that are induced by β_2-stimulants is at least partly due to the differences in β_2-receptor density among term-pregnant human myometria (Sakakibara *et al.*, 2002).

Other drugs

There are a few studies on the electrophysiological action of other drugs on the human myometrium. Prostaglandin $F_{2\alpha}$ ($PGF_{2\alpha}$) and methylergometrine maleate (methergin) potentiate the plateau part of the action potential and contraction of the myometrium of pregnant women.[63,64] The action of methergin is not inhibited by phentolamine (an α-blocker). Plateau enhancement may be the main effect. Both oxytocin and $PGF_{2\alpha}$ potentiated the spontaneous contractions by affecting the plateau part of action potentials; spike-type configurations became plateaus. However, high dosages of both the drugs were required to obtain consistent excitatory effects *in vitro*. In obstetric practice, on the other hand, uterine contractions can be induced by low doses of these drugs. The pharmacological application of oxytocin or $PGF_{2\alpha}$ might only play a triggering role in uterine contractions at induction or augmentation of labor, and complex interactions might be involved in the initiation and potentiation of contractions *in vivo*.[63]

Conclusion

The myometrium has spontaneously active and highly excitable membrane with many voltage-dependent ion channels. Contractility of the myometrium is regulated by the electrical activity of this membrane. The main external controlling factors are sex steroid hormones. The balance of estrogen and progesterone, and the changes during the course of the menstrual cycle, pregnancy and parturition, changes the resting membrane potential, the pattern of action potentials and the effects of drugs, such as catecholamines and oxytocin. Hormones also affect the conduction of excitation and produce morphological changes of cell size. All of these changes lead to synchronized contractions that are effective in expulsion of the fetus. It is particularly important for the fetus that the periodicity of the phasic contractions is strictly maintained.

Acknowledgment

The author is grateful to Aki Ueno and Sayako Kawarabayashi, a daughter of mine, for typing the manuscript.

REFERENCES

1. Nakajima A. Action potention of human myometrial fibers. *Am J Obstet Gynecol* 1971;111:266–9.
2. Inoue Y, Nakao K, Okabe K, *et al.* Some electrical properties of human pregnant myometrium. *Am J Obstet Gynecol* 1990;162: 1090–8.
3. Kuriyama H, Suzuki H. Changes in electrical properties of rat myometrium during gestation and following hormonal treatments. *J Physiol* 1976;260:315–33.
4. Anderson GF, Kawarabayashi T, Marshall JM. Effect of indomethacin and aspirin on uterine activity in pregnant rats: Comparison of circular and longitudinal muscle. *Biol Reprod* 1981; 24:359–72.
5. Pressman EK, Tucker JA Jr, Anderson NC Jr, Young RC. Morphologic and electrophysiologic characterization of isolated pregnant human myometrial cells. *Am J Obstet Gynecol* 1988;59;1273–9.
6. Kanda S, Kuriyama H. Specific features of smooth muscle cells recorded from the placental region of the myometrium of pregnant rats. *J Physiol* 1980;299:127–44.
7. Osa T. Effect of removing the external sodium on the electrical and mechanical activities of the pregnant mouse myometrium. *Jpn J Physiol* 1971;21:607–25.
8. Masahashi T, Tomita T. The contracture produced by sodium removal in the non-pregnant rat myometrium. *J Physiol* 1983;334: 351–63.
9. Kawarabayashi T. The effects of phenylepinephrine in various ionic environments on the circular muscle of mid-pregnant rat myometrium. *Jpn J Physiol* 1978;28:627–45.
10. Sims SM, Daniel EE, Garfield RE. Improved electrical coupling in uterine smooth muscle is associated with increased numbers of gap junctions at parturition. *J Gen Physiol* 1982;80:353–75.
11. Cole WC, Garfield RE. Ultrastructure of the myometrium. In Wynn RM, Jollie WP, eds. *Biology of the Uterus.* New York: Plenum Press, 1989:455–504.
12. Tsukamoto T, Kawarabayashi T, Kaneko Y, Kumamoto T, Sugimori H. Intracellular calcium of longitudinal muscles isolated from pregnant rat myometrium. *Cell Biol Int Rep* 1991;15:637–44.
13. Kawarabayashi T, Marshall JM. Factors influencing circular muscle activity in the pregnant rat uterus. *Biol Reprod* 1981;24:373–9.
14. Kawarabayashi T, Osa T. Comparative investigation of alpha-and beta-effects on the longitudinal and circular muscles of the pregnant rat myometrium. *Jpn J Physiol* 1976;26:403–16.
15. Kawarabayashi T, Ikeda M, Sugimori H, Nakano H. Spontaneous electrical activity and effects of noradrenaline on pregnant human myometrium recorded by the single sucrose-gap method. *Acta Physiol Hung* 1986;67:71–82.
16. Kawarabayashi T, Kishikawa T, Sugimori H. Effects of external calcium and calcium antagonist, diltiazem, on isolated segments of pregnant human myometrium. *Asia Oceania J Obstet Gynaecol* 1986;12:409–17.
17. Marshall JM. The physiology of the myometrium. In *The Uterus.* Baltimore: Williams & Wilkins, 1973:89–109.
18. Reiner O, Marshall JM. Action of prostaglandin PGF_{2a} on the uterus of the pregnant rat. *Naunyn Schmiedeberg Arch Pharmacol* 1976; 292:243–50.
19. Okabe K, Inoue Y, Kawarabayashi T, Kajiya H, Okamoto F, Soeda H. Physiological significance of hyperpolarization-activated inward currents (I_h) in smooth muscle cells from the circular layers of pregnant rat myometrium. *Pflugers Arch* 1999; 439:76–85.
20. Kawarabayashi T, Ikeda M, Sugimori H, Nakano H. Effects of magnesium and catecholamines on spontaneous contraction of pregnant human isthmic myometrium. *Asia Oceania J Obstet Gynaecol* 1984;10:357–84.
21. Kawarabayashi T, Kishikawa T, Sugimori H. Characteristics of action potential and contractions evoked by electrical-field stimulation of pregnant human myometrium. *Gynecol Obstet Invest* 1988;25:73–9.
22. Kawarabayashi T, Kishikawa T, Sugimori H. Effects of external calcium, magnesium, and temperature of spontaneous contractions of pregnant human myometrium. *Biol Reprod* 1989;40: 942–8.
23. Bolton TB. Mechanisms of action of transmitters and other substances on smooth muscle. *Physiol Rev* 1979;59:609–718.
24. Ohkubo T, Inoue Y, Kawarabayashi T, Kitamura K. Identification and electrophysiological characteristics of isoforms of T-type calcium channel $Ca_v3.2$ expressed in pregnant human myometrium, in press.
25. Young RC, Herndon-Smith L, Anderson NC Jr. Passive membrane properties and inward calcium current of human uterine smooth muscle cells. *Am J Obstet Gynecol* 1991;164:1132–9.
26. Ohya Y, Sperelakis N. Fast Na+ and slow Ca^{2+} channels in single uterine muscle cells from pregnant rats. *Am J Physiol* 1989;257: C408–12.
27. Young RC, Herndon-Smith L. Characterization of sodium channels in cultured human uterine smooth muscle cells. *Am J Obstet Gynecol* 1991;64:175–81.
28. Coleman HA, Parkington HC. Single channel Cl- and K-currents from cells of uterus not treated with enzymes. *Pflugers Arch* 1987;410:560–2.
29. Kihara M, Matsuzawa K, Tokuno H, Tomita T. Effects of calmodulin antagonists of calcium-activated potassium channels in pregnant rat myometrium. *Br J Pharmacol* 1990;100:353–9.
30. Toro L, Stefani E, Erulkar S. Hormonal regulation of potassium currents in single myometrial cells. *Proc Natl Acad Sci USA* 1991;87: 2892–5.
31. Toro L, Ramos-Franco J, Stefani E. GTP-dependent regulation of myometrial K-Ca channels incorporated into lipid bilayers. *J Gen Physiol* 1990;96:373–94.

32. Parkington HC, Coleman HA. Excitability in uterine smooth muscle. In Smith R, ed. *The Endocrinology of Parturition. Basic Science and Clinical Application.* Basel: Karger, 2001:179–200.
33. Wallner M, Mccra P, Ottolia M, *et al.* Characterization of and modulation by a beta-subunit of a human maxi K_{Ca} channel cloned from myometrium. *Receptors Channels* 1995;3:185–99.
34. Miyoshi H, Urabe T, Fujiwara A. Electrophysiological properties of membrane currents in single myometrial cells isolated from pregnant rats. *Pflugers Arch* 1991;419:386–93.
35. Knock GA, Smirnov SV, Aaronson PI. Voltage-gated K^+ currents in freshly isolated myocytes of the pregnant human myometrium. *J Physiol* 1999;518:769–81.
36. Hamada Y, Nakaya Y, Hamada S, Kamada M, Aono T. Activation of K^+ channels by ritodrine hydrochloride in uterine smooth muscle cells from pregnant women. *Eur J Pharmacol* 1994;288:45–51.
37. Osa T, Fujino T. Electrophysiological comparison between the longitudinal and circular muscles of the rat uterus during the estrous cycle and pregnancy. *Jpn J Physiol* 1978;28:197–209.
38. Maruta K, Osa T. Blockage by cycloheximide of the prepartum changes in membrane activity and adrenergic response of the circular muscle of rat uterus. *Jpn J Physiol* 1986;36:971–83.
39. Parkington HC, Coleman HA. The role of membrane potential in the control of uterine motility. In Carsten ME, Miller JD, eds. *Uterine Function: Molecular and Cellular Aspects.* New York: Plenum Press, 1990:95–248.
40. Morishita F, Kawarabayashi T, Sakamoto Y, Shirakawa K. Role of the sodium–calcium exchange mechanism and the effect of magnesium on sodium-free and high-potassium contractures in pregnant human myometrium. *Am J Obstet Gynecol* 1995;172:186–95.
41. Nakahara H, Kawarabayashi T, Ikeda M, Uchiumi Y, Sugimori H, Nakano H. Synchronization of uterine contractions recorded by guard-ring tocodynamometer. *Asia Oceania J Obstet Gynaecol* 1986;12:137–42.
42. Shinmoto M, Kawarabayashi T, Ikeda M, Sugimori H. Qualitative evaluation of uterine contractions recorded by a double guard-ring tocodynamometer. *Am J Obstet Gynecol* 1991;165:1282–6.
43. Kawarabayashi T, Kuriyama K, Kishikawa I, Sugimori H. Clinical features of small contraction wave recorded by an external tocodynamometer. *Am J Obstet Gynecol* 1988;158:474–8.
44. Miller SM, Garfield RE, Daniel EE. Improved propagation in myometrium associated with gap junctions during parturition. *Am J Physiol* 1989;256:C130–41.
45. Garfield RE. Control of myometrial function in preterm versus term labor. *Clin Obstet Gynecol* 1984;27:572–91.
46. Garfield RE, Hayashi RH. Appearance of gap junctions in the myometrium of women during labor. *Am J Obstet Gynecol* 1981;140:254–60.
47. Mironneau J. Excitation–contraction coupling in voltage clamped uterine smooth muscle. *J Physiol* 1973;233:127–41.
48. Bengtsson B, Chow EHM, Marshall JM. Calcium dependency of pregnant rat myometrium: Comparison of circular and longitudinal muscle. *Biol Reprod* 1984;30:869–78.
49. Osa T, Kawarabayashi T. Effects of ions and drugs of the plateau potential in the circular muscle of pregnant rat myometrium. *Jpn J Physiol* 1977;27:111–21.
50. Osa T, Ogasawara T. Effects of magnesium on the membrane activity and contraction of the circular muscle of rat myometrium during late pregnancy. *Jpn J Physiol* 1983;33:485–95.
51. Ohya Y, Sperelakis N. Tocolytic agents act on calcium channel current in single smooth muscle cells of pregnant rat uterus. *J Pharmacol Exp Ther* 1990;253:580–5.
52. Kawarabayashi T, Kobayashi M, Akahane M, Ajisawa Y. Comparison of in vitro and in vivo inhibitory effects of peptide and nonpeptide oxytocin antagonists on radioligand binding and uterine contractility of rats during pregnancy. *Am J Obstet Gynecol* 1996;175:1348–55.
53. Kobayashi M, Akahane M, Minami K, *et al.* Role of oxytocin in the initiation of term and preterm labor in rats: Changes in oxytocin receptor density and plasma oxytocin concentration and the effect of an oxytocin antagonist, L-366,509. *Am J Obstet Gynecol* 1999;180:621–7.
54. Kawarabayashi T, Kishikawa T, Sugimori H. Effects of oxytocin on spontaneous electrical and mechanical activities in pregnant human myometrium. *Am J Obstet Gynecol* 1986;55:671–6.
55. Nakao K, Inoue Y, Okabe K, Kawarabayashi T, Kitamura K. Oxytocin enhances action potentials in pregnant human myometrium – A study with microelectrodes. *Am J Obstet Gynecol* 1997;177:222–8.
56. Kawarabayashi T, Tsukamoto T, Shojo H, Nakamura S, Sugimori H. Changes in responsiveness of freshly isolated longitudinal muscle cells from rat uterus towards oxytocin during gestation: Contractility and calcium signaling. *Mol Cell Endocrinol* 1997;128:77–84.
57. Kawarabayashi T, Izumi H, Ikeda M, Ichihara J, Sugimori H, Shirakawa K. Modification by magnesium of the excitatory effect of oxytocin in electrical and mechanical activities of pregnant human myometrium. *Obstet Gynecol* 1990;76:183–8.
58. Kawarabayashi T, Kuriyama K, Nakashima T, Kiyihara T, Sugimori H. Oxytocin modulates oxytocin neurons in the paraventricular nuclei of female rats throughout pregnancy and parturition. *Am J Obstet Gynecol* 1993;168:969–74.
59. Kishikawa T. Alterations in the properties of the rat myometrium during gestation and post partum. *Jpn J Physiol* 1981;31:515–36.
60. Bulbring E, Tomita T. Catecholamine action on smooth muscle. *Pharmacol Rev* 1987;39:49–96.
61. Kawarabayashi T, Tsukamoto T, Kaneko Y, Ikeda M, Sugimori H, Shirakawa K. Changes in beta-adrenergic receptors under long-term application of ritodrine in pregnant-rat myometrium. *Gynecol Obstet Invest* 1993;35:136–9.
62. Kobayashi M, Takeda K, Murata S, *et al.* Pharmacological characterization of KUR-1246, a selective uterine relaxant. *J Pharmacol Exp Ther* 2001;297:666–71.
63. Kawarabayashi T, Sugimori H. Effects of oxytocin and prostaglandin $F_{2\alpha}$ on pregnant human myometrium recorded by the single sucrose-gap method – Comparison of an in vitro experiment and an in vivo trial. *Asia Oceania J Obstet Gynaecol* 1985;11:247–53.
64. Kawarabayashi T, Kishikawa T, Sugimori H. Effects of methylergometrine maleate (methergin) on electrical and mechanical activities of pregnant human myometrium. *Gynecol Obstet Invest* 1990;29:246–9.
65. Ohkubo T, Kawarabayashi T, Inoue Y, Kitamura K. Differential expression of L- and T-type calcium channels between longitudinal and circular muscles of the rat myometrium during pregnancy. *Gynecol Obstet Invest* 2005;59:80–5.
66. Okabe K, Terada K, Kitamura K, Kuriyama H. Features of 4-amniopyridine sensitive outward current observed in single smooth muscle cells from the rabbit pulmonary artery. *Pflugers Arch* 1987;409:561–8.

56 Animal studies of fetal maturation

N. Shinozuka

Introduction

In the field of perinatal research, we investigate a continuously growing organism that is adjusting and developing its vital functions from womb to extrauterine life.[1] In clinical terms 'the matured fetus' is a fetus that has reached a certain stage of functional growth and development, where it obtains an ability to live outside the womb alone. In a fetal physiological study, unlike in others, we must emphasize this special feature of the fetus. The following must be taken into account in fetal studies: fetal status continuously changes as pregnancy progresses. The gestational age is an important factor in development. The environment of the fetus is affected by both maternal and fetal factors. The fetus responds to the insults from outside with a variety of reactions. Glucocorticoids play an important role in development and maturation throughout the fetal life.[2–5] Thus, when we study a fetal physiological response at a certain gestational age, the result means the degree of the developmental or maturational stage of the fetus.

The respiratory, cardiovascular and neurological functions are the major functions that support life. The development of lung function was described in another section. The following issues related to studies in fetal cardiovascular and neurological maturation are outlined:

1. Animal studies in fetal physiology. Methodology using chronic animal model.
2. Animal studies in normal developmental and maturational course of cardiovascular function.
3. Chronic fetal stressed model to study fetal reaction for investigating maturation.

Animal studies in fetal physiology. Methodology using chronic animal model

For a clinician in perinatal medicine, the major concern in animal studies could be the interpretation of the results to human fetal physiology. Dynamic changes in fetal developmental course, namely maturation, have been the targets for our research.

The chronic fetal study, which is a more complicated and invasive method compared with acute model, is an essential procedure for animal experiments for investigating 'maturation'. A lot of basic research has been carried out to establish a chronic state animal model of the fetus. At the beginning of fetal physiological research, an acute fetal preparation procedure had been used.[6–8] From the 1960s, a sheep fetal preparation procedure has been applied for the chronic study model. In the 1970s and the 1980s, this methodology of fetal chronic preparation, namely 'unanesthetized fetus *in utero*',[9–12] was established as the standard procedure for investigating fetal physiology.[13–17] No objection could be raised that an ideal animal model for perinatal research purposes should be a non-human primate model, such as a baboon or a rhesus monkey. However, a non-human primate fetal study requires a lot of complicated systems such as a special cage, a tether system to connect cables and catheters for maintaining preparation, special animal care and so on, and, above all, a great deal of expense. In contrast, when we consider the availability of pregnant ewes, the total cost, ease of animal care, surgical preparation and management, the advantage of the sheep chronic experiment is clear even if the physiological difference between species is taken into account. Thus, fetal preparation using pregnant ewes has been a widely approved basic procedure for investigating fetal physiology.

The chronic preparation of the sheep fetus

The term of the fetal sheep is around 145–150 days of gestation (dGA). Birth weight at term is around 4.0–4.5 kg in the Rambouillet–Columbia sheep. Depending on the study protocol, the fetal preparation is usually done at around 100–125 dGA. The size of sheep fetus is appropriate for surgical preparation (approximately 2.0 kg at around 110 dGA).

The techniques have been described in detail elsewhere, and only a brief outline of the procedure is given in this section.[18–22]

Usually, ewes mated on only a single occasion and carrying a fetus of known gestational age are used for experiments. The gestational age is counted from the mating period and confirmed by ultrasound later. Prior to the surgery, the ewe is housed in a metabolic stall in a room with controlled light/dark cycles. Surgery is performed under halothane general anesthesia.

The uterus is exposed through a midline abdominal incision. Hysterotomy is performed and fetuses are fixed with several catheters and electrodes. The polyvinyl vascular catheters are placed via the carotid artery and jugular vein and/or femoral artery and vein. An amniotic cavity catheter is also placed. For recording fetal biophysical and neurological activities, several electrodes are attached. For recording an electrocardiogram, usually the steel electrodes are placed at the chest wall. For exploring fetal neurological activity the electorocorticogram (ECoG) electrodes using stainless wires terminating in metal pins or screws are placed bilaterally through the fetal cranial frontal bone to touch the dura mater. The ECoG signals are characteristically low voltage, low frequency and noisy bioelectric signals. To obtain high-quality ECoG signals, some techniques such as application of sealed cables (e.g., coaxial cables), placement of an indifferent and a ground electrode are required. For recording myometrial activities (uterine contraction) several wire electrodes are sewn to the myometrium. Following surgical preparation of the ewe and fetus, all fetal catheters and leads are grouped to exit the lateral abdominal wall of the ewe at a single point. Surgical closure is accomplished in layers. During and the days following surgery, antibiotics are given to the ewe and the fetus.

Maintenance

A heparin solution (10 units/ml of physiological saline) was continuously infused at a rate around 0.5 ml/h into each vascular catheter to ensure that it remained open. Fetal condition, i.e., its well-being, is usually checked by using fetal arterial blood gas data. Other fetal biophysical data such as ECoG or fetal heart rate (FHR) are also the parameters for assessing fetal well-being.

Data acquisition

The biological signals have been recorded using analog recording charts. In recent years, all data are usually recorded by means of computer-assisted data acquisition systems (DAS) that are equipped with biological amps, frequency filters, analog to top digital converters and so on. Fetal blood pressure is measured using the pressure transducer and the actual fetal pressure values are calibrated by amniotic cavity pressure. All data are stored digitally for further analysis. Sheep experiments are shown in Figures 56.1 and 56.2.

Studies in normal developmental and maturational course of cardiovascular function

The conceptual schema of fetal maturation with gestational age is shown in Figure 56.3. The degree of functional maturation must be represented as an exponential growth curve as reported for the variation in cortisol level with gestational age[4,23] (Figure 56.4). Basic research on sheep experiments suggests that the

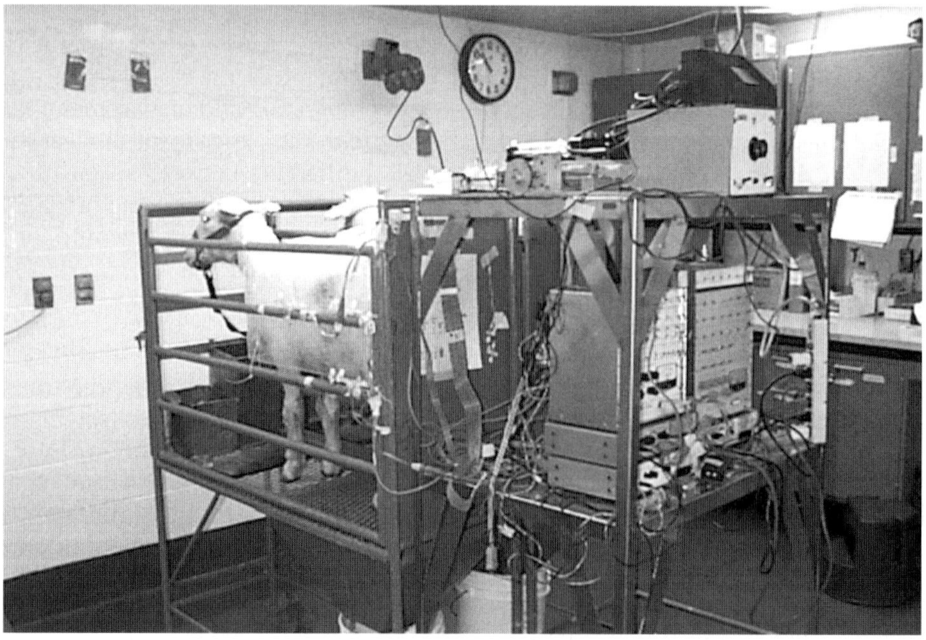

Figure 56.1 The sheep experiments. Several catheters and electrodes are fixed to the fetus.

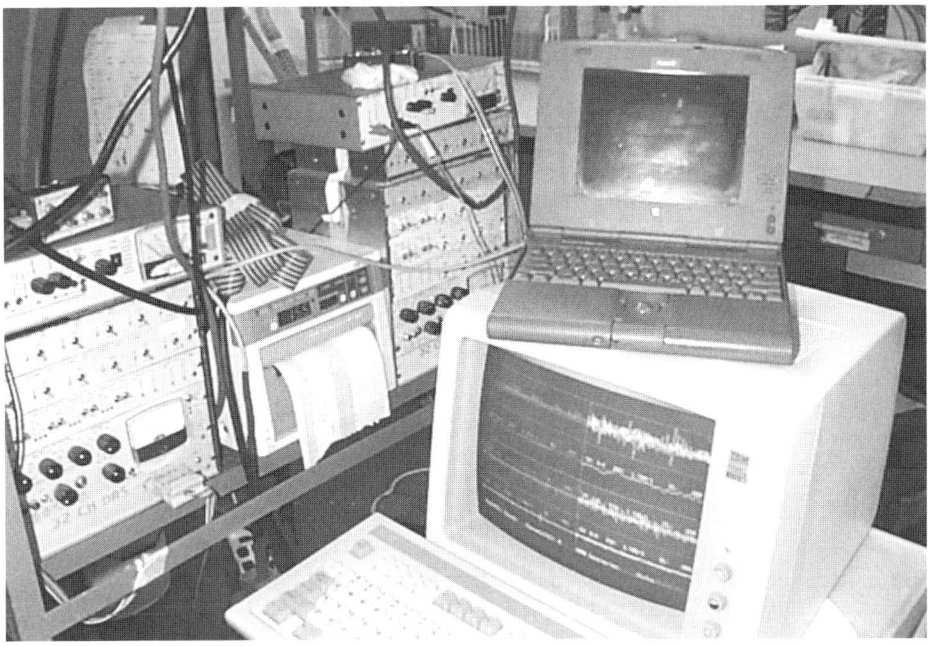

Figure 56.2 Example of a data acquisition system. The biological signals from the fetus are recorded digitally to the computer aided system for further analysis.

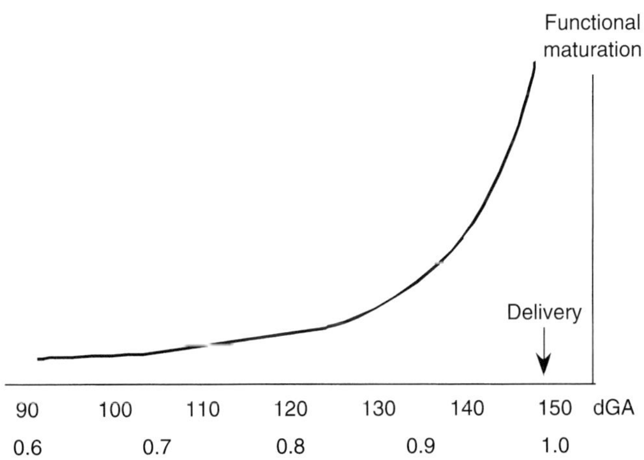

Figure 56.3 The conceptual schema of fetal maturation with gestational age. Example of sheep (term at around 145–150 dGA).

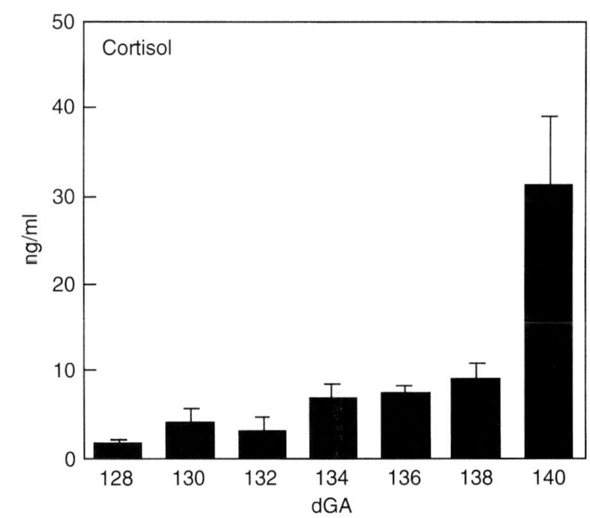

Figure 56.4 The cortisol level at fetal sheep plasma.

fetal organic maturation is accelerated around 120 dGA.[24–30] Although the developmental stage of 120 dGA, which means 80% development, does not simply translate to that of 32 weeks for the human fetus, the process of functional development and maturation should be similar.

Cardiovascular maturation

In the sheep fetus during late gestation, arterial blood pressure (BP) increases steadily and fetal heart rate (FHR) deceases steadily.[26,27,30–32] Typical changes in fetal blood pressure and heart rate with gestational age in sheep are shown in Figure 56.5. It has been assumed that the BP increase during the end of gestation is a result of both an increase in cardiac output and a rise in peripheral vascular resistance; whereas the decrease in FHR has been attributed to the baroreflex function as a result of increased BP. The baroreflex is induced by increased parasympathetic function via the vagus on basal FHR.

It has been shown that influences of sympathetic and parasympathetic activity on baseline FHR in the sheep fetus. The hormones that have stimulatory effects on the fetal cardiovascular system increase with gestational age.[26,27,30–32] The roles of the fetal endocrine, autonomic nerve system and baroreflex control on the fetal cardiovascular system have not

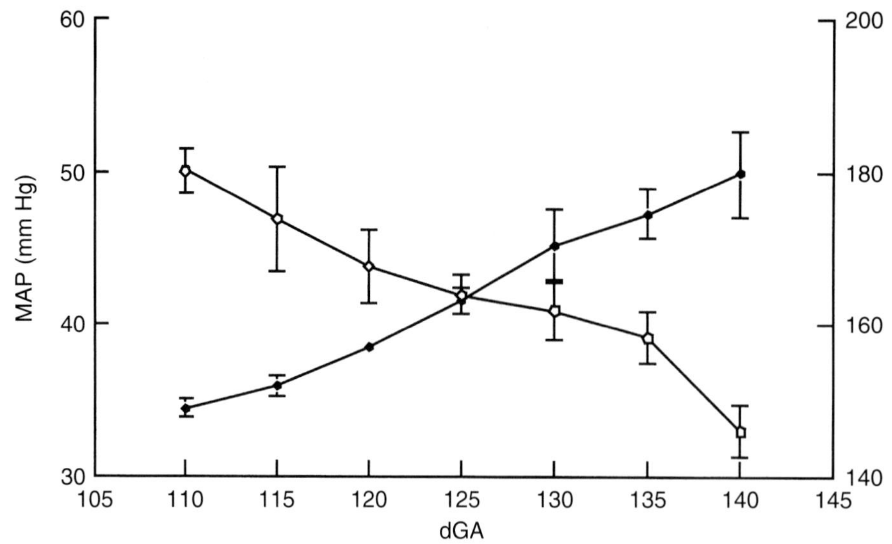

Figure 56.5 Mean fetal arterial blood pressure (MAP) and fetal heart rate (FHR). MAP increased from 110 to 140 days gestation (dGA), whereas FHR decreased steadily from 110 to 140 dGA. bpm: beats/min).

yet been characterized. In clinical medicine, FHR monitoring is an important procedure for fetal management. However, to understand the physiological meaning of FHR, we must consider the biophysical background factors, i.e., the degree of development, gestational age, intrauterine environment and so on.

Previous animal studies have reported the specification of fetal cardiovascular developments as follows: (1) Cardiac output increased in proportion to fetal gestational age and fetal weight.[33–35] (2) The cardiac output in the fetus is controlled almost solely by alteration of the heart rate.[34,36] (3) The fetal heart operates near the upper limit of the Frank–Starling curve.[37,38] (4) The fetal heart has a limited ability to change stroke volume (inotropic action).[33–35] (5) Baroreflex has been shown to operate in late gestation and plays an important role in regulating variability of arterial pressure and heart rate.[26,39] For these reasons, the ontogenic changes in baroreflex function in fetal cardiovascular maturation must be characterized. In this section, study related to the ontogenic changes in baroreflex function in fetal sheep is introduced.

Study design

1. Ontogenic changes on baroreflex function: Twenty fetal sheep were fitted with instruments and the following baroreflex protocol was carried from 110 to 140m dGA with 5-day interval.
2. Cardiovascular changes on steroid administration to the fetus: Starting at 133±1 dGA, saline (control group, CNTL) or betamethasone (Beta) was administered to the fetal jugular vein at a rate of 10 μg/h over the next 48 h. Betamethasone infusion was started at 18:00 hours. Baroreflex protocol was carried out after 40 h of Beta infusion.

Baroreflex study protocol[40,41]

Since baroreflex has been shown to play an important role during late gestation in sheep, many studies have been reported on the control of the fetal circulation. Several methods have been used for evoking the baroreflex response of the fetus. The sensitivity of the baroreflex response elicited depends on the method used. We used sodium nitroprusside (SNP) for inducing hypotension and phenylephrine (PE) for inducing hypertension. SNP is known to act as a vasodilator of both arterial and venous vessels, resulting in reduced peripheral vascular resistance and venous return.[42] PE acts as an alpha agonist that increases the force of contraction and vascular smooth muscle contraction, increases peripheral resistance and reduces heart rate by vagal reflex.[43] The baroreflex function was analyzed by adding both hypotension and hypertension trial data with the mathematical model of logistic procedure.[44] The detailed procedure is as follows:

1. Hypotension: After 1 h basal recording, SNP (10 μg/ml) was infused intravenously to the fetus at 0.1–6.4 ml/min with 2 min interval at each increment. Infusion was stopped when fetal blood pressure (FBP) had decreased by 30% or FHR fell below 100 bpm or arrhythmia appeared. Fetal arterial blood samples were taken at –5 min, end of infusion and +10 min.
2. Hypertension: After at least 1 h of recovery period from the above hypotension experiment, fetuses received PE (25 μg/ml) intravenously at 0.1–1.6 ml/min with 2 min interval at each increment, until FBP increased 30% or FHR fell below 100 bpm or arrhythmia appeared. Fetal arterial blood samples were taken at – 5 min, end of infusion and +10 min.

FBP and electrocardiogram (EKG) data were recorded with DAS at 250 Hz sampling rate. Mean

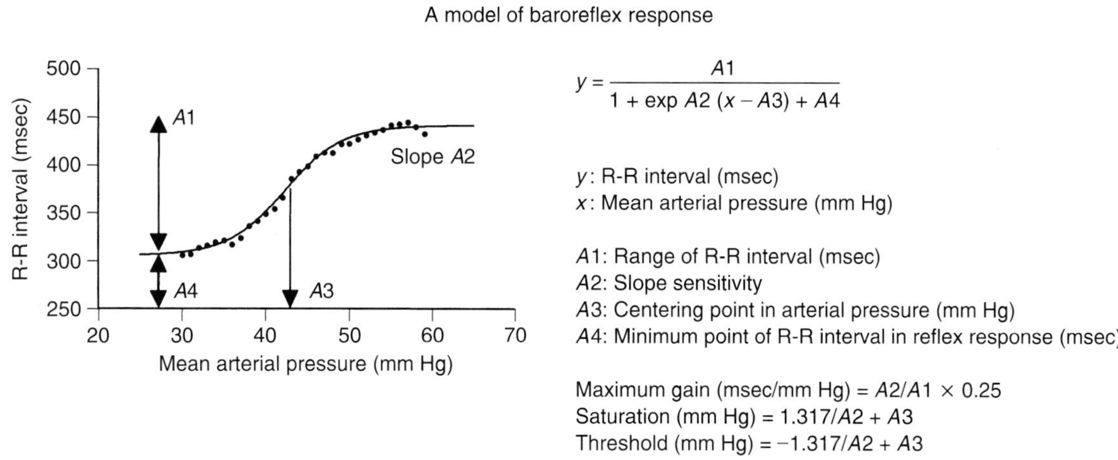

Figure 56.6 Mathematical model in analyzing baroreflex response. Using a logistic model, maximum gain, saturation and threshold are assessed as indices of baroreflex function.

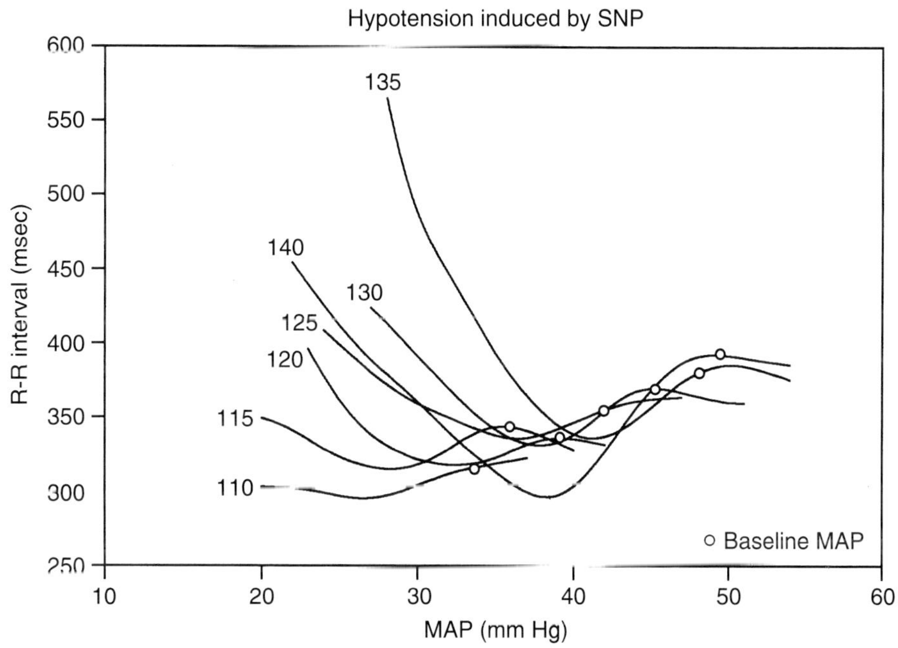

Figure 56.7 Hypotension by SNP. Open circle shows baseline (starting point). Initial reaction of SNP infusion is increase in FHR (shortening of R–R interval) against FBP fall. Compensatory tachycardia was reversed as SNP dosage increased. Then, the breakdown bradycardia caused by decreased volume in venous return and vagal activity appeared. This phenomenon of breakdown bradycardia appeared after 120 dGA and is most ominous at 135 dGA.

arterial pressure (MAP) and R–R interval from EKG signals were used for later analysis. The baroreflex function was analyzed using the logistic model shown in Figure 56.6.[44]

Ontogenic changes in baroreflex function

Hypotension induced by SNP

An initial baroreflex action during hypotension induced by SNP was to increase FHR (shortening of R–R interval) against dropping FBP due to vasodilatation. Increase in FHR by FBP fall is a sympathetic activity.

Compensatory tachycardia was reversed as SNP dosage increased. This phenomenon is not clear until 115 dGA, is distinguished at 120 dGA and is most ominous at 135 dGA. This breakdown bradycardia is assumed to be caused by decreased volume in venous return and vagal activity. The difference in response to SNP infusion at each gestational age suggests a developmental degree and a balance between sympathetic and parasympathetic control of cardiac function. However, since cardiac output is defined by stroke volume and heart rate, the factor of inotropic function, even if it is limited, must be taken into consideration. The significant difference in response between 135 and 145 dGA must be caused by the inotropic function. Moreover, this result suggests that 135 dGA is the most critical period of baroreflex development. The vagal reflex is most sensitive and the breakdown bradycardia is easily induced (Figure 56.7).

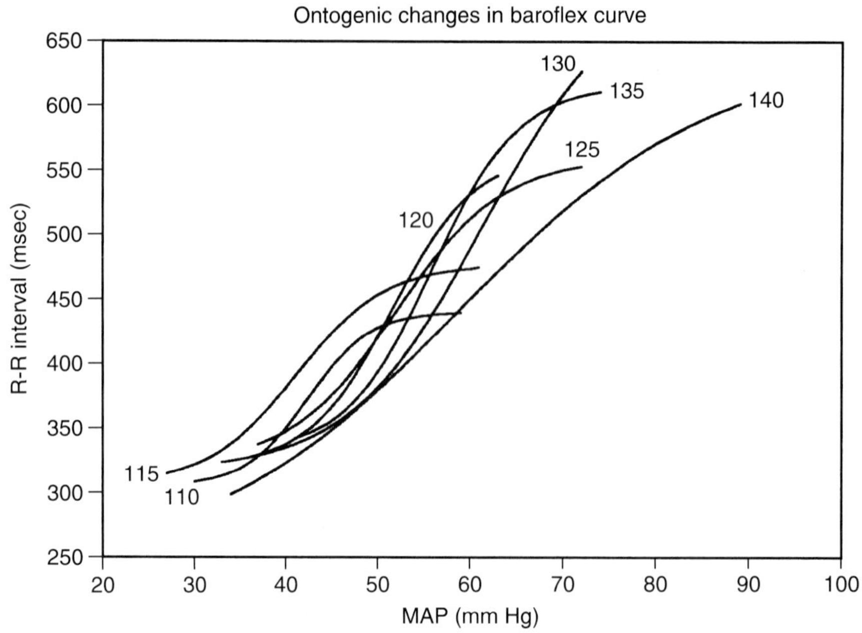

Figure 56.8 Ontogenic changes in baroreflex curve. The apparent difference in range and slope of baroreflex curves at each gestational age is found.

Hypertension induced by PE

During PE-induced hypertension trial, R–R interval increased linearly according to FBP rise. PE acts mainly as an alpha agonist, and heart rate fall is induced by vagal reflex. The difference in baroreflex slope might be a result of the activity and sensitivity in pressure of the vagal function. Significantly higher FBP achieved against similar FHR at slope saturation during late gestation suggests the development of cardiac contractility function and this must also be considered.

Analysis of baroreflex function (ontogenic study)

The baroreflex curve was studied using the data obtained from SNP-induced hypotension and PE-induced hypertension (Figure 56.8). When we look at the speculation in range and slope of baroreflex curves at each gestational age, the character of maturational course is clear. A summary of the developmental changes in baroreflex function are shown in Figure 56.9. Two critical points at 115–120 and 135–140 dGA were distinguished in baroreflex development. Significant changes in maximum gain were observed at 135–140 dGA, in saturation at both 115–120 and 135–140 dGA, and in thresholds at 115–120 dGA. As stated above, these critical points at maturational course might be caused by the degree of developmental activity, sensitivity, and balance between sympathetic and parasympathetic nerves, peripheral vessel activity, as well as the inotropic action (contractility of the heart).

Effect of gulcocorticoids on cardiovascular function

Previous studies showed that glucocorticoid administration to the sheep fetus increases both FBP and femoral vascular resistance. However, precise effects of cardiovascular baroreflex response to glucocorticoids have not yet been clarified. An example of studies on betamethasone effect on the fetal baroreflex function at 135 dGA is shown.

FBP and FHR changes on betamethasone infusion

FBP showed a constant increase after betamethasone (Beta) infusion to the fetuses. In the Beta group, FBP was statistically higher after 7 h of infusion compared with the baseline FBP of the past 24 h before infusion. FBP was also statistically higher in the Beta group after 8 h of infusion compared with the control (CNTL) group. In contrast to the fetuses in CNTL, which showed nominal 24 h variation in FHR, Beta fetuses showed significant decrease in FHR after betemethasone infusion. FHR fall in Beta fetuses from 5 to 9 h after infusion was significant compared to the baseline FHR of the past 24 h before infusion. FHR from 5 to 12 h after infusion in Beta fetuses was significantly lower compared with CNTL fetuses (Figure 56.10). After 12 h of infusion, FHR in Beta fetuses gradually recovered to the baseline FHR level. No statistical difference was found after 24 h of infusion between Beta and CNTL fetuses.

Baroreflex function at 40 h after Beta administration

Beta fetuses showed a much wider range of FBP change with relatively narrower range of FHR change. Namely, the baroreflex curve shifted to the right and the handling range was expanded. All parameters of baroreflex function were significantly altered by betamethasone (Figure 56.11).

Recent studies have reported an elevation of FBP after infusion of glucocorticoids directly to the

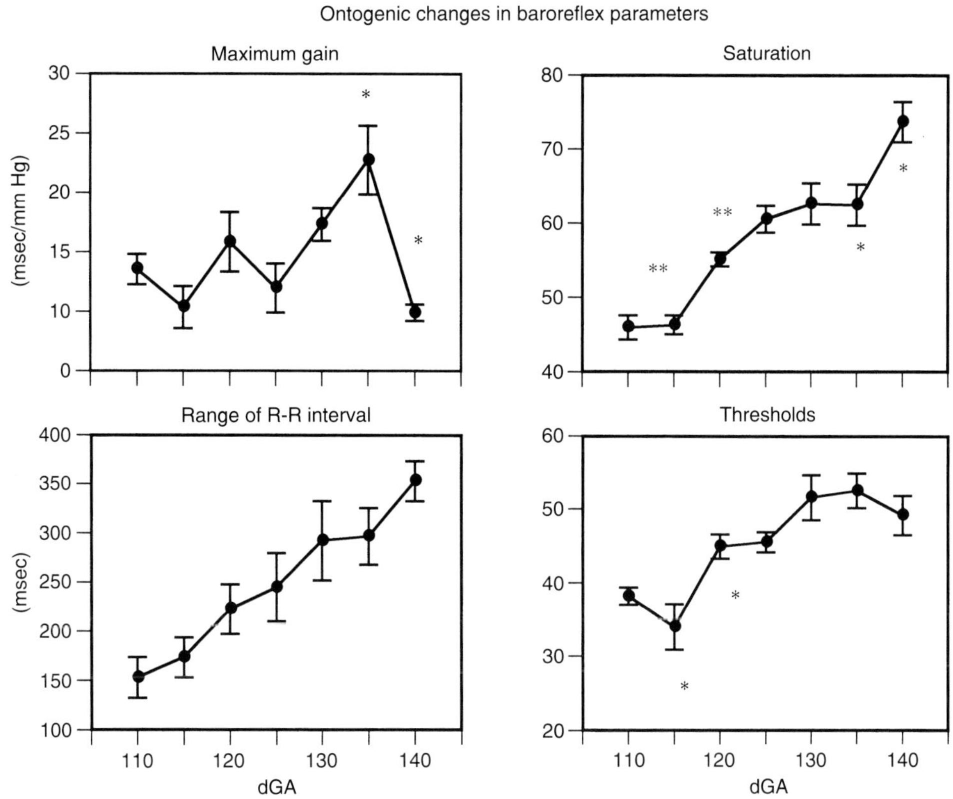

Figure 56.9 Summary of ontogenic changes in baroreflex function. Two critical points of 115–120 and 135–140 dGA were found in baroreflex development. Significant changes in max gain at 135–140 dGA, in saturation at both 115–120 and 135–140 dGA, and thresholds at 115–120 dGA. ** Difference at saturation figure. $*p<0.05$.

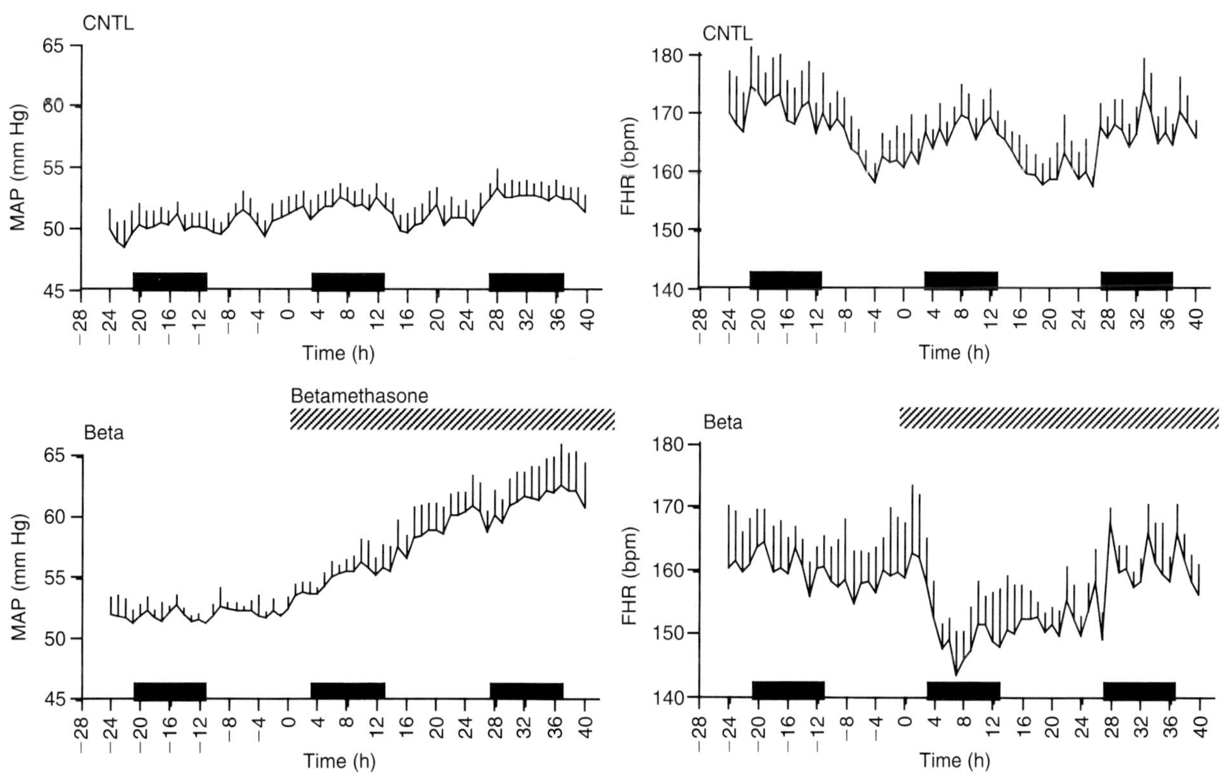

Figure 56.10 Changes in MAP and FBP by betamethasone administration on fetus. Starting at 133±1 dGA, saline (control group: CNTL) or betamethasone (Beta,) was administered to the fetal vein at a rate of 10 µg/h over the next 48 h. Hourly fetal blood pressure (FBP), fetal heat rate (FHR) in the control group (CNTL) and betamethasone-treated (Beta) fetuses. Values shown are means ± SEM for every hour. Time 0 was settled at the beginning of vehicle or betamethasone infusion. Filled bar represents hours of darkness (21:00–07:00 hours). Shadowed bar represents the infusion periods.

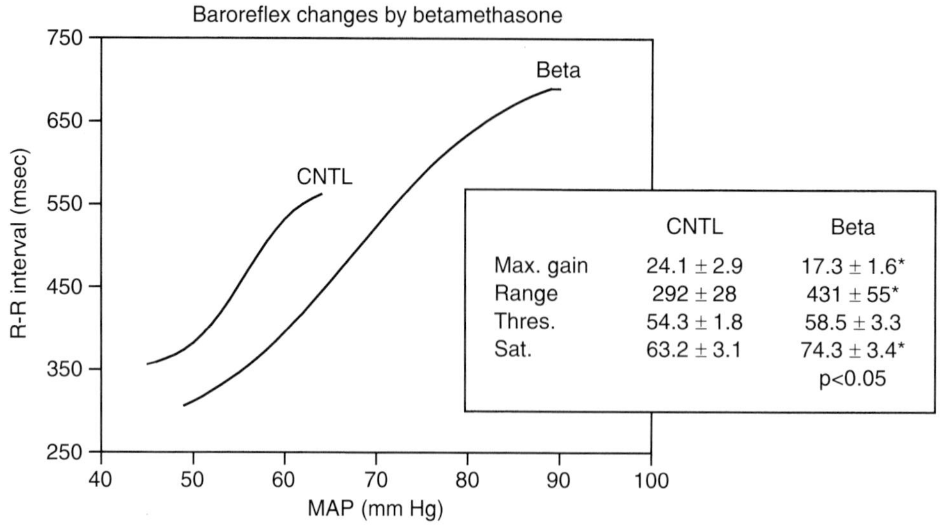

Figure 56.11 Baroreflex changes by betamethasone. Significant changes in each parameters of baroreflex function are found. The curve shifted to the right and expanded the range of handling.

fetus.[45–49] The mechanisms producing an increase in FBP during betamethasone infusion have been discussed in terms of mediation of an increase in fetal total peripheral vascular resistance and/or fetal cardiac output.[45–49]

Betamethasone may accelerate fetal cardiovascular maturation. Chronological FHR changes in Beta fetuses suggest that there are at least two steps of process ware involved in cardiovascular alterations induced by betamethasone. Initial cardiovascular response to increased FBP and significant decrease in FHR in the first 12 h of betamethasone infusion might be caused by basic baroreflex response to the rise in FBP. The second step of FHR recovery against FBP rise may be mainly caused by resetting of the baroreflex response including sympathetic and parasympathetic autonomic nervous activity. In addition, at this stage, changes in cardiac output by betamethasone must be taken into account. The newborn lamb's heart has the ability to alter the inotropic state. Thus, near-term fetus must have the ability to use inotropic action of the heart, even if it is limited, and the magnitude of the inotropic ability would indicate the degree of maturation of the fetal heart function. Another study using betamethasone-treated fetuses showed that fetal femoral blood flow and femoral vascular resistance tend to recover at the end of 48 h after betamethasone infusion.[46–49] Therefore, the second step cardiovascular alteration is also mediated by betamethasone administration to the fetuses.

The above results suggest that there are several important periods of gestational age in the course of cardiovascular maturation and that the process of maturation is mediated and modified by glucocorticoids. One of the major current concepts of programming cardiovascular system states that the precise timing and sequence of maturational events during fetal life are fundamental to normal development.

Chronic fetal stressed model to study fetal reaction for investigating maturation

From a clinical viewpoint, the major interest in fetal physiology has been fetal hypoxia. A lot of studies have been carried out to clarify the variety of reactions of the fetus to acute hypoxia insult *in utero*. Much knowledge related to biophysical background in perinatal medicine such as deceleration in heart rate monitoring, behavioral state alterations and so on have been obtained from animal experiments. Recent epidemiological studies, as Baker stated,[68–70] indicate that an adverse intrauterine environment affects fetal physiological development and may be the origin of later disease. Hence much attention has been focused on the fetal environment in the womb. Do the chronic changes in environment, in other words, the chronic stress to the fetus really alter the fetal maturational course and beyond? Restricted maternal nutrition has been shown to have an apparent effect on fetal cardiovascular function. Animal studies in rats and sheep have demonstrated hypertensive offspring induced by maternal nutrient restriction and differences in fetal growth were associated with changes in cardiovascular control.

Several chronic stressed fetal models have been reported. As an altered fetal environment model, prolonged hypoxia in chronic sheep studies[50–55] has demonstrated long- and short-term effects on fetal cardiovascular function. A long-term fetal placental embolization model[56–58] has demonstrated that umbilical blood flow and heart rate pattern alterations cause hypertension and myocardial hypertrophy. A repeated cord occlusion model[59,60] has reported the response alteration in hormonal and cardiovascular

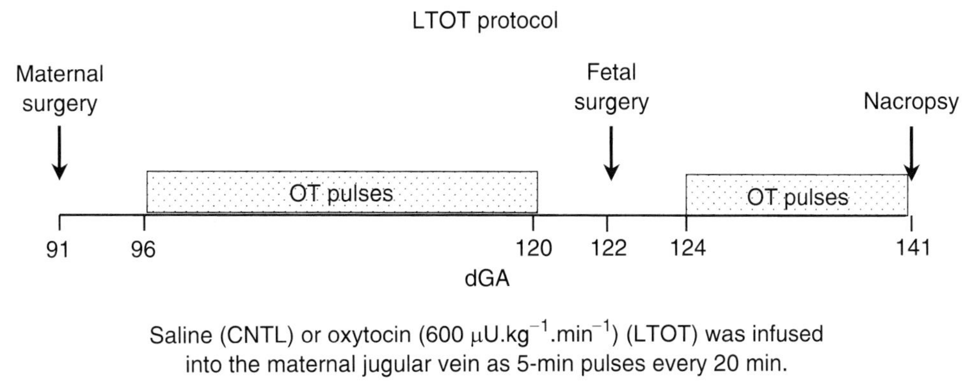

Figure 56.12 LTOT protocol. Ewes received ether saline (control group: CNTL) or oxytocin (600 μU/kg/min; long-term oxytocin group: LTOT) infusions into maternal jugular vein at 0.033 ml/min as 5-min pulses starting at 96 dGA. Oxytocin pulse infusion was stopped 1 day before fetal surgery and recommenced 2 days after fetal surgery.

responses. However, a few studies have been reported related to the experimental model of long-term environmental alteration/stress to the fetus.

In this section we introduce a long-term light stressed fetal model by means of increased uterine activity of oxytocin (LTOT model).

LTOT model[41,61–63]

Myometrial contractures are characterized by long-lasting low amplitude myometrial contractility occurring throughout pregnancy in sheep. Contractures induce a fall in fetal arterial oxygen pressure (PO_2), a decrease in uterine blood flow, and also produce mechanical stress to the fetus by compression. A previous study has shown that oxytocin (OT) induced contractures in late gestation sheep altered fetal pituitary-adrenal[61,62] functions and might accelerate neurological development as revealed by the ECoG voltage amplitude.[64,65] Since fetal hypothalamic-pituitary-adrenal axis plays an important role in ovine parturition, this kind of neuroendocrine alteration by increased myometrial contractures should be associated with alteration of physiologic function. We hypothesized that long-term increased myometrial contracture frequency, namely long-term frequent light stress to the fetus, would alter fetal physiological development and fetal responses to acute stress episodes. We therefore exposed pregnant sheep with repeated pulses of oxytocin from 96 to 131 dGA. OT dose did not cross the ovine placenta, therefore no direct effects of OT on the fetus are responsible for any fetal changes.[66]

The LTOT protocol is shown in Figure 56.12. Ewes received ether saline (control group: CNTL), or oxytocin (600 μU/kg/min; long-term oxytocin group: LTOT) infusions into the maternal jugular vein at 0.033 ml/min as 5 min pulses starting at 96 dGA. Oxytocin pulse infusion was stopped 1 day before fetal surgery and recommenced 2 days after fetal surgery. By this procedure of oxytocin pulses, myometrial contracture frequency increased by slightly over 100% ewes in LTOT compared with CNTL ewes (Table 56.1).

Table 56.1 Effect of oxytocin pulses (LTOT) or vehicle control (CNTL) on the number of contractures per hour

	CNTL	LTOT
126–130 dGA	1.35±0.13*	3.34±0.06*
131–135 dGA	1.45±0.09*	3.21±0.07*
136–140 dGA	1.52±0.13*	3.13±0.06*

Contracture frequency was counted every day and averaged in each animal to obtain representative values for each period.

Mean±SEM, * $p<0.01$.

Using the LTOT model, the following issues were studied:

1. Hormonal environment (cortisol and ACTH)
2. Blood and arterial blood gas environment
3. Response to acute fetal hypoxemia (1 h) induced by administering nitrogen to the ewe through 131±1 dGA
4. Ontogenic cardiovascular changes and baroreflex alteration
5. Behavioral alterations

Hormonal environment

Basal fetal plasma ACTH and cortisol values obtained during the study period are presented in Figure 56.13. There were no significant differences in ACTH and cortisol values between CNTL and LTOT. However, cortisol/ACTH ratios (ng/pg) were significantly lower in LTOT at 128–132 dGA (CNTL, 0.13±0.02, 0.24±0.09, 0.21±0.08; LTOT, 0.06±0.03, 0.08±0.04, 0.08±0.04). Cortisol is higher at 140 dGA in both CNTL and LTOT groups.

Blood and arterial blood gas environment

Fetal arterial blood gas values are summarized in Table 56.2. PO_2 was lower in LTOT at 126–135 dGA and O_2 content was higher in LTOT at 131–140 dGA.

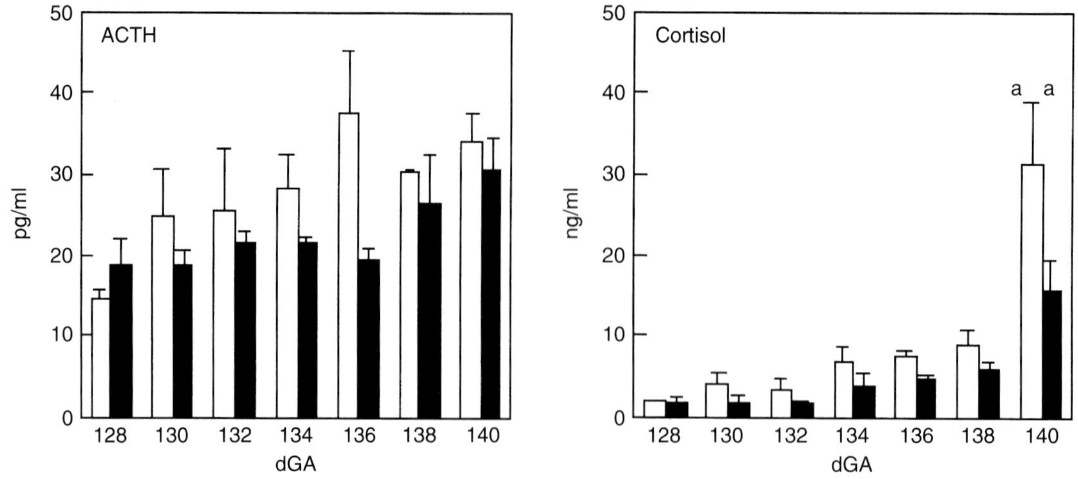

Figure 56.13 Fetal plasma ACTH and cortisol concentrations in CNTL (□) and LTOT (■). Mean ± SEM, a: $p < 0.05$ compared with 128–138 dGA.

Table 56.2 Arterial blood gas values of CNTL and LTOT during study period

		CNTL	LTOT
126–130 dGA	pH	7.36±0.001	7.36±0.001
	PCO_2 (mmHg)	47.3±0.23	48.6±0.09
	PO_2 (mmHg)	24.3±0.09*	22.4±0.17*
	Hb (μg/dl)	10.8±0.07	11.1±0.07
	O_2 sat. (%)	64.5±0.33	62.9±0.37
	O_2 content (ml/dl)	9.3±0.05	9.5±0.05
131–135 dGA	pH	7.35±0.001	7.35±0.001
	PCO_2 (mmHg)	47.5±0.23	49.9±0.09
	PO_2 (mmHg)	22.4±0.09*	20.6±0.18*
	Hb (μg/dl)	11.3±0.07	12.2±0.07
	O_2 sat. (%)	57.2±0.33	59.2±0.38
	O_2 content (ml/dl)	8.6±0.05*	9.8±0.05*
136–140 dGA	pH	7.34±0.001	7.35±0.001
	PCO_2 (mmHg)	48.7±0.28	48.5±0.16
	PO_2 (mmHg)	20.9±0.06	20.1±0.21
	Hb (μg/dl)	12.6±0.07	13.1±0.12
	O_2 sat. (%)	52.7±0.49	55±0.34
	O_2 content (ml/dl)	8.7±0.07*	9.6±0.05*

Blood samples were taken at 9:00–10:00 every day. Data were averaged in each animal to obtain representative values for each period. Mean ± SEM, *$p < 0.05$ CNTL vs. LTOT.

Response to acute fetal hypoxemia

Acute fetal hypoxemia insult was induced at 131 ± 1 dGA by administering nitrogen to the ewe through a tracheal tube for 1 h, beginning at the start of oxytocin or saline pulse. Maternal and fetal arterial blood samples (0.5 ml) were taken at −60, −15, −5, 5, 10, 20, 30, 40, 60 and 120 min. Blood samples were measured using a blood gas analyzer. Oxygen saturation (%) and hemoglobin (μg/dl) were measured with a hemoximeter. O_2 content (ml/dl) was calculated from the hemoglobin (Hb), O_2 saturation and PO_2 values.

Fetal PO_2 was significantly lower and O_2 content was significantly higher in LTOT at baseline. No difference was found in maternal blood gas and pH values at baseline (Table 56.3). At the end of 60 min hypoxemia, fetal pH, O_2 saturation, O_2 content were significantly higher in LTOT, although PO_2 did not differ between the two groups (Table 56.4). At 120 min (60 min after acute hypoxemia insult), blood gas values in both groups returned to normal value and no difference was found between the two groups (Table 56.5).

Table 56.3 Baseline fetal and maternal blood gas data (mean±SD)

	CNTL	LTOT	
Fetus			
pH	7.359±0.015	7.363±0.014	N.S.
PCO_2 (mmHg)	47.4±5.6	48.8±4.2	N.S.
PO_2 (mmHg)	23.6±2.8	21.8±2.3	$p<0.05$
Hb (g/dl)	11.3±1.3	12.0±1.5	N.S.
Sat O_2 (%)	60.0±6.5	60.2±5.4	N.S.
O_2 content (ml/dl)	8.9±0.8	9.8±1.2	$p<0.05$
Mother			
pH	7.476±0.026	7.465±0.021	N.S.
PCO_2 (mmHg)	34.8±3.5	33.8±4.4	N.S.
PO_2 (mmHg)	108.5±12.8	117.4±11.2	N.S.
Hb (g/dl)	10.4±1.8	9.8±1.2	N.S.
Sat O_2 (%)	96.6±2.3	97.7±2.4	N.S.
O_2 content (ml/dl)	13.7±2.2	12.8±1.6	N.S.

Table 56.4 Fetal blood gas data at the end of 60 min acute hypoxemia (mean±SD)

Fetus	CNTL	LTOT	
pH	7.355±0.029	7.384±0.006	$p<0.05$
PCO_2 (mmHg)	42.3±1.3	42.2±3.1	N.S.
PO_2 (mmHg)	14.1±1.0	14.3±2.8	N.S.
Hb (g/dl)	11.7 ±1.5	11.3±2.1	N.S.
Sat. O_2 (%)	29.4±3.8	38.7±7.2	$p<0.05$
O_2 content (ml/dl)	4.6±0.7	5.8±1.1	$p<0.05$

Table 56.5 Fetal blood gas data at 120 min (60 min after acute hypoxemia insult) (mean ± SD)

Fetus	CNTL	LTOT	
pH	7.355±0.018	7.372±0.012	N.S.
PCO_2 (mmHg)	47.6±2.6	46.6±1.8	N.S.
PO_2 (mmHg)	21.1±2.8	20.8±2.3	N.S.
Hb (g/dl)	11.0±0.7	112±1.1	N.S.
Sat. O_2 (%)	55.4±10.5	58.0±6.4	N.S.
O_2 content (ml/dl)	8.2±1.5	8.8±1.2	N.S.
O_2 content (ml/dl)	8.2±1.5	8.8±1.2	N.S.

Relationship between maternal and fetal PO_2 and O_2 content showed lower PO_2 but higher O_2 content at the same maternal oxygen delivery in LTOT. Linear model analysis showed statistically significant LTOT effect ($p < 0.001$; Figure 56.14).

O_2 content at PO_2 was significantly higher in LTOT and O_2 saturation at PO_2, which expressed an O_2 dissociation curve, was obviously shifted to the left in LTOT (Figure 56.15). Linear model analysis proved that the model of the same slope with different intercepts – whether or not of LTOT – was the best fitting model and the effect of LTOT was statistically significant ($p < 0.001$).

During hypoxemia and recovery period, fetal pH tended to shift higher and its variability was less in LTOT compared with CNTL (pH variability expressed as coefficient of variation (CV): CNTL, 0.33±0.15; LTOT, 0.12±0.06, mean±SD, $p<0.05$) (Figure 56.16).

Ontogenic cadiovascular changes and baroreflex alteration

FBP was significantly higher from 126 to 128 dGA in the fetuses of LTOT ewes compared with the fetuses of CNTL. FHR was significantly lower in the fetuses of LTOT from 126 to 131 dGA (Figure 56.17). The slope of daily FBP changes (CNTL, 0.76±0.21; LTOT, 0.27±

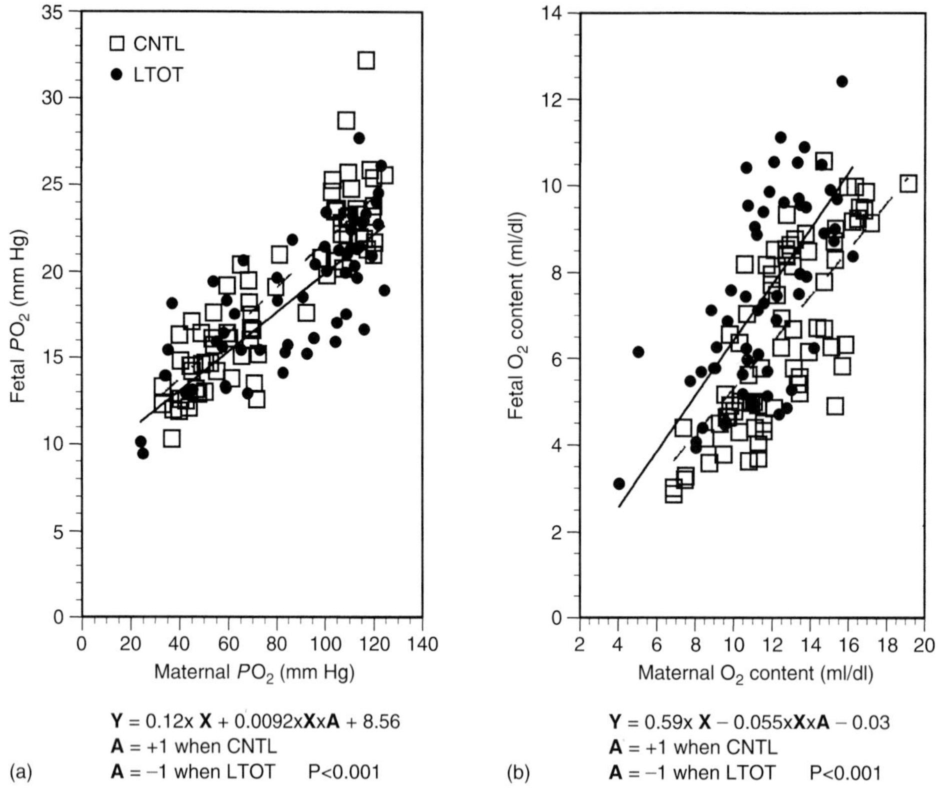

Figure 56.14 Fetal and maternal PO_2 (A) fetal and maternal O_2 content (B) before and during hypoxemia. □ CNTL; ● LTOT. (a) $Y = 0.12 \times X + 0.0092 \times X \times Z + 8.56$ (CNTL $Z = +1$: dashed line, LTOT $Z = -1$: straight line, $p < 0.001$). (b) $Y = 0.59 \times X - 0.055 \times X \times Z - 0.03$ (CNTL $Z = +1$: dashed line; LTOT $Z = -1$: straight line; $P < 0.001$).

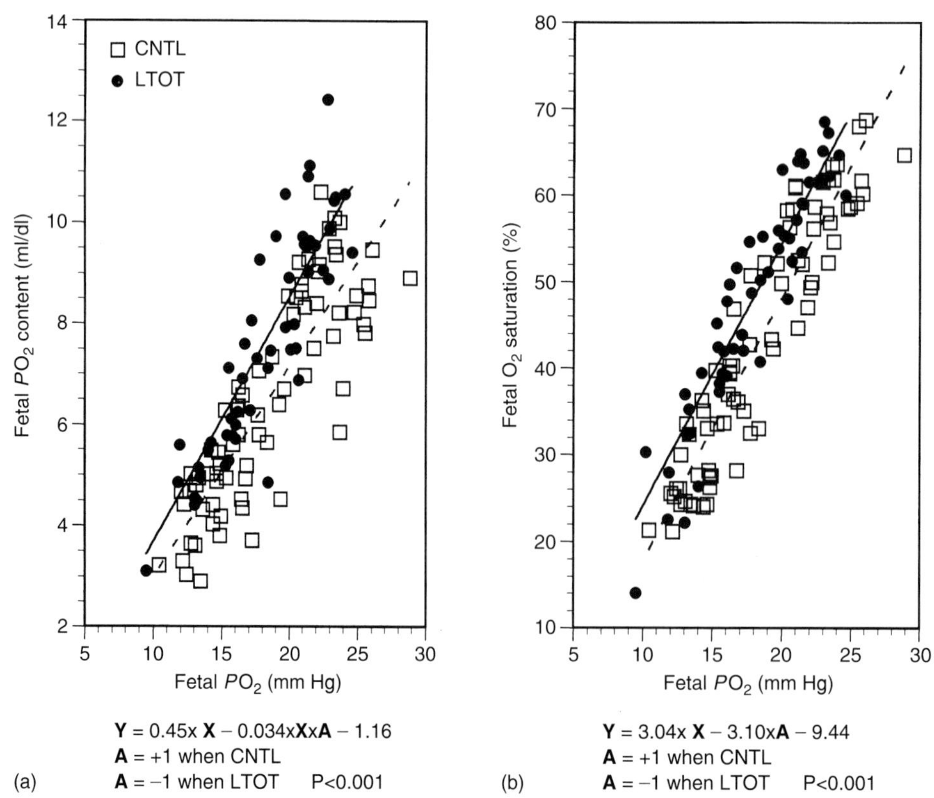

Figure 56.15 Fetal O_2 saturation (a) and fetal O_2 content (b) in relation to fetal PO_2 before and during hypoxemia. □ CNTL; ● LTOT. (a) $Y = 3.04 \times X - 3.10 \times Z - 9.44$ (CNTL $Z = +1$: dashed line; LTOT $Z = -1$: straight line; $p < 0.001$). (b) $Y = 0.45 \times X - 0.034 \times X \times Z - 1.16$ (CNTL $Z = +1$: dashed line; LTOT $Z = -1$: straight line; $p < 0.001$).

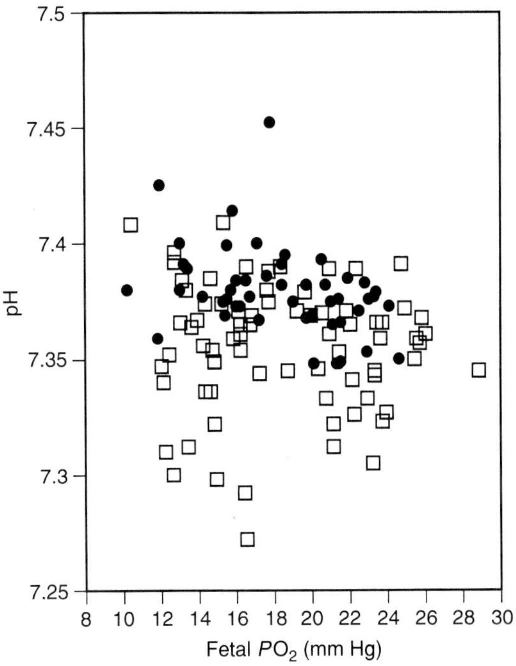

Figure 56.16 Fetal pH values before and during acute hypoxemia. □ CNTL; ● LTOT.

0.06 mmHg/dGA) and FHR (CNTL, −1.91±0.20; LTOT, −0.70±0.41 bpm/dGA) was significantly lower in LTOT (Figure 56.18).

There was no difference in the fall in FBP at the end of SNP infusion. FBP dropped by 31–37%. However, total SNP dosage (adjusted by fetal weight) required to produce this fall in FBP was significantly higher in LTOT (CNTL, 21.1±3.7; LTOT, 34.7±4.6 μg/kg). Initially, the fetus tries to compensate for the fall in FBP by increasing the FHR. In contrast, CNTL fetuses tend to show early breakdown of compensatory reaction and fall into bradycadia. The breakdown point to fall into bradycardia was significantly different between CNTL and LTOT (CNTL, 41.6±0.6bpm, 328±10 ms; LTOT, 38.7±1.4 bpm, 328±16 msec) (Figure 56.18). PO_2 and O_2 saturation values were significantly lower at the end of SNP infusion in CNTL. No difference was found in blood gas during the experiment in LTOT fetuses (Table 56.6). ACTH and cortisol responses to hypotension showed attenuated response (Figure 56.19). However, no differences were found in cortisol/ACTH ratios (ng/pg) between CNTL and LTOT groups.

The baroreflex curve was shifted to the right and showed a mature pattern in LTOT fetuses. Maximum gain (ms/mmHg) was significantly different between CNTL and LTOT (CNTL, 24.4±2.7; LTOT, 16.6±2.3) (Figure 56.20).

Behavioral alterations

ECoG has been used for analyzing fetal neurological activity. Examples of analog ECoG recording are shown in Figure 56.21. ECoG activity represents basic

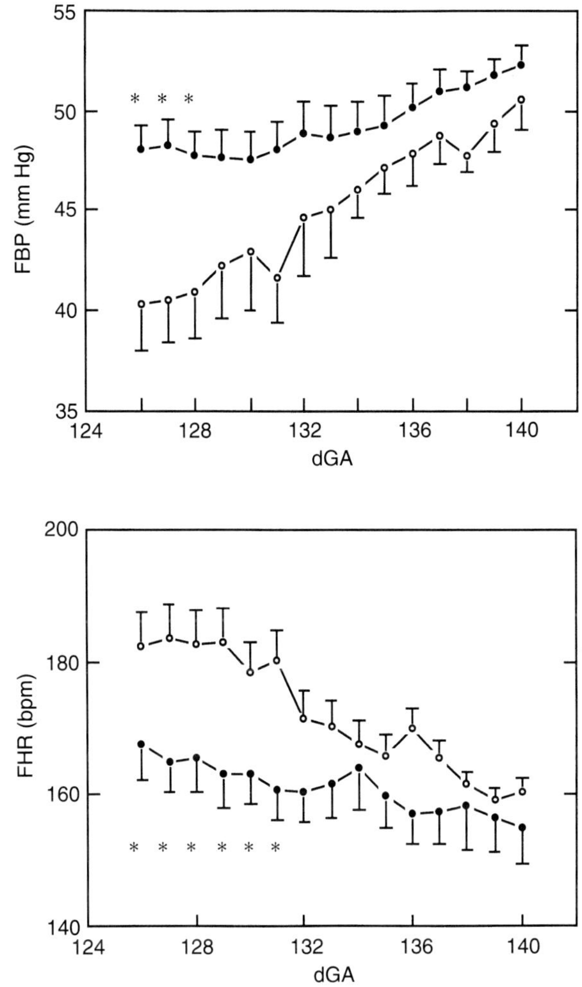

Figure 56.17 Ontogenic changes in FBP and FHR in CNTL and LTOT. CNTL (○) and LTOR (●), mean ± SEM; $p < 0.05$ compared with CNTL.

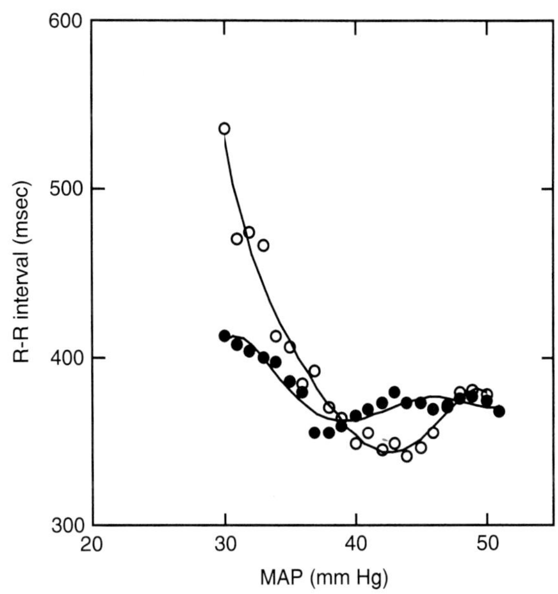

Figure 56.18 Hypotension by SNP. The breakdown point to fall into bradycardia was significantly different between CNTL and LTOT iCNTL, 41.6 ± 0.6 bpm, 328 ± 10 ms; LTOT, 38.7 ± 1.4 bpm, 328 ± 16 ms LTOT fetus showed resistive reaction to hypotension insults.

Table 56.6 Arterial blood gas values of CNTL and LTOT during SNP-induced hypotension

		CNTL	LTOT
Baseline (–5 min)	pH	7.34±0.002	7.33±0.01
	PCO_2 (mmHg)	48.4±3.4	49.2±1.1
	PO_2 (mmHg)	22.6±1.4	21.1±1.9
	Hb (μg/dl)	12.0±0.5	12.6±0.8
	O_2 sat. (%)	58.7±3.2	57.9±4.4
	O_2 content (ml/dl)	9.4±0.3	9.5±0.5
End of infusion	pH	7.34±0.005	7.34±0.01
	PCO_2 (mmHg)	50.9±0.8	50.5±1.2
	PO_2 (mmHg)	18.9±1.3*	21.2±2.0
	Hb (μg/dl)	12.1±1.1	12.8±1.2
	O_2 sat. (%)	46.3±2.3	49.6±5.3
	O_2 content (ml/dl)	7.59±0.9*	8.3±0.7
+10 min	pH	7.34±0.003	7.34±0.01
	PCO_2 (mmHg)	50.1±0.5	47.0±1.4
	PO_2 (mmHg)	21.1±1.5	22.9±2.0
	Hb (μg/dl)	12.3±1.1	12.3±0.9
	O_2 sat (%)	54.1±4.6	55.4±6.2
	O_2 content (ml/dl)	8.8±0.6	8.9±0.7

Mean±SEM, * $p<0.05$ compared with baseline (–5 min).

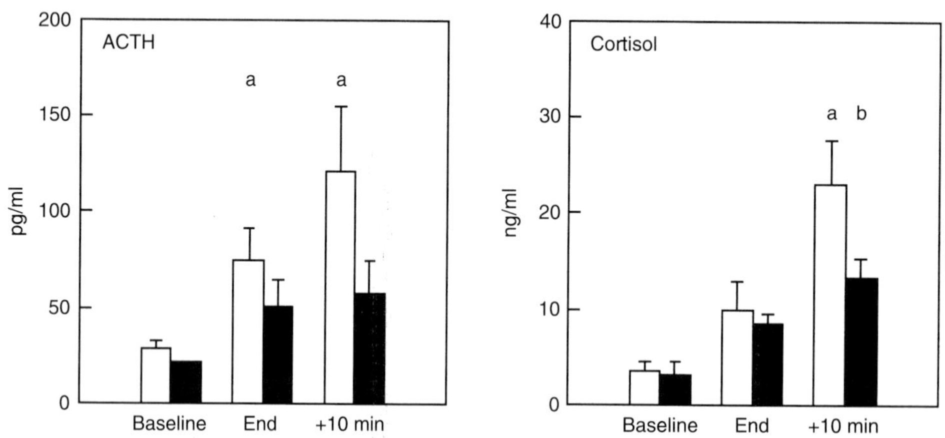

Figure 56.19 ACTH and cortisol response during SNP infusion. CNTL (□) and LTOT (■). Mean ± SEM; (a) $p < 0.05$ compared with base line; (b) $p < 0.05$ CNTL vs. LTOT.

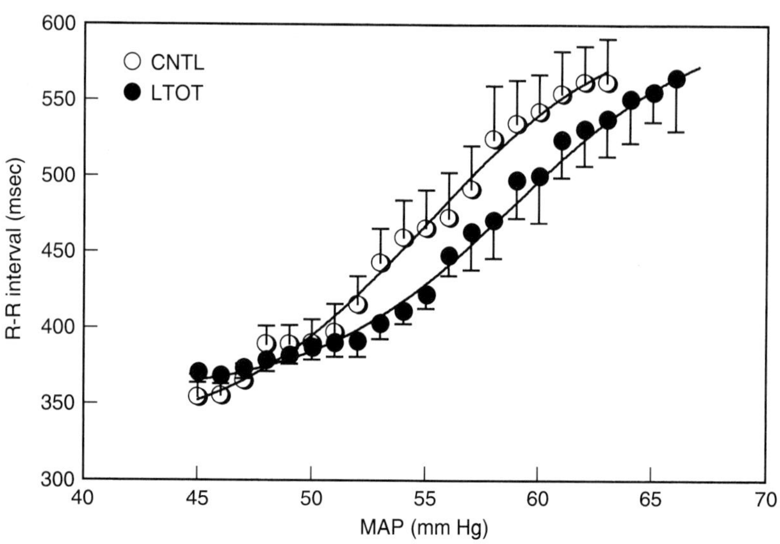

Figure 56.20 Baroreflex alteration by LTOT. Baroreflex curve was shifted to the right and showed mature pattern in LTOT fetuses.

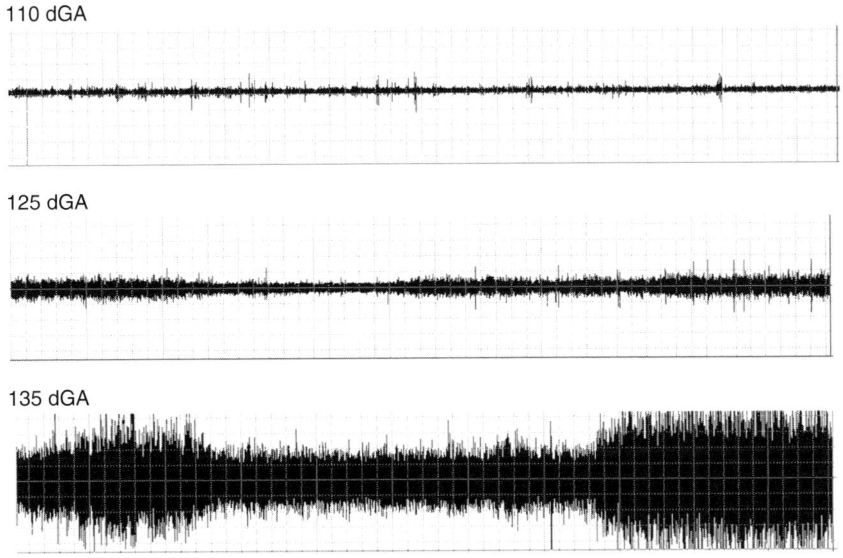

Figure 56.21 Typical ECoG recording at 110, 125 and 135 dGA.

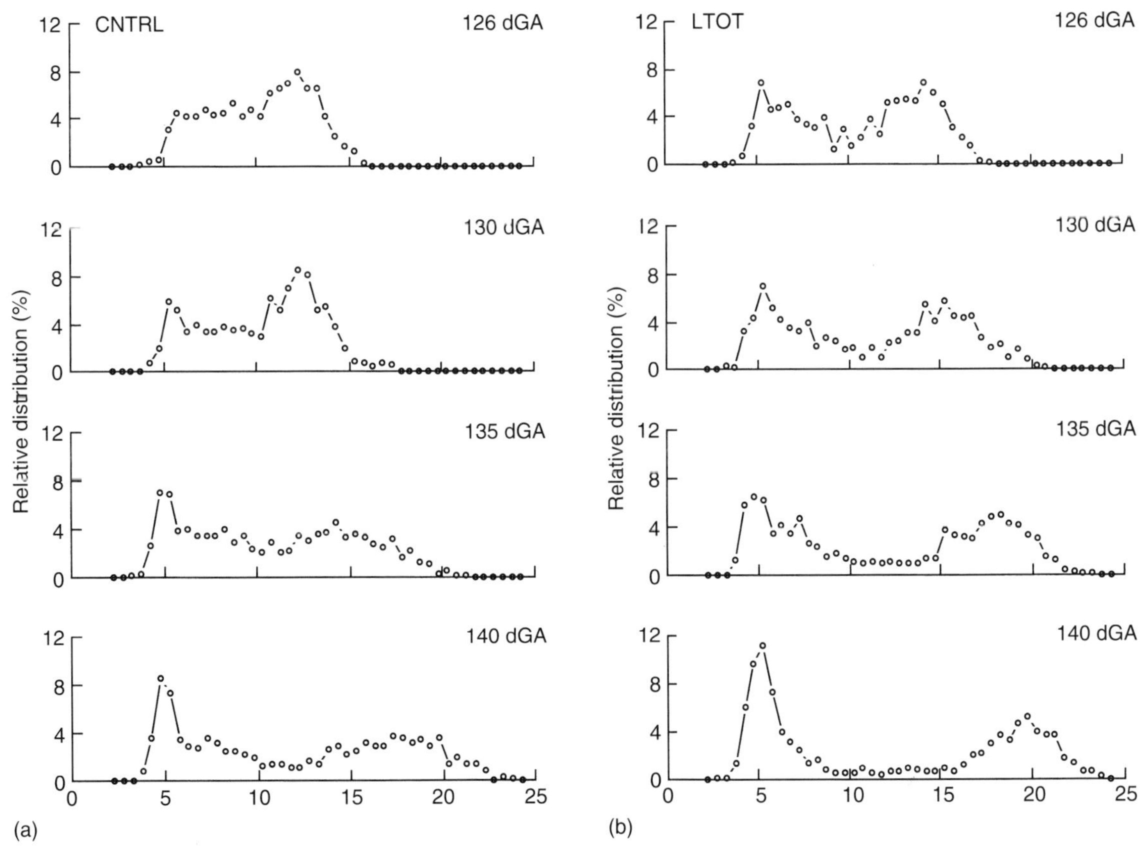

Figure 56.22 ECoG spectral edge frequency at each gestational age. ECoG power spectra analysis by calculation spectral edge frequency distribution showed apparent distinction between low- and high-frequency peaks in LTOT (Figure 56.2). In LTOT, high spectral edge frequency was statistically higher in LTOT at 126–140 dGA and low frequency was statistically lower at 126 and 130 dGA. Difference of the HV and LV peaks.

behavioral rhythm; little is known about diurnal variation of ECoG pattern. Characteristic ECoG patterns have been discussed with alternation between low-voltage fast-activity (LV) state and high-voltage slow-activity (HV) state. As pregnancy progresses the amplitude increases and the difference between the HV and LV states becomes clear.

The ECoG characteristic changes were analyzed by means of ECoG power spectral distribution analysis. Three-hour raw ECoG data sampled at 250 Hz were

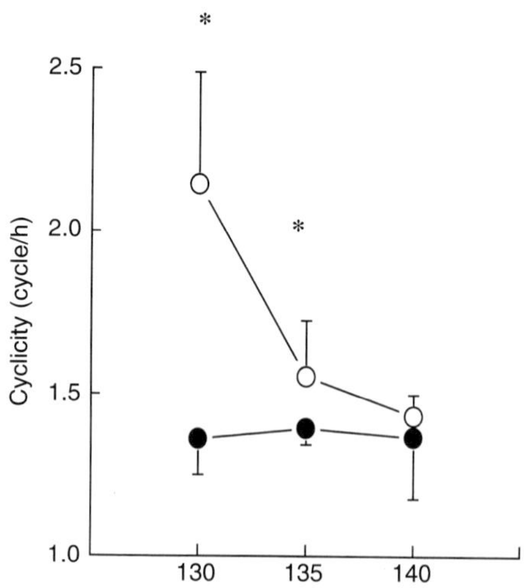

Figure 56.23 Peak HV–LV cycle frequency (cycle/hr) at 130, 135, 140 dGA CNTL ○ and LTOT ● Mean ± SEM $*p < 0.05$.

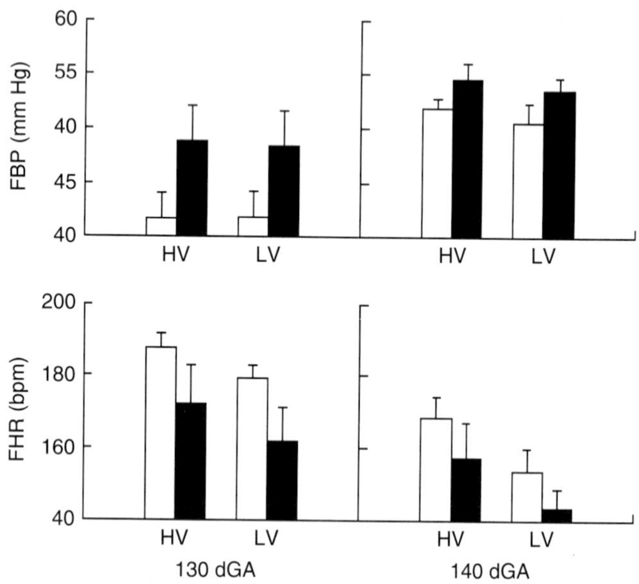

Figure 56.24 FBP and FHR in HV and LV states at 130 and 140 dGA.

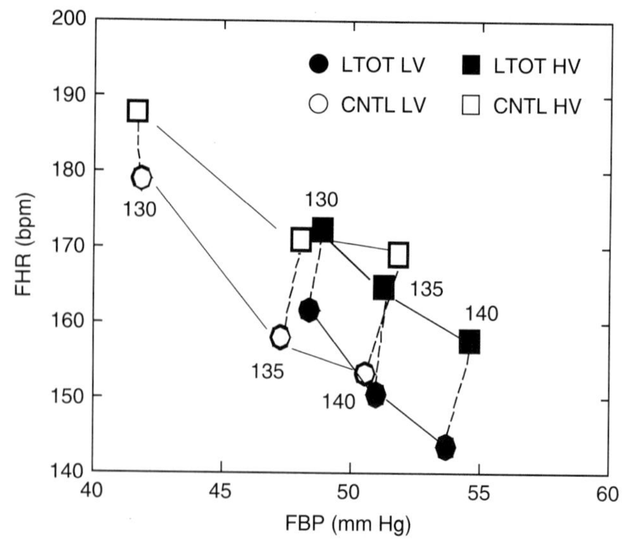

Figure 56.25 LV and HV state difference in FBP and FHR in CNTL and LTOT. The pattern of cardiovascular changes in behavioral state is shifted to the right in LTOT fetus suggesting acceleration of maturation in LTOT.

analyzed using conventional fast Fourier transform (frequency resolution at 0.04 Hz, range 0–41.6 Hz). Spectral edge frequency (90%) was calculated. Three-hour data (recorded at 10:00–14:00) at 126, 130, 135, 140 dGA were studied (Figure 56.22). ECoG power spectra analysis by calculation spectral edge frequency distribution[73,74] showed apparent distinction between low- and high-frequency peaks in LTOT (Figure 56.22). In LTOT, high spectral edge frequency was statistically higher in LTOT at 126–140 dGA and low frequency was statistically lower at 126 and 130 dGA. The mature pattern in ECoG spectra was found in LTOT fetus.

In addition, HV–LV ECoG cyclicity analysis[21] was done using the following procedures: (1) denoising by wavelet transform filtering; (2) HV–LV ECoG cyclicity by periodogram analysis. Hourly peak cycle and cycle were calculated by using period gram. Daily data at 130, 135 and 140 dGA were studied (Figure 56.23). Peak HV–LV cycle frequency in CNTL was changed to lower values by gestational age whereas that in LTOT was already low at 130 dGA and no difference was found by gestational age. Peak HV–LV cycle frequency was statistically lower in LTOT at 130 and 135 dGA.

FBP and FHR in each HV and LV state at 130 and 140 dGA are shown in Figure 56.24. Mean FBP was significantly higher and FHR was significantly lower in both HV and LV states in LTOT compared with CNTL.

FHR was increased in HV state from 130 dGA. Both FBP and FHR were increased in HV state at 140 dGA. The difference in state characteristics becomes apparent by plotting on one chart. The difference between LV and HV states with respect to FBP and FHR in CNTL and LTOT is summarized in Figure 56.25. The pattern of cardiovascular changes in behavioral state is shifted to the right in LTOT fetus suggests acceleration of maturation in LTOT.

In the LTOT studies, no difference was found at necropsy in body weight, organ weight and placenta between CNTL and LTOT.

What happens on long-term light stress to the fetus?

A single contracture produced in response to a single pulse of OT administered to the pregnant ewe in late gestation stimulates the release of fetal ACTH. A longer period of fetal exposure to contractures at an earlier stage of maturation altered the sensitivity of the fetal adrenal to ACTH both under basal and following exposure to hypoxemia, hypotension and hypertension. In the LTOT study, fetal PO_2 was lower and O_2 content higher in LTOT fetuses than in CNTL fetuses. This finding indicates that LTOT fetuses were not hypoxemic. They adapted to repeated mild stress and developed compensatory mechanisms by altering oxygenation accompanied by a shift of the oxygen dissociation curve to the left.

We also found an alteration in cardiovascular ontogenic change and baroreceptor response in LTOT fetuses. The baroreflex curve in LTOT showed a right shift and mature pattern as indicated in previous ontogenic studies. From the results obtained, we speculate that LTOT fetuses have more ability of isotropic function than CNTL fetuses. Fetal cardiovascular maturation during the final month of pregnancy is characterized by a rise in FBP and a fall in FHR. Higher FBP and lower FHR in LTOT fetuses compared with gestation matched controls suggest an acceleration of fetal cardiovascular maturation.

ECoG is one of the main indices of fetal neurological function. Biological variation is dependent upon behavioral states in late gestation. Difference in FBP and FHR in each HV–LV state indicates the degree of state maturation. The alteration of ontogenic changes in the relationship of FBP and FHR to fetal ECoG states (HV/LV states) following LTOT suggests an acceleration of fetal neurological maturation.[67,68]

Considering all results, we speculate that the altered intrauterine environment induced by increased uterine contracture activity accelerates endocrinological, neurological and functional maturation either by altered fetal oxygenation, glucocorticoid activity and/or physical stimulation of the fetus.

Fetal maturation, adaptation or adjustment by various stresses to the fetus

From the above-mentioned animal studies, a hypothesis arises that any stress to the fetus, environmental or congenital, could induce an acceleration of functional maturation. Initial compensatory response of the fetus to the environmental stress would be the acceleration of the maturation process.

An adequate stress such as uterine contracture must be a necessary factor for fetal stimulation. For the clinician, not only the gestational age but the maturational age also must be a desirable index to assess fetal well-being. Further basic research is required to answer these questions.

There is currently much interest in the effects of the quality of the intrauterine environment. Recent epidemiological studies indicate that an adverse intrauterine environment affects fetal physiological development and may be at the origin of later adult disease.[18,69–72] Restricted maternal nutrition has been shown to have an apparent effect on fetal cardiovascular function. Animal studies have demonstrated that hypertensive offspring is induced by maternal nutrient restriction and differences in fetal growth were associated with changes in cardiovascular control. Barker's hypothesis,[69,70] shows that fetal origins of adult disease is an important keyword in perinatal biomedical science. This concept has been called fetal programming, which means that an early environmental stimulation changes the developmental course and induces later physiological alteration. The environmental interactions in early development lead to changes in the physiological and physical phenotype of the developing embryo or fetus in expectation of future advantage in a particular predicted adult environment. The word 'programming' sounds as if the biological process is commanded and coded. Gluckman and Hanson use the term 'predictive adaptive responses' (PARs) to describe environmental responses.[71]

In the period before birth, environmental factors play an important role in the biological process of fetal maturation and some aspects of future life is possibly defined. By studying fetal maturation and its alteration by environmental stimulation, we can learn about the future process in development and health.[18,71,72] For these reasons, much attention should be paid to the investigation of fetal physiology and biomedical sciences.

REFERENCES

1. Stave U. Maturation, adaptation, and tolerance. In: Stave U, ed. *Perinatal Physiology*. New York: Plenum Publishing, 1970.
2. Liggins GC. Premature delivery of foetal lambs infused with glucocoticoids. *J Endocrinol* 1969;45:515–23.
3. Liggins GC, Fairclough RJ, Grieves SA, Kendall JZ, Knox DS. The mechanism of initiation of parturition in the ewe. *Recent Prog Horm Res* 1973;29:111–59.
4. Challis JRG, Lye SJ. Perturition. In: Knobil E, Neill JD, eds. *The Physiology of Reproduction*, 2nd edn. New York: Raven Press, 1994.
5. Challis JRG, Patrick JE. Fetal and maternal estrogen concentrations throughout pregnancy in the sheep. *Can J Physiol Pharmacol* 1981;59:970–8.
6. Dawes GS. Changes in the circulation at birth. *Br Med Bull* 1961; 17:148–53.
7. Dawes GS. The umbilical circulation. *Am J Obstet Gynecol* 1962;84:1634–48.
8. Dawes GS. Placental development and umbilical blood flow. *J Obstet Gynaecol Br Emp* 1962;69:815–17.
9. Natale R, Clewlow F, Dawes GS. Measurement of fetal forelimb movements in the lamb in utero. *Am J Obstet Gynecol* 1981;140: 545–51.
10. Clewlow F, Dawes GS, Johnson BM., Walker DW. Changes in breathing, electrocortical and muscle activity in unanesthetized fetal lamb. *J Physiol* 1983;341:463–76.
11. Day MA, Darby P, Hagin S. Autoradiographic analysis of regional brain glucose utilization in chronically monitored unanesthetized fetal sheep. *Brain Res* 1983;313:133–6.
12. Szeto HH. Effects of narcotic drugs on fetal behavioral activity: Acute methadone exposure. *Am J Obstet Gynecol* 1983;146:211–16.

13. Soma LR, White RJ, Kane PB. Surgical preparation of a chronic maternal–fetal model in pregnant sheep: A technique for the measurement of middle uterine blood flow, umbilical blood flow, and fetal sampling in the awake sheep. *J Surg Res* 1971;11:85–94.
14. Gresham EL, Rankin JH, Makowski EL, Meschia G, Battaglia FC. An evaluation of fetal renal function in a chronic sheep preparation. *J Clin Invest* 1972;51:149–56.
15. Dawes GS. Fetal circulation and breathing. *Clin Obstet Gynaecol* 1974;1:139–49.
16. Dawes GS. Fetal breathing movements and sleep in sheep. *Ann Rech Vet* 1977;8:413–17.
17. Dawes GS. The central control of fetal breathing and skeletal muscle movements. *J Physiol* 1984;346:1–18.
18. Nathanielsz PW, Bailey A, Poore ER, Thorburn GD, Harding R. The relationship between myometrial activity and sleep state and breathing in fetal sheep throughout the last third of gestation. *Am J Obstet Gynecol* 1980;138:653–9.
19. Robinson SR, Wong CH, Robertson SS, Nathanielsz PW, Smotherman WP. Behavioral responses of the chronically instrumented sheep fetus to chemosensory stimuli presented in utero. *Behav Neurosci* 1995;109:551–62.
20. Derks JB, Giussani DA, Jenkins SL *et al.* A comparative study of cardiovascular, endocrine and behavioral effects of betamethasone and dexamethasone administration to fetal sheep. *J Physiol* 1997;499(1):217–66.
21. Shinozuka N, Nathanielsz PW. Electrocortical activity in fetal sheep in th last seven days of gestation. *J Physiol* 1998;513(1): 273–81.
22. Unno N, Wong CH, Jenkins SL *et al.* Blood pressure and heart rate in the ovine fetus: Ontogenic changes and effects of fetal adrenalectomy. *Am J Physiol* 1998;276:H248–56.
23. Magyar DM, Fridshal D, Elsner CW *et al.* Time-trend analysis of plasma cortisol concentrations in the fetal sheep in relation to parturition. *Endocrinology* 1980;107:155–9.
24. Hyman AI, Haworth G, Bowe ET, Daniel SS, James LS. Effects of sympathetic blockade on the fetal responses to asphyxia. *Biol Neonate* 1972;21:1–8.
25. Vappavouri EK, Shinebourne EA, Williams RL, Heymann MA, Rudolph AM. Development of cardiovascular responses to autonomic blockade in intact fetal and neonatal lambs. *Biol Neonate* 1973;22:177–88.
26. Hanson MA. The control of heat rate and blood pressure in the fetus: theoretical considerations. In: Hanson MA, Spencer JAD, Rodeck CH, eds. *Fetus and Neonate: Physiology and Clinical Applications*, vol. 1. Cambridge, UK: Cambridge University Press, 1993.
27. Hanson MA. The importance of baro- and chemoreflexes in the control of the fetal cardiovascular system. *J Dev Physiol* 1988;10:491–511.
28. Dawes GS, Fox HE, Leduc BM, Liggins GC, Richards RT. Respiratory movements and rapid eye movement sleep in the foetal lamb. *J Physiol* 1972;220:119–43.
29. Clewlow F, Dawes GS, Johnston BM, Walker DW. Changes in breathing, electrocortical and muscle activity in unanaesthetized fetal lambs with age. *J Physiol* 1983;341:463–76.
30. Boddy K, Dawes GS, Fisher R, Pinter S, Robinson JS. Foetal respiratory movements, electrocortical and cardiovascular responses to hypoxaemia and hypercapnia in sheep. *J Physiol* 1974;243: 599–618.
31. Dawes GS. The control of fetal heart rate and its veiability in lambs. In: Kunzel W, ed. *Fetal Heart Rate Monitoring*. Berlin: Springer-Verlag, 1985.
32. Unno N, Wong CH, Jenkins SL, *et al.* Blood pressure and heart rate in the ovine fetus: Ontogenic changes and effects of fetal adrenalectomy. *Am J Physiol* 1999;276:H248–56.
33. Rudolph AM, Heymann MA. Cardiac output in the fetal lamb. The effect of spontaneous and induced changes of heart rate on right and left ventricular output. *Am J Obstet Gynecol* 1976;124: 183–92.
34. Rudolph AM, Heymann MA. Fetal and neonatal circulation and respiration. *Ann Rev Phyisol* 1974;36:187–207.
35. Rudolph AM, Heymann MA. Circulatory changes during growth in the fetal lamb. *Circ Res* 1970;26:289–99.
36. Rudolph AM. Organization and control of the fetal circulation. In: Jones CT, Nathanielsz PW, eds. *The Physiological Development of the Fetus and Newborn*. New York: Academic Press, 1985.
37. Walker AM, Fleming J, Smolich R, Struden R, Horne R, Maloney J. Fetal oxygen consumption, umbilical circulation and electorocortical activity transitions in fetal lambs. *J Dev Physiol* 1984;6: 267–74.
38. Girbert RD. Control of the fetal cardiac output during changes in blood volume. *Am J Physiol* 1980;238:H80–6.
39. Itskoviz J, LaGamma EF, Rudolph AM. Baroreflex control of the circulation in chronically instrumented fetal lambs. *Circ Res* 1983;52:589–96.
40. Shinozuka N, Yen A, Nathanielsz PW. Increased myometrial contracture frequency produced by pulse administration of oxytocin to the pregnant ewe from 96 to 131 days' gestation alters fetal oxygenation and responses to acute hypoxemia. *Am J Obstet Gynecol* 1999;180:1202–8.
41. Shinozuka N, Yen A, Nathanielsz PW. Increased myometrial contracture frequency at 96–140 days accelerates fetal cardiovascular maturation. *Am J Phyiol* 2000;278:H41–9.
42. Benowitz NL. Antihypertensive agents. In: Katzung BG, ed. *Basic & Clinical Pharmacology*, 7th edn. Stamford: Appleton & Lange, 1998.
43. Hoffman BB. Adrenoceptor-activating and other sympathomimetic Drugs. In: Katzung BG, ed. *Basic & Clinical Pharmacology*, 7th edn. Stamford: Appleton & Lange, 1998.
44. Kent BB, Drane JW, Blumenstein B. Mathematical model to access changes in barorecepter reflex. *Cardiology* 1976;57:295–310.
45. Wood CE, Cheung CY, Brace RA. Fetal heart rate arterial pressure, and blood volume response to cortisol infusion. *Am J Physiol* 1987;253:R904–9.
46. Derks JB, Mulder EJH, Visser GHA. The effect of maternal betamethasone administration on the fetus. *Br J Obstet Gyneacol* 1995;102:40–6.
47. Derks JB, Giussani DA, Van Dam LM, *et al.* Differential effects of betamethasone and dexamethasone fetal administration of parturition in sheep. *J Soc Gynecol Invest* 1996;3:336–41.
48. Dodic M, Wintour EM. Effects of prolonged (48 h) infusion of cortisol on blood pressure, renal function and fetal fluids in the immature ovine foetus. *Clin Exp Pharmacol Physiol* 1994;21: 971–80.
49. Tangalakis K, Lumbers ER, Moriz KM, Towstoless MK, Wintour EM. Effect of cortisol on blood pressure and vascular reactivity in the ovine fetus. *Exp Physiol* 1992;77:709–17.
50. Kitanaka T, Gilbert RD, Longo LD. Maternal responses to long-term hypoxemia in sheep. *Am J Physiol* 1989;256:R1340–7.
51. Kitanaka T, Alonso JG, Gilbert RD, Siu BL, Clemons GK, Longo LD. Fetal responses to long-term hypoxemia in sheep. *Am J Physiol* 1989;256:R1348–54.
52. Alonso JG, Okai T, Longo LD, Gilbert RD. Cardiac function during long-term hypoxemia in fetal sheep. *Am J Physiol* 1989;257:H581–9.
53. Longo LD, Dale PS, Gilbert RD. Uteroplacental Os uptake: Continuous measurements during uterine quiescence and contractions. *Am J Physiol* 1986;250:R1099–107.
54. Allen WW, Power GG, Longo LD. Fetal O_2 changes in response to hypoxic stress: a mathematical model. *J Appl Physiol Respir Environ Exerc Physiol* 1977;42:179–90.
55. Ueno N, Zhao Y, Zhang L, Longo LD. High altitude-induced changes in alpha1-adrenergic receptors and Ins(1,4,5)P3 responses in cerebral arteries. *Am J Physiol* 1997;272:R669–74.
56. Murotsuki J, Bocking AD, Gagnon R. Fetal heart rate patterns in growth-restricted fetal sheep induced by chronic fetal placental embolization. *Am J Obstet Gynecol* 1997;176:282–90.
57. Gagnon R, Murotsuki J, Challis JR, Fraher L, Richardson BS. Fetal sheep endocrine responses to sustained hypoxemic stress after chronic fetal placental embolization. *Am J Physiol* 1997;272: E817–23.
58. Gagnon R, Johnston L, Murotsuki J. Fetal placental embolization in the late-gestation ovine fetus: alterations in umbilical blood flow and fetal heart rate patterns. *Am J Obstet Gynecol* 1996; 175:63–72.
59. Giussani DA, Unno N, Jenkins SL, *et al.* Dynamics of cardiovascular responses to repeated partial umbilical cord compression in late-gestation sheep fetus. *Am J Physiol* 1997;273:H2351–60.
60. Giussani DA, Spencer JAD, Moore PJ, Bennet L, Hanson MA. Afferent and efferent components of the cardiovascular reflex response to acute hypoxia in term fetal sheep. *J Physiol* 1993; 461:431–49.
61. Owiny JR, Sadowsky DW, Zareczny S, Nathanielsz PW. Effect of pulsatile intravenous oxytocin administration to the pregnant sheep over the last third of gestation on fetal ACTH and cortisol response to acute hypotension. *J Soc Gynecol Invest* 1995;2:13–18.
62. Owiny JR, Jenkins SL, Sadowsky DW, Nathanielsz PW. Effect of pulsatile oxytocin administration to the pregnant ewe in the last third of gestation on fetal ACTH and cortisol response to acute hypoxemia. *J Soc Gynecol Invest* 1995;2:673–7.

63. Shinozuka N, Yen A, Nathanielsz PW. Alteration of fetal oxygenation and responses to acute hypoxemia by increased myometrial contracture frequency produced by pulse administration of oxytocin to the pregnant ewe from 96 to 131 days' gestation. *Am J Obstet Gynecol* 1999;180:1202–8.
64. Sadowsky DW, Martel JK, Jenkins SL, Poore MG, Cabalum T, Nathanielsz PW. Pulsatile oxytocin administered to ewes at 120 to 140 days gestational age increases the rate of maturation of the fetal electrocorticogram and nuchal activity. *J Dev Physiol* 1992; 17:175–81.
65. Sadowsky DW, Martel J, Cabalum T, Poore MG, Nathanielsz PW. Oxytocin given in a pulsatile manner to the ewe at 120 to 140 day's gestational age increases fetal plasma cortisol. *Am J Obstet Gynecol* 1992;166:200–5.
66. Glatz TH, Weitzman RE, Nathanielsz PW, Fisher DA. Metabolic clearance rate and transplacental passage of oxytocin in the pregnant ewe and fetus. *Endcrinology* 1980;106:1006–11.
67. Wakatsuki A, Murata Y, Ninomiya N, Masaoka JG, Tayner JG, Kutty KK. Autonomic nervous system regulation of baseline heart rate in fetal lamb. *Am J Obstet Gynecol* 1992;167:519–23.
68. Wakatsuki A, Murata Y, Ninomiya N, Masaoka JG, Tayner JG, Kutty KK. Physiologic barorecepter activity in fetal lamb. *Am J Obstet Gynecol* 1992;167:820–7.
69. Barker DJP. Fetal origins of coronary heart disease. *Br Med J* 1995;311:171–4.
70. Barker DJP. Fetal nutrition and cardiovascular disease in later life. *Br Med Bull* 1997;53:96–108.
71. Gluckman PD, Hanson M. *The Fetal Matrix Evolution, Development and Disease*. Cambridge, UK: Cambridge University Press, 2005.
72. Nathanielsz PW, Berghorn KA, Derks JB, *et al.* Life before birth: Effects of cortisol on future cardiovascular and metabolic function. *Acta Paediatr* 2003;92:766–72.
73. Szeto HH, Hinmann DJ. Prenatal development of sleep-wake patterns in sheep. *Sleep* 1985;8:347–55.
74. Szeto HH. Spectral edge frequency as a simple quantitative measure of maturation of electrocortical activity. *Pediatric Research* 1990;27:289–92.

57 Basic background of congenital anomalies: NTD

K. Fujimori and A. Sato

Introduction

Neural tube defects (NTDs) are the second most common class of congenital anomalies after cardiac defects. A worldwide incidence of isolated (i.e. non-syndromic) NTDs is 1.4–2.0 per 1000 live births.[1] They can also occur as part of a genetic syndrome or constellation of abnormalities. They are a major cause of stillbirth, neonatal and infant death, and lifelong severe handicap. Anencephaly accounts for one half of all cases of NTDs and is incompatible with life. With treatment, 80–90% of infants with isolated spina bifida survive with varying degrees of handicap. Factors that influence eventual neurological function include the size and location of the defect, trauma to exposed neural tissue, timing of surgical closure, degree of associated ventriculomegaly, and occurrence of complication such as infection. It is well known that NTDs are among the few preventable birth defects. Preconceptional counseling and folic acid supplementation are very important.

Embryology and types of NTDs

The neural folds in the brain and spinal cord regions fuse in the midline, converting the neural tube by days 26–28 of embryonic life (Figure 57.1).[2] Recent data indicate that closure occurs in separate regions that then fuse.[3] Clinical data suggest five possible closure sites. NTDs likely result from either failure of closure in one or more sites, or failure of two sites to meet. Neural tube closure is normally complete by the end of the fourth week after conception (6 weeks after the last menstrual period), a time when many women do not yet realize they are pregnant.

The most common types of NTDs are listed in Table 57.1.[4] Anencephaly is the most severe defect, in which the forebrain, meninges, vault of the skull, and scalp all fail to form. It is lethal, resulting in stillbirth or early neonatal demise. Spina bifida involves failure of fusion of the caudal portion of the neural tube, usually of three to five contiguous vertebrae and

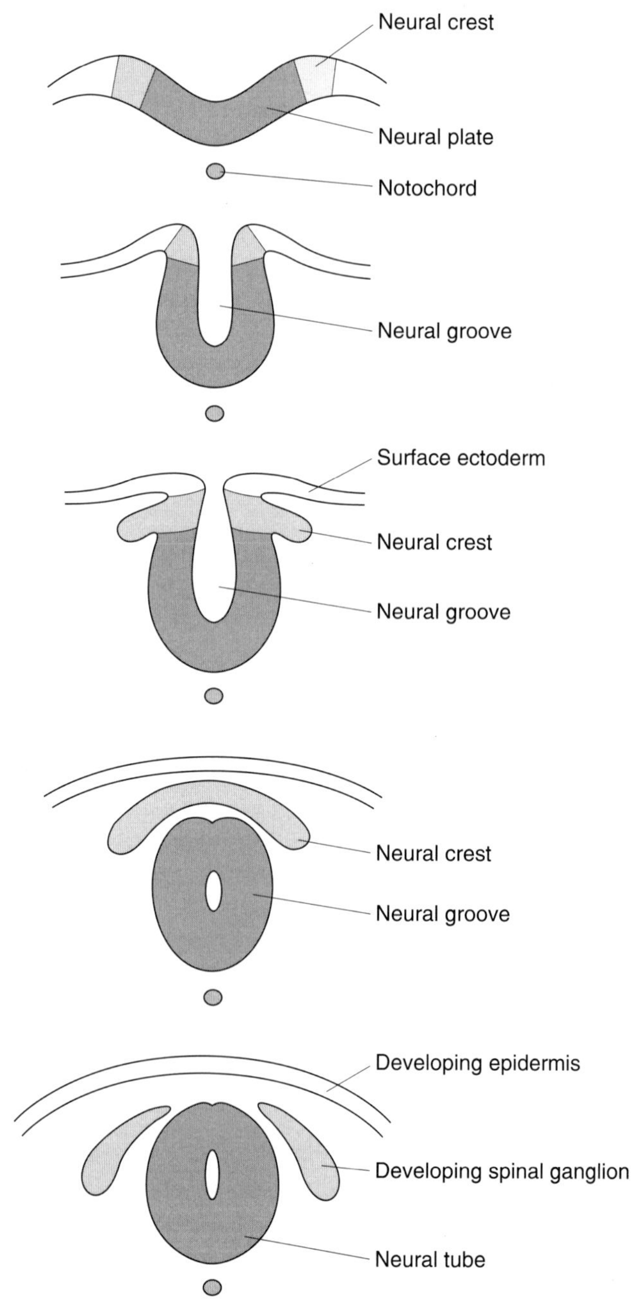

Figure 57.1

Table 57.1 Neural tube defect pathophysiology

Neural Tube Defect	Malformation
Cranial	
Anencephaly	Failure of fusion of cephalic portion of neural folds; absence of all or part of brain, neurocranium, and skin
Exencephaly	Failure of scalp and skull formation; exteriorization of abnormally formed brain
Encephalocele	Failure of skull formation; extrusion of brain tissue into membranous sac
Iniencephaly	Defect of cervical and upper thoracic vertebrae; abnormally formed brain tissue and extreme retroflexion of upper spine
Spinal	
Spina bifida	Failure of fusion of caudal portion of neural tube, usually of 3–5 contiguous vertebrae; spinal cord or meninges or both exposed to amniotic fluid
Meningocele	Failure of fusion of caudal portion of neural tube; meninges exposed
Meningomyelocele	Failure of fusion of caudal portion of neural tube; meninges and neural tissue exposed
Myeloschisis	Failure of fusion of caudal portion of neural tube; flattened mass of neural tissue exposed
Holorachischisis	Failure of fusion of vertebral arches; entire spinal cord exposed
Craniorachischisis	Co-existing anencephaly and rachischisis

spinal cord or meninges or both exposed to amniotic fluid. Meningocele is the protrusion of the meninges and cerebrospinal fluid into a sac covered by epithelium. Myleomeningocele is most common and involves serious defects that include the spinal cord, nerve roots, meninges, and cerebrospinal fluid. It occurs mostly in the lumbar area. As meninges or neural tissue plus meninges are exposed to the amniotic fluid and eventually to the environment, neural tissue is damaged, causing the structures supplied by the damaged nerves to be dysfunctional. Lesions in the lumbosacral area can lead to paraplegia and lack of bowel or bladder control. The level of the lesion is usually reflected in the severity of the clinical deficit, with higher lesions having more pronounced deficits.

Open defects are often associated with ventriculomegaly or hydrocephaly as a result of a block to cerebrospinal fluid circulation. The increased intracranial pressure may cause pressure atrophy of the developing brain, although neurological dysfunction cannot be reliably estimated from the thickness of the compressed cortical mantle. Rachischisis describes the situation in which none of the vertebral arches fuse, and the entire spine is open. This condition is generally incompatible with life.

Etiology

Many risk factors of NTDs are known, including family history, exposure to certain environmental agents, genetic syndromes, and racial or ethnic groups. Main and Mennuti presented the recognized causes of neural tube defects, as listed in Table 57.2.[5]

Family history is the most important risk factor for NTDs. Because they are multifactorial in inheritance, the risk to a first-degree relative is approximately 2–3%. While this is lower than the risk of autosomal dominant or recessive disorder, it is 20–30 times higher than the risk of NTDs in the general population. The level of risk is directly related to the number of affected relatives and their degree of relatedness of the fetus.[6,7] However, only 5% of NTDs occur in families with a positive family history.[8] More than 90% occur in families with no prior history.[9]

Exposure to certain environmental agents has been implicated in NTD formation. Exposure must occur during the first 28 days of gestation when the neural tube is developing. Hyperglycemia from insulin-dependent diabetes increases the risk of NTD.[9] Although this may inhibit fetal glycolysis, functional deficiency of arachidonic acid or myoinositol in the developing embryo, or alterations in the yolk sac,[10] the exact mechanism is unknown. Hyperthermia (high maternal body temperature) during neural tube formation has also been implicated in causing defects. Maternal fever and sauna baths have both been reported to increase the relative risk up to sixfold.[11]

Anticonvulsants, most notably valproic acid and carbamazepine, induce NTDs. Especially, fetuses exposed to valproic acid in the first trimester have a 1–2% risk of spina bifida.[12] This is because valproic acid acts as an antagonist and impairs folate absorption. Aminopterin and isotretinoin also have been associated with anencephaly or encephalocele.

Some inherited syndromes known to include NTDs are Meckel–Gruber, Roberts SC phocomelia, Jarco–Levin, and Harde syndrome, as well as trisomy 13, trisomy 18, and triploidy. These autosomal recessive diseases have 25% recurrence risk, and trisomies 13 and 18 and triploidy have a 1% recurrence risk.[13] Cloacal extrophy and sacrococcygeal teratoma may be associated with spina bifida, and amniotic bands may cause spina bifida or anencephaly.[13]

Some geographic regions and racial or ethnic groups are associated with NTDs. The UK has the highest frequency of NTDs, with an incidence of almost 1% compared with 0.2% in the USA.[14]

Table 57.2 Recognized causes of neural tube defects

Multifactorial inheritance—anencephaly, meningomyelocele, meningocele, and encephalocele
Single mutant genes
- Meckel syndrome—autosomal recessive (phenotype includes occipital encephalocele and rarely anencephaly)
- Median-cleft face syndrome—possible autosomal dominant (phenotype includes anterior encephalocele)
- Robert syndrome—autosomal recessive (phenotype includes anterior encephalocele)
- Syndrome of anterior sacral meningomyelocele and anal stenosis—dominant, either autosomal or X-linked
- Jarco-Levin syndrome—autosomal recessive (phenotype includes meningomyelocele)
- HARDE syndrome—autosomal recessive (phenotype includes encephalocele)

Chromosome abnormalities
- 13 trisomy
- 18 trisomy
- Triploidy
- Other abnormalities, such as unbalanced translocation and ring chromosome

Probably hereditary, but mode of transmission not established
- Syndrome of occipital encephalocele, myopia, and retinal dysplasia
- Anterior encephalocele among Bantus and Thais

Teratogens
- Valproic acid (phenotype includes spina bifida)
- Aminopterin/amethopterin (phenotype includes anencephaly and encephalocele)
- Thalidomide (phenotype includes, rarely, anencephaly and meningomyelocele)

Maternal predisposing factors
- Diabetes mellitus (anencephaly more frequent than spina bifida)

Specific phenotypes, but without known cause
- Syndrome of craniofacial and limb defects secondary to aberrant tissue bands (phenotype includes multiple encephaloceles)
- Cloacal exstrophy (phenotype includes myelocystocele)
- Sacrococcygeal teratoma (phenotype includes meningomyelocele)

China, Egypt, and India also have a very high incidence of NTDs. The reasons for these high incidences are considered to be related to both the ethnic (genetic) background of the inhabitants and the environmental influences, such as diet. For example, Sikhs living in India have more than twice the incidence of NTDs as Sikhs living in Canada.[7]

Certain ethnic and racial groups also appear to be at high risk. For example, a study using population-based data from California found that incidence of NTDs of Hispanic women was higher than Caucasian women (1.12 vs. 0.96 per 1000). African-American and Asian women were at low risk (0.75 and 0.75 per 1000).[15]

Several investigators reported that obese women had a two- to threefold risk for NTDs as well as other anomalies.[16–18] Subsequently, Shaw *et al.* found a significant twofold increased incidence of NTDs in women whose body mass index (BMI) was 30 or higher.[19,20]

Although there is no firm evidence that influenza virus causes congenital malformation,[21] Lynberg *et al.* reported in a case–control study that children born to women with influenza early in pregnancy had a threefold risk of NTDs. This may be related to be associated with hyperthermia.[22]

The most important environmental influence in NTDs formation appears to be related to the dietary intake of folic acid, because pregnancies complicated by a fetal NTD have lower maternal plasma levels of folate than pregnancies that are unaffected. Recently, a specific gene defect associated with folic acid metabolism has been implicated. A thermolabile variant of 5,10-methylenetetrahydrofolate reductase (MTHFR) has the mutation 677CT, which results in a substitution of valine for alanine. This variant enzyme has reduced activity leading to altered homocysteine metabolism. Hyperhomocystinemia increases the risk for fetal NTDs, atherosclerosis, thromboembolism, and recurrent miscarriage.[23] Several studies have shown that parents who have had a pregnancy complicated by an NTD and their affected offspring are more likely to carry a mutation in the gene encoding the enzyme MTHFR than the unaffected population. For example, in The Netherlands, 14–16% of mothers, 10–15% of fathers, and 13–18% of children with spina bifida are homozygous for the MTHFR mutation compared with 5% of the general population.[24–26] Other mutations in this enzyme with similar effects also have been reported.[26] Therefore, it seems possible that folic acid supplementation helps to overcome the effects of this enzyme mutation, resulting in more normal levels of homocysteine and adequate production of methionine. The Medical Research Council Vitamin Study Research Group published the results of a large, prospective, randomized, double-blind study of folic acid supplementation conducted at 33 centers in seven countries.[27] The results showed that folic acid supplementation reduced NTD recurrences by 70%.[27] Czeizel and Dudas subsequently showed that periconceptional folic acid supplementation decreased the risk of first occurrence of an NTD.[28] But, folic acid supplementation does not prevent all cases, other unknown genes or factors are presumed to cause some cases. Recently, Rothenberg *et al.* showed that autoantibodies against folate receptors were present in sera from women whose pregnancies are complicated by an NTD. They hypothesized that autoantibodies against folate receptors in women could be associated with pregnancy complicated by an NTD.[29]

Diagnosis

Alpha-fetoprotein

Prior to the late 1970s, there was no way to identify NTDs during pregnancy, but then it was discovered that amniotic fluid and maternal serum alpha-fetoprotein (MSAFP) was a marker for pregnancy of NTDs. AFP is a fetal-specific globulin similar to albu min in molecular weight and is synthesized early in gestation by the yolk sac and subsequently by the gastrointestinal tract and fetal liver. The kidney and placenta also produce trace amounts of AFP. The level of fetal plasma AFP peaks between 10 and 13 weeks of gestation and declines exponentially from 14 to 32 weeks and then more sharply until term. AFP enters the fetal urine and is excreted into the amniotic fluid. Peak levels of amniotic fluid AFP (AFAFP) are reached between 12 and 14 weeks of gestation, decline between 10% and 15% per week during the second trimester, and are almost non-detectable at term.[30] AFP passes into the maternal circulation by diffusion across the placental membranes and may also be transported via the placental circulation.[31] AFP levels in maternal plasma or serum rise above non-pregnant levels as early as the seventh week of gestation. Although maternal serum levels are significantly lower than amniotic fluid levels, these increase during gestation.[32] When there is a fetal abnormality such as an opening uncovered by epithelium in the body or a number of other problems, then the maternal AFP serum levels are increased. Brock and Sutcliffe showed that amniotic fluid AFP levels were much higher in pregnancies complicated by fetal anencephaly.[33] Subsequently, Brock *et al.* demonstrated that maternal serum AFP levels were also elevated in affected pregnancies.[34] The first large prospective trial for maternal serum AFP screening was the UK Collaborate Study on Alpha-fetoprotein in Relation to Neural Tube Defects.[35] Subsequently, other investigators confirmed the effect of screening for NTDs.[36–38]

Maternal serum AFP (MSAFP) screening for NTDs is ideally performed between 16 and 18 weeks of gestation. MSAFP is measured in nanograms per liter and reported as a multiple of median (MoM) of the unaffected population. MoM is used because AFP levels do not follow a Gaussian distribution, and because it aids in comparison of results from different laboratories and populations. Cutoffs between 2.0 and 2.5 MoM (for most laboratories) as upper limits indicate an increased risk for a fetal NTD of other structural anomaly (and warrants further evaluation). It is considered that the detection rates are almost 100% for anencephaly and 85–92% for open spina bifida, with a false-positive rate between 2% and 5%.[39] A number of factors can influence the interpretation of an MSAFP value. The most important factor for efficient MSAFP screening is the accuracy of the gestational age determination. Consequently, a first-trimester ultrasound (especially measurement of crown–rump length, CRL) is the preferable means of documenting gestational age, and femur length and biparietal diameter should be measured to confirm gestational age for AFP screening. Maternal weight affects the MSAFP concentration. The heavier the women, the lower the MSAFP value as a result of dilution in the larger blood volume. Maternal ethnicity may also alter the interpretation of an MSAFP level, because black women have a 10–15% higher MSAFP than non-blacks.[40] This is important because the incidence of NTDs in blacks is lower. Pregnant women with insulin-dependent diabetes mellitus have MSAFP values that are significantly lower than the non-diabetic women in the second trimester, which require adjustments in the interpretation.[41,42] This is critical because there is up to a 10-fold higher frequency of NTDs in the offspring of these patients. MSAFP must also be altered in multiple gestations. Because the maternal serum AFP level is approximately doubled in normal twin pregnancy, different cutoffs are needed to interpret this test in multiple gestations. When a 2.5 MoM cutoff in twin pregnancy is used, 99% of cases of anencephaly and 89% of open NTDs are detected but generate a 30% false-positive rate.[43] Raising the twin cutoff to 5.0 MoM decreases the false-positive rate to 3% but also decreases the detection of anencephaly to 83% and of open NTDs to 39%. Wapner *et al.* reported a detection rate of 50–85% and a false-positive rate of 5% using a cutoff of 4.5 MoM.[44] Because serum screening for fetal abnormalities in multiple gestation will always be limited by the inability to confirm which fetus is affected, many centers do not offer serum screening in multiple gestation even for NTDs.

Women with MSAFP levels higher than the cutoff level of 2–2.5 MoM should be referred for genetic counseling and consideration of a diagnostic test. The diagnostic test offered to women with a positive MSAFP test result is genetic amniocentesis. If the AFAFP level is elevated, an assay is performed to determine the presence or absence of acetylcholine-esterase. Acetylcholine-esterase is predominantly neuronally derived, giving it additional specificity for nervous system lesions. Therefore, elevated AFAFP levels together with the presence of acetylcholine-esterase are considered diagnostic for a fetal NTD. A combined use AFP and acetylcholine-esterase identified 100% of cases of anencephaly, 100% of cases of open spina bifida, and 20% of ventral wall defects, with a false-positive rate of 2.2 per 1000 amniocentesis.[45] One advantage of amniocentesis is that amniotic fluid can also be obtained for determination of the fetal karyotype. In pregnancies complicated by an elevated MSAFP level, the incidence of fetal aneuploidy is 0.61% in ultrasonographically determined normal fetuses and 16% in abnormal fetuses.[46,47]

Women already known to be at high risk of having a fetus with an NTD because of a previously affected pregnancy, a positive family history, medication exposure, diabetes, or other risk factors can be offered a diagnostic test directly. Performing a genetic amniocentesis in all these women would result in a 98% detection rate for NTDs and a 100% detection rate for aneuploidy. However, all high-risk women for NTDs would undergo amniocentesis unnecessarily. Although second-trimester amniocentesis is a relatively safe procedure, it is associated with a post procedure pregnancy loss rate of approximately 1 in 200.[48]

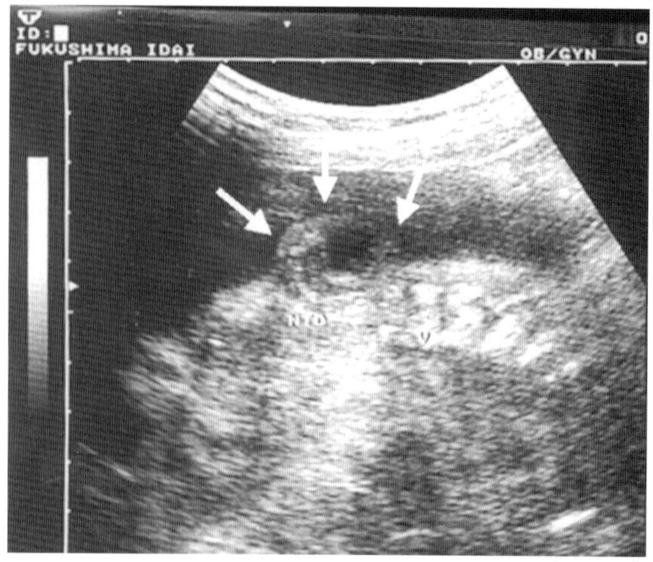

Figure 57.2 A sagittal scan of the spine revealing a meningomyelocele (arrows) overlying a spinal defect.

Ultrasound

The ultrasound diagnosis of NTDs is based on soft tissue and bone findings with the recognition of associated abnormalities in the skull and brain. The soft tissue findings include absence of skin covering the defect and presence of a round sac (Figure 57.2) that may correspond to a meningocele or myelomeningocele. The bone findings are derived from the vertebral abnormalities associated with spina bifida.

Spina bifida is associated with a variety of typical intracranial abnormalities, including ventriculomegaly (Figure 57.3) and hypoplasia of the posterior fossa structures. The associated abnormalities include frontal bone scalloping (lemon sign; Figure 57.4)[49] and obliteration of the cisterna magna with either an absent cerebellum or abnormal anterior curvature of the cerebellar hemispheres (banana sign; Figure 57.5).[49] The fruit signs are very helpful for early diagnosis of the open spina bifida.

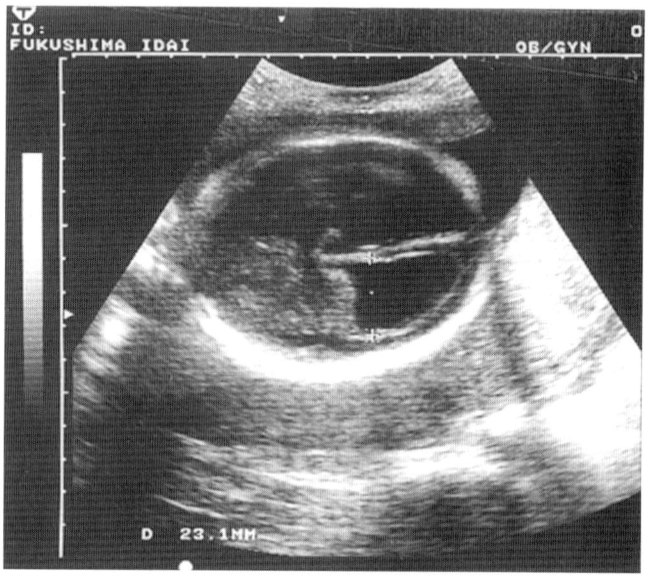

Figure 57.3 Severe ventriculomegaly in the 30th week of gestation is present on the transverse view of the head with meningomyelocele

There are three main scanning sections used in the evaluation of the spine: sagittal, transverse, and coronal (see Romero *et al.*,[50] pp. 36–43). In the sagittal section, the normal spine appears as two parallel lines converging in the sacrum. Sagittal scans are also useful for evaluating the spinal curvatures of which exaggeration may be an indirect sign of spina bifida. In the coronal section, the normal spine appears as either two or three parallel lines. Spina bifida is typically characterized by a widening of the two external lines due to a divergent separation of the lateral processes of the vertebrae (Figure 57.6). Sagittal and coronal views are most useful in this evaluation. In the transverse section, the neural canal appears as a closed circle. In the presence of a defect, the posterior laminae are typically absent, and the lateral processes are set apart (Figure 57.7).[51] The presence of a sac is certainly helpful in the diagnosis of the spinal defect whereas the absence of a sac can make detection difficult. This myelomeningocele sac should not be confused for a skin-covered defect. It is a common belief that indirect signs of spina bifida, such as paralysis of the lower extremities and bladder distention, can be useful in the diagnosis of the lesion.

The accuracy in the diagnosis of spina bifida depends on the experience of the sonographer, the quality of the equipment, and the amount of time dedicated to the scan. It is believed that the accuracy of referral centers should be close to 100%, in large part due to recognition of associated cranial findings.

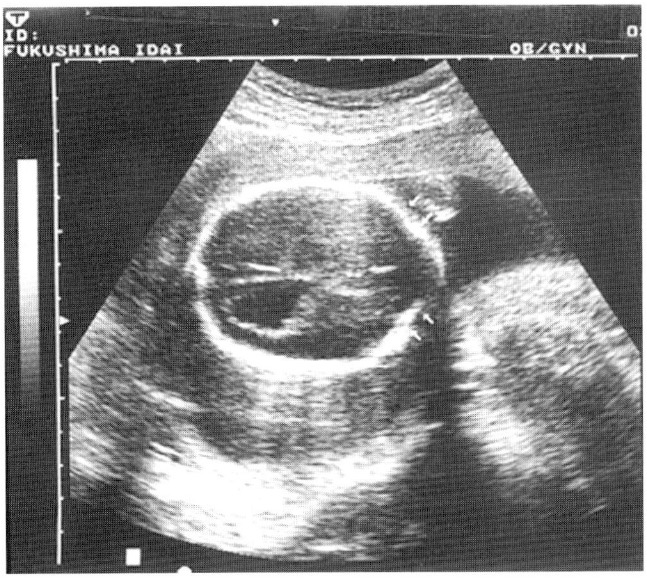

Figure 57.4 Axial ultrasound in the fetal head demonstrated bifrontal deformity of the calvaria (arrows) (lemon sign)

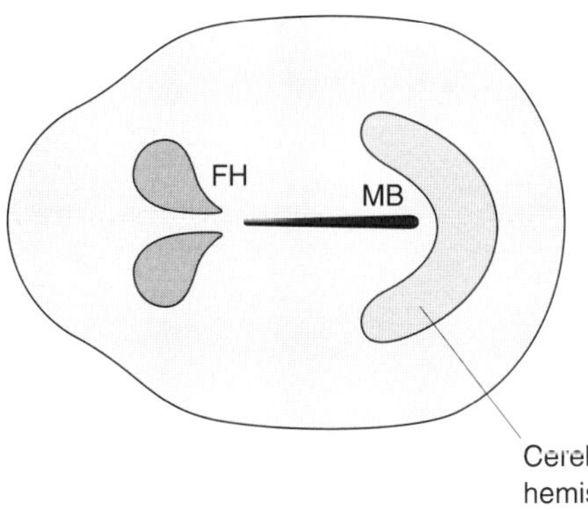

Figure 57.5 Obliteration of the cisterna magna with either absent cerebellum or abnormal anterior curvature of the cerebellar hemispheres (banana sign)

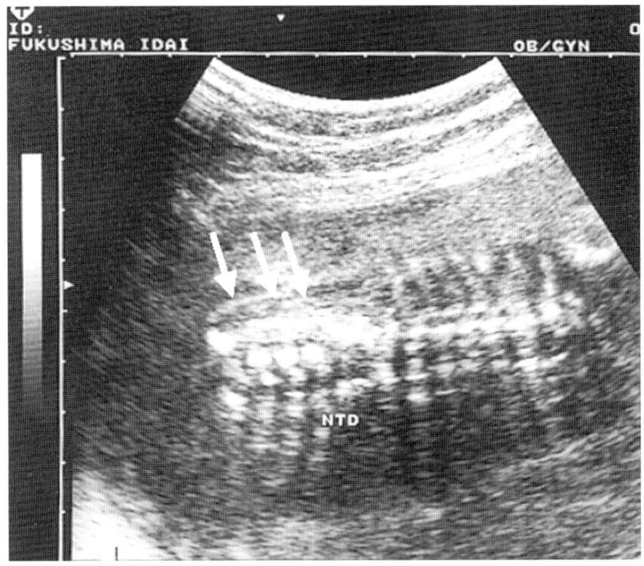

Figure 57.6 Coronal plane demonstrating lateral splaying of the lateral process with widening of the spinal canal (arrows).

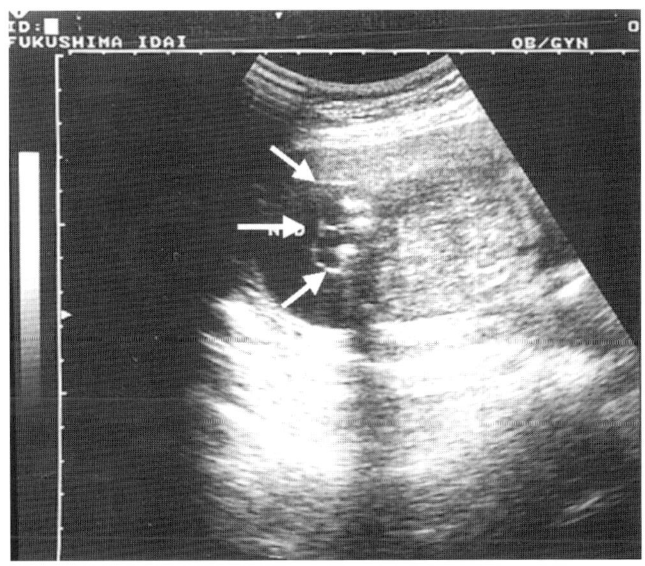

Figure 57.7 Transverse scan of the body of a fetus affected by a large spinal defect (arrows). The cystic and irregular echoes arising posteriorly from the defect suggested the presence of meningomyelocele.

The accuracy of routine non-targeted examinations is uncertain. In the RADIUS (routine antenatal diagnostic imaging with ultrasound) trial, in which routine ultrasound was performed in conjunction with maternal AFP screening, the sensitivity was 80%.[52] In a survey of European centers, Boyd *et al.* reported overall sensitivity of 75%, but a large variation between centers from 33% to 100%.[53] In one retrospective study conducted in Great Britain, the estimated sensitivity was marginally higher for serum AFP screening, 84–92%, than for ultrasound screening, 70–84%.[54] In all these studies, it is unclear whether the cranial signs of fetal spina bifida were systematically researched. In a more recent retrospective multicentric study using the cranial signs, the sensitivity of ultrasound was 85%.[55] Careful scanning of the rest of the fetus should be performed to exclude associated abnormalities.

Several authors have reported on the accuracy of the prenatal diagnosis of spina bifida by ultrasound. Table 57.3 shows the results of the three largest series available for study (see Romero *et al.*,[50] pp. 36–43).

Regarding the diagnosis of other NTDs using ultrasound, anencephaly was the first congenital anomaly identified *in utero*.[56] The diagnosis relies on the failure to demonstrate the cranial vault. The anencephalic fetus has a typical frog-like appearance and usually has a short neck (Figure 57.8). The diagnosis can probably be made within 10 weeks of gestation by transvaginal ultrasound.

Cephalocele is also to be diagnosed by transvaginal ultrasound within 10 weeks of gestation. Specific

Table 57.3 Accuracy of ultrasound in the prenatal diagnosis of spina bifida[50]

	n	Prevalence (%)	Sensitivity (%)	Specificity (%)	PPV	NPV
Allen et al.	374	2.1	87	99	87	99
Persson et al.	10,147	0.1	40	100	100	99
Roberts et al.	1261	1.4	30	96	92	99
Roberts et al.	1991	1.7	80	99	80	99

PPV, positive predictive value; NPV, negative predictive value.

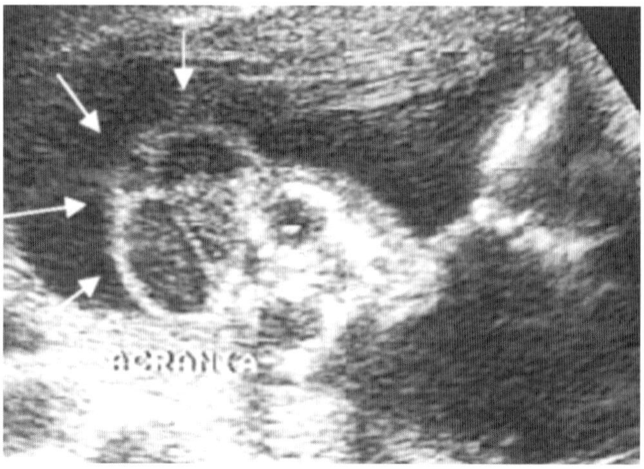

Figure 57.8 Acrania/anencephaly. Transvaginal scan in coronal plane shows protruding brain (arrows) with absent calvaria. This has a 'Mickey mouse' shape on coronal scans.

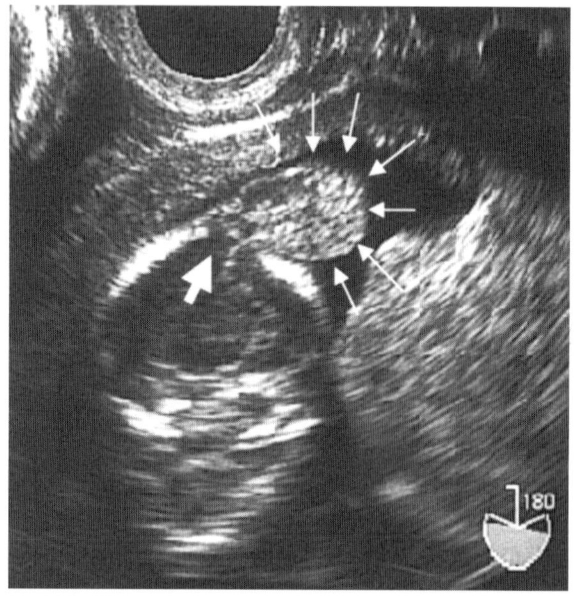

Figure 57.9 Encephalocele. Transvaginal scan of cranium shows large amount of brain protruding posteriorly (thin arrows) and a bony defect (big arrow).

findings in diagnosis of the cephalocele are to identify the soft tissue masses from scalp and the skull defect (Figure 57.9). The helpful findings for differential diagnosis are: (1) cephaloceles are often associated with hydrocephaly, (2) brain tissue can be seen in some cephaloceles, (3) cystic hygromas with multiple septa are often associated with other signs of hydrops and have a paracervical origin, and (4) severe scalp edema can be confused with a cephalocele, but usually a sagittal scan can identify an intact skull and the diffuse nature of the condition (see Romero *et al.*,[50] pp. 36–43).

Route of delivery

NTDs remain controversial as to whether the route of delivery influences outcome. Theoretically, a vaginal delivery may be further damaged by the mechanical forces of labor and by amniotic fluid contamination of the cerebrospinal fluid because of exposed neural tissue during labor. In the early 1980s, Chervenak *et al.* reported that infants with NTDs delivered by elective cesarean section (CS) have a better outcome in a small series of infants.[57] However, in a retrospective study of children with spina bifida, significant differences in any of several neurologic functions were not noted regardless of the route of delivery. In the early 1990s, two papers published conflicting results from large populations of affected infants. A prospective series in 1991 by Luthy *et al.* compared infants with spina bifida delivered by CS before labor, CS after labor, and vaginal delivery.[58] The level of motor deficit was assessed for each child as their motor level in relation to their radiologically determined anatomic level with degree of deficit and then evaluated across delivery categories. A significantly greater degree of motor loss, regardless of the anatomic level of the lesion, was noted in children delivered after labor, either by CS or vaginally. The greatest preservation of motor skills was noted in children delivered by CS before the onset of labor. In contrast, another review of outcomes in a similar, relatively large series of infants with NTDs did not reveal significant differences among routes of delivery.[59] As endpoints, this study assessed neurologic level and method of community locomotion. Infants were broadly grouped into functional neurologic levels of L2, L3–4, and below L5 levels. Although vaginal delivery initially seemed to be more neurologically deleterious to breech infants, even this significance was lost on follow-up of these infants. However, as breech presentation, resulting from neurologic dysfunction of hydrocephalus with an enlarged head, is common in pregnancies complicated by fetal spina bifida, cesarean delivery is standard for the breech fetus with an NTD.[59] The best delivery route for the vertex fetus remains controversial. No prospective randomized trial of vaginal delivery vs. cesarean delivery for vertex fetuses with spina bifida has been performed. All studies of vaginal vs. cesarean delivery are retrospective and all suffer from various biases.[58,60,61] Theoretically, cesarean delivery possibly avoids mechanical trauma and infection of the fetal spine.

As it is still not clear whether or how the method of delivery significantly affects neurologic outcome in these infants, the American College of Obstetricians and Gynecologists recommends that decisions about the timing and route of delivery should be made individually in consultation with personal experience and knowledge of such complications, which may include maternal–fetal medicine specialists, neonatologists, and pediatric neurosurgeons.[4]

Generally, delivery at term is optimal. However, rapidly increasing ventriculomegaly may prompt delivery before term so that a shunting procedure can be performed.

The fetus with spina bifida should be delivered at a hospital with neonatal intensive care facilities and personnel capable of managing the spine defect and any immediate complications.[62] Because individuals with an NTD are at risk of developing a severe, potentially life-threatening allergy to latex, clinicians handling tho infant should wear latex-free gloves.[63]

Fetal surgery (*in utero* repair)

Isolated open spina bifida often results in permanent neurological damage. Observations are consistent with a two-hit hypothesis in these fetuses. The first 'hit' is the defect itself, and the second comes from continued exposure to amniotic fluid.[64] An experimental evidence from both animal and human studies suggests that early gestational repair of open spina bifida may help preserve neurological function that might be lost due to *in utero* mechanical and chemical trauma. Animal studies involving primates, rats, and pigs have demonstrated that, compared to an untreated group, surgical closure successfully preserved neurologic function.[65–67]

Moreover, several investigators theorized that antenatal closure or coverage of the spine defect might prevent some of the neurological damage. Recently, both open surgical closure and laparoscopic techniques are being evaluated. Harrison's group, by using the fetal sheep model, has shown that repair of induced fetal spine defects prevent tissue damage and improve neurological function.[68] Bruner *et al.* described four human fetuses whose open lower spine defects were covered endoscopically with a maternal skin graft at 22–24 weeks.[69] It was hoped that this would prevent herniation of the hindbrain into the foramen magnum with obstruction and ventriculomegaly, the Arnold–Chiari malformation. They also compared 10 fetuses that underwent open surgical repair at 26–30 weeks with 20 fetuses without antenatal repair.[70] The surgically treated fetuses had a significantly decreased need for ventriculoperitoneal shunt placement after delivery. Johnson *et al.* at the Children's Hospital of Philadelphia (CHOP) also suggests that a reversal of the hindbrain herniation and a decreased incidence of neonatal ventriculoperitoneal shunting for hydrocephaly can be achieved.[71]

Open maternal–fetal surgery for NTD was initially undertaken at four centers in the USA as an investigative procedure under the guidance of institutional review boards. Many centers believe the procedure to be an innovative therapy that should not be ethically withheld. However, a survey of almost 1000 members of the Society for Maternal–Fetal Medicine indicated that 56% felt the procedure has still not been validated.[72]

Fetal surgical repair of open spina bifida exposes the mother to the risks of anesthesia, hemorrhage, chorioamnionitis and sepsis, thrombosis, tocolytic induced pulmonary edema, and uterine rupture. Additionally, preterm labor, preterm premature rupture of membranes, and oligohydramnios may occur in up to 50% of the patients.[73] Because of concerns about the safety and unproven benefits, fetal surgery for the correction of open spina bifida should be considered investigational. This surgery should only be conducted in a collaborative research setting in highly specialized centers.[74] The randomized trial has begun in the face of strong physician and patient belief that maternal–fetal surgery for NTD is a proved and beneficial technique. If clinical outcomes are not improved by the intervention, future open surgical procedures for this condition should be abandoned.[75] It also remains controversial because spina bifida is not a lethal defect.

Management

Although recent reports indicate that NTDs *in utero* repair may improve neurologic function and reduce morbidity from hydrocephalus and the Arnold–Chiari malformation by reversal of the hindbrain herniation component, the treatment of NTDs has been performed by postnatal surgical management. Postnatal surgery is aimed at covering the exposed spinal cord, preventing infection, and treating hydrocephaly with a ventricular shunt. Steinbok *et al.* reported a 91% shunt rate in 101 children after minimum follow-up period of 8.6 years.[76] The CHOP published shunt rates among 189 children treated for spina bifida between 1983 and 2000.[77] One hundred percent (35/35) of children with thoracic level lesions received shunts, compared with 88% (100/114) of children with lumbar lesion and only 68% (27/40) of children with lesions confined to the sacrum. In recently treated patients, the upper level of the spina bifida lesion appears to be a major determinant of the need for shunt placement. Fewer neurosurgeons are automatically placing shunts at the same time as the spinal lesion is closed.

Prevention

The risk of having an NTD pregnancy can be reduced by raising folic acid consumption around the time of conception.[78–80] But how much folic acid supplementation is enough to prevent NTDs is still controversial. Women in Western countries typically have a baseline folate level of 5 ng/ml (normal range, 6–20 ng/ml).[81] The Food and Drug Administration in the USA established standard fortifying cereal and grain products such as cereal, bread, rice, and pasta with folic acid. By putting 140 μg of folic acid into each 100 g of grain products, it was established that the folic acid intake would increase 100 g per day.[82] Although women of reproductive age should be advised to ingest a diet that includes folate-rich foods, several studies have shown that diet alone is not effective in increasing serum folate levels. Therefore, folic acid supplementation should be encouraged.

The ingestion of supplement 0.2 mg of folic acid each day would reduce the incidence of NTDs by only 20%.[81] These calculations are supported by data from the US Public Health Service that confirm that since the grain fortification began the incidence of NTDs in the USA has decreased by only 19%.[83] It is recommended that women of reproductive age take 0.4 mg of folic acid supplement each day. This would reduce the incidence of NTDs by 36%. Intake of a 4 mg supplemental dose is recommended for women with high risk for an offspring with NTDs. For example, if previous pregnancy has been complicated by an NTD, the mother's intake of folic acid supplement should be 4 mg per day in the next pregnancy, starting at least 4 weeks before conception and continuing through the first 3 months of pregnancy.[84] This would reduce the incidence of NTDs by 82%. A 5-mg/day supplement dose is predicted to reduce the incidence of NTDs by 85%.[81] Although folic acid is considered non-toxic even at very high doses and is rapidly excreted in the urine, there seems to be minimal risk associated with a high supplementation of 5 mg of folic acid per day. Supplementation of folic acid could mask the symptoms of pernicious anemia. However, folic acid cannot mask the neuropathy typical of this diagnosis. Currently, 12% of patients with pernicious anemia present with neuropathy alone.[85] With folic acid supplementation, this proportion may be increased, but there is no evidence that initiating treatment after the development of a neuropathy results in irreversible damage.[86]

The March of Dimes contracted the Gallop Organization to conduct a random-digit-detailed telephone survey of a national sample of 2001 women aged 15–45 years to assess knowledge about folic acid use.[87] Less than one-third of women of childbearing age consume a daily supplement containing folic acid. Only 13% of women knew that folic acid helps prevent birth defects, and only 7% knew that folic acid should be taken before pregnancy.

Without folic acid supplementation, the empirical recurrence risk after one affected child is 3–4%, and after two affected children it is 10%. With supplementation, the risk after one affected child is less than 1%.[14]

In humans, the only source of folic acid is the diet, and absorption occurs primarily in the proximal jejunum. Before folic acid can be absorbed, it must be reduced to the monoglutamate form.[88] Pancreatic conjugates within the intestine are responsible for this process. The activity of conjugate is decreased by anticonvulsants, oral contraceptives, alcohol, and sulfa drugs. So, women taking antiepileptic agents have decreased absorption of folic acid resulting in folic acid deficiency.[89–91]

Folic acid supplementation may not decrease the risk of NTDs in women with high first-trimester blood glucose levels, or high first-trimester maternal temperature, or in women who take valproic acid. In women with high glucose levels and high maternal temperature, the exact mechanism is unknown. First-trimester valproic acid use results in a 1–2% risk of having a fetus with spina bifida, but the mechanism may be different from that of other antiepileptic agents.[92] Fetuses with aneuploidy or genetic syndromes may have NTDs as a result of their specific generic abnormality. These NTDs are not prevented by folic acid.

Prognosis and outcome

About 23% of the estimated NTD pregnancy is aborted.[93,94] Despite aggressive intervention, nearly 14% of all spina bifida neonates do not survive past 5 years of age, with the mortality rate rising to 35% in those with symptoms of brainstem dysfunction secondary to the Arnold–Chiari malformation.[95] Mothers who choose to continue the pregnancy must be prepared for a child who needs significant care and may incur high medical expenses. Unfortunately, many healthcare professionals have considered that the fetus with spina bifida would be mentally retarded, never walk, and suffer bladder and bowel incontinence. Recently, Mirzai *et al.* commented that the majority of children with myelomeningocele could have a normal IQ and a socially acceptable degree of continence, and be able to walk.[96] The greatest concern is whether the child with spina bifida will ever walk. In a 25-year follow-up of 71 patients treated at birth in an aggressive, non-selective manner, Bowman *et al.* observed that 46% of young adults (33/71) ambulated the majority of the time (75–100%).[62] An additional 13% (9/71) ambulated 25–50% of the time. Forty-one percent (29/71) ambulated only with the aid of a wheelchair. When stratified by lesion level, patients with lower defects were more likely to ambulate the majority of the time. The next problem of the fetus with spina bifida is intelligence. Bowman *et al.* reported that 85% of the 71 young adults followed by their group were attending or had graduated from high school and/or college, and 63% attended regular classes.[62] Forty-five percent were actively employed, and almost 10% worked as volunteers. Most of the 71 patients lived with their parents, although 11 lived independently and two were married. Mirzai *et al.* noted that 60% of their young adults had normal IQ and development.[96] However, a normal IQ was seen in 76% without hydrocephaly. McLaurin *et al.* reported that 70% of myelomeningocele had a normal IQ.[97] Steinbok *et al.* observed that 58% of their cohort attended public school, and were in the appropriate grade for their age.[76] So, most children with spina bifida are not mentally retarded. Regarding bladder and bowel incontinence, Bowman *et al.* noted that 85% of their young adults (60/71) used clean intermitted catheterization (CIC), and 90% of them (54/60) performed their own catheterization. For those patients on CIC, 15% always had urinary continence, 68% were dry the majority of the time (75–100%), and 7% were dry 50% of the time. Fifty-two percent of the young adults reported bowel control the majority of the time, and 52% reported 100% social bowel continence.[62] Steinbok *et al.* reported 75% social continence of urine, defined as the ability to remain dry and odor-free without the use of a diaper, and 86% social continence of bowel.[76]

It should be obvious from these reports that most affected children will grow into young adults with normal intelligence, walking, and with social continence of both bladder and bowel. Bruner and Tulipan emphasized that, although a small number of affected children would experience devastating sequelae, equal number would be apparently normal, and prenatal imaging is becoming increasingly sophisticated in identifying the extent of disease and likely long-term outcomes.[98]

Table 57.4 Estimated incidence of neural tube defects based on specific risk factors in the United States[53]

Population	Incidence per 1000 Live births
Mother as reference	
General incidence	1.4–1.6
Women undergoing amniocentesis for advanced maternal age	1.5–3.0
Women with diabetes mellitus	20
Women on valproic acid in first trimester	10–20
Fetus as reference	
1 sibling with NTD	15–30
2 siblings with NTD*	57
Parent with NTD	11
Half sibling with NTD	8
First cousin (mother's sister's child)	10
Other first cousins	3
Sibling with severe scoliosis secondary to multiple vertebral defects	15–30
Sibling with occult spina dysraphism	15–30
Sibling with sacrococcygeal teratoma or hamartoma	≤15–30

NTD = neural tube defect.
*Risk is higher in British studies. Risk increases further for three or more siblings or combinations of other close relatives.

Recurrence risk

Several types of NTDs appear to have a unique recurrence risk. Hall *et al.* reported 7.8% recurrence risk with high spina bifida, 0.7% with low spina bifida, 2.2% with anencephaly, and no increase risk for craniorachischisis, encephalocele, or multiple defects.[99] Main and Mennuti reported the estimated incidence of NTDs based on specific factors in the USA (Table 57.4).[5] The common risk factor, family history, varies with the underling population risk. The recurrence risk was more than 10 times greater than the rate in the general population.

REFERENCES

1. Crapan JD, Roberts HE, Edmonds LD, *et al.* Surveillance for anencephaly and spina bifida and the impact of prenatal diagnosis – United States, 1985–1994. *MMWR CDC Surveill Summ* 1995;44:1–13.
2. Moore KL. *Before We Are Born.* Philadelphia: Saunders, 1977:46.
3. Golden JA, Chernoff GF. Multiple site of anterior neural tube closure in humans: Evidence from anterior neural tube defects (anencephaly). *Pediatrics* 1995;95:506–10.
4. American College of Obstetricians and Gynecologists, Committee on Practice Bulletin. Neural tube defects, No. 44, July 2003.
5. Main DM, Mennuti MT. Neural tube defects: Issues in perinatal diagnosis and counseling. *Obstet Gynecol* 1986;67:1–16.
6. Bonaiti-Pellie C, Smith C. Risks tables for genetic counseling in some common congenital malformations. *J Med Genet* 1974; 11:374–7.
7. Nussbaum RL, McInnes RR, Willard HF. Genetics of disorders with complex inheritance. In *Thompson and Thompson Genetics in Medicine*, 6th edn. Philadelphia: WB Saunders, 2001: 289–310.
8. Aitken DA, Crossley JA, Spencer K. Prenatal screening for neural tube defects and aneuploidy. In Rimsui DL, Connor JM, Pyeritz RE, Kort BE, eds. *Emery and Rimoin's Principles and Practice of Medical Genetics*, 4th edn. New York: Churchill and Livingstone, 2002:763–801.

9. Becerra JE, Khoury MJ, Cordero JF, Erickson JD. Diabetes mellitus during pregnancy and the risks for specific birth defects: A population based study. Pediatrics 1990;85:1–9.
10. Reece EA, Hobbins JC. Diabetic embryopathy: Pathogenosis prenatal diagnosis and prevention. *Obstet Gynecol Surv* 1986; 41;325–35.
11. Milunsky A. *Genetic Disorders and the Fetus: Diagnosis, Prevention and Treatment,* 3rd edn. Balimore: Johns Hopkins University Press, 1992:1–12.
12. Robert E, Robert JM, Lopras C. Is valproic acid teratogenic? *Rev Neural* 1983;139:445–7.
13. Jones KL. *Smith's Recognizable Pattern of Human Malformation,* 5th edn. Philadelphia: Saunders, 1997.
14. Cunningham FG, Gant NF, Leveno KJ, *et al.* eds. *Williams Obstetrics: Prenatal Diagnosis and Fetal Therapy.* New York: McGraw-Hill, 2001:973–1004.
15. Feuchtboum LB, Currier RJ, Riggle S, Roberson M, Lorey FW, Cunningham GC. Neural tube defect prevalence in California (1990–1994): Eliciting patterns by type of defect and maternal race/ethnicity. *Genet Test* 1999;3:265–72.
16. Mikail LN, Mittendorf R,Walker CK. The association of maternal obesity and isolated mayor fetal congenital cardiac anomalies in African-American woman. *Am J Obstet Gynecol* 1996;174:446.
17. Waller DK, Mills JL, Simpson JL, *et al.* Are obese woman at higher risk for producing malformed offspring? *Am J Obstet Gynecol* 1994;170:541–8.
18. Werler MM, Louik C, Shapiro S, Mitchell AA. Pregnant weight in relation to risk of neural tube defects. *J Am Med Assoc* 1996; 275:1089–93.
19. Shaw GM, Velie EM, Schaffer D. Risk of neural tube defect affected pregnancies among obese women. *J Am Med Assoc* 1996;275:1093–6.
20. Shaw GM, Todoroff K, Schaffer DM, Selvin S. Maternal height and prepregnancy body mass index as risk factors for selected congenital anomalies. *Paediatr Perinat Epidemiol* 2000;14:234–9.
21. Korones SB. Uncommon virus infections of the mother, fetus, and newborn: Influeza, mumps and measles. *Clin Perinatol* 1988;15;259–72.
22. Lynberg MC, Khoury HJ, Lu X, Cocian T. Maternal flu, fever, and the risk of neural tube defects: A population-based case–control study. *Am J Epidemiol* 1994;140:224–55.
23. Lockwood CJ. Heritable coagulopathies in pregunancy. *Obstet Gynecol Surv* 1999;54:754–65.
24. Van der Put MN, Steegers-Theunissen RP, Frosst P, *et al.* Mutated methylenetetrahydrofolate reductase as a risk factor for spina bifida. *Lancet* 1995;346:1070–1.
25. Van der Put MN, Eskes TK, Blom HJ. Is the common 677C T mutation in the methylenetetrahydrofolate reductase gene a risk factor for neural tube defects? A meta analysis. *QJM* 1997;90:111–5.
26. Van der Put MN, Blom HJ. Neural tube defects and a disturbed folate dependent homocysteine metabolism. *Eur J Obstet Gynecol Reprod Biol* 2000;92:57–61.
27. Prevention of neural tube defects results of the Medical Research Council Vitamin Study. *Lancet* 1991;338:131–7.
28. Czeizel AE, Dudas I. Prevention of the first occurrence of neural tube defects by periconceptional vitamin supplementation. *N Engl J Med* 1992;327:1832–5.
29. Rothenberg SP, da Costa MP, Sequeria JM, *et al.* Autoantibodies against folate receptors in women with a pregnancy complicated by a neural-tube defect. *N Engl J Med* 2004;350:134–42.
30. Burton BK. Elevated maternal serum alpha-fetoprotein (MSAFP): Interpretation and follow-up. *Clin Obstet Gynecol* 1988;31: 293–305.
31. Brumfield CG, Clovd GA, Davis RO, Finley SC, Hauth JC, Boots L. The relationship between maternal serum and amniotic fluid alpha-fetoprotein in women undergoing early amniocentesis. *Am J Obstet Gynecol* 1990;163:903–6.
32. Roberts NS, Dunn LK, Weiner S, Godmilow L, Miller R. Midtrimester amniocentesis: Indication, technique, risk and potential for prenatal diagnosis. *J Reprod Med* 1983;28:167–88.
33. Brock JH, Sutcliffe RG. Alpha-fetoprotein in the antenatal diagnosis of anencephaly and spina bifida. *Lancet* 1972;ii:197–9.
34. Brock DJH, Bolton AE, Monaghan JM. Prenatal diagnosis of anencephaly through maternal serum-alphafetoprotein measurement. *Lancet* 1973;ii:923.
35. UK Collaborative Study on Alpha-fetoprotein in Relation to Neural tube Defects. Maternal serum-alpha-fetoprotein measurement in antenatal screening for anencephaly and spina bifida in early pregnancy. *Lancet* 1977;ii:1323–32.
36. Burton BK, Sowers SG, Nelson LH. Maternal serum a-feto-protein screening in North Carolina: Experience with more than twelve thousand pregnancies. *Am J Obstet Gynecol* 1983;146:439–44.
37. Haddow JE, Kloza EM, Smith DE, Knight GJ. Data from an alphafetoprotein pilot screening program in Maine. *Obstet Gynecol* 1983;62:556–60.
38. Milunsky A, Alpert E, Neff RK, Frigoletto FD Jr. Prenatal diagnosis of neural tube defects. IV. Maternal serum alpha-fetoprotein screening. *Obstet Gynecol* 1980;55:60–6.
39. Jenkins TM, Wapner RJ. Prenatal diagnosis of congenital disorders. In Creasy RK Resnik R, eds. *Maternal–Fetal Medicine, Principles and Practice,* 5th edn. Philadelphia: Saunders, 2004:245.
40. O'Brien JE, Dverin E, Drugan A, Tohnson MP, Yaron Y, Evans MI. Race-ethnicity-specific variation in multiple-marker biochemical screening: Alpha-fetoprotein, HCG, and estoriol. *Obstet Gynecol* 1997;89:355–8.
41. Wold NJ, Cukle H, Boreham J, Stirrat GM, Turnbull AC. Maternal serum alpha-fetoprotein and diabetes mellitus. *Br J Obstet Gynecol* 1979;86:101–5.
42. Crossley JA, Berry E, Aitken DA, Conner JM. Insulin-dependent diabetes mellitus and prenatal screening results: Current experience from a regional screening programme. *Prenat Diagn* 1996;16:1039–42.
43. Cuckle H, Wold N, Stevenson JD, *et al.* Maternal serum alphafetoprotein screening for open neural tube defects in twin pregnancies. *Prenat Diagn* 1990;10:71–7.
44. Wapner RJ, Johnson A, Davis G. Prenatal diagnosis in twin gestations: A comparison between second trimester amniocentesis and first trimester chorionic villus sampling. *Obstet Gynecol* 1993;82:49–56.
45. Loft AG, Hogdall E, Larsen SO, Norgood-Pedersen B. A comparison of amniotic fluid alpha-fetoprotein and acotulchalineestrase in the prenatal diagnosis of open neural tube defects and anterior abdominal wall defects. *Prenat Diagn* 1993;13: 93–109.
46. Watoson WJ, Chescheir NC, Katz VL, Seeds JW. The role of ultrasound in evaluation of patients with elevated maternal serum alpha-fetoprotein: A review. *Obstet Gynecol* 1991;78: 123–8.
47. Harmon JP, Hiett AK, Palmer CG, Golochowski AM. Prenatal ultrasound detection of isolated neural tube defects: Is cytogenetic evaluation warranted? *Obstet Gynecol* 1995;86: 595–9.
48. Gardner RJ, Sutherland GR, eds. Prenatal diagnostic procedures. In *Chromosome Abnormalities and Genetic Counseling.* Oxford Monographs on Medical Genetics, No. 29, 2nd edn. New York: Oxford University Press, 1996:336–44.
49. Nicolaides KH, Campbell S, Gabbe SG, Guidetti R. Ultrasound screening for spina bifida: Cranial and cerebellar signs. *Lancet* 1986;2:72–4.
50. Romero R, Pilu G, Jeanty P, *et al.,* eds. Spina bifida. In *Perinatal Diagnosis of Congenital Anomalies.* New York: Appleton and Lange, 1988:36–43, 46–50.
51. Campbell S. Early prenatal diagnosis of neural tube defects by ultrasound. *Clin Obstet Gynecol* 1977;20:351–9.
52. Crane JP, LeFevre ML, Winborn RC, *et al.* A randomized trial of prenatal ultrasonographic screening: Impact on the detection, management, and outcome of anomalous fetuses. The RADIUS Study Group. *Am J Obstet Gynecol* 1994;171:392–9.
53. Boyd PA, Wellesley DG, de Walle HEK, *et al.* Evaluation of the prenatal diagnosis of neural tube defects by fetal ultrasonographic examination in different centres across Europe. *J Med Screen* 2000;7:169–74.
54. Williamson P, Alberman E, Rodeck C, Fiddler M, Church S, Harris R. Antecedent circumstances surrounding neural tube defect births in 1990–91. The Steering Committee of the National Confidential Enquiry into Counseling for Genetic Disorders. *Br J Obstet Gynaecol* 1997;104:51–5.
55. Sebire NJ, Noble PL, Thorpe-Beeston JG, Snijders RJM, Nicolaides KH. Presence of the "lemon" sign in fetuses with spina bifida at the 10–14-week scan. *Ultrasound Obstet Gynecol* 1997;10:403–7.
56. Campbell S, Johnstone FD, Holt EM, May P. Anencephaly: Early ultrasonic diagnosis and active management. *Lancet* 1972;2: 1226–7.
57. Chervenak FA, Berkowitz R, Tortora M, Hobbins JC. The management of fetal hydrocephalus. *Am J Obstet Gynecol* 1985; 151:933–42.
58. Luthy DA, Wordinsky T, Shurtleff DB, *et al.* Cesarean section before onset of labor and subsequent motor function in infants

with myelomeningocele diagnosed antenatally. *N Engl J Med* 1991;324:662–6.

59. Cochrane D, Aronyk K, Sawatzky B, Wilson D, Steinbok P. The effects of labor and delivery on spinal cord function and ambulation in patients with meningomyelocele. *Childs Nerv Syst* 1991;7:312–5.
60. Bensen JT, Dillard RG, Burton BK. Open spina bifida: Does cesarean section delivery improve prognosis? *Obstet Gynecol* 1988;71:532–4.
61. Sakala EP, Andree I. Opimal route of delivery for meningomyelocele. *Obstet Gynecol Surv* 1990;45:209–12.
62. Wilkins-Haug L. Consideration for delivery of infants with congenital abnormalities. *Obstet Gynecol Clin North Am* 1999; 26:399–412.
63. Bowman RM, Mclone DG, Grant JA, Tomita T, Ito JA. Spina bifida outcome: A 25-year prospective. *Pediatr Neurosurg* 2001; 34:114–20.
64. Heffez DS, Aryanpur J, Hutchins GM, Freeman JM. The paralysis associated with myelomeningocele: Clinical and experimental data implicating a preventable spinal cord injury. *Neurosurgery* 1990;26:987–92.
65. Michejda M. Intrauterine treatment of spina bifida: Primate model. *Z Kinderchir* 1984;39:259–61.
66. Heffez DS, Aryanpur J, Rotellini NA, Hutchis G, Freeman JM. Intrauterine repair of experimental surgically created dysraphism. *Neurosurgery* 1993;32:1005–10.
67. Meuli M, Meuli-Simmen C, Hutchins GM, *et al.* In utero surgery rescues neurological function at birth in sheep with spina bifida. *Nat Med* 1995;1:342–7.
68. Meuli M, Meuli-Simmen C, Yingling CD, *et al.* In utero repair of experimental myelomeningocele saves neurological function at birth. *J Pediatr Surg* 1996;31:397–402.
69. Bruner JP, Richards WO, Tulipan NB, Arney TL. Endoscopic coverage of fetal myelomeningocele in utero. *Am J Obstet Gynecol* 1999;180:153–8.
70. Bruner JP, Walsh WF, Boehm FH, *et al.* Open fetal repair of myelomeningocele improves neurologic outcome in the neonate. 19th Annual Meeting of the Society for Maternal–Fetal Medicine. *Am J Obstet Gynecol* 1999;180:831.
71. Johnson MP, Sutton LN, Rintoul N, *et al.* Fetal myelomeningocele repair: Short-term clinical outcomes. *Am J Obstet Gynecol* 2003;189:482–7.
72. Lyerly AD, Cefalo RC, Socol M, Fogarty L, Sugarman J. Attitudes of maternal–fetal specialists concerning maternal–fetal surgery. *Am J Obstet Gynecol* 2001;185:1052–8.
73. Bruner JP, Tulipan N, Paschall RL, *et al.* Fetal surgery for myelomeningocele and the incidence of shunt-dependent hydrocephalus. *J Am Med Assoc* 1999;282:1819–25.
74. ACOG Committee Opinion. No. 252. Fetal surgery for open neural tube defects. March 2001.
75. Moise KJ. Maternal–fetal surgery for spina bifida: On the brink of new era? *Am J Obstet Gynecol* 2003;189:311.
76. Steinbok P, Irvine B, Cochrane DD, Irwin BJ. Long-term outcome and complications of children born with meningomyelocele. *Childs Nerv Syst* 1992;8:92–6.
77. Rintoul N, Sutton LN, Hubbard AM, *et al.* A new look at myelomeningoceles: Functional level, vertebral level, shunting and the implications for fetal intervention. *Pediatrics* 2002;109: 409–13.
78. Wald N, Sneddon J, Densem J, Frost C, Stone R. Prevention of neural tube defects: Results of the MRC Vitamin Study. *Lancet* 1991;338:132–7.
79. Botto LD, Moore CA, Khoury MJ, Erickson JD. Neural-tube defects. *N Engl J Med* 1999;341:1509–19.
80. Wald N. Folic acid and the prevention of neural tube defects: Maternal nutrition and pregnancy outcome. *Ann N Y Acad Sci* 1993;678:112–29.
81. Wald NJ, Law HR, Morris JK, Wald DS. Quantifying the effect of folic acid. *Lancet* 2001;358:2069–73.
82. Food standards: Amendment of identify for enriched grain products to require standards of addition of folic acid FDA. Final rule. *Fed Reg* 1996;61:8781–97.
83. Honein MA, Paulozzi LJ, Mathews TJ, Ericson JD, Wong LY. Impact of folic acid fortification of the US food supply on the occurrence of neural tube defects. *J Am Med Assoc* 2001;285: 2981–6.
84. American College of Obstetricians and Gynecologists. Folic acid for the prevention of recurrent neural tube defects. ACOG Committee Opinion 120.Washington, DC: ACOG, 1993.
85. Lindenbaum J, Healton EB, Savage DG, Brust JC, Garrett TJ, Podell ER. Neuropsychiatric disorders caused by cobalamin deficiency in the absence of anemia or macrocytosis. *N Engl J Med* 1988;318:1720–8.
86. Wald NJ, Bower C. Folic acid, pernicious anemia, and prevention of neural tube defects. *Lancet* 1994;343:307.
87. Centers for Disease Control and Prevention. Knowledge and use of folic acid by woman of childbearing age – United States, 1995–1998. *MMWR Morb Mortal Wkly Rep* 1999;48:325–7.
88. Herbent V, Colman N, Spivack M, *et al.* Folic acid deficiency in the United States: Folate assays in a prenatal clinic. *Am J Obstet Gynecol* 1975;123;175–9.
89. Pritchard JA, Whalley PL, Scott DE. Infants of mothers with megaloblastic anemia due to folate deficiency. *J Am Med Assoc* 1970;211;1982–4.
90. Iyengar L, Babu S. Folic acid absorption in pregnancy. *Br J Obstet Gynecol* 1975;82:20–3.
91. Johan E, Magnus EM. Plasma and red blood cell folate during normal pregnancy. *Acta Obstet Gynecol Scand* 1981;60:247–51.
92. Lindhout D, Omtzigt JG, Cornel MC Spectrum of neural tube defects in 34 infants prenatally exposed to antiepileptic drugs. *Neurology* 1992;42(Suppl 5):111–8.
93. Roberts HE, Moore CA, Cragan JD. Impact of prenatal diagnosis on the birth prevalence of neural tube defects. Atlanta 1990–1991. *Pediatrics* 1995;96:880–3.
94. Velie EM, Shaw GM. Impact of prenatal diagnosis and elective termination on prevalence and risk estimates of neural tube defects in California, 1989–1991. *Am J Epidemiol* 1996;144:473–9.
95. Worley G, Schuser JM, Oakes WJ. Survival at 5years of a cohort of newborn infants with myelomeningocele. *Dev Med Child Neurol* 1996;38:816–22.
96. Mirzai H, Ersahim Y, Mutluer S, Kayahan A. Outcome of patients with meningomylocele. *Childs Nerv Syst* 1998;14:120–3.
97. McLaurin RL. Myelomeningocele: Outcome and large complication. In Section of Pediatric Neurosurgery of the American Association of Neurological Surgeons, eds. *Pediatric Neurosurgery: Surgery of the Developing Nervous System*, 2nd edn. Philadelphia: Saunders, 1989:53–70.
98. Bruner JP, Tulipan N. Tell the truth about spina bifida. *Ultrasound Obstet Gynecol* 2004;24:595–6.
99. Hall JG, Friedman JM, Kenna BA, Popkin J, Jawanda M, Arnold W. Clinical, genetic, and epidemiological factors in neural tube defects. *Am J Hum Genet* 1988;43:827–37.

58 Basic background of congenital anomalies: congenital heart diseases and lung diseases

T. Kanzaki

Epidemiology

Congenital heart disease (CHD) is the most common severe congenital abnormality with an incidence of about 8.8 in 1000 live births. Epidemiologic studies that have excluded patent ductus arteriosus in premature infants have suggested an overall lower incidence of CHD (3.7 in 1000 live births).

Table 58.1 Comparison of disease seen in infant and fetal series

Diagnosis	Brompton (%)	NERICP (%)	Fetal (%)
Ventricular septal defect	15.4	15.7	5
Complete transposition	10.4	9.9	2
Tetralogy of Fallot	9.9	8.9	3
Coarctation	10.5	7.5	3
HLHS	3.7	7.4	11
Mitral atresia	0	0	5
Critical aortic stenosis	1.1	1.9	4
AVSD	3.9	5.0	17.5
Pulmonary stenosis/atresia	4.9	6.4	5
Atrial septal defect	0.5	2.9	0
TAPVC	3.6	2.6	< 1
Cardiomyopathy	2.7	2.6	4
Tricuspid atresia	4.7	2.6	4
Double-inlet ventricle	4.3	2.4	2
Double-outlet ventricle	3.0	1.5	3
Trunk	2.1	1.4	1.5
Ebstein's malformation	0	0	7
Tumor	0	0	1
Corrected transposition	0.8	0.9	< 1
Miscellaneous	11.3	10.4	< 1

AVSD, atrioventricular septal defect; Brompton, Royal Brompton Hospital, London; HLHS, hypoplastic left heart syndrome; NERICP, New England Infant Cardiac Care Program; TAPVC, totally anomalous pulmonary venous connection

Table 58.2 Risk factors for CHD

Fetal
Chromosomal abnormalities
Extracardiac anatomic abnormalities
Non-immune hydrops fetalis
Fetal cardiac arrhythmia
Maternal
Family history of CHD
Maternal metabolic disorders
Maternal teratogen exposure

A clear difference in the proportion of individual anomalies between the fetus and the infant can be seen in Table 58.1.[1] This is because these are all lesions readily detectable during the screening four-chamber scan. In contrast, the rate of detection of ventricular septal defects, complete transposion and teratology of Fallot is lower than in infancy because these lesions are not readily detectable on routine scan. Nevertheless, CHD remains the most common severe abnormality in the newborn. Its prenatal diagnosis allows for better pregnancy counseling and improved neonatal outcome.

CHD and chromosomal abnormalities

Traditionally, the etiology of most congenital heart defects has been considered multifactorial, with interaction between genetic and environmental factors. Only about 10–15% of all congenital heart defects have been attributed to known chromosomal abnormalities, genetic syndromes, and teratogenic embryopathies. The risk factors for CHD can be grouped into two main categories, fetal and maternal (Table 58.2).

The frequency of chromosomal abnormalities in infants with CHD has been estimated as 5–10% from postnatal data. Some studies have suggested that up to 39% of fetuses with congenital heart defects diagnosed by fetal echocardiogram at 18–20 weeks' gestation have a chromosomal anomaly, although chromosomal anomalies account for only 5% of congenital heart defects in liveborns. This discrepancy is attributed to *in utero* losses of aneuploid fetuses.

Cardiac defects tend to be specific common chromosomal abnormalities and their associated congenital cardiac defects (Table 58.3).[2] In general, malformations of the right side of the heart are rarely associated with karyotypic abnormalities. The diagnosis of transposition of the great vessels and tricuspid atresia is not usually associated with chromosomal abnormalities. On the other hand, atrio-ventricular septal defect, perimembranous ventricular defect, tetralogy of Fallot, double-outlet right ventricle, and hypoplasitic left heart syndrome are associated with chromosomal abnormalities.

Table 58.4 is a list of the most common chromosomal abnormalities and their associated congenital cardiac defects.[2] Data obtained from postnatal studies suggest that the incidence of cardiac defects is 40–50% in trisomy 21, 25–45% in Turner's syndrome, and more than 90% in trisomies 13 and 18.

Single-gene disorders associated with CHD

Although the etiology of many syndromes remains unknown, approximately 3% of congenital heart defects are attributed to single-gene defects. Table 58.5 is a list of the more common genetic syndromes of unknown etiology and their associated cardiac and extracardiac features.[3]

Table 58.3 Congenital heart disease and associated chromosomal abnormalities

Cardiac defect	Fetuses, total	Aneuploid fetuses	Infants, total	Aneuploid infants
Atrioventricular septal defect	193	75	186	133
Ventricular septal defect	70	34	542	47
Hypoplastic left heart syndrome	168	10	108	3
Pulmonary atresia/stenosis	61	3	201	1
Transposition of the great arteries	22	0	119	0
Aortic atresia/stenosis	42	2	73	3
Tricuspid atresia	46	2	19	0
Truncus arteriosus	15	2	68	1
Coarctation of aorta	114	33	132	11
Tetralogy of Fallot/ Double-outlet right ventricle	86	19	159	20

Table 58.4 Incidence and type of congenital heart disease in chromosomal aneuploidy

Chromosomal abnormality	Incidence at live birth	Associated cardiac abnormality (%)	Common cardiac abnormalities
Trisomy 21	1:800	40–50	Atrioventricular septal defect, ventricular septal defect
Trisomy 18	1:8,000	> 90	Ventricular septal defect, double-outlet right ventricle
Trisomy 13	1:20,000	> 80	Ventricular septal defect, atrial septal defect
45,X	1:10,000	25–45	Coarctation of aorta, bicuspid aortic valve

Table 58.5 Single-gene disorders associated with congenital heart defects

Syndrome	Associated cardiac defects	Other anomalies detected prenatally	Inheritance
Holt–Oram	Septal defect, coarctation of the aorta, HLHS	Absent thumb, upper-extremity phocomelia, syndactyly	AD, sporadic
Noonan	Septal defect, pulmonary stenosis, patent ductus arteriosus	Cystic hygroma, micrognathia	AD
CATCH-22	Conotruncal heart defect	Cleft lip, cleft palate, microcephaly	AD
Ellis–van Creveld	Atrial septal defect, single atrium	Cleft lip, postaxial polydactyly, Dandy–Walker malformation	AR
Treacher–Collins	Septal defects, patent ductus arteriosus	Micrognathia	AD
Kartagener	Dextrocardia	Situs inversus, communicating hydrocephalus	AR
Kippel–Feil	Ventricular septal defect	Sacral agenesis	AD, sporadic
Williams	Aortic stenosis, septal defects	Unilateral renal agenesis, IUGR	AD, sporadic

AD, autosomal dominant; AR, autosomal recessive; HLHS, hypoplastic left heart syndrome; IUGR, intrauterine growth retardation

Table 58.6 Empiric estimation of recurrence risk for congenital heart defects

	Individual(s) affected			
Defect	One sibling	Two siblings	Mother	Father
Ventricular septal defect	3	10	6–10	2
Patent ductus arteriosus	3	10	4	2.5
Atrial septal defect	2.5–3.2	8	4–4.5	1.5
Tetralogy of Fallot	2.5	8	2.5	1
Pulmonary stenosis	2	6	4–6.5	1.5
Coarctation of the aorta	2–8	6	2	2
Aortic stenosis	2	6	13–18	3
Transposition of the great vessels	1.5	5		
Endocardial cushion defects	3	10		
Hypoplastic left heart	2	6		
Ebstain anomaly	1	3		
Pulmonary atresia	1	3		

Recurrence risk

In general, recurrence risk of 1–5% is estimated for the majority of congenital cardiac abnormalities. For the majority of cases the exact cause of the congenital heart defect is unknown, making it difficult to precisely predict whether the anomaly will occur again in a future pregnancy. Large population studies of isolated defects provide the most practical recurrence risks, though they may not always be applicable and their limitation should be outlined to the patients. In general, recurrence risks are higher in the child of the affected rather than the siblings, and increase significantly with each additional affected relative. Affected mothers are also at a higher risk of having affected offspring than affected fathers. These data are summarized in Table 58.6.[4]

REFERENCES

1. Allan LD, *et al.* Prospective diagnosis of 1,006 consecutive cases of congenital disease in the fetus. *J Am Coll Cardiol* 1994;23:1452–8.
2. Abuhamad A. *A Practical Guide to Fetal Echocardiography*. Philadelphia, PA: Lippincott-Raven, 1997.
3. *Online Mendelian Inheritance in Man*. http://www.ncbi.nlm.nih.gov/Omim/.
4. Welch KK, *et al.* The role of genetic counseling in the management of prenatally detected congenital heart defects. *Semin Perinat* 2000;24:373–9.

59 Clinical and genetical approach to skeletal dysplasia

K. Ozono, N. Namba, Y. Miyoshi, K. Wada and T. Michigami

Introduction

Skeletal dysplasias comprise more than 200 diseases and are not infrequent as a whole. However, each of the skeletal dysplasias is rather rare and many pediatricians are unfamiliar with the recent advances in understanding of the pathogenesis and the medical management of these diseases. Skeletal dysplasias are clinically important, especially for the neonatologist since the respiratory complications sometimes result in neonatal death. Recent advances in the research on bone and cartilage metabolism have shed light on the molecular mechanisms of skeletal diseases and made a great contribution to the management of patients with skeletal dysplasia.[1–3] The identified genes responsible for skeletal dysplastic diseases are increasing in number (Table 59.1).[4–8] Importantly, several new techniques have been developed for diagnosis and treatment of patients with skeletal dysplasias.

Bone formation or skeletogenesis consists of two different pathways, membranous bone formation and enchondral bone formation. The former process is direct bone formation from mesenchymal cells without a cartilage mold. The skull is the representative bone formed via membranous bone formation. In contrast, most bones including long bones and vertebrae are formed by enchondral bone formation. Several important factors have been identified as being involved in this process and some of them are reviewed in this chapter.[1–7] Moreover, the defects of these factors lead to skeletal dysplastic diseases.

The manifestations of skeletal dysplasia are numerous. *In utero*, polyhydroamnios and growth retardation of fetus is often associated with skeletal dysplasias. After birth, respiratory difficulty is the primary issue to be solved in patients with severe skeletal dysplasias. Characteristic faces and disproportionate short stature are often the hallmarks of skeletal dysplasias in childhood. Extraskeletal features including hypoplastic hair, skin legions and immunological abnormality imply specific skeletal dysplasia.

The wide variation in phenotypic severity is one of the features of skeletal dysplasia. Sometimes the names of diseases are distinct to describe the difference in phenotype even when the same gene is responsible for the diseases. Such diseases are allelic and have similar features, although the severity and the survival rate are quite different. For example, mutations of the FGF receptor 3 (FGFR 3) gene are associated not only with achondroplasia, the most common chondrodysplasia, but also with thanatophoric dysplasia and hypochondroplasia.[9] Another example is the case of the defects in the type II collagen gene including hypochondrogenesis, spondyloepiphyseal dysplasia, Kniest and Stickler diseases.[10]

In general, phenotype is severe in patients with skeletal dysplasias found in the perinatal period, and long survival is not achieved in many of them mainly due to respiratory problems. Elucidation of the relationship between the skeletogenesis and lung development may lead to better treatments for severe forms of skeletal dysplasias. In contrast, the treatments for childhood cases of skeletal dysplasias have been improved such as growth hormone for achondroplasia, bisphosphonate for osteogenesis imperfecta and bone marrow transplantation for malignant osteopetrosis. Thus, the opportunity has increased for pediatricians to treat patients with skeletal dysplasia.

In this manuscript, we take an overview of some of the key players in the enchondral bone formation and their implication in skeletal diseases. We aim to help clinicians to manage patients with skeletal dysplasia with better understanding of the diseases. At first, molecular mechanisms of the proliferation and differentiation of chondrocytes in growth plate are reviewed. Then, recent advances in genetics and clinical aspects are described in several representative skeletal dysplastic diseases. Clinical approach to skeletal dysplasia is mentioned in the last part of the manuscript.

Table 59.1 Skeletal dysplasia and its responsible gene

1. *FGF receptor or FGF*	
Achondroplasia	FGFR3 (G1138A,C)
Hypochondroplasia	FGFR3 (C1659A,G; C1620A)
Thanatophoric dysplasia	FGFR3 (I, C742T; II, A1948G)
Pfeiffer syndrome	FGFR1 (C755G); FGFR2 (T1036C; G1037A)
Crouzon syndrome	FGFR2 (G1037A; T1036C,A; C1073G, etc.)
Jackson–Weiss syndrome	FGFR2
Apert syndrome	FGFR2 (C934G; C937G)
Beare–Stevenson cutis gyrata syndrome	FGFR2
Muenke craniosynostosis	FGFR3 (C749G)
Hypophosphatemic rickets, AD	FGF23
2. *Collagen*	
Osteogenesis imperfecta	COL1A1; COL1A2
Achondrogenesis type II	COL2A1
Hypochondrogenesis	COL2A1
Spondyloepiphyseal dysplasia	COL2A1
Kniest dysplasia	COL2A1
Stickler dysplasia	COL2A1; COL11A2
Stickler dysplasia type 2	COL11A1
Spondyloepimetaphyseal dysplasia (Strudwick type)	COL2A1
Multiple epiphyseal dysplasia type 2	COL9A2
Metaphyseal dysplasia (Schmid)	COL10A1
3. *Matrix protein*	
Pseudoachondroplasia	COMP
Multiple epiphyseal dysplasia	COMP
Shprintzen–Goldberg syndrome	FBN1
Keutel syndrome	MGP
Multiple epiphyseal dysplasia	MATN3
4. *Hormone, hormone receptor, signal transducer*	
Metaphyseal dysplasia (Jansen)	PTH/PTHrP receptor (gain)
Blomstrand chondrodysplasia	PTH/PTHrP receptor (loss)
Albright osteodystrophy	Gsα
McCune–Albright syndrome	Gsα
Vitamin D dependency type I	1-α-hydroxylase

Table 59.1 Continued

Vitamin D dependency type II	Vitamin D receptor
Osteoporosis-pseudoglioma	LRP5 (loss)
High bone mass	LRP5 (gain)
Familial expansile osteolysis	TNFRSF11A
Juvenile Paget's disease	OPG
5. *Enzyme*	
Hypophosphatasia	TNS alkaline phosphatase
Osteopetrosis	Carbonic anhydrase II, TCIGR1, CLCN7, GL
Pycnodysostosis	Cathepsin K
Smith–Lemli–Opitz syndrome	δ^7-sterol reductase
Mucopolysaccharidoses	Lysosome enzyme (Hurler, Morquio)
X-linked recessive chondrodydplasia punctata	Arylsulfatase E
Rhizomelic chondrodysplasia punctata	PEX7
Coffin–Lowry syndrome	RSK-2
Noonan syndrome	PTPN11
SEMD Pakistani type	PAPSS2
Osteolysis Torg type	MMP2
Wolcott–Rallison syndrome	EIF2AK3
OLEDAID	NEMO
6. *Transcription factors*	
Boston-type craniosynostosis	MSX2
Campomelic dysplasia	SOX9
Cleidocranial dysplasia	CBFA1
Saethre–Chotzen syndrome	TWIST
Polysyndactyly type II	HOXD-13
Greig syndrome	GLI3
Polydactyly type A	GLI3
Ulnar-mammary syndrome	TBX3
Holt–Oram syndrome	TBX5
Townes–Brocks syndrome	SALL1
Nail–patella syndrome	LMX1B
Tricho-rhino-phalangeal dysplasia type 1	TRPS1
Ellis–van Creveld	EVC
EEC syndrome	p63
Trichodentooseeous syndrome	DLX3
Leri–Weill dyschondrostosis	SHOX
7. *Others*	
Diastrophic dysplasia	Sulfate transporter (DTDST)
Achondrogenesis type IB	Sulfate transporter (DTDST)

Table 59.1 Continued

Atelosteogenesis type 2	Sulfate transporter (DTDST)
Craniometaphseal dysplasia	Pyrophosphate transporter (ANK)
Chondrodysplasia	Growth/differentiation factor-5
(Hunter–Thompson, Grebe)	(CDMP-1)
Osteosclerosis	SOST
Brachydactyly type C	CDMP-1
Camurati–Engelmann	TGFB1
SED tarda	SEDL (ER-Golgi transport)
Cartilage–hair hypoplasia	RMRP
Kenny–Caffey syndrome	TBCE (chaperone protein)
Multiple synostosis syndrome	Noggin
Spondylocostal dysostosis	DLL3
Brachydacyly A1	IHH
Progressive pseudorheumatoid dysplasia	WISP3
Brachydacyly B2	ROR2
Dyggve–Melchior–Clausen dysplasia	FLJ90130
Shwachman–Diamond	SBDS

Common mutations are described in parentheses.

Development of cartilage and bone

Enchondral bone formation is a multistep process where chondrocytes proliferate and differentiate step by step, resulting in layered structure, namely resting, proliferating, hypertrophic and calcifying zones (Figure 59.1).[3] After the extracellular matrix is calcified, bone tissue (primary spongiosa) replaces cartilage. During the chondrocytic differentiation, the main components of the matrix are changed from collagen type II to collagen type I via collagen type X. Recently, many molecules including SOX9, FGF receptor 3 (FGFR3) and parathyroid hormone-related peptide (PTHrP) have been found to play important roles in the process.[1–3] These integrated networks of such bioactive factors tightly control enchondral bone development in the limb. Moreover, the genes encoding these molecules are responsible for several types of skeletal dysplasias. The process of chondrocytic differentiation is terminated by the death of hypertrophic chondrocytes, followed by blood vessel invasion, which promotes replacement of the cartilaginous matrix by the primary spongiosa.

The first step of chondrocytic differentiation or chondrogenesis is the mesenchymal cell condensation of undifferentiated progenitor cells. The differentiation of mesenchymal precursor cells into chondrocytes requires a transcription factor, Sox9.[11,12] Sox9 is a member of the Sox family of transcription factors that contain high mobility group (HMG)-box DNA-binding domain. Sox9 upregulates the expression of characteristic cartilaginous matrix genes such as collagens type II, IX, and XI, and aggrecan. In humans, haploinsufficiency of the Sox9 gene causes campomelic dysplasia (MIM 114290), which is characterized by deformities of long bones.[13] Most affected neonates die from respiratory failure due to hypoplastic tracheal and rib cartilage. Interestingly, some XY patients with campomelic dysplasia exhibit male-to-female sex reversal because Sox9 is involved not only in chondrogenesis but also in mammalian sex determination as a downstream regulator of the transcription factor, SRY.

FGFR3, as the other FGFRs, is a membrane bound protein, consisting of three immunoglobulin-like domains in the extracellular portions, a transmembrane domain and two tyrosine kinase domains in the intracellular portion.[14] FGFR3 is expressed in the proliferating chondrocytes. Its ligands, most importantly FGF18, bind to the FGFR3 and activate the receptor by its autophosphorylation and the phosphorylation of other substrate proteins.[15] The major signaling pathways of FGFR3 are thought to be the mitogen activating protein kinase (MAPK) pathway and the STAT-1 pathway. These signals mediate the inhibitory effects of FGFs on the proliferation and differentiation of chondrocytes.

The importance of FGF signaling in skeletal development was first revealed with the discovery that a point mutation in the transmembrane domain of FGFR3 causes achondroplasia (MIM 100800).[14] The abnormality of the FGFR3 gene is also associated with hypochondroplasia (MIM 146000), thanotophoric dysplasia (MIM 187600), and severe achondroplasia with developmental delay and acanthosis nigricans (SADDAN) syndrome.[16]

PTHrP was initially discovered as a causal factor of humoral hypercalcemia of malignancy.[17] However, gene-targeting experiments have revealed that PTHrP plays an important role in chondrogenesis via a local action.[18] PTHrP-null mice, for example, exhibit a severe disorder of enchondral bone formation, characterized by shortened bones and premature maturation and ossification of the cartilaginous tissues.[19] Mice lacking the parathyroid hormone (PTH)/PTHrP receptor exhibit similar phenotypes. PTHrP and PTH, the latter of which is one of the main regulators of calcium and bone metabolism share the PTH/PTHrP receptor. Therefore, the PTH/PTHrP receptor mediates both the endocrine actions of PTH and the auto/paracrine actions of PTHrP. The PTH/PTHrP receptor is mainly expressed in the transitional zone between proliferating and hypertrophic cells (i.e., the prehypertrophic zone) in growth plate. PTHrP regulates the transition from proliferation to differentiation in chondrocytes.

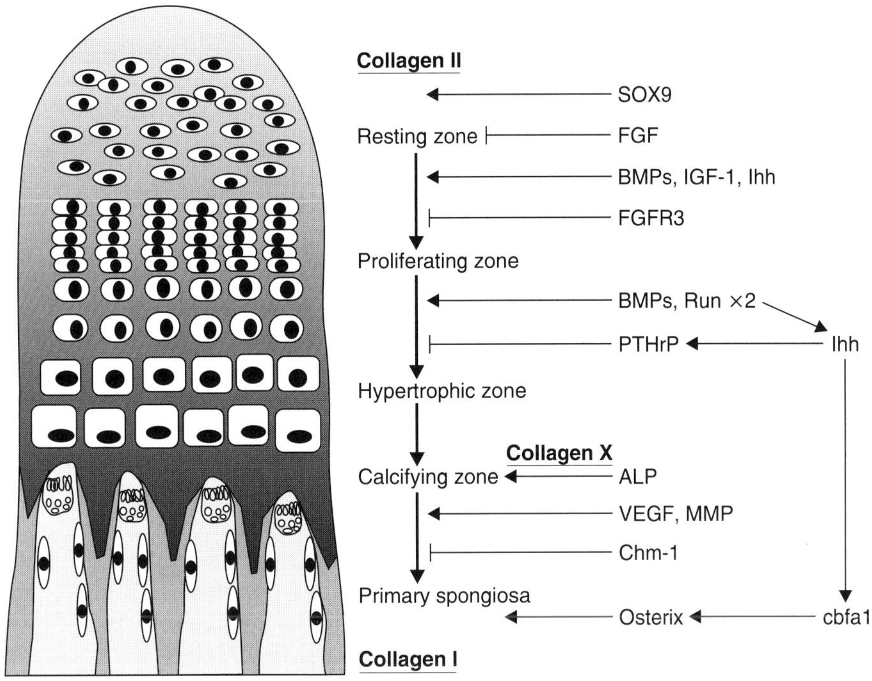

Figure 59.1 Enchondral bone formation. Chondrocytes form the layer structure according to the stage of differentiation in growth plate and eventually cartilage is replaced by bone matrix, primary spongiosa. In the process of the enchondral bone formation, chondrocytes proliferate and differentiate into hypertrophic chondrocytes, then matrix is calcified. The main matrix proteins which are underlined are changed from collagen type II to collagen type I via collagen type X. Many molecules including SOX9, PTHrP, and FGFR3 have been found to play an important role in the process as shown in the figure. FGF, fibroblast growth factor; BMP, bone morphogenic protein; IGF-1, insulin-like growth factor; Ihh, Indian hedgehog; FGFR3, FGF receptor 3; PTHrP, PTH-related peptide; ALP, alkaline phosphatase; VEGF, vascular endothelial growth factor; MMP, matrix metaroproteinase; Chm-1, chondromodulin-1.

Indian hedgehog (Ihh), a member of a family of proteins that are important for embryonic patterning, is highly expressed in the prehypertrophic zone and in the upper hypertrophic chondrocytes.[20,21] Actually, Ihh is secreted by prehypertrophic and early hypertrophic chondrocytes. The mice Ihh–/– show abnormal chondrocytic differentiation and a failure to specify appendicular perichondrial cells to the osteoblast lineage.[22] Ihh induces the expression of PTHrP and inhibits differentiation of hypertrophic chondrocytes followed by the delay of the mineralization of cartilage matrix. This effect of Ihh on chondrocytic differentiation is mediated by increasing PTHrP production in the growth plate. Because PTHrP keeps chondrocytes in the proliferative pool and suppresses Ihh production, PTHrP and Ihh establish a negative-feedback loop that maintains a balance of chondrocyte proliferation and differentiation.[22] Ihh is also a potent stimulator of chondrocyte proliferation, and conversely an inhibitor of chondrocyte maturation.[23] In this sense, Ihh has the positive effect on normal chondrocyte proliferation in a PTHrP-independent manner. Heterozygous missense mutations in the Ihh gene have been recently identified as a cause of autosomal dominant form of brachydactyly type A1 (MIM 112500).[24] This type of brachydactyly is characterized by the shortening or the absence of middle phalanges.

Runx2, also called cbfa1, belongs to the Runt transcription factor family.[25–27] Runx2 was initially discovered as an essential molecule for osteoblast differentiation.[25–27] It has been shown that inactivating mutations of one allele of the human Runx2 gene cause cleidocranial dysplasia (MIM 119600).[25] However, further experiments revealed that Runx2 is also expressed in chondrocytes, and severe delay of chondrocyte maturation is found in genetically manipulated mice lacking this factor.[28]

Hypertrophic chondrocytes are the most characteristic in shape and produce the specific matrix protein, collagen type X. Then, the matrix is calcified and replaced by bone tissue. In other words, an avascular cartilage template is reconstructed into highly vascularized bone tissue. In contrast to immature chondrocytes which secrete angiogenic inhibitors, hypertrophic chondrocytes produce angiogenic stimulators such as vascular endothelial growth factor (VEGF) and FGF, and become a target for capillary invasion.[29] The invasion of blood vessels is critical in the last stage of chondrocyte maturation. The mammalian growth plate is highly hypoxic and expresses the transcription factor hypoxia-inducible factor 1 (HIF-1), which belongs to the PAS subfamily of bHLH (basic helix–loop–helix) transcription factors and is known to induce the VEGF expression in many tissues and cells.[30] HIF-1 is not sufficient to induce VEGF expression in cartilage or other factor(s) block the inducible activity of HIF-1 before the maturation of chondrocytes becomes complete.

The degradation of calcified cartilage matrix is another important event for enchondral bone formation. During hypertrophic change, chondrocytes synthesize type X collagen, which is associated with denaturation and loss of type II collagen resulting from increased collagenase activity. The transcription factor Cbfa1 has been shown to regulate expression of matrix metalloproteinase (MMP) 13 (collagenase-3).[31] MMP-9 is also an important enzyme for matrix degradation.[32] Remarkably, inactivation of matrix metalloproteinase-9 (MMP-9) resulted in bone phenotype similar to that found in VEGF-knockout mouse, suggesting the involvement of proteinases as well as VEGF in the processes of vascular invasion in growth plate and endochondral ossification. Indian hedgehog plays an important role in skeletal angiogenesis and calcification of cartilage.[33]

As described in this section, enchondral bone formation is elaborately regulated by many factors such as transcription factors, growth factors, enzymes and matrix proteins. Moreover, the defect in the regulation leads to dysplastic bone and cartilage formation both in humans and mice.

Clinical and genetical aspects of skeletal dysplasias

Skeletal dysplasias associated with FGFR abnormality

The abnormality of FGFR3 gene is associated with achondroplasia, hypochondroplasia, thanatophoric dysplasia and the most rare form, SADDAN.[14–16] Its cognate ligand remains unclear, but FGF18, 17 and 8 are likely to elicit its signal via binding to the FGFR3.[15] These ligands are produced in the perichondrium. The FGF family of proteins consists of at least 23 structurally related polypeptides that play a critical role in a variety of biological processes. The FGFRs represent a family of four tyrosine kinase receptors (FGFR1–4) that bind FGFs with variable affinity.

Achondroplasia is the most common form of rhizomeric dwarfism with a rate of 1 per 15,000–30,000 births. The disease is inherited in an autosomal dominant manner, but more than 90% of the cases are sporadic. Advanced paternal age is reported in sporadic cases. Its clinical features are short stature caused by rhizomelic shortening of the limbs, characteristic faces with frontal bossing and mid-face hypoplasia, exaggerated lumbar lordosis, and trident hand. As typical radiologic features, caudal narrowing of the interpediculate distance, rather than the normal caudal widening, and a notch-like sacroiliac groove are found in children with achondroplasia. Interestingly, the same mutation of the FGFR3 gene is the cause of achondroplasia in almost all patients (G to A transition at nucleotide 1138).[34,35] This mutation causes the substitution of amino acid 380 (Gly380Arg), and can be recognized by polymerase chain reaction (PCR) followed by digestion with restriction enzyme SfcI. The same mutation of FGFR3 was also found in Japanese patients with achondroplasia. The detection of this mutation is especially helpful in the diagnosis of neonatal patients with this disease. Other minor mutations are also reported (G to C at nucleotide 1138 and G to T at nucleotide 1123).

In our experience, some patients with achondroplasia are not recognized prenatally even when routine examination with ultrasonography is undertaken. This is partly because the disproportion develops more prominently after birth. In our study in which the relationship between age and clinical data (height, arm span and measurements of skeletal radiographs) were statistically analyzed in 27 achondroplasia patients with the G380R genotype, the height standard deviation score decreased with age. In making a clinical diagnosis of achondroplasia in early infancy, it should be noted that short stature and squared pelvis deformity are not prominent in some cases.[36]

To treat the short stature of patients with achondroplasia, recombinant human growth hormone (GH) has been administered. First-year response is typically a 2–3 cm increase in growth velocity in prepubertal children.[37] However, the effect of GH treatment on the final adult height is not conclusive so far. GH treatment, at least in the prepubertal period, seems to influence the degree of disproportion. The activating mutation of FGFR3 promotes apoptosis of chondrocytes. Insulin-like growth factor (IGF)-I, which is a mediator of GH, may reduce apoptosis of chondrocytes expressing mutated FGFR3.[38] More recently, it has been reported that c-type natriuretic peptide is effective to prevent shortening of long bones in the mice model for achondroplasia.[39]

Achondroplasia can be associated with respiratory difficulty in early infancy and childhood, although the degree of the difficulty is usually not so severe. One of the respiratory difficulties is manifested as sleep apnea syndrome.[40,41] Although a large-scale study on sleep apnea syndrome in achondroplasia is lacking, but approximately 30% of patients with achondroplasia suffer from sleep apnea syndrome. In a serious situation, sleep apnea syndrome leads to hypoxia, pulmonary hypertension, heart failure and sudden death. The causes of sleep apnea syndrome in achondroplasia are both obstruction of airway and failure of central control of respiration. The obstructive sleep apnea is derived from the small oral cavity with a relatively large tongue, hypertrophy of tonsilla and adenoid as well as weakness of trachea. Neurological problems including hydrocephalus and compression of the spinal cord due to a small foramen magnum are relatively common in achondrolasia and may cause central sleep apnea syndrome. Polysomnography is used

	Telephone receiver (femur)	Cloverleaf skull
Type I	+	+ or –
Type II	–	+

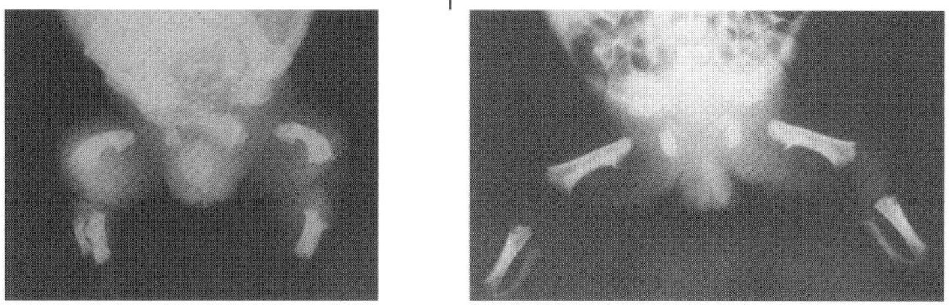

Type I Type II

Figure 59.2 Two types of thanatophoric dysplasia. Thanatophoric dysplasia types 1 and 2 are characterized by telephone receiver-like bended femur and straight femur, respectively as x-ray figures are shown in the bottom. Cloverleaf skull is often associated with type 2 and sometimes with type 1.

to make a diagnosis of sleep apnea syndrome. Symptomatic patients require tonsillectomy, adenoidectomy or continuous positive airway pressure therapy.

Thanatophoric dysplasia, a lethal form of dwarfism, is also caused by mutations of the FGFR3 gene. In histological analyses, the most characteristic feature in thanatophoric dysplasia is the protrusion of perichondrium into the growth plate. The growth plate is irregular and narrow, as in other chondrodysplasias. An anomaly of the brain (abnormal fissure in the temporal lobe) is also observed. Thanatophoric dysplasia is divided into two subtypes according to the finding of the shape of the femur (I, curved femur; II, straight femur) (Figure 59.2). A cloverleaf-like deformity of the skull is often associated with type II but may also be present in type I. The most common mutations in type I and II of thanatophoric dysplasia were reported to be Arg248Cys and Lys650Glu, respectively.

Hypochondroplasia is a relatively mild disease, manifested as short stature. The head is not affected. The spinal canal narrows in its caudal portion as is true in achondroplasia. Fingers are short, although hands are not of the trident type. Asn540Leu is reported to be the most common mutation found in this disease.

The other form in this family is called SADDAN, which stands for severe achondroplasia with developmental delay and acanthosis nigricans. The patients with SADDAN survive infancy without prolonged life-support measures. The FGFR3 mutation (A1949T, Lys650Met) occurs at the nucleotide adjacent to the TD type II (TD2) mutation (A1948G: Lys650Glu) and results in a different amino acid substitution in the kinase domain activation loop.

All these disorders are autosomally dominant, mainly sporadic, and are caused by gain-of-function mutations, leading to a constitutively active FGFR3. The degree of activation of FGFR3 correlates well with the severity of the chondrodysplasia; the mutated FGFR3 found in thanatophoric dysplasia is the most activated form. This relationship provides the first evidence for negative regulation of chondrogenesis by FGFR3. Several animal models have established that FGFR3 negatively regulates chondrocyte proliferation. MAPK is a major downstream effecter of FGFR3 activity. Indeed, chondrocytes expressing a constitutively active form of MEK, the MAPK activator, present an achondroplasia phenotype similar to that observed with constitutively active FGFR3. Conversely, blockade of MAPK activation rescues achondroplasia obtained with constitutively active FGFR3. In addition, it has been shown that FGFR3 represses chondrocyte proliferation through activation of the transcription factor STAT1 by a yet unknown mechanism.

Collagenopathy

Type I collagen is the most abundant protein in bone. This type of collagen is synthesized as the heterotrimer of procollagens a1(I) and a2(I). Heterozygous mutations in the two genes for procollagen a1(I) and a2(I). (*COL1A1* and *COL1A2*) have been found in patients with osteogenesis imperfecta (MIM 166200, 166210, 166220, 166230).[42,43] These mutations cause a change either in the structure of the protein or in the number of collagen molecules made. The severe forms of osteogenesis imperfecta are reported to have a glycine substitution within the Gly-X-Y amino acid repeat. Mutated collagens interfere with the formation of collagen fibrils. In contrast, null mutations of *COL1A1* cause the mild form of osteogenesis imperfecta.[44]

Osteogenesis imperfecta is characterized by low bone mineral density (BMD) with fragility, and frequent bone fracture leads to deformity of long bones and chronic bone pain. It was classified into four forms by Sillence *et al.*[45]: a dominant form with blue sclerae, type I; a perinatally lethal OI syndrome, type II; a progressively deforming form with normal sclerae, type III; and a dominant form with normal sclerae, type IV. However, type IV is rather heterogeneous and includes patients with a moderate to severe disease who do not fit type I or III. Thus, other types of OI (V, VI, and VII) without identifiable collagen type I mutations have been recently described.[43]

There is no curative treatment for osteogenesis imperfecta. However, the therapy using pamidronate, a derivative of bisphosphonate, has recently been developed and has successfully alleviated symptoms in children with OI. In short, cyclic intravenous administration of pamidronate improved BMD and reduced the frequency of bone fracture. However, there are few studies reporting the outcome measures of bisphosphonate therapy in children with OI. Glorieux *et al.* observed that in patients with severe osteogenesis imperfecta aged 3–16 years, intravenous pamidronate (mean annual dose 6.8 mg/kg) increased lumbar vertebral BMD by an average of 42% per year.[46] The same group also demonstrated that in children with OI types III or IV less than 2 years of age, a 12-month treatment with pamidronate at a mean dose of 12.4 mg/kg increased lumbar vertebral BMD by 86% to 227%. Recently, Astrom and Soderhall reported that monthly infusions of pamidronate for 2–9 years resulted in gradual increase in total body and lumbar spine bone density in children with OI.[47]

As another novel treatment for patients with severe osteogenesis imperfecta, transplantation of bone marrow cells containing adult mesenchymal stem cells has been attempted.[48] Mesenchymal stem cells can differentiate into multiple cell types present in several tissues, including bone, fat, cartilage, and muscle, making them ideal candidates for cell-based therapies. More recently, mesenchymal cell therapy using isolated mesenchymal stem cells has been reported.[49] In the report, donor marrow-derived mesenchymal cells were administered to treat six children who had undergone standard bone marrow transplantation for severe osteogenesis imperfecta. Five of six patients showed engraftment in one or more sites, including bone, skin, and marrow stroma, and had an acceleration of growth velocity during the first 6 months postinfusion.

Adult stem cells can be used after the *ex vivo* genetic manipulation to correct genetical disorders. For osteogenesis imperfecta, one study in which adeno-associated viral vectors were used to disrupt dominant-negative mutant *COL1A1* collagen genes in mesenchymal stem cells from patients with a severe form of osteogenesis imperfecta was reported.[50] It seems that the gene was successfully targeted in adult human stem cells.

Collagen types II, IX, X and XI are expressed in the cartilaginous tissue. Collagen type II specific to cartilage matrix is synthesized as the homotrimer of collagen $\alpha 1$(II). Mutations in the single gene for type II procollagen have been found in patients with type II achondrogenesis (MIM 200610)-hypochondrogenesis, spondyloepiphyseal dysplasia (MIM 183900), Kniest dysplasia (MIM 156550) and Stickler (hereditary arthro-ophthalmopathy) syndrome (MIM 108300).[51] The platyspondylic lethal skeletal dysplasias (PLSD), Torrance type (MIM 151210) was found to be caused by *COL2A1* mutations.[52] The platyspondylic lethal skeletal dysplasias is a heterogeneous group of chondrodysplasias characterized by severe platyspondyly and shortening of limbs. Interestingly, the most common form of PLSD is thanatophoric dysplasia (TD), which is caused by mutations in the *FGFR3* as described previously.

Type X collagen is a homotrimeric, short-chain, nonfibrillar extracellular matrix component. The expression of type X collagen is restricted to hypertrophic chondrocytes. The mutation in the *COL10A1* is associated with Schmid metaphyseal chondrodysplasia (MIM 156500).[53] It is reported that Stickler syndrome type 2 with a different vitreo-retinal phenotype from that of type 1 is caused by a mutation in the *COL11A1* (MIM 604841). Multiple epiphyseal dysplasia (MIM 132400) is caused by a mutation in the *COL9A1* or the *COMP* gene.[54,55] The *COMP* gene is also responsible for pseucoachondroplasia (MIM 177170), which is one of the most frequent skeletal dysplasias and resembles achondroplasia except for head and face.[55]

Other chondrodysplasias

The chondrodysplastic disease, achondrogenesis is characterized by severely impaired chondrogenesis with extremely short limbs and narrow thorax, leading to the perinatal death of patients with this disease. Fetal hydrops and hydroamnios are also associated with achondrogenesis. Although achondrogenesis has been subtyped in several ways, the definition reported by Borochowitz *et al.*, based on detailed analyses of clinical, radiological and morphological studies, seems to have received consensus: type I (MIM 200600) A (Houston–Harris), IB (Fraccaro) and type II (Langer–Saldino, MIM 200610). A histological analysis of cartilaginous tissue is very helpful, especially to make the diagnosis of achondrogenesis type IB.[56] Achondrogenesis type IB is caused by the mutations of the diastrophic dysplasia (*DTDST*) gene.[57]

The *DTDST* gene encodes a sulfate transporter, which is required for the synthesis of sulfated proteoglycans in cartilage with other name, *SLC26A2*.[58] It is not surprising that defects of this gene result in a chondrodysplasia phenotype, although the precise mechanism whereby the impaired sulfation of proteoglycans causes abnormal enchondral ossification remains to be elucidated. Several mutations of the *DTDST* gene were reported in patients with achondrogenesis type IB, the most severe form, atelosteogenesis type II or neonatal osseous dysplasia (MIM 256050), an intermediate form and the mildest form of the diseases, diastrophic dysplasia (MIM 222600). The recessive multiple epiphyseal dysplasia (MIM 226900) is also caused by the mutations of *DTDST*. Homozygous mutant mice for the gene were characterized by growth retardation, skeletal dysplasia and joint contractures, thereby recapitulating the essential aspects of the diastrophic dysplasia phenotype in humans. The skeletal phenotype included reduced toluidine blue staining of cartilage, chondrocytes of irregular size, delay in the formation of the secondary ossification center and osteoporosis of long bones.

The cartilage hair hypoplasia (CHH, MIM 250250) or spondylometaphseal dysplasia McKusick type is characterized by disproportionate short stature, hypoplastic hair, ligamentous laxity, defective immunity, hypoplastic anemia, and neuronal dysplasia of the intestine (Hirschsprung disease). CHH was found to be caused by mutations in the ribonuclease mitochondrial RNA processing gene (*RMRP*).[59] The untranslated *RMRP* gene encodes the RNA component of a ribonucleoprotein endoribonuclease. Normally the RNase MRP complex is involved in multiple cellular and mitochondrial functions.

The difference between the Japanese and other ethnic groups is remarkable in terms of the mutations and polymorphisms in *RMRP* gene. Four novel mutations were reported in two patients with typical and atypical CHH.[60] A patient with typical CHH had a 17-bp duplication at +3 and a *de novo* 182G > A, 218A.G. The other patient with atypical CHH had a 17 bp insortion at −20 and a 218A ? C.

The X-linked spondyloepiphyseal dysplasia tarda (SEDT; MIM 313400) has the features consisting of disproportionately short trunk, short stature, characteristic radiological findings of the spine (posterior hump, end plate sclerosis, and disk space narrowing) and the hips (short and thick femoral necks), and positive family history. The linkage analyses revealed that the *SEDL* gene on the X chromosome is responsible for the disease.[61] The *SEDL* gene product, known as sedlin is a 140 amino-acid protein with a putative role in endoplasmic reticulum-to-Golgi transport. However, function of sedlin in bone and mineral metabolism remains to be characterized.

Leri–Weill dyschondrosteosis (LWD) (OMIM 127300) is caused by the haploinsufficiency of the short stature homeobox-containing (*SHOX*) gene.[62,63] LWD is an autosomal dominant form of mesomeric dysplasia first described by Leri and Weill in 1929. Patients with this condition demonstrate short stature due to shortening of the lower legs and Madelung deformity of the forearm. The abnormality of the *SHOX* gene also causes Turner skeletal features and a certain proportion of idiopathic short stature. The *SHOX* gene was cloned from the pseudoautosomal region of the sex chromosome (Xp22 and Yp11.3) and affects the adult height. It is exclusively expressed in the first and second pharyngeal arches and in the developing distal limb bones of the human embryo. The expression of SHOX is in the hypertrophic zone and less intensely in the proliferating zone in growth plate. Although the function of SHOX in growth plate is to be elucidated, it may be involved in the fusion of growth plate and affect the growth at the pubertal stage.

Abnormality in PTH/PTHrP receptor or G protein

The family of G protein has many members, and Gsα is the representative protein which has been shown to cause bone diseases.[64] G protein is a signal effector molecule, typically forming heterotrimeric guanine nucleotide-binding proteins. Mutations in Gsα protein are divided into two groups, gain of function mutation and loss of function one. McCune–Albright syndrome and Albright osteodystrophy combined with pseudohypoparathyroidism are the diseases caused by these mutations, respectively.[65]

The PTH/PTHrP receptor is a G protein-coupled membrane-bound receptor and its best-characterized second messenger is cAMP. Although cAMP activates protein kinase A (PKA) as a downstream of PTHrP receptor, it is still not clear what molecules responsible for delay of chondrocytes maturation serve as the substrates of PKA. In the growth plate, the PTH/PTHrP receptor mRNA is expressed in prehypertrophic chondrocytes at higher levels. The critical role of the PTH/PTHrP receptor in endochondral bone development is highlighted by the discovery that two rare forms of chondrodysplasias, Blomstrand lethal chondrodysplasia (MIM 215045) and Jansen's metaphyseal chondrodysplasia (MIM 156400) are caused by mutations of this receptor. Blomstrand lethal chondrodysplasia is caused by inactivating mutations of the PTH/PTHrP receptor, while the mutated receptors found in Jansen's metaphyseal chondrodysplasia are constitutively active.[66,67] The former disease is characterized by prenatal lethality, premature and abnormal bone mineralization and ossification, and shortened limbs. Endochondral bone formation is markedly advanced in fetuses with Blomstrand chondrodysplasia, and the columnar proliferative layer in the mutant growth plate is virtually absent. The disease appears to have an autosomal recessive pattern of inheritance. Jansen's metaphyseal chondrodysplasia is an autosomal dominant disorder characterized by short-limbed dwarfism secondary to severe abnormalities of the growth plate and hypercalcemia. The laboratory findings in patients with Jansen's metaphyseal chondrodysplasia are reminiscent of primary hyperparathyroidism. According to the original report, the genomic DNA from 10 JMC patients has been examined: seven patients had the H223R heterozygous nucleotide exchange, and three patients had distinct heterozygous mutations in the PTH/PTHrP receptor (T410P, T410R, and I458R).

When chondrocytes are forced to express either PTHrP or an activated form of its receptor, cartilage maturation is dramatically inhibited and bone formation delayed. Mice lacking either PTHrP or its receptor, in contrast, exhibit dwarfism of their long bones due to premature chondrocyte maturation. Therefore, PTHrP signaling negatively regulates the switch from a proliferative immature chondrocyte to a postproliferative mature hypertrophic chondrocyte.

More recently, a heterozygous missense mutation Arg150Cys has been identified in the PTH/PTHrP receptor gene of two patients with enchondromatosis or Ollier and Maffucci diseases (MIM 166000). Enchondromas are common benign cartilage tumors of bone that can occur as solitary lesions or, in enchondromatosis, multiple lesions. This type of mutated receptor is constitutively active *in vitro*. However, others reported that no mutations of the PTH/PTHrP receptor gene were found in patients with enchondromatosis.

Pseudohypoparathyroidism, especially type Ia, is associated with the loss of function-type mutations in the Gsa gene (*GNAS1*).[65] In patients with the disease, no response to PTH is observed in the excretion of phosphate and cAMP. In contrast to McCune–Albright syndrome, the mutations are scattered along the entire gene, including missense mutations and deletions. This disease is inherited in a dominant fashion, and the mutation is found in a single allele. Albright hereditary osteodystrophy (AHO), which consists of short stature, shortening of the fourth and fifth metacarpals, round face, obesity and ectopic calcification is associated with pseudohypoparathyroidism type Ia (MIM 103580). Since the *GNAS1* gene is an imprinted gene, the transmission of the disease to the next generation is characteristic. Maternal transmission of Gsa mutations leads to AHO associated with resistance to parathyroid hormone (pseudohypoparathyroidism type Ia), while paternal transmission leads only to the AHO phenotype (pseudopseudohypoparathyroidism). Pseudohypoparathyroidism type Ib (MIM 603233) has the resistance to PTH only in kidney, and a region responsible for the disease is also associated with the *GNAS1* locus. PHP-Ib is caused by heterozygous mutations disrupting a long-range imprinting control element. Recently, deletions that remove the differentially methylated region encompassing exon NESP55 and exons 3 and 4 of the antisense transcript, those are located near *GNAS1* region. Thus, it is confirmed that epigenetic defects in the imprinted *GNAS1* cluster are associated with pseudohypoparathyroidism type Ib.[68]

McCune–Albright syndrome is characterized by three major symptoms, café au lait pigmentation, multiple fibrous dysplasia and endocrine disorders including precocious puberty, hyperthyroidism, autonomous adrenal hyperplasia and growth hormone secreting pituitary adenoma. This syndrome is caused by the somatic mutation in the *GNAS1* gene, leading to elevated levels of cyclic AMP in cells. This gene has a hot spot of mutation at Arg of codon 201 (Arg201His or Arg201Cys).[69] Since these mutations are somatic, mosaicism for a mutation in the *GNAS1* gene is found in patients with McCune–Albright syndrome. Cells obtained from the lesions with fibrous dysplasia secreted a significant amount of interleukin (IL)-6 and exhibited an impaired response of IL-6 secretion to IL-1 in patients with McCune–Albright syndrome.[70] In response to the elevation of cAMP, IL-6 is produced perhaps through the cAMP response element of the IL-6 gene promoter. Fibrous dysplasia is a focal and benign fibrous bone lesion, which is caused by the activating mutation in the *GNAS1* gene. Hypophosphatemic rickets is sometimes observed as a complication of McCune–Albright syndrome. Two hypotheses have been put forward to explain the pathogenesis of hypophosphatemic rickets associated with McCune–Albright syndrome. One of them supposes the hypersensitivity to PTH in the renal tubules due to the mutation in the *GNAS1* gene, based on the inhibitory effect of PTH via cAMP on phosphate transport in the kidney. The other hypothesizes humoral factor(s) from the bone lesions which inhibit(s) phosphate reabsorption. In fact, Riminucci *et al.* recently reported the elevated plasma FGF-23 levels in patients with McCune–Albright syndrome.[71]

Hypophosphatasia

Hypophosphatasia (MIM 146300, 171760, 241500, 241510) is characterized by the hypomineralization of bone associated with the impaired activity of tissue-nonspecific alkaline phosphatase (TNSALP).[72] Hypophosphatasia has diverse phenotypes, and is usually classified into five subtypes based on the age of onset and clinical features; perinatal, infantile, childhood, adult type, and odontohypophosphatasia.[73] The severity of the disease is generally well correlated with the onset of the disease, except for odontohypophosphatasia, where only the teeth are affected. The patients with the perinatal type of hypophosphatasia almost always die around birth due to impaired development of the lung and the severe hypomineralization of their bones. However, the classification of these subgroups is not definite, and there is diversity in the phenotype which forms so-called spectrum. For example, we have previously reported a patient who achieved long-term survival without respiratory failure in spite of having fetal onset.[74] Since these patients survive longer despite their fetal onset, we should pay more attention to take care of them and to genetic counseling. The presence of such a case may depend on the development of a diagnosis procedure or on the specificity of the genotype. However, this benign form of hypophosphatasia found in the Japanese patients is surmised to be associated with a specific mutation, F310L, whose product retained approximately 70% of its enzymatic activity. The relatively high activity of the mutant enzyme may contribute to this relatively mild form.

On the other hand, mutations found in the severe form of the disease do not tend to be associated with restricted positions, although the three-dimensional model study showed that most of the severe missense mutations were localized in crucial domains, such as the active site.[75] Elucidation of the molecular heterogeneity underlying hypophosphatasia may contribute to our understanding of the clinical heterogeneity observed in hypophosphatasia and the improvement of treatment, especially in patients with severe forms of hypophosphatasia.

The patients with the classical perinatal form of hypophosphatasia almost always die *in utero* or during the neonatal period. Therefore, the perinatal form is a synonym for the lethal form. The second most severe form, the infantile type of the disease, is still associated with high mortality because of the impairment of respiratory function and hypercalcemia.[76] The patients with other types of hypophosphatasia usually do not suffer from life-threatening complications.

To date, more than a hundred mutations have been reported in the TNSALP gene in patients with hypophosphatasia, mainly in Caucasians and Japanese.[77] However, the mutations are scattered in the whole coding region, and only a few mutations have been recognized to occur frequently in the gene. Moreover, although the relationship between the clinical features and the mutation of the corresponding gene has also been analyzed, only a few reports detected the positive correlation between the mutations and severity.[75] The mutations responsible for mild hypophosphatasia may not cause a complete loss of ALP function, suggested by several reconstruction experiments in which mutated ALP activity was examined.

Although hypophosphatasia is usually inherited in an autosomal recessive manner, autosomal dominant inheritance is also recognized in some families with the mild form of the disease. Interestingly, the mutations in these families have been reported to show the dominant negative effect on the wild-type ALP activity, as one of the remarkable results of the recent progress in molecular biology.[78]

The mechanism for which the defect of ALP activity causes hypomineralization is not fully understood. There are three main assumptions for the role of ALP in mineralization process. First, ALP increases local phosphate concentration, leading to the acceleration of mineralization. Second, ALP decreases the concentration of local pyrophosphate, a substrate of ALP and an inhibitor of mineralization. Finally, ALP controls gene expression including osteopontin through the increase in intracellular phosphate concentration and affects the mineralization.

In patients with the infantile form of hypophosphatasia, bone marrow cell transplantation was tried to avoid the expected poor prognosis.[79] The patient was given T-cell-depleted, haplo-identical marrow from her healthy sister. Chimerism in peripheral blood and bone marrow became 100% donor. The patient survived and some clinical improvement was observed. More experience with transplantation of bone marrow or mesenchymal stem cells is necessary before the cell-based therapy becomes standard as treatment of severe hypophosphatasia.

Craniometaphyseal dysplasia

Craniometaphyseal dysplasia (MIM 123000) is a genetic syndrome characterized by the sclerotic change of cranial and tubular bones that commonly present at a young age, often with facial abnormalities and otolaryngologic manifestations such as a conductive hearing loss. Craniometaphyseal dysplasia is defective in ANK, the pyrophosphate transporter.[80] Thus, this disease supports the inhibitory role of pyrophosphate in mineralization.

Diseases with high or low bone mineral density

BMD is determined by both genetic and environmental factors. The genetical approach has shown that multiple genes have effects on BMD. Recent developments in molecular genetics and genomics have dramatically increased a power to identify genes which affect BMD. The sclerosing bone dysplasias can be classified into two groups such as increased trabecular bone density (osteosclerosis) and a cortical bone thickening (hyperostosis). There are several diseases which belong to sclerosing bone dysplasias, e.g., osteopetrosis, pycnodysostosis, and osteopoikilosis.

Osteopetrosis characterized by a marked increase in bone mass is a heterogeneous disorder of the skeleton in several animal species.[81] In humans, the disease is inherited as either an autosomal dominant or autosomal recessive trait. The autosomal dominant form exhibits mild symptoms only in adults (McKusick MIM 166600). The autosomal recessive form consists of three types; a mild type (MIM 259710), a lethal type (MIM 259720) which is rare, and infantile malignant osteopetrosis (MIM 259700) characterized by severe symptoms such as diffuse osteosclerosis of all bones, extramedullary hematopoiesis associated with bone marrow failure, and sensorineurogenic impairment in infancy. It is caused by defects in bone resorption by osteoclasts, resulting in increased bone mass and narrowing of the bone marrow cavity. Impaired bone resorption, as seen in the various forms of autosomal recessive osteopetrosis (MIM 259700), can be due to mutations in a subunit of the vacuolar H^+ pump (*TCIRG1* gene) or to mutations in the chloride channel *CLCN7* gene in humans.[82,83] Another form of osteopetrosis is caused by carbonic anhydrase II deficiency, and is associated with renal tubular acidosis and cerebral calcification (MIM 259730).[84] Very recently, mutation in the *GL* gene, the gene responsible for spontaneous mouse gray-lethal whose phenotype is a coat color defect and severe autosomal recessive form of osteopetrosis, leads to severe recessive osteopetrosis in humans.[85] X-linked recessive anhidrotic ectodermal dysplasia with immunodeficiency, osteopetrosis, and lymphoedema (OL-EDA-ID, MIM300301) is caused by hypomorphic mutations in NEMO, the regulatory subunit of the IKK (IkappaB kinase) complex encoded in the *IKBKG* gene.[86] Germline loss-of-function mutations in *IKBKG* are lethal in male fetuses.

Hematopoietic stem cell transplantation seems to be the most effective and rational therapy for malignant osteopetrosis at the moment, because it provides normal osteoclast precursors.[87] However, several kinds of treatment including high dose of active vitamin D and long-term therapy with interferon gamma (IFN-g), also have been reported to be effective.

Cathepsin K has been cloned as an osteoclast-specific cysteine protease. The abnormalities in this gene were reported in patients with pycnodysostosis (MIM 265800).[88] The characteristic features of this disease are disproportionate short stature, front-occipital prominence, high-arched palate, proptosis, a pointed nose, and sclerotic bones.

In addition to impaired bone resorption, increased bone formation can result in sclerosing bone disorders. Recently, it is reported that the increased TGF-β signaling results in Camurati–Engelmann disease (MIM 131300).[89] The increased bone formation in sclerosteosis (SOST MIM 269500)[90] and in Van Buchem disease (MIM 239100) turned out to be due to loss-of-function mutations of the *SOST* gene, most likely increasing bone morphogenetic protein signaling. In addition, osteoprotegerin and receptor activator of NF kappa B (RANK), whose gene is TNFRSF11A, are responsible for juvenile Paget's disease and familial expansile osteolysis.[91,92]

Infantile cortical hyperostosis (Caffey disease, MIM114000) is characterized by radiological evidence of cortical hyperostosis, soft tissue swellings, fever, and irritability.[93] Caffey disease was first reported in 1945 by Caffey and Silverman. Its principal features include acute inflammatory manifestations and the early onset time, usually in the first year of life. The cause of the disease remains unclear and the disease is self-limiting.

Further, it was recently shown that the gene encoding the low-density lipoprotein receptor related protein 5 (LRP5) is one of the regulators of peak bone mass in vertebrates.[94] The autosomal recessive osteoporosis pseudoglioma (OPPG) syndrome (MIM 259770), a disorder causing both skeletal and eye abnormalities, is due to inactivating mutations in the *LRP5* gene.[95] Besides the neonatal blindness, children with OPPG have a very low bone mass and are very sensitive to fractures and skeletal deformities. The disease is not caused by abnormal collagen matrix, and this differentiates it from the severe osteogenesis imperfecta, although it shares similar phenotype with osteogenesis imperfecta. Of interest, obligate carriers of OPPG mutations show an increased incidence for osteoporotic fractures, indicating a dominant effect of this gene on bone mass. Targeted disruption of the *LRP5* gene in mice also produces osteoporosis postnatally. On the other hand, in a family that includes phenotypically normal individuals with exceptionally dense bones (high bone mass MIM 601884), a gain-of-function mutation (G171V) in the *LRP5* gene has been described.[96] The same mutation was found in another kindred with other phenotypic abnormalities, such as torus palatinus and a wide, deep mandible in addition to high bone density. LRP5 acts as a coreceptor for Wnt proteins and is expressed in osteoblasts, where it is required for the osteoblast proliferation and functions in a Runx2-independent manner. These findings demonstrate that the LRP5 signaling pathway plays an important role in the regulation of bone mass in vertebrates.

LRP6 is another coreceptor of canonical Wnt pathway. Thus, it is interesting whether LRP6 is involved in bone metabolism, although a human disease caused by the abnormality of LRP6 has not been identified. Lrp6-null mice is embryonic lethal and not suitable for the analysis of bone metabolism. We found that a novel spontaneous mutation, *ringelschwanz* (*rs*) in the mouse is in the *Lrp6* gene.[97] While heterozygous rs animals appear normal, homozygous *rs* mutants show malformations in the vertebral column, digits and the neural tube as in *Lrp6*-null mutants, these phenotypes are less severe as compared to those in null mutants. The *rs* mutation is regarded as a hypomorphic allele of *Lrp6*. The Lrp6 dysfunction in *rs* leads to a delay in ossification at birth and to a low bone mass phenotype in adults. Thus, LRP6 is certainly involved in bone metabolism as well as LRP5.

Noonan syndrome

Noonan syndrome (MIM 163950) is an autosomal dominant disorder characterized by a variable phenotype comprising proportional short stature, congenital heart defects, and minor facial anomalies.[98] The main facial findings of Noonan syndrome are hypertelorism with down-slanting palpebral fissures, ptosis, and low-set posteriorly angulated ears with a thickened helix. Cardiovascular diseases including valvular pulmonary stenosis, atrial septal defect, and hypertrophic cardiomyopathy (HCM) are observed in 50–80% of patients with Noonan syndrome. Other symptoms are webbed neck, chest deformity, mild mental retardation, cryptorchidism, feeding difficulties, bleeding diathesis, and lymphatic dysplasias. The incidence of Noonan syndrome is estimated to be between 1/1000 and 1/2500 live births.

Recently, heterozygous missense mutations in the *PTPN11* gene, located on chromosome 12 (12q24), have been identified in 33–60% of affected familial or sporadic cases of Noonan syndrome.[99–102] The product of the *PTPN11* gene, SHP-2, is widely expressed in various tissues and is involved in several signal transduction pathways in cooperation with growth factors, cytokines, and hormones. Thus, mutations in the *PTPN11* gene could cause the wide range of clinical features in Noonan syndrome. SHP-2 is composed of two tandemly arranged src homology 2 domains, N-SH2

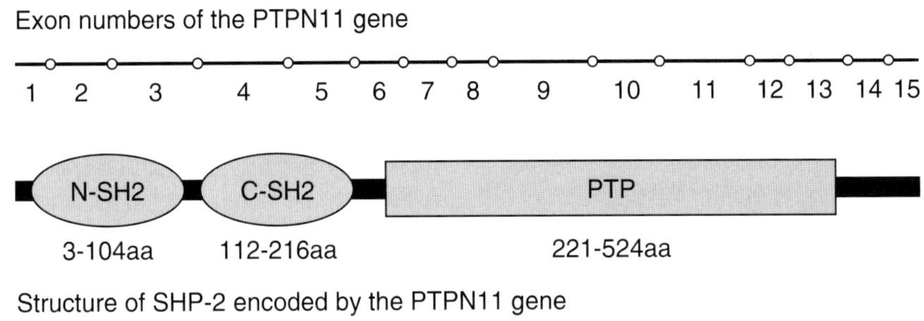

Figure 59.3 (modification of figure in Tartaglia *et al., Nature Genet* 2001) The structure of the PTPN11 gene and functional domain structure of SHP-2. The gene consists of 15 exons and the function domains of the SHP-2 protein comprise two tandemly arranged SH2 domains at the N terminus (N-SH2 and C-SH2) followed by a protein tyrosine phosphatase (PTP). The frequent mutations associated with Noonan syndrome are detected in exons 3, 8, and 13 in the gene.

and C-SH2, at the amino terminus, a single central phosphatase domain (PTP) and a carboxy-terminal tail (Figure 59.3). In the steady state, N-SH2 domain binds to PTP domain and suppresses its phosphatase activity. In contrast, the binding of both domains is loose and PTP exerts its activity in mutant SHP-2 found in Noonan syndrome. In other words, gain-of-function type mutation is found in the *PTPN11* gene in patients with Noonan syndrome. The structure of the *PTPN11* gene corresponding to the functional domain structure of SHP-2 is also depicted in the Figure 59.3. The gene consists of 15 exons. The frequent mutations are detected in exons 3, 8, and 13 in the gene.

To date, more than 70 mutations in the *PTPN11* gene have been described. Tartaglia *et al.* reported patients with *PTPN11* mutations were associated with pulmonary stenosis, while those without *PTPN11* mutations were with HCM.[103] Two other reports support the conclusion that HCM is found more frequently in patients with Noonan syndrome without *PTPN11* mutation. However, Sarkozy *et al.* showed LEOPARD syndrome (MIM 151100) with HCM was highly related to the mutations in exon 7 or 12 of the *PTPN11* gene,[102] suggesting that HCM could be associated with *PTPN11* mutations.

As mentioned above, SHP-2 is widely expressed in various tissues and cell types, and has been implicated in diverse signaling pathways including those initiated by growth factors, cytokines and hormones. SHP-2 has compound signaling functions. For instance, SHP-2 directly interacts with growth factor and cytokine receptors when its ligand induces rapidly tyrosine phosphorylation. It can also interact with a variety of signaling intermediates such as Grb2, and Gab1 and 2. As a PTP, SHP-2 is believed to function by dephosphorylation of its associated signaling molecules, thus diminishing local signals. However, the ultimate effect of SHP-2 in most signaling pathways is to enhance the signal transduction, for example, it activates the Ras-Raf-MAP kinase cascade. In most circumstances, SHP-2 plays a positive role in transducing signals relayed from tyrosine kinase-containing receptors.[103]

Perinatal period

Skeletal dysplasia, lethal type

The study in the St. John Hospital in Rome reported 14 cases of constitutional osteochondrodysplasias out of 2120 cases of newborns hospitalized (0.66%).[104] Among them, four patients (28.27%) belong to the group considered by the European Society of Pediatric Radiology as lethal. Representative lethal types of skeletal dysplasia and the corresponding causal genes are described in Table 59.2. The genes responsible for osteogenesis imperfecta, thanatophoric dysplasia, and hypophosphatasia are type I collagen gene, FGFR3 gene, and tissue non-specific ALP gene, respectively, which are essential for the development of cartilage and bone, as described in the previous section. Other important molecules in enchondral bone formation such as SOX9 and PTHrP receptor are also responsible for lethal type chondrodysplasia. Patients with campomelic dysplasia caused by SOX9 mutations often have respiratory difficulties. Other lethal forms of short limb dwarfism consist of a lethal form of arthrogryposis multiplex congenita (MIM 108110), platyspondylic lethal osteochondrodysplasia, short rib syndrome, and atelosteogenesis. Atelosteogenesis type 2 (AO2) (MIM 256050) is a neonatally lethal chondrodysplasia characterized by severe limb shortening and deficient ossification of parts of the skeleton. The disease is caused by mutations of the *DTDST* gene and its phenotypic overlap with nonlethal diastrophic dysplasia. The heterogeneous group of platyspondylic lethal skeletal dysplasias (PLSD) originally included thanatophoric dysplasias (TD1/2: MIM 187600, 187100) as the most common forms of this condition, as well as TD variants San Diego type (PLSD-SD: MIM 270230) and Torrance–Luton type (PLSD-TL: MIM 151210). The *FGFR3* gene mutations have been identified in TD1/2 and PLSD-SD, while PLSD-TL is caused by *COL2A1*. The metatropic dysplasia group includes fibrochondrogenesis, Schneckenbecken dysplasia, and various forms metatropic dysplasia.[105] The perinatally lethal metatropic group of conditions consists of lethal metatropic dysplasia (type 2) or hyperchondrogenesis, lethal

Table 59.2 Skeletal dysplasia, lethal type and responsible genes

Disease	Gene
Osteogenesis imperfecta type II	COLI
Thanatophoric dysplasia	FGFR3
Hypophosphatasia lethal type	TNSALP
Achondrogenesis	COLII
Hypochondrogenesis	COLII
Achondrogenesis IB	DTDST
Camptomelic dysplasia	SOX9
Blomstrand chondrodysplasia	PTHR1
Short rib syndrome	?

hyperplastic metatropic dysplasia (type 1) and fibrochondrogenesis. In our experience, osteogenesis imperfecta and thanatophoric dysplasia were the most frequent lethal skeletal diseases.

Amnionic fluid

Clinical analysis of patients with skeletal dysplasias, lethal type revealed several characteristic phenotypes in each disease. For example, polyhydramnios is known as one of the features in patients with congenital anomaly. However, osteogenesis imperfecta and thanatophoric dysplasia were quite different in terms of association with polyhydraminios in our patients. In 11 patients with osteogenesis imperfecta, no polyhydramnios was observed. In contrast, nine out of 11 patients with thanatophoric dysplasia were complicated with polyhydramnios.

Intrauterine growth retardation

Intrauterine growth retardation (IUGR) is often observed in fetuses with severe skeletal dysplasia. Short limb associated with skeletal dysplasia tends to underestimate the expected body weight of the fetus. In contrast, hydrops, sometimes associated with achondrogenesis and thanatophoric dysplasia, affects the weight. Patients with osteogenesis imperfecta are often skinny and show IUGR.

Bone age or calcification of bones in the fetus

In the fetus, bone age can be estimated by the number of calcified bones whose calcification occurred during the gestational period. They consisted of talus, os calcis, ishium, os pubis, sternum, vertebral bodies (coccygeal and fifth sacral), lumbar transverse processes, proximal epiphysis of tibia, and distal epiphysis of femur. We previously reported the relationship between the number of calcified bones and the gestational week. In hypophosphatasia, achondrogenesis and some forms of chondrodyplasia, calcification of bones is extremely delayed. In contrast, a mild decrease in number or normal development of calcified bones is observed in patients with osteogenesis imperfecta and thanatophoric dysplasia. These results suggest the difference in the pathogenesis of each skeletal dysplasia.

Closing comments

Due to the limitation of length, this review cannot provide readers a whole picture accounting for the recent development of investigations on skeletal dysplasia. Apparently, identification of genes responsible for skeletal dysplasia contributes to better understanding of the process in which chondrocytes, osteoblasts, and osteoclasts proliferate, differentiate, and interact with each other. Because the opportunity for the pediatrician to take care of patients with skeletal dysplasia has increased, the pediatrician should understand the biological and developmental aspects of bone and chondrocytes as well as clinical advance of treatment of patients with skeletal dysplasia.

Acknowledgments

We thank Drs Masahiro Nakayama, Osaka Medical Center and Research Institute for Maternal and Child Health. We also thank Drs Hitomi Okabe, Kunihiko Takahashi, Shigetoyo Kogaki, and Shigeo Nakajima, Osaka University Graduate School of Medicine.

REFERENCES

1. Provot S, Schipani E. Molecular mechanisms of endochondral bone development. *Biochem Biophys Res Commun* 2005;328:658–65.
2. Stains JP, Civitelli R. Cell-to-cell interactions in bone. *Biochem Biophys Res Commun* 2005;328:721–7.
3. de Crombrugghe B, Lefebvre V, Behringer RR, *et al.* Transcriptional mechanisms of chondrocyte differentiation. *Matrix Biol* 2000;19:389–94.
4. Unger S. A genetic approach to the diagnosis of skeletal dysplasia. *Clin Orthop* 2002;401:32–8.
5. van der Eerden BC, Karperien M, Wit JM. Systemic and local regulation of the growth plate. *Endocr Rev* 2003;24:782–801.
6. Hagenas L, Hertel T. Skeletal dysplasia, growth hormone treatment and body proportion, comparison with other syndromic and non-syndromic short children. *Horm Res* 2003;60(Suppl 3):65–70.
7. Cohen MM Jr. Some chondrodysplasias with short limbs, molecular perspectives. *Am J Med Genet* 2002;112:304–13.
8. Superti-Furga A. Growing bone knowledge. *Clin Genet* 2004;66:399–401.
9. Horton WA. Fibroblast growth factor receptor 3 and the human chondrodysplasias. *Curr Opin Pediatr* 1997;9:437–42.
10. Freisinger P, Bonaventure J, Stoess H, *et al.* Type II collagenopathies, are there additional family members? *Am J Med Genet* 1996;63:137–43.

11. Bi W, Huang W, Whitworth DJ, *et al.* Haploinsufficiency of Sox9 results in defective cartilage primordia and premature skeletal mineralization. *Proc Natl Acad Sci USA* 2001;98:6698–703.
12. Kawakami Y, Tsuda M, Takahashi S, *et al.* Transcriptional coactivator PGC-1a regulates chondrogenesis via association with Sox9. *Proc Natl Acad Sci USA* 2005;102:2414–9.
13. Sock E, Pagon RA, Keymolen K, *et al.* Loss of DNA-dependent dimerization of the transcription factor SOX9 as a cause for campomelic dysplasia. *Hum Mol Genet* 2003;12:1439–47.
14. Ornitz DM, Marie PJ. FGF signaling pathways in endochondral and intramembranous bone development and human genetic disease. *Genes* 2002;16:1446–65.
15. Vajo Z, Francomano CA, Wilkin DJ. The molecular and genetic basis of fibroblast growth factor receptor 3 disorders, the achondroplasia family of skeletal dysplasias, Muenke craniosynostosis, and Crouzon syndrome with acanthosis nigricans. *Endocr Rev* 2000;21:23–39.
16. Bellus GA, Bamshad MJ, Przylepa KA, *et al.* Severe achondroplasia with developmental delay and acanthosis nigricans (SADDAN), phenotypic analysis of a new skeletal dysplasia caused by a Lys650Met mutation in fibroblast growth factor receptor 3. *Am J Med Genet* 1999;85:53–65.
17. Suva LJ, Winslow GA, Wettenhall RE, *et al.* A parathyroid hormone-related protein implicated in malignant hypercalcemia, cloning and expression. *Science* 1987;237:893–6.
18. Karaplis AC, Luz A, Glowacki J, *et al.* Lethal skeletal dysplasia from targeted disruption of the parathyroid hormone-related peptide gene. *Genes Dev* 1994;8:277–89.
19. Karaplis AC. PTHrP, novel roles in skeletal biology. *Curr Pharm Des* 2001;7:655–70.
20. Karp SJ, Schipani E, St-Jacques B, *et al.* Indian hedgehog coordinates endochondral bone growth and morphogenesis via parathyroid hormone related-protein-dependent and -independent pathways. *Development* 2000;127:543–8.
21. St-Jacques B, Hammerschmidt M, McMahon AP. Indian hedgehog signaling regulates proliferation and differentiation of chondrocytes and is essential for bone formation. *Genes Dev* 1999;13:2072–86.
22. Long F, Chung UI, Ohba S, *et al.* Ihh signaling is directly required for the osteoblast lineage in the endochondral skeleton. *Development* 2004;131:1309–18.
23. Juppner H. Role of parathyroid hormone-related peptide and Indian hedgehog in skeletal development. *Pediatr Nephrol* 2000; 14:606–11.
24. Gao B, Guo J, She C, *et al.* Mutations in IHH, encoding Indian hedgehog, cause brachydactyly type A-1. *Nat Genet* 2001;28: 386–8.
25. Otto F, Thornell AP, Crompton T, *et al.* Cbfa1, a candidate gene for cleidocranial dysplasia syndrome, is essential for osteoblast differentiation and bone development. *Cell* 1997;89; 765–71.
26. Komori T, Yagi H, Nomura S, *et al.* Targeted disruption of Cbfa1 results in a complete lack of bone formation owing to maturational arrest of osteoblasts. *Cell* 1997;89:755–64.
27. Ducy P, Zhang R, Geoffroy V, *et al.* Osf2/Cbfa1, a transcriptional activator of osteoblast differentiation. *Cell* 1997;89:747–54.
28. Ueta C, Iwamoto M, Kanatani N, *et al.* Skeletal malformations caused by overexpression of Cbfa1 or its dominant negative form in chondrocytes. *J Cell Biol* 2001;153:87–100.
29. Gerber HP, Vu TH, Ryan AM, *et al.* VEGF couples hypertrophic cartilage remodeling, ossification and angiogenesis during endochondral bone formation. *Nat Med* 1999;5:623–8.
30. Schipani E, Ryan HE, Didrickson S, *et al.* Hypoxia in cartilage, HIF-1alpha is essential for chondrocyte growth arrest and survival. *Genes Dev* 2001;15:2865–76.
31. Stickens D, Behonick DJ, Ortega N, *et al.* Altered endochondral bone development in matrix metalloproteinase 13-deficient mice. *Development* 2004;131:5883–95.
32. Vu TH, Shipley JM, Bergers G, *et al.* MMP-9/gelatinase B is a key regulator of growth plate angiogenesis and apoptosis of hypertrophic chondrocytes. *Cell* 1998;93:411–22.
33. Colnot C, de la Fuente L, Huang S, *et al.* Indian hedgehog synchronizes skeletal angiogenesis and perichondrial maturation with cartilage development. *Development* 2005;132: 1057–67.
34. Rousseau F, Bonaventure J, Legeai-Mallet L, *et al.* Mutations in the gene encoding fibroblast growth factor receptor-3 in achondroplasia. *Nature* 1994;371:252–4.
35. Shiang R, Thompson LM, Zhu YZ, *et al.* Mutations in the transmembrane domain of FGFR3 cause the most common genetic form of dwarfism, achondroplasia. *Cell* 1994;78:335–42.
36. Matsui Y, Kawabata H, Ozono K, *et al.* Skeletal development of achondroplasia, analysis of genotyped patients. *Pediatr Int* 2001; 43:361–3.
37. Kanaka-Gantenbein C. Present status of the use of growth hormone in short children with bone diseases (diseases of the skeleton). *J Pediatr Endocrinol Metab* 2001;14:17–26.
38. Koike M, Yamanaka Y, Inoue M, *et al.* Insulin-like growth factor-1 rescues the mutated FGF receptor 3 (G380R) expressing ATDC5 cells from apoptosis through phosphatidylinositol 3-kinase and MAPK. *J Bone Miner Res* 2003;18:2043–51.
39. Yasoda A, Komatsu Y, Chusho H, *et al.* Overexpression of CNP in chondrocytes rescues achondroplasia through a MAPK-dependent pathway. *Nat Med* 2004;10:80–6.
40. Tasker RC, Dundas I, Laverty A, *et al.* Distinct patterns of respiratory difficulty in young children with achondroplasia, a clinical, sleep, and lung function study. *Arch Dis Child* 1998;79:99–108.
41. Mogayzel PJ Jr, Carroll JL, Loughlin GM, *et al.* Sleep-disordered breathing in children with achondroplasia. *J Pediatr* 1998;132: 667–71.
42. Cole WG. Advances in osteogenesis imperfecta. *Clin Orthop* 2002;401:6–16.
43. Roughley PJ, Rauch F, Glorieux FH. Osteogenesis imperfecta – clinical and molecular diversity. *Eur Cell Mater* 2003;5:41–7.
44. Korkko J, Ala-Kokko L, De Paepe A, *et al.* Analysis of the COL1A1 and COL1A2 genes by PCR amplification and scanning by conformation-sensitive gel electrophoresis identifies only COL1A1 mutations in 15 patients with osteogenesis imperfecta type I, identification of common sequences of null-allele mutations. *Am J Hum Genet* 1998;62:98–110.
45. Sillence DO, Senn A, Danks DM. Genetic heterogeneity in osteogenesis imperfecta. *J Med Genet* 1979;16:101–16.
46. Glorieux FH, Bishop NJ, Plotkin H, *et al.* Cyclic administration of pamidronate in children with severe osteogenesis imperfecta. *N Engl J Med* 1998;339:947–52.
47. Astrom E, Soderhall S. Beneficial effect of long term intravenous bisphosphonate treatment of osteogenesis imperfecta. *Arch Dis Child* 2002;86:356–64.
48. Chamberlain JR, Schwarze U, Wang PR, *et al.* Gene targeting in stem cells from individuals with osteogenesis imperfecta. *Science* 2004;303:1198–201.
49. Millington-Ward S, Allers C, Tuohy G, *et al.* Validation in mesenchymal progenitor cells of a mutation-independent ex vivo approach to gene therapy for osteogenesis imperfecta. *Hum Mol Genet* 2002;11:2201–6.
50. Horwitz EM, Gordon PL, Koo WK, *et al.* Isolated allogenic bone marrow-derived mesenchymal cells engraft and stimulate growth in children with osteogenesis imperfecta, implications for cell therapy of bone. *Proc Natl Acad Sci USA* 2002;99:8932–7.
51. Wilkin DJ, Bogaert R, Lachman RS, *et al.* A single amino acid substitution (G103D) in the type II collagen triple helix produces Kniest dysplasia. *Hum Mol Genet* 1994;3:1999–2003.
52. Nishimura G, Nakashima E, Mabuchi A, *et al.* Identification of COL2A1 mutations in platyspondylic skeletal dysplasia, Torrance type. *J Med Genet* 2004;41:75–9.
53. Warman ML, Abbott M, Apte SS, *et al.* A type X collagen mutation causes Schmid metaphyseal chondrodysplasia. *Nat Genet* 1993;5:79–82.
54. Czarny-Ratajczak M, Lohiniva J, Rogala P, *et al.* A mutation in COL9A1 causes multiple epiphyseal dysplasia. Further evidence for locus heterogeneity. *Am J Hum Genet* 2001;69:969–80.
55. Briggs MD, Mortier GR, Cole WG, *et al.* Diverse mutations in the gene for cartilage oligomeric matrix protein in the pseudoachondroplasia-multiple epiphyseal dysplasia disease spectrum. *Am J Hum Genet* 1998;62:311–9.
56. Cai G, Nakayama M, Hiraki Y, *et al.* Mutational analysis of the DTDST gene in a fetus with achondrogenesis type 1B. *Am J Med Genet* 1998;78:58–60.
57. Hästbacka J, de la Chapelle A, Mahtani MM, *et al.* The diastrophic dysplasia gene encodes a novel sulfate transporter: Positional cloning by fine-structure linkage disequilibrium mapping. *Cell* 1994;78:1073–87.
58. Rossi A, Superti-Furga A. Mutations in the diastrophic dysplasia sulfate transporter (DTDST) gene (SLC26A2), 22 novel mutations, mutation review, associated skeletal phenotypes, and diagnostic relevance. *Hum Mutat* 2001;17:159–71.

59. Ridanpää M, van Eenennaam H, Pelin K, *et al.* Mutations in the RNA component of RNase MRP cause a pleiotropic human disease, cartilage-hair hypoplasia. *Cell* 2001;104:195–203.
60. Nakashima E, Mabuchi A, Kashimada K, *et al.* RMRP mutations in Japanese patients with cartilage-hair hypoplasia. *Am J Med Genet A* 2003;123:253–6.
61. Gedeon AK, Colley A, Jamieson R, *et al.* Identification of the gene (SEDL) causing X-linked spondyloepiphyseal dysplasia tarda. *Nature Genet* 1999;22:400–4.
62. Shears DJ, Vassal HJ, Goodman FR, *et al.* Mutation and deletion of the pseudoautosomal gene SHOX cause Leri–Weill dyschondrosteosis. *Nat Genet* 1998;19:70–3.
63. Belin V, Cusin V, Viot G, *et al.* SHOX mutations in dyschondrosteosis (Leri–Weill syndrome). *Nat Genet* 1998;19:67–9.
64. Weinstein LS, Yu S, Warner DR, *et al.* Endocrine manifestations of stimulatory G protein alpha-subunit mutations and the role of genomic imprinting. *Endocr Rev* 2001;22:675–705.
65. Bastepe M, Juppner H. Pseudohypoparathyroidism. New insights into an old disease. *Endocrinol Metab Clin North Am* 2000;29: 569–89.
66. Schipani E, Kruse K, Juppner H. A constitutively active mutant PTH-PTHrP receptor in Jansen-type metaphyseal chondrodysplasia. *Science* 1995;268:98–100.
67. Jobert AS, Zhang P, Couvineau A, *et al.* Absence of functional receptors for parathyroid hormone and parathyroid hormone-related peptide in Blomstrand chondrodysplasia. *J Clin Invest* 1998; 102:34–40.
68. Bastepe M, Frohlich LF, Linglart A, *et al.* Deletion of the NESP55 differentially methylated region causes loss of maternal GNAS imprints and pseudohypoparathyroidism type Ib. *Nat Genet* 2005;37:25–7.
69. Weinstein LS, Shenker A, Gejman PV, *et al.* Activating mutations of the stimulatory G protein in the McCune–Albright syndrome. *N Engl J Med* 1991;325:1688–95.
70. Yamamoto T, Ozono K, Kasayama S, *et al.* Increased IL-6 production by cells isolated from the fibrous bone dysplasia tissues in patients with McCune–Albright syndrome. *J Clin Invest* 1996; 98:30–5.
71. Riminucci M, Collins MT, Fedarko NS, *et al.* FGF-23 in fibrous dysplasia of bone and its relationship to renal phosphate wasting. *J Clin Invest* 2003;112:683–92.
72. Whyte MP. Hypophosphatasia and the role of alkaline phoshatase in skeletal mineralization. *Endocr Rev* 1994;15:439–61.
73. Mornet E. Hypophosphatasia, the mutations in the tissue-nonspecific alkaline phosphatase gene. *Hum Mutat* 2000;15: 309–15.
74. Cai G, Michigami T, Yamamoto T, *et al.* Analysis of localization of mutated tissue-nonspecific alkaline phosphatase proteins associated with neonatal hypophosphatasia using green fluorescent protein chimeras. *J Clin Endocrinol Metab* 1998;83:3936–42.
75. Zurutuza L, Muller F, Gibrat JF, *et al.* Correlations of genotype and phenotype in hypophosphatasia. *Hum Mol Genet* 1999;8: 1039–46.
76. Mochizuki H, Saito M, Michigami T, *et al.* Severe hypercalcemia and respiratory insufficiency associated with infantile hypophosphatasia caused by two novel mutations of the TNSALP gene. *Eur J Pediatr* 2000;159:375–9.
77. Spentchian M, Merrien Y, Herasse M, *et al.* Severe hypophosphatasia, characterization of fifteen novel mutations in the ALPL gene. *Hum Mutat* 2003;22:105–6.
78. Müller HL, Yamazaki M, Michigami T, *et al.* Asp361Val mutant of alkaline phosphatase found in patients with dominantly inherited hypophosphatasia inhibits the activity of the wild-type enzyme. *J Clin Endocrinol Metab* 2000;85:743–7.
79. Whyte MP, Kurtzberg J, McAlister WH, *et al.* Marrow cell transplantation for infantile hypophosphatasia. *J Bone Miner Res* 2003;18:624–36.
80. Nürnberg P, Thiele H, Chandler D, *et al.* Heterozygous mutations in ANKH, the human ortholog of the mouse progressive ankylosis gene, result in craniometaphyseal dysplasia. *Nat Genet* 2001;28:37–41.
81. Tolar J, Teitelbaum SL, Orchard PJ. Osteopetrosis. *N Engl J Med* 2004;351:2839–49.
82. Frattini A, Orchard PJ, Sobacchi C, *et al.* Defects in TCIRG1 subunit of the vacuolar proton pump are responsible for a subset of human autosomal recessive osteopetrosis. *Nat Genet* 2000;25:343–6.
83. Kornak U, Kasper D, Bosl MR, *et al.* Loss of the ClC-7 chloride channel leads to osteopetrosis in mice and man. *Cell* 2001; 104:205–15.
84. Sly WS, Whyte MP, Sundaram V, *et al.* Carbonic anhydrase II deficiency in 12 families with the autosomal recessive syndrome of osteopetrosis with renal tubular acidosis and cerebral calcification. *N Engl J Med* 1985;313:139–45.
85. Chalhoub N, Benachenhou N, Rajapurohitam V, *et al.* Grey-lethal mutation induces severe malignant autosomal recessive osteopetrosis in mouse and human. *Nat Med* 2003;9:399–406.
86. Doffinger R, Smahi A, Bessia C, *et al.* X-linked anhydrotic ectodermal dysplasia with immunodeficiency is caused by impaired NF-kappaB signaling. *Nat Genet* 2001;27:277–85.
87. Wilson CJ, Vellodi A. Autosomal recessive osteopetrosis, diagnosis, management, and outcome. *Arch Dis Child* 2000;83:449–52.
88. Gelb BD, Shi GP, Chapman HA, *et al.* Pycnodysostosis, a lysosomal disease caused by cathepsin K deficiency. *Science* 1996; 273:1236–8.
89. Kinoshita A, Saito T, Tomita H, *et al.* Domain-specific mutations in TGFB1 result in Camurati–Engelmann disease. *Nat Genet* 2000;26:19–20.
90. Brunkow ME, Gardner JC, Van Ness J, *et al.* Bone dysplasia sclerosteosis results from loss of the SOST gene product, a novel cystine knot-containing protein. *Am J Hum Genet* 2001;68:577–89.
91. Whyte MP, Obrecht SE, Finnegan PM, *et al.* Osteoprotegerin deficiency and juvenile Paget's disease. *N Engl J Med* 2002; 347:175–84.
92. Hughes AE, Ralston SH, Marken J, *et al.* Mutations in TNFRSF11A, affecting the signal peptide of RANK, cause familial expansile osteolysis. *Nat Genet* 2000;24:45–8.
93. Faure C, Beyssac JM, Montagne JP. Predominance of exclusive orbital and facial involvement in infantile cortical hyperostosis (de Toni–Caffey's disease). Report of four cases and a review of the literature. *Pediatr Radiol* 1977;6:103–6.
94. Westendorf JJ, Kahler RA, Schroeder TM. Wnt signaling in osteoblasts and bone diseases. *Gene* 2004;341:19–39.
95. Gong Y, Slee RB, Fukai N, *et al.* LDL receptor-related protein 5 (LRP5) affects bone accrual and eye development. *Cell* 2001; 107:513–23.
96. Boyden LM, Mao J, Belsky J, *et al.* High bone density due to a mutation in LDL-receptor-related protein 5. *N Engl J Med* 2002; 346:1513–21.
97. Kokubu C, Heinzmann U, Kokubu T, *et al.* Skeletal defects in ringelschwanz mutant mice reveal that Lrp6 is required for proper somitogenesis and osteogenesis. *Development* 2004;131: 5469–80.
98. Jongmans M, Sistermans EA, Rikken A, *et al.* Genotypic and phenotypic characterization of Noonan syndrome: New data and review of the literature. *Am J Med Genet A* 2005;134(2): 165–70.
99. Bertola DR, Pereira AC, de Oliveira PS, *et al.* Clinical variability in a Noonan syndrome family with a new PTPN11 gene mutation. *Am J Med Genet A* 2004;130A:378–83.
100. Zenker M, Buheitel G, Rauch R, *et al.* Genotype–phenotype correlations in Noonan syndrome. *J Pediatr* 2004;144:368–74.
101. Yoshida R, Hasegawa T, Hasegawa Y, *et al.* Protein-tyrosine phosphatase, nonreceptor type 11 mutation analysis and clinical assessment in 45 patients with Noonan syndrome. *J Clin Endocrinol Metab* 2004;89:3359–64.
102. Sarkozy A, Conti E, Seripa D, *et al.* Correlation between PTPN11 gene mutations and congenital heart defects in Noonan and LEOPARD syndromes. *J Med Genet* 2003;40:704–8.
103. Tartaglia M, Niemeyer CM, Shannon KM, *et al.* SHP-2 and myeloid malignancies. *Curr Opin Hematol* 2004;11:44–50.
104. Gugliantini P, Maragliano G, Piscione M, *et al.* Constitutional osteochondrodysplasias identifiable at birth. A short review on the state of the art in radiodiagnosis in the late 20th century. *Radiol Med (Torino)* 1999;97:116–20.
105. Hall CM, Elcioglu NH. Metatropic dysplasia lethal variants. *Pediatr Radiol* 2004;34:66–74.

60 Implantation

S. Saito

Introduction

Human pregnancy represents a semiallograft to the maternal host.[1] However, the semiallogeneic embryo/fetus is not rejected by the mother. When a donated embryo is transplanted to a surrogate mother, the fetus is an allograft to the mother, but the allogeneic fetus is not rejected by the mother. Pregnancy is thus a mysterious biological phenomenon. Recent studies suggest that endometrial (maternal) lymphocytes play some role in the maintenance of pregnancy via immune mediators such as cytokines.[2] It has been postulated that tolerance to paternal antigens (Ags) must be present during pregnancy. Some regulatory lymphocytes and regulatory cytokines play a very important role in preventing allograft rejection. However, these mechanisms are not so rigid. The absence of these regulatory factors is involved in multiple implantation failure, pregnancy loss and pre-eclampsia. The low rate of successful implantation in humans suggests that the expression of these cytokines and their biologic signals should be optimal, precise and synchronized. In recent years, accumulating evidence has emerged that many factors, including cytokines, growth factors and maternal lymphocytes, contribute to the success of embryo implantation and maintenance of pregnancy.

Table 60.1 Proposed mechanism for maintenance of pregnancy

Absence of classical MHC class I and class II molecules on trophoblasts
Expression of HLA-C, HLA-G and HLA-E on trophoblasts
Expression of complement regulatory proteins on trophoblasts (CD46, CD55 and CD59)
Fas L, Fas receptor system
Immunosuppressive factors [α2 glycoprotein, alpha-fetoprotein (AFP) and TGF-β]
uNK (CD16–CD56 bright NK cells) [granulated metrial gland (GMG) cells in mice]
Cytokines (Th2-type cytokines) and hormones
Treg cells (CD4 + CD25 + T cells, Th3, Tr1)
Regulatory NK cells (NK3, NKr1)

Unique human leukocyte antigen (HLA) expression on trophoblasts

The mechanism for maintenance of pregnancy has been proposed (Table 60.1). Cytotoxic T cells, which induce rejection, recognize antigeneic peptides expressed on major histocompatibility (MHC) Ag class I or class II on target cells. Interestingly, villous trophoblasts lack MHC class I and class II molecules on their surface. As a result, villous trophoblasts cannot be recognized by maternal T cells, resulting in prevention of rejection.

Natural killer (NK) cells are lymphocytes of the innate immune system that are involved in the early defenses against foreign cells.[3] NK cell activation is controlled by a dynamic balance between complementary and antagonistic pathways. NK cells express an array of activating cell surface receptors that can trigger cytolytic programs, as well as cytokine or chemokine secretion. NK cells also express cell surface inhibitory receptors that antagonize activating pathways through protein tyrosine phosphatases. The classical MHC class I molecules HLA-C and the non-classical class I molecules HLA-E and HLA-G interact with inhibitory receptors, such as killer-cell immunoglobulin-like receptors and CD94/NKG2. A wide range of MHC class I molecules such as HLA-G also bind ILT2 and ILT4, which are members of the immunoglobulin-like transcript (ILT) family. Interestingly, extravillous trophoblasts, which invade the uterus, express HLA-C, HLA-E and HLA-G.[3] Maternal NK cell-cytotoxic activity is suppressed by inhibitory receptors resulting in the fetus being protected from maternal NK cell attack. A unique characteristic of HLA-G is the generation of multiple spliced variants. Alternative splicing of the HLA-G messenger RNA yields different membrane-bound and soluble isoforms. Interestingly, soluble HLA-G, which is produced by villous trophoblasts, is an immunosuppressive molecule inducing apoptosis of activated $CD8^+$ T cells and down-modulating $CD4^+$ T cell proliferation.[4]

Therefore, soluble HLA-G probably plays a very important role in the maintenance of pregnancy at the feto–maternal interface. Soluble HLA-G may also contribute to the control of implantation. It has been reported that human implantation was strictly related to soluble HLA-G secretion by preimplantation embryos.[5] Fuzzi *et al.* reported that after *in vitro* fertilization or intracytoplasmic sperm injection, only transfer of embryos secreting HLA-G could lead to pregnancies. In contrast, no pregnancy occurred after transfer of soluble HLA-G-negative embryos. Soluble HLA-G appears to be a key molecule at the time of implantation, and in early and late placentation.

Expression of complement regulatory proteins on trophoblasts

Activation of a complement promotes cell lysis mediation by the membrane attack complex. Complements also bind and attack self tissues, especially in areas of inflammation. However, cells are protected from the deleterious effects of complement activation by complement regulatory proteins such as CD46 (MCP), CD55 (DAF), CD59 and Crry. Crry, present only in rodents, regulates the deposition of activated C3 and C4 on the surface of autologous cells. Decreased expression of complement regulatory molecules has been found in different inflammatory disorders. Complement activation is regulated by excessive expression of complement regulatory proteins on trophoblasts. However, complement deposition is recognized at the feto–maternal interface in miscarriage cases. Survival of $Crry^{-/-}$ embryos was compromised because of complement deposition and concomitant placental inflammation.[6] Interestingly, breeding with $C3^{-/-}$ mice rescued $Crry^{-/-}$ mice from lethality, suggesting that the regulation of complements is critical in fetal control of the maternal process that mediates tissue damage.[6]

In humans, antiphospholipid syndrome (APS) is characterized clinically by fetal loss and thrombosis and serologically by the presence of auto-antibodies to lipid-binding protein. Recent data suggested that complement activation, especially C5a and C5R interaction, is necessary for thrombosis of the placental vasculature.[7] APS is generally treated with anticoagulation therapy. Recent studies demonstrated that treatment with heparin prevented complement activation *in vivo* and *in vitro* and protected mice from pregnancy complications induced by antiphospholipid antibodies.[8] These data suggest that inhibition of complement activation is essential for maintenance of pregnancy.

Fas/Fas ligand (Fas L) system

The Fas/Fas L pathway plays a critical role in promoting apoptosis and regulation of immune responses. The Fas/Fas L system appears to contribute to the immune privilege of the maternal–fetal interface. The maternal decidua and fetal trophoblasts express Fas L, and expression might prevent trafficking of reactive maternal cells into the fetal circulation and vice versa. T cells specific for fetal Ags decrease in an Ag-specific manner during pregnancy, consistent with clonal deletion in the maternal immune system. Placental trophoblasts that express Fas L can induce Fas-mediated death of maternally activated T cells, and this clonal deletion is one mechanism of tolerance to the fetal allograft.[9] The Fas/Fas L system also plays an important role in implantation. Embryonic trophoblasts and maternal decidua produce conticotropin-releasing hormone (CRH) and CRH induces Fas L expression.[10] Female rats treated with a CRH receptor type 1 antagonist, antalarmin, showed a marked decrease in implantation sites and live embryos, along with diminished endometrial Fas L expression. Embryos from mothers that lacked T cells or from syngeneic matings were not rejected when the mothers were given antalarmin.[11] These data suggest that locally produced CRH promotes implantation and maintenance of early pregnancy by killing activated T cells.

Th1/Th2 balance during pregnancy

The blastocyst and maternal endometrium develop an exquisite dialog during the implantation window. Successful embryo implantation requires the synchronization of embryo development and uterine preparation. In mice, this period begins at day 3 and is completed by day 5 (Figure 60.1). Pseudopregnancy at day 2 in mice does not represent the receptive phase for implantation of embryos. Takabatake *et al.* reported that in recipient pseudopregnant mice injected intravenously with splenocytes or culture supernatant on day 2, blastocyst transfer was performed on day 2.[10] The successful implantation rate was markedly higher in the pregnancy day 4- and day 8-splenocytes-injected groups. They further clarified that a significant increase in the implantation rate was observed when pregnancy day 4-$CD4^+$ T cells were injected into the uterus. These data suggest that $CD4^+$ T cells during early pregnancy could contribute to changing the implantation window and increase the chance of implantation.

T cells can be classified into $CD4^+$ T cells and $CD8^+$ T cells by their surface markers (Figure 60.2). $CD4^+$ T cells are also classified into Th1 cells, which produce interleukin (IL) 2, interferon (IFN) γ and tumor necrosis factor β, and Th2 cells, which produce IL-4, IL-5 and IL-13. Th1 cells are involved in cellular immunity such as rejection of cytotoxic T cell responses. On the other hand, Th2 cells are involved in immunoglobulin production. Based on these findings, Wegmann *et al.* hypothesized that physiological protection from maternal rejection is due to a Th2-type response at

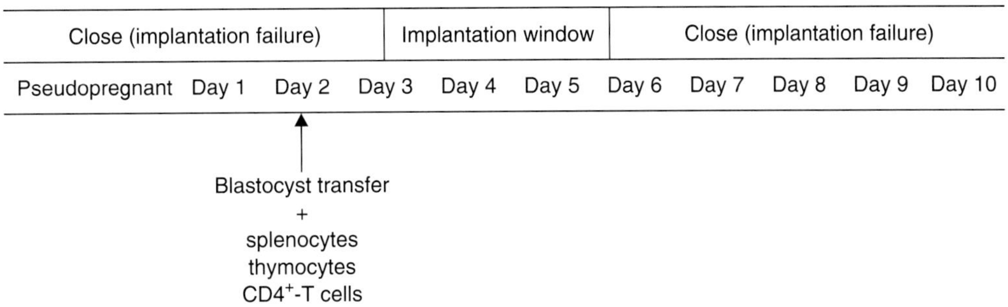

Figure 60.1 Implantation window in mice.

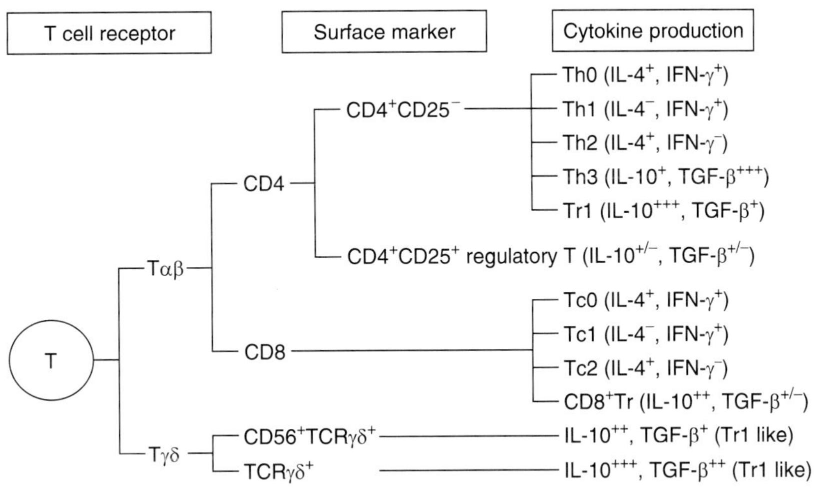

Figure 60.2 T cell subsets classified by their surface markers and cytokine profiles.

the materno–fetal interface.[12] In a mouse model, Th1 cells induced miscarriage and implantation failure. However, in humans, the peripheral blood Th1/Th2 balance in normal pregnancy is controversial, because the amplitude of this balance is very small in peripheral blood. On the other hand, the Th1/Th2 ratios in the endometrium or decidua change dramatically during the menstrual cycle and pregnancy. For example, it has been reported that the Th1/Th2 ratio was 147.5 during the proliferative phase of the endometrium, 37.4 during the secretory phase and 1.3 in early pregnancy deciduas.[13] Furthermore, the numbers and population of Th2 cells are increased at the decidua basalis compared to those at the decidua parietalis, suggesting that Th2 cells accumulate at the implantation site.[14]

Hill *et al.* first reported that Th1-type immunity is present in women with recurrent pregnancy loss, and Piccinni *et al.* first reported defective production of Th2 cytokines by decidual T cells in unexplained recurrent spontaneous abortions. Michimata *et al.* first reported decreased Th2 cells in the decidua basalis in recurrent spontaneous abortions with normal embryo, although accumulation of Th2 cells was observed in the decidua basalis in recurrent spontaneous abortions with abnormal chromosomal content.[15] These data suggested that accumulation of Th2 cells at the decidua basalis is important in maintaining pregnancy.

Regulatory T (Treg) cells in pregnancy

Recent data demonstrated that immunoregulatory activity specific for donor alloantigens is enriched in the $CD4^+CD25^+$ Treg cell population (Figure 60.2). $CD4^+CD25^+$ Treg cells play a critical role in peripheral tolerance, transplantation tolerance and maternal tolerance to the fetus. The population of $CD4^+CD25^+$ Treg cells increases in iliac lymph nodes, in inguinal lymph nodes, in the spleen, in decidua and in blood, and these cells suppress alloreactive proliferation *in vitro*.[16,17] Alubihare *et al.* injected 2×10^7 lymphocytes or an equal number of cells from a CD25-depleted cell preparation ($CD25^-$) into BALB/C nu/nu mice that lacked T cells.[16] All recipient BALB/C nu/nu female mice were mated with C57BL/6 male mice on the day after adoptive transfer. As a result, all the fetuses were aborted in allogeneic pregnancy when $CD25^-$ cells were injected, while this treatment did not induce fetal resorption in syngeneic pregnancy. These findings suggest that $CD25^+$ cells, perhaps $CD4^+CD25^+$ T cells, mediate maternal tolerance to the fetus.

In human pregnancy, $CD4^+CD25^{bright}$ Treg cells are increased in the early pregnancy decidua, but this elevated $CD4^+CD25^{bright}$ Treg cell ratio decreases to a non-pregnancy level in miscarriage cases.[17] Therefore, $CD4^+CD25^+$ Treg cells are crucial to the maintenance of tolerance in pregnancy. Recently, Polanczyk *et al.* reported that estrogen augmented Foxp3 expression, which is an essential factor for the development of $CD4^+CD25^+$ Treg cells, and that treatment with estrogen increased the $CD4^+CD25^+$ Treg cell number in mice.[18] Estrogen might promote maternal tolerance to the fetus by increasing the number of $CD4^+CD25^+$ Treg cells.

Indoleamine 2,3-dioxygenase (IDO) expression during pregnancy

IDO is an enzyme for tryptophan catabolism and it is expressed in the blastocysts, syncytiotrophoblasts, extravillous trophoblasts, macrophages and endometrial gland cells. Pharmacologic inhibition of IDO activity resulted in dramatically decreased rates of successful allogeneic pregnancy due to maternal T cell response to fetal alloantigens.[19] IDO is a key immunosuppressive mechanism in normal pregnancies, although IDO-deficient mice can become pregnant and do not abort.

Cytotoxic T lymphocyte-associated Ag 4 (CTLA-4) plays a critical role in peripheral tolerance, and it is well known that $CD4^+CD25^+$ Treg cells express CTLA-4 on their surfaces. Interestingly, CTLA-4 induces IDO enzyme activity in dendritic cells and regulates tryptophan catabolism.[20] These findings suggest that decidual $CD4^+CD25^+$ Treg cells, which express CTLA-4 on their surface, interact with dendritic cells. As a result, these signals enhance IDO activity, resulting in maintenance of pregnancy. The cross talk between $CD4^+CD25^+$ Treg cells and the IDO enzyme may induce successful pregnancy.

Cytokine profile in decidual NK cells

The Th1/Th2 paradigm has been further developed. T cell subsets that produce the immunoregulatory cytokines IL-10 and transforming growth factor (TGF) β have been clarified. Th3 cells predominantly produce TGF-β, while Tr1 cells predominantly produce IL-10. They achieve immunoregulation via

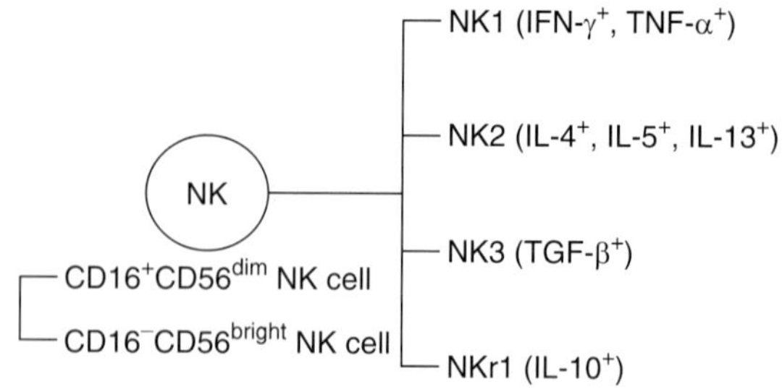

Figure 60.3 NK cell subsets by their cytokine profiles.

their cytokine production. NK cells are also classified into NK1, NK2, NK3 and NKr1 cells by their cytokine profiles (Figure 60.3).

It is well known that NK cells are the main population of lymphocytes in early pregnancy decidua. NK cells can be classified into $CD16^+CD56^{dim}$ NK cells and $CD16^-CD56^{bright}$ NK cells. The main population of peripheral blood NK cells is $CD16^+CD56^{dim}$ NK cells, whereas the main population of endometrial and decidual NK cells is $CD16^-CD56^{bright}$ NK cells. In the peripheral blood of non-pregnant subjects, IFN-γ-producing $CD16^+CD56^{dim}$ NK cells and $CD16^-CD56^{bright}$ NK cells are the main populations. After pregnancy, the populations of IL-10-producing NKr1 cells in peripheral blood $CD16^+CD56^{dim}$ NK cells and $CD16^-CD56^{bright}$ NK cells increase, although these populations decrease in miscarriage cases.[21] In the early pregnancy decidua, the main populations of $CD16^+CD56^{dim}$ NK cells and $CD16^-CD56^{bright}$ NK cells are TGF-β-producing NK3 cells, and NK3 cells in decidua are decreased in miscarriage cases.[21] Decidual $CD16^-CD56^{bright}$ NK cells produce a variety of cytokines such as granulocyte macrophage colony stimulating factor (GM-CSF), M-CSF, G-CSF, leukemia inhibitory factor (LIF) and angiotoietin. M-CSF and GM-CSF induce the DNA synthesis of trophoblasts, and LIF is an essential cytokine for implantation. Angiopoietin plays an important role in angiogenesis. These findings suggest that NK cells in the decidua play an important role in the maintenance of pregnancy by regulation of maternal immune function, placental growth and angiogenesis at the feto–maternal interface.

Conclusion

The immune environment, including the cytokine profile or lymphocyte subsets in the endometrium, clearly changes during implantation and pregnancy. These dramatic and synchronized changes are present at the local implantation site. A better understanding of these sequential events could improve clinicians' ability to treat disorders related to these processes, including infertility and early pregnancy loss.

REFERENCES

1. Medawar PB. Some immunological and endocrinological problems raised by the evolution of viviparity in vertebrates. *Symp Soc Biol* 1953;7:320–38.
2. Saito S. Cytokine cross-talk between mother and the embryo/placenta. *J Reprod Immunol* 2001;52:15–33.
3. Moffett-King A. Natural killer cells and pregnancy. *Nat Rev Immunol* 2002;2:656–63.
4. Bouteiller PL, Legrand-Abravanel F, Solier C. Soluble HLA-G1 at the materno-foetal interface. *Placenta* 2003;24(Suppl A):S10–5.
5. Fuzzi B, Rizzo R, Criscuoli L, *et al.* HLA-G expression in early embryos is a fundamental prerequisite for the obtainment of pregnancy. *Eur J Immunol* 2002;32:311–5.
6. Xu C, Mao D, Holers VM, Palanca B, Cheng AM, Molina H. A critical role for murine complement regulator Crry in fetomaternal tolerance. *Science* 2000;287:498–501.
7. Girardi G, Berman J, Redecha P, *et al.* Complement C5a receptors and neutrophils mediate fetal injury in the antiphospholipid syndrome. *J Clin Invest* 2003;112:1644–54.
8. Girardi G, Redecha P, Salmon JE. Heparin prevents antiphospholipid antibody-induced fetal loss by inhibiting complement activation. *Nat Med* 2004;10:1222–6.
9. Jiang SP, Vacchio MS. Multiple mechanisms of peripheral T cell tolerance to the fetal "allograft". *J Immunol* 1998;160:3086–90.
10. Takabatake K, Fujiwara H, Goto Y, *et al.* Intravenous administration of splenocytes in early pregnancy changes the implantation window in mice. *Hum Reprod* 1997;12:583–5.
11. Makrigiannakis A, Zoumakis E, Kalantaridou S, *et al.* Corticotropin-releasing hormone promotes blastocyst implantation and early maternal tolerance. *Nat Immunol* 2001;2:1018–24.
12. Wegmann TG, Lin H, Guilbert L, Mosmann TH. Bidirectional cytokine interactions in the maternal–fetal relationship: Is successful pregnancy a TH2 phenomenon? *Immunol Today* 1993;14:353–6.
13. Saito S, Tsukaguchi N, Hasegawa T, *et al.* Distribution of Th1, Th2 and Th0 and the Th1/Th2 cell ratios in human peripheral and endometrial T cells. *Am J Reprod Immunol* 1999;42:240–5.
14. Michimata T, Tsuda H, Sakai M, *et al.* Accumulation of CRTH2-positive T-helper 2 and T-cytotoxic 2 cells at implantation sites of human decidua in a prostaglandin D_2-mediated manner. *Mol Hum Reprod* 2002;8:181–7.
15. Michimata T, Sakai M, Miyazaki S, *et al.* Decrease of T-helper 2 and T-cytotoxic 2 cells at implantation sites occurs in unexplained recurrent spontaneous abortion with normal chromosomal content. *Hum Reprod* 2003;18:1523–8.
16. Alubihare VR, Kallikourdis M, Betz AG. Regulatory T cells mediate maternal tolerance to the fetus. *Nat Immunol* 2004;5:266–71.
17. Sasaki Y, Sakai M, Miyazaki S, Higuma S, Shiozaki A, Saito S. Decidual and peripheral blood $CD4^{+}CD25^{+}$ regulatory T cells in early pregnancy subjects and spontaneous abortion. *Mol Hum Reprod* 2004;10:347–53.
18. Polanczyk MJ, Carson BD, Subramanian S, *et al.* Estrogen drives expansion of the CD4+CD25+ regulatory T cell compartment. *J Immunol* 2004;173:2227–30.
19. Munn DH, Zhou M, Attwood JT, *et al.* Prevention of allogeneic fetal rejection by tryptophan catabolism. *Science* 1998;281:1191–3.
20. Grohmann U, Orabone C, Fallarino F, *et al.* CTLA-4-Ig regulates tryptophan catabolism in vivo. *Nat Immunol* 2002;3:1097–101.
21. Higuma-Myojo S, Sasaki Y, Miyazaki S, *et al.* Cytokine profile of natural killer cells in early human pregnancy. *Am J Reprod Immunol*, 2005;54:21–9.

61 Endocrinological aspects

N. Sagawa

The production of steroid and protein hormones by human trophoblasts is the largest in amount and diversity among endocrine organs in all mammalians. A unique and obligatory interrelationship is present between the hyperestrogenic state of human pregnancy and the fetal adrenal secretion of a large amount of C_{19} steroids, which serve as precursors for estrogen synthesis in the placenta. Human syncytiotrophoblast takes up maternal plasma low-density lipoprotein (LDL) cholesterol as a substrate for progesterone biosynthesis in the placenta.

The human placenta also synthesizes an enormous amount of protein and peptide hormones including human chorionic gonadotropin (hCG), human chorionic somatomammotropin (hCS), chorionic adrenocorticotropin (ACTH), and others.

Steroidogenesis in the fetoplacental unit

Steroid formation

Estrogen

The placenta is an incomplete steroid-producing organ. It must rely on precursors reaching it from the fetal and maternal circulations. The unique interdependence of fetus, placenta, and mother gave rise to the concept of an integrated fetoplacental–maternal unit.[1] The individual adult steroid-producing glands are capable of forming progestins, androgens, and estrogens, but this is not true of the placenta. There is a constant interplay of fetus, placenta, and mother to form the bulk of the sex steroids in pregnancy.[1] For estrogen formation by the placenta to occur, precursors must reach it from both the fetal and maternal compartments, whereas placental progesterone formation is accomplished in large part from circulation of maternal low-density lipoprotein cholesterol.[2] In the placenta, cholesterol is first converted to pregnenolone and then rapidly and efficiently to progesterone.[3] Production of progesterone reaches approximately 250 mg/day by the end of pregnancy, when the circulating levels are on the order of 130 ng/ml.[4] The placenta also produces estrogens by aromatization of circulating androgens. The major precursor in placental estrogen formation is dehydroepiandrosterone sulfate (DHEA-S), mainly from the fetal adrenal gland. The abundant sulfatase enzyme in the placenta converts DHEA-S to free (unconjugated) DHEA, when it reaches the placenta. DHEA is further converted to androstenedione, thereafter to testosterone, and finally to estrone and 17β-estradiol. However, the major estrogen formed in the human pregnancy is neither estrone nor estradiol but another estrogen, estriol. Estriol is not secreted by the ovary of non-pregnant women but constitutes more than 90% of the known estrogen in pregnancy urine. Concentrations increase with advancing gestation and reach 35–45 mg/24 h at term.[5] Estriol is also found in the amniotic fluid and maternal circulation.[6] The concentration of estriol in the maternal circulation is between 8 and 13 ng/ml at term.[7]

Estriol is produced by a unique biosynthetic process, which forms the interdependence of three compartments, fetus, placenta, and mother (Figure 61.1). Maternal cholesterol is transported as LDL cholesterol to the placenta. Cholesterol is converted to pregnenolone in the placenta and fetal adrenal. Fetal adrenal further metabolizes pregnenolone to dehydroepiandrosterone sulfate (DHAS), which is metabolized to 16α-hydroxy DHAS by 16α-hydroxylase in the fetal liver. DHAS and 16α-hydroxy DHAS are hydrolyzed by placental sulfatase in the placenta and the resulting DHA is further metabolized to estrone and estradiol, and 16α-hydroxy DHA to estriol by placental aromatase. The precursor of placental estrone and estradiol is derived from both maternal and fetal adrenals. In contrast, the precursor of estriol, 16α-hydroxy DHAS is predominantly originated from fetus reflecting fetal adrenal and liver function. Thus, increase in the maternal plasma estriol concentration in late pregnancy is the reflection of total functions and development of fetal adrenal, fetal liver, and the placenta.

Sulfatase deficiency occurs in male babies at an incidence of 1/15,000 pregnancies, whereby 16α-hydroxy DHAS is not hydrolyzed and is not further converted to estriol. The infant with sulfatase deficiency later develops X-linked ichthyosis.[8] Anencephalus-lacking

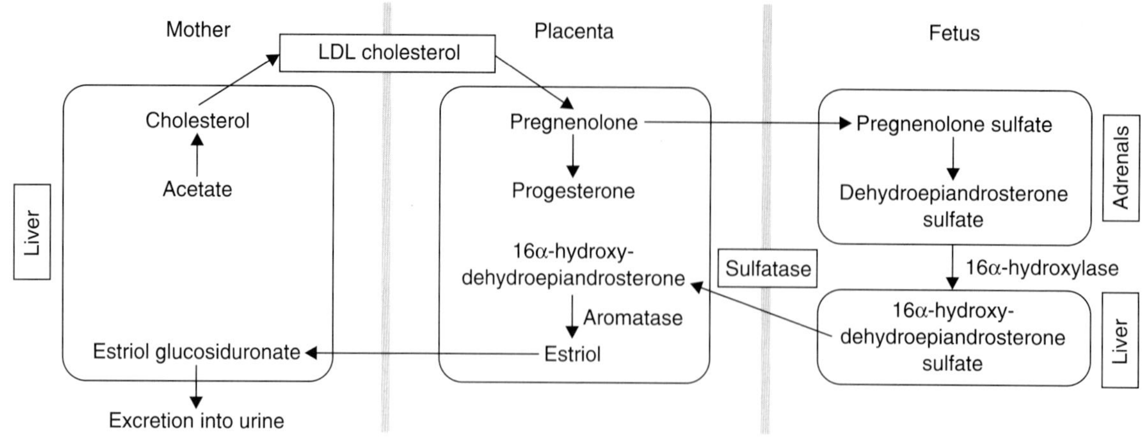

Figure 61.1 Estriol biosynthesis in fetoplacental-maternal unit.

pituitary does not secrete ACTH and estriol production is very low, approximately 10% of the normal fetus. When the fetus dies *in utero* the precursor of estriol is not provided from fetal adrenal and the estriol levels decline significantly.[1] However, changes in the maternal plasma or urinary estriol levels are too slow and do not reflect real-time fetal viability. In Down's syndrome, maternal plasma unconjugated estriol levels are low, because the production of precursor of estriol synthesis in the fetal adrenal is not adequate. Based on this fact, serum estriol levels in the late first trimester are utilized as one of the serum markers of Down's syndrome. Glucocorticoid administration suppresses placental estrogen synthesis because glucocorticoid suppresses ACTH secretion in both mother and fetus and consequently decreases DHAS secretion from both maternal and fetal adrenals.

Progesterone

The placenta is the main source of progesterone in the maternal plasma.[9] The precursor of progesterone synthesis, cholesterol, is predominantly derived from maternal plasma LDL cholesterol, since cholesterol synthesizing enzymes are not expressed in the placenta. Thus, progesterone synthesis is dependent on maternal and placental bioactivities but not on fetal viability.[10] This is the reason why the progesterone levels in maternal sera do not reflect acute fetal compromise as compared to that of estrogen. Placenta does not metabolize progesterone. A major part of placental progesterone is secreted to fetal circulation and further metabolized to glucocorticoids such as cortisol and aldosterone. The rest of the placental progesterone is secreted to maternal plasma. Plasma concentration of progesterone in the late first trimester is approximately 30–40 ng/ml and further increases to 130 ng/ml (secretion: 250 mg/day), which is approximately 10 times of corpus luteum production. Progesterone production in the syncytiotrophoblast during the early first trimester is still low and is not enough to maintain the pregnancy. Thus, corpus luteum is necessary for the maintenance of pregnancy until 6–7 weeks of gestation. Half-life of progesterone is much more shorter than that of hCG. Therefore, plasma level of progesterone decreases much earlier than that of hCG when spontaneous termination of pregnancy occurs in early pregnancy.

Corticoids

Progesterone produced in the placenta is metabolized to either cortisol or aldosterone because fetal adrenal lacks 3b-hydroxysteroid dehydrogenase (3bHSD). Cortisol is further converted to cortisone by 11b-hydroxysteroid dehydrogenase (11bHSD) in the placenta. Cortisol level in the amniotic fluid increases as fetus maturate due to cortisol excretion into fetal urine. Maternal plasma cortisol level increases secondary to the increase in cortisol binding globulin (CBG) in maternal plasma. When uteroplacental blood flow decreases in the pregnant women, complicated with pre-eclampsia, chronic hypertension or severe diabetes mellitus, blood flow in the placental intervillous space decreases resulting in the diffusion of placental steroid hormone to the fetus, increase in the steroid hormone levels in the umbilical cord. The increased cortisol might accelerate fetal lung maturation in case of fetal compromise associated with impaired uteroplacental perfusion.

Biological function of steroid

Estrogens

The functional role of placental estriol in pregnancy has caused a great deal of speculation. In many biologic systems, estriol is a weak estrogen. Its potency is approximately 0.01 times of estradiol and 0.1 times of estrone on a weight basis. However, estriol is reported to be as effective as other estrogens in one function: its ability to increase uteroplacental blood flow. Therefore, this may be a primary function of a large amount of placental estriol. Its relatively weak estrogenic function on other organ systems may be beneficial to specifically increase urteroplacental blood flow. Although acute administration of estriol is ineffective as an estrogen and does not demonstrate extensive binding to estrogen receptors, prolonged exposure to estriol does produce estrogen effects and binding occurs. Estrogens exert their biological effect on blood flow by stimulating prostaglandin biosynthesis.[11]

Estradiol stimulates protein synthesis, cell proliferation in the endometrium, myometrium, and mammary gland. It is also involved in the regulation of vascular permeability and fluid balance. The increase in blood volume and extracellular fluid volume is mediated by estrogen. Fetus is also the target of placental estrogen and its growth and development are affected by estrogen.

Estrogens are also important for initiation of parturition at an appropriate time. Estrogen stimulates phospholipid synthesis and turnover, prostaglandin production and lysosome formation in the uterine endometrium, and modulates adrenergic mechanisms in uterine myometrium, thereby contributing to the onset of labor.[12]

Progesterone

Progesterone induces the secretory endometrium, which is required for implantation. Progesterone is also important in maintaining uterine quiescence during pregnancy by suppressing uterine smooth muscle contractility.[13] It also inhibits prostaglandin synthesis in the uterus.[14] Progesterone has also been proposed as an essential hormone of mammalian pregnancy because it inhibits T lymphocyte cell-mediated responses involved in tissue rejection.[15] In this theory, it is suggested that a high local (intrauterine) concentration of progesterone can effectively block cellular immune responses to foreign antigens. Therefore, progesterone has been aptly called the 'hormone of pregnancy' because it appears to be essential for maintenance of pregnancy in all mammals examined, and its presence has been detected in species representing all classes of vertebrates. The essential nature of progesterone for pregnancy maintenance has been demonstrated by experiments in which abortion was induced after the administration of drugs that either inhibit progesterone synthesis or compete with progesterone for receptor binding or the administration of progesterone antibodies. The specificity of the abortifacient effect was demonstrated by the concurrent administration of progesterone in some of those experiments.

Human chorionic gonadotropin

hCG is the earliest product of the cells that form the embryo, representing the first signal of the embryo even prior to implantation.[16] hCG is a glycoprotein of heterodimer with molecular weight of 36.7 kDa. It is composed of two subunits, a 92-amino acid α-subunit and a 145-amino acid β-subunit. The α-subunit is homologous to thyroid-stimulating hormone (THS), luteinizing hormone (LH), and follicle-stimulating hormone (FSH). The α-subunit gene is localized to chromosome 6. The β-subunit is similar to LH and the β-subunit gene is located on chromosome 19, fairly close to the LH-β gene. In contrast to LH, hCG contains sialic acid residues, which account for its half-life (24 h) being longer than that of LH (2 h).

Clinically, hCG can be detected in either the serum or urine 7–8 days after fertilization and is the earliest biochemical marker for pregnancy. Studies during *in vitro* fertilization cycle suggest that embryos expressed hCG mRNA as early as the eight-cell stage but that intact hCG was not present until 8 days after egg retrieval. The increase in hCG levels between days 5 and 9 after ovum collection is principally due to free β-hCG production, while by day 22 most of the circulating hCG is in the dimmer form. After implantation, hCG is produced principally by the syncytiotrophoblast layer of chorionic villi and is secreted into the intervillous space. Cytotrophoblasts also can produce hCG.

These observations are in accordance with the *in vitro* studies that suggest dimmer hCG synthesis is controlled in a two-phase manner through a supply of subunits. In contrast to LH secretion in the pituitary gland, hCG is secreted constitutively as subunits are available, and it is not stored in secretory granules as in the case of pituitary LH.[17] The immature syncytiotrophoblast produces free β-hCG subunit while the ability to produce the α-subunit by cytotrophoblast appears to lag by several days.[18] As the trophoblast matures, the ratio of α-subunit to β-subunit reaches a 1:1 ratio, and the hCG concentration reaches a peak value of 100,000 mIU/ml around 9–10 weeks of pregnancy. The placenta produces more α-subunits as gestation advances, and the ratio of α-subunit to hCG is approximately 10:1 at term.[19]

The doubling time of serum hCG levels during early gestation is approximately 30 h.[20] The hCG doubling time has been utilized as a clinical marker to differentiate normal from abnormal pregnancies such as ectopic pregnancy or spontaneous abortions. When vaginal ultrasonography cannot detect the intrauterine gestational sac even after the hCG levels reach 1100–1500 mIU/ml, an ectopic pregnancy is strongly suggested. On the other hand, higher hCG levels suggest the presence of molar pregnancy or multiple gestations.

The major biologic function of hCG during early pregnancy is to rescue the corpus luteum from its premature demise while maintaining progesterone production. Until the luteal-placental shift in progesterone synthesis occurs at the seventh week of pregnancy, hCG is required for rescue and maintenance of the corpus luteum. This is supported by the report that immunoneutralization of hCG results in early pregnancy failure.[21] In the explant experiment with first-trimester chorionic tissue, intermittent administration of gonadotropin-releasing hormone (GnRH) enhanced the pulsatile secretion of hCG from the explant tissue, implicating placental GnRH as a paracrine regulator of hCG secretion.[22] When pregnancy is not established, the corpus luteum is preprogrammed to undergo luteolysis. hCG also stimulates the production of estradiol, 17-hydroxyprogesterone and other peptides, such as relaxin and inhibin from corpus luteum.

Ovarian progesterone is essential for maintenance of early pregnancy. When progesterone action is blocked with a competitive progesterone antagonist, such as mifepristone (RU 486), pregnancy is terminated. Removal of corpus luteum before, but not after the seventh week of gestation resulted in subsequent abortion.[23,24] Removal of corpus luteum after the ninth week of pregnancy had little or no influence on the pregnancy. Thus, progesterone supplementation is required when corpus luteum function is compromised prior to the ninth to tenth weeks of pregnancy. During later pregnancy, progesterone production in the placenta is sufficient for the maintenance of pregnancy.

hCS, human placental lactogen (hPL)

hCS was initially isolated in 1962 as hPL.[25] hCS has structural similarity to both pituitary human growth hormone (hGH) and prolactin (PRL). hCS is composed of 191 amino acids with a molecular weight of approximately 22 kDa and contains two disulfide bonds. It shares up to 96% homology with hGH and 67% homology with PRL.[26,27] hCS and hGH genes locate on the same portion of chromosome 17, which consists of five genes, two coding for hGH and three coding for hCS.[28] hCS is produced only in the syncytiotrophoblast and at a constant rate throughout gestation.[29,30] Consequently, serum hCS concentration correlates well with placental mass and viability. At term, the placenta produces hCS approximately 1–4 g/day and maternal serum hCS levels range from 5 to 15 μg/ml.

Despite the large amount of production during pregnancy, the physiological function of hCS has not been fully clarified. hCS has been suggested to have a major metabolic effect on the mother to ensure that the nutritional demands of the fetus are met, functioning as a growth hormone of pregnancy.[31] During pregnancy, maternal plasma glucose levels are decreased, plasma free fatty acids (FFAs) are increased, and insulin secretion is increased with resistance to endogenous insulin as a consequence of the GH-like and contra-insulin effects of hCS. Peripheral glucose uptake is suppressed in the mother but it crosses the placenta freely by a facilitated diffusion mechanism. Amino acids are transported across the placenta by an active transport mechanism against the concentration gradient. Transplacental passage of fatty acids is slow. Consequently, when the mother is in the unfed or starved state, glucose should be reserved largely for the fetus and free fatty acids would be used preferentially by the mother. Insulin and other protein hormones do not cross the placenta.

Regulation of placental secretion of hCS is poorly understood. Factors that regulate pituitary GH secretion are not effective in placenta. Although hCS has structural homology to hGH and PRL, it does not have growth promoting or lactogenic activity in humans.[31] There are several case reports on the healthy newborn from hCS-deficient pregnancy.[32,33] Thus, it is possible that hCS is not essential for pregnancy but may serve as an evolutionary redundancy for pituitary GH and PRL. However, it remains to be clarified whether pregnancies without hCS production would have a good outcome even in the state of nutritional deprivation.

Other placental protein hormones

Chorionic ACTH

A protein similar to pituitary ACTH has been isolated from the placenta. ACTH, lipotropin, and β-endorphin are recovered from the placental extract, presumably from the same or similar 31-kDa precursor proopiomelanocortin (POMC).[34] It is also reported that ACTH is secreted from dispersed placental cells.[35] Dexamethasone treatment does not alter the production of ACTH in the placenta.

The physiological significance of placental ACTH is unclear. ACTH plasma levels during pregnancy are lower than in non-pregnant women; nonetheless, the concentration increases as gestation advances.[36] Placenta secretes ACTH into both maternal and fetal circulations, but it does not cross the placenta. The administration of dexamethasone to pregnant women does not suppress urinary free cortisol levels as effectively as it does in men or non-pregnant women. Corticotropin-releasing hormone stimulates the synthesis and release of ACTH from chorionic tissue *in vitro*.[37]

Parathyroid hormone-related protein (PTH-rP) and other protein hormones

PTH-rP is synthesized in various tissues including the pregnant uterus, myometrium, endometrium, and placenta. The rate of PTH secretion by the adult parathyroid is modulated by plasma Ca^{2+} concentration. PTH-rP secretion from the placenta is regulated by calcium concentration.[38]

Relaxin is also expressed in the human placenta.[39] Relaxin is synthesized as a single 105-amino acid preprorelaxin which is cleaved to form two chains A and B. Relaxin is structurally similar to insulin and nerve growth factors. Relaxin acts on myometrial smooth muscle to stimulate adenylate cyclase and to promote uterine relaxation.

The placenta produces chorionic thyrotropin, but its biological significance in normal human pregnancy is yet to be clarified.

Growth hormone-variant (hGH-V) is expressed in the placenta but not in the pituitary.[40] The gene is located in the growth hormone–prolactin gene cluster. The variant of hGH, sometimes referred to as placental growth hormone, is a 191-amino acid protein that differs in 15 amino acids from hGH. hGH-V is synthesized in the placenta, presumably in the syncytiotrophoblasts. hGH-V is present in the maternal plasma by 21–26 weeks of pregnancy, increases in concentration to about 36 weeks of pregnancy, and remains relatively constant thereafter. The maternal plasma levels of hGH-V correlate well with those of insulin-like growth factor-1. Secretion of hGH-V from trophoblast is inhibited by glucose in a dose-dependent manner.[41] The biological activity of hGH-V is similar to that of hCS.

Hypothalamic-like releasing hormones

Gonadotropin-releasing hormone (GnRH)

Placenta secretes a relatively large amount of GnRH.[42] GnRH is present only in the cytotrophoblast but not in the syncytiotrophoblast. Placental GnRH is suggested to act as an hCG-releasing hormone.[43] First-trimester chorionic tissue secretes hCG in response to GnRH much more than that of term placenta.[44] The receptor for GnRH is expressed in both cytotrophoblast and syncytiotrophoblast. Trophoblast secretes inhibin and activin and regulates GnRH production in a paracrine manner. Human placenta can also synthesize thyrotropin-releasing hormone (TRH) *in vitro*.[45,46]

Corticotropin-releasing hormone (CRH)

The same CRH gene expressed in hypothalamic tissues is also expressed in the trophoblast, amnion, chorion leave, and decidua. Plasma levels of CRH in non-pregnant women are 15 pg/ml. Maternal plasma CRH levels increase to 250 pg/ml at early third trimester, and to 1000 pg/ml abruptly during the last 5–6 weeks of pregnancy.[47] After onset of labor, maternal plasma CRH levels increase further about two- to threefold.[48] The biological function of uterine CRH including placental CRH is not clear yet. Receptors for CRH are present in many tissues including fetal adrenal, placenta, and myometrium. Only a very small amount of placental CRH can enter fetal circulation, suggesting a relatively insignificant role in fetal adrenal steroidogenesis. A large amount of CRH is secreted into maternal circulation; however, there is also a large amount of CRH-binding protein in maternal plasma. The bound form of CRH is biologically inactive and targeted for degradation. The possible biological function of placental CRH is the relaxation of both uterine and vascular smooth muscles and immunosuppression. The physiological reverse of CRH function, the induction of myometrial contraction (i.e. the initiation of parturition by CRH), has been proposed.[49] CRH increases prostaglandin synthesis in placenta, amnion, chorion leave, and decidua.[50] In the hypothalamus, glucocorticoids inhibit CRH release; however, in the trophoblast, glucocorticoids do stimulate the expression of the CRH gene, two- to threefold increases in CRH mRNA, and protein expression after treatment of human trophoblast in culture.[51] Thus, in the placenta, a positive feedback loop of CRH, ACTH, and glucocorticoids is proposed.[37]

Growth hormone-releasing hormone (GHRH)

The mRNA for GHRH has been identified in the human placenta.[52] The biological function of placental GHRH is not known.

Other placental peptide hormones

Neuropeptide Y (NPY)

NPY, a 36-amino acid peptide, is originally isolated in the brain. It also is present in sympathetic neurons innervating the cardiovascular, respiratory, gastrointestinal, and genitourinary systems. NPY is also expressed in the placenta and localized in cytotrophoblasts.[48] Receptors for NPY are also present in the placenta, which secrete CRH by stimulation with NPY.

Inhibin and activin

Inhibin is a glycoprotein hormone that acts on the pituitary and inhibits FSH release. Inhibin is a heterodimer with dissimilar α- and β-subunits. The inhibin β-subunit is composed of one of two distinct peptides, βA or βB. Activin is closely related to inhibin and is formed by the combination of two β-subunits. This peptide hormone is produced by various tissues including testis, granulosa cells of the ovary, and corpus luteum. The placenta can produce inhibin α-, βA-, and βB-subunits at the maximal rate at term.[53,54] Placental inhibin, in conjunction with a large amount of sex steroid hormones produced in the placenta, may serve to inhibit FSH secretion and thereby block ovulation during pregnancy. Serum activin levels decline rapidly after delivery.[55] Receptors for activin are present in the placenta and amnion. Inhibin may act via GnRH to regulate hCG production in the placenta.[53]

Natriuretic peptides

Atrial natriuretic peptide (ANP), a 28-amino acid peptide, is predominantly produced in the atrial myocytes, but is also produced in the placental trophoblast.[56] Brain natriuretic peptide (BNP), predominantly produced in the heart, is also secreted from amnion cells.[57] These natriuretic peptides induce natriuresis, diuresis, and relaxation of smooth muscle. The receptors for natriuretic peptides are also expressed

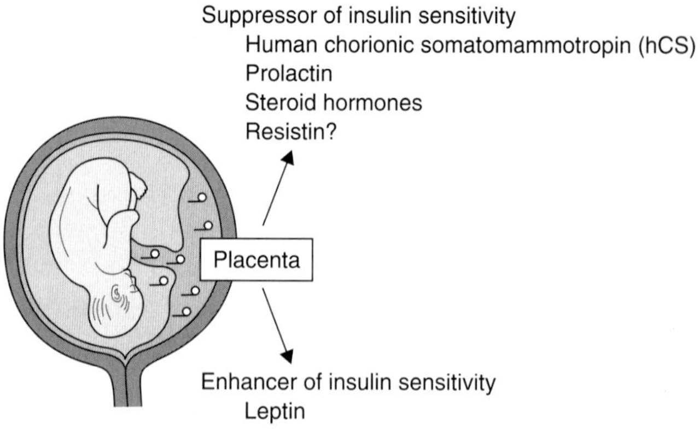

Figure 61.2 Regulation of maternal insulin sensitivity by placental hormones.

in the human placenta as well as in the myometrium, suggesting a possible role of ANP and BNP in uterine relaxation during pregnancy.[58]

Leptin

Maternal insulin sensitivity is regulated by various factors including placenta-derived hormones (Figure 62.2). Several placenta-derived hormones, such as prolactin, hCS or hPL, and steroid hormones, have been considered to decrease insulin sensitivity.[59] Placental production of these hormones is increased in accordance with the increasing size of the placenta. Recently, novel peptide hormones, leptin and resistin, originally identified as adipocytokines and regulating glucose and energy metabolism, have been reported to express in the human placenta.[60,61]

Leptin is initially identified as an adipocyte-derived hormone that decreases food intake and body weight via its receptor in the hypothalamus.[62] Subsequent animal studies revealed various physiological functions of leptin.[63,64] Leptin plays an essential role in reproduction by regulating GnRH secretion from the hypothalamus.[65,66] It also modulates glucose metabolism by increasing insulin sensitivity and activates the sympathetic nervous system.[67,68] In humans, leptin is also produced by placental trophoblasts and is secreted into both maternal and fetal circulations.[60] Leptin production in the placenta is increased in pregnancies complicated with several pathologic conditions.[69–71] Plasma leptin levels are significantly elevated in molar pregnancy.[69] Leptin gene expression in the placenta is augmented in severe pre-eclampsia, and maternal plasma leptin levels in severe pre-eclampsia are significantly higher than those in normotensive pregnant women.[70] Leptin production in the placenta is also increased in diabetic pregnancy with insulin treatment.[71] Leptin is also proposed to play a functional role in implantation by virtue of its stimulatory effect on matrix metalloproteinase expression in cytotrophoblast.[72]

Resistin

Resistin is a newly identified adipocyte-derived hormone that decreases insulin sensitivity and increases plasma glucose concentration, thus contributing to the development of type II diabetes mellitus.[73] Resistin is proposed to link obesity to insulin resistance.[74] Adipocyte secretes various substances that modulate insulin sensitivity, such as free fatty acid, TNF-α, and leptin. Resistin was recently cloned by Steppan *et al.*[73] as a substance whose expression in the adipose tissue decreases by treatment with thiazolidinedione, an antidiabetic drug. Thus, resistin is proposed to be a major factor that induces insulin resistance and hyperglycemia in obese persons.

Northern blot analysis revealed resistin mRNA expression in term placenta as well as in the amniotic membrane.[61] Resistin mRNA expression was also detected in a trophoblastic cell line (BeWo cells) and a very faint band was detected in decidua vera tissue. *In situ* hybridization and immunohistochemistry suggest the expression of resistin in placental villi, mainly in syncitiotrophoblast. Resistin protein was secreted from cultured placental tissue.[61] Resistin gene expression in term placental tissue was significantly larger than that in chorionic villous tissue in the first trimester. By contrast, the resistin gene was expressed to a lesser degree in adipose tissue than in term placental tissue. Moreover, resistin gene expression in the adipose tissue of pregnant women at term did not differ from that of non-pregnant women. As resistin is supposed to induce insulin resistance and increase the plasma glucose level,[73,74] it is possible that placental resistin may contribute to regulation of maternal glucose metabolism in concert with various placental hormones including leptin (Figure 62.2).

However, the regulatory mechanism of resistin gene expression in the human placenta is not yet elucidated. Further investigation on the effects of these hormones on the maternal glucose metabolism and insulin sensitivity may provide a better understanding of the placental role in maternal energy metabolism and fetal growth.

REFERENCES

1. Jaffe RB. Neroendocrine – metabolic regulation of pregnancy. In Yen SSC, Jaffe RB, and Barbieri RL, eds. *Reproductive Endocrinology – Physiology, Pathophysiology, and Clinical Management*, 4th edn. Philadelphia, PA: WB Saunders Company, 1999:751–84.
2. Carr BR, Parker CR Jr, Madden JD, MacDonald PC, Porter JC. Maternal plasma adrenocorticotropin and cortisol relationship throughout human pregnancy. *Am J Obstet Gynecol* 1981;139:416–21.
3. Pion R, Jaffe RB, Erickson G, *et al.* Studies on the metabolism of C-21 steroids in the human feto-placental unit: 1. Formation

of α,β-unsaturated 3-ketones in mid-term placentas perfused in situ with pregnenolone and 17a-hydroxypregnenolone. *Acta Endocrinol (Copenh)* 1965;48:234–41.

4. Johanson ENB. Plasma levels of progesterone in pregnancy measured by a rapid competitive protein binding technique. *Acta Endocrinol (Copenh)* 1979;61:607–15.
5. Frandsen VA, Stakeman G. The clinical significance of oestriol estimators in late pregnancy. *Acta Endocrinol (Copenh)* 1963;44: 183–91.
6. Schindler AE, Siiteri PK. Isolation and quantitation of steroids from normal human amniotic fluid. *J Clin Endocrinol Metab* 1968;28: 1189–95.
7. Goebelsmann U, Chen LC, Saga M, *et al.* Plasma concentration and protein binding of oestriol and its conjugates in pregnancy. *Acta Endocrinol (Copenh)* 1973;74:592–8.
8. Bradshaw KD, Carr BR. Placental sulfatase deficiency: Maternal and fetal expressions of steroid sulfatase deficiency and X-linked ichthyosis. *Obstet Gynecol Surv* 1986;68:505–9.
9. Simpson ER, NacDonald PC. Endocrine physiology of the placenta. *Ann Rev Physiol* 1981;43:163–85.
10. Liu JH and Rebar RW. Endocrinology of pregnancy. In Cresy RK, Resnik R, eds. *Maternal–Fetal Medicine*, 4th edn. Philadelphia, PA: WB Saunders Company, 1999:379–91.
11. Resnik R, Killam AP, Battablia FC, Makowski EL, Meshia G. Stimulation of uterine blood flow by various estrogens. *Endocrinology* 1974;94:1192–8.
12. Casey ML, Winkel CA, Porter JC, MacDonald PC. Endocrine regulation of the initiation and maintenance of parturition. *Clin Perinatol* 1983;10:709–25.
13. Roberts JM, Lewis VL, Riemer RK. Hormonal control of uterine adrenergic response. In Bottari J, Thomas P, Vokser A, Vokser R, eds. *Uterine Contractility*. New York: Masson, 1984:161–85.
14. Cane EM, Villee CA. The synthesis of prostaglandin F by human endometrium in organ culture. *Prostaglandins* 1975;281–90.
15. Siiteri PK, Ferbers F, Clemens LE, Chang RJ, Gondos B, Stites D. Progesterone and maintenance of pregnancy: Is progesterone nature's immunosuppression ? *Ann N Y Acad Sci* 1977;286: 384–98.
16. Hay DL, Lopata A. Chorionic gonadotropin secretion by human embryo in vitro. *J Clin Endocrinol Metab* 1988;67:1322–9.
17. Muyan M, Boime I. Secretion of chorionic gonadotropin from human trophoblast. *Placenta* 1997;18:237–43.
18. Hay DL. Discordant and variable production of human chorionic gonadotropin and its free alpha- and beta-subunits in early pregnancy. *J Clin Endocrinol Metab* 1985;61:1195–9.
19. Takemori M, Nishimura R, Ashitaka Y, Tojo S. Release of human chorionic gonadotropin (hCG) and its alpha-subunit (hCGa) from perifused human placenta. *Endocrinol Jpn* 1981;28:757–63.
20. Lenton EA, Woodward AJ. The endocrinology of conception cycles and implantation in women. *J Reprod Fertil* 1988;36(Suppl):1–12.
21. Stevens VG. Antifertility effects from immunization with intact subunits and fragments of hCG. In Edwards RG, Johnson MG, eds. *Physiological Effects of Immunity against Reproductive Hormones*. London: Cambridge University Press, 1975:249–64.
22. Barnea ER, Kaplan M, Naor Z. Comparative stimulatory effect of gonadotropin-releasing hormone (GnRH) and GnRH agonist upon pulsatile human chorionic gonadotropin secretion in superfused placental explants: Reversable inhibition by a GnRH antagonist. *Hum Reprod* 1991;6:1063–9.
23. Csapo AI, Pulkkinen MO, Wiest WG. Effect of luteectomy and progesterone replacemant therapy in early pregnant patients. *Am J Obstet Gynecol* 1973;115:756–62.
24. Csapo AI, Pulkkinen MO. Indispensability of the human corpus luteum in the maintenance of early pregnancy: Luteectomy evidence. *Obstet Gynecol Surv* 1978;33:69–75.
25. Josinovich JB, MacLaren JA. Presence in the human placenta and term serum of a highly lactogenic substance immunologically related to pituitary growth hormone. *Endocrinology* 1962;71:209–16.
26. Bewley TA, Dixon JS, Li CH. Sequence comparison of human pituitary growth hormone, human chorionic somatomammotropin, and ovine pituitary growth and lactogenic hormones. *Int J Pept Protein Res* 1972;4:281–9.
27. Cooke NE, Coit D, Shine J. Human prolactin cDNA structural analysis and evolutionary comparisons. *J Biol Chem* 1981;256: 4007–15.
28. Owerbach D, Rutter WJ, Martial JA. Genes for growth hormone chorionic somatomammotropin and growth hormone-like gene on chromosomes 17 in humans. *Science* 1980;209:289–95.
29. McWilliams D, Boime I. Cytological localization of placental lactogen messenger ribonucleic acid in syncytiotrophoblast layers of human placenta. *Endocrinology* 1980;107:761–9.
30. Hoshina M, Boothby M, Boime I. Cytological localization of chorionic gonadotropin a and placental lactogen mRNAs during development of the human placenta. *J Cell Biol* 1982;93:190–8.
31. Grumbach MM, Kaplan SL, Abrams CL, Bell JJ, Conte FA. Plasma free fatty acid response to the administration of chorionic 'growth hormone-prolactin'. *J Clin Endocrinol Metab* 1996;26:476–85.
32. Nielsen PV, Pedersen H, Kampmann EM. Absence of human placental lactogen in an otherwise uneventful pregnancy. *Am J Obstet Gynecol* 1984;135:322–54.
33. Parks JS, Nielsen PV, Sexton LA, Jorgensen EH. An effect of gene dosage on production of human chorionic somatomammotropin. *J Clin Endocrinol Metab* 1985;60:994–8.
34. Odagiri E, Sherrill BJ, Mount CD, Nicholson WE, Orth DN. Human placental immunoreactive corticotropin, lipotropin, and β-endorphin: Evidence for a common precursor. *Proc Natl Acad Sci USA* 1979;16:2027–35.
35. Liotta A, Osathanondh R, Ryan KJ, Krieger DT. Presence of corticotropin in human placenta: Demonstration of in vitro synthesis. *Endocrinology* 1977;101:1552–8.
36. Carr BR, Simpson ER. Cholesterol synthesis in human fetal tissues. *J Clin Endocrinol Metab* 1982;55:447–52.
37. Riley SC, Walton JC, Herlick JM, Challis IJG. The localization and distribution of corticotropin-releasing hormone in the human placenta and fetal membranes throughout gestation. *J Clin Endocrinol Metab* 1991;72:1001–8.
38. Hellman P, Ridefelt P, Juhlin C, Akerstrom G, Rastad J, Gylfe E. Parathyroid-like regulation of parathyroid hormone-related protein release and cytoplasmic calcium in cytotrophoblast cells of human placenta. *Arch Biochem Biophys* 1992;293:174–81.
39. Bogic LV, Mandel M, Bryant-Greenwood GD. Relaxin gene expression in human reproductive tissues by in situ hybridization. *J Clin Endocrinol Metab* 1995;80:130–9.
40. Cunningham FG, Gant NF, Leveno KJ, *et al.* The placental hormones. In *Williams Obstetrics*, 21st edn. New York: McGraw-Hill, 2001:chap 6, 109 28.
41. Patel N, Alsat E, Igout A, *et al.* Glucose inhibits human placenta GH secretion, in vitro. *J Clin Endocrinol Metab* 1995;80:1743–50.
42. Siler-Khodr TM. Chorionic peptides. In McNellis D, Challis JRG, MacDonald PC, Nathanielsz PW, Roberts JM, eds. *The Onset of Labor: Cellular and Integrative Mechanisms. An NICHD Workshop*. Ithaca: Perinatology Press, 1988:213–31.
43. Siler-Khodr TM. Hypothalamic-like peptides of the placenta. *Semin Reprod Endocrinol* 1983;1:321–40.
44. Currie WD, Steele GL. Luteinizing hormone-releasing hormone (LHRH) and LHRH-stimulated human chorionic gonadotropin secretion from perfused first trimester placental cells. *Recent Prog Horm Res* 1993;97:71–4.
45. Gibbons JM, Mitnick M, Chieffo V. In vitro biosynthesis of THS- and LH-releasing factors by human placenta. *Am J Obstet Gynecol* 1975;121:127–31.
46. Khodr GS, Siler-Khodr TM. Placental luteinizing hormone-releasing factor and its synthesis. *Science* 1980;207:315–20.
47. Goland RS, Wardlaw SL, Blum M, Tropper PJ, Stark RI. Biologically active corticotropin-releasing hormone in maternal and fetal plasma during pregnancy. *Am J Obstet Gynecol* 1988; 159:884–90.
48. Petraglia F, Calza L, Giardino L, *et al.* Identification of immunoreactive neuropeptide-(gamma) in human placenta: Localization, secretion, and binding sites. *Endocrinology* 1989;124:2016–20.
49. Wadhwa PD, Porto M, Garite TJ, Chcz-DeMet A, Sandman CA. Maternal corticotropin-releasing hormone levels in the early third trimester predict length of gestation in human pregnancy. *Am J Obstet Gynecol* 1998;179:1079–85.
50. Jones SA, Challis JRG. Local stimulation of prostaglandin production by corticotropin-releasing hormone in human fetal membranes and placenta. *Biochem Biophys Res Commun* 1989;159:192–9.
51. Robinson BG, Emanuel RL, Frim DM, Majzoub JA. Glucocorticoid stimulates expression of corticotropin-releasing hormone gene in human placenta. *Proc Natl Acad Sci USA* 1988;85:5244–50.
52. Berry SA, Srivastava CH, Rubin LR, Phipps WR, Pescovtz OH. Growth hormone releasing hormone-like messenger ribonucleic acid and immunoreactive peptide are present in human testis and placenta. *J Clin Endocrinol Metab* 1992;75:281–8.
53. Petraglia F, Sawchenko P, Lim AT, River J, Vale W. Localization, secretion, and action of inhibin in human placenta. *Science* 1987; 237:187–91.

54. Petraglia F, Garuti GC, Calza L, *et al.* Inhibin subunits in human placenta: Localization and messenger ribonucleic acid levels during pregnancy. *Am J Obstet Gynecol* 1991;165:750–55.
55. Petraglia F, Gallinelli A, De-Vita D, Lewis K, Mathews L, Vale W. Activin at parturition: Changes of maternal serum levels and evidence for binding sites in placenta and fetal membranes. *Obstet Gynecol* 1994;84:278–82.
56. Lim AT, Gude NM. Atrial natriuretic factor production by the human placenta. *J Clin Endocrinol Metab* 1995;80:3091–6.
57. Itoh H, Sagawa N, Hasegawa M, *et al.* Brain natriuretic peptide is present in the human amniotic fluid and is secreted from amnion cells. *J Clin Endocrinol Metab* 1993;76:907–11.
58. Itoh H, Sagawa N, Hasegawa M, *et al.* Expression of biologically active receptors for natriuretic peptides in the human uterus during pregnancy. *Biochem Biophys Res Commun* 1994;203:602–7.
59. Abrams B, Pickett KE. Maternal nutrition. In Creasy RK, Resnik R, eds. *Maternal–Fetal medicine*, 4th edn. Philadelphia, PA: WB Saunders Company, 1999:122–31.
60. Masuzaki H, Ogawa Y, Sagawa N, *et al.* Nonadipose tissue production of leptin: Leptin as a novel placenta-derived hormone in humans. *Nat Med* 1997;3:1029–33.
61. Yura S, Sagawa N, Itoh H, *et al.* Resistin is expressed in the human placenta. *J Clin Endocrinol Metab* 2003;88:1394–7.
62. Zhang Y, Proenca R, Maffei M, Barone M, Leopold L, Friedman JM. Positional cloning of the mouse *obese* gene and its human homologue. *Nature* 1994;372:425–32.
63. Campfield LA, Smith FJ, Guisez Y, Devos R, Burn P. Recombinant mouse OB protein: Evidence for a peripheral signal linking adiposity and central neural networks. *Science* 1995;269:546–9.
64. Halaas JL, Gajiwala KS, Maffei M, *et al.* Weight-reducing effects of the plasma protein encoded by the *obese* gene. *Science* 1995; 269:543–6.
65. Chehab FF, Lim ME, Lu R. Correction of the sterility defect in homozygous obese female mice by treatment with the human recombinant leptin. *Nat Genet* 1996;12:318–20.
66. Yura S, Ogawa Y, Sagawa N, *et al.* Accelerated puberty and late onset hypothalamic hypogonadism in female transgenic skinny mice overexpressing leptin. *J Clin Invest* 2000;105:749–55.
67. Ogawa Y, Masuzaki H, Hosoda K, *et al.* Increased glucose metabolism and insulin sensitivity in transgenic skinny mice overexpressing leptin. *Diabetes* 1999;48:1822–9.
68. Shek EW, Brands MW, Hall JE. Chronic leptin infusion increases arterial pressure. *Hypertension* 1998;31(Pt 2):409–14.
69. Sagawa N, Mori T, Masuzaki H, Ogawa Y, Nakao K. Leptin production by hydatidiform mole. *Lancet* 1997;350:1518–9.
70. Mise H, Sagawa N, Matsumoto T, *et al.* Augmented placental production of leptin in preeclampsia: Possible involvement of placental hypoxia. *J Clin Endocrinol Metab* 1998;83:3225–9.
71. Lepercq J, Cauzac M, Lahlou N, *et al.* Overexpression of placental leptin in diabetic pregnancy – A critical role for insulin. *Diabetes* 1998;47:847–50.
72. Castellucci M, Matteis R, Meisser A, *et al.* Leptin modulates extracellular matrix molecules and metalloproteinases: Possible implications for trophoblast invasion. *Mol Hum Reprod* 2000;6:951–8.
73. Steppan CM, Bailey ST, Bhat S, *et al.* The hormone resistin links obesity to diabetes. *Nature* 2001;409:307–12.
74. Flier JS. The missing link with obesity? *Nature* 2001;409:292–3.

62 Regulation of extravillous trophoblast differentiation

K. Fukushima, K. Tsukimori and H. Nakano

During early development, cytotrophoblast (CT) differentiation contributes to the organization of the feto–maternal interface. One layer of the differentiated trophoblast, which is marked by an invasive phenotype, is called extravillous trophoblast (EVT). EVT invades decidual tissue and the maternal uterine wall. Recent evidence shows that EVT invasion has a crucial role in organizing and maintaining feto-placental circulation. In this chapter, we focus on interstitial and endovascular invasion and their regulatory mechanisms during EVT differentiation.

Differentiation of CT

During the early phase of human pregnancy, CT cells are derived from trophectodermal cells of the blastocyst and contribute to organization of the feto–maternal interface through cell proliferation and differentiation. Differentiation of CT proceeds by two pathways that result in morphologically and functionally distinct trophoblast populations (Figure 62.1). One population consists of multinucleated, non-replicating syncytiotrophoblast cells (ST), beneath which lie immature, replicating, mononuclear villous CT. After the blastocyst attaches to the endometrium, mononuclear CT cells that surround the embryonic disk fuse to ST to form a syncytial layer. This layer covers the intravillous space and transports nutrients, wastes, and gases between fetal and maternal blood.[1]

The other population is the EVT, and these cells have invasive properties. EVT cells leave the cellular column to intrude into the decidua and uterine wall, and they are observed as cytokeratin-positive cells in the decidua, the intima of the spiral arteries, and the proximal third of the myometrium. It is thought that interstitial invasion of the placental bed by EVT promotes placental anchorage. Interstitial invasion is accompanied by endovascular invasion, in which some invading EVT cells interact, resulting in replacement of endothelium and the muscular tunica of maternal vessels, including the spiral arteries. This replacement substantially decreases vascular resistance and results in increased blood flow toward the intervillous space.[2,3]

Alteration of adhesion molecules during interstitial invasion

Examination of tissue sections of human placental bed biopsies shows that EVT cells switch integrin phenotype during differentiation and invasion.[4] The CT stem cells, which are anchored to the basement membrane, express α6b4 integrin. Formation of the cell column is accompanied by $\alpha5\beta1$ up-regulation, and as EVT cells intrude into the uterine wall they express the $\alpha1\beta1$ subunit as well as the $\alpha5\beta1$ subunit. Generally, α6b4 staining is weak and discontinuous at the uterine wall.[4] During this normal trophoblast invasion, the extracellular matrix (ECM) undergoes a transition from laminin (Ln) to fibronectin (Fn) and collagen type IV (C4). Ln is abundant in the superficial areas that face the villous trophoblast. In contrast, C4 and Fn are more abundant at deeper sites.[4,5] Thus, it can be assumed that EVT cells alter their integrin expression in parallel with the variation in ECM distribution during invasion. Not only integrin adhesion receptors, but also E-cadherin expression are altered during the invasive pathway.[6] Expression of E-cadherin, the cell–cell adhesion molecule, is strong in CT stem cells and weak in differentiating and invading EVT cells.[7] These findings are summarized in Figure 62.2.[7,8]

EVT invasion is a biochemically active process because invading cells have to secrete proteases including serine protease, cathepsin, and metalloproteinases. Matrix metalloproteinases (MMPs) have 15 family members that are classified by substrates and structured into four subgroups. The MMPs are inactivated by tissue inhibitor of metalloproteinases (TIMP). The TIMP family consists of four members: TIMP-1, -2, -3, and -4. Among all of these enzymes,

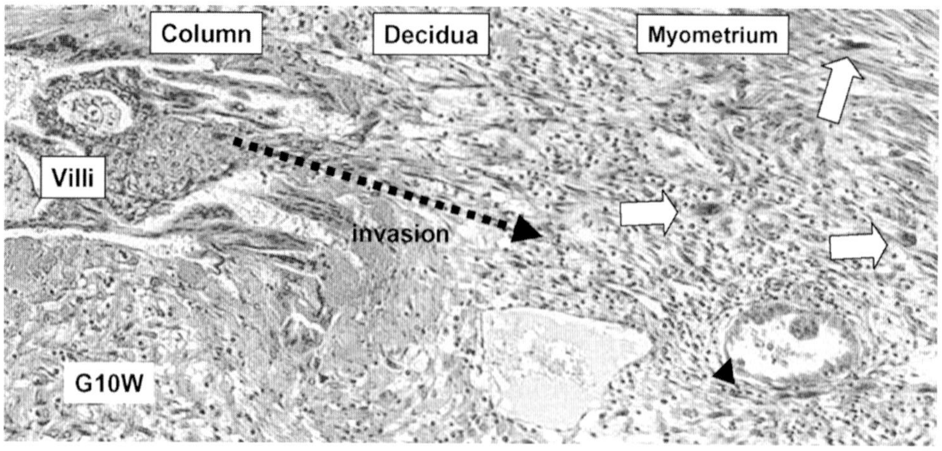

Figure 62.1 Microscopic appearance of extravillous trophoblast in placenta in early gestation during invasion. H&E stained placental tissue from patients with cervical cancer who underwent radical hysterectomy at 10 weeks of gestation. Arrow, invaded extravillous trophoblast; arrow head, maternal vessel replaced by trophoblast.

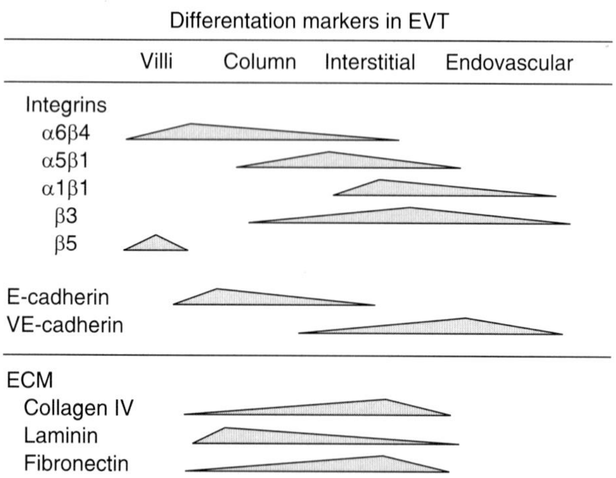

Figure 62.2 Alteration of adhesion molecules expressed in EVT during invasion. Scheme of the alteration of integrin and cadherin expression and distribution of extracellular matrix at each placental site during invasion. Modified from Zhou *et al.*[8,16]

MMP-2 and MMP-9 are considered to be the most important for EVT invasion.[9,10] Several pieces of evidence have shown that ECM and integrin can affect the activity of MMPs and behavior of EVT cells.[11,12] MMP-9 is up-regulated at deeper sites as in the case of integrin $\alpha1\beta1$.[13] Damsky *et al.*[5] investigated the effect of integrin–ECM interaction on EVT invasive properties using antibody inhibition to matrigel invasion assay. Antibodies against Ln and C4 blocked EVT invasion. The anti-$\alpha6$ antibody did not inhibit EVT invasion, whereas anti-$\beta1$ antibody did inhibit invasion. When combined, these antibodies acted synergistically. In contrast, anti-Fn antibodies stimulated rather than blocked invasion. Thus, the EVT–ECM interaction that subsequently arouses integrin conversion seems to be important in controlling EVT phenotype.

The significance of normal placentation of CT differentiation is highlighted by the fact that in pre-eclampsia, in which both interstitial and endovascular invasion are abnormally shallow, CT cells show significant defects in differentiation.[8,13–15] Furthermore, CT cells in women with pre-eclampsia increase expression of the $\alpha5\beta1$ subunit, but fail to both up-regulate $\alpha1\beta1$ and down-regulate α6b4.[5,15] Thus, the cells appear arrested in their differentiation and express an ECM receptor phenotype that may not be optimal for invasion.[16] Taking all these findings together, it is likely that expression of these integrin subunits is involved in the regulation of normal EVT differentiation.

Alteration of adhesion molecules during endovascular invasion

Angiogenesis plays a crucial role in both normal physiological and pathological conditions including placental development. During invasion, EVT finally replaces the endothelial cells in uterine vessels. Moreover, EVT cells also intrude into the vascular muscles. This endovascular differentiation induces remodeling of spiral arteries to increase blood flow toward the intervillous space, which is covered by ST, the other form of differentiated CT. As in the case of interstitial invasion, integrin subunits expressed in EVT dramatically change. Along with endovascular differentiation, the adhesion molecule repertories change in a comprehensive manner that mimics the pattern for endothelial cells.[16] Zhou *et al.*[16] reported that EVT *in vivo* showed reduced staining for adhesion receptors characteristic of stable monolayer epithelial cells and showed enhanced staining for adhesion molecules characteristic of endothelial cells. CT in cell columns show reduced E-cadherin staining and express VE-cadherin, PECAM-1, VCAM-1, and α4-integrins. EVT cells in the uterine interstitium and maternal vessels start to express $\alpha V\beta 3$ integrin. These molecules ($\alpha V\beta 3$ and VE-cadherin) enhance CT invasiveness.[16] In a later report, Zhou *et al.* showed that pre-eclamptic CT does not stain for most of the endothelial-type adhesion molecules that are expressed by control CT cells.[17] Inhibitors of $\alpha V\beta 3$ or $\alpha V\beta 5$ show anti-angiogenic activity in many models.[18] Indeed, a humanized version of LM609, a monoclonal antibody that blocks $\alpha V\beta 3$ signaling, has entered clinical trials for use in treatment.[19] Although genetic studies in mice have provided several controversial points, it is believed that these integrins play an important role in angiogenesis.[20] Thus, these endothelial-cell-related molecules are considered to play an important role in endovascular differentiation in EVT.

The vascular endothelial growth factor (VEGF) family members and their receptors (VEGFR) seem to have important actions during the initial stages of angiogenesis.[21] EVT cells in early gestation express VEGF-A, VEGF-C, placental growth factor (PlGF), VEGFR-1, and VEGFR-3. When binding of VEGF-A, PlGF, and VEGF–PlGF heterodimer to VEGFR-1 is inhibited, tube-like formation on matrigel is impaired and expression of integrin $\alpha 1\beta 1$ is decreased. This effect is enhanced when VEGF-C binding to endogenous VEGFR-3 is blocked. This result suggests that the signal from VEGFR1/3 is involved in the alteration of integrin switching. The same research group also reported that CT responds to VEGF ligands by the autocrine system.[22] Dunk *et al.*[23] reported that angiopoietin 1 and angiopoietin 2 can act as a mitogen and stimulate nitric oxide release from first trimester trophoblast, as well as VEGF.[23–26] These angiogenic factors also influence the angiogenic state of maternal blood vessels.[27]

Effect of cytokines and growth factor on EVT invasion (Table 62.1)

Interleukins

Interleukin-1 (IL-1) increases MMP-9 secretion and stimulates MMP-9 activities.[28,29] IL-1 or its receptors are important for implantation of the blastocyst.[30] Thus, IL-1 is a positive regulator of trophoblast differentiation along the invasive pathway.[31] IL-6 activates MMP-2 and MMP-9 in trophoblasts.[32] Circulating levels of IL-6 are increased in patients with pre-eclampsia.[33,34] IL-10 down-regulates MMP-9 activity and EVT invasiveness. IL-15 increases ETV invasion and migration, as well as MMP-1 production by Jeg-3 cells.[35] IL-10 and IL-15 seem to regulate trophoblast invasiveness by autocrine mechanisms.[35–37] Wang *et al.* reported lower levels of expression of IL-8 and IL-15 in pre-eclamptic placentas.[38]

Transforming growth factor

Transforming growth factor beta (TGFβ) stimulates the synthesis of matrix glycoproteins[39] and TIMP secretion through down-regulation of urokinase, plasmin, and plasminogen activator.[40–42] TGFβ inhibits cellular proliferation and migration,[37,43,44] whereas TGFα promotes EVT differentiation through the invasive pathway.[42]

Tumor necrosis factor alpha (TNFα)

TNFα levels are elevated in patients with pre-eclampsia,[45,46] and TNFα has been shown to regulate progesterone, estradiol, and human chorionic gonadotropin (hCG) production in CTs.[47] TNFα stimulates trophoblastic MMP-9, MMP-1, and MMP-3 production in human chorionic cells,[48] whereas TNFα decreases TIMP secretion.[32,49] TNFα induces apoptosis,[50] integrin subunit conversion, and functional activation in EVT cell lines.[51]

Insulin-like growth factors and relatives

Insulin-like growth factor (IGF)-II promotes trophoblast differentiation along the invasive pathway. Hamilton *et al.*[52] showed that IGF-II promotes cell migration. IGFBP-1 increases trophoblast cell migration,[42] invasion,[52] TIMP-1 secretion, and gelatinolytic activity.[53]

Other soluble factors

Leukemia inhibitory factor (LIF) is important for implantation of the blastocyst.[30] LIF inhibits the gelatinolytic activity of trophoblasts bearing an Ln receptor.[54]

TNF, VEGF, and ECM as collaborative regulators in EVT differentiation

As discussed above, many growth factors and cytokines have been shown to have an ability to produce certain effects on trophoblast function; however, the mechanism to regulate integrin subunit conversion has been unclear. Fukushima *et al.*[51] reported that TNFα suppressed α6 integrin expression and enhanced α1 integrin expression in a dose-dependent manner in a human EVT cell line; TNFα also induced apoptosis, which is suppressed by signals via integrin β1, with aggregation also induced by TNFα (Figure 62.3). Because integrins comprise a large family of cell surface receptors that recognize a variety of ECM components,[55] these results suggest that TNFα and ECM might collaboratively regulate EVT differentiation through integrin signaling (Figure 62.4). EVT cells alter their integrin expression in parallel with varied ECM distribution during invasion.[4,5] Thus, it has been

Table 62.1 Summary of biological effects of soluble factors on cytotrophoblast

	Biological effect on cytotrophoblast (and/or EVT)	References
IL-1	Promotes invasion	Lala and Lysiak,[31] Librach *et al.*[29]
	Increases MMP9 secretion	Meisser *et al.*[28]
	Promotes differentiation in invasive pathway	
IL-6	Increases circulating level in pre-eclamptic patients	Conrad and Benyo,[33] Conrad *et al.*[34]
	Activates MMP2 and 9	Meisser *et al.*[32]
IL-8	Lower level of expression in pre-eclamptic placenta	Wang *et al.*[38]
IL-10	Inhibits invasion	Roth *et al.*,[36] Roth and Fisher[37]
IL-15	Lower level of expression in pre-eclamptic placenta	Wang *et al.*[38]
	Increases invasiveness	Zygmunt[35]
TNF	Progesterone, hCG, estradiol synthesis	Li *et al.*[47]
	Stimulates MMP1, 3, 9, decrease TIMP	So *et al.*,[48] Takahashi *et al.*,[49] Meisser *et al.*[32]
	Induces integrin subunit conversion	Fukushima *et al.*[51]
	Induces apoptosis	Levy and Nelson[50]
	Elevates circulating level and expression in pre-eclamptic patients and placenta	Hamai *et al.*,[45] Rinehart *et al.*[46]
TGFβ	Stimulates matrix glycoproteins	Feinberg *et al.*[39]
	Inhibits cellular proliferation and migration	Graham *et al.*,[43] Khoo *et al.*,[44] Roth and Fisher[37]
	Stimulates TIMP secretion by down-regulation of urokinase, plasmin, plasminogen activator	Graham and Lala,[40] Graham *et al.*,[41] Irving and Lala[42]
TGFα	Promotes differentiation	Irving and Lala[42]
LIF	Inhibits gelatinolytic activity	Bischof *et al.*[54]
IGF2	Stimulates differentiation and migration	Irving and Lala[42]
IGFBP1	Increases cell migration, invasion, TIMP-1 secretion and gelatinolytic activity	Irving and Lala,[42] Hamilton *et al.*,[52] Bischof *et al.*[53]
VEGF	Increases proliferation and NO release	Charnock-Jones *et al.*,[18] Athanassiades *et al.*,[25] Ahmed *et al.*[26]
	Involves in tube-like formation in matrigel (VEGFR)	Zhou *et al.*[22]
Ang2	Increases proliferation and NO release	Dunk *et al.*[23]

IL, interleukin; TNF, tumor necrosis factor; TGF, transforming growth factor; LIF, leukemia inhibitory factor; IGF, insulin-like growth factor; IGFBP, IGF binding protein; VEGF, vascular endothelial growth factor; Ang, angiopoietin.

suggested that the alteration of integrin expression during differentiation of EVT may be responsible for mediating distinct signals to EVT upon adhesion to ECM. In other words, ECM regulates EVT differentiation; however, at the same time, this is an adaptation for EVT.

We should note physiological microenvironments surrounding EVT during early pregnancy. Hypoxia and oxidative stress caused by hypoperfusion and transient ischemia affect cytokine production.[56–58] Placental VEGF expression is up-regulated by hypoxia.[59] Hypoxia also induces proinflammatory cytokines including TNFα.[60] TNFα plays a pivotal role in pregnancy[61] and seems to be necessary for fetal development because it is expressed in normal tissues of a wide range of organs in the human fetus.[62] Zhou *et al.*[22] suggested that the signal from VEGF–VEGFR is involved in the alteration of integrin switching. We have found that TNFα and VEGF induce integrin $\alpha V\beta3$ expression and aggregation in an immortalized human EVT cell line.[63] It might be assumed that signals via $\alpha V\beta3$ integrin receptor and VEGFR are involved in endovascular differentiation. TNFα induces expression of VEGF in several kinds of cells.[64,65] Thus, there could be sequential and synergistic effects between TNFα and VEGF together with ECM in the physiological regulation of EVT differentiation. This hypothesis might explain biological communication between the maternal microenvironment and fetal trophoblast. As an immunological defending response, maternal cells secrete TNFα. Although some trophoblast cells are eliminated by apoptosis, at the same time, ECM could act as a survival factor for trophoblast cells through

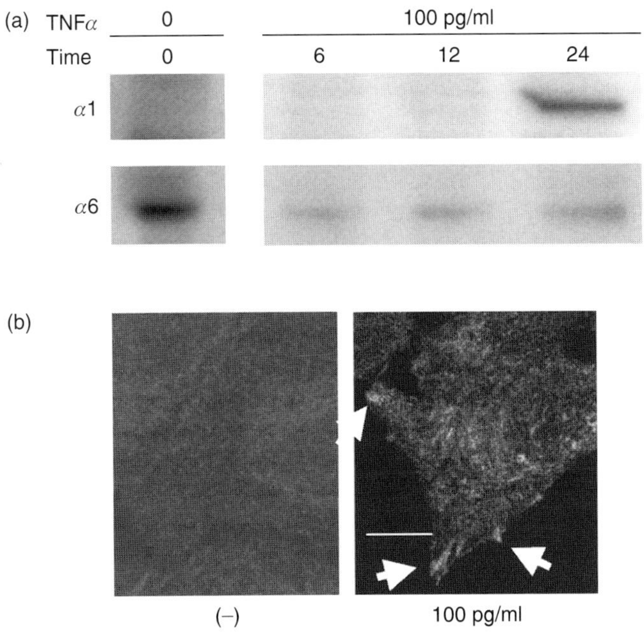

Figure 62.3 TNF induces integrin subunit switching in TCL1 cells. (a) Immunoblot analysis using anti-1 and -6 integrin subunits. TCL1 cells were seeded and grown at 37°C. After 1 day of incubation, the medium was replaced with fresh, complete medium containing 10% fetal calf serum and 20 or 100 pg/ml TNF for the indicated times. Cellular proteins were extracted and then analyzed by immunoblotting. Reproduced from Ref. 51. (b) TNF strengthens integrin adhesive functions. TCL1 cells were seeded on collagen type I-coated coverslips. The cells were incubated with or without 100 pg/ml TNF for 24 h. Cells were then fixed and stained with an anti-1 integrin subunit monoclonal antibody. The white arrows indicate integrin 1 subunit aggregation. Reproduced from Fukushima *et al.*[51]

integrin signaling if they can successfully convert phenotype. TNFα also enhances the formation of a number of endothelial cell molecules.[66] If excessive hypoxia and/or inflammation develop, such regulation might be impaired with induction or failure of both cellular survival and EVT differentiation. Indeed, when cultured under hypoxic conditions, CT cells fail to differentiate.[67]

In this chapter, we have presented research findings along with EVT invasion, which has been implicated as one of the 'key phenomena' in the normal placentation and hypothec paradigm. TNFα together with VEGF-systems might be key players in this differentiation adaptation with ECM. Of course, there have been suggestions that many other soluble factors could be involved in the regulation of trophoblast phenotype, and there are probably other key molecules that are essential for invasive phenotype, e.g. regulation of MMP secretion and activity. It is necessary to take into account cross talk among these molecules in the course of a normal pregnancy. Much more data are needed in order to integrate the current pieces of research evidence for this very interesting field.

Acknowledgment

This work was supported in part by a grant-in-aid from the Ministry of Education, Japan (16790609), Kanzawa Medical Research Foundation, and Inamori Foundation.

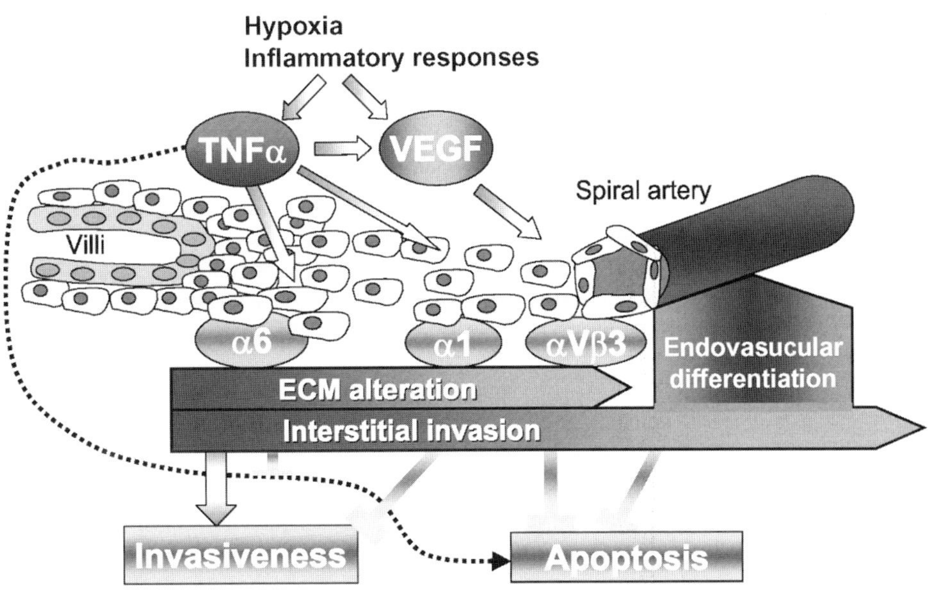

Figure 62.4 A hypothetical paradigm for TNF/VEGF/ECM collaboration during EVT differentiation. See text for details. ECM, extracellular matrix.

REFERENCES

1. Vicovac L, Aplin JD. Epithelial–mesenchymal transition during trophoblast differentiation. *Acta Anat* 1996;156:202–16.
2. Brosens IA, Robertson WB, Dixon HG. The role of spiral arteries in the pathogenesis of preeclampsia. *Obstet Gynecol Annu* 1972; 1:177–91.
3. Robertson WB, Brosens IA, Dixon HG. Placental bed vessels. *Am J Obstet Gynecol* 1973;117:294–5.
4. Damsky CH, Fitzgerald ML, Fisher SJ. Distribution patterns of extracellular matrix components and adhesion receptors are intricately modulated during first trimester cytotrophoblast differentiation along the invasive pathway, in vivo. *J Clin Invest* 1992;89: 210–22.
5. Damsky CH, Librach C, Lim KH, *et al.* Integrin switching regulates normal trophoblast invasion. *Development* 1994;120:3657–66.
6. Damsky CH, Sutherland AE, Fisher SJ. Adhesive interactions in early mammalian embryogenesis, implantation, and placentation. *FASEB J* 1993;7:1320–9.
7. Fisher SJ, Cui T-Y, Zhang L, *et al.* Adhesive and invasive interactions of human cytotrophoblast cells in vitro. *J Cell Biol* 1989; 109:891–902.
8. Zhou Y, Damsky CH, Fisher SJ. Preeclampsia is associated with abnormal expression of adhesion molecules by invasive cytotrophoblast cells. *J Clin Invest* 1993;91:950–60.
9. Bischof P, Meisser A, Campana A. Involvement of trophoblast in embryo implantation: Regulation by paracrine factors. *J Reprod Immunol* 1998;39(1–2):167–77.
10. Bischof P, Meisser A, Campana A. Paracrine and autocrine regulators of trophoblast invasion – A review. *Placenta* 2000;21:S55–60.
11. Werb Z, Tremble PM, Behrendtsen O, Crowley E, Damsky CH. Signal transduction through the fibronectin receptor induces collagenases and stromelysin gene expression. *J Cell Biol* 1989; 109:877–89.
12. Kliman HJ, Feinberg RF. Human trophoblast – extracellular matrix (ECM) interactions in vitro. ECM thickness modulates morphology and proteolytic activity. *Proc Natl Acad Sci USA* 1990;87:3057–61.
13. Lim KH, Zhou Y, Janatpour M, *et al.* Human cytotrophoblast differentiation/invasion is abnormal in pre-eclampsia. *Am J Pathol* 1997;151(6):1809–18.
14. Genbacev O, DiFederico E, McMaster M, Fisher SJ. Invasive cytotrophoblast apoptosis in preeclampsia. *Hum Reprod* 1999;14: 56–66.
15. Redline RW, Patterson P. Preeclampsia is associated with an excess of proliferative immature intermediate trophoblasts. *Hum Pathol* 1995;26:594–600.
16. Zhou Y, Fisher SJ, Janatpour M, *et al.* Human cytotrophoblasts adopt a vascular phenotype as they differentiate. A strategy for successful endovascular invasion? *J Clin Invest* 1997;99:2139–51.
17. Zhou Y, Damsky CH, Fisher SJ. Preeclampsia is associated with failure of human cytotrophoblasts to mimic a vascular adhesion phenotype. One cause of defective endovascular invasion in this syndrome? *J Clin Invest* 1997;99:2152–64.
18. Charnock-Jones DS, Sharkey AM, Boocock CA, *et al.* Localization and activation of the receptor for vascular endothelial growth factor on human trophoblast and choriocarcinoma cells. *Biol Reprod* 1994;51:524–30.
19. Vuckovic M, Ponting J, Terman BI, Niketic V, Seif MW, Kumar S. Expression of vascular endothelial growth factor receptor, KDR, in human placenta. *J Anat* 1996;188:361–6.
20. Hynes RO. A reevaluation of integrins as regulators of angiogenesis. *Nat Med* 2002;8:918–21.
21. Shibuya M. Structure and function of VEGF/VEGF-receptor system involved in angiogenesis. *Cell Struct Funct* 2001;26:25–35.
22. Zhou Y, McMaster M, Woo K, *et al.* Vascular endothelial growth factor ligands and receptors that regulate human cytotrophoblast survival are dysregulated in severe preeclampsia and hemolysis, elevated liver enzymes, and low platelets syndrome. *Am J Pathol* 2002;160:1405–23.
23. Dunk C, Shams M, Nijjar S, *et al.* Angiopoietin-1 and angiopoietin-2 activate trophoblast Tie-2 to promote growth and migration during placental development. *Am J Pathol* 2000;156:2185–99.
24. Charnock-Jones DS, Sharkey AM, Boocock CA, *et al.* Localisation and activation of the receptor for vascular endothelial growth factor on human trophoblast and choriocarcinoma cells. *Biol Reprod* 1994;51:524–30.
25. Athanassiades A, Hamilton GS, Lala PK. Role of vascular endothelial growth factor (VEGF) in human extravillous trophoblast proliferation, migration and invasiveness. *Placenta* 1998;19:465–73.
26. Ahmed A, Dunk CE, Kniss D, Wilkes M. Role of VEGF receptor (Flt-1) in mediating calcium dependent nitric oxide release and limiting DNA synthesis in human trophoblast cells. *Lab Invest* 1997;76:779–91.
27. Zhou Y, Bellingard V, Feng KT, McMaster M, Fisher SJ. Human cytotrophoblasts promote endothelial survival and vascular remodeling through secretion of Ang2, PlGF, and VEGF-C. *Dev Biol* 2003;263(1):114–25.
28. Meisser A, Chardonnens D, Campana A, Bischof P. Effects of tumour necrosis factor alpha, interleukin-1 alpha, macrophage colony stimulating factor and transforming growth factor beta on trophoblastic matrix metalloproteinases. *Mol Hum Reprod* 1999; 5:252–60.
29. Librach CL, Feigenbaum SL, Bass KE, *et al.* Interleukin-1 beta regulates human cytotrophoblast metalloproteinase activity and invasion in vitro. *J Biol Chem* 1994;269:17125–31.
30. Simon C, Frances A, Lee BY, *et al.* Immunohistochemical localization, identification and regulation of the interleukin-1 receptor antagonist in the human endometrium. *Hum Reprod* 1995;10: 2472–7.
31. Lala P, Lysiak J. Role of locally produced growth factors in human placental growth and invasion with special reference to transforming growth factors. New York: Springer-Verlag, 1994.
32. Meisser A, Cameo P, Islami D, Campana A, Bischof P. Effects of interleukin-6 (IL-6) on cytotrophoblastic cells. *Mol Hum Reprod* 1999;5:1055–8.
33. Conrad KP, Benyo DF. Placental cytokines and the pathogenesis of preeclampsia. *Am J Reprod Immunol* 1997;37:240–9.
34. Conrad KP, Miles TM, Benyo DF. Circulating levels of immunoreactive cytokines in women with preeclampsia. *Am J Reprod Immunol* 1998;40:102–11.
35. Zygmunt M, Hahn D, Kiesenbauer N, Munstedt K, Lang U. Invasion of cytotrophoblastic (Jeg-3) cells is up-regulated by interleukin-15 in vitro. *Am J Reprod Immunol* 1998;40:326–31.
36. Roth I, Corry DB, Locksley RM, Abrams JS, Litton MJ, Fisher SJ. Human placental cytotrophoblasts produce the immunosuppressive cytokine interleukin 10. *J Exp Med* 1996;184:539–48.
37. Roth I, Fisher SJ. IL-10 is an autocrine inhibitor of human placental cytotrophoblast MMP-9 production and invasion. *Dev Biol* 1999; 205:194–204.
38. Wang Y, Baier J, Adair CD, *et al.* Interleukin-8 stimulates placental prostacyclin production in preeclampsia. *Am J Reprod Immunol* 1999;42:375–80.
39. Feinberg RF, Kliman HJ, Wang CL. Transforming growth factor beta stimulates trophoblast oncofetal fibronectin synthesis in vitro: Implications for trophoblast implantation in vivo. *J Clin Endocrinol Metab* 1994;78:1241–8.
40. Graham CH, Lala PK. Mechanism of control of trophoblast invasion in situ. *J Cell Physiol* 1991;148:228–34.
41. Graham CH, Connelly I, MacDougall JR, Kerbel RS, Stetler-Stevenson WG, Lala PK. Resistance of malignant trophoblast cells to both the anti-proliferative and anti-invasive effects of transforming growth factor beta. *Exp Cell Res* 1994;214:93–9.
42. Irving JA, Lala PK. Functional role of cell surface integrins on human trophoblast cell migration: Regulation by TGF beta, IGF-II, and IGFBP-1. *Exp Cell Res* 1995;217:419–27.
43. Graham CH, Lysiak JJ, McCrae KR, Lala PK. Localization of transforming growth factor-beta at the human fetal–maternal interface: Role in trophoblast growth and differentiation. *Biol Reprod* 1992;46:561–72.
44. Khoo NK, Zhang Y, Bechberger JF, Bond SL, Hum K, Lala PK. SV40 Tag transformation of the normal invasive trophoblast results in a premalignant phenotype. II. Changes in gap junctional intercellular communication. *Int J Cancer* 1998;77:440–8.
45. Hamai Y, Fujii T, Yamashita T, *et al.* Evidence for an elevation in serum interleukin 2 and tumor necrosis factor levels before the clinical manifestations of preeclampsia. *Am J Reprod Immunol* 1997;38:89–93.
46. Rinehart BK, Terrone DA, Lagoo-Deenadayalan S, *et al.* Expression of the placental cytokines tumor necrosis factor , interleukin 1 and interleukin 10 is increased in preeclampsia. *Am J Obstet Gynecol* 1999;181:915–20.

47. Li Y, Matsuzaki N, Masuhiro K, *et al.* Trophoblast-derived tumor necrosis factor-alpha induces release of human chorionic gonadotropin using interleukin-6 (IL-6) and IL-6-receptor-dependent system in the normal human trophoblasts. *J Clin Endocrinol Metab* 1992;74:184–91.
48. So T, Ito A, Sato T, Mori Y, Hirakawa S. Tumour necrosis factor stimulates the biosynthesis of matrix metalloproteinases and plasminogen activator in cultured human chorionic cells. *Biol Reprod* 1992;46:772–8.
49. Takahashi S, Sato T, Ito A, *et al.* Involvement of protein kinase C in the interleukin 1 alpha induced gene expression of matrix metalloproteinases and tissue inhibitor 1 of metalloproteinases (TIMP-1) in human uterine cervical fibroblasts. *Biochim Biophys Acta* 1993;57–65.
50. Levy R, Nelson DM. To be, or not to be, that is the question. Apoptosis in human trophoblasts. *Placenta* 2000;21:1–13.
51. Fukushima K, Miyamoto S, Komatsu H, *et al.* TNF-alpha-induced apoptosis and integrin switching in human extravillous trophoblast cell line. *Biol Reprod* 2003;68(5):1771–8.
52. Hamilton GS, Lysiak JJ, Han VK, Lala PK. Autocrine–paracrine regulation of human trophoblast invasiveness by insulin-like growth factor (IGF)-II and IGF-binding protein (IGFBP)-1. *Exp Cell Res* 1998;10:147–15.
53. Bischof P, Meisser A, Campana A, Tseng L. Effects of deciduas conditioned medium and insulin-like growth factor binding protein-1 on trophoblast matrix metalloproteinases and their inhibitors. *Placenta* 1998;19:457–46.
54. Bischof P, Haenggeli L, Campana A. Effect of leukemia inhibitory factor on human cytotrophoblast differentiation along the invasive pathway. *Am J Reprod Immunol* 1995;34:225–30.
55. Yamada KM, Geiger B. Molecular interactions in cell adhesion complexes. *Curr Opin Cell Biol* 1997;9:187.
56. Wang Y, Walsh SW, Kay HH. Placental lipid peroxides and thromboxane are increased and prostacyclin is decreased in women with preeclampsia. *Am J Obstet Gynecol* 1992;167:946–9.
57. Walsh SW, Wang Y, Jesse R. Peroxide induces vasoconstriction in the human placenta by stimulating thromboxane. *Am J Obstet Gynecol* 1993;169:1007–12.
58. Nelson DM, Johnson RD, Smith SD, Anteby EY, Sadovsky Y. Hypoxia limits differentiation and up-regulates expression and activity of prostaglandin H synthase 2 in cultured trophoblast from term human placenta. *Am J Obstet Gynecol* 1999;180:896–902.
59. Shore VH, Wang TH, Wang CL, Torry RJ, Caudle MR, Torry DS. Vascular endothelial growth factor, placenta growth factor and their receptors in isolated human trophoblast. *Placenta* 1997;18: 657–65.
60. Chung IB, Yelian FD, Zaher FM, *et al.* Expression and regulation of vascular endothelial growth factor in a first trimester trophoblast cell line. *Placenta* 2000;21:320–4.
61. Hunt JS, Chen HL, Miller L. Tumor necrosis factors: Pivotal components of pregnancy? *Biol Reprod* 1996;54:554–62.
62. Yui J, Garcia-Lloret M, Wegmann TG, Guilbert LJ. Cytotoxicity of tumour necrosis factor-alpha and gamma-interferon against primary human placental trophoblasts. *Placenta* 1994;15:819–35.
63. Fukushima K, Miyamoto S, Tsukimori K, Kobayashi H, Seki H, Takeda S, Kensuke E, Ohtani K, Shibuya M, Nakano H. Tumor necrosis factor and vascular endothelial growth factor induce endothelial integrin repertories, regulating endovascular differentiation and apoptosis in a human extravillous trophoblast cell line. *Biol Reprod* 2005;73:172–9.
64. Yoshida S, Ono M, Shono T, *et al.* Involvement of interleukin-8, vascular endothelial growth factor, and basic fibroblast growth factor in tumor necrosis factor alpha-dependent angiogenesis. *Mol Cell Biol* 1997;17:4015–23.
65. Ko Y, Totzke G, Gouni-Berthold I, Sachinidis A, Vetter H. Cytokine-inducible growth factor gene expression in human umbilical endothelial cells. *Mol Cell Probes* 1999;13:203–11.
66. Doukas J, Pober JS. IFN-gamma enhances endothelial activation induced by tumor necrosis factor but not IL-1. *J Immunol* 1990; 145:1727–33.
67. Genbacev O, Zhou Y, Ludlow JW, Fisher SJ. Regulation of human placental development by oxygen tension. *Science* 1997;277: 1669–72.

63 Trophoblast dysfunction and maternal endothelial cell dysfunction in the pathogenesis of pre-eclampsia

K. Tsukimori, K. Fukushima and H. Nakano

The etiology and pathogenesis of pre-eclampsia remain poorly understood. Several investigators have suggested that poor placentation is an important predisposing factor of pre-eclampsia and that endothelial cell dysfunction underlies disease manifestations.[1–4] In response to reduced placental perfusion due to poor placentation, the placenta may promote the release of various factors that initiate systemic endothelial cell dysfunction, leading to an increase in both vascular resistance and arterial pressure and activation of the coagulation cascade associated with pre-eclampsia. In this chapter, we focus on functional abnormalities of the placenta and trophoblast in pre-eclampsia, as well as the potential cellular and molecular mechanisms that contribute to the maternal endothelial cell dysfunction seen in this disorder.

Poor placentation

During early pregnancy, cytotrophoblast (CT) cells invade the uterus and its spiral arteries (in interstitial and endovascular invasion, respectively). As a result of endovascular invasion, CT cells replace the endothelial layers of spiral arteries with destruction of the medial elastic, muscular, and neural tissue. This replacement substantially decreases vascular resistance, resulting in increased blood flow toward the intervillous space.[5,6] In pre-eclampsia, extravillous trophoblast (EVT) cell invasion of the uterus is shallow, and endovascular invasion does not progress beyond the terminal portion of the spiral arteries (Figure 63.1).[5] Myometrial segments of these arteries remain anatomically intact and undilated; in addition, adrenergic nerve supply to the spiral arteries is not affected. The mean external diameters of the uterine spiral arteries in women with pre-eclampsia are less than one-half the diameters of similar vessels from uncomplicated pregnancies. The failure of EVT invasion in pre-eclampsia results in a reduction in uteroplacental perfusion. Because the process of EVT invasion of spiral arteries is normally completed by weeks 20–22 of gestation,[7] a critical underlying lesion in pre-eclampsia is the failure of EVT to invade the myometrial portion of the muscular spiral arteries.

Normal trophoblast invasion requires meticulously regulated expression of specific adhesion molecules for both cell–cell interactions as well as cell–extracellular matrix (ECM) interactions.[8] In pre-eclampsia, CT cells increase expression of adhesion molecules present in the initial proliferative phenotype, $\alpha5\beta1$, but fail both to upregulate adhesion molecules that promote invasion, $\alpha1\beta1$, and to down-regulate molecules that inhibit invasion, $\alpha6\beta4$ (Table 63.1).[9–12] Thus, the cells appear arrested in their differentiation and express an ECM receptor phenotype that may not be optimal for invasion.[12] In addition, endovascular invasion seems to require the ability of endovascular trophoblast cells to alter phenotype to resemble vascular endothelial cells.[13] In pre-eclampsia, trophoblast cells in decidual vessels do not express the endothelial antigens vascular adhesion molecule-1 (VCAM-1) and platelet endothelial adhesion molecule-1 (PECAM-1).[12] When these data are considered together, this overall dysfunctional expression of adhesion molecules may be responsible for the pathological findings of impaired interstitial and endovascular invasion in pre-eclampsia.

Factors involved in poor placentation

Hypoxic environment

Several studies suggest that oxygen tension can modulate trophoblast differentiation. Fox and Path

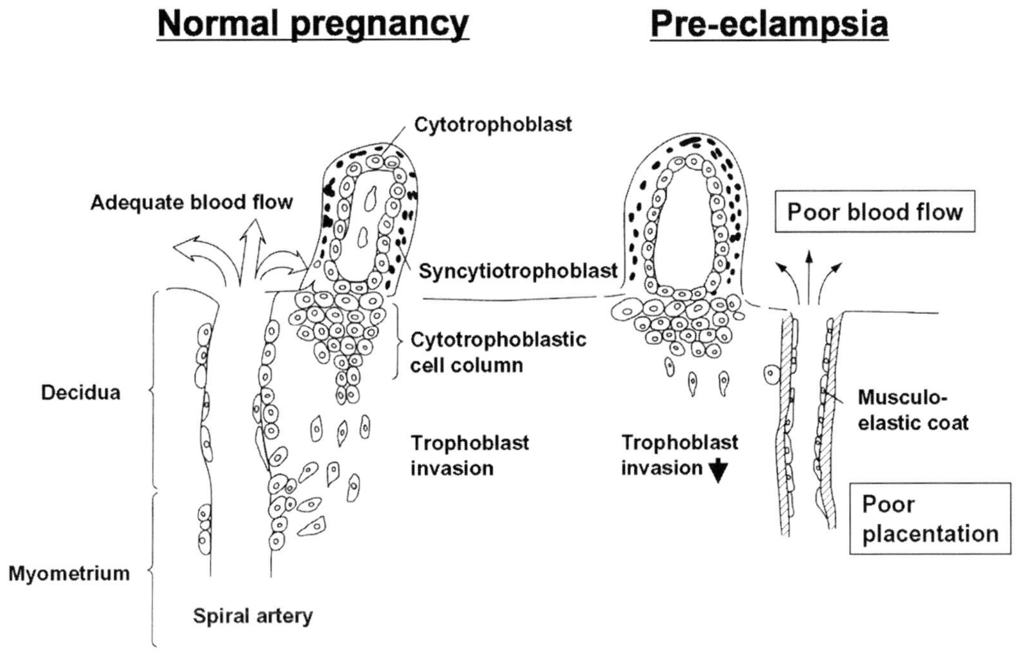

Figure 63.1 Trophoblast invasion in normal and pre-eclamptic pregnancies. Modified from Saito *et al.*[23] with permission.

Table 63.1 Integrin expression by cytotrophoblast cells in normal and pre-eclamptic pregnancies (modified from Zhou et al.[12])

Integrin receptor	ECM ligands	Functional link	Change from villus to placental bed: Normal pregnancy	Pre-eclampsia
$\alpha 6/\beta 4$	BM ligand (Ln ?)	Inhibit invasion	Down-regulated	Unchanged
$\alpha 5/\beta 1$	Fn	Initial proliferation	Upregulated	Up-regulated
$\alpha 3/\beta 1$	Ln, Fn, Col	Proliferation	Uniformly expressed	Uniformly expressed
$\alpha 1/\beta 1$	Ln, Col IV, Col I	Promote invasion	Up-regulated	Not expressed (weakly expressed)

ECM, extracellular matrix; BM, basement membrane; Ln, laminin; Fn, fibronectin; Col, collagen

reported that placental villi cultured under hypoxic conditions showed variable syncytial degeneration and a marked increase in the number and growth-promoting activity of CT cells.[14] More recently, using an *in vitro* organ culture model, CT maintained under hypoxic conditions failed to express integrin $\alpha 1$ and VE-cadherin.[15,16] These findings suggest that under hypoxic conditions CT cells enter a proliferative pathway and do not differentiate to the invasive phenotype. The adhesion molecule phenotype of these cells mimics that of CT from women with pre-eclampsia.[12]

In vitro, hypoxia stimulates the production of inflammatory cytokines and other mediators such as tumor necrosis factor-α (TNF-α), Interleukin (IL)-1α, IL-1β,[17] and transforming growth factor-β (TGFβ)[18] by trophoblasts. TNF-α induces apoptosis,[19] integrin subunit conversion, and functional activation in an EVT cell line.[20] TGFβ also inhibits cellular proliferation and migration.[21–23] In addition, trophoblasts under hypoxic conditions increase production of soluble fms-like tyrosine kinase 1 (sFlt-1), an antagonist for both vascular endothelial growth factor (VEGF) and placental growth factor (PlGF).[24] The enzyme sFlt-1 is involved in an alteration of integrin switching that decreases cell invasiveness.[25] In placentas from women with pre-eclampsia, there is increased production of TNF-α,[17] TGFβ,[18] and sFlt-1,[25,26] as well as decreased production of VEGF.[25] Taken together, this evidence suggests that hypoxia induces production of inflammatory cytokines and/or growth factors and then modulates cytotrophoblast differentiation and adhesion antigen expression, resulting in the inadequate invasion seen in pre-eclampsia.

Immunologic factors

Epidemiological evidence indicates that first pregnancy, change of partner, donor insemination, and use of barrier contraceptives all increase the risk of pre-eclampsia, suggesting that a prior immune response to foreign or paternal antigens protects against development of pre-eclampsia.[27–29] In pre-eclampsia, human leukocyte antigen (HLA)-G, a surrogate auto-antigen known to prevent recognition by natural killer (NK) cells, is not expressed in trophoblasts.[30,31] HLA-G down-regulates NK cell-mediated cytotoxicity[32] and suppresses IL-2–induced cell damage.[33] The soluble HLA-G1 isoform also down-regulates CD8-positive T cell (cytotoxic T cell) reactivity.[34] These findings suggest that invasive trophoblast lacking HLA-G is attacked by NK cells and cytotoxic T cells, resulting in the inadequate trophoblast invasion seen in pre-eclampsia. Recently, Saito and colleagues reported that pre-eclampsia is associated with a Th1 predominant immunity.[35] Th1-type cytokines such as IL-2, IFN-γ, TNF-α, and TNF-β activate cytotoxic T cells and NK cells. Activated cytotoxic T cells and NK cells can attack invading trophoblasts, causing a failure of trophoblast invasion.

Genetic factors

There is evidence of an increased incidence of pre-eclampsia among sisters, mothers, and daughters. Some studies have implicated several genes as risk factors for pre-eclampsia including angiotensin,[36] endothelial nitric oxide synthase (eNOS),[37] TNF-α,[38] the factor Leiden mutation,[39] and hyperhomocysteinemia.[40] Recent data focused on fetoplacental rather than maternal acting genes suggest that fetoplacental genes may carry an associated risk. These could be genes encoding factors associated with CT invasion. The risk of pre-eclampsia increases with a change in partner,[41] implying the importance of paternal genes. By following both men and women who were products of pre-eclamptic pregnancy, it has been suggested that both maternally and paternally inherited genes play a contributory role,[42] possibly by contributing to the genetic constitution of the placenta.

Biological changes of placental function

Poor placentation causes a reduction in uteroplacental perfusion, causing placental ischemia/hypoxia. Placental ischemia/hypoxia is known to induce several mediators such as reactive oxygen species (ROS) and inflammatory cytokines. Several biochemical abnormalities have been reported in placentas obtained from women with pre-eclampsia (Table 63.2).

Increased oxidative stress

Increased superoxide (O_2^-) synthesis rates have been noted in placentas from women with pre-eclampsia.[43,44] The expression of xanthine oxidase, which is an important source of O_2^- generation, is also enhanced in placentas from women with pre-eclampsia.[45] As an indirect indication of excessive generation of ROS, nitrotyrosine content, a stable marker for peroxinitrite ($ONOO^-$), is increased in placentas from women with pre-eclampsia.[46,47] When oxygen free radicals are not eliminated by antioxidants, lipid peroxide formation is induced.[48] Placental levels of lipid peroxidation products, as well as other markers of oxidative stress such as malondialdehyde (MDA),[49,50] 8-iso-PGF2α,[51] and protein carbonyl[52] are increased. *In vitro* production of lipid peroxides is also increased in trophoblasts from women with pre-eclampsia.[51,53,54] Placental antioxidant levels such as vitamin E, as well as the activities of glutathione peroxidase,[55] and both mRNA expression and enzyme activity for Cu/Zn-superoxide dismutase (SOD), are decreased in pre-eclampsia.[44] Thus, the placenta represents a state of oxidative stress in pre-eclampsia.

Altered cytokine production

Expression of inflammatory cytokines such as TNF-α and IL-1β is increased in pre-eclamptic placentas.[56,57] However, Benyo and colleagues failed to observe increased mRNA levels of both TNF-α and IL-1β in pre-eclamptic placenta.[58] Placental levels of IL-8,[59] IL-10,[60] and IL-15[61] are decreased in pre-eclampsia. Thus, although the picture is not entirely clear, placental cytokine production is altered in pre-eclampsia.

Increased vasoconstriction

Placental thromboxane production is increased, whereas placental PGI_2 production is decreased in pre-eclampsia.[62,63] Endothelin (ET)-1 expression and production are increased in trophoblasts obtained from women with pre-eclampsia.[64,65] Regarding nitric oxide (NO) production, Napolitano and colleagues reported that inducible nitric oxide synthase (iNOS) expression, which represents the main source of NO, is decreased; conversely, endothelial nitric oxide synthase (eNOS) expression is increased in trophoblasts obtained from women with pre-eclampsia.[64] In contrast, other investigators have failed to observe increased eNOS activity[66] and eNOS immunostaining levels.[67] Page and colleagues reported that expression of neurokinin (NK) B is increased in trophoblasts from women with pre-eclampsia.[68] Thus, in pre-eclampsia placental vasoconstrictor production is increased, whereas placental vasodilator production is decreased.

Table 63.2 Biological changes in pre-eclamptic placenta

Marker or activity	Location	Reference no(s).
Increased oxidative stress		
Increased superoxide synthesis	Placental tissue and trophoblast cells	43, 44
Increased xanthine oxidase expression	Invasive cytotrophoblast	45
Increased nitrotyrosine immunostaining	Invasive cytotrophoblast	46, 47
Increased MDA level	Placental homogenate	49, 50
Increased 8-isoprostane level and production	Placental tissue pieces	51
Increased protein carbonyl level	Placental and decidual homogenate	52
Increased lipid peroxide production	Trophoblast cells and villous tissue	51, 53, 54
Decreased glutathione peroxidase activity	Placental homogenate	55
Decreased vitamin E level	Placental homogenate	55
Decreased Cu/Zn-SOD activity and mRNA expression	Trophoblast cells	44
Altered cytokine production		
Increased TNF-α production and mRNA expression	Placental tissue	56, 57
Increased IL-1β mRNA expression	Placental tissue	56
No change for inflammatory cytokine (TNF-α, IL-1α, IL-1β, IL-6) mRNA expression	Placental homogenate	58
Decreased IL-8 production	Placental villous tissue	59
Decreased IL-10 immunostaining	Villous trophoblast cells	60
Decreased IL-15 production	Placental tissue and trophoblast cells	61
Increased vasoconstriction		
Increased thromboxane production	Placental tissue and cytotrophoblast	62, 63
Increased ET-1 production and mRNA expression	Trophoblast cells	64, 65
Increased NKB mRNA expression	Outer syncytiotrophoblast	68
Decreased prostacyclin production	Placental tissue and cytotrophoblast	62, 63
Decreased iNOS mRNA expression	Trophoblast cells	64

MDA, malondialdehyde; TNF, tumor necrosis factor; IL, interleukin; ET, endothelin; NKB, neurokinin B; iNOS, inducible nitric oxide synthase

Maternal endothelial cell dysfunction in pre-eclampsia

Several pieces of evidence indicate that adverse changes in structure and function of the maternal vascular endothelium account for the altered vascular reactivity, activation of the coagulation cascade, and multisystem damage that occurs in pre-eclampsia.[69,70] Pathologic changes in endothelial cells that line the renal glomerular capillaries (glomerular endotheliosis) are a consistent feature in women with pre-eclampsia.[71–73] Structural changes of the endothelium have been found in uteroplacental vessels.[74] In addition, functional evidence of endothelial alteration has been reported. The level of the endothelial prostanoid prostacyclin (PGI_2) is reduced weeks before as well as during clinically evident pre-eclampsia.[75–77] Vessels removed from women with pre-eclampsia manifest reduced endothelial-mediated vasodilator function.[78–80] A variety of substances indicative of endothelial dysfunction are increased in the blood of women with pre-eclampsia including cellular fibronectin (cFN),[81–83] von Willebrand factor,[84,85] thrombomodulin,[86,87] and VCAM-1.[88,89] Many of these substances including serum soluble VCAM-1[90] and cFN[83] are elevated weeks before pre-eclampsia becomes clinically evident.

Linkage between placental dysfunction and maternal endothelial dysfunction

To link placental dysfunction with the generalized endothelial dysfunction seen in pre-eclampsia, the existence of factor X, released from the placenta into the maternal circulation, was proposed. Indeed, we and other investigators have reported that serum from women with pre-eclampsia has a cytotoxic effect on cultured endothelial cells.[91,92] The factor seems to modulate endothelial cell function rather than damage the cells directly. In response to serum or plasma from women with pre-eclampsia, production of PGI_2[93,94] and NO[95–97] is altered, and increases are seen in cFN production,[98,99] mitogenic activity,[100,101] uptake of fatty acids,[102] and expression of platelet-derived growth factor (PDGF).[103] Many of these activities are not only elevated weeks before pre-eclampsia becomes clinically evident, but, as with the clinical signs of the syndrome, they disappear shortly after delivery.[91,99–101] Initially, Factor X was thought to be a single factor, but increasing evidence suggests the presence of several interacting factors. Several candidate factors have been proposed, including oxidative damage products, proinflammatory cytokines, syncytiotrophoblast microvesicles (STBM), and angiogenic factors.

Oxidative damage products

Circulating levels of lipid peroxidation products such as MDA[104–106] and 8-iso-PGF2α[50,107] are increased in pre-eclampsia. As described above, these products are elevated in concentration in trophoblasts from women with pre-eclampsia. Increased lipid peroxidation increases endothelial monolayer permeability to protein[108] and increases incorporation of fatty acids into endothelial cell membranes.[109] Free 8-iso-PGF2α is also a biologically active vasoconstrictor *in vivo*.[110] Nitrotyrosine staining, a stable marker for $ONOO^-$ is increased in sera from women with pre-eclampsia[111] and in pre-eclamptic placenta.[46,47] The free radical $ONOO^-$ is one of the most potent reactive species, and it can lead to increases in lipid peroxides and direct or indirect cellular damage.[112]

Proinflammatory cytokines

Proinflammatory cytokines such as TNF-α and IL-1β can produce endothelial dysfunction either directly or by activating maternal leukocytes.[3,113,114] In pre-eclampsia, circulating levels of IL-6, TNF-α,[115–117] and its two soluble receptors (p55 and p75 TNF-R)[117] are increased. Expression of placental cytokines including TNF-α and IL-1β is also increased in pre-eclampsia.[56,57] In contrast, Benyo and colleagues demonstrated that placental levels of inflammatory cytokines (e.g., TNF-α, IL-1α, IL-1β, and IL-6) are not altered,[58] suggesting that tissues other than the placenta, such as activated leukocytes or endothelium, may be involved in the elevation of inflammatory cytokines found in the circulation of women with pre-eclampsia. Hung and colleagues reported that hypoxia–reoxygenation of placental tissue *in vitro* increases production of TNF-α and causes endothelial dysfunction,[118] suggesting that a local inflammatory response can induce systemic endothelial dysfunction either directly or by activating maternal leukocytes during their passage through the placenta.

Syncytiotrophoblast microvesicles (STBM)

Circulating STBM are detected in the plasma of normal pregnant women, but they are present in significantly increased amounts in women with pre-eclampsia.[119] STBM induce ultrastructural endothelial cell injury[120,121] and reduce endothelial cell-mediated vasodilation in isolated human arteries.[122] Hung and colleagues reported that *in vitro* hypoxia–reoxygenation stimulates apoptotic changes within syncytiotrophoblasts in normal third-semester placentas, suggesting that aponecrotic processes secondary to reduced placental perfusion can lead to deportation of STBM into the maternal circulation.[123]

Angiogenic factors

VEGF is a well-known promoter of angiogenesis, and it also induces nitric oxide and vasodilatory prostacuclins in endothelial cells suggesting a role in decreasing vascular tone and blood pressure.[124,125] Decreased concentrations of circulating free VEGF have been noted in women with clinical pre-eclampsia,[26] and decreases have even been detected before clinically evident pre-eclampsia developed.[126,127] Recent studies have demonstrated that sFlt-1, an antagonist for VEGF, is increased in serum[26,128–130] and placenta[25,26] from women with pre-eclampsia. Levine and colleagues reported that increased levels of sFlt-1 predict subsequent development of pre-eclampsia.[129] In addition, animal model experiments have recently demonstrated that exogenous sFlt-1 administered to pregnant rats induces hypertension, proteinuria, and glomelural endotheliosis.[26] Nagamatsu and colleagues reported that trophoblasts under hypoxic conditions *in vitro* increase production of sFlt-1.[24] Interestingly, recent evidence suggests that TNF-α also stimulates the release of sFlt-1 from placental explants.[131]

Maternal and placental interactions in pathogenesis of pre-eclampsia

Abnormal placentation is not uniquely associated with pre-eclampsia. For example, infants with intrauterine growth restriction[132] and one third of infants with preterm birth[133] manifest abnormal features of placentation identical to those seen in pre-eclampsia. It has been proposed that abnormal placentation must interact with maternal factors to cause the clinical features of pre-eclampsia. Maternal constitutional factors, such as genetic, behavioral, and environmental factors would predispose to pre-eclampsia. These constitutional factors, likely influenced by the unique physiological changes of pregnancy, would interact with placental factors induced by placental ischemia/hypoxia to bring about the pathophysiological changes of pre-eclampsia.[1,134]

Constitutional factors

Preexisting hypertension, diabetes, obesity, and increased insulin resistance, as well as African descent

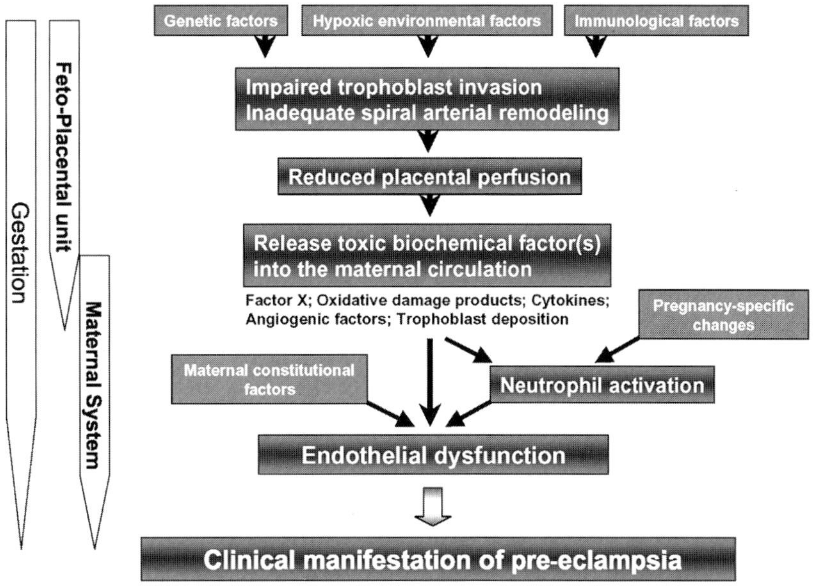

Figure 63.2 Proposed linkage between poor placentation and maternal endothelial dysfunction in pathogenesis of pre-eclampsia. See text for detail.

and increased blood homocysteine concentration, are already known to be predisposing factors.[135] Interestingly, these are also risk factors for other endothelial diseases, in particular atherosclerosis. The concept of common risk factors for the two disorders is supported by the relationship of pre-eclampsia to cardiovascular disease in later life.[136,137] In addition, pre-eclampsia and atherosclerosis share common alterations of lipid profile including elevated triglycerides,[104] reduced HDL-cholesterol,[138] and increased small dense LDL-cholesterol.[139] LDL particles are smaller than those of normal controls, which may facilitate their oxidation.[140,141]

Pregnancy-specific changes

It is well known that a neutrophilic leukocytosis occurs in pregnancy.[142] Sacks and colleagues used whole blood flow cytometric techniques to report that normal third-trimester pregnancy is characterized by remarkable activation of peripheral blood leukocytes, an activation that is further increased in pre-eclampsia.[143] We and other investigators have demonstrated that isolated neutrophils from women with pre-eclampsia synthesize more superoxide than those of normotensive pregnant women.[144-146] In an investigation of the mechanism of extreme neutrophil activation in pre-eclampsia, Aly and colleagues demonstrated that STBM, which are present in blood in elevated levels in pre-eclampsia,[119] lead to activation of maternal neutrophils.[147] Maternal neutrophils could also be locally activated during passage of maternal blood through the placenta.[117,148] In addition, we have reported that sera from women with pre-eclampsia enhance superoxide production of neutrophils *in vitro*.[144] The interaction of these activated neutrophils with endothelium would then result in the release of reactive oxygen species and endothelial injury.[149] Taken together, this evidence suggests that activated neutrophils, occurring as a usual component of maternal response to pregnancy, could provide a link between the placental dysfunction and maternal endothelial cell dysfunction seen in pre-eclampsia.

Conclusion

The two central pathophysiological themes of pre-eclampsia are placental trophoblast dysfunction and endothelial cell dysfunction within the maternal systemic vasculature. As discussed above, it has been proposed that multiple factors (e.g., hypoxic environmental, genetic, and immunological factors) may lead to impaired trophoblast invasion and inadequate spiral arterial remodeling (Figure 63.2). This, in turn, results in reduced placental perfusion. In response to this ischemic and/or hypoxic state, affected placentas secrete or elaborate substances into the maternal circulation that directly or indirectly cause systemic vascular endothelial cell dysfunction. In addition, pregnancy-specific changes (e.g., activation of neutrophils) combined with maternal constitutional factors (e.g., genetic disposition and circulating lipoproteins) are also involved in development of pre-eclampsia. It is necessary to clarify the mechanisms involved in placental and maternal endothelial dysfunction and to identify the factor(s) connecting them in order to understand, treat, and eventually prevent pre-eclampsia.

Acknowledgment

This work was supported in part by a grant-in-aid from the Japanese Ministry of Education (16790609 and 16591666).

REFERENCES

1. Roberts JM, Lain KY. Recent insights into the pathogenesis of pre-eclampsia. *Placenta* 2002;23:359–72.
2. Redman CWG, Sargent IL. Pre-eclampsia, the placenta and the maternal systemic inflammatory responses – A review. *Placenta* 2003;24:S21–7.
3. Roberts JM, Hubel CA. Is oxidative stress the link in the two-stage model of pre-eclampsia? *Lancet* 1999;354:788–9.
4. Wang Y, Alexander JS. Placental pathophysiology in preeclampsia. *Pathophysiology* 2000;6:261–70.
5. Brosens IA, Robertson WB, Dixon HG. The role of spiral arteries in the pathogenesis of preeclampsia. *Obstet Gynecol Annu* 1972;1:177–91.
6. Robertson WB, Brosens IA, Dixon HG. Placental bed vessels. *Am J Obstet Gynecol* 1973;117:294–5.
7. Pijnenborg R, Robertson WB, Brosens I, Dixon G. Trophoblast invasion and the establishment of haemochorial placentation in man and laboratory animals. *Placenta* 1981;2:71–92.
8. Damsky CH, Fitzgerald ML, Fisher SJ. Distribution patterns of extracellular matrix components and adhesion receptors are intricately modulated during first trimester cytotrophoblast differentiation along the invasive pathway, in vivo. *J Clin Invest* 1992;89:210–22.
9. Damsky CH, Librach C, Lim KH, *et al.* Integrin switching regulates normal trophoblast invasion. *Development* 1994;120:3657–66.
10. Redline RW, Patterson P. Preeclampsia is associated with an excess of proliferative immature intermediate trophoblasts. *Hum Pathol* 1995;26:594–600.
11. Zhou Y, Damsky CH, Chiu K, Roberts JM, Fisher SJ. Preeclampsia is associated with abnormal expression of adhesion molecules by invasive cytotrophoblasts. *J Clin Invest* 1993;91:950–60.
12. Zhou Y, Damsky CH, Fisher SJ. Preeclampsia is associated with failure of human cytotrophoblasts to mimic a vascular adhesion phenotype – One cause of defective endovascular invasion in this syndrome? *J Clin Invest* 1997;99:2152–64.
13. Zhou Y, Fisher SJ, Janatpour M, Genbacev O, Dejana E, Wheelock M, Damsky CH. Human cytotrophoblasts adopt a vascular phenotype as they differentiate. A strategy for successful endovascular invasion? *J Clin Invest* 1997;99:2139–2151.
14. Fox H, Path MC. Effect of hypoxia on trophoblasts in organ culture. A morphologic and autoradiographic study. *Am J Obstet Gynecol* 1970;107:1058–64.
15. Genbacev O, Zhou Y, Ludlow JW, Fisher SJ. Regulation of human placental development by oxygen tension. *Science* 1997;277: 1669–1672.
16. Zhou Y, Genbacev O, Damsky CH, Fisher SJ. Oxygen regulates human cytotrophoblast differentiation and invasion – implications for endovascular invasion in normal pregnancy and in pre-eclampsia. *J Reprod Immunol* 1998;39:197–213.
17. Benyo DF, Miles TM, Conrad KP. Hypoxia stimulates cytokine production by villous explants from the human placenta. *J Clin Endocrinol Metab* 1997;82:1582–8.
18. Caniggia I, Grisaru-Gravnosky S, Kuliszewsky M, Post M, Lye SJ. Inhibition of TGF-beta 3 restores the invasive capability of extravillous trophoblasts in preeclamptic pregnancies. *J Clin Invest* 1999;103:1641–50.
19. Levy R, Nelson DM. To be, or not to be, that is the question. Apoptosis in human trophoblasts. *Placenta* 2000;21:1–13.
20. Fukushima K, Miyamoto S, Komatsu H, Tsukimori K, Kobayashi H, Seki H, Takeda S, Nakano H. TNF-alpha-induced apoptosis and integrin switching in human extravillous trophoblast cell line. *Biol Reprod* 2003;68:1771–8.
21. Graham CH, Lysiak JJ, McCrae KR, Lala PK. Localization of transforming growth factor-beta at the human fetal–maternal interface: Role in trophoblast growth and differentiation. *Biol Reprod* 1992;46:561–72.
22. Khoo NK, Zhang Y, Bechberger JF, Bond SL, Hum K, Lala PK. SV40 Tag transformation of the normal invasive trophoblast results in a premalignant phenotype. II. Changes in gap junctional intercellular communication. *Int J Cancer* 1998;77:440–8.
23. Roth I, Fisher SJ. IL-10 is an autocrine inhibitor of human placental cytotrophoblast MMP-9 production and invasion. *Dev Biol* 1999;205:194–204.
24. Nagamatsu T, Fujii T, Kusumi M, *et al.* Cytotrophoblasts up-regulate soluble fms-like tyrosine kinase-1 expression under reduced oxygen: An implication for the placental vascular development and the pathophysiology of preeclampsia. *Endocrinology* 2004;145:4838–45.
25. Zhou Y, McMaster M, Woo K, *et al.* Vascular endothelial growth factor ligands and receptors that regulate human cytotrophoblast survival are dysregulated in severe preeclampsia and hemolysis, elevated liver enzymes, and low platelets syndrome. *Am J Pathol* 2002;160:1405–23.
26. Maynard SE, Min JY, Merchan J, *et al.* Excess placental soluble fms-like tyrosine kinase 1 (sFlt1) may contribute to endothelial dysfunction, hypertension, and proteinuria in preeclampsia. *J Clin Invest* 2003;111:649–58.
27. Robillard P-Y, Hulsey TC. Association of pregnancy induced hypertension, pre-eclampsia, and eclampsia with duration of sexual cohabitation before conception. *Lancet* 1996;347:619.
28. Robillard PY, Dekker GA, Hulsey TC. Primipaternities in families – Is the incidence of pregnancy-induced hypertensive disorders in multigravidas an anthropological marker of reproduction. *Aust N Z J Obstet Gynaecol* 1998;38:284–7.
29. Smith GN, Walker M, Tessier JL, Millar KG. Increased incidence of preeclampsia in women conceiving by intrauterine insemination with donor versus partner sperm for treatment of primary infertility. *Am J Obstet Gynecol* 1997;177:455–8.
30. Colburn GT, Chiang MH, Main EK. Expression of the nonclassic histocompatibility antigen HLA-G by preeclamptic placenta. *Am J Obstet Gynecol* 1994;170:1244–50.
31. Lim KH, Zhou Y, Janatpour M, *et al.* Human cytotrophoblast differentiation/invasion is abnormal in preeclampsia. *Am J Pathol* 1997;151:1809–18.
32. Marchal-Bras-Goncalves R, Rouas-Freiss N, Connan F, *et al.* A soluble HLA-G protein that inhibits natural killer cell-mediated cytotoxicity. *Transplant Proc* 2001;33:2355–9.
33. Hamai Y, Fujii T, Yamashita T, *et al.* The expression of human leukocyte antigen-G on trophoblasts abolishes the growth-suppressing effect of interleukin-2 toward them. *Am J Reprod Immunol* 1999;41:153–8.
34. Solier C, Aguerre-Birr M, Lenfant F, *et al.* Secretion of pro-apoptotic soluble HLA-G1 by human villous trophoblast. *Eur J Immunol* 2002;32:3576–86.
35. Saito S, Sakai M. Th1/Th2 balance in preeclampsia. *J Reprod Immunol* 2003;59:161–73.
36. Ward K, Hata A, Jeunemaitre X, *et al.* A molecular variant of angiotensinogen associated with preeclampsia. *Nat Genet* 1993;4:59–61.
37. Arngrimsson R, Hayward C, Nadaud S, *et al.* Evidence for a familial pregnancy-induced hypertension locus in the enos gene region. *Am J Hum Genet* 1997;61:354–62.
38. Masse J, Giguere Y, Kharfi A, Girouard J, Forest JC. Pathophysiology and maternal biologic markers of preeclampsia. *Endocrine* 2002;19:113–25.
39. Morgan T, Ward K. New insights into the genetics of preeclampsia. *Semin Perinatol* 1999;23:14–23.
40. Dekker GA, de Vries JI, Doelitzsch PM, *et al.* Underlying disorders associated with severe early-onset preeclampsia. *Am J Obstet Gynecol* 1995;173:1042–8.
41. Trupin LS, Simon LP, Eskenazi B. Change in paternity: A risk factor for preeclampsia in multiparas. *Epidemiology* 1996;7:240–4.
42. Esplin MS, Fausett MB, Fraser A, *et al.* Paternal and maternal components of the predisposition to preeclampsia. *N Engl J Med* 2001;344:867–872.

43. Sikkema JM, van Rijn BB, Franx A, *et al.* Placental superoxide is increased in pre-eclampsia. *Placenta* 2001;22:304–8.
44. Wang Y, Walsh SW. Increased superoxide generation is associated with decreased superoxide dismutase activity and mRNA expression in placental trophoblast cells in pre-eclampsia. *Placenta* 2001; 22:206–12.
45. Many A, Hubel CA, Fisher SJ, Roberts JM, Zhou Y. Invasive cytotrophoblasts manifest evidence of oxidative stress in preeclampsia. *Am J Pathol* 2000;156:321–31.
46. Myatt L, Rosenfield RB, Eis AL, Brockman DE, Greer I, Lyall F. Nitrotyrosine residues in placenta: Evidence of peroxynitrite formation and action. *Hypertension* 1996;28:488–93.
47. Norris M, Todeschini M, Cassis P, *et al.* L-Arginine depletion in preeclampsia orients nitric oxide synthase toward oxidant species. *Hypertension* 2004;43:614–22.
48. Walsh SW. The role of fatty acid peroxidation and antioxidant status in normal pregnancy and in pregnancy complicated by preeclampsia. *World Rev Nutr Diet* 1994;76:114–8.
49. Cester N, Staffolani R, Rabini RA, *et al.* Pregnancy-induced hypertension: A role for peroxidation in microvillous plasma membranes. *Mol Cell Biochem* 1994;131:151–5.
50. Gratacos E, Casals E, Deulofeu R, Cararach V, Alonso PL, Fortuny A. Lipid peroxide and vitamin E patterns in pregnant women with different types of hypertension in pregnancy. *Am J Obstet Gynecol* 1998;178:1072–6.
51. Walsh SW, Vaughan JE, Wang Y, Roberts LJ. Placental isoprostane is significantly increased in preeclampsia. *FASEB J* 2000;14:1289–96.
52. Zusterzeel PL, Rutten H, Roelofs HM, Peters WH, Steegers EA. Protein carbonyls in decidua and placenta of pre-eclamptic women as markers for oxidative stress. *Placenta* 2001;22:213–9.
53. Walsh SW, Wang Y. Secretion of lipid peroxides by the human placenta. *Am J Obstet Gynecol* 1993;169:1462–6.
54. Walsh SW, Wang Y. Trophoblast and placental villous core production of lipid peroxides, thromboxane, and prostacyclin in preeclampsia. *J Clin Endocrinol Metab* 1995;80:1888–93.
55. Wang Y, Walsh SW. Antioxidant activities and mRNA expression are increased in preeclamptic placentas. *J Soc Gynecol Investig* 1996;3:179–84.
56. Rinehart BK, Terrone DA, Lagoo-Deenadayalan S, *et al.* Expression of the placental cytokines tumor necrosis factor α, interleukin 1β, and interleukin 10 is increased in preeclampsia. *Am J Obstet Gynecol* 1999;181:915–20.
57. Wang Y, Walsh SW. TNFα concentrations and mRNA expression are increased in preeclamptic placentas. *J Reprod Immunol* 1996; 32:157–69.
58. Benyo DF, Smarason A, Redman CW, Sims C, Conrad KP. Expression of inflammatory cytokines in placentas from women with preeclampsia. *J Clin Endocrinol Metab* 2001;86:2505–12.
59. Wang Y, Baier J, Adair CD, *et al.* Interleukin-8 stimulates placental prostacyclin production in preeclampsia. *Am J Reprod Immunol* 1999;42:375–80.
60. Hennessy A, Pilmore HL, Simmons LA, Painter DM. A deficiency of placental IL-10 in preeclampsia. *J Immunol* 1999;163:3491–5.
61. Agarwal R, Loganath A, Roy AC, Wong YC, Ng SC. Expression profiles of interleukin-15 in early and late gestational human placenta and in pre-eclamptic placenta. *Mol Hum Reprod* 2001;7:97–101.
62. Walsh SW. Preeclampsia: An imbalance in placental prostacyclin and thromboxane production. *Am J Obstet Gynecol* 1985;152:335–40.
63. Ding ZQ, Rowe J, Sinosich MJ, Saunders DM, Gallery ED. In-vitro secretion of prostanoids by placental villous cytotrophoblasts in pre-eclampsia. *Placenta* 1996;17:407–11.
64. Napolitano M, Miceli F, Calce A, *et al.* Expression and relationship between endothelin-1 messenger ribonucleic acid (mRNA) and inducible/endothelial nitric oxide synthase mRNA isoforms from normal and preeclamptic placentas. *J Clin Endocrinol Metab* 2000; 85:2318–23.
65. Ding Z, Rowe J, Sinosich MJ, Saunders DM, Hawkins T, Gallery ED. Serum from women with preeclampsia partially corrects the abnormal in vitro prostacyclin secretion of preeclamptic villous cytotrophoblasts but not that of prostaglandin E2 or endothelin-1. *Am J Obstet Gynecol* 1997;177:1491–5.
66. Conrad KP, Davis AK. Nitric oxide synthase activity in placentae from women with pre-eclampsia. *Placenta* 1995;16:691–9.
67. Ghabour MS, Eis AL, Brockman DE, Pollock JS, Myatt L. Immunohistochemical characterization of placental nitric oxide synthase expression in preeclampsia. *Am J Obstet Gynecol* 1995;173:687–94.
68. Page NM, Woods RJ, Gardiner SM, *et al.* Excessive placental secretion of neurokinin B during the third trimester causes pre-eclampsia. *Nature* 2000;405:797–800.
69. Roberts JM, Taylor RN, Musci TJ, Rodgers GM, Hubel CA, McLaughlin MK. Preeclampsia: An endothelial cell disorder. *Am J Obstet Gynecol* 1989;161: 1200–4.
70. Taylor RN, Roberts JM. Endothelial cell dysfunction. In Lindheimer M, Roberts J, Cunningham F, eds. *Chesley's Hypertensive Disorders in Pregnancy*. New York: Appleton & Lange, 1999:395–429.
71. Fisher KA, Lluger A, Spargo BH, Lindheimer MD. Hypertension in pregnancy: Clinical–pathological correlations and remote prognosis. *Medicine* 1981;60:267–76.
72. McCartney CP, Spargo BH, Larincz AB, Lefebure Y, Newton RE. Renal structure and function in pregnant patients with acute hypertension. *Am J Obstet Gynecol*.1964;90:579–90.
73. Spargo B, McCartney C, Winemuller R. Glomerular capillary endotheliosis in toxemia of pregnancy. *Arch Pathol* 1959;68: 593–9.
74. Shanklin DR, Sibai BM. Ultrastructural aspects of preeclampsia. I. Placental bed and uterine boundary vessels. *Am J Obstet Gynecol* 1989;161:735–41.
75. Fitzgerald DJ, Entman SS, Mulloy K, Fitzgerald GA. Decreased prostacyclin biosynthesis preceding the clinical manifestation of pregnancy-induced hypertension. *Circulation* 1987;75:956–63.
76. Mills JL, DerSimonian R, Raymond E, *et al.* Prostacyclin and thromboxane changes predating clinical onset of preeclampsia: A multicenter prospective study. *J Am Med Assoc* 1999;282: 356–62.
77. Remuzzi G, Marchesi D, Zoja C, *et al.* Reduced umbilical and placental vascular prostacyclin in severe pre-eclampsia. *Prostaglandins* 1980;20:105–10.
78. Ashworth JR, Warren AY, Baker PN, Johnson DM. A comparison of endothelium-dependent relaxation in omental and myometrial resistance arteries in pregnant and nonpregnant women. *Am J Obstet Gynecol* 1996;175:1307–12.
79. McCarthy AL, Woolfson RG, Raju SK, Poston L. Abnormal endothelial cell function of resistance arteries from women with preeclampsia. *Am J Obstet Gynecol* 1993;168:1323–30.
80. Pascoal I, Lindheimer M, Nalbaltian-Brandt C, Umans J. Preeclampsia selectively impairs endothelium-dependent relaxation and leads to oscillatory activity in small omental arteries. *J Clin Invest* 1998;101:464–70.
81. Friedman SA, deGroot CJM, Taylor RN, Heilbron DC, Roberts JM. Plasma cellular fibronectin as a measure of endothelial involvement in preeclampsia and intrauterine growth retardation. *Am J Obstet Gynecol* 1994;170:838–41.
82. Lockwood C, Peters J. Increased plasma levels of ED1+ cellular fibronectin precede the clinical signs of preeclampsia. *Am J Obstet Gynecol* 1990;162:358–62.
83. Taylor RN, Crombleholme WR, Friedman SA, Jones LA, Casal DC, Roberts JM. High plasma cellular fibronectin levels correlate with biochemical and clinical features of preeclampsia but cannot be attributed to hypertension alone. *Am J Obstet Gynecol* 1991;165:895–901.
84. Redman CWG, Denson KWE, Beilin LJ Factor-VIII consumption in preeclampsia. *Lancet* 1977;2:1249.
85. Thorp J, White G, Moake J, Bowes WA. von Willebrand factor multimeric levels and patterns in patients with severe preeclampsia. *Obstet Gynecol* 1990;75:163–7.
86. Boffa MC, Valsecchi L, Fausto A, *et al.* Predictive value of plasma thrombomodulin in preeclampsia and gestational hypertension. *Thromb Haemost* 1998;79:1092–5.
87. Minakami H, Takahashi T, Izumi A, Tamada T. Increased levels of plasma thrombomodulin in preeclampsia. *Gynecol Obstet Invest* 1993;36:208–10.
88. Lyall F, Greer IA, Boswell F, Fleming R. Suppression of serum vascular endothelial growth factor immunoreactivity in normal pregnancy and in pre-eclampsia. *Br J Obstet Gynaecol* 1997; 104:223–8.
89. Higgins JR, Papayianni A, Brady HR, Darling MRN, Walshe JJ. Circulating vascular cell adhesion molecule-1 in pre-eclampsia, gestational hypertension, and normal pregnancy – Evidence of selective dysregulation of vascular cell adhesion molecule-1 homeostasis in pre-eclampsia. *Am J Obstet Gynecol* 1998;179: 464–9.
90. Krauss T, Kuhn W, Lakoma C, Augustin HG. Circulating endothelial cell adhesion molecules as diagnostic markers for the early identification of pregnant women at risk for development of preeclampsia. *Am J Obstet Gynecol* 1997;177:443–9.

91. Rogers GM, Taylor RN, Roberts JM. Preeclampsia is associated with a serum factor cytotoxic to human endothelial cells. *Am J Obstet Gynecol* 1988;159:908–14.
92. Tsukimori K, Maeda H, Shingu M, Koyanagi T, Nobunaga M, Nakano H. The possible role of endothelial cells in hypertensive disorders during pregnancy. *Obstet Gynecol* 1992;80:229–33.
93. Baker PN, Davidge ST, Barankiewicz J, Roberts JM. Plasma of preeclamptic women stimulates and then inhibits endothelial prostacyclin. *Hypertension* 1996;27:56–61.
94. deGroot DJM, Davidge ST, Friedman SA, McLaughlin MK, Roberts JM, Taylor RN. Plasma from preeclamptic women increases human endothelial cell prostacyclin production without changes in enzyme activity or mass. *Am J Obstet Gynecol* 1995; 172:976–85.
95. Baker PN, Davidge ST, Roberts JM. Plasma from women with preeclampsia increases endothelial cell nitric oxide production. *Hypertension* 1995;26:244–8.
96. Davidge ST, Baker PN, Roberts JM. NOS expression is increased in endothelial cells exposed to plasma from women with preeclampsia. *Am J Physiol* 1995;269:H1106–12.
97. Davidge ST, Signorella AP, Hubel CA, Lykins DL, Roberts JM. Distinct factors in plasma of preeclamptic women increase endothelial nitric oxide or prostacyclin. *Hypertension* 1996;28: 758–64.
98. Roberts JM, Edep ME, Goldfine A, Taylor RN. Sera from preeclamptic women specifically activate human umbilical vein endothelial cells in vitro: Morphological and biochemical evidence. *Am J Reprod Immunol* 1992;27:101–8.
99. Taylor RN, Casal DC, Jones LA, Varma M, Martin JN Jr, Roberts JM. Selective effects of preeclamptic sera on human endothelial cell procoagulant protein expression. *Am J Obstet Gynecol* 1991;165:1705–10.
100. Musci TJ, Roberts JM, Rodgers GM, Taylor RN. Mitogenic activity is increased in the sera of preeclamptic women before delivery. *Am J Obstet Gynecol* 1988;159:1446–51.
101. Taylor RN, Heilbron DC, Roberts JM. Growth factor activity in the blood of women in whom preeclampsia develops is elevated from early pregnancy. *Am J Obstet Gynecol* 1991;163: 1839–44.
102. Endresen MJ, Morris JM, Nobrega AC, Buckley D, Linton EA, Redman CWG. Serum from preeclamptic women induces vascular cell adhesion molecule-1 expression on human endothelial cells in vitro – A possible role of increased circulating levels of free fatty acids. *Am J Obstet Gynecol* 1998;179:665–70.
103. Taylor RN, Musci TJ, Rodgers GM, Roberts JM. Preeclamptic sera stimulate increased platelet-derived growth factor mRNA and protein expression by cultured human endothelial cells. *Am J Reprod Immunol* 1991;25:105–8.
104. Hubel CA, McLaughlin MK, Evans RW, Hauth BA, Sims CJ, Roberts JM. Fasting serum triglycerides, free fatty acids, and malondialdehyde are increased in preeclampsia, are positively correlated, and decrease within 48 hours post partum. *Am J Obstet Gynecol* 1996;174:975–82.
105. Hubel CA. Dyslipidemia, iron, and oxidative stress in preeclampsia: Assessment of maternal and feto-placental interactions. *Semin Reprod Endocrinol* 1998;16:75–92.
106. Wang Y, Walsh SW, Guo J, Zhang J. The imbalance between thromboxane and prostacyclin in preeclampsia is associated with an imbalance between lipid peroxides and vitamin E in maternal blood. *Am J Obstet Gynecol* 1991;165:1695–700.
107. Barden A, Beilin LJ, Ritchie J, Croft KD, Walters BN, Michael CA. Plasma and urinary 8-iso-prostane as an indicator of lipid peroxidation in pre-eclampsia and normal pregnancy. *Clin Sci* 1996;91:711–18.
108. Granger DN, Rutili G, McCord JM. Superoxide radicals in feline intestinal ischemia. *Gastroenterology* 1981;81:22–9.
109. Endresen MJ, Lorentzen B, Henriksen T. Increased lipolytic activity and high ratio of free fatty acids to albumin in sera from women with preeclampsia leads to triglyceride accumulation in cultured endothelial cells. *Am J Obstet Gynecol* 1992;167:440–7.
110. Roberts LJ, Morrow JD. The isoprostanes: Novel markers of lipid peroxidation and potential mediators of oxidant injury. *Adv Prostaglandin Thromboxane Leukot Res* 1995;23:219–24.
111. McCord N, Ayuk PT, Sargent IL, Redman CWG, Boyd CAR. Evidence of increased oxidative stress in preeclampsia. *Placenta* 2002;23(A39):114.
112. Lowe DT. Nitric oxide dysfunction in the pathophysiology of preeclampsia. *Nitric Oxide* 2000;4:441–58.
113. Pober JS, Cotran RS. Cytokines and endothelial cell biology. *Physiol Rev* 1990;70:427–51.
114. Redman CWG, Sucks GP, Sargents IL. Preeclampsia, an excessive maternal inflammatory response to pregnancy. *Am J Obstet Gynecol* 1999;180:499–506.
115. Conrad KP, Benyo DF. Placental cytokines and the pathogenesis of preeclampsia. *Am J Reprod Immunol* 1997;37:240–9.
116. Conrad KP, Miles TM, Benyo DF. Circulating levels of immunoreactive cytokines in women with preeclampsia. *Am J Reprod Immunol* 1998;40:102–11.
117. Vince GS, Starkey PM, Austgulen R, Kwiatkowski D, Redman CWG. Interleukin-6, tumour necrosis factor and soluble tumour necrosis factor receptors in women with pre-eclampsia. *Br J Obstet Gynaecol* 1995;102:20–5.
118. Hung TH, Charnock-Jones DS, Skepper JN, Burton GJ. Secretion of tumor necrosis factor-alpha from human placental tissues induced by hypoxia–reoxygenation causes endothelial cell activation in vitro: A potential mediator of the inflammatory response in preeclampsia. *Am J Pathol* 2004;164:1049–61.
119. Knight M, Redman CWG, Linton EA, Sargent IL. Shedding of syncytiotrophoblast microvilli into the maternal circulation in preeclamptic pregnancies. *Br J Obstet Gynaecol* 1998;105:632–40.
120. Smarason AK, Sargent IL, Starkey PM, Redman CWG. The effect of placental syncytiotrophoblast microvillous membranes from normal and pre-eclamptic women on the growth of endothelial cells in vitro. *Br J Obstet Gynaecol* 1993;100:943–9.
121. Smarason AK, Sargent IL, Redman CWG. Endothelial cell proliferation is suppressed by plasma but not serum from women with preeclampsia. *Am J Obstet Gynecol* 1996;174:787–93.
122. Cockell AP, Learmont JG, Smarason AK, Redman CW, Sargent IL, Poston L. Human placental syncytiotrophoblast microvillous membranes impair maternal vascular endothelial function. *Br J Obstet Gynaecol* 1997;104:235–40.
123. Hung TH, Skepper JN, Charnock-Jones DS, Burton GJ. Hypoxia–reoxygenation: A potent inducer of apoptotic changes in the human placenta and possible etiological factor in preeclampsia. *Circ Res* 2002;90:1274–81.
124. Morbidelli L, Chang CH, Douglas JG, Granger HJ, Ledda F, Ziche M. Nitric oxide mediates mitogenic effect of VEGF on coronary venular endothelium. *Am J Physiol* 1996;270:H411–15.
125. He H, Venema VJ, Gu X, Venema RC, Marrero MB, Caldwell RB. Vascular endothelial growth factor signals endothelial cell production of nitric oxide and prostacyclin through flk-1/KDR activation of c-Src. *J Biol Chem* 1999;274:25130–5.
126. Polliotti BM, Fry AG, Saller DN, Mooney RA, Cox C, Miller RK. Second-trimester maternal serum placental growth factor and vascular endothelial growth factor for predicting severe, early-onset preeclampsia. *Obstet Gynecol* 2003;101:1266–74.
127. Taylor RN, Grimwood J, Taylor RS, McMaster MT, Fisher SJ, North RA. Longitudinal serum concentrations of placental growth factor: Evidence for abnormal placental angiogenesis in pathologic pregnancies. *Am J Obstet Gynecol* 2003;188:177–82.
128. Koga K, Osuga Y, Yoshino O, *et al.* Elevated serum soluble vascular endothelial growth factor receptor 1 (sVEGFR-1) levels in women with preeclampsia. *J Clin Endocrinol Metab* 2003;88: 2348–51.
129. Levine RJ, Maynard SE, Qian C, *et al.* Circulating angiogenic factors and the risk of preeclampsia. *N Engl J Med* 2004;350: 672–83.
130. Tsatsaris V, Goffin F, Munaut C, *et al.* Overexpression of the soluble vascular endothelial growth factor in preeclamptic patients: Pathophysiological consequences. *J Clin Endocrinol Metab* 2003;88:5555–63.
131. Ahmad S, Ahmed A. Elevated placental soluble vascular endothelial growth factor 1 receptor-1 inhibits angiogenesis in preeclampsia. *Circ Res* 2004;95:884–91.
132. Khong TY, De Wolff, Robertson WB, Brosens I. Inadequate maternal vascular response to placentation in pregnancies complicated by pre-eclampsia and by small-for-gestational age infants. *Br J Obstet Gynaecol* 1986;93:1049–59.
133. Arias F, Rodriquez L, Rayne SC, Kraus FT. Maternal placental vasculopathy and infection: Two distinct subgroups among patients with preterm labor and preterm ruptured membranes. *Am J Obstet Gynecol* 1993;168:585–91.
134. Ness RB, Roberts JM. Heterogeneous causes constituting the single syndrome of preeclampsia: A hypothesis and its implications. *Am J Obstet Gynecol* 1996;175:1365–70.
135. Roberts JM, Cooper DW. Pathogenesis and genetics of preeclampsia. *Lancet* 2001;357:53–6.

136. Chesley LC, Annitto JE, Cosgrove RA. The remote prognosis of eclamptic women: Sixth periodic report. *Am J Obstet Gynecol* 1976;124:446–59.

137. Sibai B, El-Nazer A, Gonzalez-Ruiz A. Severe preeclampsia eclampsia in young primigravid women: Subsequent pregnancy outcome and remote prognosis. *Am J Obstet Gynecol* 1986; 155:1011–16.

138. Kaaja R, Tikkanen M, Viinikka L, Ylikorkala O. Serum lipoproteins, insulin, and urinary prostanoid metabolites in normal and hypertensive pregnant women. *Obstet Gynecol* 1995;85:353–6.

139. Sattar N, Bendomir A, Berry C, Shepherd J, Greer IA, Packard CJ. Lipoprotein subfraction concentrations in preeclampsia: Pathogenic parallels to atherosclerosis. *Obstet Gynecol* 1997;89: 403–8.

140. Hubel CA, Shakir Y, Gallaher MJ, Mclaughlin MK, Roberts JM. Low density lipoprotein particle size decreases during normal pregnancy in association with triglyceride increases. *J Soc Gynecol Invest* 1998;5:244–50.

141. Ogura K, Miyatake T, Fukui O, Nakamura T, Kameda T, Yoshino G. Low-density lipoprotein particle diameter in normal pregnancy and preeclampsia. *J Atheroscler Thromb* 2002;9:42–7.

142. Brinkman CR. Biological adaptation of pregnancy. In Creasy RK, Resnik R, eds. *Maternal Fetal Medicine*. 2nd edn. Philadelphia, PA: WB Saunders, 1989:734–45.

143. Sacks GP, Studena K, Sargent K, Redman CWG. Normal pregnancy and preeclampsia both produce inflammatory changes in peripheral blood leukocytes akin to those of sepsis. *Am J Obstet Gynecol* 1998;179:80–6.

144. Tsukimori K, Maeda H, Ishida K, Nagata H, Koyanagi T, Nakano H. The superoxide generation of neutrophils in normal and preeclamptic pregnancies. *Obstet Gynecol* 1993;81:536–40.

145. Crocker IP, Wellings RP, Fletcher J, Baker PN. Neutrophil function in women with pre-eclampsia. *Br J Obstet Gynaecol* 1999; 106:822–8.

146. Lee VM, Quinn PA, Jennings SC, Ng LL. Neutrophil activation and production of reactive oxygen species in pre-eclampsia. *J Hypertens* 2003;21:395–402.

147. Aly AS, Khandelwal M, Zhao J, Mehmet AH, Sammel MD, Parry S. Neutrophils are stimulated by syncytiotrophoblast microvillous membranes to generate superoxide radicals in women with preeclampsia. *Am J Obstet Gynecol* 2004;190:252–8.

148. Mellembakken JR, Aukrust P, Olafsen MK, Ueland T, Hestdal K, Videm V. Activation of leukocytes during the uteroplacental passage in preeclampsia. *Hypertension* 2002;39:155–60.

149. Palluy O, Morliere L, Gris JC, Boone C, Modat G. Hypoxia/reoxygenation stimulates endothelium to promote neutrophil adhesion. *Free Radic Biol Med* 1992;13:21–30.

64 Basic aspects of trophoblastic disease

N. Wake, K. Asanoma, T. Matsuda and H. Kato

Genetics of hydatidiform moles

Hydatidiform moles that have grossly swollen villi are divisible into two entities: the classical complete mole and the partial mole. The complete mole presents as a rapidly progressing hydatidiform change affecting the whole placenta, with widespread and gross trophoblastic hyperplasia in the absence of an embryo and its covering amnion. The majority of complete moles have a 46, XX karyotype. Inspection of the karyotype of a mole and its parents readily reveals that both members of chromosome pairs of the complete mole are traceable to one paternal chromosome. Thus, these moles result from duplication of a paternal haploid set in a functionally empty ovum, a process called androgenesis. Most probably, these moles develop from fertilization of an empty ovum by a haploid sperm followed by the duplication of its chromosomes.[1–6] The maternal nuclear complement is either eliminated or inactivated in an empty ovum. This mechanism would account for the preponderance of XX moles, because their YY counterparts are probably lost during early cleavage stages.

The rare 46, XY moles can also be found.[7–9] Estimates of the total number of these moles range from 4% to 20% in a small series. Southern blots of polymerase chain reaction (PCR) products clearly demonstrate that both alleles shown in the mole derive from the two paternal alleles in some gene loci, whereas the allele derives from one of two paternal alleles in the remaining loci. The genetic features shown in these moles are compatible with fertilization of an empty egg by two spermatozoa. Dispermy would result in an XX, XY or YY sex chromosome constitution, in a 1:2:1 ratio. Again, YY moles are lethal.

In addition to androgenesis, occasional complete moles that are diploid but biparental in origin have been described. While androgenetic complete moles are usually sporadic, biparental complete moles are associated with a predisposition to recurrent molar pregnancies and frequently occur in more than one member of a family. Women with a biparental complete mole have a much greater risk of having more complete moles than women with an androgenetic complete mole or partial mole, and have an appreciable risk of persistent trophoblastic disease. The biparental complete mole arises from an unusual pregnancy associated with a failure to set maternal imprints within the ovum. The gene, mutated in the woman with a biparental complete mole, shows an autosomal recessive mode of inheritance and has been mapped to chromosome 19q 13.4.

In the partial moles there is a slow hydatidiform change that affects only some of the villi. There is focal, moderate, trophoblastic hyperplasia, irrespective of the survival of the embryo. An accumulation of cytogenetic data has shown that dispermic triploids that were products of an intact ovum fertilized by two spermatozoa were responsible for these partial moles.[10–13] We have encountered unusual cases of partial moles in the course of systematic cytogenetic studies of partial moles, each with a tetraploid karyotype. These rare partial moles result from the combination of a haploid ovum with three paternal haploid sets as a result of trispermic fertilization.[14–16] The majority of partial moles result from dispermic triploids. Tetraploids with one maternal and three paternal haploid sets provide unequivocal morphological examples of partial moles. In addition to these, complete moles that involve the whole placenta in hydatidiform changes are androgenetic in origin. These findings illustrate an intriguing correlation between a molar phenotype and the ratio of paternal to maternal genome in the conceptus. In this connection, the fact that benign ovarian teratomas are parthenogenetic in origin leads to the possibility that the maternal and paternal genomes are not functionally equivalent. The teratoma that consists of embryonic tissue elements in the absence of extraembryonic tissues has two maternally derived haploid sets. These findings point to some dependence of the extraembryonic tissues, notably trophoblast, on the paternal genome, while some maternal genes are apparently required for the development of the embryo proper. Only male plus female diploid combinations of pronuclei would give rise to normal embryos. Particular sets of genes undergo a separate specific imprinting during oogenesis and spermatogenesis. Most probably, disruption of imprinted regulation for a particular set of genes in complete and partial moles contributes to the formation of molar phenotypes, but these remain to be identified. Histopathological criteria to differentiate between partial and complete moles are inconsistent among countries. In addition, histological features overlap significantly between these moles, especially when the moles are evaluated in the early gestational stage. These indicate the necessity of genetic demonstration of each class of moles.

Malignant trophoblastic neoplasms with different modes of origin

It is well known that the complete mole has a propensity to malignancy. However, there has been no direct proof in the majority of patients that choriocarcinoma indeed derived from a complete mole. The androgenetic origin of complete moles provides us with a method for determining the origin of choriocarcinomas. The genome of choriocarcinoma should reflect that of the pregnancy from which the tumor arose. After a live birth or spontaneous abortion, both maternal and paternal contributions to the genome should be present in the tumor genome. Choriocarcinoma after complete mole conceptions should carry only the paternal genome. The absence of a paternal contribution in the tumor genome is a feature of non-gestational choriocarcinoma. Based on these genetic backgrounds, a small number of choriocarcinomas have been examined so far.[17–23] However, the number of cases reported is too small to show whether there is a predominant association of complete mole with choriocarcinoma or not. Thus, we examined the genetic origin of a relatively large number of trophoblastic tumors in order to demonstrate the propensity to malignancy of the complete mole.

Genomic DNAs obtained from 24 fresh or paraffin-embedded tumors were successfully amplified by PCR.[24] Based on pregnancy history, these tumors included (1) 9 postmolar trophoblastic tumors, (2) 12 tumors preceded by live birth or abortion and (3) 3 non-gestational tumors. PCR polymorphism data revealed the absence of a maternal genome in eight postmolar trophoblastic tumors (Table 64.1). This was contrasted with the presence of a maternal genome in all 12 tumors preceded by live birth or abortion and in the three non-gestational tumors. Thus, these eight postmolar trophoblastic neoplasms developed from malignant transformation of complete moles. Six tumors were homozygous at three or more gene loci in which the partners were heterozygous. A female sex chromosome constitution was anticipated because PCR failed to amplify any fragment specific to the *SRY* (which is specific to the Y chromosome) gene sequence in these tumors. These genetic features may be compatible with those of the complete mole that results from fertilization of an empty egg by an X-bearing sperm. The heterozygosity was recognized in two tumors at a few gene loci. The 240-base-pair (bp) PCR product specific to the *SRY* gene sequence was present in one tumor but not in the other. It seemed likely that the two tumors originated from an XX or XY dispermic, androgenetic mole (Figure 64.1).

The remaining choriocarcinoma contained an allele derived from the patient at a few gene loci. This finding is compatible with the assumption that the tumor did not arise from a complete mole. A full-term delivery prior to a complete mole conception would explain this tumor development.

All 12 tumors in class (2) had alleles of both paternal and maternal contribution. However, discordance of sex between the antecedent pregnancy product and the tumor was recognized in three choriocarcinomas. The absence of a paternal contribution suggested a parthenogenetic origin for the three non-gestational choriocarcinomas. The findings that PCR polymorphisms were either homozygous in certain loci or heterozygous in others may mean that the tumor was derived from a germ cell after meiosis I. As a result, at least three subtypes with different modes of origin were demonstrated in the 24 trophoblastic tumors. Although more than half of the trophoblastic tumors collected here had a maternal contribution to their genomes, the data still support the suggestion that of all forms of pregnancy that predispose patients to choriocarcinoma, the most likely is the complete mole.

Molecular mechanisms associated with trophoblastic diseases

Gene expression profile in complete moles

Kato *et al.*[25] used microarray analysis to investigate the expression profiles of 589 genes committed to cell growth control, in order to characterize the regulatory circuitry for cell proliferation in complete moles. Complete moles are characterized by hyperplastic trophoblasts and have a high propensity to cause choriocarcinoma. Characteristic alterations in gene expression profiles were observed when compared with normal villi. A total of 57 genes were significantly up-regulated in complete moles. These involved the Ras/mitogen-activated protein kinase III, Janus kinase/STAT5 and Wnt signal pathways, implicating growth factor- or cytokine-mediated signal pathways in the trophoblastic hyperplasia of complete moles.

Table 64.1 PCR-polymorphism analysis of choriocarcinomas and invasive mole (antecedent pregnancies were complete moles) and parents

Patients	DNA	D1S80	ApoB	D5S107	DRB	D9S43	RB	D17S30	DMD	SRY
1	P	f/g	a/–	a/b	4/–	a/–	a/b	c/–	(+)	(+)
	T	f/g	a/c	b/c	4/12	a/b	a/b	c/–		
	M	e/f	b/c	b/c	9/12	b/–	b/–	c/–		
2	P	**b/d**	**a/c**	a/b	2/3,6	a/c	**a/b**	**c/f**	(+)	(–)
	T	**b/d**	**a/c**	a/–	2/–	a/–	**a/b**	**c/f**		
	M	a/–	a/c	b/c	2/4	a/–	b/–	a/e		
3	P	b/g	a/b	c/d	4/–	b/–	a/–	b/e	(+)	(–)
	T	b/–	a/–	d/–	4/–	b/–	a/–	b/–		
	M	a/g	a/c	c/d	2/4	c/d	a/b	e/f		
4	P	d/h	a/c	c/–	2/3,6	a/b	c/–	c/e	(+)	(–)
	T	d/–	a/–	c/–	ND	b/–	c/–	e/–		
	M	c/–	a/c	e/f	3,6/–	b/c	a/b	d/–		
5	P	a/b	a/b	e/f	4/–	c/d	a/b	d/f	(+)	(–)
	T	a/–	b/–	f/–	4/–	c/–	b/–	d/–		
	M	d/e	b/–	b/d	2/–	d/e	a/d	f/g		
6	P	i/–	a/–	b/d	4/2	b/f	c/–	d/–	ND	ND
	T	i/–	a/–	b/–	4/–	b/–	c/–	d/–		
	M	i/j	a/–	b/c	3,6/–	b/g	a/b	c/d		
8	P	a/b	a/–	a/b	1/–	f/g		d/f	(+)	(–)
	T	b/–	a/–	a/–	1/–	g/–	ND	f/–		
	M	c/d	a/c	c/–	4/12	h/–		a/b		
9	P	h/i	a/–	a/b	11/9			b/–	(+)	(–)
	T	h/–	a/–	a/–	11/–	ND	ND	b/–		
	M	h/–	a/c	b/–	4/9			b/c		
10*	P	d/–	a/c	a/b	**4/8**	b/h	a/–	**b/d**	(+)	(+)
	T	d/–	a/–	b/–	**4/8**	b/–	a/–	**b/d**		
	M	a/b	a/c	a/b	4/9	b/f	a/–	a/–		

P, paternal DNA; T, tumor DNA; M, maternal DNA; ND, not determined. Bold type indicates a heterozygous pattern in the tumor DNA.
*Invasive mole

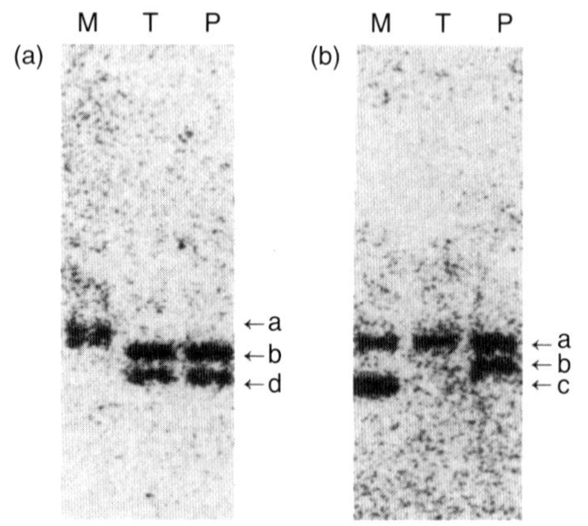

Amplified gene(locus)	MCT118 (D1S80)	3-beta (ApoB)
Location	1p36-p35	2p24-p23
Technique	VNTR	VNTR

Figure 64.1 PCR–polymorphism of two chonocarcinomas. The tumor showed two bands that were absent in maternal DNA, suggesting an androgenic origin. P, PCR products from paternal DNA; T, PCR products from tumor DNA; M, PCR products from maternal DNA; VNTR, variable number of tandem repeats.

Several genes associated with antiapoptosis, cell structuring and/or cell attachment were also up-regulated in complete moles. In contrast, relatively fewer genes were down-regulated and these involved insulin growth factor binding proteins, Versican, interleukin-1, tumor necrosis factor receptor, CD44 and Rad 52. The genes identified as being up- or down-regulated may help to elucidate the regulation mechanisms of trophoblastic proliferation and the mechanisms causing a pathological phenotype in complete moles (Figure 64.2).[25]

Silencing of NECC1/Hop expression in choriocarcinoma

Choriocarcinoma is a highly invasive tumor consisting of markedly anaplastic trophoblasts totally lacking in residual villous structures. Demonstration of a predominant association between a complete mole and choriocarcinoma suggests that the molecular events of mole and choriocarcinoma development are related, since the putative forerunner carries unique genetic features (as mentioned previously). The

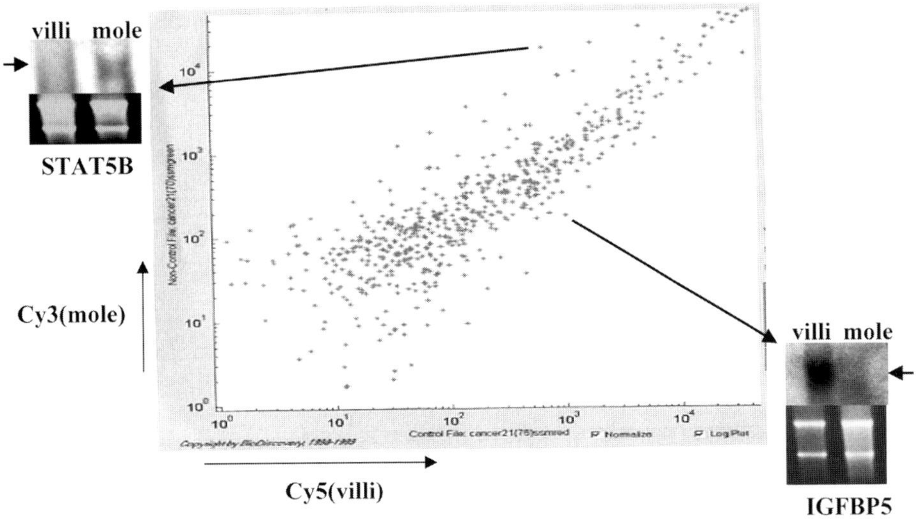

Figure 64.2 A log plot of a microarray experiment demonstrating distribution of 425-gene expression in normal and molar villi. Fluorointensity of Cy-3, which is labeled to mRNA from a complete mole, is plotted vertically. Fluorointensity of Cy-5, from normal villi, is plotted horizontally. Up-regulation of STAT5B expression and down-regulation of 1GFBP5 expression in mole are shown. *x*: Control file: mole red Cy3; *y*: non-control file: norma, villi green Cy5.

monoallelic contribution shown in the complete mole would render a certain gene susceptible to functional inactivation by 'one-hit' kinetics. Alternatively, uniparental transmission of genes that are subject to parental imprinting in humans would impair their regulation. Thus, the features exhibited by a complete mole would be associated with inactivation of particular tumor suppressor genes, contributing to the propensity to malignancy.

Many tumor suppressor genes are inactivated by intragenic mutations in one allele, accompanied by the loss of a chromosomal region containing the remaining allele; this is termed loss of heterozygosity. Mapping of such deleted regions has been used to idontify sequences involved in malignancies. However, the monoallelic contribution exhibited by the complete mole and its transformant would mask the chromosomal region where the allelic loss frequently occurs. To resolve this difficulty, Asanoma *et al.*[26] constructed a PCR-subtracted fragmentary cDNA library between normal placenta villi and the choriocarcinoma cell line (CC1) and isolated a candidate choriocarcinoma suppressor gene. This gene comprised an open reading frame of 219 nucleotides encoding 73 amino acid residues and contained a homeodomain as a consensus motif, being identical with homeodomain-only protein (HOP), which is essential for cardiomyocyte development.[27,28] This gene, designated as *n*ot *e*xpressed in *c*horiocar*c*inoma clone 1 (*NECC1*),[26] is located on human chromosome 4q11–q12. *NECC1* expression is ubiquitous in the brain, placenta, lung, smooth muscle, uterus, bladder, kidney and spleen. Normal placental villi expressed *NECC1*, but all of the choriocarcinoma cell lines examined and most of the surgically removed choriocarcinoma tissue samples failed to express it. Asanoma *et al.*[26] transfected this gene into choriocarcinoma cell lines and observed remarkable alterations in cell morphology and suppression of *in vivo* tumorigenesis. Induction of chorionic somatomammotropin hormone 1 (CSH1) and a remarkable alteration in cell morphology including multinucleation by *NECC1* expression suggested the differentiation of choriocarcinoma cells to syncytiotrophoblasts (Figure 64.3).

The tumor suppressive ability of *NECC1* does not require the third/fourth helix and the C-terminal domain. The inhibitory effect of mutant *NECC1*, which deletes the third/fourth helix and the C-terminal domain, on choriocarcinoma cell growth properties is analogous to that of wild-type *NECC1*. The results imply that the DNA binding capability of *NECC1* is not required for choriocarcinoma cell differentiation and the resultant tumorigenic suppression. This unexpected finding may be supported by the previously reported evidence that several homeobox genes exhibit their biological functions in the absence of DNA binding. The data suggest that loss of *NECC1* expression is involved in the malignant conversion of placental trophoblasts.

Human chromosome 7 carries a putative tumor suppressor gene involved in choriocarcinoma

To determine which chromosome carries a putative tumor suppressor gene, microcell hybrids were isolated following fusion of choriocarcinoma cells with

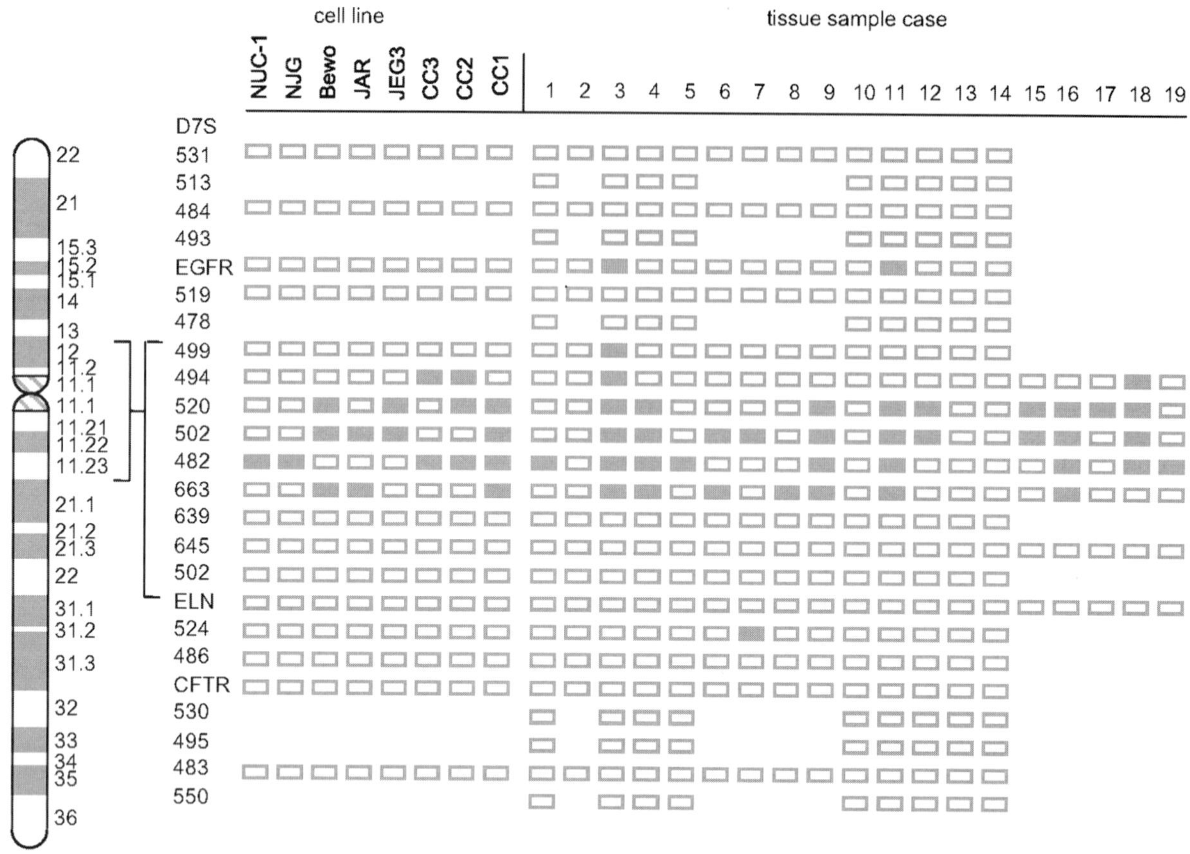

Figure 64.3 Map of homozygous deletions on chromosome 7. Close squares represent homozygous deletions. Open squares indicate the retention of a single or both alleles.

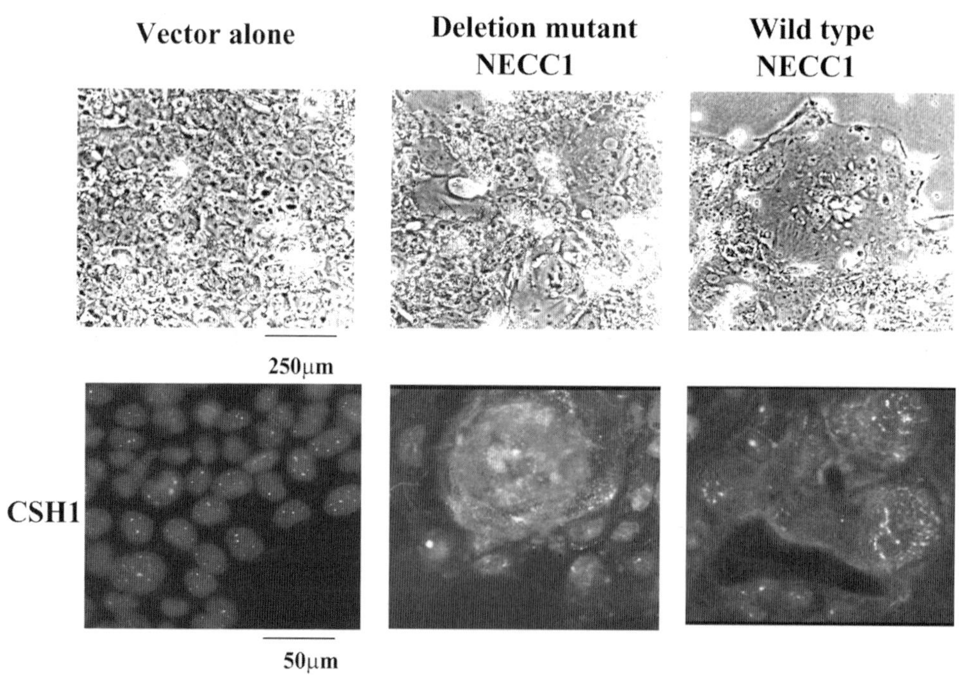

Figure 64.4 Morphology and immunofluorescent staining of NECC1 transfected BeWo cells. BeWo cells transfected with vector only, deletion mutant NECC1, and wild-type NECC1 were photographed using phase-contrast microscopy at 40. Lower photographs are immunofluorescent staining of CSH1. NECC1 deletion mutant and wild-type transfectants expressed abundant CSH1. CSH1, choriomammotropin hormone 1.

microcells from mouse A9 cells containing a single human chromosome, 1, 2, 6, 7, 9 or 11. Microcell hybrids with the introduction of chromosome 7 were suppressed or modulated for tumorigenicity and exhibited altered *in vitro* growth properties. Introduction of chromosomes 1, 2, 6, 9 or 11 had no effect. Tumorigenic revertants isolated from microcell hybrids with the introduced chromosome 7 contained reduced numbers of chromosome 7. These findings suggest that chromosome 7 contains a putative tumor suppressor gene for choriocarcinoma. Changes in the phenotypes seen in microcell hybrids were not associated with the presence of either the *ERV3* or the *H-plk* locus on the introduced chromosome 7, indicating that the putative tumor suppressor gene is outside the *ERV3* and *H-plk* gene loci. Furthermore, we obtained evidence for defining a critical region on chromosome 7 (7p12–7q11.23) that was frequently lost in surgically removed choriocarcinoma tissues and cell lines. Using a panel of microsatellite markers, biallelic deletions were observed, which strongly suggests the presence of a tumor suppressor gene within this critical region (Figure 64.4).[29]

Genome imprinting

It has been clearly established that both paternal and maternal contributions are necessary for maintaining a balanced development of both embryonic and extraembryonic tissues, and the disruption of such a balance may lead to hyperplastic proliferation of the trophoblast, which characterizes molar pregnancies. Based on this hypothesis, it is likely that genomic imprinting, which is disrupted in the androgenetic mole, may play a pivotal role in the development of choriocarcinoma. *H19* and *IGF2* are two classic examples of related imprinted genes. A high level of *H19* expression, in contrast to a considerably lower level of *IGF2* expression, was demonstrated in choriocarcinoma.[30] *P57*^{KIP2} may also play a role in the pathogenesis of gestational trophoblastic disease (GTD).[31] *P57*^{KIP2} is a cyclin-dependent kinase inhibitor and is imprinted with the maternal allele being expressed. *P57*^{KIP2} was found to be highly expressed in proliferating trophoblasts of the normal placenta, but was expressed at a low level in the complete mole and choriocarcinoma. This is in accordance with what is expected on the basis of the imprinting of the maternal allele. However, at present, their exact role and diagnostic usefulness are not clear.

Other molecular events involved in trophoblastic diseases

Malignant transformation in the hydatidiform mole is a multistep process involving the accumulation of several genetic events, including activation of oncogene and/or loss of tumor suppressor genes. A small number of oncogenes and tumor suppressor genes have been found to play putative roles in the pathogenesis of GTD. For example, the oncogenes *c-myc*, *c-erb-B-2*, *bcl-2* and *mdm-2*,[32] the guanosine triphosphatase-activating protein genes, *p53*, *p21 WAF1/KIP1* and *Rb* and the tumor suppressor gene *DOC-2/hDab2*[33] have all been listed as candidates.

There are reports of increased *c-fms* RNA in the complete mole compared with the normal placenta[34] and *c-myc* and *ras* RNA in choriocarcinomas.[35] The significance of such simple quantitative changes in proto-oncogene expression by abnormal trophoblast is hard to evaluate since several proto-oncogenes are already expressed at high levels in normal placentas.

Epidermal growth factor receptors (EGFR) are expressed more strongly in molar placentas than in normal placentas of similar gestational age. Tumors with a histological diagnosis of invasive mole and choriocarcinoma show very strong binding of EGFRs. EGFR expression has been associated with the secretion of human chorionic gonadotrophin. Following exposure to chemotherapy, EGFR binding sites have been noted to be diminished in choriocarcinoma cells.[36]

Summary

The complete mole is androgenetic in origin. The vast majority of complete moles result from the fertilization of an egg devoid of nuclei (an empty egg) by a haploid spermatozoon. Fertilization of an empty egg by two spermatozoa is responsible for a rare class of complete mole. The genome of choriocarcinoma should reflect that of the pregnancy from which the tumor arose. Thus, the predominant association of the complete mole with choriocarcinoma suggests that the molecular events for the formation of a complete mole and the malignant conversion of trophoblasts are related. The monoallelic contribution shown in the complete mole would render a certain gene susceptible to functional inactivation by ‘one-hit’ kinetics. Alternatively, uniparental transmission of genes that are subject to parental imprinting in humans would impair their regulation. Loss of *NECC1* expression, biallelic deletions at the critical (7p12–7q11.23) region and enhanced *H19* expression in choriocarcinoma would reflect the genetic features exhibited by the putative forerunner, the complete mole. In addition, alterations in gene expression profiles accompanied by malignant conversion of trophoblasts would facilitate choriocarcinogenesis from the complete mole. In the future, identification of molecular targets down- or upregulated in choriocarcinoma will provide us with the management tools for GTDs.

REFERENCES

1. Kajii T, Ohama K. Androgenetic origin of hydatidiform mole. *Nature* 1977;268:633–4.
2. Wake N, Takagi N, Sasaki M. Androgenesis as a cause of hydatidiform mole. *J Natl Cancer Inst* 1978;60:51–7.
3. Wake N, Shina Y, Ichinoe K. A further cytogenetic study of hydatidiform mole, with reference to its androgenetic origin. *Proc Jpn Acad* 1978;54:533–7.
4. Lawler SD, Pickthall VI, Fisher RA, *et al.* Genetic studies of complete and partial hydatidiform moles. *Lancet* 1979;2:580.
5. Yamashita K, Wake N, Araki T, *et al.* Human lymphocyte antigen expression in hydatidiform mole: Androgenesis following fertilization by a haploid sperm. *Am J Obstet Gynecol* 1979;135: 597–600.
6. Jacobs PA, Wilson CM, Sprenkle JA, *et al.* Mechanism of origin of complete hydatidiform moles. *Nature* 1980;268:714–6.
7. Ohama K, Kajii T, Ikamoto E, *et al.* Dispermic origin of XY hydatidiform moles. *Nature* 1981;292:551–2.
8. Wake N, Seki T, Fujita H, *et al.* Malignant potential of homozygous and heterozygous complete moles. *Cancer Res* 1984;44: 1226–30.
9. Wake N, Fujino T, Hoshi S, *et al.* The propensity to malignancy of dispermic heterozygous moles. *Placenta* 1987;8:319–26.
10. Vassilakos P, Riotton G, Kajii T. Hydatidiform mode: Two entities. A morphologic and cytogenetic study with some clinical considerations. *Am J Obstet Gynecol* 1977;127:167–70.
11. Szulman AE, Surti U. The syndromes of hydatidiform mole. I. Cytogenetic and morphologic correlations. *Am J Obstet Gynecol* 1978;131:665–71.
12. Szulman AE, Philippe E, Bou'e JG, Bou'e A. Human triploidy: Association with partial hydatidiform moles and non molar conceptuses. *Hum Pathol* 1981;12:1016–21.
13. Lawler SD, Fisher RA, Pickthall VJ, *et al.* Genetic studies on hydatidiform moles. I. The origin of partial moles. *Cancer Genet Cytogenet* 1982;5:309–20.
14. Sheppard DM, Fisher RA, Lowler SD, Povey S. Tetraploid conceptus with three paternal contributions. *Hum Genet* 1982;62:371–4.
15. Sutri U, Szulman AE, Waquer K, *et al.* Tetraploid partial hydatidiform moles: Two cases with a triple paternal contribution and a 92, XXXY karyotype. *Hum Genet* 1986;72:15–21.
16. Vejerslev LO, Ficher RA, Surti U, Wake N. Hydatidiform mole: Cytogenetically unusual cases and their implications for the present classification. *Am J Obstet Gynecol* 1987;157:180–4.
17. Wake N, Tanaka K, Chapman, *et al.* Chromosomes and cellular origin of choriocarcinoma. *Cancer Res* 1981;41:3137–43.
18. Fisher RA, Lawler SD, Povey S, *et al.* Genetically homozygous choriocarcinoma following pregnancy with hydatidiform mole. *Br J Cancer* 1988;58:788–92.
19. Chaganti RSK, Koduru PRK, Chakraborty R, Jones WB. Genetic origin of a trophoblastic choriocarcinoma. *Cancer Res* 1990;50: 6330–3.
20. Fisher RA, Paradinas FJ, Newland ES, Boxer GM. Genetic evidence that placental site trophoblastic tumours can originate from a hydatidiform mole or a normal conceptus. *Br J Cancer* 1992;65:355–8.
21. Fisher RA, Newlands ES, Jeffreys AJ, *et al.* Gestational and nongestational trophoblastic tumours distinguished by DNA analysis. *Cancer* 1992;69:839–45.
22. Arima T, Imamura T, Amada S, *et al.* Genetic origin of malignant trophoblastic neoplasms. *Cancer Genet Cytogenet* 1994;73:95–102.
23. Sasaki S, Katayama PK, Roesler M. Cytogenetic analysis of choriocarcinoma cell lines. *Acta Obstet Gynecol Jpn* 1982;34:2253–6.
24. Arima T, Imamura T, Sakuragi N, *et al.* Malignant trophoblastic neoplasms with different modes of origin. *Cancer Genet Cytogenet* 1995;85:5–15.
25. Kato H, Terao Y, Ogawa M, *et al.* Growth-associated gene expression profiles by microarray analysis of trophoblast of molar pregnancies and normal villi. *Int J Gynecol Pathol* 2002;21:255–60.
26. Asanoma K, Matsuda T, Konda H, *et al.* NECC1, a candidate choriocarcinoma suppressor gene that encodes homeodomain consensus motif. *Genomics* 2003;81:15–25.
27. Shin CH, Liu ZP, Passier R, *et al.* HOP, an unusual homeodomain protein. *Cell* 2002;110:725–35.
28. Chen F, Kook H, Milewski R, *et al.* Hop is an unusual homeobox gene that modulates cardiac development. *Cell* 2002;110:713–23.
29. Matsuda T, Sasaki M, Kato H, *et al.* Human chromosome carries a putative tumour suppressor gene(s) involved in choriocarcinoma development. *Oncogene* 1997;15:2773–81.
30. Arima T, Matsuda T, Takagi N, *et al.* Association of IGF2 and H19 imprinting with choriocarcinoma development. *Cancer Genet Cytogenet* 1997;93:39–47.
31. Chilosi M, Piazzola E, Lestani M, *et al.* Differential expression of $p57^{KIP2}$, a maternally imprinted cdk inhibitor, in normal human placenta and gestational trophoblastic disease. *Lab Invest* 1998; 78:269–76.
32. Fulop V, Mok SC, Genest DR, *et al.* c-myc, c-erbB-2, c-fms and bcl-2 oncoproteins. Expression in normal placenta, partial and complete mole, and choriocarcinoma. *J Reprod Med* 1998;43:101–10.
33. Fulop V, Colitti CV, Genest D, *et al.* DOC-2/hDab2, a candidate tumor suppressor gene involved in the development of gestational trophoblastic diseases. *Oncogene* 1998;17:419–24.
34. Maruo T, Mochizuki M. Immunohistochemical localization of epidermal growth factor receptor and myc oncogene product in human placenta: Implication for trophoblast proliferation and differentiation. *Am J Obstet Gynecol* 1987;156:721–7.
35. Cheung AN, Srivastava G, Pittaluga S, *et al.* Expression of c-myc and c-fms oncogenes in trophoblastic cells in hydatidiform mole and normal human placenta. *J Clin Pathol* 1993;46:204–7.
36. Sarkar S, Kacinski BM, Kohorn EI, *et al.* Demonstration of myc and ras oncogene expression by hybridization in situ in hydatidiform mole and in the BeWo choriocarcinoma cell line. *Am J Obstet Gynecol* 1986;154:390–3.

65 The placenta

K. Benirschke

The normal placenta

In the idealized menstrual cycle of 28 days, fertilization takes place on day 14, the developing blastocyst develops in the fallopian tube, travels through the tube to the endometrial cavity and implants on approximately day 6.[1] It usually implants on the anterior or the posterior surface of the upper endometrium, invades the decidualizing endometrium by ingesting its cells through trophoblastic activity and becomes interstitially implanted, that is to say, it becomes completely surrounded by the endometrium. At first, mostly trophoblastic proliferation takes place around a large cavity, the blastocystic cavity that contains a gel and the tiny embryo. From the gradually developing embryo, the three layers (ectoderm, mesoderm and endoderm) develop; the mesoderm expands into the future umbilical cord, and then comes to line the blastocystic cavity, thus making it the future chorionic membrane, and hence the mesoderm proliferates into the gradually developing villi, from inside outward. The trophoblast, initially polyploid, differentiates into cytotrophoblast from which the syncytiotrophoblast develops on the villous surfaces. The cytotrophoblast differentiates into two components, the villous cytotrophoblast (also called 'Langhans' layer') that underlies the syncytium, and the extravillous trophoblast. It is the latter group of cells that assume the infiltrative arm of the expanding shell; it infiltrates the decidua and, somewhat later, the endometrial (spiral) arterioles. This infiltration stops before the myometrium is reached, thus it normally leaves a thin layer of decidua basalis to remain between the villi and myometrium. It is at this interface where the Nitabuch and Rohr fibrinoid layers are produced, eosinophilic substances that are produced by the extravillous trophoblast. The latter cells, because of their formerly uncertain origin (maternal or fetal), have also been called the 'X-cells'; they often produce small cysts containing major basic protein (MBP). The MBP is similar to that found in the granules of eosinophilic polymorphonuclear cells, and it is secreted into the maternal circulation, like the human chorionic gonadotropin. Its function is completely unknown.

The embryo then lengthens and folds. From the edges of its ectodermal plate the amnionic cavity forms, which then gradually fills with clear fluid. As the embryo folds in all directions, the edges of the ectoderm and amnion come to meet over the developing umbilical cord mesenchyme and the amnion fuses with this mesenchyme tightly. As the amnion fills with fluid (perhaps derived from that contained in the extraembryonic coelom), it expands and gradually becomes passively attached to the inner surface of the chorionic membrane. It completely fuses with this membrane at about 12 weeks of gestation.[2] Prior to that fusion, it is being held in position by the gel of the extraembryonic coelom (Figure 65.1).

It is important to realize that the amnion has an inner epithelial layer that rests on a complex connective tissue layer, but it does not contain blood vessels. Moreover, the amnion can usually be dislodged from the chorionic surface of the placenta

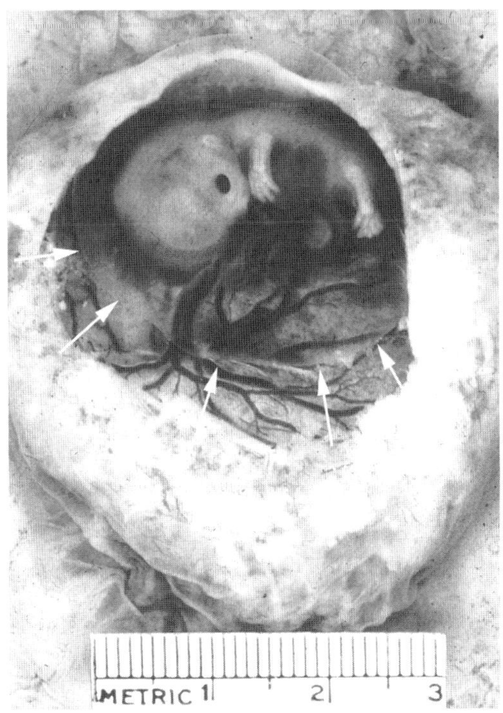

Figure 65.1 Eight weeks conceptus *in utero*. The arrows denote the edge of the expanding amnion. Note that the dome of the placental membranes is not attached to the opposite side of the uterus.

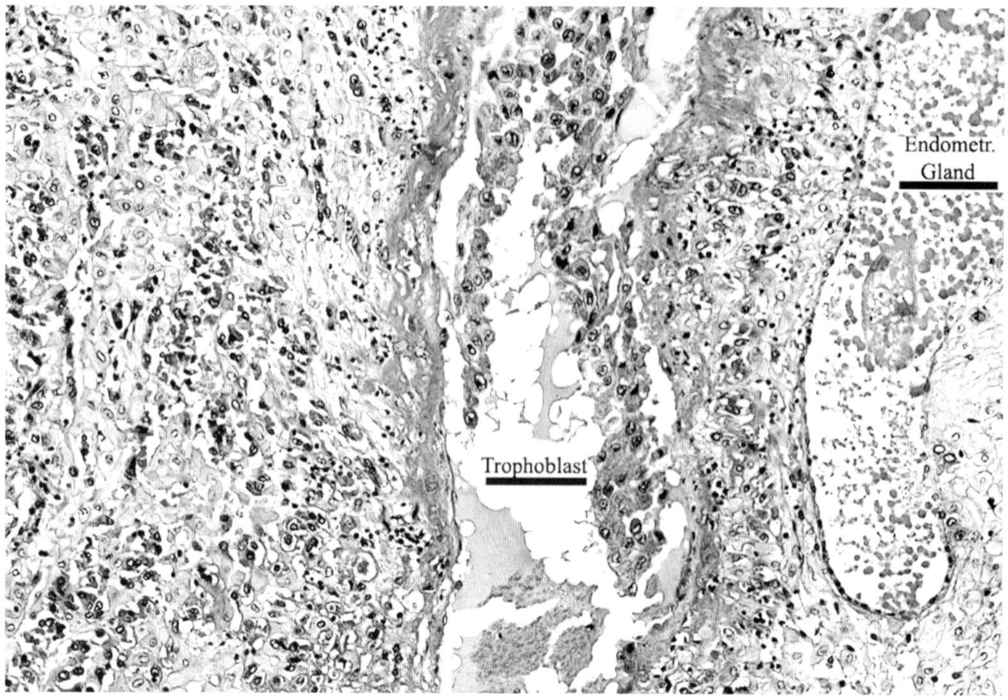

Figure 65.2 Extravillous trophoblast growing within a decidual spiral arteriole.

and is thus often disrupted by the manipulations at delivery. Furthermore, if the amnion were to disrupt prior to becoming affixed to the chorion (before 12 weeks), then amnionic bands may form, which ultimately can disrupt parts of the fetus.[3]

From the endodermal layer of the embryo develops the yolk sac. Its epithelium provides the precursors for liver, hematopoietic cells and germ cells, apart from producing the intestines after the embryo has folded. Having folded, the rotation of the intestines inside the embryo gradually pulls the yolk sac into the fetal abdominal cavity; there, it is connected to the possible remains of Meckel's diverticulum. Also from the distal part of the yolk sac, a small, temporary extension develops into the developing umbilical cord, the primitive allantoic diverticulum. It is very transitory in humans while a true sac develops in many other mammals and serves as a receptacle for fetal urine. In human placentation, the fetal urine accumulates in the amnionic cavity. Blood vessels infiltrate the villi and establish the fetal circulation somewhat later in the expansion of the villous tissue. It is not quite certain whether these vessels also differentiate *in situ* in the placental villi or whether they progress only from the fetus toward the periphery. Thus, ultimately two umbilical arteries progress from the fetus through the umbilical cord to the villous circulation, ramifying over the chorionic plate of the placenta. They are readily distinguished as arteries or veins by their position: the major arterial branches pass over the veins. They are virtually indistinguishable histologically. The vessels can be followed toward the periphery, where they are seen to dip into the villous tissue and, generally, a single vein returns to the same location as the arterial branch. Each such branch establishes a single fetal cotyledonary district whose circulation does not merge with the adjacent cotyledons.[4]

The extravillous cytotrophoblast arrodes the maternal arterioles, grows into them and there causes the 'physiologic change', altering these maternal arterial blood vessels by removing their musculature and depositing fibrinoid. At first, thick columns virtually occlude the lumens, later they hollow out and the complete intervillous circulation is then established (Figures 65.2 and 65.3). Needless to say, fetal and maternal circulations are separated by the trophoblast and a thin layer of connective tissue.

Gross examination

The placenta should be inspected after the baby is delivered and some minimal observations should be charted. It is our practice also to save the placenta in a refrigerator for several days, as its examination may be valuable for pathologists in cases where the infant is abnormal or fails to thrive. The important observations to be made at the time of delivery are the following features: (1) the length and insertion of the umbilical cord should be ascertained; (2) the presence or absence of retroplacental clot (abruptio placentae) needs to be looked for; (3) the color of the fetal surface (meconium staining or opacification from chorioamnionitis) needs to be charted and (4) the color of the villous tissue should be inspected. The last

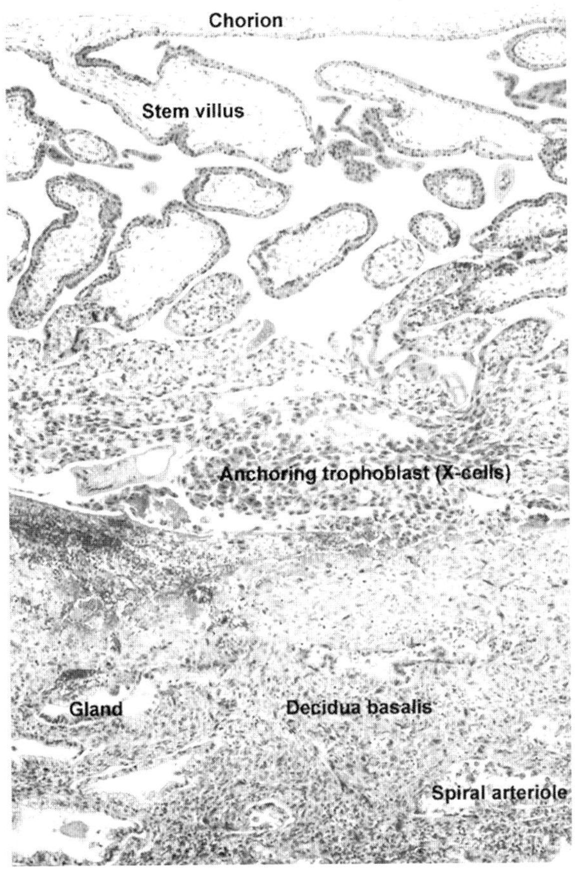

Figure 65.3 The placental floor in early implantation. The darker cells are extravillous trophoblast that intermingles with the decidual cells.

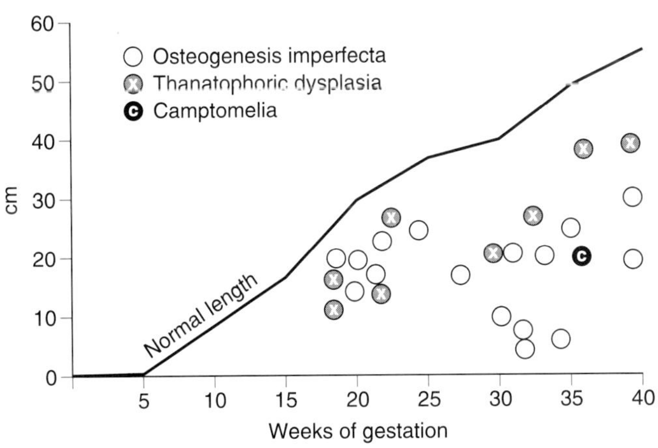

Figure 65.4 Length of umbilical cord in excessively short cord syndromes. The line represents the normal length.

observation is important as it can denote whether a baby has lost blood through transplacental hemorrhage. The color of the villous tissue is almost totally a reflection of the fetal hemoglobin content. Thus, an anemic neonate has a very pale villous tissue that may reflect erythroblastosis, parvovirus B19 infection, hemoglobinopathy or, importantly, significant fetal blood loss. If it is unusually pale (and the obstetrician of course needs to be acquainted with the normal colors), then a maternal blood film should be made immediately, which needs to be studied by the Kleihauer–Betke technique.[3] If infarcts or other unusual findings are made, the placenta should be sent for pathologic examination. Special circumstances are to be observed in multiple pregnancy and these are discussed in a subsequent section.

Umbilical cord

The normal cord insertion is somewhere near the center of the placental disk. In about 5% of normal gestations it inserts at the placental margin, and in ~1% of placentas it is located in the membranes ('velamentous insertion'). The latter is of significance in that it is often a cause of fetal growth restriction and also because the fetal vessels ramifying in the membranes have lost their protection by Wharton's jelly and may become disrupted, leading to massive fetal hemorrhage. The length of the umbilical cord is important and it can rarely be reassessed after the placenta is sent for study. Thus, it should at least be estimated, if not measured, at the time of delivery. In the normal-term gestation, the umbilical cord is approximately 55 cm long, and 85% have a counterclockwise (left) twist. The reason for this 'chirality' is unknown, but I suspect that it relates to the fetal movements because immobile fetuses, such as those found with osteogenesis imperfecta cases, have usually no twists. The cord in those cases is also unusually short (Figure 65.4). In contrast, when knots in the cord exist or when there are nuchal cords, it is often significantly lengthened. This may be the result of excessive fetal movements. It is also important to ascertain in unusually long cords whether there is excessive twisting of the cord on the surface of the fetus, the place where it inserts on the abdomen. It is not uncommon that excessive twisting leads to fetal demise, even abortions (Figure 65.4). In addition, one may find 'false knots' which represent redundancies of vessels or excess Wharton's jelly, unimportant features.

The normal umbilical cord contains three blood vessels, two arteries and one vein. In some 1% of neonates only one artery is found [single umbilical artery (SUA)] and this is frequently associated with congenital anomalies (~45%) and also with fetal trisomies. While the presence of SUA may signal the neonatologist that special attention should be paid to possible internal anomalies (heart, kidney), it is important to realize that many babies with SUA are entirely normal. True knots in the umbilical cord usually form early during development and they are now often recognized sonographically. They may lead to complete obstruction of blood flow and to fetal demise. In other cases, true knots have so impeded the venous (oxygenated blood) return from the placenta that surface thrombi will be observed on the placenta, which can even be calcified. Obviously, such features may determine whether major sequelae develop in the fetus, such as central nervous system (CNS) destruction and cerebral palsy.

The membranes

The free membranes are referred to as the chorion laeve but, in the older placental literature, all of the placenta and its membranes were referred to as the membranes or 'secundines'. The 'free' membranes as we know them now have an outer layer of deciduas capsularis, which is followed by atrophied villi in between extravillous trophoblast, then comes the chorion and innermost is the amnion. When the membranes have a measurable portion between the site of rupture and the placental disk, then it cannot have been a placenta previa if it is delivered vaginally. At the site of rupture one often finds blood clot and some inflammation can occur here from the processes of labor. Histologically, there is then deciduitis, and thrombosis may be present in the decidual blood vessels. While this may be grossly interpreted as representing an abruptio placentae, that is not quite correct, as the blood is accumulated only behind the membranes, not behind the villous tissue. Of course, since chorioamnionitis is so much more common in immature placentas, these features are much more frequently found in such births. For the pathologist, the study of the deciduas capsularis is best undertaken when a membrane roll is made so as to increase the chances of finding abnormalities. These are principally findings of 'atherosis' (alterations of decidual arteries in pre-eclampsia to be discussed below) aside from the inflammation. Since atherosis is so frequently found in these vessels, this has raised the question of where the vascular supply of the deciduas capsularis originates. It is usually assumed that the expanding membranes are merely pressed against the deciduas vera of the opposite side of the uterus and that there is perhaps no ingrowth of decidua vera into the decidua capsularis, but definitive studies have not been made. Macroscopic findings of early placentas negate this suggestion of true ingrowth from the deciduas vera (Figure 65.1).

It is important for the pathologist to recognize that the amnion consists of a single layer of epithelial cells (that occasionally have patches of squamous metaplasia) that are situated on a dense, avascular connective tissue membrane. When the amnion disrupts spontaneously before it attaches to the chorion in early pregnancy, the amnion fails to grow subsequently and may become entangled in fetal extremities when the fetus moves about. This is the mechanism for amnionic bands and its many complications, primarily digital amputations. The cause of such disruptions is unknown but does not usually relate to trauma or any antecedent event that has been elucidated. In such cases, one can invariably find a rim of amnion at the reflection of the umbilical cord, as it is here firmly affixed to the mesenchyme of the cord. Amnion nodosum is the other pathological condition worthy of note. In the absence of amnionic fluid (as in renal agenesis, polycystic kidneys, urethral obstruction, etc.) fetal urine fails to fill the sac and focal degeneration of the amnionic epithelium takes place. Amnion nodosum is most pronounced on the placental disk, never on the cord and only rarely on the free membranes. At the sites of this epithelial disruption, vernix caseosa embeds and forms microscopic nodules, the amnion nodosum. This is of course possible only after the fetus has made sufficient vernix to be embedded, and it is thus not found in very immature fetuses with renal agenesis (Figure 65.5).

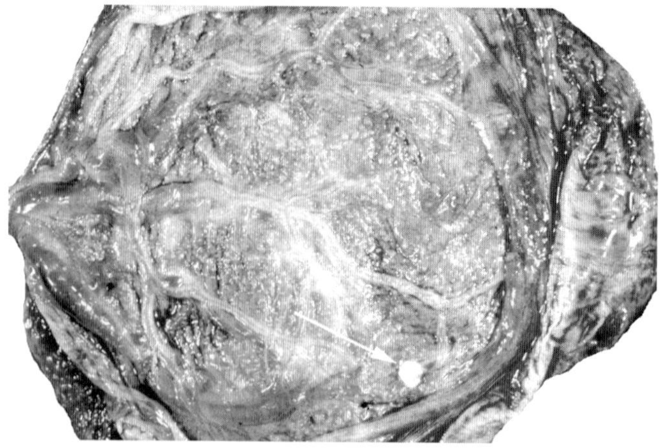

Figure 65.5 Placental surface in renal agenesis with amnion nodosum; at the arrow is the degenerated, calcified remains of the yolk sac (a normal feature).

Meconium staining of the membranes is common. It occurs in nearly 15% of our placentas and is usually the result of post-term gestations. Numerous clinical impressions have suggested that meconium discharge is the result of fetal hypoxia, but other studies indicate that this may not be so. For instance, most stillborn fetuses, assuredly having died from hypoxia, are not stained. Moreover, elevated levels of motilin (the gastrointestinal hormone that regulates bowel movements) are present. Meconium can be recognized histologically in the macrophages of amnion and chorion by their yellow pigmentation and enlargement. It must be cautioned also that this pigment disappears quickly when slides are exposed to light. Slides must thus be examined soon after their preparation. Moreover, the pigment may also be due to hemosiderin from chronic bleeding somewhere in the gestational sac; it must therefore be critically appraised.

Villous tissue

The villous tissue changes with the maturation of the placenta. In young organs, the villi are relatively

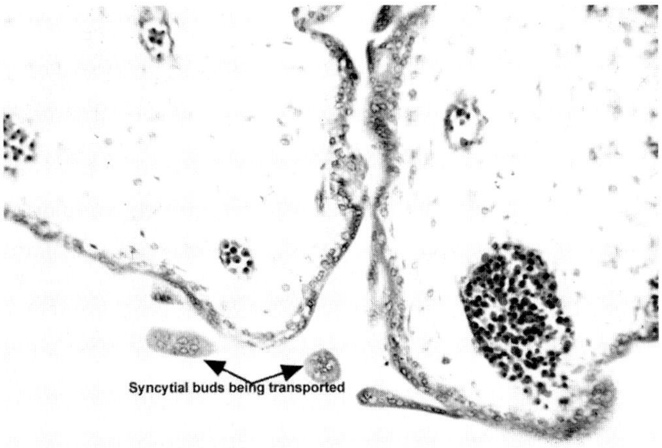

Figure 65.6 Immature villi with numerous NRBCs within the capillaries. The stroma is 'loose' and appears edematous, but that is normal. A few syncytial buds are in the process of detaching. The cytotrophoblastic Langhans' layer is visible beneath the superficial syncytium.

large, have numerous cells and the fetal capillaries are dispersed peripherally beneath the trophoblast. The villi look 'edematous' and this changes with maturity as more villi sprout peripherally (Figure 65.6). In the term placenta then the most peripheral villi are small and contain mostly three to four capillaries with few connective tissue elements. There are also some macrophages within the villi, the so-called Hofbauer cells, which are more readily seen in immature organs. They are important cells in the elimination of antigens and assist in the removal of focal hemorrhage as they occur, for instance, in cytomegalovirus (CMV) infections. They may then contain hemosiderin.

The surface of the villi is covered by trophoblast. There is an inner layer of cytotrophoblast (Langhans layer) in which mitoses occur, which produce the cytoplasm and the nuclei for the covering syncytiotrophoblast. The syncytium, however, is the actual organ of exchange. It is a single, uninterrupted membrane covering all villi, has no cell borders and the nuclei have become incapable of mitosis. The syncytiotrophoblast has a fine brush border of microvilli and its cytoplasm possesses numerous transport vesicles, and its surface has many receptor sites for nutrient exchange. Importantly, the syncytium expresses no human leukocyte antigen (HLA) antigens that could potentially excite a maternal rejection process. So far as is now known, only HLA-G is expressed and this is not antigenic to the mother. The cytotrophoblast is easily visible in young placentas, but it is difficult to recognize these cells at term, although they are always there when studied by the electron microscope. Since cytotrophoblast continues to produce new syncytium, the cells and cytoplasm of the latter bunch up and form the so-called knots, or sprouts. These increase in number toward term and then they are recognized on about 30% of peripheral villi. They also often detach and are carried away in the intervillous (maternal) circulation and swept to the maternal lung. Here they die, as they have no reproductive capacity. When the villi shrink, as is the case in pre-eclampsia, because of deficient water transfer to the fetus, there is more 'buckling' of the syncytium and more knots are found; this is referred to as the 'Tenney–Parker' change.

A number of conditions cause histologically recognizable changes in villi, the most important and frequent of which is infarction. Death of villi, usually of larger districts, is caused by the obliteration of spiral (decidual) arterioles. This occurs most commonly in pre-eclampsia and may be associated with abruption of the placenta from bleeding into the deciduas basalis. But infarcts are also common at the edge of the placenta and then they are usually without consequence. Edema of villi is a frequent finding in fetal anemia (erythroblastosis, hemoglobinopathy) and of course in hydatidiform moles. In addition, one may find inflammatory cells within the villi in the condition known as 'villitis of unknown etiology' (VUE), in CMV infections and in syphilis.

Finally, there may be too many capillaries within the terminal villi. This condition, known as chorangiosis, is seen in chronic hypoxia (e.g. in placentas from high altitude), in the Beckwith–Wiedemann syndrome, associated with chorangiomas, and a few other conditions (diabetes). When such alterations are found, one should also look for the presence of nucleated red blood cells (NRBCs) in the fetal capillaries; they are not present in placentas after about 25 weeks and, when present, they may also signal prolonged intrauterine hypoxic states.

Infections

One of the most important aspects of obstetrics today is the ascending infection with chorioamnionitis and premature birth ensuing. This is an especially important feature for the 20–30-week gestations as the often associated severe prematurity may lead to fetal infection and, most importantly, to CNS damage with cerebral palsy, the outcome. Chorioamnionitis is common and it often recurs in subsequent pregnancies. I believe that it results mainly from the deficiency of endocervical mucus that normally protects the intrauterine environment from vaginal organisms. This, in turn, probably reflects severe chronic endocervicitis. While septic distribution of some maternal organisms occurs (listeriosis, cytomegalovirus infection, toxoplasmosis), these are, numerically speaking, unimportant entities.

The endocervical canal produces copious amounts of dense mucus in normal pregnancy that contains abundant antibodies and protective immunocytes. The canal is also normally closed and narrow till labor commences. When organisms are allowed to cause endocervicitis and proliferate here, the inflammatory process generates enzymes (mainly a phospholipase)

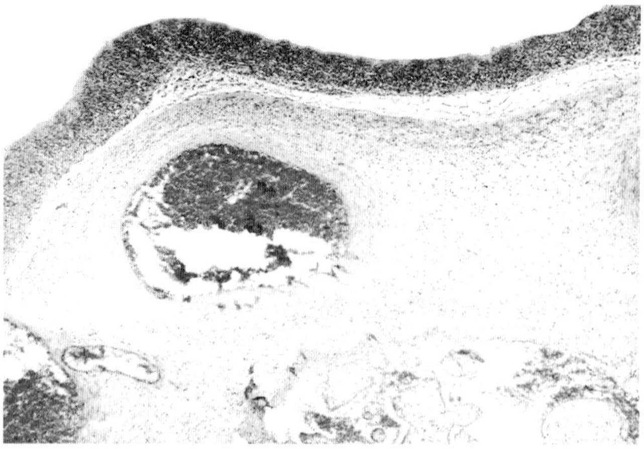

Figure 65.7 Placental surface in marked, long-standing chorioamnionitis. The dense leukocytic infiltrate is seen beneath the amnion.

that lead to the local production of prostaglandins with dilatation of the cervix followed by lower uterine segment. This, in turn, leads to deciduitis of the 'forelying' decidua capsularis and the organisms may enter the amnionic cavity, with or without the rupture of membranes. Once they are in the amnionic cavity, the leukotactic property of the organisms leads to a series of inflammatory sequelae, first on the surface of the placenta, then on the umbilical cord and, when inhaled, the infection may cause fetal pneumonia (Figure 65.7). The first effect is the emigration of maternal leukocytes from the intervillous space beneath the chorionic surface of the placenta; then inflammation of surface vessels follows; thereafter, umbilical phlebitis and finally umbilical arteritis take place. This pus that obscures the fetal surface of the placenta and makes it to be 'cloudy' (opaque) is thus of mixed origin, maternal and fetal. Studies of gastric aspirates and lung exudate have shown this admixture definitively. In time, after days of aspiration of this infective material, the fetal lung reacts with infiltration of a lymphocytic response. Often, it is possible to identify some bacterial organisms, but this is generally uncommon. The reason for our inability to recognize organisms histologically lies in the nature of the inciting antigens. They are frequently not visible in histologic sections (such as *Trichomonas*, *Mycoplasma*, *Ureaplasma*, *Chlamydia*) but they can be cultured if efforts are made. An exception is found in the infections with group B streptococci. Because of their toxins (hemolytic and cytolytic), one may identify numerous organisms, but only relatively little inflammation is found with this common infection.

Numerous attempts have been made to treat this ascending infection when it is recognized by a dilating cervix or by maternal fever, but that is usually too late in the course of the disease. Moreover, most efforts to treat the fetus *in utero* with administration of antibiotics to the mother have been unsuccessful. Thus, it becomes more important to anticipate the infection, especially its recurrent nature, and treat with antibiotics prior to the dilatation of the cervix. The pathologist observes placentas with an opacified (cloudy) fetal surface and, histologically, by the presence of numerous polymorphonuclear leukocytes in chorion and amnion (Figure 65.7). Later, there is exudation from the umbilical vein and then the arteries. The remainder of the placenta, especially its villous structures, is entirely normal, but usually immature. The membranes, however, are markedly altered. The deciduitis and often decidual necrosis are severest near the point of membrane rupture, which is very close to the endocervical canal. There may be a fresh clot attached at this site and it is occasionally mislabeled as representing an abruption. In twin gestations, it is invariably twin A, lying closest to the endocervix that has the infection and severest inflammation. Chlamydial organisms are the commonest cause of genital infection nowadays, causing urethritis, salpingitis (with infertility ensuing), cervicitis and occasionally a disseminated infection. Since this organism is not visible in routine preparations of histologic slides, it must be considered when chorioamnionitis is present.

Disseminated infections represented by lesions in the placenta are found in listeriosis. This gram-positive coccobacillus causes maternal sepsis and disseminates into the fetus most commonly via abscess formation in the placenta. Numerous epidemics have been described, which have usually been of a food-borne origin, as the organism is widespread and proliferates well in the refrigerated state. The placenta may show small abscesses and many organisms are commonly found on the placental surface. When the fetus is thus infected, the condition known as 'granulomatosis infantiseptica' may result with disseminated abscesses, meningitis, dermatitis and other sequelae. Since the organism is highly susceptible to ampicillin, early diagnosis is essential.

Toxoplasma organisms of placenta and fetus are commonly acquired parenterally from the fecal contamination originating from cats. In felines, the intestines propagate the organism and, when feces are dry and subject to dust contamination, the pregnant mother may become infected. That is an important reason for cleaning litter boxes while the fecal material is still moist. Toxoplasma cysts of a congenital infection may be seen in the chorion and even more commonly in Wharton's jelly of the umbilical cord, but they are sparse. The fetus may develop hydrocephalus and a variety of other pathologic states. The infection is easily preventable but difficult to treat once it is diagnosed.

CMV infection is also common and it may be sexually transmitted at times. It infects the villi of the placenta and can then disseminate into the fetus. The outcome is highly variable, but is often associated with growth restriction, cerebral manifestations, jaundice and other complications. The usually small placenta may show characteristic changes. In early infections, one finds inclusion bodies within villi, thrombosis of capillaries and occasional villous hemorrhages. Plasma cells that are otherwise very unusual features of normal placentas then infiltrate; eventually, the villus atrophies and hemosiderin pigment deposit in Hofbauer cells. The antigen is easily demonstrated with modern techniques of antibody-marked histologic staining, as is of course the case also with the determination of serum antibodies. When the infection is longstanding and when it is severe, thrombi may develop even in the larger surface vessels (Figure 65.8), and these may be calcified as well.

Only a few other disseminated infections are of importance. Thus, varicella infection has been described rarely, hepatitis antigens can cross the placenta, Coxsackie viruses have been transmitted with few placental lesions visible and the placenta may also contain numerous intervillous malaria organisms during a malaria attack. Transmission to the fetus transplacentally, however, of the widespread malaria infection is extremely rare.

A final comment must be made about a reasonably common condition known as VUE. This condition is frequently found in the placenta of growth-restricted fetuses and in stillbirths. Worse, it often recurs in subsequent pregnancies. When large districts of the placenta are so affected, fetal demise is common but there are no abnormal findings of any infectious nature in the fetal tissues. The villi in VUE are probably infiltrated by maternal T-cells and macrophages. They here cause an obliteration of the capillary beds and the restrictive cause of fetal growth is therefore readily understood. But the precise cause of why the maternal lymphocytes invade the placenta is as yet unknown. It has been speculated that this is akin to a 'rejection' phenomenon, but why the fetal HLA type should be recognized by the mother's immune cells is so far obscure.

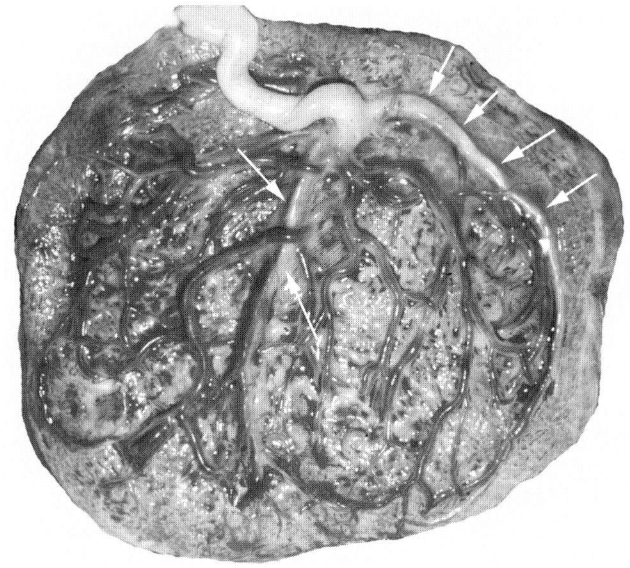

Figure 65.8 Placenta in severe CMV infection with extensive venous thromboses at arrows. The thrombi were at least partially calcified.

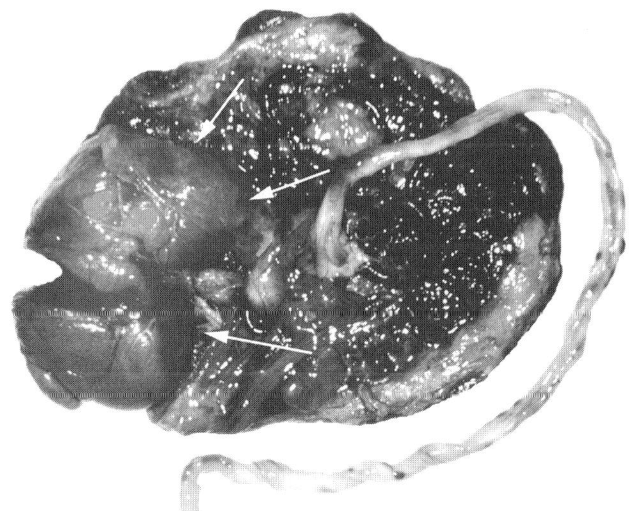

Figure 65.9 Large chorioangioma bulging from the placental surface at left.

Tumors and microchimerism

The commonest tumor of the placenta is the chorangioma.[6] It is frequently found only accidentally in sections prepared at random. Angiomas occur in villi as an expansion of the fetal capillary and mesenchymal cells; they form nodules that can be seen grossly and which are easily shelled out of their beds. Interestingly, their surface is usually covered by a single layer of trophoblast that suggests the expansion of fetal vessels being very focal in nature. Chorangiomas occur more frequently at high altitude and are often also associated with 'chorangiosis', an increase of the normal number of capillaries in the peripheral villi. They are benign tumors despite their frequently great cellularity. In fact, chorangiomas have been mislabeled in the past as being sarcomas, mesenchymomas or have been assigned other appellations, but they have never metastasized. Large chorangiomas may protrude on the fetal surface (Figure 65.9); they may be one cause of hydramnios and they may also infarct from thrombosis resulting in cessation of the hydramnios. Recent studies have shown that they are at least in part the result of increased angiopoietin expression.[7] On rare occasions, the angioma may be associated with an excessive degree of trophoblastic proliferation. This condition has been labeled 'chorangiocarcinoma', but its true nature and degree of malignancy are still poorly defined.

Maternal tumors have also been found to have set metastases in the placenta occasionally, perhaps most commonly the carcinoma of the breast. They may focally destroy placental tissue but most of them do not disseminate into the fetus. This only contrasts with the occasional metastatic melanomas, which can travel into the fetus, but here the metastases are usually rejected in neonatal life. Maternal B-cell lymphomas have been described recently as having disseminated into villi and they have caused neonatal deaths from tumor dissemination. Most maternal leukemias, however, do not spread to villi or to fetus. The situation differs with fetal cells disseminating into the mother transplacentally. It is now recognized that fetal cells often traverse the placenta in small numbers. These are mostly RBCs, but nucleated elements have also reached the maternal circulation, perhaps even fetal stem cells. In the maternal organism, these elements may live for many years and, perhaps as determined by their antigenic expression, they may be destroyed in the mother. Recent studies, however, have also shown that some of these fetal cells themselves may impart an antibody/rejection response against the mother. This microchimerism is now thought to be the cause of some maternal autoimmune diseases, such as systemic sclerosis and postpartum thyroiditis. Indeed, it has been shown that the maternal thyroid epithelium may on occasion be replaced by fetal cells when postpartum thyroiditis has occurred.

Choriocarcinoma *in situ* has been described a few times in otherwise normal placentas and this tumor has even been disseminated into the mother. Macroscopically, such tumors have given the impression of being infarcts, and only histologic preparations have shown them to be malignant neoplasms. In some cases, the tumor has caused villous destruction with exsanguination of the fetus into the mother. This entity is completely unrelated to the usual cause of choriocarcinoma that may follow the presence of a hydatidiform mole, and its chromosomes have not yet been studied. The reason for their occurrence is obscure.

Moles

When the villi swell up with much fluid from the intervillous space by transport through the syncytium, they swell and may become so swollen as to take on a grape-like configuration that is grossly visible. We refer to this as hydatid swelling and it is doubtlessly related to the deficient movement of the accumulated fluid to the fetus because the fetus has died and the fetal placental circulation has ceased. The result is the formation of (a) 'hydatid degeneration' of the placenta in abortion and (b) hydatidiform moles (mole merely means mass). Because the entire placental tissue may not have become transformed into grape-like masses, we speak of 'partial hydatidiform moles' (PHM) and also of 'complete hydatidiform moles' (CHM). The former may represent a variety of conditions; triploidy of the conceptus is the commonest antecedent condition, but PHM may also be due to a set of twins, the placenta of one having become truly molar, i.e. a CHM.

The differentiation of these two types of moles is not always easy, but it should be attempted. When two separate masses or a distinctly divided placenta is present, twinning is the most likely origin. But the differentiation of PHM and CHM may often present difficulties for the pathologist and a strong recommendation has been made to submit some of the abnormal tissue for ploidy analysis that is most efficiently done by flow cytometry, or for cytogenetic study. Flow cytometry is the easiest and the quickest way for this differential diagnosis. It quickly identifies triploidy ($3n$) from diploidy ($2n$) and this is relevant primarily because triploid moles are only exceptionally rarely followed by gestational trophoblastic neoplasms (GTNs).

Partial moles (PHM) are most commonly the result of fertilization of one oocyte by two spermatozoa. This imbalance leads to defective fetal development and, usually, the embryo dies early while the placenta continues to grow and accumulates fluid. It is much less common that a polar body (two maternal components – gynogenic) provides the additional set of chromosomes. In such pregnancies, there is considerably better fetal development. Nevertheless, the embryo develops somewhat abnormally and shows numerous anomalies that are invariably lethal soon after birth. One of the more characteristic anomalies is the fusion of two fingers and often also of toes. The placentas of PHM are enlarged, irregularly molar and the villi have scalloped borders that often lead to trophoblastic inclusions. These inclusions are not truly invasive features, but represent tangential sections through infolded surfaces.

The CHM is similarly enlarged but more uniformly (Figure 65.10). The distension is mostly within the terminal villi and these can often be traced to thinner and firmer structures represented by the former stem villi that do not participate so much in the swelling. The amount of trophoblastic development varies greatly in CHM; at times it is massive and suspicious of tumor development. But the former method of 'grading moles', depending on the amount and nature of trophoblastic proliferation, has been abandoned as it has proven to have little prognostic significance. The villi of CHM have no capillaries, in contrast to what is often the case in PHM. Since the revolutionary insight gained by Kajii and Ohama,[8] it is now accepted that CHM is 'androgenetic'. That is to say, their chromosomes are derived only from the spermatozoon. They are also $2n = 46$,XX because a Y-bearing sperm would lead to a $2n = 46$,YY conceptus and those cells are not viable. Thus, one can easily understand the development of a CHM by visualizing the fertilization by an X-bearing spermatozoon of an 'empty' egg, i.e. an oocyte that has lost its nucleus. The 23,X chromosomes (from the spermatozoon) of

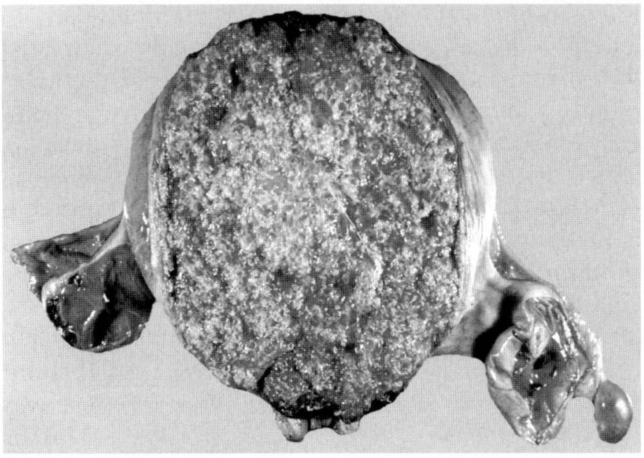

Figure 65.10 Uterus filled with a CHM. The ovaries are enlarged because of gonadotropin stimulation.

the newly fertilized oocyte would then duplicate. But, because of imprinting features, an ovum fertilized by only male chromosomes does not develop a functional embryo; it can only produce a placenta. When early complete moles have been carefully examined, diminutive embryos are found occasionally; they are severely stunted and would soon have vanished. Thus, CHMs have generally no fetus and no vasculature, and there is also no recognizable amnionic cavity. For the sake of completeness, it must be mentioned that a few exceptions have been reported. Thus, a rare gynogenic mole has been found; also rarely, a diploid spermatozoon has led to the formation of moles and, equally amazing, a small number of CHMs fertilized by two sperms were found to be $2n = 46,XY$. These aberrations from the usual, however, have not had different sequelae.

Because the swelling of terminal villi and the enlargement of a molar placenta obviously take time to develop, really early CHMs may be difficult to identify; they may appear to be spontaneous abortions, i.e. 'blighted ova'. In addition, spontaneous intermixtures of normal villi and molar villi have been observed in chimeras. However, all of these are uncommon features. They merely indicate that detailed study may be needed to unravel what is otherwise a great biologic complexity. Furthermore, nobody has described an empty egg, which we hypothesize as being the starting point for molar development. We thus assume that some abnormality in the maternal oocyte nucleus exists that prevents it from participating in embryonic development. What this is, is being studied. Occasional chromosomal errors and genetic defects have thus been identified, but that is in a minority of cases so far. We may need more information on the reasons for the great geographic/racial differences in the occurrence of CHMs to attain a better understanding of its real causes. Genetic errors have been identified on occasion as the basis for familial moles. But why it is that CHMs occur in European/American stock with a frequency of ~1:2000 and in the Japanese population, for instance, as commonly as in ~1:350 is not known now.

Trophoblastic tumors

Choriocarcinoma is the most malignant, albeit uncommon, outcome of hydatidiform moles. But other neoplastic entities are now recognized (epithelioid trophoblastic tumor; placental site nodule; exaggerated placental site) so that they have now all been grouped as GTNs. Nevertheless, the choriocarcinoma is the best recognized and the most frequent of these tumors. It is composed solely of trophoblast, cytotrophoblast and syncytiotrophoblast, and most commonly it follows complete moles. Because the choriocarcinoma continues to produce chorionic gonadotropin, it is easily screened for and the follow up of moles is usually undertaken with serial determination of gonadotropin levels. The other unusual feature of these tumors, especially the choriocarcinoma, is that it is highly susceptible to methotrexate and actinomycin D therapy. Even metastatic lesions are mostly treated successfully now when they are recognized early enough.

While choriocarcinoma most commonly follows a CHM, it may also arise from abortions, even from ectopic pregnancies. It may be present accidentally in an otherwise normal placenta and is then referred to a choriocarcinoma *in situ*. It then looks like some bland infarct, but may of course have serious sequelae. What causes choriocarcinoma to develop is uncertain, although it would appear that excessive proliferation of trophoblast is a precursor, as it is engendered often in moles. The tumor is usually very hemorrhagic and metastases occur anywhere but they are most feared when they occur in the brain.

The other tumorous lesions referred to above are more characteristically produced by the extravillous trophoblast, the X-cells whose main purpose is the invasion of the uterus and the modulation of the uterine vessels. By and large, these tumors are much less common; they usually behave in a less malignant fashion and can often be treated by excision.

Multiple pregnancies

Twinning is common and monozygotic (MZ) – 'identical' – and dizygotic (DZ) – 'fraternal' – twins occur (Figure 65.11). When higher than twin multiple pregnancies take place, MZ and DZ multiples may be admixed. In order to understand the placenta of monozygotic twins it is necessary that one visualizes the stages at which the 'splitting' of the developing embryo can occur (Figure 65.12). Thus, when segregation of blastomeres takes place very early (during the first 3 days), then the two entirely separate placentas

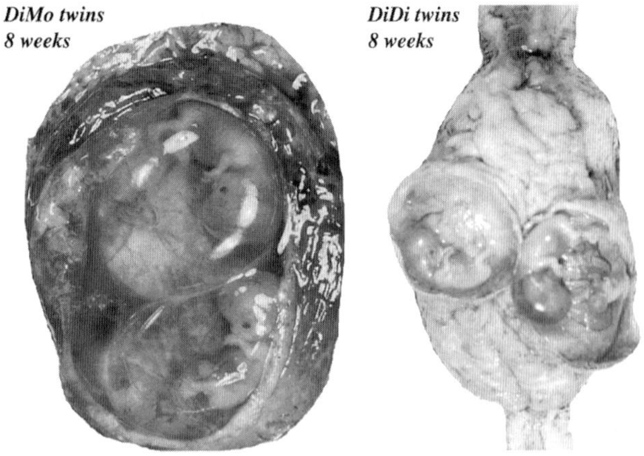

Figure 65.11 Two uteri within which are 8-week-old twin fetuses. At the left are monochorionic (identical) twins with their amnionic sacs. At the right are two fraternal, dichorionic twins within adjacent placental implantations.

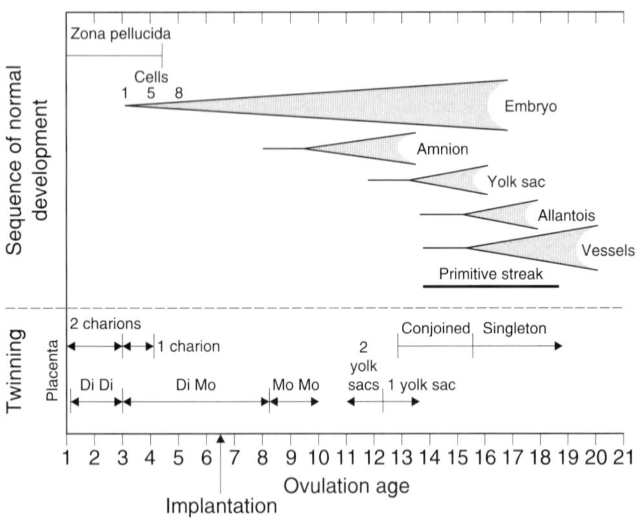

Figure 65.12 Conceptual drawing of early splitting of embryos/placentas in the process of producing monozygotic twins.

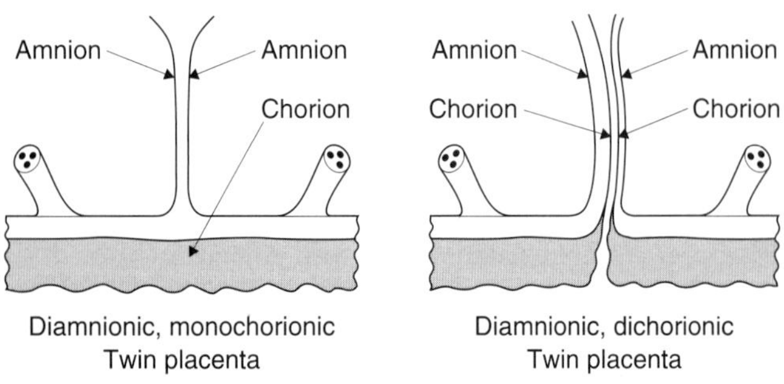

Figure 65.13 Diagram to show the membrane relationship in monochorionic twin placentas (left) and dichorionic twin placentas (right).

may develop; but when it occurs later, a single chorion and two amnions develop; and when it occur later still, a monoamnionic sac can be produced. Eventually, after 13 days of development, twinning becomes impossible or else conjoined twins would develop. Therefore, the placenta of MZ twins may be dichorionic (20%) or monochorionic (80%). This is what is actually found and it is important as the classification of twins may depend on this; and so does the formation of blood vessels that may connect the two fetal circulations. The anastomotic connections then occur only in MZ and monochorionic twins; DZ twins virtually never have such anastomoses and are worthy of being reported.

The frequency of DZ twins depends largely on the genetic factors that control polyovulation. Polyovulation is controlled by maternal FSH levels; it is very high in the Nigerian Yoruba tribe, but much lower in Oriental people. Therefore, the percentage of MZ twins is much higher in Japan than it is in African or European populations. The consequences of this are significant also as most problems in the placentation of twins occur with monochorionic (MZ) twins.

The placenta of dichorionic twins is easy to understand (Figures 65.11 and 65.13). The two blastocysts implant either side by side in the uterus or on opposite surfaces. Two fused placentas may thus arise, having a diamnionic, dichorionic 'dividing membrane'. Sonographically, this is commonly recognized by the thickness of the membrane and by a small elevation of the placental tissue at the meeting point of the chorionic surface. The pathologist observes that these membranes are thicker, less translucent and that atrophied blood vessels may be apparent in the dividing membranes. Anastomoses between the two fetal circulations do not occur or are so rare that they warrant a case report. The umbilical cords of both types of twins are much more often marginally (or membranous–velamentous) inserted. That is also the case of occasional singleton placentas, but in twins it may be the consequence of competition for space in an expanding placenta. Alternatively, it may be the result of improper early central implantation but the precise mechanics are undetermined. Importantly, such abnormal cord insertion may also be found on the dividing membranes and the velamentous vessels then represent a danger of disruption when these are ruptured during delivery.

Monochorionic placentas in contrast nearly always have blood vessel connections on the fetal surface. These take essentially three forms: most common is an artery-to-artery communication (Figure 65.14); the next most common are artery-to-vein connections and vein-to-vein anastomoses are least often found. The connections are readily identified in the delivered placenta. One may stroke blood back and forth in an artery–artery (AA) anastomosis; the recognition of artery–vein (AV) connections is much more difficult and it is also the most important and troublesome

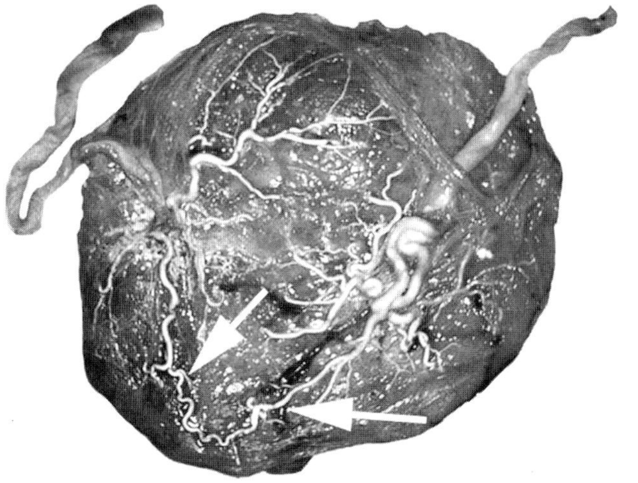

Figure 65.14 Monochorionic twin placenta with a single large artery-to-artery anastomosis (at arrows).

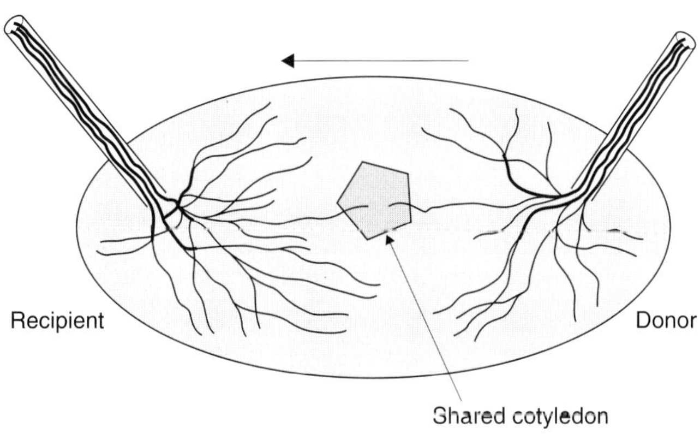

Figure 65.15 Drawing to show the shared cotyledon in a monochorionic twin placenta with the TTTS.

connection. Injection with milk or other fluids makes it easy to recognize the type of anastomosis, and it is usually necessary to undertake such injections if the AV anastomosis of the twin-to-twin-transfusion syndrome (TTTS) is to be understood. As has been said earlier, arteries generally cross over the veins, especially in the larger vessels. They are thus easily recognized and their course can be followed by careful gross inspection. Generally speaking, in the normal placenta an arterial branch distributes blood to a single cotyledon. When this branch is followed to its end, the artery suddenly stops, bends down into the villous and then perfuses one cotyledon. Nearby, a vein emerges from this cotyledon and sends blood back to the umbilical vein. In the TTTS, however, this vein sends blood back to the other twin, thus establishing the basis for the TTTS. One needs to inject these suspect terminal arterial branches, fill the cotyledon completely and see the injected material emerge in the vein of the 'recipient' twin in order to establish the basis for the TTTS. There may be several such 'common districts' (they have been referred to as the 'third circulation') and they may even have different directions. Their net size determines the severity of the TTTS; it is generally held now that the coexistence of an AA communication prevents this syndrome in its worst states.

In such monochorionic twin placentas (the majority are diamnionic, monochorionic – DiMo), the dividing membranes are composed of two amnions; they are translucent and lack the remnants of former vessels.

The most important and frequent complication of MZ twinning is the TTTS. It comes about by the presence of a single 'shared (common) cotyledon' (Figure 65.15). An artery from the donor enters one cotyledon and this is drained to the recipient who becomes fluid-overloaded and because of excessive urination develops hydramnios. That is how the syndrome usually becomes symptomatic, most frequently between 20 and 30 weeks of gestation. The donor urinates little or not at all and becomes the 'stuck twin'. Hydramnios usually terminates the pregnancy unless it is treated by the modern method of laser obliteration of the offending vessels. In order to do this surgery, one requires considerable knowledge of the vascular features of the placental surface and it should not be attempted unless this detailed knowledge is acquired. It must also be appreciated that even large intertwin anastomoses may have other serious sequelae. Thus, when one DiMo twin dies *in utero*, blood may be transferred rapidly from the surviving twin back into the now dead fetus. This can lead to an at least temporary deficient CNS perfusion in the survivor and thus, cerebral palsy in one of the surviving twins is relatively common. Such a mechanism is also implored in understanding the death of the later-dying original 'Siamese' twin pair (Eng).

Monoamnionic twins are always monochorionic (MZ) and thus suffer the possibility of entangling of their umbilical cords. Complex knots may develop early in fetal life and they may become constrictive and cause fetal demise (Figure 65.16). At times, one finds thrombi in such umbilical cords or in blood vessels of the chorionic surface from the chronically restricted blood flow during intrauterine life. Moreover, chorangiosis is often observed in such placentas.

Acardiac twins occur in many forms; some are nearly perfectly formed babies, but most are severely abnormal and they may even grossly appear as though they were skin-covered teratomas. Most acardiacs also have a single umbilical artery. They are always MZ, or identical, although they represent the worst possible congenital abnormality imaginable. The formation of acardiacs is best explained by the presence of both an AA and a VV anastomosis in the surface of the placenta (Figure 65.17). We believe that in very early embryonic development, the normal twin causes a

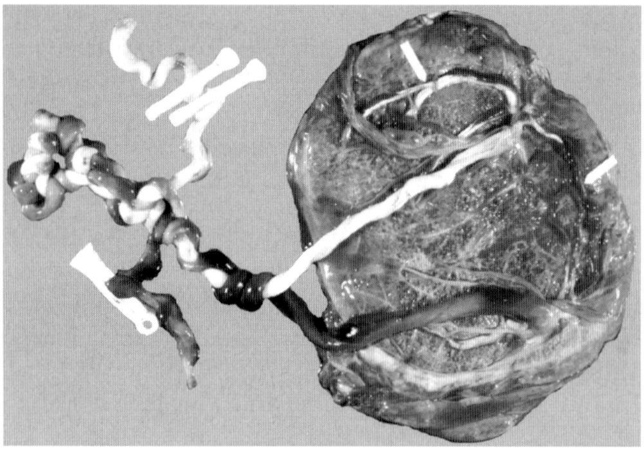

Figure 65.16 Monoamnionic twin placenta with extensive entangling of umbilical cords that led to fetal demise.

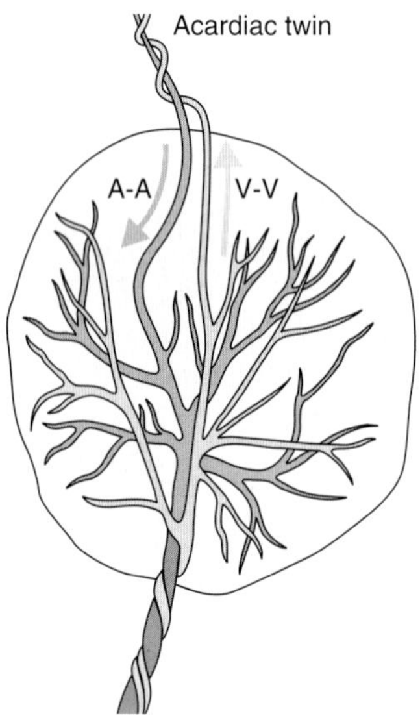

Figure 65.17 Drawing to show the setup of the vascular connections that lead to the development of an acardiac twin.

reversal of blood flow through the AA connection and the VV, thus returning the blood in the opposite direction; perhaps, they were then already of different sizes. Because blood from the artery now enters the developing acardiac fetus at its abdomen, the legs develop more adequately, while the cephalic end is usually most deficiently developed. And, because of the reversal of flow, the heart of the acardiac develops poorly (it may be two-chambered) or not at all. These acardiac fetuses are chromosomally generally normal and of the same sex as the cotwin. It might be mentioned also that such acardiacs have been reported quite accidentally in many different species.

When many more fetuses are implanted, a condition that is now much more common with the practice of 'assisted reproductive technology' (ART), the placentas may be closely packed and have no blood vessel connections. They generally have abnormal cord insertions and, depending on their number, many are born prematurely. It has also been our observation that frequently one or more of the fetuses are surgically eliminated by KCl injection and a fetus papyraceus is then found in the membranes with a markedly atrophied placenta. What is amazing in such specimens is the marked spiraling of their cords, as this must have originated very early in development. Finally, the placentas of such ART pregnancies present challenging problems in that more fetuses and placentas may be found than embryos originally implanted into the uterus. Thus, monochorionic twins are admixed and can only be explained by assuming that one embryonic precursor has split early in gestation. Perhaps, the practice of embryonic culture *in vitro* for several days is responsible for this spontaneous MZ twinning event.

Abortions

Spontaneous abortions are very common in human development. They are much more common than in most species that have been studied in detail. The vast majority occurs during the first 3 months of gestation and the majority is due to chromosomal errors. Generally, a deformed or macerated embryo is found on examination of the specimen but equally often, especially in the earliest abortions, the amnionic sac is empty and the fetal vasculature of the placenta has atrophied; these specimens are often referred to as blighted ovum. The placenta is otherwise atrophied and may have focal hydatid changes of the villi. The trophoblast is unremarkable or atrophied. Occasional retroplacental hemorrhages accompany these specimens. A frequent cause of spontaneous abortion is the presence of an excessively long umbilical cord with severe twisting (Figure 65.18). The causes of the twisting and excessive length of the cord are unknown but I speculate that this is the result of excessive movements in early life. It often leads to severe twisting on the surface of the umbilical cord insertion on the abdominal surface, which must be observed to understand this cause of embryonic demise.

Placental and fetal hydrops

The placenta of hydropic fetuses is much enlarged and most often very waterlogged. The villi are swollen and often contain prominent Hofbauer cells (macrophages). There are many causes for hydrops and depending on their nature, the histopathology differs. In erythroblastosis and in the placentas of the fetal thalassemias, the capillaries contain NRBCs in profusion. In transplacental infection with parvovirus B19, one may find characteristically nuclear inclusion bodies that are found most often within the nucleated red cells. But, at later stages, they may be

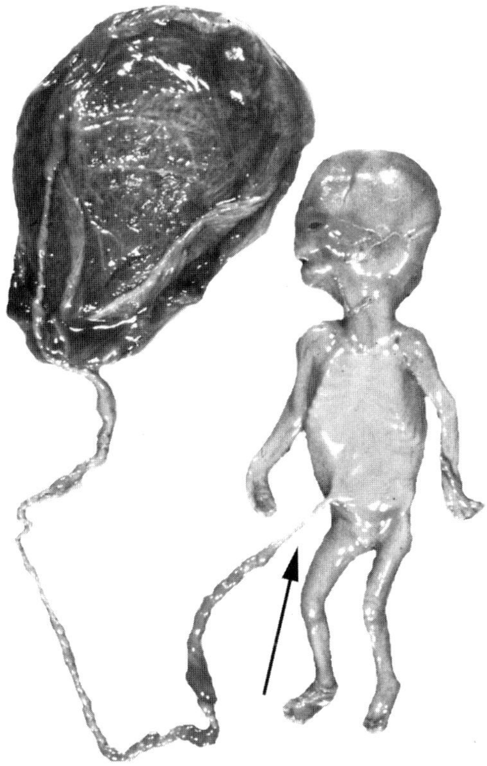

Figure 65.18 Abortus with an excessively long and heavily twisted umbilical cord and the even more excessive twisting on the abdominal surface of the fetus.

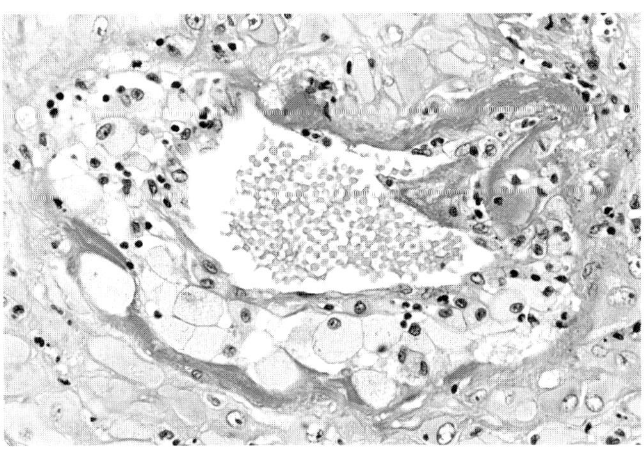

Figure 65.19 Atherosis in the spiral arteriole of a patient with severe pre-eclampsia.

inconspicuous and identification of the etiology of hydrops will commonly depend on serologic findings or on staining the tissue with specific antibodies. When the hydrops is caused by fetal anomalies, such as left heart hypoplasia, cystic adenomatous malformation of the lung, sacrococcygeal teratoma, etc., the placenta is merely large, edematous and pale. Some of the other fetal conditions that lead to hydrops are summarized below.

Maternal and fetal diseases affecting the placenta

Pre-eclampsia

The cause of pre-eclampsia [or pregnancy-induced hypertension (PIH)] is still unknown, but speculations about its origin abound. Less controversial are the placental sequelae in PIH. Generally speaking, the placenta is smaller and exhibits what is called 'advanced maturation'. This is a misnomer, however, and merely applies to the histologic features of such placentas as having smaller villi; they appear to be more mature than would be expected at the usually immature gestational age. The villi are not only smaller but also have less mesenchymal fluid content. As a consequence, the superficial cover of trophoblast buckles and more knots or 'sprouts' of syncytium become apparent. This is referred to as the Tenney–Parker change, after the first authors to describe this feature. This increased number of sprouts (more than 30% of terminal villi) also leads to their more frequent deportation in the maternal circulation and was thus witnessed as a peculiarity of women dying in eclampsia as they had more such elements in their pulmonary capillaries.

Pre-eclampsia is associated characteristically with the presence of atherosis in the maternal, decidual spiral arterioles. It is conceived that the normal transformation of these blood vessels does not occur because of inadequate extravillous trophoblastic infiltration in early development. The atherosis is reasonably characteristic for PIH and may be found in the decidua basalis and also (often easiest) in the decidua capsularis of the membranes. But, not in all cases of even severe PIH can one find this change; it can also be associated with thrombosis. Atherosis affects only the maternal arterial bed; it spares the veins. Characteristically, it consists of the deposition of foam cells (cholesterol-laden macrophages) in the lumen and wall of the arterioles (Figure 65.19). This lesion may obstruct blood flow, as thrombosis would also do and thereby lead to placental/fetal hypoxia and typically to placental infarcts. When infarcts are of recent origin, they still have fetal blood remaining and they are red. As infarcts age, they lose the fetal hemoglobin and become pale and, eventually white. They are firm and sharply delimited from the spongy adjacent placenta tissue. In contrast to the more common marginal infarcts seen in normal placentas, infarcts of PIH are distributed centrally. They also may surround focal intervillous thrombi, which are characterized by a laminated appearance due to the 'lines of Zahn' in a thrombus. The occlusion of maternal spiral arterioles also causes the degeneration of decidua basalis and destruction of maternal veins. This may lead to hemorrhages and the condition is known as abruptio placentae (Figure 65.20). While abruption is commonest in PIH, it also can occur in traumatic injuries to the placenta. For instance,

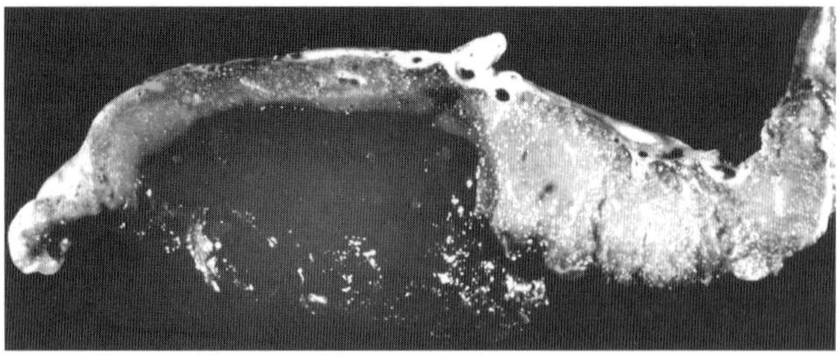

Figure 65.20 Abruptio placentae with fetal demise in pre-eclampsia. Note the compression of nearly one-half of the placenta. Infarcts are also present.

amniocentesis occasionally needs to be done by trespassing the placental tissue and that can disrupt major blood vessels. More common though is abruption of the placenta in automobile accidents, for instance, when a seat belt injures the pregnant uterus. Very rarely, an abruption was caused by external version of a breech presentation; thus, it needs to be borne in mind that this can occur when versions are attempted. It is not uncommon that small retroplacental hematomas are found on careful examination, especially adjacent to placental infarcts. When they are as large and sudden as shown in Figure 65.20, however, they are lethal for the fetus.

One feature of placental infarcts differs from infarcts occurring in other organs (e.g. the kidney), namely, the dead tissue does not become 'organized' in the usual sense. That is to say, blood vessels from the adjacent tissues do not enter the infarct and the dead tissue is also not removed by macrophage activity.

Placenta percreta

It is normal for placentation that a small amount of decidua basalis separates the villi from the myometrium. It is not fully understood why it is that the trophoblast stops invading or destroying the endometrium at that point, as one can readily find X-cells in the myometrium underlying most placental sites and they are found in myometrial blood vessels beneath the placenta. Only when there is insufficient decidua present does the villous portion of the placenta attach itself to the myometrium and then form a placenta accreta. I believe that this occurs most commonly because prior disease (e.g. tuberculosis or chronic endometritis) has destroyed the endometrium and endometrial repair does not take place by lateral growth of endometrium. Thus, when a placenta implants over a prior curettage site, the development of focal placenta accreta may occur. It is generally witnessed only by the disruption of the placental floor when the placenta is examined or clinically by postpartum bleeding. Thus, when placental tissue remains attached to a focus of myometrium, a placental 'polyp' may form, which is composed of fragments of placental tissue enmeshed in blood clot and is occasionally accompanied by inflammation. Also, because of insufficient decidualization of the higher endocervical canal, placenta previa is often associated with focal placenta accreta.

When deeper infiltration of the myometrium by placental tissue has occurred, we speak of placenta increta and when it has penetrated, we refer to it as placenta percreta. These terms are frequently misinterpreted to mean that the placenta has actually invaded the myometrium to destroy it and 'grow through the endometrium', to emerge on the peritoneal surface. This is really true only of ectopic pregnancies in the fallopian tube. When they rupture, this is due to placenta percreta but primarily so because there is only minimal or absent decidualization, thus ensuring that a placenta percreta can form; and because of the thinness of the tubal wall, rupture may occur when the conceptus enlarges. It must be said, however, that ever so rarely a full-term gestation takes place in the tube. Moreover, all abdominal implantations are placentas accreta and it is for that reason that the placenta will not detach on delivery. It has also recruited an enormous blood supply from the neighborhood.

Placenta percreta has become more common in recent years and it is now often diagnosed sonographically. Virtually, invariably this is the result of a prior cesarean section. When the uterus is sutured, usually by a single layer of resorbable fibers, the edges of the prior incision are poorly aligned and since there is no new growth of myometrium to connect the edges, repair occurs by connective tissue. When a new pregnancy takes place, this scar widens and thins; when a placenta is attached directly over the site, it may appear as though it has penetrated the uterus, but that occurs only by separating the myometrial edges from the prior cesarean section. Thus, having implanted on connective tissue (instead of the normal decidua), the placenta may even attach itself to the posterior surface of the urinary bladder. On occasion, some bladder wall is removed at the excision of such specimens and it appears as though a true invasion has taken place. But that is no more than the usual infiltration of extravillous trophoblast into the uterine musculature that occurs in all pregnancies. In other words, while it is theoretically possible that an occasional placenta may truly invade, the common placenta percretas are the result of insufficient healing of a prior section scar. It might be mentioned parenthetically that, when a pathologist has the opportunity to examine the hysterectomy specimens of such percretas, the endocervical canal is tough to cut, it is firmly closed and it is filled with that sticky mucus that normally prevents ascending infection of the amnionic cavity.

Fetal storage diseases

Numerous storage diseases of the fetus, the so-called 'errors of metabolism', affect the placental morphology.

One of the first to be recognized was 'I-cell disease' in which the trophoblastic cells show diffuse vacuolation. The same is true for many other storage diseases and, to differentiate among them, it is necessary to undertake enzyme studies. Fetal leukemia occurs occasionally and can be recognized by the circulating nucleated cells, but care must be taken not to overinterpret these as they may be a transitory phenomena, for instance, in Down's syndrome. More important are fetal neuroblastoma and sacrococcygeal teratoma; both may present as hydrops with typical swelling and edema of the villi. In neuroblastoma, however, the neuroblasts are seen to plug many capillaries and occasional rosettes may be identified.

REFERENCES

1. Hertig AT. *Human Trophoblast*. Springfield: Charles C Thomas, 1968.
2. Boyd JD, Hamilton WJ. *The Human Placenta*. Cambridge: W Heffer, 1970.
3. Benirschke K, Kaufmann P, Baergen R. *The Pathology of the Human Placenta*, 5th edn. New York: Springer-Verlag, 2006.
4. Wigglesworth JS. Vascular anatomy of the human placenta and its significance for placental pathology. *J Obstet Gynaecol Br Commonw* 1969;76:979.
5. Landing BH. Amnion nodosum: A lesion of the placenta apparently associated with deficient secretion of fetal urine. *Am J Obstet Gynecol* 1950;60:1339.
6. Benirschke K. Recent trends in chorangiomas, especially those of multiple andrecurrent chorangiomas. *Pediatr Dev Pathol* 1999;2:264.
7. Guschmann M. Solitary and multiple chorangiomas – Clinical consequences, expression of growth factors and differences in the growth rate. *Z Geburtsh Neonatol* 2003;207:6.
8. Kajii T, Ohama K. Androgenetic origin of hydatidiform mole. *Nature* 1977;268:633.

66 Clinically significant pathology of the placenta

B. Hargitai and T. Marton

Introduction

Histopathological examination of the placenta can contribute to the determination of the causes of fetal demise, growth restriction, or neonatal condition. Recently, several guidelines[1–3] and books have been published in the subject of placental pathology.[4,5] The ever-growing evidence-based knowledge requires recapitulation of the clinicopathological correlation. The benefits of placental examination include recognition of maternal conditions having an effect on subsequent pregnancies (autoimmune disease, antiphospholipid syndrome, thombophylia) or that may have medicolegal implications (e.g. concerning the etiology of long-term neurodevelopmental sequelae or the approximate timing of an intrauterine death.[6,7] Timing of the lesions and fetal damage can be estimated and possibly vital clues obtained concerning the etiology of the fetal or neonatal condition. Many features of the placenta can be judged only in the clinicopathological context, partly because of the occasionally loose correlation between the histological changes and the clinical symptoms and partly because of the large reserve capacity of the placenta. It is also apparent that satisfactory clinical information improves the rate of recognized histological features, which underlines the importance of the clinical information submitted to the pathologist.[8]

This chapter attempts to highlight clinicopathological associations bearing great importance in everyday obstetrical and neonatal care.

Placenta referral to the histopathology laboratory

The increased workload of perinatal pathology departments would not allow examination of all placentas, which is not even necessary, except those well-defined conditions when placenta referral is indicated. This 'minimal list' can be extended in selected centers with specific research project. Referral is decided at the delivery suit. The indications of placenta referral are as follows.[1]

Fetal conditions, when referral is indicated

Intrauterine growth restriction (IUGR) (birth weight below 2.5 kg or third percentile), prematurity (less than 37 weeks of gestation), placental abruption, fetal hydrops, fetal developmental abnormality, chromosome aberration, stillbirth, severe fetal distress requiring admission to neonatal unit, rhesus (and other) isoimmunization, morbidly adherent placenta, twins/other multiple pregnancy (complicated or uncomplicated), abnormal placental shape (if clinically relevant, including placental tumors) or other postnatally diagnosed disorders of the placenta (hematoma, too large or too small placenta, infarction, discoloration of membranes), umbilical cord containing two vessels, premature rupture of membranes (PROM) (more than 36 h).

Diseases of the neonate with possible intrauterine origin

These include neonatal infection (pneumonia, or sepsis within 72 h) and neonates with neurological signs.

It is also recommended to examine the placentas from pregnancies with maternal diseases that might have consequences in the neonate. These are maternal pyrexia and maternal group B streptococcus, pre-eclampsia, hypertension, severe diabetes, including gestational diabetes, maternal thrombopathies–thrombophilias, other metabolic disease, maternal autoimmune disease, maternal tumor and storage disease.

Generally, referral *is not indicated for* cholestasis of pregnancy (with no further complication), hepatitis B, HIV infection (seropositivity with no manifest disease), other maternal disease with normal pregnancy outcome, normal pregnancy, placenta previa, postpartum hemorrhage.

In the pathology laboratory, placentas are selected for pathological examination

A full examination of the placenta includes macrosocopic and histological examination of representative samples of the placenta, membrane and umbilical cord. The indications for examination of the placentas are as follows.[1]

Rhesus isoimmunization with admission to the neonatal unit, in any intrauterine death/stillbirth (even if a postmortem examination of the baby does not take place), anemia requiring intrauterine transfusion, morbidly adherent placenta, maternal pyrexia, neonatal infection, prematurity (<34 weeks and not PET/IUGR), severe fetal distress, any admission to the neonatal unit, IUGR, prematurity (<34 weeks) due to PET/IUGR, severe PET, abruption, hydrops and fetal anomaly. The goal in this group is to demonstrate the placental consequences of the clinical condition, in other instances to identify the etiology.

The rest of the placentas belong to a risk group for neonatal disease, so storage is recommended (in unfixed state, for 2 weeks, 4°C, urgent examination on clinical request). These placentas are from pregnancies with PROM, prematurity (34–36 weeks), uncomplicated gestational diabetes, rhesus negative mother, maternal group B streptococcus and uncomplicated pre-eclampsia.

The normal placenta

Normal human placenta has a range of features that are dependent on many factors including maternal size, ethnic origin, geographic area, age, parity, etc.

All placentas are examined at the delivery suit after birth macroscopically.

The *membranes* can lose their transparency, become mat/murky and thickened in chorioamnionitis, subchorionic hemorrhage. Small, white-gray granular nodules appear in oligohydramnios and this alteration is referred to as amnion nodosum, which can be confused with squamous metaplasia macroscopically, but the latter is a normal variant.

Circumvallate placenta presents with a yellow-whitish rim on the fetal surface. Its significance is uncertain, some correlate it with IUGR.

The normal *placenta* is ovoid, and the fetus to placenta weight ratio is 7 at term, growing gradually from 1 at 14/40 weeks of gestation. Normal thickness is approximately 1.5–2.5 cm. Irregular placental shape, multilobed placenta can be a sign of disturbed implantation, or developmental abnormality of the uterus. The placental weight correlates with the fetal weight and a small placenta is prone to result in placental insufficiency and subsequent fetal demise. A large placenta is usually associated with fetal overgrowth syndromes and genetic disorders (Beckwith–Wiedemann syndrome, congenital nephrosis syndrome of the fetus). Other underlying conditions are maternal diabetes, maternal and fetal anemia and fetoplacental hydrops.[9]

The fetal surface has to be searched for vessels leaving the disk, but not returning to it, because that can be a sign of a retained cotyledon. Generally, the fetal surface reflects the changes that can be seen in the membrane or on the subchorionic surface. The color of the normal placenta varies between red and dark red, which depends on the time of clipping the umbilical cord. In a normal placenta, palpation is spongy and homogenous and does not suggest any focal lesions (except for small, peripheral infarcts or perivillous fibrin deposition in term placentas).

After turning the placenta, the maternal side has to be checked for completeness. The *umbilical cord* length is 40–70 cm at term, with one coil over 5 cm on an average.[10] The normal umbilical cord has three vessels and is inserted on the placental disk, preferably in central or paracentral position.

Twin placentas

It is essential to determine the chorionicity of twin placentas, because of the increased morbidity and mortality rate of the monochorionic gestation. The commonest type is the dichorionic placenta. It can have a single disk (either fused or non-separated) or two separated disks. While dichorionic twins can be both di- and monozygotic, monochorionic twins are always monozygotic. Monochorionic, diamniotic twins represent the second most frequent twinning. There is always a single placental disk. Chorionicity can be easily identified with the help of two forceps: the septum needs to be separated into two layers. In case of two thin, equally translucent webs the twin placenta is monochorionic, whereas in uneven separation, having one smooth, opaque, thin layer and a thicker one with uneven surface, the pregnancy is dichorionic.

The rarest finding is the monochorionic, monoamniotic twin placenta (with a single placental disk).

Clinicopathological correlations

Umbilical cord

The umbilical cord is short by definition if it measures less than 40 cm. A short umbilical cord carries an increased risk for fetal/neonatal morbidity or mortality and there is an increased rate of neurological abnormality. The cord is considered to be long if it is longer than 70 cm. A long umbilical cord has a correlation with maternal factors, such as systemic diseases, delivery complications and increased maternal age. According to Baergen *et al.*, fetal factors included non-reassuring fetal status, respiratory distress, vertex presentation, cord entanglement, male sex and increased birth weight. Other frequently observed placental features were increased placental weight, overcoiled cord, true knots and congestion. Cord prolapse causing fetal distress also occurred more often with a long umbilical cord.[11]

Marginal cord insertion shows correlation with IUGR, stillbirth, neonatal death, premature birth and low birth weight. A possible explanation is that a disturbed implantation is behind the atypical cord insertion. The same is true for velamentous cord insertion.

Over- or undercoiling of the cord has an increased risk for fetal demise, fetal intolerance to labor, IUGR, and chorioamnionitis.[10] It is apparent that an extremely overcoiled umbilical cord has an elevated vascular resistance, and vascular obstruction is often behind the fetal loss in these cases.

A true knot can cause fetal death (associated with perinatal mortality of 10%), whereas a loose knot *per se* does not cause harm to the fetus (Figure 66.1). Long umbilical cord is a risk factor for both knot and increased coiling.

Single umbilical artery[12] has an association with fetal malformation and chromosome aberration in 25–50%. In normally formed infants, IUGR is frequent and there is also an increased perinatal mortality.

Thrombosis of the umbilical vessels has a very poor prognosis,[4] but survival can also occur.

Besides the well-known consequences of intrauterine infection (see below), umbilical cord vessel vasculitis and funisitis are associated with cord vessel thrombosis and vasospasm of cord vessels.[5] Necrotizing funisitis is a rare form of umbilical inflammation usually seen with acute chorioamnionitis. Candida, streptococci, herpes and syphilis are reported to play a role in the pathogenesis of necrotizing funisitis (Figure 66.2).[4]

Membranes

Acute chorioamnionitis (including 'subchorial intervillositis') has a strong association with premature rupture of the membranes and preterm delivery.[13] Fetal intrauterine infection may occur. Maternal pyrexia and tachycardia are described as maternal effects, but may be asymptotic. Recently, chorioamnionitis has been implicated as a risk factor for periventricular leukomalacia and cerebral palsy.[14]

Chronic chorioamnionitis has been observed in prolonged rupture of membrane and herpes virus infection.[4]

Amnion epithelial vacuolization can be artifact, but lipid containing droplets in the epithelium are specific for gastroschisis.[4]

In contrast to the common belief, pigmented macrophages and the presence of meconium staining are not necessarily associated with adverse fetal outcome. Meconium staining indicates the danger of meconium aspiration and with other histological signs of fetal distress may underline the diagnosis. Vasospasm of cord vessels and fetal chorionic vessels are reported as a consequence of meconium exposure.[15]

Acute and chronic deciduitis and decidual necrosis in the parietal decidua are frequently associated with ascending infiltrations of the placental membranes, which may be non-significant in isolation. In retroplacental hematoma, severe, necrotizing acute deciduitis is a common finding. The significance of chronic deciduitis with scattered infiltration of lymphocytes is uncertain.[4]

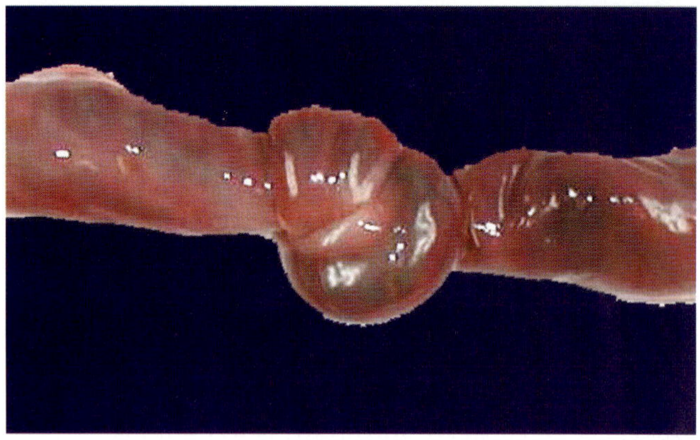

Figure 66.1 Tight knot of the umbilical cord.

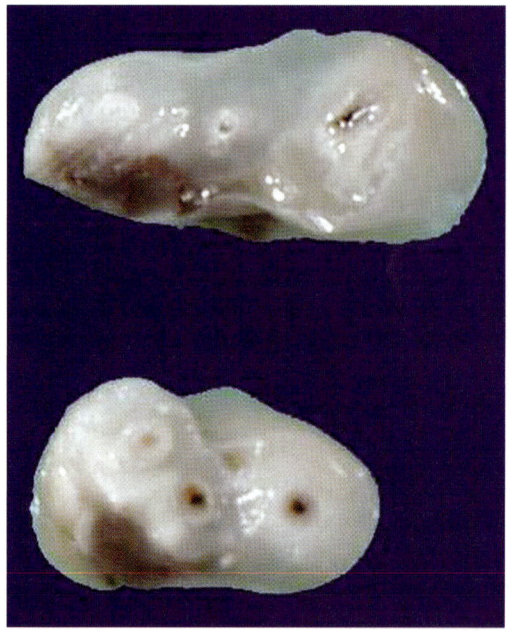

Figure 66.2 Necrotizing funisitis. See the whitish necrotic areas in the umbilical cord.

Placenta

Macroscopic alterations of the placenta

Low placental weight, below the 10th percentile for gestational age occurs in IUGR, pre-eclampsia, increased intervillous fibrin deposition, villitis of unknown origin and trisomies.[9] Placental weight shows correlation with the fetal weight; a small fetus has a generally smaller placenta than a large fetus, but a small placenta may lead to growth restriction.

The placenta is thin (the medical term is placenta annulare or placenta membranacea) by definition if the average thickness is less than 2 cm and the placenta has a large membranous area. While the fetal outcome is usually favorable, there is a risk of maternal bleeding, placenta previa, placenta accreta. Often premature delivery occurs and possibly it is more frequent in IUGR.[16]

The hemorrhages of the placenta include retroplacental hematoma. A large retroplacental hematoma causes a crater (Figure 66.3) and extensive infarction involving a sufficient proportion of villous tissue with secondary fetal hypoxia and/or perinatal death. An early separation (placental abruption) can be lethal if extensive. An elevated maternal serum alpha-fetoprotein level can be associated with old hematomas.

Subchorionic hematoma (Figure 66.4) usually has no clinical significance when patchy, focal or present as a thin diffuse layer. Although rarely, in extreme cases, a massive hematoma (massive subchorial thrombosis, Breus' mole) can result in abortion.

Placenta previa is usually diagnosed by ultrasound before delivery. If undetected and if it causes bleeding, it can be life threatening for both mother and fetus.

Placenta accreta, increta and percreta are potentially life-threatening clinical conditions, causing uterine rupture, and massive postpartum hemorrhage, or leading to cesarean section if prenatally diagnosed. Placenta creta is often an indication of postpartum hysterectomy because of the excessive bleeding. To make the pathological diagnosis of a placenta accreta, examination of the entire uterus is necessary as a posthysterectomy specimen.

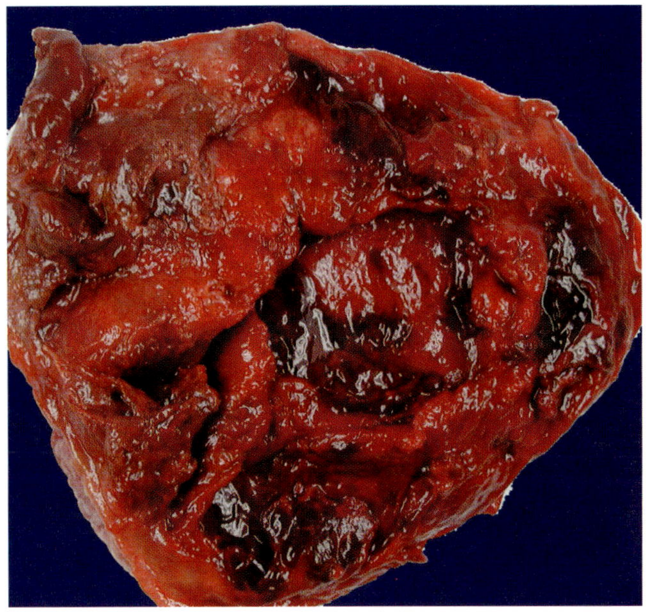

Figure 66.3 The crater in the middle of the placenta was caused by a retroplacental hemorrhage.

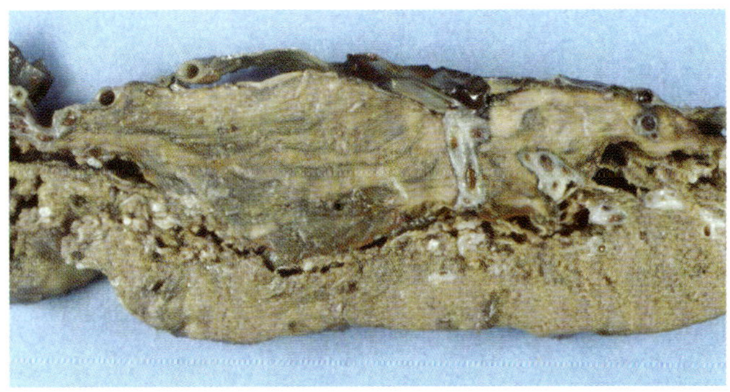

Figure 66.4 Lamellated, large subchorionic hematoma can be seen on the fetal surface of this placenta.

Microscopic alterations of the placenta

- Abnormalities of the placental chorionic villi, the intervillous space and chorionic vessels that result in a reduced functional capacity of the placenta:
  (1) A *placental infarct* (Figure 66.5a and b) has no significance if it is single, marginal and/or involves less than about 5% of the villous tissue. If a placental infarction involves more than 10% of the placental volume it is regarded as extensive infarct and can have serious clinical consequences such as fetal hypoxia, IUGR, stillbirth, pregnancy-induced hypertension, abruptio placentae, neurological abnormalities because of the reduced size villous tree.[4]
  (2) *Extensive perivillous fibrin deposition*, involving more than 20–30% of the villous tissue and functional placenta, is an important histological entity, associated with IUGR and fetal death. In these cases often 70–80% of villous population is enveloped by fibrin. The maternal serum AFP can be extremely elevated.[17,18]
- There are two special patterns of the fibrin deposition: massive basal plate perivillous fibrin deposition is termed as '*maternal floor infarct*' and is known to be associated with high mortality and IUGR.[4,5,19,20]
- The massive perivillous fibrin deposition in a net-like pattern (Figure 66.6a and b) is the '*gitter infarct*'. 'Gitter infarct' and 'maternal floor infarct' are historical names, none of them a true infarct, but a special type of perivillous fibrin deposition.
  (3) *Abnormalities of the fetal vessels*: Fetal chorionic vessels and fetal stem vessels of the placenta may contain fresh or organized thrombus. The organized thrombus can calcify, or contains small vascular spaces if recanalized. Obstruction of fetal vessels (Figure 66.7) is associated with groups or fields of hyalinized, *avascular villi*. These villi cannot take part in the blood gas exchange for the complete lack of capillaries. Presence of extensive avascular villi (Figure 66.8), due to fetal vessel thrombosis, was reported in association with stillbirth, IUGR, maternal and fetal coagulopathy and fetal thromboembolic disease leading to cerebral palsy.[7] *Intimal fibrin cushion*, a non-symmetric intimal swelling with endothelial disruption, is described in neonatal asphyxia, in association with disseminated capillary thrombi of fetal vessels. The severity of the fetal

(a)

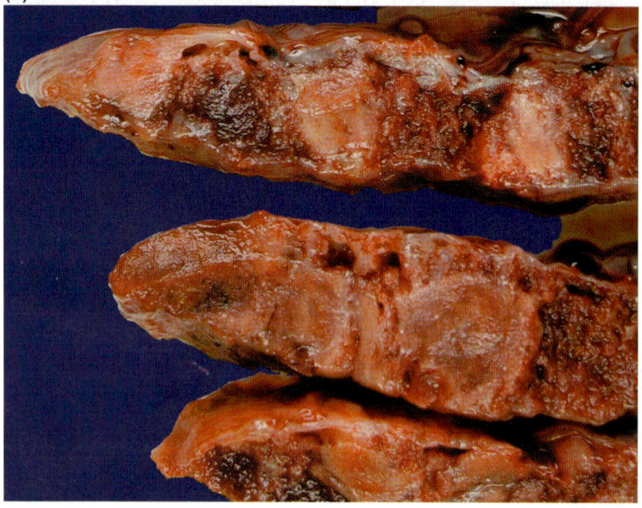

(b)

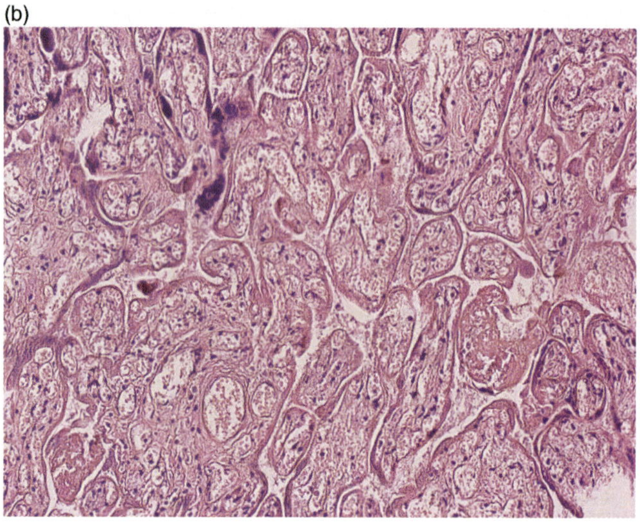

Figure 66.5 Multiple fresh infarcts in a term placenta: (a) macroscopic picture and (b) microscopic image representing necrotic villi.

consequences depends more on the accompanying vascular lesions, mainly on fetal vessel thrombosis.[15] If there are large areas of avascular villi, the prognosis is dependent on the proportion of the placenta as described above.

- *Hemorrhagic endovasculitis* (HEV) is a controversial entity, which was reported to be a postmortem artifact and was doubted as being a specific disease. The histological appearance is characterized by thrombotic-recanalized stem vessels and extravasated, fragmented red blood cells (Figure 66.8). HEV was found to be associated with meconium staining and postmaturity. Earlier report revealed association with stillbirth, IUGR, neurological disability and maternal hypertension. HEV was reported also in livebirths, associated with perinatal complications, fetal distress and IUGR.
- Interlesional relationships exist between thrombotic, chronic inflammatory and chronic vaso-occlusive lesions.[4]

(a)

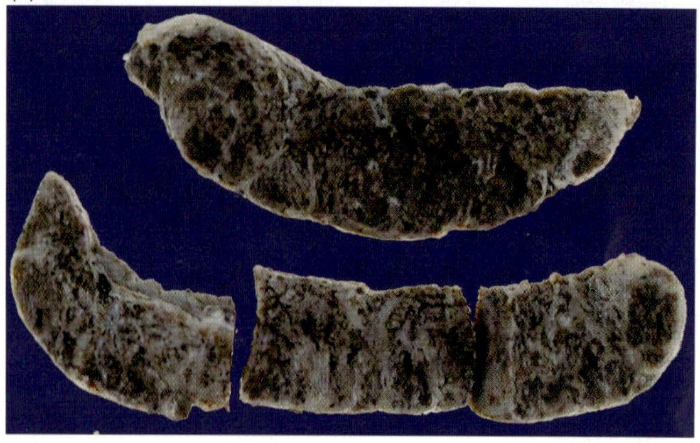

(b)

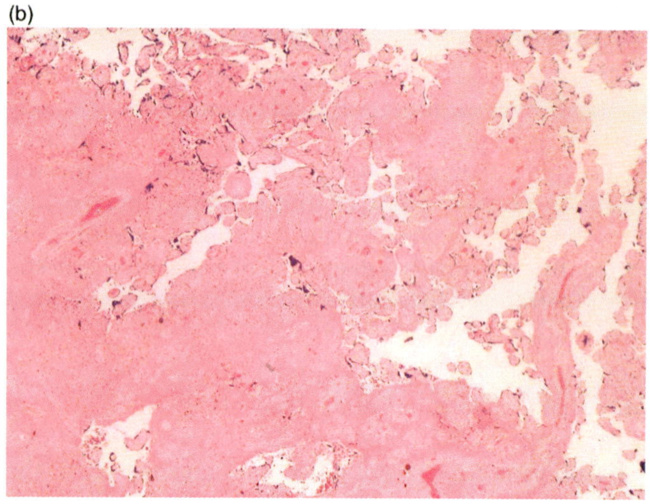

Figure 66.6 Net-like fibrin deposition in the placenta: (a) macroscopic picture and (b) microscopic image shows villi entrapped by fibrin.

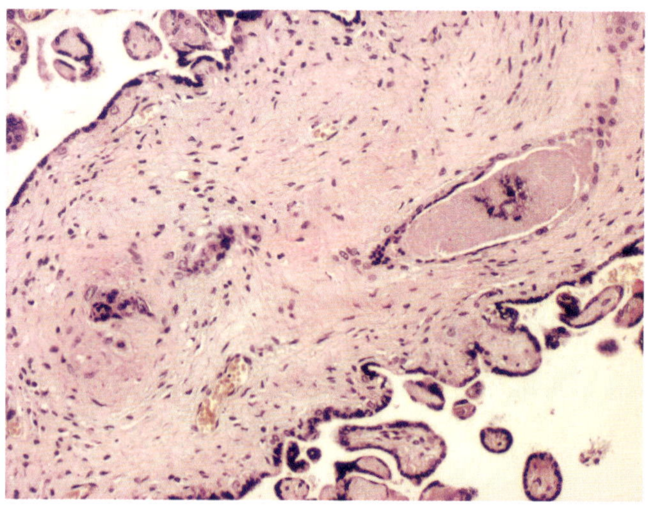

Figure 66.7 Stem vessel occlusion with small avascular villi.

(4) Most frequently, *intervillous hemorrhage* and *thrombus* are related to maternal vessel lesion and are of maternal origin. Small and focal lesions have no clinical importance. Large and multiple lesions may cause fetal compromise or demise depending on the functional placental

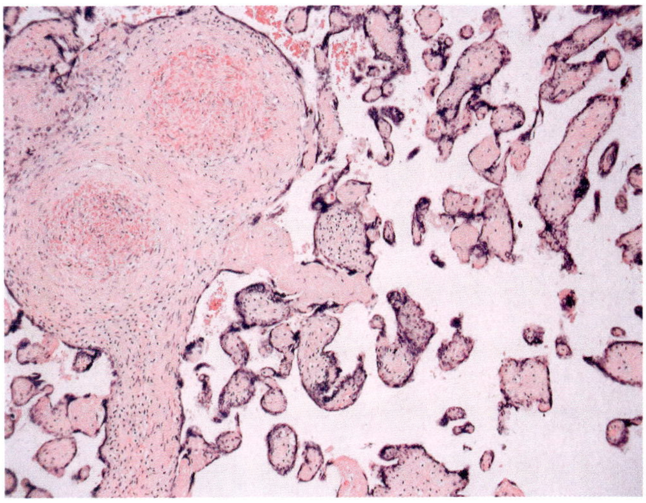

Figure 66.8 A group of avascular villi around a stem villus. The stem villi show hemorrhagic endovasculitis.

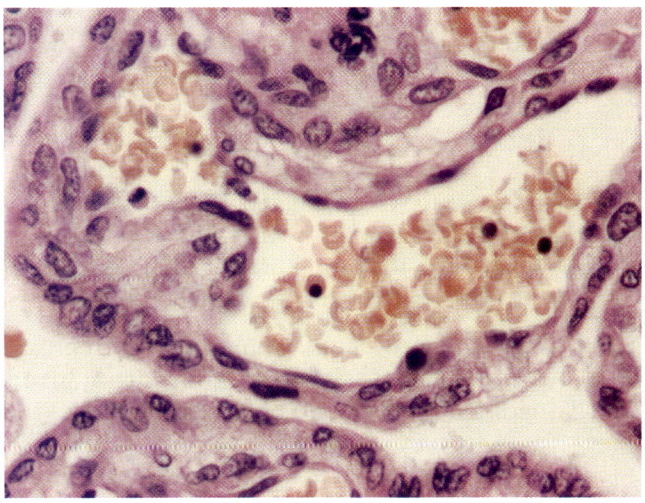

Figure 66.9 Nucleated red blood cells in a fetal capillary.

parenchyma loss and the rest of the unaffected placenta. Quite often they can be seen in pre-eclampsia and is surrounded by infarct as a rim. In some cases intervillous hemorrhage and thrombus are signs of fetal bleeding into the maternal circulation as described by Kline. Only a minority of these alterations leads to a large amount of fetal blood loss and stillbirth or severe anemia followed by ischemic lesions of parenchymal organs.

- Changes of the chorionic villi secondary to pre-eclampsia, intrauterine hypoxia or fetal conditions and maternal spiral artery changes:

(1) Increased number of *syncytial knots* occurs in pre-eclampsia, hypertension, diabetes mellitus, maternal anemia and pregnancy at high altitude. It can also be seen in a thick histological section (artifact). Despite the fact that it occurs

(a)

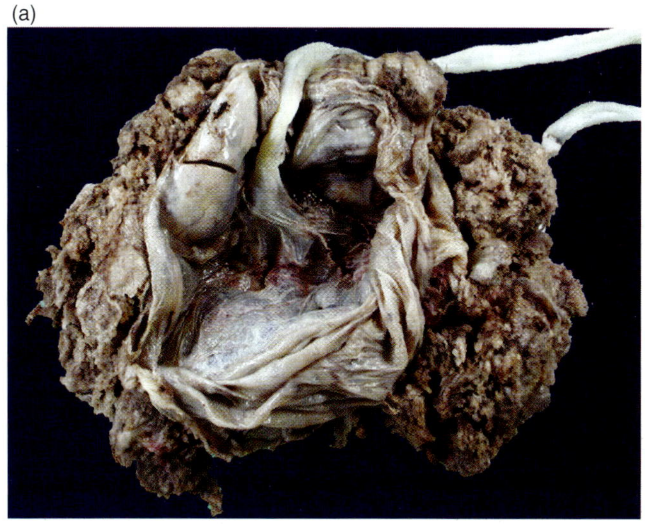

(b)

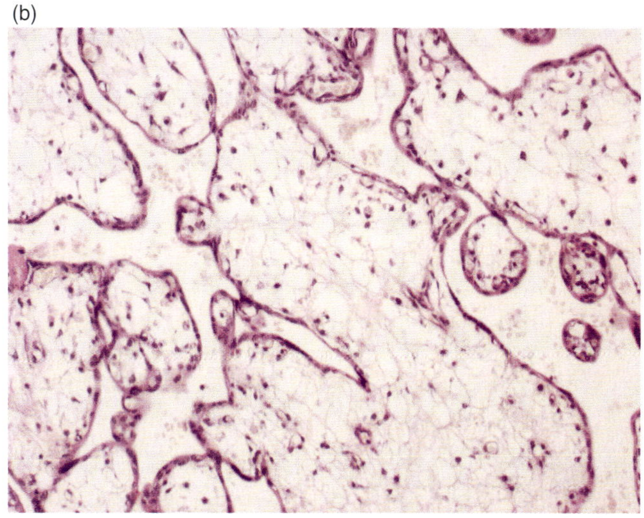

Figure 66.10 Placental edema: (a) macroscopic picture – the bulky placenta and (b) edematous terminal villi.

in pre-eclampsia, the correlation between increased syncytial knotting and fetal hypoxia has not been proved. Excessive increase of syncytial knotting may be due to reduced fetal perfusion and placental hypoxia or can be the sign of accelerated maturation if the duration of pregnancy was less than 40 weeks.

(2) *Elevated number of nucleated red blood cells* (NRBCs) may occur in many causes of chronic hypoxia (Figure 66.9), IUGR, stillbirth, acute and chronic fetal blood loss or anemia, maternal diabetes and erythroblastosis fetalis.[4]

(3) An increase of vasculo-syncytial membrane (VSM) is described in pregnancies at high altitude, pre-eclampsia, maternal heart failure and maternal anemia. *VSM deficiency* was reported in pre-eclampsia, materno-fetal rhesus incompatibility, maternal diabetes, low birth weight and stillbirths.[4,5]

(4) *Extensive stromal fibrosis* occurs in terminal villous deficiency, in IUGR, and in avascular villi due to fetal stem vessel thrombosis.

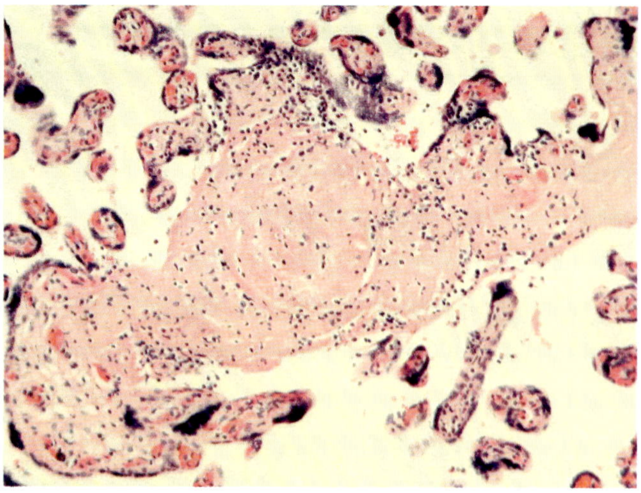

Figure 66.11 Villitis of unknown etiology (VUE). Chronic inflammatory cells infiltrate the villus, the chorionic epithelium is damaged.

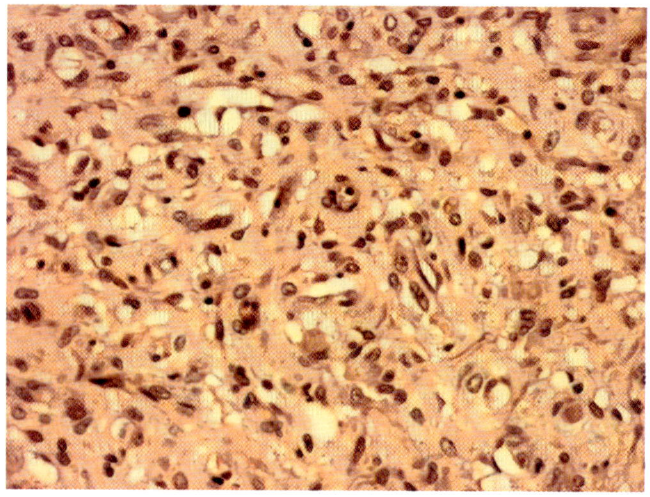

Figure 66.12 Microscopic appearance of chorangioma with small capillary-like vessels and sinusoids.

(5) Placentas from pregnancies with hydrops fetalis may show a combination of immaturity and edema. *Villous edema* occurs also in infections (syphilis, CMV, toxoplasma, parvovirus) (Figure 66.10a and b) and in hydatidiform moles. Edema may be within normal limits, when focal.[4]

(6) A *failure of villous maturation* was found to be associated with fetal hypoxia, IUGR, maternal diabetes and materno–fetal rhesus incompatibility. Maturation failure may lead to intrauterine death.[5,21]

(7) *Accelerated villus maturation* (maturitas precox)[4] can be observed in prematurely delivered placentas in pre-eclampsia and the features are related to chronic ischemia.

(8) *Abnormalities of the maternal vessels* are usually associated with pre-eclamptic toxemia. *Uteroplacental* or *decidual arteriopathy* is a failure of physiological adaptation of maternal vessels. Uteroplacental vessel fibrinoid necrosis, acute atherosis and uteroplacental vessel thrombosis are closely related with pregnancy-induced hypertension, maternal essential hypertension, pre-eclampsia resulting in fetal complications such as IUGR, SGA and stillbirth. It is associated with APA, systemic lupus erythematosus and thrombophilia.[4,5,22]

- Inflammatory processes involving the placental villi or intervillous space:

(1) *Acute villitis* is usually associated with severe maternal infection, preterm delivery and might lead to intrauterine infection and intrauterine death (IUD).[4]

(2) The etiology of *chronic villitis* is usually not known (villitis of unknown origin, VUO, or villitis of unknown etiology, VUE) (Figure 66.11). In about 15% of cases CMV, toxoplasma and syphilis infection are the underlying causes of chronic villitis.

- Chronic villitis is associated with IUGR and/or stillbirth. Chronic villitis of unknown etiology is associated with IUGR and preterm birth, and tends to recur during subsequent pregnancies.[4]

(3) *Chronic histiocytic intervillositis* (chronic perivillositis) is characterized by dense histiocytic intervillous infiltrate, and is reported in association with elevated maternal serum AFP, recurrent abortion, IUGR and preterm delivery. Malarial infection should be excluded.[23]

- Miscellaneous conditions of the chorionic villi:

(1) *Mesenchymal dysplasia* is the hallmark of Beckwith–Wiedemann syndrome.[24]

(2) Perinatal death, congenital malformation and cerebral palsy were found to be associated with *chorangiosis* as a response to low-grade tissue hypoxia. Although others have supported this observation, the question still remained as to how chronic hypoxia results in increased vascularization. The significance of this alteration needs further investigation.[25]

(3) *Chorangioma* is a tumor-like lesion, resembling infantile hemangiomas (Figure 66.12). It is most likely of hyperplastic origin, arising from the subtrophoblastic reticular tissue of the immature stem villi. Large lesions can lead to cardiac failure, hydrops and death of the fetus due to high-output cardiac failure. Other possible complications are transplacental bleeding, and feto–maternal transfusion leading to anemia. Chorangioma was reported to be associated

with pre-eclampsia, multiple gestation, premature delivery, fetal thrombocytopenia and fetal angiomas (Kasabach–Merritt syndrome).[4]

(4) *Umbilical cord hemangioma* is a rare entity and its complications are related to the size of the lesion. It can be associated with elevated AFP level; fetal disseminated intravascular coagulation, fetal hydrops as well as fetal demise have been described.[26]

Conclusion

In conclusion, we would like to emphasize the importance of placental referral to the pathology laboratory and the placenta examination. We would also like to encourage communication between clinicians and pathologists to discover further clinicopathological correlations for the benefit of the patients.

REFERENCES

1. Hargitai B, Marton T, Cox PM. Examination of the human placenta. Best practice No 178. *J Clin Pathol* 2004;57(8):785–92.
2. Khong TY. A topographical and clinical approach to examination of the placenta. *Pathology* 2001;33(2):174–86.
3. Langston C, Kaplan C, Macpherson T, *et al.* Practice guideline for examination of the placenta: Developed by the Placental Pathology Practice Guideline Development Task Force of the College of American Pathologists. *Arch Pathol Lab Med* 1997; 121(5):449–76.
4. Benirschke K, Kaufmann P. *Pathology of the Human Placenta*, 4th edn. New York: Springer-Verlag, 1999.
5. Fox H. *Pathology of the Placenta*, 2nd edn. London: W.B. Saunders, 1997.
6. Altshuler G. Placenta within the medicolegal imperative. *Arch Pathol Lab Med* 1991;115(7):688–95.
7. Kraus FT. Cerebral palsy and thrombi in placental vessels of the fetus: Insights from litigation. *Hum Pathol* 1997;28(2):246–8.
8. Redline RW, Boyd T, Campbell V, *et al.* Maternal vascular underperfusion: Nosology and reproducibility of placental reaction patterns. *Pediatr Dev Pathol* 2004;7(3):237–49.
9. Naeye RL. Do placental weights have clinical significance? *Hum Pathol* 1987;18(4):387–91.
10. Machin GA, Ackerman J, Gilbert-Barness E. Abnormal umbilical cord coiling is associated with adverse perinatal outcomes. *Pediatr Dev Pathol* 2000;3(5):462–71.
11. Baergen RN, Malicki D, Behling C, Benirschke K. Morbidity, mortality, and placental pathology in excessively long umbilical cords: Retrospective study. *Pediatr Dev Pathol* 2001;4(2):144–53.
12. Chow JS, Benson CB, Doubilet PM. Frequency and nature of structural anomalies in fetuses with single umbilical arteries. *J Ultrasound Med* 1998;17(12):765–8.
13. Gibbs RS, Romero R, Hillier SL, Eschenbach DA, Sweet RL. A review of premature birth and subclinical infection. *Am J Obstet Gynecol* 1992;166(5):1515–28.
14. Wu YW, Colford JM Jr. Chorioamnionitis as a risk factor for cerebral palsy: A meta-analysis. *J Am Med Assoc* 2000;284(11):1417–24.
15. Altshuler G. Some placental considerations related to neurodevelopmental and other disorders. *J Child Neurol* 1993;8(1): 78–94.
16. Ahmed A, Gilbert-Barness E. Placenta membranacea: A developmental anomaly with diverse clinical presentation. *Pediatr Dev Pathol* 2003;6:201–3.
17. Redline RW, O'Riordan MA. Placental lesions associated with cerebral palsy and neurologic impairment following term birth. *Arch Pathol Lab Med* 2000;124(12):1785–91.
18. Görbe É, Rigó J Jr, Marton T, Kõhalmi B, Csabay L, Csapó ZS. Maternal floor infarct, gleichzeitiges Auftreten von intrauteriner Fetusretardierung und hohem mütterlichen AFP-Spiegel. *Z Geburtshilfe Neonatol* 1999;203(5):218–20.
19. Bane AL, Gillan JE. Massive perivillous fibrinoid causing recurrent placental failure. *Br J Obstet Gynaecol* 2003;110(3):292–5.
20. Naeye RL. *Disorders of the Placenta, Fetus and Neonate: Diagnosis and Clinical Significance*. St Louis: Mosby Year Book, 1992.
21. Stalmach T, Hebisch G, Meier K, Dudenhausen JW, Vogel M. Rescue by birth: Defective placental maturation and late fetal mortality. *Obstet Gynecol* 2001;97(4):505–9.
22. Magid MS, Kaplan C, Sammaritano LR, Peterson M, Druzin ML, Lockshin MD. Placental pathology in systemic lupus erythematosus: A prospective study. *Am J Obstet Gynecol* 1998;179(1): 226–34.
23. Boyd TK, Redline RW. Chronic histiocytic intervillositis: A placental lesion associated with recurrent reproductive loss. *Hum Pathol* 2000;31(11):1389–96.
24. Jauniaux E, Nicolaides KH, Hustin J. Perinatal features associated with placental mesenchymal dysplasia. *Placenta* 1997;18:701–6.
25. Altshuler G. Chorangiosis. An important placental sign of neonatal morbidity and mortality. *Arch Pathol Lab Med* 1984;108(1):71–4.
26. Kamitomo M, Sueyoshi K, Matsukita S, Matsuda Y, Hatae M, Ikenoue T. Hemangioma of the umbilical cord: Stenotic change of the umbilical vessels. *Fetal Diagn Ther* 1999;14(6):328–31.

SECTION VII

Fetal diagnosis and therapy

Section Editors: **W. Holzgreve and M. Evans**

67 Non-invasive prenatal diagnosis: maternal blood

O. Lapaire, B. Zimmermann, X. Yan Zhong, S. Hahn and W. Holzgreve

Abstract

One of the major topics of prenatal research today is the genetic analysis of fetal cells or fetal DNA/RNA, which can be accumulated from the blood of pregnant women. It is the intention of the clinician and scientists of the laboratory to offer a risk-free diagnostic method for pregnant women in order to reduce the number of invasive interventions [e.g. amniocentesis (AC), chorionic villi sampling (CVS)] and the procedure-related risk of fetal loss, as well as to provide additional markers for prenatal screening programs and for prenatal diagnosis. Until now the technical problems of cell enrichment has prevented routine use of fetal cell sampling. In contrast, cell-free fetal DNA in maternal plasma can now be used for the extremely reliable identification of fetal genetic traits, clearly distinguished from maternal sequences (e.g. the fetal rhesus status) or inherited polymorphism. Only recently, a new field of investigation has been opened by the demonstration of the cell-free form of fetal RNA in maternal plasma, which is surprisingly stable and holds promise for non-invasive screening for fetal aneuploidies or pregnancy-associated disorders.

Introduction

Routine clinical prenatal diagnosis with a view to identify fetal genetic disorders was started in the 1970s. Since its inception, the reason for prenatal diagnosis is the detection of fetal aneuploidy and malformations. The overall risk of fetal chromosomal disorders is continuously rising due to the increasing average age of pregnant women in the Western world, especially in Europe. The maternal age alone as a screening marker has a low sensitivity of 30–40% for trisomy 21 (M. Down), dependent on the age distribution of the studied population. Down's syndrome is the most common chromosomal abnormality among live births and is the most frequent form of mental retardation caused by a chromosomal aberration. Prenatal protocols for Down's syndrome screening have been introduced for several reasons:

- Trisomy 21 has a high prevalence (1 in 700 births in the absence of prenatal intervention)
- The high morbidity and mortality in affected fetuses and the consecutive socioeconomic costs
- The area-wide availability of diagnostic tests to detect this chromosomal abnormality
- The availability of safe and accessible interventions to introduce abortions of affected fetuses

As a whole, the society desires Down's syndrome screening to be done as early as possible in pregnancy, despite the effectiveness of second-trimester serum screening. First- or early second-trimester diagnosis of fetal abnormalities allows more time for decision making, greater privacy and safer methods of pregnancy termination. However, a number of issues must be addressed before earlier screening can be offered on a general population basis. These issues include the availability and acceptability of early invasive diagnostic methods (e.g. chorionic villus sampling and amniocentesis), as well as clinical effectiveness.

Three screening markers, two serum and one fetal ultrasound marker have been shown to be effective for first-trimester screening for Down's syndrome.[2,3] The two serum markers in combination with the maternal age constitute a first-trimester maternal serum screening test that achieves a sensitivity of 63% at a 5% false-positive rate.[2]

An improved performance can be attained by the addition of sonographic analysis for increased fetal nuchal translucency (NT) (Figure 67.1). NT by itself is a strong marker of Down's syndrome and is associated with detection rates between 60% and 70% at a 5% false-positive rate.[4] When it is combined with the pregnancy-associated plasma protein A (PAPP-A),

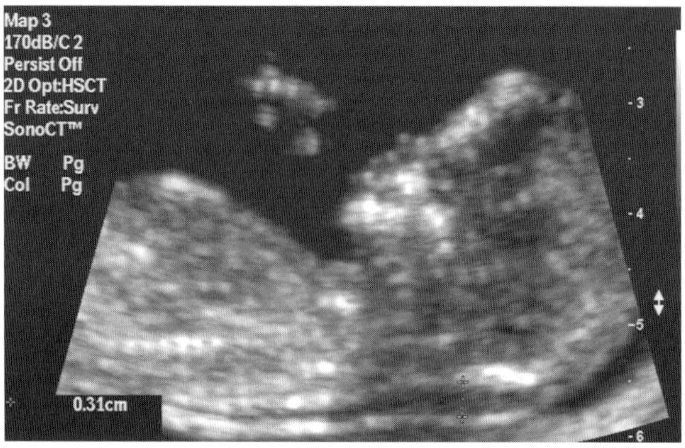

Figure 67.1 Transabdominal measurement of the fetal nuchal translucency (3.1 mm) at the end of the first trimester.

free beta-human chorionic gonadotrophin (beta-hCG), and the maternal age, an overall sensitivity rate of approximately 85% at a 5% false-positive rate can be obtained.[5–7]

The combination of serum and ultrasound markers at the end of the first trimester is better than any of the second-trimester serum tests that are nowadays available and, at least in a hypothetical model, are more cost-effective (screening plus liveborn costs).[8] However, the performance of NT as a screening marker has not been consistent from study to study, probably because of the variability of the operator's experience and training.[9] Further studies as well as proper training and ongoing quality management are necessary before a widespread use of this screening regimen can be implemented.[10]

In case of a suspicious result (in Switzerland: overall risk for trisomy 21 >1:380), invasive testing, with either amniocentesis (AC) or CVS, is advised during a profound genetic counseling. AC is the commonly used ultrasound-guided technique for withdrawing amniotic fluid from the uterine cavity, using a needle via a transabdominal approach. CVS refers also to the invasive procedures for prenatal diagnosis of genetic disorders, in which small specimens of the placenta are achieved for chromosome or DNA analysis. Two approaches are available for obtaining chorionic tissue, a transcervical and a transabdominal CVS, depending on the routine of the performer and the location of the placenta. However, due to the procedure-related risk of fetal loss, which is estimated to be 0.5–1% of all interventions, a rising percentage of pregnant women opt not to have any invasive diagnostic procedures. Thus, the rate of procedure-related unaffected fetal loss is estimated to be 44–45 per 100,000 women screened when either first-trimester screening (NT, free beta-hCG, and PAPP-A) or a second-trimester quadruple test has been performed.

For that reason international projects have been set up in the field of prenatal medicine research for effective, risk-free, and reliable alternative methods and additional markers. The object of the research is to obtain fetal tissue, with either the enrichment of fetal cells or cell-free DNA, and recently RNA, extracted from the maternal blood. Fetal cells have been found in the maternal blood, though in very low quantities. Therefore, the primary step was their detection, enrichment, and characterization with molecular biologic methods.[11] Besides fetal cells, cell-free fetal DNA and fetal RNA, independent of fetal gender and genetic polymorphism status, were found in the maternal plasma. With the progress in prenatal research and technical advances, some results of non-invasive prenatal medicine research have already come into the clinical setting: as a diagnostic tool, fetal DNA, extracted from maternal plasma, can now be used for the extremely reliable identification of fetal genetic traits that are absent in the maternal genome (e.g. the fetal rhesus status or patients with an elevated risk for X-chromosomal inherited disorders, e.g. hemophilia, fragile X-syndrome).

To examine fetal DNA, nowadays a polymerase chain reaction (PCR) is normally used as the first step in the vast majority of DNA analyses. In a few hours, an automated PCR can amplify a single DNA molecule a millionfold. The greatly amplified target DNA is subsequently analyzed via other techniques.

The recent detection of fetal RNA in the plasma of pregnant women has led to new opportunities. Unlike fetal DNA, quantitative analysis of fetal RNA with PCR methods has the advantage of being applicable to all gravidae, irrespective of fetal gender and genetic polymorphism.[12]

To analyze fetal RNA, a reverse-transcriptase PCR (RT-PCR) is used for transforming messenger RNA (mRNA) into complementary DNA (cDNA) by an RNA-dependent DNA polymerase, specified as RT. The cDNA complex is then changed into a double stranded DNA, thus becoming the template for a subsequent PCR reaction.

The main source of fetal RNA is thought to be the placenta. Fetal RNA is surprisingly stable in the maternal plasma. Data indicate that the measurement of circulating placental RNA may provide a new method for non-invasive prenatal diagnosis and monitoring. The future clinical application of this technology would be the application of RNA as an additional screening tool for chromosomal aneuploidies and other pregnancy-associated disorders.

Non-invasive clinical diagnostics using fetal cells in maternal blood samples

A long sought goal of prenatal medicine has been the reduction of invasive diagnostic procedures for fetal cell sampling, and its procedure-related risk of miscarriage, by isolating fetal cells from the maternal blood.

In the 1990s, the first report about successful enrichment of fetal cells, extracted from maternal blood, was published. The cells could be analyzed for possible aneuploidies by fluorescent *in situ* hybridization (FISH).[13] FISH can identify different chromosomal mutations including deletions, duplications, aneuploidy, and the presence of derivative chromosomes with specific DNA probes. However, small mutations, including small deletions and insertions as well as point mutations, cannot be identified with the FISH technique. When the DNA probes are designated with a fluorochrome, fast detection of the fluorescent signal is possible via fluorescence microscopy. The main difficulty of this method has been the very low concentration of fetal cells in the maternal serum. It could be shown that only two to six cells per milliliter of maternal blood are present.[14] Fetal cells can be found in the blood of pregnant women from the first trimester on. However, a rapid, simple, and consistent procedure for their isolation for prenatal non-invasive testing has not been found. Almost any procedure available in experimental cell research for cell enrichment has been used to isolate fetal cells out of maternal blood. For the multistep enrichment, the density gradient centrifugation is always used as the first step,[15] fluorescence-activated cell sorting (FACS)[16] or magnetic activated cell sorting (MACS) (see Figure 67.2)[17] follow as the second step after the attachment of magnetically labelled or flourescent antibodies for specific fetal cell surface markers. A major effort has been made during the last years to standardize and validate these processes among different laboratories.

The latter method is easy to perform and has a higher turnover of samples, as well as a higher sensitivity than FACS (see Figure 67.3). The third step includes FISH, culture, or PCR. However, the cell culture, with or without enrichment, as well as the multistep enrichment procedure itself requires many manipulations in which a certain amount of cells may be lost. New methods, such as automatic scanning, are needed to install the cell enrichment in the routine clinical use. Different populations of fetal cells can be enriched from the maternal blood; CD34 + hematopoietic progenitor cells and cells from the trophoblast are used.[17] Each of these cell lines has some specific disadvantages. For example, it is not possible to cultivate nuclear erythrocytes. This fact does not allow a metaphase analysis for chromosomal testing. On the other hand CD34 + cells can be cultivated. However, they persist postpartum in the maternal blood circulation and make a prenatal testing in the next pregnancy more difficult. Furthermore, cells are not constantly present in the maternal circulation. The isolated cells have been investigated using cytochemistry, soret band absorption microscopy, monoclonal antibodies for ε- and γ-chain-hemoglobin, monoclonal antibody for i-antigen, and FISH. In summary, the enrichment of fetal cells from the maternal blood is too laborious to be a serious alternative in the clinic and to supersede prenatal invasive diagnostic procedures. Today, the international research has partially turned its attention to the cell-free fetal DNA and RNA.

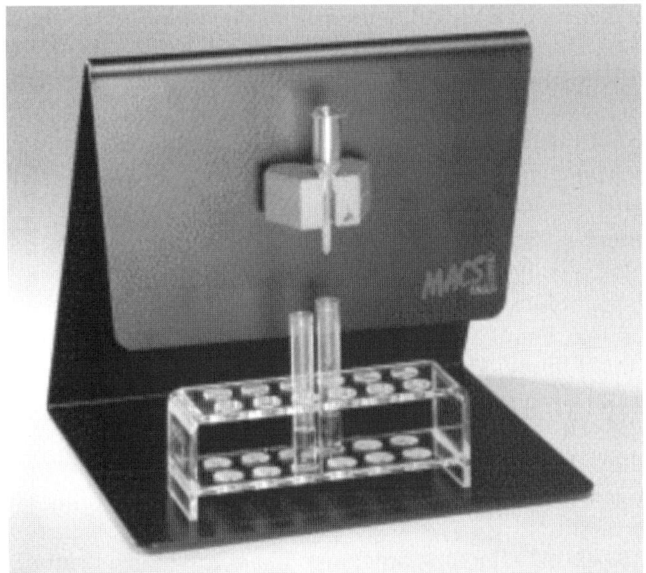

Figure 67.2 Aspect of a MACS system, used in our laboratory.

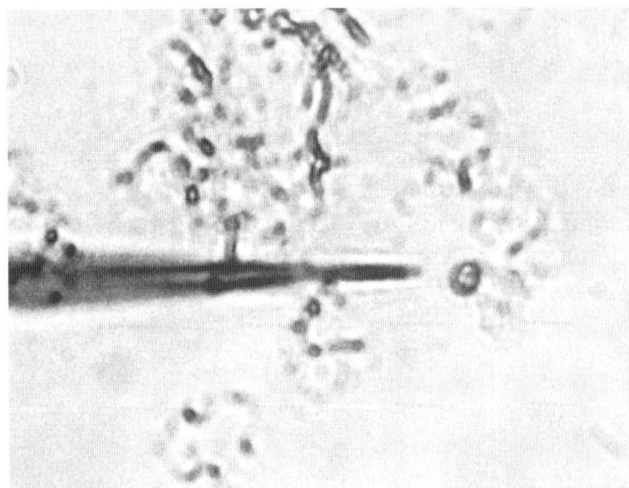

Figure 67.3 Micromanipulation of a single fetal erythroblast.

Non-invasive prenatal diagnostic tests with fetal DNA

The first publication about cell-free fetal DNA, extracted from maternal blood, dated from 1997.[18] Quantitative investigations showed that the concentration of fetal DNA during pregnancy is much higher than that of fetal cells.[18] Quantitative levels can be measured with real-time PCR. Real-time PCR has several advantages over conventional PCR: the data collection is done during amplification. The accumulation of PCR products over time is measured directly, without post-PCR modifications. Therefore, it is less prone to contamination, as the results are analyzed automatically without having to open the PCR reaction vessel, and there is no post-PCR work. It also permits the rapid analysis of numerous samples in one analytic run and is therefore better for automation.

The quantitation of fetal DNA may provide additional knowledge regarding the outcome of pregnancy. Fetal DNA is elevated in specific pregnancy-associated disorders like pre-eclampsia,[19] hyperemesis gravidarum,[20] or trisomy 21.[21] In case of pre-eclampsia, it could be demonstrated that the severity of the disease correlates with the level of cell-free fetal DNA in the blood of affected pregnant women.[22] Furthermore, cell-free fetal DNA can be used as an additional marker for Down's syndrome. Although its sensitivity is lower than that of other biochemical screening-markers, like alphafetoprotein (AFP), unconjugated estriol (uE3), hCG or Inhibin A, predominantly due to its width of distribution, it shows a 21% detection rate (with a set 5% false positive rate), when cell-free fetal DNA from maternal plasma/serum is singularly used as marker for Down's syndrome.[23] These studies suggested that an elevated concentration of fetal DNA may be a valuable marker for pregnancy-associated diseases.[23] As the majority (more than 90%) of free DNA in maternal serum is derived from the mother, it is difficult to differentiate the origin. Previously, it was possible only to examine genetic traits that are not present in the maternal genome. However, with this non-invasive and risk-free method it is now possible to detect Y-specific sequences in pregnancies with an elevated risk for X-chromosomal inherited disorders (e.g. hemophilia, fragile X-syndrome). Approximately, 15% of Caucasian pregnancies are potentially at risk of severe intrauterine hemolytic disease, mainly due to rhesus D incompatibility. The need to know the rhesus constellation, as well as the large number of X-linked disorders, has prodded several groups to develop non-invasive risk-free methods for diagnostic tests.

With the highly specific real-time PCR method, it is nowadays possible to detect these fetal genetic traits with an almost 100% sensitivity and specificity. A few laboratories offer routinely the detection of the fetal rhesus status. This is a success in the 15-year-old international research on this topic.

A recently published work of our laboratory demonstrated that fetal DNA can be separated from maternal DNA, due to the difference in its size.[24] A majority of fetal DNA has a size of <0.3 kb, whereas the maternal DNA, which constitutes more than 90% of the amount of circulating DNA in the maternal blood, shows a size of >1 kb.[25] The difference in size may account for the different origin. Fetal DNA derives predominantly from the placenta, whereas maternal DNA has its main origin in the hematopoietic system.[26,27] After size separation of the fetal DNA, it is possible to detect fetal microsatellite markers with fluorescent PCR.[24] Until now, this new technology has been used for the determination of many disorders like myotonic dystrophy,[28] achondroplasia,[29] and beta-thalassemia.[30]

Non-invasive prenatal screening tests with fetal DNA

The current focus in research on fetal DNA investigates its use as a maternal serum marker in the second trimester for fetal Down syndrome and other pregnancy-associated disorders. The quantitative measurement of fetal DNA could complement the second-trimester serum markers. By increasing the specificity of the screening, it could help to prevent a considerable amount of unnecessary invasive procedures. The median of fetal DNA concentration is reported to be approximately twofold higher in pregnancies with Down's syndrome, compared with unaffected pregnancies, but the data are disputed by other reports and larger sample numbers, and meticulously accurate, standardized quantification are demanded to allow final conclusions.

In order to use the fetal DNA as a screening marker, a gender-independent fetal DNA marker that can be assayed by real-time PCR is needed. Polymorphic sequences are presently used in the clinical samples that are investigated for fetal rhesus status to ascertain the presence of adequate amounts of fetal DNA. Although a number of sequences have to be examined in each pregnancy to ascertain distinction between fetal and maternal DNA, this approach is still relatively easy to implement.

The presence of fetal DNA in maternal plasma has revealed significant clinical potential for the prenatal diagnosis of fetal genetic diseases and pregnancy-associated complications.

A caveat of the approach is that the DNA present in the circulation is predominantly of maternal origin and interferes with molecular analysis of the fetal DNA. Hence, paternally inherited fetal loci that are clearly different from maternal genomic sequences can be readily examined. Paternally inherited mutant genes in compound heterozygous genetic disorders may also be detected if the paternal mutation is dissimilar from the maternal allele. In general, the detection of fetal single gene disorders is at least cumbersome and sometimes impossible with current methods. Our group was able to detect four paternal inherited mutations of the β-globin[31]. The detection rate was 86%, 100%, 100% and 81%, respectively. Only one false positive result was seen in one of the four examined point mutations. The continuing use of mass-spectroscopy will allow the detection of specific alleles, point mutations or even differences in single nucleotides (single-nucleotide polymorphism).

Most studies generate data from pregnancies with male fetuses as sequences on the Y chromosome are unique DNA markers, which are absent in the maternal genome. This approach is only applicable to approximately 50% of the pregnancies, but is straightforward to perform. An impediment in the generation of accurate data is the low number of fetal sequences in the plasma, such that the samples quantified by the real-time PCR have copy numbers close to the detection limit and therefore the results of a study may be limited by this fact.

Non-invasive prenatal diagnosis and screening with fetal RNA from maternal plasma, expressed from the placenta

A new development in prenatal screening research constitutes the measurement of fetal RNA in the maternal blood. It gives the possibility to screen for sex-unspecific disorders.[12] Fetal RNA in maternal plasma is surprisingly stable and holds promise for non-invasive gene expression profiling.[32–34] Unlike fetal DNA, extracted from maternal serum or plasma, fetal RNA can be used for prenatal testing irrespective of fetal gender and genetic polymorphism status. To date, only a few reports present quantitative data on this phenomenon. They indicate that fetal RNA extracted from maternal plasma represents a gender independent marker, which may be used for non-invasive gene-expression profiling and may be a suitable additional screening tool for pregnancy associated pathologies. In the case of preeclampsia, not only elevated levels of cell-free fetal DNA, but also elevated levels of fetal RNA were detectable in maternal plasma.[35] The presence of fetal RNA in maternal plasma/serum gives the possibility of investigating the expression of certain genes in analogy with the presently used RNA markers in oncology.[36]

The fast progress and success in non-invasive prenatal research may give a future prospect for valuable alternatives in regard to invasive prenatal diagnostic tests.

REFERENCES

1. Stranc LC, Evans JA, Hamerton JL. Chorionic villus sampling and amniocentesis for prenatal diagnosis. *Lancet* 1997;349:711–4.
2. Canick JA, Kellner LH. First trimester screening for aneuploidy: Serum biochemical markers. *Semin Perinatol* 1999;23:359–68.
3. Wald NJ, Hackshaw AK. Combining ultrasound and biochemistry in first-trimester screening for Down's syndrome. *Prenat Diagn* 1997;17:821–9.
4. Stewart TL, Malone FD. First trimester screening for aneuploidy: Nuchal translucency sonography. *Semin Perinatol* 1999;23: 369–81.
5. Crossley JA, Aitken DA, Cameron AD, McBride E, Connor JM. Combined ultrasound and biochemical screening for Down's syndrome in the first trimester: a Scottish multicentre study. *BJOG* 2002;109:667–76.
6. Wapner R, Thom E, Simpson JL, Pergament E, Silver R, Filkins K, Platt L, Mahoney M, Johnson A, Hogge WA, Wilson RD, Mohide P, Hershey D, Krantz D, Zachary J, Snijders R, Greene N, Sabbagha R, MacGregor S, Hill L, Gagnon A, Hallahan T, Jackson L. First-trimester screening for trisomies 21 and 18. *N Engl J Med* 2003;349:1405–13.
7. Muller F, Benattar C, Audibert F, Roussel N, Dreux S, Cuckle H. First-trimester screening for Down syndrome in France combining fetal nuchal translucency measurement and biochemical markers. *Prenat Diagn* 2003;23:833–6.
8. Cusick W, Buchanan P, Hallahan TW, Krantz DA, Larsen JW Jr, Macri JN. Combined first-trimester versus second-trimester serum screening for Down syndrome: A cost analysis. *Am J Obstet Gynecol* 2003;188:745–51.
9. Haddow JE, Palomaki GE, Knight GJ, Williams J, Miller WA, Johnson A. Screening of maternal serum for fetal Down's syndrome in the first trimester. *N Engl J Med* 1998;338:955–61.
10. Mennuti MT, Driscoll DA. Screening for Down's syndrome – Too many choices? *N Engl J Med* 2003;349:1471.
11. Holzgreve W, Hahn S. Prenatal diagnosis using fetal cells and free fetal DNA in maternal blood. *Clin Perinatol* 2001;28:353–65.
12. Poon LL, Leung TN, Lau TK, Lo YM. The presence of fetal RNA in maternal plasma. *Clin Chem* 2000;46:1832–4.
13. Hahn S, Sant R, Holzgreve W. Fetal cells in maternal blood: Current and future perspectives. *Mol Hum Reprod* 1998;4:515–21.
14. Krabchi K, Gros-Louis F, Yan J, Bronsard M, Masse J, Forest JC, Drouin R. Quantification of fetal nucleated cells in maternal blood between the 18th and 22nd weeks of pregnancy using molecular cytogenetic techniques. *Clin Genet* 2001;60:145–150
15. Oosterwijk JC, Mesker WE, Ouwerkerk MC. Fetal cell detection in maternal blood: A study of 236 samples using erythroblasts morphology. DAB and HbF staining, and FISH analysis. *Cytometry* 1998;32:178–85.
16. Bianchi DW, Williams JM, Sullivan LM, Hanson FW, Klinger KW, Shuber AP. PCR quantification of fetal cells in maternal blood in normal and aneuploid pregnancies. *Am J Hum Genet* 1997;61:822–9.
17. Gaenshirt AD, Burschy M, Garritsen HS, *et al.* Magnetic cell sorting and the transferrin receptor as potential means to prenatal diagnosis from maternal blood. *Am J Obstet Gynecol* 1992;166: 1350–6.
18. Lo YMD, Corbetta N, Chamberlain PF, Rai V, Sargent IL, Redman CW, Wainscoat JS. Presence of fetal DNA in maternal plasma and serum. *Lancet* 1997; 350:485–7.
19. Hahn S, Kiefer V, Brombacher V, Troeger C, Holzgreve W. Fetal cells in maternal blood: An update from Basel. *Eur J Obstet Gynecol Reprod Biol* 1999;85:101–4
20. Sugito Y, Sekizawa A, Farina A, Yukimoto Y, Saito H, Iwasaki M. Relationship between severity of hyperemesis gravidarum and fetal DNA concentration in maternal plasma. *Clin Chem* 2003; 49:1667–9.
21. Zhong XY, Burk MR, Troeger C, Jackson LR, Holzgreve W, Hahn S. Fetal DNA in maternal plasma is elevated in pregnancies with aneuploid fetuses. *Prenat Diagn* 2000;20:795–8.
22. Swinkels DW, de Kok JB, Hendriks JC, Wiegerienck E, Zusterzeel PL, Steegers EA. Hemolysis, elevated liver enzymes, and low platelet count (HELLP) syndrome as a complication of preeclampsia in pregnant women increases the amount of cell-free fetal and maternal DNA in maternal plasma and serum. *Clin Chem* 2002;48:650–3.
23. Farina A, LeShane ES, Lambert-Messerlian GM, Canick JA, Lee T, Neveux LM, Palomaki GE, Bianchi DW. Evaluation of fetal cell free DNA as a second-trimester marker of Down syndrome pregnancy. *Clin Chem* 2003;49:239–42

24. Li Y, Zimmermann B, Rusterholz C, Kang A, Holzgreve W, Hahn S. Size separation of circulatory DNA in maternal plasma permits ready detection of fetal DNA polymorphisms. *Clin Chem* 2004;50:1002–11.
25. Lo YM, Tein MS, Lau TK, Haines CJ, Leung TN, Poon PM. Quantitative analysis of fetal DNA in maternal plasma and serum: Implications for non-invasive prenatal diagnosis. *Am J Hum Genet* 1998;62:768–775.
26. Guibert J, Benachi A, Grebille AG, Ernault P, Zorn JR, Costa JM. Kinetics of SRY gene appearance in maternal serum: Detection by real time PCR in early pregnancy after assisted reproductive technique. *Hum Reprod* 2003;18:1733–6.
27. Lui YY, Chik KW, Chiu RW, Ho CY, Lam CW, Lo YM. Predominant hematopoietic origin of cell free DNA in plasma and serum after sex-mismatched bone marrow transplantation. *Clin Chem* 2002;48:421–7.
28. Amicucci P, Gennarelli M, Novelli G, Dallapicolla B. Prenatal diagnosis of myotonic dystrophy using fetal DNA obtained from maternal plasma. *Clin Chem* 2000;46:301–2.
29. Saito H, Sekizawa A, Morimoto T, Suzuki M, Yanaihara T. Prenatal DNA diagnosis of a single-gene disorder from maternal plasma. *Lancet* 2000;356:1170.
30. Chiu RW, Lau TK, Leung TN, Chow KC, Chui DH, Lo YM. Prenatal exclusion of beta thalassaemia major by examination of maternal plasma. *Lancet* 2002;360:998–1000.
31. Ying L, Di Naro E, Vitucci A, Zimmermann B, Holzgreve W, Hahn S. Detection of paternally inherited fetal point mutations for β-Thalassemia using size-fractioned cell free fetal DNA in maternal plasma. *JAMA* 2005;293:843–9.
32. Tsui NB, Ng EK, Lo YM. Stability of endogenous and added RNA in blood specimens, serum, and plasma. *Clin Chem* 2002; 48:1647–53.
33. Ng EK, Tsui NB, Lau TK, *et al.* mRNA of placental origin is readily detectable in maternal plasma. *Proc Natl Acad Sci USA* 2003;100:4748–53.
34. Lo YMD, Chiu RWK. The biology and diagnostic applications of plasma RNA. *Ann N Y Acad Sci* 2004;1022:135–9.
35. Ng EK, Leung TN, Tsui NB, *et al.* The concentration of circulating corticotrophin-releasing hormone mRNA in maternal plasma is increased in preeclampsia. *Clin Chem* 2003;49:727–31.
36. Hasselmann DO, Rappl G, Rossler M, Ugurel S, Tilgen W, Reinhold U. Detection of tumour-associated circulating mRNA in serum, plasma and blood cells from patients with disseminated malignant melanoma. *Oncol Rep* 2001;8:115–8.

68 Multiple gestations: pregnancy evaluation by ultrasonography

S. Tercanli, D. V. Surbek, R. Zanetti-Dällenbach, I. Hösli and W. Holzgreve

Introduction

Since the introduction of ultrasound in prenatal medicine, the prognosis of multiple pregnancies has improved dramatically. Early and appropriate diagnosis of multiplicity and chorionicity, detection of discordant fetal growth, evaluation of fetal well-being by biophysical scoring and Doppler sonography as well as planning of delivery mode by determination of fetal presentation are some of the most important diagnostic advances that represent the basis of adequate clinical management. Multiple pregnancies are at increased risk for several complications during pregnancy and childbirth like prematurity, fetal growth retardation, twin–twin transfusion syndrome (TTS), pre-eclampsia, stillbirth and malpresentation. Therefore, early diagnosis of multiple pregnancies and in particular determination of chorionicity is mandatory for the appropriate assessment of risk factors, for intensive prenatal care and early detection as well as for treatment options of complications. Before the introduction of prenatal ultrasound, detection rate of twin pregnancies before delivery was lower than 50%,[1] while in countries where routine ultrasound in pregnancy is performed, the rate is close to 100%.[2] Consequently, this has led to decreased perinatal morbidity and mortality in twin and higher multiple gestations in the past 30 years.

In the following chapter we will give an overview of the most important clinical issues of multiple pregnancy where ultrasonography plays a major role in the diagnostic procedure.

Early diagnosis of multiple pregnancies

Why should a multiple pregnancy be diagnosed early? First, the number of fetuses, which can be confirmed by ultrasound, is a strong determinator of prognosis of a pregnancy, which is generally best for singletons and gets worse with higher-order multiplicity. As in singleton pregnancies, gestational age can be confirmed by an early ultrasound during the first trimester using growth charts of crown–rump length corresponding to gestational age.[3] In the first and second trimesters of pregnancy, growth charts for singleton pregnancies can be used appropriately for twin pregnancies.[4] More importantly, early ultrasound allows for definitive diagnosis of chorionicity, which itself is also a strong predictor of fetal outcome.

Usually, early diagnosis of multiple pregnancy by transvaginal sonography is easy.[5] After the fifth week of pregnancy (from the last menstrual period), different gestational sacs are visible in multichorionic gestations, whereas in monochorionic twins only one chorionic cavity is visible. From the sixth or seventh week of pregnancy, it is possible to identify the number of embryos and yolk sacs in multichorionic as well as monochorionic gestations (Figure 68.1a and b). As soon as two or more embryos with heart activity are discernible, the diagnosis of multiple gestations is confirmed. Although a false diagnosis of a singleton pregnancy may be made if a hurried scan is performed by an inexperienced examiner, the diagnosis at this stage is virtually error-free. Possible pitfalls may be chorial hematomas or a decidual pseudosac mimicking a second or third gestational sac, or conjoined twins mimicking a singleton pregnancy (Figure 68.2a and b).

Another issue in early diagnosis is the phenomenon of vanishing twins, which seems to occur in a significant proportion of twin gestations[6,7] and might be the reason for discordant diagnosis in subsequent ultrasound examinations. This phenomenon of 'vanishing embryos' is especially well established from *in vitro* programs such as those shown in Table 68.1, which summarizes data obtained in pregnancies after *in vitro* fertilization (IVF) where intact heart action of the embryos was the intake criterion for the prospective study. Vanishing embryos is the spontaneous abortion of a multiple gestation member in the first trimester either by expulsion or – more often – by complete resorption of the embryo (Figure 68.3). In many cases it remains asymptomatic, though sometimes it is accompanied by vaginal bleeding.

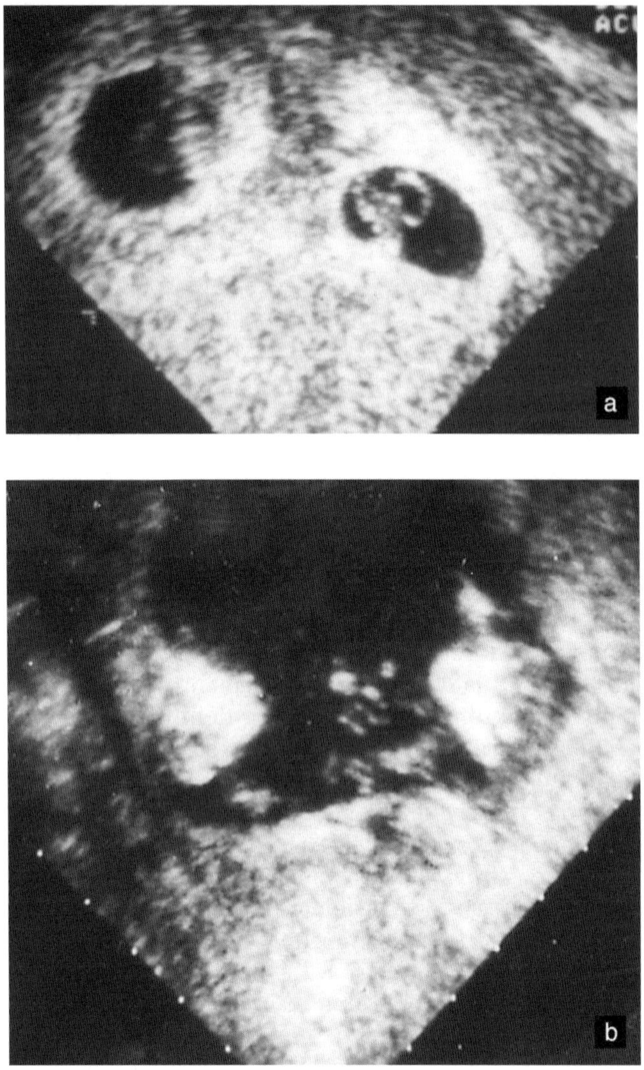

Figure 68.1 Transvaginal sonograms of pregnancies in the first trimester. (a) Dichorionic twin pregnancy with clear separation of the chorionic cavities. (b) Monochorionic twin pregnancy with both embryos anencephalic.

Prognosis for the surviving twin seems excellent, although recently it has been hypothesized that unexplained cerebral palsy might be the consequence in the survivor of a vanishing twin pair.[8,9]

Prenatal diagnosis of zygosity, chorionicity and amnionicity

Dizygotic twinning results in dichorionic–diamniotic pregnancies, even though the placentae may be fused (Figure 68.4). In contrast, monozygotic twinning may result in dichorionic–diamniotic, monochorionic–diamniotic or monochorionic–monoamniotic placentation, depending on the age of division. The division of the embryo results in the following constellations: from day 1 to day 3 after fertilization, dichorionic–diamniotic twins; from day 4 to day 6, dichorionic–monoamniotic twins; from day 7 to day 9, monochorionic–monoamniotic twins. If the division takes place after day 9,

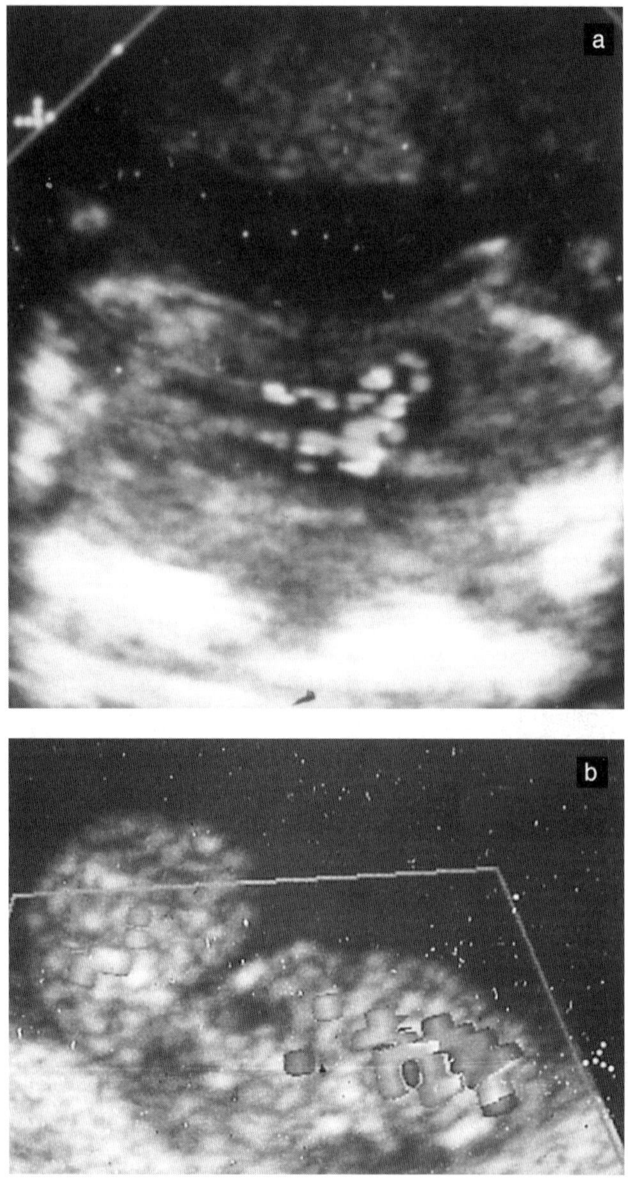

Figure 68.2 Conjoined twins mimicking a singleton pregnancy. Color-coded Doppler sonography. (a) A common fetal heart. (b) Two independent fetal hearts.

Table 68.1 Vanishing embryos in pregnancies with multiples. The 'intake criterion' was intact heart action. All pregnancies are from the *in vitro* fertilization program of Dr. Robert Fischer, Hamburg

Initial scan	Cases	Second trimester
Twins	52	34 twins 18 singletons
Triplets	22	8 triplets 11 twins 3 singletons
Quadruplets	4	2 quadruplets 2 triplets

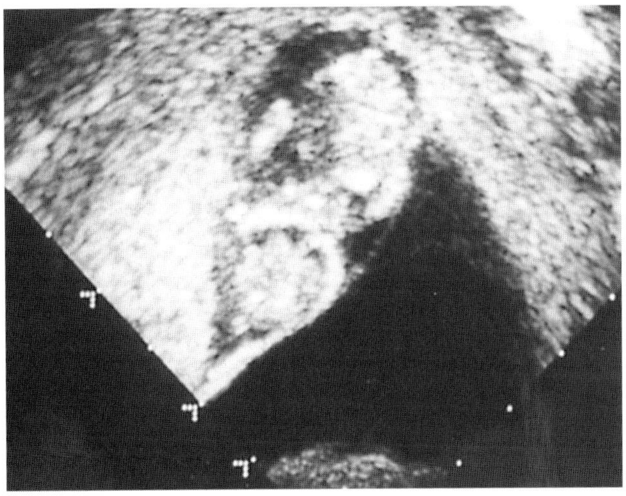

Figure 68.3 Dichorionic twin pregnancy with a 'vanishing embryo'. After spontaneous abortion of the twin in the upper left corner of the uterus, the amniotic fluid in this sac has almost disappeared and the embryo is getting almost 'resorbed'.

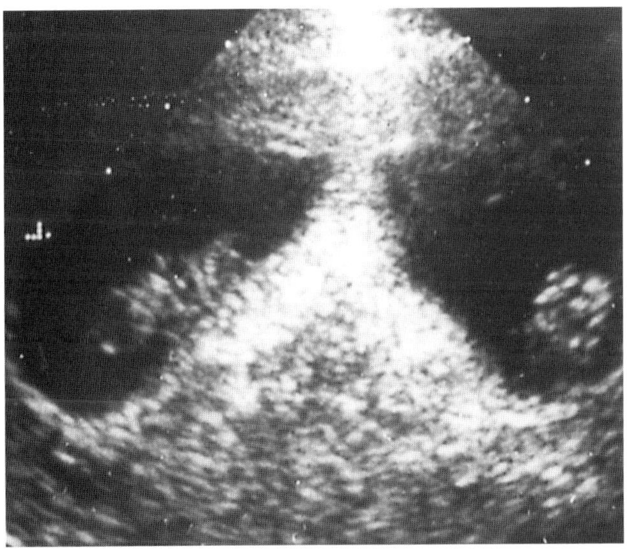

Figure 68.4 Dichorionic twin pregnancy where both chorion frondosum areas are so close to one another that the two placentae seems to be 'fused'.

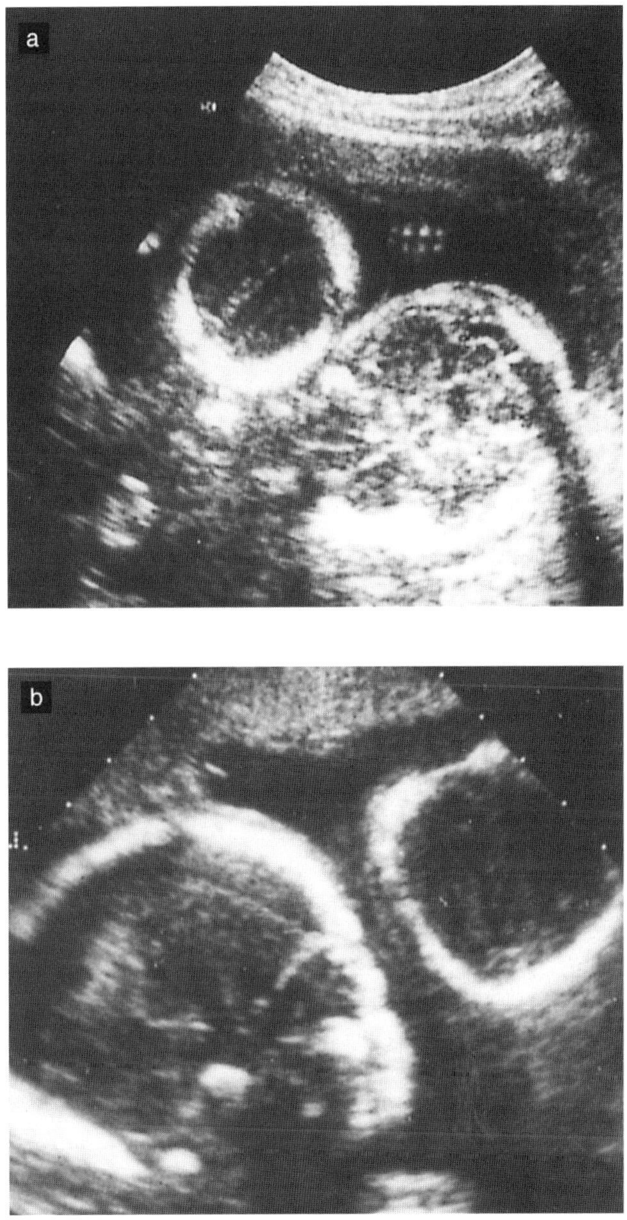

Figure 68.5 Twin pregnancy with (a) discordant growth and (b) intrauterine fetal demise. The sonogram shows the head of the survivor in the lower left and the dead fetus in the upper right corner.

conjoined twins result. Dichorionic placentation is found in 30% of monozygotic pregnancies.[10] As a rule, dizygous twins are always dichorionic, although this dogma has recently been disproven.[11,12]

Virtually all monochorionic twins, which represent about 20% of all twin pregnancies, have vascular anastomoses in the placenta, whereas almost none of the dichorionic (fused) placentas shows such cross-circulation.[13] These vascular shunts usually remain balanced, but occasionally they might become functional, leading to typical monochorionic twin complications like discordant growth (Figure 68.5a) and TTS.[14] Alternatively, in situations with one intrauterine fetal demise (Figure 68.5b) complications from vascular anastomoses might arise in the surviving twin. These include severe conditions like multicystic encephalomalacia and renal infarctions. In earlier publications, several authors postulated that embolization of thromboplastin-like material across the shared circulation followed by disseminated intravascular coagulation is the cause of this phenomenon, which is also called the twin disruption syndrome. More recent evidence, however, suggests another pathophysiological mechanism, which is based on the assumption that a sudden blood pressure gradient may occur at the moment of fetal demise, followed by severe hypotension and exsanguinations in the surviving fetus, leading to acute hypoxic organ damage predominantly in the brain in

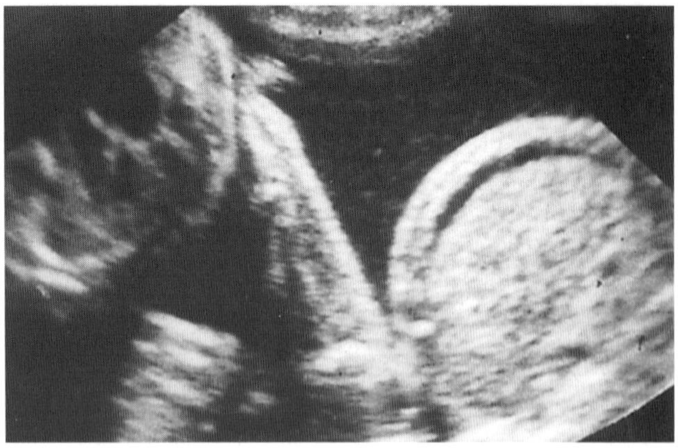

Figure 68.6 Twin–twin transfusion sequence in monochorionic and monoamniotic twin pregnancy. The right fetus has a beginning ascites in the abdomen as a sign of cardiac failure.

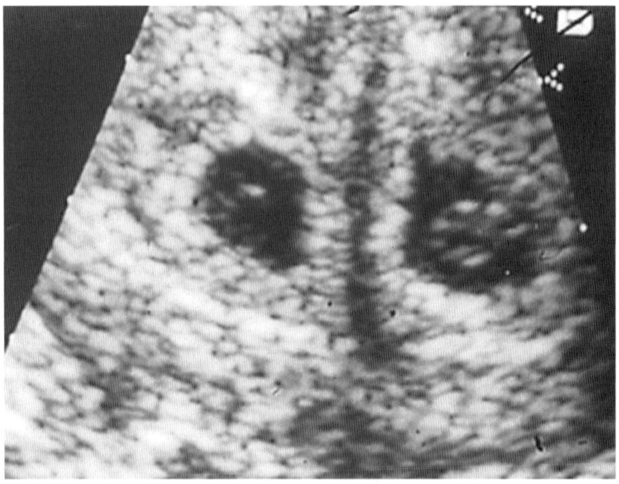

Figure 68.7 Dichorionic twin pregnancies. The two sacs are clearly separated.

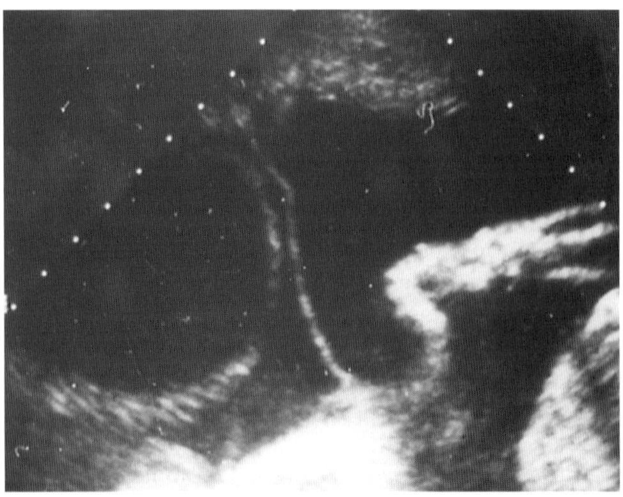

Figure 68.8 Biamniotic twin pregnancy with two discernable amniotic membranes surrounding the embryo.

up to 20% of survivors.[15] This phenomenon could be called an acute TTS.[16]

These complications occur only in monochorionic gestations (Figure 68.6). In particular, the fetal loss rate in monochorionic pregnancies is up to four times higher as compared to dichorionic twin pregnancies. Chorionicity is thus the most important factor influencing the outcome of twin pregnancies. Consequently, accurate prenatal diagnosis of chorionicity is of predominant importance for the clinical management of twin pregnancies.

As outlined above, monochorionic twins usually have a separating membrane, and thus are diamniotic. Fewer than 2% of twins are monoamniotic. Besides complications of monochorionicity, these pregnancies are at high risk for cord accidents during pregnancy and birth, resulting in an extremely high fetal loss rate of 50–75%. Delivery by early elective cesarean section is therefore one of the most important features of the management of monoamniotic twins.

Determination of chorionicity and amnionicity before birth is done by ultrasonography. In early pregnancy during the first trimester, it is usually easy to differentiate the type of placentation by transvaginal sonography. If two gestational sacs with two embryos are identified, the diagnosis of dichorionic twins can be made with certainty (Figure 68.7). On the other hand, if there is only one gestational sac with two embryos, monochorionic twins are diagnosed. To separate monoamniotic from diamniotic gestation, it is necessary to discern two amniotic membranes surrounding the embryos (Figure 68.8), or, at a later stage, to identify a partition membrane between the fetuses (Figure 68.9). If there is no membrane visible, the sonographer has to be cautious as a separating membrane might exist but might be hardly visible on ultrasound scan (Figure 68.10a), particularly in cases of severe oligohydramnios or anhydramnios of one twin combined with polyhydramnios in the other (Figure 68.10b), as it is typically present in TTS ('stuck twin').

Later in the first trimester, from about 10 to 14 weeks' gestation, the key to the differentiation of mono- and dichorionic–diamniotic twins is the 'twin peak' sign or lambda sign (Figure 68.11) used to predict dichorionic twins if present.[17] The latter finding consists of chorionic tissue extending between layers of the interfetal septum close to the placenta.

In the second or third trimester of gestation, other criteria become important in the determination of chorionicity. A reliable diagnosis of chorionicity can only be made if the fetuses are of opposite sex (dizygotic) or there are clearly two separated placentae visible, which is often not the case in dichorionic twins (Figure 68.12). Entanglement of umbilical cords represents a reliable sign confirming the presence of a single amniotic cavity in monoamniotic gestation.[18] In cases with the same fetal sex, with one non-separated placenta and with a dividing membrane between the fetuses, determination of chorionicity is difficult after

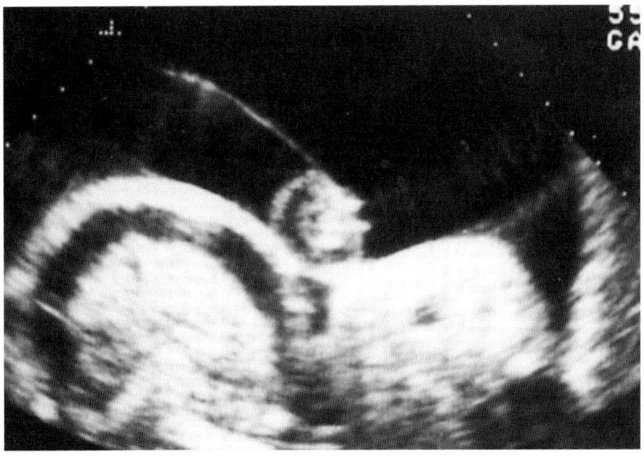

Figure 68.9 Biamniotic twin pregnancies with the partition membrane between the fetuses. A twin–twin transfusion syndrome is indicated by severe ascites in the left twin.

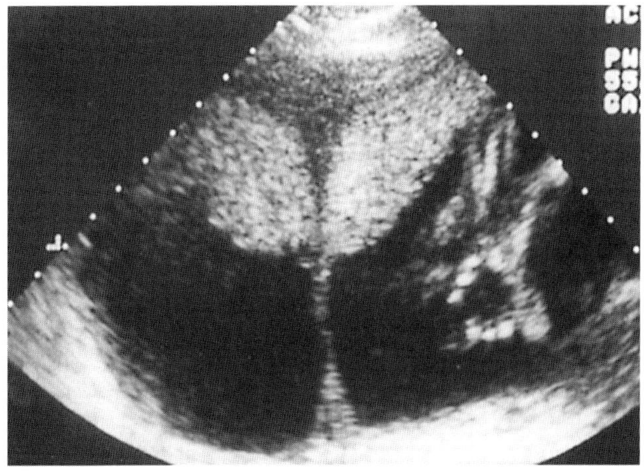

Figure 68.11 'Twin peak' sign in a dichorionic twin pregnancy.

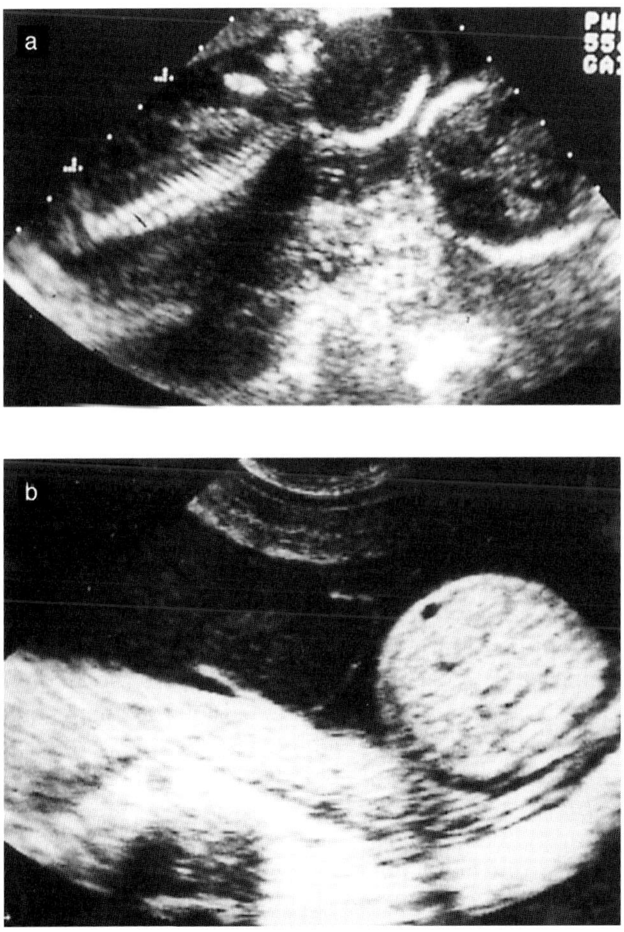

Figure 68.10 Biamniotic twin pregnancies. (a) The separating membrane can hardly be seen on top of the head of the left, smaller fetus. (b) Polyhydramnios is visible in the left, oligohydramnios in the right sac.

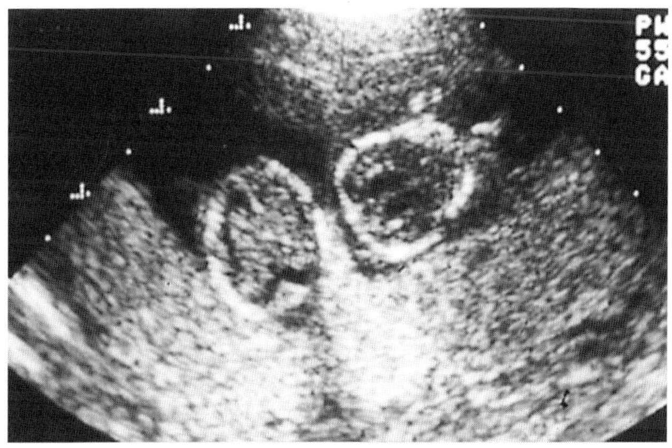

Figure 68.12 Dichorionic twin pregnancies. Although the two placentae are in close proximity to one another, they are separated.

the first trimester of gestation and requires other criteria. Thickness of the dividing membrane (Figure 68.13) measured by ultrasound is one criterion that is able to predict chorionicity, using a cutoff level of 2 mm.[19] Another important sonographic feature is the number of layers identified in the dividing membrane.[20] While not always technically possible, it remains a reliable criterion of dichorionic placentation if three or more layers are present. Probably the best approach is the combination of these criteria, reaching excellent predicting values in the determination of chorionicity.[21]

Fetal malformations and chromosomal anomalies in multiple pregnancy

Twins, above all monozygotic twins, are known to be at increased risk for malformations – not only because the presence of two fetuses in one pregnancy doubles the chance of a defect.[22] The incidence of malformations is higher in monochorionic than in dichorionic twins and the highest in monoamniotic twins. Furthermore, the incidence of chromosomal aneuploidy seems to be higher in twin gestations as compared to singletons.[23,24] A detailed study of fetal morphology in

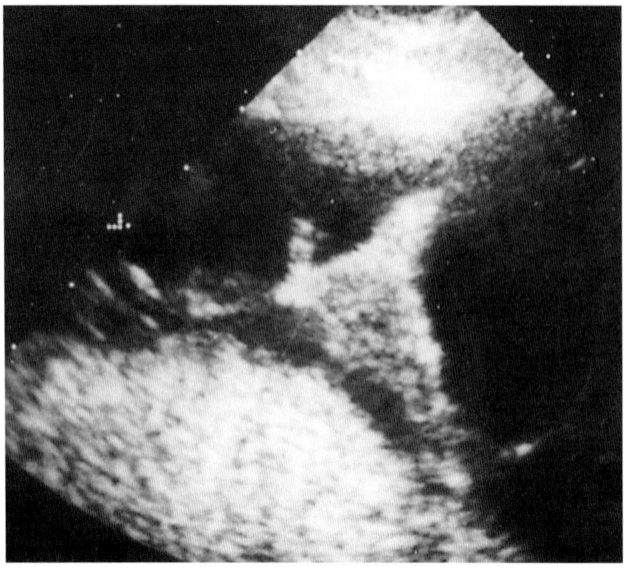

Figure 68.13 Dichorionic twin pregnancies. The thickness of the dividing membrane is more than 2 mm.

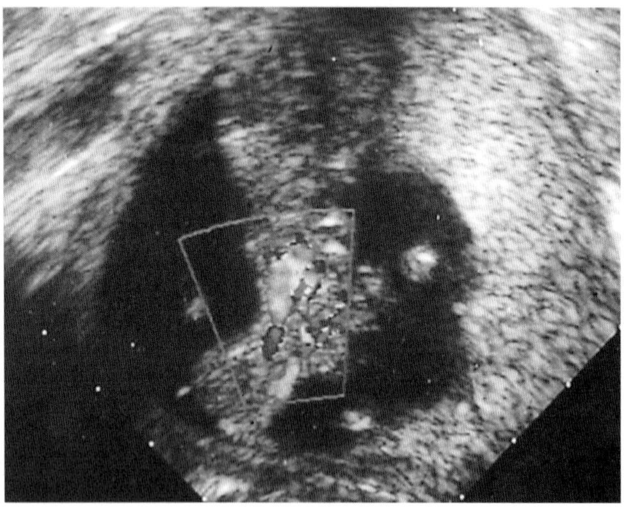

Figure 68.14 Sonogram of conjoined twins with two separate hearts.

multiple pregnancy by ultrasound is time-consuming and sometimes much more difficult than in singletons, but it should be done during routine ultrasound surveillance. Emphasis should be put not only on typical anomalies unique to the twinning process, but also on other anomalies known to be increased in twin pregnancies.

Congenital anomalies specific to multiple gestation occur infrequently but are usually severe. The rate of conjoined twins (Figure 68.14) is 1 in 50,000 births.[25] Prenatal diagnosis by ultrasonography including determination of type of anomaly and of shared organs (Figure 68.15) is important for the optimal management of those pregnancies in terms of appropriate determination of prognosis and plan of delivery route (cesarean section) and postnatal care. In severe cases diagnosed early, termination of pregnancy is an option that many parents choose. Ultrasonographic criteria for the detection of conjoined twins have been proposed: a missing separating membrane, a fixed position of the twins toward each other and a lack of separate visualization of the fetuses in a specific anatomical region. Different patterns of physical joining exist, resulting in different prognosis of the pregnancies. The symmetric complete form of conjoined twinning is present when two fetuses are anatomically almost 'complete' except the part of the body where they share a certain amount of tissue. These 'diplopagi' are described after the body structure that is joined, namely, craniopagi, thoracopagi (accounting for 57% of diplopagi, Figure 68.16), omphalopagi and pygopagi. Postnatal separation is often possible in diplopagi except in cases where gross parts of the heart or central nervous system are shared. The symmetric incomplete forms are represented by twins with one trunk and a single lower part of the body together with two heads (dicephalus) or by twins with one head and upper trunk and a double lower body (dipygus). Asymmetric forms are conjoined twins, one of which is severely malformed and often rudimentary (parasitic twin) while the other is normally developed.

An extreme form of twin-specific asymmetric malformation is the so called acranius–acardius, also known as chorangiopagus parasiticus, or twin reversed arterial perfusion (TRAP) sequence. Numerous theories about pathogenesis of this syndrome, which occurs in a frequency of 1 in 35,000 births, have been subject to discussion in the literature. Typical features are functional vascular anastomoses between not-joined twins with reverse arterial perfusion of the lower part of the malformed twin leading to varying degrees of upper body reduction including acardia and acranius.[26] Doppler sonography may be helpful in identifying cardiac structures, reversed perfusion and vascular anastomoses.[27] A different theory of pathogenesis is the primary existence of acranius–acardius malformation, which is supported by the fact that the malformed twin has been found to have a high prevalence of chromosomal anomalies. Mortality in the reversely perfused twin is 100%. The other fetus, the so-called 'pump-twin', is usually severely compromised by a high-output heart failure, which leads to a mortality of 50%. An intervention might be necessary and indicated, which includes ligation/coagulation of the cord or of intra-abdominal blood vessels of the acranius–acardius twin.

Congenital anomalies not specifically related to multiple gestations have the same ultrasonographic features as in singleton pregnancies. These malformations affect mainly the tracheoesophageal anatomy, the genitourinary and central nervous systems (e.g. neural tube defects), and the cardiovascular system.

Chromosomal anomalies are also increased in multiple gestations. The risk of chromosomal anomalies

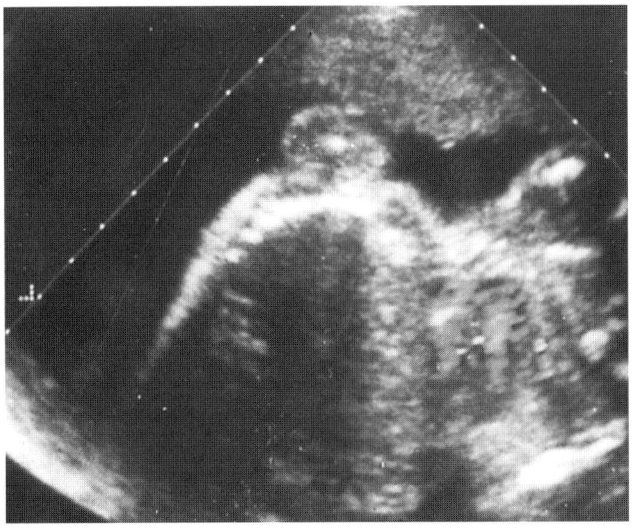

Figure 68. 15 Sonogram of conjoined twins with one heart.

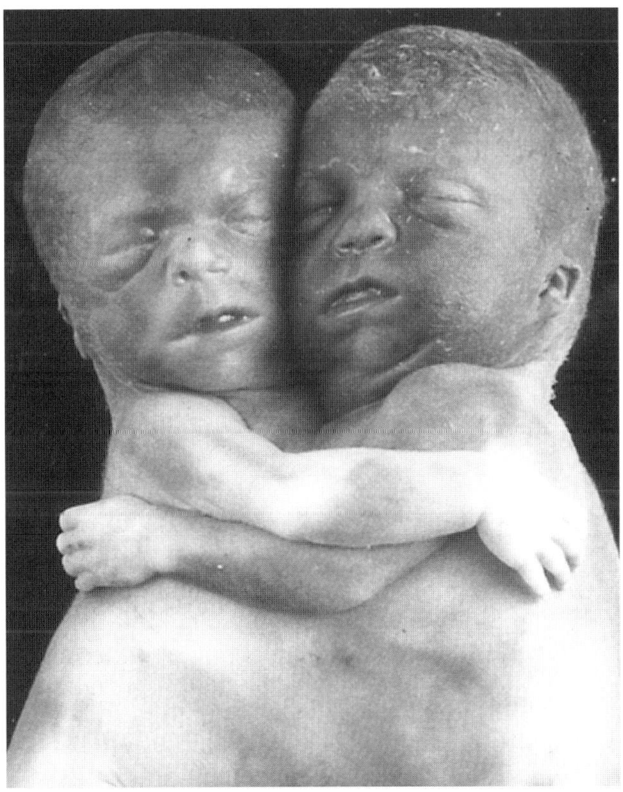

Figure 68.16 Almost completely conjoined twins. Thoracopagus anomaly.

in a twin pregnancy can be calculated using maternal age, zygosity and nuchal translucency of the twin fetuses. In dichorionic twins, the detection rate of nuchal translucency measurements for chromosomal anomalies is similar to that in singletons, whereas in monochorionic twins there are more false positives due to placentation-specific alterations of the nuchal translucency. In particular, care must be taken if a large difference in nuchal translucency is found in monochorionic twins because this could be an early manifestation of TTS and not of a karyotype anomaly. In monozygous twins, the karyotype is the same in both twins, and calculations are used for both. In dizygous twins, the risk must be calculated separately for each of the twins. Biochemical parameters such as free β-HCG and PAPP-A (in the first trimester) or α-fetoprotein, free β-HCG, estriol and inhibin (in the second trimester) can be used but are less useful, yielding a lower detection rate of chromosomal anomalies in twins.[28] Simple use of normative values from singleton pregnancies is not possible as medians are different. Current studies are evaluating the validity of twin pregnancy-adjusted normative values.

If the parents want prenatal karyotyping, chorionic villus sampling (CVS) or amniocentesis (AC) can be performed as possible options.[29–32] The parents must be informed in detail about the difficulties and risks of karyotyping in multiple pregnancies. The procedure might be technically difficult, leading to incomplete results (i.e. karyotyping of only one fetus in twins). On the other hand, difficulties might arise if one fetus turns out to be healthy while the other is affected by a severe chromosomal anomaly. In multiple gestations, CVS imposes specific problems due to a missing safeguard in proving that identical karyotypes represent monozygotic twins rather than sampling from the same chorion frondosum. In multichorionic gestations, the placentas might be close to each other, leading to difficulties in separate sampling (Figure 68.17). Furthermore, contamination of one sample with the villi of the other might happen. If fetal sex is different, it could be safely determined that both fetuses have been karyotyped. When suspicion arises, 'follow-up' amniocentesis should be offered. Consequently, CVS in twins should only be performed if individual samples can be guaranteed. Amniocentesis is the alternative procedure, often preferred in multiple gestation. After the puncture and retrieval of amniotic fluid of one amniotic sac, indigo carmine is injected before the needle is retracted. In the following puncture of the second amniotic cavity, the aspirated amniotic fluid is checked in color to exclude re-entry of the amniotic cavity of the same fetus. With this technique, amniocentesis in twins with a correct diagnosis of fetal karyotypes is feasible in most twin pregnancies[33] and has a somewhat lower loss rate as CVS. As a rule, the higher the risk for chromosomal anomaly in a twin, the earlier the diagnosis should be made, ideally by CVS. The reason for this is that if one twin is affected and the parents opt for selective termination, the risk of the latter procedure for the surviving twin is lower, the earlier the selective feticide of the co-twin is performed.

If in a multiple pregnancy one child is proven by prenatal diagnosis to be affected with an untreatable condition, e.g. trisomy 18 or 13 or a severe malformation, a selective feticide can be performed by applying KCl directly to the fetal heart.[34] This technique, however, may exclusively be used if monochorionic

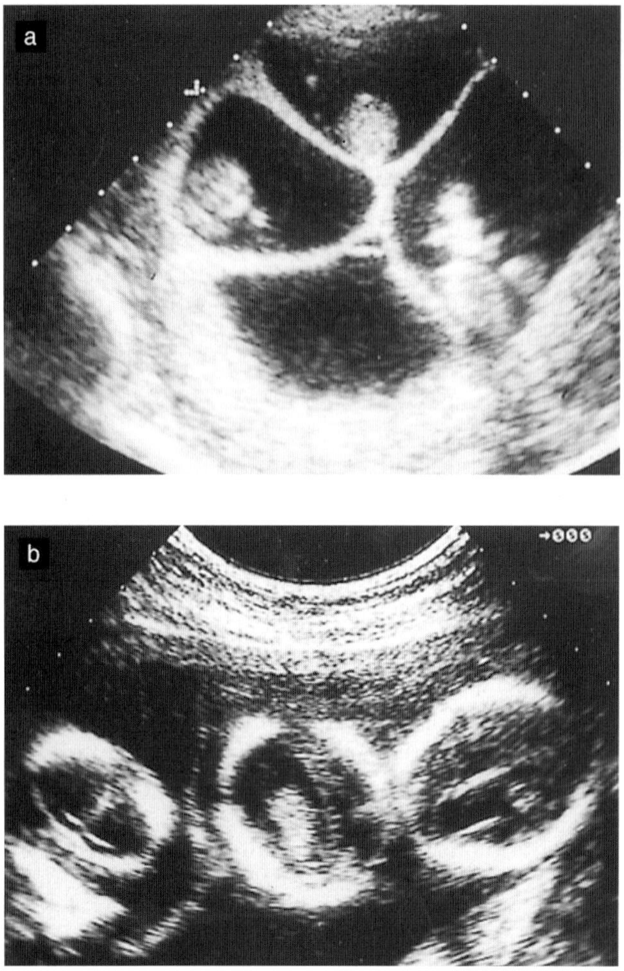

Figure 68.17 High multiple pregnancies. (a) Quadruplet pregnancy in the first trimester. The placentae are so close to each other that they cannot be easily sampled separately. (b) Triplet pregnancy in the third trimester. The separating membranes are more difficult to be seen than in the first trimester.

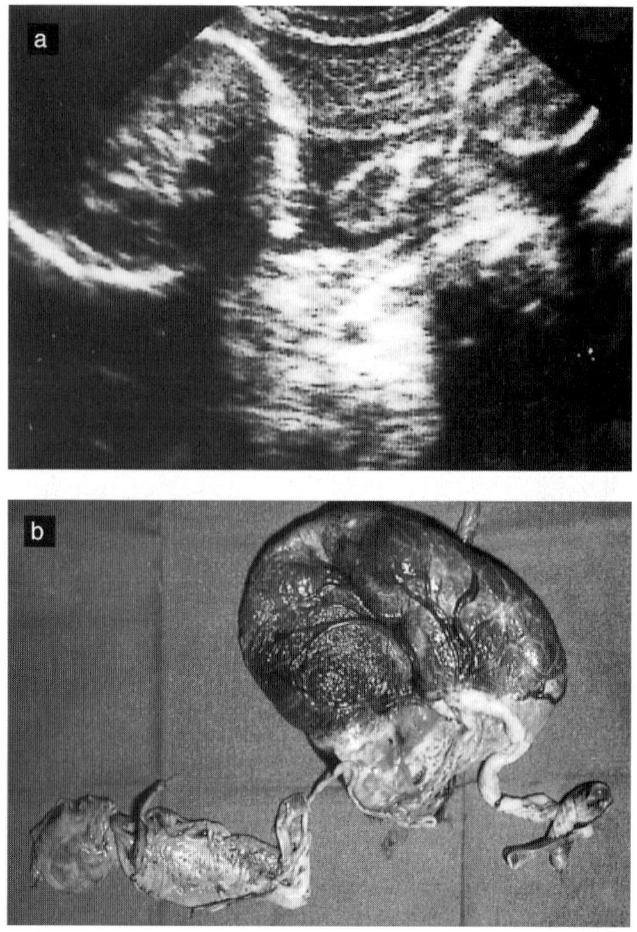

Figure 68.18 Situation after selective feticide. (a) Sonogram shows the small dead fetus in the upper right corner of the picture. (b) After delivery the 'fetus papyraceus' and the 'dead part' of the placenta can easily be seen.

placentation is excluded. The selective fetocide is ethically not much different from a termination of a whole pregnancy in singletons, except for the fact that the pregnancy *per se* continues and the dead fetus usually follows after the livebirth of the co-twin together with the placenta (Figure 68.18a and b).[35]

In pregnancies with very high multiples, e.g. octuplet pregnancies (Figure 68.19a and b), this would be bound to fail (Figure 68.20a and b), so that a 'reduction' of the number of living fetuses has been performed in order to avoid loss of the whole pregnancy spontaneously or through termination. This procedure is called multifetal pregnancy reduction and is performed by intracardiac injection of KCl in 'multiple-chorionic' multiples; again, monochorionicity must be excluded. The outcome of the pregnancy after this procedure depends significantly on the starting number of fetuses, the finishing number and the operator's experience.[36] The primary aim, however, must be to avoid iatrogenic higher-order multiple pregnancy, e.g. by controlled use of ovulation inducing drugs or by restriction of the number of transferred embryos to two during IVF procedure.

Fetal growth in multiple pregnancies

As in all pregnancies, the appropriate dating of pregnancy is important in terms of determination of fetal growth to differentiate growth restriction from normal growth. Dating is best done in the first or early second trimester by combining the date of the last menstrual period with fetal ultrasound measurements.

We mentioned before that in twin pregnancies, growth charts of singletons can be used at least up to the beginning of the third trimester, because normal growth in twins is the same as in singletons. Only after 28–30 weeks of pregnancy does intrauterine growth gradually decrease compared to singletons.[4,37] It has been estimated that after 32 weeks of pregnancy, weight gain of both fetuses in twin pregnancy equals the weight gain of one singleton.

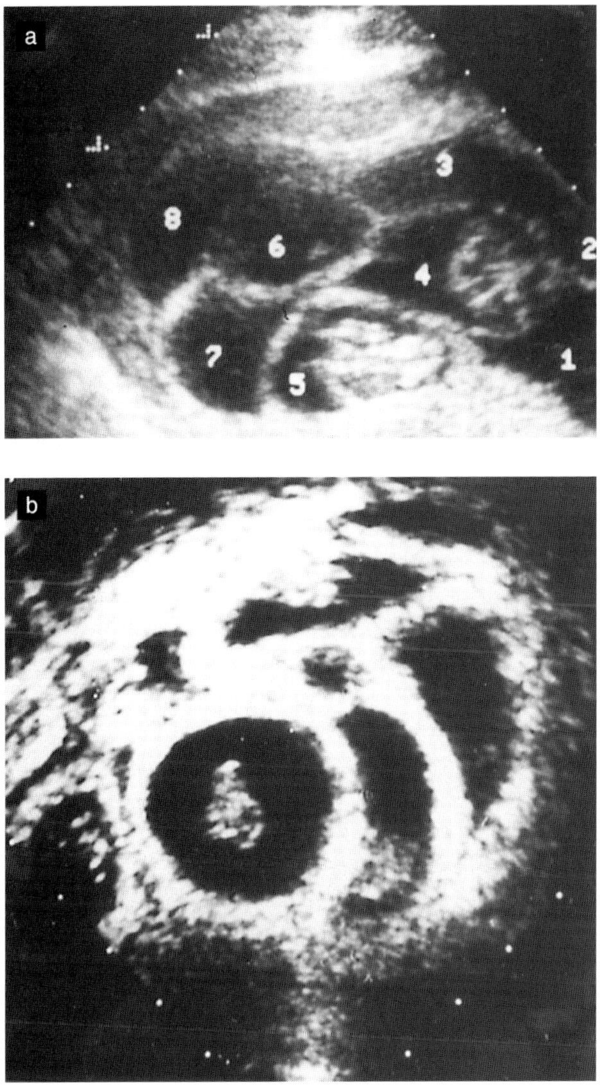

Figure 68.19 (a, b) Two independent octuplet pregnancies which both occurred after ovulation induction by gynecologic practitioners.

Assessment of fetal growth in twin pregnancies has been performed initially by measurements of biparietal diameter,[38] though it has been shown later that biparietal diameter is not an appropriate measurement for detection of discordance in twins.[39] Possible explanations for these difficulties might be different fetal positions and overlaying fetal parts of the other twin. Better estimates of fetal growth and prediction of discordance are accomplished by femur length and abdominal circumference,[40–43] where technical difficulties in measuring seem to be of minor importance.

If discordant growth in twin pregnancy (defined by an estimated weight difference of 20–25% between the fetuses) is diagnosed by prenatal ultrasound, several possibilities exist. The most common cause for the weight discordance is a constitutional weight difference in normal dizygotic twins. In contrast, pathologic causes might result in often severe growth difference between twins. The prevalence of intrauterine growth restriction is up to 10 times higher in twins than in singletons, in particular in monochorionic twins. Pathologic conditions include intrauterine growth retardation affecting one or both twins, because of local uteroplacental factors (which might happen in dichorionic or monochorionic pregnancies) or TTS (Figure 68.21a and b). In some cases, congenital anomaly of only one

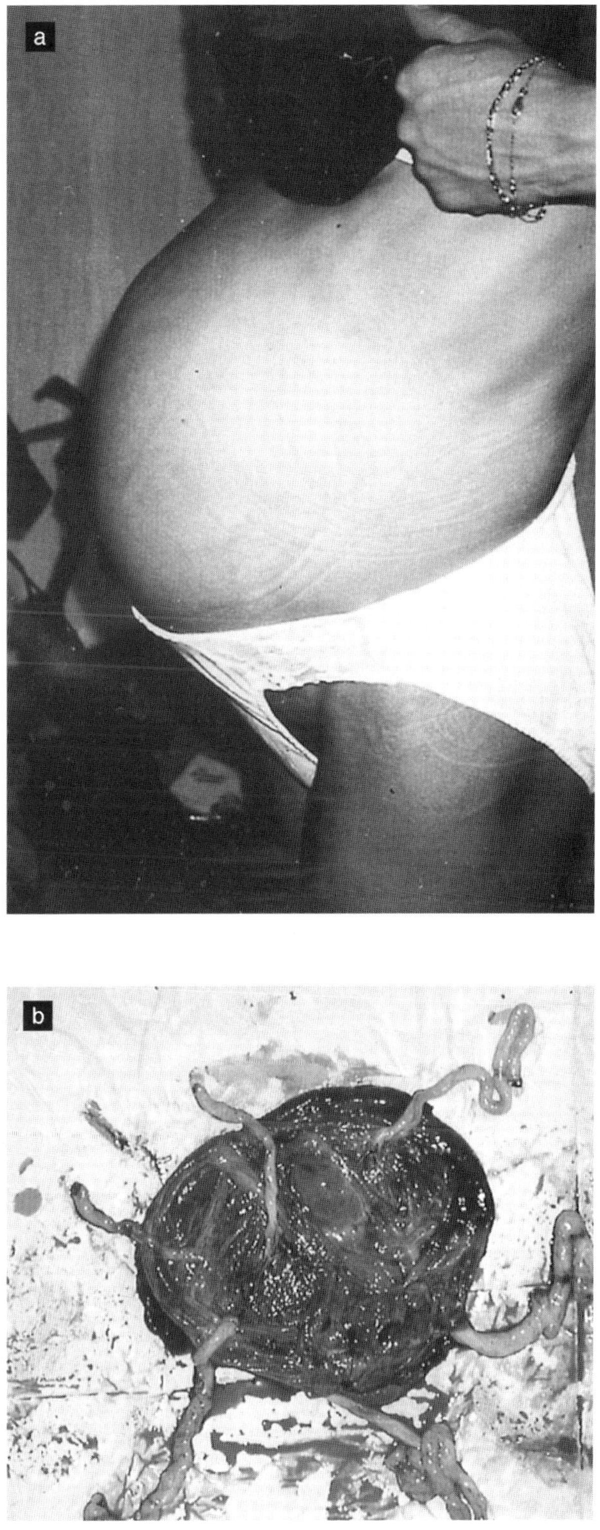

Figure 68.20 Complication of high multiple pregnancies. (a) Triplet pregnancy at 26 weeks of gestation. (b) Placenta of sextuplet pregnancy after spontaneous abortion.

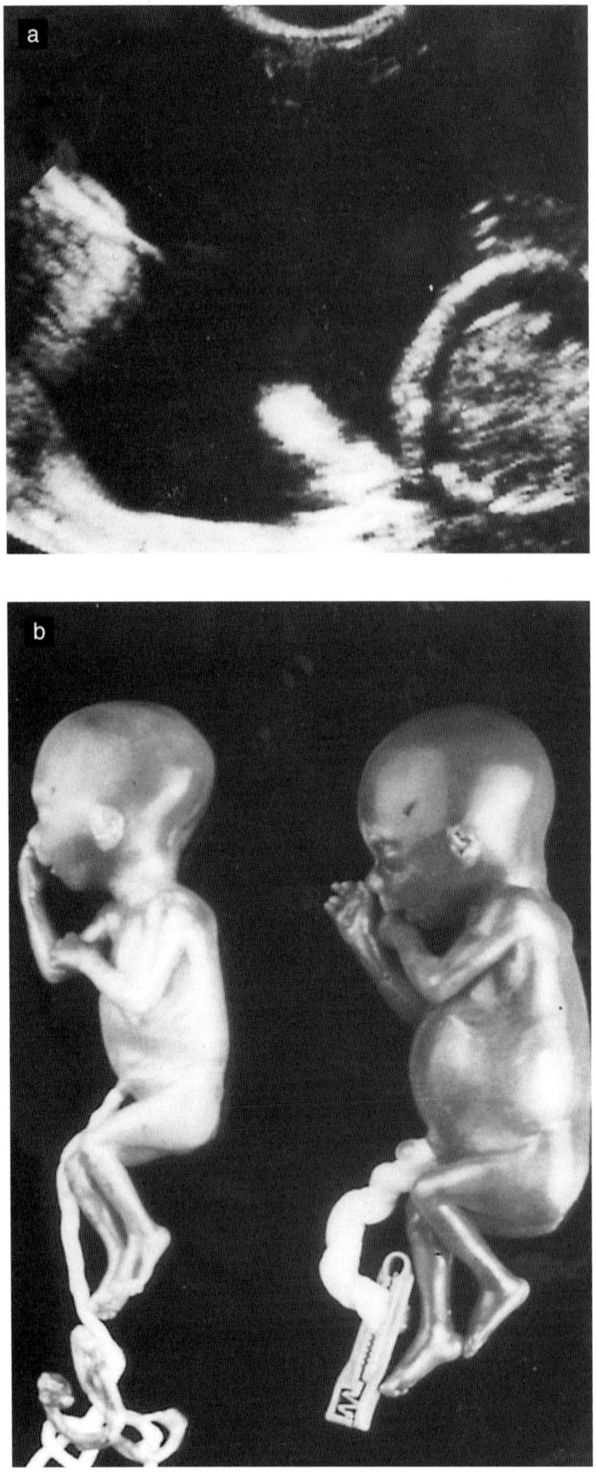

Figure 68.21 Twin–twin transfusion syndrome. (a) Sonogram showing severe polyhydramnios and non-immune hydrops in the recipient twin. (b) Fetus after spontaneous abortion. The right one is plethoric, whereas the left one (donor twin) is anemic and smaller.

fetus might also lead to discordant growth. An important question in discordant twins is chorionicity and amniotic fluid amount. Overall, perinatal morbidity and mortality besides later intellectual sequelae are increased in twin pregnancies, irrespective of the underlying cause.[44]

Doppler velocimetry has proved to be predictive of fetal hypoxia in growth-retarded singletons.[45] Similarly, this technique might be used in twins as an additional measure for detection of growth discordance and fetal compromise.[46,47] Furthermore, with color Doppler, placental anastomoses in twin–twin transfusin syndrome can be detected, which might be helpful for intrauterine treatment by fetoscopic laser ablation of placental vessels (see below).[48]

As in singletons, an individual biophysical profile including non-stress testing should be applied in both twins in growth restricted twin pregnancies as an important tool for assessment of fetal well-being.[49]

Twin–twin transfusion syndrome

TTS is a condition that develops in about 10–25% of monochorionic twin pregnancies. The underlying cause for this syndrome is imbalance of vascular anastomoses between the placental circulation of both twins within the single (monochorionic) placenta. This imbalance leads to decreased feto-placental blood volume in the donor and increased volume in the recipient. The definition of TTS includes the polyhydramnios–oligohydramnios sequence (POS). Typical sonographic features include in the donor fetus oligohydramnios or anhydramnios ('stuck twin' phenomenon), small or absent bladder and growth restriction, whereas the recipient shows polyhydramnios and a large bladder. In both twins, the condition can lead to cardiac decompensation, detectable by ultrasound (including tricuspid regurgitation and negative ductus venosus A-wave in the recipient, pericardial effusion and hydrops). Doppler flow measurements in umbilical arteries can be pathologic in both twins (absent or reversed end-diastolic flow). Ultimately, fetal death in one or both twins can occur. Severe TTS has a 90% mortality and a high rate of neurologic long-term morbidity (handicap) in survivors if untreated.

The severity of TTS can be assessed by ultrasound, which correlates with the prognosis. Several criteria for classification have been proposed, the Quintero staging system being the most widely used.[50]

Management options depend on severity of TTS, gestational age and women's preference and include expectant management with close follow-up (in mild TTS), repetitive amniodrainage, needle septostomy or endoscopic laser coagulation of anastomoses. Cohort studies[51] and a recent multicenter randomized trial[52] suggest that laser treatment in severe TTS is superior to repetitive amniodrainage regarding neonatal mortality as well as morbidity. With regard to the current evidence, laser treatment seems to be the treatment of choice in severe TTS, but the long-term neurologic outcome results of the randomized trial are still awaited.

Ultrasonography for prediction of preterm deliveries in multiple pregnancies

Twin gestations are known to have a significantly increased risk of preterm delivery as compared to singletons. Early diagnosis of preterm contractions and individual preterm delivery risk assessment is therefore particularly important. Cervical ultrasound has recently been shown to be predictive of preterm delivery. Initial studies measuring cervical length by transabdominal ultrasonography found a significant correlation of a shortened cervix with preterm delivery. As shown by different examiners, transabdominal measurement of cervical length has the disadvantage of being biased by the degree of bladder filling, which led to the increased use of transvaginal ultrasound probes in pregnancy.[53] Besides the cervical length, dilatation of the internal cervical os, protrusion of membranes in the cervical canal, length of funneling and thickness of the wall of the lower uterine segment have been used more or less successfully to diagnose cervical incompetence and to predict preterm birth. Ultrasonographic determination of cervical morphology has been shown to be superior to digital examination of the cervix for the prediction of preterm birth if there is no overt cervical dilatation of 2 cm or more. While some studies have used transvaginal ultrasound for the prediction of the likelihood of preterm delivery in patients with preterm labor, a recent multicenter study proved a correlation of cervical length measured in the second trimester in asymptomatic patients with the risk of preterm delivery.[54] A major finding in this study was that cervical length did seem to be a continuous variable rather than a dichotomous variable, suggesting that cervical function might be a continuum, in contrast to the earlier belief that the cervix is either 'competent' or 'incompetent'. Other studies have shown that ultrasonography of the cervix might be used as well in the follow-up after cervical cerclage, measuring the distance between the cerclage suture and the internal cervical os.[55]

Though some of these studies have excluded multiple pregnancies, others have specifically determined the predictive value in twin pregnancies.[56] One may conclude that ultrasonographic determination of the cervix and the lower part of the uterus is an important additional tool in predicting preterm delivery in multiple gestations, where the risk of prematurity is especially high.

Intrapartum ultrasonography in multiple gestation

There is considerable controversy in the literature around intrapartum management of multiple gestations.[57] Multiple pregnancies of higher order are usually delivered by cesarean section. In twins, the single most important question is the route of delivery in different subsets of twins and, additionally, in different clinical situations like prematurity, growth retardation or pre-eclampsia. Above all, the management plan for delivery has to take presentation of the twins into consideration, which includes all possible combinations of vertex, breech, transverse and oblique presentation of the first and second twins.[58] Ultrasonography can be reliably used for detection of these different presentations before onset of labor, during labor, after delivery of the first twin or after interventions like external or internal version of the second twin. Again, ultrasound examination is the most important tool in the peripartum management of twin pregnancies.

Conclusions

The aim of this chapter was to discuss the most important clinical applications of ultrasonography in multiple gestations. Beginning with early gestation, diagnosis of multiplicity, zygosity, chorionicity and amnionicity are predominant tasks for determination of the risk of complications later in pregnancy. Typical complications of monochorionic twins with vascular anastomoses are being explained. Fetal congenital anomalies in multiple gestations are different in many ways from singletons and represent another problem of primary importance in routine medical care. Multiple gestation-specific anomalies like conjoining can be discerned from non-specific congenital malformations, which exist as well in singletons. Invasive procedures for prenatal chromosomal analysis are briefly discussed, which are more difficult than in singletons as one has to deal with more than one maternal and one fetal karyotype.

Discordant fetal growth is a major complication in multiple gestations. The diagnosis is usually confirmed by ultrasonography; at the same time, the underlying pathology like growth restriction based on fetal malformation of one twin or TTS might be evaluated. Cervical change assessed by vaginal ultrasonography has been shown to be predictive of spontaneous preterm delivery in singletons; similarly this might be applicable in multiple gestations. Finally, peripartum ultrasonography for the detection of presentation is crucial in planning delivery and possible intrapartum intervention in twins.

REFERENCES

1. Grennert L, Persson PH, Gennser G, Kullander S. Ultrasound and human-placental-lactogen screening for early detection of twin pregnancies. *Lancet* 1976;1(7949):4–6.
2. Wenstrom KD, Gall SA. Incidence, morbidity and diagnosis of twin gestations. *Clin Perinatol* 1988;15:1–11.
3. Daya S. Accuracy of gestational age estimation using fetal crown–rump length measurements. *Am J Obstet Gynecol* 1993;168:903–8.
4. Reece EA, Yarkoni S, Abdalla M, Gabrielli S, Holford T, *et al.* A prospective longitudinal study of growth in twin gestations compared with growth in singleton pregnancies I. The fetal head. II. The fetal limbs. *J Ultrasound Med* 1991;10:439–43.
5. Holzgreve W, Westendorp J, Tercanli S. First trimester ultrasound. In Evans MI, ed. *Reproductive Risks and Prenatal Diagnosis.* Norwalk: Appleton & Lange, 1992:121–50.
6. Sampson A, de Crespigny LC. Vanishing twins: The frequency of spontaneous fetal reduction of a twin pregnancy. *Ultrasound Obstet Gynecol* 1992;2(2):107–9.
7. Newton R, Casabonne D, Johnson A, Pharoah P. A case–control study of vanishing twins as a risk factor for cerebral palsy. *Twin Res* 2003;6(2):83–4.
8. Benirschke K, Kim CK. Multiple pregnancy. *N Engl J Med* 1973;288:1276–84, 1329–36.
9. Souter VL, Kapur RP, Nyholt DR, *et al.* A report of dizygous monochorionic twins. *N Engl J Med* 2003;349(2):154–8.
10. Robertson EG, Neer KJ. Placental injection studies in twin gestation. *Am J Obstet Gynecol* 1983;147:170–4.
11. Blickstein I. The twin–twin transfusion syndrome. *Obstet Gynecol* 1990;76:714–22.
12. Pharoah PO, Adi Y. Consequences of in-utero death in a twin pregnancy. *Lancet* 2000;355(9215):1597–602.
13. Fusi L, McParland P, Fisk N, *et al.* Acute twin–twin transfusion: A possible mechanism for brain damages survivors after intrauterine death of a monochorionic twin. *Obstet Gynecol* 1991;78:517–20.
14. Finberg HJ. The twin peak sign: Reliable evidence of dichorionic twinning. *J Ultrasound Med* 1992;11:571–7.
15. Nyberg DA, Filly RA, Golbus MS, Stephens JD. Entangled umbilical cords: A sign of monoamniotic twins. *J Ultrasound Med* 1984;3:29–32.
16. Townsend RR, Simpson GF, Filly RA. Membrane thickness in ultrasound prediction of chorionicity of twin gestations. *J Ultrasound Med* 1988;7:326–32.
17. D'Alton ME, Dudley DK. The ultrasonographic prediction of chorionicity in twin gestation. *Am J Obstet Gynecol* 1989;160:557–61.
18. Scardo JA, Ellings JM, Newman RB. Prospective determination of chorionicity, amnionicity and zygosity in twin gestations. *Am J Obstet Gynecol* 1995;173:1376–80.
19. Bryan E, Little J, Burn J. Congenital anomalies in twins. *Baillières Clin Obstet Gynecol* 1987;1:697–721.
20. Lubs HA, Ruddle F. Chromosomal abnormalities in the human population: Estimation of rates based on New Haven newborn study. *Science* 1970;169:495–7.
21. Hanson JW. Incidence of conjoined twinning. *Lancet* 1975;2(7947)1257.
22. Ash K, Harman CR, Gritter H. TRAP sequence – Successful outcome with indomethacin treatment. *Obstet Gynecol* 1990;76; 960–62.
23. Pretorius DH, Leopold GR, Moore TR, *et al.* Acardiac twin. Report of Doppler sonography. *J Ultrasound Med* 1988;7:413–6.
24. Spencer K, Nicolaides KH. Screening for trisomy 21 in twins using first trimester ultrasound and maternal serum biochemistry in a one-stop clinic: A review of three years experience. *BJOG* 2003;110(3):276–80.
25. Jackson LG, Wapner RJ, Barr MA. Safety of chorionic villus biopsy. *Lancet* 1986;1(8462)674–5.
26. Librach CL, Doran TA, Benzie RJ, Jones JM. Genetic amniocentesis in seventy twin pregnancies. *Am J Obstet Gynecol* 1984; 148:585–91.
27. Wapner RJ, Johnson A, Davis G, Urban A, Morgan P, Jackson L. Prenatal diagnosis in twin gestations: A comparison between second-trimester amniocentesis and first-trimester chorion villous sampling. *Obstet Gynecol* 1993;82:49–56.
28. Pruggmayer MRK, Jahoda MGJ, Van der Pol JG, *et al.* Genetic amniocentesis in twin pregnancies: Results of a multicenter study of 529 cases. *Ultrasound Obstet Gynecol* 1992;2:6–10.
29. Westendorp A, Holzgreve W, Miny P. Selective fetocide of a twin with trisomy 18 by intracardial KCL application. *Arch Gynecol* 1988;244:59–62.
30. Evans MI, Goldberg JD, Dumez Y, *et al.* Efficacy of second trimester selective termination (ST) for fetal abnormalities: International collaborative experience among the world's largest centers. *Obstet Gynecol* 1993;82:61–6.
31. Evans MI, Berkowitz RL, Wapner RJ, *et al.* Improvement in outcomes of multifetal pregnancy reduction with increased experience. *Am J Obstet Gynecol* 2001;184(2):97–103.
32. McKeown T, Record RG. Observations on fetal growth in multiple pregnancy in man. *J Endocrinol* 1952;8:386–401.
33. Grennert L, Persson PH, Genser G. Intrauterine growth of twins judged by BPD measurements. *Acta Obstet Gynecol Scand* 1978;78:28–32.
34. Erkkola R, Ala-Mello S, Piiroinen O, *et al.* Growth discordancy in twin pregnancies. A risk factor not detected by measurements of biparietal diameter. *Obstet Gynecol* 1985;66:203–6.
35. Brown CE, Guzick DS, Leveno KJ, *et al.* Prediction of discordant twins using ultrasound measurement of biparietal diameter and abdominal perimeter. *Obstet Gynecol* 1987;70:677–81.
36. Babson SG, Phillips DS. Growth and development of twins dissimilar in size at birth. *N Engl J Med* 1973;289:937–40.
37. Soothill PW, Nicolaides KN, Bilardo CM, Campbell S. Relation of fetal hypoxia in growth retardation to mean blood velocity in the fetal aorta. *Lancet* 1986;2(8516):1118–20.
38. Giles WB. Doppler assessment in multiple pregnancy. *Semin Perinatol* 1987;11:369–71.
39. DeLia JE, Cruikshank DP, Keye WR. Fetoscopic neodymium:YAG laser occlusion of placental vessels in severe twin–twin transfusion syndrome. *Obstet Gynecol* 1990;75:1046–53.
40. Lodeiro JG, Vintzileos AM, Feinstein SJ, *et al.* Fetal biophysical profile in twin gestations. *Obstet Gynecol* 1986;67:824–7.
41. Quintero RA, Morales WJ, Allen MH, Bornick PW, Johnson PK, Kruger M. Staging of twin–twin transfusion syndrome. *J Perinatol* 1999;19:550–5.
42. Hecher K, Plath H, Bregenzer T, Hansmann M, Hackeloer BJ. Endoscopic laser surgery versus serial amniocenteses in the treatment of severe twin–twin transfusion syndrome. *Am J Obstet Gynecol* 1999;180:717–24.
43. Senat MV, Deprest J, Boulvain M, Paupe A, Winer N, Ville Y. Endoscopic laser surgery versus serial amnioreduction for severe twin-to-twin transfusion syndrome. *N Engl J Med* 2004;351(2): 136–44.
44. Andersen HF, Nugent CE, Wanty SD, Hayashi RH. Prediction of risk of preterm delivery by ultrasonographic measurement of cervical length. *Am J Obstet Gynecol* 1990;163:859–67.
45. Iams JD, Goldenberg RL, Meis PJ, *et al.*, the National Institute of Child Health and Human Development Maternal Fetal Medicine Unit Network. The length of the cervix and the risk of spontaneous premature delivery. *N Engl J Med* 1996;334:567–72.
46. Guzman ER, Houlihan C, Vintzileos A, Ivan J, Benito C, Kappy K. The significance of transvaginal ultrasonographic evaluation of the cervix in women treated with emergency cerclage. *Am J Obstet Gynecol* 1996;175:471–6.
47. Vayssiere C, Favre R, Audibert F, *et al.* Cervical length and funneling at 22 and 27 weeks to predict spontaneous birth before 32 weeks in twin pregnancies: A French prospective multicenter study. *Am J Obstet Gynecol.* 2002;187(6):1596–604.
48. Cetrulo C. The controversy of mode of delivery in twins: The intrapartum management of twin gestation. *Semin Perinatol* 1986;10:39–43.
49. Chervenak FA, Youcha S, Hobbins JC, Berkowitz RL. Intrapartum management of twin gestation. *Obstet Gynecol* 1985;65(1):119–24.

69 Chromosomal abnormality screening

M. I. Evans, J. N. Macri, R. Snijders and R. S. Galen

Introduction

Principles of screening tests

Screening for any disease process requires a fundamental understanding of the differences between diagnostic and screening tests. Diagnostic tests are meant to give a definitive answer to the question – Does the patient have this particular problem? They are often complex and require sophisticated analysis and interpretation. They are usually performed only on patients felt to be 'at risk'. Because they tend to be expensive, in contrast, screening tests are typically performed on healthy patients and are often offered to the entire relevant population. They, therefore, need to be cheap, easy to use, and interpretable by everyone; their function is only to help define who, among the low risk group, is, in fact, at high risk (Table 69.1). Screening test results are, by definition, not pathonomonic for the disease.[1] Their role is to delineate who needs further testing.

There are four key measures used in the evaluation of screening tests (sensitivity, specificity, positive predictive value, and negative predictive value) (Figure 69.1). Sensitivity and specificity fundamentally address the question from an epidemiologic viewpoint. For example, of all the people with the disease, what percentage was identified by the test? This is the definition of sensitivity. Specificity is the converse, i.e. of all the people who do not have the disease process, what percentage of the patients test negative? Physicians are generally more interested in different questions, however, because only after a positive test does the patient usually get interested. Of all patients who have a positive test, what percentage of them actually have the disease? This is the positive predictive value. The negative predictive value is just the opposite, i.e. of all the people who have a negative test, what percentage of them are actually negative?

A key point to remember is that, in general, sensitivity and specificity do not vary as a function of prevalence, unless there is an influence of other factors on the equation. However, positive and negative predictive values do vary (Figures 69.3 and 69.4). In a population in which the prevalence is very low, the proportion of positives that will be false positive will be much higher than in a population in which the prevalence is very high. In the former case the vast

Table 69.1 Screening tests vs. diagnostic tests

Diagnostic tests
Performed only on 'at risk' population
Commonly expensive
Commonly have risk
Give definitive answer
Screening tests
Offered to general population of patients
Healthy patients
Cheap
Easy
Reliable
Quick
Define 'at risk' population
Do not give definitive answer

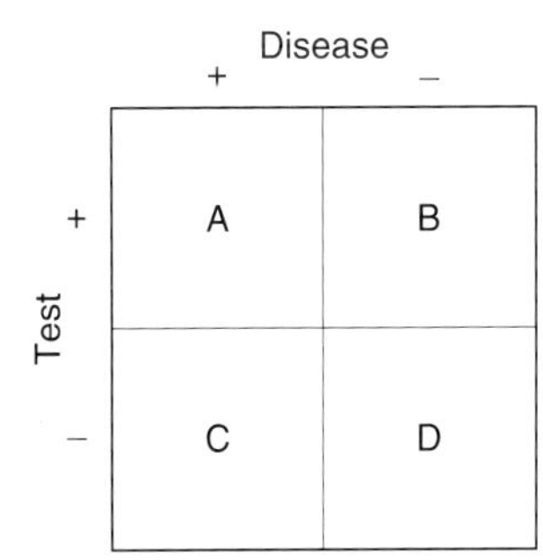

Sensitivity A/A + C
Specificity D/B + D

Positive predictive value A/A + B
Negative predictive value D/C + D

Figure 69.1 Two-by-two table of disease and tests.

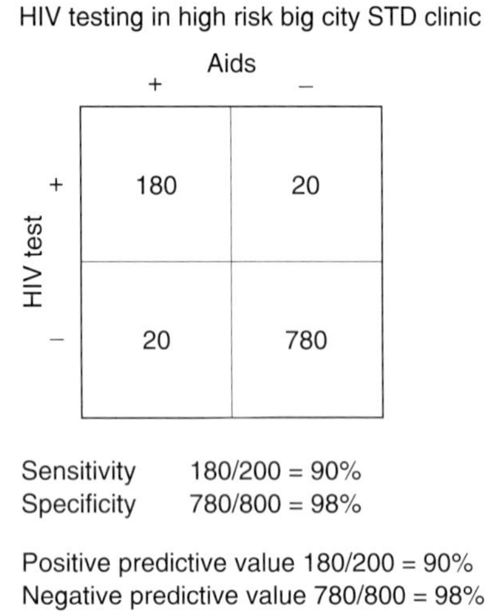

Figure 69.2 Two-by-two table in high-risk population for sensitivity and predictive values.

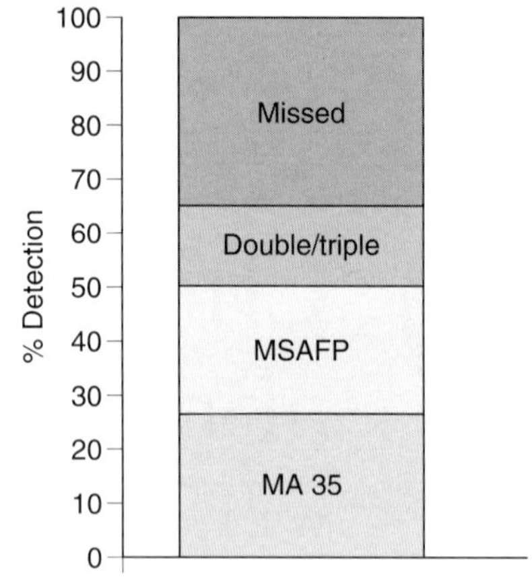

Figure 69.4 Maternal age 35 identifies about 25% of Down's syndrome pregnancies. Low AFP brings the total to about 50%. Double or triple screening raises that number to about 60%. Half of the 80% of cases occurring in women under 35 are detectable.

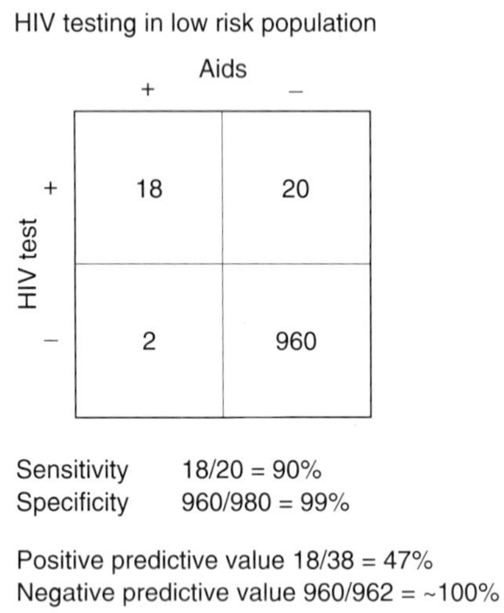

Figure 69.3 Two-by-two table in low-risk population for sensitivity and predictive values.

majority of positives will, in fact, be false positives. In both high and low prevalence areas, the sensitivity and specificity of the tests should be the same. However, the positive and negative predictive values will be widely different. If a test is absolutely useless (no better than chance), then the predictive value after testing will be the same as the population risk (prevalence) before testing. When this occurs, the test performs no better than a coin flip, and the sensitivity and specificity add to 100%.

The past few years have seen continued advancement in attempts to refine the sensitivity and specificity of chromosomal screening, and to reduce the overall costs of the screening programs *per se*.[2,3] The goal is to reduce the need for expensive costs of invasive testing that follow a positive screening, and also, although not commonly mentioned, to reduce the cost of the care of abnormal newborns who might as a result of screening be detected and terminated at the wishes of the parents.[1–5]

Screening for chromosome abnormalities

Merkatz *et al.* first published the association of low maternal serum alpha-fetoprotein (AFP) with an increased risk of chromosome abnormalities, particularly Down's syndrome in 1984.[6] Subsequently, there was a gradual acceptance of the association, as well as an eventual understanding that Down's syndrome is not the only aneuploid condition association with low maternal serum AFP. For example, trisomy 18 usually has even lower AFP values.[7]

The adoption of wide scale screening with maternal serum AFP effectively doubled the potential detection of chromosome abnormalities in the population. Before the massive explosion of infertility therapies, only about 20% of Down's syndrome babies were born to women over age 35 (Figure 69.5). More recent data suggest that the proportion of births to women over 35 has gone from about 5% to nearly 15%, and the proportion of Down's syndrome cases in women over 35 is now more than 30%.[8] The addition of a well-coordinated maternal serum AFP screening program as developed in the late 1980s could detect approximately 30% of the 75% of cases that are born to women under age 35. The detailed mechanics of biochemical screening, i.e. with adjustments for gestational age, race, diabetic status, multiple gestation status, maternal weight, and adjustments via a different database or correction factors for maternal race, have been published previously and will not be repeated here.[9]

In 1988, Wald *et al.* suggested that a combination of parameters including AFP, beta-human chorionic gonadotrophin (β-hCG), and unconjugated estriol (uE3) could significantly increase the detection frequency of Down's syndrome to approximately 60% of the total.[10] Multiple studies have corroborated the increased efficacy of multiple marker screening as opposed to AFP alone in detecting chromosome abnormalities, particularly Down's syndrome.[11–14]

Despite overwhelming data and recommendations of national organizations such as the American College of Obstetricians and Gynecologists that multiple numbers be offered, by the millennium still nearly 20% of patients in the United States who had screening were still just having AFP alone (M. I. Evans, unpublished data).

Evans *et al.* have investigated many of the 'dogmas' of three decades of biochemical screening and found that many of these are no longer valid. We believe that the wide variance in results reported from around the world is largely due to subtle, and sometimes not so subtle, differences in laboratory methodologies.[15–19] For example, the bitter arguments about double vs. triple screening are in part explained by wide differences in assays among laboratories that particularly affect estriol. When the methods are 'standardized', much of the variability disappears and will allow for an 'apples vs. apples' as opposed to 'apples vs. oranges' comparison.[19] Similarly, much of the other reported variations in the literature likewise disappear with standardization, and the diabetic correction factor becomes unnecessary with proper accounting for the fact that diabetic patients are of higher maternal weight,[15] and maternal weight correction, *per se*, continues to be important.[16,17]

Over the past several years there have been numerous papers that have attempted to refine methodologies of sample collection[20,21] and more precisely explored the impact of various factors such as more precise dating or the efficacy of Down's syndrome detection rates.[22,23] Likewise with an ever increasing proportion of pregnancies resulting from infertility therapies, questions have risen as to whether modifications of risk or screening strategies are required.[24]

A number of papers have suggested dimeric inhibin A as an excellent marker that may raise the sensitivity by 3–7% for a given screen positive rate.[25–28] Out of this data have come calls for 'quadruple' screening, and various combinations of biochemical and biophysical (ultrasound) data. There are also paradigms that include different parameters at different times combined. While preliminary data do suggest a high sensitivity with improved specificity,[29,30] hiding results from patients for up to a month is ethically problematic in our opinion. No doubt there will be multiple approaches to screening that emerge, and there will be no one uniform standard approach.[31]

A two-step approach has been the so- called 'integrated' test.[28–31] This is a combination of first-trimester blood and ultrasound. The first-trimester results are not communicated to the patient, who then waits for second-trimester blood results before a risk assessment is completed. Two studies, the 'SURUSS' trial and the 'FASTER' trial have data that suggest a reduced false-positive rate for comparable sensitivity, but the trade-off is the need for patients to wait as much as 6 weeks for start to finish of the screening process.[29,30] For patients who do not particularly care about the results, the delay may be fine, but our experience suggests that many anxious patients would find such a delay intolerable.[32–35]

As reproductive techniques have dramatically increased the proportions of multiple pregnancies, questions about the efficacy of screening tests have emerged. We and others have debated the data of biochemical screening on twins or more. There have been several papers that have promoted 'pseudo risks' for twins by biochemical data. We continue to be concerned about the accuracy of these tests and believe that in multiple pregnancies biophysical data are more likely to be accurate.[36–39]

First trimester

The future of screening for Down's syndrome (and other anomalies) lies in the first trimester. Substantial evidence now shows that free βHCG is reliably elevated and PAPP-A is diminished in Down's pregnancies.[39,40] Data from multiple laboratories have been consistent in suggesting 70% to even 90% detection rates. In combination with ultrasound nuchal translucency (NT) measurements, almost all publications in which the ultrasound component was performed in a technically sound fashion have shown at least a 70% sensitivity.[41]

Several large-scale studies – particularly the King College group in London and the NICHD funded 'BUN' and 'FASTER' trials – all essentially confirmed that first-trimester data will be at least equal to routine second-trimester double or triple screening.[29,40]

Measurement of fetal NT thickness

Guidelines for measurement of fetal NT thickness have been drafted by the Fetal Medicine Foundation (FMF). More than 300 centers around the world have adopted the FMF guidelines and they take part in the quality control scheme. Quality control of ultrasound scans involves assessment of the distribution of NT measurements and assessment of randomly selected images in terms of magnification, section (sagittal or oblique), caliper placement, skin line (nuchal only or nuchal and back), and visualization of the amnion separate from the nuchal membrane.[34]

The ability to measure NT and obtain reproducible results improves with training; good results are achieved after 80 scans for the transabdominal route and 100 scans transvaginally.[41] The ability to achieve a reliable measurement of NT is dependent on the motivation of the sonographer. Results were compared from hospitals that used NT in clinical practice

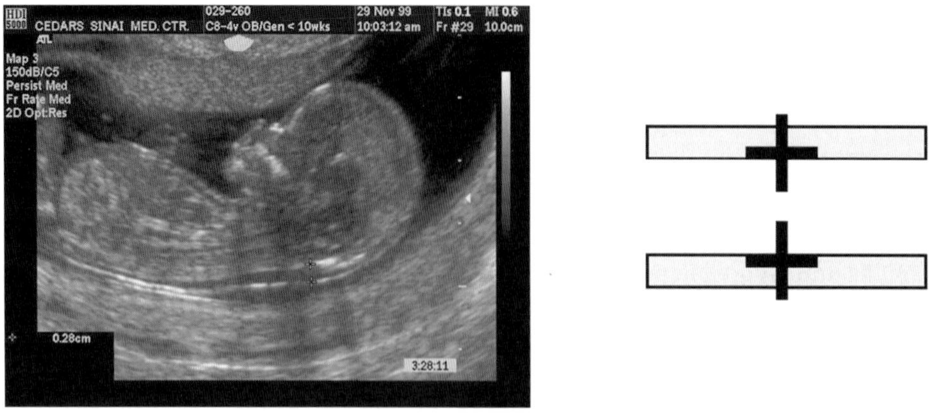

Figure 69.5 Ultrasound measurement of the fetal neck at 12 weeks.

(interventional) to those obtained in hospitals that recorded the measurements but did not act on the results (observational). In the interventional group, successful measurement of NT was achieved in 100% of cases and the measurement was >2.5 mm in 2.3% of cases; the respective percentages in the observational group were 85% and 12%.[42,43]

Guidelines

- Equipment to measure up to 0.1 mm and time allocated for each scan at least 10 min.
- Transabdominal or transvaginal route. The transabdominal route gives a success rate of 95%; in 5% of cases it is necessary to perform vaginal sonography.
- Gestational age between 10^{+3} and 13^{+6} weeks [crown–rump length (CRL) 38–84 mm, biparietal diameter <27 mm]. At these gestations the success rate for obtaining a measurement is more than 98%. From 14 weeks onward the fetal position (vertical) makes it more difficult to obtain measurements.[44]
- Good sagittal section of the fetus, as for measurement of fetal CRL. An optimal measurement is obtained when the fetus is in a neutral position (neither in flexion nor in extension).
- Magnification so that the fetus occupies at least three-quarters of the screen and that each increment in the distance between callipers is only 0.1 mm.
- Distinguish between fetal skin and amnion (both appear as thin membranes!) by waiting for spontaneous fetal movement away from the amniotic membrane. Alternatively, the fetus may be bounced off the amnion by asking the mother to cough and/or by tapping the maternal abdomen.
- Measure the maximum thickness of the subcutaneous translucency between the skin and the soft tissue overlying the cervical spine by placing the calipers on the lines as shown in Figure 69.5.

The umbilical cord may be round the fetal neck in 5–10% of cases and this can produce an increased NT as it adds about 0.8 mm to the measurement.[45] Measurements of NT above and below the cord will be different and in the calculation of risk it is appropriate to use the smaller measurement. It is well established that NT normally increases with gestational age.[46–51] Therefore, the difference from the normal median for gestation is used to determine the factor by which the age-related risk is adjusted.

Increased NT and chromosome defects

Studies that report on first-trimester fetal NT thickness and chromosome defects can be divided into four groups. Initial observational studies examined the prevalence of chromosome defects in fetuses with increased NT. Subsequent observational studies examined in (high risk) pregnancies prior to invasive testing the proportion of Down's syndrome and normal fetuses that present with increased NT. Implementation studies then reported on the feasibility of introducing screening by NT in routine practice and, finally, centers that introduced the test reported experience with screening based on the combination of maternal age, gestational age, and fetal NT thickness.

Observational studies

In the early 1990s, several reports on fetuses with increased NT demonstrated a possible association between NT and chromosome defects in the first trimester of pregnancy (Table 69.2).[52–65] The mean prevalence of chromosome defects in 14 series involving 1457 patients was 28%. However, the percentage ranged from 19% to 88%. This variation in results presumably reflects differences in the maternal age distributions and differences in the definition of minimum thickness of the abnormal translucency, ranging from 2 to 10 mm.

In subsequent studies NT thickness was assessed immediately before fetal karyotyping, mainly for advanced maternal age (AMA). Detection rates for trisomy 21 varied from 30% to 84% (Table 69.3)[66–71] with false-positive rates ranging from 1% to 6%. Detection rates were relatively low if measurements were taken before 10 weeks of gestation, and/or machines measured whole millimeters only.[49,50]

Table 69.2 Summary of reported series on first-trimester fetal nuchal translucency (NT) providing data on gestational age (GA) in weeks, criteria for diagnosis of increased NT thickness, and the presence of associated chromosome defects (T21 = trisomy 21, T18 = trisomy 18, T13 = trisomy 13)

				Abnormal karyotype					
Author	GA (weeks)	NT (mm)	*N*	Total	T21	T18	T13	45,X	Other
Johnson *et al.*[52]	10–14	≥ 2.0	68	41 (60%)	16	9	2	9	5
Hewitt *et al.*[53]	10–14	≥ 2.0	29	12 (41%)	5	3	1	2	1
Shulman *et al.*[54]	10–13	≥ 2.5	32	15 (47%)	4	4	3	4	0
Nicolaides *et al.*[55]	10–13	≥ 3.0	88	33 (38%)	21	8	2	0	2
Pandya *et al.*[56]	10–13	≥ 3.0	1,015	193 (19%)	101	51	13	14	15
Szabo and Gellen[57]	11–12	≥ 3.0	8	7 (88%)	7	0	0	0	0
Wilson *et al.*[58]	8–11	≥ 3.0	14	3 (21%)	0	0	0	1	2
Ville *et al.*[59]	9–14	≥ 3.0	29	7 (28%)	4	3	1	0	0
Trauffer *et al.*[60]	10–14	≥ 3.0	43	21 (49%)	9	4	1	4	3
Nadel *et al.*[61]	10–15	≥ 4.0	63	43 (68%)	15	15	1	10	2
Schulte-Vallentin and Schindler[62]	10–14	≥ 4.0	8	7 (88%)	7	0	0	0	0
Van Zalen-Sprock *et al.*[63]	10–14	≥ 4.0	18	5 (28%)	3	1	0	1	1
Cullen *et al.*[64]	11–13	≥ 6.0	29	15 (52%)	6	2	0	4	3
Suchet *et al.*[65]	8–14	≥ 10.0	13	8 (62%)	0	0	0	7	1
			1457	413 (28%)	198	100	24	56	35

Table 69.3 Summary of reported series on first-trimester fetal NT before amniocentesis or CVS providing data on gestational age (GA) in weeks, criteria for diagnosis of increased NT thickness, false-positive rate (FPR), detection rate (DR), and odds of an affected pregnancy (OAP) for trisomy 21

Author	GA (weeks)	NT cutoff	*N*	FPR (%)	DR trisomy 21	OAP trisomy 21
Nicolaides *et al.*[66]	10–13	≥ 3 mm	1273	4	84% (21/25)	1 in 4
Zimmerman *et al.*[67]	10–13	≥ 3 mm	1151	2	67% (2/3)	1 in 12
Hewitt *et al.*[53]	10–14	≥ 3 mm	1312	4	57% (12/21)	1 in 5
Comas *et al.*[68]	9–13	≥ 3 mm	487	1	57% (4/7)	1 in 13
Savoldelli *et al.*[69]	9–12	≥ 3 mm	1400	<1	54% (15/28)	1 in 2
Borell *et al.*[70]	10–13	≥ 3 mm	479	6	44% (8/18)	1 in 5
Haddow *et al.*[50]	9–15	95th percentile	3308	5	31% (18/58)	1 in 10
Brambati *et al.*[51]	8–15	≥ 3 mm	1819	2	30% (8/26)	1 in 7
Scott *et al.*[71]	9–13	95th percentile	445	5	30% (3/10)	1 in 8

Increased NT and normal karyotype

Souka *et al.*[72] recently presented findings in 4116 chromosomally normal fetuses with increased NT together with a review of the literature. There are at least five conditions that may underlie increased NT and these include heart defects or heart failure, intathoracic compression, altered composition of the dermis, abnormal lymphatic system, and neuromuscular abnormalities.

Heart defects

Two fetal echocardiographic studies at 10–16 weeks of gestation reported that 16 (80%) of the 20 fetuses with cardiac defects had an abnormal collection of nuchal fluid.[72,73] In addition, a study of 29,154 pregnancies demonstrated that the prevalence of cardiac defects increases with increasing NT. In fetuses with an NT < 95th percentile, it was 0.8 per 1000 compared to 15 per 1000 in the group with increased NT

Table 69.4 Prevalence of major cardiac defects in chromosomally normal fetuses with increased NT thickness

NT thickness	*N*	Cardiac defects
< 95th percentile	27,332	0.8/1000 (~1 in 1250)
95th percentile–3.4 mm	1507	5/1000 (~1 in 200)
3.5–4.4 mm	208	29/1000 (~1 in 35)
4.5–5.4 mm	66	91/1000 (~1 in 10)
≥ 5.5 mm	41	195/1000 (~1 in 5)
Total	29,154	1.7/1000

thickness (Table 69.4).[74,75] Examination of chromosomally normal pregnancies with an NT of 3.5 mm or more (1% of the population) at 15–20 weeks by an echocardiographer identifies approximately 40% of significant cardiac defects.

Public policy

Why then has not first-trimester screening already replaced the second-trimester testing? The answers are complex, but can be divided into several different categories. First, many patients do not come for prenatal care until the second trimester. It is well known that there are universal correlations between socioeconomic status and gestational age at the first visit for prenatal care. No matter how good a first-trimester test is, it does no good for a patient first seen at 24 weeks.[76]

Second, even in 2001 with voluminous articles and college opinions touting multiple markers, 20% of patients were still getting the 1980s model of AFP alone (M. I. Evans, unpublished data). Significant professional education will be needed to leapfrog the practice in first-trimester screening.

Third, until immediate invasive testing is readily available and accepted, first-trimester screening results would be worse than no screening if the patient then had to wait a month to have an amniocentesis for a definitive answer.[34–65] We see this as very problematic for the 'integrated' test that combines first- and second-trimester laboratory results and ultrasound. Chorionic villus sampling (CVS) has long since proven to be safe and effective in experienced hands. As the so-called limb reduction defect scare has been shown to be false at appropriate gestational ages, hopefully, the availability of CVS and acceptance will swing the pendulum back toward the desire for first-trimester screening for testing, which has many advantages for the patient. We actually expect the concept of maternal age as a stand-alone variable to be phased out over the next several years.[76]

Trisomy 18

Although screening has generally focused on trisomy 21, our data and those of others have always shown a varied pattern of anomalies detected by screening.[77] A different pattern of analyte levels has been observed in trisomy 18. The values of AFP, hCG, and uE3 appear to be very low.[78] This suggests a different pathophysiology than for Down's syndrome. In Down's syndrome, the low AFP and uE3, and high hCG can be explained as reflecting inappropriate immaturity or dysmaturity of the fetus, i.e. all values are consistent with a younger gestational age. In trisomy 18, however, that explanation does not work.[79] We have previously shown that there are different patterns of genomically directed intrauterine growth retardation in different aneuploidies[77] but how this translates into serum markers is unclear. Nevertheless, some reports have shown that an algorithm can be used to identify the majority of trisomy 18 cases while adding about 0.75% to the population being offered amniocentesis.[79,80]

The end of AMA

The association of AMA with increasing risks of chromosomal abnormalities, particularly Down's syndrome, has been appreciated for decades.

The choice of age 35 at least in the United States was an arbitrary compromise determined in part by naivety in data collection. Cohorts of Down's syndrome risk were usually reported in 5-year groupings, and there was clearly a big jump from the 30–34 to 35–39 age group. It was only later when data were reported on a year–age-specific curve that the slope of the curve was shown to be changing before age 35. Furthermore, the difference from one year to the next was obviously nowhere as dramatic as suggested in the 5-year cohorts.[9]

Another dramatic development of the 1970s was changing laws in the United States concerning a woman's right to end a pregnancy. New York and California were among the first states to repeal laws that made abortion virtually impossible to obtain legally. In 1973 the US Supreme Court ruled that in the first trimester a state had very little right to interfere with a woman's defined right of privacy in terminating a pregnancy.[81,82] In the second trimester the state's interests were primarily only in ensuring the safety of the procedure. It was only in the third trimester that the state could exert a compelling interest in protecting the 'rights' of the fetus over the mother's wishes.

The combination of new technology plus the ability to terminate abnormal pregnancies led to a surge of interest in prenatal diagnosis. As with most new technologies, utilization was initially highest among patients of upper socioeconomic status who had the knowledge of the availability of the technology as well as the means to travel to far-off centers to obtain such services.[83]

The evidence that first-trimester screening followed by first-trimester diagnosis by CVS can bring about a substantially higher sensitivity and specificity within the same time frame than CVS in AMA is overwhelming. The question thus reduces to how and when to update the accepted 'culture' in the United States to be consistent with the current scientific knowledge base.

There has to be the understanding that age is not being discarded, but will merely become one of a number of variables that can be assessed to give the most accurate assessment of risk possible. With education, the ultrasound portion of the equation will become more standardized to laboratory levels of quality assurance. Non-profit organizations such as the Fetal Medicine Foundation in London and the Fetal Medicine Foundation in America, as well as others, will certainly help coordinate the transition and training needed to make such a reality.

It is also not realistic to expect a shift of 'standards' and practice to change on a single day. Thus, there will have to be a short phase-in period, under which either the old or the new approach will be considered acceptable. However, it is also reasonable to expect the insurance companies, which will have to pay for such tests, to vociferously and clearly articulate to their subscribers and physicians that they are not about to vastly increase the number of patients having tests. Thus, the right will be likely the 'right' to pay out of one's own pocket for testing for AMA, *per se*.

It is time for AMA, as a stand-alone criterion for having invasive testing, to go the way of the buggy whip. The principal objection to screening as entry to testing has been removed. It can all now be done in the first trimester. The science has evolved. It is now time for the culture and the standards to follow.

REFERENCES

1. Evans MI, Krivchenia EL, Yaron Y. Screening in Evans MI and Bui: Genomic revolution and obstetrics and gynecology. *Baillieres Clin Obstet Gynecol* 2002;16:645–58.
2. Evans MI, Chik L, O'Brien JE, *et al.* MOMs and DADS: Improved specificity and cost effectiveness of biochemical screening for aneuploidy with DADS. *Am J Obstet Gynecol* 1995;172:1138–47.
3. Evans MI, Chik L, O'Brien JE, *et al.* Logistic regression generated probability estimates for trisomy 21 outcomes from serum AFP and BHCG: Simplification with increased specificity. *Matern Fetal Med* 1996;5:1–6.
4. Evans MI, Sobecki MA, Krivchenia EL, *et al.* Parental decisions to terminate/continue following abnormal cytogenetic prenatal diagnosis: "What" is still more important than "when". *Am J Med Genet* 1996;61:353–5.
5. Pryde PG, Odgers AE, Isada NB, Johnson MP, Evans MI. Determinants of parental decision to abort or continue for non-aneuploid ultrasound detected abnormalities. *Obstet Gynecol* 1992;80:52–6.
6. Merkatz IR, Nitowsky FM, Macri JN, Johnson WE. An association between low maternal serum alpha-fetoprotein and fetal chromosome abnormalities. *Am J Obstet Gynecol* 1984;148:886–94.
7. Nyberg DA, Kramer D, Resta RG, *et al.* Prenatal monographic findings of trisomy 18: Review of 47 cases. *J Ultrasound Med* 1993;2:103–13.
8. Martin JA, Hamilton BE, Ventura SJ, *et al.* Births: Final data for 2001. *National Vital Statistics Report 51*, #2. Hyattsville, MD: National Center for Health Statistics, 2002.
9. Evans MI, Krivchenia EL, Yaron. Screening. In Evans MI, Bui TH, eds. *The Genome Revolution and Obstetrics and Gynecology. Balliere's Best Practice and Research in Clinical Obstetrics and Gynecology.* London: Harcourt Brace Publishing Co., 2002;16:624–57.
10. Wald NJ, Cuckle HS, Densem JW, *et al.* Maternal serum screening for Down syndrome in early pregnancy. *Br Med J* 1988;297:883–7.
11. Cheng EY, Luthy DA, Zebelman AM, Williams MA, Lieppman RE, Hickok DE. A prospective evaluation of a second-trimester screening test for fetal Down syndrome using maternal serum alpha-fetoprotein, hCG, and unconjugated estriol. *Obstet Gynecol* 1993;81:72–7.
12. Aitken DA, McCaw G, Crossley JA, *et al.* First-trimester biochemical screening for fetal chromosome abnormalities and neural tube defects. *Prenat Diagn* 1993;13:681–3.
13. Wald N, Densem J, Stone R, Cheng R. The use of free 1993, β-hCG in antenatal screening for Down's syndrome. *Br J Obstet Gynaecol* 1993;100:550–7.
14. Goodburn SF, Yates JRW, Raggatt PR, *et al.* Second-trimester maternal serum screening using alpha-fetoprotein, human chorionic gonadotrophin, and unconjugated oestriol: Experience of a regional programme. *Prenat Diagn* 1994;14:391–402.
15. Evans MI, Harrison HH, O'Brien JE, *et al.* Correction for insulin dependent diabetes in maternal serum alpha fetoprotein testing has outlived its usefulness. *Am J Obstet Gynecol* 2002;187: 1084–6.
16. Evans MI, Harrison HH, O'Brien JE, *et al.* Maternal weight correction for alpha fetoprotein: Mathematical truncations revisited. *Genet Test* 2002;6:221–3.
17. Spencer K, Bindra R, Micolaides KH. Maternal weight correction of maternal serum PAPP-A and free beta-hCG MoM when screening for trisomy 21 in the first trimester pregnancy. *Prenat Diagn* 2003;23(10):851–5.
18. Evans MI, O'Brien JE, Dvorun E, *et al.* Standardization of methods reduces variability: Explanation for the historical discrepancies in biochemical screening. *Genet Test* 2003;7:81–3.
19. Spencer K. The influence of different sample collection types on the levels of markers used for Down's syndrome screening as measured by the Kryptor immunosassay system. *Ann Clin Biochem* 2003;40(Pt 2):166–8.
20. Spencer K, Crossley JA, Aitken DA, Nix AB, Dunstan FD, Williams K. Temporal changes in maternal serum biochemical markers of trisomy 21 across the first and second trimester of pregnancy. *Ann Clin Biochem* 2002;39(Pt 6):567–76.
21. Ghisoni L, Ferrazzi E, Castagna C, Levi Setti PE, Masini AC, Pigni A. Prenatal diagnosis after ART success: The role of early combined screening tests in counseling pregnant patients. *Placenta* 2003; Suppl:S99–S103.
22. Donnenfeld AE, Icke KV, Pargas C, Dowman C. Biochemical screening for aneuploidy in ovum donor pregnancies. *Am J Obstet Gynecol* 2002;187(5):1222–5.
23. Canick JA, Saller DN Jr, Lambert-Messerlian GM. Prenatal screening for Down syndrome: Current and future methods. *Clin Lab Med* 2003;23(2):395–411.
24. Silver HM, Lambert-Messerlian GM, Reis FM, Diblasio AM, Petraglia P, Canick JA. Mechanism of increased maternal serum total activin a and inhibin a in preeclampsia. *J Soc Gynecol Investig* 2002;9(5):308–12.
25. Wald NJ, Huttly WJ, Hackshaw AK. Antenatal screening for Down's syndrome with the quadruple test. *Lancet* 2003;8:835–6.
26. Benn PA, Fang M, Egan JF, Horne D, Collins R. Incorporation of inhibin-A in second-trimester screening for Down syndrome. *Obstet Gynecol* 2003;102(2):413(author reply 413–4).

27. Spencer K, Liao AW, Ong CY, Geerts L, Nicolaides KH. Maternal serum levels of dimeric inhibin A in pregnancies affected by trisomy 21 in the first trimester. *Prenat Diagn* 2001;21(6):441–4.
28. Malone *et al.* Faster trial. *New Engl J Med*, in press.
29. Wald NJ, Rodeck C, Hackshaw AK, Walters J, Chitty L, Mackinson AM. First and second trimester antenatal screening for Down's syndrome: The results of the Serum, Urine and Ultrasound Screening Study (SURUSS). *J Med Screen* 2003;10(2):56–104.
30. Cuckle HS. Growing complexity in the choice of Down's syndrome screening policy. *Ultrasound Obstet Gynecol* 2002; 19:323–6.
31. Souter VL, Nyberg DA, Benn PA, Zebelman A, Luthardt F, Luthy DA. Correlation of second-trimester sonographic and biochemical markers. *J Ultrasound Med* 2004;23(4):505–11.
32. Cusick W, Buchanan P, Hallahan TW, Krantz DA, Larsen JW Jr, Macri JN. Combined first-trimester versus second-trimester serum screening for Down syndrome: A cost analysis. *Am J Obstet Gynecol* 2003;188(3):745–51.
33. Muller F, Benattar C, Audibert F, Roussel N, Dreux S, Cuckle H. First-trimester screening for Down syndrome in France combining fetal nuchal translucency measurement and biochemical markers. *Prenat Diagn* 2003;23(10):833–6.
34. Nicolaides KH, Bindra R, Heath V, Cicero S. One-stop clinic for assessment of risk of chromosomal defects at 12 weeks of gestation. *J Matern Fetal Neonatal Med* 2002;12(1):9–18.
35. Crossley JA, Aitken DA, Cameron AD, McBride E, Connor JM. Combined ultrasound and biochemical screening for Down's syndrome in the first trimester: A Scottish multicentre study. *BJOG* 2002;109(6):667–76.
36. Drugan A, O'Brien JE, Dvorin E, *et al.* Multiple marker screening in multifetal gestations: Prediction of adverse pregnancy outcomes. *Fetal Diagn Ther* 1996;11:16–19.
37. O'Brien JE, Dvorin E, Yaron Y, *et al.* Differential increases in AFP, HCG, and uE3 in twin pregnancies: Impact upon attempts to quantify Down syndrome screening calculations. *Am J Med Genet* 1997;73:109–112.
38. Wald N, Cuckle H, Wu TS, George L. Maternal serum unconjugated oestriol and human chorionic gonadotrophin levels in twin pregnancies: Implications for screening for Down's syndrome. *Br J Obstet Gynaecol* 1991;98(9):905–8.
39. Cuckle H. Down's syndrome screening in twins. *J Med Screen* 1998;5(1):3–4.
40. Wald NJ, Rish S, Hackshaw AK. Combining nuchal translucency and serum markers in prenatal screening for Down syndrome in twin pregnancies. *Prenat Diagn* 2003;23(7):588–92.
41. Wapner R, Thom E, Simpson JL, *et al.* First trimester maternal serum biochemistry and fetal nuchal translucency screening (BUN) study group. First-trimester screening for trisomies 21 and 18. *N Engl J Med* 2003;349(15):1405–13.
42. Braithwaite JM, Morris RW, Economides DL. Nuchal translucency measurements: Frequency distribution and changes with gestation in a general population. *Br J Obstet Gynaecol* 1996;103:1201–4.
43. Bower S, Chitty L, Bewley S, *et al.* First trimester nuchal translucency screening of the general population: Data from three centres (abstract). *The 27th British Congress of Obstetrics and Gynaecolology*, 1995.
44. Roberts LJ, Bewley S, Mackinson AM, Rodeck CH. First trimester fetal nuchal translucency: Problems with screening the general population 1. *Br J Obstet Gynaecol* 1995;102:381–5.
45. Whitlow BJ, Economides DL. The optimal gestational age to examine fetal anatomy and measure nuchal translucency in the first trimester. *Ultrasound Obstet Gynecol* 1998;11:258–61.
46. Schaefer M, Laurichesse-Delmas H, Ville Y. The effect of nuchal cord on nuchal translucency measurement at 10–14 weeks. *Ultrasound Obstet Gynecol* 1998;11(4):271–3.
47. Pandya PP, Goldberg H, Walton B, *et al.* The implementation of first trimester scanning at 10–13 weeks' gestation and the measurement of fetal nuchal translucency thickness in two maternity units. *Ultrasound Obstet Gynaecol* 1995;5:20–5.
48. Pajkrt E, de Graaf IM, Mol BW, van Lith JM, Bleker OP, Bilardo CM. Weekly nuchal translucency measurements in normal fetuses. *Obstet Gynecol* 1998;91(2):208–11.
49. Yagel S, Anteby EY, Rosen L, Yaffe E, Rabinowitz R, Tadmor O. Assessment of first-trimester nuchal translucency by daily reference intervals. *Ultrasound Obstet Gynecol* 1998;11:262–5.
50. Haddow JE, Palomaki GE, Knight GJ, Williams J, Miller WA, Johnson A. Screening of maternal serum for fetal Down's syndrome in the first trimester. *N Engl J Med* 1998;338:955–61.
51. Brambati B, Cislaghi C, Tului L, *et al.* First-trimester Down's syndrome screening using nuchal translucency: A prospective study. *Ultrasound Obstet Gynecol* 1995;5:9–14.
52. Johnson MP, Johnson A, Holzgreve W, *et al.* First-trimester simple hygroma: Cause and outcome. *Am J Obstet Gynecol* 1993;168:156–61.
53. Hewitt BG, de Crespigny L, Sampson AJ, Ngu AC, Shekleton P, Robinson HP. Correlation between nuchal thickness and abnormal karyotype in first trimester fetuses. *Med J Aust* 1996;165(7): 365–8.
54. Shulman LP, Emerson D, Felker R, Phillips O, Simpson J, Elias S. High frequency of cytogenetic abnormalities with cystic hygroma diagnosed in the first trimester. *Obstet Gynecol* 1992;80:80–2.
55. Nicolaides KH, Azar G, Snijders RJM, Gosden CM. Fetal nuchal oedema: Associated malformations and chromosomal defects. *Fetal Diagn Ther* 1992;7:123.
56. Pandya PP, Altman D, Brizot ML, Pettersen H, Nicolaides KH. Repeatability of measurement of fetal nuchal translucency thickness. *Ultrasound Obstet Gynaecol* 1995;5:334–7.
57. Szabo J, Gellen J. Nuchal fluid accumulation in trisomy-21 detected by vaginal sonography in first trimester. *Lancet* 1990; 336:1133.
58. Wilson RD, Venir N, Faquharson DF. Fetal nuchal fluid – Physiological or pathological? – In pregnancies less than 17 menstrual weeks. *Prenat Diagn* 1992;12:755–63.
59. Ville Y, Lalondrelle C, Doumerc S, *et al.* First-trimester diagnosis of nuchal anomalies: Significance and fetal outcome. *Ultrasound Obstet Gynecol* 1992;2:314–6.
60. Trauffer PL, Anderson CE, Johnson A, Heeger S, Morgan P, Wapner RJ. The natural history of euploid pregnancies with first-trimester cystic hygromas. *Am Obstet Gynecol* 1994;170: 1279–84.
61. Nadel A, Bromley B, Benacerraf BR. Nuchal thickening or cystic hygromas in first- and early second-trimester fetuses: Prognosis and outcome. *Obstet Gynecol* 1993;82:43–8.
62. Schulte-Vallentin M, Schindler H. Non-echogenic nuchal oedema as a marker in trisomy 21 screening. *Lancet* 1992; 339:1053.
63. Van Zalen-Sprock MM, Van Vugt JMG, Van Geijn HP. First-trimester diagnosis of cystic hygroma – Course and outcome. *Am J Obstet Gynecol* 1992;167;94–8.
64. Cullen MT, Gabrielli S, Green JJ, *et al.* Diagnosis and significance of cystic hygroma in the first trimester. *Prenat Diagn* 1990; 10:643–51.
65. Suchet IB, Van der Westhuizen NG, Labatte MF. Fetal cystic hygromas: Further insights into their natural history. *Can Assoc Radiol J* 1992;6:420–4.
66. Nicolaides KH, Azar G, Byrne D, Mansur, Marks K. Fetal nuchal translucency: Ultrasound screening for chromosomal defects in first trimester of pregnancy. *Br Med J* 1992;304:867–69.
67. Zimmerman R, Hucha A, Savoldelli G, Binkert F, Acherman J, Grudzinskas JG. Serum parameters and nuchal translucency in first trimester screening for fetal chromosomal abnormalities. *Br J Obstet Gynaecol* 1996;103:1009–14.
68. Comas C, Martinez JM, Ojuel J, *et al.* First-trimester nuchal edema as a marker of aneuploidy. *Ultrasound Obstet Gynecol* 1995;5:26–9.
69. Savoldelli G, Binkert F, Achermann J, Schmid W. Ultrasound screening for chromosomal anomalies in the first trimester of pregnancy. *Prenat Diagn* 1993;13:513–8.
70. Borell A, Costas D, Martinez JM, Delgado RD, Farguell T, Fortuny A. Criteria for fetal nuchal thickness cut-off: A re-evaluation. *Prenat Diagn* 1997;17:23–9.
71. Scott F, Boogert A, Sinosich M, Anderson J. Establishment and application of a normal range for nuchal translucency across the first trimester. *Prenat Diagn* 1996;16:629–34.
72. Souka AP, Nicolaides KH. Diagnosis of fetal abnormalities at the 10–14 week scan. *Ultrasound Obstet Gynecol* 1997;10: 429–42.
73. Souka AP, Snijders RJM, Novakov A, Soares W, Nicolaides KH. Defects and syndromes in chromosomally normal fetuses with increased nuchal translucency thickness at 10–14 weeks of gestation. *Ultrasound Obstet Gynecol* 1998;11:391–400.
74. Gembruch U, Knopfle G, Bald R, Hansmann M. Early diagnosis of fetal congenital heart disease by transvaginal echocardiography. *Ultrasound Obstet Gynecol* 1993;3:310–317.
75. Achiron R, Rotstein Z, Lipitz S, Mashiach S, Hegesh J. First-trimester diagnosis of fetal congenital heart disease by transvaginal ultrasonography. *Obstet Gynecol* 1994;84:69–72.

76. Hyett J, Perdu M, Sharland G, Snijders R, Nicolaides KH. Using fetal nuchal translucency to screen for major congenital cardiac defects at 10–14 weeks of gestation: Population based cohort study. *Br Med J* 1999;318:81–5.
77. Hyett JA, Perdu M, Sharland GK, Snijders RS, Nicolaides KH. Increased nuchal translucency at 10–14 weeks of gestation as a marker for major cardiac defects. *Ultrasound Obstet Gynecol* 1997;10(4):242–6.
78. Evans MI, Macri JN, Galen RS, Drugan A. Biochemical screening. In Evans MI, Johnson MP, Yaron Y, Drugan A, eds. *Prenatal Diagnosis*. New York: McGraw Hill, in press.
79. Johnson MP, Barr M Jr, Qureshi F, Drugan A, Evans MI. Symmetrical intrauterine growth retardation is not symmetrical: The ontogeny of organ specific gravimetric deficits in mid-trimester and neonatal trisomy 18. *Fetal Diagn Ther* 1989;4: 110–19.
80. Drugan A, Dvorin E, Koppitch FC, Greb A, Krivchenia EL, Evans MI. Counseling for low maternal serum alpha-fetoprotein should emphasize all chromosome anomalies, not just Down syndrome! *Obstet Gynecol* 1989;73:271–4.
81. Palomaki GE, Haddow JE, Knight GJ, *et al*. Risk-based prenatal screening for trisomy 18 using alpha-fetoprotein, unconjugated estriol, and human chorionic gonadotropin. *Prenat Diagn* 1995;15:713.
82. Leporrier N, Herrou M, Morello R, Leymarie P. Fetuses with Down's syndrome detected by prenatal screening are more likely to abort spontaneously than fetuses with Down's syndrome not detected by prenatal screening. *BJOG* 2003;110(1):18–21, 2003.
83. US Supreme Court. Roe vs. Wade 410 US, 113, 1973.
84. US Supreme Court. Doe vs. Bolton 410 US, 179, 1973.
85. Evans MI, Hanft RS. The introduction of new technologies. *ACOG Clin Semin* 1997;2:1–3.

70 Amniocentesis

S. Tercanli, P. Miny and W. Holzgreve

Introduction

Midtrimester amniocentesis is the most commonly performed invasive technique in prenatal diagnosis. Valenti *et al.* reported the first successful diagnosis of Down's syndrome in 1968.[1] Since that time the number of midtrimester amniocentesis has increased dramatically and amniocentesis is nowadays an established standard tool in the assessment of pregnancies that are at risk for a variety of chromosomal disorders, single gene defects, biochemical analysis and fetal infections. Chromosome analysis and tests related to risk screening for aneuploidy remain by far the most common laboratory procedures in prenatal diagnosis worldwide. Conventional chromosome analysis has maintained its role as a gold standard for the primary exclusion of aneuploidy from amniotic fluid cells. Frequent indications listed in Table 70.1 for offering second-trimester amniocentesis are pregnancies considered to be at an increased risk.

Prior to any prenatal invasive test, patients should be counseled. The risks and benefits of all invasive and non-invasive tests must be discussed as well as the limitations of any procedure. In the case of specific risk factors or abnormal ultrasound findings the information should be as complete and appropriate as possible. Considering the current developments in prenatal diagnosis by performing advanced methods for individual risk calculation, e.g. nuchal translucency measurement and biochemical serum marker screening, counseling of pregnant women will become more and more important. It can be assumed that in this context a more selective approach to invasive testing may result in the next few years. One of the significant problems in counseling pregnant women is still how to explain to women (e.g. socioeconomic, ethical and cultural variability) the complex implications of risk calculation. Our own experiences showed that appropriate individual counseling is more time-consuming and requires more appropriate methods.

Table 70.1 Common indications for amniocentesis

Advanced maternal age (=35 years)
Family history for chromosome anomalies, single gene defects, etc.
Abnormal maternal serum screening in the second trimester
Increased risk for chromosomal anomalies following first trimester screening – if chorionic villus sampling is not available
Abnormal ultrasound findings
Maternal infections potentially affecting the fetus

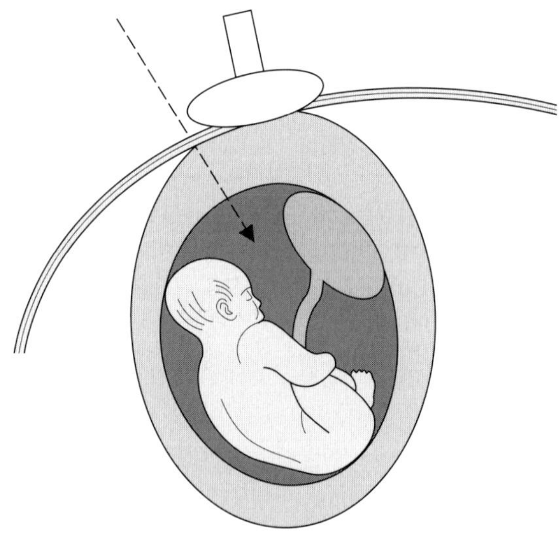

Figure 70.1 Diagram of amniocentesis. Transplacental perforation should be avoided if possible.

Technique

Midtrimester amniocentesis is commonly performed between 15 and 16 weeks of gestation (Figures 70.1 and 70.2). Prior to the procedure of ultrasound, evaluation of the uterus (e.g. exclusion of fibroids), the fetus, amniotic fluid volume and position of the placenta is recommended, because the failure rate can be reduced by avoiding the removal of bloody fluid or multiple injections.[2–4] Patients' anxiety may be reduced if adequate information is given to them during the procedure at each step. After disinfection of the maternal abdomen, amniocentesis is performed under direct ultrasound guidance generally using an

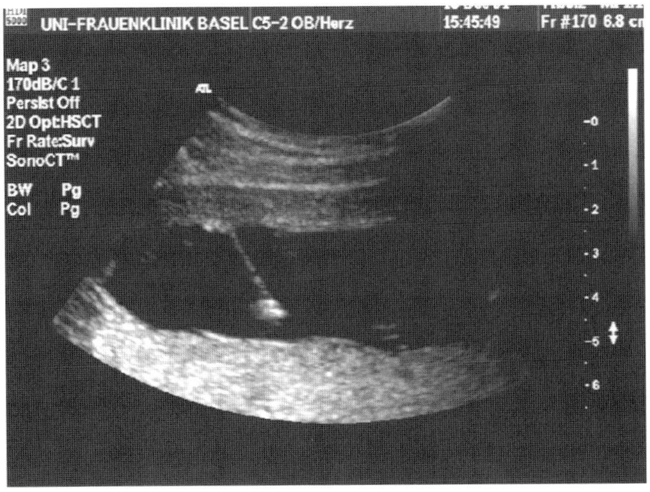

Figure 70.2 Second-trimester amniocentesis under ultrasound guidance.

18–20-gauge needle. The amniotic fluid volume obtained should not be more than 1 ml per gestational week. The first 2 ml of amniotic fluid should be rejected in order to avoid maternal cell contamination. If bloody amniotic fluid is aspirated, the analysis of the chromosomes from cultured cells will take a longer time and there might be a slightly higher risk of misdiagnosis due to the risk of culturing maternal cells from any tissue other than blood cells. In women with Rh-negative blood group Rh-immune globulin must be administered, if the father of the child is Rh-positive or his blood group is unknown. Following the procedure it seems helpful to demonstrate the fetus again to the mother by ultrasound evaluation. There is no clear evidence in the literature that ultrasound guidance itself will reduce the fetal loss rate, but it may reduce the maternal fears. In contrast, it is assumed that the abortion rate increases if the placenta is perforated.[5] Operator experience may also prejudice the fetal loss rate but this has not been definitively determined.[6] However, there is a general agreement that the operators performing genetic amniocentesis need to be trained, and maintaining stable ongoing expertise is recommended.[7–9] Especially in multiple pregnancies, amniocentesis should be performed by trained investigators. Amniocentesis in twin pregnancies consists in obtaining of amniotic fluid from both cavities. As recommended in the past, dye injection into the first punctured sac was performed routinely.[10] Advanced ultrasound technology allows the evaluation of both fetuses and makes dye injection obsolete in experienced hands. Controversy is ongoing whether both amniotic sacs should be injected in cases of monochromic diamniotic twins. In diachronic twins a single needle insertion technique is often favored, but may result in cytogenetic problems. On the other hand it is not known whether a single-needle technique may induce rupture of the membrane.

Cytogenetic aspects

Compared to other methods for prenatal karyotyping, the benefits of an amniocentesis are the simplicity of the implementation of the procedure and the convenience of the analysis for the cytogenetic laboratory. In clinical practice the level of alpha-fetoprotein (AFP) in amniotic fluid is determined routinely. Currently, it is debated that these may no longer be needed because high-resolution ultrasound is able to detect neural tube defects and abdominal wall defects. However, the detection of spina bifida depends on the experiences of the sonographer. Therefore, evaluation of AFP in the amniotic fluid is still recommended.

Cell culture as a prerequisite for conventional chromosome analysis on amniocytes causes a turnaround time of at least 1 week. In practice, the average processing time is probably close to 2 weeks in most of the laboratories. Ongoing trends in prenatal diagnosis aim at early and rapid diagnosis as well as at the improvement of risk screening for aneuploidy. Fluorescent *in situ* hybridization (FISH) on interphase amniocytes and quantitative fluorescence polymerase chain reaction (QF-PCR) are efficient tools for the rapid exclusion of selected aneuploidies.[11] Regarding the overall detection rate of unbalanced chromosome anomalies, the same limitations apply for both techniques with current approaches. It is suggested that QF-PCR is advantageous at least in all centers with access to the necessary hardware or those with large sample numbers. We believe, however, that for rapid karyotyping, if available, direct preparation from chorionic villi should be the method of first choice when there is an increased risk of unbalanced chromosome anomalies, i.e. after the ultrasound diagnosis of fetal malformations. This method carries a false-negative rate of below 1% as compared to up to 35% with interphase FISH or QF-PCR.[13] In conclusion, it can be stated that FISH and QF–PCR should be used as additional tests.

Particularly in blood-stained probes, maternal cell contamination of amniotic fluid cell is a rare but well-known cause of diagnostic error in the prenatal diagnosis of fetal disorders (<3/1000).[14] Using fluorescent-labeled microsatellites permits the differentiation between maternal and fetal cells. Mosaicism is one other remaining problem and is seen in 1/1000 of samples.[15]

Complications

The risks that may be associated with second-trimester amniocentesis include leakage of amniotic fluid, vaginal bleeding, contractions, chorioamnionitis, failure to obtain a sample, pregnancy loss and, possibly, fetal injury.[5,16–23]

Actual fetal loss rates related to genetic amniocentesis vary among randomized studies and may be comixed

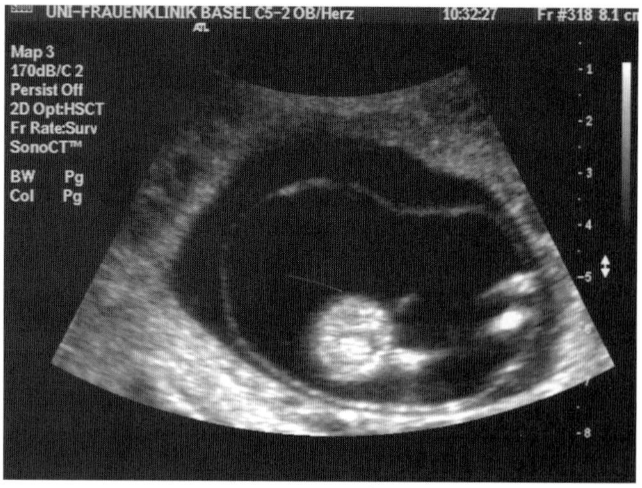

Figure 70.3 Gestational and amniotic sac at 12 weeks demonstrating absence of fusion between amniotic membranes and the surrounding cavity.

by transplacental needle passage, multiple-needle insertion and use of larger needles sizes.[17–19]

The total fetal loss rate related to the procedure is often calculated to be around 0.5%.[24] But in many studies the source for this reported level of risk was non-distinctive, and the background risk of miscarriage was unaccounted for. In the three larger multicenter studies the risk of fetal loss following amniocentesis was approximately 1%, but bias due to selection cannot be excluded.[3,7,22] These results were comparable with the former findings in the only randomized controlled trial reported by Tabor.[5] Recently, Seeds reviewed 68,119 amniocenteses from both controlled and uncontrolled studies providing straightforward arguments for several conclusions.[25]

Currently, midtrimester amniocentesis under ultrasound guidance is associated with a procedure-related rate of excess pregnancy loss of 0.33% (95% CI, 0.09–0.56). Among only controlled studies, the risk is 0.6% (95% CI, 0.31–0.90). Adding the natural risk of loss of about 1.08% among control groups the total rate of losses can be determined to be around 1.6%.

Application of ultrasound guidance may reduce the number of injections and may also lower the incidence of blood-stained fluid. Analysis of only controlled studies shows that this trend remains, but is not statistically significant.

Injury of the fetus is rare and cannot be completely prevented by using ultrasound guidance, but may occur more frequently.

The earlier reported experience of higher risks due to placental perforation does not support an increased rate of miscarriage. As shown in the comprehensive overview, other complications (such as vaginal bleeding and infection or leakage of amniotic fluid) could not be analyzed due to the limited number of described terms or were not comparable.

Following the improvement in the technique and the laboratory methods there have been attempts in bringing forward the time of amniocentesis in the past by performing early amniocentesis, which is technically more demanding (Figure 70.3). Both the randomized studies designed to assess the safety and cytogenetic accuracy of early amniocentesis showed an increased rate of fetal losses as well as a higher rate of talipes, equinovarus and oligohydramnios. Also, more multiple-needle insertions were performed in early pregnancies compared to midtrimester amniocentesis. The rate of laboratory failures following early investigations was increased. Comparing early vs. late amniocentesis, it is suggested that the procedure in the second trimester is more favorable.[26,27]

REFERENCES

1. *Valenti C, Schutta EJ, Kehaty T.* Prenatal diagnosis of Down's syndrome. *Lancet* 1968;2(7561):220.
2. Romero P, Jeanty EA, Reece P, *et al.* Sonographically monitored amniocentesis to decrease intraoperative complications. *Obstet Gynecol* 1985;65:426–30.
3. Simpson NE, Dallaire L, Miller JR, *et al.* Prenatal diagnosis of genetic disease in Canada: Report of a collaborative study. *Can Med Assoc J* 1976;115:793–6.
4. NICHD National Registry for Amniocentesis Study Group. Midtrimester amniocentesis for prenatal diagnosis. Safety and accuracy. *J Am Med Assoc* 1976;236:1471–6.
5. Tabor A, Madsen M, Obel E, Philip J, Bang J, Norgaard-Pedersen B. Randomized controlled trial of genetic amniocentesis in 4606 low-risk women, *Lancet* 1986;1:1287–93.
6. Blessed WB, Lacoste H, Welch RA. Obstetrician-gynecologists performing genetic amniocentesis may be misleading themselves and their patients. *Am J Obstet Gynecol* 2001;184(7):1340–2.
7. NICHD National Registry for Amniocentesis Study Group. Midtrimester amniocentesis for prenatal diagnosis: Safety and accuracy. *J Am Med Assoc* 1976;236:1471–6.
8. Mennuti MT, Brummond W, Crombleholme WR, Schwartz RH, Arvon DA. Fetal-maternal bleeding associated with genetic amniocentesis. *Obstet Gynecol* 1980;55:48–54.
9. Porreco RP, Young PE, Resnik R, Cousins L, Jones OW, Richards T, *et al.* Reproductive outcome following amniocentesis for genetic indications. *Am J Obstet Gynecol* 1982;143:653–60.
10. Pijpers L, Jahoda MG, Vosters RP, Niermeijer MF, Sachs ES. Genetic amniocentesis in twin pregnancies. *Br J Obstet Gynaecol* 1988;95(4):323–6.
11. Kuo WL, Tenjin H, Segraves R, *et al.* Detection of aneuploidy involving chromosomes 13, 18 or 21 by fluorescence in situ hybridization (FISH) to interphase and metaphase amniocytes. *Am J Hum Genet* 1991;49:112–9.
12. Fauth C, Speicher MR. Classifying by colors: FISH-based genome analysis. *Cytogenet Cell Genet* 2001;93:1–10.
13. Miny P, Tercanli S, Holzgreve W. Developments in laboratory techniques for prenatal diagnosis. *Curr Opin Obstet Gynecol* 2002;14(2):161–8.
14. Benn PA, Hsu LYF. Maternal cell contamination of amniotic fluid cell cultures: Results of a US nationwide survey. *Am J Med Genet* 1983;15:297–305.
15. Bui T-H, Iselius L, Lindsten J. European collaborative study on prenatal amniotic fluid cell cultures. Prenat Diagn 1984;4:145–62.
16. Jeanty P, Rodesch F, Romero R, Venus I, Hobbins JC. How to improve your amniocentesis technique, *Am J Obstet Gynecol* 1983;146:593–6.

17. Carpenter RJ, Hinkley CM, Carpenter AF. Midtrimester genetic amniocentesis: Use of ultrasound direction vs. blind needle insertion, *J Reprod Med* 1983;28:35–40.
18. Williamson RA, Varner MW, Grant SS. Reduction in amniocentesis risks using a real-time needle guide procedure. *Obstet Gynecol* 1985;65:751–5.
19. Romero R, Jeanty P, Reece EA, *et al.* Sonographically monitored amniocentesis to decrease intraoperative complications. *Obstet Gynecol* 1985;65:426–30.
20. Simpson NE, Dallaire L, Miller JR, *et al.* Prenatal diagnosis of genetic disease in Canada: Report of a collaborative study, *Can Med Assoc J* 1976;115:739–46.
21. Philip J, Bang J. Outcome of pregnancy after amniocentesis for chromosome analysis. *Br Med J* 1978;2:1183–4.
22. United Kingdom Medical Research Council. An assessment of the hazards of amniocentesis: Report of the MRC Working Party on amniocentesis. *BJOG* 1978;85(Suppl 2):1–41.
23. Antsaklis A, Papantoniou N, Xygakis A, Mesogitis S, Tzortzis E, Michalas S. Genetic amniocentesis in women 20–34 years old: Associated risks. *Prenat Diagn* 2000;20:247–50.
24. Centers for Disease Control and Prevention. Chorionic villus sampling and amniocentesis: Recommendations for prenatal counseling, *MMWR Morb Mortal Wkly Rep* 1995;44:1–4.
25. Seeds JW. Diagnostic midtrimester amniocentesis: How safe? *Am J Obstet Gynecol* 2004;191(2):607–15.
26. CEMAT. Randomised trial to assess safety and fetal outcome of early and midtrimester amniocentesis. The Canadian Early and Midtrimester Amniocentesis Trial (CEMAT) Group. *Lancet* 1998; 51(9098):242–7.
27. Sundberg K, Bang J, Smidt-Jensen S, *et al.* Randomised study of risk of fetal loss related to early amniocentesis versus chorionic villus sampling. *Lancet* 1997;350(9079):697–703.

71 Cordocentesis

C. P. Weiner

The development of high-resolution ultrasound made it feasible to clearly image the umbilical cord. In the early 1980s, Daffos performed the first intentional percutaneous umbilical blood sampling (cordocentesis) under ultrasound guidance spurred by a desire to accurately diagnose fetal toxoplasmosis.[1] The procedure rapidly gained favor with demonstration of its safety[2–4] and directly spurred the development of fetal medicine. A wide range of fetal norms (hematological, endocrinological, immunological, biochemical, and biophysical[5]) were developed, a crucial step in the evolution of fetal medicine. And while many early indications for cordocentesis have been supplanted by less invasive techniques, there remain several indications for fetal blood sampling. The most common presently are assessment and treatment of red cell and platelet alloimmunization, antenatal diagnosis of inherited blood or metabolic diseases, rapid karyotyping of malformed or severely growth-restricted fetuses in some countries, and rarely the determination of fetal acid–base status.

Methods

Cordocentesis is performed in the outpatient setting by a single operator with or without an assistant. There is no benefit of maternal fasting, sedation, prophylactic antibiotics, or tocolysis. Though it is technically more difficult prior to 20 weeks, and the loss rate is much higher prior to 16 weeks, cordocentesis can be performed as early as 12 weeks. The patient's partner is encouraged to attend both the counseling session preceding the procedure, and the procedure itself. The limitations and potential complications must be stated unambiguously before written informed consent is obtained, and a targeted ultrasound examination performed.

There are two methods for cordocentesis: freehand and the use of a fixed needle guide. The preferred location for umbilical cord puncture is the placental origin where it is relatively fixed regardless of technique. The first few centimeters of the fetal origin of the umbilical cord are innervated, and puncture there causes pain. The umbilical vein is the preferred target rather than the umbilical artery because of its lower association with complications discussed subsequently. A 'no touch' philosophy is essential. If you do not touch the shaft of the needle, you cannot contaminate it.

The freehand technique employs a 18–20-gauge spinal needle 8–12 cm long.[1] The subcutaneous and deep layers are infiltrated with a local anesthetic agent. The needle course is tracked by imaging the tip and shaft with the ultrasound transducer held either in the opposite hand of the operator or by the assistant. Since the needle is not fixed, the tip can move several centimeters in all axes should either the site of insertion be suboptimal or the fetus move during the procedure. The operator secures the needle after the vessel has been punctured and the assistant aspirates a series of 1-ml syringes. Preheparinization of the syringe is unnecessary unless a fetal blood gas is needed. The freehand technique remains most popular because of the flexibility it allows the operator.

I, however, prefer to perform cordocentesis using a fixed needle guide[2] attached to the base of the ultrasound transducer. Typically, the transducer is held by the operator's assistant. The predicted course of the needle, which can travel only in the vertical plane, is displayed on the ultrasound screen, allowing the operator to select a precise target for puncture. Deviation from the predicted path occurs when there is an abrupt change in the relationship between the puncture site in the maternal abdominal wall and the uterus as the needle traverses between the two. The most common causes are abrupt patient movement or inspiration and failure to hold the transducer surface flat against the maternal abdomen. Fetal movement is rarely an issue because of the speed of the procedure. A smaller-gauge needle such as a 22 or 25 is used because lateral movement of the needle is not possible. I prefer to target the umbilical cord longitudinally at the 'easiest' site for a direct approach. More than 50% of the time I target a free loop. Placental puncture is avoided whenever possible when the indication is alloimmunization (RBC or platelet) just as for amniocentesis. Local anesthesia is unnecessary for diagnostic procedures using a 22-gauge needle. A local anesthetic should be used when the procedure is lengthy (e.g.

intravascular transfusion). Prophylactic antibiotics are not indicated for either cordocentesis or intravascular transfusion. In my experience, amnionitis complicates less than 1 in 800 diagnostic procedures when the 'no touch' philosophy is rigorously adhered to and a needle guide is used (1 in 1200 procedures).

Fetal movement while the needle is intraluminal increases the risk of umbilical cord trauma; it may also either prevent a successful puncture or shorten the access time available regardless of technique. I keep prepared a neuromuscular antagonist such as pancuronium (0.3 mg/kg estimated fetal weight) on the sterile field for every procedure, and routinely use it to eliminate fetal movement when performing a mid-loop puncture. The pancuronium is given either intramuscularly into the fetal buttock, or preferably, intravenously as soon as the vein is punctured; the effect here is evident within seconds. Vercuronium is preferred over pancuronium for simple diagnostic procedures because its shorter half-life allows a more rapid return of fetal movement and heart rate variability.[6] In contrast, pancuronium is preferred for fetal transfusion because it maintains fetal cardiac output despite the volume load.

The volume of blood removed depends on the gestation and indication for sampling. Five milliliters is typical, and adequate for a karyotype, umbilical venous blood gas, and complete blood profile with Kleihauer–Betke testing, with 2 ml remaining for use.

Table 71.1 Complications of cordocentesis

Complications
Bradycardia or asystole
Premature rupture of membranes
Premature labor
Umbilical hemorrhage
Placental hemorrhage
Chorioamnionitis
Umbilical thrombosis
Fetal to maternal hemorrhage

Table 71.2 Risk factors for cordocentesis

Risk factors
Umbilical artery puncture (associated with bradycardia)
Fetal hypoxemia (associated with bradycardia)
Technique – freehand vs. needle guide
Gestational age – prior to 20 weeks, both techniques
Number of punctures (freehand technique only)
Duration of procedure (freehand technique only)
Experience (freehand technique only, presumably because of #4, 5)

Major complications and risk factors for cordocentesis

The major complications of cordocentesis are listed in Table 71.1. They include all complications associated with amniocentesis plus fetal bradycardia, umbilical cord laceration, and thrombosis. Risk factors for cordocentesis are noted in Table 71.2.

Bradycardia is the major complication of cordocentesis. Essentially, all emergency cesarean deliveries and most perinatal losses are associated with a fetal bradycardia. Umbilical artery puncture and hypoxia are the major risk factors for bradycardia. In the absence of profound anemia or fetal heart failure, fetal hypoxia is associated with an elevated umbilical artery resistance index and it can be used as a risk marker. The incidence of bradycardia with absent and/or reversed diastolic flow approaches 25%. Umbilical artery puncture increases the risk of fetal bradycardia 5- to 10-fold.[3,7,8] The presence of either oligohydramnios or a two-vessel cord increases the risk of arterial puncture.

The observation that the bradycardia is associated with an elevated resistance index in one but not both umbilical arteries suggests localized vasospasm is the cause. Pancuronium reduces the prevalence of bradycardia in appropriately grown but not growth-restricted fetuses.[8] It is possible some episodes of bradycardia occur when fetal movement tugs on the umbilical cord causing needle trauma and irritation to the underlying vascular smooth muscle. Bradycardia after umbilical vein puncture may reflect disruption of the adjacent umbilical artery smooth muscle as the tip traverses the cord.

In the event of a bradycardia, vigorous fetal stimulation by palpation is beneficial as the heart will speed up and then slow again if the manual stimulation is stopped too early. A variety of chronotropes (e.g. atropine) and bicarbonate have also been given as part of the fetal resuscitation without predictable effect.

Umbilical cord laceration and thrombosis are associated with freehand procedures and are not reported to date when a needle guide was used.[7] Though bleeding from the umbilical puncture site is common, prolonged bleeding with sequelae is uncommon.

Even when performed at a midloop, the fetus does 'react' to the cordocentesis. Umbilical artery resistance typically declines after either a diagnostic procedure or a fetal intravascular transfusion.[9] The higher the 'normal' baseline resistance index, the greater the decline. The decrease is associated with prostacyclin release from the vascular endothelium.[10,11] Endothelial adaptation to hypoxia also explains why hypoxemia is a risk factor for bradycardia.[8] Rizzo *et al.* demonstrated that endothelin is released upon umbilical vein puncture of growth-restricted but not appropriately grown fetuses.[12] Fetuses who develop bradycardia release more endothelin.

It was generally accepted that the technique selected was a matter of operator preference and had no impact on outcome. There is now evidence to challenge this concept. The first line of evidence is indirect. The often stated 'advantage' of the freehand technique, its flexibility, may also increase risk. Analogous to a lever, a small movement at the hub of the needle amplifies the distance the tip moves. In association with this inescapable fact, freehand cordocentesis produces a significantly greater increase in the MSAFP than amniocentesis after controlling for placental puncture.[13] In contrast, the incremental change in MSAFP when a needle guide is used is similar to amniocentesis.[14] Further, the association between fetal thrombocytopenia and bleeding from the umbilical puncture site after a freehand cordocentesis is high enough to have prompted a recommendation that all fetuses at risk for alloimmune thrombocytopenia receive a prophylactic platelet transfusion at cordocentesis.[15] Yet, there is no relationship between the fetal platelet count and the bleeding time from the puncture site when a needle guide is used.[16] The latter may reflect either less lateral movement of the needle after puncture or the thinner gauge needle, or both. The loss rates reported after second trimester amniocentesis are lower when thinner needles are used.[17] Not surprisingly, there are also reports that suggest that an amniocentesis performed with a needle guide is safer than one performed freehand.[18]

Though no single center has adequate volume for a randomized trial, and comparisons of loss rates sustained by groups using the freehand and needle guide techniques are problematic since it is hard to separate procedure-related losses from those secondary to the natural progression of disease, there is evidence to suggest many losses are technique-dependent. I examined the role of technique by combining our experience with that of Professor Okamura of Tokohu University, who also uses a fixed needle guide for all procedures.[7] Over 25 operators with varying levels of experience performed 1260 diagnostic cordocenteses at a mean gestational age of 29 weeks. The umbilical vein (confirmed by the blood pressure reading) was punctured in 90% demonstrating that the desired vessel can be targeted. A procedure-related loss was defined as any loss within 2 weeks of the procedure except those resulting from elective pregnancy termination. Overall, there were 12 losses (0.9%) (Table 71.3).

Table 71.3 Frequency of major complications of cordocentesis when a needle guide is used

Final diagnosis	GA (weeks) at cordocentesis	Percent emergency delivery*	Percent death within 2 weeks**
RBC alloimmunization	28 ± 4	0.2	0.2
Uteroplacental dysfunction	32 ± 4	5.0	0.9
Chromosome abnormality	29 ± 6	7.7	9.9
All others	28 ± 6	0.3	0.2

*From Weiner, unpublished; **from Weiner and Okamura;[7] fetuses with a chromosome abnormality delivered by cesarean section were delivered before the karyotype was completed

Though there are more recent studies, Ghidini *et al.* provided adequate information for stratification and that the low level of experience reported by the involved centers may be more reflective of today's reality.[19] After deleting my experience from the analyses, the overall loss rate was 7.2% (96/1328) with the freehand method.[19] This rate was significantly higher than the overall loss rate when a needle guide was used (0.9%, 12/1260; $P < 0.00001$). But this is a superficial comparison.

To exclude the contribution of the underlying pathology to the loss rate, procedures may be divided into high and low risk with the latter excluding chromosomal abnormalities, non-immune hydrops, intrauterine growth restriction (IUGR), and fetal infection. Such exclusions virtually eliminate all abnormal fetuses that might be at risk for a loss *unrelated* to the procedure. The perinatal loss rate for these low-risk procedures using the freehand technique was 3% (20/660). This rate is 15 times the needle guide rate (0.2%, 2/1021; $P < 000001$), which *includes* fetuses with infection, hydrops, and structural malformations.

Donner et al. reported 759 diagnostic cordocenteses *with a known outcome* using the freehand technique.[20] Acknowledging several limitations (final diagnoses were not necessarily reported and 87% (34/39) of their perinatal losses were excluded as being unrelated to the procedure), their stated loss rate was 0.8% including 94 therapeutic terminations in the denominator. Subtracting the terminations from their total yields a loss of 1.1% (7/665). Of these pregnancies, 160 were sampled because of severe early IUGR. We can identify their low-risk group by excluding the IUGR fetuses and assuming that all fetuses with chromosomal abnormalities were either in the growth-restriction group, therapeutic termination group, or the one fetus with trisomy 18 noted in the paper. This leaves a low-risk group of 504 in which there were six fetal/neonatal losses (1.2%). This rate is significantly higher than that achieved in a similar group using a needle guide ($P = 0.03$).

These findings strongly suggest that many of the procedure-related losses associated with cordocentesis are technique-dependent. And while a few skilled operators might duplicate the results obtained with a needle guide, the majority of practitioners who perform only a few cordocenteses per year would benefit from the use of a guide.

Indications and applications for cordocentesis

Antenatal diagnosis of blood disorders

The use of recombinant DNA techniques on placental biopsy material in the first trimester of pregnancy or amniocytes in the second for the diagnosis has supplanted cordocentesis for the diagnosis of many of these conditions.[21] Cordocentesis is still needed for a phenotype diagnosis, in those patients requiring confirmation of normality based on a linked probe, those who lack key affected relatives, those who are not informative by any of the available probes, and those in whom DNA analysis is not feasible because of late referral.

Antenatal diagnosis of metabolic disorders

Antenatal diagnosis of over 100 of these disorders is now possible by the analysis of amniotic fluid, placental tissue, or fetal blood. Cordocentesis is particularly useful when the gestational age is close to the local limit for abortion, as with late prenatal care or after failed chorionic villus or amniotic fluid techniques.

Red blood cell alloimmunization

Cordocentesis is not indicated in most instances of maternal RBC alloimmunization for fetal blood typing. Accurate typing can now be accomplished by applying polymerase chain reaction to either trophoblast or amniocytes obtained in the early second trimester when the risk of exacerbating sensitization is lower.[22,23]

Fetal blood sampling made it possible to better understand the pathophysiology of this disease and allows for an improved method of assessment and treatment.[24–29] The net result of improved understanding is an improved perinatal outcome. The most important advancement in the non-invasive management of RBC alloimmune disease was the recognition that most severely anemic fetuses have an elevated peak flow velocity in the middle cerebral artery.[30,31] Previously, the severity of fetal hemolysis was estimated from: (1) the history of previously affected pregnancies; (2) the level of maternal hemolytic antibodies in a first sensitized pregnancy; (3) the amniotic fluid bilirubin concentration; (4) the altered morphometry of fetus and placenta; and (5) the presence of pathological fetal heart rate (FHR) patterns. However, the scatter of values around the regression lines describing the relationships between fetal anemia and the data obtained from these indirect methods of assessment was wide.[32] And though the vast majority of fetuses with an elevated peak velocity in the middle cerebral artery are anemic, a sizable percentage of anemic fetuses have normal velocities, and the relationship between velocity and the magnitude of the hemoglobin deficit varies greatly among fetuses.

The only accurate method for determining severity is blood sampling by cordocentesis with the measurement of fetal hemoglobin concentration, reticulocyte count, blood type, strength of the direct Coombs test and total bilirubin concentration. However, the timing of the first cordocentesis remains less than concrete. Invasive procedures should be minimized not only because of the fetal risk, but also because transplacental puncture enhances the risk of fetomaternal hemorrhage,[14,33] increases maternal antibody titer, and worsens disease. I prefer to avoid cordocentesis until the peak middle cerebral artery flow velocities are abnormal in those pregnancies under 20 weeks' gestation. However, since as many as half the fetuses with mild to moderate anemia have normal velocities, it is reasonable depending on referral patterns and distances to consider sampling all women with a history of severe disease, those with high antibody titers, and fetuses with pathological FHR patterns.

A fetal blood sample is obtained, the hemoglobin concentration measured, and an intravascular blood transfusion given as necessary.[34] The goal of the first transfusion is to correct the hemoglobin deficit completely unless there is hydrops. Immune hydrops in the human fetus is almost always characterized by an elevated umbilical venous pressure (UVP), which is consistent with high output heart failure or left ventricular dysfunction perhaps secondary to the low oxygen carrying capacity.[35] These fetuses tolerate the first intravascular transfusion poorly, and should be corrected initially to a hemoglobin level of no more than 8–9 g/dl. (We routinely monitor the fetal UVP to avoid over-transfusion.) The second transfusion is performed a few days later at which time the target hemoglobin for this and all subsequent transfusions is 18 g/dl. Subsequent transfusions are given at 3- to 4-week intervals until 34 to 36 weeks' gestation, their timing based on the findings in the middle cerebral artery and the knowledge that following a fetal blood transfusion the mean rate of decrease in fetal hemoglobin is approximately 0.3 g/dl/day.[34] Currently, the survival rate of red cell isoimmunized pregnancies treated with cordocentesis exceeds 90% in experienced hands, and virtually all losses are associated with immune hydrops fetalis.[34] Importantly, we have demonstrated normal long-term neurodevelopment despite the profound anemia prior to treatment.[36]

How often to repeat cordocentesis in the occasional affected fetus which is not anemic is determined by the change in the peak flow velocity in the middle cerebral artery and by the 'hemolysis pattern' determined at the first sampling.[37] This prospectively validated grading scheme is based on the reticulocyte count and the strength of the positive direct Coombs test. Most fetuses do not require a second sampling. That said, non-anemic sensitized fetuses remain at risk for postnatal hyperbilirubinemia that is in direct correlation to their antenatal bilirubin levels.[38,39]

Platelet alloimmunization

Immune thrombocytopenia (ITP) is not an indication for cordocentesis.[40] The assumed risk of fetal intracranial hemorrhage during labor is not supported by the aggregate experience of the last two decades. There is no more than one *fetal* loss documented in the literature secondary to an intrapartum fetal hemorrhage.[40] Most losses attributed to ITP were associated with a maternal connective tissue disorder or a neonatal bleed. In almost all other instances, either the cause of death or the timing of death is either not stated or not known. ITP is the most common autoimmune disorder of reproductive age women; if true, there should be no controversy that thrombocytopenia secondary to ITP posed a significant fetal risk during labor. Yet, the loss rate from cordocentesis in the best hands for a 'low risk' fetus is 0.2%.[7] Further, there is no direct or indirect evidence that cesarean section for autoimmune thrombocytopenia improves neonatal outcome.

There has been significant progress in the management of severe fetal alloimmune thrombocytopenia.[41,42] It is clear that medical therapy consisting of primarily high doses of intravenous gammaglobulin (1–2 g/kg/week) with a prednisone rescue for suboptimal responders is an effective treatment for the majority of affected pregnancies.[43] At-risk pregnancies begin the weekly infusion between 10 and 20 weeks depending on past history. Most undergo a single cordocentesis around 28 weeks to confirm normal platelet counts. When secondary to Pl(A1) platelet antigen incompatibility, fetuses with platelet counts >20,000 at the initiation of therapy are predicted to maintain their platelet count at the second fetal blood sampling at >20,000. The history of the previous sibling does not predict the initial fetal blood sampling, the second fetal blood sampling, or the response to treatment.[44] Even suboptimal fetal responders have a dramatic decrease in the risk of antenatal hemorrhage. Fetal platelet transfusion is associated with a high loss rate when used for primary therapy (up to 17%[45]). Its role is now secondary, indicated for those fetuses with extremely low platelet counts or those with a count <50,000 prior to a planned vaginal delivery. There is no relationship between the fetal platelet count and bleeding from the puncture site when a needle guide is used.[16]

Evaluation of non-immune hydrops fetalis

Cordocentesis is central to the complete evaluation of non-immune hydrops since it allows the separation of cardiac from non-cardiac etiologies.[46] The UVP is a surrogate for the central venous pressure. Studies of human fetuses[47] indicate that it is very similar to right-sided heart pressure. An elevated UVP is consistent with myocardial dysfunction whether caused by anemia (e.g. parvovirus infection, hemolytic disease), myocarditis, or obstructed cardiac return (thoracic mass effect). Successful treatment of cardiogenic hydrops is associated with normalization of the UVP before the hydrops resolves. Hydrops that is responsive to shunting is caused by a shift of the mediastinum, which then obstructs cardiac return. An elevated UVP also predicts that the fetus with hydrothorax and hydrops will be cured by a thoracoamniotic shunt. If the UVP is neither elevated nor normalizes after draining the chest, a shunt will not help. The underlying problem lies elsewhere.

Miscellaneous

Not yet accepted but a likely valid indication for cordocentesis is presence of maternal thyroid stimulating antibody (TSiG) or active maternal Graves disease.[48,49] Emerging evidence suggests even mild degrees of thyroid dysfunction is associated with impaired long-term neurodevelopment.[50–52] While there is a relationship between the degree of maternal and fetal thyroid suppression with such agents as propylthiouracil (PTU), it is common to find the fetus being significantly over- or under-treated despite the mother being euthyroid. For fetal hyperthyroidism, the maternal PTU dose is increased and the woman is given thyroxine replacement. For hypothyroidism, the fetus can be given thyroxine intra-amniotically on a weekly basis.[53] Women with a history of Graves disease who have undergone thyroid ablation should be screened for the presence of TSiG. The fetus is at minimal risk if the TSiG study is negative.

REFERENCES

1. Daffos F, Capella-Pavlovsky M, Forestier F. A new procedure for fetal blood sampling in utero: Preliminary results of fifty-three cases. *Am J Obstet Gynecol* 1983;146:985–7.
2. Weiner CP. Cordocentesis for diagnostic indications – two years experience. *Obstet Gynecol* 1987;70:664–8.
3. Daffos F. Access to the other patient (review). *Semin Perinatol* 1989;13:252–9.
4. Maxwell DJ, Johnson P, Hurley P, Neales K, Allan L, Knott P. Fetal blood sampling and pregnancy loss in relation to indication. *Br J Obstet Gynaecol* 1991;98:892–7.
5. Ramsay MM, James DK, Steer PJ, Weiner CP, Gonik B, eds. *Normal Values in Pregnancy*, 3rd edn. Philadelphia: WB Saunders, 2005.
6. Mouw RJC, Hermans J, Brandenburg HCR, Kanhai HHH. Effects of pancuronium or atracurium on the anemic fetus during and directly after intrauterine transfusion (IUT): A double blind randomized study. *Am J Obstet Gynecol* 1997;176(2): S18.
7. Weiner CP, Okamura K. Diagnostic fetal blood sampling – technique related losses. *Fetal Diagn Ther* 1996;11:169–75.

8. Weiner CP, Wenstrom KD, Sipes SL, Williamson RA. Risk factors for cordocentesis and fetal intravascular transfusions. *Am J Obstet Gynecol* 1991;165:1020–3.
9. Weiner CP, Anderson T. The acute effect of cordocentesis with or without fetal curarization and of intravascular transfusion upon umbilical artery waveform indices. *Obstet Gynecol* 1989;73: 219–24.
10. Weiner CP, Robillard JE. Effect of acute intravascular volume expansion upon human fetal prostaglandin concentrations. *Am J Obstet Gynecol* 1989;161:1494–7.
11. Capponi A, Rizzo G, Pasquini L, Turri E, Arduini D, Romanini C. Indomethacin modifies the fetal hemodynamic response induced by cordocentesis. *Am J Obstet Gynecol* 1997;176(2):S19.
12. Rizzo G, Capponi A, Rinaldo D, Arduini D, Romanini C. Release of vasoactive agents during cordocentesis: Differences between normally grown and growth-restricted fetuses. *Am J Obstet Gynecol* 1996;175:563–70.
13. Nicolini U, Kochenour NK, Greco P, *et al.* Consequences of fetomatemal hemorrhage after intrauterine transfusion. *Br Med J* 1988; 297:1379–81.
14. Weiner CP, Grant SS, Hudson J, Williamson RA, Wenstrom KD. Effect of diagnostic and therapeutic cordocentesis upon maternal serum alpha fetoprotein concentration. *Am J Obstet Gynecol* 1989;161:706–8.
15. Paidas MJ, Lynch L, Lockwood CJ, Alvarez MA, Bussel J, Berkowitz RL. Alloimmune thrombocytopenia: Fetal and neonatal losses related to fetal blood sampling. *Am J Obstet Gynecol* 1995;172: 475–9.
16. Weiner CP. Fetal blood sampling and fetal thrombocytopenia. *Fetal Diagn Ther* 1995;10:173–7.
17. Tabor A, Philip J, Bang J, Madsen M, Obel EB, Norgaard-Pedersen B. Needle size and risk of miscarriage after amniocentesis (letter). *Lancet* 1988;1(8578):183–4.
18. Weiner CP, Williamson RA, Varner MW, Grant S. Safety of second trimester amniocentesis. Lancet 1986;ii:226.
19. Ghidini A, Sepulveda W, Lockwood CJ, Romero R. Complications of fetal blood sampling. *Am J Obstet Gynecol* 1993;168: 1339–44.
20. Donner C, Simon P, Karioun A, Avni F, Rodesch F. Experience of a single team of operators in 891 diagnostic funipunctures. *Obstet Gynecol* 1994;84:827–31.
21. Boehm CD, Kazazian HH. Examination of fetal DNA for hemoglobinopathies. In Alter BP, ed. *Perinatal Hematology.* New York: Churchill Livingstone, 1989:30–63.
22. Yankowitz J, Li S, Murray JC. Polymerase chain reaction determination of RhD blood type: An evaluation of accuracy. *Obstet Gynecol* 1995;86:214–7.
23. Yankowitz J, Li S, Weiner CP. Polymerase chain reaction determination of RhC, Rhc, and RhE blood types: An evaluation of accuracy and clinical utility. *Am J Obstet Gynecol* 1997; 176:1107–11.
24. Berkowitz RL, Chitkara U, Goldberg JD, *et al.* Intrauterine transfusion in utero: The percutaneous approach. *Am J Obstet Gynecol* 1986;154:622.
25. Grannum PAT, Copel JA, Plaxe SC, *et al.* In utero exchange transfusion by direct intravascular injection in severe erythroblastosis fetalis. *N Engl J Med* 1986;314:1431.
26. Nicolaides KH, Rodeck CH, Kemp J, *et al.* Have Liley charts outlived their usefulness? *Am J Obstet Gynecol* 1986;155:90.
27. Nicolaides KH. Studies on fetal physiology and pathophysiology in rhesus disease. *Semin Perinatol* 1986;13:328.
28. Weiner CP, Robillard JE. Atrial natriuretic factor, digoxin-like immunoreactive substance, norepinephrine, epinephrine, and plasma renin activity in human fetuses and their alteration by fetal disease. *Am J Obstet Gynecol* 1988;159(6):1353–60.
29. Soothill PW, Lestas AN, Nicolaides KH, *et al.* 2,3-Diphosphoglycerate in normal, anaemic and transfused human fetus. *Clin Sci* 1988;74:527.
30. Mari G, Moise KJ Jr, Deter RL, Carpenter RJ Jr. Flow velocity waveforms of the umbilical and cerebral arteries before and after intravascular transfusion. *Obstet Gynecol* 1990;75:584–9.
31. Mari G, Deter RL, Carpenter RL, *et al.* Noninvasive diagnosis by Doppler ultrasonography of fetal anemia due to maternal red-cell alloimmunization. Collaborative Group for Doppler Assessment of the Blood Velocity in Anemic Fetuses. *N Engl J Med* 2000;342:9–14.
32. Nicolaides KH, Sadovsky G, Cetin E. Fetal heart rate patterns in red blood cell isoimmunized pregnancies. *Am J Obstet Gynecol* 1989;161:351.
33. Nicolini U, Kochenour NK, Greco P. Consequences of fetomaternal haemorrhage after intrauterine transfusion. *Br Med J* 1988;297:1379.
34. Weiner CP, Williamson RA, Wenstrom KD, *et al.* Management of fetal hemolytic disease by cordocentesis. II. Outcome of treatment. *Am J Obstet Gynecol* 1991;165:1302–7.
35. Weiner CP, Pelzer GD, Heilskov J, Wenstrom KD, Williamson RA. The effect of intravascular transfusion on umbilical venous pressure in anemic fetuses with and without hydrops. *Am J Obstet Gynecol* 1989;161:1498–501.
36. Swingle HM, Harper DC, Bonthius D, Weiner CP, Widness JA, Aylward GA. *Long-term Neurodevelopmental Follow-up and Brain Volumes of Children following Severe Fetal Anemia with Hydrops.* Los Angeles: American Academy of Cerebral Palsy and Developmental Medicine, 2004;9/29–10/1.
37. Weiner CP, Williamson RA, Wenstrom KD, Sipes SL, Grant SS, Widness JA. Management of fetal hemolytic disease by cordocentesis. I. Prediction of fetal anemia. *Am J Obstet Gynecol* 1991;165(3):546–53.
38. Weiner CP, Wenstrom KD. Outcome of alloimmunized fetuses managed solely by cordocentesis but not requiring antenatal transfusion. *Fetal Diagn Ther* 1994;9(4):233–8.
39. Weiner CP. Human fetal bilirubin levels and fetal hemolytic disease. *Am J Obstet Gynecol* 1992;166(5):1449–54.
40. Weiner CP. Why fuss over diagnosing fetal thrombocytopenia secondary to ITP? Contemp Ob/Gyn 1995;40:45–50.
41. Radder CM, Brand A, Kanhai HH. Will it ever be possible to balance the risk of intracranial haemorrhage in fetal or neonatal alloimmune thrombocytopenia against the risk of treatment strategies to prevent it? *Vox Sang* 2003;84(4):318–25.
42. Bussel JB. Alloimmune thrombocytopenia in the fetus and newborn. *Semin Thromb Hemost* 2001;27(3):245–52.
43. Bussel JB, Berkowitz RL, Lynch L, *et al.* Antenatal management of alloimmune thrombocytopenia with intravenous gamma-globulin. A randomized trial of the addition of low-dose steroid to intravenous gamma-globulin. *Am J Obstet Gynecol* 1996;174(5): 1414–23.
44. Gaddipati S, Berkowitz RL, Lembet AA, Lapinski R, McFarland JG, Bussel JB. Initial fetal platelet counts predict the response to intravenous gammaglobulin therapy in fetuses that are affected by PLA1 incompatibility. *Am J Obstet Gynecol* 2001;185(4): 976–80.
45. Overton TG, Duncan KR, Jolly M, Letsky E, Fisk NM. Serial aggressive platelet transfusion for fetal alloimmune thrombocytopenia: Platelet dynamics and perinatal outcome. *Am J Obstet Gynecol* 2002;186(4):826–31.
46. Weiner CP. Umbilical venous pressure measurement in the evaluation of nonimmune hydrops. *Am J Obstet Gynecol* 1993; 168:817–23.
47. Weiner Z, Efrat Z, Zimmer EZ, Iskovitz-Eldor J, Copel JA. Direct measurement of central venous pressure in human fetuses. *Am J Obstet Gynecol* 1997;176:S19.
48. Wenstrom KD, Weiner CP, Williamson RA, Grant SS. Prenatal diagnosis of fetal hyperthyroidism using funipuncture. *Obstet Gynecol* 1990;75:1–5.
49. Yankowitz J, Weiner CP. Medical fetal therapy. *Clin Obstet Gynaecol* 1995;9:553–70.
50. Salerno M, Di Maio S, Militerni R, Argenziano A, Valerio G, Tenore A. Prognostic factors in the intellectual development at 7 years of age in children with congenital hypothyroidism. *J Endocrinol Invest* 1995;18:774–9.
51. Kooistra L, van der Meere JJ, Vulsma T, Kalverboer AF. Sustained attention problems in children with early treated congenital hypothyroidism. *Acta Paediatr* 1996;85:425–9.
52. Weber G, Siragusa V, Rondanini GF, *et al.* Neurophysiologic studies and cognitive function in congenital hypothyroid children. *Pediatr Res* 1995;37:736–40.
53. Van Loon AJ, Derksen JT, Bos AF, Rouwe CW. In utero diagnosis and treatment of fetal goitrous hypothyroidism, caused by maternal use of propylthiouracil. *Prenat Diagn* 1995;15:599–604.

72 Perinatal Rh hemolytic disease and other alloimmunizations: screening and treatment

L. S. Voto

Severe hemolytic disease due to rhesus (Rh) incompatibility still constitutes a source of concern for obstetricians and pediatricians. In Argentina, as well as in most developing countries, this disease is one of the main causes of fetoneonatal morbidity and mortality due to the lack of appropriate prophylaxis with postpartum anti-D γ-globulin and inadequate prenatal control.[1]

Perinatal hemolytic disease (PHD) represents one of the most significant examples in medicine of successful management of a disease and adequate prophylaxis.

By the first half of the century, PHD accounted for 45% of all perinatal deaths. Nowadays, this rate has significantly decreased to 5%, as a result of in-depth understanding of the etiology and pathogenesis of the disease, the advances in perinatal technology, the creation of sophisticated centers for high-risk perinatal care and, mainly, from its prophylaxis.

The Rh blood group antigens

Biochemistry and molecular genetics

A group of non-glycosylated hydrophobic transmembrane proteins of 30–32 kDa are known to carry the Rh blood antigens (D, Ce, and Ee series). These proteins, which are not found in the red cells of rare Rh_{null} individuals with membrane defects, are erythroid-specific and have a distinctive sequence homology. The Rh_D and non-D proteins show 92% sequence identity and a similar predicted membrane topology.

The Rh proteins D and Cc/Ee are encoded by the RHD and RHCE genes, respectively. These genes are arranged in tandem on chromosome 1p34–p36 and probably result from the duplication of a common ancestral gene.

The human RH locus is considered a two-gene model where all Rh-D positive haplotypes have two structural genes (namely, RHD and RHCE) and most Rh-D negative ones have only one structural gene (namely, RHCE). D protein is encoded by the RHD gene, whereas the C/c and E/e proteins are encoded by the RHCE gene. The relationship between blood group D epitopes and the amino acid polymorphisms of the Rh proteins still remains unclear, but it has been found that the molecular basis for the C/c (Ser→Pro) and E/e (Pro→Ala) specificities result from amino acid polymorphisms at positions 103 and 226, respectively. In the Rh system, polymorphism and gene diversity seem to be produced mainly by gene conversion. But cases of gene deletion have also been observed in the Rh system. Rh_{null} phenotypes have been found to be caused by a mechanism of transcriptional regulation, which has not been clearly described yet.

In the cells of the Rh_{null} individuals, morphological and functional abnormalities of cation transport as well as phospholipid asymmetry have been observed and are thought to lead to severe clinical conditions. Also, Rh proteins and other glycoproteins (such as Rh50 glycoprotein, CD47, glycophorin B, Duffy, LW) are either not present, or their quantity is markedly lower in the Rh_{null} individuals' cells, which might mean that Rh proteins form a multimeric complex with these glycoproteins.[2]

Etiology and pathogenesis of Rh–Hr incompatibility

The antigens of the Rh system are located on the surface of the erythrocyte, although they are also thought to be part of the trophoblast.[3]

Rh system's anti-D antibodies are responsible for the majority of clinically detectable PHD cases. This situation is observed in Rh-negative mothers whose husbands are Rh-positive, and whose immunization occurred during pregnancy, abortion, postpartum or incompatible transfusion.

There are other Rh–Hr system's antibodies that are capable of producing a clinical disease. They are listed in order of frequency as follows: anti-c (of Hr), anti-C (of Rh), anti-e (of Hr) or the combination of any of them with factor D.

In Argentina, 13% of couples are Rh-incompatible, and it is estimated that there is 1 PHD case every 150 deliveries. On the other hand, according to different statistics, the immunization rate is between 7% and 14%.

Rh sensitization mechanism

The passage of fetal red blood cells to maternal circulation is considered normal during pregnancy. Using the Kleihauer–Betke technique, it was established that the passage of fetal red blood cells is not higher than 0.1–0.2 ml. In this case the competent immunological system would not be activated; however, the chances of it being stimulated are much higher if transplacental hemorrhage is greater than the established values.

There are certain obstetric events that can increase the risk, such as placenta previa, ruptured placental membranes, external version, cesarean section, manual removal of placenta, and – in the early stages of pregnancy – abortion, and ectopic pregnancy.

All invasive procedures during pregnancy cause passage of fetal red blood cells. Chorionic villus sampling performed during the first trimester of pregnancy, which is frequently used nowadays, has been associated with very severe cases of hemolytic disease even with hydrops. Amniocentesis causes fetomaternal hemorrhage in 2–3% of the cases. Spontaneous or induced abortion is also associated with transplacental hemorrhage.

Antigen D has already developed by the 35th to 45th day of gestation, which explains why 4–5% of postabortion patients may become sensitized. Intravenous drug abuse can also lead to isoimmunization.

When an Rh-negative person receives Rh-positive blood, an immunologic response takes place in 50% or more of the cases.

The primary immunologic response is usually weak. The initial antibodies are of immunoglobulin M (IgM) nature, with a high molecular weight and are unlikely to cross the placenta. As a result, they do not produce fetal hemolysis labely in pregnancy, the IgG antibodies cross the placenta and produce hemolysis.

The IgG antibodies involved in the etiology and pathogenesis of PHD due to anti-D are mainly subtypes IgG1 and IgG3. The former crosses the placenta early in pregnancy, and therefore have a role in the most severe cases of PHD.

In our experience, the frequency of immunization in Rh-negative patients during their second pregnancy with compatible Rh-positive fetuses is 12–15%.

ABO incompatibility in an Rh-negative patient provides partial protection against primary anti Rh-isoimmunization, but not against a secondary immunologic response. In the former, the anti-A or anti-B incompatibility immunized blood cells are captured by the liver, which is not an immunologically active organ and does not produce anti-Rh antibodies. On the other hand, in a secondary immunologic response, the spleen receives the blood cell stroma and produces anti-Rh antibodies. Therefore, there is a higher incidence of Rh hemolytic disease in children whose parents are HBO compatible.

Pathogenesis and physiopathology of perinatal hemolytic disease

According to different studies, the rate of active transport of human IgG varies in the course of normal gestation; before 12 weeks of pregnancy this transfer is very low, but it has been demonstrated that, in severe Rh disease, the direct antiglobulin test on the fetal (Rh-positive) red cells may be positive as early as 6–10 weeks. The IgG antibodies rise exponentially until term. Sometimes, IgG levels in the infants could be higher than in the mother. The placental transport of IgG1 and IgG3 in women with Rh (D) immunizations is not diminished compared with normal pregnancy. The placental transport of IgG3 is significantly higher in pregnancies at risk of hemolytic disease of the newborn with IgG3 concentrations in normal pregnancy.[4]

The pathogenesis of PHD lies in the hemolysis of fetal erythrocytes caused by maternal antibodies. Hemolysis then results in fetal anemia.

According to the severity of hemolysis, PHD will be anemic, icteroanemic, or hydropic. In hydropic PHD, the hepatic parenchyma is replaced partially with secondary erythropoiesis tissue, which causes a portal and umbilical venous hypertension syndrome, as well as alterations in the metabolism of proteins, and decreased albumin. Both clinical conditions cause edema and ascitis, which are characteristic of hydrops.

Frequently, fetal cardiac failure secondary to severe anemia is observed. The other two forms of PHD, anemic and icteroanemic, are the result of a less severe hemolysis that does not compromise either the cardiocirculatory system or the protein metabolism.

Early fetal gene diagnosis

The use of polymerase chain reaction (PCR) for detection of the RHD gene can measure the RHD gene status for unborn babies at risk for hemolytic disease of the newborn. The occurrence of D gene variants has led to errors in prenatal typing. The effectiveness of using PCR in a clinical setting has been reported. It verifies the importance of testing more than one region of the gene and also the need for a testing strategy where both maternal and paternal testing for RHD gene dosages are performed.[5]

In the present time, it is possible to determine the fetal DNA in maternal serum during the first trimester of pregnancy. The advantage of this method is its non-invasive nature.[6]

Follow-up of the Rh-negative patient

The anamnesis will focus on relevant data such as: number of previous deliveries, history of anti-D prophylaxis, history of perinatal morbidity and mortality attributable to hemolysis, history of previous transfusions, and history of neonatal exchange transfusions or luminotherapy in previous deliveries.

If an indirect Coombs test does not detect anti-D antibodies, it should be repeated every 4 weeks until immediate puerperium.

If the test is positive we will proceed as follows:

- Study of husband's zygosity. If he is heterozygous, the fetus might not be Rh-positive
- Serial titration of anti-D antibodies every 3 weeks with the purpose of drawing a curve
- Serial ultrasonographic follow-up to evaluate fetal growth or detect characteristic signs of the disease: polyhydramnios, hepatomegalia, ascitis, soft tissue edema
- Doppler measurement of middle cerebral artery (MCA) peak systolic velocity provides a non-invasive modality for determining moderate or severe fetal anemia. The sensitivity of an increased peak systolic velocity in the MCA for the prediction of moderate or severe fetal anemia is 100% either in the presence or the absence of hydrops fetalis, and the false-positive rate is 12%.[7,8] The study of amniotic fluid (AF) is another very good predictive tool in the evaluation of fetal anemia.[9]

Many methods have been used to evaluate AF by detecting fetal hemolysis. Liley plotted curves of AF ΔOD450 values based on gestational age and derived three zones of severity of fetal disease. Therefore, from the Liley curves, fetal condition can be predicted based on the AF ΔOD450 value:[10,11]

- AF spectrophotometry, in accordance with a previous history of Rh disease and levels of anti-D antibodies in relation to the patient's gestational age
- If the patient's antibody titer is just at the critical level and the patient has not had a baby with PHD, the initial amniocentesis can be done at 28–29 weeks' gestation. If the titer or the history suggests that the PHD may be more severe, then amniocentesis can be performed earlier. In this way, a fetus that needs an intrauterine transfusion can be identified.

  Many methods have been used to evaluate AF by detecting fetal hemolysis. Liley plotted of AF ΔOD450 values based on gestational age and derived three zones of severity of fetal disease. Therefore, from the Liley curves, fetal condition can be predicted according to the AF ΔOD450 value[10,11]

  At present, however, Doppler measurement of middle cerebral artery peak systolic velocity constitutes the method of choice for the follow-up of fetal anemia
- Cordocentesis for the prediction of the severity of fetal anemia through the analysis of fetal blood started to be used when high-resolution ultrasound was developed. However, cordocentesis is currently not recommended for the evaluation of fetal anemia. It should be used as a route for transfusional therapy. Cordocentesis is only indicated in cases either requiring assessment of fetal anemia < 26 weeks gestation (anti-D titers $> 1/128$) or showing AF spectrophotometric analysis in the Upper Zone B or Zone C of Liley's chart, anterior placenta, and a poor obstetric history[12]
- Antenatal fetal monitoring as soon as it is reliable to assess fetal vitality and specially sinusoid patterns.

Treatment of severe maternal–fetal Rh-incompatibility

In 1963, Liley described intrauterine transfusion as the only possible way to prevent intrauterine fetal death of severely affected Rh-positive fetuses. When pregnancy interruption is indicated, fetal prematurity becomes an aggravating factor, which conspires against successful results.

The purpose of all the procedures described below is to allow the fetus to reach viability.

Intrauterine fetal transfusion

Intraperitoneal route

It is estimated that the total amount of blood transfused into the peritoneal cavity flows into the fetal bloodstream within 7–10 days after being injected.

This technique relies on the absorption capability of the fetal peritoneum and subdiaphragmatic lymphatic system, and it is not usually indicated before the 24th week of gestation. Ultrasound plays an essential role in this procedure: it locates the fetal abdomen and shows the precise point of entry.

The inferior portion of the peritoneal cavity is then accessed, considering the bladder as a reference point to prevent injury to the liver or spleen.

Type O, Rh-negative blood – compatible with maternal blood – with a hematocrit concentration not less than 75% should be transfused. Blood should have been recently extracted (not more than 48 h before the procedure).

Ascites, if present, should be evacuated before the procedure, although in this case the intravascular route is always preferred.

The use of uterine inhibitors is recommended, and the administration of antibiotics in order to prevent possible infections is controversial.

The procedure should be repeated, according to the patient's evolution, every 14 days or more, until fetal viability is achieved.

The amount of blood to be transfused should be estimated as follows: gestational age in weeks minus 20, multiplied by 10. For example, in a 28 week pregnancy, $(28-20) \times 10=80$, a total of 80 ml of erythrocytes should be transfused.

Intravascular fetal transfusion

Indications to use this approach are especially in case of fetal hydrops or very severe fetal anemia. This technique, which may be used as from 18 weeks of pregnancy, involves access to an umbilical vessel near its placental insertion, in the intrahepatic portion of the umbilical vein, or in the fetal heart (fetal rescue operation).

Nowadays, this procedure is superior to the former because it allows the immediate reversal of fetal anemia as it is possible to obtain a sample of fetal blood and determine its hematocrit and hemoglobin values. Also, a faster remission of fetal hydrops is observed in most of the cases.

The amount of blood to be transfused depends on the patient's gestational age, and blood donor's and fetal blood's hematocrit. The procedure should be repeated according to post-transfusion hematocrit values, until fetal extraction is indicated.

If no complications occur, this technique allows the lengthening of intrauterine fetal life until the fetus is viable, which results in a marked decrease in perinatal mortality rates.

High-dose intravenous IgG for the treatment of severe Rh alloimmunization

Intrauterine fetal transfusion, either by the intraperitoneal or intravascular routes, has shown to be an effective treatment of Rh-hemolytic disease. However, some fetuses are already severely compromised at an early stage when it is technically impossible to indicate the procedure.

In agreement with other authors, we have found that repeated invasive techniques result in an important increase in anti-D titers owing to the variable amounts of fetomaternal bleeding inevitably caused by the procedure itself. As a result of this, a moderate Rh disease in a present pregnancy can often become a severe one in the subsequent gestation.

It has been reported that transfusional therapy before 32 weeks of gestation is associated with a higher fetal mortality rate.[13] The early treatment in the first weeks of pregnancy would reduce the severity of fetal anemia, decreasing the fetal morbidity and mortality. That is why we started a protocol of treatment with high doses of γ-globulin.[1]

The use of high doses of intravenous immunoglobulin (IVIG) in the treatment of immunologic diseases both in children and adults and recurrent intrauterine fetal loss has been frequently reported in the literature with varying degrees of effectiveness.

Although the mechanisms of action of IVIG remain unclear, several explanations have been proposed during pregnancy: feedback inhibition of antibody synthesis, competition for macrophage or Fc receptors of target cells, and blockade of Fc-mediated antibody placental transport. We have used IVIG therapy in a prospective study in order to analyze its effectiveness in the antenatal treatment of severe Rh-hemolytic disease.

The only immunoglobulin that is transferred into the fetal circulation is IgG; the other classes of maternal immunoglobulins are either not transferred or only cross the placenta in small quantities. The mechanisms involved in the active transfer of IgG across the human placenta are not yet known. Brambell *et al.*'s studies in rabbits suggest that the transport of IgG molecules across the placenta is mediated through a receptor for the Fc part of the molecule. Further studies have clarified the role of Fc as a placental Fc receptor for IgG. This receptor has been demonstrated on the surface of the trophoblast at 10 weeks and at term.

The mechanisms of placental transfer of exogenous IgG infused into the mother are still to be elucidated. It must be emphasized that transplacental IgG transfer is a slow process and requires an intact Fc portion of the IgG molecule. Gitlin *et al.*'s studies demonstrated that when labeled IgG was injected into pregnant women at various intervals before delivery, even after 12 days, the concentration in the infant's serum was only about 40% of that in the mother. Studies performed by Contractor *et al.* about IgG transport in perfused placentas suggest that the trophoblast absorbs a substantial amount of human IgG and all bovine IgG, both broken down into small fractions by a mechanism of non-specific endocytosis, and transmits these fragments to the fetal circulation. A small amount of human IgG, however, would escape this process of lysosomal destruction by diverse protective mechanisms, and would be released intact on the fetal side.

There are very few cases in the literature reporting the treatment of severe Rh-hemolytic disease with high doses of IVIG and the findings are too dissimilar to allow for conclusive generalizations. Rewald and Berlin *et al.* obtained satisfactory results with the combined use of plasmapheresis and IVIG in 4 cases of severe Rh-hemolytic disease. De la Cámara *et al.* reported the successful treatment of two cases with repeated doses of IVIG throughout gestation. Scott *et al.*, on the other hand, used a combined protocol of IVIG and repeated intrauterine transfusions in one case of hemolytic disease.

We have administered IVIG as the only treatment in 24 severely Rh-sensitized patients with a previous history of affected fetuses and/or neonates, with elevated anti-D titers, and a high degree of intrauterine hemolysis. Patients in group 1 (< 20 weeks, $n = 8$) fulfilled the first two of these inclusion criteria, whereas in groups 2 (20–28 weeks, $n=7$) and 3 (> 28 weeks, $n=9$), IVIG treatment was indicated on the basis of intrauterine hemolysis.

IVIG was infused at a daily dose of 0.4 g/kg maternal body weight for 4–5 consecutive days, and repeated every 21 days until delivery.

Group 3 also included those patients who attended the antenatal clinic very late in pregnancy; as a consequence of this delay, the fetuses in these cases were highly compromised because of the advanced stage of the hemolytic disease, and they evidenced major neonatal depression and severe fetal anemia at birth, requiring – in almost all cases – exchange transfusions.

Initial mean anti-D level was significantly higher in group 1 (25.9 ± 12.9 IU/ml) than in the other two groups, whose values were, however, higher than 10 IU/ml. AF total bilirubin levels before the onset of therapy were pathologic and in 55% of the cases they coincided with Zone 3 of Liley's chart. Hydrops fetalis at the onset of treatment accounted for the only three fetal deaths in groups 1 and 2. None of the fetuses developed hydrops during treatment. Six of the nine neonates in group 3 were depressed at birth (1-min Apgar below 7). However, at 5 min only one newborn showed an Apgar below 7. Mean birth weight was over 2500 g in all the cases. Neonatal hematological condition in group 2 (50% of the babies required only phototherapy) was better than in the other two groups (transfusional therapy).

The decrease in pre- vs. post-treatment anti-D antibody quantification, the reduction in intrauterine hemolysis and the strongly positive direct antiglobulin test in all neonates may indicate that the mode of action of high doses of IVIG in Rh-hemolytic disease is (1) feedback inhibition of antibody synthesis and (2) partial blockade of Fc-mediated antibody transport across the placenta. No adverse effects from the drug were observed in the mother or neonate.

Our findings show that IVIG treatment was effective in both groups 1 and 2, where IVIG was administered before the 28th week of gestation and the fetuses were not hydropic at the onset of therapy. In group 3, however, where fetal anemia was already advanced at the time of treatment, intrauterine transfusions and prompt fetal extraction should have been the treatment of choice.

The analysis of the series including only the 13 most severely affected cases as judged by their history of fetal/neonatal death, demonstrated again the effectiveness of IVIG treatment. It can be inferred from the results in this particular group of patients that (1) after 28 weeks' gestation the administration of IVIG does not elicit significant reductions in anti-D titers and intrauterine hemolysis, thus intrauterine transfusion is the therapy of choice, and (2) IVIG treatment is not indicated in case of hydrops fetalis. Except for these two indications, it is in this series with the poorest history, the highest antibody level and failure of transfusional therapy in previous gestations, where we find the most encouraging therapeutical results of IVIG treatment.

The high cost of IVIG therapy is immediately outweighed by the highly satisfactory perinatal results obtained in our population of extremely severe Rh-sensitized patients. Moreover, babies born after treatment with intrauterine transfusions, as well as those prematurely delivered because of their severe disease, require a prolonged stay in the neonatal intensive care unit (a mean of 60 days in the latter case), the cost of which greatly exceeds that of IVIG therapy.

To conclude, the results of our study, which to the best of our knowledge is the largest reported in the literature, show the value of high doses of IVIG in the treatment of severe Rh incompatibility when administered repeatedly before 28 weeks' gestation and in the absence of hydrops fetalis.

High-dose γ-globulin (IVIG) followed by intrauterine transfusions: a new alternative for the treatment of severe fetal hemolytic disease

Intrauterine fetal transfusion (IUT) is currently the therapy of choice in cases of severe anti-D isoimmunization. However, its efficacy is reduced in patients with early severe hydrops fetalis due to the technical difficulties in performing this procedure before 20 weeks' gestation and because the fetuses are already anemic at that time.

The purpose of this study was to determine whether early onset of high-dose γ-globulin therapy followed by IUTs is more effective than IUTs alone in the treatment of very severe isoimmunized fetuses.

The population studied in this retrospective clinical research was assigned to one of the following two groups: (1) Gamma group: 30 patients receiving γ-globulin therapy before 21 weeks' gestation and IUTs after 20 weeks or (2) IUT group: 39 patients receiving IUT treatment starting at a gestational age of 20–25 weeks.

Both groups were statistically similar regarding history of perinatal deaths and anti-D antibody titers. The number of hydropic fetuses at the first IUT and of fetal deaths were significantly higher in the IUT than in the Gamma group. No significant differences were observed between the groups in fetal hematocrit at first IUT and at birth. However, the percentage of severely anemic fetuses was higher in the IUT group. Fetal mortality rate was 36% less in the Gamma group.

In summary, in very severe cases of Rh-isoimmunization:

(1) the development of fetal hemolysis in the first 20 weeks of gestation increases the risk of fetal death;
(2) the early onset of invasive fetal therapy is only partially effective and potentially harmful; and

(3) according to the present study, those patients who received high-dose intravenous γ-globulin in the first 20 weeks of pregnancy seem to have a better fetal outcome.

Our results show that high-dose γ-globulin therapy followed by IUTs improves fetal survival in these severe cases.[14] Conventional treatment has also been modified by the administration of immunoglobulin to the neonate.[15]

Neonatal treatment

Our studies suggest that the frequency of neonatal transfusion therapy can be reduced by a combination of conventional phototherapy with HDIVIG. Further studies are needed to determine the optimum timing and dosage of HDIVIG therapy.[16]

Other studies show that intravenous immunoglobulin is effective in decreasing the maximum bilirubin levels and the need for repeated exchange transfusions in Rh hemolytic disease of the newborn. There is, however, an increased need of blood transfusions for late anemia in the babies treated with IVIG.[17]

Other alloimmunizations

Routine antibody screening of Rh (D)-positive women is probably not warranted from a clinical cost–benefit perspective.[18]

Anti-c isoimmunization follow-up is similar to that of anti-D and, together with anti-E, they are the next in order of frequency as a cause of perinatal alloimmunization.[19]

The treatment for anti-E sensitization is similar to that of anti-D. AF is a weak indicator of the result, that is why the management of the disease remains questionable. It is not clear yet if the presence of anti-E implies the accummulation of a hemolytic effect with other antibodies.

Pregnancy follow-up in anti-Kell alloimmunization

It is identified by the presence of anti-Kell antibodies in maternal serum or previous fetal anemia. The search for hemolysis in AF through bilirubin concentration is not useful as the pathogenesis responds to fetal anemia due to the inhibition of erythroid progenitor and not to the destruction of the Kell-positive erythroid by the antibodies.

Therefore, cordocentesis should be chosen to obtain fetal blood and, in this way, be able to detect fetal anemia and make the Kell-serotyping by studying the fetal DNA when the father is K1 heterozygous.

Other studies show that fetal anemia due to anti-Kell isoimmunization might be due in part to erythropoietic suppression, but it is still largely a hemolytic process. The methods based on a hemolytic process, including use of a critical maternal serum titer of 1:32, serial AF analyses when the titer was in excess and liberal use of funipuncture, were successful in identifying severely affected fetuses.[20]

Natural and monoclonal anti-Kell antibodies inhibit the growth in the Kell-positive erythroid progenitor.

Fetal hematology

It shows just a few reticulocytosis and normoblasts compared to fetuses affected by anti-D, which suggests that erythroid suppression would be the mechanism responsible for fetal anemia, a mechanism that has been proved by Vaughan's studies.[21]

The treatment is similar to that of the anti-D. Needless to say, an ultrasound follow-up is very important.

Summary: steps to follow

Rh-isoimmunization: patients with no maternal and/or perinatal history of the disease

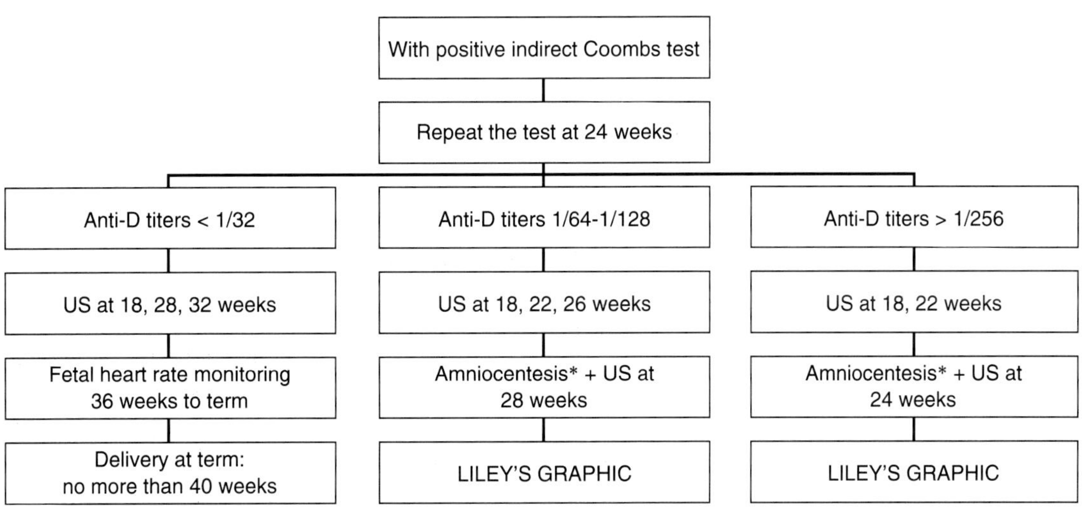

*And/or MCA peak systolic velocity and conventional ultrasound

Rh-isoimmunization: patients with no maternal and/or perinatal history of the disease

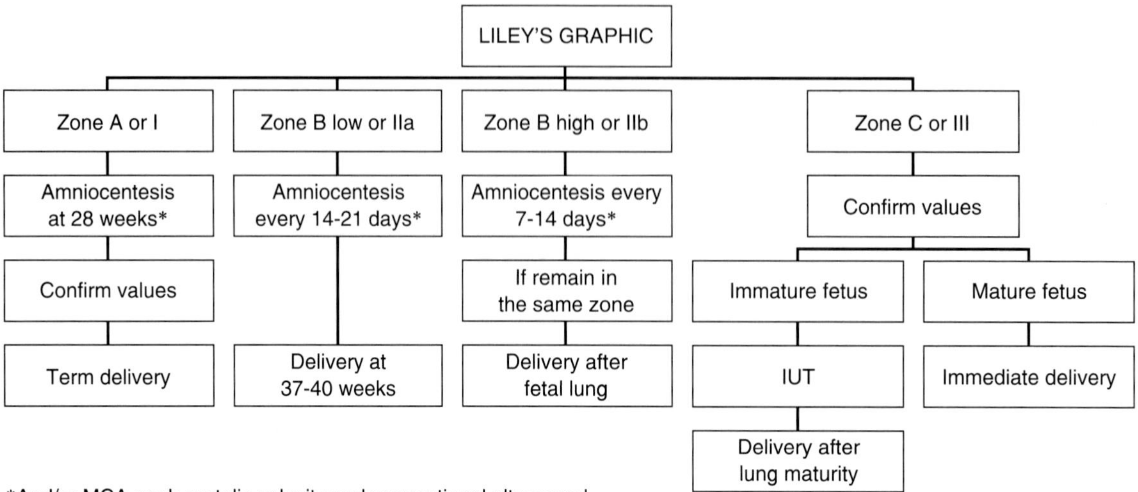

*And/or MCA peak systolic velocity and conventional ultrasound

Rh-isoimmunization: patients with maternal and/or perinatal history of the disease

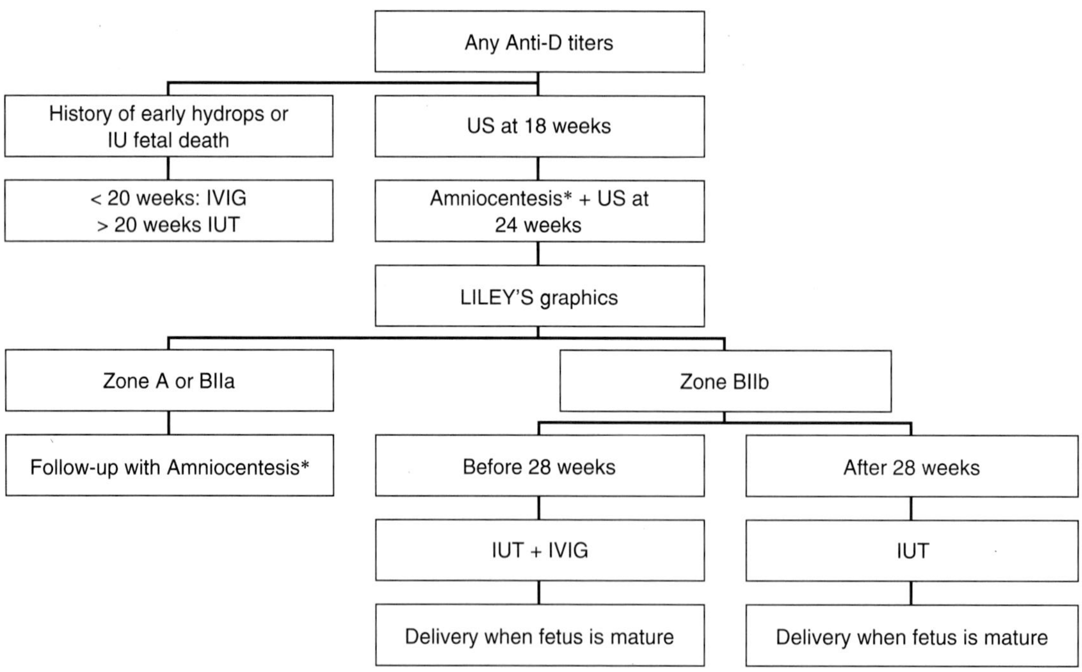

*And/or MCA peak systolic velocity and conventional ultrasound

Prophylaxis

In 40–50% of pregnancies, the passage of fetal red blood cells to maternal circulation usually takes place during the last trimester. In the majority of the cases the amount of blood transferred is less than 0.1 ml.[22]

In 1977, there were 110 cases of stillbirths or postnatal deaths due to anti-D hemolytic disease in the UK. In 1992, the figure decreased to only nine cases. This decrease came as a result of the introduction of anti-D γ-globulin prophylaxis since 1969 but it is also subject to the application of public health policies for perinatal care, especially in developing countries.[23]

In 1969, the prophylaxis protocol consisted of anti-D γ-globulin administration only after the birth of an Rh-positive child, or after certain pregnancy events such as antepartum hemorrhage. Most of the deaths resulted from maternal sensitization between 28 and 40 weeks of the first pregnancy (third trimester) and during postpartum.

Further studies have determined that the percentage of sensitization decreases from 1.2% to 0.28% if antenatal prophylaxis is carried out.

In practice, the combination of antenatal and postnatal prophylaxis will prevent immunization in 96% of the high-risk cases. The remaining 4% corresponds to the absence or inappropriate administration of immunoglobulin when it is indicated.

Due to the fact that isoimmunization during pregnancy is caused by transplacental hemorrhage,[24] the risk of immunization increases after the following procedures:

(1) Spontaneous or induced abortion
(2) Amniocentesis
(3) Chorion villus sampling
(4) Cordocentesis
(5) Ectopic pregnancy
(6) Fetal manipulation: external version
(7) Antepartum hemorrhage
(8) Antepartum fetal death
(9) Positive blood transfusion

The standard postpartum dose of 300 μg contains enough anti-D to neutralize at least 15 ml of fetal red blood cells.

There are different methods to detect excessive fetomaternal hemorrhage:

- Kleihauer–Betke technique is, if carried out correctly, a very sensitive and specific method, but it is subject to laboratory and technological errors.
- Flow cytometry is also a very sensitive method, but difficult to perform and too expensive.
- The Rosette method is easy to carry out and very sensitive, but has low specificity and its results must be confirmed by Kleihauer–Betke method or flow cytometry.
- A gel technology method has been reported for the assessment of fetomaternal hemorrhage and determination of minimum necessary dose of RhIG. This technique works well in determining the appropriate dose of anti-D required to treat D patients with D+ newborns. There are potential cost savings in decreased use of RhIG, less direct technical time required and more rapid availability of results.[25]

Anti-D γ-globulin has very few adverse effects. Some fetuses yield with a slightly positive direct Coombs test at birth after antenatal administration. The presence of anemia or hyperbilirubinemia is very rare. All plasma involved in the production of anti-D immunoglobulin is carefully checked for infectious diseases.

There have not been any HIV cases due to contaminated plasma.

The American College of Obstetricians and Gynecologists recommends both typifying the pregnant patient and looking for antibodies in her first visit, and again at 24–28 weeks, offering anti-D γ-globulin to all Rh-negative, non-sensitized patients.

It has been found that transplacental hemorrhage occurs in 3%, 12%, and 45% of the cases during the first, second, and third trimesters, respectively.

The capacity of an antibody to eliminate D-red cells *in vivo* depends both on its avidity, and to a lesser degree, on its affinity for the D-antigen. Absorption is also a limiting factor.

Even though antepartum γ-globulin administration offers many additional benefits, some authors argue that, as the incidence of isoimmunization is relatively small, it makes medication 16 times less cost-effective than postpartum prevention programs. The *Cochrane Review* states that anti-D, given within 72 h after childbirth, reduces the risk of RhD alloimmunization in Rh-negative women who have given birth to an Rh-positive infant. However, the evidence on the optimal dose is limited.[26]

Unit equivalents

50 μg	250 IU
100 μg	500 IU
300 μg	1500 IU
225 μg	1250 IU

Route of administration

The route of administration is intramuscular through the deltoides muscle. In the gluteal area, it only penetrates to the subcutaneous tissue, thus absorption is prolonged.

Anti-D IgG use recommendations

- Dose: 500 IU or 100 μg every 4 ml of fetal red blood cells in maternal circulation.
- Indications
  - Postpartum, within the first 72 h = 300 μg
  - Prenatal
    - First trimester: abortion, ectopic pregnancy, chorionic villus sampling, or amniocentesis
    - Second trimester: suspected fetomaternal hemorrhage, invasive procedures
    - Third trimester: prophylactic: 500 IU at 28 and 34 weeks or only one dose of 300 μg between the above-mentioned weeks[27]

General and future management of RhD isoimmunization

Future therapy will involve selective modulation of the maternal immune system, turning the need for intrauterine transfusions into a rarity.[28]

When Rh_D sensitization occurs, careful follow-up of these mothers and judicious intervention can result in good outcomes for most pregnancies. Both Doppler assessment of middle cerebral artery peak systolic velocity and spectral analysis of AF at 450 nm (△OD450) are useful in the diagnosis and management of fetal anemia.[29]

REFERENCES

1. Margulies M, Voto LS, Mathet E, Margulies M. High-dose intravenous IgG for the treatment of severe alloimmunization. *Vox Sang* 1991;61:181–9.
2. Carton JP. Defining the Rh blood group antigens. Biochemistry and molecular genetics. *Blood Rev* 1994;8:199–212.
3. Hohlfeld P, Wirthner D, Tissot JA. Perinatal hemolytic disease: Physiopathology. *J Gynecol Obstet Biol Reprod* 1998;27(2):135–43.
4. Palfi M, Hilden JO, Gottvall T, Selbing A. Placental transport of maternal immunoglobulin G in pregnancies at risk of Rh (D) hemolytic disease of the newborn. *Am J Reprod Immunol* 1998;39(5):323–8.
5. Chan FY, Cowley NM, Wolter L, *et al.* Prenatal RHD gene determination and dosage analysis by PCR: Clinical evaluation. *Prenat Diagn* 2001;21(4):321–6.
6. Costa JM, Giovangrandi Y, Ernault P, *et al.* Fetal RHD genotyping in maternal serum during the first trimester of pregnancy. *Br J Haematol* 2002;119(1):255–60.
7. Mari G, Deter RL, Carpenter RL, *et al.* Noninvasive diagnosis by Doppler ultrasonography of fetal anemia due to maternal red-cell alloimmunization. *N Engl J Med* 2000;342:9–14.
8. Queenan JT. Rh isoimmunization. *Contemporary OB/GYN Archive.* Washington DC: Georgetown University School of Medicine, 2002:April 15.
9. Nishie EN, Brizot ML, Liao AW, Carvalho MH, Toma O, Zugaib M. A comparison between middle cerebral artery peak velocity and amniotic fluid optical density at 450 nm in the prediction of fetal anemia. *Am J Obstet Gynecol* 2003;188(1):214–9.
10. Liley AW. Liquor amnii analysis in the management of the pregnancy complicated by rhesus sensitization. *Am J Obstet Gynecol* 1961;82:1359.
11. Liley AW. Errors in the assessment of haemolytic disease from amniotic fluid. *Am J Obstet Gynecol* 1969;86:485.
12. Voto LS. Ultrasonography in Rh hemolytic disease. Maternal–Fetal Medicine Department, Juan A. Fernández Hospital, University of Buenos Aires, School of Medicine, Buenos Aires, Argentina.
13. Klumper FJ, van Kamp IL, Vandenbussche FP, *et al.* Benefits and risks of fetal red-cell transfusion after 32 weeks gestation. *Eur J Obstet Gynecol Reprod Biol* 2000;92(1):91–6.
14. Voto LS, Mathet ER, Zapaterio JL, Orti J, Lede RL, Margulies M. High-dose gammaglobulin (IVIG) followed by intrauterine transfusions (IUTs): A new alternative for the treatment of severe fetal hemolytic disease. *J Perinat Med* 1997;25:85–8.
15. Porter TF, Silver RM, Jackson GM, Branch DW, Scott JR. Intravenous immune globulin in the management of severe RhD hemolytic disease. *Obstet Gynecol Surv* 1997;52(3):193–7.
16. Voto LS, Sexer H, Ferreiro G, *et al.* Neonatal administration of high-dose intravenous immunoglobulin in rhesus hemolytic disease. *J Perinat Med* 1995;23:443–51.
17. Mukhopadhyay K, Murki S, Narang A, Dutta S. Intravenous immunoglobulins in rhesus hemolytic disease. *Indian J Pediatr* 2003;70(9):697–9.
18. Lurie S, Eliezer E, Piper I, Woliovitch I. Is antibody screening in Rh (D)-positive pregnant women necessary? *J Matern Fetal Neonatal Med* 2003;14(6):404–6.
19. Hackney DN, Knudtson EJ, Rossi KQ, Krugh D, O'Shaughnessy RW. Management of pregnancies complicated by anti-c isoimmunization. *Obstet Gynecol* 2004;103(1):24–30.
20. McKenna DS, Nagaraja HN, O'Shaughnessy R. Management of pregnancies complicated by anti-Kell isoimmunization. *Obstet Gynecol* 1999;93(5, Pt 1):667–73.
21. Vaughan JI, Warwick R, Letsky E, Nicolini U, Rodeck CH, Fisk NM. Erythropoietic suppression in fetal anemia because of Kell alloimmunization. *Am J Obstet Gynecol* 1994;171:247–52.
22. Jorgensen J. Fetal–maternal bleeding during pregnancy and delivery. *Acta Obstet Gynecol Scand* 1977;56:487–90.
23. Joseph KS, Kramer MS. The decline in Rh hemolytic disease: Should Rh prophylaxis get all the credit? *Am J Public Health* 1998;88(2):209–15.
24. Quartier P, Floch C, Meier F, Fruchart MF, Brossard Y, Lejeune C. Massive fetomaternal hemorrhage and prevention of fetomaternal rhesus incompatibility. The failure of our present system of prevention. *J Gynecol Obstet Biol Reprod (Paris)* 1993;22(5): 517–9.
25. Fernandes JR, Chan R, Coovadia AS, Reis MD, Pinkerton PH. A gel technology system to determine postpartum RhIG dosage. *Immunohematology* 2000;16(3):115–9.
26. Crowther C, Middleton P. Anti-D administration after childbirth for preventing Rhesus alloimmunization. *Cochrane Rev* 2004;4. The Cochrane Library, Chichester, UK: John Wiley & Sons, Ltd.
27. Hartwell EA. Use of Rh immune globulin: ASCP practice parameter. *Am J Clin Pathol* 1998;110(3):281–92.
28. Moise KJ Jr. Management of rhesus alloimmunization in pregnancy. *Obstet Gynecol* 2002;100(4):833.
29. Harkness UF, Spinnato JA. Prevention and management of RhD isoimmunization. *Clin Perinatol* 2004;31(4):721–42.

73 Prenatal therapy of endocrine and metabolic disorders

G. Rosner, S. B. Shachar, Y. Yaron and M. I. Evans

Introduction

Our understanding of molecular and genetic basis of disease is ever-increasing. This has resulted in more and better ways for primary prevention. This is often achieved by prenatal diagnosis and termination of affected pregnancies and more recently, preimplantation genetic diagnosis. Some metabolic and endocrine disorders however, such as congenital adrenal hyperplasia and cardiac arrhythmias are amenable to pharmacological interventions.[1,2] This chapter describes different modes of intrauterine pharmacological therapy in the fetus with an endocrine or metabolic disorder. The use of folic acid supplementation for the prevention of neural tube defects will also be discussed.

Endocrine disorders

Adrenal disorders

Congenital adrenal hyperplasia

Treatment of congenital adrenal hyperplasia (CAH) in the fetus is an excellent example of pharmacological therapy during pregnancy. CAH is a group of autosomal recessive metabolic disorders characterized by an enzymatic defect in the steroidogenetic pathway. As a result of the enzymatic deficiency, there is a compensatory increase in adrenocorticotropic hormone (ACTH) secretion in order to maintain cortisol production. This leads to overproduction of the steroid precursors in the adrenal cortex, causing adrenal hyperplasia. The most common abnormality, responsible for > 90% of patients with CAH is caused by a deficiency of the 21-hydroxylase (21-OH) enzyme. Other, less common causes for CAH include deficiencies in 11β-hydroxylase, 17α-hydroxylase, and 3β-hydroxysteroid-dehydrogenase. Decreased 21-OH activity results in accumulation of 17-hydroxyprogesterone (17-OHP) which is converted via androstenedione to androgens, the levels of which increase by as much as several hundred-fold (Figure 73.1). The excess androgens cause virilization of the undifferentiated female external genitalia. The degree of virilization may vary from mild clitoral hypertrophy to complete formation of a phallus and scrotum. In contrast, genital development in males is normal. The excess androgens cause postnatal virilization in both genders and may manifest in precocious puberty.

The 'classical' form of CAH involves a severe enzyme deficiency or even a complete block of enzymatic activity, which is associated in more than half of the cases with a life-threatening salt-losing form. The classical form is easy to recognize in female newborns but may be overlooked in males, who may present at a later stage with severe dehydration and even demise. The 'nonclassical' attenuated form of 21-OH deficiency results in partial blockade of enzymatic activity and results in simple virilization in women only later in life. It is estimated to occur in ~3.5% in Ashkenazi Jews and ~2% in Hispanics.[3]

The gene for 21-OH is in close linkage to the human leukocyte antigen (HLA) major histocompatability complex on the short arm of chromosome 6.[4] The gene for 21-OH (CYP21B) has now been mapped, allowing direct mutation analysis in informative families.[5]

In the past, diagnosis of CAH was made by the finding of elevated levels of 17-OHP in the amniotic fluid. With the development of chorionic villus sampling (CVS) in the 1980s, linkage-based molecular diagnosis in the first trimester became available. Since the discovery and mapping of the gene, direct DNA mutation analysis has become the routine approach.

The fetal adrenal gland can be pharmacologically suppressed by maternal administration of dexamethasone.[6] The suppression can prevent masculinization of affected female fetuses in carrier couples. In the first attempt to prevent female genital birth defects in 1982, Evans *et al.* administered dexamethasone to a carrier mother beginning at 10 weeks of gestation.[6] Serial maternal estriol and cortisol levels indicated that adrenal gland suppression had been achieved. The female fetus was born at 39 weeks' gestation with normal external genitalia. Forrest and David then

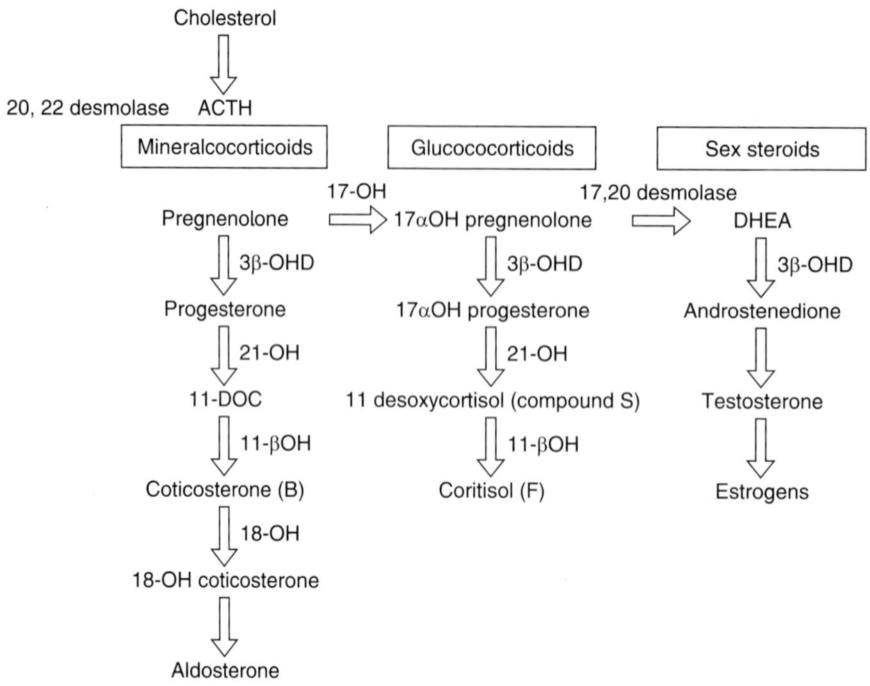

Figure 73.1 Steroidogenic pathway: androgen production in 21-hydroxylase deficiency (congenital adrenal hyperplasia).

employed a similar protocol beginning at 9 weeks' gestation to treat several fetuses at risk for CAH.[7] Female fetuses subsequently confirmed to be affected with severe CAH were spared masculinization of the external genitalia. Several hundred pregnant women and their fetuses have since been treated with prevention of masculinization in more than 85% of affected females.[8]

The differentiation of the external genitalia begins at about 7 weeks of gestation. Thus, diagnosis by amniocentesis or even CVS is too late to prevent masculinization. Therefore for carrier parents, pharmacological therapy has to be initiated prior to prenatal diagnosis: Therapy is administered to all patients at risk, despite the fact that the chance of an affected female fetus for carrier parents is only 1 in 8 (i.e., 1/4 affected × 1/2 female). Following molecular diagnosis, by CVS, in seven out of eight patients, therapy is discontinued if the diagnosis of a male is made or if CAH is ruled out. However, if the fetus is an affected female, therapy is continued throughout gestation. Stress-dose corticosteroids should be given to the mother during labor and tapered gradually postpartum.

No consistent untoward effects on fetuses have been reported. Greater weight gain, edema and striae were noticed in treated mothers but no increased risk of hypertension or gestational diabetes was noted.[8]

Inclusion criteria of the European Society for Paediatric Endocrinology and Wilkins Pediatric Endocrine Society[9] for prenatal treatment of CAH include: (1) a previously affected sibling or first-degree relative with known mutation causing classical CAH proven by DNA analysis; (2) reasonable expectation that the father is the same as the proband's; (3) availability of rapid and quality genetic analysis; (4) therapy started less than 9 weeks following the last menstrual period; (5) lack of intent for therapeutic abortion; and (5) reasonable expectation of patient's compliance.

There is an agreement that the treatment requires a professional team that includes an expert high-risk obstetrician, a pediatric endocrinologist, genetic counselor and a molecular genetic laboratory.

Thyroid disorders

Hypothyroidism

Congenital hypothyroidism affects about 1:3000 to 1:4000 infants.[10] About 85% of the cases are the result of thyroid dysgenesis, a heterogeneous group of developmental defects characterized by inadequate amount of thyroid tissue. Congenital hypothyroidism is only rarely associated with errors of thyroid hormone synthesis, thyroid-stimulating hormone (TSH) insensitivity, or absence of the pituitary gland. Fetal hypothyroidism may not necessarily manifest in a goiter before birth since maternal thyroid hormones may cross the placenta. Congenital hypothyroidism presenting with a goiter can be found in only about 10–15% of cases, with an estimated prevalence of 1:30,000–1:50,000 live births.[11] Fetal goiterous hypothyroidism is caused in most instances by maternal exposure to thyrostatic agents used to treat maternal hyperthyroidism.[12] These drugs include propylthiouracil (PTU), the inadvertent use of radioactive ^{131}I in the pregnant women or iodide exposure. Maternal ingestion of amiodarone (antiarrhythmic drug) or lithium (drug for people with mood disorders) may also cause hypothyroidism in the fetus. Finally, fetal hypothyroidism may result from transplacental passage of maternal blocking antibodies (known as TBIAb or TBII) or rarely due to rare defects in fetal thyroid hormone biosynthesis.[11]

Fetal goiterous hypothyroidism may lead to severe fetal and neonatal consequences. An enlarged goiter may cause esophageal obstruction which may lead to polyhydramnios, which may result in preterm delivery or premature rupture of membranes. Rarely, a goiter may even lead to high-output heart failure due to high vascular flow in the goiter.[13] A large fetal goiter can cause extension of the fetal neck leading to dystocia in labor. The effects of the fetal hypothyroidism itself may be devastating. Without treatment, postnatal growth delay and severe mental retardation may ensue. Even with immediate diagnosis and treatment at birth, long-term follow up of children with congenital hypothyroidism has demonstrated that they have lower scores on perceptual-motor, visuospatial, and language tests.[14]

In suspicious cases, an extensive maternal and family history should be obtained. In patients with a positive history, maternal thyroid hormone levels, as well as blocking immunoglobulin levels should be measured. In addition, all women with a history of any thyroid disease (both hypothyroidism and hyperthyroidism) are advised to have monthly fetal ultrasound scans to screen for fetal goiter, polyhydramnios, or fetal tachycardia.[15]

Occasionally, fetal goiterous hypothyroidism may be identified by an ultrasound scan performed due to increased uterine size caused by polyhydramnios secondary to esophageal obstruction and impaired swallowing. Sometimes, a fetal goiter may incidentally be discovered on a routine scan. Before the advent of cordocentesis, amniotic fluid levels of TSH and FT4 (free thyroxine) were used as potential indicators of fetal thyroid function. However, these proved to be inconsistent.[16] With cordocentesis, fetal thyroid status can be directly and accurately evaluated; fetal response to therapy can therefore be reliably measured using available appropriate nomograms for fetal serum levels of FT4, total T4 (thyroxine), free T3 (triiodothyronine), total T3, and TSH.[15,17] *In utero* treatment was initially suggested by Van Herle *et al.* using intramuscular injection of levothyroxine sodium.[18] Subsequent studies however, have indicated that intra-amniotic administration of thyroxine may be superior and can lead to resolution of the polyhydramnios as well. The dose of the injected drug may be refined using the fetal thyroid profile in the amniotic fluid and the thyroid size.[19] The doses commonly used for treatment range from 200 to 500 mg intra-amniotic every week. With this regimen, fetal goiters have been shown to regress, the hyperextension of the fetal head have been shown to resolve and fetal and newborn TSH levels have normalized.[19]

Hyperthyroidism

Neonatal hyperthyroidism is rare with an incidence of 1:4000 to 1:40,000 live births.[10] Fetal thyrotoxic goiter is usually secondary to maternal autoimmune disease, principally Graves' disease or Hashimoto's thyroiditis. As many as 12% of infants of mothers with a known history of Graves' disease are affected with neonatal thyrotoxicosis, which may occur even if the mother is euthyroid.[20] As with hypothyroidism, inherent to the underlying mechanism is the transplacental passage of maternal IgG antibodies. In this case the antibodies, known as TSAb or (TSI), are predominantly directed against the TSH receptor.

Usually, the investigation of fetal hyperthyroidism begins only after the discovery of fetal goiter. Often, the goiter is diagnosed on ultrasound in patients referred due to elevated thyroid stimulating antibodies. In some cases, fetal goiters are realized serendipitously on routine ultrasonography. Others may be discovered in patients referred for scan because of polyhydramnios. Beside the risks related to the goiter itself, untreated fetal hyperthyroidism may be associated with a mortality rate of 12–25% due to high-output cardiac failure.[21] Once a fetal goiter is identified, biochemical evaluation is indicated. Historically, amniotic fluid levels of TSH and FT4 were used as potential indicators of fetal thyroid function. These, however, proved inconsistent in that amniotic fluid levels of these hormones do not always correlate with their serum levels. Some controversy still exists regarding their use, however, they may be of some benefit in centers that do not have available cordocentesis.[16] As stated previously, cordocentesis allows reliable assessment of fetal thyroid status TSH,[15,17] and treatment can be planned accordingly.

Once the diagnosis of fetal hyperthyroidism is confirmed, fetal treatment should be initiated. Authors have attempted treating fetal hyperthyroidism with maternally administered antithyroid drugs. Porreco and Bloch have reported maternal treatment of fetal thyrotoxicosis with the antithyroid drug propylthiouracil (PTU), which lead to a good outcome.[22] The initial dose used was 100 mg PO three times a day, which was later decreased to 50 mg PO three times a day. Wenstrom *et al.* described a favorable outcome using maternal methimazole to treat fetal hyperthyroidism in a patient who could not tolerate PTU.[21] Hatjis also treated fetal goiterous hyperthyroidism with a maternal dose of 300 mg PTU. This patient, however, required supplemental synthroid to remain euthyroid. There was good fetal outcome in this case as well.[23]

Inborn errors of metabolism

Methylmalonic acidemia

The methylmalonic acidemias (MMAs) are a group of enzyme-deficiency diseases inherited in an autosomal recessive manner resulting from one of several genetically distinct etiologies. Some cases are caused by mutations in the gene encoding methylmalonyl-coenzyme A mutase while others are due to a defect that catalyzes the biosynthesis of adenosylcobalamin from vitamin B_{12}. The disease is characterized by a wide clinical spectrum ranging from a benign condition to a fatal neonatal disease. In the severe form, MMA is characterized by severe metabolic acidosis, developmental delay and biochemical abnormalities that include methylmalonic aciduria, long chain ketonuria and intermittent hyperglycinemia. Patients with defects in adenosylcobalamin biosynthesis may respond to administration of large doses of vitamin B_{12}, which may enhance the amount of active holoenzyme (mutase apoenzyme plus adenosylcobalamin). A proposed mechanism for the neurological abnormalities observed in methylmalonic acidemia was suggested by a group of Brazilian investigators who administered methylmalonic acid to rats during the first month of their life.[24] A significant diminution of myelin content and of ganglioside *N*-acetylneuraminic acid were noted in the cerebrum.

More than 20 years ago, Ampola and colleagues were the first to attempt prenatal diagnosis and treatment of a B_{12}-responsive variant of MMA.[25] They followed the pregnancy of a patient who had previously suffered the loss of a child to severe acidosis and dehydration at the age of 3 months. The diagnosis of MMA was made posthumously by chemical analysis of blood and urine. In the subsequent pregnancy, amniocentesis at 19 weeks revealed elevated methylmalonic acid in the amniotic fluid. Cultured amniocytes also demonstrated defective propionate oxidation and undetectable levels of adenosylcobalamin. When adenosylcobalamin was added, normal succinate oxidation and methylmalonyl-coenzyme A mutase activity were noted. These studies established that the fetus also suffered from MMA apparently due to deficient synthesis of adenosylcobalamin. It was already known that fetal MMA is associated with increased methylmalonic acid excretion in the maternal urine. Indeed, Ampola *et al.*[25] documented increased methylmalonic acidemia in maternal urine at 23 and 25 weeks gestation. Late in the pregnancy, cyanocobalamin (10 mg/day) was orally administered to the mother in divided doses. The treatment only marginally altered the maternal serum B_{12} level. However, there was a slight reduction of maternal urinary methylmalonic acid excretion that remained several fold above normal. At approximately 34 weeks gestation, 5 mg of cyanocobalamin per day was administered intramuscularly. The maternal serum B_{12} level then rose gradually to more than sixfold above normal and was accompanied by a progressive decrease in urinary methylmalonic acid excretion. Maternal urinary methylmalonate was only slightly above the normal range when delivery occurred at 41 weeks. Amniotic fluid methylmalonic acid concentrations were three times the normal mean at 19 menstrual weeks and four times the normal mean at term, despite prenatal treatment. Postnatally, the diagnosis of methylmalonic acidemia was confirmed. The infant suffered no acute neonatal complications and had an extremely high serum B_{12} level. Long-term postnatal management involved protein restriction; however, no continuous B_{12} treatment was required. In this instance prenatal treatment certainly improved the fetal and, secondarily, the maternal biochemistry. Whether there was any significant clinical benefit to the fetus by *in utero* treatment cannot be assessed adequately. It seems likely that reducing the fetal burden of methylmalonic acid should have some beneficial effect on fetal development and could reduce the risks in the neonatal period.

Andersson *et al.*[26] followed a cohort of eight children with MMA for an average of 5.7 years. Congenital malformations were described, reinforcing the deleterious effects of prenatally abnormal cyanocobalamin metabolism. Growth was significantly improved in most cases after initiation of therapy postnatally and in one case microcephaly resolved. However, developmental delay of variable severity was always present regardless of treatment onset. These data suggest that prenatal therapy of MMA may be effective and perhaps ameliorate some of the prenatal effects. Evans *et al.* have documented the changing dose requirements necessary over the course of pregnancy to maintain adequate levels of B_{12}. They sequentially followed maternal plasma and urine levels in a prenatal treated pregnancy.[27] Data such as these suggest that modulation of maternal-fetal pharmacological interchange of therapeutic drugs will be difficult to precisely control.

Multiple carboxylase deficiency

Biotin-responsive multiple carboxylase deficiency is an inborn error of metabolism caused by diminished activity of the mitochondrial biotin-dependent enzymes (pyruvate carboxylase, propionyl-coenzyme A carboxylase and α-methylcrotonyl-coenzyme A carboxylase). The condition may arise from mutations in the holocarboxilase synthetase (HCS) gene on chromosome 21q22.1 or the biotinidase gene localized to chromosome 3p25.[28–32] Affected patients present as newborns or in early childhood with dermatitis, severe metabolic acidosis, and a characteristic pattern of organic acid excretion. It has been demonstrated that metabolism in patients or in their cultured cells can be restored toward normal levels by biotin supplementation. Prenatal diagnosis can be made by demonstration of elevated levels of typical organic acids (3-hydroxyisovalerate, methylcitrate) in the amniotic fluid or in the chorionic villi. However, the existence of a mild form of HCS deficiency can complicate prenatal diagnosis as organic acids level in amniotic fluid might be normal.[33] Therefore, prenatal diagnosis must be performed by enzyme assay in cultured fetal cells in biotin-restricted medium.

Roth and colleagues treated a fetus without the benefit of prenatal diagnosis in a case in which two previous siblings had died of multiple carboxylase deficiency.[34] The first had died within 3 days of birth and in the second, the diagnosis of biotin-responsive carboxylase deficiency was made posthumously. Since the mother was first seen at 34 weeks gestation, prenatal diagnosis was not attempted. Because of severe neonatal manifestations in previous offspring and due to the probable harmlessness of biotin – oral administration was begun at a dose of 10 mg/day. There were no apparent untoward effects; maternal urinary biotin excretion increased by a factor of approximately 100 during biotin administration. Nonidentical twins were subsequently delivered at term. Cord blood and urinary organic acid profiles were normal, and cord blood biotin concentrations were four to seven times greater than normal. The neonatal course for both twins was unremarkable. Subsequent study of the cultured fibroblasts of both twins indicated that the cells of twin B (but not of twin A) had virtually complete deficiency of all three carboxylase activities. Genetic complementation studies confirmed that despite the normal clinical presentation during the newborn period, twin B was homozygous for the disease mutation. Packman and colleagues have also reported prenatal diagnosis and treatment of biotin-responsive multiple carboxylase deficiency for a mother who had previously given birth to a male with the neonatal-onset form of this disease.[35] In the subsequent pregnancy, maternal urine organic acid profiles were normal. Carboxylases activities were assayed in cultured amniotic fluid cells obtained by amniocentesis at 17 menstrual weeks. In biotin-restricted medium, the amniotic cells demonstrated the characteristic severe reduction in carboxylase activities. Since these initial reports of prenatal administration of biotin to fetuses affected with this disorder, other cases have been published,[33,36,37] further providing compelling evidence that biotin administration antenatally is effectively taken up by the fetus and prevents functional deficiency of the carboxylases in an affected newborn. No toxicity from treatment was observed. However, because experience with this treatment is confined to a small number of cases, it is reasonably to carry out prenatal diagnosis and only then to initiate treatment with biotin in any affected fetus.

Smith–Lemli–Optiz syndrome

Smith–Lemli–Optiz syndrome (SLOS) is a dysmorphological syndrome first reported in 1964.[38] Features include characteristic facies, growth and mental retardation, and anomalies of the heart, kidneys, central nervous system, and limbs. Cleft palate, postaxial polydactyly, 2–3 syndactyly of the toes and cataracts are often seen in affected patients. The 2–3 syndactyly of the toes is very specific for this disorder and is seen in > 90% of affected patients. Affected patients typically present with a narrow forehead, ptosis, anteverted nares, low-set ears, and micrognathia.

Males may present with ambiguous genitalia. In contrast with CAH, patients with SLOS are deficient in cholesterol and therefore lack steroid precursors. This leads to the lack of androgens, which results in under-masculinization of the male genitalia. Patients with the severe form of the syndrome present not only with these dysmorphological findings but also with a high rate of neonatal mortality.[39] The incidence of SLOS is estimated to be 1:20,000–1:40,000 live births,[40] and it appears to be most common in Caucasians population of North European origin, with an estimated carrier frequency of 1:70.[41] In 1993, the etiology of SLOS was discovered to be an inborn error of cholesterol biosynthesis due to a deficiency of the enzyme 7-dehydrocholesterol-Δ^7 reductase.[38,41–44] The gene for 7-dehydrocholesterol-Δ^7 reductase has been localized to chromosome 11q12–13.[44]

As a result of this enzymatic defect, there is a characteristic biochemical pattern of reduced cholesterol levels and elevated 7- and 8-dehydrocholesterol levels (7-DHC and 8-DHC, respectively) in all body fluids and tissues including red blood cells, fibroblasts, amniotic fluid and chorionic villi. The values observed in affected patients may be extremely variable. The diagnosis is made primarily by the presence of the cholesterol precursor, 7-DHC, and not by the deficiency of cholesterol. Unaffected individuals have levels of 7-DHC and 8-DHC of less than 1 mg/dl whereas patients with SLOS usually have levels of 7–20 or greater. Clinical manifestations correlate with cholesterol levels. Severely affected patients have very low levels of total cholesterol (usually <10–15 mg/dl), while those with more mild manifestations may present with levels of 40–70 mg/dl. Prenatal diagnosis of SLOS has been available since 1994 by either amniocentesis or chorionic villus sampling.[45–47]

Since identification of the cholesterol metabolic defect in SLOS, a treatment protocol has been attempted providing exogenous cholesterol. This form of therapy has now been provided to many patients with SLOS for the past several years in many centers in the United States and internationally,[48–50] with the goal of raising cholesterol levels and decrease the precursors, 7-DHC and 8-DHC. It has been shown that dietary cholesterol supplementation can restore a normal growth pattern in children and adolescents with SLOS, alleviate behavioral abnormalities and improve general health.[48–50]

Fetal therapy strategies may theoretically include providing cholesterol to the mother or to the fetus. The former, however, is not possible because cholesterol does not cross the placenta well in the second trimester and there is lack of evidence that it crosses the placenta in the third trimester. Moreover, cholesterol is available only in a crystalline form, which cannot be given intravenously or intramuscularly. Furthermore, it is impractical to inject cholesterol into the amniotic fluid because it would precipitate.

However, cholesterol can be given to the fetus by giving fresh frozen plasma in the form of low-density lipoprotein (LDL)-cholesterol. The group at Tufts University has attempted treatment antenatally in several affected fetuses. In cases where treatment was started late in pregnancy, the results were inconclusive. Although few descriptions of fetal therapy for SLOS exist, the latest report of antenatal treatment comes from that same group of investigators.[51] Therapy was begun at 34 weeks of gestation and resulted in increased fetal cholesterol levels and red blood cell mean corpuscular volume with subtle improvement in fetal growth, as assessed by consequent fetal weight plots. However, no significant change in 7-DHC and 8-DHC levels was observed, further emphasizing the inconclusiveness of that treatment. However, the main point is that since significant development of the central nervous system and myelination occurs prior to birth it is a reasonably to assume that providing cholesterol to the fetus, as early as possible would result in the most clinical benefit.

Galactosemia

Galactosemia is an inborn error of metabolism caused by the diminished activity of the enzyme galactose-1-phosphate uridyltransferase (GALT). This causes a defective metabolism of the sugar galactose which is the constituent of lactose, the main carbohydrate of milk, resulting in accumulation of galactose in the bloodstream. It is inherited in an autosomal recessive manner and results in cataracts, mental deficiency, growth deficiency, and ovarian failure. Clinical symptoms appear in the neonatal period and can be largely ameliorated by elimination of galactose from the diet. Cellular damage in galactosemia is thought to be mediated by accumulation of galactose-l-phosphate intracellularly and of galactitol in the lens. The *GALT* gene, localized to chromosome 9p13, is the only known gene to be associated with galactosemia. Several disease-causing mutations are commonly encountered in classical galactosemia, the most frequently observed is the Q188R classical mutation. Mutational analysis is available usefully for the six classical galactosemia alleles (Q188R, S135L, K285N, L195P, Y209C, F171S) and for the N314D Durate variant mutation.[52] In cases in which disease causing mutation are not identified (as observed in 10–29% of classic galactosemia), GALT sequence analysis may be performed to detect private mutations. Galactosemia can be diagnosed prenatally by study of cultured amniocytes and chorionic villi.

There are suggestions that even the early postnatal treatment of galactosemic individuals with a low galactose diet may not be sufficient to ensure normal development. Some have speculated that prenatal damage to galactosemic fetuses could contribute to subsequent abnormal neurological development and to lens cataract formation. Furthermore, it has been recognized that female galactosemics, even when treated from birth with galactose deprivation, have a high frequency of primary or secondary amenorrhea because of ovarian failure. This is because oocytes have already been damaged irreversibly long before birth. There also may be some subtle abnormalities of male gonadal function.

Exposure to a high-galactose diet has been considered to represent an animal model for human galactosemia. Chen and colleagues have observed a reduction in the oocyte content of rat ovaries after prenatal exposure to a 50% galactose diet.[53] No analogous alterations in the testes were observed in prenatally treated males. Experiments in rats suggest that toxicity to the female gonads from galactose or its metabolites is most obvious during the premeiotic stages of ovarian development. Recently, impaired germ cell migration leading to the development of gonads with deficient initial pools of germ cells was proposed as the causal link between galactosemia and premature ovarian failure.[54]

These observations in animals and human beings have led to speculation that galactose restriction during pregnancy may be desirable if the fetus is affected with galactosemia. In the human female, ovarian meiosis begins at 12 and is complete by 28 menstrual weeks. Thus, ovarian damage, and perhaps neurological or lens abnormalities, might occur prior to the usual time when prenatal diagnosis by amniocentesis can be accomplished. Thus, anticipatory treatment in pregnancies at risk for having a galactosemic fetus might best be initiated very early in gestation or even preconceptually.

Despite these experiments and speculations, we are unaware of studies that adequately assess the impact of prenatal administration of a low-galactose diet to galactosemic fetuses. However, such data, especially controlled, will be difficult to obtain. Nevertheless, prenatal galactose restriction is probably desirable in galactosemia and should be harmless. There is little reason to suppose that galactose restriction would have adverse consequences, since galactosemic and normal fetuses are both capable of some endogenous galactose synthesis.

Multifactorial disorders

Neural tube defects

Neural tube defects (NTDs) are malformations secondary to abnormal neural tube closure between the third and fourth weeks of gestational age. The etiology is complex and imperfectly understood with both genetic and environmental factors involved. Animal studies suggest that NTDs can arise from a variety of vitamin or mineral deficiencies. There are historical data in humans suggesting increased NTD frequencies in subjects with poor dietary histories or with intestinal bypasses. Biochemical evidence of suboptimal nutrition is present in some women bearing infants with NTDs. Analysis of recurrence patterns within families and of twin–twin concordance data provides evidence of a genetic influence in nonsyndromal cases, although factors such as socioeconomic status, geographic area, occupational exposure, and maternal use of antiepileptic drugs are also associated with variations in the incidence of NTDs.[55] In 1980, Smithells *et al.* suggested that vitamin supplementation containing 0.36 mg folate can reduce the frequency of NTD recurrence by sevenfold in women with one or more prior affected children.[56,57] For almost a decade, there has been a great deal of controversy regarding the benefit of folate supplementation for the prevention of NTDs.[58–61] Finally, in 1991, a randomized double-blinded trial designed by the Medical Research Council Vitamin Study Research Group demonstrated that preconceptual folate reduces the risk of recurrence in high-risk patients.[62] Subsequently, it was shown that preparations containing folate and other vitamins also reduce the occurrence of first time NTDs.[63] In response to these findings, guidelines were issued calling for consumption of 4.0 mg/day folic acid by women with a prior child affected with a NTD, for at least 1 month prior to conception through the first 3 months of pregnancy. In addition, 0.4 mg/day folic acid is recommended to all women planning a pregnancy to be taken preconceptually. The data on NTD recurrence prevention is now very well established, and became routine for high-risk cases. As of January, 1998, the United States Food and Drug Administration has mandated that breads and grains be supplemented with folic acid. The impact of food fortification with folic acid on birth prevalence of NTDs during the years 1990–1999 was evaluated by assessing birth certificate reports before and after mandatory fortification.[64] It was found that the birth prevalence of NTDs reported decreased by 19%. It is important to note that the continuing decline in NTDs rates are estimated to be due to the introduction and increased utilization of prenatal diagnosis, recommendations for multivitamin use in women of childbearing age, and the population-wide increases in blood folate levels since food fortification was mandated.[65]

Folate plays a central part in embryonic and fetal development because of its role in nucleic acid synthesis mandatory for the widespread cell division that takes place during embryogenesis. Folate deficiency can occur because of low dietary folate intake or because of increased metabolic requirement as seen in particular genetic alterations such as the polymorphism of the thermolabile enzyme methyltetrahydrofolate reductase (MTHFR). A metabolic effect of folate deficiency is homocysteine elevation in blood. As mentioned, the thermolabile variant of MTHFR 677TT, is a known risk factor for NTDs. However, evidence regarding a second polymorphism in the same gene, 1298A→C, does not support its role in NTDs.[66] Additionally, numerous studies analyzing MTHFR variants have resulted in positive associations with increased NTD risk only in certain populations, suggesting that these variants are not large contributors to the etiology of NTDs.[67] Therefore, it seems less likely to advise parents prospectively to test for MTHFR variants. Reinforcement to the assumption that additional candidate genes other than MTHFR may be responsible for an increase risk to NTDs comes from the NTD collaborative group of Duke University.[68] A total of 175 American Caucasian NTD patients and their families were examined for the thermolabile variant of MTHFR. Although a significant association has been found comparing patients and controls, no such association was found in patients' parents. Two other key enzymes in the metabolic pathway of homocysteine are methionine synthase (MTR) and methionine synthase reductase (MTRR). Recently reported, MTR and a specific (A66G) MTRR polymorphisms have been found to be associated with increased risk for NTDs. Interestingly, the NTDs risk was not influenced by maternal preconception folic acid intake at doses of 0.4 mg/day. However, due to limited sample size further studies are needed in order to draw meaningful inferences.[69] Other candidate genes suggested as risk factor for NTDs (mainly spina bifida), are polymorphisms in the mitochondrial membrane transporter gene UCP2.[70] Despite previous studies suggesting zinc deficiency to play a role in the etiology of NTDs,[71,72] further studies found this observation inconclusive.[73,74] Methionine deficiency might be involved in NTDs as 30%-55% reduction in the risk of having NTD associated pregnancy was reported when methionine intake was greater then the lowest quartile of intake, with further reduction in risk with greater methionine intake.[75] In conclusion, preconception intake of folic acid alone or as multivitamin supplementation reduces the risk of recurrence and first time NTDs. Additionally, folic acid-multivitamin supplementation reduces the occurrence of other congenital anomalies such as seen in the urinary tract (e.g., vesicorenal reflux, horshoe kidney, and others), in the cardiovascular system (e.g., conotruncal heart defects), and anomalies involving the limbs and face (orofacial clefting).

Pharmacologic approaches

It might be appropriate to consider suppressing excessive cholesterol production prenatally in severe hypercholesterolemia when a safe and effective agent for accomplishing this becomes available (although there is no clear evidence for hypercholesterolemic prenatal damage). If cysteamine or related agents were to prove an effective treatment for lethal variants of cystinosis, prenatal therapy might be considered, because excessive and possibly harmful cystine accumulation is evident even in cystinotic fetuses. Cysteamine levels have been detected in chorionic villi, and significant elevations even at 10 weeks' gestation have been hypothesized.

Inhibitors of gamma-glutamyl transpeptidase, if safe, would elevate intracellular glutathione levels and inhibit oxoproline production in glutathione synthase deficiency, thereby averting the characteristic neonatal acidosis. In theory, it would be desirable to minimize copper accumulation in Wilson disease as early as possible. If and when reliable prenatal diagnosis of Wilson disease is possible, cautious administration of penicillamine prenatally might be considered. This would be a double-edged sword, however, as the teratogenic potential of penicillamine would demand careful evaluation. Batshaw and colleagues[76] have treated certain urea cycle defects by administering arginine and benzoate. Since hyperammonemia in some of these entities develops very acutely after birth, it might be desirable to consider pretreating the fetus with these compounds just prior to or during labor to minimize postnatal hyperammonemia.[76] Conversely, it may be desirable to consider drug avoidance as an approach to fetal treatment. For example, fetuses with glucose-6-phosphate dehydrogenase deficiency are sensitive to a variety of drugs that induce hemolysis. It would probably be appropriate to avoid administering such agents to women carrying or known to be at risk for carrying fetuses deficient in glucose-6-phosphate dehydrogenase.

Umbilical cord catheterization under ultrasound guidance may lead to the development of other types of fetal treatment.[77] Systems such as gene replacement are being developed for certain lysosomal storage disorders. Progress is being made in postnatal experimental models on administration of thymic cells for certain immune deficiency states, bone marrow transplantation for a variety of genetic disorders, and gene transfer. The development of better and earlier techniques for prenatal treatment will be complex, especially with regard to gene transfer; but progress will be made, and access to the fetal vasculature may be required for these methods to have a chance for success.

Bone marrow transplantation or thymic cell infusion is actually only a specialized example of organ transplantation. In the future, fetal organ transplantation may become possible and may open many prospects for surgical treatment of certain biochemical genetic disorders.

One can also speculate about the therapeutic possibilities involving compounds administered directly into the amniotic fluid or into the fetal intestinal tract. It might be possible, for example, to administer thyroid hormone in this fashion or to prevent meconium ileus in cystic fibrosis by instilling not yet determined enzymes into the fetal intestinal tract.

Conclusion

While a multitude of metabolic disorders exist, prenatal treatment for most has never been attempted or considered. The discovery of new disease associated genes and prenatal carrier testing may in the future allow preconceptual carrier detection, without the tragedy of first having an affected child. This may provide targeted therapy in families who chose to continue the pregnancy and offer the prospect of improved outcome by ameliorating at least some of the prenatal deleterious effects of the metabolic disease.

REFERENCES

1. Evans MI, Pinsky WW, Johnson MP, Schulman JD. Medical fetal therapy. In: Evans MI, ed. *Reproductive Risks and Prenatal Diagnosis*. Norwalk: Appleton & Lange, 1992;236.
2. Johnson MP, Evans MI, Quintero RA, Flake AW. In utero therapy of the fetus. In: Gleisher N, Buttino L Jr, Elkayam U, Evans MI, Galbraith RM, Gall SA, Sibai BM, eds. *Principles and Practice of Medical Therapy in Pregnancy*, 3rd edn. Norwalk: Appleton & Lange, Chap. 25.
3. Speiser PW, Dupont B, Rubinstein P, Piazza A, Kastelan A, New MI. High frequency of nonclassical steroid 21-hydroxylase deficiency. *Am J Hum Genet* 1985;37:650–67.
4. Dupont B, Oberfield SE, Smithwick EM *et al.* Close genetic linkage between HLA and congenital adrenal hyperplasia (21-hydroxylase deficiency). *Lancet* 1977;2:1309–12.
5. White PC, Grossberger D, Onufer BJ *et al.* Two genes encoding steroid 21-hydroxylase are located near the genes encoding the fourth component of complement in man. *Proc Natl Acad Sci USA* 1985;82:1089–93.
6. Evans MI, Chrousos GP, Mann DL *et al.* Pharmacologic suppression of the fetal adrenal gland in utero: attempted prevention of abnormal external genital masculinization in suspected congenital adrenal hyperplasia. *J Am Med Assoc* 1985;253:1015–20.
7. Forest M, David M. Prenatal treatment of congenital adrenal hyperplasia due to 21-hydroxylase deficiency. *7th International Congress of Endocrinology*, Quebec, Canada, 1984, Abstract y11.
8. New MI, Carlson A, Obeid J *et al.* Prenatal diagnosis for congenital adrenal hyperplasia in 532 pregnancies. *Clin Endocrinol Metab* 2001;86:5651–7.
9. Clayton PE, Miller WL, Oberfield SE, Ritzen EM, Sippell WG, Speiser PW, ESPE/LWPES CAH Working Group. Consensus statement on 21-hydroxylase deficiency from the European Society for Paediatric Endocrinology and the Lawson Wilkins Pediatric Endocrine Society. *Horm Res* 2002;58:188–95.
10. Fisher DA, Neonatal thyroid disease of women with autoimmune thyroid disease. *Thyroid Today* 1986;9:1–7.
11. Fisher DA, Klein AH. Thyroid development and disorders of thyroid function in the newborn. *N Engl J Med* 1981;304:702–12.
12. Volumenie JL, Polak M, Guibourdenche J *et al.* Management of fetal thyroid goitres: A report of 11 cases in a single perinatal unit. *Prenat Diagn* 2000;20:799–806.
13. Morine M, Takeda T, Minekawa R *et al.* Antenatal diagnosis and treatment of a case of fetal goitrous hypothyroidism associated with high-output cardiac failure. *Ultrasound Obstet Gynecol* 2002; 19:506–9.
14. Rovet J, Ehrlich R, Sorbara D. Intellectual outcome in children with fetal hypothyroidism. *J Pediatr* 1987;110:700–4.
15. Thorpe-Beeston JG, Nicolaides KH, McGregor AM. Fetal thyroid function, *Thyroid* 1992;2:207–17.
16. Sack J, Fisher DA, Hobel CJ, Lam R. Thyroxine in human amniotic fluid. *J Pediatr* 1975;87:364–8.
17. Ballabio M, Nicolini U, Jowett T, Ruiz de Elvira MC, Ekins RP, Rodeck CH. Maturation of thyroid function in normal human fetuses. *Clin Endocrinol* 1989;31:565–71.
18. Van Herle AJ, Young RT, Fisher DA, Uller RP, Brinkman CR III. Intra-uterine treatment of a hypothyroid fetus. *J Clin Endocrinol Metab* 1973;40:474–7.

19. Gruner C, Kollert A, Wildt L, Dorr HG, Beinder E, Lang N. Intrauterine treatment of fetal goitrous hypothyroidism controlled by determination of thyroid-stimulating hormone in fetal serum. A case report and review of the literature. *Fetal Diagn Ther* 2001;16:47–51.
20. Bruinse HW, Vermeulen-Meiners C, Wit JM. Fetal treatment for thyrotoxicosis in non-thyrotoxic pregnant women. *Fetal Ther* 1988;3:152–7.
21. Wenstrom KD, Weiner CP, Williamson RA, Grant SS. Prenatal diagnosis of fetal hyperthyroidism using funipuncture. *Obstet Gynecol* 1990;76:513–17.
22. Porreco RP, Bloch CA. Fetal blood sampling in the management of intrauterine thyrotoxicosis. *Obstet Gynecol* 1990;76:509–12.
23. Hatjis CG. Diagnosis and successful treatment of fetal goitrous hyperthyroidism caused by maternal Graves' disease. *Obstet Gynecol* 1993;81:837–9.
24. Brusque A, Rotta L, Pettenuzzo LF *et al.* Chronic postnatal administration of methylmalonic acid provokes a decrease of myelin content and ganglioside *N*-acetylneuraminic acid concentration in cerebrum of young rats. *Braz J Med Biol Res* 2001;34:227–31.
25. Ampola MG, Mahoney MI, Nakamura E *et al.* Prenatal therapy of a patient with vitamin B responsive methylmalonic acidemia. *N Engl J Med* 1975;293:313.
26. Andersson HC, Marble M, Shapira E. Long term outcome in treated combined methylmalonic acidemia and homocysteinemia. *Genet Med* 1999;1:146–50.
27. Evans MI, Duquette DA, Rinaldo P *et al.* Modulation of B12 dosage and response in fetal treatment of methylmalonic aciduria (MMA). Titration of treatment dose to serum and urine MMA. *Fetal Diagn Ther* 1997;12:21–23.
28. Leon Del Rio A, Leclerc D, Gravel RA. Isolation of a cDNA encoding human holocarboxylase synthetase by functional complementation of a biotinauxotroph of *E. coli. Proc Natl Acad Sci USA* 1995;92:4626–30.
29. Suzuki Y, Akoi Y, Ishida Y *et al.* Isolation and characterization of mutations in the holocarboxylase synthetase cDNA. *Nat Genet* 1994;8:122–8.
30. Akoi Y, Suzuki Y, Sakamoto O *et al.* Molecular analysis of holocarboxylase synthetase deficiency: a missense mutation and a single base deletion are predominant in Japanese patients. *Biochim Biophys Acta* 1995;1272:168–74.
31. Dupuis L, Leon-Del-Rio A, Leclerc D *et al.* Clustering of mutations in the biotin-binding region of holocarboxilase synthetase in biotin responsive multiple carboxylase deficiency. *Hum Mol Genet* 1996;5:1011–16.
32. Popmponio RJ, Hymes J, Reynolds TR *et al.* Mutation in the human biotinidase gene that cause profound biothinidase deficiency in symptomatic children: molecular, biochemical, and clinical analysis. *Pediatr Res* 1997;42:840–8.
33. Suormala T, Fowler B, Jakobs C *et al.* Late onset holocarboxylase synthetase deficiency: Pre- and post-natal diagnosis and evaluation of effectiveness of antenatal biotin therapy. *Eur J Pediatr* 1998;157:570–5.
34. Roth KS, Yang W, Allen L *et al.* Prenatal administration of biotin: biotin responsive multiple carboxylase deficiency. *Pediatr Res* 1982;16:126–9.
35. Packman S, Cowan MJ, Golbus MS *et al.* Prenatal treatment of biotin responsive multiple carboxylase deficiency. *Lancet* 1982;1:1435–8.
36. Thuy LP, Belmont J, Nyhan W. Prenatal diagnosis and treatment of holocarboxylase synthetase deficiency. *Prenat Diagn* 1999;19: 108–12.
37. Thuy LP, Jurecki E, Nemzer L *et al.* Prenatal diagnosis of holocarboxylase synthetase deficiency by assay of the enzyme in chorionic villus material followed by prenatal treatment. *Clin Chim Acta* 1999;284:59–68.
38. Smith DW, Lemli L, Opitz JM. A newly recognized syndrome of multiple congenital anomalies. *J Pediatr* 1964;64:210–17.
39. Curry CJR, Carey JC, Holland JS. Smith–Lemli–Opitz syndrome – type II: Multiple congenital anomalies with male pseudohermaphroditism and frequent early lethality. *Am J Med Genet* 1987; 26:45–57.
40. Opitz JM. RSH-SLO ("Smith–Lemli–Opitz") syndrome: Historical, genetic, and development considerations. *Am J Med Genet* 1994;50:344–6.
41. Kelley RI. Diagnosis of Smith–Lemli–Opitz syndrome by gas chromatography/mass spectrometry of 7-dehydrocholesterol in plasma, amniotic fluid and cultured skin fibroblasts. *Clin Chim Acta* 1995;236:45–58.
42. Kelley RI. A new face for an old syndrome. *Am J Med Genet* 1997;65:251–6.
43. Tint GS, Irons M, Elias E *et al.* Defective cholesterol biosynthesis associated with the Smith–Lemli–Opitz syndrome. *N Engl J Med* 1994;330:107–13.
44. Waterham HR, Wijburg FA, Hennekam RCM *et al.* Smith–Lemli–Opitz is caused by mutations in the 7-dehydrocholesterol reductase gene. *Am J Hum Genet* 1998;63:329–38.
45. Gelman-Kohan Z, Nisani R, Chemke J, Appelman Z, Rappaport S, Hegesh E. Prenatal detection of recurrent SLOS type 2. *Am J Hum Genet* 1990;47:A57.
46. Hobbins JC, Jones OW, Gottesfeld MD, Persutte W. Transvaginal ultrasonography and transabdominal embryoscopy in the first-trimester diagnosis of Smith–Lemli–Opitz syndrome, type II. *Am J Obstet Gynecol* 1994;171:546–9.
47. Sharp P, Haan E, Fletcher JM, Khong TY, Carey WF. First trimester diagnosis of Smith–Lemli–Opitz syndrome. *Prenat Diagn* 1997; 17(4):355–61.
48. Irons M, Elias E, Tint GS *et al.* Abnormal cholesterol metabolism in the Smith–Lemli–Opitz syndrome: Report of clinical and biochemical findings in 4 patients and treatment in 1 patient. *Am J Med Genet* 1994;50:347–52.
49. Irons M, Elias ER, Abuelo D *et al.* Treatment of Smith–Lemli–Opitz syndrome: Results of a multicenter trial. *Am J Med Genet* 1997; 68:311–14.
50. Elias ER, Irons MB, Hurley AD, Tint GS, Salen G. Clinical effects of cholesterol supplementation in six patients with the Smith–Lemli–Opitz syndrome (SLOS). *Am J Med Genet* 1997;68:305–10.
51. Irons MR, Nores J, Stewart TL *et al.* Antenatal therapy of Smith–Lemli–Opitz syndrome. *Fetal Diagn Ther* 1999;14:133–7.
52. Elsas LJ. Prenatal diagnosis of galactos-1-phosphate uridyltransferase (GALT) deficient galactosemia. *Prenat Diagn* 2001;21: 302–3.
53. Chen YT, Mattison DR, Feigenbaum L *et al.* Reduction in oocyte number following prenatal exposure to a high galactose diet. *Science* 1981;314:1145–7.
54. Bandyopadhyay S, Chakrabarti J, Banerjee S *et al.* Prenatal exposure to high galactose adversely affects initial gonadal pool of germ cells in rats. *Hum Reprod* 2003;18:276–82.
55. Frey L, Hauser WA. Epidemiology of neural tube defects. *Epilepsia* 2003;44(Suppl 3):4–13.
56. Smithells RW, Nevin NC, Seller MJ *et al.* Further experience of vitamin supplementation for prevention of neural tube defect recurrences. *Lancet* 1983;1:1027–31.
57. Smithells RW, Sheppard S, Schorah CJ *et al.* Possible prevention of neural tube defects by preconceptual vitamin supplementation. *Lancet* 1980;1:339–40.
58. Younis JS, Granat M. Insufficient transplacental digoxin transfer in severe hydrops fetalis. *Am J Obstet Gynecol* 1987;157:1268–9.
59. Mills JL, Rhoads GG, Simpson JL *et al.* The absence of a relation between the periconceptional use of vitamins and neural-tube defects. *N Engl J Med* 1989;321:430–5.
60. Mulinare J, Cordero JF, Erickson JD, Berry RJ. Periconceptional use of multivitamins and the occurrence of neural tube defects. *J Am Med Assoc* 1988;260:3141–5.
61. Schulman JD. Treatment of the embryo and the fetus in the first trimester: current status and future prospects. *Am J Med Genet* 1990;35:197–200.
62. MRC Vitamin Study Research Group. Prevention of neural tube defects: results of the MRC vitamin study. *Lancet* 1991;338: 132–7.
63. Czeizel AE, Dudas I. Prevention of the first occurrence of neural-tube defects by preconceptional vitamin supplementation. *N Engl J Med* 1992;327:1832–5.
64. Honein MA, Paulozzi LJ, Mathews TJ, Erickaon JD, Wong LY. Impact of folic acid fortification of the US food supply on the occurrence of neural tube defects. *J Am Med Assoc* 2001;285: 2981–6.
65. Olney RS, Mulinare J. Trends in neural tube defect prevalence, folic acid fortification, and vitamin supplement use. *Semin Perinatol* 2002;26:277–85.
66. Parle-McDermott A, Mills JL, Kirke PN *et al.* Analysis of MTHFR 1298A→C and 677 C→T polymorphisms as risk factor neural tube defects. *J Hum Genet* 2003;48:190–3.
67. Finnell RH, Shaw GM, Lammer EJ, Volcik KA. Does prenatal screening for 5,10-methylenetetrahydrofolate reductase (MTHFR) mutations in high-risk neural tube defect pregnancies make sense? *Genet Test* 2002;6:47–52.

68. Rampersaud E, Melvin EC, Siegel D *et al.* Updated investigations of the role of methylenetetrahydrofolate reductase in human neural tube defects. *Clin Genet* 2003;63:210–14.
69. Zhu H, Wicker NJ, Shaw GM *et al.* Homocysteine remethylation enzyme polymorphisms and increased risks for neural tube defects. *Mol Genet Metab* 2003;78:216–21.
70. Volocik KA, Shaw GM, Zhu H *et al.* Risk factors for neural tube defects: associations between uncoupling protein 2 polymorphisms and spina bifida. *Birth Defects Res Part A Clin Mol Teratol* 2003; 67:158–61.
71. Sever LE. Zinc deficiency in man. *Lancet* 1973;I:887.
72. McMichael AJ, Dreosti IE, Gibson GT. A prospective study of serial maternal serum zinc levels and pregnancy outcome. *Early Hum Dev* 1982;7:59–69.
73. Stoll C, Dott B, Alembik Y, Koehl C. Maternal trace elements, vitamin B12, vitamin A, folic acid, and fetal malformations. *Rep Toxicol* 1999;13:53–7.
74. Hambidge M, Hackshaw A, Wald N. Neural tube defects and serum zinc. *Br J Obstet Gynaecol* 1993;100:746–9.
75. Shoob HD, Sargent RG, Thompson SJ *et al.* Dietary methionine is involved in the etiology of neural defect-affected pregnancies in humans. *J Nutr* 2001;131:2653–8.
76. Batshaw M, Brusilow S, Waber L *et al.* Treatment of inborn errors of urea synthesis: activation of alternative pathways of waste nitrogen synthesis and excretion. *N Engl J Med* 1982;306: 1387–92.
77. Nicolaides KH, Thorpe-Beeston JG, Noble P. Cordocentesis. In: Eden RD, Boehm H, eds. *Assessment and Care of the Fetus: Physiological, Clinical and Medicolegal Principles.* Norwalk: Appleton & Lange, 1990:291.

74 Fetal surgical interventions

M. R. Harrison and M. I. Evans

Introduction

Over the last two decades, fetal therapy has evolved into four major areas: open surgical approaches, 'closed' endoscopic surgical approaches, pharmacologic therapy, and stem cell/gene therapy. Advances in the field have been characterized by dramatic successes, but also intense frustration at technical challenges and moving targets as ancillary therapies change risk/reward equations.[1]

If something can be treated safely postnatally, then there is no justification for prenatal intervention. However, for the conditions discussed below, profound and irreparable damage occurs before birth, making fetal intervention the best or sometimes only way to ameliorate the damage. Some procedures have been quite rare. Others are more common, but the expectation is that with improvements and increasing utilization of prenatal diagnosis, more women will consider the opportunities to treat fetuses before birth.[2]

Surgical therapy

In utero closed fetal surgery

The most efficacious percutaneous *in utero* fetal surgery has been for the evaluation and treatment of obstructive uropathy. Lower urinary tract obstruction (LUTO) is a heterogenous entity that affects 1:5000–8000 newborn males. Posterior urethral valves or urethral atresias are the most common causes for LUTO, although other etiologies, such as stenosis of the urethral meatus, anterior urethral valves, ectopic insertion of a ureter and tumors of the bladder, have been observed. LUTO can result in massive distention of the bladder with compensatory hypertrophy and hyperplasia of the smooth muscle within the bladder wall, leading to loss of compliance and elasticity and poor postnatal function generally requiring surgical reconstruction.[3] Elevated intravesicular pressures prevent urine inflow from the ureters and eventual distortion of the ureterovesicle angles contributes to reflux hydronephrosis. Progressive pyelectasis and calyectasis compress the delicate renal parenchyma within the encasing serosal capsule, leading to functional abnormalities within the medullary and eventually the cortical regions. Focal compressive hypoxia likely contributes to the progressive fibrosis and perturbations in tubular function resulting in urinary hypertonicity, which is observed. Obstructive processes can eventually lead to type IV cystic dysplasia and renal insufficiency.[4–7]

The effects extend beyond the genitourinary tract. Progressive oligo/anhydramnios leads to compressive deformations as seen in Potter sequence, including extremity contractures and facial dysmorphology. Absence of normal amniotic fluid volume also interferes with pulmonary growth and development. Constant compressive pressure on the fetal thorax leads to restriction of expansion of the chest through normal physiologic 'breathing movements'. Babies born with LUTO generally die secondary to pulmonary complications and not renal failure.

The prenatal sonographic diagnosis of LUTO includes dilated and thickened walls of the bladder, hydronephrosis, and oligohydramnios. (Figure 74.1) Urethral strictures or atresia, urethral agenesis, megalourethra, ureteral reflux, and cloacal anomalies may be present and have a very similar appearance on ultrasound. The typical 'keyhole sign' of proximal urethral dilation is secondary to urethral obstruction present in PUV or atresia. However, the precise diagnosis can only be made after birth.[7]

The prenatal evaluation and management of fetuses with the sonographic findings of LUTO are complex.[4–6] Ruling out other congenital anomalies, such as cardiac and neural tube defects, is necessary before intervention can be considered.

Karyotyping is needed to confirm a normal male chromosomal status, as cases of LUTO have an increased incidence of aneuploidy. Female fetuses almost always have more complex syndromes of cloacal malformations, which do not benefit from *in utero* shunt therapy. Because of the presence of oligo/anhydramnios, we commonly obtain karyotypes by transabdominal chorionic villus sampling, which gives reliable results within 5 days during which the remainder of the prenatal evaluation is under way. Fluorencence *in situ* hybridization can be used to get rapid status of chromosomes 13, 18, 21, X, and Y.[8]

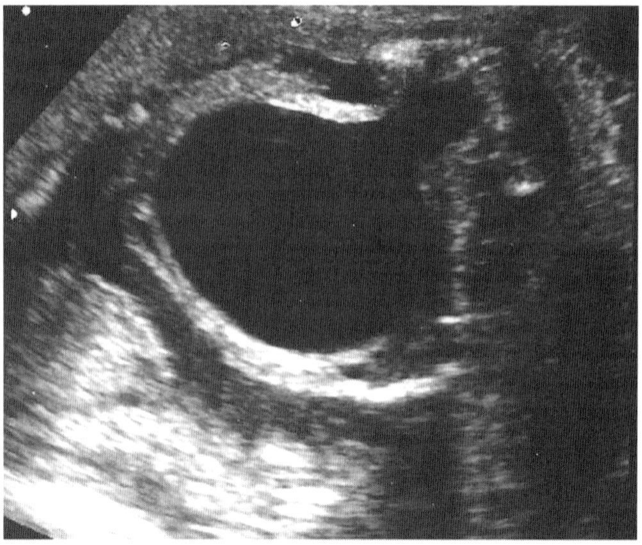

Figure 74.1 Oligohydramnios and dilated bladder in a fetus at 17 weeks with good electrolytes.

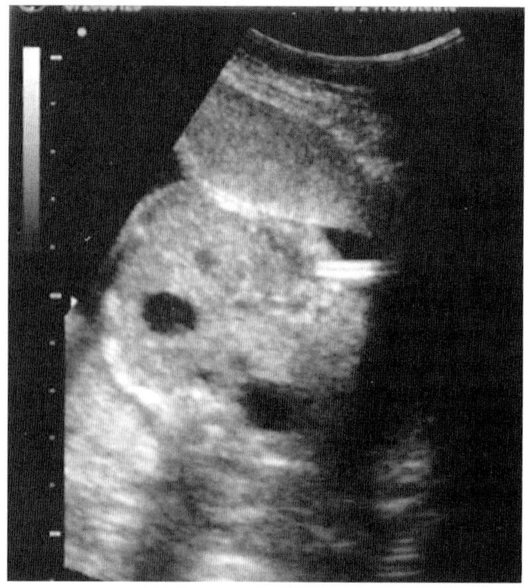

Figure 74.2 Vesicoamniotic shunt with the proximal portion lying within the fetal bladder while the distal portion lies within the amniotic fluid space allowing diversionary draining of urine into the appropriate space.

Essential to the prenatal workup is the evaluation of underlying renal status in the fetus. Over the past 15 years, we have developed a multicomponent approach for the analysis of fetal urine that evaluates proximal tubular and possible glomerular status using sodium, chloride, osmolality, calcium, β-2 microglobulin, albumin, and total protein concentrations.[5] Predictive reliability has been shown to be significantly improved by sequential samplings at 48–72-h intervals.[6] Using such an approach, one can directly correlate the degree of impaired renal function and damage with the extent of urinary hypertonicity and proteinuria. As such, the ability to counsel patients about the renal status of their fetus and the long-term prognosis has been dramatically improved.

Table 74.1 Upper threshold values for selecting fetuses that might benefit from prenatal intervention

Sodium	< 100 mg/dl
Chloride	< 90 mg/dl
Osmolality	< 190 mOsm/l
Calcium	< 8 mg/dl
β-2 microglobulin	< 6 mg/l
Total protein	< 40 mg/dl

Vesicoamniotic catheter shunts bypass the urethral obstruction diverting the urine into the amniotic space to allow appropriate drainage of the upper urinary tract and prevention of pulmonary hypoplasia and physical deformations. (Figure 74.2) In fetuses with isolated LUTO, a normal male karyotype, and progressively improving urinary profile that meet threshold parameters (Table 74.1), intervention has been very successful in salvaging fetuses using percutaneous vesicoamniotic shunt therapy.

Experience in humans has been widely variable and appears to be related to the extent of prenatal evaluation prior to shunt placement, as well as the etiology of obstruction. Freedman *et al.* confirmed that Prune Belly infants, without complete urethral obstructions, have very good renal outcomes following vesicoamniotic shunt therapy.[7] They have also found significant improvement in survival and renal function in infants with posterior urethral valves treated by shunting; however, many have mild to moderate renal insufficiency at birth and several of these have progressed to renal failure, dialysis, and transplantation. The worst group of infants appears to be those with urethral atresia. However, there have been survivors with urethral atresia following early shunt intervention. These findings support animal studies, which indicated that early-onset complete obstructions resulted in more severe renal damage than later-onset or partial obstructions. Such data emphasize the necessity for early diagnosis, evaluation, and intervention in such cases.

More recently, data from our experience over the past 15 years suggest that patients having bladder shunts had a 91% survival rate, but that long-term renal function was not guaranteed. Just under half had 'normal renal function', and about a quarter had mild impairments. The experience depended highly on the exact etiology of the disorder with posterior urethral value having the best outcomes and urethral atresia the worst. The experience suggests that close pediatric urologic/renal function assessment is essential. The Paris group has found that about 25% of children had serious, long-term renal impairments and about 15% actually developed end-stage renal disease requiring transplant. (M. Dommergues and F. Mueller, unpublished data).

Although vesicoamniotic shunting has clearly improved survival and renal function in cases of early obstructive uropathy, complications of this procedure remain unacceptably high. We found in the 1980s and 1990s that in 40% of our cases the shunts became physically displaced into the amniotic or intraperitoneal space, or became obstructive with loss of drainage function, necessitating replacement. On balance, intervention for LUTO has saved fetuses that would otherwise have surely died. Many have normal to moderately impaired renal function. A carefully balanced approach in counseling is required for patients to determine what is right for them.

Other shunts

In the late 1970s, shunting was attempted for obstructive hydrocephalus.[9] Attempts in the late 1970s and early 1980s at *in utero* ventriculoperitoneal shunting were nearly uniformly disastrous. However, in retrospect, most of the operated patients were, in fact, very poor candidates for intervention. Many had multisystem syndromic disorders, including aneuploidy, and hopeless congenital anomalies, such as holoprosencephaly.

Accordingly, ventriculoamniotic shunts were abandoned since the early 1980s. With a better understanding of the poor natural history of the anomaly, and better, more accurate diagnostic techniques, we have speculated that there may eventually be limited applications for prenatal neurologic shunting in cases of early-onset, isolated, progressive obstructive hydrocephaly.

The other use of percutaneously placed shunts has been for thoracic abnormalities.[10,11] The macrocystic form of congenital cystic adenomatous malformation can present with a very large intrathoracic mass with a dominant macrocyst that causes cardiac and mediastinal shift and comes with its potential hemodynamic changes, as well as pulmonary compression and risk of lung hypoplasia. Such dominant cysts can be approached using pleuroamniotic shunts to chronically drain these structures, reducing their volume, and diminishing their space-occupying effects within the thoracic cavity.

Isolated pleural effusions can also accumulate to the point of causing hemodynamic changes and onset of generalized hydrops as well as pulmonary compression, which interferes with normal lung development increasing the risk of hypoplasia. Small, unilateral effusions generally do not warrant intervention, but must be followed closely as they have the potential for rapid progression and development of generalized hydrops.[11]

As with all fetal interventions, prenatal evaluation prior to intervention is critical for appropriate case selection. Seemingly isolated effusions may be the first sign of a cardiac malformation, aneuploidy, anemia, or an infectious process. Thoracoamniotic shunting is effective in carefully evaluated cases when the risk of pulmonary hypoplasia from large effusions early in gestation is present, or early signs of progressive hydrops (unilateral–bilateral effusion, skin or scalp edema, ascites, pericardial effusion) appear. Fetal anemia, *per se*, is not an indication for thoracoamniotic effusion shunting, as hydropic changes will usually resolve with timely fetal transfusion therapy. Also, if one waits to intervene until the fetus develops significant ascites, the prognosis even with successful shunt intervention diminishes considerably.[11] However, several cases with suddenly progressive pleural effusions and the onset of generalized hydrops (skin/scalp edema, pericardial effusion, and moderate ascites) have been treated with complete resolution of all hydropic complications and normal postnatal infants.

Open surgical approaches

For a limited number of indications, open fetal surgery has been performed for about 20 years.[2] Appropriate concerns for maternal risk, rigorous selection criteria, and somewhat frustrating results have limited its use. There have been continuing innovation and development of instruments and techniques motivated by the clinical necessity to improve the safety of open fetal surgery for both the fetus and the mother.

Congenital diaphragmatic hernia (CDH)

The fetal approach to CDH has undergone continuous evolution since the first attempted CDH repair in 1986 and the first success in 1989.[12–15] Definitive repair of CDH by reduction of viscera from the chest, diaphragmatic patch placement, and abdominal silo construction (to reduce intra-abdominal pressure) had unacceptable mortality, particularly after a clinical trial showed open fetal repair was no better than postnatal repair, when the liver was herniated into the chest.[16,17] The definitive repair was abandoned as an option for CDH; *in utero* tracheal occlusion took its place.[17–24] (Figure 74.3) Tracheal occlusion leads to an increase in lung size through accumulation of pulmonary secretions, which reduces the herniated viscera from the chest and decreases the risk of lung hypoplasia. The technique of achieving reliable, complete and reversible trachael occlusion has evolved. Initially, it could only be accomplished by open fetal surgery and fetal neck dissection (taking care to avoid the recurrent laryngeal nerves) and placement of occlusive hemoclips. Next, a fetoscopic technique was developed to accomplish the same neck dissection and tracheal clip (the Fetendo Clip Procedure).[21,22] While successful, it proved difficult with a significant learning curve. Attempts to simplify the procedure by developing an appropriate polymer to

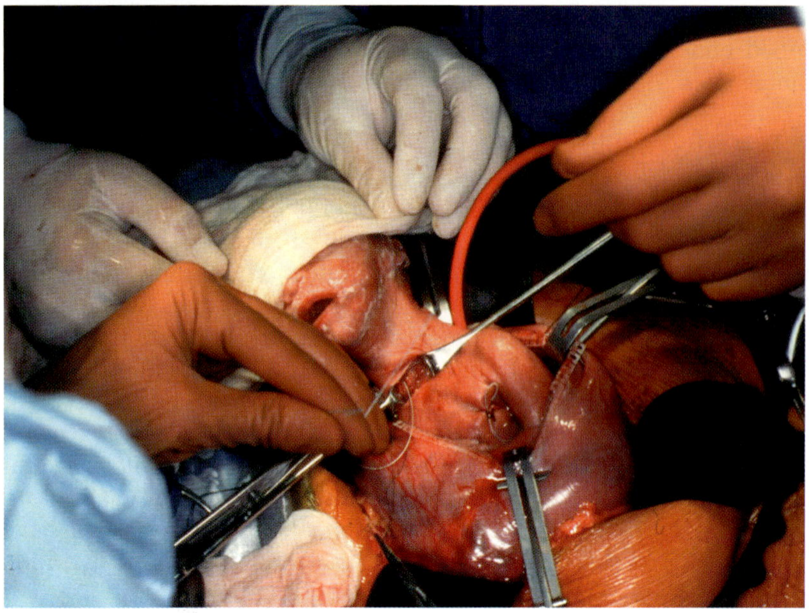

Figure 74.3 Surgical isolation of the fetal trachea prior to placement of hemoclips in a tracheal occlusion procedure for CDH.

use as a tracheal plug inserted through the fetal mouth were unsuccessful. Experience quickly showed that unless there was complete occlusion, the pulmonary secretions would leak, thereby defeating the purpose of the plug. Finally, a relatively simple technique was developed in which a fetoscope passed through a single port is advanced into the fetal trachea (fetal bronchoscopy) and a detachable silicone balloon is inflated to occlude the trachea.

CDH has been a classic example of rapid changes in technology clouding any simple attempts to understand the role for fetal surgery. With increasing sophistication of the surgical approach as well as concomitant improvements in neonatal care using extracorporeal membrane oxygenation, it was impossible to accurately determine the relative benefits of each approach without a prospective, randomized comparison that held all other details constant. Thus, after much debate, a randomized trial of surgery for CDH vs. optimal postnatal care was funded by the National Institute of Child Health and Human Development.[17] The principle component of the trial was that patients in the postnatal care (control) arm would receive the same neonatal care by the same center as the surgical arm.

It was originally expected that patients undergoing surgery would have a survival rate of about 70% as compared to the best data on controls expecting about 35%. The surgically treated patients achieved expected survival. However, the trial was stopped prematurely, when by having the controls cared for at the same tertiary specialty centers as the surgical group, survival in the controls was essentially the same as the surgical group. Such data show conclusively the principle of 'the moving target' and how our use of technology must continually adapt to changing conditions.[23]

Congenital cystic adenomatoid malformation (CCAM)

CCAM is a space-occupying congenital cystic lesion of the lung, which may grow and induce hydrops by causing mediastinal shift and compromise venous return to the heart. When fetuses with CCAM develop hydrops, the fetal mortality approaches 100%[25–27] (Figure 74.4). Fetal resection of CCAM reverses hydrops and has improved survival dramatically.[25–27] The fetal operation is performed by exposure of the arm and chest wall on the side of the lesion through the maternal hysterotomy. A large muscle sparing thoracotomy is performed through the midthorax of the fetus and the lobe containing the CCAM is isolated. The attachments of the lobe to the adjacent lung tissue are bluntly divided and the lobar hilum is divided by the use of a TIA stapler or a bulk ligature. During the remainder of the pregnancy, the remaining normal lung shows compensatory growth that fills the space left, showing mass removal.

Sacrococcygeal teratoma (SCT)

Fetal SCT arises from the presacral space, which may grow to massive proportions and in some fetuses induce high-output failure from tumor vascular steal. Fetal SCT with high-output physiology with associated placentomegaly or hydrops uniformly result in fetal demise[28,29] (Figure 74.5). The pathophysiologic rationale for fetal surgery is to ligate the vascular connections to the tumor, remove the vascular 'sin', and reverse the high-output physiology. The fetal operation is performed by exteriorization of the fetal buttocks with attached tumor.[28] Every attempt is made to keep the head, torso, and lower extremities of the fetus in the uterus. Since the tumor can sometimes be larger than the fetus, a significant loss of uterine

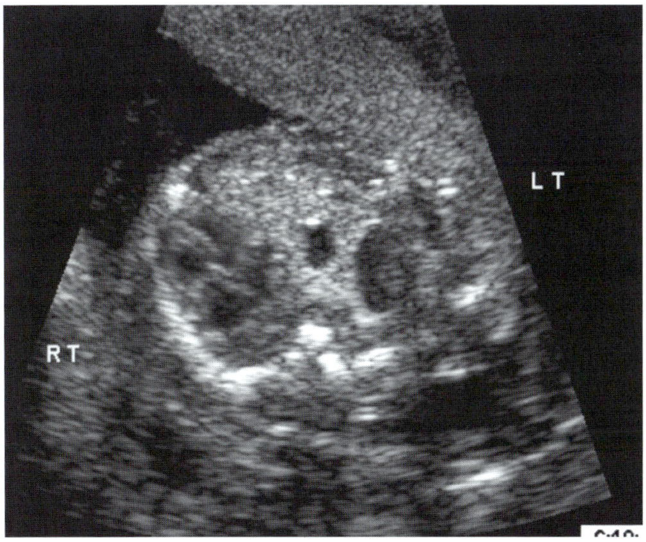

Figure 74.4 Microcystic congenital cystic adenomatous malformation (microcystic) with the beginnings of hydrops.

volume occurs, and the uterus may contract, increasing the risk of placental abruption, placental dysfunction because of compression, or postoperative preterm labor. Once exteriorized, the anus is identified and the fetal skin incised posterior to the anorectal sphincter complex to avoid injury to the continence mechanism. A tourniquet is then applied to the base of the tumor and brought down gradually as the tumor is finger fractured down to its vascular pedicle. The vascular pedicle is then ligated with suture ligatures or TIA device stapled depending on the width of the pedicle. The entire fetal procedure can be performed in less than 15 min with minimal blood loss. Because of the increase in afterload following ligation of the low resistance tumor circuit, the fetal hemodynamic status must be monitored by fetal echocardiography during and in the immediate period following the ligation.

ex utero intrapartum treatment (EXIT) procedure

The EXIT procedure is a modified cesarean delivery and may be applied to deliver fetuses after fetal surgical procedures, such as tracheal ligation, or for fetuses with difficult airway problems, such as massive cervical teratomas or cystic hygromas.[30,31] The most important component of the EXIT procedure is the maintenance of uteroplacental perfusion until the fetal airway is secured and ventilation is established. In direct contrast to cesarean section where uterine contraction for hemostasis is encouraged, uterine relaxation is maintained by deep general anesthesia. The fetal manipulations are then performed with maternal support via the placenta. Clips can be removed, chest masses removed, bronchoscopy performed, and stable airway access established in otherwise very difficult circumstances with this approach. Once the fetus is ready for transport to the nursery or adjacent operating suite following these preliminary

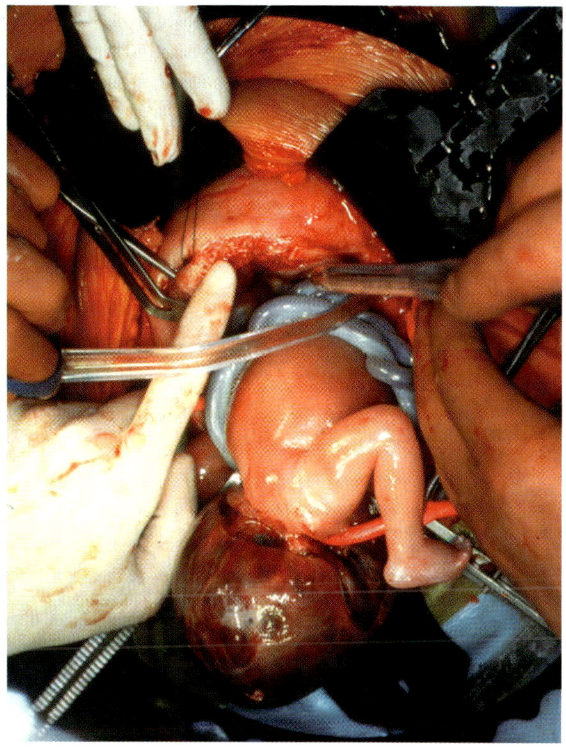

Figure 74.5 Saccrococcygeal teratoma in a fetus.

steps, the cord is clamped and cut and the cesarean delivery completed.

Meningomyelocele

Babies with myelingomyloceles have impaired lower motor function and loss of bowel and bladder control. A significant percentage develop obstructive hydrocephalus which requires ventriculoperitoneal shunting.[32] Experience from the 1970s and 1980s showed that babies with meningomyelocele delivered atraumatically by cesarean section had a better level of motor function for the given level of anatomic defect, than those babies delivered through the vaginal canal.[33] Such data suggest that compression and trauma to the cord in the delivery process can have permanent long-term sequelae to motor function. It therefore follows that trauma to the spinal cord *in utero*, either from banging into the uterine wall, or the toxic effects of the amniotic fluid in the third trimester, *per se*, could be detrimental to the function of the spinal cord. Furthermore, the traditional dogma that the pathogenesis of meningomyelocele was that an abnormally developed spinal cord, which did not in turn, engender the proper development of the bony spinal column, may not be the whole story. It is possible that the primary defect is in the bony spinal column, which exposes a presumptively undamaged spinal cord. The cord is then damaged by the toxic affects of amniotic fluid and trauma from the uterine environment and repeated contact with the uterine wall. Thus, the rationale for attempts to cover and protect the spinal cord in utero, to minimize the sequelae.[34]

Three groups have done most of the work in this area and have attempted to repair meningomyeloceles in utero, both as an open surgical procedure and endoscopically, with the stated attempt to reduce long-term morbidity and mortality.[35,36,37]

The principal benefit of the surgery is likely secondary, i.e. a significant reduction in the number of babies requiring ventriculoperitoneal shunting for obstructive hydrocephalus.[38,39] There is still much controversy surrounding the data.[32] A randomized, prospective trial comparing fetal to postnatal neurosurgical closure began in 2003, but will take several years to be completed. A major milestone of this trial has been the agreement among the participating centers not to perform any cases outside the trial, and other centers around the country have agreed not to start programs until the trial is completed.

Conclusion

There are an increasing number of congenital and genetic abnormalities for which *in utero* treatment is possible, and in some cases, now relatively routine. Advances in therapies have progressed at different paces for different disorders, but there is a great hope and enthusiasm that progress will continue to expand the number of disorders for which therapy can be effective.

REFERENCES

1. Evans MI, Bui TH, eds. *The Genome Revolution and Obstetrics and Gynecology. Balliere's Best Practice and Research in Clinical Obstetrics and Gynecology*. London: Harcourt Brace Publishing Co., 2002;16.
2. Harrison MR, Evans MI, Adzick NS, Holzgrove W. *The Unborn Patient*. Philadelphia, PA: W. B. Saunders, 2000.
3. Johnson MP, Flake AW, Quintero RA, Evans MI. Shunt procedures. In Evans MI, Johnson MP, Moghissi KS, eds. *Invasive Outpatient Procedures in Reproductive Medicine*. New York: Raven Press, 1997.
4. Evans MI, Sacks AL, Johnson MP, Robichaux III AG, May M, Moghissi KS. Sequential invasive assessment of fetal renal function, and the in utero treatment of fetal obstructive uropathies. *Obstet Gynecol* 1991;77(4):545–50.
5. Wilson RD, Johnson MP. Prenatal ultrasound guided percutaneous shunt for obstruction, uropathy and thoracic disease. *Semin Pediatr Surg* 2003;12:182–9.
6. Johnson MP, Corsi P, Bradfield W, *et al.* Sequential fetal urine analysis provides greater precision in the evaluation of fetal obstructive uropathy. *Am J Obstet Gynecol* 1995:173:59–65.
7. Freedman AL, Bukowski TP, Smith CA, Evans MI, Johnson MP, Gonzalez R. Fetal therapy for obstructive uropathy: Specific outcomes diagnosis. *J Urol* 1996;156:720–4.
8. Feldman B, Aviram-Goldring A, Evans MI. Interphase FISH for prenatal diagnosis of common aneuploidies. *Methods Mol Biol* 2002;204:219–41.
9. Drugan A, Krause B, Canady A, Zador IE, Sacks AJ, Evans MI. The natural history of prenatally diagnosed ventriculomegaly. *J Am Med Assoc* 1989;261:1785–8.
10. Ahmad FK, Sherman SJ, Hagglund KH, Johnson MP, Krivehcnia EL. Isolated unilateral pleural effusion: The role of sonographic surveillance and in utero therapy. *Fetal Diagn Ther* 1996;11: 383–89.
11. Nicolaides KH, Azar GB. Thoracoamniotic shunting. *Fetal Diagn Ther* 1990;5:153–64.
12. Adzick N, Harrison M, Flake A, Glick P, Bottles K. Automatic uterine stapling devices in fetal surgery: Experience in a primate model. *Surg Forum* 1985;XXXVI:479–81.
13. Jennings RW, Adzick NS, Longaker MT, Lorenz HP, Estes JM, Harrison MR. New techniques in fetal surgery. *J Pediatr Surg* 1992;27:1329–33.
14. Jennings RW, Adzick NS, Longaker MT, Lorenz HP, Harrison MR. Radiotelemetric fetal monitoring during and after open fetal operation. *Surg Gynecol Obstet* 1993;176:59–64.
15. Harrison MR, Longaker MT, Adzick NS, *et al.* Successful repair in utero of a fetal diaphragmatic hernia after removal of herniated viscera from the left thorax. *N Engl J Med* 1990;322:1582–4.
16. Harrison MR, Adzick NS, Flake AW, *et al.* Correction of congenital diaphragmatic hernia in utero: VI. Hard-learned lessons. *J Pediatr Surg* 1993;28:1141–7; discussion 1417–8.
17. Harrison MR, Keller RL, Hawgood SB, *et al.* A randomized trial of fetal endoscopic tracheal occlusion for severe fetal congenital diaphragmatic hernia. *N Engl J Med* 2003;349:1916–24.
18. Harrison MR, Sydorak RM, Farrell JA, Kitterman JA, Filly RA, Albanese CT. Fetoscopic temporary tracheal occlusion for congenital diagphragmatic hernia: Prelude to a randomized, controlled trial. *J Pediatr Surg* 2003;38(7):1012–20.
19. Heerema AE, Rabban JT, Sydorak RM, Jarrison MR, Jones KD. Lung pathology in patients with congenital diaphragmatic hernia treated with fetal surgical intervention, including tracheal occlusion. *Pediatr Dev Pathol* 2003.
20. Sydorak RM, Harrison MR. Congenital diaphragmatic hernia: Advances in prenatal therapy. *Clin Perinatol* 2003;30(3):465–79.
21. Danzer E, Sydora RM, Harrison MR, Albanese CT. Minimal access fetal surgery. *Eur J Obstet Gynecol Reprod Biol* 2003;108(1):3–13.
22. Evans MI, Harrison MR, Flake AW, Johnson MP. Fetal therapy. *Best Pract Res Clin Obstet Gynaecol* 2002;16(5):671–83.
23. Paek BW, Coakley FV, Lu Y, *et al.* Congenital diaphragmatic hernia: Prenatal evaluation with MR lung volumetry. *Preliminary Experience* 2000;220(1):63–7.
24. Wenstrom KD. Fetal surgery for congenital diaphragmatic hernia. *N Engl J Med* 2003;349(20):1887–8.
25. Adzick NS, Kitano Y. Fetal surgery for lung lesions, congenital diaphragmatic hernia, and saccrococcygeal teratoma. *Semin Pediatr Surg* 2003;12:154–67.
26. Adzick NS, Harrison MR, Crombleholme TM, *et al.* Fetal lung: Management and outcome. *Am J Obstet Gynecol* 1998;179:884–9.
27. Crombleholme TM, Coleman BG, Howell LJ, *et al.* Elevated cystic adenomatoid malformation volume (CVR) outcome in prenatal diagnosis of cystic adenomatoid malformation of the lung. *J Pediatr Surg* 2002;37:331–8.
28. Hotterman AX, Filiatrault D, Lallier M, *et al.* The natural history of sacrococcygeal teratomas diagnosed through routine obstetric sonogram: A single institution experience. *J Pediatr Surg* 37:331–8.
29. Paek B. Vaezy S, Fujimoto V, *et al.* Tissue ablation using high-intensity focused ultrasound: Potential for fetal treatment. *Am J Obstet Gynecol* 2003;189:703–5.
30. Liechty KW, Crombleholme TM, Flake AW, *et al.* Intrapartum airway management for giant neck masses. The EXIT (ex utero intrapartum treatorus procedure). *Am J Obstet Gynecol* 1997;177:870–4.
31. Hedrick HL. Ex utero intrapartum therapy. *Semin Perinatol* 2003; 12:190–5.
32. Meningomyelocele: Prenatal diagnosis, pathophysiology & management. *Semin Perinatol* 2003;12:168–174.
33. Lemire RJ. Neural tube defects. *J Am Med Assoc* 1988;259: 558–62.
34. Meuli M, Meuli-Simmen C, Hutchins GM, *et al.* In utero surgery rescues neurological function at birth in sheep with spina bifida. *Nature Med* 1995;1:342–6.
35. Bruner JP, Tulipan N, Paschall RL, *et al.* Fetal surgery for myelomeningocele and the incidence of shunt-dependent hydrocephalus. *J Am Med Assoc* 1999;282(19):1819–25.
36. Sutton LN, Adzick NS, Bilaniuk LT, Johnson MP, Crombleholme TM, Flake AW. Improvement in hindbrain herniation demonstrated by serial fetal magnetic resonance imaging following fetal surgery for myelomeningocele. *J Am Med Assoc* 1999;282:1826–31.
37. Tulipan N, Hermanz-Schulman M, Bruner JP. Reduced hindbrain herniation after intrauterine myelomingocele repair. A report of four cases. *Pediatr Neurosurg* 1998;29:274–8.
38. Bruner JP, Tulipan N, Paschall RL, *et al.* Intrauterine repair of myelomingocele, "hindbrain herniation", and the incidence of shunt dependent hydrocephalus. *J Am Med Assoc* 1999;282: 1819–25.
39. Johnson MP, Adzick WS, Rintoul N, *et al.* Fetal menyongocele repair: Short term outcomes. *Am J Obstet Gynecol* 2003;189:482–7.

SECTION VIII

Screening and risk assessment

Section Editors: **G. Monni and S. Chasen**

75 First-trimester ultrasound screening for fetal malformations

S. T. Chasen

The most significant advance in first-trimester ultrasound screening has been the recognition of nuchal translucency (NT) as a potent marker for fetal aneuploidy.[1] Abnormal NT in a euploid fetus is also associated with structural fetal abnormalities that can be diagnosed in the second-trimester.[2] Thus, measurement of NT can lead to earlier and targeted screening in the second trimester.

While abnormal NT can suggest the possibility of a structural abnormality, advances in ultrasound imaging have made the direct diagnosis of some anomalies possible.[3,4] Evaluation of other anatomic structures in the first trimester can diagnose anomalies or identify useful markers for anomalies that may be diagnosed later in pregnancy. As more women will be presenting for NT measurement at 11–14 weeks' gestation, it is important to consider other anatomic structures amenable to evaluation at this time.

Evaluation of first-trimester anatomy

Fetal head

Structures that can be well visualized in the first trimester include the calvarium and portions of the developing brain. Midline structures, including a falx cerebri and thalamic bodies, are easily visualized. Choroid-filled lateral ventricles can be identified as well. The cavum septum pellucidum and structures in the posterior fossa cannot be reliably evaluated in many cases, though visualization becomes more likely by 14 weeks.

Fetal face

The profile is well imaged in most fetuses from 11 to 14 weeks, and this has led to the use of nasal bone evaluation in Down's syndrome screening.[5] The orbits can be identified as well. While the lips can be seen at these gestational ages in some fetuses, they cannot be reliably evaluated in a significant proportion of cases.

Fetal spine

The cervical and cervical spines can be evaluated in the first trimester. Unfortunately, the lumbar and sacral spines, in which spina bifida are much more likely to occur, are often not well imaged prior to the second trimester.

Fetal heart

Aside from cardiac axis, the structure of the fetal heart is generally not well evaluated at 14 weeks' gestation or earlier. Four-chamber view, outflow tracts, ductus arteriosus, and the aortic arch cannot be evaluated in many cases at these gestational ages.[6]

Abdomen

An intact diaphragm and stomach bubble are visible at 11–14 weeks in most cases. The umbilical cord insertion in the ventral wall and the urinary bladder just below the site of cord insertion can be seen in the vast majority of fetuses as well. The kidneys can usually be identified, though this is not possible in a small proportion of cases.

Extremities

By 11 weeks, high-resolution ultrasound can document the presence of all long bones in the extremities in most fetuses. Reference ranges for limb measurements early in pregnancy have been published.[7] The hands and feet are usually easily identified. Evaluation of the fingers is possible, though this may be limited prior to the second trimester.

Diagnosis of fetal anomalies at 11–14 weeks

While we can identify many structures by the end of the first trimester, sonographic diagnosis of abnormalities in these structures is limited. Although first-trimester sonographic diagnosis has been reported for a wide variety of anomalies,[4,8–10] relatively few can be reliably diagnosed or excluded with confidence. The following anomalies can be reliably diagnosed or excluded sonographically in most cases at the 11–14 weeks' scan.

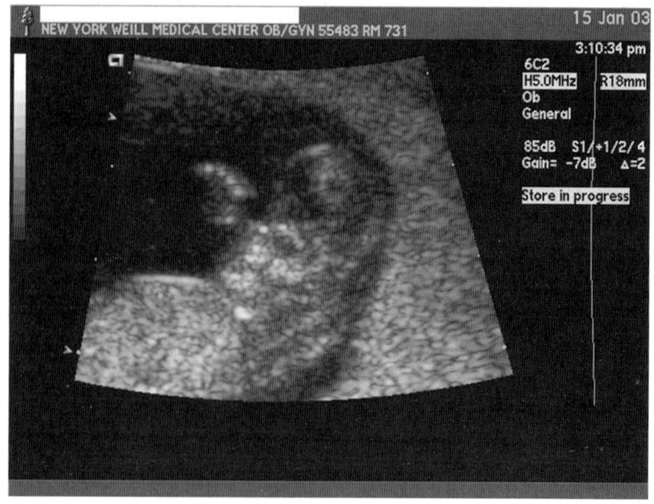

Figure 75.1 Acrania at 11 weeks' gestation. No bony structures are seen above the level of the orbits. Brain tissue can be seen. This would not be visualized in the case of anencephaly.

Anencephaly/acrania

Anencephaly and acrania are characterized by the absence of a cranial vault. Both conditions are easily identified or excluded after 10 weeks' gestation.[11] While anencephaly is characterized by absence of the cranial vault and the cerebral cortex, the latter structure can be seen in acrania (Figure 75.1). Both conditions are uniformly lethal. While there is some controversy as to whether acrania is due to failed closure of the rostral portion of the neural tube (as is anencephaly), women should be counseled to take high doses of folic acid starting prior to conception in future pregnancies to prevent open neural tube defects.

Holoprosencephaly

This condition is due to the failure of the forebrain to cleave into hemispheres early in gestation. Alobar holoprosencephaly, in which no midline structures are noted and only a single ventricle is present, is the most severe variant. This condition should be strongly suspected when two separate choroid plexuses are not seen in a transverse view through the fetal brain. Alobar holoprosencephaly can be diagnosed or excluded after 10 weeks' gestation[12] (Figure 75.2). Semilobar and lobar holoprosencephaly, in which some form of midline division has occurred, cannot always be detected prior to the second trimester.

While not lethal in all cases, alobar holoprosencephaly is associated with virtual absence of cognitive function. Cytogenetic studies are indicated, as this abnormality is associated with trisomy 13 as well as other less common forms of aneuploidy. As holoprosencephaly has been described to have autosomal recessive inheritance in some families,[13] recurrence can be excluded with identification of normal midline structures by the end of the first trimester.

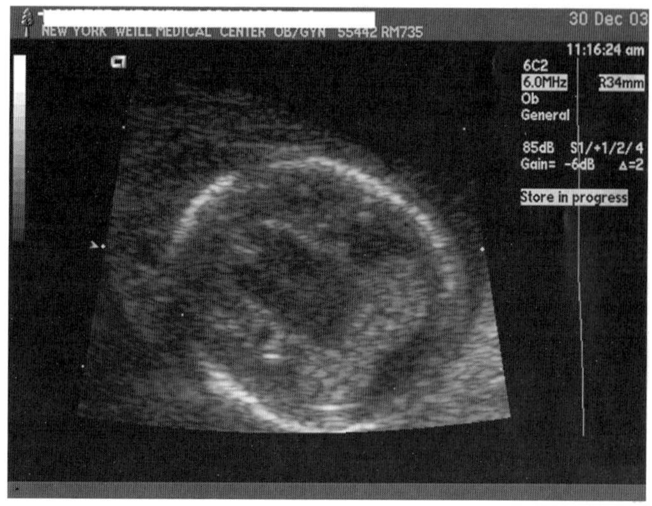

Figure 75.2 Alobar holoprosencephaly at 12 weeks' gestation. A single, small crescent-shaped holoventricle is seen anteriorly. The thalami are large, and not divided by a third ventricle. Separate choroid plexuses are not seen.

Cephalocele

Cephalocele is characterized by a defect in the skull, with protrusion of the meninges. In most cases, there will be brain tissue in the meningeal sac (encephalocele). Most midline cephaloceles are open neural tube defects, though they are much less common than either anencephaly or spina bifida. When a non-midline cephalocele is detected, amniotic band syndrome may be present.

Ultrasound can detect cephalocele at 11–14 weeks (Figure 75.3). Large cephaloceles are easily identified, though smaller ones may not be seen early in pregnancy. In patients with a prior fetus with Meckel–Gruber syndrome, which is characterized by cephalocele, multicystic kidneys, and polydactyly, first-trimester ultrasound can be used to detect early signs of recurrence of this autosomal recessive condition.[14]

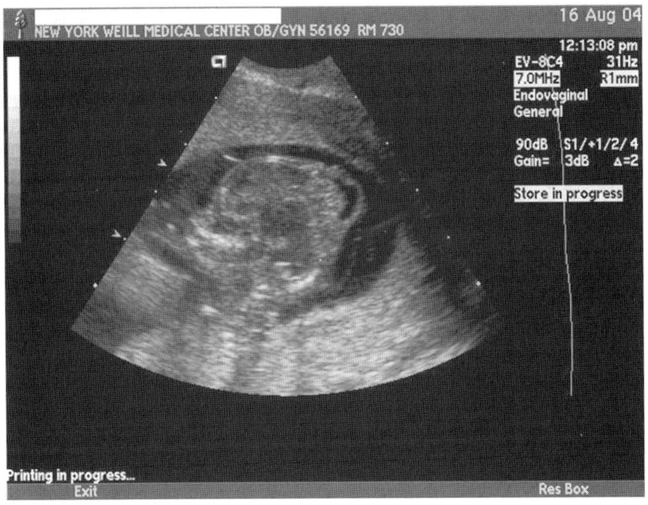

Figure 75.3 Encephalocele at 12 weeks' gestation. In this profile view, a midline skull defect is seen above the level of the occiput.

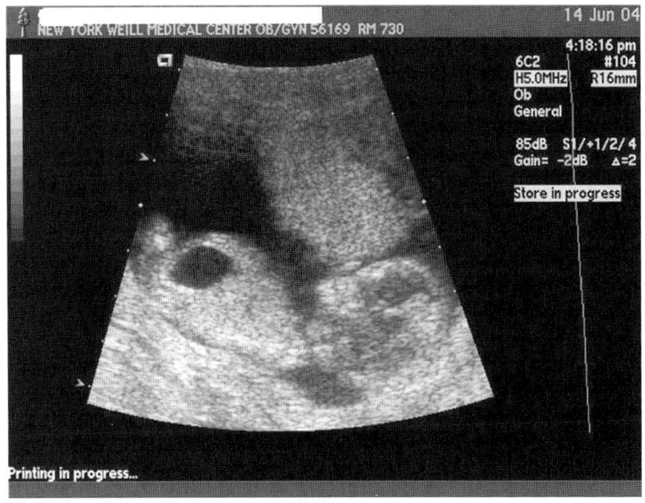

Figure 75.5 Megacystis at 11 weeks' gestation. A cystic midline mass is seen in the pelvis.

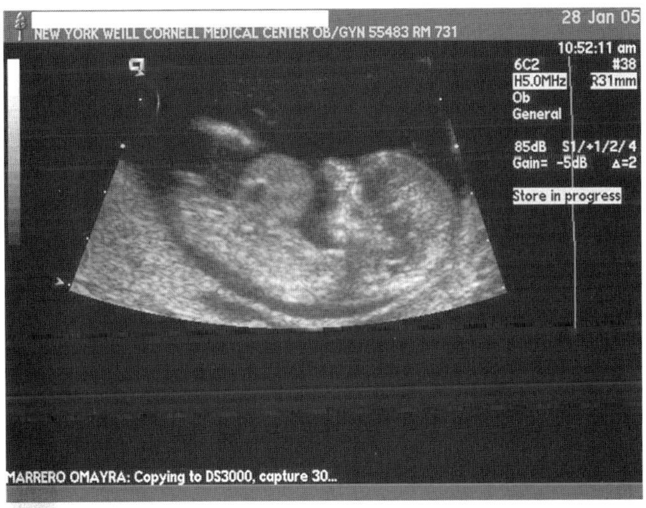

Figure 75.4 Omphalocele at 13 weeks' gestation. A large sac containing bowel and liver is seen.

Omphalocele

Omphalocele is a midline ventral wall defect. All layers of the abdominal wall are absent at the site of the umbilical cord insertion, and a sac can be seen protruding from this site. The sac usually contains bowel and stomach. In larger lesions, liver may be present. The umbilical cord can be seen inserting into the sac.

It is important not to confuse physiologic midgut herniation, which occurs prior to 11–12 weeks' gestation, with omphalocele.[15] After 12 weeks' gestation, omphalocele, particularly if a large defect is present, is easily identified (Figure 75.4). Omphalocele is frequently associated with trisomy 18 or trisomy 13.

Skeletal defects

Though fetal long bones can be identified and measured late in the first trimester, most skeletal dysplasias that are characterized by abnormal limb growth cannot be reliably detected or excluded early in pregnancy.[16] Limb reduction defects, which occur sporadically, are characterized by the absence of all or a large part of an extremity, which can be identified at the 11–14 weeks' scan.

Megacystis

In this condition, the fetal urinary bladder is markedly enlarged (Figure 75.5). A longitudinal diameter of > 7 mm has been suggested to establish the diagnosis.[17] While the presence of megacystis does not indicate a specific diagnosis, high rates of fetal aneuploidy (especially when NT is abnormal) and obstructive uropathy have been reported.[18] The presence of megacystis is an indication to evaluate the genitourinary tract for obstructive uropathy early in the second trimester.

Approach to screening

In patients who present for ultrasound late in the first trimester, evaluation of fetal anatomy can provide valuable information. This information can be obtained in a relatively short amount of time in most patients.[4,6] While certain findings (such as nuchal edema or megacystis) are not diagnostic and require second-trimester follow-up, some conditions can be diagnosed or excluded at this stage in pregnancy. This may be especially useful to those at high risk of having a fetus with malformations detectable in the first trimester.

Studies evaluating the detection rates for anomalies in the first trimester suggest that the majority of major structural anomalies can be identified or suspected.[4,8,9] As these studies have been done in large perinatal centers, however, it is not clear that similar outcomes can be achieved outside this setting. The experience of the examiner is important, as a learning curve for prenatal diagnosis in the first trimester has been demonstrated.[9]

While evaluation of anatomy at 11–14 weeks is recommended when NT is measured, this examination cannot replace routine second-trimester ultrasound. Comparison of detection rates of fetal anomalies demonstrates higher sensitivity at 16–20 weeks.[9] This is particularly true for cardiac abnormalities, the most common category of malformations.

Conclusion

With the emergence of first-trimester risk assessment for aneuploidy, many patients will be undergoing ultrasound late in the first trimester. If the sole objective of this examination is to measure NT, the opportunity to assess fetal anatomy will be lost. With experience, examination of the fetus at 11–14 weeks' gestation can be accomplished in a short period of time, and patients will have the benefit of early diagnosis of certain anomalies.

REFERENCES

1. Nicolaides KH. Nuchal translucency and other first-trimester sonographic markers of chromosomal abnormalities. *Am J Obstet Gynecol* 2004;191:45–67.
2. Hyett JA. Increased nuchal translucency in fetuses with a normal karyotype. *Prenat Diagn* 2002;22:864–8.
3. Whitlow BJ, Chatzipapas IK, Lazanakis ML, Kadir RA, Economides DL. The value of sonography in early pregnancy for the detection of fetal abnormalities in an unselected population. *Br J Obstet Gynaecol* 1999;106:929–36.
4. Souka AP, Nicolaides KH. Diagnosis of fetal abnormalities at the 10–14-week scan. *Ultrasound Obstet Gynecol* 1997;10:429–42.
5. Cicero S, Curcio P, Papageorghiou A, Sonek J, Nicolaides K. Absence of nasal bone in fetuses with trisomy 21 at 11–14 weeks of gestation: An observational study. *Lancet* 2001;358:1665–7.
6. Timor-Tritsch IE, Bashiri A, Monteagudo A, Arslan AA. Qualified and trained sonographers in the US can perform early fetal anatomy scans between 11 and 14 weeks. *Am J Obstet Gynecol* 2004;191:1247–52.
7. Zorzoli A, Kustermann A, Caravelli E, *et al.* Measurements of fetal limb bones in early pregnancy. *Ultrasound Obstet Gynecol* 1994;4:29–33.
8. Chen M, Lam YH, Lee CP, Tang MH. Ultrasound screening of fetal structural abnormalities at 12 to 14 weeks in Hong Kong. *Prenat Diagn* 2004;24:92–7.
9. Taipale P, Ammala M, Salonen R, Hiilesmaa V. Learning curve in ultrasonographic screening for selected fetal structural anomalies in early pregnancy. *Obstet Gynecol* 2003;101:273–8.
10. Dugoff L. Ultrasound diagnosis of structural abnormalities in the first trimester. *Prenat Diagn* 2002;22:316–20.
11. Johnson SP, Sebire NJ, Snijders RJ, Tunkel S, Nicolaides KH. Ultrasound screening for anencephaly at 10–14 weeks of gestation. *Ultrasound Obstet Gynecol* 1997;9:14–6.
12. Sepulveda W, Dezerega V, Be C. First-trimester sonographic diagnosis of holoprosencephaly: Value of the "butterfly" sign. *J Ultrasound Med* 2004;23:761–5.
13. Barr M Jr, Cohen MM Jr. Autosomal recessive alobar holoprosencephaly with essentially normal faces. *Am J Med Genet* 2002; 112:28–30.
14. Tanriverdi HA, Hendrik HJ, Ertan K, Schmidt W. Meckel–Gruber syndrome: A first trimester diagnosis of a recurrent case. *Eur J Ultrasound* 2002;15:69–72.
15. van Zalen-Sprock RM, Vugt JM, van Geijn HP. First-trimester sonography of physiological midgut herniation and early diagnosis of omphalocele. *Prenat Diagn* 1997;17:511–8.
16. Gabrielli S, Falco P, Pilu G, Perolo A, Milano V, Bovicelli L. Can transvaginal fetal biometry be considered a useful tool for early detection of skeletal dysplasias in high-risk patients? *Ultrasound Obstet Gynecol* 1999;13:107–11.
17. Sebire NJ, Von Kaisenberg C, Rubio C, Snijders RJ, Nicolaides KH. Fetal megacystis at 10–14 weeks of gestation. *Ultrasound Obstet Gynecol* 1996;8:387–90.
18. Sepulveda W. Megacystis in the first trimester. *Prenat Diagn* 2004;24:144–9.

76 Fetal nasal bone in screening for Down's syndrome

S. Cicero, J. D. Sonek, G. Rembouskos and K. H. Nicolaides

Introduction

Chromosomal abnormalities represent a major cause of perinatal death and childhood disabilities. Prenatal diagnosis of chromosomal defects necessitates invasive testing. All of the commonly used invasive techniques such as chorionic villus sampling, amniocentesis, and cordocentesis, are associated with a risk of fetal loss risk of about 1%. For this reason, invasive procedures are reserved for pregnancies considered to be at high risk for chromosomal defects. The methods of screening to identify the high-risk group are described in Table 76.1. Screening using ultrasound is based on the fact that most fetuses with chromosomal abnormalities deviate phenotypically from euploid fetuses and many of these deviations can be detected by prenatal ultrasound.

Improvements in ultrasound resolution have allowed us to evaluate and measure very minute fetal structures with a concomitant decrease in the room for error. If they are to be included in prenatal screening protocols, their evaluation must be done with a high degree of precision and accuracy. This can be accomplished only through strict standardization of the fetal image and with appropriate training and an ongoing quality assurance. It is only by strictly adhering to these principles that ultrasound markers can be incorporated into any screening protocol.

Calculation of the individual patient-specific risk of chromosomal defects requires the incorporation of several factors. The first is the background risk, which is based on the maternal age, gestational age, and historical factors such as a previous offspring with aneuploidy. The background risk is then modified by multiplying it by a series of likelihood ratios, which are based on the results of screening tests (ultrasound and biochemical) carried out during the course of the pregnancy. A series of likelihood ratios can be used in such a fashion to adjust the risk of aneuploidy either at the same time in pregnancy (combined screening) or at different times in pregnancy[1] (disclosure and nondisclosure sequential screening).

Table 76.1 The screening performance of the various tests is compared by examining the detection rate (DR) for a fixed screen positive rate of 5%

Screening test	DR (%)
MA (≥37 years)	30
Maternal serum biochemistry at 16 weeks (AFP and β-hCG and uE3)	65
NT at 12 weeks	80
NT and β-hCG and P-APPA at 12 weeks	90
NT and NB and β-hCG and P-APPA at 12 weeks	96

MA, maternal age; AFP, α-fetoprotein; β-hCG, free β-human chorionic gonadotropin; uE3, unconjugated estriol; NT, nuchal translucency; PAPP-A, pregnancy-associated plasma protein-A; NB, nasal bone.

Background

The physical characteristics of individuals affected by trisomy 21 were initially described by Langdon Down[2] in 1866. He reported that their skin is too large for their body, their face is flat, and the nose is small.[2] In recent years it has become possible to observe these features by ultrasound examination even as early as in the third month of intrauterine life. Extensive studies over the last 15 years have demonstrated that the most effective sonographic marker of trisomy 21, and other chromosomal abnormalities, is increased nuchal translucency (NT) at $11–13^{+6}$ weeks' gestation. Another promising marker for trisomy 21, which has been extensively studied over the past 5 years, is the absence and hypoplasia of the fetal nasal bones (NB).

This chapter reviews evidence for the association between absence or hypoplasia of the fetal nasal bones and Down's syndrome in the first and second trimester of pregnancy, and examines the value of incorporating this novel marker in screening policies.

Development of the nasal bones

During the fourth week of gestation, collections of neural crest cells undergo proliferation, forming the nasal placodes. In the sixth week, the nasal placodes of the frontonasal prominence invaginate to form the nasal pits and the lateral and medial processes. The medial nasal processes eventually fuse with the nasofrontal process to form the nasal septum, which in turn grows toward the forming palate, defining the left and right nasal cavities. The cartilaginous frame of the nose is developing at the same time. During the eighth week, initial centers of ossification of the NB appear in the membrane covering the cartilaginous nasal capsule.[3–7]

In 1994 Sandikcioglu *et al.*[8] established standards for the normal prenatal development of the NB. This study showed that the left and right NBs appear as a thin bony contour ventral to the cartilaginous nasal septum in the sagittal plane, and change gradually during growth to wedge-shaped bones. The initial appearance of the NB occurred at different developmental stages in normal fetuses. The smallest crown–rump length (CRL) at which NB was observed histologically was 42 mm corresponding to approximately 10.9 weeks' gestation. Furthermore, the NB was noted to increase in length with advancing gestation and its morphology changes, being overall wider and coming to a sharp point at the anterior tip in the most mature specimens.[8]

Anthropometric and radiological studies

An anthropometric study of 105 patients with Down's syndrome at 7 months to 36 years of age reported that the nasal root depth was abnormally short in about 50% of cases.[9] Keeling *et al.*[10] investigated the abnormal development of the NB in aborted Down's syndrome fetuses. They examined the development of the axial skeleton in 31 human trisomy 21 aborted fetuses at 12–24 weeks' gestation and found a 60% incidence of either NB absence (26%) or NB hypoplasia (34%).[10] Stempfle *et al.*[11] conducted a radiological study and found that the NB was absent in 23% of the 60 Down's syndrome aborted fetuses between 15 and 40 weeks' gestation. The authors also observed that, when present, the NB in the Down's syndrome fetuses was short.[11]

Sonographic, radiological, and histological correlation

Tuxen *et al.*[12] conducted a postmortem radiological study to investigate the presence of the NB in 33 aborted Down's syndrome fetuses at 14–25 weeks' gestation. They found that 30% (10 of 33) of fetuses had either bilateral or unilateral absence of NB. They also performed a histological evaluation of the specimens, which confirmed a complete NB absence in 7 of 10 fetuses. Histological evaluation was not performed in the remaining three, including the two that had unilateral absence of the NB. Presence of an NB was confirmed in all 23 fetuses that had a radiological evidence of NB formation.[12]

Minderer and his colleagues[13] compared prenatal sonographic evaluations of the NB in 17 Down's syndrome fetuses between 11 and 14 weeks' gestation, to those obtained by histological study performed after termination of pregnancy. In this report, the NB could not be examined sonographically in 1 of the 17 cases, due to fetal position, and in the remaining 16 cases the NB was either absent or hypoplastic. By contrast, the histological evaluation of the NB area showed evidence of NB formation in 16 of the 17 cases. Armed with the knowledge of the results of the histological evaluation, the investigators reviewed the ultrasound images of the fetuses originally classified as having an absent NB. They claimed that they were able to now detect evidence of an NB albeit 'smaller, less distinct, and less echogenic'.[13]

A study by Larose *et al.*[14] compared sonographic and radiological findings on the NB in 21 aborted fetuses with trisomy 21. The ultrasonographic evaluations were done between 11^{+3} and 13^{+5} weeks' gestation. The subsequent radiological studies on the aborted fetuses were performed between 13 and 25^{+5} weeks' gestation. Interestingly, the incidence of NB absence on ultrasound was very similar to the one noted on x-ray. However, the ultrasound and x-ray findings were discordant in 9 of the 21 cases (43%). Four of the cases where the NB was present on ultrasound showed no evidence of an NB on x-ray, indicating a possible wrong assessment of the fetal profile by ultrasound. In the other five cases where the NB was noted to be absent on ultrasound, an NB was seen on the x-ray. However, radiological examinations were performed at a later gestational age than that of the ultrasound examination,[14] allowing time between the two examinations for further NB development.

The apparent discrepancies in the NB identification among the three modalities (ultrasound, radiology, and histology) have a number of possible explanations. It is likely that small areas of calcification can be seen on histological evaluation even if those cannot be detected on either ultrasonography or x-ray. The likelihood of picking these up will depend on the number of sections done. Different types of staining were used in the two studies[12,13] mentioned above possibly contributing to the contradictory results. In the study by Larose *et al.*,[14] the ultrasounds and the x-rays were done at very different gestational ages (11^{+3}–13^{+5} weeks for ultrasound and 13–25^{+5} weeks for x-ray). Since the prevalence of NB absence changes with gestational age, they are not truly comparable. Just as is the case with the ultrasound examination, controlling for the gestational age and standardization of the technique for both the radiological and the histological examinations is crucial.

Sonographic studies

The observation that in fetuses affected by trisomy 21 sonographic examination may reveal absence of the NB was only made at the beginning of 2001. In the initial description by Sonek and Nicolaides,[15] three Down's syndrome fetuses were evaluated in the second trimester. Two of them had no identifiable NB and one had a hypoplastic NB. A review of the videotaped exam from the first trimester examination of one of the fetuses at the time of the NT evaluation revealed that the NB could not be identified at that point in pregnancy.[15] Armed with this information, observational studies were undertaken to investigate the role of NB examination in screening for Down's syndrome.

First trimester: the 11–13^{+6}-week scan

Several studies have demonstrated that the fetal NB can be visualized by sonography in the first trimester of pregnancy, and that there is a high association between absent NB at 11–13^{+6} weeks and trisomy 21, as well as other chromosomal abnormalities.[16–25]

Cicero *et al.*[16] reported for the first time on the absence of the NB in trisomy 21 fetuses in the first trimester of pregnancy. In this observational study, ultrasound was used to determine the presence or absence of the NB in 701 fetuses at 11–13^{+6} weeks' gestation following screening by maternal age and NT, and immediately before chorionic villus sampling. The NB was noted to be absent in 73% (43 of 59) of Down's syndrome fetuses and in only 0.5% (3 of 603) of chromosomally normal fetuses. In this initial study, presence or absence of the NB was found to be independent of other fetal and maternal variables. It became clear that incorporation of the examination of the NB into screening for trisomy 21 by maternal age and NT could increase the sensitivity of the test and reduce the false positive rate.[16]

In an extended series[18] of 5918 fetuses undergoing prenatal diagnosis by chorionic villous sampling at 11–13^{+6} weeks, the fetal profile was successfully examined in 5851 (98.9%) cases. The NB was absent in 129 of 5223 (2.5%) chromosomally normal fetuses, in 229 of 333 (68.8%) fetuses with trisomy 21 and in 95 of the 295 (32%) with other chromosomal defects. An additional important finding of this study is that the prevalence of NB absence was higher in fetuses of Afro-Caribbean origin than in Caucasians (Table 76.2). The prevalence was also noted to decrease as the gestational age increased (Table 76.3) and to increase as the NT measurement increased beyond the normal range (Table 76.4). Consequently, in the calculation of an individual patient-specific risk for trisomy 21 it is necessary to take into account these demographic and ultrasound findings.[18]

The fact that ethnic origin of the mother may play a role on the evaluation of the fetal NB, was also suggested by Prefumo *et al.*[26] The authors conducted a prospective study in 4492 fetuses and demonstrated that having a mother of African origin is significantly associated with an increased likelihood of absent fetal NB compared with Caucasians, even after correcting for maternal age, parity, and CRL.

There are seven additional studies[19–25] that support the high association between trisomy 21 and absent NB at 11–13^{+6} weeks. In their combined data on 12,315 fetuses the fetal profile was successfully examined in about 97% of cases. The NB was absent in

Table 76.2 Prevalence of absent nasal bone (NB) in chromosomally normal and trisomy 21 fetuses and likelihood ratio (LR) according to ethnic group (from Cicero *et al.*[18])

			LR (95% CI) for trisomy 21	
Ethnic group	**Trisomy 21; *n* (%)**	**Normal karyotype; *n* (%)**	**NB absent**	**NB present**
Total (*n*=5851)	229/333 (68.8)	129/5223 (2.5)	27.8 (23.1–33.5)	0.32 (0.27–0.37)
Caucasian (*n*=5384)	207/303 (68.3)	105/4811 (2.2)	31.3 (25.5–38.4)	0.32 (0.27–0.38)
Afro-Caribbean (*n*=170)	11/14 (78.6)	13/145 (9.0)	8.8 (4.7–15.5)	0.24 (0.08–0.52)
Asian* (*n*=201)	10/14 (71.4)	9/179 (5.0)	14.2 (6.8–28.4)	0.30 (0.12–0.58)
Chinese/Japanese (*n*=69)	1/2 (50.0)	2/61 (3.3)	15.3 (2.1–73.4)	0.52 (0.10–0.94)
Mixed (*n*=27)	—	0/27 (—)	—	—

*People originating from India, Pakistan, Bangladesh, Sri Lanka and Philippines.

Table 76.3 Prevalence of absent nasal bone (NB) in chromosomally normal and trisomy 21 fetuses and likelihood ratio (LR) according to crown–rump length (CRL) (from Cicero *et al.*[18])

			LR (95% CI) for trisomy 21	
CRL (mm)	Trisomy 21; *n* (%)	Normal karyotype; *n* (%)	NB absent	NB present
Total (*n*=5851)	229/333 (68.8)	129/5223 (2.5)	27.8 (23.1–33.5)	0.32 (0.27–0.37)
45–54	41/49 (83.7)	32/675 (4.7)	17.6 (12.3–25.2)	0.17 (0.09–0.30)
55–64	78/118 (66.1)	63/1850 (3.4)	19.4 (14.7–25.5)	0.35 (0.27–0.44)
65–74	85/118 (72.0)	25/1805 (1.4)	52.0 (34.8–77.8)	0.28 (0.21–0.37)
75–84	25/48 (52.1)	9/893 (1.0)	51.8 (25.8–102.8)	0.48 (0.35–0.62)

Table 76.4 Prevalence of absent nasal bone (NB) in chromosomally normal and trisomy 21 fetuses and likelihood ratio (LR) according to nuchal translucency thickness (NT) (from Cicero *et al.*[18])

			LR (95% CI) for trisomy 21	
NT (mm)	Trisomy 21 *n* (%)	Normal karyotype; *n* (%)	NB absent	NB present
Total (*n*=5851)	229/333 (68.8)	129/5223 (2.5)	27.8 (23.1–33.5)	0.32 (0.27–0.37)
≤95th	23/38 (60.5)	53/3245 (1.6)	37.1 (25.0–52.5)	0.40 (0.26–0.56)
> 95th–3.4	48/83 (57.8)	40/1500 (2.7)	25.1 (16.7–37.4)	0.45 (0.34–0.56)
3.5–4.4	49/67 (73.1)	16/294 (5.4)	13.4 (8.2–22.1)	0.28 (0.19–0.41)
4.5–5.4	26/41 (63.4)	5/84 (6.0)	10.7 (4.6–25.3)	0.39 (0.25–0.55)
≥5.5	83/104 (79.8)	15/100 (15.0)	5.3 (3.4–8.7)	0.24 (0.16–0.34)

about 1% of chromosomally normal fetuses and in 67% of the fetuses with trisomy 21.

Malone *et al.*[27] reported the results of a multicenter study which included 6316 fetuses scanned at 10–14 weeks' gestation. The nasal bone could be evaluated in only 75.9% of the cases. The NB was apparently present in all nine of the trisomy 21 fetuses where the NB could be evaluated. Their results contrast with the above published studies in a number of ways. The fact that the fetal nose could be examined only in 75.9% of the cases bring up questions regarding the level of training involved in this study and the fact that the NB was reported as being present in all nine trisomy 21 fetuses bring up questions regarding the technique. Furthermore, images published by the lead authors of this study suggest that their technique may not be consistent with that used by others.[28] Similarly, De Biasio and Venturini,[29] who retrospectively examined the images obtained for measurement of NT, reported that the NB was present in all five fetuses with trisomy 21. However, the five images that they published did not meet accepted criteria for either the measurement of NT or for examination of the NB.

Based on the vast majority of the currently available data (Table 76.5), it can be concluded that at 11–13^{+6} weeks the fetal profile can be successfully examined in about 98% of cases. The NB is absent in about 65% of trisomy 21 fetuses but only in about 1% of chromosomally normal fetuses.[16–25] Consequently, absence of the NB is an important marker of trisomy 21. However, appropriate adjustments need to be made on the basis of maternal ethnic origin, fetal CRL and NT when calculation of individual patient-specific risk for trisomy 21 is performed.[18]

Second trimester: 15–24-week scan

Absence or hypoplasia of the NB represents a new ultrasound marker in the second trimester of pregnancy as well, and it is likely to have a major impact on screening for trisomy 21 during the 16–24-week scan. Its benefit has now been confirmed in large trials.

Bromley *et al.*[30] assessed the NB using ultrasound in 239 fetuses between 15 and 20 weeks' gestation. Six (37%) of the 16 Down's syndrome fetuses had no

Table 76.5 Summary of studies reporting on the prevalence of absent nasal bone in first-trimester trisomy 21 fetuses

			Absent nasal bone	
Author(s)	**Study**	**Successful examination; n (%)**	**Normal; n (%)**	**Trisomy 21; n (%)**
Cicero *et al.* (2001)[16*]	Pre-CVS	701/701 (100)	3/603 (0.5)	43/59 (72.9)
Otano *et al.* 2002[19]	Pre-CVS	183/194 (94.3)	1/175 (0.6)	3/5 (60.0)
Zoppi *et al.* 2003[20]	Screening	5525/5532 (99.8)	7/3463 (0.2)	19/27 (70.0)
Orlandi *et al.* (2003)[21]	Screening	1027/1089 (94.3)	10/1000 (1.0)	10/15 (66.7)
Viora *et al.* (2003)[22]	Screening	1752/1906 (91.9)	24/1733 (1.4)	8/10 (80.0)
Senat *et al.* (2003)[23]	Retrospective	956/1040 (91.9)	4/944 (0.4)	3/4 (75)
Wong *et al.* (2003)[24]	Pre-CVS	119/143 (83.2)	1/114 (0.9)	2/3 (66.7)
Cicero *et al.* (2003)[17*]	Pre-CVS	3788/3829 (98.9)	93/3358 (2.8)	162/242 (67)
Cicero *et al.* (2004)[18]	Pre-CVS	5851/5918 (98.9)	129/5223 (2.5)	229/333 (68.8)
Orlandi *et al.* (2005)[25]	Screening	2411/2411 (100)	9/2396 (0.4)	8/15 (53.3)
Total		17,824/18,133 (98.3)	185/15,048 (1.2)	282/412 (68.4)

*Included in Cicero *et al.* (2004)[18].

detectable NB. Among the fetuses with a normal karyotype, absence of the NB had a prevalence of 0.5%. In this study, absence of the NB was associated with a likelihood ratio for Down's syndrome of 83. Interestingly, in 2 of the 16 (13%) Down's syndrome fetuses, NB absence was the only abnormal finding. In addition, the NB length was found to play an important role. Biparietal diameter (BPD) to NB length (NBL) ratio was generated to control for the gestational age and the size of the fetus. This ratio increases as the NB becomes shorter. Using the BPD/NBL ratio of 10 or greater as a cut off in screening for Down's syndrome gives this test sensitivity of 81% with a false positive rate of 11%. This study confirmed that NB length increases linearly with gestation in chromosomally normal fetuses. However, the NB length in Down's syndrome fetuses was found to be uniform over the gestational age investigated (3.5 ±0.47 mm) suggesting the possibility that a single cut-off value for NB length may be appropriate in Down's syndrome screening in the first half of the second trimester.[30]

Such approach was used in another study[31] looking at the utility of NB evaluation in the second trimester (15–22 weeks). The authors examined the fetal profile in 1046 singleton pregnancies undergoing amniocentesis for fetal karyotyping at 15–22 weeks. The NB was absent or hypoplastic (< 2.5 mm) in 21 of the 34 (61.8%) fetuses with Down's syndrome, in 12 of 982 (1.2%) chromosomally normal fetuses, and in 1 of the 30 (3.3%) with other chromosomal defects. It was noted that the prevalence of NB hypoplasia was higher in the euploid Afro-Caribbean population (8.8%) in comparison to the Caucasian population (0.5%), suggesting for the first time that adjustments based on ethnicity may need to be made when using the NB for screening in the second trimester as well. Furthermore, the overall likelihood ratio for trisomy 21 for hypoplastic NB was 50.5 (95% CI 27.1–92.7) and for present NB it was 0.38 (95% CI 0.24–0.56).[31]

Bunduki *et al.*[32] looked at the utility of NB measurement in the second trimester (16–24 weeks' gestation) in 1631 patients. The association between hypoplasia of the NB and Down's syndrome was also demonstrated. Using the 5th percentile of the normal curves generated in the same study as a cut off for screening for trisomy 21, a sensitivity of 59% was achieved.[32]

Vintzileos *et al.*[33] looked retrospectively at profiles of 29 Down's syndrome fetuses between 17.7 and 20.7 weeks' gestation. The NB was absent in 12 of the 29 (41%) fetuses with trisomy 21 and in none of the 102 chromosomally normal fetuses.[33]

A prospective study involving ultrasound evaluation of the fetal NB between 19 and 22 weeks' gestation[34] also looked at the utility of NB length and its presence or absence in screening for Down's syndrome. The normal NB ranges were based on examinations of 1913 fetuses. All five Down's syndrome fetuses in the study had either an absent NB or a NB length below the 2.5th percentile. None of the fetuses with other chromosomal abnormalities had a short or absent NB.[34]

It is premature to speculate on the precise detection rates that could be achieved in the second trimester by a combination of maternal age, serum biochemistry, and ultrasound examination for the fetal NB and other sonographic markers. Nevertheless, on the basis of currently available data, nasal hypoplasia is likely to be the single most sensitive and specific second trimester marker of trisomy 21.

Ultrasound examination of the nasal bone: technique

Ultrasound evaluation of the NB requires strict adherence to standard criteria and it is essential that the operators performing this examination undergo adequate training and gain extensive experience.[35,36]

The need for adequate training is highlighted by a study published in 2003,[37] which looked at the extent of training needed for 15 sonographers experienced in measuring fetal NT, to become competent in examining the fetal NB at 11^{+0}–13^{+6} weeks' gestation. The study demonstrated that the number of supervised scans required to achieve proficiency is on average 80 with a range of 40–120. However, evaluation of the NB does not appear to significantly impact the length of the ultrasound examination.[37]

This was confirmed in a study of 501 consecutively scanned fetuses by experienced sonographers. The authors reported that the fetal NB could be successfully examined and measured in all cases without extending the length of time required for scanning.[38]

With a few minor exceptions, the method of NB evaluation is very similar in both the first and second trimesters of pregnancy. The NB should be seen as an echogenic line within the nasal bridge, i.e., underneath the nasal skin. This is usually not a difficult task in the second trimester. The following is a description of the technique at 11–13^{+6} weeks' gestation:

1. The fetal CRL should be 45–84 mm. There is no value on examining the fetal NB before this gestational age, as the NB first appears at a CRL of 42 mm.[8]
2. The image should be magnified so that the head and the upper thorax only are included in the screen (Figures 76.1 and 76.2).
3. A mid-sagittal view of the fetal profile should be obtained with the ultrasound transducer held in parallel to the direction of the nose (i.e., ultrasound beam perpendicular to longitudinal axis of the NB). The ultrasound transducer should then be gently tilted from side to side to ensure that the NB is seen separate from the nasal skin. The fetus should be facing the transducer.
4. When the correct view is obtained, three distinct lines will be visualized: the first two lines, which are close to the forehead, are horizontal and parallel to each other resembling an 'equal sign' (Figure 76.1). The top line represents the skin and the bottom one, which is usually thicker and more echogenic than the overlying skin, represents the NB. Therefore, it is the absence of the bottom line of the 'equal sign' that represents absence of the NB (Figure 76.2). A third line located distally to the 'equal sign' and at a slightly higher level, represents the tip of the nose.
5. If the bottom line of the 'equal sign' is completely absent, the diagnosis of NB absence is fairly straightforward. Occasionally, a line that is thinner and less echogenic than the skin line is noted within the nasal bridge. This may either represent a NB that is not yet ossified or an unusually prominent cartilage. Either way, this finding should also be classified as nasal bone absence. Similarly, the

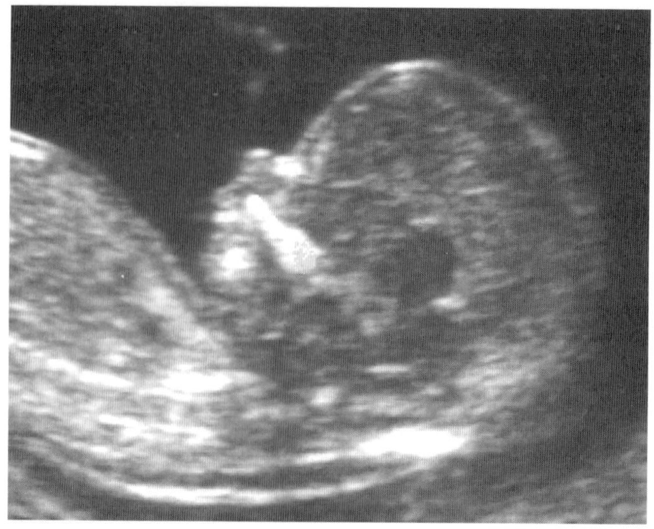

Figure 76.1 Fetal profile at 12 weeks of gestation in a normal fetus showing the nasal bone.

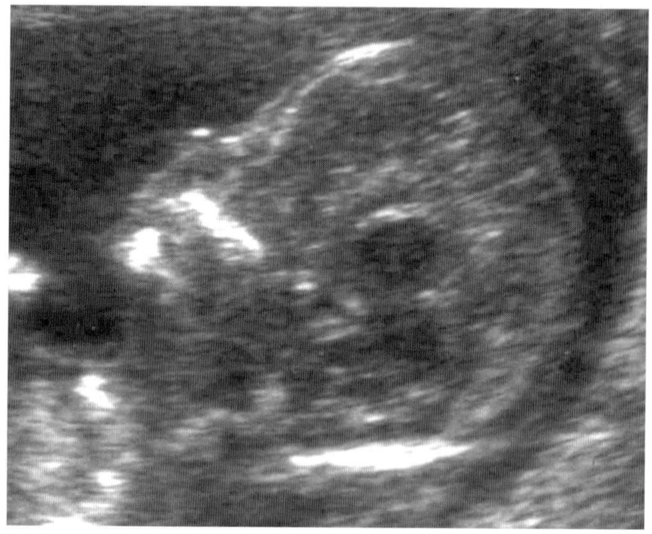

Figure 76.2 Fetal profile at 12 weeks of gestation in a trisomy 21 fetus showing absence of the nasal bone.

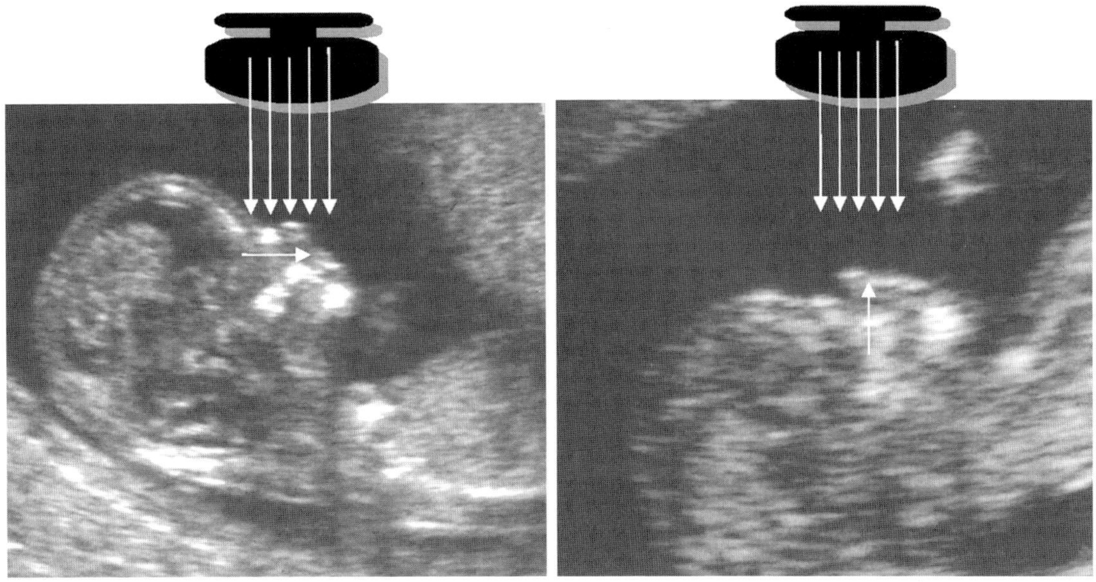

Figure 76.3 The best angle of insonation to assess the nasal bone in the first trimester is 90° to the longitudinal axis of the nasal bone (i.e., the beam of the ultrasound perpendicular to the longitudinal axis of the nasal bone) (left). Evaluation of the nasal bone should not be attempted with either a 0° or 180° angle of insonation (i.e., with the ultrasound beam parallel to the longitudinal axis of the nasal bone) (right).

presence of a tiny echogenic dot that can occasionally be seen in the area of the nasal bone should not be interpreted as NB presence.

6. If the NB is noted to be absent at $11–11^{+6}$ weeks' gestation, it is our recommendation to repeat the examination 1–2 weeks later because of the relatively high false positive rate at this early gestational age. Risk assessment is based on the results of the repeat examination.

Two techniques for caliper placement have been employed to measure the NB in the first trimester of pregnancy: measuring the central hyperechogenic region only or including the entire length of the echogenic line.[21,39]

The angle of insonation used to evaluate the NB is extremely important. The best angle of insonation used to simply differentiate between the presence and the absence of the NB is 90° to the longitudinal axis of the NB (i.e., the beam of the ultrasound perpendicular to the longitudinal axis of the NB) (Figure 76.3). Evaluation of the NB should not be attempted with either a 0° or 180° angle of insonation (i.e., with the ultrasound beam parallel to the longitudinal axis of the NB) (Figure 76.3). At this angle, the NB is insonated at its thinnest dimension and the lateral resolution of the ultrasound equipment available today is not sufficient to reliably detect the NB in this view. When the transducer is adjusted to an angle of insonation approaching 45° or 135°, the lateral scatter at the ends of the NB is reduced rendering the NB ends as more sharply delineated (Figure 76.4). This is helpful in the second trimester to improve the accuracy of NB length measurement. Figures 76.5–76.7 show absence, hypoplasia, and presence of NB in the mid-second trimester.

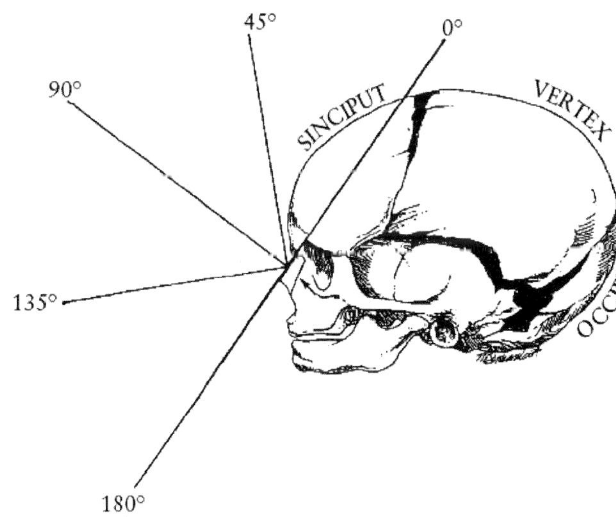

Figure 76.4 Diagrammatic representation of the bony structures of the fetal face with angles of insonation. Reprinted and adapted with permission from O'Brien W, Cefalo R. Simpson J, eds. *Obstetrics: Normal and Problem Pregnancies,* 3rd edn. New York: Churchill Livingstone, 1996:393.

Several factors make the ultrasound examination challenging; the foremost of these are maternal habitus and an unfavorable fetal position, such as hyperextension or vertical position. Others factors, such as large uterine fibroids or, early in pregnancy, retroflection of

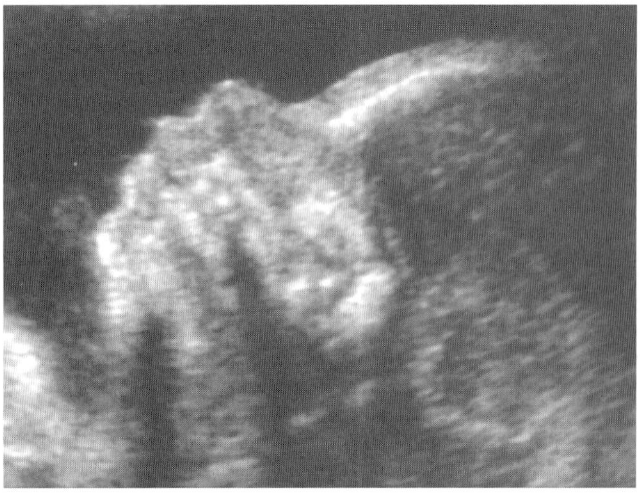

Figure 76.5 Fetal profile at 20 weeks of gestation in a trisomy 21 fetus showing absence of the nasal bone.

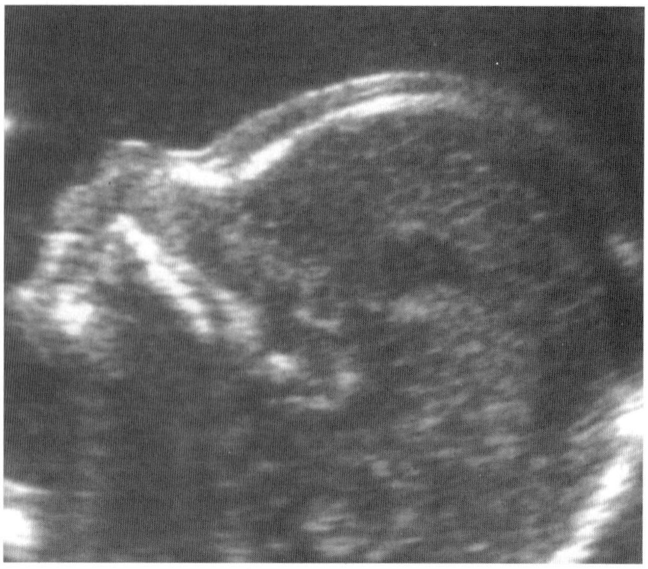

Figure 76.7 Fetal profile at 20 weeks of gestation in a normal fetus showing presence of the nasal bone.

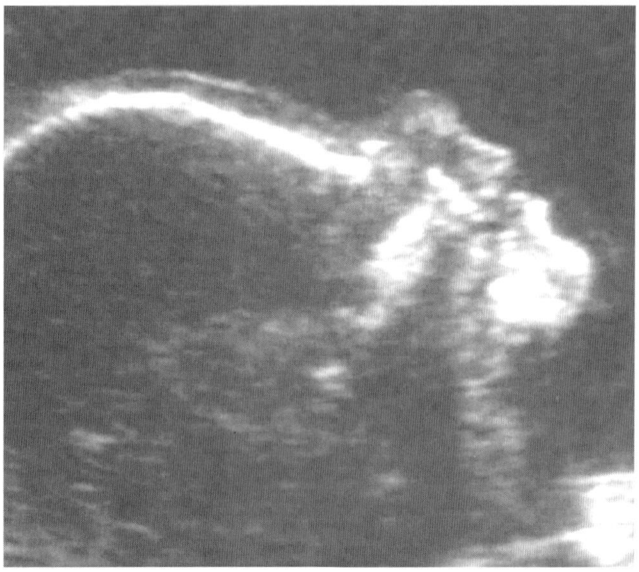

Figure 76.6 Fetal profile at 20 weeks of gestation in a trisomy 21 fetus showing absence of the nasal bone.

the uterus can also make the examination difficult. Fetal small parts, especially the hand, often lie in close proximity to the fetal face, especially early in gestation. This can lead to erroneous results in two ways. If the digits are actually resting on the fetal face they can mimic the NB. Small parts in front of the fetal face, but not actually resting on it, can produce an obscuring effect and may create an erroneous impression of NB absence. Finally, fetal face contains other echogenic structures, which are located laterally to the NB, which can give the incorrect impression that the NB is present if the correct technique is not followed. These structures include the medial aspect of the orbis oculi and the maxilla. Being able to demonstrate either the presence or the absence of the NB from several different angles will make the correct diagnosis more certain.

Occasionally, the addition of transvaginal sonography can be a helpful adjunct. However, the directions and angles with which the fetus can be viewed using this approach are limited. Rarely, the patient may need to be asked to return for a follow-up if the initial examination is not satisfactory.

Three-dimensional assessment of the nasal bones

The role of three-dimensional (3D) sonography and its potential benefit in the assessment of the fetal NB, has been investigated in the last 2 years in the first, second, and third trimesters of pregnancy. The published studies have focused on trying to overcome the technical difficulties encountered during routine two-dimensional (2D) sonography, and on further investigating aspects of the NB development, by using different techniques such as multiplanar imaging and 3D rendering of the facial bones.

First trimester of pregnancy

The two major technical problems in the assessment of the fetal NB during the $11–13^{+6}$-week scan are the need to obtain a mid-sagittal view of the fetal profile and the need for the angle between the ultrasound beam and the fetal profile to be about 45° (i.e., ultrasound beam perpendicular to the NB). In the acquired

3D volume, multiplanar imaging permits to view a true mid-sagittal section of the fetus using the optimal angle. However, in the first study published on 3D assessment of the NB in the first trimester of pregnancy, Rembouskos *et al.*[40] found that the optimal visualization of the fetal NB in a reconstructed view of the nasal bridge by 3D multiplanar imaging, is entirely dependent on the initial 2D section. In this study, the authors demonstrated that in order to obtain a good quality volume, the initial section should be taken with a sagittal view of the fetal profile facing upwards, and that the angle between the fetal profile and the ultrasound beam should be in a range of 30–60°, with maximum quality at 45°. In volumes obtained in any other initial 2D view, the visualization of the fetal NB was poor at this gestation, and could lead to an erroneous diagnosis of absent NB. Consequently, the inability to examine the NB by 2D scanning because of the fetal position cannot be overcome by 3D ultrasound.[40]

In correctly acquired volumes, 3D multiplanar mode permits further assessment of both NBs. Peralta *et al.*[41] used this technique to examine the gap between the two NBs at $11–13^{+6}$ weeks of gestation, and compared the 3D findings to those obtained following 2D examination. The authors found that a gap between the NB is present in about 20% of the fetuses examined by 3D. When the gap measured 0.6 mm or more (40% of cases), it was possible to obtain a perfect mid-sagittal plane where the NB could erroneously be considered absent. By contrast, in all cases in which the gap was less than 0.6 mm, the NB was visualized in the perfect mid-sagittal plane. These findings can be explained by the limit of the lateral resolution of the ultrasound equipment. However, none of the cases with a gap was associated with a diagnosis of absent NB when the examination was performed with the 2D scan, and therefore the false positive rate would not increase. Furthermore, the authors observed that, when using the multiplanar mode, unilateral or bilateral absence of the NB could be demonstrated in about 1% of the chromosomally normal fetuses, and in 61% of the fetuses with trisomy 21. In about 10% of trisomy 21 fetuses only one of the two NB was absent. However, all the cases with unilateral absence demonstrated with the 3D scan, were classified as 'absent' NB during the 2D ultrasound examination, and therefore the sensitivity of the test, when performed by 2D sonography, would not decrease.[41]

In the original description of the technique for examination of the fetal NB by 2D ultrasound,[16] it was suggested that, once obtained the mid-sagittal section of the fetus, the transducer should be gently tilted from one side of the fetal profile to the other, in order to adequately examine the NB. Therefore, by using this technique, it is extremely unlikely that the presence of a gap can lead to a false positive diagnosis of absent NB when 2D sonographic assessment of the NB is undertaken.[16]

Second and third trimesters of pregnancy

The role of multiplanar imaging and 3D rendering of the NB have also been evaluated in the second and third trimesters of pregnancy. It has been suggested that 3D ultrasonography allows a better description of normal, absent, hypoplastic and unilaterally absent NB.[42–44]

Lee *et al.*,[42] used the multiplanar mode to evaluate the NB of 20 fetuses with Down's syndrome and 20 fetuses with normal karyotype, between 16 and 30 weeks' gestation. Two examiners independently evaluated the same images. The prevalence of absent NB in the fetuses with Down's syndrome was 40% (8 of 20) and 45% (9 of 20) by examiner #1 and examiner #2, respectively. These results were similar to those observed by 2D sonography. However, the prevalence of absent NB in the normal population was 20% (4 of 20) and 10% (2 of 20) by examiner #1 and examiner #2, respectively. These prevalences are much higher than those reported using 2D sonography during this gestational time period (< 1.3%). These data suggest that routine application of 3D assessment of the NB in screening for trisomy 21 could increase the false positive rate.[42]

More recently, Benoit and Chaoui[44] assessed the unilateral absence of NB by using 3D rendering of the facial bones in the second and third trimesters. Out of the 20 fetuses with Down's syndrome, 9 (45%) had nasal bone absence noted on the 2D ultrasound. Six had bilateral nasal bone absence documented on the 3D ultrasound and three had unilateral absence with the discernible nasal bone being hypoplastic in two fetuses and normal in length in one. None of the 18 euploid fetuses evaluated had an absent nasal bone on 2D ultrasound and all had both nasal bones present on 3D. In this study, similarly to what Peralta *et al.*[41] found in the first trimester, in all Down's syndrome fetuses with unilateral absent NB, that the 2D assessment of the nasal bridge was consistent with an 'absent' NB.[44] It appears that unilateral nasal bone absence does not increase the false negative rate.

Integrated first-trimester sonographic and biochemical screening

A retrospective case–control study,[45] comprising 100 trisomy 21 and 400 chromosomally normal singleton pregnancies at $11–13^{+6}$ weeks of gestation, and a subsequent study which extended this series of data[46] looked at the feasibility of combining the NB evaluation the NT measurement and maternal serum free β-hCG and PAPP-A in screening for Down's syndrome. Firstly, it was concluded that the presence or absence of the NB is independent of the serum biochemistries. Secondly, it was estimated that combining all four markers and maternal age would yield a Down's syndrome detection rate of 96% for a false positive rate of 5%.[45,46]

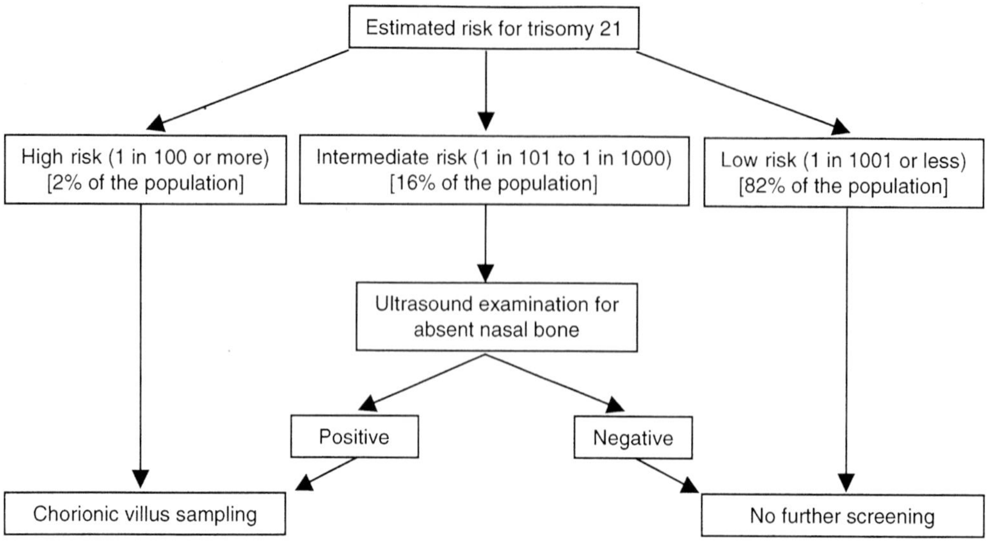

Figure 76.8 New individual risk orientated two-stage approach to first-trimester screening, (Nicolaides *et al.*[50]). Screening by maternal age, fetal nuchal translucency and maternal serum free β-human chorionic gonadotropin and pregnancy-associated plasma protein-A.

Nasal bone reference ranges by ultrasound

First trimester

Cicero *et al.*[39] reported that in the chromosomally normal group the fetal NB length increases significantly with CRL from a mean of 1.3 mm at a CRL of 45 mm to 2.1 mm at CRL of 84 mm. The Down's syndrome fetuses with a detectable NB tended to have a shorter NB than the chromosomally normal fetuses. However, the difference in the NB lengths was not sufficiently great to be of clinical utility.[39]

Second trimester

Guis *et al.*[47] published reference ranges for NB lengths, based on 376 cases, between 14 and 34 weeks' gestation. Sonek *et al.*[48] provided reference range based on a larger number of patients (3547) and for a wider gestational range (11–40 weeks) using the ultrasound technique described above was published in 2003.

Impact of the nasal bone evaluation in screening for trisomy 21 in the first trimester of pregnancy

This chapter reviews studies to date, which overwhelmingly support the significant contribution which NB evaluation makes to ultrasound screening for Down's syndrome. The clinical implementation of this method may take form in essentially two ways. The optimal approach would be for operators who perform NT screening to be also proficient in NB evaluation. However, since the preliminary data indicate that NB evaluation may require more expertise and experience than NT evaluation an alternative approach was recently proposed by Nicolaides *et al.*[50] Their proposed policy involves a two-stage screening approach (Figure 76.8). The first stage consists of screening using the combination of maternal age, fetal NT, and maternal serum free β-hCG and PAPP-A at $11–13^{+6}$ weeks' gestation. The results of the initial screen would be then divided into three categories: high risk (risk estimate of 1:100 or greater), intermediate risk (risk estimate of 1:101 to 1:1000), and low risk (risk estimate of 1:1001 or less). The authors proposed that the high-risk group should be offered chorionic villus sampling and that the low-risk group can be reassured that their fetus is unlikely to have a chromosomal abnormality. The intermediate group would undergo further ultrasound evaluation to determine the presence or absence of NB. The patients where the fetus is noted to have an absent NB would be offered chorionic villus sampling and those with a present nasal bone would be reassured. The authors modeled the performance of this approach on their prospective experience with combined screening in 75,821 singleton pregnancies and their published experience with NB evaluation. They estimated that using this approach the detection rate for an overall false positive rate of 2% would be approximately 92%. This compares favorably to using the combined screen alone where the detection rate is approximately 80% for the same false positive rate.[50–53]

Conclusion

Trisomy 21 is the most common chromosomal abnormality found at birth, with an incidence of about 1:600. However, the sonographic appearance of individuals with Down's syndrome, is often quite similar to those with normal karyotype, making screening for Down's syndrome more difficult compared to that of other chromosomal abnormalities. Hence the importance of a continued search for markers, that would accurately discriminate between affected and unaffected fetuses.

The sonographic appearance of increased NT and absent/hypoplastic NB could be due to connective tissue abnormalities.[54–56] The increased thickness of subcutaneous tissues in association with Down's syndrome has lead to the development of screening based on the NT measurement between 11 and 13^{+6} weeks of gestation, which is the most sensitive and specific ultrasound marker for this condition.[57]

Several studies have demonstrated that the best screening test for trisomy 21 in the first trimester of pregnancy is based on the combination of maternal age, fetal NT thickness, and maternal serum free β-hCG and PAPP-A. This test allows a detection rate of 90% for a false positive rate of 5%.[5,34,50] By adding the ultrasonographic evaluation of the NB, a sensitivity of over 90% could be achieved for a false positive rate of about 2%.[45,46,50] In the second trimester, the finding of an absent NB yields likelihood ratios for Down's syndrome of 51–83.[30,31]

Although extensive studies have demonstrated that absence of the NB is a highly sensitive and specific marker of trisomy 21, its examination in the first trimester requires highly skilled operators. Therefore, incorporation of this marker into the 11–13^{+6}-week scan can come about only after extensive training and experience. It may be that this sonographic marker will be primarily used in specialized centers to reevaluate the risk in patients with an intermediate risk level category after an initial screening using fetal NT and maternal serum biochemistry as a part of a two-stage screening method.[50]

The introduction of individual risk-orientated two-stage screening for trisomy 21,[50] which includes examination of the fetal NB in those women with a individual risk between 1:101 to 1:1000, could increase the detection rate to more that 90%, and the false positive rate could be decreased to about 2%. This is important for three main reasons: firstly, the low false positive rate reduces the number of miscarriages of chromosomally normal fetuses associated with invasive testing;[58,59] secondly, the decrease in the number of invasive tests results in a reduction of economic costs; thirdly, this approach provides an early reassurance to pregnant women and, for those with an affected fetus, allows the possibility of an early termination of pregnancy.

In order to reproduce these results, it is imperative that sonographers receive appropriate training and adhere to a standard technique for the measurement of NT and the assessment of the NB. Furthermore, the success of a screening program necessitates the presence of a system for regular audit of results and continuous assessment of the quality of images such as the one established by the Fetal Medicine Foundation.[60]

REFERENCES

1. Snijders RJM, Nicolaides KH. *Assessment of Risk. Ultrasound Markers for Fetal Chromosomal Defects*. Carnforth, UK: Parthenon Publishing, 1996.
2. Down LJ. Observations on an ethnic classification of idiots. *Clin Lect Rep London Hosp* 1866;3:259–62.
3. Enlow DH. *Facial Growth*, 3rd edn. Philadelphia, PA: WB Saunders, 1990.
4. Beck JC, Sie KCY. The growth and development of the nasal airway. *Funct Reconstr Rhinoplasty* 1999:257–62.
5. Larsen WJ. *Human Embryology*, 3rd edn. London: Churchill Livingstone, 2001;368.
6. Sperber GH. *Craniofacial Embryology*, 4th edn, London: Wright, Butterworths, 1989;104–24.
7. Williams PL, Warwick R, Dyson M, Bannister L. *Gray's Anatomy*, 37th edn. London: Churchill Livingstone, 1989;386.
8. Sandikcioglu M, Molsted K, Kjaer I. The prenatal development of the human nasal and vomeral bones. *J Craniofac Genet Dev Biol* 1994;14:124–34.
9. Farkas LG, Katic MJ, Forrest CR, Litsas L. Surface anatomy of the face in Down's syndrome: linear and angular measurements in the craniofacial regions. *J Craniofac Surg* 2001;12:373–9.
10. Keeling JW, Hansen BF, Kjaer I. Pattern of malformation in the axial skeleton in human trisomy 21 fetuses. *Am J Med Genet* 1997;68:466–71.
11. Stempfle N, Huten Y, Fredouille C, Brisse H, Nessmann C. Skeletal abnormalities in fetuses with Down's syndrome: A radiologic postmortem study. *Pediatr Radiol* 1999;29:682–8.
12. Tuxen A, Keeling JW, Reintoft I, Fischer Hansen B, Nolting D, Kjaer I. A histological and radiological investigation of the nasal bone in fetuses with Down syndrome. *Ultrasound Obstet Gynecol* 2003;22:22–6.
13. Minderer S, Gloning KP, Henrich W, Stoger H. The nasal bone in fetuses with trisomy 21: Sonographic versus pathomorphological findings. *Ultrasound Obstet Gynecol* 2003;22:16–21.
14. Larose C, Massoc P, Hillion Y, Bernard JP, Ville Y. Comparison of fetal nasal bone assessment by ultrasound at 11–14 weeks and by postmortem X-ray in trisomy 21: A prospective observational study. *Ultrasound Obstet Gynecol* 2003;22:27–30.
15. Sonek J, Nicolaides K. Prenatal ultrasonographic diagnosis of nasal bone abnormalities in three fetuses with Down syndrome. *Am J Obstet Gynecol* 2002;186:139–41.
16. Cicero S, Curcio P, Papageorghiou A, Sonek J, Nicolaides K. Absence of nasal bone in fetuses with trisomy 21 at 11–14 weeks of gestation: An observational study. *Lancet* 2001;358:1665–7.
17. Cicero S, Longo D, Rembouskos G, Sacchini C, Nicolaides KH. Absent nasal bone at 11–14 weeks of gestation and chromosomal defects. *Ultrasound Obstet Gynecol* 2003;22:31–5.
18. Cicero S, Rembouskos G, Vandecruys H, Hogg M, Nicolaides KH. Likelihood ratio for trisomy 21 in fetuses with absent nasal bone at the 11–14 weeks scan. *Ultrasound Obstet Gynecol* 2004;23: 218–23.
19. Otano L, Aiello H, Igarzabal L, Matayoshi T, Gadow EC. Association between first trimester absence of fetal nasal bone on ultrasound and Down's syndrome. *Prenat Diagn* 2002;22:930–2.

20. Zoppi MA, Ibba RM, Axiana C, Floris M, Manca F, Monni G. Absence of fetal nasal bone and aneuploidies at first-trimester nuchal translucency screening in unselected pregnancies. *Prenat Diagn* 2003;23:496–500.
21. Orlandi F, Bilardo CM, Campogrande M *et. al.* Measurement of nasal bone length at 11–14 weeks of pregnancy and its potential role in Down syndrome risk assessment. *Ultrasound Obstet Gynecol* 2003;22:36–9.
22. Viora E, Masturzo B, Errante G, Sciarrone A, Bastonero S, Campogrande M. Ultrasound evaluation of fetal nasal bone at 11 to 14 weeks in a consecutive series of 1906 fetuses. *Prenat Diagn* 2003;23:784–7.
23. Senat MV, Bernard JP, Boulvain M, Ville Y. Intra- and interoperator variability in fetal nasal bone assessment at 11–14 weeks of gestation. *Ultrasound Obstet Gynecol* 2003;22:138–41.
24. Wong SF, Choi H, Ho LC. Nasal bone hypoplasia: Is it a common finding amongst chromosomally normal fetuses of southern Chinese women? *Gynecol Obstet Invest* 2003;56:99–101.
25. Orlandi F, Rossi C, Orlandi E *et al.* First-trimester screening for trisomy-21 using a simplified method to assess the presence or absence of the fetal nasal bone. *Am J Obstet Gynecol* 2005;192: 1107–11.
26. Prefumo F, Sairam S, Bhide A, Penna L, Hollis B, Thilaganathan B. Maternal ethnic origin and fetal nasal bones at 11–14 weeks of gestation. *Br J Obstet Gynaecol* 2004;111:109–12.
27. Malone FD, Ball RH, Nyberg DA *et al.*; FASTER Research Consortium. First-trimester nasal bone evaluation for aneuploidy in the general population. *Obstet Gynecol* 2004;104:1222–8.
28. Welch KK, Malone FD. Nuchal translucency-based screening. *Clin Obstet Gynecol* 2003;46:909–22.
29. De Biasio P, Venturini PL. Absence of nasal bone and detection of trisomy 21. *Lancet* 2002;13:1344.
30. Bromley B, Lieberman E, Shipp T, Benaceraff B. Fetal nasal bone length: A marker for Down syndrome in the second trimester. *J Ultrasound Med* 2002;21:1387–94.
31. Cicero S, Sonek J, McKenna D, Croom C, Johnson L, Nicolaides K. Nasal bone hypoplasia in fetuses with trisomy 21. *Ultrasound Obstet Gynecol* 2003;21:15–18.
32. Bunduki V, Ruano J, Miguelez J, Yoshizaki C, Kahhale S, Zugaib M. Fetal bone length: Reference range and clinical application in ultrasound screening for trisomy 21. *Ultrasound Obstet Gynecol* 2003;21:156–60.
33. Vintzileos A, Walters C, Yeo L. Absent nasal bone in the prenatal detection of fetuses with trisomy 21 in a high-risk population. *Obstet Gynecol* 2003;101:905–8.
34. Gamez F, Ferreiro P, Salmean JM. Ultrasonographic measurement of fetal nasal bone in a low risk population at 19–22 gestational weeks. *Ultrasound Obstet Gynecol* 2003;22:152–3.
35. Bouley R, Sonek J. Fetal nasal bone: The technique. *Down's Screening News* 2003;10:33–4.
36. Sonek JD, Cicero S. Ultrasound evaluation of the fetal nasal bone: The technique (an update). *Down's Screening News* 2004;11:25.
37. Cicero S, Dezerega V, Andrade E, Scheier M, Nicolaides KH. Learning curve for sonographic examination of the fetal nasal bone at 11–14 weeks. *Ultrasound Obstet Gynecol* 2003;22:135–7.
38. Kanellopoulos V, Katsetos C, Economides DL. Examination of fetal nasal bone and repeatability of measurement in early pregnancy. *Ultrasound Obstet Gynecol* 2003;22:131–4.
39. Cicero S, Bindra R, Rembouskos G, Tripsanas C, Nicolaides K. Fetal nasal bone length in chromosomally normal and abnormal fetuses at 11–14 weeks of gestation. *J Matern Fetal Neonatal Med* 2002;11:400–2.
40. Rembouskos G, Cicero S, Longo D, Vandecruys H, Nicolaides KH. Assessment of the fetal nasal bone at 11–14 weeks of gestation by three-dimensional ultrasound. *Ultrasound Obstet Gynecol* 2004;23:232–6.
41. Peralta CF, Falcon O, Wegrzyn P, Faro C, Nicolaides KH. Assessment of the gap between the fetal nasal bones at 11 to 13 + 6 weeks of gestation by three-dimensional ultrasound. *Ultrasound Obstet Gynecol* 2005;25:464–7.
42. Lee W, DeVore GR, Comstock CH *et al.* Nasal bone evaluation in fetuses with Down syndrome during the second and third trimesters of pregnancy. *J Ultrasound Med* 2003;22:55–60.
43. Goncalves LF, Espinoza J, Lee W *et al.* Phenotypic characteristics of absent and hypoplastic nasal bones in fetuses with Down syndrome: Description by 3-dimensional ultrasonography and clinical significance. *J Ultrasound Med* 2004;23:1619–27.
44. Benoit B, Chaoui R. Three-dimensional ultrasound with maximal mode rendering: A novel technique for the diagnosis of bilateral or unilateral absence or hypoplasia of nasal bones in second-trimester screening for Down syndrome. *Ultrasound Obstet Gynecol* 2005;25:19–24.
45. Cicero S, Bindra R, Rembouskos G, Spencer K, Nicolaides KH. Integrated ultrasound and biochemical screening for trisomy 21 using fetal nuchal translucency, absent fetal nasal bone, free beta-hCG and PAPP-A at 11 to 14 weeks. *Prenat Diagn* 2003;23: 306–10.
46. Cicero S, Spencer K, Avgidou K, Faiola S, Nicolaides KH. Maternal serum biochemistry at 11–13$^{(+6)}$ weeks in relation to the presence or absence of the fetal nasal bone on ultrasonography in chromosomally abnormal fetuses: an updated analysis of integrated ultrasound and biochemical screening. *Prenat Diagn* 2005; 25:977–83.
47. Guis F, Ville Y, Doumerc S, Pons J, Frydman R. Ultrasound evaluation of the length of the fetal nasal bones throughout gestation. *Ultrasound Obstet Gynecol* 1995;5:304–7.
48. Sonek J, McKenna D, Webb D, Croom C, Nicolaides K. Nasal bone length throughout gestation: Normal ranges based on 3537 fetal ultrasound measurements. *Ultrasound Obstet Gynecol* 2003;21:152–5.
49. Snijders RMJ, Noble P, Sebire N, Souka A, Nicolaides KH. UK multicentre project on assessment of risk of trisomy 21 by maternal age and fetal nuchal translucency thickness at 10–14 weeks of gestation. *Lancet* 1998;351:343–6.
50. Nicolaides KH, Spencer K, Avgidou K, Faiola S, Falcon O. Multicenter study of first-trimester screening for trisomy 21 in 75821 pregnancies: Results and estimation of the potential impact of individual risk-orientated two-stage first-trimester screening. *Ultrasound Obstet Gynecol* 2005;25:221–6.
51. Spencer K, Souter V, Tul N, Snijders R, Nicolaides KH. A screening program for trisomy 21 at 10–14 weeks using fetal nuchal translucency, maternal serum free ß-human chorionic gonadotropin and pregnancy-associated plasma protein-A. *Ultrasound Obstet Gynecol* 1999;13:231–7.
52. Bindra R, Heath V, Liao A, Spencer K, Nicolaides KH. One stop clinic for assessment of risk for trisomy 21 at 11–14 weeks: A prospective study of 15030 pregnancies. *Ultrasound Obstet Gynecol* 2002;20:219–25.
53. Spencer K, Spencer CE, Power M, Dawson C, Nicolaides KH. Screening for chromosomal abnormalities in the first trimester using ultrasound and maternal serum biochemistry in a one stop clinic: A review of three years prospective experience. *Br J Obstet Gynaecol* 2003;110:281–6.
54. von Kaisenberg CS, Krenn V, Ludwig M, Nicolaides KH, Brand-Saberi B. Morphological classification of nuchal skin in human fetuses with trisomy 21, 18, and 13 at 12–18 weeks and in a trisomy 16 mouse. *Anat Embryol* 1998;197:105–24.
55. von Kaisenberg CS, Brand-Saberi B, Christ B, Vallian S, Farzaneh F, Nicolaides KH. Collagen type VI expression in the skin of trisomy 21 fetuses. *Obstet Gynecol* 1998;91:319–23.
56. Bohlandt S, von Kaisenberg CS, Wewetzer K, Christ B, Nicolaides KH, Brand-Saberi B. Hyaluran in the nuchal skin of chromosomally abnormal fetuses. *Human Reprod* 2000;15:1155–8.
57. Nicolaides KH. Nuchal translucency and other first-trimester sonographic markers of chromosomal abnormalities. *Am J Obstet Gynecol* 2004;191:45–67.
58. Tabor A, Philip J, Madsen M, Bang J, Obel EB, Norgaard-Pedersen B. Randomised controlled trial of genetic amniocentesis in 4,606 low-risk women. *Lancet* 1986;1287–93.
59. Smidt-Jensen S, Permin M, Philip J *et al.* Randomised comparison of amniocentesis and transabdominal and transcervical chorionic villus sampling. *Lancet* 1992;340:1238–44.
60. Fetal Medicine Foundation. Down's screening at 11–14 weeks. Last accessed: May 14, 2005. Available from: http://www.fetalmedicine.com.

77 Second-trimester ultrasound screening of fetal anomalies

L. Yeo and A. M. Vintzileos

Introduction

It is an unfortunate fact that birth defects sometimes occur in human development.

In fact, they are the single most common cause of perinatal mortality in many countries. It is important to detect fetal congenital anomalies prior to birth for various reasons, such as delivering at a tertiary care center, offering prenatal surgical correction, giving the option of invasive testing, and appropriately and accurately counseling parents.

While there are varying modalities that currently exist to screen for fetal anomalies (such as magnetic resonance imaging and fetoscopic examination), the most accepted method is ultrasonographic imaging. The concept of prenatal ultrasonography as a screening tool has received widespread acceptance among both physicians and patients. Unlike biochemistry screening, ultrasound is a very tangible and realistic tool that provides a visible assessment for patients. Accordingly, the second trimester is often utilized because fetal anatomic structures are readily assessed at this time of pregnancy. Once sonographic screening in the second trimester reveals the presence of abnormalities, further diagnostic testing may be offered to the patient such as amniocentesis or percutaneous umbilical blood sampling. Although the advantage of performing sonography in patients at high risk for fetal structural anomalies is clear, the benefits and cost-effectiveness of routine ultrasound screening in low-risk pregnant patients are not as clear.

This chapter focuses on the components of a normal fetal anatomic survey, second-trimester sonographic markers for aneuploidy, and describes the value of sonographic second-trimester screening.

Second-trimester fetal anatomic survey and its contents

Because ultrasonography utilizes sound waves to provide imaging capability, it has rapidly become the most commonly used method for imaging during pregnancy. Its major advantages include lack of adverse fetal effects,[1] the ability to view the fetus in real-time mode (with capabilities of observing and studying fetal behavior/movements), and most recently the ability to acquire a volume of data to generate three-dimensional imaging. With the introduction of two-dimensional static scanning in the early 1970s, physicians were allowed to view the fetus for the first time. Subsequently, in the late 1970s and early 1980s, real-time B-mode imaging became widespread as a clinical tool. However, despite its many technological advancements over the years, many in the USA still believe that the appropriate use of fetal sonography should be limited to only where there is an indication. This is despite the fact that detailed examination of the fetus for both aneuploidy markers and structural abnormalities has become a true reality. In contrast, many European countries perform ultrasound examinations routinely during pregnancy.

In order to screen for fetal abnormalities on a second-trimester ultrasound, the sonographer must be able to recognize normal fetal anatomy first. Accordingly, we will describe the features of a targeted, complete fetal anatomic survey on ultrasound. There are many possible indications to undergo an obstetrical exam, such as estimating gestational age and/or growth, vaginal bleeding, multiple gestation, history or prior congenital anomaly or syndrome, placental localization, adjunct to interventional or invasive procedures, biophysical profile, and evaluation of amniotic fluid quantity. In most cases, ultrasonography will provide reassurance of a normal and healthy fetus. Because most anomalies are sporadic and often occur in otherwise low-risk women, we believe that all patients regardless of risk should have uniform access to obstetrical sonography in the second trimester. Most importantly, this should be performed with a high level of expertise, since both false-positive and false-negative information can have a detrimental impact. A systematic fetal anatomic survey is able to detect the majority of fetal malformations,[2] and can also evaluate fetal growth, amniotic fluid, placenta, and cervix. To be effective, the sonographic exam should be performed systematically, and with complete thoroughness.

Recently, we examined the value (from the patient's perspective) of a targeted ultrasound performed after an abnormal karyotype was discovered.[3] All patients valued the ultrasound because it provided visualization of anomalies, and this additional information influenced pregnancy management. Interestingly, all patients thought that the impact of sonography was superior to chromosomal diagnosis alone, and all believed that sonography should be utilized in patients facing likewise clinical situations. These patients found sonography invaluable because it provided more information and helped them to accept the diagnosis of fetal aneuploidy.

Published guidelines exist that describe the components of a complete obstetrical ultrasound. This involves both biometric measurements, which reflect gestational age, growth or size, and evaluation of specific organ structures for the absence/presence of anomalies. In 1994, the American Institute of Ultrasound in Medicine published standards for the performance of obstetrical ultrasound.[4] In the first trimester, the requirements include evaluation of the uterus, adnexa, cul-de-sac, gestational sac, crown–rump length, fetal number, and presence/absence of cardiac activity. In the second and third trimesters, the requirements include fetal life/number/presentation/activity (with multiple gestations requiring additional documentation), amniotic fluid, placental location/appearance/relationship to the internal os, fetal biparietal diameter (BPD) or head circumference (HC), limb measurement, estimated fetal weight (requires abdominal diameter or circumference), uterus, cervix, adnexa, cerebral ventricles, posterior fossa, four-chamber view of the heart and position, spine, stomach, kidneys, bladder, abdominal cord insertion site, and umbilical cord.

However, in order to increase the diagnostic sensitivity for fetal anomalies, a more comprehensive exam above and beyond what is required by the American Institute of Ultrasound in Medicine should be performed. Table 77.1 depicts the components of a second-trimester fetal anatomic survey that we routinely perform via ultrasonography. Of course, to carry out this task, other criteria should also be met. For instance, proper sonographic equipment and transducers with the highest-frequency probe should be utilized to maximize fetal anatomic resolution. The sonographers should be adequately and appropriately trained to ensure that these detailed exams are performed at the highest level. To properly recognize fetal anomalies, one must be familiar with normal fetal anatomy, normal variants, and the various sonographic landmarks.

Factors that can limit the ability to adequately examine the fetus sonographically in the second trimester include sonographer expertise, quality of

Table 77.1 Components of second-trimester sonographic fetal anatomic survey (at Robert Wood Johnson Medical School)

Anatomic structures
Head
Cranial shape, degree of mineralization
Cerebral hemispheres, cavum septum pellucidum, thalami, cerebral peduncles, lateral ventricles, choroid plexus, third and fourth ventricles, cerebellum and vermis, cisterna magna
Face/neck
Orbits, nasal bone, lips/palate, profile, nuchal fold, ear length
Thoracic cavity
Lungs
Configuration of bony thorax, including ribs and clavicles
Heart
Four-chamber views (apical and subcostal), both outflow tracts, aortic and ductal arches, inferior and superior vena cavae, valves, atria and ventricular septums
Abdominal
Situs
Stomach
Liver, gallbladder, spleen
Umbilical vein, portal vein
Bowel
Wall/cord insertion site
Genitourinary system
Kidneys
Bladder
Genitalia
Spine
Extremities
Upper (including bilateral hands)
Lower (including bilateral feet)
Umbilical cord
Number of umbilical arteries
Placental insertion site
Biometry measurements
Biparietal diameter
Head circumference
Atria of lateral ventricles, cisterna magna, nuchal fold (when applicable)
Cerebellum
Thoracic circumference (when applicable)
Abdominal circumference
Femur lengths, humerus lengths, radius and ulna lengths, tibia and fibula lengths
Foot length
Nasal bone length
Orbital diameters
Other
Estimation of dates or evaluation of growth
Number of fetuses, position
Placenta
Amniotic fluid
Cervix/lower uterine segment

ultrasound equipment, length of time spent scanning, incompletely filled or overfilled maternal bladder, maternal habitus, depth of penetration, tissue density, and other scanning characteristics, fibroids, early or advancing gestational age, ossification of fetal bony structures (later in the second trimester), fetal position, and amniotic fluid abnormalities (increased or decreased). Techniques that can improve fetal visualization include using various probes (including transvaginal scanning, for instance, in the obese patient) and changing maternal position (which effectively changes the fetal position).

The timing of scans in the second trimester may vary, depending on the scanning center, indication for the exam (amniocentesis), or physician preference. Later scans (for example, 23–24 weeks) can improve visualization of certain fetal anatomic structures such as the heart and improve overall sensitivity. However, scanning later in the second trimester of pregnancy may limit the window of opportunity for patients who desire termination of pregnancy for various reasons. On the other hand, patients who desire amniocentesis testing may choose to undergo a sonographic survey earlier, such as 16–17 weeks of gestation. Some patients who have had a previous child affected with structural anomalies or genetic syndromes may choose to undergo an initial early scan for some reassurance, and then a more detailed repeat exam later in the pregnancy. At our own center, we schedule fetal anatomy surveys around 18–21 weeks in order to optimize anatomy assessment, and yet still provide patients the opportunity for amniocentesis if necessary. Some studies suggest that among low-risk women, second-trimester ultrasound screening is easier to perform and less likely to require an additional scan at 20–22 weeks than at 18 weeks.[5] Fetal echocardiograms are best performed between 22 and 24 weeks when cardiac structures are large enough, and better visualization and assessment are possible.

With multiple gestations, not only should the fetal anatomy be evaluated, but the number, position of fetuses, and type of dividing membrane should be delineated. In addition, when screening for fetal anomalies sonographically, the placenta and amniotic fluid volume must also always be assessed. Placental appearance, thickness, echogenicity, location, and characteristics should be examined, along with amniotic fluid volume, to rule out polyhydramnios, oligohydramnios, or anhydramnios. These structures can provide clues to a potential anomalous fetus. For instance, polyhydramnios is associated with esophageal atresia, anyhydramnios is associated with renal agenesis, and a thickened placenta can be seen with fetal hydrops.

At the beginning of the examination, the entire uterus should be imaged both transversely and longitudinally to assess fetal position, amniotic fluid volume, and placental location. Determining the right and left sides of the fetus is crucial. Situs solitus is the term used when there is the usual arrangement of organs and vessels within the fetal body. Finally, examination of the lower uterine segment and cervix is important.

The examination of the fetal intracranial anatomy is extremely important since the presence of central nervous system abnormalities can have a major and devastating impact on perinatal morbidity and mortality. From the late first trimester until delivery, the calvarium can be identified. Thus, the BPD and HC can be readily measured. The calvarium should not be hypomineralized (which can indicate a skeletal dysplasia), and should be elliptical in shape. Reverberation artifact from properly mineralized bone will usually obscure the proximal hemisphere. 'Strawberry'- or 'lemon'-shaped heads can indicate the presence of trisomy 18 or neural tube defects, respectively. Brachycephaly (anteroposterior shortening) can also be a sign of fetal trisomy 21 or trisomy 18 ('strawberry' head). Dolicocephaly (elongation of the anteroposterior length) can be a normal variant, or secondary to decreased amniotic fluid and compression of the fetal head. Tangential imaging through the fetal calvarium may identify cranial sutures (hypoechoic spaces between bones), which are best visualized early in gestation since ossification progresses with time. In certain syndromes (such as craniosynostosis and skeletal dysplasias), premature closure of the sutures can be seen.

The transthalamic view (Figure 77.1) is an axial view through the cranium at the level of the thalami. At this level, the BPD and HC are obtained. Because of excessive variation in the BPD shape which can occur, when the head is either brachycephalic or dolicocephalic, the HC is the preferred measurement. The BPD is obtained with the cranial bones perpendicular to the ultrasound beam, and is measured from the outer margin of the near-calvarium to the inner margin of the far-calvarium. The HC is measured circumferentially at the outer margin of the calvarium. Other anatomic structures that should be assessed in the transthalamic view are the cavum septum pellucidum (fluid-filled midline structure anterior to the thalami and between the lateral ventricles), midline falx, third ventricle (located between the thalami), and frontal horns of the lateral ventricles. Visualization of the cavum septum pellucidum implies proper formation of midline intracranial structures. Its absence can be a sign of agenesis of the corpus callosum, holoprosencephaly, or other brain anomalies.

The transventricular view (Figure 77.2) is found just superior to the transthalamic view, and is marked by the lateral ventricles, which contain sonolucent cerebrospinal fluid. Within this system is the echogenic choroid plexus, which normally fills the body of the lateral ventricle extending into the atrium. The frontal horns are seen as prominent sonolucent anterior components of the lateral ventricles. Through an axial plane of the atrium, the cerebral ventricle is measured.

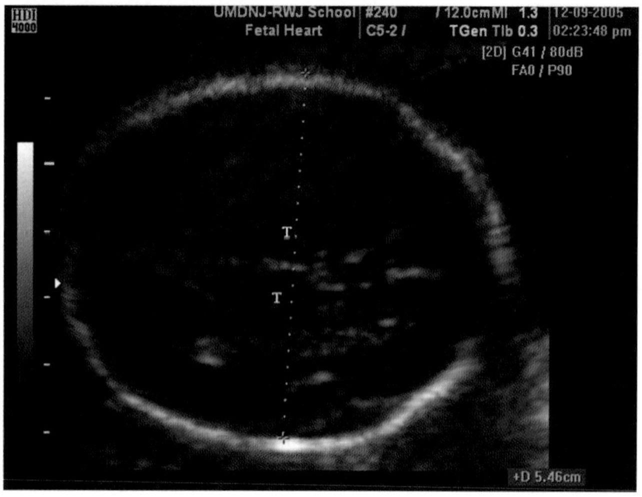

Figure 77.1 Axial view through the fetal head with calipers demonstrating measurement of the biparietal diameter. This is also the view for measurement of the head circumference. Both thalami (T) are also depicted.

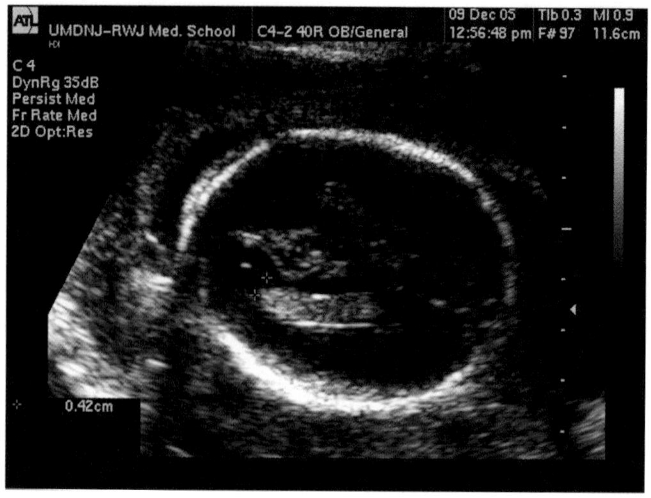

Figure 77.2 Transventricular view of the fetal head demonstrating measurement of the atria of the lateral ventricle (0.42 cm) and the echogenic choroid plexus.

To rule out ventriculomegaly/hydrocephalus, normally it should be < 10 mm.

The transcerebellar view (Figure 77.3) contains the biconvex cerebellar hemispheres and midline vermis, cisterna magna (between the dorsum of cerebellar hemispheres and inner calvarium), and nuchal fold. Importantly, the transcerebellar diameter can also be measured and utilized as a one-point estimate of gestational age. The transcerebellar view is obtained by angling the scan plane down posteriorly from the transthalamic view. This area is of vital importance in ruling out open spina bifida, since obliteration of the cisterna magna and a 'banana' shape of the cerebellum may be seen with this disorder. Other anomalies that can be ruled out in this view include Dandy–Walker malformation/variant, cerebellar agenesis/hypoplasia, and occipital encephaloceles. The cisterna magna normally ranges from 3 to 9 cm.[6] On occasion, this measurement may be increased, but is a usually normal finding if the transcerebellar diameter is normal for gestational age and the vermis is well seen and intact. An incorrect scan plane can lead to a false-positive appearance of Dandy–Walker variant or to an abnormally large measurement of the cisterna magna.[7] An increased nuchal fold (6 mm or greater) may be secondary to fetal aneuploidy (especially Down's syndrome, DS) or may be falsely thickened due to breech presentation. In certain clinical scenarios, the intracranial major vessels (such as middle cerebral artery) can be identified with color and/or power Doppler imaging (Figure 77.4). This information may be quite useful in assessing for anemia (Rh isoimmunization, parvovirus infection) or intrauterine fetal growth restriction. On occasion, the fetal head may be low in the pelvis that it prohibits an adequate examination of the intracranial anatomy; transvaginal scanning may be quite useful and solve this dilemma.

Although examination of the fetal face is not required, we believe it should be examined routinely because it can add tremendous information when discriminating between genetic disorders/syndromes, including aneuploidy, and it completes the full examination of the fetus. Three distinct planes can be examined: axial, coronal (Figure 77.5), and sagittal (profile) (Figure 77.6) although a combination of these planes is the most optimal. In evaluating for cleft lip/palate (anterior palate), both axial and coronal images toward the anterior surface of the nose/upper lips provide the best visualization. The posterior or hard palate cannot be imaged sonographically, since it is obscured by overlying osseous structures. Other anatomic structures that should be evaluated include the chin (to rule out micrognathia), nasal bone (Figure 77.6), nose, lower lips, tongue, orbits (and diameters if necessary, to exclude hyper/hypotelorism), and ear length (which can be shortened in both aneuploid and non-aneuploid fetuses). Multiple studies have found sonographically absent or short fetal nasal bone in both the first and second trimesters to be sensitive for the detection of DS.[8–10] Structures in the anterior neck that may have to be examined on occasion include the fetal thyroid, and the fluid-filled trachea and hypopharynx.

Examination of the fetal spine should be performed in three planes: sagittal, transverse, and coronal. Each vertebral segment is composed of three echogenic ossification centers (two posteriorly and one anteriorly, which is the vertebral body), which are positioned in a symmetric triangular-shaped configuration in the transverse plane. In this plane, the posterior processes are also oriented toward the midline like the roof of a house. When these processes appeared splayed, a neural tube defect must be ruled out. Transverse imaging of the spine is perhaps the most sensitive method of examination for a spinal defect, since it allows a

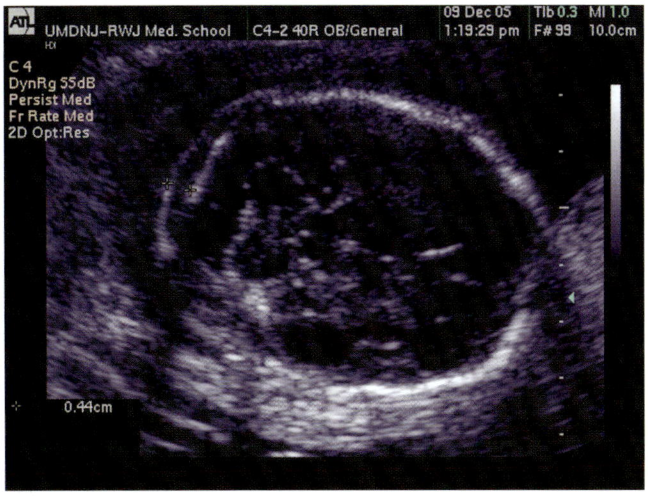

Figure 77.3 Transcerebellar view demonstrating cerebellar hemispheres, cisterna magna, and nuchal fold measurement (0.44 cm, normal).

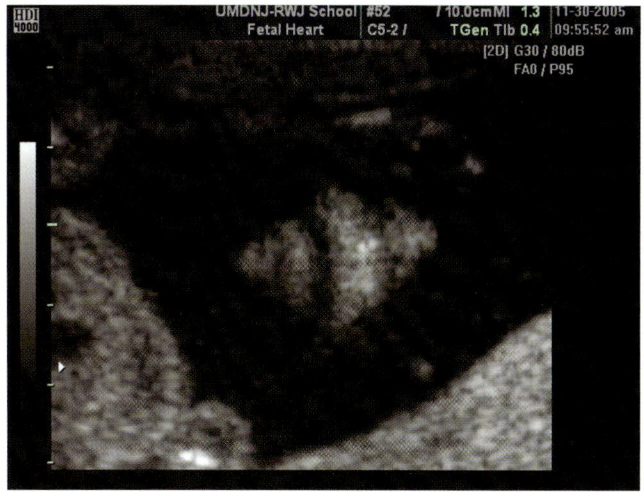

Figure 77.5 Coronal view of fetal face showing nose, upper and lower lips.

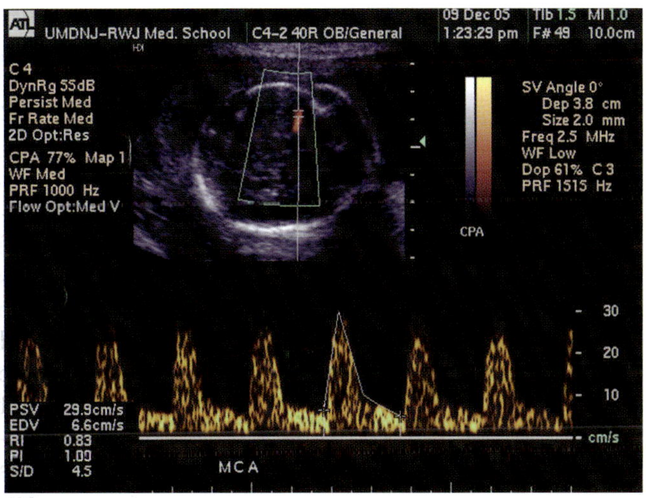

Figure 77.4 Normal middle cerebral artery Doppler waveform. The systolic/diastolic ratio is high (4.5), consistent with normal high-resistance pattern.

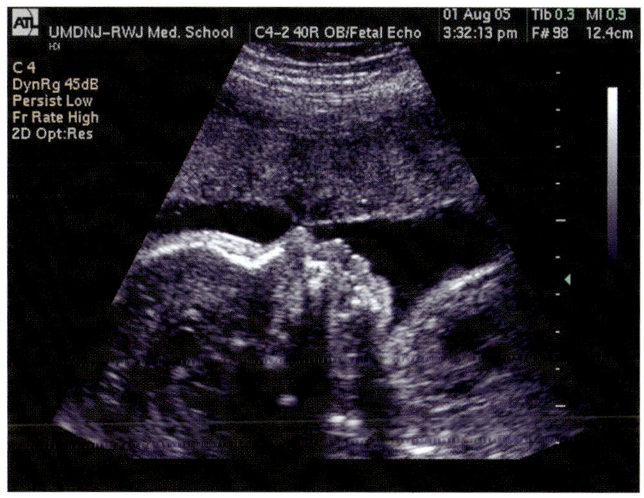

Figure 77.6 Normal sagittal profile of fetus showing nasal bone.

simultaneous examination of posterior ossification centers and overlying soft tissue. Sagittal imaging of the fetal spine (Figure 77.7) should show two rows of approximately parallel ossification centers with overlying intact skin. Both sagittal and coronal views are useful to observe this ‘lining up’ of the ossification centers, and should be able to rule out scoliosis or hemivertebrae (which can cause disorganization or absence of ossification centers). The sacrum normally should curve slightly upward. The overlying skin and soft tissues should also be examined carefully to rule out masses/tumors, or open spina bifida.

In examining the fetal thorax, the scapulae, clavicles, and ribs should be assessed, especially when ruling out certain types of skeletal dysplasias. Abnormal lung tissue and echogenicity (such as bronchopulmonary sequestration, cystic adenomatoid malformations), diaphragm, pleural effusions, and thoracic circumference (to rule out pulmonary hypoplasia) should all be examined.

Performing an adequate and detailed fetal cardiac examination on ultrasound can be one of the most difficult and challenging tasks, since it is dynamic, complex, and can depend significantly on fetal position. First, the situs should be established along with the presence of a normal cardiac rate and rhythm. In a transverse image of the fetal chest, the heart should occupy about one-third of the fetal thorax, and its normal axis and position should be verified (apex points to the left, bulk of the heart occupies left side of chest, $45 \pm 20°$ angle of the heart relative to the midline). Any alterations in position, axis, or both can suggest intrinsic malposition or an intrathoracic mass. In order to sufficiently rule out cardiac defects,

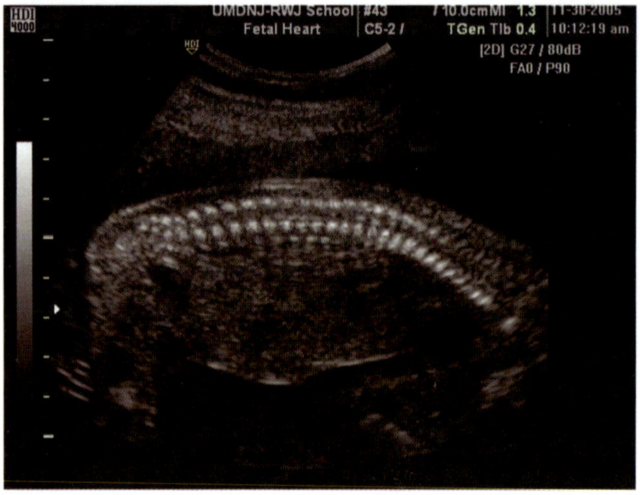

Figure 77.7 Normal sagittal view of fetal spine. Note the overlying skin is intact, and the parallel features of the spinal centers.

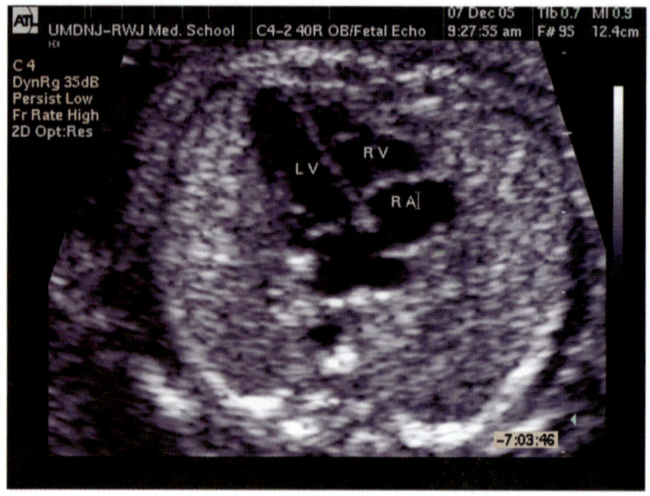

Figure 77.8 Apical four-chamber view of the fetal heart, demonstrating left atrium and left ventricle (LV) and right atrium and ventricle (RA, RV).

multiple planes and views (in addition to the four-chamber view) should be examined in real-time imaging. A single static four-chamber view is no longer acceptable or adequate to completely examine the heart. Both outflow tracts should be evaluated to increase the sensitivity for cardiac defects, such as tetralogy of Fallot, transposition of the great vessels, truncus arteriosus, etc. In screening second-trimester fetuses, we advocate visualization of the four-chamber apical (Figure 77.8) and subcostal views, both outflow tracts, longitudinal parasternal arches (aortic and ductal), inferior/superior vena cava, valves, and the atria/ventricular septa. All chambers should have approximately equal sizes, the great vessels should cross each other, the pulmonary veins should be seen entering the left atrium, and there should be no pericardial effusion. Depending on the indication or clinical scenario, color, M-mode, or pulsed Doppler sonography can also be performed of the fetal heart and its great vessels. In about 3–4% of normal second-trimester fetuses,[11] an echogenic intracardiac focus can be seen, usually located in the left ventricle. It is caused by specular reflection from the papillary muscle and chordae tendinae. However, some studies have also confirmed an association between this and fetal DS in high-risk populations.[12]

Fetal abdominal organs that can be identified on second-trimester ultrasonography include liver (majority of the upper abdomen), gallbladder (right upper quadrant at inferior edge of the liver and 'teardrop'-shaped), spleen (solid organ posterior to stomach), stomach, bowel, umbilical vein, and cord insertion site/adjacent anterior abdominal wall. The abdominal circumference (AC) is taken at the transverse level where stomach and spine are visualized, and the umbilical vein joins the right portal venous system, which should curve away from the stomach (Figure 77.9). If, however, the curve is toward the stomach, persistence of the right umbilical vein should be suspected. The AC has its greatest value in evaluating fetal growth later in pregnancy, and also comprises a parameter used for fetal dating. This is because AC deviations are a result of changes in both liver size and subcutaneous fat. The stomach should always be located below the diaphragm as a fluid-filled structure in the left upper quadrant. An absent or small stomach in the usual location despite prolonged scanning to allow for filling can be indicative of esophageal atresia with or without tracheoesophageal fistula, or diaphragmatic hernia (stomach located within the chest). The rest of the abdomen is filled with bowel, with the appearance changing with advancing gestational age. In the second trimester, the fetal bowel appears as midlevel to increased echogenicity filling the abdominal cavity; when using higher-frequency transducers, it often appears mildly echogenic when compared to the liver.[13] True hyperechoic bowel is diagnosed when its echogenicity is similar to that of bone. It can be a normal variant, or associated with aneuploidy, infection, cystic fibrosis, fetus swallowing blood, intrauterine growth restriction, and bowel malformations/atresias. To exclude ventral wall defects such as omphalocele or gastroschisis, the umbilical cord insertion site into the abdominal wall (Figure 77.10) must be evaluated to confirm the cord penetrating the abdomen, with the adjacent abdominal wall intact. No fetal ascites or hydrops should be seen under normal circumstances.

The fetal genitourinary tract is a common site for fetal anomalies. The kidneys appear as bilateral, hypoechoic, paraspinal structures that contain the urine-filled renal pelvis and can sometimes be difficult to visualize. Dilation of the renal pelvis/calyx or ureter, renal masses, hyperechogenicity, parenchymal cysts, or enlargement/absence of the kidneys may reflect anomalies. To delineate the renal arteries, color

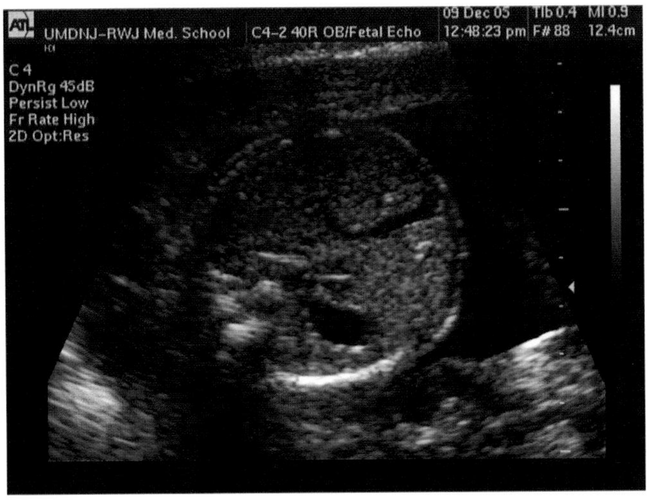

Figure 77.9 Correct view of taking the abdominal circumference measurement.

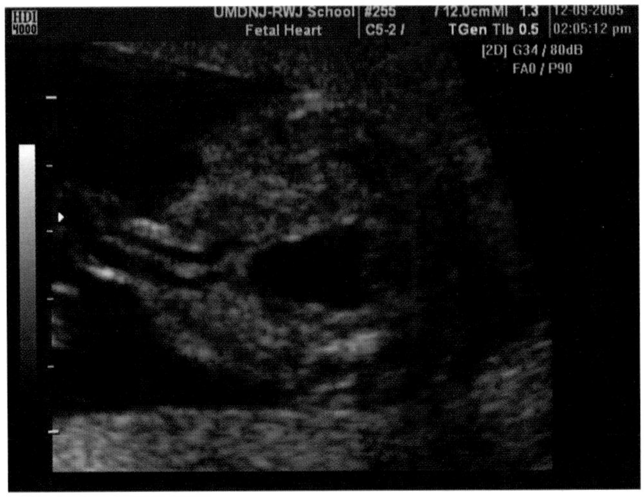

Figure 77.10 Transverse view of fetus depicting abdominal wall cord insertion site. The sonolucent bladder is also visualized with each of the two umbilical arteries starting to course around its periphery.

or power Doppler imaging is frequently used. The fetal adrenals can be seen cephalad to their kidneys. While the right adrenal lies immediately posterior to the inferior vena cava, the left adrenal lies lateral to the aorta. The fetal bladder is sonolucent (contains urine) and located in the midline, anteriorly, and low in the pelvis (Figure 77.10). Absence of the bladder may be secondary to recent voiding or bladder/cloacal exstrophy, while a very enlarged bladder may be a sign of lower obstructive uropathy. Male genitalia is confirmed only if penis and scrotum are seen. Occasionally, the hypoechoic umbilical cord lying between the thighs can be mistaken for the solid penis. Also, a prominent clitoris seen during the early second trimester can also sometimes be confused for a penis. The echogenic testicles usually do not descend into the scrotum until the seventh month. Female genitalia are identified by the presence of several parallel linear echoes, which represent the margins of the labia, and not by the observed absence of penis/scrotum. One should never forget that ambiguous genitalia may also be present.

Although routine evaluation of all fetal upper and lower extremities is not a part of routine obstetrical sonographic guidelines, it is our opinion that a complete survey of all extremities (including hands/feet) may provide important diagnostic information and can screen for abnormalities. Both the hands should contain five fingers, should be open (full extension of all fingers in the same plane as the metacarpals), have normal movement and tone, and the middle phalanx of the fifth digit must be visualized (Figure 77.11). The presence of clenched hands with overlapping digits is a highly sensitive (95%) sonographic marker of trisomy 18.[14] All the long bones (femur, humerus, radius, ulna, tibia, fibula) should be present and there should not be demineralized, shortened, fractured, contracted, or bowed bones. The ulna normally extends farther into the elbow, and the tibia extends farther into the patella. Routinely on our second-trimester surveys, we measure all long bone lengths. These measurements should be obtained with the long bone located horizontally within the image, since vertical measurements can falsely 'shorten' the actual length (Figure 77.12). Also, only the ossified portions of the bone should be measured, with the hypoechoic cartilaginous epiphyses excluded. Both lower extremities should not be clubbed, nor the plantar surface appear 'rocker-bottom'. Five toes should be present, and they should not appear dysplastic. Foot length (Figure 77.13) is also another biometric parameter than can be obtained.

Normally, the umbilical cord is comprised of three vessels: two smaller umbilical arteries and one larger umbilical vein; this can be confirmed by directly imaging the cord or by observing the umbilical arteries coursing around the fetal bladder. Depending on the clinical situation, an umbilical artery Doppler waveform can be obtained (Figure 77.14). Its flow is a reflection mainly of the placental resistance, and to a certain extent, of the fetal systemic circulation. Once the umbilical vein enters the fetal abdomen, it turns superiorly, enters the liver, and communicates with the portal vein. The umbilical vein also continues into the ductus venosus, and then the inferior vena cava and right atrium.

Sonographic aneuploidy markers in the second trimester

Aneuploid fetuses account for approximately 6–11% of all stillbirths and neonatal deaths.[15] Prenatal ultrasonography can often detect many abnormalities in fetuses with aneuploidy. These can include major structural defects or other 'soft' sonographic markers

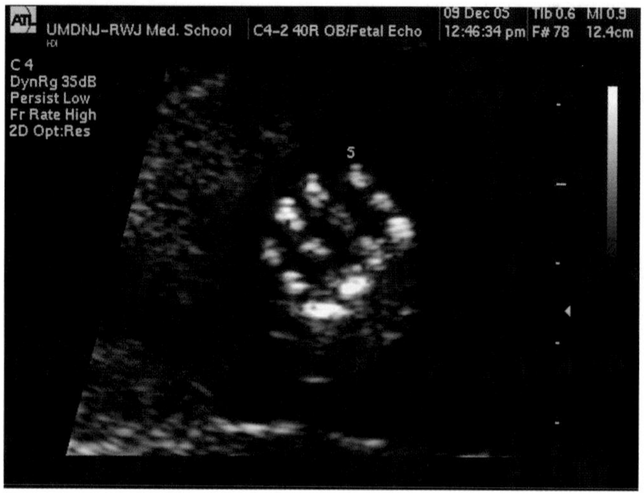

Figure 77.11 Fetal hand demonstrating echogenic phalanges of four fingers, including the fifth digit.

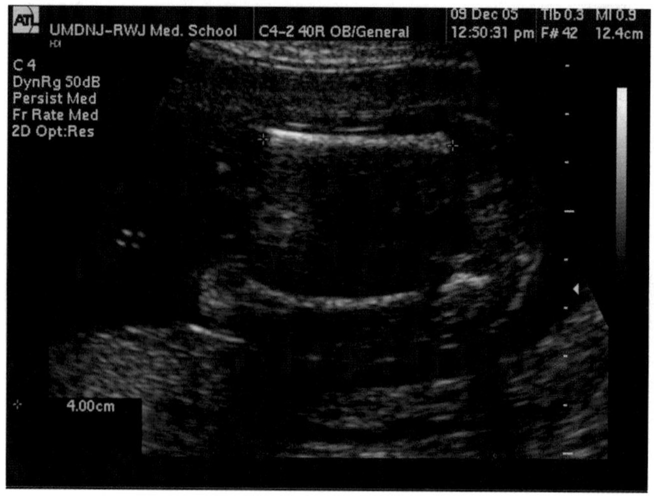

Figure 77.12 Femur length measured from proximal end to distal metaphysis, including only the ossified portions. Note the other femur lying parallel and directly below the measured femur length.

of aneuploidy. Aneuploidy 'soft' markers are usually non-specific, most commonly seen in normal fetuses, are often transient (such as choroid plexus cysts), and may not be significantly linked to perinatal outcome. The aneuploidy markers that we use in our institution include shortened long bones, pyelectasis, increased nuchal fold thickening, hyperechoic bowel, choroid plexus cysts, hypoplastic middle phalanx of the fifth digit, clinodactyly, sandal gap (wide space between first and second toes), two-vessel cord, echogenic intracardiac focus, short ear length, and absent nasal bone. Each marker alone has only low to moderate sensitivity for detecting fetal DS. Many of these sonographic findings when found in isolation in low-risk patients do not necessarily increase the risk for aneuploidy. However, when found in the context of multiple other sonographic abnormalities or markers (in low-risk patients), or when isolated markers are seen in high-risk patients, the risk for fetal aneuploidy may increase. In general, as the number of markers present increases, the risk for chromosomal abnormality also increases directly.

The presence of most fetal congenital abnormalities will increase the risk for underlying aneuploidy except for some disorders felt to be 'acquired' (rather than inherent) from tissue or vascular disruption. Such disorders include hydranencephaly, gastroschisis, tumors, amniotic band syndrome, limb–body wall complex, etc. Examples of specific structural anomalies that can be associated with fetal aneuploidy are cerebral ventriculomegaly, holoprosencephaly, agenesis of the corpus callosum, Dandy–Walker malformation/cerebellar hypoplasia, spina bifida, cleft lip/palate, ocular abnormalities, craniofacial anomalies, cystic hygroma, non-immune hydrops, cardiac abnormalities, diaphragmatic hernia, duodenal atresia, omphalocele, genitourinary anomalies, clubfeet, and extremity malformations.

The most common autosomal trisomy in liveborn infants is DS. Because only 25% of DS fetuses in the second trimester have a sonographically detectable major anomaly (unlike trisomies 18 and 13 where the majority will have anomalies visualized), several investigators have been searching to find aneuploidy ultrasonographic markers in order to increase the sensitivity for fetal DS.[16] Genetic sonography is performed in the second trimester, ideally between 18 and 20 weeks. It is a specific, targeted exam for fetal aneuploidy (most specifically for trisomy 21) where the examiner evaluates for abnormal fetal biometry, fetal structural anomalies, and other markers of aneuploidy. By combining multiple aneuploidy markers, the sensitivity for DS can be increased to >80%, with false-positive rates of 10–15% (by defining as abnormal the ultrasound exam with at least one abnormal marker present). Information derived from a normal genetic sonogram is used to generate an adjusted (lower) DS risk to guide a high-risk woman's decision on genetic amniocentesis. Thus far, many studies have been published that examine the accuracy of genetic sonography for detecting DS in high-risk populations.[17] By defining as abnormal the ultrasound with at least one abnormal marker, the overall sensitivity is 77% (50–93%) and the false-positive rate is 13% (7–17%).[17] In 1998, a large multicenter collaborative study involving 11 centers (including our own) examined the sensitivity of sonography in detecting fetal DS.[18] They found that 85% of DS fetuses ($n=241$) had at least one abnormal finding on ultrasound. In 2003, an eight-center study (including our own) evaluated the utility of second-trimester genetic sonography among high-risk pregnancies, including 176 DS fetuses.[19] The sensitivity for DS was 72%, with a range from 64% to 80% at the various sites. Significantly, about half (47%) of DS fetuses had a thickened nuchal fold of 5 mm or

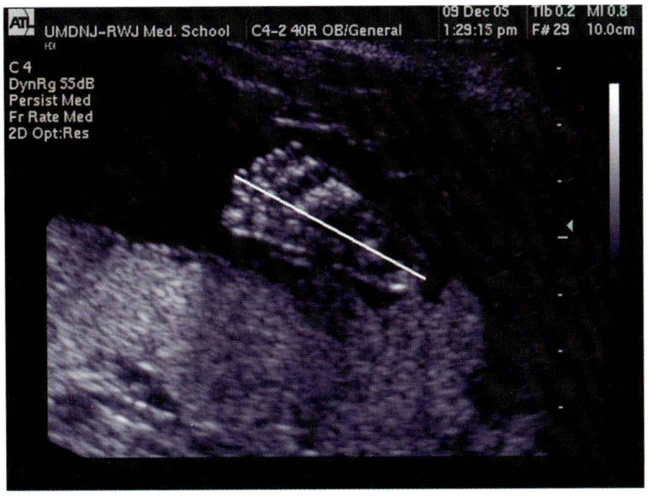

Figure 77.13 Measurement of second-trimester fetal foot length, with all five toes demonstrated.

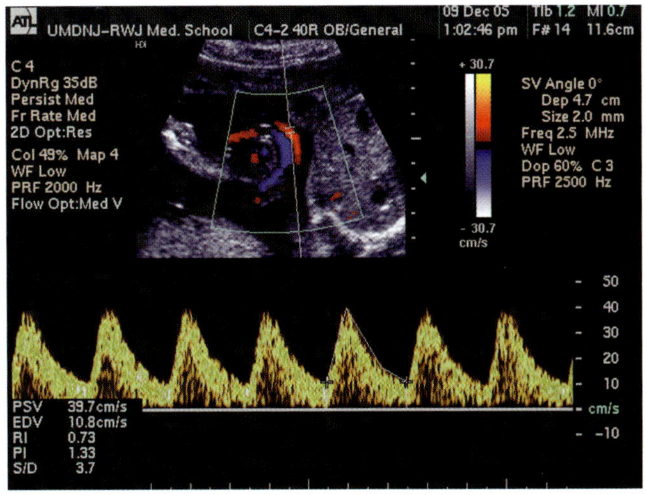

Figure 77.14 Normal Doppler waveform of umbilical artery in a second-trimester fetus. The systolic/diastolic ratio is 3.7.

more, making this marker the one with the highest sensitivity.

Nuchal fold thickening is the single most sensitive and specific marker for fetal DS (sensitivity 40% and false-positive rate of 0.1%),[20] although absent nasal bone has also recently been shown by us to have a 41% sensitivity and 100% specificity for fetal DS.[8] Short femur length (measured to expected length <0.91) has been found in 24% of DS fetuses,[21] while a short humerus (measured to expected length <0.90) identified 50% of DS fetuses, with a false-positive rate of 6.25%.[22] Unfortunately, there tends to be a large overlap in bone measurements between affected and normal fetuses. The sensitivity for pyelectasis (anteroposterior diameter renal pelvis >4 mm in second trimester) for DS is 25%.[22] Echogenic bowel has a reported sensitivity of 7–12.5%, while echogenic intracardiac focus has a sensitivity of 18%.[22] Recently, we examined the sensitivity for fetal DS by sonographic ear length.[23] We found that of 51 DS fetuses, 41% ($n=21$) had ear length ≤10th percentile. However, short ear length was not as sensitive a marker for DS as it was for trisomies 18 (96%) and 13 (100%). Although an association between choroid plexus cysts and trisomy 18 has been established,[24] the association with fetal DS has been controversial, especially when isolated. When the choroid plexus cyst(s) are isolated, obstetrical management should not be altered in the absence of any other high-risk factors.[25] Single umbilical artery has been found to be associated with aneuploidy and congenital malformations. The risk for fetal aneuploidy depends on the presence of associated anomalies: the greater the number of anomalies the greater the chances for aneuploidy. In a low-risk patient, an isolated single umbilical artery on ultrasound is probably not an indication for fetal karyotyping, provided that a search for additional malformations is negative.

In 1996, our group was the first to publish data on using second-trimester genetic sonography to guide clinical management of women at high-risk for fetal DS.[26] Subsequently, once we analyzed our 1999 data, in the presence of a normal genetic ultrasound, we counseled patients that the likelihood for fetal DS was reduced by at least 80% from the *a priori* risk (triple or quadruple screen, or if unavailable, maternal age).[17] Over almost a 10-year period (since November 1992), we have evaluated 5299 fetuses by genetic sonography; the overwhelming majority (85%) had no markers seen (normal scan), 12% had one abnormal marker present, and 3% had two or more markers present. When one or more abnormal sonographic markers were present, the sensitivity, specificity, positive and negative predictive values for DS were 87% (52/60), 91% (4395/4831), 11% (52/488), and 99.8% (4395/4403), respectively. Approximately two-thirds of DS fetuses had two or more abnormal sonographic markers seen.

Second-trimester ultrasound screening for fetal abnormalities

While there are numerous acceptable indications for performing a second-trimester sonographic exam during pregnancy, perhaps one of the most common indications is to rule out the presence of fetal abnormalities. While the advantages of performing a screening ultrasound in the pregnancies at high risk for fetal anomalies is clear, the benefits and cost-effectiveness of routine sonographic screening in pregnancy are not as obvious. In the USA, approximately 60–70% of all pregnant women undergo an ultrasound at various times in the gestation.[27] However, the efficacy of routine sonographic screening for fetal abnormalities varies widely. One of the first studies to determine the diagnostic accuracy of ultrasonography in high-risk pregnancies was performed during the late 1970s and early 1980s in the UK.[28] It was around this time that real-time imaging became widespread as a clinical tool. This study found that 95% of malformations were correctly diagnosed.[28] Other published sensitivities have ranged broadly anywhere from 13.3% to 82.4%,[29] with the average collaborative world experience being 50%.[30] After reviewing these extremely wide and different detection rates, it becomes apparent why the reliability and utility of sonographic screening for fetal abnormalities have become very controversial in some countries. Even for those who already advocate routine sonographic screening, when to perform scans and the number of sonographic exams are debatable and inconsistent. Since 75% of patients with abnormal fetuses will be 'low risk', it is reasonable to review data in the literature that assess the impact of routine screening sonography.[29]

Diagnosing fetal anomalies prior to birth can provide many advantages. Prenatal sonographic diagnosis can lead to further diagnostic testing (such as amniocentesis), prepare parents for an adverse pregnancy outcome, alert the clinician to the possibility of other abnormalities, and determine appropriate management choices (such as intrauterine therapy, early delivery, delivery at a tertiary care center, or termination of pregnancy). However, all these advantages are achieved only if the ultrasound exam is performed by qualified, knowledgeable individuals, who possess expertise performing ultrasonographic exams. Sonographic screening done by individuals who are inexperienced and unqualified may not only increase the costs of health care, but can create high false-negative and false-positive results with significant consequences.

There are a multitude of biases and problems that can account for the sensitivity variation across various studies.[29] Fetal abnormalities that resolve, technical factors (obesity, fetal positioning), quality of sonographic equipment, and undetectability of certain anomalies comprise some of the reasons. In addition, each center has differing criteria and interpretations as to what exactly constitutes a detailed sonographic exam. There is no doubt that the less detailed the exam, the higher the chances are for having a lower diagnostic accuracy. Selection bias can also play an important role in affecting diagnostic accuracy, depending on whether the patient source is a hospital, or office practice-based. Perhaps the most important bias is the variation in sonographic skills, capability, and experience of individuals performing the ultrasound examination. In the Helsinki study that incorporated patient populations from two hospitals, the ultrasonographic sensitivity for detecting anomalies was more than twofold higher in the university hospital than in the city hospital (77% vs. 36%).[31] A study in Vienna examined the influence of the experience of the investigator on the rate of sonographic diagnosis of fetal malformations.[32] Of 323 cases of fetal malformations, obstetricians in private offices detected 22%, hospital examiners detected 40%, and examiners in the prenatal diagnosis and therapy center detected 90% of all fetal malformations.[32] The selection of pregnant women is also significant. Screening high-risk women is likely to be much more effective. In this scenario, the chances of discovering an anomaly is higher, and the sonographers may be more attentively focused. For instance, in one study they found that the average sensitivity in low-risk populations is 55%, while in high-risk populations it is 92%.[29]

The gestational age at the time of ultrasound screening also impacts sensitivity, since various anomalies are manifested at differing gestational weeks or may be easier to visualize/detect, and some anomalies may present only later in gestation (duodenal atresia). In general, the more sonographic exams a patient undergoes during the pregnancy, the higher the rate of anomaly detection. Levi found that the average sensitivity from studies including scans performed once before 20 weeks was 45%; when scanning was done several times during the pregnancy, the sensitivity rose to 60%.[29] The prevalence of specific malformations within a given population may also have a significant impact on the overall sensitivity of ultrasound. A low frequency of anomalies in a certain population can introduce bias in diagnostic accuracy. Studies that exclude certain anomalies because they are felt to be 'minor' or undetectable may have dramatically different sensitivities than when all fetal anomalies are included. In 1996, one study found that the sensitivity of sonography for diagnosing both minor/major anomalies was only 8.7%; however, if only major anomalies detectable by ultrasound were included, the sensitivity was increased up to 75%.[30] Finally, other factors that can affect the reported fetal abnormality detection rates in sonographic screening may be related to ascertainment biases, such as lack of autopsies (considered the 'gold standard'), suboptimal or incomplete neonatal evaluation at birth, and insufficient length of neonatal follow-up since some abnormalities may not express themselves immediately after birth and can take time to manifest.[29]

In the USA, the RADIUS (Routine Antenatal Diagnostic Imaging with Ultrasound) study was the first randomized clinical trial of second-trimester ultrasound.[33] This trial was performed to determine the benefits, if any, of routine sonograms among pregnant women at low risk. It compared routinely scanned pregnant women to those having ultrasounds only when indicated. An additional ultrasound exam was performed in the early third trimester in the study group. Although the identification rate of anomalies was found to be three times better with routine ultrasound vs. indicated ultrasound (35% vs. 11%, respectively), the sensitivity in detecting anomalies by ultrasound performed between 15 and 22 weeks was extremely low (17%). A possible source of bias was that practice-based patients were utilized, which may have created an inadvertent selection bias (rather than a community or hospital-based population). This study reported a relative detection rate of 2.7 (95% CI, 1.3–5.8) in tertiary vs. non-tertiary ultrasound units.[33] Within a subgroup evaluated at tertiary care centers, the detection rate of anomalous fetuses was 35% vs. 13% in non-tertiary centers. This trial found that sonographic screening did not significantly influence the management or outcome of pregnancies complicated by congenital malformations. A 1998 study at a tertiary care center found that the sensitivity of anomaly detection in women at risk for anomalies was very high (89.7%).[34] In the screening group, or lower-risk population, although the sensitivity was less (47.6%), it was still sufficient to ensure cost-effectiveness for their patients.[34]

In 1999, the Eurofetus study was designed to evaluate the sensitivity of routine sonographic screening for fetal malformations.[35] In the largest among screening studies, ultrasound screening was applied to almost 200,000 pregnant women in 60 hospital laboratories and 14 European countries. They found a sensitivity rate of 64% (2363/3685), which at first glance, was much higher compared to the RADIUS study. However, for various reasons these two studies may not be exactly comparable. For example, patients studied in the RADIUS trial were low risk (and probably not relevant to the average population), since very strict exclusion criteria had been applied prior to patient recruitment. The criteria used to designate major fetal anomalies (gold standard) were also very liberal, and both of these facts could have lowered the sensitivity. On the other hand, in the Eurofetus study, all patients were studied regardless of their risk status, and only 'truly' major abnormalities were considered as endpoints. This could have artificially raised the sensitivity of the sonographic screening.

The Helsinki trial had patients undergo one ultrasound screening exam within the second trimester; 40% of major fetal anomalies were detected.[36] Although screening did detect most anomalies of the central nervous system, genitourinary system, and cases with multiple anomalies, it was less satisfactory in detecting cardiac and gastrointestinal tract anomalies.[36] The Belgian Multicentric Study found that of 381 structurally abnormal fetuses, 154 were correctly detected by ultrasound (sensitivity 40%).[37] The specificity, positive and negative predictive values were 99.9%, 95%, and 98.6%, respectively.

In 2002, we examined the value of our aforementioned complete anatomic sonographic survey in detecting fetal abnormalities, and correlated our sonographic findings with perinatal autopsy results.[38] Autopsy findings were considered the 'gold standard'. Of 88 abnormal autopsies, 85 fetuses had one or more abnormal structural sonographic findings, for a sensitivity of 97% (for anomalous fetuses). From autopsy, a total of 372 separate abnormalities were found; of the 299 major and 73 minor abnormalities, prenatal ultrasonography detected 75% and 18%, respectively. Thus, we found that the sensitivity for detecting minor abnormalities was poor, even when utilizing a complete sonographic survey. We found either complete agreement or only minor differences between sonographic and autopsy findings in 65% of the cases.[38]

In examining the literature, it is evident that there is a wide range in sensitivity of ultrasonography to detect fetal anomalies, and it depends highly on the clinical setting in which the exam is performed, along with the varying skills, expertise, and experience of those performing the sonographic exam. Therefore, there appears to be insufficient evidence to comment on a single estimate of the sensitivity of routine ultrasound in screening for fetal anomalies. However, in many studies, the specificity of a fetal anatomic survey has been found to exceed 99%.[33,39–41] This fact indicates that in the low-risk population, sonography may be helpful in ruling out abnormalities and detecting the normal, but may not be equally reliable in detecting abnormalities. It is expected that with time, the sensitivity of sonographic screening programs should improve. This can be partly attributable to improvements in equipment quality, training, and experience of sonographers, along with the emergence of new technological advances such as three- and four-dimensional sonography. It is thought that uniform and detailed training for practitioners is the best guarantee for an efficient screening program.[29] In addition, standardization of the scanning process for each and every scan should also improve overall sensitivity. In a 1996 review article, Seeds argues that the diagnostic sensitivity of the screening obstetrical ultrasound examination appears to be highest in high-risk patients examined by highly specialized and experienced personnel.[42] However, diagnostic sensitivity may be quite good even in low-risk patients with a basic or routine examination if recognized guidelines for content are followed and referral to experienced referral resources for unclear or suspicious images is liberally practiced.[42]

A common and often touted benefit of the prenatal detection of fetal abnormalities, especially those that are life-threatening, is the delivery of these infants in tertiary care centers that are capable of providing immediate and appropriate care. A valid and legitimate question often asked is whether routine sonography improves the survival rates of anomalous neonates. Ten years ago, the RADIUS study examined this question.[33] Screening ultrasound was not found to have any impact on the detection, management, and outcome of fetuses with anomalies. Although survival rates for fetuses with anomalies were not affected by sonographic screening, in an analysis of infants with life-threatening anomalies, 75% (21/28) in the routinely screened group survived, vs. 52% (11/21) in the routine-care group.[33] While this difference did not reach statistical significance, this may be attributed in part to the small sample sizes.

At present, there is insufficient evidence to either refute or support the benefit of routine sonography in reducing mortality of those neonates with life-threatening anomalies, although this may not be intuitively apparent to those families affected with these problems. It is clear that further studies are required to address this issue.

A significant question regarding routine ultrasonography is whether this improves overall perinatal morbidity and mortality. It is known that routine diagnostic sonography can lead to accurate determination of gestational age, multiple gestations, and placental abnormalities, thus theoretically improving perinatal risk. Three trials have examined perinatal morbidity and mortality in patients undergoing routine ultrasonography. In both the RADIUS and Stockholm trials, perinatal mortality rates were similar between the routine sonography and control groups.[27,43] However, the Helsinki trial found that the perinatal mortality rate was significantly improved in the routine ultrasound group (4.6/1000 vs. 9.0/1000); this 49.2% reduction was mainly attributable to improved early detection of major malformations, which led to termination of pregnancy.[31] In all three trials, no differences were found between the study and control groups in terms of perinatal morbidity.[27,31,43] Perinatal morbidity was defined as admission to the neonatal unit,[31,43] moderate morbidity (neonatal sepsis, grade I or II intraventricular hemorrhage, stay of > 5 days in neonatal unit), or severe morbidity (ventilation > 48 h, stay of > 30 days in neonatal unit).[27] In terms of birth weight and number of low birth weight (< 2500 g) infants, the RADIUS and Helsinki trials found a similar birth weight distribution between the routine ultrasound and control groups.[27,31] However, the Stockholm trial found fewer births of < 2500 g (2.5% vs. 4%) in the routine ultrasound group.[43] Finally, this same trial found that for women smokers, there was a higher mean birth weight (3413 vs. 3354 g) in the routine ultrasound group, and the authors surmised that this improvement could be attributed to healthier maternal behaviors after women visualized their fetuses on ultrasound.[43] The RADIUS trial investigators concluded that adopting sonographic screening in the USA would increase health-care costs without either improving perinatal outcome or providing any measurable benefit from early detection of fetal anomalies. In contrast, however, another group found that routine abnormality screening improves perinatal outcome by leading to termination of pregnancies for certain anomalies, and selected delivery at tertiary care centers for life-threatening malformations.[34]

An important issue to examine is the cost–benefit analysis of routine second-trimester sonography. Our group recently performed a cost–benefit analysis based on the RADIUS results, and compared a policy of routine second-trimester sonography in low-risk pregnant women vs. not offering such screening.[44] We concluded that routine second-trimester sonographic screening is associated with net benefits only if the ultrasound was performed in tertiary care centers. Another tertiary center also assessed the cost-effectiveness of anomaly screening in their patient population, and found that routine screening appeared cost-effective.[34] Leivo and associates demonstrated that a one-stage second-trimester screening ultrasound was co[illegible] effective, and was associated with fewer perinat[illegible] deaths.[45] In the UK, a prospective study was performed to evaluate the cost–benefit of changing from selective to routine ultrasound screening for fetal anomaly.[46] They found that routine sonography was the sole method of detection for 11 major and 18 less severe congenital abnormalities found in low-risk pregnancies, which would not previously have qualified for selective ultrasound. They felt that routine fetal anomaly ultrasound would seen to be economically justifiable.[46] In 2002, Roberts reviewed evidence from the literature and found a need for more data on the costs and cost-effectiveness of routine sonographic screening for fetal anomalies.[47]

All published trials have shown that more twin pregnancies are diagnosed earlier with routine ultrasound. The Helsinki trial found that with the routine ultrasound group, 100% of twins were detected prior to 21 weeks, compared with 76% in the control group.[31] In addition, they found that the perinatal mortality for the twins was 27.8/1000 vs. 65.8/1000, respectively. The RADIUS trial also performed subgroup analyses for small for gestational age infants and neonates born at 42 weeks.[27] The data did not show improvement in overall outcome for these conditions when routing sonography was performed.

In conclusion, examination of the available evidence shows that in low-risk pregnancies, routine ultrasonography may reduce perinatal mortality because of induced abortions following the detection of fetal abnormalities. In the USA, the current standard of care remains at performing ultrasound only for specific indications. However, some would argue that every obstetrical patient should have an ultrasound examination only if it is competently performed, properly recorded, and if the patient is aware of appropriate goals and limitations.[42]

Although ultrasonographic screening for fetal abnormalities may have widely varying sensitivities depending on the particular unit, in our opinion it still offers great value to both patients and physicians that may not be quantifiable. Psychological reassurance, referrals, genetic counseling, antepartum management, and preparation of families and health care providers are just some examples of the possible advantages. Overall, these reasons may outweigh the 'risks' of ultrasound, such as false-positive diagnoses. If patients are given the choice and counseled regarding the diagnostic capabilities of present-day sonography, most would choose to undergo fetal anomaly screening. It is important to remember that pregnant women often do not perceive ultrasonography as a 'test', but rather utilize it as a tool to evaluate their fetus as a patient. We concur with this philosophy, and would also argue that examining the fetus as a patient via ultrasound should be offered routinely, as in all other aspects of adult medicine.

Conclusions

Second-trimester sonographic screening for fetal anomalies and prenatal diagnosis is performed for many reasons. It can provide useful information and knowledge for patients, may give them reassurance regarding their pregnancy and the health of their fetus, provides the opportunity for further diagnostic testing such as amniocentesis, provides counseling regarding prognosis, and can modify management (such as location and method of delivery, termination, fetal surgery). Some patients will utilize this information to prepare ahead of the delivery date by consulting geneticists, pediatric surgeons, neonatologists, and other specialists. In addition, for the physician, information regarding specific abnormalities or aneuploidy can optimize pregnancy management, along with the labor and delivery process. Importantly, knowledge of anomalies can raise the possibility of genetic syndromes, can impact future pregnancies, and can influence counseling regarding genetics and prognosis. Therefore, because of its many advantages, it is our opinion that all patients should have access to sonographic screening within the second trimester of pregnancy, and a complete, targeted, and thorough exam should be performed to increase sensitivity.

REFERENCES

1. American College of Obstetricians and Gynecologists. New ultrasound output display standard. *2003 Compendium of Selected Publications*, 2003:69–70.
2. Grandjean H, Larroque D, Levi S. The performance of routine ultrasonographic screening of pregnancies in the Eurofetus Study. *Am J Obstet Gynecol* 1999;181(2):446–54.
3. Yeo L, Vintzileos AM, Guzman ER, Day-Salvatore D, Farren-Chavez D. Targeted ultrasound after an abnormal karyotype: The patient's persepctive. *Am J Obstet Gynecol* 2001;185:S233.
4. The American Institute of Ultrasound in Medicine. *Standards for Performance of the Antepartum Obstetrical Ultrasound Examination*. Laurel, MD: American Institute of Ultrasound in Medicine, 1994.
5. Schwarzler P, Senat MV, Holden D, Bernard JP, Masroor T, Ville Y. Feasibility of the second-trimester fetal ultrasound examination in an unselected population at 18, 20 or 22 weeks of pregnancy: A randomized trial. *Ultrasound Obstet Gynecol* 1999;14(2):92–7.
6. Mahony BS, Callen PW, Filly RA, Hoddick WK. The fetal cisterna magna. *Radiology* 1984;153:773–6.
7. Laing FC, Frates MC, Brown DL, Benson CB, DiSalvo DN, Doubilet PM. Sonography of the fetal posterior fossa: False appearance of mega-cisterna magna and Dandy–Walker variant. *Radiology* 1994;192:247–51.
8. Vintzileos A, Walters C, Yeo L. Absent nasal bone in the prenatal detection of fetuses with trisomy 21 in a high-risk population. *Obstet Gynecol* 2003;101:905–8.
9. Cicero S, Bindra R, Rembouskos G, Tripsanas C, Nicolaides KH. Fetal nasal bone length in chromosomally normal and abnormal fetuses at 11–14 weeks of gestation. *J Matern Fetal Neonatal Med* 2002;11:400–2.
10. Bromley B, Liberman E, Shipp TD, Benacerraf BR. Fetal nose bone length; a marker for Down syndrome in the second trimester. *J Ultrasound Med* 2002;21:1387–94.
11. Levy DW, Mintz MC. The left ventricular echogenic focus: A normal finding. *AJR Am J Roentgenol* 1988;150(1):85–6.
12. Sepulveda W, Cullen S, Nicolaidis P, Hollingsworth J, Fisk NM. Echogenic foci in the fetal heart: A marker of chromosomal abnormality. *Br J Obstet Gynaecol* 1995;102(6):490–2.
13. Vincoff NS, Callen PW, Smith-Bindman R, Goldstein RB. Effect of ultrasound transducer frequency on the appearance of the fetal bowel. *J Ultrasound Med* 1999;18(12):799–803.
14. Yeo L, Guzman ER, Day-Salvatore D, Walters C, Chavez D, Vintzileos AM. Prenatal detection of fetal trisomy 18 through abnormal sonographic features. *J Ultrasound Med* 2003;22:581–90.
15. Alberman ED, Creasy MR. Frequency of chromosomal abnormalities in miscarriages and perinatal deaths. *J Med Genet* 1977;14: 313–5.
16. Vintzileos AM, Egan JF. Adjusting the risk for trisomy 21 on the basis of second trimester ultrasonography. *Am J Obstet Gynecol* 1995;172:837–44.
17. Yeo L, Vintzileos AM. The use of genetic sonography to reduce the need for amniocentesis in women at high-risk for Down syndrome. *Semin Perinatol* 2003;27:152–9.
18. Persutte WH, Hobbins JC, Nyberg DA, *et al.* Trisomy 21 multicenter collaborative project (abstract). *Am J Obstet Gynecol* 1998; 178:S22.
19. Hobbins JC, Lezotte DC, Persutte WH, *et al.* An eight center study to evaluate the utility of mid-term genetic ultrasounds among high-risk pregnancies. *J Ultrasound Med* 2003;22:33–8.
20. Benacerraf BR, Barss BA, Laboda LA. A sonographic sign for the detection in the second trimester of the fetus with Down's syndrome. *Am J Obstet Gynecol* 1985;151:1078–9.
21. Nyberg DA, Resta RG, Hickok DE, *et al.* Femur length shortening in the detection of Down syndrome: Is prenatal screening feasible? *Am J Obstet Gynecol* 1990;162:1247–52.
22. Bromley B, Benacerraf BR. The genetic sonogram scoring index. *Semin Perinatol* 2003;27:124–9.
23. Yeo L, Guzman ER, Ananth CV, *et al.* Prenatal detection of fetal aneuploidy by sonographic ear length. *J Ultrasound Med* 2003; 22:565–76.
24. Gross SJ, Shulman LP, Tolley EA, *et al.* Isolated fetal choroid plexus cysts and trisomy 18: A review and meta-analysis. *Am J Obstet Gynecol* 1995;172:83–7.
25. Chitty LS, Chudleigh P, Wright E, Campbell S, Pembrey M. The significance of choroid plexus cysts in an unselected population: Results of a multicenter study. *Ultrasound Obstet Gynecol* 1998;12:391–7.
26. Vintzileos AM, Campbell WA, Rodis JF, *et al.* The use of second-trimester genetic sonogram in guiding clinical management of patients at increased risk for fetal trisomy 21. *Obstet Gynecol* 1996;87:948–52.
27. Ewigman BG, Crane JP, Frigoletto FD, LeFevre ML, Bain RP, McNellis D. Effect of prenatal ultrasound screening on perinatal outcome. RADIUS Study Group. *N Engl J Med* 1993;329:821–7.
28. Campbell S, Pearce JM. The prenatal diagnosis of fetal structural anomalies by ultrasound. *Clin Obstet Gynecol* 1983;10:475–506.
29. Levi S. Ultrasound in prenatal diagnosis: Polemics around routine ultrasound screening for second trimester fetal malformations. *Prenat Diagn* 2002;22:285–95.
30. Skupski DW, Newman S, Edersheim T, *et al.* Fetus–placenta–newborn: The impact of routine obstetric ultrasonographic screening in a low-risk population. *Am J Obstet Gynecol* 1996;175:1142–5.
31. Saari-Kemppainen A, Karjalainen O, Ylostalo P, Heinonen OP. Ultrasound screening and perinatal mortality: Controlled trial

systematic one-stage screening in pregnancy. The Helsinki Ultrasound Trial. *Lancet* 1990;336:387–91.

32. Bernaschek G, Stuempflen I, Deutinger J. The influence of the experience of the investigator on the rate of sonographic diagnosis of fetal malformations in Vienna. *Prenat Diagn* 1996;16: 807–11.
33. Crane JP, LeFevre ML, Winborn RC, *et al.* A randomized trial of prenatal ultrasonographic screening: Impact on the detection, management, and outcome of anomalous fetuses. The RADIUS Study Group. *Am J Obstet Gynecol* 1994;171:392–9.
34. VanDorsten JP, Hulsey TC, Newman RB, Menard MK. Fetal anomaly detection by second-trimester ultrasonography in a tertiary center. *Am J Obstet Gynecol* 1998;178:742–9.
35. Grandjean H, Larroque D, Levi S, the Eurofetus team. The performance of routine ultrasonographic screening of pregnancies in the Eurofetus study. *Am J Obstet Gynecol* 1999;181:446–54.
36. Saari-Kemppainen A, Karjalainen O, Ylostalo P, Heinonen OP. Fetal anomalies in a controlled one-stage ultrasound screening trial. A report from the Helsinki Ultrasound Trial. *J Perinat Med* 1994;22:279–89.
37. Levi S, Hyjazi Y, Schaapst JP. Sensitivity and specificity of routine antenatal screening for congenital anomalies by ultrasound: The Belgian Multicentric Study. *Ultrasound Obstet Gynecol* 1991; 1:102–10.
38. Yeo L, Guzman ER, Shen-Schwarz S, Walters C, Vintzileos AM. Value of a complete sonographic survey in detecting fetal abnormalities: Correlation with perinatal autopsy. *J Ultrasound Med* 2002;21:501–10.
39. Chitty LS, Hunt GH, Moore J, Lobb MO. Effectiveness of routine ultrasonography in detecting fetal structural abnormalities in a low risk population. *Br Med J* 1991;303:1165–9.
40. Levi S, Schaaps JP, De Havay P, Coulon P, Defoort P. End-result of routine ultrasound screening for congenital anomalies: The Belgium Multicentric Study 1984–92. *Ultrasound Obstet Gynecol* 1995;5:366–71.
41. Shirley IM, Bottomley F, Robinson VP. Routine radiographer screening for fetal abnormalities by ultrasound in an unselected low risk population. *Br J Radiol* 1992;65:564–9.
42. Seeds JW. The routine or screening obstetrical ultrasound examination. *Clin Obstet Gynecol* 1996;39:814–30.
43. Waldenstrom U, Axelsson O, Nilsson S, *et al.* Effects of routine one-stage ultrasound screening in pregnancy: A randomized controlled trial. *Lancet* 1988;2:585–8.
44. Vintzileos AM, Ananth CV, Smulian JC, Beazoglou T, Knuppel RA. Routine second-trimester ultrasonography in the United States: A cost benefit analysis. *Am J Obstet Gynecol* 2000;182:655–60.
45. Leivo T, Tuominen R, Saari-Kemppainen A, Ylostalo P, Karjalainen O, Heinonen OP. Cost-effectiveness of one-stage ultrasound screening in pregnancy: A report from the Helsinki ultrasound trial. *Ultrasound Obstet Gynecol* 1996;7:309–14.
46. Long G, Sprigg A. A comparative study of routine versus selective fetal anomaly ultrasound scanning. *J Med Screen* 1998;5:6–10.
47. Roberts T, Henderson J, Mugford M, Bricker L, Neilson J, Garcia J. Antenatal ultrasound screening for fetal abnormalities: A systematic review of studies of cost and cost effectiveness. *Br J Obstet Gynaecol* 2002;109:44–56.

78 First-trimester maternal serum markers of fetal anomalies

D. A. Krantz, T. W. Hallahan and J. N. Macri

Historically, prenatal screening for Down's syndrome and other chromosomal abnormalities had been conducted in the second trimester of pregnancy with results available between 16 and 18 weeks of pregnancy. Such screening can detect 60–70% of Down's syndrome cases with a false-positive rate of 5%.[1] Now, first-trimester Down's syndrome screening has become an important option for prospective parents providing risk information as early as 11–12 weeks of pregnancy and detecting up to 90% of Down's syndrome cases at the same 5% false-positive rate.[2–16]

The advantages of first-trimester screening are that most patients (95%) receive very early reassurance that they are at low risk, the test provides a significantly higher detection efficiency compared to most second-trimester screening methods, patients have more time and more diagnostic options to consider, and in cases where patients choose to terminate an affected pregnancy safer procedures are available in the first trimester. Further, pregnancies that may have ended in an unexplained fetal loss may now have karyotype information available.

First-trimester Down's syndrome and trisomy 18 screening includes the biochemical analysis of free beta human chorionic gonadotropin (free beta hCG) and pregnancy-associated plasma protein A (PAPP-A) combined with the ultrasound evaluation of nuchal translucency. This protocol has been studied extensively, and the first-trimester risk estimates have been validated.[17]

Free beta hCG

During normal pregnancy free beta hCG rises to peak levels at 8–9 weeks of pregnancy and then steadily declines to about 20 weeks when concentrations begin to level off. In second-trimester Down's syndrome pregnancies, free beta hCG is significantly elevated with a median MoM (multiple of the median) of 2.64.[18] By contrast, free alpha hCG has been observed to be unchanged (median MoM = 0.99)[19] or marginally elevated (median MoM = 1.31)[20] in cases of Down's syndrome. This proportionally higher increase observed in the beta subunit relative to the alpha subunit observed at the protein level is reflected at the mRNA level. Indeed, Eldar-Geva *et al.* demonstrated that the beta subunit MRNA content was proportionally increased compared to the alpha subunit in cultured second-trimester trophoblasts.[21] This suggests that the increase of the beta subunit in maternal serum may be due in part to increased synthesis. More recently, beta subunit MRNA has been detected in maternal serum and has also been demonstrated to be elevated in cases of Down's syndrome.[22]

In the first trimester, free beta hCG is significantly elevated in Down's syndrome pregnancies and is the only Down's syndrome marker that is effective in both first- and second-trimester screening. In two recent studies the median free beta hCG MoM in Down's syndrome increased with increasing gestational age from about 1.5 MoM at 9 weeks' gestation to 2.1 MoM at 13 weeks 6 days' gestation.[23,24] In the Serum, Urine and Ultrasound Screening Study (SURUSS) case–control study the median MoM of free beta hCG in Down's syndrome cases increased from 1.6 MoM at 10 weeks' gestation to 2.6 MoM at 13 weeks 6 days.[25] Therefore, free beta hCG becomes more effective with increasing gestational age. In trisomy 18 affected pregnancies, a study of 28 cases showed the median free beta hCG MoM to be 0.18 in the first trimester representing an 80% reduction from normal pregnancies.[7]

Pregnancy-associated plasma protein-A

Pregnancy-associated plasma protein-A (PAPP-A) is a 750 kDa zinc metalloproteinase. It is produced by the trophoblast and exists in maternal circulation as a disulfide bridged dimeric glycoprotein and as a 2:2 complex with the proform of eosinophil major basic protein (proMBP). Circulating levels are detectable as early as 4 weeks in pregnancy and double approximately every 6 days throughout the first trimester. PAPP-A concentrations rise exponentially in the second trimester to reach approximately 50 mg/l in the third trimester.

In the first trimester, PAPP-A is significantly decreased in Down's syndrome pregnancies. The discrimination between unaffected and Down's syndrome pregnancy is greatest earlier in pregnancy. Our own data on 163 cases of Down's syndrome showed a median MoM of 0.3 at 9 weeks and 0.8 MoM at 13 weeks 6 days.[23] Spencer *et al.*[24] showed a median MoM of 0.37 at 9 weeks and 0.70 at 13 weeks 6 days while the SURUSS study showed a median MoM of 0.29 at 9 weeks and 0.62 at 13 weeks 6 days.[25] Therefore, PAPP-A becomes less effective with increasing gestational age and by the second trimester is no longer a marker for Down's syndrome. In trisomy 18 pregnancies, the median first trimester level of PAPP-A is 0.33 representing a 2/3 reduction from normal levels.[7]

Table 78.1 Impact of training and quality review of nuchal translucency measurements on first-trimester Down's syndrome screening detection rates

Study	Snidjers *et al.*[28]	Haddow *et al.*[29]
Training and quality review	Yes	No
Centers	22	11
Patients	96,127	3991
False-positive rate	5%	5%
Detection rate	77%	31%

Results based on nuchal translucency only without biochemistry

Combining free beta hCG and PAPP-A

The levels of both free beta hCG and PAPP-A in Down's syndrome affected pregnancies tend to increase with increasing gestational age. As a result, with increasing gestational age free beta hCG becomes more effective while PAPP-A becomes less effective. These two trends tend to offset each other, such that the combination is effective in screening for Down's syndrome between 9 weeks and 13 weeks 6 days. However, the combined performance of free beta hCG and PAPP-A is optimized in the earlier gestations. For example, at a 5% false-positive rate, the detection rate is 69% if the blood is drawn at 10 weeks while it is 63% if the blood is drawn at 13 weeks.[26] These detection rates are as good as or better than those seen with second-trimester triple test.

Dried blood collection

Maternal serum screening has largely involved venepuncture collection of whole blood into red-top tubes. Recently, whole blood sample collection using finger-stick lancets and filter paper has become more common. The ease of collection and transport of dried blood specimens allows for greater flexibility in screening logistics. Since no phlebotomist is required, the simple finger-stick procedure can easily take place in the physician's office, ultrasound lab or ultimately in the patient's home. Quantitative analysis of prenatal screening markers in dried blood samples is highly correlated with liquid serum samples.[27] In addition, dried blood technology stabilizes serum proteins and therefore provides better overall analyte precision leading to both higher detection rates and lower false-positive rates.

Combined biochemistry and ultrasound screening

In addition to maternal serum markers, the evaluation of fetal nuchal translucency in ultrasound has been demonstrated to be a highly effective marker for Down's syndrome.[28] As a result, for the first time, biochemical and biophysical markers are combined in a single screening protocol for the detection of Down's syndrome. The challenge has been to introduce nuchal translucency assessment in a standardized, quality-controlled fashion to allow for efficient population screening. Laboratories perform a significant number of quality control procedures prior to releasing the results of biochemical tests to the clinician. Nuchal translucency, as a quantitative marker in the screening process must meet similar standards of quality control as biochemical markers. Therefore, sonographers must be specifically trained to perform nuchal translucency measurement using a standardized methodology and their results audited on a regular basis. The improved effectiveness of nuchal translucency screening when a quality control program is in place is dramatic (Table 78.1). In the study of Snidjers *et al.*,[28] in which sonographers underwent training and quality review, nuchal translucency detected 77% of Down's syndrome cases while in the study of Haddow *et al.*,[29] in which there was no specific training or quality control, the detection was only 31%.

Currently, the standard first-trimester Down's syndrome and trisomy 18 screening protocol combines the biochemical analysis of free beta hCG and PAPP-A with the ultrasound evaluation of nuchal translucency. A summary of 15 studies encompassing over 80,000 patients using the free beta hCG, PAPP-A and nuchal translucency protocol demonstrates a

Table 78.2 Summary of first-trimester Down's syndrome screening studies using free beta hCG, PAPP-A and nuchal translucency

Study	*N*	FPR	Down's syndrome cases		Detection rate (%)
			Number detected	Total	
Orlandi *et al.*[2]	744	5.0	6	7	86
Biagiotti *et al.*[3]	232	5.0	24	32	75
De Biasio *et al.*[4]	1467	3.3	11	13	85
De Graaf *et al.*[5]	300	5.0	31	37	84
Spencer *et al.*[6]	1156	5.0	187	210	89
Krantz *et al.*[7]	5718	5.0	30	33	91
Niemimaa *et al.*[8]	1602	5.4	4	5	80
Schucter *et al.*[9]	4939	5.0	12	14	86
Von Kaisenberg *et al.*[10]	3864	6.6	16	19	84
Bindra *et al.*[11]	15030	5.0	74	82	90
Wapner *et al.*[12]	8514	5.0	48	61	79
Spencer *et al.*[13]	10458	5.0	23	25	92
Sheffield *et al.*[14]	18140	5.0	60	64	94
Borrell *et al.*[15]	2780	3.3	7	8	88
Stenhouse *et al.*[16]	5084	5.9	14	15	93
Total	80,028	5.0	547	625	88

FPR, false-positive rate

Table 78.3 Relative contribution of biochemistry and nuchal translucency (NT) in first-trimester Down's syndrome screening at a 5% false-positive rate (reprinted from Krantz *et al.*[7])

Initial protocol	PAPP-A + NT	Free beta hCG + NT	Free beta hCG + PAPP-A	NT
A. % detected	81%	80%	63%	74%
B. % undetected	19%	20%	37%	26%
Additional marker(s)	Free beta hCG	PAPP-A	NT	Free beta hCG + PAPP-A
C. Combined detection (%)	91%	91%	91%	91%
D. Extra detection with inclusion of additional marker(s) = (C − A)	10%	11%	28%	17%
E. % of remaining undetected cases detected with inclusion of additional marker(s) = (D ÷ B)	53%	55%	76%	65%

88% detection rate for Down's syndrome at a 5% false-positive rate (Table 78.2).[2–16]

Combined biochemical and biophysical screening significantly improves the detection and false-positive rates for Down's syndrome compared to either mode alone. The study by Krantz *et al.*,[7] for example, showed the additional detection rate attributable to each marker in the protocol. In that study, free beta hCG added 10%, PAPP-A added 11% and nuchal translucency added 28% detection beyond that achieved by the corresponding other two markers alone (Table 78.3). Therefore to reach the optimal detection rate it is necessary to include all of these markers in the analysis.

Combined screening is also highly effective in detecting trisomy 18 and other chromosomal abnormalities. Using an independent algorithm for the calculation of patient specific trisomy 18 risk detects 97% of trisomy 18 cases with only an additional 1.2% false-positive rate.[7] In the biochemistry and ultrasound nuchal (BUN) translucency study, all 11 cases of trisomy 18 and 16 of 29 (55%) cases of other chromosomal abnormalities were detected.[12] Spencer *et al.* have shown that triploidy is associated with abnormal combined screening results with triploidy types I and II having different patterns of marker levels.[30] Type I triploidy, in which the additional chromosome is of paternal origin is associated with extremely high free beta hCG, mildly decreased PAPP-A and increased nuchal translucency. Type II triploidy, in which the additional chromosome is of maternal origin is associated with extremely low free beta hCG, extremely low PAPP-A and normal nuchal translucency.

Other perinatal risks

Abnormal free beta hCG and PAPP-A are both associated with increased perinatal risk. Low levels of PAPP-A are associated with increased risk of intrauterine growth restriction.[31–37] For example, Krantz *et al.*[31] found that PAPP-A values less than the 1st percentile were associated with a 5.4-fold increase in the odds of intrauterine growth restriction with a positive predictive value of 24.1%. Krantz *et al.*[31] also found that free beta hCG values less than the 1st percentile were associated with a 2.7-fold increase in the odds of intrauterine growth restriction with a positive predictive value of 14.3% while other studies that evaluated less extreme cut-offs for free beta hCG or treated free beta hCG as a continuous variable did not find an association with intrauterine growth restriction.[32,33,36–39] Goetzl *et al.*[40] have found that low levels of both free beta hCG and PAPP-A are associated with increased risk of spontaneous abortion. Free beta hCG levels below the 1st percentile were associated with an 8.5-fold increase in the odds of spontaneous abortion while levels below the 5th percentile were associated with a 4.3-fold increase in the odds ratio. PAPP-A levels below the 1st percentile were associated with a 5.4-fold increase, while PAPP-A levels below the 5th percentile were associated with a 2.4-fold increase in the odds of spontaneous abortion. Most importantly, patients with normal free beta hCG, PAPP-A and nuchal translucency (i.e., those with levels between the 5th and 95th percentiles) had a very low risk of fetal loss before 20 weeks (0.36%). Yaron *et al.*[34,38] found a similar association between free beta hCG and PAPP-A with fetal loss.

Maternal factors

As with second-trimester screening, maternal factors play a role in first-trimester Down's syndrome screening. Several studies have shown that patients with increased maternal weight tend to have lower free beta hCG and PAPP-A levels.[41–43] Spencer *et al.*[42] showed that there can be a twofold difference in Down's syndrome risk estimates if maternal weight is not accounted for. The effect on trisomy 18 risk can be even greater since heavier patients would have lower levels of both free beta hCG and PAPP-A which would increase the trisomy 18 risk based on both markers.

Ethnic differences in biochemical results have also been observed.[43] After weight adjustment, free beta hCG levels are higher for African Americans (15%) and Asians (6%) but lower for Hispanics (11%) compared to Caucasians. For PAPP-A, African Americans have 30% higher levels than Caucasians after weight adjustment.

The effect of assisted reproduction techniques on first-trimester combined ultrasound and biochemical Down's syndrome screening is minimal. Orlandi *et al.*[44] found that the false-positive rate for intracytoplasmic sperm injection (ICSI) (5.2%) and IVF pregnancies (4.2%) was only slightly higher than the false-positive rate in naturally conceived pregnancies (3.3%). Similarly, Liao *et al.*[45] found that the false-positive rate increased by only 1.2 percentage points in IVF pregnancies. Wojdemann *et al.*[46] found no significant difference in the false-positive rates among a group of naturally conceived pregnancies (4.9%), in vitro fertilization (IVF) pregnancies (4.7%) and ovulation induction pregnancies (5.1%).

Screening in twin pregnancy

First-trimester screening of twin pregnancies offers a distinct advantage over second-trimester screening in that it can be used to evaluate the risk of each individual fetus. In second-trimester screening, which is based on biochemical markers alone, the risk is pregnancy specific. For monozygotic twins, in which either both are affected or both are unaffected, second-trimester detection efficiencies can be expected to be similar to that observed in singleton pregnancies. However, 67% of naturally conceived and 93% of assisted reproduction twin conceptions are dizygotic, and therefore the majority of Down's syndrome affected twin pregnancies can be expected to be discordant. In such cases, since the observed maternal serum marker levels are the sum contributions from each fetus, not only is it impossible to determine which fetus is contributing abnormal analyte levels but the detection efficiency will be decreased due to a dilution effect from the contribution of the normal fetus. Indeed the detection of Down's syndrome in twins by second-trimester maternal serum screening is estimated at about 50%, significantly lower than that expected in singletons at a 5% false-positive rate.[47]

In first-trimester screening, nuchal translucency, a biophysical marker, is fetus specific. Fetus-specific risks can be calculated based on nuchal translucency and the detection rate should be similar to that observed in singleton pregnancy. However, each fetus will carry an approximate 5% false-positive rate and therefore the false-positive rate per twin pregnancy based on nuchal translucency only is significantly greater than in singleton pregnancy. For example, in a study by Sebire *et al.*,[48] 7.3% of fetuses had an increased nuchal translucency. However, among pregnancies, 11.6% had at least one twin with an increased nuchal translucency.

Incorporating biochemistry into the first-trimester protocol along with nuchal translucency can reduce the false-positive rate. In our own data on a group of 212 twin pregnancies the false-positive rate was reduced from 13.2% using maternal age and nuchal translucency to 6.6% by also including the biochemistry.[49] Detection efficiency in twin pregnancy is difficult to document because Down's syndrome affected twin pregnancies are rare. However, modeling indicates that combining free beta hCG and PAPP-A with nuchal translucency can result in 80% detection rate for a 7% false-positive rate in twin pregnancy.[49] Therefore it is feasible to screen twin pregnancies for Down's syndrome in the first trimester. However until larger datasets of affected twin pregnancy are available a caution that risk estimates in twin pregnancy are less precise than in singleton pregnancy should be indicated on patient reports.

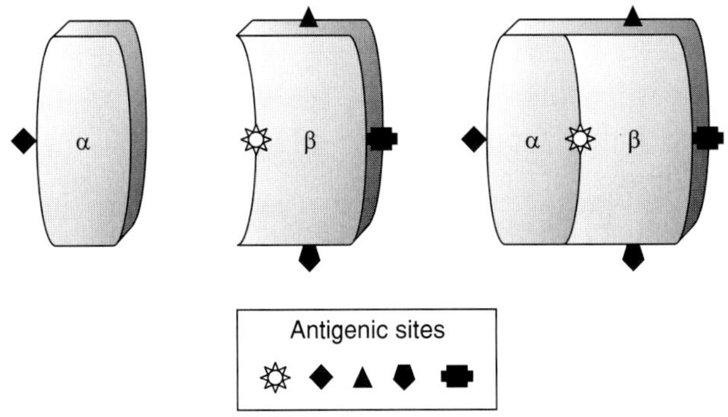

Figure 78.1 Schematic representation of hCG and its free subunits.

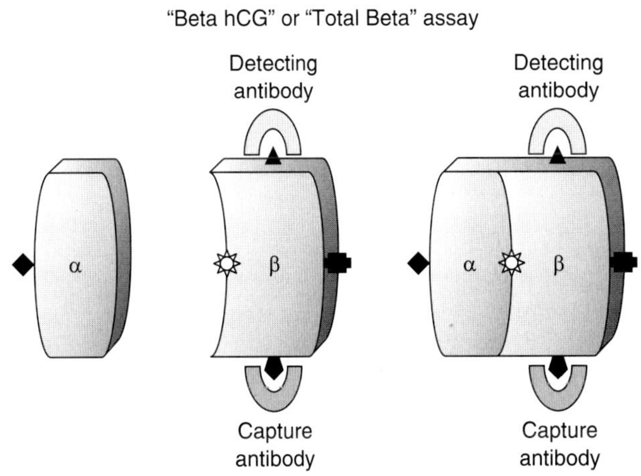

Figure 78.2 Schematic representation of assay commonly used to measure intact hCG.

Free beta hCG vs. intact hCG

HCG is a noncovalently bound heterodimeric glycoprotein consisting of an alpha and beta subunit. It exists in maternal circulation predominantly as the biologically active intact dimer. It is also found in the unbound state as both the free alpha and free beta subunits (Figure 78.1). The genes for the alpha and beta subunits of hCG are separate and distinct with the alpha subunit located on chromosome 6 and the beta subunit located on chromosome 19.[50] The separate synthesis and unbalanced secretion of subunits provides the rationale for monitoring levels of hCG subunits in obstetrical and gynecological disorders. Thus, assays for free beta hCG and intact hCG measure distinct proteins in the maternal blood.

Assays used to measure intact hCG are commonly called 'total beta' or simply 'beta hCG' assays. These assays use a capture antibody directed to the beta subunit of hCG and a detecting antibody directed to another epitopic site on the beta subunit (Figure 78.2). As a consequence, these assays detect both intact hCG and free beta hCG. However, since the intact molecule is present in a 200-fold molar excess relative to the free beta subunit, these assays reflect the concentration of intact hCG. During pregnancy intact hCG is measurable as early as 5 weeks in pregnancy making it an excellent indicator of pregnancy. An immediate and steep increase is observed with hCG levels peaking at about 120 IU/ml at 9 weeks followed by a steady decline to about 20 weeks when concentrations level off at 10–20 IU/ml.

Free beta hCG exists in maternal blood at a level of about 1/200th that of intact hCG. Assays that measure free beta hCG utilize an epitopic site that is located at the interface with the alpha subunit such that it is covered in the intact hCG molecule (Figure 78.3). As a result, antibodies directed toward this site capture free beta hCG but not intact hCG which is washed away in the assay procedure.

Prior to the prospective evaluation of the first-trimester combined screening protocol free beta hCG and intact hCG were evaluated in a number of studies.[29,51–76] Overall, it was seen that intact hCG was not an effective marker in the first trimester of pregnancy with a median MoM in 463 cases of Down's syndrome of just 1.30 while free beta hCG was an effective marker with a median MoM of 2.0 based on 858 cases of Down's syndrome (Tables 78.4 and 78.5). Hallahan *et al.*,[64] summarized seven case–control studies[57–60,64–66] in which both intact hCG and free beta hCG were measured in the same samples and showed that free

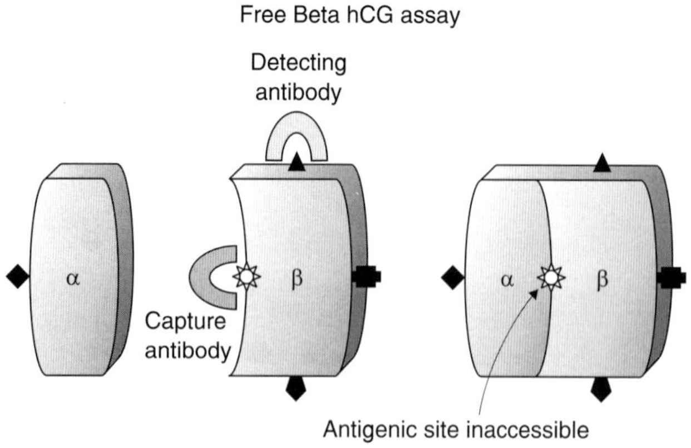

Figure 78.3 Schematic representation of free beta hCG assay.

Table 78.4 Median first-trimester intact hCG multiples of the median (MoM) values in Down's syndrome cases

Study	Cases	Median Down's syndrome MoM
Cuckle *et al.*[51]	22	1.10
Bogart *et al.*[52]	6	1.14
Brock *et al.*[53]	21	1.43
Johnson *et al.*[54]	11	0.91
Kratzer *et al.*[55]	17	1.23
Van Lith[56]	24	1.19
Aitken *et al.*[57]	16	0.97
Macintosh *et al.*[58]	20	1.45
Biagiotti *et al.*[59]	41	1.12
Brizot *et al.*[60]	41	1.50
Forest *et al.*[61]	12	1.83
Cassals *et al.*[62]	19	1.35
Aitken *et al.*[63]	8	1.05
Wald *et al.*[64]	77	1.23
Jauniaux *et al.*[65]	17	0.96
Haddow *et al.*[29]	48	1.54
Hallahan *et al.*[66]	63	1.37
Overall	463	1.30

beta hCG detected nearly twice as many cases of Down's syndrome as intact hCG (Table 78.6). On the basis of these results prospective first-trimester screening studies using the combined protocol have all included free beta hCG.

Recently, Spencer *et al.*[24,26] have suggested that the evaluation of all the Down's syndrome markers should be conducted on a week by week basis since the performance of the markers varies by gestational age. Spencer *et al.* showed that the combination of free beta hCG and PAPP-A had detection rates that were

Table 78.5 Median first-trimester free beta hCG MoM in Down's syndrome cases

Study	*N*	Median Down's syndrome MoM
Spencer *et al.*[67]	13	1.85
Aitken *et al.*[57]	16	1.96
Macri *et al.*[68]	38	2.20
Brambati *et al.*[69]	13	1.13
Macintosh *et al.*[58]	21	2.10
Biagiotti *et al.*[59]	41	2.00
Brizot *et al.*[60]	41	2.00
Noble *et al.*[70]	102	2.13
Forest *et al.*[61]	12	1.60
Krantz *et al.*[71]	22	2.09
Scott *et al.*[72]	8	2.00
Wald *et al.*[64]	77	1.79
Jauniaux *et al.*[65]	17	1.46
Berry *et al.*[73]	47	1.99
Spencer *et al.*[74]	22	1.72
Haddow *et al.*[29]	48	2.08
Wheeler and Sinosich[75]	17	2.06
Spencer *et al.*[76]	210	2.15
Hallahan *et al.*[66]	63	1.89
Overall	828	2.00

7–11% better than the combination of intact hCG and PAPP-A at each gestational week from 10 to 13 weeks at a corresponding 5% false-positive rate (Table 78.7).

In a case–control study, Wald *et al.*[25] modeled the performance of free beta hCG and PAPP-A in combination with nuchal translucency. The model indicated that free beta hCG significantly outperformed intact hCG within the combined protocol at 10 and 11 weeks' gestation but that at 12 weeks the two markers had similar performance and that at 13 weeks intact hCG performed better. However, Krantz *et al.*[77] determined that a more appropriate analysis would show that free beta hCG was better than intact hCG at 10, 11 and 12 weeks and that the two markers only appear similar in the model at 13 weeks. In response, Wald *et al.*[78] concluded that their data at 13 weeks were probably due to chance and that there was an advantage to using free beta hCG compared to intact hCG in the first trimester. An analysis[79] combining the results from Spencer *et al.*[72] and Wald *et al.*[23] demonstrated that using free beta hCG was better than intact hCG in a protocol that includes PAPP-A and nuchal translucency at 10–13 weeks. When false-positive rates were evaluated the difference between the two markers was even more apparent. For example at 10 weeks, the false-positive rate with free beta hCG was half that of intact hCG (Table 78.8).

Table 78.6 Meta-analysis of intact hCG vs. free beta hCG in case–control studies in which both analytes were measured in the same sample set (reprinted from Hallahan *et al.*[66])

Study	*N*		Intact hCG					Free beta hCG				
			Unaffected		DS cases			Unaffected		DS cases		
	Unaffected	DS	Median	SD	Median	SD	%DS* > 95th percentile	Median	SD	Median	SD	%DS* > 95th percentile
Aitken *et al.*[57]	320	16	1.0	0.2190	0.97	0.3150	11.8%	1.0	0.2580	1.96	0.2560	30.3%
Macintosh *et al.*[58]	258	21	1.0	—	1.45	0.4512	—	1.0	—	2.10	0.4280	—
Biagiotti *et al.*[59]	246	41	1.01	0.2458	1.12	0.2555	8.2%	1.0	0.2208	2.00	0.2294	39.3%
Brizot *et al.*[60]	394	41	1.0	0.2054	1.50	0.1939	20.2%	1.0	0.2911	2.00	0.3168	28.7%
Wald *et al.*[64]**	383	77	1.0	—	1.23	0.1957	13.0%	1.0	0.2833	1.79	0.2870	22.9%
Jauniaux *et al.*[65]	51	17	1.0	0.2375	0.96	0.1347	0.0%	1.0	0.3474	1.46	0.1673	0.1%
Hallahan *et al.*[66]	400	63	1.0	0.1697	1.37	0.2158	25.5%	1.0	0.2157	1.89	0.2322	36.8%
Overall	2052	276	1.0	0.2083	1.27	0.2421	16.2%	1.0	0.2545	1.89	0.2782	30.4%

DS, Down's syndrome; SD, standard deviation
*Based on normal distribution parameters
**Author provided observed %DS cases > 95th percentile for intact hCG
— indicates data was not available

Table 78.7 Comparison of the performance of free beta hCG vs. intact hCG in combination with PAPP-A and maternal age in first-trimester screening using an overall 5% false-positive rate (data from Spencer *et al.*[26])

Gestational age (weeks)	Intact hCG+PAPP-A		Free beta hCG+PAPP-A	
	FP	DR	FP	DR
10	4.7	58	4.7	69
11	4.9	56	4.8	67
12	5.1	56	5.0	65
13	5.2	56	5.3	63

FP, false positive; DR, detection rate

Screening strategies

First-trimester screening is usually conducted between 11 weeks 1 day and 13 week 6 days' gestation. In general, the patient comes in for an ultrasound exam, crown–rump length (CRL) is measured for accurate gestational dating and a nuchal translucency value is obtained. At the time of the ultrasound exam a blood specimen is collected and forwarded to the laboratory along with the ultrasound information. The biochemical analytes are analyzed in the laboratory and risk results based on free beta hCG, PAPP-A and nuchal translucency are available usually within a few days.

One-stop clinic for the assessment of risk

The one-stop clinic for the assessment of risk (OSCAR) approach represents a procedural variation of first-trimester screening in which the blood sample is collected and analyzed on a rapid assay instrument during the patient's ultrasound appointment. The advantage of this modality is that the biochemical result is ready during the patient's visit allowing her to have her combined risk result immediately with the option of having chorionic villus sampling (CVS) the same day. This screening strategy is currently practiced very effectively in many European clinics.[11,13] The disadvantage is that in order to analyze the biochemistry specialized equipment and personnel are required at the ultrasound center. Therefore, this strategy is best suited for settings with high volume in order for the biochemical screening to be cost effective. The rapid assays needed to provide a blood result in under a half hour have not yet been approved by the Food and Drug Administration (FDA) and are therefore not currently available in the United States. Even with the rapid assays the total time required to interview the patient, draw a blood specimen, allow time for clotting and centrifugation, perform the biochemical assays and conduct the ultrasound examination could easily last more than 1 h. Further, the burdens of data entry, quality control and risk assessment in this modality are all the responsibility of the ultrasound clinic.

Table 78.8 Free beta hCG vs. intact hCG within a Down's syndrome protocol including PAPP-A and nuchal translucency and maternal age

Gestational age (weeks)	Detection rate at a 5% false-positive rate		False-positive rate at a fixed 85% detection rate	
	Intact hCG	Free beta hCG	Intact hCG	Free beta hCG
10	84%	88%	6.0%	3.1%
11	83	86	6.7	4.1
12	82	86	6.9	4.3
13	85	85	5.1	4.7

Analysis[79] performed using results from Spencer *et al.*[24,26] and Wald *et al.*[25]

Finger-stick blood collection with instant risk assessment

Instant risk assessment (IRA) is a variation of the OSCAR approach that takes advantage of the simplified blood collection and transport of dried blood. In this approach, patients draw their own blood at home about 1 week before their ultrasound appointment using a sterile lancet and a dried blood collection card. The sample is mailed to the laboratory and the biochemical results are ready in time for the ultrasound exam. Like the OSCAR approach the risk results are available immediately at the conclusion of the ultrasound exam but with IRA the ultrasound center has no need for specialized equipment and personnel. Additional time is not required for drawing blood and waiting for a biochemical result. That time may be better spent performing more detailed ultrasound evaluations such as ductus venosus, nasal bone and tricuspid valve regurgitation for those specific patients that have a borderline risk.

Independent sequential screening

The first-trimester combined screening test with free beta hCG, PAPP-A and nuchal translucency can detect approximately 90% of Down's syndrome pregnancies with a 5% false-positive rate. In sequential testing both first-trimester screening and second trimester multiple marker screening are performed independently. In this case, the false-positive rate in first trimester is additive with the false-positive rate in second trimester. For example, in the BUN study, a group that contained about 50% advanced maternal age patients, 9.9% of patients had increased risk results in the first trimester and another 9.0% had increased risk results in the second trimester.[80] Thus, the overall false-positive rate for the screening program using data in both trimesters was nearly doubled.

Modified sequential screening

Alternatively, the Down's syndrome risk can be calculated based on both the first- and second-trimester markers. Such an approach can reduce the increase in the false-positive rate compared to the independent sequential approach described above. However, sophisticated software is required to ensure that the patient's results in the second trimester are appropriately matched with those from the first trimester.

The modified sequential screening approach requires 95% of the population to return for second-trimester multiple marker screening. A refinement to this approach could be to offer second-trimester screening only to those patients with a borderline result.[81] For example, those patients with very high risks (e.g., greater than 1 in 100) in the first trimester can be immediately offered CVS. Those patients with low risk (e.g., less than 1 in 1500) can be reassured that no further screening is necessary. Patients with borderline first-trimester risks (e.g., between 1 in 100 and 1 in 1500) could be offered second-trimester multiple marker screening and have their final risk calculated based on the marker results in both the first and second trimester. This so-called 'contingency' screening approach has the advantage of reducing by as much as 75% the number of second-trimester screening tests that are performed, reducing the overall cost of the screening program and minimizing the number of added false positives generated by second-trimester testing.[81]

The sequential screening approaches outlined above have been described with respect to multiple marker serum screening in the second trimester. Nyberg *et al.*[82] and Bromley *et al.*[83] have determined likelihood ratios for second-trimester ultrasound markers. Any of the sequential screening methodologies described above could be conducted by substituting the second-trimester serum markers with second-trimester ultrasound markers. More data is needed to determine whether one approach is superior to the other. However, in settings where a second-trimester anomaly scan is common practice, use of the ultrasound screen may provide significant logistical advantages.

Future improvements

Future goals are to improve upon the already excellent screening performance while still maintaining screening in the first trimester. The most promising advancement may be the inclusion of ultrasound assessment of fetal nasal bone. Cicero *et al.*[84] observed that 73% of Down's syndrome cases had absent nasal bone while only 0.5% of unaffected cases had absent nasal bone in the first trimester of pregnancy. The results of Cicero *et al.* have been confirmed in several studies.[23,85–90] but one study by Malone *et al.*[91] had divergent results. The promising results with the nasal bone marker open up the possibility of significantly reducing the false-positive rate of first-trimester Down's-syndrome screening while maintaining a 90% detection rate or alternatively increasing the detection rate to better than 95%.

Conclusion

One of the first questions that expectant parents ask after discovering they are pregnant is 'Will my baby be normal?' Although there are no guarantees that a baby will be healthy, screening can reassure the vast majority of couples that they are not likely to have a baby with a major birth defect. Along with the benefits of early reassurance and diagnosis, first-trimester screening with free beta hCG, PAPP-A and nuchal translucency has raised the standards in terms of detection efficiency. As a result, the ability to screen for Down's syndrome and trisomy 18 in the first trimester of pregnancy represents the most significant advancement in prenatal screening in the past 10 years.

REFERENCES

1. Wald NJ, Huttly WJ, Hackshaw AK. Antenatal screening for Down's syndrome with the quadruple test. *Lancet* 2003;361: 835–6.
2. Orlandi F, Damiani G, Hallahan TW, Krantz DA, Macri JN. First-trimester screening for fetal aneuploidy: biochemistry and nuchal translucency. *Ultrasound Obstet Gynecol* 1997;10(6):381–6.
3. Biagiotti R, Brizzi L, Periti E, d'Agata A, Vanzi E, Cariati F. First trimester screening for Down's syndrome using maternal serum PAPP-A and free beta-hCG in combination with fetal nuchal translucency thickness. *Br J Obstet Gynaecol* 1998; 105(8):917–20.
4. De Biasio P, Siccardi M, Volpe G, Famularo L, Santi F, Canini S. First-trimester screening for Down syndrome using nuchal translucency measurement with free beta-hCG and PAPP-A between 10 and 13 weeks of pregnancy – the combined test. *Prenat Diagn* 1999;19(4):360–3.
5. de Graaf IM, Pajkrt E, Bilardo CM, Leschot NJ, Cuckle HS, van Lith JM. Early pregnancy screening for fetal aneuploidy with serum markers and nuchal translucency. *Prenat Diagn* 1999; 19(5):458–62.
6. Spencer K, Souter V, Tul N, Snijders R, Nicolaides KH. A screening program for trisomy 21 at 10–14 weeks using fetal nuchal translucency, maternal serum free beta-human chorionic gonadotropin and pregnancy-associated plasma protein-A. *Ultrasound Obstet Gynecol* 1999;13(4):231–7.
7. Krantz DA, Hallahan TW, Orlandi F, Buchanan P, Larsen JW Jr, Macri JN. First-trimester Down syndrome screening using dried blood biochemistry and nuchal translucency. *Obstet Gynecol* 2000;96(2):207–13.
8. Niemimaa M, Suonpaa M, Perheentupa A, *et al.* Evaluation of first trimester maternal serum and ultrasound screening for Down's syndrome in Eastern and Northern Finland. *Eur J Hum Genet* 2001;9(6):404–8.
9. Schuchter K, Hafner E, Stangl G, Metzenbauer M, Hofinger D, Philipp K. The first trimester 'combined test' for the detection of Down syndrome pregnancies in 4939 unselected pregnancies. *Prenat Diagn* 2002;22(3):211–15.
10. von Kaisenberg CS, Gasiorek-Wiens A, Bielicki M, *et al.* Screening for trisomy 21 by maternal age, fetal nuchal translucency and maternal serum biochemistry at 11–14 weeks: A German multicenter study. *J Matern Fetal Neonatal Med* 2002;12(2):89–94.
11. Bindra R, Heath V, Liao A, Spencer K, Nicolaides KH. One-stop clinic for assessment of risk for trisomy 21 at 11–14 weeks: a prospective study of 15 030 pregnancies. *Ultrasound Obstet Gynecol* 2002;20(3):219–25.
12. Wapner R, Thom E, Simpson JL, *et al.* First-trimester screening for trisomies 21 and 18. *N Engl J Med* 2003;349(15):1405–13.
13. Spencer K, Spencer CE, Power M, Dawson C, Nicolaides KH. Screening for chromosomal abnormalities in the first trimester using ultrasound and maternal serum biochemistry in a one-stop clinic: A review of three years prospective experience. *Br J Obstet Gynecol* 2003;110(3):281–6.
14. Sheffield LJ, Williamson R, Halliday JL, *et al.* SLAMDUNC-a very successful new community program for first trimester combined screening for Down syndrome. *Am J Hum Genet* 2003;73(Suppl 5):593.
15. Borrell A, Casals E, Fortuny A, *et al.* First-trimester screening for trisomy 21 combining biochemistry and ultrasound at individually optimal gestational ages. An interventional study. *Prenat Diagn* 2004;24(7):541–5.
16. Stenhouse EJ, Crossley JA, Aitken DA, Brogan K, Cameron AD, Connor JM. First-trimester combined ultrasound and biochemical screening for Down syndrome in routine clinical practice. *Prenat Diagn* 2004;24(10):774–80.
17. Spencer K. Accuracy of Down syndrome risks produced in a first-trimester screening programme incorporating fetal nuchal translucency thickness and maternal serum biochemistry. *Prenat Diagn* 2002;22:244–6.
18. Macri JN, Spencer K, Garver K, *et al.* Maternal serum free beta hCG screening: results of studies including 480 cases of Down syndrome. *Prenat Diagn* 1994;14:97–103.
19. Spencer K. Free alpha-subunit of human chorionic gonadotropin in Down syndrome. *Am J Obstet Gynecol* 1993;168:132–5.
20. Wald NJ, Densem JW, Smith D, Klee GG. Four-marker serum screening for Down's syndrome. *Prenat Diagn* 1994;14:707–16.
21. Eldar-Geva T, Hochberg A, deGroot N, Weinstein D. High maternal serum chorionic gonadotropin level in Down's syndrome pregnancies is caused by elevation of both subunits messenger ribonucleic acid level in trophoblasts. *J Clin Endocrinol Metab* 1995;80:3528–31.
22. Ng EK, El-Sheikhah A, Chiu RW, *et al.* Evaluation of human chorionic gonadotropin beta-subunit mRNA concentrations in maternal serum in aneuploid pregnancies: A feasibility study. *Clin Chem* 2004;50:1055–7.
23. Orlandi F, Rossi C, Orlandi E, *et al.* Optimization of first trimester Down syndrome screening with simplified nasal bone assessment. *Am J Obstet Gynecol*, in press.
24. Spencer K, Crossley JA, Aitken DA, Nix AB, Dunstan FD, Williams K. Temporal changes in maternal serum biochemical markers of trisomy 21 across the first and second trimester of pregnancy. *Ann Clin Biochem* 2002;39(Pt 6):567–76.
25. Wald NJ, Rodeck C, Hackshaw AK, Walters J, Chitty L, Mackinson AM. First and second trimester antenatal screening for Down's syndrome: The results of Serum, Urine and Ultrasound Screening Study (SURUSS). *Health Technol Assess* 2003;7(11):1–87.
26. Spencer K, Crossley JA, Aitken DA, Nix ABJ, Dunstan FDJ, Williams K. The effect of temporal variation in biochemical markers of trisomy 21 across the first and second trimesters of

pregnancy on the estimation of individual patient-specific risks and detection rates for Down's syndrome. *Ann Clin Biochem* 2003;40:219–31.

27. Macri JN, Anderson RW, Krantz DA, Larsen JW, Buchanan PD. Prenatal maternal dried blood screening with alpha-fetoprotein and free beta-human chorionic gonadotropin for open neural tube defect and Down syndrome. *Am J Obstet Gynecol* 1996;174: 566–72.
28. Snijders RJ, Noble P, Sebire N, Souka A, Nicolaides KH. UK multicentre project on assessment of risk of trisomy 21 by maternal age and fetal nuchal-translucency thickness at 10–14 weeks of gestation. Fetal medicine foundation first trimester screening group. *Lancet* 1998;352:343–6.
29. Haddow JE, Palomaki GE, Knight GJ, Williams J, Miller WA, Johnson A. Screening of maternal serum for fetal Down's syndrome in the first trimester. *N Engl J Med* 1998;338:955–61.
30. Spencer K, Liao AW, Skentou H, Cicero S, Nicolaides KH. Screening for triploidy by fetal nuchal translucency and maternal serum free beta-hCG and PAPP-A at 10–14 weeks of gestation. *Prenat Diagn* 2000;20:495–9.
31. Krantz D, Goetzl L, Simpson JL, *et al.* Association of extreme first-trimester free human chorionic gonadotropin-beta, pregnancy-associated plasma protein A, and nuchal translucency with intrauterine growth restriction and other adverse pregnancy outcomes. *Am J Obstet Gynecol* 2004;191:1452–8.
32. Ong CYT, Liao AW, Spencer K, Munim S, Nicolaides KH. First trimester maternal serum free beta human chorionic gonadotrophin and pregnancy associated plasma protein A as predictors of pregnancy complications. *Br J Obstet Gynaecol* 2000;107: 1265–70.
33. Tul N, Pusenjak S, Osredkar J, Spencer K, Novak-Antolic Z. Predicting complications of pregnancy with first-trimester maternal serum free beta hCG, PAPP-A and inhibin A. *Prenat Diagn* 2003;23:990–6.
34. Yaron Y, Heifetz S, Ochshorn Y, Lehavi O, Orr-Urteger A. Decreased first trimester PAPP-A is a predictor of adverse pregnancy outcome. *Prenat Diagn* 2002;22:778–82.
35. Pedersen JF, Sorensen S, Ruge S. Human placental lactogen and pregnancy-associated plasma protein A in first trimester and subsequent fetal growth. *Acta Obstet Gynecol Scand* 1995;74:505–8.
36. Smith GCS, Stenhouse EJ, Crossley JA, Aitken DA, Cameron AD, Connor JM. Early pregnancy origins of low birth weight. *Nature* 2002;417:916.
37. Smith GCS, Stenhouse EJ, Crossley JA, Aitken DA, Cameron AD, Connor JM. Early pregnancy levels of pregnancy-associated plasma protein A and the risk of intrauterine growth restriction, premature birth, preeclampsia, and stillbirth. *J Clin Endocrinol Metab* 2002;87:1762–7.
38. Yaron Y, Ochshorn Y, Heifetz S, Lehavi O, Sapir Y, Orr-Urtreger A. First trimester maternal serum free human chorionic gonadotropin as a predictor of adverse pregnancy outcome. *Fetal Diag Ther* 2002;17:352–6.
39. Morssink LP, Kornman LH, Hallahan TW, *et al.* Maternal serum levels of free beta hCG and PAPP-A in the first trimester of pregnancy are not associated with subsequent fetal growth retardation or preterm delivery. *Prenat Diagn* 1998;18:147–52.
40. Goetzl L, Krantz D, Simpson JL, *et al.* Pregnancy-associated plasma protein A, free beta-hCG, nuchal translucency, and risk of pregnancy loss. *Obstet Gynecol* 2004;104:30–6.
41. de Graaf IM, Cuckle HS, Pajkrt E, Leschot NJ, Bleker OP, van Lith JM. Co-variables in first trimester maternal serum screening. *Prenat Diagn* 2000;20:186–9.
42. Spencer K, Bindra R, Nicolaides KH. Maternal weight correction of maternal serum PAPP-A and free beta-hCG MoM when screening for trisomy 21 in the first trimester of pregnancy. *Prenat Diagn* 2003;23:851–5.
43. Krantz D, Hallahan T, Macri J. Weight correction and ethnic differences for first trimester Down syndrome biochemical markers. *Am J Hum Genet* 2003;73(Suppl):411.
44. Orlandi F, Rossi C, Allegra A, *et al.* First trimester screening with free beta-hCG, PAPP-A and nuchal translucency in pregnancies conceived with assisted reproduction. *Prenat Diagn* 2002;22:718–21.
45. Liao AW, Heath V, Kametas N, Spencer K, Nicolaides KH. First-trimester screening for trisomy 21 in singleton pregnancies achieved by assisted reproduction. *Hum Reprod* 2001;16:1501–4.
46. Wojdemann KR, Larsen SO, Shalmi A, Sundberg K, Christiansen M, Tabor A. First trimester screening for Down syndrome and assisted reproduction: no basis for concern. *Prenat Diagn* 2001;21:563–5.
47. Spencer K, Salonen R, Muller F. Down's syndrome screening in multiple pregnancies using alpha-fetoprotein and free beta hCG. *Prenat Diagn* 1994;14:537–42.
48. Sebire NJ, Snijders RJ, Hughes K, Sepulveda W, Nicolaides KH. Screening for trisomy 21 in twin pregnancies by maternal age and fetal nuchal translucency thickness at 10–14 weeks of gestation. *Br J Obstet Gynaecol* 1996;103:999–1003.
49. Orlandi F, Krantz DA, Hallahan TW, Buchanan PD, Larsen JW. First-trimester Down syndrome screening in twins. *Am J Hum Genet* 2000;67(Suppl): Abstact 155.
50. Naylor SL, Chin WW, Goodman HM, Lalley PA, Grzeschik KH, Sakaguchi AY. Chromosome assignment of genes encoding the alpha and beta subunits of glycoprotein hormones in man and mouse. *Somatic Cell Genet* 1983;9:757–70.
51. Cuckle HS, Wald NJ, Barkai G, *et al.* First-trimester biochemical screening for Down syndrome. *Lancet* 1988;2:851–2.
52. Bogart MH, Golbus MS, Sorg ND, Jones OW. Human chorionic gonadotropin levels in pregnancies with aneuploid fetuses. *Prenat Diagn* 1989;9:379–84.
53. Brock DJ, Barron L, Holloway S, Liston WA, Hillier SG, Seppala M. First-trimester maternal serum biochemical indicators in Down syndrome. *Prenat Diagn* 1990;10:245–51.
54. Johnson A, Cowchock FS, Darby M, Wapner R, Jackson LG. First-trimester maternal serum alpha-fetoprotein and chorionic gonadotropin in aneuploid pregnancies. *Prenat Diagn* 1991;11: 443–50.
55. Kratzer PG, Golbus MS, Monroe SE, Finkelstein DE, Taylor RN. First-trimester aneuploidy screening using serum human chorionic gonadotropin (hCG), free ahCG and progesterone. *Prenat Diagn* 1991;11:751–63.
56. Van Lith JMM. First-trimester maternal serum human chorionic gonadotrophin as a marker for fetal chromosomal disorders. The Dutch Working Party on Prenatal Diagnosis. *Prenat Diagn* 1992;12:495–504.
57. Aitken DA, McCaw G, Crossley JA, *et al.* First-trimester biochemical screening for fetal chromosome abnormalities and neural tube defects. *Prenat Diagn* 1993;13:681–9.
58. Macintosh MCM, Iles R, Teisner B, *et al.* Maternal serum human chorionic gonadotrophin and pregnancy associated plasma protein A, markers for fetal Down syndrome at 8–14 weeks. *Prenat Diagn* 1994;14:203–8.
59. Biagiotti R, Cariati E, Brizzi L, Dagata A. Maternal serum screening for Down's syndrome in the first trimester of pregnancy. *Br J Obstet Gynaecol* 1995;102:660–2.
60. Brizot ML, Snijders RJ, Butler J, Bersinger NA, Nicolaides KH. Maternal serum hCG and fetal nuchal translucency thickness for the prediction of fetal trisomies in the first trimester of pregnancy. *Br J Obstet Gynaecol* 1995;102:127–32.
61. Forest JC, Masse J, Rousseau F, Moutquin JM, Brideau NA, Belanger M. Screening for Down syndrome during the first and second trimesters: impact of risk estimation parameters. *Clin Biochem* 1995;28:443–9.
62. Casals E, Fortunoy A, Grudzinskas JG, *et al.* First-trimester biochemical screening for Down syndrome with the use of PAPP-A, AFP, and beta-hCG. *Prenat Diagn* 1996;16:405–10.
63. Aitken DA, Wallace EM, Crossley JA, *et al.* Dimeric inhibin A as a marker for Down's syndrome in early pregnancy. *N Engl J Med* 1996;334:1231–6.
64. Wald NJ, George L, Smith D, Densem JW, Petterson K. Serum screening for Down's syndrome between 8 and 14 weeks of pregnancy. International Prenatal Screening Research Group. *Br J Obstet Gynaecol* 1996;103(5):407–12.
65. Jauniaux E, Nicolaides KH, Nagy AM, Brizot M, Meuris S. Total amount of circulating human chorionic gonadotrophin alpha and beta subunits in first trimester trisomies 21 and 18. *J Endocrinol* 1996;148:27–31.
66. Hallahan T, Krantz D, Orlandi F, *et al.* First trimester biochemical screening for Down syndrome: free beta hCG versus intact hCG. *Prenat Diagn* 2000;20:785–9.
67. Spencer K, Macri JN, Aitken DA, Connor JM. Free beta-hCG as first-trimester marker for fetal trisomy. *Lancet* 1992;339:1480.
68. Macri JN, Spencer K, Aitken DA, *et al.* First-trimester free beta (hCG) screening for Down syndrome. *Prenat Diagn* 1993;13:557–62.
69. Brambati B, Tului L, Bonacchi I, Shrimaker K, Suzuki Y, Grudzinskas JG. Serum PAPP-A and free beta hCG are first trimester screening markers for Down syndrome. *Prenat Diagn* 1994;14:1043–7.
70. Noble PL, Abraha HD, Snijders RJ, Sherwood R, Nicolaides KH. Screening for fetal trisomy 21 in the first trimester of pregnancy:

maternal serum free beta-hCG and fetal nuchal translucency thickness. *Ultrasound Obstet Gynecol* 1995;6:390–5.

71. Krantz DA, Larsen JW, Buchanan PD, Macri JN. First-trimester Down syndrome screening: free beta-human chorionic gonadotropin and pregnancy-associated plasma protein A. *Am J Obstet Gynecol* 1996;174:612–6.
72. Scott F, Wheeler D, Sinosich M, Boogert A, Anderson J, Edelman D. First trimester aneuploidy screening using nuchal translucency, free beta human chorionic gonadotropihin and maternal age. *Aust NZ J Obstet Gynaecol* 1996;36:381–4.
73. Berry E, Aitken DA, Crossley JA, Macri JN, Connor JM. Screening for Down's syndrome: Changes in marker levels and detection rates between first and second trimester. *Br J Obstet Gynaecol* 1997;104:811–7.
74. Spencer K, Noble PL, Snijders RJM, Nicolaides KH. First-trimester urine free beta hCG, beta core, and total oestriol in pregnancies affected by Down's syndrome: Implications for first-trimester screening with nuchal translucency and serum free beta hCG. *Prenat Diagn* 1997;17:525–38.
75. Wheeler DM, Sinosich MJ. Prenatal screening in the first trimester of pregnancy. *Prenat Diagn* 1998;18:537–43.
76. Spencer K, Souter V, Tul N, Snijders R, Nicolaides KH. A screening program for trisomy 21 at 10–14 weeks using fetal nuchal translucency, maternal serum free beta human chorionic gonadotropin and pregnancy associated plasma protein-A. *Ultrasound Obstet Gynecol* 1999;13:231–7.
77. Krantz DA, Hallahan TW, James Macri V, Macri JN. Statistical flaw in SURUSS model (letter). *Prenat Diagn* 2004;24:753–4.
78. Wald N, Rodeck C, Hackshaw A, Rudnicka A. Correlations between nuchal translucency and serum markers in SURUSS (letter). *Prenat Diagn* 2004;24:835–6.
79. Bloom P, ed. Free beta or intact hCG. *DS News* 2004;11:37.
80. Platt LD, Greene N, Johnson A, *et al.* Sequential pathways of testing after first-trimester screening for trisomy 21. *Obstet Gynecol* 2004;104:661–6.
81. Wright D, Bradbury I, Benn P, Cuckle H, Ritchie K. Contingent screening for Down syndrome is an efficient alternative to non-disclosure sequential screening. *Prenat Diagn* 2004;24:762–6.
82. Nyberg DA, Souter VL, El-Bastawissi A, Young S, Luthhardt F, Luthy DA. Isolated sonographic markers for detection of fetal Down syndrome in the second trimester of pregnancy. *J Ultrasound Med* 2001;20:1053–63.
83. Bromley B, Lieberman E, Shipp TD, Benacerraf BR. The genetic sonogram: A method of risk assessment for Down syndrome in the second trimester. *J Ultrasound Med* 2002;21:1087–96.
84. Cicero S, Curcio P, Papageorghiou A, Sonek J, Nicolaides K. Absense of nasal bone in fetuses with trisomy 21 at 11–14 weeks of gestation: An observational study. *Lancet* 2001;358:1665–7.
85. Cicero S, Rembouskos G, Vandecruys H, Hogg M, Nicolaides KH. Likelihood ratio for trisomy 21 in fetuses with absent nasal bone at the 11–14 week scan. *Ultrasound Obstet Gynecol* 2004;23: 218:223.
86. Orlandi F, Bilardo CM, Campogrande M, *et al.* Measurement of nasal bone length at 11–14 weeks of pregnancy and its potential role in Down syndrome risk assessment. *Ultrasound Obstet Gynecol* 2003;22:36–9.
87. Otano L, Aiello H, Igarzabal L, Matayoshi T, Gadow EC. Association between first trimester absence of fetal nasal bone on ultrasound and Down syndrome. *Prenat Diagn* 2002;22:930–2.
88. Viora E, Masturzo B, Errante G, Sciarrone A, Bastonero S, Campogrande M. Ultrasound evaluation of fetal nasal bone at 11 to 14 weeks in a consecutive series of 1906 fetuses. *Prenat Diagn* 2003:23;784–7.
89. Zoppi MA, Ibba RM, Axianna C, Floris M, Manca F, Monni G. Absense of fetal nasal bone and aneuploidies at first-trimester nuchal translucency screening in unselected pregnancies. *Prenat Diagn* 2003;23:496–500.
90. Cicero S, Bindra R, Rembouskas G, Spencer K, Nicolaides KH. Integrated ultrasound and biochemical screening for trisomy 21 using fetal nuchal translucency, absent fetal nasal bone, free beta hCG and PAPP-A at 11–14 weeks. *Prenat Diagn* 2003;23:306–10.
91. Malone FD, Ball RH, Nyberg DA, *et al.* First-trimester nasal bone evaluation for aneuploidy in the general population. *Obstet Gynecol* 2004;104:1222–8.

79 Influence of ethnicity on prenatal screening

F. Sethna and B. Thilaganathan

Introduction

With each passing day, the Western world becomes increasingly multicultural, multiethnic, and multilingual. Statistics from the last census (2001) carried out in the UK revealed that 7.9% of the population (4.6 million people) were from a minority background, with the majority being from the Indian subcontinent or Africa and the Caribbean.[1] In comparison, in the USA, approximately 28% of the population at the present time are from a minority background (African Americans, Hispanics, Asians, Pacific Islanders, Native Americans, and Alaskan Natives representing the majority).

It is anticipated that immigrants and their descendents will continue to shape and alter the demographic landscape for several years to come. Consequently, it can be predicted that women from the ethnic minorities will form a growing proportion of the obstetric populations of many health districts. As clinicians assume responsibility for caring for an increasingly diverse population, genetic and ethnic connections to disease will become clearer. All health professionals must be prepared to meet the challenges such diversity will pose, if a uniform standard of health care is to be provided for all patients. It is important to be aware of the variations in need between individuals within similar communities, and not just across the population as a whole.

Prenatal screening allows women to make informed decisions about their reproductive choices. The vast majority of structural and chromosomal abnormalities arise in pregnancies without any risk factors. Therefore, aneuploidy and anomaly screening is offered to all women. However, certain genetic disorders occur with an increased frequency, or are confined to certain ethnic groups, and in these cases screening will be targeted at these individuals. It is important to ensure that prenatal screening is available and accessible equally to all women regardless of their background. In this chapter, we will be examining the influence of ethnicity on screening methods within the field of prenatal diagnosis, targeted screening in ethnic groups and finally the effect of ethnicity on uptake of screening.

Effects of ethnicity on screening methods

Down's syndrome

Down's syndrome is the commonest congenital cause of severe mental retardation.[2] In developed countries, there are approximately 100,000 deliveries per year, per 10,000,000 of the population. The birth incidence of trisomy 21 is about 1 in 500, and therefore, in such a population the total number of affected neonates is about 200.[3] The incidence of Down's syndrome rises sharply with increasing maternal age;[4] however, as the majority of children are born to women in their 20s and early 30s, 75% of babies with Down's syndrome are born to women in this age group. Screening women of all ages for Down's syndrome is now common practice in the West.

There is substantial variation in screening services for Down's syndrome throughout the world. Options for screening include nuchal translucency measurement (alone, in combination with first-/second-trimester biochemistry, fetal nasal bone assessment or ductus venous Doppler measurement), maternal serum screening in the second trimester or ultrasound for the detection of fetal defects and markers at 16–23 weeks. The influence of ethnic origin on screening efficacy by each of these modalities will now be examined in turn.

Nuchal translucency

Babies born with Down's syndrome show a distinct set of physical characteristics. Langdon Down first reported in 1866 that the skin of individuals with trisomy 21 appeared to be too large for their bodies.[5] This excess skin, in the form of nuchal translucency thickness, has formed the basis of one of the main non-invasive prenatal tests for this disorder since the early 1990s. Since this time, the association between increased nuchal translucency at 11–14 weeks' gestation and chromosomal abnormality has been well established and documented.[6–8] For an invasive testing rate of 5%, about 75% of trisomic pregnancies can be identified using this method of screening alone. Two studies have shown that nuchal translucency screening can be effectively and equitably delivered to a multiethnic population. Thilaganathan *et al.* performed an observational study in a district general hospital with a large multiethnic population serving African, Asian, Caribbean, and Caucasian women.[9] In comparison, Chen *et al.* examined the effect of ethnic origin on nuchal translucency in a multiethnic Asian population comprising Chinese, Indian, Pakistani, Nepalese, and Filipino women.[10] Significant differences in the nuchal translucency measurement were obtained between the different ethnic groups in both studies. The magnitude of the differences was small, ranging from 0.08 to 0.22 mm. However, when compared to reported nuchal translucency intraobserver and interobserver variabilities of 0.54 and 0.62 mm, respectively,[11] the differences are clinically insignificant. No correction for ethnic origin is, therefore, required when first-trimester nuchal translucency screening for Down's syndrome is performed in multiethnic populations.

Ductus venosus

There is a clear association between abnormal Doppler flow in the ductus venosus (absence/ reversed) and fetal aneuploidy. The use of ductus venosus Doppler velocimetry in combination with nuchal translucency is better than either test alone, since it increases the sensitivity in the detection of Down's syndrome to 94% and decreases the likelihood ratio of a negative test to 0.08.[12] Although, the effect of ethnicity on ductus venosus Doppler indices are unknown, this screening method is so technically demanding that it is only likely to be performed on selected high-risk populations.

Nasal bone

In 2001 Cicero and colleagues demonstrated the possibility of using absence of the nasal bone at 11–14 weeks as a marker for Down's syndrome. They examined 701 routine ultrasound scans performed on women about to undergo prenatal diagnosis because of positive results on nuchal translucency screening.[13] The same group subsequently reported that nasal bones were absent in about 3% of chromosomally normal fetuses, in two-thirds of those with trisomy 21, and in about one-third of babies with other chromosomal defects.[14] The estimated likelihood ratio for trisomy 21 in the latter study was over 120 when the nasal bone cannot be seen. Given the significance of this ratio, and before nasal bone assessment is integrated into routine screening programs, knowledge about how to correct for ethnicity is required if this test is to be used equitably in multiethnic populations.

Table 79.1 The prevalence of absent nasal bones (NB) in normal and aneuploid pregnancies and their associated likelihood ratios (LR) for trisomy 21 (from Cicero *et al.*[18])

	Caucasian	Afro-Caribbean	Asian
Number	5284	170	201
Absent NB in aneuploid fetuses (%)	68.3	78.6	71.4
Absent NB in normal fetuses (%)	2.2	9.0	5.0
LR for trisomy 21 with absent NB	31.3	8.8	14.2
LR for trisomy 21 with NB	0.32	0.24	0.3

It is known that morphometry of the splanchnocranium, and of nasal bones in particular, differs between adults of various ethnic origins.[15] Likewise, ethnicity is known to influence whether the nasal bones are seen in second-trimester fetuses. It has been shown that second-trimester nasal bone hypoplasia is commoner in fetuses of Afro-Caribbean mothers than in Caucasian mothers.[16] More recently, studies have demonstrated a similar significant difference in the rate of visualization of the fetal nasal bones in the first trimester in chromosomally normal fetuses in mothers of different ethnic origins.[17]

In 2004 Cicero *et al.* produced data to update the likelihood ratio for trisomy 21 in fetuses with absent nasal bone at the 11- to 14-week scan. They examined 5918 pregnancies undergoing first-trimester karyotyping and found that the incidence of absent nasal bone was higher in fetuses of Afro-Caribbean and Asian origin than in Caucasians; it decreased with increasing fetal crown–rump length and increased with increased fetal nuchal translucency.[18] The authors provided data on the incidence of absent nasal bone in chromosomally normal and trisomy 21 fetuses and likelihood ratios according to ethnic group (see Table 79.1).

These data suggest that appropriate corrections may be applied for maternal ethnic origin and the absence of the nasal bones. However, as both parents contribute to a baby's phenotypic appearance, it remains to be determined whether any correction is also required for the father's ethnic origin.

Second-trimester maternal serum screening

In 1984, a major advancement in screening for chromosomal defects was made by Merkatz *et al.* who reported low levels of maternal serum alpha-fetoprotein (AFP) in trisomy 21 pregnancies.[19] Since this time, prenatal screening for trisomy 21 based on the analysis of biochemical markers in maternal serum between 15 and 22 weeks of pregnancy has become an established part of obstetric practice. The principal markers found to be of value are AFP, total human chorionic gonadotrophin (hCG) (or its individual subunits: free β-hCG and free α-hCG), unconjugated estriol (uE_3) and dimeric inhibin-A. On average, in Down's syndrome affected pregnancies, the AFP and uE_3 levels are about three-quarters that of an unaffected pregnancy (multiple of the median, MoM < 0.84), whereas inhibin-A and free β-hCG levels are about double (MoM > 1.3 and > 1.6, respectively). Most screening programs use multiple markers in combination with maternal age to generate a risk. Performance is known to vary according to the choice of markers used and whether ultrasound has been used to determine the gestational age. When the latter is used in combination with maternal age, the detection rate for a 5% false-positive rate is estimated to be 59% for the double test (AFP and either total hCG or free β-hCG), 69% for the triple test (AFP, total hCG, and uE_3), and 76% for the quadruple test (AFP, hCG, uE_3, and inhibin-A).

The results of second-trimester maternal serum biochemistry are expressed as MoM values for gestation. MoM values normalize results for gestation to provide an equivalent measure between laboratories. The majority of published population data used to derive median values for the individual markers relate to European and American Caucasian populations. The degree of risk to an individual pregnant woman relies on combining the results with maternal age in a complex mathematical algorithm using commercially available software programs. The test is interpreted as positive or negative according to whether or not risk exceeds a fixed cut-off point. It is known that smoking, maternal weight, parity, previous pregnancy results, multiple pregnancy, and insulin-dependent diabetes can influence the concentration of the markers. It has been proposed that adjusting the risk algorithm, by taking into account these factors, can lead to an improvement in detection efficiency, although to what extent is not clear.

Another factor known to have an impact on the biochemical marker levels is ethnic origin. Gilbert *et al.*[20] raised the issue that racial differences existed in both age ranges for Down's syndrome and in the medians for biochemical markers. They proposed that outcome data on serum screening should be collected by ethnic groups, so that validated risk estimations could be formed, thereby making serum screening in ethnic groups more effective.

There have been several publications documenting differences in the marker levels in Afro-Caribbean, South Asian, Oriental, and Hispanic women compared to Caucasian women. Maternal serum AFP and hCG levels have been shown to be approximately 10–15% higher in black women compared to Caucasian women. In contrast, uE_3 levels hardly differ, and dimeric inhibin-A levels are about 8% lower in pregnancies in African Women. One of the largest published studies[21] evaluated data from more than 21,000 pregnancies to determine the extent of race-specific differences in median concentrations of analytes used in the triple test. This study found that at most gestational ages, median AFP, hCG, and uE_3 values for Caucasian, Afro-Caribbean, Hispanic, and other patients were all significantly different. Further, these differences remained significant even after the data were corrected for patient weight. For the individual analytes the extent of the variation was not the same at different gestational ages. It is important that screening laboratories follow the literature to keep abreast of new findings to ensure that they continue to provide the best possible screening service for women from minority backgrounds.

Correcting for ethnic origin has a small overall effect on screening performance. The detection rate increases by about 0.5% for a false-positive rate of 5%.[22] Having said that, the adjustment is worthwhile because it does not require resources and because of its established value in screening for open neural tube defects (NTDs) using serum AFP, where the false-positive rate is higher in Asian and Afro-Caribbean women compared to white women for a fixed AFP cut-off level. In fact, The American College of Medical Genetics recommends that a correction be made when screening for NTD also.[23] If Down's screening is being carried out in isolation and there is no risk of NTD for the mother, it could be argued that an adjustment for ethnicity need not be made because of the counterbalancing effect of the different analytes used in combination. For example, a Hispanic patient was screened at 16 weeks with median values (1.00 MoM) of AFP, hCG, and uE_3 when interpreted against a Hispanic patient-derived data set. If a primary Caucasian population data set had been used, her AFP value would have remained the same, hCG would have been 1.06 MoM and the uE_3 value 1.12 MoM. Although the higher hCG MoM would increase the Down's risk, the higher uE_3 MoM value would counteract to reduce the risk.

First-trimester maternal serum screening

All the serum markers used or considered in the second trimester have been assessed in Down's syndrome and unaffected pregnancies during the first trimester. Only two serum markers have stood out as being useful in screening at 11–14 weeks, namely, pregnancy-associated plasma protein-A (PAPP-A) and free β-hCG. Maternal serum PAPP-A levels are lower in pregnancies affected by trisomy 21, with the difference in PAPP-A levels between trisomy 21 and normal pregnancies decreasing with increasing gestational age. In comparison, the maternal serum-free β-hCG level is higher in trisomy 21 pregnancies, and the difference in levels between unaffected and affected pregnancies increases with advancing gestation.[24]

The consensus estimate of screening performance by using PAPP-A and free β-hCG in combination with maternal age is a 60% detection rate with a 5% false-positive rate. This is similar to the screening performance of second-trimester double markers, but not as good as the screening performance of second-trimester triple or quadruple markers. However, there is a significant improvement in screening efficiency when biochemistry analysis is combined with ultrasound in the first trimester. This form of screening can be provided in the setting of a one-stop clinic for assessment of risk (OSCAR), and is associated with a detection rate of about 90%, when the fetal nuchal translucency is also measured.

In 2000, Spencer *et al.* examined the influence of ethnic origin on first-trimester biochemical markers of chromosomal abnormalities. It was seen that the median maternal serum marker MoMs for free β-hCG and PAPP-A were 19% and 48% higher in Afro-Caribbean women, and 19% and 35% higher in Asian women compared to Caucasian women. Correcting for maternal weight made very little difference to the Afro-Caribbeans (21% and 57% higher after weight correction), but reduced the effect in Asians (4% and 17% higher after weight correction). Correcting first-trimester biochemical markers for maternal ethnicity and weight has little impact at the population level for detection rates (an increase in the overall detection rate by a mere 1.4%). However, the effect on the individual patient-specific risk can be substantial (up to a twofold increase), and can certainly make a difference to the patient's decision on whether to have an invasive test. For example, in a 67-kg, 25-year-old Afro-Caribbean, with an uncorrected free β-hCG of 2.10 MoM, and a PAPP-A of 0.65 MoM, the risk of trisomy 21 without correction for weight and ethnicity would be 1 in 540. After correction, the free β-hCG MoM would be 1.73, while the PAPP-A MoM would be 0.41, with a corrected screening risk of 1:260.[25]

It would appear that ethnic origin has a greater impact on first-trimester biochemical markers than second-trimester biochemical markers. However, further larger data sets are required to develop robust methods of correcting for ethnic origin and to assess the biological significance of such marker production between various ethnic groups.

Sixteen to twenty-three weeks' ultrasound scan

If the midtrimester 16- to 23-week scan demonstrates major structural defects, it is advisable to offer fetal karyotyping, even if these defects are isolated. The prevalence of these defects is low and therefore the financial cost implications are relatively small. Even if the defect is potentially correctable by surgery, such as exomphalos, it would seem appropriate to exclude an underlying chromosomal abnormality. The management policy for major fetal structural abnormality is unlikely to require changing on an ethnic basis. The same does not follow for the so-called 'minor' markers of chromosomal abnormality.

Minor defects or markers are common and they are not usually associated with any handicap, unless there is an associated chromosomal abnormality. Most practitioners adopt an individualized approach to the assessment of risk depending on the marker identified either using the appropriate likelihood ratio or a genetic sonogram score.[3] In high-risk populations as defined by advanced maternal age or positive maternal serum biochemistry, this approach has been shown to maintain a high sensitivity for fetal aneuploidy without significantly increasing the invasive prenatal testing rate.

However, routine karyotyping of all low-risk pregnancies with these markers would have major implications, in terms of both miscarriage and financial costs. As a general concern, this process of sequential screening assumes the unproven independence between the findings of different screening results. For example, second-trimester intracardiac echogenic foci are known to increase in prevalence when first-trimester nuchal translucency measurements are elevated in fetuses of normal karyotype.[26] Hence, prior screening test results should be followed until data evaluating the interdependence of such markers become available.

Additionally, only a few have attempted to evaluate ethnic variation in such minor markers for fetal aneuploidy. Despite this, they have all invariably established significant ethnic variations in prevalence of the markers such as nasal bone, intracardiac echogenic foci, humeral, and femoral length.[27–33] Hence, if these markers are to be used for modulating the risk of fetal chromosomal abnormality, the ethnic influence of the exact markers used need to be evaluated. In the long term, it would seem more reliable to use first-trimester nuchal translucency and maternal serum biochemistry, where corrections are not required or are easily made.

Neural tube defects

NTDs have a complex etiology in which both genetic and environmental factors appear to be involved. Analysis of recurrence patterns within families and of twin-concordance data provides evidence of a genetic influence in sporadic cases, but factors such as socio-economic status and geographic area (independent of race or ethnicity) are also associated with variations in the incidence of NTDs. Furthermore, exposure during pregnancy to various drugs, most commonly antiepileptics, are associated with increased risk of NTDs. Recently, Rothenberg *et al.* demonstrated the increased prevalence of autoantibodies against folate receptors in serum of women with a current or previous pregnancy complicated by a fetal NTD.[34,35] It remains to be established whether there is a causative relationship between the presence of these antibodies and the development of NTDs.

Screening by midtrimester ultrasound appears to be superior to maternal serum AFP assessment, but the latter modality is still widely used as a prior screening modality before detailed ultrasound assessment. The ethnic variation in AFP levels are well established and corrective formulas may be applied to produce accurate risks for NTDs in various ethnic groups as recommended by the American College of Medical Genetics guidelines for the screening of NTDs.[23]

Targeted screening in ethnic groups

There are certain inherited disorders that occur more frequently in every ethnic, demographic, or racial group, than in the general population. Small genetic differences are known to exist between individuals from different ethnic groups. Certain ethnic groups have a higher risk of certain genetic conditions, especially autosomal recessive disorders, than the general population. Prenatal diagnosis is available for many genetic conditions, and a growing number of women are seeking advice regarding prenatal testing for a present or planned pregnancy. Knowledge of a patient's ethnicity can, therefore, help make a diagnosis, or help to identify individuals or couples at an increased risk of having a child with a specific genetic condition. The American College of Obstetricians and Gynecologists (ACOG) recommends genetic counseling for couples at increased risk of birth defects. Counseling enables the couple to become more informed about the disorders involved, the current availability of prenatal and postnatal testing, the accuracy and limitations of such testing, and their reproductive options.[36]

"Jewish" genetic disorders

The "Jewish" genetic disorders are a group of disorders that occur at a higher frequency among Jews compared to the general population, yet are not exclusive to the Jewish population. There is no official list of conditions; however, it is known that Mendelian disorders and diseases associated with predisposition genes have a higher incidence in an individual of Ashkenazi or Sephardic ancestry. As different Jewish groups are at risk of different disorders, it is important to establish not only a patient's religion, but also their ethnicity and ancestral countries of origin.

Ancestors of the Ashkenazi Jews lived in Central and Eastern Europe (Germany, Poland, Lithuania, and Russia). Approximately 95% of Jews living in North America are Ashkenazi. This population are more likely to carry genes for Tay–Sachs disease, Canavan disease, familial dysautonomia, Niemann–Pick (type A) disease, Fanconi anemia (group C), Bloom syndrome, Gaucher disease (the non-neuronopathic type), mucolipidosis type IV, and cystic fibrosis (CF; see Table 79.2). As these conditions can be severely incapacitating, tragically debilitating, or lead to death in infancy or early childhood, some orthodox communities encourage the use of premarital carrier screening to discourage the marriage of two carriers.

Table 79.2 Common genetic disorders and carrier frequency in the Ashkenazi Jewish population

Disease	Carrier frequency
Tay–Sachs disease	1 in 26
Canavan disease	1 in 38
Familial dysautonomia	1 in 30
Niemann–Pick disease (type A)	1 in 70
Fanconi anemia (group C)	1 in 89
Bloom syndrome	1 in 110
Gaucher disease	1 in 10
Mucolipidosis IV	1 in 100
Cystic fibrosis	1 in 25

In comparison, the Sephardic Jews ancestry can be traced to Spain, Portugal, North Africa (Morocco and Tunisia), and the Middle East. This Jewish population is more likely to be carriers for beta-thalassemia, familial Mediterranean fever, glucose-6-phosphate dehydrogenase (G6PD) deficiency, and Type III glycogen storage disease.

The Ashkenazi Jewish community is a unique and ideal population that provides screening of multiple diseases because detection rates are high (> 95%) when tested for a limited number of mutations. The ACOG recommends screening couples with European-Jewish ancestry at a minimum for Tay–Sachs disease, Canavan disease, and CF.[37,38] No standards of care have been set for the Sephardic population.

Hemoglobinopathies

Hemoglobinopathies are the commonest single gene recessive disorders in the world. They occur as a result of mutations in the globin gene and are primarily seen in populations whose ancestors are from Africa, the Middle East, the Caribbean, the Mediterranean, Asia, and the Far East. These disorders have appeared in the West due to global migration. In the UK, the NHS Sickle Cell and Thalassaemia Screening Programme are working toward a policy of universal antenatal screening that will allow the offer of sickle cell and thalassemia screening to all women as an integral part of early antenatal care.

The population of Cyprus (both Greek and Turkish) has one of the highest rates of beta-thalassemia carriers in the world, and in the past one of every 158 infants was born with the condition. Today in Cyprus, antenatal screening for thalassemia has been almost totally superseded by premarital screening. The religious authorities had ethical objections to screening during pregnancy, on the grounds that it excluded most options other than termination of affected pregnancies.

The church in Cyprus, therefore, insists on testing as a formal prerequisite to church weddings. The certificate required states merely that the partners have been tested and appropriately advised. In this way, the confidentiality of the test result is preserved and the couple can exercise an informed choice about reproduction. This societal approach to inherited genetic disorders is to be applauded, and it would be a suitable model for other communities to adapt.

Cystic fibrosis

CF is a common inherited condition that affects many systems in the body, most often resulting in chronic, progressive lung disease, problems with digestion, and subsequent malnutrition. CF is the most commonly inherited disease in Caucasians, affecting approximately 1:2500 individuals, but it has been identified in people of all races and ethnicities around the world. The incidence in other ethnic groups varies from 1:15,000 for African Americans to 1:90,000 in Asians. In 2001, the ACOG and the American College of Medical Genetics[38] recommended that CF carrier screening be offered to all Caucasian couples who are pregnant, or are considering pregnancy. These groups additionally recommended that carrier screening be made available to other ethnic populations with the understanding that the likelihood of being a CF carrier may be much lower in non-Caucasian populations (see Table 79.3).[39]

Although there have been over 1000 mutations identified that cause CF, only 25 have been recommended for carrier screening as additional mutations are rare, not well understood, and have minimal impact on the overall probability of affecting a child. Mutations of the CF also vary with ethnicity. The ΔF508 mutation accounts for 70% of the CF mutations in Caucasians of Northern European descents but only 30% of CF mutations in individuals of Ashkenazi Jewish descent. A different mutation, W1282X, is more common in the Ashkenazi Jews.

Glucose-6-phosphate dehydrogenase deficiency

G6PD deficiency is the most common human enzyme deficiency. G6PD deficiency can result in the rapid destruction of blood cells in the presence of infection or certain drugs. Different populations have different types of mutations, but within a specific population, common mutations are usually shared. There are a wide variety of normal genetic variants of the enzyme G6PD. The main races affected are in West Africa, the Mediterranean, the Middle East, and South East Asia. The degree of deficiency varies, often being mild in black Africans, more severe in Orientals, and most severe in Mediterraneans. Severe deficiency also occasionally occurs in Caucasians. Antenatal screening is available for at-risk patients.

Table 79.3 The detection rate for the cystic fibrosis ΔF508 mutation test in various populations, including carrier frequency before and after a negative ΔF508 mutation test[39]

Ethnicity	Detection rate (%)	Before test	After negative test
Ashkenazi Jewish	97	1/29	1/934
Caucasian (northern European)	90	1/25	1/241
Caucasian (southern European)	70	1/25	1/81
African American	69	1/65	1/207
Hispanic American	57	1/46	1/105
Asian	30	1/90	1/128

This is a pooled set of data based on ΔF508 deletion and requires additional information to accurately predict risk of specific Hispanic populations. Residual carrier risk after a negative test is further modified by the presence of a positive family history of CF and/or by mixed ethnicity

Effects of screening on ethnicity

Knowledge

The uptake of any screening test is influenced by knowledge of the condition being screened for. Parents need appropriate knowledge of Down's syndrome, what it is, and how it affects the child and adult, both mentally and physically. They also need appropriate knowledge of the screening test, together with the limitations of the test, so they can decide whether they wish to be screened. A study by Chilaka *et al.*[40] at Leicester General Hospital in the UK looked at the knowledge of Down's syndrome amongt pregnant women from different ethnic groups. The study showed that racial groups other than Caucasian had a poorer understanding of Down's syndrome. Fifty-one percent of Caucasians in the study had a good knowledge of Down's syndrome compared to 8% of Asians born outside the UK. The factors affecting knowledge included the quality of spoken English, knowing an affected child, parity, and religion. Only five women in the study could not speak English; however, none of these women had any reasonable knowledge of Down's syndrome compared to those who could speak English. The importance of the study results are highlighted by its main finding that knowledge of the condition was the most influential factor in the decision making process about accepting or declining a Down's syndrome screening test. In addition, information retention about prenatal screening also varies significantly by ethnicity and level of education.[41]

Access and equity

Women from ethnic minorities can experience financial, linguistic, and cultural barriers to access health care services, limiting utilization of genetic and other maternal child health services. Genetic conditions may go undetected with deleterious impact during prenatal, perinatal, and newborn periods. Society has an ethical obligation to ensure equitable access to health care for all, yet there remains a persistence of health disparities across race, income, and ethnicity.

The extent and quality of prenatal care is important for the health of women and their babies. Early prenatal care can encourage healthy habits during pregnancy, help to identify potential medical problems, facilitate screening and involvement with parenting support, nutrition, and other educational resources. Women from ethnic groups have been shown to use antenatal services less intensely with a high proportion booking too late for screening to be useful. Although the percentage of women receiving prenatal care during the first 3 months of pregnancy has increased over the past two decades for white, black, Asian, and Hispanic women, white women are still the most likely to receive prenatal care in their first trimester. Sadly, a significant proportion of women from the ethnic minorities still receive no care until the third trimester.

In some countries in the world, a substantial barrier to health care access for some people is the lack of either public or private health insurance. Another difficulty in accessing health services is the problem of communication and language barriers. The difficulties for the patient, if English is not the first language, with respect to screening can be divided into problems of recruitment into a screening program, of giving the patients enough information to allow informed consent, and of problems arising if detailed information needs to be provided in follow up. To counter language difficulties interpreters may be used and information leaflets can be produced in different languages. Interpreting skills continue to be a scarce resource in any health service. One way to cope with this problem has been the setting up of a language service, which enables remote interpreting via a shared telephone line. Another is by asking relatives to act as interpreters. However, this can be problematic as it is often assumed that they are knowledgeable in all aspects of both languages, and this may place them under a great deal of stress. Also, patients may feel uncomfortable with even close relatives knowing about their medical conditions, as it may have profound cultural implications such as impacting on marriage prospects for themselves or their close family.

In many cultures, the concept of having to go outside the family for health education or infant care is an alien concept, and would indicate an unacceptable lack of respect for the older women in the family who traditionally are an important part of the child care system, and who expect to instruct the young mother in the care of her baby. To be obliged to seek such education from members of another culture whose values and beliefs are different from one's own is almost bizarre. However, if the concept of instruction in parentcraft by a midwife is accepted, the actual attendance at parentcraft may present considerable difficulties. The 'usual' inhibitions to attendance experienced by young women, e.g. child care, the need to take time off work, may be further complicated by the need for a young woman to be escorted (particularly in the evenings), or by difficulties with communication or socioeconomic issues.

Despite these constraints, with an ethnically sensitive strategy, it is still possible to provide equal access to prenatal screening. For example, in a previous study on ethnic differences in nuchal translucency measurement, it was noted that the ethnic balance of the population accepting and declining prenatal Down's syndrome screening was not significantly different in an obstetric population from one of the most socially deprived regions of the UK, where over 15% of the women did not speak English.[42]

Culture and religion

Understanding and valuing cultural diversity is critical to ensure the best possible care. For example, a woman is likely to decline prenatal screening and diagnosis because of fears that she may be divorced by her partner or shunned by her in-laws in the event that a fetal abnormality is diagnosed. The difficulties such attitudes create are further amplified by the fact that such women may well have a poorer understanding of the local language, be financially insecure, and be reliant on their partner for right of residency in the country. This maternal perception, often unbeknown to the clinician, may be interpreted by health care workers as denial or lack of knowledge.

It is also important not to make the assumption that all women from a particular community follow the same customs and religion. For example, attitudes to termination vary even within the Muslim community. Some Muslim parents do not see termination as 'halal' (permitted) but as 'haram' (not permitted). They know their child is diseased but they choose to keep it believing that God's will (inshaallah) created that child and they expect to get their rewards in heaven. Even when termination of pregnancy is acceptable, there are different interpretations of the gestation up to which such a procedure may be carried out.[43]

Clinicians, therefore, need to develop an appreciation and respect for cultures and religions that differ hugely from their own. This may be often impossible to attain unless members of the local ethnic and religious communities are co-opted into health service delivery as health care workers of aides.

Consanguinity

In the West our knowledge and understanding of consanguinity is limited. While marriages between close biological kin are preferred in many parts of the world, such unions are not commonplace in the West. First-cousin marriages are legal in countries such as the UK and Australia, but are against the law in others. The 1981 marriage law of the People's Republic of China prohibits marriage between couples related as first cousins or closer, and in the USA, consanguineous unions are prohibited in 30 States. Irrespective of prevailing legislation, a future decline in the prevalence of consanguineous unions can be predicted, accompanying the expected reduction in family sizes. Regardless, it is important that health care providers have an understanding of the potential genetic consequences of such unions. This was recognized by the National Society of Genetic Counselors (NSGC) in America, who developed guidelines providing recommendations on counseling and screening for consanguineous couples defined as being second cousins or closer.[44]

Most of the genetic fall-out of consanguinity is in the form of autosomal recessive disorders, which in fact adversely affect only a minority of such families. The more closely two people are related, the more genes they share, and the more likely that both will carry a copy of the same recessive mutation, thereby increasing their chances of having a child affected by that disorder. Although it is not possible to come up with one number for all populations of consanguineous couples, the risk is not as high as was previously envisaged. It is estimated that the additional risk of significant birth defects, including mental retardation or genetic disorders, above the general population risk is about 1.7–2.8% for first-cousin unions. The consensus from the NSGC is that beyond a thorough medical family history, with follow-up of significant findings, no additional preconception screening is recommended for consanguineous couples. Consanguineous couples should be offered similar genetic screening as suggested for any couple of their ethnic group.

Conclusions

Ethnic differences in the delivery of health care are prevalent across various domains of health, including mortality, morbidity, behavior, and utilization of health services. This chapter highlighted some areas of ethnic differences and potential inequalities in access to prenatal testing. The elimination of health inequality will first require a reliable assessment of the disparity in care provision as well as a clear understanding of differences across populations identified in terms of race/ethnicity. Further research is required to improve our understanding of why testing may not be offered, the reasons for failure to take up testing when offered, and to identify whether there are other social inequalities in the access to prenatal testing.

REFERENCES

1. Office of National Statistics. Census, 2001.
2. Matilainen R, Airasksinen E, Mononen T, Launiala K, Kaariainen R. A population-based study on the causes of mild and severe mental retardation. *Acta Paediatr* 1995;84(3):261–6.
3. Nicolaides KH. Screening for chromosomal defects. *Ultrasound Obstet Gynecol* 2003;21:313–21.
4. Hook EB. Rates of chromosome abnormalities at different maternal ages. *Obstet Gynecol* 1987;94:387–402.
5. Down LJ. Observations on an ethnic classification of idiots. *Clin Lect Rep Lond Hosp* 1866;3:259–62.
6. Nicolaides KH, Brizot ML, Snijders RJM. Fetal nuchal translucency: ultrasound screening for fetal trisomy in the first trimester of pregnancy. *Br J Obstet Gynaecol* 1994;101:782–6.
7. Pandya PP, Brizot ML, Kuhn P, Snijders RJM, Nicolaides KH. First trimester fetal nuchal translucency thickness and risk for trisomies. *Obstet Gynaecol* 1994;84:420–3.
8. Pandya PP, Snijders RJM, Johnson SP, Brizot ML, Nicolaides KH. Screening for fetal trisomies by maternal age and fetal nuchal translucency thickness at 10–14 weeks of gestation. *Br J Obstet Gynaecol* 1995;102:957–62.
9. Thilaganathan B, Khare M, Williams B, Wathen NC. Influence of ethnic origin on nuchal translucency screening for Down syndrome. *Ultrasound Obstet Gynecol* 1998;12(2):112–4.
10. Chen M, Lam YH, Tang MH, *et al.* The effect of ethnic origin on nuchal translucency at 10–14 weeks of gestation. *Prenat Diagn* 2002;22(7):576–8.
11. Pandya PP, Altman DG, Brizot ML, Pettersen H, Nicolaides KH. Repeatability of measurement of fetal nuchal translucency thickness. *Ultrasound Obstet Gynecol* 1995;5(5):334–7.
12. Mavrides E, Sairam S, Hollis B, Thilaganathan B. Screening for aneuploidy in the first trimester by assessment of blood flow in the ductus venosus. *Br J Obstet Gynecol* 2002;109(9):1015–9.
13. Cicero S, Curuio P, Papageorghiou A, Soneik J, Nicolaides KH. Absence of nasal bone in fetuses with trisomy 21 at 11–14 weeks of gestation: An observational study. *Lancet* 2001;358:1665–7.
14. Cicero S, Longo D, Rembouskos G, Sacchini C, Nicolaides KH. Absent nasal bone at 11–14 weeks of gestation and chromosomal defects. *Ultrasound Obstet Gynecol* 2003;22(1):31–5.
15. Otodile FA. Nasal bones and pyriform apertures in Blacks. *Ann Plast Surg* 1994;32(1):21–6.
16. Cicero S, Sonek JD, McKenna DS, Croom CS, Johnson L, Nicolaides KH. Nasal bone hypoplasia in trisomy 21 at 15–22 weeks' gestation. *Ultrasound Obstet Gynecol* 2003;21(1):15–8.
17. Prefumo F, Sairam S, Bhide A, Penna L, Hollis B, Thilaganathan B. Maternal ethnic origin and fetal nasal bones at 11–14 weeks of gestation. *Br J Obstet Gynecol* 2004;111(2):109–12.
18. Cicero S, Rembouskos G, Vandecruys H, Hogg M, Nicolaides KH. Likelihood ratio for trisomy 21 in fetuses with absent nasal bone at the 11–14-week scan. *Ultrasound Obstet Gynecol* 2004;23(3): 218–23.
19. Merkatz IR, Nitowsky HM, Macri JN, Johnson WE. An association between low maternal serum alpha-fetoprotein and fetal chromosomal abnormalities. *Am J Obstet Gynecol* 1984;148(7):886–94.
20. Gilbert L, Nicholl J, Alex S, *et al.* Ethnic differences in the outcome of serum screening for Down syndrome. *Br Med J* 1996;312:94–5.
21. Benn PA, Clive JM, Collins R. Medians for second-trimester maternal serum alpha-fetoprotein, human chorionic gonadotropin, and unconjugated estriol; differences between races or ethnic groups. *Clin Chem* 1997;43(2):333–7.
22. Watt HC, Wald NJ, Smith D, Kennard A, Densem J. Effect of allowing for ethnic group in prenatal screening for Down syndrome. *Prenat Diagn* 1996;16(8):691–8.
23. American College of Medical Genetics. *Standards and Guidelines for Clinical Genetics Laboratories.* American College of Medical Genetics, 2004.
24. Spencer K, Souter V, Tul N, Snijders R, Nicolaides KH. A screening program for trisomy 21 at 10–14 weeks using fetal nuchal translucency, maternal serum free β-human chorionic gonadotropin and pregnancy-associated plasma protein-A. *Ultrasound Obstet Gynecol* 1999;13(4):231–7.

25. Spencer K, Ong CYT, Liao AWJ, Nicolaides KH. The influence of ethnic origin on first trimester biochemical markers of chromosomal abnormalities. *Prenat Diagn* 2000;20(6):491–4.
26. Prefumo F, Presti F, Thilaganathan B, Carvalho JS. Association between increased nuchal translucency and second trimester cardiac echogenic foci. *Obstet Gynecol* 2003;101(5, Pt 1):899–904.
27. Rebarber A, Levey KA, Funai E, Monda S, Paidas M. An ethnic predilection for fetal echogenic intracardiac focus identified during targeted midtrimester ultrasound examination: A retrospective review. *BMC Pregnancy Childbirth* 2004;4(1):12.
28. Shipp TD, Bromley B, Lieberman E, Benacerraf BR. The frequency of the detection of fetal echogenic intracardiac foci with respect to maternal race. *Ultrasound Obstet Gynecol* 2000;15(6):460–2.
29. Zelop CM, Borgida AF, Egan JF. Variation of fetal humeral length in second-trimester fetuses according to race and ethnicity. *J Ultrasound Med* 2003;22(7):691–3.
30. Mastrobattista JM, Pschirrer ER, Hamrick MA, *et al.* Humerus length evaluation in different ethnic groups. *J Ultrasound Med* 2004;23(2):227–31.
31. Kovac CM, Brown JA, Apodaca CC, *et al.* Maternal ethnicity and variation of fetal femur length calculations when screening for Down syndrome. *J Ultrasound Med* 2002;21(7):719–22.
32. Borgida AF, Zelop C, Deroche M, Bolnick A, Egan JF. Down syndrome screening using race-specific femur length. *Am J Obstet Gynecol* 2003;189(4):977–9.
33. Shipp TD, Bromley B, Mascola M, Benacerraf B. Variation in fetal femur length with respect to maternal race. *J Ultrasound Med* 2001;20(2):141–4.
34. Rothenberg SP, Da Costa MP, Sequeira JM, *et al.* Autoantibodies against folate receptors in women with a pregnancy complicated by a neural-tube defect. *N Engl J Med* 2004;350(2):134–42.
35. Rothenberg SP, Da Costa MP, Sequeira JM, *et al.* Autoantibodies against folate receptors in women with a pregnancy complicated by a neural tube defect. *Obstet Gynecol Surv* 2004;59(6):410–1.
36. Driscoll DA, Wenstrom KD, Williams J. Third ACOG Committee on Genetics. ACOG Technology Assessment in Obstetrics and Gynecology. Number 1, July 2002. Genetics and molecular diagnostic testing. *Obstet Gynecol* 2002;100:193–211.
37. ACOG Committee on Genetics. Screening for Tay–Sachs disease – ACOG Committee Opinion 162. *Int J Gynaecol Obstet* 1996; 52(3):311–2.
38. American College of Obstetricians and Gynecologists, American College of Medical Genetics. Preconception and prenatal carrier screening for cystic fibrosis. In *Clinical and Laboratory Guidelines*. ACOG, American College of Medical Genetics, 2001
39. Grody WW, Cutting GR, Klinger KW, Richards CS, Watson MS, Desnick RJ. Laboratory standards and guidelines for population-based cystic fibrosis carrier screening. *Genet Med* 2001;3(2): 149–54.
40. Chilaka VN, Konje JC, Stewart CR, Narayan H, Taylor DJ. Knowledge of Down syndrome in pregnant women from different ethnic groups. *Prenat Diagn* 2001;21(3):159–64.
41. Browner CH, Preloran M, Press NA. The effects of ethnicity, education and an informational video on pregnant women's knowledge and decisions about a prenatal diagnostic screening test. *Patient Educ Couns* 1996;27(2):135–46.
42. Thilaganathan B, Sairam S, Michalidis G, Wathen NC. First trimester nuchal translucency: Effective routine screening for Down's syndrome. *Br J Radiol* 1999;72(862):946–8.
43. Zlotogora J. Parental decisions to abort or continue a pregnancy with an abnormal finding after an invasive prenatal test. *Prenat Diagn* 2002;22(12):1102–6.
44. Bennett RL, Motulsky AG, Bittles A, *et al.* Genetic counseling and screening of consanguineous couples and their offspring: Recommendations of the National Society of Genetic Counselors. *J Genet Counsel* 2002;11(2):97–119.

80 Ultrasound screening of congenital heart defects

R. Chaoui

Introduction

Congenital heart defects (CHD) are one of the most common anomalies in human fetuses (5/1000 livebirths) and are the leading cause of death due to malformations in the first year of life. Heart abnormalities and soft markers are present in a substantial amount in fetuses with chromosomal aberrations and fetal echocardiography and are thus an intrinsic part of the genetic scan.[1]

A prenatal diagnosis can be reliably achieved by means of ultrasound during pregnancy and the accurate prenatal diagnosis improves in many conditions of the fetal outcome by delivering the baby at a specialized tertiary center. In this chapter the examination of the fetal heart is reviewed, focusing on the role of screening and how to imply the heart into the genetic scan.

Examination techniques of the fetal heart

No organ in the fetus can be examined with as many diagnostical techniques as the heart. Detailed information on structure, function and time-related events has become available thanks to the development of sophisticated tools.[1] However, this has not been accompanied by a significant increase in prenatal detection rate of anomalies, but rather in the increasing reliability of precise diagnosis.

Real-time gray-scale ultrasound and two-dimensional (2D) echocardiography

Gray-scale 2D ultrasound is still the gold standard for the structural evaluation of the fetal heart. Resolution has continuously increased over the last two decades in step with the huge progress in the development of computer technology and fast processors. In most sophisticated (and expensive) ultrasound machines there is an ideal setting for fetal heart examination, which is based on a high image resolution (using scan heads with 250-1012 acoustic lines), a high frame rate and good penetration. Visualization of very tiny structures like the coronary arteries using real-time ultrasound has become possible as well as of other structures such as the fetal thymus that has not been seen before. The increased resolution using 5–7-MHz transducers has also led to the identification of new details like the echogenic intracardiac focus with the discussion on whether or not it is associated with chromosomal or other anomalies (see below).

Two main features, however, have facilitated enormously the fetal heart examination and are now standard even on mid- to low-range machines: the cine-loop and the zoom functions. The magnification of the image allows better assessment of the structures of interest and visualization of the different cardiac cycle phases image by image facilitates assessment of the structures during systole and diastole. In recent years, image resolution in gray scale was increased by completing the native image with harmonic and/or compound imaging.

Time motion or M-mode

Time motion application in the fetus was not possible until simultaneous real-time visualization became available. Cardiac biometry first performed with M-mode was very soon abandoned since such measurements became easier using cine-loop technique to image selectively diastole and systole.[2,3] Two main fields of interest are still in the domain of M-mode: one is the classification of fetal arrhythmia and the other is the calculation of indices used in cardiology to assess contractility, e.g. shortening fraction, ejection fraction, etc.

Spectral Doppler flow velocity waveform

Doppler ultrasound enables a non-invasive quantification of perfusion across different fetal cardiac valves and vessels. Peak velocities can be assessed and indices calculated. By measuring the area of a valve the perfusion can then be calculated either as stroke volume or involving the heart frequency as cardiac output. The advent of color Doppler enabled a more reliable use over spectral Doppler across the known valves, but also the evaluation of more difficult otherwise not assessable regions, as pulmonary arteries and veins, ductus arteriosus, foramen ovale and even coronary vessels.

Color Doppler

In addition to the gray-scale examination of the fetal heart, color Doppler is now considered as the second part of a complete cardiac evaluation. The method allows rapid orientation within the fetal heart and completes the evaluation supplied by gray-scale information. Once abnormal flow is suspected, quantification becomes mandatory using spectral Doppler. The advent of color Doppler did not contribute to a huge increase in detection rate of CHD but increased the reliability of screening when routinely applied and in the detailed fetal echocardiography in suspected heart diseases.

We described a few years ago how most congenital heart anomalies could be detected in only three planes using color Doppler: the four-chamber view, the five-chamber view and the three-vessel-trachea view.[4] The exact examination in gray scale completed by the expected typical flow in color Doppler became the basis of diagnosis of fetal CHD.

Three-dimensional fetal echocardiography

As soon as the first 3D ultrasound equipment became available, an attempt to examine the fetal heart was undertaken. It was hoped that 3D information of the fetal heart could facilitate understanding of orientation, especially the assessment of the great vessels' anatomy, which is difficult for many examiners. However, since the heart is beating the main challenge is still the gating of the signals and the acquisition of information during systole or diastole.[5] The advent of spatio-temporal image correlation (STIC) technology a few years ago allowed a reliable acquisition of a 3D with systole and diastole as off-line 4D fetal echo.[6] STIC can be used in gray scale[6] or in combination with color or power Doppler mode.[7] A detailed description of 3D of heart and vessels is described elsewhere in this book and I refer to the reader to this chapter. The technique is however too new to be evaluated for its role in screening for fetal heart defects or in genetic scan.

Screening of the fetal heart or targeted examination based on indications

CHD have a multifactorial etiology and therefore prenatal detection cannot be achieved solely by concentrating on the high-risk population defined by patient history. Therefore, seeking for heart abnormalities should be part of the midtrimester ultrasound screening. In many countries such a general screening is not established (no insurance or mother care coverage), but is often performed either on indication of risk or because of the willingness of the patient.

Signs of cardiac disease are often subtle, necessitating careful targeted examination. In the 1980s, the four-chamber view was proposed as the most important plane for screening, allowing a greater detection rate for anomalies. Recently, however, incorporation of views of the great vessels has been recommended as part of the routine screening examination.

Many studies in the last 10 years have emphasized the importance of cardiac screening, but they have achieved widely divergent results, with reported detection rates varying from 5 to 92%.[8] However, it should be noted that these studies employed different approaches and are therefore not directly comparable (see Chaoui [8] for details).

There is a list of indications, generally accepted as referral reason for fetal echocardiography, which are presented in another chapter. The percentage of detection of heart anomalies within single groups (the yield) differs from 3–5% (i.e. diabetes, drugs and genetic ultrasound) to more than 50% (i.e. suspicious four-chamber view). In some indications fetal echocardiography is performed to calm the pregnant woman (low recurrence risk in positive family history) and in other conditions to seriously rule out a heart anomaly (non-immune hydrops and extracardiac malformations).

Fetal cardiac examination in a low-risk population and targeted fetal echocardiography in a high-risk population

It is generally agreed that the 'four-chamber view' should be part of every routine ultrasound in pregnancy. However, there are different reasons why this plane was not successful in improving the detection rate of CHD in the recent past. In order to achieve an accurate assessment of this plane we recommend following a step-by-step checklist on every single cardiac examination, including the list in Table 80.1.

It is agreed further that the assessment of the great vessels belongs rather to an extended fetal cardiac examination. We expect, however, that in future this will be part of a basic cardiac examination as well, since many anomalies of the great vessels are not detectable in the simple four-chamber-screening and their detection has been demonstrated to improve the outcome in various CHD. Whereas the four-chamber view can be examined in a single plane, the great vessels can be only assessed by a dynamic scan, i.e. by tilting and moving the transducer.[9] The checklist for assessing the great vessels will include the list as presented in Table 80.2.

Table 80.1 Checklist for the basic cardiac examination and the targeted fetal echocardiography for the four-chamber view

	Basic Examination	Targeted Fetal Echo
Upper Abdomen	Stomach and heart on the same side of the fetus	Same
Descending aorta/ Inferior Vena cava		– Aorta on the left side of the spine – Normal arrangement of Aorta and Inferior vena cava in the upper abdomen
Heart Size	about 1/3 of the thoracic cavity	Same
Heart Position	2/3 of the heart is in the left hemithorax	Same
		Same
Heart Axis	septum at an angle of about 45° to the midline	Same
Heart rhythm	120–180 Beats/min, no arrhythmia	Same
Ventricles	Two equally contracting ventricles, of approximately equal cavity size and wall thickness	Right Ventricle is shorter than the left and has the moderator band at the apex. Heart apex is build by the left ventricle
Atria	Two atria of approximately equal size with foramen ovale defect in middle third of atrial septum	Same
Valves	Two opening atrioventricular valves	Same
Crux of heart	Intact	Intact and slightly lower insertion of the tricuspid valve than to the mitral valve
Ventricular septum	Intact from apex to crux	Same
Pulmonary vein(s)		at least one should be seen by colour flow mapping connecting to the left atrium
Color Doppler flow shows		– antegrade perfusion across atrioventricular valves – no aliasing (turbulences) – no regurgitation – no crossing over the ventricular septum

Targeted fetal echocardiography should be performed by those familiar with the prenatal diagnosis of CHD and the wide spectrum of possible anomalies. In this chapter I cannot recommend whether the examiner should be an obstetrician or a pediatric cardiologist, as this may be decided by the local specificities of the country. I recommend, however, a close cooperation between both groups, especially while counseling a pregnant woman with a suspected heart anomaly in the fetus.

Often the expectations are bigger and therefore the time, equipment and expertise needed for an examination are greater. In these conditions the use of color and pulsed Doppler techniques increases the accuracy of the examination. In cases of arrhythmia M-mode or pulsed Doppler should be used to demonstrate the relationship between atrial and ventricular contractions.

The checklist in these conditions is longer and the dynamic examination of the heart in different planes[9] is mandatory, as shown in Tables 80.1 and 80.2.

Fetal echocardiography and the detection of a congenital heart defect

There are two steps in the detection of a fetal heart defect, namely, first, the suspicion of an abnormality and second, the detailed precise description and classification of the heart defect. Generally, the first is easily achieved when the examiner is able to get the four-chamber view and the great vessels in nearly all patients as described in Tables 80.1 and 80.2 and he/she knows the typical hints for an abnormal heart in these planes. The second step can be solved chiefly by getting experience of many CHD and knowing the spectrum of the different diseases. In many countries the latter examination is either achieved together with a pediatric cardiologist or by referring the pregnant woman to a pediatric cardiologist specialized in fetal echo examination.

Table 80.2 Examination of the great arteries as part of an extended basic cardiac examination or as targeted fetal echocardiography

	Extended Basic Examination	Targeted Fetal Echo
Aorta	arises from the left ventricle	arises from the left ventricle continues toward the aortic arch
Ventricular septum	continuous with ascending aorta	Same
Pulmonary trunk	– arises from the RV – is slightly larger than aorta – crosses over the ascending aorta – bifurcates to give the left and right pulmonary arteries – connects to the ductus arteriosus	Same
Duct and aortic arch		– are of approximately equal size – point to the left side of the spine – the trachea is on the right of both vessels – Thymus is present – No left superior vena cava on the left of the pulmonary trunk
Color flow shows		– antegrade perfusion across both semilunar valves – no aliasing (turbulences) except in the ductus region in third trimester – no regurgitation – no reverse flow in either the ductus arteriosus or the aortic arch

Table 80.3 Common suspicions leading to referral to targeted fetal echocardiography

Common suspicions in the four-chamber view	Cardiomegaly Arrhythmia Heart to the right/heart-stomach on different site Single ventricle One small ventricle (right or left) Discrepant size of the ventricles Defect in the ventricular septum, AV-junction One common AV-valve Echogenic focus in the LV Tumors in the heart
Common suspicions in the great vessels assessment	Perimembraneous VSD in the five-chamber view VSD with overriding aorta Dilated aortic root Discrepant calibre of ascending aorta and pulmonary trunk Hypoplastic or non-continuing aorta or pulmonary trunk Parallel great vessels arrangement One single vessel only visualized Aortic arch on the right side of the spine (and trachea)

It is important to know the most common 'abnormalities' detected during fetal cardiac scan and leading to a referral. In my experience the most common signs detected in the four-chamber view and the great vessel planes are summarized in Table 80.3. The differential diagnosis of most common suspicions of referrals is summarized in Table 80.4.

Fetal echocardiography in genetic scan

Fetal examination allows detection of fetuses at high risk for chromosomal aberrations owing to malformations or signs called soft markers.[10] The latter

Table 80.4 Differential diagnoses of some common suspicions

Suspicion	Differential diagnoses
Single ventricle	Mitral atresia Tricuspid atresia Double inlet ventricle Large Atrioventricular septal defect
Small left ventricle	Hypoplastic left heart syndrome Coarctation of the aorta Mitral atresia with VSD Double outlet right ventricle
Small right ventricle	Pulmonary atresia with intact septum Tricuspid atresia with VSD
Ventricular Septum Defect	Isolated VSD Atrioventricular septal defect Double inlet ventricle Interrupted aortic arch Aortic coarctation Conotruncal anomalies (see overriding aorta)
Overriding aorta over the VSD	Tetralogy of Fallot Pulmonary atresia with VSD Truncus arteriosus communis Absent pulmonary valve syndrome Double outlet right ventricle
Parallel Vessels	Double outlet right ventricle Complete Transposition of the great arteries Congenitally corrected Transposition of the great arteries
Tiny ascending aorta	Hypoplastic left heart syndrome Aortic coarctation Tubular hypoplasia of the aortic arch Interruption of the aortic arch
Two normal appearing ventricles, but one single great vessel recognized	Double outlet right ventricle (vessels over each other) Transposition of the great arteries (vessels over each other) Truncus arteriosus communis Dilated Aorta (in pulmonary atresia with VSD)

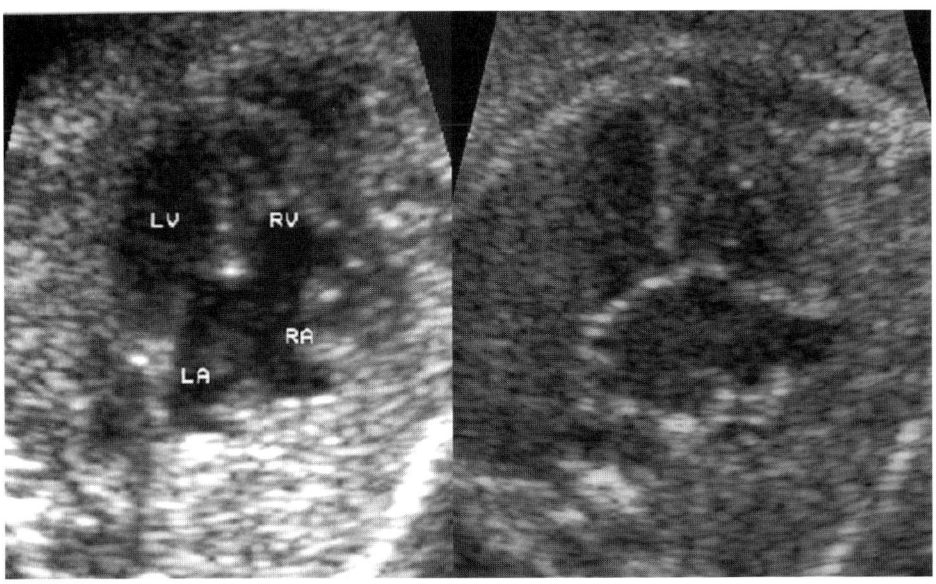

Figure 80.1 Fetuses with atrioventricular septal defect during diastole (left) and systole (right). In the left image the gap in the crux of the heart is easily recognized. On the right side on the one hand both AV valves are linear and on the other the measurement of atrial to ventricular length reveals a ratio 0.6 suspicious for an AVSD.

increases the risk to a specific malformation, without being obligatorily *per se* a structural malformation. The fetal heart belongs to the organs often evaluated carefully when looking for a chromosomal anomaly, either the common numerical aberrations such as trisomy 21, 18, 13 or monosomy X or more specific deletions such as the microdeletion 22q11 involving often the heart. In numerical aberrations except

Down's syndrome, the other anomalies have many extracardiac signs leading to an invasive procedure independent from the heart finding.

Structural heart anomaly

Atrioventricular septal defect (AVSD) (Figure 80.1) is the most common heart anomaly associated with a chromosomal aberration, mainly trisomy 21 and 18. The diagnosis can be achieved by detecting the gap in the crux of the heart (the combination of defects within the interventricular and interatrial septa). The association with trisomy 21 or 18 is between 50 and 80%; however, when in AVSD the left ventricle is small as in combination with aortic coarctation, the rate of aneuploidy is lower (10% or less) and if there are signs of isomerism (i.e. stomach on the right side) there is no association with chromosomal aberrations.

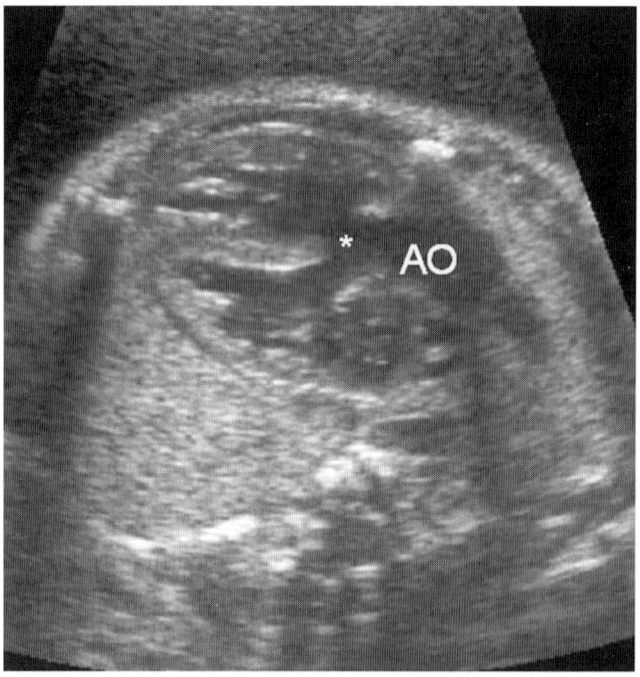

Figure 80.2 This is an overriding of the aorta over a VSD (*), which can be detected in the visualization of the five-chamber view. This is a sign and its differential diagnosis is listed in Table 80.4.

We proposed recently a new simple cardiac measurement the atrial to ventricular length (AVL) ratio,[11] in order to increase the detection rate for AVSD on routine scan. After a standardized four-chamber view, the ratio of the atrial length to the length of the ventricle in the midline is measured. Whereas the normal AVL-ratio during the second trimester is constant around 0.5, almost all fetuses with AVSD had a ratio exceeding 0.6.[11]

Other anomalies that are found in association with trisomy 21 are the ventricular septal defect (VSD) and the tetralogy of Fallot. Typical anomalies for trisomy 18 are besides the VSD and AVSD, the overriding of the aorta (Figure 80.2) with or without the pulmonary stenosis, a double-outlet right ventricle and occasionally a left outflow tract obstruction. Trisomy 13 cardiac anomalies are besides the VSD, left outflow tract obstructions such as aortic coarctation of the aorta and occasionally a hypoplastic left heart syndrome (HLHS). Turner syndrome has in almost all cases been detected prenatally, generally in combination with a cystic hygroma, also the left ventricular outflow tract obstruction, typically the aortic coarctation, and also occasionally the HLHS.

Cardiac soft markers

Intracardiac echogenic focus

The debate on this unspecific sign will not be discussed in this chapter. There are controversial data in the literature supporting the echogenic focus (EF) as a sign for Down's syndrome[10] as well as a benign sign with no relationship to chromosomal anomalies.

As most cases (around 90%) are found as isolated EF in the left ventricle (Figure 80.3), it is to be emphasized that EF in the right ventricle or two EF in the left

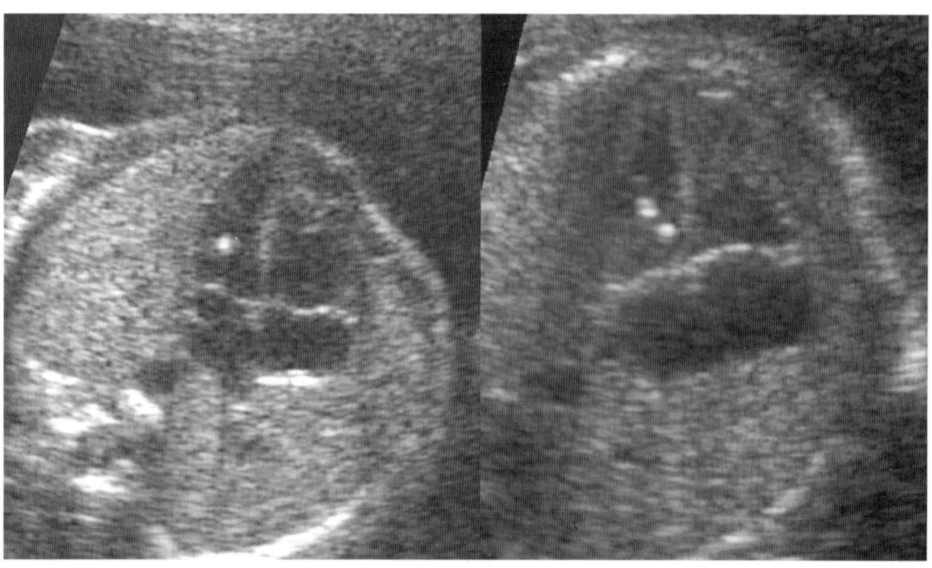

Figure 80.3 Two fetuses with echogenic foci. On the left the echogenic focus is present in the left ventricle and is the most common condition found. In the right figure two echogenic foci are present in the left ventricle. This fetus had a heart defect associated with a del.22q11.

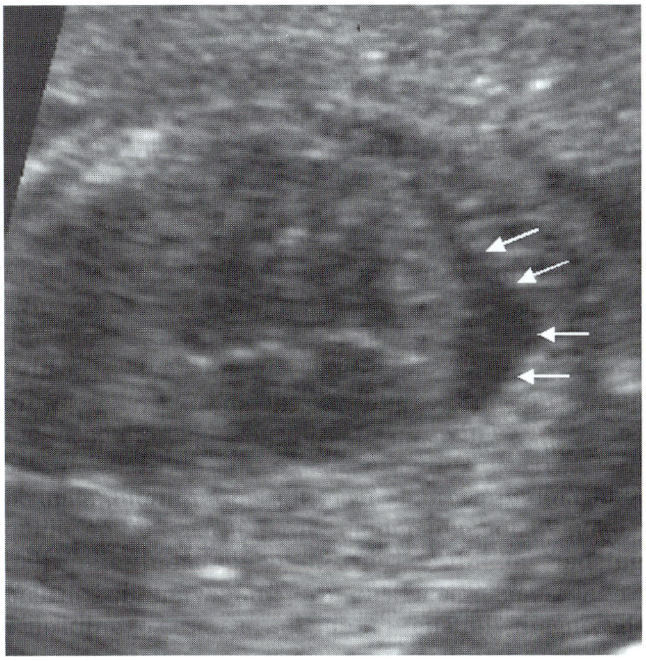

Figure 80.4 In this fetus with Down's syndrome there is a pericardial effusion at 20 weeks.

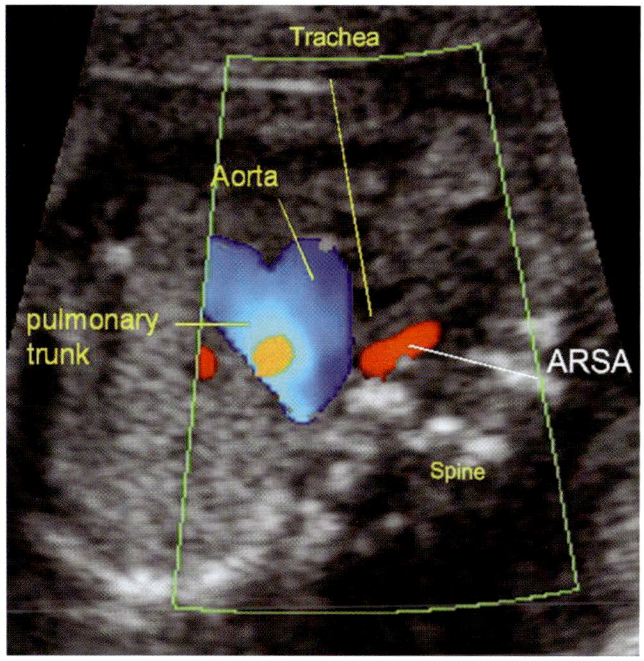

Figure 80.5 In this fetus with Down's syndrome at 20 weeks, an aberrant right subclavian artery (ARSA) is present. It is demonstrated in the three-vessel-tracheal view as a vessel with a course behind the trachea toward the right arm.

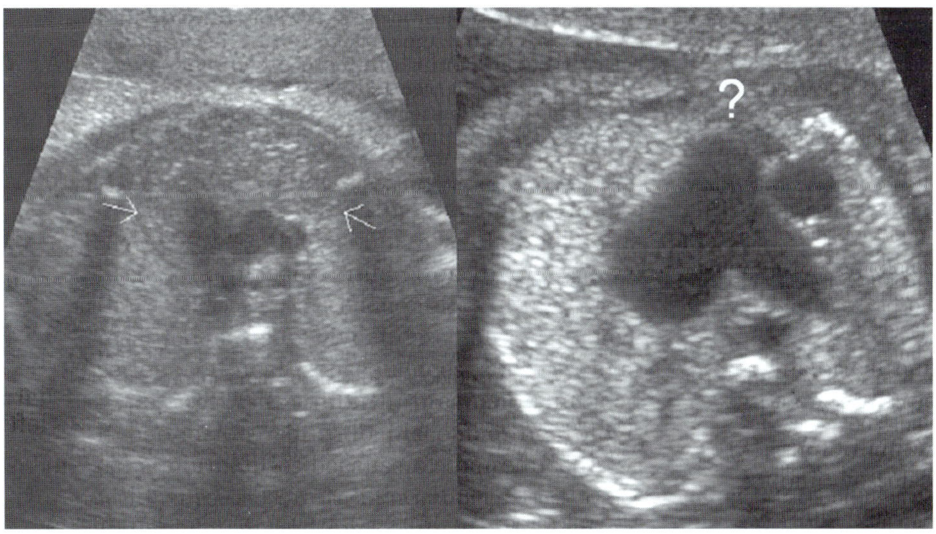

Figure 80.6 Thymus sign in predicting fetuses with del.22q11. In the left figure the thymus is recognized (arrows) as a slightly echogenic structure in front of the three-vessels and behind the sternum. In the right figure the fetus had an absent pulmonary valve syndrome with gross dilated pulmonary arteries. No thymus was visualized between the vessels and sternum (?) and FISH technique revealed the suspected del.22q11.

(Figure 80.3), right or both ventricles increase significantly the risk for chromosomal anomalies. The isolated EF in the left ventricle was accepted in the past year as increasing the background risk of a factor of 1.5 or even only 1. This led recently to a debate whether the findings of an EF should be told to younger women or not.[12,13]

In an observation of a series with CHD we found that 11% of all cardiac defects were associated with an EF,[14] some with malformations not detectable in the four-chamber plane such as the tetralogy of Fallot or a transposition of the great arteries (TGA). A total of 50% of all the cases were, however, not isolated left ventricular EF. Therefore, not only chromosomal anomalies but also cardiac defects should be ruled out in fetuses with a detected EF.

As the use of nuchal translucency (NT) in the risk assessment for chromosomal anomalies, the importance of second-trimester soft markers is reduced, especially the EF.

Discrepant LV/RV width

Devore[15] described an increased risk for trisomy 21 in early second-trimester fetuses with a narrow left ventricle compared with the right ventricle, without the additional signs of an aortic coarctation.

Tricuspid regurgitation

Isolated tricuspid regurgitation detected by the routine use of color Doppler is present in ca. 4% of all normal fetuses at the 20–22-week scan.[16] Tricuspid regurgitation was, however, also discussed as associated with Down's syndrome when detected at 16–18 weeks[15] or at the 11–14-week scan.[17]

Pericardial effusion

An isolated pericardial effusion was described to increase the risk of association with Down's syndrome (Figure 80.4).[18] It is not known whether in these cases, the effusion is the remaining of early hydrops with a thickened NT in early pregnancy. This sign was unfortunately not evaluated in recent years in the age of NT measurement.

Linear insertion of the AV valves

This is an interesting new sign presented by a French group a few years ago. Fredouille *et al.*[19] found on autopsy specimens of hearts from fetuses with Down's syndrome that in some cases, even with the absence of structural heart anomalies both atrioventricular valves (AV valves) inserted at the same level and not the tricuspid valve inserting lower in the right ventricle as under normal conditions. This is a very subtle and interesting sign, used also in the detection of AV-septal defect, but it should be evaluated by other groups.

Aberrant right subclavian artery (ARSA): the new cardiac sign for Down's syndrome

The normal right subclavian artery arises as a first vessel from the brachiocephalic artery and courses ventral of the trachea. An aberrant right subclavian artery (ARSA) arises separately from the aortic arch in the region of the junction of the aortic arch and the ductus arteriosus. It courses to the right arm behind the trachea and is thus detectable with color Doppler in the three-vessels-trachea view[20] (Figure 80.5).

In a few pediatric cardiology studies it was described that an ARSA (also called lusorian artery) is found in 1% of the normal population but is as high as 35% in persons with Down's syndrome with or without heart defects.

We were the first to describe this sign in fetuses with Down's syndrome in a paper published recently,[20] where we found that 5/14 (36%) of consecutive fetuses with Down's syndrome had this aberrant vessel, which we detected prenatally. Only one had it as an isolated sign, three in association with an EF in addition to extracardiac signs, and in only one case was it associated with an AVSD.

Personal experience and communication from pathologists support the fact that this sign is also common in trisomy 13, 18 and recent reports emphasized the occurrence in Turner syndrome and in microdeletion 22q11.

Further observations from other groups are necessary to confirm our new finding.

Cardiac signs for microdeletion 22q11

The del.22q11 is reported to have a frequency of 1:4000 livebirths and is considered to be after trisomy 21 the second most common chromosomal anomaly in liveborn children with a CHD. The earlier used and now abandoned acronym CATCH-22 summarizes the combination of finding in these patients: C = cardiac anomaly, A = abnormal facies, T = thymus hypo or aplasia, C = cleft palate, H = hypercalcemia and 22 for del.22q11. Prenatally, the clinical features of an abnormal facies are generally very subtle and we can mainly rely on the heart anomaly and, as we showed a few years ago, also on the thymus sign.

Among the heart anomalies, conotruncal and aortic arch malformations are the leading defects permitting a concrete suspicion of a del.22q11. The occurrence of this deletion is present in ca. 50% of all cases with interrupted aortic arch, 40% of absent pulmonary valve syndrome, 30% of Truncus arteriosus communis, 20% of pulmonary atresia with VSD, 15% with tetralogy of Fallot, and in around 5% in other anomalies such as complex transpositions, double-outlet right ventricle and others.[21]

A few years ago we examined a group of 147 fetuses with CHD, including 76 with conotruncal defects. In this study we examined the role of analyzing the absence or hypoplasia of the thymus in predicting a del.22q11. Ten of the 147 cases had a del.22q11, all being in the group with conotruncal anomaly. Nine of the 10 fetuses with microdeletion had an abnormal thymus detected prenatally (sensitivity 90%, specificity 98.5%). In our experience the examination of the thymus region helps in defining a group at high risk for del.22q11[21] (Figure 80.6).

According to other studies additional signs were described to increase the risk of 22q11 (in predefined high-risk groups) and some of these are increased NT in early pregnancy, intrauterine growth retardation, polyhydramnios, renal or facial abnormality, right aortic arch, aberrant right subclavian artery, aberrant pulmonary artery, etc.[22,23]

REFERENCES

1. Chaoui R. Fetal echocardiography: State of the art of the state of the heart. *Ultrasound Obstet Gynecol* 2001;17:277–84.
2. Sharland GK, Allan LD. Normal fetal cardiac measurements derived by cross-sectional echocardiography. *Ultrasound Obstet Gynecol* 1992;2:175–81.
3. Chaoui R, Heling KS, Bollmann R. Ultrasound measurements of the fetal heart in the 4-chamber image plane. *Geburtsh Frauenheilk* 1994;54:92–7.
4. Chaoui R, McEwing R. Three cross-sectional planes for fetal color Doppler echocardiography. *Ultrasound Obstet Gynecol* 2003;21:81–93.

5. Chaoui R, Kalache KD, Hartung J. Application of three-dimensional power Doppler ultrasound in prenatal diagnosis. *Ultrasound Obstet Gynecol* 2001;17:22–9.
6. Devore GR, Falkensammer P, Sklansky MS, Platt LD. Spatio-temporal image correlation (STIC): New technology for evaluation of the fetal heart. *Ultrasound Obstet Gynecol* 2003;22:380–7.
7. Chaoui R, Hoffmann J, Heling KS. Three-dimensional (3D) and 4D color Doppler fetal echocardiography using spatio-temporal image correlation (STIC). *Ultrasound Obstet Gynecol* 2004;23: 535–45.
8. Chaoui R. The four-chamber-view: four reasons why it seems to fail in screening for cardiac abnormalities and suggestions to improve detection rate. *Ultrasound Obstet Gynecol* 2003;22:3–10.
9. Chaoui R. The examination of the normal fetal heart using two-dimensional echocardiography. In Yagel S, Silvermann N, Gembruch U, eds. London: Martin Dunitz, *Fetal Cardiology* 2003: 141–9.
10. Bromley B, Lieberman E, Shipp TD, Benacerraf BR. The genetic sonogram – A method of risk assessment for Down syndrome in the second trimester. *J Ultrasound Med* 2002;21:1087–96.
11. Machlitt A, Heling KS, Chaoui R. Increased cardiac atrial-to-ventricular length ratio in the fetal four-chamber view: A new marker for atrioventricular septal defects. *Ultrasound Obstet Gynecol* 2004 24:618–22.
12. Filly RA, Benacerraf BR, Nyberg DA, Hobbins JC. Choroid plexus cyst and echogenic intracardiac focus in women at low risk for chromosomal anomalies. *J Ultrasound Med* 2004;23:447–9.
13. Doubilet PM, Copel JA, Benson CB, Bahado-Singh RO, Platt LD. Choroid plexus cyst and echogenic intracardiac focus in women at low risk for chromosomal anomalies: The obligation to inform the mother. *J Ultrasound Med* 2004l;23:883–5.
14. Chaoui R, Bierlich A. Intracardiac echogenic focus and fetal heart defects (abstract). *Ultrasound Obstet Gynecol* 2000;16:13–4.
15. Devore GR. The role of fetal echocardiography in genetic sonography. *Semin Perinatol* 2003;27:160–72.
16. Respondek ML, Kammermeier M, Ludomirsky A, Weil SR, Huhta JC. The prevalence and clinical significance of fetal tricuspid valve regurgitation with normal heart anatomy. *Am J Obstet Gynecol* 1994;171:1265–70.
17. Huggon IC, DeFigueiredo DB, Allan LD. Tricuspid regurgitation in the diagnosis of chromosomal anomalies in the fetus at 11–14 weeks of gestation. *Heart* 2003;89:1071–3.
18. Sharland G, Lockhart S. Isolated pericardial effusion: An indication for fetal karyotyping? *Ultrasound Obstet Gynecol* 1995;6:29–32.
19. Fredouille C, Piercecchi-Marti MD, Liprandi A, *et al.* Linear insertion of atrioventricular valves without septal defect: A new anatomical landmark for Down's syndrome? *Fetal Diagn Ther* 2002;17:188–92.
20. Chaoui R, Heling KS, Sarioglu N, Schwabe M, Dankof A, Bollmann R. Aberrant right subclavian artery (lusorian artery) as a new cardiac sign in second and third trimester fetuses with Down syndrome. *Am J Obstet Gynecol* 2005;192:257–63.
21. Chaoui R, Kalache KD, Heling KS, Tennstedt C, Bommer C, Korner H. Absent or hypoplastic thymus on ultrasound: A marker for deletion 22q11.2 in fetal cardiac defects. *Ultrasound Obstet Gynecol* 2002;20:546–52.
22. Boudjemline Y, Fermont L, Le Bidois J, Lyonnet S, Sidi D, Bonnet D. Prevalence of 22q11 deletion in fetuses with conotruncal cardiac defects: A 6-year prospective study. *J Pediatr* 2001;138:520–4.
23. Volpe P, Marasini M, Caruso G, *et al.* 22q11 deletions in fetuses with malformations of the outflow tracts or interruption of the aortic arch: impact of additional ultrasound signs. *Prenat Diagn* 2003; 23:752–7.

81 Ultrasound screening of chromosomal abnormalities by nuchal translucency

M. A. Zoppi and G. Monni

Introduction

Nuchal translucency (NT) is the term that has been used for 10 years to describe the echo-free space behind the fetal neck visible by ultrasound in almost all fetuses at 10–14 weeks[1] (Figure 81.1). Before this gestational age the NT is not clearly evident in all cases and after 14 weeks the NT reduces, becoming less transonic and turning into the nuchal fold space visible in the second trimester.

The NT is in fact the ultrasound image of some soft tissues that cover the occipital bone and cervical spine (muscles, connective tissue, lymphatic vessels, subcutaneous tissues and cutis).

In physiological condition these tissues can accumulate more or less fluids and as a result the thickness of the NT is expected to differ among normal fetuses.

Moreover, during the 11–14-week period, the thickness of the NT increases with the crown–rump length (CRL) and with the age of the fetus. Tables of reference for NT thickness in normal fetuses have been generated by cross-sectional studies. Some studies have calculated the ranges by using linear regression formula; however, the quadratic regression approach seems to better fit the trend of nuchal thickness.[2–5]

Other studies have shown that longitudinal assessments of NT in the same fetus showed a tendency toward increase of the thickness to a peak that is reached individually and differently by each fetus, mostly around 12 weeks, followed by a decrease.[6]

It is evident that due to local contingent conditions (operators, machines, approach to the ultrasound technique and ethnicity), there are subtle differences among different centers that perform the measurement of the NT. Therefore, it has been suggested that local reference ranges for normal NT be preferred to assess the thickness whenever it is possible.[7]

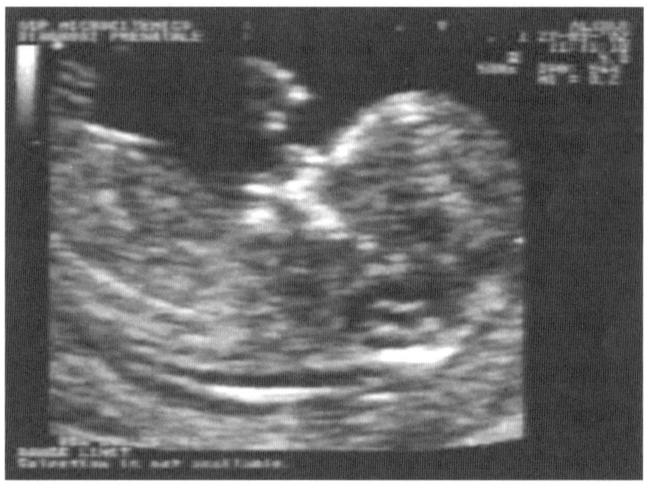

Figure 81.1 Nuchal translucency.

At 10 weeks, essentially, the NT thickness in normal fetuses most frequently measures around 1–1.2 mm, and at 13–14 weeks, around 1.7–1.9 mm.

The visualization and measurement of the NT is not included among the main identified objectives of first-trimester ultrasound as recommended in most guidelines issued by ultrasound scientific societies. Ascertaining the presence of the gestational sac in the uterine cavity, the number of fetuses, the embryonic or fetal heartbeat and the duration of pregnancy is usually done in the first-trimester scan.[8–10]

Therefore, during the first-trimester ultrasound examination, only if it is specifically requested is a normal NT visualized and measured. Because of the implications that the measurement of the NT can carry for the pregnancy (reducing or increasing the risk of chromosomal abnormalities, opening a scenario for invasive prenatal diagnosis), it is advisable to perform the measurement only in the correct setting (by a skilled operator and in a certified screening program, after a request for screening by the informed patient).[11]

The enlarged nuchal translucency

Sometimes there can be a surplus accumulation of fluid in the nuchal tissues (Figure 81.2). The accumulation of nuchal fluid can be caused by either an increased amount of fluid directed in the nuchal region or some difficulty in the drainage of the normal quantity of fluid present in the neck.

Regardless of the underlying cause of the accumulation of fluids, what is apparent on the ultrasound is the increased thickness of the echo-free space behind the fetal neck, which has been labeled 'enlarged NT'.[12] This space can be absolutely transonic or faintly echogenic, and can be limited to the neck or extended the whole length of the fetus as a 'space suit'[13] (Figure 81.3).

When the NT is very enlarged at 10–14 weeks, it can easily be visualized during the scan without especially looking for it. This is a situation comparable with that which occurs with some soft markers for chromosomopathies in the second trimester (hyperechogenic focus, hyperechogenic bowel, dilated renal pelvis, etc.),[14] when these signs are evident, without our having to look for them. Although these signs are not malformations, and they can be visible during an ultrasound examination, which does not have the finality of chromosomopathy screening, the guidelines of some scientific societies that have faced this problem recommend disclosing the presence of evident soft markers to the patient, in order to offer the opportunity for adequate genetic counseling.[8]

It has been noticed since the early 1990s that fetuses with trisomy 21 can show an enlarged NT at first-trimester examination[15] (Figure 81.4).

When an ultrasound scan is performed with the specific intention of measuring the NT, it is essential to correctly visualize the fetus and to perform the NT measurement in an adequate way in order to compare the actual measurement with the reference values. The range of NT thickness varies with CRL, so that the 95th percentile for a CRL of 45 mm is quite different from that for a CRL of 82 mm, and it is evident that a fixed cutoff for NT measurement cannot be used efficiently to assess the enlargement of an NT.[16]

It has been noted that the majority of fetuses with trisomy 21 show an NT greater than the 95th percentile of ranges obtained for normal fetuses with a standard technique of NT measurement. Fetuses with chromosomal abnormalities other than trisomy 21 (trisomy 18, trisomy 13, Turner syndrome, Klinefelter syndrome and triploidy) can have an enlarged NT[16] (Figures 81.5–81.7).

In fetuses with normal and abnormal chromosomes the enlarged NT is frequently a transient sign. In an early study of trisomies 21, at the beginning of the second trimester, a reabsorption of the nuchal edema

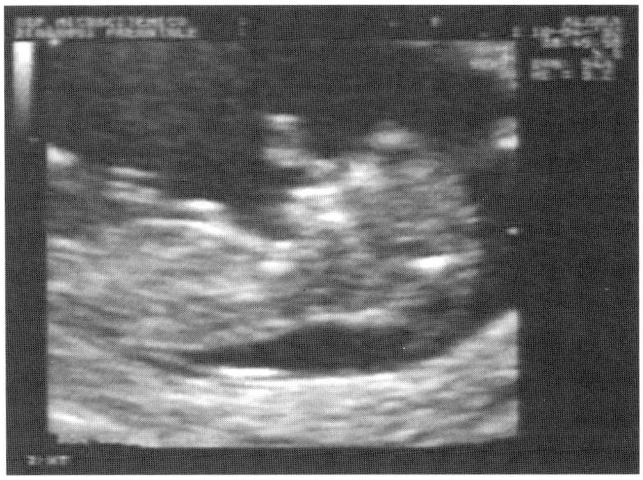

Figure 81.2 Enlarged NT.

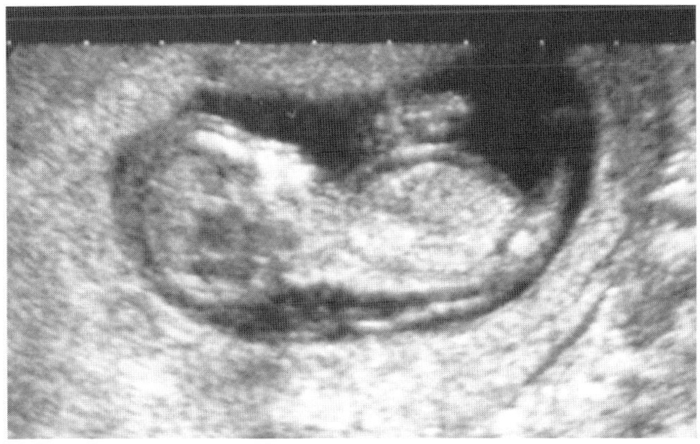

Figure 81.3 'Space suit' nuchal translucency

has been longitudinally described in six cases.[17] A study of the evolution of enlarged NT during the first trimester described a decrease in the thickness that occurred in both chromosomally normal and abnormal fetuses. In the second measurement performed in the same fetus, the frequency of decreasing NT was greater in the normal than in the abnormal karyotype fetuses.[18]

In fetuses with Turner syndrome the evolution of first-trimester enlarged NT is frequently described as a cystic hygroma (cystic malformation of the lymphatic system) in the second trimester[19] (Figure 81.8).

Pathophysiology of enlarged NT

The term 'enlarged NT in the first trimester' that is used in ultrasound practice may indicate many different background conditions.

An accumulation of fluids in the neck is presumed to come from either an abnormal local composition of the tissues that tend to capture more fluids or a situation of hampered reabsorption of a normal quantity of fluids regularly passed from the vessel to the

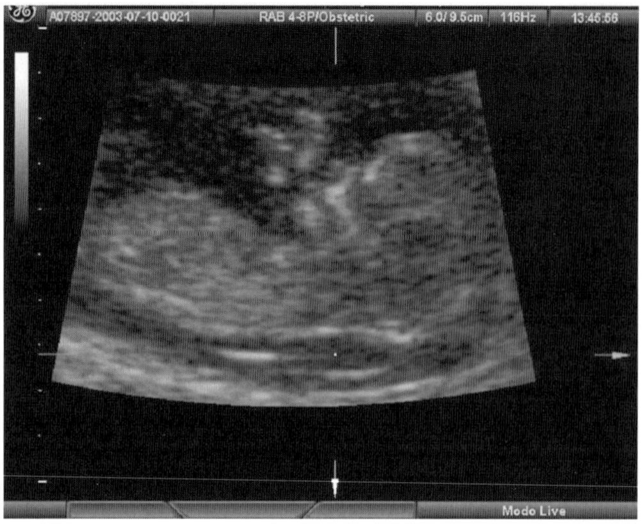

Figure 81.4 Trisomy 21 fetus with enlarged nuchal translucency.

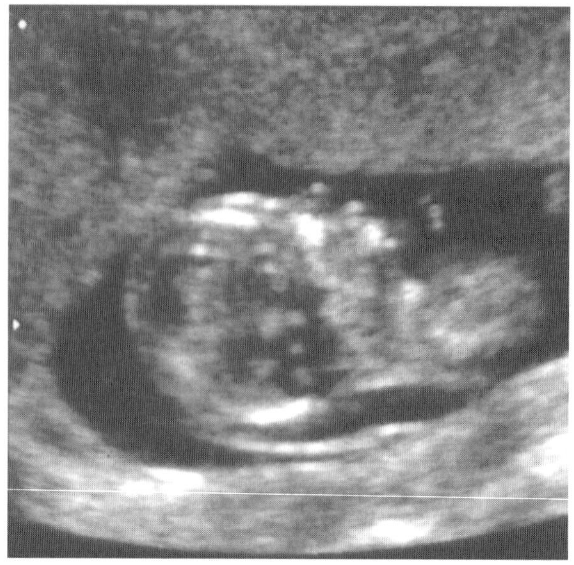

Figure 81.6 Trisomy 13 with enlarged NT.

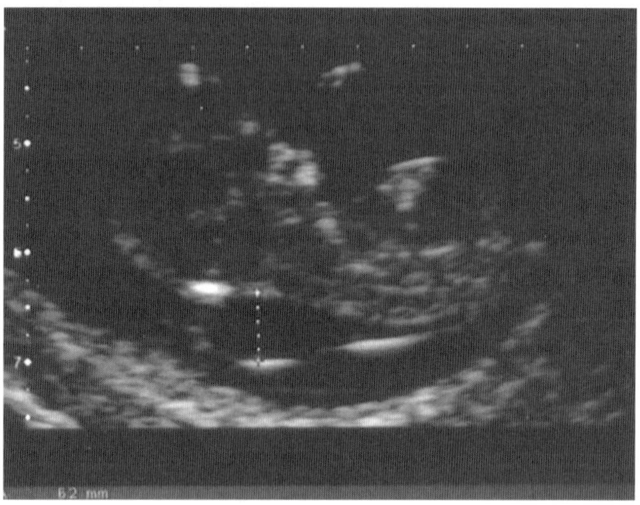

Figure 81.5 Trisomy 18 with enlarged NT.

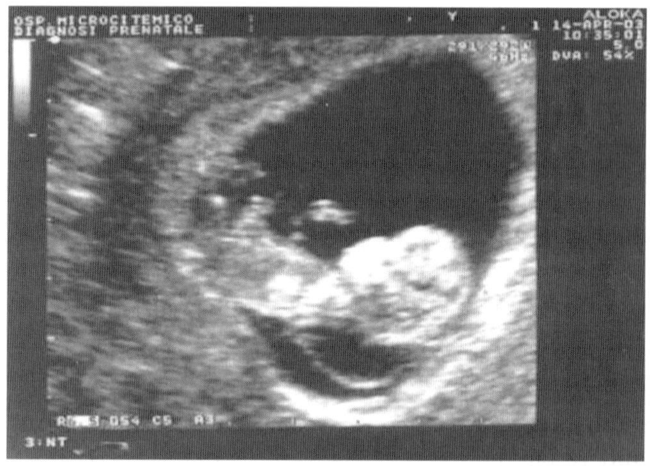

Figure 81.7 Turner syndrome with enlarged NT.

interstitial spaces, or from a condition of increased passage of fluids from the vessel to the connective, due to an abnormal hydrostatic pressure as a consequence of impairment of the arterial or venous circulation.[20–26]

In trisomy 21, some alteration in the composition of the skin, with an increased expression of type VI collagen and a rise in the quantity of hyaluronic acid, could justify an increased entrapment of liquids that for reasons not yet explained, in the first-trimester fetus, is evident only in the nuchal region.[23,24] An extra accumulation of fluid that exceeds the normal capacity of the mechanism deputed for drainage may be the cause of enlarged NT in trisomy 21 fetuses.[26]

In Turner syndrome, the accumulation of fluid in the nuchal region seems to be related to a failure in the drainage by the lymphatic system, because of an abnormal structure that involves the minor lymphatic vessels in the skin, and the greater vessel, with a lack

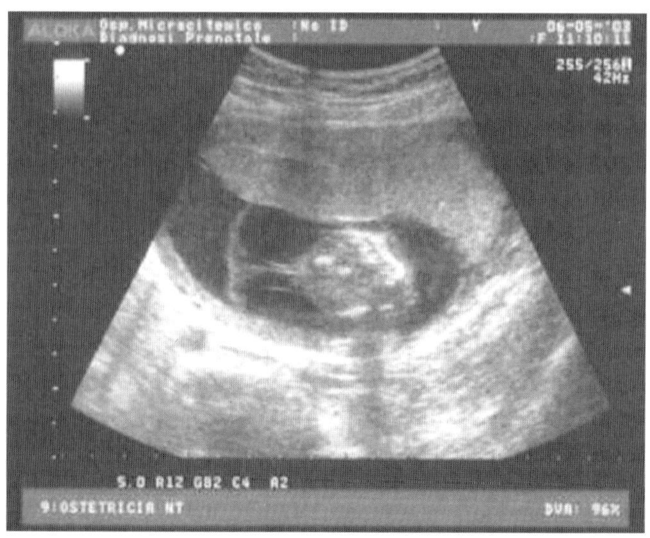

Figure 81.8 Turner syndrome fetus at 16 weeks.

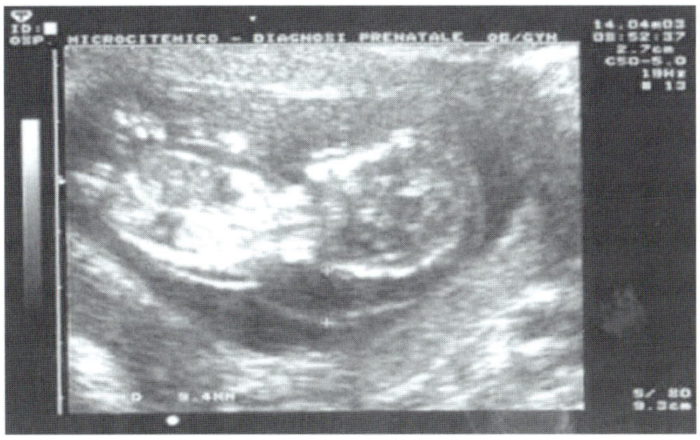

Figure 81.9 Turner syndrome fetus at 12 weeks.

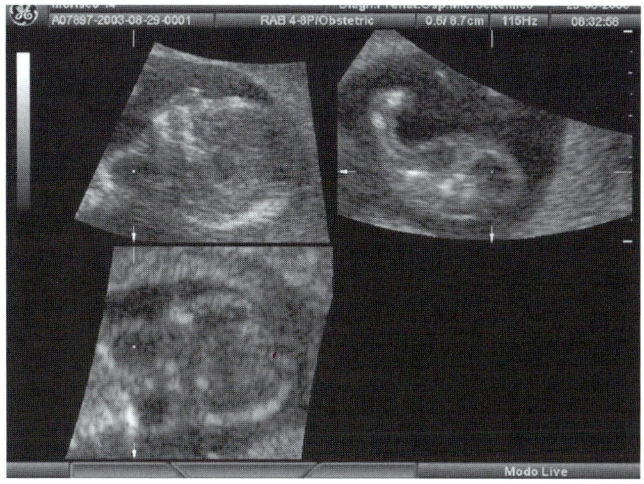

Figure 81.10 Multiplanar view of a trisomy 21 fetus with enlarged jugular lymphatic sacs.

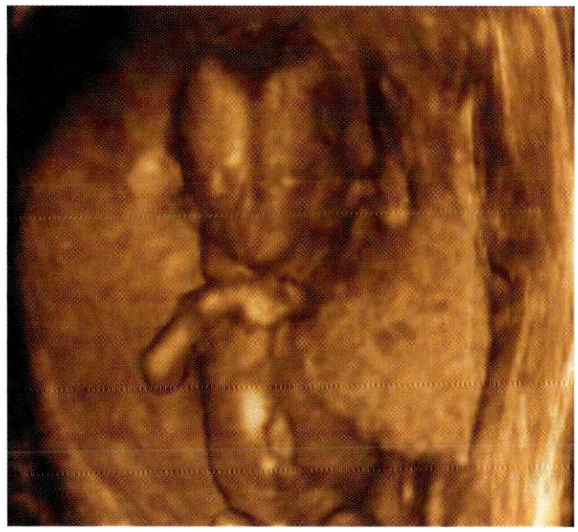

Figure 81.11 Three-dimensional surface rendering of a trisomy 21 fetus with enlarged jugular lymphatic sacs.

of definitive connections between the jugular lymphatic sacs and jugular veins system, as an expression of a failure in the development of the lymphatic system, due to the underlying karyotype anomaly[22,26] (Figure 81.9). In fetuses with Turner syndrome, the first-trimester translucencies are typically large, bilateral and septated, occupying the lateral and posterior regions of the neck of the fetus. In Turner syndrome, the first-trimester NT is in fact often not transient, with a tendency to evolve into a second-trimester 'cystic hygroma colli'.[26]

A different mechanism related to a temporary lymphatic failure due to a delay in the connection with the venous system has been considered in trisomy 21 and normal fetuses. In these cases, the evolution toward a reabsorption in the second trimester is frequent.[26]

Pathological studies carried out on fetuses with enlarged NT with normal karyotype and trisomies 21 and 18 have in fact shown in the posterior side of the neck of the fetus, exactly where the NT is visualized by ultrasound, the presence of some cavities, negative for immunohistochemical markers for lymphatic vessel endothelium and arteries. These cavities seem to be the result of coalescence of edematous mesenchymal spaces (due to an edematous mesenchymal). In these cases, a lymphatic distension of jugular lymphatic sacs in the lateral side of the neck has been shown to occur prior to the manifestation of the nuchal edema (Figures 81.10 and 81.11). The hypothesis was that the first occurrence would be the delay in the lymphatic drainage, which may then cause the accumulation of mesenchymal fluid and nuchal edema. At 14 weeks, when the jugular lymphatic sacs are fully developed, making definitive connections with the venous system, both nuchal edema and dilatation of lymphatic sacs finally resolve.[26–27]

In trisomy 21 another mechanism has been postulated to cause the accumulation of fluids and enlargement of the NT, due to an increase of the perfusion of the vessel directly to the neck and the upper part of the fetus. In pathology studies, a narrowing of the isthmus of the aorta, associated with a dilatation of the supravalvular portion of the vessel, has been described. An increased passage of fluids into the connective tissue due to an increase in hydrostatic pressure could be involved in the enlargement of the NT.[28]

An accumulation of extravascular liquids, as it is present in adults with an impairment of cardiac function, can also be present in fetuses with chromosomal abnormalities or normal karyotype fetuses with structural heart abnormality. The subcutaneous edema depends on an impaired reabsorption of fluids due to an increase of the hydrostatic pressure in the venous system. A wide spectrum of heart defects has been described to be present in fetuses with chromosomal abnormalities and normal fetuses with enlarged NT, but a clear connection between specific cardiac diseases and the development of the enlarged NT in the

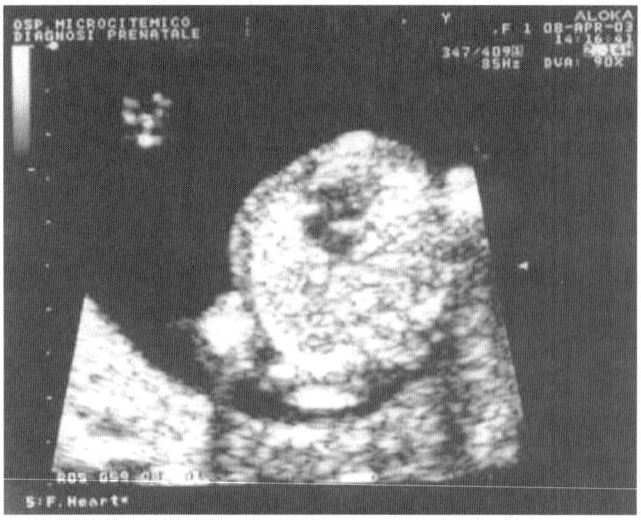

Figure 81.12 Heart defect in a first-trimester fetus with normal karyotype and enlarged NT.

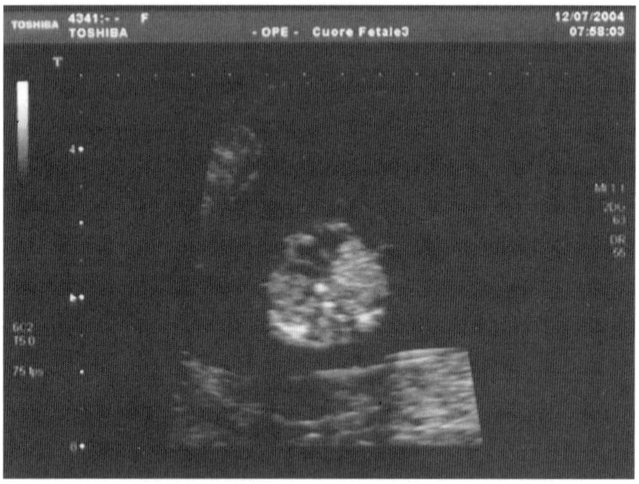

Figure 81.13 Heart defect in a first-trimester fetus with trisomy 21 and enlarged NT.

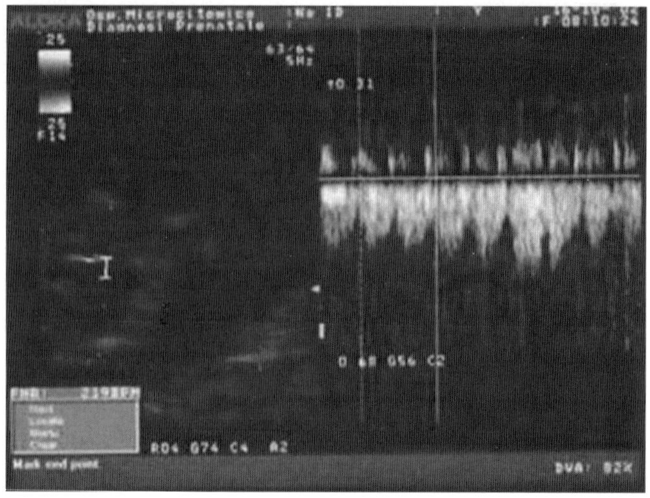

Figure 81.14 First-trimester tachycardia in a first-trimester fetus with normal karyotype and enlarged NT.

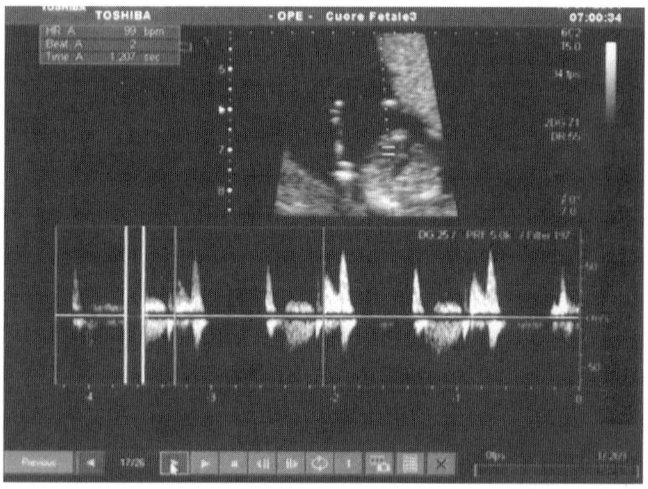

Figure 81.15 First-trimester second-degree heart block in a normal karyotype fetus with enlarged NT.

first trimester of pregnancy has not been demonstrated[28,29] (Figures 81.12–81.15).

A relationship between an impaired diastolic function and enlarged NT has been hypothesized on the grounds of some alteration signs on the velocimetry of the ductus venosus in fetuses with abnormal karyotype, cardiac defects and NT thickness.[30–31] The ductus venosus is a vessel that connects the umbilical circulation with the right atrium. In the first trimester of pregnancy the pulsed Doppler waveform of this vessel is characterized by a forward flow with a peak during systole, a second peak in diastole and a forward velocity during atrial contraction (Figure 81.16). In cases where the pressure in the atrium at the end of the diastolic phase is increased (which could be a sign of cardiac dysfunction due to several factors, including some structural malformations of the heart), the velocity during the atrial contraction in the ductus venosus decreases: it can be zero or reversed (Figure 81.17–81.18). In fetuses with chromosomal abnormalities that are suspected to have a greater occurrence of cardiac abnormalities and that show frequently an enlarged NT, the velocimetry of the ductus venosus is frequently altered (70–90%), with an absent or reversed atrial contraction velocity.

Another parameter that has been used to evaluate the alteration of the velocimetry in the ductus venosus is the pulsatility of the wave form, which in chromosomal abnormalities appears increased.[32] If there is a single cause that determines at the same time two parallel consequences such as the altered ductus venosus flow and the enlarged nuchal thickness, or if there is a consequential connection between the two findings, which of these findings occurs first needs to be demonstrated.

An impairment in the diastolic function has been shown in fetuses with enlarged NT in the first

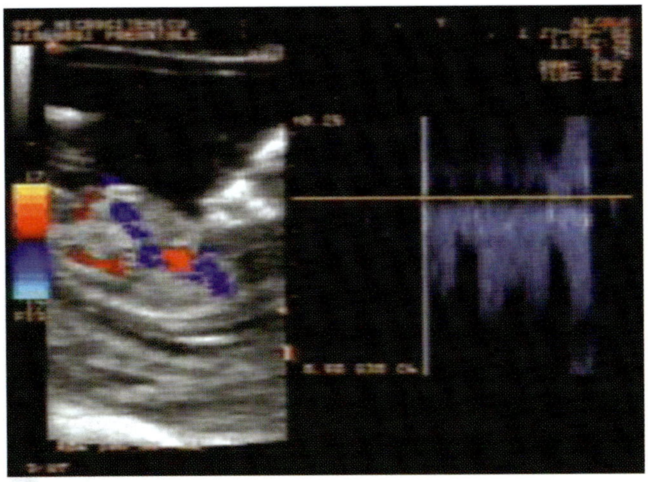

Figure 81.16 Normal velocity flow in the ductus venosus in a first-trimester fetus.

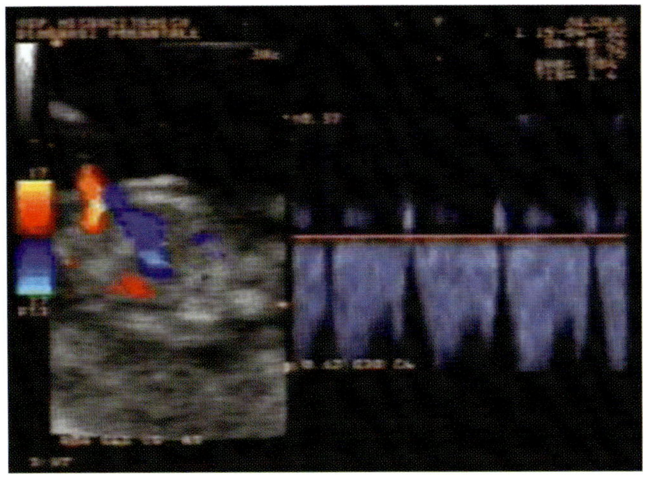

Figure 81.18 Reversed velocity during atrial contraction in the ductus venosus.

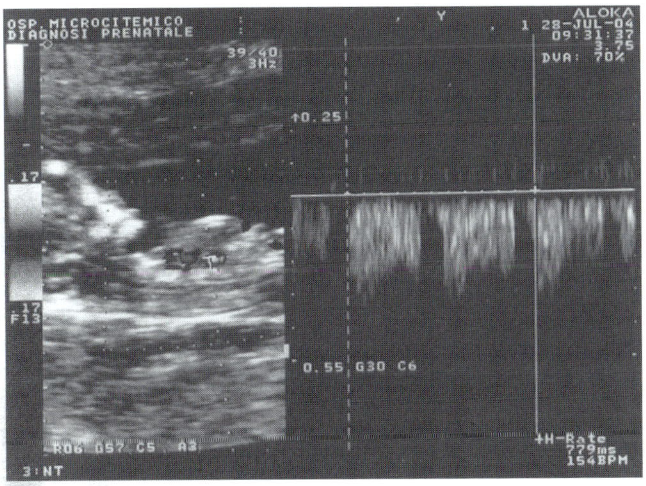

Figure 81.17 Absent velocity during atrial contraction in the ductus venosus.

trimester and normal karyotype, which persists in the second trimester, and this is demonstrated by an alteration of the velocimetry of the atrium-ventricular valves.[33]

In fetuses with enlarged NT, no impairment in the ventricular systolic function has been described. In fact, no difference of umbilical pulsatility index in the first trimester has been shown in normal karyotype fetuses with normal and enlarged NT and in trisomy 21 fetuses with enlarged NT.[34]

A mechanism of increased hydrostatic pressure in the thorax has been postulated to be involved in cases of first-trimester enlarged NT and venous congestion as in cases of diaphragmatic hernia and skeletal dysplasias.[21]

Enlarged NT for trisomy 21 screening

Amniocentesis and chorionic villus sampling (CVS) are invasive prenatal diagnosis techniques for fetal karyotype analysis, which carry a procedure-related risk of abortion of about 1%. Since the introduction of invasive prenatal diagnosis, karyotype analysis has been offered only to high-risk cases due to medical and financial reasons, and the maternal age-related risk of Down's syndrome was the older and most commonly used approach to prenatal screening. The aim of the screening is to select those women who are at high enough risk of Down's syndrome to justify an invasive prenatal diagnosis procedure.[35]

In the last 20 years, prenatal ultrasound examination has been able to identify some of the malformations in trisomy 21 fetuses and other aneuploidies, and some of the anatomical features that differ slightly from those of normal fetuses. The ultrasound approach has been proposed for identification of cases at a higher risk.[14] In the mid-1980s the first finding of trisomy 21 that has been identified by ultrasound as a marker for trisomy 21 was the increased nuchal fold thickness in the second-trimester fetuses.[36] Later, in the mid-1990s, the association between first-trimester increased NT thickness and trisomy 21 and other chromosomal abnormalities was described.[1]

For NT, an algorithm for the calculation of individualized risk and a specific quality control for the test have been proposed since its introduction, while for serum markers for trisomy 21 this is a consolidated approach, for ultrasound in prenatal diagnosis was relatively new.[2]

Frequencies of trisomy 21 cases and normal fetuses were compared for the deviation of the measured NT from the normal expected values, in order to calculate likelihood ratios.[2] Two principal methods have been used to calculate the deviation from the normal: the Delta value and the multiple of the median (MoM).[2,37] The Delta value approach is considered to give some advantages.[38] Delta value in millimeters indicates the difference between the measured NT and the expected median of NT calculated for normal fetuses

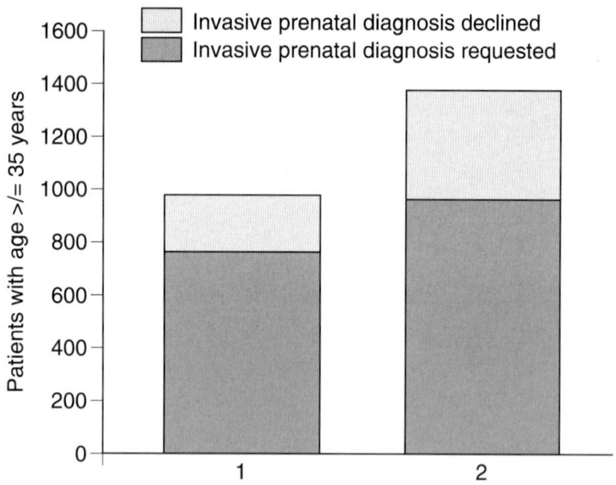

(1) In 1995 genetic counselling without NT screening
(2) In 1999 genetic counselling after NT screening in Cagliari center (44)

Figure 81.19 Acceptance of invasive prenatal diagnosis.

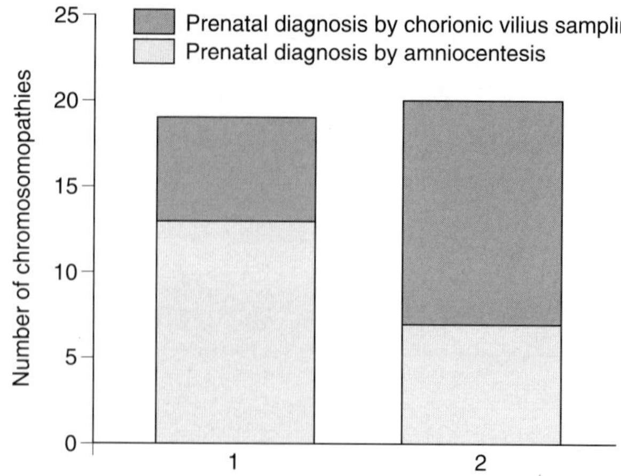

(1) In 1995 genetic counselling without NT screening
(2) In 1999 genetic counselling after NT screening in Cagliari center (44)

Figure 81.20 Procedure used for prenatal diagnosis of chromosomopathies.

for a given CRL. An estimate of the risk for trisomy 21 was calculated by multiplying the maternal age-related risk for trisomy 21 by the likelihood ratios obtained from the NT thickness, giving a new individual numerical risk.[16] The risk estimate for trisomy 21 based on the ultrasound measurement of NT is based on a few but important principles. First of all, the maternal background risk is the essential factor of the screening test for trisomy 21, and each time it needs to be considered in the calculation. Second, the results are not given as 'tested positive' or 'tested negative' on the ground of an arbitrarily chosen cutoff, but the patient is faced with a numerical result, on which she can base her decision according to her wishes and anxieties. Third, a quality control method is applied to ultrasound measurement (this is new for this field of medicine, although it has been used for decades, e.g. laboratory serum markers). There is evidence that the NT test is reliable, because the interoperator and intercenter variability can be reduced and comparable results are obtained, in cases where the measurement is performed according to a defined technique, with adequate training of operators and constant audit of the results.[39] Using this approach, in a multicentric study (22 centers involved), performed over 100,000 cases, with an average maternal age of 28 years, for a risk greater than or equal to 1 in 300, the sensitivity for trisomy 21 has been estimated to be 82%, with a false-positive rate of 8%.[40] With these performance results the NT test was considered to be the most effective prenatal screening to identify cases at risk of trisomy 21. Comparable results were obtained by other centers where guidelines for NT screening were observed.[5]

Fetuses at higher risk of trisomy 21 because of enlarged NT were at the same time found to be at higher risk of other chromosomopathies such as trisomies 18 and 13, triploidy and sex aneuploidies.[40]

Clinical importance of NT screening

The availability of an accurate screening test in the first trimester, such as NT, is useful to recognize cases at a higher risk of trisomy 21 at an early stage, in order to offer an early invasive prenatal diagnosis that could be performed preferably by CVS. It is true that when the performance of NT test is considered, the spontaneous intrauterine mortality of affected fetuses from the first trimester to term has to be taken into account. A number of those fetuses identified to be at high risk in the first trimester, and on which an invasive prenatal diagnosis procedure is performed, would be spontaneously demised in the uterus before birth, without all the trouble and anxiety that the prenatal screening procedure can carry. About 30% of trisomy 21 fetuses that are detected by first-trimester NT screening are destined to die during the pregnancy. This percentage is about 10% greater than the lethality of fetuses detected by a second-trimester screening test, which is about 20% to term.[41]

However, there is evidence that for pregnant women there are some aspects of prenatal screening that are of value. A test that gives the result early in pregnancy, and that obviously has at the same time a low rate of false negatives and false positives, with a reduced number of invasive procedures and fetal demises due to procedure-related risk, is considered to be better.[42,43] Enlarged first-trimester NT could identify, at the same time, fetuses at higher risk of abnormalities other than chromosomopathies. Cardiac defects, some structural abnormalities and genetic syndromes can occur more frequently in fetuses with enlarged NT than in the general population.[29]

Women at high risk of trisomy 21 because of advanced age can gain some advantage from having the NT test done. In fact, a more precise estimate of individual risk for trisomy 21 can be made, with the opportunity to decide about prenatal diagnosis with more autonomy. Reduction in requests for invasive prenatal diagnosis in women aged 35 years or over and earlier detection of cases at risk by first-trimester CVS are the chief advantages of the NT screening test over invasive prenatal diagnosis due to maternal age[44] (Figures 81.19 and 81.20).

NT screening can be used for screening of chromosomal abnormalities with the same accuracy in twin and multiple pregnancies.[45,46]

Recent developments in NT screening

At its introduction in clinical practice, it was proposed that the NT screening test be performed from 10 weeks 3 days (a CRL of 38 mm). With evidence that at around 12 weeks a better evaluation of fetal anatomy could in most cases be achieved, it was suggested that screening be performed after the CRL reaches 45 mm, so that at the same time, structural abnormalities can be detected early.[47]

In order to decrease the false negatives and the rate of invasive testing, the risk obtained by maternal age and NT has been combined with other markers, which occur more frequently in trisomy 21 cases than in normal fetuses, but are not related to the increase of the thickness of first-trimester NT. First-trimester maternal serum markers, pregnancy associated plasma protein-A (PAPR-A) and free beta human chorionic gonadotropin, combined with the NT test, increase the sensitivity to 90% and decrease the false-positive rate to about 3%.[48]

The combination of NT test with the sign of absent nasal bone in the first trimester is still under assessment.[49,50] The integration of the NT test with maternal screening markers of the first and second trimesters has been shown to improve the accuracy of the test, but it is necessary to wait until the second trimester to disclose the result and eventually to offer the diagnosis.[51]

With the possibility of combining and integrating different tests, a new scenario for prenatal screening for trisomy 21 is now emerging. Different tests can be performed at different times (one stop, two step, one step), the results can be disclosed after every single test or integrated, successive tests can be performed only in established cases, for example, only in borderline cases (contingent test), and each test could obtain different performances.[35] Some tests carry a greater sensitivity, others a greater specificity. There are many options to screen for trisomy 21, but the choice of the direction in which to move is delicate. If the screening test for trisomy 21 is performed on a financial basis, and the national health care system is the purchaser, it can offer a policy of screening that is more cost-effective after a rigorous cost–benefit analysis.

When a screening program concerns a disease for which the definitive diagnosis exposes a human being to a potential lethal risk, and, in case of ascertained disease, there is no cure as there is for trisomy 21 at prenatal diagnosis, many ethical problems come to light and they put doctors and patients in a great dilemma.

In this specific case of screening, the principle of self-determination for the patient, for decades applied to the field of invasive prenatal diagnosis, should be the fundamental issue of the entire process, and should be the goal to be achieved.[11] From the start, all the steps of the screening procedure should be accurately considered, leaving nothing to chance, such as, for example, the first apparently innocent question about how old she is, that everyone asks a completely unaware (about prenatal screening troubles) prospective mother.

REFERENCES

1. Nicolaides KH, Azar G, Byrne D, Mansur C, Marks K. Fetal nuchal translucency screening for chromosomal defects in first trimester of pregnancy. *Br Med J* 1992;304:867–9.
2. Pandya PP, Snijders RJM, Johnson SP, Brizot ML, Nicolaides KH. Screening for fetal trisomies by maternal age and fetal nuchal translucency thickness at 10 to 14 weeks of gestation. *Br J Obstet Gynaecol* 1995;102:957–62.
3. Snijders RJM, Nicolaides K. *Ultrasound markers for chromosomal defects*. London: Pathenon Publishing, 1996.
4. Braithwaite JM, Morris RW, Economides DL. Nuchal translucency measurements: Frequency distribution and changes with gestation in a general population. *Br J Obstet Gynaecol* 1996;103(12):1201–4.
5. Zoppi MA, Ibba RM, Floris M, Monni G. Fetal nuchal translucency screening in 12,495 pregnancies in Sardinia. *Ultrasound Obstet Gynecol* 2001;18:649–51.
6. Pajkrt E, De Graaf IM, Mol BWJ, van Lith JMM, Bleker OP, Bilardo CM. Weekly nuchal translucency measurements in normal fetuses. *Obstet Gynecol* 1998;91:208–11.
7. Logghe H, Cuckle H, Sehmi I. Centre-specific ultrasound nuchal translucency medians needed for Down syndrome screening. *Prenat Diagn* 2003;23:389–92.
8. SIEOG (Società Italiana Ecografia Ostetrica e Ginecologica). *Linee Guida*. Cento (FE), Italy: Editeam Publishing, 2002.
9. National Collaborating Centre for Women's and Children's Health. Antenatal Care Routine Care for the Healthy Pregnant Woman. Clinical Guideline. London: RCOG Press, 2003.
10. American Institute of Ultrasound in Medicine. *Practice Guidelines for the Performance of an Antepartum Obstetric Ultrasound Examination*. AIUM, 2003.
11. Chasen ST, Skupsi DW, McCullogh LB, Chervenak FA. Prenatal informed consent for sonogram: The time for first trimester nuchal translucency has come. *J Ultrasound Med* 2001;20:1147–52.
12. Nicolaides KH. *The 11–14 Weeks Scan*. London: Fetal Medicine Foundation, 2004.
13. Shulman LP, Phillips OP, Emerson DS, Felker RE, Tharapel AT. Fetal 'space-suit' hydrops in the first trimester: Differentiating risk for chromosome abnormalities by delineating characteristics of nuchal translucency. *Prenat Diagn* 2000;20(1):30–2.
14. Benacerraf BR. The second-trimester fetus with Down syndrome: Detection using sonographic features. *Ultrasound Obstet Gynecol* 1996;7:147–55.
15. Szabo J, Gellen J. Nuchal fluid accumulation in trisomy-21 detected by vaginosonography in first trimester. *Lancet* 1990; 336(8723):1133.
16. Nicolaides KH, Subire NJ, Snijders RJM, Souka AP. *The 11–14 Week's Scan Book*. London: Pathenon Publishing, 2001.
17. Pandya PP, Snijders RJM, Johnson S, Nicolaides K. Natural history of trisomy 21 fetuses with increased nuchal translucency thickness. *Ultrasound Obstet Gynecol* 1995;5:381–83.
18. Zoppi MA, Ibba RM, Floris M, Axiana C, Manca F, Monni G. Changes in nuchal translucency thickness in normal and abnormal karyotype fetuses. *Br J Obstet Gynaecol* 2003;110:584–8.

19. Fukada Y, Yasumizu T, Takizawa M, Amemiya A, Hoshi K. The prognosis of fetuses with transient nuchal translucency in the first and early second trimester. *Acta Obstet Gynecol Scand* 1997;76:913–16.
20. Moscoso G. Fetal nuchal translucency: A need to understand the physiological basis. *Ultrasound Obstet Gynecol* 1995;5:6–8.
21. Von Kaisenberg CS, Brand-Saberi B, Jonat W, Nicolaides KH. Pathophysiology of increased nuchal translucency in chromosomally abnormal fetuses. *Prenat Neonat Med* 1999;4:431–40.
22. von Kaisenberg CS, Krenn V, Ludwig M, Nicolaides KH, Brand Saberi B. Morphological classification of nuchal skin in human fetuses with trisomy 21, 18, and 13 at 12–18 weeks and in a trisomy 16 mouse. *Anat Embryol* 1998;197:105–24.
23. von Kaisenberg CS, Brand-Saberi B, Christ B, Vallian S, Farzaneh F, Nicolaides KH. Collagen type VI gene expression in the skin of trisomy 21 fetuses. *Obstet Gynecol* 1998;91:319–23.
24. Bohlandt S, von Kaisenberg CS, Wewetzler K, Christ B, Nicolaides KH, Brand-Saberi B. Hyaluronan in the nuchal skin of chromosomally abnormal fetuses. *Hum Reprod* 2000;15:1155–8.
25. Haak MC, van Vugt JMG. Pathophysiology of increased nuchal translucency: A review of the literature. *Hum Reprod Update* 2003;2:175–84.
26. Haak MC, Bartelings MM, Jackson DG, Webb S, van Vugt JM, Gittenberger-de Groot AC. Increased nuchal translucency is associated with jugular lymphatic distension. *Hum Reprod* 2002; 17:1086–92.
27. Castelli E, Todros T, Mattutino G, Torre C, Panattoni G. Light and scanning electron microscope study of nuchal translucency in a normal fetus. *Ultrasound Obstet Gynecol.* 2003;21:514–6.
28. Hyett J, Moscoso G, Nicolaides K. Abnormalities of the heart and great arteries in first trimester chromosomally abnormal fetuses. *Am J Med Genet* 1997;17:207–16.
29. Hyett J, Perdu M, Sharland G, Snijders R, Nicolaides KH. Using fetal nuchal translucency to screen for major congenital cardiac defects at 10–14 weeks of gestation: Population based cohort study. *BMJ* 1999;318:70–1.
30. Matias A, Montenegro N. Ductus venosus blood flow in chromosomally abnormal fetuses at 11–14 weeks of gestation. *Semin Perinatol* 2001;25:32–7.
31. Zoppi MA, Putzolu M, Ibba RM, Floris M, Monni G. First trimester ductus venosus velocimetry in relation to nuchal translucency thickness and fetal karyotype. *Fetal Diagn Ther* 2002;17:52–7.
32. Antolin E, Comas C, Torrents M, *et al.* The role of ductus venosus blood flow assessment in screening for chromosomal abnormalities at 10–16 weeks of gestation. *Ultrasound Obstet Gynecol* 2001;17:295–300.
33. Rizzo G, Muscatello A, Angelini E, Capponi A. Abnormal cardiac function in fetuses with increased nuchal translucency. *Ultrasound Obstet Gynecol* 2003;21(6):539–42.
34. Zoppi MA, Ibba RM, Putzolu M, Floris M, Monni G. First trimester umbilical artery pulsatility index in fetuses presenting enlarged nuchal translucency. *Prenat Diagn* 2000;20:701–4.
35. Cuckle HS. Growing complexity in the choice of Down's syndrome screening policy. *Ultrasound Obstet Gynecol* 2002;19:323–6.
36. Benacerraf BR. Barss VA, Laboda LA. A sonographic sign for the detection in the second trimester of the fetus with Down's syndrome. *Am J Obstet Gynecol* 1985;151:1078–9.
37. Biagiotti R, Periti E, Brizzi L, Vanzi E, Cariati E. Comparison between two methods of standardization for gestational age differences in fetal nuchal translucency measurement in first-trimester screening for trisomy 21. *Ultrasound Obstet Gynecol* 1997;9(4):248–52.
38. Spencer K, Bindra R, Nix AB, Heath V, Nicolaides KH. Delta-NT or NT MoM: Which is the most appropriate method for calculating accurate patient-specific risks for trisomy 21 in the first trimester? *Ultrasound Obstet Gynecol* 2003;22(2):142–8.
39. Monni G, Zoppi MA, Ibba RM, Floris M. Fetal nuchal translucency test for Down's syndrome. *Lancet* 1997;350:1631.
40. Snijders RJM, Noble P, Sebire N, Souka A, Nicolaides KH. UK multicentre project on assessment of risk of trisomy 21 by maternal age and fetal nuchal- translucency thickness at 10–14 weeks of gestation. *Lancet* 1998;352:343–6.
41. Snijders RJM, Sundberg K, Holzgreve W, Henry G, Nicolaides KH. Maternal age and gestation-specific risk for trisomy 21. *Ultrasound Obstet Gynecol* 1999;13:167–70.
42. Monni G, Ibba RM, Zoppi MA. Antenatal screening for Down's syndrome. *Lancet* 1998;352:1631–2.
43. Mulvey S, Zachariah R, McIlwaine K, Wallace EM. Do women prefer to have screening tests for Down syndrome that have the lowest screen-positive rate or the highest detection rate? *Prenat Diagn* 2003;23(10):828–32.
44. Zoppi MA, Ibba RM, Putzolu M, Floris M, Monni G. Nuchal translucency and the acceptance of invasive prenatal chromosomal diagnosis in women aged 35 and older. *Obstet Gynecol* 2001;97:916–20.
45. Sebire NJ, Snijders RJ, Hughes K, Sepulveda W, Nicolaides KH. Screening for trisomy 21 in twin pregnancies by maternal age and fetal nuchal translucency thickness at 10–14 weeks of gestation. *Br J Obstet Gynaecol* 1996;103:999–1003.
46. Monni G, Zoppi MA, Ibba RM, Putzolu M, Floris M. Nuchal translucency in multiple pregnancies. *Croat Med J* 2000;41:266–9.
47. Souka AP, Krampl E, Bakalis S, Heath V, Nicolaides KH. Outcome of pregnancy in chromosomally normal fetuses with increased nuchal translucency in the first trimester. *Ultrasound Obstet Gynecol* 2001;18:5–8.
48. Spencer K, Souter V, Tul N, Snijders R, Nicolaides A screening program for trisomy 21 at 10–14 weeks using fetal nuchal translucency, maternal serum free beta-human chorionic gonadotropin and pregnancy-associated plasma protein-A. *Ultrasound Obstet Gynecol* 1999;13:231–7.
49. Cicero S, Curcio P, Papageorghiou A, Sonek J, Nicolaides KH. Absence of nasal bone in fetuses with trisomy 21 at 11–14 weeks of gestation: an observational study. *Lancet* 2001;358:1665–7.
50. Monni G, Zoppi MA, Ibba RM. Absence of nasal bone and detection of trisomy 21. *Lancet* 2002;359:1343.
51. Wald NJ, Watt HC, Hackshaw AK. Integrated screening for Down's syndrome on the basis of test performed during the first and second trimesters. *N Engl J Med* 1999;12:461–7.

82 First-trimester ultrasound screening for Down's syndrome in multiple gestations

G. Monni and M. A. Zoppi

Introduction

In the last decades, the older maternal age at conception and the more frequent use of assisted reproductive techniques have moved to a constant increased rate of multiple pregnancies. Some specific prenatal and perinatal problems make these pregnancies at higher risk.[1–4] Neonatal mortality and morbidity are higher in multiple pregnancies, and maternal complications are more frequent.

Moreover, mostly because of the advanced maternal age, multiple pregnancies are at higher risk for chromosomal defects. At the same time, as these pregnancies (frequently obtained after years of infertility) are especially precious to the prospective parents, there is no unanimous acceptance of the need of invasive prenatal diagnostic procedures, which are more difficult to perform than in singleton pregnancies.[5,6]

Non-invasive screening tests for chromosomal abnormalities in multiple pregnancies are more acceptable. Maternal serum biochemistry for trisomy 21 in multiple pregnancies has been proposed.[7,8] However, interpretation may be difficult because of the interference between serum marker concentrations and assisted reproductive therapies, and the identification of which of the fetuses is positive at the biochemical test is of great concern.

For invasive prenatal diagnosis, the risk of miscarriage related to the procedure is increased, depending mostly on the number of needle insertions.[9,10] Prenatal diagnosis of a chromosomal abnormality in multizygotic multiples allows an informed decision about the management of the pregnancy. Therefore, an accurate estimate of individual fetal risk for chromosomal abnormality is advisable in multiple pregnancies.

Ultrasound screening for trisomy 21 by first-trimester nuchal translucency (NT) measurement is correctly applicable for twins and multiples.[11–13] The test gives an individual risk for each fetus and it is comparable in the accuracy to the screening test for trisomy 21 in singleton pregnancies.[14–17]

Type of multiples

Zygosity depends on the type of conception.

Monozygotic pregnancies originate from the division of a single zygote, and account for about 30% of twin pregnancies. The frequency of monozygotic pregnancy is stable in the world and among different populations at around 1 in 250 deliveries. The origin of monozygotic pregnancy is unknown. Next to the theory of an accidental event, a delay in the implantation of the zygote, with a reduction of oxygen transport, has been hypothesized.[18]

Multizygotic pregnancies originate from the fertilization of two or more oocytes by two or more spermatozoa (Figure 82.1). Dizygotic pregnancies account for about 70% of the total twin pregnancies. The frequency of dizygotic pregnancy varies among population, and the origin appears to be multifactorial. High levels of follicle stimulating hormone (FSH), advanced maternal age, high grade of parity, tall maternal stature and proportionate maternal weight (reflecting a good nutritional maternal status and probably higher levels of FSH), ethnical and familiar inherited factors, seasonality (peak of those kind of conceptions in summer), the application of technologies of assisted reproduction and the use of drugs for the induction of ovulation support an increased frequency of multiple conceptions.[1,2,18] The *in vitro* manipulation of embryos in techniques of assisted reproduction and the use of special culture mediums seem to induce a greater frequency of iatrogenic monozygotic pregnancies.[19] (Figure 82.2).

The chorionicity depends on the type of placentation. Dizygotic and multizygotic pregnancies are always dichorionic and multichorionic (Figure 82.3).

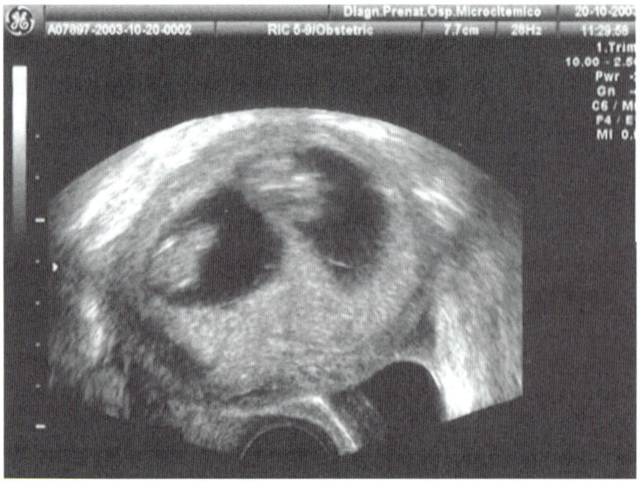

Figure 82.1 A dichorionic diamniotic twin pregnancy at 9 weeks.

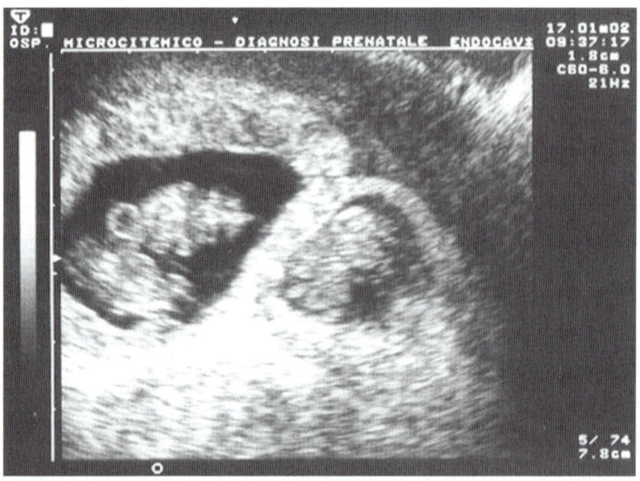

Figure 82.2 A dichorionic triamniotic triplet pregnancy obtained by *in vitro* fertilization.

Monozygotic pregnancies can be dichorionic or monochorionic, and the chorionicity depends on the time of the division of the conceptus (Figure 82.4).

If the division occurs by the third day from fertilization (and this happens in about 30% of monozygotic pregnancies), two placentas are generated. If the division occurs between the fourth and the eighth days from fertilization (and this happens in about 70% of monozygotic pregnancies), the placenta will be single with two amniotic cavities (monochorionic, diamniotic pregnancy). If the division occurs between the 9th and 13th days from fertilization (it happens in less than 1% of monozygotic pregnancies), the placenta and the amniotic cavity will be only one (monochorionic, monoamniotic pregnancy). In very rare cases, the division occurs between the 14th and 16th days from conception, and the result is conjoined twins.

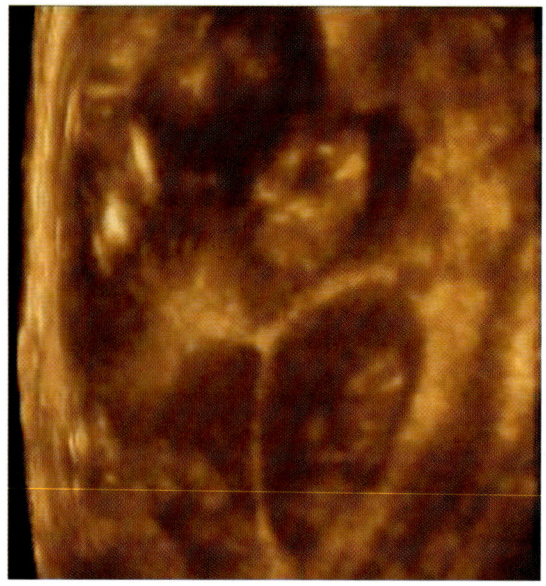

Figure 82.3 3D rendering of a multizygotic pregnancy (nine fetuses).

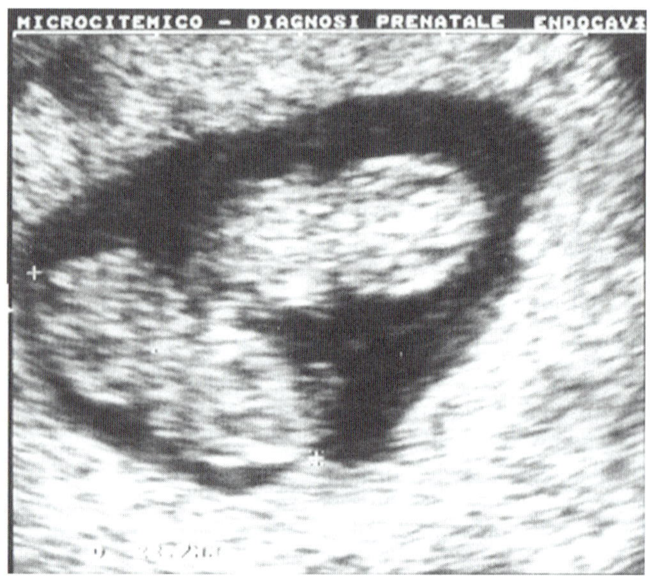

Figure 82.4 A monochorionic diamniotic pregnancy at 9 weeks.

Monozygotic twins are at higher risk for structural anomalies than multizygotic ones because of higher potential errors in the division of the zygote and pre-embryo.[1]

Prenatal ultrasound determination of chorionicity

Prenatal diagnosis of chorionicity can be made easier by ultrasound in the first trimester. By transvaginal ultrasound, gestational sacs can be seen at 5 weeks of gestation (from 4 weeks plus 2 or 3 days), and the

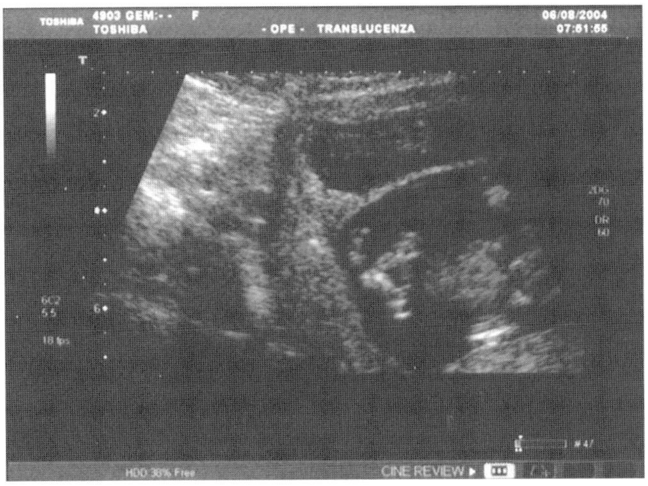

Figure 82.5 First-trimester lambda sign in a dichorionic pregnancy.

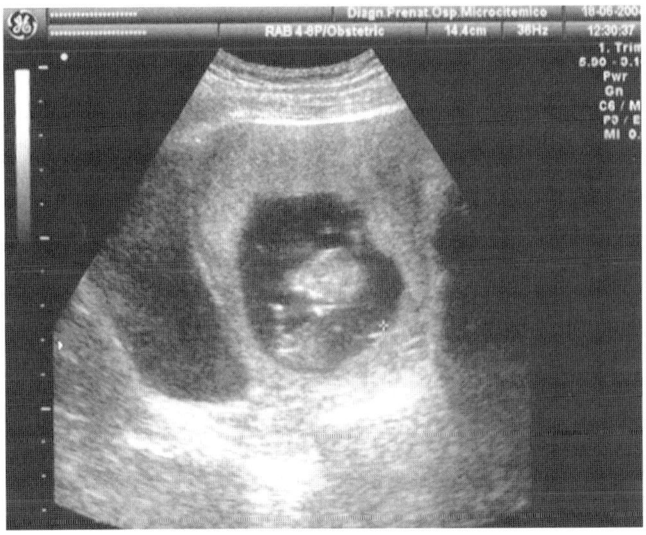

Figure 82.6 Absence of lambda sign (T sign) in a monochorionic twin pregnancy.

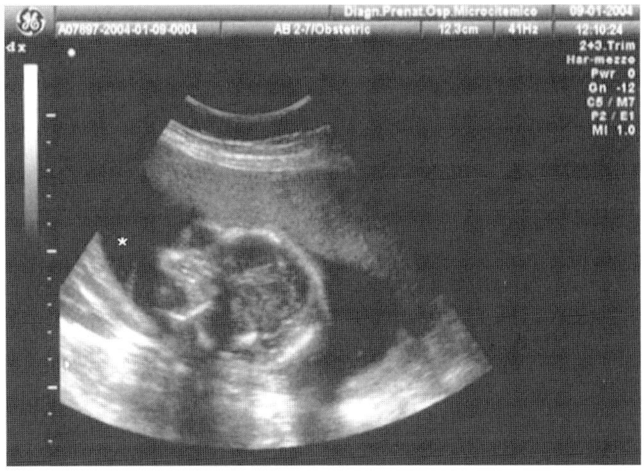

Figure 82.7 Second-trimester dichorionic pregnancy: the lambda sign has disappeared.

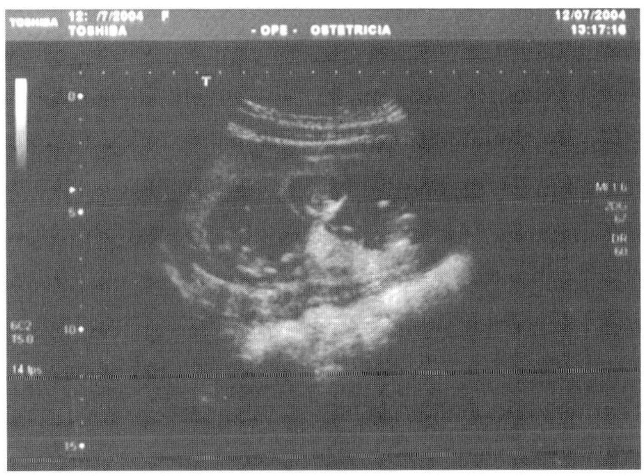

Figure 82.8 The ipsilon sign in a trichorionic pregnancy.

number of sacs indicates the number of placentas (monochorionic, dichorionic, trichorionic, etc.). As the gestation proceeds, the septum between the sacs become thinner, and only a triangular structure, the 'lambda sign' or 'twin-peak sign' remain from 10 to 14 weeks (Figure 82.5). In monochorionic pregnancy there is no chorionic tissue between the two amniotic sacs, and the joint of membranes to the chorionic sac is called the 'T sign' (Figure 82.6). In dichorionic pregnancies, later in pregnancy, the 'lambda sign' is difficult to visualize in all cases, and it can completely disappear around 20 weeks (Figure 82.7).[20]

The visualization of the 'lambda sign' is an unequivocal sign of dichorionicity, while the absence in the second trimester is not sufficient to exclude the presence of two placentas. In triplet trichorionic pregnancies, the junction of interfetal membranes is called 'ipsilon zone' (Figure 82.8).[21]

The accurate identification of chorionicity is one of most important goals of obstetric ultrasound in multiple gestations, and in all cases it should be ideally performed in the first trimester so that the risk of each individual pregnancy can be assessed.

Monochorionic pregnancies are at higher risk than dichorionic pregnancies for prenatal and perinatal problems, as they are monozygotic and because of the occurrence of specific problems due to transplacental circulation imbalance, which is the twin-to-twin transfusion syndrome. This complication occurs in about 20% of monochorionic pregnancies and frequently manifests itself at 16–22 weeks, by polyhydramnios in one sac and oligoanhydramnios in the other sac. If untreated, the mortality is about 90%. Amniodrainage or laser coagulation of arterovenous connections in the placenta is the therapy proposed in the second trimester, allowing a survival of about 50% of cases.[22]

Risk of chromosomal abnormalities in multiples

To calculate the risk of chromosomal abnormalities in multiple pregnancies, it is fundamental to estimate the zygosity.

For monozygotic pregnancies, if cases with mitotic non-disjunction that determine 'heterokaryotypia' are excluded, the karyotype in both fetuses would be the same.[23] Fetuses can be discordant for anomalies that are generated by the splitting phenomenon, but are concordant for anomalies genetically determined. Both fetuses have the same karyotype either normal or abnormal.

For multiple pregnancies derived from multizygotic conception, discordant karyotypes are expected. Therefore, prenatal sonographic estimation of zygosity is fundamental in the process of risk calculation.[9,24] In prenatal life, ultrasonographic evaluation of the placentas can give information in this direction. DNA analysis of the fetal or neonatal sampling allows a definitive diagnosis of zygosity.

When a monochorionic pregnancy is diagnosed by prenatal ultrasound (whether monoamniotic or diamniotic), monozygosity can be supposed, and an equal risk for trisomy 21 for both fetuses, similar to the maternal age-related risk, can be calculated. When dichorionic or multiple placentas are evidenced, a little probability of monozygotic pregnancy cannot be excluded, but the most frequent condition is multizygotic pregnancy. If the assessment is made in a period when it is possible to define by ultrasound the fetal gender, and the placentas are multiple, in cases with discordant sex, the probability of multizygosity is validated. The risk for the pregnancy of having one fetus with trisomy 21 is calculated by the sum of the risk for each fetus. For example, in a triplet trizygotic pregnancy, if the maternal trisomy 21 background risk is 1 in 150, the final risk for the entire pregnancy is 1 in 150 + 1 in 150 + 1 in 150. For calculations, risks can be expressed as odds (that is 1:149 + 1: 149 + 1:149), that is about 3:149 or 1:47, for a final risk for the pregnancy to have one fetus with trisomy 21 of 1 in 48. In multichorionic pregnancies, the risk for all fetuses to have trisomy 21 is very rare, this being calculated by multiplying the maternal age risk for one fetus by the risk of the other. For example, in a dichorionic and 'hypothetical' dizygotic pregnancy, where the maternal age risk for trisomy 21 is 1 in 150, the background risk of the entire pregnancy is calculated by multiplying 1:149 × 1:149, then 1:22,201, that is a risk of 1 in 22,202.

A sort of uncertainty is originated by the presence of those cases of monozygotic dichorionic pregnancies that are unrecognized in prenatal life, where the background risk of the pregnancy would be the same as the age-related risk for trisomy 21 of the pregnant woman.

Invasive prenatal diagnosis procedures for karyotype analysis in multiples

When a multiple pregnancy is discovered, extra counseling is due regarding procreative risks, pregnancy-related risk for the mother, prenatal management of the pregnancy, screening and prenatal diagnosis of fetal anomalies and chromosomal abnormalities.[9,10]

When an invasive procedure for prenatal diagnosis is planned, whatever be the approach considered (chorionic villus sampling, amniocentesis, fetal blood sampling), some fundamental conditions should be fulfilled.

The knowledge of the type of placentation is imperative (mono- or multichorionic placenta). Each sample obtained from a distinct twin should be defined (or checked by biological tests that analyze the fetal phenotype or genotype); each fetus should be mapped carefully by ultrasound during the procedure to later allow the precise identification when the result from diagnosis becomes available. We should consider the increased risk of procedure-related abortions, of invasive diagnosis in multiples, compared to singles, which depends among others factors mostly on multiple needle entrances through the uterus.

When the operators are faced with invasive procedures in multiple pregnancies, a specific experience and skill in this particular field of prenatal diagnosis is required.

Selective fetocide and multifetal embryo reduction

The diagnosis of a single affected twin after a procedure of invasive prenatal diagnosis can lead to consent to plan a selective termination of the affected fetus and to continue the pregnancy of the normal fetus.

Multifetal embryo reduction is an option that could be considered for therapeutical options in cases of high-order multiple pregnancies. Maternal and fetal risks (related to high prematurity) are increased in these pregnancies. The neonatal and pregnancy outcome have been shown to improve in cases of four or higher multiples reduced to twin, because of a significant increase of the gestational age at delivery and a better maternal outcome. At present, the role of embryo reduction for the management of triplet pregnancies is under discussion.[25,26]

Embryo reduction is usually performed in the first trimester, because it carries fewer complications than in the second, by intrathoracic or intracardiac injection of potassium chloride at 11–13 weeks, under ultrasonographic continuous guidance. When the number of fetuses is high, it is preferable to perform the reduction by steps.

At the beginning, when performing this procedure, the choice as to which fetus to reduce was based fundamentally on technical considerations (the fetus nearest to the uterine surface or the one easier to reduce for the operator). The likelihood of reducing a normal fetus while maintaining some abnormal cases (affected by structural anomalies or chromosomopathies) was considered. Therefore, it was proposed to offer invasive prenatal diagnosis for karyotype by chorionic villus sampling in all cases before performing embryo reduction.[27] Because of the difficulties and costs of such invasive prenatal diagnosis in multiples, and the greater risk of miscarriage related to the numerous procedures carried out, this approach has not been universally approved and performed.

To avoid a non-selective reduction and to decrease the use of invasive procedures, NT screening before embryo reduction has been considered. In fact, the finding of an enlarged NT, allowing the possibility of calculating the individual risk for trisomy in each fetus, can identify cases at higher risk for chromosomal abnormalities and for structural malformation in multiple pregnancies.[28]

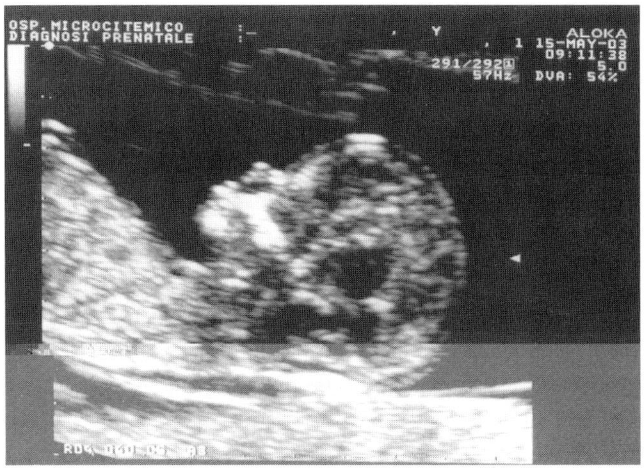

Figure 82.9 Nuchal translucency.

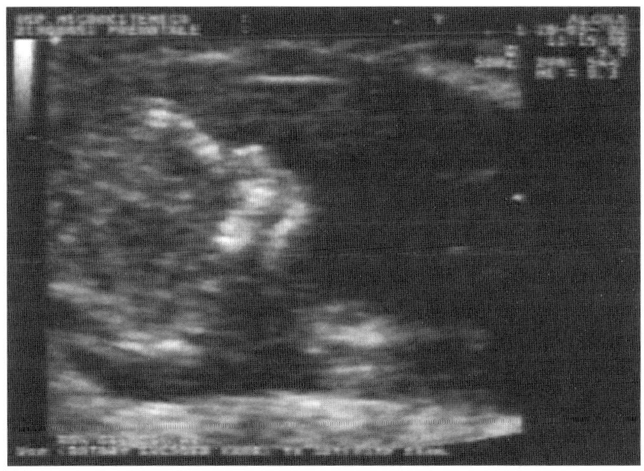

Figure 82.10 Absent nasal bone in a trisomy 21 fetus.

NT in multiples

The ultrasound measurement of the soft tissues behind the fetal neck (NT thickness or NT) (Figure 82.9), and the combination of the likelihood ratios obtained with the maternal background risk for trisomy 21, is a valid test of screening to identify fetuses with chromosomal abnormalities.

In multiple pregnancies an individual risk for trisomy 21 can be calculated for each fetus, and, as for the background risk due to maternal age, the risk for the entire pregnancy can be considered.

In twin and multiple pregnancies, screening for chromosomal abnormalities by NT can be performed and it is as accurate as in singleton pregnancies.[14–17]

In a large collaborative study on 448 twin pregnancies, Sebire *et al.* have found an enlarged NT in 7.3% of all cases and in seven out of eight cases of trisomy 21.[15]

NT measurement can be used in high-order multiple pregnancies and in those cases obtained by assisted reproductive technologies because no evident difference has been found in the rate of enlarged NT than in spontaneous multichorionic pregnancies, and the sensitivity was the same.[17]

The increased accumulation of fluid in the fetal nuchal, leading to the ultrasound finding of an enlarged NT, can be determined by several different mechanisms: cardiac failure, abnormal or delayed development of the lymphatic vessels, altered composition of the connective tissue of the skin or venous congestion due to an increased pressure in the fetal thorax.[29,30]

The presence of an enlarged NT is associated with an increased rate of chromosomal abnormalities, but the risk for structural malformations and mostly cardiac defects in fetuses with normal karyotype is increased.[31,32]

It has to be considered that a higher frequency of fetal malformation per pregnancy is expected in multifetal pregnancies than in singleton pregnancies, and in a dizygotic twin pregnancy there is a slight chance of a double risk per pregnancy for fetal malformations (because of the independent probability that is carried by each fetus).

In multiple pregnancies, the absence of nasal bone visualization, which is another accurate soft marker for trisomy 21 in the first trimester, can be used with the same efficiency as in singleton pregnancies (Figure 82.10). About 70% of trisomy 21 and an important percentage of other chromosomal abnormalities such as trisomy 18 and 13, 45, X0, can manifest the sign of the absent nasal bone at ultrasound examination performed at 11–14 weeks[33,34] (Figures 82.11–82.13).

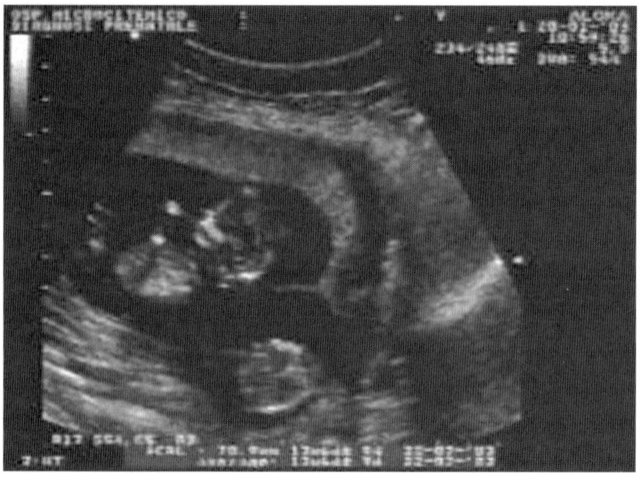

Figure 82.11 Dichorionic pregnancy with a normal fetus and a fetus with trisomy 21.

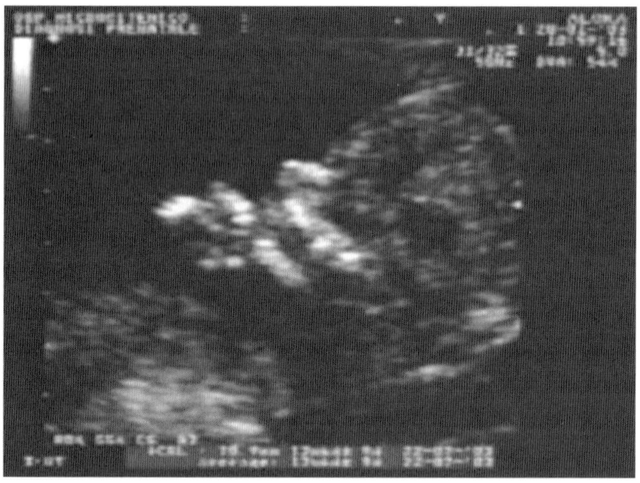

Figure 82.12 Dichorionic pregnancy: the fetus with normal karyotype with normal NT and present nasal bone.

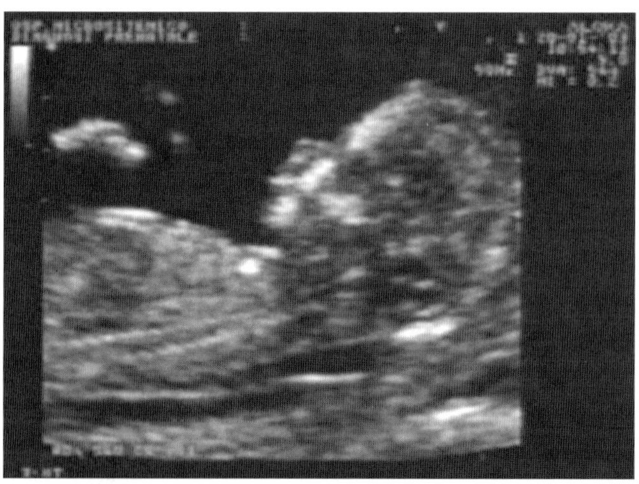

Figure 82.13 Dichorionic pregnancy: the fetus with trisomy 21 with enlarged NT and absent nasal bone.

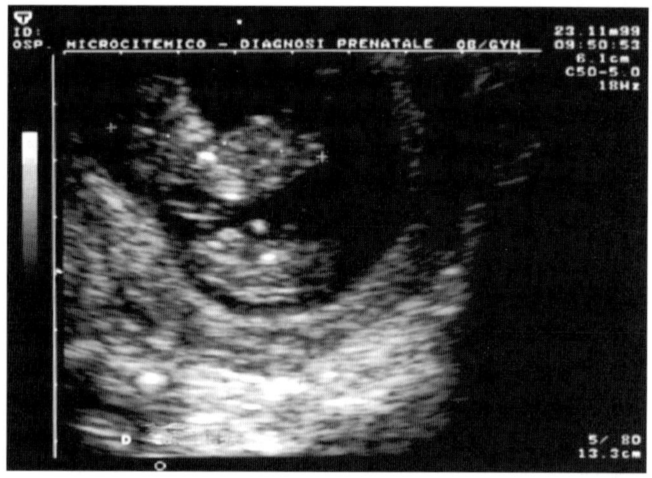

Figure 82.14 Discordant NT in a monochorionic diamniotic twin pregnancy.

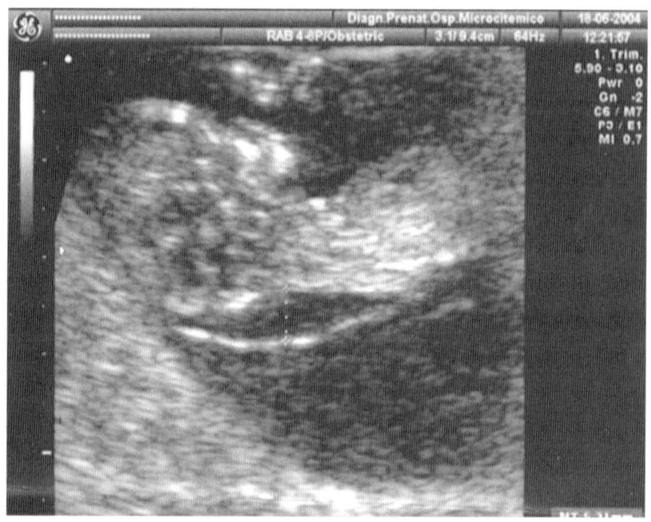

Figure 82.15 The fetus with enlarged NT in another monochorionic diamniotic twin pregnancy with discordant NT.

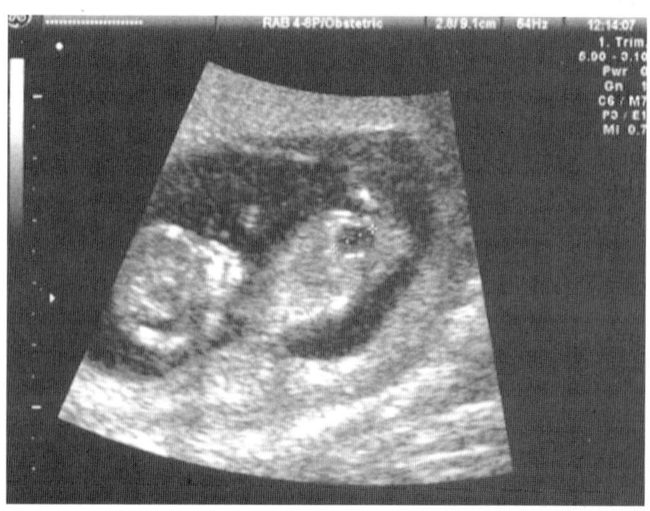

Figure 82.16 The same fetus with enlarged NT in the monochorionic diamniotic twin pregnancy with discordant NT showed an enlarged bladder.

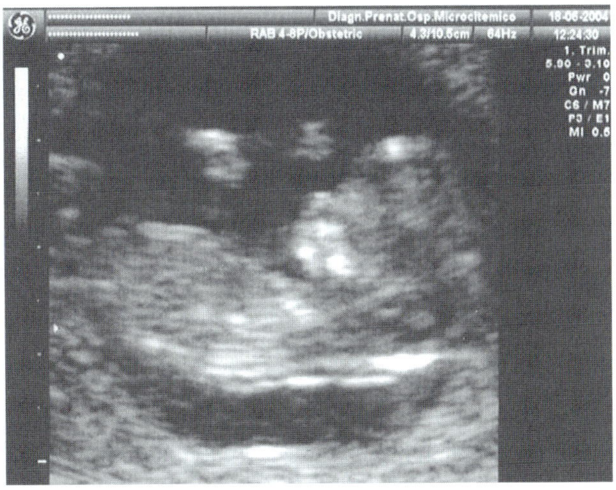

Figure 82.17 The fetus with normal NT in the monochorionic diamniotic twin pregnancy with discordant NT.

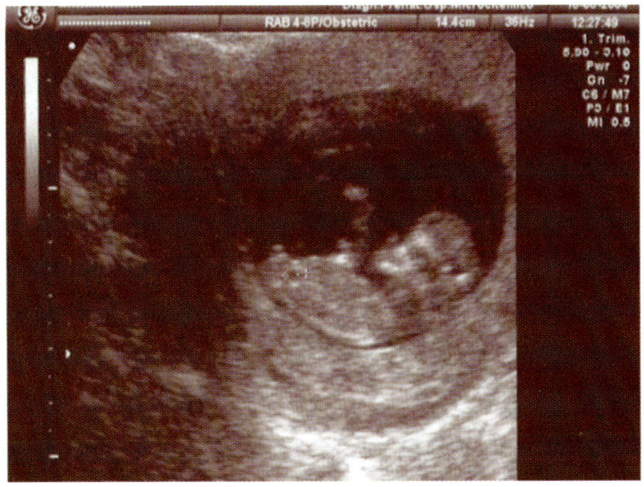

Figure 82.18 The same fetus with enlarged NT in the monochorionic diamniotic twin pregnancy with discordant NT showed a normal bladder.

The case of enlarged NT in monochorionic pregnancies

In monozygotic pregnancies the rate of Mendelian disorders and chromosomal abnormalities are identical to those of singleton pregnancies, while there is an increased risk of structural malformations. Malformations due to disruption mechanisms such as midline facial, heart and abdomen anomalies are more frequent.

A higher rate of enlarged NT has been described in monochorionic pregnancies. The enlarged NT has been described in both fetuses or in one. The enlarged NT in monochorionic pregnancies can indicate fetuses at higher risk for chromosomal abnormalities or structural defects or can be a possible early manifestation of heart failure due to twin-to-twin transfusion.[35]

When in a monochorionic pregnancy, the NT is discordant between fetuses, a consideration should be made (Figures 82.14–82.18). An enlarged NT in only one fetus may indicate a greater risk for chromosomal abnormality for the entire pregnancy. The chromosomal abnormality if present, should be present in both fetuses (in the fetus with enlarged NT and in the fetus with normal NT). In fact, excluding the extremely rare case of heterokaryotypia, due to a mitotic non-disjunction, where a normal karyotype can co-exists with a 45, X0 or a trisomy fetus, it should be considered that the two fetuses of the monochorionic diamniotic pregnancy have the same karyotype, either normal or abnormal.

However, in the same pregnancy, there is evidence of a fetus that shows a normal NT, that gives a very small risk for chromosomal abnormality, for the entire pregnancy. To rule out this kind of problem, it has been recently suggested in monochorionic pregnancies with discordant NT, to calculate the risk for Down's syndrome by using the average NT measured in the two fetuses.[36]

Moreover, it should be considered that an enlarged NT could be indicative for a structural anomaly that could be present in only one of the monozygotic fetuses, both with normal karyotype. Concordance for the most common structural abnormalities that occur in monochorionic-monozygotic twins is rare.

In monochorionic diamniotic pregnancy, an enlarged nuchal translucency could be caused by placental circulation problems, rather than chromosomal abnormalities. This early imbalance of fluids between the fetuses can anticipate in the first trimester the inter-twin-to-twin transfusion, that manifest the most important diagnostic sign after only 16 weeks.

REFERENCES

1. Snijders RJM, Nicolaides K. *Ultrasound Markers for Chromosomal Defects*. London: Parthenon Publishing, 1996.
2. Nicolaides KH, Sebire NJ, Snijders RJM, Souka AP. *The 11–14 Week's Scan Book*. London: Parthenon Publishing, 2001.
3. Dunn A, MacFarlane A. Recent trends in the incidence of multiple births and associated mortality in England and Wales. *Arch Dis Child* 1996;75:10–9.
4. Callahan T, Hall J, Ettner S, Christiansen C, Greene M, Crowley W. The economic impact of multiple-gestation pregnancies and the contribution of assisted-reproduction techniques to their incidence. *N Engl J Med* 1994;331:244–9.
5. Meschede D, Lemcke B, Stussel J, Louwen F, Horst J. Strong preference for non-invasive prenatal diagnosis in women pregnant through intracytoplasmic sperm injection. *Prenat Diagn* 1998;18:700–5.
6. Monni G, Cau G, Lai R, Demontis G, Usai V. Intracytoplasmic sperm injection and prenatal invasive diagnosis. *Prenat Diagn* 1999;19:389–90.

7. Neveux LM, Palomaki GE, Knight GJ, Haddow JE. Multiple marker screening for Down syndrome in twin pregnancies. *Prenat Diagn* 1996;16:29–34.
8. Spencer K. Screening for trisomy 21 in twin pregnancies in the first trimester using free beta-hCG and PAPP-A, combined with fetal nuchal translucency thickness. *Prenat Diagn* 2000;20:91–5.
9. Wapner RJ. Genetic diagnosis in multiple pregnancies. *Semin Perinat* 1995;19:351–62.
10. Monni G, Ibba RM. Invasive procedures in multiple pregnancies. In Weiner S, Kurjak A, eds. *Interventional Ultrasound.* New York: The Parthenon Publishing Group, 1999:105–15.
11. Nicolaides KH, Azar G, Byrne D, Mansur C, Marks K. Fetal nuchal translucency screening for chromosomal defects in first trimester of pregnancy. *Br Med J* 1992;304:867–9.
12. Monni G, Zoppi MA, Ibba RM, Floris M. Fetal nuchal translucency test for Down's syndrome. *Lancet* 1997;350:1631.
13. Snijders RJM, Noble P, Sebire N, Souka A, Nicolaides KH. UK multicentre project on assessment of risk of trisomy 21 by maternal age and fetal nuchal-translucency thickness at 10–14 weeks of gestation. *Lancet* 1998;352:343–6.
14. Pandya PP, Hilbert F, Snijders RJM, Nicolaides KH. Nuchal translucency thickness and crown–rump length in twin pregnancies with chromosomally abnormal fetuses. *J Ultrasound Med* 1995;14:565–8.
15. Sebire NJ, Snijders RJM, Hughes K, Sepulveda W, Nicolaides KH. Screening for trisomy 21 in twin pregnancies by maternal age and fetal nuchal translucency thickness at 10–14 weeks of gestation. *Br J Obstet Gynaecol* 1996;103:999–1003.
16. Maymon R, Dreazen E, Tovbin Y, Bukovsky, Weinraub Z, Herman A. The feasibility of nuchal translucency measurement in higher order multiple pregnancies achieved by assisted reproduction. *Hum Reprod* 1999;14:2102–5.
17. Monni G, Zoppi MA, Ibba RM, Putzolu M, Floris M. Nuchal translucency in multiple pregnancies. *Croat Med J* 2000;41: 266–9.
18. Keith LG, Papiernik E, Keith DM, Luke B, eds. *Multiple Pregnancy, Epidemiology, Gestation and Perinatal Outcome.* New York: The Parthenon Publishing Group, 1995.
19. Wenstrom KD, Syrop CH, Hammitt DG, Van Voorhis BJ. Increased risk of monochorionic twinning associated with assisted reproduction. *Fertil Steril* 1993;60:510–4.
20. Sepulveda W, Sebire NJ, Hughes K, Odibo A, Nicolaides KH. The lambda sign at 10–14 weeks of gestation as a predictor of chorionicity in twin pregnancies. *Ultrasound Obstet Gynecol* 1996;7:421–3.
21. Sepulveda W, Sebire NJ, Odibo A, Psarra A, Nicolaides KH. Prenatal determination of chorionicity in triplet pregnancy by ultrasonographic examination of the ipsilon zone. *Obstet Gynecol* 1996;88:855–8.
22. Senat MV, Deprest J, Boulvain M, Paupe A, Winer N, Ville Y. Endoscopic laser surgery versus serial amnioreduction for severe twin-to-twin transfusion syndrome. *N Engl J Med* 2004;351(2):136–44.
23. Machin GA. Some causes of genotypic and phenotypic discordance in monozygotic twin pairs. *Am J Med Genet* 1996;61:216–28.
24. Rodis JF, Egan JFX, Craffey A, Ciarleglio L, Greenstein RM, Scarza W. Calculated risk of chromosomal abnormalities in twin gestations. *Obstet Gynecol* 1990;76:1037–41.
25. Evans MI, Berkowitz RL, Wapner RJ, *et al.* Improvement in outcomes of multifetal pregnancy reduction with increases experience. *Am J Obstet Gynecol* 2001;184.7–103.
26. Dodd JM, Crowther CA. Reduction of the number of fetuses for women with triplet and high order multiple pregnancies (Cochrane Review). In *The Cochrane Library 2003,* issue 4. Chichester, UK: John Wiley & Sons, 2003.
27. Eddleman KA, Stone JL, Lynch L, Berkowitz RL. Chorionic villous sampling before multifetal pregnancy reduction. *Am J Obstet Gynecol* 2000;183:1078–81.
28. Monni G, Zoppi MA, Cau G, Lai R, Baldi M. Importance of nuchal translucency in multifetal pregnancy reduction. *Ultrasound Obstet Gynecol* 1999;13:377–8.
29. Moscoso G. Fetal nuchal translucency: A need to understand the physiological basis. *Ultrasound Obstet Gynecol* 1995;5:6–8.
30. Von Kaisenberg CS, Brand-Saberi B, Jonat W, Nicolaides KH. Pathophysiology of increased nuchal translucency in chromosomally abnormal fetuses. *Prenat Neonat Med* 1999;4:431–40.
31. Souka AP, Snijders RJ, Novakov A, Soares W, Nicolaides KH. Defects and syndromes in chromosomally normal fetuses with increased nuchal translucency thickness at 10–14 weeks of gestation. *Ultrasound Obstet Gynecol* 1998;11:391–400.
32. Hyett J, Perdu M, Sharland G, Snijders R, Nicolaides KH. Using fetal nuchal translucency to screen for major congenital cardiac defects at 10–14 weeks of gestation: Population based cohort study. *Br Med J* 1999;318:81–5.
33. Cicero S, Curcio P, Papageorghiou A, Sonek J, Nicolaides KH. Absence of nasal bone in fetuses with trisomy 21 at 11–14 weeks of gestation: An observational study. *Lancet* 2001;358:1665–7.
34. Monni G, Zoppi MA, Ibba RM Absence of nasal bone and detection of trisomy 21. *Lancet* 2002;359:1343.
35. Sebire NJ, D'Ercole C, Hughes K, Carvalho M, Nicolaides KH. Increased nuchal translucency thickness at 10–14 weeks of gestation as a predictor of severe twin-to-twin transfusion syndrome. *Ultrasound Obstet Gynecol* 1997;10:86–9.
36. Vandecruys H, Faiola S, Auer M, Sebire N, Nicolaides KH. Screening for trisomy 21 in monochorionic twins by measurement of fetal nuchal translucency thickness. *Ultrasound Obstet Gynecol* 2005;25:551–3.

SECTION IX

Fetal and maternal physiology

Section Editors: **B. Arabin and D. W. Skupski**

83 Maternal hemodynamic changes of pregnancy

J. Nizard

Introduction

Adaptation to pregnancy begins rapidly after conception. Most probably, all described modifications of maternal hemodynamics are triggered early every menstrual cycle, before conception, but are too small to be detected. These modifications are reversible, either at the end of the cycle with menstruations, or within the first weeks or months after delivery. Physiological modifications are only detectable when the amplitude of changes is sufficient, thus most of the time at the end of the first trimester of pregnancy. Functional as well as anatomical changes are observed in most systems, of which the cardiovascular and volume homeostasis systems are among the most important.

These changes in maternal physiology are asymptomatic in normal pregnant women, resulting from an adapted process. They are nevertheless important to know for their implications in pathology and its treatment. Most data we have derive from radioactive molecules and cells, or dye techniques previously used in pregnant women. Modern non-invasive techniques do not provide the same reliability. If echocardiography, for instance, can replace invasive measurements of cardiac output, we still lack non-invasive techniques for parameters, such as plasma volume.

Cardiovascular system

Blood volume

Plasma volume increase starts as early as 6 weeks and reaches a maximum volume of 5200 ml by the end of the third trimester, which represents an increase of 1200–1600 ml or 45% from non-pregnant values.[1,2] Although absolute volume values vary from individual to individual, and among studies, the overall percentage of increase is constant, between 45% and 50%.[3] It is not clear whether the importance of plasma volume is constant for an individual.[2,3] or depends on parity.[4,5] Interestingly, plasma volume increases throughout pregnancy, even when indexed to weight.[2]

The plasma volume increase is greater in multiple gestations and the increase is proportional to the number of fetuses.[6–8] More fetuses also means more placental volume. It is probable that the amplitude of these changes is proportional to placenta volume, since the plasma volume increase is greater, on average, in cases of molar pregnancy.[9] In the study of Pritchard on hemodilution in patients with molar pregnancies, after accounting for blood loss associated with the pathology, he describes in five out of eight patients anemia associated with significant hypervolemia.[9] The increase in blood volume ranged from 25% to 51% at 9–24 weeks when compared with non-pregnant values in the same patients. This is consistent with the increase in cases of multiple pregnancy or increased fetal weight, where placenta volume is proportionally increased.

On the other hand, in cases where placenta volume is likely to be decreased, such as pre-eclampsia and intrauterine growth restriction, plasma expansion is reduced.[10–12]

What happens at the very end of the third trimester of pregnancy is largely debated in the literature. Contradictory data on whether maternal plasma volume declines in the last month of pregnancy seem to be related to maternal positioning. The increase in plasma volume seems to continue even in the last month of pregnancy when mothers are in the left lateral position, at least in twin pregnancies. According to some authors, plasma volume reaches a plateau at around 32 weeks in singleton pregnancies, but continues to increase in twin pregnancies.[6] This peculiarity explains the increased risks of pulmonary edema in twin pregnancies when using β-mimetics or plasma expansion in the third trimester.

Why does plasma volume expand?

There are several theories to explain why plasma volume expands during pregnancy

- *Hyperaldosteronism*: Physiologic hyperaldosteronism during pregnancy can be responsible for plasma increase. Primary hyperaldosteronism is responsible for hypervolemia in non-pregnant

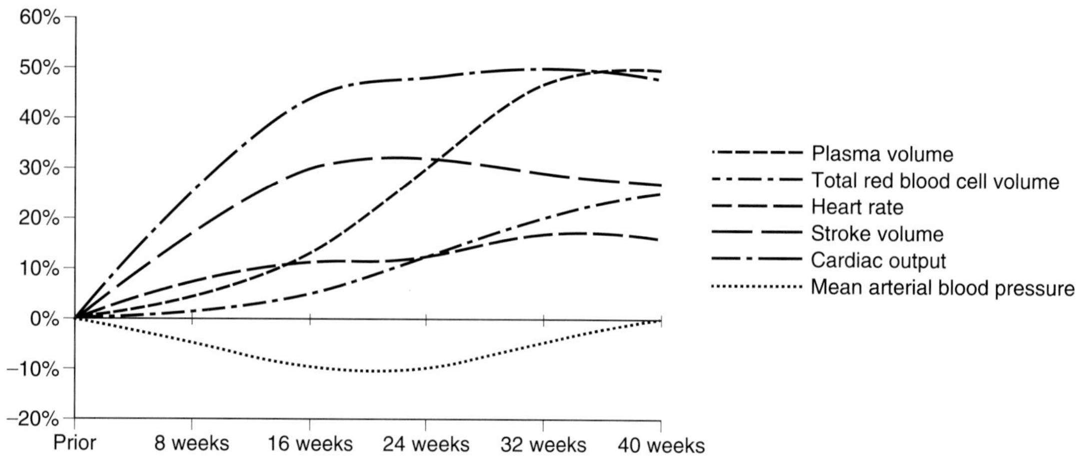

Figure 83.1 Evolution of different parameters throughout pregnancy. Adapted from Ayala *et al.*,[40] Capeless and Clapp,[36] Robson *et al.*,[33] Thomsen *et al.*,[8] and Pitkin.[17]

patients, with an increase in plasma volume of 48% and 76% in the two cases described by Briglier and Forsham, with no changes in total red blood cell volume.[13]

- *Influence of estrogens*: Estrogens affect plasma volume in many circumstances. Plasma volume expansion has been described in women using oral contraception or hormonal replacement therapy (i.e. estrogens in postmenopausal women).[14,15] Estrogens are responsible for an increase in renin levels, which are responsible for an increase in aldosterone level.
- Placental growth hormones implications are uncertain.
- *Placental circulation*: The placenta acts like a low-pressure maternal arterio–venous shunt, affecting arterial blood pressure and cardiac output. Placental circulation could thus explain part of the plasma expansion by induced hyperaldosteronism.

Red blood cells

Total red blood cell mass increases by 20–40% by term, which represents an absolute increase of 250–450 ml. The rise is the consequence of greater production of red blood cells, not longer lifetime, since iron supplementation increases even more the red blood cell mass.[1] The increase in total red blood cell volume is proportional to the weight gain in singleton pregnancies as opposed to plasma volume, which increases more than the weight gain.[2] The lesser increase in total red blood cell volume than the physiologic plasma volume expansion is responsible for pseudoanemia (Figure 83.1). Biologically, women have hemoglobin values at one standard deviation below the mean, but the value should always be above 10.5 g/dl.[16] Hematocrit can physiologically go as low as 33%.[17] The increase in red blood cell mass starts, or is detectable, later than plasma volume, by the end of the first trimester. Twin pregnancy is responsible for an increase in total red blood cell mass, but is not as proportional to weight gain as in singleton pregnancy. This increase in erythropoiesis is probably influenced by placental secretion of placental chorionic somatomammotropin, progesterone, or prolactin.[18] This increase in erythropoiesis increases maternal needs for iron by about 500 mg.[18] Moreover, maternal hemoglobin, by an increase in 2,3-diphosphoglycerate concentrations in red blood cells, has less affinity for oxygen to facilitate dissociation across the placenta to the fetus.[19]

This hemodilution, as a result of a greater increase in plasma volume than total red blood cell mass, has beneficial effects:

- It limits hemoglobin loss in cases of prepartum or postpartum hemorrhage
- It facilitates heart function by limiting blood viscosity
- It facilitates placental microcirculation by limiting blood viscosity
- It facilitates venous circulation to limit thromboembolic events[16,20]
- It limits impaired venous return, reduction in cardiac output, and hypotension in the supine position.

Heart anatomical changes

Ventricles

End-diastolic ventricular volume and ventricular mass increase throughout pregnancy. These modifications, which include anatomical modification of the maternal heart during pregnancy, take place without end-systolic volume or end-diastolic pressure increasing.[21,22] The combination of increasing end-diastolic ventricular volume and stable end-systolic volumes and end-diastolic pressure are the consequences of an increased compliance of the myocardium. It is not clear when cardiac compliance starts to increase during pregnancy.

Ventricular mass increases as soon as the first trimester[23] and the end-diastolic volume increase is detectable only in the second trimester,[21] and although the changes are not detected at the same moment, they are part of a continuum.

Atria

Left atrial diameter increases during pregnancy to reach a plateau at around 30 weeks.[24] Left atrial diameter is related to vascular filling. The increase in left atrial diameter during pregnancy is in relation with physiologic plasma volume expansion.

Vessels

Changes are observed in large vessels during pregnancy. Aortic compliance increases, which, combined with decreasing vascular tone, results in lower afterload and enhanced left ventricular performance.[25] Venous distensibility increases throughout pregnancy from the first trimester.[26] Increasing capacity of the venous system is essential to the physiological adaptation to plasma volume increase. It allows stability in venous pressure and protects the right heart from too high preload pressure. The fall in vascular resistance occurs at the same time as increasing compliance of large arteries and veins as early as the fifth week of gestation.[27] The causal relation between increased vascular compliance, fall in vascular resistance, physiologic plasma volume expansion, and increasing cardiac output during pregnancy are yet to be determined.

Cardiac output

Cardiac function was initially studied using invasive techniques. It has even been used in term pregnancies more recently.[28] Echocardiography combined with pulse- or continuous-wave Doppler measurements of cardiac output was validated against invasive techniques in non-pregnant patients.[29] These techniques were later validated in pregnant women.[30,31] Since then, most available data collected have used non-invasive techniques.

Cardiac output depends on heart rate and stroke volume. Stroke volume increases throughout pregnancy as demonstrated by the mid-20th-century invasive procedures and more recent non-invasive ultrasound examinations.[32–34] The major causes responsible for stroke volume increase are:

- A moderate increase in preload and greater venous return
- A decreased afterload, increased arterial compliance, and fall in vascular resistance
- An increased cardiac compliance and an intrinsic myocardial contractility increase that is independent of loading conditions.[35]

Cardiac output increases by 30–50% during pregnancy.[28,30,32–35] The increase in cardiac output is detectable as early as the fifth week of gestation. Early in pregnancy, the cardiac output increase is mostly the result of a stroke volume increase.[33,36] Heart rate increase occurs later in pregnancy and contributes, then, to the increase in cardiac output observed in the second half of pregnancy[33,37] (Figure 83.1).

Caval syndrome in pregnancy was described by Holmes in 1960.[38] Maternal position influences hemodynamics. When in the supine position, the uterus compresses the inferior vena cava, affecting venous return to the right atrium. The reduction in preload affects all hemodynamic parameters. Ueland *et al.* compared stroke volume, heart rate, and cardiac output at three different intervals in pregnancy, 20–24 weeks, 28–32 weeks, and 38–40 weeks.[39] They performed their measurements in the supine, lateral decubitus, and sitting position. Their main findings were:

- In the lateral decubitus, there is a fall in cardiac output by the end of the third trimester, as a result of the fall in stroke volume.
- In the supine position, cardiac output values at the very end of pregnancies are lower than non-pregnant values, as a result of a major fall in stroke volume partly compensated by an increase in heart rate.

Evolution of cardiac output in late pregnancy was not clearly described in the literature. This issue seems settled by the work of Clark *et al.* in 1989.[28] In a study on 10 healthy singleton pregnant patients between 36 and 38 weeks of gestation, using invasive central hemodynamic assessment, they found a 44% increase in cardiac output, with a 17% increase in heart rate and 27% increase in stroke volume.[28] They concluded that cardiac output does not fall in late pregnancy. Therefore, the variations in cardiac output measurements in late pregnancy observed in older studies were probably related to maternal positioning during measurements.

Blood pressure

Arterial blood pressure

Arterial blood pressure declines from the seventh week.[36]

Using 24-h mean blood pressure measurements in normal pregnancies, Ayala *et al.* found a steady decrease of systolic blood pressure, diastolic blood pressure, and mean arterial pressure up to the 21st week of gestation, followed by an increase to near non-pregnant values by the end of pregnancy[40]

(Figure 83.1). When the circadian variations of blood pressure were studied, the lowest pressures were measured at 4–5 h, and the highest at 12–21 h.[41] The magnitude of the difference between the highest and the lowest blood pressure within the same circadian period is maximal in the second trimester. These modifications in blood pressure are influenced by maternal age, but not by parity.[42]

Vascular systemic resistance

The total vascular resistance drop early in pregnancy is probably due to the low-resistance placental vascularization. It seems actually to be the first parameter to be significantly modified in early pregnancy.[43] Duvekot *et al.* performed serial weekly measurements from 5 to 8 weeks of gestation. They unfortunately did not have non-pregnant values and compared the results with the 5 weeks' gestation data. It is not clear if this drop in total vascular resistance, due to the placental low-resistance effect on the maternal circulation, is a cause or a consequence of plasma expansion and hyperaldosteronism. The only significant changes observed from the sixth to the eighth week of gestation compared to the fifth week were a rise in plasma 17-estradiol and a drop in plasma 17β-hydroxyprogesterone. Interestingly, Walters and Lim described in 1969 a fall in total vascular resistance when estro-progestative contraceptives were given to women.[15] The total vascular resistance remains low throughout pregnancy and is still 21% lower than non-pregnant values at 36–38 weeks of gestation.[28]

Conclusion

Pregnancy is characterized by early modifications in most hemodynamic parameters. These modifications are a consequence of normal adaptation to pregnancy and serve as control values for inadequate adaptation of pathologic pregnancies.

REFERENCES

1. Pritchard JA. Changes in the blood volume during pregnancy and delivery. *Anesthesiology* 1965;26:393–9.
2. Lund CJ, Donovan JC. Blood volume during pregnancy. Significance of plasma and red cell volumes. *Am J Obstet Gynecol* 1967;98:394–403.
3. Pritchard JA, Rowland RC. Blood volume changes in pregnancy and the puerperium. III. Whole body and large vessel hematocrits in pregnant and nonpregnant women. *Am J Obstet Gynecol* 1964; 88:391–5.
4. Adams JQ. Cardiovascular physiology in normal pregnancy: Studies with the dye dilution technique. *Am J Obstet Gynecol* 1954;67:741–59.
5. Pirani BB, Campbell DM, MacGillivray I. Plasma volume in normal first pregnancy. *J Obstet Gynaecol Br Commonw* 1973; 80:884–7.
6. Rovinsky JJ, Jaffin H. Cardiovascular hemodynamics in pregnancy. I. Blood and plasma volumes in multiple pregnancy. *Am J Obstet Gynecol* 1965;93:1–15.
7. MacGillivray I, Campbell D, Duffus GM. Maternal metabolic response to twin pregnancy in primigravidae. *J Obstet Gynaecol Br Commonw* 1971;78:530–4.
8. Thomsen JK, Fogh-Andersen N, Jaszczak P. Atrial natriuretic peptide, blood volume, aldosterone, and sodium excretion during twin pregnancy. *Acta Obstet Gynecol Scand* 1994;73:14–20.
9. Pritchard JA. Blood volume changes in pregnancy and the puerperium. IV. Anemia associated with hydatidiform mole. *Am J Obstet Gynecol* 1965;91:621–9.
10. Salas SP, Rosso P, Espinoza R, Robert JA, Valdes G, Donoso E. Maternal plasma volume expansion and hormonal changes in women with idiopathic fetal growth retardation. *Obstet Gynecol* 1993;81:1029–33.
11. Duvekot JJ, Cheriex EC, Pieters FA, Peeters LL. Severely impaired fetal growth is preceded by maternal hemodynamic maladaptation in very early pregnancy. *Acta Obstet Gynecol Scand* 1995; 74:693–7.
12. Brown MA, Gallery ED. Volume homeostasis in normal pregnancy and pre-eclampsia: Physiology and clinical implications. *Baillieres Clin Obstet Gynaecol* 1994;8:287–310.
13. Biglieri EG, Forsham PH. Studies on the expanded extracellular fluid and the responses to various stimuli in primary aldosteronism. *Am J Med* 1961;30:564–76.
14. Luotola H, Pyorala T, Lahteenmaki P, Toivanen J. Haemodynamic and hormonal effects of short-term oestradiol treatment in postmenopausal women. *Maturitas* 1979;1:287–94.
15. Walters WA, Lim YL. Cardiovascular dynamics in women receiving oral contraceptive therapy. *Lancet* 1969;2:879–81.
16. Koller O. The clinical significance of hemodilution during pregnancy. *Obstet Gynecol Surv* 1982;37:649–52.
17. Pitkin RM. Nutritional support in obstetrics and gynecology. *Clin Obstet Gynecol* 1976;19:489–513.
18. Jepson JH, Lowenstein L. Role of erythropoietin and placental lactogen in the control of erythropoiesis during pregnancy. *Can J Physiol Pharmacol* 1968;46:573–6.
19. Bille-Brahe NE, Rorth M. Red cell 2,3-diphosphoglycerate in pregnancy. *Acta Obstet Gynecol Scand* 1979;58:19–21.
20. Peeters LL, Verkeste CM, Saxena PR, Wallenburg HC. Relationship between maternal hemodynamics and hematocrit and hemodynamic effects of isovolemic hemodilution and hemoconcentration in the awake late-pregnant guinea pig. *Pediatr Res* 1987;21:584–9.
21. Rubler S, Damani PM, Pinto ER. Cardiac size and performance during pregnancy estimated with echocardiography. *Am J Cardiol* 1977;40:534–40.
22. Laird-Meeter K, van de Ley G, Bom TH, Wladimiroff JW, Roelandt J. Cardiocirculatory adjustments during pregnancy – An echocardiographic study. *Clin Cardiol* 1979;2:328–32.
23. Thompson JA, Hays PM, Sagar KB, Cruikshank DP. Echocardiographic left ventricular mass to differentiate chronic hypertension from preeclampsia during pregnancy. *Am J Obstet Gynecol* 1986; 155:994–9.
24. Vered Z, Poler SM, Gibson P, Wlody D, Perez JE. Noninvasive detection of the morphologic and hemodynamic changes during normal pregnancy. *Clin Cardiol* 1991;14:327–34.
25. Hart MV, Morton MJ, Hosenpud JD, Metcalfe J. Aortic function during normal human pregnancy. *Am J Obstet Gynecol* 1986; 154:887–91.
26. Sakai K, Imaizumi T, Maeda H, *et al.* Venous distensibility during pregnancy. Comparisons between normal pregnancy and preeclampsia. *Hypertension* 1994;24:461–6.
27. Spaanderman ME, Willekes C, Hoeks AP, Ekhart TH, Peeters LL. The effect of pregnancy on the compliance of large arteries and veins in healthy parous control subjects and women with a history of preeclampsia. *Am J Obstet Gynecol* 2000;183:1278–86.
28. Clark SL, Cotton DB, Lee W, *et al.* Central hemodynamic assessment of normal term pregnancy. *Am J Obstet Gynecol* 1989;161:1439–42.
29. Loeppky JA, Hoekenga DE, Greene ER, Luft UC. Comparison of noninvasive pulsed Doppler and Fick measurements of stroke volume in cardiac patients. *Am Heart J* 1984;107:339–46.
30. Easterling TR, Carlson KL, Schmucker BC, Brateng DA, Benedetti TJ. Measurement of cardiac output in pregnancy by Doppler technique. *Am J Perinatol* 1990;7:220–2.
31. Easterling TR, Watts DH, Schmucker BC, Benedetti TJ. Measurement of cardiac output during pregnancy: Validation of

Doppler technique and clinical observations in preeclampsia. *Obstet Gynecol* 1987;69:845–50.

32. Bader RA, Bader ME, Rose DF, Braunwald E. Hemodynamics at rest and during exercise in normal pregnancy as studies by cardiac catheterization. *J Clin Invest* 1955;34:1524–36.
33. Robson SC, Hunter S, Boys RJ, Dunlop W. Serial study of factors influencing changes in cardiac output during human pregnancy. *Am J Physiol* 1989;256:H1060–5.
34. Walters WA, MacGregor WG, Hills M. Cardiac output at rest during pregnancy and the puerperium. *Clin Sci* 1966;30:1–11.
35. Gilson GJ, Samaan S, Crawford MH, Qualls CR, Curet LB. Changes in hemodynamics, ventricular remodeling, and ventricular contractility during normal pregnancy: A longitudinal study. *Obstet Gynecol* 1997;89:957–62.
36. Capeless EL, Clapp JF. Cardiovascular changes in early phase of pregnancy. *Am J Obstet Gynecol* 1989;161:1449–53.
37. Mabie WC, DiSessa TG, Crocker LG, Sibai BM, Arheart KL. A longitudinal study of cardiac output in normal human pregnancy. *Am J Obstet Gynecol* 1994;170:849–56.
38. Holmes F. The supine hypotensive syndrome. Its importance to the anaesthetist. *Anaesthesia* 1960;15:298–306.
39. Ueland K, Novy MJ, Peterson EN, Metcalfe J. Maternal cardiovascular dynamics. IV. The influence of gestational age on the maternal cardiovascular response to posture and exercise. *Am J Obstet Gynecol* 1969;104:856–64.
40. Ayala DE, Hermida RC, Mojon A, *et al.* Blood pressure variability during gestation in healthy and complicated pregnancies. *Hypertension* 1997;30:611–8.
41. Hermida RC, Ayala DE, Mojon A, *et al.* Blood pressure patterns in normal pregnancy, gestational hypertension, and preeclampsia. *Hypertension* 2000;36:149–58.
42. Ayala DE, Hermida RC. Influence of parity and age on ambulatory monitored blood pressure during pregnancy. *Hypertension* 2001; 38:753–8.
43. Duvekot JJ, Cheriex EC, Pieters FA, Menheere PP, Peeters LH. Early pregnancy changes in hemodynamics and volume homeostasis are consecutive adjustments triggered by a primary fall in systemic vascular tone. *Am J Obstet Gynecol* 1993;169:1382–92.

84 Pathophysiology of pre-eclampsia

T. Podymow, P. August and D. Skupski

Pre-eclampsia is a hypertensive condition unique to pregnancy with both maternal and fetal manifestations. The maternal disease is characterized by vasospasm, endothelial dysfunction, activation of the coagulation system and high blood pressure. The maternal pathophysiologic changes are mainly ischemic, affecting the vasculature of the placenta, kidney, liver and brain. Pre-eclampsia is diagnosed in a woman with new onset of hypertension >140/90 mmHg after the 20th gestational week accompanied by proteinuria >300 mg/day. Other common clinical and laboratory abnormalities include facial and peripheral edema, thrombocytopenia, elevated uric acid levels (greater than 5.5 mg/dl or 327 mmol/L) and elevated transaminase levels (greater than twice the normal). The greatest concern is that pre-eclampsia can progress to eclampsia, which is life-threatening convulsions associated with cerebral hemorrhage, or to hemolysis, elevated liver enzymes and low platelets (HELLP) syndrome. Eclampsia is frequently preceded by severe headaches, visual disturbance (halos or auras) and hyper-reflexia, while HELLP syndrome is frequently preceded by right upper quadrant or epigastric pain. The consequences of pre-eclampsia for the fetus are a result of decreased placental perfusion and include intrauterine growth restriction and fetal loss. Delivery is the only definitive cure of pre-eclampsia/eclampsia, and in order to prevent serious maternal complications premature delivery is often necessary; as such hypertensive disorders in pregnancy are the leading cause of indicated premature delivery. In this chapter, the pathophysiology of pre-eclampsia and the pathogenesis of these manifestations will be examined.

Pathophysiology

The pathophysiology of pre-eclampsia has been described divided into two stages:[1] alterations in placental perfusion (stage 1) and the maternal syndrome (stage 2).

Placenta – Stage I

The pathophysiology of pre-eclampsia begins with abnormalities in the development of the placenta, leading to the production of abnormal vasculogenic substances, which upon reaching the maternal circulation produce the maternal clinical syndrome. There is considerable evidence for the importance of the placenta in the pathogenesis of pre-eclampsia; pre-eclampsia can develop without a fetus in the case of molar pregnancies (a rapidly growing placenta with trophoblastic tissue) and in multiple gestations (increased placental mass). There are also case reports of twin pregnancies where pre-eclampsia is reversed upon termination of the severely growth-restricted twin and involution of the pathologic placenta.[2]

In normal gestation, the uterine artery's terminal branches, the spiral arteries, invade the placenta and are transformed from muscular arteries into relaxed flaccid vessels to accommodate an eventual 10-fold increase in uterine blood flow. This transformation is dependent on the placental trophoblasts that invade and surround the uterine spiral artery's vascular walls.[3] The placental trophoblasts, normally epithelial cells, replace their adhesion molecules with those of endothelial cells to assume vascular endothelial cell phenotype prior to invading the uterine arteries,[4] a process termed pseudovasculogenesis. This vascular remodeling results in increased blood flow and supply of nutrients and oxygen to the fetus by the end of the first trimester. In pre-eclampsia, pseudovasculogenesis is defective; cytotrophoblast invasion from the placenta is shallow, the arteries remain small and muscular[5] and the ensuing placental ischemia is thought to trigger the release of placenta-derived factors (Figure 84.1). Of considerable interest is the increased incidence of pre-eclampsia in women with medical conditions associated with microvascular disease such as hypertension, diabetes and collagen vascular disease, as the impaired placental perfusion leading to ischemia may be the common source of this disease.[1]

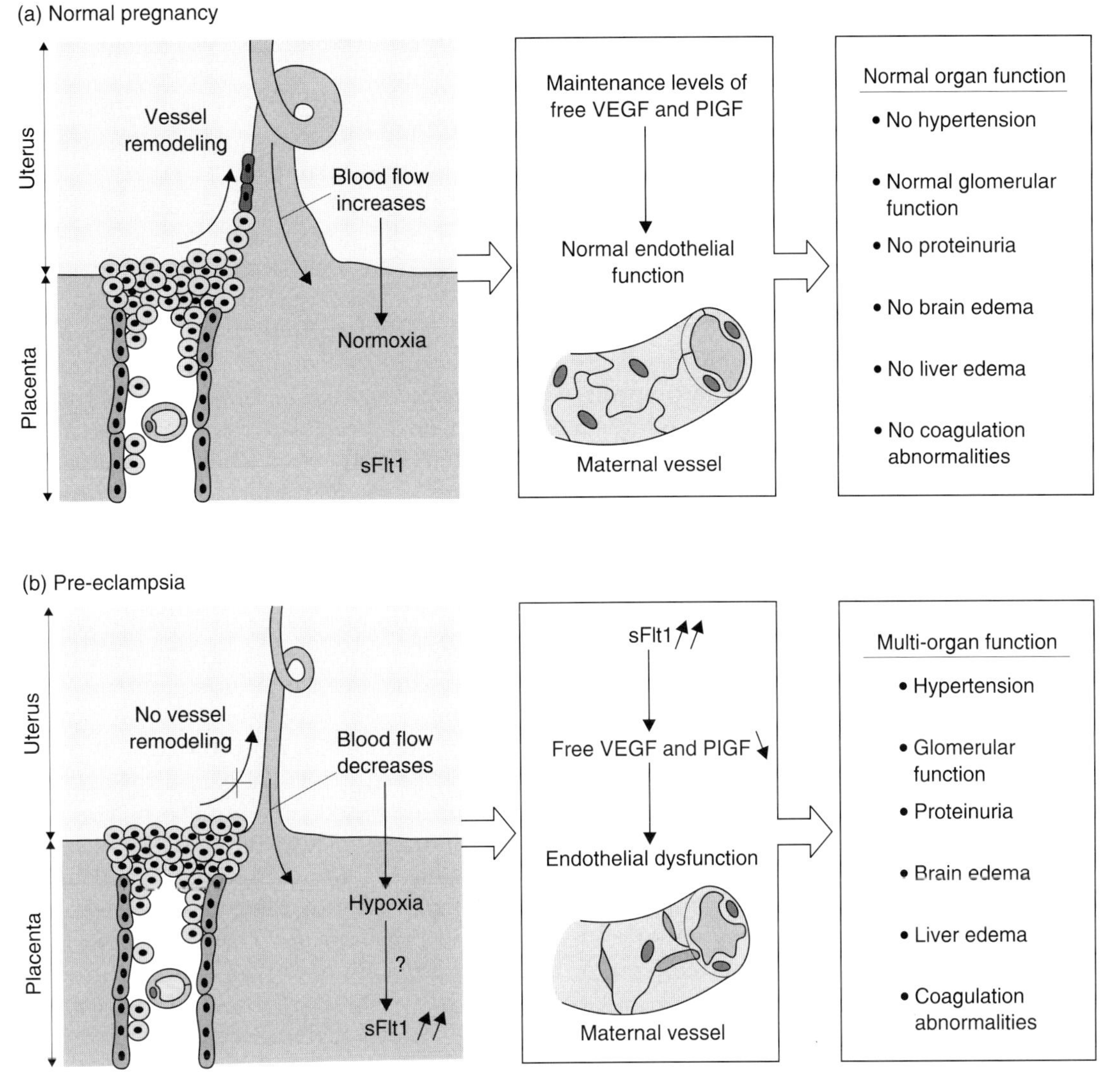

Figure 84.1 Hypothesis on the role of sFlt-1 in pre-eclampsia. (a) During normal pregnancy, the uterine spiral arteries are infiltrated and remodeled by endovascular invasive trophoblasts, thereby increasing blood flow significantly in order to meet the oxygen and nutrient demands of the fetus. (b) In the placenta of pre-eclamptic women, trophoblast invasion does not occur and blood flow is reduced, resulting in placental hypoxia. In addition, increased amounts of soluble Flt1 (sFlt-1) are produced by the placenta and scavenge VEGF and PlGF, thereby lowering circulating levels of unbound VEGF and PlGF. This altered balance causes generalized endothelial dysfunction, resulting in multi-organ disease. It remains unknown whether hypoxia is the trigger for stimulating sFlt-1 secretion in the placenta of pre-eclamptic mothers and whether the higher sFlt-1 levels interfere with trophoblast invasion and spiral artery remodeling. Adapted from Luttun and Carmeliet[8] with permission.

The idea that impaired placental perfusion leads to release of 'factors' into the maternal circulation to cause the clinical manifestations of pre-eclampsia is not new, although the precise nature of these 'factors' awaits ultimate description. The placenta-derived pre-eclampsia factors causing systemic endothelial dysfunction have for decades been elusive. Maynard *et al.* have reported that angiogenic proteins such as placental growth factor (PlGF) and vascular endothelial growth factor (VEGF) are both required for normal angiogenesis and endothelial function in pregnancy, and are reduced in women with pre-eclampsia. Recent studies report elevated maternal serum levels of a protein, which in pre-eclampsia appears to scavenge these factors and induce endothelial dysfunction: a soluble fms-like tyrosine kinase 1 (sFlt-1) (also called soluble vascular endothelial growth factor receptor 1, sVEGFR-1). This molecule is a circulating modified VEGF receptor, whose function is to neutralize VEGF and PlGF, and is found in excess quantities in both the placenta and the serum of pre-eclamptic women[6,7]. When administered to pregnant rats, sFlt-1 has been shown to induce a pre-eclampsia-like phenotype with albuminuria, hypertension and renal pathologic changes of glomerular endotheliosis.[6] In human studies, increased serum levels of sFlt-1 and reduced levels of PlGF have been found to predict the subsequent development of pre-eclampsia,[7] and decreased urinary PlGF in the early second trimester is strongly associated with subsequent early development of pre-eclampsia.[9] The mechanism for the upregulation of sFlt-1 and whether normalization of VEGF and PlGF levels might halt progression of pre-eclampsia are yet unknown.

Other factors that may be derived from the placenta and are postulated to be related to pre-eclampsia are substances that increase oxidant stress, leptin and a variety of cytokines including tumor necrosis factor α. Oxidative stress due to hypoxia-driven free-radical generation at the fetal–maternal interface has been suggested as a cause of pre-eclampsia. The by-products of increased oxidative stress, possibly released by the placenta in response to hypoxia or ischemia, have been implicated in endothelial cell damage in pre-eclampsia.[10,11] Small studies using antioxidants to prevent pre-eclampsia have been encouraging and vitamins E and C are under study in larger trials to determine their potential role in prevention.[12]

Pathologically, the lesion of the placenta in pre-eclampsia is termed acute atherosis and is characterized by an accumulation of fat-laden macrophages and infiltrates in the arteries not invaded by trophoblast cells. In a study of 400 placentas from pre-eclamptic women, vascular lesions in the placenta correlated with the severity of clinical disease.[13] Pre-eclampsia is also associated with a greater degree of placental infarction than in normal gestation; however, the placenta has considerable reserve, explaining why some infants are growth-restricted or die but more often are normal for gestational age.

Pathophysiology of the maternal syndrome of pre-eclampsia – Stage II

Blood pressure in pre-eclampsia

High blood pressure in pre-eclampsia is due mainly to a reversal of the vasodilatation of normal pregnancy, replaced by a marked increase in peripheral vascular resistance.[14] Pre-eclamptics do not develop overt hypertension until late gestation (after 20 weeks, and usually not until the third trimester), but vasoconstrictor influences may be present much earlier. For instance, longitudinal and epidemiologic surveys show that women destined to develop pre-eclampsia have slightly higher 'normal' blood pressure (e.g. diastolic levels >70 mmHg) as early as the second trimester.[15–17]

The precise mechanism of pre-eclamptic hypertension is obscure. During normal pregnancy the renin–angiotensin system is stimulated, most likely in response to vasodilatation and lower blood pressure. In contrast with normal pregnancy, women with pre-eclampsia have suppressed plasma renin activity, aldosterone, urinary aldosterone excretion and angiotensin II levels. There is evidence that the renin–angiotensin system is stimulated early in pregnancy in women who later develop pre-eclampsia and that the developing vasoconstriction and hypertension turn off renin secretion. This decrease in renin has been used as a screening test to identify gravidas in midgestation who are at risk for the development of pre-eclampsia.[18]

Blood pressure in pre-eclampsia is also characteristically labile, and exaggerated responses to norepinephrine and angiotensin despite normal plasma levels have been noted.[19] There is a reversal of the normal circadian rhythm, with blood pressures often being higher at night.[20] In addition, increases in peripheral vascular resistance and blood pressure that characterize pre-eclampsia have been found to be mediated partly by a substantial increase in sympathetic vasoconstrictor activity, which reverts to normal after delivery.[21] These observations lend mechanistic support for the use of methyldopa, which is metabolized to α-methylnorepinephrine and replaces norepinephrine to decrease sympathetic tone centrally.

Changes in eicosanoid metabolism occur in normal pregnancy, particularly prostacyclin (PGI_2) and thromboxane (TXA_2) production, and further alterations arise in pre-eclampsia. Prostaglandins such as PGI_2 are increased in normal pregnancy, particularly vasodilatory prostanoids (mostly PGI_2) by vascular endothelial cells,[22] and this may contribute to the generalized vasodilatation characteristic of pregnancy. Reduced PGI_2, but not TXA_2, has been found to occur months before the clinical onset of pre-eclampsia.[23,24] There is substantial literature suggesting that alterations in prostaglandin metabolism underlie the pathogenesis of pre-eclampsia.[22–26] Manifestations such as increments in vascular reactivity and blood pressure, as well as intravascular coagulation, have been proposed to be due to an imbalance between PGI_2 and TXA_2 synthesis, resulting in a relative or absolute PGI_2 deficiency. These findings are consistent with evidence that pre-eclampsia is characterized by generalized vascular endothelial cell dysfunction, leading to diminished production of PGI_2, as well as other vasodilatory endothelial cell products.

In spite of the large body of evidence supporting a role for alterations in prostaglandin metabolism in pre-eclampsia, it is important to emphasize that these substances are difficult to measure, and act locally, so measurements from peripheral blood may not reflect local effects. Nevertheless, the notion that pre-eclampsia is characterized by a deficiency of PGI_2 with stable or increased TXA_2 production has been the basis of several large multicenter randomized trials evaluating low-dose aspirin (which inhibits platelet TXA_2 generation but spares vascular PGI_2 production) in the prevention of pre-eclampsia. Despite early, relatively small studies that reported striking reductions in the risk of pre-eclampsia in women treated with low-dose aspirin, a recent Cochrane review including data from 36,500 women did not reveal the overall beneficial effect of aspirin on pregnancy outcome.[27]

Endothelial cell function

In recent years, the role of the vascular endothelial cells in the modulation of vascular smooth muscle contractile activity, as well as in coagulation and regulation of blood flow, has increased the understanding of endothelial cell function in the pathophysiology of pre-eclampsia and other chronic cardiovascular conditions, such as atherosclerosis and essential hypertesion. Endothelial cells, which have receptors for numerous vasodilators and constrictors, produce hormones, autacoids, and mitogenic cytokines, including PGI_2, nitric oxide and endothelin. The pathophysiologic changes of pre-eclampsia, particularly those present before clinically apparent disease, support the hypothesis that altered endothelial function contributes to many of the changes observed in the pre-eclamptic syndrome.[28] Women with pre-eclampsia manifest increased circulating markers of endothelial activation (von Willibrand Factor, cellular fibronectin, thrombomodulin, endothelin, V-CAM).[29] Pre-eclamptic blood vessels demonstrate reduced endothelial-mediated vasodilation *in vitro*,[29] and *in vivo* studies have shown that flow-mediated (endothelium-dependent) dilatation is impaired in women with previous pre-eclampsia.[26] Most recently, raised plasma concentrations of asymmetric dimethylarginine (ADMA), the endogenous inhibitor of endothelial nitric oxide synthase, has been shown to be elevated in women with evidence of abnormal endothelial function prior to the development of pre-eclampsia.[30]

There are numerous reports of a hypertensive syndrome produced by inhibiting nitric oxide synthase in various experimental models of gestation, with some features similar to human pre-eclampsia.[31,32] Results from women with pre-eclampsia are conflicting, with reports of increased as well as decreased serum and urinary metabolites of nitric oxide in pre-eclampsia.[33–35]

Endothelins represent other vasoconstrictors postulated to play a role in pre-eclampsia.[36–39] In this respect, circulating levels of endothelin-1 are generally (but not universally) reported as increased in this disorder, but it is unclear if such levels have pathogenic significance or are a by-product of endothelial damage.

The evidence for endothelial cell dysfunction in the pathogenesis of the maternal manifestations of pre-eclampsia is strong, and its cause continues to be actively investigated. As mentioned, circulating factors of placental origin, e.g. sFlt-1, are likely involved. Indeed, sera from women destined to develop pre-eclampsia have the capacity to alter endothelial cell function or cause endothelial cell activation *in vitro* (assessed by nitric oxide and PGI_2 generation).[40] Sera from pre-eclamptic patients are also mitogenic and increase messenger RNA for, as well as production of, the platelet-derived growth factor β in culture.[41] There is also a growing body of evidence implicating increased lipid peroxides as well as by-products of increased oxidative stress, possibly released by the placenta in response to hypoxia or ischemia, in the genesis of endothelial cell damage in pre-eclampsia.[10,42–44]

Metabolic disturbances in pre-eclampsia

Hyperinsulinemia, obesity, glucose intolerance and dyslipidemia (e.g. increased triglycerides, reduced high-density lipoproteins) are associated with cardiovascular disease and essential hypertension. Insulin resistance and hyperinsulinemia (mediated by hormonal changes) are also characteristic of normal pregnancy, and are maximal in the third trimester.[45] Several laboratories have reported exaggerated metabolic disturbances in patients with pre-eclampsia, including hypertriglyceridemia, increased levels of free fatty acids, decreased levels of lipoprotein a, increased insulin levels, and glucose intolerance.[46–50] These observations are intriguing, particularly because they may be related to the evidence for increased oxidative stress in pre-eclampsia (lipid abnormalities may result in increased oxidative stress.

Obesity remains an important risk factor for pre-eclampsia, with strong positive association between maternal prepregnancy body mass index and the risk of pre-eclampsia.[51] Early pregnancy dyslipidemia[52] and gestational diabetes[53] are also associated with an increased two- to threefold risks of pre-eclampsia. At this time it is uncertain if these are the cause or markers for endothelial dysfunction, or if they may represent oxidative stress in pre-eclampsia.

Cardiac function in pre-eclampsia

Blood pressure normally declines in early pregnancy, systolic pressure changes little, while diastolic pressure falls by 10 mmHg at 13–20 weeks and then rises again to prepregnancy levels in the third trimester. Normal pregnancy is characterized by primary vasodilatation and increased cardiac output is due in part to the decreased afterload. As noted, high blood pressure in pre-eclampsia is due mainly to a reversal of the vasodilatation of normal pregnancy, replaced by marked increases in peripheral vascular resistance. Most studies of cardiovascular hemodynamics in women with pre-eclampsia have been performed in women with established disease and may be confounded by ongoing treatment. Invasive hemodynamic monitoring of untreated pre-eclamptics as well as limited careful echocardiographic studies demonstrate that women with pre-eclampsia have either normal or slightly decreased cardiac output in association with increased systemic vascular resistance and increased afterload. Serial echocardiographic studies throughout gestation have shown that in women who eventually developed pre-eclampsia, increased cardiac output and decreased peripheral vascular resistance were found early in pregnancy followed by high-resistance low cardiac output states when pre-eclampsia developed.[54] Other studies of nulliparous gravidas with pre-eclampsia in the third trimester using pulmonary artery catheter, show decreased cardiac output in pre-eclamptic patients compared with controls.[14,55] Peripheral vascular resistance was increased and pulmonary capillary wedge pressure was below normal. This has been confirmed in other studies, and amounts to a normal ventricle contracting normally against a markedly increased afterload.[56] Peripartum heart failure can occur in this setting, though it is usually a complication of pre-existing heart disease.[57]

Plasma volume and red blood cell mass are increased in normal pregnancy, as physiologic vasodilatation leads to stimulation of the renin–angiotensin system, and volume retention ensues. In pre-eclampsia, however, plasma volume is decreased, which is documented by measurement with Evans blue dye.[58,59] The decrease in plasma volume may be secondary to vasoconstriction and hypertension, although there are some reports that decreases in plasma volume may precede hypertension.[58,60,61] These latter reports have led to the use of volume expansion therapy with vasodilator drugs in the treatment of pre-eclampsia. In view of the suppressed renin–angiotensin system in pre-eclampsia, the decreased plasma volume seems likely secondary to vasoconstriction and a 'smaller' intravascular compartment. Reports that the decreased plasma volume may have preceded hypertension[61] led to the experimental use of volume expansion therapy, although in Cochrane analysis, this treatment remains unproven.[62]

Renal changes in pre-eclampsia

Consistent with the effects of pre-eclampsia on the endothelium, the renal lesion characteristic of pre-eclampsia is glomerular endotheliosis.[19,63,64] The glomeruli are enlarged and swollen but not hypercellular, due primarily to hypertrophy of the intracapillary cells (mainly endothelial but mesangial as well), which encroach on the capillary lumina, giving the appearance of a bloodless glomerulus. The basement membrane is usually not thickened and foot processes are usually well preserved, even when severe proteinuria is present. Interestingly, sFlt-1, which is elevated in women with pre-eclampsia, has been administered to pregnant rats and induces hypertension, proteinuria and glomerular endotheliosis, the classic lesion of pre-eclampsia.[6] Similarly, these renal alterations are also observed in experimental models that are characterized by reduced VEGF levels in the case of VEGF knockout mice.[65]

Localized lesions resembling those of focal and segmental glomerulosclerosis (FSGS) are present in about 20% of women with pre-eclampsia. The significance of this finding is not clear; some consider it to be a sequelae of pre-eclampsia, a form of secondary FSGS, whereas others consider that it may be a manifestation of pre-existing subclinical nephrosclerosis.

In pre-eclampsia, both glomerular filtration rate and renal blood flow decrease, the former more so than the latter, leading to a decrease in filtration fraction.[19] The decrement is usually modest (25%) even when morphologic changes are pronounced. Because renal function normally rises 35–50% during pregnancy, creatinine levels are usually still below the upper limits of normal. The basis for the altered renal hemodynamics is not certain and renal histological and hormonal changes are probably involved. Recent evidence suggests that the hormone relaxin, a natural vasodilator produced by the corpus luteum and placenta, is reduced in women with pre-eclampsia and may contribute to the renal changes observed.[66,67] Fractional urate clearances decrease, often before overt disease is apparent, with a uric acid level greater than 5.5 mg/dl (327 mmol/L) being an important marker of pre-eclampsia. This appears to be a sensitive marker of decreased renal clearance and glomerular filtration. Proteinuria > 0.3 g/day (but in some cases nephrotic range, i.e. > 3 g/day), is another hallmark that may appear late in the clinical course of the disease. Rarely, renal insufficiency may develop due to acute tubular or cortical necrosis associated with pre-eclampsia.[68]

Sodium excretion appears to be impaired in pre-eclampsia, documented in studies of renal excretory ability after saline infusion,[69] though the reduction in intravascular volume and decreased placental perfusion are major reasons to avoid diuretics in pre-eclampsia.[19] Renal handling of calcium is also abnormal in pre-eclampsia, with hypocalciuria, low plasma 1,25-dihydroxyvitamin D3 and high parathyroid hormone noted.[70,71]

Coagulation system

Pregnancy is associated with an increase in hemostatic factors and decrease in fibrinolytic proteins; factors II, VII, X, VIII, XII and fibrinogen increase 20–200% whereas the fibrinolytic protein S has a 40% decrease during pregnancy.[72] The inherited coagulopathies are major causes of thromboembolic disease in both pregnant and non-pregnant individuals; the most common are autosomal dominant deficiencies of antithrombin III, protein C, protein S, as well as activated protein C resistance due to the factor V Leiden mutation, and a function-enhancing mutation in the prothrombin gene (prothrombin G20210A) and hyperhomocystinemia. The pregnancy-associated changes in hemostatic and fibrinolytic proteins exacerbate the clinical effect of heritable coagulopathies. A postulated mechanism for pre-eclampsia in relation to the coagulopathies is the development of microthrombi in the placental circulation, with decreased placental perfusion leading to pre-eclampsia, hypertension and proteinuria.[73] Factor V Leiden mutation is the most common heritable coagulopathy, affecting 5–9% of European populations, though it is rare in Asian and African populations.[74,75] A recent meta-analysis suggests that factor V Leiden is associated with a twofold increased risk for pre-eclampsia.[76] The risk of the prothrombin 202210 polymorphism though suggestive as a risk factor is less clearly so, and the MTHFR genotype (leading to hyperhomocystinemia) does not appear to confer an increased risk.[76] Increased incidence of pregnancy-related complications including pre-eclampsia has been found for deficiencies in protein C, protein S, antithrombin III, but determination of the specific odds of developing pre-eclampsia with these thrombophilias is ongoing.[77] Clinically, some advocate screening for thrombophilias in women with early (< 34 weeks) or severe (> 160/110 mmHg) pre-eclampsia with consideration of heparin treatment in those found to be positive. Primary preventive treatment for women with known thrombophilic mutations but no clotting history is less certain until more trial data are available.

Falling platelet counts are a known manifestation of pre-eclampsia. The precise mechanism is unclear, but it appears that microangiopathy and endothelial cell damage stimulate platelet activation and consumption.[78,79] When severe, this may lead to disseminated intravascular coagulation.[80] Platelet activation may lead to increased generation of TXA_2, which may in turn increase vasoconstriction and platelet aggregation.[81] Increased release of platelet products such as serotonin may also contribute to vasoconstriction, and pharmacologic agents that inhibit serotonin such as ketanserin have been used successfully in the treatment of pre-eclampsia.[82]

Hepatic abnormalities

The liver dysfunction that may accompany pre-eclampsia is correlated to the histological findings, which include periportal hemorrhages, ischemic lesions and fibrin disposition. These are consistent with both endothelial damage and activation of the coagulation system leading to some amount of liver tissue edema or necrosis. Involvement may range from mild enzyme abnormalities to HELLP with markedly elevated transaminase levels, to subcapsular bleeding or hepatic rupture. HELLP syndrome is well described in the clinical literature[83] and requires the presence of hemolysis on peripheral smear and platelet counts below 100,000/mm^3 and transaminase levels greater than twice the normal for diagnosis. Liver involvement in pre-eclampsia generally signifies more serious disease and is associated with an increased risk of maternal complications compared to pre-eclampsia alone.[84]

Central nervous system

Eclampsia and seizures in pre-eclampsia that cannot be attributed to another cause are the most common central nervous system complication and are responsible for the most maternal deaths in this disease. In one small series, seizures were preceded by headache in 64% and by visual changes in 32%.[85] Visual disturbances include blurred vision, scotomas and, rarely, reversible cortical blindness (reversible posterior leukencephalopathy). In these cases, CT and MRI studies showed extensive bilateral white-matter abnormalities suggestive of vasogenic edema without infarction in the occipital and posterior parietal lobes of the cerebral hemispheres.[86,87]

Postmortem pathologic specimens of eclampsia reveal hemorrhages and petechiae, vasculopathy and ischemia with microinfarcts.[88] The cause of cerebral hemorrhage is debated; vasospasm, thrombosis and rupture have been postulated and transcranial Doppler studies document increased cerebral blood flow velocity consistent with vasospasm in women with pre-eclampsia and eclampsia.[89–91] Convulsions have been observed in women with only mild to moderate hypertension; the mechanisms for the seizures are not known, though by computed tomography and magnetic resonance imaging[92,93] cerebral edema has been described, as have hemorrhage and edema in the vascular watershed areas of the posterior hemispheres.[94] Predominance of posterior lesions may explain the increased incidence in pre-eclampsia–eclampsia of visual disturbances. Rarely, hemorrhages may be major and associated with permanent neurologic sequelae. Cerebral edema observed on some computed tomography studies may be a consequence of excess administration of fluids in patients with low oncotic pressure due to hypoalbuminemia. Rarely, reversible posterior leukoencephalopathy may develop in patients with eclampsia, which is transient blindness that resolves completely in most cases.[86] The findings on neuroimaging are characteristic of subcortical edema without infarction.

Long-term sequelae of pre-eclampsia

The pathophysiologic changes of pre-eclampsia appear to confer a long-term risk for cardiovascular disease in the mother. In an analysis of follow-up of over 30,000 hypertensive pregnant women, gestational hypertension, mild pre-eclampsia and severe pre-eclampsia were associated with 2.8-, 2.2- and 3.3-fold greater risks for premature cardiovascular events;[95] a magnitude of excess risk that is on par with smoking. Severe pre-eclampsia was also associated with a 2.3-fold greater risk for thromboembolic events[95] and in a separate study the rate ratio for later death from stroke for the pre-eclampsia/eclampsia group was 3.59.[96] Whether this is a result of permanent endothelial injury or if pre-eclampsia is a manifestation of an underlying predisposition to vascular disease is not known.

REFERENCES

1. Roberts JM, Pearson G, Cutler J, Lindheimer M. Summary of the NHLBI working group on research on hypertension during pregnancy. *Hypertension* 2003;41(3):437–45.
2. Heyborne KD, Porreco RP. Selective fetocide reverses preeclampsia in discordant twins. *Am J Obstet Gynecol* 2004;191(2): 477–80.
3. Pijnenborg R, Dixon G, Robertson WB, Brosens I. Trophoblastic invasion of human decidua from 8 to 18 weeks of pregnancy. *Placenta* 1980;1(1):3–19.
4. Zhou Y, Damsky CH, Chiu K, Roberts JM, Fisher SJ. Preeclampsia is associated with abnormal expression of adhesion molecules by invasive cytotrophoblasts. *J Clin Invest* 1993;91(3):950–60.
5. Brosens IA, Robertson WB, Dixon HG. The role of the spiral arteries in the pathogenesis of preeclampsia. *Obstet Gynecol Annu* 1972;1:177–91.
6. Maynard SE, Min JY, Merchan J, *et al.* Excess placental soluble fms-like tyrosine kinase 1 (sFlt1) may contribute to endothelial dysfunction, hypertension, and proteinuria in preeclampsia. *J Clin Invest* 2003;111(5):649–58.
7. Levine RJ, Maynard SE, Qian C, *et al.* Circulating angiogenic factors and the risk of preeclampsia. *N Engl J Med* 2004;350(7): 672–83.
8. Luttun A, Carmeliet P. Soluble VEGF receptor Flt1: The elusive preeclampsia factor discovered? *J Clin Invest* 2003;111:600–2.
9. Levine RJ, Thadhani R, Qian C, *et al.* Urinary placental growth factor and risk of preeclampsia. *J Am Med Assoc* 2005;293(1): 77–85.
10. Poranen AK, Ekblad U, Uotila P, Ahotupa M. Lipid peroxidation and antioxidants in normal and pre-eclamptic pregnancies. *Placenta* 1996;17(7):401–5.
11. Barden A, Ritchie J, Walters B, *et al.* Study of plasma factors associated with neutrophil activation and lipid peroxidation in preeclampsia. *Hypertension* 2001;38(4):803–8.
12. Roberts JM, Speer P. Antioxidant therapy to prevent preeclampsia. *Semin Nephrol* 2004;24(6):557–64.
13. Ghidini A, Salafia CM, Pezzullo JC. Placental vascular lesions and likelihood of diagnosis of preeclampsia. *Obstet Gynecol* 1997;90(4, Pt 1):542–5.
14. Visser W, Wallenburg HC. Central hemodynamic observations in untreated preeclamptic patients. *Hypertension* 1991;17(6, Pt 2): 1072–7.
15. Fallis NE, Langford HG. Relation of second trimester blood pressure to toxemia of pregnancy in the primigravid patient. *Am J Obstet Gynecol* 1963;87:123–5.
16. Page EW, Christianson R. The impact of mean arterial pressure in the middle trimester upon the outcome of pregnancy. *Am J Obstet Gynecol* 1976;125(6):740–6.
17. Kyle PM, Clark SJ, Buckley D, *et al.* Second trimester ambulatory blood pressure in nulliparous pregnancy: A useful screening test for pre-eclampsia? *Br J Obstet Gynaecol* 1993;100(10):914–9.
18. August P, Helseth G, Cook EF, Sison C. A prediction model for superimposed preeclampsia in women with chronic hypertension during pregnancy. *Am J Obstet Gynecol* 2004;191(5):1666–72.
19. Lindheimer M, Katz A. *Renal Physiology and Disease in Pregnancy*, 2nd edn. New York: Raven Press; 1992.
20. Ayala DE, Hermida RC, Mojon A, Fernandez JR, Iglesias M. Circadian blood pressure variability in healthy and complicated pregnancies. *Hypertension* 1997;30(3, Pt 2):603–10.
21. Schobel HP, Fischer T, Heuszer K, Geiger H, Schmieder RE. Preeclampsia – A state of sympathetic overactivity. *N Engl J Med* 1996;335(20):1480–5.
22. Fitzgerald D, Fitzgerald G. Eicosanoids in the pathogenesis of preeclampsia. In Laragh JH, Brenner BH, eds. *Hypertension: Pathophysiology, Diagnosis, and Management.* New York: Raven Press, 1990:1789–807.
23. Fitzgerald DJ, Entman SS, Mulloy K, Fitzgerald GA. Decreased prostacyclin biosynthesis preceding the clinical manifestation of pregnancy-induced hypertension. *Circulation* 1987;75(5):956–63.
24. Mills JL, DerSimonian R, Raymond E, *et al.* Prostacyclin and thromboxane changes predating clinical onset of preeclampsia: A multicenter prospective study. *J Am Med Assoc* 1999;282(4): 356–62.
25. Fitzgerald DJ, Rocki W, Murray R, Mayo G, FitzGerald GA. Thromboxane A2 synthesis in pregnancy-induced hypertension. *Lancet* 1990;335(8692):751–4.
26. Chambers JC, Fusi L, Malik IS, Haskard DO, De Swiet M, Kooner JS. Association of maternal endothelial dysfunction with preeclampsia. *J Am Med Assoc* 2001;285(12):1607–12.
27. Duley L, Henderson-Smart DJ, Knight M, King JF. Antiplatelet agents for preventing pre-eclampsia and its complications. *Cochrane Database Syst Rev* 2004;1:CD004659.
28. Roberts JM, Taylor RN, Musci TJ, Rodgers GM, Hubel CA, McLaughlin MK. Preeclampsia: An endothelial cell disorder. *Am J Obstet Gynecol* 1989;161(5):1200–4.
29. Sibai BM, Kustermann L, Velasco J. Current understanding of severe preeclampsia, pregnancy-associated hemolytic uremic syndrome, thrombotic thrombocytopenic purpura, hemolysis, elevated liver enzymes, and low platelet syndrome, and postpartum acute renal failure: Different clinical syndromes or just different names? *Curr Opin Nephrol Hypertens* 1994;3(4):436–45.
30. Savvidou MD, Hingorani AD, Tsikas D, Frolich JC, Vallance P, Nicolaides KH. Endothelial dysfunction and raised plasma concentrations of asymmetric dimethylarginine in pregnant women who subsequently develop pre-eclampsia. *Lancet* 2003;361(9368): 1511–7.
31. Baylis C, Beinder E, Suto T, August P. Recent insights into the roles of nitric oxide and renin–angiotensin in the pathophysiology of preeclamptic pregnancy. *Semin Nephrol* 1998;18(2):208–30.
32. Molnar M, Suto T, Toth T, Hertelendy F. Prolonged blockade of nitric oxide synthesis in gravid rats produces sustained hypertension, proteinuria, thrombocytopenia, and intrauterine growth retardation. *Am J Obstet Gynecol* 1994;170(5, Pt 1):1458–66.
33. Seligman SP, Buyon JP, Clancy RM, Young BK, Abramson SB. The role of nitric oxide in the pathogenesis of preeclampsia. *Am J Obstet Gynecol* 1994;171(4):944–8.
34. Begum S, Yamasaki M, Mochizuki M. Urinary levels of nitric oxide metabolites in normal pregnancy and preeclampsia. *J Obstet Gynaecol Res* 1996;22(6):551–9.
35. Silver RK, Kupferminc MJ, Russell TL, Adler L, Mullen TA, Caplan MS. Evaluation of nitric oxide as a mediator of severe preeclampsia. *Am J Obstet Gynecol* 1996;175(4, Pt 1):1013–7.
36. Taylor RN, Varma M, Teng NN, Roberts JM. Women with preeclampsia have higher plasma endothelin levels than women with normal pregnancies. *J Clin Endocrinol Metab* 1990; 71(6):1675–7.
37. Nova A, Sibai BM, Barton JR, Mercer BM, Mitchell MD. Maternal plasma level of endothelin is increased in preeclampsia. *Am J Obstet Gynecol* 1991;165(3):724–7.
38. Clark BA, Halvorson L, Sachs B, Epstein FH. Plasma endothelin levels in preeclampsia: Elevation and correlation with uric acid levels and renal impairment. *Am J Obstet Gynecol* 1992;166(3): 962–8.
39. Benigni A, Orisio S, Gaspari F, Frusca T, Amuso G, Remuzzi G. Evidence against a pathogenetic role for endothelin in preeclampsia. *Br J Obstet Gynaecol* 1992;99(10):798–802.
40. Davidge ST, Signorella AP, Hubel CA, Lykins DL, Roberts JM. Distinct factors in plasma of preeclamptic women increase endothelial nitric oxide or prostacyclin. *Hypertension* 1996;28(5): 758–64.
41. Taylor RN, Casal DC, Jones LA, Varma M, Martin JN Jr, Roberts JM. Selective effects of preeclamptic sera on human endothelial cell procoagulant protein expression. *Am J Obstet Gynecol* 1991; 165(6, Pt 1):1705–10.
42. Hubel CA, Roberts JM, Taylor RN, Musci TJ, Rogers GM, McLaughlin MK. Lipid peroxidation in pregnancy: New perspectives on preeclampsia. *Am J Obstet Gynecol* 1989;161(4): 1025–34.
43. Barden A, Beilin LJ, Ritchie J, Croft KD, Walters BN, Michael CA. Plasma and urinary 8-iso-prostane as an indicator of lipid peroxidation in pre-eclampsia and normal pregnancy. *Clin Sci (Lond)* 1996;91(6):711–8.
44. Serdar Z, Gur E, Develioglu O, Colakogullari M, Dirican M. Placental and decidual lipid peroxidation and antioxidant defenses in preeclampsia. Lipid peroxidation in preeclampsia. *Pathophysiology* 2002;9(1):21.
45. Seely EW, Solomon CG. Insulin resistance and its potential role in pregnancy-induced hypertension. *J Clin Endocrinol Metab* 2003;88(6):2393–8.
46. Sattar N, Bendomir A, Berry C, Shepherd J, Greer IA, Packard CJ. Lipoprotein subfraction concentrations in preeclampsia:

Pathogenic parallels to atherosclerosis. *Obstet Gynecol* 1997; 89(3):403–8.

47. Murai JT, Muzykanskiy E, Taylor RN. Maternal and fetal modulators of lipid metabolism correlate with the development of preeclampsia. *Metabolism* 1997;46(8):963–7.
48. Lorentzen B, Birkeland KI, Endresen MJ, Henriksen T. Glucose intolerance in women with preeclampsia. *Acta Obstet Gynecol Scand* 1998;77(1):22–7.
49. Long PA, Abell DA, Beischer NA. Importance of abnormal glucose tolerance (hypoglycaemia and hyperglycaemia) in the aetiology of pre-eclampsia. *Lancet* 1977;1(8018):923–5.
50. Solomon CG, Graves SW, Greene MF, Seely EW. Glucose intolerance as a predictor of hypertension in pregnancy. *Hypertension* 1994;23(6, Pt 1):717–21.
51. O'Brien TE, Ray JG, Chan WS. Maternal body mass index and the risk of preeclampsia: A systematic overview. *Epidemiology* 2003;14(3):368–74.
52. Enquobahrie DA, Williams MA, Butler CL, Frederick IO, Miller RS, Luthy DA. Maternal plasma lipid concentrations in early pregnancy and risk of preeclampsia. *Am J Hypertens* 2004;17(7): 574–81.
53. Ostlund I, Haglund B, Hanson U. Gestational diabetes and preeclampsia. *Eur J Obstet Gynecol Reprod Biol* 2004;113(1): 12–6.
54. Easterling TR, Benedetti TJ, Schmucker BC, Millard SP. Maternal hemodynamics in normal and preeclamptic pregnancies: A longitudinal study. *Obstet Gynecol* 1990;76(6):1061–9.
55. Groenendijk R, Trimbos JB, Wallenburg HC. Hemodynamic measurements in preeclampsia: Preliminary observations. *Am J Obstet Gynecol* 1984;150(3):232–6.
56. Lang RM, Pridjian G, Feldman T, Neumann A, Lindheimer M, Borow KM. Left ventricular mechanics in preeclampsia. *Am Heart J* 1991;121(6, Pt 1):1768–75.
57. Cunningham FG, Pritchard JA, Hankins GD, Anderson PL, Lucas MJ, Armstrong KF. Peripartum heart failure: Idiopathic cardiomyopathy or compounding cardiovascular events? *Obstet Gynecol* 1986;67(2):157–68.
58. Brown MA, Zammit VC, Mitar DM. Extracellular fluid volumes in pregnancy-induced hypertension. *J Hypertens* 1992;10(1):61–8.
59. Silver HM, Seebeck M, Carlson R. Comparison of total blood volume in normal, preeclamptic, and nonproteinuric gestational hypertensive pregnancy by simultaneous measurement of red blood cell and plasma volumes. *Am J Obstet Gynecol* 1998;179(1):87–93.
60. Chesley L. *Hypertensive Disorders in Pregnancy*. New York: Appleton-Century-Crofts, 1978.
61. Gallery ED, Hunyor SN, Gyory AZ. Plasma volume contraction: A significant factor in both pregnancy-associated hypertension (pre-eclampsia) and chronic hypertension in pregnancy. *Q J Med* 1979;48(192):593–602.
62. Duley L, Williams J, Henderson-Smart DJ. Plasma volume expansion for treatment of women with pre-eclampsia. *Cochrane Database Syst Rev* 2000;2:CD001805.
63. Packham DK, Mathews DC, Fairley KF, Whitworth JA, Kincaid-Smith PS. Morphometric analysis of pre-eclampsia in women biopsied in pregnancy and post-partum. *Kidney Int* 1988;34(5): 704–11.
64. Gaber L, Lindheimer M. Hypertensive disorders in pregnancy. Stanford: Appleton and Lange, 1999.
65. Eremina V, Sood M, Haigh J, *et al.* Glomerular-specific alterations of VEGF-A expression lead to distinct congenital and acquired renal diseases. *J Clin Invest* 2003;111(5):707–16.
66. Jeyabalan A, Novak J, Danielson LA, Kerchner LJ, Opett SL, Conrad KP. Essential role for vascular gelatinase activity in relaxin-induced renal vasodilation, hyperfiltration, and reduced myogenic reactivity of small arteries. *Circ Res* 2003;93(12):1249–57.
67. Davison JM, Homuth V, Jeyabalan A, *et al.* New aspects in the pathophysiology of preeclampsia. *J Am Soc Nephrol* 2004;15(9): 2440–8.
68. Pertuiset N, Grunfeld JP. Acute renal failure in pregnancy. *Baillieres Clin Obstet Gynaecol* 1994;8(2):333–51.
69. Brown MA, Gallery ED, Ross MR, Esber RP. Sodium excretion in normal and hypertensive pregnancy: A prospective study. *Am J Obstet Gynecol* 1988;159(2):297–307.
70. Taufield PA, Ales KL, Resnick LM, Druzin ML, Gertner JM, Laragh JH. Hypocalciuria in preeclampsia. *N Engl J Med* 1987;316(12): 715–8.
71. August P, Marcaccio B, Gertner JM, Druzin ML, Resnick LM, Laragh JH. Abnormal 1,25-dihydroxyvitamin D metabolism in preeclampsia. *Am J Obstet Gynecol* 1992;166(4):1295–9.
72. Delorme MA, Burrows RF, Ofosu FA, Andrew M. Thrombin regulation in mother and fetus during pregnancy. *Semin Thromb Hemost* 1992;18(1):81–90.
73. Preston FE, Rosendaal FR, Walker ID, *et al.* Increased fetal loss in women with heritable thrombophilia. *Lancet* 1996;348(9032):913–6.
74. Lockwood CJ. Heritable coagulopathies in pregnancy. *Obstet Gynecol Surv* 1999;540(12):754–65.
75. Ridker PM, Miletich JP, Hennekens CH, Buring JE. Ethnic distribution of factor V Leiden in 4047 men and women. Implications for venous thromboembolism screening. *J Am Med Assoc* 1997; 277(16):1305–7.
76. Lin J, August P. Genetic thrombophilias and preeclampsia: A meta-analysis. *Obstet Gynecol* 2005;105(1):182–92.
77. Kupferminc MJ, Eldor A, Steinman N, *et al.* Increased frequency of genetic thrombophilia in women with complications of pregnancy. *N Engl J Med* 1999;340(1):9–13.
78. Ballegeer VC, Spitz B, De Baene LA, Van Assche AF, Hidajat M, Criel AM. Platelet activation and vascular damage in gestational hypertension. *Am J Obstet Gynecol* 1992;166(2):629–33.
79. Konijnenberg A, Stokkers EW, van der Post JA, *et al.* Extensive platelet activation in preeclampsia compared with normal pregnancy: Enhanced expression of cell adhesion molecules. *Am J Obstet Gynecol* 1997;176(2):461–9.
80. Letsky EA. Disseminated intravascular coagulation. *Best Pract Res Clin Obstet Gynaecol* 2001;15(4):623–44.
81. Malatyalioglu E, Adam B, Yanik FF, Kokcu A, Alvur M. Levels of stable metabolites of prostacyclin and thromboxane A2 and their ratio in normotensive and preeclamptic pregnant women during the antepartum and postpartum periods. *J Matern Fetal Med* 2000;9(3):173–7.
82. Steyn DW, Odendaal HJ. Randomised controlled trial of ketanserin and aspirin in prevention of pre-eclampsia. *Lancet* 1997;350(9087):1267–71.
83. Sibai BM. Diagnosis, controversies, and management of the syndrome of hemolysis, elevated liver enzymes, and low platelet count. *Obstet Gynecol* 2004;103(5, Pt 1):981–91.
84. Martin JN Jr, Rinehart BK, May WL, Magann EF, Terrone DA, Blake PG. The spectrum of severe preeclampsia: Comparative analysis by HELLP (hemolysis, elevated liver enzyme levels, and low platelet count) syndrome classification. *Am J Obstet Gynecol* 1999;180(6, Pt 1):1373–84.
85. Katz VL, Farmer R, Kuller JA. Preeclampsia into eclampsia: Toward a new paradigm. *Am J Obstet Gynecol* 2000;182(6): 1389–96.
86. Hinchey J, Chaves C, Appignani B, *et al.* A reversible posterior leukoencephalopathy syndrome. *N Engl J Med* 1996;334(8): 494–500.
87. Chambers KA, Cain TW. Postpartum blindness: Two cases. *Ann Emerg Med* 2004;43(2):243–6.
88. Richards A, Graham D, Bullock R. Clinicopathological study of neurological complications due to hypertensive disorders of pregnancy. *J Neurol Neurosurg Psychiatry* 1988;51(3):416–21.
89. Riskin-Mashiah S, Belfort MA, Saade GR, Herd JA. Transcranial doppler measurement of cerebral velocity indices as a predictor of preeclampsia. *Am J Obstet Gynecol* 2002;187(6):1667–72.
90. Ohno Y, Kawai M, Wakahara Y, Kitagawa T, Kakihara M, Arii Y. Transcranial assessment of maternal cerebral blood flow velocity in patients with pre-eclampsia. *Acta Obstet Gynecol Scand* 1997;76(10):928–32.
91. Qureshi AI, Frankel MR, Ottenlips JR, Stern BJ. Cerebral hemodynamics in preeclampsia and eclampsia. *Arch Neurol* 1996; 53(12):1226–31.
92. Dahmus MA, Barton JR, Sibai BM. Cerebral imaging in eclampsia: Magnetic resonance imaging versus computed tomography. *Am J Obstet Gynecol* 1992;167(4, Pt 1):935–41.
93. Moodley J, Bobat SM, Hoffman M, Bill PL. Electroencephalogram and computerised cerebral tomography findings in eclampsia. *Br J Obstet Gynaecol* 1993;100(11):984–8.
94. Drislane FW, Wang AM. Multifocal cerebral hemorrhage in eclampsia and severe pre-eclampsia. *J Neurol* 1997;244(3):194–8.
95. Kestenbaum B, Seliger SL, Easterling TR, *et al.* Cardiovascular and thromboembolic events following hypertensive pregnancy. *Am J Kidney Dis* 2003;42(5):982–9.
96. Wilson BJ, Watson MS, Prescott GJ, *et al.* Hypertensive diseases of pregnancy and risk of hypertension and stroke in later life: Results from cohort study. *Br Med J* 2003;326(7394):845.

85 Physiological changes of the uterine cervix during pregnancy and delivery

V. N. A. Breeveld-Dwarkasing and F. K. Lotgering

Introduction

During most of human pregnancy, the uterine cervix is a dynamic anatomical structure that serves as a barrier between the fetus in its intrauterine environment and the vagina as the portal to the outside world. In the prelude to parturition a process called ripening takes place in which the cervix changes from a structure that is firm and rigid to one that is soft and elastic that can be pulled open by uterine contractions, allowing passage of the fetus. It functions reliably, but is not foolproof: in preterm delivery the cervix opens prematurely and in cervical dystocia it may fail to dilate adequately. Recent work has improved our understanding of the mechanisms that underlie these changes, but current knowledge still cannot truly explain its dysfunctions. From the many factors and cells that are involved, it is now concluded that cervical ripening and softening are caused by an inflammatory-like mechanism. In this chapter we summarize what is known and not known about the physiological changes of the uterine cervix in pregnancy and delivery, with emphasis on the remarkable remodeling of its viscoelastic properties.

Anatomy

The cervix is positioned between the muscular body of the uterus and the vagina, connecting the uterine cavity with the vagina through its canal, which can dilate during delivery. The cervix consists predominantly of fibrous connective tissue (collagen 80% of total protein content) and 10–15% smooth muscle fibers.[1] The proportion of smooth muscle cells is higher near the myometrium (28%) than near the vagina (6%).[1] Through most of gestation the cervix is a firm structure but the fibrous tissue which is responsible for this has to change its structure to become soft and pliable during delivery. This process of cervical ripening is characterized by a gradual phase which starts in the early third trimester, preparing the cervix for the second phase (during delivery) in which it becomes soft and pliable in a few hours time. During the first phase of cervical ripening, both collagen synthesis and denaturation increase, with denaturation dominating the process. During this stage the cervix may already feel soft to the touch but the highly denatured collagen network still provides sufficient resistance against uterine contractions. During dilatation further digestion of denatured collagen leads to loss of collagen and, consequently, of firmness.[2] The cervical ripening takes place mainly in the deep stromal layer of the cervix, a fact that emphasizes the importance of tissue sampling sites in biochemical studies of cervical ripening.

The cervix receives its blood supply primarily from the cervical branch of the uterine artery and anastomoses with the vaginal arteries are common. Blood flow increases markedly in the first trimester, when blood flow of the portio vaginalis uteri in healthy pregnant women was found to be increased to 69 ml/min/100 g.[3] The cervix contains abundant autonomic and sensory nerves, and they are derived from the hypogastric (T13-L4), splanchnic (L6-S2) and vagus nerves.[4] The sensory information transmitted through the vagus nerves includes pain and other reflex information from the cervix during labor and delivery that seems to bypass the spinal cord.[5] In addition, afferent unmyelinated C-fibers of these nerves which are associated with cervical vasculature and smooth muscle cells produce neuropeptides that play a role in the local neurogenic inflammatory processes associated with cervical ripening such as causing the vasculature to leak, edema and migration of inflammatory immune cells.[4] However, the cervix apparently functions normally to retain the fetuses during pregnancy even in the absence of neuronal connections, as in the transplanted uterus in the mouse,[6] and in women with a preexisting spinal cord lesion.

Clinical considerations

The readiness of the uterine cervix to dilate not only after pharmacological induction of labor, but also in spontaneous preterm or term labor, is traditionally assessed with the use of the modified Bishop score.[7] The score takes into account the dilatation, length, consistency, and position of the cervix. The ripeness of the cervix increases with advancing dilatation, reduction in length, progressive softening, and a more anterior position of the cervix. These changes are the result of the changes in viscoelastic properties, uterine contractions, and descent of the fetus. Although clinicians use these variables to predict the risk of preterm delivery and/or the chance of successful induction, the subjectivity of the assessment and interobserver variability limit their predictive value. As a consequence, investigators have sought methods to measure the same variables objectively.

Cervical dilatation has been measured with the use of ultrasound crystals attached to the vaginal surface of the cervix, close to the cervical canal in humans[8,9] and in cows.[10] Because the propagation velocity of the ultrasound pulse in cervical tissue is approximately 1500 m/s and remains constant, the distance between the two ultrasound crystals can be calculated from the time it takes for the pulse to travel from one to another. The method is somewhat limited in that it measures dilatation at the external opening of the cervix, instead of at the internal os where softening and opening (funneling) may begin. Both species demonstrate a similar picture, as represented in Figure 85.1 for nulliparous women.

Initially, during the latent phase, uterine contractions do not result in an increase in distance between the crystals attached to the vaginal cervix. The first measurable response, during the early dilatation phase, is an increase in distance during a contraction followed by an almost complete rebound after the contraction. During the acceleration phase, the distance increases with each contraction and does not return to its prior position, thus resulting in progressive dilatation. A deceleration phase, as originally reported by Friedman,[12] does not normally occur.[8,13] The initial cervical response to a uterine contraction as well as the onset of the acceleration phase occur at a smaller cervical diameter in parous than in nulliparous women. The initial response in parous women occurs at 2.9 cm and in nulliparous women it occurs at 3.6 cm. The onset of acceleration begins at 3.4 cm in parous and at 4.8 cm in nulliparous women.[8] As a consequence, calculated myometrial work per cm of cervical dilatation in parous parturients is less than in nulliparous parturients, which means that less force is needed to dilate the cervix in parous than in nulliparous women.

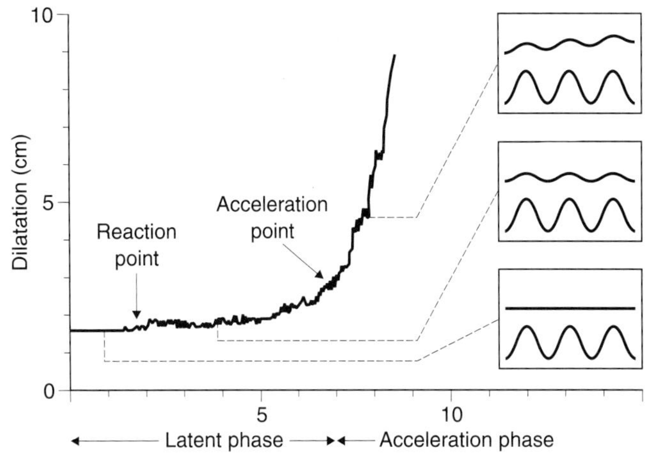

Figure 85.1 Cervical dilatation in women as measured with ultrasound crystals attached to the cervix. In the early latent phase the cervix does not respond to contractions by dilatation, in the late latent phase dilatation increases temporarily with contractions, in the acceleration phase the cervix dilates progressively with contractions. From van Dessel[11] with permission.

Cervical length has been measured extensively in recent years with the use of transvaginal ultrasound transducers. The method is limited in that there is substantial intra- and interobserver variability in measurements of cervical length, even when experienced observers perform the measurements under standardized conditions.[14] In singleton pregnancies, the uterine cervix on average is 40 ± 7 mm at mid-gestation and only slightly less at 30 weeks' gestation.[15] A short cervical length in asymptomatic women before 20 gestational weeks is a successful predictor of preterm delivery before 34 weeks' gestation, with a likelihood ratio of a positive test (cervical length < 25 mm) of 6.3 (CI 3.3–12.0) and that of a negative test of 0.8 (CI 0.65–0.95).[16] Likewise, a short cervical length is a useful predictor of successful labor induction, with a total rate of cesarean sections of 21% in women with a cervical length of ≤ 25 mm and 43% in women with a longer cervix.[17] Transvaginal sonographically measured cervical length itself was found to be a better predictor of successful labor induction than the traditional Bishop score,[17] with the notion however, that the differences were significant only in those women with an unripe cervix (Bishop score ≤ 5), which suggests that other factors, including the viscoelastic properties, are also important.

Softening of the cervix has been difficult to quantitate. However, light-induced fluorescence (LIF) of collagen has been used to investigate the changes in collagen content of the cervix during gestation and following labor induction with sodium nitroprusside, a nitric oxide donor, in the guinea pig[18] and in humans.[19] Collagen fluorescence decreased towards delivery and increased gradually postpartum, and treatment with sodium nitroprusside caused a significant reduction in fluorescence. Collagen gives a characteristic fluorescence spectrum with a peak around 390 nm. One of the major cross-links of collagen, pyridinoline, is believed to be the intrinsic fluorophor. A decreased fluorescence suggests a reduction in collagen cross-links, associated with cervical ripening.

In the unripe cervix the cervical lips are positioned against the posterior fornix, and while ripening and softening, the cervix gradually moves forward so that the cervical canal lines up with the vagina. It has been attempted to study the position of the cervix with transvaginal ultrasound. However, the anterior cervical angle was found not to be either a useful predictor of induction success (sensitivity 22%, positive predictive value 40%) or of preterm birth.[20,21]

The cervix is always involved in cases of preterm delivery, even if the primary cause is not the cervix. In the case of cervical insufficiency, or cervical incompetence, a preexistent weak cervix is unable to retain a pregnancy in the absence of uterine contractions. Historically, cervical incompetence is a clinical diagnosis based on a history of two or more second-trimester pregnancy losses, after painless dilatation up to 4 cm.[22] The incidence of cervical incompetence has been estimated as 2/1000 births in Denmark.[23] Such an intrinsic weakness of the cervix may be surgically treated by a cerclage. Cervical incompetence may be suspected in case of Mullerian abnormalities [cervical hypoplasia, as with *in utero* diethylstilbestrol (DES) exposure], surgical trauma as in prior late abortion, cone excision, trachelectomy, obstetrical trauma, or in the case of connective tissue disease (Ehlers–Danlos syndrome). A cervix which appears to be short by transvaginal sonography is also a risk factor for preterm delivery, but is not always caused by cervical incompetence. Therefore, the entities that could lead to preterm delivery should not be used interchangeably with cervical incompetence. Cervical incompetence may vary in degree and it may be expressed differently in subsequent pregnancies and although a short cervix may indicate a higher risk for preterm delivery it does not discriminate between underlying pathologies.[24] In normal pregnancies the cervix also shortens progressively between the 10th and the 40th week.[25] That is why the American College of Obstetricians and Gynecologists recommends not to screen women at low risk routinely and to perform serial cervical length measurements only in women with a historical risk factor for preterm delivery.[26] These, include bacterial vaginosis, placental and intra-amniotic infections, extreme uterine distension as in multiple pregnancies, blunt abdominal trauma leading to placental abruption, diabetes, and smoking. When these causes lead to preterm delivery, irrespective of the etiology, a common biochemical pathway has to become active that will lead to cervical effacement and dilatation just as in normal delivery. Strategies to prevent preterm deliveries that are less invasive than cerclage, such as reduction of physical activities or even the application of vaginal pessaries are likely to be effective in the mere presence of risk factors, when clinical symptoms or a typical obstetrical history are absent.[27]

The change in cervical function from retaining the fetus *in utero* during pregnancy to allowing the fetus a smooth passage during delivery requires an extensive and intriguing remodeling of the viscoelastic properties of the cervix, as we will discuss in greater detail.

Tissue remodeling

Proper timing of the tissue remodeling in the cervix may make the difference between a severely premature, a healthy term, or a postterm infant, and between spontaneous delivery, a cesarean section, or a failed induction. Our understanding of the intriguingly complex mechanisms that underlie this remodeling process is still far from complete. We will first describe the physiological changes that occur in the extracellular matrix (ECM) which is responsible for both the strength and plasticity of the cervix, subsequently the cellular events that are responsible for the changes in the ECM, and finally the hormonal changes that induce the invasion of cells and regulate the actions of both the resident and the invasive cells.

Extracellular matrix

The cervix is not a static tissue but a dynamic organ and the ECM plays a major role in the dynamic changes in strength and plasticity of the cervix during pregnancy and parturition and the different phases of the menstrual cycle. The ECM constitutes collagens, proteoglycans, and elastin, which are synthesized by the smooth muscle cells and fibroblasts that represent the majority of the cells that are usually present in the cervix. During ripening the structural integrity of the ECM changes as a result of structural changes in the collagen network, a shift in the composition of the total proteoglycan content and possibly a change in the arrangement of elastin fibers. During ripening the resident cells are mostly involved in releasing inflammatory mediators and proteolytic enzymes, while during labor an additional number of neutrophils and macrophages invade the cervix and release the enzymes stored in their granules, which are responsible for the much faster softening. We will discuss the dynamic regulation of collagen, elastin, and other constituents of the ECM in more detail.

Collagen

The fibrous connective tissue of the cervix consists largely of collagen type I (70%) and type III (30%), and taken together they represent 80% of the total protein content of the cervix. Collagen molecules are three stranded molecules typically arranged in a triple helical configuration. Their strands are bound together by disulfide bridges and the molecules are

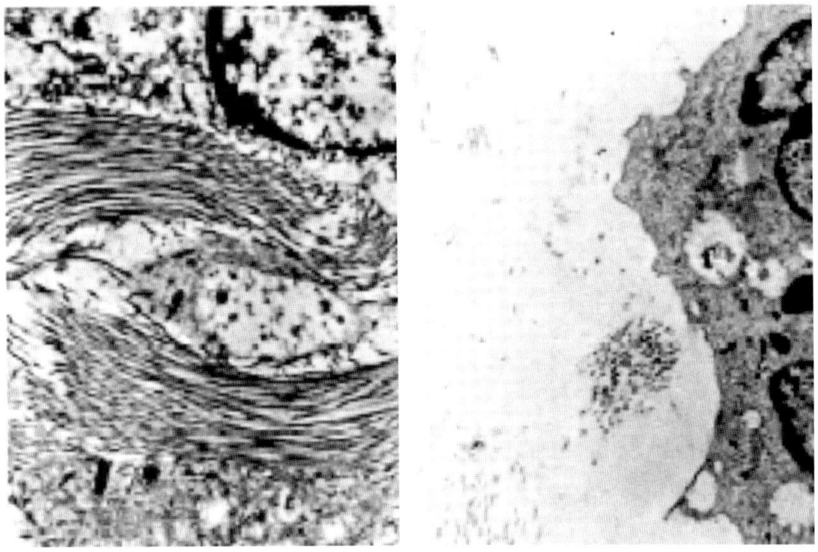

Figure 85.2 Electron micrographs of the cervix of pregnant guinea pigs obtained before term (left) and following ripening at term (right). Note the large number of collagen fibers present during early pregnancy and the decrease in fibers during ripening. From Garfield *et al.*[31] with permission.

cross-linked by pyridinoline side chains to form strong nonextendable fibers. The synthesis of collagen triple helices is complex in that it requires co-translational and posttranslational steps in addition to the protein synthesis *per se*. Two relevant co-factors are vitamin C and copper. Copper is a co-factor for peptidyl-lysine oxidase, an enzyme involved in the cross-linking of collagen fibers that is inhibited by smoking.[28] Normally, the synthesis and degradation of collagen are in a dynamic balance, depending on the stage of pregnancy.

In the nonpregnant state, the collagen bundles are densely packed together. During pregnancy the collagen is gradually remodeled, during the process of ripening that prepares the cervix for labor and dilatation. Yet, even during the first trimester of pregnancy the collagen fibers become less tightly packed.[29] Through these changes, the pregnant cervix feels softer than the non pregnant cervix, while a more parallel alignment of the fibers assures proper closing function.

As long as the helical conformation of the molecule remains intact, collagen is not readily accessible for proteolytic enzymes. Even when the collagen molecules are denatured, they can still maintain their three-dimensional network conformation through cross-bridges and still offer considerable resistance to physical stress, as is the case during cervical ripening.[2] Unwound, denatured, collagen is subject to further digestion by proteolytic enzymes, including collagenases which may result in a greater solubility of collagen,[30] and this could be responsible for the decreased collagen content of the cervix shortly before delivery as observed in cows.[2] In pathologic conditions, including cervical incompetence and *in utero* diethylstilbestrol exposure, a too extensive ripening process may occur in mid-pregnancy.[29] The difference between an unripe and a maximally ripened cervix are clearly demonstrated in Figure 85.2. Subsequently, during parturition macrophages and neutrophils progressively invade the cervix, release their catabolic enzymes that dissolve the dispersed collagen fibers, and allow the cervix to dilate within hours.

Immediately after delivery, the involution of the cervix is accompanied by a two- to threefold increase in the synthesis of collagens I and III,[32] thereby starting the repair that will allow the successful carrying of a subsequent pregnancy.

Elastin

Although elastin constitutes only 1% of the total connective tissue and its content does not appear to change with the stage of pregnancy, it is an important component of the ECM of the cervix.[33] Elastin does not offer the same resistance against the mechanical forces of uterine contractions and the fetal presenting part as collagen does,[34] but it adds to the cervix the quality of elasticity. Added to the strength of the collagen, the elastic component may serve to keep the cervix closed during pregnancy, while allowing it to dilate during labor. But maybe even more importantly, it may enable the cervix to bounce back to its original diameter after delivery. Elastin is localized to specific regions of the cervix and is not dispersed through the cervical stroma. Elastin seems to be concentrated at the external os and from there on it spreads to the periphery in a band upwards to the internal os where it becomes sparse in the muscular area below the internal os.[33] The elastin fibers of the cervix are made up of membranes and fibrils which are organized in a fishnet-like structure[34] so they can be stretched in any direction. They are likely to be responsible for the

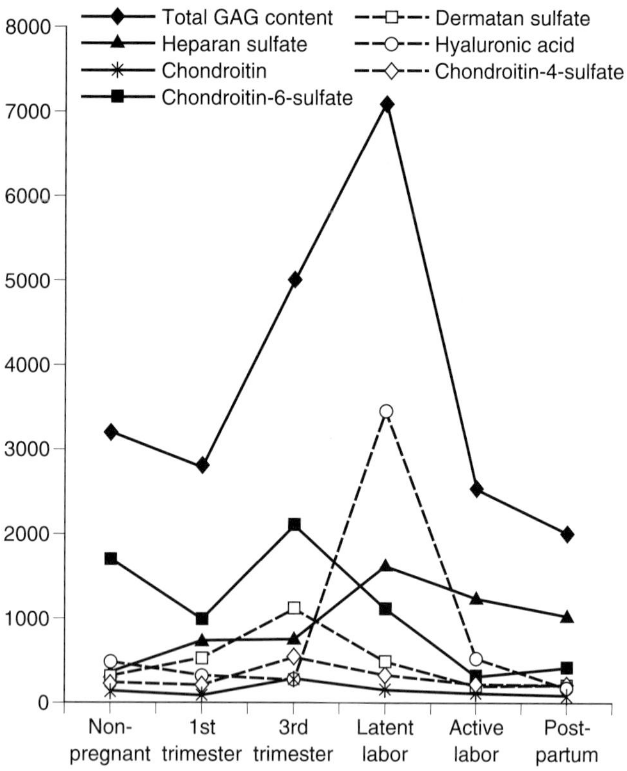

Figure 85.3 Pregnancy-induced changes in the total glycosaminoglycans (GAG) content and the content of the individual GAGs (nmol/g dry weight) in the cervix of pregnant women at delivery and postpartum. Adapted from Osmers *et al.*[37] with permission.

dynamic changes in cervical length and temporary funneling at the internal os of the cervical canal that occur during pregnancy in response to maternal positional changes, fetal movements and uterine contractions as observed by ultrasound.[35] Biopsies from incompetent cervices have shown a reduction in total elastin, fragmented fibers and an abnormal arrangement of the elastin compared with those of uncomplicated term pregnancies.[36]

Proteoglycans and hyaluronic acid

Proteoglycans play an important but complex role in the spatial arrangements and stabilization of the ECM. In addition, they regulate the induction of cytokines. Proteoglycans are glycoproteins that contain one or more glycosaminoglycan (GAG) side chains in addition to a protein core. In the past, the nomenclature of the proteoglycans was based on these side-chains and studying the changes in content of the various GAGs during pregnancy showed a complex pattern (Figure 85.3).

The changes in GAG concentrations (nmol/g dry weight) are most pronounced during late gestation and labor. The change in total GAGs content is already pronounced in the third trimester and is caused predominantly by an increase in chondroitin-6-sulfate, while the further increase during labor is largely caused by an increase in hyaluronic acid. From a functional point of view, however, the relevance of these changes in total and individual GAG concentrations may be questioned as the complete proteoglycan molecule and its spatial arrangement rather than the content of side chains is important with regard to their role as building blocks of the ECM. Thanks to modern gene technology, a new appreciation of the molecular design has lead to a new and simplified nomenclature based on homologies of the protein core and to the grouping of distinct gene families and subfamilies, often with similar or identical structural and functional relationships.[38] Members of at least two proteoglycan subfamilies are present in the cervix, i.e., the small leucine-rich proteoglycans (formerly called small dermatan-sulfate proteoglycans) that include decorin and biglycan,[32,39] and the hyalectan (hyaluronan and lectin interacting) proteoglycans that include versican (a large chondroitan/dermatan sulfate proteoglycan), aggrecan (a chondroitin sulfate proteoglycan), and a large (220 kDa) keratan sulfate proteoglycan.[40] Decorin seems relevant as it coats and stabilizes the collagen fibrils through a tight alignment of the fibrils, by binding its protein core with different sites of the collagen fibrils. The decorin concentration is lower in the cervix of term and parturient women than in nonpregnant and early pregnant women[41] and the decorin to collagen ratio correlates inversely with the softness of the cervix. This suggests that the dispersion of collagen near term is in part mediated by loss of decorin. Biglycan interacts with collagen via its GAG side chains and like decorin its concentration decreases during cervical ripening.[32] The hyalectans probably enhance the water binding capacity of hyaluronic acid. The concentrations of versican and the large keratin sulfate proteoglycan increase in the ECM during labor,[32,40] when a significant increase in the hyaluronic acid content also occurs.[37] Hyaluronic acid is a glycosaminoglycan which is produced by fibroblasts; it is hydrophilic and attracts water to the ECM, and helps to disrupt the collagen. In addition, it is involved in PGE_2 synthesis and cytokine production,[42] while its breakdown products have angiogenic, inflammatory, immune-stimulating, antiapoptotic and heat-shock protein-inducing properties,[43] all of which may contribute to accelerated ripening of the cervix in early labor. In the immediate postpartum period, uterine involution and cervical retraction are associated with a two- to threefold increase in mRNA not only for collagen I and III but also of the small leucine-rich proteoglycans, including decorin and biglycan, as part of the repair process.[32]

Mediators

Matrix metalloproteinases

Matrix metalloproteinases (MMPs) are the primary mediators of ECM degradation in the cervix during pregnancy and parturition.[44–47] These zinc-dependent enzymes have been divided into four subgroups, collagenases, gelatinases, membrane type MMPs (MT-MMPs), and stromelysins. They are capable of degrading collagen and elastin, as well as other ECM components, including proteoglycans. All cell types present in the cervix are capable of producing MMPs. The physiologically important collagenases MMP-1 and MMP-8 are produced by the resident fibroblasts (MMP-1) and the invading neutrophils (MMP-8). They cleave the triple helices of the intact undenatured collagen, degrading it into smaller fragments. MMP-1 preferentially cleaves type III collagen, and MMP-8 type I collagen.[48] MMP expression is regulated at several levels, including gene transcription, gene translation, latent enzyme secretion, pro-enzyme activation and, importantly, inactivation by endogenous inhibitors. Some MMPs, e.g., MMP-1 are synthesized on demand in response to hormones, cytokines, growth factors, and physical stress.[49] They may be secreted as latent enzymes into the ECM, or bound to the cell surface and become activated by proteinases, including other MMPs.[50] Other MMPs such as MMP-8 are synthesized by leucocytes, such as neutrophils and macrophages and stored in their granules as latent enzymes to be released when these cells are stimulated. At the onset of labor, neutrophils are attracted to the ECM. The MMPs present in neutrophil granules as well as in the ECM are activated, in response to increased cytokine activity resulting from hormone induction. As a consequence, during labor, MMP concentrations are increased both in the cervical tissue and in the circulation.

The ECM degrading activity of the MMPs is counterbalanced by the activity of tissue inhibitors of metalloproteinases (TIMPs). These inhibitors are present in the cervix throughout gestation[29] and prevent it from becoming too severely damaged by the MMPs. The synthesis of TIMPs varies with the level of MMP activity, which in turn is dependent of the stage of cervical ripening and dilatation.[51] Other suppressive factors of MMP expression include TGF-β and glucocorticoid.[52]

Cytokines

Cytokines, including the interleukins (ILs) IL-1 (α and β), IL-6, and IL-8, are causally linked to preterm and term labor. Cytokines attract neutrophils to the cervix, stimulate their extravasation, and the subsequent release of MMPs from their granules and also stimulate fibroblasts to synthesize and secrete MMPs. IL-1α stimulates MMP-1 secretion by human cervical fibroblasts and iNOS mRNA expression in these cells,[53] while IL-1β, IL-6, IL-8, and tumor necrosis factor alpha (TNFα) expression is linked to invading neutrophils.[54] When IL-1β or IL-8 are administered intracervically, they induce premature ripening and delivery.[55,56] IL-1β, IL-6, and IL-8 are also found to be increased during bacterial vaginosis or intra uterine infections, and then they play a causal role in early cervical ripening and premature delivery.[57] Interleukin-levels in the lower uterine segment,[58] placental blood, maternal serum, and amnionic fluid[59] are also found to increase progressively with the increase of the cervical diameter in normal labor at term.

TGF-β is an immunosuppressant and a potent chemo-attractant for monocytes and neutrophils.[60] It stimulates fibroblasts to synthesize collagen and proteoglycans. TGF-β increases after delivery,[32] and may thereby contribute to the involution of the cervix.

Nitric oxide

Nitric oxide (NO) is a short-lived free radical gas that is produced by nitric oxide synthases (NOS) in a reaction in which arginine, oxygen, and NADPH are converted into citrulline, NO, and NADP. There are three forms of NOS, all of them have been identified in the cervix. They are the constitutive calcium-dependent isoforms bNOS (brain NOS) and eNOS (endothelial NOS) and an inducible Ca-independent isoform (iNOS).

An important effect of NO is smooth muscle relaxation and therefore it is believed to aid in myometrial relaxation during pregnancy and possibly in cervical relaxation during delivery,[61] as may be concluded from the observations in rats, where during active labor NO production is upregulated manifold in the cervix, it is simultaneously downregulated in the myometrium.[62] Interestingly, the relaxing effect of NO on the myometrium appears to be mediated through an effect on calcium-activated potassium channels and not through cGMP as has been previously assumed.[63,64]

The increase in cervical NO during labor is mediated mainly by the increased expression of inducible nitric oxide synthase (iNOS)[65] in cervical stromal cells and invading neutrophils, macrophages, and mast cells.[66] In addition to being a smooth muscle relaxant, and probably functionally more important, NO is also involved in the regulation of several inflammatory mediators that induce cervical softening. NO-donors such as sodium nitroprusside induce a rapid and significant softening of the cervix in early pregnant women, when it is applied into the cervical canal.[67] Sodium nitroprusside given intracervically to term pregnant guinea pigs induced changes in the ECM that were similar to those observed in guinea pigs that delivered spontaneously.[18] NO stimulates the release of prostaglandin (PG) E2 and PGF2α by human cervical fibroblast, through stimulating cyclo-oxygenase. It also stimulates the synthesis of proteoglycans, probably through a PGE2-dependent pathway. NO increases the production of MMP1 in human fibroblasts.[53] High concentrations in the cervical tissues may cause cell death.[68] The view that NO is actively involved in the pathways that lead to ECM degradation which contributes to cervical ripening is supported by the observation in pregnant rats that the NOS-synthesis inhibitor L-NAME significantly reduces the distensibility of the cervix.[62]

Endothelial NOS (eNOS) and brain NOS (bNOS) provide low background levels of NO in the cervix. The concentration of bNOS is significantly increased in active labor[69] while reports with regard to eNOS concentrations are contradictory. Both constitutive isoforms are believed to be more involved in smooth muscle relaxation, while the massive increase in NO synthesis which is caused through the greatly increased iNOS expression may be more important for its involvement in immune and inflammatory response.

Cellular compartment

The cervix contains epithelial cells, smooth muscle cells, and fibroblasts, as well as a variable population of migratory cells, neutrophils, macrophages, and mast cells. All the various cell types in the cervix participate in one way or the other in the process of cervical ripening. The epithelial cells not only provide local protection against invading organisms, but secrete inflammatory modulators, including iNOS.[66] The resident fibroblasts and smooth muscle cells in the cervix are not only the source for collagens and proteoglycans and several growth factors, they also take part in the inflammatory-like response of the ripening cervix through the secretion of cytokines and proteolytic tissue-degrading enzymes. Early in gestation, smooth muscle cells and fibroblasts proliferate. Late in gestation, especially in early labor, the rate of proliferation is reduced, physiologic cell death (apoptosis) increases, and neutrophils and macrophages are attracted to the cervical stroma. Most of the information about the contribution of the individual cell types to the process of cervical ripening has been derived from *in vitro* studies, i.e., cell cultures and in a lesser amount from immunohistochemical or *in situ* hybridization studies, so the possible effect of interactions between different cell types in most cases cannot be specified. Based on these studies, hormones or inflammatory mediators given to patients may not always induce the desired effect. In the following sections we will discuss what is known about the cellular components of the cervical stroma and their role in the physiological changes that occur during pregnancy and delivery.

Stromal cells

Smooth muscle cells are present in the muscular outer layer of the cervix and in the stroma. Smooth muscle cells in the cervix may have two functions, one of muscle contraction and one of secretion of catabolic enzymes. Although the literature does not offer any clear guidance in this matter, it may be perceived as logical that muscle contractions may be the more important function in the outer layer, because of the arrangement of muscle fibers in bundles while in the stroma the more dispersed smooth muscle cells may contribute to the inflammatory-like mechanisms of the cervix. However, these two functions may not be completely separated because of the observation that an electromyogram (EMG) derived from the cervix is higher in women with a clinically unripe compared to a ripe cervix.[70,71] During parturition contractile activity of the cervix diminishes in response to increased levels of NO.[72]

The proposed mechanism by which NO exerts its relaxing effect on the myometrial smooth muscle cells has recently been revised. Previously it was thought that the relaxing effect of NO was mediated through soluble guanylyl cyclase (sGC) activation and cGMP accumulation, like in vascular and gastrointestinal smooth muscle cells. More recent studies, however, have shown that NO-induced relaxation is independent of this pathway.[64] It has been proposed that the NO-induced relaxation in the myometrium is mediated through the activation of calcium-activated potassium-[63] or PKG-independent regulation of myosin phosphatase.[64] Although it has been reported that an analog of the cGMP inhibits contractile activity of the cervix,[73] further studies are clearly needed to determine just how NO exerts its effect on cervical smooth muscle relaxation.

Besides contributing to the ECM by synthesizing collagens and proteoglycans,[38] cervical smooth muscle cells also participate in the inflammatory-like mechanism that leads to degradation of the ECM. They do so through the production of cytokines, including IL-1β and TNF-α, which in turn, induce expression of MMP-1 and MMP-9.[74] They also produce IL-8, upon lipopolysaccharide- and cytokine-stimulation, which stimulates neutrophil invasion and degranulation and, consequently, the release of proteolytic enzymes, including MMPs.[75]

In some aspects cervical fibroblasts are similar to cervical smooth muscle cells in that they both contribute to the ECM by synthesizing collagens and proteoglycans and they are both capable of producing cytokines, proteolytic enzymes such as MMPs and proteolytic enzyme inhibitors such as TIMPs. However, there are some fundamental differences in the way they react to stimulation by pro-inflammatory cytokines. For example, both cervical smooth muscle cells and fibroblasts increase their gene expression of MMP-1 and not of MMP-2 when stimulated by IL-1β or TNF-α, but fibroblasts also react by increasing TIMP expression, and cervical smooth muscle cells do not.[74] So fibroblasts have the primary function to provide the cervix with strength through the secretion of collagen and proteoglycans. Upon proper stimulation, they produce MMP-1, MMP-2, and MMP–9 as well as cytokines, including IL-6 and IL–8,[76,77] which are effective on the other side of the balance. Cultured human cervical fibroblasts respond to mechanical stress or the administration of PG-F2α, IL-1α, or NO with the production or secretion of MMP-1.[49,53]

Invading cells

Inflammatory cells of all kinds are present in cervical stroma throughout gestation[41] as they are in all organs that are in contact with the exterior. Shortly before the onset of labor the cervix is invaded by a large number of neutrophils, and to a lesser extent by macrophages. They contribute to the increased levels of NO, cytokines, and MMPs that are actively involved in cervical ripening and dilatation.

In pregnant women, neutrophils are thought to be the main source of the increased levels of collagenolytic enzymes, including MMPs.[78] During labor, neutrophilic infiltration of the lower uterine segment increases with cervical dilatation, as do the concentrations of MMP-8 and IL-8. At 2–3 cm dilatation, neutrophils are present close to the endothelium of the blood vessels but have not yet invaded the tissue. When dilatation progresses, the process of neutrophil invasion is associated with increased expression of adhesion molecules, including intercellular adhesion molecule-1, endothelial leucocyte adhesion molecule-1 and vascular cell adhesion molecule-1.[79] Shortly after delivery, the neutrophil concentration shows a marked further increase, and with it the expression of IL-1β and IL-8.[80] This may represent an anti-infectious property rather than being associated with cervical involution.

Macrophages are present in somewhat higher numbers in the cervical stroma of women during parturition,[80] while other inflammatory cells, including mast cells, T-cells, and plasma cells that are present in small numbers during gestation, do not increase appreciably during labor.[41] Mast cells play a role in angiogenesis during the first half of gestation, through mast cell degranulation that causes the release of vascular endothelial growth factor (VEGF), basic fibroblast growth factor (bFGF), IL-1, and IL-6.[81] Macrophages and mast cells do not seem to play an important role in the initiation of labor.

Hormonal regulation

Progesterone and estrogen

Progesterone keeps the myometrium from contracting and the cervix from softening. Spontaneous labor is preceded by a reduction in the circulating concentration of progesterone and/or an increase in estrogen in several but not in humans, and premature labor can be induced successfully by estrogen injection in sheep.[82] This underlines the concept that progesterone dominance is important to maintain uterine quiescence, while estrogen dominance would lead to labor. The fact that parturition in humans is not preceded by a drop in serum progesterone concentration or a shift in serum progesterone/estrogen balance does not necessarily mean that the concept of the progesterone/estrogen balance is invalid in humans as circulating hormone concentrations are only part of the picture in which receptor quantity and sensitivity also plays a role. In the guinea pig, progesterone receptor expression decreases shortly before parturition, whereas estrogen receptor-α (ER-α) remains high throughout late gestation and parturition.[83] Humans seem to be similar to guinea pigs in that the responsiveness of their cervix to progesterone and estrogen is likely not to be mediated through changes in circulating blood levels but by changes at the receptor level. The fact that progesterone antagonists effectively induce cervical ripening and labor in women supports the functional importance of progesterone blockade in the onset of labor.[84,85] In addition, progesterone may upregulate the production of TIMPs,[51] and inhibit the IL1- (α and β) mediated induction of MMP-9 in cervical fibroblasts of term pregnant rabbits,[86] by which it blocks the MMP-induced degradation of the ECM. Estrogen stimulates the infiltration of eosinophils in the rat[87] and the enzymatic activity of the procollagenases in cell cultures from the guinea pig cervix.[88,89] Furthermore, estrogens enhance the cytokine-induced attraction of neutrophils to the cervix, an effect that is blocked by progesterone,[90,91] and the presence of ER-β in neutrophils suggests that estrogens may attribute to the release of MMPs from the neutrophils in the cervix.[92] Overall, the progesterone to estrogen ratio at the tissue and cellular level is likely to be of major importance for uterine quiescence and cervical closure during pregnancy as well as for the initiation of cervical ripening and delivery.

Prostaglandins

Prostaglandins (PGs) are unsaturated cyclic fatty acids derived from arachidonic acid in a reaction catalyzed by cyclo-oxygenase (COX)-1 and COX–2. COX-1 is expressed constitutively and COX-2 is induced by cytokines and growth factors.

Local (vaginal and intracervical) application and systemic administration of PGs (PGE_1, PGE_2, and $PGF_{2\alpha}$) and their synthetic analogs induce clinical ripening of the cervix and the onset of labor. In current obstetrical practice PGE_2-gel applied vaginally is routinely used to induce cervical softening. Collagen extractability from cervical biopsies of women treated with PG increased significantly compared to the cervix of nonpregnant women[93] or term pregnant women with an unfavorable cervix.[94] However, incubating biopsy samples with PGE_2 from pregnant women at different stages of pregnancy revealed that pregnancy stage has a major influence on the response of cervical tissues to PGE_2. For example, in the early first-trimester collagen synthesis is stimulated, and proteoglycan synthesis is decreased, by PGE_2. In cervical tissues obtained from late first-trimester pregnancy until term the effect of PGE2 on the synthesis of proteoglycans and collagen is reversed, while in tissues obtained at the start of labor, incubation with PGE_2 causes a decrease in both collagen and proteoglycan synthesis.[95]

Several mechanisms are activated by PGs. PGE_2 enhances the effect of IL-8, a potent neutrophil chemoattractant,[96] which is abundantly present in the cervix and whose concentration in this tissue increases progressively with cervical dilatation.[97]

If endogenous PGs play a role in the physiological ripening and dilatation of the cervix it is to be expected that PG levels should rise in cervical tissue at late gestation and labor. However, analysis of cervical mucus samples shows no increase in PGE_2 and $PGF_{2\alpha}$ content during the period of cervical ripening.[98] This suggests that if PGE_2 and $PGF_{2\alpha}$ are active during normal labor, their levels are under tight temporal and spatial control and that they would be synthesized locally in the tissues, acting in a paracrine way. Incubated cervical tissues obtained from patients during the first trimester of pregnancy produced PGs and prostaglandin metabolites, an effect that may at least in part be mediated by NO.[99] Functional LH and hCG receptors have been localized in the cervix of women and treatment of endocervical tissue with hCG induced a significant decrease in COX-2 expression and thus could inhibit PG synthesis. During the last few days prior to labor in the baboon, PGE_2 receptor expression in the cervix increases and thereby sensitizes the cervix to PGE_2.[100] The PGE_2 receptor, EP_4 is also present in human cervical fibroblasts and seems to mediate GAG synthesis.[101] PGE_2 may also cause an increase in cervical MMP-9 concentration in rats, by a cAMP-dependent mechanism.[102] Oxytocin infusion is widely used to augment labor by stimulating increased frequency and intensity of myometrial contractions, although in two randomized clinical studies intravenous infusion of low doses of oxytocin seemed to be as effective as local application of PGE_2 gel in inducing cervical effacement.[103,104] In cows, oxytocin-receptor expression in the cervix increases markedly during late gestation, predominantly in the mucosal cells.[105] In sheep, cervical oxytocin receptor levels during pregnancy are low [106] and remain low during late gestation and labor.[107] However, in sheep oxytocin is able to induce marked cervical softening in the estrus period because the oxytocin receptor is maximally present. The observations in sheep and the fact that in clinical practice oxytocin infusion is not always as effective in prelabor ripening of the cervix of pregnant women, suggests that high oxytocin receptor levels are necessary to make the cervix sensitive to oxytocin. In cows it has been shown that oxytocin stimulates COX expression and by this way the release of PGE_2.[108] It could be possible that in women the effect of oxytocin is generated through an increased PGE_2 synthesis at the uterine level since oxytocin receptor expression in the uterus is increased during labor.[109] Preinduction with PGE_2, which is commonly practiced when oxytocin infusion is used to induce labor, may overcome the critical period when oxytocin receptors at the uterine or the cervical level have not yet increased to sufficiently high levels to induce endogenous PGE_2.

The conclusion is that although prostaglandins and oxytocin are able to induce cervical softening when used in labor induction, their role in cervical ripening and softening during physiological spontaneous deliveries at the cervical level is still disputed as the mechanisms that could possibly be involved have not yet been clearly established.

Conclusion

Since the concept of cervical ripening as a local inflammatory reaction has been introduced by Liggins,[110] the intriguingly complex remodeling of the uterine cervix in the onset of labor has shown to be an exciting field for continued research. Although many factors and mechanisms that could be involved in this process have been identified, mostly from animal models and *in vitro* studies, and have led to new concepts and ideas, not all of them have been shown to actually occur in the cervix of women that give normal birth. We have made a selection of those factors of which the clinical relevance is evident or could prove to be promising targets for pharmacological or mechanical interventions to prevent preterm and postterm delivery as well as failure of ripening and dilatation in response to pharmacological induction of labor.

REFERENCES

1. Rorie DK, Newton M. Histologic and chemical studies of the smooth muscle in the human cervix and uterus. *Am J Obstet Gynecol* 1967;99:466–9.
2. Breeveld-Dwarkasing VN, te Koppele JM, Bank RA, van der Weijden GC, Taverne MA, Dissel-Emiliani FM. Changes in water content, collagen degradation, collagen content, and concentration in repeated biopsies of the cervix of pregnant cows. *Biol Reprod* 2003;69:1608–14.
3. Zubek L, Monos E, Csepli J. Significance of blood flow measurement in the cervix uteri in the 1st trimester of pregnancy. *Zentralbl Gynakol* 1986;108:900–5.
4. Collins JJ, Usip S, McCarson KE, Papka RE. Sensory nerves and neuropeptides in uterine cervical ripening. *Peptides* 2002;23: 167–83.
5. Whipple B, Komisaruk BR. Brain (PET) responses to vaginal–cervical self-stimulation in women with complete spinal cord injury: Preliminary findings. *J Sex Marital Ther* 2002;28:79–86.
6. El Akouri RR, Kurlberg G, Dindelegan G, Molne J, Wallin A, Brannstrom M. Heterotopic uterine transplantation by vascular anastomosis in the mouse. *J Endocrinol* 2002;174.
7. Bishop EH. Pelvic scoring for elective induction. *Obstet Gynecol* 1964;24:266–8.
8. Van Dessel HJ, Frijns JH, Kok FT, Wallenburg HC. Ultrasound assessment of cervical dynamics during the first stage of labor. *Eur J Obstet Gynecol Reprod Biol* 1994;53:123–7.
9. Eijskoot F, Storm J, Kok F, Wallenburg H, Wladimiroff J. An ultrasonic device for continuous measurement of cervical dilation during labor. *Ultrasonics* 1977;15:183–5.

10. Breeveld-Dwarkasing VN, Struijk PC, Lotgering FK *et al.* Cervical dilatation related to uterine electromyographic activity and endocrinological changes during prostaglandin F(2alpha)-induced parturition in cows. *Biol Reprod* 2003;68:536–42.
11. Van Dessel HJHM. The behavior of the uterine cervix during labor. Doctoral thesis, Erasmus University, Rotterdam, 1992.
12. Friedman EA. Graphical analysis of labor. *Am J Obstet Gynecol* 1954;68:1568–75.
13. Zhang J, Troendle JF, Yancey MK. Reassessing the labor curve in nulliparous women. *Am J Obstet Gynecol* 2002;187:824–8.
14. Valentin LBI. Intra- and interobserver reproducibility of ultrasound measurements of cervical length and width in the second and third trimesters of pregnancy. *Ultrasound Obstet Gynecol* 2002;20:256–62.
15. Dijkstra K, Janssen H, Kuczynski E, Lockwood C. Cervical length in uncomplicated pregnancy: A study of sociodemographic predictors of cervical changes across gestation. *Am J Obstet Gynecol* 1999;180:639–44.
16. Honest H, Bachmann LM, Coomarasamy A, Gupta JK, Kleijnen J, Khan KS. Accuracy of cervical transvaginal sonography in predicting preterm birth: A systematic review. *Ultrasound Obstet Gynecol* 2003;22:305–22.
17. Gabriel R, Darnaud T, Chalot F, Gonzalez N, Leymarie F, Quereux C. Transvaginal sonography of the uterine cervix prior to labor induction. *Ultrasound Obstet Gynecol* 2002;19:254–7.
18. Fittkow CT, Shi SQ, Bytautiene E, Olson G, Saade GR, Garfield RE. Changes in light-induced fluorescence of cervical collagen in guinea pigs during gestation and after sodium nitroprusside treatment. *J Perinat Med* 2001;29:535–43.
19. Maul H, Olson G, Fittkow CT, Saade GR, Garfield RE. Cervical light-induced fluorescence in humans decreases throughout gestation and before delivery: Preliminary observations. *Am J Obstet Gynecol* 2003;188:537–41.
20. Novakov-Mikic A, Ivanovic L, Dukanac J. Transvaginal ultrasonography of uterine cervix in prediction of the outcome of labour induction. *Med Pregl* 2000;53:569 78.
21. Arabin B, van Eyck J. Sonographic diagnosis of cervical incompetence for prevention and management. *Ultrasound Rev* 2001;3: 1–10.
22. Harger JH. Cerclage and cervical Insufficiency: An evidence-based analysis. *Obstet Gynecol* 2002;100:1313–27.
23. Lidegaard O. Cervical incompetence and cerclage in Denmark 1980–1990. A register based epidemiological survey. *Acta Obstet Gynecol Scand* 1994;73:35–8.
24. Althuisius S, Dekker G, Hummel P, Bekedam D, Kuik D, van Geijn H. Cervical Incompetence Prevention Randomized Cerclage Trial (CIPRACT): Effect of therapeutic cerclage with bed rest vs. bed rest only on cervical length. *Ultrasound Obstet Gynecol* 2002;20(2):163–7.
25. Gramellini D, Fieni S, Molina E, Berretta R, Vadora E. Transvaginal sonographic cervical length changes during normal pregnancy. *J Ultrasound Med* 2002;21:227–32.
26. ACOG. ACOG Practice Bulletin Number 48. Cervical insufficiency. *Obstet Gynecol* 2003;102:1091–9.
27. Arabin B, Halbesma JR, Vork F, Hubener M, van Eyck J. Is treatment with vaginal pessaries an option in patients with a sonographically detected short cervix? *J Perinat Med* 2003;31:122–33.
28. Kleissl HP, van der RM, Naftolin F, Glorieux FH, de Leon A. Collagen changes in the human uterine cervix at parturition. *Am J Obstet Gynecol* 1978;130:748–53.
29. Ludmir J, Sehdev HM. Anatomy and physiology of the uterine cervix. *Clin Obstet Gynecol* 2000;43:433–9.
30. Uldbjerg N, Ekman G, Malmstrom A, Olsson K, Ulmsten U. Ripening of the human uterine cervix related to changes in collagen, glycosaminoglycans, and collagenolytic activity. *Am J Obstet Gynecol* 1983;147:662–6.
31. Garfield RE, Maul H, Shi L *et al.* Methods and devices for the management of term and preterm labor. *Ann N Y Acad Sci* 2001;943: 203–24.
32. Westergren-Thorsson G, Norman M, Bjornsson S *et al.* Differential expressions of mRNA for proteoglycans, collagens and transforming growth factor-beta in the human cervix during pregnancy and involution. *Biochim Biophys Acta Mol Basis Dis* 1998;1406: 203–13.
33. Leppert PC, Cerreta JM, Mandl I. Orientation of elastic fibers in the human cervix. *Am J Obstet Gynecol* 1986;155:219–24.
34. Leppert PC, Yu SY. Three-dimensional structures of uterine elastic fibers: Scanning electron microscopic studies. *Connect Tissue Res* 1991;27:15–31.
35. Yost NP, Bloom SL, Twickler DM, Leveno KJ. Pitfalls in ultrasonic cervical length measurement for predicting preterm birth. *Obstet Gynecol* 1999;93:510–16.
36. Leppert PC, Yu SY, Keller S, Cerreta J, Mandl I. Decreased elastic fibers and desmosine content in incompetent cervix. *Am J Obstet Gynecol* 1987;157:1134–9.
37. Osmers R, Rath W, Pflanz MA, Kuhn W, Stuhlsatz HW, Szeverenyi M. Glycosaminoglycans in cervical connective-tissue during pregnancy and parturition. *Obstet Gynecol* 1993;81:88–92.
38. Iozzo RV. Matrix proteoglycans: From molecular design to cellular function. *Ann Rev Biochem* 1998;67:609–52.
39. Norman M, Ekman G, Malmstrom A. Changed proteoglycan metabolism in human cervix immediately after spontaneous vaginal delivery. *Obstet Gynecol* 1993;81:217–23.
40. Fischer DC, Kuth A, Winkler M *et al.* A large keratan sulfate proteoglycan present in human cervical mucous appears to be involved in the reorganization of the cervical extracellular matrix at term. *J Soc Gynecol Invest* 2001;8:277–84.
41. Winkler M, Rath W. Changes in the cervical extracellular matrix during pregnancy and parturition. *J Perinat Med* 1999;27:45–60.
42. Kobayashi H, Sun GW, Terao T. Production of prostanoids via increased cyclo-oxygenase-2 expression in human amnion cells in response to low molecular weight hyaluronic acid fragment. *Biochim Biophys Acta Gen Subj* 1998;1425:369–76.
43. Stern R. Devising a pathway for hyaluronan catabolism: Are we there yet? *Glycobiology* 2003;13:105R–115R.
44. Ledingham MA, Denison FC, Riley SC, Norman JE. Matrix metalloproteinases-2 and -9 and their inhibitors are produced by the human uterine cervix but their secretion is not regulated by nitric oxide donors. *Hum Reprod* 1999;14:2089–96.
45. Lenhart JA, Ryan PL, Ohleth KM, Palmer SS, Bagnell CA. Relaxin increases secretion of matrix metalloproteinase-2 and matrix metalloproteinase-9 during uterine and cervical growth and remodeling in the pig. *Endocrinology* 2001;142:3941–9.
46. Lenhart JA, Ryan PL, Ohleth KM, Palmer SS, Bagnell CA. Relaxin increases secretion of tissue inhibitor of matrix metalloproteinase-1 and -2 during uterine and cervical growth and remodeling in the pig. *Endocrinology* 2002;143:91–8.
47. Stygar D, Wang H, Vladic YS, Ekman G, Eriksson H, Sahlin L. Increased level of matrix metalloproteinases 2 and 9 in the ripening process of the human cervix. *Biol Reprod* 2002;67: 889–94.
48. Balbin M, Fueyo A, Knauper V *et al.* Collagenase 2a (MMP-8) expression in murine tissue-remodeling processes. Analysis of its potential role in postpartum involution of the uterus. *J Biol Chem* 1998;273:23959–68.
49. Yoshida M, Sagawa N, Itoh H *et al.* Prostaglandin F2{alpha}, cytokines and cyclic mechanical stretch augment matrix metalloproteinase-1 secretion from cultured human uterine cervical fibroblast cells. *Mol Hum Reprod* 2002;8:681–7.
50. Curry TG, Osteen KG. The matrix metalloproteinase system: Changes, regulation, and impact throughout the ovarian and uterine reproductive cycle. *Endocr Rev* 2003;24:428–65.
51. Imada K, Ito A, Itoh Y, Nagase H, Mori Y. Progesterone increases the production of tissue inhibitor of metalloproteinases-2 in rabbit uterine cervical fibroblasts. *FEBS Lett* 1994;341:109–12.
52. Szabo KA, Ablin RJ, Singh G. Matrix metalloproteinases and the immune response. *Clin Appl Immunol Rev* 2004;4:295–319.
53. Yoshida M, Sagawa N, Itoh H *et al.* Nitric oxide increases matrix metalloproteinase-1 production in human uterine cervical fibroblast cells. *Mol Hum Reprod* 2001;7:979–85.
54. Young A, Thomson AJ, Ledingham M, Jordan F, Greer IA, Norman JE. Immunolocalization of proinflammatory cytokines in myometrium, cervix, and fetal membranes during human parturition at term. *Biol Reprod* 2002;66:445–9.
55. El Maradny E, Kanayama N, Halim A, Maehara K, Sumimoto K, Terao T. Interleukin-8 induces cervical ripening in rabbits. *Am J Obstet Gynecol* 1994;171:77–83.
56. Chwalisz K, Benson M, Scholz P, Daum J, Beier HM, Hegele-Hartung C. Cervical ripening with the cytokines interleukin 8, interleukin 1 beta and tumour necrosis factor alpha in guinea-pigs. *Hum.Reprod* 1994;9:2173–81.
57. Ito A, Hiro D, Ojima Y, Mori Y. Spontaneous production of interleukin-1-like factors from pregnant rabbit uterine cervix. *Am J Obstet Gynecol* 1988;159:261–5.
58. Maul H, Nagel S, Welsch G, Schafer A, Winkler M, Rath W. Messenger ribonucleic acid levels of interleukin-1 beta, interleukin-6 and interleukin-8 in the lower uterine segment increased significantly at final cervical dilatation during term parturition,

while those of tumor necrosis factor alpha remained unchanged. *Eur J Obstet Gynecol Reprod Biol* 2002;102:143–7.
59. Hebisch G, Grauaug AA, Neumaier-Wagner PM, Stallmach T, Huch A, Huch R. The relationship between cervical dilatation, interleukin-6 and interleukin-8 during term labor. *Acta Obstet Gynecol Scand* 2001;80:840–8.
60. Parekh T, Saxena B, Reibman J, Cronstein BN, Gold LI. Neutrophil chemotaxis in response to TGF-beta isoforms (TGF-beta 1, TGF-beta 2, TGF-beta 3) is mediated by fibronectin. *J Immunol* 1994; 152:2456–66.
61. Ekerhovd E, Brannstrom M, Weijdegard B, Norstrom A. Nitric oxide synthases in the human cervix at term pregnancy and effects of nitric oxide on cervical smooth muscle contractility. *Am J Obstet Gynecol* 2000;183:610–16.
62. Buhimschi I, Ali M, Jain V, Chwalisz K, Garfield RE. Differential regulation of nitric oxide in the rat uterus and cervix during pregnancy and labour. *Hum Reprod* 1996;11:1755–66.
63. Shimano M, Nakaya Y, Fukui R *et al.* Activation of Ca^{2+}-activated K^+ channels in human myometrium by nitric oxide. *Gynecol Obstet Invest* 2000;49:249–54.
64. Buxton ILO, Kaiser RA, Malmquist NA, Tichenor S. NO-induced relaxation of labouring and non-labouring human myometrium is not mediated by cyclic GMP. *Br J Pharmacol* 2001;134:206–14.
65. Ledingham MA, Thomson AJ, Young A, Macara LM, Greer IA, Norman JE. Changes in the expression of nitric oxide synthase in the human uterine cervix during pregnancy and parturition. *Mol Hum Reprod* 2000;6:1041–8.
66. Tschugguel W, Schneeberger C, Lass H *et al.* Human cervical ripening is associated with an increase in cervical inducible nitric oxide synthase expression. *Biol Reprod* 1999;60:1367–72.
67. Facchinetti F, Piccinini F, Volpe A. Chemical ripening of the cervix with intracervical application of sodium nitroprusside: A randomized controlled trial. *Hum Reprod* 2000;15:2224–7.
68. Allaire AD, D'Andrea N, Truong P, McMahon MJ, Lessey BA. Cervical stroma apoptosis in pregnancy. *Obstet Gynecol* 2001; 97:399–403.
69. Bao S, Rai J, Schreiber J. Brain nitric oxide synthase expression is enhanced in the human cervix in labor. *J Soc Gynecol Investig* 2001;8:158–64.
70. Rudel D, Pajntar M. Active contractions of the cervix in the latent phase of labour. *Br J Obstet Gynaecol* 1999;106:446–52.
71. Pajntar M, Verdenik I. Electromyographic activity in cervices with very low Bishop score during labor. *Int J Gynaecol Obstet* 1995; 49:277–81.
72. Ekerhovd E, Brannstrom M, Weijdegard B, Norstrom A. Nitric oxide synthases in the human cervix at term pregnancy and effects of nitric oxide on cervical smooth muscle contractility. *Am J Obstet Gynecol* 2000;183:610–16.
73. Ekerhovd E, Brannstrom M, Delbro D, Norstrom A. Nitric oxide mediated inhibition of contractile activity in the human uterine cervix. *Mol Hum Reprod* 1998;4:915–20.
74. Watari M, Watari H, DiSanto ME, Chacko S, Shi GP, Strauss JF III. Pro-inflammatory cytokines induce expression of matrix-metabolizing enzymes in human cervical smooth muscle cells. *Am J Pathol* 1999;154:1755–62.
75. Watari M, Watari H, Fujimoto T *et al.* Lipopolysaccharide induces interleukin-8 production by human cervical smooth muscle cells. *J Soc Gynecol Invest* 2003;10:110–17.
76. Sugano T, Narahara H, Nasu K, Arima K, Fujisawa K, Miyakawa I. Effects of platelet-activating factor on cytokine production by human uterine cervical fibroblasts. *Mol Hum Reprod* 2001;7: 475–81.
77. Sugano T, Nasu K, Narahara H, Kawano Y, Nishida Y, Miyakawa I. Platelet-activating factor induces an imbalance between matrix metalloproteinase-1 and tissue inhibitor of metalloproteinases-1 expression in human uterine cervical fibroblasts. *Biol Reprod* 2000;62:540–6.
78. Osmers R, Rath W, Adelmann-Grill BC *et al.* Origin of cervical collagenase during parturition. *Am J Obstet Gynecol* 1992;166: 1455–60.
79. Winkler M, Kemp B, Fischer DC, Ruck P, Rath W. Expression of adhesion molecules in the lower uterine segment during term and preterm parturition. *Microsc Res Tech* 2003;60:430–44.
80. Osman I, Young A, Ledingham MA *et al.* Leukocyte density and pro-inflammatory cytokine expression in human fetal membranes, decidua, cervix and myometrium before and during labour at term. *Mol Hum Reprod* 2003;9:41–5.
81. Varayoud J, Ramos JG, Bosquiazzo VL, Munoz-de-Toro M, Luque EH. Mast cells degranulation affects angiogenesis in the rat uterine cervix during pregnancy. *Reproduction* 2004;127:379–87.
82. Wu WX, Ma XH, Coksaygan T *et al.* Prostaglandin mediates premature delivery in pregnant sheep induced by estradiol at 121 days of gestational age. *Endocrinology* 2004;145:1444–52.
83. Rodriguez HA, Kass L, Varayoud J *et al.* Collagen remodelling in the guinea-pig uterine cervix at term is associated with a decrease in progesterone receptor expression. *Mol Hum Reprod* 2003;9: 807–13.
84. Stjernholm YM, Sahlin L, Eriksson HA, Bystrom BE, Stenlund PM, Ekman GE. Cervical ripening after treatment with prostaglandin E2 or antiprogestin (RU486). Possible mechanisms in relation to gonadal steroids. *Eur J Obstet Gynecol Reprod Biol* 1999;84: 83–8.
85. Rechberger T, Abramson SR, Woessner JF. Onapristone and prostaglandin E(2) induction of delivery in the rat in rate pregnancy: A model for the analysis of cervical softening. *Am J Obstet Gynecol* 1996;175:719–23.
86. Imada K, Ito A, Sato T, Namiki M, Nagase H, Mori Y. Hormonal regulation of matrix metalloproteinase 9/gelatinase B gene expression in rabbit uterine cervical fibroblasts. *Biol Reprod* 1997;56: 575–80.
87. Luque EH, Ramos JG, Rodriguez HA, Munoz de Toro MM. Dissociation in the control of cervical eosinophilic infiltration and collagenolysis at the end of pregnancy or after pseudopregnancy in ovariectomized steroid-treated rats. *Biol Reprod* 1996;55: 1206–12.
88. Rajabi MR, Solomon S, Poole AR. Biochemical evidence of collagenase-mediated collagenolysis as a mechanism of cervical dilatation at parturition in the guinea pig. *Biol Reprod* 1991;45: 764–72.
89. Rajabi MR, Dodge GR, Solomon S, Poole AR. Immunochemical and immunohistochemical evidence of estrogen-mediated collagenolysis as a mechanism of cervical dilatation in the guinea pig at parturition. *Endocrinology* 1991;128:371–8.
90. Tanaka K, Nakamura T, Takagaki K, Funahashi M, Saito Y, Endo M. Regulation of hyaluronate metabolism by progesterone in cultured fibroblasts from the human uterine cervix. *FEBS Lett* 1997;402:223–6.
91. Ramos JG, Varayoud J, Kass L *et al.* Estrogen and progesterone modulation of eosinophilic infiltration of the rat uterine cervix. *Steroids* 2000;65:409–14.
92. Stygar D, Wang H, Vladic YS, Ekman G, Eriksson H, Sahlin L. Co-localization of oestrogen receptor {beta} and leukocyte markers in the human cervix. *Mol Hum Reprod* 2001;7:881–6.
93. Norman M, Ekman G, Malmstrom A. Prostaglandin E(2)-induced ripening of the human cervix involves changes in proteoglycan metabolism. *Obstet Gynecol* 1993;82:1013–20.
94. Ekman G, Malmstrom A, Uldbjerg N, Ulmsten U. Cervical collagen: An important regulator of cervical function in term labor. *Obstet Gynecol* 1986;67:633–6.
95. Noström, A. Influence of prostaglandin E_2 on the biosynthesis of connective tissue constituents in the pregnant human cervix. *Prostaglandins* 1982;23:361–7.
96. Kelly RW. Pregnancy maintenance and parturition: The role of prostaglandin in manipulating the immune and inflammatory response. *Endocr Rev* 1994;15:684–706.
97. Sennstrom MB, Ekman G, Westergren-Thorsson G *et al.* Human cervical ripening, an inflammatory process mediated by cytokines. *Mol Hum Reprod* 2000;6:375–81.
98. Hertelendy F, Zakar T. Prostaglandins and the myometrium and cervix. *Prostaglandins Leukot Essent Fatty Acids* 2004;70:207–22.
99. Ledingham MA, Denison FC, Kelly RW, Young A, Norman JE. Nitric oxide donors stimulate prostaglandin F2{alpha} and inhibit thromboxane B2 production in the human cervix during the first trimester of pregnancy. *Mol Hum Reprod* 1999;5:973–82.
100. Smith GCS, Wu WX, Nathanielsz PW. Effects of gestational age and labor on the expression of prostanoid receptor genes in pregnant baboon cervix. *Prostaglandins Other Lipid Mediat* 2001;63: 153–63.
101. Schmitz T, Dallot E, Leroy MJ, Breuiller-Fouche M, Ferre F, Cabrol D. EP4 receptors mediate prostaglandin E2-stimulated glycosaminoglycan synthesis in human cervical fibroblasts in culture. *Mol Hum Reprod* 2001;7:397–402.
102. Lyons CA, Beharry KD, Nishihara KC *et al.* Regulation of matrix metalloproteinases (type IV collagenases) and their inhibitors in the virgin, timed pregnant, and postpartum rat uterus and cervix by prostaglandin E(2)-cyclic adenosine monophosphate. *Am J Obstet Gynecol* 2002;187:202–8.
103. Jackson GM, Sharp HT, Varner MW. Cervical ripening before induction of labor: A randomized trial of prostaglandin E2 gel versus low-dose oxytocin. *Am J Obstet Gynecol* 1994;171:1092–6.

104. Magann EF, Perry KG Jr, Dockery JR Jr, Bass JD, Chauhan SP, Morrison JC. Cervical ripening before medical induction of labor: A comparison of prostaglandin E2, estradiol, and oxytocin. *Am J Obstet Gynecol* 1995;172:1702–6.
105. Fuchs AR, Ivell R, Balvers M, Chang SM, Fields MJ. Oxytocin receptors in bovine cervix during pregnancy and parturition: gene expression and cellular localization. *Am J Obstet Gynecol* 1996; 175:1654–60.
106. Wathes DC, Smith HF, Leung ST, Stevenson KR, Meier S, Jenkin G. Oxytocin receptor development in ovine uterus and cervix throughout pregnancy and at parturition as determined by in situ hybridization analysis. *J Reprod Fertil* 1996;106:23–31.
107. Wu W, Nathanielsz PW. Changes in oxytocin receptor messenger RNA in the endometrium, myometrium, mesometrium, and cervix of sheep in late gestation and during spontaneous and cortisol-induced labor. *J Soc Gynecol Invest* 1994;1:191–6.
108. Shemesh M, Dombrovski L, Gurevich M, Shore LS, Fuchs AR, Fields MJ. Regulation of bovine cervical secretion of prostaglandins and synthesis of cyclooxygenase by oxytocin. *Reprod Fertil Dev* 1997;9:525–30.
109. Fuchs AR, Fuchs F, Husslein P, Soloff MS. Oxytocin receptors in the human uterus during pregnancy and parturition. *Am J Obstet Gynecol* 1984;150:734–41.
110. Liggins CG. Cervical ripening as an inflammatory reaction. In: Ellwood DA, Andersen ABM, eds. *The Cervix in Pregnancy and Labour: Clinical and Biochemical Investigations.* Edinburgh: Churchill Livingstone, 1981.

86 Physiology of maternal sleep in pregnancy

K. Biedermann and R. Huch

Introduction

Pregnancy involves fundamental readjustment of the maternal organism, often associated with unpleasant changes, notably fatigue and reduced energy.[1,2] It is popularly believed to impair sleep. Pregnant women try to sleep more, but are still often tired and perform less efficiently.[3] Those affected tend to account for their residual fatigue in terms of progressive sleep deprivation, due to altered and fragmented sleep in pregnancy.[4] By means of a questionnaire on wrist actimetry in daily life and polysomnography in the sleep laboratory, we investigated the changes in sleep habit and quality in pregnancy and assessed their relationship to fatigue.

Background

Methods of sleep research

Polysomnography – a combination of electroencephalography (EEG), electromyography (EMG) and electrooculography (EOG) – is the gold standard for sleep investigation and arbiter of sleep stage division into rapid eye movement (REM) sleep and non-REM (NREM) sleep, which is itself subdivided into four stages of differing depths.[5]

The sleep EEG is the sum curve of the electrical vectors on the scalp produced by the discharge of thousands of neurons. This neuron activity consists of waves differing in frequency and amplitude. The sum curve is broken down by Fourier analysis into individual frequency bands. The proportion of waves at a given frequency (power density) is deduced from this spectrum; in particular, the slow waves (1–12 Hz frequency band) indicative of deep sleep are differentiated from intermediate (13–17 Hz, α-rhythm of the resting waking state) and rapid waves (18–25 Hz), which occur in NREM sleep stages 1 and 2. Whole-night spectral analysis shows waves of the whole frequency spectrum in all sleep stages, but with different power densities in the different frequency bands.

Figure 86.1 shows the different sleep stages (sleep structure) combined with Fourier analysis of the sleep EEG. The sleep stages are shown along the top, above the waves at different frequency bands over the entire sleep episode. Long-wave sleep (1–4 Hz) shows a marked increase in the first sleep cycles, with the maxima falling in NREM sleep stages 3 and 4. In the later sleep cycles long-wave activity decreases continuously until it eventually disappears almost completely.

Sleep stages and sleep control

NREM sleep

In stage 1 sleep, there is a decrease in the high-frequency EEG waves, but muscle tone and autonomic function (blood pressure, heart rate and respiration) remain at their waking levels or only decrease insignificantly. Dream-like experiences occur frequently and mostly relate to the thought content of the preceding waking stage. Stage 2 sleep follows after approximately 5 min. The EEG shows the characteristic spindles and spontaneous and evoked K-complexes. Muscle tone is markedly reduced, the eyes are quiet, and movement artifacts absent. Autonomic function decreases further compared to stage 1; the arousal threshold is raised. Consciousness and receptivity to external events are absent. Stage 2 NREM sleep accounts for over 50% of total sleep time and is hence the chronologically dominant sleep stage. This protracted stage is followed by the transition to deep sleep (stages 3 and 4), with the first occurrence of distinct σ-waves (0.5–4 Hz). Muscle tone is lower than in stage 2; tendon reflexes are preserved. The eyes are actively closed; eye movement is absent. Consciousness is extinguished and autonomic function further reduced. Low-frequency σ-waves dominate stage 4 NREM sleep (50%), and the EMG shows minimal muscle tone. Arousal from the deepest stage of sleep requires the strongest stimuli.

REM sleep

REM sleep, characterized by salvoes of REMs[6] is also termed paradoxical sleep because the EEG is dominated by high-frequency waking waves. However,

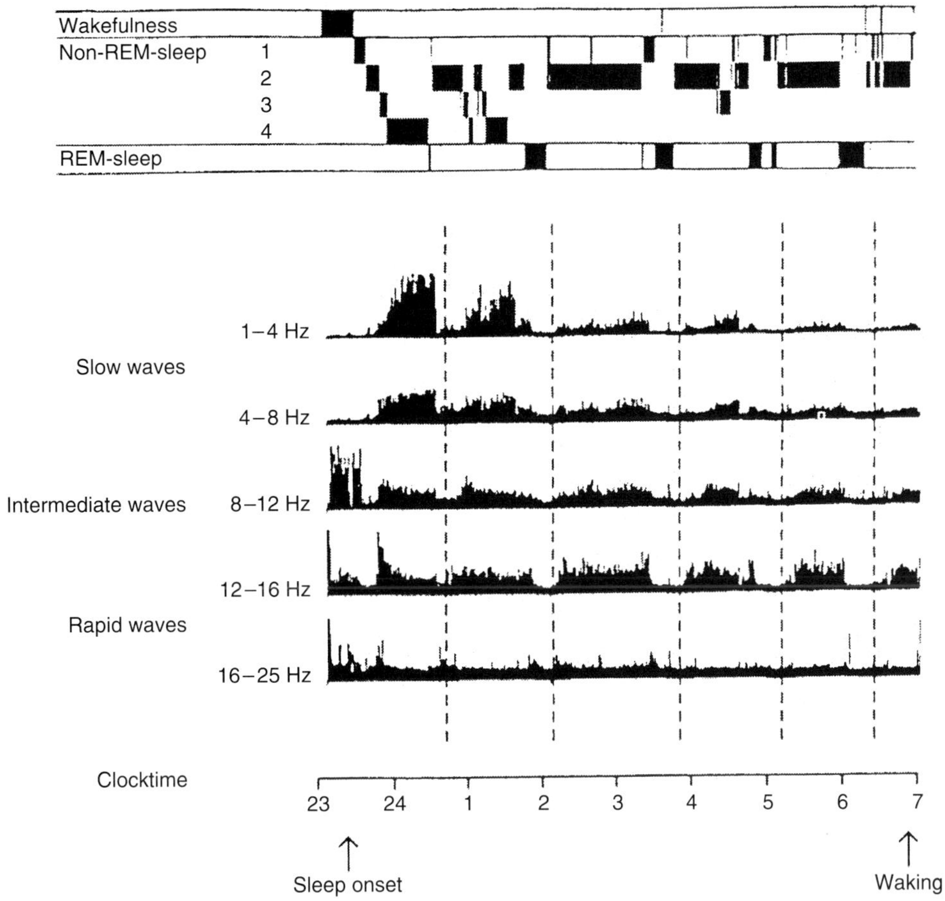

Figure 86.1 Sleep stages (sleep structure) (top) and spectral analysis (sleep architecture) in a whole-night polysomnogram (bottom).

muscle tone is almost entirely absent. REM sleep is dream intensive and altogether accounts for approximately 20% of the total sleep time, its share tending to decrease as the sleep episode progresses.

Internal clock

Like many physical functions, the sleep–wake cycle is subject to a circadian rhythm. Under normal conditions, this is set to a 24-h-day, but it also operates in experimental isolation, where it is set to a 25-h-day.[7] Animal experiments have identified the oscillator of the internal clock as a small neuron nucleus lying above the optic chiasma: the suprachiasmatic nucleus.

Sleep factors

Several sleep factors have been discovered to date, e.g. S factor,[8] sleep promoting substance,[7] σ-sleep-inducing peptide,[9,10] prostaglandin D_2,[11] immune polypeptides, such as interleukin-1, interferon and tumor necrosis factor, and neurosteroids.[12,13] None has yet been shown to play a central role. Sleep modulation and control is thus presumed to be multifactorial.[14]

Sleep and fatigue in pregnancy

Fatigue has been defined as a subjective and objective decrease in energy with respect to various spontaneous activities.[15] It is primarily the result of physical activity, or more precisely of inadequate recovery from such activity. Many other factors can cause or increase fatigue, e.g. psychological[16] and hormonal influences, in addition to anemia, hypotension, obesity, magnesium deficiency and infectious disease. Fatigue in pregnancy is multifactorial, involving psychological and emotional factors, marked hormonal changes and obvious biological determinants, such as weight gain, pregnancy anemia and the tendency to hypotension.

Sleep disturbance and decreased drive are the common complaints throughout pregnancy, present in 20% and 40% of women, respectively, in the first trimester, and increasing to 70% in the case of sleep disturbance at term.[17] A survey of 100 pregnant women at term found that mean sleep time increased in the first trimester and again in the third trimester; sleep was increasingly shallow and interrupted, while birth and baby themes came to dominate dream content at the expense of daytime experience.[18]

Clinical study

Structure and methods

A total of 189 women attending the Zurich University Hospital Obstetric Outpatients Clinic were recruited

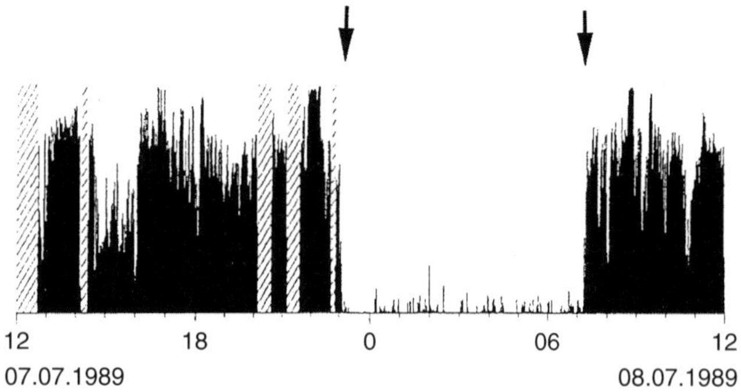

Figure 86.2 Printout of modified 24-h (noon–noon) activity data files. Arrows, onset and end of sleep; hatched areas, erased recording phases (excluded from analysis).

over 2.2 years. The inclusion criteria, in addition to informed consent, were a normal singleton pregnancy and the absence of sleep disturbance and relevant psychological or somatic complaints. At the booking visit, subjects were questioned by a (female) physician about their lifestyle and occupation and sleep behavior before pregnancy. At the end of each trimester and 6 weeks postpartum, they were reinterviewed about any changes. The questionnaires were drafted with the aid of the Institute of Pharmacology, Zurich University, and psychologists.

Activity was monitored in 70 of the subjects using wrist actigraphy:[19–21] a wrist-worn matchbox-sized monitor (Gähwiler Electronics, Zurich) converts movement to electrical signals via a piezoelectric transducer; the signals release an impulse if they exceed a set threshold (0.1 $g\,m/s^2$). Epochs were set to 1 min for optimal movement resolution compatible with the device's 1-week storage capacity. Subjects were asked to wear the monitor as far as possible continuously for 1 week on the wrist of the non-dominant hand, once per trimester and postpartum. They were also asked to record sleep times together with specific activities, e.g. driving, in a sleep and activity diary to enable blank phases and passive vibration to be excluded from the analysis. Monitors were downloaded onto an IBM PC and the raw data, comprising 10,080 measurements over the 7 days, were edited according to the diary entries. It was these modified data sets that were then analyzed (Figure 86.2).

In addition to interview and actigraphy, 10 subjects also underwent polysomnography (Grass, with online Fourier analysis) for two consecutive nights in each trimester (weeks 10, 20 and 30), commencing at lights out. Subjects could get up at their own discretion and were woken at the time they requested. The polygraphic data were manually scored according to the criteria of Rechtschaffen and Kales[5] for 20-s epochs and fed into the computer as data files for combined analysis of sleep stages and EEG spectra, in addition to conventional sleep stage analysis.

The Mann–Whitney U rank test and Wilcoxon's signed rank test were used for statistical analysis, and the significance level for longitudinal changes through pregnancy adjusted with Bonferroni's correction. The chi-squared test and Fisher's exact test were used for multiple comparisons.

Sleep study results

Population

The median age was 28 years (range 15–45 years). A total of 87 women (46.0%) were expecting their first child, 161 (85.2%) were married and 47.1% were in full-time employment at the start of the pregnancy. Median booking visit body weight was 56 kg (range 40–93 kg); median weight gain during pregnancy was 13.9 kg (range –4 to +28.5 kg), equivalent to 25.4% of baseline body weight (range –9% to +53%).

Of the women 37.6% had smoked until their pregnancy; 20% smoked more than 10 cigarettes daily. The remaining 62.4% described themselves as nonsmokers. Forty percent consumed virtually no alcohol before their pregnancy, while 11% had a weekly alcohol intake equivalent to 180 ml of 100% alcohol, for example, in 1.5 l wine, 4.5 l beer or 0.5 l spirits, assuming a medium alcohol content (12%, 4% and 36%, respectively).

Sleep times

The most reliable sleep–time data were obtained by actigraphy. These values were compared with the questionnaire answers provided by the same women and with control data for 20–40-year-old women from a representative 1983 Swiss population survey.[22]

Mean actigraphic time in bed in pregnancy was 8 h 22 min on weekdays and 8 h 42 min at weekends (Table 86.1). These values deviated somewhat from the questionnaire responses: Weekday time in bed was underestimated by 14 min, while weekend time in bed was overestimated by 25 min. The actigraphic weekday–weekend difference was only 20 min (8.42 vs. 8.22) vs. a subjective estimate of 59 min. Pregnant women reported 20 min more sleep during weekdays, and only 12 min more sleep during weekends, than the reference population. When averaged over the week, time in bed was longer in pregnancy by 18 min/night (+3.3%). This difference is slight and illustrates the fact that pregnant women, like their non-pregnant counterparts, adjust their sleep time to their occupational and social commitments. A general finding was that the pregnant women generally went late to bed, thereby failing to use a possible means of sleep compensation.(Table 86.1)

Sleep times showed no significant changes during pregnancy, but actigraphic time in bed tended to be longer in the first trimester, due to an earlier bedtime than later in pregnancy (Table 86.2). Bedtime differed significantly between the first and third trimesters ($P < 0.01$). It was surprising that many women (47.1%) were still working in the first trimester; their

Table 86.1 Whole pregnancy weekend and weekday bedtime (BT), rising time (RT) and time in bed (TIB) (h:min; mean ±SD) in the actigraphy population (n=70) vs. age-matched non-pregnant controls[19]

	Weekends			Weekdays		
	BT	RT	TIB	BT	RT	TIB
Self-rating	23:38 (1:14)	8:45 (1:17)	9:07 (1:13)	22:47 (0:52)	6:55 (1:00)	8:08 (0:59)
Actigrapy	23:31 (0:45)	8:14 (0:50)	8:42 (0:46)	23:00 (0:43)	7:21 (0:50)	8:22 (0:40)
Non-pregnant controls	22:50 (1:53)	8:38 (1:33)	8:55 (1:23)	22:02 (1:35)	6:36 (0:56)	7:48 (1:07)

Table 86.2 Actigraphic bedtime, rising time and time in bed (h:min; mean ±SD; n=70) during and after pregnancy

	Trimester			
	First	Second	Third	Postpartum
Bedtime	22:59 (0:46)	23:08 (0:45)	23:15 (0:59)	23:14 (0:50)
Rising time	7:34 (0:51)	7:34 (0:57)	7:44 (0:59)	7:37 (0:56)
Time in bed	8:37 (0:50)	8:26 (0:47)	8:29 (0:46)	8:23 (0:49)

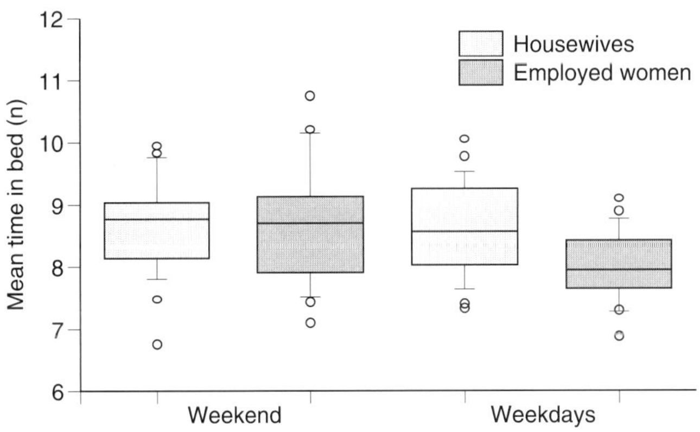

Figure 86.3 Mean time in bed in housewives (n=21) and full-time employees (n=24) on weekdays and weekends. Housewives spent longer in bed than employees on weekdays (P=0.008, Mann–Whitney test). Boxes: 25th, 50th and 75th centiles; T bars: 10th and 90th centiles.

proportion decreased progressively during pregnancy (20% in the third trimester). Rising time, on the other hand, did not change during pregnancy, ranging from 07:34 to 07:44 h.

Employment affected the total sleep time. On weekdays, housewives slept almost 1 h longer than employed women ($P < 0.001$), went to bed at the same time but sleeping some 40 min longer in the morning (Figure 86.3). However, they reported fatigue with the same frequency as their employed counterparts. At weekends, employed women slept on average only 11 min longer than housewives (9 h 30 min vs. 9 h 19 min; not significant).

Dreams

Dream activity is typically more intense in pregnancy, centered on themes of pregnancy, birth and baby,[18] and frequently tinged with anxiety.[23] A total 22% of women reported more intense dreaming in the first trimester, rising to 30% in the second and third trimesters, and returning to prepregnancy levels days after delivery. The increase in dream activity in pregnancy and postpartum was unrelated to energy levels, despite nightmares being a frequent cause of waking in pregnancy. Pregnancy dream content is non-prognostic for pregnancy outcome or quality of subsequent mother–infant bonding.[24]

Daytime naps

Before pregnancy, only 37% of the women took an occasional or regular daytime nap. During pregnancy the proportion increased to 41% in the first trimester (mean 42.6 min) and 50% in the third trimester (mean 31.3 min). Only 26% took no nap at any time during their pregnancy. Napping had little effect on sleep behavior. In fact, total sleep time in 24-h periods that included a daytime sleep was approximately 1 h longer than in identical periods with no nap; nocturnal sleep times were therefore unchanged. Naps were more often associated with nocturnal sleep onset problems (21.7% vs. 10.0%, $P < 0.05$). Napping had no effect on nocturnal motor activity (mean nil phase time and motor latency). Employment had no effect on napping.

Sleep quality

Women reported sleep changes in early pregnancy in 85% of the cases. Increases in sleep time and sleep latency were reported by 43% and 36%, respectively. Sleep was shallower (44%) and also disturbed by arousal stimuli, which had not caused waking before pregnancy. In the second trimester, 68% reported improved sleep quality, followed by further deterioration in the third trimester when sleep was more easily disturbed (52%) and more fragmented. These data were confirmed by very similar values in a Japanese study.[25] The main causes of sleep disturbance are bathroom trips,[26] unaccustomed sleep position,[27,28] back pain,[29] fetal movement,[3] nightmares, hunger and thirst.

Sleep quality ran only partly in parallel with sleep time during pregnancy. Often the changes were mutually contradictory, greater fatigue being reported despite longer sleep or subjects describing themselves as more rested despite shorter sleep. Approximately 90% of women reported fatigue during pregnancy, from the first trimester onward; self-rated energy was lowest in the first and third trimesters, unaffected by the usual amplitude of sleep changes, and unrelieved by longer sleep. Fetal sex did not affect maternal sleep behavior or energy. Hypnotics were taken only in exceptional cases (0.5%, mostly benzodiazepines); approximately 10% of the women took 'natural' hypnotics (valerian, candy).

Sleep latency. Sleep latency (the interval between lights out and the first stage 2 sleep) can only be determined by polysomnography. However, we found a significant correlation between subjective sleep onset time and polysomnographic sleep latency. Difficulty in falling asleep was one of the commonest sleep disturbances, reported by 29%, including almost 10% reporting sleep latency exceeding 30 min. However, the great majority (63.7%) fell asleep in less than 10 min. Sleep latency decreased with increasing sleep pressure, i.e. the longer subjects had been awake the more quickly they fell asleep. Mean time in bed was longer in women taking a longer time to fall asleep: women falling asleep in $\leq$10 min slept 23 min less than those falling asleep in > 10 min (8 h 43 min vs. 8 h 20 min, $P < 0.01$). The time taken to fall asleep showed only small changes throughout pregnancy, but was longest (not significantly) at term.

Actigraphic motor latency was defined similarly as sleep latency as the interval between lights out and the first nil activity phase lasting $\geq$5 min. It was longer in pregnancy than postpartum (6 vs. 5 min, $P < 0.01$), but unchanged during pregnancy itself. It was also longer on weekdays than at weekends (7 vs. 6 min, $P < 0.01$), probably due to the earlier bedtime. Restless sleep was associated with a longer motor latency as motor activity in women with restless sleep was also increased during sleep onset.

Nocturnal waking. Sleep in pregnancy was fragmented by nocturnal waking, reported by at least 40% of subjects once per night even before pregnancy. The most frequent causes were 'internal', e.g. bathroom trips or thirst (58%), external factors, e.g. noise and temperature (40%), and nightmares (21%); 9% had no explanation.

In pregnancy, the proportion of women generally waking at night increased to 78% in the first trimester, fell to 69% in the second trimester and increased again to 79% in the third trimester (vs. 23% postpartum). The proportion of women waking up more than once increased steadily from 30% in the first trimester to 52% in the third trimester. Employed women awoke less often than housewives (1.4 vs. 1.7 times per night, $P < 0.05$) who more frequently already had a young child to look after.

Nocturnal rising. Rising at night ran in parallel with waking at night during pregnancy, following 59–66% of waking episodes. Both sets of values were thus largely similar. Getting up at least once a night even before pregnancy was reported by 42.1% of women. In contrast to other studies,[16,30] this had no detectable impact on sleep quality. In the first and second trimesters, 58% and 51% of women rose at least once per night, respectively (increases of 15% and 8%, respectively); the proportion then increased in the third trimester to 76% ($P < 0.0001$). Improvement was only partial after delivery when, mainly because of the baby, rising was still more frequent than in the first and second trimesters (Figure 86.4). Bathroom trips were the commonest cause of rising at night even before pregnancy (43.8%), followed by caring for a small child (24.4%), hunger and thirst (14.6%) and uncomfortable environmental temperature and nervousness (Table 86.3). Bathroom trips remained the major cause throughout pregnancy, cited by 69.6% in the third trimester (Table 86.3), with a proportionate decrease in risings caused by a small child. The baby was, as expected, the dominant cause after pregnancy.

Fatigue and energy. Fatigue has been defined as the subjective and objective decrease in energy.[15] Fatigue and energy thus represent opposite poles of the same spectrum, describing the same reality in inversely proportional terms. Only 26% of women reported feeling rested on waking even before pregnancy; a good third described themselves as 'tired' on waking. Physical and mental energy is known to be decreased early in pregnancy. A total of 70.9% of women reported fatigue/decreased energy at the end of the first trimester; 18.5% reported feeling marked fatigue/markedly reduced energy (Table 86.4). Only a minority (3.7%) felt more energy in the first trimester than before pregnancy. Fatigue/decreased energy was thus a common complaint in early pregnancy, decreasing transiently to 34.6% in the second trimester before reascending in the third trimester to 65%. It improved postpartum in two-thirds of subjects, but was still reported in 31.6%.

Mean fatigue scores (1 = very tired, 6 = very energetic) were determined in 70 subjects throughout

Table 86.3 Causes of nocturnal rising (%) before, during and after pregnancy in 70 patients (over 1690 nights)

		Trimester			
Cause	Prepregnancy*	First ($n=422$)	Second ($n=459$)	Third ($n=438$)	Postpartum ($n=371$)
Bathroom trips	43.8	58.0	67.4	69.6	12.5
Child, breastfeeding**	24.4	24.2	19.5	13.6	80.5
Hunger/thirst	14.6	10.1	8.1	5.1	1.3
Miscellaneous	17.2	7.7	5.0	11.7	5.7

*Booking visit data; **from a previous pregnancy

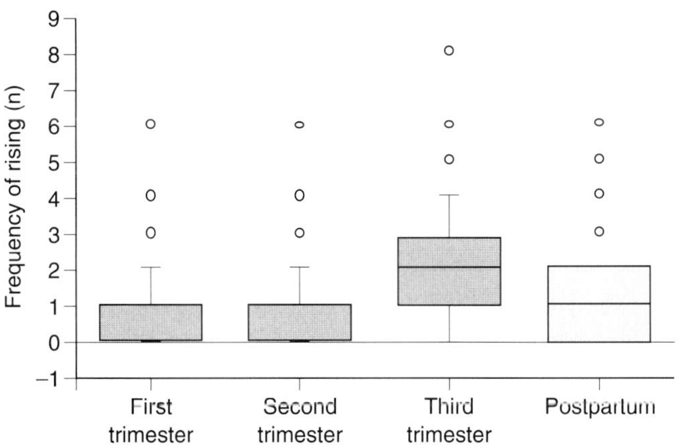

Figure 86.4 Mean frequency of nocturnal rising in pregnancy and postpartum ($n=70$), showing an increase from the second to third trimester ($P<0.0001$).

pregnancy and were used to divide the population into three groups. Sleep parameters and clinical findings were then analyzed separately for the three groups. Only one sleep parameter (bedtime) and two clinical parameters (basal hemoglobin and minimal diastolic blood pressure) correlated significantly with fatigue in pregnancy (Table 86.5).

The mean difference in bedtime between tired and energetic women was 23 min ($P=0.026$) (Table 86.5). There were no differences in rising time or time in bed. Nocturnal activity [nil activity time, percentage nil activity and mean nil phase length (mNPL)] and nocturnal waking were unrelated to fatigue. Motor latency appeared longer (not significantly) in the tired group. Daytime napping was equally frequent in all three groups.

The reasons advanced as possible causes of fatigue on waking differed throughout pregnancy and postpartum (Table 86.6): the most frequent were bathroom trips, inadequate sleep or rest, evening coffee or tea, workload, personal problems, unaccustomed sleeping position, fetal movement and pregnancy complaints. Interestingly, pregnancy-specific effects on fatigue were not given; the causes were mostly those known to cause fatigue even outside pregnancy.

Employment had little impact on the fatigue reported by approximately 60% of housewives and employed women alike. Energy was not therefore increased by a reduction in workload. Instead, work was adjusted to energy as decreased energy in pregnancy leads to workplace stress and feelings of inadequacy. The increased emotional vulnerability in pregnancy also led many pregnant women to avoid such conflict by leaving their employment. The proportion of full-time employees fell from 47.1% in the first trimester to 20% in the third; the proportion of part-time employees stayed constant throughout pregnancy at 25%.

It is also interesting that performance was not improved by more sleep. Fatigue/decreased energy was no less frequent in women sleeping longer in the first trimester vs. before pregnancy than in those not sleeping longer. The fact that pregnancy fatigue was not made good by longer sleep indicates that sleep disturbance was not the cause, provided it remained within the usual limits. Other complaints, e.g. nervousness, irritability and headache, were also often attributed to sleep disturbance, although they may themselves also be its cause.

Pregnant women are often worried that their decreased energy could affect the course of pregnancy, birth or the baby. These fears can be allayed; prematurity, birth weight and neonatal adjustment were identical in women with markedly decreased energy and those with high or only slightly reduced energy. Duration of labor and spontaneous delivery rates were also identical in both the groups. We failed to confirm the association reported between birth weight and mean sleep time during pregnancy,[31] but confirmed the finding that employment does not affect the course of pregnancy or delivery.[32]

Motor activity during sleep. Like time in bed, the nocturnal nil activity time, i.e. the sum of minute measurement units showing nil activity, also remained largely unchanged throughout pregnancy (median 6 h 50 min). Individual fluctuation during pregnancy was slight, ±18% in 80% of all subjects.

The percentage of nil activity of time in bed was 75–85% in most subjects, but fluctuated markedly (56–93%) in individual cases. It increased from the first to the second trimester ($P<0.01$), evidencing more restless sleep in the first trimester. Other

Table 86.4 Number of pregnant women (%) reporting self-rated energy changes

	Trimester			
Change in energy	**First**	**Second**	**Third**	**Postpartum**
None	13 (6.9)	36 (19.5)	50 (27.3)	2 (1.1)
Slight decrease	134 (70.9)	34 (18.4)	72 (39.3)	48 (27.1)
Severe decrease	35 (18.5)	30 (16.2)	47 (25.7)	8 (4.5)
Increase	7 (3.7)	85 (45.9)	14 (7.7)	199 (67.2)
Total	189 (100)	185 (100)	183 (100)	177 (100)

Table 86.5 Self-rated and clinical determinants of sleep quality in pregnancy and postpartum

Parameter	**Tired (n=23)**	**Indifferent (n=24)**	**Rested (n=23)**	**p***
Bedtime (h:min)	23:19	23:03	22:56	0.026
Booking hemoglobin (g %)	12.25	12.45	12.9	0.02
Minimal diastolic blood presure (mmHg)	55.5	58.0	59.5	0.02

Tired, fatigue score < 4; indifferent, fatigue score 4–4.9; rested, fatigue score ≥5; *tired vs. rested (Mann–Whitney *U* test)

Table 86.6 Number of reported causes (%) of decreased energy in pregnancy and postpartum excluding those reported by < 20% of subjects (n=189 per data point)

	Trimester			
Cause	**First**	**Second**	**Third**	**Postpartum**
Bathroom trips	118 **(62.4)**	135 **(73.0)**	134 **(72.8)**	5 (19.7)
Not enough sleep	74 **(39.2)**	66 **(35.7)**	93 **(50.5)**	49 (27.5)
Evening coffee/tea	64 **(33.9)**	76 **(41.1)**	75 (40.8)	62 **(34.8)**
Nervousness/anxiety	58 (30.7)	65 (35.1)	71 (38.6)	32 (18.0)
Workload	42 (22.2)	57 (30.8)		68 **(38.2)**
Personal problems	40 (21.2)			
Unaccustomed sleep position		53 (28.6)	89 (48.4)	
Pain, illness		49 (26.5)	79 (42.9)	
Fetal movement			90 **(48.9)**	
Crying child				113 **(63.5)**

Bold type, the three most frequent causes per interval

intertrimester comparisons showed no differences. The percentage of nil activity did not differ between weekdays and weekends, or between housewives and employed women.

The number of nocturnal nil phases (intervals of uninterrupted nil activity) was maximal (median 57) in the first trimester, then decreased in the second trimester (median 54) ($P < 0.001$), remaining unchanged (median 55) in the third trimester before falling to a minimum postpartum (median 44). The postpartum value was lower than the pregnancy values ($P < 0.0001$). Since total nil activity time remained unchanged

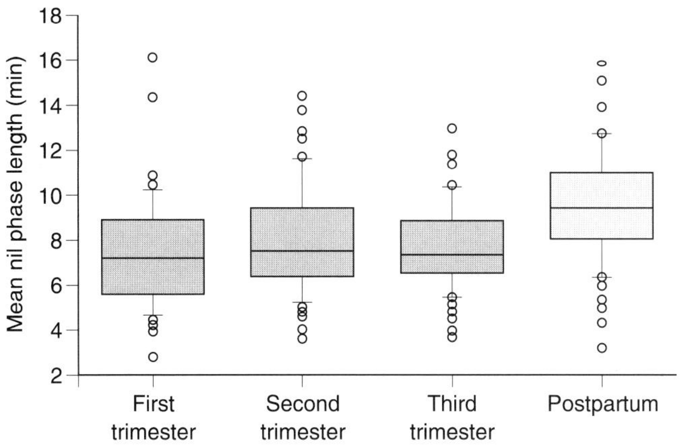

Figure 86.5 mNPL in pregnancy and postpartum (n=70), showing a longer mNPL postpartum than in any trimester (P< 0.0001, Wilcoxon's test with Bonferroni's correction for multiple comparisons).

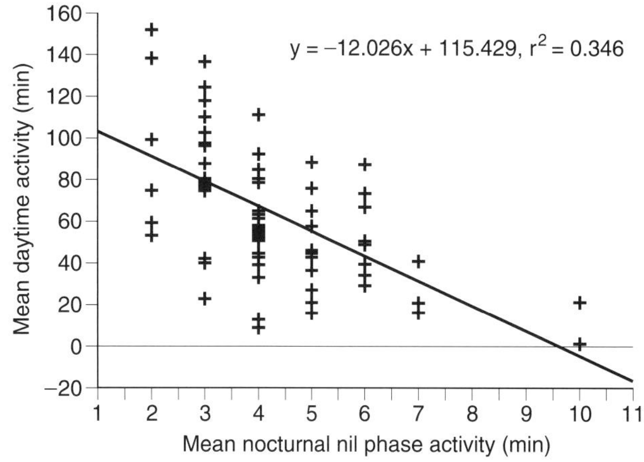

Figure 86.6 Median daytime activity vs. mean nocturnal nil phase length in first-trimester pregnancies (n=63), r=0.6.

Table 86.7 Mean sleep parameters (SE) during pregnancy

Parameter	Trimester (min) First	Second	Third	Change from first to third trimester (s)
Time in bed	451.2 (13.7)	456.1 (15.5)	476.8 (10.7)	+25.6 (5.7)
Total sleep time	388.6 (8.2)	400.8 (12.0)	382.1 (11.8)	−6.5 (1.7)
Sleep latency	20.1 (4.2)	21.7 (8.4)	25.0 (4.0)	+4.9 (24.4)
Rapid eye movement sleep latency (from stage 2)	78.7 (8.1)	70.1 (2.6)	64.7 (3.2)	−14 (17.8)
Waking after sleep onset	32.5 (9.6)	22.8 (5.0)	58.3*† (6.1)	+25.8 (79.4)
Stage 1	33.7 (4.2)	31.1 (4.0)	36.1 (5.2)	+2.4 (7.1)
Stage 2	214.9 (13.8)	234.3 (17.4)	220.9 (14.1)	+6.0 (2.8)
Stage 3	40.0 (3.5)	39.2 (2.8)	36.3 (3.3)	−3.7 (9.3)
Stage 4	20.4 (4.4)	23.8 (5.3)	18.2 (6.0)	−2.2 (10.8)
Slow-wave sleep (stages 3 and 4)	60.3 (7.2)	63.0 (6.9)	54.6 (8.8)	−5.7 (9.5)
Rapid eye movement sleep	79.7 (2.4)	72.5 (2.7)	70.5* (5.9)	−9.2 (11.5)
Movements in sleep	10.0	10.8	11.3	+1.3 (11.3)
Sleep efficiency (%)	86.5	88.1	79.9*†	−6.6

Significant changes (p< 0.05)* vs. first trimester; †vs. second trimester

throughout pregnancy, it was broken during pregnancy into more individual nil activity phases by more frequent interruptions. Sleep was at its most restless and fragmented in the first trimester.

The increased number of nocturnal nil phases in pregnancy resulted in a shorter mNPL (Figure 86.5) in pregnancy vs. postpartum (7.36–7.59 min vs. 9.56 min, P< 0.0001). In addition, the increase in mNPL from the first to the second trimester was significant (P=0.0002), but not that to the third trimester (P=0.27). Women with a low nocturnal percentage of nil activity had, as expected, a shorter mNPL (P=0.0001), also indicative of more restless sleep.

This means that during sleep in pregnancy, especially in the first trimester, motor activity was more frequent than in non-pregnancy. However, such increased motor activity had no effect on sleep quality. Motor latency was also significantly increased throughout pregnancy, indicating increased motor activity during sleep onset.

Daytime activity decreased continuously during pregnancy, in parallel with nocturnal activity, reaching a minimum postpartum, which differed significantly from the first trimester. Women with high daytime activity had higher night-time motor activity. There was a negative correlation between median daytime activity and mean night-time nil phase length (r=0.6), illustrated in Figure 86.6 (first trimester) and present in all recording periods.

Polysomnography

Conventional sleep analysis. Sleep structure, i.e. sleep stage distribution, remained largely unchanged over pregnancy (Table 86.7). The only significant

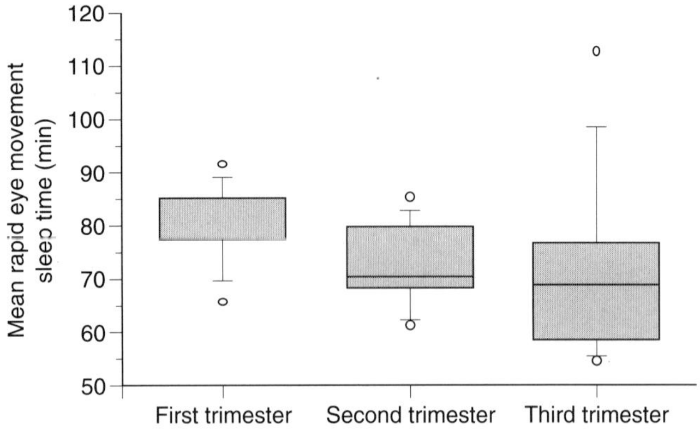

Figure 86.7 Mean REM sleep time in two nights per trimester (78, 70 and 69 min in trimesters 1, 2 and 3, respectively) in nine subjects, showing a significant decrease from the first to the third trimester ($P < 0.05$).

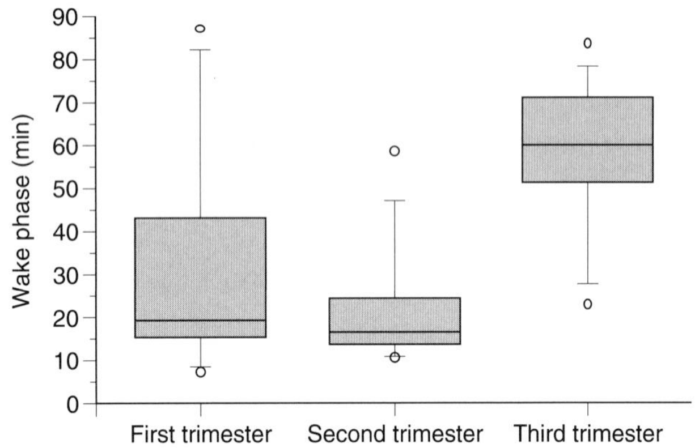

Figure 86.8 Wake phase after sleep onset (mean of two nights) per trimester in nine subjects, showing a longer wake phase in the third vs. the first and second trimesters ($P < 0.05$, Wilcoxon's test).

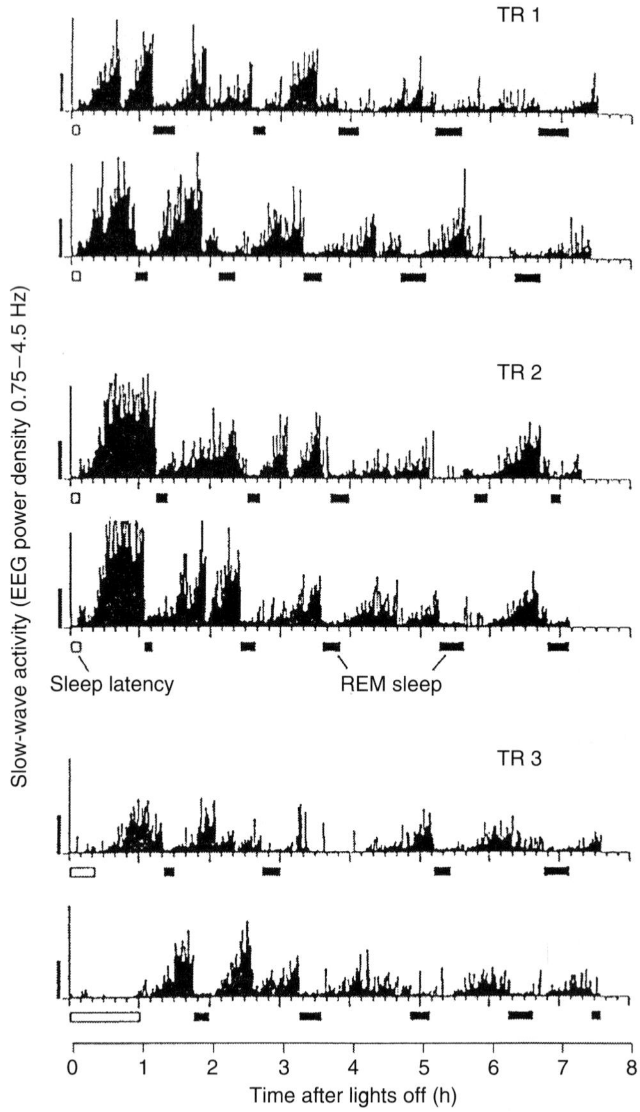

Figure 86.9 Power density of slow-wave activity (0.75–4.5 Hz) over six nights in the same pregnant woman (two nights per trimester, chronological order from top to bottom) showing decrease of slow-wave activity during pregnancy. TR1, first trimester; TR2, second trimester; TR3, third trimester; REM, rapid eye movement. From Levine *et al.*[30]

changes from the first to the third trimester were an increase in nocturnal wake phase time (from 32.5 to 58.3 min) – hence a decrease in sleep efficiency, defined as time asleep/time in bed (from 86.5 to 79.9%) – and a decrease in REM sleep time (from 79.7 to 70.5 min) (Figure 86.7).[33]

The same changes – decreased REM sleep and increased wake phase – have been found in previous studies.[34,35] An earlier report of an increase in paradoxical sleep during pregnancy[36] was based on the sleep staging criteria of Dement and Kleitman,[6] which differ from the Rechtschaffen and Kales criteria[5] in current use.

Median wake-phase time after sleep onset was longer in the third than in the first or second trimesters (60 vs. 20 min, respectively; $P < 0.05$) (Figure 86.8).

Median sleep efficiency decreased significantly from 88.6% in the first trimester and 90.5% in the second trimester to 79.9% in the third trimester, i.e. in the third trimester more than one-fifth of the time in bed was spent awake. These changes in sleep structure were of secondary significance as causes of fatigue in pregnancy. There was no difference in terms of time in bed, distribution of NREM and REM sleep, waking after sleep onset or nocturnal rising, between nights from which subjects awoke tired and those from which they awoke refreshed. The remaining sleep parameters (time

Table 86.8 Non-rapid eye movement (NREM) and rapid eye movement (REM) sleep frequency bands (Hz) showing significant power density changes during pregnancy

Trimester	NREM sleep	REM sleep
1–2	10–11	
	14–17	
2–3	1–12	3–4
	13–16	5–6
		9–11

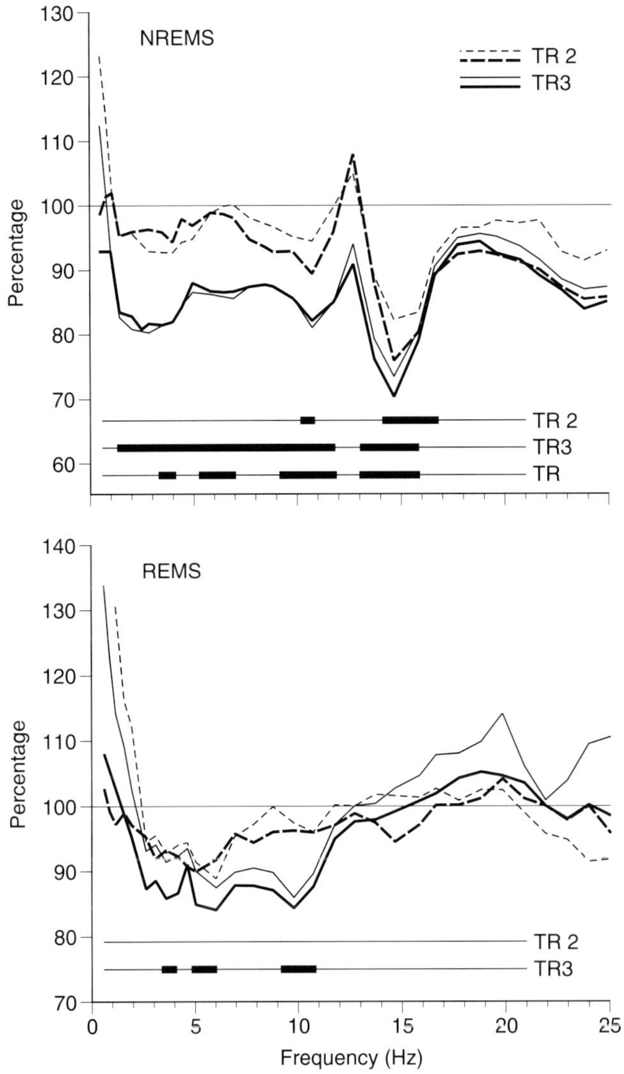

Figure 86.10 Changes (collective mean % deviation per trimester from first trimester baseline (100%) in power density in NREM sleep and REM sleep in nine pregnant women. Bold, frequency bands with significant changes; TR2, second trimester; TR3, third trimester. From Levine *et al.*[30]

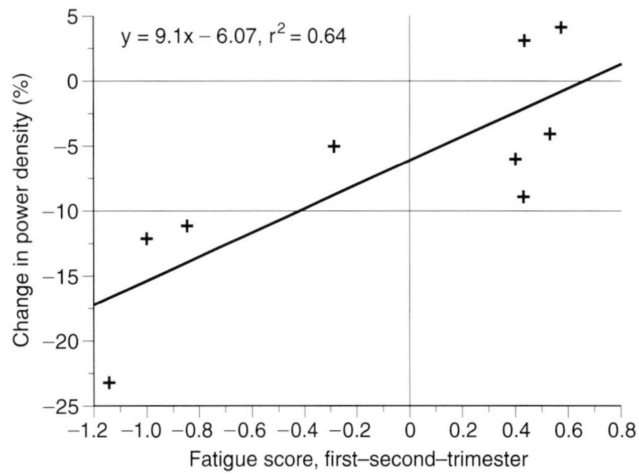

Figure 86.11 Correlation between fatigue and decrease in power density in 10.5 Hz frequency band from first to second trimester. $r=0.8$.

in bed, sleep latency, total sleep time, REM latency, REM sleep, stage 1 sleep, and sleep efficiency) also had no effect on the recuperative value of sleep. This indicates that sleep time and sleep stage distribution have little effect on fatigue in pregnancy, at least where the differences observed in this normal population are concerned. The same conclusion may not apply to larger differences in sleep parameters.

Whole-night spectral analysis. Sleep architecture analysis was focused on slow-wave EEG activity (0.75–4.5 Hz) as a measure of sleep depth. Slow-wave activity also occurs outside deep sleep, but is not recorded by conventional sleep staging. The contribution of whole-night spectral analysis is that it records power densities in the different frequency bands independently of the conventional sleep stages.

Power density decreased significantly from the first to the third trimester in the long-wave frequency band in NREM and REM sleep[33] (Figure 86.9), i.e. sleep was shallower overall in the third trimester vs. the first, even though the proportion of deep sleep was unchanged in the third trimester.

The first-trimester power density at each frequency band was used as the baseline (100%) in expressing the values in each subject during pregnancy; subsequent values were expressed as percentage deviations from this baseline. The collective deviations in the second and third trimesters (the mean of both nights in each trimester in nine subjects) are shown in Figure 86.10, which also shows the significant changes in power spectra during pregnancy as thick bars in the appropriate frequency band (Table 86.8).

There was a clear correlation between the decrease in power density at 10.5 Hz in NREM sleep and fatigue on waking from the first to the second trimester (Figure 86.11). Thus, women with a decrease in power density at 10.5 Hz of 10% all reported greater fatigue in the second vs. the first trimester, while all those feeling less tired in the second trimester showed a smaller decrease, or in some cases an increase, in power density in the same frequency band.

Hormonal effects on fatigue

The central depressant effect of progestagens causes symptoms such as fatigue, apathy, drowsiness, decreased libido, decreased drive, fluctuating mood, depressive mood and decreased energy,[37] i.e. many of the complaints typical of early pregnancy. But as serum progesterone levels up to 10 weeks' gestation do not differ significantly from luteal values,[38,39] additional mechanisms must be involved, notably changes in brain hormone metabolism (steroids in particular) and/or receptor status.

Neuroactive steroids, or neurosteroids, are progesterone derivatives, which bind not to the cytoplasmic steroid receptor of the typical end organ but to neuron

Table 86.9 Fatigue and maternal serum neurosteroid positivity in pregnancy

Fatigue	Neurosteroid positivity n/N	Neurosteroid positivity %	Pregnanolone equivalents (nmol/l)
None	0/8	0	–
Mild–moderate	1/6	17	185
Severe	6/9	66*	435 (255)†
Total	7/23	30	

n/N, fraction of pregnant women investigated: *p=0.02 vs. no and mild–moderate fatigue (Fisher's exact test): non-significant vs. mild–moderate fatigue; expressed as mean (SD)

γ-amino butyric acid ($GABA_A$) receptors where they exert benzodiazepine-like activity.[40,41] The result is marked fatigue, shown with several steroid hormones.[13,42–44] We used a binding assay [with the ionophore ligand (^{35}S)-*t*-butyl-bicyclophospho-rothionate] to screen for neurosteroids in a pilot study in 23 pregnant women between 10 and 40 weeks' gestation.[45] The results showed a correlation between severe fatigue in pregnancy and the presence of neurosteroids in peripheral venous blood throughout pregnancy (Table 86.9): neurosteroid binding was present in six out of nine pregnant women with severe fatigue vs. none out of eight women without fatigue. The correlation requires confirmation in further studies.

The sleep EEG changes seen toward the end of pregnancy – a significant decrease in power density in the slow-wave frequency band – have also been described in association with benzodiazepine use.[46–48] The physiological function of endozepines (diazepam binding inhibitors or endogenous ligands of the benzodiazepine receptors) remains to be elucidated, though they have a demonstrated role in some disease processes, such as idiopathic recurring stupor[49] and hepatic encephalopathy.[50] No blood samples in the above neurosteroid pilot study showed any evidence of endozepine binding, making this an improbable explanation for pregnancy fatigue.[45]

Progesterone also contributes to the sleep changes in pregnancy. Experimental progesterone administration in men was associated with more frequent waking, decreased deep (stage 4) sleep and increased sleep latency.[51,52]

Pregnancy fatigue can be interpreted as a biological signal to the expectant mother to take things easy physically. Reduced physical activity reduces uterine contractions and increases uteroplacental blood flow.

Clinical impact of sleep impairment

Pregnancy, sleep and fatigue

The effects of pregnancy on sleep and fatigue can be summarized as follows:

(1) Sleep changes during pregnancy. These changes show little relationship with fatigue. Some sleep parameters correlate with fatigue: later bedtime, increased waking after sleep onset, decreased power density in the low-frequency band.
(2) As pregnancy fatigue does not respond to longer sleep or less work, sleep time and workload do not appear to be its principal determinants. More plausible candidates are endocrine causes, as in the case of neurosteroids.[45]
(3) Sleep disturbance and fatigue do not affect the course of pregnancy. The most frequent pregnancy complications – prematurity, low birth weight for gestational age, intrapartum asphyxia and cesarean section rate – were no more frequent in the women with severely disturbed sleep or excessive fatigue than in the overall population.

Sleep disturbance in pregnancy: management guidelines

Pregnant women who complain about fatigue and sleep problems should be made aware that such complaints are not only frequent but also have no demonstrable impact on the pregnancy or baby and are best viewed as the body's invitation to take things easy.

Symptomatic management is required for pregnancy complaints that may often cause sleep problems, e.g. restricted respiration (increase the number of pillows to leave the chest free), obstructed nasal respiration (humidifiers, vasoconstrictor nasal drops) or nocturnal carpal tunnel syndrome (splinting of the wrist overnight). Early morning nausea can be managed with drugs [vitamin B6, suppositories of meclozine dihydrochloride, pyridoxine hydrochloride and caffeine (Itinerol®, Vifor, Switzerland)], and nocturnal calf cramps with magnesium supplements. Nocturia may respond to compression stockings, which reduce dependent fluid accumulation during the day, and hence the diuretic response to recumbency.[53] Fatigue due to anemia can be treated with prophylactic iron.

Falling asleep and remaining asleep can also be assisted by further measures, such as discussing psychosocial problems and sensitizing the patient to the increased emotional vulnerability in pregnancy. A talk with the partner or employer may also be of benefit.

Tips for active sleep preparation include a regular bedtime, preceded by a short walk in the fresh air. Evening coffee and tea should be avoided, together with heavy meals and alcohol. It is also best to go to bed only when tired; otherwise, reading or a similar activity can be recommended and/or a warm bath.

Patients can also be helped by correcting their ideas about 'enough' sleep. They need to understand that the body basically gets the sleep it needs, if not today then tomorrow or the day after.[54] It must be emphasized that it is not sleep so much as rest that is important.

Some non-drug remedies have been shown to be harmless in pregnancy, e.g. valerian drops, which have a documented hypnotic action,[55] herbal tea (e.g. lemon balm), alcohol-free beer and milk and honey mixtures.

If none of the above are effective, a hypnotic can be prescribed in exceptional cases. All medication is contraindicated in principle during the first trimester. In the second or third trimester, benzodiazepines or barbiturates can be used as short-term symptomatic therapy. Both may have adverse neuropsychological effects on the child, especially with protracted use.[56–60] To reduce the risk of neonatal hemorrhage, vitamin K supplementation is recommended in the last three weeks of pregnancy in patients on long-term barbiturates (e.g. epileptics) because of increased vitamin K turnover due to hepatic enzyme induction.[61]

The fundamental message to get across is that women should be receptive and ready to respond positively to the signals, which their bodies emit during pregnancy. The sleep problems and fatigue associated with pregnancy are transient in all cases and resolve shortly after birth.

Summary

The main pregnancy-associated changes in sleep are a decrease in depth and an increase in fragmentation, primarily due to nocturnal bathroom trips. Some 50–75% of study women got up at night during pregnancy vs. only 8.5% of controls.[22] On average, pregnant women sleep approximately 18 min longer per night than non-pregnant women and do so throughout pregnancy with certain individual fluctuations. Yet despite longer sleep, significantly more pregnant than non-pregnant women rated their sleep quality as poor or very poor (40% and 27%, respectively, vs. 4%).

More intense dream activity was reported by approximately one-fifth of the women in early pregnancy vs. before pregnancy, and by one-third in the further course of pregnancy. Dream content frequently revolved around birth and baby themes often tinged with apprehension.

Sleep fragmentation was also shown by actigraphy. Nocturnal nil activity duration did not change through pregnancy; however, the number of nocturnal nil activity phases increased and the mean nil activity phase length decreased. Motor latency was also significantly increased throughout pregnancy, confirming the more-marked motor activity during sleep onset. However, increased motor activity had no effect on the recuperative value of sleep.

Daytime sleep, reported by only 37% of women before pregnancy, increased during pregnancy to a maximum of 58% in the third trimester. Women who took a daytime nap did not differ from the others in sleep times or employment status. Daytime napping was not associated with the quality of waking or sleep fragmentation by waking and rising. In summary, there was no evidence that daytime napping was a response to poor nocturnal sleep quality; rather, it was taken if the opportunity arose.

Sleep structure showed two significant changes during pregnancy: first, a decrease in REM sleep (from 79.7 to 70.5 min) and, second, an increase in nocturnal waking after sleep onset (from 32.5 to 58.3 min). The longer waking phase reduced sleep efficiency, from 86.5 to 79.9%, i.e. one-fifth of the total time in bed was spent awake, with α-EEG activity. The main casualty of the increased waking phase was REM sleep; NREM sleep stages did not change during pregnancy. Recuperative deep sleep decreased in pregnancy by approximately 10% (not significantly). These changes in sleep structure were only observed in late pregnancy and cannot account for fatigue in early pregnancy.

Whole-night spectral analysis during pregnancy showed a significant decrease in power density in the slow-wave frequency band (1–12 Hz) and intermediate band (13–17 Hz) in both REM and NREM sleep. The decrease in power density at 10.5 Hz in NREM sleep (from first to second trimester) correlated with increased fatigue. From the second to the third trimester, we found a correlation between decreased power density in the 13–16-Hz frequency band and increased fatigue. These sleep changes need to be qualified by the fact that fatigue was already present early in the first trimester. The low-grade sleep changes cannot explain the often marked fatigue. However, the correlation between fatigue and the decrease in power density in the slow-wave band suggests that changes in sleep architecture may be at least partial determinants of fatigue.

In our study population of 189 pregnant women, 89.4% complained of definite fatigue and decreased energy in the first trimester. The fatigue involved not just physical energy but also concentration ability and memory. Such complaints are common even before women know that they are pregnant, thereby largely excluding purely psychological causes triggered by the awareness of pregnancy onset.

Workload was reduced through to the third trimester by some 58% of full-time employees largely independently of fatigue. Fatigue did not decrease after the workload was reduced, indicating that the latter is not the major determinant of pregnancy fatigue. Complaints of fatigue were as frequent in housewives, despite being able to adjust their workload more easily, and sleep a mean 27 min longer than their employed counterparts.

Pregnancy fatigue thus appears multifactorial and largely independent of sleep. Later bedtime, low basal hemoglobin and low diastolic blood pressure showed an individually significant association with fatigue. Frequent rising at night, restless sleep and increased weight gain in pregnancy were not significantly associated with fatigue. Only the endocrine changes can account for early pregnancy fatigue. Neurosteroids may play a major role in this regard,[44,45] in addition to the recognized sedative effects of progesterone.

Acknowledgments

This study was supported by a grant of the Hartmann-Müller-Foundation (Zurich). The polysomnographies were carried out in the Institute of Pharmacology of the University of Zurich (Professor A.A. Borbely).

REFERENCES

1. Reeves N, Potempa K, Gallo A. Fatigue in early pregnancy. An exploratory study. *Nurse Midwifery* 1991;36:303–9.
2. Sahota PK, Jain SS, Dhand R. Sleep disorders in pregnancy. *Curr Opin Pulm Med* 2003;9:477–83.
3. Williams B. Sleep needs during the maternity cycle. *Nurs Outlook* 1967;15:53–5.
4. Hedman C, Pohjasvaara T, Tolonen U, Suhonen-Malm AS, Myllyla VV. Effects of pregnancy on mother's sleep. *Sleep Med* 2002;3:37–42.
5. Rechtschaffen A, Kales A. *A Manual of Standardized Terminology, Techniques and Scoring System for Sleep Stages of Human Subjects* (Publication No. 204). Washington, DC: National Institutes of Health, US Government Printing Office, 1968.
6. Dement WC, Kleitman N. Cyclic variations in EEG during sleep and their relation to eye movements, body motility and dreaming. *Electroencephalogr Clin NeuroPhysiol* 1957;9:673–90.
7. Borbely AA. *Das Geheimnis des Schlafs. Neue Wege und Erkenntnisse der Forschung.* Ullstein-Sachbuch No. 34761. Frankfurt: Verlag Ullstein, 1991.
8. Pappenheimer JR. Sleep factor in CSF, brain and urine. *Front Horm Res* 1982;9:173–8.
9. Schneider-Helmert D, Schönenberger GA. Effects of DSIP in man. Multifunctional psychophysiological properties besides induction of natural sleep. *Neuropsychobiology* 1983;9:197–206.
10. Schoenenberger G, Maier PF, Tobler HJ, Monnier HJ. A naturally occurring delta-EEG enhancing nonapeptide in rabbits. Final isolation, characterization and activity test. *Pflügers Arch* 1977;369: 99–109.
11. Hayaishi O. Molecular mechanisms of sleep-wake regulations: Roles of prostaglandins D2 and E2. *FASEB J* 1991;5:2575–81.
12. McNeil RG, Gee KW, Bolger MB, *et al.* Neuroactive steroids that act at GABA-A receptors. *Drug News Perspect* 1992;5:145–52.
13. Selye H. Anaesthetic effect of steroid hormones. *Proc Soc Exp Biol Med* 1941;46:116–21.
14. Borbely AA, Tobler I. Endogenous sleep-promoting substances and sleep regulation. *Physiol Rev* 1989;69:605–70.
15. Koella WP. *Die Physiologie des Schlafes.* Stuttgart: Gustav Fischer Verlag, 1988.
16. Lavidor M, Weller A, Babkoff H. How sleep is related to fatigue. *Br J Health Psychol* 2003;8:95–105.
17. Schorsch E, Müller-Neff E. Psychiatrische Untersuchung an Wöchnerinnen. In Bürger-Prinz H, Fischer PA, eds. *Psychiatrie und Neurologie der Schwangerschaft.* Stuttgart: Enke Verlag, 1968:98.
18. Schweiger MS. Sleep disturbance in pregnancy. *Am J Obstet Gynecol* 1972;114:879–82.
19. Borbely AA, Neuhaus HU, Mattmann P, Waser PG. Langzeitregistrierung der Bewegungsaktivität: Anwendungen in Forschung und Klinik. *Schweiz Wschr* 1981;111:730–5.
20. Mullaney DJ, Kripke DF, Messin S. Wrist-actigraphic estimation of sleep time. *Sleep* 1980;3:83–92.
21. Sadeh A, Alster J, Urbach D, Lavie P. Actigraphically based automatic bedtime sleep-wake scoring: Validity and clinical applications. *J Ambul Monit* 1989;2:209–16.
22. Borbely AA. Schlafgewohnheiten, Schlafqualität und Schlafmittelkonsum der Schweizer Bevölkerung. *Schweiz Aerztezeitung* 1984;65:1606–13.
23. Karacan I, Williams R, Webb WB, Agnew H, Ross J. Sleep and dreaming during late pregnancy and postpartum. *Psychophysiology* 1968;4:378.
24. Gillman RD. The dreams of pregnant women and maternal adaptation. *Am J Orthopsychiatr* 1968;38:688–92.
25. Suzuki S, Dennerstein L, Greenwood KM, Armstrong SM, Satohisa E. Sleeping patterns during pregnancy in Japanese women. *Psychosom Obstet Gynaecol* 1994;15:19–26.
26. Lee KA, De Joseph JF. Sleep disturbances, vitality and fatigue among a select group of employed childbearing women. *Birth* 1992;19:208–13.
27. Feinsilver SH, Hertz G. Respiration during sleep in pregnancy. *Clin Chest Med* 1992;13:637–44.
28. Ogita S, Imanaka M, Takebayashi T, *et al.* Significance of exercise and bed rest in pregnancy – Study on the lying postures of gravidas during sleep. 2. *Ann Physiol Anthropol* 1990;9:93–8.
29. Fast A, Hertz G. Nocturnal low back pain in pregnancy: Polysomnographic correlates. *Am J Reprod Immunol* 1992;28:251–3.
30. Levine B, Roehrs T, Stepanski E, Zorick F, Roth T. Fragmenting sleep diminishes its recuperative value. *Sleep* 1987;10:590–9.
31. Rabkin CS, Anderson HR, Bland JM, Brooke OG, Chamberlain G, Peacock JL. Maternal activity and birth weight: A prospective, population-based study. *Am J Epidemiol* 1990;131:522–31.
32. Schramm WF, Stockbauer JW, Hoffman HJ. Exercise, employment, other daily activities, and adverse pregnancy outcomes. *Am J Epidemiol* 1996;143:211–18.
33. Brunner DP, Münch M, Biedermann K, Huch R, Huch A, Borbely AA. Changes in sleep and sleep EEG across pregnancy. *Sleep* 1994;17: 576–82.
34. Driver HS, Shapiro CM. A longitudinal study of sleep stages in young women during pregnancy and postpartum. *Sleep* 1992;15: 449–53.
35. Hertz G, Fast A, Feinsilver SH, Albertario CL, Schulman H, Fein AM. Sleep in normal late pregnancy. *Sleep* 1992;15:246–51.
36. Branchey M, Petre-Quadens O. A comparative study of sleep parameters during pregnancy. *Acta Neurol Belg* 1968;68: 453–9.
37. Kane FJ, Daly RJ, Ewing JA, Keeler MH. Mood and behavioural changes with progestational agents. *Br J Psychiatr* 1967;113: 265–8.
38. Yannone ME, McCurdy JR, Goldfien A. Plasma progesterone levels in normal pregnancy, labor and the puerperium. *Am J Obstet Gynecol* 1968;101:1058–61.
39. Lee KA, Zaffke ME. Longitudinal changes in fatigue and energy during pregnancy and the postpartum period. *J Obstet Gynecol Neonatal Nurs* 1999;28:183–91.
40. Baulieu EE. Neurosteroids: Synthesis and function. In Barnard EA, Costa E, eds. *Transmitter Amino Acid Receptors: Structures, Transduction and Models for Drug Development.* Stuttgart: Thieme Verlag, 1991:185–201.
41. Simmonds MA. Modulation of the $GABA_A$ receptor by steroids. *Semin Neurosci* 1991;3:231–9.
42. De Feudis FV. Modulation of GABA-A receptors by pregnane steroids – A new lead for developing anesthetics and anticonvulsants. *Drug News Perspect* 1989;2:278–80.
43. Majewska MD, Ford-Rice F, Falkay G. Pregnancy-induced alterations of $GABA_A$ receptor sensitivity in maternal brain. An antecedent of post-partum 'blues'? *Brain Res* 1989;482:397–401.
44. Marker RE, Kamm O, McGrew RV. Isolation of epipregnanol-3-one-20 from human pregnancy urine. *J Am Chem Soc* 1937;59: 616–8.
45. Biedermann K, Schoch P. Do neurosteroids or endozepines cause fatigue in pregnancy? *Eur J Obstet Gynecol Reprod Biol* 1995;58: 15–8.
46. Borbely AA, Mattmann P, Loepfe M, *et al.* A single dose of benzodiazepine hypnotics alters the sleep EEG in the following drug-free night. *Eur J Pharmacol* 1983;89:157–61.
47. Borbely AA, Mattmann P, Loepfe M, Strauch I, Lehmann D. Effect of benzodiazepine hypnotics on all-night sleep EEG spectra. *Hum Neurobiol* 1985;4:189–94.
48. Kubicki ST, Haag-Wüsthof C, Römmel J, Herrmann WM, Scheuler W. The pharmacodynamic influence of three bendzodiazepines on rapid eye movements, K-complexes and sleep spindles in healthy volunteers. *Hum Psychopharmacol* 1988;3: 247–55.
49. Rothstein JD, Guidotti A, Tinuper P, *et al.* Endogenous benzodiazepine receptor ligands in idiopathic recurring stupor. *Lancet* 1992;340:1002–4.
50. Mullen KD, Szauter KM, Kaminsky-Russ K. 'Endogenous' benzodiazepine activity in body fluids of patients with hepatic encephalopathy. *Lancet* 1990;336:81–3.
51. Heuser G, Kaies A, Jacobson A. Human sleep patterns after progesterone administration. *Psychophysiology* 1968;4:378.
52. Kotorii T, Nokaka K, Nakazawa Y, *et al.* Effects of medroxyprogesterone acetate on sleep of healthy young male adults. *Jpn J Psychol Neurol* 1987;41:261–7.
53. Biedermann K, Faisst K, Huch A, Huch R. Compression stocking prevention of pregnancy nocturia (letter). *Prenat Neonat Med* 1996;1:159.

54. Schumacher W. Schlafstörungen in der Schwangerschaft. Ihre Diagnostik und Therapie aus psychiatrischer Sicht. *Gynäkologe* 1987;20:176–81.
55. Balderer G, Borbely AA. Effect of valerian on human sleep. *Psychopharmacology* 1985;87:406–9.
56. Bergman U, Rosa FW, Baum C, Wiholm BE, Faich GA. Effects of exposure to benzodiazepine during fetal life. *Lancet* 1992;340: 694–6.
57. Blumenthal I, Lindsay S. Neonatal barbiturate withdrawal. *Postgrad Med J* 1977;53:157–8.
58. Fishman RH, Yanai J. Long-lasting effects of early barbiturates on central nervous system and behaviour. *Neurosci Biobehav Rev* 1983;7:19–28.
59. Gillberg C. 'Floppy infant syndrome' and maternal diazepam. *Lancet* 1977;2:244.
60. Weber LWD. Benzodiazepines in pregnancy – Academical debate or teratogenic risk? *Biol Res Pregnancy* 1985;6:151–67.
61. Janz D. Antiepileptic drugs and pregnancy: Altered utilization patterns and teratogenesis. *Epilepsia* 1982;23:53–63.

87 Immunology at the maternal–fetal interface

S. Scherjon and F. Claas

Introduction

The maternal acceptance of the semiallogeneic fetus seems to ignore the concepts of transplantation immunology. Elucidating the mechanism leading to this unique phenomenon is essential for our understanding of processes leading to normal and abnormal pregnancy, and may also result in important concepts in the field of transplantation, autoimmunity and, possibly, neoplasia control.

In 1953, Medawar explained the 'immunological paradox of pregnancy' by considering pregnancy a state of 'immunological neutrality'.[1] One of the three possible mechanisms he proposed was based on the idea that the fetus is antigenically immature. However, the idea of a complete absence of human leukocyte antigens (HLA) on fetal tissues appeared to be too simplistic. Billingham (a student of Medawar) showed in 1964 that non-classical transplantation (HLA) antigens could be found on embryonic tissue from very early gestational ages onward.[2] It was later understood that the presence of these non-classical HLA on trophoblasts are essential for the mother to recognize trophoblastic cells as 'self' and to prevent the normal immune response to non-self tissues.[3,4] Non-classical HLA were demonstrated – in direct contact with the deciduas – both on extravillous trophoblast (EVT) and on the (amnion) chorion. The second possible explanation by Medawar was based on a diminished maternal responsiveness to pregnancy. A decreased ability to elicit both a humoral and a cell-mediated immune response should lead to the acceptance of the 'foreign' fetus. Indeed, antibody titers do decrease during pregnancy, but this decrease is caused by the physiological hemodilution occurring especially during the first trimester of pregnancy. The variety of the antibody profile remains unchanged during pregnancy. On the other hand, cellular immune responses seem to be decreased during pregnancy,[5] as reflected by the improvement in some T-cell-mediated autoimmune diseases and an increased incidence of infections. In contrast, the innate defense mechanism is more prominent during pregnancy.[6] This increase in the function of the native immune system may be a compensatory mechanism for the decrease in specific T-cell reactivity.[7] Wegmann challenged the idea of a systemic immune suppression in pregnant women and suggested that cellular interactions within the placenta lead to a local immune response.[8] Also, a third possible explanation, that the uterus and especially the decidua is an immunologically privileged site, where mother and child are completely separated, cannot be the (only) explanation as even term pregnancies can be found outside the uterus with no decidua in place. Furthermore, it is now evident that during pregnancy there is cellular trafficking over the fetal–maternal interface.

Already very early after fertilization, there is direct contact between the blastocyst and the maternal decidua. From those very early days onward the immunological balance between mother and fetus has to be established and maintained as there is no doubt that the maternal immune system is certainly able to recognize the paternal antigens inherited by the fetus.[9,10] The lack of a destructive immune response mounted by the mother seems to be related to the presence of an active immune process essential for normal pregnancy. This concept is supported by findings that an increase in the number of HLA differences between mother and child reduces the chance of getting certain complications of pregnancy. Sharing of HLA between mother and fetus is associated with increased incidence of pre-eclampsia and fetal growth retardation. This was confirmed by others, suggesting that in women with a history of pre-eclampsia an unusually high degree of immunological compatibility with the fetus was found.[11–13] HLA-DR sharing between pre-eclamptic women and their partners is a risk factor for pre-eclampsia[14] and is also associated with a reduced birth weight, on average 200 g less.[15] Supporting this hypothesis is the observation that with more maternal–fetal HLA class II disparities, an improvement in rheumatoid arthritis during pregnancy and in the period thereafter was found.[16] This improvement cannot be directly explained by the increase in Th2 cytokine bias occurring during normal pregnancy.[17] Also, priming of the mother by paternal antigens, e.g. by semen, might induce an immunological hyporesponsiveness, essential for the process of maternal acceptance of her 'foreign' fetus.[18,19] The studies by Robillard[20,21] showed that the immunological response to trophoblastic invasion is dependent on earlier confrontation with paternal antigens during sexual intercourse, suggesting that certain pregnancy complications might be related to 'primi-paternity'. Mucosal alloimmunization via repeated exposure to HLA occurring during unprotected sexual intercourse generates an active immune tolerance to paternal antigens.

It has become evident that in the immunological acceptance of the semiallogeneic or even fully allogeneic fetus – after oocyte donation – local immunomodulation at the maternal–fetal interface is of key importance.

Implantation

The endometrium has through every menstrual cycle a surprisingly high regenerating capacity. It constitutes many cell types including glandular epithelium, stromal (mesenchymal) cells and endothelial cells. Decidualization of the endometrium during the menstrual cycle implies the change of stromal cells of the endometrium into decidual cells. Although already in the 19th century William Hunter had given the first description of the *membrane decidua*, it was only recently accepted that the decidua is actually a maternal membrane surrounding the (two) fetal membranes.[22] The process of decidualization, initiated by the action of progesterone on estrogens induced endometrium, facilitates the apposition of the blastocyst and the acceptance and outgrowth of trophoblastic villi. Trophoblast cells by their production of human chorionic gonadotropin support the persistence of the corpus luteum and by that the production of progesterone by the ovary. This system is also supported by the production of prolactin by the pituitary and by estrogen, inducing leukemia inhibiting factor (LIF), which enhances the effect on progesterone production.[23] From 8 weeks onward the main source of progesterone production becomes the syncythiotrophoblast. Although decidualization is essential for implantation, it is independent of the blastocyst itself. The process depends on progesterone, but also cytokines such as transforming growth factor beta (TGF-β) and insulin-like growth factor binding protein (IGFBP)[24,25] play a critical role in decidualization.[26]

Trophoblastic cells can be divided into two subtypes, villous trophoblast and EVT. Villous trophoblast is located around the villi and is in direct contact with maternal blood in the intervillous space. The cytotrophoblastic cells form the inner layer and are stem cells for the syncythiotrophoblast, which forms the outer layer of the villous. EVT has a proliferative and a migratory phenotype.[27] It invades the decidua and the uterine wall and forms the anchoring cytotrophoblast. At the decidual layer behind the placenta, the decidua basalis, there is direct contact between the ingrowing trophoblast, forming the anchor villi (interstitial trophoblast), and the endometrium surrounding the endometrial capillaries. The trophoblast that replaces the smooth muscle (intramural trophoblast) and endothelial cells (intra-arterial trophoblast) of these capillaries is called endovascular trophoblast.[27] At the other site of the developing fetus, villous structures will gradually disappear as the growing fetus and amniotic cavity will obliterate the endometrial cavity and the chorion will attach to the decidua, which at that side is called the decidua parietalis. The decidua is also considered of essential importance in the limitation of trophoblastic growth, which is necessary to prevent the occurrence of clinical features such as placenta accreta and percreta.

Many biochemical active compounds are involved in the implantation process. Cytokines such as interleukin 1β (IL-1β) induce the synthesis of prostaglandins and IGFBP-1, both needed for sufficient trophoblastic invasion. Invasion is also dependent on cell adhesion molecules, such as integrins,[27,28] and on matrix metalloproteinases (MMPs).[29] The latter are produced by trophoblast cells. Fibronectin, produced upon promotion by TGF-β by the EVT and detectable in the extracellular matrix of the deciduas, plays a critical role in the attachment of trophoblast cells to the decidua and supports the formation of cytotrophoblastic cell columns.[30]

Implantation and the non-classical major histocompatibility complex (MHC) I molecules

King and Loke described in 1991 an attractive model for a controlled permission of trophoblastic invasion – and also for limiting this invasion – into the endometrium and myometrium of the uterus.[31] Trophoblastic cells express, besides the classical HLA class I molecule HLA-C, only the non-classical class I antigens HLA-G, HLA-E and HLA-F, which have a very limited polymorphism. MHC class II antigens are completely absent on trophoblasts.[32] HLA-G is expressed only on the invading extravillous cytotrophoblast and is not present on villous syncytiotrophoblast.[33,34] By the expression of the non-classical HLA molecules, fetal trophoblastic cells, in their interaction with decidual leukocytes, are recognized as 'self' and do not evoke an immunological response by natural killer (NK) cells. This allows the EVT to invade the uterus. HLA-G is expressed in five different spliced, membrane-bound or soluble isoforms.[35]

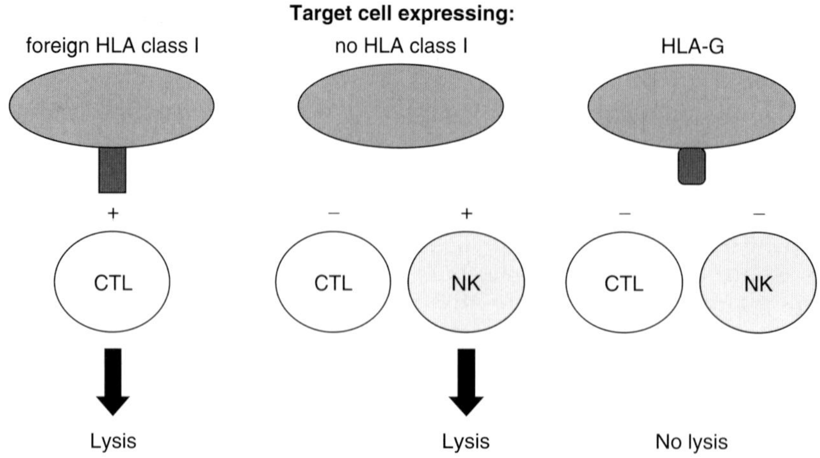

Figure 87.1 Cytotoxic T cells will react against HLA-mismatched target cells. Downregulation of the surface expression of the foreign HLA molecules will prevent this reactivity but will lead to activitation of NK cells that are triggered by the lack of HLA class I molecules on the target cell. Expression of HLA-G will prevent activation of NK cells by its interaction with KIR receptors.

Soluble HLA-G (sHLA-G) is secreted by the syncytio- and cytotrofoblast. HLA-G has the ability to present peptides derived from classical HLA class I molecules and other intracellular molecules. Although some data suggest that HLA-G expression at the maternal–fetal junction is decreased in pre-eclampsia,[36,37] this is not confirmed by others.[38]

Decidua infiltrating cells

The decidua contains many different types of (immune) cells, of which the frequency changes throughout the menstrual cycle and during pregnancy.

Uterine NK (uNK) cells

In the early proliferative phase of the endometrium, many small, round agranular cells with very little cytoplasm are found, which enlarge and become more granulated during the secretory phase. These cells, formerly called *uterine large granular lymphocytes*, turned out to be a special form of NK lymphocytes, uNK cells, with a different phenotype than NK cells found in peripheral blood. These cells do not express the classical NK marker CD16, while the CD56 surface density of these cells is more than 20 times higher compared to peripheral blood NK cells.[39,40] These uNK cells are bone marrow derived and replicate *in situ* in the endometrium.[41] Their number is maximal around ovulation and remains high around the period of implantation, accounting for at least 70% of the uterine lymphocytes.[40] uNK cells produce cytokines, like TGF-β, macrophage colony stimulating factor, tumor necrosis factor alpha (TNF-α), interferon gamma (IFN-γ), vascular endothelial growth factor, angiopoietin 1 (Ang1), Ang2, IL-3 and LIF, which are essential in trophoblast invasion and tissue remodeling.[42,40,43] On the other hand, appreciable amounts of granulocyte macrophage colony stimulating factor and IFN-γ are produced by uNK cells, possibly stimulated by IL-2, a factor related to trophoblast apoptosis, limiting the invasiveness of trophoblast cells.[44] Although there is a significant decrease of the uNK cells during the second trimester of pregnancy, at term age uNK cells are still present in appreciable amounts in the endometrium.[45]

sHLA-G is able to block uNK cell function and cytolytic T lymphocyte action, the latter possibly by an increase in apoptosis of activated CD4$^+$ and CD8$^+$ T cells.[35] By this effect on uNK cells and harmful CD8$^+$ T cells, trophoblast invasion is facilitated and endothelial cell reactivity is diminished.[46] In this context, it is essential to realize the principle difference in allorecognition between CD8$^+$ T cells and NK cells. CD8$^+$ T cells are activated by foreign HLA, while NK cells are programmed to lyse cells that lack self HLA molecules. The absence of classical HLA would be a trigger for NK cells, but the interaction of HLA-G with KIR receptors on NK cells prevents such reactivity (Figure 87.1).[47,48]

The interaction between uNK cells and HLA-G is basic for a normal, successful pregnancy, although it has been reported that women with a homozygous deletion in the HLA-G gene can have completely normal pregnancies. HLA-C is also expressed by the EVT cells and interacts with NK cells possibly in the same way as HLA-G. Although the existence of a specific receptor for HLA-G on the uNK cell is still discussed, HLA-C – and most probably HLA-G also – is recognized by receptors belonging to the KIR family, e.g. ILT3 and KIR2DL1.[49] HLA-G might, via binding of these receptors, influence cytokine secretion by T cells and modulate the Th1/Th2 balance.[46] HLA-E, also expressed by the EVT, is recognized by the NK cell by its CD94/NKG2A receptor. This interaction prevents cellular toxicity against the trophoblast.[50] It seems that HLA-E coexpression is at least necessary for the prevention of trophoblast lysis.[51] KIR receptors are expressed besides by uNK cells and also by $\gamma\delta$T cells.[52]

It seems that for implantation the cytokines produced as a result of the interaction between trophoblastic cells and uterine lymphocytes – especially uNK cells – are essential. The process has many features in common with an inflammation-like process, where cytokines play a pivotal role as well. In early pregnancy, the role of specific T cells is marginal as they seem not to be involved in the implantation process.

B and T cells

B cells and plasma cells are considered irrelevant for the regulation of trophoblast invasion as they are almost absent in the deciduas.[40] T cells form around 10% of the decidual leukocytes.[40] The number of CD8+ T cells and CD4+ (helper) T cells may change during pregnancy.[53] Recently, it was found that activated T cells are present at the placental site (decidua basalis)[40] and are even more numerous in the decidua aligning the fetal membranes (decidua parietalis).[54] Further functional characterization of T cells present in the decidua parietalis and basalis[45] should elucidate whether these cells play an active role in the (down) regulation of the maternal alloimmune response to the fetus.

Most *in vitro* studies of T cells isolated from maternal blood show a diminished T-cell activity and a concomitant increase in B-cell function. These findings are in line with clinical observations demonstrating an increased incidence of viral infections during pregnancy and the amelioration of T-cell-mediated autoimmune diseases such as rheumatoid arthritis. In contrast, the severity of antibody-mediated autoimmune diseases such as systemic lupus erythemathosus shows an increase during pregnancy.

In peripheral blood a reduction of T-helper (Th) 1 cells is demonstrated, which is partly caused by progesterone, associated with a downregulation of nuclear factor (NF) κB, which has an inhibitory effect on Th1 cell differentiation.[17] The consequence of this is that the balance of Th cells is shifted to a Th2 bias, which is the reason why normal pregnancy is characterized by a dominance of the anti-inflammatory Th2-type cytokines such as IL-4, -6, -10 and -13. The Th1 proinflammatory cytokines such as IL-2, IFN-γ and TNF-α, which activate cytotoxic T cells, are thought to have a detrimental effect on the development of pregnancy. However, the relevance of a Th2 bias in pregnancy was disputed from the beginning as it cannot be excluded that the cytokines, beneficial for processes important during implantation like spiral artery development and local tissue remodeling, are detrimental later during pregnancy.[55] Th1 cytokines especially, such as IFN-γ, are involved in the local inflammatory response during implantation.[56] Moreover, in the mouse IL-10 (Th2) knockout model, no negative effect on pregnancy outcome, pregnancy rate, litter size or birth weight was observed. In contrast, uNK cell knockout mice showed that a maternal uNK cell-deficient decidua is associated with fetal demise and a reduction in birth weight.[57] These postpartum findings were related to abnormalities in the arterial and microvascular architecture of decidual vessels. Transplantation of these mice with normal bone marrow led to the development of uNK cells preventing this pathology, whereby the decidual arterioles looked normal and the placental became larger again. uNK cells probably exert these effects in vascular modification (dilatation, elongation and branching) via the production of specific cytokines like IFN-γ[41] The complex network of cytokines and the cells contributing to this balance during pregnancy still have to be investigated, whereby it has to be considered that not only T cells, but also uNK cells produce these cytokines.

During pregnancy the adaptive immune system is activated, as shown by the development in 30% of the pregnancies of long-persisting antibodies against paternal HLA and the activation of cytotoxic T lymphocytes specific for these HLA.[58] In the decidual environment T cells may be primed by paternal antigens, but the normally expected T-cell-mediated cytotoxicity of trophoblastic cells does not occur. Through both elimination and suppression of fetus-reactive T-cell clones and also because paternal antigens are presented via non-classical HLA, the balance of Th cells is shifted to a Th2 bias. For a successful pregnancy the immunological acceptance of the fetus is essential. This acceptance is considered more and more an active process leading to the induction of immunological regulation, whereby the fetus is not attacked. The development of blocking antibodies may play a protective role by inhibiting the effect of HLA antibodies and potential fetus-reactive maternal lymphocytes. From the term placenta, activated alloreactive T cells can be isolated.[59] Locally at the level of the placenta, these activated T cells are probably downregulated by regulatory T cells. With a high level of HLA compatibility between partners, this downregulation might be less effective, explaining the higher incidence of pregnancy complications in these couples.

Macrophages

Macrophages are the second most numerous type of leukocytes present at the interface and are found in greater numbers in the decidua basalis as compared to the decidua parietalis.[45] They are the main producers of cytokine and growth factors and contribute to an adequate balance between Th1 and Th2 cytokines in the placenta, either by producing cytokines such as IL-4, IL-10 and IFN-γ or by indirectly stimulating the IFN-γ production by uNK cells.[60] Placental apoptosis, orchestrated by macrophages, is a normally occurring phenomenon in the placenta. Apoptosis is higher in third-trimester placentas compared to first-trimester placentas and it might also be higher in abnormal pregnancies, complicated by intrauterine growth restriction and/or pre-eclampsia.[61] Apoptosis is essential for the tissue remodeling occurring during implantation. The clearance of these apoptotic bodies is essential for placental homeostasis, preventing the release of potentially proinflammatory intracellular contents and of proteins that are foreign to the maternal immune system. The clearance of apoptotic debris is associated with the release of the anti-inflammatory TGF-β and possibly of other Th2-associated cytokines.

Recent evidence suggests that an even more important role for uNK cells lies in the production of cytokines (or other active substances), which prevent cytolytic actions by T cells, although these T cells are already present in an activated state.[54] LIF, and also IL-10, might control the transcription of HLA-G. In mouse, the absence of LIF is associated with total pregnancy failure. Also, human data support a pivotal role for LIF.

Apoptosis of EVT is related to the number of CD56$^+$ NK cells, while the number of uNK cells declines in parallel with apoptotic cells. The massive apoptosis of EVT is suggested to be the mechanism reducing invasiveness of the trophoblast.[62]

Fas-ligand (FasL) induced apoptosis

FasL expression on the trophoblast induces apoptosis of T cells or NK cells via their Fas receptors. In the trophoblast villi, FasL was found only on the cytotrophoblast, while the syncytiotrophoblast, which is in direct contact with the maternal blood, showed no expression of FasL. This FasL–Fas receptor interaction eliminates maternal lymphocytes specific for fetal/paternal antigens.[63–66]

The active process of tolerance induction

Several mechanisms may lead to an active downregulation of a destructive alloimmunity by the maternal immune system toward the fetus.

Dendritic cells (DCs) and regulatory T cells

DCs are important in the regulation of the immune response and have the unique opportunity to coordinate the innate and adaptive immune system. One can consider the endometrium as a mucosal surface, where DCs are confronted with trophoblastic antigens during pregnancy. DCs process and present these antigens to the maternal immune system for the induction of regulatory cells (Treg),[67] which may lead to the induction of regulatory T cells and may explain some of the findings of specific maternal tolerance to paternal antigens during pregnancy.[68] In humans in early first-trimester deciduas, DCs with a myeloid phenotype have been isolated,[69] although at a low frequency (1%). The dominance of plasmacytoid DCs in the decidua might be essential for polarizing the T-cell immune response to a Th2 bias.[70] DCs have been shown to produce TGF-α and also the T-cell inhibiting factor indoleamine 2,3-dioxygenase (IDO)[71] (see further). In the mouse model, immature DCs isolated from the decidua contain predominantly the pregnancy protective cytokine IL-10 and small amounts of the Th1 type cytokine IL-12.[72]

The family of regulatory T cells consists of the naturally occurring CD4$^+$CD25$^+$ T-regulatory cells (Treg) and the induced secondary Th3 cells and Treg type1 (T_R1) cells.[73,74] Treg cells are present in early pregnancy decidua.[75] Treg cells may develop after antigenic stimulation, under non-inflammatory conditions. Treg cells inhibit CD4$^+$ T cells to produce IL-2 and convert them into IL-10 producing T_R1-like cells and can also induce TGF-β producing Th3-like cells. This suppression is an important factor in the Th2 bias occurring during pregnancy.[76,77] IL-10 might be functional in three ways: suppression of cytotoxic T cells and their cytokines (IL-12 and IFN-γ), induction of regulatory T cells and inhibition of the maturation process of DCs leading to a more tolerogenic type of DC. Also, IL-6 and IL-1β are produced by these cells.[78,79] TGF-β is involved in the inhibition of trophoblast invasion by downregulation of collagenases and inhibition of metalloproteinases and integrins.[25,40] TGF-α is supposed to be a stimulator of trophoblast invasion. Some of these Th cells express the regulatory T-cell marker CTLA4[80] and have already been shown to induce the production of IDO by DCs after interaction between CD80 and CD86.[81] In the mouse, Treg cells, carrying the transcription factor FoxP3, are substantially increased in uterine tissue during pregnancy.[7] In venous blood during pregnancy, a doubling of CD4$^+$CD25$^+$ cells was found, which were increasing in parallel with the duration of pregnancy.[76] These expanding cells in the pregnant endometrium (both in mice and in humans) are pivotal for the suppression of the maternal immune reaction against fetal derived paternal antigens.[7,82]

Indoleamine 2,3-dioxygenase

Recently, a role for IDO regulating T-cell immunity during pregnancy has been suggested.[83] As a mechanism to prevent trophoblast lysis, IDO secreted by EVT, decidual macrophages and possibly DCs inhibits lymphocyte proliferation and survival via a decrease in extracellular tryptophan.[71,83,84] Its immunosuppressive effect might be exerted not only by a decrease of tryptophan but also by an increase of the tryptophane kynurenine metabolites. These metabolites might have a selective apoptotic effect on Th1 cells. IDO expression is induced by IFN-γ[85,86] and further stimulated by CTLA-4 expressing Treg cells.[76] It was shown that placental tissue, with a particularly high expression of IDO, made maternal $CD8^+$ T cells specifically tolerant for paternal class I MHC.[83]

Crry protein

Crry protein, a murine protective cell surface protein and a component of the natural immunity system, is also expressed on trophoblast. This protein suppresses the ongoing complement activation, especially C3, after its deposition on the membranes at the feto–maternal interface. Complement activation, promoting inflammatory reactions to the placenta, resulting in embryonic lethality, is inhibited by the expression of the Crry protein.[87] It was shown in the Crry protein knockout mice, that Crry is necessary for embryonic development.[88] In human placenta, three other complement regulators, decay accelerating factor (CD 55), membrane cofactor protein (CD 46) and CD 59, are present in high concentrations. These regulators have the same function as Crry, preventing complement activation and placental inflammation at the interface.

Progesterone

Progesterone has immune modulatory activity because of its blocking effect on T-cell activity.[89] Peripheral T cells from pregnant women have a much higher progesterone sensitivity compared to non-pregnant women, due to an increased number of progesterone receptors (PR).[90] There is an overlap between the PR-positive T cells and $\gamma\delta$T cells.[91] PR receptors also exist on uNK cells.[92] PR-positive lymphocytes and uNK cells produce, on binding with progesterone, a progesterone inhibiting binding factor (PIBF). PIBF inhibits NK cell cytotoxicity by a failure in degranulation, to release perforin and granzymes,[93] and it might also induce the secretion of IL-10 by already activated lymphocytes.

Progesterone may also play an essential role in the local regulation of invasion. It regulates the genes, effecting an increase of factors essential for the local regulation of invasion like amphiregulin, IGFBP-3[25] and immune response gene-1.[23]

In animals, medroxyprogesterone rather than progesterone had the best anti-inflammatory properties by reducing the upregulation of type 2 cyclooxygenase (COX-2) messenger RNA.[94] COX-2 is essential for the production of the labor-associated prostaglandins. Also, other labor-associated genes are downregulated by progesterone: e.g. IL-1β, IL-8, NF-κB[94] and MMP8 and MMP9.

Recently, it has been shown that progesterone treatment results in a more than 40% reduction in the incidence of preterm delivery in a high-risk group.[95] Increased NF-κB levels have been found in preterm deliveries even without signs of an infection, whereas IL-10 has an inhibiting function on prostaglandin production. Even term delivery is associated with this inflammatory-like process.[96] There is no doubt that prolactin is produced by the decidua, partly controlled by the action of progesterone. Prolactin might have an immune modulatory role via receptors shown to be present on immunocompetent cells, e.g. the uNK cell.[97,98]

Cellular trafficking

There is a very intensive and reciprocal fetal–maternal trafficking, both actively and passively, of many different substances and cells through the placenta. This process is important for the maintenance of and maternal adaptation to pregnancy and also for the maternal recognition and immunological acceptance of pregnancy. The placental supply of maternal blood, via the endometrial/decidual spiral arteries to the intervillous space, bathes the fetal syncythiotrophoblast and its constituent immunocompetent cells. Fetal villous tissue and fetal cells within the villous capillaries are only separated from the maternal blood by the capillary endothelial wall, the mesenchyme within the villous trophoblast and the syncytiotrophoblast. Also, at other locations there is a very close cell-to-cell contact. At the decidua parietalis there is direct contact between the fetal membranes – e.g. the chorion leave – and the maternal decidua. The consideration that fetal and maternal circulations, and through them the cells of the fetus and mother, are completely separated during pregnancy has been challenged by the fact that chimerism, defined as the long-term persistence of a small number of allogeneic cells, both within the mother (maternal microchimerism) and within the fetus (fetal microchimerism), is a regularly occurring process. Chimerism is known to occur after solid organ transplantation, but especially after hematopoietic cell transplantation, where it can result in a (chronic) graft-vs.-host disease, a disorder that has a profound resemblance to autoimmune diseases.

During pregnancy, these trafficking cells have a haematopoietic progenitor cell character.[99] In the third trimester 80–90% of the mothers will have circulating fetal cells, with a proportion of around 1 fetal cell in 1000 maternal cells. The occurrence of cellular trafficking over the feto–maternal interface results from a cellularly imperfect placental barrier. This cellular trafficking confronts the mother with paternal antigens, resulting in activation of alloreactive T cells and HLA antibody formation, and possibly also the induction of tolerance. HLA compatibility between mother and fetus supports the persistence of fetal cells in the maternal circulation. The migration of these cells into maternal tissues like thyroid and bone marrow have possible long-standing consequences.[100,101] The suggestion has been made that the long-term persistence of fetal cells is associated with the development of autoimmune diseases including sclerodermia, rheumatoid arthritis, thyroiditis, primary biliary cirrhosis, Sjögren syndrome, systemic lupus erythematosus and neonatal lupus syndromes. However, microchimerism might also have positive effects. The induction of tolerance to non-inherited maternal HLA (NIMA) during pregnancy[102] leads to a better acceptance of NIMA-mismatched transplanted organs[103] and a lower incidence of graft-vs.-host disease.[104]

Also, a neonatally occurring tolerogenic effect of soluble maternal HLA resulting from breast-feeding was shown.[105] The presence of chimerism might be used therapeutically, e.g. in bone marrow transplantation, where non-T-cell-depleted stem cells from haploidentical family donors are successfully used for transplantation provided that chimerism can be demonstrated.[106,107]

Conclusions

There are many immune mechanisms playing together at the fetal–maternal interface. These mechanisms are characterized by their redundancy and complexity. Any cytokine can be both down- and upregulated. The absence of B cells and the relative small numbers of T cells in the first-trimester decidua suggest that the adaptive immune system is not as important in that period of gestation as the innate system. NK cells and macrophages, representing the innate system, are more apparent in this period. As the number of NK cells in interaction with non-classical HLA (HLA-G) decreases substantially during pregnancy, other mechanisms resulting in maternal acceptance must become more important while pregnancy progresses.[108] Although trophoblast carries no HLA class II and no HLA-A and HLA-B, the mother and fetus might interact via HLA-C, as suggested by the distribution of particular HLA-C allotypes and specific KIR receptors in the population.[109]

However, it is important to realize that a successful pregnancy cannot be based on only one mechanism. In a murine model with class I expression on trophoblast and the absence of FasL, a normal tolerance to histoincompatible pregnancies was shown, without an adverse effect on pregnancy outcomes.[110] Also, the recognition of HLA-G by the NK cell is not essential for reproduction.[111] As Chaouat *et al.*[112] have stated, for a successful pregnancy, it is essential that there are 'sequential windows and extreme complexity mixed with very precise timing and tuning'.

The classical immunological model of the fetus being an allograft, which is not rejected, is less appropriate and newer models must be considered based on local immune regulation operating in parallel for the acceptance of the (semi) allogeneic fetal allograft.

REFERENCES

1. Medawar P. Some Immunological and Endocrinological Problems Raised by the Evolution of Viviparity in Vertebrates. In Pringle J, ed. Cambridge: Cambridge University Press, 1953:320–38.
2. Billingham RE. Transplantation immunity and the maternal–fetal relation. *N Engl J Med* 1964;270:667–72.
3. Head JR, Drake BL, Zuckermann FA. Major histocompatibility antigens on trophoblast and their regulation: Implications in the maternal–fetal relationship. *Am J Reprod Immunol Microbiol* 1987;15:12–8.
4. Bazer FW, Vallet JL, Roberts RM, Sharp DC, Thatcher WW. Role of conceptus secretory products in establishment of pregnancy. *J Reprod Fertil* 1986;76:841–50.
5. Krause PJ, Ingardia CJ, Pontius LT, Malech HL, LoBello TM, Maderazo EG. Host defense during pregnancy: Neutrophil chemotaxis and adherence. *Am J Obstet Gynecol* 1987;157:274–80.
6. Sacks G, Sargent I, Redman C. An innate view of human pregnancy. *Immunol Today* 1999;20:114–8.
7. Aluvihare VR, Kallikourdis M, Betz AG. Regulatory T cells mediate maternal tolerance to the fetus. *Nat Immunol* 2004;5:266–71.
8. Wegmann TG. Foetal protection against abortion: Is it immunosuppression or immunostimulation? *Ann Immunol (Paris)* 1984;135D:309–12.
9. van Rood JJ, Eernisse JG, van Leeuwen A. Leucocyte antibodies in sera from pregnant women. *Nature* 1958;181:1735–6.
10. Verdijk RM, Kloosterman A, Pool J, *et al.* Pregnancy induces minor histocompatibility antigen-specific cytotoxic T cells: Implications for stem cell transplantation and immunotherapy. *Blood* 2004;103:1961–4.
11. Scott JS, Jenkins DM, Need JA. Immunology of pre-eclampsia. *Lancet* 1978;1:704–6.
12. de Luca Brunori I, Battini L, Simonelli M, *et al.* Increased HLA-DR homozygosity associated with pre-eclampsia. *Hum Reprod* 2000;15: 1807–12.
13. Daunter B. Immunology of pregnancy: Towards a unifying hypothesis. *Eur J Obstet Gynecol Reprod Biol* 1992;43:81–95.
14. de Luca Brunori I, Battini L, Simonelli M, *et al.* HLA-DR in couples associated with preeclampsia: Background and updating by DNA sequencing. *J Reprod Immunol* 2003;59:235–43.
15. Ober C, Simpson JL, Ward M, *et al.* Prenatal effects of maternal–fetal HLA compatibility. *Am J Reprod Immunol Microbiol* 1987;15:141–9.
16. Jansson R, Dahlberg PA, Winsa B, Meirik O, Safwenberg J, Karlsson A. The postpartum period constitutes an important risk for the development of clinical Graves' disease in young women. *Acta Endocrinol (Copenh)* 1987;116:321–5.
17. McCracken SA, Gallery E, Morris JM. Pregnancy-specific down-regulation of NF-kappaB expression in T cells in humans is essential for the maintenance of the cytokine profile required for pregnancy success. *J Immunol* 2004;172:4583–91.
18. Robertson SA, Bromfield JJ, Tremellen KP. Seminal 'priming' for protection from pre-eclampsia – A unifying hypothesis. *J Reprod Immunol* 2003;59:253–65.
19. Dekker G. The partner's role in the etiology of preeclampsia. *J Reprod Immunol* 2002;57:203–15.
20. Robillard PY, Hulsey TC, Perianin J, Janky E, Miri EH, Papiernik E. Association of pregnancy-induced hypertension with duration of sexual cohabitation before conception. *Lancet* 1994;344:973–5.
21. Clark DA. Does immunological intercourse prevent pre-eclampsia. *Lancet* 1994;344:969.
22. Wewer UM, Faber M, Liotta LA, Albrechtsen R. Immunochemical and ultrastructural assessment of the nature of the pericellular basement membrane of human decidual cells. *Lab Invest* 1985;53:624–33.
23. Sherwin J, Freeman T, Stephens R, *et al.* Identification of genes regulated by leukaemia inhibitory factor in the mouse uterus at the time of implantation. *Mol Endocrinol* 2004;18(9):2185–95.
24. Ruoslahti E, Pierschbacher MD. New perspectives in cell adhesion: RGD and integrins. *Science* 1987;238:491–7.
25. Bell SC. Decidualization and insulin-like growth factor (IGF) binding protein: Implications for its role in stromal cell

differentiation and the decidual cell in haemochorial placentation. *Hum Reprod* 1989;4:125–30.
26. Casey ML, MacDonald PC. The endothelin-parathyroid hormone-related protein vasoactive peptide system in human endometrium: Modulation by transforming growth factor-beta. *Hum Reprod* 1996;11(Suppl 2):62–82.
27. Kaufmann P, Castellucci M. Extravillous trophoblast in the human placenta – A review. *Trophoblast Res* 2004;10:21–65.
28. Librach CL, Werb Z, Fitzgerald ML, *et al.* 92-kD type IV collagenase mediates invasion of human cytotrophoblasts. *J Cell Biol* 1991;113:437–49.
29. Frenette PS, Wagner DD. Adhesion molecules – Part 1. *N Engl J Med* 1996;334:1526–29.
30. Feinberg RF, Kliman HJ, Lockwood CJ. Is oncofetal fibronectin a trophoblast glue for human implantation? *Am J Pathol* 1991; 138:537–43.
31. King A, Loke YW. On the nature and function of human uterine granula lymphocytes. *Immunol Today* 1991;12:432–5.
32. Zuckermann FA, Head JR. Expression of MHC antigens on murine trophoblast and their modulation by interferon. *J Immunol* 1986;137:846–53.
33. Loke YW, King A, Burrows T, *et al.* Evaluation of trophoblast HLA-G antigen with a specific monoclonal antibody. *Tissue Antigens* 1997;50:135–46.
34. Trundley A, Moffett A. Human uterine leukocytes and pregnancy. *Tissue Antigens* 2004;63:1–12.
35. Le Bouteiller P, Legrand-Abravanel F, Solier C. Soluble HLA-G1 at the materno–foetal interface – A review. *Placenta* 2003;24(Suppl A):S10–5.
36. Hara N, Fujii T, Yamashita T, Kozuma S, Okai T, Taketani Y. Altered expression of human leukocyte antigen G (HLA-G) on extravillous trophoblasts in preeclampsia: Immunohistological demonstration with anti-HLA-G specific antibody "87G" and anti-cytokeratin antibody "CAM5.2". *Am J Reprod Immunol* 1996;36:349–58.
37. Colbern GT, Chiang MH, Main EK. Expression of the nonclassic histocompatibility antigen HLA-G by preeclamptic placenta. *Am J Obstet Gynecol* 1994;170:1244–50.
38. Datema G, van Meir CA, Kanhai HH, van den Elsen PJ. Pre-term birth and severe pre-eclampsia are not associated with altered expression of HLA on human trophoblasts. *Am J Reprod Immunol* 2003;49:193–201.
39. Moffett-King A. Natural killer cells and pregnancy. *Nat Rev Immunol* 2002;2:656–63.
40. Loke YW, King A, Burrows TD. Decidua in human implantation. *Hum Reprod* 1995;10(Suppl 2):14–21.
41. Croy BA, Chantakru S, Esadeg S, Ashkar AA, Wei Q. Decidual natural killer cells: Key regulators of placental development (a review). *J Reprod Immunol* 2002;57:151–68.
42. Li XF, Charnock-Jones DS, Zhang E, *et al.* Angiogenic growth factor messenger ribonucleic acids in uterine natural killer cells. *J Clin Endocrinol Metab* 2001;86:1823–34.
43. Saito S, Morii T, Enomoto M, *et al.* The effect of interleukin 2 and transforming growth factor-$\beta 2$ (TGF-$\beta 2$) on the proliferation and natural killer activity of decidual $CD16^{-}CD56^{bright}$ natural killer cells. *Cell Immunol* 1993;152:605–13.
44. Jokhi PP, King A, Loke YW. Production of granulocyte-macrophage colony-stimulating factor by human trophoblast cells and by decidual large granular lymphocytes. *Hum Reprod* 1994;9:1660–9.
45. Sindram-Trujillo AP, Scherjon SA, van Hulst-van Miert PP, *et al.* Differential distribution of NK cells in decidua basalis compared with decidua parietalis after uncomplicated human term pregnancy. *Hum Immunol* 2003;64:921–9.
46. Le Bouteiller P, Pizzato N, Barakonyi A, Solier C. HLA-G, pre-eclampsia, immunity and vascular events. *J Reprod Immunol* 2003;59:219–34.
47. van der Meer A, Lukassen HG, van Lierop MJ, *et al.* Membrane-bound HLA-G activates proliferation and interferon-gamma production by uterine natural killer cells. *Mol Hum Reprod* 2004;10:189–95.
48. King A, Hiby SE, Verma S, Burrows T, Gardner L, Loke YW. Uterine NK cells and trophoblast HLA class I molecules. *Am J Reprod Immunol* 1997;37:459–62.
49. Rouas-Freiss N, Goncalves RM, Menier C, Dausset J, Carosella ED. Direct evidence to support the role of HLA-G in protecting the fetus from maternal uterine natural killer cytolysis. *Proc Natl Acad Sci USA* 1997;94:11520–5.
50. Huddleston H, Schust DJ. Immune interactions at the maternal–fetal interface: A focus on antigen presentation. *Am J Reprod Immunol* 2004;51:283–9.
51. Llano M, Lee N, Navarro F, *et al.* HLA-E-bound peptides influence recognition by inhibitory and triggering CD94/NKG2 receptors: Preferential response to an HLA-G-derived nonamer. *Eur J Immunol* 1998;28:2854–63.
52. Parham P. Killer cell immunoglobulin-like receptor diversity: Balancing signals in the natural killer cell response. *Immunol Lett* 2004;92:11–3.
53. Luppi P. How immune mechanisms are affected by pregnancy. *Vaccine* 2003;21:3352–7.
54. Sindram-Trujillo A, Scherjon S, Kanhai H, Roelen D, Claas F. Increased T-cell activation in decidua parietalis compared to decidua basalis in uncomplicated human term pregnancy. *Am J Reprod Immunol* 2003;49:261–8.
55. Chaouat G, Ledee-Bataille N, Zourbas S, *et al.* Implantation: Can immunological parameters of implantation failure be of interest for pre-eclampsia? *J Reprod Immunol* 2003;59:205–17.
56. Chaouat G, Ledee-Bataille N, Dubanchet S, Zourbas S, Sandra O, Martal J. TH1/TH2 paradigm in pregnancy: Paradigm lost? Cytokines in pregnancy/early abortion: Reexamining the TH1/TH2 paradigm. *Int Arch Allergy Immunol* 2004;134:93–119.
57. Croy BA, Ashkar AA, Minhas K, Greenwood JD. Can murine uterine natural killer cells give insights into the pathogenesis of preeclampsia? *J Soc Gynecol Investig* 2000;7:12–20.
58. van Kampen CA, Versteeg-van der Voort Maarschalk MF, Langerak-Langerak J, van Beelen E, Roelen DL, Claas FH. Pregnancy can induce long-persisting primed CTLs specific for inherited paternal HLA antigens. *Hum Immunol* 2001;62: 201–7.
59. Sindram-Trujillo AP, Scherjon SA, van Hulst-van Miert PP, Kanhai HHH, Roelen DL, Claas FHJ. Comparison of decidual leukocytes following spontaneous vaginal delivery and elective cesarean section in uncomplicated human term pregnancy. *J Reprod Immunol* 2003;62:125–37.
60. Lidstrom C, Matthiesen L, Berg G, Sharma S, Ernerudh J, Ekerfelt C. Cytokine secretion patterns of NK cells and macrophages in early human pregnancy decidua and blood: Implications for suppressor macrophages in decidua. *Am J Reprod Immunol* 2003;50:444–52.
61. Abrahams VM, Kim YM, Straszewski SL, Romero R, Mor G. Macrophages and apoptotic cell clearance during pregnancy. *Am J Reprod Immunol* 2004;51:275–82.
62. von Rango U, Krusche CA, Kertšchanska S, Alfer J, Kaufmann P, Beier HM. Apoptosis of extravillous trophoblast cells limits the trophoblast invasion in uterine but not in tubal pregnancy during first trimester. *Placenta* 2003;24:929–40.
63. Jiang SP, Vacchio MS. Multiple mechanisms of peripheral T cell tolerance to the fetal "allograft". *J Immunol* 1998;160:3086–90.
64. Hunt JS, Vassmer D, Ferguson TA, Miller L. Fas ligand is positioned in mouse uterus and placenta to prevent trafficking of activated leukocytes between the mother and the conceptus. *J Immunol* 1997;158:4122–8.
65. Guller S, LaChapelle L. The role of placental Fas ligand in maintaining immune privilege at maternal–fetal interfaces. *Semin Reprod Endocrinol* 1999;17:39–44.
66. Hammer A, Blaschitz A, Daxbock C, Walcher W, Dohr G. Fas and Fas-ligand are expressed in the uteroplacental unit of first-trimester pregnancy. *Am J Reprod Immunol* 1999;41:41–51.
67. Sallusto F, Lanzavecchia A. Mobilizing dendritic cells for tolerance, priming, and chronic inflammation. *J Exp Med* 1999;189: 611–4.
68. Tafuri A, Alferink J, Möller P, Arnold B. T cell awareness of paternal alloantigens during pregnancy. *Science* 1995;270:630–3.
69. Gardner L, Moffett A. Dendritic cells in the human decidua. *Biol Reprod* 2003;61:1438–46.
70. Ueda Y, Hagihara M, Okamoto A, *et al.* Frequencies of dendritic cells (myeloid DC and plasmacytoid DC) and their ratio reduced in pregnant women: Comparison with umbilical cord blood and normal healthy adults. *Hum Immunol* 2003;64:1144–51.
71. Mellor AL, Munn DH. Tryptophan catabolism and T-cell tolerance: Immunosuppression by starvation? *Immunol Today* 1999;20:469–73.
72. Blois SM, Alba Soto CD, Tometten M, Klapp BF, Margni RA, Arck PC. Lineage, maturity, and phenotype of uterine murine dendritic cells throughout gestation indicate a protective role in maintaining pregnancy. *Biol Reprod* 2004;70:1018–23.
73. Sakaguchi S, Sakaguchi N, Shimizu J, *et al.* Immunologic tolerance maintained by CD25 + CD4 + regulatory T cells: Their common role in controlling autoimmunity, tumor immunity, and transplantation tolerance. *Immunol Rev* 2001;182:18–32.

74. Rutella S, Lemoli RM. Regulatory T cells and tolerogenic dendritic cells: From basic biology to clinical applications. *Immunol Lett* 2004;94:11–26.
75. Sasaki Y, Sakai M, Miyazaki S, Higuma S, Shiozaki A, Saito S. Decidual and peripheral blood CD4+CD25+ regulatory T cells in early pregnancy subjects and spontaneous abortion cases. *Mol Hum Reprod* 2004;10:347–53.
76. Somerset DA, Zheng Y, Kilby MD, Sansom DM, Drayson MT. Normal human pregnancy is associated with an elevation in the immune suppressive CD25+ CD4+ regulatory T-cell subset. *Immunology* 2004;112:38–43.
77. Ling EM, Smith T, Nguyen XD, *et al.* Relation of CD4+CD25+ regulatory T-cell suppression of allergen-driven T-cell activation to atopic status and expression of allergic disease. *Lancet* 2004;363: 608–15.
78. Nagaeva O, Jonsson L, Mincheva-Nilsson L. Dominant IL-10 and TGF-beta mRNA expression in gammadeltaT cells of human early pregnancy decidua suggests immunoregulatory potential. *Am J Reprod Immunol* 2002;48:9–17.
79. Costeas PA, Koumouli A, Giantsiou-Kyriakou A, Papaloizou A, Koumas L. Th2/Th3 cytokine genotypes are associated with pregnancy loss. *Hum Immunol* 2004;65:135–41.
80. Tilburgs T, Roelen DL; van der Mast BJ, van Schip JJ, Kleijburg C, de Groot-Swings GM, Kanhai HHH, Claas FHJ, Scherjon S. Distribution of $CD4^{+}CD25^{bright}$ and $CD8^{+}CD28^{-}$ T cells in decidua and maternal blood during human pregnancy. *Placenta* (in press)
81. Grohmann U, Orabona C, Fallarino F, *et al.* CTLA-4-Ig regulates tryptophan catabolism in vivo. *Nat Immunol* 2002;3:1097–101.
82. Heikkinen J, Mottonen M, Alanen A, Lassila O. Phenotypic characterization of regulatory T cells in the human decidua. *Clin Exp Immunol* 2004;136:373–8.
83. Munn DH, Zhou M, Attwood JT, *et al.* Prevention of allogeneic fetal rejection by tryptophan catabolism. *Science* 1998;281:1191–3.
84. Grohmann U, Fallarino F, Puccetti P. Tolerance, DCs and tryptophan: Much ado about IDO. *Trends Immunol* 2003;24:242–8.
85. Kudo Y, Hara T, Katsuki T, *et al.* Mechanisms regulating the expression of indoleamine 2,3-dioxygenase during decidualization of human endometrium. *Hum Reprod* 2004;19:1222–30.
86. Kudo Y, Boyd CA, Spyropoulou I, *et al.* Indoleamine 2,3-dioxygenase: Distribution and function in the developing human placenta. *J Reprod Immunol* 2004;61:87–98.
87. Xu C, Mao D, Holers VM, Palanca B, Cheng AM, Molina H. A critical role for murine complement regulator crry in fetomaternal tolerance. *Science* 2000;287:498–501.
88. Xu C, Mao D, Holers VM, Palanca B, Cheng AM, Molina H. A critical role for murine complement regulator crry in fetomaternal tolerance. *Science* 2000;287:498–501.
89. Mori T, Kobayashi H, Nishimoto H, Suzuki A, Nishimura T, Mori T. Inhibitory effect of progesterone and 20 alpha-hydroxypregn-4-en-3-one on the phytohemagglutinin-induced transformation of human lymphocytes. *Am J Obstet Gynecol* 1977;127:151–7.
90. Szekeres-Bartho J, Hadnagy J, Pacsa AS. The suppressive effect of progesterone on lymphocyte cytotoxicity: Unique progesterone sensitivity of pregnancy lymphocytes. *J Reprod Immunol* 1985;7:121–8.
91. Barakonyi A, Polgar B, Szekeres-Bartho J. The role of gamma/delta T-cell receptor-positive cells in pregnancy: Part II. *Am J Reprod Immunol* 1999;42:83–7.
92. van den HM, McBey BA, Hahnel AC, Croy BA. An analysis of the uterine lymphocyte-derived hybridoma cell line GWM 1-2 for expression of receptors for estrogen, progesterone and interleukin 2. *J Reprod Immunol* 1996;31:37–50.
93. Polgar B, Kispal G, Lachmann M, *et al.* Molecular cloning and immunologic characterization of a novel cDNA coding for progesterone-induced blocking factor. *J Immunol* 2003;171:5956–63.
94. Loudon JA, Elliott CL, Hills F, Bennett PR. Progesterone represses interleukin-8 and cyclo-oxygenase-2 in human lower segment fibroblast cells and amnion epithelial cells. *Biol Reprod* 2003;69: 331–7.
95. Meis PJ, Klebanoff M, Thom E, *et al.* Prevention of recurrent preterm delivery by 17 alpha-hydroxyprogesterone caproate. *N Engl J Med* 2003;348:2379–85.
96. Simpson KL, Keelan JA, Mitchell MD. Labor-associated changes in interleukin-10 production and its regulation by immunomodulators in human choriodecidua. *J Clin Endocrinol Metab* 1998;83: 4332–7.
97. Pellegrini I, Lebrun JJ, Ali S, Kelly PA. Expression of prolactin and its receptor in human lymphoid cells. *Mol Endocrinol* 1992;6: 1023–31.
98. Gubbay O, Critchley HO, Bowen JM, King A, Jabbour HN. Prolactin induces ERK phosphorylation in epithelial and CD56(+) natural killer cells of the human endometrium. *J Clin Endocrinol Metab* 2002;87:2329–35.
99. Bianchi DW, Zickwolf G, Weil G, Sylvester S, DeMaria MA. Male fetal progenitor cells persist in maternal blood as long as 27 years postpartum. *Proc Natl Acad Sci* 1996;93:705–8.
100. Srivatsa B, Srivatsa S, Johnson KL, Bianchi DW. Maternal cell microchimerism in newborn tissues. *J Pediatr* 2003;142:31–5.
101. O'Donoghue K, Chan J, de la Fuente J. Long-term consequences of pregnancy: The persistence of fetal cells in maternal organs. *J Soc Gynecol Invest* 2004;11:193A.
102. Claas F, Gijbels Y, VanderVelden-DeMunck J, VanRood J. Induction of B cell unresponsiveness to noninherited maternal HLA antigens during fetal life. *Science* 1988;241:1815–7.
103. Burlingham W, Grailer A, Heisey D, *et al.* The effect of tolerance to noninherited maternal HLA antigens on the survival of renal transplants from sibling donors. *N Engl J Med* 1998;339:1657–64.
104. van Rood JJ, Loberiza FR Jr, Zhang MJ, *et al.* Effect of tolerance to noninherited maternal antigens on the occurrence of graft-versus-host disease after bone marrow transplantation from a parent or an HLA-haploidentical sibling. *Blood* 2002;99:1572–7.
105. Molitor ML, Haynes LD, Jankowska-Gan E, Mulder A, Burlingham WJ. HLA class I noninherited maternal antigens in cord blood and breast milk. *Hum Immunol* 2004;65:231–9.
106. Yoshihara T, Morimoto A, Inukai T, *et al.* Non-T-cell-depleted HLA haploidentical stem cell transplantation based on feto–maternal microchimerism in pediatric patients with advanced malignancies. *Bone Marrow Transplant* 2004;34(4):373–5.
107. Monaco AP. Prospects and strategies for clinical tolerance. *Transplant Proc* 2004;36:227–31.
108. Le Bouteiller P, Solier C, Proll J, Aguerre-Girr M, Fournel S, Lenfant F. Placental HLA-G protein expression in vivo: Where and what for? *Hum Reprod Update* 1999;5:223–33.
109. Hiby SE, Walker JJ, O'Shaughnessy KM, *et al.* Combinations of maternal KIR and fetal HLA-C genes influence the risk of preeclampsia and reproductive success. *J Exp Med* 2004;200:957–65.
110. Rogers AM, Boime I, Connolly J, Cook JR, Russell JH. Maternal–fetal tolerance is maintained despite transgene-driven trophoblast expression of MHC class I, and defects in Fas and its ligand. *Eur J Immunol* 1998;28:3479–87.
111. Gomez-Lozano N, de Pablo R, Puente S, Vilches C. Recognition of HLA-G by the NK cell receptor KIR2DL4 is not essential for human reproduction. *Eur J Immunol* 2003;33:639–44.
112. Chaouat G, Zourbas S, Ostojic S, *et al.* A brief review of recent data on some cytokine expressions at the materno–foetal interface which might challenge the classical Th1/Th2 dichotomy. *J Reprod Immunol* 2002;53:241–56.

88 Fetal behavior

J. G. Nijhuis

Introduction

For many years, the fetus has been considered to be developing in a relatively safe surrounding. However, this view changed dramatically when the accessibility of the human fetus increased with the introduction of ultrasonography. This was the start of an avalanche of fetal behavioral research.[1] Increasing insight into the developing human fetus made it clear that the growing fetus could only be judged properly if one took gestational age into account, and it also became clear that intrauterine life was not so safe as one had always assumed: 'After all, the fetus is but a human being, just as prone as a child or adult to have an accident, a disease or an iatrogenic problem!'[2]

In this chapter, we will review the most important data on fetal behavioral variables and behavioral states and then discuss the clinical consequences of this knowledge.

Basic studies

Fetal heart rate patterns

Electronic monitoring of the fetal heart rate in combination with contractions, if present, is used worldwide for the assessment of fetal condition (cardiotocography, CTG). The technique was introduced for intrapartum use by Caldeyro-Barcia *et al.* in 1966,[3] Hammacher and Werners in 1968[4] and Hon in 1968.[5] In 1969, Kubli *et al.*[6] also introduced the technique for antepartum use. Although the intra- and interobserver variability is still large, the specificity is such that clinicians rely on the method.[7,8] The sensitivity, however, is rather poor. In general, good bandwidth or beat-to-beat variability in the presence of accelerations is indicative of a good fetal condition, a silent pattern (small bandwidth, no accelerations) is indicative of fetal distress, certainly in the presence of late decelerations. One of the problems is that many scores that were developed to improve the interpretation of the CTG did not take the age of the fetus into account, while Visser *et al.*[9] had already shown a clear developmental trend during gestation in the amplitude and duration of the accelerations. Timor-Tritsch *et al.*[10] pointed out that the fetal heart rate pattern (FHRP) was dependent on the fetal behavioral state. In 1982, we defined four different FHRPs, A, B, C and D, which were then used to define behavioral states in combination with the presence or absence of body and eye movements[11] (Figure 88.1). It was also found that not only the form of the accelerations changed during gestation but also during gestation the length of silent heart rate patterns (FHRP A) increased, i.e. without any sign of fetal distress.[11,13] More recently, automated antepartum baseline fetal heart rate determination and detection of accelerations and decelerations has been introduced.[14]

Fetal body movements

'and the children struggled together within her'

Bible, Genesis 25:22

This is probably one of the first descriptions of fetal movements. In 1976, Reinold[15] was the first to show that the fetus was already moving spontaneously in the first trimester of pregnancy. He also showed that absence of body movements might indicate impending fetal death, while the presence of body movements is very reassuring. With modern ultrasound techniques the very first 'fetal activity' that can be observed is the fetal heart rate.[16] In 1982, de Vries *et al.*[17] published their results on the observation of fetal somatic activity in the first half of pregnancy. They introduced a categorization of movement patterns and described how the individual movements were performed in terms of speed, force and amplitude. This work clearly shows that the majority of the repertoire of movements that can be distinguished in the third trimester and after birth are already present at 14 weeks' gestation.[17]

In the second and third trimesters, much attention has been paid to the presence of gross body movements,[18] but only in the last weeks of pregnancy does the fetus exhibit quite clearly prolonged periods of presence and absence of fetal movements. As gestational age progresses, the periods during which body

(a)	State criteria			
State criteria	State 1F	State 2F	State 3F	State 4F
Body movements	Incidental	Periodic	Absent	Continuous
Eye movements	Absent	Present	Present	Present
Heart rate pattern	A	B	C	D

(b)

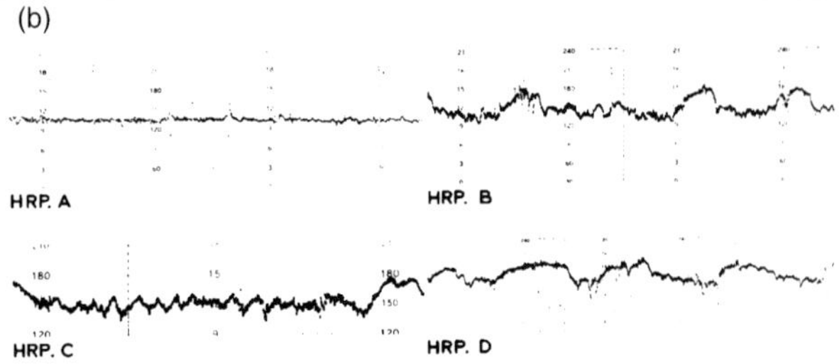

Figure 88.1 (a) Definition of the four behavioral states. (b) Examples given for each of the fetal heart rate patterns (HRP) A–D, at a recording speed of 3 cm/min. Reproduced from van Vliet *et al.*[12] with permission.

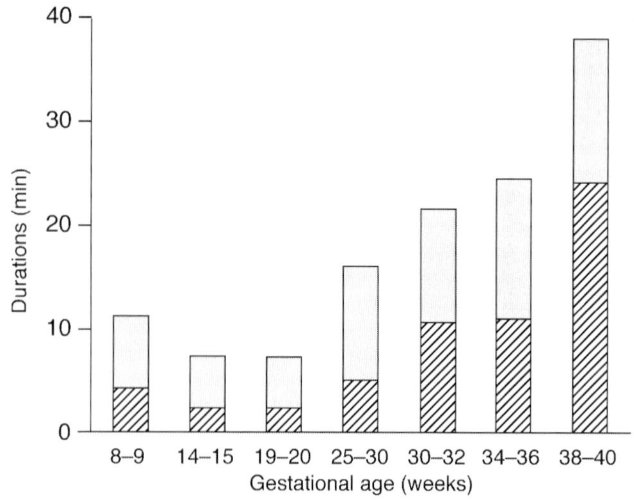

Figure 88.2 Maximum and median duration (in minutes) of periods in which body movements can be absent at different gestational ages.

movements can be absent increase dramatically. This is nicely illustrated in Figure 88.2.

This observation emphasizes again that the fetal age should be taken into account: what is normal in a fetus at 20 weeks may be abnormal in the same fetus at 38 weeks! Over the past decade it has also become clear that counting the number of movements is not very useful: even the mildly hypoxic growth-retarded fetus will still make body movements. It seems to be of much more importance to look at the quality of the movements, the speed and amplitude, etc. De Vries *et al.*[17,19] started to use the concept of quality in the first trimester and Bekedam *et al.*[20] looked for this aspect in 10 intrauterine growth-retarded fetuses between 29 and 35 weeks.

Fetal eye movements

Bots *et al.*[21] published their first observation on fetal eye movements using ultrasound and they recorded them by means of M-mode ultrasonography in 1981. Their findings were confirmed in the same year by Birnholz.[22] The possibility of observing and recording eye movements created a change allowing the study of fetal motility in relation to a new variable. Of course, at this stage fetal and neonatal data appeared to be rather similar. It is, however, not always possible to compare the fetal data with those of the neonate, because in the neonate it is not the eye movements that are used in behavioral studies but rather the criterion 'eyes open' or 'eyes closed'.[23]

Fetal breathing movements

It was Ahlfeld[24] in Germany who published the first observation of fetal breathing movements in 1888. His observations were almost unanimously neglected until the issue was reintroduced by Dawes *et al.*[25] in 1970, who described breathing movements in fetal lambs, and by Boddy and Robinson[26] in 1971 in the human fetus. Bots *et al.*[27] published a detailed analysis of human fetal breathing movements and described them as 'paradoxic' because the ribcage made an inward movement during 'inspiration' when the diaphragm made a downward movement. Originally, it was thought that breathing movements could be used as a perfect indicator for the detection of fetal distress, but soon it became apparent that breathing movements are not continuously present and are influenced by many conditions. A postprandial increase in breathing movements has already been described from 20 to 22 weeks onward,[28] and Nijhuis *et al.*[29] showed an increase after glucose intake by the mother at 24 weeks. Furthermore, smoking diminishes the incidence of fetal breathing and breathing is not only much more likely to be absent during fetal rest periods,[30] but also much more regular.[31,32] During the last weeks of pregnancy, the incidence of fetal breathing decreases and breathing movements are absent during labor.[33] The duration of periods in which breathing movements can be absent increases enormously during pregnancy, and near term it is not unusual for breathing movements to be absent for as long as 120 min.[34] In general, for behavioral studies, fetal breathing should not be studied as an independent variable but always in combination with other variables and preferably under highly standardized conditions.

Fetal mouth movements

With modern ultrasonographic equipment, the fetal mouth is easy to visualize. Specific mouthing or sucking behaviors can be observed: recurrent clusters of 'regular mouthing movements' can be observed during quiet states (state 1F), while during state 3F 'sucking movements' can be observed (for an overview, see van Woerden and van Geijn[35]). Both activities, regular mouthing and sucking, are able to entrain a fairly specific heart rate pattern, which may confuse the clinicians.[36,37]

Fetal behavior

Certainly in the second half of pregnancy, the observation of fetal activity can be combined with the simultaneous recording of the fetal heart rate and such a combined recording is then called the registration of 'fetal behavior'. In the beginning, it is as if all sorts of movements occur more or less independently of one another and they do not elicit specific FHRP. However, with the increase of gestational age, an increasing linkage can be observed between periods with 'absence of eye movements', and periods with 'absence of movements' and with a silent heart rate pattern, FHRP A.[38] This increasing linkage, which has been noticed by Drogtrop *et al.*[39] at 25–30 weeks and by Visser *et al.*[40] at 30–32 weeks, is crucial for the development of recognizable behavioral states.

Behavioral states in the neonate

'Behavioral states are constellations of physiological and behavioral variables (e.g. eyes closed, regular breathing and no movements: quiet sleep) which are stable over time and recur repeatedly, not only in the same infant, but also in similar forms in all infants' (modified from Prechtl *et al.*[23]). In the neonate, Prechtl *et al.*[23] defined five behavioral states: state 1 [quiet sleep, similar to non-rapid eye movement (REM)-sleep], state 2 (active sleep, similar to REM-sleep), state 3 (quiet awake), state 4 (active awake) and state 5 (vocalization). Three major requirements have to be fulfilled before a behavioral state can be recognized. First of all, a specific combination of certain variables must occur at the same time ('coincidence', 'linkage'), e.g. presence of body movements, eyes open and irregular breathing for state 2. Second, to be able to recognize this combination, it should be stable over time (by definition at least 3 min). Third, it must be possible to see a clear change from one state into another, a 'state transition'. If the transitional periods become too long (i.e. longer than 3 min of 'no coincidence'), it is no longer possible to clearly distinguish behavioral states.[13]

Fetal behavioral states

Following the concept of behavioral states in the neonate, Nijhuis *et al.*[11] described four fetal behavioral states. They recorded fetal behavior with two ultrasound scanners and a simultaneous registration of the FHRP. To emphasize the similarity with the neonatal states they were called 1F ('F' for fetal) to 4F, respectively.

State 1F (similar to state 1 in the neonate): Quiescence, which can be regularly interrupted by brief gross body movements, mostly startles. Eye movements are absent. The FHRP A is a stable pattern with a small oscillation bandwidth and no accelerations, except in combination with a startle (Figure 88.1).

State 2F (similar to state 2 in the neonate): Frequent and periodic gross body movements – mainly stretches and retroflexions – and movements of the extremities. Eye movements are present. FHRP B has a wider oscillation bandwidth and frequent accelerations during movements (Figure 88.1).

State 3F (similar to state 3 in the neonate): Gross body movements are absent. Eye movements are present. FHRP C is stable but with a wider oscillation bandwidth than FHRP A and no accelerations (Figure 88.1).

State 4F (similar to state 4 in the neonate): Vigorous, continual activity including many trunk rotations. Eye movements are present. FHRP D is unstable, with large and long-lasting accelerations, often fused into a sustained tachycardia (Figure 88.1).

After the introduction of the definitions, many other research groups were able to confirm the same findings.[41–43] The introduction of the concept of states had a great influence on the research that was performed in both animal and human research. As an example, it appeared to be the case that breathing movements were largely absent during state 1F,[30] but if they were present they were much more regular.[32] Therefore, to study the influence of a certain stimulus on breathing, it is now clear that such a study needs to be standardized for states. Otherwise one might think that the stimulus used abolishes breathing while, in fact, only a state transition from 2F (with breathing) into 1F (without breathing) has been induced.

Following the description of fetal behavior under normal conditions, many studies have been looking for changes in behavior in growth-retarded fetuses,[20,44,45] fetuses of diabetic mothers[46] and of mothers who used antiepileptic drugs,[47] cocaine,[48] methadone[49] and corticosteroids.[50] For reviews see Richardson,[51] Groome and Watson,[52] Koyanagi *et al.*[53] and Romanini and Rizzo.[54] Furthermore, Doppler measurements in several fetal vessels also appeared to be state related, although in compromised fetuses this state dependency plays a minor role.[55]

Clinical experiences

Studying fetal behavior is very time-consuming. This means that a behavioral study will only be performed if simpler techniques do not answer the question that is posed. Fetal heart rate monitoring is the most frequently used method, but insight into fetal behavior has had a certain influence on the interpretation of CTGs. The two most important examples are the

Table 88.1 Differential diagnosis and proposed management in silent heart rate pattern and sinusoidal heart rate pattern

Differential diagnosis	Management
Silent heart rate pattern	
State 1F	Extension of recording time
Effect of drugs	Exclusion of use of drugs
Tachycardia	Inspection of baseline
Anomalies	Ultrasonographic examination, behavioral study
Hypoxia	Contraction stress test
Brain death	Cordocentesis
Sinusoidal heart rate pattern	
Fetal mouth movements	
Sucking ('major' or 'marked')	Behavioral study
Regular mouthing ('minor')	Behavioral study
Effect of drugs	Exclusion of use of drugs
Congenital anomalies	Ultrasonographic examination
Fetal asphyxia	Biophysical profile testing
Fetal anemia	Cordocentesis

'silent' heart rate pattern and the 'sinusoidal' heart rate pattern. Obviously, a silent FHRP may indicate fetal distress, but it may also reflect a physiological behavioral state 1F. It is therefore of crucial importance that one considers a differential diagnosis if a silent heart rate pattern is recorded[56] (Table 88.1). The most extreme example of a silent heart rate pattern is entrained by the 'intrauterine brain death syndrome'. In such a case the FHRP is silent over a long period of time, with a somewhat elevated baseline and the fetus does not move (Figure 88.3). At birth – mostly via a cesarean section due to 'fetal distress' – a floppy infant is born and artificial ventilation will be needed. An electroencephalogram will be isoelectric and a diagnosis of 'brain death' will then finally be made.[56,57] This 'intrauterine coma' is probably the consequence of a hypoxic accident that is mostly not recorded. Hence, there has been a period of severe asphyxia during which the fetus almost died, but then recovered. In such a situation a cordocentesis would reveal a normal pH value.

We have already mentioned that a fetus makes regular mouthing movements during state 1F,[58] while sucking movements can be seen during 3F.[36,37] Both categories of mouth movements may entrain a 'sinusoidal-like' FHRP, a heart rate pattern that can also be recorded in combination with severe fetal anemia. Again, also for this FHRP, a differential diagnosis can be made (Table 88.1). We have only made a beginning

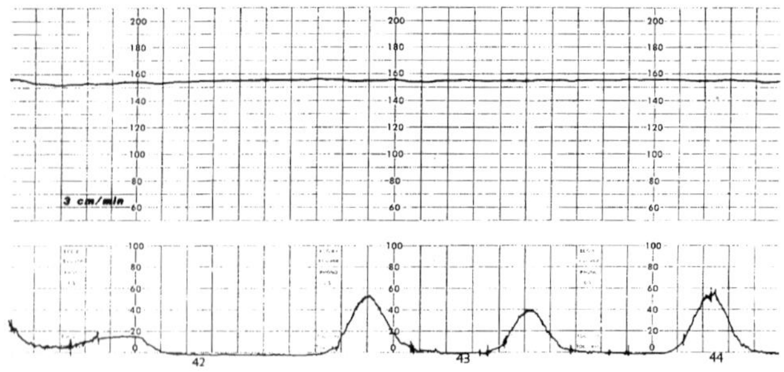

Figure 88.3 An example of a persistently silent fetal heart rate pattern without decelerations, and absence of fetal activity. Note the relatively high baseline of 155 bpm, this recording indicates fetal brain death. Reproduced with permission from Nijhuis *et al.*[56]

with the understanding of the human fetus in its natural environment, but these examples make perfectly clear how important it is to be aware of these behavioral states.

Another step forward was made by Mulder *et al.*,[50] who showed a clear effect of betamethasone on fetal behavior. This drug, which is used for the stimulation of lung maturation, decreases heart rate variability and the number of movements. Dexamethasone seems to have a similar effect, but to a much lesser degree.[59]

Visser *et al.*[60] have considered the change of consecutive variables in a deteriorating fetal condition, and proposed that changes in fetal behavior and quality of fetal movements are among the first signs, while a terminal heart rate pattern is of course the final step.

Future clinical aspects

In normal post-term pregnancies, van de Pas *et al.*[61] showed that the fetus continues to mature further, similar to the neonate already born. In the post-term fetus, the amount of states 3F and 4F increased significantly at the expense of state 2F, implying that the fetus is more 'awake' *in utero*. If one accepts that the fetus exhibits clear behavioral states, similar to the neonate, then it is perfectly understandable that birth by itself does not seem to alter the developmental pathway of this output of the central nervous system. However, most neonatal tests are not applicable for the fetus. It has already been noticed that fetuses with congenital anomalies may show bizarre behavior[62] or dissociation of heart rate and movements.[63] Other authors have been studying state transitions rather than behavioral states,[64] but still it is difficult to draw conclusions from a single behavioral recording in a single fetus. Perhaps, it would be more promising if we could develop a 'neurological examination' for the fetus, knowing that we have limited possibilities. A first step has been made by Tas *et al.*,[65] who were able to evoke an intercostal-to-phrenic inhibitory reflex (IPIR): compression of the ribcage results in apnea. In a second series of experiments, they were not able to find a different result in a group of growth-retarded fetuses, defined as growth below the 10th percentile.[66] Another possible approach is the study of fetal habituation, i.e. the fetal learning pattern. A normal fetus will habituate to a certain stimulus, which means that it will cease to respond to repeated exposure to the stimulus. For example, Hepper and Shahidullah[67] demonstrated that fetuses with Down's syndrome take longer to habituate than normal fetuses. Recently, Leader[68] concluded in a commentary, 'It seems likely that no single, isolated aspect of behavior alone will evolve but rather a combination of behaviors to form a prenatal neurological examination'.[68]

Summary

The study of fetal behavior also plays an important role in the understanding of normal fetal well-being and in the evaluation of the possibly compromised fetus. It has introduced a completely different way of looking at the developing human being. It also has become more apparent that birth by itself is not the major cause for the neonatal neurological morbidity. Morbidity does not, in the majority of cases, originate from an (hypoxic) accident during birth, but rather from an (hypoxic) accident somewhere during gestation, or it may even be genetic. Most of these mild cases will not be detected at birth and may therefore be attributed to a difficult birth, which is seldom the real cause.[69] It may well be that 'difficult birth in itself in certain cases is merely a symptom of deeper effects that influenced the development of the fetus' (Sigmund Freud[70]).

The study of fetal behavior is still very time-consuming and therefore mostly used in research protocol. In the forthcoming years, we should aim at the development of a more appropriate way to analyze fetal behavior because there is a definite need to get a better insight into the condition of the fetus before birth and in particular the condition of the fetal central nervous system. The development of an adequate and practical intrauterine neurological examination should have high priority in clinical perinatology. The fetus can no longer be regarded as a 'growing organism' that will react independently of age and state. If one wants to say something about the condition of the fetus or to learn something about its development in its intrauterine environment, then one should start to do so under standardized conditions with respect to fetal age, time of the day, relation to maternal meals, etc. and last but not least, certainly in the last trimester one should be aware of fetal behavioral states.

REFERENCES

1. Nijhuis JG, ed. *Fetal Behaviour, Developmental and Perinatal Aspects*. Oxford: Oxford University Press, 1992.
2. Nijhuis JG. Physiological and clinical consequences in relation to the development of fetal behavior and fetal behavioral states. In Krasnegor NA, Lecanuet P, Fifer WP, *et al.*, eds. *Fetal Development: A Psychobiological Perspective*. New Jersey: Lawrence Erlbaum, 1995:67–82.
3. Caldeyro-Barcia R, Mendez-Bauer C, Poseiro JJ, *et al.* Control of human fetal heart rate during labor. In Cassels DE, ed. *The Heart Rate and Circulation in the Newborn and Infant*. New York: Grune and Stratton, 1966:122–8.
4. Hammacher K, Werners PH. Über die Auswertung und Dokumentation von CTG-Ergebnissen. *Gynaecologia* 1968;166: 410–23.
5. Hon EH. *An Atlas of Fetal Heart Rate Patterns*. New Haven: Harty Press Inc., 1968.
6. Kubli FW, Kaeser O, Hinselmann M. Diagnostic management of chronic placental insufficiency. In Pecile A, Finzi C, eds. *The Foeto-placental Unit*. Amsterdam: Excerpta Medica Foundation, 1969:323–39.
7. Trimbos JB, Keirse MJCN. Observer variability in assessment of antepartum cardiotocograms. *Br J Obstet Gynaecol* 1978;85:900–6.
8. Lotgering FK, Wallenburg HCS, Schouten HJA. Interobserver and intraobserver variation in the assessment of antepartum cardiotocograms. *Am J Obstet Gynecol* 1982;144:701–5.
9. Visser GHA, Dawes GS, Redman CWG. Numerical analysis of the normal human antenatal fetal heart rate. *Br J Obstet Gynaecol* 1981;88:792–802.
10. Timor-Tritsch IE, Dierker LJ, Hertz RH, Deagan C, Rosen MG. Studies of antepartum behavioural states in the human fetus at term. *Am J Obstet Gynecol* 1979;132:524–8.
11. Nijhuis JG, Bots RSGM, Martin CB Jr, Prechtl HFR. Are there behavioural states in the human fetus? *Early Hum Dev* 1982;6: 177–95.
12. van Vliet MAT, Martin CB, Nijhuis JG, Prechtl HFR. The relationship between fetal activity and behavioral states and fetal breathing movements in normal and growth-retarded fetuses. *Am J Obstet Gynecol* 1985;153:582–8.
13. Nijhuis JG, Martin CB Jr, Prechtl HFR. Behavioural states of the human fetus. In Prechtl HFR, ed. *Continuity of Neural Functions from Prenatal to Postnatal Life. Clinics in Developmental Medicine*. Oxford: Blackwell Scientific Publications Ltd., 1984: 65–79.
14. Mantel R, Ververs I, Colenbrander G, *et al.* Automated antepartum baseline FHR determination and detection of accelerations and decelerations. In Van Geijn HP, Copray FJA, eds. *A Critical Appraisal of Fetal Surveillance*. Amsterdam: Elsevier Science BV, 1994:333–48.
15. Reinold E. Beobachtung fetaler Aktivität in der ersten Hälfte der Gravidität mit dem Ultraschall. *Pädiatr Pädol* 1976;6:274–9.
16. van Heeswijk M, Nijhuis JG, Hollanders JMG. Fetal heart rate in early pregnancy. *Early Hum Dev* 1990;22:151–6.
17. de Vries JIP, Visser GHA, Prechtl HFR. The emergence of fetal behaviour. I. Qualitative aspects. *Early Hum Dev* 1982;7:301–22.
18. Visser GHA. The second trimester. In Nijhuis JG, ed. *Fetal Behaviour, Developmental and Perinatal Aspects*. Oxford: Oxford University Press, 1992:17–26.
19. de Vries JIP, Visser GHA, Prechtl HFR. The emergence of fetal behaviour. II. Quantitative aspects. *Early Hum Dev* 1985;12: 99–120.
20. Bekedam DJ, Visser GHA, de Vries JJ, *et al.* Motor behaviour in the growth-retarded fetus. *Early Hum Dev* 1985;12:155–65.
21. Bots RSGM, Nijhuis JG, Martin CB Jr, *et al.* Human fetal eye movements: Detection *in utero* by ultrasonography. *Early Hum Dev* 1981;5:87–94.
22. Birnholz JC. The development of human fetal eye movement patterns. *Science* 1981;213:679–81.
23. Prechtl HFR, Weinmann HM, Akiyama Y. Organization of physiological parameters in normal and neurologically abnormal infants. *Neuropädiatrie* 1969;1:101–29.
24. Ahlfeld F. Ueber intrauterine Athembewegungen des Kindes. *Ver Dsch Ges Gynäk* 1888;2:203–10.

25. Dawes GS, Leduc HE, Liggins GC, *et al.* Respiratory movements and paradoxal sleep in the foetal lamb. *J Physiol* 1970;210:47–8.
26. Boddy K, Robinson JS. External method for detection of fetal breathing *in utero*. *Lancet* 1971;2:1231–3.
27. Bots RSGM, Broeders GHB, Farman DJ, *et al.* Fetal breathing movements in the normal and growth-retarded fetus: A multiscan/M-mode echofetographic study. *Eur J Obstet Gynecol Reprod Biol* 1978;8:21–9.
28. de Vries JIP, Visser GHA, Mulder EJH, *et al.* Diurnal and other variations in fetal movement, and heart rate patterns at 20–22 weeks. *Early Hum Dev* 1987;15:333–48.
29. Nijhuis JG, Jongsma HW, Crijns IJMJ, *et al.* Effects of maternal glucose ingestion on human fetal breathing movements at weeks 24, and 28 of gestation. *Early Hum Dev* 1986;13:183–8.
30. van Vliet MAT, Martin CB Jr, Nijhuis JG, *et al.* The relationship between fetal activity, and behavioural states and fetal breathing movements in normal and growth-retarded fetuses. *Am J Obstet Gynecol* 1985;153:582–8.
31. Timor-Tritsch IE, Dierker LJ, Hertz RH, *et al.* Regular and irregular human fetal respiratory movements. *Early Hum Dev* 1980;4: 315–24.
32. Nijhuis JG, Martin CB Jr, Gommers S, *et al.* The rhythmicity of fetal breathing varies with behavioural state in the human fetus. *Early Hum Dev* 1983;9:1–7.
33. Carmichael L, Campbell K, Patrick J. Fetal breathing, gross fetal body movements, and maternal and fetal heart rates before spontaneous labor at term. *Am J Obstet Gynecol* 1984;148:675–9.
34. Patrick J, Campbell K, Carmichael L, *et al.* Patterns of human fetal breathing during the last 10 weeks of pregnancy. *Obstet Gynecol* 1980;56:24–30.
35. van Woerden EE, van Geijn HP. Heart-rate patterns and fetal movements. In Nijhuis JG, ed. *Fetal Behaviour, Developmental and Perinatal Aspects.* Oxford: Oxford University Press, 1988: 41–56.
36. Nijhuis JG, Staisch KJ, Martin CB Jr, *et al.* A sinusoidal-like fetal heart-rate pattern in association with fetal sucking – Report of 2 cases. *Eur J Obstet Gynecol Reprod Biol* 1984;16:353–8.
37. van Woerden EE, van Geijn HP, Caron FJM, *et al.* Fetal mouse movements during behavioural states 1F and 2F. *Eur J Obstet Gynecol Reprod Biol* 1988;29:97–105.
38. Nijhuis JG, van de Pas M. Behavioural states and their ontogeny: Human studies. *Semin Perinatol* 1992;16:206–10.
39. Drogtrop AP, Ubels R, Nijhuis JG. The association between fetal body movements, eye movements, and heart rate patterns between 25 and 30 weeks of gestation. *Early Hum Dev* 1990;23: 67–73.
40. Visser GHA, Poelman-Weesjes G, Cohen TMN. Fetal behaviour at 30 to 32 weeks of gestation. *Pediatr Res* 1987;22:655–8.
41. van Vliet MAT, Martin CB Jr, Nijhuis JG, *et al.* Behavioural states in fetuses of nulliparous women. *Early Hum Dev* 1985;12: 121–35.
42. van Woerden EE, van Geijn HP, Caron FJM, *et al.* Automated assignment of fetal behavioural states near term. *Early Hum Dev* 1989;19:137–46.
43. Arduini D, Rizzo G, Giorlandino C, *et al.* The fetal behavioural states: An ultrasonic study. *Prenat Diagn* 1985;5:269–76.
44. van Vliet MAT, Martin CB Jr, Nijhuis JG, *et al.* Behavioural states in growth retarded human fetuses. *Early Hum Dev* 1985;12: 183–97.
45. Arduini D, Rizzo G, Romanini C. Growth retardation. In Nijhuis JG, ed. *Fetal Behaviour, Developmental and Perinatal Aspects.* Oxford: Oxford University Press, 1992:181–208.
46. Mulder EJH, Leiblum DM, Visser GHA. Fetal breathing movements in late diabetic pregnancy: Relationship to fetal heart rate patterns and Braxton Hicks' contractions. *Early Hum Dev* 1995;43:225–32.
47. van Geijn HP, Swartjes JM, van Woerden EE, *et al.* Fetal behavioural states in epileptic pregnancies. *Eur J Obstet Gynecol Reprod Biol* 1986;21:309–14.
48. Hume RF Jr, O'Donnell KJ, Stanger CL, *et al. In utero* cocaine exposure: Observations of fetal behavioural state may predict neonatal outcome. *Am J Obstet Gynecol* 1989;161:685–90.
49. Archie CL, Milton IL, Sokol RJ, *et al.* The effects of methadone treatment on the reactivity of the nonstress test. *Obstet Gynecol* 1989;74:254–5.
50. Mulder EJH, Derks JB, Zonneveld MF, *et al.* Transient reduction in fetal activity and heart rate variation after maternal betamethasone administration. *Early Hum Dev* 1994;36:49–60.
51. Richardson BS. Fetal behavioural states. *Semin Perinatol* 1992; 16:4.
52. Groome LJ, Watson JE. Assessment of *in utero* neurobehavioural development. I. Fetal behavioural states. *J Matern Fetal Invest* 1992;2:183–94.
53. Koyanagi T, Nabekura J, Nakano H. Brain function *in utero* unique to the developing fetus. *Fetal Matern Med Rev* 1995;7:129–41.
54. Romanini C, Rizzo G. Fetal behaviour in normal and compromised fetuses. An overview. *Early Hum Dev* 1995;43:117–31.
55. van Eyck J, Wladimiroff JW. Doppler flow measurements. In Nijhuis JG, ed. *Fetal Behaviour, Developmental and Perinatal Aspects.* Oxford: Oxford University Press, 1992:227–41.
56. Nijhuis JG, Crevels AJ, van Dongen PWJ. Fetal brain death: The definition of a fetal heart rate pattern and its clinical consequences. *Obstet Gynecol Surv* 1990;46:229–32.
57. Nijhuis JG, Kruyt N, van Wijck JAM. Fetal brain death. Two case reports. *Br J Obstet Gynaecol* 1988;95:197–200.
58. van Woerden EE, van Geijn HP, Swartjes JM, *et al.* Fetal heart rhythms during behavioural state 1F. *Eur J Obstet Gynecol Reprod Biol* 1988;28:29–38.
59. Mulder EJH, Derks JB, Visser GHA. Antenatal corticosteroid therapy and fetal behaviour: A randomized study of the effects of betamethasone and dexamethasone. *Br J Obstet Gynaecol* 1997; 104:1239–48.
60. Visser GHA, Ribbert LSM, Bekedam DJ. Sequential changes in Doppler waveform, fetal heart rate and movements patterns in IUGR fetuses. In Van Geijn HP, Copray FJA, eds. *A Critical Appraisal of Fetal Surveillance.* Amsterdam: Elsevier Science, 1994:193–200.
61. van de Pas M, Nijhuis JG, Jongsma HW. Fetal behaviour in uncomplicated pregnancies after 41 weeks of gestation. *Early Hum Dev* 1994;40:29–38.
62. Pillai M, Garrett C, James D. Bizarre fetal behaviour associated with lethal congenital anomalies: A case report. *Eur J Obstet Gynecol Reprod Biol* 1991;39:215–18.
63. Tas BAPJ, Nijhuis JG. Consequences for fetal monitoring. In Nijhuis JG, ed. *Fetal Behaviour, Developmental and Perinatal Aspects.* Oxford: Oxford University Press, 1992:258–69.
64. Arduini D, Rizzo G, Massacesi M, *et al.* Longitudinal assessment of behavioural transitions in healthy fetuses during the last trimester of pregnancy. *J Perinat Med* 1991;1:67–72.
65. Tas BAPJ, Nijhuis JG, Lucas AJ. The intercostal-to-phrenic inhibitory reflex in the human fetus near term. *Early Hum Dev* 1990;22:145–9.
66. Tas BAPJ, Nijhuis JG, Nelen W, *et al.* The intercostal-to-phrenic inhibitory reflex in normal and intra-uterine growth-retarded (IUGR) human fetuses from 26 to 40 weeks of gestation. *Early Hum Dev* 1993;32:177–82.
67. Hepper P, Shahidullah S. Abnormal fetal behaviour in Down's syndrome fetuses. *Q J Clin Psychol* 1992;44B:305–17.
68. Leader LR. Studies in fetal behaviour. *Br J Obstet Gynaecol* 1995; 102:595–7.
69. Nelson KB, Ellenberg JH. Intrapartum events and cerebral palsy. In Kubli F, Patel, N, Schmidt W *et al.*, eds. *Perinatal Events and Brain Damage in Surviving Children.* Heidelberg: Springer-Verlag, 1988:139–48.
70. Freud S. Die infantile Cerebrallähmung. In Nothnagel H, ed. *Specielle Pathologie und Therapie.* Vienna: Holder, 1897:1–327.

89 Fetal and neonatal hearing

B. Arabin and H. L. M. van Straaten

Introduction

The phenomenon that the sensory development of the prenate is a quiet process of gradually responding to the extrauterine world has been anticipated by mythological and religious stories, artists, writers and many philosophers since ancient times.[1] Aristotle argued that the individual first acquires sensation during pregnancy and might experience the extrauterine environment. However, doubts remained about prenatal sensory capabilities. Jean Jacques Rousseau referred to the fetus as a 'witless tadpole' and even the first scientific approaches by Preyer[2] in 1885 led to doubtful conclusions about fetal hearing capacities.

Hearing is one of the primary modalities of human beings for communicating and a prerequisite for the development of language. Serious efforts to explore prenatal recognition began in the 1920s and 1930s. Peiper[3] performed sonic stimulation with the aid of a car horn to study movement responses of the fetus. Forbes and Forbes[4] were able to acknowledge the amodal link between movement and sound by stimulating a pregnant mother lying in a water bath which was struck with a metal object. Ray[5] attempted to measure fetal reactions to the smacking of two boards together. All these authors reported habituation responses following the stimulus presentations.

Habituation and conditioning became more focal as researchers attempted to tighten scientific controls for analysis. Sontag and Wallace[6] tried to experiment with increased numbers and greater control of the involved variables orientated to a stimulus– response method by measuring physical responses towards external stimuli. It became obvious that auditory maturation does not solely function in isolation but is part of an integrated development. The hypothesis was put forward that intrauterine conditioning accounts for certain behavioral characteristics of the newborn and the refractory times of the habituation–dehabituation processes were studied.[7] Fetal movement (FM) responses to sound stimulation were observed as one major focus for fetal conditioning.[8–10] New methods of perinatal medicine such as Doppler registration of fetal heart rate (FHR) and FM, as well as ultrasound, became extremely helpful to objectify fetal responses to external stimuli.

The unborn is involved in a perceptual world with increasing specification and differentiation. During the first trimester self-generated movements are combined with somatosensory awareness resulting in coordination of early FM patterns. Later sensory challenges may derive from two environments. The 'intrauterine world' includes the emotional state and daily rhythms of the mother, touch with the umbilical cord, the uterine wall and acoustic stimuli caused by maternal circulation, digestion, movements, breathing and, finally, her voice. As birth approaches, stimuli from the 'extrauterine world' are increasingly responded to. Neurological development allowing preparatory interaction involves a considerable number of genetic actions, which might be autoregulatory as well as activated or inhibited by positive- or negative-feedback mechanisms.

Different disciplines have therefore become interested in the field of prenatal maturation of the auditory system such as embryology, genetics, neurophysiology, psychoanalysis and developmental psychology. Since pregnant mothers and most of the current methods used to register immediate responses are in the hands of obstetricians, research and clinical investigations in perinatal medicine have been directed towards this field.

Embryology and developmental anatomy

The special status of the ear is supported by the observation that the ossicles in the middle ear are of adult size by 8 months of gestation,[11] and thus the only bones to attain their final form in the prenatal period.[12] Conventionally, the ear is described in terms of the outer, middle and inner ear. Knowledge about the complex development of the ear helps in understanding its integrated function and disturbances of the auditory system.[13–28]

External ear and tympanic membrane

The external ear is divided into the pinna and the external auditory canal. From 4 weeks' gestation onwards the mesoderm from the first and second branchial

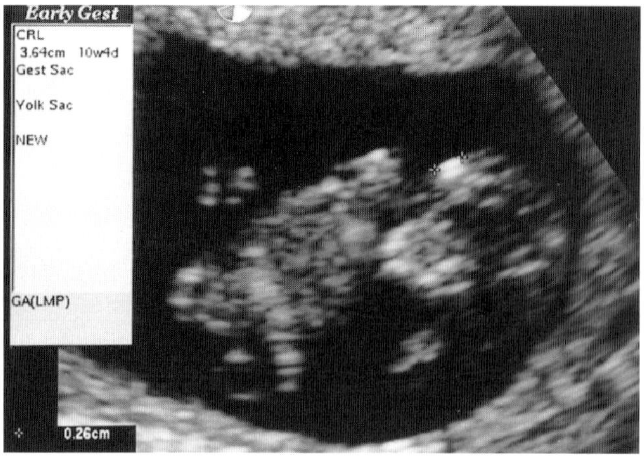

Figure 89.1 Embryo of 10 weeks with a crown–rump length of 36 mm and an 'ear length' of 2.6 mm.

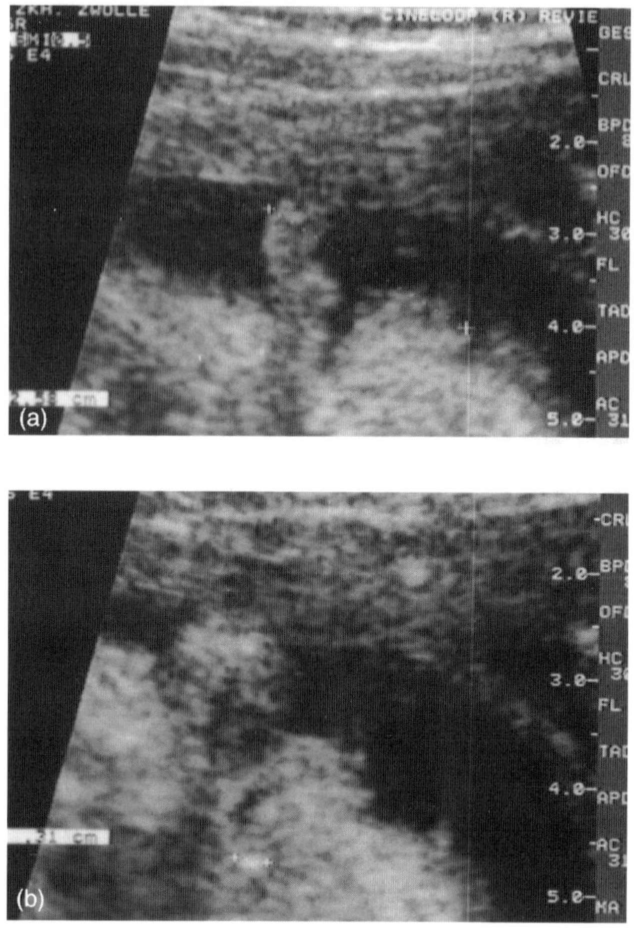

Figure 89.2 (a) Pinna of a fetal ear at 34 weeks (2.6 cm) with external auditory canal. (b) The same external auditory canal obtained by scanning towards the midline with the tympanic membrane (ring) at the central end of 31 mm.

arch gives rise to six outgrowths, the hillocks of His, condensing by 12 weeks to form the pinna. From 10 weeks onwards the future ear can be visualized (Figure 89.1). The external auditory canal develops from the first branchial groove. At 8 weeks the cavum conchae deepens, growing towards the middle ear which can be demonstrated by ultrasound in advanced pregnancy (Figure 89.2). Adult size of the external auditory canal is reached only by 9 years of age.

The tympanic membrane develops from structures associated with both the external and the middle ear. The completed tympanic membrane has three layers: an outer epithelial layer, a middle fibrous layer and an inner mucosal layer, continuous with the lining of the tympanic cavity. The tympanic membrane inserts into the tympanic ring which is complete at 16 weeks, and can be visualized by ultrasound at the end of the external auditory canal (Figure 89.2). The maximal diameter is of adult size in the term fetus.

Middle ear, temporal bone and facial nerve

The middle ear consists of the tympanic cavity, three ossicles (malleus, incus and stapes), the tensor tympani and the stapedius, tendons and the Eustachian tube.

The ossicles develop between 4 and 6 gestational weeks from the mesenchyme of the mandibular and the hyoid arches; full size is reached by 18 weeks. Only then do they become ossified and might be visualized located cranially of the mandible (Figure 89.3a). Extension of the first and second pharyngeal pouch, lined with endoderm, forms the tubotympanic recess. At week 7, constriction of the mid-portion leads to the formation of the Eustachian tube and the tympanic cavity. During further development the tympanic cavity is filled with mucoid mesenchymal tissue becoming vacuolated. By 30–34 weeks the tympanic cavity is pneumatized.

The temporal bone derives from four separate elements: the tympanic bone, the squamous portion, the styloid process and the petromastoid. Only the first three parts have formed and ossified at birth. Postnatally, there is still no complete bony ear canal and no mastoid process. The facial nerve derives from the second branchial arch. At the end of the third gestational week the acousticofacial ganglion can be identified; by the end of the embryonic period its neuroblasts form the main trunk of the facial nerve and the chorda tympani nerve. The fully developed facial nerve transverses the internal acoustic meatus, the middle ear and, finally, exits superficially from the stylomastoid behind the tympanic membrane, where it can be injured by obstetric manipulations.

Inner ear and auditory nerve

The inner ear lies in the petrous portion of the temporal bone consisting of a membranous labyrinth inside a bony labyrinth. The bony labyrinth includes the cochlea, three semicircular canals, the vestibule enclosing the utricle, the saccule and part of the cochlear duct, as well as the perilymphatic spaces. Development of the bony labyrinth occurs in three stages: cartilage formation, the formation of the perilymphatic spaces, the calcification and ossification. By 24 weeks, all centers

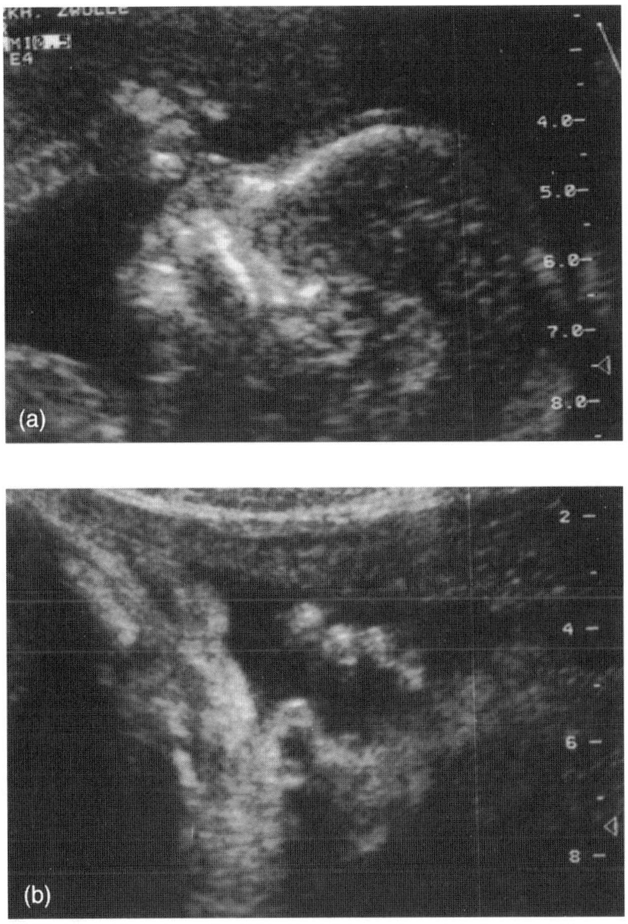

Figure 89.3 (a) Sagittal view of a fetus. Note the three ossicles superior of the mandible in front of the pinna. (b) Frontal view of a fetus 'attempting to listen', in spite of amniotic fluid in the outer ear canal, sound attenuation and internal background noise.

have fused to form a complete bony capsule. Ossification of the inner ear does not occur until each portion has attained adult size. The configuration of the membranous labyrinth is recognizable by 10 weeks and completed at around 24 weeks. Its neurosensory elements develop from the ectodermal otic placode in the 23-day-old human embryo giving rise to the otocyst. The differentiation of the vestibular and cochlear end organs takes place during the second month of pregnancy.

Light microscopy demonstrates that the first sign of differentiation of the organ of Corti in the wall of the cochlear duct starts at 10 gestational weeks. At 14 weeks, rows of inner and outer hair cells can be observed. At around 20 weeks, the human cochlear morphology is similar to what is considered the stage corresponding to the onset of cochlear function. The organ of Corti contains sensory and supporting cells. Ultrastructural development includes hair cell differentiation of inner and outer hair cells, synaptogenesis and ciliogenesis.

The eighth nerve ganglion also derives from the otocyst. After 4 weeks these cells form the auditory ganglion, dividing later into superior and inferior branches of the vestibular nerve and the cochlear nerve. The nerve cells remain bipolar throughout life, the peripheral processes terminating in the sensory areas of the inner ear and the central processes in the brainstem.

Auditory pathways

In the auditory system the second neuron is the brainstem. Structures in the human auditory pathway, from the proximal end of the cochlear nerve to the inferior colliculus, undergo myelination between 26 and 29 gestational weeks. The density of myelination increases in all pathways up to 1 year of age. Though code transmission is improved in myelinated pathways, myelination is not prerequisite for transmission. Primary and secondary crossed and uncrossed pathways ensure that each ear is represented on both sides of the brain.

In mammals the pathway proceeds to the auditory center in the cerebral cortex. The auditory pathway in human beings transforms the code represented by a mechanical response of the ear into a signal which can be utilized by higher centers. The codes are changed from level to level. Through maturation infants develop an information-processing capacity, the development of which has not yet been sufficiently studied. This knowledge, however, is essential for understanding how speech and language develop, and may have implications concerning auditory behavior, reaction to sound and diagnostic testing.

Physiological basis of hearing, encoding and transmission

Sound is created by a vibratory source that causes molecules to be displaced. It is designed for gaseous and liquid media, while oscillation in solids is mostly referred to as vibration. The quantification of sound requires measurement of the amplitude and the frequency. The amplitude is measured in units of sound pressure called pascals (Pa) proportional to the acoustic intensity or loudness. The measurement of sound pressure levels is given in decibels (dB), which are logarithmic numbers favored due to the inherent compression of the linear scales. The frequency of sound is measured in cycles per second, namely Hertz (Hz). The range of 20–20,000 Hz is accepted as the bandwidth of human hearing. Beyond these limits high sound pressure levels are required to evoke auditory responses and there is also decreased discrimination ability. Frequency and magnitude components of sound form what is called spectrum analysis.

Physiological acoustics

Knowledge of physiological acoustics can be obtained from selected references,[29–34] whereby most information is drawn from invasive recordings in nonhuman species.

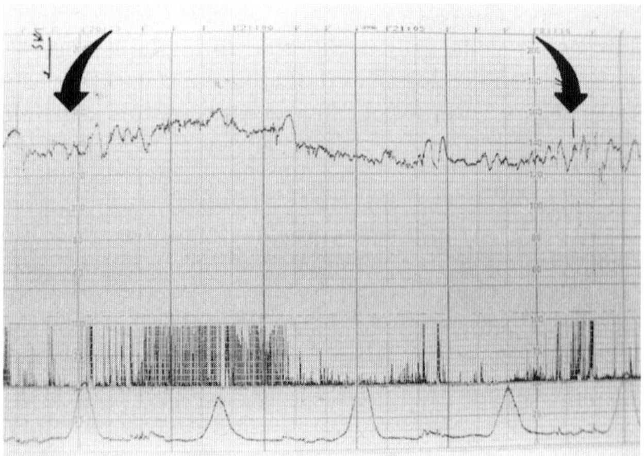

Figure 89.4 Fetal heart rate (FHR, above)/fetal movement (FM, below) tracing after vibroacoustic stimulation in an anencephalic fetus of 34 weeks. There is a long reaction (> 60 s) with increased FM and FHR after the first stimulation (first arrow) and a weaker reaction after the second stimulation (second arrow).

The overall role of the outer ear is to collect sound energy and to shape it by the resonances of the concha and the external auditory canal towards the tympanic membrane. Acoustic energy is transformed into mechanical energy as vibrations of the tympanic membrane and the ossicular chain in the middle ear air, providing an energy gain of around 30 dB due to area differences between the tympanic membrane and the footplate of the stapes. The middle ear also protects the inner ear from high sound pressures.

The role of the cochlea and structures of the inner ear is to couple the vibratory energy delivered to the oval window by the stapes footplate to the hair cells. It was postulated in 1965 by Davis[35] that the binding of the sensory hairs of the organ of Corti depolarizes the hair-cell membrane by altering its resistance. The basis of the frequency-related regional displacement of the entire cochlear partition was revealed by the classic Nobel laureate von Bekesy[36] who described it as 'traveling waves'; this was verified later by sophisticated methods.[37] The links between hair-cell receptors and the auditory system are primary auditory neurons with selective sensitivities for frequencies. With the entry of the acoustic nerve into the brainstem auditory neurons multiply. The frequency-to-place code is equally representative for the organization of central nuclei and the auditory cortex.[38,39] Many auditory abilities are attributable to subcortical processing. Decorticated animals are capable of detecting the intensity and frequency of sounds[40–42]; anencephalic fetuses demonstrate behavioral reactions to external stimuli (Figure 89.4). Central neurons are sensitive to frequency modulation and sound features.[43] An efferent auditory pathway varies the input sensitivity at the level of the hair cells.[44]

Special conditions relating to the fetus

Although perinatologists can occasionally observe gestures familiar from adult life (Figure 89.3), intrauterine hearing conditions are specific for the prenate. Information on fetal hearing has been obtained from invasive experiments on sheep or measurements in pregnancies with ruptured membranes.

Sound conduction

Vibrational direct excitation of skin and tissue is more effective for developing an acoustic field than transmission across the air–skin interface.[45,46] The external auditory canal and the fetal middle ear are filled with amniotic fluid; prenatally, the interface at the stapes footplate is a fluid medium as compared to an air medium postnatally. Sound pressures with the same phase are present at the two windows, which may reduce hair-cell activity. On the other hand, impedance similarities may cause pressure variations to be fairly well transformed.[47]

A bone conduction route is assumed for prenatal hearing based on measurements with round-window electrodes implanted after open fetal surgery in sheep. Cochlear microphonic recordings were registered towards broadband noise delivered by a loudspeaker and compared to input/output functions in the same lamb after delivery.[48] Sound energy is slightly diminished (10–20 dB) for frequencies < 250 Hz, yet significantly reduced for frequencies > 500 Hz (40–50 dB).[48,49] One reason for this 'sound isolation' is the route of sound energy 'underwater', described by bone conduction for adult and fetus.[50,51]

The effectiveness of sound transmission (outer and middle ear versus bone transmission) was tested by sheep experiments, proving that when the fetal head is covered with sound attenuating material, even though the pinna and the ear canal remain uncovered, sound levels must be greater than those necessary to evoke the same response from the bare head.[51] Both cochleae are equally stimulated, so that only one auditory image is likely to be formed.[52,53] This might have implications for lateralization in speech development.[54]

Sound attenuation

A second reason for sound isolation is the sound pressure attenuation described for externally delivered pure tones.[55] A loudspeaker in a rubber annulus was attached to the maternal abdomen, a microphone placed *in utero* near the cervix. Transmission losses ranged from 39 dB at 500 Hz to 85 dB at 5000 Hz,[56] and were 70 dB for frequencies above 2000 Hz.[57] Since an impedance mismatch may bias the results, hydrophones (underwater microphones) were used in humans[58,59] and animals.[46,60–63]

It was shown that the mother's voice in the sheep uterus is louder when picked up by a hydrophone than by a microphone placed by the abdominal wall[62] and that sound attenuation decreases during the last weeks of gestation.[61,62] Further results were obtained by placing a pregnant ewe in a sound field produced by stereo speakers[46,63] recording simultaneous measurements with a microphone in the air and a hydrophone within the uterine cavity. There was sound enhancement of broadband noises *in utero* for frequencies below 250 Hz; transmission loss increased to an average of 20 dB at 4 kHz. The overall transmission loss was 6.7 dB for broadband noise, and 10–15 dB for pure tone at 1–10 kHz. In humans, exterior sound of at least 65–70 dB was transmitted to the intrauterine cavity with attenuation of 30 dB reduction in sound pressure levels for tones up to 12 kHz; frequencies below 200 Hz were enhanced.[58,59] All in all the results of hydrophone experiments were comparable in sheep and humans.

Sound environment

The sound environment *in utero* might have an 'imprinting' and a masking effect on external sounds as studied in humans[55,57–60,64,65] and in sheep.[61,62] Measurements in sheep have demonstrated that the basal noise is increased during labor.[62] Data in humans, all gathered after rupture of membranes, might underestimate the emergence of external sounds or overestimate background noise described as pulsations of uterine vessels,[66] intervillous injections,[67] or sounds associated with digestion,[68] maternal body movements and with the mother's breath and voice (see below). The intrauterine sound environment is dominated by frequencies below 500 Hz with mean sound pressures of 90 dB at 250 Hz.[58,59]

Sound intelligibility

Intelligibility is based on the ability to distinguish complex sounds and thereby provide speech communication and musical abilities. The auditory sensitivity and prenatal sound attenuation characteristics are similar in sheep and humans.[60,68–70] Language signals are comparable[50] as proven by simultaneous recordings from microphone, fetal cochlear microphone and intrauterine hydrophone recordings in sheep. Music and voices are distinguishable from the basal noise by 8–12 dB for exterior voices and 24 dB for the mother's voice, if all had an intensity of 60 dB. The male voice with an average frequency of 125 Hz is better transmitted, but emerges in the range where internal noise is highest. Female voices with an average frequency of 220 Hz receive a greater attenuation, but emerge in a range where internal noise is low.[58]

The fetus might detect speech and music, ideally low-frequency components below 500 Hz, when the airborne signals exceed 60 dB. Intrauterine sound levels of the mother's voice were enhanced by an average of 5.2 dB. Differences are not dependent on maternal abdominal wall thickness or amniotic fluid volume.[69] Intelligibility of directly transmitted maternal voice compared to airborne maternal, female or male voices did not differ if tapes from intrauterine devices were offered to adult observers.[47] While consonants are indistinguishable, vowel sounds, rhythms and melodic timbre of voices are recognizable. Though attenuation varies with frequency, a variety of music is easily recognized from intrauterine recordings.[64,71]

Prenatal auditory responsiveness under normal conditions

To demonstrate the existence of prenatal sensory perception, one can empirically study electrophysiological, motor and cardiac auditory responsiveness.

Studies of fetal response to sound have chosen a variety of stimuli not always with apparent rationale such as car horns,[3] bicycle bells,[64] electric toothbrushes,[72] or pure tones of 100–2000 Hz, sound pressure levels from 80 to 120 dB measured in air and with various durations.[73] Studies using airborne sounds should be differentiated from studies using vibroacoustic stimuli providing vibration and airborne sound. More recent studies have used the electronic artificial larynx with a vibrating disc attached to the maternal abdomen. It is portable and designed to propagate sound pressure more efficiently, matching impedances between tissue and fluid. The electronic artificial larynx output spectrum was measured by hydrophone fixed near to a lamb's ear *in utero*.[46] Most frequencies were between 0.5 and 1 kHz with multiple harmonics up to 15,000 Hz in air. When the device was placed directly over the hydrophone, sound pressure levels averaged 135 dB, which was greater than predicted in humans.[65,74] In lambs with bilateral cochlear ablation no reactions towards vibroacoustic stimulation could be registered even with high intensities, indicating that in fetal sheep the auditory apparatus is necessary for the FHR and FM responses.[75]

Prenatal responsiveness by means of electrophysiological methods

Recordings of electrical potentials from levels of the auditory system by means of noninvasive techniques are based on compound potentials representing the activity of many cells. Noninvasive methods to investigate the effects of early auditory stimulations are the stimulus-related electroencephalographic (EEG) and magnetoencephographic (MEG) methods. Human EEG responses towards acoustic signals[76–78] have been performed, with one exception,[77] only after ruptured membranes using scalp electrodes.[76,78]

In MEG recordings sensitive magnetic field detectors are used to measure neuromagnetic auditory brainstem responses, which can be performed prenatally with intact membranes.[79,80] Short auditory stimuli like clicks of 1 kHz and a duration of 100 ms up to 100 dB are performed, in a room guaranteeing electrical radiofrequency shielding, to evoke the activity of

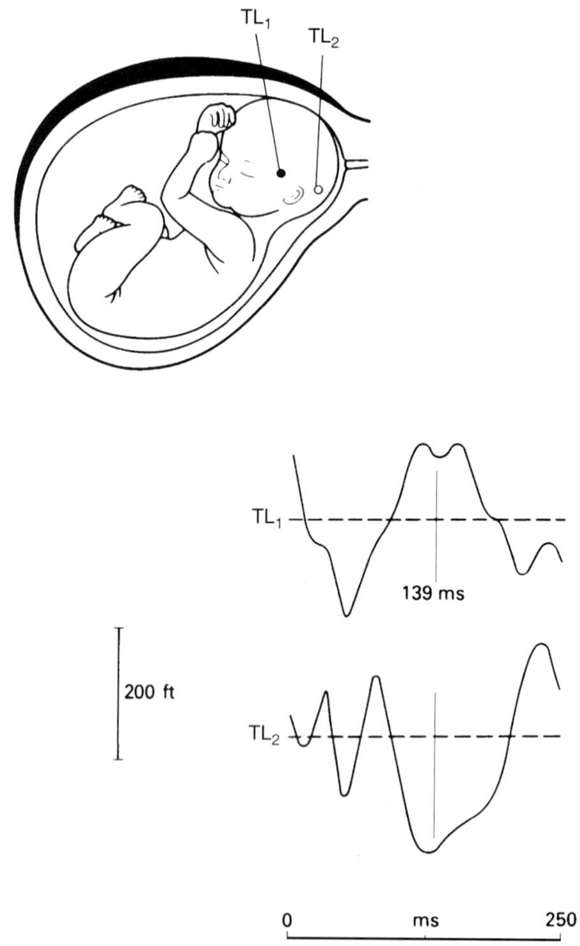

Figure 89.5 Typical waveforms obtained from brainstem after click stimulation at 34 weeks by one-channel magnetoencephalography.[79,80] TL_1, temporal $lateral_1$; TL_2, temporal $lateral_2$; Ft, fentotesla.

electromagnetic sources located in nuclei of the brainstem. In an experimental setting, we succeeded in recording stimulus-related auditory-evoked neuromagnetic fields through the mother's abdomen at 34 weeks by using a one-channel superconducting quantum interference device (SQUID) magnetometer (Figure 89.5).[79,80] The tracings were comparable with postnatal recordings. Latency shifts of brainstem components are proposed to reflect early brain maturation[81] and decrease with advancing age. Although electromagnetic methods are more precise than indirect methods in reflecting the occurrence and latency of reactions, at this moment, the methods are not yet sufficiently developed to allow systematic conclusions to be drawn.

Prenatal behavioral responsiveness

The association of evoked potentials with heartbeat and motor responses implies the reception of the auditory signals up to subcortical levels (Figure 89.4).[82] Due to the present lack of routine technology to record neural activity directly in the womb, fetal sensory abilities are examined by observing behavioral reactions. Appropriate methodology has to be used to ensure that stimulus and response are correlated. Problems arise when the fetus does not react, since we cannot say that the stimulus is not sensed.

Onset of responsiveness

Relating to the onset of immediate fetal responses it was supposed that reactions towards acoustic stimuli do not occur before 24 weeks.[74,83] Using ultrasound, blink responses were first detectable between 24 and 25 weeks, becoming consistent after 28 weeks.[74] Recently, responsiveness to sound was even described at 16 weeks of gestation.[1,84,85] Developmental origins were systematically examined using 80–2000 broadband stimuli between 15 and 25 gestational weeks. When changing the stimulus from a single sound to a series of ten 2-s pulses, an increased number of FM was found after stimulation at 20 weeks. Interpretation refers to hypotheses about the developing neural system prior to the formation of specific receptor cells as described for first reactions towards touch. Ultrasound observations also allow definition of motor responses such as body, head, arm and leg movements.[86] The methodology can be simplified by using Doppler services for the detection of FM which whilst unable to differentiate qualities of responses can differentiate quantities of FM responses with a high sensitivity and specificity.[87] Using this method to record fetal responses and external artificial larynx for stimulation we observed a first fetal reaction (FM) in singletons at 25 weeks[88] and simultaneous reactions of FM of both members of a twin pair at 27 weeks.

Developmental aspects

FM and FHR responses may be classified in immediate reactions such as startles, twinkling, accelerations or decelerations ('reflexes') as well as long-term changes of either FM, FHR baseline or variability ('changes of behavioral patterns'). FHR/FM patterns including breathing movements were studied during 1h after vibroacoustic stimulation.[89,90] Close company changes the development of reactions towards vibroacoustic stimuli in twins compared to singletons. Reactions of longer duration become more frequent in twins compared to singletons (Figure 89.6). With increasing gestational age, an increasing number of FM combined with FHR accelerations is observed in singletons and twins. Among reactions of long duration (> 60 s) FHR baseline changes more dramatically than FHR variability. We also found an increasing number of extreme changes from a very passive to a very active FHR/FM pattern in twin pregnancies. This is in accordance with findings in singletons that after vibroacoustic stimulation unusual changes of state 1F–4F occur, which rarely occur spontaneously.[91] More 'physiologic' state changes from state 1F to 2F were found using a 100-Hz square-wave vibratory stimulus.[92] In any case, vibroacoustic stimulation with the external

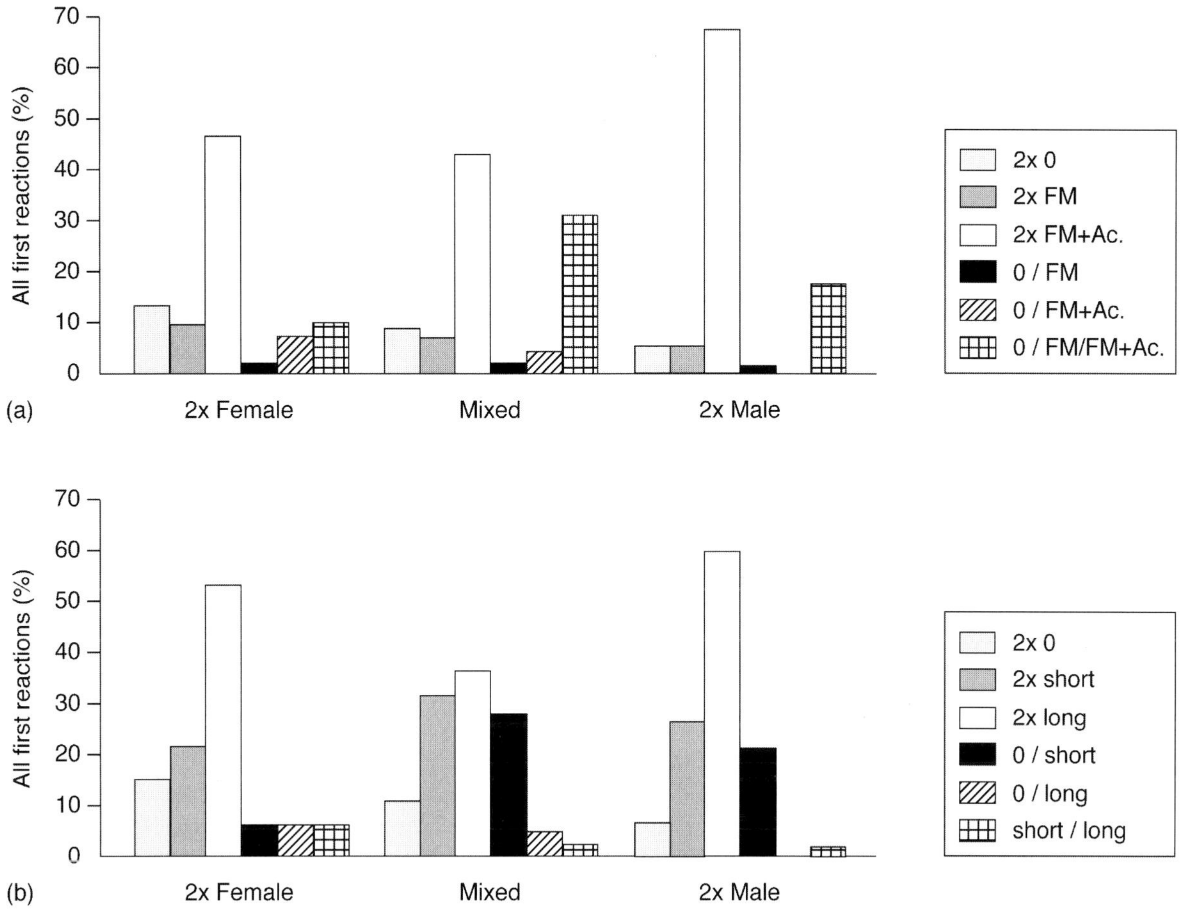

Figure 89.6 Distribution of short (< 60 s) and long (> 60 s) behavioral reactions towards vibroacoustic stimuli in 74 healthy singletons (a) and 64 healthy twins (b) obtained by longitudinal weekly measurements between 26 and 36 weeks. Note that there are significant changes with gestational age, Pearson χ^2 test $p < 0.0005$, and differences between twins and singletons, Pearson χ^2 test $p < 0.0005$.

artificial larynx must have some quite dramatic influence on the fetus, since some gynecologists have even recommended it to induce a change of fetal position to improve visualization of fetal echocardiography[93].

Quality of stimulus

Both the onset and development of auditory responsiveness also depend on qualities of the stimulus. Fetuses from 19 weeks onwards were presented with pure-tone frequencies of 100–3000 Hz. First responsiveness was detected at 23 weeks at 500 Hz, by 27 weeks responsiveness was found to 100, 250 and 500 Hz and only at 31 weeks were responses observed to 1000 and 3000 Hz.[94] It was interpreted that the delayed responsiveness to high frequency is related to the development of phase-locked firing describing a cooperation of nerve fibers to encode high-frequency sound.[95] The sound pressure level required to elicit a response at 35 weeks is 20–30 dB less than at 23 weeks, indicating that the fetal auditory system becomes more sensitive with prenatal age.[94] However, changes in attenuation, maturing behavior and sensomotor neural connections might also have an impact. Even fetal intelligibility has developmental aspects.[95] Using a habituation–dishabituation technique, fetuses aged 35 weeks could discriminate between frequencies of 250 and 500 Hz and between different speech sounds, whereas fetuses of 27 weeks were unable to make this differentiation, although they were able to differentiate between a 250-Hz tone and 80–2000-Hz broadband sound.

Specific or momentary disposition

Additional factors influence fetal acoustic responsiveness such as behavioral state before the stimulus,[96] gender,[72] position *in utero* and individual disposition (own data). Fetal responses to speech stimuli consisting of syllables ('ee' or 'ah') were studied in healthy pregnancies at 26–34 weeks' gestation. During periods of low FHR variability, a decrease in FHR and an increase in the standard deviation of heart rate were found.[97] This is the only demonstration of prenatal responses to speech stimuli whereby the response is dependent on FHR variability which is the primary determinant of fetal state.[98] Female fetuses seem to respond earlier than males.[72] In our experience, twins are ideal models to differentiate further the simultaneous influence of activity state before stimulation, individual disposition (zygosity), position and sex of

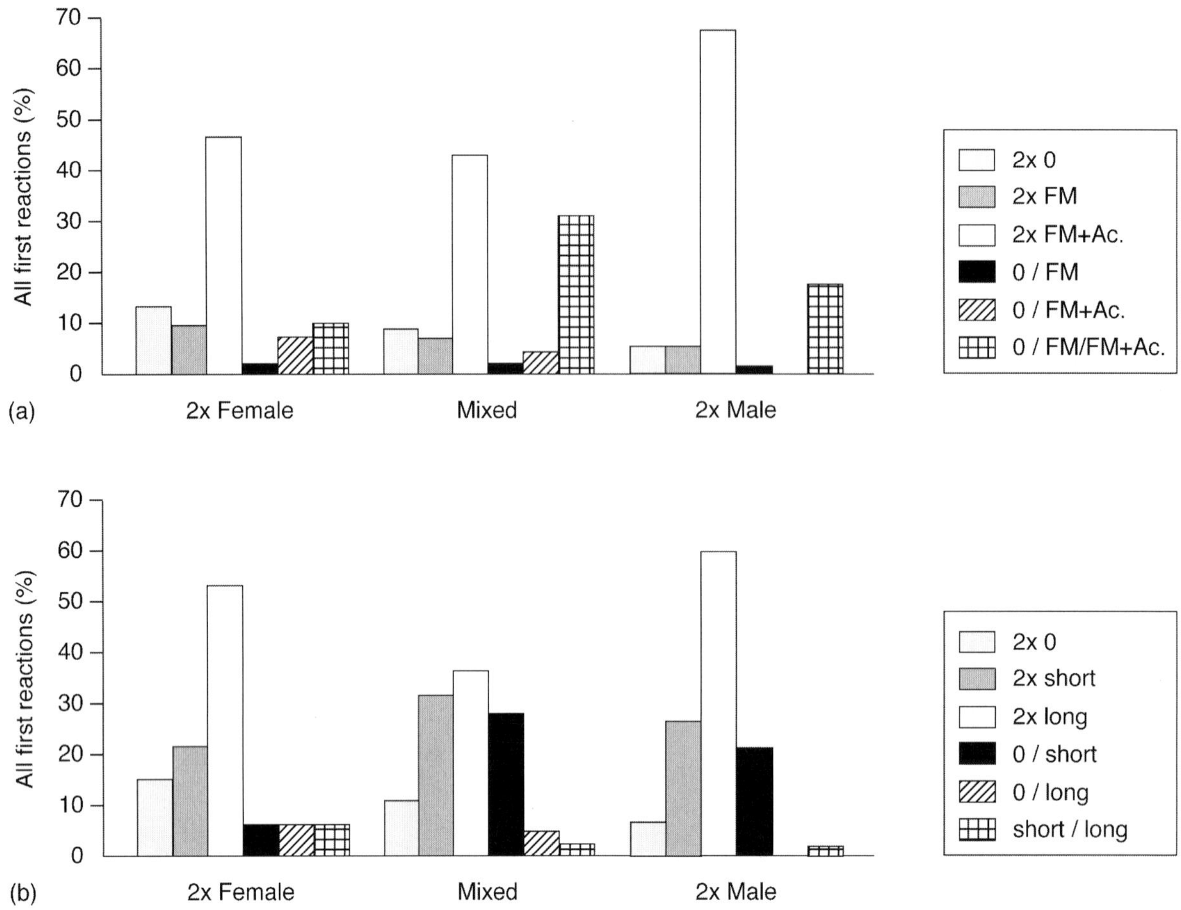

Figure 89.7 Distribution of combinations of 390 fetal heart rate (FHR)/fetal movement (FM) reactions towards vibroacoustic stimuli within 32 twin pairs. (a) Classified relating to first short reactions, (b) classified relating to duration of reactions (0, no reaction; Ac, acceleration; long, > 60 s; short, < 60 s). Note the significantly higher intertwin differences (lighter columns) in twin pairs of different sex, Pearson χ^2 test $p < 0.0001$.

the prenates by analyzing intertwin differences of FHR/FM patterns towards external artificial larynx (Figure 89.7). Similar reactions towards external artificial larynx were significantly increased in twins with the same sex and differences between sex-alike male compared to female groups can be calculated. If all parameters are analyzed by multivariate analysis, age-dependent determinants of fetal responsiveness can be evaluated.

Postnatal auditory responsiveness under normal conditions

After delivery sound conduction and environment change significantly and the newborn is more directly accessible to behavioral[98,99] and electrophysiological examinations.[30–32,99]

Postnatal responsiveness assessed by electrophysiological methods

Auditory-evoked potentials reflect electrical activity from different anatomic levels of the auditory system: the earlier components from peripheral and brainstem levels, the later ones from midbrain and cortical levels. The cochlear (0–4 ms) and early components (4–12 ms) are used for assessing peripheral hearing in children by electrocochleography and auditory brainstem response. Whereas electrocochleography can only be used under anesthesia, auditory brain response has become the method of choice to estimate hearing sensitivity in newborns since it was first described.[100,101] It reflects the integrity of the outer, middle and inner ear and the auditory pathway,[102,103] as described by Davis,[35] and is free from the effects of medication or state. Via headphones click stimuli are performed and short-latency electroencephalographic waveforms are recorded by skull electrodes (Figure 89.8). The detection of cortical potentials and auditory brainstem response as early as 25 weeks indicates functional maturity of the auditory pathway.[104] Electrophysiological responses from the cochlea, the eighth nerve and the auditory brainstem are similar to those in the adult by 32–36 gestational weeks.[103,105] The responses continue to develop in wave components, shape and latency with myelinization[103,106] until the second year. The auditory brainstem response does not necessarily depend

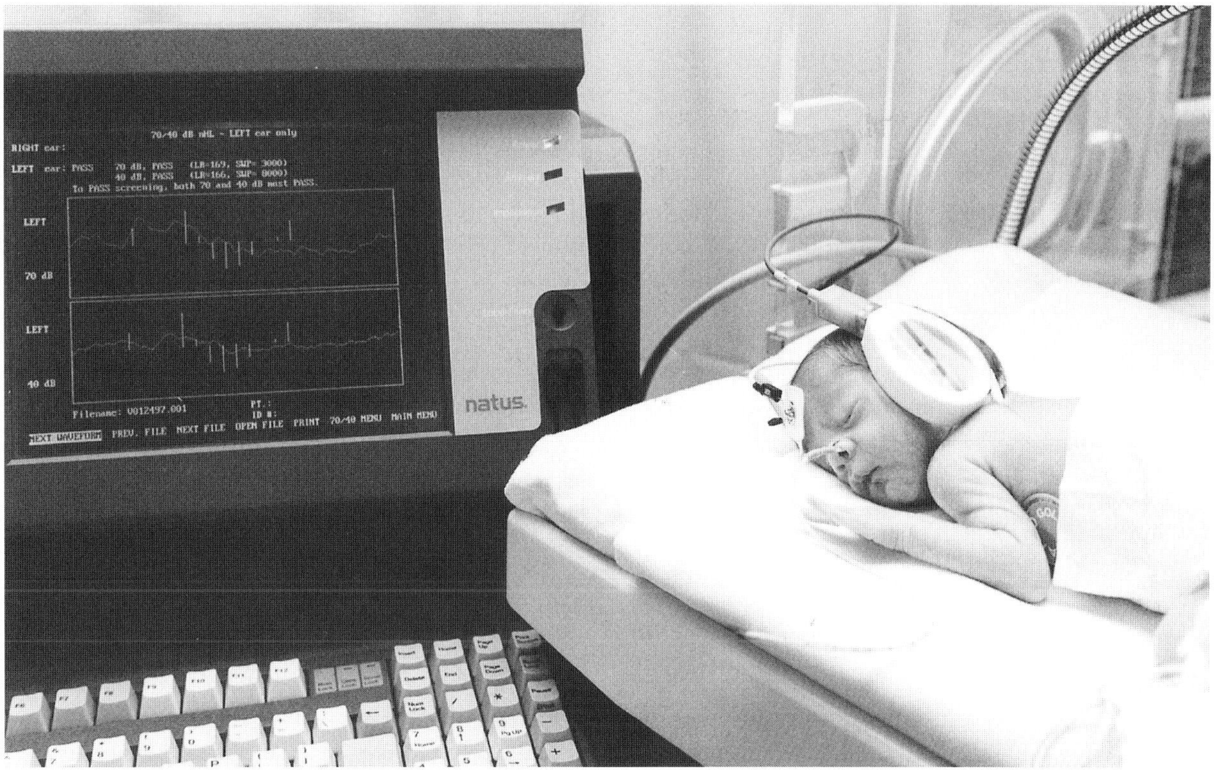

Figure 89.8 Hearing screening in a preterm infant at the NICU with an automatic version (ALGO-1E automated auditory brainstem response infant hearing screener, Natus Medical, Inc.) detecting auditory brainstem responses.

on the same neural events that are essential for perception of auditory capabilities.

Von Bekesy[36] postulated that some sound energy must be emitted from the cochlea back to the external auditory canal ('feedback from the inner ear'). Transiently evoked otoacoustic emissions can be measured, e.g., sounds generated and emitted by the outer hair cells of the cochlea in response to acoustic stimulation.[107] A small probe is placed in the external auditory canal and click stimuli are presented. Otoacoustic emission methods are candidates for application in the newborn permitting the acquisition of frequency-specific information which can be drawn later from audiometry.

Postnatal behavioral responsiveness

Behavioral reactions towards acoustic stimuli are less suitable for preterm neonates, but they are of value to learn about what babies hear and about possible positive or negative influences. Responses and alertness to voices, bells and rattles, or the neonate's ability to shut down aversive reactions due to habituation towards repeated stimuli are used to score infants according to their 'abilities'.[97] Broadband sounds (speech) are more likely than narrowband sounds to elicit responses[108] which also depend on physiological states of hunger and sleep/wakefulness.[98] A newborn infant can differentiate bandwidth, duration, interstimulus interval, frequency and sound pressure level.[109,110] Signals <4 kHz evoke responses three times more often than signals in the higher range. Lower frequencies generally evoke gross motor activity, high frequencies evoke freezing reactions. The newborn can respond to gross right–left changes, although sound localization is not purely auditory. Even soon after birth a blind infant is less likely to localize sound than a sighted infant. After 2 months infants integrate auditory and visual space (e.g., voice and facial movements).[111]

Some methods have been introduced to objectify behavioral responsiveness. The auditory response cradle compares reactions with and without sound by a pressure sensitive mattress and a monitor for head movements. As in prenatal life high intensities of up to 85 dB are needed to elicit motor responses.[112] The observer-based psychoacoustic procedure controls for observer bias by documenting behavioral changes towards acoustic stimuli while the observer is 'blinded' by earphones for all signals.[113] Using the observer-based psychoacoustic procedure infants of 2–5 weeks showed thresholds at 500 and 4000 Hz of 55- and 60-dB sound pressure levels, respectively.[114]

Effects of prenatal hearing on postnatal development

By correlating morphological and neurofunctional results with perinatal observations, conclusions might be drawn for sensomotory, cognitive and emotional development.

Recognition or 'memorization'

Considerable attention is given by parents to the possibility that the fetus forms memories of speech and music that may influence the abilities postnatally. Habituation has primarily been described by Peiper[3] who reported a decrease in FM after repeated stimulation with a car horn. Since then a number of studies have demonstrated a decrement in response to repeated stimulation while using FHR/FM or ultrasound documentation. Habituation may be distinguished from adaptation or fatigue by several criteria, the most important being the recovery of response on presentation of a new stimulus ('dishabituation') and faster habituation upon re-presentation of the stimulus.[115] The intensity of the stimulus influences habituation time (faster habituation to more intense stimuli).[115]

While habituation reflects short-term memory, there is also proof of long-term memory from pre- to postnatal life. To demonstrate the existence of prenatal sensory perception, one can indirectly study behavioral modifications of a neonate presented with stimuli she or he has been confronted with during prenatal life ('memorization').[47] Prenatal sound experience might have an influence on postnatal sound preference and fine tune the developing auditory system.[116] Neonates have been taught that if they produce a specific sucking pattern they could listen to their mother's voice. Newborn babies showed a strong preference for the voice of their mother over that of other male or female talkers. Using the specially designed baby's dummy connected to a tape recorder, newborns are even able to distinguish between their mother speaking in her native vs. in an unfamiliar language[117] (sucking with higher frequency). Using this 'high-amplitude sucking procedure', 3-day-old newborns prefer a lullaby read twice a day by the mother during the last weeks of pregnancy to a new story.[118] All this suggests the possibility of prenatal acquisitions and antenatal discrimination, however elementary it might be.

Prenatal stimulation has an impact on temperament behavior. Settings of talking, music and meditation were performed during pregnancy and correlated with behavioral outcome.[119] Talking had a 65%, music a 34% and mediation a 31% correlation with all behaviors. For talking only 58% of behavioral variables were identified as positive (e.g., the child being easily comforted, contentment), 16% as ambiguous and 26% as negative (e.g., crying for obscure reasons, needing constant supervision). Music and meditation, however, correlated in 90% and 100%, respectively, with positive attitudes. Talking is known not only to express care, but also irritability, anger or anxiety experienced in pregnancy. It is speculated that not only variations of timbre, but also hormonal or physiological changes associated with the content of speech, may evoke associations in the infant. This hypothesis is supported by a study of infants whose excessive crying was in association with their mothers' depression scores.[120]

Implications for language development and musical expression

Hearing has a close relation to the kinetic system, i.e., 'auditory–vocal–kinetic channel'.[121] From embryology we know that the origins and innervation of hearing and language function are in close proximity, suggesting that there is also 'crying *in utero*' – only we have not yet become sensitive for it. Vocal expression can be heard in fetuses from around 20 weeks onwards. Uterine crying has been proposed following unpleasant maneuvers such as attaching electrodes, versions or catheter insertions.[122–124] The newborn's phonation is based on laryngeal coordination reflecting maturation processes and training. Newborn 'cryprints' are as unique as fingerprints, and characterized by specific features such as fundamental frequency and variation in time ('vibrato') using voice-signal recording.[125]

We suppose influences of nature and nurture on prespeech development. Monozygotic twins have synchronous cry patterns at birth.[126] By listening to the mother's speech the fetus obviously stores her speech features. Early spectrography of the first cries proved that even newborns born at 28 weeks had similar voice performance features to their mothers.[127,128] How far genetic influences or experience of the same sound environment are responsible for first hearing and cry patterns remains to be determined. Babies as young as 12-h-old react to rhythms of human speech.[129] This also might imply that learning of language begins soon after or even before birth. Newborns are able to distinguish between phones in any language and make all sounds of any language.[130] By 6 months linguistic experience has resulted in language-specific phonetic prototypes.[131] Adults can no longer distinguish between phones used in unfamiliar languages. In this context, experience seems paradoxically to diminish auditory skills. Somehow, babies even stimulate adults to speak to them in a stylized way.[132]

Music exists in the passage of time and cross-culturally. It is supposed that musicality is structured by an ensemble of protorhythms of biological inheritance.[133] The hypothesis that music has prenatal origins does not explain the survival value of music,[134] but might clarify its nature with cross-cultural features of rhythm and dancing comparable to rhythmic elements *in utero*, e.g., movements of maternal vessels felt and heard by the prenate. A summary of the up-to-date knowledge on the influence of music during pregnancy is meanwhile published by the main author.[135]

Prenatal acoustical responsiveness as a test for fetal well-being

The understanding of pathophysiology has led to improvements in interpretation of behavioral and hemodynamic mechanisms. Fetal hypoxia is the condition studied most intensively. An arrest of muscular activity to reduce oxygen consumption and a redistribution of fetal blood flow to maintain oxygen delivery to essential organs were primarily described in sheep experiments[136,137] and later in humans.[138–140] Meanwhile, correlations with antenatal blood gases have been performed.[141,142] Fetal activity and blood-flow redistribution have an impact on FHR patterns. FHR variability and the presence of FHR accelerations with FM are recognized as indicators of fetal health by noninvasive and invasive studies.[142,143] In this context, (vibro)acoustic stimulation was proposed mainly for the assessment of fetal well-being and to discriminate between 'nonreactive' nonstress tests (NSTs) due to hypoxia or just to quiet state.[144,145] Using Medline we found more than 150 studies on vibroacoustic stimulation as a test of fetal well-being from 1980 to date; here we focus only on selected aspects.

Increase of 'efficiency' of non-stress testing and biophysical profile

To compare results, the frequency, duration and intensity of the stimulus as well as gestational age, FHR/FM criteria, habituation time and behavioral states in association with the response have to be analyzed. In general, a 3-s sound stimulus is adequate for a shift to an 'awake' state.[146] In a review of 61 studies, the ability of vibroacoustic stimulation to elicit FHR accelerations has been established, decreasing false-positive rates of nonreactive NSTs.[147] Pregnancies with early-onset intrauterine growth retardation (IUGR) were studied after vibroacoustic stimulation between 26 and 32 weeks' gestation. Accelerations, FHR variability and FM were reduced compared with age-matched normal fetuses.[148] The conclusion that nutritional deprivation is associated with delayed sensory maturation is not necessarily true, since similar FHR and FM patterns are recognizable in early NSTs. The result only proves that there is no reaction, though the stimulus might well be received. Vibroacoustic stimulation was performed in patients with low biophysical profile scores after 15 min. The results of patients whose biophysical profile score improved to normal were compared to normal scores without stimulation. Vibroacoustic stimulation was found to 'improve' an abnormal or equivocal biophysical profile score to normal in 82% of cases without increasing obstetric or neonatal complication rates or the false-negative rate of biophysical profile scores.[149]

Comparative observational studies and clinical trials

Some observational studies compare the vibroacoustic stimulation test concurrently with other tests. In most studies the prediction of poor outcome was comparable with results of the NST.[150,151] In the prediction of an abnormal contraction stress test (CST), a nonreactive vibroacoustic stimulation test had a sensitivity of 100% and a specificity of 91%; therefore vibroacoustic stimulation was slightly better able to diagnose fetal distress compared to the CST in pregnancies with a nonreactive NST at term.[152] After the introduction of Doppler velocimetry of fetal redistribution it has become possible to differentiate ambiguous results of NSTs noninvasively. Thus we compared the clinical value of NST, Doppler ratio of cerebral vs. umbilical blood flow, vibroacoustic stimulation test and CST to predict poor outcome using different cut-off values for all tests separately for IUGR and post-term pregnancies. Doppler velocimetry and NSTs had better prognostic capacities than vibroacoustic stimulation tests and CSTs (Figure 89.9).[153,154] We therefore do not use CST or vibroacoustic stimulation tests in clinical routine, while Doppler studies, computerized FHR analysis, or real-time ultrasound of fetal behavior and amniotic fluid analysis can be performed without 'unnatural stress' for mother and fetus. We admit that in units where skills in ultrasound examinations or sophisticated equipment are not available, vibroacoustic stimulation or CST might be of value. Clinical trials demonstrate that the introduction of vibroacoustic stimulation in combination with the NST[155] or with amniotic fluid assessment[156] has not led to an increased rate of mortality. Since in the Western world all of the currently used forms of antenatal surveillance are combined with low mortality rates, it is unlikely that vibroacoustic stimulation will ever lower perinatal mortality in any randomized or historic trial.[157] In the only controlled clinical trial, where vibroacoustic stimulation test was compared to NST,[145] false-positive tests were slightly lowered and performance reduced from a mean of 27 to 23 min. Although it has been proven that vibroacoustic stimulation does at least not increase catecholamine release[158] or meconium passage in healthy fetuses,[159] the question remains whether 4 min justify frightening – or even awakening – an innocently sleeping fetus (it is recommended that vibroacoustic stimulation is performed during quiet sleep!). In other words: which parents would appreciate this postnatally?

Vibroacoustic stimulation during labor

The same holds true for studies during labor, where vibroacoustic stimulation was primarily applied to test attenuation via hydrophones. Data suggest that an intrauterine threshold of 94-dB sound pressure level is necessary to produce a consistent FHR response during active labor.[160] At the first stage of labor vibroacoustic stimulation was studied possibly to improve interpretation of ominous spontaneous FHR testing. Undoubtedly, nonreactive responders to vibroacoustic stimulation were at significantly greater risk of subsequent abnormal FHR patterns, meconium staining and fetal distress; however, transient FHR decelerations occurred in 25% where fetal outcome was not impaired.[161] Although it was concluded that vibroacoustic stimulation differentiated compromised from non-compromised fetuses, we think that it might also

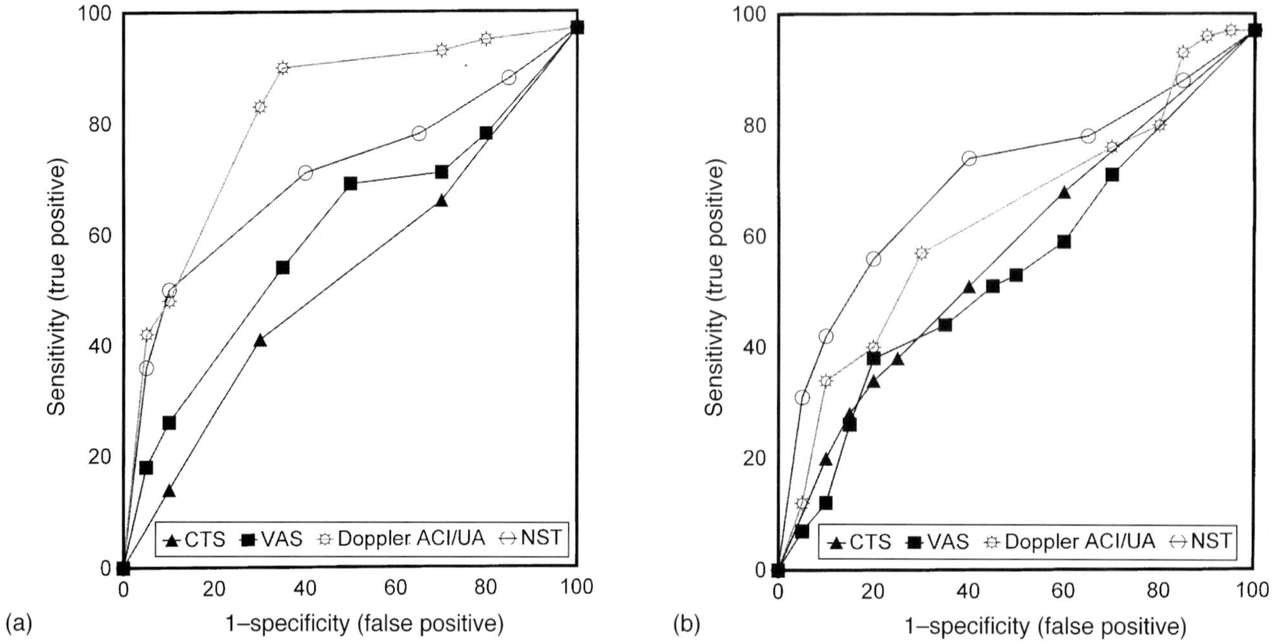

Figure 89.9 Receiver–operator characteristics of antepartum tests to predict fetal distress requiring operative delivery (measurements 1–3 days antepartum; CTS, contraction stress test; VAS, vibroacoustic stimulation; Doppler ACI/UA, resistance index ratio of arteria carotis communis/umbilical artery; NST, nonstress test) in 103 intrauterine growth retarded (IUGR) (a) and 110 post-term (b) pregnancies.[142,143]

confuse inexperienced staff. At the second stage of labor fetal blood sampling (FBS) has been correlated with vibroacoustic stimulation testing: vibroacoustic stimulation had a sensitivity of 100%, a specificity of 59.6% and a positive predictive value of 27.6% for the detection of fetal acidosis.[162] Although it was evident that mean fetal blood pH values obtained within 30 min of vibroacoustic stimulation were higher in reactive compared with decelerative or nonresponders, acidotic pH values were also found in fetuses with reactive FHR patterns after vibroacoustic stimulation.[163] In recent studies it was concluded that the FHR response after vibroacoustic stimulation does not predict neonatal outcome and might not replace FBS.[164,165] There are even warning hints about using vibroacoustic stimulation as a routine procedure, such as an unknown influence on cerebral blood flow in quiet sleep,[166] false-negative results in fetal sepsis,[167] activation of swallowing[168] or micturation[169] and provocation of unnecessary pathological FHR patterns in cases with nuchal cord.[170]

We conclude that many studies do not address the physiological changes of fetal responsiveness or habituation time by gestational age or standardize FHR/FM patterns before or after vibroacoustic stimulation. Appropriate implementation of vibroacoustic stimulation tests requires appropriate questions. In twin studies we have found that prenatal reactiveness – either to touch of the co-twin or to external stimulation – is combined with larger interindividual variations than spontaneous behavior. For the time being, we recommend vibroacoustic stimulation as a challenge test only under controlled conditions, but not for routine use just to simplify antenatal surveillance. This has been proposed by other authors.[171]

Early hearing disturbances

Compared with the vestibular part, the auditory system is phylogenetically young with a greater demand for oxygen and glucose and can therefore be selectively damaged.

Early hearing is prerequisite for speaking and for intellectual, social and emotional development.[172] Even a relatively mild hearing loss of 35–40 dB near hearing level means that a child misses approximately 50% of normal conversation.[173] Severe congenital hearing impairment affects 0.1% of live-born infants[104,174] and 1–4% of graduates of neonatal intensive care units (NICUs).[174,175] The prognosis is improved when the diagnosis is made early.[176] The fitting of hearing aids within the first 6 months improves speech and language development compared with placement at a later age. However, the age at diagnosis of hearing impairment was at least 18–30 months,[177] even in countries with a nationwide behavioral screening program starting at 9 months of age. However, the age of diagnosis is rapidly changing in those countries with a nationwide neonatal screening program. Using high-risk registers 50–75% of infants with hearing loss are identifiable.[178] Both the American Joint Committee on Infant Hearing and the European Consensus Development Conference postulated that universal hearing screening should be implemented within 3 months of life.[179,180] Habilitation should be started before

Table 89.1 Indicators associated with sensorineural and/or conductive hearing loss in the newborn (indications for hearing tests when universal screening is not available)

Indications
Positive family history or hereditary childhood sensoneural hearing loss
Congenital infections (toxoplasmosis, cytomegalovirus, rubella, syphilis, herpes)
Craniofacial anomalies including those with morphological anomalies of pinna and ear canal
Admission for ≥48 h to a neonatal intensive care unit
Stigmata or other findings associated with a syndrome known to include hearing loss

6 months of age. In those countries with limited financial facilities neonatal hearing screening may be limited to high-risk groups for hearing loss (Table 89.1). All infants admitted to neonatal intensive care units should be screened for hearing loss prior to discharge.

Electrophysiological measurements for screening

Auditory brainstem responses

The conventional auditory brainstem response (ABR), e.g., the ability to evoke and record a short-latency electroencephalographic waveform in response to a click stimulus is considered to be the gold standard in detecting the neonatal hearing threshold,[105,181,182] though it is not yet widely used because it is costly and time-consuming. The click-evoked ABR may occur as early as at 25 gestational weeks but typically appears during the 27th week. Development of the infant ABR is usually complete by the end of the second year of life.

Automated ABR infant hearing screeners have been introduced as an alternative.[183] Based on a statistical model for the detection of a response (auditory brainstem response algorithm) and a dual artifact rejection system for environmental noise and myogenic artifacts, the equipment provides a pass/fail outcome. Stimulation via headphones with 35 dB near hearing level clicks with frequencies of 700–5000 Hz can be performed even under NICU conditions (Figure 89.8). No special training is necessary. Clinical trials proved the concordance between an automated version and conventional auditory brainstem response screening,[184] whereby a sensitivity of 100% and a specificity of 98.7%[185] was detected. Follow-up results support the value of automated auditory brainstem response screening.[185] The mean time needed to perform a screening has been reduced to 8 min.[186] To avoid ambiguous results in preterms, screening is advised from a postconceptional age of 30 weeks onwards.[185]

Otoacoustic emissions

In transiently evoked otoacoustic emissions (TEOAE) measurements, 'a pass' has been defined as the presence of emitted energy of at least 3 dB signal/noise ratio between 1.6 and 4 kHz,[187] but until now no objective pass/fail criteria have been established. The response is frequency specific and does not provide an indication of audiometric threshold. Depending on the stimulus, TEOAE can be detected in up to 98% of humans with normal hearing and are absent in hearing impairment of 20–40 dB. TEOAE takes 7–9 min and can be administered by a trained nurse.[187,188] In NICU infants screened with TEOAE at 3 months, there is a sensitivity of 93% and a specificity of 84% to detect absent auditory brainstem response.[189] Hypoxia or infection may result in a reversible reduction of the TEOAE spectrum. Children with hearing loss primarily due to involvement of the auditory pathway or CNS may have normal evoked otoacoustic emissions as a result of a normal functioning cochlea.[190]

Otoacoustic emissions (OAE) screening is less suitable for use on a NICU because of the ambient noise and the difficulty of placing the ear probe in preterms.[191] Besides, children with nonorganic hearing loss or hearing loss primarily due to involvement of the auditory pathway or central nervous system may have completely normal OAEs as a result of a functioning cochlea.[192] Therefore, children at risk for auditory neuropathy should be screened with ABR methods.

Several other types of OAE have been identified. These include spontaneous OAE, clicked evoked OAE, and distortion product OAE. With future research and automated analysis, each of these methods will become increasingly available for hearing screening, especially in term neonates.

Behavioral screening

Behavioral hearing screening methods such as the auditory response cradle and the crib-o-gram have been developed for term infants. Although easy to perform, they are not suitable for screening preterm or sick neonates and detect only severe hearing impairment. The sensitivity (75%) and specificity (71%) are too low compared to neurofunctional methods.[193] Behavioral observations remain the basis of the investigation of the harmful influences of high-intensity noise in neonatal intensive care units; prematures wearing earmuffs spent more time in quiet sleep states and had higher mean oxygen saturation levels compared to controls.[194]

Information about pediatric auditory research projects are available on the Internet.[195]

Possible damage from environmental hazards during pregnancy

Children who have been exposed *in utero* to vibroacoustic stimulation for the assessment of fetal well-being have been evaluated at 4 years of age by auditory tests of 20–25 dB at frequencies between 500 and 8000 Hz in Sweden ($n=460$)[196] and the United States ($n=465$).[197] No hearing damage or neurodevelopmental abnormalities that could be connected to the vibroacoustic stimulation were found. Fetal noise-induced hearing loss has been a matter of concern regarding the working and living conditions of pregnant women.[198,199] Epidemiological and animal research suggest that noise can adversely change fetal hearing; however, studies in humans still lack control groups. Auditory brainstem response changes were examined in sheep suggesting that noise sources with low-frequency components and high-intensity impulses have temporary effects on auditory brainstem response waves, whereas long-term effects are still unknown.[200] In summary, the Committee on Hearing, Bioacoustics and Biomechanics,[201] attempting to protect fetal hearing, suggested that pregnant women should avoid noise exposures greater than 90 dB.

Direction of future research

The phenomenon of prenatal perception and the implications for future life represent a wealth for ongoing and future research.

Methodological aspects

Prenatal hearing reflects the complex neurological development of the early brain. Evaluation of fetal brain function is one of the most important objectives of basic and clinical research in perinatology. Imaging of the fetal brain only demonstrates a small part of its function and most functional approaches have been indirect. The introduction of magnetoencephalography in perinatal medicine was a pioneer step to evaluate prenatal brain function directly,[79,80] though the single-channel magnetometer did not allow high-quality auditory-evoked signals. By using multichannel MEG[202] or detectors specifically designed for the prenate, the window of observation of early gestational age and various indications might be expected to be extended. The method might be used in newborns[203]; examinations in twins would enhance our knowledge about hereditary or environmental influences. The sophisticated method might have implications for prenatal neuroscience and clinical use. Prenatal training of laryngeal coordination is likely to occur during mouthing or breathing movements. Doppler combined with real-time ultrasound examinations might elucidate how far this is performed at a special rhythm. Correlations with postnatal cry spectroscopy might be of interest.

Aspects of using early sensation for developmental support

Health is understood as the physical, mental and social well-being that goes further than just the absence of illness. As important as it is to teach children abilities at certain times creating integrated stimulations for the unborn might favor development or prevent sensory retardation. This should be a matter of concern in public health projects. In Venezuela, a program was introduced including weekly lectures to pregnant mothers about adequate stimulation and nutrition. Significant improvement was found at the 2nd and 25th days in orientation and autonomic stability of the infants in the experimental compared to the control group.[204] Perinatal auditory stimulation programs need the knowledge of critical developmental phases. Pilot studies have demonstrated an immediate reduction of fetal breathing and an increase of FM when mothers only listen to a preferred type of music via earphones,[205] or a reduction of fetal activity if fetuses only listen to rhythmic music.[64] The first study is proof that integrated programs for mother and fetus may even be regarded as conditioning (e.g., 'music, mother relaxed'). Is the unborn more affected by the mother's preferences of listening – the same holds true for singing and talking to the unborn – than by the sound alone? Postnatal conditioning has a larger scale, e.g., sound stimulations recalling intrauterine noise can not only lull the newborn to sleep,[67] but also serve as a reinforcer during sucking.[206] Similarly, feeding may be enhanced by background music. The perception of music as pleasant might even be a process of conditioning from the parents.[71] Singing lullabies and simultaneously rocking cradles have been used to soothe babies by simultaneous stimulation of the vestibular and acoustic sensory system. The experience of rhythmic stimulations by a 'breathing teddy bear' adapted to the child's individual breathing frequency has proven to facilitate neurobehavioral development.[207] Further studies relating to supportive perinatal conditioning are necessary whereby music stimulation might play an essential part.[135]

Aspects for pathological development

Working groups in Western countries are planning protocols for the evaluation of early hearing screening. Thereby it is a major goal of the Maternal Child Health grant in the United States to establish universal neonatal screening, to identify specific hearing loss by 3 months, to institute intervention by 6 months and to measure the impact of early identification on developmental outcome. Average costs were given as $25 per test,[208] and as $43,785 to identify a child with sensorineural hearing loss.[209] Considering the given incidence of hearing impairment further programs are needed. Future research of the use of acoustic therapy and shelter may provide measures positively to alter the critically ill newborn's environment.

Conclusions

Encouragement and avoidance of sound have to be considered and balanced in future analytical and interventional projects according to critical developmental phases. Whether we go so far as to found prenatal universities, as in California, is of secondary importance as long as we strive to understand the physiology and pathophysiology of early hearing and to create designs of adequate stimulation suitable to induce a comprehensive expression of our genetic potential, prevent unnecessary illness and to detect hearing loss as early as possible.

REFERENCES

1. Hepper PG. Fetal psychology: an embryonic science. In Nijhuis JG, ed. *Fetal Behaviour, Developmental and Perinatal Aspects*. Oxford: Oxford Medical Publications, 1992:129–56.
2. Preyer W. *Spezielle Physiologie des Embryo*. Leipzig: Grieben, 1885.
3. Peiper A. Sinnesempfindungen der Kinder vor seiner Geburt. *Monat Kinderheilkd* 1925;29:237–41.
4. Forbes HS, Forbes HB. Fetal sense reaction: hearing. *J Comp Psychol* 1927;7:353–5.
5. Ray W. A preliminary report on a study of fetal conditioning. *Child Dev* 1932;3:175–7.
6. Sontag W, Wallace R. The movement response of the human fetus to sound stimuli. *Child Dev* 1939;6:253–8.
7. Spelt D. The conditioning of the human fetus *in utero*. *J Exp Psychol* 1948;3:338–46.
8. Salk L. Mothers' heartbeat as an imprinting stimulus. *Trans New Acad Sci* 1961/62;24:753–63.
9. Bench RJ. Sound transmission to the human fetus through the abdominal maternal wall. *J Gen Psychol* 1968;113:86–7.
10. Sakabe N, Arayama T, Suzuki T. Human fetal evoked responses to acoustic stimulation. *Acta Otolaryngol* 1969;252(Suppl):29–36.
11. Bast TH, Anson BJ. *The Temporal Bone and the Ear*. Springfield, Il: Charles C. Thomas, 1949.
12. Anson BJ, Winch T. Vascular channels in the auditory ossicles. *Ann Otol Rhinol Laryngol* 1974;83:142–58.
13. Anson BJ, Davies J, Duckert LG. Embryology of the ear. In Paparella MM, Shumrick DA, Gluckman JL *et al.*, eds. *Otolaryngology*, 3rd edn. Philadelphia, PA: WB Saunders, 1991: 3–22.
14. Gasser RF, Shigihara S, Shimada K. The development of the facial nerve in man. *Ann Otol Rhinol Laryngol* 1967;76:37–56.
15. Gasser RF, Shigihara S, Shimada K. Three-dimensional development of the facial nerve path through the ear region in human embryos. *Ann Otol Rhinol Laryngol* 1994;103:395–403.
16. Pearson AA. Developmental anatomy of the ear. In English GM, ed. *Otolaryngology*, revised. New York: Harper Medical, 1988: 1–68.
17. Gulya AJ. Developmental anatomy of the ear. In Glasscock ME, Shambaugh GE Jr, eds. *Surgery of the Ear*, 4th edn. Philadelphia, PA: WB Saunders, 1990:5–33.
18. Kenna MA. Embryology and developmental anatomy of the ear. In Bluestone CD, Stool SE, Kenna ME, eds. *Pediatric Otolaryngology*. Philadelphia, PA: WB Saunders, 1996;1:113–26.
19. Wright A. Anatomy and ultrastructure of the human ear. In Kerr AG, Groves J, eds. *Scott-Brown's Otolaryngology*, 5th edn. London: Butterworths, 1987:1–46.
20. Schulknecht HF, Gulya AJ. Phylogeny and embryology. In Schulknecht HF, Gulya AJ, eds. *Anatomy of the Temporal Bone with Surgical Implications*. Philadelphia, PA: Lea & Febiger, 1986: 235–73.
21. Bredberg G. Cellular pattern and nerve supply of the human organ of Corti. *Acta Otolaryngol (Stockh)* 1986;236(Suppl):1.
22. Pujol R, Lavigne-Rebillard M. Early stages of innervation and sensory cell differentiation in the human organ of Corti. *Acta Otolaryngol* 1985;423(Suppl):43–50.
23. Pujol R, Uziel A. Auditory development: peripheral aspects. In Meisami E, Tiniacas TS, eds. *Handbook of Human Growth and Developmental Biology*. Boca Raton, FL: CRC Press, 1988;1(Part 2): 109–30.
24. Pujol R, Hilding DA. Anatomy and physiology of the onset of auditory function. *Acta Otolaryngol* 1973;76:1–10.
25. Lavigne-Rebillard M, Pujol R. Hair cell innervation in the human cochlea. *Acta Otolaryngol* 1988;105:398–402.
26. Lavigne-Rebillard M, Pujol R. Development of auditory hair cell surface in human fetuses: A scanning electron microscopic study. *Anat Embryol* 1986;174:369–72.
27. Moore JK, Perazzo LM, Braun A. Time course of axonal myelination in the human brainstem auditory pathway. *Hear Res* 1995; 87:21–31.
28. Shido Y, Zhimin Q, Ningshen Z. Ultrastructure of the secondary tympanic membrane in the human fetus. *Acta Anat* 1988;131: 332–7.
29. Fisch L. Integrated development and maturation of the hearing system. A critical review article. *Br J Audiol* 1983;17:137–54.
30. Durrant JD, Lovrinic JH. *Basis of Hearing Science*, 2nd edn. Baltimore, MD: Williams & Wilkins, 1984.
31. Haggard MP, Evans EF. Hearing. *Br Med Bull* 1987;43:775–1042.
32. Jahn AF, Santos-Sacchi J. *Physiology of the Ear*. New York: Raven Press, 1988.
33. Ryan A, Dallos P. Physiology of the cochlea. In Northern JJ, ed. *Hearing Disorders*, 2nd edn. Boston, MA: Little, Brown, 1984: 253–66.
34. Oliver CC. Sound and vibration transmission in tissues. *Semin Perinatol* 1989;13:3554–61.
35. Davis H. A model for transducer action in the human cochlea. *Cold Spring Harb Symp Quant Biol* 1965;30:181–93.
36. von Bekesy G. Experiments in hearing. In Wever EG, ed. *McGraw Hill Series in Psychology*. New York: McGraw Hill, 1960:745–55.
37. Rhode WS. Basilar membrane motion: results of Mossbauer motions. *Scand Audiol Suppl* 1986;25:7–15.
38. Brugge JF, Geisler CD. Auditory mechanisms of the lower brainstem. *Annu Rev Neurosci* 1978;1:363–94.
39. Merzenich MM, Knight PL, Roth GL. Representation of cochlea within primary auditory cortex in the cat. *J Neurophysiol* 1975; 38:231–49.
40. Canforth JL. Auditory cortex lesions and interaural intensity and phase-angle discrimination in cats. *J Neurophysiol* 1979;42: 1518–26.
41. Cassaday JH, Neff WD. Auditory localization: role of auditory pathways in brain stem of the cat. *J Neurophysiol* 1975;38: 842–58.
42. Massopust LC, Wolin L, Frost V. Frequency discrimination thresholds following auditory cortex ablations in the monkey. *J Audiol Res* 1971;11:227–34.
43. Keidel WB. Information processing in higher parts of the auditory pathway. In Zwicker E, Terhardt E, eds. *Facts and Models in Hearing*. New York: Springer, 1974:216.
44. Warr WB, Guinan JJ. Efferent innervation of the organ of Corti: Two separate systems. *Brain Res* 1979;173:152–5.
45. Busnel MC, Granier-Deferre C, Lacanuet JP. Fetal audition. In Turkewitz G, ed. *Developmental Psychology*. New York: New York Academy of Science, 1992:175–88.
46. Gerhardt KJ. Characteristics of the fetal sheep sound environment. *Semin Perinatol* 1989;13:362–70.
47. Querleu D, Xavier R, Boutteville C, *et al.* Hearing by the human fetus? *Semin Perinatol* 1989;13:409–20.
48. Gerhardt KJ, Otto R, Abrams RM, *et al.* Cochlear microphonics recorded from fetal and newborn sheep. *Am J Otolaryngol* 1992; 13:226–33.
49. Gerhardt KJ, Abrams RM. Fetal hearing: characterisation of the stimulus and response. *Semin Perinatol* 1996;20:11–20.
50. Hollien H, Feinstein S. Contribution of the external auditory meatus to auditory sensitivity underwater. *J Acoust Soc Am* 1975;57: 1488–92.
51. Gerhardt KJ, Huang X, Arringtom KE, *et al.* Fetal sheep *in utero* hear through bone conduction. *Am J Otolaryngol* 1995;17:374–9.
52. Dirks DD. Bone conduction threshold testing. In Katz J, ed. *Handbook of Clinical Audiology*, 4th edn. Baltimore, MD: Williams & Wilkins, 1994:132–46.
53. Peters AJM, Gerhardt KJ, Abrams RM, *et al.* Three-dimensional intraabdominal sound pressures in sheep produced by airborne stimuli. *Am J Obstet Gynecol* 1993;169:1304–15.

54. Previc FH. A general theory concerning the prenatal origins of cerebral lateralizations in humans. *Psychol Rev* 1991;98: 299–334.
55. Bench RJ. Sound transmission to the human foetus through the maternal abdominal wall. *J Gen Psychol* 1968;113:85–7.
56. Grimwalde JC, Walker D, Wood C. Sensory stimulation of the human fetus. *Aust J Ment Ret* 1970;2:63–4.
57. Walker DW, Grimwalde JC, Wood C. Intrauterine noise: a component of the fetal environment. *Am J Obstet Gynecol* 1971; 109:91–5.
58. Querleu D, Renard X, Crepin G. Preception auditive et reactivite foetale aux stimulations sonores. *J Gynaecol Obstet Biol Reprod (Paris)* 1981;10:207–14.
59. Querleu Q, Xavier R, Fabienne V. Fetal hearing. *Eur J Obstet Gynecol Reprod Biol* 1988;29:191–212.
60. Armitage SE, Baldwin BA, Vince MA. The fetal sound environment in sheep. *Science* 1980;208:1173–4.
61. Vince MA, Armitage S, Baldwin BA. The sound environment in fetal sheep. *Behavior* 1982;81:296–315.
62. Gerhardt KJ, Abrams RM, Oliver CC. Sound environment of the fetal sheep. *Am J Obstet Gynecol* 1990;162:282–7.
63. Vince MA, Billing AE, Baldwin BA, *et al.* Maternal vocalisations and other sounds in fetal lamb's sound environment. *Early Hum Dev* 1985;11:179–90.
64. Saling E, Arabin B. Untersuchungen über akustische Einflüsse auf den Fetus. In Stauber M, Diedrichs P, eds. *Psychosomatische Probleme in der Gynäkologie und Geburtshilfe.* Berlin: Springer, 1987:19–28.
65. Benzaquen S, Gagnon R, Hunse C, *et al.* The intrauterine sound environment of the human fetus during labor. *Am J Obstet Gynecol* 1990;163:484–90.
66. Henshall WR. Intra-uterine sound levels. *Am J Obstet Gynecol* 1971;112:576–8.
67. Wollak CH. The auditory activity of the sheep (*ovis aries*). *J Audiol Res* 1963;3:121–32.
68. Murooka H, Koie Y, Suda M. Analyse des sons intrauterins et leurs effects tranquillisants sur le nouveau-né. *J Gynecol Obstet Biol Reprod* 1976;5:367–76.
69. Richards DS, Frentzen B, Gerhardt KJ, *et al.* Sound levels in the human uterus. *Obstet Gynecol* 1992;80:186–90.
70. Querleu D, Renard X, Versyp F, *et al.* La transmission intra-amniotique des voix humaines. *Rev Fr Gynecol Obstet* 1988;83:43–50.
71. Woodward SC, Guidozzi F. Intrauterine rhythm and blues? *Br J Obstet Gynaecol* 1992;99:787–90.
72. Leader LR, Baille P, Martin B, Vermeulen E. The assessment and significance of habituation to a repeated stimulus by the human fetus. *Early Hum Dev* 1982;7:211–19.
73. Hepper PG, Shahidullah S. Habituation in normal and Down's syndrome fetuses. *Q J Exp Psychol* 1992;44B:105–17.
74. Birnholz J, Benacerraf B. The development of fetal hearing. *Science* 1983;222:516–18.
75. Parkes MJ, Moore PJ, Moore DR, Fisk NM, Hanson MA. Behavioral changes in fetal sheep caused by vibroacoustic stimulation: the effects of cochlear ablation. *Am J Obstet Gynecol* 1991;164:1336–43.
76. Barden TP, Peltzman P, Graham T. Human fetal electroencephalic response to intrauterine acoustic signals. *Am J Obstet Gynecol* 1968;100:1128–34.
77. Sakabe N, Arayama T, Suzuki T. Human fetal evoked response to acoustic stimulation. *Acta Otolaryngol Suppl* 1969;252:29–36.
78. Scribetta JJ, Rosen MG, Hochberg CJ, Chik L. Human fetal brain responses to sound during labor. *Am J Obstet Gynecol* 1971; 109:82–5.
79. Blum T, Saling E, Bauer R. First magnetoencephalographic recordings of the brain activity of a human fetus. *Br J Obstet Gynaecol* 1985;92:1224–9.
80. Blum T, Bauer R, Arabin B, Reckel S, Saling E. Prenatally recorded auditory evoked neuro-magnetic fields of the human fetus. In Barber C, Blum T, eds. *Evoked Potentials III.* Boston, MA: Butterworths, 1987;3:136–42.
81. Wilson LA, Wilson KS, Boros SJ. Gestational age as a factor in neonatal AEP screening. In Nodar RH, Barber C, eds. *Evoked Potentials II.* Boston, MA: Butterworths, 1984:520–6.
82. Tuber D, Berntson CD, Brachman DS, *et al.* Associative learning in premature hydranecephalic and normal twins. *Science* 1980;210:1035–7.
83. Crade M, Lovet S. Fetal response to sound stimulation: preliminary report exploring use of sound stimulation in routine obstetrical ultrasound examination. *J Ultrasound Med* 1988;7:499–503.
84. Hepper PG, White R, Shahidullah S. The development of fetal responsiveness to external auditory stimulation. *Br Psychol Soc* 1991:Abstr 30.
85. Shahidullah S, Hepper PG. The developmental origins of fetal responsiveness to an acoustic stimulus. *J Reprod Infant Psychol* 1993;11:135–41.
86. Arabin B, Riedewald S. An attempt to quantify characteristics of behavioral states. *Am J Perinatol* 1992;9:115–19.
87. Arabin B, Riedewald S, Zacharias C, Saling E. Quantitative analysis of fetal behavioural patterns by means of real time sonography and the actocardiograph. *Gynecol Obstet Invest* 1988;26:211–18.
88. Arabin B, Zacharias C, Riedewald S, Blücher U, Saling E. Analyse fetaler Reaktionen auf akustische Reize mit unterschiedlicher Registriertechnik. *Geburtsh Frauenheilkd* 1989;49:653–7.
89. Gagnon R, Hunse C, Carmichael L, Fellows F, Patrick J. Effects of vibratory acoustic stimulation on human fetal breathing and gross fetal body movements near term. *Am J Obstet Gynecol* 1986;155: 1227–30.
90. Gagnon R, Hunse C, Patrick J. Fetal responses to vibratory acoustic stimulation: Influence of basal heart rate. *Am J Obstet Gynecol* 1988;59:835–9.
91. Visser GHA, Mulder HH, Wit HP. Vibro-acoustic stimulation of the human fetus: Effect on behavioural state organization. *Early Hum Dev* 1989;19:285–96.
92. Gagnon R, Hunse C, Foerman J. Human fetal behavioural states after vibratory stimulation. *Am J Obstet Gynecol* 1989;161: 1470–6.
93. Lazebnik N, Hill LM, Costanino JP, Many A, Martin JG. Vibroacoustic stimulation enhances visualization of the four-chamber cardiac view in the third trimester. *Ultrasound Obstet Gynecol* 1996;8:309–14.
94. Hepper PG, Shahidullah S. Development of fetal hearing. *Arch Dis Child* 1994;71:81–7.
95. Shahidullah S, Hepper PG. Frequency discrimination by the fetus. *Early Hum Dev* 1994;36:13–26.
96. Devoe LD, Murray C, Faircloth D, Ramos E. Vibroacoustic stimulation and fetal behavioral state in normal term human pregnancy. *Am J Obstet Gynecol* 1990;163:1156–61.
97. Zimmer EZ, Fifer WP, Kim YI, Rey HR, Chao CR, Myers MM. Response of the premature fetus to stimulation by speech sounds. *Early Hum Dev* 1993;33:207–15.
98. Brazelton TB, Nugent KT. *Neonatal Behavioral Assessment Scale,* 3rd edn. Cambridge, UK: Cambridge University Press, 1995.
99. Peck JE. Development of hearing. 3. Postnatal development. *J Am Acad Audiol* 1995;6:113–23.
100. Sohmer H, Feinmesser M. Cochlear action potentials recorded from the external ear in man. *Ann Otol Rhinol Laryngol* 1967; 76:427–35.
101. Jewett DI, Romano MN, Williston JS. Human auditory evoked potentials: possible brain stem components detected on the scalp. *Science* 1970;167:1517–18.
102. Despland PA, Galambos R. The auditory brain stem response (ABR): A useful diagnostic tool in the intensive care nursery. *Pediatr Res* 1980;15:154–8.
103. Starr A, Achor IJ. Auditory brain stem responses in neurological disease. *Arch Neurol* 1975;32:761–6.
104. Martin WH, Schwegler JW, Gleeson AL, Shi YB. New techniques of hearing assessment. *Otolaryngol Clin North Am* 1994;27: 487–510.
105. Galambos R, Wilson MJ, Silva PD. Identifying hearing loss in the intensive care nursery: a 20-year summary. *J Am Acad Audiol* 1994;5:151–6.
106. Hecox KE. Neurologic application of the auditory brainstem response to the pediatric age group. In Jacobson JE, ed. *The Auditory Brain Stem Response.* San Diego, CA: College Hill Press, 1985:287–95.
107. Kemp DT. Stimulated acoustic emissions from within the human auditory system. *J Acoust Soc Am* 1978;64:1386–91.
108. Eisenberg R. *Auditory Competence in Early Life.* Baltimore, MD: University Park Press, 1976.
109. Eisenberg RB. Auditory behaviour in the human neonate. 1. Methodological problems and the logical design of research procedures. *J Audiol Res* 1965;5:159–77.
110. Eisenberg RB. Auditory behaviour in the human neonate. Functional properties of sound and their ontogenetic implications. *Int Audiol* 1969;9:34–45.
111. Muir DW. The development of infants' auditory spatial sensitivity. In Trehub SE, Schneider BS, eds. *Auditory Development in Infancy.* New York: Plenum, 1985:51–83.

112. Tucker SM, Bhatacharia J. Screening of hearing impairments in the newborn using the auditory response cradle. *Arch Dis Child* 1992;67:911–19.
113. Olsho LW, Koch EG, Halpin CR, Carter EA. An observer based psychoacoustic procedure for use with young infants. *Dev Psychol* 1987;23:627–40.
114. Werner LA, Gillenwater JM. Pure-tone sensitivity of 2–5 week old infants. *Infant Behav Dev* 1990;13:355–75.
115. Jeffrey WE, Cohen LB. Habituation in the human infant. *Adv Child Dev Behav* 1971;6:63–97.
116. De Caspar AJ, Fifer WP. Of human bonding: newborns prefer their mothers' voices. *Science* 1980;208:1174–6.
117. Mehler J, Jusczyk PW, Lambertz G, Halsted N, Bertoncini J, Amile-Tison C. A precursor of language acquisition in young infants. *Cognition* 1988;29:143–78.
118. Spence MJ, de Caspar AJ. Prenatal experience with low-frequency maternal voice sounds influence neonatal perception of maternal voice samples. *Infant Behav Dev* 1987;10:133–42.
119. Sallenbach WB. A theoretical framework on prenatal cognition and bonding. *Int J Prenat Perinat Stud* 1991;3:273–81.
120. Zuckerman B, Bauchner H, Parker S, Carpral H. Maternal depressive symptoms during pregnancy and newborn irritability. *J Dev Behav Paediatr* 1990;11:190–4.
121. Fisch L. The probability of response to test sounds in young children. *Sound* 1971;5:7–10.
122. Ryder GH. Vagitus uterinus. *Am J Obstet Gynecol* 1943;46: 867–72.
123. Russell PMG. Vagitus uterinus: crying *in utero*. *Lancet* 1957;1: 137–8.
124. Blair RG. Vagitus uterinus: crying *in utero*. *Lancet* 1965;2:1164–5.
125. Mende W, Wermke K, Schindler S, Wilzopolski K, Hoek S. Variability of the cry melody and the melody spectrum as indicators for certain CNS disorders. *Early Child Dev Care* 1990;65: 96–107.
126. Wermke K, Mende W, Borschberg H, Ruppert R. Voice characteristics of prespeech vocalisations of twins during the first year of life. In Powell TW, ed. *Pathologies of Speech and Language*. New Orleans, LA: ICPLA Publication of the International Clinical Phonetics and Linguistics Association, 1996:1–7.
127. Truby HM, Lind J. Cry motions of the newborn infant. *Acta Paediatr Scand* 1965;163(Suppl):61–92.
128. Truby HM. Prenatal and neonatal speech, pre-speech and an infantile speech lexicon. *Child Lang* 1975;27:1–3.
129. Condon WS, Sander WE. Neonate movement is synchronized with adult speech: interactional participation and language acquisition. *Science* 1974;183:99–101.
130. Werker JF. Becoming a native listener. *Am Sci* 1989;77:54–9.
131. Kuhl PK, Williams KA, Lacerda F, Stevens KN, Lindblom B. Linguistic experience alters phonetic perception in infants by 6 months of age. *Science* 1992;225:606–8.
132. Fernald A. Human maternal vocalisations to infants as biologically relevant signals: an evolutionary perspective. In Barkow HJ, Cosmides L, Toby J, eds. *The Adapted Mind: Evolutionary Psychology and the Generation of Culture*. New York: Oxford University Press, 1992:391–428.
133. Fridman R. Proto-rhythms: music in prenatal and postnatal life. In Blum T, ed. *Prenatal Perception, Learning and Bonding*. Berlin: Leonardo Publishers, 1993:247–52.
134. Roederer JG. The search for a survival value of music. *Music Perception* 1984;1:350–6.
135. Arabin B. Music during pregnancy. *Ultrasound Obstet Gynecol* 2002;20:425-30.
136. Natale R, Clelow F, Dawes GS. Measurement of fetal forelimb movements in lambs *in utero*. *Am J Obstet Gynecol* 1981;140: 545–51.
137. Cohn HE, Sacks EJ, Heyman MA, Rudolph AM. Cardiovascular responses to hypoxemia and acidemia in fetal lambs. *Am J Obstet Gynecol* 1974;120:817–24.
138. Manning FA, Platt DA, Sipos L. Antenatal fetal evaluation. Development of a fetal biophysical profile. *Am J Obstet Gynecol* 1980;136:787–95.
139. Wladimiroff JW, Wijngaard JAGW, Degani S, Noordam MZ, Van Eyck J, Tonge HM. Cerebral and umbilical blood flow velocity waveform in normal and growth-retarded pregnancies. *Obstet Gynecol* 1987;69:705–9.
140. Arabin B, Bergmann PL, Saling E. Simultaneous assessment of blood flow velocity waveforms in uteroplacental vessels, the umbilical artery, the fetal aorta and the fetal common carotid artery. *Fetal Diagn Ther* 1987;2:17–26.
141. Bilardo CM, Nicolaides KH, Campbell S. Doppler measurements of fetal uteroplacental circulations. Relationship with umbilical venous blood gases measured at cordocentesis. *Am J Obstet Gynecol* 1990;162:115–20.
142. Visser GHA, Sadovsky G, Nicolaides KH. Antepartum heart rate patterns in small-for-gestational age third trimester fetuses. Correlations with blood gas values obtained at cordocentesis. *Am J Obstet Gynecol* 1990;62:698–703.
143. Arabin B, Rüttgers H, Lorenz U, Kubli F. Course and predictive value of heart rate parameters from the 27th to the 42nd week of gestation. *Am J Perinatol* 1989;5:272–7.
144. Read JA, Miller FC. Fetal heart rate acceleration in response to acoustic stimulation as a measure of fetal well-being. *Am J Obstet Gynecol* 1977;149:512–17.
145. Smith CV, Phelan JP, Platt LD, Broussard P, Paul RHL. Fetal acoustic stimulation testing. 2. A randomized clinical comparison with non-stress test. *Am J Obstet Gynecol* 1986;155:131–4.
146. Pietrantoni M, Angel JL, Parsons MT, McClain L, Arango HA, Spellacy WN. Human fetal response to vibroacoustic stimulation as a function of stimulus duration. *Obstet Gynecol* 1991;78: 807–11.
147. Zimmer EZ, Divon MY. Fetal vibroacoustic stimulation. *Obstet Gynecol* 1993;81:451–7.
148. Gagnon R, Hunse C, Carmichael L, Patrick J. Vibratory acoustic stimulation in 26- to 32-week, small-for-gestational-age fetus. *Am J Obstet Gynecol* 1989;160:160–5.
149. Inglis SR, Druzin ML, Wagner WE, Kogut E. The use of vibroacoustic stimulation during the abnormal or equivocal biophysical profile. *Obstet Gynecol* 1993;82:371–4.
150. Trudinger MB, Boylan P. Antepartum fetal heart rate monitoring: value of sound stimulation. *Obstet Gynecol* 1980;55:263–8.
151. Jensen OH. Fetal heart rate response to a controlled sound stimulation as a measure of fetal well-being. *Acta Obstet Gynecol Scand* 1984;63:97–101.
152. Schiff E, Lipitz S, Sivan E, Barkai G, Mashiach S. Acoustic stimulation as a diagnostic test: comparison with oxytocin challenge test. *J Perinat Med* 1992;20:275–9.
153. Arabin B, Becker R, Entezami M, Mohnhaupt A, Weitzel HK. Prediction of fetal distress and poor outcome combined with intrauterine growth retardation using FHR monitoring and Doppler ultrasound. *Fetal Diagn Ther* 1993;8:234–40.
154. Arabin B, Becker R, Mohnhaupt A, Vollert W, Weitzel HK. Prediction of fetal distress and poor outcome combined with prolonged pregnancy using FHR and Doppler monitoring. *Fetal Diagn Ther* 1994;9:1–6.
155. Smith CV, Phelan JP, Nguyen HN. Continuing experience with the fetal acoustic stimulation test. *J Reprod Med* 1988;33:365–8.
156. Clark SL, Sabey P, Jolley K. Nonstress testing with acoustic stimulation and amniotic fluid volume assessment. *Am J Obstet Gynecol* 1989;160:694–7.
157. Richards DS. The fetal vibroacoustic stimulation test: an update. *Semin Perinatol* 1990;14:305–10.
158. Fisk NM, Nicolaidis PK, Arulkumaran S, *et al*. Vibroacoustic stimulation is not associated with sudden fetal catecholamine release. *Early Hum Dev* 1991;25:11–17.
159. Zimmer EZ, Talmon R, Makler-Shiran E, Jakobi P. Effect of vibroacoustic stimulation on fetal meconium passage in labor. *Am J Perinatol* 1996;13:81–3.
160. Gagnon R, Benzaquen S, Hunse C. The fetal sound environment during vibroacoustic stimulation in labor: effect on fetal heart rate response. *Obstet Gynecol* 1992;79:950–5.
161. Sarno AP, Ahn MO, Phelan JP, Paul RH. Fetal acoustic stimulation in the early intrapartum period as a predictor of subsequent fetal condition. *Am J Obstet Gynecol* 1990;162:762–7.
162. Ingemarsson I, Arulkumaran S. Reactive fetal heart rate response to vibroacoustic stimulation in fetuses with low scalp blood pH. *Br J Obstet Gynaecol* 1989;96:562–5.
163. Umstad M, Bailey C, Permezel M. Intrapartum fetal stimulation testing. *Aust NZ J Obstet Gynaecol* 1992;32:222–4.
164. Anyaegbunam AM, Ditchik A, Stoical R, Mikhail MS. Vibroacoustic stimulation of the fetus entering the second stage of labor. *Obstet Gynecol* 1994;83:963–6.
165. Irion O, Stuckelberger P, Moutquin JM, Morabia A, Extermann P, Beguin F. Is intrapartum vibratory acoustic stimulation a valid alternative to scalp pH determination? *Br J Obstet Gynaecol* 1996;103:642–7.
166. Wladimiroff JW, Cheung K. Vibratory acoustic stimulation and the flow velocity waveform in the fetal internal carotid artery. *Early Hum Dev* 1989;19:61–6.

167. Barford D. Fetal death from sepsis following a reassuring intrapartum fetal acoustic stimulation test [Letter]. *Obstet Gynecol* 1990;75:307–8.
168. Petrikovsky BM, Schifrin B, Diana L. The effect of fetal acoustic stimulation on fetal swallowing and amniotic fluid index. *Obstet Gynecol* 1993;81:548–50.
169. Zimmer EZ, Chao CR, Guy GP, Marks F, Fifer WP. Vibroacoustic stimulation evokes human fetal micturition. *Obstet Gynecol* 1993;81:178–80.
170. Sherer DM, Abramowicz JS, Hearn-Stebbins B, Woods JR. Sonographic verification of a nuchal cord following VAS-induced severe variable FHR decelerations with abdominal delivery. *Am J Perinatol* 1991;8:345–6.
171. Romero R, Mazor M, Hobbins HJ. A critical appraisal of fetal acoustic stimulations as an antenatal test for fetal well-being. *Obstet Gynecol* 1988;71:781–6.
172. Elliott LL, Armbruster VB. Some possible effects of the delay of early treatment of deafness. *J Speech Hear Res* 1967;10:209–24.
173. Bebout JM. Pediatric hearing aid fitting: a practical overview. *Hear J* 1989;42:13–15.
174. Curnock DA. Identifying hearing impairment in infants and young children. *Br Med J* 1993;307:1225–6.
175. Veen S, Sassen ML, Schreuder AM, *et al.* Hearing loss in very preterm and very low birth weight infants at the age of 5 years in a nationwide cohort. *Int J Pediatr Otorhinolaryngol* 1993;26: 11–28.
176. Yoshinaga-Itano C, Sedey AL, Coulter DK, Mehl AL. Language of early- and later-identified children with hearing loss. Pediatrics 1998;102:1161–71.
177. Robertson C, Aldridge S, Jarman F, Saunders K, Poulakis Z, Oberklaid F. Late diagnosis of congenital sensorineural hearing impairment: why are detection methods failing? *Arch Dis Child* 1995;72:11–15.
178. Mauk GW, White KR, Mortensen LB, Behrens TR. The effectiveness of screening programs based on high-risk characteristics in early intervention of hearing impairment. *Ear Hear* 1991;12: 312–19.
179. Joint Committee on Infant Hearing. Year 2000 Position Statement: Principles and Guidelines for Early Hearing Detection and Intervention Programs. *Am J Audiol* 2000;9:9–29.
180. Oudesluys-Murphy AM, van Straaten HLM, Bholasingh R, van Zanten GA. Neonatal hearing screening. *Eur J Pediatr* 1996;155: 429–35.
181. Jacobson JT, Jacobson CA, Spahr RC. Automated and conventional ABR screening technics in high-risk infants. *J Am Acad Audiol* 1990;1:187–95.
182. Cox LC. The current status of auditory brainstem response testing in neonatal populations. *Pediatr Res* 1984;18:780–3.
183. Peters JG. An automated infant screener using advanced evoked response technology. *Hear J* 1986;9:1–4.
184. Herrmann BS, Thornton AR, Jospeh JM. Automated infant hearing screening using the ABR: development and validation. *Am J Audiol* 1995;4:6–14.
185. Van Straaten HLM, Hille ET, Kok JH, Verkerk PH. Dutch NICU Neonatal Hearing Screening Working Group. Implementation of a nation-wide automated auditory brainstem response hearing screening program in neonatal intensive care units. *Acta Paediatr* 2003;92:332–8.
186. Hall JW, Lamb MM, Freeman SD, Beeker J. Infant hearing screening with automated ABR in the NICU. Presented at the *XXIII International Congress of Audiology*, Bari, Italy, May 1996.
187. Vohr BR, Maxon AB. Screening infants for hearing impairment. *J Pediatr* 1996;128:710–14.
188. Kennedy CR, Kimm L, Cafarelli Dees D, *et al.* Otoacoustic emissions and auditory brainstem responses in the newborn. *Arch Dis Child* 1991;66:1124–9.
189. Stevens JC, Webb HD, Hutchins J, Connell J, Smith MF, Buffin JT. Click evoked otoacoustic emissions in neonatal screening. *Ear Hear* 1990;11:128–33.
190. Baldwin M, Watkin P. The clinical application of oto-acoustic emissions in paediatric audiological assessment. *J Laryngol Otol* 1992;106:301–6.
191. Kok MR, Zanten GA, van Brocaar MP, Jongejan HTM. Click-evoked oto-acoustic emissions in very-low-birth-weight infants: A cross-sectional data analysis. *Audiology* 1994;33:152–64.
192. Doyle KJ, Sininger Y, Starr A. Auditory neuropathy in childhood. *Laryngoscope* 1998;108:1374–7.
193. Prager DA, Stone DA, Rose DN. Hearing loss screening in the neonatal intensive care unit: auditory brainstem response versus Crib-O-Gram; a cost effectiveness analysis. *Ear Hear* 1987;8: 213–16.
194. Zahr LK, de Traversay J. Premature infant responses to noise reduction by earmuffs: Effects on behavioural and physiologic measures. *J Perinatol* 1995;15:448–55.
195. Sininger Y. Pediatric auditory research projects: http://www.hei.org/pneonat.htm 1996.
196. Nyman M, Barr M, Westgren M. A four-year follow-up of hearing and development in children exposed *in utero* to vibro-acoustic stimulation. *Br J Obstet Gynaecol* 1992;99:685–8.
197. Arulkumaran S, Skurr B, Tong H, Kek LP, Yeoh KH, Ratnam SS. No evidence of hearing loss due to fetal acoustic stimulation test. *Obstet Gynecol* 1991;78:283–5.
198. Moss N, Carver D. Pregnant women at work. *Am J Ind Med* 1992;23:1–7.
199. Pierson LL. Hazards of noise exposure on fetal hearing. *Semin Perinatol* 1996;20:21–9.
200. Griffiths SK, Pierson LL, Gerhardt KJ, Abrams RM, Peters AJM. Noise induced hearing loss in fetal sheep. *Hear Res* 1994;74: 221–30.
201. Joint Committee on Infant Hearing Position Statement. ASHA 1982;24:1017.
202. Wakai RT, Leuthold AC, Martin CB. Fetal auditory evoked responses detected by magnetoencephalography. *Am J Obstet Gynecol* 1996;174:1484–6.
203. Reite M, Scheuneman D, Gilger JW, Teale P, Goldstein L, Boccia M. Auditory magnetic source localization in twins. *Brain Res Bull* 1992;28:641–4.
204. Manrique B, Contasi M, Avarado MA, *et al.* Nurturing parents to stimulate their children from prenatal stage to three years of age. In Blum T, ed. *Prenatal Perception, Learning and Bonding*. Berlin: Leonardo Publishers, 1993:153–86.
205. Zimmer EZ, Divon MY, Vilensky A, Sarna Z, Petretz BA, Paldie E. Maternal exposure to music and fetal activity. *Eur J Obstet Gynecol Reprod Biol* 1982;13:209–13.
206. De Caspar AJ, Sigafoos AD. The intrauterine heartbeat: A potent reinforcer. *Infant Behav Dev* 1983;6:19–23.
207. Thoman EB, Ingersoll EW, Acebo C. Premature infants seek rhythmic stimulation and the experience facilitates neurobehavioural development. *J Dev Behav Paediatr* 1991;12:11–18.
208. Downs MP. Universal newborn hearing screening. *Int J Pediatr Otorhinolaryngol* 1995;32:257–60.
209. Maxon AB, White KR, Behrens TR, Vohr BR. Referral rates and cost efficiency in a universal newborn hearing screening program using transient evoked otoacoustic emissions. *J Am Acad Audiol* 1995;6:271–7.

90 Fetal responses to placental insufficiency

M. L. Kush and A. A. Baschat

Introduction

The placenta forms the interface for nutrient, fluid and gas exchange between the mother and the fetus. Successful placental development is of critical importance as it is permissive for the normal development of an individual. While the fetal growth potential is genetically predetermined[1] the ultimate neonatal weight, proportions and condition at birth are dependent on placental development, fetal health and maternal health. Normal placentation of a genetically normal fetus in a healthy mother is therefore most likely to end in fulfillment of the growth potential. However, if any of these factors is deficient a number of fetal and maternal adverse outcomes may be the consequence. Of these placental insufficiency is of particular interest because it may lead to fetal growth restriction (IUGR), a condition that is associated with an increased risk for adverse health events that manifest in fetal life and extend all the way into adult life.[2–6] There are several conditions that are associated with fetal growth restriction (Figure 90.1). Of these, placental vascular insufficiency is clinically the most relevant since it is most prevalent and potentially derives a benefit from intervention.

Because of its diverse impacts placental disease has been a constant research focus for decades. However, it is the multidisciplinary approach of multiple medical subspecialties that has elevated our level of understanding to a point where the diverse impacts of placental dysfunction on fetal health are being appreciated. While traditional antenatal surveillance examines a relatively narrow spectrum of fetal responses, utilization of more sophisticated research tools has uncovered responses in almost every organ system. Before expanding on these multiple effects of placental insufficiency an understanding of the normal maturational process of the placenta and fetus is essential.

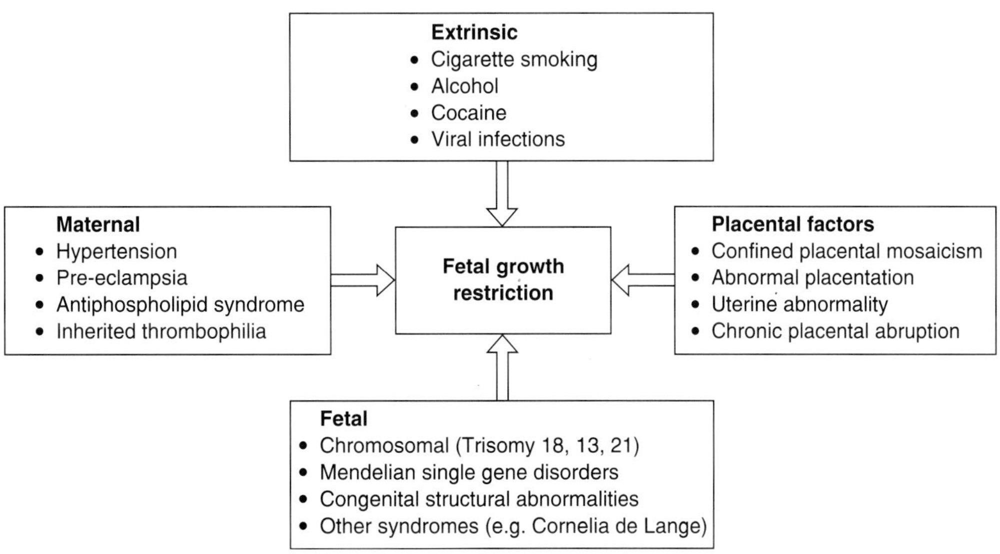

Figure 90.1 The principal causes and most common conditions that are associated with fetal growth restriction.

Placental development

Fetal growth is regulated at multiple levels, and requires successful placentation for the coordination of key components in the maternal, placental and fetal compartments for adequate maternal–fetal exchange throughout gestation. Successful placental adherence in the first trimester initiates a series of important milestones in the three overlapping gestational epochs. First-trimester initiation of placental vascular development permits nutrient and oxygen delivery to the growing trophoblast beyond the capacity of simple diffusion. Maternal adaptations to pregnancy predominate in this epoch. Differentiation of placental transport mechanisms and paracrine and endocrine signaling pathways between the mother, placenta and fetus then continue throughout the second trimester. Successful initiation of these steps allows placental growth and establishment of efficient and coordinated nutrient transfer, waste and gas exchange by the second trimester. This is a prerequisite for exponential fetal growth and differentiation in the third trimester in preparation for extrauterine life.

Following fertilization, the cytotrophoblast migrates to form anchoring sites through controlled breakdown of the extracellular matrix by metalloproteinases and localized expression of adhesion molecules. Placental adherence between the decidua and uterus is established by the formation of these anchoring villi that connect the decidua and uterus. Angiogenesis produces vascular connections to the maternal circulation that establish maternal blood supply to the intervillous space. This high level of nutrient and oxygen supply is required to support the growing embryo and trophoblast.[7,8] With this nutritional and vascular support in place, the villous trophoblast, consisting of a maternal microvillous and fetal basal layer, is formed.[9] Increasing placental synthetic activity is now sufficiently supported and results in the appearance of several secretory substances in the maternal circulation (e.g., human chorionic gonadotrophin and placental lactogen). Some of these substances promote postprandial hyperglycemia, increased fasting levels of free fatty acids, triglycerides and cholesterol, fat deposition, maternal intravascular volume expansion and relative refractoriness to vasoactive agents. These maternal adaptations increase substrate availability and steadiness of nutrient delivery to the placenta and are permissive for ongoing placental development.[10] Several paracrine signaling substances also appear in the placenta (e.g., nitric oxide, endothelin) and active cellular transport systems for major nutrient classes (glucose, aminoacids, and fatty acids) differentiate. Initiation of fetal cardiac activity allows for the active distribution of nutrients between fetus and placenta and completes the functionality of the feto-placental unit.[11] Ongoing development in the maternal and fetal compartments results in the formation of the villous trophoblast that consists of a maternal microvillous and fetal basal layer and is the primary site of exchange. The efficiency of maternal–fetal exchange depends on four principal factors: (1) the thickness that has to be traversed by diffusible substances; (2) the vascular throughput from the maternal and fetal circulations; (3) the surface area available for exchange; and (4) the elaboration of active transport mechanisms.

By the 16th week the villous trophoblast has progressively thinned down to 4 μm providing little resistance to diffusion. Vascular throughput through the placenta increases in both vascular compartments. Extravillous cytotrophoblast infiltration of the maternal spiral arteries results in progressive loss of the musculoelastic media, first in the decidual, then in the myometrial portion of these vessels.[12] This process is paralleled in the fetal compartment by continuous villous vascular branching.[13] Significant reduction in vascular resistance and a rapid increase in the exchange area are achieved by 26 weeks and then continue at a slower rate towards term. Through concurrent increases in fetal cardiac output, villous blood flow increases exponentially through the third trimester.[9,11] Under normal circumstances in the term placenta up to 600 ml/min of maternal cardiac output are delivered to an exchange area of up to 12 m^2. In the fetal compartment this is matched with a blood flow volume of 200–300 ml/Kg/min throughout gestation.[9,14,15] This magnitude of maternal blood flow is necessary since maintenance of placental function is energy intensive and consumes as much as 40% of O_2 and 70% of glucose supplied to the uterus.[16–18] Perfusion matching between the maternal and fetal compartments is further modulated and optimized through placental autoregulation, which is probably mediated through local paracrine factors such as nitric oxide (NO), endothelin, red blood cell (RBC) adenosine or cyclic guanosine monophoshate and fetal atrial natriuretic peptide (ANP). Optimal fetal growth and development is achieved when nutrient and oxygen delivery is sufficient to allow ideal fetal substrate utilization. This is only possible when the magnitude of maternal nutrient and oxygen delivery to the uterus exceeds placental demands leaving sufficient surplus for the fetus and when perfusion matching between the maternal and fetal compartments is optimized through placental autoregulation. While these developments significantly enhance the efficiency of exchange for diffusible substances other substances such as glucose, amino acids, and fatty acids that cannot efficiently pass this bilayer by simple diffusion require additional elaboration of active transport mechanisms.

Transplacental transport systems optimize the transfer of glucose, amino acids, and fatty acids.[19–21] Transmembrane ion pumps such as the Na/H^+ pump also develop, maintaining cellular homeostasis and normal cellular function.[22] Each of the nutrient classes has different roles in the fetus. Glucose is the

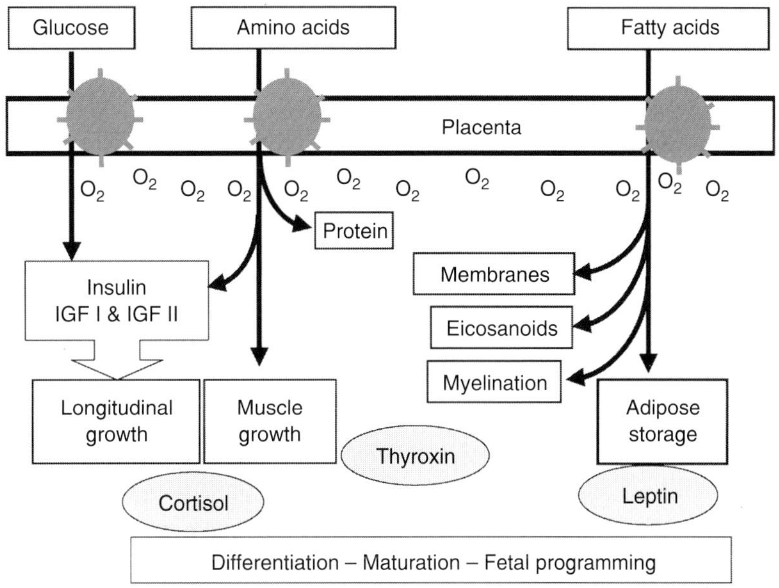

Figure 90.2 In the presence of adequate oxygenation, normal functioning of transplacental transport mechanisms for glucose, amino acids and fatty acids ensure availability of substrate for the fetus. Glucose and amino acids are the main stimulants of the insulin, IGF growth axis and stimulate longitudinal fetal growth. In addition, amino acids are utilized for protein synthesis and contribute to muscle bulk. Fatty acids have roles at many levels serving as precursors for eicosanoids and structural components of cell membranes and myelin sheaths. In the third trimester accumulation of adipose stores provides a reservoir for essential fatty acids. Endocrine axes – including hormones such as cortisol, thyroxin and leptin – modulate fetal maturation and differentiation according to substrate availability and may have significant impacts on adult life through fetal programming.

primary oxidative fuel while amino acids are incorporated into proteins. Fetal glucose and amino acids are the primary stimulants of insulin-like growth factors (IGF) I and II, and therefore stimulate longitudinal growth and differentiation.[23] Amino acids as major contributors to protein synthesis and are also laid down as muscle bulk.[23] Fatty acids are precursors for bioactive compounds including prostaglandins, thromoboxanes, leukotrienes and are also necessary for maintenance of cell membrane fluidity and permeability. In addition, long chain polyunsaturated fatty acids such as arachidionic and docosahexanoic acids are essential for normal brain and retinal development. Leptin coregulates transplacental amino acid and fatty acid transport and thereby modulates fetal body fat content and proportions.[24,25] With advancing gestation the magnitude and efficiency of transfer of these substances increases significantly to provide for placental and fetal growth requirements (Figure 90.2).

Concurrent development of the fetal circulation as a conduit for nutrient and waste delivery is an important cofactor in the fetal growth process. With establishment of a functional circulation, nutrient- and oxygen-rich blood from the primitive villous circulation enters the fetus via the umbilical vein. The arrangement of the fetal circulation allows further preferential streaming of these nutrients. The ductus venosus is the first vascular conduit encountered. Through modulations in shunting through the ductus venosus, 68–82% of umbilical venous blood continues to the liver, while the remainder is distributed to the heart.[26] Differential directionality of blood streams entering the right atrium ensures that nutrient rich blood is distributed to the left ventricle, myocardium, and brain, while low-nutrient venous return is distributed to the placenta for re-oxygenation and nutrient and waste exchange.[27] In addition to this overall distribution of left and right-sided cardiac output, several organs can modify local blood flow to meet oxygen and nutrient demands by autoregulation.[28]

With achievement of these milestones the prerequisites for normal placental and fetal growth are met. The metabolic and vascular status of the mother promotes a steady and enhanced nutrient delivery to the uterus and placental transport mechanisms allow for efficient bidirectional exchange of nutrient and waste. Under these circumstances placental and fetal growth remain closely related throughout gestation.[29] Their growth process across the three trimesters is characterized by sequential cellular hyperplasia, hyperplasia plus hypertrophy, and lastly hypertrophy alone. Placental growth follows a sigmoid curve that plateaus in midgestation preceding exponential third trimester growth of the fetus.[30,31]

During this exponential fetal growth phase of 1.5% per day initial weight gain is due to longitudinal growth and muscle bulk and therefore correlates with glucose and amino acid transport. Throughout gestation essential fatty acids are deposited in the developing brain and retina and account for up to 50% of dry brain weight.[32] After 20 weeks' gestation a notable increase in fatty acid transport and utilization initiate the deposition of significant fetal adipose tissue. From 24 weeks onward exponential fetal growth and adipose tissue deposition coincide with increasing conversion of glucose into fat, as well as increased utilization of fatty acids.[32,33] From 32 weeks to term fat stores increase from 3.2% of fetal body weight to 16% accounting for the significant reduction in body water content.[34,35] Throughout gestation, relative serum concentrations of free fatty acids remain related to maternal dietary intake. However, enhanced transplacental transport of essential polyunsaturated fatty acids and especially their storage in adipose tissue occurs during the period of exponential fetal growth. Therefore third trimester increase in fetal size is characterized by longitudinal growth accompanied by accumulation of essential body stores in preparation for extrauterine life.

Mechanisms of placental insufficiency

The mechanisms by which various diseases affect placental function are the subject of much inquiry. In maternal hypertensive disorders, increased syncytial knot formation indicates premature placental aging and apoptosis. Occlusive vasculopathy affects both the maternal and fetal circulatory compartments of the placenta, and is most pronounced in antiphospholipid syndromes. Fetal causes may exert their effects on growth at multiple levels. Placental causes may result in decreased placental blood flow and/or altered transport mechanisms with resultant abnormal placental cellular homeostasis.

The majority of IUGR pregnancies are the result of conditions that interfere with placental vascular development.[36] Depending on the gestational age and on the extent of interference with placental development, various clinical scenarios may occur within the maternal, placental, and fetal compartments. If interference with angiogenesis occurs early in the first trimester, successful placental adherence is unlikely to transpire and will likely result in miscarriage. If sufficient supply to the placenta can be established and maintained despite suboptimal vascular development, further placental differentiation is possible. However, suboptimal maternal pregnancy adaptation and deficient nutrient delivery pose limitations to placental metabolic and synthetic activity, which ultimately interfere with the differentiation of endocrine feedback loops and active transport mechanisms. If the trophoblast invasion remains confined to the decidual portion of the myometrium maternal spiral and radial arteries fail to undergo the physiologic transformation into low resistance vessels.[37,38] Altered expression of vasoactive substances may increase vascular reactivity, and if hypoxia-stimulated angiogenesis cannot overcome these challenges, placental autoregulation becomes deficient. Eventually loss of this placental autoregulation promotes vascular occlusion, infarction and permanent structural damage.[39] Maternal placental floor infarcts, fetal villous obliteration and fibrosis both increase placental blood flow resistance, producing maternal–fetal placental perfusion mismatch that decreases the effective exchange area.[39–42] With progressive vascular occlusion fetoplacental flow resistance is increased throughout the vascular bed and eventually the metabolically active placental mass is reduced. If adaptive mechanisms permit ongoing fetal survival early onset growth restriction with its many fetal manifestations develops.

The balance of compensatory and decompensatory responses determines the spectrum and degree of fetal manifestations in various organ systems. If compensatory mechanisms are unsuccessful, permanent fetal damage, or stillbirth results. With successful compensation, the consequences of nutrient shortage may remain largely subclinical, only to be unmasked through the restrictive effect on exponential fetal growth in the second to third trimester. In these cases, vascular manifestations may be less pronounced and physical characteristics more apparent. A decrease in adipose tissue or abnormal body proportions at birth may be the only indication that placental insufficiency occurred. In addition, a sizeable proportion of subtle third-trimester IUGR neonates may escape detection, particularly if population based, rather than customized, weight references are used.[43] An appreciation of the multiple manifestations of placental insufficiency provides the basis for the development of a uniform diagnostic approach to fetuses with suspected IUGR.

Fetal metabolic responses

In the setting of mild placental insufficiency, placental glucose and oxygen utilization initially remains unaffected, while fetal demands have to be met by increased fractional extraction. Only when uterine oxygen delivery falls below a critical value (0.6 mmol/min/kg fetal body weight in sheep} is fetal oxygen uptake and glucose transfer reduced.[44] When the levels of glucose transferred to the fetus fall, hypoglycemia ensues which results in a blunting of pancreatic insulin responses and allows gluconeogenesis from hepatic glycogen stores to begin.[45–48] A proportion of fetal glucose and lactate is then redirected to the placenta for nutrition. Since fetal hepatic glycogen stores are minimal, persistent, or progressive nutrient scarcity results in worsening fetal hypoglycemia. Subsequently, the ability to maintain fetal oxidative metabolism and placental nutrition becomes limited.

At this point, the downregulation of active placental transport mechanisms and the fetal need to recruit other energy sources, result in widespread metabolic responses. Limitation of amino acid transfer and breakdown of endogenous muscle protein to obtain gluconeogenic amino acids results in depletion of branched chain and other essential amino acids.[49–51]

Simultaneously, lactate accumulates due to the limited capacity for oxidative metabolism. The placental transfer capacity for fatty acids remains unaltered, unless there is a considerable loss of placental substance. However, despite maintaining the ability to transfer fatty acids, the selectivity of the transport mechanisms, especially for essential fatty acids, may decline. In the fetal circulation, free fatty acid and triglyceride levels increase secondary to reduced fetal utilization, which results in a failure to accumulate adipose stores. In this setting of advanced malnutrition, the liver metabolizes the majority of accumulating lactate. However, the fetal brain and heart can switch their primary nutrient source from glucose to lactate and ketones[52] – cardiac metabolism has the capacity to remove up to 80% of the circulating lactate.[53,54] Acid–base balance can be maintained as long as acid production is met by sufficient buffering capacity of fetal hemoglobin and a matching removal rate by these organs.

These increasing degrees of metabolic compromise have been documented through cordocentesis in human fetuses. Hypoglycemia and hypoxemia with decreased levels of essential amino acids occurs first. As the placental dysfunction worsens, progressive hypoxemia and increasing lactate production are exponentially correlated to the degree of acidemia. Overt hypoaminoacidemia, hypercapnia, hyperlacticemia, and triglyceridemia accompany the development of acidemia.[51,55–57]

Amniotic fluid elevation of the glycine/valine ratio and ammonia levels are additional indicators of this state of protein energy malnutrition (Table 90.1).[58,59] This degree of metabolic deterioration is associated with elevated transaminases as evidence of hepatic dysfunction, and may be precipitated by a significant decline of hepatic blood flow as a result of excessive shunting at the level of the ductus venosus.[60,61] Fetuses that manifest growth restriction early in gestation are more likely to have greater and broader metabolic derangements as compared to fetuses that manifest growth restriction in the third trimester which are more likely to have less severe metabolic and acid–base disturbance and only subtle changes in lipid metabolism.[62]

Fetal endocrine responses

The immediate effect of decreased fetal glucose and amino acid levels is the downregulation of the principal endocrine growth axis involving Insulin, IGF I, IGF II, and transforming factor beta.[63,64] This may be further exacerbated by pancreatic cellular dysfunction that is evident through a decreased insulin/glucose ratio and impaired fetal glucose tolerance.[51,65] Elevations in serum glucagon and stimulation of the fetal adrenal axis promote the mobilization of hepatic glycogen stores and peripheral gluconeogenesis.[66] Corticotropin releasing hormone (CRH), Adreonocorticotrophic hormone (ACTH) and cortisol levels are significantly elevated relating both to the level of hypoglycemia and the degree of placental vascular compromise.[51,67,68] However, elevations of cortisol downregulate IGF I activity and may therefore have additional negative impacts on linear growth as well as the potential to limit the capacity for postpartum catch-up growth.[69,70] In addition to the glucocorticoid axis, significant elevations of adrenaline and noradrenaline levels are also found in IUGR fetuses, while aldosterone levels appear unchanged.[71–73]

Disturbances at all stages of thyroid function have been documented in IUGR fetuses and correlate with the degree of hypoxemia.[74,75] Glandular dysfunction, as denoted by low levels of thyroxine and T3 despite elevated thyroid stimulating hormone (TSH) levels,

Table 90.1 Summary of metabolic responses to placental insufficiency

Substrate	Change
Glucose	Decreased proportional to the degree of fetal hypoxemia
Amino acids	Significant decrease in branched-chain amino acids (valine, leucine, isoleucine) as well as lysine and serine. In contrast hydroxyproline is elevated.The decrease in essential amino acids is proportional to the degree of hypoxemia
	Elevated amniotic fluid glycine to valine ratio
	Elevations in amniotic fluid ammonia with a significant positive correlation to the ponderal index
Fatty acids and triglycerides	Decrease in long-chain polyunsaturated fatty acids (docosahexanoic and arachidonic acid). Decrease in overall fatty acid transfer only with significant loss of placental substance
	Hypertriglyceridemia due to decreased utilization
	Lower cholesterol esters
Oxygen and CO_2	Degree of hypoxemia proportional to villous damage and correlates significantly with hypercapnia, acidemia, hypoglycemia and hyperlacticemia

may develop. In other cases, central production of TSH may be responsible for fetal hypothyroidism.[76] Finally, downregulation of thyroid hormone receptors may limit the biologic activity of circulating thyroid hormones in specific target tissues such as the developing brain.[77]

IUGR fetuses also show evidence of disturbed endocrine regulation of bone formation. Serum levels of active vitamin D and osteocalcin are appreciably decreased and may be responsible for decreased bone mineralization as well as decreased bone growth.[78,79]

Hematologic responses

Erythropoietin release and stimulation of RBC production, through both medullary and extramedullary sites, is triggered by fetal hypoxemia and results in polycythemia.[80–83] Extramedullary hematopoiesis may be physiologic until 28 weeks, but can occur in older fetuses by being induced by prolonged tissue hypoxemia and/or acidosis. Extramedullary sites have larger capillary fenestrations that permit the escape of large nucleated red blood cells (NRBC). Thus, elevated NRBC counts correlate with metabolic and cardiovascular status and are independent markers for poor perinatal outcome.[84–87] With advancing compromise complex hematologic abnormalities suggest dysfunctional erythropoiesis. Fetal anemia despite increased NRBC release in conjunction with an overt decrease in red cell progenitors could reflect downregulation of pro-erythropoietic cytokines, Vitamin B12, and ferritin deficiency or a combination of these.[88–91]

Coinciding with the abnormalities in red cell indices, platelet counts also decrease. Although platelet-activating factor is inhibited,[92] abnormal villous vasculature as indicated by umbilical artery absence or reversal of end-diastolic velocities (AREDV) may pose an overwhelming stimulus for placental platelet activation and aggregation.[93] Under these circumstances the incidence of thrombocytopenia increases 10-fold.[94] As the anemia and hypoxemia progress, they become independent risk factors for declining platelet counts.[95] Elevation of whole blood viscosity,[96,97] decrease in RBC membrane fluidity,[98] and platelet aggregation may be important cofactors for accelerating placental vascular occlusion and progressive dysfunction.

IUGR fetuses also show evidence of immune dysfunction at the cellular and humoral level. Decreases in immunoglobulin and absolute B-cell counts have long been recognized.[99] Reduction in total white blood cell counts and neutrophil, monocyte, and lymphocyte subpopulations occur.[100] Selective suppression of T-helper and cytotoxic T-cells has been observed.[101] The extent of these abnormalities is related to the degree of acidemia and can explain the greater susceptibility to infection these fetuses experience as neonates.

Fetal vascular responses

Doppler ultrasound allows the assessment of vascular effects of placental dysfunction in the maternal (uterine arteries) and fetal (umbilical arteries) compartments. The presence of an early diastolic notch in the uterine arteries at 12–14 weeks is the earliest evidence of delayed trophoblast invasion of the maternal spiral arteries.[102] When the 'notching' persists beyond 24 weeks of gestation, poor trophoblast invasion is almost certain.[38] These findings represent persistent elevated blood flow resistance in the maternal compartment, thus jeopardizing uterine perfusion. In the fetal circulation changes in blood flow are related to placental blood flow resistance, fetal oxygenation, organ autoregulation, and vascular reactivity. A reduction of umbilical venous blood flow volume may be the earliest Doppler sign of subtle decreases in fetal villous perfusion.[103] Abnormal villous branching or progressive villous vascular occlusion results in elevated blood flow resistance that is reflected in the umbilical artery waveform. A decrease of the umbilical artery end-diastolic velocity becomes apparent when approximately 30% of the fetal villous vasculature is abnormal.[104] AREDV can occur after 60–70% of the villous vascular tree is damaged.[105] Progression of Doppler abnormalities in the maternal compartment identifies patients at risk for pre-eclampsia, abruption and IUGR,[106] while abnormal umbilical flow indicate increased risk for hypoxemia and acidemia proportional to the severity of Doppler abnormality (Figures 90.3 and 90.4).[107,108]

Fetal circulatory responses to placental insufficiency can be subdivided into early and late responses corresponding to the degree of fetal compromise.[109,110] These circulatory responses are in part passive and due to the effects of placental afterload on the distribution of cardiac output and in part due to active organ autoregulation. Through modulations in ductus venosus shunting, umbilical venous blood increasingly bypasses the liver and is preferentially directed toward the heart. At the same time, elevated placental blood flow resistance increases right ventricular afterload. Because of the parallel arrangement of the fetal circulation, changes in cardiac afterload determine how this increased blood volume is distributed in the downstream circulation.[111–113] The result is a relative increase in left-sided cardiac output.[112,113] Consequently, blood (and nutrient) supply to the coronary circulation and brain increase. This redistribution of cardiac output can be documented by a decrease in the ratio of Doppler indices in cerebral and umbilical arteries (cerebroplacental Doppler ratio).[114] This redistribution is achieved in two principal ways. First of all, peripheral arterial vasoconstriction in the fetal trunk in conjunction with elevated placental blood flow resistance lead to elevations in thoracic and descending aortic Doppler resistance indices ('hind limb reflex') and therefore increased

(a)
(b)
(c)
(d)

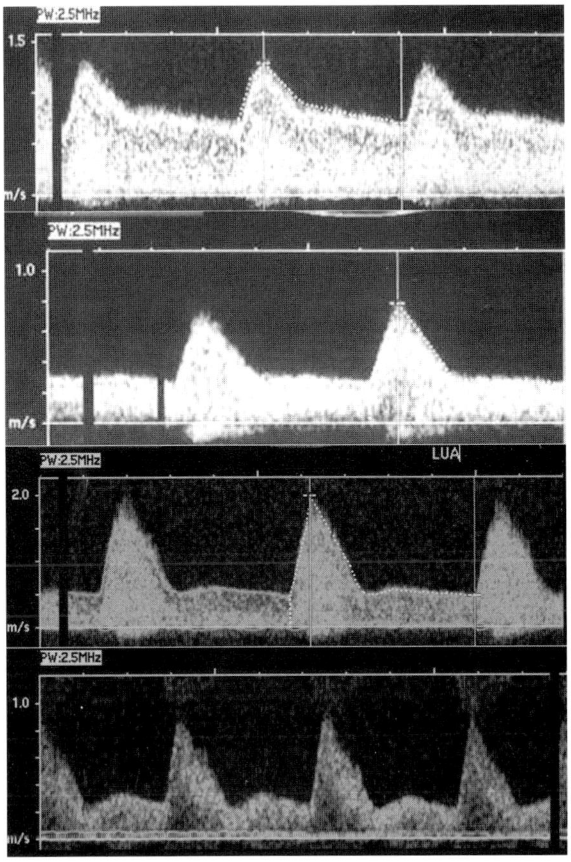

Figure 90.3 Flow velocity waveforms obtained from the uterine artery beyond 24 weeks gestation. In the first patient (a) high volume diastolic flow is established indicating successful trophoblast invasion. Elevated placental vascular resistance is associated with a decline in diastolic velocities and a subsequent rise in the Doppler index (b). Persistence of an early diastolic notch in the uterine artery flow velocity waveform is evidence of increased spiral artery blood flow resistance. Frequently, 'notching' is more subtle beyond 32 weeks (c) than in the late second or early third trimesters (d).

right ventricular afterload.[115,116] Next, cerebral blood flow may be actively enhanced during periods of perceived hypoxemia by a decrease in cerebral blood flow resistance with a subsequent decline in left ventricular afterload. This results in a decrease of the Doppler index in one of the cerebral vessels ('brain sparing) (Figure 90.5).[117,118] Fetuses that show these early Doppler changes are at increased risk for hypoxemia, while the pH is usually maintained in the normal range.[116,118,119] The shifting balance between right and left ventricular afterload accounts for the decline of the cerebroplacental Doppler index ratio and the measurable decline in end-diastolic velocities in the aortic isthmus.[120,121] At the same time, blood flow resistance in the peripheral pulmonary arteries,[122] celiac axis,[123] mesenteric vessels,[124,125] renal,[126,127] femoral and iliac arteries[128] may become elevated. Individual vital organs such as the adrenal glands[129] and spleen[130] may show evidence of enhanced blood flow. The overall impact of these changes is an improved distribution of well-oxygenated blood to the heart and brain with preferential streaming of descending aortic blood flow to the placenta for re-oxygenation (Table 90.2). These circulatory derangements are associated with elevations of endothelin, vasoactive intestinal peptide, vasopressin and renin–angiotensin levels.[131–133] A decrease of the thromboxane to prostacyclin ratio provides evidence of endothelial dysfunction, while elevations in NO production indicate a compensatory response.[134,135] It is likely that the degree of vascular reactivity is not only responsible for the high complication rate following invasive procedures, but also contributes to the clinical progression by impacting on blood flow resistance in many vascular beds.[136–139]

Late Doppler changes appear with further metabolic deterioration. Under these circumstances declining forward cardiac function, abnormal organ autoregulation, and ductus venosus shunting away from the liver occur. The shunting of flow away from the liver may compromise hepatic perfusion to a degree that interferes with organ function. In this condition, steep elevation in blood lactate and transaminases, as well as sudden compensatory hepatic artery vasodilatation have been reported.[60,61,140] When the increased metabolic demands of cardiac function cannot be met, myocardial dysfunction occurs. Declining cardiac function results in a failure to accommodate venous return and leads to increased venous Doppler indices indicating evidence of increased central venous pressure.[141] The venous flow velocity waveform is triphasic, and therefore more complex than the arterial waveform. It consists of systolic and diastolic peaks (the S- and D-waves) that are generated by the descent of the AV-ring during ventricular systole and passive diastolic ventricular filling, respectively. The sudden increase in right atrial pressure with atrial contraction in late diastole causes a variable amount of reverse flow producing a second trough after the D-wave (the a-wave) (Figure 90.6). In extreme cases, atrial pressure waves may be transmitted all the way back into the free umbilical vein resulting in pulsatile flow.

When venous Doppler indices become elevated, a significant rise in ANP occurs, probably as a compensatory mechanism to regulate blood volume.[142,143] When forward cardiac function declines significantly, coronary vasodilatation becomes exaggerated to recruit all the available coronary blood flow reserve.[144] If these adaptations fail to support myocardial nutrition sufficiently, the amount of cardiac dysfunction may become critical. Cardiac dilatation with holosystolic tricuspid regurgitation and loss of cerebral autoregulation (normalizing cerebral Doppler indices) are observed at this level of compromise and indicate loss of cardiovascular homeostasis.[145] Elevations of troponin I, S100B protein levels and transaminases provide evidence of cellular damage in the myocardium, brain, and liver.[146–148] An increased risk for necrotizing enterocolitis in survivors has been attributed to bowel injury secondary to chronic underperfusion.[149] If the

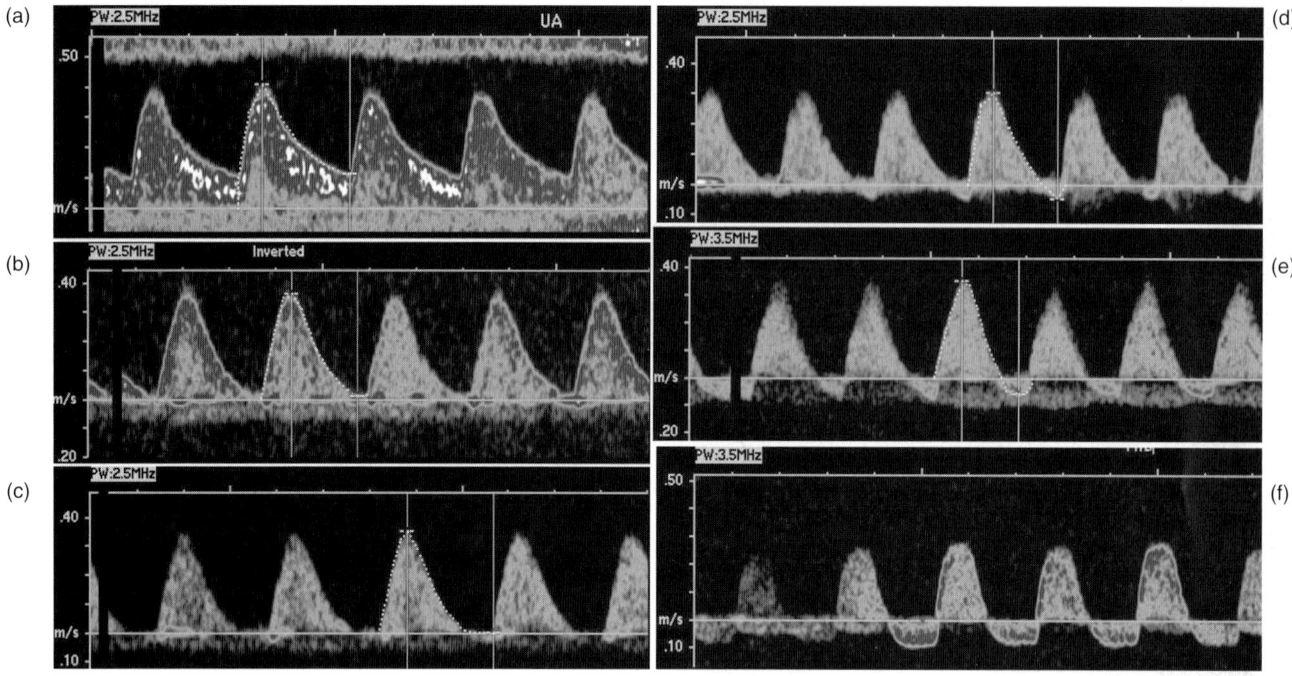

Figure 90.4 The normal umbilical artery flow velocity waveform has marked positive end-diastolic velocity that increases in proportion to systole towards term (a). Moderate abnormalities in the villous vascular structure raise the blood flow resistance and are associated with a decline in end-diastolic velocities (b). When a significant proportion of the villous vascular tree is abnormal (50–70%), end-diastolic velocities may be absent (c) or even reversed (d). Depending on the magnitude of placental blood flow resistance and the fetal cardiac function reversal of end-diastolic velocities may be minimal (d), moderate (e) or severe (f). In the latter case precordial venous flows were universally abnormal.

Table 90.2 Summary of fetal vascular responses to placental insufficiency

Response	Features	Doppler evidence
Hind limb reflex	Diversion of blood flow away from the carcass at the expense of the lower body. Achieved through increase in right ventricular afterload proximal to the umbilical arteries as well as increased blood flow resistance distally. In addition to centralization (see below) descending aortic blood flow is also preferentially distributed to the placenta	Elevation of blood flow resistance in the thoracic aorta and iliac artery
Centralization	A measurable shift in the relationship between right and left ventricular afterload, which results in redistribution of cardiac output in favor of the left ventricle (i.e., the heart and brain)	Decrease in the cerebroplacental Doppler ratio. Direct measurement of cardiac output. Reversal of end-diastolic velocity in the aortic isthmus. Inferred through absence or reversal of umbilical artery end-diastolic velocity
Brain sparing	Cerebral vasodilatation in response to perceived hypoxemia	Decrease in the carotid-, or middle cerebral artery Doppler index
Liver sparing	Preferential arterial blood supply to the fetal liver invoked when increased diversion of umbilical venous blood through the ductus venosus jeopardizes hepatic perfusion	Measured dilation of the ductus venosus with elevated Doppler index accompanied by a decreased hepatic artery Doppler index
Adrenal sparing	Enhanced adrenal perfusion is triggered as part of the fetal stress response to chronic or acute-on-chronic malnutrition	Decreased Doppler index in the adrenal artery flow velocity waveforms
Heart sparing	Marked augmentation of coronary blood flow in situations of acute on chronic hypoxemia that is achieved through upregulation of coronary vascular reserve and vasodilatation	Sudden ability to visualize and measure coronary blood flow in a setting of deteriorating venous Doppler indices in a premature IUGR fetus

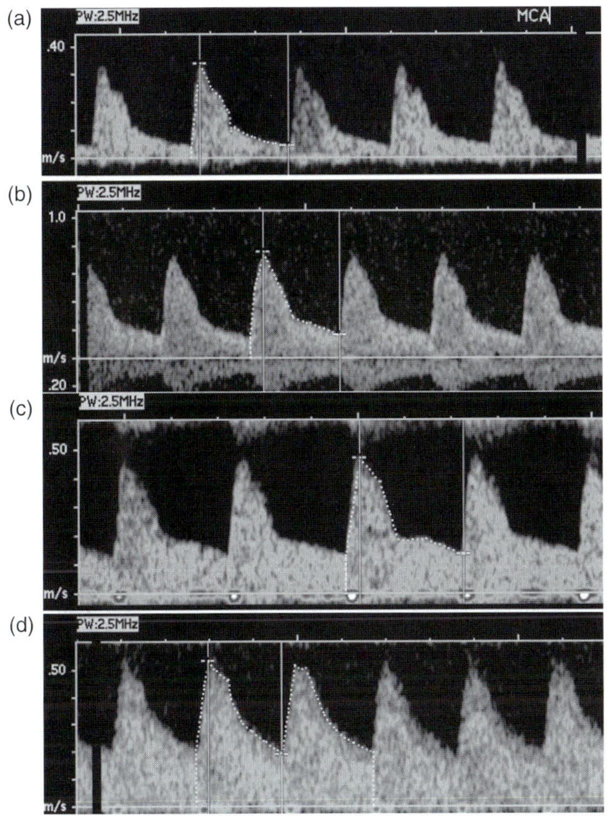

Figure 90.5 The normal middle cerebral artery flow pattern has relatively little diastolic flow (a). With elevation of placental blood flow resistance the changes in the middle cerebral artery waveform may be subtle, although the cerebroplacental ratio may become abnormal (b). With progressive placental dysfunction there may be increase in the diastolic velocity resulting in a decrease in the Doppler index (brain sparing, c). With marked brain sparing the systolic down slope of the waveform becomes smoother so that the waveform almost resembles that of the umbilical artery (d). The associated rise in the mean velocity results in a marked decline in the Doppler index.

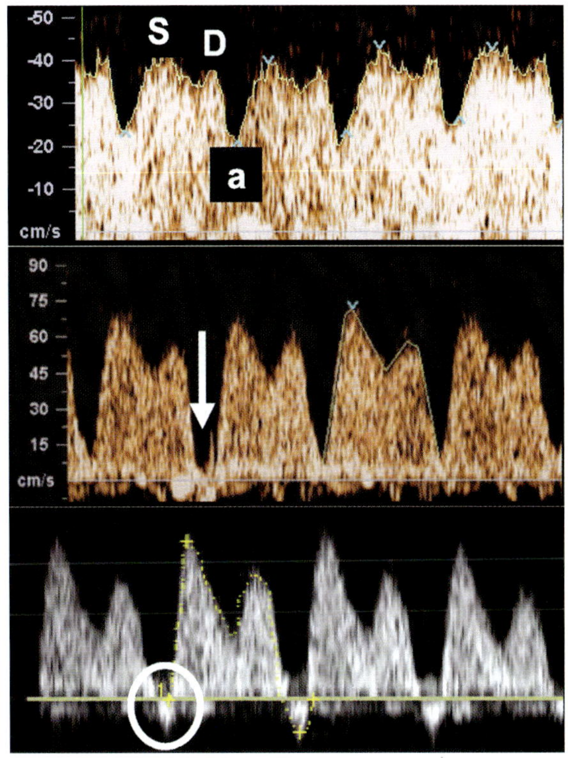

Figure 90.6 (Top panel) In the venous Doppler waveform systolic and diastolic peaks (the S- and D-waves) are generated by the descent of the AV-ring during ventricular systole and passive diastolic ventricular filling, respectively. A second late diastolic trough after the D-wave is the consequence of sharply increasing right atrial pressures during atrial systole (the a-wave). (Middle panel) With declining forward cardiac function forward velocity during atrial systole (arrow) and to a lesser degree during diastole decreased. This is associated with an increase in venous Doppler indices. (Bottom panel) When ductus venosus Doppler indices escalate, absence or reversal of forward flow during atrial systole (circle) may be observed as the most marked Doppler abnormality.

fetus remains undelivered, spontaneous late decelerations of the fetal heart rate and stillbirth ensue.[150,151]

Fetal biophysical responses

Normal fetal behavioral development proceeds sequentially with the appearance of movement, coupling, cycling of behavior, and finally the integration of movement patterns into stable behavioral states. Autonomic reflexes originating from the brainstem are superimposed on intrinsic cardiac activity and determine fetal heart rate characteristics. As gestation advances, the interaction between the nervous system and the heart becomes more refined and is modulated by ambient oxygen tension, signals from higher brain centers and the reticular activating system as well as peripheral sensory inputs. Successful maturation of these connections is reflected by decreasing baseline heart rate, increasing heart rate variability and variation, coupling of episodic accelerations with fetal movement and the superimposed impact of behavioral states. This level of central integration of fetal heart rate characteristics with fetal behavior is normally accomplished by 28 weeks of gestation.[152]

IUGR fetuses with chronic hypoxemia exhibit a delay in all aspects of central nervous system (CNS) maturation which probably relates to altered myelination as well as changes in central neurotransmitter availability.[153–157] The delayed development of behavioral milestones and their central integration with the fetal heart rate are primary determinants of lower short- and long-term variation (on computerized analysis), delayed decline in heart rate baseline and delayed development of heart rate reactivity in IUGR fetuses.[158–162] Despite the maturational delay of some aspects of CNS function, several centrally regulated responses to acid-base status are preserved.

Once fetal hypoxemia is perceived, a decline in global fetal activity precedes the loss of individual biophysical variables and is often also accompanied by a gradual decline in amniotic fluid volume.[163,164]

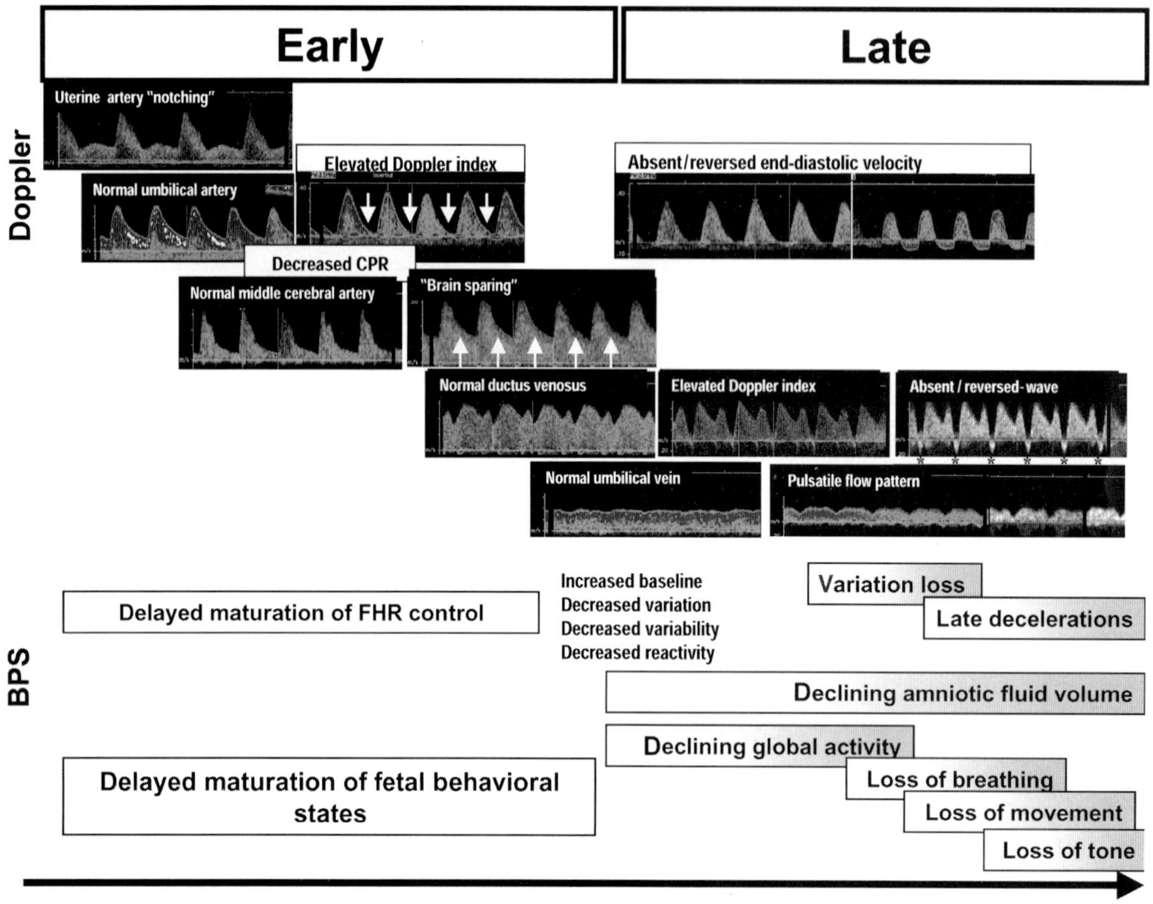

Figure 90.7 This figure summarizes the early and late responses to placental insufficiency. Doppler variables in the placental circulation precede abnormality in the cerebral circulation. Biophysical parameters (BPS) are still normal at this time and computerized analysis of fetal behavioral patterns is necessary to document a developmental delay. With progression to late responses venous Doppler abnormality in the fetal circulation is characteristic often preceding the sequential loss of fetal dynamic variables and frequently accompanying the decline in amniotic fluid volume. The * in the ductus venosus flow velocity waveform marks reversal of blood flow during atrial systole (a-wave). The decline in biophysical variables shows a reproducible relationship with acid base status. If adaptation mechanisms fail stillbirth ensues.

With increasing hypoxemia, fetal breathing movement ceases. Gross body movements and tone decrease further and are lost as acidemia deepens.[165] Abnormal fetal heart rate patterns are generally also observed at this time (Figure 90.7).[166,167] The effects of hypoxemia and vascular status on renal perfusion and fetal urine production affect amniotic fluid volume. As progressive deterioration of acid–base and vascular status occurs; a progressive decline in amniotic fluid volume is observed. The decline of these biophysical variables is determined by the central effects of hypoxemia/acidemia independent of the cardiovascular status.[168–171]

The biophysical profile score (BPS) as a composite score applies categorical cut-offs for fetal tone, breathing movement, gross body movement, amniotic fluid volume as well as traditional fetal heart rate analysis. Although a gradual decline in all of these parameters precedes an overtly abnormal BPS, analysis of the percentage change in these variables offers no advantage in the prediction of academia.[163] The five-component BPS shows a reliable and reproducible relationship with the fetal pH irrespective of the underlying pathology and gestational age.[166,172] Concurrent evaluation of fetal cardiovascular and biophysical variables indicates that Doppler deterioration precedes an abnormal BPS in the majority of IUGR fetuses.[164] When the relationship between the various testing modalities and fetal acid–base status is compared, biophysical parameters show a closer relationship with the pH while Doppler parameters have a wider variance (Figure 90.8).

An integrated approach to diagnosis and management of fetal growth restriction

The many etiologies and presentations of fetal growth restriction require a diagnostic approach that integrates information from several diagnostic modalities. Only a complete evaluation of the maternal history and the fetal, placental, and amniotic fluid characteristics can

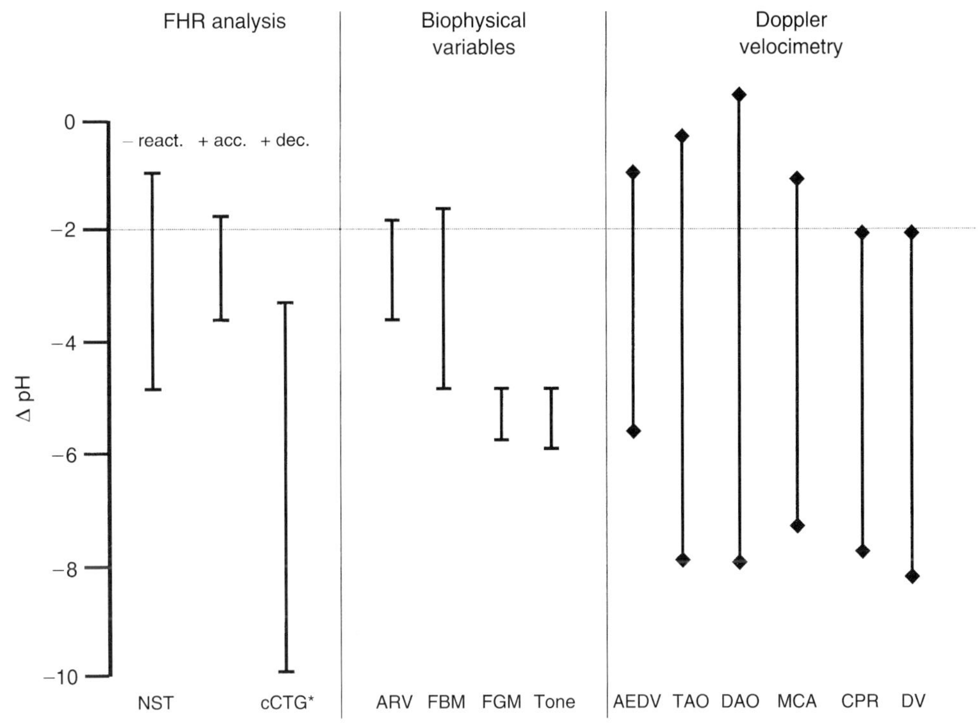

Figure 90.8 This figure displays a diagrammatic representation of pH deviation from the gestational age mean (ΔpH) with abnormal test results in various antenatal tests. These include fetal heart rate (FHR) analysis using traditional nonstress testing (NST, – react = nonreactive) and the computerized cardiotocogram (cCTG, +acc = accelerations present, +dec = obvious decelerations present). Biophysical variables (AFV, amniotic fluid volume; FBM, fetal body movement; FGM, fetal gross movement). The same relationships are expressed for umbilical artery absent end-diastolic velocity (AEDV) and deviation of the arterial or venous Doppler index > 2SD from the gestational age mean for the thoracic aorta (TAO), descending aorta (DAO) the middle cerebral artery (MCA), cerebroplacental ratio (CPR) and the ductus venosus (DV). Reproduced from Baschat[120] with permission.

direct an appropriate diagnostic workup and perinatal management. The accurate identification of fetuses that are truly at risk for adverse outcome requires exclusion of small fetuses that are normally grown and those in whom IUGR is due to an underlying condition not amenable to intervention. Conditions such as aneuploidy (especially trisomy 18, 13, and 21), skeletal dysplasia, nonaneuploid syndromes and viral infections should always be placed high on the list of differential diagnoses. Gray-scale ultrasound is the primary diagnostic tool allowing for a detailed fetal anatomic survey, biometric assessment of fetal growth, assessment of amniotic fluid volume and placental appearance. Although ultrasound provides important clues to the presence of IUGR the liability of preterm delivery and iatrogenic complications is large if the diagnosis and management is based only on biometry.[173] It is the complementary use of fetal biometry and Doppler assessment which creates the best available tool for the identification of small fetuses who are at risk for adverse outcome due to placental insufficiency.[174–177]

A detailed anatomic survey is mandatory in any fetus with suspected IUGR. Critical evaluation for aneuploidy markers such as echogenic bowel, nuchal thickening, abnormal hand positioning is necessary. Important anomalies that are associated with IUGR include gastroschisis, omphalocele, diaphragmatic hernia, and congenital heart defects. Assessment of the thoracic shape may suggest the presence of a skeletal dysplasia. Markers for viral infection are nonspecific, but may include echogenicity and calcification in organs such as the brain and liver. Occasionally, hydrops may be present.[178] The amniotic fluid volume should be assessed at the same time as the fetal anatomic survey. The regulation of amniotic fluid volume is complex, but by the third trimester primarily dependent on fetal urine production. Placental dysfunction and fetal hypoxemia both may cause fetal oliguria and consequently oligohydramnios. However, the accuracy of ultrasound in the assessment of amniotic fluid volume is poor[179] and serves as a poor screening tool for the prediction of IUGR and fetal acidosis.[180,181] Nonetheless, assessment of amniotic fluid volume by any method such as the four quadrant amniotic fluid index (AFI) and maximum vertical pocket), especially if performed serially, provides an important diagnostic as well as prognostic tool. In the setting of small fetal size, abundant amniotic fluid volume is an indicator of aneuploidy or fetal infection while normal or decreased amniotic fluid is more compatible with placental insufficiency.

The actual quantification of growth is based on fetal biometry. Since almost all fetal measurements change with gestation, an accurate assessment of gestational age is a prerequisite for the calculation of percentile ranks of absolute measurements. An estimated date of confinement (EDC) is ideally based on a sure last menstrual period when the sonographic estimate of gestational age is within the predictive error (7 days in the first and 14 days in the second trimester, and 21 days in the third trimester). Once the EDC is set by this method or a first-trimester ultrasound, it should not be changed. Later adjustments to the EDC will interfere with the ability to diagnose fetal growth abnormalities. Once the EDC has been assigned, selection of appropriate reference ranges that are based on uncomplicated pregnancies delivered at term is of importance. Individualized reference ranges of growth potential that account for maternal, ethnic, and fetal variables provide the most accurate reference.[1,182] Once gestational age is assigned, the interpretation of the ultrasound examination is based on the fetal anatomic survey, amniotic fluid volume, percentile rank of fetal size measurements, the interval growth since the last study, and a functional assessment of the feto-placental unit with Doppler ultrasound.

Of all fetal biometric measurements the abdominal circumference (AC) is related to the liver size as a major indicator of fetal glycogen storage and therefore the single best measurement with the highest sensitivity and negative predictive value for the detection of IUGR.[183–185] Its sensitivity is further enhanced by serial measurements at least 14 days apart.[186] The most accurate AC is the smallest directly measured circumference obtained at the level of the hepatic vein between fetal respirations.[187] Using a reference range based on healthy women delivering appropriately nourished neonates at term, an AC <10th percentile for gestational age is consistent with IUGR. If cross-sectional population references including small, appropriately grown, preterm and term newborns are used the 2.5th percentile is more appropriate.[188] Compared to the AC, the biparietal diameter, head circumference (HC) and transverse cerebellar diameters are poor tools for the detection of IUGR. This is in part due to the inherent physiologic variation in skull shape[189] and the relative sparing of the head growth and therefore delayed manifestation of placental insufficiency.[190] Ratios of fetal measurements do not improve the detection of growth delay, but may be helpful pointers towards underlying aneuploidy.[191–193] Concurrent measurement of the HC, AC, and femur length allows calculation of the sonographically estimated fetal weight (SEFW). An SEFW below the 10th percentile for gestational age has a lower sensitivity than the AC (85% vs. 98%) but a higher positive predictive value (51% vs. 36%).[185]

The next step in the diagnostic assessment of the suspected IUGR fetus is the evaluation of feto-placental vascular function. Randomized trials and meta-analyses confirm that the use of umbilical artery Doppler in suspected IUGR results in a significant reduction in perinatal mortality and iatrogenic intervention since documentation of placental vascular insufficiency effectively separates constitutionally small fetuses from those in need for surveillance and possible intervention.[194–196] A more complete assessment of feto-placental vascular status can be achieved if the uterine and middle cerebral arteries are examined in addition to the umbilical artery. For qualitative waveform analysis presence of uterine artery notching and umbilical artery end-diastolic velocity (positive, absent, or reversed) should be noted. For clinical Doppler waveform analysis angle independent indices are used. Of these, the pulsatility index offers the advantage of a smaller measurement error, narrower reference limits and the possibility for ongoing numerical analysis even when end-diastolic velocity is absent.[197,198] In fetuses presenting with IUGR due to placental insufficiency before 34 weeks' gestation the umbilical artery Doppler waveform is frequently abnormal. Beyond this gestational age the umbilical artery Doppler waveform may be normal. At the same time cerebral artery Doppler responses to placental insufficiency still occur.[176,199] Therefore the middle cerebral–umbilical artery Doppler ratio (cerebroplacental ratio) may be abnormal in fetuses with mild placental disease.[174,200] Beyond 34 weeks' gestation a decrease in the middle cerebral artery Doppler index or the cerebroplacental ratio should therefore heighten suspicion for IUGR even if the umbilical artery blood flow is normal (Figure 90.9).

Once the suspicion of IUGR is confirmed, fetal karyotyping should be offered and further specialized tests such as maternal serology (TORCH), thrombophilia studies, or amniotic fluid viral DNA testing, may be indicated. Once nontreatable underlying fetal conditions and chromosome abnormalities have been ruled out further antenatal surveillance should be instituted based on the severity of the maternal and/or fetal condition.

An integrated approach to surveillance in fetal growth restriction

Antenatal surveillance in IUGR gestations aims to provide longitudinal assessment that is tailored to the severity of the fetal condition and is predictive of critical outcomes. Since there are no effective therapies for *in utero* treatment of IUGR, management options include increasing the frequency of monitoring and delivery when fetal testing suggests that the intrauterine risks exceed neonatal risks of adverse outcomes. It is increasingly becoming apparent that IUGR fetuses are at particularly high risk for prematurity related complications and adverse outcomes, especially below 32 weeks' gestation.[4,201] Therefore the delivery threshold is highest between viability and 32 weeks, placing the greatest demands on the precision of fetal assessment. This requirement for detailed assessment

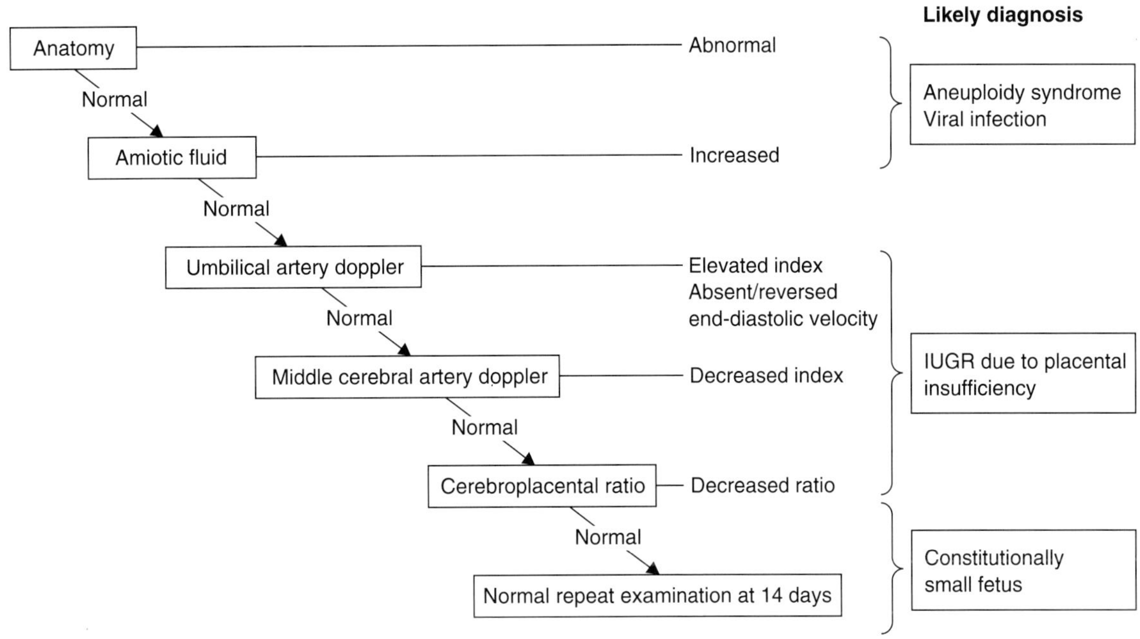

Figure 90.9 This figure displays a decision tree following the evaluation of fetal anatomy, amniotic fluid volume, umbilical and middle cerebral artery Doppler. The most likely clinical diagnosis is presented on the right hand side. A high index of suspicion for aneuploidy, viral and nonaneuploid syndrome needs to be maintained. IUGR, intrauterine growth restriction.

is offset by the need for practicability in order to facilitate generalized application. Utilizing knowledge about the fetal responses to placental insufficiency and the limitations of antenatal testing modalities helps formulate an appropriate monitoring approach to IUGR fetuses at highest risk. In this context several principles are important.

In pregnancies that present with IUGR prior to 34 weeks' gestation, umbilical artery blood flow changes usually precede other cardiovascular responses.[200,202] Once the diagnosis of IUGR has been made by biometry and Doppler evaluation, continuing surveillance for deterioration of fetal cardiovascular status requires examination of the cerebral circulation and the precordial veins. When brain sparing develops, venous Doppler indices are frequently normal and biophysical abnormalities are generally not clinically observed. Development of abnormal venous Doppler indices indicates an acceleration of the deterioration.[203,204] At this time, abnormalities in biophysical parameters become clinically apparent. However, since the BPS is a composite of five variables the overall result may deteriorate relatively late in the disease process.[164] When Doppler and biophysical parameters show abnormalities, the information gained through their concurrent evaluation is complementary and offers the best prediction of fetal status and outcome.[119]

Taking these principles into account, a surveillance approach to pregnancies with IUGR due to placental disease that combines Doppler ultrasound and biophysical profile scoring (integrated fetal testing) has been devised. The testing is always supplemented with maternal assessment of fetal movement ('kick counts'). Doppler examination includes evaluation of the umbilical artery, middle cerebral artery, ductus venosus, and free umbilical vein flow velocity waveform. The traditional nonstress test component of the BPS is supplemented by computerized fetal heart rate analysis. Monitoring frequencies are adjusted to the fetal condition. Before 28 weeks, fetuses with isolated elevation of the umbilical artery Doppler index are followed with weekly biophysical profile scoring and repeat Doppler every fortnight. If umbilical artery end-diastolic velocity disappears, MCA Doppler meets criteria for centralization or amniotic fluid volume declines all testing (Doppler and biophysical profile score) are repeated every 3–4 days. In patients with elevated ductus venous Doppler index with umbilical venous pulsations complete testing is repeated every 24 h (Figure 90.10).

The issue of optimal delivery timing for IUGR fetuses remains unresolved. In principle the decision for delivery always weighs fetal vs. neonatal intensive care unit (NICU) risks. Typically, decline in neonatal mortality is greatest between 24 and 28 weeks while morbidity declines progressively thereafter towards 32 weeks.[201] Perinatal mortality and morbidity is greatest among IUGR fetuses with abnormal venous Doppler indices irrespective of the umbilical artery Doppler waveform.[201,203] Therefore, basing delivery decision on the umbilical artery waveform alone appears no longer appropriate.[205] In preterm IUGR fetuses, we consider abnormal venous Doppler indices and/or and abnormal BPS as indicators for delivery. Beyond 34 weeks where the frequency of dramatically abnormal Doppler is lower reliance on BPS and obstetrical factors should guide delivery.

IUGR unlikely		
Normal AC, AC growth rate and HC/AC ratio UA, MCA Doppler, BPS and AFV normal	Asphyxia extremely rare Low risk for intrapartum distress	Deliver for obstetric, or maternal factors only, follow growth

IUGR		
AC<5th, low AC growth rate, high HC/AC ratio abnormal UA +/ or CPR; normal MCA and venous Doppler, BPS ≥ 8/10, AFV normal	Asphyxia extremely rare Increased risk for intrapartum distress	Deliver for obstetric, or maternal factors only, fortnightly Doppler Weekly BPS
With blood flow redistribution		
IUGR diagnosed based on above criteria, low MCA, normal venous Doppler, BPS ≥ 8/10, AFV normal	Hypoxemia possible, asphyxia rare Increased risk for intrapartum distress	Deliver for obstetric, or maternal factors only, weekly Doppler BPS 2 times per week
With significant blood flow redistribution		
UA A/REDV, normal venous Doppler, BPS ≥ 6/10, oligohydramnios	Hypoxemia common, acidemia or asphyxia possible Onset of fetal compromise	>34 weeks: deliver 32-34 weeks: consider delivery <32 weeks: antenatal steroids repeat all testing daily
With proven fetal compromise		
Significant redistribution present Increased DV pulsatility BPS ≥ 6/10, oligohydramnios	Hypoxemia common, acidemia or asphyxia likely	>32 weeks: deliver <32 weeks: admit, steroids, individualize testing daily vs. tid.
With fetal decompensation		
Compromise by above criteria Absent or reversed DV a-wave, pulsatile UV BPS < 6/10, oligohydramnios	Cardiovascular instability, metabolic compromise, stillbirth imminent, high perinatal mortality irrespective of intervention	Deliver at tertiary care center with the highest level of NICU care

Figure 90.10 The management algorithm for pregnancies complicated by fetal growth restriction is based on the ability to perform arterial and venous Doppler as well as a full five component biophysical profile score. AC, abdominal circumference; AFV, amniotic fluid volume; A/REDV, absent/reversed end-diastolic velocity; BPS, biophysical profile score; CPR, cerebroplacental ratio; DV, ductus venosus; HC, head circumference; MCA, middle cerebral artery; NST, nonstress test; NICU, neonatal intensive care unit; tid, three times daily, UA, umbilical artery.

Since the outlined surveillance approach requires multivessel Doppler as well as biophysical profile scoring it can only be performed at centers that are familiar with both techniques. Modifications of this surveillance protocol should address the limitations of such an approach. For example, the BPS alone offers little in the prediction of longitudinal progression. Thus, if biophysical profile scoring is the only surveillance tool, daily testing may be required to assure a good outcome.[206]

Further investigation and evaluation of nutritional, metabolic, endocrine, and hematologic responses at birth in growth restricted neonates and their relationship to fetal proportions, Doppler and behavioral parameters will refine our understanding of this condition. Neonatal management will become optimal when knowledge of the fetal status and an appreciation of the spectrum of fetal consequences of placental insufficiency are integrated to guide their evaluation and management. A uniform prenatal diagnostic standard and a comprehensive integrated management approach that bridges fetal and neonatal periods is most likely to impact on adult health focusing on the small fetus at risk and sparing normally developed babies from iatrogenic interventions.

REFERENCES

1. Gardosi J, Chang A, Kalyan B, *et al.* Customised antenatal growth charts. *Lancet* 1992;339:283–7.
2. Lubchenco LO, Hansman C, Boyd E. Intrauterine growth as estimated from live born birth-weight data at 24–42 weeks of gestation. *Pediatrics* 1963;32:793.
3. Battaglia FC, Lubchenco LO. A practical classification of newborn infants by weight and gestational age. *J Pediatr* 1967;71:159–63.
4. Bernstein IM, Horbar JD, Badger GJ, *et al.* Morbidity and mortality among very-low-birth-weight neonates with intrauterine growth restriction. The Vermont Oxford Network. *Am J Obstet Gynecol* 2000;182:198–206.
5. Schreuder AM, McDonnell M, Gaffney G, *et al.* Outcome at school age following antenatal detection of absent or reversed end diastolic flow velocity in the umbilical artery. *Arch Dis Child Fetal Neonatal Ed* 2002;86:F108–14.
6. Barker DJ. Fetal growth and adult disease. *Br J Obstet Gynaecol* 1992;99:275–6.
7. Aplin J. Maternal influences on placental development. *Semin Cell Dev Biol* 2000;11:115–25.
8. Pardi G, Marconi AM, Cetin I. Placental–fetal interrelationship in IUGR fetuses – A review. *Placenta* 2002;23(Suppl A): S136–41.

9. Kaufmann P, Scheffen I. Placental development. In Polin RA, Fox WW, eds. *Fetal and Neonatal Physiology*. Philadelphia, PA: WB Saunders, 1998:59–70.
10. Cunningham FG, Gant NF, Leveno KJ, Gilstrap LC, Hauth JC, Wenstrom KD (eds). Maternal adaptation to pregnancy. *Williams Obstetrics*. New York: McGraw Hill, 2001:167–200.
11. Kingdom JC, Burrell SJ, Kaufmann P. Pathology and clinical implications of abnormal umbilical artery Doppler waveforms. *Ultrasound Obstet Gynecol* 1997;9:271–86.
12. Pijnenborg R, Bland JM, Robertson WB, Brosens I. Uteroplacental arterial changes related to interstitial trophoblast migration in early human pregnancy. *Placenta* 1983;4:397–413.
13. Castellucci M, Kosanke G, Verdenelli F, Huppertz B, Kaufmann P. Villous sprouting: fundamental mechanisms of human placental development. *Hum Reprod Update* 2000;6:485–94.
14. Maini CL, Rosati P, Galli G, Bellati U, Bonetti MG, Moneta E. Non-invasive radioisotopic evaluation of placental blood flow. *Gynecol Obstet Invest* 1985;19:196–206.
15. Luckhardt M, Leiser R, Kingdom J, Malek A, Sager R, Kaisig C, Schneider H. Effect of physiologic perfusion-fixation on the morphometrically evaluated dimensions of the term placental cotyledon. *J Soc Gynecol Invest* 1996;3:166–71.
16. Meschia G. Placenta respiratory gas exchange and fetal oxygenation. In Creasy RK, Resnik R, eds. *Maternal Fetal Medicine: Principles and Practice*, 1st edn. Philadelphia, PA: WB Saunders, 1987:274–85.
17. Meschia G, Battaglia FC, Hay WW, Sparks JW. Utilization of substrates by the ovine placenta in vivo. *Fed Proc* 1980;39:245–9.
18. Carter AM. Placental oxygen consumption. Part I: In vivo studies – A review. *Placenta* 2000;21:S31–7.
19. Battaglia FC, Regnault TR. Placental transport and metabolism of amino acids. *Placenta* 2001;22:145–61.
20. Haggarty P. Placental regulation of fatty acid delivery and its effects on fetal growth – A review. *Placenta* 2002;23:S28–38.
21. Illsely NP. Glucose transporters in the human placenta. *Placenta* 2000;21:14–22.
22. Sibley CP, Glazier JD, Greenwood SL, *et al.* Regulation of placental transfer: The Na(+)/H(+) exchanger – A review. *Placenta* 2002; 23:S39–46.
23. Reece EA, Wiznitzer A, Le E, Homko CJ, Behrman H, Spencer EM. The relation between human fetal growth and fetal blood levels of insulin-like growth factors I and II, their binding proteins, and receptors. *Obstet Gynecol* 1994;84:88–95.
24. Hoggard N, Haggarty P, Thomas L, Lea RG. Leptin expression in placental and fetal tissues: does leptin have a functional role? *Biochem Soc Trans* 2001;29:57–66.
25. Jansson N, Greenwood SL, Johansson BR, Powell TL, Jansson T. Leptin stimulates the activity of the system A amino acid transporter in human placental villous fragments. *J Clin Endocrinol Metab* 2003;88:1205–11.
26. Kiserud T. The ductus venosus. *Semin Perinatol* 2001;25:11–20.
27. Rudolph AM. Distribution and regulation of blood flow in the fetal and neonatal lamb. *Circ Res* 1985;57:811–21.
28. Guyton AC, Cowley AW Jr, Young DB, Coleman TG, Hall JE, DeClue JW. Integration and control of circulatory function. *Int Rev Physiol* 1976;9:341–85.
29. Bonds DR, Mwape B, Kumar S, Gabbe SG. Human fetal weight and placental weight growth curves. A mathematical analysis from a population at sea level. *Biol Neonate* 1984;45(6):261–74.
30. Molteni RA, Stys SJ, Battaglia FC. Relationship of fetal and placental weight in human beings: Fetal/placental weight ratios at various gestational ages and birth weight distributions. *J Reprod Med* 1978;21:327–34.
31. Heinonen S, Taipale P, Saarikoski S. Weights of placentae from small-for-gestational age infants revisited. *Placenta* 2001;22: 399–404.
32. Herrera E, Amusquivar E. Lipid metabolism in the fetus and the newborn. *Diabetes Metab Res Rev* 2000;16:202–10.
33. Sparks JW, Girard JR, Battaglia FC. An estimate of the caloric requirements of the human fetus. *Biol Neonate* 1980;38(3–4): 113–19.
34. White DR, Widdowson EM, Woodard HQ, Dickerson JW. The composition of body tissues (II). Fetus to young adult. *Br J Radiol* 1991;64:149–59.
35. Ziegler EE, O'Donnell AM, Nelson SE, Fomon SJ. Body composition of the reference fetus. *Growth* 1976;40:329–41.
36. Kingdom J, Huppertz B, Seaward G, Kaufmann P. Development of the placental villous tree and its consequences for fetal growth. *Eur J Obstet Gynecol Reprod Biol* 2000;92:35–43.
37. Brosens I, Dixon HG, Robertson WB. Fetal growth retardation and the arteries of the placental bed. *Br J Obstet Gynaecol* 1977; 84:656–63.
38. Meekins JW, Pijnenborg R, Hanssens M, *et al.* A study of placental bed spiral arteries and trophoblast invasion in normal and severe pre-eclamptic pregnancies. *Br J Obstet Gynaecol* 1994; 101:669–74.
39. Sebire NJ, Talbert D. The role of intraplacental vascular smooth muscle in the dynamic placenta: a conceptual framework for understanding uteroplacental disease. *Med Hypotheses* 2002;58: 347–51.
40. Aardema MW, Oosterhof H, Timmer A, *et al.* Uterine artery Doppler flow and uteroplacental vascular pathology in normal pregnancies and pregnancies complicated by pre-eclampsia and small for gestational age fetuses. *Placenta* 2001;22:405–11.
41. Ferrazzi E, Bulfamante G, Mezzopane R, *et al.* Uterine Doppler velocimetry and placental hypoxic-ischaemic lesion in pregnancies with fetal intrauterine growth restriction. *Placenta* 1999;20: 389–94.
42. Kingdom JC, McQueen J, Connell JM, *et al.* Fetal angiotensin II levels and vascular (type I) angiotensin receptors in pregnancies complicated by intrauterine growth retardation. *Br J Obstet Gynaecol* 1993;100:476–82.
43. Clausson B, Gardosi J, Francis A, Cnattingius S. Perinatal outcome in SGA births defined by customized versus population-based birthweight standards. *Br J Obstet Gynaecol* 2001;108:830–4.
44. Jones CT, Ritchie JW, Walker D. The effects of hypoxia on glucose turnover in the fetal sheep. *J Dev Physiol* 1983;5:223–35.
45. Nicolini U, Hubinont C, Santolaya J, Fisk NM, Coe AM, Rodeck CH. Maternal–fetal glucose gradient in normal pregnancies and in pregnancies complicated by alloimmunization and fetal growth retardation. *Am J Obstet Gynecol* 1989;161:924–7.
46. Economides DL, Nicolaides KH. Blood glucose and oxygen tension levels in small-for-gestational-age fetuses. *Am J Obstet Gynecol* 1989;160:385–9.
47. Hubinont C, Nicolini U, Fisk NM, Tannirandorn Y, Rodeck CH. Endocrine pancreatic function in growth-retarded fetuses. *Obstet Gynecol* 1991;77:541–4.
48. Van Assche FA, Aerts L, DePrins FA. The fetal endocrine pancreas. *Eur J Obstet Gynecol Reprod Biol* 1984;18:267–72.
49. Cetin I, Marconi AM, Corbetta C, *et al.* Fetal amino acids in normal pregnancies and in pregnancies complicated by intrauterine growth retardation. *Early Hum Dev* 1992;29:183–6.
50. Cetin I, Corbetta C, Sereni LP, *et al.* Umbilical amino acid concentrations in normal and growth-retarded fetuses sampled in utero by cordocentesis. *Am J Obstet Gynecol* 1990;162:253–61.
51. Economides DL, Nicolaides KH, Campbell S. Metabolic and endocrine findings in appropriate and small for gestational age fetuses. *J Perinat Med* 1991;19:97–105.
52. Vannucci RC, Vannucci SJ. Glucose metabolism in the developing brain. *Semin Perinatol* 2000;24:107–15.
53. Fisher DJ, Heymann MA, Rudolph AM. Fetal myocardial oxygen and carbohydrate consumption during acutely induced hypoxemia. *Am J Physiol* 1982;242:H657–61.
54. Spahr R, Probst I, Piper HM. Substrate utilization of adult cardiac myocytes. *Basic Res Cardiol* 1985;80 (Suppl 1):53–6.
55. Soothill PW, Nicolaides KH, Campbell S. Prenatal asphyxia, hyperlacticaemia, hypoglycemia, and erythroblastosis in growth retarded fetuses. *Br Med J* 1987;294:1051–3.
56. Owens JA, Falconer J, Robinsin JS. Effect of restriction of placental growth on fetal uteroplacental metabolism. *J Dev Physiol* 1987;9:225–38.
57. Paolini CL, Marconi AM, Ronzoni S, *et al.* Placental transport of leucine, phenylalanine, glycine, and proline in intrauterine growth-restricted pregnancies. *J Clin Endocrinol Metab* 2001;86: 5427–32.
58. Wolfe HM, Sokol RJ, Dombrowski MP, Bottoms SF, Norman GS. Increased neonatal urinary ammonia: A marker for in utero caloric deprivation? *Am J Perinatol* 1989;6:4–7.
59. Bernstein IM, Silver R, Nair KS, Stirewalt WS. Amniotic fluid glycine–valine ratio and neonatal morbidity in fetal growth restriction. *Obstet Gynecol* 1997;90:933–7.
60. Roberts A, Nava S, Bocconi L, Salmona S, Nicolini U. Liver function tests and glucose and lipid metabolism in growth-restricted fetuses. *Obstet Gynecol* 1999;94:290–4.
61. Battaglia FC. Clinical studies linking fetal velocimetry, blood flow and placental transport in pregnancies complicated by intrauterine growth retardation (IUGR). *Trans Am Clin Climatol Assoc* 2003;114:305–13.

62. Spencer JA, Chang TC, Crook D, *et al.* Third trimester fetal growth and measures of carbohydrate and lipid metabolism in umbilical venous blood at term. *Arch Dis Child Fetal Neonatal Ed* 1997; 76:F21–5.
63. Fant ME, Weisoly D. Insulin and insulin-like growth factors in human development: implications for the perinatal period. *Semin Perinatol* 2001;25:426–35.
64. Ostlund E, Tally M, Fried G. Transforming growth factor-beta1 in fetal serum correlates with insulin-like growth factor-I and fetal growth. *Obstet Gynecol* 2002;100(3):567–73.
65. Nicolini U, Hubinont C, Santolaya J, Fisk NM, Rodeck CH. Effects of fetal intravenous glucose challenge in normal and growth retarded fetuses. *Horm Metab Res* 1990;22:426–30.
66. Hubinont C, Nicolini U, Fisk NM, Tannirandorn Y, Rodeck CH. Endocrine pancreatic function in growth-retarded fetuses. *Obstet Gynecol* 1991;77:541–4.
67. Goland RS, Jozak S, Warren WB, Conwell IM, Stark RI, Tropper PJ. Elevated levels of umbilical cord plasma corticotropin-releasing hormone in growth-retarded fetuses. *J Clin Endocrinol Metab* 1993;77:1174–9.
68. Giles WB, McLean M, Davies JJ, Smith R. Abnormal umbilical artery Doppler waveforms and cord blood corticotropin-releasing hormone. *Obstet Gynecol* 1996;87:107–11.
69. Cianfarani S, Germani D, Rossi L, *et al.* IGF-I and IGF-binding protein-1 are related to cortisol in human cord blood. *Eur J Endocrinol* 1998;138:524–9.
70. Spencer JA, Chang TC, Jones J, Robson SC, Preece MA. Third trimester fetal growth and umbilical venous blood concentrations of IGF-1, IGFBP-1, and growth hormone at term. *Arch Dis Child Fetal Neonatal Ed* 1995;73(2):F87–90.
71. Weiner CP, Robillard JE. Atrial natriuretic factor, digoxin-like immunoreactive substance, norepinephrine, epinephrine, and plasma are in activity in human fetuses and their alteration by fetal disease. *Am J Obstet Gynecol* 1988;159:1353–60.
72. Greenough A, Nicolaides KH, Lagercrantz H. Human fetal sympathoadrenal responsiveness. *Early Hum Dev* 1990;23:9–13.
73. Ville Y, Proudler A, Kuhn P, Nicolaides KH. Aldosterone concentration in normal, growth-retarded, anemic, and hydropic fetuses. *Obstet Gynecol* 1994;84:511–14.
74. Thorpe-Beeston JG, Nicolaides KH. Fetal thyroid function. *Fetal Diagn Ther* 1993;8:60–72.
75. Thorpe-Beeston JG, Nicolaides KH, Snijders RJ, Felton CV, Vyas S, Campbell S. Relations between the fetal circulation and pituitary-thyroid function. *Br J Obstet Gynaecol* 1991;98:1163–7.
76. Nieto-Diaz A, Villar J, Matorras-Weinig R, Valenzuela-Ruiz P. Intrauterine growth retardation at term: Association between anthropometric and endocrine parameters. *Acta Obstet Gynecol Scand* 1996;75:127–31.
77. Kilby MD, Gittoes N, McCabe C, Verhaeg J, Franklyn JA. Expression of thyroid receptor isoforms in the human fetal central nervous system and the effects of intrauterine growth restriction. *Clin Endocrinol (Oxford)* 2000;53:469–77.
78. Verhaeghe J, Van Herck E, Bouillon R. Umbilical cord osteocalcin in normal pregnancies and pregnancies complicated by fetal growth retardation or diabetes mellitus. *Biol Neonate* 1995;68: 377–83.
79. Namgung R, Tsang RC, Specker BL, Sierra RI, Ho ML. Reduced serum osteocalcin and 1,25-dihydroxyvitamin D concentrations and low bone mineral content in small for gestational age infants: Evidence of decreased bone formation rates. *J Pediatr* 1993;122: 269–75.
80. Weiner CP, Williamson RA. Evaluation of severe growth retardation using cordocentesis – Hematologic and metabolic alterations by etiology. *Obstet Gynecol* 1989;73:225–9.
81. Thilaganathan B, Athanasiou S, Ozmen S, Creighton S, Watson NR, Nicolaides KH. Umbilical cord blood erythroblast count as an index of intrauterine hypoxia. *Arch Dis Child Fetal Neonatal Ed* 1994;70:F192–4.
82. Maier RF, Gunther A, Vogel M, Dudenhausen JW, Obladen M. Umbilical venous erythropoietin and umbilical arterial pH in relation to morphologic placental abnormalities. *Obstet Gynecol* 1994;84:81–7.
83. Snijders RJM, Abbas A, Melby O, Ireland RM, Nikolaides KH. Fetal plasma erythropoetin concentration in severe growth retardation. *Am J Obstet Gynecol* 1993;168:615–19.
84. Thilaganathan B, Nicolaides KH. Erythroblastosis in birth asphyxia. *Ultrasound Obstet Gynecol* 1992;2:15–17.
85. Baschat AA, Gembruch U, Reiss I, Gortner L, Harman CR, Weiner CP. Neonatal nucleated red blood cell counts in growth-restricted fetuses: Relationship to arterial and venous Doppler studies. *Am J Obstet Gynecol* 1999;181:190–5.
86. Bernstein PS, Minior VK, Divon MY. Nucleated red blood cell counts in small for gestational age fetuses with abnormal umbilical artery Doppler studies. *Am J Obstet Gynecol* 1997;177: 1079–84.
87. Baschat AA, Gembruch U, Reiss I, Gortner L, Harman CR. Neonatal nucleated red blood cell count and postpartum complications in growth restricted fetuses. *J Perinat Med* 2003;31:323–9.
88. Stallmach T, Karolyi L, Lichtlen P, *et al.* Fetuses from preeclamptic mothers show reduced hepatic erythropoiesis. *Pediatr Res* 1998;43:349–54.
89. Hiett AK, Britton KA, Hague NL, Brown HL, Stehman FB, Broxmeyer HE. Comparison of hematopoietic progenitor cells in human umbilical cord blood collected from neonatal infants who are small and appropriate for gestational age. *Transfusion* 1995;35:587–91.
90. Rondo PH, Abbott R, Rodrigues LC, Tomkins AM. Vitamin A, folate, and iron concentrations in cord and maternal blood of intra-uterine growth retarded and appropriate birth weight babies. *Eur J Clin Nutr* 1995;49:391–9.
91. Abbas A, Snijders RJ, Nicolaides KH. Serum ferritin and cobalamin in growth retarded fetuses. *Br J Obstet Gynaecol* 1994; 101:215–19.
92. Ohshige A, Yoshimura T, Maeda T, Ito M, Okamura H. Increased platelet-activating factor-acetylhydrolase activity in the umbilical venous plasma of growth-restricted fetuses. *Obstet Gynecol* 1999; 93:180–3.
93. Trudinger B, Song JZ, Wu ZH, Wang J. Placental insufficiency is characterized by platelet activation in the fetus. *Obstet Gynecol* 2003;101:975–81.
94. Baschat AA, Gembruch U, Reiss I, Gortner L, Weiner CP, Harman CR. Absent umbilical artery end-diastolic velocity in growth-restricted fetuses: A risk factor for neonatal thrombocytopenia. *Obstet Gynecol* 2000;96:162–6.
95. Van den Hof MC, Nicolaides KH. Platelet count in normal, small, and anemic fetuses. *Am J Obstet Gynecol* 1990;162:735–9.
96. Drew JH, Guaran RL, Grauer S, Hobbs JB. Cord whole blood hyperviscosity: Measurement, definition, incidence and clinical features. *J Paediatr Child Health* 1991;27:363–5.
97. Steel SA, Pearce JM, Nash G, Christopher B, Dormandy J, Bland JM. Correlation between Doppler flow velocity waveforms and cord blood viscosity. *Br J Obstet Gynaecol* 1989;96:1168–72.
98. Lemery DJ, Beal V, Vanlieferinghen P, Motta C. Fetal blood cell membrane fluidity in small for gestational age fetuses. *Biol Neonate* 1993;64:7–12.
99. Singh M, Manerikar S, Malaviya AN, Premawathi, Gopalan R, Kumar R. Immune status of low birth weight babies. *Indian Pediatr* 1978;15:563–7.
100. Davies N, Snijders R, Nicolaides KH. Intra-uterine starvation and fetal leucocyte count. *Fetal Diagn Ther* 1991;6:107–12.
101. Thilaganathan B, Plachouras N, Makrydimas G, Nicolaides KH. Fetal immunodeficiency: A consequence of placental insufficiency. *Br J Obstet Gynaecol* 1993;100:1000–4.
102. Harrington K, Carpenter RG, Goldfrad C, Campbell S. Transvaginal Doppler ultrasound of the uteroplacental circulation in the early prediction of pre-eclampsia and intrauterine growth retardation. *Br J Obstet Gynaecol* 1997;104:674–81.
103. Rigano S, Bozzo M, Ferrazzi E, Bellotti M, Battaglia FC, Galan HL. Early and persistent reduction in umbilical vein blood flow in the growth-restricted fetus: A longitudinal study. *Am J Obstet Gynecol* 2001;185:834–8.
104. Morrow RJ, Adamson SL, Bull SB, Ritchie JW. Effect of placental embolization on the umbilical artery velocity waveform in fetal sheep. *Am J Obstet Gynecol* 1989;161:1055–60.
105. Wilcox G, Trudinger B, Cook CM, Wilcox W, Conelly A. Reduced fetal platelet counts in pregnancies with abnormal Doppler umbilical flow waveforms. *Obstet Gynecol* 1989;73:639–43.
106. Papageorghiou AT, Yu CK, Cicero S, *et al.* Second-trimester uterine artery Doppler screening in unselected populations: A review. *J Matern Fetal Neonatal Med* 2002;12:78–88.
107. Weiner CP. The relationship between the umbilical artery systolic/diastolic ratio and umbilical blood gas measurements in specimens obtained by cordocentesis. *Am J Obstet Gynecol* 1990;162:1198–202.
108. Bilardo CM, Nicolaides KH, Campbell S. Doppler measurements of fetal and uteroplacental circulations: Relationship with umbilical venous blood gases measured at cordocentesis. *Am J Obstet Gynecol* 1990;162:115–20.

109. Ferrazzi E, Bozzo M, Rigano S, *et al.* Temporal sequence of abnormal Doppler changes in the peripheral and central circulatory systems of the severely growth-restricted fetus. *Ultrasound Obstet Gynecol* 2002;19:140–6.
110. Hecher K, Bilardo CM, Stigter RH, *et al.* Monitoring of fetuses with intrauterine growth restriction: A longitudinal study. *Ultrasound Obstet Gynecol* 2001;18:564–70.
111. Rizzo G, Arduini D. Fetal cardiac function in intrauterine growth retardation, *Am J Obstet Gynecol* 1991;165:876–82.
112. Reed KL, Anderson CF., Shenker L. Changes in intracardiac Doppler flow velocities in fetuses with absent umbilical artery diastolic flow. *Am J Obstet Gynecol* 1987;157:774–779.
113. Al Ghazali W, Chita SK, Chapman MG, Allan LD. Evidence of redistribution of cardiac output in asymmetrical growth retardation. *Br J Obstet Gynaecol* 1987;96:697–704.
114. Gramellini D, Folli MC, Raboni S, *et al.* Cerebral–umbilical Doppler ratio as a predictor of adverse perinatal outcome. *Obstet Gynecol* 1992;79:416–20.
115. Griffin D, Bilardo K, Masini L, *et al.* Doppler blood flow waveforms in the descending thoracic aorta of the human fetus. *Br J Obstet Gynaecol* 1984;91:997–1006.
116. Akalin-Sel T, Nicolaides KH, Peacock J, Campbell S. Doppler dynamics and their complex interrelation with fetal oxygen pressure, carbon dioxide pressure, and pH in growth-retarded fetuses. *Obstet Gynecol* 1994;84:439–44.
117. Wladimiroff JW, Tonge HM, Stewart PA. Doppler ultrasound assessment of cerebral blood flow in the human fetus. *Br J Obstet Gynaecol* 1986;93:471–5.
118. Arbeille P, Maulik D, Fignon A, *et al.* Assessment of the fetal PO2 changes by cerebral and umbilical Doppler on lamb fetuses during acute hypoxia. *Ultrasound Med Biol* 1995;21:861–70.
119. Baschat AA. Integrated fetal testing in growth restriction: Combining multivessel Doppler and biophysical parameters. *Ultrasound Obstet Gynecol* 2003;21:1–8.
120. Fouron JC, Skoll A, Sonesson SE, Pfizenmaier M, Jaeggi E, Lessard M. Relationship between flow through the fetal aortic isthmus and cerebral oxygenation during acute placental circulatory insufficiency in ovine fetuses. *Am J Obstet Gynecol* 1999;181: 1102–7.
121. Makikallio K, Jouppila P, Rasanen J. Retrograde net blood flow in the aortic isthmus in relation to human fetal arterial and venous circulations. *Ultrasound Obstet Gynecol* 2002;19:147 52.
122. Rizzo G, Capponi A, Chaoui R, Taddei F, Arduini D, Romanini C. Blood flow velocity waveforms from peripheral pulmonary arteries in normally grown and growth-retarded fetuses. *Ultrasound Obstet Gynecol* 1996;8:87–92.
123. Gamsu HR, Vyas S, Nicolaides K. Effects of intrauterine growth retardation on postnatal visceral and cerebral blood flow velocity. *Arch Dis Child* 1991;66:1115–18.
124. Mari G, Abuhamad AZ, Uerpairojkit B, Martinez E, Copel JA. Blood flow velocity waveforms of the abdominal arteries in appropriate- and small-for-gestational-age fetuses. *Ultrasound Obstet Gynecol* 1995;6:15–18.
125. Rhee E, Detti L, Mari G. Superior mesenteric artery flow velocity waveforms in small for gestational age fetuses. *J Matern Fetal Med* 1998;7:120–3.
126. Veille JC, Kanaan C. Duplex Doppler ultrasonographic evaluation of the fetal renal artery in normal and abnormal fetuses. *Am J Obstet Gynecol* 1989;161:1502–7.
127. Arduini D, Rizzo G. Fetal renal artery velocity waveforms and amniotic fluid volume in growth-retarded and post-term fetuses. *Obstet Gynecol* 1991;77:370–3.
128. Mari G. Arterial blood flow velocity waveforms of the pelvis and lower extremities in normal and growth-retarded fetuses. *Am J Obstet Gynecol* 1991;165:143–51.
129. Tekay A, Jouppila P. Fetal adrenal artery velocimetry measurements in appropriate-for-gestational age and intrauterine growth-restricted fetuses. *Ultrasound Obstet Gynecol* 2000;16:419–24.
130. Abuhamad AZ, Mari G, Bogdan D, Evans AT 3rd. Doppler flow velocimetry of the splenic artery in the human fetus: Is it a marker of chronic hypoxia? *Am J Obstet Gynecol* 1995;172:820–5.
131. Karsdorp VH, Dekker GA, Bast A, *et al.* Maternal and fetal plasma concentrations of endothelin, lipidhydroperoxides, glutathione peroxidase and fibronectin in relation to abnormal umbilical artery velocimetry. *Eur J Obstet Gynecol Reprod Biol* 1998;80: 39–44.
132. Harvey-Wilkes KB, Nielsen HC, D'Alton ME. Elevated endothelin levels are associated with increased placental resistance. *Am J Obstet Gynecol* 1996;174:1599–604.
133. Rizzo G, Montuschi P, Capponi A, Romanini C. Blood levels of vasoactive intestinal polypeptide in normal and growth retarded fetuses: Relationship with acid–base and haemodynamic status. *Early Hum Dev* 1995;41:69–77.
134. Saldeen P, Olofsson P, Marsal K. Lack of association between Doppler velocimetry and synthesis of prostacyclin and thromboxane in umbilical cord vessels from growth retarded fetuses. *Acta Obstet Gynecol Scand* 1995;74:103–8.
135. Lyall F, Greer IA, Young A, Myatt L. Nitric oxide concentrations are increased in the feto-placental circulation in intrauterine growth restriction. *Placenta* 1996;17:165–8.
136. McQeen J, Kingdom JC, Connell JM, Whittle MJ. Fetal endothelin levels and placental vascular endothelin receptors in intrauterine growth retardation. *Obstet Gynecol* 1993;82:992–8.
137. Kingdom JC, McQueen J, Connell JM, Whittle MJ. Fetal angiotensin II levels and vascular (type I) angiotensin receptors in pregnancies complicated by intrauterine growth retardation. *Br J Obstet Gynaecol* 1993;100:476–82.
138. Parboosingh J, Lederis K, Ko D, Singh N. Vasopressin concentration in cord blood: Correlation with method of delivery and cord pH. *Obstet Gynecol* 1982;60:179–83.
139. Rizzo G, Capponi A, Rinaldo D, Arduini D, Romanini C. Release of vasoactive agents during cordocentesis: Differences between normally grown and growth-restricted fetuses. *Am J Obstet Gynecol* 1996;175:563–70.
140. Kilavuz O, Vetter K. Is the liver of the fetus the 4th preferential organ for arterial blood supply besides brain, heart, and adrenal glands? *J Perinat Med* 1999;27:103–6.
141. Hecher K, Campbell S. Characteristics of fetal venous blood flow under normal circumstances and during fetal disease. *Ultrasound Obstet Gynecol* 1996;7:68–83.
142. Capponi A, Rizzo G, De Angelis C, Arduini D, Romanini C. Atrial natriuretic peptide levels in fetal blood in relation to inferior vena cava velocity waveforms. *Obstet Gynecol* 1997;89:242–7.
143. Ville Y, Proudler A, Abbas A, Nicolaides K. Atrial natriuretic factor concentration in normal, growth-retarded, anemic, and hydropic fetuses. *Am J Obstet Gynecol* 1994;171:777–83.
144. Baschat AA, Gembruch U, Reiss I, Gortner L, Diedrich K. Demonstration of fetal coronary blood flow by Doppler ultrasound in relation to arterial and venous flow velocity waveforms and perinatal outcome – the 'heart-sparing effect'. *Ultrasound Obstet Gynecol* 1997;9:162–72.
145. Arduini D, Rizzo G, Romanini C. Changes of pulsatility index from fetal vessels preceding the onset of late decelerations in growth-retarded fetuses. *Obstet Gynecol* 1992;79:605–10.
146. Chaiworapongsa T, Espinoza J, Yoshimatsu J, *et al.* Subclinical myocardial injury in small-for-gestational-age neonates. *J Matern Fetal Neonatal Med* 2002;11:385–90.
147. Gazzolo D, Marinoni E, di Iorio R, Lituania M, Bruschettini PL, Michetti F. Circulating S100beta protein is increased in intrauterine growth-retarded fetuses. *Pediatr Res* 2002;51:215–19.
148. Roberts A, Nava S, Bocconi L, Salmona S, Nicolini U. Liver function tests and glucose and lipid metabolism in growth-restricted fetuses. *Obstet Gynecol* 1999;94:290–4.
149. Hackett GA, Campbell S, Gamsu H, Cohen-Overbeek T, Pearce JM. Doppler studies in the growth retarded fetus and prediction of neonatal necrotising enterocolitis, haemorrhage, and neonatal morbidity. *Br Med J* 1987;294:13–16.
150. Rizzo G, Arduini D. Fetal cardiac function in intrauterine growth retardation. *Am J Obstet Gynecol* 1991;165:876–82.
151. Rizzo G, Capponi A, Pietropolli A, *et al.* Fetal cardiac and extracardiac flows preceding intrauterine death. *Ultrasound Obstet Gynecol* 1994;4:139–42.
152. Manning FA. Fetal biophysical profile. *Obstet Gynecol Clin North Am* 1999;26:557–77.
153. Arduini D, Rizzo G, Romanini C, Mancuso S. Computerized analysis of behavioral states in asymmetrical growth retarded fetuses. *J Perinat Med* 1988;16:357–63.
154. Arduini D, Rizzo G, Caforio L, Boccolini MR, Romanini C, Mancuso S. Behavioral state transitions in healthy and growth retarded fetuses. *Early Hum Dev* 1989;19:155–65.
155. Nijhuis IJ, ten Hof J, Nijhuis JG, *et al.* Temporal organisation of fetal behavior from 24-weeks gestation onwards in normal and complicated pregnancies. *Dev Psychobiol* 1999;34:257–68.
156. Vindla S, James D, Sahota D. Computerised analysis of unstimulated and stimulated behavior in fetuses with intrauterine growth restriction. *Eur J Obstet Gynecol Reprod Biol* 1999;83:37–45.
157. Romanini C, Valensise H, Ciotti G, Arduini D, Giorgi P. Tryptophan availability and fetal behavioral states. *Fetal Ther* 1989;4:68–72.

158. Nijhuis IJ, ten Hof J, Mulder EJ, *et al.* Fetal heart rate in relation to its variation in normal and growth retarded fetuses. *Eur J Obstet Gynecol Reprod Biol* 2000;89:27–33.
159. Henson G, Dawes GS, Redman CW. Characterization of the reduced heart rate variation in growth-retarded fetuses. *Br J Obstet Gynaecol* 1984;91:751–5.
160. Ribbert LS, Snijders RJ, Nicolaides KH, Visser GH. Relation of fetal blood gases and data from computer-assisted analysis of fetal heart rate patterns in small for gestation fetuses. *Br J Obstet Gynaecol* 1991;98:820–3.
161. Smith JH, Anand KJ, Cotes PM, *et al.* Antenatal fetal heart rate variation in relation to the respiratory and metabolic status of the compromised human fetus. *Br J Obstet Gynaecol* 1988;95:980–9.
162. Longo LD, Packianathan S. Hypoxia-ischemia and the developing brain: Hypotheses regarding the pathophysiology of fetal neonatal brain damage. *Br J Obstet Gynaecol* 1997;104:652–62.
163. Ribbert LS, Nicolaides KH, Visser GH. Prediction of fetal acidaemia in intrauterine growth retardation: Comparison of quantified fetal activity with biophysical profile score. *Br J Obstet Gynaecol* 1993;100:653–6.
164. Baschat AA, Gembruch U, Harman CR. The sequence of changes in Doppler and biophysical parameters as severe fetal growth restriction worsens. *Ultrasound Obstet Gynecol* 2001;18:571–7.
165. Ribbert LS, Visser GH, Mulder EJ, *et al.* Changes with time in fetal heart rate variation, movement incidences and haemodynamics in intrauterine growth retarded fetuses: A longitudinal approach to the assessment of fetal well being. *Early Hum Dev* 1993;31:195–208.
166. Manning FA, Snijders R, Harman CR, *et al.* Fetal biophysical profile score. VI. Correlation with antepartum umbilical venous fetal pH. *Am J Obstet Gynecol* 1993;169:755–63.
167. Vintzileos AM, Fleming AD, Scorza WE, *et al.* Relationship between fetal biophysical activities and umbilical cord blood gas values. *Am J Obstet Gynecol* 1991;165:707–13.
168. Ribbert LS, Visser GH, Mulder EJ, Zonneveld MF, Morssink LP. Changes with time in fetal heart rate variation, movement incidences and haemodynamics in intrauterine growth retarded fetuses: A longitudinal approach to the assessment of fetal well being. *Early Hum Dev* 1993;31:195–208.
169. Pillai M, James D. Continuation of normal neurobehavioural development in fetuses with absent umbilical arterial end-diastolic velocities. *Br J Obstet Gynaecol* 1991;98:277–81.
170. Rizzo G, Arduini D, Pennestri F, Romanini C, Mancuso S. Fetal behavior in growth retardation: Its relationship to fetal blood flow. *Prenat Diagn* 1987;7:229–38.
171. Arduini D, Rizzo G, Capponi A, Rinaldo D, Romanini C. Fetal pH value determined by cordocentesis: An independent predictor of the development of antepartum fetal heart rate decelerations in growth retarded fetuses with absent end-diastolic velocity in umbilical artery. *J Perinat Med* 1996;24:601–7.
172. Ribbert LS, Snijders RJ, Nicolaides KH, *et al.* Relationship of fetal biophysical profile and blood gas values at cordocentesis in severely growth-retarded fetuses. *Am J Obstet Gynecol* 1990;163:569–71.
173. Zeitlin J, Ancel PY, Saurel-Cubizolles MJ, *et al.* The relationship between intrauterine growth restriction and preterm delivery: An empirical approach using data from a European case–control study. *Br J Obstet Gynaecol* 2000;107:750–8.
174. Ott WJ. Intrauterine growth restriction and Doppler ultrasonography. *J Ultrasound Med* 2000;19:661–5.
175. Strigini FA, De Luca G, Lencioni G, *et al.* Middle cerebral artery velocimetry: Different clinical relevance depending on umbilical velocimetry. *Obstet Gynecol* 1997;90:953–7.
176. Hecher K, Spernol R, Stettner H, *et al.* Potential for diagnosing imminent risk for appropriate- and small for gestational fetuses by Doppler examination of umbilical and cerebral arterial blood flow. *Ultrasound Obstet Gynecol* 1995;5:247–55.
177. Severi FM, Bocchi C, Visentin A, *et al.* Uterine and fetal cerebral Doppler predict the outcome of third-trimester small-for-gestational age fetuses with normal umbilical artery Doppler. *Ultrasound Obstet Gynecol* 2002;19:225–8.
178. Baschat AA, Towbin J, Bowles NE, *et al.* Is adenovirus a fetal pathogen? *Am J Obstet Gynecol* 2003;189:758–63.
179. Magann EF, Chauhan SP, Barrilleaux PS, *et al.* Amniotic fluid index and single deepest pocket: Weak indicators of abnormal amniotic volumes. *Obstet Gynecol* 2000;96:737–40.
180. Chamberlain PF, Manning FA, Morrison I, *et al.* Ultrasound evaluation of amniotic fluid volume. I. The relationship of marginal and decreased amniotic fluid volumes to perinatal outcome. *Am J Obstet Gynecol* 1984;150:245–9.
181. Chauhan SP, Sanderson M, Hendrix NW, *et al.* Perinatal outcome and amniotic fluid index in the antepartum and intrapartum periods: A meta-analysis. *Am J Obstet Gynecol* 1999;181:1473–8.
182. Bukowski R. Fetal growth potential and pregnancy outcome. *Semin Perinatol* 2004;28:51–8.
183. Sabbagha RE. Intrauterine growth retardation. In Sabbagha RE, ed. *Diagnostic Ultrasound Applied to Obstetrics and Gynecology*, 2nd edn. Philadelphis, PA: JB Lippincott Co, 1987:112–31.
184. Tamura RK, Sabbagha RE. Percentile ranks of sonar fetal abdominal circumference measurements. *Am J Obstet Gynecol* 1980;138:475.
185. Baschat AA, Weiner CP. Umbilical artery Doppler screening for detection of the small fetus in need of antepartum surveillance. *Am J Obstet Gynecol* 2000;182:154–8.
186. Divon MY, Chamberlain PF, Sipos L, *et al.* Identification of the small for gestational age fetus with the use of gestational age-independent indices of fetal growth. *Am J Obstet Gynecol* 1986;155: 1197–201.
187. Tamura RK, Sabbagha RE, Pan WH, *et al.* Ultrasonic fetal abdominal circumference: Comparison of direct versus calculated measurement. *Obstet Gynecol* 1986;67:833.
188. Weiner CP, Robinson D. The sonographic diagnosis of intrauterine growth retardation using the postnatal ponderal index and the crown heel length as standards of diagnosis. *Am J Perinatol* 1989;6:380–3.
189. Hadlock FP, Deter RL, Carpenter RJ, Park SK. Estimating fetal age: Effect of head shape on BPD. *AJR Am J Roentgenol* 1981;137:83.
190. Smith PA, Johansson D, Tzannatos C, *et al.* Prenatal measurement of the fetal cerebellum and cisterna cerebellomedullaris by ultrasound. *Prenat Diagn* 1986;6:133.
191. Warsof SL, Cooper DJ, Little D, *et al.* Routine ultrasound screening for antenatal detection of intrauterine growth retardation. *Obstet Gynecol* 1986;67:33.
192. Sarmandal P, Grant JM. Effectiveness of ultrasound determination of fetal abdominal circumference and fetal ponderal index in the diagnosis of asymmetrical growth retardation. *Br J Obstet Gynaecol* 1990;97:118.
193. Hadlock FP, Deter RL, Harrist RB, *et al.* A data-independent predictor of intrauterine growth retardation: Femur length/abdominal circumference ratio. *AJR Am J Roengenol* 1983;141:979.
194. McGowan LM, Harding JE, Roberts AB, *et al.* A pilot randomized controlled trial of two regimens of fetal surveillance for small-for-gestational age fetuses with normal results of umbilical artery Doppler velocimetry. *Am J Obstet Gynecol* 2000;182:81–6.
195. Neilson JP, Alfirevic Z. Doppler ultrasound for fetal assessment in high risk pregnancies (Cochrane review). In *The Cochrane Library*, Issue 1. Oxford: Update Software, 2002.
196. Westergaard HB, Langhoff-Roos J, Lingman G, *et al.* A critical appraisal of the use of umbilical artery Doppler ultrasound in high-risk pregnancies: Use of meta-analyses in evidence-based obstetrics. *Ultrasound Obstet Gynecol* 2001;17:466–76.
197. Gosling R.G., King D.H. Ultrasound angiology. In Marcus AW, Adamson L, eds. *Arteries and Veins*, 2nd edn. Edinburgh: Churchill Livingstone, 1975:61–98.
198. Thompson RS, Trudinger BJ, Cook CM. Doppler ultrasound waveform indices: A/B ratio, pulsatility index and Pourcelot ratio. *Br J Obstet Gynaecol* 1988;95:581–8.
199. Hershkovitz R, Kingdom JC, Geary M, *et al.* Fetal cerebral blood flow redistribution in late gestation: Identification of compromise in small fetuses with normal umbilical artery Doppler. *Ultrasound Obstet Gynecol* 2000;15:209–12.
200. Bahado-Singh RO, Kovanci E, Jeffres A, *et al.* The Doppler cerebroplacental ratio and perinatal outcome in intrauterine growth restriction. *Am J Obstet Gynecol* 1999;180:750–6.
201. Baschat AA, Galan HL Bhide A, *et al.* Viability in early onset IUGR: Is it time to reconsider intervention thresholds? *Am J Obstet Gynecol* 2003;189:S216.
202. Harrington K, Thompson MO, Carpenter RG, *et al.* Doppler fetal circulation in pregnancies complicated by pre-eclampsia or delivery of a small for gestational age baby: 2. Longitudinal analysis. *Br J Obstet Gynaecol* 1999;106:453–66.
203. Bilardo CM, Wolf H, Stigter RH, *et al.* Relationship between monitoring parameters and perinatal outcome in severe, early intrauterine growth restriction. *Ultrasound Obstet Gynecol* 2004; 23:119–25.
204. Baschat AA. Doppler application in the delivery timing of the preterm growth-restricted fetus: Another step in the right direction. *Ultrasound Obstet Gynecol* 2004;23:111–18.
205. Karsdorp VH, van Vugt JM, van Geijn HP, *et al.* Clinical significance of absent or reversed end diastolic velocity waveforms in umbilical artery. *Lancet* 1994;344:1664–8.
206. Divon MY, Girz BA, Lieblich R, *et al.* Clinical management of the fetus with markedly diminished umbilical artery end-diastolic flow. *Am J Obstet Gynecol* 1989;161:1523–7.

SECTION X

Nutrition and metabolism

Section Editors: **P. D. Gluckman and H. N. Winn**

91 The role of essential fatty acids and antioxidants in neurovascular development and complications of prematurity

K. Ghebremeskel, Y. Min, B. Thomas and M. A. Crawford

Introduction

Membrane integrity and function are dependent on the incorporation of appropriate amounts of arachidonic (20:4n-6, AA) and docosahexaenoic (22:6n-3, DHA) acids, and antioxidant protection. AA and DHA are highly unsaturated and therefore must be protected from peroxidative damage. There is an interdependence between membrane AA and DHA, and membrane-bound antioxidant enzymes. Optimum activity of the enzymes is dependent on the physical integrity of the membranes. At the same time, the membrane fatty acids require the antioxidant enzymes for protection. Paradoxically, it has also been shown that n-3 polyunsaturated fatty acids exert protective effects against injury caused by oxidative stress. In the very low birth weight baby, tissue maturation, structural integrity, function and protection are closely intertwined; hence, there is a need to consider both polyunsaturated fatty acids and antioxidants together.

Our proposition is that low AA and DHA, sub-optimal antioxidant protection and the immature anatomy in an alien oxygen radical-generating environment predispose the very low birth weight babies to serious disorders often described as the complications of prematurity. This hypothesis of *synergistic insufficiency* brings together the concepts of free-radical damage and structural integrity, consistent with the proposition of Saugstad[1] that the various complications of prematurity are 'facets of one disease'.

Essential fatty acids

The term *essential fatty acids* originated from the discovery that absence of certain fatty acids, which are not synthesized *de novo* by animals, in the diet leads to clinical abnormalities. They are vital for reproduction, normal growth, development and function of all tissues. There are two families of essential fatty acids, namely, the n-3 and n-6 families. Linoleic (18:2n-6, LA) and α-linolenic (18:3n-3, ALA) acids are the parent compounds of the n-6 and n-3 families, respectively. By convention the formula for fatty acids is abbreviated as *X*:*Y*n-*M*. *X* refers to the number of carbon atoms, *Y* to the number of double bonds, and *M* the position of the first double bond counting from the terminal methyl (CH_3) group (Figure 91.1).

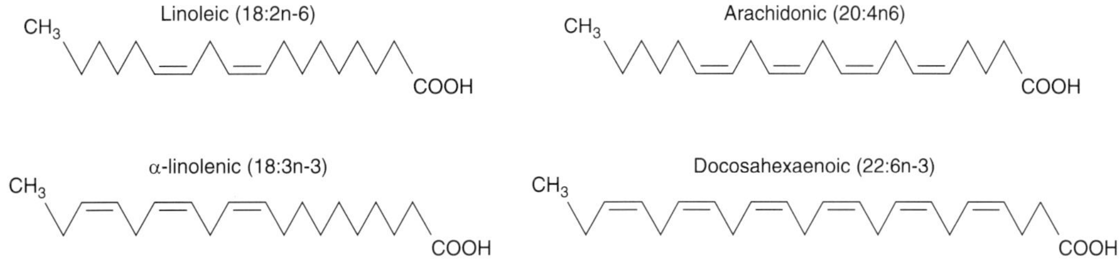

Figure 91.1 Structural formula of linoleic, α-linolenic, arachidonic and docosahexaenoic acids.

N-6 family

$18{:}2 \xrightarrow{\Delta 6} 18{:}3 \rightarrow 20{:}3 \xrightarrow{\Delta 5} 20{:}4 \rightarrow 22{:}4 \rightarrow 22{:}5$

(LA) (GLA) (AA)

N-3 family

$18{:}3 \xrightarrow{\Delta 6} 18{:}4 \rightarrow 20{:}4 \xrightarrow{\Delta 5} 20{:}5 \rightarrow 22{:}5 \rightarrow 24{:}5 \xrightarrow{\Delta 6} 24{:}6 \rightarrow 22{:}6$

(ALA) (EPA) (DHA)

LA, linoleic; GLA, γ-linolenic; AA, arachidonic;
ALA, α-linolenic; EPA, eicosapentaenoic; DHA, docosahexaenoic
Δ6, Δ6 desaturation; Δ5, Δ5 desaturation

Figure 91.2 Metabolic pathway of the synthesis of n-6 and n-3 polyunsaturated fatty acids.

Animals cannot synthesize either LA or ALA. However, they can add double bonds and carbon atoms to LA and ALA. This metabolic process produces long-chain derivatives with 20 and 22 carbon atoms, and 3, 4, 5 and 6 double bonds (Figure 91.2). The two most important members of the n-6 and n-3 families in cell membrane, which are often regarded as essential, are AA and DHA.

Dietary sources of essential fatty acids

Fruits, seeds and vegetable oils such as sunflower, safflower, soybean, cottonseed and corn are the predominant source of LA.[2] ALA is a minor constituent of most vegetable oils except in linseed, soybean and rapeseed oil; it is a major fatty acid in green leafy vegetables.[3,4] Gamma-linolenic acid (18:3n-6, GLA) is found in evening primrose, borage and blackcurrant seed oils. AA is found in eggs, lean meat and offal such as liver, brain and entrails. It is also found in substantial proportions in tropical fish and shellfish.[5–7] Fish, shellfish and fish oils are the main source of eicosapentaenoic acid (20:5n-3, EPA) and DHA. Fish caught in Northern latitudes (> 30°N) have, on average, seven times as much n-3 fatty acids as n-6 fatty acids.[5,7]

Distribution in tissues and the brain

Long-chain fatty acids, both of the n-3 and n-6 families, are vital components of cell membrane lipids (Figure 91.3). AA is present in all biological membranes and represents up to 15% of the total fatty acids in polar phospholipids. DHA is more specifically present at very high levels in the retina, brain, testis and sperm.[3] In the cerebral gray matter, DHA makes up to one-third of the total fatty acid content of ethanolamine and serine phosphoglycerides.[8,9] Among subcellular fractions of brain tissue, the highest levels of DHA are found in synapotosomes, synaptic vesicles, mitochondria and microsomes where there is evidence of selective incorporation.[10] In the photoreceptor outer segments, the level of DHA is as high as 60% of total fatty acids.[11] White matter and its myelin fractions contain low levels of AA and DHA and high levels of saturated and monounsaturated fatty acids.[12]

Essentiality of n-3 and n-6 fatty acids

Essential fatty acids are required for the structure and function of membranes.[13–15] They are also converted to eicosanoids, which are regulators and coordinators of local multicellular function. n-6 fatty acids were recognized as essential over 60 years ago.[16,17] However, it is only in the last two decades that the essentiality of the n-3 fatty acid has been conclusively established. Although AA and DHA can be formed from LA and ALA as described above, Δ6 desaturase, the enzyme required for the first and last metabolic steps, is rate limiting. In some species such as the cat, the activity of this enzyme is too low to measure hence AA and DHA are essential fatty acids and must be provided in the diet.[18] Fat-free diets or those deficient in n-6 and n-3 polyunsaturated fatty acids produce reproductive failure, retarded growth and abnormal changes in many organs such as the skin, liver and kidney in many species including the human infant.[16,17,19,20]

In experimental animals, membrane structural alterations resulting from changes in the AA and DHA composition leads to loss of cellular integrity and functions.[21–23] Deficits of the essential n-3 fatty acids cause cerebral hemorrhage in chicks,[24] and learning and visual impairment in rats.[25–27] Polydipsia, visual impairment and abnormal electroretinogram are manifested in non-human primates deficient in n-3 fatty acids.[20,28]

In addition to their structural and functional properties, some fatty acids, namely, dihommo-γ-linolenic acid (20:3n-6, DHGLA), EPA and AA are precursors of hormone-like compounds known as eicosanoids. These are a complex group of highly biologically active compounds, which are involved in the control and regulation of blood flow, intraocular pressure, cell-mediated immunity and inflammation, renal function, insulin release and reproduction.[29] Recently, it has been demonstrated that DHA is the precursor of a novel brain protective messenger, 10,17S-docosatriene, which inhibits ischemia–reperfusion-mediated leukocyte infiltration and pro-inflammatory gene expression.[30]

Essential fatty acids and pregnancy

During pregnancy, there is a high demand for AA and DHA for the development of fetal brain and other vital tissues. Consequently, in the third trimester the accretion of total n-6 and n-3 fatty acids by the fetal brain increases progressively.[31,32] It is estimated that the fetus accumulates about 70 mg/day of long-chain n-3 fatty acids, primarily DHA, during the third trimester.[32,33] The fetus has the ability to synthesize AA and DHA

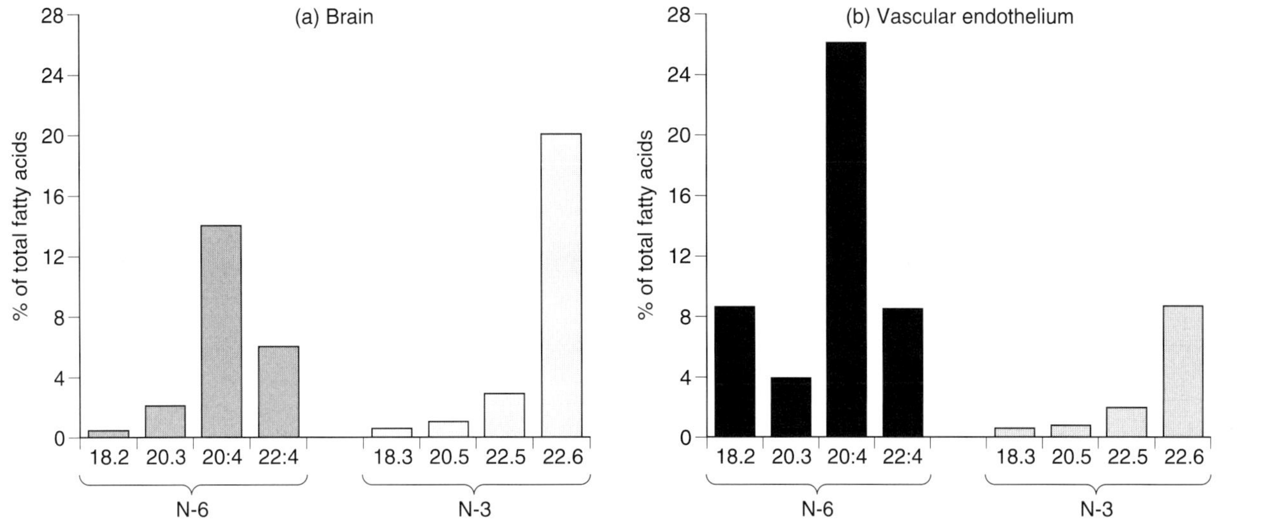

Figure 91.3 n-6 and n-3 fatty acid composition of the inner cell membrane phospholipid (ethanolamine phosphoglycerides) of the brain and vascular endothelium.

from their respective parent compounds LA and ALA.[34] However, the rate of synthesis is not fast enough to meet requirements and hence, these fatty acids are obtained from maternal circulation by placental selection and extraction. This selective transfer is reflected in a significant decrease in the blood level of AA and DHA in healthy pregnant women[35,36] and a concomitant increase in the fetus (Figure 91.4). Fish-eating populations with a raised intake of long-chain n-3 fatty acids have prolonged pregnancies and reduced incidence of both pregnancy-induced hypertension and preterm deliveries.[37] Maternal supplementation with n-3 fatty acids during prognancy, and pregnancy and lactation are associated with cerebral maturation of the newborn[38] and mental development at 4 years of age,[39] respectively.

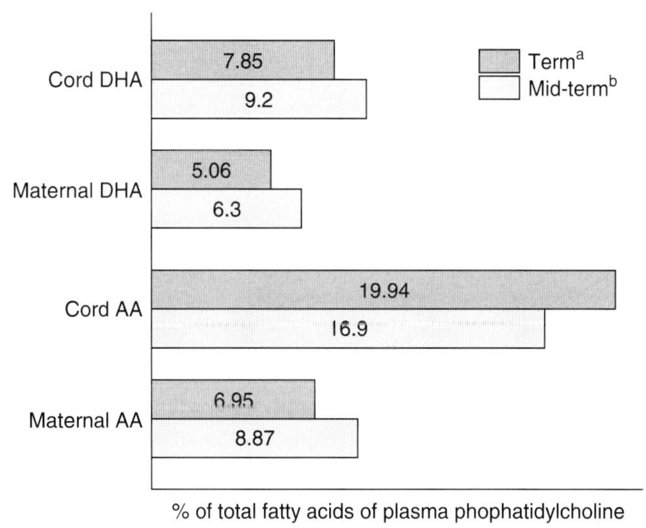

[a]Term data are from normal deliveries at 39-42 gestation weeks and birth weight >3.0 kg.
[b]Mid-term data are derived from mid-term elective abortion.

Figure 91.4 Maternal and fetal (cord blood) arachidonic (AA) and docosahexaenoic (DHA) acids in plasma choline phosphoglycerides at mid-term and term.

Essential fatty acids in the human neonates

Appropriately grown term babies of healthy mothers are born with high levels of AA and DHA due to placental enrichment. This selective placental transfer of AA and DHA from the mother to fetus would be reduced if the mothers have chronic disease such as diabetes[40–42] (Figure 91.5), impaired fatty acid metabolism or placental infarction. Babies born to mothers with marginal or low AA and DHA status because of insufficient intake prior to, and during, pregnancy will also be expected to have depressed levels of these essential fatty acids at birth.

Preterm and low birth weight babies are born with depressed levels of AA and DHA.[43–45] Our study on maternal and cord blood phosphoglycerides showed that low concentrations of AA and DHA were associated with low birth weight and gestational age, respectively, and low levels of AA and DHA, independently and together, were associated with reduced head circumference.[46,47] A parallel investigation of umbilical arteries over a wide birth weight range demonstrated that the triene/tetraene ratio (20:3n-9/20:4n-6), an index of essential fatty acid deficiency, and the 22:4n-6/22:5n-6 ratio, an index of DHA insufficiency, were abnormal in low birth weight babies.[43] In addition, it has been shown that intrauterine growth restriction is associated with changes in fetal–maternal polyunsaturated fatty acid relationship[48] and reduced levels of AA and DHA at birth.[49] Moreover, Zhang[50] has demonstrated that treatment with LA and ALA increases bi-parietal diameter and weight in the intrauterine-restricted fetus.

Subsequent to birth, in the human preterm infant, the plasma levels of AA decrease substantially, despite a threefold increase in its precursor LA

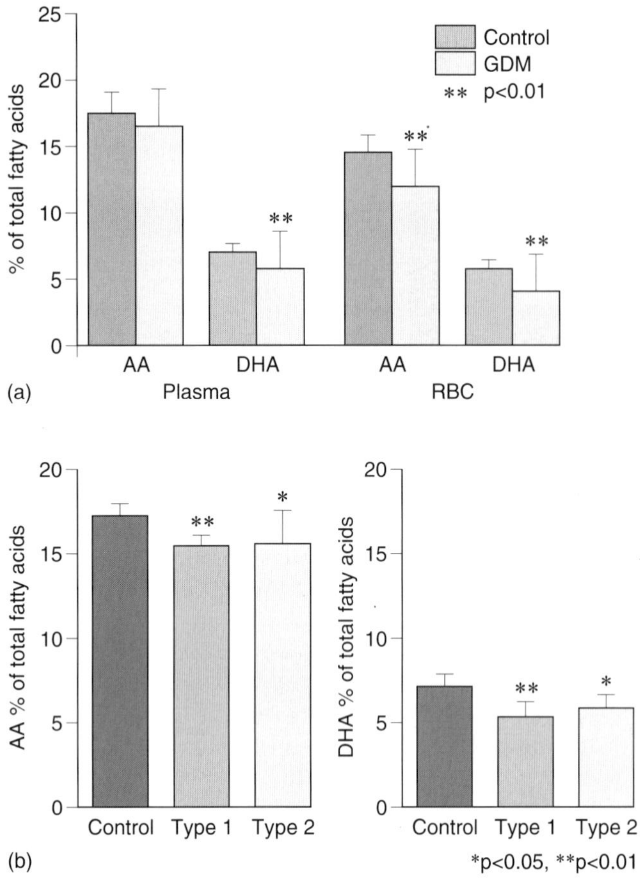

Figure 91.5 Neonates of diabetic mothers have reduced blood levels of arachidonic (AA) and docosahexaenoic (DHA) acids.

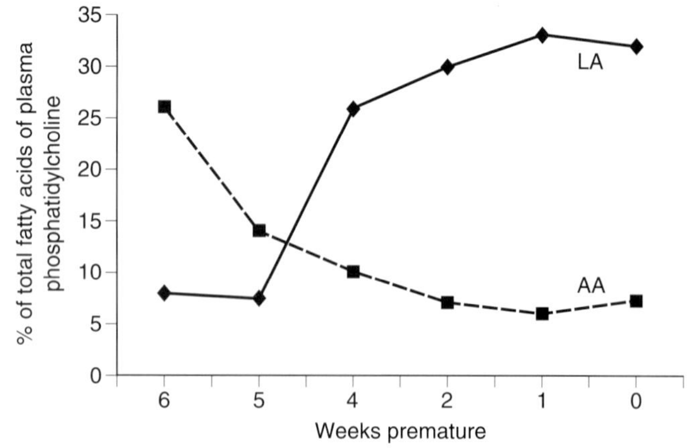

Figure 91.6 The diagram illustrates the scale and speed of loss of arachidonic acid (AA) from plasma choline phosphoglycerides of preterm babies between birth and the expected date of delivery (LA is the precursor of AA).

(Figure 91.6). A similar fall in DHA is also reported.[45,47] In preterm babies fed formula milk containing LA and ALA but devoid of AA and DHA, the plasma levels of AA and DHA decline by 47% and 23%, respectively, between birth and postnatal day 15.[51] This indicates that the rate of neonatal synthesis[52,53] is unable to meet the AA and DHA demand for growth and development.[54] Koletzko *et al.*[55] estimated that endogenous synthesis contributed only about 23% of total plasma AA by day 4 in term infants.

Postnatally, suboptimal nutritional management compounds the prenatal nutrient deficit of AA and DHA when infants are fed on artificial milks devoid of these two nutrients. Predictably, this is reflected in alterations in membrane composition. Term and preterm babies fed on conventional infant formula without AA and DHA have depressed levels of DHA in the blood[51,56,57] and in brain tissue compared with babies fed on breast milk which does contain AA and DHA.[58,59]

An insufficiency of polyunsaturated fatty acids has a profound impact on neurovisual development in term and preterm infants[60–66] that is shown to be long lasting. Infants fed on formula milk devoid of DHA had lower visual acuity and cognitive scores compared with those fed breast milk. Supplementation of formula with DHA is related to enhanced visual acuity[60–64] and discriminative learning.[67] Bjerve *et al.*[68] have reported lower psychomotor performance scores associated with low levels of plasma DHA at 1 year of age. At 3 years of age term babies who have been fed on formula milk without DHA, had significantly lowered visual and stereo acuity and letter matching compared with babies fed on breast milk.[61,66] Eight-year-old children previously fed on formula milk as preterm babies had an eight point lower IQ score compared with those fed on breast milk.[69] Lanting *et al.*[70] reported a neurodevelopmental disadvantage in a 9-year-old children who had been fed breast milk compared with those fed on formula milks.

Some reports on term infants have demonstrated improved visual acuity with formula milk containing DHA[71] while others have not.[72] In the latter study, the range of DHA in human milk is quoted as 0.1–0.9% of the fatty acids and yet the amount of DHA used was 0.02% above the lowest level. Bearing in mind that maternal diet and health will influence milk DHA,[73] one wonders as to the validity of choosing such low levels, which reflect the lowest nutritional status in the range, reported. Unfortunately, few workers select mothers for the study of human milk based on sound evidence of good health and nutritional status.

Human milk, lipid and fatty acids

In human milk, the lipid fraction provides about 60% of the energy for the infant. It mainly consists of triglycerides, which account for about 96% and phosphoglycerides for about 2–3%. The concentration of lipid in human milk is variable and is influenced by length of gestation (term or preterm), length of lactation, time of day, duration of individual feeds (low in fore and high in hind milk) and most of all maternal diet.[74,75] In contrast to lipid concentration, the fatty acid composition of mature human milk changes little with the duration of the feed, the time of the day and length of lactation.[73,76] Colostrum contains higher levels of AA and DHA than mature milk.[76,77] Similarly, very preterm and preterm human milk contain higher levels of the two fatty acids compared with term milk.[78]

Although it seems that milk AA and DHA are resistant to dietary change, they do respond to maternal diet, which is the most important determinant of fatty acid composition of human milk. Comparisons of vegetarian and non-vegetarian women show that the milk essential fatty acids reflect the diet.[79] Greenland Eskimos, North Canadian Inuit and Japanese islanders have high intakes of seals, fish and other seafoods. Consequently, breast milk from these communities is high in the n-3 fatty acids, namely, EPA and DHA.[80,81] Mothers from countries where fat provides greater than 35% of the daily energy (high fat intakes) have lower short-chain and higher long-chain fatty acid concentrations. Conversely, those from countries where the habitual diet is relatively low in fat (less than 15% of the energy) have high proportions of short-chain and AA and DHA.[73,82] It is intriguing why breast milk DHA of western (European and American) women, who are supposed to be 'well nourished', is invariably very low ($< 0.2\%$) in contrast to milk of inadequately nourished women from Africa and Asia ($> 0.4\%$). Since plant-based foods are the major sources of dietary lipids of the latter group, their intake of saturated fat would be less than 5%, which is well below the amount consumed by Western women (range: 15–25%). Hence, it is plausible that high total and saturated fat intakes reduce the relative proportions of DHA in breast milk of Western women. This proposition is consistent with our recent experimental study[83] that showed suckling pups born to dams fed high total and saturated fat diet, akin to western foods, during pregnancy and lactation had about 25% lower DHA in liver choline and ethanolamine phosphoglycerides compared with the controls indicating that the metabolism of DHA is adversely influence by saturated fat.

Breast milk and artificial formulations, which simulate breast milk, with respect to DHA, appear to enhance DHA status, cognitive development and visual functions of the preterm baby. Nevertheless, it is questionable whether these feeds meet the AA and DHA requirement for optimum development of preterm babies. The current AA and DHA recommendation for infants, and the consequential formulation, which is modeled on milk of Western women, is also questionable. It is legitimate to argue that breast milk evolved to support the postnatal development of the term neonate born with appropriately developed and functional systems. The preterm baby, who is born with immature anatomy and metabolic systems, will have to continue its interrupted prenatal development under neonatal conditions. This can only be done if the infant is provided with the appropriate nutrients in the right amounts. What the preterm baby requires in the immediate neonatal period is a surrogate placenta that provides enriched AA, DHA and other essential nutrients rather than mammary glands, which generate breast milk for the normal birth weight term baby.

Antioxidants

Membrane integrity and function are dependent on the incorporation of appropriate amounts of the highly unsaturated fatty acids, AA and DHA, which are susceptible to peroxidation unless protected by antioxidants. There is an interdependence between membrane AA and DHA and membrane-bound antioxidant enzymes. Optimum activity of the enzymes is dependent on the physical integrity of the membrane. At the same time, the membrane fatty acids require the antioxidant enzymes for protection. It has been shown that the activity of mitochondrial manganese-superoxide dismutase (Mn-SOD) is influenced by dietary essential fatty acids, while the activity of cystosolic Cu/Zn-SOD remains unaffected.[84]

Reduced competence of the antioxidant defense may lead to damage to the structural membrane of the brain, retina, lungs and other tissues, particularly in a hyperoxic environment. Indeed Saugstad[85] and Sullivan[86] postulated that oxygen radical injury may be a common pathogenic mechanism in the neonatal diseases bronchopulmonary dysplasia, hemolytic anemia, intraventricular hemorrhage and retinopathy of prematurity.

In the chicken model of intraventricular hemorrhage, we have been able to induce hemorrhage in the cerebellum between 10 and 28 days after hatching. The window of susceptibility corresponds to the time of rapid growth of the cerebellum and acquisition of long-chain polyunsaturated fatty acids. Provision of vitamin E, or ALA without vitamin E arrests the disease.[24,87] This model illustrates the importance of considering both the membrane structure and its protection together.

Research into the role of antioxidant vitamins and fatty acids in non-human primates demonstrates that these nutrients provide protection against oxidative stress. Laboratory-bred marmosets had a high hydrogen peroxide-induced erythrocyte hemolysis *in vitro*,[88] which correlated negatively with levels of vitamin E and LA.[88,89] The high erythrocyte hemolysis skin lesions and alopecia manifested in these animals were ameliorated by an increased intake of vitamin E and the correction of membrane n-6/n-3 balance.[90] Similarly, other studies[91–94] have reported that dietary n-3 fatty acids exert a protective effect against injury caused by oxidative stress.

Animal studies show reduced activities of the antioxidant enzymes in the lung and kidney of those delivered before term. These studies indicate that functionally protective enzymes are being put in place towards the end of gestation in preparation for a normal term delivery.[95,96] Similarly, the activities of superoxide dismutase, glutathione peroxidase and catalase are low in preterm and low birth weight babies.[97–99]

Preterm and low birth weight infants are born with low circulating and hepatic levels of vitamins A and E.[100–102] Reports suggest a protective effect of vitamin A against bronchopulmonary dysplasia,[103] and of vitamin E against retinopathy of prematurity[104,105] and intra/periventricular hemorrhage.[106–108]

Conclusion

All these data show that the preterm baby is born disadvantaged because of the loss of the placental input of structural fatty acids and immature endogenous peroxidative defense systems. Moreover, these premature-birth-induced disadvantages persist postnatally. Blood antioxidant protection remains depressed and the proportions of plasma structural fatty acids fall precipitously. These babies are indeed a mirror of the chicken model of brain hemorrhage caused by a combined deficit of antioxidants and structural fatty acids.

REFERENCES

1. Saugstad OD. Mechanism of tissue injury by oxygen radicals: Implications for neonatal disease. *Acta Paediatr* 1996;85:1–4.
2. Gunstone F, Norris FA. *Lipids in Foods.* Oxford: Pergamon Press, 1983.
3. Tinoco J. Dietary requirements and functions of alpha-linolenic acid in animals. *Prog Lipid Res* 1982;20:1–45.
4. Budowski P. Omega-3 fatty acids in health and disease. *World Rev Nutr Diet* 1988;57:214–74.
5. Ackman RG. Fatty acid composition of fish oils. In Barlow SM, Stansby ME, eds. *Nutritional Evaluation of Long-Chain Fatty Acids in Fish Oils.* London: Academic Press, 1982:25–88.
6. Ackman RG. Unsaturated fatty acids and health. *Omega-3 News* 1990;4:1–4.
7. O'Dea K, Sinclair AJ. High arachidonic acid content in Australian fish caught off the coast at 17°S. *Am J Clin Nutr* 1982;36:868–72.
8. O'Brian JS, Sampson EL. Fatty acid and fatty acid aldehyde composition of the major brain lipids in normal human gray matter, white matter and myelin *J Lipid Res* 1965;6:545–51.
9. Svennerholm L. Distribution of fatty acid composition of phosphoglycerides in normal human brain. *J Lipid Res* 1968;9:570–9.
10. Suzki H, Manable S, Wada O, *et al.* Rapid incorporation of docosahexaenoic acid from dietary sources into brain microsomal, synaptosomal and mitochondrial membranes in adult mice. *Int J Vit Res* 1997;67:272–8.
11. Fliesler SJ, Anderson RE. Chemistry and metabolism of lipids in the vertebrate retina. *Prog Lipid Res* 1983;22:79–131.
12. Fleischer S, Rouser G. Lipids of sub-cellular particles. *J Am Oil Chem Soc* 1965;42:588–607.
13. Salem N Jr, Kim H-Y, Yergey JA. Docosahexaenoic acid: Membrane function and metabolism. In Simopoulos AP, Kifer RR, Martin RE, eds. *Healthy Effects of Polyunsaturated Fatty Acids in Seafoods.* Orlando, FL: Academic Press, 1986:263–317.
14. Bazan NG. Supply of n-3 polyunsaturated fatty acids and their significance in the central nervous system. In Wurtman RJ, Wurtman JJ, eds *Nutrition and the Brain.* New York: Raven Press, 1990:1–4.
15. Anderson RE, O'Brian PJ, Weigand RD, *et al.* Conservation of docosahexaenoic acid in the retina. *Adv Exp Med Biol* 1992;86: 587–621.
16. Burr GO, Burr MM. A new deficiency disease produced by the rigid exclusion of fat from the diet. *J Biol Chem* 1929;82:345–67.
17. Holman RT. Essential fatty acid deficiency. *Prog Chem Fat* 1968;9: 275–348.
18. Rivers JPW, Sinclair AJ, Crawford MA. Inability of the cat to desaturate essential fatty acids. *Nature* 1975;258:171–3.
19. Holman RT, Johnson SB, Hatch TG. Human linoleic acid deficiency. *Prog Lipid Res* 1982;25:29–39.
20. Neuringer M, Anderson GJ, Connor WE. The essentiality of n-3 fatty acids for the development and function of the retina and the brain. *Ann Rev Nutr* 1988;8:517–41.
21. Clausen J, Moller D. Allergic encephalomyelitis induced by brain antigen after deficiency polyunsaturated fatty acids during myelination. *Acta Neurol Scand* 1967;43:375–88.
22. Crawford MA, Sinclair AJ. Nutritional influences in the evolution of mammalian brain. In Elliot K, Knight J, eds. *Lipids, Malnutrition and the Developing Brain.* Ciba Foundation Symposium. Amsterdam: Elsevier, 1972:267–92.
23. Galli C, Socini A. Dietary lipids in pre- and post-natal development. In Perkins EG, Visek WJ, eds. *Dietary Fats and Health.* Proceedings of American Oil Chemists Society Conference, Chicago, IL, 1983;16:278–301.
24. Budowski P, Leighfield MJ, Crawford MA. Nutritional encephalomalacia in the chick: An exposure of the vulnerable period for cerebellar development and the possible need for both $\omega 6$ and $\omega 3$ fatty acids. *Br J Nutr* 1987;58:511–20.
25. Wheeler TG, Benolken RM, Anderson RE. Visual membranes: Specificity of fatty acid precursors for the electrical response to illumination. *Science* 1975;188:1312.
26. Bourre JM, Marianne FJ, Youyou A, *et al.* The effects of dietary alpha-linolenic acid on the composition of nerve membranes, enzymatic activity, amplitude of electrophysiological parameters, resistance to poisons and electrophysiological parameters, resistance to poisons and performance of learning tasks in rats. *J Nutr* 1989;19:1880–91.
27. Yamamoto M, Saitoh M, Moriuchi A, *et al.* Effect of dietary alpha-linolenate/linoleate balance on brain lipid composition and learning ability in rats. *J Lipid Res* 1987;28:144–51.
28. Connor WE, Neuringer M, Reisbick S. Essential fatty acids: The importance of n-3 fatty acids in the retina and brain. *Nutr Rev* 1992;50:21–9.
29. British Nutrition Foundation. *The Report of the British Nutrition Foundation's Task Force on Unsaturated Fatty Acids.* London: Chapman & Hall, 1992.
30. Marcheselli VL, Hong S, Lukiw WJ, *et al.* Novel docosanoids inhibit brain ischemia-reperfusion-mediated leukocyte infiltration and pro-inflammatory gene expression. *J Biol Chem* 2003; 278(44):43807–17.
31. Clandinin MT, Chappel JE, Leong S, *et al.* Intrauterine fatty acid accretion in human brain: Implications for fatty acid requirements. *Early Hum Dev* 1980;4:120–9.
32. Martinez M. Tissue levels of polyunsaturated fatty acids during early human development. *J Pediatr* 1992;120:S129–38.
33. Clandinin MT, Chappell JE, Leong S, *et al.* Intrauterine fatty acid accretion in human brain: Implications for fatty acid requirements. *Early Hum Dev* 1980;4:131–8.
34. Chambaz J, Ravel D, Manier MC, *et al.* Essential fatty acids interconversion in the human feta liver. *Biol Neonate* 1985;47:136–40.
35. Holman RT, Johnson SB, Ogburn PL. Deficiency of essential fatty acids and membrane fluidity during pregnancy and lactation. *Proc Natl Acad Sci USA* 1991;88:4835–9.
36. Hornstra G, Al M, Houwelingen AC, *et al.* Essential fatty acids in pregnancy and early human development. *Eur J Obstet Gynecol Reprod Biol* 1995;61:57–62.
37. Olsen SF, Sorensen TIA, Secher NJ, *et al.* Intake of marine fat rich in (n-3) polyunsaturated fatty acids may increase birth-weight by prolonging gestation. *Lancet* 1986;2:367–9.
38. Helland IB, Saugstad OD, Smith L, *et al.* Similar effects on infants of n-3 and n-6 fatty acids supplementation to pregnant and lactating women. *Pediatr* 2001;108:E82–92.
39. Helland IB, Smith L, Saarem K, *et al.* Maternal supplementation with very long chain n-3 fatty acids during pregnancy and lactation augments children IQ at 4 years of age. *Pediatrics* 2003;111: 1–10.

40. Ghebremeskel K, Thomas B, Min Y, *et al* Fatty acids in pregnant diabetic women and neonates: Implications for pre-natal and post-natal development. *Prostaglandins Leukot Essent Fatty Acids* 1997;57:190.
41. Ghebremeskel K, Thomas B, Lowy C, *et al.* Type 1 diabetes compromises plasma arachidonic and docosahexaenoic acids in newborn babies. *Lipids* 2004;39(4):335–42.
42. Min Y, Lowy C, Ghebremeskel K, *et al.* Fetal erythrocyte membrane lipids modification: Preliminary observation of an early sign of compromised insulin sensitivity in the offspring of gestational diabetics. *Diabet Med* 2005;22(7):914–20.
43. Crawford MA, Costeloe K, Doyle W, *et al.* Potential diagnostic value of the umbilical artery as a definition of neural fatty acid status of the fetus during its growth. *Biochem Soc Trans* 1990;18:761–6.
44. Koletzko B, Braun M. Arachidonic acid and early human growth: Is there a relation? *Ann Nutr Metab* 1991;35:128–31.
45. Leaf AA, Leighfield MJ, Costeloe KI, *et al.* Long chain polyunsaturated fatty acids and fetal growth. *Early Hum Dev* 1992;30:183–91.
46. Crawford MA, Doyle W, Drury PJ, *et al.* N-6 and n-3 fatty acids during early human development. *J Intern Med* 1989;225(Suppl 1): 159–69.
47. Leaf AA, Leighfield MJ, Costeloe KI, *et al.* Factors affecting long-chain polyunsaturated fatty acid composition of plasma choline phosphoglycerides in preterm infants. *J Pediatr Gastroenterol Nutr* 1992;14:300–8.
48. Cetin I, Giovanni N, Alvino G, *et al.* Intrauterine growth restriction is associated with changes in polyunsaturated fatty acid fetal–maternal relationship. *Pediatr Res* 2002;52:750–5.
49. Vilbergsson G, Wennergreen M, Samsioe G, *et al.* Essential fatty acid status is altered in pregnancies complicated by intrauterine growth retardation. *World Rev Nutr Diet* 1994;76:105–9.
50. Zhang L. The effects of essential fatty acid preparation in the treatment of intrauterine growth retardation. *Am J Perinatol* 1997;14: 535–7.
51. Ghebremeskel K, Leighfield M, Leaf A, *et al.* Fatty acid composition of plasma and red cell phospholipids of preterm babies fed on breast milk and formulae. *Eur J Pediatr* 1995;154:46–52.
52. Poisson JP, Dupuy RP, Sarda P, *et al.* Evidence that liver microsomes of human neonates desaturates essential fatty acids. *Biochim Biophys Acta* 1993;1167:109–13.
53. Sauerwald TU, Hachey DL, Jensen CL, *et al.* Intermediates in endogenous synthesis of C22:6 omega-3 and 20:4 omega 6 by term and preterm infants. *Pediatrics* 1997;41:183–7.
54. Food and Agriculture Organisation/World Health Organisation. *The Role of Dietary Fats and Oils in Human Nutrition.* Report of a Joint Expert Consultation. Rome: Food and Nutrition, Paper 57, 1993.
55. Koletzko B, Decsi T, Demmelmair H. Arachidonic acid supply and metabolism in human infants born at full term. *Lipids* 1996; 31:79–83.
56. Crawford MA, Hassam AG, Williams G, *et al.* Essential fatty acids and fetal brain growth. *Lancet* 1976;1:452–3.
57. Carlson SE, Rhodes PG, Ferguson MG. Docosahexaenoic acid status of preterm infants at birth and following feeding with human milk or formula. *Am J Clin Nutr* 1986;44:798–804.
58. Farquharson J, Cockburn F, Patrick AW, *et al.* Infant cerebral cortex phospholipid fatty acid composition and diet. *Lancet* 1992;340:810–3.
59. Makrides M, Neumann MA, Byard RW, *et al.* Fatty acid composition of brain, retina, and erythrocytes in breast and formula-fed infants. *Am J Clin Nutr* 1994;60:189–94.
60. Birch EE, Birch DG, Hoffman D, *et al.* Dietary essential fatty acid supply and visual acuity development. *Invest Ophthalmol Vis Sci* 1993;33:3242–53.
61. Birch EE, Birch DG, Hoffman D, *et al.* Breast-feeding and optimal visual development. *J Pediatr Ophthalmol Strabismus* 1993;30: 33–8.
62. Carlson SE, Werkman SH, Rhodes PJ, *et al.* Visual acuity development in healthy preterm infants: Effect of marine oil supplementation. *Am J Clin Nutr* 1993;58:35–42.
63. Carlson SE, Werkman SH, Peeples JM, *et al.* Arachidonic acid status correlates with first year growth in preterm infants. *Proc Natl Acad Sci USA* 1993;90:901–7.
64. Uauy R, Birch E, Birch D, *et al.* Visual and brain function measurements in studies of n-3 fatty acid measurements in studies of n-3 fatty acid requirements of infants. *J Pediatr* 1992;120:S168–80.
65. Vavy R, Peirano P, Hoffman D, *et al.* Role of essential fatty acids in the function of the developing nervous system. *Lipids* 1996;31: 5167–76.
66. Makrides M, Simmer K, Goggin M, *et al.* Erythrocyte docosahexaenoic acid correlates with visual response of healthy term infants. *Pediatr Res* 1993;34:425–7.
67. Wainwright PE. Do essential fatty acids play a role in brain and behavioural development? *Neurosci Biobehav Rev* 1992;16: 193–205.
68. Bjerve KF, Thoresen L, Bonaa K, *et al.* Clinical studies with alpha-linolenic acid and long chain n-3 fatty acids. *Nutrition* 1992;8: 130–2.
69. Lucas A, Morley R, Cole TJ, *et al.* Breast milk and subsequent intelligence quotient in children born preterm. *Lancet* 1992;339:261–4.
70. Lanting CI, Fidler V, Huisman M, *et al.* Neurological difference between 9-year old children fed breast milk or formula milk as babies. *Lancet* 1994;344:1319–22.
71. Carlson SE, Ford AJ, Werkman SH, *et al.* Visual acuity and fatty acid status of term infants fed human milk and formulas with and without docoahexaenoate and arachidonate from egg yolk lecithin. *Pediatr Res* 1996;30:882–8.
72. Auestad N, Montalto MB, Hall RT, *et al.* Visual acuity erythrocyte fatty acid composition, and growth in term infants fed formulas with long chain polyunsaturated fatty acids for one year. Ross Pediatrics Lipid Study. *Pediatr Res* 1997;41:1–10.
73. Drury P, Crawford MA. Essential fatty acids in human milk. In Dobbing J, Gracey M, Santerre J, eds. *Clinical Nutrition of the Young Child.* New York: Raven Press Ltd, Nestec Ltd, 1990:289–312.
74. Hall B. Changing composition of human milk and early development of an appetite control. *Lancet* 1975;1:779–81.
75. Jensen RG. *The Lipids of Human Milk.* Boca Raton, FL: CRC Press, 1989.
76. Gibson RA, Kneebone GM. Fatty acid composition of human colostrum and mature breast milk. *Am J Clin Nutr* 1981;34:252–7.
77. Crawford MA, Sinclair AJ, Msuya PM, *et al.* Structural lipids and their polyenoic constituents in human milk. In Galli C, Jacini G, Pecile A, eds *Dietary Lipids and Postnatal Development.* New York: Raven Press, 1973:41–56.
78. Bitman J, Wood DL, Hamosh M, *et al.* Comparison of the lipid composition of breast milk from mothers of term and preterm infants. *Am J Clin Nutr* 1984;38:300–13.
79. Finley DA, Lonnerdal B, Dewy KG, *et al.* Breast milk composition: Fat content and fatty acid composition of vegetarians and non-vegetarians. *Am J Clin Nutr* 1985;41:787–800.
80. Innis SM, Kuhnlein HV. Long-chain n-3 fatty acids in breast milk of Inuit women consuming traditional foods. *Early Hum Dev* 1988;18:185–9.
81. Wang L, Shimizu Y, Kaneko S, et al. Comparison of the fatty acid composition of total lipids and phospholipids in breast milk from Japanese women. *Pediatr Int.* 2000;42(1):14–20.
82. Crawford MA, Hall B, Laurance BM, *et al.* Milk lipids and their variability. *Curr Med Res Opin* 1976;4:33–43.
83. Ghebremeskel K, Bitsanis D, Koukkou E, *et al.* Maternal diet high in fat reduces docosahexaenoic acid in liver lipids of the newborn and suckling pups. *Br J Nutr* 1999;81:395–404.
84. Phylactos AC, Harbidge LS, Crawford MA. Essential fatty acids alter the activity of manganese-superoxide dismutase in rat heart. *Lipids* 1994;29:111–5.
85. Saugstad OD. Hypoxanthine as an indicator of hypoxia: Its role in health and diseases through free radical production. *Pediatr Res* 1988;23:143–50.
86. Sullivan JL. Iron plasma antioxidants, and the 'oxygen radical disease of prematurity'. *Am J Dis Child* 1988;142:1341–4.
87. Budowski P, Hawkey CM, Crawford MA. The protective effect of alpha-linoleic acid on encephalomalacia in chicks. *Ann Nutr Anim* 1980;34:389–400 (in French).
88. Ghebremeskel K, Williams G, Harbige L, *et al.* Plasma vitamins A and E and hydrogen peroxide-induced *in vitro* erythrocyte haemolysis in common marmosets (*Callithrix jacchus*). *Vet Rec* 1990;126:429–31.
89. Harbige LS, Ghebremeskel K, Willliams G, *et al.* N-3 and N-6 fatty acids in relation to *in vitro* erythrocyte haemolysis induced by hydrogen peroxide in captive common marmosets (*Callithrix jacchus*). *Comp Biochem Physiol* 1990;97B:167–70.
90. Ghebremeskel K, Harbige L, Williams G, *et al.* The effect of dietary change on *in vitro* erythrocyte haemolysis, skin lesions and alopecia in common marmosets (*Callithrix jacchus*). *Comp Biochem Physiol* 1991;100A:891–6.
91. Lands WE, Miller JF Jr, Rich SM. Influence of dietary fish oil on plasma lipid hydroxperoxides. *Adv Prostagl Thrombox Leukotriene Res* 1987;17B:876–9.

92. Sosenko IRS, Innis SM, Frank L, Menhaden fish oil n-3 polyunsaturated fatty acids and protection of new born rats from oxygen toxicity. *Pediatr Res* 1989;25:399–404.
93. Ellis EF, Police RJ, Dodson LY, *et al.* Effect of dietary n-3 fatty acids on cerebral micro-circulation. *Am J Physiol* 1992;262:H1379–86.
94. Lehr H-A, Huebner C, Finckh B, *et al.* Dietary fish oil reduces leukocyte/endothelium interaction following system administration of oxidatively modified low density lipoprotein. *Circulation* 1991;84:1725–31.
95. Frank L, Sosenko IRS. Prenatal development of lung antioxidant enzymes in four species. *J Pediatr* 1987;110:106–10.
96. Hayashibe H, Assyama K, Dobashi K, *et al.* Prenatal development of antioxidant enzymes in rat lung, kidney, and heart: Marked increase in immunoreactive superoxide dismutate, glutathione peroxidase and catalase in the kidney. *Pediatr Res* 1990;27:472–5.
97. Autor AP, Frank L, Roberts RJ. Developmental characteristics of pulmonary superoxide dismutase: A relationship to idiopathic respiratory distress syndrome. *Pediatr Res* 1976;10:154–8.
98. Ripalda MJ, Rudolph N, Wong SL. Developmental patterns of antioxidant defence mechanisms in human erythrocytes. *Pediatr Res* 1989;26:366–9.
99. Phylactos AC, Leaf AA, Costeloe K, *et al.* Erythrocyte cupric/zinc superoxide dismutase exhibits reduced activity in preterm and low birthweight infants at birth. *Acta Paediatr* 1995;84:1421–5.
100. Johnson LH, Schaffer DB, Boggs TR Jr. The premature infant vitamin E deficiency and retrolental fibroplasias. *Am J Clin Nutr* 1974;27:1158–73.
101. Shenai JP, Chytil F, Jhaveri A, *et al.* Plasma vitamin A and retinal-binding protein in premature and term neonates *J Pediatr* 1981;99:302–5.
102. Ghebremeskel K, Burns, L, Burden TJ, *et al.* Vitamin A and related essential nutrients in cord blood: Relationship with anthropometric measurements at birth. *Early Hum Dev* 1994;39:177–88.
103. Shenai JP, Kennedy KA, Chytil F, *et al* Clinical trial of vitamin A supplementation in infants susceptible to bronchopulmonary dysplasia. *J Pediatr* 1987;111:269–77.
104. Finer NN, Schindler RF, Grant G, *et al.* Effect of intramuscular vitamin E on frequency and severity of retrolental fibroplasia. *Lancet* 1982;1:1087–91.
105. Hittner HM, Godio LB, Speer ME, *et al.* Retrolental fibroplasia: Further clinical evidence and ultrastructural support for efficiency of vitamin E in the preterm infant. *Pediatrics* 1983;71:423–32.
106. Chiswick ML, Johnson M, Woodhall C, *et al.* Protective effect of vitamin E (DL-alpha-tocopheral) against intraventricular haemorrhage in premature babies. *Br Med J* 1983;287:81–4.
107. Chiswick ML, Gladman G, Sinha S, *et al.* Vitamin E supplementation and periventricular hemorrhage in the newborn. *Am J Clin Nutr* 1991;53:370S–2S.
108. Speer ME, Blifield C, Rudolph AJ, *et al.* Intraventricular haemorrhage and vitamin E in the very low-birth-weight infant: Evidence for efficacy of early intramuscular vitamin E administration. *Pediatrics* 1984;74:1107–12.

92 Maternal inherited metabolic disease

R. Floyd, F. Cockburn and B. J. Clark

Introduction

Recombinant DNA technology with the mapping of the human genome has made possible the localization, identification and isolation of disease-related genes which, in turn, have improved disease diagnosis and prediction and identified inherited defects underlying many common metabolic disorders affecting adults. Inherited metabolic disease may be diagnosed prenatally, in infancy, or may present as an adult-onset disease, particularly in diseases not generally associated with a detectable chromosome aberration or a clear Mendelian pattern of inheritance. Many of these metabolic disorders have been called polygenic or multifactorial even though it is not usually known how many genetic loci are involved or how they interact with environmental factors. Diabetes mellitus and essential hypertension are examples though the genetics of both of these disease processes are currently being illuminated. There are many perturbations of maternal metabolism which can adversely affect growth and development of the human embryo and fetus. The purpose of this chapter will be to review those maternal inherited metabolic disorders which can result in failure of implantation, early loss of implanted ova and congenital malformations or metabolic disorder in the newborn infant.

The number of autosomal and X-linked chromosomal disorders identified continues to grow daily, many of which result in metabolic diseases or disorders. The development of management strategies to alleviate or correct these inherited disease processes has encouraged early detection with screening programs. Table 92.1 gives the frequency of some inborn errors of metabolism for which screening tests are available.[1] Although we now have considerable information about phenylketonuria in relation to pregnancy management and outcome there are many other inherited metabolic disorders affecting young women which carry a risk to the developing embryo and fetus.

Table 92.1 Frequency of some inborn errors of metabolism for which neonatal screening tests are available

Disorder	Average frequency in liveborn infants*
Cystic fibrosis	1 in 2500
Cystinuria	1 in 6000
Phenylketonuria	1 in 10,000
α_1 Antitrypsin deficiency	1 in 8,000
Histidinemia	1 in 10,000
Hartnup disorder	1 in 26,000
Galactosemia	1 in 60,000
Biotinidase deficiency	1 in 60,000
Maple syrup urine disease	1 in 200,000
Homocystinuria	1 in 200,000

*These frequencies vary widely between ethnic groups, e.g. phenylketonuria 1 in 7000 in Scotland and 1 in 200 000 in Japan.

Maternal metabolic disorders and pregnancy

Diabetes mellitus

It has long been known that the infant of the poorly controlled diabetic mother is at increased risk of congenital malformation, fetal overgrowth and neonatal hypoglycemia.[2] With improved care of pregnant diabetic women, these complications and perinatal mortality for the infant have been reduced.[3–7] There is a recognized higher prevalence of diabetes mellitus in children born to diabetic parents. A higher incidence of non-insulin-dependent diabetes or gestational diabetes is found in children born to diabetic mothers than when the father is diabetic.[8] There is also a higher incidence of diabetes in offspring from diabetic maternal great-grandmothers but not paternal ones.[9] Genomic imprinting is a possible explanation for these findings.[10–12] In HLA-DR4-positive diabetics, there is evidence of a gene or genes affecting the HLA region on chromosome 6p21 and the region of 11p15 where the genes for insulin and insulin-like growth factor-2 are located.[13]

A further interesting observation has been that systematic treatment of diabetic mothers during pregnancy, results in a decreased incidence of diabetes in their children.[14,15] This implies that the abnormal intrauterine environment may have as much if not more effect in determining susceptibility to subsequent diabetes in later childhood than do the genetic predisposing factors. Mechanisms for the predisposition to diabetes in the infant of a diabetic mother may be related to an intrauterine influence on the effective development of islet β-cells in the fetal pancreas or to an alteration in the numbers or sensitivity of insulin receptors in muscle, liver and other body tissues.

Cystic fibrosis

This is an autosomal recessive condition in which there is an abnormality of transmembrane protein function rather than a defect or deficiency of an enzyme which characterizes the majority of inherited metabolic disorders. Although there are problems of infertility in both females and males there is no evidence of embryopathy or fetal disorder given an adequate maternal nutritional status during pregnancy.[16]

Histidinemia

Maternal histidinemia is probably benign to the fetus. At least 61 children from 23 histidinemic mothers, most of whom were normal, have been reported.[17] No adverse outcomes secondary to this disorder have been noted.[17–21]

Hartnup disorder

Hartnup disease, a disorder of neutral amino acid transport in the intestinal epithelium, is inherited in an autosomal recessive manner. Maternal Hartnup disorder is also probably benign to the fetus. At least 14 children of women with the condition are known and almost all are normal. Therapy requires nicotinamide replacement and a high protein diet. Pregnancy does not appear to have any clinical impact on these families.[22]

Homocystinuria

Homocystinuria is an autosomal recessive disorder that is characterized by increased concentrations of homocystine and methionine in blood and urine and physical features such as mental retardation, epilepsy, ectopia lentis, osteoporosis, skeletal anomalies, fatty liver and thrombotic vascular disease. These findings are secondary to a deficiency of the enzyme cystathionine β-synthase. The disorder is responsive to B6 cofactor and a low methionine diet in about 50% of patients.[23] Pregnancies have been reported in both pyridoxine responsive and non-responsive mothers with a normal outcome.[24–26] An adequate intake of pyridoxine should be ensured as treatment with pyridoxine appears to significantly lower the risk of fetal loss.

Heterozygotes are at an increased risk for multiple thromboses, coronary artery disease and other vascular disease.[27] Third-trimester complications similar to those with other inherited coagulopathies and postpartum thrombotic deaths have been reported which suggest the use of anticoagulation therapy may be indicated.[28–30]

Folate metabolism disorders

A genetic defect in 5,10-methylenetetrahydrofolate reductase in young women has been shown to be a risk factor for neural tube defect.[31–33] This enzyme is involved in the conversion of 5,10-methylenetetrahydrofolate to 5-methyltetrahydrofolate which is involved in the conversion of homocysteine to methionine (Figure 92.1). The common mutation of 677CT defect is found in 5–7% of the European population and homozygosity for this mutation results in elevated homocysteine levels, elevated red cell folate and lowered plasma folate concentrations. Periconceptual folate administration reduces neural tube birth prevalence by over 60%.[33–36] Altered folate and vitamin B_{12} metabolism has been found in families with infants with spina bifida.[37] This study did not support a major involvement of methionine synthase in the etiology of neural tube defect but favored the involvement of genetic variation at loci coding for the formation of 5-methyltetrahydrofolate. A relatively mild biochemical defect in folate metabolism, requiring a higher nutritional folate intake, may become of major importance during pregnancy. Whether there would be value in detecting those individuals heterozygous for the known defects is questionable as universal prenatal folate supplementation is so effective. These patients have also been noted to have an increase in complications in the third trimester consistent with those seen in patients with an inherited coagulopathy and the use of anticoagulation should be considered in those patients with a history of thrombosis or poor pregnancy outcome.

Isovaleric acidemia

Maternal isolaveric acidemia has minimal impact on pregnancy and vice versa and has no ill effect on the offspring.[38] Treatment of the mother should be instituted prior to conception with protein restriction and additional glycine 0.5 g/day and L-carnitine 1 g/day to reduce the risk of metabolic acidosis in the mother and thus reduce potential hazards to the embryo and fetus. Vomiting in early pregnancy must be actively managed with a high carbohydrate intake, if necessary by nasogastric tube or parenterally, to avoid a catabolic state.

Urea cycle defects

The urea cycle defects include citrullinemia, argininosuccinic aciduria (ASLD), ornithine trancarbamylase deficiency (OTC), carbamoylphosphate synthetase

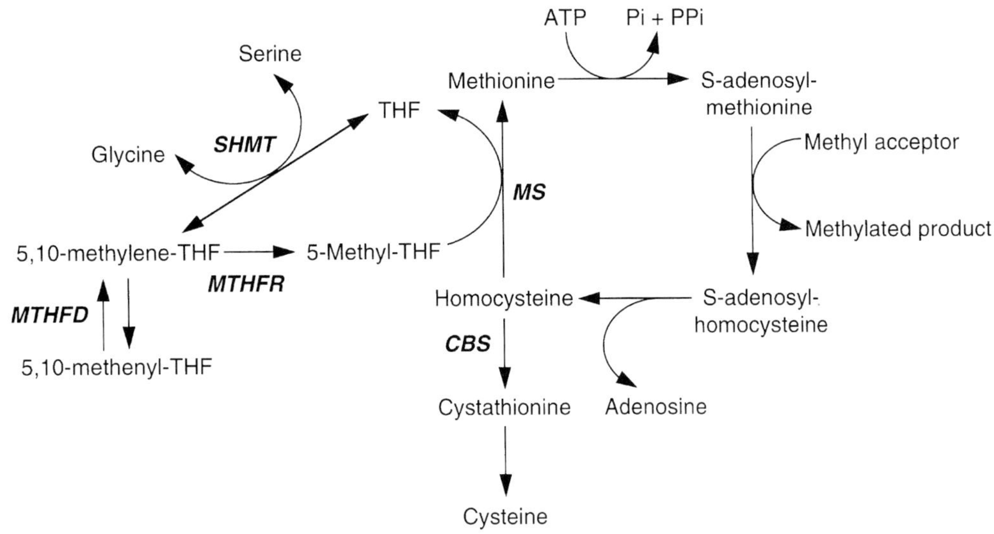

Figure 92.1

deficiency and N-acetyl glutamate synthase deficiency.[39] There are very few reports in the literature as to the effects of these disorders on pregnancy and infants. Heterozygotes for OTC deficiency, the only X-linked disorder of the urea cycle, are known to be at risk for the development of hyperammonemic coma in the peripartum period, possibly due to increased tissue catabolism.[40] It has been reported that a woman with carbamoyl phosphate synthetase I deficiency developed hyperammonemic coma and died in the postpartum period.[41]

ASLD due to argininosuccinate lyase deficiency usually presents at birth with poor feeding, lethargy, hypotonia, irritability, apnea and occasionally death in the neonatal period.[42] More often there is a chronic presentation which involves mental retardation, with or without intermittent episodes of vomiting, lethargy and irritability. Trichorrhexis nodosa is a frequent occurrence, probably because of a relative deficiency of arginine.[39] Early treatment of patients with partial ASLD can result in normal intellectual and psychomotor development and as a result some patients are now surviving into adulthood and considering pregnancy. In females affected with argininosuccinate lyase deficiency, careful clinical and biochemical monitoring of pregnancy will minimize the risk of metabolic decompensation in the perinatal period. There is one report of a 'successful' pregnancy with no evidence that the argininosuccinate was teratogenic. The mother had been treated with a low protein diet and arginine supplements but her compliance with the arginine supplementation was suboptimal. When reviewed at 3 months of age, the baby was mildly dysmorphic with hypertelorism, a broad nasal bridge and down-slanting palpebral fissures but was developing normally.[43]

In all the urea cycle defects it is essential to ensure an adequate energy intake throughout pregnancy and if vomiting occurs enteral and/or parenteral therapy with carbohydrate should be given immediately.

Glycogen storage disorders

The glycogen storage disorders result from an inborn error of glycogen metabolism secondary to mutations in the genes coding for the enzymes involved in glycogen storage. These disorders have a variable age of onset from birth to adulthood and are categorized by number based upon the chronology of recognition of the responsible enzyme defect. Only those with a reasonable likelihood of presence during and potential impact upon pregnancy are discussed.

Glucose-6-phosphate deficiency (type I glycogen storage disease) is an autosomal recessive disorder involving mutations in the genes for glucose-6-phosphate hydrolase located at 17q21 (type 1a) and glucose-6-phosphate translocase located at 11q23 (type 1b,c,d). The incidence of specific mutations varies with ethnicity.[44,45] Affected patients typically present in early infancy with hepatomegaly, hypoglycemia and lactic acidosis.[46] The majority of patients will also have hyperuricemia and marked hyperlipidemia.[46] Platelet dysfunction is common and liver adenomas often develop in older children and adults with malignant transformation in approximately 10%.[47] Patients with type 1b also have chronic or intermittent neutropenia and neutrophil dysfunction.

Maintenance of physiologic levels of glucose is the mainstay of therapy. This becomes markedly more difficult during pregnancy and provision of frequent meals high in carbohydrate content and supplementation with uncooked cornstarch during the day and prior to bedtime can usually accomplish this goal. In some cases, the use of continuous infusion of glucose solution via nasogastric tube or additional doses of cornstarch in the early morning hours may be necessary.

Multivitamins and calcium should supplement the diet and fructose and galactose restricted. Intravenous glucose and platelet transfusion may be used for abnormal bleeding; the use of allopurinol and vasopressin during pregnancy are currently proscribed.[48]

Pregnancy outcomes with adequate glucose supplementation appear to be good in most cases. The incidence of growth restriction may be increased and monitoring the fetus with serial ultrasound measurements in the third trimester should be considered. Patients with type 1b should be monitored for evidence of subclinical infection (upper respiratory, urinary tract) due to the potential for neutrophil dysfunction. Delivery at or near term should be anticipated. The intrapartum glucose levels should be closely monitored and appropriate supplementation provided.[49,50]

Type III glycogen storage disease is inherited as an autosomal recessive trait and is specifically a mutation in the gene that encodes for the debrancher enzyme amyloglucosidase. This gene is located at 1p21 and again, specific mutations vary with ethnic background.[51,52] Clinical features of the disease include liver and muscle involvement with hepatomegaly, hypotonia, weakness and muscle wasting as well as cardiac involvement. Hepatomegaly and liver function typically improve with age and muscle weakness is the primary finding in adults. Involvement of the liver alone occurs in approximately 15% of patients.[53–55]

Case reports of maternal type III glycogen storage disease relate the potential for life-threatening complications, specifically cardiac decompensation.[56] Evaluation of cardiac anatomy prior to and during pregnancy (at 28 weeks) and postpartum should be obtained. Management includes supplementation of glucose as described for type I glycogen storage disease.

Type V glycogen storage disease (McArdle's disease) is a disorder caused by mutations in the single gene encoding the muscle isoform of phosphorylase.[57] This gene is located at 11q13.[58] Phosphorylase catalyzes the removal of 1,4-glucosyl residues from the outer branches of the glycogen molecule liberating glucose-1-phosphate. This myophosphorylase deficiency results in accumulation of glycogen in skeletal muscle and reduction in ATP generation. Clinically, this manifests as muscle fatigue and cramping with strenuous exercise. There is no heart or liver involvement. Case reports of pregnancy outcomes relate no deterioration or exacerbation of symptoms.[59] Limiting activity during pregnancy will control the symptoms associated with the disorder and the only complication of labor reported is that of forearm cramping secondary to the use of an automatic blood pressure cuff.

Hyperglycinemia

Hyperglycinemia is a non-specific feature of several organic acidurias and is usually associated with intermittent ketosis. Non-ketotic hyperglycinemia is a specific disorder of glycine catabolism caused by a defect in the glycine cleavage system.[60] The disorder usually presents in the first week of life with somnolence, lethargy and lack of spontaneous movement and apneic episodes. There may be seizures and exaggerated reflexes. Milder forms of the disorder are found with non-specific mental retardation in adult life. The diagnosis is made on the basis of finding hyperglycinemia and hyperglycinuria in the absence of a disorder of organic acid metabolism. The diagnosis is usually confirmed by the finding of high cerebrospinal fluid concentrations of glycine. In the milder forms of the disorder administration of large doses of sodium benzoate has been shown to reduce CSF glycine and the frequency of seizures. The authors have experience of three pregnancies in one non-ketotic hyperglycinemic mother managed with oral sodium benzoate. The control of plasma glycine levels in the mother was relatively easy during the pregnancy and indeed was less troublesome than during the non-pregnancy phase. The three infants were normally grown and have thrived with normal subsequent development.

Galactosemia

Galactosemia is the term used to describe disorders of galactose metabolism. The disorder is actually three distinct disorders caused by defects in galactose-1-phosphate uridyl transferase, galactokinase and uridine diphosphate galactose-4-epimerase.[61] The only form discussed here is that caused by defective galactose-1-phosphate uridyl transferase in which conversion of galactose to glucose is impaired. Accumulation of galactose-1-phosphate, galactitol, galactonate and uridine diphosphate (UDP) galactose is thought to be the cause of the complications of galactose ingestion. In the newborn period, ingestion of galactose leads to vomiting and diarrhea with progression to hyperbilirubinemia, hepatomegaly, liver dysfunction and cirrhosis, hemolysis, and sepsis. Cataracts rapidly develop in the first week of life. Despite early therapy these patients still manifest developmental delay, poor growth, mental deficiency and premature ovarian failure. Up to 75% of affected females over 14 years of age will experience ovarian dysfunction. Pregnancies in affected females appear to proceed normally without adverse fetal affects.[62,63] Breast feeding is contraindicated due to effects on the mother. The production of galactose-1-phosphate from the breakdown of endogenous lactose produced in the mammary glands is problematic, leading to accumulation of galactose-1-phosphate, galactitol, galactonate and UDP-galactose.[64]

Phenylketonuria

Early treatment of phenylketonuria has resulted in a markedly improved outlook for survival with good intellect. In recent years there has been some concern that the withdrawal of dietary therapy in later life may be associated with neurological disorder and gross cerebral changes shown by magnetic resonance imaging.[65]

Charles Dent was probably the first investigator who noted the association of fetal abnormality and maternal phenylketonuria in 1956.[66] Since that time there have been many reports of fetal abnormalities associated with uncontrolled or poorly controlled maternal phenylketonuria.[67–72] Abnormalities reported in untreated phenylketonuria, when the intrapartum maternal plasma phenylalanine concentration exceeded 1.5 mmol/l, include mental retardation in 92%, microcephaly in 72%, intrauterine growth delay in 40% and congenital heart malformation in 12% of the offspring.[69] Phenylalanine is transported across the placenta by an active transport process which results in higher plasma concentrations of phenylalanine in the fetus than in the mother. The ratio of fetal to maternal plasma concentrations of phenylalanine varies throughout pregnancy with a higher ratio in the earlier months. The observed average ratio of fetal to maternal plasma phenylalanine is 1.48 with a range of 1.13–2.91.[73] Any increase in maternal plasma phenylalanine is therefore magnified within the embryonic and fetal tissues. The embryopathy affects the cardiovascular and central nervous systems causing the clinical features described.

Fortunately, fetal defects can be prevented by appropriate maternal dietary management to ensure reasonable plasma concentrations of phenylalanine from before the time of conception.[69–72,74] Two Medical Research Council Working Party reports have summarized the present recommendations for the dietary management of phenylketonuria and expressed the hope that there will be a molecular genetic treatment and prevention program for phenylketonuria.[75,76] Good management of maternal phenylketonuria prevents a variety of dangers and dilemmas for the mother and her medical advisers.[77] Dietary problems are related to the palatability, bulk and osmolality of available amino acid mixtures and the palatability and nutrient value of the permissible low-protein foods. In spite of the dangers to the developing embryo and fetus there is enormous reward for the families and health care providers for having a healthy baby by achieving good maternal dietary control. Until there is a safe effective method for the substitution of the defective gene or phenylalanine hydroxylase or both in the affected individuals, there continues to be a need to achieve prenatal and perinatal control of phenylalanine and tyrosine concentrations in mothers with phenylketonuria.

Conclusions

Perhaps the most important aspect of maternal inherited metabolic disorders is the need to have clinicians informed and aware of the wide range of maternal disorders which can predispose to embryonic, fetal and neonatal problems. For optimal pregnancy outcome, most of these conditions must be identified and metabolic control achieved preconceptually. This review does not address the effect of abnormal pharmacogenetics on maternal drug metabolism and the potential consequence to the fetus. An inherited predisposition to folate disorder will certainly alter the response to drugs that interfere with folate metabolism and maternal alcoholism is influenced by defects in alcohol dehydrogenases.[78,79] A high degree of clinical awareness and effective management would improve the outcome of infants born to mothers with metabolic disorders.

REFERENCES

1. Scriver CR, Beaudet AL, Sly WS, *et al. The Metabolic and Molecular Bases of Inherited Disease*, 7th edn. New York: McGraw-Hill, 1995.
2. Farquhar JW. The influence of maternal diabetes in foetus and child. In Gairdner D, ed. *Recent Advances in Paediatrics*, 3rd edn. London: Churchill, 1965:121–53.
3. Fuhrmann K, Reiher H, Semmler K, *et al.* Prevention of congenital malformations in infants of insulin-dependent diabetic mothers. *Diabetes Care* 1983;6:219–23.
4. Damm P, Molsted-Pedersen L. Significant decrease in congenital malformations in newborn infants of an unselected population of diabetic women. *Am J Obstet Gynecol* 1989;161:1163–7.
5. Goldman GA, Dickerd D, Feldberg D, *et al.* Pregnancy outcome in patients with insulin-dependent diabetes mellitus with preconceptual diabetic control: A comparative study. *Am J Obstet Gynecol* 1986;155:193–7.
6. Steel JM, Johnstone FD, Hepburn DA, *et al.* Can pre-pregnancy care of diabetic women reduce the risk of abnormal babies? *Br Med J* 1990;301:1070–4.
7. Kitzmiller JL, Gavin LA, Gin GD, *et al.* Pre-conception management of diabetes through early pregnancy prevents the excess of major congenital anomalies of infants of diabetic mothers. *J Am Med Assoc* 1991;265:731–6.
8. Martin AO, Simpson JL, Ober C, *et al.* Frequency of diabetes mellitus in probands with gestational diabetes: Possible maternal influence on the predisposition to diabetes. *Am J Obstet Gynecol* 1985;151:471–3.
9. Dorner G, Plagemann A, Reinagel H. Familial diabetes aggregation in Type II diabetics: Gestational diabetes as apparent risk factor for increased diabetes susceptibility in the offspring. *Exp Clin Endocrinol* 1987;89:84–90.
10. Razin A, Cedar H. DNA methylation and genomic imprinting. *Cell* 1994;77:473–6.
11. Efstratiadis A. Parental imprinting of autosomal mammalian genes. *Curr Opin Genet Dev* 1994;4:265–80.
12. Barlow DP. Imprinting: A gamete's point of view. *Trends Genet* 1994;10:194–9.
13. Julier C, Hyer RN, Davies J, *et al.* Insulin-IGF2 region on chromosome 11p encodes a gene implicated in HLA-DR4-dependent diabetes susceptibility. *Nature* 1991;354:155–9.
14. Dorner G, Steindel E, Thoelke H, *et al.* Evidence for decreasing prevalence of diabetes mellitus in childhood apparently produced by prevention of hyperinsulinism in the foetus and newborn. *Exp Clin Endocrinol* 1984;84:134–42.
15. Pettit DJ, Aleck KA, Baird HR, *et al.* Congenital susceptibility to NIDDM role of intrauterine environment. *Diabetes* 1988;33: 622–8.
16. Cohen LF, di Sant'Agenese PA, Friedlander J. Cystic fibrosis and pregnancy. A national study. *Lancet* 1980;2:842–4.
17. Lyon ICT, Gardner RJM, Veale AMO. Maternal histidinaemia. *Arch Dis Child* 1974;49:581.
18. Neville BGR, Harris RF, Stern DJ, Stern J. Maternal histidinemia. *Arch Dis Child* 1971;46:119.
19. Armstrong MD. Maternal histidenemia. *Arch Dis Child* 1975; 50:830.
20. Matsuda I, Nagata N, Endo F. A family with histidinemic parents. *J Pediatr* 1983;103:169.

21. Levy HL, Benjamin R. Maternal histidinemia: Study of families identified by routine cord blood screening. *Pediatr Res* 1985;19:210A.
22. Mahon BE, Levy HL. Maternal hartnup disorder. *Am J Med Genet* 1986;24:513.
23. Gaull GE, Rassin DK, Struman JA. Pyridoxine dependency in homocystinuria (letter). *Lancet* 1968;2:1302.
24. Bittle AH, Carson NAJ. Tissue culture techniques as an aid to prenatal diagnosis and genetic counselling in homocystinuria. *J Med Genet* 1973;10:120–1.
25. Kurczynski TW, Muir WA, Fleisher LD, *et al.* Maternal homocystinuria: Studies of an untreated mother and fetus. *Arch Dis Child* 1980;55:721–3.
26. Rassin DK, Fleisher LD, Muir A, *et al.* Fetal tissue amino acid concentrations in argininosuccinic aciduria and in maternal homocystinuria. *Clin Chim Acta* 1979;94:101–8.
27. Wouters BE, Goers GH, Blom HJ, *et al.* Hyperhomocystinemia: A risk factor in women with unexplained recurrent early pregnancy loss. *Fertil Steril* 1993;60(5):820.
28. Newman G, Mitchell JR. Homocystinuria presenting as multiple arterial occlusions. *Q J Med* 1984;210:251–8.
29. Schulman JD, Mudd SH, Shulman NR, Landvater L. Pregnancy and thrombophlebitis in homocystinemia. *Blood* 1980;56:326.
30. Constantine G, Green A. Untreated homocystinemia: A maternal death in a woman with four pregnancies, a case report. *Br J Obstet Gynecol* 1987;94:803.
31. Put van der NMJ, Steegers-Theunissen RPM, Frosst P, *et al.* Mutated methylenetetrahydrofolate reductase as a risk factor for spina bifida. *Lancet* 1995;346:1071–2.
32. Whitehead AS, Gallagher P, Mills JL, *et al.* A genetic defect in 5,10-methylenetetrahydrofolate reductase in neural tube defects. *Q J Med* 1995;88:763–6.
33. Smithells RW, Sheppard S, Schorah CJ, *et al.* Possible prevention of neural-tube defects by periconceptional vitamin supplementation. *Lancet* 1980;1:339–40.
34. Smithells RW, Sheppard S, Wild J, *et al.* Prevention of neural-tube recurrences in Yorkshire, the final report. *Lancet* 1989;2:498–9.
35. Medical Research Council Vitamin Study Research Group. Prevention of neural-tube defects; results of the Medical Research Council Vitamin Study. *Lancet* 1991;338:131–7.
36. Czeizel AE, Dudas I. Prevention of the first occurrence of neural-tube defects by periconceptional vitamin supplementation. *N Engl J Med* 1992;327:1832–5.
37. Put van der NMJ, Thomas CMJ, Eskes TKAB, *et al.* Altered folate and vitamin B12 metabolism in families with spina bifida offspring. *Q J Med* 1997;90:505–10.
38. Shih VE, Aubrey RH, De Grande G, *et al.* Maternal isovaleric acidemia. *J Pediatr* 1984;105:77.
39. Brusilow SW, Horwich AL. Urea cycle enzymes. In Scriver CR, Beaudet AL, Sly WS, *et al.*, eds. *The Metabolic and Molecular Bases of Inherited Disease*, 7th edn. New York: McGraw-Hill, 1995;32:1187–232.
40. Arn PH, Hauser ER, Thomas GH, *et al.* Hyperam-moninemia in women with a mutation at the ornithine carbamoyl transferase locus: A cause of postpartum coma. *N Engl J Med* 1990;322:1652–5.
41. Wong LJ, Craigen WJ, O'Brien WE. Postpartum coma and death due to carbamoyl-phosphate sythetase I deficiency. *Ann Intern Med* 1994;120:216–7.
42. Widhalm K, Koch S, Scheibenreiter S, *et al.* Long-term follow-up of 12 patients with the late-onset variant of argininosuccinic acid lyase deficiency: No impairment of intellectual and psychomotor development during therapy. *Pediatrics* 1992;89:1182–4.
43. Worthington S, Christodoulou J, Wilcken B, *et al.* Pregnancy and argininosuccinic aciduria. *J Inher Metab Dis* 1996;19:621–3.
44. Gerin I, Viega-da-Cunha M, Achouri Y, et al. Sequence of a putative glucose-6-phosphate translocase, mutated in glycogen storage disease type 1b. *FEBS Lett* 1997;419:235.
45. Lei KJ, Chen YT, Chen H, *et al.* Genetic basis of glycogen storage disease type 1a: Prevalent mutations at glucose-6-phosphatase locus. *Am J Hum Genet* 1995;57:766.
46. Matern D, Seydewitz HH, Bali D, Lang C. Glycogen storage disease type 1: diagnosis and phenotype/genotype correlation. *Eur J Pediatr* 2002;161(Suppl 1):S10.
47. Bianchi L. Glycogen storage disease type 1 and hepatocellular tumours. *Eur J Pediatr* 1993;152(Suppl 1):S63.
48. Johnson MP, Compton A, Drugan A, *et al.* Metabolic control of von Gierke disease (glycogen storage disease type 1a) in pregnancy: Maintenance of euglycemia with cornstarch. *Obstet Gynecol* 1990;75:507.
49. Farber M, Knuppel R, Binkiewicz, *et al.* Pregnancy and von Gierke's disease. *Obstet Gynecol* 1976;47:226.
50. Ryan IP, Havel RJ, Laros RK. Three consecutive pregnancies in a patient with glycogen storage disease type 1a (von Gierke's disease). *Am J Obstet Gynecol* 1994;170:1687.
51. Yang-Feng T, Zheng K, Yu J, *et al.* Assignment of the human glycogen debrancher gene to chromosome 1p21. *Genomics* 1002;13:931.
52. Bao Y, Denison TL, Chen YT. Human glycogen debranching enzyme gene (AGL): Complete structural organization and characterization of the 5′ flanking region. *Genomics* 1992;38:155.
53. Labrune P, Trioche P, Duvalier I, *et al.* Hepatocellular adenomas in glycogen storage disease type I and III: A series of 43 patients and review of the literature. *J Pediatr Gastroenterol Nutr* 1997;24:276.
54. Murase T, Ikada H, Muro T, *et al.* Myopathy associated with type 3 glygenolysis. *J Neurol Sci* 1973;20:287.
55. Moses S, Gadoth N, Bashan N, *et al.* Neuromuscular involvement in glycogen storage disease type III. *Acta Pediatr Scand* 1986;75:289.
56. Olsen LJ, Reeder GS, Noller KL, *et al.* Cardiac involvement in glycogen storage disease III: Morphologic and biochemical characterization with endomyocardial biopsy. *Am J Cardiol* 1984;59:980.
57. McArdle B. Myopathy due to a defect in muscle glycogen breakdown. *Clin Sci* 1951;10:13.
58. Lebo R, Gorin F, Fletterick R, *et al.* High-resolution chromosome sorting and DNA spot-blot analysis assign McArdle's syndrome in chromosome 11. *Science* 1984;225:57.
59. Dinauro S, Breslin N. Phosphorylase deficiency. In Engel A, Baker B, eds. *Myology*. New York: McGraw-Hill, 1986:1585.
60. Nyhan WL. Metabolism of glycine in the normal individual and in patients with non-ketotic hyperglycinaemia. *J Inherit Metab Dis* 1982;5:105–10.
61. Segal S, Berry G. Disorders of galactose metabolism. In Scriver CR, et al., eds. *The Metabolic and Molecular Bases of Inherited Disease*, 7th edn. New York: McGraw-Hill, 1995:967.
62. Roe T, Hallatt J, Donnell G, *et al.* Child-bearing by galactosemic women. *J Pediatr* 1971;78:1026.
63. Tedesco TA, Marrow G, Mellman WJ. Normal pregnancy and childbirth in a galactosemic woman. *J Pediatr* 1972;81:1158.
64. Brivet M, Raymond JP, Konopka P, *et al.* Effect of lactation in a mother with galactosemia. *J Pediatr* 1989;115:280–2.
65. Thompson AJ, Smith I, Brenton D, *et al.* Neurological deterioration in young adults with phenylketonuria. *Lancet* 1990;336:602–5.
66. Dent CE. *Report of 23rd Ross Conference*. Columbus, OH: Ross Laboratories, 1956.
67. Mabry CC, Denniston JC, Nelson TL, *et al.* Maternal phenylketonuria: A cause of mental retardation in children without the metabolic defect. *N Engl J Med* 1963;269:1404–8.
68. Allen JD, Brown JK. Maternal phenylketonuria. In Holt KS, Coffey VP, eds. *Some Recent Advances in Inborn Errors of Metabolism*. Edinburgh: E & S Livingston Ltd, 1968:14–38.
69. Lenke RR, Levy HL. Maternal phenylketonuria and hyperphenylalaninemia. An international survey of untreated and treated pregnancies. *N Engl J Med* 1980;303:1202–8.
70. Koch R, Friedman EG, Wenz E, *et al.* Maternal phenyl-ketonuria. *J Inherit Metab Dis* 1986;9(Suppl 2):159–68.
71. Drogari E, Beasley M, Smith I, *et al.* Timing of strict diet in relation to fetal damage in maternal phenylketonuria. *Lancet* 1987;2:927–30.
72. Clark BJ, Cockburn F. Maternal diet in inherited metabolic disease. *Acta Pediatr Scand* 1991;373:43–52.
73. Cockburn F, Farquhar JW, Forfar JO, *et al.* Maternal hyperphenylalaninaemia in the normal phenylketonuric mother and its influence on maternal plasma and fetal fluid aminoacid concentrations. *J Obstet Gynaecol Br Commonw* 1972;79:698–707.
74. Hanley WB, Clarke JTR, Schoonkeyt W. Maternal phenylketonuria (PKU) – A review. *Clin Biochem* 1987;20:149.
75. Medical Research Council Working Party on Phenyl-ketonuria. Phenylketonuria due to phenylalanine hydroxylase deficiency: An unfolding story. *Br Med J* 1993;306:115–9.
76. Medical Research Council Working Party on Phenyl-ketonuria. Recommendations on the dietary management of phenylketonuria. *Arch Dis Child* 1993;68:426–7.
77. Cockburn F, Clark BJ, Byrne A, *et al.* Maternal phenyl-ketonuria – Diet, dangers and dilemmas. *Int Pediatr* 1992;7:67–74.
78. Cockburn F. Fetal metabolism. In Reed GB, Claireaux AE, Cockburn F, eds. *Diseases of the Fetus and Newborn*, 2nd edn. London: Chapman & Hall Medical, 1995;81:1267–79.
79. Veghelyi PV. Fetal abnormality and maternal alcohol metabolism. *Lancet* 1983;11:53–4.

93 Fetal and neonatal nutrition – lipid and carbohydrate requirements and adaptations to altered supply at birth

H. Budge and M. E. Symonds

Introduction

The maintenance of a balanced and continuous supply of nutrients from the mother to the conceptus is critical in maintaining both a healthy and viable embryo as well as ensuring fetal growth and development is optimal throughout gestation. In this respect, a deficit in nutrient intake by the mother not only has a detrimental effect on the reproductive process itself but can also contribute to long-term ill health in the resulting offspring.[1,2] Even prior to conception, it is important that maternal dietary intake is adequate to ensure normal development of the egg.[3] Inadequate maternal nutrition before ovulation can potentially contribute to a range of clinical conditions including neural tube defects[4] in the fetus and even result in premature labour.[5,6]

There are seven distinct, but inter-related, stages between ovulation and weaning in which inadequate, or an imbalanced, supply of nutrition can have deleterious effects on the conceptus. These can be summarized as follows:

(1) Periconceptionally during the time of egg development
(2) Fertilization and subsequent period of embryogenesis and elongation
(3) Implantation and placental establishment
(4) Period of rapid placental growth
(5) Period of rapid fetal growth and mammary development
(6) Birth and separation of the fetus from the placenta
(7) Lactation and the period of postnatal growth.

In order to enable the newborn to establish independent life it undergoes a range of pronounced metabolic, endocrine and functional adaptations at birth.[7,8] These are vital in enabling the infant to commence independent breathing, thermoregulation and nutrient intake. Nutrient supply to the fetus is primarily regulated at the level of the placenta which effectively acts as the fetal gut. Then, after birth and the onset of breast feeding, the neonatal bowel takes on this role. There are some similarities between the function of the placenta before birth and the neonatal gut which acts to ensure that nutrient supply is maintained and then increased to meet the much higher postnatal metabolic requirements as growth accelerates.[9]

The fetus grows in a hypoxic environment in which a reduction in supply of both macronutrients, which include oxygen and micronutrients, can have adverse consequences.[10] Fetal arterial blood has a PaO_2 of around 2.8 kPa (21 mmHg) compared with ~12 kPa (90 mmHg) in the adult. The fetus adapts to this lower PaO_2 by maintaining a minimal metabolic rate,[11] ensuring available nutrients can be utilized to promote tissue growth rather than be partitioned toward metabolism. Nevertheless, even when fetal growth rate is maximal, it is usually slower than after birth.[12,13] In conjunction with this relatively low growth rate, cell division, rather than an increase in cell size, primarily contributes to fetal tissue growth. Thereafter, following birth, there is pronounced hypertrophy as nutrient supply is no longer constrained by placental exchange capacity, maternal intake and body stores. One tissue in which this adaptation is most apparent is adipose tissue.[14] Lipid synthesis has a much higher energetic requirement (i.e. 39 MJ/kg) compared with carbohydrate or protein (15–25 MJ/kg), so it is not surprising that fat deposition is normally low in the fetus and is highly dependent on fetal nutrition.[15]

Fetal fat deposition principally occurs over the final third of gestation[16] but, in contrast with all other organs, fat cells can continue increasing in size for the remainder of an individual's life. It is, therefore, not unexpected that in nutritional and environmental conditions of excess feed availability, reduced physical and metabolic activity and raised ambient temperatures, there is an increasing propensity for obesity to occur earlier and in more people.[17] The extent to which predisposition to later obesity is determined by the *in utero* environment remains an area of significant scientific interest.[18]

In this chapter, we will focus on the acquisition of fat and fatty acids by the fetus and neonate and consider their roles in brain and adipose tissue development. For the fetus, as in the adult, fat represents a storage site in which excess energy intake is stored to be mobilized in times of later nutrient deficiency.[18] The other major energy storage is glycogen which is deposited in the fetal liver and skeletal muscle.[19] We will, therefore, consider the regulation of carbohydrate metabolism within the fetus as this is the precursor for both stored glycogen and the primary metabolic substrate for fetal lipid synthesis.

Comparative requirements between humans and other mammalian species

The use of other animals has greatly added to our understanding of fetal and neonatal lipid and carbohydrate metabolism and its impact on brain and fat development. It is, therefore, important to appreciate both the differences and similarities between respective animal models which have enabled us to make substantial advances in our knowledge of fetal nutrition and physiology that would not be possible within the pronounced limitations of human studies. As a consequence of the substantial differences in length of gestation in various animal species, together with the degree of maturity of the newborn at birth, the impact of compromised placental function, as opposed to poor lactational performance, can have very different outcomes on the resulting offspring.

The most notable difference between human newborn infants and nearly all other mammals is their much higher total fat content (150 g/kg body tissue) compared with most domestic species and laboratory mammals (< 10 g/kg body tissue)[20] except the newborn guinea pig (70 g/kg body tissue). The high fat content of the human fetus reflects the dramatic increase in subcutaneous fat deposition that occurs over the final 10 weeks of gestation. This is largely white fat which has an important insulatory role in the newborn as well as providing a large energy store that can be mobilized over the first few days of neonatal life before lactation is fully established. In the latter respect, the human differs from many other mammalian species in which lactation rapidly commences at birth to ensure survival. For example, in sheep, failure to rapidly establish lactation leads to starvation, hypothermia and death within a few hours of birth.[21]

Newborn sheep, like humans,[22] also possess brown adipose tissue which is characterized as possessing a unique uncoupling protein that when maximally activated is able to produce up to 300 W/kg tissue of heat compared with 1–2 W/kg tissue by most other tissues.[23] The amount of brown fat, located around the internal organs, in newborn sheep and humans is comparable at about 2% of birth weight.[24,25] This contrasts with rats and mice in which minimal fat is present at birth and in whom brown fat is located in the interscapular region and is recruited postnatally.[26] In contrast, pigs are born with some subcutaneous fat but do not possess any brown fat.[27]

Fetal brain growth relative to adult brain weight is appreciably greater in the human than all other species for which comparable data are available (Figure 93.1). In addition, its growth rate is normally maintained for the whole of pregnancy so that the weight of the brain in the newborn is ~13% of birth weight.[28] Subsequently, as growth of all other tissues accelerates after birth, brain weight, as a fraction of total body weight, gradually declines to the adult value of ~2%, which is the typical value found in most other large animal species at birth.[29]

These pronounced differences in fetal brain growth are reflected in the ability of non-esterified free fatty acids (NEFAs) to cross the placenta. In the chorioallantoic (hemochorial) placenta of humans, although the fetal endothelium and chorionic epithelium separate the maternal and fetal circulations, NEFA can pass relatively freely from mother to fetus.[30] This contrasts with the placentae of species that have a distinct maternal layer (such as the pig and sheep) and are impermeable to NEFA.[31] Small laboratory mammals which

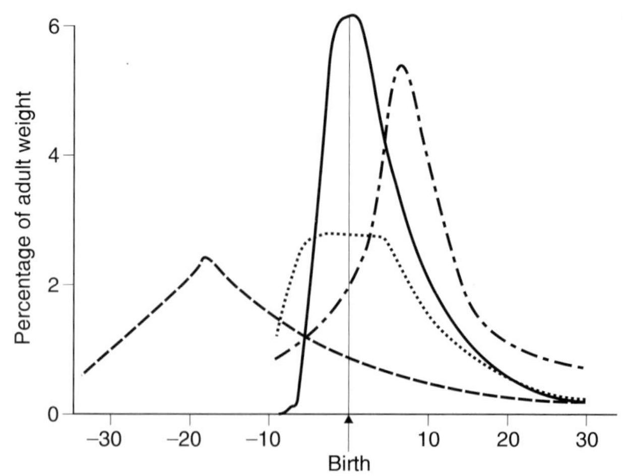

Figure 93.1 Diagrammatic summary of the rate of fetal and postnatal brain growth (wet weight) in the human compared with other species. Developmental age for each species is represented as follows: human (continuous line) in months; guinea pigs (dotted line) in days; pig (dashed line) in weeks and rat (dotted and dashed line) in days. Adapted from Dickerson[29] with permission.

have a very short gestation further differ from humans in that the offspring have an immature hypothalamic–pituitary axis at birth with brain and fat growth occurring primarily after birth.[32] This has several major functional consequences, both for organ development and nutritional requirements. The major source of energy in rat milk is lipid and the mother devotes up to 80% of her time suckling the young whose weight doubles in a week.[33] By the time of weaning, brain growth is complete and the neonate has maximized glucose production necessary to maintain the brain's high metabolic requirements compared with the rest of the body.[34] It is not until weaning that glycogen is laid down as an energy reserve for possible later food deprivation. This process of events is in marked contrast to long gestation species in which these developments all occur *in utero*. Not surprisingly, appreciable differences in milk composition between species, likely to reflect the degree of maturity of the offspring at birth, are also apparent. Humans and large mammals, such as the sheep and cow, produce milk with a lower relative fat and protein content compared with that of small mammals, such as rats and mice, that have a lower relative carbohydrate content.[33]

Lipid and carbohydrate requirements for placental and fetal growth

Dietary availability, in conjunction with the ability to mobilize maternal body tissue stores, determines nutrient supply to the conceptus and, therefore, both placental and fetal growth.[35] A reduction in maternal energy stores either before, or during gestation, can have substantial effects on fetal energy deposition[15] and these can be exaggerated in the term human infant because it possesses large stores of both lipid and carbohydrate in comparison with most other mammals.[36] Such effects are amplified because the fetus has limited ability to synthesize glucose[37] or essential fatty acids including long-chain polyunsaturated fatty acids (LCPUFAs).[38] It is, therefore, not surprising that infants with poor energy reserves at birth can have long-term deficits in their metabolic control mechanisms.[39] Indeed, such effects may be compounded by the need to mobilize energy supplies during the sometimes lengthy period of parturition[40] up to the time of full establishment of lactation.[41]

The placenta – development and function as the site of nutrient supply

The human hemochorial placenta is a fetal organ and is regulated by fetal genes. It separates the fetal and maternal circulations by a barrier composed of fetal endothelium and chorionic epithelium. The primary site of nutrient exchange is the chorionic villi which are supported by the syncytiotrophoblast and are surrounded by maternal blood.[42] They act as a lipoidal membrane across which nutrients, dissolved gases, waste products and other substances occur. Like the adult gut, this site of the placenta has a very large surface area which increases from 0.83 m^2 in week 3 of gestation to peak at ~12.5 m^2 at term.[42] At the same time, the maternal–fetal diffusion distance decreases from 55 to 4.8 mm, thereby facilitating nutrient exchange. The syncytiotrophoblast is also being continuously renewed from the underlying villous cytotrophoblast.

The placenta has a range of transport mechanisms and/or transporters which can limit or promote uptake of specific nutrients including fatty acids,[38] glucose[43] and amino acids.[44] Their abundances can be developmentally regulated and are normally reduced in the placentae of growth-retarded infants. In addition to its role in nutrient transfer, the placenta acts as an important endocrine organ secreting hormones into both the maternal and fetal circulations and, thereby, exerting direct effects on maternal metabolism and nutrient supply to the fetus.[45]

Placental requirements for growth and metabolism

Normal growth and development of the placenta is critical in ensuring that a healthy, appropriately sized fetus is born at term. The placenta grows exponentially during gestation, weighing ~6 g at week 3 of gestation and ~470 g at term. Maximal growth of the placenta precedes that of the fetus[46] but nutritional exchange capacity increases with gestational age in conjunction with structural maturation of the placenta[47] as the fetus grows and its overall metabolic rate rises.[48] At term, placental and fetal weights are positively correlated with placental weight, normally being between 10% and 15% of newborn body weight.[49]

Not surprisingly, given the diverse functions of the placenta and its rapid growth, a constant and plentiful source of energy is required. The human placenta derives energy from both glucose[43] and NEFA by glycolysis and β-oxidation,[50] respectively. It utilizes glucose as its major energy source and there are multiple glucose transporters present in the placenta.[43] Enzymes involved in glycolysis and the citric acid cycle are also active within the placenta. Indeed, it has been suggested that adequate glucose supply can prevent NEFA uptake and oxidation within the placenta by inhibiting the enzymes (e.g. carnitine palmitoyltransferase type 1) involved in this process.[51] This is not always the case, as appreciable activities of a number of enzymes involved in β-oxidation (e.g. acyl and hydroxyacyl-CoA dehydrogenases) have been detected although activity decreases with gestational age.[50] The utilization of fatty acids as a metabolic fuel may, therefore, decline as gestation progresses with glucose becoming more important.[52]

As the placenta utilizes both glucose and NEFA, abnormalities in the metabolism of either can be associated with adverse outcomes in pregnancy.[50] Diabetes during pregnancy, in which both the transfer of glucose and NEFA across the placenta are increased, causes placental and fetal macrosomia.[53] Maternal liver diseases of pregnancy may also be the result of a placental defect in NEFA oxidation,[54] with maternal symptoms worsening in late gestation when the higher metabolic demands of the fetus[55] result in increased fat mobilization and a concomitant rise in lipoprotein lipase activity.[54] Defective fatty acid oxidation in the placenta results in placental accumulation of abnormal metabolic precursors (e.g. hydroxyacylcarnitines and dicarboxylic acids)[56] that may further contribute to the intra-uterine growth retardation seen in such clinical conditions as pre-eclampsia.[57]

Fetal requirements for brain growth and neural development

As with all fetal organs, the most rapid period of brain cell division is during the period of embryonic growth. Normally, by the end of the second month of gestation, the majority of neurons have migrated within the cerebral cortex forming the gray matter.[58] At this stage of development, approximately 50% of the embryo is made up of the fetal head, with the brain utilizing up to 70% of available energy provided by the placenta. The brain has a very high lipid requirement and content, of which 60% is structural. The majority (85%) of this is present in the cerebrum. Of the latter, 65% of total lipids are phospholipids with cerebral cortical neuronal membranes being made up of phosphatidylcholine, ethanolamine, serine and inositol.[58]

The structural and metabolic functions of fatty acids in the fetus and placenta are primarily undertaken by PUFA.[59] These fatty acids with double bonds plus three (n-3) or six (n-6) carbons from the n terminus cannot be synthesized in the human body. They must, therefore, be obtained from dietary sources primarily in the form of linoleic, a n-6 fatty acid, or α-linolenic, a n-3 fatty acid.[38] LCPUFAs are also essential for neural, brain and retinal development as they are not only integral components of the membrane but also act as intracellular signals and contribute to triacylglycerol stores. The primary LCPUFAs are arachidonic acid (20 carbons:4n-6) and docosahexaenoic acid (22 carbons:6n-3) which are amongst the most metabolically active in the cell. They are not normally limited in the diet but, because of the increased demands by the fetus, their supply may become limited during pregnancy.[60] Interestingly, although the fetal brain has relatively high concentrations of docosahexaenoic acid, the absolute rate of accretion is low (e.g. 50-fold lower than in adipose tissue[38]). Although it is only during late gestation that fetal requirements appear to exceed maternal dietary intake,[38] the amount of fatty acids in the diet may have a significant effect on outcome as a reduced dietary intake has been associated with both intrauterine growth retardation and premature birth.[61]

The precise trigger for parturition remains a matter of debate. In humans, it is determined in part by the size constraints and metabolic demands of the fetal brain.[29] As the greatest period of brain growth occurs *in utero*, there is a definite maternal limitation determined by the dimensions of the pelvic outlet. At the same time, a mismatch between fetal nutrient requirements and placental supply capacity may trigger a centrally coordinated cascade of endocrine signals that initiates parturition.[62]

Fetal requirements for adipose tissue deposition

Adipose tissue is primarily laid down during the final third of gestation with the majority (~80%) being deposited as subcutaneous fat that can constitute as much as 16% of birth weight in a normally grown term infant.[63] Its major component is lipid which is primarily found in unilocular cells, although internal fat depots which have a high mitochondrial content also possess a large number of multilocular cells[64] in which the brown adipose tissue-specific uncoupling protein 1[26] is located. The combination of brown fat plus large lipid stores means that heat production within fat is sufficient to provide up to three quarters of total energy requirements at birth.[19]

Fat is not only transferred directly from the mother to the fetus but is also synthesized *in utero* primarily from glucose and also from lactate and short-chain volatile fatty acids.[65] An increase in both glucose and fatty acid supply from the mother to the fetus such as during pregnancies complicated with diabetes results in substantially more fetal fat deposition.[66] Conversely, preterm infants, as well as those with intrauterine growth retardation, are born with depleted fat stores. These individuals may, however, have an increased propensity to lay down more fat in later life.[67]

Fetal deposition of carbohydrate in the liver

Glucose is the primary nutrient utilized by the fetus for oxidative metabolism with up to two-thirds of fetal glucose being oxidized to carbon dioxide and the remaining third stored as glycogen.[68] As in the adult, glucose utilization is largely regulated by the pancreatic hormones insulin and glucagon with the adaptation that, because of the higher insulin to glucagon ratio, glycogen synthesis is stimulated whereas glycogenolysis inhibited.[69] Indeed, except under conditions of extreme nutrient deficiency, the fetal liver has minimal capacity to synthesize glucose.[37] At the same time, other counter metabolic hormones such as growth hormone do not appear to have a role in glucose homeostasis, as the fetus is normally growth hormone insensitive.[70] The fetus is usually exposed to very high circulating growth hormone concentrations[71] and its growth hormone insensitivity is most likely due to the lack of adult growth hormone receptors in the liver.[72]

Glycogen is stored primarily not only in the fetal liver, but also in skeletal muscle, and can be utilized to maintain plasma glucose concentrations during periods of reduced nutrient availability.[34] The main factor determining the content of glycogen in fetal tissues is the rate of glucose supply from the mother to the fetus which, in turn, is dependent on the maternal blood concentration.[68] Maternal and fetal blood glucose are usually very closely correlated along a glucose gradient to the fetus with fetal blood glucose being 30% lower than that of the mother.[73] Glycogen accumulation commences from 9 weeks gestation but, as for adipose tissue, it is primarily synthesized in the last third of gestation.[40]

Nutrient supply to the fetus: maintenance of a continuous supply

Lipid supply from the mother to the fetus

As a consequence of their large size and high molecular weight, lipids do not directly cross the placenta.[38] Lipids, carried in the maternal circulation by the carrier protein albumin,[74] must first be hydrolyzed to NEFAs before they can be transferred across the placenta. This hydrolysis to NEFAs is performed by the enzyme lipoprotein lipase which is abundant in the human placenta.[75] In addition, intact triacylglycerols and phospholipids can also not be transferred across the placenta.[76] Consequently, as fetal requirements increase with gestation, there is a linear rise in the plasma concentration of triglycerides in maternal blood,[77] whereas plasma NEFAs only rise in late gestation coincident with the mobilization of maternal fat stores.[78]

NEFA transfer across the placenta

The placenta has the capacity to transfer NEFAs both to, or from, the fetus with the net rate of transfer determined by the relative concentrations of NEFAs and their carrier protein, albumin, in the maternal and fetal circulations.[79] Normally, it is the concentration of albumin, which is ~20% higher in fetal than maternal blood, which determines the rate of exchange whereas plasma NEFAs can be up to three times higher in the maternal compared with fetal circulation.[80] Consequently, the plasma NEFA to albumin ratio is 30% lower in the fetus than mother and this gradient promotes fetal uptake of NEFAs. Conditions which result in an increase in maternal plasma NEFAs, such as food deprivation,[81] will result in an enhanced transfer of NEFAs to the fetus.

When NEFAs have permeated the microvillous membrane they cross the two lipid bilayers within the syncytiotrophoblast either by simple diffusion[82] or via fatty acid-binding proteins.[83] A number of these plasma membrane-associated proteins have been identified including:

(1) The plasma membrane fatty acid-binding protein which functions as an extracellular fatty acid acceptor.
(2) Fatty acid transfer proteins that span the lipid bilayer and function as such.[84]

Interestingly, the plasma membrane fatty acid-binding protein exhibits a hierarchy of binding affinities for the range of LCPUFAs that make up NEFAs in the order of docosahexaenoic acid $\geq$ arachidonic acid $\gg$ linoleic $>$ α-linolenic $\gg$ oleic acid.[85] Furthermore, the finding that this hierarchy is only found on the maternal side of the placenta may have the effect of selectively promoting the enrichment of LCPUFAs within the NEFAs that are subsequently taken up into the placental syncytiotrophoblast[86] and then transported across to the placenta.

Glucose supply from the mother to the fetus

As stated earlier, maternal blood glucose concentration is the main determinant of fetal glucose supply.[68] Glucose crosses the placenta by facilitative diffusion across specific glucose transporters (GLUT) with the fetal glucose concentration gradient from the mother increasing in late gestation as fetal demands become maximal.[52] Glucose transporters ensure that the rate of glucose transfer occurs at a greater rate than if its transfer was only dependent on simple diffusion. Two glucose transporters are present in the human placenta, GLUT1 and GLUT3,[87] and their relative abundance can change with gestational age.[43] The peak in GLUT3 abundance in late gestation, in conjunction with its higher affinity for glucose compared with GLUT1, indicates its greater contribution in facilitating placental glucose in late gestation[88] than GLUT1.

Cessation of nutrient supply: the environmental challenge to the newborn at birth

At birth, in conjunction with separation of the infant from the placenta, there is a rapid transition in metabolic homeostasis. The newborn must rapidly establish independent respiration, thermoregulation and nutrition. At the same time, there is a profound change in the composition of feed supplied to the infant. During fetal life, the primary metabolic nutrient supplied is glucose.[68] In contrast, once the infant commences suckling, it no longer receives a diet in which the main energy source is carbohydrate. Instead, the newborn consumes a diet that is rich in both lipids and carbohydrates, with half of the required energy coming from triacylglycerols and the other half from lactose.[89] As lactation is established, both the concentration and volume of lipid and lactose produced in milk increases in line with the greater demands of the infant. The change in nutrient supply and availability is accompanied by the onset of gluconeogenesis within the liver and glucose absorption across the gut.[90] This means that, in addition to the substantial changes in lung function and metabolism[91] around the time of birth, there is also a dramatic change in function of the gut and liver[7]

Table 93.1 Summary of the major adaptations at birth within the liver and gut which are necessary to enable the newborn to adapt to separation from the placenta and successfully commence suckling.

Tissue	Nutritional influences	Function
Liver	Glycogen synthesis	Energy storage depot that can be mobilized at birth
	Induction of gluconeogenic enzymes	Initiation of gluconeogenesis at birth
	Protein synthesis	Hormone receptors and binding proteins that promote tissue sensitivity to the postpartum hormones surges at birth
Gut	Maturation of gut morphology	Enables the gut to have maximal digestive capacity after birth
	Induction of digestive enzyme activity	Necessary for the breakdown and absorption of milk after birth
	Onset of digestive capacity	Facilitates the digestion of milk

(Table 93.1) in conjunction with the mobilization and activation of brown and white adipose tissue.[92]

Preparation and adaptation for life after birth

Over the final weeks and days of gestation, there is a gradual process of maturation of the majority of organ systems within the fetus that mean it can rapidly and effectively adapt to the extrauterine environment. The gradual increase in fetal plasma cortisol has a primary role in this process and is important in promoting growth of the gut mucosa,[7] promoting acid secretion, the induction of digestive enzyme activity and hormone secretion by the gut.[93] In the liver, cortisol promotes glycogen deposition, induces the expression of gluconeogenic enzymes,[7] and stimulates hormone and receptor gene expression.[94]

The occurrence of both structural and functional changes within the proximal areas of the gut ensures that ingested nutrients become digested and absorbed soon after birth. It is not uncommon for the intake of milk to be less than requirements for several days after birth.[95] Over this period, energy is largely provided by the mobilization of both fat and glycogen stores which can become greatly depleted. For example, 90% of hepatic and 60% of muscle glycogen stores can be utilized within 24 h of birth.[96] In order to promote these responses, the enzymes essential for glycogenolysis, gluconeogenesis and lipolysis are greatly stimulated. All these processes may be delayed or reduced in preterm infants in which both lipid and glycogen stores are much lower than in term infants. Not unexpectedly, such infants are at much greater risk of hypoglycemia and hypothermia.[97]

The primary role of fat in the newborn relates to protection and maintenance of a normal body temperature.[92] In the infant, this function is achieved both as a result of the production of very large amounts of heat following rapid activation of the brown adipocyte-specific uncoupling protein 1 in central fat depots,[98] or by the insulatory properties provided by subcutaneous fat.[99] It is also the main source of a rapidly mobilized energy-rich substrate in the form of lipid from which NEFAs are released.[100] The instantaneous activation of thermogenesis at birth, coincident with a near maximal metabolic rate that is seldom matched throughout the rest of the life cycle, is an important example of the very different function of fat in fetal compared with adult life. This adaptation is mediated by the rapid increase in the plasma concentrations of a number of metabolic hormones at birth, including glucocorticoids, thyroid hormones, leptin, catecholamines, insulin, glucagon and growth hormone.[92] These are also important in the range of changes in the lung, gut and liver that are critical for ensuring life after birth (see Table 93.1).

Nutrient supply to the neonate: establishment of lactation and adaptation to increased supply

Following birth, the rapid and continuous maintenance of lactation is essential in ensuring that nutrient supply to the newborn does not become limited. Over this period, as nutrient supply increases with requirements, the infant has a greater capacity to meet its full growth potential. The composition of milk and its rate of digestion is very different between breast- and bottle-fed infants.[101] Type of feeding adopted also leads to substantial differences in waking and sleeping activity cycles that will further impact on growth and metabolic requirements.[9] When the infant is fed *ad libitum* and on demand, sleep–wake activity cycles may be limited to 3–4 h at most. Ideally, feeding should be on demand which results in a feeding frequency in the neonate being every 1–2 h compared with longer gaps between feeds in older infants.[102] An environment in which such a pattern of maternal–infant interaction is permitted could be considered to have the greatest beneficial outcome for infant health, growth and mental development.[103] Indeed, human breast milk is sufficient as the sole source of energy and nutrients for the infant until around 6 months after birth.[102]

Structure and function of the neonatal gut

As in the adult, the neonatal gut has a range of functions that are all necessary in maintaining metabolic homeostasis as well as regulating appetite. It, therefore, promotes digestion and absorption of nutrients in conjunction with secretory, motility and immunological functions. The neonatal gut is, however, specifically adapted to utilizing a milk diet, the composition of which varies through lactation, over the course of a feed[95] and with maternal diet and health.

As a consequence of the pronounced growth and maturation of the fetal gut during the final third of gestation, it is normally well adapted to absorb the nutrients it receives in milk after birth.[104] Glucose and NEFA are absorbed across the small intestine, whose surface area is substantially increased compared with the remainder of the gut, as a result of substantial number of valvulae connivantes, villi and crypts, together with the microvilli that form the luminal surface of enterocytes.

Gut function in the infant is not only coordinated by counterregulatory hormones secreted by the central and peripheral endocrine glands but possibly by hormones present in milk.[105] In addition, milk contains a range of trophic factors, anti-inflammatory and anti-infective agents, plus digestive enzymes which will enhance gut development and nutrient exchange. One important difference between the transfer of nutrients across the placenta and their transfer across the mammary gland in milk production is the necessity for the nutritional components of milk to be concentrated and packaged so as to survive transfer across the alveoli of the breast and subsequent exposure to the acidic environment of the small intestine.[106]

Fatty acid supply and utilization

The fat content of the milk does not appear to be greatly influenced by maternal diet or fat stores. Fat constitutes 3.9–4.4 g per 100 ml of milk.[33] Digestion and absorption of fat in the neonatal gut is similar to adults involving four phases: emulsification, hydrolysis, solubilization and mucosal transfer. The enzymes which digest fat are termed lipases of which three are abundant in the neonatal digestive tract, namely lingual, gastric and pancreatic lipase.[89] Of these, lingual lipase secreted from von Ebner's glands in the tongue is the most important in promoting fat digestion, and its activity decreases with age.[107] In contrast, because of the low concentrations of bile salts in the neonatal duodenum, pancreatic lipase is much less important in fat digestion than in later life.[108] The low activity of pancreatic lipases is partially overcome by the presence of bile-salt stimulated lipase (BSSL) found in milk. This is activated by primary bile salts (cholate and chenodeoxycholate) and amino acids (taurine and glycine) that are present in the small intestine.[109] BSSL completely hydrolyses triacylglycerols to glycerol and NEFAs into micellar forms.[110] These combine with the aggregated bile acids or micelles to form mixed micelles which, subsequently, transport the solubilized lipids to the brush border of the gut lining for uptake into the circulation and, thereafter, uptake and utilization by the liver. This process utilizes a fatty acid-binding protein, with triacylglycerol being resynthesized in the endoplasmic reticulum and the formation of chylomicrons.[111]

Not surprisingly, preterm infants in which gut development is immature have a lower rate of fat absorption than term infants.[112] Interestingly, the commercial addition of LCPUFAs to preterm milk formulas can have beneficial effects on long-term IQ, suggesting a direct effect on brain development.[113]

Carbohydrate supply and utilization

As in the fetus, glucose is a major oxidative fuel for many organs in the infant with the brain having an obligatory requirement. The main sugar in milk is lactose which is hydrolyzed to glucose and galactose by the enzyme lactase that is secreted from the apical membrane of the small intestine.[114] Both of these sugar products are then actively transported across the small intestinal epithelium by glucose transport systems that are similar to those present in the placenta with the principal GLUTs present in the gut being GLUT1, 2, 5 and 12.[115] These transporters are all sodium independent and only GLUT 12 has been shown to be insulin responsive.[116] In contrast, another type of GLUT found in the small intestine forms part of the Na^+-dependent family of transporters.[115] The latter transport sugars by a secondary active transport mechanism rather than by facilitative diffusion. This ensures glucose can be transported into cells across its concentration gradient via the Na^+-electrochemical gradient provided by Na^+,K^+-ATPase pump.[117]

The primary factor which determines glucose supply to the infant is the quality and quantity of milk consumed, which is, in turn, dependent on the nutrient intake and health of the mother.[102] It is not, therefore, surprising that many of the adverse effects of inadequate nutrition *in utero* can be overcome after birth. These may, however, have much longer-term consequences. Infants who have developed a 'thrifty phenotype'[118] as an adaptation to an adverse *in utero* environment may suffer later adverse health effects when exposed to the mismatch of a comparatively plentiful nutrient supply after birth. It must be noted that such adaptations will be in response to a very different nutrient intake from the diet than that to which the fetus is exposed *in utero*. In this respect, inappropriate accelerated postnatal growth appears to be deleterious with substantial adverse long-term outcomes. By promoting adiposity,[67] inappropriate accelerated postnatal growth compounds cardiovascular risk[119–122] and obesity.[123,124]

REFERENCES

1. Barker DJP. In Fetal programming and public health. O'Brien PMS, Wheeler T, Barker DJP, eds. *Fetal Programming: Influences on Development and Disease in Later Life.* London: RCOG Press, 1999:3–11.
2. Rhind SM, Rae MT, Brooks AN. Effects of nutrition and environmental factors on the fetal programming of the reproductive axis. *Reproduction* 2001;122:205–14.
3. Symonds ME, Clarke L. Nutrition–environment interactions in pregnancy. *Nutr Res Rev* 1996;9:135–48.
4. Lumley J, Watson L, Watson M, Bower C. Periconceptional supplementation with folate and/or multivitamins for preventing neural tube defects. *The Cochrane Database of Systematic Reviews,* Issue 3. Art. No.: CD001056. DOI: 10.1002/14651858.CD001056, 2001.
5. Edwards LJ, McMillen IC. Impact of maternal undernutrition during the periconceptional period, fetal number, and fetal sex on the development of the hypothalamo-pituitary adrenal axis in sheep during late gestation. *Biol Reprod* 2002;66:1562–9.
6. Bloomfield FH, Oliver MH, Hawkins P, *et al.* A periconceptional nutritional origin for noninfectious preterm birth. *Science* 2001;300:606.
7. Fowden AL, Li J, Forhead AJ. Glucocorticoids and the preparation for life after birth: Are there long-term consequences of the life insurance? *Proc Nutr Soc* 1998;57:113–22.
8. Symonds ME, Bird JA, Clarke L, Gate JJ, Lomax MA. Nutrition, temperature and homeostasis during perinatal development. *Exp Physiol* 1995;80:907–40.
9. Symonds ME. In Metabolism and growth during neonatal and postnatal development. Hanson MA, Spencer JAD, Rodeck CH, eds. *The Fetus and Neonate. Volume 3. Growth.* Cambridge: Cambridge University Press, 1995:117–35.
10. Symonds ME, Budge H, Stephenson T, McMillen IC. Fetal endocrinology and development – Manipulation and adaptation to long term nutritional and environmental challenges. *Reproduction* 2001;121:853–62.
11. Hay WW. Nutrient and metabolic needs of the fetus and a very small infant: A comparative approach. *Biochem Soc Trans* 1998; 26:75–8.
12. Fry AG, Bernstein IM, Badger GJ. Comparison of fetal growth estimates based on birth weight and ultrasound references. *J Matern Fetal Neonatal Med* 2002;12:247–52.
13. Freeman JV, Cole TJ, Chinn S, Jones PR, White EM, Preece MA. Cross sectional stature and weight reference curves for the UK, 1990. *Arch Dis Child* 1995;73:17–24.
14. Clarke L, Buss DS, Juniper DS, Lomax MA, Symonds ME. Adipose tissue development during early postnatal life in ewe-reared lambs. *Exp Physiol* 1997;82:1015–7.
15. Symonds ME, Pearce S, Bispham J, Gardner DS, Stephenson T. Timing of nutrient restriction and programming of fetal adipose tissue development. *Proc Nutr Soc* 2004;63:397–403.
16. Vernon RG. In The growth and metabolism of adipocytes. Buttery PJ, Haynes NB, Lindsay DB, eds. *Control and Manipulation of Animal Growth.* London: Butterworths, 1986:67–83.
17. Jolliffe D. Continuous and robust measures of the overweight epidemic: 1971–2000. *Demography* 2004;41:303–14.
18. Symonds ME, Gardner DS. In Development of obesity. Gluckman PD, Hanson MA, eds. *Developmental Origins of Health and Disease.* Cambridge: Cambridge University Press, 2005:397–403.
19. Mellor DJ, Cockburn F. A comparison of energy metabolism in the new-born infant, piglet and lamb. *Q J Exp Physiol* 1986;71:361–79.
20. Widdowson EM, Dickerson JWT. In Comar CL, Bronner F, eds. *Mineral Metabolism.* New York: Academic Press, 1964:1–217.
21. Alexander G. Energy metabolism in the starved new-born lamb. *Aust J Agric Res* 1961;11:144–64.
22. Lean MEJ. Brown adipose tissue in humans. *Proc Nutr Soc* 1989; 48:243–56.
23. Power G. Biology of temperature: The mammalian fetus. *J Dev Physiol* 1989;12:295–304.
24. Merklin RJ. Growth and distribution of human fetal brown fat. *Anat Rec* 1974;178:637–46.
25. Alexander G, Bell AW. Quantity and calculated oxygen consumption during summit metabolism of brown adipose tissue in newborn lambs. *Biol Neonate* 1975;26:214–20.
26. Cannon B, Nedergaard J. Brown adipose tissue: Function and significance. *Physiol Rev* 2004;84:277-359.
27. Trayhurn P, Temple NJ, Van Aerde J. Evidence from immunoblotting studies on uncoupling protein that brown adipose tissue is not present in the domestic pig. *Can J Physiol Pharmacol* 1989;67: 1480–5.
28. Davison AN, Dobbing J. Myelination as a vulnerable period in brain development. *Br Med Bull* 1966;22:40–4.
29. Dickerson JWT. In Growth, development and the clinical composition of the body. Morgan JB, Dickerson JWT, eds. *Nutritional in Early Life: Concepts and Practice.* Chichester: Wiley & Sons, 2003:1–38.
30. Hull D, Elphick MC. Evidence for fatty acid transfer across the human placenta. *Ciba Found Symp* 1978;63:75–91.
31. Hull D, Elphick MC, Broughton Pipkin F. The transfer of fatty acids across the sheep placenta. *J Dev Physiol* 1979;1:31–45.
32. Symonds ME, Budge H, Stephenson T. In Physiological and nutritional aspects of the placenta. Morgan JB, Dickerson JWT, eds. *Nutrition in Early Life: Concepts and Practice.* Chichester: Wiley & Sons, 2003:91–121.
33. Prentice AM, Prentice A. Evolutionary and environmental influences on lactation. *Proc Nutr Soc* 1995;54:391–400.
34. Girard J, Ferre P, Pegorier JP, Duee PH. Adaptations of glucose and fatty acid metabolism during perinatal period and suckling–weaning transition. *Physiol Rev* 1992;72:507–62.
35. Widdowson EM. Nutrition from conception to extreme old age. *Food Nutr* 1982;8:32–40.
36. Widdowson EM. Chemical composition of newly born animals. *Nature* 1950;116:626–8.
37. Sadava D, Frykman P, Harris E, Majerus D, Mustard J, Bernard. B. Development of enzymes of glycolysis and gluconeogenesis in human fetal liver. *Biol Neonate* 1992;62:89–95.
38. Haggarty P. Effect of placental function on fatty acid requirements during pregnancy. *Eur J Clin Nutr,* 2004;1559–70.
39. Eriksson JG, Forsen T, Tuomilehto J, Osmond C, Barker DJP. Early growth and coronary heart disease in later life: Longitudinal study. *Br Med J* 2001;322:949–53.
40. Clarke L, Bryant MJ, Lomax MA, Symonds ME. Maternal manipulation of brown adipose tissue and liver development in the ovine fetus during late gestation. *Br J Nutr* 1997;77:871–83.
41. Ferre P, Decaux JF, Issad T, Girard J. Changes in energy metabolism during the suckling and weaning period in the newborn. *Reprod Nutr Dev* 1986;26:619–31.
42. Kaufmann P, Scheffen I. In Placental development. Polin RA, Fox F, eds. *Fetal and Neonatal Physiology.* New York: W. B. Saunders, 1998:47–56.
43. Illsley NP. Glucose transporters in the human placenta. *Placenta* 2000;21:14–22.
44. Cetin I. Amino acid interconversions in the fetal-placental unit: The animal model and human studies *in vivo. Pediatr Res* 2001;49:148–54.
45. Reitman ML, Bi S, Marcus-Samuels B, Gavrilova O. Leptin and its role in pregnancy and fetal development – An overview. *Biochem Soc Trans* 2001;29:68–72.
46. Heasman L, Clarke L, Dandrea J, Stephenson T, Symonds ME. Correlation of fetal number with placental mass in sheep. *Contemp Rev Obstet Gynaecol* 1998;10:275–80.
47. Stegmann JHJ. Placental development in sheep. *Bijdragen tot de Dierkunde* 1974;44:4–72.
48. Schneider H. Ontogenic changes in the nutritive function of the placenta. *Placenta* 1996;17:15–26.
49. Broughton Pipkin F, Hull D, Stephenson TJ. In Fetal physiology. Lamming GE, ed. *Marshall's Physiology of Reproduction,* 4th edn. *'Pregnancy and Lactation', Part 2 Fetal Physiology, Parturition and Lactation.* London: Chapman & Hall, 1994;3:767–861.
50. Shekhawat P, Bennett MJ, Sadovsky Y, Nelson DM, Rakheja D, Strauss AW. Human placenta metabolizes fatty acids: Implications for fetal fatty acid oxidation disorders and maternal liver diseases. *Am J Physiol* 2003;284:E1098–105.
51. Prip Buss C, Pegorier JP, Duee PH, Kohl C, Girard J. Evidence that the sensitivity of carnitine palmitoyltransferase I to inhibition by malonyl-CoA is an important site of regulation of hepatic fatty acid oxidation in the fetal and newborn rabbit. *Biochem J* 1990; 269:409–15.
52. Molina RD, Meschia G, Battaglia FC, Hay WW. Gestational maturation of placental transfer of glucose. *Am J Physiol* 1991;261: R697–704.
53. Evers IM, Nikkels PG, Sikkema JM, Visser GH. Placental pathology in women with type 1 diabetes and in a control group with normal and large-for-gestational-age infants. *Placenta* 2003;24: 819–25.

54. Ibdah JA, Bennett MJ, Rinaldo P, *et al.* A fetal fatty-acid oxidation disorder as a cause of liver disease in pregnant women. *N Engl J Med* 1999;340:1723–31.
55. Herrera E. Metabolic adaptations in pregnancy and their implications for the availability of substrate to the fetus. *Eur J Clin Nutr* 2000;54(Suppl 1):S47–51.
56. Ibdah JA, Zhao Y, Viola J, Gibson B, Bennett MJ, Strauss AW. Molecular prenatal diagnosis in families with fetal mitochondrial trifunctional protein mutations. *J Pediatr* 2001;138:396–9.
57. Broughton Pipkin F, Roberts JM. Hypertension in pregnancy. *J Hum Hypertens* 2000;14:705–24.
58. Dobbing J. In The later development of the brain and its vulnerabililty. Davis JA, Dobbing J, eds. *Scientific Foundations of Pediatrics*, 2nd edn. London: Heinemann, 1981.
59. Crawford MA, Hassam AG, Stevens PA. Essential fatty acid requirements in pregnancy and lactation with special reference to brain development. *Prog Lipid Res* 1981;20:30–40.
60. Clandinin MT, Chappell JE, Heim T, Swyer PR, Chance GW. Fatty acid accretion in fetal and neonatal liver. Implications for fatty acid requirements. *Early Hum Dev* 1981;5:355–66.
61. Olsen SF, Secher NJ. Low consumption of seafood in early pregnancy as a risk factor for preterm delivery: Prospective cohort study. *Br Med J* 2002;324:447.
62. Warnes K, Morris MJ, Symonds ME, Phillips ID, Owens JA, McMillen IC. Effects of gestation, cortisol and maternal undernutrition on hypothalamic neuropeptide Y mRNA levels in the sheep fetus. *J Neuroendocrinol* 1998;10:51–7.
63. Ziegler EE, O'Donnell AM, Nelson SE, Forman SJ. Body composition of the reference fetus. *Growth* 1976;40:329–41.
64. Yuen BS, Owens PC, Muhlhausler BS, *et al.* Leptin alters the structural and functional characteristics of adipose tissue before birth. *FASEB J* 2003;17:1102–4.
65. Vernon RG, Clegg RA, Flint DJ. Aspects of adipose tissue metabolism in foetal lambs. *Biochem J* 1981;196:819–24.
66. Greco P, Vimercati A, Hyett J, *et al.* The ultrasound assessment of adipose tissue deposition in fetuses of "well controlled" insulin-dependent diabetic pregnancies. *Diabet Med* 2003;20:858–62.
67. Dietz WH. Critical periods in childhood for the development of obesity. *Am J Clin Nutr* 1994;59:955–9.
68. Hay WW. Current topic: Metabolic interrelationships of placenta and fetus. *Placenta* 1995;16:19–30.
69. Jones CT, Rolph TP. Metabolic events associated with the preparation of the fetus for independent life. *Ciba Found Symp* 1981; 86:214–33.
70. Gluckman PD, Gunn AJ, Cutfield WS, Guilbaud O, Wilton P. Congenital idiopathic growth hormone deficiency associated with prenatal and early postnatal growth failure. *J Pediatr* 1992;121: 920–3.
71. Bauer MK, Breier BH, Harding J, Veldhuis JD, Gluckman PD. The fetal somatotrophic axis during long term maternal undernutrition in sheep; evidence of nutritional regulation in utero. *Endocrinology* 1995;136:1250–7.
72. Li J, Gilmour RS, Saunders JC, Dauncey MJ, Fowden AL. Activation of the adult mode of ovine growth hormone receptor gene expression by cortisol during late fetal development. *FASEB J* 1999;13:545–52.
73. Edwards LJ, Symonds ME, Warnes K, *et al.* Responses of the fetal pituitary-adrenal axis to acute and chronic hypoglycaemia during late gestation in the sheep. *Endocrinology* 2001;142:1778–85.
74. Stephenson TJ, Stammers JP, Hull D. Placental transfer of free fatty acids: Importance of fetal albumin concentration and acid base status. *Biol Neonate* 1993;63:273–80.
75. Mallov S, Alousi AA. Lipoprotein lipase activity of rat and human placenta. *Proc Soc Exp Biol Med* 1965;119:301–6.
76. Elphick MC, Filshie GM, Hull DT. The passage of fat emulsion across the human placenta. *Br J Obstet Gynaecol* 1978;85:610–8.
77. Darmady JM, Postle AD. Lipid metabolism in pregnancy. *Br J Obstet Gynaecol* 1982;89:211–5.
78. McDonald RG, Young M, Hytten FE. Changes in plasma non-esterified fatty acids and serum glycerol in pregnancy. *Br J Obstet Gynaecol* 1975;82:460–6.
79. Lafond J, Simoneau L, Savard R, Gagon MC. Linoleic acid transport by human placental syncytiotrophoblast membranes. *Eur J Biochem* 1994;226:707–13.
80. Benassyag C, Rigourd V, Mignot TM, *et al.* Does high polyunsaturated free fatty acid level at the feto-maternal interface alter steroid hormone message during pregnancy? *Prostaglandins Leukot Essent Fatty Acids* 1999;60:393–9.
81. Symonds ME, Bryant MJ, Lomax MA. Lipid metabolism in shorn and unshorn pregnant sheep. *Br J Nutr* 1989;62:35–49.
82. Kamp F, Zakim D, Zhang F, Noy N, Hamilton JA. Fatty acid flip-flop in phospholipid bilayers is extremely fast. *Biochemistry* 1995;34:11928–37.
83. Glatz JFC, Luiken JJFP, vanNieuwenhoven FA, vanderVusse GJ. Molecular mechanisms of cellular uptake and intracellular translocation of fatty acids. *Prostaglandins Leukot Essent Fatty Acids* 1997;57:3–9.
84. Glatz JFC, vanderVusse GJ. Cellular fatty acid-binding proteins: Their function and physiological significance. *Prog Lipid Res* 1996;35:243–82.
85. Dutta-Roy AK. Transport mechanisms for long-chain polyunsaturated fatty acids in the human placenta. *Am J Clin Nutr* 2000;71:315S–22S.
86. Campell FM, Bush PG, Veerkamp JH, Dutta-Roy AK. Detection and cellular localization of plasma membrane-associated and cytoplasmic fatty acid-binding proteins in human placenta. *Placenta* 1998;19:409–15.
87. Barros LF, Yudilevich DL, Jarvis SM, Beauminont N, Baldwin SA. Quantitation and immunlocalisation of glucose transporters in the human placenta. *Placenta* 1995;16:623–33.
88. Ehrhardt RA, Bell AW. Developmental increases in glucose transporter concentration in the sheep placenta. *Am J Physiol* 1997; 273:R1132–41.
89. Innis SM. Human milk and formula fatty acids. *J Pediatr* 1992; 120:S56–61.
90. Shirazi-Beechley SP. Molecular biology of intestinal glucose transport. *Nutr Res Rev* 1995;8:27–41.
91. Symonds ME, Clarke L. Influence of thyroid hormones and temperature on adipose tissue development and lung maturation. *Proc Nutr Soc* 1996;55:567–75.
92. Symonds ME, Mostyn A, Pearce S, Budge H, Stephenson T. Endocrine and nutritional regulation of fetal adipose tissue development. *J Endocrinol* 2003;159:293–9.
93. Trahair JF, Sangild P. Systemic and luminal influence on the perinatal development of the gut. *Equine Vet J* 1997;24:S40–50.
94. McMillen IC, Houghton DC, Phillips ID. Maturation of cytokine-receptors in preparation for birth. *Biochem Soc Trans* 2001;29: 63–8.
95. Weaver LT, Prentice A. In Nutrition in infancy. Morgan JB, Dickerson JWT, eds. *Nutrition in Early Life: Concepts and Practice.* Chichester: Wiley & Sons, 2003:205–32.
96. Shelley HJ. Glycogen reserves and changes at birth. *Br Med Bull* 1961;17:137–43.
97. King C, Harrison M. In Nutrition of the low-birth-weight and very low-birth-weight infant. Morgan JB, Dickerson JWT, eds. *Nutritional in Early Life: Concepts and Practice.* Chichester: Wiley & Sons, 2003:257–90.
98. Clarke L, Heasman L, Firth K, Symonds ME. Influence of route of delivery and ambient temperature on thermoregulation in newborn lambs. *Am J Physiol* 1997;272:R1931–9.
99. Symonds ME, Mostyn A, Stephenson T. Cytokines and cytokine-receptors in fetal growth and development. *Biochem Soc Trans* 2001;29:33–7.
100. Alexander G, Williams D. Shivering and nonshivering thermogenesis during summit metabolism in young lambs. *J Physiol London* 1968;198:251–76.
101. Sritharan N, Morgan J. In Complementary feeding for the full-term infant. Morgan JB, Dickerson JWT, eds. *Nutrition in Early Life: Concepts and Practice.* Chichester: Wiley & Sons, 2003:233–56.
102. Lawson, M. In Practical advice on food and nutrition for the mother, infant and child. Morgan JB, Dickerson JWT, eds. *Nutritional in Early Life: Concepts and Practice.* Chichester: Wiley & Sons, 2003:324–65.
103. McKenna JJ, Mosko S, Dungy C, McAninch J. Sleep and arousal patterns of co-sleeping human mother/infant pairs. A preliminary physiological study with implications for the study of sudden infant death syndrome. *Am J Phys Anthropol* 1990;83:331–47.
104. Weaver LT. In Anatomy and embryology of the gastrointestinal tract. Walker WA, Durie PR, Hamilton JR, Walker-Smith JA, eds. *Pediatric Gastrointestinal Disease.* St Louis, MO: Mosby, 1996:9–14.
105. Grosvenor CE, Picciano MF, Baumrucker CR. Hormones and growth factors in milk. *Endocr Rev* 1993;14:710–28.
106. Weaver LT. Egg, placenta, breast and gut: Comparative strategies for feeding the young. *Endocr Regul* 1993;27:95–104.
107. Sarles J, Morean H, Verger R. Human gastric lipase: Ontogeny and variations in children. *Acta Paediatr* 1992;81:511–3.
108. Hamosh M, Scanlon JW, Ganot D, Likel M, Scanlon KB, Hamosh P. Fat digestion in the newborn. *J Clin Invest* 1981;67:838–46.
109. Jensen RG, Clark RM, de Jong FA, Hamosh M, Liao TH, Mehta NR. The lipolytic triad: Human lingual, breast milk and pancre-

atic lipases: Physiological implications of their characteristics in digestion of dietary fats. *J Pediatr Gastroenterol Nutr* 1982;1: 243–55.

110. Hernell O, Blackberg L. Human milk bile salt-stimulated lipase: Functional and molecular aspects. *J Pediatr* 1994;125:S56–61.
111. Havel RJ. Postprandial lipid metabolism: An overview. *Proc Nutr Soc* 1997;56:659–66.
112. Hamosh M. Digestion in the premature infant: The effects of human milk. *Semin Perinatol* 1994;18:485–96.
113. Wainwright PE. Dietary essential fatty acids and brain function: A developmental perspective on mechanisms. *Proc Nutr Soc* 2002;61:61–9.
114. Naim HY, Sterchi EE, Levitz MJ. Biosynthesis and maturation of lactase-phlorizin hydrolase in the human small intestinal epithelial cells. *Biochem J* 1987;241:427–34.
115. Wood IS, Trayhurn P. Glucose transporters (GLUT and SGLT): Expanded families of sugar transport proteins. *Br J Nutr* 2004; 89:3–9.
116. Rogers S, Macheda ML, Docherty SE, *et al.* Identification of a novel glucose transporter-like protein-GLUT-12. *Am J Physiol* 2002;282:E733–8.
117. Joost HG, Thorens B. The extended GLUT-family of sugar/polyl transport fascilators: Nomenclature, sequence characteristics, and potential function of its novel members. *Mol Membr Biol* 2001;18:247–56.
118. Hales CN, Barker DJP. Type 2 (non-insulin-dependent) diabetes mellitus: The thrifty phenotype hypothesis. *Diabetologia* 1992;35: 595–601.
119. Forsén T, Eriksson JG, Tuomilehto J, Teramo K, Osmond C, Barker DJP. Mother's weight in pregnancy and coronary heart disease in a cohort of Finnish men: Follow up study. *Br Med J* 1997;315: 837–40.
120. Cianfarani S, Germani D, Branca F. Low birthweight and adult insulin resistance: The "catch-up growth" hypothesis. *Arch Dis Child* 1999;81:F71–3.
121. Eriksson JG, Forsen T, Tuomilehto J, Winter PD, Osmond C, Barker DJ. Catch-up growth in childhood and death from coronary heart disease: Longitudinal study. *Br Med J* 1999;318:427–31.
122. Ong KK, Ahmed ML, Emmett PM, Preece MA, Dunger DB. Association between postnatal catch-up growth and obesity in childhood: Prospective cohort study. *Br Med J* 2000;320: 967–71.
123. Rogers I, Group E-BS. The influence of birthweight and intrauterine environment on adiposity and fat distribution in later life. *Int J Obes* 2003;27:755–77.
124. Parsons TJ, Power C, Manor O. Fetal and early life growth and body mass index from birth to early adulthood in 1958 British cohort: Longitudinal study. *Br Med J* 2001;323:1331–5.

SECTION XI

Early pregnancy

Section Editors: **L. T. Mercé and S. Kupesic**

94 Contributions of 3D ultrasonography to the study of embryonic development

R. M. Sabatel López, L. Martínez-Cortés, J. C. Prados Salazar and J. L. Cuadros López

The massive changes a fertilized oocyte undergoes from the time of fertilization up to its transformation into a fetus were hidden from the human eye *in vivo* for many centuries. Thus, most of our knowledge is derived from the microscopic study of anatomical and pathological samples taken from gestating uteruses or aborted specimens.[1–3]

The evolution of ultrasound imaging and the advent of the transvaginal probe enabled the development of sonembryology, thus making available to us the development of the embryo *in vivo*.[4] From the embryological standpoint, this period includes the first 56 days of development.

We have learnt a great deal with conventional diagnostic ultrasound scans, Doppler techniques, and the use of color and power Doppler, but the advent of 3D diagnostic ultrasound techniques is changing our understanding tremendously. The opportunity to observe the volumetric morphology of the embryo and its annexa from the very beginning of gestation is clearly of immense importance in understanding the events taking place in this key period of human development.

First to third week of embryonic development

Conventional diagnostic ultrasound can detect the gestational sac in the endometrium as a round structure with a non-echogenic central area surrounded by a more refringent 2-mm ring (4 weeks and 3 days). 3D diagnostic ultrasound makes it possible to obtain images much earlier: on the 27th day of the cycle (13 days after fertilization) we can already see the outline of an eccentric structure proximal to the bottom of the endometrium, which corresponds to the gestational sac. Four days later we can easily see the yolk sac,[5] which is barely 1 mm in size. In a 2D ultrasound scan, this can hardly be identified (Figure 94.1).

Placental organogenesis begins on the ninth day postfertilization; villi formation begins on day 13, and on day 21 the intervillous circulation appears.[6] Whereas in 2D diagnostic ultrasound, trophoblastic proliferation is identified by the increase in thickness; in 3D ultrasound imaging we can even see the irregularities trophoblastic development confers on the surface of the gestational sac (Figure 94.2).

In the third week of development, the embryo attains a size of 2 mm and appears sonographically as a hyper-refringent area located on the yolk sac.[7] From an embryological point of view it is a highly complex structure: by the 21st day postfertilization the development of the notochordal process changes from 'disk shaped' to 'sandal shaped'. This process, which cannot be visualized with 2D ultrasound scanning, can be seen with 3D ultrasound imaging (Figure 94.3).

Toward days 21–22, the cardiac tube begins to beat. At this stage, the embryo is actually located between the amniotic cavity and the yolk sac, fixed to the trophoblast by a connecting stalk, which can only be verified with 3D sonography (Figure 94.4).

Folding of the embryo

The rapid growth of the nervous system induces and conditions the longitudinal folding of the embryo. At the same time, cross-embryonic growth conditions ventral folding, so that by day 28 the cephalic pole has completely bypassed the cardiac area and by day 35 the embryo has adopted a totally incurved shape.[8–12]

Embryonic folding is another process that can only be observed in three dimensions; initially, this shows the embryo and the yolk sac in different planes. Subsequently, we can identify the embryonic head and tail, not only in different planes, but also joined by a curved nervous system (Figure 94.5).

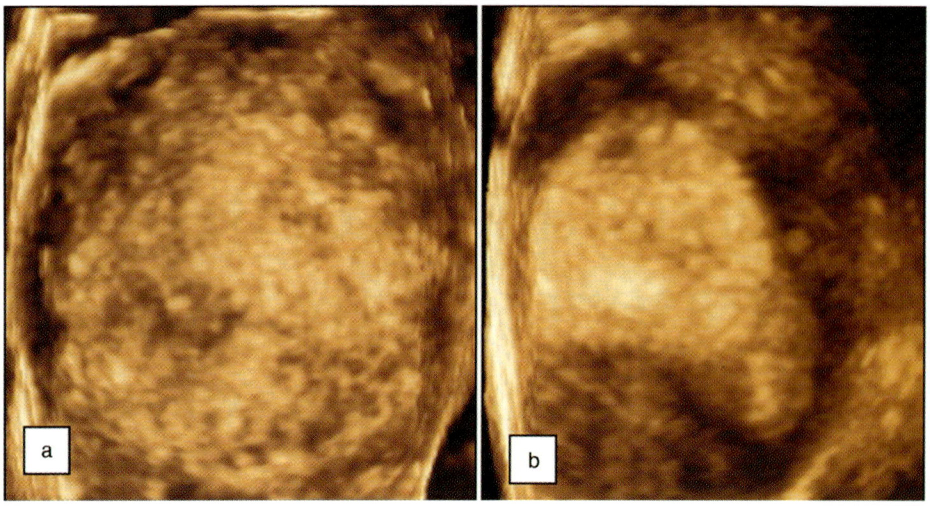

Figure 94.1 (a) Gestational sac on day 13 postfertilization. (b) Gestational sac with yolk sac in the fourth week and third day.

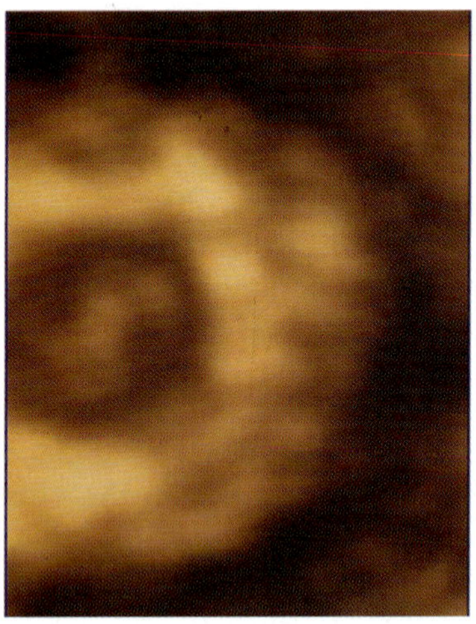

Figure 94.2 Trophoblast in the fifth week of gestation.

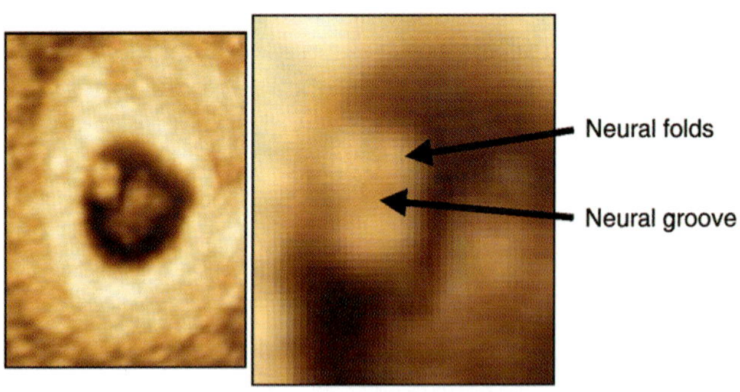

Figure 94.3 Changes in the shape of the embryo as a consequence of the notochordal process.

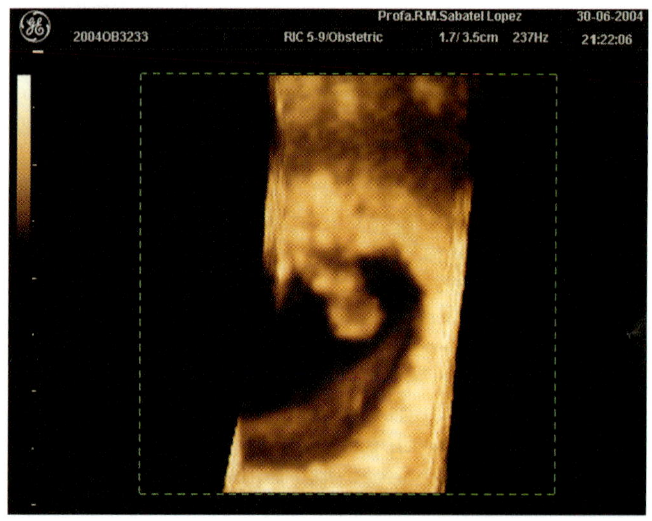

Figure 94.4 Embryo between amniotic cavity and yolk sac, with visible connecting stalk.

Development of the limbs

The development of limbs is another process unavailable to conventional diagnostic ultrasound techniques, but is visible with 3D sonography. Toward days 26–27 postfertilization we see the buds from which the arms will eventually develop, and then later the buds of the lower limbs appear. During the fourth week of development, the upper limbs adopt the form of a paddle, due to the appearance of the hand plates, whereas the lower limbs look like flippers. By the end of the fifth week the feet plates appear, and in the sixth week the flexure of the elbows. In the seventh week of embryonic development the hand and footplates face each other, and the ridges of the fingers will begin to differentiate, so that by the end of the embryonic phase, the fingers of the hand are visible (Figures 94.6 and 94.7).

Development of facial structures

Due to the curvature of the ventral area, the changes in facial morphology are not appreciable via 3D diagnostic ultrasound until the sixth week of embryonic

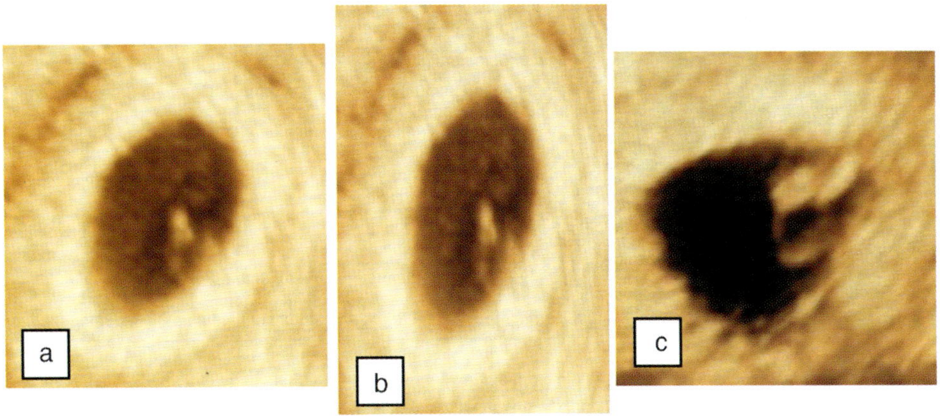

Figure 94.5 Folding of the embryo: (a, c) longitudinal folding and (b) ventral folding.

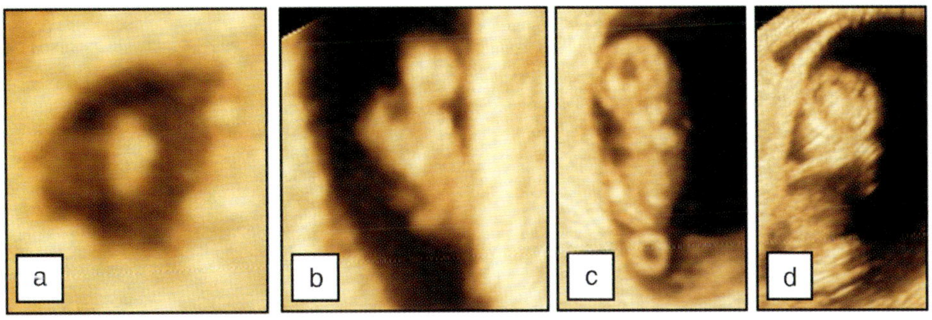

Figure 94.6 Upper limb development. (a) Bud of the arms. (b) Paddle-like arms. (c) The flexure at the elbows permits the placement of the forearm over the thorax. (d) Fingers of the hand at the eighth week of development.

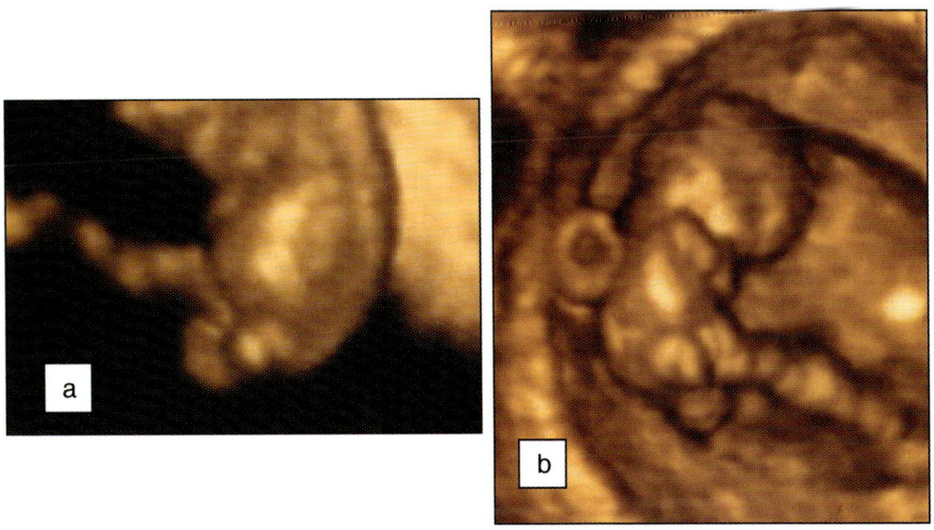

Figure 94.7 3D view of lower limb development. (a) In the seventh week the footplates face each other. (b) Knee and footplate in the eighth week of development.

development. By looking at the cephalic pole laterally, we can see the lens placode, the prominences made by the pharyngeal arches, and the auricular hillocks in whose center we see the exit for the auditory channel. A frontal view shows the mandibular and maxillary prominences of the first pharyngeal arch, the nasal pits, and the wide mouth of the embryo. At the eighth week, the frontal view makes it possible to visualize a completely closed palate and the internal configuration of the nose (Figure 94.8).

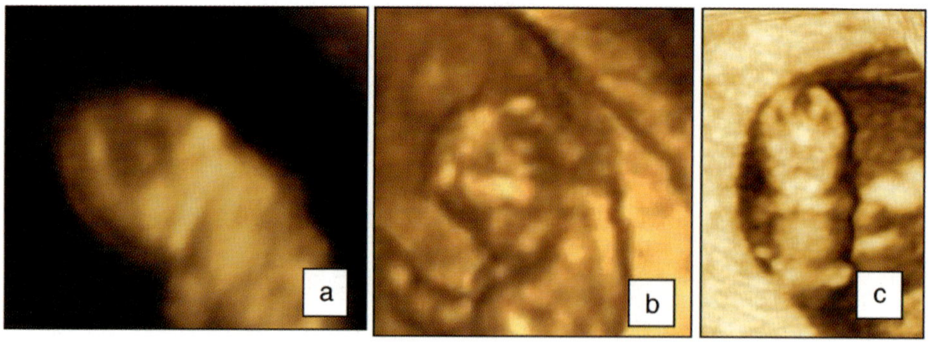

Figure 94.8 Facial structures observed with 3D ultrasound imaging. (a) Lateral view of the face at the sixth week. We can see the lens pits and the prominences of the pharyngeal arches. (b) Frontal view of the face at the sixth week. We can see the mandibular and maxillary prominences as well as the nose pits and the mouth. (c) The frontal view at the eighth week shows the nasal septum, nares, and palate.

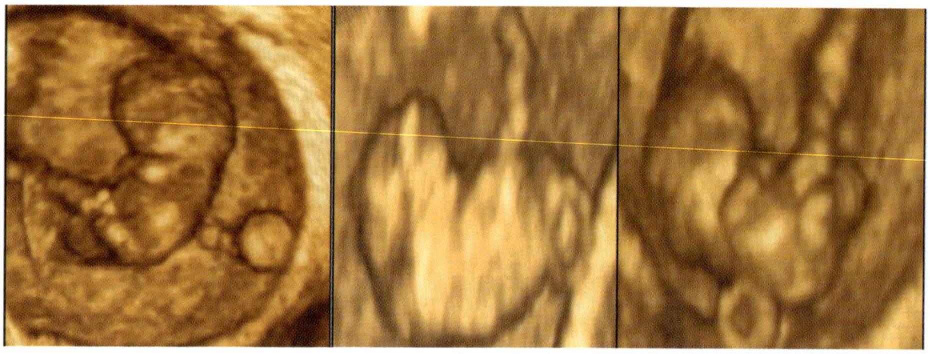

Figure 94.9 Physiological umbilical hernia with 3D sonography.

Abdominal wall

The ventral folding of the embryo makes the yolk sac independent and contributes to the progressive closing of the abdominal wall. By the seventh week, the wall is almost closed except for the area corresponding to where the umbilical will attach. This, together with the rapid intestinal development, influences two sonographically visible facts. First, communication between the primitive intestine and yolk sac becomes reduced to a very fine cord, which allows greater separation between the sac and the embryo. Second, part of the intestine remains in the proximal side of the umbilical cord and, therefore, is outside the abdominal cavity. This is called the 'physiological umbilical hernia', which is visible until the 12th to 13th week of gestation (Figure 94.9).

The spine

In the fifth week of development, the spine presents chondrification centers, visible in 3D at the sixth week of development. Between days 50 and 56 we find three ossification centers in the spine – two lateral centers corresponding to vertebral processes and a central one corresponding to the vertebral body. With 3D ultrasound imaging it is possible to locate the body of the vertebra (greater size) and even the ossification of the vertebral processes of the ribs, which have also begun to evolve during this week (Figure 94.10).

Development of the heart

Toward days 20–21, once the two cardiac tubes fuse into one, the heart begins to beat. At the end of the third week, this single tube bends giving rise to the appearance of the primitive atrium and ventricle, separated by a constriction area: the atrioventricular canal. With 3D PW, we cannot only identify the heart in the fourth week of development, but also identify its external morphology (Figure 94.11).

The complex embryology of the heart develops between the fourth and the fifth weeks. By the end of this stage the septa begin to grow, thus separating the atrioventricular canal. Some of the atrioventricular valves also begin to develop. In the heart of an 11-mm embryo it is possible to differentiate the atria from the ventricles. The former are separated by the primum septum and the ventricles are partially separated by the interventricular septum, which still has an orifice for communication between them. In tandem with

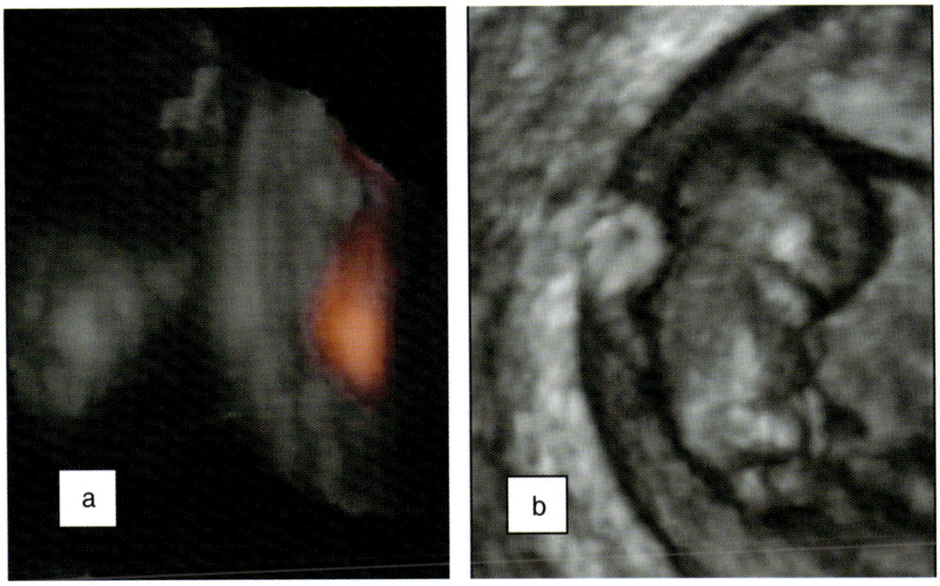

Figure 94.10 The spine (a) in the chondrification phase, sixth week of development, and (b) in the ossification phase, eighth week of development.

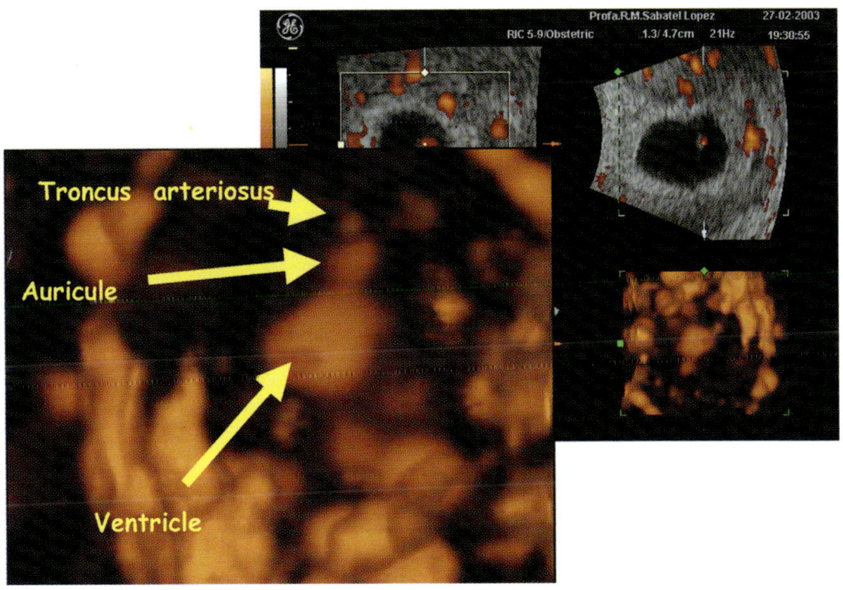

Figure 94.11 Morphology of the heart at the fourth week of development with 3D PW Doppler.

the process of separation of the four cavities, the aorto-pulmonary partition undergoes spiral rotation. With 3D color Doppler sonography we can see the four cavities, and with body capture imaging how they rotate (Figure 94.12).

In the seventh week, the ventricles are totally separated because the orifice existing in the previous week is now closed. Using 3D PW Doppler, it can be seen that the external morphology is very similar to that of the fetal heart (Figure 94.13).

We cannot state that the closing of the interventricular partition – and what this implies for the evolution of the heart conduction system – is the cause of a functional change also observed at this time: the peak embryonic heart rate, which takes place at this time. In the ninth week of amenorrhea, seventh week of development, the heart rate curve reaches its highest peak, with an average of 170 beats/min, which in some cases can reach nearly 190 beats/min. From this point onward, the heart rate decreases until it reaches a plateau by the 14th or 15th week of amenorrhea. These values are maintained during the whole gestation period. This heart rate curve is constant, independent of the number of cases investigated.[13,14]

Development of the nervous system

During the fourth week, the closing of the neural tube has occurred and its differentiation into brain and

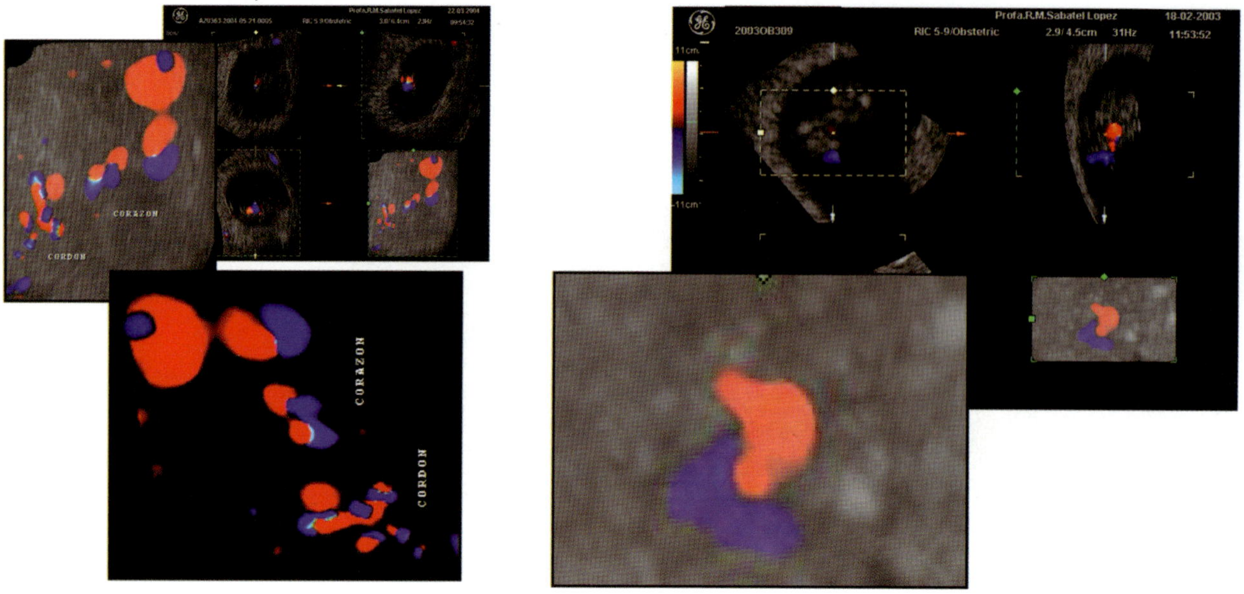

Figure 94.12 Embryonic heart at the sixth week of development.

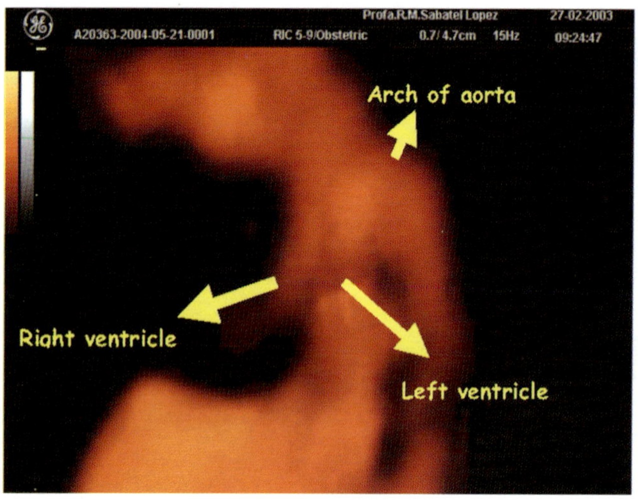

Figure 94.13 External morphology of the heart at the seventh week of development.

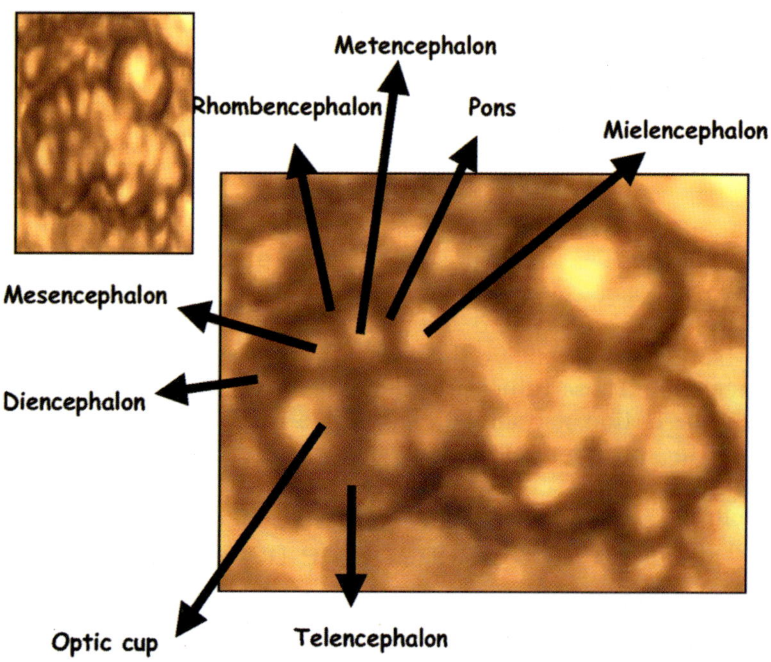

Figure 94.14 Embryo cerebral vesicles of size 14 mm viewed with 3D sonography.

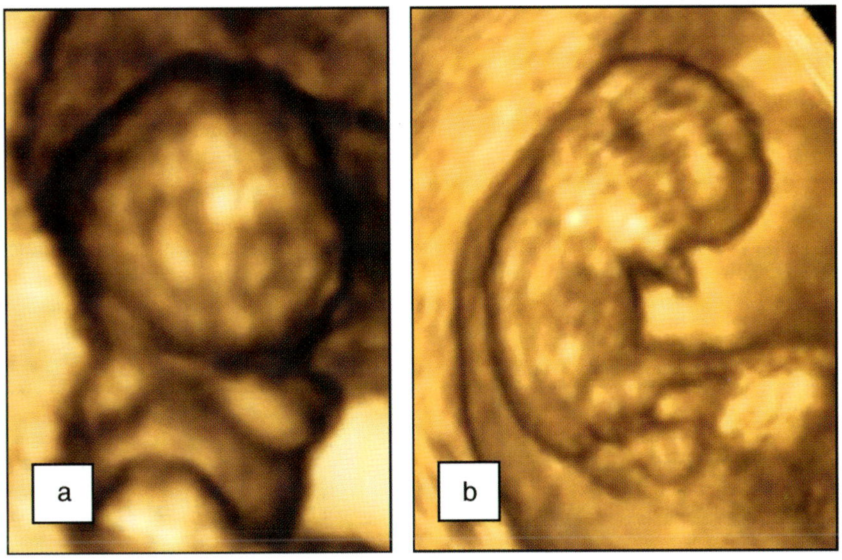

Figure 94.15 Cerebral ventricles at the eighth week of development: (a) lateral ventricles with chorioid plexuses and (b) lateral ventricle, third and fourth ventricles.

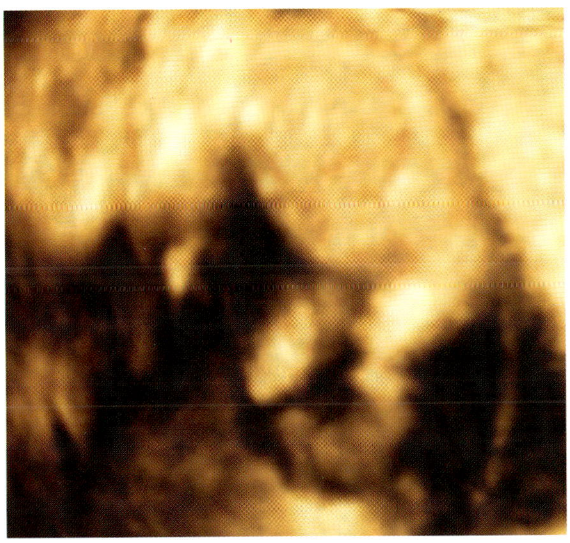

Figure 94.16 Eighth week of development: right lung views with 3D sonography.

spinal cord has begun. By the beginning of the fifth week, the three primary vesicles appear, anterior or prosencephalon, middle or mesencephalon, and posterior or rhombencephalon, and two flexures: one folding the anterior and middle vesicles, and the cervical flexure. By the end of the week, there are five cerebral vesicles: telencephalon, diencephalon, mesencephalon, telencephalon, and myelencephalon. The pontine flexure also appears. The increase in size during the fifth week permits their identification with 3D sonography (Figure 94.14).

These structures are hollow and each of them bulges to give rise to different ventricles, which by the seventh week are in clear development. By the end of this week, the chorioid plexuses begin to develop inside the lateral ventricles (Figure 94.15).

Lung development

In such small embryos, it is practically impossible to follow the development of viscera sonographically due to their small size and the density of the different tissue layers. However, the lungs are different. By the eighth week of development, the bronchial tree is made up of two main bronchi buds (the left and the right, the latter being larger), secondary bronchi and segmentary or tertiary bronchi. From a histological standpoint, the lung is at the pseudoglandular stage. With 3D diagnostic ultrasound, we can identify the embryonic lung, the lobes, and even a section of the bronchi (Figure 94.16).

This review of the first 56 days of development with a 3D ultrasound scanner reveals the real potential of the technique: understanding normal embryological processes that are not visible with 2D sonography and that are clearly necessary to detect early morphological alterations.

REFERENCES

1. Carnegie Institution of Washington. *Reports of the Director of the Department of Embryology. Yearbook.* Washington, DC: Carnegie Institution, 1926–1947;25,28,29,31,38,46.
2. Hertig AT, Rock J. Two human ova of the pre-villous satge, having an ovulation age of about 11–12 days respectively. *Carnegie Contrib Embryol* 1941;29:127–56.
3. Boyd JD, Hamilton WJ. *The Human Placenta*. New York: MacMillan Press, 1975:78–113.
4. Timor-Tritsch IE, Farine D, Rosen MG. A close look at early embryonic development with the high-frequency transvaginal transducer. *Am J Obstet Gynecol* 1988;159:676–81.
5. Sabatel RM, Galera Martinez R. Diagnostico de gestación precoz mediante la ecografía 3D. *Rev Esp Ultrasonidos Obstet Ginec* 2003;1 (Electronic Publication, www.sego.es).
6. Wilkin P. *Pathologie du Placenta. Étude Clinique et Anatomique*. Paris: Masson et Cie, 1965.
7. Laing FC, Frates MC. Ultrasound evaluation during the first trimester of pregnancy. In Callen PW, ed. *Ultrasonography in Obstetrics and Gynecology*, 4th ed. Philadelphia: W. B. Saunders Company, 2000:105–45.
8. Moore KL, Persaud TVN. *The Developing Human: Clinically Oriented Embriology*, 6th ed. Philadelphia: W. B. Saunders Company, 1998.
9. Genis Galvez JM. *Biologia del Desarrollo*. Barcelona: Espaxs, 1970.
10. Sabatel RM, Cuadros Lopez JL. Periodo embrionario: Ecografía de las 8 primeras semanas del desarrollo. Aportaciones de la ecografía 3D. Premio Clínica Abril. Granada: Real Academia de Medicina, 2003.
11. Jiraseckb JE. *An Atlas of the Human Embryo and Fetus*. Lancashire: Parthenon Publishing, 2001:29–39.
12. Sadler TW. *Lagmann Embriología Médica*, 6th ed. Editorial Médica Panamericana, 1993.
13. Hertzberg BS, Mahony BS, Bowie JD. First trimester fetal cardiac activity: Sonographic documentation of a progressive early rise in heart rate. *J Ultrasound Med* 1988;7:573–5.
14. Sabatel RM, Cuadros Lopez JL, *et al.* Behaviour of the embryonic–foetal heart rate in the first half of gestation. *XIV European Congreso of Gynaecologists and Obstetricians*, 1999.

95 Two- and three-dimensional power Doppler ultrasound: from ovulation to implantation

L. T. Mercé, M. J. Barco, S. Kupesic and A. Kurjak

Introduction

The ovarian cycle has two main purposes: first, the liberation of a mature oocyte through the ovulatory process; second, the production of a proper hormonal secretion to prepare the endometrium for the embryo implantation. All these processes require and involve great changes affecting the ovarian and uterine blood flows. The follicular growth, the corpus luteum formation and the endometrial development are physiological processes in which angiogenesis takes place in a natural way, thus providing the blood flow supply.

The uterine and ovarian blood flow changes taking place along the menstrual cycle were known basically from invasive experimental results out of different animal species. Doppler ultrasound examination, especially transvaginal color Doppler, has allowed the noninvasive approach to the importance of the blood flow in natural and artificial human reproduction. Recently, three-dimensional (3D) power Doppler and one sophisticated measurement software makes it possible to calculate the number of vessels and the blood flowing through them. This technique has greatly increased our knowledge about the uterine and ovarian vascularity.

In the present chapter, the blood flow changes taking place in the ovary and endometrium are analyzed from ovulation to implantation through the different examination techniques previously named. Currently, some of the parameters evaluated are those used in daily practice as oocyte quality and endometrial receptivity markers. Therefore, the different Doppler modalities become an essential technique to investigate the menstrual cycle physiology and a source of diagnostic and prognostic parameters about the outcome of assisted reproductive technologies.

From ovulation

The ovarian and uterine blood flow changes have different physiological and clinical implications during the menstrual cycle, so from a practical point of view, we will separate their study.

Ovarian blood flow

Doppler studies have demonstrated the ovarian blood flow participation in the recruitment and selection of the dominant follicle during the *early follicular phase* of the ovarian cycle.[1,2] Our investigations confirm that in the beginning, the intraovarian vascular resistance is correlated with the number of recruited follicles. On the contrary, when a follicle reaches 10 mm of diameter it becomes 'dominant' and the intraovarian vascular resistance decreases despite the disappearance of the follicles cohort.[3,4] This relationship between the number of follicles and the intraovarian blood flow supports the utility of these parameters as indicators of the ovarian response to the gonadotrophin stimulation treatment (Figure 95.1).

The number of follicles after pituitary suppression is a better *marker of the ovarian response* than the age of the patient and the ovarian volume.[5] This parameter predicts the number of retrieved oocytes irrespective of age and serum follicle stimulating hormone (FSH) levels.[6] The total number of antral follicles is the best predictor of the ovarian response followed by basal FSH, body mass index and the age of the woman.[7]

The blood flow of the ovarian stroma also predicts the ovarian response. The stromal peak systolic velocity during the early follicular phase is better related to the number of retrieved oocytes than the age of the

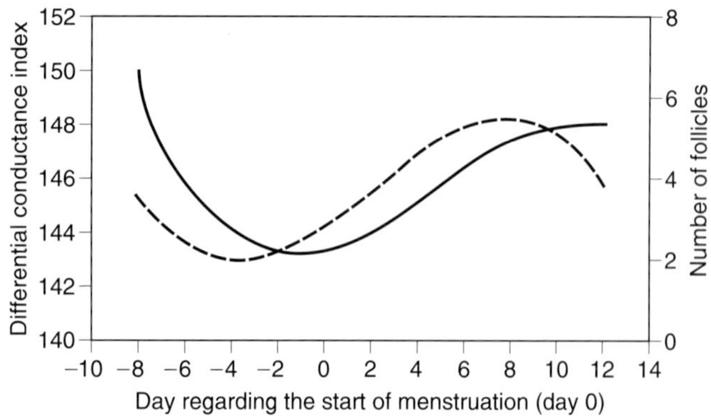

Figure 95.1 Relationship between the number of recruited follicles (red line) and stromal flow, as assessed by its differential conductance index (blue line), during the transitional luteal–follicular period in 22 normal ovulatory cycles.

patient, the basal levels of FSH and estradiol.[8] A diminished stromal blood flow is responsible for a low ovarian response whereas when it rises over 10 cm/s a high number of oocytes and a better pregnancy rate are achieved (Figure 95.2a).[9]

Three-dimensional ultrasound and power Doppler angiography make the estimation of the number of antral follicles and the stromal blood flow much easier without disturbing the patients.[10] Kupesic and Kurjak proved that the number of antral follicles and the index of stromal flow are the best predictors of a favorable outcome in *in vitro* fertilization (IVF).[10] An increased or decreased stromal blood flow can explain a high or low response in IVF cycles.[11,12] Nevertheless, some authors believe that 3D Doppler indices do not offer additional information to predict the ovarian response to gonadotrophin stimulation during IVF cycles (Figure 95.2b).[13]

Our experience in the assessment of 3D power Doppler ultrasound as a marker of the ovarian response comes from a study of 60 patients undergoing their first IVF cycle. A total of 119 ovaries have been separately evaluated because hypothetically the ovarian response could be mediated by the local vascular factors. The number of follicles $\geq$10 mm the day of human chorionic gonadotrophin (hCG) injection and the number of oocytes retrieved are considered as indicators of the ovarian response. A significant correlation ($P < 0.01$) has been observed between the ovarian volume, the number of antral follicles greater than 2 mm, ovarian vascularization index (VI), ovarian flow index (FI) and ovarian vascularization-flow index (VFI) to the number of recruited follicles and the number of retrieved oocytes (Table 95.1). Nevertheless, when a multiple regression is applied, only the number of follicles and the ovarian volume reach a statistical significance.

During the follicular phase the arterial and venous blood flow increase in the active or dominant ovary.[14–18] The color signal at the wall of the dominant follicle increases progressively to almost encircling it. This is due to the intense angiogenesis produced along with the follicular development. The blood flow also increases progressively at the vessels of the ovarian stroma, the ovarian hilum arteries,[16,17] and the venous circulation.[18] On approaching ovulation, the blood flow increases significantly compared to the contralateral or inactive ovary (Figure 95.3).

Several studies of animal experimentation deduce that blood flow increase during the follicular phase is basically due to the growth of the dominant follicle.[5] Our study, along with those of other authors,[19,20] proves this assumption by confirming a significant correlation between the diameter of the dominant follicle and the venous and arterial perifollicular maximum systolic velocity.[21] A high correlation between the dominant follicle size and the serum estradiol is classically acknowledged;[22] nevertheless a significant correlation between the follicular blood flow and the estradiol blood levels has not been proven until now.

The blood flow reaches its maximum values in the *preovulatory follicle* just prior to the follicular rupture. The maximum blood flow velocity increases from 29 h before the follicular rupture, maintaining a peak until at least 72 h after the corpus luteum appearance (Figure 95.4a).[23] The blood flow is similar in every part of the preovulatory follicle before the luteinizing hormone (LH) peak. After the LH peak the maximum systolic velocity increases at the base of the follicle and decreases significantly, almost disappearing, at the apical zone.[24] Three-dimensional power Doppler shows the preovulatory follicular wall has a number of vessels (VI) and an amount of blood flowing through them (FI) significantly increased as compared with the same ovary (Figure 95.4b).[25]

Electronic microscopy has shown the preovulatory follicular walls as having a great amount of sinusoidal dilated vessels and avascular zones due to ischemia and arteriovenous shunts.[26] These findings support the vascular mechanism of ovulation and would explain the blood flow velocity increase by the presence of shunts and the apical disappearance of Doppler signals caused by thrombosis and ischemia phenomena.

The process of angiogenesis, development and vasodilatation of the perifollicular vascular network culminates at the *ovulation*. From the follicular rupture onward, the theca vessels begin the invasion of the granulosa cells showing an intense angiogenesis and wide arteriovenous shunts. Moreover, the growth in size of the ovary leads to a straightening of the spiral arteries which compromise the hemodynamic stability of the whole system producing an increase in the turbulence of the blood flow.[3,4] This flow increase associated with changes in the spectral Doppler signal is named 'luteal conversion' and is of great help to the diagnosis of ovulation (Table 95.2). The luteal conversion is independent of the sonographic visualization or appearance of the corpus luteum. In the luteinized unruptured follicle (LUF) syndrome the follicular

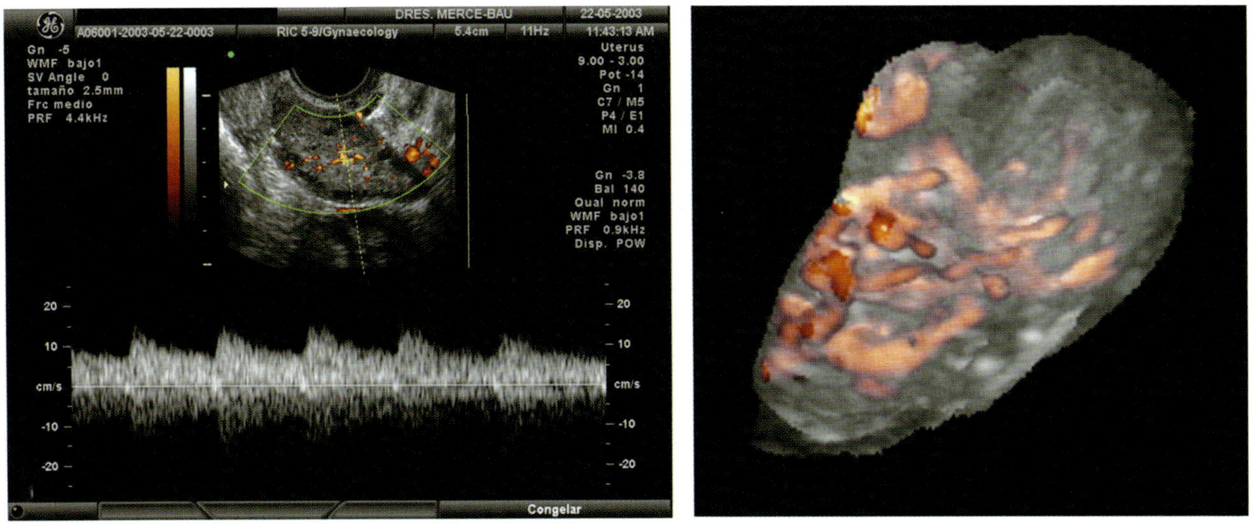

(a) (b)

Figure 95.2 Sonographic markers of the ovarian response. (a) Recording of the ovarian stromal flow velocity wave (FVW) after pituitary suppression by GnRh analogs. The peak systolic velocity is a good predictor of the number of follicles to grow. (b) Three-dimensional ultrasonography and power Doppler angiography allow the assessment of all the sonographic and Doppler parameters involved in the prediction of the ovarian response.

Table 95.1 Correlation coefficients of the sonographic parameters and power Doppler indices after pituitary supression, with the number of recruited follicles and the number of retrieved oocytes in 65 IVF cycles

	No. of follicles on hCG day	No. of retrieved oocytes
Ovarian volume	0.46	0.41
Number of follicles	0.52	0.53
Vascularization index	0.36	0.31
Flow index	0.30	0.27
Vascularization flow index	0.34	0.30

All correlation coefficients are significant ($P < 0.01$)

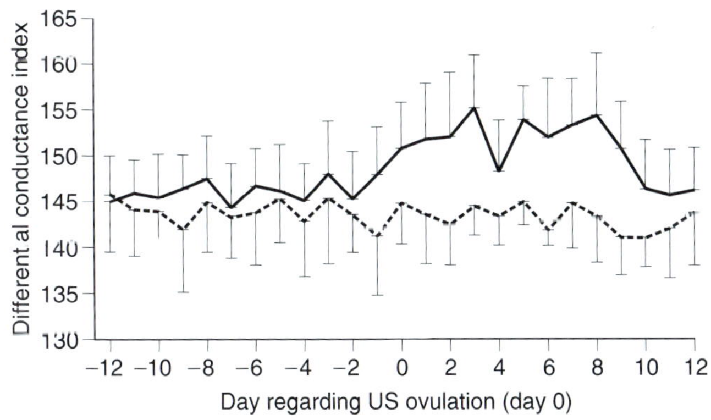

Figure 95.3 Differential conductance index of the dominant or active ovary (blue line) and the contralateral or inactive ovary (red line) during the ovarian cycle. Luteal values of the dominant ovary are significantly increased compared to those of the follicular phase or those from the luteal phase of the inactive ovary.

rupture does not take place so the luteal conversion is not present.[15] Therefore, the luteal conversion is a very reliable parameter of ovulation.

The corpus luteum has a greater arterial and venous blood flow than the preovulatory follicle.[3,4,14–18] The helical arteriole of the corpus luteum presents the highest systolic velocities with a small variability.[27] The luteal vascularity can be depicted with a great accuracy by 3D power Doppler (Figure 95.5). The luteal vascularization, flow and vascularization flow indices calculated from 3D angiography are significantly superior to the follicular ones (Table 95.3). During the luteal phase the blood flow increases in the stromal and hilum arteries of the active ovary[16,17] and also in the utero-ovarian and ovarian ipsilateral arteries.[3]

This increase in the amount of blood flow is essentially caused by the development of new vessels in the ovary carrying the corpus luteum but it should be controlled by local and systemic mediators. An inverse and significant relationship has been proven between the vascular density of the corpus luteum and its pulsatility index.[28] Color Doppler studies confirm that the arterial[17,29,30] and venous[18] blood flow of the corpus luteum is correlated with progesterone secretion. The cycles with luteal or secretory deficiency show an increase in the luteal vascular resistance[29,30] and a decrease in the venous flow velocity[18] In the LUF syndrome the blood flow remains unchanged after the LH peak. During the 'false' luteal phase, the vascular resistance is similar to that of the

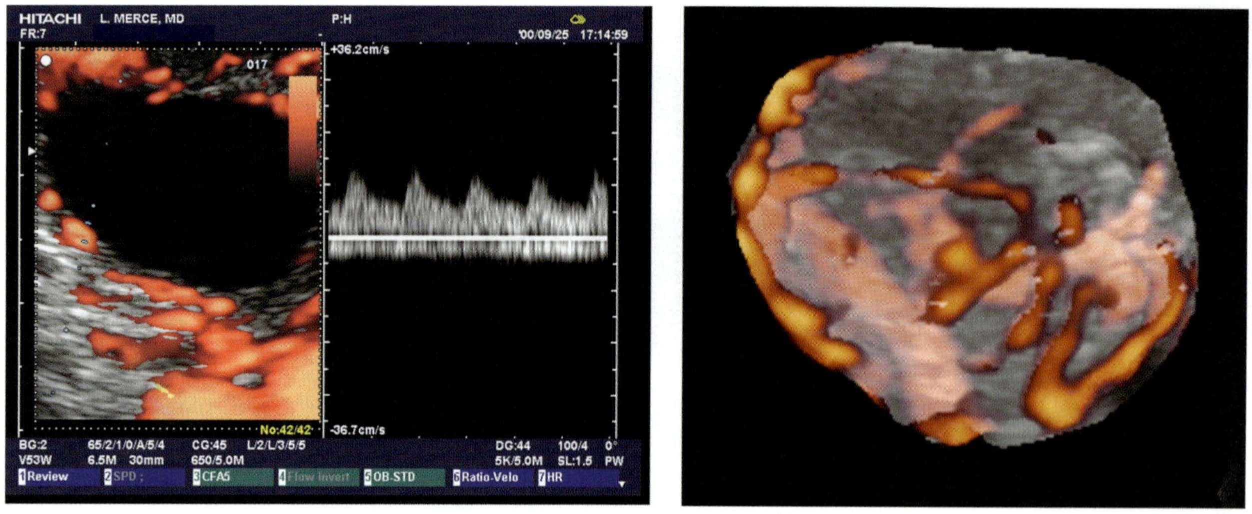

(a) (b)

Figure 95.4 Study of the preovulatory follicle blood flow by Doppler technology. (a) Color signal and FVW arterial and venous in the wall of a 20 mm follicle. Look at the absent pulsatility of the venous signal. (b) Vascular network of a preovulatory follicle by 3D power Doppler angiography.

Table 95.2 Characteristics of the 'luteal conversion' of the intraovarian vascularization

Color signal
Area increase
Intensity increase
Increase of Doppler 3D indices
Spectral signal
Velocimetry
Increase of systolic velocity
Increase of venous velocity
Decrease of resistance
Morphology
Intensity increase
Dispersion of velocities
Superposition of waves
Notch absence
Easily recorded

follicular phase without detectable differences between them (Figure 95.6).[15,18,31]

Uterine and endometrial blood flow

The blood flow of the uterine arteries and their radial branches does not experience significant changes during the early and middle follicular phase.[16,30] The findings on blood flow during the periovulatory period are contradictory. Whereas some authors[32,33] find an increasing uterine and endometrial (uterine, radial and spiral arteries) blood flow from the LH peak onward, others[16,34,35] find a decreasing blood flow until past ovulation. By means of 3D power Doppler it has been recently proven that the endometrial and subendometrial blood flow and vascularity indices increase from the middle follicular phase to attain their maximum values three days prior to ovulation. After that, these indices decrease until reaching their nadir 5 days after ovulation to increase progressively again during the middle and late luteal phases (Figure 95.7).[36]

During the luteal phase the blood flow in the whole uterine vascular tree, from the uterine arteries to the endometrial spiral arteries, increases significantly compared to that of the follicular phase.[16,32,33] As the menstrual cycle advances but especially during the luteal phase, the color signals from the intramyometrial and endometrial vessels grow in number and intensity.

When no pregnancy is achieved, the blood flow in all the utero-ovarian vascular network decreases and menstruation begins a new cycle.

To implantation

Implantation is a dynamic process requiring a true dialog between mother and embryo. The assisted reproductive technologies (ARTs) have demonstrated that success in achieving implantation and a normal ongoing pregnancy depends essentially upon the embryo quality and endometrial receptivity. Since many years, sonographic and Doppler parameters have been sought to be used as 'implantation markers'.[37,38]

The follicular size and perifollicular vascularization have been proposed as ultrasound markers of

Table 95.3 Vascularization index (VI), flow index (FI) and vascularization flow index (VFI) in the preovulatory follicle, corpus luteum and luteinized unruptured follicle (LUF) assessed by 3D power Doppler angiography (mean ± SD)

Parameter	Preovulatory follicle (n=8)	Corpus luteum (n=6)	LUF (n=3)
VI	4.24 ± 2.91	29.91 ± 14.82*,**	2.35 ± 1.10*
FI	35.46 ± 6.48	47.67 ± 3.98*,**	34.00 ± 3.65*
VFI	1.59 ± 1.27	14.72 ± 8.17*,**	0.83 ± 0.48

*$P < 0.001$ with regard to the preovulatory follicle
**$P < 0.005$ with regard to LUF
No significant differences between LUF and preovulatory follicle

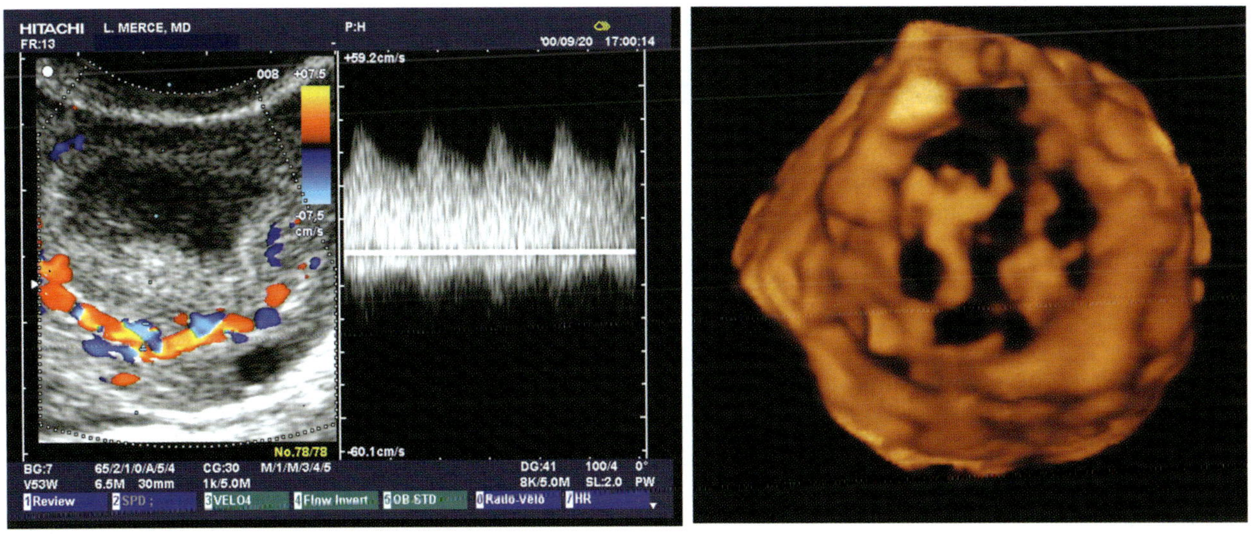

(a) (b)

Figure 95.5 Corpus luteum blood flow study by Doppler technology. (a) Color mapping and FVW during the mesoluteal phase of a normal ovulatory cycle. 'Luteal conversion' is observed. (b) Vascular network of the corpus luteum assessed by 3D power Doppler angiography.

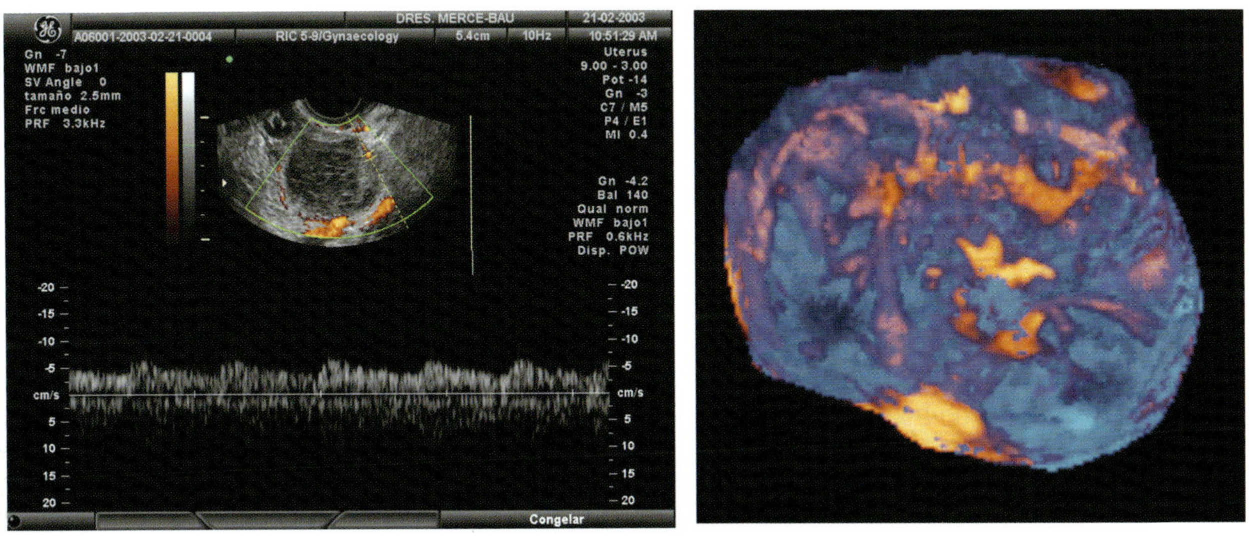

(a) (b)

Figure 95.6 Doppler investigation in the lutenized unruptured follicle (LUF). (a) Three-dimensional angiographic rendering. (b) Arterial and venous FVW. 'Luteal conversion' is not present and venous and arterial velocities are very low.

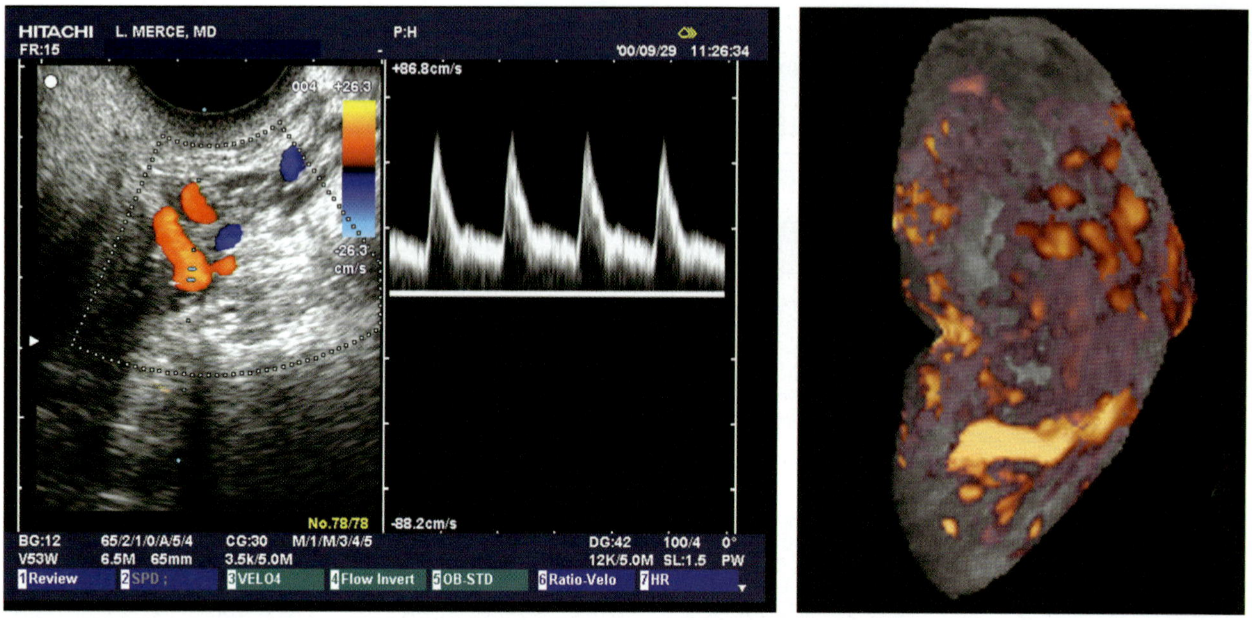

(a) (b)

Figure 95.7 Blood flow assessment of the uterine and endometrial circulations. (a) Uterine artery FVW. (b) Three-dimensional Doppler angiography representation of the endometrial vascularity during the middle luteal phase.

oocyte quality and competence. The endometrial pattern and thickness have been also evaluated as indicators of endometrial receptivity.

Follicular blood flow

The intrafollicular oxygen concentration determines a normal embryo development. Oocytes with cytoplasmatic defects and embryos with multinucleated blastomeres come mainly from follicles with severe hypoxia causing an abnormal arrangement of chromosomes.[39] On the other hand, a defective development of the perifollicular vascular network has been implicated in the origin of intrafollicular hypoxia.[40] The embryonic triploidies rate is significantly raised in the poorly vascularized follicles.[41] On the contrary, the best vascularized follicles are those showing the highest oxygen concentrations.[39] Given that similar size follicles can contain different oxygen concentrations, perifollicular vascularity is an independent marker of the follicular diameter.[42]

The follicular blood flow can be assessed by the maximum systolic velocity in the perifollicular arteries.[43,44] This technique assumes that the blood flow in a single artery represents all the follicular blood flow. The perifollicular color mapping with power Doppler is an easier and reliable technique to assess the follicular blood flow.[41,42,45,46] This procedure assumes that the color signal coming from a single perifollicular vascular plane represents all the follicular blood flow. Three-dimensional power Doppler evaluates all the perifollicular vessels and determines the vascularization index (number of vessels) and flow (flow intensity) from the whole follicular volume. Therefore it is the only method directly assessing the entire follicular blood flow (Figure 95.8).

In accordance with the percentage of color area from the perifollicular power Doppler mapping, follicles have been classified as: grade 0, when no color can be depicted[45]; grade I, less than 25% of the follicular circumference; grade II, between 26% and 50%; grade III, between 51% and 75%; and grade IV, between 76% and 100% (Figure 95.9).[41,42,46] The number of retrieved oocytes, mature and fertilized is significantly higher from the well vascularized follicles (grades III and IV) than from those showing poor vascularization (grades I and II.[41] According to our results, perifollicular vascularization determines specially the maturity and fertilization indices in follicles < 15 mm, being significantly higher in those well vascularized. The recovery rate is independent from vascularization and shows rates higher than 50% (Table 95.4).

We have evaluated a single IVF/ICSI cycle in 80 infertile women by 3D power Doppler ultrasonography. We studied the relationship between the sonographic parameters (ovarian volume, number of follicles > 10 mm and total follicular volume) and 3D power Doppler indices (vascularization index, flow index and vascularization-flow index) on the day of hCG administration with the laboratory biological parameters (number of retrieved oocytes, number of mature oocytes, number of fertilized oocytes, number of embryos on transfer day, number of Grade 1 embryos on transfer day and cumulative embryo score of all the embryos on transfer day). As you can see in Table 95.5, all the sonographic and vascularity

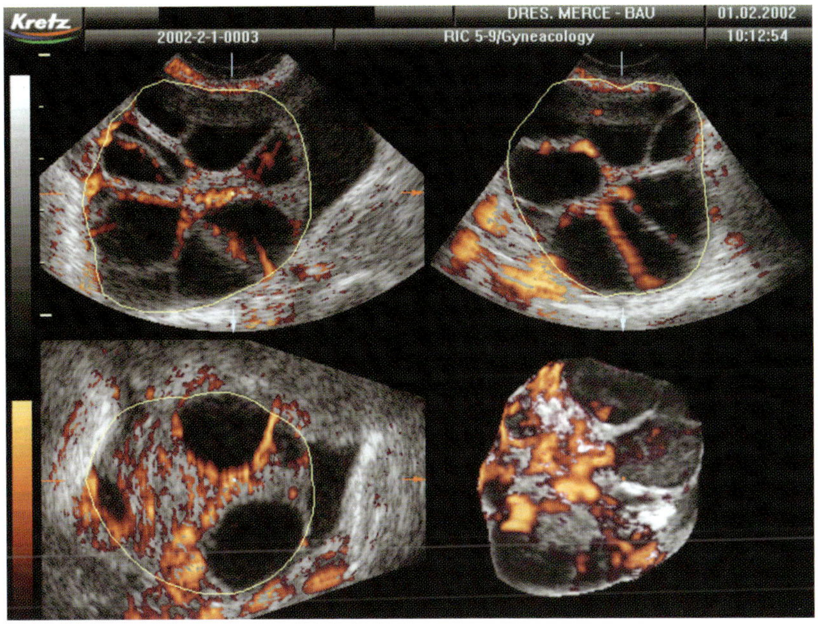

Figure 95.8 Three-dimensional power Doppler angiography rendering of the perifollicular vasculature in an IVF cycle at the day of hCG administration.

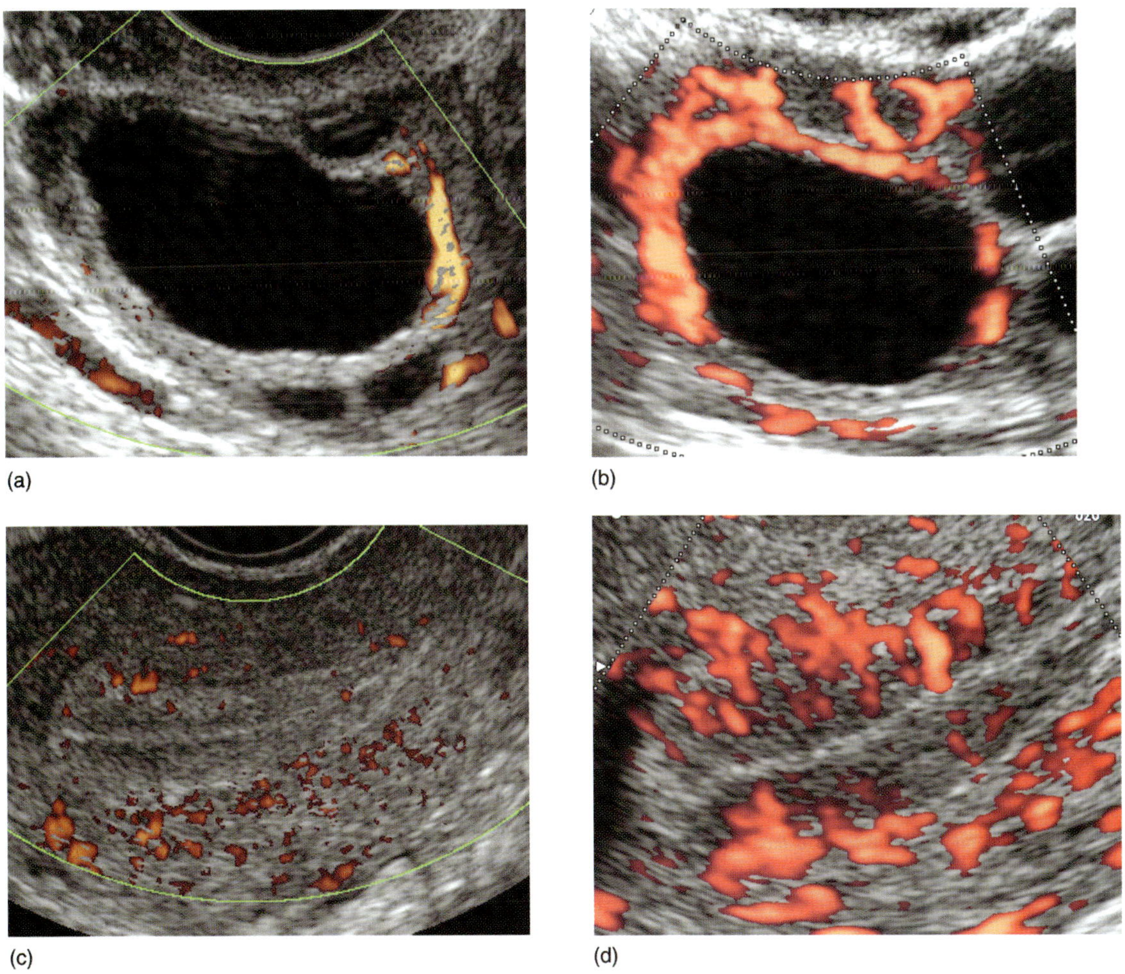

Figure 95.9 Power Doppler mapping of the follicular and endometrial blood flow. (a) Grade I, color mapping encircles less than 25% of the follicular circumference. (b) Grade IV, Doppler signal occupies 76–100% of follicular perimeter. (c) Type I endometrial mapping or peripheral flow, with color signal is visible at myometrium and only reaches outer hyperechogenic endometrial layer. (d) Type III endometrial mapping or central flow, as the color mapping is distributed through the whole endometrial thickness.

Table 95.4 Recovery, maturity and oocyte fertilization rates in follicles < 15 mm according to the percentage of vascularization on day of hCG administration in 32 IVF cycles

Rates	0–25% color		26–50% color		> 50% color	
	n	%	*n*	%	*n*	%
Recovery*	8/13	61.5	12/21	57.1	9/19	47.4
Maturity**	2/8	25	6/12	50	7/9	77.8
Fertilization†	1/7	14.3	7/11	63.6	7/7	100

*$\chi^2=0.708$; $P=0.702$
**$\chi^2=4.749$; $P=0.09$
†$\chi^2=10.823$; $P<0.005$

Table 95.5 Correlation coefficients of 3D ultrasonography and power Doppler angiography parameters on the HCG day with biological parameters and laboratory data in 80 IVF/ICSI cycles

	OV (ml)	NF	TFV (ml)	VI	FI	VFI
No. of retrieved oocytes	0.747	0.862	0.808	0.340	0.334	0.352
No. of mature oocytes	0.626	0.659	0.708	0.321	0.279*	0.337
No. of fertilized oocytes	0.558	0.564	0.628	0.379	0.295	0.395
No. of embryos on transfer day	0.544	0.554	0.595	0.345	0.272*	0.364
No. of Grade 1 embryos on the transfer day	0.386	0.449	0.407	0.442	0.368	0.464
CES of all the embryos on transfer day	0.564	0.661	0.618	0.306	0.299	0.333

OV, ovarian volume; NF, number of follicles > 10 mm; TFV, total follicular volume; VI, vascularization index; FI, flow index; VFI, vascularization-flow index; CES, cumulative embryo score. All other correlation coefficients are significant at $P<0.01$; *$P<0.05$.

parameters are significantly correlated with the laboratory data. Nevertheless, a multiple regression analysis has demonstrated that the vascularization index and the number of follicles are the only independent predictors of the number of Grade I embryos developed on the embryo transfer day. Therefore, the embryo quality depends not only of the number of follicles but of the ovarian vascularization index as well.

The transfer of an embryo from a well-vascularized follicle implies a significantly high pregnancy rate, whereas the pregnancy loss rate is increased when the embryos transferred come from low vascularized follicles.[41,46] The probability of pregnancy has been observed to be higher if at least one follicle shows a peak systolic velocity ≥10 cm/s.[45] According to our results,[38] the transfer of at least one embryo from one follicle with a vascularity ≥75% or with a peak systolic velocity ≥10 cm/s has a positive predictive value of pregnancy greater than 55%. That means that the application of this marker could improve results significantly, almost doubling the pregnancy rate (32% in this series).

Kupesic and Kurjak[10] studied 56 patients with 3D power Doppler after pituitary suppression. When the average stromal flow index from both ovaries was greater than 11, they observed a fertilization rate of 89% and a pregnancy rate of 50%. When this index was between 11 and 13 the fertilization and pregnancy rates were 75.2% and 47.2%, respectively. However, if the average flow index from both ovaries was below 11 the fertilization rate fell to 64.3% and no pregnancy was achieved. Our results are shown in Table 95.6, where significant differences between pregnant and non-pregnant patients for the majority of IVF evaluated parameters can be appreciated. Although the number of transferred embryos was similar, the biological quality was greater in the pregnant group. Three-dimensional power Doppler indices are significantly increased in the pregnant group. Ovarian flow index lower than 60 is significantly associated with a lower pregnancy rate and to a greater number of miscarriages (14.3% and 50% respectively). On the contrary, a flow index higher than 70 is significantly related to a higher pregnancy rate and to a lower rate of pregnancy loss (74.1% and 5% respectively). When the flow index was between 60 and 70 the pregnancy rate was 41% and the miscarriage rate was 37.5%.

Table 95.6 Clinical, sonographic, angiographic and biological parameters in relation to outcome in 80 IVF/ICSI cycles

Parameter	Pregnant (n=38)	Non-pregnant (n=42)	P
Age (years)	33.87±3.36	34.12±3.59	0.749
Estradiol on hCG day (pg/ml)	2852.21±1161.51	2369.64±1058.08	0.055
Ovarian volume (ml)	62.89±21.31	51.37±21.22	0.020
No. of follicles	14.39±6.28	11.71±6.28	0.070
Total follicular volume (ml)	35.76±11.60	30.14±11.76	0.035
Vascularization index	24.73±8.11	18.44±10.25	0.003
Flow index	68.65±8.39	62.20±9.93	0.003
Vascularization-flow index	8.82±3.15	6.44±3.75	0.003
No. of retrieved oocytes	11.21±5.05	8.24±5.11	0.011
No. of mature oocytes	8.18±3.71	5.55±4.17	0.004
No. of fertilized oocytes	5.89±2.85	4.00±3.35	0.008
No. of embryos on transfer day	5.71±2.78	4.00±3.21	0.014
No. of transferred embryos*	2 (1–3)	2 (1–3)	0.351
No. of transferred Grade 1 embryos*	2 (0–2)	1 (0–1)	0.001
CES of the transferred embryos	45.18±26.36	31.59±20.11	0.013

CES, cumulative embryo score. Data are presented as mean ± standard deviation or *median (range).

Table 95.7 Cut-off values for the uterine artery pulsatility index in patients undergoing assisted reproduction techniques

Authors	Treatment	Day (d)	Parameter	Limit
Steer *et al.*[48]	An+CC+hMG	Transfer-d	Mean PI	3
Zaidi *et al.*[49]	An+hMG	HCG-d	PI	3
Tsai *et al.*[50]	CC+hMG	HCG-d	Mean PI	3
Coulam *et al.*[51]	Natural	Ovulation-d	Mean PI	3.3
Coulam *et al.*[52]	Gn	Retrieval-d+transfer-d	Mean PI	3.3
Bustillo *et al.*[53]	An+HRT	15-d	Mean PI	3.3
Favre *et al.*[54]	An+hMG	Transfer-d	PI	3.55
Tekay *et al.*[55]	?	?	PI	4
Deichert *et al.*[56]	?	?	PI	4

hMG, human menopausal gonadotropin; CC, clomiphene citrate; An, gonadotropin releasing hormone analog; HRT, hormone replacement therapy; Natural: nonstimulation treatment; hCG, human chorionic gonadotropin

Uterine and endometrial blood flow

Goswany *et al.*[47] demonstrated that the uterine receptivity improved after increasing the uterine arteries blood flow under hormonal replacement therapy. The optimal uterine receptivity seems to appear when the average pulsatility index from both uterine arteries ranges from 2 to 3.[48–50] The implantation and pregnancy rates decrease significantly when the pulsatility index is greater than 3 or 4[48–56] or when no diastolic flow is registered in the Doppler signal (Table 95.7).[55,56]

According to these limits, a diminished blood flow in the uterine arteries would prevent implantation (NPV = 88–100%) but a good uterine perfusion will not always guarantee a pregnancy (PPV = 44–56%).

Table 95.8 Pregnancy rate according to endometrial blood flow mapping on the hCG administration day in 40 IVF cycles

Endometrial blood flow	No. of cases, *n* (%)	Pregnancy rate, *n* (%)
Type 0	5 (12.5%)	1(20%)
Type I	17 (42.5%)	6 (35%)
Type II	12 (30%)	5 (42%)
Type III	6 (15%)	4 (67%)

The endometrial blood flow should reflect more properly the uterine receptivity given that the endometrium is the place for the embryo implantation.[38] In accordance with the color mapping four types of endometrial blood flow can be distinguished[38,57–59]: Type 0 or negative endometrial blood flow, when only vessels from the surrounding myometrium without reaching the endometrium can be depicted; Type I or peripheral endometrial blood flow, if the color signal reaches the hyperecogenic endometrial border; Type II or intermediate endometrial blood flow, when the color map occupies the external half of the endometrial thickness; and Type III or central endometrial blood flow when vessels come to the endometrial cavity invading the entire endometrial thickness (Figure 95.9). It is more convenient to apply power Doppler to detect the signal from vessels showing low velocity blood flow, thus avoiding the loss of signal due to a perpendicular incidence of the beam, as it occurs with conventional color Doppler.[38]

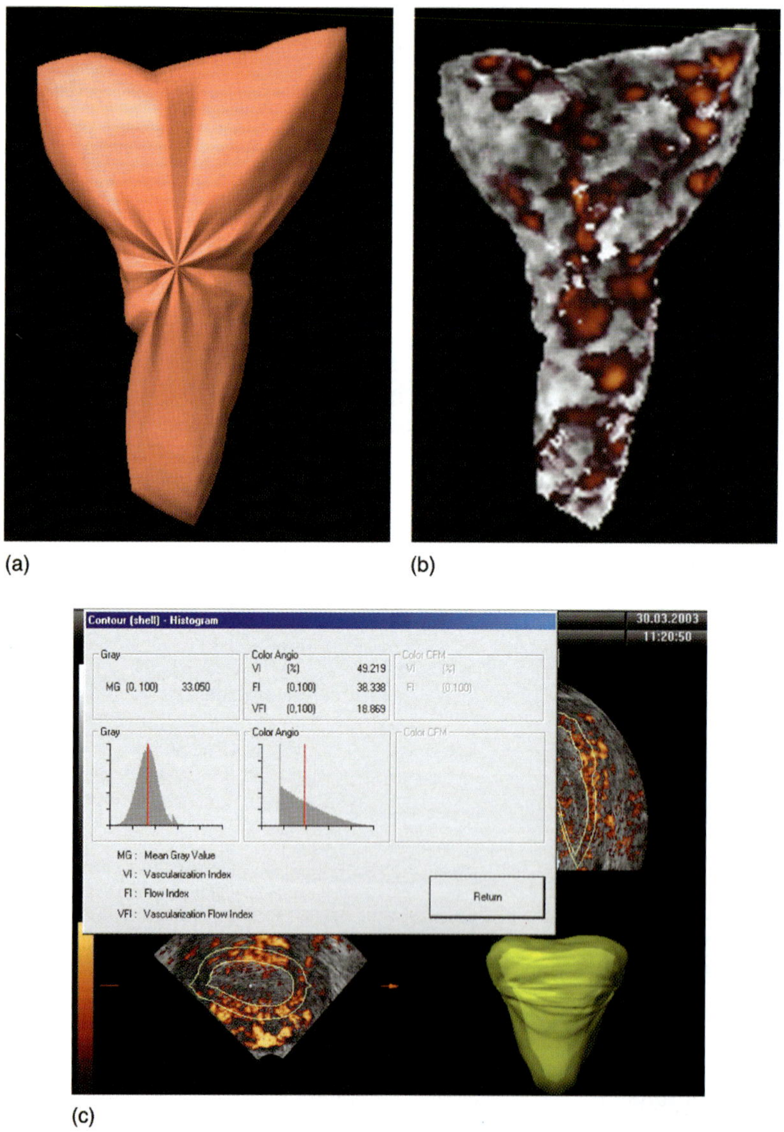

Figure 95.10 Three-dimensional ultrasound and power Doppler angiography of the endometrium and its vascularity on the day of hCG administration. (a) Endometrial volume by 'skin' rendering. (b) Three-dimensional power Doppler mapping of the endometrial vasculature. (c) Technique of 'shell' to calculate subendometrial 3D power Doppler vascularity indices.

The absence of a color map at the endometrial and myometrial subendometrial levels implies a complete failure[57] or significant decrease[60,61] of implantation, whereas the pregnancy rate increases when vessels reach the subendometrial halo and the endometrium.[57,60] In a study of about more than 600 cycles with color Doppler, the day of embryo transfer, the implantation and pregnancy rates were 24.2% and 47.8%, respectively when endometrial and subendometrial blood flow was detected; 15.8% and 29.7% if there was only subendometrial flow; and 3.5% and 7.5% when no flow was present.[60] Women showing a large endometrial blood flow area by power Doppler have a greater pregnancy rate, whereas a value below 5 mm^2 means that it is very difficult to achieve implantation despite a proper endometrial thickness.[62] Our results from 40 IVF cycles show that the pregnancy rate increases along with vascularity improvement, reaching a 67% when the color signal arrives at the endometrial cavity (Table 95.8).

Ultrasonography and 3D power Doppler have the advantage to assess the endometrial volume and the endometrial and sub-endometrial blood flow at the same time (Figure 95.10). The subendometrial flow index the day of embryo transfer is greater in the group of patients achieving pregnancy.[63] A subendometrial vascularization-flow index above 0.24 showed a 83.3% sensitivity, a specificity of 88.9%, PPV of 93.8% and NPV of 72.3% to predict gestation when it is evaluated the day of hCG administration in IVF cycles.[64]

Table 95.9 Pregnancy rate according to subendometrial 3D power Doppler indices on the hCG administration day in 40 IVF cycles

Doppler indices		No. of cases, n (%)	Pregnancy rate, n (%)
Vascularization	<10	5 (12.5%)	0 (0%)
	10–35	18 (45%)	11 (61.1%)
	>35	17 (42.5%)	5 (29.4%)
Flow	<28	12 (30%)	1 (8.3%)
	28–34	20 (50%)	12 (60%)
	>34	8 (20%)	3 (37.5%)
Vascularization-flow	<6	10 (25%)	1 (10%)
	6–12	17 (42.5%)	10 (58.8%)
	>12	13 (32.5%)	5 (38.5%)

According to our results, an intermediate vascularization, flow and vascularization-flow indices are associated to a high pregnancy rate. On the contrary, when the vascularization index is below 10 no pregnancy is achieved. When the blood flow is very high, the pregnancy rate decreases without significant differences (Table 95.9).

REFERENCES

1. Taylor KJW, Burns PN, Wells PNT, Conway DI, Hull MGR. Ultrasound Doppler flow studies of the ovarian and uterine arteries. *Br J Obstet Gynaecol* 1985;92:240–6.
2. Vrtacnik-Bokal E, Meden-Vrtovec H. Utero-ovarian arterial blood flow and hormonal profile in patients with polycystic ovary syndrome. *Hum Reprod* 1998;13:815–21.
3. Mercé LT. Velocimetría Doppler durante el ciclo ovárico normal. In Mercé LT, ed. *Ecografía Doppler en Obstetricia y Ginecología*. Madrid: Interamericana-McGraw-Hill, 1993:113–28.
4. Mercé LT, Bau S. Velocimetría Doppler del ciclo ovárico. In Bajo Arenas JM, ed. *Ultrasonografía y Reproducción*. Barcelona: Prous Science 1996:37–66.
5. Tomás C, Nuojua-Huttunen S, Martikainen H. Pretreatment transvaginal ultrasound examination predicts ovarian responsiveness to gonadotrophins in in-vitro fertilization. *Hum Reprod* 1997;12:220–3.
6. Chang MY, Chiang CH, Hsieh TT, Soong YK, Hsu KH. Use of the antral follicle count to predict the outcome of assisted reproductive technologies. *Fertil Steril* 1998;69:505–10.
7. Ng EH, Tang OS, Ho PC. The significance of the number of antral follicles prior to stimulation in predicting ovarian responses in an IVF programme. *Hum Reprod* 2000;15:1937–42.
8. Zaidi J, Barber J, Kyei-Mensah A, Bekir J, Campbell S, Tan SL. Relationship of ovarian stromal blood flow at the baseline ultrasound scan to subsequent follicular response in an in vitro fertilization program. *Obstet Gynecol* 1996;88:779–84.
9. Engmann L, Sladkevicius P, Agrawal R, Bekir JS, Campbell S, Tan SL. Value of ovarian stromal blood flow velocity measurement after pituitary suppression in the prediction of ovarian responsiveness and outcome of in vitro fertilization treatment. *Fertil Steril* 1999;71:22–9.
10. Kupesic S, Kurjak A. Predictors of IVF outcome by three-dimensional ultrasound. *Hum Reprod* 2002;17:950–5.
11. Pan HA, Wu MH, Cheng YC, Wu LH, Chang FM. Quantification of ovarian Doppler signal in hyperresponders during in vitro fertilization treatment using three-dimensional power Doppler ultrasonography. *Ultrasound Med Biol* 2003;29:921–7.
12. Pan HA, Wu MH, Cheng YC, Wu LH, Chang FM. Quantification of ovarian stromal Doppler signals in poor responders undergoing in vitro fertilization with three-dimensional power Doppler ultrasonography. *Am J Obstet Gynecol* 2004;190: 338–44.
13. Jarvela IY, Sladkevicius P, Kellly S, Ojha K, Campbell S, Nargund G. Quantification of ovarian power Doppler signal with three-dimensional ultrasonography to predict response during in vitro fertilization. *Obstet Gynecol* 2003;102:816–22.
14. Kurjak A, Kupesis-Urek S, Schulman H, Zalud I. Transvaginal color Doppler in the assessment of ovarian and uterine blood flow in infertile women. *Fertil Steril* 1991;56:870–3.
15. Mercé LT, Garcés D, Barco MJ, de la Fuente F. Intraovarian Doppler velocimetry in ovulatory, dysovulatory and anovulatory cycles. *Ultrasound Obstet Gynecol* 1992;2:197–202.
16. Sladkevicius P, Valentin L, Marsál K. Blood flow velocity in the uterine and ovarian arteries during the normal menstrual cycle. *Ultrasound Obstet Gynecol* 1993;3:199–208.
17. Tan SL, Zaidi J, Campbell S, Doyle P, Collins W. Blood flow changes in the ovarian and uterine arteries during the normal menstrual cycle. *Am J Obstet Gynecol* 1996;175:625–31.
18. Mercé LT, Bau S, Bajo JM. Doppler study of arterial and venous intraovarian blood flow in stimulated cycles. *Ultrasound Obstet Gynecol* 2001;18:505–10.
19. Weiner Z, Thaler I, Levron J, Lewit N, Itskovitz-Eldor J. Assessment of ovarian and uterine blood flow by transvaginal color Doppler in ovarian-stimulated women: correlation with the number of follicles and steroid hormone levels. *Fertil Steril* 1993;59:743–9.

20. Balakier H, Stronell RG. Color Doppler assessment of folliculogenesis in in vitro fertilization patients. *Fertil Steril* 1994;62: 1211–16.
21. Mercé LT. Doppler de los cambios ováricos y endometriales preimplantatorios. In Kurjak A, Carrera JM, eds. *Ecografía en Medicina Materno-Fetal*. Barcelona: Masson, 2000:87–104.
22. Hackelöer BJ, Fleming R, Robinson HP, Adam AH, Coutts JRT. Correlation of ultrasonic and endocrinologic assessment of human follicular development. *Am J Obstet Gynecol* 1979;135:122–8.
23. Campbell S, Bourne TH, Waterstone J, *et al*. Transvaginal color blood flow imaging of the periovulatory follicle. *Fertil Steril* 1993;60:433–438.
24. Brännström M, Zackrisson U, Hagström H-G, *et al*. Preovulatory changes of blood flow in different regions of the human follicle. *Fertil Steril* 1998;69:435–42.
25. Jarvela IY, Sladkevivius P, Kelly S, Ojha K, Nargund G, Campbell S. Three-dimensional sonographic and power Doppler characterization of ovaries in late follicular phase. *Ultrasound Obstet Gynecol* 2002;20:281–5.
26. Kitai H, Yoshimura Y, Wright KH, Santulli R, Wallch EE. Microvasculature of preovulatory follicles: comparison of *in situ* and *in vitro* perfused rabbit ovaries following stimulation of ovulation. *Am J Obstet Gynaecol* 1985;152:889–95.
27. Parsons AK. Imaging the human corpus luteum. *J Ultrasound Med* 2001;20:811–9.
28. Ottander U, Solensten NG, Bergh A, Olofsson JI. Intraovarian blood flow measured with color Doppler ultrasonography inversely correlates with vascular density in the human corpus luteum of the menstrual cycle. *Fertil Steril* 2004;81:154–9.
29. Gloock JL, Brumsted JR. Color flow pulsed Doppler ultrasound in diagnosing luteal phase defect. *Fertil Steril* 1995;64:500–4.
30. Kupesic S, Kurjak A, Vujisic S, Petrovic Z. Luteal phase defect: comparison between Doppler velocimetry, histological and hormonal markers. *Ultrasound Obstet Gynecol* 1997;9:105–12.
31. Kupesic S, Kurjak A. The assessment of normal and abnormal luteal function by transvaginal color Doppler sonography. *Eur J Obstet Gynecol Biol Reprod* 1997;72:83–7.
32. Kupesic S, Kurjak A. Uterine and ovarian perfusion during the periovulatory period assessed by transvaginal color Doppler. *Fertil Steril* 1993;60:439–43.
33. Bourne TH, Hagström HG, Granberg S, *et al*. Ultrasound studies of vascular and morphological changes in the human uterus after a positive self-test for the urinary luteinizing hormone surge. *Hum Reprod* 1996;11:369–75.
34. Steer CV, Campbell S, Pampiglione JS, Kingsland CR, Mason BA, Collins WP. Transvaginal colour flow imaging of the uterine arteries during the ovarian and menstrual cycles. *Hum Reprod* 1990;5:391–5.
35. Hsieh Y-Y, Chang C-C, Tsai H-D. Doppler evaluation of the uterine and spiral arteries from different sampling sites and phases of the menstrual cycle during controlled ovarian hyperstimulation. *Ultrasound Obstet Gynecol* 2000;16:192–6.
36. Raine-Fenning NJ, Campbell BK, Kendall NR, Clewes JS, Jonson IR. Quantifying the changes in endometrial vascularity throughout the normal menstrual cycle with three-dimensional power Doppler angiography. *Hum Reprod* 2004;19:330–8.
37. Mercé LT, Kupesic S, Kurjak A. Color Doppler assessment of implantation and early placentation. *Prenat Neonat Med* 1999;4:49–112.
38. Mercé LT. Ultrasound markers of implantation. *Ultrasound Rev Obstet Gynecol* 2002;2:110–23.
39. Van Blerkom J, Antczak M, Schrader R. The developmental potential of the human oocyte is related to the dissolved oxygen content of follicular fluid: Association with vascular endothelial growth factor levels and perifollicular blood flow characteristics. *Hum Reprod* 1997;12:1047–55.
40. Gaulden M. Maternal age effect: the enigma of Down syndrome and other trisomic conditions. *Mutua Res* 1992;296:69–88.
41. Bhal PS, Pugh ND, Chui DK, Gregory L, Walker SM, Shaw RW. The use of transvaginal power Doppler ultrasonography to evaluate the relationship between perifollicular vascularity and outcome in in-vitro fertilization treatment cycles. *Hum Reprod* 1999;14:939–45.
42. Chui DKC, Pugh ND, Walker SM, Gregory L, Shaw RW. Follicular vascularity-the predictive value of transvaginal power Doppler ultrasonography in an in-vitro fertilization programme: a preliminary study. *Hum Reprod* 1997;12:191–6.
43. Nargund G, Doyle PE, Bourne TH, *et al*. Ultrasound derived indices of follicular blood flow before hCG administration and the prediction of oocyte recovery and preimplantation embryo quality. *Hum Reprod* 1996;11:2512–7.
44. Ozaki T, Hata K, Xie H, Takahashi K, Miyazaki K. Utility of color Doppler indices of dominant follicular blood flow for prediction of clinical factors in in vitro fertilization–embryo transfer cycles. *Ultrasound Obstet Gynecol* 2002;20:592–6.
45. Coulam CB, Goodman C, Rinehart JS. Colour Doppler indices of follicular blood flow as predictors of pregnancy after in-vitro fertilization and embryo transfer. *Hum Reprod* 1999;14:1979–82.
46. Bhal PS, Pugh ND, Gregory L, O'Brien S, Shaw RW. Perifollicular vascularity as a potential variable affecting outcome in stimulated intrauterine insemination treatment cycles: A study using transvaginal power Doppler. *Hum Reprod* 2001;16:1682–9.
47. Goswany RK, Williams G, Steptoe PC. Decreased uterine perfusion – A cause of infertility. *Hum Reprod* 1988;8:955–9.
48. Steer CV, Campbell S, Tan SL, *et al*. The use of transvaginal color flow imaging after *in vitro* fertilization to identify optimum uterine conditions before embryo transfer. *Fertil Steril* 1992;57: 372–6.
49. Zaidi J, Pittrof R, Shaker A, Kyei-Mensah A, Campbell S, Tan SL. Assessment of uterine artery blood flow on the day of human chorionic gonadotropin administration by transvaginal color Doppler ultrasound in an *in vitro* fertilization program. *Fertil Steril* 1996;65:377–81.
50. Tsai Y-C, Chang J-C, Tai M-J, Kung F-T, Yang L-C, Chang S-Y. Relationship of uterine perfusion to outcome of intrauterine insemination. *J Ultrasound Med* 1996;15:633–6.
51. Coulam CB, Bustillo M, Soenksen DM, Britten S. Ultrasonographic predictors of implantation after assisted reproduction. *Fertil Steril* 1994;62:1004–10.
52. Coulam CB, Stern JJ, Soenksen DM, Britten S, Bustillo M. Comparison of pulsatility indexes on the day of oocyte retrieval and embryo transfer. *Hum Reprod* 1995;10:82–4.
53. Bustillo M, Krysa LW, Coulam CB. Uterine receptivity in an oocyte donation programme. *Hum Reprod* 1995;10:442–5.
54. Favre R, Bettahar K, Grange G, *et al*. Predictive value of transvaginal uterine Doppler assessment in an *in vitro* fertilization program. *Ultrasound Obstet Gynecol* 1993;3:350–3.
55. Tekay A, Martikainen H, Jouppila P. The clinical value of transvaginal colour Doppler ultrasound in assisted reproductive technology procedures. *Hum Reprod* 1996;11:1589–91.
56. Deichert U, Albrand-Thielman C, van de Sandt M. Dopplersonographic pelvic blood flow measurements and their prognostic value in terms of luteal phase and implantation. *Hum Reprod* 1996;11:1591–3.
57. Zaidi J, Campbell S, Pittrof R, Tan SL. Endometrial thickness, morphology, vascular penetration and velocimetry in predicting implantation in an *in vitro* fertilization program. *Ultrasound Obstet Gynecol* 1995;6:191–8.
58. Applebaum M. The menstrual cycle, menopause, ovulation induction, an in vitro fertilization. In Copel JA, Reed KL, eds. *Doppler Ultrasound in Obstetrics and Gynecology*. New York: Raven Press, 1995:71–86.
59. Battaglia C, Artini PG, Giulini S, *et al*. Colour Doppler changes and thromboxane production after ovarian stimulation with gonadotrophin-releasing hormone agonist. *Hum Reprod* 1997; 11:2477–82.
60. Chien LW, Au HK, Chen PL, Xiao J, Tzeng CR. Assessment of uterine receptivity by the endometrial-subendometrial blood flow distribution pattern in women undergoing in vitro fertilization–embryo transfer. *Fertil Steril* 2002;78:245–51.
61. Maugey-Laulom B, Commenges-Ducos M, Jullien V, Papaxanthos-Roche A, Scotet V, Commenges D. Endometrial vascularity and ongoing pregnancy after IVF. *Eur J Obstet Gynecol Reprod Biol* 2002;104:137–43.
62. Yang J-H, Wu M-Y, Chen C-D, Jiang M-C, Ho H-N, Yang Y-S. Association of endometrial blood flow as determined by a modified colour Doppler technique with subsequent outcome of in-vitro fertilization. *Hum Reprod* 1999;14:1606–10.
63. Kupesic S, Bekavac I, Bjelos D, Kurjak A. Assessment of endometrial receptivity by transvaginal color Doppler and three-dimensional power Doppler ultrasonography in patients undergoing in vitro fertilization procedures. *J Ultrasound Med* 2001;20: 125–34.
64. Wu HM, Chiang CH, Huang HY, Chao AS, Wang HS, Soong YK. Detection of the subendometrial vascularization blood flow by three-dimensional ultrasound may be useful for predicting the pregnancy rate for patients undergoing in vitro fertilization-embryo transfer. *Fertil Steril* 2003;79:507–11.

96 Implantation and the yolk sac

S. Kupesic and A. Kurjak

Introduction

Recent advances in perinatal technology have increased tremendously our understanding of early human development. This, in turn, has led investigators to ask numerous searching questions about both maternal and fetal placental hemodynamics.

The early beginning of embryonic life is a gestational period of important hemodynamic changes, mainly characterized by establishment of a continuous maternal blood flow in the intervillous space. In this development process, the maternal vascular bed and spiral arterioles form the basis for perfusion of the placenta. Current anatomical knowledge has largely been based on the classical studies of earlier investigators. In many instances, their theories have been confirmed by new information, but, in others, initial errors in observation or conclusion have been brought to light necessitating revision or replacement of the original concepts.

Many questions are presently directed to the intervillous space, probing in particular its size and form, its source of blood supply and the mechanism of circulation within it. In 1962, in an excellent review article[1] on circulation in the intervillous space Ramsey wrote: 'Old ideas die hard, however, even when their validity has been challenged, and it is well known that they frequently maintain their position in textbooks for some time after they have been discarded by workers in the forefront of the field. Old ideas also have a tendency to leave fragments of themselves, as a complicating legacies, incorporated in the theories which finally replace them'.

How little has changed in a period of more than 34 years! We are still searching for satisfactory answers to many of the queries on the intervillous circulation. However, a good deal of data are already available, especially as a result of recent research on Doppler proofs of the continuous blood flow in intervillous space. In our effort to facilitate a better understanding of the present concepts on intervillous circulation, a brief recapitulation of anatomy and embryology will be included in the subsequent sections of this chapter. It is our intention to synthesize and clear out the chronology and factography of the controversial data and theories about the establishment of intervillous circulation and yolk sac morphology and function.

The 'classic' embryological concept of the early uteroplacental circulation

The labyrinthine series of cavities, which together constitute the intervillous space in the placenta, was first identified by William and John Hunter in the 18th century. However, there is still uncertainty regarding many of its features.[2]

The first week of embryonal development is the preimplantation stage. By the end of day 5, blastocyst is formed consisting of the trophoblast and embryoblast (inner cell mass).[3]

After this period begins the implantation period, the process whereby the blastocyst attaches to and erodes through the endometrial epithelium. One of the earliest modifications of the endometrium after fertilization is an increase in vascular permeability. The other changes of the endometrium include increased vascularity, edema and thickening (i.e. decidual reaction). Trophoblast produces proteolytic enzymes that facilitate the penetration in the endometrium and erodes adjacent maternal capillaries.

By the end of the first week, the blastocyst is superficially implanted in the endometrium. Trophoblast and embryoblast start to develop along different lines.[4,5] In the seventh day after fertilization (Carnegie stage 5a) the trophoblast rapidly differentiates into two layers – an inner layer of mononuclear cytotrophoblastic cells and an outer layer of multinucleated syncytiotrophoblast. The syncytiotrophoblast comes into direct contact with the endometrial stroma. The endometrial glands in contact with the trophoblast show degenerative changes; in some instances the glandular epithelium has disappeared and the trophoblast plugs the glandular lumen.[2]

By the eighth day after fertilization, the blastocyst is completely embedded within the endometrial stroma. At the embryonic pole, the primitive syncytiotrophoblast on the surface has some deep indentations, which contain maternal blood cells.

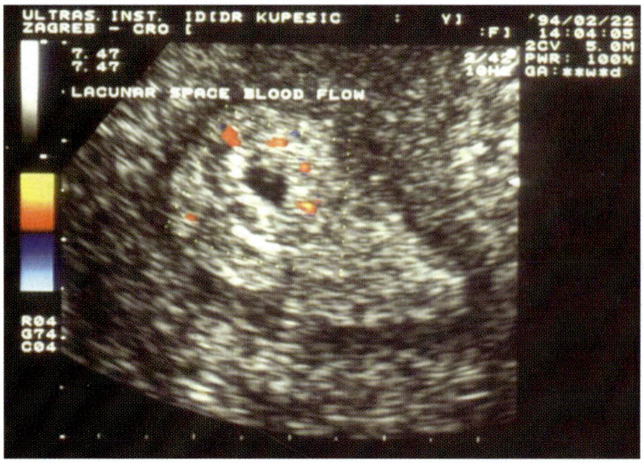

Figure 96.1 Lacunar space blood flow at the periphery of an early gestational sac as seen by color Doppler ultrasound.

The ninth day of development (Carnegie stage 5b) is named the lacunar or previllous stage. At this stage the inner cell mass (embryoblast) is differentiated into a bilaminar embryonic disk.[3]

From the eighth day after fertilization, intercommunicating fluid-filled spaces of lacunae appear in the rapidly enlarging syncytiotrophoblast. Between the 10th and 13th days (Carnegie stage 5c), lacunae convert the syncytiotrophoblast into a sponge-like structure. The lacunae are incompletely separated from each other by trabecular columns of syncytiotrophoblast. The lacunae open into several maternal sinusoids, which have probably arisen from endometrial capillaries. The lacunae become confluent. With further extensions of the maternal sinusoids and more dilatation of the endometrial blood vessels, the supply of blood to the lacunae comes largely from venous sinusoids. The lacunae rapidly become filled with a combination of maternal blood and secretion from eroded endometrial glands.[6] At this stage there is no evidence for direct arterial communication with the lacunae. It would seem that the earliest maternal blood that enters the developing lacunae is not arterial but is derived from the capillaries and venules that dilate to form sinusoids.[2] Using transvaginal color Doppler, venous signals can be clearly obtained from these spaces (Figure 96.1).

With continuing trophoblastic invasion, the maternal vessels disappear progressively back to the level of the spiral arteries and their venules, permitting a true circulation. The trabeculae are called 'primary villous stems'. They are not true villi but serve as the framework from which villi later develop. They are arranged radially and divide lacunae into a labyrinth at the 14th day after fertilization. The placenta at this stage of development is a labyrinthine rather than a villous organ.[7]

Primary chorionic villi develop between 13 and 15 days of development (Carnegie stages 6a and 6b). The trabeculae have a central cellular core produced by proliferation of the cytotrophoblastic cells. At the same time the formation of the first blood vessels starts in the extraembryonic mesoderm of the yolk sac, the connecting stalk and the chorion. The cytotrophoblastic cells extend distally toward the attachment of the syncytiotrophoblast to the endometrium. These cells from the villous tips break through syncytiotrophoblast and expand laterally to fuse with adjacent columns to form a cytotrophoblastic shell. The shell is completed by the 15th day after fertilization. Villi that are attached to the maternal tissue via the cytotrophoblastic shell are 'stem' or 'anchoring villi'. The villi that grow from the sides of the stem villi are 'branch villi'.

Days 15–21 are a period of intensive trophoblastic growth. By the 15th day, the maternal circulation becomes fully functional, when the syncytial lacunae become confluent and connected with endometrial capillaries.[8] The trabeculae, which are at first unoriented, gradually become more regularly arranged. The number of initial villi is determined by the number of trabeculae that are invaded by proliferating cytotrophoblast. On the 16th day, the extraembryonal mesenchyme appears and extends toward the villous distal end. Primary chorionic villi gradually convert into secondary villi.[3] By the 18th day, the villous mesenchymal cells begin to differentiate into blood capillaries forming an arteriocapillary venous network, which is completed by 20 days after fertilization. The villi are called 'tertiary villi'. The villous vessels become connected with the embryonic heart tube via vessels differentiated in the chorion and the connecting stalk.[6]

The establishment of the trophoblastic shell allows rapid circumferential growth of the developing placenta. This leads to the expansion of the intervillous space into which sprouts extend from the primary villous stems. The placenta is, by the 21st day of gestation, a vascularized villous organ.[7] The extensive system of venous sinusoids around the implantation site constitutes venous connections between the intervillous space and the maternal circulation.

In the fourth week of development, the cytotrophoblastic shell is thinner than in the earlier stages. At the junctions of the shell with the decidua, there are many clefts and spaces. Some of them open into the adjacent intervillous space. The 21st day after fertilization (Carnegie stage 10) the primitive embryonal heart begins to beat, and embryonal blood circulates through villous capillaries.[6] The communications with the terminal branches of the spiral arteries have not yet been completely established.[2] There are six to eight endometrial spiral arteries opening directly to the decidua basalis. They possess a wide lumen. The media of the vascular wall becomes attenuated and finally disappears completely. The lining endothelium is surrounded only by a layer of reticular and collagen fibers. As a result of these changes, it is often difficult to identify the spiral arteries and to establish their relationship to the intervillous space. From this region several narrow clefts penetrate the shell to enter to the intervillous space.

There are two types of non-villous migratory trophoblasts: (1) the interstitial or stromal trophoblast, which invades the decidua and myometrium and (2) the endovascular trophoblast, which migrates into spiral arteries and modifies them into uteroplacental arteries. The endovascular trophoblast is closely linked to the development of the trophoblastic shell.[9] It is the key factor for physiological modifications of spiral arteries. These gestational changes are needed for the development of hemochorial placentation.

Migrating trophoblast penetrates the uterine wall and invades venous sinusoids of increasing size and superficial arterioles during the fourth week. The extravillous cytotrophoblastic cells expand from the tips of the anchoring villi into the lumina of the spiral arteries. They convert the thick-walled muscular arteries into flaccid sac-like uteroplacental vessels, which can passively dilate to accommodate the greatly increased maternal blood flow required for fetal oxygenation and growth.[10]

Trophoblastic cells can be found within the spiral arteries in about the sixth week after fertilization. The trophoblastic disruption of the muscular cells and elastic fibers of the spiral arteries has two effects. Increasing blood flow causes progressive distension of these arteries into the uteroplacental arteries capable of accommodating the increasing blood supply. Uteroplacental arteries are not responsive to change within the autonomic nervous system.[6]

In the second lunar month, as a result of the extensive branching villi the intervillous space increases. During the second month many terminal parts of spiral arteries near the intervillous space contain plugs of cytotrophoblastic cells. By the end of this period of development, centrally placed communications between the decidual veins are numerous and large. After 40 days (crown–rump length 15 mm) numerous spiral arteries show direct openings into the intervillous space.[2]

The cytotrophoblastic cells appear within the lumina of the spiral arteries. The maternal blood reaches the intervillous space through the gaps between the cells of the endovascular trophoblast. The persistence of the cytotrophoblastic plugs in the lumina of the spiral arteries suggests that the blood pressure in them is not very high, otherwise the plugs would be dislodged.[2] Maximal trophoblastic activity occurs at the center of the placental bed and then extends centrifugally toward its periphery.

During the third month of gestation, in the lumina of the terminal segments of most of the spiral arteries the cytotrophoblastic plugs are always present. None of the spiral arteries open freely into the intervillous space. Later in this period of development the plugs are more loosely arranged and they are probably then less able to impede maternal blood flow into the intervillous space.[2]

Up to the end of the fourth month of gestation, the chorion frondosum develops into the definitive placenta. The chorionic villi associated with the decidua capsularis degenerate and the associated intervillous space disappears. The smooth avascular chorion laeve forms.[6] There is regression in the trophoblastic shell where the cytotrophoblastic cell columns degenerate. The trophoblastic infiltration of the myometrium occurs between 8 and 18 weeks of development.[10] The endovascular cytotrophoblast partially replaces the endothelium and invades the muscular cells of the myometrial vessels. The result is a progressive distension of these myometrial vessels.

The uteroplacental circulatory system is a low-pressure one because of progressive increase in the diameter of the vessels as they approach their entry into the intervillous space. There is a considerable drop in pressure from the proximal non-dilated portions of the uteroplacental arterioles to the distal dilated portions and full arterial pressure is not transmitted to the intervillous space.[7]

The 'heretic' concept of separation of villous tissue from the maternal circulation

This classic concept of establishment of the intervillous circulation was challenged in 1987 and 1988 by the experiments of Hustin and Shaaps.[11,12] They examined slice radiographs of hysterectomy specimens with pregnancy *in situ* collected at 7, 8 and 9 weeks of gestation and found no contrast medium in the intervillous space. When the examination was performed at 13 weeks of gestation, the placenta was rapidly filled with contrast medium. Histological examination of these hysterectomy specimens showed occlusion of the uteroplacental arteries by trophoblastic cells up to 12 weeks of gestation. Reconstruction of serial spiral arterial sections was also suggestive of the absence of the intervillous circulation before 12 weeks of gestation. At 13 weeks, on the other hand, the uteroplacental arteries were free of trophoblastic plugs, and contrast medium was found in the intervillous space, encircling the chorionic villi. This was partially confirmed *in vivo* by means of hysteroscopy, examination of chorionic villous sampling material and transvaginal sonography. These results suggest that early placenta is bathed predominantly by fluid derived from maternal plasma and uterine gland secretions. The authors believed that blood flow in the intervillous space is absent or incompletely developed before 12 weeks of gestation. Transformation of spiral arteries continues during the first trimester, when they widen progressively. Around 12 weeks of gestation, all trophoblastic plugs are eventually loosened and dislocated. This allows free entry of maternal blood to the intervillous space and establishment of a fully developed placental circulation.

Further support has been supplied by a more recent study[13] using a polarographic oxygen electrode inserted under ultrasound guidance, which demonstrated that

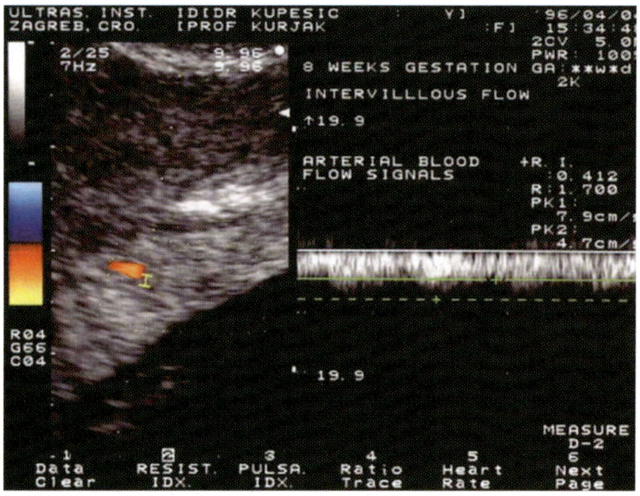

Figure 96.2 Arterial blood flow velocity waveforms from the intervillous space at 10 weeks' gestation demonstrate low impedance (RI = 0.41). Note typical spiky outline of the arterial signal.

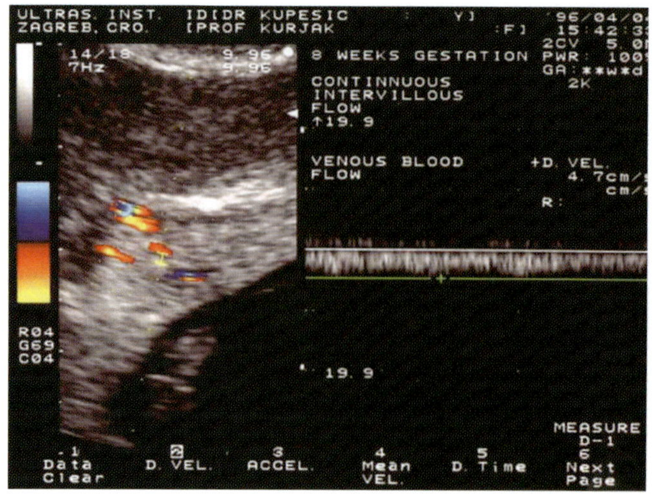

Figure 96.3 Continuous flow of a venous type in the same patient as in Figure 96.2; venous blood flow is easily detectable from the intervillous space.

between 8 and 10 weeks of gestation placental pO_2 levels were significantly lower compared with endometrial pO_2 levels, while between 12 and 13 weeks, the levels were similar. Intraplacental pO_2 levels increased significantly from 8–10 to 12–13 weeks of gestation. These results suggest that the increase of placental pO_2 may be related to the establishment of continuous maternal blood flow in the intervillous space at the end of the first trimester.

The advent and development of transvaginal color Doppler has enabled *in vivo* hemodynamic investigation of almost all segments embryonic/fetal and uteroplacental circulation.[14–21]

In 1991 and 1992, Jauniaux *et al.*[22,23] and Jaffe *et al.*[24] were unable to detect 'intraplacental' flow before 12 weeks of gestation using the transvaginal color Doppler. They found the appearance of intraplacental flow at around 14 weeks of gestation to coincide with the appearance of pandiastolic flow in the umbilical artery and with an abrupt increase in uterine artery peak systolic velocity (PSV). In agreement with the theories of Hustin and Shaaps,[11,12] they hypothesized that the simultaneous appearance of intraplacental flow, pandiastolic umbilical artery flow and abrupt increase in uterine artery blood flow velocity was to be explained by sudden loosening and disappearance of the trophoblastic plugs in the spiral arteries. By this time Kurjak *et al.*[25] were unable to demonstrate an abrupt change in the uteroplacental circulation between 12 and 14 weeks of gestation.

Hi-tech evidences of the 'classic' theory: the circle is closed

It must be emphasized that color Doppler measurements in the studies mentioned above were performed on devices of relatively moderate capability in the detection of low velocities. After the introduction of the new generation of far more sensitive color Doppler devices in the last few years, several authors reported a positive finding of intervillous circulation during first trimester of pregnancy (Figures 96.2 and 96.3).

In 1995, Kurjak *et al.*[26] presented the first report on a combined Doppler and morphopathological study of intervillous circulation. Using a transvaginal color Doppler, continuous intervillous flow of two types was detected in all examined patients: pulsatile arterial-like (Figure 96.2) and continuous venous-like flow (Figure 96.3). Parallel histological study has shown that the lumen of spiral arteries was never completely obstructed by the trophoblastic plugs. These data indicate that establishment of the intervillous circulation is a continuous process rather than an abrupt event at the end of the first trimester. One should note that arterial-like blood flow signals have shown lower resistance and pulsatility index (PI) values than those obtained in spiral arteries.

Shortly after, several other groups of authors reported similar findings. Valentin *et al.*[27] performed a combined study of uteroplacental and luteal flow with pathomorphologic analysis. Color Doppler measurements revealed positive finding of intervillous circulation from the sixth week of normal pregnancy (Figure 96.4). The same two types of Doppler signals, the pulsatile and continuous, were detected and measured with a visualization rate of more than 90% on 64 pregnancies from 5 to 11 weeks of gestation. The authors stated that the high blood velocities recorded from the subchorionic arteries were not compatible with these arteries being completely occluded by trophoblastic plugs. On pathomorphologic analysis, trophoblast plugging of the spiral arteries was incomplete, allowing passage of red blood cells. They concluded that the intervillous circulation was present as early as the first trimester.

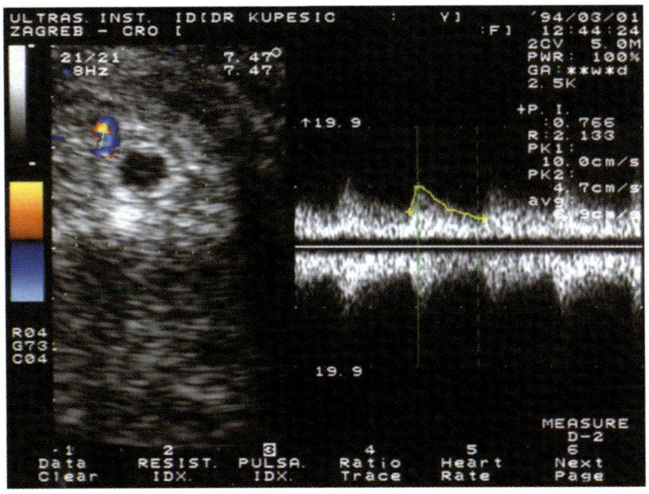

Figure 96.4 Transvaginal power Doppler imaging of a gestational sac at 5/6 weeks' gestation. This technique easily depicts blood flow surrounding the gestational sac.

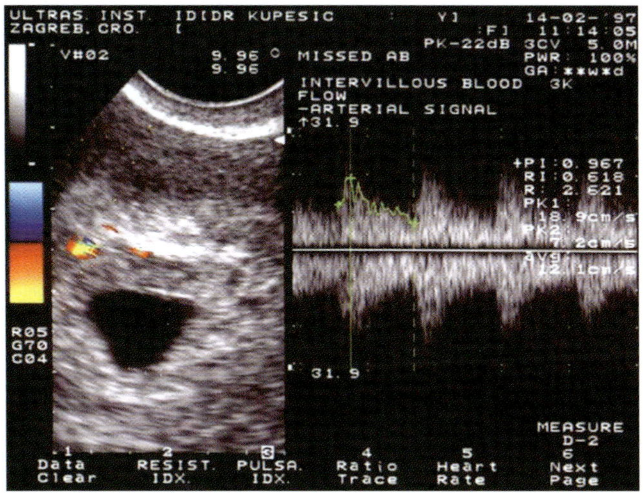

Figure 96.5 A transvaginal scan of the missed abortion at 12 weeks' gestation. Note increased RI value (0.62) of the arterial-like signal from the intervillous space.

Merce *et al.*[28] reported similar results on the group of 108 normal singleton pregnancies of 4–15 gestational weeks. They were able to detect intervillous flow from 5 weeks 6 days of gestation. It was a slightly undulating venous-like signal with tendency of increasing velocity throughout the first trimester. They also recorded arterial signals in retrochorionic segments of uteroplacental vasculature. The conclusion was that their results were in accordance with the classic embryological concept of establishment of the intervillous flow from four to seven weeks of gestation. According to Merce *et al.*,[28] uteroplacental circulation is the earliest to be affected in pregnancy, with pronounced changes from week 4 onward. Intervillous circulation and primitive umbilical blood flow were identified from week five on.

In more recent publications, Kurjak *et al.*[29,30] studied a group of 60 normal pregnancies of gestational age from 6 to 12 weeks and, for the first time, a group of 34 pathological early pregnancies: 22 cases of missed abortion (Figure 96.5) and 12 cases of anembryonic pregnancy (Figure 96.6) between 7 and 12 weeks of gestation. The same Doppler features were detected in the intervillous space of all pregnancies: pulsatile arterial-like signals with characteristic spiky outline and venous-like continuous signals. There was no difference in Doppler parameters between the group with missed abortion and the group of normal pregnancy. However, lower impedance (measured in resistance and PIs) was detected in the group with anembryonic pregnancies. These results are significantly different from those published by Jauniaux *et al.*[31] who found increased intervillous blood flow in 70% of abnormal pregnancies before 12 weeks of gestation. In these cases, a histopathologic examination showed that the trophoblastic shell was discontinuous and thinner, and that the intervillous space had been massively infiltrated by maternal blood. The

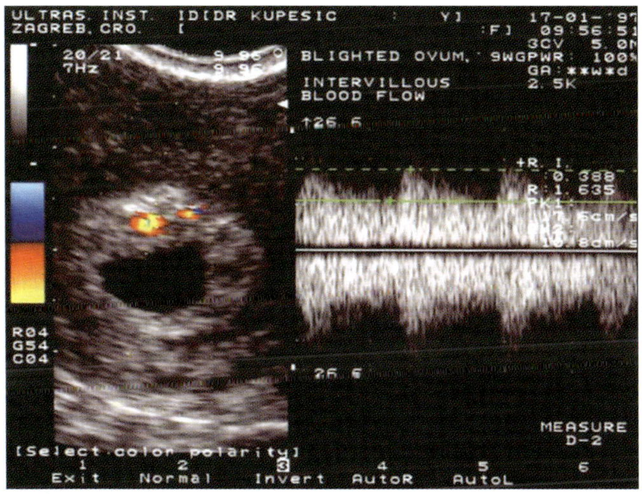

Figure 96.6 The transvaginal scan demonstrates anembryonic pregnancy. Note spiky outline and low vascular resistance (RI = 0.39) of the arterial-like signals obtained from the intervillous space of an anembryonic pregnancy.

authors hypothesized that trophoblast plugs in the spiral arteries restrict the maternal blood to flow in the intervillous space, protecting vulnerable villi from the high pressure of arterial blood. By this concept the premature entry of maternal blood in the intervillous space can disrupt the maternoembryonic interface, causing the separation of early placenta and, eventually, abortion.

In the research on placental development and formation of the uteroplacental circulation system, of crucial importance was experimental work with animal models, particularly with non-human primates, mostly with *Macaca* species. The classical work by Elisabeth Ramsey on the circulation in the intervillous space of the primate placenta is the base for all contemporary research in this field.[1,32] Recently, Nimrod *et al.*[33,34]

Table 96.1 Resistance index (RI), pulsatility index (PI), peak systolic velocity (PSV), end-diastolic velocity (EDV) and temporal averaged maximum velocity (TAMV) obtained from the intervillous space and in the spiral arteries in different gestational age groups (from Kurjak *et al.*,[41] with permission)

	Intervillous blood flow					Spiral artery blood flow				
Gestational weeks	RI (SD)	PI (SD)	PSV (SD)	EDV (SD)	TAMV (SD)	RI (SD)	PI (SD)	PSV (SD)	EDV (SD)	TAMV (SD)
7–9	0.48 (0.05)	0.71 (0.09)	28 (10)	18 (7)	25 (9)	0.58 (0.06)	0.88 (0.11)	31 (16)	22 (12)	26 (15)
10–12	0.41 (0.06)	0.61 (0.11)	28 (12)	21 (9)	26 (10)	0.51 (0.07)	0.73 (0.09)	36 (14)	20 (16)	31 (15)
13–15	0.34 (0.07)	0.43 (0.08)	35 (14)	22 (10)	30 (15)	0.43 (0.05)	0.55 (0.11)	41 (21)	26 (15)	37 (15)
16–22	0.29* (0.06)	0.34* (0.09)	40 (19)	35 (17)	37 (19)	0.41* (0.06)	0.55* (0.12)	37 (16)	23 (15)	32 (15)
23–28	0.30 (0.07)	0.36 (0.10)	36 (20)	30 (14)	32 (16)	0.40 (0.06)	0.52 (0.11)	42 (15)	26 (11)	34 (13)
29–36	0.25 (0.06)	0.29 (0.08)	36 (12)	26 (9)	32 (10)	0.34 (0.07)	0.42 (0.10)	31 (9)	21 (6)	26 (7)
37–42	0.27 (0.06)	0.31 (0.09)	32*** (14)	23** (10)	27*** (12)	0.37 (0.09)	0.48 (0.15)	30*** (12)	19 (9)	25*** (11)

SD, standard deviation
$^{*}P<0.01$; $^{**}P<0.05$; $^{***}P<0.07$

reported about the assessment of the early uteroplacental circulation in cynomolgus monkey (*Macaca fascicularis*) by color Doppler technique. They were able to detect the intervillous circulation from 18 days postconception. Regardless of the known differences in the depth of trophoblastic invasion of the spiral arteries between human and monkey, this finding can be considered as an additional evidence of early establishment of intervillous circulation in all primate placentas, although the 'argument by analogy' must be used with caution.

Publication of similar, if not the same, results obtained by few independent groups and published in prestigious journals usually produces a respectful attention of the scientific community. However, a recent editorial by Jauniaux,[35] repeating most of the facts known from his previous papers, did not appreciate enough the early reports on continuous intervillous flow. Although Jauniaux admitted that using a new equipment he was able to detect flow in some areas of intervillous space during the first trimester of pregnancy, his concern, was whether these signals originated from the intervillous space of the definitive placenta or from the chorion laeve area, because very often the areas of detectable color and spectral Doppler signals were visible near the margins of the placenta. From our own experience, we do support this observation; however, there are also signals obtained from below the center of early placenta that are, by no means, signals belonging to the area of chorion laeve. One can speculate that these signals could be from the tips of spiral arteries in the decidua under the early placenta or chorion frondosum. It is our opinion, and it is in concordance with papers by Valentin *et al.*[27] and Merce *et al.*,[28] that the relatively high velocities of blood flow detected in these vessels or vascular spaces are not compatible with complete occlusion by trophoblastic plugs unless there are arteriovenous shunts in the decidual portion of the choriodecidual junction. Their existence in the myometrium is still controversial. Hustin *et al.*[12] found some evidence while Laurini has not (personal communication). Hustin *et al.*[36] postulate that myometrial arteriovenous shunts exist and are functional, serving to limit considerably the entry of maternal blood in the intervillous space. Even more, they postulate without further explanation that the pressure in the intervillous space is temporarily higher than at the uteroplacental artery level, and thus maintains the intravascular trophoblastic plugs in place. This statement can be an objective for further investigation.

Jauniaux speculated that the finding of focal intervillous flow in the first trimester was a sign of consecutive formation of echo-poor areas as an early sign of pregnancy complications.[37,38] If this is true, how could one explain the high rate of visualization of these signals in normal pregnancies reported by our group[30,39,40,41] (Table 96.1) and Malmo group.[27] It is hard to believe that all these pregnancies were destined to fail. According to Jauniaux *et al.*[31] continuous flow in the intervillous space during the first trimester is a highly pathologic event, causing the disruption of the maternoembryonic interface by high-pressure blood flow and consequent spontaneous abortion. In his opinion,[35] this fact is the most striking evidence in favor of Hustin's concept.[11] In fact, we also do believe that the high pressure of arterial blood can disrupt the maternoembryonic interface and cause spontaneous abortion. However, this fact is not opposite to the finding of a continuous intervillous flow during the first trimester of pregnancy. This means that there are some areas where trophoblastic plugs in spiral arteries are loosened allowing the intervillous circulation of blood. In the beginning, there are only a few areas of such a flow giving enough oxygen and nutrients for the progression of pregnancy. At this stage, the intervillous space is not undisrupted like in the mature placenta. There are parts with active continuous intervillous flow and parts in which such a flow has not yet been established and nutrients and oxygen diffuse through the intercellular fluid.[42] The number of areas with the established intervillous flow is increasing with embryonic and placental growth in order to keep a state of metabolic balance. This process ends with a fully formed intervillous space under the mature placenta. Such a hypothesis can be in concordance with findings of lower oxygen levels in the placental tissue than in the endometrium between 8 and 10 weeks of pregnancy.[13] Also, it can be in concordance with the fact that in cases of inappropriate trophoblastic plugging of spiral arteries the uncontrolled pressure of arterial blood can mechanically disrupt the maternoembryonic interface.[43–52]

Mercé *et al.*[53] recently reported that the abnormal Doppler patterns, such as the increase of retrochorial vascular resistance and the presence of intervillous flow in pregnancies with gestational sac measuring less than 12 mm, has a greater incidence of miscarriage. However, intervillous flow was also detectable in pregnancies with normal outcome but in a smaller proportion than in those ending with miscarriage (11% vs. 53%). This finding confirms that intervillous circulation does exist throughout early pregnancy, but at the same time limitation of the amount and pressure of incoming maternal blood seems to be of essential importance for normal pregnancy development.

There are numerous data provided by histological and color Doppler studies proving that the intervillous circulation begins early in normal pregnancy, which is in accordance with classical embryological theories. This is possible because the trophoblastic invasion is a progressive process and although some of the spiral arteries are totally occluded, the majority of them are opened or only partially occluded. In this way, the inflow of the blood in the intervillous space is controlled and increased progressively during the first trimester. These changes are complementary to the progressive loss of the endovascular trophoblast and coherently explain the increase in blood flow within the vascular territory of the uteroplacental arteries, a universal finding in all Doppler studies, and are very difficult to explain if these arterial lumens are plugged up with the trophoblast. It is probable that changes occurring in the trophoblast in spontaneous abortions can alter the blood perfusion in both the uteroplacental arteries and intervillous space. However, the importance of these findings in the genesis or in the mechanism of miscarriage has not yet been sufficiently documented.

Furthermore, recent ultrasound technology in terms of three-dimensional (3D) power Doppler angiography offers numerous advantages in the evaluation of intervillous space (Figure 96.7), which have to be clinically tested in future.

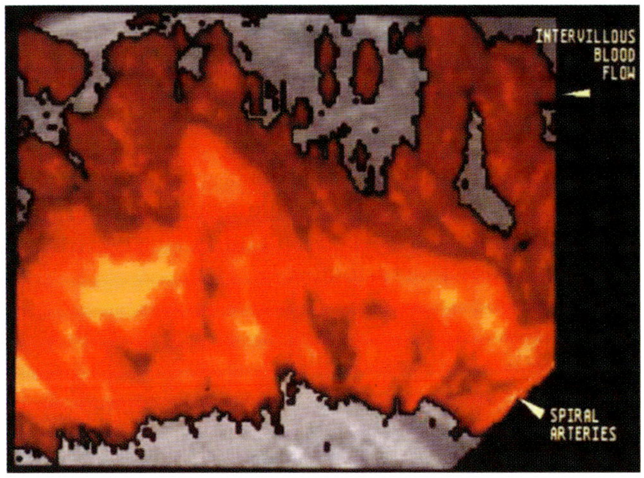

Figure 96.7 Demonstration of the intervillous circulation by three-dimensional power Doppler.

Yolk sac development

The embryonic vascular system includes the heart, the blood and the lymphatic vessels. It is the first functional organ system in the body that pumps blood through the embryonic and extraembryonic vessels to provide nutrition for rapid growth and removal of the waste products.[54] The circulatory system of an embryo is much larger when compared to the body size, and plays an important role during the early embryonic development.

Development of the vascular system begins in the mesoderm of the yolk sac close to the endoderm, at about 17 days after fertilization.[54] It is believed that there are some endodermally produced factors that stimulate the mesoderm to differentiate in this way. The first evident form of the vascular system are aggregations of the cells called blood islands. The central cells will differentiate into red blood cells and the outer cells into flattened endothelial layer. These elements of vascular system are perceptible as red spots in the mesoderm of the yolk sac wall. The blood islands fuse to form primitive vascular networks.

Precursors of the heart and the major paired blood vessels are formed in the mesoderm of intraembryonic coelom. The course of events is analogous with those occurring in the mesoderm of the yolk sac. A very similar process of creating a vascular system occurs in the chorionic mesoderm. Blood vessels formed in this way are dorsal aortae, cardinal veins and the major umbilical arteries and veins.

At first, blood washes back and forth in this primitive network of blood vessels, but eventually it takes on a patterned flow. It seems that these dynamic fluid effects are very important because they stimulate primitive blood vessels to differentiate further and take their own definitive form. If there is an obstruction to the blood flow, it bypasses the blocked vessel and passes through the surrounding small vessels. In time, one of these vessels will become a major blood vessel and will overtake the role of the blocked one. This sometimes vitally needed ability survives in the adult and leads to anastomoses.

Vitelline blood vessels

The heart begins to beat at about 21 days after fertilization. It pumps blood dorsally through blood vessels called branchial arches.[54] Blood enters the dorsal aortae (paired at this stage) from which the precursors of the internal carotid artery separate and run forward to supply the head. The main direction of blood in the dorsal aortae is toward the tail. It runs through the intersegmental arteries, which are branches of dorsal aortae, and are situated between the developing somites. Furthermore, at the level of the gut, there is an arterial complex of branches separating from dorsal aortae and running toward the site of blood formation in the yolk sac wall. In time, this arterial complex of branches will represent vitelline arteries.

Toward the tail dorsal aortae a plexus is formed from which one single blood vessel branches off and runs into the connecting stalk to the chorionic wall, where the placenta is developing. This single blood vessel is the umbilical artery.

Blood returns from the placenta through the paired umbilical veins, which also pick up blood from the yolk sac. The connection between the yolk sac vascular network and the umbilical veins is a venous complex of branches, which will become vitelline veins. The head veins, which lie just lateral to the neural tube, pick up blood from the head region. Finally, blood enters the sinus venosus and reaches the heart. This is the moment when the circle of the blood circulation around the embryonal body is closed.

The vitelline and umbilical veins have a very important role in further embryonal development. Initially, the liver bud lies between the vitelline veins. Since it enlarges, it comes to incorporate the vitelline and umbilical veins. These blood vessels form a common plexus of sinusoid vessel running through the liver. In time, the vitelline veins and left umbilical vein are converted into the hepatic portal vein. The right umbilical vein decreases in size and forms the ductus venosus, which carries blood to the right side of the heart.[54]

Hematopoiesis in human embryos begins in the yolk sac at about the middle of the third week of embryogenesis. Later, it appears in the liver and bone marrow in the fourth and fifth weeks and the eighth week, respectively.[55,56] At about the 10th to 12th week, hematopoietic tissues are found distributed evenly in the bone marrow throughout the body.[56–58] Maturation of blood cells is considered to take place extravascularly. With occasional exceptions, the blood cells in the endodermal layers are the most immature and maturation appears to proceed as the cells migrate to the mesenchymal layers and further into the blood vessels.

Color Doppler studies of the yolk sac and vitelline duct

Circulation in normal pregnancy

Little is known about a transitory subject such as the yolk sac, an organ that is active only during the first few weeks of embryonic life. The description of the formation of the human yolk sac has proven surprisingly controversial over the years.

Recently, interesting results have been published on the assessment of yolk sac vascularization in normal pregnancy. Kurjak *et al.*[21] performed transvaginal color Doppler study on 105 patients whose gestational age ranged from 6 to 10 weeks from the last menstrual period. Transvaginal color and pulsed Doppler examination was performed before the termination of pregnancy for psychosocial reasons.

The first color and pulsed signals from the yolk sac were obtained between 5 and 6 weeks of gestation. The visualization rate of the yolk sac vessels in the sixth week of gestation was 33.33%, and it increased to a value of 85.71% during the seventh and eighth weeks of gestation. As the functional activity of the yolk sac progressively declined, the visualization rate of 78.26% for 9 weeks' gestation and 61.11% for 10 weeks' gestation paralleled this process (Table 96.2). The overall visualization rate for yolk sac vessels was 72.38%. The highest visualization rates were obtained in the seventh and eighth weeks of gestation, reaching the value of 85.71%. A characteristic waveform profile included low velocity (5.8 ± 1.7 cm/s) and absence of diastolic flow (Figures 96.8 and 96.9). The PI showed a mean value of 3.24 ± 0.94 without significant changes between subgroups ($P > 0.05$). The distribution of mean PI values for yolk sac vascularity is shown in Table 96.2.

Vitelline stalk vessels (Figure 96.10) showed similar PSV (5.4 ± 1.8 cm/s) and PI values (3.14 ± 0.91) ($P > 0.05$) to those obtained from the yolk sac (Figures 96.8 and 96.9). The distribution of the vitelline artery PI values is demonstrated in Table 96.3. The overall visualization rate for vitelline arteries was 66.67%. Color and pulsed Doppler signals could be obtained from the vitelline duct during the seventh week of gestation in 85.71% of patients. The peak of visualization (89.28%) occurred during the eighth week of gestation (Table 96.3). The process of elongation of the vitelline duct together with the removal of the yolk sac from the body wall is paralleled with the decreased rate of vitelline duct visualization during the ninth (73.91%) and tenth (55.55%) weeks of gestation. Furthermore, progressive decrease of the yolk sac

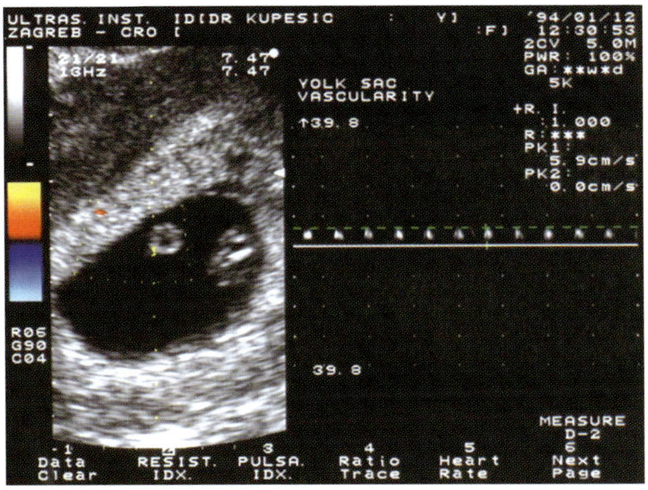

Figure 96.8 A transvaginal sonogram of a gestational sac at the sixth week of gestation. Note regular contours of the yolk sac. Pulsed Doppler signals obtained from the wall of the yolk sac demonstrate low velocity and absence of diastole (RI = 1.0).

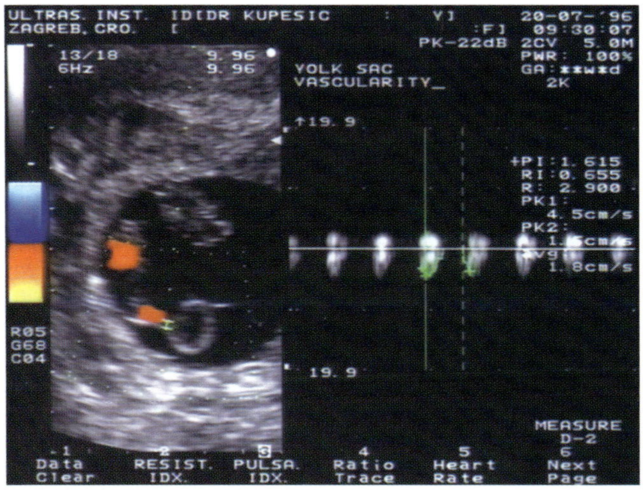

Figure 96.9 A color image of the yolk sac at 7 weeks' gestation. Pulsed Doppler signals isolated from the connection of the yolk sac and vitelline duct show absence of diastolic flow.

Table 96.2 Visualization rate of yolk sac vascularity between 6 and 10 weeks of gestation (from Kurjak *et al.*,[21] with permission)

Gestational age (weeks)	*N*	Visualization rate No.	%	PI ± SD
6	15	5	33.33	3.42 ± 0.58
7	21	18	85.71	3.14 ± 0.82
8	28	24	85.71	3.10 ± 0.94
9	23	18	78.26	3.12 ± 0.85
10	18	11	61.11	3.45 ± 0.72
Total	105	76	72.38	3.24 ± 0.94

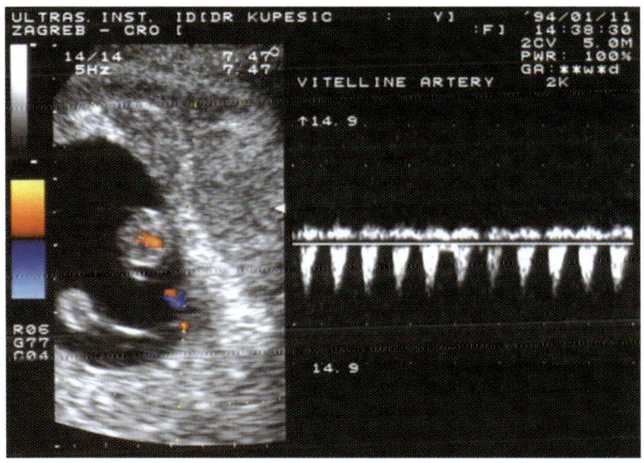

Figure 96.10 Color Doppler signals are easily obtainable from the vitelline stalk.

vascularity at the end of the first trimester coincides with the visualization of more prominent blood flow within the intervillous space.[59]

All these findings will surely help in better understanding the early development of both blood cells and blood vessels.

Vascularization of the yolk sac in abnormal pregnancies

Kurjak *et al.*[21,59] recently performed a research analyzing the vascularization of yolk sac in abnormal pregnancies. The authors analyzed 48 patients with missed abortion between 6 and 12 weeks of gestation. Yolk sac blood flow was detected in 18.54% of missed abortions. They obtained three types of abnormal vascular signals from the yolk sac in these patients: irregular

Table 96.3 Visualization rate of the vitelline duct vascularity between 6 and 10 weeks' gestation (from Kurjak *et al.*,[21] with permission)

Gestational age (weeks)	N	Visualization rate No.	%	PI ± SD
6	15	—	—	—
7	21	18	85.71	3.02 ± 0.92
8	28	25	89.28	3.05 ± 0.89
9	23	17	73.91	3.08 ± 0.91
10	18	10	55.55	3.38 ± 0.82
Total	105	70	66.67	3.14 ± 0.92

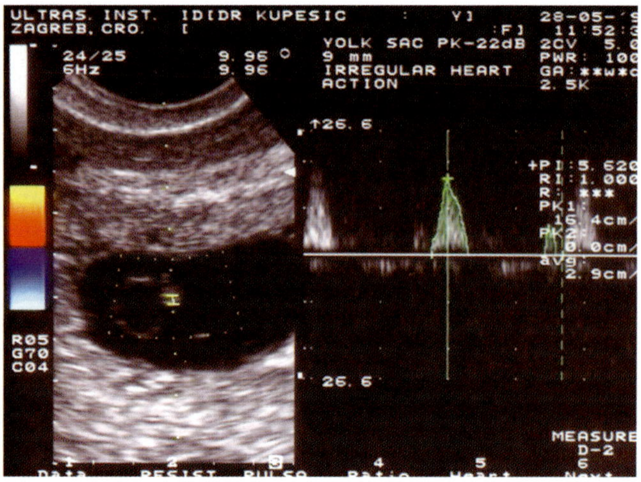

Figure 96.11 Pulsed Doppler signals derived from the yolk sac in a patient with missed abortion. Note larger diameter (7 mm) of the yolk sac and irregular blood flow signals at its periphery.

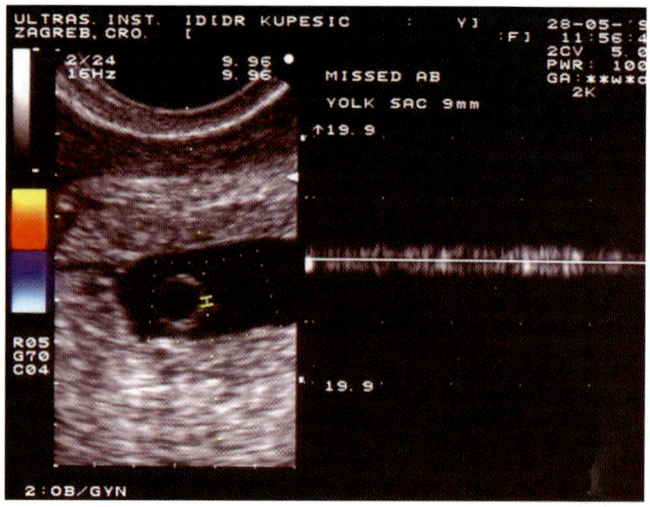

Figure 96.13 Venous blood flow signals obtained from the yolk sac at 8 weeks' gestation in a patient with missed abortion.

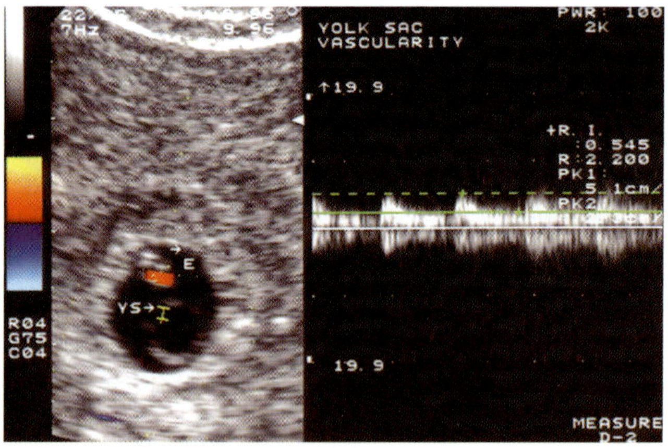

Figure 96.12 The transvaginal scan of a 9 weeks' gestation, complicated by bleeding. The pulsed Doppler waveform analysis indicates continuous blood flow. A few days after examination was completed spontaneous abortion occurred.

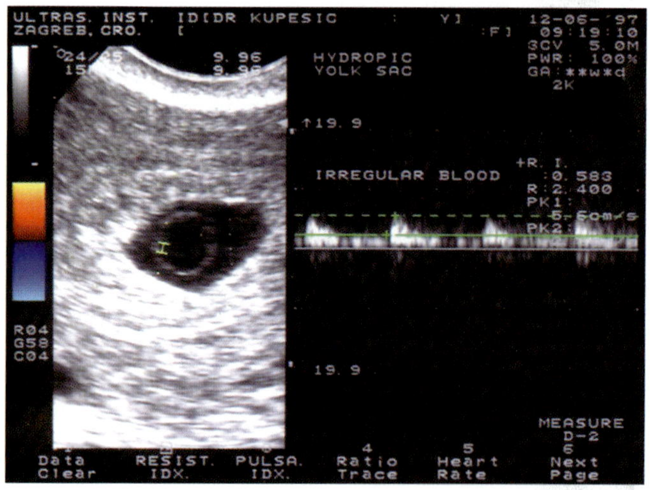

Figure 96.14 A transvaginal sonogram of a hydropic yolk sac at 6 weeks' pregnancy. Continuous diastolic flow is easily obtained from the hydropic yolk sac (RI = 0.58). Patient aborted in 1 week and karyotyping of the residual products of conception revealed trisomy 21.

blood flow (Figure 96.11), permanent diastolic flow (Figure 12) and venous blood flow signals (Figures 96.13 and 96.14).

Changes in vascularization of the yolk sac noticed in missed abortions in this study are probably a consequence of embryonic death and reabsorption of the embryo through the vitelline duct. Abnormal patterns of the yolk sac vascularity can be related to decreased vitelline blood flow, which may cause progressive accumulation of nutritive secretions not utilized by the embryo. This process ends with enlargement of the yolk sac indicative of an early pregnancy failure. Indeed, we were able to detect yolk sac vascularity in 28.57% (6/21) of missed abortions with large diameter of the yolk sac (Figure 96.14), and 20.00% (3/15) of those with normal yolk sac diameter. Sometimes, a careful ultrasonographer can visualize double yolk sac (Figure 96.15) and color Doppler ultrasound may observe abnormal Doppler patterns in these cases.

Cases with echogenic yolk sac walls ($N=7$) were characterized by the absence of blood flow. Yolk sac calcification was reported to result from the typical dystrophic changes that occur in non-viable cellular material.[60] Since studies in lower animals demonstrated that yolk sac endoderm bounds calcium, one can postulate that a derangement in the calcium transport mechanism may lead to accumulation of calcium in the yolk sac cells in humans as well. Therefore, recognition of a calcified yolk sac without blood flow signals suggests long-standing demise in the first trimester, which directs the clinician to further diagnostic workup (Figures 96.16 and 96.17).

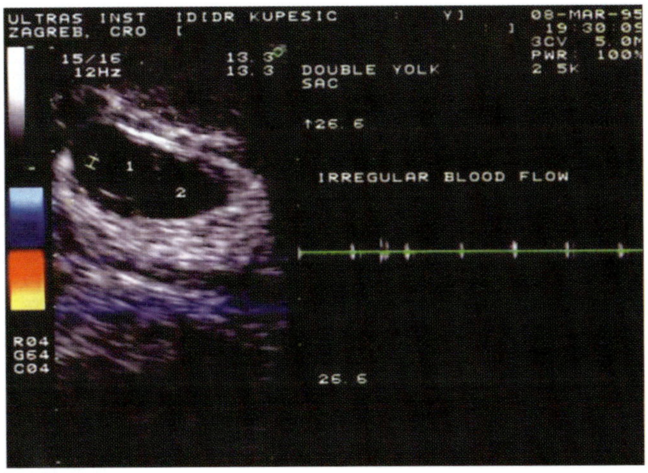

Figure 96.15 A transvaginal color Doppler scan of a gestational sac containing a double yolk sac with irregular blood flow signals.

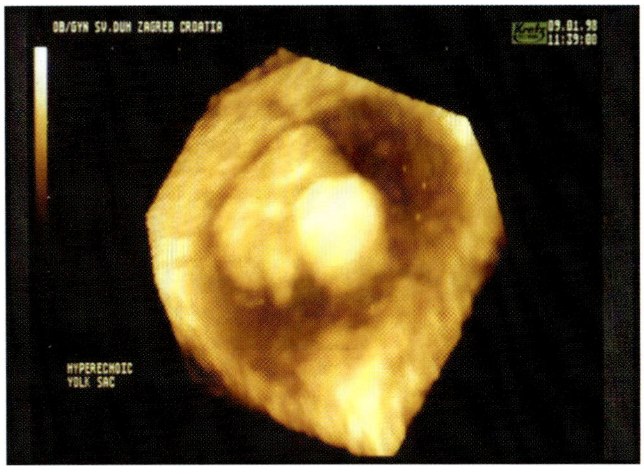

Figure 96.17 Three-dimensional scan of the hyperechogenic yolk sac.

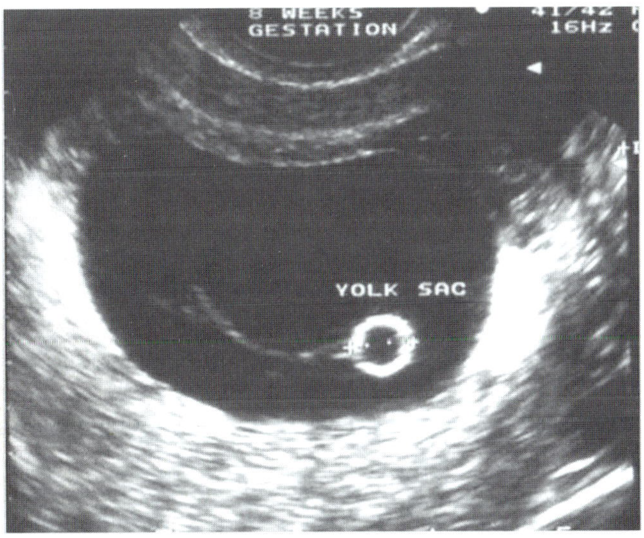

Figure 96.16 Transvaginal two-dimensional image of the hyperechogenic yolk sac.

These data indicate that there is an interaction between the yolk sac vascularity and intervillous circulation in patients with missed abortion. In patients with long-standing demise, vascular signals could not have been extracted from the hyperechoic walls of the yolk sac. Parallel assessment of the intervillous circulation in this subgroup ($N=7$) demonstrated numerous color-coded areas within the intervillous space indicating low mesenchymal turgor and progressive disruption of the maternoembryonic interface. Therefore, the changes in the intervillous circulation noticed in some missed abortions are rather the consequence of embryonic death and inadequate drainage than the primary cause of early pregnancy failure. This is contrary to the statement of Jaffe *et al.*[61] and Jauniaux *et al.*[62] who found that increased continuous intervillous flow during the first trimester of pregnancy is associated with adverse pregnancy outcome. According to their results, increased flow pressure in the spiral arteries may dislocate the thin trophoblastic shell causing the loss of villi to forceful arterial flow, which may result in miscarriage.[63] However, independent Doppler studies from three institutions using sensitive conventional and power Doppler velocimetry found that continuous and pulsatile blood flow can be extracted from intervillous space in both normal pregnancies and those with adverse outcome.[17–21,28,64]

Data presented in this study support the concept that establishment of the intervillous circulation is a progressive process during the first trimester of pregnancy. Between the sixth and tenth weeks of gestation, relatively slow blood flow in the intervillous space is detected. Simultaneously, clear blood flow signals are derived from the walls of the yolk sac supporting the hypothesis that this fragile structure is responsible for optimal delivery of nutrients and oxygen to the developing embryo up to 10 weeks of gestation. Progressive decrease of the yolk sac vascularity coincides with visualization of more prominent color-coded areas within the intervillous space demonstrating the increased metabolic needs of the developing pregnancy.

Volume of the yolk sac – correlation with blood flow studies

It is well known that the prognostic significance of the yolk sac diameter as determined by ultrasound is not clearly established. Most of the abnormal pregnancies were demonstrated to have normal yolk sac measurements,[65–67] while only a minority of abnormal early pregnancies presented either 'too small' or 'too big' yolk sac dimensions.[68,69]

Recently, we performed a study on 80 women with uncomplicated singleton pregnancy (between 5 and 12 weeks of gestation).[70] The volumes of the

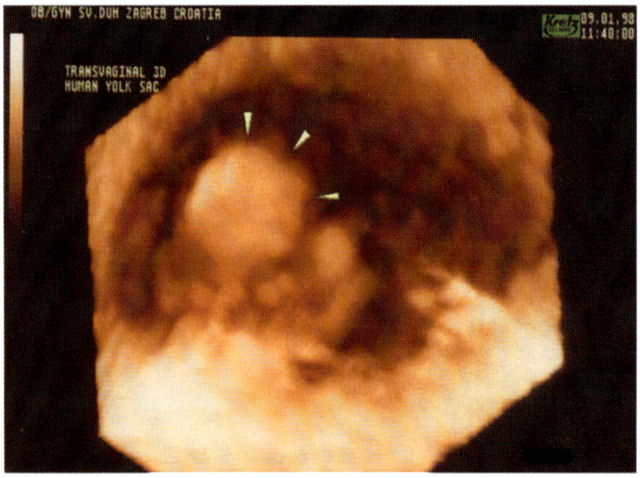

Figure 96.18 Three-dimensional scan of the yolk sac at 8 weeks' gestation. Note the regular echogenicity and contours of the yolk sac.

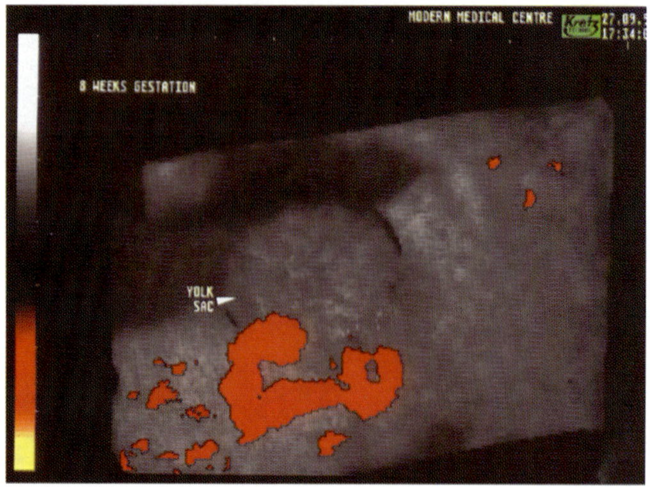

Figure 96.19 Three-dimensional power Doppler demonstrates turgescent blood vessels above the surface of the yolk sac.

gestational and yolk sacs were measured by 3D ultrasound (Voluson 530, Kretztechnik, Austria). Regression analysis revealed exponential growth of the gestational sac volume. The yolk sac volume was found to increase gradually from 5 to 10 weeks of gestation. However, when the yolk sac reaches its maximum size and volume at around 10 weeks, it has already started to degenerate (Figure 96.18), which can be proved by a significant reduction in visualization rates of the yolk sac vascularity (Figure 19). This suggests that the evaluation of the biological function of the yolk sac by measuring the diameter and/or the volume is limited. Therefore, the combination of functional and volumetric studies is necessary to point out some of the important moments during the early pregnancy:[71]

(1) Simultaneous beginning of yolk sac angiogenesis and vascular development of the embryo
(2) Non-invasive evaluation of the functional capacity of the yolk sac
(3) Definition of the shift from embryo-vitelline to embryo-placental circulation[7]
(4) 3D ultrasound studies of the direct connection between the yolk sac and the embryonic gut
(5) Evaluation of the yolk sac degeneration and location by 3D ultrasound at the end of the first trimester

The fact that blood vessels first develop in the secondary yolk sac may be related to the important role of this structure in the process of early embryonic nutrition. Further Doppler studies analyzing large cohort of patients with both normal and abnormal pregnancies will probably answer some of the numerous questions on the role of yolk sac vascularity in early embryonic development. The introduction of 3D ultrasound coupled with power Doppler imaging has produced more accurate information on implantation and the yolk sac and we look forward to the future developments in this field.

REFERENCES

1. Ramsey EM. Circulation in the intervillous space of the primate placenta. *Am J Obstet Gynecol* 1962;84:1649–63.
2. Boyd JD, Hamilton WJ. *The Human Placenta*. Cambridge: Heffer & Sons, 1970.
3. Sadler TW. *Langman's Medical Embryology*, 7th edn. Baltimore, MD: Williams & Wilkins, 1995.
4. O'Rahilly R. *Developmental Stages in Human Embryos. Part A: Embryos of the First Three Weeks (Stages 1 to 9)*. Washington, DC: Carnegie Institute of Washington, 1973:631.
5. Gasser RF. *Atlas of Human Embryos*. New York: Harper & Row, 1975.
6. Khong TY, Pearce JM. Development and investigation of the placenta and its blood supply. In Lavery JP, ed. *The Human Placenta. Clinical Perspectives*. Rockville: Aspen Publishers, 1987:25–45.
7. Fox H. *Pathology of the Placenta*. London: W.B. Saunders, 1978.
8. Padykula HA. The human placenta. In Weiss L, ed. *Cell and Tissue Biology*, 6th edn. Baltimore: Urban/Schwarzenberg, 1983:901–27.
9. Bulmer JN, Johnson PM. Antigen expression by trophoblast populations in the human placenta and their possible immunobiological relevance. *Placenta* 1985;6:127–40.
10. Fox H. Current topic: Trophoblastic pathology. *Placenta* 1991; 12:479–86.
11. Hustin J, Shaaps JP. Echographic and anatomic studies of the maternotrophoblastic border during the first trimester of pregnancy. *Am J Obstet Gynecol* 1987;157:162–8.
12. Hustin J, Shaaps JP, Lambotte R. Anatomical studies of the uteroplacental vascularization in the first trimester of pregnancy. *Troph Res* 1988;3:49–60.
13. Rodesch F, Simon P, Donner C, Jauniaux E. Oxygen measurements in endometrial and trophoblastic tissues during early pregnancy. *Obstet Gynecol* 1992;80:283–5.
14. Kurjak A, Zalud I, Salihagic A, Crvenkovic G, Matijevic R. Transvaginal color Doppler in the assessment of abnormal early pregnancy. *J Perinat Med* 1991;19:155–65.
15. Kurjak A, Predanic M, Kupesic S, Zudenigo D, Matijevic R, Salihagic A. Transvaginal color Doppler in the study of early

normal pregnancies and pregnancies associated with uterine fibroids. *J Matern Fetal Invest* 1992;3:81–5.
16. Kurjak A, Kupesic S, Predanic M, Salihagic A. Transvaginal color Doppler assessment of the uteroplacental circulation in normal and abnormal early pregnancy. *Early Hum Dev* 1992;29:385–9.
17. Kurjak A, Predanic M, Kupesic S, Funduk-Kurjak B, Demarin V, Salihagic A. Transvaginal color Doppler study of middle cerebral artery blood flow in early normal and abnormal pregnancy. *Ultrasound Obstet Gynecol* 1992;2:424–8.
18. Kurjak A, Zudenigo D, Funduk-Kurjak B, Shalan H, Predanic M, Sosic A. Transvaginal color Doppler in the assessment of the uteroplacental circulation in normal early pregnancy. *J Perinat Med* 1993;21:25–34.
19. Kurjak A, Zudenigo D, Predanic M, Kupesic S. Recent advances in the Doppler study of early fetomaternal circulation. *J Perinat Med* 1994;22:419–39.
20. Kurjak A, Zudenigo D, Predanic M, Kupesic S, Funduk-Kurjak B. Transvaginal color Doppler study of fetomaternal circulation in threatened abortion. *Fetal Diagn Ther* 1994;9:341–7.
21. Kurjak A, Kupesic S, Kostovic LJ. Vascularization of yolk sac and vitelline duct in normal pregnancies studied by transvaginal color Doppler. *J Perinat Med* 1994;22:433–40.
22. Jauniaux E, Jurkovic D, Campbell S. In vivo investigations of anatomy and physiology of early human placental circulations. *Ultrasound Obstet Gynecol* 1991;1:435–45.
23. Jauniaux E, Jurkovic D, Campbell S, Hustin J. Doppler ultrasonographic features of the developing placental circulation: Correlation with anatomic findings. *Am J Obstet Gynecol* 1992; 166:585–7.
24. Jaffe R, Warsof SL. Transvaginal color Doppler imaging in the assessment of uteroplacental blood flow in the normal first-trimester pregnancy. *Am J Obstet Gynecol*, 1991;164, 781–5.
25. Kurjak A, Predanic M, Kupesic-Urek S. Transvaginal color Doppler in the assessment of placental blood flow. *Eur J Obstet Gynecol Reprod Biol* 1993;49:29–32.
26. Kurjak A, Laurini R, Kupesic S, Kos M, Latin V, Bulic K. A combined Doppler and morphopathological study of intervillous circulation. *Ultrasound Obstet Gynecol* 1995;6(Suppl 2):116.
27. Valentin L, Sladkevicius P, Laurini R, Sodeberg H, Marsal K. Uteroplacental and luteal circulation in normal first trimester pregnancies: Doppler ultrasonographic and morphologic study. *Am J Obstet Gynecol* 1996;174:768–75.
28. Mercé LT, Barco MJ, Bau S. Color Doppler sonographic assessment of placental circulation in the first trimester of normal pregnancy. *J Ultrasound Med* 1996;15:135–42.
29. Kurjak A, Kupesic S, Kos M, Latin V, Zudenigo D. Early hemodynamics studied by transvaginal color Doppler. *Prenat Neonat Med* 1996;1:38–49.
30. Kurjak A, Kupesic S. Doppler assessment of the intervillous blood flow in normal and abnormal early pregnancy. *Obstet Gynecol* 1997;89:252–6.
31. Jauniaux E, Zaidi J, Jurkovic D, Campbell S, Hustin J. Comparison of color Doppler features and pathohistological finding in complicated early pregnancy. *Hum Reprod* 1994;9: 2432–7.
32. Ramsey EM, Chez RA, Doppman JL. Radioangiographic measurement of the internal diameters of the uteroplacental arteries in rhesus monkeys and man. *Contrib Embryol Carnegie Inst Wash* 1979;38:59–70.
33. Nimrod C, Simpson N, De Vermette R, Fournier J. Placental and early fetal haemodynamics: The suitability of the monkey model (abstract). *XII International Congress on The Fetus as a Patient*, Grado, Italy, May 23–25, 1996:68.
34. Nimrod C, Simpson N, Hafner T, *et al.* Assessment of early placental development in the cynomolgus monkey (*Macaca fascicularis*) using colour and pulsed wave Doppler sonography. *J Med Primatol* 1996;25:106–11.
35. Jauniaux E. Intervillous circulation in the first trimester: The phantom of the color Doppler obstetric opera (editorial). *Ultrasound Obstet Gynecol* 1996;8:73–6.
36. Hustin J, Kadri R, Jauniaux E. Spontaneous and habitual abortion – A pathologists point of view. *Biol Med* 1996;2:85–9.
37. Jaffe R, Dorgan A, Abramowicz A. Color Doppler imaging of uteroplacental circulation in the first trimester: Value in predicting pregnancy failure or complication. *AJR Am J Roentgenol* 1995,164.1255–8.
38. Jauniaux E, Nicolaides KH. Placental lakes, absent umbilical artery diastolic flow and poor fetal growth in early pregnancy. *Ultrasound Obstet Gynecol* 1996;7:141–4.
39. Kurjak A, Kupesic S. Doppler proof of the presence of intervillous circulation (letter). *Ultrasound Obstet Gynecol* 1996; 7:463–4.
40. Kurjak A, Kupesic S, Hafner T, Kos M, Kostovic-Knezevic LJ, Grbesa B. Conflicting data on intervillous circulation in early pregnancy. *J Perinat Med* 1997;25:225–36.
41. Kurjak A, Dudenhausen JW, Hafner T, Kupesic S, Latin V, Kos M. Intervillous circulation in all three trimesters of normal pregnancy assessed by color Doppler. *J Perinat Med* 1997;25: 373–80.
42. Kurjak A, Kupesic S, Hafner T, Latin V, Kos M, Harris RD. Intervillous blood flow in patients with missed abortion. *Croat Med J* 1998;39:41–4.
43. Burchell RC. Arterial blood flow into the human intervillous space. *Am J Obstet Gynecol* 1967; 98;303–11.
44. Karimu AL, Burton GJ. Star volume estimates of the intervillous clefts in the human placenta: How changes in umbilical arterial pressure might influence the maternal placental circulation. *J Dev Physiol* 1993;19:137–42.
45. Salafia CM, Minor VK, Pezzullo JC, Popek EJ, Rosenkrantz TS, Vintzileos AM. Intrauterine growth restriction in infants of less than thirty two weeks gestation: Associated placental pathologic features. *Am J Obstet Gynecol* 1995;173:1049–57.
46. Jackson MR, Walsh AJ, Morrow RJ, Mullen JB, Lye SJ, Ritchie JW. Reduced placental villous tree elaboration in small-for-gestational-age pregnancies: Relationship with umbilical artery Doppler waveforms. *Am J Obstet Gynecol* 1995;172:518–25.
47. Arabin B, Jimenez E, Vogel M, Weitzel HK. Relationship of utero- and fetoplacental blood flow velocity waveforms with pathomorphological placental findings. *Fetal Diagn Ther* 1992;7: 173–9.
48. Harris JWS, Ramsey EM. The morphology of human uteroplacental vasculature. *Contrib Embryol* 1966;38:43–58.
49. Brosens I, Robertson WB, Dixon HG. The role of the spiral arteries in the pathogenesis of pre-eclampsia. *Obstet Gynecol Annu* 1972;1:177–91.
50. Khong TY, DeWolf F, Robertson WB, Brossens I. Inadequate maternal vascular response to placentation in pregnancies complicated by pre-eclampsia and small-for-gestational age infants. *Br J Obstet Gynaecol* 1986;93:1049–59.
51. Boyd PA, Scott A. Quantitative structural studies on human placentas associated with pre-eclampsia, essential hypertension and intrauterine growth retardation. *Br J Obstet Gynaecol* 1985; 92:714–21.
52. Fleischer A, Schulman H, Farmakides G, *et al.* Uterine artery Doppler velocimetry in pregnant women with hypertension. *Am J Obstet Gynecol* 1986;154:806–13.
53. Mercé LT, Barco MJ, Bau S. Color Doppler sonography of the retrochorionic and intervillous circulation: predictive value in small gestational sacs. *Med Imag Internat* 1997;7:16–9.
54. McLachlan J. The vascular system. In *Medical Embryology*. McLachlan J, ed. New York: Addison-Wesley Publishing Company, 1994:105–15.
55. Fukuda T. Fetal hemopoiesis – electronic microscopic studies on human yolk sac hemopoiesis. *Virchows Arch* 1973;14: 197–213.
56. Zamboni L. Electronic microscopic studies of human blood embryogenesis in human. II. The hemopoietic activity in the fetal liver. *J Ultrastruct Res* 1965;12:525–41.
57. Fukuda T. Fetal hemopoiesis. II. Electron microscopic studies on human hepatic hemopoiesis. *Virchow Arch* 1974;16:249–70.
58. Fukuda T. Ultrastructure of fetal hemopoiesis. *Acta Haematol Jpn* 1978;41:1204.
59. Kurjak A, Kupesic S. Parallel Doppler assessment of yolk sac and intervillous circulation in normal pregnancy and missed abortion. *Placenta* 1988;196:19–23.
60. Harris RD, Vincent LM, Askin FB. Yolk sac calcification: A sonographic finding associated with intrauterine embryonic demise in the first trimester. *Radiology* 1988;166:109–16.
61. Jaffe R, Warsof SL. Color Doppler imaging in the assessment of uteroplacental blood flow in abnormal first trimester intrauterine pregnancies: An attempt to define etiologic mechanisms. *J Ultrasound Med* 1992;11:41–4.
62. Jauniaux E, Zaidi J, Jurkovic D, Campbell S, Hustin J. Comparison of color Doppler features and pathologic findings in complicated early pregnancy. *Hum Reprod* 1994;9:2432–7.
63. Jaffe R, Jauniaux E, Hustin J. Maternal circulation in the first trimester human placenta – Myth or reality? *Am J Obstet Gynecol* 1997;176:695–705.

64. Valentin L, Sladkevicius P, Laurini R, Soderberg H, Marsal K. Uteroplacental and luteal circulation in normal first-trimester pregnancies: Doppler ultrasonographic and morphologic study. *Am J Obstet Gynecol* 1996;174:768–75.
65. Crooij MJ, Westhuis M, Schoemaker J, Exalto N. Ultrasonographic measurements of the yolk sac. *Br J Obstet Gynaecol* 1982;89:931–4.
66. Reece EA, Sciosca AL, Pinter E, *et al.* Prognostic significance of the human yolk sac assessed by ultrasonography. *Am J Obstet Gynecol* 1988;159:1191–4.
67. Goldstein SR, Kerenyi T, Scher J, Papp C. Correlation between karyotype and ultrasound findings in patients with failed early pregnancy. *Ultrasound Obstet Gynecol* 1996;8:314–17.
68. Jauniaux E, Jurkovic D, Henriet Y, Rodesch F, Hustin J. Development of the secondary human yolk sac. Correlation of sonographic and anatomical features. *Hum Reprod* 1991;6:1160–6.
69. Lindsay DJ, Lyons EA, Levi CS, Zheng XH. Endovaginal appearance of the yolk sac in early pregnancy: Normal growth and usefulness as a predictor of abnormal pregnancy outcome. *Radiology* 1992;83:115–22.
70. Kupesic S, Kurjak A. Volume and vascularity of the yolk sac studied by three-dimensional ultrasound and color Doppler. *J Perinat Med* 1999;27:91–6.
71. Kurjak A, Azumendi G, Solak M. Clinical application of four-dimensional sonography in perinatal medicine. In Kurjak A, Jackson D, eds. *An Atlas of Three- and Four Dimensional Sonography in Obstretrics and Gynecology.* Boca Raton: Taylor & Francis, 2004:127–46.

97 First-trimester ultrasound

N. Montenegro and A. Matias

Introduction

In obstetrics, ultrasound has been used for many years and, from the beginning, investigators have been interested in changes in the uterus and its contents in early pregnancy.[1]

Moreover, in recent years, the introduction of higher-resolution equipment and transvaginal endosonography has brought new possibilities for the study of early gestational events.[2–4]

Nowadays, ultrasound is increasingly used in early pregnancy, either as a routine procedure or selectively for specific clinical indications. Routine ultrasonography during the first trimester is used for accurate pregnancy dating, early diagnosis of major malformations, characterization of multiple pregnancy and screening of chromosomal anomalies.[5–18]

Although the quality of images obtained during the first trimester seems to be superior when using the transvaginal approach, transabdominal ultrasonography is still widely used in this period of gestation for cultural and practical reasons.[19,20]

The use of diagnostic ultrasound during pregnancy is considered to be safe for both the mother and the fetus. Even in critical periods of development and using high-frequency transvaginal transducers, no adverse bioeffects have been demonstrated.[21–23] The benefits to patients exposed to the ultrasound intensities used at present outweigh the risks, if any.

This chapter will review the main applications of ultrasound examination during early pregnancy, relying on the experience of the authors together with that reported in the literature. Special emphasis will be placed on embryonic development during the first weeks, gestational age determination, characterization of multiple pregnancy and screening and diagnosis of fetal anomalies. In the text, gestational age will be expressed as complete weeks from last menses.

Embryonic development: ultrasound findings

The decidual thickening (Figure 97.1) is the first indirect sign of pregnancy that can be disclosed by ultrasound.[24,25] Although it is seen more often in the early phases of an intrauterine pregnancy, this hyperechogenic mantle filling the uterine cavity can also coexist with an ectopic pregnancy. As the same pattern can be found in the late luteal-phase endometrium, it should be considered as a non-specific sign.

A few days after the expected menses, a typical image of a hyperechogenic ring inside the uterine cavity can be identified by transvaginal ultrasound (Figure 97.2). This corresponds to the gestational sac, the echogenic ring being the chorionic villi surrounding the chorionic cavity. At this time, the mean level of the β-subunit of human chorionic gonadotropin (β-hCG) is found to be about 500 mIU/ml (second reference standard).[26] Thereby, the diagnosis of intrauterine pregnancy can be confirmed and a chorionic sac internal diameter of 2–6 mm will be found, corresponding to a menstrual age of 4 weeks.

During the fifth week, the chorionic sac measures 7–10 mm. When this diameter reaches 9 mm, the yolk sac can always be identified as a round, fluid-filled and eccentric structure with a diameter of 3 mm (Figure 97.3). In the authors' experience, this 9- to 10-mm diameter of the chorionic sac represents an early discriminatory value for the diagnosis of a blighted ovum. At some time during the end of the fifth week, pulsations can be visualized on real-time imaging, close to the wall of the yolk sac and within a 2- to 3-mm echogenic line corresponding to the embryo. After this time, the heart rate can be measured using simultaneous M-mode.

At 6 weeks, the echogenic line corresponding to the developing embryo is always close to the yolk sac and measures 4–6 mm (Figure 97.4). Cardiac motion can be clearly seen and the mean heart rate (Figure 97.5) at this gestational week is about 118 bpm.[26] The amnion is not yet clearly seen, so the embryo and the yolk sac are apparently free-floating in the chorionic cavity, although eccentrically fixed by the connecting body stalk.

During the seventh week, the embryonic length is 7–12 mm and the yolk sac, with a diameter of 5 mm, separates from the embryo, probably owing to the growth of the vitelline duct (Figure 97.6). At this time, the cephalic pole becomes distinguishable and an apparent single hypoechoic cavity can be seen, corresponding to a part of the primitive cerebral ventricle

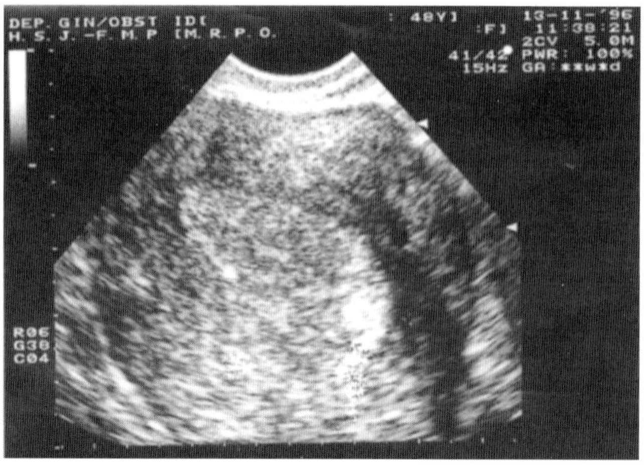

Figure 97.1 Decidual thickening.

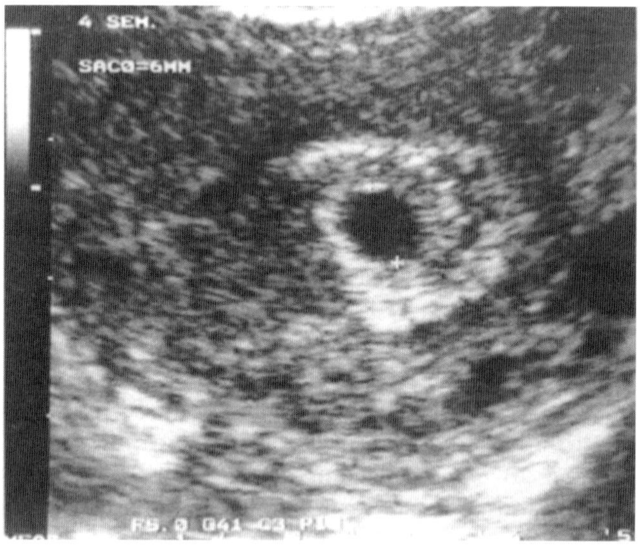

Figure 97.2 Chorionic sac at 4 weeks (last menses).

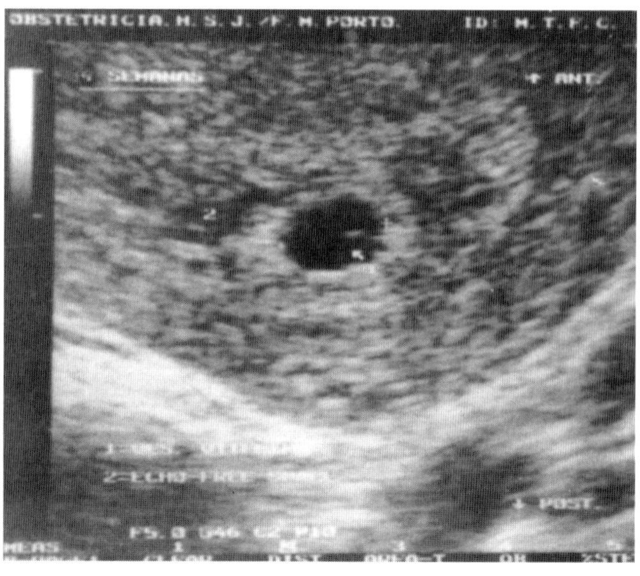

Figure 97.3 Chorionic sac with yolk sac visible at 5 weeks (two echo-free space).

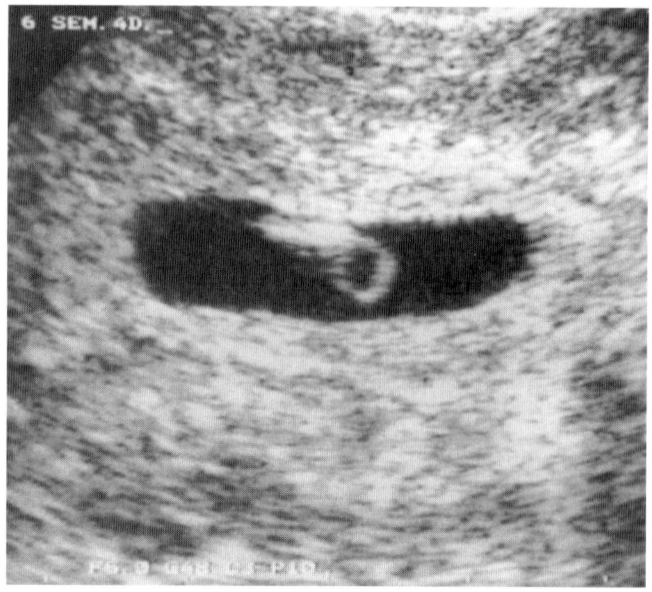

Figure 97.4 Chorionic sac at 6 weeks: echogenic line representing the embryo (+ +) and yolk sac can be identified.

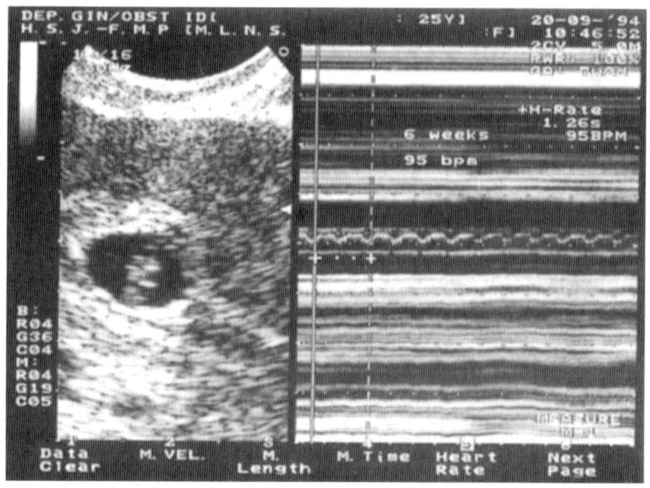

Figure 97.5 Embryonic heart rate measurement at 6 weeks (M-mode).

in the rhombencephalic area, probably the future fourth ventricle.[20–24]

At 8 weeks (Figure 97.7), the embryonic length is 12–18 mm and the upper and lower limb buds are now visible. The folding of the hypoechoic cerebral vesicle limits the lateral recesses of the rhombencephalic cavity.[27–30] The placental site can even be identified, following the umbilical cord from the abdominal wall of the embryo. Discrete undulating body movements can be sporadically seen on real-time imaging at the end of the eighth week.

During the ninth week, the embryo assumes a typical C-shaped curvature (Figure 97.8) and the crown–rump length (CRL) will be more than 2 cm (21–31 mm).[31] As landmarks, the head represents

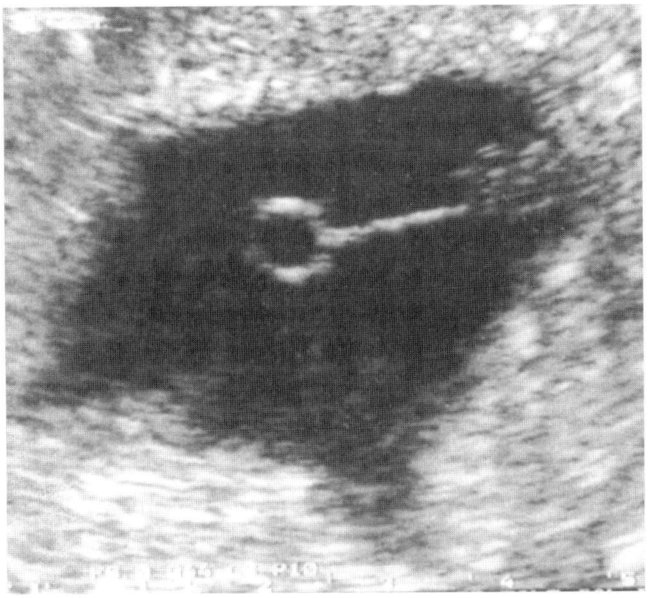

Figure 97.6 Vitelline duct and yolk sac at 7 weeks.

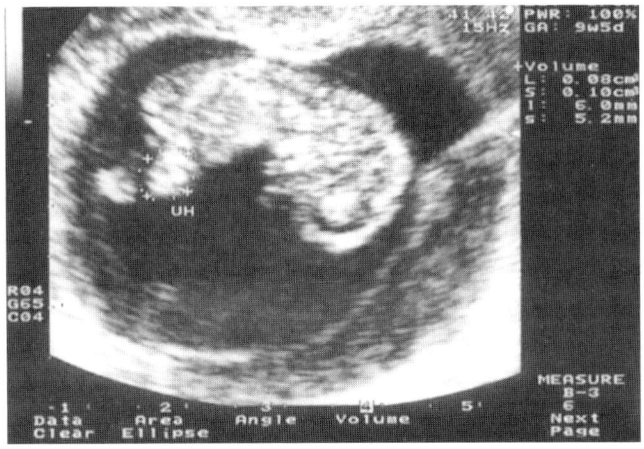

Figure 97.8 A 9-week embryo with typical C-shaped curvature and physiological umbilical hernia (UH).

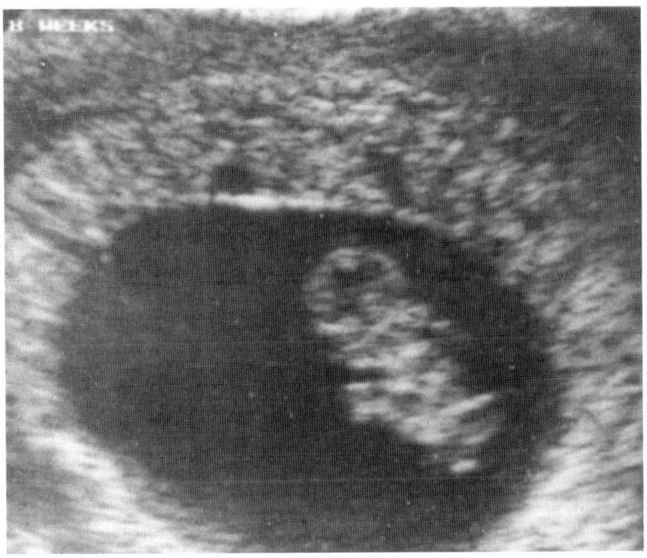

Figure 97.7 An 8-week embryo with the upper and lower limb buds visible: note, in cephalic pole, folding of ventricular cavity.

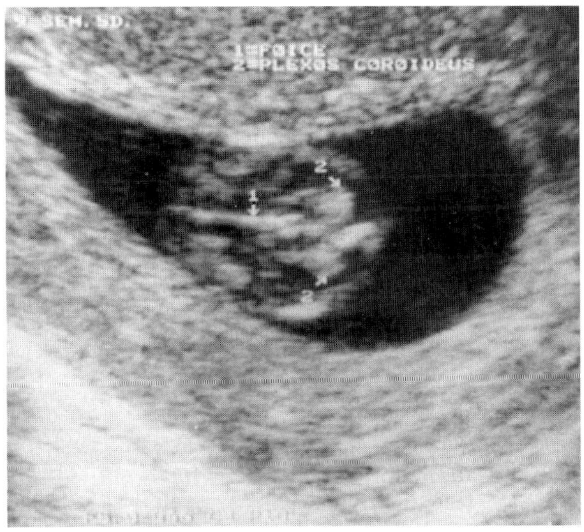

Figure 97.9 Choroid plexuses in a 9-week embryo.

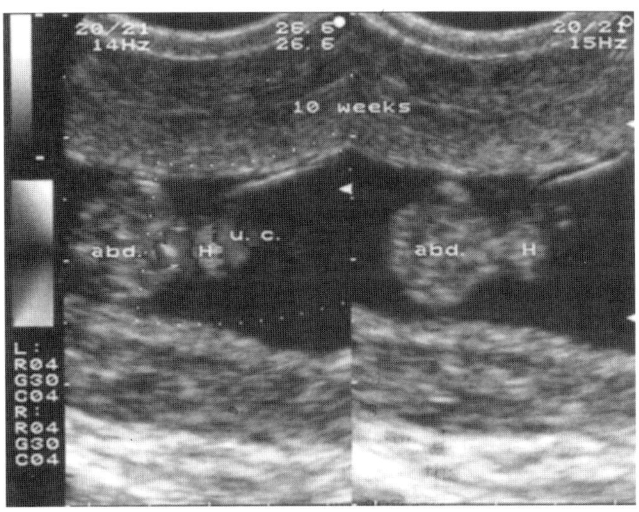

Figure 97.10 Physiological midgut herniation at 10 weeks (abd, abdomen; H, hernia; UC, umbilical cord).

one-third of the entire body and, inside the head, the hyperechoic falx and choroid plexuses and a hypoechoic heart-shaped structure corresponding to the cerebral peduncles are visible (Figure 97.9). The physiological midgut herniation, which can be identified close to the anterior abdominal wall, will persist until the end of the 11th week (Figure 97.10). Body movements are now more frequently seen.

Between 8 and 10 weeks, the amnion surrounding the embryo is always clearly seen, the yolk sac being outside in the exocelomic/chorionic cavity (Figure 97.11).[26,32]

At 10 weeks' gestation (Carnegie stages 20–23), the CRL is 32–41 mm and the embryo is slightly more

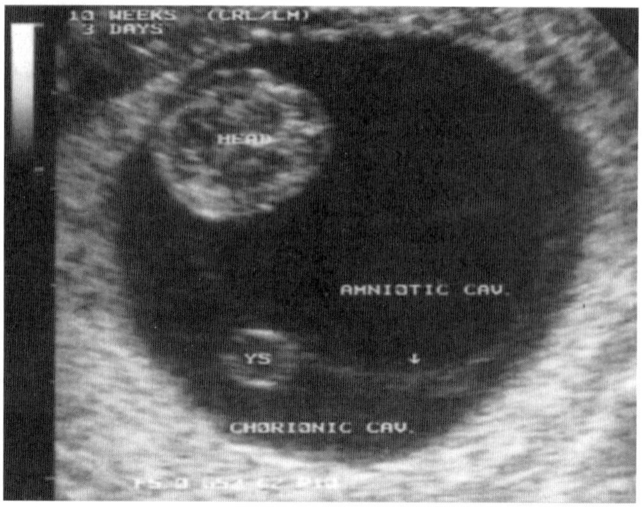

Figure 97.11 Amnion surrounding embryo: note yolk sac outside amniotic cavity.

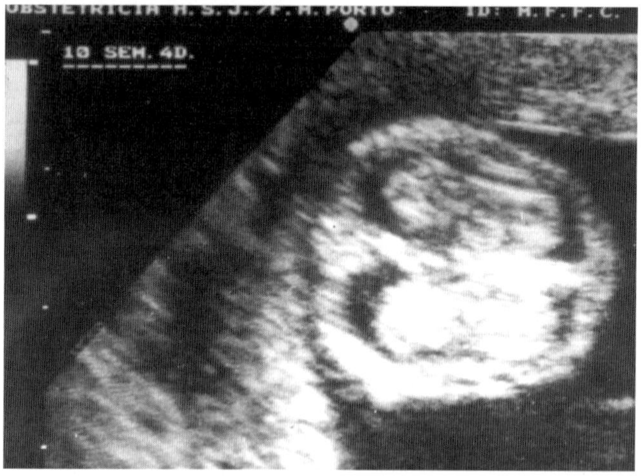

Figure 97.12 Lateral ventricles and choroid plexuses in a 10-week embryo.

curved. The choroid plexuses fill the lateral ventricles completely, and are the most prominent structures in the cephalic pole (Figure 97.12). In the posterior fossa, the cisterna magna and cerebellum can be identified, though the development process of the posterior fossa will only be concluded by 16 weeks (Figure 97.13).

In the trunk, the cardiac valvular apparatus can sometimes be distinguished inside the heart by the end of the 10th week, although more accurately from the 11th week onward. Also at the end of the 10th week, the stomach filled with a small amount of liquid, can sometimes be identified in the abdomen (Figure 97.14).

The three segments of the upper and lower limbs are clearly identified with both hands and feet in the midline. The first trimester of pregnancy is the best period to assess the number of fingers as normally the hands are wide open. Abduction of the lower limbs with lateral rotation of the hips is typically encountered between 10 and 13 weeks (Figure 97.15).

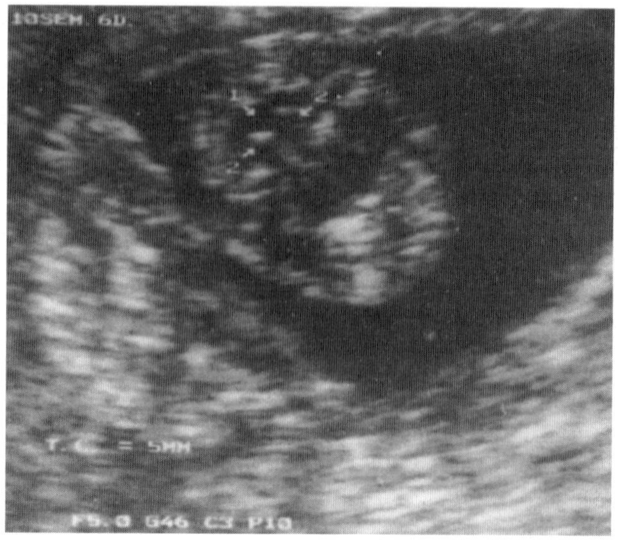

Figure 97.13 Cisterna magna (1) and cerebellum (2) in a 10-week embryo.

Body and even isolated limb movements are often identified on real-time imaging.

At 11 weeks, the fetus (no longer the embryo) acquires a human appearance and the CRL will be greater than 42 mm, reaching 76 mm at 13 weeks. From now on, a more detailed anatomical survey can be obtained, including the cerebral and cardiovascular systems and the digestive and urinary tracts.[33] The midgut is no longer herniated and can be seen as a hyperechoic round image inside the celomic cavity and situated in the median region of the lower abdomen (Figure 97.16).

Between 11 and 14 weeks of gestation, that is, between 45 and 84 mm CRL, a subcutaneous translucency behind the neck region can be disclosed in a sagittal section of the fetus. The maximum thickness between the skin and the soft tissue overlying the cervical spine can be measured, and was called nuchal translucency (NT).[13] Initially the normal values have been reported as less than 3 mm. After the prospective study of 100,000 pregnancies by Snijders and coworkers, increased NT has been defined as the value higher than the 95th centile for gestational age.[34] Increased NT has been found in association with major chromosomal anomalies and cardiac defects, and has been proposed, together with maternal age, as an efficacious screening procedure during the first trimester of pregnancy.[34]

More recently, the first reports on the use of three-dimensional ultrasound in the first trimester of pregnancy suggest its potential for early-pregnancy anatomic survey.[35]

Gestational age determination

Gestational age assignment is one of the most important issues in perinatal medicine for both clinical and research purposes. In addition to an indication of

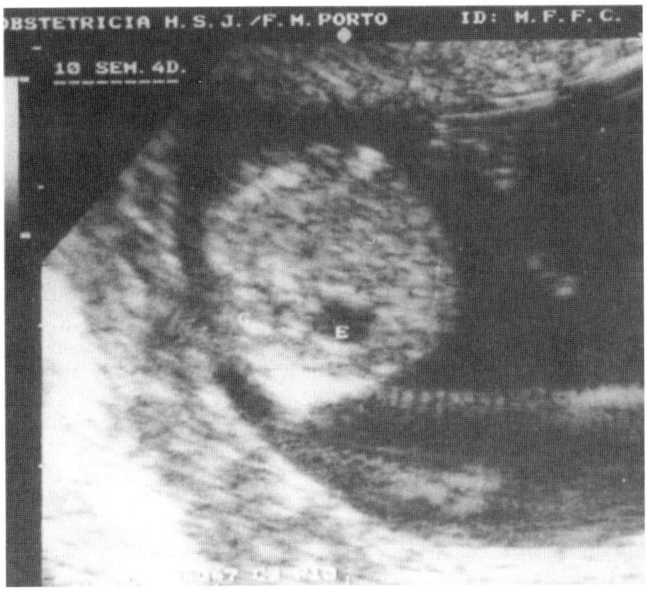

Figure 97.14 Stomach (E) in a 10-week embryo.

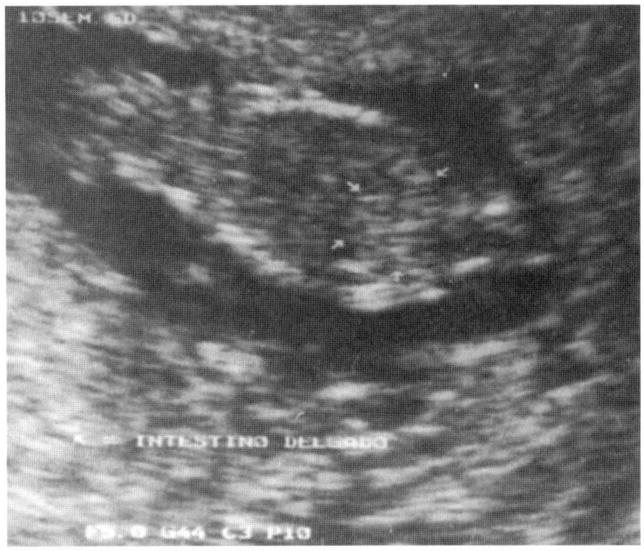

Figure 97.16 Coronal view of lower abdomen showing a hyperechoic image compatible with the gut completely inside the tummy.

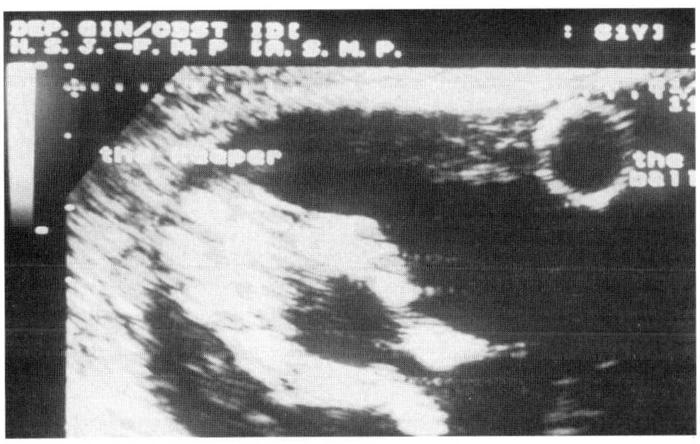

Figure 97.15 Upper and lower limbs at 11 weeks. Note the abduction of lower limbs.

medical problems, it could result in serious personal and social implications for the parents.

Even today, worldwide, the last menstrual period (LMP) is still the basis for calculation of gestational age and expected day of confinement. Nevertheless, in clinical practice, health professionals are frequently confronted by difficulties concerning the exact estimation of the LMP, incorrect reporting, cycle irregularities and the recent use of oral contraceptives. It has been estimated that about one-third of women attending antenatal care fall into one of these categories.[11]

Even in the population of women with certain dates and regular cycles, reliable biological correspondence between LMP and ovulation or fertilization is still difficult to obtain. In addition to long-available information about this phenomenon, recent studies in this field provide the confirmation that conception can occur within a 6-day period from intercourse ending at the day of ovulation.[36]

In very early pregnancies, gestational age determination by ultrasound scan is a little inaccurate, and is based on chorionic sac mean or maximum diameters. At the beginning of the fourth week, the diameter is 2–3 mm, reaching 9–10 mm when the yolk sac can be identified.[25] Once the embryo is visible, embryonic length should be measured.

As reported by Goldstein, before 10 weeks' gestation, it is really the embryonic length rather than the CRL that is being measured.[31] On the other hand, operator errors are more frequent below than above 10 weeks.[37]

A large number of reference tables for CRL measurements are available, all showing identical mean values to those originally reported in the literature, despite variations in ultrasound machines, ethnic groups and methodological aspects[31,38–42] (Figure 97.17). However, in a trisomy-18 fetus or in a fetus with triploidy, the CRL is smaller than normal, while in other major chromosomal anomalies, the CRL is not significantly different from normal.[43]

Furthermore, several studies have been reported dealing with the validity and benefits of routine ultrasound examination in the first half of pregnancy, having reduced perinatal morbidity and mortality as end points.[44,45] One of the major goals was improving the determination of gestational age. The ultrasonographic measurement of CRL before 13 weeks' or the biparietal and transverse cerebellar diameters between 14 and 22 weeks' gestation, respectively, have been widely used for this since the beginning of the 1970s.[37–50]

When comparing the accuracy of menstrual dates and ultrasonography in the first half of pregnancy, for calculating the expected date of delivery, dating by ultrasonographic biometry was more predictive than the former or even the combination of both

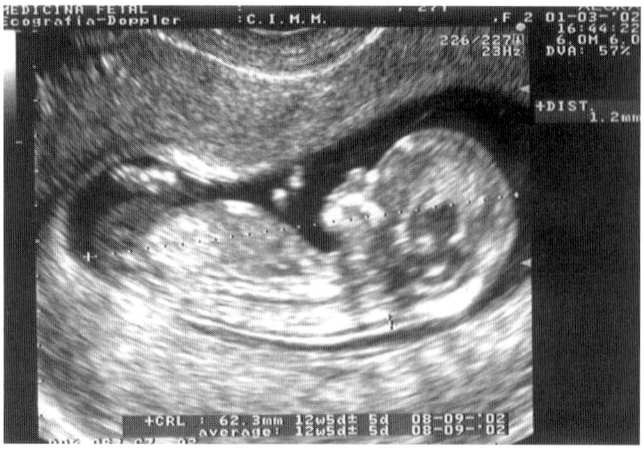

Figure 97.17 Crown–rump length, the gold standard for dating pregnancy.

methods.[12–46] Therefore, even with known menstrual dates, most authors would rather use ultrasound biometry, namely, measurement of the CRL and biparietal diameter (BPD), than the LMP for estimation of gestational age or expected date of confinement.

Clinical and ethical considerations support the medical value of routine ultrasonography in the first half of pregnancy as a standard of obstetric care.[49] If there is a tendency toward an ideal policy in such a field, some of the above-quoted reasons point to the late first trimester as the best gestational age period for a routine ultrasound examination.

Multiple pregnancy

Today, mainly as a result of the expanded use of assisted reproductive methods, multiple pregnancy is more frequently found in antenatal clinics all over the world. In the United States over the past 20 years, births of twins have increased at twice the rate, and multiple births of triplets or more have increased sevenfold faster than births of singletons.[51]

Meanwhile, higher perinatal morbidity and mortality in such pregnancies can be reduced by accurate pregnancy dating, by avoiding unnecessary prolongation of gestation and from determination of chorionicity.[52,53] It is chorionicity rather than zygosity that determines several aspects of antenatal management and perinatal outcome. Antepartum death of one twin is three times more frequent in monochorionic than in dichorionic gestation.[54]

Today, management protocols in multiple pregnancies include successful intrauterine treatments and single invasive diagnostic tests for monozygotic twins, and multifetal reduction in higher-order gestations.[55–58]

Antenatal determination of chorionicity by ultrasound is much easier in the early first trimester when two or more separate gestational sacs and embryos are identified (Figure 97.18). It is also accurate to perform an ultrasound scan between 10 and 14 weeks, relying on

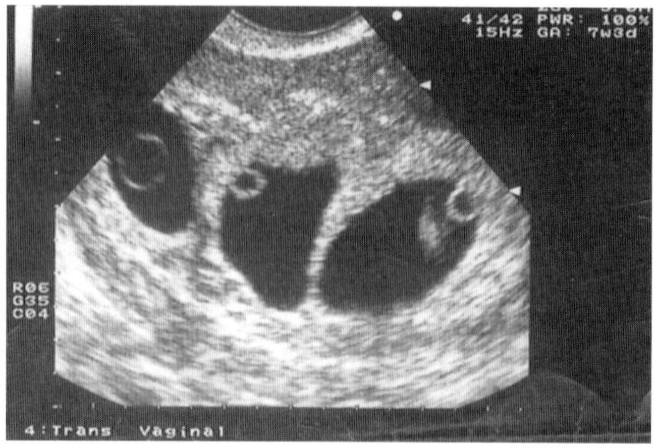

Figure 97.18 Triple pregnancy at 7 weeks' gestation.

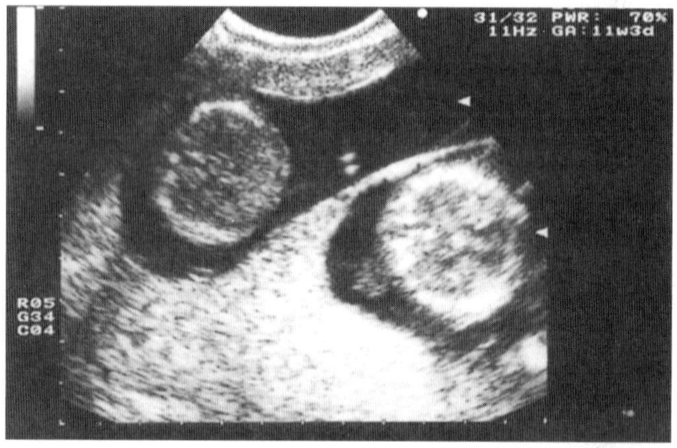

Figure 97.19 Dichorionic diamniotic twin pregnancy with clear lambda sign.

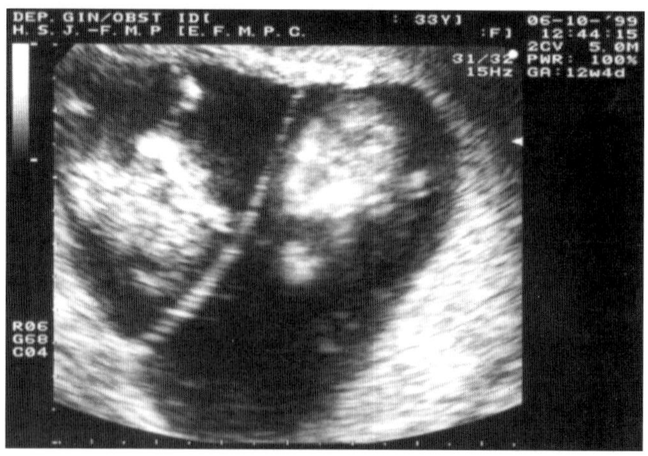

Figure 97.20 Monochorionic diamniotic twin pregnancy with the T-sign.

the demonstration of the lambda sign (Figure 97.19)[47] for dichorionic (with a positive predictive value of 100% for dichorionicity) or the T-sign (Figure 97.20) for monochorionic twin pregnancies. In the second or third trimesters of pregnancy, dividing membranes can be seen (Figure 97.21).[53] Other criteria such as

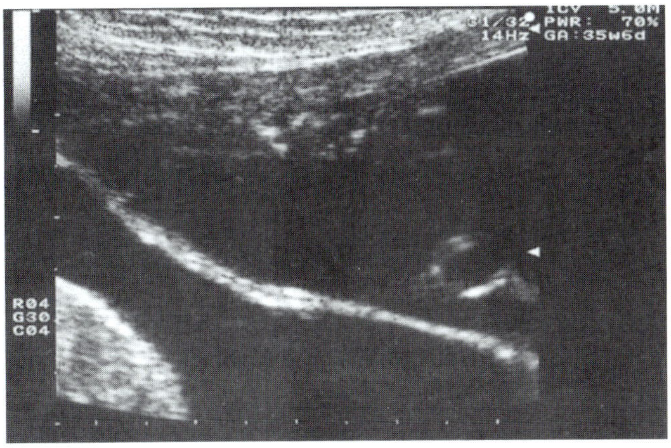

Figure 97.21 Dividing membrane in a 35-week dichorionic twin pregnancy.

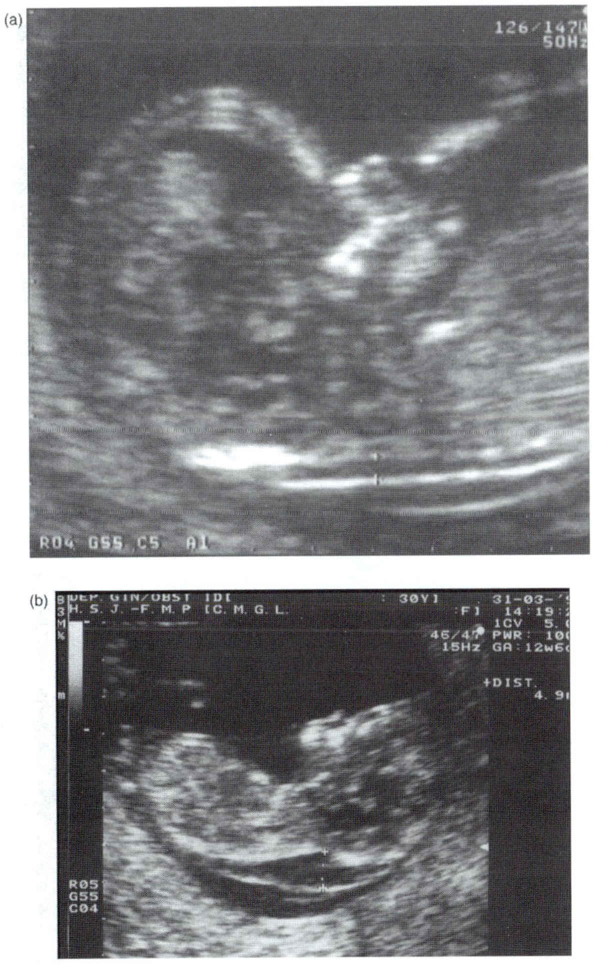

Figure 97.22 (a) Sagittal plane of a 12-week fetus showing the adequate plane for measuring nuchal translucency. (b) Increased nuchal translucency (NT=4 mm) in a 12-week fetus with Down's syndrome.

number of placentas and fetal gender are unreliable, as fused placentas and identical sex are often found in dichorionic twins.

For all these reasons, it seems relevant to advise a routine ultrasound scan at 10–14 weeks' gestation. An earlier examination, although eventually more reliable for the determination of chorionicity, will be

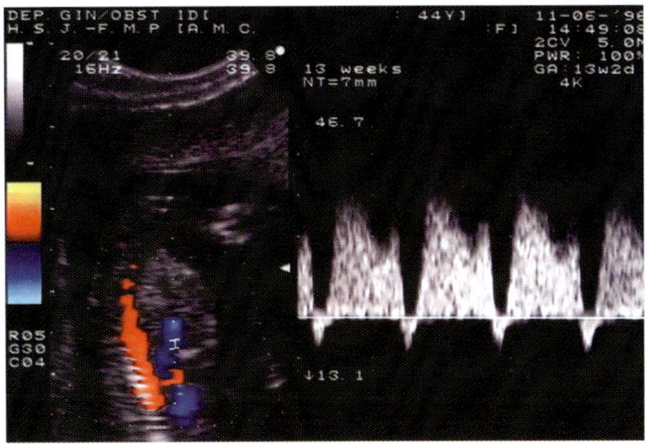

Figure 97.23 Abnormal ductus venosus blood flow in a 12-week fetus with trisomy 21.

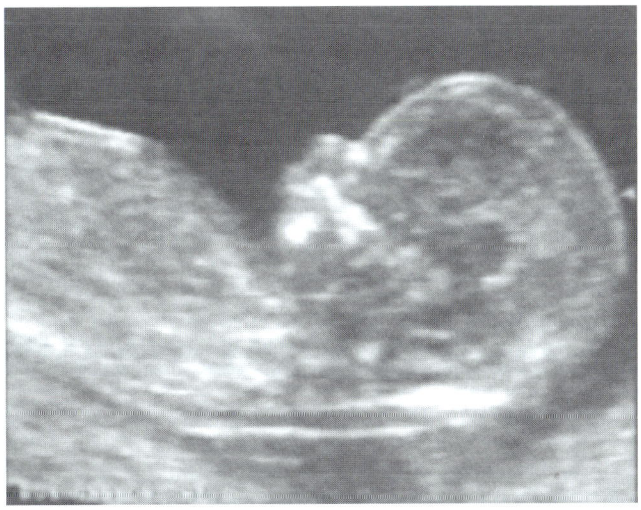

Figure 97.24 Ultrasound image of nasal bones in a 12-week fetus with normal karyotype.

less accurate for pregnancy dating.[38] Furthermore, at 10–14 weeks, it will encompass the common event of the vanishing twin, either in spontaneous or in *in vitro* fertilization pregnancies.[58]

Fetal anomalies: screening and diagnosis

The ultrasonographic fetal examination in the late first trimester is useful for both screening and diagnostic purposes.

Concerning chromosomal defects, NT thickness determination between 11 and 14 weeks' gestation was the first marker to be incorporated in first-trimester routine ultrasound examination as a screening procedure.[13,34] Increased NT has been found in association with major chromosomal defects (Figure 97.22b), namely trisomies 13, 18 and 21, Turner syndrome and triploidy as with cardiac defects, other malformations and genetic syndromes.[59,60]

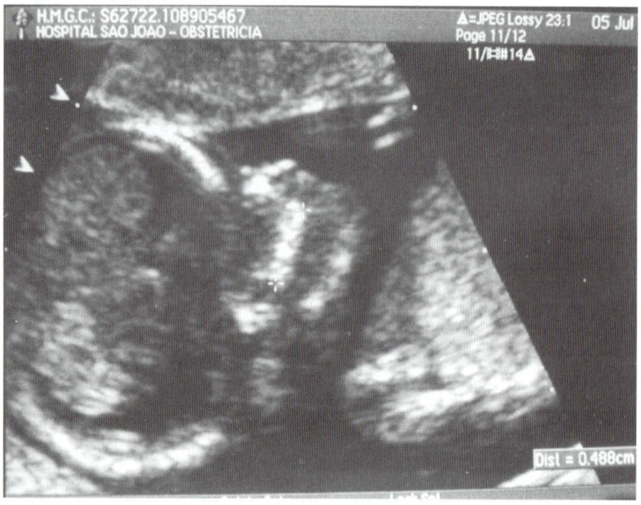

Figure 97.25 Ultrasound image of a 12-week fetus demonstrating the measurement of the maxillary bone measurement in a normal fetus.

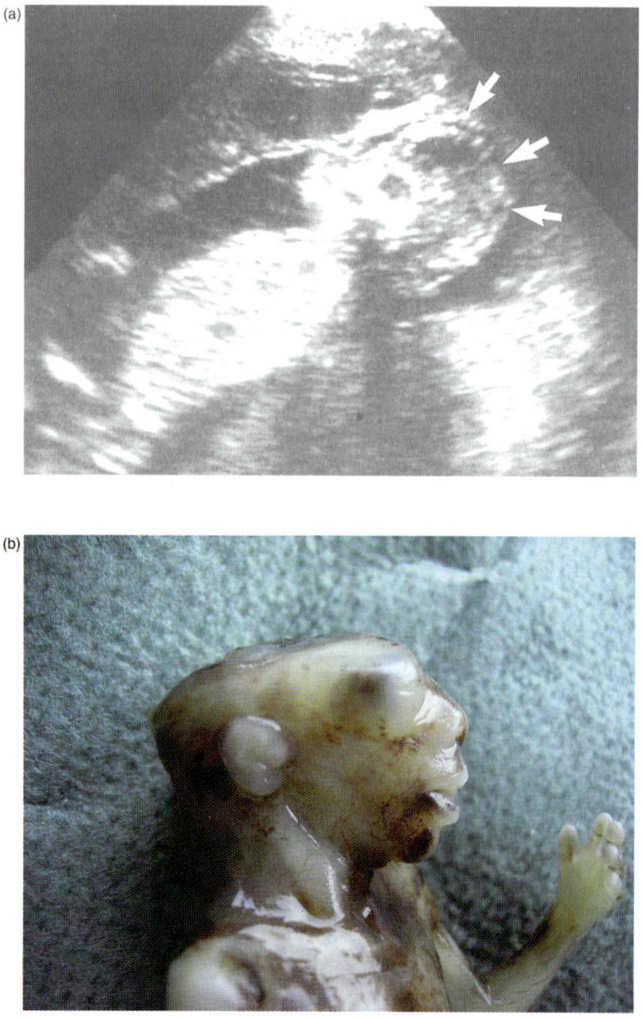

Figure 97.26 (a) Ultrasound image of an exencephaly/acrania detected at 13 weeks of gestation, showing the the absence of cranial bones. (b) Necropsic specimen of the same fetus after termination of pregnancy, confirming the prenatal diagnosis.

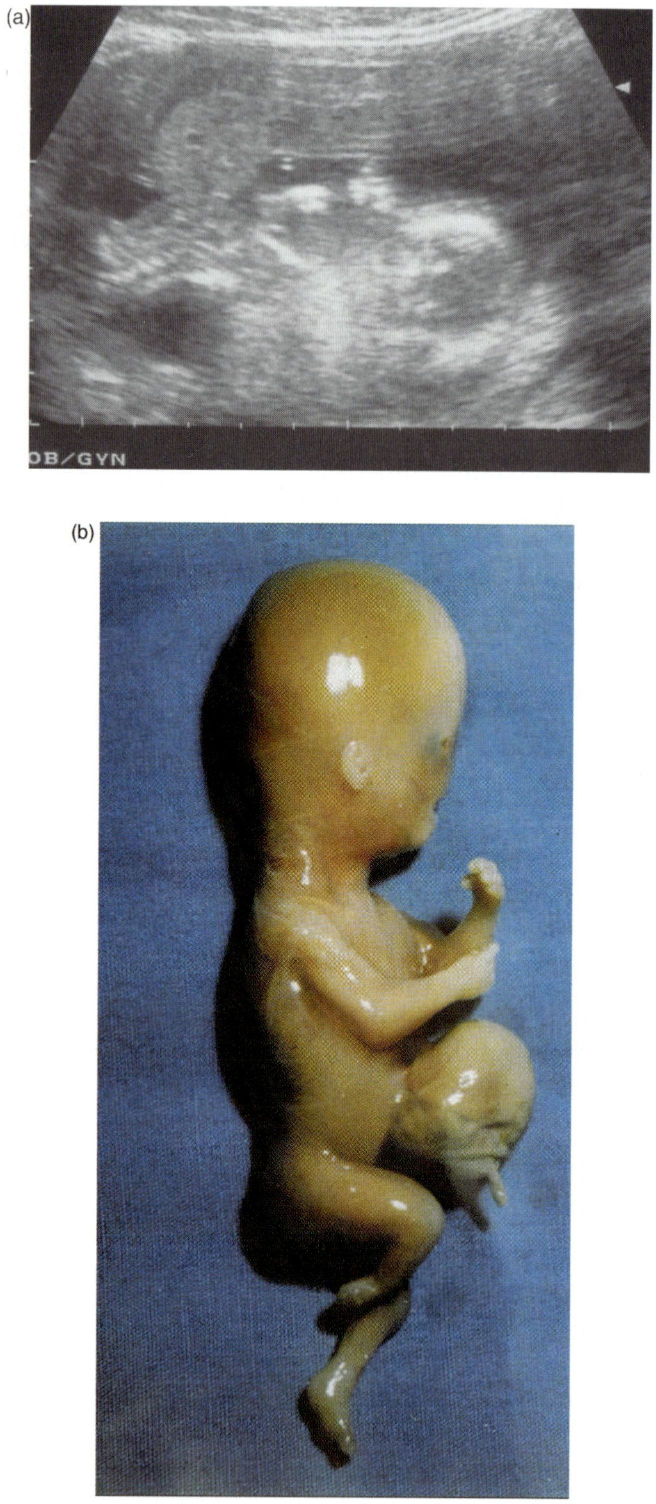

Figure 97.27 (a) Ultrasound image of an omphalocele detected at 12 weeks of gestation, showing the outbulging liver and a pronounced lordosis. (b) Necropsic specimen of the same fetus after termination of pregnancy, confirming the prenatal diagnosis.

If increased NT is combined with maternal age and factors concerning trisomy 21, the detection rate for chromosomal anomalies will be 80% with a false-positive rate of 5%. When fetal heart rate or maternal serum-free β-hCG and pregnancy-associated plasma

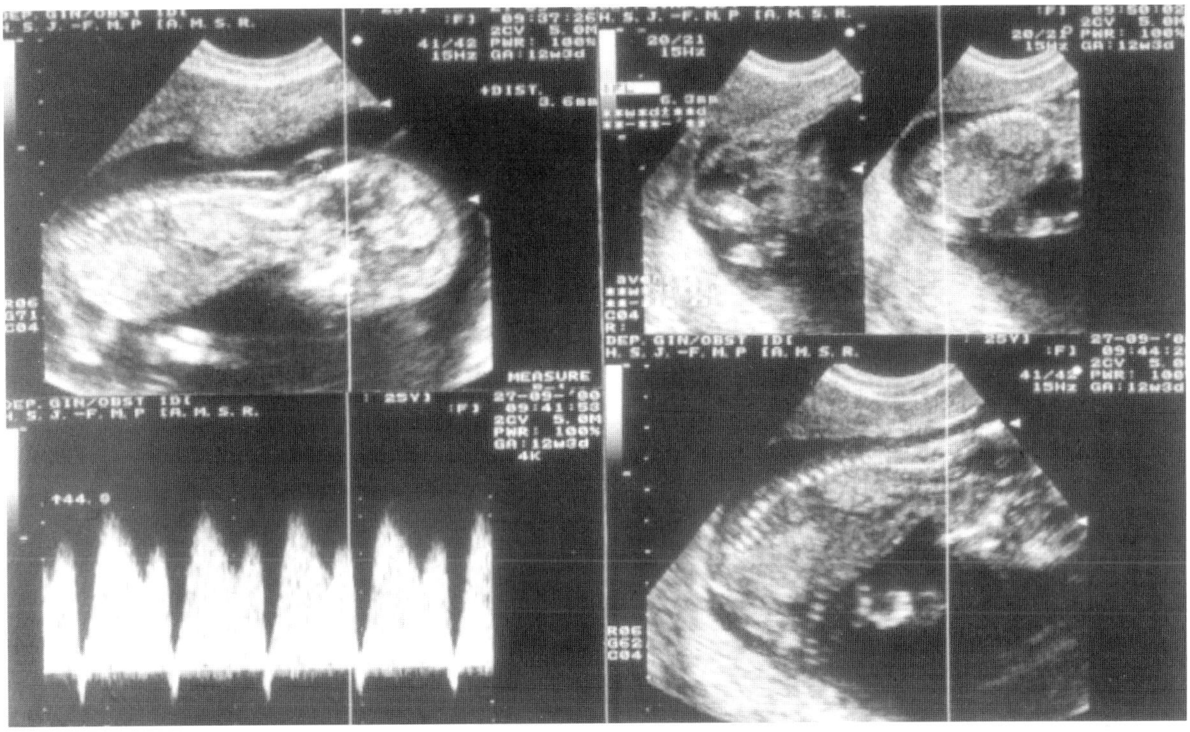

Figure 97.28 Sonographic aspects of a osteochondrodysplasia diagnosed at 12 weeks of gestation, showing short limbs, increased nuchal translucency and abnormal flow in the ductus venosus.

protein A (OSCAR clinic) are also incorporated at 11–14 weeks, detection rates will be 83 and 90%, respectively.[61,62]

The pathogenic basis of increased NT is still obscure, in spite of published work reporting an association of such an increase with cardiac defects/dysfunction.[63–66] Investigational work from our group clearly demonstrated abnormal ductus venosus (DV) blood flow in the majority of fetuses with increased NT and abnormal karyotype[15] and/or cardiac defects.[16] The combination of maternal age, NT and DV evaluation yielded a similar detection rate of NT alone, but decreased significantly the invasive testing rate.[15]

Still emphasizing the importance of ultrasound screening in the first trimester, when we adopt the same sagittal plane used for NT, other sonographic markers can be obtained and have recently been proposed to improve the detection rate for trisomy 21: ductus blood flow evaluation[15,16,63–69] (Figure 97.23), fetal nasal bones[17] (Figure 97.24) and maxillary bone length[18] (Figure 97.25). Preliminary data suggest that combining sonographic and biochemical markers in the first trimester of pregnancy could result in a detection rate of 97% for a false-positive rate of 5%, or a detection of 95% for a false-positive rate of 2%.[62]

Detailed assessment of fetal anatomy in the late first trimester is possible using either transabdominal or higher-resolution transvaginal sonography.[27,70] Therefore, potentially, the antenatal diagnosis of the majority of structural anomalies in this period of gestation can be carried out. Good examples of first-trimester diagnosis of major malformations are exencephaly/acrania (Figure 97.26), omphalocele (Figure 97.27) and osteochondrodysplasia (Figure 97.28).

After the first report of an early ultrasonic diagnosis of anencephaly in the 1970s,[71] many case reports have been published in the literature.

Following the 'natural history of fetal anomalies', the IRONFAN registry has been able to demonstrate how early anomalies can be diagnosed, in particular those that are potentially lethal, such as those occurring in the central nervous and cardiovascular systems, urinary tract and abdominal wall.[72] To date, more than 2000 anomalies, diagnosed between 9 and 15 weeks' of gestation, have been reported.

We consider that the policy of routine ultrasound examination in the second trimester will be reviewed within the next few years, once most, if not all, the lethal defects are able to be diagnosed and managed earlier in pregnancy. Furthermore, late first-trimester scan has other advantages, already discussed above, as a more accurate method of gestational age determination and for sufficiently early characterization of multiple pregnancy.

Conclusions

During recent years, interest in first-trimester pregnancy has been reinforced by the achievement of detailed imaging of early human intrauterine life using high-resolution ultrasound equipment, namely, transvaginal ultrasonography.

It is now possible to look at intrauterine events from the beginning of pregnancy, close to the time of implantation.

Acquired experience of first-trimester ultrasound examination either as a routine procedure or complementary to clinical evaluation demonstrates its essential role in obstetrical care.

Accurate gestational age determination, sufficiently early characterization of multiple pregnancy, early diagnosis of lethal anomalies and screening of chromosomal defects are important end points to be taken into account by health authorities and to recommend routine ultrasound examination in the late first trimester of pregnancy.

REFERENCES

1. Donald I. Diagnostic uses of sonar in obstetrics and gynaecology. *J Obstet Gynaecol Br Commonw* 1965;72:907–19.
2. Timor-Tritsch IE, Farine D, Mortimore GR. A close look at early embryonic development with the high-frequency transvaginal transducer. *Am J Obstet Gynecol* 1988;159:676–81.
3. Fossum GT, Davayan V, Keltzky OA. Early detection of pregnancy with transvaginal ultrasound. *Fertil Steril* 1988;49: 788–91.
4. De Crespigny LC. Early diagnosis of pregnancy failure with transvaginal ultrasound. *Am J Obstet Gynecol* 1988;159:408–9.
5. Persson PH, Kullander S. Long-term experience of general ultrasound screening in pregnancy. *Am J Obstet Gynecol* 1983; 146: 942–6.
6. Eik-Nes SH, Okland O, Aure JC. Ultrasound screening in pregnancy: A randomized controlled trial. *Lancet* 1984;1:1347.
7. Cochlin D. Effect of two ultrasound scanning regimens on the management of pregnancy. *Br J Obstet Gynaecol* 1984;91:885–8.
8. Lilford R, Chard T. The routine use of ultrasound. *Br J Obstet Gynaecol* 1985;92:434–7.
9. Neilson J, Grant A. Ultrasound in pregnancy. In Enkin M, Keirse MJN, Chalmers I, eds. *A Guide to Effective Care in Pregnancy and Childbirth*. New York: Oxford University Press, 1989:48–56.
10. Belfrage P, Fernstrom I, Hallenberg G. Routine or selective ultrasound examinations in early pregnancy. *Obstet Gynecol* 1991;69:747–81.
11. Geirsson RT. Ultrasound instead of last menstrual period as the basis of gestational age assignment. *Ultrasound Obstet Gynecol* 1991;1:212–19.
12. Todros T, Ronco G, Lombardo D, *et al.* The length of pregnancy: An echographic reappraisal. *J Clin Ultrasound* 1991;19:11–14.
13. Nicolaides KH, Azar G, Byrne D, *et al.* Fetal nuchal translucency: Ultrasound screening for chromosomal defects in first trimester pregnancy. *Br Med J* 1992;304:435–9.
14. Achiron R, Tadmor O. Screening for fetal anomalies during the first trimester of pregnancy: Transvaginal versus transabdominal sonography. *Ultrasound Obstet Gynecol* 1991;1:186–91.
15. Matias A, Gomes C, Flack N, Montenegro N, Nicolaides KH. Screening for chromosomal abnormalities at 10–14 weeks: The role of ductus venosus blood flow. *Ultrasound Obstet Gynecol* 1998;12:380–4.
16. Matias A, Huggon I, Areias JA, Montenegro N, Nicolaides KH. Cardiac defects in chromosomally normal fetuses with abnormal ductus venosus blood flow at 10–14 weeks. *Ultrasound Obstet Gynecol* 1999;14:307–10.
17. Cicero S, Curcio P, Papageorghiou, Sonek J, Nicolaides KH. Absence of nasal bone in fetuses with trisomy 21 at 11–14 weeks of gestation: An observational study. *Lancet* 2001;358:1665–7.
18. Cicero S, Curcio P, Rembouskos G, Sonek J, Nicolaides KH. Maxillary length at 11–14 weeks of gestation in fetuses with trisomy 21. *Ultrasound Obstet Gynecol* 2004;24:19–22.
19. Kossof G, Griffiths KA, Dixon CE. Is the quality of transvaginal images superior to transabdominal ones under matched conditions? *Ultrasound Obstet Gynecol* 1991;1:29–35.
20. Pennell RG, Needleman L, Pajak T. Prospective comparison of vaginal and abdominal sonography in normal early pregnancy. *J Ultrasound Med* 1991;10:63–7.
21. Gershoni-Baruch R, Scher A, Itskovitz J, *et al.* The physical and psychomotor development of children conceived by IVF and exposed to high-frequency vaginal ultrasonography (6.5 MHz) in the first trimester of pregnancy. *Ultrasound Obstet Gynecol* 1991;1:21–8.
22. Kossof G. Contentious issues in safety of diagnostic ultrasound: Editorial. *Ultrasound Obstet Gynecol* 1997;10:151–5.
23. EFSUMB (Clinical Safety Statement for Diagnostic Ultrasound). efsumb@compuser.co, 1998.
24. Montenegro N. First trimester ultrasound. Presented at the *Euro-Team Early Pregnancy 2nd Post-Graduate Course*, Porto, Portugal, June 1993.
25. Gruboeck K, Zosmer N, Jurkovic D. Ultrasound features of early pregnancy development. In Jurkovic D, Jauniaux E, eds. *Ultrasound and Early Pregnancy*. New York: Parthenon Publishing, 1996:41–52.
26. Montenegro N, Beires J, Campos I, *et al.* The human development along the first trimester of intra-uterine life. The contribution of transvaginal endosonography. *Prog Diagn Prenat* 1994;6:24–44.
27. O'Rahilly R, Muller F. Ventricular system and choroid plexuses of the human brain during the embryonic period proper. *Am J Anat* 1990;189:285–302.
28. Larsen WJ. *Human Embryology*. New York: Churchill Livingstone, 1993:375–418.
29. Achiron R, Achiron A. Transvaginal ultrasonic assessment of the early fetal brain. *Ultrasound Obstet Gynecol* 1991;1:336–44.
30. Blaas HG, Eik-Nes SH, Kiserud T, *et al.* Early development of the hindbrain: A longitudinal ultrasound study from 7–12 weeks of gestation. *Ultrasound Obstet Gynecol* 1995;5:151–60.
31. Goldstein SR. Embryonic ultrasonographic measurements: Crown–rump length revisited. *Am J Obstet Gynecol* 1991;165: 497–501.
32. Exalto N. Early human nutrition. *Eur J Obstet Gynecol Reprod Med* 1995;61:3–6.
33. Braithwaite JM, Amstrong MA, Economides L. Assessment of fetal anatomy at 12 to 13 weeks of gestation by trans-abdominal and transvaginal sonography. *Br J Obstet Gynaecol* 1996;103: 82–5.
34. Snijders RJM, Noble P, Sebire N, Souka A, Nicolaides KH. UK multicentre project on assessment of risk of trisomy 21 by maternal age and fetal nuchal translucency thckness at 10–14 weeks of gestation. *Lancet* 1998;351:343–346.
35. Bonilla-Musoles F. Three-dimensional visualization of the human embryo: A potential revolution in prenatal diagnosis. *Ultrasound Obstet Gynecol* 1996;7:393–7.
36. Wilcox AJ, Weinberg CR, Baird DD. Timing of sexual intercourse in relation to ovulation. *N Engl J Med* 1995;333:1517–21.
37. Vollebergh JHA, Jongsma HW, van Dongen PWJ. The accuracy of ultrasonic measurement of fetal crown–rump length. *Eur J Obstet Gynecol Reprod Med* 1989;30:253–6.
38. Robinson HP, Fleming JEE. A critical evaluation of sonar crown–rump length measurements. *Br J Obstet Gynaecol* 1975; 82:702–10.
39. Lasser DM, Peisner DB, Vollebergh JHA, *et al.* First trimester fetal biometry using transvaginal sonography. *Ultrasound Obstet Gynecol* 1993;3:104–8.
40. Daya S. Accuracy of gestational age estimation by means of fetal crown–rump length measurement. *Am J Obstet Gynecol* 1993;168:903–8.
41. Parker AJ, Davies P, Newton JR. Assessment of gestational age of the Asian fetus by the sonar measurement of crown–rump length and biparietal diameter. *Br J Obstet Gynaecol* 1982;89:836–8.
42. Wisser J, Dirschedl P, Krone S. Estimation of gestational age by transvaginal sonographic measurement of greatest embryonic length in dated human embryos. *Ultrasound Obstet Gynecol* 1994;4:457–62.
43. Kuhn P, Brizot ML, Pandya PP, *et al.* Crown–rump length in chromosomally abnormal fetus at 10 to 13 weeks' gestation. *Am J Obstet Gynecol* 1995;172:32–5.

44. Eik-Nes SH, Okland O, Aure JC, *et al.* Ultrasound screening in pregnancy: A randomized controlled trial. *Lancet* 1984;1:347–54.
45. Gomez KJ, Copel JA. Routine ultrasound screening. *Curr Opin Obstet Gynecol* 1994;6:426–9.
46. Mongelli M, Wilcox M, Gardosi J. Estimating the date of confinement: Ultrasonographic biometry versus certain menstrual dates. *Am J Obstet Gynecol* 1996;174:278–81.
47. Campbell S, Newman GB. Growth of the fetal biparietal diameter during normal pregnancy. *J Obstet Gynaecol Br Commonw* 1971;78:513–19.
48. Levi S, Smets P. Intra-uterine fetal growth studied by ultrasonic biparietal measurements. *Acta Obstet Gynecol Scand* 1973;52: 193–8.
49. Skupski DW, Chervenak FA, McCullough LB. A clinical and ethical evaluation of routine obstetric ultrasound. *Curr Opin Obstet Gynecol* 1994;6:435–9.
50. Montenegro N, Pereira Leite L. Fetal cerebellar measurements in second trimester ultrasonography – Clinical value. *J Perinat Med* 1989;17:365–9.
51. Luke B. The changing pattern of multiple births in the United States: Maternal and infant characteristics, 1973 and 1990. *Obstet Gynecol* 1994;84:101–6.
52. Minakami H, Sato I. Reestimating date of delivery in multifetal pregnancies. *J Am Med Assoc* 1996;275:1432–4.
53. Sepulveda W, Sebire NJ, Hughes K, *et al.* The lambda sign at 10–14 weeks of gestation as a predictor of chorionicity in twin pregnancies. *Ultrasound Obstet Gynecol* 1996;7:421–3.
54. Embom JA. Twin pregnancy with intrauterine death of one twin. *Am J Obstet Gynecol* 1985;152:424–8.
55. Nicolaides KH, Pettersen H. Fetal therapy. *Curr Opin Obstet Gynecol* 1994;6:468–71.
56. Evans MI, Dommergues M, Johnson MP, *et al.* Multifetal pregnancy reduction and selective termination. *Curr Opin Obstet Gynecol* 1995;7:126–9.
57. D'Alton M.E, Dudley DK. The ultrasonographic prediction of chorionicity in twin gestation. *Am J Obstet Gynecol* 1989; 160:557–61.
58. Sampson A, de Crespigny LC. Vanishing twins: The frequency of spontaneous fetal reduction of a twin pregnancy. *Ultrasound Obstet Gynecol* 1992;2:107–9.
59. Souka A, Snijders RJM, Novakov A, Soares W, Nicolaides KH. Defects and syndromes in chromosomally normal fetuses with increased nuchal tarslucency at 10–14 weeks of gestation. *Ultrasound Obstet Gynecol* 1998;11:391–400.
60. Hyett JA, Noble PL, Snijders RJM, *et al.* Fetal heart rate in trisomy 21 and other chromosomal abnormalities at 10–14 weeks of gestation. *Ultrasound Obstet Gynecol* 1996;7:239–44.
61. Bindra R, Heath V, Liao A, Spencer K, Nicolaides KH. One-stop clinic for assessment of risk of trisomy 21 at 11–14 weeks: A prospective study of 15030 pregnancies. *Ultrasound Obstet Gynecol* 2002;20:219–25.
62. Nicolaides KH. Nuchal translucency and other first-trimester sonographic markers of chromosomal abnormalities. *Am J Obstet Gynecol* 2004;191:45–67.
63. Hyett JA, Moscoso G, Papapanagiotou G, *et al.* Abnormalities of the heart and great arteries in chromosomally normal fetuses with increased nuchal translucency thickness at 11–13 weeks of gestation. *Ultrasound Obstet Gynecol* 1996;7:245–50.
64. Montenegro N, Matias A, Areias JC, *et al.* Ductus venosus revisited: A Doppler blood flow evaluation in the first trimester of pregnancy. *Ultrasound Med Biol* 1997;23:171–6.
65. Montenegro N, Matias A, Areias JC, *et al.* Early cardiac failure as a putative pathogenic mechanism for increased nuchal translucency. *Ultrasound Obstet Gynecol* 1996;8(Suppl 1):111.
66. Montenegro N, Matias A, Areias JC, *et al.* Increased fetal nuchal translucency: Possible involvement of early cardiac failure. *Ultrasound Obstet Gynecol* 1997;10:265–8.
67. Murta CG, Moron AF, Avila MA, Weiner CP. Application of ductus venosus Doppler velocimetry for the detection of fetal aneuploidy in the first trimester of pregnancy. *Fetal Diagn Ther* 2002;17:308–14.
68. Zoppi MA, Putzolu M, Ibba RM, Floris M, Monni G. First trimester ductus venosus velocimetryin relation to nuchal translucency thickness and fetal karyotype. *Fetal Diagn Ther* 2002;17:52–7.
69. Toyama JM, Brizot ML, Liao AW, *et al.* Ductus venosus blood fow assessment at 11 to 14 weeks of gestation and fetal outcome. *Ultrasound Obstet Gynecol* 2004;23:341–5.
70. Timor Tritsch IE, Monteagudo A, Peisner DB. High-frequency transvaginal sonographic examination for the potential malformation assessment of the 9-week to 14-week fetus. *J Clin Ultrasound* 1992;20:231–8.
71. Campbell S, Johnstone FD, Holt EM, *et al.* Anencephaly: Early ultrasonic diagnosis and active management. *Lancet* 1972;2: 1226–7.
72. Rottem S. IRONFAN A sonographic window into the natural history of fetal anomalies. *Ultrasound Obstet Gynecol* 1995;5: 361–3.

98 Hemodynamic assessment of early pregnancy

L. T. Mercé, M. J. Barco, S. Kupesic and A. Kurjak

Introduction

By 'hemodynamic assessment of early pregnancy' we refer to the study of the changes in the utero-placental, intervillous, fetal-placental, embryo-fetal and luteal ovarian circulations during the first trimester of normal pregnancies.

Although several invasive methods have been applied to experimental animal models for the study of early gestation hemodynamics, in the human species it has only been possible since the arrival of Doppler examination. This method has experienced great technological improvements from the continuous and pulsed Doppler to the 3D power Doppler angiography (PDA).

The transvaginal color Doppler has proven to be a highly efficient technique in the assessment of the placental, embryo-fetal and luteal circulations during the first trimester. Nevertheless, the theoretical risk of adverse biological effects on the embryo has restricted significantly its use during this pregnancy period. The 3D Doppler angiography represents a new technological advance that applies the ALARA principle (As Low As Reasonably Achievable), since the acquisition time of the angiograph volumes is shorter. Moreover, it is a process available only in high-technology equipment that fulfills precisely all the international regulations on ultrasound safety. In any case, it seems necessary to have at our disposal new reports that guarantee the possibility of a careful but more liberal use of this new method during early pregnancy.

Utero-placental blood flow

The utero-placental circulation is composed of the uterine vessels and their intramyometrial branches: arcuate, radial and spiral endometrial arteries. The spiral arteries will become utero-placental arteries under the trophoblastic invasion process during the first half of pregnancy.

The utero-placental blood flow increases progressively during the first trimester of normal gestations to accomplish the great demands imposed during the organogenesis period.[1] The invasion of the radial and spiral arteries by the cytotrophoblast is the mechanism to secure the progressive increase of utero-placental perfusion. These arteries lose their autoregulation ability and increase their diameters to become the utero-placental arteries.[2]

The spiral and radial arteries are those showing the greatest and most significant changes under Doppler examination as they are the target vessels of the trophoblastic invasion.[3–7] From the ultrasonographic detection of the gestational sac it is possible to depict a color signal coming out of it and getting inside the myometrium, which was named the 'comet sign'[5–7] (Figure 98.1). The flow velocity waveform (FVW) of these arteries shows a low vascular resistance and usually the protodiastolic notch is absent.

The proximity of the spiral and radial arteries in the placental basal plate rends its differentiation impossible. For this reason we call them retrochorionic arteries. Other authors use the term subchorionic and peritrophoblastic arteries.[8,9] Out of the placental site the radial arteries are placed at the myometrial internal third. The arcuate arteries run along the myometrial external third near the serosa. From the seventh week onward it is possible to identify through transvaginal color Doppler the spiral, radial and arcuate signals in 100% of the examinations.[10,11] The uterine arteries can be explored on both sides of the cervical isthmus. The FVW of the uterine arteries shows a high resistance with a protodiastolic notch usually present (Figure 98.2).

There is a gradual increase in the blood flow in the retrochorionic arteries during the normal first trimester of gestation. The resistance index diminishes from 0.52 ± 0.03 in the 4th week to 0.31 ± 0.05 in the 15th week (Figure 98.3), whereas the systolic and diastolic velocities increase progressively.[5,6] Changes at the placental vascular bed will affect in a retrograde way the entire utero-placental vascular tree. The blood flow will also increase in the radial, arcuate and uterine arteries. The vascular resistance decreases

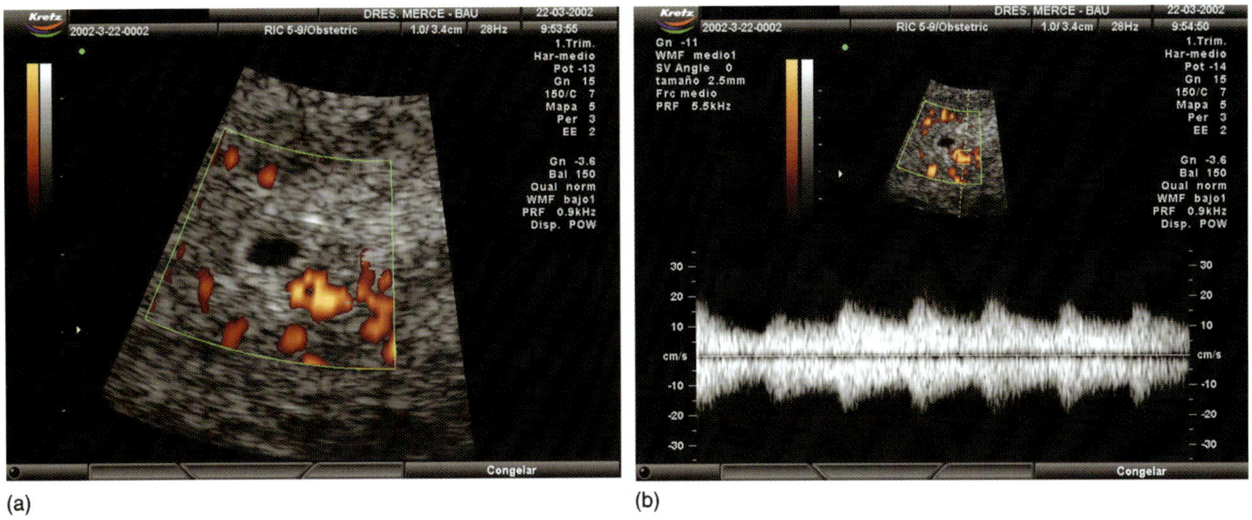

Figure 98.1 (a) Color map of the retrochorionic circulation of a gestational sac of 4 mm. The blood flow increase in the spiral and radial arteries depicts the 'comet sign'. (b) FVW of the retrochorionic circulation in the same gestational sac.

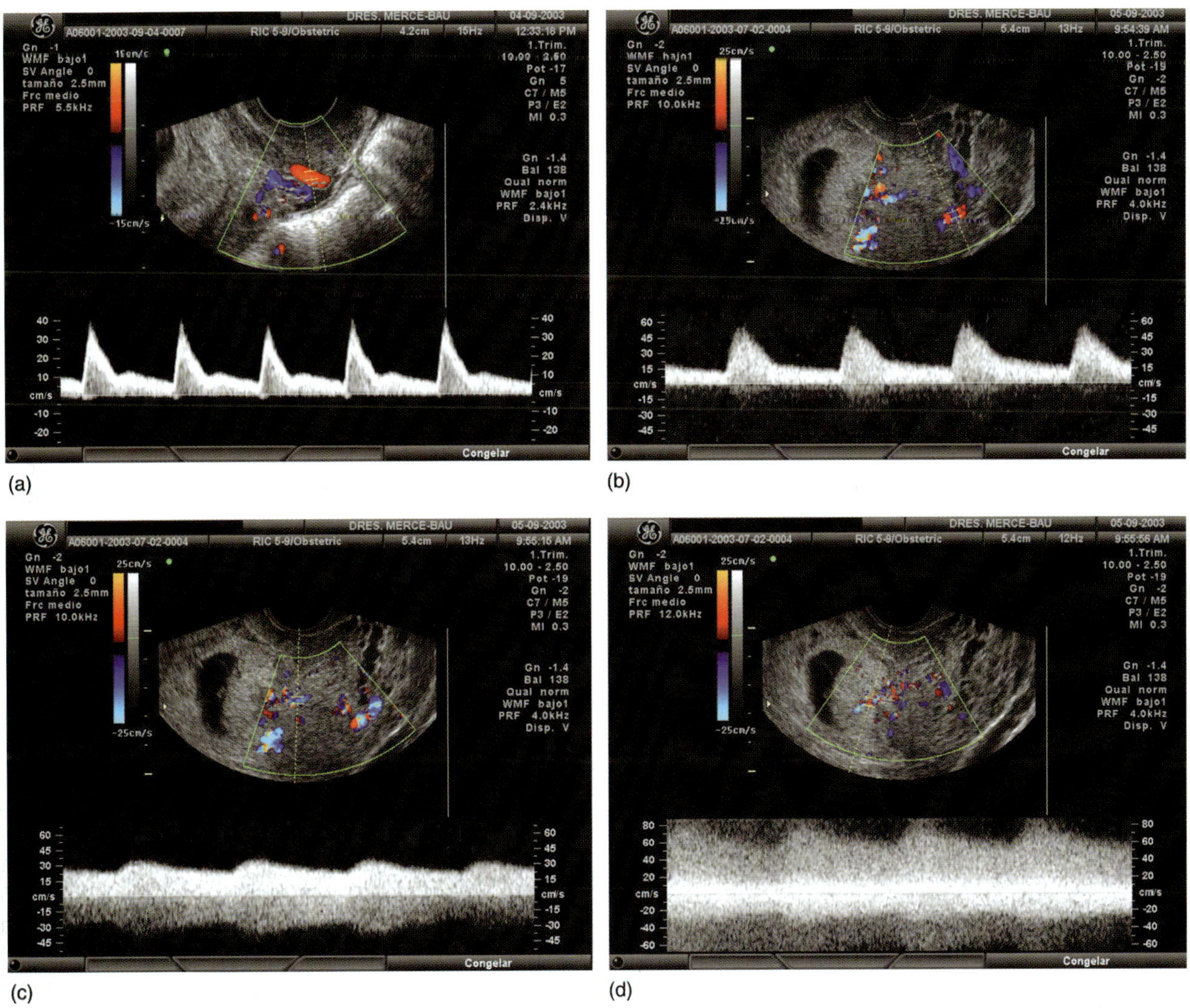

Figure 98.2 FVW of the uterine artery in a normal gestation of 8 weeks of amenorrhea (a), arcuate artery (b), radial artery (c) and spiral or utero-placental arteries (d). The vascular resistance increases as the distance from the placental insertion site increases.

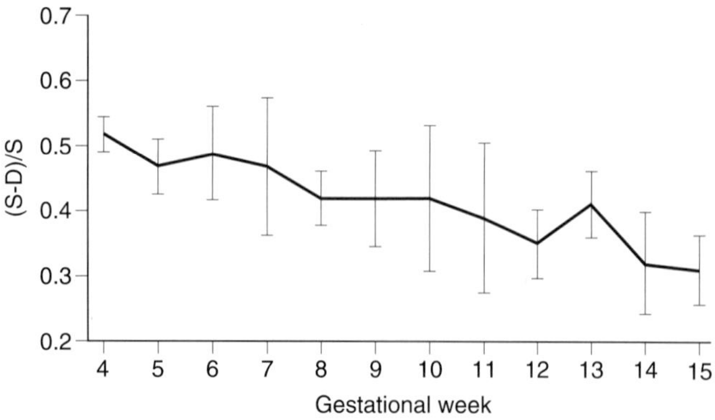

Figure 98.3 Resistance index of the retrochorionic arteries (spiral–radial) during early gestation (mean ±SD).

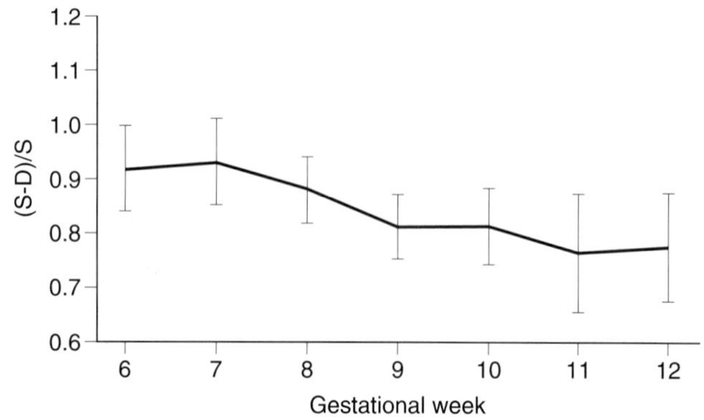

Figure 98.4 Average resistance index from both uterine arteries during early pregnancy (mean ±SD).

gradually in all the utero-placental vessels during the normal first trimester of pregnancy, but it increases along with the distance from the chorionic implantation site[8–15] (Figure 98.2). The average resistance index of the uterine arteries falls from 0.94 ±0.08 in the 5th week to 0.76 ±0.09 in the 12th week, while the maximum systolic velocity increases from 43.67 ±16.72 cm/s to 79.13 ±26.33 cm/s in the same period of time[3,4] (Figure 98.4). The protodiastolic notch is always present at the beginning but it will disappear in the second trimester.

The utero-placental blood flow, as evaluated by the retrochorionic vascular resistance, increases to 36% during the first trimester of normal pregnancies. This percentage is greater than the 30% observed throughout the remainder of pregnancy and doubles the 16% attributed to the second trophoblastic wave between the 15th and 20th weeks[16] (Figure 98.5). This fact demonstrates the importance of the vascular changes taking place in this gestational period and its unquestionable value for a successful pregnancy outcome.

Intervillous blood flow

From an embryological point of view, the intervillous circulation seems to be initiated around the 12th day

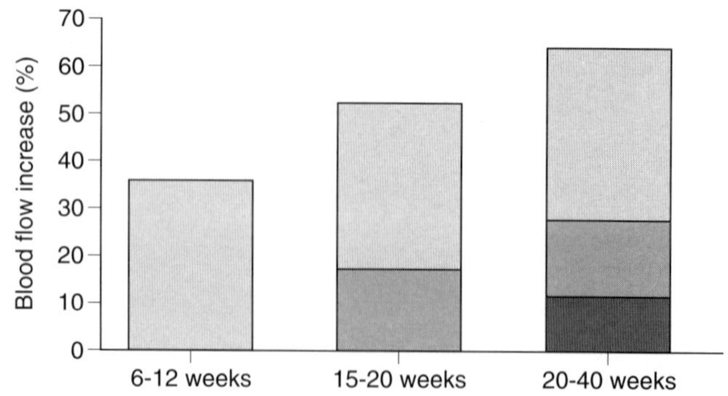

Figure 98.5 Percentage of blood flow increase at the placental site at different stages of normal pregnancy. During the first trimester a decrease in the vascular resistance takes place, which is greater than the rest of gestation.

of embryo development, when the maternal blood flows inside the syncitiotrophoblastic lacunae.[17] Nonetheless, Doppler studies have produced conflicting results.

Jauniaux *et al.*[18,19] and Jaffe and Woods[20] using transvaginal color Doppler did not find intervillous blood flow before 12 gestational weeks. Trophoblastic plugs would occlude the spiral arteries lumen[21,22] to maintain a relatively hypoxic environment to favor embryo development.[23] The intervillous blood flow was only present in miscarriages.[24,25]

Kurjak and Kupesic,[26] Valentín *et al.*[14] and Mercé *et al.*[5,6] using a similar technology were able to detect the intervillous blood flow from the sixth normal pregnancy week onward. Two patterns of flow have been registered: a continuous venous type and a pulsatile arterial type, the latter probably next to the entrance to the utero-placental arteries (Figure 98.6).

The maximum venous velocities in the intervillous space (IVS) are low and increase gradually throughout the first trimester from 2 ±0.77 cm/s at 6 weeks to 5.12 ±2.23 at 12 weeks[5,6] (Figure 98.6). For some authors[27] that increase from the 10th week occurs simultaneously with the decline in the vitelline circulation (Figure 98.7). The arterial FVW in the IVS does not experience significant changes during the first trimester.[14,26,27]

Our recent experience with 3D PDA confirms our previous results with transvaginal color Doppler. The virtual organ computer aided analysis (VOCAL) technology allows the differentiation of the IVS and retrochorionic circulations and their independent assessment (Figure 98.8). We have observed a progressive and significant increase in the vascularization, flow and vascularization-flow indices between the 6th and 12th weeks in normal pregnancies (Figure 98.9).

These findings are in accordance with a gradual disappearance of the trophoblastic plugs from the spiral arteries during the first trimester. It would produce an increase in the Doppler signals at the chorion frondosum (vascularization index) and an increase in

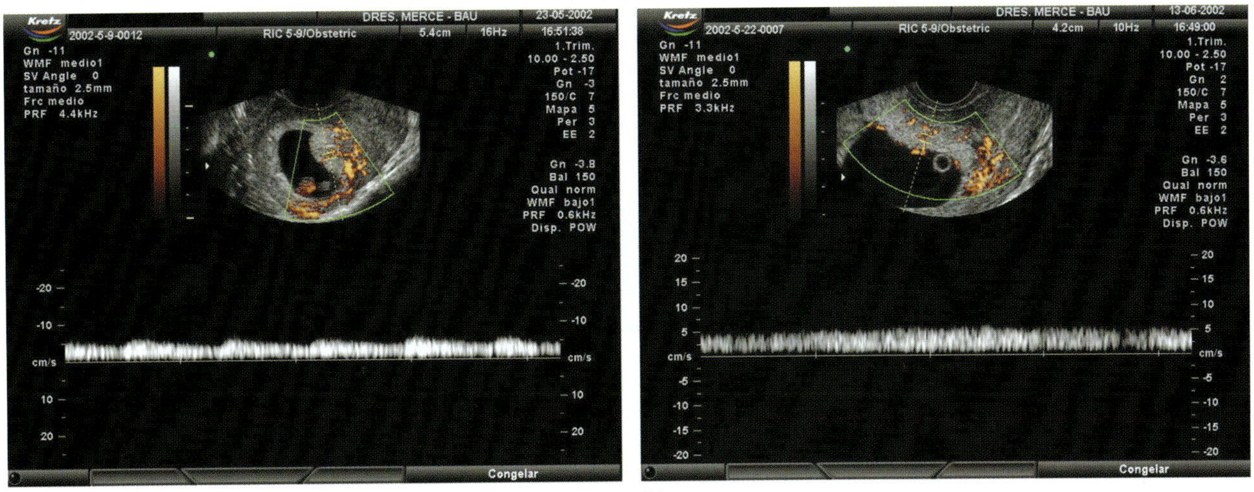

(a) (b)

Figure 98.6 Doppler signal from the intervillous circulation of arterial type (a) in the seventh week and venous type (b) in the ninth week.

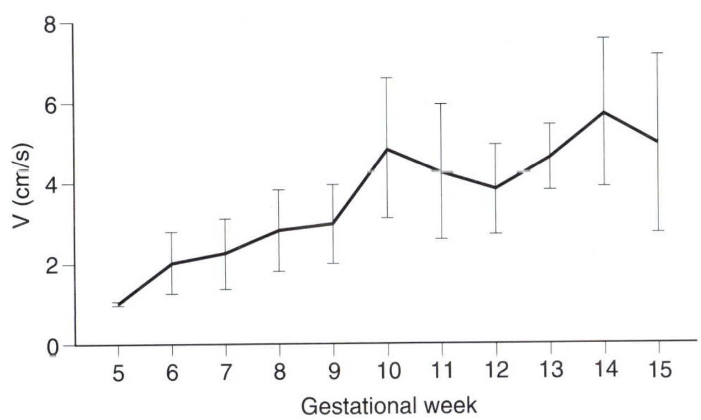

Figure 98.7 Venous maximum velocity of the intervillous circulation during normal early pregnancy (mean ± SD).

their intensity (flow index) that constitute the increase in the IVS blood flow in this period. Jauniaux *et al.*[28] in their last publication seem to admit this possibility that we are defending for more than 10 years.

Blood flow in the yolk sac

The circulation in the yolk sac precedes the fetal-placental or umbilical circulations in embryonic development.[17]

The yolk sac circulation can be detected by Doppler from the fifth week of amenorrhea onward.[29–31] It is feasible to integrate the Doppler signal in the 44[3]–67%[27] of normal gestations. During the sixth week it could be difficult to differentiate from the initial umbilical signal.[30] Its FVW is of arterial type without diastolic flow (Figure 98.10). The blood flow in the yolk sac is characterized by low velocities (between 3 and 7 cm/s) and a pulsatility index ranging from 2.19 to 4.78.[30] The yolk sac blood flow diminishes from the 10th week onward, together with the size of the sac, and coincides with the blood flow increase to the IVS.[27]

Fetal-placental blood flow

The fetal-placental or umbilical circulation links the villous vascular system with the embryo-fetal vascular system. The umbilical artery Doppler signal is detected at the end of the fifth or the beginning of the sixth week of amenorrhea, when the embryo begins to be sonographically detectable. The umbilical artery FVW is characterized by not showing a diastolic component until the 10th week of amenorrhea. The umbilical diastolic flow appears in a small percentage of cases from the 11th week onward and will be constantly present from the 14th week onward[5,6,8,30,32–34] (Figure 98.11).

From the seventh week onward it is possible to register the umbilical vein signal. The umbilical venous blood flow shows a characteristically undulated profile during the first trimester (Figure 98.11). The umbilical vein pulsations are physiological in this period of pregnancy and will disappear from the 11th week onward.[35,36]

The umbilical artery blood flow increases significantly alongside the entire first trimester of normal gestations.[5,6,8,30,32–34] Between the 6th and 14th weeks the maximum systolic velocity is increased from 5.63 ± 2.26 cm/s at 6 weeks to 21.28 ± 4.6 cm/s at 14 weeks, whereas the pulsatility index falls from 4.4 ± 1.1 to 1.38 ± 0.34 (Figure 98.12).

The decrease in the umbilical artery resistance during the first 12 weeks of gestation is essentially due to the maturation of the villous vascular tree. The appearance of diastolic velocities would explain this fact. The beginning of the fetal period will lead to

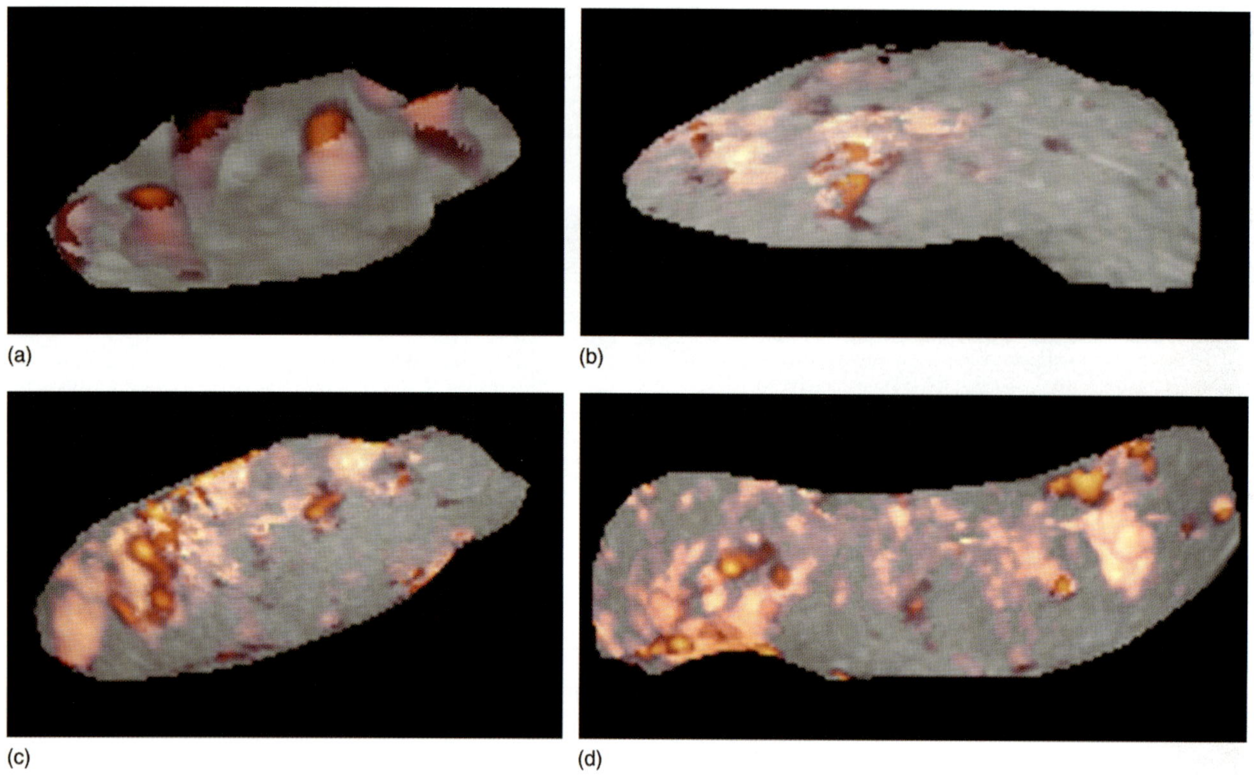

Figure 98.8 3D power Doppler angiography of the intervillous flow at 6 weeks (a), 8 weeks (b), 10 weeks (c) and 12 weeks (d) of normal pregnancies.

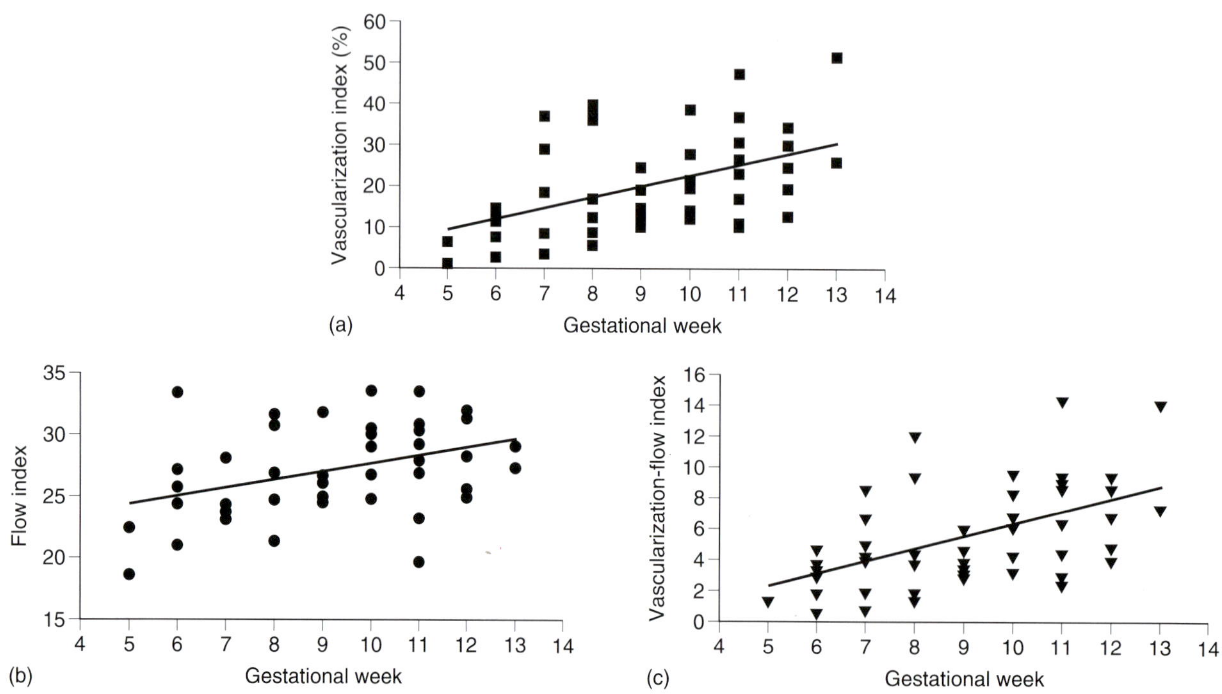

Figure 98.9 Vascularization index (a), flow index (b) and vascularization-flow index (c) of the intervillous circulation during the normal first trimester of pregnancy.

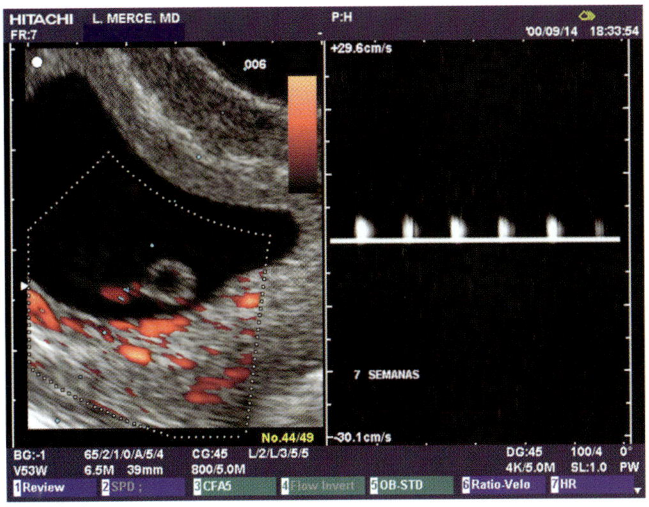

Figure 98.10 Doppler signal from the yolk sac circulation in the seventh week of pregnancy.

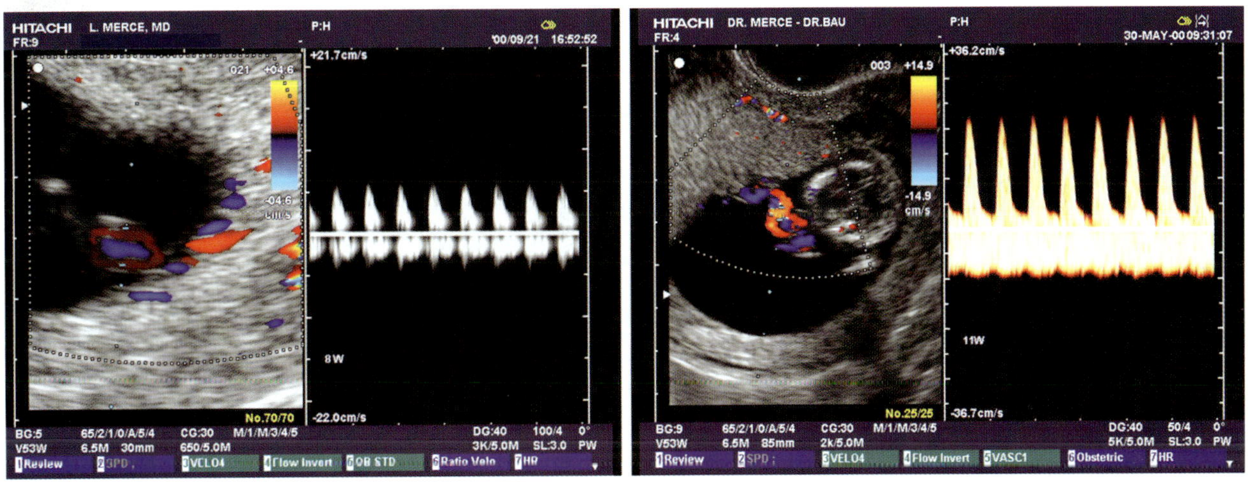

(a) (b)

Figure 98.11 Umbilical artery Doppler in the 8th (a) and 11th (b) gestational weeks. At the inferior channel, the undulating profile of the umbilical venous signal can be appreciated.

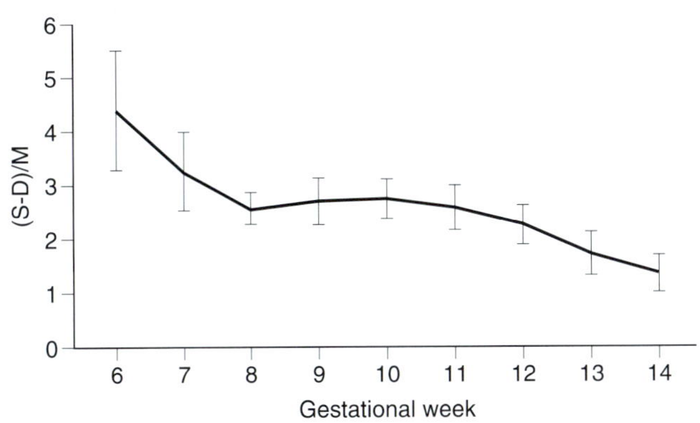

Figure 98.12 Umbilical artery pulsatility index during early pregnancy (mean ±SD).

increasing demands of oxygen and nutrients that will be supplied by an improvement in the villous transfer.

Embryo-fetal blood flow

Transvaginal color Doppler allows the evaluation of the whole intraembryonic circulation, but only the blood flow in the aorta, cerebral arteries and ductus venosus has been studied.

The trajectory of the aorta can be clearly visualized from the seventh gestational week onward. As it occurs in the umbilical artery, its Doppler signal is characterized by the absence of diastolic velocities,

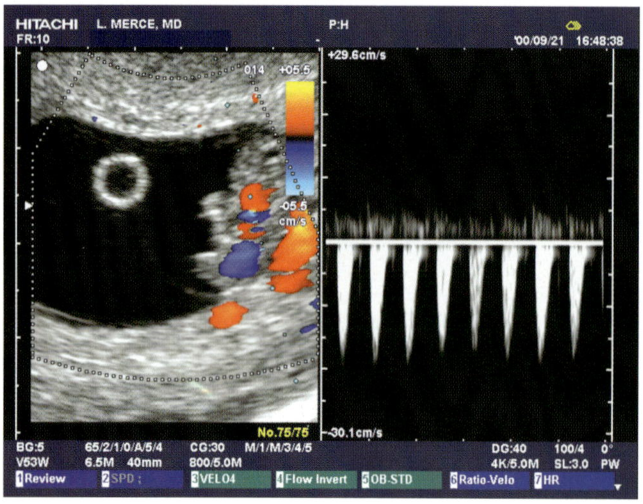

Figure 98.13 Color signal and FVW of the embryonic aorta in the ninth gestational week.

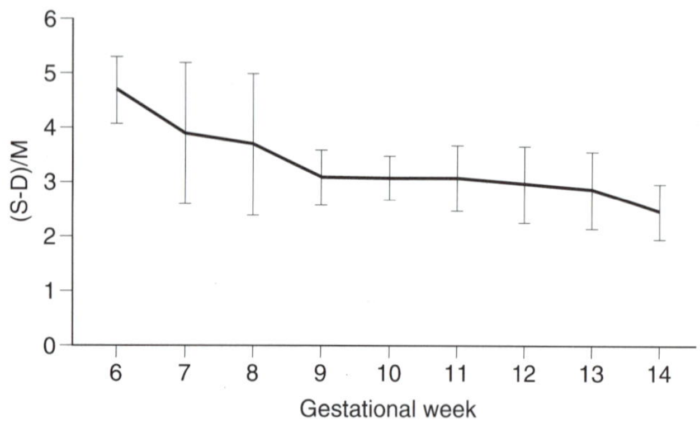

Figure 98.14 Pulsatility index of the embryonic aorta during normal first trimester of pregnancy.

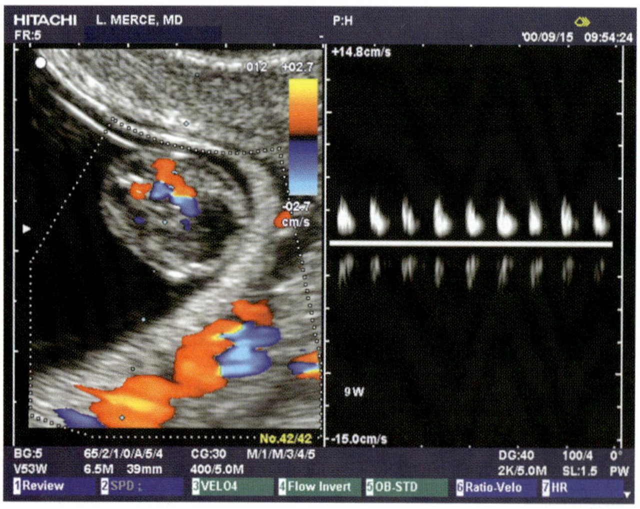

Figure 98.15 Mean cerebral artery FVW in a normal pregnancy of 9 weeks.

that begin to appear around the 13th week, being always present at the 14th and 15th weeks[8,30,33,34] (Figure 98.13). The aortic blood flow increases progressively during the whole first trimester, as proven by

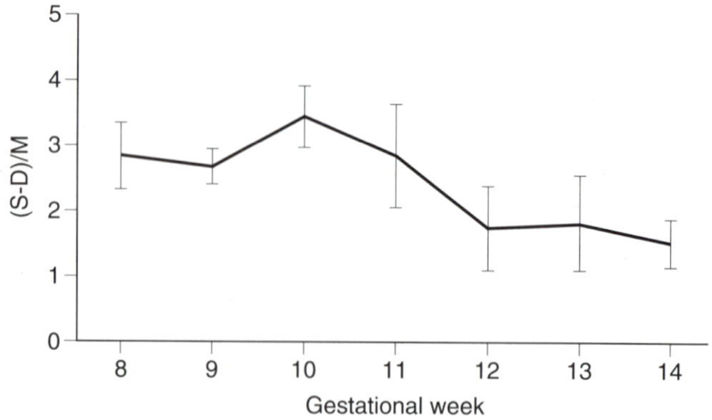

Figure 98.16 Pulsatility index of the mean cerebral artery during normal early pregnancy (mean ± SD).

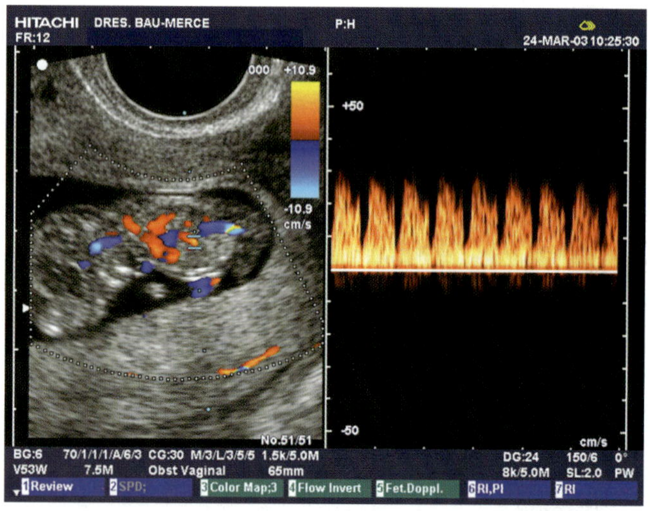

Figure 98.17 Normal Doppler recording of the ductus venosus in the 11th week.

the augmentation of systolic velocity and the reduction of the pulsatility index[8,30,33,34] (Figure 98.14).

Intracerebral signals can be registered by transvaginal color Doppler in the eighth week of amenorrhea. However, the centrifuge trajectory of the mean cerebral arteries can be depicted only from the 10th week. The cerebral blood flow increases between the 8th and 14th pregnancy weeks. Systolic velocities are present from the 11th week onward. They are visible in 80% of the 12th-week registers and are constantly present during the following weeks (Figure 98.15). The maximum systolic velocity is 4.97 cm/s at the eighth week, rising to 19.08 ± 5.21 at the 14th. The pulsatility index decreases steadily from 2.86 ± 0.49 in the eighth week to 1.49 ± 0.37 in the 14th week (Figure 98.16).

The cerebral arteries show diastolic velocities from the 11th week onward, in contrast to their absence in the umbilical and aorta arteries. The ratio between the umbilical and cerebral pulsatility indices is usually

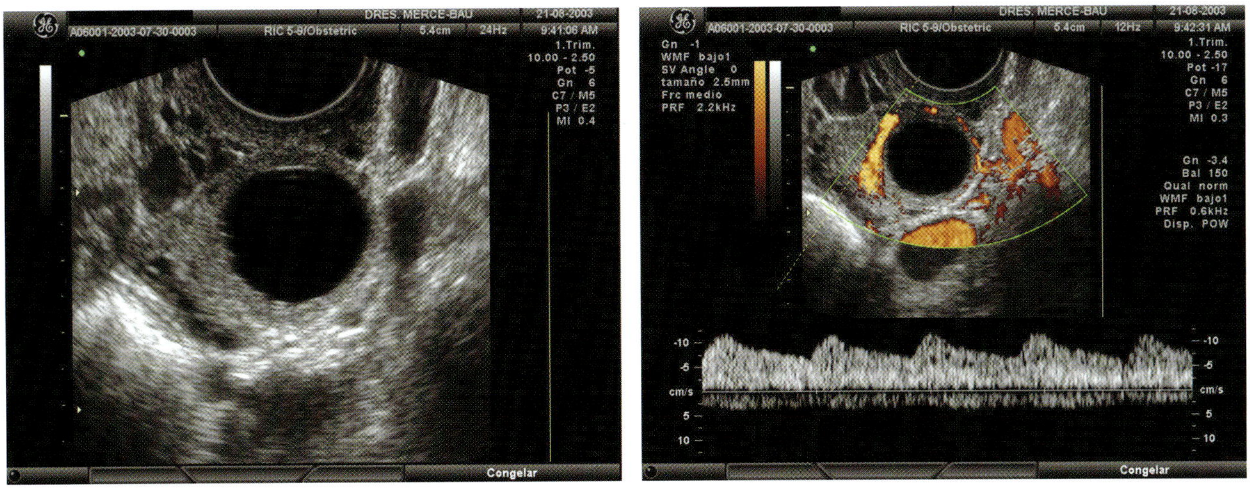

Figure 98.18 Sonolucent corpus luteum image (a) and color signal and FVW (b) in a normal fifth week of gestation.

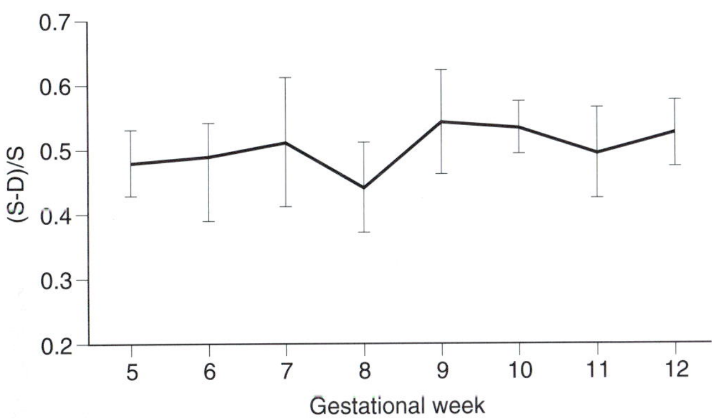

Figure 98.19 Resistance index of the normal corpus luteum vascularity during the first trimester of normal gestations (mean ±SD).

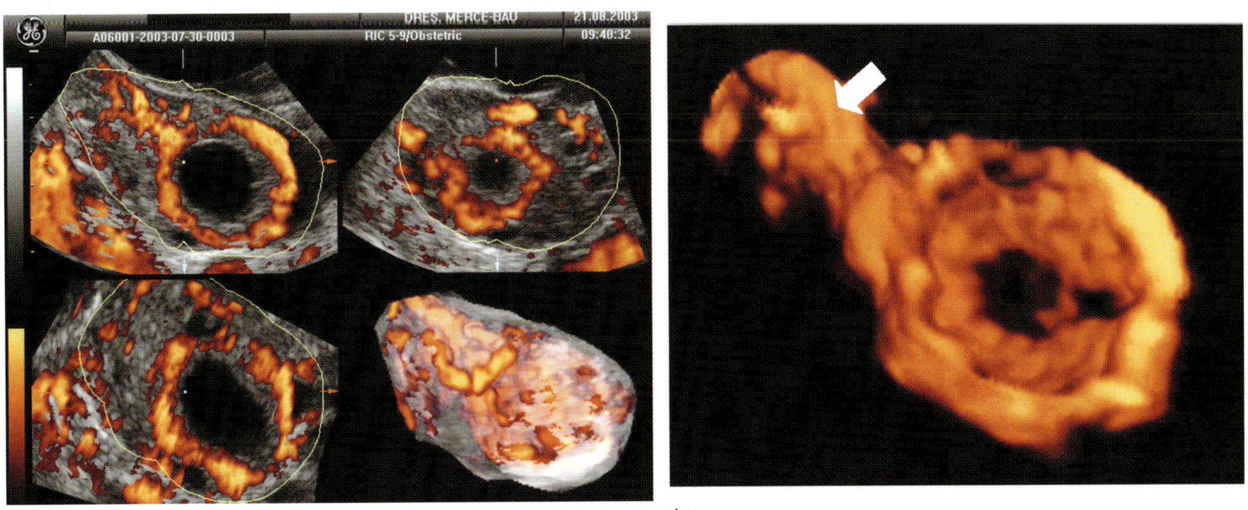

Figure 98.20 Luteal circulation assessment during early pregnancy by 3D power Doppler angiography. (a) Acquisition technique applying the VOCAL software. (b) Three-dimensional angiographic rendering of the vascular network in a gestational corpus luteum. The arrow points to the helical artery.

inferior to 1 during the first trimester.[37] These data suggest that the cerebral blood flow is independent of the vascular changes taking place in the aorta and the villous network. This autoregulation mechanism of the cerebral circulation during early pregnancy should aim to secure a proper blood supply to the growing fetal brain.

The ductus venosus is a circulatory shunt connecting the umbilical vein with the inferior cava vein. The Doppler signal shows a forward flow and triphasic morphology with three components: ventricular systole, early diastole with passive ventricular filling and late diastole with a nadir in the signal that reflects the active ventricular filling due to the atrial contraction. Although all three components of the ductus venosus FVW can be identified from the ninth week onward,[36] its visualization is more constant from the 12th to 15th week onward[36,38] (Figure 98.17). The blood flow increases progressively in the ductus from the ninth week onward throughout the rest of the pregnancy. Blood flow velocities increase as the vascular resistance decreases.[36–40]

The pulsatility increase in the ductus venosus at the end of the first trimester could indicate the presence of a fetal chromosomal anomaly associated or not associated to a congenital cardiac malformation.[41,42] It has been suggested as a marker for chromosomal abnormalities independent of the nuchal translucency,[43] and in association with it, could increase the specificity by maintaining an adequate detection rate.[44]

Luteal ovarian blood flow

The luteal function is essential during early gestation, given that its hormonal secretion sustains the pregnancy until the functional takeover of the placenta. During the first 12 gestational weeks the luteal blood flow can be easily evaluated by transvaginal color Doppler.

The corpus luteum is visualized from 66%[37] up to 100% of pregnancies.[45] In the majority of cases it has an anechogenic appearance (77%), which can hinder the differential diagnosis with a persistent follicle.[37] The Doppler examination confirms the gestational corpus luteum when it shows a 'luteal conversion' of the FVW, quite similar to that of the second half of the ovarian cycle[16] (Figure 98.18).

The luteal blood flow during early pregnancy is similar to that of the luteal phase of the ovarian cycle and there are no significant differences in the velocimetric parameters.[16,46,47] Maximum systolic velocities are usually high.[46–48] The helical or nutricia artery shows the highest systolic velocities and a low variability.[48] The resistance index ranges from 0.48 ± 0.05 in the 5th week to 0.52 ± 0.05 in the 12th week, with a slight tendency to an increase in the intraovarian vascular resistance[16] (Figure 98.19).

Lately, the 3D PDA allows the representation of the luteal angiogenesis and the study of the blood flow in a more real and precise way (Figure 98.20).

REFERENCES

1. Greiss FC Jr, Anderson SG. Uterine blood flow during early ovine pregnancy. *Am J Obstet Gynecol* 1970;106:30–8.
2. Reynolds SRM. Gestation mechanisms. *Ann N Y Acad Sci* 1959;75:691–9.
3. Mercé LT, Barco MJ, de la Fuente F. Doppler velocimetry measured in retrochorionic space and uterine arteries during early human pregnancy. *Acta Obstet Gynecol Scand* 1989;8:603–7.
4. Mercé LT. Velocimetría Doppler en la gestación precoz normal y patológica: Estudio del proceso de placentación. In Carrera JM, ed. *Doppler en Obstetricia. Hemodinamia perinatal.* Barcelona: Masson-Salvat Medicina, 1992:127–45.
5. Mercé LT, Bau S, García del Real E. Estudio Doppler en el diagnóstico prenatal precoz. *Prog Diagn Prenat* 1994;6:63–77.
6. Mercé LT, Barco MJ, Bau S. Color Doppler sonographic assessment of placental circulation in the first trimester of normal pregnancy. *J Ultrasound Med* 1996;15:135–42.
7. Mercé LT, Kupesic S, Kurjak A. Color Doppler assessment of implantation and early placentation. *Prenat Neonat Med* 1999; 4:94–112.
8. Kurjak A, Crvenkovic G, Salihagic A, Zalud I, Miljan M. The assessment of normal early pregnancy by transvaginal color Doppler ultrasonography. *J Clin Ultrasound* 1993;21:3–8.
9. Jaffe R, Woods JR. Color Doppler imaging and in vivo assessment of the anatomy and physilogy of the early uteroplacental circulation. *Fertil Steril* 1993;60:293–7.
10. Predanic M, Zudenigo D, Funduk-Kurjak B, Kurjak A, Takeuchi H. Assessment of early normal pregnancy. In Kurjak A, ed. *An Atlas of Transvaginal Color Doppler.* London: The Parthenon Publishing Group, 1994:51–69.
11. Kurjak A, Zudenigo D. Circulación maternofetal incipiente visualizada mediante Doppler color transvaginal. In Carrera JM, Kurjak A, eds. *Medicina del embrión.* Barcelona: Masson, 1997: 77–84.
12. Jurkovic D, Jauniaux E, Kurjak A, Hustin J, Campbell S, Nicoliades K. Transvaginal color Doppler assessment of the uteroplacental circulation in early pregnancy. *Obstet Gynecol* 1991;77:365–9.
13. Coppens M, Loquet P, Kollen M, De Neubourg F, Buytaert PH. Longitudinal evaluation of uteroplacental and umbilical blood flow changes in normal early pregnancy. *Ultrasound Obstet Gynecol* 1996;7:114–21.
14. Valentín L, Sladkevicius P, Laurini R, Söderberg H, Marsal K. Uteroplacental and luteal circulation in normal first-trimester pregnancies: Doppler ultrasonographic and morphologic study. *Am J Obstet Gynecol* 1996;174:768–75.
15. Makikallio K, Tekay A, Jouppila P. Uteroplacental hemodynamics during early human pregnancy. *Gynecol Obstet Invest* 2004; 58:49–54.
16. Mercé LT. Velocimetría Doppler durante la gestación precoz. In Mercé LT, ed. *Ecografía Doppler en Obstetricia y Ginecología.* Madrid: Interamericana McGraw-Hill, 1993:145–60.
17. Sadler TW. *Langman-Embriología Médica,* 7th edn. Madrid: Panamericana/Williams and Wilkins, 1996.
18. Jauniaux E, Jurkovic D, Campbell S. *In vivo* investigations of the anatomy and the physiology of early human circulation. *Ultrasound Obstet Gynecol* 1991;1:435–45.
19. Jauniaux E, Jurkovic D, Campbell S, Hustin J. Doppler ultrasonographic features of the developing placental circulation: Correlation with anatomic findings. *Am J Obstet Gynecol* 1992; 166:585–7.
20. Jaffe R, Woods JR. Color Doppler imaging and *in vivo* assessment of the anatomy and physiology of the early uteroplacental circulation. *Fertil Steril* 1993;60:293–7.
21. Hustin J, Schaaps JP. Echocardiographic and anatomic studies of the maternotrophoblastic border during the first trimester of pregnancy. *Am J Obstet Gynecol* 1987;157:162–8.
22. Hustin J, Schaaps JP, Lambotte R. Anatomical studies of the utero-placental vascularization in the first trimester of pregnancy. *Trophoblast Res* 1988;3:49–60.
23. Rodesch F, Simon P, Donner C, Jauniaux E. Oxygen measurements in endometrial and trophoblastic tissues during early pregnancy. *Obstet Gynecol* 1992;80:283–5.
24. Jauniaux E, Zaidi J, Jurkovic D, Campbell S, Hustin J. Comparison of colour Doppler features and pathological findings in complicated early pregnancy. *Hum Reprod* 1994; 9:2432–7.
25. Jaffe R, Dorgan A, Abramowicz JS. Color Doppler imaging of the uteroplacental circulation in the first trimester: Value in predicting

pregnancy failure or complication. *AJR Am J Roentgenol* 1995; 164:1255–8.

26. Kurjak A, Kupesic S. Doppler assessment of the intervillous blood flow in normal and abnormal early pregnancy. *Obstet Gynecol* 1997;89:252–6.
27 Kurjak A, Kupesic S. Parallel Doppler assessment of yolk sac and intervillous circulation in normal pregnancy and missed abortion. *Placenta* 1998;19:619–23.
28. Jauniaux E, Greenwold N, Hempstock J, Burton GJ. Comparison of ultrasonographic and Doppler mapping of the intervillous circulation in normal and abnormal early pregnancies. *Fertil Steril* 2003;79:100–6.
29. Kurjak A, Kupesic S, Kostovic L. Vascularization of yolk sac and vitelline duct in normal pregnancies studied by transvaginal color and pulsed Doppler. *J Perinat Med* 1994;12:433–40.
30. Van Zalen-SprocK, MM, van Vugt JMG, Colenbrander GJ, van Geijn HP. First-trimester uteroplacental and fetal blood flow velocity waveforms in normally developing fetuses: A longitudinal study. *Ultrasound Obstet Gynecol* 1994;4:284–8.
31. Makikallio K, Tekay A, Jouppila P. Yolk sac and umbilicoplacental hemohynamics during early human embryonic development. *Ultrasound Obstet Gynecol* 1999;14:175–9.
32. Arduini D, Rizzo G. Umbilical artery velocity waveforms in early pregnancy: A transvaginal color Doppler study. *J Clin Ultrasound* 1991;19:335–9.
33. Huisman TWA, Stewart PA, Wladimiroff JW. Doppler assessment of the normal early fetal circulation. *Ultrasound Obstet Gynecol* 1992;2:300–5.
34. Alcázar JL, Laparte C, López-García G. Estudio de la circulación embrio-fetal en la gestación precoz normal mediante Doppler pulsado transvaginal. *Prog Diagn Prenat* 1997;9:456–66.
35. Rizzo G, Arduini D, Romanini C. Umbilical vein pulsations: A physiologic finding in early gestation. *Am J Obstet Gynecol* 1992;166:675–7.
36. Van Splunder P, Huisman TWA, De Ridder MAJ, Wladimiroff JW. Fetal venous and arterial flow velocity waveforms between eight and twenty weeks of gestation. *Pediatr Res* 1996;40: 158–62.
37. Mercé LT. Estudio Doppler durante la gestación precoz. In Kurjak A, Carrera JM, eds. *Ecografía en Medicina Materno-Fetal.* Barcelona: Masson, 2000:199–212.
38. Huisman TWA, Steward PA, Wladimiroff JW, Stijnen T. Flow velocity waveforms in the ductus venosus, umbilical vein and inferior vena cava in normal fetuses at 12–15 weeks of gestation. *Ultrasound Med Biol* 1993;19:441–5.
39. Kiserud T, Eik-Ness SH, Hellevik LR, Blaas H-G. Ductus venosus: A longitudinal Doppler velocimetric study of the human fetus. *J Matern Fetal Invest* 1992;2:5–11.
40. Huisman TWA, Stewart PA, Wladimiroff JW. Ductus venosus flow velocity waveforms in the human fetus: A Doppler study. *Ultrasound Med Biol* 1992;18:33–7.
41. Montenegro N, Matias A, Areias JC, Castedo S, Barros H. Increased fetal nuchal translucency: Possible involvement of early cardiac failure. *Ultrasound Obstet Gynecol* 1997;10:265–8.
42. Matias A, Gomes C, Flack N, Montenegro N, Nicolaides KH. Screening for chromosomal abnormalities at 10–14 weeks: The role of ductus venosus blood flow. *Ultrasound Obstet Gynecol* 1998;12:380–4.
43. Borrell A, Antolín E, Costa D, Farre MT, Martínez JM, Fortuny A. Abnormal ductus venosus blood flow in trisomy 21 fetuses during early pregnancy. *Am J Obstet Gynecol* 1998;179:1612–7.
44. Antolín E, Comas C, Torrents M. The role of ductus venosus blood flow assessment in screening for chromosomal abnormalities at 10–16 weeks of gestation. *Ultrasound Obstet Gynecol.* 2001;17:295–300.
45. Durfee SM, Frates MC. Sonographic spectrum of the corpus luteum in early pregnancy: Gray-scale, color, and pulsed Doppler appearance. *J Clin Ultrasound* 1999;27:55–9.
46. Zalud I, Kurjak A. The assessment of luteal blood flow in pregnant and non-pregnant women by transvaginal color Doppler. *J Perinat Med* 1990;18:215–21.
47. Alcázar JL, Acosta MJ, Laparte C, Ruiz ML. Assessment of luteal blood flow in normal early pregnancy. *J Ultrasound Med* 1996; 15:53–6.
48. Parsons AK. Imaging the human corpus luteum. *J Ultrasound Med* 2001;20:811–9.

99 Ultrasonographic signs of miscarriage

J. M. Bajo Arenas and T. Perez-Medina

Introduction

Recent advances in ultrasonographic technology along with the availability of high-frequency transvaginal transducers allow for more precise diagnosis. For every sonographist, the decision to inform the patient about the results of sonographic examination in relation to an interrupted pregnancy or embryonic death represents a challenge. The greater the experience, the earlier it can be confirmed that a pregnancy is actually not viable. It is not appropriate to confirm a diagnosis of miscarriage if any doubts exist, when most patients can wait without risk to their health. Nonetheless, it is good practice to write the suspected diagnosis in the clinical history to avoid unpleasant situations at the next sonographic examination. It is preferable to repeat the scan a few days later, to confirm that the pregnancy is 'not viable' if the diagnosis is not absolutely straightforward.

The problems for sonographists, especially for the less experienced ones, arise when they are required to reach definitive conclusions in the presence of signs corresponding to a pregnancy of less size than expected for the last menstrual period (LMP) without the aid of a previous sonographic examination. It needs to be decided if the pregnancy is of shorter duration or aborted. Some of the data that can be obtained will help in performing a diagnosis, and in other situations, enough information should be provided by the first sonographic examination to reach a definitive diagnosis; that is to say does not require confirmation with a subsequent sonographic examination. Repetition of the sonographic examination, 7–10 days later, should allow, in most of the cases, a definitive diagnosis to be reached.

Normal development of the pregnancy in the first trimester

If we know the chronology of appearance of the visible embryonic structures from sonography and its variations, it is possible to know whether the pregnancy is correctly evolving or not.

When findings that do not correspond to the gestational age are detected, the first thing to do should be to assess the possibility that an error exists in the LMP or that ovulation has not occurred on the 14th day of the cycle. In this situation, when the embryo is alive (positive heart beat) the only requirement is to correctly date the pregnancy in most cases. The LMP is calculated from the crown–rump length (CRL) and the date of the conception and the probable date of the childbirth are obtained. This is especially true when the pregnancy is of a longer duration than that corresponding to the LMP. When the data from the sonographic examination correspond to a pregnancy of shorter duration, that is to say, retarded ovulation, the approach is different, since finding a smaller embryo than expected is a risk factor for poor pregnancy outcome.

A useful adjunct to ultrasonography is the plasmatic determination of the β-hCG (hCG, human chorionic gonadotrophin) hormone (mIU/ml) between the fourth and eighth weeks of pregnancy. This determination is, among all those that can be performed during this period, the one from which the best clinical outcome has been obtained. Although there are wide variations from one pregnancy to another, it can be very useful. Normal course pregnancies duplicate the β-hCG levels in a period from 2 to 3 days, while abnormal pregnancies (ectopic or interrupted) usually show as irregular increases or, even, decreases. Simultaneous biochemical and sonographic data permit a useful perspective on the expected outcome in normal pregnancies. Essentially, it is necessary to know the β-hCG measurement system used in each one's own laboratory and adapt it to the medium.

Based on the capacity of sonography to predict the actual gestational age of different structures (the diameter of the gestational sac, the yolk sac and the CRL) within a 1-week margin, the diameter and growth of each structure from the moment of appearance are reflected in many tables by different authors.

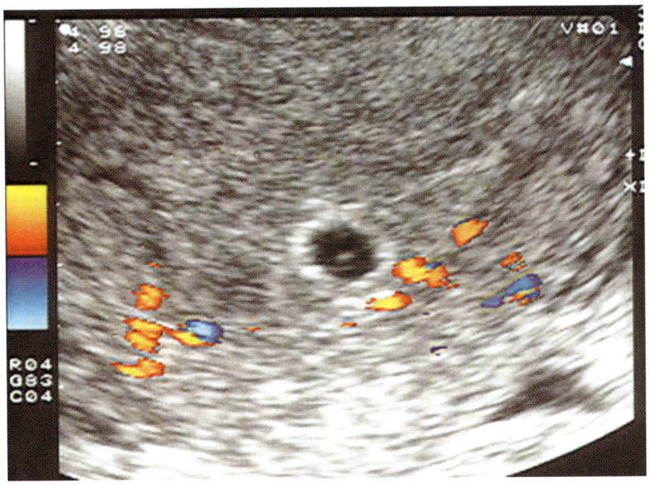

Figure 99.1 Gestational sacs more than 3–4 mm in diameter can be usually seen.

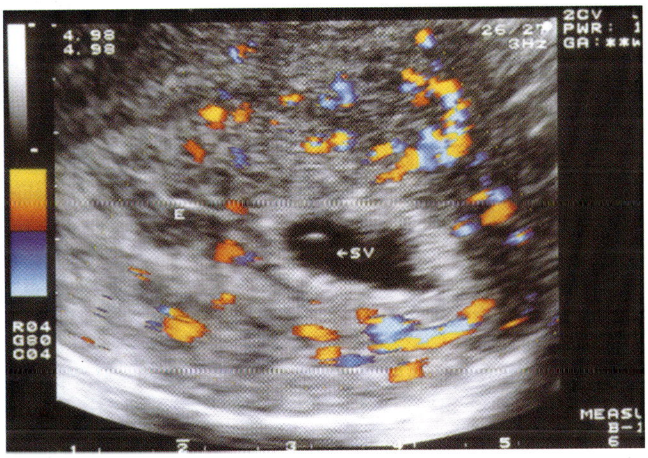

Figure 99.2 The yolk sac can be observed and measures 2–3 mm.

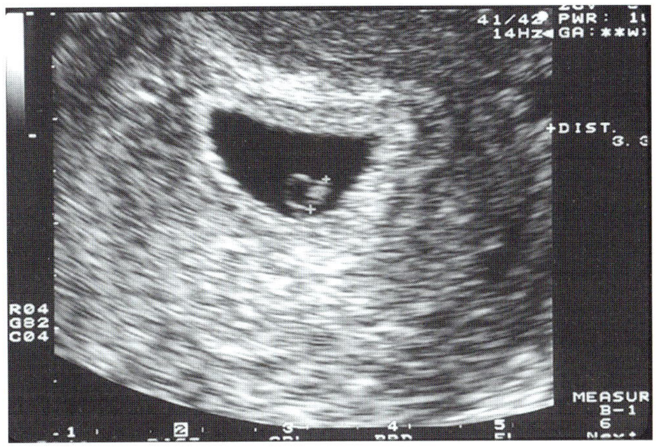

Figure 99.3 A 2–4 mm CRL embryo may be seen in the exploration.

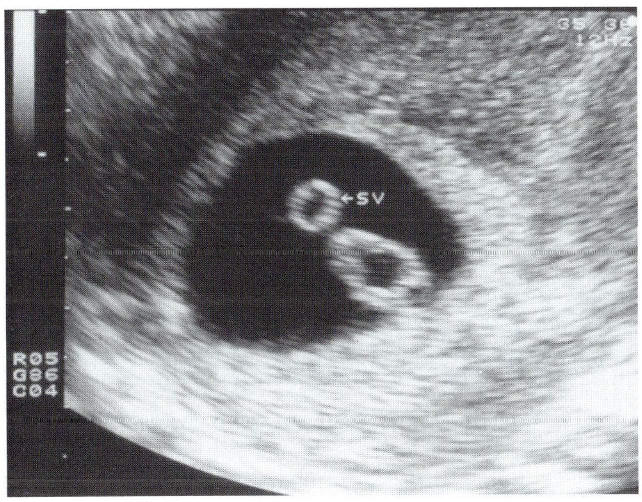

Figure 99.4 The amniotic vesicle is usually observed at the same time that the yolk sac (double bled sign).

Generally, a gestational sac of 3–4 mm average diameter can usually be seen (Figure 99.1). The size of the yolk sacs is 2–3 mm (Figure 99.2) and embryos have a CRL of 2–4 mm (Figure 99.3). The amniotic vesicle is usually identified at the same time as the yolk sac, and is known as the double-bled sign (Figure 99.4). The heart beat can be detected starting from a CRL of 3–4 mm in most cases (Figure 99.5), and is frequently detected before the embryonic echoes. Goldstein[1] states that the heart beat is present in the embryo a few days before detection by sonographic examination.

All the data obtained correspond to what is possible to visualize in normal pregnancies in patients in whom conception began 14 days after the LMP. Normal pregnancies that have begun before or after this will have differences with regard to the prospective findings, but the rhythm of change among successive sonographic examinations will be the same. So, after two sonographic examinations performed at least 1 week apart, starting from the moment when a gestational sac 5–10 mm in diameter has been visualized, a definitive diagnosis of the viability of the pregnancy can be obtained.

More than 80% of the sonographic examinations performed in the first trimester of pregnancy, in asymptomatic women without risk factors, will be normal. The earlier the first sonographic examination is performed, the higher will be the probability that we will find abnormal data or uncertain diagnoses, and the greater the probability that repetition of the sonographic examination will confirm normality. A pregnancy of 2 weeks less, in the 10th week will allow us to see a normal sac and a live embryo with 16 mm CRL, but if the sonographic examination is performed in the seventh week a small gestational sac of 8 or 10 mm diameter will probably be the only finding. The confirmation that a pregnancy is evolving correctly with a predicted of good outcome (low abortion probability) is only obtained when a live embryo is visualized and a history of associated risks does not

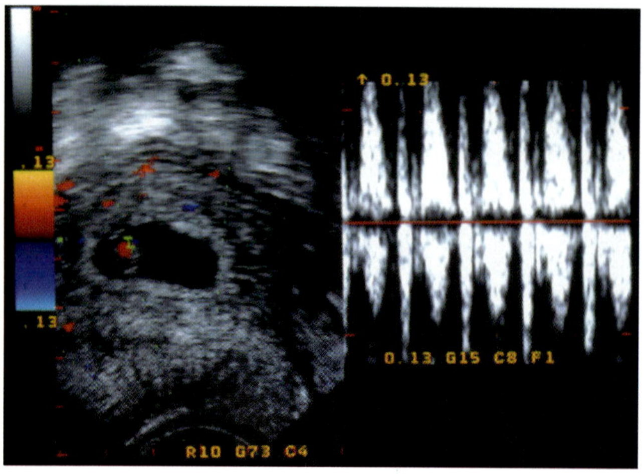

Figure 99.5 The heart motion can be detected in most cases starting from a 3–4 mm CRL embryo.

exist. On the other hand, confirmation that a pregnancy has been interrupted can only be made when an embryo is visualized of a certain size without heart beat. When there is no embryo, except in cases when the gestational sac has reached a large size, another sonographic examination 7–10 days later should be performed.

Spontaneous interruptions of the development of conception

The frequency of spontaneous interruptions of the reproductive development process is very high, especially when considered from the earliest stages. It is calculated that of each 100 potential pregnancies only 31 will carry to term with a live fetus.[2,3] The frequency of miscarriage, considered as the spontaneous interruption of the pregnancy before the fetus has reached viability, depends therefore on the approach that we use to define pregnancy. When considering pregnancies reaching implantation (biochemical pregnancy), the miscarriage frequency ranges from 30% to 40%.[4,5] On reaching the clinical diagnosis of pregnancy, the frequency is reduced to 10–15%. If the pregnancy progresses until the 12th week, the probability of abortion decreases to 3–4%. When the embryo is alive in the 12th week, the abortion rate until the 20th week is only 2%.[6]

Siddiqi *et al.*[7] report that in pregnancies under 12 weeks, controls had 5.2% of miscarriages, while cases that presented with bleeding had 16.4%. Also, when the patient is older than 34 years, the frequency increased to 11.1%, in comparison with patients under 35 years, in whom the frequency was only 4.4%. Levi *et al.*[8] found a 24% rate of abortions when positive heart beat existed but the embryo has a CRL less than 5 mm.

Table 99.1 Probability of spontaneous abortion according to the sonographic findings (from Goldstein[9])

Structure visualized	Probability of abortion (%)
Gestational sac	11.5
Yolk sac	8.5
Embryo CRL < 5 mm	7.2
Embryo CRL 6–10 mm	3.3
Embryo CRL > 10 mm	0.5

Goldstein[9] presents his data with great clinical applicability, allowing us to assess the probability of miscarriage as a function of the sonographic findings, as shown in Table 99.1.

Choong *et al.*,[10] in a series of 322 pregnant women, conclude that the most discriminatory test for predicting spontaneous miscarriage of a live embryo is a personalized multivariate analysis model, constructed with the LMP, CRL, embryonic heart rate, mean sac diameter and maternal age as the variables, with an area under the curve equal to 0.87 in their receiver operating characteristic (ROC) curve.

Embryonic and fetal causes, basically chromosomal anomalies, are the most frequent causes of miscarriage.[11] The different rates reported depend on the approaches used (whether only clinical pregnancies are considered or not). In the first weeks they can account for 80–90% of the cases. After the 12th week, the chromosomal anomalies and malformations are less relevant, although they continue to be an important cause. From this time on, maternal and environmental causes acquire more importance.

Knowledge of the frequency of spontaneous miscarriage, from the very beginning, along with theoretical knowledge of the causes of the abortion, should provide a perspective to the obstetrician who, when performing a sonographic examination, finds parameters not corresponding to a normal pregnancy. Earlier sonographic examinations in the pregnancy will allow diagnosis of many more cases of spontaneous interruptions in pregnancy.

Poor prognosis of pregnancy. Sonographic findings (Table 99.2)

Some circumstances, when present in a sonographic examination performed in the first trimester of the pregnancy, indicate a poor prognosis. Although they do not allow a definitive diagnosis of 'interruption of development,' they indicate that the prognosis for normal outcome is reduced. In the days prior to their detection, some phenomena are usually observed.

However, none of them are sufficiently reliable to give a definitive diagnosis. To be able to diagnose an abortion, or embryonic death, it is necessary to check the existence of an embryo of 5 mm CRL minimum in which heart beat is lacking.

Anomalies of the gestational sac

The gestational sac and the CRL develop simultaneously. It is possible to check whether, between the 6th and the 10th weeks, the difference usually overcomes the 15–20 mm limit. Other authors[12,13] report that when the difference between the diameter of the gestational sac and CRL is less than 5 mm (*precocious oligoamnion*), miscarriage occurs in 95% of cases (Figure 99.6). Dickey *et al.*[14] report that when the difference between these two measures was less than 5 mm, miscarriage occurred in 80% of the cases; when the difference was between 5 and 7.9 mm, miscarriage occurred in 26.5% of cases, and when the difference was more than 8 mm, miscarriage occurred in only 10.6% of cases.

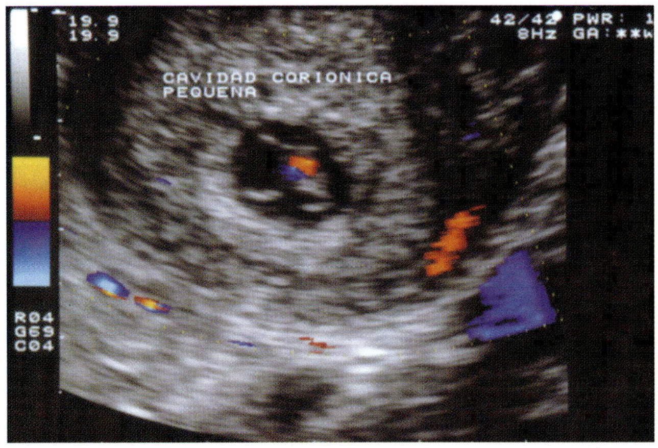

Figure 99.6 Gestational sac showing precocious oligoamnion; a good predictor for abortion.

Anomalies of the heart frequency interpreted as a function of the gestational age or CRL

Bradycardia or relative bradycardia

Increase in the fetal heart rate (FHR) until the 10th week is characteristic; it rises from 90 beats per minute (bpm) in the first weeks of visualization up to 180–190 bpm in the 12th week. From this time, FHR diminishes progressively until it reaches 140–150 bpm in the 20th week. However, important variations exist in the frequency reported by different authors in every week of pregnancy. Merchiers *et al.*[15] give importance to the observation that a decrease of the heart frequency occurs in two successive sonographic examinations. For Laboda *et al.*[16] a FHR under 85 bpm indicates a very poor prognosis, since in their series all the embryos that presented this finding, ended in miscarriages. May and Sturtevant[17] also associate poor prognosis with this finding: 6 out of 11 cases with FHR under 85 bpm between the 4.5th and the 7.3rd week miscarried.

Benson[18] sets the limit as 90 bpm for the whole first trimester to indicate a poor prognosis. In his series, all cases that had a FHR under 70 bpm ended in abortion; between 70 and 79 bpm, 91% had abortions, and between 80 and 89 bpm, 70% had abortions. Doubilet and Benson[19] suggest that a FHR more than 100 bpm until the 6.2nd week and more than 120 bpm between the 6.3rd and the 7th week, are signs of a good prognosis. They consider it a sign of a poor prognosis if a FHR of less than 110 bpm in the 7th and 8th weeks is observed. Stefos *et al.*[20] report in their series that when there is a FHR under 85 bpm between the sixth and eighth week, it is unlikely any fetus will survive. For these authors, when the FHR is between 116 and 125 bpm between the sixth and the seventh week, the prognosis is good, as it is when the FHR is more than 146 bpm between the eighth and the ninth week. No finding, except the absence of heart beat, provides a definitive diagnosis of embryonic death. However, the scientific evidence allows a more precise diagnosis. In general, heart frequencies under 85 bpm until the seventh week and under 100 bpm from this time on, are associated with an adverse result and high probability of abortion.

Anomalies of the yolk sac (size, shape, ecogenicity)

The yolk sac is the first extraembryonic structure that appears and it is visible in practically all pregnancies between the 5th and the 12th weeks. The yolk sac can be observed initially when the diameter of the gestational sac reaches 3.7 mm, on the 36th day from the LMP and is reliably observed when the diameter is 6.7 mm, on the 40th day of amenorrhea. Furthermore, according to Levi *et al.*[8] the yolk sac should always be observed when the diameter of the gestational sac is more than 8 mm (corresponding to 33 days), so that its absence would mean a better approach for gestational loss.

The importance of the visibility of the yolk sac for ecographists arises from the fact that it is the first identifiable structure in the gestational sac, preceding by 4–7 days visualization of the embryo. Its characteristic feature is an ecogenic circle that defines a sonoluscent area inside an extra-amniotically located chorionic cavity.

Some anomalies are described in their initial development as shape and volume alterations.[21,22]

In general, it is difficult to make important clinical decisions (such as diagnosing a pregnancy interruption) based on findings related to the yolk sac. This is a structure with important variations with regard to its size and dimensions. Visualization is also not absolutely safe, even in pregnancies of normal course. The alterations at this level are usually late, and it is believed that they are a consequence of the process that determines the miscarriage, not the cause. However, several publications have reported their measurement, the assessment of their characteristics, and the analysis of their association with a poor pregnancy outcome.

Lindsay *et al.*[23] report that the existence of a yolk sac of more than 2 standard deviations (SD) above that expected for the gestational age indicates a poor prognosis. All cases evolved unfavorably when a yolk sac bigger than 5.6 mm was observed before the 10th week in their series (Figures 99.7–99.9). This agrees with the data from Kupesic and Kurjak,[24] who report a poor prognosis with yolk sacs with abnormal size and abnormal Doppler vascularization. Perez-Medina *et al.*[25] report the changes in the yolk sac with respect to size, shape or the echogenicity are parameters that guide the normal or pathological development of the pregnancy. Of the 100 patients in their series, 87 (87%) had a normal development and evolved correctly until the end of the first trimester (control group); 13 (13%) had an abnormal course of the pregnancy (study group). Of the 87 patients with correct development, three had a yolk sac diameter of more than 1 SD. Of the 13 patients with abnormal course, six had a yolk sac diameter greater than 1 SD. They conclude that the sensitivity of the size of the yolk sac to predict an abnormal course of the pregnancy is 92.3%, the specificity is 66.6%, the positive predictive value (PPV) is 96.5% and the negative predictive value (NPV) is 46%; and when some of these anomalies appear, it is necessary to follow the pregnancy closely.

The regressive yolk sac is sonographically observed by a progressive increase of refrigency until a more extreme form that would indicate calcification of the sac (Figure 99.10).

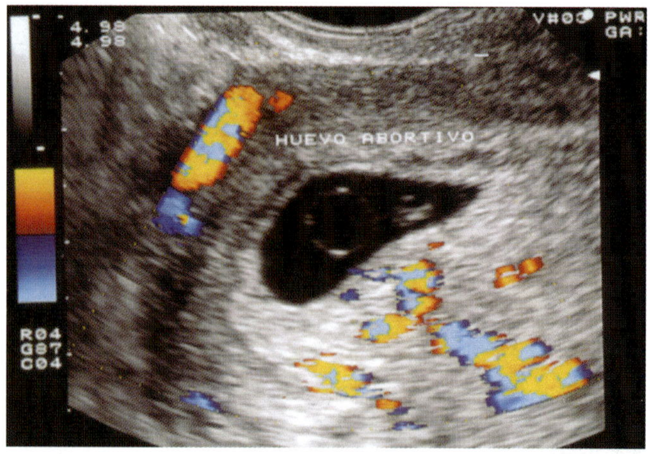

Figure 99.7 Yolk sac of 8 mm (more than 2 standard deviations for the gestational age).

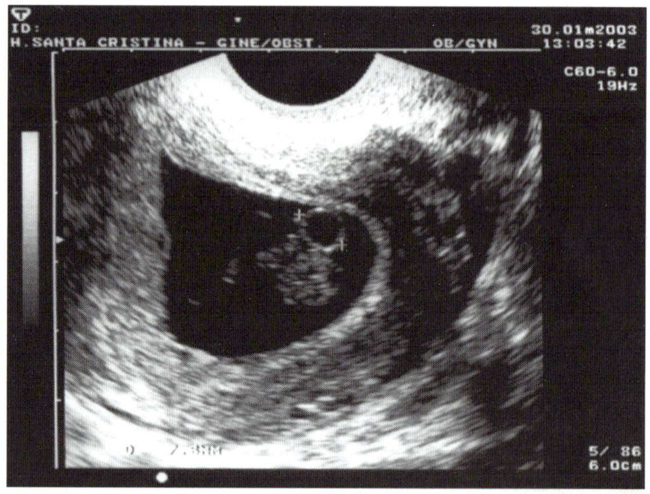

Figure 99.8 Giant yolk sac, a sign that is rapidly and easily appreciated in the sonographic examination.

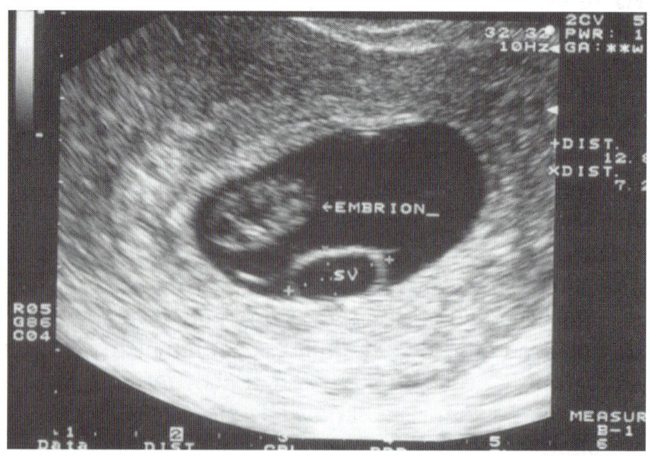

Figure 99.9 Gestational sac of 9 mm. This is a very sensitive marker for abortion.

Trophoblastic thickness at the embryonic implantation site

Bajo and colleagues[26] describe the trophoblastic thickness at the embryonic implantation site in a prospective, observational study in 592 normal pregnancies in whom serial ultrasound scans were performed from the 5th to the 12th week of pregnancy. Trophoblastic thickness was measured at the embryonic implantation site to determine the significance of the difference between the gestational age in weeks and the trophoblastic thickness in millimeters. A difference of more than 3 was highly predictive of a poor pregnancy outcome (Figure 99.11). The sensitivity of this sign in the prediction of spontaneous abortion was 82%, the specificity was 93%, the positive predictive value was 63% and the negative predictive value was 97%.

Intra-uterine bleeding. Subchorionic and retroplacental hematomas

The existence of liquid collections, mainly in subchorionic locations, is a relatively frequent finding in the sonographic examinations performed during the first trimester of pregnancy (Figure 99.12). From some of these images it is evident that some have a huge size and coincide with clinical symptomatology

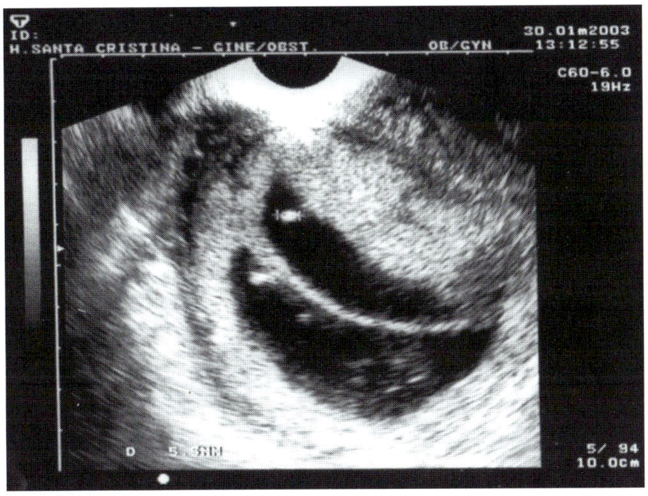

Figure 99.10 The regressive yolk sac is observed when there is a progressive increase of the internal refrigency as seen in both yolk sacs of this double pregnancy.

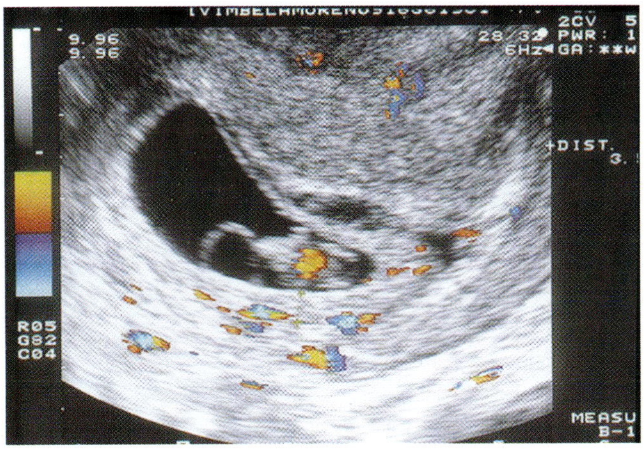

Figure 99.12 The existence of subchorionic liquid collections is a frequent finding in examinations performed in the first trimester.

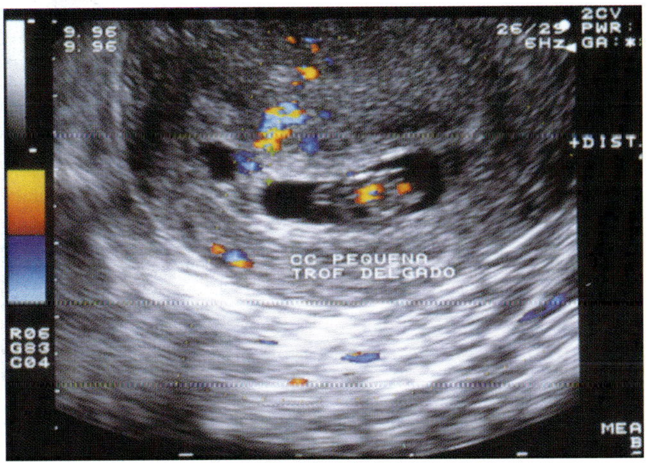

Figure 99.11 A thin trophoblast is observed. A difference of more than 3 between gestational age (weeks) and the trophoblastic thickness (mm) is highly predictive of a poor pregnancy outcome.

(vaginal bleeding), while others are casual findings in asymptomatic women and have a minimum volume. Discrepancies exist with regard to the risks and their association with abortion when used for the diagnosis of intra-uterine hemorrhage. Dickey *et al.*[27] demonstrated using Doppler color that in 37% of sonographic examinations in the first trimester subchorionic bleeding exists, and that in 47% of cases, subchorionic liquid is detected. They conclude that the liquid and the subchorionic bleeding are frequent findings during early pregnancy and are not associated with embryonic death unless accompanied by vaginal bleeding. Stabile *et al.*[28] state that the existence of small subchorionic hematomas (less than 16 ml) in women with genital bleeding does not increase the risk of miscarriage in comparison with women with bleeding without hematoma.

With regard to the diagnosis from the size and the localization of the hematoma, Glavind *et al.*[29] do not find a relationship between the size of the hematoma and the week of pregnancy in which the diagnosis was performed. For these authors retrochorionic or subplacental localization have a worse prognosis than subchorionic localization (Figure 99.13). According to Kurjak *et al.*[30] subchorionic hematomas influence abortion frequency (17% in a study group vs. 6.5% in a control group). Neither has a significant influence on the size of the hematoma, the localization being more important. Hematomas in the uterine corpus or fundus have a worse prognosis than those located near the uterine cervix (Figure 99.14). In another report, Kurjak *et al.*[31] find a higher RI of the spiral arteries in cases with retrochorionic hematoma than in controls, due to compression from the hematoma.

According to Ball *et al.*[32] it is not clear if the subchorionic bleeding is the cause or simply an underlying process that produces negative effects. They present an interesting study in which the patients are divided into three groups: the first is formed of women who present with subchorionic bleeding; the second is a control group of women without hematoma, and the third is another control group without hematoma but with vaginal bleeding. When these authors perform comparisons with controls without bleeding, an odds ratio (OR) 2.8 is obtained for abortion, 4.5 for stillbirth, 11.2 for abruptio placentae and 2.6 for preterm birth. When compared with controls with bleeding all the ORs increase except that for abortion. The weight at birth is diminished when compared with the two control groups. Genital bleeding by itself is able to increase the risk of miscarriage. Bennet *et al.*[33] compare the abortion frequency in women with genital bleeding and subchorionic hemorrhage. When the hematoma is big, the frequency of abortions is 18.8%; if medium, 9.2%; and if small 7.7%. When the

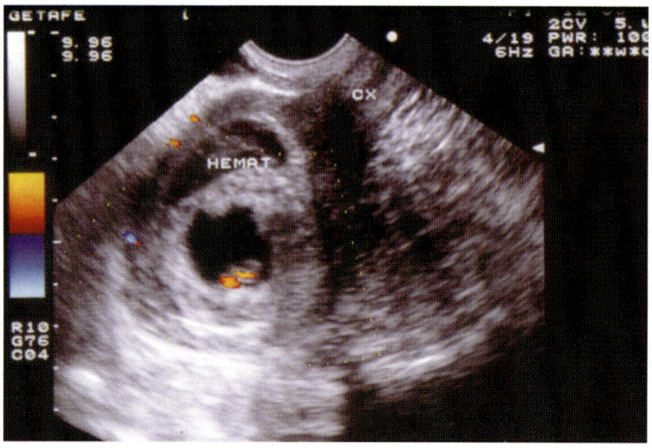

Figure 99.13 Retrochorionic or subplacental localization has a worse prognosis than subchorionic localization.

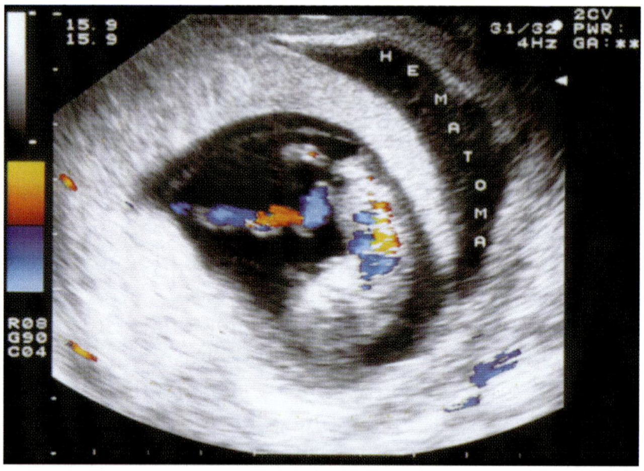

Figure 99.14 Hematomas located in the uterine corpus or fundus have a worse prognosis than those located near the uterine cervix.

woman is older than 35 years, the abortion rate is 13.8%, in comparison with 7.3% in women younger than 35 years. When the bleeding appeared before the eighth week, the frequency was 13.7%, while if it appeared later than the eighth week, the rate was reduced to 5.9%.

The presence of a small quantity of retrocorial liquid has fewer implications, when it is observed as an isolated finding, and in the context of a normal sonographic examination in a pregnancy of normal course. The existence of a subchorionic hemorrhage, especially when associated with vaginal bleeding, increases the abortion risk and requires another sonographic examination a few days later. New sonographic examinations are justified when small or moderate hemorrhages exist. The worst prognosis comes with large-sized hematomas (more than 40–50 ml), especially if located next to the uterine cervix, in the uterine corpus or fundus. Retrochorionic or subplacental hematomas, especially if moderate or big, always carry a poor diagnosis.

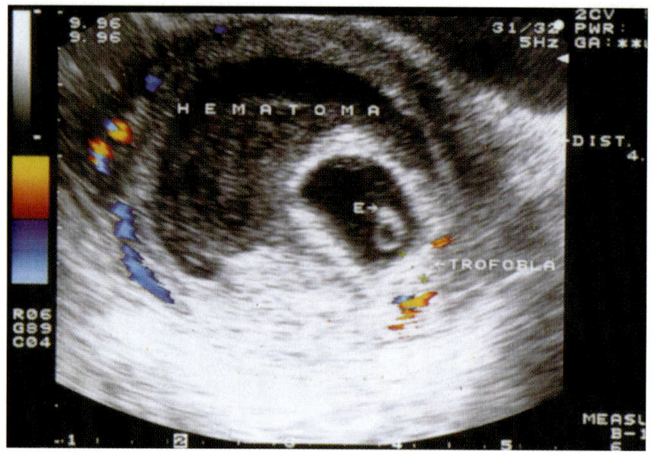

Figure 99.15 Large hematoma causing distortion in the gestational sac.

The frequency of visualization of these images is low, probably because a rapid corial detachment develops leading to the miscarriage, with bleeding and expulsion of debris. Another uncommon type of hematoma or intra-uterine bleeding is the preplacental bleeding that appears after invasive techniques that require the introduction of a needle into the uterine cavity. In general, these hematoma are moderate and evolve favorably although threatened miscarriage in the first trimester is associated with an increased incidence of adverse pregnancy outcome, independent of the presence of an intrauterine hematoma.[34] Nagy *et al.*[35]compared perinatal outcome in 187 pregnant women with intrauterine hematoma and 6488 controls in whom hematomas were not detected in the first trimester. They conclude that the sonographic presence of an intrauterine hematoma during the first trimester identifies a population of patients at increased risk for adverse pregnancy outcome.[35] On other occasions they reach such a volume that they result in occupation of the chorionic cavity, with the end effect of fetal death because of the compression (Figure 99.15).

Small CRL for the gestational age

In general, when a small-for-gestational-age CRL with positive heart beat embryo is observed, a pregnancy of shorter duration is the first diagnosis to exclude. This is frequent in women with long or irregular cycles. However, sometimes this may be observed in women with normal cycles. First of all, the date of conception should be corrected, but data that allow the association of this alteration with a higher risk of poor pregnancy outcome exist (Figure 99.16).

Koornstr and Exalto[36] report that 22.7% of embryos from women with regular cycles have a lower CRL in 1 week or more than expected from the LMP. On analyzing the results it is observed that among these embryos a rate of abortions of 16% existed, in comparison with only 5% in the embryos with a correct LMP.

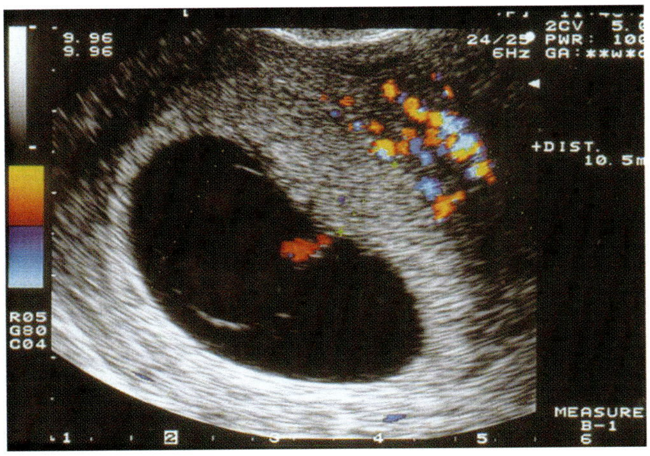

Figure 99.16 Small CRL for the gestational age, as referred to the gestational sac.

Leelapatana *et al.*[37] report that a small CRL for gestational age during the first trimester of pregnancy could be associated with tryploidies, but not with trisomy 18 and 21. Later, Bessho *et al.*[38] reported that fetuses ending in miscarriage had a quotient of measured CRL/ expected CRL of 0.74, in comparison with the 0.98 observed in fetuses that did not miscarry. These authors did not find differences in the quotient among chromosomally normal and abnormal fetuses. This result has also been confirmed in the series from Coulam *et al.*[39] who found no differences in the frequency of blighted ovum and small CRL for gestational age among chromosomally normal and abnormal fetuses.

Pattern of fetal movements

Along with the sonographic chronology of findings in a normal pregnancy, the existence and verification of fetal movements should be observed.

In a classic publication by Anderson[40] the results presented were obtained in a series of 149 cases of threatened abortion and of more than 7 weeks of gestational age. Only 2 of 65 pregnancies that later aborted presented fetal movements. On the other hand, 64 of 72 normal pregnancies presented fetal movements. So the absence of fetal movements after a relatively long period of sonographic examination, especially after the eighth week, should also be considered as a sign of poor prognosis.

Doppler flow alterations

The number of publications during the few last few years regarding the Doppler velocimetry in the first stages of normal and pathological pregnancies is large. The data that the investigators have contributed has enormously improved our knowledge of the phenomena that exist in the placentation process and development of the embryo. Kurjak and Kupesic[41] report that the process of trophoblastic invasion of the decidua is progressive, mediated by the action of proteolytic enzymes that facilitate the penetration and maternal erosion of the capillary arteries and the formation of lagoons. There are flow changes that can be measured in the uterine, retrochorionic and intervillous arteries during the first trimester of pregnancy (Figure 99.17). This is the reason why the pulsatility index (PI) and high resistance index (RI) in the first trimester should not be interpreted as a bad result, as it would be in the second trimester, as Jaffe *et al.*[42] report. Jaffe and Woods[43] explain how the intervillous circulation persists until the late first trimester. In complicated pregnancies, analyzed early, the utero-placental circulation is different from that in normal pregnancies. In these abnormal pregnancies the intervillous flow is increased. The hypothesis, based on other studies, is that the embryo of a pregnancy of normal course favors an atmosphere with a low concentration of tissular oxygen in placental tissues. Martin *et al.*[44] explain that the increased impedance to flow in the uterine arteries in the first trimester is associated with the development of pre-eclampsia and intrauterine growth retardation (likelihood ratios of 5 and 2, respectively).

Mercé *et al.*[45] measured the velocity of systolic peak, PI and RI in retrochorionic arteries and the fetal umbilical artery in 108 pregnancies between the 4th and 15th weeks. The earliest sign in the retrochorionic circulation was obtained in the 4.5th week, and the earliest in the umbilical artery at the end of the 5th week. Their results indicate that, as gestational age increases, the systolic peak of the retrochorionic, intervillous and umbilical arteries increase, while PI and RI diminish. Kurjak and Kupesic[46] assessed yolk sac morphology and vascularity, and intervillous blood flow in normal early pregnancy and missed abortion, in a prospective analysis of 87 normal pregnancies and 48 missed abortions between 6 and 12 weeks' gestation. They concluded that progressive decrease of the yolk sac vascularity coincides with visualization of more prominent color-coded areas within the intervillous space. In patients with missed abortion, such changes do not occur.

In general, most authors do not find differences in the Doppler indexes among normal outcome pregnancies and those ending in miscarriage. Jauniaux *et al.*[47] compared 30 confirmed abortions with 30 normal pregnancies. The PI of the uterine artery was higher in the abortions than in the normal pregnancies. Differences were not observed in RI and systolic peak of the uterine artery, nor in PI nor RI of spiral arteries among abortions and normal pregnancies. These authors concluded that the velocity of abnormal flow found in some complicated pregnancies with embryonic death could be related to a defective placentation and 'dislocation' of the trophoblastic wall, after which embryonic death follows. The premature access of maternal blood to the intervillous space could break

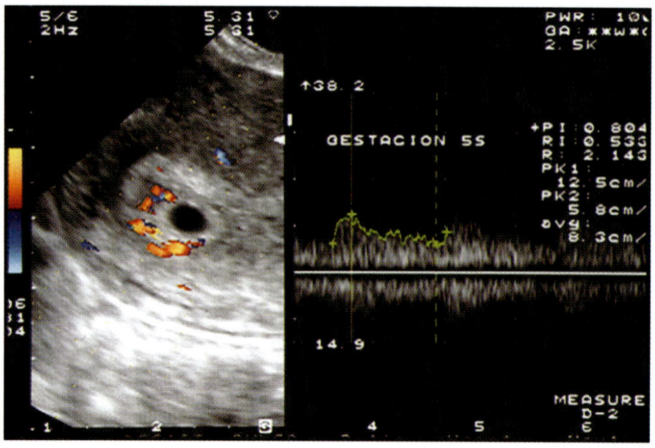

Figure 99.17 Doppler flows can be obtained in the retrochorionic and intervillous arteries in the first trimester of pregnancy.

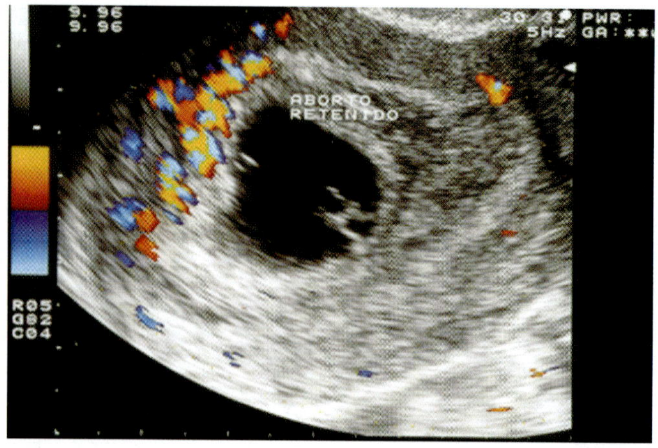

Figure 99.19 The use of transvaginal color Doppler is not helpful for predicting pregnancy outcome in living embryos.

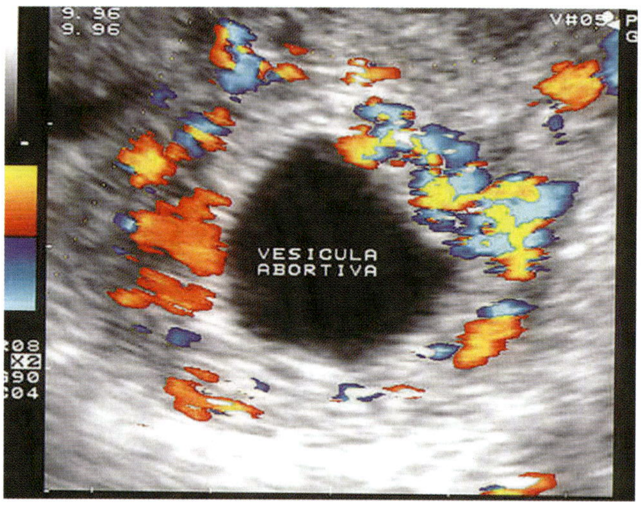

Figure 99.18 The premature access of maternal blood to the intervillous space has broken the embryonic–maternal interface, probably the cause of abortion.

the embryonic–maternal interface, and could be the cause of miscarriage (Figure 99.18). Alcazar and Ruiz-Perez[48] report that no apparent alteration occurs in the early uteroplacental circulation in patients with threatened abortion with a living embryo. So the use of transvaginal color Doppler ultrasound is not helpful for predicting pregnancy outcome in cases of threatened abortion (Figure 99.19).

Salim *et al.*[49] measured PI and RI at the level of the corpus luteum. The pregnancies with threatened abortion or ending in abortion show higher values than normal pregnancies. However, they did not observe differences when comparing data from ectopic pregnancies, hydatidiform moles, or anembryonic pregnancies. Alcazar *et al.*[50] measured the flows at the level of the corpus luteum, and did not find differences among controls, threatened abortion or blighted ovum. In pregnancies with confirmed miscarriage, the values of RI are higher.

Other factors to consider (clinical factors)

- Maternal age more than 35–40 years
- Presence of uterine bleeding
- Time of commencement of uterine bleeding
- Hormonal dynamics determination (β-hCG)
- Reproductive history (one or more previous miscarriages)
- Existence of associate pathology (multiple myomas or submucosos, uterine malformations).

Sonographic findings to diagnose an interrupted pregnancy (Table 99.3)

The two types of spontaneous interruptions of pregnancy in patients without bleeding are, from a practical point of view, deferred or missed abortions, and the blighted ovum or anembryonic pregnancies. Academically, *deferred* abortions were considered as those in which the measured CRL corresponded to 6 weeks less than that expected in an embryo lacking heart beat (Figure 99.20). Nowadays, due to the greater availability of initial sonographic examination, the diagnosis is made before the bleeding begins. Therefore, this kind of miscarriage, when the interruption is recent and bleeding has not begun, is called *missed* abortion. With regard to the anembryonic pregnancies, their frequency is much lower than is thought from a clinical point of view. There could be pregnancies initially with an embryo, that died precociously and was reabsorbed, so was not sonographically visualized. Not all gestational sacs in which an amniotic or a yolk sac is observed, although an embryo is not seen, correspond to anembryonic pregnancies, since these structures require the development of an embryo if they are to appear (Figure 99.21).

The false positive diagnoses, the really important fails, are of two types. The first is when the sonographist is not able to detect the heart beat in an embryo that actually has heart motion. This can be

Table 99.2 Ultrasonographic signs of a poor prognosis for embryonic viability

Anomalies of the gestational sac	Precocious oligoamnion: when the difference between the diameter average of the gestational sac and the CRL is smaller than 5 mm, poor prognosis
	Very thin decidual reaction (mm) for the corresponding gestational age (weeks) (difference > 3)
	Low implantation
	Distorted aspect
Alterations of the heart frequency	Bradycardia is always a sign of poor prognosis. It should be interpreted as a function of the gestational age
	Frequencies under 85 bpm until the 7th week and under 100 bpm from then on indicate poor diagnosis
Small live embryo for the LMP	Especially in women with regular cycles, the visualization of a CRL smaller by at least 1 week to that corresponding to the LMP, increases the risk for abortion
Anomalies of the yolk sac	Alterations in size (big vesicles, more than 6 mm in diameter) increase the risk
	Alterations in the structure (hyperecogenic vesicle), poor prognosis
Reverse implantation	Risk of abortion increases
Intra-uterine bleeding (hematomas)	Big hematomas, mainly retrochorionic, maximum risk. Subchorionic hematomas located in corpus or fundus, more risk than next to the uterine cervix
	If no vaginal bleeding or small size of hematoma, low risk
Fetal movements	Absence of fetal movements, starting from the 8th week
Doppler	Poor color map around the gestational sac
	Values of Doppler flow in uterine, radial, arcuata, spiral, retrochorial and intervillous arteries, as well as the umbilical artery in the first trimester of pregnancy have limited clinical applicability
Other factors	Existence of associated pathology: myomas, malformations
	Uterine hemorrhage
	Maternal age over 35 years
	History of one or more abortions (more abortions, more risk)
	Serial hormonal determinations. Two β-hCG determinations separated by2–3 days

Table 99.3 Ultrasonographic signs in the interrupted pregnancy

Embryonic death (deferred or missed miscarriage)	Absence of heart beat in embryo of minimum 5 mm CRL (even in the first sonographic examination)
Blighted ovum or anembryonic pregnancy	Gestational sac of 25 mm or more without embryo (even in the first sonographic examination)
	For some authors, gestational sac of 20 mm or more without yolk sac
	Gestational sac of 16 mm or more with yolk sac and amniotic vesicle without embryo ('empty amnion')
Interrupted pregnancy	Successive sonographic examinations: absence of significant changes in two sonographic examinations separated by 7–10 days when in the first sonographic examination a gestational sac of 15–20 mm minimum has been visualized

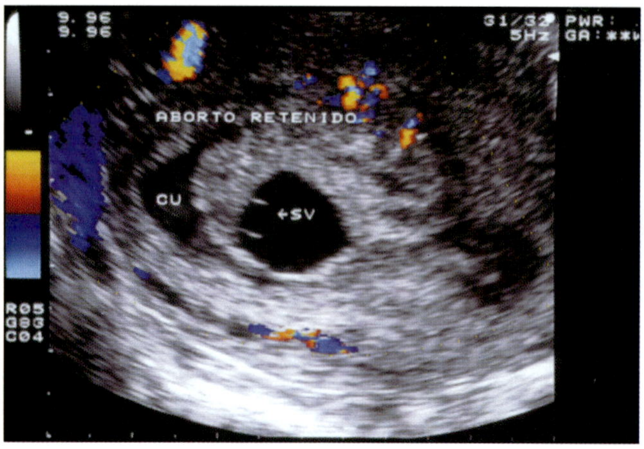

Figure 99.20 Deferred abortion.

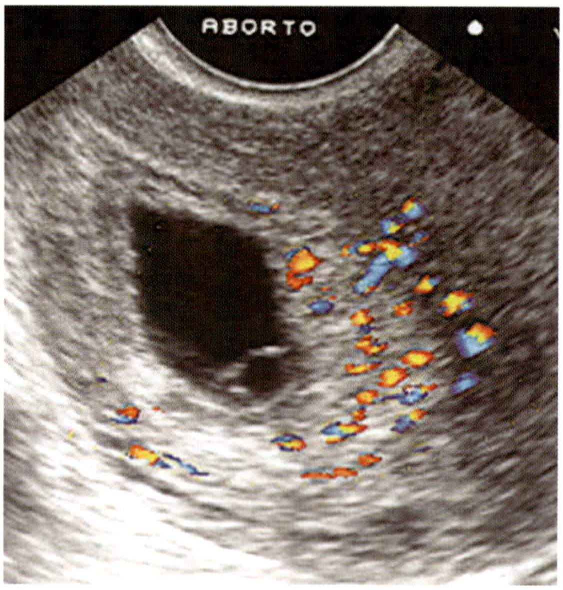

Figure 99.21 A gestational sac with a yolk sac but lacking embryo corresponding to a missed abortion.

caused by a small size of the embryo, inadequate or obsolete equipment, or suboptimal visualization due to patient's characteristics. The other type of error would be to consider that before a certain size of gestational sac an embryo must be seen. This error is caused by the selection of a low level from which to diagnose anembryonic pregnancy, and this level could correspond to the highest range in normality. In the first case, for instance, in an embryo of 4–5 mm in which one had not seen a heart beat, after one week one might see it when measured at 9–10 mm. In the second case, in a 21 mm diameter vesicle, in which the embryo was not seen, after 1 week a 5–6 mm CRL and positive heart beat embryo may be observed.

According to Daya *et al.*[51] an embryo is not seen until the gestational sac measures 8.3 mm diameter, coincident with the 41st day of amenorrhea. However, it is always observed when the gestational sac reaches 14 mm in diameter, on the 46th day of amenorrhea (6 weeks and 4 days). Goldstein *et al.*[52] report that when the pregnancy is correctly developing, the gestational sac is reliably observed in the fifth week. When the sac measures 20 mm in diameter, the embryo is observed in 100% of the cases. At 6 weeks and 4 days (46th day of amenorrhea) a heart beat is observed in 100% of cases, and when the diameter is 30 mm, in 100% of the normal cases, embryonic movements are already present (8 weeks).

Norwitz *et al.*[53] confirm the importance of examination at the very beginning of the pregnancy. To confirm the diagnosis of 'embryonic death' at the first sonographic examination, the CRL should be longer than 10 mm. Levi *et al.*[8] consider all gestational sacs of more than 8 mm diameter without yolk sac and of 16 mm or more without embryo as 'not viable'. They diagnose embryonic death when the embryo is between 4 and 5 mm CRL. Several cases with CRL smaller than 4 mm in which heart beat was not detected evolved correctly in their series.

Brown *et al.*[54] recommends waiting until the CRL is 5 mm to confirm embryonic demise if a heart beat is not detected. Bernard and Cooperberg,[55] in differentiation among blighted ovum and 'viable precocious pregnancy', consider that although the visualization of sacs with 20 mm or more without embryo is a sign of poor prognosis, definitive signs do not exist, and so recommend repeating the sonographic examination after 1–2 weeks. Nyberg *et al.*[56] wait to observe a gestational sac of more than 20 mm in diameter without yolk sac or a sac of 25 mm diameter with distorted aspect without embryo before considering a pregnancy as not viable.

McKenna *et al.*[57] report that between the 6th and the 10th week, the amniotic cavity is similar to the size of the embryo, and the visualization of an amniotic cavity without embryo corresponded to an 'empty amnion' and diagnosed interrupted pregnancy. These authors report that before the gestational sac reaches 16 mm or more, when the yolk sac is identified and neither embryo nor heart beat are detected, and an empty amniotic sac is seen, an interrupted pregnancy can be diagnosed.

In conclusion, to diagnose embryonic death, it is essential to wait to see an embryo lacking heart beat with a CRL of 5 mm minimum. For the diagnosis of blighted ovum or anembryonic pregnancy at a first sonographic examination, it seems reasonable to wait till the gestational sac reaches 25 mm, equivalent to 7 weeks pregnancy with conception on the 14th day of the cycle. This corresponds to a pregnancy in which, in 100% of cases, a live embryo would be visualized if correctly developed. In all other cases, the sonographic examination must be repeated after 7–10 days. In the great majority of cases, the second examination will allow us to confirm a normal or interrupted pregnancy.

REFERENCES

1. Goldstein MR. Significance of cardiac activity on endovaginal ultrasound in very early embryos. *Obstet Gynecol* 1992;80: 670–2.
2. Barri PN. Pérdidas embrionarias preimplantatorias. In Carrera JM, Kurjak A, eds. *Medicina del Embrión*. Barcelona: Masson, 1996:143–8.
3. Leridon H. *Human Fertility*. Chicago, IL: Chicago Press, 1977.
4. De la Fuente P. Aborto espontáneo. In Fabre E, ed. *Manual de Asistencia a la Patología Obstétrica*. Zaragoza: INO Reproducciones, 1997:73–87.
5. Knudsen UB, Hansen V, Juul S, Secher NJ. Prognosis to new pregnancy following previous spontaneous miscarriages. *Eur J Obstet Gynecol Reprod Biol* 1991;39:31–6.
6. Cashner KA, Christopher CR, Dysert GA. Spontaneous fetal loss after demonstration of to live fetus in the first trimester. *Obstet Gynecol* 1987;70:827–30.
7. Siddiqi TA, Caligaris JT, Miodovnik M, Holroyde JC, Mimouni F. Rate of spontaneous abortion after first trimester sonographic demonstration of fetal cardiac activity. *Am J Perinatol* 1988;5:1–4.
8. Levi CS, Lyons EA, Zheng XH, Lindsay DJ, Holt SC. Endovaginal US: Demonstration of cardiac activity in embryos of less than 5.0 mm in crown-rump length. *Radiology* 1990;176:71–4.
9. Goldstein MR. Embryonic death in early pregnancy: A new look at the first trimester. *Obstet Gynecol* 1994;84:294–7.
10. Choong S, Rombauts L, Ugoni A, Meagher S. Ultrasound prediction of risk of spontaneous miscarriage in live embryos from assisted conceptions. *Ultrasound Obstet Gynecol* 2003;22: 571–7.
11. Phillip T, Phillip K, Reiner A, Beer F, Kalousek DK. Embryoscopic and cytogenetic analysis of 233 missed abortions: Factors involved in the pathogenesis of developmental defects of early failed pregnancies. *Hum Reprod* 2003;18:1724–32.
12. Bromley B, Harlow BL, Laboda LA, Benacerraf BR. Small sac size in the first trimester: A predictor of poor fetal outcome. *Radiology* 1991;178:375–7.
13. Paspulati RM, Bhatt S, Nour S. Sonographic evaluation of first trimester bleeding. *Radiol Clin North Am* 2004;42:297–314.
14. Dickey RP, Olar TT, Taylor SN, Curole DN, Matulich EM. Relationship of small gestational sac and crown–rump length differences to abortion and abortus karyotypes. *Obstet Gynecol* 1992;79:554–7.
15. Merchiers EH, Dhont M, Of Sutter PA, Beghin CJ, Vandekerckhove DA. Predictive value of early embryonic cardiac activity for pregnancy outcome. *Am J Obstet Gynecol* 1991; 165:11–14.
16. Laboda LA, Estroff JA, Benacerraf BR. First trimester bradycardia. A sign of impending fetal loss. *J Ultrasound Med* 1989;8:561–3.
17. May DA, Sturtevant NV. Embryonal heart rate ace to predictor of pregnancy outcome: A prospective analysis. *J Ultrasound Med* 1991;10:591–3.
18. Benson S. Slow embryonic heart rate in early first trimester: Indicator of poor pregnancy outcome. *Radiology* 1994;192: 343–4.
19. Doubilet PM, Benson CB. Embryonic heart rate in the early first trimester: What rate normal is? *J Ultrasound Med* 1995;14: 431–4.
20. Stefos TI, Lolis OF, Sotiriadis AJ, Ziakas GV. Embryonic heart rate in early pregnancy. *J Clin Ultrasound* 1998;26:33–6.
21. Kücük T, Duru NK, Yenen MC, Dede M, Ergun A, Baser I. Yolk sac size and shape are predictors of poor pregnancy outcome. *J Perinat Med* 1999;27:316–20.
22. Stampone C, Nicotra M, Muttinelli C, Cosmi EV. Transvaginal sonography of the yolk sac in normal and abnormal pregnancy. *J Clin Ultrasound* 1996;24:3–9.
23. Lindsay DJ, Lovett IS, Lyons EA, *et al.* Yolk sac diameter and shape at endovaginal US: Predictors of pregnancy outcome in the first trimester. *Radiology* 1992;183:115–8.
24. Kupesic S, Kurjak A. Volume and vascularity of the yolk sac assessed by three-dimensional and power Doppler ultrasound. *Early Pregnancy* 2001;5:40–1.
25. Pérez-Medina T, Haya J, Soto E, et al. Alteración ecográfica del saco vitelino como predictor de mal pronóstico de la gestación. Actualidad Obstétrico Ginecológica 2002;14:94–7.
26. Bajo J, Moreno-Calvo FJ, Martinez-Cortés L, Haya FJ, Rayward J. Is trophoblastic thickness at the embryonic implantation site a new sign of negative outcome in first trimester pregnancy? *Hum Reprod* 2000;15:1629–31.
27. Dickey RP, Olar TT, Curole DN, Taylor SN, Matulich EM. Relationship of first-trimester subchorionic bleeding detected by color Doppler ultrasound to subchorionic flows, clinical bleeding, and pregnancy outcome. *Obstet Gynecol* 1992;80: 415–20.
28. Stabile I, Campbell S, Grudzinskas JG. Threatened miscarriage and intrauterine haematomas. Sonographic and biochemical studies. *J Ultrasound Med* 1989;8:289–92.
29. Glavind K, Nohr S, Nielsen PH, Ipsen L. Intra-uterine hematoma in pregnancy. *Eur J Obstet Gynecol Reprod Biol* 1991;40:7–10.
30. Kurjak A, Schulman H, Zudenigo D, Kupesic S, Kos M, Goldenberg M. Subchorionic hematomas in early pregnancy: clinical outcome and blood flow patterns. *J Fetal Matern Med* 1996;5:41–4.
31. Kurjak A, Zalud I, Predanic M, Kupesic S. Transvaginal colour and pulsed Doppler study of uterine blood flow in the first and early second trimesters of pregnancy: Normal versus abnormal. *J Ultrasound Med* 1994;13:43–7.
32. Ball RH, Ade CM, Schoenborn JA, Crane JP. The clinical significance of ultrasonographically detected subchorionic haemorrhages. *Am J Obstet Gynecol* 1996;174:996–1002.
33. Bennett GL, Bromley B, Lieberman Y, Benacerraf BR. Subchorionic bleeding in first-trimester pregnancies: prediction of pregnancy outcome with sonography. *Radiology* 1996;200: 803–6.
34. Johns J, Hyett J, Jauniaux E. Obstetric outcome after threatened miscarriage with and without a hematoma on ultrasound. *Obstet Gynecol* 2003;102:483–7.
35. Nagy S, Bush M, Stone J, Lapinski RH, Gardo S. Clinical significance of subchorionic and retroplacental haematomas detected in the first trimester of pregnancy. *Obstet Gynecol* 2003;102:94–100.
36. Koornstra G, I Exalto N. Echography in the first pregnancy trimester has prognostic value. *Ned Tijdschr Geneeskd* 1991; 135:2231–5.
37. Leelapatana P, Garrett WJ, Warren PS. Early growth retardation in the first trimester: Is it characteristic of the chromosomally abnormal fetus? *Aust NZ J Obstet Gynaecol* 1992;32:95–7.
38. Bessho T, Sakamoto H, Shiotani T, Komori S, Koyama K. Fetal loss in the first trimester after demonstration of cardiac activity: Relation of cytogenetic and ultrasound findings. *Hum Reprod* 1995;10:2696–9.
39. Coulam CB, Goodman C, Dorfmann A. Comparison of ultrasonographic findings in spontaneous abortions with normal and abnormal karyotypes. *Hum Reprod* 1997;12:823–6.
40. Anderson SG. Management of threatened abortion with real-cheats sonography. *Obstet Gynecol* 1980;55:259–2.
41. Kurjak A, Kupesic S. Doppler assessment of the intervillous blood flow in normal and abnormal early pregnancy. *Obstet Gynecol* 1997;89:252–6.
42. Jaffe R, Jauniaux AND, Hustin J. Maternal circulation in the first-trimester human placenta – Myth or reality? *Am J Obstet Gynecol* 1997;176:695–705.
43. Jaffe R, Woods JR. Doppler velocimetry of intraplacental fetal vessels in the second trimester: Improving the prediction of pregnancy complications in high-risk patients. *Ultrasound Obstet Gynecol* 1996;8:262–6.
44. Martin AM, Bindra R, Curcio P. Screening for preeclampsia and fetal growth restriction by uterine artery Doppler at 11–14 weeks of gestation. *Ultrasound Obstet Gynecol* 2001;18:583–6.
45. Mercé LT, Barco MJ, Bau S. Color Doppler sonographic assessment of placental circulation in the first trimester of normal pregnancy. *J Ultrasound Med* 1996;15:135–42.
46. Kurjak A, Kupesic S. Parallel Doppler assessment of yolk sac and intervillous circulation in normal pregnancy and missed abortion. *Placenta* 1998;19:619–23.
47. Jauniaux AND, Johnson MR, Jurkovic D, Ramsay B, Campbell S, Meuris S. The role of relaxin in the development of the uteroplacental circulation in early pregnancy. *Obstet Gynecol* 1994;84:338–42.
48. Alcazar JL, Ruiz-Perez ML. Uteroplacental circulation in patients with first-trimester threatened abortion. *Fertil Steril* 2000;73:130–5.
49. Salim A, Zalud I, Farmakides G, Schulman H, Kurjak TO, Latin V. Corpus luteum blood flow in normal and abnormal early

pregnancy: Evaluation with transvaginal color and pulsed Doppler sonography. *J Ultrasound Med* 1994;13:971–5.

50. Alcazar JL, Laparte C, Lopez-Garcia G. Corpus luteum blood flow in abnormal early pregnancy. *J Ultrasound Med* 1996;15:645–9.
51. Daya S, Woods S, Ward S, Lappalainen R, Caco C. Early pregnancy assessment with transvaginal ultrasound scanning. *Can Med Assoc J* 1991;144:441–6.
52. Goldstein I, Zimmer EA, Tamir A, Peretz BA, Paldi E. Evaluation of normal gestational sac growth: Appearance of embryonic heartbeat and embryo body movements using the transvaginal technique. *Obstet Gynecol* 1991;77:885–8.
53. Norwitz ER, Scust DJ, Fisher SJ. Implantation and the survival of early pregnancy. *N Engl J Med* 2001;345:1400–8.
54. Brown DL, Emerson DS, Felker RE, Cartier MS, Smith WC. Diagnosis of early embryonic demise by endovaginal sonography. *J Ultrasound Med* 1990;9:631–6.
55. Bernard KG, Cooperberg PL. Sonographic differentiation between blighted ovum and early viable pregnancy. *AJR Am J Roentgenol* 1985;144:597–602.
56. Nyberg DA, Mack THE, Laing FC, Patten RM. Distinguishing normal from abnormal gestational sac growth in early pregnancy. *J Ultrasound Med* 1987;6:23–7.
57. McKenna KM, Feldstein VA, Goldstein RB, Filly RA. The empty amnion: The sign of early pregnancy failure. *J Ultrasound Med* 1995;14:117–21.

100 2D and 3D Doppler assessment of abnormal early intrauterine pregnancy

J. L. Alcázar, L. T. Mercé and M. García-Manero

Introduction

The introduction of transvaginal ultrasound allowed assessing *in vivo* and non-invasively an, until then, unexplored area: early gestation. This technique revolutionized the evaluation and management of many clinical situations during this period of pregnancy. The advent of color and power Doppler ultrasound, as a further step, allowed the assessment of early pregnancy hemodynamics. Traditionally, two-dimensional (2D) color and pulsed Doppler has been applied to evaluate early human pregnancy hemodynamics during the last 15 years.[1] In recent years, a new technological advance has been introduced: 3D power Doppler ultrasonography. This new technique allows a more objective and global assessment of organ vasculature.[2]

The scope of the present chapter is to address the assessment of ovarian, uteroplacental, yolk sac and embryo-fetal hemodynamic changes in abnormal early intrauterine pregnancy by means of 2D and 3D transvaginal color and power Doppler ultrasonography. We shall review missed abortion and anembryonic pregnancy, threatened abortion and complete/incomplete abortion.

Hemodynamic changes in normally developing pregnancy have been dealt with in another chapter in this book, so we shall address specifically what happens in abnormal early pregnancy.

Abnormal early pregnancy

Missed abortion and anembryonic pregnancy

Luteal circulation

Three studies have found that luteal blood flow resistance was increased in missed abortion.[3–5] This finding may be a consequence rather than a cause of missed abortion, because missed abortion consists of a failure of early pregnancy to develop, in which the production of human chorionic gonadotropin is impaired, which in turn could have a negative effect on luteal function. However, Frates *et al.* did not find any difference between missed abortions and normal pregnancies.[6]

Regarding anembryonic pregnancies, Alcázar *et al.*[3] and Salim *et al.*[4] did not find any differences in luteal blood flow as compared with normal developing pregnancies. This could be explained by the fact that in an anembryonic pregnancy trophoblastic activity continues for a time without the presence of the embryo. Furthermore, some studies have demonstrated that luteal activity in anembryonic pregnancy, as assessed by progesterone serum levels, does not differ from normal pregnancies but is impaired in missed abortions.[7]

Uteroplacental circulation

Several authors have investigated uteroplacental circulation in abnormal early pregnancies. In the case of missed abortion and anembryonic pregnancy, most studies did not find significant differences as compared with normal pregnancies in uterine, arcuate, radial and spiral arteries or retrochorionic arteries.[8–13]

Regarding intervillous flow conflicting data have been reported. According to embryological studies, uteroplacental circulation is established around day 12 of embryo development, when maternal blood flows into the syncytiotrophoblast lacunae. Therefore, actual blood flow in the intervillous space begins around days 14–15 of embryonic development (fourth week of amenorrhea) and never later than day 40 (7 weeks + 5 days).[14,15]

However, Hustin and Schaaps challenged this concept and brought up a new theory.[16] They stated that intervillous blood flow does not actually exist until the 12th week. Their theory was based on the findings from *in vitro* studies using four placentas perfused with barium sulfate and hysteroscopic

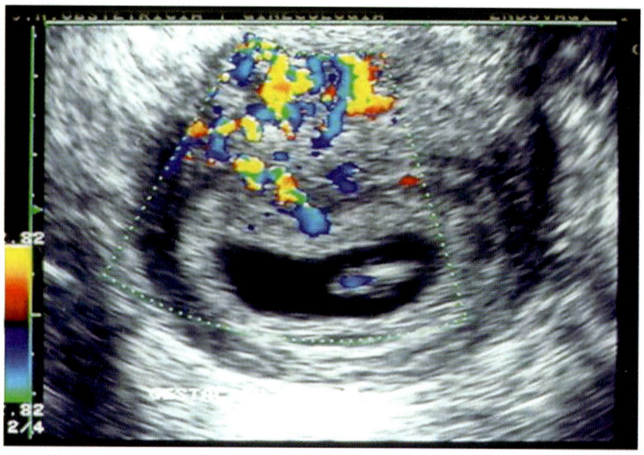

Figure 100.1 Intervillous blood flow in early pregnancy. Vessels penetrating the chorion can be clearly seen.

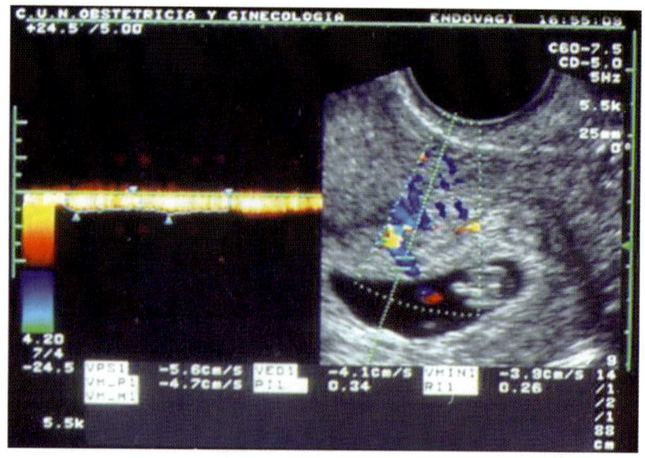

Figure 100.3 Arterial-like FVW from intervillous space.

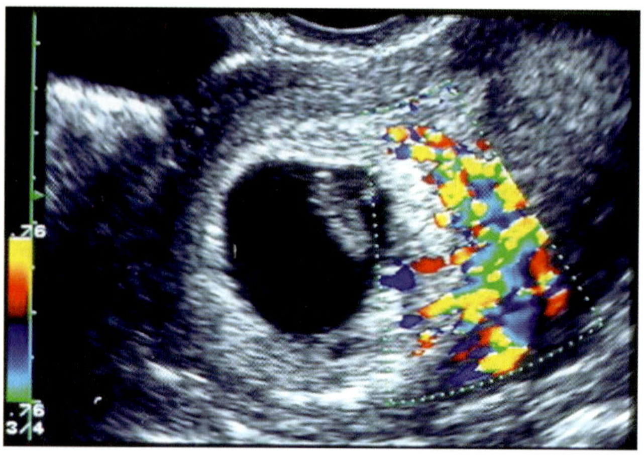

Figure 100.2 Intervillous flow in early pregnancy.

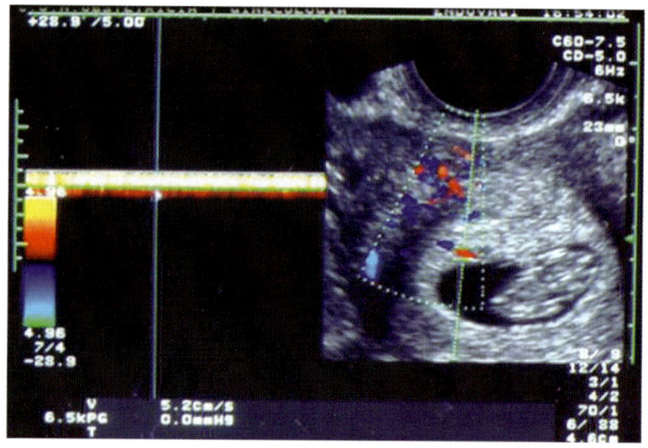

Figure 100.4 Venous-like FVW from intervillous space.

studies in 10 patients. Using transvaginal color Doppler, Jauniaux,[17] Jaffe and Woods[18] and Coppens *et al.*[19] supported this theory because they did not detect intervillous flow until the 12th week.

However, several studies have reported that intervillous flow can be detected from the sixth week onward in normal early pregnancy.[20–23] This agrees with our findings (Alcázar, unpublished data) (Figures 100.1 and 100.2). We agree with Mercé *et al.*[20] and Kurjak and Kupesic[21] that two types of intervillous flow can be found: pulsating arterial (Figure 100.3) and continuous venous (Figure 100.4).

In abnormal pregnancies, Jauniaux *et al.* found that 70% of complicated pregnancies showed intervillous flow as compared with 0% in normal developing pregnancy.[24] However, a more recent study from this group showed that intervillous flow may be detected in around 60% of normally developing pregnancies between the 7th and 13th weeks,[25] being a progressive phenomenon (36% at 8–9 weeks, 60% at 10–11 weeks and 90% at 12–13 weeks). They found that in abnormal pregnancy, the number of cases in which intervillous flow could be detected were higher than in normal pregnancies at 8–9 and 10–11 weeks, but not later. They did not discriminate between missed abortions and anembryonic pregnancies. They speculated that a premature entry of maternal blood in the intervillous space disrupts the materno–embryonic interface and is probably the final mechanism causing abortion. Similar findings have been reported by Jaffe and Warsoff.[26]

Kurjak and Kupesic found that a significant increase of venous peak velocity in the intervillous flow occurs in normal pregnancies from the 11th week onward. This change does not occur in missed abortion or anembryonic pregnancy.[21] These authors did not find differences in arterial intervillous flow between normal and abnormal pregnancies.[21,27]

Yolk sac circulation

Analyzing yolk sac hemodynamics, Kurjak and Kupesic reported that yolk sac blood flow was detected only in 19% of patients with missed abortion as compared with 67% in normal pregnancies.[27]

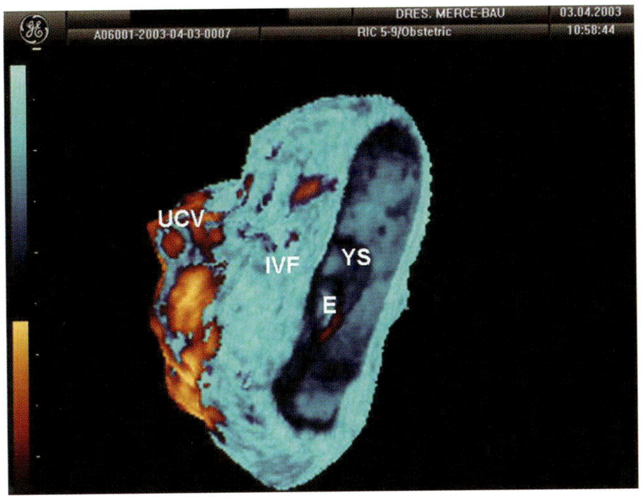

Figure 100.5 Rendering of uterochorionic vessels (UCV) and intervillous blood flow (IVF) by power Doppler three-dimensional angiography in a 7-week normal pregnancy. YS, yolk sac; E, embryo.

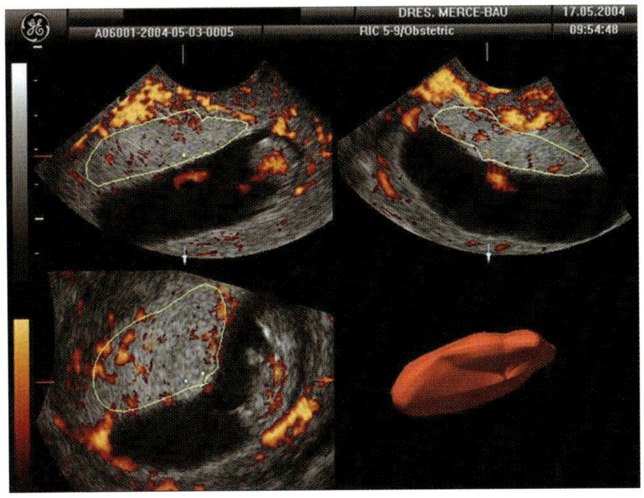

Figure 100.6 Intervillous blood flow assessment by VOCAL software during early pregnancy.

Threatened abortion

Those studies addressing hemodynamic changes in missed abortion or anembryonic pregnancy are interesting from a pathophysiologic point of view but may not be relevant to clinical practice because diagnosis can be made with B-mode ultrasound and assessment of the uteroplacental circulation does not add clinical or prognostic information. However, this situation is different in patients with threatened abortion, even more if a living embryo is identified.

Luteal circulation

Salim *et al.*, analyzing luteal blood flow found a significantly higher mean RI in threatened abortion.[4] However, we did not find any difference in luteal blood flow in threatened abortion as compared with normal developing pregnancies.[3] This difference regarding our results might be explained by the fact that all cases of threatened abortion in our study had an uneventful outcome, indicating that luteal function might be normal. Frates *et al.* reported similar findings to ours. They did not find any relationship between luteal blood flow and first-trimester pregnancy outcome.[6]

Uteroplacental circulation

Most studies assessing uteroplacental blood flow in threatened abortions conclude that Doppler assessment does not provide prognostic information because no significant differences between pregnancies with normal outcome and those that ended in abortion were found.[28–31]

Some authors have evaluated the predictive value for abnormal outcome of uteroplacental blood flow assessment in early pregnancy. Jaffe *et al.* found that an abnormally high RI (cutoff RI = 0.55) in the spiral arteries was associated with a higher probability of spontaneous abortion.[32] Leible *et al.* showed that a discordant uterine artery pulsatility index (PI) (> 1.1) would predict a subsequent miscarriage in otherwise normally developing pregnancies during the first trimester (odds ratio: 2.9, 95% CI: 1.5–5.8).[33]

On the other hand, uteroplacental blood flow assessment seems to be useless to predict pregnancy outcome in women with recurrent spontaneous abortion.[34]

Regarding intervillous flow, Mercé *et al.* observed an increase in venous velocity in 64% of spontaneous abortions before embryo death.[35]

We have evaluated the role of 3D power Doppler ultrasound in assessing intervillous flow in normal pregnancy (Figures 100.5–100.7). This technique has been shown to be reproducible,[2] overcoming one of the main problems of 2D color or power Doppler ultrasound and allowing an assessment of the entire chorion and early placenta. We found that flow index was significantly higher in pregnancies that ended in spontaneous abortion as compared with those that had normal outcome (Figure 100.8). No differences were found in vascularity and vascularity-flow indexes (Figures 100.9 and 100.10). This finding is very interesting because the flow index reflects flow velocity, thus confirming the previous finding by Mercé *et al.*[35]

Yolk sac circulation

Makikallio *et al.* have reported that yolk sac hemodynamics is not affected in cases of threatened abortion with or without retrochorionic hematoma.[36]

Embryo-fetal circulation

The assessment of embryo-fetal circulation in abnormal early pregnancy is unique to threatened abortion with a living embryo. Assessment of embryo-fetal circulation has been focused in three arterial vessels: umbilical artery, abdominal aorta and cerebral vessels.

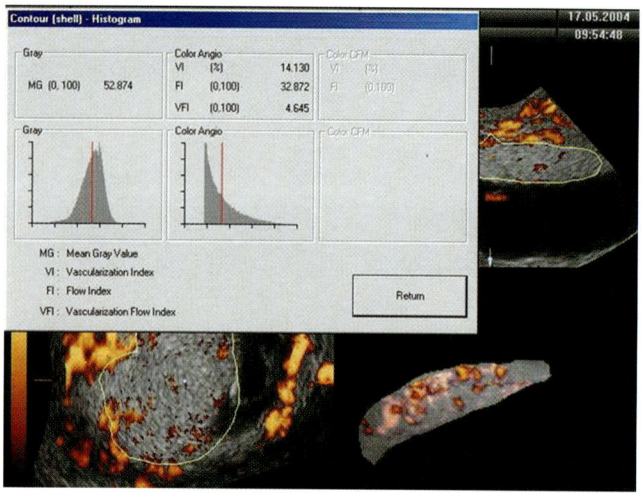

Figure 100.7 Vascularization index (VI), flow index (FI) and vascularization-flow index (VFI) are useful to evaluate intervillous blood flow during normal and abnormal early pregnancy.

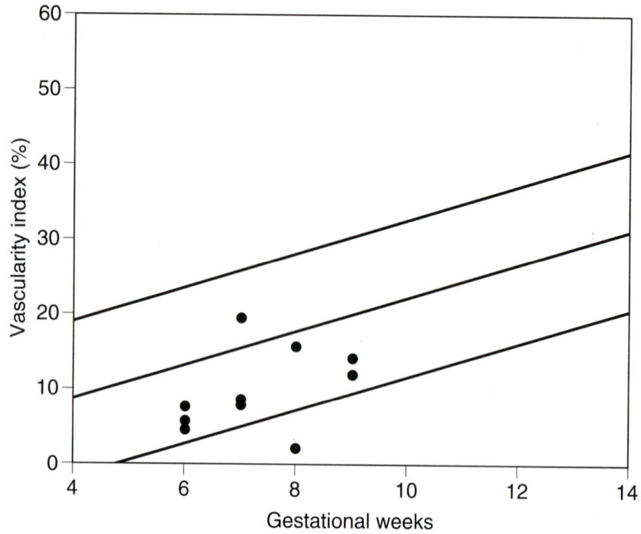

Figure 100.9 Vascularity index in cases of spontaneous abortion (closed circles). Regression line for normal pregnancies: $y=7.018+2.892$ (gestational age), $R^2=0.28$. It can be seen how most cases of spontaneous abortion are within the normal range.

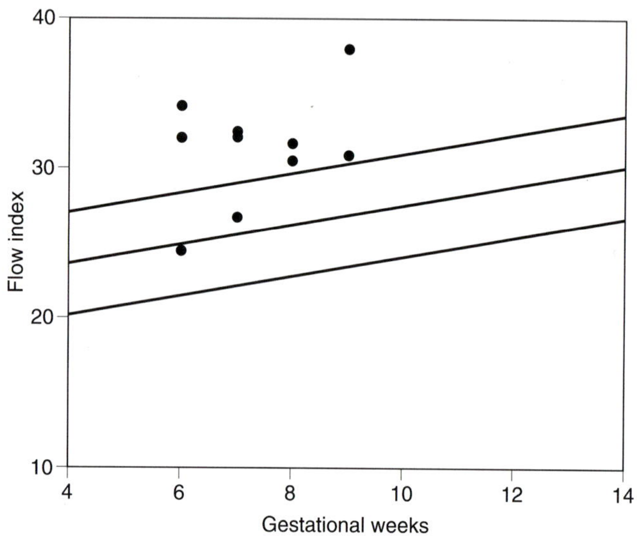

Figure 100.8 Flow index in cases of spontaneous abortion (closed circles). Regression line for normal pregnancies: $y=21.050+0.659$ (gestational age), $R^2=0.16$. It can be seen how most cases of spontaneous abortion are outside the normal range.

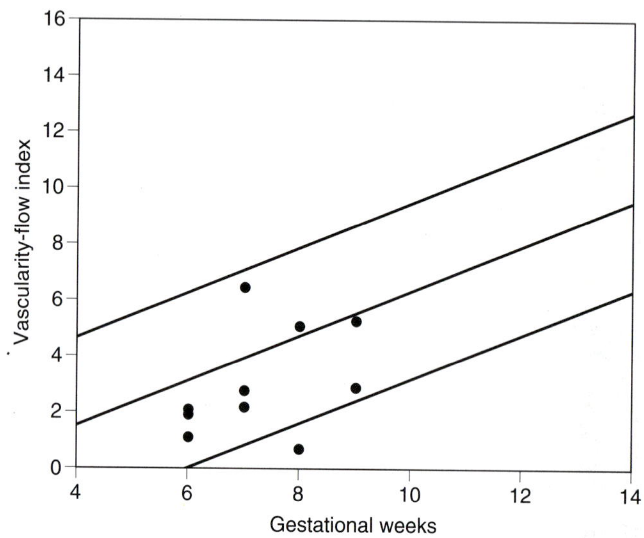

Figure 100.10 Vascularity low index in cases of spontaneous abortion (closed circles). Regression line for normal pregnancies: $y=2.383+0.859$ (gestational age), $R^2=0.29$. It can be seen how most cases of spontaneous abortion are within the normal range.

Some authors have evaluated the role of fetal hemodynamics assessment for predicting pregnancy outcome in cases of threatened abortion with retrochorionic hematoma. All studies concluded that fetal circulation assessment is not useful to predict pregnancy outcome.[29,37,38]

Complete and incomplete abortion

Differentiating between incomplete and complete spontaneous abortion is one of the most difficult tasks that a clinician has to deal with. Management may be quite different if the presence of retained tissue can be ruled out.

The use of transvaginal color Doppler ultrasonography for detecting retained products of conception after spontaneous first-trimester abortion has not been extensively evaluated to date. In our experience, this technique can be useful to detect retained trophoblastic tissue in patients with suspected incomplete abortion.[39] The presence of focal areas highly vascularized within the myometrium just beneath the endometrium or even within the endometrium (Figure 100.11) with flow velocity waveforms (FVWs) characterized by high peak systolic velocity and low impedance (Figure 100.12) was associated with the presence of retained tissue in the vast majority of the

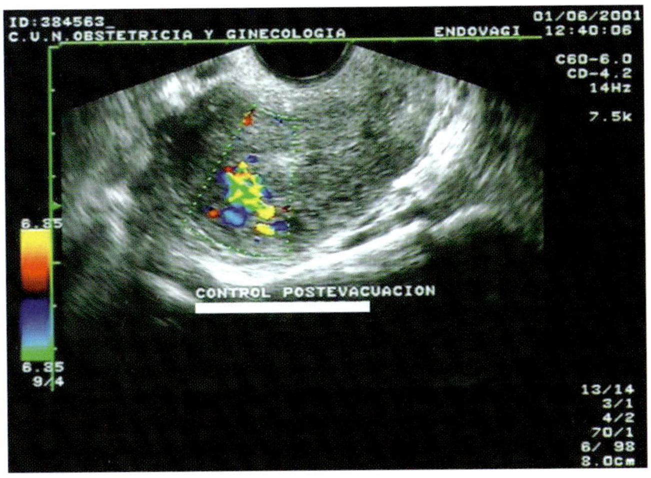

Figure 100.11 Transvaginal color ultrasound after D&C and persistent spotting. This figure shows a focal area of vascularization at the level of fundus and posterior myometrium. Retained tissue was found after D&C.

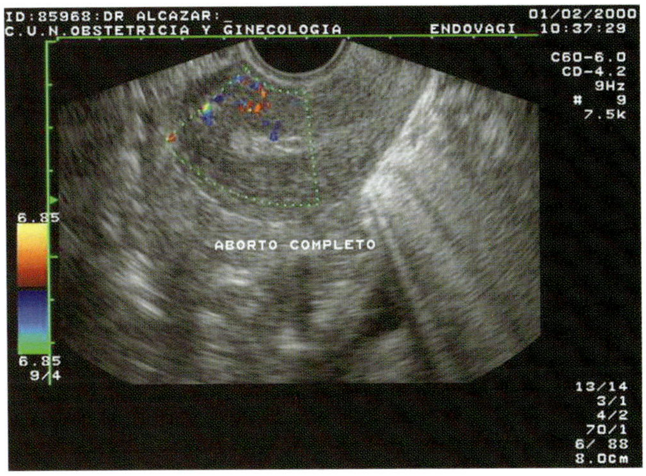

Figure 100.13 Transvaginal color Doppler ultrasound after heavy vaginal bleeding in first trimester. Scanty flow was found, suggestive of no retained tissue.

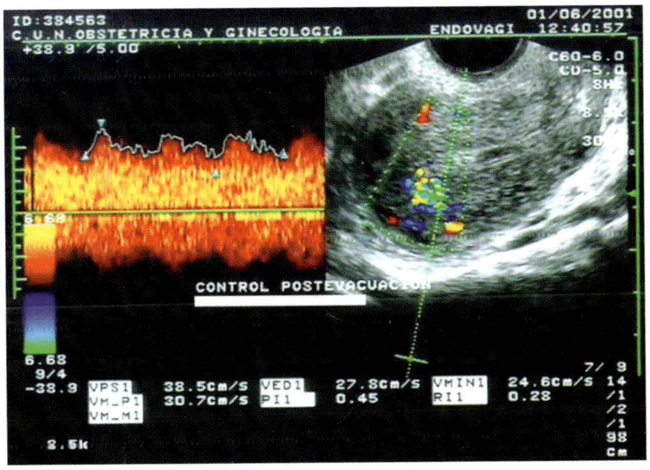

Figure 100.12 Same patient as in Figure 100.11. A low-resistance and high-velocity FVW, suggestive of trophoblastic flow is clearly found.

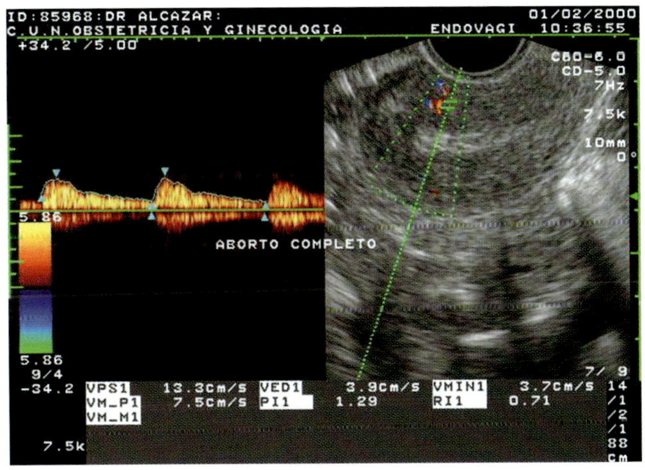

Figure 100.14 FVW from an arterial vessel in the case of Figure 100.13. High-velocity and high-resistance flow was found. Typical in absence of retained tissue.

cases. On the contrary, the absence of color signals or the presence of scanty color signals (Figure 100.13) with high-resistance blood flow (Figure 100.14) was associated with the absence of retained tissue. In our study, the sensitivity and specificity of color Doppler ultrasound in detecting retained tissue was 93.3% and 96%, respectively.

We have evaluated prospectively the role of transvaginal color Doppler ultrasonography in the management of first-trimester spontaneous abortion and we found this technique quite useful to rule out retained trophoblastic tissue.[40] Similar results have been reported by other authors.[41]

Conclusion

Transvaginal color and power Doppler allows the assessment of abnormal early pregnancy hemodynamics. The results of most published studies reveal that 2D Doppler assessment of luteal, uteroplacental and yolk sac circulations are conflicting or conclude that this assessment has a low clinical value, except for discriminating complete from incomplete abortion.

3D power Doppler ultrasonography provides promising results and opens a formidable new field of research.

REFERENCES

1. Mercé LT, Barco MJ, de la Fuente F. Doppler velocimetry measured in retrochorionic space and uterine arteries during early human pregnancy. *Acta Obstet Gynecol Scand* 1989;68:603–7.
2. Mercé LT, Barco MJ, Bau S. Reproducibility of the study of placental vascularization by three-dimensional power Doppler. *J Perinat Med* 2004;32:228–33.
3. Alcázar JL, Laparte C, López García G. Corpus luteum blood flow in abnormal early pregnancy. *J Ultrasound Med* 1996;15:645–9.
4. Salim A, Zalud I, Farmakides G, *et al.* Corpus luteum blood flow in normal and abnormal early pregnancy: Evaluation with transvaginal color and pulsed Doppler sonography. *J Ultrasound Med* 1994;13:971–5.
5. Kurjak A, Zudeningo D, Predanic M, *et al.* Recent advances in the Doppler study of early fetomaternal circulation. *J Perinat Med* 1994;22:419–39.
6. Frates MC, Doubilet PM, Durfee SM, *et al.* Sonographic and Doppler characteristics of the corpus luteum: Can they predict pregnancy outcome? *J Ultrasound Med* 2001;20:821–7.
7. Al-Sebai MAH, Kingsland CR, Diver M. The role of a single progesterone measurement in the diagnosis of early pregnancy failure and prognosis of fetal viability. *Br J Obstet Gynecol* 1995;102:364–7.
8. Alfirevic Z, Kurjak A. Transvaginal colour Doppler ultrasound in normal and abnormal early pregnancy. *J Perinat Med* 1990;18:173–80.
9. Kurjak A, Zalud I, Crvenkovic G, *et al.* Transvaginal color Doppler in the assessment of abnormal early pregnancy. *J Perinat Med* 1991;19:155–65.
10. Kurjak A, Kupesic-Urek S, Predanic M, Salihagic A. Transvaginal color Doppler assessment of uteroplacental circulation in normal and abnormal early pregnancy. *Early Hum Dev* 1992;29:385–9.
11. Jaffe R. Investigations of abnormal first-trimester gestations by color Doppler imaging. *J Clin Ultrasound* 1993;21:521–6.
12. Kurjak A, Zalud I, Predanic M, *et al.* Transvaginal color Doppler study of uterine blood flow in the first and early second trimesters of pregnancy: Normal versus abnormal. *J Ultrasound Med* 1994;13:43–7.
13. Giacobbe M, Zeferino LZ, Franzin C, *et al.* Uteroplacental circulation during the first trimester of normal and abnormal pregnancy. *Reprod Biomed Online* 2001;4:60–5.
14. Haufmann P. Entwicklung der plazenta. In Becker V, Schiebler TH, Kubli F, eds. *Die Plazenta des Menschen.* Stuttgart: Georg Thieme Verlag, 1981:37–64.
15. Mercé LT, Kupesic S, Kurjak A. Color Doppler assessment of implantation and early placentation. *Prenat Neonat Med* 1999;4:94–112.
16. Hustin J, Schaaps JP. Echographic and anatomic studies of the maternotrophoblastic border during the first trimester of pregnancy. *Am J Obstet Gynecol* 1987;157:162–8.
17. Jauniaux E. Intervillous circulation in the first trimester: The phantom of the color Doppler obstetric opera. *Ultrasound Obstet Gynecol* 1996;8:73–6.
18. Jaffe R, Woods JR. Color Doppler imaging and in vivo assessment of the anatomy and physiology of the early uteroplacental circulation. *Fertil Steril* 1993;60:293–7.
19. Coppens M, Loquet P, Kollen M, *et al.* Longitudinal evaluation of uteroplacental and umbilical blood flow changes in normal early pregnancy. *Ultrasound Obstet Gynecol* 1996;7:114–21.
20. Mercé LT, Barco MJ, Bau S. Color Doppler sonographic assessment of placental circulation in the first trimester of normal pregnancy. *J Ultrasound Med* 1996;15:135–42.
21. Kurjak A, Kupesic S. Doppler assessment of the intervillous blood flow in normal and abnormal early pregnancy. *Obstet Gynecol* 1997;89:252–6.
22. Alouini S, Carbillon L, Perrot N, *et al.* Intervillous and spiral artery flows in normal pregnancies between 5 and 10 weeks of amenorrhea using color Doppler ultrasonography. *Fetal Diagn Ther* 2002;17:163–6.
23. Makikallio K, Tekay A, Jouppila P. Uteroplacental hemodynamics during early human pregnancy. *Gynecol Obstet Invest* 2004;58:49–54.
24. Jauniaux E, Zaidi J, Jurkovic D, *et al.* Comparison of colour Doppler features and pathological findings in complicated early pregnancy. *Hum Reprod* 1994;9:2432–7.
25. Jauniaux E, Greenwold N, Hempstock J, *et al.* Comparison of ultrasonographic and Doppler mapping of the intervillous circulation in normal and abnormal early pregnancies. *Fertil Steril* 2003;79:100–6.
26. Jaffe R, Warsoff SL. Color Doppler imaging in the assessment of uteroplacental blood flow in abnormal first-trimester intrauterine pregnancies: An attempt to define etiologic mechanisms. *J Ultrasound Med* 1992;11:41–4.
27. Kurjak A, Kupesic S. Parallel Doppler assessment of yolk sac and intervillous circulation in normal and missed abortion. *Placenta* 1998;19:619–23.
28. Kurjak A, Schulman H, Zudenigo D, *et al.* Subchorionic hematomas in early pregnancy: Clinical outcome and blood flow patterns. *J Matern Fetal Med* 1996;5:41–4.
29. Kurjak A, Zudenigo D, Predanic M, *et al.* Assessment of fetomaternal circulation in threatened abortion by transvaginal color Doppler. *Fetal Diagn Ther* 1994;9:341–7.
30. Alcázar JL, Ruiz-Pérez ML. Uteroplacental circulation in patients with first-trimester threatened abortion. *Fertil Steril* 2000;73:130–5.
31. Pellizzari P, Pozzan C, Marchiori S, *et al.* Assessment of uterine artery blood flow in normal first-trimester pregnancies and in those complicated by uterine bleeding. *Ultrasound Obstet Gynecol* 2002;19:366–70.
32. Jaffe R, Dorgan A, Abramowicz JS. Color Doppler imaging of the uteroplacental circulation in the first trimester: Value in predicting pregnancy failure or complication. *AJR Am J Roentgenol* 1995;164:1255–8.
33. Leible S, Cumsille F, Walton R, *et al.* Discordant uterine artery velocity waveforms as a predictor of subsequent miscarriage in early viable pregnancies. *Am J Obstet Gynecol* 1998;179:1587–93.
34. Frates MC, Doubilet PM, Brown DL, *et al.* Role of Doppler ultrasonography in the prediction of pregnancy outcome in women with recurrent spontaneous abortion. *J Ultrasound Med* 1996;15:557–62.
35. Mercé LT, Barco MJ, Bau S. Color Doppler sonography of the retrochorionic and intervillous circulation: Predictive value in small gestational sacs. *Med Imag Int* 1997;7:16–9.
36. Makikallio K, Tekay A, Jouppila P. Effects of bleeding on uteroplacental, umbilicoplacental and yolk-sac hemodynamics in early pregnancy. *Ultrasound Obstet Gynecol* 2001;18:352–6.
37. Rizzo G, Capponi A, Seregaroli M, *et al.* Early fetal circulation in pregnancies complicated by retroplacental hematoma. *J Clin Ultrasound* 1995;23:525–9.
38. Alcázar JL. Assessment of fetal circulation in patients with retrochorionic hematoma during the first trimester of pregnancy. *Prenat Neonat Med* 1998;3:458–63.
39. Alcázar JL. Transvaginal ultrasonography combined with color velocity imaging and pulsed Doppler to detect residual trophoblastic tissue. *Ultrasound Obstet Gynecol* 1998;11:54–8.
40. Alcázar JL, Ortiz C. Transvaginal color Doppler ultrasonography in the management of first-trimester spontaneous abortion. *Eur J Obstet Gynecol Reprod Biol* 2002;102:83–7.
41. Zalel Y, Gamzu R, Lidor A, Goldenberg M, Achiron R. Color Doppler imaging in the sonohysterographic diagnosis of residual trophoblastic tissue. *J Clin Ultrasound* 2002;30:222–5.

101 Ultrasonography of ectopic pregnancy

S. Iniesta, F. Salazar and J. M. Bajo

Definition

The term *ectopic pregnancy* is applied to pregnancy following implantation of the fertilized ovum on any tissue other than the uterus endometrium.

The tubal presentation is the most common one, especially if it is in its distal third portion or the middle third one (both of them constitute nearly 95–97% of all ectopic pregnancies). Occasionally, it can appear in the interstitial portion (cornual pregnancy, 2–5%) and exceptionally in the ovary (0.5–1%), the cervix (0.1–0.15%) or the abdomen (1.4%).[1,2]

The common denominator in this group of patients is delay in the transport of the ovum fertilized in the ampulla of the tube to the normal implantation site in the uterus.

Incidence

The incidence of ectopic pregnancy has been increasing during the last few years.[3–5] Although it is difficult to estimate, it is nearly 0.94–2.6% of all pregnancies. This increased incidence is due to the use of reproduction treatments, the use of some contraceptive methods and pelvic inflammatory disease.

Day by day, with the development of vaginal ultrasound and the earlier detection of beta-subunit human chorionic gonadotropin (β-HCG) by radioimmunoassay, the diagnosis of ectopic pregnancies is improving, and it is possible to recognize an ectopic pregnancy in earlier stages (days or weeks earlier) than a few years ago, including some cases that had earlier occurred unnoticed.

Etiology

Although the etiology of ectopic pregnancy is still unknown, there are several risk factors that can be associated to ectopic pregnancy.[3,6]

- Previous pelvic inflammatory disease.[7] This is the most important cause of ectopic pregnancy and increases its incidence by 4. The presence of circulating *Chlamydia* antibodies alone increases its incidence by 2.[8]
- Previous tubal surgery (for infertility, because of previous ectopic pregnancies, bipolar tubal coagulation in the sterilization context, etc.) or any other kind of surgery in the inferior hemiabdomen that may cause tubal adhesions as well.
- Other organic tubal alterations: tubal tumors, endometriosis, peritubal adhesions, etc.
- Reproduction treatments (some factors have been associated, such as ovulation induction treatments, assisted hatching, etc.).[9]
- Contraception failures. Intrauterine devices do not increase the incidence of ectopic pregnancy by themselves, but once the pregnancy is established, the possibility of its becoming ectopic is much higher. The lowest ectopic pregnancy rates are observed with the high-copper-dose intrauterine devices, instead of the ones with low copper dose or the ones that release progesterone, which have the highest rates of ectopic pregnancy. Nevertheless, the levonorgestrel intrauterine devices result in a low rate, similar to those with high-dose copper loads.[10] Failures of tubal coagulation techniques also increase the risk of ectopic pregnancies because they may cause tubal fistulas.[11]
- Previous ectopic pregnancies.
- Tobacco.
- Infertility.

All these factors could be involved in the transportation of the fertilized ovum to the uterus, although there are also some embryonic factors that can be responsible for ectopic pregnancy and, more or less, a third of them involve chromosomal abnormalities.

Symptoms and signs

Physical findings are quite variable, and the clinical presentation has changed considerably over the past few years because of earlier diagnosis. Although the incidence of ectopic pregnancy has increased, the frequency of its complications (such as ectopic pregnancy rupture, tubal abortion, etc.) is decreasing at a very significant rate because the greater exactitude of the diagnosis methods allows detection of ectopic pregnancy in asymptomatic women and in precocious phases of the process.[12,13]

This has also allowed development of different protocols for non-surgical treatment of ectopic pregnancy, as well as less invasive surgical procedures.

Clinical situations of ectopic pregnancy

- Asymptomatic women.
- Vague abdominal pain, without any specific findings, in unruptured cases. Sometimes we can find vaginal bleeding, usually in scanty amounts. The classic clinical triad of ectopic pregnancy is *pain, vaginal bleeding* and *amenorrhea*, although the amenorrhea is sometimes difficult to assess because of the vaginal bleeding.
- Acute hemorrhagical accident, generally caused by tubal rupture or by tubal abortion with peritoneal hemorrhage. In this case, patients will present all the symptoms and signs of acute abdominal (positive Blumberg, peritoneal defense) and hypovolemic signs (extreme pallor of the skin and mucous membranes, tachycardia, hypotension, etc.).

The first symptom noticed by patients is likely to be a 1 or 2 weeks' delay in menstruation, followed by slight bleeding, which persists, with perhaps only a scant show of blood, almost every day. Although this spotting type of bleeding is rather characteristic, not infrequently the bleeding may be somewhat freer, but it is rarely so profuse as in an incomplete abortion. Instead of the menstrual period being delayed, there may be an apparent anticipation of the flow by a few days.

Pain is an early symptom, although it is sometimes very slight. In the beginning there may be only a vague tenderness in the affected side of the pelvis, but often the patient complains of sharp colicky pain occurring from time to time. When rupture or tubal abortion takes place, the pain may be very severe, and it may be associated with faintness or actual syncope and often nausea and vomiting. These symptoms are the result of the peritoneal reaction produced by the escape of blood from the tube.

Diagnosis

The clinical image of ectopic pregnancy is so typical in many cases that diagnosis is very easy, but often errors occur, so we always have to keep in mind the possibility of ectopic pregnancy if we do not want to make a wrong diagnosis.[14,15]

The diagnosis is actually based on:

- Anamnesis, insisting on the classic clinical triad and on the investigation of ectopic pregnancy risk factors.
- Abdominal and pelvic examination.
- Pregnancy test.
- Ultrasonography.

Some recent studies[16] describe novel placental and nonplacental serum markers in ectopic pregnancies, such as PAPP-A, SP-1 and human placental lactogen (HPL), but these factors have to be further studied.

If we have a positive pregnancy test and any gestational vesicle within the uterine cavity is observed by transvaginal ultrasonography, it is necessary to determine the β-hCG levels in maternal serum.

The hCG is a glucoprotein composed of two subunits, alpha and beta, joined by non-covalent unions by disulfide bonds. The alpha subunit is composed of 92 amino acids and the beta subunit, 145. The latter is responsible for the biological activity and it is the one that allows the production of some highly specific antibodies very important for radioimmunoassay detection.

The hCG is produced in the syncytiotrophoblast and its detection in maternal serum is possible 1 day after the blastocyst implantation.

In a normal gestation (non-ectopic one), the circulating β-hCG level at the time of the first delay of menstruation is, approximately, 100 UI/l, and it reaches its maximum (50,000–100,000 UI/l) between the 8th and 10th gestational weeks. Later, it decreases to around 10,000–20,000 UI/l at 18–20 weeks and remains more or less constant until the end of pregnancy.[17]

On the other hand, the β-hCG levels in an ectopic pregnancy can be very variable; cases of ectopic pregnancies with β-hCG levels as low as 14 UI/l have been documented, as well as others with 100,000 UI/l. Thus, a single determination of β-hCG level is often of little use for the diagnosis of ectopic pregnancy. Nevertheless, consecutive determinations of β-hCG levels allow differentiation between a normal gestation and an ectopic one, since the increase of the β-hCG levels is different in both.

In an intrauterine pregnancy of normal course, the serum β-hCG concentration follows a linear pattern in the first 6 weeks and it is duplicated in 2 days when its level is lower than 10,000 UI/l.

The trophoblast tissue in an ectopic pregnancy usually produces less hCG than in an intrauterine pregnancy and, therefore, its increase in the same period of time is usually smaller.

Nevertheless, some cases of ectopic pregnancy with the same increased levels of β-hCG as in intrauterine pregnancy have been described (nearly 13%), at least for a period of time. In addition, 10% of the

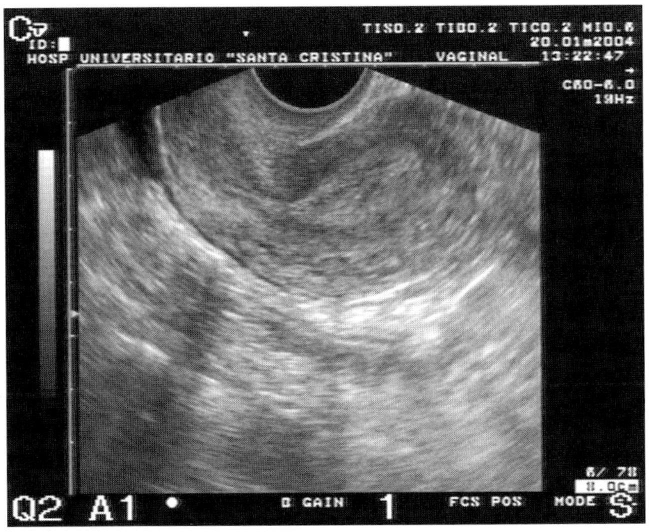

Figure 101.1 Decidual reaction of the endometrium. Positive β-hCG. Ectopic pregnancy with a tubal gestational sac.

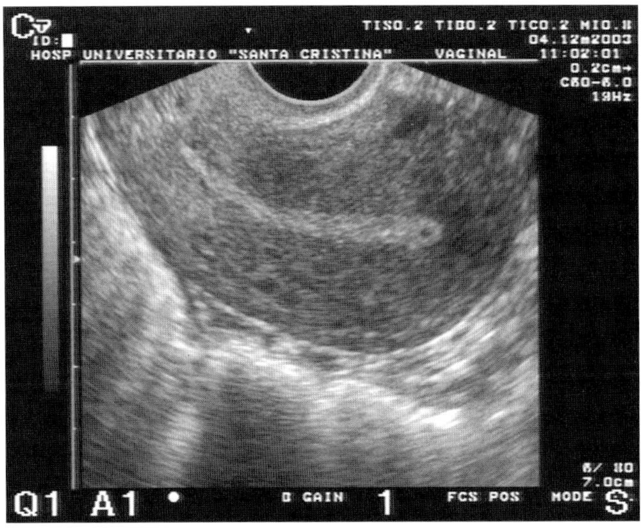

Figure 101.2 Pseudosac image inside the endometrium.

normal intrauterine pregnancies can present alterations in the increase of the β-hCG.

Some studies, during the past few years, have tried to predict the tubal rupture, the possibility of resolution or the possibility of hemorrhage by using β-hCG levels or other factors.[18,19] Although some authors have found good results by using β-hCG levels to predict tubal rupture,[20] considering that its occurrence is not probable with values lower than 2000 UI/l, with a predictive value of 80%, other authors have observed this complication with levels as low as 100 UI/l and even lower.[21–24] Therefore, occurrence of hemorrhage is not probable, although it is not impossible, with low levels of β-hCG, and its decreasing levels do not guarantee that rupture cannot take place. However, most of the authors find a statistically significant difference in the values of β-hCG between ruptured and non-ruptured ectopic pregnancies.

The decreasing levels of β-hCG combined with ultrasonography findings allow us to avoid surgical treatment in non-ruptured cases, although a very careful follow-up is needed because, as we have just discussed, the possibility of rupture exists even with decreasing levels of β-hCG. This situation can occur if the trophoblast is separated from the tubal wall, which may cause intratubal bleeding with accumulation of intratubal clots, which increase the pressure, and may cause distension and necrosis.

With transvaginal ultrasound an intrauterine gestational sac can be identified with 1000 UI/l of β-hCG ('discriminatory level'),[25] which is usually observed after 1 week of delay of menstruation. In a twin gestation this discriminatory level can be slightly higher and an ultrasonography control must be carried out within 2 or 3 days to try to find the gestational vesicle.

Once we have determined the β-hCG levels, if we do not find any gestational vesicle, we must consider two situations: the first takes place when we find a β-hCG level below 1000 UI/l, and the second when it is higher than 1000 UI/l.

β-hCG < 1000 UI/l without intrauterine gestational sac

In asymptomatic patients or with those with slight symptoms, the ultrasonography, as well as determination of β-hCG level, must be repeated in 1 week. At this time, it will be possible to find a β-hCG level higher than 1000 UI/l and also to observe an intrauterine gestational sac.[26]

Nevertheless, it is necessary to keep in mind that ectopic pregnancies produce in the endometrium some changes very similar to those induced by normal intrauterine pregnancies:[27]

- In 50% of ectopic pregnancies it is possible to observe a deciduate endometrium that appears ultrasonographically as a thickened and hyperrefringent endometrium (Figure 101.1).
- In 10–20% of ectopic pregnancies it is possible to observe a gestational pseudosac[28] (Figure 101.2), which appears as an echogenic image, located centrally in the endometrium and surrounded by a single echogenic ring. This image really corresponds to the presence of liquid in the deciduate endometrium. In a real gestational sac, a double echogenic ring is seen, composed of the vera decidua and the capsularis decidua, which form two concentric rings around the gestational sac (*double decidua sign*). This sign can be observed between the fifth and ninth gestational weeks and its presence makes the differential diagnosis easier.

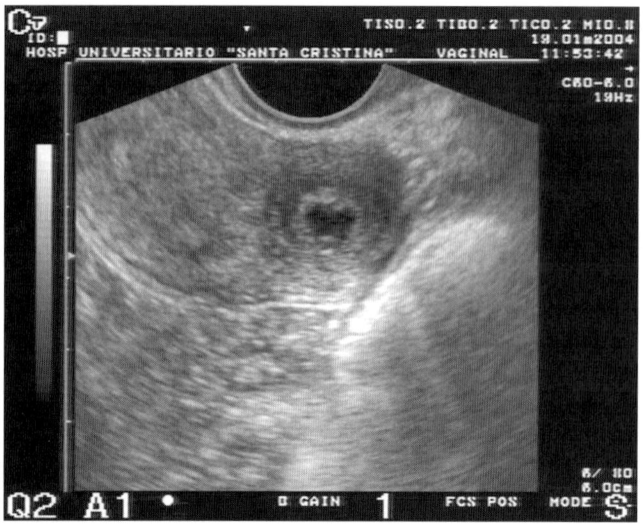

Figure 101.3 Ectopic pregnancy with ultrasound findings type 1. Outside the uterus and inside the tube an anechoic formation is visible, corresponding to the gestational vesicle.

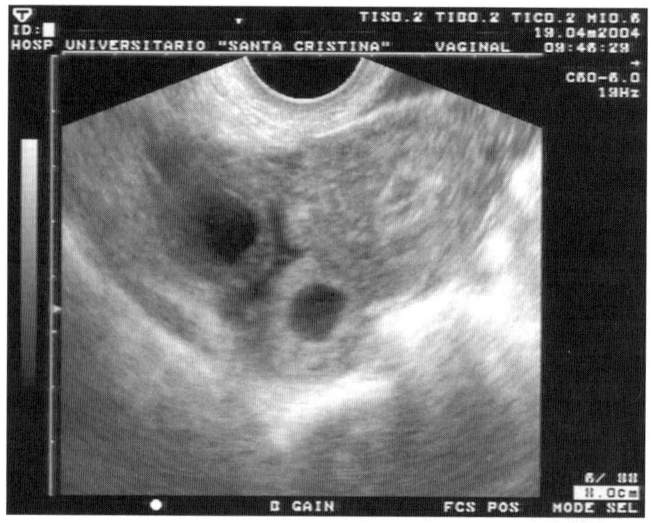

Figure 101.4 Ectopic pregnancy with ultrasound findings type 1. The corpus luteum closse to the gestational vesicle and the tube wall are visible.

- The color Doppler can also contribute to the diagnosis. An intrauterine gestational sac shows peritrophoblast vascular signals with a low resistance index (0.40–0.45). The pseudosac does not present an increase of the local flow and its resistance index may be higher (> 0.55).[29–32]

Another common problem when making the diagnosis is to differentiate the ectopic pregnancy from a complete or incomplete abortion. In the latter, ultrasonography shows a hyperechogenic image inside the uterine cavity that corresponds to clots or retained abortion rests. These findings can delay diagnosis in nearly 21% of the patients.

Also, the possibility of differentiating an ectopic pregnancy from a spontaneous abortion according to the reduction pattern of β-hCG levels in a period of time more than 48 h has been investigated. Some authors diagnose a complete abortion when the average life of the β-hCG is less than 1.4 days, whereas if it is more than 7 days, the ectopic pregnancy diagnosis is much more probable. Similarly, a plateau level of β-hCG (which has been defined as a duplication of its levels equal or higher in 7 days) is very suggestive of ectopic pregnancy.

The simultaneous presence of an intrauterine pregnancy and an ectopic one (heterotropic gestation) is not frequent at all, although its incidence is higher in pregnancies induced by reproductive techniques. It occurs in nearly 1 out of 100 of these pregnancies, which suggests a much higher frequency than the one referred historically (1 out of 30,000).[33,34]

β-hCG > 1000 UI/l without intrauterine gestational sac

In this situation a high suspicion of ectopic pregnancy exists, and the gestational sac must be looked for outside the uterus, considering that the most common location is the tube. Ultrasound findings can be categorized, depending on the visible structures, into five types:

(1) *Ultrasound image type 1*: A vesicle within the tube is visualized. The yolk sac and the embryo are not visible. The size of the gestational sac is over 3 mm (ultrasound resolution limit). It appears as a clear formation, in the parauterine region, with a central echogenic area surrounded by a hyperechogenic ring (Figures 101.3 and 101.4) that corresponds to the trophoblastic tissue, which presents an abundantly colored map because of its significant retrochorionic vascularization proliferation (Figure 101.5). The Doppler signals show a low or medium resistance index, which is very different from that found in normal tube walls, which show a high resistance. It is usual to find an average decrease of 15.5% in the ectopic pregnancy side with respect to the contralateral one. This ultrasound image is not easy to find and sometimes the gestational vesicle has less relevance than the corpus luteum that appears close to it, which we have to differentiate.

(2) *Ultrasound image type 2*: It is possible to obtain the same findings as in the previous type, but inside the gestational vesicle, the yolk sac can be visualized (Figure 101.6). The finding of the yolk sac is not a trivial matter because it makes the diagnosis easier, making possible to characterize the gestational vesicle, which is very difficult to see, especially when it is small. The presence of the yolk sac alone clarifies everything, and there is now no doubt about the presence of an ectopic pregnancy. The fact that the embryo cannot be seen does not mean that it does not exist, because we know that it is the embryo that induces the formation of the yolk sac. In the yolk sac

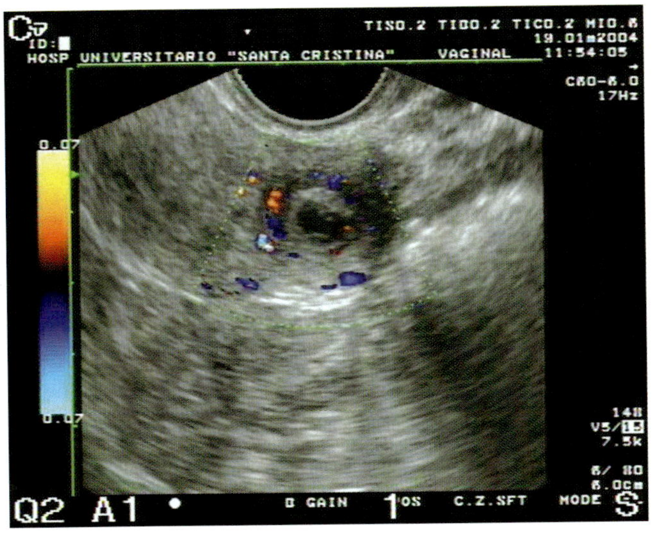

Figure 101.5 Ectopic pregnancy with ultrasound findings type 1. There is a significant vascularization around the gestational coat that corresponds to the trophoblast.

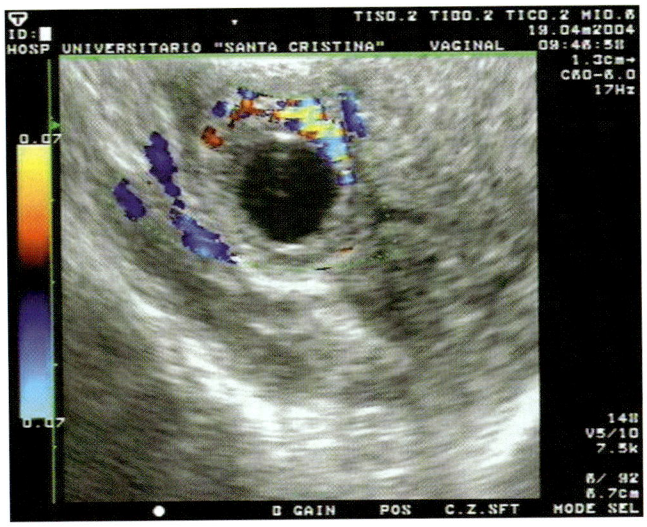

Figure 101.7 Ectopic pregnancy with ultrasound findings type 2. It's possible to see the yolk sac. The trophoblastic vascularization is also visible.

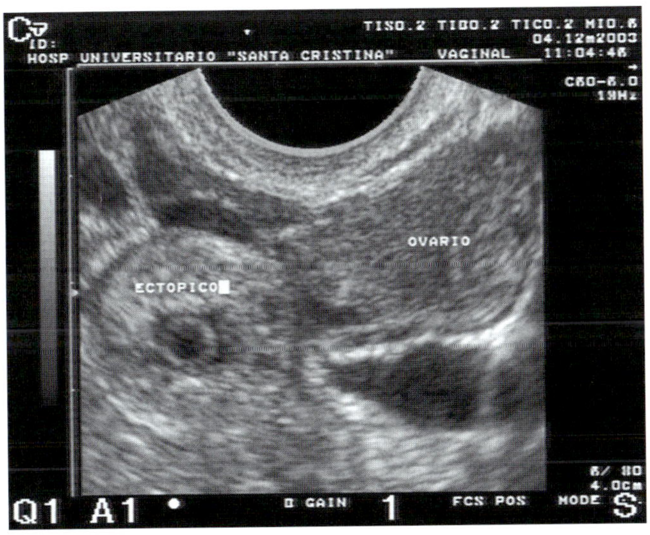

Figure 101.6 Ectopic pregnancy with ultrasound findings type 2. The gestational sac has the yolk sac inside.

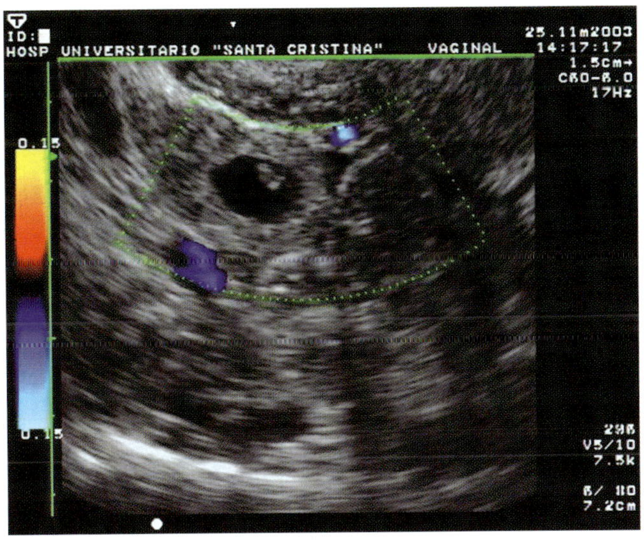

Figure 101.8 Ectopic pregnancy with ultrasound findings type 3. Gestational sac with the yolk sac and an embryo of very small size inside, in which the heartbeat is still not seen.

surroundings it is possible to observe blood flows with abundant Doppler signal and low resistance index as well as in the type 1 image (Figure 101.7).

(3) *Ultrasound image type 3*: It is possible to visualize the gestational vesicle, the yolk sac and also the embryo, but not its heart beating (Figures 101.8 and 101.9). The size of the embryo usually is not very big (Figure 101.10). It seems like it is going to start a reabsorption process and soon it disappears or is confused with the gestational sac.

(4) *Ultrasound image type 4*: The typical image of a gestational vesicle with the yolk sac and the embryo is visualized, but this time with visible cardiac beat inside the embryo. It is very easy to see the beat by using the color map or the flow wave (Figures 101.11 and 101.12). When this image appears, the diagnosis of ectopic pregnancy is made. With an abdominal probe it is possible to visualize this image in only 10% of the cases, but with the transvaginal one, in 21% of all the ectopic pregnancies.

(5) *Ultrasound image type 5*: This image corresponds with tubal rupture or with tubal abortion. In these cases the acute accident is present and the symptoms and signs are usually important. The most important sign is the hemoperitoneum (Figure 101.13), and the patient may present

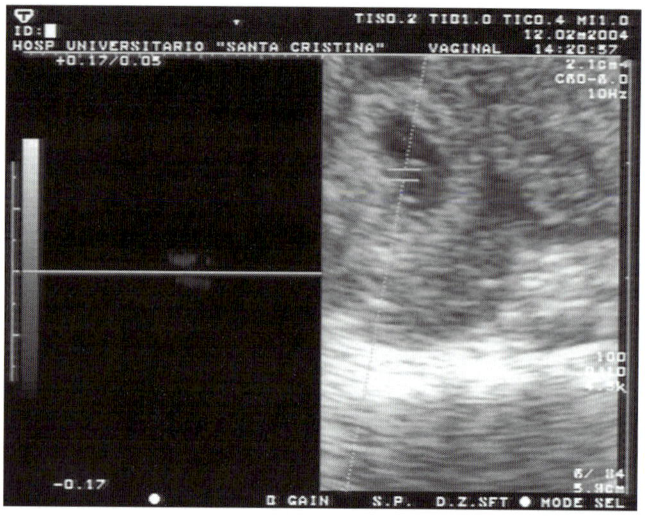

Figure 101.9 Ectopic pregnancy with ultrasound findings type 3. Inside the gestational sac, the yolk sac and also an embyo with no visible heart activity are seen.

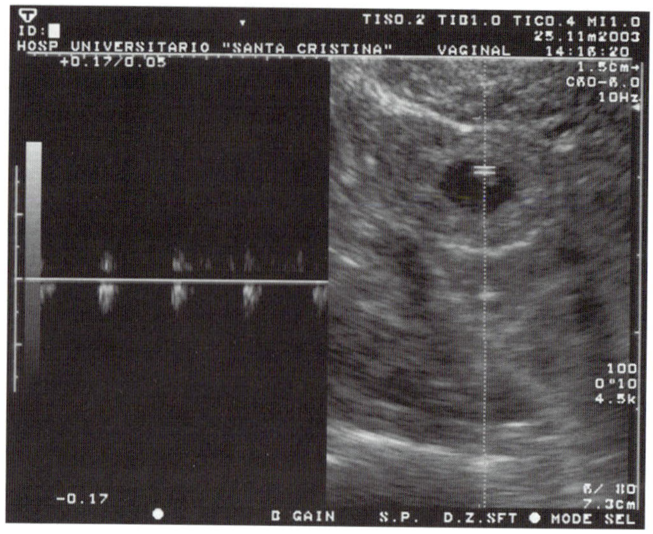

Figure 101.11 Ectopic pregnancy with ultrasound findings type 4. Inside the gestational sac the yolk sac and a live embryo are visible. The heart activity is shown by using the color signal.

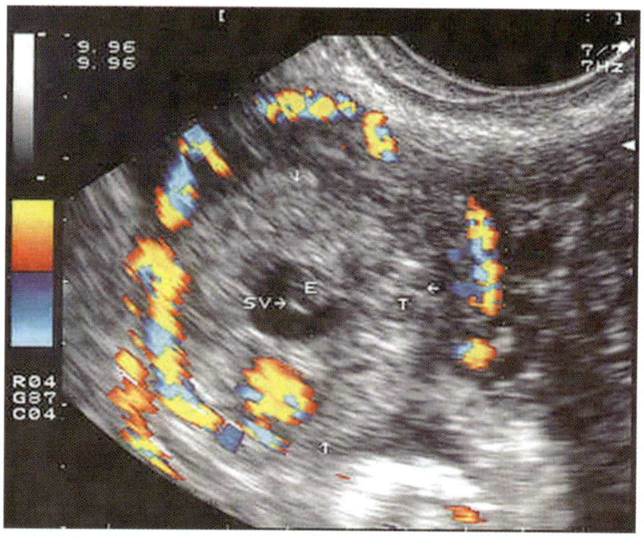

Figure 101.10 Ectopic pregnancy with ultrasound findings type 3. The yolk sac is visible inside the gestational sac and also an embryo with no visible heart activity. The Doppler signal is captured only on the peritubal trophoblast.

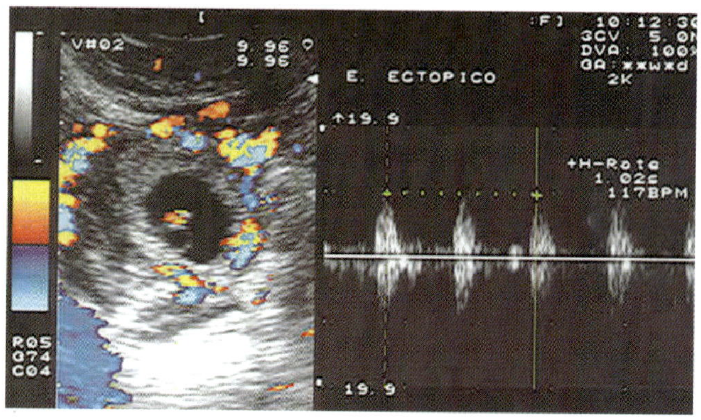

Figure 101.12 Ectopic pregnancy with ultrasound findings type 4. Inside the gestational sac the yolk sac is visible, and also an embryo with its heart beating.

hypotension and anemia. A large amount of fluid may be visible in the abdomen, in the flanks and in the cul-de-sac if a tubal rupture is present. These fluid collections may be presented as free fluid or as organized blood clots in the cul-de-sac lateral and cranial to the uterus. The clots exhibit the sonographic features of solid masses, appearing homogenous and contrasting poorly with the surrounding tissues. The tube appears refringent ultrasonographically, thickened or included in a mass of blood clots. In some cases the tube appears normal, and the blood located around it draws it, showing its shape and the fimbrias.

The mere presence of fluid in the cul-de-sac is not a specific sign of ectopic pregnancy.[35] It is present in nearly 40–83% of all ectopic pregnancies but small collections of free fluid may be seen under normal conditions in non-gravid patients, especially during the periovulatory period, and also in 20% of intrauterine pregnancies and in some other pathologies.

The total absence of ultrasonographic findings in the adnexal area does not exclude the ectopic pregnancy diagnosis. In these cases it is necessary to determine the β-hCG level again, to establish its decreasing or increasing pattern, and to repeat the ultrasonography to look for the gestational vesicle in

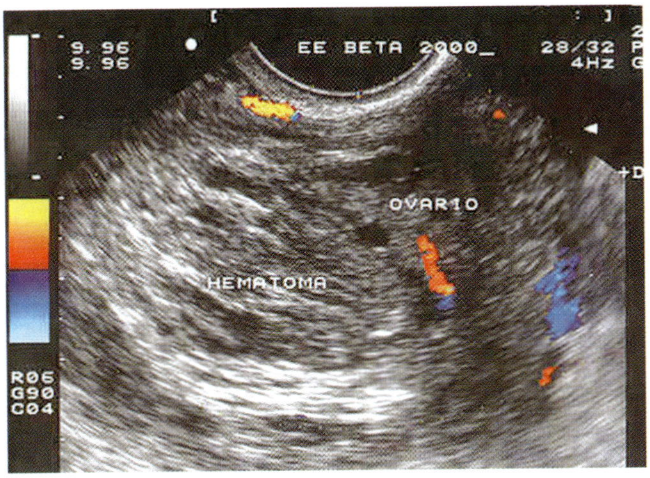

Figure 101.13 Rupture of an ectopic pregnancy (ultrasound findings type 5). An important hemoperitoneum is visible, with clots.

any location. If the patient is stable, we should not undertake laparoscopy so early, since the initial phases of ectopic pregnancy have been described with absolutely normal laparoscopy.

Generally, in all previous assumptions, the existence of a corpus luteum can be observed. It is visualized as a round hypoechogenic structure, surrounded by a ring of ovarian tissue. It can appear in the contralateral ovary in 13–23% of the cases. The transvaginal ultrasound sensitivity for the ectopic pregnancy diagnosis is very high, nearly 99%, with 98% of specificity, 98% of positive predictive value and 99% of negative predictive value.

Ultrasonography aid to conservative treatment

Ultrasound is useful as a diagnostic tool in the observation of a gestational sac inside or outside the uterus.

At present, the precocious diagnosis of ectopic pregnancy allows treatment possibilities other than surgical boarding, which was the only option considered traditionally.[36–38] These treatment possibilities are:

- expectant handling
- systemic methotrexate administration
- local methotrexate administration.

The surgical handling can be performed by laparoscopy or by laparotomy.

Expectant handling

With a precocious diagnosis of the ectopic pregnancy, before symptoms appear, and adopting a more conservative attitude, it has been possible to see that the spontaneous regression of the tubal ectopic pregnancy is a phenomenon much more common that we thought previously. This fact means that there is a high percentage of ectopic pregnancies that are resolved with no need of treatment, and that is why expectant handling has a place in the management of ectopic pregnancy.[39,40]

The main advantages of expectant handling are that it avoids the risks of surgery, general anesthesia and the potential indirect effects of the drugs used in the treatment of ectopic pregnancy.

The great difficulty in expectant handling is to select suitable patients for it. The selection criteria used differ for different authors, but in most cases there are some common aspects; the most outstanding ones are:

- Asymptomatic patient, clinically stable.
- Size: maximum diameter of the ectopic pregnancy of 2–4 cm, according to the authors.
- Absence of embryonic cardiac beat (ultrasonography finding types 1, 2 or 3).
- Decreasing values of β-hCG levels (also variable according to the authors, but at least a decrease of 2% in two determinations with a delay of at least 24 h).
- Little amount of free fluid in cul-de-sac.

Patients will have to be under periodic ambulatory control with multiple determinations of β-hCG levels and with an ultrasound following, three times a week in the beginning, and later once a week, according to the different protocols.[41] The signs that orient to a reabsorption and therefore to a spontaneous resolution of the problem are:

- β-hCG decreasing levels: it is important to be aware that sometimes it takes 70 days for the β-hCG value to become negative because of the trophoblast persistence. Serially monitored β-hCG results after conservative treatment of ectopic pregnancy may show plateaued values without indicating failure of treatment.[42]
- The gestational vesicle, the yolk sac and all the embryonic structures are wrapped into a reabsorption process, becoming increasingly small (Figure 101.14), refringent (Figure 101.15) and finally disappearing, replaced by a solid complex image (Figure 101.16).
- The color map inside the trophoblast is smaller each time (Figure 101.17), with a slight Doppler signal, which is sometimes very difficult to find.
- The resistance and pulsatility indexes inside the trophoblastic vessels are increased and, in the end, it is impossible to identify anything objectively.

The percentage of success of the expectant handling varies between 57% and 100%, although in the studies with more cases it is estimated around 70%. The best results are observed when the β-hCG levels are below 2000 UI/l.

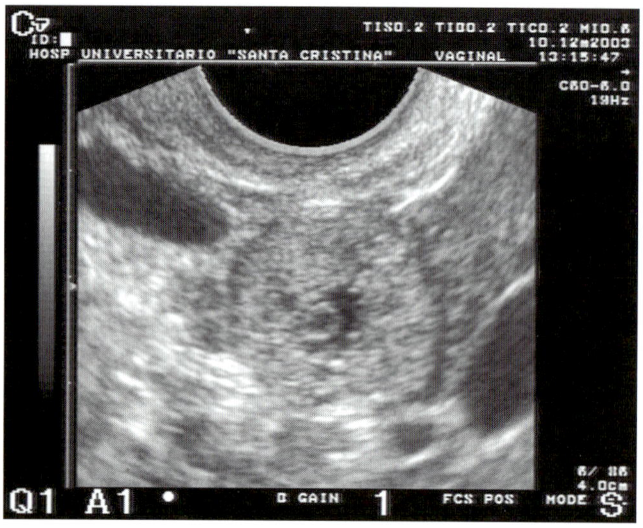

Figure 101.14 Ectopic pregnancy with spontaneous reabsorption. A yolk sac less visible and a refringent ring around it are visible.

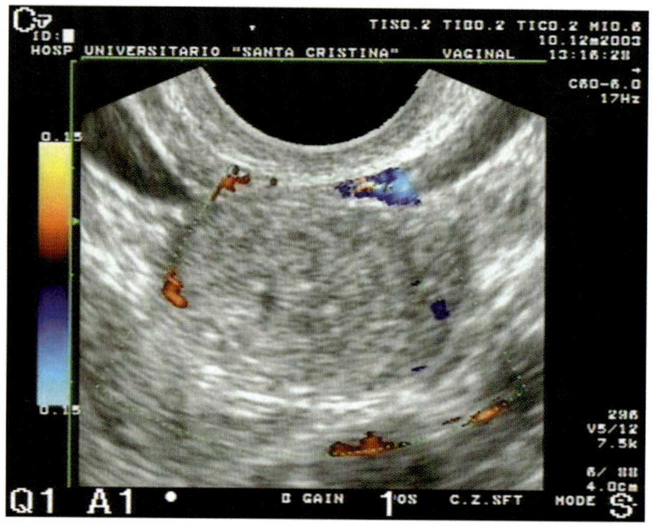

Figure 101.16 Ectopic pregnancy with spontaneous reabsorption.The yolk sac has disappeared and has been replaced by a refringent area that shows the tube more compact.

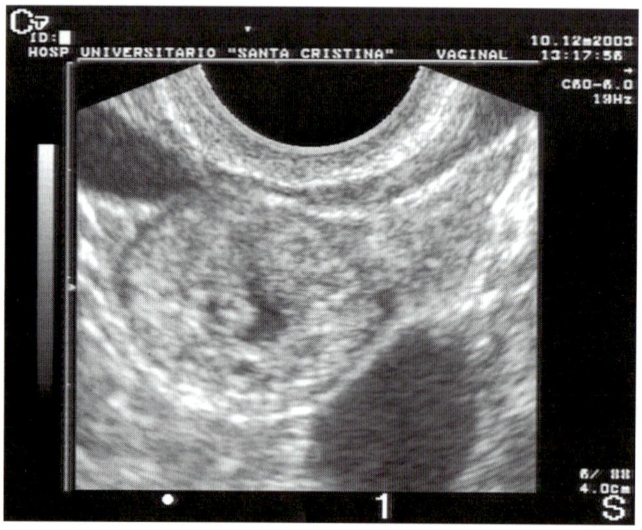

Figure 101.15 Ectopic pregnancy with spontaneous reabsorption. The yolk sac has nearly disappeared.

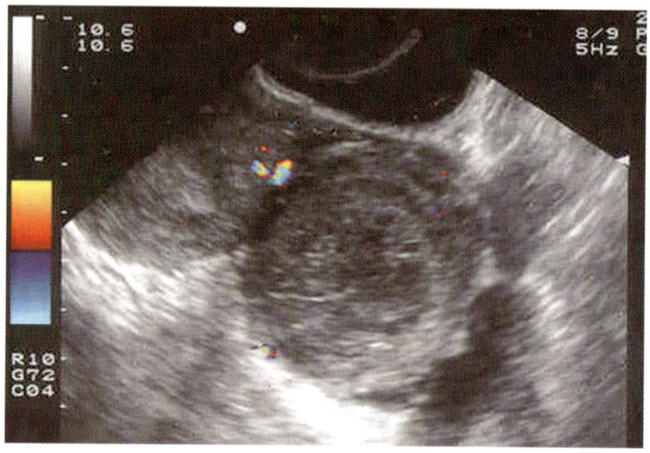

Figure 101.17 Ectopic pregnancy with spontaneous reabsorption. Color map progressively fades away.

The following are the most important indications for surgery in the cases in which expectant handling fails: abdominal pain, β-hCG levels increased or similar to the previous ones, appearance or increase of the liquid in the Douglas sac and increase of the size of the adnexal formation.

Among the disadvantages of expectant handing, it is necessary to mention, on the one hand, the prolonged period of follow-up that patients have to be put under, and on the other, the possibility of persistence of trophoblast tissue inside the tube, which could cause adhesions and great tubal damage. Nevertheless, when comparing the reproductive results of patients under expectant handling with those of patients under conservative surgery, there are no differences between the two groups in subsequent gestations, either intrauterine or ectopic rates.

Finally, it is very important to point out that this kind of treatment can be applied only if ultrasounds are used to make the diagnosis.[43]

Systemic methotrexate administration

The most common drug used in the treatment of ectopic pregnancy is methotrexate, which interferes in trophoblastic development.

Methotrexate inhibits the reduction of folic acid to tetrahydrofolic acid. Because tetrahydrofolic acid is essential in the transfer of one-carbon fragments in the synthesis of DNA, methotrexate effectively blocks DNA synthesis, inhibiting cell replication.

In the 1960s, methotrexate was used for the treatment of persistent trophoblastic tissues after an abdominal pregnancy. In 1982 it was used, for the first time, in the treatment of ectopic pregnancy.

As with expectant handling, administration of methotrexate depends on the patient's profile. The selection criteria are different for several authors, but most of them agree in using methotrexate in hemodynamic stable patients, with a non-ruptured ectopic pregnancy, with a small amount of liquid in the Douglas sac and with less than 4-cm diameter of tubal affection, with ultrasonography finding types 1, 2 or 3.

The presence of embryonic heart movements is for some authors an absolute contraindication for this kind of treatment, because results in these cases are worse and it would be better to recommend surgical treatment.

Before methotrexate administration, a complete hemogram (including platelet count) and some biochemical values to ensure that hepatic and renal functions are normal are needed.

The doses of methotrexate that have been used in different studies are quite variable. The most usual dose is 1 mg/kg, intramuscularly, every 48 h, until a total of four doses are completed or until a reduction of β-hCG levels in two consecutive days is observed. Methotrexate is usually combined with folinic acid (0.1 mg/kg) on alternate days.

At present, a single dose of 50 mg/m^2 of methotrexate is being used, and has proved to be as effective as the multiple-dose therapy. This model does not need the combination with folinic acid, and it has fewer secondary effects.

The β-hCG levels can increase during the first 3 days after the treatment, but they must be lower on the seventh day. If this reduction is smaller than 15%, it is necessary to repeat the methotrexate administration (which is necessary in nearly 8% of the cases).

Oral administration has also been used, but its results are not as good as with intramuscular administration.

Toxicity to methotrexate frequently involves the mucous membranes, with stomatitis, esophagitis, vaginitis and, occasionally, gastrointestinal ulcerations, but these are not very common, and are dose-dependent. Bone narrow suppression with granulocytopenia and thrombocytopenia is common, but generally not severe. Skin rashes and alopecia are uncommon, but they do occur; nephrotoxicity, hepatotoxicity and pulmonary fibrosis are very rare.

After 3 or 4 days of methotrexate administration, the presence of abdominal pain of variable intensity is common, described in 60% of the patients. It is usually a side effect that disappears spontaneously in 1 or 2 days, although sometimes a visit to the hospital is needed to rule out hemodynamic instability and possible rupture.

The success rate is 83–100% according to different studies.

Periodical ultrasonography and control of β-hCG levels are needed after the conservative treatment. The ultrasonographic image of the ectopic pregnancy can continue to be observed when the β-hCG values are negative. The persistence of this negative value does not have to be interpreted as a failure of treatment, and it can even take months to disappear.[44]

Asymptomatic tube ectopic pregnancy with live embryo

If the gestational sac is visualized inside the tube and we can see an embryo with positive heart movements, there are two treatment options: laparoscopic extirpation and transvaginal punction with methotrexate injection inside the gestational sac, which is used only in selected cases.[45]

One of the most important indications for local methotrexate administration is the presence of embryo heart activity. In these cases, with the local punction, we have the methotrexate local action and the blast effect of the needle. With this direct administration it is possible to reduce the dose of the drug, diminishing therefore its side effects.

The gestational sac punction has to be guided by transvaginal ultrasonography or carried out by laparoscopy. After the punction, the first thing that we have to do is to aspirate the sac content and after that to inject the methotrexate. The methotrexate dose used is variable in different studies, but it is around 10–50 mg.

After the punction, a very refringent image is visible (Figures 101.18–101.19), which changes very slowly in some cases, as described before, during reabsorption.

The success rate is nearly 85–100%, according to different authors.

Some other substances have been used for local administration instead of methotrexate (such as prostaglandins, potassium chloride, hyperosmotic glucose, etc.) for the treatment of ectopic pregnancy, but their use has now been discontinued because of their considerable secondary effects and their minimal action.

The local or systemic administration of methotrexate is also indicated in cornual or cervical ectopic pregnancies, to avoid surgical treatment, in an attempt to preserve fertility.

If the tube has not been blown apart by rupture, it can be preserved by making a longitudinal incision along the antimesenteric border of the tube and suturing the incision with fine material.

Treatment of acute rupture of tubal ectopic pregnancy

If the intraperitoneal bleeding is very profuse, symptoms of shock occur and it is obvious that surgical attention is required.

The treatment in this case consists of evacuating the hemoperitoneum and excising the ectopic pregnancy

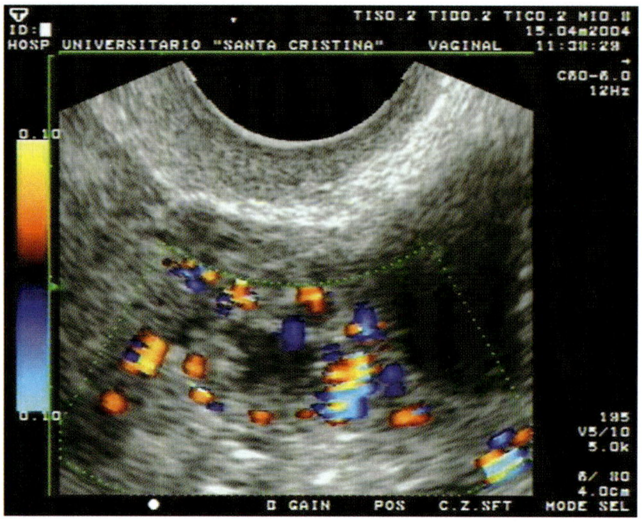

Figure 101.18 Ectopic pregnancy treated successfully with methotrexate. The reabsorption process of the tubal formation is visible.

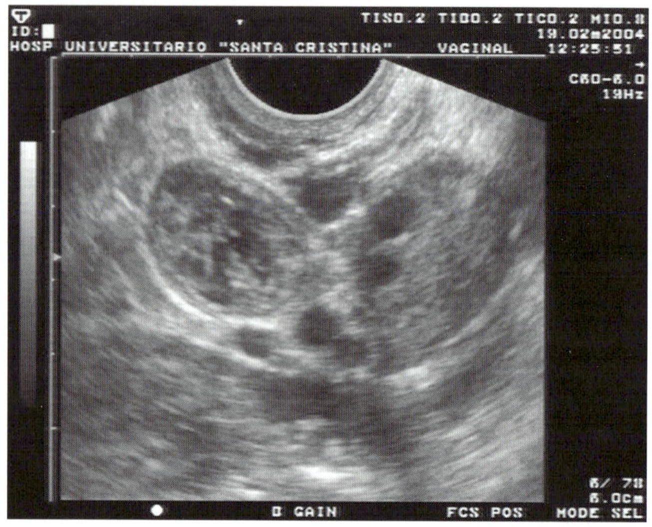

Figure 101.19 Ectopic pregnancy after intrasac methotrexate injection. Both the gestational vesicle and the embryo have been transformed into a refringent structure that will initiate the same process of reabsorption that happens when it does it spontaneously.

by laparoscopy or laparotomy, once the patient is in a stable state.

Treatment of abdominal ectopic pregnancy

The treatment in these cases consists of evacuating the fetus outside the abdominal cavity with ligation of the umbilical cord. It is not necessary to remove the placenta, which may be firmly fixed to the mesentery and the abdominal viscera. Profuse hemorrhage can occur on manipulation, and the placenta, if left *in situ*, resorbs without sequelae in most instances.

In these cases, it is also possible to use the methotrexate intramuscularly and to perform ultrasonography and control of β-hCG levels after it. Some authors have suggested the use of methotrexate to facilitate devascularization and absorption of any unremoved placenta.

Ultrasonography makes it possible to monitor the placenta left *in situ* after removing the fetus,[46] whose image can be seen inside the abdomen for a long time.

REFERENCES

1. Speroff L, Glass RH, Kase NG. Ectopic pregnancy. In Speroff L, Glass RH, Kase NG, eds. *Clinical Gynecologyc Endocrinology and Infertility*. London: Williams and Wilkins, 1999:1149–67.
2. Bouyer J, Coste J, Fernandez H, Pouly JL, Job-Spira N. Sites of ectopic pregnancy; A 10 year population-based study of 1800 cases. *Hum Reprod* 2002;17:3224–30.
3. Coste J, Bouyer J, Ughetto S, *et al*. Ectopic pregnancy is again on the increase. Recent trends in the incidence of ectopic pregnancies in France (1992–2002). *Hum Reprod* 2004;19:2014–8.
4. Boufous S, Quartararo M, Mohsin M, Parker J. Trends in the incidence of ectopic pregnancy in New South Wales between 1990–1998. *Aust N Z J Obstet Gynaecol* 2001;41:436–8.
5. Rajkhowa M, Glass MR, Rutherford AJ, *et al*. Trends in the incidence of ectopic pregnancy in England and Wales from 1966 to 1996. *BJOG* 2000;107:369–74.
6. Strandell A, Thorburn J, Hamberger L. Risk factors for ectopic pregnancy in assisted reproduction. *Fertil Steril* 1999;2:282–6.
7. Kamwendo F, Forslin L, Bodin L, Danielson D. Epidemiology of ectopic pregnancy during a 28 year period and the role of pelvic inflammatory disease. *Sex Transm Infect* 2000;76:28–32.
8. Barlow RE, Cooke ID, Odukoya O, Heatley MK, Jenkins J, Narayansingh G, *et al*. The prevalence of *Chlamydia Trachomatis* in fresh tissue specimens from patients with ectopic pregnancy or tubal factor infertility as determined by PCR and *in situ* hybridisation. *J Med Microbiol* 2001;50:902–8.
9. Jun SH, Milki AA. Assisted hatching is associated with a higher ectopic pregnancy rate. *Fertil Steril* 2004;81:1701–3.
10. Bouyer J, Rachou E, Germain E, *et al*. Risk factors for extrauterine pregnancy in women using an intrauterine device. *Fertil Steril* 2000;74:899–908.
11. Dahiya K, Khosla AH. Ectopic pregnancy after sterilization. *Trop Doct* 2004;34:255.
12. Wong E, Suat SO. Ectopic pregnancy – A diagnostic challenge in the emergency department. *Eur J Emerg Med* 2000;7:189–94.
13. Shalev E, Yarom I, Bustan M, Weiner E, Bon-Schlomo I. Transvaginal sonography as the utimate diagnosis tool for the management of ectopic pregnancy: experience with 840 cases. *Fertil Steril* 1998;69:62–5.
14. Hertzberg BS, Kliewer MA. Ectopic pregancy: Ultrasound diagnosis and interpretive pitfalls. *South Med J* 1995;88: 1191–8.
15. Chan LY, Fok WY, Yuen PM. Pitfalls in diagnosis of interstitial pregnancy. *Acta Obstet Gynecol Scand* 2003;82:867–70.
16. Mueller MD, Raio L, Spoerri S, *et al*. Novel placental and nonplacental serum markers in ectopic versus normal intrauterine pregnancy. *Fertil Steril* 2004;81:1106–11.
17. Shepherd RW, Patton PE, Novy MJ, Burry KA. Serial beta-hCG measurements in the early detection of ectopic pregnancy. *Obstet Gynecol* 1990;75:417–20.
18. Roussos D, Panidis D, Matalliotakis I, *et al*. Factors that may predispose to rupture of tubal ectopic pregnancy. *Eur J Obstet Gynecol Reprod Biol* 2000;89:15–7.
19. da Costa Soares R, Elito J Jr, Han KK, Camano L. Endometrial thickness as an orienting factor for the medical treatment of

unruptured tubal pregnancy. *Acta Obstet Gynecol Scand* 2004;83:289–92.
20. Laurie S, Insler V. Can the serum beta hCG level reliably predict likelihood of a ruptured tubal pregnancy? *Isr J Obstet Gynecol* 1992;3:152–544.
21. Bozoklu S, Bozoklu E, Ciftci A, Coskun T. Ruptured ectopic pregnancy with indetectable beta-hCG levels coexisting with acute appendicitis. *Acta Obstet Gynecol Reprod Scand* 1997;76:181–2.
22. Lurie S, Katz Z, Weissman A, Zaley Y, Caspi B. Declining beta-human chorionic gonadotropin level may provide false security that tubal pregnancy will not rupture. *Eur J Obstet Gynecol Reprod Biol* 1994;53:72–3.
23. Tulandi T, Hemmings R, Khalifa F. Rupture of ectopic pregnancy in woman with low and declining serum beta-human chorionic gonadotropin concentrations. *Fertil Steril* 1991;56:786–7.
24. Weston G, Kashyap R. Failed conservative management of cervical pregnancy despite falling beta-HCG. *Aust N Z J Obstet Gynaecol* 2001;41:346–7.
25. Peisner DB, Timor-Tritsch IE. The discriminatory zone of beta hCG for vaginal probes. *J Clin Ultrasound* 1990;18:280–5.
26. Counselman FL, Shoar S, Heller RA, King DK. Quantitative beta-hCG levels less than 1000 mIU/mL in patients with ectopic pregnancy: pelvic ultrasound still useful. *J Emerg med* 1998;16:699–703.
27. Albayram F, Hamper UM. First-trimester obstetric emergencies: Spectrum of sonographic findings. *J Clin Ultrasound* 2002;30:161–77.
28. Hill LM, Kislak S, Martin JG. Transvaginal sonographic detection of the pseudogestational sac associated with ectopic pregnancy. *Obstet Gynecol* 1990;75:986–8.
29. Jurkovic D, Bourne TH, Jauniaux E, Campbell S, Collins WP. Transvaginal color Doppler study of blood flow in ectopic pregnancies. *Fertil Steril* 1992;57:68–73.
30. Dillon EH, Feyock AL, Taylor KJW. Pseudogestational sacs: Doppler US differentiation from normal or abnormal intrauterine pregnancies. *Radiology* 1990;176:359–64.
31. Tekay A, Jouppila P. Color Doppler flow as an indicator of trophoblastic activity in tubal pregnancies detected by transavaginal ultrasound. *Obstet Gynecol* 1992;80:995–9.
32. Wherry KL, Dubinsky TJ, Waitches GM, Richardson ML, Reed S. Low-resistance endometrial arterial flow in the exclusion of ectopic pregnancy revisited. *J Ultrasound Med* 2001;20:335–42.
33. Breyer MJ, Constantino TG. Heterotopic gestation: another possibility for the emergency bedsite ultrasonographer to consider. *J Emerg Med* 2004;26:81–4.
34. Kumor S, Vimala N, Dadhwal V, Mittal S. Heterotopic cervical and intrauterine pregnancy in a spontaneous cycle. *Eur J Obstet Gynecol Reprod Biol* 2004;112:217–20.
35. Dart R, McLean SA, Dart L. Isolated fluid in the cul-de-sac. How well does it predict ectopic pregnancy? *Am J Emerg Med* 2002;20:1–4.
36. Yao M, Tulandi T. Current status of surgical and non-surgical management of ectopic pregnancy. *Fertil Steril* 1997;67:421–33.
37. Tulandi T, Sammour A. Evidence-based management of ectopic pregnancy. *Curr Opin Obstet Gynecol* 2000;12:289–92.
38. Canis M, Savary D, Pouly JL, Wattiez A, Mage G. Ectopic pregnancy: criteria to decide between medical and conservative surgical treatment? *J Gynecol Obstet Biol Reprod* 2003;32:54–63.
39. Atri M, Chow CM, Kintzaen G, *et al*. Expectant treatment of ectopic pregnancies: clinical and sonographic predictors. *AJR Am J Roentgenol* 2001;176:123–7.
40. Atri M, Bret PM, Tulandi T. Spontaneous resolution of ectopic pregnancy: Initial appearance and evolution at transvaginal US. *Radiology* 1993;186:83–86.
41. Ylostalo P, Cacciatore B, Sjoberg J, *et al*. Expectant management of ectopic pregnancy. *Obstet Gynecol* 1992;80:345–8.
42. Thompson GR, O'Shea RT, Harding A. Beta hCG levels after conservative treatment of ectopic pregnancy: is a plateau normal? *Aust N Z J Obstet Gynaecol* 1994;34:96–8.
43. Turan C, Ugur M, Dogan M, Ekici E, Vicdan K, Gokmen O. Transvaginal sonographic findings of chronic ectopic pregnancy. *Eur J Obstet Gynecol reprod Biol* 1996;67:115–9.
44. Tekay A, Martikainen H, Heikkinen H, *et al*. Disappearance of the trophoblastic blood flow in tubal pregnancy after methotrexate injection. *J Ultrasound Med* 1993;12:615–8.
45. Venezia R, Zangara C, Comparetto G, Cittadini E. Conservative treatment of ectopic pregnancy using a single echo-guided injection of methotrexate into the gestational sac. *Ultrasound Obstet Gynecol* 1991;1:132–5.
46. Bajo JM, García FA, Huertas MA. Sonographic follow-up of a placenta left *in situ* after delivery of the fetus in abdominal pregnancy. *Ultrasound Obstet Gynecol* 1996;7:285–8.

Volume 2

Textbook of Perinatal Medicine

Dedication

This textbook is dedicated to the pioneers from throughout the world who created perinatal medicine

Volume 2

Textbook of Perinatal Medicine

Second Edition

Edited by

Asim Kurjak MD
Professor and Chairman
Department of Obstetrics and Gynecology
Medical School University of Zagreb
Croatia

and

Frank A. Chervenak MD
Given Foundation Professor and Chairman
Department of Obstetrics and Gynecology
Weill Medical College of Cornell University
New York Presbyterian Hospital
USA

informa
healthcare

First published in the United Kingdom in 1998
by The Parthenon Publishing Group Ltd

Second edition published in the United Kingdom in 2006 by Informa UK Ltd
4 Park Square, Milton Park, Abingdon, Oxon OX14 4RN. Informa Healthcare is a trading division of Informa UK Ltd. Registered Office: 37/41 Mortimer Street, London WIT 3JH. Registered in England and Wales Number 1072954.

Tel: +44 (0)20 7017 6000
Fax: +44 (0)20 7017 6699
E-mail: info.medicine@tandf.co.uk
Website: www.tandf.co.uk/medicine

A CIP record for this book is available from the British Library.

Library of Congress Cataloging-in-Publication Data
Data available on application

ISBN10 1 84214 333 6 (2-volume set)
ISBN13 978 1 84214 333 9

Distributed in North and South America by
Taylor & Francis
6000 Broken Sound Parkway, NW (Suite 300)
Boca Raton, FL 33487, USA

Within Continental USA
Tel: 1(800) 272 7737; Fax: 1(800) 374 3401
Outside Continental USA
Tel: (561) 994 0555; Fax: (561) 361 6018
E-mail: orders@crcpress.com

Distributed in the rest of the world by
Thomson Publishing Services
Cheriton House
North Way
Andover, Hampshire SP10 5BE, UK
Tel: +44 (0)1264 332424
E-mail: tps.tandfsalesorder@thomson.com

Composition by Keyword Group Ltd, Great Yarmouth, Norfolk, UK
Printed and bound in India by Replika Press Pvt. Ltd

Contents for Volume 1 and 2

List of principal contributors

A. Adra Department of Obstetrics & Gynecology, American University of Beirut Medical Center, Beirut, Lebanon

J. L. Alcázar Department Obstetrics & Gynecology, Clinica Universitaria de Navarra, Pamplona, Spain

Z. Alfirevic University Department of Obstetrics & Gynaecology, Liverpool Women's Hospital, Liverpool, UK

M. M. Anceschi Institute of Gynecology, Perinatology & Child Health, University of Rome "La Sapienza", Rome, Italy

A. Antsaklis Department of Fetal-Maternal Medicine, Alexandra Maternity Hospital, Athens, Greece

Z. Appelman Institute of Genetics, Kaplan Medical Center, Rehovot, Israel

B. Arabin Department of Perinatology, Isala Clinics, 8025 AB Zwolle, The Netherlands

J. Babnik Department of Obstetrics & Gynecology, University Medical Center, Ljubljana, Slovenia

J. M. Bajo Arenas Department of Obstetrics & Gynecology, Getafe University Hospital, Madrid, Spain

L. S. Bakketeig Department of Epidemiology, University of Southern Denmark, Odense, Denmark

R. Baraibar Department of Pediatrics, Institute Universitari Dexeus, Barcelona, Spain

Y. Baytur Celal Bayar University, Medical School, Department of Obstetrics and Gynecology, Manisa, Turkey

A. Beke First Department of Obstetrics & Gynecology, Semmelweis University Medical School, Budapest, Hungary

G. Benagiano Department of Gynecological Sciences, Perinatology & Child Care, University "la Sapienza", Rome, Italy

K. Benirschke University of California, San Diego, CA, USA

K. Biedermann Department of Obstetrics & Gynaecology, Kantonales Frauenspital Fontana Lürlibadstr. 118, CH-7000 Chur, Switzerland

D. J. Birnbach Department of Anesthesiology, University of Miami School of Medicine, Miami, Florida, USA

I. Blickstein Department of Obstetrics & Gynecology, Kaplan Medical Center, Rehovot, Israel

F. Bonilla-Musoles Department of Obstetrics & Gynecology, Valencia School of Medicine, Valencia, Spain

R. Bracci Institute of Preventive Pediatrics and Neonatology, University of Siena, Siena, Italy

B. Brambati Center of Prenatal Diagnosis, Milan, Italy

V. N. A. Breeveld-Dwarkasing Department of Pathobiology, Division of Veterinary Anatomy & Physiology, Faculty of Veterinary Medicine, Utrecht University, Utrecht, The Netherlands

B. Breyer University of Zagreb, Faculty of Electrical Engineering and Computing, Zagreb, Croatia

H. Budge Centre for Reproduction and Early Life, Institute of Clinical Research, University Hospital, Nottingham, UK

P. Buekens School of Public Health & Tropical Medicine, Tulane University, New Orleans, LA, USA

F. Carmona Institut Clinic de Ginecologis, Obstetricia i Neonatologia, Hospital Clinic-University of Barcelone, Catalonia, Spain

M. R. G. Carrapato Department of Paediatrics & Neonatology, Hospital de São Sebastiao, Santa Maria da Feira, Portugal

J. M. Carrera Fetal Medicine Service, Departamento de Obstetricia y Ginecologia, Instituto Universitario Dexeus, Barcelona, Spain

R. Chaoui Center for Prenatal Diagnosis & Human Genetics, Berlin, Germany

S. T. Chasen Weill College of Cornell University, New York, NY, USA

F. A. Chervenak The New York Presbyterian Hospital, Weill Medical College of Cornell University, NY, USA

S. Cicero Fetal Medicine Foundation, London, UK

W. R. Cohen Department Obstetrics & Gynecology, Weill Medical College of Cornell University, New York, NY, USA

C. Comas Prenatal Diagnosis Unit, Centro Gutenberg, Malaga, Spain

L. Cornette The Peter Congdon Neonatal Unit, Leeds General Infirmary, Leeds, UK

E. V. Cosmi Institute of Gynecology, Perinatology & Child Health, University of Rome "La Sapienza", Rome, Italy

L. de Crespigny Murdoch Children's Research Institute, Royal Children's Hospital, University of Melbourne, Victoria, Australia

A. Csaba First Department of Obstetrics & Gynecology, Semmelweis University Medical School, Baross, Budapest, Hungary

V. D'Addario Fetal Medicine Unit, Department Obstetrics & Gynecology, University of Bari, Italy

F. Daffos Département de Diagnostic Prénatal et de Foetologie, Institut de Puériculture de Paris, Paris, France

M. Dan Unit of Infectious Diseases, Wolfson Medical Center, Holon, Israel

J. E. Deaver Women's Health Research, Jamaica Hospital Medical Center, New York, NY, USA

R. Derom Association de Soutien a la Recherche Scientifique au Profit des Naissances Multiples, Destelbergen, Belgium

G. C. di Renzo Centre of Perinatal & Reproductive Medicine, University of Perugia, Perugia, Italy

E. Domenech Department Pediatrics, Faculty of Medicine of La Laguna, University Hospital of the Canary Islands, Tenerife, Spain

S. M. Donn Division of Neonatal-Perinatal Medicine, CS Mott Children's Hospital, University Michigan Health System, Ann Arbor, MI, USA

A. Drazancic Division of Neonatal-Perinatal Medicine, CS Mott Children's Hospital, University Michigan Health System, Ann Arbor, MI, USA

J. W. Dudenhausen Department Obstetrics, Charite Campus Virchow-Klinikum, Berlin, Germany

S. J. English The Peter Congdon Neonatal Unit, Clarendon Wing, Leeds General Infirmary, Leeds, UK

A. K. Ertan Department of Obstetrics & Gynecology, Saarland University Medical School, Homburg, Germany

J. Espinoza Perinatology Research Branch, National Institute of Child Health and Human Development, NIH, DHHS, Bethesda, Maryland and Department of Obstetrics and Gynecology, Wayne State University School of Medicine, Detroit, Michigan, USA

M. I. Evans Institute for Genetics, Mt Sinai School of Medicine, New York, NY, USA

E. Fabre Department of Obstetrics and Gynecology, Hospital Clinico Universitario, Avda. San Juan Bosco, 15, 50009 Zaragoza, Spain

S. J. Fasouliotis Department of Obstetrics & Gynecology, Hebrew University Ein-Kerem, Hadassah Medical Centre, Jerusalem, Israel

R. Floyd Department Obstetrics, Gynecology & Women's Health, University of Missouri-Columbia, School of Medicine, Columbia, Missouri, USA

M. Foley Department Obstetrics & Gynecology, National Maternity Hospital, Dublin, Ireland

J. A. Fortney Heilbrunn Department of Population and Family Health, Columbia University, New York 10032, USA

E. A. Friedman Obstetrics & Gynecology, Albert Einstein College of Medicine, New York, NY, USA

K. Fujimori Department of Obstetrics & Gynecology, School of Medicine, Fukushimas Medical University, Fukushima-City, Fukushima, Japan

K. Fukushima Department of Obstetrics & Gynecology, Graduate School of Medical Sciences, Kyushu University, Higashi-Ku, Fukuoka, Japan

K. Ghebremeskel Institute of Brain Chemistry and Human Nutrition, London Metropolitan University, London, UK

P. D. Gluckman National Research Centre for Growth and Development, Liggins Institute, University of Auckland, Auckland, New Zealand

F. Goffinet Research Epidemiology Unit for Perinatal & Women's Health, Port Royal Maternity Hospital, Paris, France

L. F. Goncalves Perinatology Research Branch, National Institute of Child Health and Human Development, NIH, DHHS, Bethesda, Maryland and Department of Obstetrics and Gynecology, Wayne State University School of Medicine, Detroit, Michigan, USA

C. Gordon Department of Rheumatology, City Hospital, Birmingham, UK

J. L. Graf Department of Pediatric Surgery, University of California, San Francisco, CA, USA

B. E. Grand Department of Fetal Medicine, Juan A. Fernández Hospital of Buenos Aires, Argentina

A. Grunebaum Weill Cornell Medical Center, New York, NY, USA

B. Hargitai First Department of Obstetrics & Gynecology, Semmelweis University Medical School, Baross, Budapest, Hungary

M. R. Harrison Department of Pediatric Surgery, University of California, CA, USA

L. Hellstrom-Westas Department of Pediatrics, University Hospital Lund, Lund, Sweden

J. Herczeg Teaching Hospital of the University of Szeged, Szeged, Hungary

P. Hilton Women's Services, Royal Victoria Infirmary, Newcastle upon Tyne, UK

W. Holzgreve Women's University Hospital Basel, Basel, Switzerland

H. Hopp Charity Clinic for Obstetics, Campus Benjamin Franklin, Berlin, Germany

T. Hosono Department of Medical Engineering, Osaka Electro-communication University, Shijo-nawate, Osaka, Japan

T. Ikeda Department of Obstetrics and Gynecology, Miyazaki Medical College, University of Miyazaki, Kihara, Kiyotake-Cho, Miyazaki, Japan

S. Iniesta Santa Cristina University Hospital, Universidad Autonoma de Madrid, Madrid, Spain

T. Kanzaki Kanzaki Lady's Clinic, Nishinomiya, Hyogo, Japan and Division Obstetrics & Gynecology, Osaka University, Osaka, Japan

I. Kassis Ichilov Hospital, University of Tel Aviv, Tel Aviv, Israel

T. Kawarabayashi Department of Obstetrics & Gynecology, School of Medicine, Fukuoka University, Fukuoka, Japan

A. Khurana The Ultrasound Laboratory, C 584 Defence Colony, New Delhi, India

T. Kimura Division of Obstetrics & Gynecology, Department of Specific Organ Regulation, Osaka University Graduate School of Medicine, Suita, Japan

D. A. Krantz NTD Laboratories Inc, East Meadow, NY, USA

I. Krause Department of Pediatrics, Schneider Children's Medical Center of Israel, Sackler School of Medicine, Tel Aviv University, Israel

S. Kupesic Department of Obstetrics & Gynecology, Zagreb University Medical School, Sveti Duh, Zagreb, Croatia

A. Kurjak Department of Obstetrics & Gynecology, University of Zagreb, Sveti Duh Hospital, Zagreb, Croatia

M. L. Kush University of Maryland School of Medicine, Department Obstetrics, Gynecology & Reproductive Sciences, Baltimore, MD, USA

H. J. Landy Division of Maternal-Fetal Medicine, Department Obstetrics & Gynecology, Georgetown University Hospital, Washington DC, USA

O. Lapaire Women's University Hospital Basel, Spitalstraae, Basel, Switzerland

M. Levene Department of Paediatrics, Leeds General Infirmary, Leeds, UK

L. Lewi Department Obstetrics & Gynecology, University Hospital Gasthuisberg, Leuven, Belgium

G. Lindmark Department of Women's and Children's Health, Uppsala University, Uppsala, Sweden

G. A. Little Dartmouth-Hitchcock Medical Center, Neonatology, Lebanon

J. A. Low Department of Obstetrics and Gynecology, Queen's University, Kingston, Ontario, Canada

R. Luzietti Centre of Perinatal & Reproductive Medicine, University of Perugia, Perugia, Italy

I. Z. MacKenzie Department of Obstetrics & Gynecolcogy, John Radcliffe Hospital, Oxford, UK

K. Maeda Department of Obstetrics and Gynecology, Tottori University, Nadamachi, Yonago, Japan

S. Maheshwari Department of Pediatric Cardiology, Narayana Hrudayalaya, Anekal Taluk, Bangalore, India

G. P. Mandruzzato Department Obstetrics & Gynecology, Istituto per l'Infanzia IRCCS "Burlo Garofolo", Trieste, Italy

T. Marton Department of Histopathology, Birmingham Women's Hospital, Edgbaston, Birmingham, UK

G. Maso Department Obstetrics & Gynecology, Istituto per l'Infanzia IRCCS "Burlo Garofolo", Trieste, Italy

A. Matias Department of Obstetrics & Gynecology, Faculty of Medicine, University Hospital of S Joao, Porto, Portugal

L. T. Mercé Assisted Reproduction Unit, International Ruber Hospital, Madrid, Spain

E. Merz Department of Obstetrics & Gynecology, Krankenhaus Nordwest, Frankfurt/Main, Germany

D. Miron Pediatric Department A, Ha'Emek Medical Center, Afula 18101, Israel

G. Monni Department of Obstetrics and Gynecology, Prenatal and Preimplantation Genetic Diagnosis, Fetal Therapy, Ospedale Microcitemico, Cagliari, Italy

N. Montenegro Department of Obstetrics & Gynecology, Faculty of Medicine, University Hospital of S Joao, Porto, Portugal

A. Morag Clinical Virology Unit, Hadassah University Hospitals, Jerusalem, Israel

C. Mortera Diagnostico Prenatal y Perinatal, Institut Dexeus, Cardio-Hemodinamica, Hospital Sant J de Deu, Barcelona, Spain

A. Mulic-Lutvica Department of Women's and Children's Health, Uppsala University, Uppsala, Sweden

Y. Murata Division of Obstetrics and Gynecology, Osaka University Graduate School of Medicine, Osaka, Japan

M. F. Murphy Department of Haematology, Oxford Radcliffe Hospitals NHS Trust, Oxford, UK

H. Nakano Department of Obstetrics & Gynecology, Graduate School of Medical Sciences, Kyushu University, Higashi-Ku, Fukuoka, Japan

L. J. Nelson Department of Philosophy, Santa Clara University, Santa Clara, CA, USA

C. Nelson-Piercy Department of Obstetrics, St Thomas's Hospital, London, UK

K. H. Nicolaides Fetal Medicine Foundation, London, UK

J. G. Nijhuis Department of Obstetrics, Academisch Ziekenhuis Maastricht, The Netherlands

J. Nizard Department of Obstetrics & Gynecology, Hôpital de Poissy-Saint-Germain en Laye, Poissy, France

Z. Novak-Antolic Department of Obstetrics & Gynecology, University Medical Center, Ljubljana, Slovenia

K. Olshtain-Pops Department of Clinical Microbiology & Infectious Diseases, Hadassah University Hospital, Jerusalem, Israel

K. Ozono Division of Obstetrics & Gynecology, Department of Specific Organ Regulation, Osaka University Graduate School of Medicine, Suita, Osaka, Japan

K. M. Paarlberg Department of Obstetrics & Gynecology, University Hospital Vrije Universiteit, Amsterdam, The Netherlands

M. Pajntar Department of Obstetrics & Gynecology, University Medical Center, Ljubljana, Slovenia

E. Papiernik University Rene Descartes, Maternite de Port Royal, Hopital Cochin, Paris, France

C. Paul Department of Obstetrics & Gynecology, King's College Hospital, Denmark Hill, London, UK

L. Pereira Maternal Fetal Medicine, Oregon Health & Science University, Portland, OR, USA

P. O. D. Pharoah FSID Unit of Perinatal and Paediatric Epidemiology, Department of Public Health, University of Liverpool, Liverpool, UK

T. Podymow Division of Nephrology & Hypertension, Weill Medical College of Cornell University, New York, NY, USA

R. K. Pooh Center for Maternal, Fetal & Neonatal Medicine, Kagawa National Children's Hospital, Zentsuji City, Kagawa, Japan

P. Prats Prenatal Diagnosis Unit, Department of Obstetrics and Gynaecology, Institut Universitari Dexeus, Barcelona, Spain

E. Quarello Department of Obstetrics and Gynecology, CHI Poissy St Germain, Universite Paris-Ouest, Poissy, France

E. J. Quilligan University California Irvine, Long Beach Memorial Hospital, Long Beach, CA, USA

R. Romero Perinatology Research Branch, National Institute of Child Health and Human Development, NIH, DHHS, Bethesda, MD, USA

G. Rosner Genetic Institute, Tel Aviv Sourasky Medical Center, Israel

P. Rozenberg Department of Obstetrics & Gynecology, Poissy-Saint Germain Hospital, Versailles-Saint Quentin University, Poissy Cedex, France

F. F. Rubaltelli Department of Neonatology, Ospedale Careggi Reparto, Florence, Italy

E. Rubinstein Section of Infectious Diseases, University of Manitoba, Winnipeg, MB, Canada

R. M. Sabatel López Department Obstetrics & Gynecology, University of Grenada, Spain

N. Sagawa Department of Obstetrics & Gynecology, Mie University Graduate School of Medicine, Tsu, Mie, Japan

S. Saito Department Obstetrics & Gynecology, Toyama Medical & Pharmaceutical University, Toyama-shi, Toyama, Japan

S. Sakamoto Toyko, Aiiku Maternal & Child Health Center, Boshi Aiiku-kai,, Minato-ku, Japan

E. Z. Saling Institut für Perinatale Medizin, Berlin, Germany

O. D. Saugstad Department of Pediatric Research, The National Hospital, Oslo, Norway

J. G. Schenker Department of Obstetrics & Gynecology, Hadassah University Hospital, Jerusalem, Israel

S. Scherjon Department of Obstetrics, LUMC, Leiden, The Netherlands

B. S. Schifrin Department of Obstetrics & Gynecology, Loma Linda University School of Medicine, Loma Linda, CA, USA

Y. Schlesinger Division of Infectious Diseases, Shaare Zedek Medical Center, Jerusalem 91031, Israel

J. J. Sciarra Department of Obstetrics and Gynecology, Northwestern University Medical School Chicago, IL, USA

N. J. Sebire Department of Histopathology, Camelia Botnar Laboratories, Great Ormond Street Hospital, London, UK

C. Sen Department of Obstetrics & Gynecology, Cerrahpasa Medical School, Istanbul, Turkey

M. Seoud Department of Obstetrics & Gynecology, American University of Beirut Medical Center, Beirut, Lebanon

B. Serra Departamento de Obstetricia y Ginecologia, Instituto Universitario Dexeus, Barcelona, Spain

F. Sethna Fetal Medicine Unit, Department Obstetrics & Gynecology, St George's Hospital NHS Trust, London, UK

M. Shapiro Department of Clinical Microbiology and Infectious Diseases, Hadassah University Hospital, Jerusalem 91120, Israel

N. Shinozuka Department of Obstetrics & Gynecology, Faculty of Medicine, Teikyo University, Japan

D. W. Skupski Division of Maternal-Fetal Medicine, New York Hospital Queens, Flushing, New York, NY, USA

D. T. Spira Department of Parasitology, Hebrew Univ, Hadassah Med School, Jerusalem, Israel

Z. Stembera WHO Collaborating Center for Perinatal Medicine and Human Reproduction, Institute for the Care of Mother and Child, Podolske Nabrezi 157m 147 10 Praha 4, Czech Republic

G. M. Stirrat Centre for Ethics in Medicine, University of Bristol, Bristol, UK

K. N. S. Subramanian Georgetown University Hospital, Washington DC, USA

G. Sylvestre The New York Presbyterian Hospital, Weill Medical College of Cornell University, New York, NY, USA

A. Tabor Copenhagen University Hospital, Department of Obstetrics & Gynaecology, Hvidovre Hospital, Hvidovre, Denmark

H. A. Tanriverdi Department Obstetrics & Gynecology, Karaelmas University Medical School, Kozlu / Zonguldak, Turkey

S. Tercanli University Women's Hospital, Basel, Switzerland

J. M. Thomas National Collaborating Centre for Women and Children's Health, London, UK

J. M. Troyano Division of US & Fetal Medicine, University Hospital of the Canary Islands, La Laguna, Tenerife, Spain

K. Tsukimori Department of Obstetrics & Gynecology, Graduate School of Medical Sciences, Kyushu University, Higashi-Ku, Fukuoka, Japan

F. A. van Assche Department of Gynecology, Catholic University of Leuven, Leuven, Belgium

P. P. van den Berg Department of Obstetrics and Gynecology, University Hospital Nijmegen, Nijmegen, The Netherlands

J. van Eyck Department of Perinatology, Isala Clinics, Zwolle, The Netherlands

H. P. van Geijn Department Obstetrics & Gynecology, University Hospital Vrije Universiteit, Amsterdam, The Netherlands

W. J. van Wijngaarden Department of Obstetrics and Gynaecology, Ziekenhuis Bronovo, Den Haag, The Netherlands

Y. Ville Department of Obstetrics & Gynecology, Poissy-Saint Germain Hospital, Versailles-Saint Quentin University, Poissy Cedex, France

L. S. Voto Fundacion Miguel Margulies, Buenos Aires, Argentina

N. Wake Department of Molecular Genetics, Medical Institute of Bioregulation, Kyushu University, Beppu, Oita, Japan

J. Walker Department of Obstetrics & Gynecology, St James University Hospital, Leeds, UK

C. P. Weiner Department Obstetrics, Gynecology & Reproductive Sciences, University of Maryland School of Medicine, Baltimore, MD, USA

S. Weiner Department of Obstetrics & Gynecology, Thomas Jefferson College of Medicine, Philadelphia, PA, USA

D. J. Williams Institute of Women's Health, University College London, Elizabeth Garrett Anderson Obstetric Hospital, London, UK

M. S. Wingate Department Maternal & Child Health, University of Alabama at Birmingham, Birmingham, Alabama, USA

D. C. Wood Jr Fetal Cardiology, Maternal Fetal Medicine, Department of Obstetrics and Gynecology Thomas Jefferson University, Philadelphia, Pennsylvania, USA

H. N. Winn Department of Obstetrics, Gynecology and Women's Health, University of Missouri-Columbia School of Medicine, Columbia, MI, USA

Y. Yaron Prenatal Genetic Diagnosis Division, Genetic Institute, Tel Aviv Sourasky Medical Center, Tel Aviv, Israel

L. Yeo Department of Obstetrics, Gynecology & Reproductive Sciences, Division of Maternal Fetal Medicine, UMDNJ – Robert Wood Johnson Medical School, New Brunswick, NJ, USA

K. A. Yunis Department of Pediatrics, American University of Beirut Medical Center, Beirut, Lebanon

P. Zalloua Department of Obstetrics & Gynecology, American University of Beirut Medical Center, Beirut, Lebanon

M. A. Zoppi Department of Obstetrics and Gynecology, Prenatal and Preimplantation Genetic Diagnosis, Fetal Therapy, Ospedale Microcitemico, Cagliari, Italy

Foreword

Perinatal medicine is among the most challenging and beautiful areas of study and practice. It deals with events before birth, when the fetus is a patient and during the immediate neonatal period. The World Association of Perinatal Medicine is dedicated to the study of all aspects of perinatal biology, physiology, screening, diagnosis, management and ethics, with the goal of continuous quality improvement in the care of maternal, fetal and neonatal patients.

This textbook is based on a previous work that was produced by the European Association of Perinatal Medicine in 1998. Because perinatal medicine is now a global area of study, it is appropriate that the current textbook is a product of the World Association of Perinatal Medicine. The bonds that link perinatologists together transcend geographic, political, religious and lingual differences, resulting in a globalization that optimizes clinical care.

This textbook consists of over 200 chapters divided into 20 sections, which span the depth and breadth of the field. Beginning with the history of perinatal medicine and ending with the challenges facing this specialty in developing countries, this book is a comprehensive text designed to provide insight and guidance to clinicians throughout the world with state of the art information, written by the world's leading perinatologists.

We are grateful to the authors of the 205 chapters and the editors of the 20 sections, who have worked so diligently with us to produce this textbook, which we believe bears testament to the importance and success of international collaboration in perinatal medicine.

Asim Kurjak
Frank A. Chervenak

SECTION XII

Prenatal diagnosis and therapy

Section Editors: **K. Nicolaides and A. Antsaklis**

102 Chorionic villus sampling

B. Brambati and L. Tului

Introduction

Chorionic villus sampling (CVS) has gained a growing popularity since its inception as a means of rapid prenatal diagnosis in early pregnancy.[1,2] The International CVS Registry provides statistics for the first 13 years of use.[3–6] The first clinical experiences were published between 1982 and 1983, and in 1 year less than 200 cases were reported by six groups from five countries, whereas in September 1996 more than 200,000 cases were registered, and more than 180 centers from the six continents were on the CVS Registry mailing list.

The ability to achieve first-trimester fetal diagnoses reduces emotional and physical stress in couples at risk, maximizes patient privacy, and permits access to termination at an earlier stage of pregnancy. Prenatal diagnosis by CVS in the first trimester, when physical awareness of the conceptus may still not be present and pregnancy is not physically apparent, is expected to have less profound psychological and behavioral effects on the mother. Reports comparing the emotional distress experienced by women undorgoing amniocentesis and CVS, respectively, have shown that the latter approach evokes less anxiety, which lasts a shorter period of time, than amniocentesis.[7] Moreover, women undergoing CVS report significantly greater attachment to the fetus than women undergoing amniocentesis.[8] Although the miscarriage rate was shown to be a determinant factor of the patient's attitude toward prenatal procedures, the great benefit of an early diagnosis prepared patients to accept the higher risk of CVS, which is up to five times that of amniocentesis.[9–11]

Several clinical trials have provided information about the comparative risks of first-trimester CVS and mid-trimester amniocentesis. In national collaborative studies, the likelihood of successful pregnancy outcome has been reported to be similar for both sampling approaches.[12–15,21] However, in the early 1990s concern arose from the publication of small early first-trimester sampling series describing clusters of limb defect cases after CVS.[16–18] Although these cases could indicate a relationship between early CVS and placental damage, no evidence of teratogenic effects has been observed by the analysis of more than 200,000 CVS cases reported to the CVS International Registry.[19] There is a general agreement that no procedure-induced limb defects are expected to follow CVS when sampling is performed after 10 completed weeks of gestation by skilled and experienced operators.

Requirements for a chorionic villus sampling program

The most important requirement for a successful CVS program is technically competent staff. CVS should be performed by an obstetrician experienced in first-trimester ultrasonography, who is an expert in the pathophysiology and clinical aspects of early pregnancy, and who is well-informed about human genetics and the laboratory methods used for genetic analysis. CVS and other sampling techniques should be performed only at centers having a high level of expertise and experience, capable of applying any sampling approach as appropriate and of following the cases to delivery.[19] Training can be performed in both experimental and diagnostic cases under direct supervision of a senior expert operator. A WHO meeting set out the following criteria for self-evaluation of the expertise of centers[19]:

(1) A sampling success rate of about 90% at the first insertion (of sampling device) and up to 98% after two insertions;
(2) Laboratory success in more than 95% of all patients sampled;
(3) Capability to utilize both transcervical and transabdominal routes for CVS;
(4) A total fetal loss rate to 28 weeks of chromosomally normal pregnancies of less than 6%. Centers with a low-risk patient population (young, economically advantaged, non-smoking, sampled close to 12 weeks) should expect to do better than this; and
(5) Data collection and surveillance programs that include follow-up to delivery and infant outcome for more than 95% of all cases.

It is to be expected that these levels would ordinarily be achieved by groups with experience of 200–250 procedures. However, expertise cannot be maintained with occasional sampling; the more cases sampled per year the better the results are likely to be.

Transabdominal continuous guidance of the sampling device by a high-quality ultrasound machine is mandatory. In principle, sector and convex probes are preferred: their small contact surface allows an optimal fitting to the maternal abdomen with a comprehensive visualization of the uterus frequently still situated near or below the pubis.

CVS is performed in an outpatient facility. No medical preparation is needed before transabdominal sampling, whereas treatment of vaginal infection might be necessary before transcervical sampling. A full bladder is not required, but some degree of filling may be required in some circumstances, for instance to straighten the angle of a pronounced anteflexion of the uterus for easier transcervical sampling, or to push intestinal loops away from the anterior uterine wall for safer transabdominal sampling in a retroverted uterus. Postoperative care includes some rest only when cramping or bleeding would otherwise appear; in cases of spotting and bleeding complications, vaginal exploration should be avoided and daily vaginal douches are recommended for cleaning the vagina and thereby avoiding bacterial proliferation as much as possible.

Sampling methods

The placenta can be reached either through the maternal abdomen by needling,[22,23] or via the cervical canal by catheter or biopsy forceps.[24–26] A transvaginal chorionic needle aspiration guided by vaginal ultrasound probe has also been developed, but it is indicated only in patients where sampling by the other conventional methods appears to be hazardous.[27]

Transcervical sampling is most frequently performed using a polyethylene cannula 26 cm long and 1.5 mm in outer diameter, with a soft stainless-steel blunt obturator.[24] Recently, CVS experiences have also been reported using round-tip curved steel forceps 1.9 mm in diameter and 25 cm in length, and flexible biopsy forceps 3 mm in outer diameter and 25 cm long.[25,28] With the patient in the lithotomy position, and after antiseptic preparation of the external genitalia, the cervix is visualized and cleaned with a broad-spectrum antiseptic solution. The cervix may be grasped with a tenaculum to straighten the cervical canal, although this usually produces discomfort and may sometimes be very painful.

Two methodological approaches for transabdominal sampling have been described.[22,23] A double coaxial needle system can be inserted percutaneously through a needle guide attached to the ultrasound probe.[23] An 18-gauge, 15-cm guide needle is first introduced and then stopped at the edge of the placenta. Thereafter, a thinner 22- or 20-gauge, 20-cm needle is passed through the outer needle and repeatedly inserted until an adequate sample is obtained. As an alternative a single 20-gauge, 9- or 12-cm spinal needle can be used and inserted by a freehand ultrasound-guided approach (Figure 102.1). In the latter case, the aspirating syringe can be mounted onto a holder to make the aspiration easier. The freehand needle-insertion technique has some advantages when compared with the two-needle system. The needle is thinner and its direction can be easily adjusted when necessitated by abdominal wall or uterine displacements. Moreover, as the needle is not in direct contact with the transducer, neither a sterile ultrasound system nor sterile contact gel are needed. In addition, the sampling procedure takes less time, and the sampling device is cheaper. However, the freehand technique is a two-person approach and demands good co-operation between the sonographer and the operator.

Contraindications

Because of the specificity of the sampling route, transabdominal and transcervical sampling techniques are expected to have different types of contraindications. Vaginismus and stenotic or tortuous cervical canal, as well as myomas of the lower uterine segment, may severely hamper the introduction of either catheter or forceps. Active vaginal infection may also be an absolute contraindication to the cervical route. In the latter condition, vaginal and cervical culture and specific treatment do not seem sufficient to remove any risk of ascending infection. Transabdominal sampling may be relatively or absolutely contraindicated when obstacles such as intestines, large myomas or the gestational sac cannot be avoided.

Some conditions may be considered common contraindications for both transabdominal and transcervical sampling, namely active vaginal bleeding and an Rh-isoimmunized patient. If bleeding is present at the time of scheduled sampling, although no specific data are available, it is advisable to postpone any sampling procedure until bleeding has stopped. Feto-maternal transfusion, frequently observed following chorionic villus biopsy,[29–33] might enhance the antibody response of isoimmunized mothers and threaten fetal outcome. The patient should be informed about this potential adverse effect of CVS, and amniocentesis or cordocentesis should be evaluated as potential alternative approaches.

Indications

At the individual level, the advantages of first-trimester CVS are evident when compared with mid-trimester amniocentesis (Table 102.1). Shorter pre- and post-test waiting periods are required, and the decision to end a pregnancy is less stressful, because by that time maternal–fetal bonding is not clearly established and the gestational process is generally not visible to those in the mother's social environment, so that the social consequences of late abortion are avoided. First-trimester voluntary abortion is expected

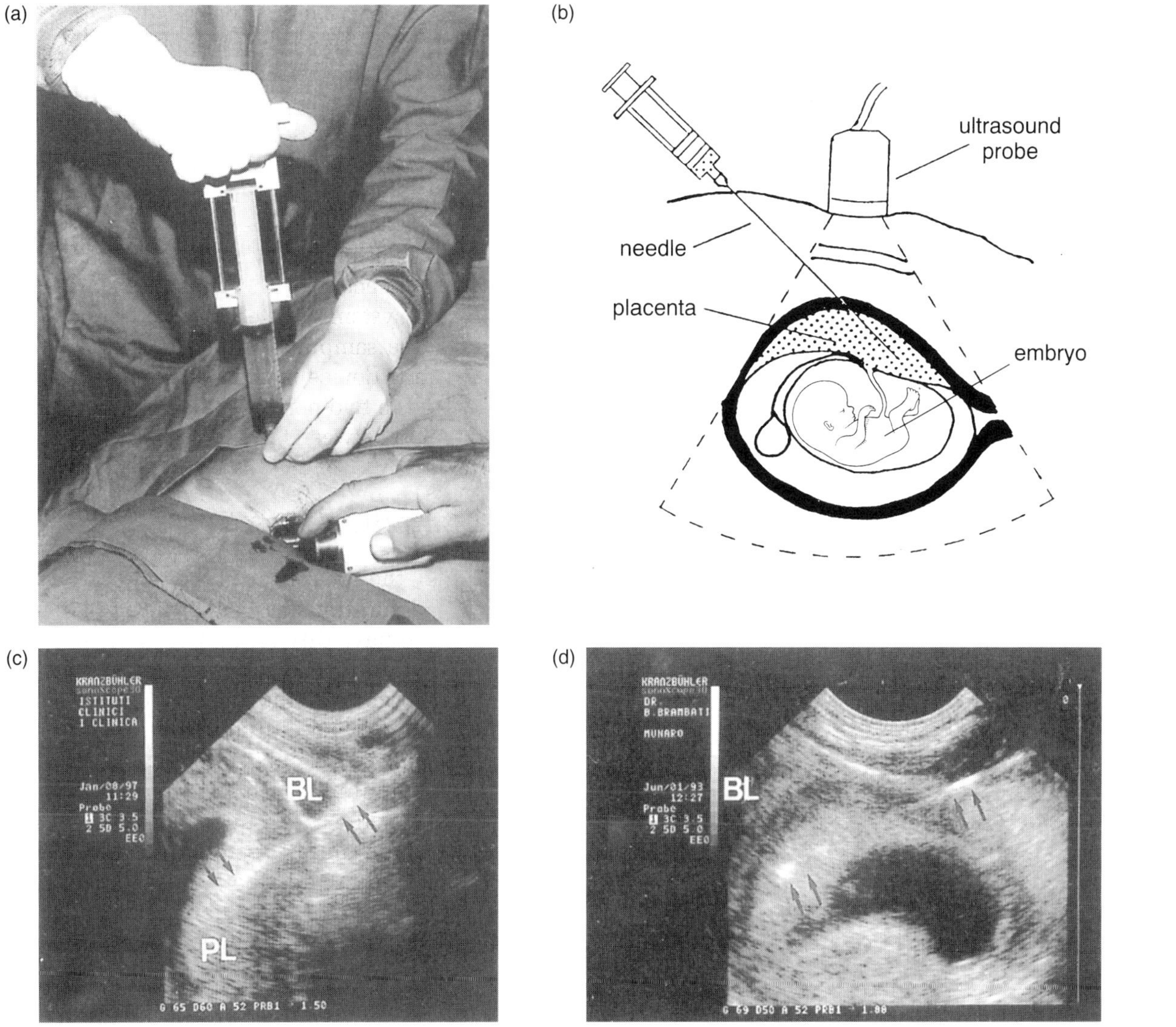

Figure 102.1 (a) Freehand needle insertion under ultrasound guidance; (b) diagram of transcervical chorionic villus sampling (CVS) by a freehand needle insertion approach; (c) transabdominal CVS in a 11.2-week pregnancy with retroflexed uterus and posterior placenta (PL). The needle (arrows) enters straight into the placenta by proceeding close to the bladder (BL) wall, thereby avoiding intestinal loops. (d) Transabdominal CVS in a 10.3-week pregnancy with antiflexed uterus and anterior placenta. The needle pathway is indicated by arrows.

to have a significantly lower rate of clinical complications. Moreover, at this time of pregnancy general anesthesia and dilatation and surgical uterine evacuation have less profound emotional effects on the patient than labor induction and delivery at about 20 weeks.

Chromosomal abnormalities are undoubtedly the most common indication for first-trimester CVS (Table 102.2). Banding of high quality can be obtained by culturing mesenchymal cells of chorionic villi, and this process usually takes 10–15 days. Rapid karyotyping may be performed by examining cytotrophoblastic cells arrested in metaphase, either immediately (a few hours) after sampling or after short-term (24–48 h) culture. However, chromosome preparations obtained by the direct method are difficult to band and would not be suitable for the detection of subtle chromosome anomalies. Moreover, false-negative results for chromosomal aberrations are expected to be about 1 per 3000 (100), whereas the rate falls to less than 1 per 10,000 if cytogenetic analysis is carried out concomitantly on long-term culture.[34,35] Placental-confined mosaicism and non-mosaic rare trisomies give rise to concern regarding proper counseling and pregnancy management. The potential adverse affects on pregnancy outcome of some chromosomal abnormalities confined to the placenta (chromosome 2, 7, 9, 14, 15, 16, 18, and 22, tetraploidy) have documented.[38,109] Whenever a high degree of mosaicism is found in both trophoblast and mesenchyme cells, uniparental disomy in the fetus with normal karyotype ascertained on amniotic or fetal blood cells should be suspected and molecular studies undertaken.[37]

Chorionic villi provide large amounts of metabolically active cytoplasm, therefore for many inherited metabolic diseases direct assay is possible, yielding diagnostic results within hours or a few days. Moreover, the amount of DNA obtained from a conventional sampling allows reliable analysis by recombinant

Table 102.1 Advantages of first-trimester chorionic villus sampling compared with mid-trimester amniocentesis

Individual and social advantages	Diagnostic advantages	Clinical advantages
Higher privacy	Rapid karyotyping	Previous cesarean section
Less emotional impact	Enzymatic assay and DNA analysis on fresh tissue	Pending cerclage
		Multiple pregnancy (and selective abortion)
Fewer legal limitations	Screening 'package' (CF, NSCD, fragile X, paternity, and so on)	General anesthesia and dilatation and curettage for voluntary abortion
Higher acceptability		Stem cell transplantation

Table 102.2 Indications for chorionic villus sampling in 10,123 cases performed at the Mangiagalli Clinic, University of Milan, and at Center for Prenatal Diagnosis, Milan[94]

Indication	No. of cases	No. of affected cases (%)
Karyotyping*		
Maternal age (years)		
<30	1146	14 (1.22)
30–34	2239	18 (0.80)
35–39	3966	77 (1.94)
=40	1966	103 (5.24)
Previous offspring with chromosome abnormality	556	17 (3.05)
Balanced parental chromosome rearrangement or parental sex chromosome aneuploidy	141	10 (7.09)
Suspicious ultrasonic findings	44	9 (20.45)
Second-trimester Down's syndrome screening	75	0
Enzymatic analysis		
Mucopolysaccharidoses	17	7 (41.2)
Lipidoses	71	19 (26.7)
Amino acid disorders	24	9 (37.5)
Carbohydrate metabolism disorders	12	4 (33.3)
Miscellaneous indications	21	4 (19.5)
DNA analysis		
Thalassemia	823	187 (22.7)
Duchenne/Becker muscular dystrophy	358	81 (22.6)
Hemophilia A/B	107	24 (22.4)
Cystic fibrosis	95	25 (26.3)
Congenital adrenal hyperplasia	33	10 (30.3)
Other monogenetic diseases	62	17 (27.4)
Infectious diseases	19	2 (10.5)
Paternity testing	19	–

*Fetal karyotyping was also performed in all the cases with primary indication other than chromosomal abnormalities

DNA technologies. This is not the case with amniotic fluid cells, which provide too little DNA, which is frequently fragmented. Chorionic tissue is therefore at present the material of choice for prenatal diagnosis of Mendelian diseases. The rapid progress of human genome research is very much broadening the range of gene defects directly detectable, and makes it possible to offer a prenatal diagnosis screening package in low-risk populations for some of the most frequent and severe conditions, e.g., cystic fibrosis (CF), non-syndromic congenital deafness (NSCD) and fragile-X mental retardation, and Rh typing in cases at risk of Rh-isoimmunization.[38,39,99]

Multiple pregnancies

Twin and higher-order multiple pregnancies are specific conditions in which first-trimester CVS can generally offer several technical advantages over mid-trimester anniocentesis. The easy evaluation of the membranes by ultrasound[40] makes both the prediction of chorionicity and amnionicity and the identification of the affected twin(s) more reliable, the use of rapid analytical methods makes substantial changes in the uterine topography very unlikely, and if same-sex dichorionic twins are diagnosed, DNA polymorphism markers may be easily checked to assure retrieval of villi from the individual placentas.[41]

Dichorionic pregnancy can easily be predicted when either two distinct placental sites are detected or, if the placentae are confluent, the septal thickness is 2 mm or more and the lambda sign is present.[40,88] Fused placentae and the presence of empty sac(s) may represent a potential source of contamination: to minimize this inconvenience the main criteria should be to guide the extremity of the aspirating device to the proximity of the umbilical cord insertion, or as far as possible from the confluence of placentas. However, in some conditions a reliable sampling could be easily achieved by the combined use of TA- and TC-CVS or, as an alternative, by using a double coaxial needle system made by a 19-gauge 9-cm-long guide needle and a 21-gauge 15-cm-long sampling needle.[88] The guide-needle is first introduced through the co-twin placenta and stopped just after reaching the placenta to be sampled, thereafter sampling is performed by passing the thinner needle through the outer one.

In the hands of experienced operators and by appropriate methodological approach, CVS has been reported to be highly effective in multiple gestations: genetic diagnosis was correct on all 338 fetuses sampled from 169 twin pregnancies,[88] while sampling was incorrect in only three out of 771 fetuses (0.4%) sampled in 424 multiple pregnancies undergoing fetal reduction to a single fetus or twins.[43] Moreover, in both experiences sampling was successfully performed in all cases by a single needle insertion. The relative risks of first-trimester CVS and mid-trimester amniocentesis have been documented in two series of 161 and 72 twins.[42] Sampling was performed at 10–12 weeks for CVS and at 16–18 weeks for amniocentesis. No differences were observed between procedures in the rates of spontaneous abortion and perinatal mortality. However, if only cases with chromosomally normal fetuses and placentae were considered, the total fetal loss rate was significantly lower in the CVS series (3.9% vs. 9.3%). In cases of twins discordant for a serious disorder, selective reduction should be considered: the advantages of the first-trimester approach include a significantly lower emotional impact and a lower risk of clinical complications.[43,44]

Timing of chorionic villus sampling

The generally accepted lowest limit of gestational age for sampling is 10 completed weeks. By that time, embryo viability is easily detectable, the placenta is clearly identifiable and adequately thick, and embryogenesis is concluded. The upper limit for transcervical sampling has been suggested to be 12–13 weeks. Indeed, by the end of the first trimester, the gestational sac becomes attached to the decidual wall. Thereafter, any attempt to insert either a catheter or a biopsy forceps entails a higher risk of indenting and damaging the membranes. These difficulties can also be accentuated by the fact that the proximal placental edge may move far from the internal cervical os.

The extension of transabdominal CVS beyond the first trimester has proven to be convenient as an alternative to amniocentesis for a prompt answer in case of late booking, suspicious ultrasonic findings, or increased risk of chromosomal abnormalities as a result of first trimester screening. Low risk and high effectiveness of transabdominal CVS in the early second trimester were clearly reported in a study[45] comparing two large series at 13–14 weeks and at 15–20 weeks with a control series al 11–12 weeks: a very low total fetal loss rate ($\leq$24 weeks) of 0.86%, 0.46%, and 1.02% was respectively observed; a trend towards lower values is apparent, although differences were not statistically significant. Sampling was successful in all cases of the three series, however a posterior and unreachable placenta was the reason for transferring to mid-trimester amniocentesis 4.2% of cases recruited for CVS at 15–20 weeks, whereas in the series at 13–14 weeks this was required in only 0.9% of cases.

The choice of route for sampling

Transcervical and transabdominal techniques appear to be comparably efficient between 8 and 12 weeks, when the overall success rate after two sampling device insertions is considered to be very near to 100%. This efficiency has been confirmed in three national randomized trials of transabdominal vs. transcervical CVS.[14,46,47] Although the data appear to confirm that the two techniques are equally effective in obtaining adequate amounts of chorionic tissue, and in two of the three randomized trials the fetal loss rate was not affected by the sampling technique,[46,47] transabdominal needling entailed a significantly smaller proportion of repeated device insertions (3.3% vs. 10.3%) and of low weight specimens (3.2% vs. 4.9%).[46] Moreover, the deviation from the allocated procedure (15.8% vs. 3.1%), due to previously undetected vaginal infection or anatomical problems, was much higher in the transcervical group.[46]

Transabdominal sampling, in our experience, has definitely become the method of choice, and our preference for this approach is based on the shorter learning time, the lower rate of immediate complications, the higher practicality and success rates at the first device insertion, the lower hazard of intrauterine infection, the opportunity to extend sampling beyond the first trimester, and the wider range of diagnostic indications. However, it is plainly advisable that a complementary approach, namely transcervical or transvaginal sampling, should be mastered for appropriate chorion biopsy in any case. Finally, the high efficiency, the absence of complications after sampling, and the very low total abortion rate observed after 12 gestational weeks, have made the use of second-trimester CVS a valuable alternative to early and mid-trimester amniocentesis, even in genetically low-risk populations.

Complications

Among early post-procedural complications, spotting within a few hours has been more frequently observed in patients undergoing transcervical rather than transabdominal CVS (3.2% vs. 1.5%, $P < 0.001$).[46] Localized peritonitis immediately after sampling occurs in very few cases, and only after transabdominal sampling, with an overall rate of 0.04%. Intrauterine infection (acute chorionamnionitis) should be considered a potential, although very rare, complication of transcervical CVS, having been reported in 0.1–0.5% of cases, and in some large series no cases at all were observed.[48] However, there is some concern about the role of less serious infection in women who experience fetal loss after transcervical CVS. Because transcervical

CVS involves passage of a cannula or forceps through the cervical canal from the perineum and vagina, microbial colonization and infection, with consequent morbidity for both mother and fetus, may result. Clinical symptoms of localized peritonitis have been reported in three cases after transabdominal CVS. Bacteria were cultured only in one of the three cases, which strongly suggested that puncture of the large intestine had caused *Escherichia coli* invasion of the peritoneum.[49] In the two other cases, the chorionic tissue culture medium was sterile, and symptoms were milder, suggesting that the peritoneal reaction resulted from bleeding from the needle puncture of the external uterine surface.

Feto-maternal transfusion has been postulated as a possible side-effect of CVS. At the end of 5 menstrual weeks, the intravillous vascular network connects with the umbilical-allantoic vessels and integrates into the general embryonic circulation. Thereafter, any disruption of villus integrity may cause fetal blood leakage. Feto-maternal hemorrhage following CVS has been demonstrated by a significant increase in maternal serum a-fetoprotein in 40–72% of cases, and in 6–18% of these the amount of blood transfused was calculated to exceed 0.1 ml.[29–31] Fetal hemorrhage should therefore be capable of initiating an immune response in RhD-negative women bearing an RhD-positive fetus. Moreover, an association between maternal serum a-fetoprotein increase and frequency of spontaneous fetal death has been suggested for the cases with the highest maternal serum a-fetoprotein levels.[32]

No increased frequency of perinatal complications, i.e. preterm birth, small-for-dates neonates, perinatal mortality and congenital malformations, have been observed both in randomized and clinical control studies.[12–15,21,48,50]

Data on pediatric follow-up of infants resulting from CVS-tested pregnancies are very scarce. Clinical evaluation was reported in 53 (9–14 years old) of 66 babies born after the earliest Chinese experience, and in 274 children in Milan evaluated at 3–5 years of age.[51,52] All the children were normally developed at the time of the study. Although these two reports seem to exclude any gross long-term effect of CVS, they lack matched controls. In the very near future, when pediatric follow-up data will be available from randomized studies comparing CVS and mid-trimester amniocentesis, it will be possible to reach more reliable conclusions about possible long-term sequelae.

Fetal loss

Several variables, both technical and biological, make it hazardous to evaluate risk based only on clinical studies. For these reasons, a randomized trial to evaluate fetal losses due to the procedure was recommended when CVS was introduced in clinical practice.[53] The overall pregnancy loss rate has been reported in a number of relatively large clinical studies, and the values range from 2.2% to 5.4%.[54–66] The data of the International CVS Registry reveal a striking difference between those centers with the largest experience and those with the least, as well as between different sampling methods.[4–6,67] In our experience,[35] in 9471 continuing pregnancies sampled by the same operator, the overall loss rate (including perinatal mortality up to 28 days after birth) was 3.38% (Table 102.3). Logistic regression analysis of the procedure-related variables showed a significant association between fetal loss rate and maternal age, the lowest rates occurring in the youngest women (1.22%) and the highest in the women of 40 years and over (odds ratio 2.52), while gestational age affected the abortion rate only at 8 weeks (3.78%), no differences in the odds ratio being present at 9–12 weeks. Sampling approach does not seem to affect fetal loss rate. No significant difference between transabdominal needling and transcervical aspiration methods resulted from two of the three randomized trials comparing techniques.[46,47] The only plausible explanation for the higher rate reported for transcervical aspiration in the Danish study[14] is the low operator experience suggested by the higher rate of complicated procedures reported for transcervical sampling. In the light of this evidence it may be inferred that, given the necessary skills, both routes are comparably safe. The number of sampling device insertions may influence pregnancy outcome: a higher fetal loss rate was demonstrated for three or more attempts in the same sampling session. This substantiates our protocol, which limits the number of device insertions in a single sampling session to 2.[13,51,55,61] Failure to obtain adequate tissue on two attempts may imply major obstacles, and the operator should reconsider the case or select a different sampling method.

Six control studies concerning risk assessment were published between 1989 and 1999.[12–15,21,50] Three of them were multicenter studies,[12,13,50] while the Danish study[14] included two single-operator centers. In the Finnish[15] as well in the Spanish[21] studies all procedure were performed at a single center by more than one operator. The sizes of four of the trials[12–14,50] were equivalent, and allowed detection of a 1% fetal loss difference between sampling methods, whereas the number of cases involved in the Finnish and Spanish studies was lower. 800 and 1011, respectively. In the US study,[13] the control group undergoing amniocentesis could not be randomized because of an almost total non-acceptance of the method. The Canadian[12] and US studies compared mid-trimester amniocentesis and transcervical CVS performed at 9–12 weeks, with the exception of 1.3% of cases performed before 9 weeks in the US study. Sampling in the Danish study was performed at 9–11 weeks, and patients were randomly assigned to amniocentesis or CVS. In the Medical Research Council (MRC) European trial,[50] the patients were recruited in the first trimester, but the range and distribution of gestational ages at CVS were not reported.

Four of the five control trials were unable to find statistical differences between first-trimester CVS and mid-trimester amniocentesis, and a significant excess of fetal losses (4.6%) was only demonstrated in the MRC European study (Table 102.4). However, a number of aspects make the latter trial unreliable. First, two of the 31 participating centers contributed more than one-third of the total number of cases, while the number of cases provided by the remaining centers ranged between 4 and 81. Second, no specifications were reported regarding the technical characteristics of the sampling devices, as well as the gestational age distribution at CVS. Lastly, the high rate of repeated insertion would suggest that the average operator skill during the study was low. The multiplicity of sampling approaches, some with potentially higher risk, and the poor technical competence of the majority of operators are confounding variables that might have caused the higher fetal loss rate in the CVS group.

In the mid-1980s, early amniocentesis (10 to 14 weeks) was offered as a safer alternative to CVS.[68–74] However expectations were not confirmed by the randomized trials comparing transabdominal CVS and early amniocentesis: fetal losses (< 20 weeks) and complications (amniotic fluid leakage, talipes equinovarus) were significantly higher for early amniocentesis;[103] fetal losses and complications were also significantly higher in the CEMA study comparing early and mid-trimester amniocentesis.[104]

Table 102.3 Outcome of 10,133 consecutive singleton pregnancies undergoing CVS at Mangiagalli Clinic, University of Milan, and at Center for Prenatal Diagnosis, Milan[35]

Voluntary abortion	
Genetic	553
Non-genetic	74
Pregnancies intended to continue	9506
Termination of pregnancy following sonographic diagnosis of malformation after CVS	35
Fetal loss (< 28 weeks)	2.69%
Stillbirth (=28 weeks)	0.32% (0.7%)
Live births	96.61%
Neonatal death (< 28 days)	0.37% (1.05%)
Premature delivery	
< 37 weeks	3.28% (9.20%)
< 32 weeks	0.59 % (0.91%)
Gestational age at birth (days)	275.2 ± 12.3
Birth weight (g)	3315.4 ± 525.2
Birth weight < 2500 g	3.70% (3.07%)
Birth weight < 1500 g	0.59% (0.85%)
Malformations	2.13% (1.9%)*
Lost to follow-up	0.41%

The figures in parentheses are for the Italian population, 1980–1983[95]
*From the Italian Birth Defects Registry[96]

The limb reduction defect controversy

In 1991, Firth *et al.*[16] reported an unusual cluster of four children with limb defects and oromandibular hypogenesis among 289 pregnancies in which CVS was performed at 8.0–9.3 weeks of gestation. Sampling was carried out by transabdominal needling, but data on technical performance were not available. Subsequently,

Table 102.4 Controlled trials of chorionic villus sampling (CVS) and amniocentesis

		No. of cases		Sampling failure (%)		Total fetal losses (%)	
Study	No. of centers	CVS	Amniocentesis	CVS	Amniocentesis	CVS	Amniocentesis
Canadian[12]	11	1169	1174	6.3	NR	7.6	7.0
American[13]	7	2235	671	1.8	NR	7.2	5.7
Danish[14]	2						
Transabdominal CVS		1180		1.8		6.2	
Transcervical CVS		1164		3.4		10.1*	
Amniocentesis			1003		0		6.3
MRC European[50]	31	1609	1594	4.8	1.8	13.6*	9.0
Finnish[15]	1	399	382	1.7	0	7.8	8.3
Spanish[21]	1	314	358	2	0	2.2	2.8

NR, not reported
*Statistically significant

Table 102.5 Frequency of limb reduction defects in clinical trials of chorionic villus sampling (CVS) and in the general population

Study	No. of CVS cases with completed follow-up*	No. of live births	Limb defect incidence (×10^4)
Jefferson Medical College, Philadelphia, and Hutzel Hospital, Detroit[105]	19,969	3.0	
Mangiagalli Clinic, University of Milan, and Center for Prental Diagnosis, Milan[48]	16,597	3.0	
Pellegrin University Hospital, Bordeaux[106]	10,144	1.0	
WHO[53]	158,774		4.9
WHO-CVS Registry[19]	208,682	5.1	
Froster-Iskenius and Baird[97]		1,213,913	5.97
Kallen *et al.*[98]		1,368,024	6.2
Italian Registry[96]		1,115,361	6.16

*Limb defects detected during pregnancy, and aborted, also included

two other clusters of four limb defect cases were published in series of about 300 cases.[17,18] In addition, five limb defect cases collected from different centers were reported in Taiwan, but no data were available on the total number of procedures, the sampling techniques, and the gestational ages at CVS.[75,76] Many reports supporting or denying any association between limb defects and CVS then followed.[77–87] However, a WHO statement based on the analysis of about 80,000 CVS cases with completed follow-up did not find any evidence (Table 102.5) to suggest an increased risk of limb defects when CVS was performed after the 8th completed gestational week.[21]

Excessive trauma to the placenta and surrounding tissues is often believed to be an important causal factor of abnormalities during the phenocritical stage of embryological development. Poor expertise and improper sampling techniques were common to the experiences reporting limb defect clusters. The analysis of the WHO-CVS Registry data was recently updated for 216,381 cases[19], respectively, and the results show no increase in the overall incidence of limb defects (Table 102.5). Firth *et al.*,[89] in a literature review, collected 75 limb defects in babies exposed to CVS, to determine the temporal relationship between CVS and limb defects, and claimed a possible inverse correlation between severity of defect and gestational age at CVS. Unfortunately, the diversity in the limb defect classification between this study and population-based studies used for comparison, and the several erroneous duplications of cases, make the conclusions of the study unreliable. The pattern of distribution of limb defects has been evaluated on 77 infants or fetuses with limb defects from 138,996 pregnancies reported to the WHO registry, and compared with the data of the population-based British Columbia Registry for malformations, using the same classification and pattern analysis.[20] The analysis of this cohort did not show any differences from the background population in the overall frequency or pattern distribution of limb defects. There was also no correlation between gestational age at CVS and severity of defects. In conclusion, these results do not indicate any increased risk of limb defects after CVS.

Conclusions

Our practice and critical analysis of the literature demonstrates that where experience and skill are available, first-trimester CVS should be considered the gold standard for prenatal diagnosis of genetic diseases: the rate of complications is very low and fetal loss rate is at least comparable with mid-trimester amniocentesis. The transabdominal sampling technique, in our experience, has become the method of choice. Our preference for this approach has been based on a number of reasons: shorter learning time,[40] lower rate of immediate complications,[48] higher practicality and success rate at the first device insertion,[46] no hazard of intrauterine infections,[107] opportunity to extend sampling beyond the first trimester.[45] Given the promising development of first-trimester screening of aneuplodies by biochemical[92] and sonographic markers,[93] the use of CVS for prompt and reliable diagnosis seems assured.[108]

REFERENCES

1. Old JM, Ward RHT, Karagozlu F, *et al.* First-trimester fetal diagnosis for haemoglobinopathies: Three cases. *Lancet* 1982;2:1414–6.
2. Brambati B, Simoni G. Fetal diagnosis of trisomy 21 in the first trimester of pregnancy. *Lancet* 1983;1:586.
3. Jackson L. *CVS Latest News*, Philadelphia, October 24, 1983.
4. Jackson L. *CVS Latest News*, Philadelphia, December 10, 1984.
5. Jackson L. *CVS Latest News*, Philadelphia, November 24, 1987.
6. Jackson L. *CVS Latest News*, Philadelphia, January 28, 1991.
7. Spencer JW, Cox DN. Emotional responses of pregnant women to chorionic villus sampling or amniocentesis. *Am J Obstet Gynecol* 1987;157:1155–60.
8. Spencer JW, Cox DN. A comparison of chorionic villus sampling and amniocentesis: Acceptability of procedure and maternal attachment to pregnancy. *Obstet Gynecol* 1988;72:714–19.
9. McCormack MJ, Rylance ME, Mackenzie WE, *et al.* Patient attitudes following chorionic villus sampling. *Prenat Diagn* 1990;10:253–6.
10. Abramsky L, Rodeck CH. Women's choices for fetal chromosome analysis. *Prenat Diagn* 1991;11:23–8.
11. Cao A, Cossu P, Monni G, *et al.* Chorionic villus sampling and acceptance rate of prenatal diagnosis. *Prenat Diagn* 1987;7:531–5.
12. Canadian Collaborative CVS-Amniocentesis Clinical Trial Group. Multicentre randomised clinical trial of chorionic villus sampling and amniocentesis. *Lancet* 1989;1:1–6.
13. Rhoads GG, Jackson LG, Schlesselman SA, *et al.* The safety and efficacy of chorionic villus sampling for early prenatal diagnosis of cytogenetic abnormalities. *N Engl J Med* 1989;320:610–17.
14. Smidt-Jensen S, Permin M, Philip J, *et al.* Randomised comparison of amniocentesis and transabdominal and transcervical chorionic villus sampling. *Lancet* 1992;340:1237–44.
15. Ammala P, Hilesmaa VK, Liukkonen S, *et al.* Randomized trial comparing first-trimester transcervical chorionic villus sampling and second-trimester amniocentesis. *Prenat Diagn* 1993;13:919–27.
16. Firth HV, Boyd PA, Chamberlain P, *et al.* Severe limb abnormalities after chorionic villus sampling at 56–66 days of gestation. *Lancet* 1991;337:762–3.
17. Burton BK, Schultz CJ, Burd LI. Limb abnormalities associated with chorionic villus sampling. *Obstet Gynecol* 1992;79:726–30.
18. Brambati B, Simoni G, Travi M, *et al.* Genetic diagnosis by chorionic villus sampling before 8 gestational weeks: Efficiency, reliability, and risks on 317 completed pregnancies. *Prenat Diagn* 1992;12:789–99.
19. WHO /PAHO Consultation on CVS. Evaluation of chorionic villus sampling safety. *Prenat Diagn* 1999;19:97–99.
20. Froster UG, Jackson L. Limb defects and chorionic villus sampling: Results from an international registry, 1992–94. *Lancet* 1996;347:489–94.
21. Borrell A, Fortuny A, Lazaro L, *et al.* First-trimester chorionic villus sampling by biopsy forceps versus mid-trimester amniocentesis: a randomized controlled trial project. *Prenat Diagn* 1999;19:1138–42.
22. Brambati B, Oldrini A, Lanzani A. Transabdominal chorionic villus sampling: A freehand ultrasound-guided technique. *Am J Obstet Gynecol* 1987;157:134–7.
23. Smidt-Jensen S, Hahnemann N. Transabdominal villus sampling for fetal genetic diagnosis. Technical and obstetrical evaluation of 100 cases. *Prenat Diagn* 1988;8:7–17.
24. Brambati B, Oldrini A, Ferrazzi E, *et al.* Chorionic villus sampling: An analysis of the obstetric experience of 1000 cases. *Prenat Diagn* 1987;7:157–69.
25. Lunshof S, Boer K, Leschot NJ, *et al.* Pregnancy outcome after transcervical CVS with flexible biopsy forceps: Evaluation of risk factors. *Prenat Diagn* 1995;15:809–16.
26. Dumez Y, Dommergues M. Chorionic villus sampling using forceps under ultrasound control. In Pescia G, Nguyen The H, eds. *Chorionic Villus Sampling CVS.* Basel: Karger, 1986:22–31.
27. Sidransky E, Black SH, Soenksen DM. Transvaginal chorionic villus sampling. *Prenat Diagn* 1990;10:583–6.
28. Borrell A, Costa D, Delgado RD, *et al.* Transcervical chorionic villus sampling beyond 12 weeks of gestation. *Ultrasound Obstet Gynecol* 1996;7:416–20.
29. Blakemore KJ, Baumgarten A, Schoenfeld-Dimaio M, *et al.* Rise in maternal alpha-fetoprotein concentration after chorionic villus sampling and the possibility of isoimmunization. *Am J Obstet Gynecol* 1986;155:988–93.
30. Brambati B, Guercilena S, Bonacchi I, *et al.* Feto-maternal transfusion after chorionic villus sampling: Clinical implications. *Hum Reprod* 1986;1:37–43.
31. Fuhrmann W, Altland K, Kohler A. Feto-maternal transfusion after chorionic villus sampling. *Hum Genet* 1988;78:83–5.
32. Mariona FG, Bhatia R, Syner FN, *et al.* Chorionic villus sampling changes maternal serum alpha-fetoprotein. *Prenat Diagn* 1986;6:69–73.
33. Smidt-Jensen S, Philip J, Zachary JM, *et al.* Implications of maternal serum alpha-fetoprotein elevation caused by transabdominal and transcervical CVS. *Prenat Diagn* 1994;14:35–45.
34. Ledbetter DH, Zachary JM, Simpson JL, *et al.* Cytogenetic results from the US Collaborative Study on CVS. *Prenat Diagn* 1992;12:317–46.
35. Brambati B, Tului L, Cislaghi C, Alberti E. First 10 000 chorionic villus samplings performed on singleton pregnancies by a single operator. *Prenat Diagn* 1998; in press.
36. Brambati B. Chorionic villus sampling. *Curr Opin Obstet Gynecol* 1995;7:109–16.
37. Kalousek DK, Langlois S, Barrett I, *et al.* Uniparental disomy for chromosome 16 in humans. *Am J Hum Genet* 1993;52:8–16.
38. Brambati B, Anelli MC, Tului L. Prenatal cystic fibrosis screening in a low-risk population undergoing chorionic villus sampling for fetal karyotyping. *Clin Genet* 1996;50:23–7.
39. Brambati B, Anelli MC, Tului L, *et al.* Fetal RhD typing by DNA amplification in chorionic villus sampling. *Lancet* 1994;344:959–60.
40. Sepulveda W, Sebire NJ, Hughes K, *et al.* The lambda sign at 10–14 weeks of gestation as a predictor of chorionicity in twin pregnancies. *Ultrasound Obstet Gynecol* 1996;7:421–3.
41. Brambati B, Tului L, Lanzani A, *et al.* First-trimester diagnosis in multiple pregnancy: Principles and potential pitfalls. *Prenat Diagn* 1991;11:767–74.
42. Wapner RJ, Johnson A, Davis G, *et al.* Prenatal diagnosis in twin gestations: A comparison between second-trimester amniocentesis and first-trimester chorionic villus sampling. *Obstet Gynecol* 1993;82:49–56.
43. Brambati B, Tului L, Camurri L, Guercilena S. First-trimester fetal reduction to a singleton infant or twins; Outcome in relation to the final number and karyotyping before reduction by transabdominal chorionic villus sampling. *Am J Obstet Gynecol* 2004;191: 2035–40.
44. Evans MI, Dommergues M, Wapner RJ, *et al.* International collaborative experience of 1789 patients having multifetal pregnancy reduction: A plateauing of risks and outcomes. *J Soc Gynecol Invest* 1996;3:23–6.
45. Brambati B, Tului L, Camurri L, Guercilena S. Early second trimester (13 to 20 weeks) transabdominal chorionic villus sampling (TA-CVS). a safe and alternative method for both high and low risk populations. *Prenat Diagn* 2002;22:907–13.
46. Brambati B, Terzian E, Tognoni G. Randomized clinical trial of transabdominal versus transcervical chorionic villus sampling methods. *Prenat Diagn* 1991;11:285–93.
47. Jackson GL, Zachary JM, Fowler SE, *et al.* A randomized comparison of transcervical and transabdominal chorionic villus sampling. *N Engl J Med* 1992;327:594–8.
48. Brambati B, Tului L. Prenatal genetic diagnosis through chorionic villus sampling. In Milunsky A, editor. *Genetic Disorders and the Fetus,* 5th ed. Baltimore and London: The Johns Hopkins University Press, 2004:179–213.
49. Brambati B, Lanzani A, Oldrini A. Transabdominal chorionic villus sampling. Clinical experience of 1159 cases. *Prenat Diagn* 1988;8:609–17.
50. MRC Working Party on the Evaluation of Chorionic Villus Sampling. Medical Research Council European Trial of chorionic villus sampling. *Lancet* 1992;337:1491–9.
51. Anguo H, Bingru Z, Hong W. Long-term follow-up results after aspiration of chorionic villus during early pregnancy. In Fraccaro M, Simoni G, Brambati B, eds. *First Trimester Fetal Diagnosis.* Berlin: Springer-Verlag, 1985:1–6.
52. Invernizzi L, Prina E, Alberti S, *et al.* Long-term follow-up of 274 children born from women who underwent first trimester CVS. In Macek M, Ferguson-Smith MA, Spala M, eds. *Early Fetal Diagnosis. Recent Progress and Public Health Implication.* Prague: Charles University Press, 1992:176–8.
53. WHO Working Group. *Report of a WHO Consultation on First Trimester Fetal Diagnosis.* Geneva: WHO, 1984: document HMG/CONS/84.5.
54. Brambati B, Lanzani A, Tului L. Transabdominal and transcervical chorionic villus sampling: Efficiency and risk evaluation of 2411 cases. *Am J Med Genet* 1990;35:160–4.

55. Hogge WA, Schonberg SA, Golbus MS. Chorionic villus sampling: Experience of the first 1000 cases. *Am J Obstet Gynecol* 1986; 154:1249–52.
56. Wade RV, Young SR. Analysis of fetal loss after chorionic villus sampling: A review of 719 patients. *Am J Obstet Gynecol* 1989; 161:513–19.
57. Jackson LG, Wapner RA, Barr MA. Safety of chorionic villus biopsy. *Lancet* 1986;1:674.
58. Green JE, Dorfmann A, Jones SL, *et al*. Chorionic villus sampling: Experience with an initial 940 cases. *Obstet Gynecol* 1988; 71:208–12.
59. Jahoda MGJ, Pijpers L, Reuss A, *et al*. Evaluation of transcervical chorionic villus sampling with a completed follow-up of 1550 consecutive pregnancies. *Prenat Diagn* 1989;9:621–8.
60. Leschot NJ, Wolf H, Van Prooijen-Knegt AC, *et al*. Cytogenetic findings in 1250 chorionic villus samples obtained in the first trimester with clinical follow-up of the first 1000 pregnancies. *Br J Obstet Gynaecol* 1989;96:663–70.
61. Miny P, Basaran S, Pawlowitzki IH, *et al*. Validity of cytogenetic analysis from trophoblast tissue throughout gestation. *Am J Med Genet* 1989;33:136–41.
62. Bovicelli L, Rizzo N, Montacuti V, *et al*. Transabdominal villus sampling: Analysis of 350 consecutive cases. *Prenat Diagn* 1988;8:495–500.
63. Smidt-Jensen S, Hahnemann N. Danish experience. In Liu DTW, Symonds EM, Golbus MS, eds. *Chorion Villus Sampling*. London: Chapman and Hall, 1987:145–8.
64. Hallak M, Johnson MP, Pryde PG, *et al*. Chorionic villus sampling: Transabdominal versus transcervical approach in more than 4000 cases. *Obstet Gynecol* 1992;80:349–52.
65. Williams J III, Wang BBT, Rubin CH, *et al*. Chorionic villus sampling: Experience with 3016 cases performed by a single operator. *Obstet Gynecol* 1992;80:1023–9.
66. Wass DM, Brown GA, Warren PS, *et al*. Completed follow-up of 1000 consecutive transcervical chorionic villus samplings performed by a single operator. *Aust N Z J Obstet Gynaecol* 1991;31:240–5.
67. Jackson L. CVS *Latest News*, Philadelphia, March 31, 1993.
68. Hanson FW, Happ RL, Tennant FR, *et al*. Ultrasonography-guided early amniocentesis in singleton pregnancies. *Am J Obstet Gynecol* 1990;162:1376–83.
69. Crandall BF, Kulch P, Tabsh K. Risk assessment of amniocentesis between 11 and 15 weeks: Comparison to later amniocentesis controls. *Prenat Diagn* 1994;14:913–19.
70. Elejalde BF, de Elejalde MM, Acuna JM, *et al*. Prospective study of amniocentesis performed between weeks 9 and 16 of gestation. *Am J Med Genet* 1990;35:188–96.
71. Penso CA, Sandstrom MM, Garber M-F, *et al*. Early amniocentesis: Report of 407 cases with neonatal follow-up. *Obstet Gynecol* 1990;76:1032–6.
72. Nevin J, Nevin NC, Dornan JC, *et al*. Early amniocentesis: Experience of 222 consecutive patients, 1987–1988. *Prenat Diagn* 1990;10:79–83.
73. Stripparo L, Buscaglia M, Longatti L, *et al*. Genetic amniocentesis: 505 cases performed before the 16th week of gestation. *Prenat Diagn* 1990;10:359–64.
74. Elias S, Simpson JL. Amniocentesis. In Simpson JL, Elias S, eds. *Essentials of Prenatal Diagnosis*. New York: Churchill Livingstone, 1993:27–44.
75. Hsieh FJ, Chen D, Tseng LH, *et al*. Limb-reduction defects and chorionic villus sampling. *Lancet* 1991;337:1091–2.
76. Hsieh F-J, Shyu M-K, Sheu B-C, *et al*. Limb defects after chorionic villus sampling. *Obstet Gynecol* 1995;85:84–8.
77. Miny P, Holzgreve W, Horst J, *et al*. Limb abnormalities and chorionic villus sampling. *Lancet* 1991;337:1423–4.
78. Mastroiacovo P, Botto LD, Cavalcanti PD, *et al*. Limb anomalies following chorionic villus sampling: A registry-based case-control study. *Am J Med Genet* 1992;44:856–64.
79. Monni G, Ibba RM, Lai R, *et al*. Limb reduction defects and chorionic villus sampling. *Lancet* 1991;337:1091.
80. Mahoney MJ. Limb abnormalities and chorionic villus sampling. *Lancet* 1991;337:1422–3.
81. Jackson LG, Wapner RJ, Brambati B. Limb abnormalities and chorionic villus sampling. *Lancet* 1991;337:1423.
82. National Institute of Child Health and Human Development. Workshop on chorionic villus sampling and limb and other defects, October 20, 1992. *Am J Obstet Gynecol* 1993;169:1–6.
83. Schloo R, Miny P, Holzgreve W, *et al*. Distal limb deficiency following chorionic villus sampling? *Am J Med Genet* 1992;42:404–13.
84. Blakemore K, Filkins K, Luthy DA, *et al*. Cook obstetrics and gynecology catheter multicenter chorionic villus sampling trial: Comparison of birth defects with expected rates. *Am J Obstet Gynecol* 1993;169:1022–66.
85. Dolk H, Bertrand F, Lechat MF. Chorionic villus sampling and limb abnormalities. *Lancet* 1992;339:876–7.
86. Gruppo Italiano Diagnosi Embriofetali (GIDEF). Transverse limb reduction defects after chorion villus sampling: A retrospective cohort study. *Prenat Diagn* 1993;13:1051–6.
87. Olney RS, Khoury MJ, Alo CJ, *et al*. Increased risk for transverse digital deficiency after chorionic villus sampling (CVS): Results of the US multistate case-control study, 1988–1992. *Teratology* 1994;49:376(Abstr.).
88. Brambati B,Tului L, Guercilena S, Alberti E. Outcome of first-trimester chorionic villus sampling for genetic investigation in multiple pregnancy. *Ultrasound Obstet Gynecol* 2001;17:209–16.
89. Firth HV, Boyd PA, Chamberlain PF, *et al*. Analysis of limb reduction defects in babies exposed to chorionic villus sampling. *Lancet* 1994;343:1069–71.
90. Delhanty JD. Preimplantation diagnosis. *Prenat Diagn* 1994; 14:1217–27.
91. Simpson JL, Elias S. Isolating fetal cells in maternal circulation for prenatal diagnosis. *Prenat Diagn* 1994;14:1229–42.
92. Brambati B, Tului L, Bonacchi I, *et al*. Serum PAPP-A and free β-hCG are first-trimester screening markers for Down's syndrome. *Prenat Diagn* 1994;14:1043–7.
93. Snijders RJM, Johnson S, Sebire NJ, *et al*. First-trimester ultrasound screening for chromosomal defects. *Ultrasound Obstet Gynecol* 1996;7:216–26.
94. Brambati B. CVS risk evaluation. *Presented at the Eighth International Conference on Prenatal Diagnosis and Therapy*, Goa, India, June 1996.
95. Parazzini F, Pirotta N, La Vecchia C, *et al*. I determinanti della mortalità perinatale ed infantile nelle Regioni italiane: 1980–1983. *Ann Obstet Gynecol Med Perinatol* 1990;111:9–146.
96. Indagine Policentrica Italiana sulle Malformazioni (IPIMC). *10 Anni di Sorveglianza sulle Malformazioni Congenite in Italia 1978–1987*. Milan: CNM Edizioni Scientifiche, 1990.
97. Froster-Iskenius UG, Baird PA. Limb reduction defects in over one million consecutive livebirths. *Teratology* 1989;39:127–35.
98. Kallen B, Rahmani TMZ, Winberg J. Infants with congenital limb reduction registered in the Swedish Register of Congenital Malformations. *Teratology* 1984;29:73–85.
99. Coviello DA, Brambati B, Tului L, *et al*. First-trimester prenatal screening for the common 35delG GJB2 mutation casing prelingual deafness, *Prenat Diagn* 2004;24:631–34.
100. Hahnemann JM, Vejerslev LO. Accuracy of cytogenetic findings on chorionic villus sampling (CVS)-Diagnostic consequences of CVS mosaicism and non-mosaic discrepancy incentres contributing to EUCROMIC 1986–1992. *Prenat Diagn* 1997;17: 801–829.
101. Nicolaides K, Brizot M de L, Patel F, Snijders R. Comparison of chorionic villus sampling and amniocentesis for fetal karyotyping at 10–13 weeks' gestation. *Lancet* 1994;344:435–39.
102. Sundberg K, Bang J, Smidt-Jensen S, *et al*. Randomised study of risk of fetal loss related to early amniocentesis versus chorionic villus sampling. *Lancet* 1997;350:697–703.
103. Philip J, Silver RK, Wilson RD, *et al*. Late first-trimester invasive prenatal diagnosis: results of an international randomized trial. *Obstet Gynecol* 2004;103:1164–73.
104. The Canadian Early and Mid-trimester Amniocentesis Trial (CEMAT) Group. Randomized trial to assess safety and fetal outcome of early and mid-trimester amniocentesis. *Lancet* 1998; 351:242–47.
105. Wapner R, Jackson L, Evans MI, Johnson MP. *Presented at 6th Annual Meeting of the Society of Perinatal Obstetricians*, February 1996; Kona, Hawaii.
106. Brun J-L, Mangione R, Gangho F, *et al*. Feasibility, accuracy and safety of chorionic villus sampling: a report of 10.741 cases. *Prenat Diagn* 2003;23:295–301.
107. Brambati B, Tului L. Chorionic Villus Sampling am amniocentesis. *Curr Opin Obstet Gynecol* 2005;17:197–201.
108. Nicolaides KH. Nuchal translucency and other first-trimester sonographic markers of chromosomal abnormalities (review article). *Am J Obstet Gynecol* 2004;191:45–67.
109. Wolstenholme J, Rooney DE, Davison EV. Confined placental mosaicism, IUGR, and adverse pregnancy outcome: a controlled retrospective U.K. collaborative survey. *Prenat Diagn* 1994;14: 345–61.

103 Amniocentesis

A. Tabor

Introduction

Amniocentesis is the method by which amniotic fluid is removed from the pregnant uterus. Amniotic fluid cell culture from second-trimester amniocentesis has been one of the primary tools of prenatal diagnosis: hundreds of thousands of pregnancies have provided extensive experience of monitoring for chromosomal disorders, as well as many hundreds of diagnoses of metabolic disorders. The vast majority of amniocenteses are carried out to diagnose cytogenetic disorders, inborn errors of metabolism and other genetic disorders using chromosome analysis, biochemical studies and recombinant DNA analysis. Therapeutic amniocentesis will not be considered here. This chapter will consider the technique of amniocentesis, the possible complications of the test, and its diagnostic accuracy.

Indications

The commonest indications for performing amniocentesis are increased risks of Down's syndrome or neural tube defects. The indications for performing fetal chromosome analysis vary slightly from country to country. In Western societies, amniocentesis is mostly offered to the following groups, considered to be at an increased risk:

(1) Increased risk of Down's syndrome, following first trimester risk assessment using nuchal translucency and double test;
(2) Maternal age above 35 years (the age limit varies between 35 and 40 years);
(3) Prior birth/abortion of a child/fetus with a chromosome abnormality;
(4) Abnormal parental karyotype; and
(5) Fetal structural abnormality detected on ultrasound scan.

During the last decade the concept of prenatal diagnosis has changed, with the discovery of biochemical and ultrasonic markers for Down's syndrome. A woman's risk of having a Down's syndrome fetus may now be estimated by combining her age-related risk with the risk attributable to the markers. It has been estimated that 90% of Down's syndrome fetuses could be detected by using the nuchal translucency scan in combination with the double test (free β-HCG and pregnancy associated plasma protein A) and maternal age at an amniocentesis rate of 5%.[1] The addition of more biochemical and ultrasonic markers may further increase the detection rate. These markers permit a more selective approach to invasive testing and may in the future be offered to all pregnant women. It should, however, be emphasized that markers can only be used as screening tests, the only diagnostic test being chorionic villus sampling or amniotic fluid cell culture. The proportion of invasive prenatal diagnostic tests being performed such as amniocentesis is increasing due to the increasing use of first trimester Down's syndrome screening. As the result of this screening is available for around 12–13 weeks, women will increasingly opt for chorionic villus sampling.

Technical aspects

Amniocentesis has been performed for prenatal diagnosis for more than 40 years. However, very few randomized controlled trials have evaluated the risks of the procedure, or assessed the optimal technique. Such studies are difficult, as they require a very large number of patients.

Ultrasonography

The failure rate of amniocentesis is reduced by using real-time ultrasound[2] (Figure 103.1). Whether ultrasonography may also reduce the abortion rate after the procedure has not been investigated.

Placental perforation

The abortion risk has been shown in some large studies[3,4] to be increased when the placenta is perforated, while in other studies this was not the case.[5,6] Although the evidence is inconclusive, it is widely agreed that placental perforation should be avoided.

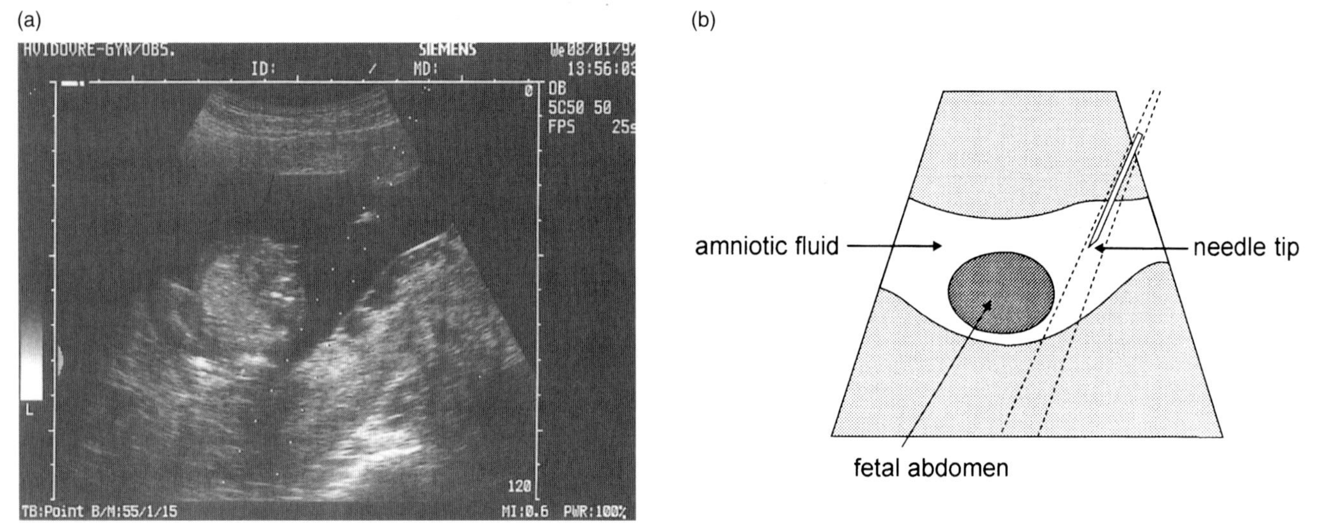

Figure 103.1 Ultrasound-guided second-trimester amniocentesis (a) on the ultrasound screen and (b) in a line drawing. The dotted line represents the needle-guide.

Needle size and number of insertions

Needles larger than 18 or 20 gauge are associated with an increased abortion rate. The risk of fetal loss increases with the number of needle insertions.[7,8]

Operator

The abortion rate[9] as well as the failure rate of amniocentesis[2] have been shown to be inversely correlated with the experience of the operator. In Denmark, the National Board of Health recommends that a gynecologist should perform 50 amniocenteses under supervision, and then 25 amniocenteses per year to keep up the routine.[10]

Timing and volume

Most amniocenteses have been performed early in the second trimester, i.e. from week 14 to 17. A maximum volume of 20 ml is removed, allowing material for polymerase chain reaction (PCR) or fluorescent *in situ* hybridization (FISH), duplicate culture flasks to be set up as well as α-fetoprotein determination. During the last decade, amniocentesis has been performed earlier in the second and even in the first trimester. The technique of early amniocentesis is similar to amniocentesis performed at later gestational ages. However, in the first trimester there are two sacs, the amniotic cavity and the extra-embryonic coelome. The incomplete fusion of the amnion and chorion in early gestation may result in tenting of the membranes, which may necessitate more needle insertions.[11] It is important to distinguish the two sacs ultrasonographically at the time of the amniocentesis, as the fluid in the extra-embryonic coelome is jelly-like, difficult to aspirate, and has a different α-fetoprotein concentration than amniotic fluid.[12] Retrieval of fluid from this sac should be avoided, as it will only rarely produce enough cells to allow a cytogenetic diagnosis. After 11 completed weeks of gestation, the sampling success rate is nearly 100%.[13]

The volume of amniotic fluid is approximately 100 ml in the 12 weeks of gestation, and it has been shown, that the abortion risk as well as the rate of talipes equinovarus is significantly increased, when amniocentesis is performed before 15 weeks.[14,15] It is therefore recommended not to perform amniocentesis before 15 weeks.

Multiple pregnancy

In order to assess whether amniotic fluid has been retrieved from both sacs in twin pregnancies, a marker (a dye or a biochemical substance) may be injected into the first sac.[17] When the second sac is punctured, the absence of the marker in the amniotic fluid indicates that both sacs have been sampled. However, real-time ultrasound allows visually-guided amniotic fluid sampling from both sacs,[18] thus making dye-injection obsolete.

Whether amniocentesis in twin pregnancies should be performed by using one or two needle insertions remains to be shown. A single needle insertion could reduce the abortion risk, but may on the contrary create the problems of amniotic band syndrome or a mono-amniotic twin pregnancy, or give rise to cytogenetic problems.[19]

In conclusion, amniocentesis should be performed after 15 weeks of gestation, under aseptic conditions, using real-time ultrasound, by a trained operator, avoiding placental perforation, using needles no larger than 20 gauge, and performing at the most two insertions on the same day.

Cytogenetic and biochemical aspects of amniocentesis

Amniotic fluid cells are derived from the fetus as well as from the extra-embryonic membranes and the trophoblast. The cells from the latter two tissues may differ in karyotype from the fetus itself, thus causing mosaicism. Viable cells in the amniotic fluid are cultured and used for karyotyping, and investigation of metabolic and biochemical disorders. Uncultured cells may be used to detect specific chromosome aberrations by using chromosome-specific probes and FISH on interphase cells,[20] but complete karyotyping is not yet possible on uncultured cells.

Culture failure

In large laboratories, culture failure occurs in less than 1% of second-trimester cases. The culture failure rate increases with decreasing gestational age: after 11 completed weeks the culture failure rate is the same as in the second trimester,[21] while in weeks 8–9 culture is unsuccessful in more than 30% of cases.[22] Culture failure seems to occur more often in cases of fetal aneuploidy,[23] emphasizing the importance of counseling, further ultrasonic investigation and secondary testing in these cases.

Maternal cell contamination

Maternal cell contamination may cause misdiagnosis, if only maternal cells are examined or mosaicism is suspected. The rate of maternal cell contamination is 1–3 per 1000 cases,[24] but this figure should probably be doubled as maternal cell contamination is only detected when the fetus is male. The contamination rate may be lowered by using a stylet in the needle when performing the amniocentesis, and by aspirating the first 2 ml in a separate syringe to be used for amniotic fluid α-fetoprotein determination.[24] Screening for maternal cell contamination may be considered in blood-stained amniotic fluid samples. An assay using fluorescent labeled microsatellites provides results quickly and seems promising.[25]

Diagnostic accuracy of amniocentesis

The level of α-fetoprotein is determined and a fetal karyotype test is performed routinely on amniotic fluid samples in most laboratories.

Amniotic fluid α-fetoprotein and acetylcholinesterase

The concentration of α-fetoprotein in amniotic fluid is increased when the fetus has an open neural tube defect. The accuracy of this test may be improved by combining it with acetylcholinesterase electrophoresis, giving a detection rate for anencephaly and spina bifida of more than 99.5%, with a false-positive rate of 0.03%.[26]

Amniotic fluid α-fetoprotein may no longer be necessary in centers where high-resolution ultrasonography is available.[27]

Accuracy of fetal chromosome analysis

A large-scale study to assess the accuracy of fetal chromosome analysis has never been performed. This would require complete follow-up on all pregnancies and chromosome analysis of live-born children as well as abortions, whether induced or spontaneous. In a literature survey of 57,921 cases, the accuracy of fetal chromosome analysis was established to be between 99.2% and 99.9%, based on the phenotype at birth.[28]

Mosaicism remains the main problem in prenatal diagnosis and is seen in 0.1% of all samples.[29] When two or more different cell lines are detected in the same amniotic fluid sample, this may reflect a true mosaic abnormality in the fetus, an abnormality in the trophoblast, or a culture artifact (pseudo-mosaicism).[30] While repeat amniocentesis cannot be recommended to solve this problem, fetal blood sampling may determine the karyotype of the fetus *per se*.[30] A 100% detection of mosaicism cannot be expected, when only a limited number of amniotic fluid cells are examined.

It may be concluded that fetal karyotyping is a test with a very high detection rate and a very high accuracy. It should, however, be remembered that false-positive results do occur, although very rarely.

Complications

Maternal

Infection

There is minimal risk to the mother. The risk of amnionitis is less than 0.1% for all procedures.[8]

Immediate complications

In the Danish randomized trial,[3] women in the study and control groups were specifically asked about bleeding, abdominal pain and amniotic fluid leakage 4 weeks after amniocentesis or ultrasonography. The complication rate was higher after amniocentesis (12.1%) than after ultrasonography (5.8%). Vaginal bleeding occurred equally often in the two groups, but amniotic fluid leakage was reported four times more often in the study group (39 vs. 10 women).

The earlier amniocentesis is performed, the higher the leakage rate.[3,15,16]

Rhesus isoimmunization

Feto-maternal hemorrhage (FMH) occurs in approximately half of all pregnant women,[31] and therefore it is not surprising that rhesus immunization may occur during normal pregnancy. The immunization incidence has been reported to be 1.1–1.6% among primigravidas and 2.2% among multigravidas.[32,33] FMH occurs during amniocentesis in one out of six women,[34] and may therefore theoretically give rise to subsequent isoimmunization.

In two retrospective studies, the immunization incidences after amniocentesis were 2.1%[35] and 3.4%.[36] In a prospective cohort study,[37] the immunization rate was 1.4% (95% confidence limits 0.2–2.6). This may be an overestimation of the immunization rate attributable to the present pregnancy, as the five immunized women were multiparous, and at least three of them had had events in a prior pregnancy which may have presensitized them. The observed 1.4% immunization rate is not different from the spontaneous immunization rate. However, due to the wide confidence interval it cannot be excluded that amniocentesis exposes the rhesus-negative woman to a slightly higher immunization risk. In a population-based study of long-term outcome after amniocentesis,[38] ABO isoimmunization was found significantly more often in the infants subjected to amniocentesis. A protective effect of anti-D immunoglobulin administration after amniocentesis was suggested by the results of the Medical Research Council (MRC) study,[2] which reported that none of 59 women who had been given anti-D were isoimmunized, as compared to three cases among untreated women.

The World Health Organization recommends that a small dose of anti-D be given at the time of amniocentesis to D-negative women.[39] Practice differs between countries regarding whether this recommendation is followed or not. In the United States and in the United Kingdom a dose of 100–125 μg is administered.

Anxiety

In Italian[40] and Danish[41] controlled studies using self-rating scales, anxiety and depression varied similarly in women having amniocentesis and in control women. The variations in anxiety level observed throughout pregnancy in both these studies correspond to those changes observed during normal pregnancy.[42] However, among women having amniocentesis due to advanced maternal age, the anxiety level was increased while awaiting the results of the test.[41,43] It seems that amniocentesis generally has little, if any, psychological impact on pregnancy.

Fetal

The risks to the fetus may either be direct, leading to subsequent abortion, or indirect secondary to removal of amniotic fluid.

Fetal loss rate

The fetal loss rate associated with amniocentesis is superimposed on a background spontaneous abortion rate, which is higher the earlier amniocentesis is performed. The 'background' risk of spontaneous abortion varies with maternal age, parity and social variables.[44,45] In ultrasonically-proven viable pregnancies, the abortion rate after week 15 varies between 1% and 2%,[3,46,47] and as many as 0.7% of women referred for amniocentesis have been shown to have had a missed abortion.[7] In studies designed to assess the fetal loss rate, it is therefore evident that comparability of study and control groups is of major importance, as well as assessment of fetal viability in both groups.

In the 1970s three large cohort studies recruited women 'at risk' to the study group, and all included a matched control group. The National Institute of Child Health and Human Development (NICHD) multicenter study[8] compared 1040 subjects having amniocentesis with 992 controls matched for age, race, parity and socioeconomic factors. The total fetal loss rate and the second-trimester abortion rate were similar in the two groups (3.5% and 2.3% in the study group, compared with 3.2% and 2.1% in the control group). Amniocentesis was performed following ultrasonography in 30% of the women, while amniocentesis was carried out blindly in the rest of the group. In the control group, assessment of fetal viability was not carried out at entry into the study.

In a Canadian multicenter study,[7] 1020 women having amniocentesis were compared to women admitted in early pregnancy. The rate of conception loss was 2.3% before the 24th week in the study group as well as in the control group. Women in the control group may however have had a higher than average risk of fetal loss, as they had been admitted due to pregnancy complications. Amniocentesis was performed following ultrasonography for 98% of the women, while no assessment of fetal viability at entry into the study was carried out in the control group.

In an English multicenter study[2] a 1.2% increased rate of spontaneous abortion was found among 2428 women having amniocentesis and as many matched controls. The main part of this study was criticized for ascertainment bias, due to methodological problems such as differences between the study and control groups regarding maternal age and gestational age at entry into the study, inclusion in the study group of women with increased levels of serum α-fetoprotein, and exclusion from the control group of women who had aborted spontaneously. However, a supplementary, methodologically correct, study confirmed the finding of an increased abortion rate following amniocentesis. Although not significantly different, the size of the risk was 1.0–1.5%. Amniocentesis was performed following ultrasonography in approximately two-thirds of the subjects, while no assessment of fetal viability at entry into the study was carried out in the control group.

The results of the above three large multicenter studies[2,7,8] may have been affected by selection. Furthermore, only the largest study detected an increased fetal loss rate after amniocentesis. In the two smaller studies, involving approximately 1000 women in both the study and the control groups, there was no difference; this could, however, be ascribed to the sample size.

In the only randomized controlled trial of amniocentesis[2] the total sample size was calculated to be

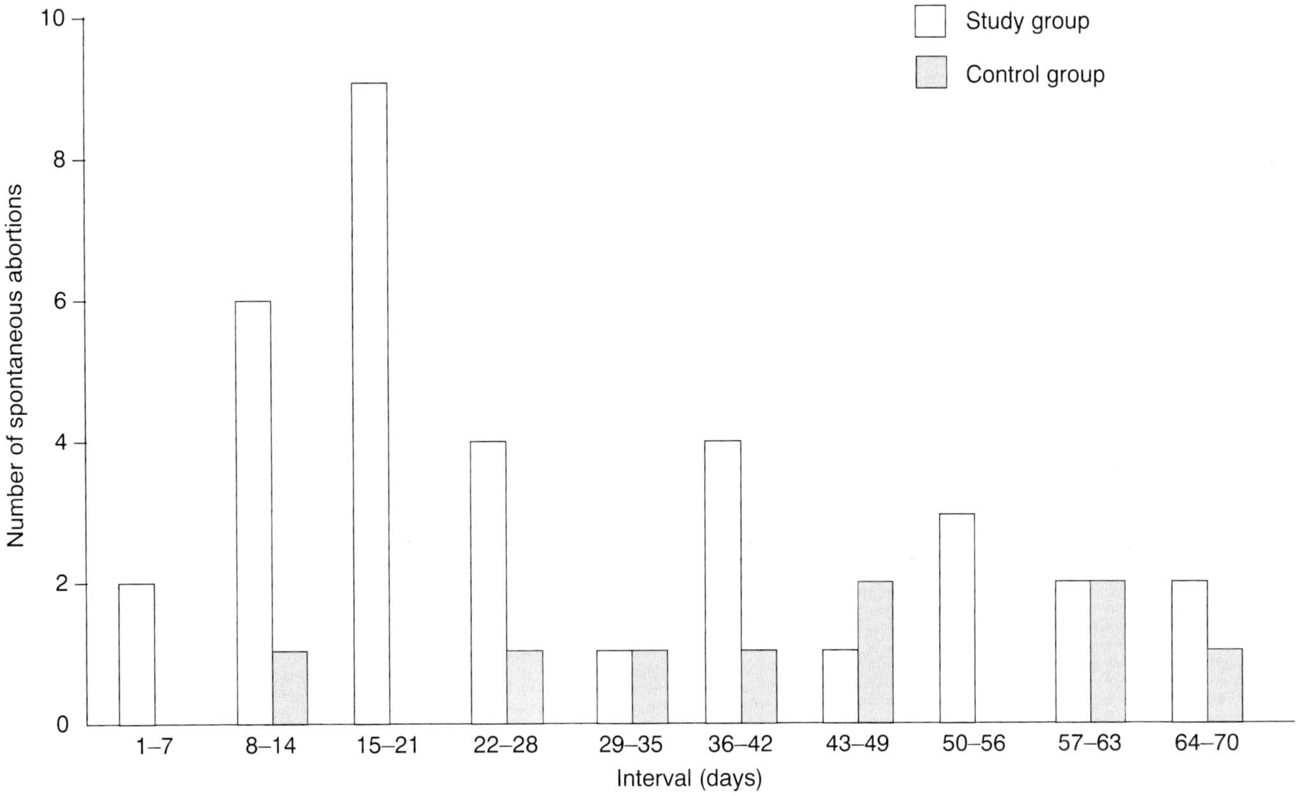

Figure 103.2 Interval between amniocentesis (study group) or ultrasound scan (control group) and spontaneous abortion.

approximately 4800 women, in order to have an 80% chance of detecting an increase in miscarriage rate from the estimated 1.5% in the general population to 2.5% following amniocentesis. The study included 4606 women aged 25–34 years, who would not otherwise have been offered genetic amniocentesis. By choosing this group of women, it was ethically possible to perform a randomized trial. Apart from the fact that women in the study group had amniocentesis and women in the control group an ultrasound scan at the same gestational age to assess fetal viability, antenatal care was similar for the two groups. Randomization achieved comparability between the study and control groups regarding age, background factors and time of entry into the study. The follow-up rate was high (99.9%), as well as the compliance (99.1% in both groups). The design and conduction of this study therefore do not seem to have been biased in any major way.

The fetal loss rate after the 16th week (mean gestational age of amniocentesis in the study group and of ultrasonography in the control group) was 1.7% in the study group and 0.7% in the control group. Amniocentesis was thus associated with an increased fetal loss rate of 1.0% (95% confidence limits 0.3–1.5%), which corresponds to a relative risk of 2.3 (1.3–4.0). There is no reason to believe that the procedure-related risk of amniocentesis should be any smaller in older women. There was a substantial increment in the number of abortions in the first 3–4 weeks after amniocentesis (Figure 103.2).

The 1.0% increased miscarriage rate may actually underestimate the true difference between the two groups, as chromosomally abnormal fetuses are at an increased risk of being aborted spontaneously.[48] Eleven pregnancies in the study group and only one in the control group were terminated due to fetal chromosome abnormality.

Women who miscarried after amniocentesis could not be distinguished from the rest of the study group by obstetrical or social variables, but they had significantly more often had transplacental taps, retrieval of miscolored amniotic fluid or an elevated level of maternal serum α-fetoprotein before amniocentesis. The last two variables are more likely to be reflections of an abnormal pregnancy than a complication of amniocentesis.

Early amniocentesis (before 15 weeks). Early amniocentesis has been compared to chorionic villus sampling (CVS) or amniocentesis in weeks 15–18, taking into account the background rates of pregnancy loss at earlier gestational ages. In the first study, which included a randomised sub-group, the fetal loss rate was significantly higher after early amniocentesis than following CVS.[14] In a larger Canadian randomised trial, the spontaneous fetal loss rate was also significantly higher following early amniocentesis as compared to traditional amniocentesis in weeks 15–18.[15] In a smaller Danish randomised trial, the spontaneous fetal loss rate was significantly higher after early filtration amniocentesis compared with transabdominal CVS.[16]

It may therefore be concluded, that amniocentesis should not be performed before 15 weeks gestation.

Multiple pregnancy. The fetal loss rate in multiple gestations has not been estimated in a controlled trial and is difficult to determine due to the increased miscarriage rate *per se* in twin pregnancies.

An increased postamniocentesis abortion rate in multiple gestations may be expected, since most operators use more than one needle insertion, a variable associated with an increased fetal loss rate. The fetal loss rate has been reported to be between 2 and 8%,[17,49,50] but most studies have small sample sizes. In the largest series of 476 twin pregnancies, the fetal loss rate was 2.7% before 28 weeks of gestation, comparable to that in the control group.[51]

We may thus conclude that the fetal loss rate following amniocentesis in weeks 16–18 is around 1.0% (95% confidence limits 0.3–1.5%) in singleton pregnancies; in twin pregnancies the fetal loss rate may be more than doubled. Amniocentesis should not be performed before 15 weeks of gestation.

Complications to the infant

Amniocentesis does not affect the preterm birth rate, the stillbirth rate or the perinatal mortality rate.[3,7,8] The mean birth weight of the infants was also independent of whether amniocentesis had been performed. In a randomized controlled trial of amniocentesis,[3] the rate of low birth weight infants (i.e. < 2500 g) was similar in the study and control groups. The number of very low birth weight infants (i.e. < 1500 g) was, however, significantly higher in the study group.

Perinatal morbidity

Lower limb malformations. In the main part of the MRC study,[2] congenital dislocation of the hip and talipes equinovarus were found more often among subject infants. This finding could not be confirmed in the methodologically more correct supplementary part of the MRC study,[2] nor in the other controlled studies.[3,7,8] Furthermore, a case–control study[52] of 1342 infants found no association between amniocentesis and talipes or hip malformations. Amniocentesis in week 16–18 thus does not seem to be associated with an increased rate of congenital malformations. In the two randomized trials of early amniocentesis,[14–16] however, the prevalence of talipes equinovarus at birth was significantly higher after amniocentesis than after CVS.

Neonatal respiratory distress. Severe unexplained respiratory difficulties at birth were found significantly more often in study group babies as compared to the controls in the MRC study.[2] This increase was most marked in those infants born between 34 and 37 weeks of gestation (8.2% in subjects and 0.9% in controls). The mortality attributable to respiratory distress was also higher among subjects than controls (0.26 compared with 0.13%).

The suggested association between amniocentesis and respiratory difficulties was confirmed in the Danish randomized trial[3]; 25 infants in the study group (1.1%) developed respiratory distress syndrome (RDS) as compared to 12 infants in the control group (0.5%). Pneumonia was also diagnosed more often in the study group (15 infants compared to six). The association between amniocentesis and RDS was independent of birth weight and of gestational age. The hypothesis that amniocentesis may produce a relative pulmonary hypoplasia in some fetuses is supported by animal studies. Structural changes were observed in the lungs of baby monkeys after amniocentesis compared with control monkeys,[53] and in guinea pigs even transient oligohydramnios led to pulmonary complications.[54] In newborn children, a lower ratio of crying vital capacity to birth weight was found in 10 infants whose mothers had had amniocentesis, in comparison with 10 infants born after uneventful pregnancies.[55] However, the two groups of mothers may not have been comparable. In another study of 39 infants born after pregnancies subjected to amniocentesis and 42 controls, the lung growth and development also seemed affected by amniocentesis.[56]

There is thus some evidence suggesting that amniocentesis may increase the rate of respiratory difficulties in the newborn. It may be that altered amniotic fluid volume after amniocentesis or subsequent chronic amniotic fluid leakage interferes with normal lung development and lung structure at term, thus giving rise to pulmonary hypoplasia and consequently to RDS in the newborn.[57] Whether these antenatal and neonatal changes have any long-term impact on lung development remains to be shown. In a large population-based study of long-term outcome after amniocentesis including 1296 cases and 3704 controls, respiratory problems were reported more often among controls.[38]

Infant follow-up

Two of the large controlled studies[2,8] followed up the infants at the age of 10–12 months, and found no difference in physical growth or neurological development between study- and control-group infants. Few studies have followed up the children beyond infancy. In a large population-based database study, no group differences were revealed at the age of 7–18 years.[38] In a prospective longitudinal follow-up study, Finegan *et al.*[58] found no difference between

91 infants whose mothers had had an amniocentesis, and 53 control infants, regarding mental and motor development, temperament or physical growth at the age of 6 months. At the ages of 4 and 7 years, there was no difference between the two groups regarding intelligence, language or physical growth.[59,60] Subject children were, however, more likely to have had an ear infection than the control infants. The size of this study may be too small to detect anything but large differences between the groups.

It may be concluded that, apart from an increased risk of developing respiratory problems, amniocentesis in weeks 16–18 does not seem to influence newborn infants. A possible long-term impact on the upper as well as on the lower respiratory tract has yet to be studied.

REFERENCES

1. Nicolaides KH. Nuchal translucency and other first-trimester sonographic markers of chromosomal abnormalities. *Am J Obstet Gynecol* 2004;191:45–67.
2. Medical Research Council Working Party on Amniocentesis. An assessment of the hazards of amniocentesis. *Br J Obstet Gynaecol* 1978;85(Suppl 2):1–41.
3. Tabor A, Philip J, Madsen M, *et al.* Randomized controlled trial of genetic amniocentesis in 4606 low-risk women. *Lancet* 1986; 1:1287–93.
4. Kappel B, Nielsen J, Hansen KB, *et al.* Spontaneous abortion following mid-trimester amniocentesis. Clinical significance of placental perforation and blood-stained amniotic fluid. *Br J Obstet Gynaecol* 1987;94:50–4.
5. Crane JP, Kopta MM. Genetic amniocentesis: Impact of placental position upon the risk of pregnancy loss. *Am J Obstet Gynecol* 1984;150:813–16.
6. Hanson FW, Tennant FR, Zorn EM, *et al.* Analysis of 2136 genetic amniocenteses: Experience of a single physician. *Am J Obstet Gynecol* 1985;152:436–43.
7. Simpson NE, Dallaire L, Miller JR, *et al.* Prenatal diagnosis of genetic disease in Canada: Report of a collaborative study. *Can Med Assoc J* 1976;115:739–46.
8. NICHD National Registry for Amniocentesis Study Group. Midtrimester amniocentesis for prenatal diagnosis. Safety and accuracy. *J Am Med Assoc* 1977;236:1471–6.
9. Leschot NJ, Verjaal M, Treffers PE. Risks of midtrimester amniocentesis: Assessment in 3000 pregnancies. *Br J Obstet Gynaecol* 1985;92:804–7.
10. National Board of Health. Guidelines for prenatal diagnosis – prenatal information, risk assessment, counselling and diagnosis. Copenhagen: Committee for Health Information, 2005:21–22.
11. Elejalde BR, de Elejalde MM, Acuna JM, *et al.* Prospective study of amniocentesis performed between weeks 9 and 16 of gestation: Its feasibility, risks, complications and use in early genetic prenatal diagnosis. *Am J Med Genet* 1990;35:188–96.
12. Wathen NC, Cass PL, Campbell DJ, *et al.* Early amniocentesis: α-fetoprotein levels in amniotic fluid, extraembryonic coelomic fluid and maternal serum between 8 and 13 weeks. *Br J Obstet Gynaecol* 1991;98:866–70.
13. Sundberg K, Smidt-Jensen S, Philip J. Amniocentesis with increased cell yield, obtained by filtration and reinjection of the amniotic fluid. *Ultrasound Obstet Gynecol* 1991;1:91–4.
14. Nicolaides K, Brizot ML, Patel F, *et al.* Comparison of chorionic villus sampling and amniocentesis for fetal karyotyping at 10–13 weeks' gestation. *Lancet* 1994;344:435–9.
15. CEMAT (The Canadian Early and Mid-trimester Amniocentesis Trial study group). Randomised trial to assess safety and fetal outcome of early and midtrimester amniocentesis. *Lancet* 1998; 351:242–7.
16. Sundberg K, Bang J, Smidt-Jensen S, Brocks V, Lundsteen C, Parner J, *et al.* Randomised study of fetal loss related to early amniocentesis versus chorionic villus sampling. *Lancet* 1997;350:697–703.
17. Pijpers L, Jahoda MGJ, Vosters RPL, *et al.* Genetic amniocentesis in twin pregnancies. *Br J Obstet Gynaecol* 1988;95:323–6.
18. Elias S, Gerbie AB, Simpson JL, *et al.* Genetic amniocentesis in twin gestations. *Am J Obstet Gynecol* 1980;138:169–73.
19. Gilbert WM, Davis SE, Kaplan C, *et al.* Morbidity associated with prenatal disruption of the dividing membrane in twin gestations. *Obstet Gynecol* 1991;78:623–30.
20. Kuo WL, Tenjin H, Segraves R, *et al.* Detection of aneuploidy involving chromosomes 13, 18 or 21 by fluorescence *in situ* hybridization (FISH) to interphase and metaphase amniocytes. *Am J Hum Genet* 1991;49:112–19.
21. Stripparo L, Buscaglia M, Logatti L, *et al.* Genetic amniocentesis: 505 cases performed before the sixteenth week of gestation. *Prenat Diagn* 1990;10:359–64.
22. Nevin J, Nevin NC, Dornan JC, *et al.* Early amniocentesis: Experience of 222 consecutive patients, 1987–1988. *Prenat Diagn* 1990;10:79–83.
23. Persutte WH, Lenke RR. Failure of amniotic fluid cell growth: Is it related to fetal aneuploidy? *Lancet* 1995;345:96–7.
24. Benn PA, Hsu LYF. Maternal cell contamination of amniotic fluid cell cultures: Results of a US nationwide survey. *Am J Med Genet* 1983;15:297–305.
25. Smith GW, Graham CA, Nevin J, *et al.* Detection of maternal cell contamination in amniotic fluid cell cultures using fluorescent labelled microsatellites. *J Med Genet* 1995;32:61–4.
26. Milunsky A, Sapirstein VS. Prenatal diagnosis of open neural tube defects using the amniotic fluid acetylcholinesterase assay. *Obstet Gynecol* 1982;59:1–5.
27. Sepulveda W, Donaldson A, Johnson RD, *et al.* Are routine α-fetoprotein and acetylcholinesterase determinations still necessary at second-trimester amniocentesis? Impact of high-resolution ultrasonography. *Obstet Gynecol* 1995;85:107–12.
28. Loft A, Tabor A. Discordance between prenatal cytogenetic diagnosis and outcome of pregnancy. *Prenat Diagn* 1984;4:51–9.
29. Bui T-H, Iselius L, Lindsten J. European collaborative study on prenatal amniotic fluid cell cultures. *Prenat Diagn* 1984;4:145–62.
30. Gosden CM, Nicolaides KH, Rodeck CH. Fetal blood sampling in investigation of chromosome mosaicism in amniotic fluid cell culture. *Lancet* 1988;1:613–17.
31. Clayton EM, Feldhaus WD, Whitacre FE. Fetal erythrocytes in the maternal circulation of pregnant women. *Obstet Gynecol* 1964;23:915–19.
32. Davey MG, Zipursky A. McMaster Conference on prevention of rhesus immunization. *Vox Sang* 1979;36:50–64.
33. Bowman JM, Chown B, Lewis M, *et al.* Rhesus iso-immunization during pregnancy: Antenatal prophylaxis. *Can Med Assoc J* 1978; 118:623–7.
34. Tabor A, Bang J, Nørgaard-Pedersen B. Feto-maternal haemorrhage associated with genetic amniocentesis: Results of a randomized trial. *Br J Obstet Gynaecol* 1987;94:528–35.
35. Golbus MS, Stephens JD, Cann HM, *et al.* Rhesus iso-immunization following genetic amniocentesis. *Prenat Diagn* 1982;2:149–56.
36. Murray JC, Karp LE, Williamson RA, *et al.* Rhesus iso-immunization related to amniocentesis. *Am J Med Genet* 1983;16:527–34.
37. Tabor A, Jerne D, Bock JE. Incidence of rhesus immunization after genetic amniocentesis. *Br Med J* 1987;293:533–6.
38. Baird PA, Yee IML, Sadovnick AD. Population-based study of long-term outcomes after amniocentesis. *Lancet* 1994;344: 1134–6.
39. WHO (World Health Organization). Prevention of rhesus sensitization. WHO Technical Report Series, 1971; no. 468.
40. Fava GA, Kellner R, Michelacci L, *et al.* Psychological reactions to amniocentesis: A controlled study. *Am J Obstet Gynecol* 1982;143:509–13.
41. Tabor A, Jonsson MH. Psychological impact of amniocentesis in low-risk women. *Prenat Diagn* 1987;7:443–51.

42. Lubin B, Gardener SH, Roth A. Mood and somatic symptoms during pregnancy. *Psychosom Med* 1975;37:136–46.
43. Beeson D, Golbus MS. *Anxiety Engendered by Amniocentesis.* Birth Defects Original Articles Series, 1979;15:191–7.
44. Harlap S, Shiono PH, Ramcharan S, *et al.* A prospective study of spontaneous fetal losses after induced abortions. *N Engl J Med* 1979;301:677–81.
45. Obel EB. Risk of spontaneous abortion following legally induced abortion. *Acta Obstet Gynecol Scand* 1980;59:131–7.
46. Gustavii B. Chorionic biopsy and miscarriage in first trimester. *Lancet* 1984;1:562.
47. MacKenzie WE, Holmes DS, Newton JR. Spontaneous abortion rate in ultrasonographically viable pregnancies. *Obstet Gynecol* 1988;71:81–3.
48. Hook EB. Chromosome abnormalities and spontaneous fetal death following amniocentesis: Further data and associations with maternal age. *Am J Hum Genet* 1983;35:110–16.
49. Anderson RL, Goldberg JD, Golbus MS. Prenatal diagnosis in multiple gestations: 20 years' experience with amniocentesis. *Prenat Diagn* 1991;11:263–70.
50. Weisz B, Rodeck CH. Invasive diagnostic procedures in twin pregnancies. *Prenat Diagn* 2005;25:751–8.
51. Yukobowich E, Anteby EY, Cohen SM, *et al.* Risk of fetal loss in twin pregnancies undergoing second trimester amniocentesis (1). *Obstet Gynecol* 2001;98:231–4.
52. Wald NJ, Terzian E, Vickers PA, *et al.* Congenital talipes and hip malformation in relation to amniocentesis: A case–control study. *Lancet* 1983;2:246–9.
53. Hislop A, Fairweather DVI. Amniocentesis and lung growth: An animal experiment with clinical implications. *Lancet* 1982;2: 1271–2.
54. Moessinger AC, Collins MH, Blanc WA, *et al.* Oligohydramnios-induced lung hypoplasia: The influence of timing and duration in gestation. *Pediatr Res* 1986;20:951–4.
55. Vyas H, Milner AD, Hopkin IE. Amniocentesis and fetal lung development. *Arch Dis Child* 1982;57:627–8.
56. Milner AD, Hoskyns EW, Hopkin IE. The effects of midtrimester amniocentesis on lung function in the neonatal period. *Eur J Pediatr* 1992;151:458–60.
57. Thompson PJ, Greenough A, Nicolaides KH. Lung volume measured by functional residual capacity in infants following first trimester amniocentesis or chorionic villus sampling. *Br J Obstet Gynaecol* 1992;99:479–82.
58. Finegan J-AK, Quarrington BJ, Hughes HE, *et al.* Infant outcome following mid-trimester amniocentesis: Development and physical status at age 6 months. *Br J Obstet Gynaecol* 1985;92: 1015–23.
59. Finegan J-AK, Quarrington BJ, Hughes HE, *et al.* Child outcome following mid-trimester amniocentesis: Development and physical status at age 4 months. *Br J Obstet Gynaecol* 1990;97:32–40.
60. Finegan J-AK, Sitarenios G, Bolan PL, *et al.* Children whose mothers had second trimester amniocentesis: Follow-up at school age. *Br J Obstet Gynaecol* 1996;103:214–18.

104 Cordocentesis: indications

F. Daffos

Cordocentesis opened the fetal vascular compartment to diagnosis and therapy.[1–3] It contributed to the notion that the fetus was a patient, and transformed the view of antenatal diagnosis from the normal/abnormal dichotomy, in which abortion was the only 'therapeutic' option, into a field in which a fine prognosis could be made and antenatal therapy envisaged. In the last 15 years fetal blood sampling has become a major diagnostic tool in a new field, namely fetal medicine, which for practical reasons is considered a part of gynecology and obstetrics, but which is in fact closer to 'antenatal pediatrics' in view of the disease conditions treated, warranting specific training.

Advances in our knowledge of fetal pathophysiology and fetal blood biology in the last 10 years mean that the indications for fetal blood sampling are no longer classified in terms of antenatal diagnosis of a given abnormality, but are integrated into a medical approach.

Fetal malformations

Fetal karyotyping

Karyotyping is always indicated when there is a malformation, regardless of its nature; the use of fetal blood has specific indications, as it can provide etiologic information according to the type of malformation.[4]

Cytogenetic analysis from amniocentesis is rarely possible in less than 8 days. In contrast, the karyotype from fetal blood is obtained within 48 h, and is therefore particularly indicated in advanced pregnancies where management decisions will depend on whether a chromosome abnormality is associated with the observed malformation.[5] In addition, long delays in obtaining results have adverse psychological effects for the mothers.

Fetal blood sampling is also indicated for karyotyping when there is mosaicism on amniotic fluid culture. The karyotype from fetal blood generally confirms that the result was due to maternal blood contamination in cases of sexual mosaicism, or due to culture artifacts in cases of autosomal mosaicism.[6,7]

Abnormalities of hands and arms

The TAR syndrome (thrombocytopenia and absence of radius) is confirmed by the presence of fetal thrombocytopenia (generally below 50,000). For the diagnosis of Fanconi's anemia, chromosome strand breaks are easier to identify on lymphocytes.

Cardiac malformations

These can be part of the Di George syndrome, in which case T lymphocytes are absent, as shown by the study of lymphocyte subpopulations. In this particular case, unsuccessful fetal blood culture for karyotyping can be a sign of Di George syndrome, as it is T cells that divide in culture.

Microdeletion of chromosome 22, found in certain familial forms of the Di George syndrome, is generally less difficult to identify on a blood karyotype which, in trained hands, is of better quality than a karyotype on fibroblasts derived from amniotic fluid.

Cerebral abnormalities

Non-specific abnormalities can result from an intracerebral hemorrhage syndrome. They are found increasingly often and can be due to auto- and especially alloimmune fetal thrombocytopenia, or to a hemorrhagic syndrome such as fetal intravascular coagulopathy which is sometimes encountered in very severe fetal infections. Thorough testing of fetal coagulation is warranted in these cases.

Infectious syndromes

Fetal blood sampling initially had a major place in the diagnosis of the main pathogenic agents interfering severely with fetal development. Prenatal diagnosis of toxoplasmosis, rubella, cytomegalovirus, parvovirus and varicella was first carried out using fetal blood. Recent progress, especially in cell culture and polymerase chain reaction (PCR) amplification, has improved the reliability of the diagnosis. In addition, pathogenic agents can be detected in amniotic fluid obtained by simple amniocentesis.[8]

In prenatal diagnosis of congenital toxoplasmosis, tests for parasite DNA by PCR on amniotic fluid have eliminated this indication for fetal blood sampling since 1993. In the same way, several publications have shown that cytomegalovirus can readily be detected by culture and PCR in amniotic fluid, perhaps more easily than in fetal blood. However, diagnosis of some infections, such as parvovirus B19, still warrants fetal blood sampling.

Diagnostic value

Congenital rubella

The drastic reduction in cases of rubella during pregnancy in the last 15 years, thanks to vaccination, has meant that research on prenatal diagnosis of this infection has waned. The diagnosis is highly reliable when specific anti-rubella immunoglobulin M (IgM) is found in fetal blood, together with acid-labile interferon and elevated total IgM.[9,10] The reliability of diagnosis based on amniotic fluid has not been studied; it should be possible but further studies are necessary.

Parvovirus B19 infection

This virus, which specifically infects fetal erythropoietic precursors, is easier to detect in fetal blood than in amniotic fluid.[11]

Prognostic value

The indications for fetal blood sampling for the diagnosis of infections have become more limited in recent years. In contrast, simple diagnosis is no longer sufficient, and an attempt must also be made to assess the prognosis according to the pathogen, gestational age and the severity of fetal disease.

Congenital toxoplasmosis

With the exception of fetal thrombocytopenia, which correlates with the severity of infection, we have found no other useful blood parameters in this setting.

Cytomegalovirus

If the infected fetus has normal laboratory values,[12,13] there is a chance that it will be a healthy carrier and have no congenital manifestations. This is generally the case. Signs of severe fetal hepatic involvement, and especially intravascular coagulopathy, are a major risk factor for severe congenital abnormalities.

Parvovirus B19

Fetal blood sampling can be used to assess the degree and severity of fetal anemia due to this virus.[14–16] In addition, the stage of the disease can be determined by counting erythroblasts and studying erythropoietic precursors. In the regenerative phase, when anemia and erythroblastosis are present, the outcome is spontaneously favorable and transfusions are unnecessary. In the non-regenerative phase, with more or less profound bone marrow aplasia, transfusions are necessary until marrow function recovers. In every case of fetal infection, severe thrombocytopenia indicates a very poor prognosis.

Anemic syndromes

The most frequent anemic syndromes are rhesus and erythrocyte alloimmunization, parvovirus infection, congenital rubella after the acute hepatic and erythroblastocytic phase, and spontaneous and traumatic feto-maternal bleeding which leads to acute anemia with signs of fetal distress (Kleihauer's test is strongly positive). In these anemic syndromes fetal blood sampling is the main tool used for diagnosis, prognosis and treatment.[17–21] The hemoglobin concentration, hematocrit, erythroblast count and mean corpuscular volume must be taken into account when assessing the type of anemia, its course and its severity. Hyperbilirubinemia, which is never very elevated (because of transplacental filtration), points to a hemolytic cause of the anemia.

The prognosis of fetal anemia depends not only on its etiology but also on the hemoglobin level and the chronic (rhesus incompatibility) or acute/subacute (parvovirus infection or feto-maternal hemorrhage) nature of the anemia. Anemia with a hematocrit below 16% (hemoglobin 5 or 6 g) is frequently accompanied by signs of fetoplacental hydrops on ultrasound. In chronic anemia, the acid–base balance and fetal pH seem to remain normal down to a hemoglobin level of approximately 3 g. In cases of such extremely severe anemia, anoxia leads to often irreversible cell damage, even when the anemia is corrected by transfusion.

The universally accepted treatment for anemia is *in utero* transfusion with specially prepared red cell concentrates. Ultrasound-guided puncture is also indispensable in this indication. It allows red cells to be transfused directly into the fetal vascular compartment, and can be used to check efficacy by measuring the hemoglobin and hematocrit at the end of the transfusion.

Anoxemic syndromes

In cases of severe intrauterine growth retardation, when ultrasound malformations have been ruled out together with infectious and chromosomal abnormalities, a diagnosis of chronic fetal distress of anoxemic origin can be made.[22–25] Without replacing the prognostic information provided by the fetal heart rate and the different items of Manning's biophysical score,[26] fetal blood sampling helps with decision-making by revealing chronic fetal distress and acute decompensation (Table 104.1). A good deal of research is being conducted to identify other biological markers.[27–30]

Fetal blood sampling has also been used to check the efficacy of experimental treatment by maternal hyperoxygenation or fetal nutrition by intra-amniotic injection of amino acids and glucose.

Table 104.1 Biological signs of acute and chronic fetal distress

Chronic fetal distress	Acute fetal distress
Stimulation of erythropoiesis	Acidosis
Rise in erythroblasts	Hypoxia
	Hypercapnia
Cell damage	
Shortened red cell lifespan	
Hepatic cytolysis	
Decrease in fat storage	
Hypertriglyceridemia	
Modification of cortisol and ACTH levels	
Rise in cortisol	
Fall in ACTH	
Change in maternal supply	
Hypoglycemia	
Fall in essential amino acids	
Modification of growth hormones	
Hypoinsulinemia	
Decrease in IgG-1	

ACTH, adrenocorticotropic hormone; IgG-1, immune gamma globulin-1

Hemorrhagic syndromes

These syndromes are far more frequent than previously realized.

Hereditary hemorrhagic syndromes

These are due to genetic clotting factor deficiency (hemophilia A or B, factor V and VII deficiency, and afibrinogenemia) or to abnormalities of the platelet count or function (May Hegglin syndrome, Glanzmann thrombasthenia, etc.).[31]

Except in cases where the gene is known and the mutation identified in the family (permitting diagnosis by molecular biology on trophoblast or amniotic fluid), these conditions are diagnosed phenotypically using fetal blood by clotting factor assays (relative to fetal standards) or by studies of fetal platelet function.

Acquired hemorrhagic syndromes

Intravascular disseminated coagulation

As in adults, this leads to a fall in fetal fibrinogen levels and platelet counts, and to the presence of fibrin products. The most frequent causes are very severe congenital infections (especially those due to cytomegalovirus and *Toxoplasma gondii*).

Immune-mediated thrombocytopenia

The most severe and earliest of these are of alloimmune origin (especially involving the PLA-1 or HPA-1a system), but fetal thrombocytopenia due to antiplatelet antibodies, e.g. idiopathic thrombocytopenic purpura, can sometimes be severe (< 50,000 platelets),[32–36] Fetal blood sampling is the only way of diagnosing these forms of thrombocytopenia, as there is no correlation between fetal and maternal platelet counts or antiplatelet antibody titers. According to the severity of the thrombocytopenia, fetal blood sampling can also be used to select the method of delivery that will be least traumatic for the fetus and therefore avoid intracerebral hemorrhage.

These hemorrhagic syndromes can be treated by *in utero* transfusion of platelet or clotting factor concentrates, whose efficacy depends on their half-life.

Other indications for fetal blood sampling

Diagnosis

Many hereditary diseases cannot be diagnosed by means of molecular biology, as the culprit gene has not yet been identified. Only studies of fetal serum or blood components can provide the antenatal diagnosis.[37–40]

Therapeutic interventions

Intravenous injection of drugs into the fetal circulation is currently limited to curare before invasive procedures (transfusion, vesical or pulmonary shunt) that necessitate complete fetal immobility. This method has occasionally been used to correct the fetal heart rate after failure of maternal treatment.[41]

Pharmacological studies

Access to the fetal blood compartment allows studies of transplacental drug passage and efficacy by simultaneous maternal and fetal blood sampling. Vitamin K1 is a good example of the complexity of antenatal pharmacology. It crosses the placental barrier very readily but has no therapeutic effect, as it does not affect vitamin K1-dependent clotting factors in the fetus.[42]

For obvious ethical reasons, prenatal pharmacology is rarely used. However, many maternal drug treatments have been studied by using fetal blood samples obtained for other purposes.

Conclusion

Fetal medicine has been transformed in the last 15 years. 'Prenatal diagnosis' is now too limited a term, as we are able not only to diagnose, but also to establish a prognosis and to treat many conditions, exactly in the same way as in adult medicine.

The place of fetal blood sampling in fetal medicine has seen a similar change. Less useful for diagnostic purposes than 10 years ago, because of advances in molecular biology (especially PCR), it remains an irreplaceable prognostic and therapeutic tool.

Fetal blood sampling has now become part of an impressive therapeutic arsenal, alongside imaging methods, invasive techniques and laboratory investigations. Its main indications now are in establishing the prognosis of infections, and in the prognosis and treatment of anemic and hemorrhagic syndromes.

REFERENCES

1. Daffos F, Capella-Pavlovsky M, Forestier F. Fetal blood sampling via the umbilical cord using a needle guided by ultrasound. Report of 66 cases. *Prenat Diagn* 1983;3:271–7.
2. Daffos F, Capella-Pavlovsky M, Forestier F. Fetal blood sampling during pregnancy with use of a needle guided by ultrasound: A study of 606 consecutive cases. *Am J Obstet Gynecol* 1985;153: 655–60.
3. Pielet B, Socol ML, MacGregor SN, *et al.* Cordocentesis: An appraisal of risks. *Am J Obstet Gynecol* 1988;159:1497–500.
4. Gosden C, Rodeck CH, Nicolaides KH, *et al.* Fetal blood chromosome analysis: Some new indications for prenatal karyotyping. *Br J Obstet Gynaecol* 1985;92:915–20.
5. Taillemite JL, Daffos F, Joyce N, *et al.* Fetal karyotyping on fetal blood obtained from the umbilical vein using ultrasound. *J Gynecol Obstet Biol Reprod* 1985;14:315–19.
6. Gosden C, Nicolaides KH, Rodeck CH. Fetal blood sampling in investigation of chromosome mosaicism in amniotic fluid cell culture. *Lancet* 1988;1:613–17.
7. Shalev E, Zalel Y, Weiner E, *et al.* The role of cordocentesis in assessment of mosaicism found in amniotic fluid cell culture. *Acta Obstet Gynecol Scand* 1994;73:119–22.
8. Holhfeld P, Daffos F, Costa M, *et al.* Prenatal diagnosis of congenital toxoplasmosis with a polymerase chain reaction test on amniotic fluid. *N Engl J Med* 1994;331:695–9.
9. Daffos F, Forestier F, Grangeot-Keros L, *et al.* Prenatal diagnosis of congenital rubella. *Lancet* 1984;2:1–3.
10. Morgan-Capner P, Rodeck CH, Nicolaides KH, *et al.* Prenatal detection of rubella-specific IgM in fetal sera. *Prenat Diagn* 1985;5:21–6.
11. Peters MT, Nicolaides KH. Cordocentesis for the diagnosis and treatment of human fetal parvovirus infection. *Obstet Gynecol* 1990;75:501–4.
12. Riviere D, Riviere MR. Prenatal diagnosis of a fetus with partial monosomy 7 (q34 Ø qter) and partial trisomy 18 (q21 Ø qter). *Prenat Diagn* 1993;13:983–8.
13. Lynch L, Daffos F, Emanuel D, *et al.* Prenatal diagnosis of fetal cytomegalovirus infection. *Am J Obstet Gynecol* 1991;165:714–18.
14. Naides SJ, Weiner CP. Antenatal diagnosis and palliative treatment of non-immune hydrops fetalis secondary to fetal parvovirus B19 infection. *Prenat Diagn* 1989;9:105–14.
15. Gloning KP, Schramm T, Brusis E, *et al.* Successful intrauterine treatment of fetal hydrops caused by parvovirus B19 infection. *Behring Inst Mitt* 1990;85:79–85.
16. Andreux JP, Renard M, Daffos F, *et al.* Erythropoietic progenitor cells in human fetal blood. *Nouv Rev Fr Hematol* 1991;33:223–6.
17. Boulot P, Cattaneo A, Taib J, *et al.* Hematologic values of fetal blood obtained by means of cordocentesis. *Fetal Diagn Ther* 1993;8:309–16.
18. Forestier F, Daffos F, Galactéros F, *et al.* Hematological values of 163 normal fetuses between 18 and 30 weeks of gestation. *Pediatr Res* 1986;20:342–6.
19. Barss VA, Benacerraf BR, Frigoletto FD, *et al.* Management of isoimmunized pregnancy by use of intravascular techniques. *Am J Obstet Gynecol* 1988;159:932–7.
20. Nicolaides KH, Soothill PW, Rodeck CH, *et al.* Rh disease: Intravascular fetal blood transfusion by cordocentesis. *Fetal Ther* 1986;1:185–92.
21. Poissonnier MH, Brossard Y, Demeideros N, *et al.* L'exsanguinotransfusion *in utero*: Une nouvelle thérapeutique pour les incompatibilités sanguines foeto-maternelles sévères. *Diagn Prise Charge Affect Foet II* 1986;xx:93–101.
22. Hambartsoumian E, Ville Y, Frydman R. Retard de croissance intra utérin d'origine vasculaire: Quelles thérapeutiques seraient possibles *in utero*? *Med Foet Echo Gynécol* 1994;18:7–15.
23. Cox WL, Daffos F, Forestier F, *et al.* Physiology and management of intrauterine growth retardation: A biologic approach with fetal blood sampling. *Am J Obstet Gynecol* 1988;159:36–41.
24. Cetin I, Marconi AM, Bozzetti P, *et al.* Umbilical amino acid concentrations in appropriate- and small-for-gestational age infants: A biochemical difference present *in utero*. *Am J Obstet Gynecol* 1988;158:120–6.
25. Nicolaides KH, Bradley RJ, Soothill PW, *et al.* Maternal oxygen therapy for intrauterine growth retardation. *Lancet* 1987;1:942–5.
26. Manning FA, Snijders R, Harman CR, *et al.* Fetal biophysical profile score. VI. Correlation with antepartum umbilical venous fetal pH. *Am J Obstet Gynecol* 1993;169:755–63.
27. Kawamura T, Power GG, Araki T. Plasma adenosine concentration in appropriate- and small-for-gestational age fetuses. *Am J Obstet Gynecol* 1994;170:684–8.
28. Schiff E, Weiner E, Zalel Y, *et al.* Endothelin-1,2 levels in umbilical vein serum of intra-uterine growth-retarded fetuses as detected by cordocentesis. *Acta Obstet Gynecol Scand* 1994;73:21–4.
29. Soothill PW, Nicolaides KH, Campbell S. Prenatal asphyxia, hyperlacticaemia, hypoglycaemia, and erythroblastosis in growth retarded fetuses. *Br Med J* 1987;294:1051–3.
30. Thieriot Prevost G, Daffos F, Forestier F, *et al.* Serum growth, promoting activity in normal and hypotrophic fetuses at midpregnancy. *Pediatr Res* 1987;22;39–40.
31. Daffos F, Forestier F, Kaplan C, *et al.* Prenatal diagnosis and management of bleeding disorders with fetal blood sampling. *Am J Obstet Gynecol* 1988;158:939–46.
32. De Carolis S, Noia G, De Santis M, *et al.* Immune thrombocytopenic purpura and percutaneous umbilical blood sampling; an open question. *Fetal Diagn Ther* 1993;8:154–60.
33. Moise KJ Jr, Carpenter RJ Jr, Cotton DB, *et al.* Percutaneous umbilical cord blood sampling in the evaluation of fetal platelet counts in pregnant patients with autoimmune thrombocytopenia purpura. *Obstet Gynecol* 1988;72:346–50.
34. Muller JY, Kaplan C, Reznikoff-Etievant MF, *et al.* *In utero* fetal sampling in neonatal alloimmune thrombocytopenia: Justification and usefulness. In *Current Studies in Hematology and Blood Transfusion*. Basel: Karger, 1988.
35. Kaplan C, Daffos F, Forestier F, *et al.* Management of alloimmune thrombocytopenia. Antenatal diagnosis and *in utero* transfusion of maternal platelets. *Blood* 1988;72:340–3.
36. Kaplan C, Morel Kopp MC, Clemenceaui C, *et al.* Fetal and neonatal alloimmune thrombocytopenia/current trends in diagnosis and therapy. *Transfus Med* 1992;2:265–71.
37. Berdoukas V, Argyle J, Cox W, *et al.* Prenatal diagnosis for hemoglobinopathies – 10 years' experience using fetal blood sampling. *Pathology* 1993;25:48–51.
38. Corney G, Whitehouse DB, Hopkinson DA, *et al.* Prenatal diagnosis of alpha-1-antitrypsin deficiency by fetal blood sampling. *Prenat Diagn* 1987;7:101–8.
39. Rosa R, Premu MO, Calvin MC, *et al.* Possibility of prenatal diagnosis of hereditary triose phosphate isomerase deficiency. *Prenat Diagn* 1986;6:231–4.
40. Lecomte MC, Feo O, Bournier O, *et al.* Premier diagnostic anténatal d'une elliptocytose héréditaire due à un défaut de tétramérisation de la spectrine (elliptocytose de type I). *Nouv Rev Fr Hematol* 1985;27:68.
41. Weiner CP, Thompson MI. Direct treatment of fetal supraventricular tachycardia after failed transplacental therapy. *Am J Obstet Gynecol* 1988;158:570–3.
42. Mandelbrot L, Guillaumont M, Leclercq M, *et al.* Placental transfer of vitamin K1 and its implications in fetal hemostasis. *Thromb Haemost* 1988;60:39–43.

105 Fetal pharmacological therapy

M. I. Evans, Y. Yaron, P. Lewis and R. F. Hume Jr

Introduction

The concept and reality of fetal therapy is now entering its fourth decade. Ever since Lilley's first attempt to treat fetal anemias in the 1960s, physicians have wondered what else could be attempted. First thoughts centered on surgical approaches, and these have been detailed elsewhere. However, medical approaches, while not as glamorous, have made significant contributions to our understanding of fetal physiology, and the process of disease.

For decades, drugs and other agents have been administered to pregnant women for treatment of fetal disorders not usually classified as metabolic in the hope of improving the capacity for postnatal adaptation. Well-known examples include exchange transfusions in Rhesus disease, the administration of corticosteroids for the prevention of respiratory distress syndrome in premature infants, and the administration of phenobarbital prior to birth in the hope of inducing liver enzymes for postnatal reduction of serum bilirubin concentration. However, there are very few examples of attempted prenatal treatment for genetically determined metabolic defects.

Errors of metabolism

Congenital adrenal hyperplasia

The most common and the best described adrenal abnormality affecting the fetus is congenital adrenal hyperplasia (CAH). This comprises a group of autosomal recessive disorders characterized by a deficiency in one or more of the enzymes required for adrenal cortisol biosynthesis. The most common abnormality, responsible for > 90% of patients with CAH, is caused by a deficiency of the enzyme 21-hydroxylase (21-OH), also known as p450c21.[1] Other, less common causes for CAH include enzyme deficiencies in 11β-hydroxylase, 17α-hydroxylase, p450scc deficiency, and 3β-OH-dehydrogenase. Diminished 21-OH activity results in accumulation of 17-hydroxyprogesterone (17-OHP) due to the decrease in its conversion to 11-deoxycorticosterone (Figure 105.1). The excess 17-OHP is then converted via androstenedione to androgens, the levels of which increase by as much as several hundred fold. The excess androgens cause masculinization of the undifferentiated female external genitalia. The degree of masculinization may vary from clitoral hypertrophy to complete formation of a phallus and scrotum. By contrast, genital formation in male fetuses is normal, but signs of androgen excess develop in childhood, and may manifest in precocious masculinization, and accelerated growth and development. The 'classical' form of CAH involves an almost complete block of enzyme activity and is clinically present at birth. The 'non-classical' form involves only partial blockade of the enzymatic activity and is usually clinically apparent later in life. 21-OH deficiency is inherited as an autosomal recessive trait in close linkage to the HLA major histocompatability complex on the short arm of chromosome 6.[2] The gene for 21-OH (CYP21B) has been mapped, allowing direct mutation analysis in informative families.[3]

Historically, in the late 1970s and early 1980s, diagnosis of CAH was made by the finding of elevated levels of 17-OHP in amniotic fluid. With the development of chorionic villus sampling (CVS) in the 1980s, linkage-based diagnosis in the first trimester became available. Since discovery and mapping of the allelic variants in the 1980s, direct DNA analysis has become the routine approach. In addition, the sonographic detection of an abnormally enlarged phallus should alert the physician to investigate for CAH.[4]

The fetal adrenal gland can be pharmacologically suppressed by maternal replacement doses of dexamethasone.[5] In an attempt to prevent female genital birth defects, Evans *et al.*[5] first administered dexamethasone at a dose of 0.25 mg *quater in die* to a mother known to be at risk for CAH, beginning at 10 weeks of gestation. Serial maternal estriol and

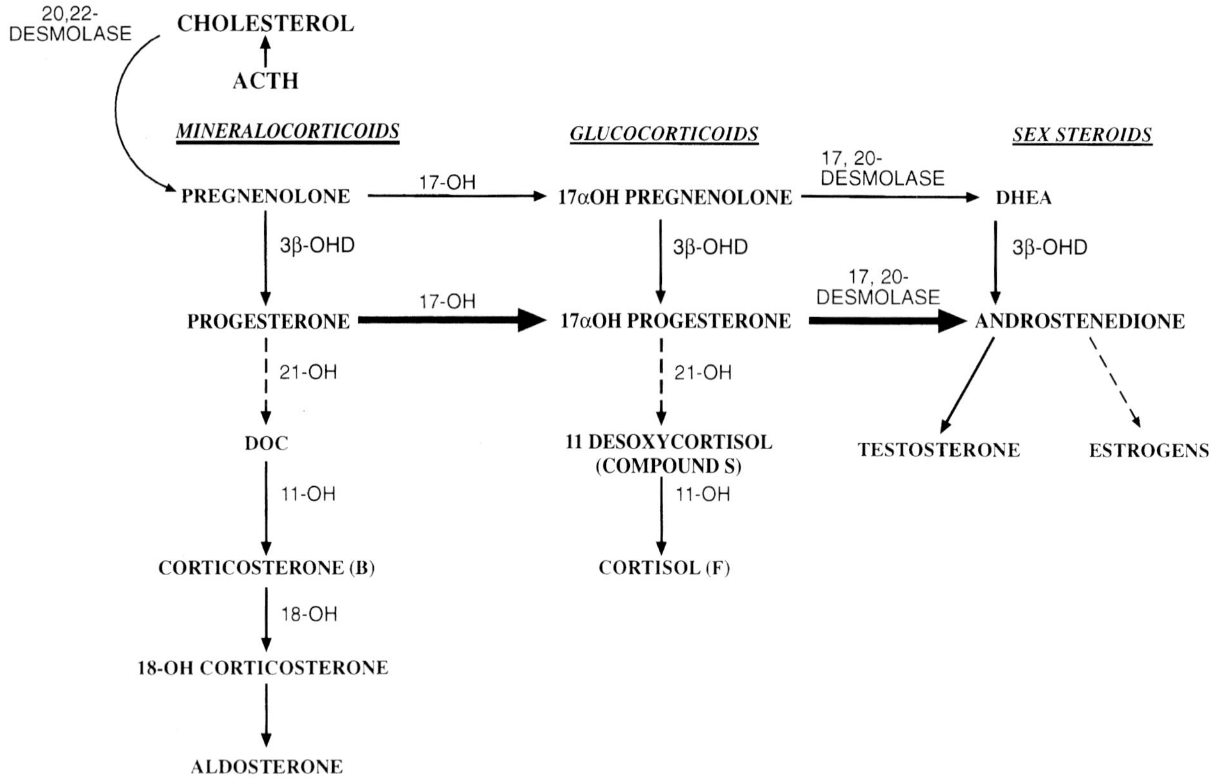

Figure 105.1 Pathway of congenital adrenal hyperplasia with blockage at 21-hydroxylase leading to excess androgens.

cortisol levels indicated that adrenal gland suppression had been achieved. The fetus, ultimately found to be affected, was born at 39 weeks of gestation with normal external genitalia. Forrest and David[6] then employed a similar protocol beginning at 9 weeks of gestation to treat several fetuses known to be at risk for CAH. Subsequently, those female fetuses confirmed to be clinically affected with the severe form of CAH were spared masculinization of the external genitalia.

Since the differentiation of the external genitalia begins at about 7 weeks of gestation, diagnosis by amniocentesis or even CVS comes too late to prevent masculinization. Thus, for patients at risk of having an affected fetus, pharmacological therapy has to be initiated prior to diagnosis. This implies that therapy needs to be administered to all patients at risk despite the fact that the chance of an affected female fetus for carrier parents is only 1 in 8 (i.e. 1/4 affected ∞ 1/2 female). Direct DNA diagnosis or linkage studies may then be performed by CVS in the first trimester. Thus, for seven out of eight patients, therapy can be discontinued as soon as the diagnosis of CAH is ruled out. If the fetus is indeed found to be an affected female, then therapy is continued throughout gestation. Stress-dose corticosteroids should be given to the mother during labor and tapered gradually postpartum. If, however, the fetus is a male, or is unaffected, the therapy is discontinued at the time of diagnosis.

To date, several infants who have inherited the classic CAH mutation, and who clearly would have been masculinized, were born with normal genitalia. In a few cases some masculinization has still been observed following this regimen beginning at 9 weeks. Our current protocol, therefore, is to begin at 7 weeks, although there have been too few cases to assess this modification.[7,8] These events represent the first prevention of a birth defect and may serve as a model for other attempts at pharmacological fetal therapy.

Although this therapy is widely accepted it is still considered experimental by some, especially insurance companies. A recently published commentary written in the *Journal of the American Medical Association* advocates Institutional Review Board approval be obtained on all patients offered this treatment. As long-term follow-up has not been documented on individuals who received *in utero* steroid treatment for CAH, a registry has been proposed by the Lawson Wilkins Pediatric Endocrine Society for studies in North America.[9] This should help to assess the long-term outcome of fetuses exposed to high-dose steroids.

Methylmalonic acidemia

Methylmalonic acidemia is related to a functional vitamin B_{12} deficiency. Coenzymatically active B_{12} is required for the conversion of methylmalonyl-coenzyme A to succinyl-coenzyme A. Several genetically determined etiologies for methylmalonic acidemia include

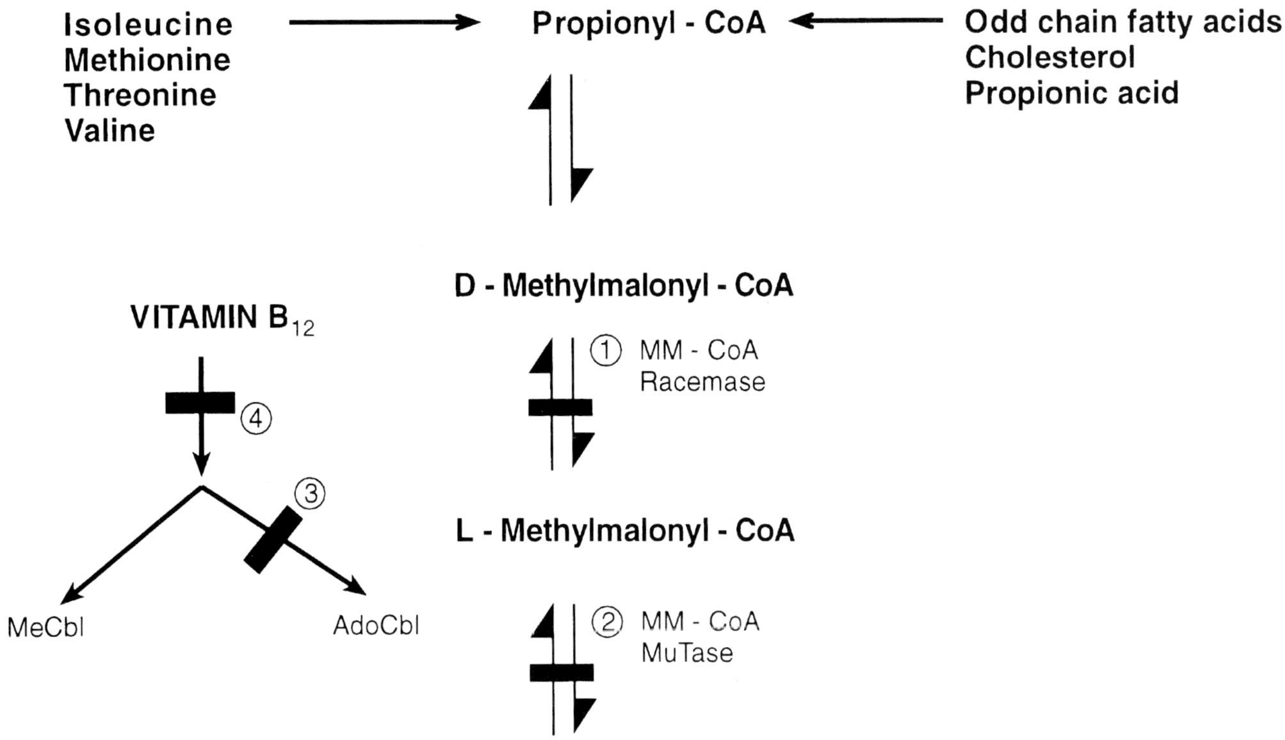

Figure 105.2 Pathway of methylmalonic aciduria and reaction driven by excess vitamin B_{12}.

defects in methylmalonyl-coenzyme A mutase or in the metabolism of vitamin B_{12} to the coenzymatically active form, adenosylcobalamin, by the converting enzyme. Some patients may respond to administration of large doses of B_{12}, which can enhance the amount of active holoenzyme (mutase apoenzyme plus adenosylcobalamin) (Figure 105.2).

It was already known that fetal methylmalonic acidemia is associated with increased methylmalonic acid excretion in maternal urine. Ampola *et al.*[10] documented increased methylmalonic acidemia in a maternal urine sample first collected at 23 weeks of gestation; the methylmalonic acid excretion per milligram of creatinine was approximately twice the upper normal limit and demonstrated a further rise by 25 weeks. Urinary methylmalonate excretion is not abnormal in heterozygous females carrying a normal fetus, as shown subsequently by these same investigators.

Very late in pregnancy, cyanocobalamin (10 mg/day) was orally administered to the mother in divided doses. The treatment only marginally altered the maternal serum B_{12} level; however, there was a slight reduction of urinary methylmalonic acid excretion that remained several-fold above normal. At approximately 34 weeks of gestation, administration of 5 mg of cyanocobalamin per day intramuscularly was begun. The maternal serum B_{12} level then rose gradually to more than six-fold above normal and was accompanied by a progressive decrease in urinary methylmalonic acid excretion. Maternal urinary methylmalonate was only slightly above the normal range when delivery occurred at 41 menstrual weeks. Amniotic fluid methylmalonic acid concentrations were three times the normal mean at 19 menstrual weeks and four times the normal mean at term, despite prenatal treatment.

Postnatally, the diagnosis of methylmalonic acidemia was confirmed. The infant suffered no acute neonatal complications and had an extremely high serum B_{12} level. Long-term postnatal management involved protein restriction; however, no continuous B_{12} treatment was required.

In this instance, prenatal treatment certainly improved the fetal and, secondarily, the maternal biochemistry. Whether there was any significant clinical benefit to the fetus by *in utero* treatment cannot be assessed adequately. It seems likely that reducing the fetal burden of methylmalonic acid should have some beneficial effect on fetal development and could reduce the risks in the neonatal period. However, this is only speculation.

Evans *et al.* have recently documented the changing dose requirements necessary over the course of pregnancy to maintain adequate levels of B_{12}. They sequentially followed maternal plasma and urine levels in a prenatally treated pregnancy.[11] Data such as these suggest that modulation of maternal–fetal pharmacological interchange of therapeutic drugs will be difficult to control precisely.

Multiple carboxylase deficiency

Biotin-responsive multiple carboxylase deficiency is an inborn error of metabolism in which the mitochondrial biotin-dependent enzymes, pyruvate carboxylase, propionyl-coenzyme A carboxylase, and β-methyl-crotonyl-coenzyme A carboxylase have diminished activity. Affected patients present as newborns or in the early childhood period with dermatitis, severe metabolic acidosis, and a characteristic pattern of organic acid excretion. Metabolism in patients or in their cultured cells can be restored toward normal levels by biotin supplementation. There have been two reports of prenatal administration of biotin to fetuses affected with this disorder.

Roth *et al.*[12] treated a fetus without the benefit of prenatal diagnosis in a case in which two siblings of the fetus had died of multiple carboxylase deficiency. The first sibling had died within 3 days of birth, and in the second the diagnosis of biotin-responsive carboxylase deficiency was made posthumously.

The patient was first seen at 34 weeks of gestation. Prenatal diagnosis was not attempted because of the late stage of pregnancy. The maternal urinary organic acid profile was normal throughout the final 4 weeks of pregnancy. Because of severe neonatal manifestations in the previous siblings and the probable harmlessness of biotin, oral administration of this compound to the mother was begun at a dose of 10 mg/day. There were no apparent untoward effects; maternal urinary biotin excretion increased by a factor of approximately 100 during biotin administration.

Non-identical twins were subsequently delivered at term. Cord blood and urinary organic acid profiles were normal, and cord blood biotin concentrations were four to seven times greater than normal. The neonatal course for both twins was unremarkable. Subsequent study of the cultured fibroblasts of both twins compared under biotin-rich and biotin-depleted growth conditions indicated that, in biotin-depleted medium, the cells of twin B (but not of twin A) had virtually complete deficiency of all three carboxylase activities. Genetic complementation studies confirmed that, despite the normal clinical presentation during the newborn period, twin B was homozygous for the disease mutation.

Packman *et al.*[13] have also reported prenatal diagnosis and treatment of biotin-responsive multiple carboxylase deficiency for a mother who had previously given birth to a male with the neonatal-onset form of this disease. In the next pregnancy, maternal urine organic acid profiles were normal. The three carboxylase activities were assayed in cultured amniotic fluid cells obtained by amniocentesis at 17 menstrual weeks. In biotin-restricted medium, the amniotic cells demonstrated the characteristic severe reduction in carboxylase activities.

The preceding two cases provide compelling evidence that biotin administration effectively prevents neonatal complications in certain patients with biotin-responsive multiple carboxylase deficiency. No toxicity from treatment was observed. At this time, it is not possible to assess definitively the relative advantages or disadvantages of prenatal treatment, although such therapy appears both effective and logical.

Galactosemia

Galactosemia is an inborn error of metabolism caused by diminished activity of the enzyme galactose-1-phosphate uridyltransferase. It is inherited in an autosomal recessive manner and results in cataracts, growth deficiency and ovarian failure. Galactosemia can be diagnosed prenatally by study of cultured amniocytes and chorionic villi. Clinical symptoms appear in the neonatal period and can be largely ameliorated by elimination of galactose from the diet. However, oocytes have already been damaged irreversibly long before birth. Cellular damage in galactosemia is thought to be mediated by accumulation of galactose-1-phosphate intracellularly and of galactitol in the lens.

There are suggestions that even the early postnatal treatment of galactosemic individuals with a low galactose diet may not be sufficient to ensure normal development. Some have speculated that prenatal damage to galactosemic fetuses could contribute to subsequent abnormal neurological development and to lens cataract formation. Furthermore, it has been recognized recently that female galactosemics, even when treated from birth with galactose deprivation, have a high frequency of primary or secondary amenorrhea because of ovarian failure. There may also be some subtle abnormalities of male gonadal function.

Exposure to a high-galactose diet has been considered to represent an animal model for human galactosemia. Chen *et al.*[14] have observed a reduction in the oocyte content of rat ovaries after prenatal exposure to a 50% galactose diet. No analogous alterations in the testes were observed in prenatally treated males. Experiments in rats suggest that toxicity to the female gonads from galactose or its metabolites is most obvious during the premeiotic stages of ovarian development.

These observations in animals and human beings have led to speculation that galactose restriction during pregnancy may be desirable if the fetus is affected with galactosemia. In the human female, ovarian meiosis begins at 12 and is complete by 28 menstrual weeks. Thus, ovarian damage, and perhaps neurological or lens abnormalities, might occur prior to the usual time when prenatal diagnosis by amniocentesis can be accomplished. Thus, anticipatory treatment in pregnancies at risk for having a galactosemic fetus might best be initiated very early in gestation or even preconceptually.

Despite these experiments and speculations, we are unaware of studies that adequately assess the impact of prenatal administration of a low-galactose diet to galactosemic infants. For obvious reasons such data, especially controlled, will be difficult to obtain. Nevertheless, prenatal galactose restriction is probably desirable in galactosemia and should be harmless. There is little reason to suppose that galactose restriction would have adverse consequences, since galactosemic and normal fetuses are both capable of some endogenous galactose synthesis.

Hypothyroidism

Fetal hypothyroidism may have severe fetal and neonatal consequences. Fetal esophageal obstruction, secondary to a goiter, can lead to polyhydramnios, and may result in preterm delivery. Furthermore, a fetal goiter can cause extension of the fetal neck leading to dystocia. Without treatment, postnatal growth delay and severe mental retardation can ensue. Even with immediate diagnosis and treatment at birth, long-term follow-up of children with congenital hypothyroidism has shown them to have lower scores on perceptual-motor, visuospatial and language tests.[15]

Maternal hyperthyroidism is often associated with fetal hypothyroidism. This may be secondary to the suppression of the fetal thyroid by maternally administered propylthiouracil. Conversely, fetal hypothyroidism may also result from transplacental passage of maternal blocking antibodies. These antibodies, known as TB1Ab (or TBII), block thyroid-stimulating hormone (TSH) binding. Occasionally, fetal hypothyroidism is the result of inadvertent use of TBII in the pregnant women, maternal ingestion of amiodarone or lithium, or excessive maternal iodine intake, sometimes in the form of vaginal douching. Fetal hypothyroidism caused by an intrinsic fetal abnormality is uncommon, occurring in 1 in 4000–5000 births.[16] The most common form of such permanent hypothyroidism in infants is thyroid dysgenesis. This may include hypoplastic and ectopic thyroid, or the total absence of thyroid tissue (athyreosis) which is associated with undetectable levels of thyroglobulin. Congenital hypothyroidism is only rarely associated with errors of thyroid hormone synthesis, TSH insensitivity or absence of the pituitary gland.

Inquiry regarding a history of maternal hypothyroidism is considered as routine. In patients with this history, routine maternal thyroid hormone levels as well as blocking immunoglobulin levels should be measured. In addition, all women with a history of any thyroid disease (both hypothyroidism and hyperthyroidism) are advised to have monthly fetal ultrasound to screen for goiter, polyhydramnios or fetal tachycardia.[17]

Fetal goiterous hypothyroidism is initially identified by ultrasound. Most commonly, the indication for the ultrasonographic scan is a fundal height greater than expected by gestational age. In such cases the increased uterine size is caused by polyhydramnios, resulting from esophageal obstruction and impaired swallowing. Sometimes, a fetal goiter is incidentally discovered on a routine scan. Finally, some cases are diagnosed on serial scans in fetuses with either known elevated maternal thyroid immunoglobulins, or maternal treatment with antithyroid medications. Before the advent of cordocentesis, amniotic fluid levels of TSH and free thyroxine (FT4) were used as potential indicators of fetal thyroid function. However, these proved inconsistent.[18] Currently, with cordocentesis, fetal thyroid status can be directly and accurately evaluated and fetal response to therapy reliably measured, using available nomograms.[17,19] Fetal hypothyroidism is diagnosed by measuring fetal serum levels of free T4, total T4, free T3, total T3 and TSH.

In utero treatment was initially suggested by Van Herle *et al.*[20] using intramuscular injection of levothyroxine sodium. Subsequent studies, however, have indicated that intra-amniotic administration of thyroxine is superior. The doses commonly used for treatment range from 200 to 500 mg intra-amniotic every week.[21] More recently, it has been recommended that the dosage be adjusted for the fetal weight using 10 mg/kg, similar to the recommended dose for neonates.[22] With this regimen, fetal goiters have been shown to regress, and fetal and newborn TSH levels have normalized.

Hyperthyroidism

Neonatal hyperthyroidism is rare with an incidence of 1:4000 to 1:40,000.[23] In these cases, fetal thyrotoxic goiter is usually secondary to maternal autoimmune disease, principally Graves' disease or Hashimoto's thyroiditis. It is estimated that as many as 12% of infants of mothers with a known history of Graves' disease are affected with neonatal thyrotoxicosis. This may even occur despite the fact that the mother may be euthyroid.[24] As with hypothyroidism, inherent to the underlying mechanism is the transplacental passage of maternal IgG antibodies. In this case the antibodies, known as TSAb (or TSI), are predominantly directed against the TSH receptor.

Usually, the investigation of fetal hyperthyroidism begins only after the discovery of fetal goiter. Often, the goiter is diagnosed on ultrasound in patients referred due to elevated thyroid-stimulating antibodies. In some cases, fetal goiters are realized serendipitously on routine ultrasonography. Others may be discovered in patients referred for scan because the fundal height measures greater than expected by gestational age. In these cases there is often polyhydramnios as a result of the goiter. Once a fetal goiter is identified, biochemical evaluation is indicated. Historically, amniotic fluid levels of TSH and FT4 were used as potential indicators of fetal thyroid function. These, however, proved inconsistent in that amniotic fluid levels of these hormones do not always correlate with their serum levels. Some controversy still exists regarding their use; however, and they may be of some benefit in centers that do not have available cordocentesis.[18] With the advent of cordocentesis, fetal thyroid status can be reliably documented[17,19] and treatment planned according to the results (Figures 105.1 and 105.2).

Once the diagnosis of fetal hyperthyroidism is confirmed, fetal treatment should be initiated. Authors have attempted treatment of fetal hyperthyroidism with maternally administered antithyroid drugs. Porreco and Bloch[25] have reported maternal treatment of fetal thyrotoxicosis with propylthiouracil which led to a good outcome. The initial dose used was 100 mg orally three times a day, which was later decreased to 50 mg orally three times a day. Wenstrom *et al.*[26] described a favorable outcome using maternal methimazole to treat fetal hyperthyroidism in a patient who could not tolerate propylthiouracil. Hatjis also treated fetal goiterous hyperthyroidism with a maternal dose of 300 mg propylthiouracil. This patient, however, required supplemental synthroid to remain euthyroid. There was good fetal outcome in this case as well.[27]

Abnormalities of mineral metabolism

Specific prenatal mineral supplementation has yet to be reported for prevention of human fetal disease. However, such additives have been used in animals with genetic deficiencies. Animal studies are of considerable interest and suggest the possibility of analogous human treatment.

Manganese

The effects of prenatal manganese supplementation on the prevention of otolith defects in mice affected with the pallid mutation have been investigated. Pallid mice have defective pigmentation, including an absence of pigment from the membranous labyrinth. This pigmentary characteristic is fully penetrant in the pallid homozygous recessive, whereas another manifestation, impaired otolith formation, is variably expressed. A significant correlation between litter size and the expression of the otolith abnormalities in the offspring have been known for decades; the otolith defect may be influenced by competition *in utero* for an unidentified substance.

Hurley and Bell[28] reported that development of the inner ear in normal rats and mice was affected by decreased manganese. In mice, experimental manganese deprivation *in utero* induced a defect of the inner ear that was morphologically and behaviorally indistinguishable from pallid, although manganese deficiency did not mimic the effect of the mutant gene on pigmentation. Subsequently, these investigators observed that manganese supplementation of pallid mice throughout gestation with a diet containing from 45 to 2000 parts per million of manganese yielded a dose-dependent decrease in the percentage of abnormal otoliths.

These data have been extended to a genetic basis for susceptibility. In several studies on prenatal manganese restriction, the percentage of otolith abnormalities was influenced by the strain of mice studied. Thus, interactions of manganese intake and genetic predisposition influence otolith development in several strains. These observations suggest that, at low or borderline levels of dietary intake of many nutrients, the genotype of the fetus can substantially alter fetal responses.

There are a number of genetic defects in animals with associated pigmentary and inner ear abnormalities. Some data suggest that manganese may play a role in modifying the expression of such defects. Hurley and Bell have suggested that a sex-linked form of ocular albinism in humans, associated with labyrinthine dysfunction, may be analogous to some of these animal models. We are unaware of any studies of manganese metabolism in human ocular albinism, or of attempts to administer manganese prenatally in the hope of ameliorating expression of any associated labyrinthine defects.

Copper

Hurley and Bell[28] have investigated possible deleterious effects of prenatal copper administration on mice with the recessive mutant 'crinkled' gene. These investigators have suggested that the 'crinkled' gene produces many phenotypic characteristics common to patients with Menkes' kinky-hair syndrome. Dietary supplementation of pregnant mice with copper sulfate partially ameliorated the effects of the crinkled gene in the offspring. Different prenatal copper regimens have resulted in varying degrees of success. Copper nitrilotracete appeared to be superior to copper sulfate in increasing postnatal survival and body copper content of the mutant offspring of heterozygous dams. Postnatal supplementation with copper did not increase survival of the mutants.

These studies may lead to insights relevant to prenatal treatment of Menkes' syndrome, a sex-linked disorder characterized by progressive degeneration of neurological function in infants. Alterations suggestive of functional copper deficiency are present in affected infants. Fibroblasts from patients with Menkes' disease accumulate excess copper probably present in an abnormally bound form. Menkes' disease has been refractory to postnatal therapy with copper, and it is conceivable that, by analogy to the crinkled mutation, prenatal treatment might be of benefit.[29]

Despite apparent responses to prenatal mineral administration of pallid and crinkled mutations, the relationships of these mutants, if any, to ocular albinism and Menkes' disease, respectively, remain speculative. Although animal studies have proved encouraging, they have not yet led to trials of prenatal mineral supplementation in genetically defective human beings.

Nutritional approaches

It might be appropriate to consider suppressing excessive cholesterol production prenatally in severe hypercholesterolemia if a safe and effective agent for accomplishing this were available (although there is no clear evidence for hypercholesterolemic prenatal damage). If cysteamine or related agents were to prove an effective treatment for lethal variants of cystinosis, prenatal therapy might be considered, because excessive and possibly harmful cystine accumulation is evident in cystinotic fetuses. Cysteamine levels have been detected in chorionic villi, and significant elevations even at 10 weeks of gestation have been hypothesized. Inhibitors of gamma-glutamyl transpeptidase, if safe, would elevate intracellular glutathione levels and inhibit oxoproline production in glutathione synthase deficiency, thereby averting the characteristic neonatal acidosis. In theory, it would be desirable to minimize copper accumulation in Wilson disease as early as possible. If and when reliable prenatal diagnosis of Wilson disease is possible, cautious administration of penicillamine prenatally might be considered. This would be a double-edged sword, however, as the teratogenic and lathyritic potential of penicillamine would demand careful evaluation. Batshaw *et al.* have treated certain urea cycle defects by administering arginine and benzoate. Since hyperammonemia in some of these entities develops very acutely after birth, it might be desirable to consider pretreating the fetus with these compounds just prior to, or during labor to minimize postnatal hyperammonemia.[30] Conversely, it may be desirable to consider drug avoidance as an approach to fetal treatment. For example, fetuses with glucose-6-phosphate dehydrogenase deficiency are sensitive to a variety of drugs that induce hemolysis. It would probably be appropriate to avoid administering such agents to women carrying or known to be at risk for carrying fetuses deficient in glucose-6-phosphate dehydrogenase.

Umbilical cord catheterization under ultrasound guidance may lead to the development of other types of fetal treatment.[31] Systems such as gene replacement are being developed for certain lysosomal storage disorders. Progress is being made in postnatal experimental models on administration of thymic cells for certain immune deficiency states, bone marrow transplantation for a variety of genetic disorders and gene transfer. The development of better and earlier techniques for prenatal treatment will be complex, especially with regard to gene transfer, but progress will be made, and access to the fetal vasculature may be required for these methods to have a chance for success.

Bone marrow transplantation or thymic cell infusion is actually only a specialized example of organ transplantation. In the future, fetal organ transplantation may become possible and may open many prospects for surgical treatment of certain biochemical genetic disorders.

One can also speculate about the therapeutic possibilities involving compounds administered directly into the amniotic fluid or into the fetal intestinal tract. It might be possible, for example, to administer thyroid hormone in this fashion or to prevent meconium ileus in cystic fibrosis by instilling not yet determined enzymes into the fetal intestinal tract.

Multifactorial disorders

Cardiac fetal therapy

Although great strides have been made in the diagnosis of fetal cardiac anatomical and functional abnormalities, *in utero* cardiac therapy currently is limited to the treatment of significant arrhythmias. In the future, treatment of some congenital anomalies, particularly valvular anomalies, may be attempted prenatally. Treatment of fetal arrhythmias is discussed elsewhere.

Neural tube defects

Animal studies suggest that neural tube defects (NTDs) can arise from a variety of vitamin or mineral deficiencies. There are historical data in humans suggesting increased NTD frequencies in subjects with poor dietary histories or with intestinal bypasses. Biochemical evidence of suboptimal nutrition is present in some women bearing infants with NTDs. In 1980, Smithells *et al.*[32,33] suggested that vitamin supplementation containing 0.36 mg folate can reduce the frequency of NTD recurrence by sevenfold in women with one or more prior affected children. For almost a decade, there has been a great deal of controversy regarding the benefit of folate supplementation for the prevention of NTDs.[34–37] Finally, in 1991, a randomized double-blinded trial designed by the Medical Research Council Vitamin Study Research Group demonstrated that preconceptual folate reduces the risk of recurrence in high-risk patients.[38] Subsequently, it was shown that preparations containing folate and other vitamins also reduce the occurrence of first-time NTDs.[39] In response to these findings, guidelines were issued calling for consumption of 4.0 mg/day folic acid by women with a prior child affected with an NTD, for at least 1 month prior to conception and through the first 3 months of pregnancy. In addition, 0.4 mg/day folic acid is recommended to all women planning a pregnancy to be taken preconceptually.

Conclusion

There are several different systems that have been clearly shown to be amenable to prenatal pharmacological intervention. For some, such as CAH and NTDs, birth defects can be prevented. For others, physiology can be altered, but the long-term consequences of earlier intervention are not yet clear and will require much more work. Nevertheless, these efforts have given us a better understanding of fetal physiology, and help us to design better approaches to treatment.

REFERENCES

1. New MI, White PC, Pang S, *et al.* The adrenal hyperplasias. In Scriver CR, Beaudet AL, Sly WS, Valle D, eds. *The Metabolic Basis of Inherited Disease*, 6th edn. New York: McGraw-Hill, 1881–917.
2. Dupont B, Oberfield SE, Smithwick EM, *et al.* Close genetic linkage between HLA and congenital adrenal hyperplasia (21-hydroxylase deficiency). *Lancet* 1977;2:1309–11.
3. White PC, Grossberger D, Onufer BJ, *et al.* Two genes encoding steroid 21-hydroxylase are located near the genes encoding the fourth component of complement in man. *Proc Natl Acad Sci USA* 1985;82:1089–93.
4. Mandell J, Bromley B, Peters CA, Benacerraf BR. Prenatal sonographic detection of genital malformations. *J Urol* 1995;153: 1994–6.
5. Evans MI, Chrousos GP, Mann DL, *et al.* Pharmacologic suppression of the fetal adrenal gland *in utero*: Attempted prevention of abnormal external genital masculinization in suspected congenital adrenal hyperplasia. *J Am Med Assoc* 1985;253:1015.
6. Forrest M, David M. Prenatal treatment of congenital adrenal hyperplasia due to 21-hydroxylase deficiency. *Presented at 7th International Congress of Endocrinology*, Quebec, Canada, 1984 (abstr y11).
7. Shulman DI, Mueller OT, Gallardo LA, Stiff D, Ostrer H. Treatment of congenital adrenal hyperplasia *in utero*. *Pediatr Res* 1989;25:2.
8. Pang S, Pollack MS, Marshall RN, Immken L. Prenatal treatment of congenital adrenal hyperplasia due to 21-hydroxylase deficiency. *N Engl J Med* 1990;22:1.
9. Seckl JR, Miller WL How safe is long-term prenatal glucocorticoid treatment? *J Am Med Assoc* 1997;13:1077–9.
10. Ampola MG, Mahoney MI, Nakamura E, *et al.* Prenatal therapy of a patient with vitamin B responsive methylmalonic acidemia. *N Engl J Med* 1975;293:313.
11. Evans MI, Duquette DA, Rinaldo P, *et al.* Modulation of B12 dosage and response in fetal treatment of methylmalonic aciduria (MMA); titration of treatment dose to serum and urine MMA. *Fetal Diagn Ther* 1997;12:21–3.
12. Roth KS, Yang W, Allen L, *et al.* Prenatal administration of biotin: Biotin responsive multiple carboxylase deficiency. *Pediatr Res* 1982;16:126.
13. Packman S, Cowan MJ, Golbus MS, *et al.* Prenatal treatment of biotin responsive multiple carboxylase deficiency. *Lancet* 1982;1: 1435.
14. Chen YT, Mattison DR, Feigenbaum L, *et al.* Reduction in oocyte number following prenatal exposure to a high galactose diet. *Science* 1981;314:1145.
15. Rovet J, Ehrlich R, Sorbara D. Intellectual outcome in children with fetal hypothyroidism. *J Pediatr* 1987;110:700–4.
16. Trainer TD, Howard PL. Thyroid function tests in thyroid and nonthyroid disease. *Crit Rev Clin Lab Sci* 1983;19:135–71.
17. Thorpe-Beeston JG, Nicolaides KH, McGregor AM. Fetal thyroid function. *Thyroid* 1992;2:207–17.
18. Sack J, Fisher DA, Hobel CJ, Lam R. Thyroxine in human amniotic fluid. *J Pediatr* 1975;87:364–8.
19. Ballabio M, Nicolini U, Jowett T, Ruiz de Elvira MC, Ekins RP, Rodeck CH. Maturation of thyroid function in normal human fetuses. *Clin Endocrinol* 1989;31:565–71.
20. Van Herle AJ, Young RT, Fisher DA, Uller RP, Brinkman CR III. Intra-uterine treatment of a hypothyroid fetus. *J Clin Endocrinol Metab* 1973;40:474–7.
21. Abuhamad AZ, Fisher DA, Warsof SL, *et al.* Antenatal diagnosis and treatment of fetal goitrous hypothyroidism: Case report and review of the literature. *Ultrasound Obstet Gynecol* 1995;6:368–71.
22. Hadi HA, Strickland RT. *In utero* treatment of fetal goitrous hypothyroidism caused by maternal Graves' disease. *Am J Perinatol* 1995;12:455–8.
23. Fisher DA. Neonatal thyroid disease of women with autoimmune thyroid disease. *Thyroid Today* 1986;9:1–7.
24. Bruinse HW, Vermeulen-Meiners C, Wit JM. Fetal treatment for thyrotoxicosis in non-thyrotoxic pregnant women. *Fetal Ther* 1988;3:152–7.
25. Porreco RP, Bloch CA. Fetal blood sampling in the management of intrauterine thyrotoxicosis. *Obstet Gynecol* 1990;76:509–12.
26. Wenstrom KD, Weiner CP, Williamson RA, Grant SS. Prenatal diagnosis of fetal hyperthyroidism using funipuncture. *Obstet Gynecol* 1990;76:513–17.
27. Hatjis CG. Diagnosis and successful treatment of fetal goitrous hyperthyroidism caused by maternal Graves' disease. *Obstet Gynecol* 1993;81:837–9.
28. Hurley LS, Bell LT. Genetic influence on response to dietary manganese deficiency in mice. *J Nutr* 1974;104:133.
29. Evans MI, Pinsky WW, Johnson MP, Schulman JD. Medical fetal therapy. In Evans MI, ed. *Reproductive Risks and Prenatal Diagnosis*. Norwalk, CT: Appleton & Lange, 1992:236.
30. Batshaw M, Brusilow S, Waber L, *et al.* Treatment of inborn errors of urea synthesis: Activation of alternative pathways of waste nitrogen synthesis and excretion. *N Engl J Med* 1982;306:1387.
31. Nicolaides KH, Thorpe-Beeston JG, Noble P. Cordocentesis. In Eden RD, Boehm FH, eds. *Assessment and Care of the Fetus: Physiological, Clinical and Medicolegal Principles*. Norwalk, CT: Appleton & Lange, 1990:291.
32. Smithells RW, Sheppard S, Schorah CJ, *et al.* Possible prevention of neural tube defects by preconceptual vitamin supplementation. *Lancet* 1980;1:399–40.
33. Smithells RW, Nevin NC, Seller MJ, *et al.* Further experience of vitamin supplementation for prevention of neural tube defect recurrences. *Lancet* 1983;1:1027.
34. Younis JS, Granat M. Insufficient transplacental digoxin transfer in severe hydrops fetalis. *Am J Obstet Gynecol* 1987;157:1268.
35. Mills JL, Rhoads GG, Simpson JL, *et al.* The absence of a relation between the periconceptional use of vitamins and neural-tube defects. *N Engl J Med* 1989;321:430.
36. Mulinare J, Cordero JF, Erickson JD, Berry RJ. Periconceptional use of multivitamins and the occurrence of neural tube defects. *J Am Med Assoc* 1988;260:3141.
37. Schulman JD. Treatment of the embryo and the fetus in the first trimester: Current status and future prospects. *Am J Med Genet* 1990;35:197.
38. MRC Vitamin Study Research Group. Prevention of neural tube defects: Results of the MRC vitamin study. *Lancet* 1991;338:132–7.
39. Czeizel AE, Dudas I. Prevention of the first occurrence of neural-tube defects by preconceptional vitamin supplementation. *N Engl J Med* 1992;327:1832–5.

106 Management of red cell isoimmunized pregnancies

K. H. Nicolaides and N. J. Sebire

In red cell isoimmunized pregnancies, the degree of severity of hemolytic disease in the infant varies from none apparent at birth to fetal hydrops and intrauterine death at as early as 17 weeks of gestation. Without any form of treatment, 45–50% of affected infants have no or mild anemia, and a further 25–30% have some degree of hepatosplenomegaly, moderate anemia and jaundice, which develops rapidly within the first 24 h of life. If appropriate treatment (exchange transfusion) is not carried out, the progressive jaundice leads to brain damage (kernicterus) which will culminate in death or severe handicap (deafness, spasticity and choreoathetosis). The remaining 20–25% become hydropic and usually die either *in utero* or in the neonatal period; in half of these the hydrops develops at between 18 and 30 weeks of gestation.[1] In the antenatal management of red cell isoimmunized pregnancies, the aim is firstly to predict whether the fetus is severely affected, and if so, at what stage of pregnancy fetal hydrops will develop or intrauterine death will occur, and secondly to correct the fetal anemia and to deliver the baby at the optimal time. There are at least 100 red cell surface antigens and the development of maternal antibodies to approximately 30 of these can lead to fetal hemolytic disease. However, the vast majority of cases are the result of either ABO incompatibility (two-thirds of cases) or rhesus incompatibility.

ABO incompatibility

Although ABO feto-maternal incompatibility occurs in about 20% of all pregnancies, fetal hemolysis occurs rarely (< 2%), and this is usually mild.[2] The condition is almost exclusively confined to group A and B infants born to group O mothers, since some group O mothers have anti-A and anti-B antibodies from the IgG class, which can cross the placenta. Group A and B individuals usually have only immunoglobulin M (IgM) anti-B and anti-A antibodies which do not cross the placenta. The reasons for the mildness of the condition are: (a) there is a small number of A and B antigenic sites on the fetal red cell membrane and full expression of these antigens does not occur until the age of 2–4 years; and (b) the A and B antigens are present in all tissues and secretions and they compete with the red cell antigens for the small number of maternal IgG antibodies entering the fetal circulation. Because of the mildness of the fetal disease, no special antenatal measures are necessary for the management of these pregnancies. After delivery the baby is tested for the development of hyperbilirubinemia, and if this occurs exchange transfusions are performed.

Rhesus incompatibility

Management of rhesus-negative women without antibodies

In rhesus-negative women, the rhesus status of the partner is determined; if he is also rhesus-negative then the fetus must necessarily be rhesus-negative and the pregnancy is therefore not at risk of rhesus isoimmunization disease. If the father is rhesus-positive then further maternal antibody screening should be undertaken at 20 weeks and at 4-weekly intervals thereafter until delivery. Following delivery, umbilical cord and maternal blood are tested. The cord blood is tested for the rhesus status of the fetus, the Coombs' test is carried out for the presence of antibodies on the fetal erythrocytes, and the hemoglobin concentration is measured. The maternal blood is tested for antibodies, and a Kleihauer test[3] is performed to estimate the degree of feto-maternal hemorrhage. If the mother has no antibodies and the baby is rhesus D-positive, anti-D IgG is given.

Prevention of rhesus D isoimmunization

Anti-D administration is effective in preventing immunization in a rhesus-negative woman, but has no effect if the woman is already isoimmunized. The administration of 100 μg anti-D IgG to a mother will neutralize at least 4 ml of rhesus D-positive fetal erythrocytes that might have entered her circulation; this is equivalent to a Kleihauer count of 80 fetal cells per 50 low-power fields. This dose of anti-D IgG should be given to all rhesus-negative, unimmunized women within 72 h of the delivery of a rhesus-positive baby. Furthermore, a Kleihauer test should be performed on the maternal blood and further anti-D given if the feto-maternal hemorrhage is greater than 4 ml. Anti-D should also be administered antenatally if abortion, antepartum hemorrhage, amniocentesis or other potentially immunizing episodes occur. In some countries there is a policy of antenatal prophylaxis for all rhesus-negative women (anti-D IgG 300 μg is given at 28 weeks, or 100 μg at 28 and 34 weeks).

Atypical blood group incompatibility

With the use of anti-D prophylaxis and the fall in incidence of rhesus D isoimmunization, an increasing proportion of isoimmunized pregnant women have either non-rhesus antibodies or rhesus antibodies other than D antibodies. The main reason for the development of these antibodies is blood transfusions. So-called compatible blood transfusions are compatible to ABO and D, but transfused red cells have many antigens that are missing in the recipient. Following blood transfusions, 1–2% of recipients develop 'atypical' antibodies. The majority of these are either IgM or very weakly immunogenic and either do not produce hemolytic disease in the fetus (e.g. anti-P) or very rarely do so (e.g. anti-M, anti-N, anti-S). Some of the antibodies, however, such as anti-C, anti-E and anti-Kell, can cause severe hemolytic disease and intrauterine death. Pregnancies complicated by the presence of these antibodies should therefore be managed in the same way as those with rhesus D incompatibility.

Pathophysiology of fetal anemia

In normal pregnancy, the fetal mean hemoglobin concentration increases linearly with gestation from 10 g/dl at 16 weeks to 15 g/dl at 40 weeks, and 1 SD is approximately 1.2 g/dl.[4] In red cell isoimmunized pregnancies the lifespan of fetal erythrocytes is reduced, because antibody-coated red cells are destroyed in the reticuloendothelial system. Moderate anemia is defined by a hemoglobin concentration deficit of 2–4 SD, and severe anemia by a deficit of more than 4 SD. The fetal blood oxygen content decreases in proportion to the degree of anemia, but the fetal blood $p\text{O}_2$, $p\text{CO}_2$ and pH usually remain within the normal ranges.[5]

The fetus compensates for anemia by hemodynamic adjustments as demonstrated by Doppler ultrasound studies.[6] Furthermore, in anemia the fetal 2,3-diphosphoglycerate concentration is increased and the consequent decrease in hemoglobin oxygen affinity presumably improves delivery of oxygen to the tissues.[7] In moderate anemia, the umbilical arterial plasma lactate concentration is increased, but this is cleared by a single passage through the placenta and normal umbilical venous levels are maintained.[8]

In severe anemia, the placental capacity for lactate clearance is exceeded and the umbilical venous concentration increases exponentially. When the hemoglobin deficit exceeds 5 SD, the functional reserve of the cardiovascular system is exhausted and hydrops fetalis develops.[4] Furthermore, with severe anemia there is concomitant occurrence of erythroblastosis.[4] Since the latter reflects recruitment of hepatic erythropoiesis, fetal hydrops may be a consequence of portal hypertension and/or hypoproteinemia due to expansion of erythropoietic tissue in the liver.[9–12]

Prediction of fetal anemia

The severity of fetal hemolysis can be predicted from (a) the history of previously affected pregnancies, (b) the level of maternal hemolytic antibodies, (c) the amniotic fluid bilirubin concentration, (d) the altered morphometry of the fetus and the placenta, (e) the presence of pathological fetal heart rate patterns, and (f) changes in the flow velocity waveforms obtained by Doppler studies of the fetal circulation. However, there is a wide scatter of values around the regression lines describing the associations between the degree of fetal anemia and the data obtained from these indirect methods of assessment.

History of previously affected pregnancies

The disease tends to be progressively more severe with successive pregnancies because of the 'boosting' effect of small feto-maternal hemorrhages during pregnancy and delivery. Thus, once a rhesus stillbirth or hydrops has occurred in a family, there is a 90% chance that the next rhesus-positive infant, if left untreated, will also die *in utero*. It has been estimated that after one previous stillbirth 50% of subsequent stillbirths occur *in utero* before 35 weeks, but after more than one stillbirth 50% die before 32 weeks of gestation.[13]

Maternal hemolytic antibody concentration

The association between maternal serum hemolytic antibody concentration and pregnancy outcome has been recognized from the 1950s, and measurement of maternal anti-D has been the main method of managing red blood cell isoimmunized pregnancies. The traditional method of detecting rhesus antibodies in the maternal serum is the indirect Coombs' test.[14] Low titers (< 1/32) correspond to mild disease in the fetus.[15,16] When the titer is >1/32 the disease may be severe. In a study of 208 rhesus isoimmunized pregnancies at 17–36 weeks of gestation, the maternal serum anti-D concentration was measured and the fetal hemoglobin concentration was determined; there was a significant association between the maternal hemolytic antibody concentration and the fetal hemoglobin concentration deficit.[17] However, there was a wide scatter of results which could be due to individual variation in the rate of transfer of antibody across the placenta, expression of antigens in fetal red cells, and fetal erythropoiesis in response to hemolysis. Nevertheless, the association allowed estimation of probabilities of different degrees of fetal anemia from measurement of maternal anti-D concentration. If the maternal anti-D concentration is =5 IU/ml there is a 97% chance that the fetus is not anemic. Levels between 5 and 14 IU/ml are associated with moderate but not severe anemia. In contrast, if the anti-D concentration is >15 IU/ml there is a 30% chance that the fetus is anemic, and in more than 5% of cases, depending on the actual level, the degree of anemia is severe and in such cases cordocentesis is indicated.

Pollock and Bowman[18] suggested that instead of measuring total IgG, a more accurate prediction of the degree of fetal anemia could be provided by examining different subclasses, since IgG3 is less likely to be associated with hydrops, while a combination of IgG1 and IgG3 is associated with the most severe disease. Similarly, *in vitro* assays of cell-mediated immune response against Rh-positive cells can be performed, but there is no clear relationship with the degree of anemia in such studies.[19–21]

Amniocentesis and cordocentesis

Measurement of the bilirubin concentration in the amniotic fluid gives an indirect indication of the degree of fetal hemolysis.[22,23] Although there are many methods for the interpretation of the amniotic fluid AOD 450,[24] the most widely employed method is that of Liley.[25,26] Amniocentesis has been recommended when the maternal antibody level is more than 4 IU/ml, or 10 weeks before the gestational age at which the patient had a previous fetal death or delivery of a severely affected baby.[27] For the third trimester of pregnancy amniocentesis and interpretation of amniotic fluid OD 450 values by the Liley method has proved to be reliable.[28] However, the validity of extrapolating the Liley charts to the second trimester has been questioned, and it has been suggested that amniocentesis does not provide more accurate information than other non-invasive tests for predicting the degree of fetal anemia.[17]

Cordocentesis provides the most direct, therefore accurate, measure of fetal anemia. In addition to fetal hemoglobin concentration, it is possible to measure other hematologic and biochemical indices which may provide further prediction of the degree of anemia. For example, the reticulocyte and nucleated red cell count may be increased,[29,30] serum bilirubin levels increased,[31] fetal erythropoietin levels increased,[32] and blood gases perturbed, although this is a late feature of the disease. All such additional results, although improving our understanding of the pathophysiology of the disease, have not been proven useful in the clinical management of affected patients.

Fetal–placental morphometry

Attempts have been made to identify by ultrasonography those fetuses whose condition is deteriorating, before the development of ascites and hydrops. These studies have assessed changes in placental, hepatic, splenic or cardiac appearance, which are logical choices considering the pathophysiology of the condition. Vintzileos *et al.*[33] suggested that an ultrasonographically-detected increase in the size of the fetal liver is an early sign of fetal anemia. DeVore *et al.*[34] proposed that enlargement of the fetal liver would compress hepatic vessels, leading to decreased venous drainage of the umbilical vein, and therefore umbilical vein dilatation. Grannum[35] suggested that an increase in placental thickness usually indicates worsening fetal anemia. Chitkara *et al.*[36] documented fetal anemia by cordocentesis and demonstrated that in moderate to severe disease the development of polyhydramnios was the earliest sonographic abnormality. DeVore *et al.*[37] found the detection of a fetal pericardial effusion using real-time-directed M-mode echocardiography to be a valuable sign, while Benacerraf and Frigoletto[38] have noted that visualization of both sides of the fetal bowel wall may be the earliest evidence of fetal ascites. Oepkes *et al.*[39] measured the fetal spleen by ultrasound and found splenomegaly in all non-hydropic anemic fetuses.

In a study investigating the relationship between placental thickness, umbilical vein diameter or fetal abdominal circumference, head-to-abdomen circumference ratio and intraperitoneal volume and the degree of fetal anemia, assessed by direct fetal blood sampling, in 50 pregnancies complicated by rhesus isoimmunization it was concluded that: (a) in the presence of hydrops the fetuses are always severely anemic; and (b) in the absence of hydrops there are no consistent ultrasonographically-detectable markers that can reliably distinguish mild from severe hemolytic disease.[40]

Fetal heart rate patterns

In red cell isoimmunized pregnancies, reports on fetal heart rate monitoring have focused on the association between fetal compromise and the sinusoidal fetal heart rate pattern. Rochard *et al.*[41] reported the presence of a sinusoidal pattern in severely compromised fetuses that are either hydropic or die in the perinatal period. Studies examining the relationship between fetal heart rate patterns and fetal blood gases and hemoglobin concentrations obtained at cordocentesis have established that: (a) severe fetal anemia or oxygen content deficit are commonly associated with a sinusoidal fetal heart rate pattern; and (b) although a non-reactive or decelerative fetal heart rate pattern is suggestive of fetal anemia, the vast majority of moderately anemic fetuses have a reactive fetal heart rate pattern.[42,43]

Doppler ultrasound

Doppler ultrasound provides a non-invasive method for the study of fetal hemodynamics. Investigation of the uterine and umbilical arteries gives information on the perfusion of the utero-placental and feto-placental circulations, respectively, while Doppler studies of selected fetal organs are valuable in detecting the hemodynamic rearrangements that occur in response to fetal hypoxemia or anemia. In red cell isoimmunization, impedance to flow in the uterine and umbilical arteries is normal. However, fetal anemia is associated with increased cardiac output, increased blood flow in the umbilical vein, and increased blood velocity in the inferior vena cava, the descending thoracic aorta, and the common carotid and middle cerebral arteries.[44–47]

Treatment

Determination of fetal blood type

Fetal blood type can be reliably determined by fetal blood sampling.[48] More recently, however, with the use of molecular biology techniques, specifically the polymerase chain reaction, it is possible to identify the rhesus D gene[49] from diverse samples including fetal blood, amniotic fluid, chorionic villus biopsy, and even nucleated fetal cells in the maternal circulation.[50–57] This information in early pregnancy may avoid unnecessary invasive testing in later pregnancy if negative, and allow planning of subsequent samplings and/or transfusions if positive. Further modifications of the technique of isolating fetal cells in the maternal circulation (to eliminate false-negatives in particular) may lead to this becoming a routine part of antenatal care in such pregnancies.

Experimental techniques for therapy

During the last 50 years, several therapeutic approaches have been undertaken in the management of red cell isoimmunized pregnancies, with the aim of ameliorating the severity of the condition and preventing intrauterine fetal death. These include (a) reduction or alteration of maternal rhesus antibodies by such measures as plasmapheresis or the injection or ingestion of material prepared from rhesus-positive red cells,[58–62] (b) prevention of fetal hemolysis by immunosuppression with corticosteroids and promethazine hydrochloride,[63–66] (c) increasing fetal red cell production by the administration of high doses of vitamin B_{12}, folic acid and other known hematinics,[67] and (d) alteration of the fetal blood group by bone marrow transplantation from rhesus-negative donors to erythroblastotic fetuses at 12–17 weeks of gestation.[67,68] However, these attempts have been mainly experimental and have not gained widespread application.

The first intrauterine intravascular fetal blood transfusions for severe rhesus disease were performed in the 1960s by cannulation of the fetal femoral artery, the saphenous vein or a chorionic plate vessel, which were exposed by hysterotomy.[69–71] These techniques of open fetal transfusion were associated with high rates of fetal mortality, mainly due to preterm delivery, and were subsequently abandoned in favor of the less invasive percutaneous intraperitoneal route.[72] Nonetheless, they had the advantage of providing accurate data regarding the degree of fetal anemia and the severity of the disease.

Intraperitoneal transfusions

During the 1960s and early 1970s the reported fetal survival rates with intraperitoneal transfusions were 24–56%, and the procedure-related fetal mortality rate was 5–10%.[73] More recently, the extensive use of ultrasonography in the assessment, treatment and follow-up of affected fetuses has contributed to a dramatic improvement in survival rates of non-hydropic fetuses. Nevertheless, the outlook for hydropic fetuses remains poor,[74] possibly because in the presence of ascites resorption of erythrocytes is impaired.

Intravascular transfusions

In the 1980s, interest in the intravascular route was renewed with the development of a technique for transfusion through an umbilical cord vessel by fetoscopy.[75,76] More recently, fetoscopy was replaced by cordocentesis[48,77,78] or needling of the intrahepatic umbilical vein.[79]

At cordocentesis, a fetal blood sample is first obtained and the hemoglobin concentration determined. If this is below the normal range, the tip of the needle is kept in the lumen of the umbilical cord vessel and fresh, packed, rhesus-negative blood compatible with that of the mother, or irradiated maternal blood, is infused into the fetal circulation. The fetal heart rate and the flow of the infused blood are monitored continually throughout the procedure by ultrasonography. At the end of the transfusion, a further fetal blood sample is aspirated for determination of the final hemoglobin concentration.

Transplacental, rather than transamniotic, entry of the umbilical cord reduces the risk of displacement of the needle by fetal movements, and avoids both leakage of amniotic fluid and intra-amniotic fetal bleeding since the amniotic membrane is not punctured.

However, feto-maternal hemorrhage is more likely, which may increase the severity of the disease.

Theoretically, the umbilical artery should be the preferred route for intravascular fetal blood transfusion, both in order to achieve oxygenation and buffering of the acidotic donor blood in the placenta before it enters the fetus, and because thrombotic occlusion of one of the two umbilical arteries rather than the single umbilical vein may not be fatal. However, in practical terms it is more advantageous to transfuse into the vein because: (a) the sonographic observation of the intravascular flow of blood provides constant reassurance that the tip of the needle has not slipped into the Wharton's jelly, where injection of even 1 ml of blood could lead to cord tamponade and fetal death; (b) fetal bradycardias occur more often and last longer when transfusing into an artery than a vein, presumably as a result of procedure-related spasm of the more muscular umbilical artery; and (c) intra-amniotic bleeding occurs more often and lasts longer after withdrawal of the needle from an artery than a vein, presumably as a result of the higher arterial than venous blood pressure.

Transfusions are given at a rate of approximately 10 ml/min without inducing fetal heart rate decelerations. The advantage of rapid 'top-up' transfusions is that the duration of transfusion and therefore the risks of procedure-related complications such as infection, or cord accidents as a result of fetal movements (tamponade, vasospasm or hemorrhage), is decreased. The volume of donor blood necessary to correct fetal anemia can be calculated by considering the pretransfusion fetal hemoglobin concentration, the hemoglobin of the transfused blood, the desired post-transfusion hemoglobin, and the normal mean feto-placental blood volume for that gestation.[80] After transfusion of the calculated volume of donor blood, the fetal hemoglobin is measured, and further blood transfused as necessary to bring the final value to around the 75th percentile of the reference range.

For patients with a previous red cell isoimmunization-affected pregnancy, an effort should be made to perform the first cordocentesis at approximately 10 weeks before the time of the earliest previous fetal or neonatal death, fetal transfusion, or birth of a severely affected baby, but not before 16–17 weeks of gestation. In our experience, from the management of more than 500 rhesus isoimmunized patients, fetal death or the development of hydrops rarely occur before this stage of gestation, presumably because the fetal reticuloendothelial system is too immature to result in massive destruction of antibody-coated erythrocytes. In patients without a previously-affected pregnancy, cordocentesis should be performed (a) if the fetus develops ultrasound features of hydrops such as ascites, (b) when the maternal hemolytic antibody level is 15 IU/ml or more, (c) if the fetal heart rate is sinusoidal or decelerative, and (d) if Doppler studies demonstrate hyperdynamic fetal circulation.

Subsequent transfusions are timed on the basis of the fetal hemoglobin achieved at the end of the previous transfusion, and the observation that following a transfusion the rate of decrease in fetal hemoglobin is approximately 0.3 g/dl per day and in fetal hematocrit is 0.01 g/dl per day.[48,81] However, although this figure is useful in timing the next transfusion, there is a wide range of results and it is therefore necessary to use additional criteria, such as weekly ultrasound scans to detect early ascites and blood velocity measurements to detect the hyperdynamic circulation of developing anemia. Transfusions are repeated up to 35–38 weeks and delivery is aimed at 34–38 weeks.

The reported overall survival rate of red cell isoimmunized pregnancies treated with intravascular transfusions is more than 85% (Table 106.1). The survival rate for non-hydropic fetuses is more than 90%, whereas in the presence of hydrops the survival rate is less than 80%.[30,78,79,81–97]

Table 106.1 Survival rates of pregnancies complicated by isoimmunization disease treated with intrauterine transfusions

Study	n	Survival (%)
Bang *et al.*[79]	1	1 (100)
DeCrespigny *et al.*[82]	4	3 (75)
Doyle *et al.*[83]	8	5 (63)
Nicolaides *et al.*[48]	18	17 (94)
Berkowitz *et al.*[84]	8	6 (75)
Socol *et al.*[85]	3	3 (100)
Grannum *et al.*[78]	26	21(81)
Orsini *et al.*[86]	15	10 (67)
Barss *et al.*[87]	13	11 (85)
Parer[88]	5	4 (80)
Ronkin *et al.*[81]	8	8 (100)
Nicolini *et al.*[89]	30	25 (83)
Lemery *et al.*[90]	15	10 (67)
Poissonnier *et al.*[91]	107	84 (79)
Pattison and Roberts[92]	20	18 (90)
Harman *et al.*[93]	44	40 (91)
Weiner *et al.*[30]	48	46 (96)
Moise[94]	20	19 (95)
Plockinger *et al.*[95]	21	18 (86)
Harman[96]	129	114 (88)
Merchant *et al.*[97]	7	7 (100)
Harris Birthright Centre	220	194 (88)
Total	770	664 (86)

Summary

The only accurate method for determining the severity of disease is blood sampling by cordocentesis and measurement of the fetal hemoglobin concentration. However, cordocentesis may result in feto-maternal hemorrhage,[98] an increase in the maternal hemolytic antibody concentration,[99] and consequent worsening of the disease. It should therefore be reserved for those patients with a history of severe disease and those with high hemolytic antibody levels, pathological fetal heart rate patterns or abnormal flow velocity waveforms.

In patients with a history suggestive of severe disease, cordocentesis should be performed 10 weeks before the time of the earliest previous fetal or neonatal death, fetal transfusion or birth of a severely affected baby. For patients with mild or no previous rhesus-affected pregnancies, the maternal hemolytic antibody levels should be determined every 2–3 weeks from 16 weeks of gestation onwards. In those pregnancies where antibody concentrations are persistently below 15 IU/ml, delivery should be allowed to occur spontaneously at term. However, if the antibody levels are $\geq$15 IU/ml, the disease may be severe and the degree of the hemolytic process in the fetus should be determined by cordocentesis.

If the fetus is not anemic, another cordocentesis should be considered if (a) the mother reports decreased fetal movements; (b) there is a sharp increase in the maternal hemolytic antibody concentration; (c) there is ultrasonographic evidence of fetal hydrops, early ascites or dilated heart with a pericardial effusion; (d) there is cardiotocographic evidence of a sinusoidal or decelerative fetal heart rate pattern; or (e) Doppler studies indicate the development of hyperdynamic fetal circulation.

At cordocentesis, the degree of fetal anemia can be defined accurately by measurement of the fetal hemoglobin concentration, and corrected by intrauterine blood transfusion. While this can be given intraperitoneally, the intravascular route is preferred.

REFERENCES

1. Bowman JM, Pollock JM. Amniotic fluid spectrophotometry and early delivery in the management of erythroblastosis fetalis. *Pediatrics* 1965;35:815–35.
2. Bowman JM. Neonatal management. In Queenan JT, ed. *Modern Management of the Rhesus Problem*, 2nd edn. Hagerstown, MD: Harper and Row, 1977.
3. Kleihauer B, Braun H, Betke K. Demonstration von fetalem haemoglobin in den erythrozyten eines blutausstriches. *Klin Wochenscenschr* 1957;35:637.
4. Nicolaides KH, Soothill PW, Clewell W, *et al*. Fetal haemoglobin measurement in the assessment of red cell isoimmunization. *Lancet* 1988;1:1073–5.
5. Soothill PW, Nicolaides KH, Rodeck CH. Fetal blood gas and acid–base parameters. In Rodeck CH, ed. *Fetal Medicine*. London: Blackwell Scientific Publications, 1989:57–89.
6. Bilardo CM, Nicolaides KH, Campbell S. Doppler studies in red cell isoimmunization. *Clin Obstet Gynecol* 1989;32:719–27.
7. Soothill PW, Lestas AN, Nicolaides KH, *et al*. 2,3-Diphosphoglycerate in normal, anemic and transfused human pregnancies. *Clin Sci* 1988;74:527–30.
8. Soothill PW, Nicolaides KH, Rodeck CH, *et al*. Relationship of fetal hemoglobin and oxygen content to lactate concentration in Rh isoimmunized pregnancies. *Obstet Gynecol* 1987;69:268–71.
9. Bowman JM. The management of Rh isoimmunization. *Obstet Gynecol* 1978;52:1–16.
10. Nicolaides KH, Warenski JC, Rodeck CH. The relationship of fetal protein concentration and haemoglobin level to the development of hydrops in rhesus isoimmunization. *Am J Obstet Gynecol* 1985;152:341–4.
11. Nicolaides KH. Studies on fetal physiology and pathophysiology in rhesus disease. *Semin Perinatol* 1989;13:328–37.
12. Grannum PAT, Copel JA. Prevention of Rh isoimmunization and treatment of the compromised fetus. *Semin Perinatol* 1988;12: 324–35.
13. Walker W. In Neumark E, ed. *Proceedings of the 7th Congress of the European Society of Haematology*, Basel, 1960:1186.
14. Coombs R, Mourant A, Race R. A new test for the detection of weak and incomplete Rh agglutinins. *Br J Exp Pathol* 1945;26: 255.
15. Allen FH, Diamond LK, Jones AR. Erythroblastosis fetalis. IX. The problems of stillbirth. *N Engl J Med* 1954;251:453.
16. Jacobs WM. Fetal survival rates in Rh-immunized gravidas: Correlation of antibody titers and past obstetric history. *Obstet Gynecol* 1962;19:806.
17. Nicolaides KH, Rodeck CH, Mibashan RS, *et al*. Have Liley charts outlived their usefulness? *Am J Obstet Gynecol* 1986;155:90–4.
18. Pollock JM, Bowman JM. Anti-Rh (D) IgG subclasses and severity of Rh hemolytic disease of the newborn. *Vox Sang* 1990;59: 176–9.
19. Nance SJ, Nelson JM, Horenstein J, *et al*. Monocyte monolayer assay: An efficient noninvasive technique for predicting the severity of hemolytic disease of the newborn. *Am J Clin Pathol* 1989;92:89–92.
20. Hadley AG, Kumpel BM, Leader KA, *et al*. Correlation of serologic, quantitative and cell-mediated functional assays of maternal alloantibodies with the severity of haemolytic disease of the newborn. *Br J Haematol* 1991;77:221–8.
21. Moise KJ, Perkins JT, Sosler SD, *et al*. The predictive value of maternal serum testing for the detection of fetal anemia in red cell alloimmunization. *Am J Obstet Gynecol* 1995;172:1003–9.
22. Bevis DC. Blood pigments in haemolytic disease of the newborn. *J Obstet Gynaecol Br Emp* 1956;63:68–75.
23. Walker AH. Liquor amnii studies in the prediction of haemolytic disease of the newborn. *Br Med J* 1957;2:376–8.
24. Queenan JT. Amniotic fluid analysis. In Queenan JT, ed. *Modern Management of the Rhesus Problem*, 2nd edn. Hagerstown, MD: Harper and Row, 1977:73–129.
25. Liley AW. Liquor amnii analysis in the management of the pregnancy complicated by rhesus sensitization. *Am J Obstet Gynecol* 1961;82:1359–70.
26. Liley AW. Errors in the assessment of hemolytic disease from amniotic fluid. *Am J Obstet Gynecol* 1963;86:485–94.
27. Whitfield CR. A 3-year assessment of an Action Line method of timing intervention in rhesus isoimmunization. *Am J Obstet Gynecol* 1970;108:1239–44.
28. Bowman JM, Pollock JM. Antenatal Rh prophylaxis: 28-week gestation service program. *Can Med Assoc J* 1978;118:627–30.
29. Nicolaides KH, Thilaganathan B, Rodeck CH, *et al*. Erythroblastosis and reticulocytosis in anemic fetuses. *Am J Obstet Gynecol* 1988;159:1063–5.
30. Weiner CP, Williamson RA, Wenstrom KD, *et al*. Management of fetal hemolytic disease by cordocentesis. I. Prediction of fetal anemia. *Am J Obstet Gynecol* 1991;165:546–53.
31. Weiner CP. Human fetal bilirubin levels and fetal hemolytic disease. *Am J Obstet Gynecol* 1992;166:1149–54.
32. Thilaganathan B, Salveson DR, Abbas A, *et al*. Fetal plasma erythropoietin concentration in red blood cell-isoimmunized pregnancies. *Am J Obstet Gynecol* 1992;167:1292–7.

33. Vintzileos AM, Campbell WA, Storlazzi, *et al*. Fetal liver ultrasound measurements in isoimmunized pregnancies. *Obstet Gynecol* 1986;68:162–7.
34. DeVore GR, Mayden K, Tortora M, *et al*. Dilation of the umbilical vein in rhesus hemolytic anemia: A predictor of severe disease. *Am J Obstet Gynecol* 1981;141:464–6.
35. Grannum PA. Ultrasound examination of the placenta. *Clin Obstet Gynaecol* 1983;10:459–73.
36. Chitkara U, Wilkins I, Lynch L, *et al*. The role of sonography in assessing severity of fetal anemia in Rh- and Kell-isoimmunized pregnancies. *Obstet Gynecol* 1988;71:393–7.
37. DeVore GR, Acherman RJ, Cabal LA, *et al*. Hypoalbuminemia: The etiology of antenatally diagnosed pericardial effusion in rhesus-hemolytic anemia. *Am J Obstet Gynecol* 1982;142:1056–7.
38. Benacerraf BR, Frigoletto FD. Sonographic sign for the detection of early fetal ascites in the management of severe isoimmune disease without intrauterine transfusion. *Am J Obstet Gynecol* 1985;152:1039–41.
39. Oepkes D, Meerman RH, Vandenbussche FP, *et al*. Ultrasonographic fetal spleen measurements in red blood cell alloimmunized pregnancies. *Am J Obstet Gynecol* 1993;169:121–8.
40. Nicolaides KH, Fontanarosa M, Gabbe SG, *et al*. Failure of six ultrasonographic parameters to predict the severity of fetal anemia in rhesus isoimmunization. *Am J Obstet Gynecol* 1988;158:920–6.
41. Rochard F, Schifrin BS, Goupil F, *et al*. Non-stressed fetal heart rate monitoring in the antepartum period. *Am J Obstet Gynecol* 1976;126:699–706.
42. Nicolaides KH, Sadovsky G, Visser GHA. Heart rate patterns in normoxemic, hypoxemic and anemic second-trimester fetuses. *Am J Obstet Gynecol* 1989;160:1034–7.
43. Sadovsky G, Visser GHA, Nicolaides KH. Heart rate patterns in fetal anemia. *Fetal Ther* 1988;3:216–23.
44. Rightmire DA, Nicolaides KH, Rodeck CH, *et al*. Midtrimester fetal blood flow velocities in rhesus isoimmunization: Relationship to gestational age and to fetal hematocrit in the untransfused patient. *Obstet Gynecol* 1986;68:233–6.
45. Copel JA, Grannum PA, Green JJ, *et al*. Fetal cardiac output in the isoimmunized pregnancy: A pulsed Doppler-echocardiographic study of patients undergoing intravascular intrauterine transfusion. *Am J Obstet Gynecol* 1989;161:361–5.
46. Nicolaides KH, Bilardo K, Campbell S. Prediction of fetal anemia by measurement of the mean blood velocity in the fetal aorta. *Am J Obstet Gynecol* 1990;162:209–12.
47. Vyas S, Nicolaides KH, Campbell S. Doppler evaluation of the middle cerebral artery in anemic fetuses. *Am J Obstet Gynecol* 1990;162:1066–8.
48. Nicolaides KH, Soothill PW, Rodeck CH, *et al*. Rh disease: Intravascular fetal blood transfusion by cordocentesis. *Fetal Ther* 1986;1:185–92.
49. Van den Veyver IB, Chong SS, Cota J, *et al*. Single cell analysis of the rhesus D blood type for use in preimplantation diagnosis in the prevention of severe hemolytic disease of the newborn. *Am J Obstet Gynecol* 1995;172:533–40.
50. Bennett PR, Kim CL, Colin Y, *et al*. Prenatal determination of fetal RhD type by DNA amplification following chorion villus biopsy or amniocentesis. *N Engl J Med* 1993;329:607–10.
51. Fisk NM, Bennet P, Warwick RM, *et al*. Clinical utility of fetal RhD typing in alloimmunized pregnancies by means of polymerase chain reaction on amniocytes or chorionic villi. *Am J Obstet Gynecol* 1994;171:50–4.
52. Williams J, Baker J, Dildy G, *et al*. Rhesus D blood typing of the fetus at risk for isoimmunization using DNA from amniotic fluid. *Presented at the 41st Annual Meeting of the Society for Gynecologic Investigation*, Chicago, IL.
53. Spence WC, Maddalena A, Demers DB, *et al*. Molecular analysis of the RhD genotype in fetuses at risk for RhD hemolytic disease. *Obstet Gynecol* 1995;85:296–8.
54. Fuhrman HC, Klink F, Grzejszczyk G, *et al*. First trimester diagnosis of Rh (D) with an immunofluorescence technique after chorionic villus sampling. *Prenat Diagn* 1987;7:17–21.
55. Geifman-Holtzman O, Bernstein IM, Berry SM, *et al*. Prenatal diagnosis of fetal rhesus (Rh) C, D and E types by polymerase chain reaction (PCR). *Am J Obstet Gynecol* 1995;172:265.
56. Kickler TS, Blakemore K, Shirey RS, *et al*. Chorionic villus sampling for fetal Rh typing: Clinical implications. *Am J Obstet Gynecol* 1992;166:1407–11.
57. Lo Y-MD, Bowell PJ, Selinger M, *et al*. Prenatal determination of fetal RhD status by analysis of peripheral blood of rhesus-negative mothers. *Lancet* 1993;341:1147–8.
58. Powell LC Jr. Intense plasmapheresis in the pregnant Rh-sensitized woman. *Am J Obstet Gynecol* 1968;101:153–70.
59. Fraser I, Bothamley JA, Bennett MO, *et al*. Intensive antenatal plasmapheresis in severe rhesus isoimmunisation. *Lancet* 1976; 1:6–9.
60. Carter B. Preliminary report of a substance which inhibits anti-Rh serum. *Am J Clin Pathol* 1947;17:646–9.
61. East EN, Mair CM. Intensive immunization of already sensitised Rh-negative women: Birth of mildly diseased baby. *J Lab Clin Med* 1949;34:983–91.
62. Bierme SJ, Blanc M, Abbal M, *et al*. Oral Rh treatment for severely immunized mothers. *Lancet* 1979;1:604–5.
63. Hunter OB Jr. Cortisone in the management of hemolytic disease of the newborn. *NY State J Med* 1955;55:1136–40.
64. Caritis S, Meuller-Heubach E, Edelstone D. Effect of betamethasone on analysis of amniotic fluid in the rhesus sensitized pregnancy. *Am J Obstet Gynecol* 1977;127:529–32.
65. Gudson JP, Witherow CC. Possible ameliorating effects of erythroblastosis by promethazine hydrochloride. *Am J Obstet Gynecol* 1973;117:1101–8.
66. Charles AG, Blumenthal LS. Promethazine hydrochloride therapy in severely Rh-sensitized pregnancies. *Obstet Gynecol* 1982;60:627–30.
67. Allen FH. Attempts at prevention of intrauterine death in erythroblastosis fetalis. *N Engl J Med* 1963;269:1344–9.
68. Linch DC, Rodeck CH, Nicolaides KH, *et al*. Attempted bone marrow transplantation in a 17-week gestation fetus. *Lancet* 1986;2:1453.
69. Freda VJ, Adamsons KJ. Exchange transfusion *in utero*. *Am J Obstet Gynecol* 1964;89:817–21.
70. Asensio SH, Figueroa-Longo JG, Pelegrina IA. Intrauterine exchange transfusion. *Am J Obstet Gynecol* 1966;95:29–33.
71. Seelen J, Van Kessel H, Eskes T, *et al*. A new method of exchange transfusion *in utero*. Cannulation of vessels on the fetal side of the human placenta. *Am J Obstet Gynecol* 1966;95:872–6.
72. Liley AW. Intrauterine transfusion of the fetus in haemolytic disease. *Br Med J* 1963;2:1107–9.
73. Bock JT. Intrauterine transfusions in severe rhesus hemolytic disease. *Acta Obstet Gynecol Scand* 1976;Suppl. 53:29–36.
74. Watts DH, Luthy DA, Benedetti TJ, *et al*. Intraperitoneal fetal transfusion under direct ultrasound guidance. *Obstet Gynecol* 1988;71:84–8.
75. Rodeck CH, Holman CA, Karnicki J, *et al*. Direct intravascular fetal blood transfusion by fetoscopy in severe rhesus isoimmunisation. *Lancet* 1981;1:625–7.
76. Rodeck CH, Nicolaides KH, Warsof SL, *et al*. The management of severe rhesus isoimmunization by fetoscopic intravascular transfusions. *Am J Obstet Gynecol* 1984;150:769–74.
77. Berkowitz RL, Chitkara U, Goldberg JD, *et al*. Intrauterine transfusion *in utero*: The percutaneous approach. *Am J Obstet Gynecol* 1986;154:622–7.
78. Grannum PA, Copel JA, Moya FR, *et al*. The reversal of hydrops fetalis by intravascular intrauterine transfusion in severe isoimmune fetal anemia. *Am J Obstet Gynecol* 1988;158:914–19.
79. Bang J, Bock JE, Trolle D. Ultrasound-guided fetal intravenous transfusion for severe rhesus haemolytic disease. *Br Med J* 1982;284:373–4.
80. Nicolaides KH, Clewell W, Rodeck CH. Measurement of human fetoplacental blood volume in erythroblastosis fetalis. *Am J Obstet Gynecol* 1987;57:50–3.
81. Ronkin S, Chayen B, Wapner RJ, *et al*. Intravascular exchange and bolus transfusion in the severely isoimmunized fetus. *Am J Obstet Gynecol* 1989;160:407–11.
82. DeCrespigny L, Robinson HP, Quinn M, *et al*. Ultrasound-guided fetal blood transfusion for severe rhesus isoimmunisation. *Obstet Gynecol* 1985;66:529–32.
83. Doyle LW, Cauchi M, DeCrespigny LC, *et al*. Fetal intravascular transfusion for severe erythroblastosis: Effects on hematology and survival. *Aust N Z J Obstet Gynaecol* 1986;26:192–5 .
84. Berkowitz RL, Chitkara U, Goldberg JD, *et al*. Intrauterine intravascular transfusions for severe red blood cell isoimmunization: Ultrasound-guided percutaneous approach. *Am J Obstet Gynecol* 1986;155:574–81.
85. Socol ML, MacGregor SN, Pielet BW, *et al*. Percutaneous umbilical transfusion in severe rhesus isoimmunization: Resolution of fetal hydrops. *Am J Obstet Gynecol* 1987;157:1369–75.
86. Orsini LF, Pilu G, Calderoni P, *et al*. Intravascular intrauterine transfusion for severe erythroblastosis fetalis using different techniques. *Fetal Ther* 1988;3:50–9.

87. Barss VA, Benaceraff BR, Frigoletto FD, *et al.* Management of isoimmunized pregnancy by use of intravascular techniques. *Am J Obstet Gynecol* 1988;159:932–7.
88. Parer JT. Severe rhesus isoimmunization – current methods of *in utero* diagnosis and treatment. *Am J Obstet Gynecol* 1988; 158;1323–9.
89. Nicolini U, Kochenour NK, Greco P, *et al.* When to perform the next intra-uterine transfusion in patients with Rh alloimmunization: Combined intravascular and intraperitoneal transfusion allows longer intervals. *Fetal Ther* 1989;4:14–20.
90. Lemery D, Urbain ME, Van Lieferinghen P, *et al.* Intra-uterine exchange transfusion under ultrasound guidance. *Eur J Obstet Gynecol Reprod Biol* 1989;33:161–8.
91. Poissonnier MH, Brossard Y, Demedeiros N, *et al.* Two hundred intrauterine exchange transfusions in severe blood incompatibilities. *Am J Obstet Gynecol* 1989;161:709–13.
92. Pattison N, Roberts A. The management of severe erythroblastosis fetalis by fetal transfusion: Survival of transfused adult erythrocytes in the fetus. *Obstet Gynecol* 1989;74:901–4.
93. Harman CR, Bowman JM, Manning FA, *et al.* Intrauterine transfusion – intraperitoneal versus intravascular approach: A case–control comparison. *Am J Obstet Gynecol* 1990;162:1053–9.
94. Moise KJ. Changing trends in the management of red cell alloimmunisation in pregnancy. *Arch Pathol Lab Med* 1994;118: 421–8.
95. Plockinger B, Strumpflen I, Deutinger J, *et al.* Diagnosis and treatment of fetal anemia due to isoimmunization. *Arch Gynecol Obstet* 1994;255:195–200.
96. Harman CR. Invasive techniques in the management of alloimmune anemia. In Harman CR, ed. *Invasive Fetal Testing and Treatment.* London: Blackwell, 1995:109–89.
97. Merchant RH, Lulla CP, Gupte SC, *et al.* Fetal outcome following intrauterine intravascular transfusion in rhesus alloimmunization. *Indian Pediatr* 1995;32:971–7.
98. Nicolini U, Kochenour NK, Greco P, *et al.* Consequences of fetomaternal haemorrhage after intrauterine transfusion. *Br Med J* 1988;297:1379–81.
99. Bowell P, Wainscoat JS, Peto TE, *et al.* Maternal anti-D concentrations and outcome in rhesus haemolytic disease of the newborn. *Br Med J* 1982;285:327–9.

107 Management of fetal and neonatal alloimmune thrombocytopenia

M. F. Murphy

Introduction

Neonatal alloimmune thrombocytopenia is the platelet equivalent of hemolytic disease of the newborn. Feto-maternal incompatibility may cause maternal alloimmunization against a fetal platelet antigen inherited from the father and absent in the mother, and fetal and neonatal thrombocytopenia may result from placental transfer of immunoglobulin G (IgG) antibodies.

Most cases are diagnosed after birth, hence the term 'neonatal alloimmune thrombocytopenia'. However, the condition develops *in utero*, and the fetus may be severely affected. It is appropriate to emphasize this through the use of alternative terminology, such as 'fetal and neonatal thrombocytopenia' or 'fetomaternal alloimmune thrombocytopenia' (FMAIT).

Considerable progress has been made in laboratory aspects of platelet immunology since FMAIT was first recognized,[1] allowing a more precise diagnosis of the condition, and there have been advances in fetal medicine and transfusion medicine resulting in considerable improvements in its antenatal and neonatal management. However, there remains a need for a better understanding of the natural history of FMAIT and for improved methods for identifying high-risk pregnancies so that antenatal intervention can be directed at those cases at greatest risk of severe thrombocytopenia and hemorrhage.

Pathophysiology

Platelet alloantigens

FMAIT is caused by the destruction of fetal platelets by maternal alloantibodies against platelet-specific alloantigens. There are a number of well-characterized biallelic platelet alloantigen systems, and a number of rare, private, or low frequency antigens have also been described (Table 107.1). Most were first discovered during the investigation of cases of FMAIT. In addition to these platelet-specific alloantigens, platelets express antigens found on many other cells, including ABO blood group and human leukocyte antigen (HLA) class I. Platelet antigens are known to be expressed from 16 weeks of gestation,[2] and placental transfer of IgG antibodies can occur from 14 weeks, so thrombocytopenia can occur very early in pregnancy.

Platelet-specific alloantigens are located on platelet membrane glycoproteins involved in hemostasis through interactions with the vascular endothelium and plasma coagulation proteins. Most of these antigens are on the GPIIb/IIIa complex, which plays a central role in platelet aggregation as a receptor for fibrinogen. Other important glycoproteins are GPIb/IX, which is the main receptor for von Willebrand factor involved in platelet adhesion to the damaged vascular endothelium, GPIa/IIa, which is involved in adhesion to collagen and CD 109 which also appears to be a collagen receptor. Congenital absence or deficiency of these glycoproteins results in bleeding disorders; for example, lack of GPIIb/IIIa causes Glanzmann's thrombasthenia and absence of GPIb/IX results in Bernard–Soulier syndrome.

Table 107.1 shows the platelet-specific antigens implicated in FMAIT according to the current human platelet alloantigen (HPA) nomenclature, in which each system is numbered consecutively (HPA-1, -2, -3, etc.) according to its date of discovery and the high-frequency allele in each system is designated 'a' and the low-frequency allele, 'b'.[3] Table 107.1 also includes the glycoprotein localization of the antigens, their frequency in a Caucasian population, and the amino acid difference on the relevant glycoprotein between the alleles in each system; for example, there is a single C–T point mutation on GPIIIa resulting in the substitution of leucine by proline in HPA-1b.[4,5] Knowledge of the genetic basis of platelet-specific antigens makes it possible to carry out molecular genotyping on whatever material is available, for example, platelet typing using fetal DNA from amniotic fluid or chorion villus

Table 107.1 HPA systems

System	Antigen	Alternative names	Phenotype frequency* (%)	Glycoprotein	Nucleotide change	Amino acid change
HPA-1	HPA-1a	Zw^a, Pl^{A1}	97.9	GPIIIa	T^{196}	Leucine^{33}
	HPA-1b	Zw^b, Pl^{A2}	28.8		C^{196}	Proline^{33}
HPA-2	HPA-2a	Ko^b	>99.9	GPIbα	C^{524}	Threonine^{145}
	HPA-2b	Ko^a, Sib^a	13.2		T^{524}	Methionine^{145}
HPA-3	HPA-3a	Bak^a, Lek^a	80.95	GPIIb	T^{2622}	Isoleucine^{843}
	HPA-3b	Bak^b	69.8		G^{2622}	Serine^{843}
HPA-4	HPA-4a	Yuk^b, Pen^a	>99.9	GPIIIa	G^{526}	Arginine^{143}
	HPA-4b	Yuk^a, Pen^b	<0.1		A^{526}	Glutamine^{143}
HPA-5	HPA-5a	Br^b, Zav^b	99.0	GPIa	G^{1648}	Glutamic acid^{505}
	HPA-5b	Br^a, Zav^a, Hc^a	19.7		A^{1648}	Lysine^{505}
HPA-6				GPIIIa	G^{1564}	Arginine^{489}
	HPA-6bw	Ca^a, Tu^a	0.7		A^{1564}	Glutamine^{489}
HPA-7				GPIIIa	C^{1267}	Proline^{407}
	HPA-7bw	Mo	0.2		G^{1267}	Alanine^{407}
HPA-8				GPIIIa	T^{2004}	Arginine^{636}
	HPA-8bw	Sr^a	< 0.01		C^{2004}	Cysteine^{636}
HPA-9				GPIIb	G^{2603}	Valine^{837}
	HPA-9bw	Max^a	0.6		A^{2603}	Methionine^{837}
HPA-10				GPIIIa	G^{281}	Arginine^{62}
	HPA-10bw	La^a	< 1.6		A^{281}	Glutamine^{62}
HPA-11				GPIIIa	G^{1996}	Arginine^{633}
	HPA-11bw	Gro^a	< 0.25		A^{1996}	Histidine^{633}
				GPIbβ	G^{141}	Glycine^{15}
HPA-12	HPA-12bw	Iy^a	0.4		A^{141}	Glutamic acid^{15}
				GPIa	C^{2531}	Threonine^{799}
HPA-13	HPA-13bw	Sit^a	0.25		T^{2531}	Methionine^{799}
				GPIIIa		
HPA-14	HPA-14bw	Oe^a	< 0.17		Δ $AAG^{1929–1931}$	Δ Lysine^{611}
	HPA-15a	Gov^b	74	CD109	C^{2108}	Serine^{703}
HPA-15	HPA-15b	Gov^a	81		A^{2108}	Tyrosine^{703}
					C^{517}	Threonine^{140}
HPA-16	HPA-16bw	Duv^a	< 1	GPIIIa	T^{517}	Isoleucine^{140}
				GPIIb/IIIa		
		Va^a	< 0.4			
		Pl^T	> 99.9	GPV		
		Vis		GPIV		
		Pe^a		GPIbα		
		Dy^a		38 kD GP		
		Mou^a	26	unknown		

*Frequencies based on studies in Caucasians.

samples. Various techniques are available, but the most commonly used is the polymerase chain reaction with sequence-specific primers (PCR-SSP).[6]

Platelet alloantibodies

Series of cases of FMAIT with detectable platelet-specific alloantibodies have shown that the commonest antibody in Caucasian women is anti-HPA-1a in 78–89% of cases, followed by anti-HPA-5b in 6–15%, and the remainder are due to other specificities.[7,8] In Japan, anti-HPA-5b and anti-HPA-4b are the most frequent antibodies. The HPA-1a/1b polymorphism is very rare in Japan and anti-HPA-1a antibodies have never been found.[9]

HLA antibodies are frequently found in pregnant women, but are not thought to cause FMAIT. This is

Table 107.2 FMAIT due to HPA-1a alloimmunization during pregnancy

Study	Number of pregnant women studied	HPA-1a-negative mothers	HPA-1a-positive fetuses (if tested)	Maternal anti-HPA-1a	Overall incidence of FMAIT
Mueller-Eckhardt *et al.* (1989)[7]	1211	26 (2.2%)	23/25	2/23 (8.7%)	2 (0.16%)
Reznikoff-Etievant *et al.* (1988)[11]	860	27 (3.1%)	16/25	0	0
Blanchette *et al.* (1990)[12]	5,000	81 (1.6%)	25/29	3/50 (6%)	1 (0.02%)
Kaplan *et al.* (1993)[13]	2,000	—	—	—	2 (0.1%)
Burrows and Kelton (1993)[14]	15,471	—	—	—	10 (0.06%)
Doughty *et al.* (1995)[15]	3,473	74 (2.2%)	—	2/22 (9.1%)	2 (0.06%)*
Williamson *et al.* (1995)[16]	24,417	618 (2.5%)	—	44/385 (11.4%)	8 (0.03%)

*Twins equally affected

because antibodies against fetal HLA are absorbed by placental HLA; only HLA antibodies against HLA not expressed by the fetus pass into the fetal circulation.[10]

Incidence

The incidence of FMAIT is between 1 in 1000 and 1 in 5000 live births (Table 107.2).[7,11–16] This is surprisingly low, considering that 2% of women are HPA-1a negative and that 98% of men are HPA-1a positive. However, only about 10% of HPA-1a-negative women develop anti-HPA-1a (Table 107.2).

Alloimmunization to HPA-1a appears to be HLA class II restricted. Reznikoff-Etievant and colleagues reported a strong association with HLA-DR3, which was present in 71–95% of women developing anti-HPA-1a.[17] It was later found that all alloimmunized women were positive for HLA-DRw52, and all responders tested by restriction fragment length polymorphism had the DRw52a allele at the DRB3 locus.[18,19] Further studies using the PCR-SSP showed that two cases previously typed as HLA-DRw52a (HLA-DR3*0101) were in fact HLA-DRw52c (HLA-DR3*0301), and one additional case out of seven new ones was found to be HLA-DRw53 (HLA-DR4*0101).[20] This means that FMAIT is not always associated with HLA-DRw52a, and that pregnancies in HPA-1a-negative women without this HLA type cannot be excluded from the group at risk of FMAIT. There is no similar association between HPA-1b alloimmunization and HLA-DRw52a,[21] but a significant association has been reported between HLA-DRw6 and alloimmunization to HPA-5b.[22]

It is important to note that the presence of platelet-specific alloantibodies does not necessarily mean that there will be fetal or neonatal thrombocytopenia (Table 107.2). The factors influencing the development of thrombocytopenia and its severity are poorly understood, and there is no obvious correlation with the titer or isotype of the IgG antibodies.

Diagnosis

Clinical aspects

The diagnosis of FMAIT is usually made on clinical grounds, but it can be discovered incidentally when a blood count is carried out routinely or for other reasons. Most frequently, a neonate who is otherwise well is observed to have widespread purpura at or soon after birth. The mother is healthy, and her first child is affected in 50% of cases.[7,23] These studies also found that 10–15% of infants had no evidence of bleeding, but the remainder had purpura, bruising, and/or more severe hemorrhage.[7,23] Intracranial hemorrhage (ICH), which is the major cause of mortality and long-term morbidity, occurred in 15–20% of cases. In the study of Kaplan and associates,[23] involving 127 cases, death due to severe hemorrhage occurred in 7% and there were neurological sequelae in 21%. Although there is a serious risk of severe hemorrhage at the time of delivery, nearly 50% of ICH cases occur *in utero*,[7] usually between 30 and 35 weeks of gestation, but sometimes even before 20 weeks.[8] There may be more unusual presentations, such as isolated fetal hydrocephalus, unexplained fetal anemia, or recurrent miscarriages.[24,25]

The first step in the diagnosis of FMAIT is confirmation of isolated thrombocytopenia, followed by exclusion of other causes of neonatal thrombocytopenia, such as infection, disseminated intravascular coagulation, maternal autoimmune thrombocytopenia, and conditions causing impaired neonatal megakaryocytopoiesis.

Laboratory investigations

A diagnosis of suspected FMAIT on clinical grounds requires laboratory confirmation. Testing is aimed at detection of a maternal platelet-specific alloantibody against the paternal platelets, which are a more convenient source of platelets expressing the relevant antigen than the baby's own platelets, and determination of the platelet antigen types of the mother and father.

The investigation is best carried out in a reference laboratory which is able to carry out the necessary tests speedily and advise on clinical management. Testing usually comprises the combination of a sensitive assay using intact platelets, such as the platelet immunofluorescence test,[26] with a glycoprotein-specific antigen capture method, such as the monoclonal antibody-specific immobilization of platelet antigens assay,[27] which allows detection of weak antibodies and mixtures of antibodies. Molecular methods, such as PCR-SSP,[6] are now used for platelet genotyping.

Investigation becomes more complicated if it is not possible to demonstrate parental incompatibility for platelet-specific alloantigens by detection of the corresponding maternal antibody. Maternal platelet-specific antibodies have been reported to be undetectable in up to 20% of cases,[23] but this may be less with improved methods for detecting antibodies, and it may now be possible to demonstrate parental incompatibility for HPA-1a or another HPA in this situation. Another cause of difficulty in laboratory investigation is if a rare private antigen is involved; the mother has an antibody against the paternal platelets, but this antibody reacts with platelets from very few or no normal donors and its specificity is not obvious.

Management

Unexpected neonatal thrombocytopenia

There is as yet no routine antenatal screening for FMAIT, so most cases will be unexpected. The need for immediate treatment depends on the presence of bleeding and the severity of the thrombocytopenia. Any delays or difficulties in the laboratory confirmation of the diagnosis of FMAIT should not prevent prompt treatment of an infant with bleeding or severe thrombocytopenia.

The best way of raising the platelet count rapidly is to transfuse compatible platelets. These can be provided by plateletpheresis of the mother, in which case the concentrate should be irradiated to prevent transfusion-associated graft-vs-host disease. Ideally, a platelet concentrate prepared from the mother should also be washed to remove platelet antibodies. However, in practice, washing platelet concentrates is technically demanding and the transfusion should not be delayed unduly, as the initial transfusion may be extremely important in minimizing the risk of postnatal hemorrhage. A better strategy for providing compatible platelets before the results of serological testing are available is to transfuse platelets from HPA-1a-negative donors. Some transfusion centers ensure that HPA-1a-negative, or HPA-1a- and -5b-negative, platelet concentrates are always available for this eventuality. Often only one transfusion of compatible platelets is sufficient, as the thrombocytopenia is self-limiting. The clinical condition of the infant should be carefully monitored and the platelet count measured at least once daily until it is obvious that it has reached a 'safe' level and is increasing spontaneously. If there has been severe thrombocytopenia, a cerebral ultrasound or nuclear magnetic resonance scan should be performed to detect clinically silent ICH.

The transfusion of platelet concentrates from random donors is unlikely to be effective. There has only been one formal study of the use of intravenous immunoglobulin for the neonatal management of FMAIT; the response rate was 75% and the increase in platelet count was delayed for 24–48 h, during which time the infants remained at risk of ICH.[28]

Antenatal management

The recurrence of FMAIT in subsequent pregnancies is very high (> 85%) and the condition tends to become more severe.[23,29] If a previous sibling has suffered ICH, the risk of antenatal ICH is high in a subsequent pregnancy, and it is easy to justify antenatal intervention. If the previous infant was thrombocytopenic, but did not have a major hemorrhage, the risk of antenatal hemorrhage is more difficult to assess. There are no non-invasive tests for the prediction of which fetuses are at greatest risk of hemorrhage. The levels of maternal platelet antibodies have not been found to be predictive of the severity of thrombocytopenia,[23,30] and cerebral ultrasound scans will be abnormal only if ICH has occurred.

The only method available at the present time for assessing the fetal platelet count is fetal blood sampling,[31] which allows the diagnosis of FMAIT *in utero* and the assessment of severity to be made with certainty. In addition, this technique provides a means for transfusing compatible platelets to severely affected fetuses. The procedure usually takes only a few minutes, and a few milliliters of pure fetal blood is obtained. Fetal platelet counts are reliable and it is unusual to have problems because of contamination of the sample with maternal blood or amniotic fluid;[32] the normal range is similar to adults and there is no significant variation with gestational age.[33]

The main risks of the procedure are severe hemorrhage from the cord puncture site and obstruction of the cord circulation due to a hematoma. The main problems are most likely to occur with the initial blood sampling at around 20–22 weeks' gestation, when the cord is small and the platelet count may be very low. Fetal blood sampling for FMAIT should be performed at referral centers, where the risk is about 1%. In one series,[34] which now extends to nearly 200 fetal blood samplings for FMAIT, there have been two fetal deaths, one due to bleeding and one due to a cord hematoma. Severe bleeding requiring fetal red cell transfusions occurred in two other pregnancies, but there was eventually a successful outcome in these pregnancies. Another group has reported five fetal

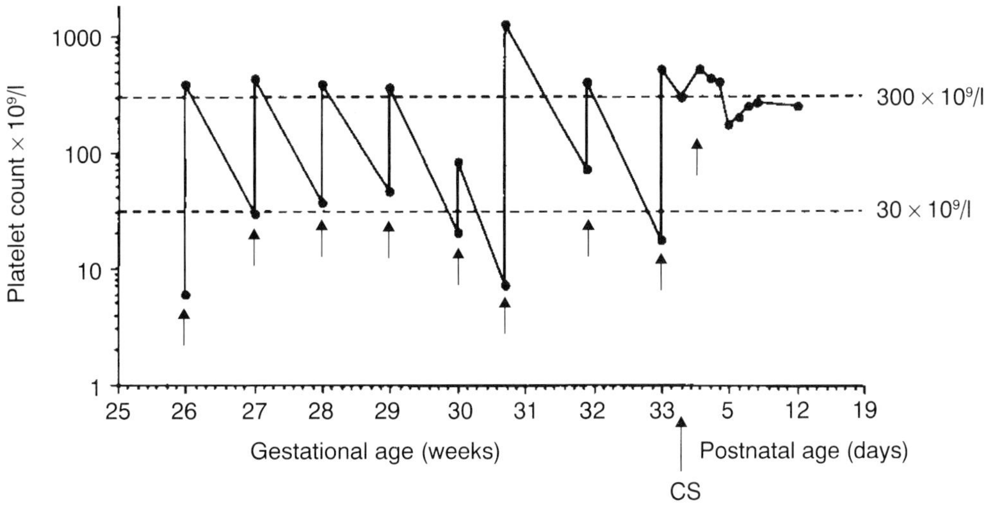

Figure 107.1 The seventh pregnancy of a patient who had already had five miscarriages. The last of these was shown to have hydrops and hydrocephalus and a platelet count of only 17×10^9/l, and the serological findings supported a diagnosis of FMAIT due to anti-HPA-1a. The fetal platelet count was less than 10×10^9/l at 25 weeks of gestation in the sixth pregnancy, and a cord hematoma developed during fetal blood sampling, resulting in fetal death. In the seventh pregnancy, prednisolone 20 mg/day and intravenous immunoglobulin 1 g/week were administered to the mother from 16 weeks until delivery. The figure shows pre- and post-transfusion platelet counts following serial fetal blood samplings and platelet transfusions (arrows). The fetal platelet count was less than 10×10^9/l at 26 weeks. The aim was to maintain the fetal platelet count above 30×10^9/l by raising the immediate post-transfusion platelet count to above 300×10^9/l after each transfusion. The fetal platelet count fell below 10×10^9/l on one occasion following a transfusion when there were problems in preparing the fetal platelet concentrate and the dose of platelets was inadequate. CS, cesarean section.

deaths due to exsanguination.[35] Because of the risk of bleeding, it has become routine practice to transfuse platelets to the fetus following fetal blood sampling for suspected FMAIT.[34,35]

The aim of antenatal management where there has been a previously affected pregnancy is to minimize the risk of severe hemorrhage such as ICH, but the optimal management remains controversial.[36] The therapeutic options being explored include maternal administration of intravenous immunoglobulin[37] and fetal platelet transfusions; early cesarean section alone is not considered to be effective in preventing antenatal or perinatal hemorrhage. Counselling of couples with an index case about the risks of severe fetal/neonatal thrombocytopenia in a subsequent pregnancy needs to be based on the severity of disease in the index case and the outcome of immunological investigations. The following should be taken into account:

- thrombocytopenia in subsequent cases is as or, generally, more severe
- the best predictors of severe fetal thrombocytopenia in a future pregnancy are the occurrence of antenatal intracranial hemorrhage and severe thrombocytopenia (platelet count $< 20 \times 10^9$/L) in a previous pregnancy
- the antibody specificity and titre do not reliably correlate with the severity of NAIT, and are of no value in the management of individual cases
- the zygosity of the partner. If the father is heterozygous for the relevant HPA e.g. HPA-1a/1b, fetal platelet typing can be performed using a fetal blood sample obtained at 18 weeks of gestation or using chorionic villus or amniotic fluid samples obtained earlier in pregnancy.

As few trials have been performed on the antenatal management of FMAIT, it is difficult to make definite recommendations. Weekly platelet transfusions by FBS have been shown to prevent ICH even in high risk cases (Figure 107.1), but are technically demanding, invasive and associated with a high mortality due to hemorrhage, cardiac dysrhythmias and premature labour.[34,38,39]

The high incidence of complications associated with FBS, and the effectiveness of maternal therapy in about 67% of cases,[39,40,41,42] suggest that treatment with IVIgG (1g/kg/week) without an initial FBS should be used as initial management.[43,44] This should be considered from or before 16 weeks' gestation in the cases where there is a history of antenatal ICH in previous pregnancies, because the earliest reports of ICH are at 16 weeks.[34] IVIgG could be started a few weeks later (20–22 weeks) for those fetuses with a sibling history of severe thrombocytopenia but no antenatal ICH. FBS may be used to monitor the effect of maternal therapy (4–8 weeks after starting IVIgG) and to indicate if alternative therapy is required. Failure with maternal therapy may potentially be rescued by the addition of oral prednisolone (0.5 mg/kg/day) and/or an increased dose of IVIgG (2g/kg/week), serial fetal platelet transfusions or by early delivery at an acceptable gestation.

Further studies are required to determine the optimal antenatal management for FMAIT.

Antenatal treatment appears to have improved the outcome of severely affected cases of FMAIT. However, there is little information on the long-term development of the children who have been treated *in utero*. All apparently successfully treated infants should probably have a cranial ultrasound or nuclear magnetic resonance scan performed after birth and developmental follow-up for at least 2 years to detect neurological impairment caused by occult ICH.

The main issues in the preparation of platelet concentrates for fetal transfusions are compatibility with maternal antibodies, adequate dosage without volume overload, and avoidance of transfusion-transmitted infections and transfusion-associated graft-vs-host disease. The mother is a convenient source of platelets for single transfusions, but use of the mother for repeated transfusions is not practical, and panels of selected donors need to be established, particularly for types HPA-lb/lb and HPA-5a/5a, as the most frequent antibodies responsible for FMAIT are anti-HPA-1a and anti-HPA-5b.[7,8] The blood group of the fetus should be determined at the first fetal blood sampling, and fetal hemolysis due to high-titer anti-A and anti-B should be avoided by testing donors for these antibodies. Maternal HLA antibodies may occasionally be responsible for the shortened survival of platelets transfused to the fetus, in which case the concentrates should be prepared from the mother or HLA-matched HPA-compatible donors.[45]

The risk of transfusion-transmitted infection should be minimized by standard microbiological screening of blood donors, who should in addition be cytomegalovirus seronegative. The concentrates should be gamma irradiated to prevent transfusion-associated graft-vs-host disease. Concentration of the platelet concentrate to a platelet count of $2500–4000 \times 10^9/l$ is essential to achieve satisfactory post-transfusion platelet counts without an unacceptably high transfusion volume. If the fetal platelet count is raised to $300–500 \times 10^9/l$ after each transfusion, it should be no lower than $30 \times 10^9/l$ 1 week later; this is thought to be a 'safe' level for the fetal platelet count, and 1 week is an acceptable interval for patients receiving serial transfusions.

In summary, the optimal antenatal management of FMAIT remains uncertain. More information is needed about the frequency and timing of ICH, and the benefits and notes of different management strategies.

Antenatal screening

Progress in the antenatal management of FMAIT in women who have had previously affected pregnancies draws attention to the issue of how to identify and manage the first affected infant.[46] The diagnosis of FMAIT in first-affected infants is usually made only after birth, by which time serious hemorrhage might have already occurred. Improvements in methods for large-scale platelet antigen typing and platelet antibody detection have raised the possibility of antenatal screening for pregnancies at risk of FMAIT alongside established programs of screening for hemolytic disease of the newborn. Recent studies in London and Cambridge, UK, have demonstrated the feasibility of such programs in determining the frequency of HPA-1a alloimmunization and its clinical sequelae.[15,16] The inclusion of typing for HLA-DR3*0101 following the initial identification of HPA-1a-negative pregnant women would focus on women most likely to develop anti-HPA-1a, but would not identify all affected pregnancies.[20]

An important obstacle to the introduction of antenatal screening is that the optimal management of women with anti-HPA-1a with no previous history of affected pregnancies is uncertain. Reliable non-invasive methods for identifying the fetuses at greatest risk of antenatal ICH are not available. Antenatal management has significant risks, which have to be balanced against those of a conservative policy with no antenatal intervention but prompt identification and treatment of affected cases after delivery, and only large scale trials will clarify this issue.

REFERENCES

1. Harrington WJ, Sprague CC, Minnich V, *et al.* Immunologic mechanisms in idiopathic and neonatal thrombocytopenic purpura. *Ann Intern Med* 1953;38:433–69.
2. Gruel Y, Boizard B, Daffos F, *et al.* Determination of platelet antigens and glycoproteins in the human fetus. *Blood* 1986;68: 488–92.
3. von dem Borne AEG, Decary F. ICSH/ISBT Working Party on Platelet Serology. Nomenclature of platelet-specific antigens. *Vox Sang* 1990;58:176.
4. Simsek S, von dem Borne AEG. Molecular genetics of human platelet antigens. *Infusionsther Transfusionsmed* 1994;21(Suppl 3): 29–33.
5. von dem Borne AEG, de Haas M, Simcek S, *et al.* Platelet and neutrophil alloantigens in clinical medicine. *Vox Sang* 1996; 70(Suppl 3):34–40.
6. Metcalfe P, Waters AH. HPA-1 typing by PCR amplification with sequence-specific primers (PCR-SSP): A rapid and simple technique. *Br J Haematol* 1993;85:227–9.
7. Mueller-Eckhardt C, Kiefel V, Grubert A, *et al.* 348 cases of suspected neonatal alloimmune neonatal thrombo-cytopenia. *Lancet* 1989;1:363–6.
8. Waters A, Murphy M, Hambley H, *et al.* Management of alloimmune thrombocytopenia in the fetus and neonate. In Nance ST, ed. *Clinical and Basic Science Aspects of Immunohaematology*. Arlington: American Association of Blood Banks, 1991:155–77.
9. Wang L, Juji T, Shibata Y, *et al.* Sequence variation of human platelet membrane glycoprotein IIIa associated with the Yuk^a/Yuk^b alloantigen system. *Proc Jpn Acad* 1991;67: 102–6.
10. Doughty RW, Gelsthorpe K. Some parameters of lymphocyte antibody activity through pregnancy and further eluates of placental material. *Tissue Antigens* 1976;8:43–8.
11. Reznikoff-Etievant MF, Kaplan C, Muller JY, *et al.* Alloimmune thrombocytopenias, definition of group at risk: A prospective study. *Curr Stud Haematol* 1988;55:119–24.

12. Blanchette VS, Chen L, de Friedberg ZS, *et al.* Alloimmunization to the PL^{A1} platelet antigen: Results of a prospective study. *Br J Haematol* 1990;74:209–15.
13. Kaplan C, Schlegel N, Durand-Zaleski I, *et al.* Anti-HPA-1a materno-fetal platelet alloimmunization: Costs and benefits of a prospective routine program. *Thromb Haemost* 1993;69:1191 (abstr. 2318).
14. Burrows RF, Kelton JG. Fetal thrombocytopenia and its relation to maternal thrombocytopenia. *N Engl J Med* 1993;329:1463–6.
15. Doughty HA, Murphy MF, Metcalfe P, *et al.* Antenatal screening for fetal alloimmune thrombocytopenia: The results of a pilot study. *Br J Haematol* 1995;90:321–5.
16. Williamson LM, Hackett GA, Rennie JM, *et al.* Determination of the natural history of neonatal alloimmune thrombocytopenia by antenatal screening. *Blood* 1995;86 (Suppl 1):538 (abstr. 2141).
17. Reznikoff-Etievant MF, Muller JY, Julien F, *et al.* An immune response gene linked to MHC in man. *Tissue Antigens* 1983;22: 312–4.
18. Valentin N, Vergracht A, Bignon JD, *et al.* HLA-DRw52a is involved in alloimmunization against PL-A1 antigen. *Human Immunol* 1990;27:73–9.
19. Decary F, L'Abbe D, Tremblay L, *et al.* The immune response to HPA-1a antigen: Association with HLA-DRw52a. *Transfusion Med* 1991;1:55–62.
20. L'Abbe D, Tremblay L, Goldman M, *et al.* Alloimmunization to platelet antigen HPA-1a (Zw^{a}): Association with HLA-DRw52a is not 100%. *Transfusion Med* 1992;2:251.
21. Kuijpers RWAM, von dem Borne AEGK, Kiefel V, *et al.* Leucine 33-proline 33 substitution in human platelet GpIIIa determines HLA-DRw52a association of the immune response against HPA-1a (Zw^{a}/PL^{A1}) and HPA-lb (Zwb/PLA2). *Hum Immunol* 1992;34: 253–6.
22. Mueller-Eckhardt C, Kiefel V, Kroll H, *et al.* HLA-DRw6, a new immune response marker for immunization against the platelet alloantigen Br^{a}. *Vox Sang* 1989;57:90–1.
23. Kaplan C, Daffos F, Forestier F, *et al.* Current trends in neonatal alloimmune thrombocytopenia: Diagnosis and therapy. In Kaplan-Gouet C, Schlegel N, Salmon C, McGregor J, eds. *Platelet Immunology: Fundamental and Clinical Aspects.* Paris: Colloque INSERM/John Libbey Eurotext, 1991:267–78.
24. Montemagno R, Soothill PW, Scarcelli M, *et al.* Detection of alloimmune thrombocytopenia as cause of isolated hydrocephalus by fetal blood sampling. *Lancet* 1994;343:1300–1.
25. Murphy MF, Hambley H, Nicolaides K, *et al.* Severe fetomaternal alloimmune thrombocytopenia presenting with fetal hydrocephalus. *Prenat Diagn* 1996;16:1152–5.
26. von dem Borne AEG, Verheugt FWA, Oosterhof F, *et al.* A simple immunofluorescence test for the detection of platelet antibodies. *Br J Haematol* 1975;39:195–207.
27. Kiefel V, Santoso S, Weisheit M, *et al.* Monoclonal antibody-specific immobilization of platelet antigens (MAIPA): A new tool for the identification of platelet-reactive antibodies. *Blood* 1987; 70:1722–6.
28. Mueller-Eckhardt C, Kiefel V, Grubert A. High-dose IgG treatment for neonatal alloimmune thrombocytopenia. *Blut* 1989;59: 145–6.
29. Shulman NR, Marder VJ, Hiller MC, *et al.* Platelet and leucocyte isoantigens and their antibodies. *Prog Hematol* 1964;4:222–304.
30. Prouix C, Filion M, Goldman M, *et al.* Analysis of immunoglobulin class, IgG subclass and titre of HPA-1a antibodies in alloimmunised mothers giving birth to babies with or without neonatal alloimmune thrombocytopenia. *Br J Haematol* 1994;87:813–7.
31. Daffos F, Forestier F, Muller JY, *et al.* Prenatal treatment of alloimmune thrombocytopenia. *Lancet* 1984;2:632.
32. Daffos F, Capella-Pavlovsky M, Forestier F. Fetal blood sampling during pregnancy with use of a needle guided by ultrasound: A study of 606 consecutive cases. *Am J Obstet Gynecol* 1985; 153:655–60.
33. Hohlfeld P, Forestier F, Kaplan C, *et al.* Fetal thrombocytopenia: A retrospective survey of 5194 fetal blood samplings. *Blood* 1994;84:1851–6.
34. Murphy MF, Waters AH, Doughty HA, *et al.* Antenatal management of fetomaternal alloimmune thrombo-cytopenia – Report of 15 affected pregnancies. *Transfusion Med* 1994;4:281–92.
35. Paidas MJ, Berkowitz RL, Lynch L, *et al.* Alloimmune thrombocytopenia: Fetal and neonatal losses related to cordocentesis. *Am J Obstet Gynecol* 1995;172:475–9.
36. Reesink HW, Engelfriet CP. International forum: Prenatal management of fetal alloimmune thrombocytopenia. *Vox Sang* 1993; 65:180–9.
37. Bussel JB, Berkowitz RL, McFarland JG, *et al.* Antenatal treatment of neonatal alloimmune thrombocytopenia. *N Engl J Med* 1988;319:1374–8.
38. Murphy MF, Pullon HWH, Metcalfe P, *et al.* Management of fetal alloimmune thrombocytopenia by weekly *in utero* platelet transfusions. *Vox Sang* 1990;58:45–9.
39. Birchall JE, Murphy MF, Kaplan C, Kroll H on behalf of the European FMAIT Study Group. European collaborative study for the antenatal management of fetomaternal alloimmune thrombocytopenia. *Br J Haematol* 2003;122:275–88.
40. Lynch L, Bussel JB, McFarland JG, et al. Antenatal treatment of alloimmune thrombocytopenia. *Obstet Gynecol* 1992;80:67–71.
41. Bussel JB, Berkowitz RL, Lynch L, *et al.* Antenatal management of alloimmune thrombocytopenia with intravenous gammaglobulin: A randomized trial of the addition of low dose steroid to intravenous immunoglobulin in 55 maternal-fetal pairs. *Am J Obstet Gynecol* 1996;174:1414–23.
42. Kaplan C, Murphy MF, Kroll H, *et al.* On behalf of the European Working Group on NAIT. Feto-maternal alloimmune thrombocytopenia: Antenatal therapy with intravenous immunoglobulin and steroids – More questions than answers. *Br J Haematol* 1998; 100: 62–5.
43. Radder CM, Brand A, Kanhai HHH. A less invasive treatment strategy to prevent intracranial hemorrhage in fetal and neonatal alloimmune thrombocytopenia. *Am J Obstet & Gynecol* 2001; 185:683–8.
44. Mackenzie F, Brennand J, Peterkin M, Cameron A. Management of fetal alloimmune thrombocytopenia – a less invasive option? *J Obstet Gynaecol* 1999;19:119–21.
45. Murphy MF, Metcalf, P, Waters AH, *et al.* Antenatal management of severe feto-maternal alloimmune thrombocytopenia: HLA incompatibility may affect responses to fetal platelet transfusions. *Blood* 1993;81:2174–9.
46. Murphy MF, Williamson LM, Urbaniak SJ. Antenatal screening for fetomaternal alloimmune thrombocytopenia: Should we be doing it? *Vox Sang* 2002;83(suppl.1):409–16.

108 Severe twin-to-twin transfusion syndrome: diagnosis and endoscopic laser coagulation

N. J. Sebire, J. Hyett and K. H. Nicolaides

In monozygotic twin pregnancies, early embryonic splitting, which occurs in approximately one-third of cases, results in dichorionic placentation and two independent placental circulations.[1,2] Splitting after the third day of fertilization is associated with monochorionic placentation, with vascular communications between the two fetoplacental circulations; if cleavage occurs after day 12 the fetuses are conjoint. The clinical entity of severe twin-to-twin transfusion syndrome (TTS) is a result of imbalance in the net flow of blood across the placental vascular anastomoses from one fetus, the donor, to the other, the recipient, and occurs in about 15% of monochorionic pregnancies.

Pathophysiology

The phenomenon of a shared circulation between monochorionic twins was first described by Schatz in 1875.[3] Although anastomoses may be arterial–arterial or veno–venous, it is the arterio–venous anastomoses that are primarily responsible for the development of TTS. These arterio–venous anastomoses are usually deep in the placenta, but almost always proceed through the cotyledonary capillary bed.[1] Mild, moderate or severe TTS may develop, depending on the net flow between these anastomoses, which are variable in size, number and direction.[1]

The precise underlying mechanisms by which a subgroup of monochorionic pregnancies with vascular communications go on to develop TTS are not fully understood. However, it has been suggested that the primary defect is abnormal development of the placenta of the donor twin, which causes increased peripheral resistance in this placental circulation, promoting shunting of blood to the recipient. The donor therefore suffers from both hypovolemia, due to blood loss, and hypoxia, due to placental insufficiency.[4,5] The recipient fetus compensates for its expanded blood volume with polyuria,[6] but since protein and cellular components remain in its circulation the consequent increase in colloid oncotic pressure draws water from the maternal compartment across the placenta. A vicious cycle of hypervolemia, polyuria and hyperosmolality is established, leading to high-output heart failure and polyhydramnios.

In contrast to neonatal TTS, studies examining fetal blood obtained by cordocentesis in pregnancies with severe TTS have reported large intertwin differences in plasma albumin and total protein concentrations,[7,8] but no consistent differences in hemoglobin concentration between donor and recipient fetuses.[4,7–9]

Diagnosis

Traditionally, the diagnosis of TTS has been made retrospectively, in the neonatal period, on the basis of an intertwin difference in birth weight of 20% or more and in hemoglobin concentration of 5 g/dl or more.[10–12] These observations were made in live births, and therefore the criteria apply only to moderate TTS, since severe cases result in miscarriage or intrauterine death. Additionally, large intertwin differences in hemoglobin and birth weight are found in some dichorionic twin pregnancies and are not pathognomonic of TTS.[13]

Severe disease manifests clinically in the early second trimester of pregnancy with the mother complaining of a sudden increase in abdominal girth associated with extreme discomfort, and occasionally respiratory distress. On examination, there is tense polyhydramnios, which is pathognomonic of TTS

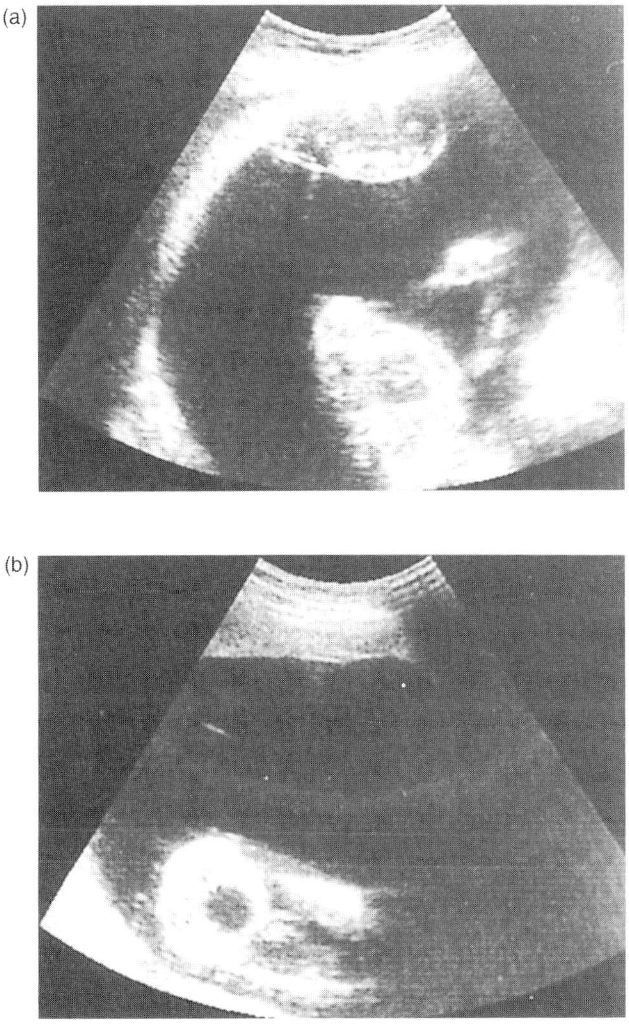

Figure 108.1 Ultrasound images demonstrating the features of TTS. (a) The 'stuck' donor fetus is in an anhydramniotic sac with no visible bladder. (b) The recipient fetus has a large bladder and polyhydramnios.

when observed at this early stage of gestation. In such cases of severe TTS, ultrasound examination will reveal a twin pregnancy with the polyhydramnios/anhydramnios sequence, with or without discordance in fetal size. However, the pathognomonic features of severe TTS are the presence of a large bladder in the polyuric recipient fetus in the polyhydramniotic sac, and a non-visualized bladder in the anuric donor that is found 'stuck' and immobile at the edge of the placenta or the uterine wall, where it is held fixed by the collapsed membranes of the anhydramniotic sac (Figure 108.1).

Other sonographic findings that may prove to be of prognostic significance include the presence of a hypertrophic, dilated and dyskinetic heart in the recipient fetus, while in the donor the heart may be dilated and the bowel hyperechogenic; these features are manifestations of hypoxia and are commonly seen in hypoxemic fetuses from pregnancies complicated by severe uteroplacental insufficiency. The donor fetus may also demonstrate ventriculomegaly and/or microcephaly secondary to hypoxia.

Color Doppler studies in severe TTS presenting with acute polyhydramnios during the second trimester of pregnancy have demonstrated the presence of several superficial vessels connecting the two circulations.[14] Additionally, the umbilical artery pulsatility index (PI) has been reported to be increased in both donor and recipient fetuses; in the former, this may be the consequence of abnormal placental development, and in the latter this may be the result of polyhydramnios-related compression.[15]

Doppler findings in the circulation of the donor fetus (decreased blood flow velocity in both the thoracic aorta and the middle cerebral artery) suggest that this fetus is compromised by severe uteroplacental insufficiency, but with the additional disadvantage imposed by chronic hemorrhage and hypovolemia.[15] In the recipient fetus, there may be a decreased PI in the middle cerebral artery and decreased velocity in the aorta, which may be the consequence of hypervolemia-related congestive heart failure, which worsens with advancing gestation.

Although Doppler abnormalities have been described in TTS, at present the use of these investigations is generally limited, because they are neither useful in the diagnosis of TTS nor do they appear to provide useful prediction of prognosis.

Screening for TTS

Although severe TTS presents in the second trimester, the underlying hemodynamic alterations must begin much earlier in the pregnancy. In a screening study involving 485 twin pregnancies with live fetuses at the 10–14-week scan, the risks of subsequent miscarriage before 24 weeks of gestation and perinatal death after 24 weeks were 2% and 1%, respectively, for dichorionic twins, and 12% and 2%, respectively, for monochorionic twins.[16] It was postulated that the high risk of fetal loss in monochorionic twins could be attributed to the development of TTS.

Early sonographic features that have been examined as possible predictors of subsequent development of TTS are large intertwin disparities in crown–rump length (CRL) and nuchal translucency thickness at the 10–14-week scan[17] and intertwin membrane folding at 15–17 weeks. We have reviewed 69 monochorionic twin pregnancies, diagnosed by ultrasound examination at 10–14 weeks of gestation; at 15–17 weeks, 18 (26%) of the cases demonstrated intertwin membrane folding with large discrepancies in amniotic fluid volume. In 10 of these cases there was subsequent development of severe TTS. In the other eight cases, large discrepancies in amniotic fluid volume and intertwin differences in size persisted throughout pregnancy, but all these cases with moderate TTS resulted in healthy live births without the need for any antenatal intervention. Similarly, the 51 pregnancies with no membrane folding resulted in live births. Large intertwin disparities in fetal CRL at the 10–14-week scan were observed only in the moderate TTS group, whereas intertwin disparities in fetal nuchal translucency thickness were observed both in the moderate and in the severe TTS groups.

Laser coagulation of the communicating placental vessels

Technique

The method of choice for treating severe TTS is endoscopic Nd:YAG laser coagulation of the placental blood vessels that connect the circulations of the two fetuses. De Lia *et al.*[18] described a technique involving general or regional anesthesia in which the endoscope was introduced into the uterus after laparotomy, hysterotomy and the insertion of a purse-string suture to control bleeding and amniotic fluid leakage. This was attempted in 30 twin pregnancies and successful laser coagulation was achieved in 26 of these; 18 of the pregnancies resulted in the delivery of at least one live baby.[19] However, despite the advantages of this approach, the technique has not gained widespread application, presumably because of its invasive nature.

Ville *et al.*[20,21] reported a sonoendoscopic technique performed under local anesthesia for the successful separation of chorioangiopagus twins. Detailed ultrasound examination, including color flow mapping, is first performed to localize the placenta, the intertwin amniotic membrane, the placental insertion of the umbilical cords and the communicating blood vessels on the chorionic plate. The appropriate site of entry on the maternal abdomen is chosen to avoid injury to the placenta or fetuses and to allow access to the suspected area of vascular communications.

Under continuous ultrasound visualization, a rigid 2-mm-diameter fetoscope (field of vision 75°) housed in a 2.7-mm-diameter cannula (KeyMed, Southend, UK) is introduced transabdominally into the amniotic cavity of the recipient twin. A 400-μm-diameter Nd:YAG laser fiber (MBB, Munich, Germany) is then passed down the sidearm of the cannula to 1 cm beyond the tip of the fetoscope. A combination of ultrasonographic and direct vision is used to examine systematically the chorionic plate along the whole length of the intertwin membrane and identify the crossing vessels, which are coagulated by the administration of a total of 1000–4500 J delivered in 3-s shots using an output of 30–50 W at a distance of 1 cm. Subsequently, amniotic fluid is drained through the fetoscope cannula over a period of 10–15 min to obtain subjective normalization of the amniotic fluid volume on ultrasonographic examination. The total procedure usually takes 30–45 min to complete.

Rationale and advantages

The aim of systematic coagulation of all superficial placental vessels that cross or are adjacent to the intertwin amniotic membrane is to interrupt the vascular communications between the circulations of the two fetuses. Arterio–venous anastomoses (which are thought to play a major role in the hemodynamic disturbance underlying feto-fetal transfusion) are found deep in common cotyledons, but their afferent and efferent branches are superficial.[1] Although the intertwin membrane does not necessarily overlie these common cotyledons,[22] coagulation of all crossing vessels will inevitably include the afferent and efferent branches of these anastomoses. In reality, the main problem with endoscopic laser surgery is that coagulation of all placental vessels that cross the intertwin membrane interrupts the vascular supply to more than the common cotyledons and this may account for many cases where the donor twin dies following the procedure. The extent to which we will be able to restrict coagulation to the common cotyledons, and the potential increase in survival without increasing handicap, remain to be determined.

Laser coagulation of the communicating vessels potentially avoids many of the complications associated with severe TTS treated by other means. Cerebral palsy with periventricular leukomalacia is a well-recognized complication of monochorionic twin pregnancies and is usually attributed to vascular accidents following the intrauterine death of one of the fetuses.[23–26] This complication is commonly seen in survivors after amniodrainage or other methods of treatment. Suggested mechanisms include a severe hypotensive episode due to hemorrhage from the survivor into the placenta of the dead fetus, or disseminated intravascular coagulation after the release of thromboplastin from the dead twin. Laser coagulation of communicating vessels should potentially avoid these complications. However, brain damage observed in association with TTS does not occur only when one of the fetuses dies, and in some cases it may be the consequence of intrauterine ischemic-hypoxic brain injury; in the donor, fetus hypoxia may be the consequence of hypovolemia and uteroplacental insufficiency, whereas in the recipient hypoxia may be due to increased blood viscosity and hypervolemia-related congestive heart failure.

Endoscopic laser coagulation was performed in our center on a total of 137 completed pregnancies. In 45 pregnancies both babies survived, in 46 one baby survived and in 46 there were no survivors. There were, therefore, 91 (67%) pregnancies with at least one survivor and the total number of babies that survived was 136 of 274 (50%). In the 136 survivors, regular examinations were carried out and 134 (98%) are developing normally. However, two of them are handicapped or will potentially become handicapped.

Alternative methods of management

Expectant management

In twin pregnancies with presumed TTS, development of acute polyhydramnios at less than 28 weeks of gestation is associated with a high perinatal mortality rate, primarily because of spontaneous abortion or very preterm delivery of growth-retarded babies or babies with hydrops. Saunders *et al.*[5] reviewed 53 such pregnancies in the literature and the fetal survival rate was only 5%. In the few babies that survive with expectant management there is a high incidence of morbidity. Brain damage may occur due to a combination of factors including intrauterine hypoxia and preterm delivery.[5,27] In addition, death of one fetus, usually the donor, may be associated with subsequent death or hypoxic/ischemic sequelae in the cotwin.[23–29]

Medical therapy

Indometacin has been used in an attempt to prevent the onset of preterm delivery, both through its tocolytic properties and through its action in reducing fetal urine production and therefore polyhydramnios. In a study reporting the administration of indometacin in three pregnancies with TTS presenting with polyhydramnios at 20–25 weeks of gestation, one patient delivered at 25 weeks and both the babies died.[30] In each of the other two pregnancies one fetus died within 4 days of the onset of treatment; the pregnancies continued to 30 and 36 weeks, respectively, and the two babies survived but one of the neonates had multicystic encephalomalacia.

Selective fetocide

The poor prognosis of untreated TTS, particularly when one of the fetuses is severely compromised, has led various groups to consider selective fetocide as a method of treatment. The rationale behind this approach is to interrupt TTS and maximize the chances of survival of one of the fetuses, mainly by potentially reducing the chance of severe preterm delivery. Several techniques have been described, including: (1) surgical removal of one fetus by hysterotomy;[31] (2) ultrasound-guided pericardial injection of saline to achieve cardiac tamponade or the intracardiac injection of potassium chloride;[7,26,32–35] (3) ultrasound-guided insertion of thrombogenic coils or fibrin into the heart or the umbilical vein of one of the fetuses[36,37] and (4) ultrasound-guided ligation of one umbilical cord.[38] In 15 pregnancies that were managed by selective fetocide at 20–26 weeks of gestation there were eight survivors (27% of the total).

Serial amniodrainage

The traditional method of treating severe TTS is by serial amniocenteses and drainage of large volumes of amniotic fluid. This treatment presumably prevents the polyhydramnios-mediated risk of spontaneous abortion or very premature delivery.[5,39–41] It is also possible that with advancing gestation and increasing fetoplacental blood volume the relative significance of the hemodynamic effects of placental anastomoses is reduced. In this respect, repeated amniocentesis may, at least in some cases, allow the fetal cardiovascular system to outgrow the deleterious effect of placental anastomoses.[5,6] In addition, amniodrainage reduces amniotic fluid pressure and may relieve the compression of the membranously inserted cord or superficial vessels, which could improve blood flow in the donor fetus.[42]

In studies published before 1992, amniodrainage was associated with survival in 30–40% of cases.[5] Subsequently, six papers from four centers have reported survival of 57–83% of fetuses, and 76–100% of the pregnancies had at least one survivor.[39,40,43–45] It is possible that the marked improvement in survival with serial amniodrainage, compared to previous studies that apparently used the same treatment protocols, presumably reflects differences in the severity of the disease. A major difference, in terms of outcome, between treatment with endoscopic laser and serial amniodrainage may be in the rate of neurological handicap in the survivors. Thus, with endoscopic surgery, both in our first series and in the current extended group, the rate of handicap is less than 5%. In contrast, in all three studies with amniodrainage that reported on rates of neurological handicap, the rate was much higher at 25%, 37% and 18%, respectively.[5,41,45]

Conclusion

Severe TTS complicates 10–15% of monochorionic twin pregnancies and characteristically presents with the oligohydramnios/polyhydramnios sequence in the second trimester. Increased fetal nuchal translucency thickness at 10–14 weeks of gestation and folding of the intertwin membrane at 15–17 weeks may be the first sonographic signs in the development of severe TTS. The most rational method of treating the condition is interruption of the placental vascular anastomoses by endoscopic laser ablation. This therapy is associated with survival of at least one baby in about 70% of pregnancies and more than 95% of survivors are healthy.

REFERENCES

1. Benirschke K, Kim CK. Multiple pregnancy. *N Engl J Med* 1973;228:1276–84.
2. Hrubec Z, Robinette D. The study of human twins in medical research. *N Engl J Med* 1984;310:435–41.
3. Schatz F. Eine besondere art von einseitiger polyhydramnie mit anderseitiger oligohydramnie bei eineiigen zwillingen. *Arch Gynakol* 1882;19:329.
4. Saunders NJ, Snijders RJM, Nicolaides KH. Twin–twin transfusion syndrome in the second trimester is associated with small intertwin hemoglobin differences. *Fetal Diagn Ther* 1991;6:34–6.
5. Saunders NJ, Snijders RJM, Nicolaides KH. Therapeutic amniocentesis in twin–twin transfusion syndrome appearing in the second trimester of pregnancy. *Am J Obstet Gynecol* 1992;166:820–4.

6. Rosen D, Rabinowitz R, Beyth Y, *et al*. Fetal urine production in normal twins and in twins with acute polyhydramnios. *Fetal Diagn Ther* 1990;5:57–60.
7. Weiner CP, Ludomirski A. Diagnosis, pathophysiology and treatment of chronic twin-to-twin transfusion syndrome. *Fetal Diagn Ther* 1994;9:283–90.
8. Berry SM, Puder KS, Bottoms SF, *et al*. Comparison of intrauterine hematologic and biochemical values between twin pairs with and without stuck twin syndrome. *Am J Obstet Gynecol* 1995; 172:1403–10.
9. Fisk NM, Borrell A, Hubinont C, *et al*. Feto-fetal transfusion syndrome: Do the neonatal criteria apply *in utero*? *Arch Dis Child* 1990;65:657–61.
10. Rausen AR, Seki M, Strauss L. Twin transfusion syndrome. *J Pediatr* 1965;66:613–28.
11. Abraham JM. Character of placentation in twins, as related to hemoglobin levels. *Clin Pediatr Phila* 1969;8:526–30.
12. Tan KL, Tan R, Tan SH, *et al*. The twin transfusion syndrome. Clinical observations on 35 affected pairs. *Clin Pediatr Phila* 1979;18:111–14.
13. Danskin FH, Neilson JP. Twin-to-twin transfusion syndrome: What are appropriate diagnostic criteria? *Am J Obstet Gynecol* 1989;161:365–9.
14. Hecher K, Ville Y, Nicolaides KH. Doppler studies of the fetal circulation in twin–twin transfusion syndrome. *Ultrasound Obstet Gynecol* 1995;5:318–24.
15. Hecher K, Ville Y, Nicolaides KH. Color Doppler ultrasound in the identification of communicating vessels in twin-to-twin transfusion syndrome and acardiac twins. *J Ultrasound Med* 1995; 14:37–40.
16. Sebire NJ, Snijders RJM, Hughes K, *et al*. The hidden mortality of monochorionic twin pregnancies. *Br J Obstet Gynaecol* 1997; 104:1203–7.
17. Sebire NJ, Snijders RJM, Hughes K, *et al*. Screening for trisomy 21 in twin pregnancies by maternal age and fetal nuchal translucency thickness at 10–14 weeks of gestation. *Br J Obstet Gynaecol* 1996;103:999–1003.
18. De Lia JE, Cruikshank DP, Keye WR. Fetoscopic neodymium:YAG laser occlusion of placental vessels in severe twin–twin transfusion syndrome. *Obstet Gynecol* 1990;75:1046–53.
19. De Lia JE, Kuhlmann RS, Harstad TW, *et al*. Fetoscopic laser ablation of placental vessels in severe previable twin–twin transfusion syndrome. *Am J Obstet Gynecol* 1995;172:1202–11.
20. Ville Y, Hecher K, Ogg D, *et al*. Successful outcome after Nd:YAG laser separation of chorioangiopagus twins under sonoendoscopic control. *Ultrasound Obstet Gynecol* 1992;2:429–31.
21. Ville Y, Hyett J, Hecher K, *et al*. Preliminary experience with endoscopic laser surgery for severe twin–twin transfusion syndrome. *N Engl J Med* 1995;332:224–7.
22. De Lia JE, Kuhlmaa RS, Cruikshank DP, *et al*. Placental surgery: A new frontier. *Placenta* 1993;14:477–85.
23. Bendon RW, Siddiqi T. Acute twin-to-twin *in utero* transfusion. *Pediatr Pathol* 1989;9:951–8.
24. Bejar R, Vigliocco G, Gramajo H, *et al*. Antenatal origin of neurologic damage in newborn infants. II. Multiple gestations. *Am J Obstet Gynecol* 1990;162:1230–6.
25. Fusi L, MacOharland P, Fisk N, *et al*. Acute twin–twin transfusion: A possible mechanism for brain-damaged survivors after intrauterine death of a monozygotic twin. *Obstet Gynecol* 1991;78: 517–22.
26. Mahone PR, Sherer DM, Abramowicz JS, *et al*. Twin–twin transfusion syndrome: Rapid development of severe hydrops of the donor following selective fetocide of the hydropic recipient. *Am J Obstet Gynecol* 1993;169:166–8.
27. Larroche JC, Droulle P, Delezoide AL, *et al*. Brain damage in monozygous twins. *Biol Neonate* 1990;57:261–78.
28. Sherer DM, Abramowicz JS, Jaffe R, *et al*. Twin–twin transfusion with abrupt onset of microcephaly in the surviving recipient following spontaneous death of the donor twin. *Am J Obstet Gynecol* 1993;169:85–8.
29. Margono F, Feinkind L, Minkoff HL. Foot necrosis in a surviving fetus associated with twin–twin transfusion syndrome and monochorionic placenta. *Obstet Gynecol* 1992;79:867–9.
30. Jones JM, Sbarra AJ, Dililklo L, *et al*. Indomethacin in severe twin-to-twin transfusion syndrome. *Am J Perinatol* 1993;10:24–6.
31. Urig MA, Simpson GF, Elliott JP, *et al*. Twin–twin transfusion syndrome: The surgical removal of one twin as a treatment option. *Fetal Ther* 1988;3:185–8.
32. Wittmann BK, Farquharson DF, Thomas WDS, *et al*. The role of fetocide in the management of severe twin transfusion syndrome. *Am J Obstet Gynecol* 1986;155:1023–6.
33. Weiner CP. Diagnosis and treatment of twin-to-twin transfusion in the mid-second trimester of pregnancy. *Fetal Ther* 1987;2:71–4.
34. Chescheir NC, Seeds JW. Polyhydramnios and oligohydramnios in twin gestations. *Obstet Gynecol* 1988;71:882–6.
35. Donnenfield AE, Glazerman LR, Cutillo DM, *et al*. Fetal exsanguination following intrauterine angiographic assessment and selective termination of a hydrocephalic, monozygotic co-twin. *Prenat Diagn* 1989;9:301–9.
36. Bebbington MW, Wilson RD, Machan L, *et al*. Selective fetocide in twin transfusion syndrome using ultrasound-guided insertion of thrombogenic coils. *Fetal Diagn Ther* 1995;10:32–6.
37. Dommergues M, Mandelbrot L, Delezoide AL, *et al*. Twin-to-twin transfusion syndrome: Selective fetocide by embolisation of the hydropic fetus. *Fetal Diagn Ther* 1995;10:26–31.
38. Lemery DJ, Vanilieferinghen P, Gasq M, *et al*. Fetal umbilical cord ligation under ultrasound guidance. *Ultrasound Obstet Gynecol* 1994;4:399–401.
39. Elliott JP, Urig MA, Clewell WH. Aggressive therapeutic amniocentesis for treatment of twin–twin transfusion syndrome. *Obstet Gynecol* 1991;77:537–40.
40. Reisner DP, Mahony BS, Petty CN, *et al*. Stuck twin syndrome: Outcome in 37 consecutive cases. *Am J Obstet Gynecol* 1993; 169:991–5.
41. Pinette MG, Pan Y, Pinette SG, *et al*. Treatment of twin–twin transfusion syndrome. *Obstet Gynecol* 1993;82:841–6.
42. Fries MH, Goldstein RB, Kilpatrick SJ, *et al*. The role of velamentous cord insertion in the etiology of twin–twin transfusion syndrome. *Obstet Gynecol* 1993;81:569–74
43. Urig MA, Clewell WH, Elliott JP. Twin–twin transfusion syndrome. *Am J Obstet Gynecol* 1990;163:1522–6.
44. Mahony BS, Petty CN, Nyberg DA, *et al*. The stuck twin phenomenon: Ultrasonographic findings, pregnancy outcome and management with serial amniocentesis. *Am J Obstet Gynecol* 1990;163:1513–22.
45. Trespidi L, Buschetto C, Caravelli E, *et al*. Serial amniocenteses in the management of twin-to-twin transfusion syndrome: When is it valuable? *Fetal Diagn Ther* 1997;12:15–20.

109 Fetal stem-cell and gene therapy

Y. Yaron, A. W. Flake, M. P. Johnson and M. I. Evans

Introduction

Surgery is the logical approach for structural problems. Medicines can replace enzymatic deficiencies, but drugs are by definition essentially palliative approaches. Gene therapy can, in theory, replace the missing substance, but at the same time give the individual the ability to make the substance itself. Gene therapies *per se* have been divided into two categories: classic gene therapy and stem-cell therapy.

Gene therapy

Gene therapy refers to the correction of a disease state by introduction of foreign nucleic acid sequences designed to target the affected tissue. The term 'gene therapy' was brought into use to avoid the negative connotations of the term 'human genetic engineering', first used at the 6th International Congress of Genetics held in 1932 to imply 'the application of genetic principles to animal and plant breeding'.[1] Any form of genetic manipulation, however, was limited to the application of Mendelian principles for breeding until the basics of molecular genetics and techniques for transfection of genes in bacteria became available in the 1960s. Several approaches for gene transfer were investigated before viral vectors were shown to be the first relatively efficient methods for gene transfer into mammalian cells in culture. By the late 1970s, transfection techniques became more efficient as a result of selection systems for cultured cells and recombinant DNA technology. The development of retroviral vectors in the 1980s further improved the efficiency of gene transfer into mammalian cells for the purpose of gene therapy.[1] Finally, the last few years have seen an explosion of experimental studies and clinical trials of gene therapy in almost every discipline of medicine. Many genetic disorders are already manifest in the newborn with irreversible organ damage: hence the attractiveness of *in utero* gene therapy. This section will review some of the advances in gene therapy in general and focus finally on the possible future applications of *in utero* gene therapy.

Therapeutic gene design

Gene therapy may be applied to all diseases that have a clear genetic cause such as the inborn errors of metabolism. There are several approaches to the treatment of different diseases by gene therapy. Not all approaches currently share the same popularity or effectiveness. However, by outlining the different approaches the reader can appreciate the tremendous opportunities that this mode of treatment presents.

Gene replacement therapy

Loss-of-function mutations are responsible for a wide range of human diseases. Such mutations result in absence, reduction or faulty production of an essential protein such as an enzyme or a receptor. Restoring the lost function can, theoretically, be achieved by introducing the normal or wild-type gene in a manner that would facilitate the production of the missing gene-product in the affected tissues at the appropriate timing. This appears to be the most useful approach for *in utero* gene therapy.

Vitally directed enzyme pro-drug therapy – suicide genes

Suicide genes encode novel non-mammalian enzymes that can convert a relatively non-toxic pro-drug into a highly toxic agent. Cells genetically transduced to express such genes essentially commit metabolic suicide in the presence of the appropriate pro-drug. Such metabolic suicide genes may include viral enzymes like the varicella zoster or herpes simplex-derived thymidine kinase (HSV-Tk1) or enzymes of bacterial origin like the *Escherichia coli*-derived cytosine deaminase.[2] Only cells transfected with these enzymes metabolize the pro-drug thereby causing cell death. This approach may be applied to the therapy of cancer or retroviral infections.[3] Insertion of HSV-Tk1 gene confers a sensitivity to the antiherpes drug ganciclovir.

The enzyme phosphorylates the non-toxic ganciclovir to a potent DNA synthesis inhibitor.[4] The selective effect of such suicide genes can further be perfected by employment of a triggering mechanism. This approach takes advantage of the unique production of embryonic and fetal molecules by some tumor types. For example, the alpha-fetoprotein (AFP) gene which is normally expressed in fetal liver is transcriptionally inactive in the adult, but is reactivated in hepatocellular carcinoma. This fact can be utilized in creating a hepatocarcinoma-specific gene-targeting mechanism. A hybrid gene can be constructed consisting of HSV-Tk1 gene under the control of the human AFP gene promoter. This hybrid gene can then be transferred into AFP-producing hepatoma cells. Although the gene construct can transfect many cell types, only AFP-producing cells will express the HSV-Tk1 gene, rendering them increasingly sensitive to ganciclovir treatment.[5] This approach is most commonly used in cancer gene therapy.

Gene suppression therapy

Another approach is the employment of foreign genes to oppose the expression of what are, usually, dominant genes that may cause diseases ranging from cancer to viral infections. This may also be used to oppose the expression of genes that are responsible for genetic diseases that are caused by a mutated protein that assumes an altered function which is responsible for the disease manifestations [i.e., sickling caused by sickle cell hemoglobin (HbS)]. Several strategies have been employed to achieve this goal.

Antisense RNA. With this approach, oligodeoxyribonucleotide sequences (oligos) are designed to target certain key regulatory elements of genes that are implicated in disease states. For example, by binding to promoter regions of certain proto-oncogenes (e.g., c-*myc*) it is possible to block the binding of regulatory molecules that activate the oncogene, thus rendering it inactive.[6] These oligos have the advantage of being relatively short sequences, several-fold smaller than whole genes, making them suitable for transfer by viral vectors.[7]

Ribozymes. It is believed that RNA molecules were, evolutionarily, the first class of molecules that possessed enzymatic activity. Ribozymes are such a class of RNA molecules that can perform catalytic activity in the absence of proteins. Specifically, they hybridize to and cleave target messenger RNA (mRNA) molecules thereby preventing their translation into specific proteins. This approach may have a therapeutic application by targeting ribozymes to specific mRNA of key proteins implicated in disease states.[8]

Gene delivery techniques

With recombinant DNA technology and the ever-increasing number of newly mapped and cloned genes, the construction of therapeutic gene sequences seems to be relatively straightforward, as outlined in the previous section. In contrast, the rate-limiting step towards gene therapy appears to be the development of safe and efficient gene delivery techniques that would bring the therapeutic gene into the target tissue where it is to be expressed. Currently employed techniques include various viral vectors, lipofection, naked plasmid DNA, gene guns, electroporation, multiple injections, ingestion or inhalation and selective organ perfusion. All these are currently in the early stages of investigation and development.

Viral vectors

By far the most widely employed techniques for gene delivery make use of viral vectors. Many protocols use an *ex vivo* approach, whereby cells are removed from the patient, genetically modified and then re-implanted. This approach, however, is both cumbersome and costly, requires high-tech facilities, and most importantly, is limited to cell that can readily be obtained and cultured such as blood cells. This approach cannot be applied to solid tissues and non-dividing cells such as muscle cells or neurons. The *in vivo* approach for gene delivery by viral vectors can greatly facilitate gene therapy protocols of the future, by enabling transfection into non-dividing cells. However, before *in vivo* gene therapy may safely be employed, some significant problems must be overcome. Ideally, therapeutic genes should be exclusively expressed only in the relevant cell type and be free of any untoward effects on healthy cells. Several different types of viral vectors have been employed for gene delivery.

Retroviruses. Retroviruses have two identical single-stranded RNA genomes packaged into a viral particle, composed of a viral-encoded envelope *env* protein which is embedded in a lipid bilayer derived from the host plasma membrane. The viral core consists of virally encoded proteins such as *reverse transcriptase* and *integrase* enzymes that are essential for viral replication and integration of viral DNA into host chromosomes. Because the genome of retroviral vectors is incorporated into the host cell genome, the transgenic cells retain the new genetic information through subsequent cell divisions. Thus, the transgene is relatively stable. Vector titers however are low, require dividing cells for effective transfection to occur and thus are unsuitable for non-dividing cells like neurons or muscle cells.

Adenoviruses. Adenoviral vectors usually do not incorporate their DNA into the genome of the host cell and generally remain within the host cell as episomes. This is of concern since it may limit the longevity of the expressed transgene. However, unlike retroviruses, they do not require actively dividing cell lines and high titers can be generated. Such vectors, therefore, would theoretically be more suitable for targeting non-dividing cells. This is especially true for the treatment of muscle cells, in particular myoblasts, since myoblasts have an abundance of $3\beta,5\beta$-integrin, which is the main component of the internalization receptor for adenoviruses (AVs). This could contribute, among other things, to the relatively high susceptibility of myoblasts to AV infection and AV-mediated gene transduction.[9]

Adeno-associated virus. Adeno-associated viral (AAV) vectors are non-pathogenic, integrating DNA vectors in which all viral genes have been removed and helper virus co-transfection is virtually eliminated. These vectors tend to persist in infected cells for prolonged periods of time, with no significant untoward effect on the host. Like AVs, AAV vectors may also persist in an episomal state. Although AAV vectors may exhibit a relative preference for actively dividing cells, they do not require host-cell proliferation. Thus, AAV is an excellent vector candidate for gene transfer in both *ex vivo* and *in vivo* gene therapy.

Non-viral vectors

Unlike the risks associated with viral transfection, non-viral gene delivery techniques appear to be as safe as conventional pharmaceutical products. Various non-viral vectors are currently being assessed in a variety of experimental studies and clinical trials of gene therapy for a variety of disorders, including cystic fibrosis, cancer and peripheral vascular disease.[10]

Lipofection. In contrast to the stable transfection of cells by some viral vectors, other gene delivery techniques may induce only a transient gene expression, a concept known as 'gene therapeutics'. An example of this approach is lipofection whereby DNA plasmids carrying the therapeutic genes are entrapped in lipid vesicles (liposomes). These liposomes act as vehicles that deliver the gene to the target cells where they are only transiently expressed. This is due to the fact that they do not incorporate into the host genome.[11] This approach is particularly promising in treatment of diseases that are manifested in the epithelial lining of various organs, making them accessible to surface delivery methods. Liposomes can also be introduced into internal organs via selective vasculature catheterization. This approach has been employed for selective delivery of recombinant genes (e.g., HLA-B7 plasmid DNA) to the lungs via the pulmonary vasculature in a patient with pulmonary metastases. The treatments were well tolerated and no adverse respiratory, cardiac, immunological or other organ toxicities were detected.[12]

Receptor-mediated endocytosis. Uptake of the therapeutic DNA by the specific target cells or tissue is a prerequisite for successful implementation of gene therapy. The physiological process of receptor-mediated endocytosis can be exploited to deliver genetic material to specific cell types. This approach uses antibodies or ligands with an affinity to a specific cell-membrane receptor (e.g., transferrin), and are known to undergo endocytosis. These are complexed with the therapeutic gene through a covalently bound polycationic linker molecule (e.g., poly-lysine). The complexes in turn bind to the cell surface receptor and are endocytosed into the cell's endosomal compartment. Certain steps must be taken to avoid degradation of the DNA, and to assist endosomal escape of the DNA into the cytosol where it is to be expressed.[13]

Gene targeting

Once introduced into the target cells, the therapeutic gene may be integrated into the host cell genome or remain as cytoplasmic episomes. Integration of novel DNA into the genome carries the potential of durable gene expression and propagation of the therapeutic gene into daughter cells. However, non-site-specific viral vectors integrate randomly into the host genome. This has the potential risk of disrupting functional genes and is known as insertional mutagenesis. This could result in a loss of gene function, defective regulation and gene expression, or an altered gene product. To overcome this problem, therapeutic genes may be designed in a manner that would ensure their integration into predetermined loci within the genome. This may be achieved by homologous recombination where the therapeutic gene is flanked by DNA sequences homologous to the genomic target locus. This approach takes advantage of the endogenous recombinational machinery of the cell which favors crossing-over between homologous sequences. This results in insertion of the therapeutic gene (if one crossover occurs) or replacement of the genomic sequence with the therapeutic gene (if two crossovers occur).[14] Another potentially effective technique (though still not widely used for gene therapy) is that of site-specific recombination. This approach employs exogenously supplied enzymes that induce recombinations (recombinases) at highly specific sites in the target DNA. Based on the number and orientation of these recombination sites, recombinase activity results in deletions, inversions or gene insertion.[15]

Experimental studies and clinical trials

Adenosine deaminase deficiency

Historically, the adenosine deaminase (ADA) gene was the first to be used in a gene therapy clinical trial aimed at achieving actual medical cure.[16] ADA deficiency is another form of fatal severe combined immunodeficiency disease with profound T-lymphocytopenia. Affected individuals have variable defects of both T- and B-lymphocyte function and greatly increased morbidity and mortality caused by frequent viral and bacterial infection, leading to death in early childhood. Classical treatments include administration of the missing enzyme linked to polyethylene glycol (PEG–ADA), as well as bone marrow transplantation. Despite its severity, the disease is genetically simple, and restoration of a functional ADA gene into the patient's lymphocytes should theoretically result in clinical improvement. In 1990, a clinical trial was initiated using retroviral-mediated transfer of the ADA gene into the T-cells of two ADA-deficient children who did not respond to conventional PEG–ADA administration.[16] Peripheral blood lymphocytes were collected, cultured *ex vivo*, infected with a retroviral vector expressing the ADA complementary DNA (cDNA), and re-infused into the patients. This procedure was repeated monthly for 2 years. Subsequently, both children have been reported to have ADA-positive circulating lymphocytes. One patient had over 50% ADA-positive lymphocytes and a normal immune state. The other patient had only 0.1–1% ADA-positive lymphocytes, but a reportedly good clinical state. Gene treatment ended after 2 years, but integrated vector and ADA gene expression in T-cells persisted.[17,18] Several other teams have tried similar approaches for treating ADA deficiency by gene therapy with varying success.[19,20]

Cystic fibrosis

Cystic fibrosis is an autosomal recessive disease caused by a mutation of the cystic fibrosis transmembrane conductance regulator (CFTR) gene. The CFTR protein is a chloride-ion transporter, regulating transmembrane voltage. Reduced or absent cAMP-mediated chloride transport in epithelial-lined organs is responsible for the clinical manifestations. The disease is characterized mainly by accumulation of mucus in the lung, predisposing it to inflammation. Other affected organs include the gastrointestinal tract and the reproductive system. Studies with experimental animals demonstrate that the human CFTR cDNA could be transferred to the airway epithelium using an adenoviral vector (Ad-CFTR), with expression of the human CFTR gene lasting for at least 6 weeks.[21] The first human trial of gene therapy for cystic fibrosis was initiated in 1993. This clinical trial included four patients with cystic fibrosis who received the adenoviral vector (Ad-CFTR) by instillation to their nasal or bronchial epithelium.[22] Both the CFTR protein and mRNA, undetectable prior to treatment, were observed in about 14% of one patient's epithelium cells, and mRNA alone in another patient for 1 week. However, after 10 days, no expression was found.[22] Liposome-mediated treatment has also been attempted in cystic fibrosis patients. The restoration rate of CFTR activity was only 20%, peaking 3 days post-treatment, and reverting to pre-treatment levels after a week.[23] Hepatobiliary disease is the second most common cause of mortality in patients with cystic fibrosis. In the liver, only the intrahepatic biliary epithelial cells express the CFTR gene. To assess the feasibility of treating the hepatobiliary component of cystic fibrosis, intrahepatic biliary ephithelial cells were isolated from cystic fibrosis patients, immortalized *in vitro*, transfected with an Ad-CFTR vector, and assayed 2–31 days later for CFTR function. Transfected cells showed CFTR function for 31 days post-transfection although the number of responsive cells decreased with time.[24] Present gene-delivery methods do not appear to induce permanent CFTR gene expression, either in lung or in intrahepatic biliary epithelial cells. For gene therapy to be effective in cystic fibrosis, repeated administrations need to be performed. This would obviously limit the use of adenoviral vectors because of their potential to induce an immune response.

Inborn errors of metabolism

Numerous experimental studies have addressed the feasibility of gene therapy for a wide variety of metabolic disorders characterized by lack or complete deficiency of essential enzymes. Most of these studies are still in the early stages of animal model and *in vitro* human cell-culture studies.

Gaucher disease. A common inherited metabolic disorder, this is an excellent candidate for targeted gene therapy using hematopoietic stem cells. The feasibility of introducing the human glucocerebrosidase gene into hematopoietic progenitors with long-term expression using a variety of retroviral vectors has been demonstrated in animal models.[25] Subsequently, it was shown that glucocerebrosidase enzyme expression can be detected in peripheral blood lymphocytes more than 12 months post-transplantation, with a transduction efficiency of up to 95% in hematopoietic stem cells (CD34 +).[26] This provides encouraging data for the future use of gene therapy for this disease.

Phenylketonuria. Classical phenylketonuria is caused by a deficiency of hepatic phenylalanine hydroxylase (PAH), resulting in mental retardation. A recombinant adenoviral vector containing the human PAH cDNA was constructed and administered to a phenylketonuria-animal model: PAH-deficient mice (strain PAHenu2).[27] The hyperphenylalaninemic phenotype was completely normalized within 1 week of treatment; however, the therapeutic effect did not persist. This study indicates that only 10–20% of normal enzymatic activity in the mouse liver is necessary to restore normal serum phenylalanine levels. These results indicate that phenylketonuria has the potential to be corrected by gene therapy once a vector system which allows long-term expression is developed.

Maple syrup urine disease. Maple syrup urine disease (MSUD) is an autosomal recessive disease caused by a deficiency of branched-chain keto acid dehydrogenase, a mitochondrial multienzyme complex responsible for the decarboxylation of leucine, isoleucine and valine.

The complex consists of three subunits (E1, E2 and E3) and mutations in any subunit result in MSUD. No satisfactory treatment for MSUD is currently available.[28] To assess the feasibility of gene therapy for this disease, a retroviral vector containing the human E2 cDNA was used to restore leucine decarboxylation activity in fibroblasts derived from a MSUD patient with a mutation in the E2 subunit. Decarboxylation activity in transduced cells was restored to 93% of the wild-type level. Correct targeting of the expressed wild-type E2 protein to mitochondria was demonstrated by comparing the immunofluorescent pattern of E2 and a mitochondrial marker protein. Stable expression of enzyme activity has been achieved for at least 7 weeks. These results demonstrate the capacity for phenotypic correction of a gene defect whose product is a part of a multienzyme complex.[28]

Metachromatic leukodystrophy. Metachromatic leukodystrophy is an autosomally recessive disease characterized by deficient activity of arylsulfatase A (ASA). This results in progressive accumulation of cerebroside sulfate in oligodendrocytes in the brain causing dysmyelination. An adenoviral vector with the ASA gene has been shown to achieve successful transduction with expression of ASA in primary fibroblasts from metachromatic leukodystrophy patients. In addition, the expressed ASA protein was correctly targeted to lysosomes and its resulting enzymatic activity was shown to be 2.3–5.0 times the activity of normal control cells.[29]

Hematological disorders

These disorders are, at least theoretically, more readily amenable to gene therapy since circulating blood cells can easily be reached for both *ex vivo* and *in vivo* gene therapy. Several studies have addressed hematological disorders as candidates for gene therapy. These include disorders of hemoglobin synthesis and coagulation defects. Mutations at the α-globin locus are a common class of mutations in humans resulting in the various forms of a-thalassemia. Deletion of all four adult α-globin genes results in the perinatal lethal condition manifested by hydrops fetalis. It has been demonstrated that introduction of a human α-globin transgene can ameliorate the severity of the disorder in a mouse thalassemia model, providing hope for gene therapy of this disorder.[30] To be relevant to the human disease, however, this treatment will have to occur prenatally with the affected fetus being treated *in utero*.

Coagulation disorders are also potential candidates for gene therapy. The need to replace deficient coagulation factors with blood-derived products that resulted in human immunodeficiency virus (HIV) infection further underlines the need for safe and effective treatments. Hemophilia B, a model of such coagulation disorders, is characterized by an X-linked deficiency of factor IX. It has previously been suggested that keratinocytes in the skin might provide a suitable target cell for delivery of factor IX to the systemic circulation in patients with hemophilia B. Experiments in transgenic mice demonstrated that human factor IX can be efficiently synthesized in the skin by keratinocytes and secreted across the epidermal basement membrane to reach the systemic circulation where significant levels can be attained.[31]

Neuromuscular disorders

Both muscle and the nervous system are affected by a myriad of genetic disorders that could potentially be treated by gene therapy. They are characterized by relatively inaccessible, non-dividing, terminally differentiated cells. This underscores the need to find efficient and safe gene delivery techniques for these cell types before any success can be achieved. The search for a gene therapy approach for Duchenne's muscular dystrophy and Parkinson's disease provides some insight into the difficulty of this task. Duchenne's muscular dystrophy, a lethal X-linked disorder, is caused by mutations in the dystrophin gene which is an exceptionally large gene (2300 kb, 79 exons) mapped to chromosome region Xp21. A lack of dystrophin results in muscle degeneration leading to progressive weakness and death by the second decade. Duchenne's muscular dystrophy demonstrates the problems associated with somatic gene therapy due to the enormous size of the gene and the large number of target cells that need to be treated. Myoblast transfer therapy and gene therapy have both been proposed as potential treatments for this disorder. Myoblast implantation has had some success in animal models but little, if any, effect on patients with Duchenne's muscular dystrophy.[32] Gene therapy based on the introduction of dystrophin gene-constructs by retroviral or adenoviral vectors has also been successful in animal models.[33] Adenoviral vectors may be a potentially effective delivery system for muscle disease, provided immature muscle cells are abundant in the muscle. This is due to the fact that myoblasts have an abundance of $\beta3,\beta5$-integrin, which is the main component of the internalization receptor for adenoviruses.[9] Unfortunately, the level of $\beta3,\beta5$-integrin is about three times lower in mature myotubes than in myoblast precursors. Another drawback of adenoviruses is that the maximal size of a gene insert is only about 7.5 kb. This is obviously not sufficient to accommodate the whole dystrophin gene, but may be enough to accommodate a dystrophin minigene (6.3 kb) that may confer partial dystrophin activity.[34] Although the minigene encodes a truncated protein, its expression has been shown in a mouse model to protect muscle fibers against the degeneration process that affects the dystrophin-deficient myofibers.[2]

Cancer

An area that sees some of the most concentrated effort towards the implementation of gene therapy is that of cancer. Insight into the mechanisms of cell development and growth regulation within cancer cells has provided researchers with multiple pathways and potential methods for genetic intervention. Different approaches for employing genes and various gene delivery methods have been attempted. Although no ideal 'cure' gene has been identified, there are several potential therapeutic genes that may alter the biological behavior of malignant cells by decreasing their malignant potential or making them sensitive to chemotherapy. With regard to *in utero* gene therapy, there is a growing number of inherited genes that are responsible for familial cancer. An example of early expression of tumor-susceptibility genes is the retinoblastoma gene that may manifest in the first year of life. Potentially, such genes may be targeted *in utero* to prevent their expression by one of the approaches described above.

Ethical issues

Germ-line gene therapy has a sparked a lively ethical discussion concerning both the technical feasibility and the ethical acceptability of human germ-line modification for the prevention of serious disease. It may be argued by some that this is a slippery slope towards the Orwellian concept of 'human genetic engineering', viewing germ-line gene therapy as having a potential for misuse in trait enhancement and 'neo-eugenics', and feeling that this raises troubling ethical concerns.[35] Conversely, others view this as merely the concept of fetal gene therapy, taken a step further.[36] Some suggest that there is merit in continuing the discussion about human germ-line intervention, so that this technique can be carefully compared with alternative strategies for preventing genetic disease.[37] There is definitely a need for development of guidelines for research and clinical practice for the coming years in order to address the ethics, safety, accuracy, cost and overall merit of pre-implantation genetics.[38] This issue is becoming more than a hypothetical one since the advent of pre-implantation genetic diagnosis.

Fetal stem-cell therapy

In utero stem-cell therapy is an important new approach to the treatment of genetic disorders in the fetus. This approach poses several significant advantages over treatment of such conditions in the neonatal period:

(1) In early gestation, the fetal immunological system is immature, and during a critical 'window of opportunity' does not recognize foreign antigens, thus obviating the need for human leukocyte antigen (HLA)-matched donors:

(2) Institution of therapeutic stem cells at an early developmental stage may facilitate their incorporation into tissue-specific 'niches'; thus, immuno-ablative therapy associated with high morbidity and mortality is not necessary;

Table 109.1 Some examples of genetic disorders that may potentially be treated by *in utero* stem-cell therapy

Hemoglobinopathies
Sickle cell anemia
Alpha and beta thalassemia major
Hemophilia
Immunodeficiency diseases
Severe combined immunodeficiency syndrome (SCID)
Chronic granulomatous disease
Agammaglobulinemia
Chediak–Higashi syndrome
Wiskott–Aldrich syndrome
Inborn errors of metabolism
Mucopolysaccharidoses
Krabbe's disease
Adrenal leukodystrophy
Metachromatic leukodystrophy
Niemann–Pick
Gaucher's disease
Neuromuscular disorders
Duchenne's muscular dystrophy
Becker's muscular dystrophy

(3) Establishment of cellular therapy at an early stage may theoretically prevent the pathological processes that cause irreversible damage;

(4) The prenatal exposure to donor antigens induces tolerance, and their recognition as 'self', allowing postnatal cellular therapy from the same donor, if needed.[39]

The conceivable scope of disorders that may potentially be treated by such an approach is tremendous. Obviously, various hematological disorders may be treated with hematopoietic stem cell; defects in liver metabolism and protein production may be treated by hepatocytes; muscular disorders may be amenable to myoblast therapy. Table 109.1 provides a partial list of genetic disorders that may potentially be treated by *in utero* stem-cell therapy.

Hematopoietic fetal stem-cell therapy

Bone marrow transplantation, a well-established therapeutic mode, is based on the observation that engraftment and proliferation of a small number of normal hematopoietic stem cells are sufficient to sustain normal hematopoiesis for a lifetime. This mode of therapy has been used for the reconstitution of bone marrow in patients with hematological malignancies (i.e., leukemia) but also in the treatment of genetic hematological conditions (thalassemias). Despite its widespread success, bone marrow transplantation has several significant limitations:

(1) Scarcity of HLA-compatible donors;
(2) The adverse effects of HLA-mismatch: graft failure and graft-vs.-host disease;
(3) The need for myeloablation to achieve successful engraftment into the bone marrow;
(4) Even with successful engraftment, some of the disease manifestation may have already caused some irreversible damage.

The lack of a suitable donor may mean choosing between two evils: postponing bone marrow transplantation, sometimes to the point where it may be too late, or choosing a partially matched donor, leading to engraftment failure or graft-vs.-host disease. The need for myeloablation requires strict isolation to prevent opportunistic infections.

Theoretically, at least, *in utero* stem-cell therapy overcomes these limitations: there is no need for a matched donor, because early in gestation, exogenous cells manifesting foreign antigens may induce immunological tolerance. Thus, multiple sources of potential donors open up. These may include fetal stem cells, cord-blood stem cells or adult-derived stem cells. With the latter, a designated donor such as an unaffected sibling or parent may be used. This allows postnatal bone marrow transplantation after tolerance to their antigens has been established, obviating the need for an HLA-matched donor. With the maturation of the T-cells, a process of negative selection takes place in the thymus. This results in deletion of T-cell clones that manifest affinity to self-antigens, and preservation of multiple T-cell clones that exhibit affinity to non-self-antigens. Introduction of foreign antigens prior to the period during which this critical process takes place will result in deletion of T-cell clones that display affinity to these foreign antigens. Eventually, the immune system will treat these antigens as 'self'. The critical 'window of opportunity' may be as early as 12–14 weeks of gestation.[40] In immunodeficiency states, however, this window of opportunity may extend even further particularly when T-cell function is abnormal.

Since the immature fetal immune system cannot mount an immune response against foreign antigens, there is a reduced likelihood of rejection. However, graft-vs.-host disease remains a significant problem that requires depleting the donor bone marrow of T-cells. There are likely more available 'niches' in the bone marrow during the fetal period; thus, myeloablation is not necessary for ensuring engraftment. This also prevents the need for isolation and, in any case, the uterine environment is an ideal sterile environment. With the current invasive diagnostic techniques such as amniocentesis and chorionic villus sampling, and the ever-expanding list of disease genes being discovered through the concerted efforts of the Human Genome Project, it is conceivable that many hematologic disorders may prove to be amenable to fetal hematopoietic stem-cell (HSC) therapy. This is further facilitated by recent technical advances in invasive fetal intervention. It is now realistic to perform chorionic villus sampling at 10 weeks' gestation, perform the necessary DNA analysis for diagnosis, and administer fetal HSC therapy at 12–14 weeks. This would allow engraftment and establishment of an adequate reconstitution of normal hematopoiesis during the period leading to delivery. This would also avoid such complications as recurrent infections, the need for multiple transfusions, and growth restriction that often accompany such disorders.

Source of donor cells

Fetal HSCs. Theoretically at least, fetal-derived HSCs may be the best source since they contain a small number of mature T-cells prior to 14 weeks' gestation. This fact eliminates the severe outcome of graft-vs.-host disease, and avoids the need for T-cell depletion, which is both cumbersome and may also adversely influence engraftment success. Other benefits of using fetal-derived HSCs may be attributed to ontologic differences in the capacity for both proliferation and differentiation of fetal vs. adult HSCs.[39] Animal studies have shown that adult-derived HSCs have a limited capacity for self-renewal compared to fetal liver-derived cells[41] and that umbilical cord blood-derived HSCs have increased replating potential compared to those derived from adult bone marrow. Furthermore, the proportion of responding cells decreases with age, when comparing HSCs purified from adult bone marrow, from umbilical cord blood and from fetal liver.[42] Fetal-derived cells appear to have a wider spectrum of lineages that they can express, when compared with adult-derived HSCs.[43] Finally, fetal cells may have better bone marrow homing ability that would improve engraftment success.

Unfortunately, the use of fetal HSCs poses great ethical and technical difficulties. Ethically, the use of normal fetuses through elective terminations of pregnancy as a potential source is likely to meet with widespread opposition. Even if the ethical obstacles were overcome, there is a serious concern regarding the sterility of fetal HSCs obtained through standard terminations of pregnancy.[44] Obviously, the contamination of transplanted HSCs with bacterial, viral or fungal pathogens may have grave consequences for the recipient fetus and/or the mother. Thus, alternative methods for obtaining contamination-free fetal HSCs need to be devised. Another technical problem has to do with the fact that the fetal liver, the rich source of HSCs, can only provide a limited supply of cells. Moreover, once this supply has been exhausted, it is not renewable. This undermines one of the alleged benefits of fetal HSC therapy, namely, the induction of tolerance to the donor cells.

Cord blood HSCs. The use of cord blood as a source for HSCs would certainly pose less of an ethical problem. Cord blood is relatively rich in circulating HSCs and cryopreservation of cord blood for autologous transfusion in the event of developing a hematopoietic malignancy is becoming widespread. Cord blood may be collected in a relatively sterile fashion, thus eliminating some of the concerns regarding possible transmission of infection. However, cord blood has a finite quantity of HSCs and it is not replenishable. Furthermore, unless the cord-blood donor is a known relative, who may become a postnatal bone marrow transplantation donor, there is no benefit gained by induction of tolerance.

Adult HSCs. Currently, adult-derived HSCs appear to be the most practical source for *in utero* fetal HSC therapy. This source would be ethically acceptable, infection-free, and most importantly, provide a readily renewable reservoir of donor cells. Thus, the induction of 'pre-immune' tolerance to donor antigens would allow the repeated administration of postnatal bone marrow transplantation from the same donor to whom tolerance has been obtained, such as a family member. There are, however, some significant limitations to the use of adult-derived HSCs. The presence of mature T-cells in adult bone marrow is responsible for graft-vs.-host disease. Unfortunately, complete depletion of T-cells often results in engraftment failure. Nonetheless, it is becoming technically possible to enrich adult bone marrow with hematogenic progenitors while reducing T-cell content to a level that would be tolerable with respect to graft-vs.-host disease, and still obtain engraftment.[45] Another concern stems from the use of a family member as a potential source of donor cells. In autosomal recessive disorders, the family member (parent or sibling) may be a heterozygous carrier, and the HSCs may not have the full therapeutic potential.

Future developments will most likely focus on the improvement of techniques for enrichment of adult bone marrow, and the discovery of ways in which HSCs can be propagated indefinitely in culture.

Diseases potentially amenable to fetal HSC therapy

The prerequisites for institution of fetal HSC therapy are:

(1) Understanding of the disease pathophysiology;
(2) The ability to perform first-trimester prenatal diagnosis;
(3) Incomplete amelioration by postnatal bone marrow transplantation.

The list of hematopoietic disorders potentially amenable to fetal HSC therapy can be divided into three general categories: hemoglobinopathies, immunodeficiency disorders and inborn errors of metabolism.

Hemoglobinopathies

The most common hemoglobinopathies are sickle cell disease and thalassemia syndromes (alpha and beta). These disorders may theoretically be diagnosed by DNA analysis in the first trimester, given previous knowledge of the specific gene mutations in the carrier parents. They can be ameliorated by postnatal bone marrow transplantation; however, some of the severe manifestations of the disorders may have already occurred by the time of delivery. Moreover, as time goes by in search of a suitable donor, additional organ damage may have occurred. Bone marrow transplantation also carries a risk of severe morbidity and mortality, and has yet to become standard treatment in these disorders. In thalassemias, the disease pathology is due to a lack of alpha or beta hemoglobin chains, and the ensuing anemia and extramedullary hematopoiesis. In sickle cell disease, the anemia is compounded by the tendency for sickling at low oxygen tension, leading to vaso-occlusive episodes. The addition of red blood cells with normal hemoglobin reduces the viscosity of the blood in a dose-dependent fashion. For successful HSC therapy of sickle cell disease, a sufficient amount of HSCs have to be transferred in order to overcome the anemia, but also to significantly alter the ratio of abnormal/normal red blood cells in order to reduce the risk of sickling. Maintaining a high proportion of red blood cells originating from transplanted HSCs may be possible in both disorders due to the longer half-life in the circulation of normal cells compared to abnormal ones.

Immunodeficiency diseases

These include a wide range of disorders with variable modes of inheritance and different molecular causes. Most of these disorders appear to be good candidates for *in utero* HSC therapy. However, those diseases in which a survival benefit exists for normal cells are likely to have the greatest likelihood of success. An example of such a disease is the severe combined immunodeficiency syndrome. More than 50% of these cases are caused by an X-linked recessive mutation of the gene encoding a common component, the cytokine receptor super-family.[46] Affected individuals suffer repeated infections due to T-cell dysfunction and diminished B-cell response. Bone marrow transplantation therapy for severe combined immunodeficiency disease with HLA-matched donors has been successful without myeloablation. This suggests that the normal HSCs have a survival advantage over the abnormal ones.[47] Even if no competitive advantage is expected for the donor HSCs, the partial reconstitution of a normal cell-line may be sufficient to ameliorate some of the clinical manifestations, and at least result in donor-specific tolerance. As predicted, immunodeficiency disorders were the first to be treated successfully with *in utero* HSC therapy, as will be outlined in the section about 'Clinical experience'.

Inborn errors of metabolism

The last group of disorders that may be treated by *in utero* HSCs are inborn errors of metabolism, that are caused by a specific defect of a lysosomal enzyme. This results in the inability to hydrolyze specific substrates, like glycogen, mucopolysaccharides or sphingolipids, which in turn accumulate and cause disease-specific tissue and organ damage. At least in some of these disorders, prenatal administration of HSCs may provide a source for normal mononuclear cells that may differentiate into tissue-specific phagocytes (Kupffer cells in the liver, macrophages in lymphatic organs, and microglia in the brain). The phagocytotic cells can theoretically dispose of the accumulating substances, thereby ameliorating some of the severe disease manifestations. The importance of initiating prenatal therapy is underlined in many of these disorders since severe and irreversible organ damage (especially in the central nervous system) may have already occurred at the time of birth in many of these disorders. In addition to early onset of central nervous system damage in some disorders such as metachromatic leukodystrophy, postnatal maturation of the blood–brain barrier may prevent the access of therapeutic HSCs into the central nervous system postnatally. It is still unclear, however, whether it is feasible to treat severe central nervous system-damaging disorders by supplying *in utero* HSCs for replacement of glial cells. More research using adequate animal models is required.

Animal models of fetal hematopoietic stem-cell therapy

The first evidence for *in utero* induction of immunological tolerance comes from well-known observations in cattle. Dizygotic cattle twins may share interplacental circulation, resulting in a state of hematopoietic chimerism. This leads to permanent tolerance for skin and organ transplantation between such siblings. Flake and coworkers demonstrated that pre-immune transplantation of allogenic fetal liver-derived hematopoietic cells results in long-term, multilineage hematopoietic chimerism in a sheep model.[48] They reported that the success of such treatments declined with increasing gestational age, supporting the concept of a 'window of opportunity' limited by immunological development for successful application of *in utero* HSC transplantation. Zanjani and colleagues also demonstrated that tolerance may be induced to xenogeneic transplantation. This was achieved by *in utero* transfer of human HSC into fetal sheep.[49] Multilineage engraftment was achieved and maintained for several years. Moreover, they were able to obtain multilineage repopulation after retransplantation into a second-generation recipient.[50] This was achieved by isolation of human HSC from a human–sheep hematopoietic chimera model, and performing *in utero* HSC transfer. However, only two of the six recipients demonstrated human HSC engraftment at birth. Nonetheless, this was taken as evidence for the engraftment of 'immortal' HSCs, confirming the potential of *in utero* HSC transplantation for lifelong reconstitution of fetuses with hematopoietic disease.

Clinical experience

There have been only a handful of reported clinical studies of *in utero* HSC therapy. Most cases, however, were unsuccessful either due to suboptimal timing, dose or source of donor cells, or due to graft-vs.-host disease.[51] Nonetheless, a few reports in the last few years have fuelled high expectations of this mode of therapy. The first successful experience has been reported by Touraine.[52] He reported successful treatment of a child with bare lymphocyte syndrome and a child with severe combined immunodeficiency disease using fetal liver-derived HSCs transfused into the umbilical cord. The child with bare lymphocyte syndrome had 10% donor lymphocytes at birth and as many as 26% at 1 year of age. More importantly, this child was free of infection. The child with severe combined immunodeficiency disease had received postnatal cell transplants, making the interpretation of the results of the prenatal treatment more difficult.

Flake and colleagues reported a successful *in utero* HSC treatment of a child diagnosed *in utero* with X-linked severe combined immunodeficiency disease. The source of the HSCs was the unaffected father's bone marrow. The donor bone marrow was enriched for CD34 + cells, and depleted of CD3 + cells. The fetus received three transplants at 16, 17.5 and 18.5 weeks' gestation, by ultrasound-guided intraperitoneal injection. Postnatal documentation of engraftment by several methods confirmed high levels of donor cell engraftment, with 100% of T lymphocytes of donor origin. Serial analyses confirmed persistence of the engraftment with progressive improvement in lymphocyte counts and humoral response, with evidence of specific response to vaccinations.[53]

Myoblast therapy

Another potential use of stem-cell therapy exists for muscular disorders with the transfer of myoblasts, which are the stem-cell precursors of muscle fibers. Duchenne's muscular dystrophy is a paradigm for such disorders. Theoretically, donor myoblasts injected into muscles of affected patients may fuse with host muscle fibers, thus contributing their nuclei, which are potentially capable of replacing the deficient dystrophin. There have been several attempts at postnatal myoblast transfer therapy for Duchenne's muscular dystrophy. Morandi and coworkers performed myoblast transplantation in three Duchenne's muscular dystrophy patients from HLA-matched donors. However, 3 months later, biopsies from the injected muscles failed to demonstrate dystrophin expression by immunocytochemistry and reverse transcriptase-polymerase chain reaction (RT-PCR).[54] Mendell and associates injected donor myoblasts once a month for 6 months into the biceps brachii muscles in 12 boys with Duchenne's muscular dystrophy. Six months after the final myoblast transfer, the presence of dystrophin was assessed with the use of specific antibodies. No significant improvement in muscle strength was noted although in one patient, 10% of muscle fibers expressed donor-derived dystrophin, three other patients had less than 1% donor dystrophin, and the remaining eight patients had none.[55] Miller and co-workers evaluated myoblast implantation in ten boys (aged 5–10 years) with Duchenne's muscular dystrophy. Using RT-PCR, evidence of myoblast survival and dystrophin mRNA expression was obtained in three patients after 1 month and in one patient after 6 months.[56] The lack of success in treatment of Duchenne's muscular dystrophy by postnatal myoblast therapy underscores the value of *in utero* myoblast cell therapy.

Conclusions

Genetic approaches, once thought to be improbable and futuristic, are now reaching reality. Stem-cell therapies are more likely to be clinically applied in the next few years but direct injection of genes will probably have a place within the next decade. It will be incumbent upon the proponents of these therapies to ensure that the ethical arguments are well developed and espoused so that public opinion will welcome such developments.

REFERENCES

1. Wolff JA, Lederberg J. An early history of gene transfer and therapy. *Hum Gene Ther* 1994;5:469–80.
2. Trinh QT, Austin EA, Murray DM, Knick VC, Huber BE. Enzyme/prodrug gene therapy: Comparison of cytosine deaminase/5-fluorocytosine versus thymidine kinase/ganciclovir enzyme/prodrug systems in a human colorectal carcinoma cell line. *Cancer Res* 1995;55:4808–12.
3. Mullen CA. Metabolic suicide genes in gene therapy. *Pharmacol Ther* 1994;63:199–207.
4. Kun LE, Gajjar A, Muhlbauer M, *et al.* Stereotactic injection of herpes simplex thymidine kinase vector producer cells (PA317-G1Tk1SvNa.7) and intravenous ganciclovir for the treatment of progressive or recurrent primary supratentorial pediatric malignant brain tumors. *Hum Gene Ther* 1995;6:1231–55.
5. Ido A, Nakata K, Kato Y, *et al.* Gene therapy for hepatoma cells using a retrovirus vector carrying herpes simplex virus thymidine kinase gene under the control of human alpha-fetoprotein gene promoter. *Cancer Res* 1995;55:3105–9.
6. Janicek MF, Sevin BU, Nguyen HN, Averette HE. Combination anti-gene therapy Targeting c-myc and p53 in ovarian cancer cell lines. *Gynecol Oncol* 1995;59:87–92.
7. Mercola D, Cohen JS. Antisense approaches to cancer gene therapy. *Cancer Gene Ther* 1995;2:47–59.
8. Sullivan SM. Development of ribozymes for gene therapy. *J Invest Dermatol* 1994;103(Suppl 5):85S–9S.
9. Acsadi G, Jani A, Huard J, *et al.* Cultured human myoblasts and myotubes show markedly different transducibility by replication-defective adenovirus recombinants. *Gene Ther* 1994; 1:338–40.
10. Alton EW, Middleton PG, Caplen NJ, *et al.* Non-invasive liposome-mediated gene delivery can correct the ion transport defect in cystic fibrosis mutant mice. *Nature Genet* 1993;5: 135–42.
11. Ledley FD. Non-viral gene therapy. *Curr Opin Biotechnol* 1994; 5:626–36.
12. Nabel EG, Yang Z, Muller D, *et al.* Safety and toxicity of catheter gene delivery to the pulmonary vasculature in a patient with metastatic melanoma. *Hum Gene Ther* 1994;5:1089–94.
13. Phillips SC. Receptor-mediated DNA delivery approaches to human gene therapy. *Biologicals* 1995;23:13–6.
14. Morrow B, Kucherlapati R. Gene targeting in mammalian cells by homologous recombination. *Curr Opin Biotechnol* 1993;4: 577–82.
15. Sauer B. Site-specific recombination: Developments and applications. *Curr Opin Biotechnol* 1994;5:521–7.
16. Culver K, Anderson F, Blaese R. Lymphocyte gene therapy. *Hum Gene Ther* 1991;2:107–9.
17. Blaese RM, Culver KW, Miller AD, *et al.* T lymphocyte-directed gene therapy for ADA-SCID: Initial trial results after 4 years. *Science* 1995;270:475–80.
18. Kohn D, Weinberg KI, Parkman P, *et al.* Gene therapy for neonates with ADA-deficient SCID by retroviral-mediated transfer of the human ADA cDNA into umbilical cord CD34+ cells (abstract). *Blood* 1993;82(Suppl 1):1245.
19. Bordignon C, Notarangelo LD, Nobili N, *et al.* Gene therapy in peripheral blood lymphocytes and bone marrow for ADA-immunodeficient patients. *Science* 1995;270:470–5.
20. Kohn DB, Weinberg KI, Nolta JA, *et al.* Engraftment of gene-modified umbilical cord blood cells in neonates with adenosine deaminase deficiency. *Nature Med* 1995;1:1017–23.
21. Korst RJ, McElvaney NG, Chu CS, *et al.* Gene therapy for the respiratory manifestatians of cystic fibrosis. *Am J Respir Crit Care Med* 1995;151(3, Pt 2):S75–S87.
22. Crystal R, McElvaney M, Rosenfeld M, *et al.* Administration of an adenovirus containing the human CFTR cDNA to the respiratory tract of individuals with cystic fibrosis. *Nature Genet* 1994;8: 42–50.
23. Caplen NJ, Alton EW, Middleton PG, *et al.* Liposome-mediated CFTR gene transfer to the nasal epithelium of patients with cystic fibrosis. *Nature Med* 1995;1:39–46.
24. Grubman SA, Fang SL, Mulberg AE, *et al.* Correction of the cystic fibrosis defect by gene complementation in human intrahepatic biliary epithelial cell lines. *Gastroenterology* 1995;108:584–92.
25. Wei JF, Wei FS, Samulski RJ, Barranger JA. Expression of the human glucocerebrosidase and arylsulfatase A genes in murine and patient primary fibroblasts transduced by an adeno-associated virus vector. *Gene Ther* 1994;1:261–8.
26. Nimgaonkar M, Bahnson A, Kemp A, *et al.* Long-term expression of the glucocerebrosidase gene in mouse and human hematopoietic progenitors. *Leukemia* 1995;9(Suppl 1):S38–S42.
27. Fang B, Eisensmith RC, Li XH, *et al.* Gene therapy for phenylketonuria: Phenotypic correction in a genetically deficient mouse model by adenovirus-mediated hepatic gene transfer. *Gene Ther* 1994;1:247–54.
28. Mueller GM, McKenzie LR, Homanics GE, Watkins SC, Robbins PD, Paul HS. Complementation of defective leucine decarboxylation in fibroblasts from a maple syrup urine disease patient by retrovirus-mediated gene transfer. *Gene Ther* 1995;2:461–8.
29. Ohashi T, Watabe K, Sato Y, Saito I, Barranger JA, Eto Y. Successful transduction of oligodendrocytes and restoration of arylsulfatase A deficiency in metachromatic leukodystrophy fibroblasts using an adenovirus vector. *Gene Ther* 1995;2:443–9.
30. Paszty C, Mohandas N, Stevens ME, *et al.* Lethal alpha-thalassaemia created by gene targeting in mice and its genetic rescue. *Nature Genet* 1995;11:33–9.
31. Alexander MY, Bidichandani SI, Cousins FM, Robinson CJ, Duffie E, Akhurst RJ. Circulating human factor IX produced in keratin-promoter transgenic mice: A feasibility study for gene therapy of haemophilia B. *Hum Mol Genet* 1995;4:993–9.

32. Pagel CN, Morgan JE. Myoblast transfer and gene therapy in muscular dystrophies. *Microsc Res Tech* 1995;30:469–79.
33. Morgan JE. Cell and gene therapy in Duchenne muscular dystrophy. *Hum Gene Ther* 1994;5:165–73.
34. Karpati G, Acsadi G. The principles of gene therapy in Duchenne muscular dystrophy. *Clin Invest Med* 1994;17:499–509.
35. Penticuff J. Ethical issues in genetic therapy. *J Obstet Gynecol Neonat Nurs* 1994;23:498–501.
36. Resnik D. Debunking the slippery slope argument against human germ-line gene therapy. *J Med Philos* 1994;19:23–40.
37. Wivel NA, Walters L. Germ-line gene modification and disease prevention: Some medical and ethical perspectives. *Science* 1993;262:533–8.
38. Pergament E, Bonnicksen A. Preimplantation genetics: A case for prospective action. *Am J Med Genet* 1994;52:151–7.
39. Flake AW, Zanjani ED. Cellular therapy. *Obstet Gynecol Clin North Am* 1997;24:159–77.
40. Blackman M, Kappler J, Marrack P. The role of the T-cell receptor in positive and negative selection of developing T-cells. *Science* 1990;248:1335–42.
41. Fleischman RA, Mintz B. Development of adult bone marrow stem cells in H-2 compatible and noncompatible mouse fetuses. *J Exp Med* 1984;159:159–69.
42. Lansdorp P, Dragowska W, Mayani H. Ontogeny-related changes in proliferative potential of human hematopoietic cells. *J Exp Med* 1993;178:787–91.
43. Ikuta K, Kina T, MacNeil I, *et al.* Developmental switch in thyn-dc lymphocyte maturation potential occurs at the level of hematopoietic stem cells. *Cell* 1990;62:863–74.
44. Rice HE, Hedrick MH, Flake AW, *et al.* Bacterial and fungal contamination of human fetal liver collected trans-vaginally for hematopoietic stem cell transplantation. *Fetal Diagn Ther* 1993; 8:74–8.
45. Srour EF, Zanjani ED, Cometta K, *et al.* Persistence of human multilineage, selfrenewing lymphohematopoietic stem cells in chimeric sheep. *Blood* 1993;82:3333–42.
46. Noguchi M, Yi H, Rosenblatt HM, *et al.* Interleukin-2 receptor gamma chain mutation results in X-linked severe combined immunodeficiency in humans. *Cell* 1993;73:147–57.
47. Buckley RH, Schiff SE, Schiff RI, *et al.* Haploidentical bone marrow stem cell transplantation in human severe combined immunodeficiency [review]. *Sem Hematol* 1993;30:92–104.
48. Flake AW, Harrison MR, Adzick NS, *et al.* Transplantation of fetal hematopoietic stem cells *in utero*: The creation of hematopoietic chimeras. *Science* 1986;233:776–8.
49. Zanjani ED, Pallavicini MG, Ascensao JL, *et al.* Engraftment and long-term expression of human fetal hemopoietic stem cells in sheep following transplantation *in utero*. *J Clin Invest* 1992;89: 1178–88.
50. Zanjani ED, Flake AW, Rice H, *et al.* Long-term repopulating ability of xenogeneic transplanted human fetal liver hematopoietic stem cells in sheep. *J Clin Invest* 1994;93:1051–5.
51. Flake AW, Zanjani ED. *In utero* transplantation of hematopoietic cells. *Crit Rev Oncol Hematol* 1993;15:35–48.
52. Touraine JL. Rationale and results of *in utero* transplants of stem cells in humans. *Bone Marrow Transplant* 1992;1:121–6.
53. Flake AW, Puck JM, Almieda-Porada G, *et al.* Successful *in utero* correction of X-linked recessive severe combined immunodeficiency (X-SCID): Fetal intraperitoneal transplantation of CD34 enriched paternal bone marrow cells (EPPBMC). *N Engl J Med* 1996;335:1806–10.
54. Morandi L, Bernasconi P, Gebbia M, *et al.* Lack of mRNA and dystrophin expression in DMD patients three months after myoblast transfer. *Neuromuscul Disord* 1995;5:291–5.
55. Mendell JR, Kissel JT, Amato AA, *et al.* Myoblast transfer in the treatment of Duchenne's muscular dystrophy [see comments]. *N Engl J Med* 1995;333:832–8.
56. Miller RG, Sharma KR, Pavlath GK, *et al.* Myoblast implantation in Duchenne muscular dystrophy: The San Francisco study. *Muscle Nerve* 1997;20:469–78.

110 Treatment of fetal arrhythmias

S. Maheshwari, J. A. Copel and C. S. Kleinman

Introduction

Technical advances have made it possible to diagnose both structural and functional heart disease prenatally. The developing fetus normally adapts to abnormal flow patterns, and is, therefore, rarely compromised by structural heart disease. In such cases, the major dilemma is whether to continue the pregnancy or not. However, in the case of fetal cardiac rhythm disturbances there are diagnostic, therapeutic and ethical dilemmas due to the potential for *in utero* therapy.

From the diagnostic point of view, in the absence of reliable transabdominal fetal electrocardiography, echocardiography and Doppler ultrasound are used to analyze cardiac rhythm by relating mechanical events to preceding electrical events. However, without an electrocardiogram some diagnoses are almost impossible to make (e.g. Wolff–Parkinson–White syndrome).

In terms of therapy, the pharmacological treatment of *in utero* arrhythmias involves the administration of potent cardiac medications to the mother. The treatment of this 'patient within a patient' therefore involves moral, ethical and even legal considerations. How much maternal risk is appropriate for a given fetal therapy? Can a mother provide informed consent that is free of subconscious coercion to provide potentially lifesaving treatment for her unborn child? Who should represent the unconsenting fetus in these deliberations?

The appropriate management of an arrhythmia requires an understanding of the precise nature, electrophysiologic mechanism and natural history of the arrhythmia, the pharmacology, pharmacokinetics and possible toxicity of the antiarrhythmic agents used in the maternal–fetal unit, and a detailed risk–benefit analysis.[1,2]

Although not all fetuses with sustained arrhythmias develop hydrops fetalis, the potential for this life-threatening complication is present for any fetus with such arrhythmias. Diastolic filling of the fetal ventricle is very dependent on atrial systole, probably due to limited compliance of the fetal myocardium compared to the ventricular myocardium of older children and adults.[3] This intrinsic 'stiffness' of fetal myocardium makes the fetal heart more prone to the deleterious effects of tachycardias, which foreshorten the diastolic filling period. The fetal heart, therefore, behaves as a heart with a limited reserve.[4] These properties of the myocardium and the unique fetal circulatory system, with the two ventricular cavities connected in parallel with one another, explains why hemodynamic compromise leads to elevated right atrial pressure, systemic venous hypertension and, ultimately, to systemic edema and hydrops fetalis.

The management of a fetus with a sustained arrhythmia begins with a risk–benefit analysis that considers whether the fetus has reached pulmonary maturity, and whether there is evidence of hydrops fetalis. If the fetus is mature, the best treatment option may be delivery and postnatal antiarrhythmic treatment, if necessary. If delivery is inadvisable due to prematurity, the presence or absence of hydrops dictates the urgency of treatment. As the mortality rate for severely hydropic infants is high (irrespective of the cause of the hydrops), vigorous attempts at *in utero* therapy are warranted.

In the fetus with sustained tachycardia but without evidence of hydrops, the therapeutic dilemma increases. In this setting, the decision regarding provision of therapy must depend on several considerations, including (1) the potential risk of developing hydrops fetalis, although determining the likelihood of this developing in a given patient may be difficult, or at times impossible; (2) the potential risks of antiarrhythmic therapy to mother and fetus and (3) individual considerations, including the wishes of the parents after an extensive discussion of benefits and risks. Such decisions must respect maternal autonomy and may be influenced by the gestational age of the fetus, and whether fetal viability imparts a limitation on maternal autonomy.

Fetal rhythm analysis and interpretation

When auscultation of the fetal heart reveals an abnormally rapid (> 160 bpm), slow (< 100 bpm) or irregular rate, the clinician is confronted with the task of accurately diagnosing the nature of the arrhythmia. The use of real-time-directed M-mode echocardiography has made this possible.[5,6] Fetal cardiac anatomy

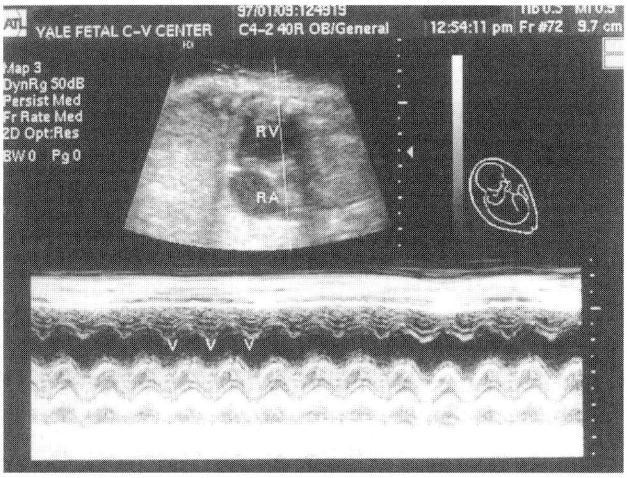

Figure 110.1 Normal M-mode recording. The M-mode cursor sweeps across the ventricle and the atrium. The ventricular wall contraction occurs at the same rate as the atrial wall motion, suggesting a normal 1:1 conduction. RV, right ventricle; RA, right atrium; V, ventricular wall; Λ, atrial wall.

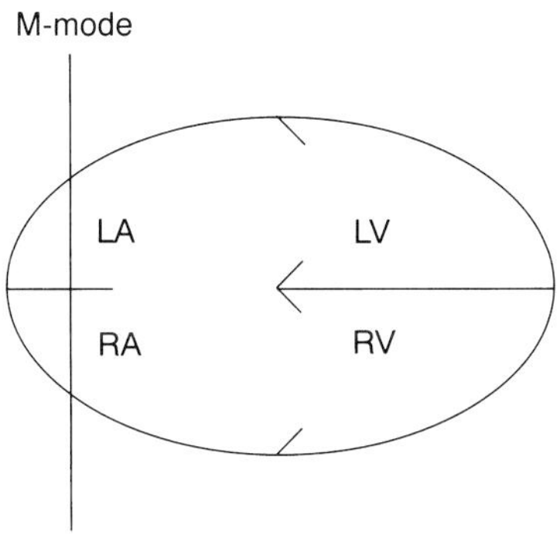

Figure 110.2 The M-mode cursor passing through both atria. Atrial systole is marked by the inward motion of the right and the left atrial walls and motion of the atrial septum primum within the left atrial cavity. LA, left atrium; LV, left ventricle; RA, right atrium; RV, right ventricle.

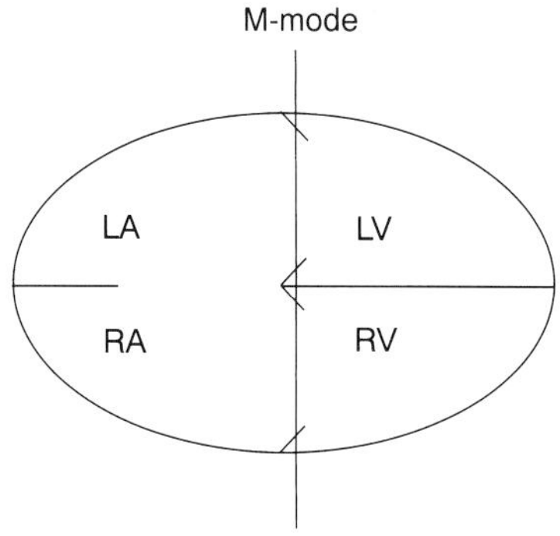

Figure 110.3 The M-mode cursor passing through the leaflets of the AV valves. The leaflets demonstrate an M-shaped motion during ventricular diastole, representing normal biphasic diastolic filling of the ventricles. Initial filling (E wave) is representative of passive early-diastolic filling, whereas atrial systole (active atrial contraction) is represented by the A wave. The onset of ventricular systole begins with inward motion of the ventricular wall. The atrial rate is the A–A interval and the ventricular rate is calculated from the V–V interval. LA, left atrium; LV, left ventricle; RA, right atrium; RV, right ventricle.

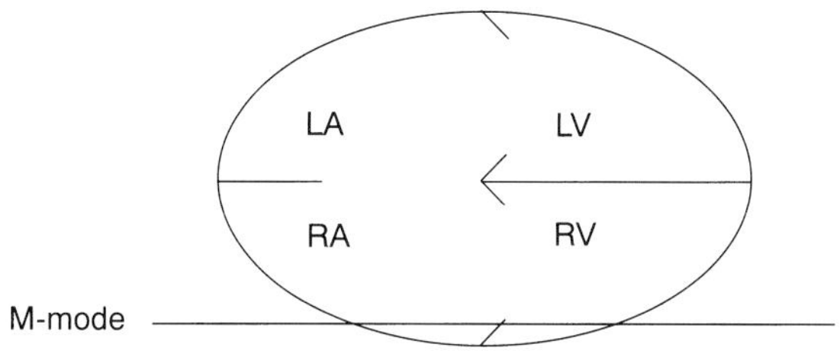

Figure 110.4 Atrial and ventricular systole is manifested by contraction of the atrial and ventricular walls, respectively. LA, left atrium; LV, left ventricle; RA, right atrium; RV, right ventricle.

is first reviewed using two-dimensional imaging. The two-dimensional image is then used to orient the position of the M-mode sampling line. M-mode echocardiographic recordings of cardiac motion against time are made to time mechanical events in the cardiac cycle (Figure 110.1). The assumption is that mechanical events reflect preceding electrical stimulation of the atrium and ventricle. Alternatively, the sample volume of a pulsed Doppler scanner may be placed within the ventricles to provide further information concerning the timing of mechanical events and their influence on ventricular diastolic filling and systolic ejection.[7–10]

For rhythm analysis, atrial and ventricular wall motion may be visualized. Depending on the position of the fetal heart in relation to the ultrasound beam, the M-mode cursor can be directed through a plane that lies perpendicular, parallel or tangential to the interventricular septum (Figures 110.2–110.5).

Fetal antiarrhythmic agents

In this section, we will review the pharmacology and pharmacokinetics of the various medications used to treat *in utero* fetal arrhythmias via either maternal or direct fetal administration. We shall not discuss drug doses in detail because most doses are determined empirically, beginning with standard adult doses, recognizing that the metabolism of many drugs is altered in pregnancy by the changes in maternal blood volume and renal and hepatic metabolism. Doses can then be titrated upward, while closely monitoring the mother and fetus for toxic effects, or until a response is seen. We hospitalize all mothers for introduction of medications so that they can be monitored closely for any untoward effects. They are maintained on continuous telemetry until stable dosing is achieved. Each drug can be used for several different indications and

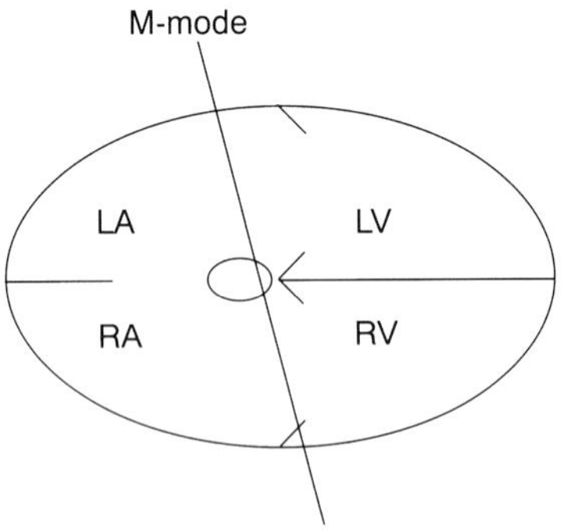

Figure 110.5 Aortic valve motion can be recorded. Ventricular systole is marked by opening of the aortic valve leaflets and/or ventricular wall contraction, whereas atrial activity is represented by atrial wall contraction. LA, left atrium; LV, left ventricle; RA, right atrium; RV, right ventricle.

this will be further considered in the section on specific fetal arrhythmias.

The antiarrhythmic agents have traditionally been classified into four groups. Class I agents act chiefly by inhibiting the fast sodium channels: class IA agents include quinidine, procainamide and disopyramide; class IB agents include lidocaine and mexiletine and class IC agents include flecainide and propafenone. Class II agents act by β-blockade (e.g. propranolol). Class III agents act by a combination of electrophysiologic mechanisms and include amiodarone and sotalol. Class IV agents are the calcium-channel blockers, such as verapamil.

Digoxin

Although digoxin is not included in the preceding classification of antiarrhythmic agents, it is the mainstay of fetal therapy. It remains the drug of first choice in the treatment of *in utero* supraventricular tachycardia (SVT).

Mechanism of action

Digoxin inhibits the Na/K–ATPase pump. This leads to an increase in intracellular sodium, which in turn promotes calcium influx by the sodium–calcium exchange mechanism. The increased cytosolic calcium ion concentration leads to enhanced myocardial contractility. This effect may be useful in treating the congestive heart failure (CHF) presumed to occur secondary to the tachyarrhythmia.

Digoxin also causes parasympathetic activation, resulting in sinus slowing and atrioventricular (AV) nodal inhibition. This leads to a slowing in AV node conduction and a prolongation of the AV refractory period. This may serve to protect the ventricle against a rapid ventricular rate in the face of a SVT. It also has a potential role in breaking reentrant SVT involving the AV node as a part of the reentry circuit. Sympathetic inhibition via inhibition of sympathetic nerve discharge may play an additional important role in the effects of digoxin in CHF.

Pharmacokinetics

Most studies demonstrate that maternal and fetal serum levels of digoxin are similar, although the ratio of fetal to maternal levels may vary from 0.6 to 1.0. The major excretion of digoxin is via the kidneys, so maternal doses have to be decreased in the presence of renal failure. On the other hand, the increased glomerular filtration rate seen in normal pregnancies results in larger doses usually being required in pregnant women.

Clinical experience suggests that transplacental passage of this agent is impaired in the presence of hydrops fetalis,[11] but many patients do respond, with termination of the tachycardia and subsequent resolution of the hydrops. Direct administration of digoxin to the fetus by periodic intramuscular injections has been used when indirect therapy via the mother has failed to control the arrhythmia.[12,13]

A digoxin-like immunoreactive substance (DLIS) may be present in the serum of pregnant women and newborn infants who have not been treated with digoxin. This DLIS appears to be biologically inactive and does not increase the toxicity of digoxin, but its presence makes the maternal, fetal and neonatal digoxin concentrations measured by radioimmunoassay difficult to interpret.[14] During the administration of digoxin we therefore monitor the mother and fetus carefully for clinical evidence of digoxin toxicity, while striving to attain maternal digoxin levels toward the upper end of the therapeutic range (1.5–2 ng/ml). To attain these levels, we have used intravenous digoxin loading (total loading dose of 1 mg) followed by rather large oral maintenance doses (0.50–0.75 mg/day), which can be titrated upward or downward depending on response and toxicity.

Drug interactions

Quinidine, flecainide, verapamil and amiodarone may increase serum digoxin levels by decreasing the renal and non-renal clearance of digoxin. The dose of digoxin therefore needs to be adjusted when any of these medications are used concurrently. Procainamide and sotalol have no pharmacokinetic interactions with digoxin.

Features of digoxin toxicity

Features of toxicity include gastrointestinal problems (anorexia, nausea, vomiting and diarrhea), neurologic problems (malaise, fatigue, confusion, facial pain, insomnia, depression, vertigo and disturbed yellow–green color vision), and cardiac symptoms. These are largely explained by increased vagal tone and include AV block and sinus bradycardia. Digoxin also increases the automaticity of junctional and His–Purkinje tissue. Accelerated atrial, junctional or ventricular arrhythmias may therefore result, and when combined with AV nodal block are highly suggestive of digoxin toxicity. Any 'new' arrhythmia appearing in a patient receiving digoxin should raise the suspicion of digoxin toxicity.

Quinidine

Quinidine is the prototype of class IA agents. It has a wide spectrum of activity against reentrant as well as ectopic atrial and ventricular tachyarrhythmias.

Mechanism of action

Quinidine, like all class I agents, blocks fast inward currents of sodium ions. It slows conduction and increases refractoriness in the retrograde limb of AV nodal tachycardias and over accessory pathways. It also has a vagolytic effect and inhibits muscarinic receptors. This can lead to sinus tachycardia or an increased ventricular rate in atrial flutter–fibrillation.

Pharmacokinetics

Quinidine is primarily metabolized by hydroxylation in the liver. Hepatic failure, therefore leads to higher blood levels. The transplacental passage of quinidine is variable. Traditionally, before quinidine is administered, a test dose of 0.2 g is given to check for drug-induced idiosyncratic reactions, including cardiovascular collapse.

Side effects

Quinidine may prolong the QT interval, which can lead to serious arrhythmias including ventricular tachycardia and torsades de pointes. This proarrhythmic effect of quinidine and of other agents in this class (e.g. procainamide and flecainide) must be discussed with parents when informed consent is sought for inclusion of this agent in the treatment regimen.

Quinidine excess is best prevented by serial measurements of QRS duration and QT interval on the electrocardiogram. If the maternal QRS duration widens by 50%, or if the total QRS duration exceeds 140 ms, or if QT or QTU prolongation occurs beyond 500 ms, the quinidine dose should either be reduced or its inclusion in therapy reassessed. Unfortunately, these parameters cannot be monitored in the fetus.

Non-cardiac side effects include diarrhea, nausea, headaches, dizziness, angioedema and tinnitus. Hypersensitivity reactions including fever, skin rash, agranulocytosis, thrombocytopenia, hepatitis, hemolytic anemia and lupus erythematosus have occurred. Neonatal thrombocytopenia has been reported with maternal use, and in view of anecdotal reports of retinal damage and intrauterine death with the use of maternal quinidine, we currently use quinidine very rarely.

Drug interactions

Concomitant use of quinidine and digoxin may lead to a twofold or a greater increase in serum digoxin levels. If quinidine is used along with other agents, such as amiodarone or sotalol, there is a much greater propensity for QT prolongation. Such combinations should, therefore, be avoided. Other agents that interact to prolong the QT interval include the macrolide antibiotics (e.g. erythromycin), the antihistamine terfenadine, certain antifungals (e.g. ketoconazole) and other type I antiarrhythmics.

Procainamide

This is another class IA agent, which is generally effective against a wide variety of supraventricular and ventricular arrhythmias, including ventricular tachycardia. Procainamide does not prolong the QT interval to the same extent as quinidine, and therefore has a relatively lower associated incidence of torsades de pointes.

Pharmacokinetics

There is rapid renal elimination (half-life 3.5 h with normal renal function). Unlike quinidine, there is no pharmacokinetic interaction with digoxin.

Side effects

Hypotension is a common side effect with intravenous administration of procainamide. In atrial fibrillation, the ventricular rate may increase as the atrial rate slows down, allowing more frequent AV nodal conduction, so that concomitant digitalization is advisable. Proarrhythmic effects, including torsades de pointes, can occur and may be dose-related, although the incidence is less than with quinidine.

Other side effects include fever and rash (early), and arthralgia, lupus and agranulocytosis (late toxicity).

Although procainamide is included here under medications used for *in utero* therapy, there have only been scattered reports of its use, with varying degrees of success. There have been reports of successful transplacental cardioversion of fetal SVT with procainamide,[15] while others have reported that procainamide is not effective in the treatment of fetal arrhythmias.[12]

Flecainide

Although flecainide continues to be used for life-threatening arrhythmias, it acquired a bad reputation because of its proarrhythmic effects in the Cardiac Arrhythmia Suppression Trial (CAST) study[16,17] of postmyocardial infarction patients.

Mechanism of action

Flecainide inhibits the fast sodium channel, and therefore depresses the upstroke of the cardiac action potential. It also has a marked inhibitory effect on His–Purkinje conduction with QRS widening.

Side effects

Cardiac side effects include aggravation of ventricular arrhythmias and the threat of sudden death (as shown in the CAST study). The proarrhythmic effect of flecainide has created controversy regarding its appropriate use.

When flecainide is used for the treatment of atrial flutter or fibrillation, it can cause a decrease in atrial rate with accelerated AV conduction and ventricular arrhythmias. It should, therefore, be coadministered with digoxin, β-blockers or verapamil to avoid accelerated AV conduction.

Extracardiac side effects are related to the central nervous system (blurred vision, dizziness, headache, nausea, paresthesias, fatigue, tremor and nervousness).

Usage

This potent antiarrhythmic has been used in the treatment of life-threatening arrhythmias of both supraventricular (including Wolff–Parkinson–White syndrome, atrial flutter, atrial fibrillation) and ventricular origin in patients without structural heart disease.

The largest study on the use of maternal flecainide for fetal therapy was by Allan *et al.*,[18] who treated 14 patients with flecainide, of whom 12 responded with termination of the arrhythmia. There was one intrauterine death. The main advantage of flecainide was that the mean time to conversion was about 48 h, and quick control of the rhythm allowed resolution of the hydrops.

Although flecainide is effective in the treatment of fetal arrhythmias,[19] its proarrhythmic effect makes it unsuitable for routine use. Its use should be confined to high-risk patients with life-threatening arrhythmias, which are refractory to treatment with other agents. It should be emphasized that while certain fetal arrhythmias may be potentially life-threatening to the fetus they are not life-threatening to the mother. Therefore, exposing her to potentially toxic medication may not be justifiable.

Propranolol

β-Blocking agents, such as propranolol, have been utilized for the treatment of fetal SVTs. Propranolol is a non-selective β-adrenergic blocker, which slows down AV nodal conduction. It also inhibits atrial ectopic activity and, therefore is useful in the prophylaxis of macro-reentrant SVT by inhibiting the initiating atrial ectopic beats.

Pharmacokinetics

The half-life of propranolol ranges from 1 to 6 h. It is metabolized primarily in the liver. Propranolol readily crosses the placenta, although the degree of transfer is variable. As propranolol has a broad therapeutic index, the maternal dose can generally be increased without untoward maternal effects in efforts to attain therapeutic fetal levels. The starting dose is 60 mg orally every 6 h, with rapid titration to 180–240 mg orally every 6 h.

Side effects

A number of fetal/neonatal adverse effects have been reported following the use of propranolol in pregnancy. These include intrauterine growth retardation (IUGR) (although a confounding factor is that most pregnant women who are prescribed propranolol are hypertensive and this is a risk factor for IUGR), hypoglycemia, bradycardia, respiratory depression at birth (these are the most common side effects), hyperbilirubinemia, hyperirritability, hypocalcemia with convulsions, thrombocytopenia and polycythemia. If propranolol is used for *in utero* therapy, the newborn should be observed for 24–48 h after delivery for any evidence of bradycardia, hypoglycemia or other symptoms of β-blockade.

Amiodarone

Amiodarone is a unique wide-spectrum antiarrhythmic agent manifesting chiefly class III activity but also with powerful class I activity and ancillary class II and class IV activity.

Mechanism of action

Amiodarone lengthens the effective refractory period by prolonging the action potential duration in all cardiac tissues, including any bypass tract that may be present. It also has powerful class I (sodium channel inhibition), class II (β-blockade) and class IV (calcium antagonism) effects. Its class IV effects might explain the bradycardia and AV nodal inhibition associated with its use, and the relatively low incidence of torsades de pointes that is seen.

Pharmacokinetics

Amiodarone undergoes variable and slow gastrointestinal absorption. The main problem associated with its use for *in utero* therapy is its long half-life of 25–110 days, and the serious toxic effects that can occur. Amiodarone is excreted by the skin, the biliary tract and the lacrimal glands.

Side effects

In higher doses, there is an unusual spectrum of toxicity, the most serious being pneumonitis, potentially leading to fatal pulmonary fibrosis.

Amiodarone may inhibit the sinoatrial or AV node, but is generally regarded as a safe drug from the hemodynamic point of view. Although torsades de pointes is relatively rare, it can occur.

Central nervous system problems include proximal muscle weakness, peripheral neuropathy and neural symptoms (headaches, ataxia, tremors, impaired memory, insomnia, dreams).

Amiodarone has a complex effect on the metabolism of thyroid hormones. It contains iodine and shares a structural similarity to thyroxine. It can, therefore, inhibit the peripheral conversion of T4 to T3 with a rise in the serum level of T4 and a fall in the level of T3. In about 3–5% of patients hypo- or hyperthyroidism may develop.

Drug interactions

The most serious interaction is an additive proarrhythmic effect with other drugs prolonging the QT interval, such as class I antiarrhythmic agents and class III agents, including sotalol. Amiodarone may increase quinidine and procainamide levels, and these combinations are therefore not advised.

Although amiodarone is a powerful antiarrhythmic agent and has been used with increasing frequency in children and adults, its appropriateness for *in utero* fetal therapy remains to be clarified. There have been several case reports documenting the successful use of amiodarone for fetal arrhythmias,[20,21] although hypothyroidism in the newborn has been reported and is of serious concern.[22]

Apart from maternal administration of amiodarone, there are reports in the literature of amiodarone injections into the umbilical vein, after maternal therapy with multiple antiarrhythmics, including amiodarone, failed to resolve the fetal arrhythmia.[21] As serious adverse effects attributable to amiodarone have been observed in the newborn, we continue to be cautious about advocating the use of amiodarone for fetal arrhythmias because of the limited data available. If it is used for refractory or life-threatening arrhythmias, it is mandatory to check thyroid function tests in the newborn period and to monitor the mother closely for any possible side effects.

Verapamil

Mechanism of action

Verapamil inhibits the action potential of the AV node, where depolarization is calcium-mediated. It thus inhibits one limb of the reentry circuit, which is believed to underlie most paroxysmal SVTs. Verapamil increases AV block and this explains the reduction in the ventricular rate in atrial flutter and fibrillation. Verapamil also has a negative inotropic effect on the heart and causes arterial dilatation, the combination of which can lead to hypotension and even cardiac arrest.

Drug interactions

Verapamil can interact with digoxin to increase serum digoxin levels. Digoxin doses should therefore be adjusted downward in order to avoid toxicity.

Side effects

Headache, facial flushing, dizziness and constipation can occur. Verapamil has a striking negative inotropic effect. Its use is contraindicated in ventricular tachycardia as it can cause myocardial depression, which may be lethal.

In infants, the use of verapamil is contraindicated as it can cause hypotension and cardiovascular collapse. It is believed that the immature myocardium, with its inherently limited systolic and diastolic reserve, is extremely calcium channel-dependent for contractile force. Administration of a profound calcium channel-blocking agent can have an extremely negative effect on the myocardium of the already stressed immature heart. Although verapamil is used for the treatment of fetal arrhythmias, it should therefore be used with caution, especially in the presence of cardiac failure and myocardial depression.

Adenosine

Adenosine is also a class IV agent that is a potassium channel opener and an indirect calcium antagonist. It inhibits the AV node and prevents reentry of electrical impulses through the AV node. The chief indication for its use is, therefore, narrow complex SVT [AV nodal reentrant tachycardia (AVNRT), AV reentrant tachycardia (AVRT) and Wolff–Parkinson–White syndrome]. Adenosine has no effect on ectopic atrial tachycardia or atrial flutter.

Adenosine is quite effective in breaking reentrant SVT, so it may be considered for inclusion early in the treatment protocol as a therapeutic/diagnostic trial. Should administration of this agent result in even a brief episode of sinus rhythm, one may be reassured regarding the accuracy of the initial electrophysiological diagnosis of the arrhythmia, and further therapy should be focused on the assumption that one is dealing with a reciprocating SVT. Adenosine may also be useful in breaking refractory SVT when transplacental therapy is unsuccessful. In that setting it should be followed by intraumbilical venous digoxin to load the fetus with a long-acting agent.

Pharmacokinetics

Adenosine has an extremely short half-life of 10–30 s. It must, therefore, be delivered directly to the fetal umbilical vein rather than to the mother for transplacental passage. The dosage should be approximately 100–200 μg/kg of estimated fetal dry weight.

Side effects

Side effects include headache, flushing, bronchoconstriction, chest pain and excess sinus or AV nodal inhibition. Since adenosine is given to the fetus rather than to the mother, none of these effects would be expected for the mother, although the electrophysiological side effects may occur in the fetus, especially with excessive dosing.

Tachyarrhythmias

Supraventricular tachycardia

The most common tachyarrhythmias identified in the fetus are SVTs. SVTs may be (1) reentrant (reciprocating), related to a 'circus' movement of electrical activity, (2) automatic (arising in an irritable ectopic focus above the bundle of His) or (3) a manifestation of atrial flutter or fibrillation.

Reentrant tachycardias

In the fetus and neonates, the most common electrical mechanism underlying SVT involves a reentrant or

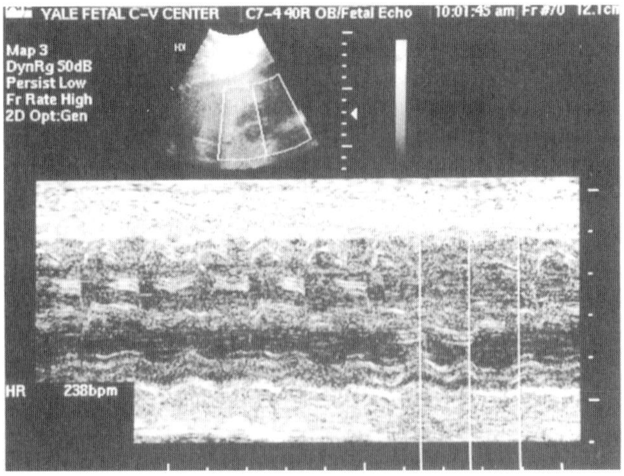

Figure 110.6 M-mode echocardiogram demonstrating a rapid atrial rate of 238 bpm secondary to SVT. The M-mode cursor is at the level of the atria.

reciprocating mechanism. An electrical impulse enters the atrium from the ventricle and develops a circular movement of repeated electrical stimulation that is faster than, and independent of, the normal sinus nodal pacemaker. Because the heart will beat at the rate of the fastest pacemaker, this electrical stimulus drives the heart at an abnormally fast and fixed rate.

The two common kinds of reentrant tachycardias are AVNRT and AVRT. In AVNRT there are two pathways with differing conduction velocities and refractory periods within the AV node itself. The usual inciting mechanism is an extra systole that encounters the fast conducting pathway (with a longer refractory period), while it is still refractory following the preceding normal sinus beat. AV conduction, therefore, occurs down the slow pathway. If the fast pathway has recovered by this point, ventriculo-atrial conduction may occur up the fast pathway to the atrium. This results in establishment of a circus movement of electrical activity.

In AV reentrant tachycardia, there is a discrete accessory conduction pathway that bypasses the usual delay within the AV node. This pathway directly connects atrial to ventricular muscle (as in the 'bundle of Kent' in the Wolff–Parkinson–White syndrome) and serves as the fast link in the reentrant pathway.

Reentrant tachycardia can be recognized by its sudden onset and sudden termination, with both events associated with precipitating extrasystoles. For fetal SVT, the typically encountered heart rate is in the 220–260-bpm range (Figure 110.6).

Therapy

As the AV node is generally a part of the reentrant circuit, any maneuver that slows down AV nodal conduction may abruptly terminate the reentrant tachycardia. An increased vagal tone caused by cord or head compression during uterine contractions has been reported to break SVT. Antiarrhythmic agents that depress conduction and prolong refractory periods in the AV node or accessory conduction tissue can disturb the reentrant circuit and may be useful for the termination of, as well as the prevention of, AVNRT or AVRT. These include the cardiac glycosides (digoxin), the class IA antiarrhythmics (quinidine, procainamide), class IC antiarrhythmics (flecainide), β-blockers (propranolol), the calcium channel-blocking agents (verapamil), and the class III antiarrhythmic agents (amiodarone).

We usually begin maternal therapy with digoxin and then add propranolol, flecainide or other agents, if necessary. It is important to note that the diagnosis of Wolff–Parkinson–White syndrome cannot be made prenatally, because its diagnosis depends on the analysis of an electrocardiogram. The use of digoxin remains controversial in the treatment of Wolff–Parkinson–White syndrome because it can increase conduction over the accessory pathway and lead to a rapid ventricular response in the presence of atrial flutter or fibrillation. Patients who are being considered for transplacental therapy of SVT with digoxin should, therefore, be informed about the potential risks associated with digoxin and the Wolff–Parkinson–White syndrome.

Atrial flutter and fibrillation

These arrhythmias are much rarer than SVT in fetal life. They can be associated with congenital cardiac malformations and can present with hydrops fetalis. In addition, therapeutic control is more difficult than with SVT. Atrial flutter results from a circuit movement of electrical energy within the body of the atrium itself. Although the typical flutter rate in the postnatal period is about 300 bpm, in the fetus monotonous atrial flutter rates of 400–500 bpm typically occur (Figure 110.7). Although postnatally, therapy aimed at decreasing the ventricular response is successful, this has unfortunately not been found to be the case prenatally. This is probably related to the relatively restrictive myocardium of the fetus, with a relatively volume-loaded right heart. Unless the atrial flutter is controlled, atrial contractions would continue against a closed AV valve, resulting in high atrial and systemic venous pressures contributing to the persistence of the hydrops. Thus, with *in utero* therapy of atrial flutter, it is imperative that the therapeutic endpoint be a resumption of 1:1 AV contraction.

Fetal therapy for atrial flutter involves (1) the control of the ventricular response rate with digoxin, verapamil or β-blockers that act at the level of the AV node and (2) the use of a class I antiarrhythmic agents, such as quinidine, procainamide or flecainide, to restore a normal atrial rhythm. Amiodarone may be used as an alternative if class I agents are ineffective or poorly tolerated.

Atrial fibrillation appears to be even rarer in the fetus than atrial flutter. Digoxin therapy can be attempted. If, however, the arrhythmia persists

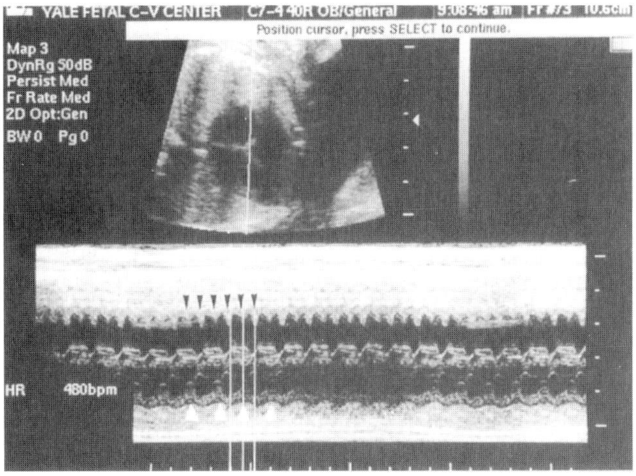

Figure 110.7 Atrial flutter with 2:1 block. Rapid and regular atrial contractions are being measured on the top panel (black arrows), while slower ventricular wall contractions are shown on the lower panel (white arrows). The atrial rate is around 480 bpm, with a ventricular response rate, which is half of that.

despite the control of the ventricular response rate, and if there is associated prematurity and/or hydrops fetalis, a class IA or IC antiarrhythmic agent is another option.

There is an increased mortality rate in patients with atrial flutter and fibrillation, which probably reflects the difficulty encountered in controlling this arrhythmia, in addition to its association with structural heart disease. It should be noted that the association of congenital heart disease with sustained fetal arrhythmias and hydrops fetalis appears to be ominous, imparting an extremely poor prognosis for survival with or without vigorous *in utero* and postnatal therapy.

Ventricular tachycardia

Fetal ventricular tachycardias are much less common than tachycardias of the supraventricular origin and they are also much more difficult to diagnose without an electrocardiogram. Many patients with this tachycardia are initially thought to have SVT. Careful examination of the M-mode echocardiographic tracings and recognition of the presence of AV dissociation (i.e. a lack of 1:1 relationship between atrial and ventricular contractions) are required to make this diagnosis. AV dissociation may also be found in junctional tachycardia, but is not found in AV reentrant tachycardias.

As fetal ventricular tachycardias are uncommon there, is not much literature available on *in utero* therapy. We have followed those fetuses with structurally normal hearts free of hydrops fetalis without any therapy. If there is evidence of right ventricular dilatation in the presence of a ventricular tachycardia and the fetus is previable, it would be reasonable to consider *in utero* therapy. Agents that could potentially be used after considering the risk–benefit ratio include β-blockers, flecainide, and perhaps, amiodarone. Although flecainide has been used with some success in the treatment of this arrhythmia, there are risks with this form of therapy, because *in utero* electrocardiograms are not available, and certain contraindications to the use of flecainide, such as a prolonged QT interval or a prolonged QRS duration, are not available for analysis before therapy is initiated. It is therefore important to inform the parents about possible risks and the limitations of *in utero* diagnosis and therapy for ventricular tachycardia, before treatment is initiated.

Bradydysrhythmias

The detection of a persistent fetal bradycardia (defined as a heart rate <100 bpm) poses an infrequent but difficult management problem. In late pregnancy, the obstetrician's initial response is to suspect fetal distress. Inappropriate premature or operative delivery may follow. It is therefore important to be able to distinguish and diagnose the various causes of bradycardia in the fetus.

Sinus bradycardia is usually of no pathological significance, and implies immaturity of the fetal conduction system if it occurs in the presence of normal cardiac structure with normal heart rate responses to fetal activity. In the absence of hydrops fetalis, moderate sinus bradycardia (heart rates between 90 and 120 bpm) does not appear to be an ominous fetal arrhythmia. It requires no treatment and usually disappears spontaneously toward term.[23]

In atrial bigeminy with block, the bradycardia is related to coupled atrial ectopic beats. The ectopic beats follow too closely on the sinus beats to initiate ventricular contraction and the ventricular rate is thus halved. Electrophysiologically the ectopic beat is so closely coupled to the previous normal sinus beat that it encounters the AV node while it is still refractory, resulting in every second beat being blocked. This is a benign variant of premature atrial contractions and usually resolves quickly.

AV block implies that conduction of sinus or atrial impulses to the ventricle is delayed or interrupted. First-degree AV block is defined as prolongation of the PR interval and is impossible to identify in a fetus because of the absence of a reliable electrocardiogram. Second-degree AV block has been traditionally characterized as Mobitz type 1 or Mobitz type 2. Mobitz type 1 AV block, also referred to as Wenckebach conduction, is characterized by progressive PR prolongation with successive cycles prior to an eventual atrial impulse that fails to conduct to the ventricles. In contrast, Mobitz type 2 AV block refers to abrupt failure of AV conduction for one or more beats and is not preceded by progressive PR prolongation. During second-degree AV block multiple atrial impulses may be blocked for each impulse conducted. Conduction may occur in a regular or irregularly recurring pattern. Regular block can be characterized by the conduction ratio as 2:1, 3:1, 4:1, etc. Mobitz type 2 AV block has

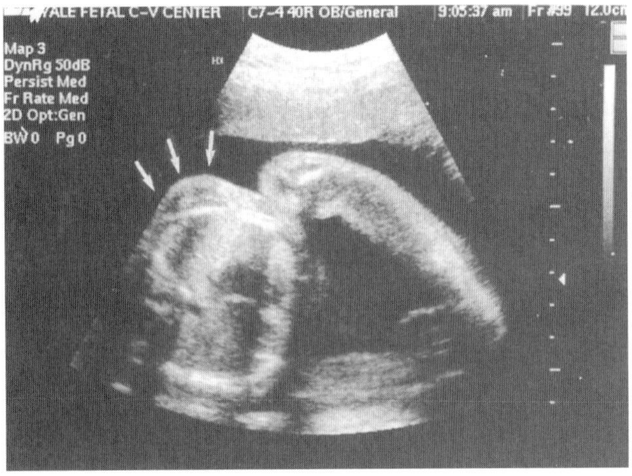

Figure 110.8 Fetal hydrops in a fetus with complete heart block. The arrows indicate the abdominal wall edema.

been reported in fetuses. Some of these may progress to complete heart block. In the presence of Mobitz type 2 AV block, we recommend testing the mother for anti-Ro and anti-La antibodies. If these are positive one may hypothesize that the fetus is developing progressive damage to the AV node on an autoimmune basis, and the use of maternal steroids to ameliorate the inflammatory autoimmune response might be reasonable.[24]

Complete AV block

In third-degree heart block, no atrial impulses conduct to the ventricles. It is diagnosed when there is AV dissociation with a regular atrial rate exceeding a slow ventricular rate.

Etiology

Complete AV block occurs in two settings, characterized by the presence or absence of major congenital and anatomic cardiac defects. Certain forms of congenital heart disease have a high association with complete heart block, particularly AV septal defects and those involving abnormalities in bulboventricular looping, such as L-transposition of the great arteries or left atrial isomerism.[25] About 30% of the newborns with complete heart block have associated cardiac malformations.[26]

Congenital complete AV block in the absence of structural heart disease occurs in 1:15,000 to 1:20,000 live births.[27] An association between maternal connective tissue disease and congenital AV block was first demonstrated in 1977.[28] This has been demonstrated to be secondary to the transplacental passage of maternal IgG antibodies, termed anti-Ro (SSA) and anti-La (SSB). Several reports have demonstrated selective binding of immune complexes to His–Purkinje tissue and to fetal myocardium.[29,30] This has been associated with the presence of inflammatory infiltrates and fibrosis in the region of the AV node and bundle of His. The immune complex binding to fetal myocardium may also account for the clinical finding of myocarditis in some of these fetuses.

Prognosis

Clinical experience has shown that complete heart block in association with structural heart disease can be associated with the development of CHF and hydrops fetalis (Figure 110.8). On the other hand, fetal complete heart block without cardiac malformations only occasionally leads to hydrops fetalis, especially at higher atrial rates. In most cases, once complete AV block develops it is irreversible. The prognosis for the fetus with complete AV block, associated structural heart disease and hydrops fetalis, is very poor. On the other hand, the fetus with complete AV block, an adequate escape rate, and no evidence of CHF can usually be followed to term with serial ultrasounds to monitor for signs of cardiac decompensation. These fetuses tend to have a relatively good prognosis. In a multicenter study,[31] fetal or neonatal death was significantly related to the presence of associated structural heart defects, hydrops, an atrial rate less than 120 bpm and a ventricular rate less than 55 bpm.

In fetuses without CHF, vaginal delivery may be attempted. Assessment of the fetal atrial rate variability is a suitable form of intrapartum monitoring, which can be performed using external Doppler devices. Internal monitoring must not be used as it only reflects the ventricular rate that does not respond to changes in fetal oxygenation or acid–base status. If, however, hydrops fetalis is present, a cesarean section should always be performed since in these cases a vaginal delivery may result in a sudden and dramatic deterioration of the fetal condition.[26]

Management

Although several different therapies have been attempted in the treatment of a fetus with complete heart block with or without myocarditis, so far there has been no universally effective prenatal therapy. Maternal administration of β-agonists to increase fetal ventricular rate, such as ritodrine or terbutaline, has been attempted. This therapy may be associated with some increase in fetal heart rate, although in our experience this does not necessarily translate to an improvement in fetal edema because AV coordination has not been reestablished. In complete heart block, there is a lack of 1:1 AV contraction. This leads to an increase in atrial pressure with a consequent rise in systemic venous pressure causing the hydrops. Unless the 1:1 AV contraction sequence is restored, any therapy aimed at increasing the ventricular response rate may not be successful in helping resolve the hydropic state.

There have been several reports on the use of maternal steroid therapy in the presence of fetal hydrops and congenital complete heart block.[24,32,33] The rationale behind this treatment is that the anti-inflammatory effect of steroids could ameliorate the fetal inflammatory reaction by reducing damage to the fetal conduction tissue and/or myocardial dysfunction caused by myocarditis. Dexamethasone has been used, as it is not metabolized by the placenta and is available to the fetus in an active form. Steroids also hasten lung maturity and their use may be associated with improved survival in premature infants. Although steroids have been shown to be effective in the treatment of the fetal myocarditis, with subsequent resolution of some of the fetal edema and improvement in the degree of block, the complete heart block itself may not necessarily be reversible.

Other prenatal therapies that are of interest, but which are not yet in standard use, include pacing of the fetal ventricle via a maternal transuterine–fetal transthoracic route.[34] At this point, we do not believe that such therapy is warranted unless studies on animal models demonstrate that ventricular pacing by itself may have a positive therapeutic effect.

Experimental therapeutic regimens, including the performance of plasmapheresis to diminish the quantity of maternal antibody that is transmitted to the fetus, have also been described.[35] Although congenital heart block persisted in the neonate described in this report, there were no signs of myocarditis at birth.

Conclusion

Fetal arrhythmias remain difficult, at times, to diagnose accurately and treat, because of the limitations of direct 'patient' accessibility. A close collaboration between obstetricians, perinatologists and pediatric cardiologists is essential to optimize patient management. Ideally, once a fetal arrhythmia is diagnosed, the mothers should be referred to tertiary care centers with specialized teams available for joint consultation and prenatal management of the problem. If the arrhythmia persists despite optimal medical therapy, delivery should preferably be at a center that has trained pediatric cardiologists experienced in dealing with arrhythmias in the neonatal period.

Although much progress has been made in the diagnosis and prenatal management of fetal arrhythmias, controversies persist. Hopefully, with time, our knowledge and experience will become more clearly defined.

REFERENCES

1. Kleinman CS, Copel JA, Weinstein ME, *et al.* *In utero* diagnosis and treatment of fetal supraventricular tachycardia. *Semin Perinatol* 1985;9:113–29.
2. Kleinman CS, Copel JA. Fetal cardiac arrhythmias – Diagnosis and therapy. In Creasy R, Resnick R, eds. *Maternal–Fetal Medicine: Principles and Practice*, 3rd edn. Philadelphia: Saunders, 1993:326–41.
3. Friedman WF. The intrinsic physiological properties of the developing heart. In Friedman WF, Lesch M, Sonnenblick EH, eds. *Neonatal Heart Disease.* New York: Grune and Stratton, 1972:87–111.
4. Kleinman CS, Donnerstein RL. Ultrasonic assessment of cardiac function in the intact human fetus. *J Am Coll Cardiol* 1985;5(Suppl 1):845–945.
5. Shime J, Bertrand M, Hagen-Ansert S, *et al.* Two-dimensional and M-mode echocardiography in the human fetus. *Am J Obstet Gynecol* 1984;148:679–85.
6. DeVore GR, Siassi B, Platt LD. Fetal echocardiography: III. The diagnosis of cardiac arrhythmias using real-time-directed M-mode ultrasound. *Am J Obstet Gynecol* 1983;146:792–9.
7. Kleinman CS, Copel JA. Fetal cardiac dysrhythmias: Diagnosis and therapy. In Chervenak FA, Isaacson GC, Campbell S, eds. *Ultrasound in Obstetrics and Gynecology.* Boston: Little Brown, 1993:939–52.
8. Friedman AH, Copel JA, Kleinman CS. Fetal echocardiography in the diagnosis and management of fetal structural heart disease and arrhythmias. In Reed GB, Claireaux AE, Cockburn F, eds. *Diseases of the Fetus and Newborn*, 2nd edn. London: Chapman and Hall Medical, 1995:955–69.
9. Kleinman CS, Donnerstein RL, Jaffe CC, *et al.* Fetal echocardiography: A tool for evaluation of *in utero* cardiac arrhythmias and monitoring of *in utero* therapy. Analysis of 71 patients. *Am J Cardiogr* 1983;51:237–43.
10. Allan LD, Anderson RH, Sullivan ID, *et al.* Evaluation of fetal arrhythmias by echocardiography. *Br Heart J* 1983;50:240–5.
11. Tounis JS, Granat M. Insufficient transplacental digoxin transfer in severe hydrops fetalis. *Am J Obstet Gynecol* 1987;157:1268–9.
12. Weiner CP, Thompson MIB. Direct treatment of fetal supraventricular tachycardia after failed transplacental therapy. *Am J Obstet Gynecol* 1989;158:570–3.
13. Hallak M, Neerhof MG, Perry R, *et al.* Fetal supraventricular tachycardia and hydrops fetalis: Combined intensive, direct and transplacental therapy. *Obstet Gynecol* 1991;78:523–5.
14. Ward RM. Maternal drug therapy for fetal disorders. *Semin Perinatol* 1992;16:12–20.
15. Dumesic DA, Silverman NH, Tobias S, *et al.* Transplacental cardioversion of fetal supraventricular tachycardia with procainamide. *N Engl J Med* 1982;307:1128–31.
16. CAST Investigators (Cardiac Arrhythmia Suppression Trial). Preliminary report: Effect of encainide and flecainide on mortality in a randomized trial of arrhythmia suppression after myocardial infarction. *N Engl J Med* 1989;321:406–12.
17. Akhtar M, Breithardt G, Camm AJ, Coumel P, *et al.* CAST and beyond. Implications of the cardiac arrhythmia suppression trial. Task force of the working group on arrhythmias of the European Society of Cardiology. *Circulation* 1990;81:1123–7.
18. Allan LD, Chita SK, Sharland GK, *et al.* Flecainide in the treatment of fetal tachycardias. *Br Heart J* 1991;65:45–8.
19. Kofinas AD, Simon NV, Sagel H, *et al.* Treatment of fetal supraventricular tachycardia with flecainide acetate after digoxin failure. *Am J Obstet Gynecol* 1991;165:630–1.
20. Arnoux P, Seyral P, Llurens M, *et al.* Amiodarone and digoxin for refractory fetal tachycardia. *Am J Cardiol* 1987;59:166–7.
21. Gembruch U, Manz M, Bald R, *et al.* Repeated intravascular treatment with amiodarone in a fetus with refractory supraventricular tachycardia and hydrops fetalis. *Am Heart J* 1989;118:1335–8.
22. Laurent M, Betremieux P, Biron Y, *et al.* Neonatal hypothyroidism after treatment by amiodarone during pregnancy. *Am J Cardiol* 1987;60:942.
23. Crawford D, Chapman M, Allan L. The assessment of persistent bradycardia in prenatal life. *Br J Obstet Gynaecol* 1985;92:941–4.
24. Copel JA, Buyon PJ, Kleinman CS. Successful *in utero* therapy of fetal heart block. *Am J Obstet Gynecol* 1995;173:1384–90.
25. Shenker L, Reed LK, Anderson FC, *et al.* Congenital heart block and cardiac anomalies in the absence of maternal connective tissue disease. *Am J Obstet Gynecol* 1987;157:248–53.
26. Gembruch U, Hansmann M, Redel DA, *et al.* Fetal complete heart block: Antenatal diagnosis, significance and management. *Eur J Obstet Gynecol Reprod Biol* 1989;31:9–22.
27. Michaels M, Engle MA. Congenital complete heart block: An international study of the natural history. *Cardiovasc Clin* 1972; 4:85–101.
28. Chameides L, Trex RC, Vetter V, *et al.* Association of maternal systemic lupus erythematosus with congenital complete heart block. *N Engl J Med* 1977;2907:1204–7.

29. Lee AL, Coulter S, Erner S, *et al.* Cardiac immunoglobulin deposition in congenital heart block associated with maternal anti-Ro autoantibodies. *Am J Med* 1987;83:793–6.
30. Litsey ES, Noonan AJ, O'Connor NW, *et al.* Maternal connective tissue disease and congenital heart block. *N Engl J Med* 1985;312: 98–100.
31. Schmidt KG, Ulmer HE, Silverman NH, *et al.* Perinatal outcome of fetal complete atrioventricular block: A multicenter experience. *J Am Coll Cardiol* 1991;17:1360–6.
32. Bierman FZ, Laxmi B, Jaffe I, *et al.* Fetal hydrops and congenital complete heart block: Response to maternal steroid therapy. *J Pediatr* 1988;112:646–8.
33. Buyon JP, Swersky SH, Fox HE, *et al.* Intrauterine therapy for presumptive fetal myocarditis with acquired heart block due to systemic lupus erythematosus. *Arthritis Rheum* 1987;30:44–9.
34. Carpenter RJ Jr, Strasburger JF, Garson A Jr, *et al.* Fetal ventricular pacing for hydrops secondary to complete atrioventricular block. *J Am Coll Cardiol* 1986;8:1434–6.
35. Barclay CS, French MAH, Ross LD, *et al.* Successful pregnancy following steroid therapy and plasma exchange in a woman with anti-Ro (SSA) antibodies. Case report. *Br J Obstet Gynaecol* 1987; 94:369–71.

111 Prenatal diagnosis and therapy: animal studies

J. L. Graf and M. R. Harrison

Introduction

During the past two decades, fetal surgery has become an option for some life-threatening and even non-lethal conditions. The advances in obstetric sonography, diagnostic imaging, and sampling techniques have allowed for the early prenatal diagnosis of some fetal anomalies. Serial prenatal ultrasounds have given us the opportunity to learn the natural history of these anomalies. This prenatal information may influence the timing, location and method of delivery, and, in highly selected cases, provides opportunity for *in utero* fetal surgery for the treatment of life-threatening anomalies.[1]

Fetal surgery is an option only if the following stringent criteria are met: (1) the natural history and pathophysiology of the disease are understood; (2) prenatal diagnosis is accurate and criteria exist to predict which fetuses have a poor enough prognosis to warrant fetal surgery; (3) maternal risk is acceptably low; and (4) in most cases, an animal model exists in which *in utero* therapy has demonstrated efficacy. Clinical studies may provide some of this information, but many of these vital questions cannot be answered without experimental studies.[2] This chapter will focus on animal studies that are used to study fetal therapy.

Animal studies

Since fetal therapy involves risk to both the mother and the fetus, before it can be offered to families the proposed fetal procedure must be technically feasible, safe, and effective in treating the anomaly. These requirements are best met through rigorous experimental animal studies. An animal model of the disease must simulate the natural history, pathophysiology and sequelae of the anomaly that is seen in human fetuses. The model must also allow for fetal intervention and provide objective criteria to determine the efficacy of the intervention. Animal models that have been used to study fetal disease processes and fetal interventions are listed in Table 111.1.

Table 111.1 Animal models for fetal studies

Sheep	Rabbit	Mouse	Monkey
Congenital diaphragmatic hernia	Esophageal ligation	Cleft lip	Congenital diaphragmatic hernia
Biliary atresia	Congenital diaphragmatic hernia	Cellular transplantation	Tocolysis
Cardiac defects	Craniosynostosis	Wound healing	Hydrocephalus
Hydrocephalus	Gastroschisis		Spina bifida
Urinary tract obstruction	Intrauterine growth retardation		Fetoscopy
Bladder exstrophy	Urinary tract obstruction		Fetal vascular access
Amniotic bands	Wound healing		Urinary tract obstruction
Myelomeningocele	Pulmonary hypoplasia		
Craniosynostosis			
Congenital cystic adenomatoid malformation			

In some instances, nature provides an animal model of a disease process that closely mimics that seen in humans. For example, intrauterine growth retardation is seen in fetal rabbits positioned in the middle of the uterine horn (a vascular 'watershed' area).[3] However, most of the disease processes that are seen in human fetuses must be created in the animal model prior to fetal intervention (e.g., creation in fetal lambs of a diaphragmatic hernia that is subsequently repaired later in gestation).[4]

The choice of an animal model takes into consideration several variables. The importance of each variable depends on the focus of the particular study. Variables include accurate time-dating of the pregnancy, seasonal availability, litter number, duration of gestation, fetal size, rate of spontaneous and intervention-induced miscarriage, susceptibility of the gravid uterus to preterm labor, operative considerations (i.e., anesthesia, instruments of appropriate size, venous access, etc.) and cost.

To demonstrate experimental fetal animal studies in different animal models, we shall discuss three models in greater depth:

(1) Congenital diaphragmatic hernia in sheep;
(2) Intrauterine growth retardation in rabbits;
(3) Hydrocephalus in monkeys.

Congenital diaphragmatic hernia in sheep

Congenital diaphragmatic hernia (CDH) is an anatomically simple defect that is correctable after birth by removing the herniated viscera from the chest and repairing the diaphragmatic defect. Unfortunately, the physiologic consequences of CDH are much more extensive and up to 60% of afflicted infants die of pulmonary insufficiency despite optimal postnatal care.[5] The pulmonary hypoplasia appears to be related to *in utero* lung compression by the herniated abdominal viscera. In theory, the *in utero* removal of abdominal viscera from the chest should allow pulmonary development to continue so that pulmonary function is adequate at birth.[6]

To test this theory, a model of CDH was developed in sheep.[7] The sheep has been used as a model for a wide variety of fetal anomalies and interventions. There are several advantages to using sheep as an animal model, including accurate time-dated pregnancies, a long gestation (gestational term 145 days), frequent twinning (provides a control fetus), a large animal to work on, reliable vascular access, stability during anesthesia, the ability to monitor the fetus non-invasively with ultrasound, and a quiescent uterus postintervention. Disadvantages include seasonal pregnancy, cost of long-term care, and a lower phylogenicity. Additionally, the quiescent postoperative uterus is not representative of a human uterus, which is exquisitely sensitive to

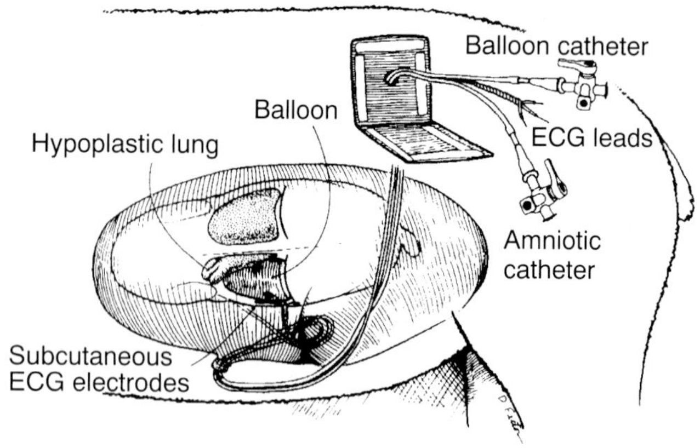

Figure 111.1 Fetal lamb model simulating congenital diaphragmatic hernia. A balloon placed in the left hemithorax is gradually inflated, simulating herniated abdominal viscera compressing the lung. ECG, electrocardiographic.

preterm labor after intervention; therefore, one may not assume that a procedure which is technically feasible in a sheep will be so in a human.

For the model of CDH the following characteristics were required: (1) a space-occupying lesion in the fetal thorax must enlarge through gestation and produce severe pulmonary hypoplasia incompatible with life after birth; (2) simulated postnatal diaphragmatic repair by removal of the space-occupying lesion; and (3) quantitative assessment of the effect of the simulated lesion and its removal on survival at birth and pulmonary vascular and parenchymal development.

All work performed at UCSF was under Institutional Review Board approval. Following 48 h of fasting, time-dated ewes at 100 days of gestation were induced with ketamine (Parke-Davis, Morris Plains, NJ, USA), intubated and maintained on a halothane–oxygen mixture on a Harvard ventilator. Antibiotics were given intravenously and into the amniotic fluid when the uterus was closed. Following a maternal midline laparotomy, a purse-string suture was placed through the uterine wall and hysterotomy performed inside the purse-string. A fetal left thoracotomy was performed and an inflatable silicone rubber balloon inserted into the left chest. Electrocardiographic (ECG) leads were tunneled subcutaneously on the fetus. The ECG leads and inflatable balloon catheter were brought out through the hysterotomy and maternal abdomen and were then tunneled to the ewe's left flank (Figure 111.1).

Twice a week the balloon had saline added for inflation while the fetal heart rate was observed. If fetal bradycardia was seen, the balloon was deflated until the heart rate stabilized, and the saline was then added more gradually and in smaller increments. The total balloon volume was 100 cm^3 at 120 days of gestation and 150 cm^3 at 140 days of gestation. This volume was calculated to be a little less than one half the total lung volume through the last trimester. After cesarean delivery, all lambs were intubated and ventilated. Frequent blood gas measurements were taken by a catheter placed in the umbilical or femoral artery. Lambs underwent deflation of the balloon to simulate postnatal surgical repair. After 2 h support was withdrawn to determine viability. Control lambs were delivered by cesarean section and were not operated on, except for one twin, which had a balloon placed but never inflated. Analysis of the lungs included weight, construction of pressure–volume curves, fixation with barium–gelatin and gluteraldehyde, and microscopic examination.

The results of this study showed that lambs with the inflated balloon catheter had reduced lung weight, flattened pressure–volume loops, and reduction in air space volume and vascular bed volume. Blood gas analysis showed acidosis, hypoxia and hypercarbia. None of the experimental lambs were viable. Simulated postnatal repair by balloon deflation did not improve viability. The histologic studies did not show any striking difference between experimental and control lambs. All of these findings simulate the clinical and pathologic findings seen in human infants with CDH. This model provided valuable knowledge regarding compression as a causative factor of the pulmonary hypoplasia seen in infants with CDH. This knowledge led to refinements in the prenatal diagnosis and management of human fetal diaphragmatic hernia, including consideration of *in utero* correction.

Intrauterine growth retardation in rabbits

One-third of low birth weight babies are small for gestational age secondary to intrauterine growth retardation (IUGR). IUGR is believed to represent fetal undernutrition and in most cases this is because placental insufficiency prevents adequate nutrient and/or oxygen transfer from mother to fetus.[8] Nutritional supplementation of the mother will not benefit the fetus because of insufficient placental function. In theory, fetal enteral feeding could provide fetal nutrition. Amniotic fluid is swallowed and absorbed by the fetus, therefore instillation of nutrients into the amniotic fluid may provide a means to improve fetal nutrition, leading to improvement in IUGR.[9,10]

Rabbits provide a natural model for IUGR.[3] By virtue of the fetal position in the uterine horn, a 'runt' in the litter is usually present. The position of this fetus is in a vascular 'watershed' between the ovarian and vaginal artery, and is consistently the third fetus from the ovary. In contrast, the first fetus from the ovary is in a 'favored' position, having an excellent blood supply. The weight ratio of the runt to the favored fetus is consistently 0.85. For this study there were several advantages to working with rabbits in addition to the natural model of IUGR. These include accurate time-dated pregnancies, enough fetuses to provide littermate controls, uterine quiescence allowing fetal manipulation without inducing abortion, short gestation (gestational term 31 days), inexpensive animal costs, and relative tameness which allows chronic intervention. Disadvantages of working with rabbits include an exquisite sensitivity to anesthetics with a very narrow margin between anesthesia and respiratory arrest, cannibalism of young, and high rates of spontaneous abortion if the rabbit is stressed by the environment (noise, movement, handling, etc.).

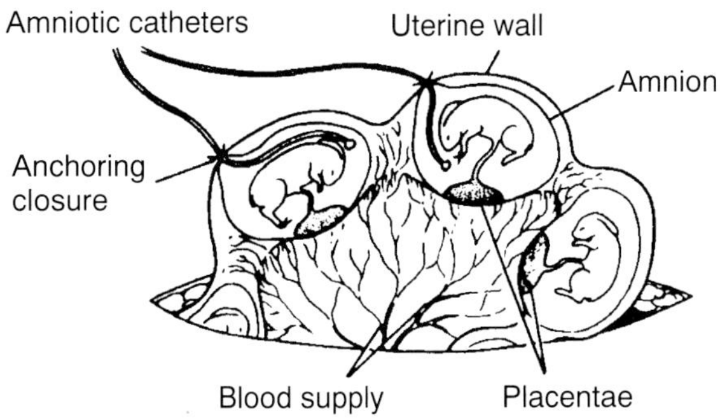

Figure 111.2 Fetal rabbit model of intra-amniotic nutrient infusion.

Time-mated rabbits were shipped to arrive 3–6 days before the planned procedure, to allow adaptation to their new environment. The does were not fasted preoperatively since they rarely vomit. At 23 days of gestation, the does received premedication with ketamine and acepromazine (Fort Dodge Laboratories Inc., Fort Dodge, IO, USA) followed by halothane–oxygen via a face mask. Preoperative antibiotics were given intramuscularly. For this relatively short procedure, intravenous access was not required. The rabbits were placed on a heating pad as they quickly become hypothermic during intra-abdominal procedures. Following a maternal midline laparotomy, the uterus was inspected to determine the litter size. The runt was identified by position in the uterine horn. A purse string was placed through the uterine wall and a hysterotomy made using electrocautery. The fetus was marked for future identification by placing a silk stitch in the fetal foot. A polyethylene catheter was placed into the amniotic cavity and secured in place when the purse-string was tied (Figure 111.2). A second catheter was placed in the amniotic cavity of the fetus in the most favored position. The catheters were led out of the incision and were tunneled subcutaneously to an exit site near the ear where they were attached to a swivel harness that allowed the rabbit to move freely about the cage. The abdominal incision was closed in layers; a subcuticular suture was used to close the maternal skin because rabbits chew out external stitches or staples.

Amniotic 'feeding' was provided to the litter runt by infusion of dextrose, dextrose and amino acid, or a lipid solution. The fetus in the ovarian position had placement of a catheter and infusion of saline. Control animals were fetuses from the opposite horn who had catheters placed but no nutrient or saline infusion. The fetuses were delivered on gestational day 30, and fetal body, liver and brain weights were recorded.

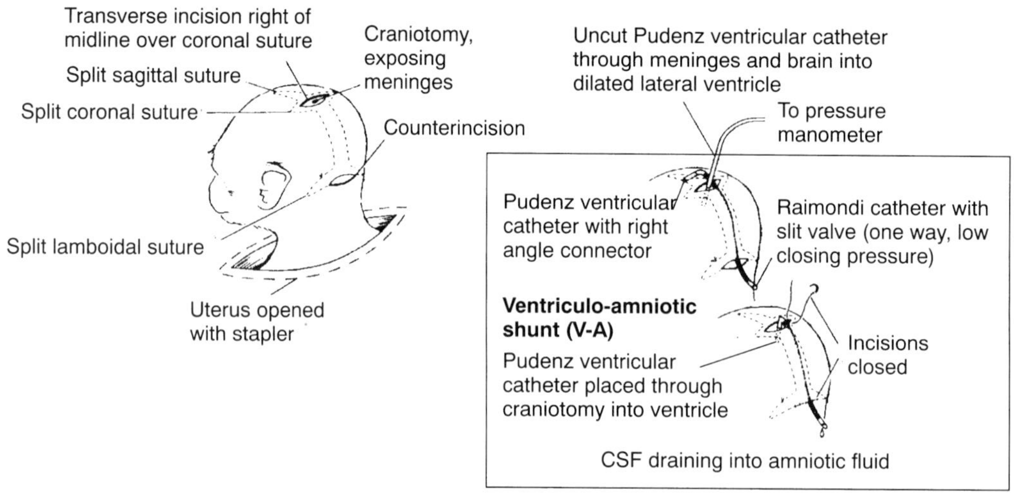

Figure 111.3 Fetal monkey model of ventriculo-amniotic shunting after subarachnoid kaolin injection. CSF, cerebrospinal fluid.

Interestingly, the results of this study showed that none of the nutrient amniotic infusions increased the weight ratio of the runt to the favored fetus. In fact, the fetus who received lipid infusion had a worsening of IUGR and lipid globules present in the fetal lungs. This study suggests that it is perhaps oxygen deficiency that leads to IUGR. The fact that nutrients did not enhance fetal growth suggests that oxygen may be the growth-limiting factor in this natural model of IUGR. Additional useful information was that substances placed into the amniotic fluid may be aspirated into the lungs. The results of this study did not support the use of transamniotic nutrient supplementation as a prenatal treatment for IUGR.[11]

Hydrocephalus in monkeys

Children born with significant hydrocephalus often have neurologic damage and a poor prognosis despite early postnatal treatment.[12] Fetal hydrocephalus may be detected by prenatal ultrasound. Given the poor prognosis after birth and the ability to detect the abnormality prenatally, the question arose as to whether prenatal treatment was possible. The consideration of fetal intervention was based on the assumptions that: (1) obstruction of cerebrospinal fluid (CSF) increases intraventricular pressure and leads to ventriculomegaly and has a deleterious effect on the developing brain; and (2) release of the obstructed CSF would allow for normal brain development. A model of hydrocephalus was developed in the monkey, based on obstruction of CSF flow and allowing for subsequent fetal intervention for CSF drainage.[13,14]

Monkeys are the most rigorous model used to test fetal surgical interventions. The gravid monkey uterus is very sensitive to preterm labor. Maintaining a pregnancy after fetal intervention has proved to be extremely challenging. Successful fetal intervention and maintenance of the pregnancy is perhaps more difficult in monkeys than in humans and thus provides an excellent and demanding model to use as a prerequisite for human fetal intervention.[15]

Rhesus monkeys with time-dated pregnancies received ketamine premedication and were then intubated, and anesthesia was maintained with halothane and nitrous oxide inhalation. In addition to providing anesthesia, halothane acts to relax the uterus. Ventilation was controlled or by hand. Intravenous access was obtained and antibiotics administered. The gravid uterus was exposed through a midline incision and the site of the placental disks determined. After a small hysterotomy was made with electrocautery, the uterus was opened using a stapling device. Kaolin (J.T. Baker Chemical Co., Phillipsburg, NJ, USA) was injected through the atlanto-occipital membrane into the subarachnoid space. The uterus was closed after removal of the uterine staples. Ultrasound was used to evaluate the fetuses postoperatively for the development of hydrocephalus. All fetuses with kaolin properly placed into the subarachnoid space developed ventriculomegaly. The fetuses were born with enlarged heads, diastasis of cranial sutures and bulging fontanels. Microscopic examination of the brains showed changes that closely parallel those seen in afflicted human neonates; there was thinning of the cortical mantle, primarily involving the white matter with preservation of the gray matter. This suggested that the structural changes induced by kaolin injection may be reversible.

The kaolin injection model of obstructive hydrocephalus in the monkey was used to evaluate the efficacy of *in utero* ventricular shunting. Kaolin was injected as described above and 14–21 days later, experimental fetuses underwent ventriculo-amniotic shunting. Non-shunted fetuses with kaolin-induced hydrocephalus served as controls. The shunting procedure is outlined in Figure 111.3. A shunt with a one-way flow valve was placed from the dilated lateral ventricle to the amniotic cavity. The results of this study were the following; ventriculo-amniotic shunting led to an increase in viability, a decrease in ventricular size to normal, and a decrease in head size.

Table 111.2 Life-threatening anomalies that may be amenable to *in utero* intervention

Anomaly	Effect on fetus	Natural history	*In utero* intervention	Animal model
Urinary obstruction	Hydronephrosis	Renal failure	Percutaneous catheter	Rabbit, sheep
	Lung hypoplasia	Pulmonary failure	Vesicostomy, open orfetoscopic	
Congenital cystic adenomatoid malformation	Lung hypoplasia, hydrops	Hydrops, death	Open pulmonary lobectomy	Sheep
Congenital diaphragmatic hernia	Lung hypoplasia	Pulmonary failure	Open complete repair, temporary endoscopic tracheal occlusion	Sheep, rabbit, monkey
Sacrococcygeal teratoma	High output cardiac failure	Hydrops, death	Tumor resection	None
Twin–twin transfusion syndrome	Vascular 'steal' through placenta	Hydrops, death	Fetectomy, cord ligation, laser ablation of communicating vessels	Sheep

However, histopathologic brain injury did not improve after shunting and there were problems with shunt occlusion. Based on these findings, we believe that knowledge of the pathophysiology of congenital hydrocephalus and the impact of fetal decompression on neurologic outcome, and improved efficacy of shunts are required before this procedure can be offered to humans. Of note, there is currently a self-imposed moratorium on fetal intervention for hydrocephalus.

Conclusion

During the past 15 years, with the availability of sophisticated prenatal diagnosis, the rationale and feasibility of prenatal intervention for a number of fetal anomalies has been investigated. Based on animal studies that have shown that *in utero* intervention may be justifiable, technically feasible and efficacious, human fetal intervention has been performed for some life-threatening conditions (Table 111.2). The use of animal studies in the field of fetal surgery has been crucial in our development of successful therapeutic strategies, and has also demonstrated strategies that were unsuccessful and need further investigation. With continuing research efforts and rigorous animal studies the applications for fetal surgical intervention should continue to expand and offer new hope for some life-threatening fetal anomalies.

REFERENCES

1. Harrison MR. Fetal surgery. *Am J Obstet Gynecol* 1996;174:1255–64.
2. Harrison MR, Golbus MS, Filly RA. *The Unborn Patient,* 2nd edn. Philadelphia, PA: W.B. Saunders, 1990.
3. Flake AW, Villa RL, Adzick NS, *et al.* Transamniotic fetal feeding. II: A model of intrauterine growth retardation using the relationship of 'natural runting' to uterine position. *J Pediatr Surg* 1987;22:816–9.
4. Harrison MR, Ross NA, de Lorimier AA. Correction of congenital diaphragmatic hernia *in utero.* III: Development of a successful surgical technique using abdominoplasty to avoid compromise of umbilical blood flow. *J Pediatr Surg* 1981;16:934–42.
5. Harrison MR, Adzick NS, Estes JM, *et al.* A prospective study of the outcome for fetuses with diaphragmatic hernia [see comments]. *J Am Med Assoc* 1994;271:382–4.
6. Harrison MR, Bressack MA, Churg AM, *et al.* Correction of congenital diaphragmatic hernia *in utero.* II: Simulated correction permits fetal lung growth with survival at birth. *Surgery* 1980;88:260–8.
7. Harrison MR, Jester JA, Ross NA. Correction of congenital diaphragmatic hernia *in utero.* I: The model: Intrathoracic balloon produces fatal pulmonary hypoplasia. *Surgery* 1980;88:174–82.
8. Creasy RK, Resnick R. Intrauterine growth retardation. In Milunsky A, Friedman EA, Gluck L, eds. *Advances in Perinatal Medicine.* New York: Plenum Press, 1981;1:117–64.
9. Pitkin RM, Reynolds WA. Fetal ingestion and metabolism of amniotic fluid protein. *Am J Obstet Gynecol* 1975;123:356–63.
10. Char VC, Rudolph AM. Digestion and absorption of carbohydrates by the fetal lamb *in utero. Pediatr Res* 1979;13:1018–23.
11. Flake AW, Villa-Troyer RL, Adzick NS, *et al.* Transamniotic fetal feeding. III: The effect of nutrient infusion on fetal growth retardation. *J Pediatr Surg* 1986;21:481–4.
12. Mealy J, Gilmor RL, Bubb MP. The prognosis of hydrocephalus overt at birth. *J Neurosurg* 1973;39:348–51.
13. Nakayama DK, Harrison MR, Berger MS, *et al.* Correction of congenital hydrocephalus *in utero.* I: The model: Intracisternal kaolin produces hydrocephalus in fetal lambs and rhesus monkeys. *J Pediatr Surg* 1983;18:331–8.
14. Glick PL, Harrison MR, Halks-Miller M, *et al.* Correction of congenital hydrocephalus *in utero.* II: Efficacy of *in utero* shunting. *J Pediatr Surg* 1984;19:870–81.
15. Harrison MR, Anderson J, Rosen MA, *et al.* Fetal surgery in the primate. I: Anesthetic, surgical, and tocolytic management to maximize fetal–neonatal survival. *J Pediatr Surg* 1982;17:115–22.

112 Fetal cells in maternal blood: diagnostic and clinical aspects

W. Holzgreve, R. Zanetti-Dällenbach, C. De Geyter, P. Miny, S. Tercanli, O. Lapaire, I. Hösli and S. Hahn

Introduction

One of the great challenges facing obstetricians and medical geneticists in this century is how to meet the increased demand for prenatal counseling and diagnosis. Due to the inherent, albeit low, risks involved with current invasive procedures for prenatal diagnosis, such as amniocentesis or chorionic villus sampling, the need has been voiced for non-invasive alternatives.[1]

Hence, the past decade has witnessed many concerted, even multinational, efforts to establish a means of performing prenatal diagnosis using risk-free non-invasive methods. The main endeavor in this respect has been the attempt to enrich fetal cells from the circulation of pregnant women, and indeed great strides have been made both in the detection of fetal aneuploidies[2–4] and also in the diagnosis of single-gene disorders.[5,6] As with all major scientific enterprises, this research has also led to unexpected findings, which themselves have become the focus of further interesting scientific questions.

In this chapter, we will highlight the most important developments regarding the diagnostic potential of fetal cells gained from the maternal periphery and how these developments have recently altered our thinking with regard to certain disorders, such as preeclampsia[7] and even autoimmune diseases such as scleroderma.[8]

Eclampsia as the initial evidence for feto–maternal cell exchange

It is more than a century since Schmorl, in 1893, reported his finding that trophoblasts could be detected in the lungs of 14 out of 17 women who had died of eclampsia.[9] This finding should have alerted researchers to the concept of feto–maternal cell exchange, with its possible immunological consequences and the likelihood that the process can be altered under pathological conditions. However, these factors have only recently been appreciated once again. The problem that confronted pioneers in the field, and which needed to be resolved first, was to determine which fetal cell was most suited for genetic analysis.

Despite the confirmation of Schmorl's initial findings in the early 1960s by Attwood and Park,[10] who reported that trophoblasts were frequently found in the lungs of patients who had died from a variety of causes during pregnancy, or immediately thereafter, and were also found to be elevated under conditions of eclampsia, trophoblasts have been found to be unsuitable for fetal cell analysis in the blood of pregnant women. This was partially due to the irregularity of trophoblast transfer into the maternal circulation;[11] although trophoblasts were present in the uterine vein, they were detectable to a much lower extent in the inferior vena cava and not at all in the peripheral circulation. This phenomenon is probably largely due to the trapping and filtering-out of these large multinucleate cells from the circulation in the lungs of pregnant women.[10]

This scarcity has been exacerbated by the apparent inability to specifically enrich these cells due to the general lack of suitable antibodies.[12–14] Furthermore, their heterogeneous genetic nature, arising on the one hand from their multinucleate status, but also from the potential mosaicism existing in the placenta,[15,16] severely restricts their use in a genetic analysis based on fluorescent *in situ* hybridization (FISH). This limitation does not apply to diagnostic approaches based on polymerase chain reaction (PCR), and indeed it was by this means that Hawes *et al.*[17] were able to correctly perform a diagnosis for paternally inherited β-thalassemias. The use of trophoblast cells may, however, be reinstituted in the semi-invasive method of cervical washings, a development that will have to await a thorough assessment of its efficacy and safety before it can be established as a possible alternative.[18]

Fetal lymphocytes and the problem of persistence

Although fetal lymphocytes have been readily identified[19] and enriched by fluorescence-activated cell sorting[20] in blood samples taken from pregnant women, the disadvantage of their use has been their potential longevity. They have been shown to persist for periods of up to 6 years postpartum in the mother's circulation.[21–25] This increases the risk of obtaining cells from previous pregnancies. These results again served to show that fetal cells migrate into the maternal periphery, where they can be enriched and identified, thereby providing the basis for a non-invasive prenatal diagnostic test. However, the results should have led researchers to raise the question of the possible immunological consequence of foreign immune effector cells persisting in a new host. As will be discussed later in this chapter, the answer to this question has recently become the focus of considerable scientific interest.

Evidence that the maternal immune system can react to the presence of semiallogeneic cells is provided by the observation that anti-human leukocyte antibodies (HLA) can be detected within the late-second/early-third trimester of a small percentage of primiparae, with a tendency that these are more frequent in multiparous women.[26,27] Although thought to be partially suppressed, or shifted to a less cytolytic TH2 phenotype,[28] maternal T-cells have been found to react to fetal cells.[29] This raises the question of how these fetal lymphocytes are able to persist for such long periods in a potentially aggressive host.

Prompted by the numerous observations that fetal lymphocytes can persist for several years after delivery in the maternal blood stream,[21,22] Bianchi *et al.*[25] readdressed this question by the fluorescence-activated cell sorting of blood from women currently pregnant, and from those who had previously borne a son, for the presence of hemopoietic stem cells, lymphoid progenitor cells, T- and B-lymphocytes. In this examination, they tested for the presence of male cells by a Y-specific PCR analysis. In the CD34-positive stem-cell-enriched fraction obtained from blood samples of women who were currently pregnant (9.5–19 weeks of gestation and prior to any invasive procedure) this group found that male DNA was detectable in 4 out of the 13 cases where the fetus was female. As extensive precautions against the danger of contamination were taken, it could be concluded that this Y-chromosome-positive material could be the result of male fetal cells persisting from previous pregnancies where these women had borne sons or had terminations. On the other hand, male DNA was only detectable in 13 out of the 19 pregnancies bearing a male fetus. This implies that this population of fetal cells may not be present in the blood of all pregnant women, or if so, then they may sometimes be below the threshold of the detection method employed. When examining blood from women who had previously borne a son and who were not currently pregnant, the observation was made that male DNA was detectable in the samples that had been enriched for lymphoid progenitor cells (CD34+ CD38+) for periods of up to 27 years after the birth of the last son. In the same analysis, male fetal T-lymphocytes were found to persist for a period of up to 6 years. This study indicated that pregnancy might lead to the establishment of a long-term microchimeric state in the mother. One possible explanation for the extended survival of lymphocytic precursor cells, in contrast to mature T-lymphocytes, is the limited amounts of HLA molecules that these progenitors express.

Are feto–maternal microchimera implicated in disease?

If fetal cells can persist for several decades after birth in the blood stream of the mother, one can ask the justifiable question of whether these cells could be involved in the establishment, or at least progression, of diseases, in particular autoimmune disorders. The reasoning for this being that women are more prone to such diseases and that the fetal cells resulting from this microchimeric state would contain immune effector cells of the type proposed to be important for the eliciting of such disorders.[30]

This facet is currently being addressed by several groups, the first report of which was recently published by Nelson *et al.*[8] These studies have focused on the autoimmune disorder scleroderma, an invariably fatal graft vs. host disease, because of the higher predilection of this disease in women, especially in the postchildbearing years. Furthermore, graft vs. host disease has been observed in blood-transfusion patients in instances where the blood was obtained from a HLA homozygous donor,[31] which implies that the microchimerism that can result after such a transfusion may be implicated in the later development of the autoimmune disorder. Hence, it seems feasible that the microchimerism of fetal cells that occurs in women after birth may play a role in the etiology of autoimmune disorders. It was this hypothesis that Nelson *et al.*[8] set out to test. They examined peripheral blood samples that had been taken from a cohort of patients with scleroderma, and where possible, from their healthy sisters and normal controls. As all of these recruited patients had borne at least one son, the authors examined the potential levels of male, and hence fetal, cells in the periphery of these women by a quantitative PCR method for Y-chromosome sequences.[32] In this study, they determined that the levels of male DNA equivalents per given blood sample were considerably higher in the instances of scleroderma than in either of the control populations (a maximum of 61 vs. 5, or a mean of 11.1 vs. 0.38 in 16 ml of whole blood). A further interesting point of this study was the observation that patients with scleroderma more frequently had a major histocompatibility complex (MHC) class II homozygous child than the controls. Although, in contrast, no such relationship was found for MHC class I alleles, these data do provide support for the proposal put forward by Artlett *et al.*,[33] whereby fetal–maternal HLA compatibility would confer susceptibility to scleroderma, by means of a graft vs. host reaction. Such HLA compatibility may also help explain the prolonged survival of potential immune effector cells in the new host, in that while maternal T-cells would normally register paternal alloantigens,[29] their clearing, at least in a murine system, is less rapid under syngeneic conditions.[34] Should this hypothesis be validated, it will be interesting to investigate the possible association of microchimeras with other autoimmune disorders such as systemic lupus erythematosus.

An interesting alternative speculation is that, although scleroderma is rare in males, microchimeras of maternal origin could be involved in the development of this disorder under similar instances of HLA compatibility. Since maternal cells can be found with significant frequency in cord blood samples,[35–37] indicating that the exchange of cells is not unilaterally restricted from fetus to mother, but is bidirectional, further supports this hypothesis.

Erythroblasts and the first successful detection of fetal aneuploidies

The conclusion gained by most researchers in the field to date from work on fetal lymphocytes is that fetal cells do traverse the placental barrier, but that care is needed to be taken to ensure that the cell chosen was of limited lifespan and self-replicative capacity. The cell that fulfills these criteria most effectively, by being easy to enrich and readily identifiable, is the erythroblast, also referred to as the nucleated red blood cell (NRBC). Consequently, most attention has been focused on this cell type.

Evidence for the presence of fetal erythrocytes in the circulation of pregnant women was first obtained by Kleihauer *et al.*,[38] who, by developing a staining procedure specific for fetal hemoglobin, were able to detect fetal erythrocytes under certain conditions such as rhesus incompatibility. These observations were confirmed by Clayton *et al.*[39] in the early 1960s, who also noted an increase in the number of these cells following terminations or amniocentesis. Since no direct genetic proof existed in these studies, such as by the identification of a Y chromosome, that the cells observed were indeed fetal, these reports were at best indicative but not conclusive: a fact that became all the more important when it emerged that the majority of erythroblasts detected in the circulation of pregnant women were not of fetal but rather of maternal origin.[7,40–42]

Evidence for fetal origin of some of these cells was first provided by Bianchi *et al.*[43] in 1990, when they enriched by fluorescence-activated cell sorting for fetal erythroblasts on the basis of their high expression of the transferrin receptor (CD71), and proved their fetal origin by the presence of male DNA. Our group was shortly thereafter able to successfully apply the then new magnetic cell sorting technology[44] to similarly enrich for fetal erythroblasts using micromagnetic beads.[45] The relative ease of these enrichment protocols no doubt facilitated the first correct determinations of fetal aneuploidies by the use of such cells, which were reported in close succession by Elias',[2] Bianchi's[3] and also our[4] groups.

These first optimistic results prompted the National Institute of Child Health and Human Development (NICHD) to extend its Fetal Cell Isolation Study (NIFTY) trial into a phase II clinical investigation. The aim of this trial is to assess the diagnostic efficacy of detecting aneuploid fetal cells in affected pregnancies.

For this study, a cohort of at least 3000 women were recruited who were considered to be at risk of bearing an aneuploid fetus: maternal age of greater than 35 years, indicative serum screening, sonographic abnormalities or previous instance of an aneuploid fetus. Furthermore, only those who were about to undergo an invasive diagnostic procedure were enrolled, as this permits a direct comparison to the experimental laboratory results obtained regarding fetal sex and ploidy. In all instances, informed consent was requested under the understanding that no experimental results were made available to the participants, nor that these results would in any way influence the lives of the mother or her baby. A further important aspect of this trial was a psychosocial study that investigated such relevant issues as social acceptance and coercion. The results of this study, following a rigorous statistical evaluation, were available in 2002.

A general observation made by the participants of this trial is that detection of fetal aneuploidies appeared to be easier than the determination of fetal sex, in that the number of aneuploid fetal cells appeared in greater numbers in the periphery of pregnant women than their normal counterparts. By the use of a quantitative PCR analysis, Bianchi *et al.*[32]

were recently able to confirm these findings, in that the quantity of male fetal DNA in maternal blood was higher in pregnancies with an aneuploid fetus, than in those with karyotypically normal fetuses. Furthermore, it has been found that the expression of CD71, the antigen commonly used for the enrichment of fetal erythroblasts, is also elevated under conditions involving an aneuploidy. It, hence, appears that the system favors the detection of fetal aneuploidies, which will be a major benefit for those wishing to develop this methodology for prenatal diagnostic purposes. Until then, however, several obstacles still need to be overcome, such as the need for automated image analysis and rapid fetal cell identification. This deficit has been noted by companies such as Applied Imaging, who are sponsoring a second similar trial that makes exclusive use of their image analysis equipment, proprietary enrichment protocols and antibodies for fetal erythroblast identification. The majority of those researchers desiring to use fetal erythroblasts for diagnostic purposes encounter the problem that, even after enrichment for fetal cells, the cells are hidden in the midst of a large population of co-enriched maternal cells. This problem is exacerbated by the fact that the majority of erythroblasts are of maternal and not of fetal origin.[7,40,42]

Ways in which this major problem may be surmounted include the use of new enrichment protocols,[47–50] more specific antibodies,[51,52] better fetal specific markers[53] and, as mentioned previously, automated scanning and detection systems.[54–58]

Recent success with the detection of single gene disorders

PCR was first used in the field, not for the detection of fetal genetic anomalies, but to provide additional evidence for the existence of fetal cells in maternal blood, a matter that had then still been the subject of considerable dispute. This was first achieved by Lo *et al.*[57,58] They were able to determine the sex of the fetus with considerable accuracy by performing a PCR analysis with primers specific for the Y chromosome directly on whole-blood samples taken from pregnant women. That such an allele-specific amplificatory approach, i.e. where the gene of interest was missing from the maternal genome, could be used diagnostically was shown by the subsequent detection of a paternally inherited hemoglobinopathy[59] and assessment of the fetal rhesus status.[60] The sensitivity of this technique for the non-invasive detection of the rhesus factor was shown to be enhanced by carrying out the examination on fetal RhD mRNA rather than on RhD DNA.[61] The rationale for this was that the number of mRNA copies is far in excess of the few fetal RhD DNA templates. This approach was followed by Al-Mufti *et al.*, who found a similar increment in sensitivity when examining RhD mRNA vs. DNA in fractions that had been enriched for fetal erythroblasts.[62]

As discussed, the main disadvantage of this method is that it is restricted to those instances where the gene of interest is absent from the maternal genome. In order to overcome this obstacle, researchers have resorted to techniques first pioneered in the examination of preimplantation embryos,[63] namely, by physically isolating single fetal cells under the microscope and then performing PCR on them. It is by these means that significant breakthroughs have been achieved, in the examination of both the fetal genotype for Duchenne's muscular dystrophy by Sekizawa *et al.*[5] and hemaglobinopathies in the laboratory of Kan.[6]

Enhanced transfer of fetal cells into the maternal periphery in pre-eclampsia

As mentioned above, the occurrence of fetal cells, in this instance trophoblasts, migrating into the maternal cell periphery was first described in patients who had died from eclampsia.[9] During our routine investigations we had previously observed a remarkable rise in the number of erythroblasts detectable in the periphery of women with pre-eclampsia.[64] Since, we at that time, were not able to determine whether these were fetal, and since, as discussed, the minority of these cells appeared to be fetal, we have recently readdressed this issue, by focusing exclusively on male singleton pregnancies.[7] In this case–control study, we examined an equal number of patients diagnosed with pre-eclampsia and an equal number of gestational-age-matched controls, who were similarly pregnant with a single male fetus, but who had not had any invasive procedure nor had the pregnancy been complicated by any hematological disorders.

With this approach, but now with the aid of FISH for the X and Y chromosomes, we were able to determine what proportion of enriched erythroblasts were male, and hence fetal, and how many were female, and therefore maternal. As before, our results indicated a clear significant increase in the number of morphologically identified erythroblasts in the pre-eclamptic patients when compared to the normal controls (a mean of 32 vs. 7). Interestingly, a comparative increase in the number of Y-chromosome-positive cells was also noted (a mean of 9 vs. 2). Although this increase in Y-chromosome-positive cells could not account for all the erythroblasts observed in the pre-eclamptic cases, this result did indicate that while not all of these erythroblasts were fetal, a significant proportion was. A further interesting feature of this examination was the linear correlation that we observed between the maternal and fetal erythroblast populations. This implies that one and the same factor, which is able to traverse the placental barrier, is responsible for the same changes in both these pools. Erythropoietin is a likely candidate for such a factor, since hypoxic conditions that are known to occur in pre-eclampsia[65–67] are known to induce an expression of this gene.[68] However, it remains to be shown whether it is indeed involved, since the placenta is thought normally to be impervious to the transfusion of such cytokines.[69] This freer exchange of both cells and cytokines across the feto–maternal barrier could, however, be brought about by the gross morphological differences in the placenta found in pre-eclampsia,[67,70] whereby the fetal syncytiotrophoblast appears to be incapable of differentiating normally and, hence, is incapable of invading the maternal arterioles successfully.[71–73]

In this respect, it is unlikely that the increase in the feto–maternal cell exchange that we have observed to occur in pre-eclampsia is causal to the disease, but is probably a reflection upon the structural changes in this barrier. The increase in both maternal and fetal erythroblast pools is probably a reflection upon the generalized hypoxic state that occurs in these individuals.

One intriguing possibility is that while this alteration in feto–maternal cell transfer may not be involved in the etiology of pre-eclampsia, the increased flow of semi-allogenic cells into the maternal periphery may contribute to other disorders, such as the associated hemolysis, elevated liver enzymes, low platelets (HELLP) syndrome, which bears certain hallmarks of an overt immune response.

Since the transfer across the placenta is bidirectional it will be interesting to observe whether the flow is also enhanced in the direction of mother to fetus. Our preliminary results do indeed indicate that a greater number of maternal cells are found in cord blood samples obtained from pregnancies affected by pre-eclampsia when compared to normal samples.

Conclusion

Great strides have been made in bringing us closer to the day when a non-invasive prenatal diagnosis using fetal cells from maternal blood will become part of the repertoire at the disposal of the modern obstetrician and geneticist. We doubt, however, that the advent of this will render current invasive practices obsolete, since other new methods, such as chorionic villus sampling with its inherent advantages of earlier gestational age, did not replace amniocentesis. It is more likely that it will become a complementary technique, with its own advantages and disadvantages. This is partially due to the current inability to obtain a full karyotype from fetal erythroblasts, and that even with the aid of five-color FISH, only the most common fetal aneuploidies are detected, namely those for chromosomes 13, 18, 21, X and Y. Although this may account for as much as 60–70% of all chromosomal aberrations routinely detected in our prenatal diagnostic facility,[1] in those instances where a full karyotype is required, it will be necessary to resort to using current invasive procedures.

An unexpected and scientifically interesting spin-off of the research carried out in this field is the new knowledge that has been gained concerning the transfer of both fetal and maternal cells across the placental barrier, and the possible roles this may have in the etiology or progression of certain disorders such as scleroderma and pre-eclampsia.

Acknowledgments

This work was supported in part by the Swiss National Science Foundation, Grant No. 3200-047112.96 and NIH (USA) Contract No. N01-HD-4-3202.

REFERENCES

1. Holzgreve W. Will ultrasound-screening and ultrasound-guided procedures be replaced by non-invasive techniques for the diagnosis of fetal chromosome anomalies? (editorial) *Ultrasound Obstet Gynecol* 1997;9:217–9.
2. Elias S, Price J, Dockter M, *et al.* First trimester prenatal diagnosis of trisomy 21 in fetal cells from maternal blood. *Lancet* 1992; 340:1033.
3. Bianchi DW, Mahr A, Zickwolf GK, Houseal TW, Flint AF, Klinger KW. Detection of fetal cells with 47,XY,+21 karyotype in maternal peripheral blood. *Hum Genet* 1992;90:368–70.
4. Gänshirt-Ahlert D, Börjesson-Stoll R, Burschyk M, *et al.* Detection of fetal trisomies 21 and 18 from maternal blood using triple gradient and magnetic cell sorting. *Am J Reprod Immunol* 1993; 30:194–201.
5. Sekizawa A, Kimura T, Sasaki M, Nakamura S, Kobayashi R, Sato T. Prenatal diagnosis of Duchenne muscular dystrophy using a single fetal nucleated erythrocyte in maternal blood. *Neurology* 1996;46:1350–3.
6. Cheung MC, Goldberg JD, Kan YW. Prenatal diagnosis of sickle cell anaemia and thalassaemia by analysis of fetal cells in maternal blood. *Nat Genet* 1996;14:264–8.
7. Holzgreve W, Ghezzi F, Di Naro E, Maymon E, Gänshirt D, Hahn S. Disturbed feto–maternal cell traffic in pre-eclampsia. *Obstet Gynecol* 1998;91(5, Pt 1):669–72.
8. Nelson JL, Furst DE, Maloney S, *et al.* Microchimersim and HLA-compatible relationships of pregnancy in scleroderma. *Lancet* 1998;351:559–62.
9. Schmorl G. *Pathologisch – anatomische Untersuchungen über Puerperaleklampsie.* Leipzig: Vogel Press, 1893.
10. Attwood HD, Park WW. Embolism to the lungs by trophoblast. *J Obstet Gynaecol Br Commonw* 1960;68:611–7.
11. Douglas GW, Thomas L, Carr M, Cullen NM, Morris R. Trophoblasts in the circulating blood during pregnancy. *Am J Obstet Gynecol* 1959;58:960–73.
12. Covone AE, Johnson PM, Mutton D, Adinolfi M. Trophoblast cells in peripheral blood of pregnant women. *Lancet* 1984;2:841–3.

13. Covone AE, Kozman R, Johnson PM, Latt SA, Adinolfi M. Analysis of peripheral maternal blood samples for the presence of placental-derived cells using Y-specific probes and mAb H315. *Prenat Diagn* 1988;5:591–607.
14. Bertero MT, Carnaschella C, Serra A, Bergui L, Caligaris-Cappio F. Circulating 'trophoblast' cells in pregnancy have maternal genetic markers. *Prenat Diagn* 1988;8:588–90.
15. Henderson KG, Shaw TE, Barret IJ, Telenius AHP, Wilson RD, Kalousek DK. Distribution of mosaicism in human placentae. *Hum Genet* 1996;97:650–4.
16. Goldberg JD, Wohlferd MM. Incidence and outcome of chromosomal mosaicism found at the time of chorionic villus sampling. *Am J Obstet Gynecol* 1997;176:1349–53.
17. Hawes CS, Suskin HA, Kalionis B, *et al.* Detection of paternally inherited mutations for β-thalassemia in trophoblast isolated from peripheral maternal blood. *Ann N Y Acad Sci* 1994;731:181–5.
18. Kingdom J, Sherlock J, Rodeck C, Adinolfi M. Detection of trophoblast cells in transcervical samples collected by lavage or cytobrush. *Obstet Gynecol* 1995;86:283–8.
19. Walknoska J, Conte FA, Grumbach MM. Practical and theoretical implication of fetal/maternal lymphocyte transfer. *Lancet* 1969; 1:1119–22.
20. Herzenberg LA, Bianchi DW, Schröder J, Cann HM, Iverson CM. Fetal cells in the blood of pregnant women: Detection and enrichment by fluorescence-activated cell sorting. *Proc Natl Acad Sci USA* 1979;76:1453–5.
21. Schroder J, Tilikainen A, de la Chapelle A. Fetal leucocytes in maternal circulation after delivery. *Transplantation* 1974;17:346–60.
22. Ciaranfi A, Curchod A, Odartchenko N. Post partum survival of fetal lymphocytes in the maternal blood. *Schweiz Med Wochenschr* 1977;107:134–8.
23. Hsieh TT, Pao CC, Hor JJ, Kao SM. Presence of fetal cells in maternal circulation after delivery. *Hum Genet* 1993;92:204–5.
24. Liou JD, Hsieh TT, Pao CC. Presence of cells of fetal origin in maternal circulation of pregnant women. *Ann N Y Acad Sci* 1994;731:237–41.
25. Bianchi DW, Zickwolf GK, Weil GJ, Sylvester S, Demaria MA. Male fetal progenitor cells persist in maternal blood for as long as 27 years postpartum. *Proc Natl Acad Sci USA* 1996;93:705–8.
26. van Rood GG, Eernisse G, van Leeuwen A. Leukocyte antibodies in sera from pregnant women. *Nature* 1958;181:1735–6.
27. Regan L, Braude PR. Is antipaternal cytotoxic antibody a valid marker in the management of recurrent abortion? *Lancet* 1987; 2:1280.
28. Wegmann TG, Lin H, Guilbert L, Mosmann TR. Bidirectional cytokine interactions in the maternal–fetal relationship: Is successful pregnancy a TH2 phenomenon? *Immunol Today* 1993;14: 353–6.
29. Tafuri A, Alferink J, Möller P, Hämmerling G, Arnold B. T cell awareness of paternal alloantigens during pregnancy. *Science* 1995;270:630–3.
30. Moller G. Models of autoimmunity. *Immunol Rev* 1993;118: 1–310.
31. McMilin KD, Johnson RL. HLA homozygosity and the risk of related-donor transfusion-associated graft versus-host disease. *Transfus Med Rev* 1993;7:37–41.
32. Bianchi DW, Williams JM, Sullivan LM, Hanson FW, Klinger KW, Shuber AP. PCR quantitation of fetal cells in maternal blood in normal and aneuploid pregnancies. *Am J Hum Genet* 1997;61:822–9.
33. Artlett CM, Welsh KI, Black CM, Jiminez SA. Fetal–maternal HLA compatibility confers susceptibility to systemic sclerosis. *Immunogenetics* 1997;47:17–22.
34. Bonney EA, Matzinger P. The maternal immune system's interaction with circulating fetal cells. *J Immunol* 1997;158:40–7.
35. Hall JM, Lingenfelter P, Adams SL, Lasser D, Hansen JA, Bean MA. Detection of maternal cells in human umbilical cord blood using fluorescence *in situ* hybridization. *Blood* 1995;86:2829–32.
36. Lo YM, Lo ES, Watson N, *et al.* Two-way cell traffic between mother and fetus: Biologic and clinical implications. *Blood* 1996;88:4390–5.
37. Scaradavou A, Carrier C, Mollen N, Stevens C, Rubinstein P. Detection of maternal DNA in placental/umbilical cord blood by locus specific amplification of the non-inherited maternal HLA gene. *Blood* 1996;88:1494–500.
38. Kleihauer E, Braun H, Betke K. Demonstration von fetalem Hämaglobin in der Erythrozyten eines Blutausstriches. *Klinische Wochenschr* 1957;35:637–8.
39. Clayton EM, Feldhaus WD, Whiteacre FE. Fetal erythrocytes in the maternal circulation of pregnant women. *Obstet Gynecol* 1964; 23:915–9.
40. Gänshirt-Ahlert D, Garritsen H, Miny P, Holzgreve W. Fetal cells in maternal circulation throughout gestation. *Lancet* 1994;343: 1038–9.
41. Slunga Tallberg A, el Rifai W, Keinanen M, *et al.* Maternal origin of nucleated erythrocytes in peripheral venous blood of pregnant women. *Hum Genet* 1995;96:53–7.
42. Slunga Tallberg A, el Rifai W, Keinanen M, *et al.* Maternal origin of transferrin receptor positive cells in venous blood of pregnant women. *Clin Genet* 1996;49:196–9.
43. Bianchi DW, Flint AF, Pizzimneti MF, Knoll JHM, Latt SA. Isolation of fetal DNA from nucleated erythrocytes in maternal blood. *Proc Natl Acad Sci USA* 1990;87:3279–83.
44. Miltenyi S, Müller W, Weichel W, Radbruch A. High gradient magnetic cell separation with MACS. *Cytometry* 1990;11:231–8.
45. Gänshirt-Ahlert D, Burschyk M, Garritsen HS, *et al.* Magnetic cell sorting and the transferrin receptor as potential means of prenatal diagnosis from maternal blood. *Am J Obstet Gynecol* 1992; 166:1350–5.
46. Bianchi DW, Simpson JL, Jackson LG, Elias S, Holzgreve W, Evans MI, Dukes KA, Sullivan LM, Klinger KW, Bischoff FZ, Hahn S, Johnson KL, Lewis D, Wapner RJ, de la Cruz F. Fetal gender and aneuploidy detection using fetal cells in maternal blood: analysis of NIFTY I data. National Institute of Child Health and Development Fetal Cell Isolation Study. Prenat Diagn.
47. Hall JM, Adams S, Williams S, Rehse MA, Layton TJ, Molesh DA. Purification of fetal cells from maternal blood using an avidin–biotin immunoaffinity column. *Ann N Y Acad Sci* 1994; 731:115–27.
48. Steele CD, Wapner RJ, Smith JB, Haynes MK, Jackson LG. Prenatal diagnosis using fetal cells isolated from maternal peripheral blood: A review. *Clin Obstet Gynecol* 1996;39:801–13.
49. Sitar G, Manenti L, Farina A, *et al.* Characterization of the biophysical properties of human erythroblasts as a preliminary step to the isolation of fetal erythroblasts from maternal blood for non invasive prenatal genetic investigation. *Haematologica* 1997;82: 5–10.
50. Wachtel SS, Sammons D, Manley M. Fetal cells in maternal blood: Recovery by charge flow separation. *Hum Genet* 1995;98:162–6.
51. Savion S, Carp H, Shepshelovich J, *et al.* Use of antibodies against the human antigen of erythroblasts for the detection of nucleated erythrocytes in the maternal circulation. *Biol Neonate* 1997;71: 126–30.
52. Zheng YL, Zhen DK, Demaria MA, *et al.* Search for the optimal fetal cell antibody: Results of immunophenotyping studies using flow cytometry. *Hum Genet* 1997;100:35–42.
53. Hengstschlager M, Bernaschek G. Fetal cells in the peripheral blood of pregnant women express thymidine kinase: A new marker for detection. *FEBS Lett* 1997;404:299–302.
54. Mignon-Godefroy K, Guillet J, Butor C. Solid phase cytometry for detection of rare events. *Cytometry* 1997;27:336–44.
55. Eigen M, Rigler R. Sorting single molecules: Application to diagnostics and evolutionary biotechnology. *Proc Natl Acad Sci USA* 1994;91:5740–7.
56. Netten H, Young IT, van Vliet LJ, Tanke HJ, Vroljik H, Sloos WCR. FISH and chips: Automation of fluorescent dot counting in interphase cell nuclei. *Cytometry* 1997;28:1–10.
57. Lo YMD, Patel P, Wainscoat JS, Sampietro M, Gillmer MDG, Fleming KA. Prenatal sex determination by DNA amplification from maternal peripheral blood. *Lancet* 1989;2:1363–5.
58. Lo YM, Patel P, Baigent CN, *et al.* Prenatal sex determination from maternal peripheral blood using the polymerase chain reaction. *Hum Genet* 1993;90:483–8.
59. Camaschella C, Alfarano A, Gottardi E, *et al.* Prenatal diagnosis of fetal hemoglobin Lepore–Boston disease on maternal peripheral blood. *Blood* 1990;75:2102–6.
60. Lo YMD, Bowell PJ, Selinger M, *et al.* Prenatal determination of fetal RhD status by analysis of peripheral blood of rhesus negative mothers. *Lancet* 1993;341:1147–8.
61. Hamlington J, Cunningham J, Mason G, Mueller R, Miller D. Prenatal detection of rhesus D genotype. *Lancet* 1997;349:540.
62. Al-Mufti R, Howard C, Overton T, *et al.* Detection of fetal mRNA in maternal blood as a strategy for non-invasive prenatal diagnosis. *Am J Obstet Gynecol* 1998;179(1):210–4.
63. Handyside AH, Delhanty JDA. Preimplatation genetic diagnosis: Strategies and suprises. *Trends Genet* 1997;13:270–5.

64. Gänshirt D, Börjesson-Stoll R, Burschyk M, *et al.* Successful prenatal diagnosis from maternal blood with magnetic-activated cell sorting. *Ann N Y Acad Sci* 1994;731:103–14.
65. Redman CWG. Hypertension in pregnancy. In Chamberlain G, ed. *Turnbull's Obstetrics.* London: Churchill Livingstone Press, 1995:441–70.
66. Witlin AG, Sibai BM. Hypertension in pregnancy: Current concepts of pre-eclampsia. *Annu Rev Med* 1997;48:115–27.
67. Roberts J. Pregnancy-related hypertension. In Creasey RK, Resnik R, eds. *Maternal–Fetal Medicine: Principles and Practice,* Philadelphia: W.B. Saunders Press, 1994:804–43.
68. Bauer C. The oxygen sensor that controls EPO production: Facts and fancies. *J Perinat Med* 1995;23:7–12.
69. Reisenberger K, Egarter C, Kapiotis S, Sternberger B, Gregor H, Husslein P. Transfer of erythropoeitin across the placenta perfused in vitro. *Obstet Gynecol* 1997;89:738–42.
70. Salafia CM, Pezzullo JC, Lopez Zeno JA, Simmens S, Minior VK, Vintzileos AM. Placental pathologic features of preterm preeclampsia. *Am J Obstet Gynecol* 1995;173:1097–105.
71. Mayhew TM. Patterns of villous and intervillous space growth in human placentas from normal and abnormal pregnancies. *Eur J Obstet Gynecol Reprod Biol* 1996;68:75–82.
72. Zhou Y, Damsky CH, Chiu K, Roberts JM, Fisher SJ. Preeclampsia is associated with abnormal expression of adhesion molecules by invasive cytotrophoblasts. *J Clin Invest* 1993;91:950–60.
73. Zhou Y, Fisher SJ, Janatpour M, *et al.* Human cytotrophoblasts adopt a vascular phenotype as they differentiate. A strategy for successful endovascular invasion? *J Clin Invest* 1997;99:2139–51.

113 Ultrasonographic soft markers for chromosomal abnormalities

A. Antsaklis

Genetic sonography

Until the mid-80s, the main indication for second-trimester genetic amniocentesis was maternal age ≥35 years at the time of delivery. Maternal serum screening triple test, was introduced in the mid-80s and today is a standard practice, in order to reduce the loss of normal fetuses from amniocentesis, since it is important to identify methods that focus on a better group of candidates for invasive procedures. Women aged 35 years and older have traditionally been offered genetic amniocentesis, because at 35 the incidence of trisomy [e.g. Down's syndrome (DS)] starts to rapidly increase. Also at this time, the risk of any aneuploidy roughly equals the risk of amniocentesis-related pregnancy loss of 1 in 200, thus justifying the test.

Using maternal age to select women for an amniocentesis and make an antenatal diagnosis of DS is associated with a low detection rate. Maternal age is a poor method of screening.

Because younger women have the majority of pregnancies, younger women give birth to the majority (65%) of all DS children. In the 1980s, it was reported that alpha fetoprotein was unusually low in pregnancies complicated by DS. Elevated serum levels of chorionic gonadotropin and decreased unconjugated estriol have been identified in pregnancies with fetuses with DS. This combination of these three analytes is more predictive than any individual analyte alone. It is termed the *triple screen*, or *multiple marker screening test*, and has become the preferred DS screening test in many centers with a 5% screen-positive rate, the multiple marker screening test identifies approximately 60% of all DS pregnancies in women under the age of 35. In women over 35 years, it detects over 75% of DS pregnancies.

Genetic sonography has been established in the last decade as a very useful examination and offers the opportunity to better select candidates for invasive prenatal diagnosis by using a series of sonographic markers that are present more frequently in aneuploid than euploid fetuses. This permits the identification of 60–80% of the affected fetuses and this applies equally well to women whose fetuses are at high and at low risk for aneuploidy. Conversely, when these sonographic markers are absent, the age-specific risk of aneuploidy can be readjusted in women at increased risk of carrying an abnormal fetus because of age.

The second-trimester sonography includes evaluation of fetal biometry, and anatomy for detection of structural and non-structural anomalies (Figures 113.1 and 113.2). Examples of anomalies associated with DS are as congenital heart defects, duodenal atresia, ventriculomegaly, hypoplasia of the middle phalanx of the fifth digit with clinodactyly, flat face with maxillary hypoplasia, macroglossia, brachycephaly, hydrops and clubbed foot. Congenital heart disease (CHD) is the most common anomaly in infants with DS (44% of the infants with DS have CHD), with 45% of these defects being atrioventricular septal defects, 35% ventricular septal defects, 8% isolated secundum atrial septal defects, 7% persistent pattern ductus arteriosus and 4% isolated tetralogy of Fallot.[1] The prenatal diagnosis of CHD carries a significant risk of fetal aneuploidy. When prenatal diagnosis of CHD is found in association with other fetal structural malformations, the incidence of fetal chromosomal abnormalities is 60–70%, while when isolated CHD is found, the incidence of aneuploidy is 15–20%.

Ninety-nine percent of newborns with trisomy 18, 90% of newborns with trisomy 13 and 50% of newborns with trisomy 21 have CHD and, especially, ventricular septal defect.

Therefore, normal cardiac ultrasound examination theoretically decreases the prior risk of the birth of a child with trisomy 21 by 50% and almost eliminates the risk of trisomy 18 or 13.

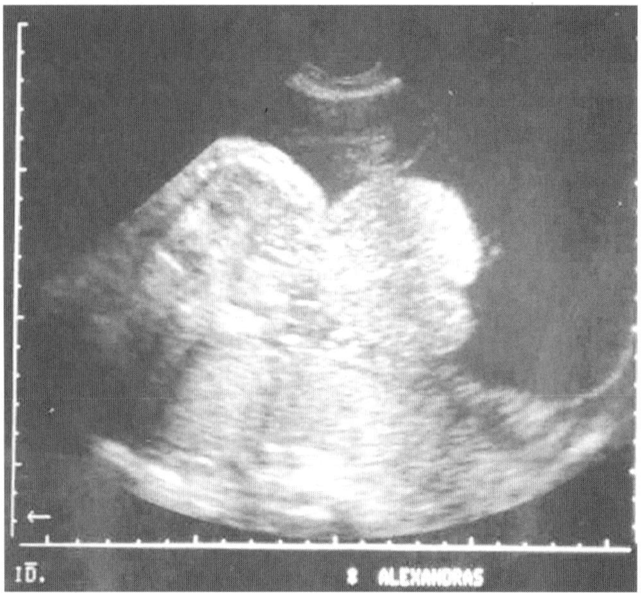

Figure 113.1 Fetal omphalocele.

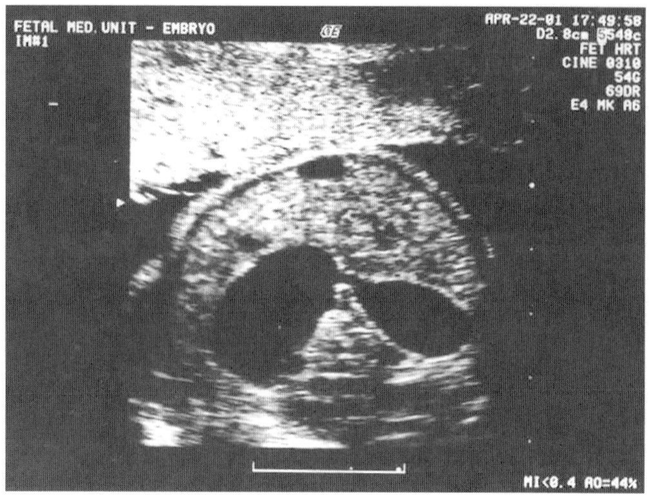

Figure 113.2 Duodenal atresia.

Non-structural markers (soft markers) included nuchal fold thickness of 6 mm or greater, renal pyelectasis (anterior–posterior diameter of renal pelvis greater than 4 mm), choroid plexus cyst (CPC), hyperechogenic bowel, echogenic intracardiac focus (EIF) and extremity shortening (humerus or femur). These markers are more common than the major structural abnormalities in fetuses with trisomy 21 and are non-specific. These markers are also present in fetuses without abnormalities, are often transient and can be readily detected during the second trimester.

Risk status is ascertained preferably by the patient's age and biochemical screening test results (triple or quadruple markers). Low risk is defined as anyone having a 'negative' biochemical screen or, in the absence of biochemical information, a maternal age younger than 35 years.

The soft markers for DS were originally described to help improve the sonographic detection of DS in high-risk women (predominantly pregnant women of advanced maternal age), who were attempting to gather more accurate risk information than that based on age alone before deciding whether to proceed to amniocentesis.

Major abnormalities are observed in fewer than 25% of affected fetuses, whereas one or more soft markers may be observed in 50% of the affected fetuses. This emphasizes the importance of soft markers for the detection of fetal trisomy 21 among high-risk women in whom high sensitivity is desirable. But the false-positive rate may be unacceptably high (13–17%) if any one of the soft markers is detected among low-risk women.

Sonographic markers are often associated with other markers or structural abnormalities and the risk of fetal DS increases with the number of markers present. Sonographic markers were considered isolated when they were not associated with the major or the other soft marker.

These sonographic markers are more common in fetuses with chromosomal defects, leading to the assumption that they might be useful in the prenatal identification of the fetus at risk of aneuploidy.

Echogenic intracardiac focus

EIF (golf ball) is defined as a small bright area within the fetal heart ventricles, generally in the left ventricle, but occasionally bilateral or right-sided located below the mitral or tricuspid valves with similar echogenicity to bone, and represents microcalcification in the papillary muscle or chordae tendinae of the fetal heart in the second trimester.[2] The majority of the cases of EIF are simple, but in some cases there is a multiple EIF in one or more chambers of the heart (Figure 113.3).

During the routine examination of the four-chamber view of the fetal heart, these foci are seen to move synchronously with the valve leaflets throughout the cardiac cycle.

Recently, it has been confirmed that EIF is caused by mineralization within the papillary muscle, but the cause of such changes remains unknown.

EIF is the most recent and the most controversial of the soft markers, because it is a subjective finding and its prevalence is influenced by a variety of factors, including the resolution of the sonographic equipment, the technique and the sonographer's experience and the maternal ethnic background.[3] The prevalence of second-trimester foci in fetuses with black mothers is 6%, in white mothers it is 10%, in Asian mothers, 30% and in mothers in whom the race is not identified, 11%.

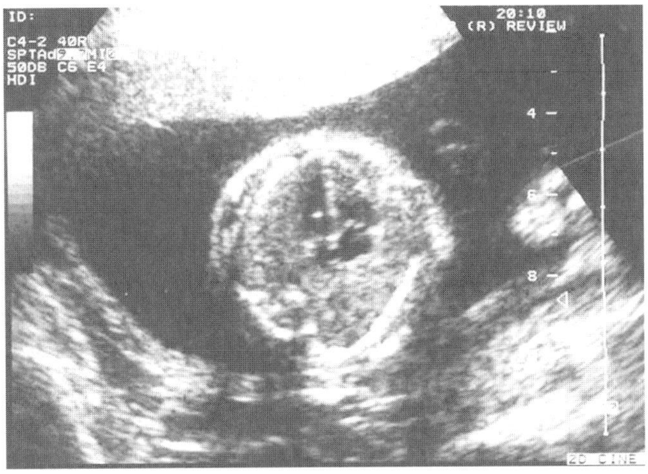

Figure 113.3 Echogenic Intracardiac focus.

It has been shown that fetuses of Asian mothers have a three- and eightfold increased incidence of EIF over fetuses of white and black mothers, respectively, and because the incidence of EIF among fetuses of Asian mothers is actually higher than it is among fetuses with DS, this particular marker cannot be used accurately to predict the risk of DS in the Asian population.[4]

Fetal position is also important and EIF is best visualized when the cardiac apex is oriented toward the transducer. The association between aneuploidy and EIF was first seen in the early 1990s and is now well established.[5,6] The EIF is considered a soft marker for trisomies 21 and 13. This finding is neither sensitive nor specific and < 20% of aneuploid fetuses as well as 5–10% of normal fetuses display this sonographic marker.

EIF is not associated with congenital heart defects in chromosomally normal fetuses. The prevalence of EIF has been quoted to be as low as 0.46% and as high as 22% in the second and third trimesters of pregnancy. The prevalence of EIF may be affected by the timing of the ultrasound examination during pregnancy, as sometimes EIF resolves or develops late, and also whether the EIF was detected in pregnancies at high risk or low risk of aneuploidy. In high risk, the prevalence of isolated EIF in the second trimester is 3.5% and in low risk it lies between 0.4 and 7.4%.

In a period of 3 years, 10,769 women had a routine detailed anomaly scan, and there were 311 cases of isolated EIF. Among these, there was only one case of trisomy 21. In the same period, there were 14 cases with DS. The sensitivity of isolated EIF for detecting trisomy 21 was 7.1% and the specificity was 97.1%. They concluded that the isolated EIF is a normal ultrasonographic finding and should not be considered as a risk factor for trisomy 21 in an unselected low-risk population.[7]

Whether low-risk woman should undergo invasive testing because of the presence of a fetal EIF remains controversial.[5] Isolated EIF carries a relative risk of twice the prior risk of the presence of DS.[8,9]

The prevalence of this marker in high- and low-risk pregnancies is between 3% and 5%, making this finding the most commonly detected ultrasound marker. The prenatal detection of EIF might be potentially significant as a marker for aneuploidy.

Nyberge *et al.* confirmed that EIF is associated with an increased risk of trisomy 21, although as an isolated marker this association just reached statistical significance. These data support a large number of other studies suggesting an association between EIF and trisomy 21, whereas some studies have failed to show this association.[10]

Two independent studies in a high-risk population showed that the risk of aneuploidy in fetuses with isolated EIF is about four times greater than the risk in those with a normal scan.[11,12]

In a total of 5480 women undergoing amniocentesis, the prevalence of EIF was 4.6% (253 cases) and trisomy 21 was diagnosed in 23 cases (9.1%) of the 253 fetuses with EIF and in 69 (1.3%) of the 5227 without EIF.[5,11,13]

In a low-risk population, there is no such association. In 9263 low-risk pregnancies 153 fetuses had EIF and none of them had trisomy 21.[6]

On the contrary, Bromley *et al.* identified 290 fetuses with EIF of whom 165 were from a low population according to the maternal age and four (2.4%) had trisomy 21, concluding that the risk of aneuploidy is also increased in the low-risk population with EIF.[14]

On the basis of the current literature, there is strong evidence to support the fact that EIF is more prevalent in fetuses with chromosomal defects, specifically trisomy 13 and trisomy 21. In the high-risk population, an isolated EIF is associated with an increased risk of trisomy 21, whereas in the low-risk population the risk is considerably lower than the risk of fetal loss associated with amniocentesis.

When a EIF is identified, a detailed scan for other signs of aneuploidy must be undertaken.

Although this finding has been reported in association with fetal chromosome abnormalities, no other major or minor anomalies were identified in this fetus. In the absence of other risk factors, this is considered a normal variation and no further evaluation is recommended. When an EIF is identified, it is necessary to evaluate for other sonographic markers of trisomy 21, such as nuchal thickness. These additional efforts will help add to the certainty that the EIF is a normal variant in a low-risk woman.[15]

In the absence of associated sonographic findings suggestive of fetal DS in low-risk women, the risk of an affected fetus when an isolated EIF is found remains lower than the risk of fetal loss associated with an amniocentesis. In an otherwise unselected healthy pregnancy with a fetus at low risk of aneuploidy, the discovery of an isolated EIF on routine detailed anomaly scanning in the second trimester is

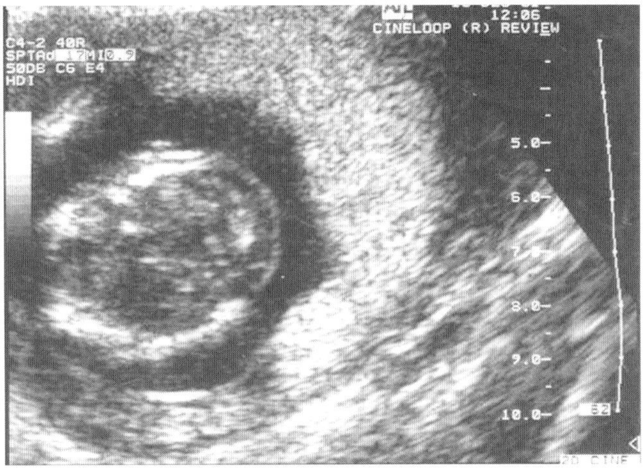

Figure 113.4 Increased nuchal thickness.

normal and should not be considered as a risk factor for trisomy 21.[7]

Nuchal fold

Nuchal thickness was the first sonographic marker associated with an increased risk of trisomy 21 in the fetus and is now accepted as the single most sensitive and specific marker for the detection of DS in the second trimester, in high- and low-risk pregnancies.

Sonographic measurements of nuchal thickness are obtained at the level of the posterior fossa on a modified transverse view of the fetal head, which includes the thalami, the cavum septi pellucidi, the cerebellum hemisphere the cicterna magna as well as the occipital bone (Figure 113.4). The soft tissue thickness posterior to the occiput is measured from the outside of the occipital bone to the outer skin edge and should be measured three times with the largest consistent measurement used for evaluation. Measurements ≥ 6 mm are considered abnormal and it has been suggested that a nuchal fold of > 6 mm was associated with a marked increase in the risk of DS.[16,17] Several investigators recommended that nuchal fold measurements become a part of every scan performed in this period of the second trimester.[18] It has been found using a 6-mm cutoff that there is an increase in sensitivity in older fetuses (19–24 weeks) vs. the fetuses between 14 and 18 weeks from 35% to 83% with a minimal corresponding decrease in specificity from 98.8% to 96.5%, and a high incidence (76%) of nuchal thickening among fetuses with DS between 14 and 18 weeks of gestation, and it has been suggested that for older fetuses, 6 mm should be used as a threshold between 19 and 24 weeks.[19] Several meta-analyses have studied the efficacy of the nuchal fold thickness measurements. Overall, Wald *et al.* in 1998 calculated a sensitivity of 38% for the efficacy of nuchal fold and a specificity of 98.7% for the diagnosis of trisomy 21.[20]

The gestational age at which the nuchal fold is measured is definitely an important issue. The nuchal fold is a transient finding, which may fluctuate even within the second trimester, and this marker does resolve over time. Nuchal fold measurements should only be used between 15 and 20 weeks. During this period, the normal measurements of nuchal fold remain remarkably constant at < 5 mm.

Furthermore, nuchal fold abnormalities can resolve on subsequent scans whether or not the fetus has DS. A thickened nuchal fold is also associated with other euploid syndromes, such as Noonan syndrome and heart defects.

A thickened nuchal fold can appear one week and be gone the next with normal follow-up measurements still resulting in a fetus with DS.

There are two recommendations. (1) Once a thickened nuchal fold is identified in the second trimester regardless of resolution in a subsequent scan, it places the patient at a high risk of fetal DS. (2) Measurements after 19 or 20 weeks are less reliable. Never use these measurements after 20 weeks in predicting the presence or the absence of DS.

Most of the nuchal thickening in fetuses with DS is thought to represent some form of lymphatic abnormality similar to cystic hygromata. Nuchal fold measurement is a useful marker for the detection of fetuses at risk of DS, and is a screening test that can alter the risk of a fetus having DS.

It has been shown that a normal nuchal fold in high-risk patients can decrease the risk of an affected fetus both in patients with abnormal triple test and in patients with advanced maternal age.[21,22]

The nuchal fold is the single most sensitive and specific finding leading the list for detecting fetuses at risk of DS, although the combination of several markers together has resulted in the most effective method for detecting affected fetuses.

Choroid plexus cyst

Cysts of the choroids plexus in the fetal brain usually are present in the second trimester as a solitary unilateral and simple round anechoic structure within the choroids plexus of the lateral ventricle (Figure 113.5). CPC is considered a marker predominantly for trisomy 18. Most of the cases are detected incidentally at routine second-trimester anomaly scan. Occasionally, they can be multiple, bilateral or complex. The prevalence of these cysts in the second trimester is approximately 1% and more than 25% disappear before 26 weeks.

The observation that most of the fetuses with CPC had trisomy 18 demonstrates that CPC can be the only marker in a trisomy 18 fetus.[23,24]

Despite the large number of cases of CPC reported, there is no consensus regarding the definitive role of this ultrasound marker in the prenatal detection of aneuploidy.[25]

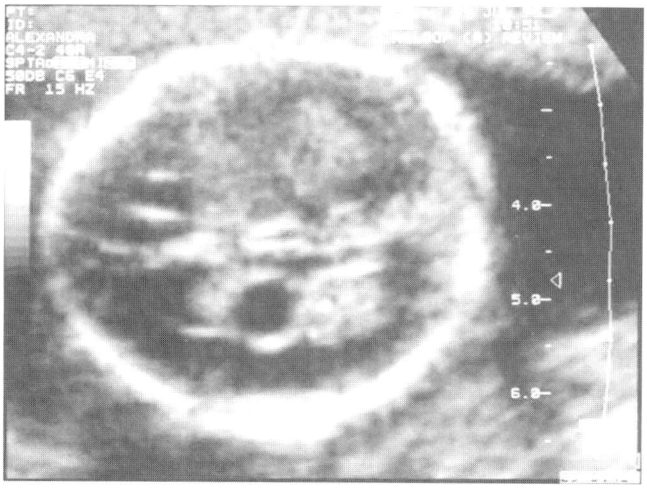

Figure 113.5 Unilateral choroid plexus cyst.

There is agreement that the ultrasound characteristics of CPC, such as bilaterality, size, number, complexity and resolution, are not related to the risk of aneuploidy. Once a CPC has been identified, a detailed fetal anatomical survey is needed including examination of the fetal hands, heart and central nervous system. Most of the controversy has been focused on whether an isolated CPC should be an indication of amniocentesis for trisomy 18.

Maternal age is an independent risk factor for trisomy 18 and in calculations of the risk of trisomy 18, this variable has to be taken into consideration.

Among fetuses with isolated CPC, the likelihood ratio for trisomy 18 is 0.03 and increases to 0.4 with one additional ultrasound finding and to 20.5 if there are two or more additional abnormalities detected by ultrasound. It was concluded that if the cyst is apparently isolated, the risk of trisomy 18 is marginally increased and maternal age should be the main factor in deciding whether or not to offer fetal karyotyping.[26] In a recently published meta-analysis, it was shown that the option of offering prenatal karyotyping to rule out trisomy 18 in cases with isolated CPC is only justified when the maternal age at delivery is 36 years or older.[27]

In a large review, 658 fetuses with CPC were identified in 101,600 births. Overall, 2.1% of these had a chromosomal abnormality. When only isolated findings of CPC were separately analyzed, 0.5% were chromosomally abnormal. If the analysis was stratified by age, 0.36% of mothers below the age of 36 years were aneuploid, whereas 2.4% were older.[28]

A review of 13 studies reporting more than 100 cases of isolated CPC revealed that the prevalence of trisomy 18, regardless of the maternal age or previous screening, was 0.6% or 1/176, which is above the population frequency of trisomy 18.[29]

It was concluded that the presence of isolated CPC, in an otherwise normal second-trimester fetus, carries an increased risk of trisomy 18. A detailed ultrasound examination of the fetus should be mandatory and if no abnormal findings are detected, maternal age and maternal serum screening results should be considered to determine whether the offering of karyotyping is advisable.[29] When a CPC is identified in a patient otherwise considered at low risk for fetal aneuploidy, it is necessary to exclude other sonographic markers of trisomy 18, such as 'clenched' hands. These efforts will help add to the certainty that CPC is a normal variant in low-risk women. Women confronted with the information that their fetus has a 'marker' for a chromosomal anomaly often have to endure a great deal of anxiety.

It has been suggested that the reporting of these two findings (the CPC and the EIF) causes more harm than good. It was recommended that when a CPC or an EIF is the only detected abnormality in a patient otherwise considered at low risk for fetal aneuploidy, it is considered a normal variant and not clinically significant and does not change her status from low to high risk and no further evaluation is needed.

Fetal echogenic bowel (FEB)

FEB is not a truly pathological condition, but rather a non-specific ultrasound feature associated with a number of fetal pathological conditions of which chromosomal defects and cystic fibrosis (CF) are the most well known (Figure 113.6).

FEB is defined as the fetal small bowel as echogenic as the surrounding bone in the second-trimester fetus.

Different pathological conditions, such as trisomy 21, CF, severe early onset of intrauterine growth restriction (IUGR), thalassemia, intramniotic bleeding, gastrointestinal obstruction, mesenteric ischemia, perinatal death and cytomegalovirus infections have been associated with second-trimester hyperchoid bowel.[19,30,31]

Poor perinatal outcome has been noted in one-third of pregnancies with FEB, including chromosomal defect in 9% of the cases, CF in 2%, congenital infection in 3% and IUGR in 8%.

The main limitation in the use of FEB as an ultrasound marker is the fact that the diagnosis is highly subjective and attempts to grade the echogenicity of fetal bowel have been abandoned due to the subjective nature of the findings.[32] The improved image resolution and the transducer frequency play a significant role in the diagnosis of this condition. The association between FEB and aneuploidy was established by Nyberg *et al.* in 1990, who reported increased bowel echogenicity in 5 (7%) of 68 second-trimester fetuses with trisomy 21. It has been estimated that the overall prevalence of chromosomal defects in cases of FEB was approximately 10% (79 out of 804) and the estimated risk of aneuploidy in cases of isolated FEB has been calculated to be between three- and fivefold greater than the background risk according to maternal age.[29,33]

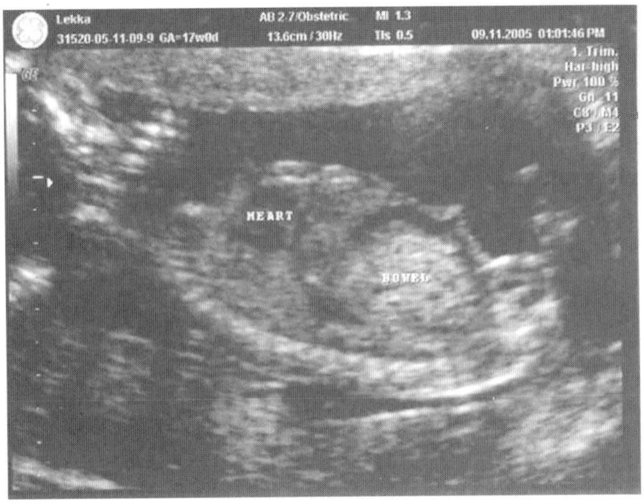

Figure 113.6 Fetal echogenic bowel.

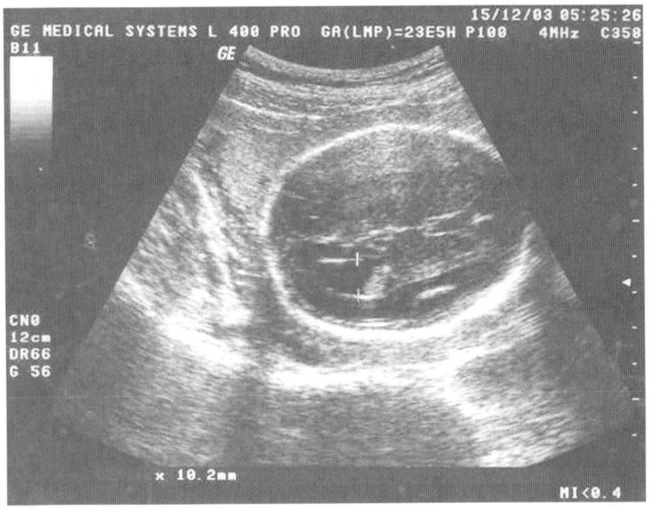

Figure 113.7 Mild ventriculomegaly.

Slotnik and Abuhamand in 1996 published a system that grades the relative echogenicity of the bowel when compared with the density of the adjacent fetal iliac crest. Of 7432 patients, 145 had fetuses with echogenic bowel. In 40 fetuses with bowel that was echogenic, but less echodense than the iliac crest, no cases of DS or CF were identified. In 81 cases where the bowel was equally echodense as the iliac crest, two cases of CF and two cases of DS were identified. When the bowel was more echodense than the fetal iliac crest, five cases of CF and six cases of DS were diagnosed out of 24 fetuses with echogenic bowel.[34]

Once the diagnosis of FEB is made, a detailed ultrasound examination of the fetus is warranted for other markers for aneuploidy to exclude intra-amniotic bleeding. If no associated findings are detected, the option of perinatal karyotyping should be discussed with the parents.[31]

Routine CF screening should also be considered, although in a low-risk population for this condition the chances seem to be low.[30]

If prenatal karyotyping is performed, fetal DNA testing for CF mutations should be considered. However, a serious limitation of CF testing is the small fraction of CF mutations currently available for screening. The diagnosis is only definitive in cases of homozygous fetuses.[35]

Routine screening for infection has not been advocated in view of the low yield and because most affected fetuses have additional findings suggestive of congenital infections. While this is not a particularly sensitive marker for DS, it is present in only 0.6% of the second-trimester fetal population; hence, the identification of this marker should lead to consideration of karyotyping, particularly if accompanied by any other sonographic findings.[2]

Mild ventriculomegaly

Mild ventriculomegaly (MV) is defined as a ventricular width of 10 mm or greater at the level of the atrium. A practical decision was made to include this as an anomaly rather than as a sonographic marker. The incidence of congenital ventriculomegaly ranges from 0.3 to 1.5 in 1000 births.

MV, including isolated MV (IMV), is the most common brain abnormality found on prenatal ultrasound (Figure 113.7). The most accepted definition of ventriculomegaly is the width of the atria of the lateral ventricles exceeding 10 mm.[36]

Progressive ventriculomegaly usually results from an excessive accumulation of cerebrospinal fluid, either because of obstructed flow or from loss of brain tissue, and is associated with CNS abnormalities, such as spina bifida, Dandy Walker complex, agenesis of the corpus callosum, congenital infections, chromosomal abnormalities and intracerebral hemorrhage.

The natural history and the etiology of MV remains unknown, much less well defined and does not appear to be associated with either obstruction or atrophy. The incidence of MV in a low-risk population is 1.48 per 1000 live births and increases to 22 per 1000 in high-risk patients. It usually involves both ventricles, but it may be unilateral or asymmetrical.[37,38]

In case of MV, a detailed genetic scan must include examination for markers of aneuploidy, fetal echocardiogram and serological tests for congenital infections should be taken, blood samples for platelet antigen typing and amniocentesis for karyotyping should be offered. IMV does not appear to be associated with raised intracranial pressure and appears to resolve in approximately 29% of the cases, remains stable in 57% and progresses in 14%.[39,40]

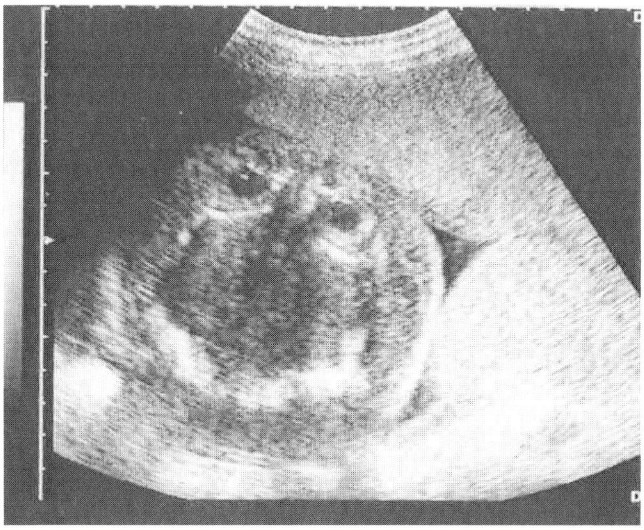

Figure 113.8 Mild dilatation of the fetal renal pelvis.

The incidence of chromosomal abnormalities varied from 3% to 12.6% (mean 9%) in cases with MV and 40% have other findings, while in cases with IMV the incidence decreased to 4%. It has been suggested that the majority of fetuses with MV and abnormal karyotyping will have additional sonographic abnormalities.[41]

The follow-up of fetuses with IMV in early childhood is good with 90% of the cases being normal. The quality of the outcome studies is poor with a small number of patients. Counseling should be based on the premise that IMV is a diagnosis of exclusion and outcome is generally good and further detailed studies are needed to document the significance of this finding.

Mild pyelectasis

Dilatation of the fetal renal pelvis (pyelectasis) was defined as an anteroposterior (AP) diameter ≥4 mm of fetal renal pelvis at 16–20 weeks, ≥5 mm at 20–30 weeks and ≥7 mm at 30–40 weeks of gestation[42] (Figure 113.8). An AP renal pelvis diameter of less than 7.0 mm was found to be predictive of a normal postnatal renal outcome. Pyelectasis may be unilateral or bilateral, but is more frequently reported as bilateral. There is also a marked sex difference with a male:female ratio of around 2:1.[43,44] The majority of cases of pyelectasis detected in the second trimester will resolve either before delivery or within the first year of postnatal life.[23] Mild pyelectasis is commonly detected in the second-trimester fetus and is associated with an increased risk of both chromosomal abnormalities and urinary tract pathologies. Thirty percent of cases with mild pyelectasis have persistent postnatal renal anomalies. The association with aneuploidy remains unclear, but it seems likely that mild pyelectasis is a marker that will alter prior risks.

Pyelectasis was described in association with trisomies 21, 13 and 18 and Benacerraf *et al.* reported seven fetuses (3.3%) with DS from a selected population of 211 fetuses with hydronephrosis. It also has been shown that the risk is higher when pyelectasis is associated with other abnormalities.[42]

In a recent study by Chudleigh *et al.* of 737 fetuses with mild pyelectasis from an unselected population of 101,600 births, it has been shown that when pyelectasis was present as an isolated finding, the risk of aneuploidy in women < 36 years of age was 0.33% and 2.2% in women > 36 years. Another approach has been to estimate the increased risk due to mild pyelectasis and adjust the prior risk by this factor.

It has been suggested that isolated mild pyelectasis confers a risk of trisomy 21 that is 1.5 times the background risk.[45]

Mild pyelectasis is a marker not sufficiently sensitive and specific to be used as an isolated finding for the detection of DS and the relative risk of DS is 1.5 times the prior risk. Mild pyelectasis is a soft marker to be used only in combination with other markers. Isolated pyelectasis in a low-risk patient should not warrant an amniocentesis.[8] The association between prenatal pyelectasis and postnatal pathologies (urinary tract obstruction and vesico-uretal reflux) is well established and 3–5% of cases of second-trimester pyelectasis may require urinary tract surgery. The sensitivity of second-trimester pyelectasis in identifying postnatal pathologies is improved by selecting those fetuses with persisting AP pelvis > 10 mm in the third trimester.

The detection of perinatal pyelectasis is an indication of detailed genetic sonogram looking for other markers of aneuploidy and for extra renal anomalies. The urogenital system should be examined carefully and care should be taken to exclude the duplex system, multicystic displastic kidney and to examine the bladder. Parents should be assured that this finding is common and the risk of serious sequelae is very small. Repeated scans should be performed early in the third trimester if the dilatation is still present or is increased; furthermore, postnatal scans and other investigations should be initiated as clinically indicated.[43]

Other sonographic markers

There are some other sonographic features of fetuses with DS. However, these may not be either sensitive or specific enough to be helpful for sonographic screening and they are difficult technically to evaluate accurately. Individuals with DS have short ears but the measurements are difficult to accomplish accurately and there is an overlap between normal and abnormal.

Hypoplastic or absence of the middle phalanx of the fifth digit is known as a finding among neonates with DS and together with clinodactyly can be demonstrated in the early second trimester. This marker is difficult to measure and the false-positive rate is as high as 18%[46] for using this finding as a screening tool for DS.

Recently, there is evidence to suggest that delayed fusion of the amnion and the chorion is associated with an increased incidence of DS.[47] This finding is rare, occurring only occasionally in fetuses with DS and in normal fetuses.

The separation of the great toe (sandal gap toe) is a morphological feature seen in infants with trisomy 21, but occasionally detected *in utero* because of the rarity of this abnormality, and regarding its power as a marker is not useful in screening for fetal DS (Figure 113.9).

Some other fetal biometric parameters have been investigated as potential indicators of fetal trisomy 21. They do not have the same efficacy of detecting DS. The femur was considered shortened when the measured to expected ratio was 0.91 or less and the overall sensitivity and specificity for detecting DS was 29% and 92%, respectively.[48] The short humerus (measured to expected ratio 0.89 or less) has a sensitivity of 31% and a specificity of 95%, whereas when the short femur and short humerus are present, there is 33% sensitivity and 95% specificity for detecting DS.

Vintzileos *et al.*[49] measured four fetal long bones and compared their length with controls standardized on the basis of gestational age. Femur, humerus, tibia and fibula were measured in 493 normal fetuses and 22 with trisomy 21. The risk of having at least one of the four bones shortened had a sensitivity of 64% and a specificity of 78%.[49]

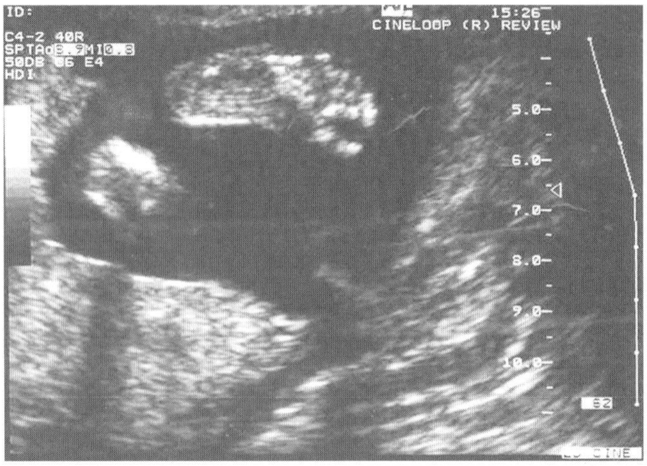

Figure 113.9 Seperation of the great toe (sandal gap toe).

Scoring index

It is clear that the use of multiple sonographic markers is a more sensitive method and improves the detection of fetal aneuploidy over the use of any simple marker. Several authors have proposed grading or scoring systems to improve risk assessment. Benacerraf *et al.* proposed a scoring system based on the major and minor abnormalitites.[50] Major fetal abnormalities and the thickened nuchal fold both have a score of 2 and even if isolated, there is a strong indication for amniocentesis. Soft markers are often present in normal fetuses and each one receives a score of 1 (short femur and humerus, pyelectasis, echogenic fetal bowel, EIF and CPC) (Table 113.1).

Table 113.1 Proposed sonographic score for the detection of DS

	Score	Likelihood ratio
Major structural anomalies	2	25
Nuchal fold	2	18.6
Short femur	1	2.5
Mild pyelectasis	1	2.2
FEB	1	1.5
Echogenic indracardiac focus EIF	1	5.5
CPC	1	2.0

From Benacerraf *et al.*[51]
If amniocentesis is performed for fetuses scoring > 2, 73% of fetuses with trisomy 21 and 85% of fetuses with trisomy 18 can be identified with a false positive of 4%. Each likelihood ratio can be multiplied by the maternal age-based risk

It has been demonstrated, that the sonographic scoring index can achieve a sensitivity of 81% for trisomy 21 and 85% for trisomy 18 with a false-positive rate of 4%, when a score ≥ 2 is used for amniocentesis.

The use of ultrasound-adjusted risks of fetal trisomy 21 is expected to decrease the number of amniocenteses in women over the age of 35 when a genetic ultrasound examination does not demonstrate any abnormal ultrasound markers, while still identifying the majority of fetuses with DS. By applying Bayes' theorem to the risk of trisomy at a given maternal age in a fetus with a sonographic score of 0, a modified risk was calculated.

In women over 35 years of age, a threshold of 1 was used as a positive criterion to optimize the identification of the affected fetuses. This results in a sensitivity of 83% and a false-positive rate of 13%, respectively. The same scoring system can be used to decrease the risk of trisomy 21 in patients at risk of having an affected fetus, either because of advanced maternal age or because of abnormal triple screening test.

Women of 40 years of age or older, with a genetic sonogram score of 0, were advised to undergo amniocentesis since the score 0 could not reduce the patient's age-specific risk below the commonly accepted threshold for offering amniocentesis. Women between the age of 35 and 39 years, however, can benefit from the genetic sonography.[52]

It has been suggested that a genetic sonogram be offered as an option for women who are at increased risk of having fetuses with aneuploidy, but who do not wish to undergo invasive testing without additional information.

Nyberg *et al.* have developed the genetic sonogram via the age-adjusted ultrasound risk assessment for DS, based on maternal age and the likelihood ratios of the various sonographic markers.[4] Major structural anomalies, nuchal thickening, echogene bowel, short humerus, short femur, EIF and pyelectasis have likelihood ratios of 25, 18.6, 5.5, 2.5, 2.2, 2.0 and 1.5, respectively. Each likelihood ratio can be multiplied by the maternal age-based risk to revise the individual risk of the woman. They found that using one or more sonographic markers allowed identification of 68% of fetuses with DS with a false-positive rate of 12.5%.[8]

Vintzileos *et al.*[49] determined that the best combination of sonographic markers for detecting affected fetuses was the thickened nuchal fold, pyelectasis and short humerus, resulting in a sensitivity of 89% with a false-positive rate of 6.7%. It also has been demonstrated that a normal ultrasound could reduce the risk of DS by a likelihood ratio of 0.4.[49]

They reported that the yearly utilization of the genetic sonogram rather than amniocentesis was 0.4% in 1993, 16.6% in 1994, 48% in 1995 and 55% in 1996. They showed that women are accepting the genetic sonogram more and over half of the women presenting to the ultrasound laboratory, because of advanced maternal age or abnormal triple test screen, choose to have the genetic sonogram before they decide whether or not to have amniocentesis.[2,22,49]

In addition to the combination of sonographic markers with maternal age, the triple biochemical screen may also add information to the specific risk that a woman has a fetus with DS, before a woman makes a decision to undergo amniocentesis.

In a study by Yagel *et al.* evaluating women less than 35 years of age with abnormal triple screen results, the sensitivity for detection of DS using sonographic markers was 80%.[53] The use of ultrasound-adjusted risks of fetal trisomy 21 is expected to decrease the number of amniocenteses in older women when a genetic ultrasound examination does not demonstrate any abnormal ultrasound markers, while still identifying the majority of fetuses with DS.

A multicenter study was undertaken to evaluate the diagnostic efficacy of the genetic sonogram. Of a total of 176 fetuses with DS, 125 (71%) had an abnormal long bone length (femur, humerus) or a major structural abnormality or a sonographic soft marker for DS. The combined diagnostic sensitivity was 71.6%. The sensitivity of individual markers varies between 3% (sandal gap) and 46.5% (nuchal fold thickness). In this eight-center study, it was concluded that the genetic sonogram can be used to better adjust the DS risk for high-risk patients.[54]

In conclusion, multivariate analysis of sonographic markers of trisomy 21 has resulted in a detection rate of DS between 75% and 90% and presents a reasonable alternative to high-risk women considering invasive testing. Multivariate analysis permits more accurate counseling and allows identification of the optional components of a genetic sonogram. This may lead to a standardization of the contents, a shorter duration of the examination with no loss of sensitivity and a decrease in the false-positive rate.[55]

REFERENCES

1. Freeman SB, Taft LF, Dooley KJ. Population-based study of congenital heart defects in Down syndrome. *Am J Med Genet* 1998;80(3):213–7.
2. Shipp TD, Benacerraf BR. Second trimester ultrasound screening for chromosomal abnormalities. *Prenat Diagn* 2002;22:296–307.
3. Achiron R, Liptiz S, Gabbay V, Yagel S. Prenatal ultrasonographic diagnosis of fetal heart echogenic foci: No correlation with Down syndrome. *Obstet Gynecol* 1997;89:945–8.
4. Shipp TD, Bromley B, Lieberman E, Benacerraf BR. The frequency of the detection of fetal echogenic intracadiac foci with respect to maternal race. *Ultrasound Obstet Gynecol* 2000;15:460–2.
5. Bromley B, Lieberman E, Laboda L, Benacerraf BR. Echogenic intracardiac focus: A sonographic sign for fetal Down syndrome. *Obstet Gynecol* 1995;86:998–1001.
6. Sepulveda W, Romero D. Significance of echogenic foci in the fetal heart. *Ultrasound Obstet Gynecol* 1998;12:445–9.
7. Lamont RF, Havutcu E, Salgia S, Adinkra R, Nicholl R. The association between isolated fetal echogenic cardiac foci on second trimester ultrasound scan and trisomy 21 in low risk unselected women. *Ultrasound Obstet Gynecol* 2004;23:346–651.
8. Nyberg DA, Luthy DA, Resta RG, Nyberg BC, Williams JA. Age adjusted ultrasound risk assessment for fetal Down's syndrome during the second trimester description of the method and analysis of 142 cases. *Ultrasound Obstet Gynecol* 1998;12:8–14.
9. Snijders RM, Nicolaides KH. *Ultrasound Markers for Fetal Chromosomal Defects.* New York: Parthenon Publishing Group, 1996.
10. Nyberg D, Souter V, El-Bastawiss A, Young S, Luthhardt F, Luthy D. Isolated sonographic markers for detection of fetal Down syndrome in the second trimester of pregnancy. *J Ultrasound Med* 2001;20:1053–63.
11. Winder TC, Anderson AM, Cheng EY, *et al.* Echogenic intracardiac focus in 2nd trimester fetuses with trisomy 21: Usefulness as a U/S marker. *Radiology* 2000;216:450–6.
12. Vibhakar NI, Budorick NE, Scioscia AL, *et al.* Prevalence of aneuploidy with cardial intraventricular echogenic focus in an at risk patients population. *J Ultrasound Med* 1999;18:265–8.
13. Manning JE, Ragavendra N, Sayre J, *et al.* Significance of fetal intracardiac echogenic foci in relation to trisomy 21: A prospective sonographic study of high-risk pregnancy women. *Am J Roentgenol* 1998;170:1083–4.
14. Bromley B, Lieberman E, Shipp TO, *et al.* Significance of an echogenic intracardiac focus in fetuses at high and low risk for aneuploidy. *J Ultrasound Med* 1998;17:127–31.

15. Filly R, Benacerraf B, Nyberg D, Hobbins J. choroid plexus cyst and echogenic intracardiac focus in women at low risk for chromosomal anomalies. *J Ultrasound Med* 2004;23:447–9.
16. Benacerraf BR, Barss VA, Laboda LA. A sonographic sign for the detection in the second trimester of the fetus with Down's syndrome. *Am J Obstet Gynecol* 1985;151:1078–9.
17. Benacerraf BR, Gelman R, Frigoletto FD Jr. Sonographic identification of second trimester fetus with Down's syndrome. *N Engl J Med* 1987;317(22):1371–6.
18. Smith-Bindman R, Hosmer W, Feldstein VA, Deeks JJ, Goldberg JD. Second trimester ultrasound to detect fetuses with Down syndrome. A meta-analysis. *J Am Med Assoc* 2001;285:1044–55.
19. Gray DL, Crane JP. Optimal nuchal skin fold thresholds based on gestational age for prenatal detection of Down syndrome. *Clin J Obstet Gynecol* 1994;171:1282–6.
20. Wald N, Kennard A, Hackshaw A. Antenatal screening for Down's syndrome. *Health Technol Assess* 1998;2:41.
21. Drugan A, Johnson MP, Reichler A, Hume RF Jr, Itskovicz-Eldor J, Evans MI. Second trimester minor ultrasound anomalies impact on the risk of aneuploidy associated with advanced maternal age. *Obstet Gynecol* 1996;88(2):203–6.
22. Bahado-Singh RO, Goldstein I, Verpairojkit B, Copel JA, Mahoney MJ, Baumgarten A. Normal nuchal thickness in the mid-trimester indicates reduced risk of Down's yndrome in pregnancies with abnormal triple-screen results. *Am J Obstet Gynecol* 1995;173(4):1106–10.
23. Nicolaides K, Snijders RJ, Gosden CM, Berry C, Cambell S. Ultrasonographically detectable markers of fetal chromosomal abnormalities. *Lancet* 1992;340:704–7.
24. Fitzsimmons J, Droste S, Shepard TH, Pascoe-Mason J, Chinn A, Mack LA. Long bone growth in fetuses with Down syndrome. *Am J Obstet Gynecol* 1989;161:1174–7.
25. Ghidini A, Strobelt N, Lacatelli A. Isolated fetal choroid plexus cysts: Role of ultrasonography in establishment of the risk of trisomy 18. *Am J Obstet Gynecol* 2000;182:972–7.
26. Snijders RJ, Shawa L, Nocolaides KH. Fetal choroid plexus cysts and trisomy 18: Assessment of risk based on ultrasound findings and maternal age. *Prenat Diagn* 1994;14:119–27.
27. Yoder PR, Sabbagha RE, Gross, SJ, Zelop CM. The second trimester fetus with isolated choroids plexus cysts: A meta-analysis of risk of trisomies 18 and 21. *Obstet Gynecol* 1999;93:869–72.
28. Chitty LS, Chydleigh P, Wright E. The significance of choroid plexus cysts in an unselected population. Results of a multicenter study. *Ultrasound Obstet Gynecol* 1998;12:39.
29. Sepulvede W, Lopez-Tenorio J. The value of minor ultrasound markers for fetal aneuploidy. *Curr Opin Obstet Gynecol* 2001; 13:183–191.
30. Yaron Y, Hassan S, Geva E, Kupferminc MJ, Yavetz H, Evans M. Evaluation of fetal echogenic bowel in the second trimester. *Fetal Diagn Ther* 1999;14:176–80.
31. Penna L, Bower S. Hyperechogenic bowel in the second trimester fetus: A review. *Prenat Diagn* 2000;20:909–13.
32. Bromley B, Donbilet P, Frigoletto FD Jr, Krauss C, Estroff JA, Benacerraf BR. Is fetal hyperechoic bowel on second trimester sonogram an indication for amniocentesis. *Obstet Gynecol* 1994;83:647–51.
33. Nyberg DA, Resta RG, Luthy DA. Prenatal sonographic findings of Down syndrome: Review of 94 cases. *Obstet Gynecol* 1990; 76:370–7.
34. Slotnik RN, Abuhamad AZ. Prognostic implications of fetal echogenic bowel. *Lancet* 1996;347:85.
35. Sepulveda W, Sebire NJ. Fetal echogenic bowel: A complex senario. *Ultrasound Obstet Gynecol* 2000;16:510–4.
36. Cardoza JD, Coldstein RB, Filly RA. Exclusion of fetal venticulomegaly with a single measurement the width of the lateral ventricular atrium. *Radiology* 1988;169:711–4.
37. Kelly E, Allen V, Seaward G, Windrim R, Ryan G. Mild venticulomegaly in the fetus, natural history, associated findings and outcome of isolated mild venticulomegaly a literature review. *Prenat Diagn* 2001;21:697–700.
38. Achiron R, Schimmel M, Achiron A, Mashiach S. Fetal mild idiopathic venticulomegaly: Is there a correlation with foetal trisomy. *Ultrasound Obstet Gynecol* 1993;3:89–92.
39. Robson S, Mc Cormak K, Rankin J. Prenatally detected mild/moderate cerebral ventriculomegaly: Associated anomalies and outcome. Northern Congenital Abnormality Survey Steering Group. *Eur J Pediatr Surg* 1998;8:70–1.
40. Senat MV, Bernard JP, Schwarzler P, Britten J, Ville Y. Prenatal diagnosis and follow-up of 14 cases of unilateral ventriculomegaly. *Ultrasound Obstet Gynecol* 1999;14:327–32.
41. Pilu G, Falco P, Gabrielli S, Perolo A, Sandri F, Bovicelli L. The clinical significance of fetal isolated cerebral borderline ventriculomegaly: Report of 31 cases and review of the literature. *Ultrasound Obstet Gynecol* 1999;14:320–6.
42. Benacerraf BR, Mandell J, Estroff JA, Harlow BL, Frigoletto FD Jr. Fetal pyelectasis: A possible association with Down syndrome. *Obstet Gynecol* 1990;76:58–60.
43. Chudleigh T. Mild pyelectasis. *Prenat Daign* 2001;21:936–41.
44. Chudleigh PM, Chitty LS, Pembrey M, Campbell S. The association of aneuploidy and mild fetal pyelectasis in an unselected population: The results of a multicenter study. *Ultrasound Obstet Gynecol* 2001;14(Suppl 1):12.
45. Pilu G, Nicolaides KH. Features of chromosomal defects. In *Diagnosis of Fetal Abnormalities: The 18-23 Week Scan.* Carnforth, UK: Parthenon Publishing Group, 1999:99–104.
46. Benacerraf BR, Harlow BL, Frigoletto FD Jr. Hypoplasia of the middle phalanx of the fifth digit: A feature of the second trimester fetus with Down's syndrome. *J Ultrasound Med* 1990; 9:389–94.
47. Appelman Z, Zalel Y, Fried S, Caspi B. Delay fusion of amnion and chorion: A possible association with trisomy 21 (letter). *Ultrasound Obset Gynecol* 1998;11:303–4.
48. Nyberg DA, Resta RG, Luthy DA, Hickok DE, Williams MA. Humerus and femur length shortening in the detection of Down's syndrome. *Am J Obstet Gynecol* 1993;168:534–9.
49. Vintzileos AM, Campbell WA, Guzman ER, Smulion JC, McLean DA, Ananth CV. Second trimester ultrasound markers for detection of trisomy 21: Which markers are best? *Obstet Gynecol* 1997;89(7):941–4.
50. Benacerraf BR, Nadel A, Bromley B. Identification of second trimester fetuses with autosomal trisomy by use of a sonographic scoring index. *Radiology* 1994;193:135–40.
51. Benacerraf BR, Nyberg D, Bromley B, Frigoletto FD Jr. Sonographic scoring index for prenatal detection of chromosomal abnormalities. *J Ultrasound Med* 1992;11(9):449–58.
52. Nadel AS, Bromley B, Frigoletto FD Jr, Benacerraf BR. Can the presumed risk of autosomal trisomy be decreased in fetus of older women following a normal sonogram? *J Ultrasound Med* 1995;14:297–302.
53. Yagel S, Anteby EY, Hochner-Celnilier D, *et al.* The role of mid-trimester targeted fetal organ screening combined with the triple test and maternal age in the diagnosis of trisomy 21: A retrospective study. *Am J Obstet Gynecol* 1998;178:40.
54. Hobbins J, Lezotte D, Pesutle W, *et al.* An 8 center study to evaluate the utility of midterm genetic sonograms among high risk pregnancies. *J Ultrasound Med* 2003;22:33–8.
55. Vergani P, Locatelly A, Piccoli MG, *et al.* Best second trimester sonographic markers for the detection of trisomy 21. *J Ultrasound Med* 1999;18:469–73.
56. Strocter AM, Snijders RJ, Carlson DE, *et al.* Fetal echogenic bowel parameters to be considered in differential diagnosis. *Ultrasound Obstet Gynecol* 2000;16:519–523.
57. Thompson MO, Thialganathan B. Effect of routine screening for Down's syndrome on the significance of isolated fetal hydronephrosis. *Br J Obstet Gynecol* 1998;105:860–864.

114 Fetal anatomy in the first trimester of pregnancy

A. Antsaklis and A. Souka

Introduction

First-trimester ultrasound scan was initially used to date the pregnancy. In the last 15 years, technological progress and, in particular, the introduction of the transvaginal approach made possible the detailed examination of the fetal anatomy in the first trimester for the diagnosis of structural defects.

In this decade, a number of studies have shown that nuchal translucency (NT) (the accumulation of fluid in the nuchal area, Figure 114.1) can be measured by ultrasound at 11–14 weeks. NT measurement is a sensitive and accurate screening test for the diagnosis of chromosomal abnormalities yielding a sensitivity of about 75% for a 5% screen positive rate.[1] The introduction of first-trimester biochemical markers free beta-human chorionic gonadotropin (beta-hCG) and pregnancy associated plasma protein A (PAPP-A) has increased the sensitivity to about 90% for the same screen positive rate.[2]

Increased NT at 11–14 weeks has been associated with structural defects and in particular cardiac defects and a wide range of genetic syndromes.[3] Possible pathophysiological mechanisms include cardiac dysfunction, venous stasis, anomalous or delayed development of the lymphatic vessels of the neck, abnormal collagen biosynthesis, fetal anemia and congenital infections.

The majority of the fetal organs can be visualized in the first trimester and transvaginal scanning has greatly increased our ability to examine the first-trimester fetus.

Using ultrasound scanning in the first trimester, we can accurately date the pregnancy, establish fetal viability and ascertain chorionicity in multiple pregnancies. At 11–14 weeks, we can estimate the risk of chromosomal defect by NT measurement and examine fetal anatomy.

The normal first-trimester fetus

Several ultrasound studies[4–28] using mainly the transvaginal approach at 4–12 weeks of gestation describe the development of the normal fetus as follows.

The fourth week

The gestational sac is visible from about 4 weeks and 3 days as a hypoechoic, ring-like 2–3 mm structure surrounded by a hyperechoic rim. Further details within the sac cannot yet be defined. The sac represents the chorionic cavity and is typically located in the upper part of the decidualized endometrium in an eccentric position.

The fifth week

The yolk sac becomes visible as the first structure within the sac at about 5 weeks and is always present at 5 weeks and 4 days. At the end of the fifth week the fetal pole measuring 2–3 mm can be seen beside the yolk sac and heart motion may be identified. At this stage the fetal heart rate is about 100 beats/min.

The sixth week

At 6 weeks, the embryo measures (crown–rump length, CRL) 4–8 mm. The fetal pole, the yolk sac and the heart motion are always visible. Heart activity should always be seen in embryos of 5 mm (6 weeks and 4 days) or more. The gestational sac contains two

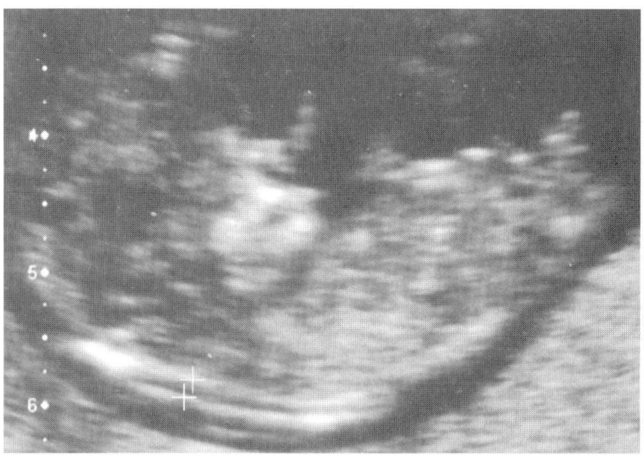

Figure 114.1 Nuchal translucency in an 11-week fetus.

fluid-filled cavities: the coelomic (chorionic) cavity with the yolk sac and the considerably smaller amniotic cavity with the fetal pole. The two cavities are separated by a thin membrane surrounding the embryo, the amniotic membrane. At the end of the sixth week the cavity of the rhombencephalon becomes visible as a small hypoechogenic area at the cephalic part of the fetal pole.

The seventh week

At 7 weeks the CRL is 9–14 mm and the mean heart rate is about 130 beats/min. The amniotic cavity starts expanding rapidly. The head can be distinguished from the body and hypoechogenic areas (brain vesicles, Figure 114.2) appear in the developing brain at the cephalic end of the embryo. The cavity of the rhombencephalon that will eventually form the pons and the cerebellum can always be identified at 7 weeks as a rhomboid, hypoechoic area at the cranial pole of the embryo. At this stage the rhombencephalon is larger than the developing hemispheres. The small cavities of the hemispheres originating from the dividing Y-shaped telencephalon, the diencephalon (that will form the thalami, hypothalamus and the third ventricle) and the mesencephalon (that will later form the nuclei and the aqueduct of Sylvius) may be identifiable.

The umbilical cord is short and appears wider and hyperechogenic at the point of the insertion in the abdomen; this is the first sign of bowel herniation into the cord. The lower limb buds can vaguely be depicted.

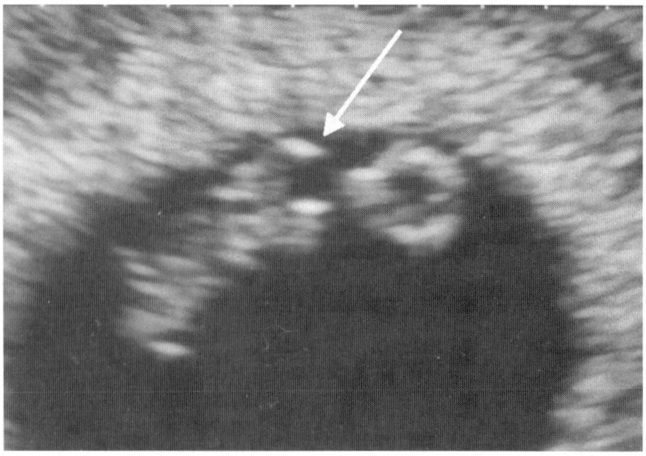

Figure 114.2 A 7-week fetus. The arrow points to the cavity of the rhombencephalon.

The eighth week

At 8 weeks, the CRL is 15–22 mm, the brain vesicles are more prominent and the choroid plexuses can be visualized as small hyperechogenic areas. The rhombencephalon is still the largest cavity lying on top of the brain. There is a broad connection between the lateral ventricles, the diencephalon and the mesencephalon. Fetal heart rate is about 160 beats/min and the heart occupies more than 50% of the thoracic cavity. Atria and ventricles are sometimes visible at the end of the eighth week. The abdominal cavity is fully occupied by the liver anteriorly and the stomach dorsally while the intestine is herniated into the umbilical cord. Fluid in the stomach can occasionally be seen toward the end of the eighth week probably as a product of the gastric epithelium, since swallowing movements only start at 11 weeks. The outlines of the skull, spine and ribs can vaguely be seen. The limbs appear as short echogenic outgrowths and the first body movements become visible during the eighth week.

The ninth week

At 9 weeks, the CRL is 23–31 mm. The amniotic cavity is now larger than the coelomic cavity and occupies most of the sac volume. The fetal body becomes ellipsoid with the head being disproportionately big and the soles of the feet touch in the midline. The choroid plexuses are obvious and occupy almost fully the lateral ventricles. The cortex is thin and hypoechoic. The cerebral hemispheres become visible and are clearly separated. The connection between the mesencephalon and the third ventricle becomes narrower. The fetal heart rate reaches a peak of about 175 beats/min. Bowel herniation is visible in all fetuses. The first ossification centers can be seen at the mandible and clavicle. Limb movements can be identified.

The postembryonic period (10–11 weeks)

During the postembryonic period, the CRL is 32–54 mm. The fetus acquires human shape and the fetal body becomes longer although the head is still disproportionately large with a prominent forehead and a flat occiput. The cerebral hemispheres start being detectable during the ninth week. Ossification starts from the occipital bone at 10 weeks. The cortex is about 1 mm thick at the end of the first trimester. The lateral ventricles occupy completely the anterior part of the head and cover the diencephalon. The mesencephalon gradually moves toward the middle of the brain, the third ventricle, after a transient increase, becomes narrow and the cerebral hemispheres fuse in the midline at 11–12 weeks. Fetal heart rate drops to about 165 beats/min at the end of the 11th week. The motion of the atrioventricular valves and the atrial and ventricular septa may be visible at 10 weeks. All cardiac structures can be visualized at the end of the 11th week. Starting from the end of the eighth week the small bowel herniates into the umbilical cord and gives the sonographic appearance of a hyperechogenic mass at the insertion of the cord. Maximum herniation of the

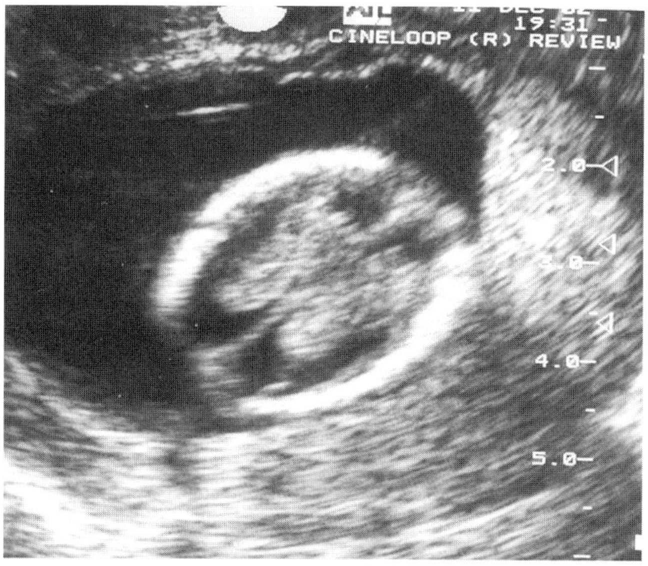

Figure 114.3 Fetal skull and brain.

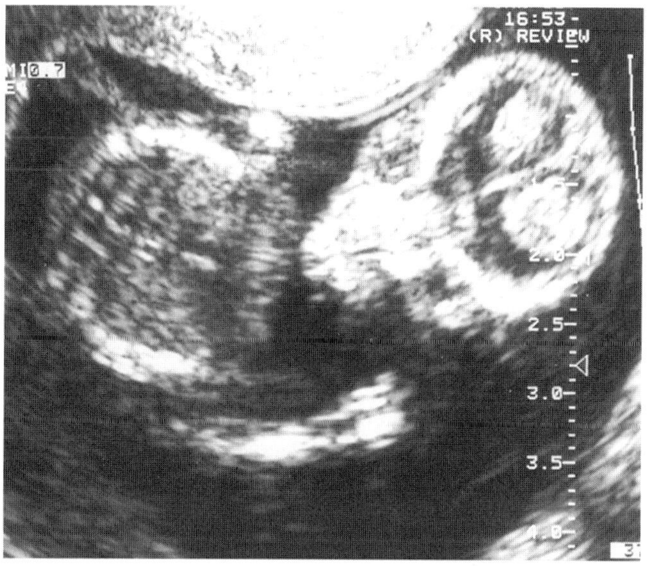

Figure 114.4 Fetal face.

bowel is detectable at the beginning of the 10th week, whereas the return of the bowel in the abdominal cavity begins at 10 weeks and 4 days and is usually completed at 11 weeks and 5 days. In 75% of embryos the stomach is visible before the 10th week. The ossification centers of the spine and the long bones start being visible at 10 weeks. The ossification of the spine begins at the level of the cervical vertebrae and spreads caudally to the thoracic and lumbosacral areas during weeks 12–13. Ossification of the metacarpals and metatarsals can be identified at 12 weeks. The digits and sometimes the toes become visible from 11 weeks.

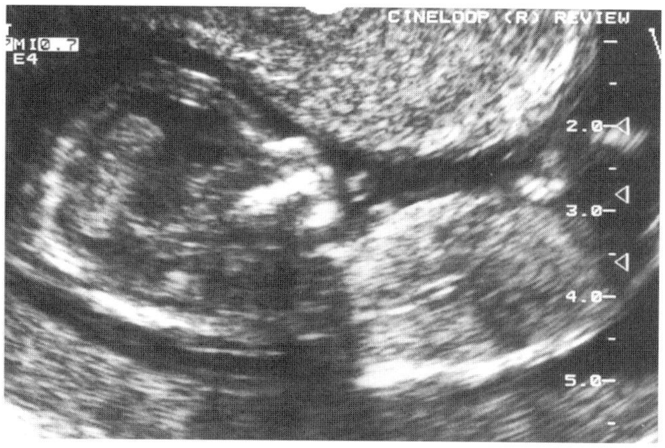

Figure 114.5 Fetal profile.

Fetal anatomy at 11–14 weeks

Although in the general population structural defects are relatively common (3–5%) and cardiac defects the commonest amongst them, few studies have addressed the issue of fetal anatomy in low-risk populations as part of the 11–14 weeks' scan.[20,29–34] Visualization of the cardiac anatomy at this gestational period has been reported from specialists in fetal echocardiography and has been mainly limited to high-risk pregnancies.[35–45]

Two studies[20,46] examining fetal anatomy at 11–14 weeks have used the following protocol:

(1) Skull and brain: examination of the completeness of the skull, the presence of the midline in the brain and the butterfly shape of the choroid plexuses (Figure 114.3).
(2) Face: examination of the orbits and lenses and the view of the fetal profile (Figures 114.4 and 114.5).
(3) Spine: examination of the alignment of the vertebrae and the skin covering the spine (Figure 114.6).
(4) Heart: examination of the four-chamber view and the great vessels (three-vessel view, Figures 114.7 and 114.8).
(5) Stomach: visualization of the stomach as a hypoechoic structure at the left upper abdomen (Figure 114.9).
(6) Abdomen: examination of the umbilical cord insertion into the abdominal wall (Figure 114.10).
(7) Kidneys: visualization of the kidneys as hyperechoic structures with a hypoechoic center lateral to the spine (Figure 114.11).
(8) Bladder: visualization of the bladder as a hypoechoic structure in the fetal pelvis (Figure 114.12).
(9) Extremities: examination of the long bones, fingers, toes and the movement and posture of the joints (Figures 114.13 and 114.14).

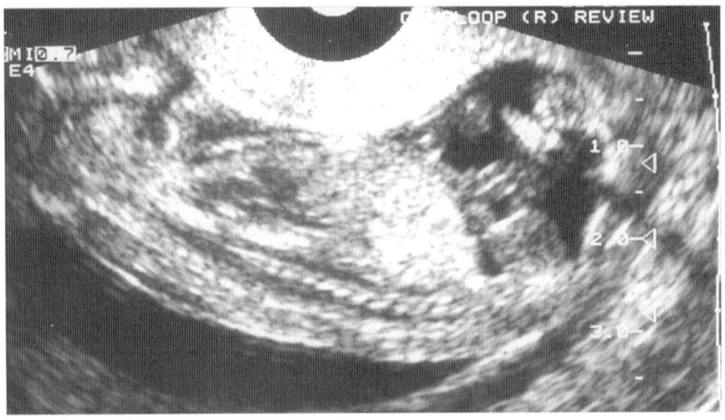

Figure 114.6 Fetal spine.

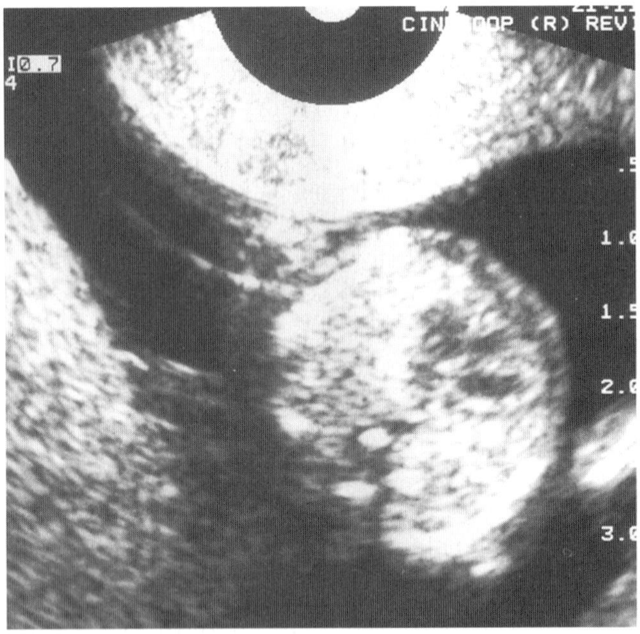

Figure 114.7 Fetal heart. The four-chamber view.

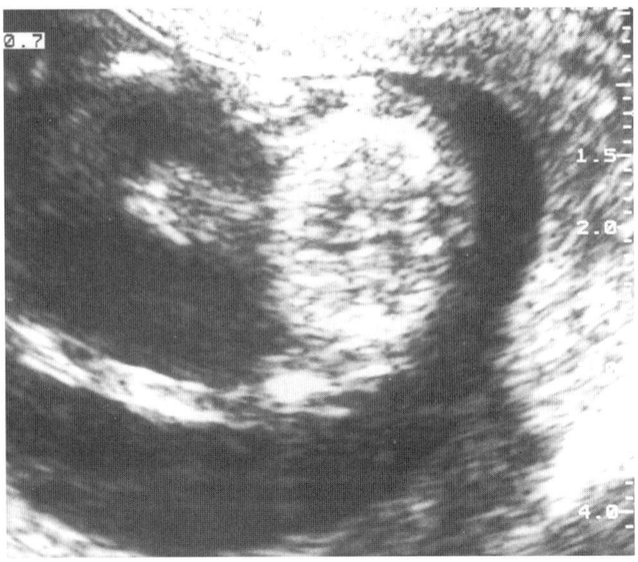

Figure 114.8 Fetal heart. The three-vessel view.

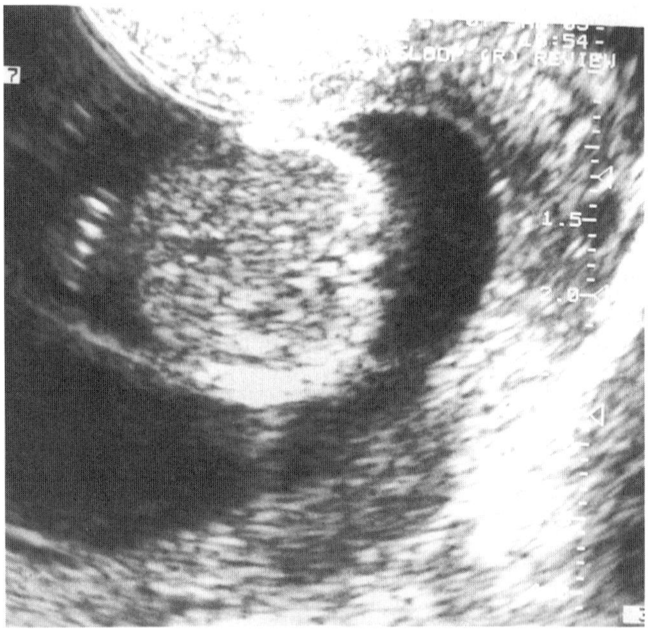

Figure 114.9 Transverse section of the abdomen (the stomach).

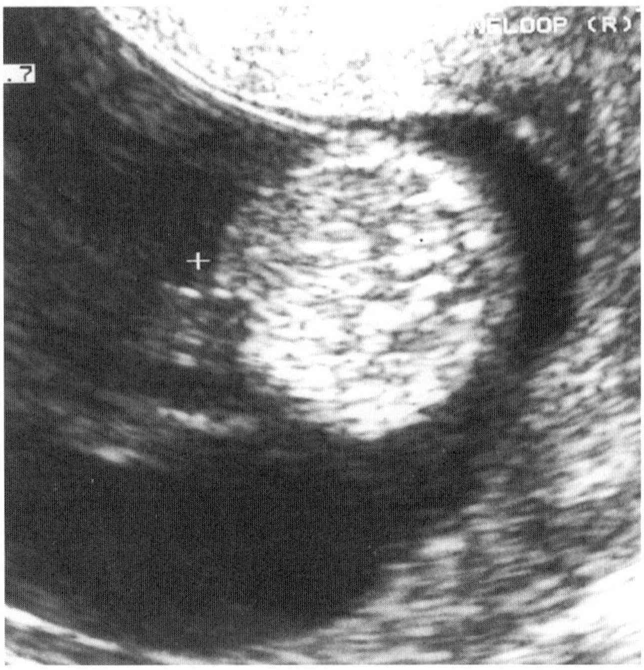

Figure 114.10 Umbilical cord insertion.

In a study of 1144 fetuses examined at 11–14 weeks with a combination of the transabdominal and transvaginal route full check of the fetal anatomy was achieved in 48% of the fetuses, whereas non-cardiac anatomy was visualized in 86% of the fetuses.[46] Successful visualization of the fetal organs depended on CRL (Table 114.1). The use of the transvaginal approach increased successful examination of the

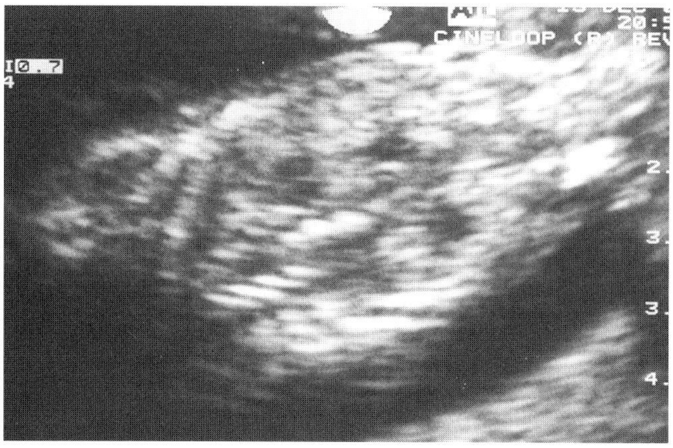

Figure 114.11 Fetal kidneys.

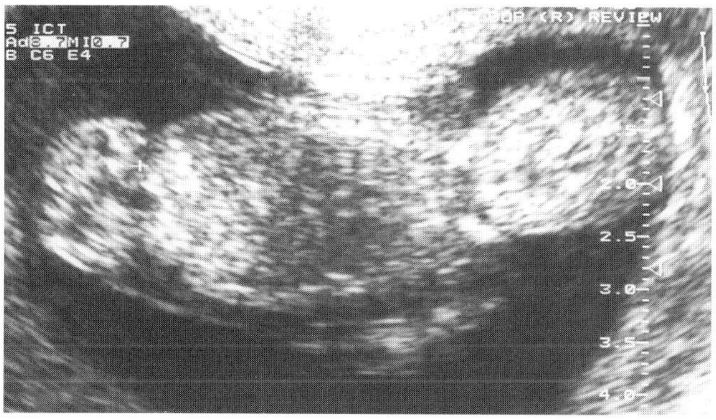

Figure 114.12 Fetal bladder.

fetal anatomy from 72% to 86% of the fetuses (Table 114.2). Transvaginal scanning was particularly helpful in examining the face, kidneys and bladder.

In a screening study for structural abnormalities at 11–14 weeks using transvaginal ultrasound, fetal anatomy (not including face and heart) was seen in 94% of the cases.[30] Similarly in an anatomical survey of 298 fetuses at 12+0 to 13+6 weeks of gestation, Braithwaite *et al.* were able to complete the examination of the fetal anatomy, including the four-chamber view, in 95% of the fetuses.[20] With the combination of the transabdominal and transvaginal route the four-chamber view of the heart was seen in 97% of the fetuses, the bladder in 98%, the head, brain and kidneys in 99% and the remaining organs (diaphragm, stomach, abdominal wall, spine and extremities) in 100% of the fetuses. The use of the transvaginal approach increased successful examination of the fetal anatomy from 72% to 95%.[20] In both studies the factors influencing visualization of the fetal organs were gestation, maternal habitus and uterine position and the authors stress the contribution of the transvaginal ultrasound in completing the examination of the fetus.

A few studies have addressed the issue of visualizing the four-chamber view and the outflow tracts at 11–14 weeks (Tables 114.3 and 114.4).[36–39,44,46,47]

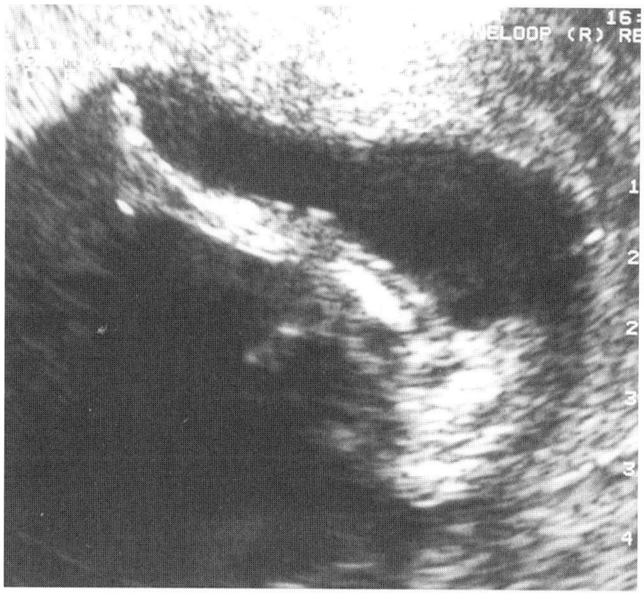

Figure 114.13 Fetal lower extremity.

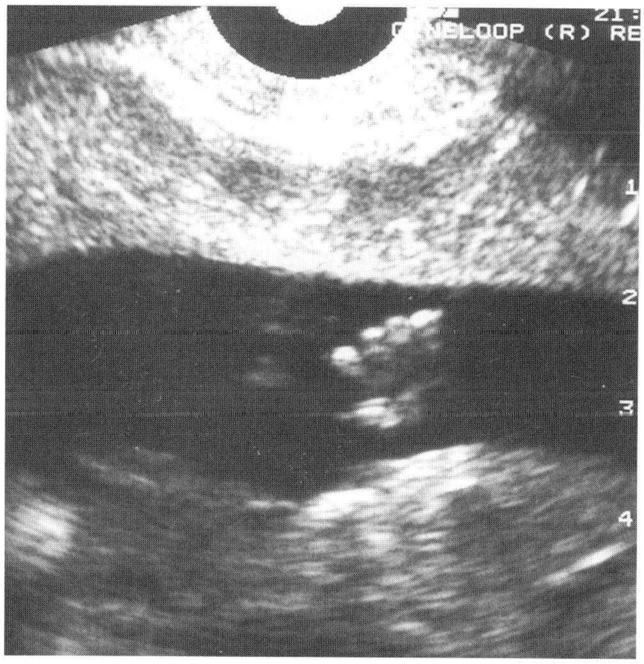

Figure 114.14 Fetal hand.

Examination of the fetal heart at this early gestation is still mainly restricted to high-risk patients and performed in specialized centers by experts in fetal echocardiography. Visualization rates of the four-chamber view improved with gestation, remaining poor before 11 weeks and increasing to more than 90% during the 12th and 13th weeks (Table 114.3). Similarly, visualization of the outflow tracts was achieved in the majority of the fetuses examined between 12+0 and 13+6 weeks of gestation. Only two studies have examined cardiac anatomy as part of

Table 114.1 Visualization of fetal anatomic structures according to crown–rump length. Anatomy Check I = includes all other organs except of the heart, Anatomy Check II = all organs including heart anatomy[46]

CRL (mm)	N	Anatomy Check I	Anatomy Check II	Head/ Brain	Face	Spine	Heart	Abdomen	Stomach	Kidneys	Bladder	Extremities
45–54	174	113 (64.94%)	38 (21.83%)	174 (100%)	171 (98.27%)	172 (98.85%)	44 (25.28%)	172 (98.85%)	166 (95.40%)	123 (70.68%)	170 (97.70%)	174 (100%)
55–64	400	337 (84.25%)	173 (43.25%)	400 (100%)	398 (99.5%)	399 (99.75%)	183 (45.75%)	400 (100%)	398 (99.50%)	341 (85.25%)	397 (99.25%)	400 (100%)
65–74	413	386 (93.46%)	233 (56.41%)	413 (100%)	409 (99.03%)	413 (100%)	238 (57.62%)	413 (100%)	412 (99.75%)	388 (93.94%)	412 (99.75%)	413 (100%)
75–82	157	150 (95.54%)	105 (66.87%)	157 (100%)	157 (100%)	157 (100%)	105 (66.87%)	157 (100%)	157 (100%)	150 (95.54%)	157 (100%)	157 (100%)
Total	1,144	986 (86.18%)	549 (47.98%)	1,144 (100%)	1,135 (99.21%)	1,141 (99.73%)	570 (49.82%)	1,142 (99.82%)	1,133 (99.03%)	1,002 (87.58%)	1,136 (99.30%)	1,144 (100%)

Table 114.2 The contribution of transvaginal scanning in visualizing fetal anatomy according to crown–rump length[46]

CRL (mm)	N	TAS	TAS + TVS
45–54	174	99 (56.89%)	113 (64.94%)
55–64	400	301 (75.25%)	337 (84.25%)
65–74	413	307 (74.33%)	386 (93.46%)
74–82	157	119 (75.79%)	150 (95.54%)
Total	1,144	826 (72.20%)	986 (86.18%)

the routine 11–14 weeks' scan.[20,46] In the first study on 298 women, examination was performed at 12 + 0 to 13 + 6 weeks and the four-chamber view was seen in 76% of fetuses transabdominally, 95% transvaginally and 97% using a combined approach. Outflow tracts were not examined.[20] In the second study, 1144 women were examined at 11 – (13 + 6) weeks of gestation (CRL 45–82 mm). Complete cardiac anatomy was seen in 50% of fetuses, with visualization of the four-chamber view in 87% of cases and of the three-vessel view in 50% of cases.

Studies on screening for structural defects by first-trimester ultrasound

Three studies on a total of 12,327 pregnancies have examined the impact of assessing fetal anatomy in the first trimester on the detection rate of structural defects (Table 114.5). The differences in the detection rates can mainly be attributed to differences in protocols, definition and postnatal ascertainment of anomalies. The study with the lowest detection rate reports on all (major and minor) anomalies; if only major anomalies were included, the first-trimester scan sensitivity would be 50.8% and the overall ultrasound scan sensitivity 78.8%.[34] Detection rates in the two other studies have been calculated excluding nuchal anomalies. The majority of abnormalities diagnosed in the second and third trimester would not be detectable in the first trimester including central nervous system defects (microcephaly, ventriculomegaly, brain atrophy, Dandy–Walker malformation, cerebellar asymmetry), cardiac defects (tetralogy of Fallot, hypoplastic left heart, ventricular septal defects), renal defects (hydronephrosis, multicystic dysplastic kidneys) and gastrointestinal defects (bowel obstruction). However, it is likely that at least some of the cases of neural tube defects and cardiac defects and probably all cases of abdominal wall defects and limb reduction defects will in the future be diagnosed in the first trimester. These studies have shown that the first-trimester scan can detect more than one-third of the major structural anomalies, including lethal anomalies or those leading to severe handicap (anencephaly, holoprosencephaly, body stalk anomaly).

In conclusion, examination of the fetal anatomy is feasible during the routine 11–14 weeks scan and the completeness of the examination mainly depends on maternal habits and gestational age. It is clear that the optimal gestation for examining both cardiac and non-cardiac anatomy starts from the beginning of the 12th week to the end of the 13th week of gestation. Access to the transvaginal approach is important in completing the examination.

With the modern trend of shifting prenatal diagnosis at the earliest possible gestation and the advancing technology, it is not difficult to see the 11–14 weeks' scan becoming the first minianomaly scan with the aim of diagnosing the severest structural anomalies, thus giving the parents earlier reassurance about the well-being of their fetus.

Table 114.3 Visualization rates of the 4-chamber view according to gestational age

	Visualization rate % (Number of fetuses examined)			
Author	**10–10^{+6} wks**	**11–11^{+6} wks**	**12–12^{+6} wks**	**13-13^{+6} wks**
Dolkart and Reimers 1991[36]	0 (8)	30 (10)	90 (10)	100 (13)
Johnson *et al.* 1992[37]	27 (26)	58 (33)	71 (51)	74 (61)
Bronshtein *et al.* 1992[38]	NE	17 (18)	36 (25)	100 (NS)
Gembruch *et al.* 1993[39]	NE	80 (15)	93 (30)	100 (51)
Gembruch *et al.* 2000[47]	56 (9)	88 (16)	93 (15)	100 (16)
Haak *et al.* 2002[44]	NE	85 (85)	97 (85)	98 (85)
Souka *et al.* 2004[46]	NE	67 (1,144)	87 (1,144)	96 (1,144)

NE: not examined, NS: not specified

Table 114.4 Visualization rates of the outflow tracts according to gestational age

		Visualization rate % (Number of fetuses examined)			
Author	**Vessel**	**10–10^{+6} wks**	**11–11^{+6} wks**	**12–12^{+6} wks**	**13–13^{+6} wks**
Dolkart and Reimers 1991[36]	Aorta	0 (10)	20 (10)	40 (10)	46 (13)
	Pulmonary	0 (10)	0 (10)	40 (10)	38 (13)
Johnson *et al.* 1992[37]	Aorta	4 (26)	24 (33)	59 (51)	62 (61)
	Pulmonary	12 (26)	21 (33)	41 (51)	51 (61)
Gembruch *et al.* 1993[39]	Combined	NE	67 (15)	80 (30)	100 (51)
Gembruch *et al.* 2000[47]	Combined	44 (9)	75 (16)	93 (15)	100 (16)
Haak *et al.* 2002[44]	Aorta	NE	33 (85)	77 (85)	95 (85)
	Pulmonary	NE	75 (85)	89 (85)	98 (85)
Souka *et al.* 2004[46]	Combined	NE	25 (1,144)	48 (1,144)	61 (1,144)

NE: not examined

Table 114.5 Screening studies of major structural abnormalities by first-trimester ultrasound

			Prenatal diagnosis	
Author	**N**	**Anomalies**	**Total**	**11–13^{+6} weeks**
Hernandi and Torocsik, 1997[30]	3,991	40	30 (75.0%)	11 (27.5%)
Economides *et al.* 1998[33]	1,632	13	10 (76.9%)	7 (53.8%)
Carvalho *et al.* 2002[34]	2,853	66	52 (78.8%)	25 (37.8%)
Drysdale *et al.* 2002[48]	960	18	15 (83.3%)	2 (11.1%)
Total	9,436	137	94 (68.6%)	58 (42.3%)

Structural defects at 11–14 weeks

Central nervous system defects

Acrania/anencephaly (birth prevalence 1 in 1000)

The diagnosis of anencephaly in the second and third trimesters of the pregnancy is based on the absence of cranium and cerebral hemispheres. Animal studies have shown that the absence of the skull leads to progressive degeneration and destruction of the brain tissue. Similarly, ultrasound studies have shown that in human embryo acrania progresses to exencephaly and anencephaly.[48–56] Acrania, meaning the absence of the skull (cranium), is the hallmark of anencephaly in the first trimester. The brain may show signs of degeneration or even appear normal. Several authors have described cases of anencephaly from as early as 9 weeks; the appearance of the brain varies from echogenic and disorganized with abnormal shape of the skull and head circumference smaller than the abdominal circumference to completely normal.[48,49,53–55] In the four screening studies for structural defects by first-trimester ultrasound, all cases of anencephaly were diagnosed in the first trimester.[30,32,34,57] In two screening studies for chromosomal abnormalities by NT measurement on a total of 6861 pregnancies, all seven anencephalic fetuses were correctly identified in the first trimester.[50,56] In another screening study of about 54,000 pregnancies there were 47 cases of anencephaly.[51] In the first phase of the study the sensitivity of the first-trimester scan for diagnosing anencephaly was 74% (23 of 31 cases) but this increased to 100% (16 of 16 cases) in the second phase when sonographers were instructed to look for the specific signs of anencephaly at this early gestation.

Holoprosencephaly (birth prevalence 1 in 5000)

This rare but severe defect covers a spectrum of conditions where there is a defect in the division of the prosencephalon, the frontal part of the brain. There are three types (lobar, semilobar, and alobar holoprosencephaly) depending on the degree of fusion of the prosencephalon. In the lobar type, the ventricles and thalami are divided but the cavum septum pellucidum is absent. In the semilobar type the lateral ventricles and thalami are only partially separated and in the alobar type there is complete fusion of the ventricles with a large monoventricle and fused thalami. The defect is strongly related to chromosomal abnormalities (particularly trisomies 13 and 18) and other structural defects (mainly facial clefts). Holoprosencephaly was present in 24% of the 46 fetuses with trisomy 13 at 10–14 weeks, as described by Snidjers *et al.*[58] The diagnosis of the alobar type has been reported in the first trimester based on the visualization of a single ventricle and the fusion of the thalami.[59–67] In the earliest report of alobar holoprosencephaly Blaas *et al.* diagnosed the defect at 9 weeks and 2 days (CRL 22 mm).[66] There was a small monoventricular endbrain behind the forehead and a proboscis. The diagnosis was confirmed a week later. In four screening studies for structural defects by first-trimester ultrasound on a total of about 9500 fetuses, there were four cases of holoprosencephaly and three were diagnosed in the first trimester.[30,33,34,46] Spina bifida (birth prevalence 1 in 1000) is the result of failed closure of the neural tube normally occurring during the sixth week, whereas the ossification of the spine begins at 10 weeks. The hallmarks of the diagnosis of spina bifida in the second trimester are the scalloping of the frontal bones of the skull (lemon sign) and the displacement of the cerebellum (Arnold–Chiari malformation, banana sign).

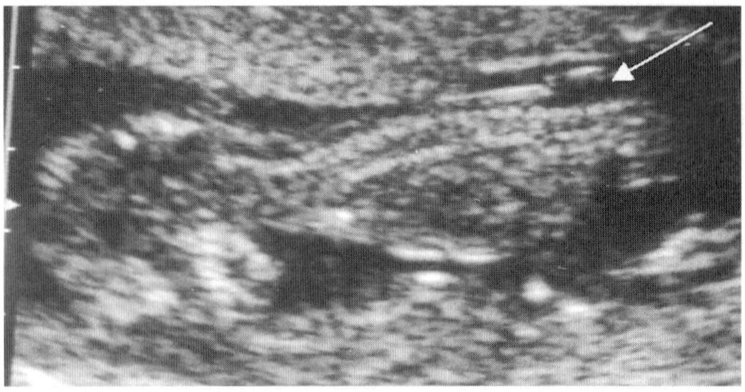

Figure 114.15 Spina bifida in a 13-week fetus.

The diagnosis of spina bifida has been reported in the first trimester from as early as 9 weeks.[68–72] Blaas *et al.* identified the defects in three embryos from high-risk pregnancies at 9 weeks of gestation (CRL 22–28 mm).[71] The authors used a combination of two- and three-dimensional transvaginal ultrasound to examine the spine. They note that the scalloping of the frontal bones and the Arnold–Chiari malformation did not occur before 12 weeks (Figure 114.15).

In four screening studies for structural defects by first-trimester ultrasound, there were 12 cases of spina bifida on a total of about 9500 fetuses and six were diagnosed in the first trimester.[30,33,34,46] It is of interest that at least in some cases the lemon sign and banana sign are present in the first trimester (Figures 114.16 and 114.17).

Heart defects

Congenital heart defects are amongst the commonest structural defects with a birth prevalence of 5–10 per 1000 births. Approximately, one half of those will need medical or surgical treatment (major defects) and the other half will be asymptomatic (minor defects). First-trimester diagnosis of several cardiac abnormalities has been reported in the first trimester, such as ectopia cordis, common truncus arteriosus, dextrocardia, monoventricular heart, Uhl disease, atrioventricular septal defect and ventricular septal defect.[73–77]

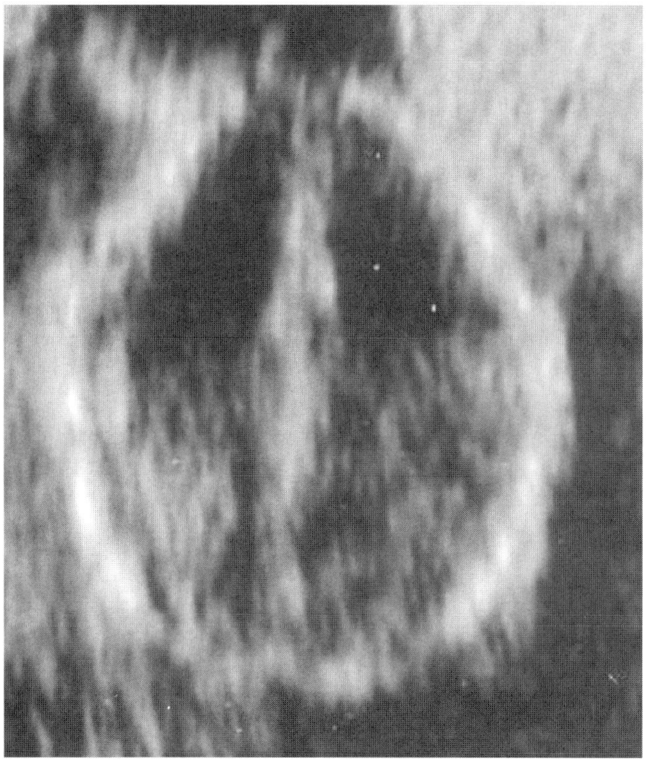

Figure 114.16 Lemon sign in a 13-week fetus.

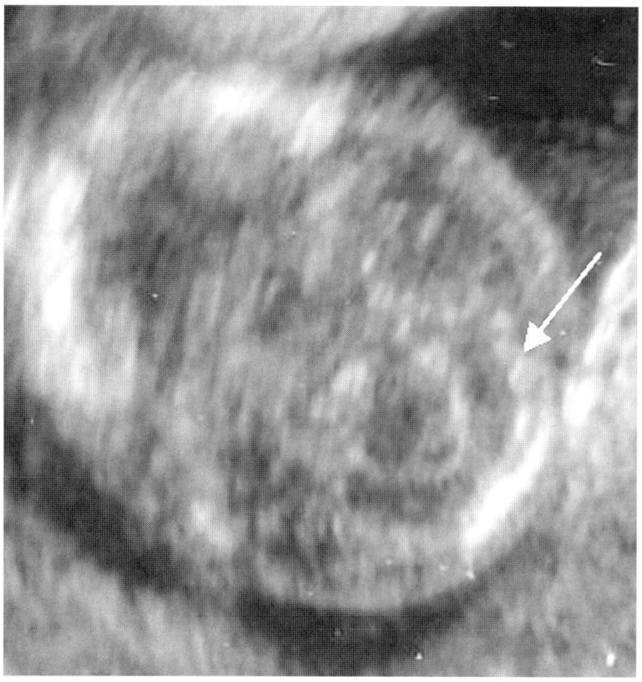

Figure 114.17 Banana sign in a 13-week fetus.

In a screening study of 114 pregnancies at risk for cardiac defects by transvaginal ultrasound at 11–16 weeks of gestation, there were six abnormal fetuses scanned at 11–14 weeks and the defect was diagnosed in five (sensitivity 83%).[78] Nuchal fluid was increased in four fetuses. In another small study of 15 high-risk fetuses scanned at 12 – (13+0) weeks,[79] the first-trimester scans were normal in 10 cases and inconclusive in four cases; one of the two cardiac anomalies (left isomerism) was identified at 12 weeks and a muscular ventricular septal defect was diagnosed postnatally (sensitivity 83%). Haak *et al.* performed first-trimester transvaginal fetal echocardiography in 54 fetuses with increased NT and reported sensitivity and specificity of 88% and 97%, respectively.[43] Another study on 241 fetuses with increased NT at 11–14 weeks (CRL 40–85 mm) identified 28 of the 37 cardiac anomalies in the first trimester (sensitivity 76%).[80]

Screening studies for heart defects have so far been limited to high-risk pregnancies defined by family history, maternal disease (diabetes, epilepsy) or increased nuchal thickness and performed in the setting of fetal echocardiography units by experts in cardiac scanning, thus explaining the high sensitivities reported. There is a strong association of increased NT with cardiac defects. A meta-analysis of screening studies reported that the detection rates for heart abnormalities were about 37% and 31% for NT cutoffs of 95th and 99th percentiles, respectively.[81] Fetal echocardiography, during the first trimester if possible, should be included in the routine follow-up of the fetuses with increased nuchal fluid.

Abdominal wall defects

Exomphalos (omphalocele, birth prevalence 1 in 4000)

In exomphalos there is midline defect of the abdominal wall through which intra-abdominal viscera herniated into a sac. The umbilical cord inserts at the apex of the sac. Herniation of the small bowel only is a normal step of the embryonic development and occurs between 8 and 10 weeks. The diagnosis of exomphalos is made if the bowel fails to return into the abdominal cavity by 11 weeks or if other viscera are herniated at any gestation.

Exomphalos is commonly associated with chromosomal abnormalities and syndromes. Chromosomal abnormalities, usually trisomy 18, are present in about half of the fetuses with exomphalos in the first trimester, one-third of cases in the second trimester and about 15% at birth. Exomphalos may be part of an extended defect in the abdominal wall development. If the abnormality involves the cephalic fold it results in pentalogy of Cantrell (exomphalos, ectopia cordis, cardiac defects, diaphragmatic hernia, sternal cleft). If it involves the caudal fold it results in bladder or cloacal exstrophy, bowel atresia and vertebral defects.

Many cases with exomphalos have been diagnosed in the first trimester, the earliest case being at 11 weeks for exomphalos containing liver.[82–87] Van Zalen-Sprock *et al.* reported on 14 cases with exomphalos at 11–14 weeks.[86] Nuchal fluid was increased in eight fetuses and seven of those were chromosomally abnormal. Exomphalos contained bowel only in fetuses with chromosomal abnormality. Liver was often present in the contents of the sac as well as bowel in the chromosomally normal ones.

In a study of 622 high-risk patients there were two cases of exomphalos diagnosed in the first trimester.[31] In four screening studies on a total of about 9500 patients there were two cases with exomphalos correctly identified in the first trimester.[30,33,34,46]

In a study screening for chromosomal defects at 10–14 weeks by NT measurement in about 1500 patients, the diagnosis of exomphalos was made at this early gestation.[56] Finally, in another screening study for chromosomal defects at 11–14 weeks by NT measurement, 15,726 fetuses were examined and there were 18 cases of exomphalos.[87] The karyotype was normal in seven fetuses; the remaining 11 fetuses had trisomies 18, 13 or triploidy. This study showed that the prevalence of exomphalos and the risk of chromosomal defects in affected fetuses is increased in the first trimester because of the strong association with lethal chromosomal anomalies.[87]

Gastroschisis (birth prevalence 1 in 4000)

In gastroschisis there is a small defect of the abdominal wall laterally and usually on the right of the umbilical cord insertion through which herniation of the viscera (usually small bowel) occurs. Although gastroschisis is as common at birth as exomphalos, there are few cases reported in the first timester.[88,89] Prenatal diagnosis is based on the visualization of loops of bowel floating in the amniotic fluid. Gastroschisis is rarely associated with chromosomal abnormalities.

Defects of the urinary tract

Megacystis

Dilatation of the urinary bladder in first-trimester fetuses has been reported in association with obstructive uropathy (usually with posterior urethral valves or urethral atresia), severe renal abnormalities and prune belly syndrome.[90–97]

Liao *et al.* studied 145 fetuses with bladder diameter more than or equal to 7 mm at 10–14 weeks of gestation.[98] Fetuses with mild and moderate megacystis (bladder diameter 7–15 mm) were chromosomally abnormal in 24% of cases; in the ones with normal karyotype spontaneous resolution occurred in 90% of cases but in 10% there was progressive evolution to obstructive uropathy and/or echogenic kidneys. Fetuses with severe bladder dilatation (more than 15 mm) were chromosomally abnormal in 11% of cases but progression to obstructive uropathy was observed in all of the remaining chromosomally normal cases.

In a study of 622 high-risk patients there were two cases of megacystis diagnosed in the first trimester.[31] In four screening studies on a total of about 9500 patients there were two cases with megacystis correctly identified in the first trimester.[30,33,34,46]

Meckel–Gruber syndrome (birth prevalence 1 in 10,000)

This is a lethal, autosomal recessive condition with variable phenotypic expression. The typical features include encephalocele, bilateral polycystic kidneys and polydactyly. Other features may be present such as growth deficiency of prenatal origin, microcephaly, cerebral and cerebellar hypoplasia, anencephaly, Dandy–Walker malformation, absence of the corpus callosum, cleft lip and palate, renal agenesis, hypoplastic bladder, obstructive uropathy, syndactyly of the fingers and toes. Phenotype may vary from isolated polydactyly, which may represent the mild expression of the heterozygote state, to the full clinical manifestation of the disease. The diagnosis is based on ultrasound examination demonstrating encephalocele, usually occipital, enlarged, dysplastic, echogenic kidneys and polydactyly.

In three studies on a total of 15 pregnancies from high-risk families all eight affected fetuses were correctly diagnosed in the first trimester.[99–101] Another case of the syndrome from a low-risk couple was identified at 13 weeks in a study screening for chromosomal abnormalities by NT measurement.[100] In four screening studies on a total of about 9500 patients there were two cases with Meckel–Gruber syndrome diagnosed in the first trimester.[30,33,34,46] These studies have shown that the phenotype of Meckel–Gruber syndrome is present from the first trimester and it is likely that the diagnosis is actually easier at this early gestation when amniotic fluid volume is still within the normal range rather than in the second trimester when oligohydramnios hinders detailed ultrasound examination.

Skeletal defects

Caudal regression syndrome (sirenomelia, birth prevalence 1 in 500,000)

This is a rare sporadic defect involving vertebral abnormalities varying from partial sacral agenesis to complete absence of the lumbosacral part of the spine. Sirenomelia, the extreme form of the syndrome presents with variable degrees of hypoplasia and fusion of the lower limbs and is associated with genitourinary, gastrointestinal and central nervous system defects. Sirenomelia is about 250 times more common in mothers with poorly controlled diabetes.

There are five cases of first-trimester diagnosis of sirenomelia, the earliest being at 9 weeks of gestation.[102–105] In one case the mother was a diabetic presenting with ketoacidotic coma.[102] Features of the syndrome identifiable in the first trimester are CRL shorter than expected for the gestation, inability to visualize independently the lower limbs and abnormal movement of the lower limbs, intra-abdominal cyst and increased nuchal tanslucecny.

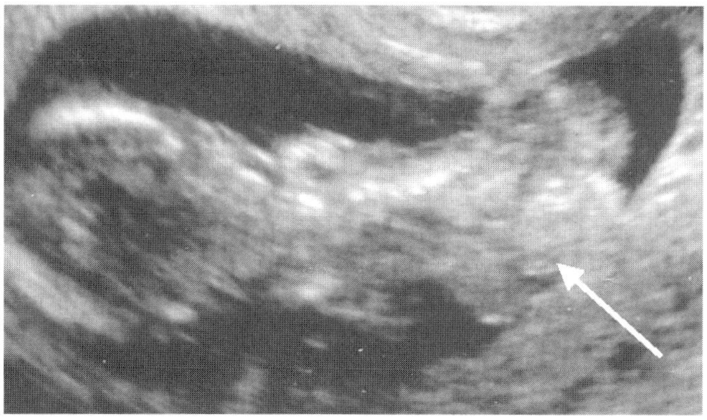

Figure 114.18 Body stalk anomaly in a 12-week fetus. The arrow points to the large abdominal wall defect. Part of the fetal body lies outside the amniotic cavity and is stuck to the uterine wall.

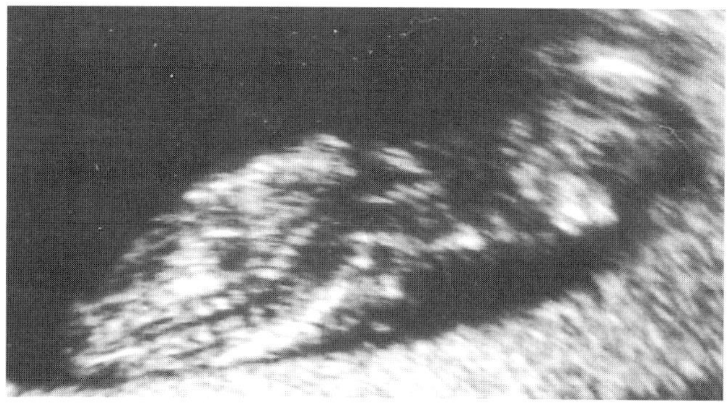

Figure 114.19 Kyphoscoliosis in a 14-week fetus.

Body stalk anomaly (birth prevalence 1 in 15,000)

This is a rare sporadic anomaly characterized by anterior wall defect, kyphoscoliosis, limb reduction and a rudimentary umbilical cord (Figure 114.19). Possible pathogenetic mechanisms included abnormal folding of the trilaminar embryo in the first 4 weeks of gestation, early rupture of the amniotic membrane and abnormal embryonic blood supply. In a study of about 106,000 pregnancies for chromosomal abnormalities by NT measurement there were 14 cases of body stalk anomaly and all were diagnosed in the first trimester.[106] In all fetuses the lower part of the body was outside the amniotic sac, in the coelomic cavity, which is possible because of early rupture of the amniotic membrane (Figure 114.17). NT was increased in about 70% of cases and the karyotype was normal in all cases. Contrary to this theory, Paul *et al.* presented a fetus with body stalk anomaly at 10 weeks of gestation (CRL 35 mm).[107] There were multiple anomalies including clefting defect of the cranium and brain, anterior wall defect, severe kyphoscoliosis and deformity of the lower limbs. The fetus was inside the amniotic sac, which appeared intact with no sonographic features of rupture. The earliest diagnosis of the defect is at 9 weeks of gestation; the fetus was partly outside the amniotic cavity, there was an abdominal wall defect and the lower limbs could not be seen.[108] In four screening studies on a total of about 9500 patients there was one fetus with body stalk anomaly diagnosed in the first trimester.[30,33,34,46]

Skeletal dysplasias

Skeletal dysplasias present with a prevalence of about 1 in 4000 (Figure 114.19). Although in some skeletal syndromes the clinical picture does not become obvious until the second or even the third trimester, there are skeletal defects that have been diagnosed in the first trimester and the commonest ultrasound features include limb shortening and bowing, limb fractures and hypomineralization of the skull and the spine and increased NT.

Achondrogenesis (birth prevalence 1 in 40,000)

Achondrogenesis type II is a lethal, autosomal recessive skeletal dysplasia usually presenting with hydrops, severe shortening of the limbs, narrow thorax, and hypomineralization of the vertebral bodies but normal mineralization of the skull. In the rarer type I of the disease there is hypomineralization of the skull and rib fractures.

There are two case reports on the first-trimester sonographic diagnosis of achondrogenesis type II in high-risk pregnancies; both fetuses had increased NT and short limbs that were abnormally positioned, with lack of movement.[109,110] There is also a report of a fetus with achondrogenesis type I presenting at 13 weeks with increased NT, short limbs, small thorax and deficient ossification of the skull, vertebral bodies and pelvic bones.[111]

Hypophosphatasia (birth prevalence 1 in 100,000)

Hypophosphatasia is a rare skeletal disease, which is clinically classified according to the age of onset of symptoms. The most severe type is perinatal hypophosphatasia, which has an autosomal recessive mode of inheritance. The perinatal form of the disease is due to abnormalities in the tissue-non-specific isoenzyme of alkaline phosphatase.

Souka *et al.*[112] reported on three pregnancies of a high-risk family. In the two affected pregnancies the diagnosis was made at 12 and 14 weeks and the features were marked hypomineralization of the skull and spine, narrowing of the chest with short ribs, shortening of all the long bones, bilateral talipes and increased NT.

Osteogenesis imperfecta type II
(birth prevalence 1 in 60,000)

This is a lethal skeletal dysplasia where the majority of cases are new mutations of the genes encoding collagen type I. Recurrence (6–7%) is usually due to parental mosaicism (somatic or germ-line), although, in a small number of families, autosomal recessive inheritance has been observed. In the second trimester, the characteristic sonographic features are short limbs and ribs with multiple fractures and hypomineralization of the skull.

Makrydimas *et al.* reported on an affected fetus presenting at 11 weeks with obvious shortening of all long bones and ribs and increased NT.[113]

Roberts syndrome

This is a rare, autosomal recessive condition characterized by symmetrical limb defects of variable severity (tetraphocomelia), facial cleft, hypertelorism, microcephaly and growth retardation.

In a fetus with Roberts syndrome, from a high-risk family, the sonographic findings at 11 weeks were increased NT and tetraphocomelia.[114]

Short-rib polydactyly syndrome

This is a rare, autosomal recessive, lethal skeletal dysplasia, characterized by short limbs, narrow thorax and postaxial polydactyly.

In a fetus with short-rib polydactyly syndrome type I, from a high-risk family, the sonographic findings at 13 weeks were increased NT, narrow chest, short limbs and polydactyly.[115]

REFERENCES

1. Snijders RJM, Noble P, Sebire N, Souka A, Nicolaides KH. UK multicentre project on assessment of risk of trisomy 21 by maternal age and fetal nuchal translucency thickness at 10–14 weeks of gestation. *Lancet* 1998;351:343–6.
2. Spencer K, Spencer CE, Power M, Dawson C, Nicolaides KH. Screening for chromosomal abnormalities in the first trimester using ultrasound and maternal serum biochemistry in a one-stop clinic: A review of three years prospective experience. *Br J Obstet Gynaecol* 2003;110(3):281–6.
3. Souka AP, Krampl E, Bakalis S, Heath V, Nicolaides KH. Outcome of pregnancy in chromosomally normal fetuses with increased nuchal translucency in the first trimester. *Ultrasound Obstet Gynecol* 2001;18:9–17.
4. Green JJ, Hobbins JC. Abdominal ultrasound examination of the first trimester fetus. *Am J Obstet Gynecol* 1988;159:165–75.
5. Timor-Tritsch IE, Farine D, Rosen MG. A close look at early embryonic development with the high-frequency transvaginal transducer. *Am J Obstet Gynecol* 1988;159:676–81.
6. Timor-Tritsch IE, Warren WB, Peisner DB, Pirrone E. First-trimester midgut herniation: A high-frequency transvaginal sonographic study. *Am J Obstet Gynecol* 1989;161:831–3.
7. Kushnir U, Shalev J, Bronshtein M, *et al.* Fetal intracranial anatomy in the first trimester of pregnancy: Transvaginal ultrasonographic evaluation. *Neuroradiology* 1989;31:222–5.
8. Brons JTJ, van Geijn HP, Bezemer PD, Nauta JPJ, Arts NFT. The fetal skeleton: Ultrasonographic evaluation of the normal growth. *Eur J Obstet Gynecol Reprod Biol* 1990;34:21–36.
9. Timor-Tritsch IE, Peisner DB, Raju S. Sonoembryology: An organ-oriented approach using a high-frequency vaginal probe. *J Clin Ultrasound* 1990;18:286–98.
10. Bree RL, Marn CS. Transvaginal sonography in the first trimester: Embryology, anatomy and hCG correlation. *Semin Ultrasound CT MR* 1990;11:12–21.
11. Timor-Tritsch IE, Monteagudo A, Warren WB. TV sonographic definition of the CNS in the first and early second trimesters. *Am J Obstet Gynecol* 1991;164:497–503.
12. Dolkart LA, Reimers FT. Transvaginal fetal echocardiography in early pregnancy: Normative data. *Am J Obstet Gynecol* 1991;165:688–91.
13. Timor-Tritsch IE, Monteagudo A, Peisner DB. High-frequency transvaginal sonographic examination for the potential malformation. Assessment of the 9-week to 14-week fetus. *J Clin Ultrasound* 1992;20:231–8.
14. Blaas HG, Eik-Nes SH, Kiserud T, Hellevik LR. Early development of the forebrain and midbrain: A longitudinal ultrasound study from 7 to 12 weeks of gestation. *Ultrasound Obstet Gynecol* 1994;4:183–92.
15. Wisser J, Dirschedl P. Embryonic heart rate in dated human embryos. *Early Hum Dev* 1994;37:107–15.
16. Wisser J, Dirschedl P, Krone S. Estimation of gestational age by transvaginal sonographic measurement of greatest embryonic length in dated human embryos. *Ultrasound Obstet Gynecol* 1994;4:457–62.
17. Zorzoli A, Kusterman A, Caravelli E, *et al.* Measurements of fetal limb bones in early pregnancy. *Ultrasound Obstet Gynecol* 1994; 4:29–33.
18. Blaas HG, Eik-Nes SH, Kiserud T, Hellevik LR. Early development of the hindbrain: A longitudinal ultrasound study from 7 to 12 weeks of gestation. *Ultrasound Obstet Gynecol* 1995;5:151–60.
19. Blaas HG, Eik-Nes SH, Kiserud T, Hellevik LR. Early development of the hindbrain: A longitudinal ultrasound study from 7 to 12 weeks of gestation. *Ultrasound Obstet Gynecol* 1995;6:240–9.
20. Braithwaite JM, Armstrong MA, Economides DL. Assessment of fetal anatomy at 12 to 13 weeks of gestation by transabdominal and transvaginal sonography. *Br J Obstet Gynaecol* 1996;103: 82–5.
21. Rosati P, Guariglia L. Transvaginal sonographic assessment of the fetal urinary tract in early pregnancy. *Ultrasound Obstet Gynecol* 1996;7:95–100.
22. Hata T, Manabe A, Makihara K, Hata K, Miyazaki K, Senoh D. Assessment of embryonic anatomy at 6–8 weeks of gestation by intrauterine and transvaginal sonography. *Hum Reprod* 1997;12: 1873–6.
23. van Zalen-Sprock RM, van Brons JTJ, van Vugt JMG, van Harten HJ, van Gijn HP. Ultrasonographic and radiologic visualization of the developing embryonic skeleton. *Ultrasound Obstet Gynecol* 1997;9:392–7.
24. Blaas HG, Eik-Nes SH, Berg S, Thorp H. In-vivo three-dimensional ultrasound reconstructions of embryos and early fetuses. *Lancet* 1998;352:1182–6.
25. Blaas HG, Eik-Nes SH, Bremnes JB. Embryonic growth. A longitudinal biometric ultrasound study. *Ultrasound Obstet Gynecol* 1998;12:346–54.
26. Hata T, Atsushi M, Aoki S, Kohji M, Yoshino K, Yamamoto K. Three-dimensional intrauterine sonography of human pregnancy: Preliminary study. *Hum Reprod* 1998;13:740–3.
27. Blaas HG, Eik-Nes SH, Berg S, Thorp H. In-vivo three-dimensional ultrasound reconstructions of embryos and early fetuses. *Lancet* 1998;352:1182–6.
28. Tanaka H, Senoh D, Yanagihara T, Hata T. Intrauterine sonographic measurement of embryonic brain vesicle. *Hum Reprod* 2000;15:1407–12.
29. Oakley GP. Frequency of human congenital malformation. *Clin Perinatol* 1986;13:545–50.
30. Hernadi L, Torocsik M. Screening for fetal anomalies in the 12th week of pregnancy by transvaginal sonography in an unselected population. *Prenat Diagn* 1997;17:753–9.
31. Cullen MT, Green J, Whetham J, Salafia C, Gabrielli S, Hobbins JC. Transvaginal ultrasonographic detection of congenital anomalies in the first trimester. *Am J Obstet Gynecol* 1990;163:466–76.
32. Whitlow BJ, Economides DL. The optimal gestational age to examine fetal anatomy and measure nuchal translucency in the first trimester. *Ultrasound Obstet Gynecol* 1998;11:258–61.
33. Economides DL, Braithwaite JM. First trimester ultrasonographic diagnosis of fetal structural abnormalities in a low risk population. *Br J Obstet Gynecol* 1998;105:53–7.
34. Carvalho MHB, Brizot ML, Lopes LM, Chiba CH, Miyadahira S, Zugaib M. Detection of fetal structural abnormalities at the 11–14 week ultrasound scan. *Ultrasound Obstet Gynecol* 2002;22:1–4.
35. D'Amelio R, Giorlandino C, Masala L, *et al.* Fetal echocardiography using transvaginal and transabdominal probes during the first

period of pregnancy: A comparative study. *Prenat Diagn* 1991;11: 69–75.

36. Dolkart LA, Reimers FT. Transvaginal fetal echocardiography in early pregnancy: Normative data. *Am J Obstet Gynecol* 1991;165: 688–91.
37. Johnson P, Sharland G, Maxwell D, Allan L. The role of transvaginal sonography in the early detection of congenital heart disease. *Ultrasound Obstet Gynecol* 1992;2:248–51.
38. Bronstein M, Siegler E, Eshcoli Z, Zimmer E. Transvaginal ultrasound measurements of the fetal heart at 11 to 17 weeks of gestation. *Am J Perinatol* 1992;9:38–42.
39. Gembruch U, Knopfle G, Bald R, Hansmann M. Early diagnosis of fetal congenital heart disease by transvaginal echocardiography. *Ultrasound Obstet Gynecol* 1993;3:310–7.
40. Carvalho JS, Moscoso G, Ville Y. First trimester transabdominal fetal echocardiography. *Lancet* 1998;351:1023–7.
41. Gembruch U, Shi C, Smrcek JM. Biometry of the fetal heart between 10 and 17 weeks of gestation. *Fetal Diagn Ther* 2000; 15:20–31.
42. Huggon IC, Ghi T, Cook AC, Zosmer N, Allan LD, Nicolaides KH. Fetal cardiac abnormalities identified prior to 14 weeks' gestation. *Ultrasound Obstet Gynecol* 2002;20:22–9.
43. Haak MC, Bartelings MM, Gittenberger-De Groot AC, Van Vugt JM. Cardiac malformations in first-trimester fetuses with increased nuchal translucency: Ultrasound diagnosis and postmortem morphology. *Ultrasound Obstet Gynecol* 2002;20:14–21.
44. Haak MC, Twisk JW, Van Vugt JM. How successful is fetal echocardiographic examination in the first trimester of pregnancy? *Ultrasound Obstet Gynecol* 2002;20:9–13.
45. Weiner Z, Lorber A, Shalev E. Diagnosis of congenital cardiac defects between 11 and 14 weeks' gestation in high-risk patients. *J Ultrasound Med* 2002;21:23–9.
46. Souka AP, Pilalis A, Kavalakis Y, Kosmas Y, Antsaklis P, Antsaklis A. Assessment of fetal anatomy at the 11–14 weeks ultrasound examination. *Ultrasound Obstet Gynecol* 2004;24(7):730–4.
47. Gembruch U, Shi C, Smrcek JM. Biometry of the fetal heart between 10 and 17 weeks of gestation. *Fetal Diagn Ther* 2000;15: 20–31.
48. Kennedy KA, Flick KJ, Thurmond AS. First-trimester diagnosis of exencephaly. *Am J Obstet Gynecol* 1990;162:461–3.
49. Bronstein M, Ornoy A. Acrania: Anencephaly resulting from secondary degeneration of a closed neural tube: Two cases in the same family. *J Clin Ultrasound* 1991;19:230–4.
50. Chatzipapas IK, Whitlow BJ, Economides DL. The "Mickey Mouse" sign and the diagnosis of anencephaly in early pregnancy. *Ultrasound Obstet Gynecol* 1998;13:196–9.
51. Johnson SP, Sebire NJ, Snidjers RJM, Tunkel S, Nicolaides KH. Ultrasound screening for anencephaly at 10–14 weeks of gestation. *Ultrasound Obstet Gynecol* 1997;9:14–6.
52. Goldstein RB, Filly RA, Callen PW. Sonography of anencephaly: Pitfalls in early diagnosis. *J Clin Ultrasound* 1989;17:397–402.
53. Souka AP, Bakalis S. Diagnosis of fetal abnormalities at the 11–14 weeks scan – Abnormal ultrasound findings. In Nicolaides KH, ed. *The 11–14 Week Scan. The Diagnosis of Fetal Abnormalities.* London: Parthenon Publishing Group, 1999:115–47.
54. Becker R, Mende B, Stiemer B, Entezami M. Sonographic markers of exencephaly at 9 + 3 weeks of gestation. *Ultrasound Obstet Gynecol* 2000;16:582–4.
55. Cuillier F. Prenatal diagnosis of exencephaly at 10 weeks gestation, confirmed at 13 weeks gestation. *J Gynecol Obstet Biol Reprod* 2001;30:706–7.
56. Pajkrt E, van Lith JMM, Mol BWJ, Bleker OP, Bilardo CM. Screening for Down's syndrome by fetal nuchal translucency measurement in a general obstetric population. *Ultrasound Obstet Gynecol* 1998;12:163–9.
57. Drysdale K, Ridley D, Walker K, Higgins B, Dean T. First-trimester pregnancy scanning as a screening tool for high-risk an abnormal pregnancies in a district general hospital setting. *J Obstet Gynecol* 2002;22:159–65.
58. Snijders RJM, Sebire NJ, Nayar R, Souka A, Nicolaides KH. Increased nuchal translucency in trisomy 13 fetuses at 10–14 weeks of gestation. *Am J Med Genet* 1999;86:205–7.
59. Toth Z, Csecsei K, Szeifert G, Torok O, Papp Z. Early prenatal diagnosis of cyclopia associated with holoprosencephaly. *J Clin Ultrasound* 1986;14:550–3.
60. Bronstein M, Wiener Z. Early transvaginal sonographic diagnosis of alobar holoprosencephaly. *Prenat Diagn* 1991;11:459–62.
61. Gonzalez-Gomez F, Salamanca A, Padilla MC, Sabatel RM. Alobar holoprosencephalic embryo detected via transvaginal sonography. *Eur J Obstet Gynecol Reprod Biol* 1992;47: 266–70.
62. Sakala EP, Gaio KL. Fundal uterine leiomyoma obscuring first trimester transabdominal sonographic diagnosis of fetal holoprosencephaly. *J Reprod Med* 1993;38:400–2.
63. Turner CD, Silva S, Jeanty P. Prenatal diagnosis of alobar holoprosencephaly at 10 weeks of gestation. *Ultrasound Obstet Gynecol* 1999;13:360–2.
64. Wong HS, Lam YH, Tang MHY, Cheung LWK, Ng LKL, Yan KW. First-trimester ultrasound diagnosis of holoprosencephaly: Three case reports. *Ultrasound Obstet Gynecol* 1999;13:356–9.
65. Tongsong T, Wanapirak C, Chanprapaph P, Siriangkul S. First trimester sonographic diagnosis of holoprosencephaly. *Int J Gynaecol Obstet* 1999;66:165–9.
66. Blaas HG, Eik-Nes SH, Vainio T, Isaksen CV. Alobar holoprosencephaly at 9 weeks gestational age visualised by two- and three-dimensional ultrasound. *Ultrasound Obstet Gynecol* 2000;15:62–5.
67. Hsu TY, Chang SY, Ou CY, *et al.* First trimester diagnosis of holoprosencephaly and cyclopia with triploidy by transvaginal three-dimensional ultrasonography. *Eur J Obstet Gynecol Reprod Biol.* 2001;96:235–7.
68. Blumenfeld Z, Siegler E, Bronshtein M. The early diagnosis of neural tube defects. *Prenat Diagn* 1993;13:863–71.
69. Sebire NJ, Noble PL, Thorpe-Beeston JG, Snidjers RJM, Nicolaides KH. Presence of the "lemon sign" in fetuses with spina bifida at the 10–14-week scan. *Ultrasound Obstet Gynecol* 1997;10: 403–5.
70. Bernard JP, Suarez B, Rambaud C, Mullet F, Ville Y. Prenatal diagnosis of neural tube defect before 12 weeks' gestation: Direct and indirect semeiology. *Ultrasound Obstet Gynecol* 1997;10:406–9.
71. Blaas HG, Eik-Nes SH, Isaksen CV. The detection of spina bifida before 10 gestational weeks using two- and three-dimensional ultrasound. *Ultrasound Obstet Gynecol* 2000;16:25–9.
72. Buisson O, De Keersmaecker B, Senat MV, Bernard JP, Moscoso G, Ville Y. Sonographic diagnosis of spina bifida at 12 weeks: Heading towards indirect signs. *Ultrasound Obstet Gynecol* 2002; 19:290–2.
73. DeVore GR, Steiger GR, Larson EJ. Fetal echocardiography: The prenatal diagnosis of a ventricular septal defect in a 14-week fetus with pulmonary artery hypoplasia. *Obstet Gynecol* 1987;69:494–7.
74. Bronshtein M, Siegler E, Yoffe N, Zimmer EZ. Prenatal diagnosis of ventricular septal defect and overriding aorta at 14 weeks' gestation, using transvaginal sonography. *Prenat Diagn* 1990;10:697–702.
75. Gembruch U, Knopfle G, Chatterjee M, Bald R, Hansmann M. First-trimester diagnosis of fetal congenital heart disease by transvaginal two-dimensional and Doppler echocardiography. *Obstet Gynecol* 1990;75:496–8.
76. Bronshtein M, Zimmer EZ, Milo S, Ho SY, Lorber A, Gerlis M. Fetal cardiac abnormalities detected by transvaginal sonography at 12–16 weeks' gestation. *Obstet Gynecol* 1991;78:374–8.
77. Achiron R, Rotstein Z, Lipitz S, Mashiach S, Hegesh J. First-trimester diagnosis of fetal congenital heart disease by transvaginal sonography. *Obstet Gynecol* 1994;84:69–72.
78. Gembruch U, Knopfle G, Bald R, Hansmann M. Early diagnosis of congenital heart disease by transvaginal sonography. *Ultrasound Obstet Gynecol* 1993;3:310–7.
79. Carvalho J, Moscoso G, Ville Y. First-trimester transabdominal fetal echocardiography. *Lancet* 1998;351:1023–7.
80. Huggon IC, Ghi T, Cook AC, Zosmer N, Allan LD, Nicolaides KH. Fetal cardiac abnormalities identified prior to 14 weeks' gestation. *Ultrasound Obstet Gynecol* 2002;20:22–9.
81. Makrydimas G, Sotiriadis A, Ioannidis JP. Screening performance of first-trimester nuchal translucency for major cardiac defects: A meta-analysis. *Am J Obstet Gynecol* 2003;189:1330–5.
82. Schmidt W, Kubli F. Early diagnosis of severe congenital malformations by ultrasonography. *J Perinat Med* 1982;10: 233–41.
83. Brown DI, Emerson DS, Shulman LP, Carson SA. Sonographic diagnosis of omphalocele during the 10th week of gestation. *Am J Radiol* 1989;153:825–6.
84. Pagliano M, Mossetti M, Ragno P. Echographic diagnosis of omphalocele in the first trimester of pregnancy. *J Clin Ultrasound* 1990;18:658–60.
85. Heydanus R, Raats AM, Tibboel D, Lost FJ, Wladimirrof JW. Prenatal diagnosis of fetal abdominal wall defects: A retrospective analysis of 44 cases. *Prenat Diagn* 1996;16:411–7.
86. van Zalen-Sprock RM, van Vugt JMG, van Geijn HP. First-trimester sonography of physiological midgut herniation and early diagnosis of omphalocele. *Prenat Diagn* 1997;17:511–8.

87. Snidjers RJM, Sebire NJ, Souka A, Santiago C, Nicolaides KH. Fetal exomphalos and chromosomal defects: Relationship to maternal age and gestation. *Ultrasound Obstet Gynecol* 1995;6:250–5.
88. Kushnir O, Izquierdo L, Vigil D, Curet LB. Early transvaginal diagnosis of gastroschisis. *J Clin Ultrasound* 1990;18:194–7.
89. Guzman ER. Early prenatal diagnosis of gastroschisis with transvaginal sonography. *Am J Obstet Gynecol* 1990;162:1253–4.
90. Bulic M, Podobnik M, Korenic B, Bistricki J. First-trimester diagnosis of low obstructive uropathy: An indicator of initial renal function in the fetus. *J Clin Ultrasound* 1987;15:537–41.
91. Stiller R. Early ultrasonic appearance of fetal bladder outlet obstruction. *Am J Obstet Gynecol* 1989;160:584–5.
92. Drugan A, Zador IE, Bhatia RK, Sacks AJ, Evans M. First trimester diagnosis and early in utero treatment of obstructive uropathy. *Acta Obstet Gynecol Scand* 1989;68:645–9.
93. Zimmer EZ, Bronshtein M. Fetal intra-abdominal cysts detected in the first and early second trimester by transvaginal sonography. *J Clin Ultrasound* 1991;19:564–7.
94. Yoshida M, Matsumura M, Shintaku Y *et al.* Prenatally diagnosed female prune-belly syndrome associated with tetralogy of Fallot. *Gynecol Obstet Invest* 1995;39:141–4.
95. Fried S, Appelman Z, Caspi B. The origin of ascites in prune belly syndrome – Early sonographic evidence. *Prenat Diagn* 1995;15: 876–7.
96. Hoshino T, Ihara Y, Shirane H, Ota T. Prenatal diagnosis of prune belly syndrome at 12 weeks of pregnancy: Case report and review of the literature. *Ultrasound Obstet Gynecol* 1998;12: 362–6.
97. Cazorla E, Ruiz F, Abad A, Monleon J. Prune belly syndrome: Early antenatal diagnosis. *Eur J Obstet Gynecol* 1997;72:31–3.
98. Liao AW, Sebire NJ, Geerts L, Cicero S, Nicolaides KH. Megacystis at 10–14 weeks of gestation: Chromosomal defects and outcome according to bladder length. *Ultrasound Obstet Gynecol* 2003; 21:338–41.
99. Pachi A, Giancotti A, Torcia F, de Prosperi V, Maggi E. Meckel–Gruber syndrome: Ultrasonographic diagnosis at 13 weeks' gestational age in an at-risk case. *Prenat Diagn* 1989;9:187–90.
100. Sepulveda W, Sebire NJ, Souka A, Snidjers RJM, Nicolaides KH. Diagnosis of the Meckel–Gruber syndrome at eleven to fourteen weeks' gestation. *Am J Obstet Gynecol* 1997;176:316–9.
101. van Zalen-Sprock RM, van Vugt JMG, van Geijn HP. First-trimester sonographic detection of neurodevelopmental abnormalities in some single-gene disorders. *Prenat Diagn* 1996;16:199–202.
102. Baxi L, Warren W, Collins M, Timor-Tritsch IE. Early detection of caudal regression syndrome with transvaginal scanning. *Obstet Gynecol* 1990;75:485–9.
103. Carbillon L, Seince N, Largilliere C, Bucourt M, Uzan M. First-trimester diagnosis of sirenomelia. A case report. *Fetal Diagn Ther* 2001;16:284–8.
104. Monteagudo A, Mayberry P, Rebarber A, Paidas M, Timor-Tritsch IE. Sirenomelia sequence: First-trimester diagnosis with both two- and three-dimensional sonography. *J Ultrasound Med* 2002;21: 915–20.
105. Schiesser M, Holzgreve W, Lapaire O *et al.* Sirenomelia, the mermaid syndrome – Detection in the first trimester. *Prenat Diagn* 2003;23:493–5.
106. Daskalakis G, Sebire NJ, Jurkovic D, Snidjers RJM, Nicolaides KH. Body stalk anomaly at 10–14 weeks of gestation. *Ultrasound Obstet Gynecol* 1997;10:416–8.
107. Paul C, Zosmer N, Jurkovic D, Nicolaides K. A case of body stalk anomaly at 10 weeks of gestation. *Ultrasound Obstet Gynecol* 2001;17:157–9.
108. Becker R, Runkel S, Entezami M. Prenatal diagnosis of body stalk anomaly at 9 weeks of gestation. Case report. *Fetal Diagn Ther* 2000;15:301–3.
109. Fisk NM, Vaughan J, Smidt M, Wigglesworth J. Transvaginal ultrasound recognition of nuchal oedema in the first-trimester diagnosis of achondrogenesis. *J Clin Ultrasound* 1991;19:586–90.
110. Soothill PW, Vuthiwong C, Rees H. Achondrogenesis type 2 diagnosed by transvaginal ultrasound at 12 weeks of gestation. *Prenat Diagn* 1993;13:523–8.
111. Meizner I, Barnhard Y. Achondrogenesis type I diagnosed by transvaginal ultrasonography at 13 weeks' gestation. *Am J Obstet Gynecol* 1995;173:1620–2.
112. Souka AP, Raymond FL, Mornet E, Geerts L, Rane S, Nicolaides KH. Hypophosphatasia associated with increased nuchal translucency: A report of three consecutive pregnancies. *Ultrasound Obstet Gynecol* 2002;20:294–5.
113. Makrydimas G, Souka AP, Skentou H, Lolis D, Nicolaides KH. Osteogenesis imperfecta and other skeletal dysplasias presenting with increased nuchal translucency in the first trimester. *Am J Med Genet* 2001;98:117–20.
114. Petrikovsky BM, Gross B, Bialer M, Solamanzadeh K, Simhaee E. Prenatal diagnosis of pseudothalidomide syndrome in consecutive pregnancies of a consanguineous couple. *Ultrasound Obstet Gynecol* 1997;10:425–8.
115. Hill LM, Leary J. Transvaginal sonographic diagnosis of short-rib polydactyly dysplasia at 13 weeks' gestation. *Prenat Diagn* 1998; 18:1198–201.

SECTION XIII

Intrauterine growth

Section Editors: **J. M. Carrera and G. P. Mandruzzato**

115 Fetal growth characteristics

J. M. Carrera, B. Serra and R. Devesa

Introduction

'Growth' is generally defined as the process whereby the body mass of a living being increases in size as a result of the increase in the number (hyperplasia) and size (hypertrophy) of its cells and intercellular matrix. 'Development', on the other hand, should be understood as the process by which organs and their regulatory mechanisms gradually assume their functions. Broadly speaking, the term 'growth' is preferred when referring to measurable anatomic changes, while 'development' is used to refer to the gradual acquisition of specific physiological functions.

From the time of conception, embryonic and fetal growth does not happen in a disorganized manner, but is governed by still poorly defined physical and chemical mechanisms, which are responsible for a perfectly modulated cellular multiplication and differentiation. Gestation is a biological process that normally develops according to a predetermined sequence from its beginning. Duration of pregnancy is also pre-established and varies in different species (in humans 266 days or 38 weeks from the time of fertilization). Major intrauterine changes take place: a 130-μm zygote weighing 10 μg multiplies its length 4000 times and its weight 200 million times. During the embryonic stage (the first 8 weeks of development), the embryo does not look like a human being, although his or her appearance and proportions change during the remaining period of gestation: the head to body length ratio increases from 1:2 at 3 months to 2:5 at 5 months and 1:3 at 9 months.

It is surprising that fetal growth has been of little interest to physicians for almost the entire history of medicine. There is no mention of the birth weight of a child in the Bible, ancient Greek, or in the writings of Roman and Arabic physicians. Cone[1] reviewed the history of weighing the newborn infant and found the earliest mention of birth weight in the fourth edition (1964) of the celebrated textbook of Françoise Mauriceau, the great French obstetrician of the 17th century. According to Mauriceau, one fetus of 9 months ordinarily weighs 13 lb (about 6 kg). However, this excessively high birth weight was, amazingly, quoted by Smellie, a Scottish obstetrician, and Lobb, an English surgeon. In 1747, Lobb stated that the mean birth weight of neonates was approximately 16 lb. The first birth weights with scientific value were provided by the German physician Roederer in 1753, who reported average weights of 6 lb 12 oz (3038 g) in male infants and 6 lb 5 oz (2841 g) in females. In 1786, Clarke published the following estimations: 7 lb 5 oz (3291 g) in males and 6 lb 11 oz (3009 g) in females. Nevertheless, scientific and systematic studies on birth weight appeared in 1835, when Quetelet, trained in statistics and mathematics, reported mean values of 3200 and 2900 g for male and female neonates, respectively.

Anatomical studies of fetal growth were initiated by Streeter[2] and Scammon and Calkins[3], who provided useful information on intrauterine growth as estimated from weights at postmortem examinations. In 1951, Thomson[4] was the first author to construct growth curves derived from fetal crown–rump length and fetal weight and in 1963, Lubchenco and colleagues[5] presented weight curves in the form of percentiles.

Nowadays, the interest of Perinatal Medicine is not only focused on clarifying the characteristics of the fetal growth and its possible anomalies, but also in the consequences that they can have all through the life. In some way, these discoveries have changed the image of obstetrics as a discipline.[6]

Mechanisms of fetal growth

A series of processes occurring simultaneously during fetal growth, i.e. organic differentiation, weight gain and development of bodily function, prepare the fetus for an extrauterine life in optimal conditions. 'Timing' in each system may be different: formation of the ear, tactile sense, urine production or circulatory changes may occur much earlier than thermoregulation, endocrine adaptations or pulmonary maturation. At present, fetuses weighing less than 500 g cannot be maintained alive. In neonates weighing more than 1000 g, current advances in technology allow us to overcome functional immaturity-related complications and to achieve excellent survival rates.

Cellular processes characteristic of fetal growth (mass growth, protein synthesis and differentiation) are still poorly understood.

Cell mass growth

Cell mass growth involves three mechanisms (i.e. an increase in the number of cells, an increase in the size of cells and an increase in the intercellular matrix) interacting with each other, especially the increase in cell number and size of cells. Cell division or multiplication (hyperplasia) is usually followed by an increase in the size of individual cells secondary to the uptake of nutrients from the outside. After a determined cell size is attained, a subsequent cell division resumes. Sinclair[7] estimated at 10^{14} the total number of cells of an adult human being that are accomplished after 45 cell generations derived from the fertilized ovum. Immediately after fertilization of the ovum, growth of the fertilized egg is characterized by simple cell division until a certain stage is reached, after which cell multiplication is accompanied by an increase in the cytoplasm. While at the beginning of the embryonic period, divisions of cells occur simultaneously (synchronism), at more advanced stages of development, cell divisions are asynchronous, i.e. in each tissue of different organs only a few cells undergo division at the same time.

It is well known that DNA forms the primary genetic material. Martell and Bertolini[8] established the following: (a) the DNA content of a determined cell lineage remains constant, whatever variations in the environmental and nutritional conditions occur; (b) the DNA content of each cell lineage is related to its functional complexity; (c) the organism as a whole shows greater DNA content and consequently more total genetic information as complexity increases and (d) all cells of different tissues in the same species show an identical composition of DNA bases, which remains unaffected by changes in the environmental or nutritional conditions.

The human haploid genome has approximately 3×10^9 base pairs, forming between 50,000 and 100,000 genes of 1000 to 200,000 base pairs each. Functionally, the genome is involved not only in the genetic code system, but also in DNA regulation and replication, as well as chromosome alignment and recombination.

The intercellular matrix, mainly composed of hyaluronic acid and water-retaining complex polysaccharides, is poorly developed in the embryonic stage, but as the fetus grows, collagen and elastic fibers become prominent (collagen fibers account for a third of the proteins of the organism).[8]

Protein synthesis

Of all substances synthesized by cells during the process of growth and development (nucleic acids, glycogen, fat, steroids, etc.), proteins are undoubtedly the most important. Briefly, transcription refers to the process by which a base sequence of messenger RNA (mRNA) is synthesized (by an RNA polymerase) on a complementary strand of DNA and translation is the rather complex process by which mRNA, transfer RNA (tRNA) and ribosomes effect the production of protein from amino acids. A set of three consecutive nucleotides (triplet or codon) provides the genetic information to code for a specific amino acid that will be incorporated into a protein chain or serves as a termination signal.

Cellular differentiation

Although all cells of the organism have the same chromosomal content, the fact that they differ in functional differentiation continues to be a mystery. It has been suggested that cellular differentiation is a process of repression and derepression.[8] However, it is highly improbable that such a large amount of repressor substances could exist, for example, to repress indefinitely the multiplication capacity of neurons. In any case, permanent inhibition of a series of cell function capacities to open the way to the development of other functions may be based on specific immunological responses and may occur through methylation of some DNA or histone bases.

Numerous studies support the concept that 'embryonic induction' is essential for the development of tissue diversity. Embryonic induction refers to the stimulation of a specific developmental pattern in specific cell groups (responding or target tissue) by other close groups (stimulating or inductor tissue). For example, vertebral bodies are formed from the notochord, whereas the halves of the vertebral arch derive from the neural tube, so that anomalies in the development of one component will produce anomalies in the other. However, the molecular basis of these interactions is poorly understood.

The diversity of substances required for each process of cellular differentiation may be simplified by the action of 'organizing substances' (molecular inductors) whose presence would only be required at a given time of development (e.g. in a particular cell lineage); from this moment on, cell division would proceed normally. This is currently the subject of extensive research. Among these molecules, growth factors have been identified in almost all animals including humans and constitute a group of proteins with primarily stimulating activity. Growth factors are also involved in tissue differentiation, e.g. transforming growth factor-β is associated with differentiation of the ectodermal layer into the mesodermal layer. Genes with the function of activating cell differentiation have also been identified (e.g. homeobox genes).

General characteristics of fetal growth

Fetal growth is primarily genetically controlled (differentiation from other species, racial differences, gender, etc.) but also considerably modified by more intangible environmental factors. Genetic factors are involved in the control of embryonic development, rate of cell division, number of cells forming each organ and tissue and 'potential' growth of fetal weight and height. The human fetus may be considered to be the result of the interaction of its genetic potential and the environment, i.e. fetal and maternal factors that limit or favor growth. This explains the high rate of variability among individuals of the same species, which is genetically and biologically necessary.

According to Elejalde and de Elejalde[9], normal fetal growth and development is proportional, symmetrical, global, temporal and controlled. Proportional growth refers to the development of different parts of the body as expected to give rise to an infant of normal weight and appearance at the end of gestation. Double organs show the appropriate symmetry. The mechanisms by which right/left and cranial/caudal symmetry and asymmetry axes are established have not been fully identified, although it seems that a genetic alteration would produce protein anomalies[10] resulting in true morphogenetic substances, the effects of which would be related to their function, spatial disposition, or simply to their gradient or concentration (right, left, cranial or caudal). Theoretically, for example, an elevated concentration on the left would place the heart in the correct site or would determine an anatomical differentiation in the formation of the right and left bronchial tree. Moreover, all organs grow following a determined rate and up to a determined time to maintain the expected proportions and symmetry. Each organ and system has its own 'timing' – a particular growth rate – although the rate of fetal growth and development during the first trimester of gestation is much faster than during the second and third trimesters. Finally, cellular growth of each organ at each moment of intrauterine life is perfectly established (with minimal and maximal ranges) in relation to the gestational age.

All these features determine that fetal growth, in reference to weight and height gain, is a dependent, constant and linear function and although all organs and tissues have different growth rates and capacities, the overall proportion of the fetus is preserved.

REFERENCES

1. Cone TE Jr. De pondere infantum recens natorum. The history of the weighing of the newborn infant. *Pediatrics* 1961;28:490–8.
2. Streeter GL. *Contrib Embryol* 1920;11:143.
3. Scammon RE, Calkins LA. *Growth in the Fetal Period.* Minneapolis: University of Minnesota Press, 1929.
4. Thomson AM. Growth curves for (A) foetal crown–rump length in mm and (B) foetal weight. *Br J Nutr* 1951;5:158–66.
5. Lubchenco LO, Hansman C, Dressler M, Boyd E. Intra-uterine growth as estimated from liveborn birthweight data at 24 to 42 weeks of gestation. *Pediatrics* 1963;32:793–800.
6. Bukowski R. Fetal growth potential and pregnancy outcome. *Semin Perinatol* 2004;28(1):51–8.
7. Sinclair D. *Human Growth after Birth.* New York: Oxford University Press, 1973.
8. Martell M, Bertolini LB. *Crecimiento y desarrollo en los dos primeros años de vida postnatal.* Publicación no. 672. Montevideo, Uruguay: Centro Latino Americano de Perinatologia, 1976.
9. Elejalde BR, de Elejalde MM. The prenatal growth of the human body determined by the measurements of bones and organs by ultrasonography. *Am J Med Genet* 1986;24:575–98.
10. Brown NA, Wolpert L. The development of handedness in left/right symmetry. *Development* 1990;109:1.

116 Regulating factors

J. M. Carrera, B. Serra, E. Scazzochio and M. Carrera

Introduction

Fetal growth can be divided into two stages, consisting of two phases each; a first stage of exponential fetal growth, in which differentiation of organs and systems occurs simultaneously, and a second stage of linear fetal growth that continues until birth, in which maturation processes predominate. Although some specific endocrinological actions can be related to certain aspects of fetal growth, in general terms the mechanisms responsible for general coordination or development of particular organs are still to be elucidated (Figure 116.1).

Fetal growth rate is primarily governed by an intrinsic fetal growth potential, which is essentially genetic in nature ('genetic regulating factor'). Genetic control of fetal growth, however, is largely modified by two superimposed intrauterine growth regulating factors: 'hormone regulating factor' (of fetal origin and of a stimulating nature) and 'environmental regulating factor' (of maternal origin and mostly restrictive in nature). Thus, the slope of the fetal growth curve throughout pregnancy, and consequently the birth weight, results from the interaction of inhibiting and stimulating factors on the fetal genotype. The human fetus may be considered as the interaction between genetic potential (its chance of 'being') and incidental factors associated with the accomplishment of this goal (the 'environment'), which may act to limit or favor this purpose.[1–7]

Whilst the genetic regulating factor predominates during the first half of pregnancy, determining a narrow range of fetal growth variability, hormone and environmental regulating factors have a marked effect during the second half of gestation, inducing a wide range of variability in fetal growth and development. In addition, other factors play a main role in fetal growth regulation, such as the bioavailability of substrates for the fetus, the nature of fetoplacental interaction, and the organization of progressive fetal maturation.

Genetic regulation of fetal growth

The mechanisms through which genetic information in the fertilized ovum controls cellular multiplication and differentiation until giving rise to a human being are purely speculative.[8] Biochemical aspects of fetal growth are also poorly defined. It is well known, however, that two cell genomes (paternal and maternal) are required for normal embryonic growth and development. Surani and colleagues[9] and Solter[10] found that parthenogenetic embryonic cells with male genome produced primarily embryonic tissues, whereas parthenogenetic embryonic cells with only genetic contribution from the female could initiate preimplantational development and even placentation, but were unable to differentiate extra-embryonic tissues properly. It has been suggested that these differences related to genetic contribution from the male and female arise from 'imprinting' during gametogenesis. Although the molecular nature of these phenomena has not been reliably demonstrated, there is

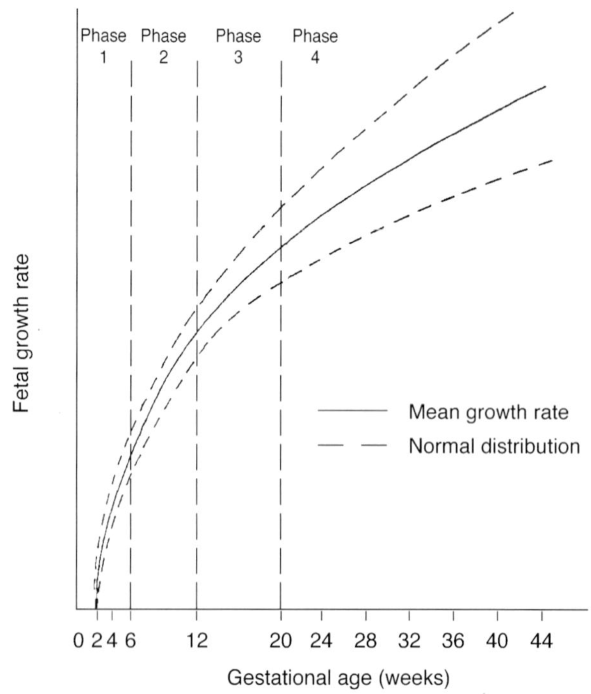

Figure 116.1 Fetal growth rate in relation to physical parameters. There is exponential growth in the first two phases (until 12 weeks' gestation) and linear growth thereafter. The normal range becomes wider as the fetal growth rate decreases, so that the accuracy of a single measurement to estimate gestational age is inversely proportional to age.

evidence that locus-specific methylation patterns are probably inherited according to predetermined paternal/maternal patterns.[11]

Holliday and Pugh[12] postulated that developing fetal cells would probably be subjected to genetic control, resembling in nature the 'modifying enzymes' of some bacteria. These enzymes would allow a precise number of cell divisions. Differentiation would be attained until a certain stage of development, by means of changing the position of some sequences of DNA bases in each cell division, inducing activation of a particular gene or genes, which, in turn, would initiate cell differentiation. Accordingly, the following issues may be explained:

(1) In the full-term fetus, the total number of cells is the result of 42 successive divisions of the fertilized ovum. The importance of this precise number is appreciated by the fact that only five more cell divisions are required to achieve the adult size. In this case, the genetic chronometer 'counts' exactly the number of cell divisions and decides, according to an established program, after which cell division, differentiation of a particular cell lineage is going to be started.
(2) A given developmental process occurs at a given gestational age. It is evident that the program is 'written' in basic sequences of DNA, which, after consecutive replications, activate particular genetic 'commutators' to induce these events.
(3) There is a time order in the formation of fetal structures. This order is obviously related to the number of cell divisions, carefully counted by the 'genetic chronometer' in the developing cells.
(4) Although cell differentiation may be induced by activation of a single gene, codification and an active enzymatic system at different genomic sites with identical control sequences are required.
(5) Differential characteristics of genetic code and DNA changes would be responsible for preserving the stability of each cell lineage.

The effect of the genetic regulating factor on fetal growth and development has been demonstrated in studies carried out in monozygotic twins whose final heights were highly correlated ($r = 0.95$), as opposed to the definitive heights of dizygotic twins.

However, fetal genotype accounts for about 15% of variations in birth weight due to certain inherited traits. These include fetal sex, racial and ethnic characteristics, and paternal and maternal genetic contributions.

Approximately 2% of variations in birth weight can be attributed to sex chromosomes.[13] The birth weight of a full-term male infant is on average 150–200 g higher than that of a female. This increase may be due to the effect of testicular hormones or to a more marked antigenic difference between the male fetus and his mother.[14] Placentas from male neonates also weigh more than those from females (2% higher at 40 weeks).

Generally speaking, Black neonates have a tendency to be smaller than Caucasian babies, although they have a faster maturation thereafter. Asian newborns are smaller than both Caucasian and Black neonates. As an example, the mean birth weight of Cheyenne newborns – tribe of North American Indians – is 3800 g, compared with 2400 g for newborns from the Luni tribe in New Guinea.[15] However, it is important to take the influence of socioeconomic conditions into consideration when comparisons between different ethnic groups are made.

Paternal influence on fetal weight is exclusively exerted through autosomal genes and sex chromosomes. From an anthropometric perspective, for each centimeter by which paternal height exceeds normal values, fetal weight at birth is increased by 9 g.[16] The maternal contribution is more complex and not only expressed through genetic material; in fact, the effect of maternal genotype on fetal growth and development is probably as important as the fetal genotype-derived influence.[17] Anthropometric data indicate that maternal weight prior to pregnancy has a greater influence than maternal height.[18]

It is therefore evident that several factors, which are considered physiological but have a genetic basis, determine the weight of a newborn child.[19] However, the majority of these factors (height and weight of the mother and the father, ethnicity, parity, etc.) are regrettably not considered in the population models used currently. The exception is the gestational age.[7] The consequence of this omission is the adoption of an inadequate classification of the newborn children. So the newborn babies, whose mothers are low weight and short height and therefore belong to an ethnic group of normally small newborn babies, are misclassified as babies subject to a growth restriction.[20]

Hormonal regulation of fetal growth

In addition to a genetic chronometer, there is no doubt that other 'endocrine chronometers', inducing hormonal secretion, must be present. The genetic chronometer is virtually immutable, whereas the endocrine chronometer(s) are theoretically susceptible to pharmacological modification.

Maternal hormones

The placenta is impermeable to many maternal hormones, especially to protein hormones and growth factors (for that reason, the fetus is substantially autonomous from an endocrinological point of view). With regard to other hormones, thyroxine and cortisol can pass through the placenta, but in practice they do not reach fetal blood because increased concentrations of thyroxine and hydrocortisone in the maternal circulation are not accompanied by significant increases in fetal blood levels of these hormones.

Although maternal hormones are not directly implicated in fetal growth, they are indirectly involved by ensuring adequate concentrations of glucose and nutrients in fetal blood. Some disorders of fetal development and endocrinological function may be explained by changes in blood glucose levels. In maternal diabetes, for example, pancreatic function of the fetus may be affected as a result of fetal hyperglycemia secondary to maternal hyperglycemia. During the first half of pregnancy, there is a noticeable maternal hyperinsulinism (due to an increase in the number and function of pancreatic cells) resulting from progestational and estrogenic stimuli, that promotes maternal anabolism but does not increase the energy supply to the fetus. By contrast, fetal anabolism predominates during the latter half of pregnancy due to an increase in a series of anti-insulin factors (an increase in insulin clearance, an increase in insulin receptor resistance and insulin antagonists of endocrine nature), resulting in a partial catabolism of maternal reserves that are directed to the fetus.

On the other hand, catecholamines, angiotensin II, aldosterone and prostaglandins play an important role in maintaining maternal cardiovascular homeostasis and uteroplacental blood flow. According to Speroff,[21] by analogy with the kidney, prostaglandins and the renin–angiotensin system would be involved in the regulation of uterine blood flow.

Placental growth factors

The placental growth is determined by the proliferation, differentiation and migration of the cytotrophoblast. The proliferation of the trophoblastic cells is closely related to the placental growth. For this reason, the progressive reduction of this proliferation, after its time of maximal activity between the eighth and ninth week of gestation, suggests that the placental invasion has been successful.[22,23] On the contrary, an increase of the proliferation rate during the last period of gestation must lead to think that there are some problems of implantation that can be associated with hypoxia conditions.

The fetal growth depends basically on the placental function. The placenta is an organ specialized in providing an appropriate fetal nutrition, but it also acts as an endocrine organ. In this sense, the specialized cells of the trophoblast produce peptide growth factors, whose function is to serve as modulators of the fetal growth.

One of these growth factors is the insulin-like growth factor (IGF), which has a fundamental role in the control of the placental and fetal growth.[24,25] Nowadays we know that it not only stimulates the production of glucose and amino acids, but also acts in the proliferation and differentiation by producing several hormones.[26] It has been shown that growth hormone-induced growth stimulation is mediated by IGFs,[27] in particular IGF-1.

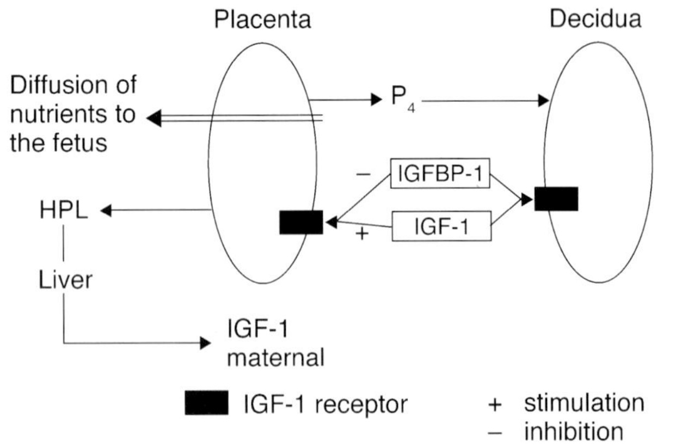

Figure 116.2 Paracrine and autocrine regulation of insulin-like growth factor-1 (IGF-1) and IGF-binding protein (IGFBP-1) in the placenta and decidua. HPL, human placental lactogen; P_4, progesterone.

For this reason, human fetal IGF levels have been associated with birth weight.[28,29] Recent studies have confirmed IGF secretion in a large variety of fetal tissue, mainly the connective tissue and mesenchymal cells, and the paracrine effects of this factor.[30] Fetal IGF-1 levels have been shown to be significantly lower in cases of growth restriction.[31] There is a statistically significant increase in maternal IGF-1 levels in the third trimester of pregnancy, which stimulates the transplacental passage of nutrients. IGF-1 action seems to be modulated by placental lactogen. On the other hand, this mechanism may be inhibited by IGF binding proteins (IGFBP-1), which bind to placental IGF receptors. Apparently, progesterone may in turn modulate this effect by regulating decidual secretion of IGFBP-1 (Figure 116.2).[32] However, further studies are warranted to define the role of growth hormone in fetal weight regulation.

On the other hand, low levels of serum IGF-1 in IUGR and preterm infants appear to predict an increased risk of retinopathy of prematurity (ROP).[33]

IGF bioavailability is modulated by specific binding proteins. Among these, IGFBP-1 is present in the decidua and at the decidua–trophoblast interface[34] and may act as a local modulator of IGF action on fetal growth. Increased IGFBP-1 has been implicated in poor placentation, potentially by reducing trophoblast invasion of the spiral arteries in early pregnancy,[35] raised serum maternal IGFBP-1 concentrations occur in pregnancies that are complicated by IUGR or pre-eclampsia.[35–37]

There is a robust relationship among the rate of increase in individual maternal IGF-1 levels after 16 weeks, placental mass, and neonatal fat mass. This does not imply causality but does indicate that mid-pregnancy changes in IGF-1 levels may be a valuable marker for anomalous fetal growth.[38]

Human placental development combines elements of tumorigenesis and vasculogenesis. The dysfunction of the vascular endothelium is now thought to be the primary factor responsible for growth anomalies.[39]

Besides IGF, also other growth factors as the vascular endothelial growth factor (VEGF) can be important. VEGF is a specific mitogen and survival factor for endothelial cells, and a crucial promoter of angiogenesis in physiological and pathophysiological conditions.[40,41] During pregnancy, VEGF is essential to the proliferation of trophoblasts, the development of embyonic vasculature, and the growth of maternal and fetal blood vessels in the uterus.[42]

Fetal vasculogenesis and angiogenesis, and vascular adaptation of the uterine circulation, are unique.[43] VEGF is a protein with antiapoptotic, mitogenic, and permeability-increasing activities specific for the vascular endothelium.

Other factors of vasculogenesis

Ashworth *et al.*[44] showed that myometrial arteries from women with pre-eclampsia have an attenuated response to the endothelium-dependent vasodilator, bradykinin. However, Ashworth *et al.* used vasopressin as a vasoconstrictor, a substance that has no known role in the myometrial vascular bed[45] and only assumes a physiological role in cases of profound shock.[46,47] Other more physiological agents, such as noradrenaline, 5-hydroxytryptamine, angiotensin II, prostaglandin F2 α and endothelin-1, do not provide such a contraction on myometrial arteries[45] and therefore cannot be used.

Ong *et al.* confirmed that myometrial arteries from women with pre-eclampsia or intrauterine growth restriction, exhibit an attenuated endothelium-dependent vasodilatory response.[48]

Fetal hormones

Recent studies also suggest that the underlying mechanisms that regulate feto-placental growth responses to changes in substrate availability involve the endocrine, paracrine, and autocrine effects of placental growth hormone, placental lactogen, insulin, the family of IGFs, and their binding proteins.

Fetal growth hormone

Fetal growth hormone concentrations are substantially higher than those found after birth (resembling growth hormone levels in patients with acromegalia) and show a peak at 20–24 weeks' of gestation.[49] However, the influence of growth hormone on the regulation of fetal growth is negligible.[50] This is probably related to the absence of growth hormone receptors in the fetal liver.[51] For example, mean growth hormone levels in anencephalic fetuses are 80% lower than those found in normal conditions, but fetal weight is not significantly reduced.[52] In cases of growth hormone familial deficiency, weight at birth is practically normal, height may be somewhat lower,[53] and there are no clinical signs of growth hormone deficiency. In animal studies, fetal growth rate was not affected by hypophysectomy[54] or decapitation.[55]

Despite this evidence, results of different studies suggest that growth hormone possibly contributes to fetal growth to some extent. Hoet[56] considered that growth hormone can increase the sensitivity of β-cells of the pancreas to plasma glucose levels. Thus, the well-known increase in the number of fetal β-cells and insulin levels that is observed in maternal diabetes does not appear in anencephalic fetuses from diabetic mothers. Fetal weight may be conditioned by insulin–growth hormone balance. In fact, the relationship between growth hormone and insulin is shown by the intrauterine diabetogenic effect of growth hormone[57] and by an inhibiting action on fetal hypoglycemia secondary to endogenous hyperinsulinism, acting as an antagonist of insulin. Some functional similarities between growth hormone and placental lactogen may be expected given that 85% of their amino acids are identical. Growth hormone promotes lipolysis and glycogen deposits in the fetal liver,[58] and exerts a direct stimulation of the adrenal glands[59] and possibly of the epiphyses of long bones.[30]

An 80% decrease in neonatal growth hormone secretion after childbirth has also been demonstrated. The fact that growth hormone levels increase in fetal plasma by the same relative proportion that growth hormone levels decrease in the hypophysis has remained unclear for many years. These findings suggest a 'defect' in the regulation of growth hormone secretion, probably due to immaturity of the fetal hypothalamus–portal system and absence of IGF3. At the end of gestation, however, this situation is reversed by maturation of the portal system and functioning of the hypothalamic negative feedback regulating system.[60]

Thyroxine

Despite the essential role attributed to thyroxine in cell metabolism, the thyroid gland does not seem to be implicated as a regulating factor of intrauterine growth. Thyroid hormones, however, are involved in antenatal maturation of the fetal lungs and skeleton. It has been shown that birth weights of hypothyroid fetuses are even higher than the average.[61] The excess of thyroxine in thyrotoxic fetuses does not accelerate fetal growth rate, and they are even susceptible to intrauterine growth retardation.[62] Fetuses from thyroidectomized rats and rabbits did not exhibit growth retardation.[8]

However, thyroxine may be involved in fetal growth as shown by results of experimental studies. Sheep fetuses undergoing thyroidectomy 7 weeks prior to delivery showed marked growth restriction.[63] This indicates that a period of time is required for thyroxine-related effects to become evident. Inconsistencies

Table 116.1 Effect of experimental manipulation of fetal insulin levels on fetal weight at term in different animal species[78]

Insulin level	Procedure	Species	Fetal weight
High	Maternal diabetes	Monkey, pig	Unchanged
		Sheep, rat	Unchanged
High	Insulin infusion	Pig, sheep	Unchanged
		Monkey, rat	↑10–25%
High	Glucose infusion	Sheep, rat	↑10–20%
Low	Pancreatectomy	Sheep, rat	→ 20–30%
	Diabetogenic drugs	Sheep, rat	→ 20–40%
		Monkey	→ 10–20%

between these results and those mentioned above may be explained by ovine placenta not being permeable to thyroxine and tri-iodothyronine,[64] whereas in humans, rats and rabbits, the placenta is slightly permeable to maternal thyroxine. It seems that small amounts of maternal hormone are sufficient to maintain normal fetal growth rates. In the absence of both maternal and fetal thyroid hormones, fetal growth restriction occurs. In rhesus monkeys, ablation of maternal and fetal thyroid tissue by means of radioactive iodine was followed by a decrease in protein synthesis, with decreased levels of total RNA, total proteins, ATPase activity, and carbonate dehydratase activity.[65] Studies on the growth of fetal guinea pigs showed decreased plasma levels of thyroxine and tri-iodothyronine in cases of intrauterine growth restriction.[66] Information based on these experiences may be relevant in humans.

Insulin

Insulin is the only fetal hormone related to intrauterine growth. Macrosomia is frequently observed in pregnancies complicated by diabetes mellitus. Given that maternal insulin cannot diffuse through the placental membrane, insulin is exclusively of fetal origin. It has been suggested that maternal hyperglycemia would induce fetal hyperglycemia, which would stimulate fetal pancreatic islet cells with an increase in the secretion of insulin.[67] Fetal hyperinsulinism mobilizes glucose deposits, increasing fetal growth. Other authors[68] have also shown that an increase in maternal amino acids causes a similar stimulating effect on fetal insulin secretion.

Clinical and experimental evidence indicates that insulin can be considered as the true 'fetal growth hormone'. High insulin levels are found in neonates of diabetic mothers.[69] There is a positive correlation between plasma insulin levels and fetal weight in a high number of animal species. A positive correlation between insulin cord levels and excessive birth weight in newborns of diabetic mothers has also been reported.[70] Low insulin levels have been consistently associated with low weight fetuses (Table 116.1).[71,72] Fetal injections of insulin in rat[73] and sheep models[74] produced an increase in birth weight with an increase in fat tissue and nitrogen content. Growth restriction was reported in fetuses of rhesus monkeys and sheep which were rendered insulin-dependent by chemical ablation of pancreatic β-cells after uterine injection of streptozocin,[75,76] and despite the induction of hyperglycemia, use and oxidation of glucose in fetal tissues was impaired. Intrauterine growth restriction has also been documented in full-term neonates with pancreatic agenesis[77] whose development seemed to be interrupted at 30–32 weeks' gestation (the time at which excessive fetal growth in maternal diabetes is documented).[76] Pancreatectomy-induced growth retardation has also been confirmed in experimental studies. In sheep fetuses,[78] pancreatectomy was followed by a 40–50% decrease of the growth index (Figures 116.3 and 116.4) that returned to normal after insulin therapy.[79] Fetal insulin concentration varied in parallel with glucose levels.[78]

Insulin effects in the antenatal and postnatal periods are substantially different. Maternal plasma glucose levels are maintained within a narrow range by maternal insulin, so that there is a relatively constant and uniform glucose perfusion to the fetus. The absence of sudden fluctuations in glucose levels is the reason for a fetal lack of requirement of pancreatic β-cells, resulting in a fetal pancreas insensitive to acute increases in glucose concentrations (to some extent a situation similar to that found in diabetics).[80] Amino acids show an even greater stimulating effect on insulin secretion than glucose. However, in cases of sustained hyperglycemia (e.g., maternal diabetes) the fetal pancreas ultimately

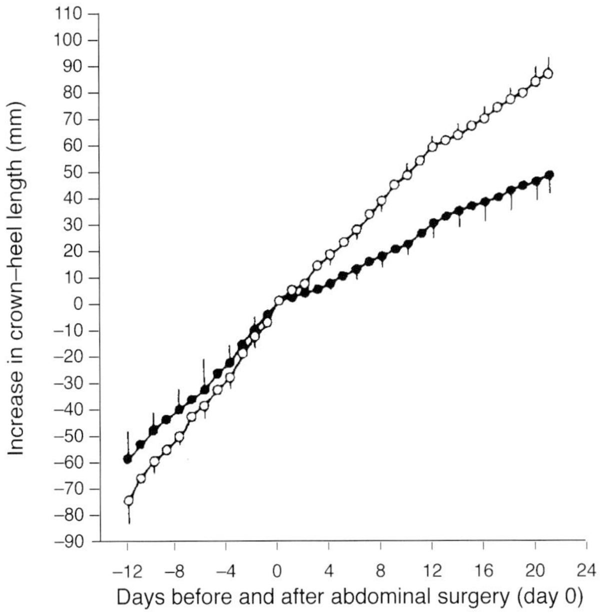

Figure 116.3 Mean ± SD crown–rump length (crown–heel) in sheep fetuses before and after pancreatectomy on day 0 (•, $n=6$) and before and after a sham operation on day 0 (○, $n=5$).[78]

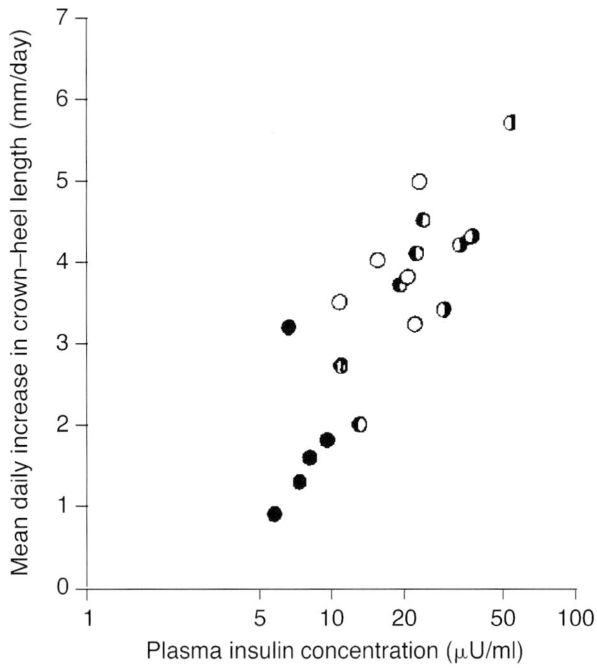

Figure 116.4 Relationship between plasma insulin concentration and daily increase in crown–rump length in sheep fetuses after a sham operation (○) or pancreatectomy and insulin replacement (•) ($y=3.97$, $\log x+1.50$; $n=19$; $r=0.847$; $p<0.001$).[78]

shows a response with hyperplasia of β-cells and an increase in insulin secretion.

An adequate supply of nutrients and uteroplacental blood flow are necessary for fetal growth stimulation by insulin. In maternal diabetes with progressive uteroplacental vascular insufficiency due to microangiopathy of villi arterioles, fetal hyperinsulinism due to β-cell hyperplasia is followed, on the contrary, by chronic hypoglycemia and growth restriction.

No insulin receptors are found during the first stages of fetal growth, so that there is a lack of response to insulin at this stage.[81] On the other hand, it seems that these receptors are not insulin-specific, as they also respond to somatomedins.[82]

In rats, plasma insulin levels decrease suddenly after birth and remain low despite proper postnatal development of the animal. Plasma levels of growth hormone also decrease. These findings may be explained by glucose being the only intrauterine fetal nutrient. After birth, insulin loses its role as a growth hormone since a nutrient (milk) poor in carbohydrates but rich in fat is supplied. The stimulating action of insulin on fetal growth is due in part to its direct anabolic effect on fetal metabolism and to an indirect stimulating effect on other growth factors, such as somatomedins (IGF-1 and IGF-2). It has been shown that the higher the fetal weight, the higher the IGF-1 levels are.[83]

Placental hormones

Human placental lactogen

Human chorionic somatomammotropin (HCS), also known as human placental lactogen (HPL) or human chorionic growth prolactin (HCGP), is the only placental hormone significantly related to fetal growth. This hormone, secreted by the placental syncytiotrophoblast, diffuses exclusively to the maternal circulation. Maternal plasma levels of HPL increase exponentially according to placental growth. HPL represents 5–10% of the total proteins synthesized and released by the placenta. The levels of HPL are closely related to placental weight, i.e., to functional trophoblastic tissue mass.[84]

Human placental lactogen is detectable in maternal plasma from weeks 6–8 of pregnancy. In normal conditions, HPL levels show an exponential increase up to a plateau of 6 ± 1 mg/ml at week 35, which is 1000-fold higher than baseline growth hormone levels. As stated above, HPL replaces growth hormone in some of its functions.

Physiological actions of HPL include a series of maternal changes (Figure 116.5).[85,86] In relation to the lipolytic activity of this hormone, HPL mobilizes fat deposits with a subsequent increase in plasma free fatty acids and triglycerides which would be therefore available to fetal needs. On the other hand, there is an increase in insulin resistance due to a peripheral antagonist effect of HPL on glycolytic activity but not on lipogenic or glycogenetic activities. HPL induces a decrease in maternal glucose consumption, thus ensuring adequate nutrients to the fetus, stimulates amino acid incorporation to proteins (an action probably synergistic with insulin), and increases circulating levels of insulin as a response to glucose overload.

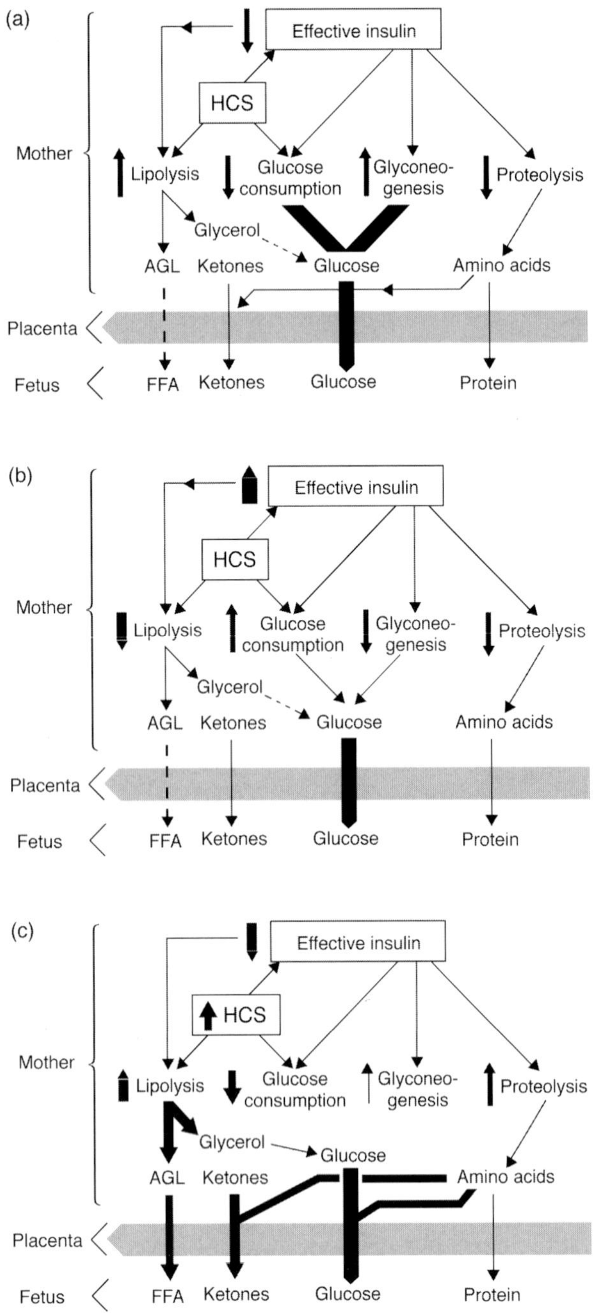

Figure 116.5 Role of human chorionic somatomammotropin (HCS) in (a) the provision of maternofetal substrate,[86] (b) the provision of maternofetal substrate and nutritional status,[86] and (c) maternofetal provision in fasting conditions.[86] FFA, free fatty acids.

Based on the knowledge of these partial functions, it may be assumed that the metabolic role of HPL in relation to fetal development consists mainly in ensuring an adequate supply of carbohydrates by inhibiting insulin glycolysis in maternal tissue, facilitating the conversion of fat into metabolic nutrients, and protecting the maternal protein supply by its synergistic effect on the protein-anabolic activity of insulin, so that lipids rather than carbohydrates are more extensively used for maternal nutrition. Since transplacental diffusion of large amounts of lipids is not possible, and given that fetal nutrients are mainly carbohydrates, this maternal metabolic condition favors fetal nutrition. This pathway is particularly important in cases of maternal malnutrition; in fact, fasting is the main stimulus for HPL secretion in pregnancy. The anti-insulin effects of HPL are only counteracted in the immediate postprandial state by peak plasma levels of insulin, which, on the other hand, allow maternal hepatic stores of glycogen and fat to be replaced. Increased insulin and HPL levels activate protein synthesis. Therefore, insulin constitutes a fluctuating modulator of HPL effects on the maternal organism.[87] Food intake increases 'effective insulin' and restores maternal substrates, whereas fasting induces a decrease in 'effective insulin', and the catabolic effects of HPL guarantee an adequate supply of nutrients to the fetus.

Sex steroids

Progesterone has catabolic and insulinogenic effects, and estrogens are antagonists of HPL effects on bone growth. It is likely that both sex steroids and hydrocortisone would also have a modulating effect on physiological actions of HPL and that HPL, in turn, may regulate the effects of some growth factors, such as IGF-1 and IGFBP-1.[32]

Eicosanoids

Recent studies have considered prostaglandin E_2 of placental origin as responsible for a reduction of fetal breathing movements occurring in hypoglycemic conditions.[88] Accordingly, the fetus would 'save' glucose to be used by other more essential processes.

Placental proteins

During the last years, several research works have linked the low levels of pregnancy-associated plasma protein A (PAPP-A) and free beta-subunit of human chorionic gonadotrophin (FβhCG) to fetal growth anomalies. However, there are still some doubts about the consistency of this association.

One study found a positive correlation between PAPP-A at 8–14 weeks and eventual birth weight[89] and an analysis of 60 *in vitro* fertilization pregnancies described lower concentrations of PAPP-A in the first trimester among eight women who eventually delivered preterm.[90] A further study of 5297 women showed lower PAPP-A and FβhCG levels at 10–14 weeks' gestation among women who miscarried, delivered babies small for gestational age and developed pre-eclampsia.[91]

The association between first-trimester biochemistry and later pregnancy complications has been examined in such a multicenter, prospective, non-interventional cohort study among a subgroup of 8839 women with singleton, karyotypically normal babies, where outcome data had been retrieved. This analysis showed strong and highly statistically significant

Table 116.2 Adjusted odds ratios for adverse perinatal outcomes associated with first-trimester PAPP-A and free hCG in the lowest 5th percentile (from Smith *et al.*[92])

	PAPP-A < 5th percentile		Free hCG < 5th percentile	
Outcome	**Adjusted odds ratio (95% CI)**	**P**	**Adjusted odds ratio (95% CI)**	**P**
Birth weight < 5th percentile	2.9 (2.0–4.1)	< 0.001	1.3 (0.9–2.0)	0.15
Delivery 24–32 weeks	2.9 (1.6–5.5)	0.001	1.1 (0.5–2.7)	0.77
Delivery 33–36 weeks	2.4 (1.7–3.5)	< 0.001	0.5 (0.3–1.0)	0.04
Pre-eclampsia	2.3 (1.6–3.3)	< 0.001	1.1 (0.7–1.8)	0.64
Stillbirth	3.6 (1.2–11.0)	0.02	2.3 (0.7–8.2)	0.18

Odds ratios adjusted for BMI, height, smoking status, ethnicity, parity, maternal age, gestational age at the time of sampling, PAPP-A and free hCG
Odds ratio for delivery week 33–36 also adjusted for interaction between age, ≥35 years and height

associations between levels of PAPP-A at 8–14 weeks and the risk of fetal growth anomalies.[92]

The association persisted in multivariate adjusting for body mass index (BMI), height, smoking status, ethnicity, parity, maternal age, gestational age at the time of sampling (Table 116.2). There was also an association between FβhCG and growth restriction across the range of deciles. However, the association between FβhCG and later outcome did not persist in multivariate analysis including the PAPP-A level.

Other studies also reflect a defect in early pregnancy placentation and later adverse outcome. For this reason, low first-trimester maternal circulation of PAPP-A, is associated with an increased risk of growth restriction.[93–97]

However, some researchers consider that this so-called association cannot be considered as proven, since some epidemiological,[98] diagnostic and methodological variables have not been taken into account (errors in dating).[99]

PAPP-A has been found to be part of the system controlling the IGFs in trophoblast. PAPP-A has been identified as a protease for IGFBP-4.[100] IGFBPs bind IGF-I and IGF-II, inhibiting their interaction with cell surface receptors and have, therefore, a key role in modulating IGF activity.[101] Because PAPP-A breaks down IGFBI[100] low levels of PAPP-A would be expected to be associated with high levels of IGFBP and, therefore, low levels of free IGF.

Environmental regulation of fetal growth

Reduction of the free rate of fetal growth due to its environment is a common and normal occurrence. In the absence of these environmental conditioning factors, it is possible that the weight at birth would be doubled. It has been postulated that fetal growth restriction may be exerted by the activation of a predetermined maternal regulating factor[102] ('environmental chronometer'), which may be triggered by the maternal genotype and by the degree to which maternal fetal growth was restricted during its own development. Therefore, it is possible that fetal weight variations may be transmitted through successive generations without forming part of the genotype. This hypothetical regulating factor would act on the 'intrauterine environment' and through the external environment where the mother lives. With regard to the intrauterine environment, it seems logical that the first mechanism of action would be related to a limiting effect on the trophoblastic activity resulting in a decrease in the exchange surface of the placenta.

On the other hand, if maternal support to fetal growth is unlimited, fetal growth rate would be linear not only until week 38, but also until the time of delivery. Gruenwald[103] considered that from week 38 onwards there is a physiological placental insufficiency due to a lack of maternal support, which limits fetal growth potential. This has been definitely confirmed by the postnatal increase in growth rate once the newborn is free from intrauterine restriction, thus achieving again the growth rate present before 38 weeks' gestation. Gruenwald[103] observed that in countries with the highest neonatal birth weights, such as Sweden, there was a delay in the flattening of the fetal growth curve (with respect to the potential fetal growth curve) as compared with communities with a worse degree of nourishment.

On the other hand, as commented on in the description of factors affecting fetal growth, the ability of the uterus to retain the fetus until maturity, and the ability to nourish the fetus properly (adequate uteroplacental blood flow, etc.) vary according to multiple factors, such as parity, maternal weight, maternal height, fetal gender, etc.

In respect of the 'external environment', the mother herself seems to act as a buffer protecting the fetus from an adverse environment. Until recently, it was considered that only substantial changes in the diet,[104] percentage of oxygen[72] or socioeconomic factors would be able to induce minor modifications of birth weight. Recent studies,[105] however, have suggested that fetal availability of macronutrients (particularly carbohydrates and amino acids), mainly during the last weeks of pregnancy, plays an important role on fetal weight at birth. An inadequate maternal nutrition during pregnancy has been associated with small fetuses.[106] In animal studies, a decrease in oxygen supply also induced fetal growth retardation.[107]

REFERENCES

1. Díaz del Castillo E. *Pediatría Prenatal.* México: Interamericana, 1974.
2. Bukowski R, Saade GR, Malone FD, *et al.* Association between impaired fetal growth potential and adverse pregnancy outcome. *Am J Obstet Gynecol* 2003;187:57.
3. Bukowski R, Zhang J, Gardosi GR, *et al.* Fetal growth potential as a predictor of neonatal morbidity (abstract). *Am J Obstet Gynecol* 2002;185:245.
4. Bukowski R, Saade GR, Cliver SP, *et al.* Impairment of the individual growth potential and intelligence at age 5 years (abstract). *Am J Obstet Gynecol* 2002;187:98.
5. Bukowski R, Saade GR, Cliver SP, *et al.* Prenatal prediction of the impairment of the individual fetal growth potential. *Am J Obstet Gynecol* 2003;187:190.
6. Bukowski R, Burgett AD, Gei A, *et al.* Impairment of fetal growth potential and neonatal encephalopathy. *Am J Obstet Gynecol* 2003;188:1011–5.
7. Bukowski R. Fetal growth potential and pregnancy outcome. *Semin Perinatol* 2004;28(1):51–8.
8. Liggins GC. The drive to fetal growth. In Beard RW, Nathanielsz PW, eds. *Fetal Physiology and Medicine.* Philadelphia, PA: W.B. Saunders Co., 1976:254–301.
9. Surani MAH, Barton SC, Howlett SK, Norris ML. Influence of chromosomal determinants on development of androgenetic and parthogenetic cells. *Development* 1988;103:171–81.
10. Solter D. Differential imprinting and expression of maternal and paternal genomes. *Ann Rev Genet* 1988;22:127–46.
11. Sapienza C, Peterson AG, Rossant J, Balling R. Degree of methylation of transgenes is dependent on gamete of origin. *Nature* 1987;238:251–4.
12. Holliday R, Pugh JE. DNA modifications mechanism and gene activity during development. *Science* 1975;187:226–32.
13. Polani PE. Chromosomal and other genetic influences on birth weight variation. In Elliot K, Knight J, eds. *Size at Birth.* Amsterdam: Associated Scientific Publishers, 1974:127–64.
14. Ounsted C, Ounsted M. Effect of Y-chromosome on fetal growth rate. *Lancet* 1970;2:857–8.
15. Meredith HC. Body weights of viable human infants. A worldwide comparative treatise. *Hum Biol* 1970;42:217–64.
16. Abdul-Karim RW, Beydoun SN. Growth of the human fetus. *Clin Obstet Gynecol* 1974;17:37–52.
17. Penrose LS. *Recent Advances in Human Genetics.* London: Churchill Livingstone, 1961:56.
18. Love EJ, Kinch RAH. Factors affecting the birth weight in normal pregnancy. *Am J Obstet Gynecol* 1965;91:342–9.
19. Gardosi J, Chang A, Kalyan B, *et al.* Customised antenatal growth charts. *Lancet* 1992;339:283–7.
20. Mongelli M, Gardosi J. Reduction of false-positive diagnose of fetal growth restriction by application of customized fetal growth standards. *Obstet Gynecol* 1996;88:844–8.
21. Speroff L. An essay: Prostaglandins and toxemia of pregnancy. *Prostaglandins* 1973;3:721–8.
22. Chan CC, Lao TT, Cheung AN. Apoptotic and proliferative activities in first trimester placentae. *Placenta* 1999;20:223–7.
23. Pardi G, Marconi AM, Cetin I. Pathophysiology of intrauterine growth retardation: Role of the placenta. *Acta Pediatr* 1997;423: 170–2.
24. Gurel D, Ozer E. Expression of IGF-IR and trophoblastic proliferative activity in placenta from pregnancies complicated by IUGR. *Pathol Res Prenat* 2003;199:803–9.
25. Holmes R, Porter H, Newcomb P, Holly JM, Soothill P. An immunohistochemical study of type I insulin-like growth factor receptors in the placentae of pregnancies with appropriately grown or growth restricted fetuses. *Placenta* 1999;20:325–30.
26. Maruo T, Murata K, Matsuo H, Samoto T, Mochizuki M. Insulin like growth factor I as a local regulator of proliferation and differentiated function of the human trophoblast in early pregnancy. *Early Pregnancy* 1995;1:54–61.
27. Froesch ER, Schmid C, Schwander J, Zapf J. Actions of the insulin-like growth factors. *Ann Rev Physiol* 1985;443–67.
28. Ashton K, Zapf J, Einschenk I, MacKenzie IZ. Insulin-like growth factors (IGF) I and II in human foetal plasma and relationship to gestational age and foetal size during mid-pregnancy. *Acta Endocrinol Scand* 1985;110:558–63.
29. Giudice LC, de Zegher F, Gargosky SE, *et al.* Insulin-like growth factors and their binding proteins in the term and preterm human fetus and neonate with normal and extremes of IUGR. *J Clin Endocrinol Metab* 1995;80:1548–55.
30. Mesiano S, Young SR, Baxter RC, Hintz RC, Browne CA, Thorburn GD. The effect of hypophysectomy with and without thyroxine replacement on growth and circulating concentrations on insulin-like growth factors I and II in the fetal lamb. *Endocrinology* 1987;l20:1821–30.
31. Bassett JM, Fletcher JM. Hormonal regulation of fetal metabolism and growth: The roles of pancreatic and adrenal hormones. In Jones CT, ed. *Biochemical Development of the Fetus and Neonate.* Amsterdam: Elsevier Biomedical Press, 1982:393–403.
32. Iwashita M, Kobayashi M, Matsuda A, *et al.* Feto-maternal interaction of IGF-I and its binding proteins in fetal growth. In Sakamoto S, Takeda Y, eds. *Advances in Perinatal Medicine.* Amsterdam: Elsevier, 1992:187–91.
33. Hellström A, Engström E, Härd A-L, *et al.* Postnatal serum insulin-like growth factor I deficiency is associated with retinopathy of prematurity and other complications of premature birth. *Pediatrics* 2003;112(5):1016–20.
34. Gratton RJ, Asano H, Han VK. The regional expression of insulin-like growth factor II (IGF-II) and insulin-like growth factor binding protein-1 (IGFBP-1) in the placentae of women with pre-eclampsia. *Placenta* 2002;23:303–10.
35. Giudice LC, Martina NA, Crystal RA, Tazuke S, Druzin M. Insulin-like growth factor binding protein-1 at the maternal–fetal interface and insulin-like growth factor-1, insulin-like growth factor-II, and insulin-like growth factor binding protein-1 in the circulation of women with severe preeclampsia. *Am J Obstet Gynecol* 1997;176:751–8.
36. Anim-Nyame N, Hills FA, Sooranna SR, Steer PJ, Johnson MR. A longitudinal study of maternal plasma insulin-like growth factor binding protein-1 concentrations during normal pregnancy and pregnancies complicated by pre-eclampsia. *Hum Reprod* 2000;15:2215–9.
37. Stone S, Langford K, Seed PT, Stat MSC. Longitudinal analysis of serum insulin-like growth factor-I and insulin-like growth factor binding protein-1 in antiphospholip syndrome and in healthy pregnancy. *Am J Obstet Gynecol* 2003;189(1):274–9.
38. Clapp JF, Schmidt S, Paranjape A, Lopez B. Maternal insulin-like growth factor-I levels (16F-I) reflect placental mass and neonatal fat mass. *Am J Obstet Gynecol* 2004;190:730–6.
39. Bosio MP, Wheeler T, Anthony F, Conroy R, O'Herlichy C, McKenna P. Maternal plasma vascular endothelial growth factor concentrations in normal and hypertensive pregnancies and their relationship to peripheral vascula resistance. *Am J Obstet Gynecol* 2002;2:146–52.
40. Dvorak HF, Brown LF, Detmar M, Dvorak AM. Vascular permeability factor/vascular endothelial growth factor, microvascular

hypermeability, and angiogenesis (Review). *Am J Pathol* 1995; 146:1029–39.
41. Ferrara N, Davis-Smyth T. The biology of vascular endothelial growth factor (Review). *Endocr Rev* 1997;18:4–25.
42. Jelkmann W. Pitfals in the measurement of circulating vascular endothelial growth factor (mini review). *Clin Chem* 2001;47(4): 617–23.
43. Vuorella P, Helske S, Horning C, Alitalo K, Weich H, Halmesmaki E. Amniotic fluid-soluble vascular endothelial growth factor receptor-1 in preeclampsia. *Obstet Gynecol* 2000;95(3):353–7.
44. Ashworth JR, Warren AY, Baker PN, Johnson IR. Loss of endotheliaum-dependent relaxation in myometrial resistance arteries in preeclampsia. *Br J Obstet Gynaecol* 1997;104:1152–8.
45. Hayman R. *Circulating Factors, The Endothelium and Pre-eclampsia.* Nottingham: University of Nottingham, 1999.
46. Smith JJ, Kampine JP. Humoral regulation of the circulation. In Smith JJ, Kampine JP, eds. *Circulatory Physiology – The Essentials.* Baltimore, MD: Williams & Wilkins, 1990.
47. Plane F, Garland CJ. Influence of contractile agonists on the mechanism of endothelium-dependent relaxation in rat isolated mesenteric artery. *Br J Pharmacol* 1996;119:191–3.
48. Ong S-S, Moore RJ, Warren AY, Crocker IP. Myometrial and placental artery reactivity alone cannot explain reduced placental perfusion in pre-eclampsia and IUGR. *Br J Obstet Gynaecol* 2003; 110:909–16.
49. Von Muhlendahl KE, Pachaly J, Schmidt-Gollwitzer M. Lack of correlation between clinical data and growth hormone concentrations in cord blood. *Biol Neonate* 1976;29:281–5.
50. Gluckman PD, Basset NS, Butler JH. The somatotropic axis in the fetus and newborn. In Albrecht E, Pepe GJ, eds. *Perinatal Endocrinology.* Ithaca, NY: Perinatology Press, 1986:1–20.
51. Basset NS, Gluckman PD, Breier BH, Ball KT. Growth hormone and insulin-like growth factors in the fetus: Regulation and role in fetal growth. In Gluckman PD, Johnston BM, Nathanielsz PW, eds. *Advances in Fetal Physiology. Research in Perinatal Medicine.* Ithaca, NY: Perinatology Press, 1989:303–14.
52. Grumbach MM, Kaplan SL. Ontogenesis of growth hormone, insulin, prolactin and gonadotropin secretion in the human fetus. In Comline RS, Cross KW, Daves GC, Nathanielsz PW, eds. *Foetal and Neonatal Physiology.* London: Cambridge University Press, 1973:462–87.
53. Laron S. The role of growth hormone on fetal development *in utero.* In Abramovici MA, Clermke A, eds. *Drugs and Fetal Development.* New York: Plenum Press, 1973:391.
54. Chez RA, Hutchinson DL, Salazar H, Mintz DH. Some effects of fetal and maternal hypophysectomy in pregnancy. *Am J Obstet Gynecol* 1970;108:643–50.
55. Harris GW, Donovan BT, eds. *The Pituitary Gland.* London: Butterworth, 1966:299–323.
56. Hoet JJ. Normal and abnormal fetal weight gain. In Wolstenholme GEW, O'Connor M, eds. *Foetal Autonomy.* London: Churchill Livingstone, 1969:186–213.
57. Parker MJ, Bassett JM. Antagonism by growth hormone of insulin action in fetal sheep. *J Endocrinol* 1985;105:379–82.
58. Stevens D, Alexander G. Lipid deposition after hypophysectomy and growth hormone treatment in the sheep fetus. *J Dev Physiol* 1986;8:139–45.
59. Devaskar UP, Devaskar SU, Voina S, Velayo N, Sperling MA. Growth hormone stimulates adrenal steroidogenesis in the fetus. *Nature* 1981;290:404–5.
60. Gluckman PD, Parsons Y. Growth hormone secretion in the fetal sheep following stereotaxic electolytic lesioning of the fetal hypothalamus. *J Dev Physiol* 1985;5:101–28.
61. Anderson HS. Studies of hypothyroidism in children. *Acta Paediatr Scand* 1961;50(Suppl 125):1–150.
62. Samsamy B, Jethwa AKN, Ferriman D. Congenital thyrotoxicosis. *Proc R Soc Med* 1970;63:577–8.
63. Hopkins PS, Thorburn GD. The effects of foetal thyroidectomy on the development of the ovine foetus. *J Endocrinol* 1972;54:55–6.
64. Erenberg A, Fisher DA. Thyroid hormone metabolism in the foetus. In Comline RS, Cross KW, Dawes GS, Nathanielsz PW, eds. *Foetal and Neonatal Phyiology.* London: Cambridge University Press, 1973:508–26.
65. Holt A, Cheek DB, Kerr GR. Prenatal hypothyroidism and brain composition in a primate. *Nature* 1973;243:413–5.
66 Jones CT, Labefer HN, Roebuck MM. Studies on the growth of the fetal guinea pig. Changes in plasma hormone concentration during normal and abnormal growth. *J Dev Physiol* 1984;6:461–72.
67. Pedersen J, Osler M. Hyperglycemia as a cause of characteristic features of the fetus and the newborn of diabetic mothers. *Dan Med Bull* 1981;8:78–82.
68. Milner RDG. Amino acids and beta cell growth in structure and function. In Merkatz IR, Adam PAJ, eds. *The Diabetic Pregnancy.* New York: Grune & Stratton, 1979:145.
69. Hill DE. Fetal effects of insulin. *Obstet Gynecol Ann* 1982;11: 133–49.
70. Beard RW, Oakley NW. The fetus of the diabetic. In Beard RW, Nathanielsz PW, eds. *Fetal Physiology and Medicine.* Philadelphia, PA: W.B. Saunders, 1976:137–57.
71. Harding J, Jones C, Robinson J. Studies on experimental growth retardation in sheep. The effects of a small placenta in restricting transport to and growth of the fetus. *J Dev Physiol* 1985;7:427–32.
72. Jones CT, Harding JE, Gu W, Lafeber HN. Placental metabolism and endocrine effects in relation to the control of fetal and placental growth. In Jensen A, Kunzel E, eds. *The Endocrine Control of the Fetus. Physiologic and Pathophysiologic Aspects.* Berlin: Springer-Verlag, 1988:213–22.
73. Picon L. Effect of insulin on growth and biochemical composition of the rat fetus. *Endocrinology* 1967;81:1419–21.
74. Liggins GC. The influence of fetal hypothalamus and pituitary on growth. In Elliot K, Knight J, eds. *Size at Birth.* Amsterdam: Associated Scientific Publisher, 1974:165.
75. Hill DE, Holt AB, Reba R, Cheek DB. Alterations in the growth pattern of fetal rhesus monkeys following the *in utero* injection of streptozotocin (abstract). *Pediatr Res* 1972;6:336.
76. Cheek DB. The growth of the brain. In Cheek DB, ed. *Fetal and Postnatal Cellular Growth.* New York: Wiley, 1975:3–22.
77. Fowden AL. Pancreatic endocrine function and carbohydrate metabolism in the fetus. In Albrecht E, Pepe GJ, eds. *Perinatal Endocrinology.* Ithaca, NY: Perinatology Press, 1985:71–90.
78. Fowden AL. The role of insulin in fetal growth. In Sakamoto S, Takeda Y, eds. *Advances in Perinatal Medicine.* Amsterdam: Elsevier, 1992:177–81.
79. Fowden AL, Comline RS, Hughes P. The effects of pancreatectomy on the sheep fetus. *Acta Physiol Pol* 1988;39:415–20.
80. Oakley NW, Beard RW, Turner RC. Effect of sustained hyperglycaemia on the fetus in normal and diabetic pregnancies. *Br Med J* 1972;1:466–91.
81. Bocek RM, Beatty CH. Effect of insulin on the carbohydrate metabolism of fetal rhesus monkey muscle. *Endocrinology* 1969;85:615–8.
82. Hintz RL, Clemmons DR, Underwood LE, Van Wyk JJ. Competitive binding of somatomedin to the insulin receptors of adipocytes, chondrocytes and liver membranes. *Proc Natl Acad Sci USA* 1972;69:2351–3.
83. D'Ercole AJ. Somatomedins/insulin-like growth factors and fetal growth. *J Dev Physiol* 1987;9:481–96.
84. Josimovich JB, Kosor B, Bocella L, Mintz DH, Hutchinson DL. Placental lactogen in maternal serun as a index of fetal health. *Obstet Gynecol* 1970;36:244.
85. Speroff L, Glass RH, Kase NG. Endocrinología del embarazo. In Speroff L, Glass RH, Kase NG, eds. *Endocrinología Ginecológica e Infertilidad,* 3rd edn. Barcelona: Ediciones Toray, 1986: 275–310.
86. Grumbach MM, Kaplan JL, Vinik A. In Berson SA, Yalow RS, eds. *Methods in Investigative and Diagnostic Endocrinology.* Amsterdam: North Holland, 1973:797.
87. Kaplan SL, Grumbach MM, Shepherd TH. The ontogenesis of human fetal hormones. *J Clin Invest* 1972;51:3080–93.
88. Fowden AL, Harding R, Ralph MM, Thorburn GD. The nutritional regulation of plasma PGE concentrations in the fetus and pregnant ewe during late gestation. *J Physiol* 1987;394:1–12.
89. Pedersen JF, Sorensen S, Ruge S. Human placental lactogen and pregnancy-associated plasma protein A in first trimester and subsequent fetal growth. *Acta Obstet Gynecol Scand* 1995;74:505–8.
90. Johnson MR, Riddle AF, Grudzinskas JG, *et al.* Reduced circulating placental protein concentrations during the first trimester are associated with preterm labour and low birth weight. *Hum Reprod* 1993;8:1942–7.
91. Ong CY, Liao AW, Spencer K, *et al.* First trimester maternal serum free beta human chorionic gonadotrophin and pregnancy associated plasma protein A as predictors of pregnancy complications. *Br J Obstet Gynaecol* 2000;107:1265–70.
92. Smith GCS, Stenhouse EJ, Crossley JA, *et al.* Early pregnancy levels of pregnancy-associated plasma protein A and the risk of intrauterine growth restriction, premature birth, pre-eclampsia and stillbirth. *J Clin Endocrinol Metab* 2002;87:1762–7.

93. Smith GCS. First trimester origins of fetal growth impairment. *Semin Perinatol* 2004;28(1):41–50.
94. Wenstrom KD, Owen J, Boots L, DuBard MB. Elevated second trimester human chorionic gonadotrophin levels in association with poor pregnancy outcome. *Am J Obstet Gynecol* 1994;171: 1038–41.
95. Benn PA, Horne D, Briganti S, Rodis JF, Clive JM. Elevated second trimester maternal serum hCG alone or in combination with elevated alpha-fetoprotein. *Obstet Gynecol* 1996;87:217–22.
96. Milunsky A, Jick SS, Bruell CL, *et al.* Predictive values, relative risks, and overall benefits of high and low maternal serum a-fetoprotein screening in singleton pregnancies: New epidemiologic data. *Am J Obstet Gynecol* 1989;161:291–7.
97. Lieppman RE, Williams MA, Cheng EY, *et al.* An association between elevated levels of human chorionic gonadotropin in the midtrimester and adverse pregnancy outcome. *Am J Obstet Gynecol* 1993;168:1852–7.
98. Spencer K. The influence of smoking on maternal serum PAPP-A and free beta hCG levels in the first trimester of pregnancy. *Prenat Diagn* 1999;19:1065–6.
99. Smith GCS, Stenhouse EJ, Crossley JA, *et al.* Development early-pregnancy origins of low birth weight. *Nature* 2002;417:916.
100. Lawrence JB, Oxvig C, Overgaard MT, *et al.* The insulin-like growth factor (IGF)-dependent IGF binding protein-4 protease secreted by human fibroblasts is pregnancy-associated plasma protein-A. *Proc Natl Acad Sci USA* 1999;96:3149–53.
101. Clemmons DR. Role of insulin-like growth factor binding proteins in controlling IGF actions. *Mol Cell Endocrinol* 1998;140:19–24.
102. Ounsted M, Ounsted C. Maternal regulation of intrauterine growth. *Nature* 1966;212:995–7.
103. Gruenwald P. Growth of the human fetus. I: Normal growth and its variation. *Am J Obstet Gynecol* 1966;94:1112–9.
104. Charlton V, Johengen M. Effects of intrauterine nutritional supplementation on fetal growth retardation. *Biol Neonate* 1985;48: 125–32.
105. Charlton V. Substrate availability *in utero* and fetal growth. In Gluckman PD, Johnston BM, Nathanielsz PW, eds. *Advances in Fetal Physiology. Research in Perinatal Medicine.* Ithaca, NY: Perinatology Press, 1989:245–62.
106. Rosso P. Nutrition and maternal–fetal exchange. *Am J Clin Nutr* 1981;34(Suppl 4):744–8.
107. Clapp J, Szeto H, Larrow R, *et al.* Fetal metabolic response to experimental placental vascular damage. *Am J Obstet Gynecol* 1981;40:446–50.

117 Dynamics of fetal growth

J. M. Carrera, F. Figueras, B. Serra and M. Carrera

Introduction

Fetal growth has been evaluated by obstetricians by observing maternal abdomen enlargement, and for many years measurement of the uterine height was practically the only method to estimate intrauterine growth. Although, after the introduction of antenatal ultrasound imaging many studies were reexamined, the only reliable method to measure the product was to do so after delivery. Neonatal anthropometry was developed under these circumstances in an attempt to measure systematically multiple variables related to gestational age of the neonate (after a pregnancy considered normal), and growth tables in relation to weight, height, head circumference, volume of different organs, etc. were developed.

Ultrasound examination has allowed the assessment of not only fetal growth as a whole but also the individual growth of all visible structures. At present, virtually all parts of the fetus have been measured cross-sectionally and longitudinally from its initial vestiges until birth, so that normal ranges of practically all fetal structures throughout the gestational period have been established. Fetal growth is a dynamic process, the evaluation of which requires at least a comparison of two measurements taken at different intervals to obtain more reliable information on how fetal growth develops.

Dynamics of fetal growth

Fetal growth has been studied by means of biochemical methods and anthropometric methods.

Biochemical methods

Biochemical studies carried out in experimental animals and in necropsy specimens from human fetuses have focused on cellular biochemical aspects, and assessment of changes in fetal biochemical composition and in the chemical composition of some individual organs.

Cellular biochemical studies

Biochemical methods for measuring the number and volume of cells were introduced by Winick.[1] Since DNA is almost exclusively limited to the nucleus, and the DNA content of a diploid nucleus in a given species is constant, the total DNA content of an organ reflects exactly the number of diploid nuclei; therefore, dividing the total DNA of an organ by the fixed DNA content of the diploid nucleus results in the actual number of cells. Similarly, weight, proteins, or RNA content of a cell can be determined by dividing total weight, total proteins, or total RNA content of an organ by the number of cells. These values, however, are not valid for organs with a high number of non-diploid nuclei (e.g. liver, testis), or multinucleated cells (e.g. pancreas). Although the time-course of fetal and placental cellular growth in pregnancy has been studied with this method, in practice, weight/DNA and protein/DNA ratios are used to estimate cell volume, and the RNA/DNA ratio is used to assess the mean RNA content of each cell.

According to data reported by Winick,[1] three growth stages are identified: a first stage consisting of proportional increases in weight, proteins, and DNA content (hyperplasia) (DNA increase occurs both in the fetus and in the different organs); a second stage, characterized by a slower increase in DNA content as compared with proteins and weight; and a third stage, in which there is an increase in neat proteins and weight, but not in DNA content (hypertrophy). This different behavior is related to a decrease in the rate of DNA synthesis.

During the first half and a large part of the second half of gestation, growth is based on cell hyperplasia, whereas by the end of pregnancy, hyperplasia is combined with hypertrophy. Therefore, malnutrition during the stage of hyperplasia causes inhibition of the cell division index, resulting in irreversible size reduction and a decrease in the number of cells of an organ. Malnutrition during the stage of cell hypertrophy causes growth deceleration, with recovery taking place once the adverse factor has been corrected, resulting in an organ of normal volume. This pattern of cellular growth is valid for organs in which regeneration is not possible. The time at which the process of cell division is interrupted, however, varies in different organs.

Changes in fetal biochemical composition

In terms of relative fetal body composition, fetal growth means constant adjustment of proportions.

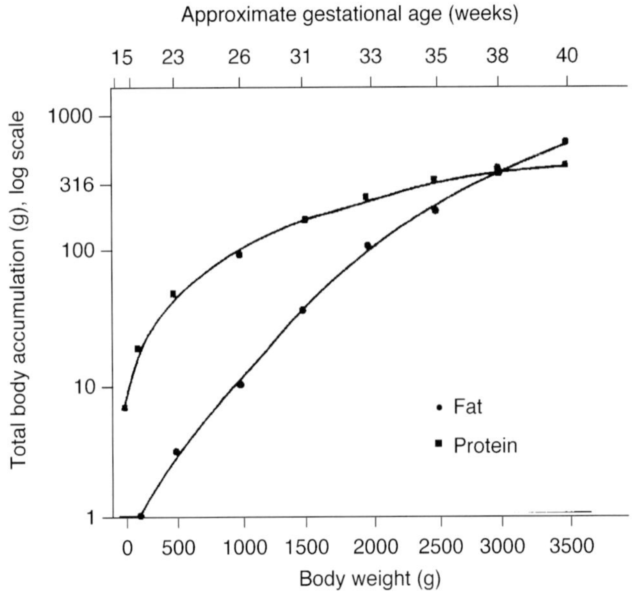

Figure 117.1 Protein and fat accumulation curve (data from Southgate and Hey[5]).

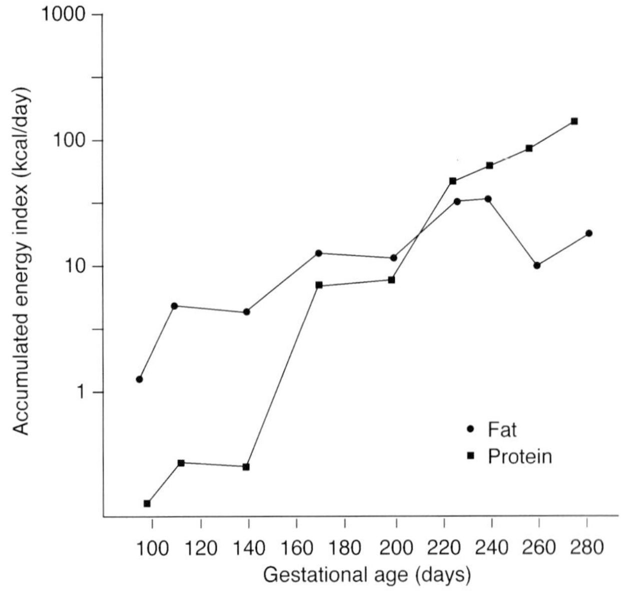

Figure 117.2 Energy stored in fetal proteins and fat (graph constructed according to calculations from Widdowson[3] and data from Southgate and Hey[5]).

Water content is about 94% in an embryo at 10 weeks and 70–80% in a full-term fetus. The percentages of extra- and intracellular water change from 65% and 15–20% during the first weeks of pregnancy to 40% and 38%, respectively, at the end of gestation, due to a progressive increase in the cellular mass by storage of substances (especially proteins) and water. High levels of hyaluronic acid, acting as a gelatinous matrix, probably play an important role in preserving the structure of fetal tissues.

The curve of protein accumulation shows a rapid increase until 26 weeks' gestation (fetal weight 1 kg), followed by slow weekly decreases and steady values starting from 35 weeks' gestation (Figure 117.1).

The rate of fat synthesis early in pregnancy is very low and probably limited to synthesis of structural lipids of cellular membranes and other structures. During the second half of gestation, fat synthesis and storage rates increase exponentially[2] and from 38 weeks' of gestation fat levels are higher than those of proteins.

Figure 117.2 shows energy rates stored in fetal proteins and fat according to the calculations of Widdowson.[3] Maximal protein-derived energy rates are found between days 220 and 260 of pregnancy (about 30 kcal/day). Storage of fat-derived energy is very low until day 140 of pregnancy (< 6 kcal/day). However, starting from day 200 and coinciding with an increase in fat synthesis, there is a marked increase in energy as strong as (100 kcal/day). Therefore, requirements of metabolizable energy are almost totally fulfilled at the end of pregnancy. This fact is very important since fetal weight decreases in cases of intrauterine growth restriction are mainly related to fat loss.[4] Fetal lipid composition remains unchanged from 6 to 32 weeks' of gestation, given that lipid metabolism is perfectly developed early in pregnancy. In relation to fat distribution, Southgate and Hey[5] reported increases in body fat of 10–80 g between day 200 and birth, whereas subcutaneous fat showed an exponential increase, from 20 to 350 g during the same period. Subcutaneous fat wasting characterizes fetal growth restriction.

Changes in chemical composition in fetal organs

Liver. Southgate and Hey[5] described that from day 100 of pregnancy, the curve of fetal liver weight is similar to that of total body weight. Fetal liver composition (Table 117.1) also remained unchanged from the second trimester.[4,5] Widdowson and colleagues[6] studied liver cell growth by measuring DNA and protein content, and found a rapid increase in DNA from week 15 to the end of gestation, while the protein/DNA ratio showed no variations between weeks 15 and 25. This suggests that in the early stages, liver growth occurs by an increase in the number of cells rather than by an increase in the volume of these.

Heart. Functional development of the heart is completed by day 31. Cardiac development is initially very fast, but from day 100 of pregnancy, the heart weight curve is similar to that of total fetal body weight. The chemical composition of this organ remains stable during the last two trimesters of pregnancy (Table 117.2). Widdowson and Dickerson[7] reported an increase in sodium concentration and a decrease in potassium concentration from week 20 to the end of gestation, apparently related to interstitial fluid loss of the cardiac muscle.

Table 117.1 Fetal liver composition (from day 100 to full term),[5] for fetuses with normal and small weights for gestational age

	Median (g/kg)	Mean (g/kg)	Range (g/kg)
Water			
Normal	811	809	780–840
Small	795	805	788–824
Total nitrogen			
Normal	19.8	19.4	12.3–22.9
Small	21.3	20.9	17.4–22.9
Proteins			
Normal	121.4	121.3	76.7–143
Small	133.1	131.5	107.8–143
Fat			
Normal	23.8	23.9	10.0–32.6
Small	22.8	23.5	16.4–32.3
Glycogen			
Normal	13.8	16.3	4.4–40
Small	15.5	17.2	4.5–38

Table 117.2 Fetal heart composition (from day 100 to full term),[5] for fetuses with normal and small weights for gestational age

	Median (g/kg)	Mean (g/kg)	Range (g/kg)
Water			
Normal	811	809	780–840
Small	331	828	798–850
Total nitrogen			
Normal	16	16.8	11.2–22.9
Small	18.9	18.8	17.0–20.3
Proteins			
Normal	100	105	69.7–142.9
Small	118	118	106.0–127
Fat			
Normal	16.8	17.6	9.9–23.9
Small	21.1	21.2	14.7–27.1
Glycogen			
Normal	6.4	11	0.8–32.8
Small	4.6	5.91	4.0–10.8

Table 117.3 Fetal kidney composition (from day 100 to full term),[5] for fetuses with normal and small weights for gestational age

	Median (g/kg)	Mean (g/kg)	Range (g/kg)
Water			
Normal	834	816	568–885
Small	842	843	774–908
Total nitrogen			
Normal	14.5	14.7	11.6–18.5
Small	15.4	16	9.5–24.6
Proteins			
Normal	90.5	91.8	72.3–115.7
Small	96.5	99.9	59.3–153.6
Fat			
Normal	19.1	18.1	12.6–24.7
Small	20.9	22	12.3–30.6
Glycogen			
Normal	6.4	11	0.8–32.8
Small	4.6	5.91	4.0–10.8

Kidney. The kidney grows and develops rapidly during the fetal period (the fetal kidney becomes functional from the ninth week). Kidney weight is variable during the first trimester of pregnancy, but from day 100 of pregnancy its growth curve is similar to that of total fetal body weight (Table 117.3). Nitrogen concentration in renal tissue increases throughout pregnancy.[7] It should be noted that small-for-dates babies have a higher renal fat content than appropriate-for-gestational age newborns.

Anthropometric methods

Neonatal anthropometry

The distinction between the constitutionally small and the growth-restricted infant is being increasingly accepted, the former being considered the low extreme of the distribution of normal neonates weight, which is not considered a pathologic condition by itself. Thus, birth weight alone has been observed to be poorly correlated with perinatal outcome.[8] On the contrary, abnormalities of neonatal constitution are believed to reflect impaired fetal nutrition and have been found to be more useful indicators of adverse perinatal and long-term outcomes.[9] The skin-fold thickness at different sites, the mid-arm circumference to occipitofrontal circumference ratio, and the ponderal index (weight (g)/height $(cm)^3$) have been suggested as useful parameters to identify growth-restricted fetuses.

Fetal anthropometry

Theoretically, fetal anthropometric studies can be carried out in the framework of different designs, which can be categorized in cross-sectional (each fetus is measured once) and longitudinally (measurements are made in the same fetus at different gestational age).[10,11] Since growth is a dynamic process, it seems biologically plausible that its quantification requires the evaluation of serial measurements. Nevertheless, longitudinal studies are more likely to result in biased estimates (e.g. high-risk fetuses and/or pregnancies are more likely to be intensively scanned). On the other hand, the high correlation between measurements on the same fetus means that the effective sample size will be nearer to the number of fetuses than to the total number of measurements. In addition, longitudinal designs require more complex statistical models than cross-sectional studies. Among the methods described to construct longitudinal curves, the most straightforward ones, as pairwise means, do not account for the regression toward the mean phenomena, which is essential to analyze growth 'velocities'. More complex methods, as multilevel models, appear to be the most appropriate methodology to derive conditional centiles, which take into account the fetus' size earlier in gestation. Software applications (packages ML-3 and ML-n) for these methods have been developed in recent years.[12–14] Although, there are preliminary clinical data suggesting that conditional centiles better predict infants with low ponderal index than unconditional centiles,[15] further studies are needed before the introduction of these reference ranges in clinical practice.

Other design drawbacks could hamper the validity of fetal anthropometric standards. Among them, inappropriate selection of cases, unclear inclusion and exclusion criteria, small sample size and unreliable gestational ages are considerably frequent.[10,11]

Fetal weight. All authors agree that fetal weight is the most sensitive indicator of fetal nutrition and growth, since fetal weight is the earliest parameter to be affected by adverse intrauterine circumstances. For this reason, however, and because of the high variability in birth weight among different population groups,[16–18] it is difficult to obtain a pattern of fetal growth exclusively based on fetal weight, particularly because there is a linear relationship between weight at birth and duration of gestation. On the other hand, the construction of tables or curves of normal fetal weight at different weeks of gestation faces several difficulties. These include the fact that data obtained in longitudinal studies are not reliable (a fetus or a neonate may be weighed only once, and previous weight variations are unknown), weights of fetuses born prematurely cannot be included in the range of normality, and comparison of different tables and curves is further complicated by the lack of uniformity in the entry of data.

In 1963, Lubchenco and coworkers[19] presented weight curves in the form of percentiles as estimated from the birth weights of 5635 liveborn Caucasian infants at 24–42 weeks of gestation. One year later, Gruenwald[20,21] estimated intrauterine growth in the form of standard deviations (Figures 117.3 and 117.4). Many other curves representing intrauterine growth have been reported thereafter. These curves, however, cannot be superimposed due to sample-inherent limitations, such as differences in socioeconomic conditions, altitude, racial features, etc. For example, fetal weight curves constructed for singleton fetuses in Spain, France, Italy, Czechoslovakia, and other countries showed fetal weights higher than the median weights of Colorado babies in the study of Lubchenco and coworkers[19] (Denver is 1584 m above sea level) which, in turn, were lower than those given by Swedish authors.[22,23] Fetal weight curves used by the authors of this chapter[24] are depicted in the form of percentiles (Figure 117.5) and standard deviations (Figure 117.6).

Most fetal weight curves can be divided into four areas of different fetal growth rates (Figure 117.7), i.e. low rate (up to 16 weeks' gestation, mean weight gain ≤10 g/week); accelerated rate (between 16 and 26–27 weeks' gestation, 85 g/week); maximal rate (between 28 and 38 weeks' gestation, 200 g/week); and decelerated rate (around 37–38 weeks' gestation, 70 g/week). Beyond 42 weeks' gestation, fetal weight shows no variation or negligible increases. A remarkable fact is that 10% of the weight at term is exclusively reached during the first half of pregnancy, and it is only after the first two trimesters of pregnancy that the fetus acquires one-third of its weight at birth. During the first half of pregnancy, however, organogenesis and progressive development and refinement of fetal structures are taking place. The most crucial period of fetal life starts at about 28 weeks of gestation, coinciding with the maximal slope of fetal weight gain (mean 200 g/week).

Fetal weight curves are somewhat different when constructed according to sex or multiple pregnancies. Values obtained in females are lower than in males, with differences of up to 300 g in some sections. In multiple pregnancies, McKeown and Record[25,26] reported that maternoplacental supply can ensure normal growth of fetuses until achievement of a determined overall weight, so that earliness of weight deficit is inversely related to the number of fetuses.

Differences in fetal weight curves. Fetal weight curves derived from data reported by different authors may be substantially different. After an extensive review of the literature, Gruenwald[27] proposed a classification of fetal weight curves into four groups (Figure 117.8). Group 1 included data on intrauterine growth as estimated from weights of dead fetuses.[28,29] These estimations were clearly beneath weight curves of the remaining groups for most weeks of gestation, given that they were based on postmortem examination of abnormal fetuses. Group 2 consisted of fetal weight curves made with corrected data of liveborn neonates. In these cases, dead fetuses, inaccurate menstrual data, liveborn neonates with anomalies, etc. have been excluded.[19,27,30] Most published fetal weight curves based on adequately corrected material are included in this group. Group 3 was formed by fetal weight curves somewhat above group 2, since, in general, uncorrected[27] or partially corrected data[28,29] were used. Group 4 included fetal weight curves based on uncorrected material or representing populations with particular racial or social characteristics[33–35] (Kaltreider, personal communication).

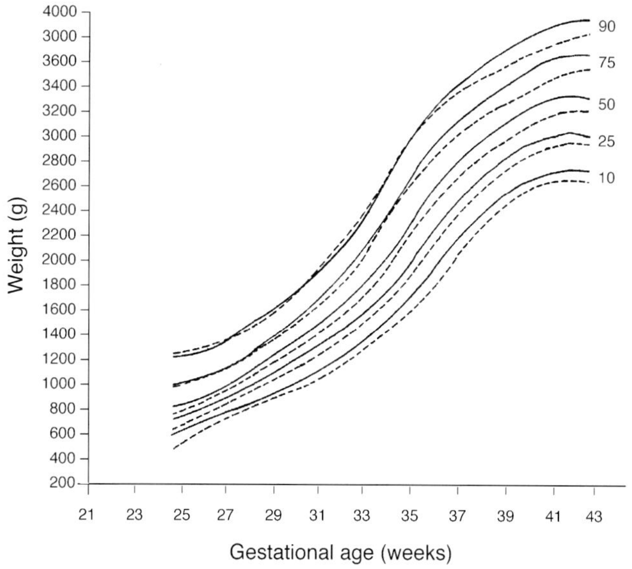

Figure 117.3 Fetal weight curves (percentiles) for males (solid lines) and females (dotted lines) (data from Clavero Salvador *et al.*[16]).

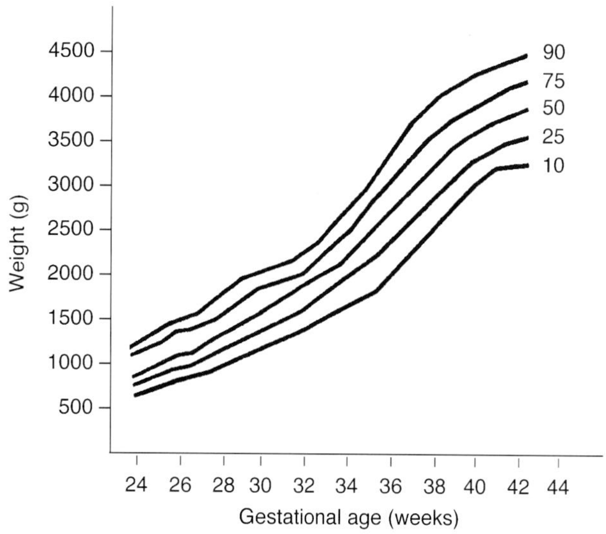

Figure 117.5 Overall fetal growth curve in percentiles.[21]

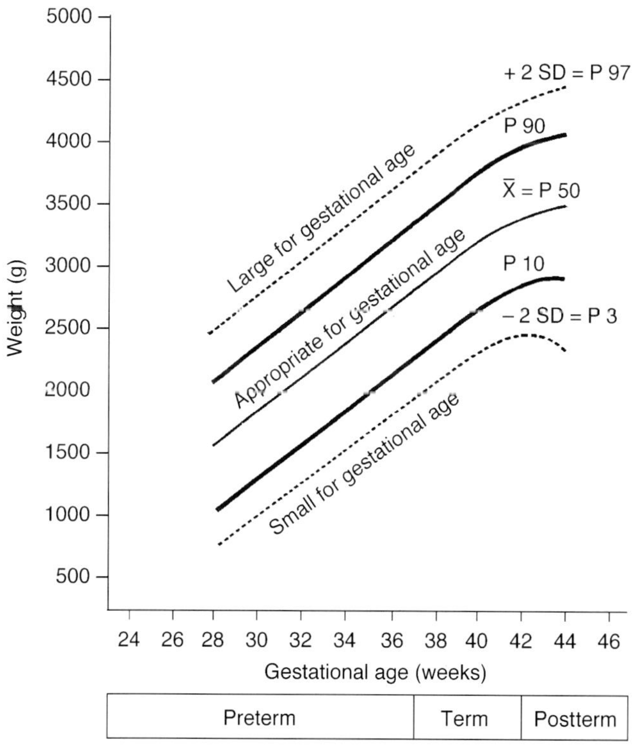

Figure 117.4 Relationship between fetal growth curves in percentiles (from Clavero Salvador *et al.*[16]), and curves constructed with standard deviations (from Alonso and Arizcun[17] and Meredith[18]).

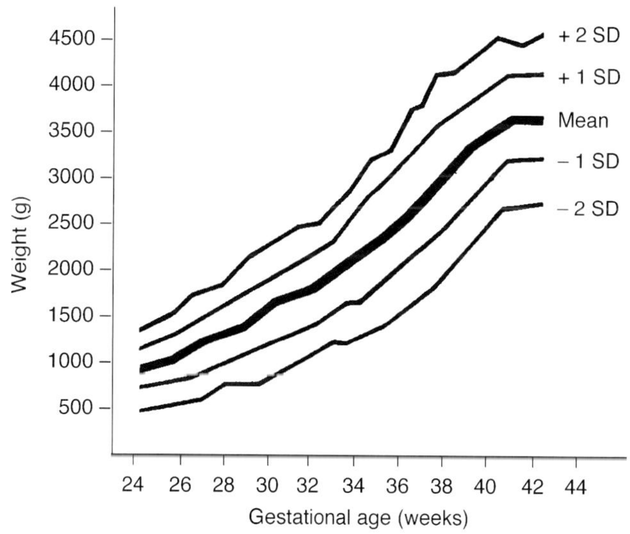

Figure 117.6 Overall fetal growth curve with standard deviations.[21]

As noted by Gruenwald,[27] all types of fetal weight curves except those based on deadborn neonates, coincide at 38 weeks of gestation because at this time the likelihood of an error in gestational age is very rare. Before this time, outstanding differences found in some cases may be attributed to information bias or inadequate correction. From 38 weeks' gestation to birth, fetal weight curves diverge again due to changes in the supply line (maternal and placental) among different population groups on which curves are based.[27] In fact, although all types of fetal weight curves stabilize at 41 weeks' gestation, heights are different according to the socioeconomic conditions of the sample. Thus, a difference of more than 500 g is found between the curve of Kaltreider, based on data from the indigent black population in Baltimore, USA (personal communication), and that of Lindell,[23] based on Swedish neonates (a tall population with high living standards). The fact that the estimations of Lubchenco and colleagues[19] were lower than those given by other authors may be attributed to the altitude of Denver.

Human fetal weight would presumably follow a straight line after term if there were no limitations to provision of nutrients, that is, if maternal and placental supply provide endless support to fetal growth.[20,21]

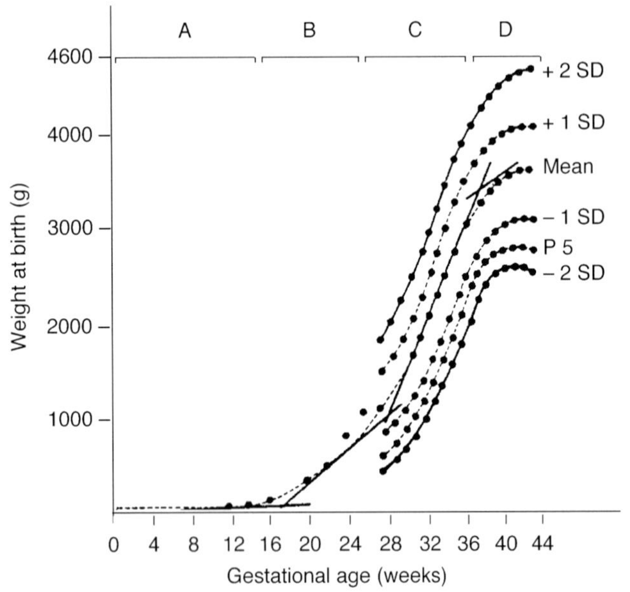

Figure 117.7 Fetal weight curve (with standard deviations) divided into four areas of low (A), accelerated (B), maximal (C), and decelerated (D) fetal growth rates.

Therefore, deviations from the ideal extrapolated curve are less evident as nutritional supply decreases.

Customized birth weight standards. Due to the fact that several maternal (height, weight, race, age, parity, etc.) and fetal (number, gender, etc.) variables play a significant role in fetal growth both in low-[36] and high-risk[37] pregnancies, population-based birth weight standards result in misclassification of a large proportion of cases.[38] Individually adjusted or customized growth charts aim to optimize the assessment of fetal growth by taking individual variation into account, and by projecting an optimal curve, which delineates the potential weight gain in each pregnancy. Customized birth weight standards increase the possibility of identification of fetuses at risk of stillbirth, neonatal death, and low Apgar score, probably due to improved identification of growth restriction.[39] Moreover, customized curves are better correlated with neonatal morphometry than population-based standards.[40] The evidence of their usefulness as well as the fact that customized charts could be used in clinical setting in a very flexible way, make customized birth weight references the current standard for evaluation of fetal growth.

Fetal height. As in the case of fetal weight, fetal height curves show a moderately sigmoid shape with an ascending trend as gestational age increases. Fetal

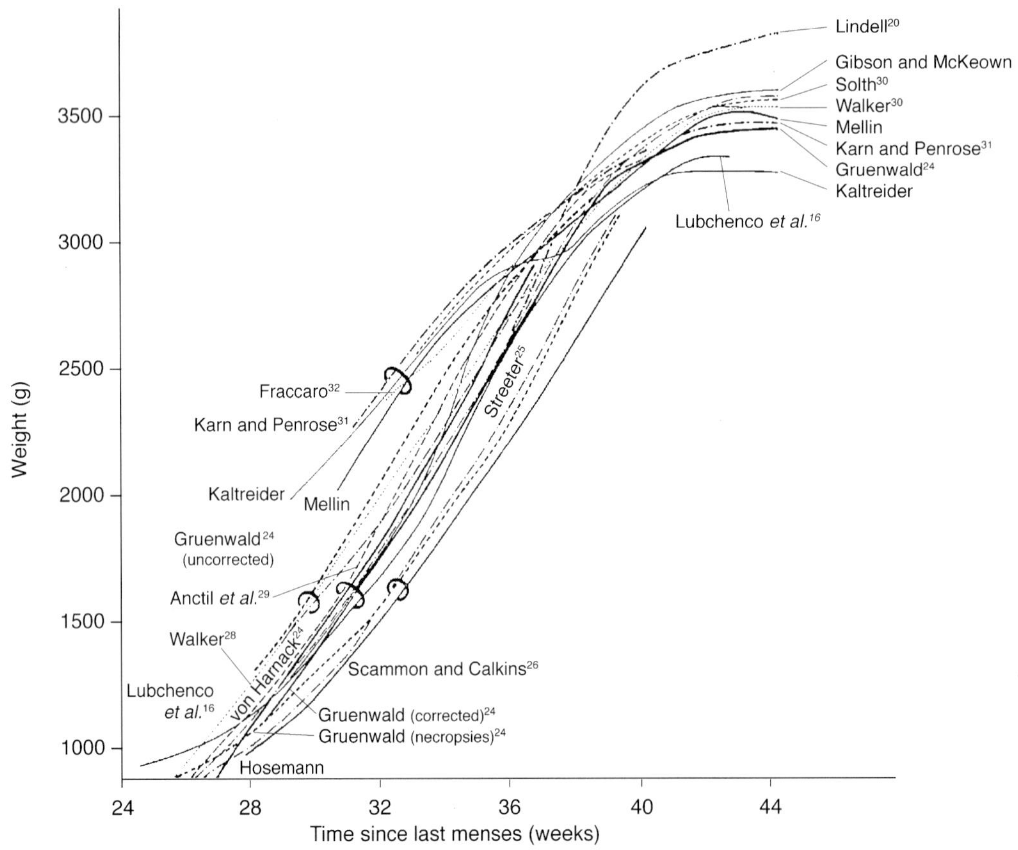

Figure 117.8 Fetal growth curves classified into four groups by Gruenwald.[24]

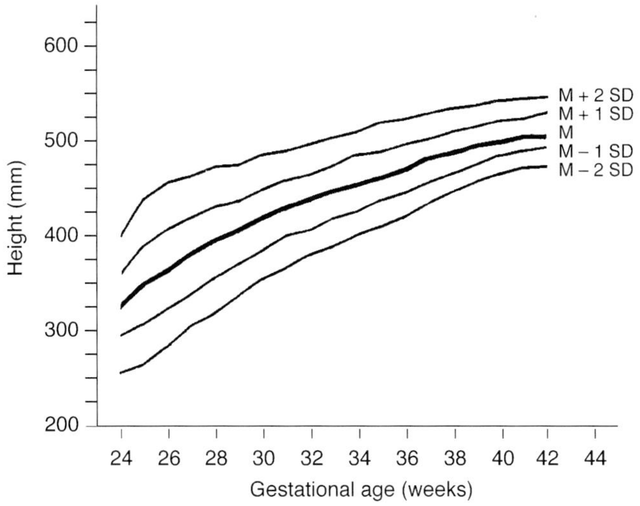

Figure 117.9 Overall fetal height curve with standard deviations.[21]

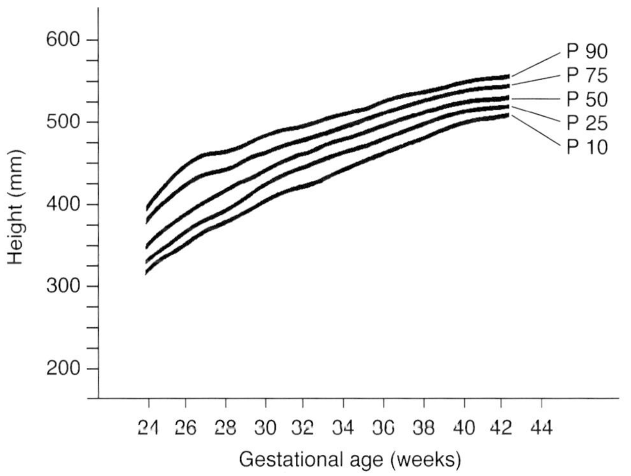

Figure 117.10 Overall fetal height curve in percentiles.

height curves from our institution (Figures 117.9 and 117.10) were based on a depurated sample of 8876 liveborn neonates at 22–42 weeks of gestation.

After fetal weight, fetal height is the second parameter that is rapidly affected by fetal macro- and microenvironmental conditions. While fetal heights recorded in Sweden[22] and in some areas of the USA[41] were taller than in Spain, our figures are, in turn, higher than those reported by others.[19,42] Fetal height has rarely been used in the past for assessing fetal growth. The anthropometric value of this parameter in association with fetal weight and head circumference to identify some fetal growth patterns has been recently established.[27,41]

Head circumference. Given that fetal brain weight is the parameter least affected by an adverse intrauterine environment (malnutrition), the importance of this measurement is considerable. Although head circumference is not a highly reliable index of fetal growth and nutritional conditions, it is a sensitive indicator of gestational age, which may be useful for comparison with the remaining parameters. Therefore, as may be expected, head-circumference curves do show large variations throughout the gestational period. The curve is almost linear with a more accentuated slope than the fetal-height curve (Figure 117.11). Interestingly, Ferrazzi *et al.*[43] found that normalization of the umbilical vein flow provided the most sensitive parameter for growth-restricted fetuses, suggesting that due to the brain-sparing effect, head circumference is preserved in placental insufficiency. Differences in the individual curves by sex were smaller than those observed in fetal height curves, and values of the fetal head circumference in twins are lower than the overall fetal growth curve. Comparatively, our values for fetal head circumference are higher than those reported by Lubchenco and colleagues,[19] but lower than those presented by Miller and Hassanein[41] and Usher and McLean.[44]

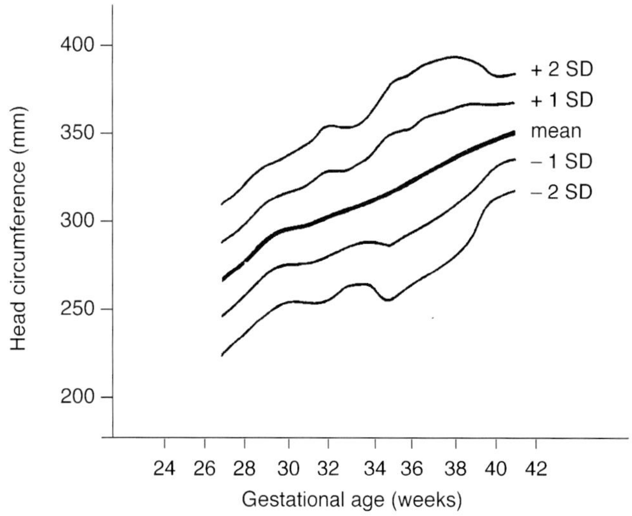

Figure 117.11 Fetal head circumference curve with standard deviations.

Three-dimensional fetal growth assessment. The advent of three-dimensional sonography has allowed a new insight into fetal growth. Calculation of organ volumes could be made reliably and in a non-invasive way using this new technology. Brain volume has been found[45] to increase from 34 ml at 18 weeks to 316 ml at 34 weeks of gestation. At the same time, brain growth demonstrates a marked slow down as expressed by a weekly increment in brain volume at 34 weeks of only one-third of the weekly increment at 19 weeks of gestation. Fetal liver is very important in determining the status of fetal growth. In uncomplicated pregnancies, mean fetal hepatic volume was 9.7 ml $\pm$4.4 at 20 weeks and 96.4 ml $\pm$8.2 at 36 weeks of gestation.[46–48] Interestingly, the fetal brain/liver volume

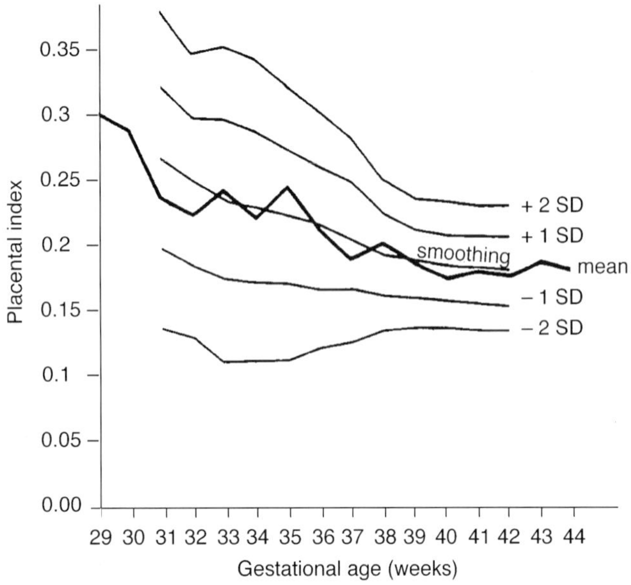

Figure 117.12 Placental index curve (fetoplacental relationship) throughout gestation (from Gruenwald[21]).

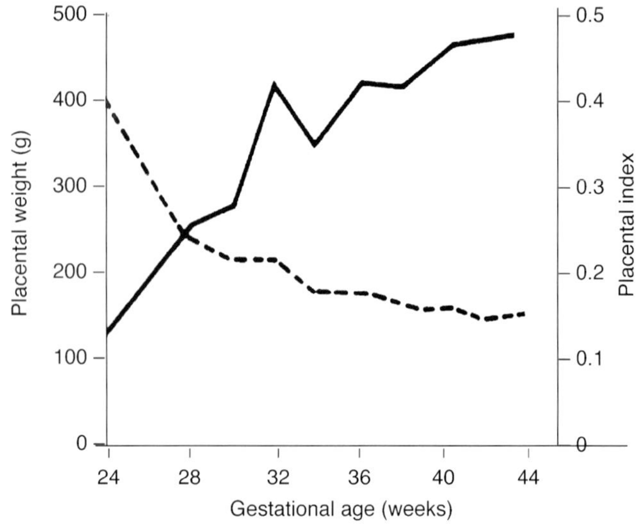

Figure 117.13 Relationship between placental index and fetal growth throughout gestation.

ratio has been described as a predictor of fetal outcome in the growth-restricted fetus. An inverse relationship exists in small-for-gestational-age fetuses between brain/liver volume ratio and fetal weight-related umbilical venous blood flow. Fetal lung volume ranged from 1.18 ml at 18 weeks to 56.26 ml at 37 weeks for the left lung, and from 1.69 ml at 17 weeks to 60.2 ml at 39 weeks for the right lung.[49–50] Fetal kidneys volume has been observed to increase linearly through the second and third trimester, ranging from 1.5 ml at 20 to 16.3 ml at 40 weeks for the right kidney, and from 1.8 ml at 20 to 17 ml at 40 weeks for the left one.[51]

Relationship between fetal anthropometry and placental biometry

The interest elicited by placental weight and its relationship with fetal weight is fully justified by the crucial role played by this organ in fetal growth and nutrition. For this reason, it is surprising that this question has been poorly addressed in studies on fetal growth published in the literature.

Analysis of placental weight at different gestational ages shows different periods similar to the evolution of fetal weight. Until 16 weeks' of gestation, placental weight is greater than fetal weight because of a more rapid growth of the placenta early in pregnancy. Placental and fetal weights are similar by 16–28 weeks' gestation. At week 27, however, the placenta has already achieved 50% of its weight at term (because of its rapid initial weight gain), whereas the fetus has only gained 30% of the weight at birth. During the period of maximal fetal growth (28–38 weeks' of gestation), placental growth rate is much lower than fetal growth rate (in relative terms placental growth is restricted with respect to fetal growth). From 38 weeks' of gestation, placental growth rate shows an accentuated deceleration as compared to fetal weight gain, which is even more apparent from week 40. Curves of the relationship between fetal and placental weights expressed as percentages of normal fetal weight at birth are particularly illustrative of this finding.

The inter-relationship between fetal and placental weights can be studied by the so-called 'fetoplacental relationship' (fetal weight/placental weight ratio), the 'placentofetal relationship' (placental weight/fetal weight ratio), also named the placental index, which is the most usual method (Figures 117.12 and 117.13). The fetoplacental relationship increases as pregnancy advances, whereas the placental index decreases. At 24 weeks' of gestation, the value of the fetoplacental relationship is 3; at week 35 it varies between 4 and 5; at term it varies between 5 and 6; and from 40 weeks' of gestation, there is no change. The placental volume is the parameter that correlates better with fetal weight.[16] In contrast, there is a poor correlation with the number of cotyledons, suggesting that by the fourth month structural development of the placenta has been completed, so that potential adverse factors acting later on in pregnancy have no effect on the number of cotyledons.

REFERENCES

1. Winick M. Changes in nucleic acid and protein content of the human brain during growth. *Pediatr Res* 1968;2:352–5.
2. Widdowson EM, Spray CM. Chemical development in utero. *Arch Dis Child* 1951;26:205–14.
3. Widdowson EM. In Assali NS, ed. *Biology of Gestation.* New York: Academic Press, 1968
4. Apte SV, Iyengar L, Nagarajan V. Effect of antenatal iron supplementation on placental iron. *Am J Obstet Gynecol* 1971;110: 350–1.
5. Southgate DAT, Hey EN. In Roberts DF, Thompson AM, eds. *The Biology of Human Fetal Growth.* London: Taylor & Francis, 1976:195.
6. Widdowson EM, Crabb DE, Milner RDG. Cellular development of some human organs before birth. *Arch Dis Child* 1972;47: 652–5.
7. Widdowson EM, Dickerson JWT. In Comar CL, Brouner F, eds. *Mineral Metabolism.* New York: Academic Press, 1963.
8. Beattie RB, Johnson P. Practical assessment of neonatal nutrition status beyond birth weight; an imperative for the 1990s. *Br J Obstet Gynecol* 1994;101:842–6.
9. Fay RA, Dey PL, Saadie CM, Buhl JA, Gebski VJ. Ponderal index: A better definition of the 'at risk' group with intrauterine growth problems than birth-weight for gestational age in term infants. *Aust N Z J Obstet Gynaecol* 1991;31:17–19.
10. Royston P, Altman DG. Design and analysis of longitudinal studies of fetal size. *Ultrasound Obstet Gynecol* 1995;6:307–12.
11. Royston P. Calculation of unconditional and conditional reference intervals for foetal size and growth from longitudinal measurements. *Stat Med* 1995;14:1417–36.
12. Goldstein H. Efficient statistical modelling of longitudinal data. *Ann Hum Biol* 1986;13:129–41.
13. Prosser R, Rasbash J, Goldstein H. *ML3 Software for Three-level Analysis. User's Guide for V.2.* London: Institute of Education, 1991.
14. Rasbash J, Woodhouse G. *MLn Command Reference. Version 1.0.* London: Institute of Education, 1995.
15. Owen P, Burton K, Ogston S, Khan KS, Howie PW. Using unconditional and conditional standard deviation scores of fetal abdominal area measurements in the prediction of intrauterine growth restriction. *Ultrasound Obstet Gynecol* 2000;16(5):439–44.
16. Clavero Salvador PA, Gilabert T, Canals MJ, Pérez Fernández A. Relación entre el desarrollo de la placenta y el feto. *Acta Ginecol* 1975;27:369–74.
17. Alonso T, Arizcun J. Antropometría perinatal. *Acta Ginecol* 1975; 27:449–66.
18. Meredith HC. Body weight at birth of viable human infants: A worldwide comparative treatice. *Hum Biol* 1970;42:217–64.
19. Lubchenco LO, Hansman C, Dressler M, Boyd E. Intrauterine growth as estimated from liveborn birthweight data at 24 to 42 weeks of gestation. *Pediatrics* 1963;32:793–800.
20. Gruenwald P. The fetus in prolonged pregnancy. *Am J Obstet Gynecol* 1964;89:503–9.
21. Gruenwald P. Infants of low birth weight among 5000 deliveries. *Pediatrics* 1964;34:157–62.
22. Sterky G. Swedish standard curves for intrauterine growth. *Pediatrics* 1970;46:7–8.
23. Lindell A. Prolonged pregnancy. *Acta Obstet Gynecol Scand* 1956;35:136–63.
24. Carrera JM. Intrauterine growth retardation. *Proceedings of VIII World Congress of Gynecology and Obstetrics (FIGO),* Mexico DF, October 17–22, 1976.
25. McKeown T, Record RG. The influence of placental size on foetal growth in man, with special reference to multiple pregnancy. *J Endocrinol* 1953;9:418–26.
26. McKeown T, Record RG. Observation of foetal growth in multiple pregnancy in man. *J Endocrinol* 1952;8:386–401.
27. Gruenwald P. Growth of the human fetus. I: Normal growth and its variation. *Am J Obstet Gynecol* 1966;94:1112–19.
28. Streeter GL. *Contrib Embriol* 1920;11:143.
29. Scammon RE, Calkins LA. *Growth in the Fetal Period.* Minneapolis, MN: University of Minnesota Press, 1929.
30. Von Harnack GA. Das übertragene, untergewichtige Neurguborene. *Monatsschr Kinderh* 1960;108:412–15.
31. Walker J. Growth of the human fetus. *Cold Spring Harb Symp* 1954;19:39.
32. Anctil AO, Joshi GB, Lucas WE, Little WA, Callagan DA. Prematurity: A more precise approach to identification. *Obstet Gynecol* 1964;24:716–21.
33. Solth K. Die Veränderung des Geburtsgewichtes in Lanfe der letzten Jahrzehnte. *Arch Gynäkol* 1950;177:678–89.
34. Karn MN, Penrose LE. Birth weight and gestation time in relation to maternal age, parity and infant survival. *Ann Eugen* 1951; 16:147–64.
35. Fraccaro M. A contribution to the study of birth weight based on an Italian sample. *Ann Hum Genet* 1956;20:282–98.
36. Mongelli M, Gardosi J. Longitudinal study of fetal growth in subgroups of a low risk population. *Ultrasound Obstet Gynecol* 1995; 6:340–4.
37. de Jong CL, Gardosi J, Baldwin C, Francis A, Dekker GA, van Geijn HP. Fetal weight gain in a serially scanned high-risk population. *Ultrasound Obstet Gynecol* 1998;11:39–43
38. Gardosi J, Chang A, Kalyan B, *et al.* Customised antenatal growth charts. *Lancet* 1992;339:283–7.
39. Clausson B, Gardosi J, Francis A, Cnattingius S. Perinatal outcome in SGA births defined by customised versus population-based birthweight standards. *Br J Obstet Gynaecol* 2001;108: 830–4.
40. Sanderson DA, Wilcox MA, Johnson IR. The individualised birthweight ratio: A new method of identifying intrauterine growth retardation. *Br J Obstet Gynaecol* 1994;101(4):310–14.
41. Miller H, Hassanein K. Fetal malnutrition in white new-born infants: Maternal factors. *Pediatrics* 1973;52:504–12.
42. Ghosh S, Bhargave S. Intrauterine growth of North Indian babies. *Pediatrics* 1971;47:826–30.
43. Ferrazzi E, Rigano S, Bozzo M, *et al.* Umbilical vein blood flow in growth-restricted fetuses. *Ultrasound Obstet Gynecol* 2000; 16(5):432–8.
44. Usher R, McLean J. Intrauterine growth of liveborn Caucasian infants at sea level: Standard obtained from measurements in seven dimensions of infants born between 25 and 44 weeks of gestation. *Pediatrics* 1969;74:901–10.
45. Pooh RK, Pool K, Nakagawa Y, Nishida S, Ohno Y. Clinical application of three-dimensional ultrasound in fetal brain assessment. *Croat Med J* 2000;41:245–51.
46. Chang FM, Hsu KF, Ko HC, Yao BL, Chang CH, Yu CH, Chen HY. Three-dimensional ultrasound assessment of fetal liver volume in normal pregnancy. *Ultrasound Med Biol* 1997;23(3):381–89.
47. Roberts AB, Mitchell JM, McCowan LM, Barker S. Ultrasonographic measurement of liver length in the small-for-gestational age fetus. *Am J Obstet Gynecol* 1999:180:643–48.
48. Kuno A, Hayashi Y, Akiyama M, Yamshiro C, Tanaka H, Yanagihara T, Hata T. Three-dimensional sonographic measurement of liver volume in the small-for-gestational-age fetus. *J Ultrasound Med* 2000;21:361–66.
49. Pöhls UG, Rempen A. Fetal lung volumetry by three-dimensional ultrasound. *Ultrasound Obstet Gynecol* 1998;11:6–12.
50. Luady JAM, Janssen MMM, Struyk PC, Stijnen T, Wladimiroff W. Three-dimensional ultrasonography of fetal lung volume: a preliminary study. *Ultrasound Obstet Gynecol* 1998;11:13–16.
51. Kinje JC, Okaro CI, Bell SC, de Cha al R, Taylor DJ. A cross-sectional study of changes in fetal renal size with gestation in appropriate -and small-for-gestational age fetuses. *Ultrasound Obstet Gynecol* 1997;9:22–6.

118 Intrauterine growth restriction: concept and epidemiology

E. Fabre, R. González de Agüero, J. L. de Agustín and A. Ezquerra

Concepts related to growth restriction

It is clear that there exists an optimal range of size at birth, within which complications are rare. The incidence of morbidity and mortality increases when there is a deviation from this optimal range. In order to specify this clinical impression we need a standard reference with which to be able to define terms like 'too small', as well as to relate to dependent variables such as mortality and morbidity rates. Considering intrauterine growth, it is important to recognize several remarkable concepts and definitions.

Growth and maturity

In any consideration about development, one may arbitrarily distinguish maturation, meaning change of structure and function, from growth in the sense of increase in mass, while realizing that the two of them are not entirely independent of each other. Growth is measured in terms of change in weight and size in relation to age. Maturation determines the functional capabilities of the organism and its parts, and thus controls such aspects as the ability of a neonate to adjust itself to extrauterine life; it is largely independent of the effects of deprivation.

Low birth weight

The term low birth weight (LBW) describes infants with a weight of less than 2500 g, regardless of gestational age[1]. To avoid confusion, the word preterm is used for infants born under 37 weeks' gestation, regardless of the birth weight. Further subdivisions of LBW have been commonly used: very low birth weight (VLBW) and extremely low birth weight (ELBW) describe infants with weights less than 1500 and 1000 g, respectively (Figure 118.1). From this point of view, LBW at first glance seems to be a simple concept: any baby below a certain threshold of weight is an LBW baby. But what is threshold? And should it be the same for babies of all types and from all populations? Are there different kinds of LBW babies?

Populations vary considerably in the size of their babies at birth. The median birth weight among infants born in India is lower than in Ireland, while the median gestational age at birth is very similar, and the percentage of LBW infants is higher in India than in Ireland (Table 118.1). The differences in the birth weight could reflect either the diversity of the human biology or the social differences among the studied populations. The election of a universal threshold below which LBW is defined will mistakenly define the Indian population of newborns as having a high incidence of a pathological condition. For a really valid comparison we therefore need a specific reference standard for the individual population under study.

A method has been suggested to adjust the differences in mean birth weight among different populations. It is based on the observation that many distributions tend to be approximately 'normal' in shape in their central portion. The effect of a shift in the mean birth weight in different populations can then be eliminated by using the percentage of births below the estimate (mean –2 SD). The result is an 'adjusted' rate for (relative) LBW occurrence, which is applicable regardless of the mean birth weight for the population (Table 118.2).[2] This procedure yields a much greater degree of uniformity for the 'adjusted' LBW percentages as compared to the unadjusted percentages. This simple technique is only applicable if the birth-weight distribution is known to be Gaussian.

Mathematically oriented studies[3] have argued that the roughly normal birth-weight curve in any population is really a mixture of two distributions, one of the normal population and the other of a pathological group of babies (referred to as the 'residual' distribution) in whom small size is a reflection of some unhealthy maternal or fetal condition. The comparison between Japanese babies and African-American

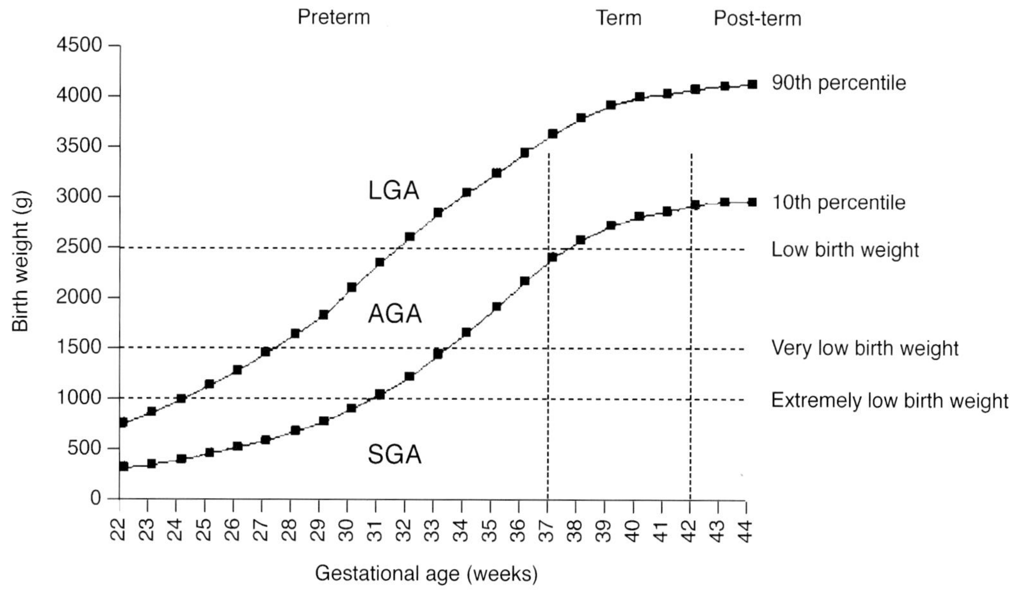

Figure 118.1 Increase in body weight of a fetus during the second half of gestation according to menstrual age and including recommended terminology. LGA, AGA and SGA, large, appropriate and small for gestational age, respectively.

Table 118.1 Comparison of birth weight and gestational age at delivery in different countries (based on data from Rooth[2])

Country	Infants weighing ≤2500g at birth (%)	Median birth weight (g)	Median gestational age at birth (weeks)
Ireland	5.9	3478	40.5
Poland	6.8	3380	40.1
Venezuela	7.9	3206	39.7
Greece	9.5	3287	39.8
Taiwan	11.3	3106	40.0
Japan	11.3	3029	40.2
Iran	14.2	3024	39.4
Philippines	14.2	2889	39.6
Malaysia	17.3	3057	40.2
India	29.0	2771	40.6

Table 118.2 Low-birth-weight percentages before and after adjustment for differences in mean birth weight (based on data from Rooth[2])

Country	Mean birth weight (g)	Mean −2 SD (g)	Low birth weight (%)	
			Unadjusted	Adjusted
Austria	3150	2200	5.7	5.5
Cuba	2900	1850	10.8	3.5
Hungary	2900	1900	10.0	5.6
Japan	2950	2150	5.3	3.3
New Zealand	3150	2200	5.2	4.0
Sweden	3205	2250	3.9	3.8
USA (six states)	3100	2100	6.0	3.5

babies illustrates this fact.[4] The mean birth weight in Japanese babies is about the same as that for American blacks, at about 3200 g. But these two populations differ markedly in the proportion of births in the residual distribution, 1.3% in Osaka and 4.3% in American black babies, who are small for presumably pathological reasons. This difference, because it is composed of infants at very high risk of death, explains why mortality is so much higher among African-American infants than among Japanese infants, even though both populations have relatively equal mean birth weights. The important point to note is that it is the pathological conditions that lead to an excess of small babies in the residual distribution that should stimulate public health action, not that part of the variation in birth weight which appears to be irrelevant to human health.

The use of a single cutoff point for birth weight when applied to a range of gestational ages will automatically result in heterogenous data. Children born with low birth weight include both the ones born preterm as well as those born at term gestation but subnormal in weight. For this reason a classification frequently used in epidemiological surveys is to take all LBW babies and to divide them arbitrarily into preterm-LBW (< 37 weeks) and term-LBW (37 weeks or more); fetuses with retarded growth would fall into the second group and preterm babies into the first. This classification does not differentiate the fetus with delay of growth and born before 37 weeks' gestation, which is identified as born preterm; therefore it ignores a substantial number of growth-retarded fetuses.

Preterm delivery and fetal growth appear to have distinct determinants, and one of the most important and little-appreciated observations about the state of our knowledge in this area is that, while we have considerable understanding of the causes of impaired fetal growth, we know next to nothing about the causes of preterm delivery. For term-LBW infants, most underlying causes (e.g. maternal smoking, weight at conception and gestational weight gain) have been identified, for preterm-LBW infants, the etiology largely remains unexplained.[5] Both concepts differ in another important way. Preterm delivery is much more important as a cause of infant mortality in developed nations. Fetal growth impairment, though not rare, does not cause the same rate of mortality as does early delivery. The long-term impact of fetal growth restriction on neurodevelopment, though more important than its effect on the newborn, is also not as pronounced as the effect of preterm birth.

For public policy purposes, a single cutoff value for low birth weight in all populations must therefore be treated with a certain amount of skepticism. It is a crude indicator, useful for making a quick and rough assessment, but one that needs more refinement if public policy initiatives are to be appropriately targeted. However, this approach has several advantages, considering that it is easy to use and offers a practical means to compare incidences worldwide and among populations of different ethnic origin and socioeconomic status, taking into account their own restrictions.

Small-for-gestational age fetuses

Intrauterine growth of the human fetus can be charted by plotting birth weight, or other birth dimensions, against the gestational age. Starting from fetal growth curves, distributions of birth weight at each gestational age, intrauterine growth anomalies have been quantitatively defined, in terms of absolute values of weight for gestational age, or standard deviations from a mean, or percentile ranking. A deficit of birth weight in relation to gestational age is evidence of fetal growth restriction. The LBW concept underestimates the magnitude of the problem since it does not include those infants whose weight at birth falls below the cutoff of weight for gestational age but who weigh more than 2500 g; these infants also have intrauterine growth restriction (IUGR).

Neonates can be categorized as appropriate (in weight) for gestational age (AGA), small for gestational age (SGA) or large for gestational age (LGA). In general, the term SGA refers to those infants below the 10th percentile of birth weight relative to a specific gestational age in representative distributions[6] (Figure 118.1). However, there is no general agreement as to what constitutes an SGA fetus. Some studies have used the third or fifth percentiles,[7,8] whereas others have used 2SD below the mean birth weight[9,10] as the cutoff point. Birth-weight distributions are affected by factors other than intrauterine nutrition, including maternal height, weight, race, parity, ethnic background and sex of the newborn. It is obvious that the use of different birth-weight percentiles, or correction of the standard for the mentioned factors have a major effect on the birth weights that define SGA fetuses. Even when the same statistical criteria are used, the limits often vary among different populations,[11–14] and hence are not always comparable (Table 118.3). For this reason infants of certain weights will be diagnosed as being small for gestational age in some studies but not others. In consequence, many of the SGA-related risk factor and infant outcome studies are not comparable, which often leads to conflicting results.[15] Although at present it remains universally accepted as the best and most standardized method for examining fetal growth and its restriction, we should look closely at its limitations.

SGA is not synonymous with fetal malnutrition; one may occur without the other. Fetal malnutrition is a clinical diagnosis and is independent of birth weight at a given gestational age, and may be present at almost any birth weight. An infant who is classified as SGA may or may not have malnutrition. Fetal malnutrition is characterized by obvious intrauterine weight loss or failure to acquire normal amounts of subcutaneous fat and muscle.[16] Weight, length and head circumference may or may not be affected. In fetal malnutrition, the subcutaneous tissue and underlying muscle are diminished and the skin of arms, legs, elbows, knees and interscapular regions is very loose. Perinatal problems and/or central nervous system sequelae occur primarily in malnourished babies, whether AGA or SGA, but not those who were simply SGA and not malnourished.

The clinical manifestations of fetal malnutrition depend, in part, on when it began during gestation. Babies whose length, head circumference and weight are significantly reduced were probably exposed to malnutrition beginning early in the second trimester. Those whose length and head circumference are less affected but are small and underweight with some loss of subcutaneous tissues and muscle probably became malnourished early in the third trimester. For babies who are significantly underweight for gestational age with obvious loss of subcutaneous tissues, but with length and head circumference within the normal range, an insufficient or unbalanced nutrient supply most likely occurred in the late third trimester. For the last two categories, weight may be above the 10th percentile for gestational age; however, signs of malnutrition may be obvious.

Intrauterine growth restriction

The phrase IUGR describes the fetus who has failed to reach its own theoretical normal growth potential.[17]

Table 118.3 Differences between definitions of small-for-gestational age neonates based on a birth weight below the 10th percentile for gestational age

Gestational age (weeks)	Birth weight (g) Lubchenco *et al.*[6]	Babson *et al.*[11]	Brenner *et al.*[12]	Naeye and Dixon[13]	Williams *et al.*[14]
28	860	695	770	967	727
32	1290	1351	1310	1534	1301
36	2050	2173	2190	2121	2229
38	2430	2602	2510	2570	2629
40	2630	2880	2750	2776	2848
42	2720	3039	2830	2778	2965

Currently, most investigators accept the SGA infant as a marker for IUGR and, in everyday usage, the term IUGR is often used synonymously with SGA, although there is little doubt that the two are not identical. The National Institute of Child Health and Human Development in the USA[18] recommends that, both for clinical and research purposes, IUGR birth should be defined as resulting in birth weight less than the 10th percentile for gestational age, using criteria appropriate to the populations under study. However, IUGR is used to denote a pathophysiological process resulting in restriction of fetal growth, while SGA refers to a statistical grouping of infants below the 10th percentile. From a practical standpoint, there may be considerable overlap of these groups, although at a conceptual level the distinction may be important.[19] Statistically, 10% of infants should fall below the 10th percentile regardless of medical intervention and this group may reflect both biological diversity as well as restriction of growth. Small infants may be constitutionally small, small secondary due to infections, toxic or congenital growth limitations, or small due to deprivation or placental insufficiency.[20] The biological variation of birth weight implies that not all SGA infants are growth-retarded and that some infants classified as AGA can be growth-retarded. A fetus that has stopped growing but is delivered before the weight crosses the 10th percentile should still be considered an infant subjected to a growth-restricting process even if the birth weight is appropriate for gestational age.

LBW and SGA are pediatric terms that refer only to the anthropometry of the newborn and mainly to birth weight. These concepts have a notable disadvantage: they are limited to the recognition at birth of an event that has already occurred, while the most important time for identification of whether or not there is growth restriction is during the antenatal period. Currently, only ultrasound is capable of providing data sufficiently accurate for assessing the fetal growth rate. IUGR may be indicated by insufficient growth rates of several fetal measures that are easily observed *in utero* regardless of birth weight. The growth restriction describes a dynamic event in which the fetus deviates progressively from a normal growth line, and hence diagnosis of true IUGR requires at least two measurements of size.[21] A single measurement will not be able to differentiate between size and growth. The observation of a fetus with small dimensions at a determined date does not confirm that there has been a change in the rhythm of growth. Although ultrasound allows the longitudinal study of fetal growth, it has not been utilized by epidemiologists to study IUGR. On the contrary, the concept and definition of SGA are still utilized in order to evaluate the utility of the ultrasonic measures. This is a paradoxical situation in which the value of a technique that studies the longitudinal growth of the fetus is mistakenly judged by a unique observation and measurement at birth.

In fetuses with IUGR, two different patterns of growth can be demonstrated by using ultrasound.[22] In the first case, growth decreases from early in pregnancy, with a sustained low rate; these infants are usually small, presenting a reduction of all of their external measures. This symmetry has important prognostic implications as it relates to whatever primary process is limiting fetal growth and the potential functional damage that may follow. Symmetric IUGR is seen with extrinsic conditions (intrauterine infections and exposure to drugs) that are active early in a pregnancy, or alternatively with intrinsic embryonic conditions (genetic causes and congenital anomalies) that act to diminish the growth potential of an affected fetus. Symmetric IUGR may be considered to represent a wide variety of conditions with a large range of prognoses. In most cases, the small size of the newborn is constitutional and not associated with abnormality. However, in many others the risk of perinatal asphyxia, serious permanent disability or non-survival accompanies the subnormal growth. In the second case, growth may be normal until early in the third trimester but then flattens. The infant is small, with the head circumference and length being relatively normal in size for gestational age, but with a reduced abdominal circumference, weight/length ratio and ponderal index. Head growth assessed sonographically by biparietal diameter or head circumference often remains normal throughout the pregnancy or only drops below the normal growth curve later. Trunk growth, conversely, as indicated by abdominal circumference, decreases earlier. The overall pattern of fetal growth in these cases is typically normal until late in the second or early in the third trimester, when the limit of the uteroplacental capacity to sustain a normal fetal growth rate is reached. Asymmetrical IUGR is mainly a result of uteroplacental insufficiency secondary to extrinsic factors like hypertension, diabetes mellitus, etc. The asymmetry is perhaps the result of predictable adaptation of the fetus to sequential deprivation, and fetal asphyxia is often the terminal event. The long-term prognosis for the infant with asymmetric IUGR is usually better than that for the infant with non-constitutional symmetric IUGR.

In summary, IUGR is defined as a pathological decrease of the fetal growth rhythm. The result is a fetus that does not reach its growth potential and has a high risk of perinatal complications. The diagnosis is difficult considering that it is not always easy to define accurately the fetal growth rhythm. In spite of this inconvenience, the definition of IUGR should be based on fetal growth and not on the birth weight or other birth dimensions. The condition of IUGR is not homogenous and similar presentations may have different etiologies and implications. IUGR does not define a homogenous population that necessarily shares a common fate, nor does it mean that those infants of similar birth weight share a common prognosis.

Epidemiology

The use of many different standards in order to define the anomalies of fetal growth is leading to statistical anarchy. Since the LBW concept was accepted as an international definition, one might think that a standard reference percentile should serve equally well as the basis of an international definition of SGA babies, thereby enabling direct comparisons to be made of data from different sources. But we seem to be a long way from any such agreement, and a locally produced standard is usually thought to be more appropriate than any general standard. Most studies on perinatal epidemiology are based on classification by birth weight because this measurement is generally readily available. Likewise, risk factors and perinatal mortality are chiefly reported in terms of birth weight. In only a few reports are populations defined in terms of birth weight and gestational age.

Epidemiological factors

Epidemiologic investigations have revealed that in developed countries, the predominant risk factors in order of importance are: (1) cigarette smoking (2) low maternal weight gain and (3) low prepregnancy weight. These three risk factors account for nearly two-thirds of growth-retarded infants.[23] Other risk factors for LBW include black race, first births, female sex, short maternal stature, maternal low birth weight, prior LBW birth, maternal illnesses, fetal infections and a variety of metabolic and genetic disorders.

Age and parity

It has become axiomatic that the age of the mother is a determinant factor that determines her reproductive efficiency. Rates of LBW are significantly higher among young mothers.[24] At the other end of the spectrum, older women are beginning to show the effects of the aging process. Consequently, the pattern of LBW related to age is a U-shaped curve, with incidence elevated below 20 and over 35 years of age. However, it is not clear if the risk of teenage childbearing is due to young maternal age or to the low socioeconomic status that often accompanies teenage pregnancy.

Socioeconomic status

LBW is closely related to socioeconomic disadvantage. Socioeconomic status is usually determined by income, occupation and education. Low educational attainment is associated with higher rates of LBW. Women with a lower education level are 50% more likely to have VLBW babies and more than twice as likely to have moderately LBW babies (between 1500 and 2500 g) than women who have graduated from college.[25] It appears unlikely that income and education by themselves account for the differences in birth weight. Rather, it is the social and physical environment that these factors represent that is exerting an effect.

Race and ethnic background

In the United States, the prevalence of LBW varies according to the ethnic background. African–American infants (13.5%) are twice as likely to be born LBW than whites (5.8%), Hispanic origin (6.2%) or Asian–American infants (6.5%).[26] Epidemiological research has shown that these ethnic group differences are not wholly explained by ethnic differences in the occurrence of various medical illness, in smoking or use of other drugs, or in the use of prenatal care, or by demographic characteristics and other lifestyle differences. This provides some evidence that poverty may not be the sole reason for the high rates of LBW births among African–Americans. While it is valuable to know what does not cause the racial group differences in LBW, more emphasis needs to be placed on studying the basic biological differences between the racial groups, which may be responsible for these disparities.

Maternal weight gain and prepregnancy weight

Maternal weight gain during pregnancy results from a variety of factors, including maternal dietary intake, prepregnancy weight and height, length of gestation and the size of the fetus. Epidemiological evidence has demonstrated a nearly linear association between maternal weight gain during pregnancy and birth weight, and an inverse relationship to the rate of LBW.[27] A meta-analysis of nine studies found that weight gain during pregnancy has a significant effect on birth weight when prepregnancy weight is low.[23] Investigators who have examined the effect of a given gestational weight gain in women with different prepregnancy weight for height status have been virtually unanimous in concluding that the two factors strongly interact. A clear tendency exists toward increasing rates of IUGR with decreasing prepregnancy weight for height among women with low gestational weight gain. The effect of gestational weight gain on fetal growth is weak, or perhaps even absent, in obese women.[28] The evidence for other effect modifiers is not nearly as strong as that for prepregnancy weight for height.

Lifestyle choices

The bulk of evidence shows a clear and consistent association between LBW (primarily due to IUGR and not preterm birth) and smoking during pregnancy. Cigarette smoking is unequivocally the largest and most important known modifiable risk factor for LBW. It accounts for up to 20% of all LBW births.[25] The result holds among women of different ages, gravidities, geographic regions, social classes and ethnic groups. It has been consistently reported that, even after controlling for other factors, women who smoke are about twice as likely to deliver an LBW baby as are women who do not smoke.[29,30] Other behaviors, such as the abuse of alcohol and other drugs, while important, do not have nearly the same impact on overall rates of LBW births as cigarette smoking. The effects of alcohol intake during pregnancy upon birth weight have also been widely studied. A prospective study of 900 pregnant women adjusted for social class and smoking demonstrated that drinking more than 100 g of alcohol per week (10 standard measures) is associated with a risk of IUGR twice as high as for those drinking less than 50 g per week. The effects of alcohol and smoking are synergistic, although it is probable that smoking is a greater risk factor for IUGR than is drinking.[31]

Prenatal care

It is unclear whether or not the observed decreased rates of LBW among women who receive prenatal care are due to its effectiveness in preventing LBW or to other differences between women who receive prenatal care and those who do not. Women who receive prenatal care are a heterogenous group, but are generally healthier, more educated, and more advantaged than women who do not receive prenatal care. Rather than preventing LBW, prenatal care may be another indication of the many health-enhancing behaviors that characterize healthy, insured women who have healthy children. Although prenatal care provides a variety of valuable medical services to pregnant women and their fetuses (for example, management of normal birth, maternal hypertension and maternal diabetes, and/or detection of congenital malformations and genetic diseases in the fetus), evidence suggests that prenatal care may not provide significant benefits with respect to LBW.

Previous LBW infants

Several studies have shown that a maternal history of previous preterm or LBW infants increases the risk of giving birth to a subsequent preterm or LBW infant. LBW is known to repeat itself in 25% of cases where no maternal high-risk factor exists,[32] although many of them are born of a low-risk pregnancy and might be constitutionally small. Bakketeig and colleagues[33] showed that birth weight and not length of gestation is the best predictor of birth weight in subsequent pregnancies, just as length of gestation is the better predictor for subsequent gestational length. Mothers whose first-born infants were LBW have a two- to three-times higher risk of having an LBW second infant than the total population of secundiparae; the tendency to repeat births of lower weight is not markedly affected by a tendency to repeat medical complications that predispose to LBW.

Assisted reproductive technology (ART)

In the last few years, the number of births after the use of ART has increased steadily around the world, especially in developed countries. However, ART has been associated with an increased number of adverse perinatal outcomes, multiple pregnancies, preterm birth, low birth weight (LBW), very low birth weight (VLBW) and perinatal death.[34] Some studies suggest that the high incidence of multiple births after the use of ART is responsible for the majority of adverse perinatal outcomes, such as preterm delivery and LBW. Schieve found that ART singletons were 2.6 times more likely to be term-LBW compared with the general population.[35] Wang found that the observed number of preterm births and LBW was 2.4 and 2.1 times higher respectively than the expected number when applying general population birth rates. The comparison between ART singletons and general population singletons suggests that ART infants have a higher risk for preterm birth and LBW. This increased risk persists even when comparing ART singletons conceived with the transfer of only one embryo with singletons in the general population.[36]

Incidence and mortality

The incidence of LBW by region ranges from 31.1% in Middle South Asia and 19.7% for Asia as a whole to 14.0% in Africa, 10.1% in Latin America, 6.8% in North America and 6.5% in Europe.[37] The LBW rate is lower in many Western European nations, while in underdeveloped countries the LBW rates are often over 10% and the incidence of LBW is four times higher than that of developed countries. The LBW rate in Europe varies from 4.1% in Finland to 9.5% in Romania (Table 118.4).[38]

The general opinion is that the incidence of LBW in developed countries is diminishing. However, researchers using time series data have observed that the LBW rate has increased in the past few years. In European Union (EU) the incidence of LBW has increased from 5.97% in 1982 to 6.87% in 2002 (Table 118.5).[38] The Spanish Perinatal Mortality Survey of the Perinatal Medicine Section of the Spanish Obstetrical and Gynecological Society recorded data

Table 118.4 Incidence of low-birth-weight (LWB) and perinatal mortality rates in European countries in 2003 (based on data from WHO Regional Office for Europe)

Country	Incidence of LWB (%)	Perinatal mortality rate per 1000 births
Albania	4.2	—
Austria	7.1	3.61
Belgium	—	—
Bulgaria	8.9	12.1
Croatia	5.15	6.35
Czech Republic	6.62	3.65
Denmark	6	4.17
Finland	4.1	3.42
France	8	—
Germany	—	5.91
Greece	—	—
Hungary	8.7	5.34
Iceland	—	3.37
Israel	8.3	—
Italy	—	—
Lithuania	4.7	5.47
Luxembourg	—	5.64
Malta	7.04	4.72
Moldova	5.2	11.42
Netherlands	—	7.37
Norway	5.1	3.87
Poland	5.94	5.6
Portugal	7.4	6.15
Romania	9.5	11.79
Russian Federation	6.1	10.33
Slovakia	6.98	6.61
Slovenia	5.9	4.34
Spain	—	—
Sweden	4.62	3.87
Switzerland	—	7
Ukraine	5.4	8.07
United Kingdom	—	8.48
European Union (EU)	6.92	6.45

from 597,585 births, with known birth weight and gestational age, at hospitals in different Spanish regions from 1980 to 1992.[39] During the period surveyed the total incidence of LBW increased from 4.8% in 1980 to 7.1% in 1992 (Table 118.6).

The contribution of LBW to perinatal deaths is very important. In the Spanish Perinatal Mortality Survey, LBW represents 66.4% of fetal deaths, 69.6% of early neonatal deaths, and 67.7% of overall perinatal deaths. The high percentage of perinatal deaths generated from a relatively low number of LBW infants should call attention to the importance of this problem. Table 118.6 shows mortality rates during the perinatal period in LBW births. In the overall period surveyed, the fetal mortality rate was 31 times higher in LBW fetuses than in those born weighing $\geq$2500 g (87.0 vs. 2.8/1000 births), the early neonatal mortality rate was 40 times higher (64.8 vs. 1.6/1000 live births) and the perinatal mortality rate was 33 times higher (146.1 vs. 4.4/1000 births) (Table 118.6).

Table 118.5 Trends in the incidence of low birth weight from 1982 to 2002 (based on data from WHO Regional Office for Europe)

	Incidence of low birth weight (%)		
Country(*)	1982	1992	2002
Finland	3.7	3.8	4.3
Romania	7.6	8.21	9
Spain	3.9	5	7.1
Eropean Union	5.97	5.99	6.87

(*)Finland and Romania have been selected because they are the countries in which the incidence of LBW is the highest and the lowest in Europe respectively.

Medical scientists have focused on two major strategies to find ways to reduce the number of perinatal deaths: improving the survival of infants, and preventing births in groups of lower weight that have a higher risk of death. In European Union (EU), during the last two decades, the overall perinatal mortality rates have declined substantially (14.86 in 1980 vs. 6.42/1000 births in 2004), while rates of LBW have increased (from 5.97% in 1982 to 6.92% in 2003).[38] How can these very highly correlated outcomes, perinatal mortality and LBW rates, have shown such different tendencies? The seemingly contradictory decline in perinatal mortality without parallel declines in LBW birth is attributed to the increasing survival of LBW infants (Table 118.7). From an epidemiologist's point of view, in a given population, the overall perinatal mortality rate depends as much on the birth-weight distribution as on the birth-weight-specific mortality rates. In European Union, the recent decrease in perinatal mortality can be attributed solely to specific mortality improvements for each birth-weight group, since the incidence of LBW has increased. This mortality pattern indicates that our response to LBW has been effective at the level of treatment but not at the level of prevention. Every year many LBW infants are now added to the population who would not previously have survived. Although the vast majority of these infants are healthy, some of them have such severe handicaps as to make their impact on the population prevalence of cerebral palsy noticeable.

An examination of the epidemiology of LBW children must therefore include consideration of whether the children were born preterm or at term gestation.

Table 118.6 Trends in the incidence of low birth weight, fetal mortality, early neonatal mortality and perinatal mortality from 1980 to 1992 (mortality rates per 1000)

Birth weight (g)	1980	1983	1986	1989	1992	1980–1992
Incidence (%)						
< 2500	4.8	5.3	6.0	6.4	7.1	6.0
Fetal mortality rate						
< 2500	127.7	97.3	91.5	75.2	63.6	87.0
≥2500	3.2	3.1	2.8	2.7	2.2	2.8
Early neonatal mortality rate						
< 2500	91.2	82.4	73.7	57.2	39.4	64.8
≥2500	2.4	1.5	1.7	1.3	1.3	1.6
Perinatal mortality rate						
< 2500	207.2	171.7	158.4	128.1	100.5	146.1
≥2500	5.6	4.7	4.4	4.1	3.6	4.4

Spanish Perinatal Mortality Survey of the Perinatal Medicine Section of the Spanish Obstetrical and Gynecological Society

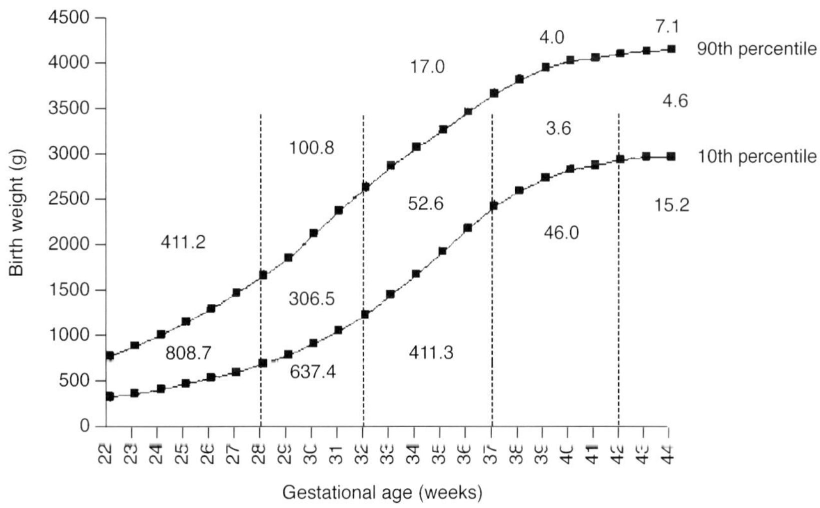

Figure 118.2 Perinatal mortality rate (per 1000 births) by birth weight and gestational age groups based on the Spanish Perinatal Mortality Survey from 1980 to 1992.

Table 118.7 Trends in the incidence and perinatal mortality rate (per 1000 births) in preterm (< 37 weeks) and term (≥37 weeks) low-birth-weight infants (< 2500 g)

	1980		1983		1986		1989		1992		1980–1992	
	Preterm	Term	Preterm	Term	Preterm	Term	Preterm	Term	Preterm	Term	Preterm	Term
Incidence (%)	3.0	1.9	3.0	2.4	3.4	2.6	3.5	2.8	4.1	2.9	3.4	2.5
Perinatal mortality rate (per 1000)	284.5	82.8	267.0	53.3	236.0	56.1	201.5	36.5	154.7	24.0	220.1	46.3

Spanish Perinatal Mortality Survey of the Perinatal Medicine Section of the Spanish Obstetrical and Gynecological Society

In developed countries, the major contributor to LBW is preterm birth, while in underdeveloped countries it is IUGR.[40] In the Spanish Perinatal Mortality Survey, when the analysis is carried out differentiating the preterm LBW births from the term LBW births, it is observed that the preterm LBW rate has increased by 37%, from 3.0% in 1980 to 4.1% in 1992, and the term LBW rate has also increased by 53%, from 1.9 to 2.9% (Table 118.7). Compared to term LBW infants, preterm LBW infants are four to five times more likely to die within the perinatal period. The perinatal mortality rate in preterm LBW infants in the overall period was 220.1/1000 births, compared to 46.3/1000 births in term LBW infants (Table 118.7). In the United States the incidence of increase in LBW from 1981 to 1991 (6.6 vs. 7.1%) resulted from the increase in preterm LBW infants (3.8 vs. 4.4%), while the term LBW rate decreased from 2.9 to 2.7% in the same period.[39] In the United States, the increased incidence of preterm LBW infants during 1981–1991 partly reflects changes in the distribution of selected maternal and infant characteristics. In particular, the percentage of births to unmarried women and women receiving no prenatal care may be markers of psychosocial and environmental risk factors for preterm deliveries.

There is evidence that the growth restriction process is associated with significant consequences to the infant. The likelihood of stillbirth or death during the first week of life is several times higher in SGA than in AGA babies, considering the corresponding gestational age (Figure 118.2). It is obvious that babies weighing less than about 1000 g are very likely to die, regardless of gestational age. The group with birth weight 1000–2000 g also has a rather high perinatal mortality rate, especially at early gestations. At all gestational ages, mortality falls steeply when birth weight increases up to about 4000 g, while the influence of gestational age at any given weight is comparatively much smaller.

REFERENCES

1. World Health Organization. Public health aspects of low birth weight. Third report of the Expert Committee on Maternal and Child Health. *World Health Organization Tech Rep Ser* 1961;217:3–16.
2. Rooth G. Low birth weight revised. *Lancet* 1980;1:639–41.
3. Wilcox AJ, Russel IT. Birth weight and perinatal mortality: I. On the frequency distribution of bith weight. *Int J Epidemiol* 1983;12:314–18.
4. Kleinman JC. Implications of difference in birthweight distribution for comparison of birthweight-specific mortality. In *Proceedings of the International Collaborative Effort on Perinatal and Infant Mortality*. Hyattsville, MD: National Center for Health Statistics, 1992;III:V28–V43.
5. Berkowitz GS, Papiernik E. Epidemiological of preterm birth. *Epidemiol Rev* 1993;15:414–43.
6. Lubchenco LO, Hansman C, Dressler M, Boyd E. Intrauterine growth as estimated from liveborn birthweight data at 24 to 42 weeks of gestation. *Pediatrics* 1963;32:793–800.
7. Fitzhardinge PM, Steven EM. The small-for-date infant. II. Neurological and intellectual sequelae. *Pediatrics* 1972;50:50–7.
8. Michaeleis R, Schulte F, Nolte R. Motor behavior of small-for-gestational age newborn infants. *Pediatrics* 1970;76:208–15.
9. Gruenwald P. Growth of the human fetus. *Am J Obstet Gynecol* 1966;94:1112–19.
10. Usher R, McLean F. Intrauterine growth of live-born Caucasian infants at sea level: Standards obtained from measurements in seven dimensions of infants born between 24 and 44 weeks of gestation. *Pediatrics* 1969;74:901–10.
11. Babson SG, Behrman RE, Lessel R. Fetal growth. Live-born birthweights for gestational age of white middle class infants. *Pediatrics* 1970;45:937–44.
12. Brenner WE, Edelman DA, Headricks CH. A standard of fetal growth for the United States of America. *Am J Obstet Gynecol* 1976;126:555–64.
13. Naeye RL, Dixon JB. Distortions in fetal growth standards. *Pediatr Res* 1978;12:1987–91.
14. Williams RL, Creasy RK, Cunningham GC. Fetal growth and perinatal viability in California. *Obstet Gynecol* 1982;59:624–32.
15. Goldenberg RL, Cutter GR, Hoffman HJ, Foster JM, Nelson KG, Hauth JC. Intrauterine growth restriction: Standards for diagnosis. *Am J Obstet Gynecol* 1989;161:271–7.
16. Metcoff J. Clinical assessment of nutritional status at birth. Fetal malnutrition and SGA are not synonymous. *Peditr Clin N Am* 1994;41:875–91.
17. Salvadori B. Poor intrauterine growth. In Scarpelli EM, Cosmi EV, eds. *Reviews in Perinatal Medicine*. New York: Raven Press, 1981;4:79–87.
18. Read MS, Catz C, Grave G, McNellis D, Warshaw JB. Introduction: Intrauterine growth restriction – Identification of research needs and goals. *Semin Perinatol* 1984;8:2–4.
19. Carrera JM. Crecimiento intrauterine retardado: Concepto y frecuencia. In Carrera JM, ed. *Crecimiento Fetal Normal y Patológico*. Barcelona: Masson SA, 1997:219–24.
20. Sedes JW. Impaired fetal growth: definition and clinical diagnosis. *Obstet Gynecol* 1984;64:303–10.
21. Altaman DG, Hytten FE. Intrauterine growth restriction; let´s be clear about it. *Br J Obstet Gynaecol* 1989;96:1127–32.
22. Kurjak A, Latin V, Polak J. Ultrasonic recognition of two types of growth restriction by measurement of four fetal dimensions. *J Perinat Med* 1978;6:102–8.
23. Kramer MS. Determinants of low birth weight: Methodological assessment and meta-analysis. *Bull World Health Organ* 1987;65:663–737.
24. National Center for Health Statics. *Advance Report of Final Natality Statistics, 1991*. Monthly Vital Statistics Report, vol.42, No. 3. Hyattsville, MD: Public Health Service, 1993;42(3).
25. Kleinman J, Madans JH. The effects of maternal smoking, physical stature, and educational attainment on the incidence of low birth weight. *Am J Epidemiol* 1985;121:832–55.
26. Kleinman J, Kessel S. Racial differences in low birth weight: Trends and risk factors. *N Engl J Med* 1987;317:749–53.
27. Luke B, Dickinson C, Petrie RH. Intrauterine growth: Correlations of maternal nutritional status and rate of gestational weight gain. *Eur J Obstet Gynecol Reprod Biol* 1981;12:113–21.
28. Abrams BG, Laros RK Jr. Pre-pregnancy weight, weight gain and birth weight. *Am J Obstet Gynecol* 1986;154:503–9.
29. Montgomery SM, Ekborn A. Smoking during pregnancy and diabetes mellitus in a British longitudinal birth cohort. *Br Med J* 2002;324:26–7.
30. Zaren B, Lindmark G, Bakketeig L. Maternal smoking affects growth more in the male fetus. *Pediatr Perinat Epidemiol* 2000;14(2):118–26.
31. Wright JL, Waterson EJ, Barrison IJ, Toplis PJ, Lewis IG, Gordon MG. Alcohol consumption, pregnancy and low birth weight. *Lancet* 1983;1:663–5.
32. Tejani NA. Recurrence of intrauterine growth restriction. *Obstet Gynecol* 1982;59:329–31.
33. Bakketeig LS, Hoffman HJ, Harley EE. The tendency to repeat gestational age and birth weight in successive births. *Am J Obstet Gynecol* 1979;135:1086–1103.
34. Petersen K, Hornnes PJ, Ellingsen S, Jensen F, Brocks V, Starup J. *et al.* Perinatal outcome after in vitro fertilization, *Acta Obstet Gynecol Scand* 1995;74:129–31.
35. Schieve LA, Meikle SF, Susan F, Ferre C, Peterson HB, Jeng G. *et al.* Low and very low birth weight in infants conceived with use of assisted reproductive technology. *N Engl J Med* 2002;346: 731–37.
36. Wang YA, Sullivan EA, Black D, Dean J, Bryant J, Chapman M. *et al.* Preterm birth and low birth weight after assisted reproductive technology-related pregnancy in Australia between 1996 and 2000. *Fertil Steril* 2005;83:1650–8.
37. United Nations. *Demographic Yearbook*. New York: United Nations Publications, 1991.
38. World Health Organization. European health for all database (database on Internet). WHO Regional Office for Europe (cited 2006 Feb 24). Available from: http://www.euro.who.int
39. Fare E, González de Agüero R, de Agustín JL, Tajada M, Repollés S, Sanz A. Perinatal mortality in term and post-term births. *J Perinat Med* 1996;24:163–9.
40. Villar J, Belizán JM. The relative contibution of prematurity and fetal growth restriction to low birth weight in developing and developed societies. *Am J Obstet Gynecol* 1982;143:793–8.

119 Etiology and pathogenesis of intrauterine growth restriction

J. M. Carrera, B. Serra and J. Mallafré

Introduction

Agents or factors supposedly associated with intrauterine growth restriction (IUGR) can be divided into intrinsic (endogenous) and extrinsic (exogenous) factors. The subject, however, is further complicated because these factors can be studied with regard to the fetus and/or the placenta, and because there are doubts about how some of these mechanisms should be classified. Therefore, we prefer to consider maternal, fetal and placental factors, although their endogenous or exogenous condition will be mentioned when describing the pathogenesis of IUGR.

Maternal factors

General and constitutional factors

Age

Evidence seems to confirm that at maternal age between 21 and 29 years, conditions for the development of normal newborns are the best, with the lowest rates of abortion, prematurity, perinatal mortality and growth restriction. At these ages, metabolic, homeostatic, nutritional, and psychological mechanisms reach a prime. Butler and Alberman[1] have shown that for equal parities, there is a significant effect of maternal age on fetal weight, i.e., the rate of growth restriction increases before and after this decade. In our experience, the incidence of infants with a birth weight < 1500 g related to both, prematurity and IUGR, in women under the age of 20 years is twofold higher than in women aged between 25 and 30 years. On the other hand, there is a higher rate of congenital defects in mothers under 15 years, especially of those (anencephalia) that are sometimes associated with IUGR. Older women experience a larger number of metabolic and vascular disorders (hypertension, diabetes mellitus) that favor poor implantation and uteroplacental insufficiency. The greater relative risk of fetal chromosomal abnormalities, frequently associated with IUGR, in women over 35 years of age is well known.

Maternal height

Some authors[2] consider that for each centimeter by which maternal height exceeds normal values, fetal weight at birth is increased by 16 g, while others[3,4] affirm that when the weight factor is corrected, maternal height has little effect on the weight of the fetus. In the opinion of Fabre and colleagues,[5] shorter women, usually with a lower weight before pregnancy, have more low birth weight infants. Other investigators, such as Abdul-Karim and Beydoum[6] found that the influence of paternal height on fetal weight is more closely correlated than maternal height. It has been argued that infants born of short-stature fathers have a mean decrease of 183 g in birth weight as compared with those born of high-stature fathers.[7] Lechtig *et al.*[8,9] and Junis *et al.*[10] observed a statistically significant association between short maternal height and the incidence of fetuses with low weight at birth (Figure 119.1). A positive association between paternal adult height and fetal growth has been described after controlling for confounding factors.[11]

Maternal weight at birth

Ounsted and Ounsted[12] have shown a statistically significant relationship between neonatal birth weight and maternal birth weight, and have suggested a potent hereditary influence on fetal variables. Many mothers of infants with IUGR have been small-for-dates themselves.[13–15] Moreover, it has been reported that women who were themselves low birth weight infants as a result of IUGR are more likely to deliver an IUGR fetus than those mothers who were low birth weight secondary to prematurity.

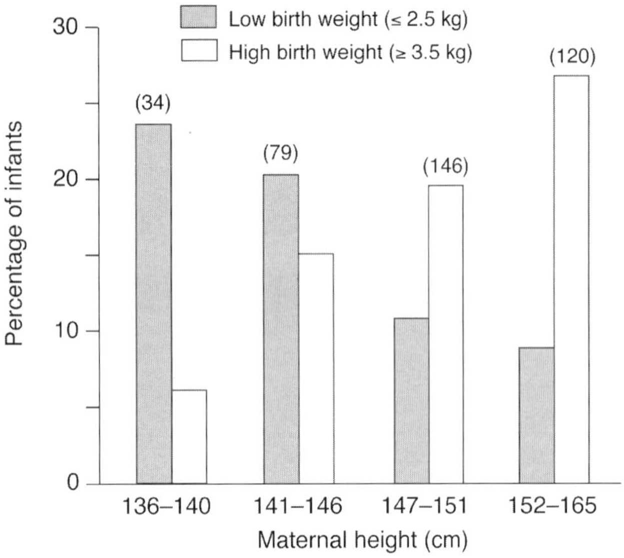

Figure 119.1 Relationship between short maternal height and percentage of infants with low birth weight.[8]

Table 119.1 Relationship between pre-pregnancy weight and neonatal weight in Caucasian and Black women[11]

Maternal pre-pregnancy weight (kg)	n		Mean neonatal birth weight (g)	
	Caucasians	Blacks	Caucasians	Blacks
<45	1293	122	3066	3057
45–53	8851	618	3215	3132
54–62	9733	806	3332	3176
63–70	3198	369	3419	3262
71–80	854	144	3431	3282
≥80	406	72	3444	3410
Total	24335		2133	

Maternal weight prior to pregnancy

Simpson and associates[16] have shown a clear association between maternal and fetal weight. Fetal growth restriction is particularly associated with mothers weighing less than 54 kg (Table 119.1). Fabre and colleagues[5] found a positive correlation between maternal body mass index and neonatal birth weight. According to the statistical analysis in this study, maternal weight prior to pregnancy would account for 11.02% of differences in birth weight. Similar results have been documented in other reports.[17–21]

Maternal weight gain during pregnancy

Low maternal weight gain in pregnancy,[22,23] in particular prior to 12 weeks' gestation,[24] may be considered an index of possible fetal malnutrition. Weight gains < 3 kg until 20 weeks' gestation or an increase < 1 kg/month in the second half of pregnancy[5] should alert to the risk of IUGR.

Maternal heart volume

Lehmann and coworkers[18] demonstrated a clear association between neonatal birth weight and maternal heart volume, with heart volumes < 600 ml in mothers of newborns with birth weights < 3000 g (Table 119.2). In cases of IUGR, Duvekot and colleagues[25] reported poor cardiovascular adaptation at the beginning of pregnancy with hypovolemia and reduced maternal heart volume.

Race

It is very difficult to find strictly comparable studies of different ethnic groups matched for social and economic status, as well as to isolate the effects of genetic factors from those related to unfavorable nutritional, socioeconomic and environmental conditions.[26] As stated by Gruenwald,[27] the actual influence of ethnic factors on fetal weight will remain unknown until diverse ethnic groups have been living under comparable conditions for a period of time, perhaps two generations. However, there is extensive information which provides evidence of ethnic differences. Thus, Indian infants are constantly smaller in different circumstances: in India as compared with general registries, in South Africa as compared with other ethnic groups, in Malaysia as compared with Chinese, and in Kenya as compared with Caucasians and Blacks. Even taking into account socioeconomic and environmental differences, it seems that there are differences in birth weight between Caucasian and Black neonates, which can be attributed in half of the cases to purely racial influences.[28] At 40 weeks' gestation, weights of White fetuses are 156 g greater on average than those of Blacks, even when the weight factor is corrected for economic level and parity (Figure 119.2).[29] Jans[30] offers a clear example of the role played by ethnic factors, finding that Bambuti pygmy babies from the Itu tropical forest have a very low mean birth weight (2635 g) with an extremely low weight variation as compared with that usually found in Caucasians. But other sudies[31] have not found statistically significant differences between White and Aboriginal population in Australia. They concluded that there is no reason to use separate fetal growth curves when examining Aboriginal fetuses.

Genetic and familial factors

Epidemiological studies have demonstrated a possible role of genetic and familial factors in determining birth weight.[32,33] Klebanov[34] found that delivery of small for gestational age infants and preterm delivery were significantly more common among women who were themselves small for gestational age and who were delivered preterm, respectively. In addition,

Table 119.2 Relationship between maternal heart volume, maternal height and weight, placental weight, and weight and height of neonates[2]

Fetal age or weight at birth	Maternal weight at birth (kg)	Maternal height (cm)	Placental weight (g)	Neonatal weight (g)	Neonatal height (cm)	Maternal heart volume (ml)	*n*
3400–3600 g	62.3	163	560	3552	50	647	15
≥4000 g	74.7	165	737	4270	53	671	25
40–41 weeks	60.6	163	475	2746	47	568	29
38–39 weeks	60.6	161	480	2632	46	597	17
36–37 weeks	61.7	162	442	2497	46	597	18

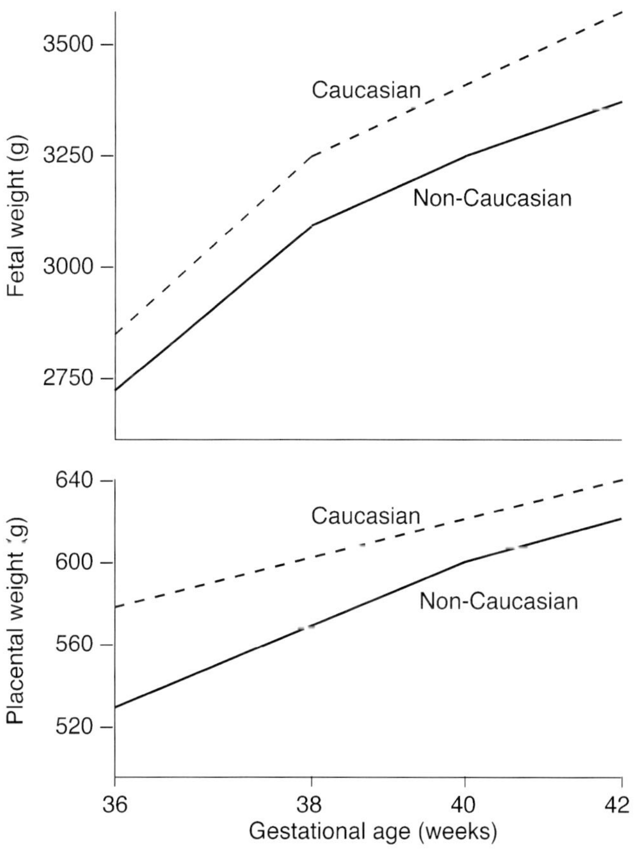

Figure 119.2 Relationship between racial group and fetal and placental weights.[29]

several studies have found that infants are more likely to have low birth weight if their mother's sisters had delivered small for gestational age infants.[35] Bakketeig[32] found that mothers whose fetus was small for gestational age are two to three times more likely to produce a small for gestational age second infant compared to the total population of mothers who had delivered their first and second infants without IUGR. These observations support the importance of genetic or environmental factors in the genesis of an infant of low birth weight. Although it is difficult to exclude familial aggregation of certain specific environmental factors such as dietary habits with any certainty, it is unlikely that in developed countries these factors have a large impact on birth weight.

Ghezzi[36] assessed the familial pattern of the IUGR condition through a detailed pedigree analysis of a selected population of women with more than one affected child, and he identified a subset of families in which the IUGR condition demonstrated vertical transmission, suggesting an autosomal pattern of inheritance. Some fetuses from different families showed an abnormal chromosome constitution and severe IUGR, indicating that more than one genetic cause may contribute to the low birth weight.

Chromosome abnormalities have been cited by several investigators as the possible genetic cause of IUGR. Moreover, placental chromosome mosaicism, favoring an abnormal segregation of imprinted regions in the fetus, has been widely described in IUGR fetuses. Ghezzi[36] postulated two further conditions where an inherited genetic cause can be identified: first, a dominant or recessive inheritance of gene mutations may disturb the correct fetal growth; second, a parental carrier of balanced chromosome abnormalities may confer a risk not only for unbalanced malformed fetuses, but also for IUGR conditions due to the anomalous segregation of the imprinted regions.

Several authors believe that the identification of the inheritance pattern of IUGR has an important clinical value because a knowledge of the family history and of the parental karyotypes may be helpful in preventing both fetal malformations and adverse neonatal morbidity in subsequent low birth weight infants.

Socioeconomic conditions

Unfavorable socioeconomic conditions markedly increase the incidence of fetuses with low weight at birth in relation to the following factors: diet, family and social environment, education and intellectual level, type of work, teenage pregnancies and marital status, among others. Women of low socioeconomic class are prone to a larger extent than their counterparts to early, frequent and numerous pregnancies, which continue to a more advanced maternal age. It

Table 119.3 Maternal education level and rate of intrauterine growth restriction (IUGR)

Maternal education	IUGR group	Control group	Total
University degree	10	19	29
Secondary education	12	61	73
Primary education	78	20	98
Total	100	100	200

has been largely recognized that fetal and neonatal risks increase significantly at the limits of age and parity, as well as in cases of repeated gestations at short intervals.[8,9,37,38]

Role of sense of control

There is limited earlier literature on the role of sense of control and pregnancy outcomes, especially IUGR. Several authors have looked at how sense of control might affect health outcomes. Taylor and Seeman[39] concluded that sense of control might act as a mediator of the effects of socioeconomic status on health, while other authors think that sense of control may have an impact on how one copes with stress, perhaps modulating how stress affects health outcomes. Literature also suggest that other measures of control may have an impact on access to health care services, health behaviors and participation on screening activities.[40–43] Durousseau[44] found no statistically significant association between IUGR and maternal pregnancy intendedness, initial happiness about becoming pregnant, and maternal sense of control.

Deficient maternal schooling

Deficient maternal schooling is associated with illiteracy and ignorance, with unawareness of the physiology of reproduction and the possibilities of contraception, and as a result, high natality rates, poor hygiene, and scarce or absent medical control of pregnancies are found among these social groups (Table 119.3).[45]

Marital status

In the study by Norska,[46] the percentage of single mothers was 1.2% in the control group vs. 6.9% in the group with IUGR.

Psychosocial factors

Few studies have examined the association between psychosocial factors and the risk of IUGR, probably due to the difficulty to separate the impact of these factors (pregnancy intendedness, initial happiness about becoming pregnant, stress, etc.) from that of other sociodemographic variables. Several limitations should be considered when assessing the results of these studies.[47–50]

Inappropriate physical work

Inappropriate or excessive physical work can exert an unfavorable effect on fetal nutrition, particularly when found in association with other factors related to a precarious economic condition. Some types of work can cause poor intrauterine fetal growth, such as those which implicate heavy physical work; jobs requiring long periods of time spent in forced or uncomfortable positions which, in addition, impair renal or uterine circulation; jobs with chemical products or accompanied by mechanical vibrations; stressful working places, causing risk of nerve-induced uterine contractions; work in the open air under unfavorable meteorological conditions, or work in poorly ventilated and highly contaminated closed spaces; or work in places far from home that require travel of several kilometers each day. In these cases, a decrease in neonatal weight may be expected.[51,52]

Maternal malnutrition

On a worldwide scale, maternal malnutrition is the most frequent cause of IUGR. One should distinguish, however, between transient nutritional deficits (of different causes, either forced or voluntary) and chronic undernutrition.

Transient malnutrition. There is evidence that when a normally well-nourished woman suffers from severe starvation for a period of time, gestation is not substantially affected. Studies carried out in The Netherlands[53,54] during wartime (1944–45), when for 27 weeks daily food intake was lower than 1000 kcal and 40 g of protein, a marked decrease in fetal weight (< 240 g) was not documented. Perinatal mortality did not increase either, and intellectual or somatic deficits did not occur in the long term. Placental abnormalities were not seen. Hammond[55] postulates that, in these cases, fetuses are able to compete with the mother for the use of nutrients due to their high metabolic rate.

Chronic malnutrition. In these cases, there is prepregnancy and pregnancy malnutrition. Gruenwald[56,57] compared the birth weight of Japanese neonates born in different decades: in a period of severe food deprivation (1945–46), birth weight was significantly lower than that of North American infants, whereas some years later (1963–64), when nutritional problems disappeared, differences between both populations were almost inappreciable (Figure 119.3). In a rural Guatemalan population, Lechtig[68] reported a higher incidence (40%) of low birth weight neonates, with a four-fold mortality rate during the first year of life among women who had been severely undernourished since childhood. After nutritional intervention, a progressive reduction in the incidence of low birth weight was observed. According to others,[59] establishment of a balanced diet during the last trimester of pregnancy could even compensate the effects of malnutrition in the first months of gestation on fetal weight.

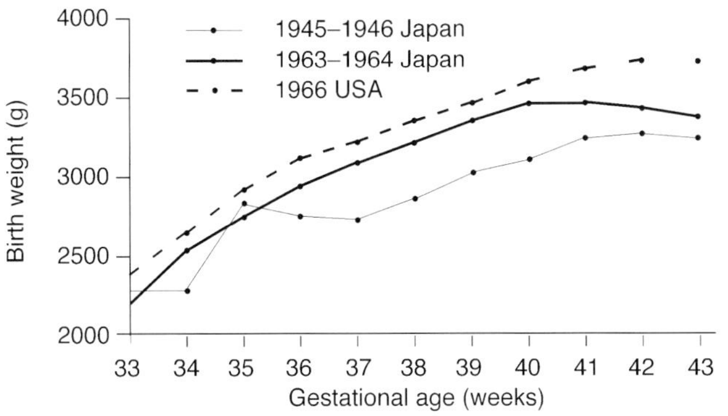

Figure 119.3 Fetal growth curves in Japanese neonates born in two different periods: 1945–46 (wartime) and 1963–64 (economic recovery), as compared with American neonates.[57]

Pathogenetic mechanisms involved in poor intrauterine fetal growth include: (a) a low nutrient supply to the placenta, which, in turn, causes a deficient turnover of amino acids and other substances in the major organs, such as the fetal liver[60]; and (b) placental abnormalities, with a marked decrease in placental weight and in the number of chorionic villi.[61,62] This indicates that the placenta is highly sensitive to the effects of malnutrition.[63]

Nutritional deficits. Long-standing unbalanced diets can be harmful for fetal growth.[64,65] Papiernik and associates[66] assessed the influence of maternal diet on fetal growth in a middle-class Parisian community. The mean caloric intake was 1689 ± 123 kcal in the study group and 1944 ± 155 kcal in the control group. In general, subjects included in the study group consumed less fat and significantly lower amounts of carbohydrates than controls. The study showed that IUGR in women with no apparent cause was associated with a lower caloric intake (300 kcal) than controls. Since protein consumption was similar in both groups, a decrease in the ingestion of carbohydrates was the presumed reason for fetal growth restriction. On the contrary, Bender and Nuñez[67] found that after adjusting for other known maternal risk factors, caloric intake did not present a direct effect on IUGR. Lechtig[9] found that protein supplementation had no effect on fetal weight, in contrast to carbohydrate supplementation, which had a positive effect on fetal weight gain. Abnormalities in blood composition caused by selective nutritional deficits (folic acid, magnesium, riboflavin and other vitamins, iron, etc.) should be included in this subgroup as well as, in a broad sense, some hypoxic states (high altitude) or disorders preventing adequate maternal nutrition. Riboflavin deficiencies in the last trimester of pregnancy cause a delay in the appearance of rapid isoenzymes of alkaline phosphatase, which, in turn, determines fetal hypotrophy. In these cases, placental alkaline phosphatase activity is dramatically reduced.

Micronutrients and fetal growth

Observational studies, recently reviewed by Ramakrishnan *et al.*[68] and Fall *et al.*[69] show for almost every vitamin and mineral, associations between poor maternal micronutrient status and IUGR or other adverse pregnancy outcomes, but most studies should be considered with caution because of methodology problems. Nevertheless, we will review available information regarding different micronutrients and its relation with fetal growth.

Fat-soluble vitamins. Trials among HIV-positive mothers in Tanzania[70] and South Africa[71] showed no effect of vitamin A alone on fetal growth. Regarding vitamin D, two studies of adequate quality have not found significant differences in fetal growth in newborns from mothers that received vitamin D supplementation during pregnancy. There is a trial of vitamin E supplementation in pregnancy focused on hypertensive disorders.[72] Women with a previous history of pre-eclampsia or with abnormal uterine artery Doppler waveforms were randomly assigned to receive vitamins C and E or placebo. The supplement was associated with a significant decrease in the incidence of pre-eclampsia and a lower number of small-for-gestational-age infants, but showed no effect on mean birth weight.

Water-soluble vitamins. Vitamin B-1 (thiamin), B-2 (riboflavin) and B-3 (niacin) are essential cofactors for energy metabolism, and therefore its deficiency might be expected to result in impaired fetal growth, but despite evidence that deficiency in pregnancy is common, there are only observational studies that focus this issue and with contradictory results.[73,74] Vitamin B-12 is derived mainly from animal sources and its deficiency is therefore more common in vegetarians, but there is no literature available regarding its relation with pregnancy. On the other hand there is a large body of literature on folic acid in pregnancy. A recent Cochrane review[75] concluded that despite a significant reduction in maternal anemia, there was only a small and non-significant effect on the incidence of low birth weight. Finally, several observational studies showed positive correlations between maternal vitamin C status and birth weight.[76,77]

Minerals. Iron. Several large studies in developed countries have shown a U-shaped relationship between maternal hemoglobin concentration and birth weight, with higher birth weights at both ends of the distribution.[78,79] This fact may be explained by maternal plasma volume expansion, which although producing anemia, probably acts as a compensatory mechanism to improve uteroplacental perfusion. Evidence from developing countries shows that maternal iron deficiency is associated with low birth weight and poor obstetric outcome,[78,79] but the previous Cochrane review[80] reveals that data from these countries are not sufficient for drawing conclusions.

Zinc deficiency states are characterized by impaired growth, and although there are numerous observational studies, most of them have an inadequate size or methodological problems.[81] Although a large, well conducted study on 580 women with low serum zinc concentrations in a developed country showed a significant increase in birth weight, recent large trials of zinc in low-income women of developing countries showed no effects on birth weight.[82,83]

Iodine. Levels of iodine in soil and therefore in plant foods are highly variable, with several deficiency areas. A non-randomized trial in Algeria[84] showed a significantly higher birth weight in iodine-supplemented mothers.

Calcium. Most trials of calcium supplementation couldn't find any effect on birth weight,[85,86] although the Cochrane metaanalysis,[87] showed a significant effect on low birth weight, probably because of prolongation of gestation rather than enhanced fetal growth.

Magnesium. The Cochrane review[88] showed a beneficial effect on low birth weight.

Other trace elements. The role of copper, selenium, chromium, manganese and molybdenum in human pregnancy remains unknown.

Geographical and climatic factors

Although in poverty-stricken areas it is difficult to differentiate geographical factors from socioeconomic conditions, there is enough evidence of the influence of altitude and temperature on birth weight of neonates.

Altitude

Chronic maternal hypoxia caused by living at high altitudes may be a restrictive factor of placental and fetal growth,[89,90] although pregnancy increases maternal ventilation and raises arterial O_2 saturation, which helps to protect against altitude-associated IUGR. On equal terms of socioeconomic status, it seems that there are differences in the weight of babies born at sea-level and at high altitudes,[91] that Moore quantifies in 100 g fall per 1000 m elevation gain.[92] Adaptations in multigenerational high-altitude populations seem to permit higher uterine artery blood flows and protect against altitude-associated IUGR.

Climatic conditions

Although an inverse correlation between mean fetal weight and mean annual temperature has been reported, these data should be interpreted with caution since many other variables (race, socioeconomic status, etc.) are associated with the effect. Toverud[93] found that babies born in summer had a greater birth weight than babies born in winter, and he explained these differences by changes in maternal energy production and tissue regeneration stimulated by rest when the weather is cold. In contrast, Prasaad[94] reported that birth weights of Indian babies were systematically lower in summer and the rainy season than in winter.

Air pollution

The association between air pollution and adverse pregnancy outcomes, among them IUGR, has been studied in several countries,[95–97] but a recent review of 12 epidemiologic studies conducted by Maisonat concluded that current scientific knowledge on the impact of air pollution on fetal growth is still limited.[98]

Toxic habits

Smoking

Cigarette smoking has been unequivocally associated with low birth weight. The first report on the reduction of fetal weight by the effect of maternal smoking was published by Simpson and Linda,[99] and thereafter extensively documented by others.[1,100,101] Different studies[102,103] have demonstrated that after excluding other variables, the weight at birth is reduced by an average of 170–200 g in infants born to mothers who smoke more than 10 cigarettes a day. The distribution curves of birth weights according to weeks of gestation confirms a displacement to the right in the curve corresponding to smoking women (Figure 119.4).[104] This factor accounts for 5% of variations in weight at birth.[5]

There is no agreement regarding the mechanism by which cigarette smoking decreases fetal weight, but some of the following have been postulated[105–111]: (a) increased fetal levels of carboxyhemoglobin[105,106]; (b) left-shift of the hemoglobin dissociation curve; (c) nicotine-related uteroplacental vasoconstriction; (d) moderate anorexia and deficient maternal nutrition, preventing fetal compensation of the high rate of fetal carboxyhemoglobin by means of an increase of hematocrit; (e) reduced plasma volume; and (f) increase in requirements for vitamin B_{12} and some amino acids which are necessary for tobacco-supplied cyanide detoxification. Given the variety of factors involved, it is not possible to establish a common pathogenetic mechanism for the effects of maternal smoking. This is the reason for which, in some cases, fetal weight is the only parameter affected, while in others fetal height and head circumference are also reduced.[101,112]

Despite this information, a lot of controversy was aroused in the 1970s, with most authors[107,108] in favor of the causative role played by cigarette smoking, and others[109] believing that maternal constitutional differences between smokers and non-smokers could be responsible for the depressant effect on fetal weight. Recently, a relationship between IUGR and an alteration of epidermal growth factor receptor in placental membranes of smokers has been suggested.[113]

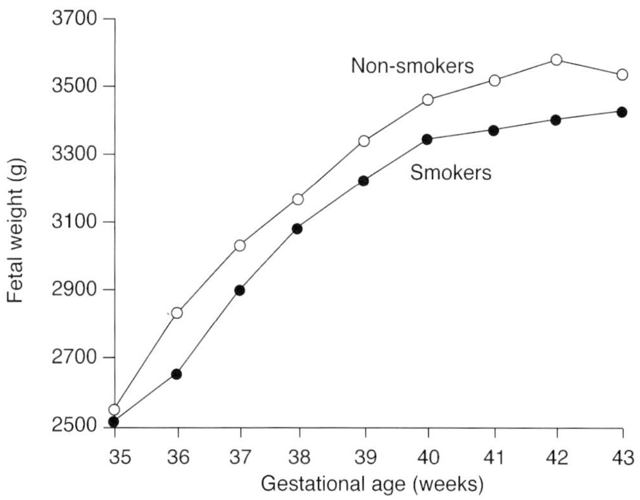

Figure 119.4 Influence of smoking habit on fetal weight.[1]

Recently, it has been discovered that offspring of mothers who smoked during pregnancy are more likely to develop type II diabetes.[114]

Zaren[115] found that the negative effect on fetal growth from maternal smoking curiously affected male fetuses proportionally more than female ones. A different hormonal milieu is suggested as possible explanation for the greater male susceptibility.

Alcohol use

Ulleland[116] reported for the first time that IUGR was particularly common among children born to alcoholic mothers. In addition to evidence of the adverse effects of alcohol on fetal weight in animal models,[117,118] there are multiple reports in humans.[119] The weight at birth is reduced by an average of 160–190 g in infants born to mothers with daily alcohol consumption >200 g. Different authors[120,121] described the characteristics of these children and established the concept of 'fetal alcoholic syndrome', in which weight, height, and head circumference of the neonates are below the 3rd percentile. Moreover, different abnormalities (skeletal, cardiac, neurological, etc.) and craniofacial stigmata are frequently observed. Frequently, alcohol consumption is accompanied by elevated caffeine, tobacco and/or cannabis consumption, complicating the epidemiological analysis of the effect of each of these substances.[122]

Caffeine

Methylxanthines, especially caffeine and theophylline, are found in numerous food products, beverages and medicines. Although a clear deceleration effect of caffeine on fetal growth has been reported in experimental animals,[123] data in pregnant women are controversial. Risks associated with maternal caffeine consumption during pregnancy and perinatal outcomes have been proved difficult to estimate. Caffeine is consumed by most of pregnant women, and small risks influence large numbers of pregnancies. The ingestion of more than seven or eight cups of coffee a day (600 mg of caffeine) apparently increases the rates of both fetal growth restriction and prematurity.[124–127] These findings, however, have not been confirmed in other studies.[128–130] It is possible that caffeine consumption and smoking interact to reduce fetal growth, but the involved mechanisms remain unclear.

Some earlier studies[131] provide reassurance that moderate caffeine consumption during pregnancy does not meaningfully influence fetal growth, but large quantities of caffeine should be avoided.

Illicit drug addiction

Babies born to heroin-addicted mothers weigh significantly less than do those born to mothers who do not consume opioids,[132–134] independently of maternal nutrition and drug use withdrawal during gestation. Low fetal weight is related both to prematurity and IUGR. An increase in fetal weight has been shown in pregnant women giving maintaining doses of methadone, although similar fetal weights than in controls were not reached.[135]

At early stages of gestation, opioids have a critical influence on fetal growth. Different mechanisms have been proposed to explain the effect of drug abuse on fetal growth, such as a significant decrease in the number of cells of different organs and in the size of the brain[132] (methadone antagonizes cell reduction by an unknown mechanism), impairment of carbohydrate fetal metabolism (methadone seems to have a hyperglycemic action), and a decrease in plasma concentrations of corticosteroids[136] (methadone may reverse a relative adrenal hypofunction, acting indirectly on carbohydrate metabolism).

With respect to the effect of cocaine on fetal weight, no conclusive evidence is available.[137,138] A recent multicenter study, however, failed to demonstrate an increased incidence of low birth weight and preterm birth among cocaine consumers, although there was a significantly higher rate of abruptio placenta.

Drug treatment

Some teratogenic drugs also have an important effect on fetal growth. Adverse effects of tetracyclines include fetal growth restriction secondary to skeletal hypoplasia when this antibiotic is administered during the first trimester of pregnancy, and permanent staining of the teeth in the second trimester. Untoward effects of anticoagulation drugs (warfarin), especially when given between 6 and 9 weeks' gestation,[139] comprise mental restriction, dysmorphisms (nasal hypoplasia), and evident IUGR. Folic acid antagonists (aminopterin and derivatives) are potentially lethal drugs for the embryo when given within 40 days before conception. The administration of these compounds during the first trimester of pregnancy can cause severe structural defects (neural tube defects, abnormalities of the limbs, ophthalmic hypoplasia, etc.) and fetal growth restriction that persists in postnatal life.[140] Hydantoin anticonvulsants are responsible for the 'fetal hydantoin syndrome' characterized by mental restriction, a number of craniofacial defects, and fetal growth restriction.[141] The 'fetal trimethadione syndrome' consists of characteristic craniofacial and cardiac defects which are almost always associated with mental and fetal growth restriction.[141] Lithium causes a number of cardiac defects (Ebstein's disease) and IUGR.

Maternal diseases

A large number of maternal disorders have been related to fetal growth restriction.

Poor adaptation of maternal circulation

There is growing evidence for poor pregestational preparation of maternal circulation (with or without uterine vascular insufficiency) as a cause of very early recurrent miscarriages and IUGR.[142] Current research is focused on color Doppler examination of the uterine arteries to detect defective placentation. Results of these studies will probably provide some keys for establishing an early prognosis of pregnancies in which this condition occurs. Immunologic aspects may also be involved in poor adaptation of maternal circulation.[143] This seems particularly plausible in very early IUGR with positive antiphospholipid antibodies (lupus anticoagulant and anticardiolipin antibodies), in which the cause may lie in an early inhibition of the production of prostacyclin at the vascular endothelium.[144]

Chronic renal disease

Chronic renal diseases most frequently associated with IUGR include chronic pyelonephritis, glomerulosclerosis, chronic glomerular disease, and lupus glomerulonephritis.[145,146] Fetal growth restriction in maternal renal disease is largely secondary to protein loss.[145] Chronic renal disease should always be suspected in patients with a history of IUGR associated with 'toxemias' and persistent proteinuria and hypertension after childbirth.

In patients with blood urea nitrogen > 60 mg/dl, fetal mortality is 80–100%. In fact, Parbooshing and Cochburn[147] reported an IUGR incidence of 100% in patients with plasma urea levels upon 60 mg/dl and/or creatinine clearance values below 60 ml/min.

Pre-eclampsia and chronic hypertension

Hypertensive disorders of pregnancy and chronic hypertension exert an unfavorable effect on fetal growth.[148–150] In patients with hypertension and proteinuria, fetal weight is decreased by 300–400 g.[151] In our experience, fetal growth restriction is initiated from 35–36 weeks of gestation, so that the birth weight of preterm infants is lower than that expected for the gestational age. It is likely that severe pre-eclampsia or serious chronic hypertension need to be present to substantially affect fetal weight.[152]

Several studies support the hypothesis that pre-eclampsia is an etiologically heterogeneous disorder that occurs in at least two separate subsets, one with normal or enhanced placental function and another involving placental dysfunction.[153–155] In the subset with placental dysfunction, IUGR fetuses often have asymmetric fetal body proportion and reduced fetal length, which is consistent with placental hypoperfusion.

Uteroplacental ischemia has been considered for many years to be the most important factor of fetal distress and hypotrophy. Vasoconstriction would account for most cases of sudden intrauterine fetal death. It seems equally proven that placental oxygen consumption is decreased in hypertensive pregnancies with hypertrophic fetuses. The involvement of coagulation disorders has been recently hypothesized based on the identification of extensive infarctions and intervillous and perivillous fibrin deposits in placentas of some small-for-date neonates from hypertensive mothers. Intervillous fibrin deposits could be explained by activation of coagulation pathways.[156,157] There is evidence of platelet activation in many cases of IUGR occurring in normotensive and hypertensive pregnancies.[158] Trudinger[159] reported depletion of platelets in maternal blood in IUGR associated with pre-eclampsia as a result of intravascular coagulation in the placenta with local deposition of fibrin and platelets. An abnormal increase in the thromboxane/prostacyclin index at the intervillous level and in the peripheral blood due to a deficient production of prostacyclins of trophoblastic origin is currently accepted as the cause of altered vascular reactivity.[160]

Elevated homocisteine is an independent risk factor for peripheral vascular thrombosis, found in 20–30% of pre-eclamptic women, that seems to act through similar mechanisms.[161] Recent reports have related elevated homocysteine plasma levels in the early second trimester with the subsequent development of pre-eclampsia,[162–164] but other studies have not observed this relation.[165]

Placental growth factor (PlGF) and vascular endothelial growth factor (VEGF) are involved in placental angiogenesis through interactions with the VEGFR-1 and VEGFR-2 receptors, and placentas of pregnancies with fetal growth restriction are characterized by abnormal angiogenic development, classically associated with hypoxia.[166] Tsatsaris[167] suggested that there are two different pathophysiological mechanisms associated with pre-eclampsia. The first one is related to an overproduction of competitive VEGFR-1 that may lead to suppression of VEGF and PlGF effects. The second one is the downregulation of its membrane bound form (VEGFR-1) in the placental bed, which may result in the defective uteroplacental development.

Maternal hyperinsulinemia

There is evidence for interrelationships between glucose, insulin and human placental lactogen (HPL) in fetal growth. Fragmentary data were obtained by three research groups. Abell and coworkers[168] found that low estriol levels and hypotrophic fetuses were associated with a higher incidence of abnormal glucose tolerance, particularly hypoglycemia, but also hyperglycemia. Frydman[169] demonstrated that insulin levels were clearly increased in many pregnant women with growth-restricted fetuses, especially in the postprandial phase, as a result of which less substrates are offered to the fetus due to excessive dispersion to maternal deposits. Grumbach[170,171] described the anti-insulin activity of HPL, and Spellacy[172] confirmed the lipolytic properties of this agent. Accordingly, postprandial maternal hyperinsulinemia due to high hormonal secretion, low tissue resistance to insulin, or impaired insulin removal by the placenta (low HPL levels) would enhance anabolism and decrease transplacental passage of carbohydrate substrates. In a group of pregnant women with IUGR, Frydman and colleagues[169] found that glucose ingestion was followed by an increase in the maximal peak of insulin, marked inhibition of HPL, and prominent reduction of free fatty acids and amino acids. This situation may be further complicated by deficient fetal insulin production. The hypothesis of the 'selfish mother' is depicted in Figure 119.5.

Long-standing, poorly controlled insulin-dependent diabetes associated with diabetic retinopathy, hypertension and nephritis may cause placental microvascular disorders that give rise to an increase in IUGR.[173] Low fetal weight is accompanied by low weight of all other fetal organs.

In pregnancies complicated by insulin-dependent diabetes, treatment with insulin and caloric restriction results in a decreased incidence of macrosomia and perinatal mortality, although fetal growth restriction may increase significantly (19.1% vs. 10.8% in the control group).[174] Fetal weight decrease may be explained by iatrogenic hyperinsulinemia and/or excessive caloric restriction with marked consumption of carbohydrate substrates, especially in the postprandial phase.[175] For this reason, there is a high percentage of newborns above the 90th percentile when maternal serum glucose levels are maintained between 100 and 150 mg/100 ml, while low birth weights are frequent when glucose concentrations are < 100 or > 150 mg/100 ml.[176]

Pregnant women with a family history of diabetes mellitus should have a glucose tolerance test, since a marked decrease in the K_1 coefficient is consequently associated with fetal weight alterations. Abnormal glucose tolerance (hyperglycemia) is especially found in old and obese women of high parity with history of miscarriages, fetal death, and newborns of unusual birth weights (low or high).[177]

Impairment of fetal growth in cases of maternal hypoglycemia secondary to unbalanced diets or relative hyperinsulinemia is related to enhanced maternal lipolysis and ketonemia[178] or catecholamine release.

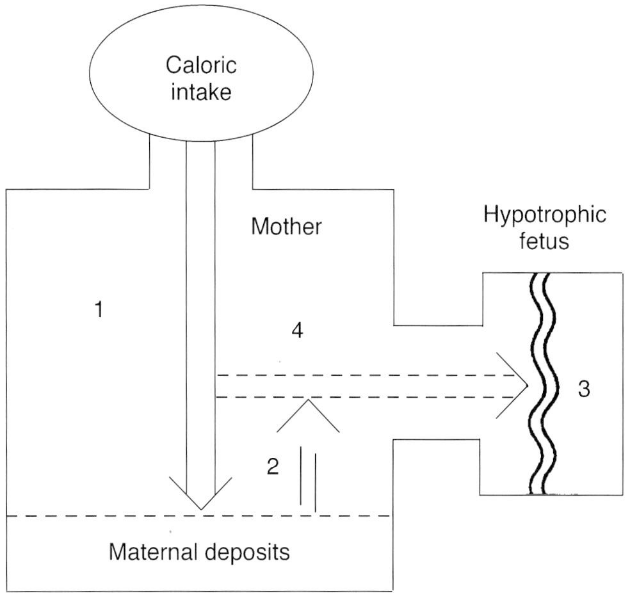

Figure 119.5 Hypothesis of the 'selfish mother' according to Frydman and colleagues.[169] Possible causes: 1, excessive insulin anabolism; 2, low tissue insulin resistance; 3, deficient fetal insulin production; 4, others.

Chronic cardiopulmonary disease

Fetal growth restriction has been reported in patients with heart or lung disease causing hypoxemia, such as coarctation of the aorta, pulmonary atresia, reduced cardiac output, bronchial asthma, bronchiectasis, etc.

Anemia

Whilst low levels of hemoglobin (<6 g/dl) are associated with an increase in perinatal mortality, moderate anemia (6–10 g/dl) is associated with a significant decrease in fetal weight.[179] This may be due to a decrease in oxygen transport (sickle cell anemia, etc.) or it may simply be related to poor maternal nutrition.

Urinary tract infection

It has been generally accepted that pyelonephritis during pregnancy causes IUGR.[145]

Autoimmune diseases

The association between systemic lupus erythematosus and IUGR is well known, although it is usually difficult to distinguish between the effects of high doses of glucocorticoids and azathioprine, and vasculitis caused by the disease.[180] On the other hand antiphospholipid (lupus-like) syndrome has been associated with an increase in the incidence of miscarriages, IUGR and intrauterine death.[144,181,182] Serum concentrations of insulin-like growth factor I (IGF-I) and insulin-like growth factor binding protein I (IGFBP-I) are abnormal in the antiphospholipid syndrome.

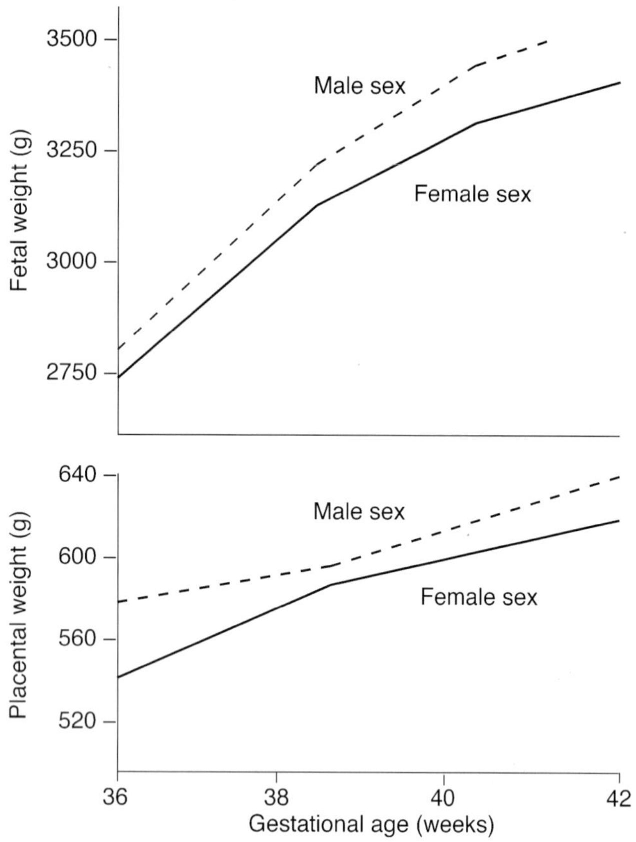

Figure 119.6 Relationship between sex of the neonate and birth weight and placental weight.[29]

Angiotensinogen mutation

Angiotensinogen is the precursor of the vasoactive hormone angiotensin II, which plays an important role in blood pressure regulation, body fluid volume, and vascular remodeling. It has been shown that mutations affecting its gene lead to failed pregnancy volume expansion and fetal growth impairment.[183–185]

Vaginal hemorrhage

North[186] reported an increase in perinatal mortality and in the incidence of small-for-dates neonates in pregnancies complicated by vaginal hemorrhage during the second trimester.

Fetal factors

Fetal sex

It is well known that the birth weight of full-term male infants is an average of 140–150 g higher than that of females (about 4% difference). Consequently, the incidence of IUGR may be higher among females if birth weight curves are not differentiated by sex (Figure 119.6).

Chromosomal abnormalities

Chromosomal abnormalities are accompanied by a high incidence of IUGR.[187,188] Chromosomal defects are identified in approximately 15% of cases of IUGR.

Autosomal abnormalities

Down's syndrome (trisomy 21). Various studies[189,190] have demonstrated that, as compared with normal babies, newborns with trisomy 21 have lower birth weights (about 450 g) and are shorter. The mean birth weight of infants with trisomy 21 is 2725 g.[187] Although the length of gestation is reduced by 7–10 days, this fact cannot account for such a large difference in fetal weight. Because in these cases placental morphology is normal, it may be concluded that IUGR in fetuses with trisomy 21 is related to a decrease in intrinsic fetal growth potential.

Edward's syndrome (trisomy 18). Fetal growth restriction is an outstanding characteristic of this syndrome, and most fetuses are below the 10th percentile at any time of gestation. The mean birth weight of neonates with trisomy 18 is 2333 g.[187]

Patau's syndrome (trisomy 13). Fetal weight is less severely affected than in trisomy 18. The mean birth weight of babies with trisomy 13 is 2400 g.[187]

Segmental chromosome imbalances

All these syndromes are accompanied by a significantly higher incidence of IUGR. Seventy percent of neonates with 5p-cri-du-chat syndrome have a birth weight below the 10th percentile. Fetal growth restriction also occurs in other syndromes, such as monosomy 21, 18p-short arm, and ring chromosome-related abnormalities.[191] Disorders caused by autosomal ruptures, such as Fanconi's anemia and Bloom's syndrome are also associated with fetal growth restriction.

Abnormalities of sex chromosomes

Turner's syndrome (45,X). About one-third of neonates with this defect weigh less than 2500 g at birth.[192] A mean birth weight of 2800 g has been reported in babies with Turner's syndrome.[193] The occurrence of IUGR apparently depends on the presence of mosaicisms in other cell lines and on the abnormal structure of the X chromosome.[194] This karyotype is found in 20% of miscarriages in the first trimester of pregnancy, and it is estimated that 90% of fetuses with Turner's syndrome are not viable.

Multiple X syndromes.

Multiple X syndromes are more frequent than monosomies, i.e., the XXX karyotype is found in 1:1125 female babies born alive, and XYY in 1:700 male infants born alive. Barlow[195] reported that for every extra X chromosome, fetal weight loss is equivalent to 300 g, and that for every extra Y chromosome, fetal weight loss is equivalent to 100 g.

Other chromosomal abnormalities that have been associated with fetal growth restriction are shown in Table 119.4.

Table 119.4 Cytogenetic anomalies that may be associated with intrauterine growth restriction

Ring 1	Ring 9
1q partial trisomy	Ring 18
4p trisomy	18p-
Ap–	18q-
5p–	Ring 21
5q–	Trisomy 22

Inherited syndromes

A variety of diseases of bone dysplasias, e.g., dwarfism (achondroplasia, hypochondroplasia, Russell–Silver syndrome etc.) and chondrodystrophies, osteogenesis imperfecta, etc. have been associated with IUGR. Placental sulfatase deficiency has also been cited in connection with IUGR. With regard to neural tube defects, most studies report low mean weight at birth in cases of both anencephalia (2117 g) and spina bifida cystica (200 to 240 g less than in the control group).[196,197]

Maternofetal radiation

Fetal pathology depends on the x-ray dose and the time of exposure. Radiation effects on fetal weight are related to a large extent to placental damage. Although there are no data for calculating the risk of fetal complications due to unintentional radiation therapy during the first trimester of pregnancy, it seems that the risk increases when the dose exceeds 10 rads. Radiation-induced IUGR may be due to chromosome ruptures, congenital malformations of the central nervous system, inhibition of cell replication, etc.

Intrauterine infection

Embryopathic infectious processes may influence intrinsic fetal growth potential in several ways, either by first affecting the mother, thereby directly affecting the fetus, or by negatively affecting both. When they directly affect the fetus during the stages of organ differentiation, they are capable of causing permanent reductions in the number of cells, thereby causing more or less severe damage to most of the fetal organs (Figure 119.7). According to Knox,[198] 10% of IUGR cases are due to transplacental infection of the fetus. Rubella and cytomegalovirus infection are the most significant, followed by herpes simplex, toxoplasmosis, paludism, congenital syphilis, and other acute bacterial infections.

Rubella infection illustrates the pathogenesis of IUGR. During primary viremia the virus affects at the placenta, causing villous placentitis and lesion of the vascular endothelium. Continued viral replication with secondary viremia may then follow.[199] Viral fetal invasion determines direct inhibition of cell replication, obliterans angiopathy, chromosomal ruptures and cytolysis. These abnormalities together with chronic ischemia derived from vascular placental lesions would explain IUGR. Sixty percent of neonates with congenital rubella have a birth weight below the 10th percentile.[200] Viral replication also affects postnatal growth. In these cases, continued viral secretion after childbirth has been documented. With regard to cytomegalovirus infection, IUGR is found in 35% of cases.[201] It seems that there is a relationship between severity of infection and frequency of fetal growth restriction.

On the contrary chlamydia pneumonia infection is unlikely to play a role in the pathogenesis of IUGR.[202]

Twin pregnancies

This is one of the most frequent causes of IUGR. In all series of IUGR, twin pregnancies account for 20% of cases.[203] The intrauterine growth curve of twin pregnancies is similar to that of singleton pregnancies until week 33 of gestation; from then on, the curve for monozygotic twins diverges whilst that of dizygotic twins does so between weeks 35 and 36. Weight discrepancy in twin pregnancies may be due to twin-to-twin transfusion (severe anemia in the 'donor' twin), but most frequently to placental problems (unequal nutritional supply due to a smaller placenta, marginal insertion of the cord, etc.). Poor perinatal outcome has been reported for the 'smaller' twin.[204,205]

Immunological factors

In 1953, Medawar,[206] a specialist in transplantation, considered for the first time the product of conception as a 'grafted' tissue and argued that a mechanism preventing rejection of the placenta by the maternal immune system has to exist to allow viviparity. The lack of normal HLA antigenic expression in the trophoblast is probably the principal mechanism. HLA-G expression protects trophoblastic cells from maternal recognition and immunological response to incompatibility.[207] From an immunological point of view, it is currently accepted that there is active signaling between embryonic and maternal tissue even before implantation of the fertilized egg. An embryonic secretion product, presumably platelet activating factor, induces the release of early pregnancy factor (a sign of immunosuppression),[208] which, in turn, stimulates the secretion of leukocytic molecules responsible for the suppression of T cell function.

In animal models, 'dwarf's syndrome' or Runt's syndrome refers to weight restriction as a result of an exacerbated host-vs.-graft reaction. In human beings it is also possible that immunological mechanisms could play an important role in some forms of IUGR. Some findings include weight restriction found in fetuses undergoing intrauterine transfusion, an

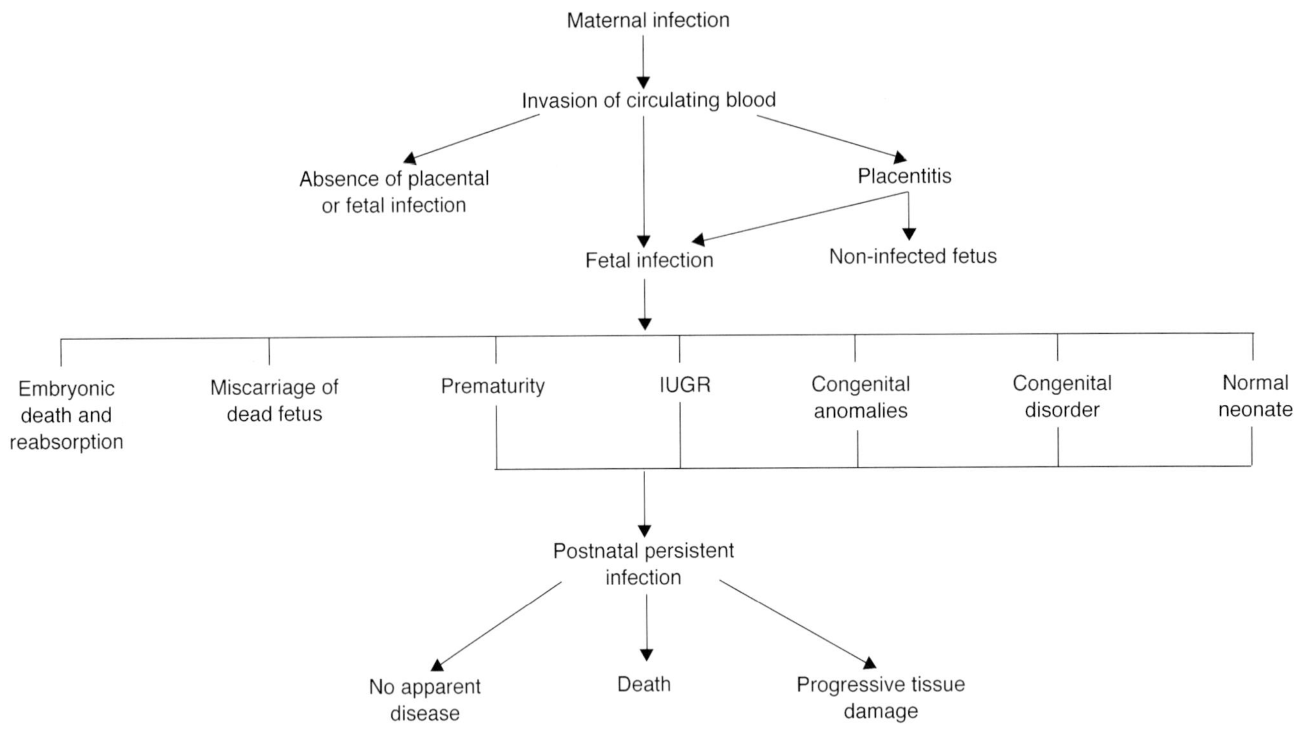

Figure 119.7 Pathogenesis and outcome of fetal infection. IUGR, intrauterine growth restriction.

increase in congenital anomalies in gestations with incompatibility against human leukocyte antigen (HL-A), and the similarity of placental histological features in some case of IUGR with those seen in animals with the dwarf's syndrome.[209]

Some findings suggest that reproduction efficacy may be affected by maternofetal 'genetic disparity'. Jones[210] indicated that mean placental weight was lower in gestations with probable genetic disparity regarding the fetus, and found a higher incidence of low weight fetuses in patients with leukoagglutinins. In contrast, larger placentas are found in male fetuses from primiparas in cases of ABO incompatibility. Billington[211] demonstrated in mice that genetic disparity in hybrid animals caused significantly larger placentas than in pure lineage animals. Findings in humans also indicate that genetic similarity may be an etiological factor of IUGR; newborns of incestuous unions and of first cousins weigh 200–300 g less than normal. The fact of a lower weight of female fetuses as compared with males has been attributed by Ounsted and Ounsted[212] to a certain antigenicity of the Y chromosome.

Based on these data, the concept originally proposed by Walton and Hammond[213] has been broadened, suggesting that intrauterine growth is mainly controlled by two variables; that is, genetic disparity between mother and fetus, and predetermined stimulus of maternal regulator. Independently of the immunological mechanism involved, signs of immune depression that may persist up to 9 months after childbirth are found in many small-for-gestational age neonates.[214,215]

Interval between pregnancies

There is a decrease in both, duration of gestation and fetal weight, when the time passed between the last delivery and the new pregnancy is less than 2 years or more than 6 years.[216] The incidence of infants with low weight at birth is higher in women with short intervals between gestations.

Fetal order at birth

Fetal growth restriction occurs more often in first-born neonates, particularly when the mother is very young or old. The second or third child of the same mother usually weighs more than the first child. Mean fetal and placental weights in multiparas are significantly higher than in primiparas (at 40 weeks, 3.4% and 2.5%, respectively). The first pregnancy may well determine a true maturation of uterine structures, especially the vessels, which become more sensitive to gestational stimuli resulting in improved local conditions in subsequent gestations. On the other hand, and according to data of Scott and Usher,[217] the probability of fetuses with IUGR increases in relation to the number of previous gestations with low birth weight neonates (Figure 119.8).

Uteroplacental factors

Uterine anomalies

Congenital uterine anomalies, in particular uterus bicornuate and septate uterus, are consistently associated

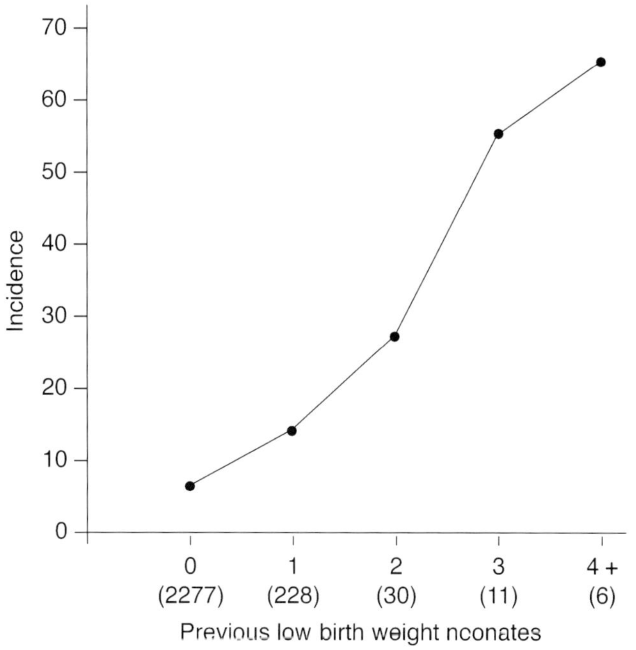

Figure 119.8 Incidence of fetal growth restriction in the current pregnancy according to number of previous gestations with low birth weight neonates. The total number of current gestations studied in each group is given in parentheses.[218]

with IUGR,[218] accounting for approximately 1–3% of cases.[219] Although Scott and Usher[217] did not find statistically significant differences in neonatal birth weight between pregnant women with and without uterine fibromyoma, other authors[219] reported uterine fibromas in 1–5% of cases of IUGR. Uterine synechiae have not been related to IUGR.[218]

Placental anomalies

Anomalous cord insertion

Sotelo-Avila and Shanklin[220,221] studied the relationship between the site of cord insertion and IUGR. The incidence of full-term small-for-dates neonates was significantly higher in cases of anomalous cord insertion. Velamentous insertion of the cord is a well-defined pathologic entity, with an 1% estimated frequency. This anomaly accounts for approximately 12% of cases of IUGR. Fetal growth restriction has also been associated with marginal and markedly eccentric insertions of the cord.

Abnormalities of placental form

The girdle placenta is the only abnormality of placental form associated with a high incidence of small-for-gestational age birth. A phenomenon of secondary placental growth to compensate for an early placental insufficiency seems to be confirmed by the observation by Shanklin and Sotelo-Avila[221] of a decreased superficial cord vasculature.

Abnormalities of placental site

It is well known that placenta previa, especially total and partial placenta previa, is associated with a higher frequency of IUGR.[222]

Tumors

Vascular tumors originating from extra-embryonic primitive mesenchyma, mainly hemangiomas and hamartomas, have been associated with an increased incidence of growth restriction.[56,220] It has been suggested that the effect on fetal growth is exerted through placental insufficiency[56,223] resulting from a considerable portion of fetal blood flow passing through the tumor rather than through functional placental tissue. However, arteriovenous shunting as a cause of IUGR and even fetal death has been proposed by other authors.[220,221,224] Although it has been insisted that there is a frequent association between these tumors and growth restriction and also with congenital anomalies, Fox[225] considered the latter improbable. In large tumors, cardiomegaly and cardiovascular insufficiency is a prominent complication in neonates due to increased peripheral resistance of the placental vasculature.

Single umbilical artery

The absence of one umbilical artery has an incidence of 1% in singleton pregnancies and up to 7–14% in twin pregnancies. Malformations are present in about 15–20% of fetuses with a single umbilical artery syndrome and can affect any organ system. They are accompanied by IUGR,[226] particularly when they are associated with trisomies. Growth restriction is caused by reduced fetoplacental blood flow.

Parabiotic syndrome

Monochorionic multiple gestations place the fetuses at risk of twin transfusion syndrome. In such cases an arteriovenous shunt is present at the placental level between the two members of the set. Under those conditions, one fetus, the donor, provides the major share of the blood supply to its co-twin. As pregnancy progresses, this major physiopathologic change in the fetal blood volume causes the donor fetus to become anemic and growth-restricted, whilst the recipient twin becomes fluid-overloaded, polycythemic and cardiomegalic.

Placental mosaicism

Numerous cases of placental aneuploidies have been described, particularly trisomies 2, 7, 9, 10, 12, 13, 15, 16 and 18,[227–230] that have been associated with miscarriages, growth restriction and fetal death, despite the fact that fetuses were chromosomally normal. Kalousek and Dill[227] have suggested that the occurrence of non-disjunction at random in the very early stages after conception could give rise to mosaicism in the placenta or in the fetus.

There is a high correlation between the number of aneuploid cells found in cultured villi and the number confirmed in studies of the placenta at term. These data are also relevant for fetal outcome. Thus, growth restriction (80% of cases) and fetal death (20–30% of cases) normally need only be feared in cases of high levels of mosaicism (more than 35% of cells involved).[231,232] For this reason, it has been suggested that, at least in part, the length of gestation and fetal survival depends upon the ratio of euploid cells to aneuploid cells in the placenta. Many other conceptions are, however, aborted before 22 weeks of gestation. There are nevertheless case reports of normal fetuses.[233,234] Fetal outcome may be related to the effect of uniparental dysomy. Some authors[235,236] have shown a threefold increase in mosaicism confined to the placenta in growth-restricted fetuses (25%) as compared with neonates with normal birth weight (8%). Placental molecular reports support the concept of a clear biological effect of chromosome mosaicism on fetal growth.[236,237]

Pathogenesis

All different etiological factors related to IUGR act through common pathogenetic mechanisms. Based on studies in animal models,[238–240] three basic etiopathogenic mechanisms are currently recognized: (a) decrease in intrinsic fetal growth potential, (b) uteroplacental vascular insufficiency, and (c) fetal malnutrition secondary to maternal malnutrition.

Decrease in intrinsic fetal growth potential

Intrinsic fetal growth potential relies upon genetic material, sex and anatomy of the fetus, and length of gestation. Different etiological factors, such as those of genetic or chromosomal origin, embryopathic infectious processes (rubella, cytomegalovirus, toxoplasmosis, syphilis, paludism, etc.), and toxic habits or radioactive agents begin to exert their influence from the time of conception, or at least from the embryonic stage, acting on fetal metabolism and organogenesis. In these circumstances, although the placental maternal blood supply remains unaffected, the fetus is unable to progress. However, genetic potential accounts for about 35–40% of variations in fetal weight.

Growth restriction may result from a single genetic defect (e.g., cystic fibrosis, phenylketonuria) or a polygenic multifactorial action, which would explain the majority of height and weight variations of 'hereditary' type. The influence of chromosomal-related factors on fetal weight is probably exerted by affecting the duration of some periods (G_1 or G_2) of the cell cycle. Studies in rats have shown that chromosomal antigenic inequality (Y trophoblast and XX decidua) would apparently explain greater trophoblastic plugs in male eggs and greater development subsequently.

Abnormalities of placental nutrients and oxygen supply

Etiopathogenic mechanisms that cause a deficient supply of oxygen and/or nutrients through the placenta are included in this section. In addition to chronic hypoxia and fetal malnutrition secondary to maternal malnutrition already mentioned, uteroplacental insufficiency deserves particular attention.

Uteroplacental insufficiency

This includes those factors capable of affecting maternal–fetal–placental exchange as a result of (a) impaired uterine perfusion due to anomalies of the terminal uterine branches, and (b) a deficient exchange surface due to villous microcirculatory anomalies.

Impaired uterine perfusion due to physiological changes. Uterine vasculature undergoes a series of modifications, that is, an increase in uterine circulation with arterial and venous hypertrophy and hyperplasia, in order to increase blood flow from 50 ml/min at 10 weeks of gestation to 600 ml/min at term. Main changes after implantation consist in the formation of the intervillous space and trophoblastic infiltration of the spiral arteries.

Trophoblastic infiltration produces fibrinoid degeneration with disruption of the musculoelastic wall,[241] and adrenergic denervation of uterine vessels with a marked decrease in sympathetic neurotransmitters.[242] These changes are accompanied by vasodilation and inhibition of platelet aggregation in relation to the effects of prostacyclin[243,244] released by placental vascular endothelial cells (Figure 119.9). Local decrease of the thromboxane/prostacyclin index as an adaptative mechanism prevents spiral artery thrombosis and subsequent placental infarction. As a consequence of trophoblastic activity, the spiral arteries are converted into a low-resistance, high-flow vascular bed. Prostacyclin also favors a phenomenon of vascular insensitivity.[245]

Partial or total replacement of the normal musculoelastic wall by fibrinoid material has the following effects: (a) widening of spiral arteries (30-fold as compared with non-pregnant women) which confers greater capacity and an infundibuliform aspect to these vessels; (b) reduced vascular resistance of the placental bed, which therefore determines a higher adaptation capacity of spiral arteries for increasing blood flow; and (c) decrease or abolition of the vasoconstriction response to stimuli of adrenergic agents (catecholamines, etc.) or to stimuli of the autonomic nervous system. Control of uteroplacental circulation is mainly exerted on radial rather than on spiral arteries.

Impaired uterine perfusion due to pathological changes. Uteroplacental insufficiency takes place during the last weeks of gestation (because of a deprived supply line according to Gruenwald[246]) that justifies a decrease in fetal growth rate around the 37th gestational week. This 'physiological' insufficiency is

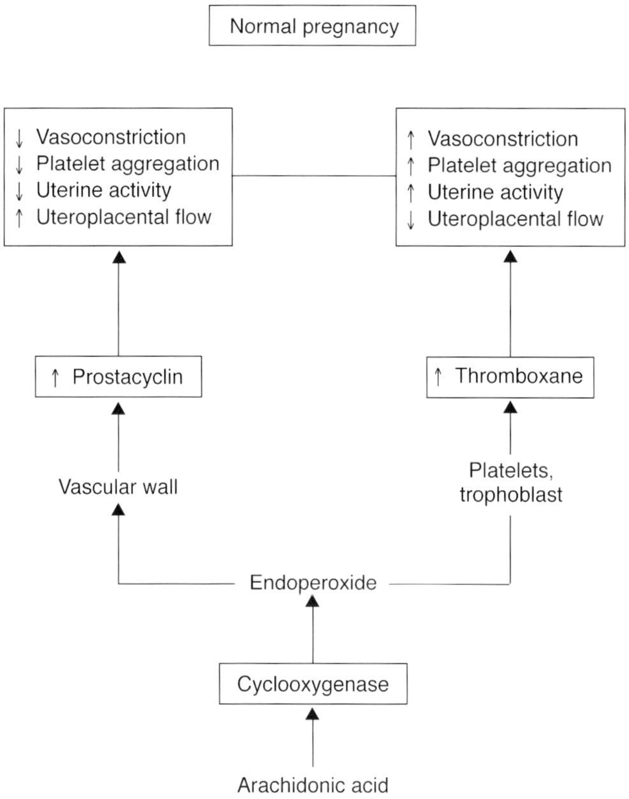

Figure 119.9 Normal gestation. A balanced thromboxane/prostacyclin index guarantees an adequate uteroplacental blood flow. As compared with pregestational status, there is a decrease of this index in the systemic circulation with a clear enhancement of prostacyclin-related vasodilation and inhibition of platelet aggregation.

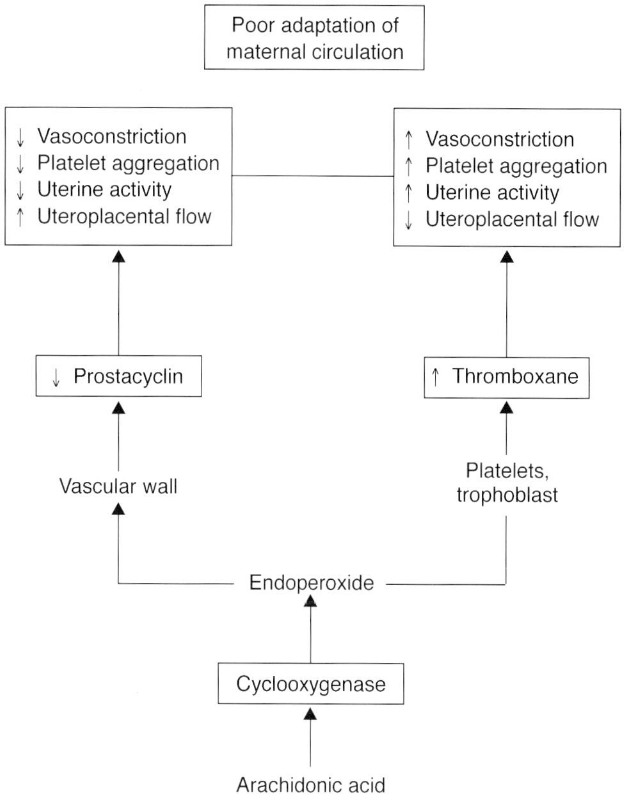

Figure 119.10 In gestations with 'poor adaptation of maternal circulation', there is a pathological increase in the thromboxane/prostacyclin index leading to an increase in systemic resistance, platelet aggregation and uterine activity, all of which cause a decrease in uteroplacental blood flow.

related to inability of the maternal environment to satisfy fetal needs despite the fetal capacity to maintain growth rate. Early or enhanced 'physiological' uteroplacental insufficiency accounts for about 35% of cases of growth restriction.[247]

The sequence of events leading to impaired uterine perfusion is probably initiated by a pathologic increase in the thromboxane/prostacyclin index in the intervillous space secondary to reduced prostacyclin production,[243] resulting in discontinuation of trophoblastic infiltration of the spiral arteries[248] and preservation of their vasomotor activity.[241,249] As a consequence of impaired trophoblastic activity there is an early reduction of uteroplacental blood flow.

Moreover, alterations in systemic maternal circulation include a decrease in prostacyclin levels and a relative increase in thromboxane (TX_2). An unbalanced thromboxane/prostacyclin index leads to an increase in vascular resistance and vasopressor sensitivity, and a reduction of plasma volume. This cascade (Figure 119.10) seems to be precipitated by a reduced prostacyclin production,[250–252] which is further supported by the finding of statistically significant decreases (50%) of prostaglandin I_2 in pre-eclampsia.[253] In addition, there is an activation of coagulation with increased platelet aggregability, thrombopenia etc., as well as general and local vasoconstriction (vasospasm, hypertension, etc.) leading to decreased systemic blood flow and, in short, to a reduction in uteroplacental blood flow and IUGR.[250,254] At the level of the uteroplacental circulation, there is also a specific decrease in prostacyclins, probably mediated by a local paracrine mechanism resulting from high epinephrine and norepinephrine concentrations in the maternal portion of the placenta.

On the other hand, specific changes in the vascular endothelium resulting from insufficient trophoblastic activity include alterations of permeability (responsible for fibrin and lipid deposits) and a decrease in the local synthesis of prostacyclin and other factors, such as endothelial-derived relaxing factor, nitric acid and C-protein (anticoagulant), with a simultaneous increase in vascular endothelial growth factor (VEGF), asymmetric dimethylargine (ADMA), an endogenous inhibitor of endothelial nitric oxide synthase,[255,256] and platelet-derived growth factor. All these factors will favor acute atherosis, vasoconstriction, and activation of coagulation. Lipid deposits are frequently accompanied by IgG, IgM and complement deposits and perivascular lymphomonocytic infiltration resulting from a maternal immunitary reaction against antigens from the endovascular trophoblastic cells (Figure 119.11).

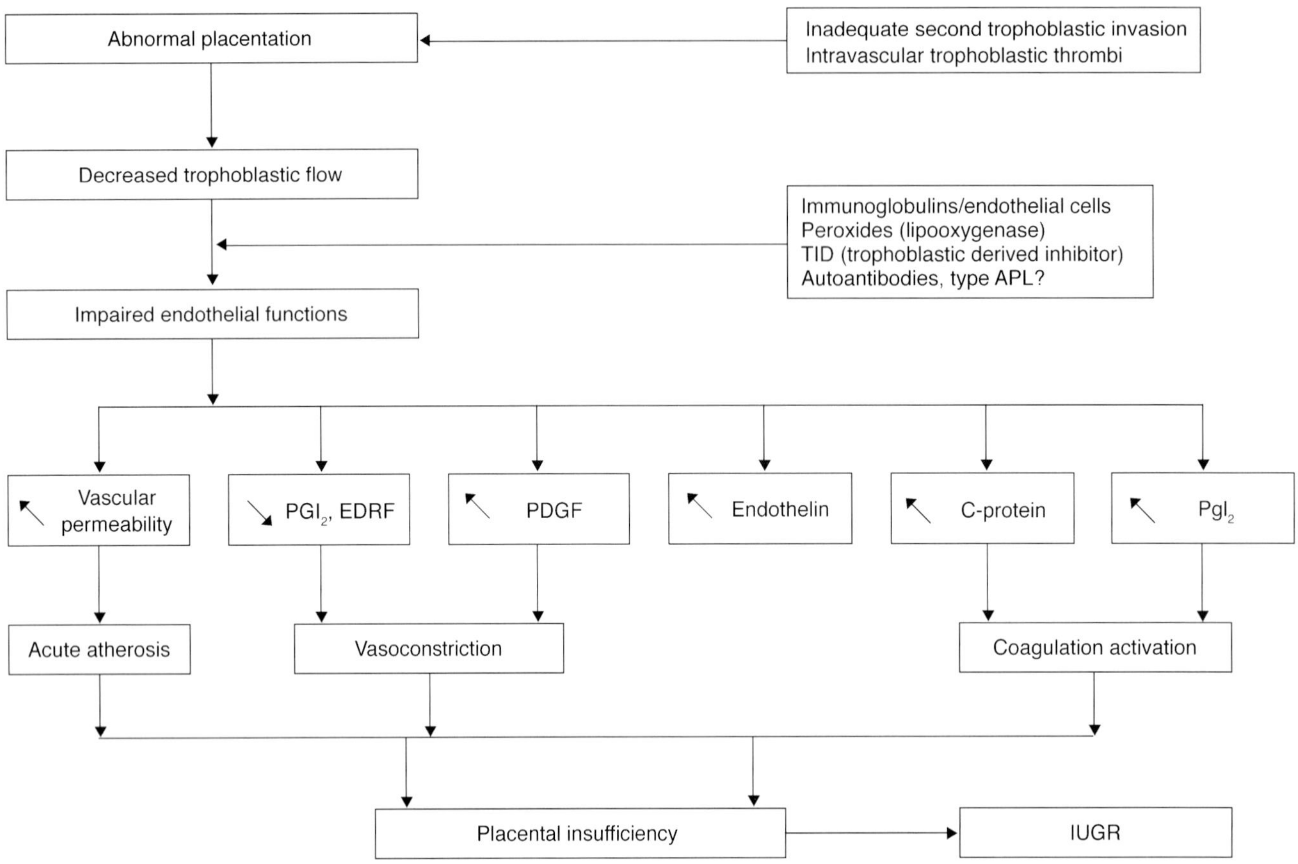

Figure 119.11 Summary of the physiopathologic hypothesis of intrauterine growth restriction (IUGR) of vascular cause. APL, antiphospholipid antibody; PGI_2, prostaglandin I_2; EDRF, endothelial-derived relaxing factor; PGDF, platelet-derived growth factor; VEGF, vascular endothelial growth; ADMA, asymmetric dimethylargine.

In cases of pre-eclampsia with or without IUGR, an immunologically mediated deficiency in trophoblast invasion of the spiral arteries of the placental bed leads to a poorly perfused fetoplacental unit. The subsequent secretion of VEGF into the maternal circulation leads to activation of the vascular endothelium. Galatzios[257] observed a correlation between raised umbilical cord serum VEGF levels and the development of pre-eclampsia, and in some circumstances of IUGR and preterm delivery. On the other hand, Sawidon[258] observed a correlation between elevated concentrations of ADMA and the same pathologies.

Subclinical placental infection may cause the release of inflammatory cytokines,[259] which, in turn, cause an overproduction of VEGF in the placenta, which may lead to IUGR.

The correlation between serum levels of antiphospholipid antibodies and fetal morbidity including IUGR has been demonstrated in different studies.[260–262] From a biological point of view, antiphospholipid antibodies increase the risk of venous and arterial thrombosis, and inhibit local synthesis of prostacyclins.

Impaired uterine perfusion finally causes hypoxic ischemia in the intervillous space, with secondary vasoconstriction of villi arterioles. In this case, changes in uterine blood flow velocity waveforms may be detected in Doppler studies before changes are detected in umbilical velocity waveforms, as occurs for example in patients with pre-eclampsia.

Deficient transplacental transport of amino acids. The level of most amino acids is higher in the fetal circulation than in maternal plasma, reflecting that there are transportation systems of amino acids through the trophoblastic cells. IUGR is associated with reduced plasma concentrations of a number of amino acids despite normal or higher maternal concentrations than in normal pregnancies.[263] Whether this is a cause or a consequence of the IUGR remains unclear, but some evidence shows that hypoxia can downregulate amino acid transporter expression and activity in cultured human trophoblastic cells.[264]

Deficient exchange surface. The main pathologic finding is a significant decrease in the number of arterioles of the tertiary villi,[265] which may be the result of two basic pathogenetic mechanisms: (a) lack of formation of arterioles, due to interference in the process of placental maturational angiogenesis,[266] or (b) obliteration, secondary to a thromboembolic or vasospastic phenomenon.[267,268] In both cases, the cause of these changes may ultimately lie in a decrease in uterine perfusion, or in the fetus itself through changes in vascular resistance mediated by poorly understood biochemical or reflex mechanisms.[267,269,270] In these cases, changes in umbilical velocity waveforms may be detected in Doppler studies whilst uterine blood flow velocity waveforms are unaffected.[271–274] The current theory is that prolonged reduction in maternal intervillus flow, and hence oxygen delivery, would result in prolonged vasoconstriction with secondary reduction in stem villus luminal diameter, increased flow resistance and vascular medial hypertrophy.[268,275–277]

Fetal malnutrition secondary to maternal malnutrition

This is one of the main causes of IUGR. Deprivation of adequate fetal nutrition alters cellular homeostasis. Limited bioavailability of amino acids for protein synthesis is the origin of a series of modifications. Nucleotides are subtracted from DNA synthesis and diverted to RNA synthesis, which is manifested by high and low activities of the enzymes RNA-polymerase and DNA-polymerase, respectively. However, despite increased RNA synthesis, total cellular concentration is low due to an increase in RNA hydrolysis, manifested by an increase in alkaline RNAase.

Because each organ has a different growth pattern, acme of cell division indexes are not synchronized, giving rise to different periods of vulnerability for each organ or system. When data obtained in rats are extrapolated to human beings, considering that human growth is mostly hyperplastic, the consequences of growth restriction appear especially discouraging, in particular for brain development. However, some differences between growth in rats and human fetuses should be mentioned. In humans, the speed of cell division is lower, so that the effects of malnutrition would be less severe during the same period of time. Neuroblastic proliferation also occurs in a highly protected period (prior to 20 weeks' gestation) when factors affecting fetal growth are not usually present. Injury late in pregnancy is associated with underdevelopment of the cerebellum, nerve cell synapses, and dendritic arborization, which may be as important as a reduction in the number of neurons.

Specific effects of malnutrition on cell growth and fetal development depend on the stage at which the adverse factor begins to affect the fetus (Figure 119.12) and the mechanisms involved. Malnutrition early in pregnancy during the stage of cell proliferation or hyperplasia causes inhibition of the cell division index. This results in irreversible size reduction and a decrease in the number of cells of an organ. Malnutrition during the stage of cell hypertrophy causes growth deceleration, with recovery taking place once the adverse factor has been corrected, resulting in an organ of normal volume. In general terms, there is an association between a high rate of cell division and the intensity of effects of the growth-limiting factor.

With regard to the mechanisms involved, evidence is based on experimental studies. Severe protein restriction in rats[278,279] produced symmetrical and harmonious growth restriction (all organs were affected, including the brain). There was a 20% decrease in the animals' weights, and a number of biochemical changes were found. These included a decrease in protein, DNA and RNA concentrations in all organs, which was proportional to the decrease in the animals' weights. A decrease in DNA-polymerase activity was followed by an increase in alkaline RNAase activity. In all brain specimens examined, there was a reduced number of neuroglial elements and neurons,[280] as well as decreased DNA concentrations. The magnitude of these biochemical and cellular changes was related to the degree of protein deprivation and the stage at which restriction began.

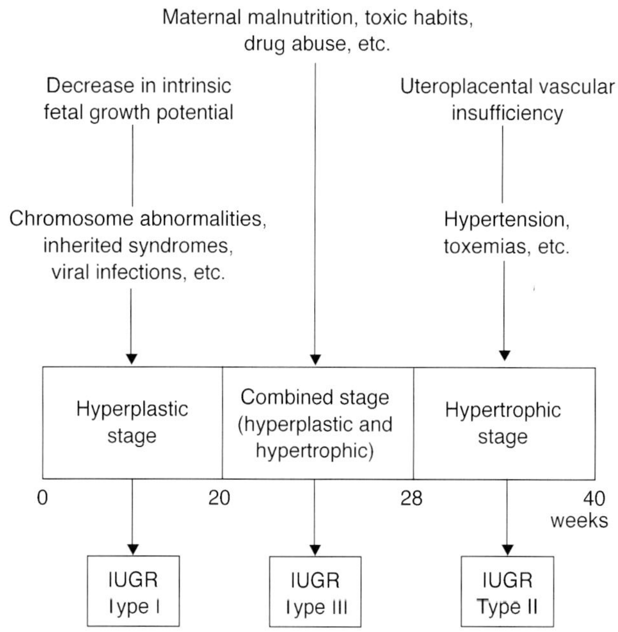

Figure 119.12 Pathogenesis and classification of intrauterine growth restriction (IUGR) (stage at which the adverse factor begins to affect the fetus, affected stages, and types of IUGR).

In studies of selectively induced uteroplacental vascular insufficiency, ligation of the uterine artery providing blood supply to the rat uterine horn produced growth restriction of fetuses implanted in that horn.[281,282] In these animals, IUGR was asymmetrical or disharmonious (not all organs were equally affected). Whilst the liver only reached half of the normal size and showed an almost complete glycogen depletion, the brain was practically unaffected. Biochemical abnormalities included marked decrease in DNA, RNA and proteins in the fetal liver, high RNAase activity both in the liver and the brain, and almost unchanged RNA concentration and negligible and transiently increased RNase activity in the brain.

Extrapolation of findings of cell growth reduction in animal models to human beings should be carried out with caution. As a matter of fact, weights of neonates (3500 g) born to women with a mean weight of 60 kg accounts for 5.8% of the maternal weight, whereas rats weighing 200 g give birth to 10 animals of 5 g each, which is 25% of the rat maternal weight. On the other hand, the length of gestation in experimental animals is significantly shorter, and the intensity of nutritional and vascular restrictions is unusual in human beings.

Two aspects, however, should be commented on. Biochemical and cellular changes found in rats with intense protein restriction and subsequent IUGR can be due to a decrease in primary fetal growth and/or caused by maternal nutritional deficiency. Since causative factors act early during the whole gestational period, symmetrical and harmonious growth restriction occur in both cases, that is, all organs are similarly affected. Differences in the intensity and course of injury would also explain moderate anthropomorphic variations between the two types of growth restriction.

Studies in humans are consistent with this interpretation. Naeye[283] reported significantly lower weights of brains from fetuses born after 33 weeks in a group of low maternal weight and poor weight gain during pregnancy as compared with a group of normal or high maternal weight and marked weight gain. By contrast, biochemical and cellular changes found in different organs in cases of IUGR derived from uteroplacental insufficiency are very similar to those described in rats undergoing ligation of the uterine artery. In these circumstances, in which the causative factor acts late in pregnancy beyond the hyperplastic stage of growth, IUGR is asymmetrical and disharmonious, and the brain is practically unaffected.

Differences in postnatal behavior between both groups are in agreement with this pathogenetic assumption. Campbell[284] found that the earlier fetal growth restriction occurred, the more affected were cephalometric parameters recorded during ultrasound scanning. At follow-up, a higher percentage of children had heights, head circumferences and weights below the 10th percentile throughout childhood as compared with normal children. When growth restriction began prior to week 26, not only was somatic growth impaired, but also in many cases intellectual development was affected, whereas in late IUGR with almost normal cephalometric profiles, postnatal somatic and intellectual development was usually normal.

REFERENCES

1. Butler NR, Alberman ED. Stillbirth and early and late neonatal mortality rates by maternal smoking habit. The second report of the British Perinatal Mortality Survey (1958). In Butler NR, Alberman ED, eds. *Perinatal Problems.* London: Churchill Livingstone, 1969.
2. Abdul-Karim RW, Beydoun SN. Growth of the human fetus. *Clin Obstet Gynecol* 1974;17:37–52.
3. Love EJ, Kinch RA. Factors influencing the birth weight in normal pregnancy. *Am J Obstet Gynecol* 1965;91:342–9.
4. Ounsted C, Ounsted M. Effect of Y chromosome on fetal growth care. *Lancet* 1970;2:857–8.
5. Fabre E, González de Agüero R, Sobreviela M. Dieta materna y crecimiento fetal. *Prog Obstet Ginecol* 1993;36(Suppl):S19–39.
6. Abdul-Karim RW, Beydoum SN. Growth of the human fetus. *Clin Obstet Gynecol* 1974;17:37–52.
7. Wilcox MA, Newton CS, Johnson IR. Paternal influences on birth weight. *Acta Obstet Gynecol Scand* 1995;74:15–8.
8. Lechtig A, Klein RE. Prenatal nutrition and birth weight: is there a casual association? In Dobbing JE, ed. *Maternal Nutrition in Pregnancy: Eating for Two?* London: Academic Press, 1981:131–56.
9. Lechtig A, Habicht JP, Delgado H, Klein RE, Yarbrourgh C, Martorell R. Effect of food supplementation during pregnancy on birth weight. *Pediatrics* 1975;56:508–20.
10. Junis KA, Beydoun H, Tiamim H. Maternal predictors of small-for-gestational-age in uncomplicated births. *Int J Gynaecol Obstet* 2002;79:33–5.
11. Pritchard CW, Sutherland HW, Carr-Hill RA. Birthweight and paternal height. *Br J Obstet Gynecol* 1983;90:156–61.
12. Ounsted M, Ounsted C. Maternal regulation of intrauterine growth. *Nature* 1968;87:777–81.
13. Leff M, Orleans M, Haverkampt AD. The association of maternal low birthweight and infant low birthweight in racially mixed population. *Paediatr Perinat Epidemiol* 1992;6:51–61.
14. Hackman E, Emanuel I, Van Belle G, Daling J. Maternal birth weight and subsequent pregnancy outcome. *J Am Med Assoc* 1983;250:2016–9.
15. Klebanov MA, Graubard BI, Kesser SS. Low birth weight across generations. *J Am Med Assoc* 1984;252:2423–7
16. Simpson JW, Lawless RW, Cameron A. Responsibility of the obstetrician to the fetus: Influence of pre-pregnancy weight and pregnancy weight gain on birth weight. *Obstet Gynecol* 1975; 45:481–7.
17. Abrams BF, Laros RK. Pre-pregnancy weight, weight gain and birth weight. *Am J Obstet Gynecol* 1986;154:503–9.
18. Lehmann V, Rotte K, Schmidt CH. The correlation between maternal heart volume, placental weight and infant's birth weight in poor intrauterine fetal growth. In Salvadori B, Bacchi-Modena A, eds. *Poor Intrauterine Fetal Growth.* Parma: Minerva Médica, 1977:123–5.
19. Scheive LA, Cogsvell ME, Scanlon KS. Maternal weight gain and preterm delivery: differential effects by body mass index. *Epidemilogy* 1999;10:141–7.
20. Wolfe HM, Zador IE, Gross TL, Martier SS, Sokol RJ. The clinical utility of maternal body mass index in pregnancy. *Am J Obstet Gynecol* 1991;164:1306–10.
21. Abrams B, Newman V, Key T, Parker J. Maternal weight gain and preterm delivery. *Obstet Gynecol* 1989;74:577–83.
22. Singer JE, Westphal M, Niswander K. Relationship of weight gain in pregnancy to birth weight and infant growth development in the first year of life. *Obstet Gynecol* 1968;31:417–23.
23. Niswander KR, Singer J, Westphal M, Weiss W. Weight gain during pregnancy and pre-pregnancy weight: association with birth weight of term gestation. *Obstet Gynecol* 1969;33:482–91.
24. Hediger ML, Scholl TO, Belsky DH, Ances IG, Salmon RW. Patterns of weight gain in adolescent pregnancy: effects on birth weight and preterm delivery. *Obstet Gynecol* 1989;74:6–12.
25. Duvekot JJ, Cheriex EC, Pieters AA, Menheere PC, Schouten HJ, Peeters LL. Maternal volume homeostasis in early pregnancy in relation to fetal growth restriction. *Obstet Gynecol* 1995;85:361–7.
26. Wilkox M, Gardosi J, Mongelli M. Birth weight from pregnancies dated by ultrasound in a multicultural British population. *Br Med J* 1993;307:588–91.
27. Gruenwald P. Chronic fetal distress and placental insufficiency. *Biol Neonate* 1963;5:215–21.
28. Naylor AF, Myrianthopoulos NC. The relation of ethnic and selected socioeconomic factors to human birth weight. *Ann Hum Genet* 1967;31:71–83.
29. Hendricks CH. Patterns of fetal and placental growth: the second half of fetal pregnancy. *Obstet Gynecol* 1964;24:357–65.
30. Polani PE. Chromosomal and other genetic influences on birth weight variations. In Elliot K, Knight E, eds. *Size at Birth.* Amsterdam: Associated Scientific Publishers, 1979:127–64.
31. Humphrey M, Holzheimer D. Fetal growth charts of aboriginal foetuses. *Aust NZ J Obstet Gynaecol* 2000;40(4):388–93.

32. Bakketeig LS, Hoffman HJ, Harley EE. The tendency to repeat gestational age and birth weight in successive births. *Am J Obstet Gynecol* 1979;135:1086–103.
33. Emanuel I, Filakti H, Alberman E, Evans SJ. Intergenerational studies of human birthweight from the 1958 birth cohort. 1. Evidence for a multigenerqational effect. *Br J Obstet Gynecol* 1992;99:67–74.
34. Klebanoff MA, Schulsinger C, Mednick BR, Secher NJ. Preterm and small for gestational age birth across generations. *Am J Obstet Gynecol* 1997;176:521–6.
35. Ounstead M, Ounstead C. Rate of intrauterine growth. *Nature* 1968;220:599–600.
36. Ghezzi F, Tibiletti MG, Raio L, Di Naro E. Idiopathic fetal IUGR: A possible inheritance pattern. *Prenat Diagn* 2003;23:259–65.
37. Birch H, Gussow J. *Disadvantaged Children: Health Nutrition and School Failure*. New York: Grune & Stratton, 1970.
38. Lechtig A, Yarbrough C, Delgado H, Martorell R, Klein RE, Behar M. Effect of moderate maternal malnutrition on the placenta. *Am J Obstet Gynecol* 1975;123:191–201.
39. Taylor SE, Seeman TE. Psychosocial resources and the SES-health relationship. *Ann N Y Acad Sci* 1999;22:210–55.
40. Gregg EW, Kriska AM, Narayan KM, Knowler W. Relationship of locus of control to physical activity among people with and without diabetes. *Diabetes Care* 1996;19:1118–21.
41. Walker LO, Cooney AT, Riggs MW. Psychosocial and demographic factors related to health behaviors in the first trimester. *J Obstet Gynecol Neonatal Nurs* 1999;28:606–14.
42. Riini CK, Dunkel-Schetter C, Wadwa PD, Sandman CA. Psychosocial adaptation and birth outcomes: the role of personal resources, stress and socio-cultural context in pregnancy. *Health Psychol* 1999;18:333–45.
43. Eggleston E, Ong A, Kotelchuk M. Unintended pregnancy and low birthweight in Ecuador. *Am J Public Health* 2001;91: 808–10.
44. Durousseau S, Chavez GF. Associations of intrauterine growth restriction among term infants and maternal pregnancy intendedness, initial happiness about being pregnant and sense of control. *Pediatrics* 2003;111:1171–5.
45. Samuelson G. Dietary habits and nutritional status in adolescents over Europe. An overview of current studies in the Nordic countries. *Eur J Clin Nutr* 2000;54:S21–8.
46. Norska J. Causes of intrauterine fetal distrophy. In Salvadori B, Bacchi-Modena A, eds. *Poor Intrauterine Fetal Growth*. Parma: Minerva Médica, 1977:137–9.
47. Aatrs MC, Vingerhoet AJ. Psychosocial factors and intrauterine fetal growth: a prospective analysis. *J Psychosom Obstet Gynecol* 1993;14:249–58.
48. Lobel M, De Vincent CJ, Kaminer A, Meyer BA. The impact of prenatal stress and optimistic disposition on birth outcomes in medically high-risk women. *Health Psychol* 200;19:544–53.
49. Sable MR, Wilkinson DS. The impact of major stress, major live events and pregnancy attitudes on low birth weight. *Fam Plann Perspect* 2000;32:288–94.
50. Stanford JB, Hobbs R, James P, De Witt MJ, Fisher RC. Defining dimensions of pregnancy intendedness. *Matern Child Health J* 2000;4:83–190.
51. Simpson JL. Are physical activity and employment related to preterm birth and low birthweight? *Am J Obstet Gynecol* 1993;168:1231–8.
52. Dye TD, Fernandez ID, Rains A, Fershteyn Z. Recent studies in the epidemiological assessment of physical activity, fetal growth and preterm delivery: A narrative review. *Clin Obstet Gynecol* 2003;45:415–22.
53. Smith CA, Steinbach HL. The effect of wartime starvation in Holland upon pregnancy and its products. *Am J Obstet Gynecol* 1947;53:599.
54. Smith CA. Effects of maternal undernutrition upon the newborn infant in Holland 1944–1945. *J Pediatr* 1947;30:229.
55. Hammond J. Physiological factors affecting birth weight. *Proc Nutr Soc* 1944;2:8.
56. Gruenwald P. Growth of the human fetus. I. Normal growth and its variation. *Am J Obstet Gynecol* 1966;94:1112–9.
57. Gruenwald P. The relation of deprivation to perinatal pathology and late sequels. In Gruenwald P, ed. *The Placenta*. Lancaster: Medical Technical Publishing Co., 1975.
58. Lechtig A, Delgado H, Yarbrough CH, Habicht JP, Martorell R, Klein RE. A simple assessment of the risk of low birth weight to select women for nutritional intervention. *Am J Obstet Gynecol* 1976;125:25–34.
59. Iyengar L, Rajalakshmi K. Effect of folic acid supplement on birth weights of infants. *Am J Obstet Gynecol* 1975;122:332–6.
60. Mund-Hoyne S, Bender G, Hünesmann B, Schander K. Uptake of i.v. administered 75-selen-methionin in various organs of non-pregnant and pregnant rats. In Salvadori B, Bacchi-Modena A, eds. *Poor Intrauterine Fetal Growth*. Parma: Minerva Médica, 1977.
61. Laga EM, Driscoll SG, Munro HN. Comparison of placentas from two socioeconomic groups. II. Biochemical characteristics. *Pediatrics* 1972;50:33–9.
62. Laga EM, Driscoll SG, Munro HN. Quantitative studies of human placenta. I. Morphometry. *Biol Neonate* 1973;23:231–59.
63. Dayton DH, Filer LJ, Canosa C. Cellular changes in placentas of undernourished mothers in Guatemala. *Fed Proc* 1969;28:488.
64. Luke B. Nutritional influences on fetal growth. *Clin Obstet Gynecol* 1994;37:538–49.
65. Pitkin RM, Kaminetzky HA, Newton M, Pritchard JA. Maternal nutrition. A selective review of clinical topics. *Obstet Gynecol* 1972;40:773–85.
66. Papiernik E, Frydman R, Hajeri H, Spira A, Bachalier M. Intrauterine growth restriction. Presented at the *5th European Congress of Perinatal Medicine*, Uppsala, Sweden, 1976.
67. Bender E, Nuñez RM. Energy intake, maternal nutritional status and IUGR. *Cat Saude Publica, Rio de Janeiro*. 2003;19(1):279–85.
68. Ramakrishnan U, Manjrekar R, Rivera J, Gonzalez-Cossio T, Martorell R. Micronutrients and pregnancy outcome: A review of the literature. *Nutr Res* 1999;19:103–59.
69. Fall CHD, Yajuik CS, Roo S, Davies AA. Micronutrients and fetal growth. *J Nutr* 2003;133(55):1747–55.
70. Fawzi WW, Msamanga G, Spiegelman D, *et al*. Randomised trial of effects of vitamin A supplements on pregnancy outcomes and T cell counts in HIV-1 infected women in Tanzania. *Lancet* 1998;351:1477–82.
71. Coutsoudis A, Pillay K, Spooner E, Kuhn L, Coovadia HM. Randomized trial testing the effect of vitamin A supplementation on pregnancy outcomes and early mother-to-child HIV-1 transmission in Durban, South Africa. South African Vitamin A Study Group. *AIDS* 1999;13:1517–24.
72. Chappell LC, Seed PT, Briley AL, *et al*. Effect of antioxidants on the occurrence of preeclampsia in women at increased risk; a randomized controlled trial. *Lancet* 1999;354:810–6.
73. Bamji MS. Enzymic evaluation of thiamin, riboflavin and pyridoxine status of parturient women and their newborn infants. *Br J Nutr* 1976;35:259–65.
74. Ramsay VP, Neumann C, Clerk V, Swenseid MF. Vitamin cofactor saturation indices for riboflavin, thiamin and piridoxine in placental tissue of Kenyan women. *Am J Clin Nutr* 1983;37: 969–73.
75. Mahomed K. Folate supplementation in pregnancy. (Cochrane Review) In *The Cochrane Library*, Issue 4:CD000183. Update Software, Oxford, 2002.
76. Mathews F, Yudkin P, Neil A. Influence of maternal nutrition on outcome of pregnancy: prospective cohort study. *Br Med J* 1999; 319:339–43.
77. Doyle W, Crawford MA, Wynn MA, Wynn SW. The association between diet and birth dimensions. *J Nutr Med* 1990;1:9–17.
78. Scholl TO, Hedinger ML. Anemia and iron deficiency anemia: compilation of data on pregnancy outcome. *Am J Clin Nutr* 1994;59:492S–501S.
79. Rasmussen KM. Is there a causal relationship between iron deficiency anemia and weight at birth, length of gestation and perinatal mortality? *J Nutr* 2001;131:590–603.
80. Mahomed K. Iron supplementation in pregnancy (Cochrane Review). In The Cochrane Library, Issue 4:CD000117. Update Software, Oxford, 2002.
81. Mahomed K. Zinc supplementation in pregnancy (Cochrane Review). In *The Cochrane Library*, Issue CD000230. Update Software, Oxford, 2002.
82. Osendarp SJ, Van Raaji JMA, Arifeen SE, Whed MA, Baqui AK, Fuchs GJ. A randomized placebo-controlled trial of the effect of zinc supplementation during pregnancy on pregnant outcome in Bangladeshi urban poor. *Am J Clin Nutr* 2000;71:114–9.
83. Caulfield LE, Zavaleta N, Figueroa A, Leon Z. Maternal zinc supplementation does not affect size at birth or pregnancy duration in Peru. *J Nutr* 1999;129:1563–8.
84. Chaouki ML, Benmiloud M. Prevention of iodine deficiency disorders by oral administration of lipiodol during pregnancy. *Eur J Endocrinol* 1994;130:547–51.
85. Prentice A. Calcium requirements in pregnancy and lactation. *NFI Bull* 1998;19:1–4.

86. Bucher HC, Guyatt GH, Cook RJ, *et al.* Effect of calcium supplementation on pregnancy-induced hypertension and preeclampsia, a meta analysis of randomized controlled trials. *J Am Med Assoc* 1996;275:1113–7.
87. Atallah AN, Hofmeyr GJ, Duley L. Calcium supplementation during pregnancy for preventing hypertensive disorders and related problems. In *The Cochrane Library,* Issue 4:CD001059. Update Software, Oxford, 2002.
88. Makrides M, Crowther CA. Magnesium supplementation in pregnancy (Cochrane Review). In *The Cochrane Library,* Issue 4: CD000937. Update Software, Oxford, 2002.
89. Krüger H, Arias-Stella J. The placenta and the newborn infant at high altitudes. *Am J Obstet Gynecol* 1970;106:586–91.
90. Keyes LE, Armaza JF, Niermeyer S, Vargas E. Intrauterine growth restriction, preeclampsia and intrauterine mortality at high altitude in Bolivia. *Pediatr Res* 2003;54(1):20–5.
91. Lichty JA, Ting RY, Buns PD, Dyar E. Studies of babies born at high altitude. Relation of altitude to birth weight. *Am Med Assoc J Dis Child* 1957;93:666–78.
92. Moore LG. Fetal growth restriction and maternal oxygen transport during high altitude pregnancy. *High Alt Med Biol* 2003; 4(2):141–56.
93. Toverud KU. The vitamin C requirements of pregnant and lactating women. *Acta Pediatr Scand* 1939;24:332.
94. Prasaad LS. Small for dates. *Indian J Pediatr* 1956;23:115.
95. Bobak M. Pregnancy outcomes and outdoor air pollution: an ecological study in districts of the Czech Republic. *Occup Environ Med* 1988;56:539–43.
96. Ritz B, Yu F, Fruin S, Chapa G. Ambient air pollution and risk of birth defects in southern California. *Am J Epidemiol* 2002;155: 17–25.
97. Liu S, Krewsk D, Shi Y, Chen Y. Association between gaseous ambient air pollutants and adverse pregnancy outcome in Vancouver, Canada. *Environ Health Perspect* 2003;111(14): 1773–8.
98. Maisonat M, Correa A, Misra D, Jaakkola JJ. A review of the literature on the effects of ambient air pollution on fetal growth. *Environ Res* 2004;95(1):106–15.
99. Simpson WJ, Linda L. A preliminary report on cigarette smoking and the incidence of prematurity. *Am J Obstet Gynecol* 1957; 73:808–15.
100. Meyer MB. How does maternal smoking affect birth weight and maternal weight gain? *Am J Obstet Gynecol* 1978;131:888–93.
101. Miller HC, Hassanein K, Hensleigh PA. Fetal growth restriction in relation to maternal smoking and weight gain in pregnancy. *Am J Obstet Gynecol* 1976;125:55–60.
102. Hasselmeyer ED, Meyer MB, Longo LD, *et al.* Pregnancy and infant health. In *The Health Consequences of Smoking in Women. A Report of the Surgeon General.* DHEW Publication no. 79–50069. Washington, DC: Government Printing Office, 1980.
103. Royal College of Physicians. *Smoking and Health Now.* London: Pitman, 1970.
104. Schwartz AL, Raw TW. Hormonal regulation of glycogen metabolism in human fetal livers. *Diabetes* 1975;24:1113.
105. Tanaka T, Harano Y, Morimura H, Mori R. Maternal smoking and fetal growth restriction. *Biochem Biophys Res Commun* 1965; 27:55–60.
106. Suzuki T, Horiguchi T, Comas-Urrutia L, Mueller Heubach E, Morishima HO, Adamsons K. Pharmacological effects of nicotine upon the fetus and mother in the rhesus monkey. *Am J Obstet Gynecol* 1971;111:1092–101.
107. Butler NR, Goldstein H, Ross EM. Cigarette smoking in pregnancy: its influence on birth weight and perinatal mortality. *Br Med J* 1972;2:127–35.
108. Astrup A, Olson HM, Trolle D, Kjeldsen K. Effect of moderate carbon monoxide exposure on fetal development. *Lancet* 1972;2:1220–2.
109. Hickey RJ, Clelland RC, Bowers EJ. Maternal smoking, birth weight, infant death and the self-selection problems. *Am J Obstet Gynecol* 1978;131:805–11.
110. Shiono PH, Klebanoff MA, Nugent RP, *et al.* The impact of cocaine and marihuana use on low birth weight and preterm birth. A multicenter study. *Am J Obstet Gynecol* 1995;172: 19–27.
111. Raymond EG, Cnattingius S, Kiely JL. Effects of maternal age, parity, and smoking on the risk of stillbirth. *Br J Obstet Gynaecol* 1994;101:301–6.
112. Di Franza JR, Lew RA. Effect of maternal cigarette smoking on pregnancy complications and sudden infant death syndrome. *J Fam Pract* 1993;40:385–94.
113. Gabriel R, Alsat E, Evain-Brion D. Alteration of epidermal growth factor receptor in placental membranes of smokers: relationship with intrauterine growth restriction. *Am J Obstet Gynecol* 1994; 170:1238–43.
114. Montgomery SM, Ekbom A. smoking during pregnancy and diabetes mellitus in a British longitudinal birth cohort. *Br Med J* 2002;324:26–7.
115. Zaren B, Lindmark G, Bakketeig L. Maternal smoking affects growth more in the male fetus. *Paediatr Perinat Epidemiol* 2000; 14(2):118–26.
116. Ulleland CN. The offspring of alcoholic mothers. *Ann N Y Acad Sci* 1972;197:167–9.
117. Abel EL, York JL. Absence of effects of prenatal ethanol on adult emotionality and ethanol consumption in rats. *J Stud Alcohol* l979;40:547–53.
118. Ellis FW, Pick JR. An animal model of fetal alcohol syndrome in beagles. *Alcoholism* 1977;4:123–34.
119. Surgeon General Advisory on Alcohol and Pregnancy. *FDA Bull* 1981:119.
120. Jones KL, Smith DW, Ulleland CN, Streissguth AP. Pattern of malformation in offspring of chronic alcoholic mothers. *Lancet* 1973;1:1267–71.
121. González-Merlo J, Mestres J, Urne J. Patrón de malfor-maciones en la descendencia de madres alcohólicas. Síndrome alcohólico fetal. In Altirriba EJ, Sabater J, Balaña F, eds. *Prevención de la Subnormalidad.* Barcelona: Salvat, 1979:313–44.
122. Fried PA, O'Conell CM. A comparison of the effects of prenatal exposure to tobacco, alcohol, cannabis and caffeine on birth size and subsequent growth. *Neurotoxicol Teratol* 1987;9:79–85.
123. Fuji T, Nishimura H. Adverse effects of prolonged administration of caffeine on the rat fetus. *Toxicol Appl Pharmacol* 1972;22: 449–57.
124. Van der Berg BJ. Epidemiological observation of prematurity. Effects of tobacco, coffee and alcohol. In Reed DM, Stanley FJ, eds. *The Epidemiology of Prematurity.* Baltimore, MD: Urban & Schwarzenberg, 1977.
125. Weathersbee PS, Olsen LK, Lodge JR. Caffeine and pregnancy: A retrospective survey. *Postgrad Med* 1977;62:64–9.
126. Eskenazi B, Stapleton AL, Kharrazi M. Associations between maternal decaffeinated and caffeinated coffee consumption and fetal growth and gestational duration. *Epidemiology* 1999;10: 242–9.
127. Vlajinac HD, Petrovic RR, Marinkovic JM. Effect of caffeine intake during pregnancy on birth weight. *Am J Epidemiol* 1997; 145:335–8.
128. Linn S, Schoenbaum S, Monson R. No association between coffee consumption and adverse outcomes of pregnancy. *N Engl J Med* 1982;306:141–5.
129. Grosso LM, Rosenberg KD, Belanger K. Maternal caffeine intake and intrauterine growth restriction. *Epidemiology* 2001;12: 447–55.
130. Cook DG, Peakock JL, Feyerabend C. Relation of caffeine intake and blood caffeine concentrations during pregnancy to fetal growth: prospective population based study. *Br Med J* 1996; 313:1358–62.
131. Brackey MB, Triche EW, Belanger K, Hellenbrand K, Leaderer BP. Association of maternal caffeine consumption with decrement in fetal growth. *Am J Epidemiol* 2003;157(5):456–66.
132. Naeye RL, Blanc W, Leblanc W, Khatamee MA. Fetal complications of maternal heroin addiction: abnormal growth, infections and episodes of stress. *J Pediatr* 1973;83:1055–61.
133. Naeye RL, Blanc W, Paul CH. Effects of maternal nutrition on the human fetus. *Pediatrics* 1973;52:494–503.
134. Brown ER, Zuckerman B. The infant of the drug-abusing mother. *Pediatr Ann* 1991;20:555–6.
135. Zelson C, Lee SJ, Casalino M. Neonatal narcotic addiction: Comparative effects of maternal intake of heroin and methadone. *N Engl J Med* 1973;289:1216–20.
136. Glass L, Rajegowda BK, Kahn EJ, Floyd MV. Effect of heroin withdrawal on respiratory rate and acid-base status in the newborn. *N Engl J Med* 1972;186:746–8.
137. Chasnoff IJ, Burns WJ, Schnoll SH, Burns KA. Cocaine use in pregnancy. *N Engl J Med* 1985;313:666–9.
138. Handler A, Kistin N, Davis F, Ferre C. Cocaine use during pregnancy: perinatal outcomes. *Am J Epidemiol* 1991;133:818–21.

139. Hall JG, Danti RM, Wilson KM. Maternal and fetal sequelae of anticoagulants during pregnancy. *Am J Med* 1980;68:1322–9.
140. Shaw EB, Steinbach HL. Aminopterin-induced fetal malformations. *Am J Obstet Gynecol* 1977;127:191.
141. Hanson JW, Myrianthoupoulas NC, Harvey MAS, Smith DW. Risks to the offspring of women treated with hydantoin anticonvulsants, with emphasis on the fetal hydantoin syndrome. *J Pediatr* 1976;89:662–8.
142. Carrera JM, Mallafré J, Otero F, Rubio R, Carrera M. Síndrome de mala adaptación circulatoria materna: bases etiopatogénicas y terapéuticas. In Carrera JM, ed. *Doppler en Obstetricia.* Barcelona: Masson-Salvat, 1992:335–9.
143. Scott JB, Rote NS, Branoh DW. Immunologic aspects of recurrent abortion and fetal death. *Obstet Gynecol* 1987;70:645–56.
144. Lubbe WF, Liggins G. Lupus anticoagulant and pregnancy. *Am J Obstet Gynecol* 1985;153:322–7.
145. Katz AI, Davison JM, Hayslett JP, *et al.* Pregnancy in women with kidney disease. *Kidney Int* 1980;18:192–203.
146. Surian M, Imbasciate E, Cosci P, *et al.* Glomerular disease and pregnancy: a study of 123 pregnancies in patients with primary and secondary glomerular disease. *Nephron* 1984;36:101–5.
147. Parbooshing J, Cochburn F. Fetal growth restriction and maternal renal disease. In Salvadori B, Bacchi-Modena A, eds. *Poor Intrauterine Fetal Growth.* Parma: Minerva Médica, 1977:103–6.
148. Donnelly JF, Flowers CHE, Creadick RN, Wells HB, Greenberg BG, Surles KB. Maternal, fetal and environmental factors in prematurity. *Am J Obstet Gynecol* 1964;88:918–31.
149. Xiao R, Sorensen TK, Williams MA, Luthy DA. Influence of preeclampsia on fetal growth. *J Matern Fetal Neonatal Med* 2003;13:157–62.
150. Odegard RA, Vatten LJ, Nilsen ST. Preeclampsia and fetal grpwth. *Obstet Gynecol* 2000;96:950–5.
151. Robson SC, Chang TC. Intrauterine growth restriction. In Reed CB, Claireaux AE, Cockburn E, eds. *Diseases of the Fetus and Newborn.* London: Chapman and Hall Medical, 1995:275–83.
152. Zuspan FO. Adrenal gland and sympathetic nervous system response in eclampsia. *Am J Obstet Gynecol* 1972;114:304–13.
153. Ness RB, Roberts JM. Heterogeneous causes constituting the single syndrome of preeclampsia: a hypothesis and its implications. *Am J Obstet Gynecol* 1996;175:1365–7.
154. Rasmussen S, Irgens LM. Fetal growth and body proportion in preeclampsia. *Obstet Gynecol* 2003;101:575–83.
155. Xiong X, Demianczuk NN, Buekens P, Saunders LD. Association of preeclampsia with high birth weight for age. *Am J Obstet Gynecol* 2000;183:148–55.
156. Frigoletto F, Tullis JL, Reid DE, Hinman J. Hyper-coagulability in the dysmature syndrome. *Am J Obstet Gynecol* 1971;111:867–73.
157. Bonnar J. Intravascular coagulation and pregnancy. *J Clin Pathol* 1974;27:514.
158. Norris LA, Sheppard BL, Burke G, Bonnar J. Platelet activation in normotensive and hypertensive pregnancies complicated by intrauterine growth restriction. *Br J Obstet Gynaecol* 1994;101: 209–14.
159. Trudinger BJ. Platelets and IUGR in pre-eclampsia. *Br J Obstet Gynaecol* 1976;83:284–6.
160. Walsh SW. Thromboxane production in placentas of women with pre-eclampsia. *Am J Obstet Gynecol* 1989;160:1535–6.
161. Graham IM, Daly LE, Refsum HM, Robinson K, Brattstorm LE. Plasma homocysteine as a risk factor for vascular disease. The European Concerted Action Project. *J Am Med Assoc* 1997;277: 1775–81.
162. Vollset SE, Refsum H, Irgens LM, Emblem BM, Tverdal A, Gjessing Monsen AL. Plasma total homocysteine, pregnancy complications, and adverse pregnancy outcomes: The homocysteine study. *Am J Clin Nutr* 2000;71:962–8.
163. Dekker JA, de Vries JI, Doelitzsch PM, Huijgens PC, von Blomberg BM, Jakobs C. Underlying disorders associated with severe early-onset preeclampsia. *Am J Obstet Gynecol* 1995; 173:1042–8.
164. Rajkovic A, Catalano PM, Malinov MR. Elevated homocysteine levels with preeclampsia. *Obstet Gynecol* 1997;90:168–71.
165. D'Anna R, Baviera G, Corrado F, Ientile R. Plasma homocysteine in early and late pregnancies complicated with preeclampsia and isolated IUGR. *Acta Obstet Gynecol Scand* 2004;83.155–8.
166. Regnavet TR, de Vrijer B, Galan HL, Davidsen MC. The relationship between transplacental O_2 difussion and placental expression of PlGF, VEGF and their receptors in a placental insufficiency model of fetal growth restriction. *J Physiol* 2003;550(Pt 2):641–56.
167. Tsatsaris V, Goffin F, Munant C, Brichant JF. Overexpression of the soluble vascular endothelial growth factor receptor in preeclamptic patients: pathophysiological consequences. *J Clin Endocrinol Metab* 2003;88(11):5555–6.
168. Abell DA, Beischer NA, Papas AJ, Willis MM. The associations between abnormal glucose tolerance (hyperglycemia and hypoglycemia) and estriol excretions in pregnancy. *Am J Obstet Gynecol* 1976;l24:388–92.
169. Frydman R, Papiernik E, Girard JR, Assan R. Intrauterine growth restriction. Presented at the *5th European Congress of Perinatal Medicine*, Uppsala, Sweden, 1976.
170. Grumbach MM, Kaplan SL. Ontogenesis of growth hormone, insulin, prolactin and gonadotropin secretion in the human fetus. In Comline RS, Cross KW, Daves GC, Nathanielsz PW, eds. *Foetal and Neonatal Physiology.* London: Cambridge University Press, 1973:462–87.
171. Grumbach MM, Kaplan JL, Vinik A. In Berson SA, Yalow RS, eds. *Methods in Investigative and Diagnostic Endocrinology.* Amsterdam: North-Holland 1973:797–805.
172. Spellacy WN. Maternal and fetal metabolic inter-relationships. In Sutherland HW, Stowers JM, eds. *Carbohydrate Metabolism in Pregnancy and the Newborn.* Edinburgh: Churchill Livingstone, 1975:42–57.
173. Pedersen J. *The Pregnant Diabetic and her Newborn*, 2nd edn. Baltimore, MD: Williams & Wilkins, 1977:127–41.
174. Branconi F, Faldi P, Mello G, *et al.* The poor endouterine growth of the fetus in treated diabetic patients. In Salvadori B, Bacchi-Modena A, eds. *Poor Intrauterine Fetal Growth.* Parma: Minerva Médica, 1977.
175. Douglas CHP. Intrauterine growth restriction. In Aladjem S, ed. *Prenatal Risk.* St. Louis, MO: Mosby Year Book, 1976.
176. Persson B. Assessment of metabolic control in diabetic pregnancy. In Elliot K, Knight J, eds. *Size at Birth.* Amsterdam: Associated Scientific Publishers, 1974:247–73.
177. Haworth JC, Dilling LA. Effect of abnormal glucose tolerance in pregnancy on infant mortality rate and morbidity. *Am J Obstet Gynecol* 1975:122:555–60.
178. Churchill JA, Berendes HW. Intelligence of children whose mothers had acetonemia during pregnancy. *Panamerican Health Org Sci Publ* 1969;85:30.
179. Kuizon M, Cheong RL, Ancheta LP, Desnacido JA, Macapinlac MP, Baens JC. Effect of anemia and other maternal characteristics on birth weight. *Clin Hum Nutr* 1985;39C:419–26.
180. Fine LG, Barnett EV, Danowitch GM. Systemic lupus erythematosus in pregnancy. *Ann Intern Med* 1981;94:667–77.
181. Branch DW, Scott JR, Kochenoor NK, Hershgold E. Obstetric complications associated with the lupus anticoagulant. *N Engl J Med* 1985;313:1322–6.
182. Lockwood CJ, Romero R, Feinberg RF, Clyne LP, Coster B, Hoobins JC. The prevalence and biological significance of lupus anticoagulant and anticardiolipin antibodies in a general obstetric population. *Am J Obstet Gynecol* 1989;161:369–73.
183. Morgan T, Craven C, lalouel JM, Ward K. Angiotensinogen Thr235 variant is associated with abnormal physiologic change of the uterine spiral arteries in first trimester decidua. *Am J Obstet Gynecol* 1999;180:95–102.
184. Ward K, Hata A, Jeunemaitre X, Helin C, Nelson L, Namikava C. A molecular variant of angiotensinogen associated with preeclampsia. *Nat Genet* 1993;4:59–61.
185. Morgan T, Craven C, Nelson L, Lalouel JM, Ward K. Angiotensinogen Thr235 expression is elevated in decidual spiral arteries. *J Clin Invest* 1997;100:1406–15.
186. North AF. Small-for-dates neonates. I. Maternal gestational and neonatal characteristics. *Pediatrics* 1966;38:1013–9.
187. Polani PE. Chromosomal and other genetic influences on birth weight variations. In Elliot K, Knight J, eds. *Size at Birth.* Amsterdam: Associated Scientific Publishers, 1974:127–64.
188. Naeye RL. Prenatal organ and cellular growth with various chromosomal disorders. *Biol Neonate* 1967;11:248–60.
189. Hall A, Fleming JEC, Abdulla V. Ultrasonic fetal cephalometry – Some improvements and future developments. *Ultrasonics* 1970;8:34–5.
190. Smith A, McKeown T. Prenatal growth of mongoloides defectives. *Arch Dis Child* 1955;30:257.
191. Chen CP, Chern SR, Chang TY, Lee CC. Prenatal diagnosis of mosaic ring chromosome 22 associated with cardiovascular

abnormalities and intrauterine growth restriction. *Prenat Diagn* 2003;23:40–3.
192. Reisman LE. Chromosome abnormalities and intrauterine growth restriction. *Pediatr Clin North Am* 1970;17:101–10.
193. Lindsten J. The nature and origin of X chromosome aberrations in Turner syndrome: A cytogenetical and clinical study of 57 patients. Stockholm: Almquist and Wiskell, 1963.
194. Bergsma D. *Birth Defects Compendium*, 2nd edn. New York: Alan R. Liss., 1979.
195. Barlow P. The influence of inactive chromosomes on human development. Anomalous sex chromosome complements and the phenotype. *Humangenetik* 1973;17:105–36.
196. Kolski R, Mane-Garzón F, Seuanez H. Estudio de 56 casos de anencefalia en el Uruguay. *Arch Pediatr Uruguay* 1977;48:209–18.
197. Wald NJ, Cuckle HS, Boreham J, Althouse R. Birth weight of infants with spina bifida cystica. *Br J Obstet Gynaecol* 1980; 87:578–81.
198. Knox GE. Influence of infection on fetal growth and development. *J Reprod Med* 1978;21:352–8.
199. Hugues WT. Infecciones y retardo de crecimiento intrauterino. *Pediatr Clin North Am (Spanish edn)* 1970;17:119.
200. Cooper JM, Soffronoff EC, Bolognese RJ. Oxytocin challenge test in monitoring high-risk pregnancies. *Obstet Gynecol* 1975:45:27–33.
201. McCracken GH, Shinefield HMR, Cobb K, Rausen AR, Dische R, Eichenwald HF. Congenital cytomegalic inclusion disease: a longitudinal study of 20 patients. *Am J Dis Child* 1969;117:522–39.
202. Baboniau C, Smith DA, Shaplaud D, Arno G. Placental infection with *Chlamydia pneumoniae* and intrauterine growth restriction. *Cardiovasc Res* 2003;60(1):165–9.
203. Fraser D, Picard R, Picard E, Leiberman JR. Birth weight discordance, intrauterine growth restriction and perinatal outcomes in twins. *J Reprod Med* 1994;39:504–8.
204. Ghai V, Vidyasagar D. Morbidity and mortality factors in twins: an epidemiologic approach. *Clin Perinatol* 1988;15:123–40.
205. McCulloch K. Neonatal problems in twins. *Clin Perinatol* 1988;15:141–58.
206. Medawar PP. Some immunological and endocrinological problems raised by the evolution of viviparity in vertebrates. *Symp Soc Exp Biol* 1953;44:320–38.
207. Sargent IL, Redman CWG, Starkey PM. Placenta como injerto. In Redman CWG, Sargent IL, Starkey PM, eds. *La Placenta Humana*. Barcelona: Masson, 1995:207–78.
208. Noonan EP, Holliday WJ, Morton H, Clunie CJA. Early pregnancy factor of immunosuppresion. *Nature* 1979;278:639–50.
209. Jones MD, Battaglia FC. Intrauterine growth restriction. *Am J Obstet Gynecol* 1977;127:540–9.
210. Jones WR. Immunological factors in human placentation. *Nature* 1968;218:480.
211. Billington WD. Immunological factors in pregnancy. *Nature* 1964;202:317–18.
212. Ounsted M, Ounsted C. Maternal regulation of intrauterine growth. *Nature* 1966;212:995–7.
213. Walton A, Hammond J. The maternal effects on growth and conformation in shire horse/shetland pony crosses. *Proc R Soc Lond* 1938;125B:311.
214. Stites DP, Carr MC, Fudenberg HH. Ontogenity of cellular immunity in the human fetus: development of responses to phytohemaglutinins and allogeneic cells. *Cell Immunol* 1974;11: 257–71.
215. Jones WR. Cord serum immunoglobulin levels in 'small-for-dates' babies. *Aust Paediatr J* 1972;8:30–2.
216. Díaz del Castillo E. *Pediatría Prenatal*. México: Nueva Editorial Interamericana, 1974:47–79.
217. Scott DE, Usher R. Fetal malnutrition. Its incidences, causes, and effects. *Am J Obstet Gynecol* 1966;94:951–63.
218. Thoulon JM, Combet A. Uterine factors in poor intrauterine fetal growth. In Salvadori B, Bacchi-Modena A, eds. *Poor Intrauterine Fetal Growth*. Parma: Minerva Médica, 1977:85–9.
219. Rousseau P, Rihm G, Wolff F, Houyet PH, Keller B, Muller P. Retard de croissance intrauterine: étude de quelques facteurs par la combinaison du poids de naissance et l'âge gestationnel. *Rev Franc Gynecol* 1971;66:31–6.
220. Sotelo-Avila C, Shanklin DR. Congenital malformations in an autopsy population. *Arch Pathol* 1967;84:272–9.
221. Shanklin DR, Sotelo-Avila C. The influence of placental lesions on the newborn infant. *Pediatr Clin North Am* 1970;17:25–42.
222. Varma TR. Prediction of delivery date by ultrasound cephalometry. *Br J Obstet Gynaecol* 1973;80:316–19.
223. De Costa EJ, Gerbie AB, Andresen RH, Gallanis TC. Placental tumors. Hemangiomas, with special reference to an associated clinical syndrome. *Obstet Gynecol* 1956;7:249–59.
224. Eitzman DV, Shanklin DR. Placental lesions. *J Reprod Med* 1968;1:27–32.
225. Fox H. Senescence of placental villi. *J Obstet Gynecol* 1967;74:881–5.
226. Matheus M, Sala MA. Intrauterine growth: evolution of the fetal length, weight of the fetus and placenta, and placental index in the second half of pregnancy. *AMB Rev Assoc Med Bras* 1977;23:88–90.
227. Kalousek DK, Dill FJ. Chromosomal mosaicism confined to the placenta in human conceptions. *Science* 1983;221:665–7.
228. Kalousek DK, Dill FJ, Pantzar JJ, McGuillivray BC, *et al.* Confined chorionic mosaicism in prenatal diagnosis. *Hum Genet* 1987;77:163–7.
229. Kalousek DK, Howard-Peebles PN, Olson SB, *et al.* Confirmation of CVS mosaicism in term placenta and high frequency of intrauterine growth restriction associated with confined placental mosaicism. *Prenat Diagn* 1991;11:743–50.
230. Holzgreve B, Exeler R, Holzgreve W, Wittwer B, Miny P. Nonviable trisomies confined to the placenta leading to poor pregnancy outcome. *Prenat Diagn* 1992;12(Suppl):95.
231. Hashish AF, Monk NA, Lovell-Smith MP, Bardwell LM, Fiddes TM, Gardner RJM. Trisomy detected at chorionic villus sampling. *Prenat Diagn* 1989;9:427–32.
232. Appelman Z, Rosensaft J, Cheuake J, *et al.* Trisomy 9 confined to the placenta: prenatal diagnosis and neonatal follow-up. *Am J Med Genet* 1991;40:464–6.
233. Tharapel T, Elias S, Shulman LP, Seely L, Emerson DS, Simpson JL. Resolved co-twin as an explanation for discrepant chorionic villus results: non mosaic 47,XX,+16 in villi (direct and culture) with normal (46,XX) amniotic fluid and neonatal blood. *Prenat Diagn* 1989;9:467–72.
234. Miny P, Hammer P, Gerlach B, *et al.* Mosaicism and accuracy of prenatal cytogenetic diagnoses after chorionic villus sampling and placental biopsies. *Prenat Diagn* 1991;11:581–9.
235. Wapner RJ, Simpson JL, Golbus MS, *et al.* Chorionic mosaicism: association with fetal loss but not with adverse perinatal outcome. *Prenat Diagn* 1992;12:347–55.
236. Wilkins-Haug L, Roberts DJ, Morton CC. Confined placental mosaicism and intrauterine growth restriction: a case–control analysis of placentas at delivery. *Am J Obstet Gynecol* 1995;172:44–50.
237. Schuring-Blom GH, Keijzer M, Jakobs ME, *et al.* Molecular cytogenetic analysis of term placentae suspected of mosaicism using fluorescence *in situ* hybridization. *Prenat Diagn* 1993;13:671–9.
238. Wigglesworth JS. Experimental growth restriction in the fetal rat. *J Pathol Bacteriol* 1964;88:1.
239. Wigglesworth JS. Morphological variations in the insufficient placenta. *J Obstet Gynaecol Br Commonw* 1964;71:871–84.
240. Van Geijn HP, Jongsma HW, De Haan J, Eskes TK, Prechtl HF. Induction of severe intrauterine growth restriction in the Sprague-Dawley rat. *Am J Obstet Gynecol* 1980;136:1061–6.
241. Gerretsen G, Huisjes HJ, Elema JD. Morphological changes of the spiral arteries in the placental bed in relation to pre-eclampsia and foetal growth restriction. *Br J Obstet Gynaecol* 1981;88:876–81.
242. O'Shaughnessy RW, Scott GD, Iams D, Zuspan FP. Plasma catecholamines in normal pregnancy and in pregnancies complicated by mild chronic hypertension. *Clin Exp Hypertens (B)* 1983;2:113–21.
243. Walsh SW. Physiology of low-dose aspirin therapy for the prevention of pre-eclampsia. *Semin Perinatol* 1990;14: 152–70.
244. Moncada S, Vane JR. Pharmacology and endogenous roles of prostaglandin endoperoxides, thromboxane A2 and prostacyclin. *Pharmacol Rev* 1979;30:293–331.
245. Sánchez-Ramos L, O'Sullivan MJ, Garrido-Calderón J. Effect of low-dose aspirin on angiotensin II pressor response in human pregnancy. *Am J Obstet Gynecol* 1987;156:193–4.
246. Gruenwald P. Pathology of the deprived fetus and its supply line. In Elliot K, Knight J, eds. *Size at Birth*. Amsterdam: Associated Scientific Publishers, 1974:2–26.
247. Dawes GS. *Fetal and Neonatal Physiology*. Chicago, IL: Year Book Medical, 1968.
248. Robertson WB, Khong TY. Pathology of the uteroplacental bed. In Sharp F, Symonds EM, eds. *Hypertension in Pregnancy*. Ithaca, NY: Perinatology Press, 1987;101–13.

249. Ramsey EM, Donner MW. *Placental Vasculature and Circulation.* Stuttgart: Georg Thieme, 1980:90.
250. Remuzzi G, Marchesi D, Zoja C, *et al.* Reduced umbilical and placental vascular prostacyclin in severe pre-eclampsia. *Prostaglandins* 1980;20:105–10.
251. Walsh SW. Thromboxane production in placentas of women with pre-eclampsia. *Am J Obstet Gynecol* 1989;160:1535–6.
252. Walsh SW, Coulter S. Increased placental progesterone synthesis may cause decreased placental prostacyclin synthesis in pre-eclampsia. *Am J Obstet Gynecol* 1989;161:1586–92.
253. Goodman RP, Killam AP, Brash AR, Branch RA. Prostacyclin production during pregnancy: Comparison of production during normal pregnancy and pregnancy complicated by hypertension. *Am J Obstet Gynecol* 1982;142:817–22.
254. Downing I, Shepherd GL, Lewis PJ. Reduced prostacyclin production in pre-eclampsia. *Lancet* 1980;2:1374.
255. Yanagisawa M, Kurihara H, Kimura S, *et al.* A novel potent vasoconstrictor peptide produced by vascular endothelial cells. *Nature* 1988;332:411–5.
256. Radunovic N, Lockwood CHJ, Alvarez M, Nastic D, Petkovic S, Berkowitz RL. Fetal and maternal plasma endothelin levels during the second half of pregnancy. *Am J Obstet Gynecol* 1995; 172:28–32.
257. Galatzios G, Papazoglou D, Giagloglou K, Vassaras G. Umbilical cord serum vascular endothelial growth factor (VEGF) levels in normal pregnancies and in pregnancies complicated by preterm delivery or preeclampsia. *Intern J Gynecol Obstet* 2004; 85:6–11.
258. Sawidov MD, Hingorani D, Tsikas D, Frölich JC. Endothelial dysfunction and raised plasma concentrations of asymmetrical dimethylarginine in pregnant women who subsequently developed preeclampsia. *Lancet* 2003;361:1511–17.
259. Romero R, Avila C, Santhanum U, Seghal PB. Amniotic fluid interleukin-6 in preterm delivery: association with infection. *J Clin Invest* 1990;85:1392–400.
260. Lockshin MD, Druzin MI, Goei S, *et al.* Antibody to cardiolipin as a predictor of fetal distress or death in pregnant patients with systemic lupus erythematosus. *N Engl J Med* 1985;313:152–6.
261. Branch DW, Scott J, Kochenour NK, Hershgold E. Obstetric complications associated with the lupus anticoagulant. *N Engl J Med* 1985:313:1322–6.
262. El-Poeiy A, Myers SA, Gleicher N. The relationship between autoantibodies and intrauterine growth restriction in hypertensive disorders of pregnancy. *Am J Obstet Gynecol* 1991;164; 1253–61.
263. Cetin I, Ronzoni S, Marconi AM, *et al.* Maternal concentrations and fetal-maternal concentration differences of plasma amino acids in normal and intrauterine growth-restricted pregnancies. *Am J Obstet Gynecol* 1996;174:1575–83.
264. Nelson DM, Smith SD, Furesz TC, Sadovsky Y. Hypoxia reduces expression and function of system A amino acid transporters in cultured term human trophoblast. *Am J Physiol Cell Physiol* 2003;284:C310–5.
265. Giles GW, Trudinger BJ, Baird PJ. Fetal umbilical artery flow velocity waveforms and placental resistance: A pathological correlation. *Br J Obstet Gynaecol* 1985;92:31–8.
266. Trudinger BJ, Cook CM. Umbilical and uterine artery flow velocity waveforms in pregnancy associated with major fetal abnormality. *Br J Obstet Gynaecol* 1985;92:666–70.
267. Meizner I, Katz M, Lunenfeld E, Insler V. Umbilical and uterine flow velocity in pregnancies complicated by major fetal anomalies. *Prenat Diagn* 1987;7:491–3.
268. Sebire NJ, Goldin RD, Regan L. Histomorphological evidence for chronic vasoconstriction of placental stem vessels in pregnancies with intrauterine growth restriction and abnormal umbilical artery Doppler velocimetry. *J Pathol* 2001;195:19A.
269. Shapiro BL. Down's symdrome: a disruption of homeostasis. *Am J Med Genet* 1983;14:241–69.
270. Jones CT. Reprogramming of metabolic development by restriction of fetal growth. *Biochem Soc Trans* 1985;13:84–91.
271. Trudinger BJ, Giles WB, Cook CM. Utero-placental blood flow velocity-time waveforms in normal and complicated pregnancies. *Br J Obstet Gynaecol* 1985;92:39–45.
272. Trudinger BJ, Giles WB, Cook CM. Flow velocity waveforms in the maternal uteroplacental and fetal umbilical placental circulation. *Am J Obstet Gynecol* 1985;152:155–63.
273. Hsieh FJ, Chang FM, Ko TM, Chen HY, Chen YP. Umbilical artery flow velocity waveforms in fetuses dying with congenital anomalies. *Br J Obstet Gynaecol* 1988;95:478–82.
274. Carrera JM, Mallafré J, López-Rodó V, Ruiz J, Torrents M, Serra B. Epidemiología del crecimiento intrauterino retardado. Etiopatogenia y tipos. *Prog Obstet Ginecol* 1993;36:52–18.
275. Van de Veen F, Fox H. The human placenta in idiopathic intrauterine growth retardation: A light and electron microscopic study. *Placenta* 1983;4:65–78.
276. Fok RY, Pavlova Z, Bernischke K, Paul RH, Platt LD. The correlation of arterial lesions with umbilical artery Doppler velocimetry in the placentas of small for dates pregnancies. *Obstet Gynecol* 1990;75:578–83.
277. Sebire NJ. Umbilical artery Doppler revisited: pathophysiology of changes in intrauterine growth restriction revealed. *Ultrasound Obstet Gynecol* 2003;21:419–22.
278. Winick M, Noble J. Cellular response in rats during malnutrition at various ages. *J Nutr* 1966;89:300–6.
279. Winick M, Noble A. Quantitative changes in ribonucleic acids and protein during normal growth of rat placenta. *Nature* 1966; 212:34–5.
280. Winick M. Crecimiento celular en la desnutrición intrauterina. *Pediatr Clin North Am* 1970;17:69–78.
281. Metz J, Heinrich D. Experimental study of poor intrauterine fetal growth by placental vascular insufficiency. In Salvadori B, Bacchi-Modena A, eds. *Poor Intrauterine Fetal Growth.* Parma: Minerva Médica, 1977:213–5.
282. Winick M. Cellular changes during placental and fetal growth. *Am J Obstet Gynecol* 1971;109:166–76.
283. Naeye RL, Blanc W, Paul CH. Effects of maternal nutrition on the human fetus. *Pediatrics* 1973;52:494–503.
284. Campbell ST. Fetal growth. *Clinics in Obstetrics and Gynaecology.* London: WB Saunders, 1974.

120 Classification of intrauterine growth restriction

J. M. Carrera, B. Serra and P. Prats

Introduction

Several researchers who have investigated intrauterine growth restriction (IUGR) over the years have suggested a whole host of classifications for this phenomenon. Now, available data regarding the physiopathology of fetal growth and the etiopathogenesis of IUGR, and the modern methods for diagnosing it, are very different from those of 20 years ago. On the other hand, the terminology and classifications used in the past have caused confusion. For example, 'fetal size' has been confused with 'fetal growth', and 'intrauterine growth restriction' has been confused with small-for-gestational age birth weights.[1] The classification of fetuses with growth restriction therefore not only implicates an attempt to understand the etiopathogenesis of the process, but also, more specifically, a way of approaching each case and establishing the appropriate prognosis and obstetric management strategy.

Attempts to classify IUGR

The first classification of IUGR which was generally used was that proposed by Winick *et al.*[2–6] This group based their research on rats (vascular ligatures, restriction of nutrients, etc.) and reached the conclusion that there are two basic types of growth restriction: (a) intrinsic IUGR, principally derived from the fetus itself and (b) extrinsic IUGR, caused either by placental vascular insufficiency (asymmetrical IUGR) or by maternal protein restriction (symmetrical IUGR). Symmetrical IUGR seems to be caused by an impairment of cellular hyperplasia, whereas the asymmetrical one would be the result of an abnormal cellular hypertrophia. This classification was adopted with slight variations by the majority of English-speaking authors.[7,8]

Campbell *et al.*[9,10] proposed a classification based on the profile of the fetal biparietal diameter (BPD) curve. These authors distinguished between: (a) restrictions with an 'early low profile' in the cephalometric curve and (b) restrictions with a downturn or 'late flattening' of this curve. This classification, which was used by most ultrasonographists, was subsequently expanded by Levi *et al.*,[11–13] who also recognized the value of the head circumference/ abdominal circumference (HC/AC) index. IUGR was thus classified as: (a) harmonious (normal HC/AC ratio) or (b) disharmonious (HC > AC). Experience went on to show that harmonious IUGR was generally intrinsic with an early low cephalometric profile, and disharmonious IUGR was, in contrast, extrinsic and characterized by a late flattening of the BPD curve.

The majority of English-speaking specialists[14] went on to adopt the classification of symmetrical and asymmetrical IUGR, with some of them adding a third type called symmetrical IUGR with 'femur sparing', characterized by a femur length appropriate for the gestational age, but disproportionate to the rest of the biometrical parameters.[15]

Several classifications have been suggested for the neonate, based on its specific characteristics (presence or absence of malformations, corporal biometry, trophism, etc.). Rosso and Winick[16] established two groups: (a) with congenital malformations and (b) without congenital malformations; the latter was subdivided into type I (extrinsic symmetrical) and type II (extrinsic asymmetrical). In 1977, Sieroszewski[17] and Holtorff[18] proposed, independently of each other, two very similar classifications. The former divided fetuses that are small-for-gestational age (SGA) into hypoplastic and hypotrophic, and the latter grouped them as eutrophic (genetically small), hypoplastic, hypotrophic or with multiple congenital malformations.

In practice, most pediatric units classify growth restriction as (a) proportionate (symmetrical), or (b) disproportionate (asymmetrical), by simply calculating the ponderal index of Rohrer. This index is obtained by dividing the neonatal weight by the cube of the neonatal length (crown–heel) and then multiplying by 100. If this index is normal (=2.20), IUGR is

Table 120.1 Integrated classification of intrauterine growth restriction (IUGR) (from Carrera[26])

	IUGR		
Parameter	**Type I**	**Type II**	**Type III**
Biometry	Alterations in weight, length and head circumference	Alterations in weight	Alterations in weight and length
Etiology	Intrinsic	Pathological extrinsic	Deficient extrinsic
Onset	Early	Late	Semiearly
Morphology	Symmetrical harmonic	Asymmetrical disharmonic	Semiharmonic
Trophism	Eutrophic	Undernourished dystrophic	Malnourished hypotrophic

symmetrical, and if it proves to be abnormally low, IUGR is considered asymmetrical.[19–23]

On behalf of the evolution of fetal growth over time, Salvadori[24] identified three theoretical types of restriction: (a) 'primary', or constant throughout gestation; (b) 'secondary', which may be early or late depending on the moment in which the factor that causes the growth restriction begins to affect the fetus and (c) 'transitory', when recovery occurs after a deceleration in fetal growth.

Gruenwald[25] and other authors have classified growth restriction as either slight, moderate or serious/severe according to the severity of the syndrome.

Integrated classification of IUGR

We first proposed this classification in 1976,[26–37] taking into account all basic features of growth restriction: onset (early or late), etiology (intrinsic, abnormal), anthropometry of the neonate (weight, length and HC), general morphology (harmonious, disharmonious or semiharmonious) and trophism (eutrophic, hypotrophic, dystrophic) (see Table 120.1). Depending on these characteristics, we differentiate three types of growth restriction: type I: intrinsic–harmonious; type II: extrinsic–disharmonious and type III: extrinsic–semiharmonious.

Type I: intrinsic–harmonious

This type is also known as 'symmetrical' or 'early'. The noxa still acts from the beginning of gestation, or at least since the embryonic phase. Due to this precocity, all three parameters usually assessed to judge fetal growth are affected: weight, length and HC. There are references in the literature to microsomatic and hypoplastic fetuses, and also to fetal hypogrowth.

The most outstanding characteristics of this group are:

(1) Neonates do not have a dystrophic appearance and their bodies are well-proportioned;
(2) There is normally no fetal hypoxia;
(3) Metabolic insufficiency is not intense and
(4) The placenta is small and usually histologically normal except in cases of infectious embryopathy.

There are basically three causes:

(1) Genetic or chromosomic causes, that include three possibilities: genetically small but 'normal' fetuses; fetuses with chromosomic alterations (e.g. trisomies) and malformed fetuses;
(2) Infectious causes: viral embryopathies (particularly rubella and cytomegalovirus), toxoplasmosis, etc. and
(3) Toxic causes or ionizing radiations, which are very uncommon.

These fetuses present some characteristics that can be identified prenatally by ultrasound:

(1) Growth restriction is early;
(2) Growth pattern is symmetrical and
(3) There are usually no signs of fetal hypoxia (Doppler studies are normal).

Neonates have sharply defined characteristics, which enable to establish the diagnosis of intrinsic IUGR at birth (Figure 120.1):

(1) Eutrophic appearance;
(2) Harmonious and well-proportioned development;
(3) HC corresponds to weight at birth, but not to gestational age;
(4) Differentiation and maturity of the organs corresponds to gestational age;
(5) The number of cells of the different organs is low (hypoplasia);
(6) Nearly 50% of the cases have serious alterations or congenital malformations, which make life difficult. The prospects for cerebral evolution are very bleak (small cerebral weight, incomplete neuronal capacity, delay in myelinization). Apart from the group of 'normal' neonates, which should be considered as a variant of normality, postnatal development is usually bad.

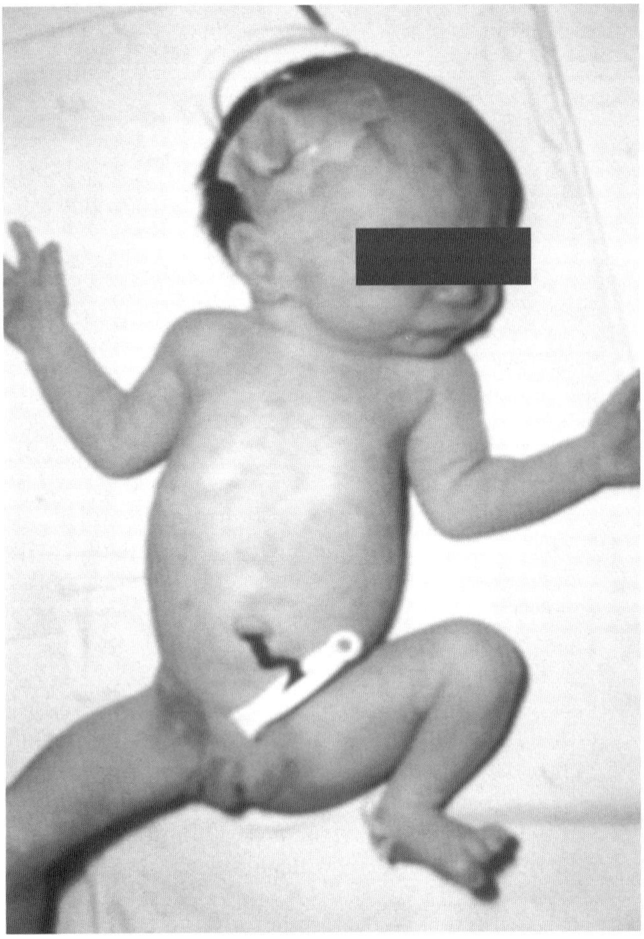

Figure 120.1 Small-for-gestational age neonate who has experienced type I intrauterine growth restriction.

From the pathogenic point of view, the primary growth potential of the fetus is inhibited or modified in these cases by the above-mentioned factors, which produce a decrease in the rate of the use of nutrients per weight unit and a permanent reduction in the number of cells (hypoplasia), by acting on the fetal metabolism and the organogenic process. Even if there is an adequate maternal diet and a satisfactory placental transfer of nutrients, the fetus is, under these circumstances, incapable of taking complete advantage of them, and this logically results in an alteration or restriction of its growth.

Type II: extrinsic–disharmonious

This type is also known as 'asymmetrical', 'late' or 'placental'. As the related factors only occur in the last trimester, only the weight is affected, while the length and HC remain normal or near normal. Its pathogeny is similar to those of IUGR produced artificially in rats by vascular deprivation (failure of nutritive supply).[38]

There are also references in the literature to prenatal dystrophy, fetoplacentary malfunctioning, preterm hypermaturity, chronic fetal distress, prenatal immaturity and placentary insufficiency.

The characteristics of this group are:

(1) Dystrophic or hypermature appearance;
(2) There is usually fetal hypoxia;
(3) The metabolic insufficiency is constant and
(4) The placenta is pathological but not small, and has an almost normal DNA content.

The basic cause lies in an insufficiency of the malfunctioning placenta determined by:

(1) A deficit in uterine perfusion or
(2) A deficit in the vascular surface area (alteration in the villous microcirculation).

Some factors are usually considered enhancing (advanced age of mother, uterine circulatory disorders, anomalies in placental insertion), while others are considered determining (pre-eclampsia, high blood pressure, diabetes, postmaturity). These factors do not usually come into play until the rapidly developing fetus needs the placental reserves (weeks 35–36). If there is a failure in the 'supply line' at this point,[39] the weight curve declines and the fetus becomes more vulnerable. Fetuses generally exhibit the following characteristics:

(1) Late growth restriction;
(2) Asymmetrical growth pattern and
(3) There are usually signs of hypoxia or fetal distress.

Neonates with extrinsic IUGR reveal the following characteristics (Figure 120.2):

(1) Dystrophic appearance; they seem to have lost weight and have an excess of skin;
(2) Disharmonious, disproportionate development;
(3) HC and length correspond better to gestational age than to weight;
(4) The number of cells in their organs is normal, although the cellular mass is reduced (especially in the liver);
(5) They frequently develop postnatal hypoglucemias and
(6) A considerable proportion suffer from neurological disorders caused by perinatal hypoxia.

Type III: extrinsic–semiharmonious or extrinsic symmetrical

This type is somewhat mixed compared with the previous two types; while the operative factor is extrinsic (malnutrition or maternal nutrient deficiency) its consequences resemble those of an intrinsic IUGR, since the noxa is usually active throughout the gestation.

The characteristics of this group are:

(1) Harmonious but undernourished appearance;
(2) Constant metabolic insufficiency;

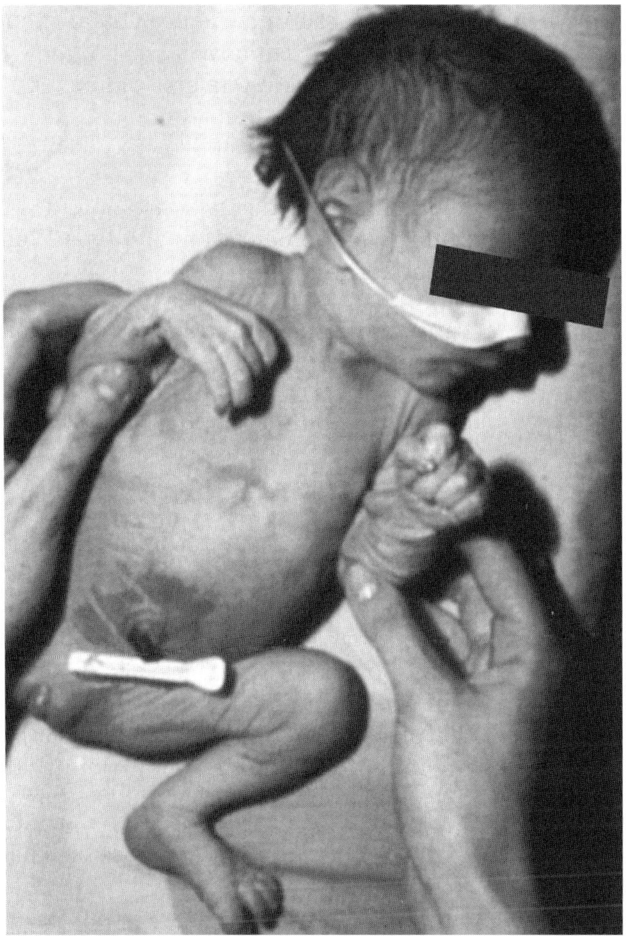

Figure 120.2 Small-for-gestational age neonate who has experienced type II intrauterine growth restriction.

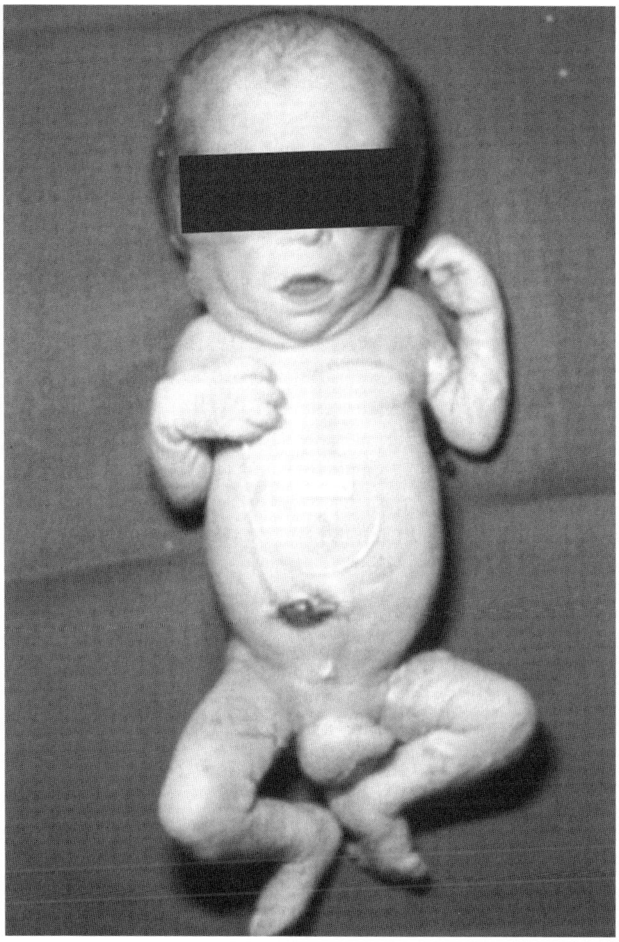

Figure 120.3 Small-for-gestational age neonate who has experienced type III intrauterine growth restriction.

(3) Respiratory insufficiency is uncommon and
(4) A small placenta, with few morphological anomalies, but with clear biochemical changes (DNA reduction).

The cause lies in a severe alteration in maternal nutrition, due to the lack of particularly important factors, such as folic acid, amino acids or other nutrients.

Babies delivered by ill-nourished mothers have been the subject of extensive anthropomorphic, biochemical and cellular studies, which have shown that (Figure 120.3):

(1) Weight, length and HC are reduced, although the reduction in the latter seems less than in intrinsic symmetrical IUGR;
(2) Although all organs are smaller, some of them, specially the liver and the spleen, are particularly small;
(3) Both the number (15–20%) and individual volume of the cells are reduced and
(4) If malnutrition continues postnatally during the cellular division period, the reduction in the number of brain cells can reach up to 60%.[6]

The pathogenesis of this group has been described in detail elsewhere in this chapter.

Factors leading to a modification of the classification

The information that has emerged in recent years has made certain modifications necessary, particularly in the characterization of type I IUGR.

Biometrical studies on SGA neonates with associated congenital defects (chromosomopathies or malformations) observed that these fetuses frequently present an asymmetrical pattern instead of an symmetrical one. Several pediatric studies have shown that a high proportion of malformed neonates and virtually all of those with chromosomopathies associated with growth restriction have a disproportionate disharmonious morphology, so that we include them in the group of asymmetrical growth restriction[19,21,23] and not in that of symmetrical growth restriction.[40] According to several authors, fetuses with symmetrical and asymmetrical IUGR show similar rates of congenital defects[41,42] and a similar degree of acid–base impairment.[43] The ponderal index of Rohrer is abnormally low in the majority of cases. However, necropsic studies on trisomic fetuses (particularly trisomies 18 and 21) reveal a significant reduction in the size and weight of the majority of organs and viscera, apart from the spleen,[44] even after making the appropriate correction for weight.[45] The exception is trisomy 13, where the weight and size of organs are normal.[46] Regarding malformed fetuses, growth restriction may have three origins:[47] (a) the nature of the malformation itself (e.g. cardiopathy) determines the growth restriction by means of hemodynamic alterations;[48] (b) the restriction creates circumstances suiting the emergence of the malformation (early growth restriction represents a state of heightened susceptibility to malformations[49] and (c) the growth restriction and the malformation are the consequence of a common etiological factor (e.g. prenatal infections such as rubella and cytomegalovirus).[48]

A decrease in umbilical perfusion has been observed in a significant proportion of IUGR fetuses with associated congenital defects (chromosomopathies and major malformations). The absence of fetal hypoxia in a type I IUGR is therefore not always true. Several researchers[50–57] have observed a pathological increase in umbilical artery resistance indexes, which could not, however, be confirmed in the uteroplacental arteries. It is still not well known why this increase in umbilical resistance, which in many cases will finally cause an asymmetrical growth restriction, appears in fetuses with congenital defects. There are, at least in theory, two possible explanations: (a) there is a process that obliterates the arteries of the placental tertiary villi,[51] secondary to a thromboembolic or angiospastic phenomenon mediated by the fetus and (b) the placental maturing process does not occur or is delayed, with the logical consequence of placental immaturity.[58] In both cases, there could be a secondary effect on the potential for fetal growth.

A significant number of fetuses with early intrinsic growth restriction and congenital defects present biochemical signs of hypoxia or acidemia. The chance to obtain fetal blood by means of funiculocentesis[59] has enabled us to assess different biochemical parameters (oxygenation, acid–base balance), which give us information on the real state of the fetus.[60] These studies have confirmed that fetuses with late extrinsic IUGR often present hypoxia and acidemia,[61–64] but also that a significant number of fetuses with early restriction, especially those with concomitant congenital defects, present biochemical parameters compatible with chronic hypoxia and even with episodes of severe hypoxia.[65] On the other hand, the mean body weight and degree of karyocytosis is higher in fetuses with triploidies than in SGA fetuses that are chromosomically normal. This makes us think that there is a general delay in hematological maturation in triploidies.[65]

Anatomopathological studies of placentas in trisomic fetuses are both histologically and functionally abnormal,[45,66–68] with a reduced vascular capacity in the tertiary villi,[67] which probably accounts for the decrease in the umbilical conduction indexes and the frequent episodes of distress observed in this type of fetuses.

Early defects in circulatory adaptation can give rise to highly precocious growth restrictions, the majority of which end in pregnancy interruptions. There is increasing evidence that poor pregestational circulatory preparation, with or without uterine vascular deficits, can cause repeated abortions, with associated growth restriction.[69] An inadequate vascular backup, either anatomically or functionally, prevents an adequate implantation, and so a defective circulatory anchorage is established. This 'poor maternal circulatory adaptation' can also have an immunological cause.[70]

Cytogenetic studies of placentas of apparently idiopathic growth restrictions reveal the presence of mosaicisms restricted to the placenta.[71]

Fetuses affected by an infectious embryopathy (rubella, cytomegalovirus) develop a mixed IUGR type.

Echographic follow-ups on some very early onset restrictions demonstrate that some fetuses with a symmetrical morphology during the first half of gestation go on to develop a clearly asymmetrical IUGR. Most of these fetuses are carriers of a congenital defect. In the past, early restrictions with congenital defects were classified as morphologically symmetrical IUGR;[29,32,33,40,72] only in recent years several researchers have refuted this view.[45,65,73] Our opinion, which is endorsed by Droste,[45] is that these cases are probably symmetrical growth restrictions with a superimposed asymmetrical IUGR. An asymmetrical IUGR, accompanied by histological and functional placental alterations, with a reduction in umbilical–placental perfusion and eventual fetal hypoxia, can thus be found in many congenital defects, whether fetal (chromosomopathies, major malformations), and/or placental (mosaicisms restricted to the placenta). However, we should probably not consider it a primary asymmetrical growth restriction, but rather a secondary asymmetrical IUGR, added or superimposed on a symmetrical IUGR due to a reduction of the intrinsic growth potential. This could explain why early echographic studies on these fetuses generally reveal a generalized delay in symmetrical growth, with the asymmetrical or disharmonious nature of fetal growth only becoming apparent later on.

For all these reasons, in recent years we have abandoned classifications based on rigid anthropometric criteria and have adopted another one that strikes us as more useful in practice and pays special attention to the etiopathogenic features of the process.

Modified integrated classification

Considering the large amount of new morphological (cytogenetic and anthropometric), echographic (biometric and Doppler studies) and hematologic (oxygenation, acid–base balance) data obtained by research, we should now adopt the following classification (Table 120.2).

Table 120.2 Modified integrated classification of intrauterine growth restriction (IUGR) (from Carrera and Serra[37])

Type I IUGR	Type II IUGR	Type III IUGR
'Normal' SGA oligohydramnios	Without embryopathies	Infectious
SGA with congenital defects	With oligohydramnios	Toxic embryopathies

SGA, small-for-gestational age

Type I IUGR

This growth restriction is brought on by a reduction in the intrinsic growth potential. The causal agent or agents act during the blastemic and/or embryonic stages. Two subtypes must be distinguished.

Normal small neonates

These neonates are characterized by early reduction in fetal growth (that could be assessed before weeks 30–32), accompanied by harmonious (symmetrical or proportionate) fetal growth and a normal trophism. The well-proportioned fetus presents a HC that corresponds to the weight at birth but not to the gestational age. These neonates are absolutely normal, apart from their delayed growth (maximum 2–3 weeks), and do not show any of the neonatal complications normally associated with IUGR. This condition must be considered as a normality variant due to a genetically low growth potential, which may run in the family.[74]

Neonates with congenital anomalies

These neonates show a very early (or ultraearly) reduction in embryonic or fetal growth with a progressively disharmonious morphology. All these cases present congenital anomalies, either chromosomic or genetic. The delayed growth can always be diagnosed before 22 weeks of gestation, but the fetal corporal asymmetry becomes more apparent as pregnancy advances. A significant number of these gestations abort. The surviving fetuses present a considerable number of deficits as a consequence of the frequent reduction in the number of brain cells.[74] At least 25% of fetuses with severe early growth restriction, which can be diagnosed with echography, are aneuploid.[73]

Type II IUGR

This is defined as delayed growth resulting from an alteration in the supply line, clinically apparent at a late stage (from 30 to 32 weeks), generally through an asymmetrical and disharmonious development of the fetus. It represents 55–75% of all growth restrictions.[9] In fact, the only confirmed reduction in weight in most of these neonates is biometrically restricted to the trunk. Length and HC correspond both more to the gestational age than to the weight. Fetuses have a markedly dystrophic appearance. The number of cells of the different organs is generally normal, although the cellular mass is reduced (especially in the liver), and a reduction in functional elements is sometimes appreciable in some organs. A substantial reduction in the number of nephrons has been demonstrated when the neonate is below the third percentile, and this could not be compensated postnatally.[75] It seems that this type of restriction could cause some pathological processes in adult life, such as cardiovascular diseases,[76] diabetes,[77–81] altered time of onset of puberty,[82] reduced size of the uterus,[83] delayed follicular development,[84] earlier menopause,[85] obesity,[86,87] arterial stiffness[88] and abnormal retinal vascular morphology.[89] This association could be explained with Barker's theory: intrauterine malnutrition leads to a reduction of energy destined to growth in order to allow survival and development of vital organs as the brain. If the availability of nutrients is insufficient to determine critical moments of fetal life, this could lead to an impaired development of the endocrine system and its posterior function.

Even when the data in the literature are contradictory, there seems to be a statistically significant association between the degree of hypoxemia and fetal acidemia and the data obtained by Doppler velocimetry from umbilical, aortic, common carotid and mean cerebral readings.[90–94]

Some authors, given that the velocimetrical data are inherently uncertain for determining the degree of asphyxia, perform a funiculocentesis when the fluxometrical study suggests a centralization of the flow.[95]

Three basic types of clinical pathogenic processes are accepted in this group:

(1) Chronic hypoxia, particularly as a result of cardiorespiratory diseases, which may induce, on a permanent basis, a low partial saturation of oxygen in the blood of the uterine artery.
(2) Maternal malnutrition, which can be due to maternal undernourishment (rare in our society) or an unbalanced maternal diet (sometimes associated with smoking). IUGR can also be caused by maternal hyperinsulinism, with an exaggerated postprandial anabolism and a dispersal of nutrients to the maternal reserves and away from the fetus. This is the so-called 'selfish mother' hypothesis of Frydman *et al.*[96] All pregnant women with baseline or postprandial hypoglucemias are suspects for this group.
(3) Uteroplacental vascular insufficiency, whether through a deficit in uterine perfusion or through a deficit in the vascular exchange surface area, due generally to an insufficient villous microcirculation.

Clinically, it is useful to classify two subgroups.

Table 120.3 Frequency of the three types of intrauterine growth restriction (IUGR) in case histories (from Carrera and Serra[37])

Type of IUGR	Frequency (%)
I	19.7
II	53.9
III	9.2
Non-classified	17.1

Type II IUGR without oligohydramnios

It is to be supposed, in these cases, that the fetal hypoxia is still moderate, since the extreme mechanisms of fetal adaptation have still not been established.

Type II IUGR with oligohydramnios

The gestation must be closely watched in these cases, since there is a fetal adaptation mechanism, which can lead to an acute decompensation.

In the past, it was thought that this kind of IUGR fetuses have an accelerated maturation due to intrauterine stress. This would make them more resistant to neonatal respiratory distress, especially if they were prematurely delivered. But Bernstein[97] has shown that this is not true. He compared the rate of respiratory distress, intraventricular hemorrhage and neonatal mortality between type II IUGR fetuses and controls of the same gestational age, and he found that all these complications were more frequent in the growth-restricted fetuses, independent of the prenatal administration of corticosteroids. Other authors have recently confirmed this observation.[98]

Type III IUGR

This is characterized by delayed growth due to mixed mechanisms, which generally act during a relatively early phase of gestation. For this reason, the fetus usually presents a semiharmonious growth with a hypotrophic appearance. Many fetuses present specific alterations related to the noxa that has produced the growth restriction. The Doppler study is generally normal, and there are no alterations in the hemodynamic parameters of fetal asphyxia. From the etiopathogenic point of view, two types can be identified:

(1) *Infectious embryopathies*: the cause usually lies in rubella, cytomegalovirus or toxoplasmosis infections.
(2) *Toxic embryopathies*: caused by medication, drugs or toxins, although it is not always possible to identify the origin.

In our recent case histories, the distribution of the different types of IUGR is as follows: 19.7% type I, 53.9% type II, 9.2% type III and 17.1% of cases that we have been unable to classify for lack of consistent data (Table 120.3).

REFERENCES

1. Altman DG, Hytten FE. Intrauterine growth restriction: Let's be clear about it. *Br J Obstet Gynaecol* 1989;96:1127–32.
2. Winick M, Noble A. Cellular response in rats during malnutrition at various ages. *J Nutr* 1966;89:300–6.
3. Winick M, Coscia A, Noble A. Cellular growth of human placenta. I. Normal placental growth. *Pediatrics* 1967;39:248–51.
4. Winick M. Changes in nucleic acid and protein content of the human brain during growth of the human brain. *Pediatr Res* 1968;2:352–5.
5. Winick M, Rosso P. Head circumference and cellular growth of the brain in normal and marasmic children. *J Pediatr* 1969;74:774–8.
6. Winick M, Brasel J, Rosso P. Nutrition and cell growth. In Winick M, ed. *Nutrition and Development*. New York: John Wiley, 1972.
7. Tajani N, Mann LI, Weiss RR. Antenatal diagnosis and management of the small-for-gestational age fetus. *Obstet Gynecol* 1976;47:31.
8. Hobbins JC. *Diagnostic Ultrasound in Obstetrics*. New York: Churchill Livingstone, 1979.
9. Campbell S, Dewhurst CJ. Diagnosis of the small-for-dates fetus by serial ultrasonic cephalometry. *Lancet* 1971;2:1002–15.
10. Campbell S, Thoms A. Ultrasound measurement of the fetal head-to-abdomen circumference ratio in the assessment of growth restriction. *Br J Obstet Gynaecol* 1977;84:165–79.
11. Levi S, Kenwez J. Poor intrauterine fetal growth classification based on intrauterine echography. In Salvadori B, Bacchi-Modena A, eds. *Poor Intrauterine Fetal Growth*. Parma: Minerva Médica, 1977:37–41.
12. Levi S. Exploration du couple foeto-placentaire par les ultrasons. *Proceedings of the XXV Congress of the Federal Society of Gynecology and Obstetrics* (in French). Montreal, 1975:165–8.
13. Levi S, Maamari R. Echographic diagnosis of poor intrauterine fetal growth. In Salvadori B, Bacchi-Modena A, eds. *Poor Intrauterine Fetal Growth*. Parma: Minerva Médica, 1977:251–4.
14. Warsof SL, Cooper DJ, Little D, Campbell S. Routine ultrasound screening for antenatal detection of intrauterine growth restriction. *Obstet Gynecol* 1986;67:33–9.
15. Clark SL. Patterns of intrauterine growth restriction. *Clin Obstet Gynecol* 1992;35(1):194–201.
16. Rosso P, Winick M. Intrauterine growth restriction. A new systematic approach based on the clinical and biometrical characteristics of this condition. *J Perinat Med* 1974;42:147–60.
17. Sieroszewski J. Poor intrauterine fetal growth. Classification system for the fetus. In Salvadori B, Bacchi-Modena A, eds. *Poor Intrauterine Fetal Growth*. Parma: Minerva Médica, 1977:31–5.
18. Holtorff J. Poor intrauterine fetal growth. An intrauterine nomenclature approach. In Salvadori B, Bacchi-Modena A, eds. *Poor Intrauterine Fetal Growth*. Parma: Minerva Médica, 1977:23–7.
19. Miller RC, Hassanein K. Diagnosis of impaired fetal growth in newborn infants. *Pediatrics* 1971;48:511–22.
20. Villar J, Belizan JM. The timing factor in the pathophysiology of the intrauterine growth restriction syndrome. *Obstet Gynecol Surv* 1982;37:499–506.
21. Balcazar H, Haas J. Classification schemes of small-for-gestational age and type of intrauterine growth restriction and its implications for early neonatal mortality. *Early Hum Dev* 1990;24:219–30.
22. Grauw TJ, Hopkins B. Severity of growth restriction and physical condition at birth in small-for-gestational age infants. *Biol Neonate* 1991;60:176–83.
23. Tudehope DI. Neonatal aspects of intrauterine growth restriction. *Fetal Med Rev* 1991;3:73–85.

24. Salvadori B. Poor intrauterine fetal growth: An attempt to make out an intrauterine classification. In Salvadori B, Bacchi-Modena A, eds. *Poor Intrauterine Fetal Growth*. Parma: Minerva Médica, 1977.
25. Gruenwald P. Chronic fetal distress and placental insufficiency. *Biol Neonate* 1963;5:215–21.
26. Carrera JM. Intrauterine growth restriction. Proceedings of the *VIII World Congress of Gynecology and Obstetrics (FIGO)*, Mexico DF, October 1976.
27. Carrera JM. Diagnóstico prenatal del retardo de creci-miento fetal. *Clín Ginecol* 1977;2.
28. Carrera JM. Diagnosis of intrauterine growth restriction. In Salvadori B, Bacchi-Modena A, eds. *Poor Intrauterine Fetal Growth*. Parma: Minerva Médica, 1977:277–81.
29. Carrera JM. Concepto, selección y clasificación de los recién nacidos pequeños por retardo de crecimiento intrauterino. *Prog Obstet Ginecol* 1978;21:197–208.
30. Carrera JM, Mallafré J. Tratamiento *in utero* del retardo de crecimiento fetal. In Esteban Altirriba J, ed. *Perinatología Clínica*. Barcelona: Salvat, 1980;3.
31. Carrera JM. Regulación del crecimiento fetal. In Carrera JM, ed. *Biología y Ecología Fetal*. Barcelona: Salvat, 1981.
32. Carrera JM. Crecimiento fetal: Sus alteraciones. *Clín Ginecol* 1981;5:1–7.
33. Carrera JM. Patogénesis del crecimiento intrauterino retardado. *Clín Ginecol* 1981;5:71–85.
34. Carrera JM, Serrat X. Crecimiento intrauterino retardado: Concepto, frecuencia y clasificación. *Clín Ginecol* 1981;5: 36–42.
35. Carrera JM. *Clasificación del crecimiento intrauterino retardado*. PhD thesis, University of Santiago de Compostela, 1981.
36. Carrera JM. Tratamiento prenatal del retraso de crecimiento fetal. In Carrera JM, ed. *Biología y Ecología Fetal*. Barcelona: Salvat, 1981.
37. Carrera JM, Serra B. Clasificación del crecimiento intrauterino retardado. *Rev Iberoam Fertil* 1993;10:21–30.
38. Wigglesworth JS. Experimental growth restriction in the fetal rat. *J Pathol Bacteriol* 1964;88:1.
39. Gruenwald P. Growth of the human fetus. I. Normal growth and its variation. *Am J Obstet Gynecol* 1966;94:1112–9.
40. Gabbe S, Niebye JR, Simpson JL. *Obstetrics: Normal and Problem Pregnancies*. New York: Churchill Livingstone, 1986:771.
41. Nyberg DA, Abuhamad A and Ville Y. Ultrasound assessment of abnormal fetal growth. *Semin Perinatol* 2004;28:3–21.
42. Vik T, Vatten L, Jacobsen G. Prenatal growth in symmetric and asymmetric small-for-gestational-age infants. *Early Hum Dev* 1997;48:167–76.
43. Blackwell SC, Moldenhauer J, Redman M. Relationship between the sonographic pattern of intrauterine growth restriction and acid–base status at the time of cordocentesis. *Arch Gynecol Obstet* 2001;263:191–3.
44. Fitz-Simmons J, Droste S, Shepard TH, Pascoe-Mason J, Fantel A. A growth failure in second trimester fetuses with trisomy 21. *Teratology* 1990;42:337–45.
45. Droste S. Fetal growth in aneuploid conditions. *Clin Obstet Gynecol* 1992;35(1):119–25.
46. Fujinaga M, Shepard TH, Fitz-Simmons J. Trisomy 13 in the fetus. *Teratology* 1990;41:233–8.
47. Khoury MJ, Erickson JD, Cordero JF, McCarthy BJ. Congenital malformations and intrauterine growth restriction: A population study. *Pediatrics* 1988;82:83–90.
48. Creasy RK, Resnick R. Intrauterine growth restriction. In Creasy RK, Resnick R, eds. *Maternal Fetal Medicine: Principles and Practice*. Philadelphia: WB Saunders, 1984:491–510.
49. Spiers PS. Does growth restriction predispose the fetus to congenital malformations? *Lancet* 1982;1:312–4.
50. Trudinger BJ, Giles WB, Cook CM, Bombardieri J, Collins L. Fetal umbilical artery flow velocity waveforms and placental resistance: Clinical significance. *Br J Obstet Gynaecol* 1985;92:23–30.
51. Meizner I, Katz M, Lunenfeld E, Insler V. Umbilical and uterine flow velocity waveforms in pregnancies complicated by major fetal anomalies. *Prenat Diagn* 1987;7:491–3.
52. Schulman H. The clinical implications of Doppler ultrasound analysis of uterine and umbilical arteries. *Am J Obstet Gynecol* 1987;156:889–93.
53. Hsieh FJ, Chang FM, Ko TM, Chen HY, Chen YP. Umbilical artery flow velocity waveforms in fetuses dying with congenital anomalies. *Br J Obstet Gynaecol* 1988;95:478–82.
54. Hata K, Hata T, Senoh D, Aoki S, Takamiya O, Kitao M. Umbilical artery blood flow velocity waveforms and association with fetal abnormality. *Gynecol Obstet Invest* 1989;27:179–82.
55. Gaziano E, Knok E, Wager GP, Bendel RP, Olson JD. Pulsed Doppler umbilical artery waveforms: Significance of elevated artery systolic/diastolic ratios in the normally grown fetus. *Obstet Gynecol* 1990;75:189–93.
56. Carrera JM, Mortera C. Estudio Doppler de los defectos congénitos. *Primer Congreso Mundial de Obstetricia y Ginecología*, London, 1991.
57. Carrera JM, Mortera C, Alegre M, *et al*. Velocimetría Doppler en el control del crecimiento fetal. In Carrera JM, ed. *Doppler en Obstetricia*. Barcelona: Masson-Salvat, 1992:309–15.
58. Trudinger BJ, Giles WB, Cook CM. Flow velocity waveforms in the maternal uteroplacental and fetal umbilical placental circulations. *Am J Obstet Gynecol* 1985;152:155–63.
59. Daffos F, Capella-Paulousky M, Forestier F. A new procedure on pure fetal blood sampling *in utero*. *Prenat Diagn* 1983;3:271–7.
60. Daffos F, Capella-Paulousky M, Forestier F. Fetal blood sampling during pregnancy with use of needle guided by ultrasound: A study of 606 consecutive cases. *Am J Obstet Gynecol* 1985;53: 655–60.
61. Soothill PW, Nicolaides KH, Campbell S. Prenatal asphyxia hyperlacticaemia, hypoglucaemia and erythroblastosis in growth-retarded fetuses. *Br Med J* 1987;294:1051–3.
62. Cox WL, Daffos F, Forestier F, Descombey D, Autrant C, Auger MC. Physiology and management of intrauterine growth restriction: A biologic approach with fetal blood sampling. *Am J Obstet Gynecol* 1988;159:36–41.
63. Nicolaides KH, Economides DL, Soothill PW. Blood gases, pH and lactate in appropriate and small-for-gestational age fetuses. *Am J Obstet Gynecol* 1989,161:996–1001.
64. Weiner CP, Williamson RA. Evaluation of severe growth restriction using cordocentesis. *Obstet Gynecol* 1989;73:225–9.
65. Nicolaides KH, Moya JMF, Snijders RJM. Cordocentesis en fetos pequeños para la edad de gestación. *Prog Diagn Prenat* 1991; 3:15–22.
66. Kuhlmann RS, Werner AL, Abramowicz J, Warsof SL, Arrington J, Levy DL. Placental histology in fetuses between 18 and 23 weeks' gestation with abnormal karyotype. *Am J Obstet Gynecol* 1990;163:1264–70.
67. Rochelson B, Kaplan C, Guzmán E, Arato M, Hansen K, Trunca C. A quantitative analysis of placental vasculature in the third trimester fetus with autosomal trisomy. *Obstet Gynecol* 1990,75.59–63.
68. Delozier-Blanchet CD. Anomalies cytogenetiques et function placentaire. *Rev Fr Gynecol Obstet* 1991;86:725–9.
69. Carrera JM, Mallafré J, Otero F, Rubio R, Carrera M. Síndrome de mala adaptación circulatoria materna: Bases etiopatogénicas y terapéuticas. In Carrera JM, ed. *Doppler en Obstetricia*. Barcelona: Masson-Salvat, 1992:335–59.
70. Scott JB, Rote NS, Branch DW. Immunologic aspects of recurrent abortion and fetal death. *Obstet Gynecol* 1987;70:645–56.
71. Kalousek DK, Howard-Peebles PN, Olson SB, *et al*. Confirmation of CVS mosaicism in term placentae and high frequency of intrauterine growth restriction association with confirmed placental mosaicism. *Prenat Diagn* 1991;11:743–50.
72. Villar J, Smeriglio V, Martorell R, Brown CH, Klein RE. Heterogeneous growth and mental development of intrauterine growth-retarded infection in the first 3 years of life. *Pediatrics* 1984;74:783–91.
73. Drugan A, Johnson MP, Isada NB, *et al*. The smaller than expected first trimester fetus is at increased risk for chromosome anomalies. *Am J Obstet Gynecol* 1992;167:1525–8.
74. Dashe JS, McIntire DD, Lucas MJ. Effects of symmetric and asymmetric fetal growth on pregnancy outcomes. *Obstet Gynecol* 2000;96(3):321–7.
75. Pollak RN, Divon MJ. Intrauterine growth restriction: Definition, classification and etiology. *Clin Obstet Gynecol* 1992;35:99–107.
76. Hinchcliffe SA, Lynch MRJ, Sargent PH, Howard CV, Van Velzen D. The effort of intrauterine growth restriction in the development of renal nephrons. *Br J Obstet Gynaecol* 1992;99:296–301.
77. Barker DJ. Fetal growth and adult disease. *Br J Obstet Gynaecol* 1992;92:275–82.
78. Phillips DIW, Barker DJP, Hales CN, Hirst S, Osmond C. Thinness at birth and insulin resistance in adult life. *Diabetology* 1994;37:150–4.
79. Kanaka-Gantenbein C, Mastorakos G, Chrousos GP. Endocrine related cancer and consequences of IUGR. *Ann N Y Acad Sci* 2003;997:150–7.

80. Ozanne SE, Fernandez-Twinn D, Hales N. Fetal growth and adult diseases. *Semin Perinatol* 2004;28:81–7.
81. Cianfarani S. Fetal origin of adult diseases: Just a matter of stem cell number? *Med Hypotheses* 2003;61(3):401–4.
82. Ibañez,L, Ferrer A, Marcos MV, Hierro FR, de Zegner F. Early puberty: Rapid progression and reduced final heights in girls with low birth weight. *Pediatrics* 2000;106:72.
83. Ibañez L, Potau N, Enriquez G, de Zegner F. Reduced uterine and ovarian size in adolescent girls born small for gestational age. *Pediatr Res* 2000;47:575–7.
84. Da Silva-Butkus P, Van den Hurk R, Velde ER, Taverne MAM. Ovarian development in IUGR and normally developed piglets originating from the same litter. *Reproduction* 2003;126:249–58.
85. Cressswell JL, Egger P, Fall CHD, Osmond C, Fraser RB, Barker DJP. Is the age of menopause determined in utero? *Early Hum Dev* 1997;49:143–8.
86. Nales CN, Ozanne SZ. The dangerous route of catch-up growth. *J Physiol* 2003;1:5–10.
87. Hack M, Schluchter M, Cartar L, Rahman M. Growth of very low birth weight infants to age 20 years. *Pediatrics* 2003;112(1):30–8.
88. Cheung YF, Wong KY, Lam BC, Tsoi NS. Relation of arterial stiffness with gestational age and birth weight. *Arch Dis Child* 2004; 89:217–21.
89. Hellström A, Dahlgren J, Marsal K, Ley D. Abnormal retinal vascular morphology in young adults following intrauterine growth restriction. *Pediatrics* 2004;113(2):77–80.
90. Pardi G, Cetin J, Marconi AM, *et al.* Diagnostic value of blood sampling in fetuses with growth restriction. *N Engl J Med* 1993; 328:692–6.
91. Nicolaides KH, Bilardo CM, Soothill PW, Campbell S. Absence of end-diastolic frequencies in the umbilical artery: A sign of fetal hypoxia and acidosis. *Br Med J* 1988;297:1026–7.
92. Bilardo CM, Nicolaides KH, Campbell S. Doppler measurement of fetal and uteroplacental circulation: Relationship with umbilical venous blood gases measured at cordocentesis. *Am J Obstet Gynecol* 1990;162:15–19.
93. Vyas S, Nicolaides KH, Bowers S, Campbell S. Middle cerebral artery flow velocity waveforms in fetal hypoxemia. *Br J Obstet Gynaecol* 1990;97:797–803.
94. Burke G, Stuart B, Crowley P, Scanaill SN, Drumm J. Is intrauterine growth restriction with normal umbilical artery blood flow a benign condition? *Br Med J* 1990;300:1044–5.
95. Campbell S, Soothill PW. Rule of fetal blood gas analysis in intrauterine growth restriction. *Lancet* 1990;336:1316–7.
96. Frydman R, Papiernik E, Girard JR, Assan R. Fetal growth. *Proceedings of the V Congreso Europeo de Medicina Perinatal,* Uppsala, 1976:203–25.
97. Bernstein IM, Horbar JD, Badger GJ. Morbidity and mortality among very low birth weight neonates with intrauterine growth restriction. The Vermont Oxford Network. *Am J Obstet Gynecol* 2000;182:198–206.
98. Gilbert WM, Danielsen BD. Pregnancy outcomes associated with intrauterine growth restriction. *Am J Obstet Gynecol* 2003;188: 1596–601.

121 Natural history of fetal compromise in intrauterine growth retardation

J. M. Carrera, C. Comas, M. Torrents, A. Muñoz, C. Mortera and B. Serra

There are a number of causes of fetal compromise in intrauterine growth retardation (IUGR), ranging from inadequate uteroplacental perfusion to compression of the umbilical cord due to oligohydramnios, insufficient placental microcirculation or a deterioration in maternal oxygenation. These phenomena can occur singly or in combination, and sooner or later they lead to hypoxemia, which triggers the fetal defense mechanisms designed to limit as far as possible the extent of asphyxia and, above all, to avoid brain damage and fetal death – sometimes, regrettably, to no avail.

Some of these mechanisms are hemodynamic, and aim to adapt the fetal circulation to the changed circumstances, but others are biochemical and seek to supply energy to the fetus under anaerobic conditions, and reduce its need for oxygen. A healthy fetus is equipped with a significant number of mechanisms and strategies for reducing the impact of asphyxia. Severe and possibly irreversible damage occurs only when the gravity of the anoxia exceeds the system's capacity to maintain the cellular mechanism within acceptable limits in specially vulnerable organs, such as the brain or the heart. On the other hand, fetal responses against such asphyxic aggression are not uniform. While some fetuses or neonates emerge neurologically undamaged from an episode of asphyxia, others acquire serious neurological and mental deficits. It goes without saying that the circumstances prior to the asphyxic accident must be evaluated with sufficient attention to explain why some are more vulnerable than others. It is therefore a mistake to consider that perinatal asphyxia causes brain damage and/or cerebral palsy in every case.[1–3]

However, although the incidence of hypoxic encephalopathy as a result of IUGR has declined considerably as a consequence of obstetric practice, which places an even greater emphasis on the interests of the fetus, it cannot by any means be considered a thing of the past. It is true that the great obstetric traumas generated by brain damage have practically disappeared, and many encephalopathies are now recognized as being secondary to genetic, infectious or metabolic processes unrelated to asphyxia, but even so a certain number of handicaps clearly do have this origin. The cerebral palsy rate in neonates at term is still 1–2 per 1000 in industrial countries.[1] According to the calculations of the American Academy of Pediatrics and the American Association of Obstetricians and Gynecologists,[4] at least 10% of these are associated with perinatal asphyxia.[5] Finally, prolonged follow-up studies[6] warn that neonates with hypoxic encephalopathy who survive the postnatal period show handicap figures at the age of 8 years between 15% and 10%, depending on whether the hypoxic encephalopathy is moderate or severe.

All this indicates the importance of studying the biophysical and biochemical mechanisms of fetal compromise and, if possible, establishing markers that allow us to identify cases of growth retardation with a poor neurological prognosis.

We shall distinguish between, on the one hand, the possibility of performing hemodynamic studies (with the use of Doppler technology) in those cases with a physiopathology primarily based on uteroplacental deterioration, and, on the other hand, fetal defensive biochemical mechanisms against hypoxia and their intrauterine study.

Hemodynamic study of fetal deterioration

The reduction in the number of functional arterioles in the tertiary villi, through the mechanisms already described in the explanation of the pathogenesis of IUGR, progressively increases the circulatory resistance in the umbilical artery, and gives rise to a decrease in the pO_2 in the umbilical vein. Both these events set into motion a phenomenon of circulatory redistribution principally characterized by the centralization of blood flow. The better-oxygenated blood goes toward the most vital organs (brain, heart, adrenals), while vasoconstriction limits the blood's arrival at the organs considered less indispensable (digestive system, lungs, skin, skeleton, etc.).

The redistribution or centralization of blood flow has been studied in animal experimentation by various researchers,[7–9] and the above-mentioned mechanical pattern has been confirmed. However, it should be stressed that when fetal hypoxemia was induced by maternal hypoxemia, not only was there an increase in cardiac and cerebral perfusion, but there was also a significant increase in the umbilical blood flow, and this was not the case when the fetal asphyxia originated from microembolization of the umbilical arteries, thus creating conditions similar to those of a human fetus with a placental lesion.[10,11]

Thanks to the Doppler technique, it is possible to recognize four periods with relatively well-defined hemodynamic, biophysical and biochemical patterns. These are (1) a silent period of increase in resistance; (2) a period with reduction in umbilical blood flow; (3) a period with centralization of the blood flow and (4) a period with decentralization of blood flow.

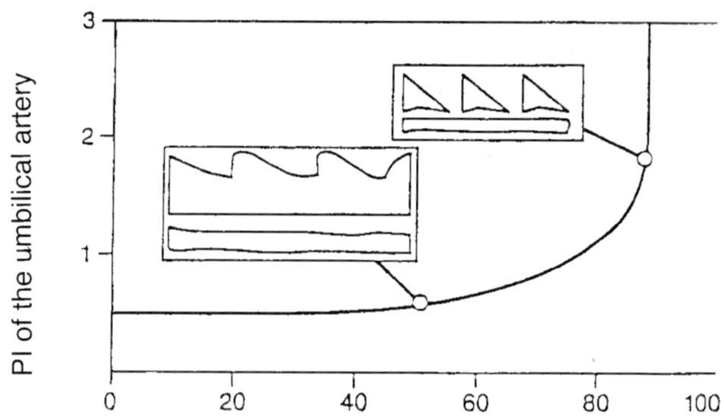

Figure 121.1 Trudinger's mathematical model,[12] relating the morphology of the flow velocity waveform of the umbilical artery (Doppler) with the resistance in the villous arteriolar system (percentage of obstructed villous arterioles). PI, pulsatility index.

Silent period of increase in resistance

Pathophysiological basis

The progressive deterioration of the villous microcirculation is reflected in the Doppler study of the umbilical artery, when the functional obstruction reaches 50% of the villous arteriolar system, and significantly modifies the pulsatility index (PI)[12] (Figure 121.1).

Before this percentage is reached, the capacity of the placental reserves covers the theoretical deficit of gaseous exchange, provided the maternal supply line remains satisfactory.[13]

Doppler hemodynamic profile

The hemodynamic profile is completely normal over a certain period (generally 3–6 weeks), and there is no pathology of any kind. The flow velocity waveform (FVW) of the umbilical artery is normal (positive blood flow over the whole cardiac cycle, with normal PIs, resistance or conductancy.[14,15] Doppler studies on the remaining vessels (aorta, common carotid and middle cerebral arteries) also prove normal. We can therefore speak of a 'normal hemodynamic pattern'.

In a Doppler study we carried out on 82 cases of growth retardation confirmed at birth, we demonstrated that 36 of them (43.9%) had a normal umbilical PI; the study of the remaining fetal vessels proved normal in all these cases (Table 121.1). For this reason, we consider it unnecessary in practice to widen the hemodynamic study of the fetus when the umbilical FVW is normal.

Biophysical correlation

Both the cardiotocography and the remaining parameters of the biophysical profile are normal.

Biochemical correlation

The study of fetal blood gases by funiculocentesis is normal. According to the limits of our current experience, such an exploration is therefore not justified when the Doppler study is normal.

Obstetric outcome

The perinatal mortality rate is not increased.

Reduction in umbilical blood flow

This is the first objective sign of the start of chronic fetal distress brought on by the placental lesion.

Pathophysiological basis

It has been demonstrated that the functional obstruction of over 50% of the villous arterioles is translated into a clear deterioration of the umbilical FVW[6] (Figure 121.1).

Although some studies claim that the umbilical artery is not always the first vessel affected,[16] in our experience and in that of other authors,[17,18] an increase in umbilical resistance is usually the first observable hemodynamic signal when there is a placental lesion affecting the villous microcirculation. In 15–20% of fetuses with growth retardation with a placental cause, the abrupt decrease in pO_2 can give rise, through the aortic and carotid chemoreceptors, to an increase in the aortic and/or cerebral PI, which exceeds and/or precedes those observed in the umbilical artery. On the other hand, it is also possible to observe pathological values of the aortic or cerebral PI before an alteration in umbilical perfusion, when the cause of fetal distress does not reside in the placenta but in a disorder in the mother's internal medium (hypoxemia through maternal cardiorespiratory pathology, an acute deficit of specific nutrients, severe anemia, etc.), or in her hemodynamics

Table 121.1 Cases of intrauterine growth retardation, grouped into four groups according to the pulsatility index (PI) results in the umbilical artery and the fetal hemodynamic profile (FHP); thoracic aorta PI, common carotid artery PI and middle cerebral artery PI. The pH of the umbilical vein was measured at birth

		Cases		Perinatal mortality		pH < 7.20	
Group	**Association**	*n*	%	*n*	%	*n*	%
I	Normal umbilical PI + normal FHP	36	43.9	0	0.0	6	16.6
II	Normal umbilical PI + abnormal FHP	0	0.0	—	—	—	—
III	Abnormal umbilical PI + normal FHP	22	26.8	0	0.0	8	36.3
IV	Abnormal umbilical PI + abnormal FHP	24	29.2	6	25.0	15	62.5
Total		82	100.0	6	7.3	29	35.3

(e.g. hypertensive crises with a renal or endocrine origin). Even in these cases, umbilical conductance may be increased.

Alternatively, there is irrefutable experimental evidence that a placental lesion is followed by a decrease in umbilical arterial perfusion. Morrow *et al.*[10,11] working with fetal sheep subjected to an embolism of the villous microcirculation (plastic micropistons 50 μm in diameter), observed gradual changes in the FVW of the umbilical artery similar to those described in human fetuses subjected to growth retardation through villous pathology (reduction in end-diastolic blood flow, zero diastole and, finally, reverse blood flow). The cause, therefore, of the deterioration of the umbilical FVW lies in the increase in microvillous vascular resistance, which while primarily inducing a deficit in the perfusion in the umbilical artery, is also the reason for a progressive decrease in the pO_2 in the umbilical vein. Hypoxemia is thus the result and not the cause of the hemodynamic umbilical–placental alteration. This is why a reduction in pO_2 without any placental lesion does not give rise to any change in the umbilical FVW,[10,11,19,20] and neither does this change occur through an increase in hematic viscosity or a rise in maternal blood pressure.[10,11]

Doppler hemodynamic profile

A moderate increase in umbilical resistance is the only finding capable of revealing the onset of chronic fetal distress for a specific period of time, the duration of which largely depends on how quickly the placental lesion takes effect. During this period, the Doppler study of the rest of the fetal circulatory system, including the aorta, is usually normal. In our experience 56% of fetuses with growth retardation presented an altered umbilical PI, but of these only 52% were accompanied by a pathological hemodynamic pattern.

The umbilical FVW presents positive flow velocities throughout the entire cardiac cycle, but the pulsatility (or conductance) indices reveal values outside the accepted limits for the gestation.

The only compensatory hemodynamic process that can be observed at this time, with the use, in particular, of color Doppler, is the reopening of the ductus venosus, the caliber of which is physiologically reduced at the end of the second trimester. This mechanism makes it possible to extract a significant amount of blood from the fetal liver, and this goes directly to the heart. This 'shunt' can delay by some weeks the need for a centralization of the blood flow, but induces the appearance of typical asymmetric growth retardation.[18]

In the cerebral circulation, it is also possible to confirm, in some cases, the existence of a decrease in the PI of the M_2 sector of the middle cerebral artery, with the M_1/M_2 index passing from below 1 (normal) to over 1 (pathological). This occurrence, secondary to the selective vasodilatation of that arterial tract, which can be considered as the subcortical sector of the artery, represents a preservation mechanism for specific areas in the brain, and precedes the authentic brain-sparing effect.

The objective of these two compensatory mechanisms is to delay as far as possible the stimulation of the aortic and carotid chemoreceptors, which will set in motion the centralization of flow.

Biophysical correlation

All the parameters of the biophysical profile, including the cardiotocographic study, are normal, as are the results of 'vibroacoustic stimulation' (VAS) tests and even the stress tests (test of strength, oxytocin test, etc.). This is because these variables are affected only when hypoxia of the fetal brain and/or heart occurs.

Biochemical correlation

The fetus is normally in normoxia. In our experience, it is not necessary to carry out diagnostic funiculocentesis in this phase if there is confirmation that centralization of the blood flow has not begun.

Obstetric outcome

There were no fetal deaths in our statistics for this group but there was a significant increase in the percentage of small-for-dates neonates. For this reason, the percentage of neonates with pH below 7.20 reached 38%. In fact, the percentage of intrapartum fetal distresses tripled, proof of a greater fetal vulnerability. The cesarean rate rose to 30–40%.

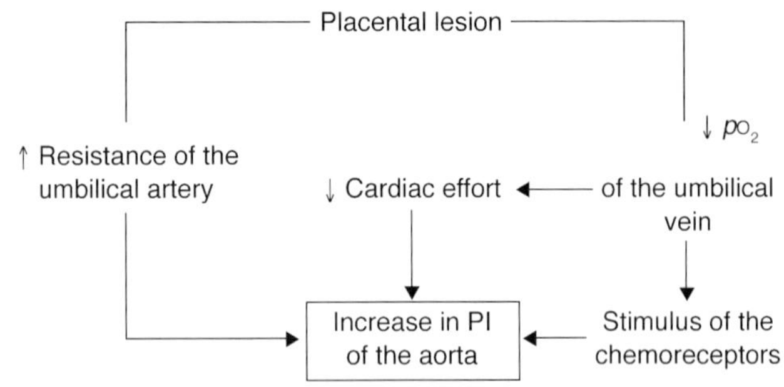

Figure 121.2 Outline of the mechanisms that influence the pulsatility index (PI) in the aorta after the placental lesion.

Centralization of blood flow

Pathophysiological basis

As the resistance in the umbilical arterial system increases, there is also a corresponding decrease in the pO_2 in the umbilical vein. This means that the fetus must carry out, in addition to a reopening of the ductus venosus, a redistribution of its blood flow once a specific pO_2 value has been reached, in order to protect its most important structures from hypoxia. As we have already explained, this redistribution consists of a circulatory centralization with selective vasodilatation of certain organs, such as the brain, the heart and the adrenals, and a vasoconstriction of other sites such as the lung, the intestine, the skin, the kidney or the skeleton. This redistribution can be seen with Doppler, which records a successive increase in the PI of the aorta and the renal artery, and a decreased PI in the common carotid artery and the intracranial vessels.

These changes in the perfusion of the various organs are primarily mediated by neuronal stimulation, whether directly by stimulation of the vagal center or through the aortic and carotid chemoreceptors. In 1969, Dawes *et al.*[21] confirmed that the aortic chemoreceptors in sheep respond to small reductions in arterial oxygen levels. However, it is very probable that these vasoconstriction phenomena are modulated by other factors, such as, for example, the direct effect of hypoxemia and acidemia on certain tissues through liberating vasoactive substances, secretion of catecholamines, or an overall increase in the activity of the autonomic nervous system.

Although the chronological pattern is not well established, it seems that the first vessel to be affected after the umbilical artery is the aorta. The increase in resistance in the descending thoracic aorta is the result of the combined action of several factors: an increase in umbilical–placental resistance, arterial vasoconstriction resulting in progressive hypoxemia and, finally, a decrease in myocardial contractility.[22] Lingman *et al.*[23] postulate an inverse relationship between myocardial contractility and the aortic and umbilical PI (Figure 121.2).

Doppler hemodynamic profile

Doppler study reveals an increase in PI, not only in the umbilical artery but also in the descending thoracic aorta and its branches, such as the renal artery.[24–28] There is a progressive loss of end-diastolic velocity in both vessels when the resistance reaches a certain level. At the same time, there is a noticeable decrease in the PI of the cerebral and common carotid arteries, evidence of a further vasodilatation process.

In our previously mentioned study, of the 82 cases of IUGR studied, 46 (56.1%) presented a pathological umbilical PI, 52% of the fetuses also had an abnormal increase in the PI of the thoracic aorta and 41.1% presented a further decrease in resistance in the common carotid and/or middle cerebral arteries.

It is often possible to recognize three phases in the centralization of blood flow.

Initial phase. The PI in the umbilical artery is high, but there are still positive values in the Doppler frequencies throughout the whole cardiac cycle, even in telediastole.

On the other hand, the FVW of the common carotid artery, which has no end-diastolic frequencies until weeks 32–34,[29] recovers its end-diastolic flow shortly after a proven moderate increase in intracranial perfusion. This suggests that the fall in the PI of the common carotid artery is due to the reduction in the resistance of the cerebral vessels.

The study of the umbilical PI/middle cerebral PI (U/C) relationship can prove particularly helpful in making a definitive assessment of centralization at this stage. Several authors[17,30,31] maintain that this is the best fluxometric index for tracing IUGR.

Advanced phase. The umbilical FVW shows zero diastole. The first to disappear were the telediastolic frequencies, but afterward the lack of blood flow affected the whole diastole. According to Trudinger,[12] this situation occurs when an 80% obstruction in the villous arteriolar system has been attained. The FVW of the aorta also loses its end-diastolic values.

In conjunction with this deterioration in the umbilical blood flow, the vasodilatation of the cerebral vessels arrives at its maximum point, which means that the PI of both the common carotid and the middle cerebral arteries attain their lowest values.

Terminal phase. In addition to an absence of end-diastolic flow, there is the onset of a reverse flow, both in the umbilical artery and in the aorta, and this obviously aggravates the prognosis. As well as the arterial hemodynamic findings already described, there are signs in this phase of cardiac insufficiency, revealed by Doppler study of the fetal venous circulation through a decrease both in the velocity peaks in the exit tracts and in the ventricular ejection force, and through a possible visualization of the coronary blood flow.[32]

As regards the venous return circulation, there are three signals:

(1) Raised reverse blood flow in the inferior vena cava, coinciding with auricular contraction. This finding, which reveals difficulties in the blood flow through the right atrium, can be due both to alterations in the fetal cardiac frequency and to deficient auricular contractility.[33–35] The reverse flow can reach up to 30% of the total blood flow (under normal conditions this does not exceed 10%).
(2) Reduction in the telediastolic velocity values in the ductus venosus (in the notch that reflects the auricular contraction). This reduction can lead to an inversion of the blood flow. This would be secondary not only to the increase in telediastolic volume determined by the increase in the peripheral resistance, but also to the reduction in the capacity for myocardial response.
(3) 'Venous' pulsation in the umbilical vein, with an apparent cyclical decrease in the venous flow, coinciding with the zero diastole of the umbilical artery.

As regards the exit blood flows, there have been reports of their progressive deterioration in this phase, with a clear reduction in their velocity peaks and decreased cardiac output.[36] The most recent observation in this respect is probably the reduction in the values of the so-called 'ventricular ejection force' (VEF).[37]

It has been demonstrated that the VEF values of both the right and the left ventricles are similar and increase throughout gestation in fetuses with normal growth. In contrast, there is a significant decrease in both ventricles, below the fifth percentile of the normality curves, in the terminal phase of the centralization of the blood flow.[37] Furthermore, there is an excellent correlation between the VEF values and the severity of the acidosis registered by funiculocentesis. It can therefore be stated that this hemodynamic finding is significantly related to a serious fetal compromise.

The visualization of the coronary blood flow, in the context of a severe uteroplacental insufficiency, must be interpreted as a very serious sign of fetal distress, probably *pre mortem*. The phenomenon is particularly visible in the diastole.

The coronary vasodilation, which makes it possible, can be the result of three different types of mechanism: (a) an attempt at compensation provoked by low myocardial oxygen pressure; (b) loss of myocardial contraction force, which causes a reduction in the pressure on the coronary arteries (especially during the diastole) and (c) decrease in the velocity of the intracardial blood flows, with the same result as in (b).

The first autoregulating mechanism described could be called a heart-sparing effect, and this has been studied in detail.[32]

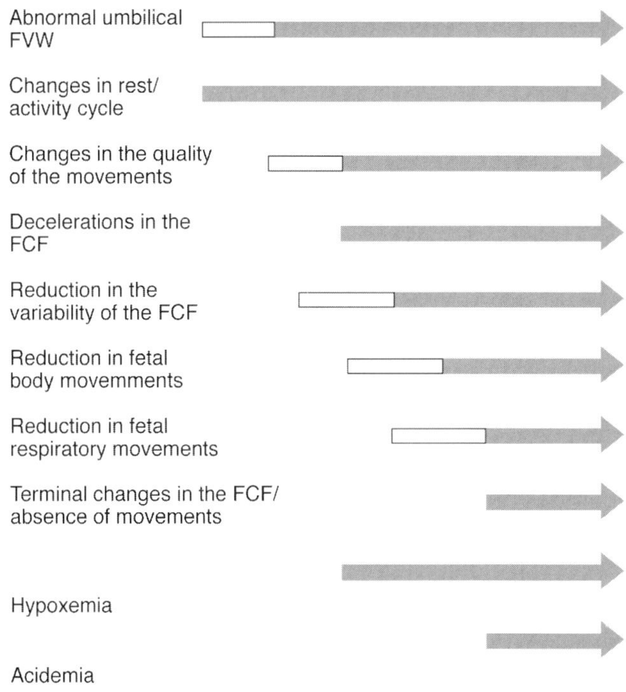

Figure 121.3 Chronological correlation (represented by the different lengths of the arrows) of the biophysical signs of fetal deterioration. The open parts of the arrows represent the silent phase whereas the hatched parts represent the detection phase. FVW, flow velocity waveforms; FCF, fetal cardiac frequency.

Biophysical correlation

In the initial phase of centralization, the cardiotocographic readings can still apparently be normal and Manning's biophysical profile proves to be unaltered or doubtful (5–7 points).

The biophysical parameters affected most early on are concerned with behavior: changes in the cyclical periods of rest/activity[38] and a decrease in multiple rolling movements (Figure 121.3).

Although there is an increase in the pathological results of the biophysical stress tests with respect to the previous stage, we have not been able to establish whether their comparative percentages are significantly different statistically.

However, in the advanced phase there is a progressive deterioration in the fetal cardiac frequency register and late decelerations appear. The time lapse from the pathological quality of the umbilical PI until the appearance of late decelerations in the register has been evaluated as between 9 and 60 days,[39,40] with a mean of 2–3 weeks.[11–13] Echographically, on the other hand, there is an ostensible decrease in fetal movements (somatic and respiratory) and in fetal tone. There can be a marked decrease in amniotic fluid; Phelan *et al.*[44] obtained indices of between 5 and 8. If all these data are marked in accordance with Manning, the biophysical profile usually attains a score of under 7. In this phase the number of positive oxytocin tests is already clearly significant, as are the force tests and the vibroacoustic stimulation. We are then confronted with the decompensation of a chronic fetal distress, which, until then, could be considered as compensated.

Finally, in the late phase, and owing to the loss of cardiac automatism, not only do apparent late decelerations appear in the cardiotocographic reading, but there is also noticeable loss of reactivity. These ominous readings do not appear until 2–3 weeks after the minimum values of the cerebral PI have been attained. In fact, this interval depends on the ability of the fetus to compensate for the reduction in its metabolic supply.[42]

The biophysical profile shows very low values, always under 5, owing to the alteration of all its parameters (severe decrease in fetal movements and tone, etc.) and an increasingly significant oligohydramnios (Phelan's index under 5).

Biochemical correlation

When the velocimetric values are altered not only in the umbilical artery, but also in the remaining fetal vessels (aorta, common carotid and middle cerebral arteries), there is a risk of low pO_2 and pH values in the fetal blood obtained by cordocentesis.[17,30,38,45,46] In fact, centralization gets under way only when the fetus is already suffering from a degree of hypoxemia and acidosis.

In the initial phase, with end-diastolic frequencies still present in both the umbilical artery and the aorta, the percentage of cases with hypoxemia does not generally exceed 25–30%.

The situation changes dramatically in the advanced phase, when the end-diastolic values of the Doppler frequency in those two vessels disappear: in this case 70–80% of the fetuses present hypoxemia, and 40–60% present acidosis.[17,30,46,47] The majority of authors[48–50] consider that the absence of end-diastolic flow signifies pathological results in the acid–base study of the fetal blood.

Finally, in the terminal phase, practically all the fetuses have a pO_2 of between 2 and 4 SD below the mean.[51]

Obstetric and neonatal outcome

A high number of deaths in fetuses (250 per 1000) and neonates are concentrated in this group, and there is a significant increase in neonates with pH under 7.20 (83.3%). A cesarean section was performed in all our cases. Furthermore, the surviving fetuses present a high number of complications (e.g. necrotizing enterocolitis and hemorrhages), which are attributable to the persistent vasoconstriction of specific organs.[52]

Various authors[14,15,53] have observed that the absence of end-diastolic values in the aorta accurately predicts neonatal morbidity.

Arduini *et al.*[54] have designed a test that determines whether fetuses will have a specially bad prognosis if they are not immediately extracted. They administer oxygen humidified at 60% to the mother, and carry out a fetal hemodynamic study using Doppler before, just after and 20 min after therapy. If the PI values are not substantially modified, the fetuses will suffer a rapid deterioration.

Decentralization of blood flow

Montenegro *et al.*[17,30] give this name (decentralization of blood flow) to the irreversible hemodynamic changes that follow on from the centralization of blood flow and that precede fetal death.

Pathophysiological basis

If the hypoxia persists, a phenomenon of generalized fetal vascular paralysis will ultimately occur.

We can probably hypothesize that the situation is similar to those described in the fetuses of monkeys[55] or sheep[56] subjected to severe and sustained hypoxemia. The appearance of cerebral edema and the resulting increase in intracranial pressure hinder the mechanism for cerebral blood perfusion. The cerebral edema is probably brought about by the local accumulation of lactic acid resulting from the sustained anaerobic metabolism, which alters the permeability of the cellular membrane, increases the osmotic intracellular pressure and ultimately leads to the edema and eventual tissue necrosis.

The result of all this is that, in addition to the hypoxemia of the cerebral centers, there is a progressively irreversible interference in the control mechanisms of the arterial tone. This situation usually occurs when the hypoxemia is extreme: more than 4 SD below the mean.[51,57,58]

Doppler hemodynamic profile

The diagnosis of decentralization of blood flow essentially rests on two findings:

(1) Confirmation of resistance in the umbilical and peripheral circulation (aorta, renal, etc.) with the presence of reverse end-diastolic flow and
(2) Increase, after a brief period of stabilization, in the PI in the intracranial arteries, the values of which can appear normal; there are even FVW without diastoles or with reverse flow.[59]

It is not known how much time can pass from the onset of this picture until *in utero* fetal death, but it is probably no more than 2–3 days, and in many cases only a few hours; this explains the remote possibility of observing it through Doppler.

Biophysical correlation

If a cardiotocographic examination is carried out at this point, it is certain that a terminal pattern will be observed, indicating the so-called 'intrauterine brain death syndrome'.[60–65] The readings invariably show a fixed fetal cardiac frequency, with no variability from one heartbeat to another and a complete absence of accelerations or decelerations, even when contractions are induced by an oxytocin test or an EVA is performed. The biophysical profile, on the other hand, will show an immobile atonic fetus, drawn in on itself and with hardly any amniotic fluid, although some authors[64,66] have described some cases with hydramnios. The score will not exceed 2 points.

Only on very rare occasions will it be possible by echography to confirm the existence of cystic periventricular cerebral lesions (porencephaly) or evident ventriculomegaly,[65,67,68] the consequence of the hypoxic necrosis.[60,67–69]

Figure 121.4 presents the probable sequence of the pathophysiological mechanisms and biophysical signals, which can be observed through exploration, in a case of IUGR through uteroplacental vascular insufficiency.

Biochemical correlation

As has already been mentioned above, a funiculocentis will confirm extreme hypoxemia (values of pO_2 −4 SD below the mean and a significant acidosis).

Obstetrical outcome

This is a situation that results in either fetal or neonatal death, especially if an emergency extraction is carried out. A cesarean section is therefore generally considered unnecessary.[65]

The role of Doppler in the decision to terminate the gestation

The decision to terminate the gestation, and the birth route, must be taken in the light of:

(1) Objective data on the fetal condition (e.g. type of IUGR, presence or absence of congenital defects, onset of centralization of blood flow);
(2) Degree of fetal pulmonary maturity and
(3) Specific clinical characteristics of the case (e.g. parity, cervical conditions).

If it is an intrinsic, harmonic IUGR, with evidence, or a high probability, that there are fetal anomalies (trisomies, malformative syndromes), it is advisable to wait for the results of the tests on pulmonary maturity, fetal hemodynamics, etc. and attempt birth by the vaginal route. If there is no confirmation of any congenital defects, the procedure should be the same as in extrinsic IUGR.

In the case of extrinsic, or disharmonic IUGR, the tests currently available for controlling a fetus should be a guide as to the appropriate time to interrupt the gestation.

Our current state of knowledge and diagnostic possibilities give us two options as regards when to extract the fetus:

(1) Interrupt the gestation when the cardiotocographic reading is abnormal and/or there are clear signs of chronic fetal distress (reduction in tone and fetal movements, oligohydramnios, observation of meconial fluid by amnioscopy), which implies high levels of asphyxia and perinatal morbidity and mortality[70,71] or
(2) Interrupt the gestation at the onset of the centralization of blood flow, thus increasing the prematurity rate.

In order to reduce the latter risk to a minimum, especially if the gestation has not reached 30 weeks, it is advisable to study the fetal blood gases by means of funiculocentesis. This step should especially be taken when the PI values in the umbilical artery and aorta are obviously altered but there is still end-diastolic flow. If the diastole is zero, and especially in cases of reverse flow, the fetal prognosis is very poor and funiculocentesis proves to be useless.

With a fetus which is mature, or in the transitional maturing phase, the decision to carry out the interruption must always be made before the disappearance of the diastolic velocities. The decision will always be somewhat late by the time that zero diastole has appeared, given the high number with acidosis (70%) and perinatal deaths in this group.

Fetal defensive mechanisms against hypoxia: biochemical study of fetal deterioration

We are well aware of the resistance and capacity for adaptation of the fetal organism, as compared with adults of the same species, when confronted by hypoxia. It is common knowledge, for example, that newborn rats survive without oxygen 30 times as long as adult rats. However, the immature fetus probably has a much less well-developed capacity for adaptation.

Fetal defense against hypoxia uses various mechanisms of widely differing teleological significance,[72] from the appearance of a polycythemia, designed to increase the transportation of oxygen through the fetal blood;[73] to the dilatation of the placental vessels, as a consequence of an excess carbon dioxide.[74] If we concentrate on the most important of these mechanisms, we could say that the preservation of life, and particularly of the brain, is the fruit of a collaboration between a mechanism for neuroendocrine regulation (paraortic and carotid ganglions, sympathetic–parasympathetic play, adrenal glands, release of catecholamines) and the

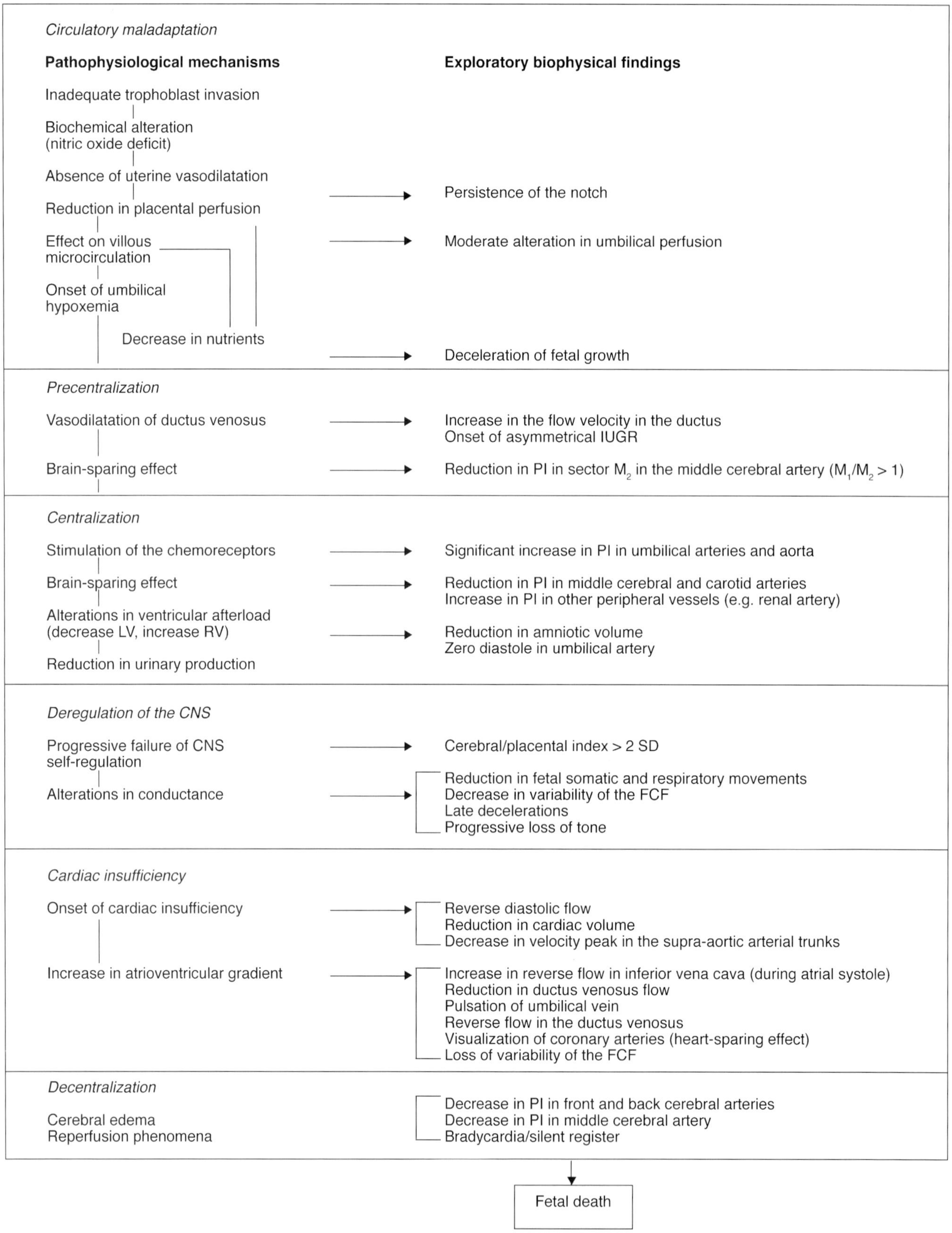

Figure 121.4 Sequence of the pathophysiological mechanisms and biophysical signals. IUGR, intrauterine growth retardation; PI, pulsatility index; LV, left ventricle; RV, right ventricle; CNS, central nervous system; FCF, fetal cardiac frequency.

mechanisms for maintaining cellular and systemic homeostasis.[75] The integrity of the various systems, especially that of the central nervous system, depends on the precise adjustments made between these biophysical and biochemical mechanisms when they show regulation among themselves, from their own genetic program of specialization.

A considerable number of mechanisms are interrelated in order to regulate the hemodynamic changes that we have described. Hypoxemia and hypercapnia induce dilatation of the cerebral blood vessels. This is attained by means of the stimulus to the chemoreceptors already alluded to, but there is also an increase in sympathetic activity (epinephrine and norepinephrine – adrenalin and noradrenalin) which, along with the release of arginine–vasopressin, increases the peripheral vascular resistance.

The fetus, unlike the adult, responds to hypoxia with bradycardia. The decrease in pO_2 in the umbilical vein stimulates the aortic and carotid chemoreceptors.[76,77] Later on, this bradycardia is maintained by peripheral vasoconstriction, which raises fetal blood pressure and stimulates the arterial baroreceptors.

From the energetic point of view, the fetus falls back on the release of energy via the biochemical energy release mechanisms under conditions of anaerobiosis. Although this recourse allows it to survive for a time, in the long run it leads to energetic failure, to the exposure of its glucogen reserves and the acidification of its internal medium.

There is relative agreement that a fetus responds to hypoxia in an ordered and systematic manner, which wavers only when the ictus is severe and has exceeded certain limits. This seems particularly to be the case when, as in uteroplacental insufficiency, the limitations both on energy and on oxygen occur progressively. Fetal deterioration is also, with some exceptions, progressive.

Owing to our current knowledge of fetal pathophysiology, it is possible to identify five stages in the process of fetal deterioration: full fetal adaptation, energy failure, hypoxia without ischemia, hypoxia with ischemia and reperfusion and death.

Full fetal adaptation stage

In this stage, which is relatively silent from the hemodynamic point of view, the most noteworthy feature is the precentralization of blood flow.

There are hardly any discernible changes on the biochemical front in this first stage of fetal adaptation to hypoxia. It is only when the situation becomes chronic that, in addition to a progressive decrease in the plasma concentration of glucose and amino acids, there is an increase in the production of erythropoietin. The generation of the latter is stimulated, both in fetuses[78,79] and in adults,[80] by chronic hypoxia, which correlates satisfactorily with growth retardation[81] and fetal metabolic problems (e.g. diabetes, preeclampsia). The raised erythropoietin values are followed, on the other hand, by an increase in the number of circulating erythroblasts, as a probable consequence of a mechanism for the premature release of red cells by the bone marrow, or of a persistence in hepatic erythropoiesis, all of which are mediated by erythropoietin.[82,83]

Energy failure stage

From the hemodynamic point of view, this stage sees the centralization of blood flow, with a selective vasodilatation of organs such as the brain, the heart or the adrenals, and a vasoconstriction of other territories, such as the lung, the intestine, the skin, the kidney or the skeleton.

On the biochemical–energetic front, anaerobic glucolysis enables the fetus momentarily to attain a substitute energy source in order to survive. However, if the conditions for fetal oxygenation do not improve, this defense mechanism will become not only inoperative but also dangerous. In effect, owing to the accumulation of lactic acid, it will lead to a fall in the pH and metabolic acidosis; there will also be a progressive depletion of energy reserves (hypoglucemia, the loss of stored glucogen, etc.) with a significant decrease in adenosine triphosphate (ATP). The ultimate consequence is energy failure.

The explanation for this lies in the fact that, while 38 mol of ATP (equivalent to more than 100,000 stored calories) is formed under normal conditions, or aerobiosis, only 2 mol of ATP (approximately 20,000 calories) is formed for every mole of glucose metabolized by the anaerobic route. Thus, the energy obtained by anaerobiosis is equivalent to 1/17 of that achieved by oxidative degradation.

The insufficiency of ATP[84,85] leads to the functional alteration of the membrane, which alters the cellular ionic homeostasis. There is an increase in intracellular sodium ions and a withdrawal of potassium ions, all of which leads to a depolarization of the membrane, with an opening up of the calcium channels.

At a certain point, the intracellular accumulation of calcium ions goes beyond the compensatory possibilities of the cell, which does not manage to maintain its ionic equilibrium. As a consequence of this, calcium turns into a cellular toxin.

Apart from the opening up of the above-mentioned channels, there are other mechanisms for increasing intracellular calcium. The reduction in ATP gives rise to the release of calcium from the endoplasmic reticulum, and the increase in intracellular sodium, resulting from the functional lesion of the cellular membrane, also stimulates the release of the calcium ion from the mitochondria.

There are also some modifications produced in this stage, which can be verified in fetal blood if cordocentesis is carried out:

(1) A decrease in the plasma concentration of glucose as a result of anaerobic glucolysis, necessary in conditions of hypoxia, in order to obtain sufficient

energy for fetal survival. The consequences of this process are a drop in the pH, metabolic acidosis, fetal hypoglucemia[86] and, finally, a depletion of the glycogen reserves, despite the low metabolic indices.

(2) A decrease in the plasma concentration of amino acids, independent of the degree of hypoxia.

(3) An increase in the viscosity of the blood, as a result of the rise in the hematocrit. Heightened viscosity interferes with the perfusion of the vital tissues. The relative blood viscosity increases logarithmically (not linearly) with the increase in platelet aggregation.

Hypoxia without ischemia stage

The hemodynamic pattern established at this stage is known as 'severe hypoxia without ischemia' with full cerebral vasodilatation. The reactive possibilities of the centralization of the blood flow have reached their maximum level, but are in their terminal phase. The Doppler study of the renal descending aorta funicular artery shows very high indices of pulsatility, with no telediastolic velocimetric values or the presence of reverse flow. In contrast, the intracranial arteries exhibit particularly low PI values.

On the biochemical front, the intracellular ionic calcium concentration goes up substantially, and this increase represents the first link in a chain of events that will lead to neuronal death.

The most outstanding event is probably the activation of phospholipases A and C, which gives rise to a phospholipidic hydrolysis of the membrane, which then ruptures, irreversibly altering its permeability. The immediate consequence is a deterioration in the cellular homeostatic balance. On the other hand, phospholipase C catalyzes the production of inositol triphosphate, which releases calcium from the endoplasmic reticulum.

Hypoxemia with ischemia stage

In recent years, it has been demonstrated that hypoxia needs ischemia to set in motion the chain of biochemical events that originates in the irreversible lesion to the cellular membrane and end up in the massive production of oxygen-derived free radicals which produce a natural death.

When the oxygen content in the fetal blood (pO_2) falls below –3 SD of the mean, the capacity of the defense mechanisms to continue protecting the fetus is eroded. Therefore, if the asphyxia is very severe there is a failure in the centralization of the blood flow and ischemia occurs, more or less irreversibly, in all the organs that had been preserved until then. When cerebral hypoxia– ischemia is produced, the blood pressure and cardiac output fall. This phenomenon is often very abrupt, and is predetermined by the fall in peripheral vasoconstriction. Cerebral self-regulation disappears and the cerebral blood flow becomes passive.

On the hemodynamic front, there is an increase in the PI values, both in the middle cerebral and carotid arteries, which can even be accompanied by reverse blood flow, proof of the appearance of ischemia, which is secondary, among other things, to progressive cerebral edema. However, this increase is not stable, for there are brief episodes of vasodilatation (a fall in PI), which may be considered attempts at reperfusion. At the same time, we can observe a complete absence of end-diastolic values and, in most cases, reverse blood flow, in the peripheral fetal vessels.

From the biochemical point of view, the increase in the intracellular concentration of calcium sets in motion other relevant mechanisms that will make an inexorable contribution to the lesion and to neuronal death:

(1) Release from the lesioned membrane of free fatty acids, especially arachidonic acid. The latter's oxidative degradation, through both cyclo-oxygenase and lipoxygenase, generates large amounts of oxygen free radicals, which inhibit the prostacyclin synthetase. The immediate consequence is a decrease in the concentration of prostacyclin and the loss of prostaglandin (PG) I_2 and thromboxane A_2 balance.

(2) Structural change of xanthine dehydrogenase into xanthine oxygenase, which, as we shall see, precipitates the formation of free radicals from hypoxanthine.

(3) Activation of the release of excitatory amino acids, which subject the neuronal receptors to a prolonged overstimulation.

Ultimately, the consequence of all this is cellular edema and neuronal death, which can be primary if it occurs at the same time as the hypoxic ictus, or secondary if it occurs in a later phase of reperfusion.

Reperfusion and death stage

It has been well established over the last 10 years that cerebral lesions related to a lack of oxygen originate not only at the time of asphyxic ictus, but also, and very particularly, in the reperfusion phases, which take place in the centralization of the blood flow's terminal phase, as well as in its decentralization phase, thus giving rise to the so-called 'secondary neuronal death'.[86] There is, in this respect, experimental proof in fetal sheep that reperfusion, after a relatively long period of ischemia, increases the production of free radicals.[87] Free radicals play a deleterious role in every case.[88–90]

From the hemodynamic point of view, the end result is a phenomenon of generalized fetal vascular paralysis with a decentralization of blood flow.

Biochemical markers of cerebral hypoxia

In theory, it is possible to study fetal homeostasis and evaluate possible hypoxia by studying the acid–base status of the fetal blood obtained by means of cordocentesis.[91–93]

The quantification of pO_2, pCO_2, pH and an excess of bases in the fetal blood will provide us with a mere snapshot of that status, without any retrospective information on the changes that the fetus has been able to overcome, and this will also be lacking in any prospective value as regards a possible cerebral lesion,[94,95] hence the interest in finding and developing authentic biochemical markers of fetal hypoxia.

The progressive understanding of the cellular mechanisms of hypoxia has led to the belief that the products generated throughout the cascade of chemical reactions, which ultimately lead to neuronal death, could be used as markers. This is the case with erythropoietin, excitatory amino acids, hypoxanthine, free fatty acids, lipidic peroxides and oxygen free radicals.

However, our current knowledge of these products largely comes from animal experimentation or studies on neonates that have been subjected to intrauterine asphyxia. Only some of these parameters, such as erythropoietin, have been studied in fetal blood or amniotic fluid. Studies attempting to determine markers for hypoxia in maternal blood are scarce, but these would be of real use in clinical practice. All this means that we are taking the first steps in this field and that it will be necessary to wait for some years before introducing any of these markers in day-to-day clinical practice.

We can speculate that these markers might be divided into three categories:

(1) Markers of chronic fetal hypoxia
(2) Markers of fetal decompensation
(3) Markers of reoxygenation and/or neuronal death.

Markers of chronic fetal hypoxia

Although the pH in the umbilical artery continues to be the most widely used indicator to evaluate fetal hypoxia, there is a great deal of evidence on its limited correlation with the neurological evolution of the newborn baby.[94,95] This is because, although it is an excellent indicator of recent acute hypoxia, it is incapable of indicating prolonged chronic hypoxia,[81] hence the interest in erythropoietin, which seems to be a good marker for chronic hypoxia during the second half of gestation.[96]

Erythropoietin is a glycoprotein, the production of which, both in the fetus and in the adult, is stimulated by hypoxia.[78,79,97,98] As it does not cross the placenta it is considered that, when found in large quantities in the fetal or neonatal blood, whether obtained by cordocentesis or postpartum in the blood of the umbilical cord, it may constitute a marker of chronic fetal hypoxia[99,100] from at least week 20 of gestation.[101] Accordingly, several researchers have found high levels of erythropoietin in umbilical cord blood in gestations with hypertension,[102,103] intrauterine growth retardation[83,103,104] (with a good correlation between the values of this parameter and the degree of fetal acidemia) and other pathologies that are accompanied by placental insufficiency,[104] even with totally normal umbilical pH values (Table 121.2). Likewise, there is no noticeable correlation in these cases between the values of erythropoietin and those of pO_2 in the umbilical artery.[81,102,105] However, when there was no acidosis there was only a limited relationship between high erythropoietin figures and the presence of meconium or an alteration in the fetal cardiac frequency (Table 121.3).

Salvesen *et al.*,[106] in a parallel study of maternal blood and fetal blood (obtained by cordocentesis), noted that, in gestations complicated by diabetes mellitus, maternal hyperglycemia is accompanied by fetal hyperglycemia and fetal acidemia, with a marked increase in erythropoietin. There is speculation that this increase can be due both to hypoxia and to hyperinsulinemia, or both, and that the rise in fetal hemoglobin can also be mediated by erythropoietin or hyperinsulinemia.

In contrast, the erythropoietin level is not modified in those pathologies that, although they affect the fetus, do not do so by means of an insufficiency in the placenta. This is the case, for example, in pyelonephritis.[107]

On the other hand, several authors[83,104] have confirmed a significant correlation between the

Table 121.2 Relationship between placental pathology and fetal erythropoietin and umbilical pH values (from Maier *et al.*[81])

		Erythropoietin (mU/ml)		Umbilical pH	
Placental findings	***n***	**Median**	**Range**	**Median**	**Range**
Fetal vasculopathy	14	85.6	23.7–119.7	7.28	7.22–7.31
Acute pathology of intervillous space	28	61.3	24.2–125.1	7.31	7.21–7.35
Chronic pathology of intervillous space	45	54.9	20.9–114.4	7.29	7.21–7.32
Chorioamnionitis with fetal reaction	60	51.3	27.7–118.7	7.30	7.24–7.34
Normality	26	35.2	19.2–48.7	7.30	7.20–7.33

Table 121.3 Erythropoietin in umbilical venous blood, according to obstetric risk and signs of fetal distress during birth (from Maier *et al.*[81])

		Erythropoietin (mU/ml)		
Group	***n***	**Mean**	**Median**	**Range**
Low risk	19	28.0	25.1	11.9–55.3
High risk	95	42.6	25.8	5.4–19.3
Meconium	12	80.6	50.6	10.7–317.6
FCF anomalies	40	110.2	44.7	78–1404.5
Meconium C abnormal FCF	10	80.2	47.8	18.7–200.4
Umbilical acidosis	24	202.4	72.6	6.1–1070.2

FCF, fetal cardiac frequency

concentration of erythropoietin and the number of circulating nucleated erythrocytes.

It seems that labor at birth with no signs of fetal distress does not raise erythropoietin levels;[108] on the contrary, some researchers[109] speculate on the possibility that the administration of β-mimetic tocolytics may stimulate the production of erythropoietin through a decrease in fetal oxygenation. They thus consider that β-sympathomimetics should be used sparingly once the fetal condition has been affected.

The determination of erythropoietin during pregnancy can be made in both fetal blood (cordocentesis) and amniotic fluid. The latter expresses the situation in the fetal serum with reasonable exactitude, although with a slight delay and somewhat lower figures.

In this way, the rise in erythropoietin levels has been confirmed in amniotic fluid (normal figures 9–12 mU/ml) in various pathologies associated with chronic placental insufficiency, but its values prove to be normal in other syndromes, such as Down's syndrome, for example.[110]

Some authors[99,100] use the determination of erythropoietin in amniotic fluid to clarify whether fetal deaths are the consequence of an acute event (normal erythropoietin), or a chronic condition (high glycoprotein values).

In practice, however, erythropoietin has principally been used as a marker of hypoxia postpartum, through the determination of its concentration in the venous cord blood.[81,108] Our experiences with this marker are collated in Table 121.4. It can be seen that its values in preeclampsia were double the normal ones in our unit, and it is confirmed that this parameter does not correlate with the values of the umbilical pH, but it does do so with the presence of meconium and anomalies of the fetal cardiac frequency, above all those that express an ectasis of the intervillous space.

Markers of fetal decompensation

The onset of severe fetal hypoxia with reactive vasodilatation of the cerebral blood vessels is accompanied by, among other chemical changes, a local increase in three markers: excitatory amino acids, hypoxanthine and free fatty acids.

Excitatory amino acids

The amino acids glutamate and aspartate, which usually play an important role as neurotransmitters, intensify their concentration in the cerebral extracellular space by up to 5–10 times the norm during episodes of hypoxia and, above all, of hypoxemia with ischemia. They are then converted into neurotoxins.

The increase in these amino acids is a consequence both of the increase in the intracellular calcium concentration in the neurons, which produce glutamate and aspartate, and the failure to absorb them on the part of the presynaptic membranes when ATP decreases.[86]

Neuronal death can occur as a consequence of two types of lesional mechanism: a ‘rapid’ mechanism, which takes place a few minutes after the hypoxic ictus, and a ‘late’ mechanism, which can begin up to 24 h after the episode. In the first case, the cellular lesion is the result of the massive entry of sodium, chlorine and water into the cell, which gives rise to an osmotic load and lysis of the cellular membrane. In the second case, in contrast, calcium ions enter through specific channels when they are stimulated by *N*-methyl-D-aspartate. This increase in the intracellular concentration of calcium perpetuates the process by gradually setting into motion the other, previously mentioned, cellular lesion mechanisms. While the rapid mechanism explains primary neuronal death, the late mechanism is more common in secondary neuronal death with successive episodes of anoxia and reoxygenation.

Table 121.4 Erythropoietin values in umbilical vessels in cases of diabetes and pre-eclampsia

			Erythropoietin (mU/ml)		
Pathology	***n***	**%**	**Mean**	**SD**	***P* value**
Diabetes	13	5.1	34.43	31.13	0.94 (NS)
Control group	240	94.9	31.72	28.58	
Pre-eclampsia	8	3.1	62.59	58.26	0.024 (S)
Control group	245	96.9	30.86	26.81	

NS, not significant; S, significant

It has been demonstrated that the levels of glutamate and aspartate in cerebrospinal fluid were, respectively, three and four times greater in animal fetuses subjected to asphyxia than in the control group,[111] and this significantly correlated with the degree of hypoxic–ischemic encephalopathy.

We can now draw on considerable information on these possible biochemical markers of hypoxia in experimentation animals (particularly sheep) and through carrying out cerebral assessments using microdialysis probes,[112,113] but there are still no studies in humans.

Hypoxanthine

During hypoxia, ATP is degraded with considerable difficulty; hence the increase in the concentration of adenosine monophosphate (AMP), which is later transformed into adenosine, inosine and, finally, hypoxanthine. The increase in these biochemical products, especially the latter, therefore represents a marker of fetal hypoxia. Thiringer[114] has demonstrated that the concentration of hypoxanthine in venous blood, during the advanced and terminal phases of the centralization of blood flow, was much greater than in arterial blood. It is possible that this is also the case in moderate hypoxia.

In the hypoxia stage with vasodilatation, hypoxanthine is successively converted into xanthine and uric acid, owing to the enzyme xanthine dehydrogenase. Its concentration in the fetal blood, like that of adenosine and inosine, is therefore only moderately intensified in this phase. Furthermore, adenosine and inosine increase cerebral blood flow, reduce carbon dioxide and modulate the neurotransmitters so that, overall, an endogenous mechanism for cerebral protection is set in motion.[115–119]

However, when ischemia ensues as a consequence of the increase in intracellular calcium, a structural change takes place, from xanthine dehydrogenase to xanthine oxygenase. The result is that the first route is blocked and uric acid is produced by means of a second route, which occasions the production of oxygen-derived free radicals. This route is the customary one in cases of reperfusion and reoxygenation after one or many episodes of neuronal hypoxia. In effect, the chronic lack of oxygen in hypoxia with stable vasodilatation avoids both the excessive stimulation of the first route and the activation of the second. However, when successive episodes of ischemia and reperfusion occur, the usual route is blocked and the 'savage route' is induced, and the concentrations of hypoxanthine and oxygen free radicals are increased.

When uterine perfusion in fetal sheep is reduced experimentally,[120] it has been noted that the highest values of hypoxanthine and xanthine in cerebrospinal fluid are found precisely in the normothermic recovery phase. These high levels of substrata facilitate the formation of oxygen free radicals, which induce encephalic lesions. After 3 days of hypoxic ictus, the necropsy on the animals showed varying degrees of edema, neuronal alterations through coagulation and necrosis, and cellular death. Such changes were especially evident in the Purkinje brain cells. These findings agree with those of several earlier studies.[121–123]

Several authors suggest, as a marker for hypoxia during pregnancy, both in animal experimentation[120,124,125] and in human clinical practice, the determination of hypoxanthine in the fetal circulation. This, they argue, could provide us with information on the gravity of the hypoxic ictus and, above all, could offer a prognosis on the subsequent fetal or neonatal encephalic cavitation (porencephaly or leukomalacia) resulting from intrauterine hypoxia/ischemia.

This marker seems to be particularly predictive in cases of periventricular leukomalacia in neonates.[126,127] Saugstad[128] and others[129,130] consider that hypoxanthine in cord blood is more specific in the evaluation and quantification of hypoxia than lactate, acid–base excess or pH, as these parameters are incapable of reflecting the intracellular energy status. The oxidation of hypoxanthine during episodes of reperfusion generates oxygen free radicals, which contribute to the destruction of the cerebral tissues and, therefore, to the genesis of leukomalacia.[127]

Some authors[131] therefore consider this parameter as a gold standard of hypoxia. There is a host of studies that relate hypoxia to high levels of this marker.[132]

Likewise, in the neonate[133] the quantity and prolongation of the urinary excretion of oxypurines (hypoxanthine and xanthine) is clearly related to the gravity of the intrauterine hypoxic episode, with its neonatal neurological consequences and an extension of the possible cerebral lesion.

Arachidonic acid

Arachidonic acid is one of the free fatty acids released after the lesion to the membrane is produced by phospholipid hydrolysis. Its release, as a result of the activity of phospholipases A and C, provokes a cascade of biochemical reactions that lead to the production of prostaglandins, thromboxane and leukotrienes. This is why, in moderate hypoxia, there is an increase in both prostacycline and thromboxane in the cerebrospinal fluid, and probably also in the fetal blood.

However, when ischemia is combined with hypoxia, the cascade of arachidonic acid alters, forming first oxygen free radicals and, later on, lipid peroxides as a by-product. These free radicals inhibit prostacycline synthetase and impede the formation of prostacycline by increasing the relative concentration of thromboxane. This imbalance precipitates vasoconstriction and excessive platelet aggregation, and produces successive episodes of ischemia and reperfusion, which considerably impair the neuronal prognosis. On the other hand, the lipid peroxides can produce vasoconstriction by directly affecting the vessels; as a result, more calcium enters smooth muscular cells of the vascular wall and endothelium-derived relaxing factor (EDRF)/nitric oxide is rendered inactive.[134]

Even when the demonstration of this imbalance of prostanoids is theoretically possible by studying the fetal blood obtained through cordocentesis, there is no published experiment that indicates that it could be useful as a marker of hypoxia.

Various researchers have shown that human neonates subjected to asphyxia during birth presented a significant rise in the majority of prostanoids investigated in the cerebrospinal fluid, especially thromboxane.[135]

Markers for reoxygenation and/or neuronal death

In this instance, we should principally mention the oxygen free radicals and their by-products.

Oxygen-derived free radicals

A free radical is any molecule that has one or more unpaired electrons (i.e. an odd number) in its outer layer. This makes them very reactive, and endows them with a strong tendency to initiate chain reactions to get rid of this extra electron, or accept another one to stabilize the unpaired electron, or join up with a non-radical molecule.

Oxygen is essential to the life of aerobic organisms. In all the cells in the organism, it is in the mitochondria (organelles which produce cellular energy or ATP) that the largest amount of oxygen is used up through being the terminal acceptor of electrons in the cellular respiration process. However, owing to its biradical nature, oxygen and its metabolites are potentially cytotoxic. The reduction of oxygen produces an oxygen superoxide radical (O_2–), hydrogen peroxide (H_2O_2) and the hydroxyl radical. The reaction between oxygen superoxide and hydrogen peroxide results in more hydroxyl radicals.

When oxygen free radicals come into contact with the restored fatty acids, the so-called lipid peroxides are formed, and these stimulate the peroxidation reactions, which are extraordinarily toxic for all the cellular elements, especially for membranes.

Of the oxygen consumed by the cell, 90% is reduced by cytochrome oxidase without any formation of oxygen free radicals. Only 10%, in both the cytoplasm and the mitochondria, is reduced by other routes, which produce free radicals. Cells are endowed with a wide range of enzymatic and non-enzymatic defenses, the radical 'scavengers', to prevent the damaging effects of these radicals.

The deleterious effect takes place when an imbalance occurs between the excessive production of free radicals and lipid peroxides and the antioxidant activity of the cellular defense systems.[88,136] Oxygen, like the god Janus, has two faces: one beneficial and life-giving and the other malevolent, a producer of deficiencies and death.

As we have already seen, the free radicals are precipitated by severe hypoxia, and they are a by-product of biochemical reactions or processes such as the synthesis of prostaglandins, the conversion of xanthine into uric acid by the 'savage route' and the auto-oxidation of catecholamines.

A cellular lesion and, ultimately, cellular death, are produced as a consequence of lipid peroxidation, the rupture of the cellular membrane and the decomposition of DNA molecules. Sooner or later this is followed by the destruction of cellular aerobic respiration, the synthesis of structural and enzymatic proteins and even the cell's genetic apparatus.

These molecules are formed above all in the reperfusion and reoxygenation stage, which arises from the failure of the centralization of blood flow and finishes with its decentralization and neuronal death.

One of the gestational pathologies in which oxygen free radicals play a leading role is preeclampsia, not only because it is a generator of placental ischemia, and therefore of fetal hypoxia, but also because it is possible that the imbalance between oxidants and antioxidants is related to the pathogenesis of pre-eclampsia.[137,138] Free radicals and lipid peroxides could be elements that link the poor immunological adaptation with the endothelial cellular ictus.[138] In fact, a significant increase in lipid peroxides has been confirmed in pre-eclampsia, with an accompanying decrease in the antioxidant capacity of the maternal blood. It is very probable that the principal source of these lipid peroxides is the placenta.

REFERENCES

1. Committee on Obstetrics, Maternal and Fetal Medicine. *Fetal and Nonatal Neurologic Injury*. ACOG Technical Bulletin 163. Washington, DC: ACOG, 1992.
2. Naeye RL, Peters EC, Barthlomew M, *et al.* Origins of cerebral palsy. *Am J Dis Child* 1989;143:1154.
3. Carter BS, Haverkamp AD, Merenstein GB. The definition of acute perinatal asphyxia. *Clin Perinatol* 1993;20:287–304.
4. American Academy of Pediatrics, American College of Obstetricians and Gynecologists. Relationship between perinatal factors and neurologic outcome. In Poland RL, Freeman RK, eds. *Guidelines for Perinatal Care*, 3rd edn. Elk Grove Village, IL: American Academy of Pediatrics, 1992:221–4.
5. Blair E, Stanley FJ. Intrapartum asphyxia: A rare cause of cerebral palsy. *J Pediatr* 1988;112:515.
6. Robertson CMT, Finer NN, Grace MGA. School performance of survivors of neonatal encephalopathy associated with birth asphyxia at term. *J Pediatr* 1989;114:753.
7. Rudolph AM, Heymann MA. The circulation of the fetus *in utero*. Methods for studying distribution of blood flow, cardiac output and organ blood flow. *Circ Res* 1967;21:163–7.
8. Johnson GN, Palahniuk RJ, Tweed WA, *et al.* Regional cerebral blood flow changes during fetal asphyxia produced by slow partial umbilical cord compression. *Am J Obstet Gynecol* 1979; 135:48–52.
9. Behrman RE, Lees MH, Peterson EN, *et al.* Distribution of the circulation in the normal and asphyxiated fetal primate. *Am J Obstet Gynecol* 1970;108:956–69.
10. Morrow RJ, Adamson SL, Bull SB, Ritchie JWK. Antenatal hypoxemia does not affect umbilical artery waveforms in sheep. *Obstet Gynecol* 1990;75:590–3.
11. Morrow RJ, Adamson SL, Bull SB, Ritchie JWK. Hypoxia acidemia, hyperviscosity and maternal hypertension do not affect the umbilical artery velocity waveforms in fetal sheep. *Am J Obstet Gynecol* 1990;163:1313–20.
12. Trudinger BJ. Doppler ultrasound study and fetal abnormality. In Drife JO, Donnan D, eds. *Antenatal Diagnosis of Fetal Abnormalities*. London: Springer-Verlag, 1991:113.
13. Gruenwald P. The relation of deprivation to perinatal pathology and late sequels. In Gruenwald P, ed. *The Placenta*. Lancaster: Medical Technical Publishing, 1975.
14. Laurin J, Marsal K, Persson PH, Lingman G. Ultrasound measurement of fetal blood in predicting fetal outcome. *Br J Obstet Gynaecol* 1987;94:940–8.
15. Laurin J, Lingman G, Marsal K, Persson PH. Fetal blood flow in pregnancies complicated by intrauterine growth retardation. *Obstet Gynecol* 1987;69:895–902.
16. Guidetti R, Luzi G, Simonazzi E, *et al.* Correlation between cerebral blood flow and umbilical blood flow in the fetus recorded with a pulsed Doppler system. *Abstract Book of the XI European Congress of Perinatal Medicine*. Rome: CIC Edizione Internazionali, 1988:252.
17. Montenegro CA. Perfil hemodinámico fetal-Diástole-Zero 'revisitada'. *J Brasileiro Ginecol* 1992;102:375–80.
18. Giorlandino G, Vizzone A. *Flussimetria ostetrica materna e fetale. Testo Atlante*. Rome: CIC Edizione Internazionali, 1993.
19. Morrow RJ, Adamson SL, Ritchie JWK, Pearce JM. The pathophysiological basis of abnormal flow velocity waveforms. In Pearce JM, ed. *Doppler Ultrasound in Perinatal Medicine*. Oxford: Oxford University Press, 1992.
20. De Haan J. Fisiopatología de los cambios de los índices de flujo Doppler en la circulación fetal. In Carrera JM, ed. *Doppler en Obstetricia*. Barcelona: Masson-Salvat, 1992.89–97.
21. Dawes GS, Duncan SL, Lewis BV, *et al.* Cyanide stimulation of the systemic arterial chemoreceptors in foetal lambs. *J Physiol* 1969; 201:117–28.
22. De Vore GR. Examination of the fetal heart in the fetus with intrauterine growth retardation using M-mode echocardiography. *Semin Perinatol* 1988;12:66–79.
23. Lingman G, Legarth J, Rahman F, Stangenberg M. Myocardial contractility in the anemic human fetus. *Ultrasound Obstet Gynecol* 1991;1:266–8.
24. Marsal K, Lingman G, Giles W. Evaluation of the carotid, aortic and umbilical blood velocity waveforms in the human fetus. *XI Annual Conference of the Society for the Study of Fetal Physiology*, Oxford. Oxford: The Nuffield Institute, 1984:C33.
25. Marsal K, Lindblad A, Lingman G, Eik-Nes SH. Blood flow in the fetal descending aorta: Intrinsic factors affecting fetal blood flow i.e. fetal breathing movements and fetal cardiac arrhythmia. *Ultrasound Med Biol* 1984;10:339–48.
26. Wladimiroff JW, Tonge HM, Stewart PA. Doppler ultrasound assessment of cerebral blood flow in the human fetus. *Br J Obstet Gynaecol* 1986;93:471–5.
27. Arabin B, Bergmann PL, Saling E. Simultaneous assessment of blood flow velocity waveforms in uteroplacental vessels, the umbilical artery, the fetal aorta and the common carotid artery. *Fetal Ther* 1987;2:17–26.
28. Arabin B, Siebert M, Jimenez E, Saling E. Obstetrical characteristic of a loss of end-diastolic velocities in the fetal aorta and/or umbilical artery using Doppler ultrasound. *Gynecol Obstet Invest* 1987;25:173–80.
29. Bilardo CM, Campbell S, Nicolaides KH. Mean blood velocity and flow impedance in the fetal descending thoracic aorta and common carotid artery in normal pregnancy. *Early Hum Dev* 1988;18:213–7.
30. Montenegro CA, Meirelles J, Fonseca AL, *et al.* Cordocentèse et evaluation du bien-étre foetal dans une population à très haut risque. *Rev Franç Gynecol Obstet* 1992;87:467–77.
31. Gramellini P, Folli MC, Raboni S, *et al.* Cerebral–umbilical Doppler ratio as a predictor of adverse perinatal outcome. *Obstet Gynecol* 1992;79:416–20.
32. Gembruch U, Baschat AA. Demonstration of fetal coronary blood flow by color-coded and pulsed wave Doppler sonography: A possible indicator of severe compromise and impending demise in intrauterine growth retardation. *Ultrasound Obstet Gynecol* 1996;7:10–6.
33. Indik JH, Chen V, Reed KL. Association of umbilical venous with inferior vena cava blood flow velocities. *Obstet Gynecol* 1991; 77:551–7.
34. Reed KL. Venous flow velocities in the fetus. In Jaffe R, Warson SL, eds. *Color Doppler Imaging in Obstetrics and Gynecology*. New York: McGraw-Hill, 1992:179.
35. Rizzo G, Arduini D, Romanini C. Inferior vena cava flow velocity waveforms in appropriate and small-for-gestational-age fetuses. *Am J Obstet Gynecol* 1992;166:127–80.
36. Rizzo G, Arduini D. Fetal cardiac function in intrauterine growth retardation. *Am J Obstet Gynecol* 1991;165:876–82.
37. Rizzo G, Capponi A, Rinaldo D, *et al.* Ventricular ejection force in growth retarded fetuses. *Ultrasound Obstet Gynecol* 1995;5: 247–55.
38. Arduini D, Rizzo G, Romanini C, Mancuso S. Are blood flow velocity waveforms related to umbilical cord acid–base status in the human fetus? *Gynecol Obstet Invest* 1989;27:183–7.
39. Reuwer PJ, Sijmons EA, Rietman GW, *et al.* Intrauterine growth retardation: Prediction of perinatal distress by Doppler ultrasound. *Lancet* 1987;2:415–8.
40. Bekedam DJ, Visser GH, Van Der Zee AG, *et al.* Abnormal velocity waveforms of the umbilical artery in growth retarded fetuses: Relationship to antepartum late heart rate decelerations and outcome. *Early Hum Dev* 1990;24:79–89.

41. Arduini D, Rizzo G, Romanini C. Changes of pulsatility index from fetal vessels preceding the onset of late decelerations in growth retarded fetuses. *Obstet Gynecol* 1992;79:605–10.
42. Arduini D, Rizzo G. Color Doppler studies of fetal circulation in intrauterine growth retardation. In Jaffe R, Warson SL, eds. *Color Doppler Imaging in Obstetrics and Gynaecology*. New York: McGraw-Hill, 1992:183.
43. Griffin DR, Bilardo K, Diaz-Recasens J, *et al.* Doppler blood flow waveforms in the descending thoracic aorta of the human fetus. *Br J Obstet Gynaecol* 1984;91:997–1002.
44. Phelan JP, Smith CV, Bronssard P, Small M. Amniotic fluid volume assessment with the four-quadrant technique at 36–42 weeks of gestation. *J Reprod Med* 1987;32:540–2.
45. Nicolaides KH, Bilardo CM, Soothill PW, Campbell S. Absence of end-diastolic frequencies in the umbilical artery: A sign of fetal hypoxia and acidosis. *Br Med J* 1988;297:1026–7.
46. Nicolaides KH, Bilardo CM, Campbell S. Prediction of fetal anaemia by measurement of mean blood velocity in the fetal aorta. *Am J Obstet Gynecol* 1990;162:209–12.
47. Hsieh FJ, Chang FM, Ko TM, *et al.* Umbilical artery flow velocity waveforms in fetuses dying with congenital anomalies. *Br J Obstet Gynaecol* 1988;95:478–82.
48. Ferrazzi E, Pardi G, Bauscaglia M, *et al.* The correlation of biochemical monitoring versus umbilical flow velocity measurements of the human fetus. *Am J Obstet Gynecol* 1988;159: 1081–7.
49. Tyrrell S, Obais AH, Lilford RJ. Umbilical artery Doppler velocimetry as a predictor of fetal hypoxia and acidosis at birth. *Obstet Gynecol* 1989;74:332–7.
50. Bilardo CM, Nicolaides KH, Campbell S. Doppler measurement of fetal and uteroplacental circulation: Relationship with umbilical venous blood gases measured at cordocentesis. *Am J Obstet Gynecol* 1990;162:115–9.
51. Vyas S, Nicolaides KH, Bower S, Campbell S. Middle cerebral artery flow velocity waveforms in fetal hypoxemia. *Br J Obstet Gynaecol* 1990;97:797–803.
52. Manning FA, Harman CR, Menticoglou S, Morrison J. Assessment of fetal well-being with ultrasound. *Obstet Gynecol Clin North Am* 1991;18:891–905.
53. Hackett GA, Campbell S, Gamsu H, *et al.* Doppler studies in the growth retarded fetus and prediction of neonatal necrotising enterocolitis haemorrhage and neonatal morbidity. *Br Med J* 1987;294:13–6.
54. Arduini D, Rizzo G, Romanini C, Mancuso S. Haemodynamic changes in growth retarded fetuses during maternal oxygen administration as predictors of fetal outcome. *J Ultrasound Med* 1989;8:193–6.
55. Myers RE, De Courtney-Myers GM, Wagner KR. Effects of hypoxia on fetal brain. In Beard RW, Nathanielsz PW, eds. *Fetal Physiology and Medicine*. London: Butterworth, 1984:419.
56. Richardson BS, Rurak D, Patrick IE, *et al.* Cerebral oxidative metabolism during sustained hypoxaemia in fetal sheep. *J Dev Physiol* 1989;2:37–43.
57. Vyas S. Pulsed Doppler examination of the normal human fetus. In Pearce JM, ed. *Doppler Ultrasound in Perinatal Medicine*. Oxford: Oxford University Press, 1992.
58. Vyas S, Campbell S. Doppler studies of the cerebral and renal circulations in small-for-gestational-age fetuses. In Pearce JM, ed. *Doppler Ultrasound in Perinatal Medicine*. Oxford: Oxford University Press, 1992:268–78.
59. Mari G, Wasserstrum N. Flow velocity waveforms of the fetal circulation preceding fetal death in a case of lupus anticoagulant. *Am J Obstet Gynecol* 1991;164:776–8.
60. Adams RD, Prod'Hom LS, Rabinowicz TH. Intrauterine brain death. *Acta Neuropathol* 1977;40:41–9.
61. Gaziano EP, Freeman DW. Analysis of heart rate patterns preceding fetal death. *Obstet Gynecol* 1977;50:578–82.
62. Van der Moer PE, Gerretsen G, Visser GHA. Fixed fetal heart rate pattern after intrauterine accidental decerebration. *Obstet Gynecol* 1985;65:125–7.
63. Nijhuis JG, Kruyt N, Van Vijck JAM. Fetal brain death. Two case reports. *Br J Obstet Gynaecol* 1988;85:197–200.
64. Nijhuis JG, Crevels AJ, Van Dongen PWJ. Fetal brain death: The definition of a fetal heart rate pattern and its clinical consequences. *Obstet Gynecol Surv* 1990;45:229–32.
65. Zimmer EZ, Jakobi P, Goldstein !, Gutterman E. Cardiotocographic and sonographic findings in two cases of antenatally diagnosed intrauterine fetal brain death. *Prenatal Diagn* 1992; 12:271–6.
66. Ellis WG, Goetzman BW, Lindenberg JA. Neuropathologic documentation of prenatal brain damage. *Am J Dis Child* 1988; 142:858–66.
67. Nwaesei CG, Pape KE, Martin DJ, *et al.* Periventricular infarction diagnosed by ultrasound: A postmortem correlation. *J Pediatr* 1984;105:106–10.
68. Hill A. Assessment of the fetus: Relevance to brain injury. *Clin Perinatol* 1989;16:413–4.
69. Larroche JCL, Droulle P, Delezoide AL, *et al.* Brain damage in monozygous twins. *Biol Neonate* 1990;57:261–78.
70. Visser GH. Abnormal antepartum fetal heart rate patterns and subsequent handicap. *Baillieres Clin Obstet Gynaecol* 1988;2:117–24.
71. Favre R, Nissand J, Messer G. Velocimetric sylvienne foetale. Critére d'extraction dans l'hypotrophic sévere. *J Gynecol Obstet Biol Reprod* 1991;20:699.
72. Himwich HE, Bernstein AO, Herrlich H, *et al.* Mechanisms for the maintenance of life in the newborn during anoxia. *Am J Physiol* 1942;135:387–91.
73. Walker JJ, Tumbull EDN. *Lancet* 1953;2:312.
74. Panigel M. *Am J Obstet Gynecol* 1962;84:1664.
75. Cohn HE, Sacks EJ, Heymann MA, *et al.* Cardiovascular responses to hypoxemia and acidemia in fetal lambs. *Am J Obstet Gynecol* 1974;120:817–24.
76. Dawes GS, Duncan SL, Lewis BV, *et al.* Cyanide stimulation of the systemic arterial chemoreceptors in fetal lambs. *J Physiol* 1969;201:1171–2.
77. Nylund L, Lagercrantz H, Lunell NO. Catecholamines in fetal blood during birth in man. *J Dev Physiol* 1979;1:427–35.
78. Zanjani ED, Mann LI, Burlington H, *et al.* Evidence for a physiologic role of erythropoietin in fetal erythropoiesis. *Blood* 1974;44:285–90.
79. Clemons GK, Fitzsimmons SI, Demanincor D. Immunoreactive erythropoietin concentrations in fetal and neo-natal rats and the effects of hypoxia. *Blood* 1986;68:892–9.
80. Eckardt KU, Boutellier U, Kurtz A, *et al.* Rate of erythropoietin formation in humans in response to acute hypobaric hypoxia. *J Appl Physiol* 1989;66:1785–8.
81. Maier RF, Böhme K, Dudenhausen JW, Obladen M. Cord blood erythropoietin in relation to different markers of fetal hypoxia. *Obstet Gynecol* 1993;81:575–80.
82. Naeye RC. Hypoxemia and the sudden infant death syndrome. *Science* 1974;186:837–8.
83. Snijders RJM, Abbas A, Melby O, *et al.* Fetal plasma erythropoietin concentration in severe growth retardation. *Am J Obstet Gynecol* 1993;168:615–9.
84. Raichle ME. The pathophysiology of brain ischemia. *Ann Neurol* 1983;13:210.
85. Palmer C, Brucklacher RM, Christensen MA, Vannucci RC. Carbohydrate and energy metabolism during the evolution of hypoxic–ischemic brain damage in the immature rat. *J Cereb Blood Flow Metab* 1990:10:227–35.
86. Kjellmer I. Mechanisms of perinatal brain damage. *Ann Med* 1991;23:675–9.
87. Bagenholm R, Nilsson UA, Gotborg CW, Kjellmer I. Free radicals are formed during perfusion after ischemia in the brain of fetal sheep. *Abstracts of the 14th European Congress of Perinatal Medicine*, Helsinki, June 1994:283.
88. Frank L, Massaro D. Oxygen toxicity. *Am J Med* 1980;69: 117–26.
89. Kontos HA. Oxygen radicals in cerebral vascular injury. *Circ Res* 1985;57:508–16.
90. Rosenberg AA, Murdaugh E, White CW. The role of oxygen free radicals in postasphyxia cerebral hypoper-fusion in newborn lambs. *Pediatr Res* 1989;26:215–9.
91. Daffos F, Capella-Paulousky M, Forestier F. A new procedure for pure fetal blood sampling *in utero*: Preliminary results of fifty-three cases. *Am J Obstet Gynecol* 1983;146:985–7.
92. Nicolaides KH, Soothill PW, Rodeck CH, Campbell S. Ultrasound guided sampling of umbilical cord and placental blood to assess fetal well-being. *Lancet* 1986;1:1065–7.
93. Nicolaides KH, Economides DC. Cordocentesis of small-for-gestational age fetuses. In Chamberlain GV, ed. *Modern Antenatal Care of the Fetus*. Oxford: Blackwell Scientific, 1990:127–49.
94. Dijxhoom MJ, Visser GHA, Fidler UI, *et al.* Apgar score, meconium acidaemia at birth in relation to neonatal neurological morbidity in term infants. *Br J Obstet Gynaecol* 1986;93:217–22.
95. Dennis J, Johnson A, Mutch L, *et al.* Acid–base status at birth and neurodevelopmental outcome at four and one-half years. *Am J Obstet Gynecol* 1989;161:213–20.

96. Fingerova H, Petrova P, Kilianova E, *et al.* Erythropoietin levels in umbilical cord blood at birth in relation to the course of postnatal adaptation. *Abstracts of the 14th European Congress of Perinatal Medicine*, Helsinki, June 1994:36.
97. Cotes PM, Canning CE, Lind T. Changes in serum immunoreactive erythropoietin during the menstrual cycle and normal pregnancy. *Br J Obstet Gynaecol* 1983;90:304–11.
98. Thomas RM, Canning CE, Cotes PM, *et al.* Erythropoietin and cord blood haemoglobin in the regulation of human fetal erythropoiedid. *Br J Obstet Gynaecol* 1983;90:795–800.
99. Teramo KA, Voutilainen P, Clemons GK, *et al.* Amniotic fluid erythropoietin levels in fetal death. Can it differentiate between acute and chronic events? *Abstracts of the 14th European Congress of Perinatal Medicine*, Helsinki, June 1994:37.
100. Teramo KA. Does erythropoietin have a role in obstetrics? *Abstracts of the 14th European Congress of Perinatal Medicine*, Helsinki, June 1994:453.
101. Thilaganathan B, Salvesen DR, Abbas A, *et al.* Fetus plasma erythropoietin concentration in red blood cell-isoimmunized pregnancies. *Am J Obstet Gynecol* 1992;167:1292.
102. Teramo KA, Widness JA, Clemons GK, *et al.* Amniotic fluid erythropoietin in normal and abnormal pregnancy. *Obstet Gynecol* 1987;69:710–6.
103. Ruth V, Fyhrquist F, Clemons G, Raivio KO. Cord plasma vasopressin, erythropoietin and hypoxanthine as indices of asphyxia at birth. *Pediatr Res* 1988;24:490–4.
104. Maier RF, Günther A, Vogel M, *et al.* Umbilical venous erythropoietin and umbilical arterial pH in relation to morphologic placental abnormalities. *Obstet Gynecol* 1994;84:81–7.
105. Widness JA, Teramo KA, Clemons GK, *et al.* Direct relationship of antepartum glucose control and fetal erythropoietin in human type I (insulin-dependent) diabetic pregnancy. *Diabetologia* 1990;33:778–83.
106. Salvesen DR, Brudeneu JM, Snijders R, *et al.* Fetal plasma erythropoietin in pregnancies complicated by maternal diabetes mellitus. *Am J Obstet Gynecol* 1993;168:88–94.
107. Cavenee MP, Cox SM, Mason R, Cunningham FG. Erythropoietin pregnancies complicated by pyelonephritis. *Obstet Gynecol* 1994;84:252–4.
108. Halevi A, Dollberg S, Manir D, *et al.* Is cord blood, erythropoietin a maker of intrapartum hypoxia? *J Perinatol* 1992;12:215–9.
109. Rouse DJ, Widness JA, Weiner CP. Effect of intravenous β-sympathomimetic tocolysis on human fetal serum erythropoietin levels. *Am J Obstet Gynecol* 1993;168:1278–82.
110. Campbell J, Wathen N, Lewis M, *et al.* Amniotic fluid erythropoietin levels in normal and Down's syndrome pregnancies. *Abstracts of the 14th European Congress of Perinatal Medicine*, Helsinki, June 1994:52
111. Hagberg H. Neuroactive compounds and perinatal brain damage. Therapeutic strategies. *Abstract Book of the 2nd World Congress of Perinatal Medicine*, Rome, September 1994:17.
112. Hagberg H, Lehman A, Sandberg M, *et al.* Ischaemia-induced shift of inhibitory and excitatory aminoacids from intra to extracellular compartments. *J Cereb Blood Flow Metab* 1985;5:413–9.
113. McDonald JW, Johnston MV. Physiological and pathophysiological roles of excitatory amino acids during central nervous system development. *Brain Res Brain Res Rev* 1990;15:4–70.
114. Thiringer K. Cord plasma hypoxanthine as a measure of foetal asphyxia. *Acta Paediatr Scand* 1983;72:231–7.
115. Corradetti R, Lo Conte G, Moroni F, *et al.* Adenosine decreases aspartate and glutamate release from rat hippocampal slices. *Eur J Pharmacol* 1983;104:19–26.
116. Hagberg H, Andersson P, Lacarewicz J, *et al.* Extracellular adenosine, inosine, hypoxantine, and xanthine in relation to tissue nucleotides and purines in rat striatum during transient ischemia. *J Neurochem* 1987;49:227–31.
117. Park TS, Van WD, Rubio R, Berne RM. Increased brain interstitial fluid adenosine concentration during hypoxia in new born piglet. *J Cereb Blood Flow Metab* 1987;7:178–83.
118. Phillis JW, Walter GA, O'Reagan MH, Stair RE. Increases in cerebral cortical perfusate adenosine and inosine concentrations during hypoxia and ischemia. *J Cereb Blood Flow Metab* 1987; 7:679–86.
119. Lloyd HG, Spence I, Johnson GA. Protective effect of adenosine against hypoxic damage. Synaptic depression and adenosine. *Trends Pharmacol Sci* 1988;9:193–4.
120. De Haan HH, Van Reempts JLH, Ules JSH, *et al.* Effects of asphyxia on the fetal lamb brain. *Am J Obstet Gynecol* 1993;169:1493.
121. Reynolds ML, Evans CAN, Reynolds EDR, *et al.* Intracranial haemorrhage in the preterm sheep fetus. *Early Hum Dev* 1979;3:163–86.
122. Ting P, Yamaguchi S, Bacher JK, *et al.* Hypoxic–ischemic cerebral necrosis in midgestational sheep fetuses: Physiopathologic correlations. *Exp Neurol* 1983;80:227–45.
123. Gunn AJ, Parer JT, Mauard EL, *et al.* Cerebral histologic and electrocortographic changes after asphyxia in fetal sheep. *Pediatr Res* 1992;31:486–91.
124. Saugstad OD, Schrader H. The determination of inosine and hypoxanthine in rat brain during normothermic and hypothermic anoxia. *Acta Neurol Scand* 1978;57:282–8.
125. Thiringer K, Blomstrand S, Hrbek A, *et al.* Cerebral arteriovenous difference for hypoxantine and lactate during graded asphyxia in the fetal lamb. *Brain Res* 1982;239:107–17.
126. Guicheney P, Zorn JR, Sureau C, Olive G. Plasma hypoxanthine in neonatal hypoxia. A comparison of two methods. *Eur J Obstet Gynecol Reprod Biol* 1978;8:89–94.
127. Russell GAB, Jeffers G, Cooke RWI. Plasma hypoxanthine: A marker for hypoxic–ischaemic induced periventricular leucomalacia? *Arch Dis Child* 1992;67:388–92.
128. Saugstad OD. Hypoxanthine as a measurement of hypoxia. *Pediatr Res* 1975;9:1958–61.
129. Bratteby LE, Swanström S. Hypoxanthine concentration in plasma during the first two hours after birth in normal and asphyxiated infants. *Pediatr Res* 1982;16:152–5.
130. Saugstad OD. Hypoxanthine as an indicator of hypoxia: Its role in health and disease through free radical production. *Pediatr Res* 1988;23:143–50.
131. Pietz J, Gutteberg N, Gluck L. Hypoxanthine: New standard for asphyxia. *Pediatr Res* 1987;21:373A.
132. O'Connors MC, Harkness RA, Simmonds RI. The measurement of hypoxanthine, xanthine, inosine and uridine in umbilical cord blood and fetal scalp blood samples as a measure of fetal hypoxia. *Br J Obstet Gynaecol* 1981;88:381–90.
133. Harkness R, Whitelaw AGL, Simmonds RJ. Intrapartum hypoxia: The association between neurological assessment of damage and abnormal excretion of ATP metabolites. *J Clin Pathol* 1982;35: 999–1007.
134. Chin JH, Azhar S, Hoffman BB. Inactivation of endothelial-derived relaxing factor by oxidized lipoproteins. *J Clin Invest* 1992;89:10.
135. Jiménez R, Vilanova JM, Figueras J. Prostaglandins and thromboxane B_2 levels in CSF of asphyxiated newborns. *Abstracts of the 14th European Congress of Perinatal Medicine*, Helsinki, June 1994:289.
136. Sies H. Oxidative stress: From basic research to clinical application. *Am J Med* 1991;91(Suppl 3C):31S–8S.
137. Wickens D, Wilkins MH, Luneyc J, *et al.* Free radical oxidation (peroxidation) products in plasma in normal and abnormal pregnancy. *Ann Clin Biochem* 1981;18:158–62.
138. Dekker GA, Bast A, Zeeman GG, *et al.* Oxygen free radicals: The link between immunological maladaptation and endothelial cell injury in preeclampsia. *Proceedings of the XIIIth European Congress of Perinatal Medicine*, Mayo 1992. Amsterdam: Elsevier, 1992:365–77.

122 Management of small-for-gestational-age fetuses: antenatal and intrapartum strategies

J. M. Carrera, F. Figueras, R. Devesa and J. Mallafré

Introduction

There is increasing opinion[1] that small-for-gestational-age (SGA) fetuses is an heterogeneous condition that includes several etiologic and clinical groups, namely (i) abnormal SGA, fetuses whose smallness is secondary to chromosomal, structural or infective abnormalities; (ii) intrauterine growth restriction (IUGR), fetuses with impaired placental function; and, by exclusion, (iii) normal SGA, fetuses that represent the lower spectrum of the weight distribution of the normal population.

Since the etiology and prognosis is different, the management of each category should also be completely different.

It seems obvious that the best treatment we can offer a fetus with growth retardation, whose circulation and homeostasis are progressively deteriorating, is extraction at the most appropriate time. A suspected delay in fetal growth confers vital importance to the management of the pregnancy to avoid as far as possible the dangers that threaten its life and well-being. The prognosis can be significantly improved by good prenatal supervision, the early identification of the growth anomaly, the diagnosis of possible congenital defects, the early detection in the fetus of phenomena of adaptation and decompensation as regards hypoxia, and the appropriate interruption of gestation where necessary.

For the correct management of SGA fetuses, the following factors must be taken into account:

(1) Gestational age and fetal maturity: not only to decide on possible interruption of the gestation, but also to use the most appropriate control procedure (for example, the use of cardiotocography before week 30 of gestation has not proved very useful).
(2) Basic or associated medical pathology. Treatment of the underlying disease can improve the fetal condition and postpone any need for extraction.
(3) Type of growth retardation (see earlier chapter).
(4) Existence or otherwise of a congenital defect. The approach to a case can be completely transformed by the existence of a (chromosomic or malformative) congenital defect, especially if it leads to a poor prognosis.
(5) Presence or otherwise of oligohydramnios, a key factor for some authors: it can indicate a significant congenital defect or placental insufficiency in the decompensation phase.
(6) Results of fetal control tests. These are governed by the preferences or facilities of each clinic (echography, cardiotocography, acoustic stimulation test, fetal movements study, umbilical Doppler, fetal hemodynamic pattern, biophysical profile, etc.).

Other authors in this book have already discussed the prenatal diagnosis of SGA, its detection in patients not at risk, along with the methods for establishing the state or condition of the fetus for the gestational age. In this chapter, we concentrate on the possibilities currently available, or under research, to improve the prognosis for these fetuses, or gain time until they become sufficiently mature to be extracted.

Over the last 20 years a host of medical and pharmacological means of theoretically improving nutrition and the fetal condition have been attempted. The concept of intrauterine treatment of growth retardation is particularly appealing, although its results have been less than convincing.

Primary prevention

Primary prevention is only achievable if the causes of the disease are understood and risk factors are likely to be manipulated.

Genuine primary preventive strategies for SGA include: smoking cessation programs, antirubella vaccination, counseling for prevention of toxoplasmosis, prenatal diagnosis programs (contributes to the early discovery of a significant number of the congenital defects associated with SGA), strategies aimed at reducing the number of multiple pregnancies in women on assisted reproductive techniques, and, finally, primary preventive strategies for pre-eclampsia-mediated IUGR (sperm exposure, prevention obesity and insulin resistance).[2]

Secondary prevention

Secondary prevention is aimed at detection and treatment of the preclinical phase of a disease. Therefore, it requires the availability of methods of early detection and means of intervention and correction of the pathophysiological changes. Maternal serum screening has proved disappointing for IUGR: elevated levels of alpha-fetoprotein and human chorionic gonadotrophin are associated with IUGR but are a very poor screening test (sensitivity about 5%).[3] Since IUGR is caused by uteroplacental insufficiency, which is considered to be secondary to the spectrum of complications caused by poor trophoblast invasion, IUGR can be associated with an increased resistance in the uterine arteries. Doppler evaluation of this vessel constitutes the most promising screening method for IUGR. Evaluation of this tool has been hampered by different criteria for growth restriction and for abnormal Doppler waveform, by discrepancies in the targeted population and by differences in instrumentation (use of color Doppler, transvaginal vs. transabdominal approach) among the studies. Nevertheless, a recent multicentric and massive population-based study[4] aimed at evaluating the role of transvaginal uterine artery at 23 weeks, has demonstrated an overall sensitivity for growth restriction of 16%. Nevertheless, when the event of interest is the occurrence of disease requiring delivery before 32 weeks (which represents the subgroup with significant perinatal morbidity and mortality), the sensitivity for pre-eclampsia-associated and no-pre-eclampsia-associated growth restriction is 93% and 56%, respectively, with specificities of 95%. It would be appealing to move the screening into early pregnancy, but despite the fact that it seems a promising strategy for pre-eclampsia, the sensitivity of uterine artery Doppler evaluation in early second trimester for growth restriction requiring delivery before 32 weeks is only 28% (12% for growth restriction without pre-eclampsia).[5] Hence, it seems that uterine artery evaluation identifies a subgroup with an increased risk for developing severe growth restriction.

Nevertheless, in order to achieve secondary prevention ways to correct this preclinical phase are required. Since the spectrum of complications caused by poor trophoblast invasion is characterized by reduced endothelial production of prostacyclin and increased production of thromboxane A2 by platelets and the enzyme cyclo-oxygenase, which plays a central role in this pathophysiological mechanism, can be inhibited by aspirin. Oral administration of low-dose aspirin might prevent or delay the onset of placental insufficiency. In recent years, clinical trials evaluating the efficacy of uterine artery based screening strategies and treatment with aspirin in pregnancies that are at risk, have yielded discouraging results both with 150 mg[6] and 100 mg,[7] with no significant reduction in the occurrence of growth restriction. Despite the lack of evidence for the usefulness of this secondary prevention strategy, identifying pregnancies at risk, may enable a closer surveillance during the late second trimester and third trimesters.

Tertiary prevention

In IUGR, tertiary prevention should be aimed to minimize the complications of this disease, namely, fetal morbidity and mortality. Proper antenatal care is the most important part of tertiary prevention. Although several physical and pharmacological strategies have been suggested, it seems obvious that the best treatment we can offer a fetus with growth retardation, whose circulation and homoeostasis are progressively deteriorating, is extraction at the most appropriate time. Tertiary preventive strategies can be roughly divided into those focused on treatment (therapeutic strategies) and those aimed at optimizing the delivery timing (obstetric management strategies).

Therapeutic strategies

Nutritive supplements to the diet

All the fetal substrates originate from the maternal circulation, which means that, in theory, the maternal administration of food supplements would be the most physiological therapy and benefit the fetus, since the supply of many nutrients depends on the concentrations in both circulations.

Nutritional supplementation is indicated whenever the usual diet of the mother is considered to be clearly deficient. In practice, this is the case when the daily intake of calories is under 2200.[8]

In contrast, nutritional supplementation is not indicated, and can not only be ineffective but even detrimental, when the supposed growth retardation is due to phenomena such as pre-eclampsia or placento-funicular malformations.

Lechtig and coworkers[9,10] observed not only an increase in maternal and fetal weight when they supplemented the inadequate diets of a group of undernourished mothers, but also a clear improvement in the proportions of growth retardations at the age of 36 months.

Other authors[11] recommend the administration of arginine, tyrosine and perhaps cysteine – all fetuses show a low capacity for compensating for their deficits – to mothers in zones where these are normally found wanting.

The administration of folic acid and vitamin B_{12} can also be suggested, owing to their involvement in the metabolism of nucleic acids.

Rahia therapy

This consists of measures based on hygiene, and particularly rest. The renal and uteroplacentary circulation increases in the prone position, and especially on the side, as the uterine contractility decreases. On the other hand, complete rest considerably reduces the expenditure of energy, and it is possible that some energy substrates normally used in muscular exertion may now be placed at the disposal of the fetus.[12]

It is important that this rest is taken in the lateral position. Goodlin[13] emphasizes that rest in the supine position can cause an aortic–caval compression and interfere in the placental circulation.[14] Mengert and coworkers[15] demonstrated that compression of the caval vein through tying or compression with the fingers (e.g., in the course of a cesarean operation) produced retroplacental hemorrhage. In contrast, complete rest in the lateral position improved the functioning of the placenta, as demonstrated by the increase in concentration of urinary estriol.[16] This is an innocuous and cheap measure that has been widely used in recent years. Hospitalization can be useful from week 30 of gestation.[17] Despite these observations, the only clinical trial[18] aimed at evaluating the effect of bed rest for suspected fetal growth restriction, which included 107 women, did not observe differences between bed rest and ambulatory management for fetal growth parameters and neonatal outcomes.

Perfusions of dextrose and amino acids

Maternal perfusion with solutions of dextrose (or glucose) has been suggested.[17,19–21] This therapy was introduced after the observation that maternal hypoglycemia was associated with an increase in the incidence of small-for-gestational-age fetuses.[22–24]

There is evidence that insulin levels are markedly increased in many mothers of fetuses with a low weight for the gestational age, especially in the postprandial phase.[25] It is highly possible that the low level of human placental lactogen (HPL) contributes, in many cases, to the excessive anabolism, considering the lipolytic properties attributed to it.

Grumbach and coworkers[26] have verified the anti-insulin activity of human chorionic somatomammotropin or HPL. The low level of placental production of HPL can therefore noticeably affect the continuous supply of glucose to the fetus and consequently its development. In this respect, Spellacy and colleagues[27] believe that a disorder in the regulation of the secretion of HPL can be considered as a factor that induces fetal growth retardation.

All these findings point to the theoretical benefit of infusions of dextrose or glucose in those patients with permanent hypoglycemia, as well as in others with relatively rhythmic hypoglycemia resulting from postprandial hyperinsulinism.[28–45]

This type of therapy is currently used less, owing to a basic pathophysiological consideration: fetuses with extrinsic growth retardation suffer not only from hypoglycemia, but also from hypoxemia and academia.[46–48] The administration of glucose to the mother (or directly to the fetus) can increase acidemia, causing further deterioration in the fetus,[43,49] and most clinics have therefore abandoned this measure.

It has been noted that plasma levels of maternal amino acids which are low during the third trimester of gestation or during birth are associated with infants with a low weight or reduced head circumference.[50,51] This has given rise to attempts to administer perfusions of amino acids to these pregnant women,[52–55] but protein supplementation also involves potential risks. High concentrations of some amino acids can be toxic: there is a proven relationship between high levels of certain amino acids in the fetus and mental retardation (maternal phenylketonuria), as well as premature births and perinatal deaths.[56]

Maternal hemodilution

Despite the fact that numerous studies on animals have demonstrated the benefits of maternal hemodilution to the uteroplacental blood flow,[57] it has only come into use relatively recently in human medicine.[58] The main arguments put forward for the introduction of this therapy in the treatment of IUGR are the following:

(1) There is a statistically significant positive correlation between the maternal plasma volume and the weights of the fetus and placenta in cases of idiopathic growth retardation.[59]
(2) Doppler study of IUGR shows that a significant decrease in the resistance indices of the uterine artery and the fetal arteries is produced in therapy with hemodilution.
(3) Maternal hemodilution produces not only an increase in plasma volume but also reduced viscosity in the blood and an antiaggregant platelet effect in some colloids.[58]

Despite its potential benefits, it must be stressed that hemodilution without complementary oxygen therapy can strikingly increase the fetal oxygen deficit by decreasing its capacity for transportation.[60] This would explain some of the failures of this technique.[61]

A Cochrane meta-analysis[62] aimed at evaluating the effectiveness of plasma expansion for the treatment of growth restriction failed to find any study which fulfilled the quality standards to be included, concluding that there is not enough evidence to evaluate the use of plasma volume expansion for suspected impaired fetal growth.

Betamimetics

It has been established that the administration of uterus-relaxing betamimetics produces effects beneficial to the uteroplacental flow and the mother–fetus exchange[63,64] and to the possibilities of postnatal survival.[65,66] These effects are probably due to various causes:

(1) Increase in maternal minute volume due to the chronotropic or positive inotropic effect,[67–70] which implies an increase in uterine flow. This justifies a greater placental output, along with the increase in circulating glucose also produced.
(2) Moderate increase in the flow in the uterine artery, with a parallel decrease in its vascular resistance, and at the same time an increase in the diastolic velocities in the umbilical artery.[71–73]
(3) Relaxation of the uterine musculature, with an increase in fetal well-being and a facilitation of exchange.[74]
(4) Vasodilatation of the villous capillaries, enabling the fetal blood to be increased in the placenta. This, along with the increase in cardiac expenditure, implies an increase in placental–fetal blood flow which enhances exchanges, especially those based on simple diffusion. Renaud and coworkers[68] observed a significant increase in cervical circulation in cases of fetal hypotrophy after using ritodrine, although there were no appreciable differences in normal cases.
(5) Raised glucose levels, both in mothers and fetuses, due to the stimulation of glycolysis. This has been repeatedly observed during childbirth.[75–78]
(6) Activation of pulmonary maturing, with a significant increase in the lecithin/sphingomyelin ratio in the amniotic fluid.[79–81] This property makes possible the (not infrequent) premature extraction of the fetus.
(7) Activation of cerebral maturing. There is growing evidence that babies born from mothers treated with betamimetics present neurological reflexes appropriate to neonates of a greater chronological age.

Despite the irrefutable scientific evidence to support this therapy, its efficacy in practice is difficult to prove. On the other hand, it has been suggested that the vasodilating effect of betamimetics could not only lower the blood pressure, but also induce a decrease in plasma volume, thus worsening the fetal situation.[59]

A Cochrane review[82] of clinical trials aimed at evaluating the effect of betamimetics in growth restriction, which included two studies of 118 women, observed that no statistically significant differences were found between the betamimetic groups and the control groups for low birth weight (relative risk 1.17, 95% confidence interval, CI 0.75–1.83), other anthropometric measures or neonatal morbidity and mortality.

Sedatives

Some experimental studies[83,84] suggest that chlorpromazine dilates the myometrial vessels. The combination of this effect with the general sedation induced in the patient, which is propitious for rest, can endorse its administration, especially in cases of toxemia. It has been suggested that this beneficial effect is due to a momentary reduction in the cerebral consumption of oxygen, which makes it more resistant to hypoxia.

Heparin and anticoagulants

The activation of the processes of coagulation has frequently been described in cases of fetal growth retardation.[85,86] At the same time, it was discovered that, in some cases of preeclampsia, intravascular coagulation and fibrin deposition were produced in various organs, as well as in the placental intervilli spaces[87–90]; some cases of fetal growth retardation associated with preeclampsia are related to a depletion in the platelet levels in the maternal blood, resulting from intravascular coagulation in the placenta, which gives rise to a localized deposit of fibrin and platelets.[91–93]

These findings led to attempts to treat growth retardation with anticoagulants.[94] Some studies showed good results after treatment with heparin,[95–97] above all when the treatment was introduced early on (between weeks 32 and 36). The results after that were always poor.

For the proponents of this treatment, heparin not only plays a preventive role, but also cures vascular parietal lesions by reducing the placenta's aggregating capacity and breaking up fibrin deposits. (Moreover, heparin has the advantage of not crossing the placental barrier.)

It is also possible to use low-molecular-weight heparins (sodium enoxaparine), which apparently do not cross the placental barrier when used in the second to third trimester of gestation, despite their low molecular weight.[98,99]

Acetylsalicylic acid

There are conclusive proofs that the reduction in uteroplacental perfusion and disturbances in the villous microcirculation are connected to an imbalance in the production of prostacyclin and thromboxane.

A host of studies over the last few years have demonstrated that acetylsalicylic acid at low doses irreversibly inhibits platelet cyclo-oxygenase, thus reducing thromboxane synthesis but without modifying the production of prostacyclin (PGI_2) of endothelial origin.[100–103] Owing to this irreversible inactivation, the inhibiting effect is accumulative with repeated doses, with the result that daily doses of 30–50 mg of aspirin provoke a complete suppression of the synthesis of platelet thromboxane in 7–10 days.[104]

A balance between thromboxane and prostacyclin is thus attained in both the maternal and the fetoplacental circulations, the vascular reactivity to the vasomotor agents is normalized and platelet aggregation is inhibited. It is still not completely known how aspirin acts.

For some authors, the reported effect depends on the dosage: low doses (100 mg) permit the inhibition of platelet cyclo-oxygenase without affecting the endothelial enzyme.[103,105] This ability to select the action is eliminated if the dose is increased.[103]

For others,[106,107] aspirin has been found to have a trophoblast-derived inhibitor action that permits the inhibition of the placental synthesis of thromboxane and the establishment of the physiological balance of prostaglandins.

Sibai and coworkers[108] and Pedersen and Fitzgerald[109] have shown that 20 mg of aspirin produces inhibition of platelet cyclo-oxygenase activity and permits the biological detection of salicylemia, but that the systemic concentrations of the salicylates induced are insufficient for stimulating the acetylation of endothelial cyclo-oxygenase.

The administration of aspirin at low doses results in:

(1) The modification of the synthesis of prostaglandins in the maternal circulation[100,101,108] and in that of the fetus[100–108];
(2) The modification of vascular sensitivity to angiotensin[105]; and
(3) The inhibition of platelet adherence to collagen, in conditions of stasis or slow blood flow.

In other studies[110,111] dipyridamol was also introduced as a complement; this inhibits phosphodiesterase, which impedes the degradation of cAMP, with an aggregant and vasodilatory effect (principally mediated by prostacyclin).

A significant decline has been noted in the incidence of delayed growth, with an increase in the weight of neonates born to mothers at high risk of IUGR,[110–112] irrespective of the use of dipyridamol. In contrast, differences were found with this treatment in the Italian study,[113] although this work is open to a number of methodological objections.

Another effect of therapy with aspirin at low doses (between 60 and 100 mg/day) is the reduction of the incidence of pre-eclampsia in women with a high risk of suffering from this, owing to their obstetric history,[114] an increased sensitivity to the pressor action of angiotensin II,[93] or anomalies in the Doppler scans of the uterine arteries.[115] However, further studies are required for definitive validation of these opinions.

A recent Finnish prospective randomized study on first-trimester low-dose aspirin administration in patients with abnormal uterine artery blood flow showed encouraging prevention of pre-eclampsia.[116] Although the rate of IUGR was not significantly affected there are several arguments that support the use of low-dose aspirin in high-risk pregnancies that are identified through abnormal uterine artery Doppler. The safety of aspirin in pregnancy has been documented in a large number of patients.[117] The severity of IUGR may be decreased[118] and a decline of maternal delivery indications for pre-eclampsia is likely to decrease the preterm delivery rate. Placental disease with severe IUGR may be the first manifestation of previously undiagnosed underlying thrombophilia.[119]

Atrial natriuretic peptide

The atrial natriuretic peptide (ANP) is an endogenous peptide with diuretic, natriuretic and vasodilatory properties.[120] It is synthesized in the right atrium. It has been reported that ANP is capable of provoking vasodilatation of the placental circulation in animals.[121]

In the animal model, the administration of ANP to guinea pigs in which IUGR was induced by the ligature of the uterine artery[122] significantly increased the blood flow to the placenta.

The concentrations of ANP in fetuses with IUGR are significantly higher than in fetuses with normal growth, suggesting an adaptive fetal response in an attempt to increase the blood flow.[123] Furthermore, it has been demonstrated that there are up to 80% fewer receptors for ANP in the arteries of placentas in IUGR compared to those of normal fetuses, which could demonstrate that an alteration in the placental receptors for ANP would be the etiopathogenic basis for some IUGR. More data should be obtained in this respect in the future.

Sexual steroids

Some obstetricians administer varying doses of progesterone and estrogens on a completely empirical basis.

Several authors[124–129] showed some years ago that progesterone reduces the excitability and contractility of the myometrium muscular fiber, thus contributing to uterine relaxation.

In fact, as Beydoun and coworkers have shown,[130] progesterone treatment on ovariectomized rabbits is capable of significantly increasing the fetal and placental weights through hyperplasia. Other studies have presented similar results with synthetase analogs.[131,132]

It must be remembered, however, that therapy with steroids can inhibit the fetal pulmonary surfactants. In fact, nowadays there is very little support for the continued use of sexual steroids for this indication.

Oxygen therapy

Oxygen is an essential component for fetal growth: a 20–40% oxidative metabolism is required to provide the energy necessary for fetal growth.[133,134] In fact, it seems that hypoxemia must be the cause of the retarded growth observed in mothers who are carriers of hemoglobinopathy, cyanotic cardiopathy and asthma, or who live at very high altitudes, as occurs in animals subject to hypobaric hypoxemia.[135–137] Those fetuses with retarded growth on whom funiculocentesis was performed[138] revealed a partial pressure of oxygen lower than that of normal fetuses.

All the available studies refer to an intermittent administration of oxygen (10–120 min), which increases fetal respiratory movements[139] and active movements[140] and provokes a notable improvement in fetal circulatory distribution[141,142] as well as lower perinatal mortality.[143]

However, no studies have been able to demonstrate that this is useful in improving fetal oxygenation during pregnancy when it is carried out discontinuously, as it inevitably has to be.[144] On the contrary, there is evidence that it can reduce oxygenation by producing a uteroplacental vasoconstriction.[145,146] This side effect could be avoided by the supplementary administration of vasoactive drugs. Betamimetics would probably perform this task. Moya and coworkers[147] reported two cases of severe neonatal depression due to the alkalosis produced by hyperventilation during anesthesia.

Further arguments against oxygen therapy are:

(1) Oxygen increases the use of glucose and therefore aggravates hypoglucemia[148];
(2) Oxygen therapy increases cerebrovascular resistance and decreases peripheral resistance, which prejudices cerebral oxygenation and hypoglycemia[142]; and
(3) There is no evidence that oxygen therapy increases fetal growth or improves the transportation of nutrients across the placenta.[141]

Nowadays the administration of oxygen is considered to be justified only in those cases in which the 'oxygen test' was positive. This test consists of observing whether velocimetric changes are produced in the fetal aorta after administration of oxygen. If there is a notable increase in the diastolic velocities, oxygen therapy is indicated.[142]

A Cochrane meta-analysis,[149] aimed at evaluating the effectiveness of oxygen therapy in growth restriction, which included three randomized studies with 94 women, observed a significant reduction in perinatal mortality (relative risk 0.5; 95% CI 0.32–0.81) when compared with placebo. Nevertheless, a greater gestational age in the treatment group might introduce a bias which could account for the differences.

Intra-amniotic therapy

Various studies have stated that the supply of nutrients to the human fetus is restricted by growth retardation; autopsies have demonstrated a decrease in the reserves of glycogen and fat similar to that in undernourished children.[150] For this reason, the intra-amniotic injection of amino acids and glucose has been suggested for attempting to improve the nutrition of the fetus.[151–156]

There has been some debate as to whether the absorption by the fetus of the products deposited in the amniotic cavity takes place through diffusion across the amnios or through deglutition, digestion and absorption in the fetal digestive tract. Even when the former route is secure, experiments in cases of anencephaly,[157] with albumins marked with ^{131}I or with ^{51}Cr[158] demonstrate that digestive absorption is probably the preferred route.[159–161]

Experimental studies in animals have demonstrated that amino acids and proteins injected into the amniotic fluid are not only consumed by the fetus through absorption in the digestive tract,[159,162–164] but also passed on through the placenta and the umbilical cord.[153,165–167] For this reason, there is a marked increase in the weight of the placenta after intra-amniotic feeding.[168]

Overall, the studies on various animal species demonstrate that the supply of amino acids and glucose to the fetus can improve the fetal prognosis, regardless of the route used (intra-amniotic, intragastric or intravenous[159,162,164,168–171]). In contrast, the provision of lipids not only fails to enhance fetal nutrition but can also prove deleterious by aggravating the IUGR and respiratory difficulties.[172]

Repeated amniotic puncture multiplies the risks and complications, even more so in the frequent cases of severe oligohydramnios. Infection and premature birth are still more problematic, as the fetus itself is at stake.

Apart from the risks inherent in the technique, the administration of an excess of glucose can provoke a decrease in the fetal arterial oxygen content,[165,166,173] owing to the fact that glucose induces an increase in the consumption of fetal oxygen, as well as provoking lactic acidosis. This risk is greater if its administration is performed directly, as discussed below.

Direct administration of nutrients to the fetus

Various studies in animals have demonstrated the efficacy of this method. The direct administration to the stomach or intestine of sheep[174,175] of glucose and amino acids by means of a catheter rapidly increased their levels in the fetal blood, and produced an increase in weight in those fetuses previously experiencing delayed growth brought on by a limited maternal diet.[171] There is also an account of direct intravenous administration[176] which correlated the fetal weight with the daily concentration of nutrients administered.

There is only one case report of direct administration of nutrients in humans. Saling[177] administered amino acids and vitamins over 9 days by means of an intraperitoneal catheter to a fetus with growth retardation at 33 weeks of gestation, after which a spontaneous birth occurred without complications.

This treatment route requires a more complete experimental basis to demonstrate its efficacy in the face of its evident drawbacks, to make its evaluation possible in humans.

Intermittent abdominal decompression

This technique, first described by Heyns and colleagues[178] and recently modified by Shimonovitz and coworkers,[179] attempts to improve uteroplacental blood flow and, as a result, fetal oxygenation.

It consists of an adjustable plastic garment on a rigid support with a decompression mechanism that induces a decrease in the pressure round the maternal abdomen. Shimonovitz and coworkers[179] reported good results with intermittent applications of a negative pressure of 70 mmHg over 30 s at 1-min intervals, for a total of 30 min twice a day. An analytical overview of the studies published on this topic up to that point[180] reported a significant reduction in perinatal mortality.

Blecher[181] measured the placental blood flow before, during and after decompression, and noted that on 50% of occasions there was an increased blood flow, and this was particularly noticeable during decompression. Other authors[182–186] have also observed an increase in blood flow in cases with placental insufficiency on the flow curves, along with improvements in various hormonal tests. This technique could therefore produce an improvement in uteroplacental blood flow that could last for a certain time afterwards, provided that the placenta is not too insufficient.

Although this procedure has been virtually discarded in Western Europe, it is still practiced in Eastern European countries in the treatment of chronic fetal afflictions.[187,188] The recommended method is as follows: treatments of 8–10 h overall, made up of applications of 30–60 min/day (2 atm).

Pharmacology of prostacyclin/thromboxane balance

The work of Clark and coworkers[189] in animal experimentation demonstrates a clear increase in the blood flow in the uterine artery after the intra-arterial administration of prostacyclin, although this has not always been confirmed afterwards.[190,191] It does not therefore seem that the administration of prostacyclin can be useful for this purpose.

As regards thromboxane synthetase inhibitors, Van Assche and coworkers[192] have used dazoxiben, a product that inhibits the production of thromboxane A_2 in some cases of pre-eclampsia. The conditions under which it was applied (small number of patients, late administration) do not make it possible to draw any conclusions.

Nitric oxide liberators

The maternal administration of glyceryl trinitrate (GTN), an agent that releases nitric oxide, is capable of improving both the uterine and the umbilical circulation; this is verified in practice by a significant reduction in the pulsatility indices of both arteries.[193,194] This pharmacological action is especially evident in the cases of growth retardation associated with pre-eclampsia.

The pathophysiological explanation lies in the fact that pre-eclampsia gives rise to a reduction in the activity and production of nitric oxide, which has negative repercussions on the uteroplacental circulation. The GTN administered to the mother exerts a direct action firstly on the uterine vasculature, provoking its vasodilation and improving the provision of oxygen and nutrients to the intervillous space, and secondly on the villous microcirculation, thus also provoking vasodilatation here. In theory, the administration of GTN would be indicated in all those cases of growth retardation associated with pre-eclampsia in which the nitric oxide test (sublingual administration of 0.3 mg of GTN) has previously proved positive (decrease at 30 min of maternal blood pressure and the pulsatility indices in uterine and umbilical arteries).[195] However, further studies are required to determine whether this therapy is free of risks and proves capable of persistently improving uteroplacental vascular insufficiency in the cases mentioned. Until such studies are undertaken, the administration of GTN can be used as a diagnostic, but not a therapeutic tool.

Immunological treatment

It is theoretically possible that the inhibition of the secreting activity of B lymphocytes or the blocking of the peripheral action of immunoglobulins could occasion an improved fetal outcome in gestations that are complicated by the presence of antiphospholipid antibodies.

Edelman[196] reported on the administration of corticoids in 22 cases and noted a normalization of the plasma levels in anticardiolipin antibodies in 80% of pregnant women. Several authors[197–199] have recorded the results obtained from the administration of intravenous gamma-globulin in pre-eclamptic patients with fetuses with growth retardation and antiphospholipid antibodies. There is no question that the treatment reduced the plasma levels of these antibodies, but it is not clear whether it improved the clinical picture. The mechanism of action of the gamma-globulins is still open to debate.

Pharmacology of cerebral observation

Barbiturates were proposed some years ago[84] as a means of momentarily reducing the cerebral consumption of oxygen and, therefore, the vulnerability of this organ to hypoxia. Since then the majority of studies have shown that these drugs have very limited value in the intrauterine prevention of cerebral lesions.[200]

Our present-day understanding of the cellular consequences of hypoxia enables us to hold out some hopes for the *in utero* prevention of posthypoxic cerebral lesions, when fetal extraction – which continues to be the most expeditious therapeutic measure – is still not possible or has to be postponed owing to other circumstances.[201]

There are four possible pharmacological strategies: the avoidance of: (1) increased intercellular calcium; (2) excessive release of amino acid exciters; (3) pathological arachidonic acid cascade; and (4) oxygen free radicals.

Increase of intercellular calcium. An increase in intercellular calcium is the first biochemical link in the chain of events leading to neuronal death. This could theoretically be avoided, although only partially, by means of the administration of calcium channel antagonists, such as nifedipine, which has proved to be effective in the avoidance of local infarcts in rabbits,[202] flunarizine, which apparently provides a certain degree of cerebral tissue protection in rat fetuses afflicted by hypoxia[203,204] and lidoflazine, which, when administered in sheep after the hypoxic ictus, improved the prognosis of these lesions.[203]

The most promising of all these drugs is apparently flunarizine, since it has the most favorable action on the cerebral circulation and crosses the placental and hematoencephalic barriers with ease. However, these findings remain to be confirmed in human species and the administration strategy needs to be determined (before, during or after the hypoxic episode).

If the blockage of the calcium channels were to prove effective, this treatment could impede the subsequent activation of the phospholipases and the amino acid exciters, as well as the release of free fatty acids.

Excessive release of amino acid exciters

The avoidance of the release of, for example, glutamate or aspartate, can be achieved by pharmacologically inhibiting the receptors of certain amino acids (competitive antagonists).

The experimental use of rats and sheep has confirmed the neuropreventive possibilities of a broad-spectrum excitatory-amino-acid receptor antagonist, kynureic acid, which attenuates the cerebral lesion by up to 35%; an *N*-methyl-D-aspartate antagonist (N-receptor), MK-801; a glutamate release inhibitor, BW1003C87, which reduces the cerebral lesion by up to 50%; and, finally, an a-amino-3-hydroxy-5-methyl-4-isoxazolepropionic acid receptor antagonist, identified as NBQX, which induced a reduction of 28%.[205,206] These antagonists can be used before or immediately after the hypoxic–ischemic ictus.[207]

Alternatively, non-competitive antagonists, such as phenciclidine, dextromethorphan or magnesium sulfate, have also been used. Propentophylline, which attenuates the excess of amino acid exciters, seems capable of reducing cerebral lesions by 28%. All these products have been used on various experimental animals (rats, cats, rabbits, sheep, lambs) with encouraging results, as already indicated, since their administration before and/or after provoked hypoxia significantly reduced neuronal lesions and the appearance of postischemic accidents.

Some of these drugs, such as BW1003C87, seem to play only a neuroprotective role if they are administered before the hypoxic ictus. The cerebral lesions in these cases are reduced from 98% to 45%.[206]

The drug with the most future appears to be MK-801 because, apart from its therapeutic actions, it easily crosses the placental and blood–brain barriers. However, more information is required on its potential toxicity[208] and its effects on the human fetus.

Pathological arachidonic acid cascade. Avoidance of this would reduce both the production of oxygen-derived radicals and the prejudicial effects of prostacyclin/thromboxane imbalance. Both these aims could theoretically be met by administering prostaglandin synthetase inhibitors and inhibiting cyclo-oxygenase with products such as indomethacin. Encouraging experiments have been carried out on adult animals (dogs, rats, cats), showing that the administration of indomethacin before the ischemic ictus improves postischemic reperfusion.[209] There are also well-known data on its gestational administration in the prophylaxis for premature births, because of its effects on the closure of the ductus arteriosus, the regulation of breathing and the reduction in amniotic fluid.

Indomethacin has recently been used at low doses as a neuropreserver in underweight neonates. It apparently achieves a significant reduction in the incidence of intraventricular hemorrhages, with no further consequences.[210] More information is required on its use in the fetus with this specific indication.

Another theoretical measure for avoiding prostacyclin/thromboxane imbalance could consist of the administration of the former at therapeutic doses. However, the studies available have not shown any appreciable benefits.[211]

Oxygen free radicals. Avoidance of these could be achieved either by eliminating their production or by eliminating their deleterious derivatives.

The first goal could be attained either by blocking xanthine oxidase, which catalyzes the degradation of hypoxanthine, or by inhibiting the lipid peroxidation that gives rise to the destruction of membranes. Alopurinol has been used in the first case, and has proved effective to some extent in the avoidance of cerebral edema in rats submitted to overall ischemia. The inhibition of peroxidation part can be attempted with 21-aminosteroids (U7400GF), although there is little information on this possibility.

The elimination of free radicals in animal experimentation has been attempted by two types of products: enzymatic antioxidants such as superoxide dismutase and catalase, and the free radical 'scavengers', a very heterogeneous group of drugs, which include methionine, mannitol, ascorbic acid and tocopherol.

The administration of the above-mentioned antioxidants before the hypoxic ictus has proved capable, in the fetuses of both dogs and rats, of improving cerebral blood flow and the somatosensory potentials.[212]

However, at the moment, the use of vitamins C, E and C+E[213] has provided no *in vitro* evidence of any effect on lipid peroxidation or placental perfusion in normal placentas and patients with pre-eclampsia.

Finally, Gutteridge's group[214,215] also highlights the extracellular antioxidants, which include metal-bound proteins (transferrin, lactoferrin, haptoglobin, hemopexin, etc.), 'iron-oxidant proteins' (ceruloplasmin) and extracellular 'scavenger' proteins[216,217] such as extracellular superoxide dismutase and glutathione peroxide. The principal function of the extracellular antioxidants seems to be the deactivation of the catalysts needed for the formation of oxygen free radicals.[218,219]

Some studies[220,221] suggest that some malformations in diabetes can have as their pathogenic mechanism the excessive generation of oxygen free radicals, activated by a high concentration of glucose. It would thus be possible, at least experimentally, to avoid the teratogenic effect by means of the administration of free radical scavengers.[221,222] However, we lack documented information on their usefulness and lack of risks, and this prevents us from attempting to administer them in human gestation.

Obstetric management strategies

The association between IUGR and increased perinatal mortality, morbidity and impaired long-term neurodevelopmental outcome has received considerable attention in recent years. There is general acknowledgement in this pathology of a sharp increase in the cases of intrapartum fetal distress, the risk of neonatal depression (low Apgar scores), meconium aspiration and acidosis.[223] On the other hand, several studies[224–228] have shown that the ante- and intrapartum fetal mortality rate is significantly greater in small-for-gestational-age fetuses than in premature fetuses matched for weight.

Finally, the respiratory distress syndrome, necrotizing enterocholitis, intraventricular hemorrhage and periventricular leukomalacia have been reported to be increased in preterm growth restricted neonates.[229]

Since there is no effective fetal therapy for growth restriction, timing of delivery is an essential issue in the management of these fetuses. Delay could increase hypoxia and affect brain development, but early delivery carries the dangers of prematurity and the associated risk of cerebral palsy. During the last 30 years, obstetricians have been searching for a tool to prenatally predict these events of critical importance.

Decision to terminate gestation

A multicentric randomized controlled trial, the Growth Restriction Intervention Trial (GRIT),[230] aimed at comparing the effect of delivering early with delaying birth for as long as possible, has been recently published. A total of 588 fetuses between 24 and 36 weeks were randomized to immediate delivery or delayed delivery until the obstetrician was no longer certain. The study observed that when obstetricians were uncertain about timing of delivery, they were prepared to vary the timing by about 4 days, and although such delay caused some stillbirths, earlier delivery resulted in an almost equal number of additional deaths. Moreover, at 2 years of age, there was a trend toward more disability in the immediate delivery group. Although this study did not provide a detailed clinical guidance on the exact point at which compromised fetuses should be delivered, it stressed the critical importance of delivery timing. Arterial and venous Doppler parameters, biophysical variables and fetal heart rate analysis are used for this purpose. In addition, others factors such as maternal complications (especially in pre-eclampsia), severity of growth restriction, neonatal resources, parental opinion and, overall, gestational age, complicate the decision-making in those fetuses. Although the order in which alteration of Doppler and biophysical parameters take place has been clarified in recent studies,[231–233] the existing wide variation in policies is not surprising.[234]

Gestations in which systematic delivery cannot be justified. Various situations can be included in this category:

(1) Gestations with fetuses that are small for gestational age but normal. As already explained, these fetuses have a moderately low genetic growth potential, but are normal. They represent the lower spectrum of growth normality. From the biometric point of view, they are found in the lower centiles but their weekly increases are satisfactory, when using appropriate longitudinal standards to evaluate growth velocity.
(2) Fetuses with malformations or chromosomal anomalies. The strategy followed depends on the type of anomaly, the gestation period and the decision of the parents. When abortion is feasible, parents must be informed of this option. If the gestation follows its course (late diagnosis, refusal to interrupt), its management must be based on observation, irrespective of the fetal maturity or the results of tests to control the fetal condition. Each case must be studied and managed on its individual merits, with the opinion of the parents taken into account.
(3) Gestations with fetuses with an apparently IUGR, but which do not present oligohydramnios and have normal tests of fetal well-being. In these cases vigilant observation should be carried out, in strict accordance with each particular unit's control criteria (twice-weekly non-stress test, weekly echographic control, Doppler umbilical examination, oxytocin or funiculocentesis test if there are any doubts).

Gestations requiring delivery. The interruption of gestation must be normal practice, provided the fetus is viable (mature fetus or in the transitional maturing phase), in the following cases:

(1) Detention of fetal growth over a period of 3 weeks (evaluated with appropiate longitudinal standards) with pathological cerebroplacental ratio and likely fetal lung maturation.
(2) Presence of oligohydramnios (echograpic examination) or meconium amniotic fluid (amnioscopy) and likely fetal lung maturation.
(3) Doppler (persistent venous abnormal flow, reversed end-diastolic flow in the umbilical artery) or biophysical (persistent altered biophysical profile, silent or decelerative cardiotocography) criteria suggesting fetal decompensation and acidosis.
(4) Study of fetal blood biochemistry (funiculocentesis) indicating an irrefutably pathological acid–base balance.

The theoretical aim of the interruption is the extraction of the fetus before the centralization of the fetal blood flow reaches an advanced phase and can injure the fetus. In this regard, it is important, if Doppler is available, to follow the evolution of the hemodynamic changes taking place in the fetus (covered in other chapters in this book).

When the fetus is immature, an attempt must be made to accelerate its maturation by the usual means (administration of corticoids, etc.). Preterm IUGR/ARED fetuses exhibit divergent cardiovascular responses to prenatal steroids. Intensive Doppler-based fetal monitoring may identify a subset of fetuses prone to decompensation after maternal steroid administration. When abnormal venous Doppler studies are found, delivery may be more appropriate than steroids.[235] It must be remembered that the risks from IUGR can be intensified with prematurity.[236] If gestation has not reached 28 weeks, the decision to expel the fetus involves risk. The decision of whether to interrupt the gestation or not must always be studied in the light of each particular case.

In contrast with the classical statement that growth-retarded fetuses have an accelerated pulmonary maturation, current observations have suggested a higher incidence of respiratory distress in those fetuses when compared with preterm neonates with normal weight.[237] The study of the amniotic fluid in these fetuses shows a high quantity of surfactants and lipidic cells. However, it is possible that in some cases there is a delay, as a result of placental insufficiency, in the maturing of type II fetal alveolar cells, which are responsible for the production of surfactants.[238,239] Furthermore, it must be remembered that labor, and even some hours with broken membranes, improve the surfactant content in the amniotic fluid.

When we studied our practice of terminating gestations in our unit, we noted that our strategy has changed substantially over the last 20 years. In the first 5 years (1976–80) the number of births with a spontaneous onset was 70.3%, but by the last period this had been reduced to less than half this figure (28%), with a parallel increase in the number of inductions, and particularly in the number of elective cesarean sections.

Management and timing

Though clear guidelines supported by strong evidence cannot be provided, protocols for management of SGA fetus may be developed according to current knowledge. Although some recent management protocols have been published,[240,241] our local protocol is as follows:

(1) SGA (estimated fetal weight below the 5th centile with normal cerebroplacental ratio and normal uterine artery Doppler flow): excluding infectious and genetic causes, the perinatal results are good. Delivery should only be indicated for obstetrics or maternal factors. Weekly BPS and fortnightly Doppler evaluation should be performed.
(2) IUGR with normal fetal well-being tests (estimated fetal weight below the 5th centile with abnormal cerebroplacental ratio or uterine artery Doppler flow): weekly Doppler and BPS 2 times /week should be performed. Delivery beyond 37 weeks or when pulmonary maturity is proven could be considered.
(3) IUGR (estimated fetal weight below the 5th centile with abnormal cerebroplacental ratio or uterine artery Doppler flow) with significant blood flow redistribution (absent or reversed end-diatolic flow in the umbilical artery):
   a. beyond 34 weeks: deliver
   b. between 32 and 34 weeks:
      i. REDV: steroids and deliver in 24–48 h
      ii. AEDV: steroids, daily Doppler and BPS
   c. below 32 weeks: steroids, daily Doppler and BPS
(4) IUGR (estimated fetal weight below the 5th centile with abnormal cerebroplacental ratio or uterine artery Doppler flow) with proven fetal compromise (persistent increased ductus venosus waveforms pulsatility, low short-term variability in cardiotocography or oligohydramnios):
   a. beyond 32 weeks: deliver
   b. below 32 weeks: hospital admission, steroids, daily Doppler and BPS/8–12 h
(5) IUGR (estimated fetal weight below the 5th centile with abnormal cerebroplacental ratio or uterine artery Doppler flow) with fetal decompensation (persistent absent or reversed a-wave in the ductus venosus or persistent pulsatile

Table 122.1 Means of initiating birth in our unit during two different periods: 1976–80 and 1990–94

	1976–80	1990–94
Spontaneous onset (%)	70.33	28.2
Induction (%)	20.00	39.8
Elective cesarean section (%)	9.06	31.9

Table 122.2 Means of terminating birth in our unit during two different periods: 1976–80 and 1990–94

	1976–80	1990–94
Vaginal route (%)	84.19	55.5
Cesarean section (%)	16.80	44.4

umbilical vein + persistent BPS < 6/10, decelerative cardiotocography): deliver at a tertiary care center. In the subgroup under 28 weeks, each case should be evaluated by a multidisciplinary committee composed by an obstetrician and a neonatologist with experience in those cases, and taking into account the opinion of the parents: expectant management could be an option is these extremely preterm and compromised fetuses.

Elective route of birth

The literature reiterates the finding that two-thirds of fetuses with growth retardation can tolerate the stress of birth perfectly well, and, therefore, they are delivered by the vaginal route. A cesarean section should be performed in only one-third of gestations.[242,243] This is true in principle (Table 122.l) but in our present experience the total number of cesarean sections is 44.4% (Table 122.2). Nowadays, in most hospitals the number of cesarean sections in this category has gone up to 30–50%.[223,242,244]

The decision between induction of the birth or a cesarean section must be made on the basis of various criteria, especially: fetal condition (phase of fetal adaptation to hypoxia, decompensation phase), special obstetric features (parity, fetal presentation, pelvic and cervical conditions) and gestational age.

Generally speaking, the following situations lead towards an elective cesarean section

(1) IUGR in the phase of fetal adaptation to hypoxia (e.g. incipient centralization of blood flow, normoamnios or moderate oligohydramnios, abnormal uterine artery waveforms) with poor obstetric conditions;
(2) IUGR in the phase of fetal decompensation irrespective of obstetric conditions;
(3) SGA fetuses with malformations capable of causing mechanical dystocia (e.g., hydrocephaly, voluminous teratomas); and
(4) Progressive deterioration of the maternal condition (e.g., cardiopulmonary diseases, kidney diseases).

A recent study,[245] aimed at evaluating the prospect of vaginal delivery of growth-restricted fetuses with abnormal umbilical artery blood flow and negative oxytocin challenge test, has observed that the vaginal delivery rate was significantly lower in the abnormal flow group compared with the normal flow group, but in cases finally destined for a trial of labor the vaginal delivery rates were similar. There was no indication that any fetus was exposed to detrimental hypoxia or distress. These results should encourage obstetricians to perform trials of vaginal delivery when there is no unanimous indication for cesarean delivery.

Means of inducing birth

Once the decision has been made to interrupt the pregnancy through induction, this must be planned in the light of the fetal condition. It must be remembered that the reserves of glycogen and fat are severely depleted in a fetus with growth retardation, which has a greater or lesser degree of uteroplacental insufficiency. The hypoxic stress derived from labor can give rise to a rapid depletion of the scanty fetal reserves. This makes it necessary to establish an anaerobic defense metabolism, with subsequent metabolic acidosis.

For this reason, the induction of birth must be meticulous and avoid any hyperstimulation. In our unit we remain loyal in these cases to induction through amniotomy and the administration of oxytocin with a continuous perfusion pump.

The induction begins with a dose of 0.5 or 1 mU/min, which is doubled every 20 min until theoretically effective uterine dynamics are attained (three to four contractions every 10 min). The dosage is stabilized at this point, but with the maintenance of the infusion rhythm necessary for maintaining satisfactory dynamics. In the event that there is no sign of fetal distress, the drip is continued for 12 h. If the active period of the birth is not reached during this time, the induction must be considered a failure and a cesarean section will be decided upon.[244,246]

The administration of intracervical prostaglandins in order to mature the neck before the instillation of the oxytocin infusion is a procedure that we rarely use in this pathology, since resorting to it can produce hyperdynamics and secondary alterations to the fetal heart rate.[244,247,248]

Over the course of the last 5 years in our unit, something over a third of the inductions in growth retardation have terminated in expedient cesarean sections, owing to intrapartum fetal distress or failed induction; these figures are similar to those reported by other authors.[249]

Intrapartum control

Owing to the frequency of placental insufficiency in fetuses with growth retardation, causing a genuinely chronic fetal distress, it is clear that birth represents an excessive stress for many of them. For this reason, labor, whether begun spontaneously or induced, must be controlled by continuous cardiotocographic monitoring, at first externally and then internally when cervical conditions permit it. Any significant anomalies in the findings must be followed up with biochemical control, as in any other high-risk gestation.

The intrauterine pressure of the contractions is similar to that of a normal gestation,[250,251] therefore any alterations in the FCF observed in growth retardations during delivery are not conditioned by anomalies in the uterine dynamics. The presence of a higher number of these anomalies can be attributed to the frequent oligohydramnios and to the higher number of inductions (with their familiar iatrogenesis).

As regards the cardiotocographic readings, in our experience there are no significant differences (with respect to a control group) in the baseline of the FCF, or in the early decelerations; in contrast, the percentage of contractions that generate late decelerations is significantly greater in the group with IUGR, above all in the dilatation period. This has been endorsed by other authors.[252] These characteristics of the outline of the FCF explain why clinical control of the birth proves insufficient, since the baseline of the FCF remains practically unaltered.

As for the determinations of pH carried out during birth in our last series, on 10% of occasions the pH was less than 7.20; on 27.5% it ranged between 7.20 and 7.25, and on the remaining occasions (62.5%) surpassed the figure of 7.25. The figures for pathological and prepathological pH easily surpass those of any control group of normal births. It must be borne in mind that we performed 31.9% of elective cesarean sections on account of abnormally low fetal respiratory reserves. These figures are also very similar to others that are on record.[252]

This acute fetal distress is mostly a simple intensification of preexisting chronic fetal distress. For this reason, extrinsic (or type II) growth retardations, which generally have a vascular uteroplacental cause, exhibit differences in behavior during birth that are statistically significant with respect to other intrinsic (or type I) retardations.

The intensification of this chronic fetal distress is probably produced by different mechanisms:

(1) Exhaustion of the placental functional reserves due to spontaneous or induced contractions;
(2) Greater fetal vulnerability through the lack of subcutaneous fat and peripheral vasoconstriction motivated by the redistribution of blood towards more vital zones; and
(3) Reduction in the quantity of Wharton's jelly in the umbilical cord, which reduces its tonicity and facilitates its prolapse and compression.

Recently, a study[253] aimed at evaluating the role of pulsioximetry in growth-restricted fetuses, have found that fetal pulse oximetry is reliable, according to umbilical cord blood measurements and Apgar scores, reducing cesarean deliveries in cases of non-reassuring cardiotocographic patterns in those fetuses.

Obstetric anesthesia

Of all the various types of anesthetic procedures, it seems to us that peridural anesthesia is the most satisfactory in cases of growth retardation. This type of anesthesia avoids the administration of analgesics, anxiolytics and spasmolytics which are capable of depressing the fetus, and it is particularly useful in the frequent cases of association of toxemia and fetal growth retardation. In addition, it makes biophysical and biochemical monitoring more tolerable for the mother.

It must be taken into account that a fetus with IUGR has greater sensitivity to general anesthesia, owing to its hypoproteinemia. This characteristic, which means that the drug does not leave the general circulation with the same speed as normal, can occasion an increase in its concentration in the central nervous system, and this is translated into an increase in the number of neonatal depressions.[242,244] Furthermore, it seems that the hepatic capacity to metabolize the drug is also diminished, and there is a degree of renal incapacity for its elimination.

It also does not seem advisable to use paracervical anesthesia, as it is well known that this increases the number of bradycardias.

REFERENCES

1. Soothill PW, Bobrow CS, Holmes R. Small for gestational age is not a diagnosis. *Ultrasound Obstet Gynecol* 1999;13:225–8.
2. Dekker G, Sibai B. Primary, secondary and tertiary prevention for pre-eclampsia. *Lancet* 2001;357:207–16.
3. Yaron Y, Ochshorn Y, Heifetz S, Lehavi O, Sapir Y, Orr Urtreger A. First trimester maternal serum free human chorionic gonadotropin as a predictor of adverse pregnancy outcome. *Fetal Diagn Ther* 2002;17:352–6.
4. Papageorghiou AT, Yu CK, Bindra R, Pandis G, Nicolaides KH. Multicenter screening for pre-eclampsia and fetal growth restriction by transvaginal uterine artery Doppler at 23 weeks of gestation. *Ultrasound Obstet Gynecol* 2001;18:441–9.
5. Martin AM, Bindra R, Curcio P, Cicero S, Nicolaides KH. Screening for pre-eclampsia and fetal growth restriction by uterine artery Doppler at 11-14 weeks of gestation. *Ultrasound Obstet Gynecol* 2001;18:583–6.
6. Yu CK, Papageorghiou AT, Parra M, Palma Dias R, Nicolaides KH. Randomized controlled trial using low-dose aspirin in the prevention of pre-eclampsia in women with abnormal uterine artery Doppler at 23 weeks' gestation. *Ultrasound Obstet Gynecol* 2003;22:233–9.

7. Subtil D, Goeusse P, Houfflin-Debarge V, *et al.* Randomised comparison of uterine artery Doppler and aspirin (100 mg) with placebo in nulliparous women: The Essai Regional Aspirine Mere-Enfant study (Part 2). *Br J Obstet Gynecol* 2003;110:485–91.
8. Frydman R, Hajeri H, Spira F, Papiernik E. Nutritional factors in poor intrauterine fetal growth. In Salvadori B, Bacchi-Modena A, eds. *Poor Intrauterine Fetal Growth.* Parma: Minerva Médica, 1977:61–3.
9. Lechtig A, Arroyave G, Habicht JP, Behar M. Maternal nutrition and fetal growth. *Arch Latinoam Nutr* 1971;21:505–30.
10. Lechtig A, Yarbrough E, Delgado H, *et al.* Effect of moderate maternal malnutrition on the placenta. *Am J Obstet Gynecol* 1975;123:191–201.
11. Lindblad BS. In Beard RW, Nathanielsz PW, eds. *Fetal Physiology and Medicine.* Philadelphia, PA: WB Saunders, 1976–80.
12. Bowes WA, Droegemueller W. Management of intrauterine growth retardation. In Reid DE, Christian CD, eds. *Controversy in Obstetrics and Gynecology.* Philadelphia, PA: WB Saunders, 1974:10.
13. Goodlin RC. Importance of the lateral position during labor. *Obstet Gynecol* 1971;37:698–701.
14. Kerr MG. The mechanical effects of the gravid uterus in late pregnancy. *Br J Obstet Gynaecol* 1965;72:513–7.
15. Mengert WF, Goodson JH, Campbell RG, Haynes DM. Observations on the pathogenesis of premature separation of the normally implanted placenta. *Am J Obstet Gynecol* 1953;66:1104–12.
16. Grene J, Dhiring JL, Smith K. Placental function test. *Am J Obstet Gynecol* 1965;92:1030–58.
17. Beischer NA, O'Sullivan EF. The effect of rest and intravenous infusion of hypertonic dextrose on subnormal estriol excretion in pregnancy. *Am J Obstet Gynecol* 1972;113:771–8.
18. Laurin J, Persson P-H. The effect of bedrest in hospital on fetal outcome in pregnancies complicated by intra-uterine growth retardation. *Acta Obstet Gynecol Scand* 1987;66:407–11.
19. Sabata V, Znamenacek K, Pribylova H, Melichar V. The effect of glucose in the prenatal treatment of small-for-date fetuses. *Biol Neonate* 1973;22:78–86.
20. Sabata V, Stembera ZK, Zidovsky I, *et al.* Glucose in the treatment of poor intrauterine fetal growth. In Salvadori B, Bacchi-Modena A, eds. *Poor Intrauterine Fetal Growth.* Parma: Minerva Médica, 1977:469.
21. Chang A, Abell DA, Beischer NA, Wood C. Trial of intravenous therapy in women with low urinary estriol excretion. *Am J Obstet Gynecol* 1977;127:793–9.
22. Abell DA, Beischer NA. The influence of abnormal glucose tolerance on pregnancy outcome when oestriol excretion is subnormal. *Br J Obstet Gynaecol* 1975;82:936–42.
23. Abell DA, Beischer NA, Wood C. Routine testing for gestational diabetes pregnancy hypoglycemia and fetus growth retardation and results of treatment. *J Perinat Med* 1976;4:197–212.
24. Abell DA, Beischer NA. The relationship between maternal glucose tolerance and fetal size at birth. *Aust NZ J Obstet Gynecol* 1976;16:1–12.
25. Frydman R, Papiernik E, Girard Jr, Assan R. Intrauterine growth retardation. Presented at the *V Congreso Europeo de Medicina Perinatal,* Uppsala, 1976:203.
26. Grumbach MN, Kaplan SL, Vinick L. Ontogenesis of growth hormone, insulin, prolactin and gonadotrophin secretion in the human foetus. In Comline KS, Cross L, eds. *Foetal and Neonatal Physiology.* Cambridge: Cambridge University Press, 1973:462–87.
27. Spellacy WN, Teoh ES, Buhi WC, *et al.* Value of human chorionic somatomammotropin in managing high risk pregnancies. *Am J Obstet Gynecol* 1971;19:588.
28. Coltart TM, Read RW, Turner RC, Oakley MW. Blood glucose and insulin relationships in the human mother and fetus before outset of labour. *Br Med J* 1969;4:17–9.
29. Liggins GC. The drive to fetal growth. In Beard RW, Nathanielsz PW, eds. *Fetal Physiology and Medicine.* Philadelphia, PA: WB Saunders, 1976:254.
30. Susa JB, McCormick KL, Widness JD, *et al.* Chronic hyperinsulinemia in the fetal rhesus monkey: Effects on fetal growth and composition. *Diabetes* 1979;28:1058–63.
31. Jones CT. Observations on the control of prenatal growth in the guinea pig. In Gluckman PD, Johnston BM, Nathanielsz PW, eds. *Advances in Fetal Physiology.* Ithaca, NY: Perinatology Press, 1989:287–302.
32. Fowden AL. The endocrine regulation of fetal metabolism and growth. In Gluckman PD, Johnston BM, Nathanielsz PW, eds. *Advances in Fetal Physiology.* Ithaca, NY: Perinatology Press, 1989:229–43.
33. Wolf H, Stubbe P, Sabata V. The influence of maternal glucose infusions on fetal growth hormone levels. *Pediatrics* 1970;45:36–42.
34. Gluckman PD, Bassett NS, Butler JH. The somatotropic axis in the fetus and newborn. In Albrecht E, Pepe GJ, eds. *Perinatal Endocrinology.* Ithaca, NY: Perinatology Press, 1986:1–20.
35. Oliver MH, Harding JE, Breier BH, *et al.* Glucose but not a mixed amino acid infusion regulates plasma insulin-like growth factor-I concentration in fetal sheep. *Pediatr Res* 1993;34:62–5.
36. Fowden AL. The role of insulin in fetal growth. *Early Hum Dev* 1992;29:177–81.
37. Takeda Y, Nakabayashi M, Iwashita M. Intrauterine treatment of the growth retarded fetuses. *J Perinatol Med* 1990;18:108.
38. Sabata V, Stembera ZK, Znamenacek K, *et al.* The possibilities of influencing energy supplies in small-for-dates fetuses and newborn infants. In Huntingford PJ, Beard RW, Hytten FE, Scopes JW, eds. *Perinatal Medicine.* London: Karger, 1971:148–51.
39. Sabata V, Paul K, Zezulakova J, Dittrichova J. The effect of prenatal therapy in pregnancies with small-for-date fetuses on psychoneurologic development of the infant. In Maros M, ed. *Prevention of Physical and Mental Congenital Defects. Part B: Epidemiology, Early Detection and Therapy, and Environmental Factors.* New York: Alan R Liss, 1985:249.
40. Ruckhaberle KE, Sabata V, Viehweg B, *et al.* Characteristics of the trophoblast in placental resorption villi after antepartum glucose infusions: Possibilities for the therapy of chronic placental insufficiency. *J Perinatol Med* 1981;9:211–8.
41. Fournie A. Possibilité de traitement *in utero* de la souffrance foetale chronique. In *Retard de croissance intra-utérin. I. Period antenatal.* Deauville, 1986:281–8.
42. Oakley NW, Beard RW, Turner RC. Effect of sustained maternal hyperglycaemia on the fetus in normal and diabetic pregnancies. *Br Med J* 1972;1:44–9.
43. Lawrence GF, Brown VA, Parsons RJ, Cooke ID. Feto-maternal consequences of high-dose glucose infusion during labour. *Br J Obstet Gynaecol* 1982;89:27–32.
44. Stembera ZK, Herzmann J. Evaluation of the DHEA-S test at an index of fetoplacental insufficiency. *J Perinatol Med* 1973;1:192–7.
45. Carrera JM, Mallafre J. Tratamiento *in utero* del retardo de crecimiento fetal. In Esteban-Altirriba J, Cabero L, eds. *Perinatología clínica 3. Retardo de crecimiento intrauterino.* Barcelona: Salvat, 1980:89–114.
46. Economides DL, Nicolaides KH. Blood glucose and oxygen tension levels in small-for-gestational-age fetuses. *Am J Obstet Gynecol* 1989;160:385–9.
47. Economides DL, Nicolaides KH, Gahl W, *et al.* Plasma amino acids in appropriate and small-for-gestational-age infants. *Am J Obstet Gynecol* 1989;161:1219–27.
48. Nicolaides KH, Economides M, Shoothill P. Blood gases, pH, and lactate in appropiate and small-for-gestational-age fetuses. *Am J Obstet Gynecol* 1989;161:996–1001.
49. Nicolini V, Hubinont C, Santolaya J, *et al.* Effect of intravenous glucose challenge in normal and growth retarded fetuses. *Horm Metab Res* 1990;22:426–30.
50. Churchill JA, Moghissi KS, Evans TN, Frohman C. Relationships of maternal amino acid blood levels to fetal development. *Obstet Gynecol* 1969,33:492–54.
51. McClain PE, Metcoff J, Crosby WM, Costiloe JP. Relationship of maternal amino acid profiles at 25 weeks of gestation to fetal growth. *Am J Clin Nutr* 1978;31:401–7.
52. Herbert WNP, Seeds JW, Bowes WA, Sweeney CA. Fetal growth response to total parenteral nutrition in pregnancy. *J Reprod Med* 1986;31:263–6.
53. Raunio A, Chandra PC, Chawla H. Parenteral hyperalimentation for fetal growth in two cases of pancreatitis in pregnancy. *Report of The Society of Perinatal Obstetrics. Annual Meeting,* San Antonio, TX, 1982:123.
54. Mesaki N, Kubo T, Iwasaki H. A study of the treatment for intrauterine growth retardation. *Acta Obstet Gynecol Jpn* 1980; 32:879–85.
55. Chimura T, Funayama T, Mitsui T, Kaneko N. Effect of infusion therapy on intrauterine fetal growth retardation. *Acta Obstet Gynecol Jpn* 1982;34:551–8.
56. Stein Z, Susser M, Rush D. Prenatal nutrition and birth weight: Experiments and quasi-experiments in the past decade. *J Reprod Med* 1978;21:287.
57. Crino JP, Harris AP, Parisi VM, Johnson TR. Effect of rapid intravenous crystalloid infusion on uteroplacental blood flow and placental implantation-site oxygen delivery in the pregnant ewe. *Am J Obstet Gynecol* 1993;168:1603–9.

58. Saveleva G, Djivelegova G, Chalina P, *et al.* Hemodilution in obstetrical pathology. *M Medicina* 1986;10:164–78.
59. Salas SP, Rosso P, Espinoza R, *et al.* Maternal plasma volume expansion and hormonal changes in women with idiopathic fetal growth retardation. *J Obstet Gynecol* 1993;81:1029–33.
60. Kempen P. Hemodilution, block and Cesarean section. Proceedings of the 21st Annual Meeting of the Society for Obstetrics Anesthesiology and Perinatology, Seattle, 1989; abstr.D–44.
61. Hambartsoumian E, Ville Y, Frydman R. Retard de croissance intra-utérin d'origine vasculaire. Quelles thérapeutiques seraient possibles *in utero*? *Med Fetale Echogr Gynecol* 1994;18:7–14.
62. Say L, Gülmezoglu AM, Hofmeyr GJ Plasma volume expansion for suspected impaired fetal growth (Cochrane Review). In *The Cochrane Library*, Issue 3. Chichester, UK: John Wiley & Sons, 2004.
63. Flynn MJ. In Esteban-Altirriba J, González-Merlo J, eds. *El feto de riesgo elevado.* Barcelona: Jims, 1970:373.
64. Joelsson I, Lunell ND, Elnäs S, *et al.* Beta-receptor stimulation, perfusion of the intervillous space and oxygenation of the fetus. *V Congreso de Medicina Perinatal*, Uppsala, 1976; abstr.52:34.
65. Schuman K, Riedel H. Effect of tocolisis on the duration of pregnancy and birth weight in twins. In Salvadori B, Bacchi-Modena A, eds. *Poor Intrauterine Fetal Growth.* Parma: Minerva Médica, 1977:509.
66. TambyRaja RL, Ratman SS. Feto pequeño: crecimiento retardado y pretérmino. *Ginecol Obstet Temas Actuales (Sp)* 1982;3:495–514.
67. Renaud R, Brettes P, Irrhann M, *et al.* A double-blind cross-over trial to assess the effect of ritodrine on uterine blood flow in normal and pathologic pregnancies. A preliminary report. In Baungarten K, Weselins de Casparis A, eds. *Proceedings of the International Symposium on the Treatment of Fetal Risk*, Baden, Austria, 1973:53.
68. Renaud R, Irrmann M, Gandar R, Flynn MJ. The use of ritodrine in the treatment of premature labor. *J Obstet Gynaecol Br Commonw* 1974;81:182–6.
69. Hiltmann WD, Wiest W. The cardiovascular side effects of the mother during treatment of fetus distress with betamimetics. In Salvadori B, Bacchi-Modena A, eds. *Poor Intrauterine Fetal Growth.* Parma: Minerva Médica, 1977:512.
70. Lippert TH, Debrandi PB, Roemer VM, Fridrich R. Hemodynamic changes in placenta, myometrium and heart after administration of the uterine relaxant ritodrine. *Int J Clin Pharmacol Ther Toxicol* 1980;18:15–20.
71. Brennan SC, MacLaughlin MK, Chez RA. Effects of prolonged infusion of beta-adrenergic agonists on uterine and umbilical blood flow in pregnant sheep. *Am J Obstet Gynecol* 1977; 128:709–15.
72. Ruckhäberle KE, Petzold J, Viehweg B, *et al.* Therapeutical effort and prenatal modification of selected disordered fetomaternal relations. *Zentrabl Gynakol* 1985;107:803–11.
73. Ingemarsson I, Arulkumarun S, Ratnam S. Single injection of terbutaline in term labor. *Am J Obstet Gynecol* 1985;153:859–65.
74. Greiss FC. Differential reactivity of the myoendometrial and placental vasculatures: Adrenergic responses. *Am J Obstet Gynecol* 1972;112:20–30.
75. Gamissans O. Preterm human pregnancy. *Proceedings of the 4th European Congress of Perinatal Medicine*, Prague, 1972.
76. Cabero L, Viscasillas P, Roses A, *et al.* Efecto de la infusión de una droga betamimética (ritodrine) a la madre sobre los niveles sanguíneos maternos y fetales de glucosa. *Clin Invest Ginecol Obstet* 1975;2:15–20.
77. Cabero L, Baro F, Escribano MI, *et al.* Modificaciones electrolíticas de la glucemia y del hematocrito tras la administración de Ritodrine para el tratamiento de la amenaza de parto prematuro. *Clin Invest Ginecol Obstet* 1983;10:93.
78. Cabero L, Viscasillas P, Roses A, *et al.* Efectos de la infusión de una droga betamimética a la madre sobres los niveles sanquíneos maternos y fetales de glucosa. *Clin Invest Ginecol Obstet* 1975;2:15.
79. Gamissans O, Corominas A, Pascual C. Effect of a corticosteroid and of a b-adrenergic drug of amniotic liquor lecithin/sphingomyelin ratio in pre-term human pregnancy. *Proceedings of the 4th European Congress of Perinatal Medicine*, Prague, 1974:3–7.
80. Lipshitz J, Broyles K, Hessler JR, *et al.* Effects of hexoprenaline in the lecithin/sphingomyelin ratio and pressure–volume relationship in fetal rabbits. *Am J Obstet Gynecol* 1981;139:726–34.
81. Cabero L, Quílez M, Escribano I, *et al.* Síndrome de distress respiratorio neonatal en casos de amenaza departo prematuro tratados con betamiméticos. *Clin Invest Ginecol Obstet* 1976;3. 169–71.
82. Say L, Gülmezoglu AM, Hofmeyr GJ. Betamimetics for suspected impaired fetal growth (Cochrane Review). In *The Cochrane Library*, Issue 3. Chichester, UK: John Wiley & Sons, 2004.
83. Cliff WJ, Martin JD, Michael CA. Fetal chronic distress. *Nature (London)* 1963;199:399.
84. Trolle D. Decrease in the mortality rates for low-birth-weight infants after phenobarbitone treatment. *Acta Obstet Gynecol Scand* 1976;55:13–20.
85. Frigoletto FD, Tullis JL, Reid DE, Hinman J. Hypercoagulability in the dysmadure syndrome. *Am J Obstet Gynecol* 1971;11:867–73.
86. Bonnar J. A review of the obstetrical aspects of haemostasis. *Br J Haematol* 1973;25:274–5.
87. Bonnar J, McNicol GP, Douglas AS. Coagulation and fibrinolytic systems in pre-eclampsia and eclampsia. *Br Med J* 1971;2:12–6.
88. Bonnar J, McNicol GP, Douglas AS. The blood coagulation and fibrinolytic systems in the newborn and the mother at birth. *Br J Obstet Gynaecol* 1971;78:355–60.
89. McKay DG. Hematologic evidence of disseminated intravascular coagulation in eclampsia. *Obstet Gynecol Surv* 1972,27:399.
90. Roberts JM, Taylor RN, Musci TJ, *et al.* Pre-eclampsia: An endothelial cell disorder. *Am J Obstet Gynecol* 1989;161:1200–4.
91. Trudinger BJ. Platelets and intrauterine growth retardation in pre-eclampsia. *Br J Obstet Gynaecol* 1976;83:284–6.
92. Howie PW, Prentice CR, McNicol GP. Coagulation, fibrinolysis and platelet function in pre-eclampsia, essential hypertension and placental insufficiency. *Br J Obstet Gynaecol* 1971;78:992–1003.
93. Kitzmiller JL, Lang JE, Yelenosky PF, *et al.* Hematologic assays in pre-eclampsia. *Am J Obstet Gynecol* 1974;118:362–7.
94. Buyse FGC, Wormgoor BA, Bernard JT, Koudstaal J. Anticoagulant therapy of patients with repeated placental infarction. *Obstet Gynecol* 1974;43:844–8.
95. Flessa HC, Kapstrom AB, Gluek HI, Will JJ. Placental transport of heparin. *Am J Obstet Gynecol* 1965;93:570–3.
96. Chupin L, Herrmann JM, Maillet R, *et al.* Effects de l'heparina dans l'hypotrophie foetale d'origine vasculaire maternelle. *J Gynecol Obstet Biol Reprod* 1978;7:849–54.
97. Hoffbauer H, Vogel M, Pett A. On the diagnosis of fetal growth retardation and its treatment with heparin. In Salvadori B, Bacchi-Modena A, eds. *Poor Intrauterine Fetal Growth.* Parma: Minerva Médica, 1977:493.
98. Daffos F, Forestin F, Capella-Paulosky M. New procedure for fetal blood sampling during pregnancy: Its application to prenatal pharmacology. *Dev Pharmacol Ther* 1984;7(Suppl):47–51.
99. Gillis S, Shushan A, Eldo A. Use of low molecular weight heparine for prophylaxis and treatment of thrombo-embolism in pregnancy. *Int J Gynecol Obstet* 1992;39:297–301.
100. Benigni A, Gingorini G, Frusca T, *et al.* Effect of low dose aspirin on fetal and maternal generation of thromboxane by platelets in women at risk of pregnancy-induced hypertension. *N Engl J Med* 1989;321:357–62.
101. Schiff E, Pelleg E, Goldenberg M, *et al.* The use of aspirin to prevent pregnancy-induced hypertension and lower the ratio of thromboxane A_2 to prostacyclin in relatively high risk pregnancies. *N Engl J Med* 1989;321:351–6.
102. Wallenburg HCS, Dekker GA, Makovitz JW, Rotmans P. Low-dose aspirin prevents pregnancy-induced hypertension and pre-eclampsia in angiotensin-sensitive primigravidae. *Lancet* 1986; 1:1–3.
103. Ylikorkala O, Mälikä UM, Kääpä P, Viinika L. Maternal ingestion of acetylsalicylic acid inhibits fetal and neonatal prostacyclin and thromboxane in humans. *Am J Obstet Gynecol* 1986;155:345–9.
104. Patrono C, Ciabattoni G, Patrignani P, *et al.* Clinical pharmacology of platelet cyclo-oxygenase inhibition. *Circulation* 1985;72: 1177–84.
105. Sánchez-Ramos L, O'Sullivan MJ, Garrido Calderón J. Effect of low dose aspirin on angiotensin II pressor response in human pregnancy. *Am J Obstet Gynecol* 1987;156:193–4.
106. Nelson DM, Walsh SW. Aspirin differentially affects thromboxane and prostacyclin production by trophoblast and villous core compartments of human placental villi. *Am J Obstet Gynecol* 1989; 161:1593–8.
107. Walsh SW. Low dose aspirin: Treatment for the imbalance of inneated thromboxane and decreased prostacyclin in pre-eclampsia. *Am J Perinatol* 1989;6:124–32.
108. Sibai BM, Mirro R, Chesney CM, Leffler C. Low dose aspirin in pregnancy. *Obstet Gynecol* 1989;74:551–6.
109. Pedersen AK, Fitzgerald GA. Dose related kinetics of aspirin. Presystemic acetylation of platelet cyclo oxygenase. *N Engl J Med* 1984;311:1206–11.

110. Wallenburg HCS, Rothmans N. Prevention of recurrent idiopathic fetal growth retardation by low-dose aspirin and dipyridamol. *Am J Obstet Gynecol* 1987;157:1230–5.
111. Uzan S, Beaufils M, Bréart G, *et al.* Prevention of fetal growth retardation with low-dose aspirin: Findings of the EPREDA trial. *Lancet* 1991;337:1427–31.
112. Trudinger BJ, Cook CM, Thompson RS, *et al.* Low-dose aspirin therapy improves fetal weight in umbilical placental insufficiency. *Am J Obstet Gynecol* 1988;159:681–5.
113. Italian Study of Aspirin in Pregnancy. Low-dose aspirin in the prevention and treatment of intrauterine growth retardation and pregnancy-induced hypertension. *Lancet* 1993;341:396–400.
114. Beaufils M, Uzan S, Donsimoni R, Colau JC. Prevention of pre-eclampsia by early antiplatelet therapy. *Lancet* 1985;1:840–2.
115. McParland P, Pearce JM, Chamberlain GVP. Doppler ultrasound and aspirin in recognition and prevention of pregnancy-induced hypertension. *Lancet* 1990;335:1552–5.
116. Vainio M, Kujansuu E, Iso-Mustajarvi M, *et al.* Low dose acetylsalicylic acid in prevention of pregnancy-induced hypertension and intrauterine growth retardation in women with bilateral uterine artery notches. *BJOG Br J Obstet Gynecol* 2002;109:161–7.
117. Kozer E, Nikfar S, Costei A, *et al.* Aspirin consumption during the first trimester of pregnancy and congenital anomalies: A meta-analysis. *Am J Obstet Gynecol* 2002;187:1623–30.
118. Harrington K, Kurdi W, Aquilina J, *et al.* A prospective management study of slow-release aspirin in the palliation of uteroplacental insufficiency predicted by uterine artery Doppler at 20 weeks. *Ultrasound Obstet Gynecol* 2000;15:13–8.
119. Kupfermine MJ, Many A, Bar-Am A, *et al.* Mid-trimester severe intrauterine growth restriction is associated with a high prevalence of thrombophilia. *Br J Obstet Gynecol* 2002;109:1373–6.
120. Goetz KI. Physiology and pathophysiology of atrial peptides. *Am J Physiol* 1988;254:1–15.
121. Reid DL, Goodfriend TL, Hollister MC, *et al.* Effects of atrial natriuretic factor on maternal ovine vascular resistance. *J Dev Physiol* 1989;11:25–8.
122. Jansson TB. Low-dose infusion of atrial natriuretic peptide in the conscious guinea pig increases blood flow to the placenta in growth-retarded fetuses. *Am J Obstet Gynecol* 1992;166:213–8.
123. Kingdom JCP, McQueen J, Connel JMC, Whittle MJ. Maternal and fetal atrial natriuretic peptide levels at delivery from normal and growth retarded pregnancies. *Br J Obstet Gynaecol* 1992;99:845–9.
124. Sammour MB, El-Kabarity H, Khalifa AS. Progesterone therapy in pre-eclamptic toxemia. *Acta Obstet Gynecol Scand* 1975;54:195–202.
125. Salvadori B. Exogenous progesterone and feto-placental function. In Salvadori B, ed. *The Therapy of Feto-placental Insufficiency.* Berlin: Springer-Verlag, 1975:304–12.
126. Salvadori B, Vadora E, Bacchi-Modena A, *et al.* Estrone, 17-•-estradiolo, Estriolo plasmatici e Estriolo 16 glicoruconato urinario dopo progesterone. *Comunicación a I Reunión del Congreso di Studio e di Ricerca in Medicina*, Parma, 11-12 May 1977.
127. Csapo AI, de Sousa filho MB, de Souza JC, de Souza O. Effect of massive progestational hormone treatment on the parturient human uterus. *Fertil Steril* 1966;17:621–36.
128. Merialdi A. Discussion of additional therapeutic technique. In Salvadori B, Bacchi-Modena A, eds. *Poor Intrauterine Fetal Growth.* Parma: Minerva Médica, 1977:481–3.
129. Torok I, Csapo AF. The effects of progesterone, prostaglandin F2? and oxytocin on the calcium activation of the uterus. *Prostaglandins* 1976;12:253–70.
130. Beydoun SN, Abaul-Karim RW, Haviland ME. The regulatory effect of estrogens on fetal growth. III. Placental deoxyribonucleic acid, ribonucleic acid and proteins. *Am J Obstet Gynecol* 1974;120:918–21.
131. Pearce JM, McParland P, Steel SA, Huiskes N. Effects of allylestrenol on deteriorating utero-placental circulation. *Lancet* 1988;2:1252.
132. Garmacheva N, Konstantinova N. Introduction into perinatal medicine. *M Medicina* 1978;5:296–317.
133. Clapp JF, Szeto HH, Larrow R, *et al.* Fetal metabolic response to experimental placental vascular damage. *Am J Obstet Gynecol* 1981;140:446–51.
134. Rudolph A. Oxygenation in the fetus and neonate—a perspective. *Semin Perinatol* 1984;8:158–67.
135. Pollack RN, Divon MY. Intrauterine growth retardation: Definition, classification and etiology. *Clin Obstet Gynecol* 1992;35:99–107.
136. Cunningham FG, MacDonald PC, Gant N, *et al. Williams Obstetrics.* Norwalk, CT: Appleton & Lange, 1993:878.
137. Chang JH, Rutledge JC, Stoops D, Abbe R. Hypobaric hypoxia-induced intrauterine growth retardation. *Biol Neonate* 1984;46:10–3.
138. Soothill PW, Nicolaides KH, Campbell S. Perinatal asphyxia, hyperlacticaemia, hypoglycaemia and erythroblastosis in growth retarded fetus. *Br Med J* 1987;294:1051–3.
139. Gagnon R, Hunse C, Vijan S. The effect of maternal hyperoxia on behavioral activity in growth retarded human fetuses. *Am J Obstet Gynecol* 1990;163:1894–9.
140. Ruedrich DA, Devoe LD, Searle N. Effect of maternal hyperoxia on the biophysical assessment of fetuses with suspected intrauterine growth retardation. *Am J Obstet Gynecol* 1989;161:188–92.
141. Nicolaides KH, Campbell S, Bradley RJ, *et al.* Maternal oxygen therapy for intrauterine growth retardation. *Lancet* 1987;1:942–5.
142. Arduini D, Rizzo G, Mancusso S, Romanini C. Short-term effects of maternal oxygen administration on blood flow velocity waveforms in healthy and growth-retarded fetuses. *Am J Obstet Gynecol* 1988;157:1077–80.
143. Battaglia C, Artini PG, D'Ambrogio G, *et al.* Maternal hyperoxygenation in the treatment of intrauterine growth retardation. *Am J Obstet Gynecol* 1992;167:430–5.
144. Romney SL, Gabe1 PV. Maternal glucose loading in the management of fetal distress. *Am J Obstet Gynecol* 1966;96:698–709.
145. Panigel M. Placental perfusion experiments. *Am J Obstet Gynecol* 1962;84:1664–83.
146. Cook CM, Trudinger B. Angiotensin sensitivity predicts aspirin benefit in placental insufficiency. *Am J Obstet Gynecol* 1993;100:46–50.
147. Moya F, Morishima HD, Shnider SM, James LS. Influence of maternal hyperventilation on the newborn infant. *Am J Obstet Gynecol* 1965;91:76.
148. Ribbert LSM, Van Lingen RA, Visser HA. Continuous maternal hyperoxygenation in the treatment of early fetal growth retardation. *Ultrasound Obstet Gynecol* 1991;1:331–5.
149. Say L, Gülmezoglu AM, Hofmeyr GJ. Administración de oxígeno materno para el retraso de crecimiento fetal presunto. En: *La Cochrane Library plus en español.* Oxford: Update Software.
150. Naeye RL. Malnutrition: Probable cause of fetal growth retardation. *Arch Pathol* 1965;79:284–301.
151. Renaud R, Vincendon G, Boog G, *et al.* Injections intra-amniotiques d'acides amines dans les cas de malnutrition foetales: premiers resultats. *J Gynecol Obstet Biol Reprod* 1972;1:231–44.
152. Renaud R, Kirschtetter L, Koehl C, *et al.* Amino-acid intra-amniotic injections. In Persianinov LS, Chervakova TV, Presl J, eds. *Recent Progress in Obstetrics and Gynecology. Proceedings of the VIIth World Congress of Obstetrics and Gynecology.* Amsterdam: Excerpta Médica, 1974:234–56.
153. Manzanilla SR, Sevilla R, Suárez Cobo M, *et al.* Alimentación fetal oral intrauterina. Investigación basica con albúmina 131-I, intraamniótica. *Ginecol Obstet Mex* 1970:27.
154. Heller L. Intrauterine amino acid feeding of the fetus. In Bode H, Warshaw J, eds. *Parenteral Nutrition in Infancy and Childhood.* New York: Plenum Press, 1974:206–13.
155. Massobrio M, Margaria E, Campogrande M, *et al.* Treatment of severe feto-placental insufficiency by means of intra-amniotic injection of amino acids. In Salvadori B, ed. *Therapy of Fetoplacental Insufficiency.* Berlin: Springer-Verlag, 1975:296–303.
156. Ranzoni S, Marconi AM, Paolini CL, *et al.* The effect of a maternal infusion of amino acids on umbilical uptake in pregnancies complicated by intrauterine growth restruction. *Am J Obstet Gynecol* 2002;187:741–6.
157. Casanova Alvarez N, Manzanilla Sevilla R, Suarez Cobo M, Maass Ecoto R. Intrauterine fetal oral feeding. Study with intra-amniotic albumin I131 in a case of anencephalia. *Gynecol Obstet Mex* 1974;35:155–63.
158. Pritchard J. Deglutition by normal and anencephalic fetuses. *Obstet Gynecol* 1965;25:289–97.
159. Pitkin RM, Reynolds WA. Fetal ingestion and metabolism of amniotic fluid protein. *Am J Obstet Gynecol* 1975;123:356–63.
160. Neubuser D, Braun R. Concerning the foetal use of amino-acids injected in amniotic fluid. Presented at the *V Congreso Europeo de Medicina Perinatal,* Uppsala, 1976;abstr.61:40.
161. Gitlin D, Kumate J, Morales C. The turnover of amniotic fluid protein in the human conceptus. *Am J Obstet Gynecol* 1972;113:632–45.
162. Jacobs DG, Wesson DE, Mago-Cao H, *et al.* Effect of oesophageal ligation on the growth of fetal rabbits. *J Pediatr Gastroenterol Nutr* 1989;8:245–51.

163. Charlton VE. Fetal nutrition supplementation. *Semin Perinatol* 1984;8:25–30.
164. Charlton VE, Johengen M. Nutrient and waste product concentration diffences in upper and lower body arteries of fetal sheep. *J Dev Phisiol* 1984;6:431–7.
165. Harding J, Owens J, Robison J. Should we try to supplement the growth retarded fetus? A cautionary tale. *Br J Obstet Gynaecol* 1992;99:707–10.
166. Harding J, Lui L, Evans S, *et al.* Intra-uterine feeding of the growth retarded fetuses: Can we help? *Early Hum Dev* 1992;29:193–7.
167. Saling E, Dudenhausen J, Kynast G. Basic investigation about intra-amniotic compensatory nutrition of the malnourished fetus. In *Recent Progress in Obstetrics and Gynecology. Proceeding of the VIIth World Congress of Obstetrics and Gynecology.* Prague: Excerpta Medica, 1974:227–33.
168. Charlton VE, Johengen M. Fetal intravenous nutritional supplementation ameliorates the development of embolization-induced growth retardation in sheep. *Pediatr Res* 1987;22:55–61.
169. Fiser R, Erenberg A, Fisher D, Oh W. Blood gas and pH changes during glucose infusion in the fetal sheep. *Am J Obstet Gynecol* 1973;115:942–5.
170. Philips J, Diamond J, Fo Kalsrud E. Fetal rabbit intestinal absorption: Implication for transamniotic fetal feeding. *J Pediatr Surg* 1990;25:909–13.
171. Charlton VE, Johengen M. Effect of intrauterine nutritional supplementation on fetal growth retardation. *Biol Neonate* 1985;48: 125–42.
172. Flake A, Villa-Troyer R, Adzick S, Harrison M. Transamniotic fetal feeding. III. The effect of nutritional infusion on fetal growth retardation. *J Pediatr Surg* 1986;21:481–4.
173. Philipps AF, Porte PJ, Stabinski S, *et al.* Effect of chronic fetal hyperglycemia upon oxygen consumption in the ovine uterus and conceptus. *J Clin Invest* 1984;74:279–86.
174. Charlton VE, Reis BL. Response of the chronically catheterized fetal lamb to intestinal administration of amino acids. *Clin Res* 1980;28:121A.
175. Charlton VE, Reis BL. Effects of gastric nutritional supplementation on fetal umbilical uptake of nutrients. *Am J Physiol* 1981;241:E178–85.
176. Young M, Soltesz G, Noakes D, *et al.* The influence of intrauterine surgery and of fetal intravenous nutritional supplements *in utero* on plasma free amino acid homeo-stasis in the pregnant ewe. *J Perinat Med* 1975;3:180–97.
177. Saling E. Versuch einer neuen kompensatorischen Versorgung des hypotrophen Feten. *Geburtsh Frauenheilk* 1987;47:90–2.
178. Heyns OS, Samson NS, Graham JAC. Influence of abdominal decompression on intra-amniotic pressure and fetal oxygenation. *Lancet* 1962:1:282–92.
179. Shimonovitz S, Yagel S, Zacut D, *et al.* Intermittent abdominal decompression: An option for the prevention of intrauterine growth retardation. *Br J Obstet Gynaecol* 1992;99:693–5.
180. Hofmeyer GJ. Abdominal decompression in pregnancy. In Chalmers I, Enkin M, Keirse MJNC, eds. *Effective Care in Pregnancy and Childbirth.* Oxford: Oxford University Press, 1989:647–52.
181. Blecher JA. The volume of the maternal placental circulation before and after abdominal decompression. *S Ag J Med Sci* 1968;33:43–8.
182. Coxon A, Haggith JW. The effects of abdominal decom-pression on vascular haemodynamics in pregnancy and labour. *J Obstet Gynaecol Br Commonw* 1971;78:49–54.
183. Müller-Tyl E, Salzer H, Altmann P, Spona J. Abdominal decompression: An aid in the management of PIFG. In Salvadori B, Bacchi-Modena A, eds. *Poor Intrauterine Fetal Growth.* Parma: Minerva Médica, 1977.
184. Turnbull AC, Anderson AB. Endocrine factors in the outset of labour. *Proc R Soc Med* 1970;63:1095–6.
185. Mac Rae DJ, Mohamedally SM, Willmot MP. Clinical and endocrinological aspects of dysmaturity and the use of intermittent abdominal decompression in pregnancy. *Br J Obstet Gynaecol* 1971;78:636–41.
186. Mac Rae DJ. Treatment of poor intrauterine fetal growth. In Salvadori B, Bacchi-Modena A, eds. *Poor Intrauterine Fetal Growth.* Parma: Minerva Médica, 1977:477–80.
187. Tchernovcha F, Abrachmanova E, *et al.* Hyperbar oxygenotherapy in the pregnancy pathology. *Akus i Ginek* 1986;6:3–8.
188. Aksenova T. Hyperbar oxygenotherapy and pregnancy with hypoxic syndrome. *Akus i Ginek* 1979;6:6–9.
189. Clark KE, Austin JE, Seeds AE. Effect of bisenoic prostaglandins and arachidonic acid on the uterine vasculature of pregnant sheep. *Am J Obstet Gynecol* 1982;142:261–68.
190. Landauer M, Phernetton TM, Parisi VM, *et al.* Ovine placental vascular response to the local application of prostacyclin. *Am J Obstet Gynecol* 1985;151:460–3.
191. Jouppila P, Kirkinen P, Koivula A, Ylikorkala O. Failure of exogenous prostacyclin to change placental and fetal blood flow in pre-eclampsia. *Am J Obstet Gynecol* 1985;151:661–5.
192. Van Assche FA, Spitz B, Vermylen J, Deckmijn H. Preliminary observation on treatment of pregnancy-induced hypertension with a thromboxane synthetase inhibitor. *Am J Obstet Gynecol* 1984;148:216–8.
193. Neri I, Di Renzo GC, Caserta G, *et al.* Impact of the L-arginine/nitric oxide system in pregnancy. *Obstet Gynecol Surv* 1995;50: 851–8.
194. Grunewald C, Kublickas M, Carlström K, *et al.* Effects of nitroglycerin on the uterine and umbilical circulation in severe pre-eclampsia. *Obstet Gynecol* 1995;86:600–5.
195. Luzy G, Caserta G, Glerici G, Di Renzo GC. Fetomaternal hemodynamic effects induced by sublingual administration of a nitric oxide donor, glyceryl trinitrate, in mild-pre-eclampsia and threatened preterm labor. In Carrera JM, ed. *Creamiento Fetal.* Barcelona: Masson, 1997;23:6446–7.
196. Edelman PH. Anticorps de specificité phospholipidique et arrêt de grossesse. Aspect clinique de l'immunologie de la reproduction. In *Progrès en Gynécologie.* Paris: Doin, 1991:165–74.
197. Katz VL, Thorp IM, Watson WJ, *et al.* Human immunoglobulin therapy for pre-eclampsia associated with lupus anticoagulant and anticardiolipin antibody. *Obstet Gynecol* 1991;76:986–8.
198. Parke A, Maier D, Wilson D, *et al.* Intravenous gammaglobulin, antiphospholipid antibodies, and pregnancy. *Ann Intern Med* 1989;110:495–6.
199. Wapner RJ, Cowchock S, Shapiro SS. Successful treatment in two women with antiphospholipid antibodies and refractory pregnancy losses with intravenous immunoglobulin infusions. *Am J Obstet Gynecol* 1989;61:1271–2.
200. Goldberg RN, Moscoso P, Bauer CR, *et al.* Use of barbiturate therapy in severe perinatal asphyxia: A randomized controlled trial. *J Pediatr* 1986;109:851–6.
201. Espinoza MI, Parer JT. Mechanisms of asphyxial brain damage, and possible pharmacologic interventions in the fetus. *Am J Obstet Gynecol* 1991;164:1582–91.
202. Meyer FB, Anderson RE, Yaksh TL, Sundt TM. Effect of nimodipine on intracellular brain pH, cortical blood flow and EEG in experimental focal cerebral ischemia. *J Neurosurg* 1986;64: 617–26.
203. Thiringer K, Hrbek A, Karlsson K, *et al.* Postasphyxial cerebral survival in newborn sheep after treatment with oxygen free radical scavengers and a calcium antagonist. *Pediatr Res* 1987;22:62–6.
204. Gunn AJ, Mydlar T, Bennet L, *et al.* The neuroprotective actions of a calcium channel antagonist, flunarizine, in the infant rat. *Pediatr Res* 1989;25:573–6.
205. Rogers MC, Kirsh JR. Current concepts in brain resuscitation. *J Am Med Assoc* 1989;261:3143–7.
206. Guilland E, Puka-Sundvall M, Andiné P, *et al.* Hypoxic-ischemia in the neonatal rat brain: Effects of pre- and post-treatment with a gentamate release inhibitor. *Abstracts of the 14th European Congress of Perinatal Medicine,* Helsinki, 1994;abstr.287:June.
207. Williams C, Mallard C, Tan WKM, *et al.* Perinatal asphyxia: Mechanisms of damage and neuroprotection. *Abstract Book of the 2nd World Congress of Perinatal Medicine,* Rome, 1993:72: September.
208. Stevens MK, Yaksh TL. Systematic studies on the effects of the NMDA receptor antagonist MK-801 on cerebral blood flow and responsivity, EEG, and blood–brain barrier following complete reversible cerebral ischemia. *J Cereb Blood Flow Metab* 1990;10:77–88.
209. Shigeno S, Fritsch KA, Shigeno T, Brock M. Effects of indomethacin on RCBF during and after focal cerebral ischemia in the cat. *Stroke* 1985;16:235–40.
210. Ment L, Oh W, Ehrenkranz RA, *et al.* Low dose indomethacin and neonatal intraventricular haemorrhage. *Abstracts of the 14th European Congress of Perinatal Medicine,* Helsinki, 1994; abstr.472:June.
211. Van Der Kerckhoff W, Hossmann KA, Hossmann U. No effects of prostacyclin on blood flow, regulation following global cerebral ischemia. *Stroke* 1983;14:724–30.
212. Liu TH, Beckman JS, Freeman BA, *et al.* Polyethysene glycol-conjugated superoxide dismutase and catalase reduce ischemic brain injury. *Am J Physiol* 1989;256:H589–93.
213. Poranen AK, Ekblad U, Votila P, Ahotopa H. Placental lipid peroxides and antioxidants in normal and pre-eclamptic pregnancies

and the effect of vitamins C and E on placental circulation and lipid peroxidation. *Abstracts of the 14th European Congress of Perinatal Medicine*, Helsinki, 1994;abstr.14:June.

214. Gutteridge JMC, Stock S. Caeruloplasmin physiological and pathological perspectives. *CRC Crit Rev Clin Lab Sci* 1981;14:257–329.
215. Gutteridge JMC. Free radical production and detoxification. In Koppe JG, Eskes TKAB, Van Geijn HP, *et al*, eds. *Care, Concern and Cure in Perinatal Medicine*. Carnforth, UK: Parthenon Publishing, 1992:341–50.
216. Marklund SL, Holme E, Hellner L. Superoxide dismutase in extracellular fluids. *Clin Chem Acta* 1982;120:41–5.
217. Maddipati KR, Marnett LJ. Characterization of the major hydroperoxide reducing activity of human placenta. *J Biol Chem* 1987;262: 17398–403.
218. Saran M, Bors W. Oxygen radicals acting as chemical messengers: A hypothesis. *Free Rad Res Commun* 1989;7:213–20.
219. Halliwell B, Gutteridge JMC. The antioxidant of human extracellular fluid. *Arch Biochem Biophysiol* 1990;280:1–8.
220. Eriksson UJ, Borg LAH. Protection by free oxygen radical scavenging enzymes against glucose-induced embryonic malformation *in vitro*. *Diabetologia* 1991;34:325–31.
221. Eriksson UJ, Borg LAH. Diabetes and embryonic malformations. Role of substrate-induced free-oxygen radical production for dysmorphogenesis in cultured rat embryos. *Diabetes* 1993;42:411–9.
222. Marinari UM, Traverso N, Macoberti G, Pronzato MA. Free radicals and fetal pathology. *J Perinat Med* 1994;22(Suppl):39–42.
223. Wright DJ, Wolfe HM, Evans MI. Intrauterine growth retardation: Intrapartum management. In Divon MY, ed. *Abnormal Fetal Growth*. New York: Chapman & Hall, 1991:217–31.
224. Scott KE, Usher R. Fetal malnutrition. Its incidence, causes and effects. *Am J Obstet Gynecol* 1966;94:951–63.
225. Butler NR. The problems low birthweight and early delivery. *J Obstet Gynecol Br Commonw* 1965;62:1001–3.
226. Butler NR. Gestational age, size maturity. In Dawkins M, MacGregor WG, eds. *Clinics in Developmental Medicine*, No.19. London: Spastics Society, Heinemann, 1965.
227. Caballero A, Carazo A, Corredera J. Crecimiento intrauterino retardado del feto. *Toko-Ginecol Pract* 1975;374:1237–70.
228. Baraibar R. Neuroepidemiología neonatal. *Bull Soc Catalana Pediatr* 1982;42:235–88.
229. Gembruch U, Gortner L. Perinatal aspects of pretem intrauterine growth restriction. *Ultrasound Obstet Gynecol* 1998;11:233–9.
230. The GRIT study group. Infant wellbeing at 2 years of age in the Growth Restriction Intervention Trial (GRIT): Multicentred randomised controlled trial. *Lancet* 2004;364(9433):513–20.
231. Hecher K, Bilardo CM, Stigter RH, *et al*. Monitoring of fetuses with intrauterine growth restriction: A longitudinal study. *Ultrasound Obstet Gynecol* 2001;18(6):564–70.
232. Baschat AA, Gembruch U, Harman CR. The sequence of changes in Doppler and biophysical parameters as severe fetal growth restriction worsens. *Ultrasound Obstet Gynecol* 2001;18(6):571–7.
233. Ferrazzi E, Bozzo M, Rigano S, *et al*. Temporal sequence of abnormal Doppler changes in the peripheral and central circulatory systems of the severely growth-restricted fetus. *Ultrasound Obstet Gynecol* 2002;19(2):140–6.
234. Fetal Compromise Group. Formal measurement of clinical uncertainty: Prelude to a trial in perinatal medicine. *Br Med J* 1994; 308:111–2.
235. Simchen MJ, Alkazaleh F, Adamson SL, *et al*. Tse fetal cardiovascular response to antenatal steroids in severe early-onset intrauterine growth restriction. *Am J Obstet Gynecol* 2004;190(2):296–304.
236. Seeds JW. Impaired fetal growth. Ultrasonic evaluation and clinical management. *Obstet Gynecol* 1984;64:577–84.
237. Spinillo A, Capuzzo E, Piazzi G, Baltaro F, Stranati M, Ornetto A. Significance of low birthweight for gestational age among very preterm infants. *Br J Obstet Gynaecol* 1997;104:668–73.
238. Fairbrother PF, Du-Toit IL, Cheifitz RL. The amniotic fluid foam test and fat cell count in malnourished and well-nourished fetuses. *Br J Obstet Gynaecol* 1975;82:182–6.
239. Dyson D, Blake M, Cassady G. Amniotic fluid lecithin/sphingomyelin ratio in complicated pregnancies. *Am J Obstet Gynecol* 1975;122:722–81.
240. Steer PH. The management of large and small for gestational age fetuses. *Semin Perinatol* 2004;28(1):59–66.
241. Baschat AA, Hecher K. Fetal growth restriction due to placental disease. *Semin Perinatol* 2004;28:67–80.
242. Alvarado A, Niz J. Crecimiento intrauterino retardado. Asistencia al parto. *Rev Iberoam Fertil* 1993;10:59–63.
243. Lin CC, Evans MI. Intrapartum management. In Lin CC, Evans MI, eds. *Intrauterine Growth Retardation*. New York: McGraw-Hill, 1984:315–51.
244. Monleón J, Mínguez J, Perales A, *et al*. Asistencia al parto en casos de crecimiento intrauterino retardado. *Prog Obstet Ginecol* 1993;36:40–8.
245. Li H, Gudmundsson S, Olofsson P. Prospect for vaginal delivery of growth restricted fetuses with abnormal umbilical artery blood flow. *Acta Obstet Gynecol Scand* 2003;82(9):828–33.
246. Monleón FJ, Díez E, Domenech A, *et al*. Características de los trazados de la FCF a lo largo del parto del recién nacido de bajo peso para la edad gestacional. *Toko-Ginecol Pract* 1976;386:693–704.
247. Miller A, Rayburn W, Smith C. Patterns of uterine activity after intravaginal prostaglandin E2 during pre-induction cervical ripening. *Am J Obstet Gynecol* 1991;165:1006–9.
248. Milliez J, Jannet D, Touboul C, *et al*. Maturation of the uterine cervix by repeated intracervical instillation of prostaglandin E_2. *Am J Obstet Gynecol* 1991;165:523–8.
249. Nieto Díaz A, Matorras R, Serra M, *et al*. Implica un mayor intervencionismo obstétrico intraparto el crecimiento intrauterino retardado asimétrico? *Rev Iberoam Fertil* 1995;12:15–9.
250. Monleón J, Mínguez J, Diez E, *et al*. Some aspects of labour in poor intrauterine fetal growth. In Salvadori B, Bacchi-Modena A, eds. *Poor Intrauterine Fetal Growth*. Parma: Minerva Médica, 1977:437–40.
251. Monleón J, Mínguez JA, Díez E, Domenech A. Control intraparto del retardo de crecimiento intrauterino. In Esteban-Altirriba J, Cabero L, eds. *Perinatología Clínica 3. Retardo del crecimiento intrauterino*. Barcelona: Salvat, 1980:131–44.
252. Lampe LG, Komaromy B, Adam B. Antenatal diagnosis, management and perinatal survival of growth retarded infants. In Salvadori B, Bacchi-Modena A, eds. *Poor Intrauterine Fetal Growth*. Parma: Minerva Médica, 1977:397–402.
253. Siristatidis C, Salamalekis E, Vitoratos N, *et al*. Intrapartum surveillance of IUGR fetuses with cardiotocography and fetal pulse oximetry. *Biol Neonate* 2003;83(3):162–5.

123 Growth-restricted newborns: characteristics and management

R. Baraibar and L. Sánchez

In order to provide correct postnatal care for low birth weight infants, it is important for the neonatologist to have adequate information on the antenatal history of a fetus affected by intrauterine growth restriction (IUGR). This includes the time at which IUGR was identified, the evolution and characteristics of cephalometric parameters, the presence of congenital anomalies or chromosome abnormalities, maternal diseases and toxic habits, uteroplacental function, hemodynamic changes (Doppler abnormalities in the umbilical or fetal circulation) and antepartum or intrapartum signs of fetal distress (characteristics of the amniotic fluid, abnormal fetal heart rate patterns or changes in blood pH).

The terms 'intrauterine growth restriction' (IUGR) and 'small-for-gestational age' (SGA) are related but not synonymous. IGUR refers to a process that causes a reduction in an expected pattern of fetal growth. This process results in an attenuation of fetal growth potential. SGA refers to an infant with a birth weight lower than a predetermined cut-off value.

Management in the delivery room and neonatal resuscitation

The birth process represents a risk situation for SGA infants, so the presence at the delivery of personnel trained in neonatal resuscitation (ideally, a neonatologist) is essential for many of these babies. The 'normal' SGA infant with smallness of a presumably genetic origin would probably not require any specialized care. The fetus would be born in good condition and the baby would remain with the mother, with the same protocols of perinatal care followed as for normal appropriate-for-gestational-age (AGA) infants.

For proper management of SGA infants with congenital defects, it is desirable that discussions are held between the parents and the obstetric team beforehand, about the possible postnatal viability of the fetus and the expected management after the birth, according to the evidence of prenatal studies (ultrasound pattern of congenital defects, fetal karyotype). It might be decided to avoid resuscitation maneuvers in cases of some chromosome abnormalities or multiple congenital anomalies associated with severe physical defects or neurological dysfunction. A complete and careful neonatal examination, however, is required to confirm morphological anomalies associated with the chromosomal defect. A thorough fetal postmortem examination would also be required.

In cases of less severe congenital defects, management will vary in relation to the characteristics of each type of malformation. In the hypotrophic SGA infant, the higher probability of perinatal asphyxia and meconium aspiration should be taken into account, as well as the early appearance of hypothermia, hypoglycemia, acidosis and anemia/polycythemia. Neonates with congenital infections may present a highly compromised clinical condition (hydrops, coagulation disorders, heart failure, liver failure, etc.) and may require aggressive resuscitation. However, others may be asymptomatic. Isolation measures will be necessary for some SGA newborns with viral infections.

Immediate neonatal examination

The SGA infant should undergo a careful physical examination, especially when reliable information on the circumstances of gestation is not available. This includes the following:

(1) Infant's weight and height, measurement of head circumference and ponderal index$_1$ with calculations on a population-based weight/gestational-age curve. It is useful also to know paternal height, because it has been shown that very low paternal height has an influence on the weight and height

of the neonate[1] [ponderal index = (weight × 100)/height[3]], where weight is in grams and height is in centimeters.
(2) Clinical evidence of malnutrition, when possible accompanied by measurement of the quadriceps skin-fold thickness and the mid-arm circumference. It is well known that the greatest severity of malnutrition produces the highest occurrence and intensity of clinical manifestations (asphyxia, hypoglycemia, hypocalcemia and polycythemia) in the neonatal period.[2–4]
(3) Description and careful recording of major and minor congenital defects. An attempt should be made to recognize clinically relevant associations, sequences or syndromes.
(4) Clinical evidence of intrauterine malnutrition: the hypotrophic SGA infant frequently appears as an 'alert' neonate – thin, dry, with soft tissue wasting, the eyes open and the skin desquamated and wrinkled and sometimes covered or impregnated with meconium. The extremities seem to be more lengthy, with large hands and feet. Occasionally, the skin color is plethoric, but in cases of perinatal asphyxia it may appear pale, owing to peripheral vasoconstriction. In all cases, data of the physical and neurological examinations in combination with reference tables,[5] should be used for assessing the gestational age of the newborn infant.

Other tests that should be considered include the following: for non-hypotrophic SGA infants, karyotyping, skeletal radiographic survey and complete ultrasound screening (heart, brain, abdomen) for SGA infants with congenital defects; serum immunoglobulins, serological tests for congenital infections, investigation of cytomegalovirus in urine and DNA testing if specific intrauterine infections are suspected (cytomegalovirus, toxoplasm). Further tests are acid–base balance, serial serum glucose levels, calcium, hemogram with erythroblast count, coagulation tests, serum creatinine and liver enzymes for hypotrophic SGA infants.

Main clinical symptoms of SGA newborns

Perinatal asphyxia

It is well known that IUGR associated with placental insufficiency causing malnutrition and chronic hypoxia places the fetus in a condition in which stress derived from even an uncomplicated birth cannot be properly supported. Lin and colleagues[6] have shown statistically significant differences in Apgar scores at 1 and 5 min and mean pH values between AGA and SGA neonates. Thornberg and coworkers[7] have reported a series of 42,203 live infants in which the population of SGA babies was clearly over-represented in the birth asphyxia group. Following the recommendations of the American Academy of Pediatrics, the American Heart Association[9] and European Resuscitation Council,[10] it is very important to ensure that all necessary equipment and personnel trained in neonatal resuscitation are present at the delivery of growth-restricted babies. It is necessary to have results available of acid–base status in umbilical cord vessels during resuscitation and glucose levels during the first minutes of life, in order to determine the exact requirements of oxygen, bicarbonate and glucose.

Although some of SGA infants requiring neonatal care suffered from postasphyxia metabolic acidosis, restoration can frequently be achieved by oxygen therapy, adequate ventilatory support and prevention of heat loss. Bicarbonate administration should be limited to patients with laboratory evidence of sustained metabolic acidosis and decreased blood pH levels. Spencer and associates[11] have shown that, in severely acidotic term newborns not requiring resuscitation, SGA infants showed less improvement than AGA babies of the same gestational age. In the SGA group, spontaneous rise of pH was slower, and there was a smaller fall of the $PaCO_2$ with no changes in base deficits. Since respiratory and heart rates did not differ between AGA and SGA infants, the clinical observation did not identify babies who were less efficient at compensating for acidemia.

Serial sampling is required for the monitoring of blood glucose. Rapid and uncontrolled infusion of hyperosmolar glucose solutions, particularly in preterm SGA babies, should be avoided. Simmons and coworkers[12] found that, in uteroplacental insufficiency states, glucose transport is differentially altered in the lung and brain of SGA fetuses. Although glucose transport was decreased in type II pneumocytes, lung fibroblasts and lung tissue, glucose transport was not altered in brain tissue and glial cells; this may contribute to the phenomenon of 'brain sparing'.

Clinical symptoms of hypoxic–ischemic damage in SGA neonates can be assessed similarly to those in AGA babies. In general, 0.26% of the SGA newborns had abnormal neurological symptoms on neonatal examination. These figures, however, may vary across studies in relation to the suitability of perinatal care. The risk of neurological sequelae correlates better with late Apgar scores and severity of neurological symptoms than with early Apgar scores. Meconial aspiration, pulmonary hypertension (secondary to asphyxia and aggravated by polycythemia), and acute hemorrhagic pulmonary edema are more common in hypotrophic SGA groups than in the general population.[13] Treatment of hypoxic–ischemic encephalopathy, pulmonary hypertension and meconial aspiration is described in Chapter 7.

Neonatal hypoglycemia

The incidence of hypoglycemia in SGA infants is extremely variable, depending on different factors, such as the severity of intrauterine malnutrition

Table 123.1 Treatment of hypoglycemia in small-for-gestational-age infants (hypoglycemia = glycemia of < 30 mg/dl in full-term infants, < 20 mg/dl in preterm infants and < 40 mg/dl in term newborns after the first 24 h of life

Asymptomatic newborn infants
(1) Attempt oral feeding (bottle, oral tube) with 5–10% dextrose solution or sugar-fortified hypoallergenic milk formula, 10 ml/kg. Control serum glucose levels at 30–60 min
(2) Remember that 10% solutions are hyperosmolar and may be poorly tolerated
(3) Consider the intravenous route initially when birth weight is < 1500 g, oral intake is poorly tolerated or there are symptoms
Symptomatic newborn infants
(1) Preferably use the intravenous route: 0.25–1 g/kg (2.5–10 ml/kg) of 10% dextrose; also: 1–4ml/kg of 25% dextrose (higher concentrations are inadequate) at a rate of 12 ml/min
(2) Continue at a rate of 4–8 mg/kg per min of 5 to 10–15% glucose solution according to fluid requirements, tolerance and infant's condition
(3) Add sodium and chloride after the first 12 h and potassium after the first 48 h when superimposed deficiencies are not present
(4) Do not give glucagon. The indication of corticoids (hydrocortisone 5 mg/kg per day orally or intravenously, or prednisone 2 mg/kg per day orally) is exceptional
Note: Measurement of blood sugar levels by means of colorimetric strips should not be used for diagnostic purposes and only for the systematic screening of infants at risk. Results obtained should be confirmed by laboratory assay of plasma or serum glucose concentrations. Glycemia in whole blood is 15 mg/dl lower than in plasma or serum

(expressed as birth weight < 3rd centile, ponderal index < 10th centile and skin-fold thickness < l0th centile); associated perinatal complications (e.g., asphyxia); suitability of clinical control of the neonate during the first hours of life; and early oral or intravenous glucose supplementation. In different studies, the incidence of neonatal hypoglycemia varied between 40% and 67% in preterm SGA infants and between 10.7% and 24% in full-term SGA babies.[14,15] Singhal and coworkers[16] demonstrated that SGA babies had a sevenfold increased risk of manifesting hypoglycemia compared with AGA babies, and approximately two-thirds of the hypoglycemic babies had one or more risk factors, including birth asphyxia (24%), diabetic mother (24%), respiratory distress (14%) and septicemia (12%). Other contributing factors are hypothermia and inadequate neonatal transport. In this study, carried out in New Delhi,[12] a total of 60% of SGA babies were asymptomatic, although it has been established that babies with few symptoms and moderate hypoglycemia may be followed by adverse neurodevelopmental outcome.[17] The most common symptom observed was lethargy (81%), jitteriness (67%), respiratory abnormalities (42%), hypotonia (40%) and seizures (30%).

The etiopathogenetic mechanism of hypoglycemia in SGA infants involves a marked decrease in the energy reserves that are the substrates of gluconeogenesis and glycogenolysis.[19] Treatment of hypoglycemia demands adequate administration of glucose (Table 123.1).[20,21] In the SGA infant, however, there is a defect in the intermediate metabolism of this substrate administered postnatally.[22] Glycerol, lactate and amino acids (alanine) are sources of glucose production in case of glycogen deficiency. In the SGA neonate, these substances are increased even in the presence of hypoglycemia; this indicates a deficiency or abnormality of gluconeogenic liver enzymes, in particular phosphoenolpyruvate carbokinase. Although other enzymatic inducers of gluconeogenesis, such as glucagon and catecholamines, may also be reduced in SGA babies, the administration of glucagon to correct low blood sugar levels is not considered appropriate in these infants with reduced glycogen stores.[23,24] Intravenous hydrocortisone, which would decrease the peripheral consumption of glucose by decreasing insulin levels and increasing alanine production, may be useful in extreme situations,[25] provided that a sufficient amount of proteins is concurrently infused.

In contrast to the hyperinsulinism found in newborns from diabetic mothers, hypoglycemia in SGA babies progresses during the first hours of life unless SGA has been accompanied by severe malnutrition, prematurity or perinatal asphyxia, in which case blood sugar levels decrease immediately and rapidly after birth. Serial sampling over the first 24–36 h is required for prompt detection of hypoglycemia and intervention. Special attention should be paid to babies being breast fed or when facilities for monitoring blood sugar are unsatisfactory or unavailable.[26] In these cases, the eventual oral intake of 5% water–dextrose supplement or sugar-fortified hypoallergic milk formulas until sufficient milk secretion is produced and normal glucose levels are attained should be recommended.

Hypocalcemia

A higher incidence of hypocalcemia in SGA infants than in AGA babies has not been clearly established.

Sator-Kulic[27] showed normal values of serum calcium ions in SGA infants on the first and the third days after birth. Only hypotrophic SGA infants or neonates who have suffered from perinatal asphyxia would have a higher incidence of low serum calcium levels. In these cases, calcemia should be determined within 12 and 24 h after birth. Routine assay of serum calcium in asymptomatic full-term SGA infants is not required.

Hypothermia

The hypotrophic SGA neonate has a greater cephalic volume and total body surface in relation to his or her weight, so that there is a greater heat loss than in the AGA baby. In the full-term SGA infant, in contrast to the preterm AGA infant, radiant and convective heat losses may be reduced by the ability to diminish body surface area by a flexion posture of the extremities. Although the term SGA infant has a greater thermogenic capacity than peers of the same weight and lower gestational age, this is established at the cost of caloric expenditure that cannot be maintained for a long time.[28] The scarce subcutaneous fat prevents correct thermal insulation, and the scarce brown fat stores prevent a correct response to the initial cold stress. Therefore, prompt and complete drying of the infant after birth, and wrapping in thermal paper after resuscitation, maintaining the baby under a radiating heat source, is crucial.

Nourishment problems: necrotizing enterocolitis

The need to feed the hypotrophic SGA infant early, together with a frequently complicated perinatal period, imposes demands on the bowel that often cannot be satisfied. Although some studies[29] have not found differences in the gastric residual volumes of breast milk between healthy preterm SGA and AGA infants with gestational age of 28–36 weeks, vomiting and regurgitation are sometimes observed in hypotrophic term SGA babies orally fed at high rates with milk or glucose.

Perinatal asphyxia causes a redistribution of blood flow to different organs with relative ischemia in some. Mesenteric ischemia together with tissue hypoxia and hyperviscosity, especially in the very early preterm hypotrophic SGA infant, predisposes to necrotizing enterocolitis (NEC). Several studies demonstrate a trend toward an increased incidence of this entity.[30,31] In the study by Kurscheid and Holschneider,[32] 30% of the 73 patients treated for NEC were SGA infants. In these cases, feeding (in the form of elementary formulas) should not be started until the achievement of a stable hemodynamic status, absence of gastric retention, normal abdominal palpation and spontaneous passage of meconium. In the Vermont Oxford Nerwork (VON) study, including 19,759 very low birth weight (VLBW) neonates prenatal corticosteroid use was not associated with decreased risks of NEC.[33]

A potential protective role against NEC of different feeding strategies, like use of breast milk or continuous vs. bolus feeding in preterm and SGA newborns has been suggested but not evidence based.[34,35]

Preterm SGA infants have higher metabolic rates than AGA babies because of their faster growth rate and larger brain size.[36] In addition, they absorb dietary nutrients less well, particularly fat and proteins. It has even been shown that, in term SGA infants,[37] serum concentrations α-lactalbumin are significantly higher than in AGA infants of similar gestational age. This indicates that IUGR causes a delayed postnatal decrease in macromolecular absorption and delayed intestinal maturation.

To satisfy caloric requirement, 150 cal/kg/day should be reached from the seventh day of life.

Studies on iron status in infants of low birth weight[38] have shown that, at birth, preterm AGA infants had higher serum ferritin concentrations than preterm SGA babies. Preterm infants who were not supplemented with iron, irrespective of their adequacy for gestational age, showed evidence of iron deficiency before 4 months of age.

With respect to the effect of IUGR on postnatal weight change in preterm infants, Bauer and associates[39] reported significantly higher weight loss and body water loss during the first week of life in preterm AGA infants than weight-matched preterm SGA babies. Loss of weight and total body water in AGA infants was accompanied by a greater diuresis than in SGA infants at the same amount of fluid intake. Fluid requirements of full-term SGA infants are 80–90 ml/kg on the first day of life, reaching 10–150 ml/kg/day after the first week. Fluid requirements in preterm SGA babies, however, should be calculated daily and individualized according to the presence of associated conditions and the type of heat source under which the baby is maintained.

Cerebral hemorrhage and ischemic brain damage

In a study of the impact of prematurity and IUGR on neonatal hemorrhagic and ischemic brain damage, carried out by Amato and colleagues,[40] a higher incidence of peri- and intraventricular hemorrhage (IVH) in the AGA group (36.8%) than in SGA babies (18.5%) was reported. In both groups, however, a significantly higher incidence of cerebral hemorrhage was found in babies of <1000 g in body weight compared with babies of >1000 g in body weight. Ischemic brain lesions (periventricular leukomalacia) were equally distributed between AGA and SGA babies (10.5% vs. 3.7%) independently of body weight category.

If only extremely low birth weight babies are considered, most of studies have demonstrated a greater incidence of IVH in SGA newborns compared to AGA ones. According to the VON data comparing SGA and AGA VLBW neonates,[33] the odds ratio in SGA was 1.13 for IVH and 1.25 for severe IVH. In this case, the prenatal use of steroids seemed to have a protective role.

Respiratory distress syndrome and other prematurity-related pathologies

Although initial studies suggested that IUGR-related fetal stress would protect SGA infants against severe respiratory distress syndrome (RDS) by stimulating fetal lung maturity,[41] recent investigations do not seem to confirm this.[30,42,43] Thompson and colleagues[44] compared neonatal ventilatory requirements and outcome in 135 very early preterm SGA infants to those from controls matched for gestation age and gender. Although there was no significant difference in the median duration of mechanical ventilation, more SGA infants required ventilation and were ventilated because of RDS. However, in a subgroup also matched for mode of delivery, differences between the two groups were not encountered. Ley *et al.* have shown a higher incidence of RDS among preterm SGA infants born before 29 weeks gestation with the use of fetal growth standards, based on ultrasonically estimated fetal weights, but not in SGA infants born between 29 and 32 weeks' gestation.[45] In the large VON cohort,[33] RDS is also slightly increased (odds ratio 1.19) in SGA born before 30 weeks of gestation compared to AGA of the same gestational age.

In the study of Schiff and colleagues,[43] 127 pre-eclamptic women who had undergone amniocentesis for pulmonary maturity assessment were matched for gestational age, sex, race and infant gender with non-hypertensive women with preterm labor who had undergone the same procedure. There were no significant differences between SGA and AGA infants born to women with pre-eclampsia in comparison with their matched controls in the incidence of an immature result and respiratory distress syndrome.

In VLBW infants (less than 1500 g or born before 30 weeks' gestation), the condition of being SGA seems to confer also an additional risk of other prematurity-related morbidities,[33–45] like ductus ligation, chronic lung disease and retinopathy of prematurity.

Polycythemia and coagulation disorders

It is well known that chronic tissue hypoxia induces an increase in plasma erythropoietin concentration in human fetal life and this response stimulates fetal erythropoiesis. Increased plasma erythropoietin concentrations in SGA fetuses have been documented as early as 26 weeks' gestation.[46] The degree of increase was significantly associated both with fetal acidemia and, more strongly, with fetal erythroblastosis. Furthermore, a more accurate assessment of tissue oxygenation in SGA newborns may be obtained by determining the erythroblast count rather than blood pH values. Perinatal asphyxia and placental vascular changes may cause disturbances in placental–fetal exchange, which may induce changes in the total blood volume and subsequent deterioration of the hemodynamic status. The risk of manifesting polycythemia (hematocrit > 65% in peripheral blood) in SGA infants was between threefold[18] and 25-fold[47] greater compared with AGA babies (0.5%). Although about one-third of polycythemic infants had one or more symptoms, on neurodevelopment follow-up the development indices of both asymptomatic and symptomatic cases were found to be comparable.[47]

In healthy preterm SGA neonates, no correlation was seen between serum levels of vitamin K_1 and plasma levels of coagulation factors II and X. After the administration of 1 mg vitamin K_1, no accelerated increase in coagulation factor activities was seen.[48]

Kupferminc and colleagues studied the increased prevalence of inherit or acquired thrombophilias in woman with mild severe IGUR. The trombophilias significantly increased were factor V Leiden mutation, prothrombin gene mutation and protein S deficiency.[49]

Biochemical, metabolic and compositional changes in SGA infants are shown in Tables 123.2 and 123.3.

Mortality

The perinatal mortality rate among IUGR infants is 10–20 times the rate among AGA infants.[58]

Compared with AGA babies, fetuses affected by IUGR have a higher risk of death antenatally, whereas SGA infants have a higher risk of death in the neonatal period. Although the perinatal mortality of SGA babies ranges between 50% and 60%, their neonatal mortality is lower than that of preterm AGA infants of the same weight. When crown–heel length was used to classify growth patterns,[59] proportionate IUGR with short crown–heel length had a significantly greater mortality than disproportionate IUGR infants with normal crown–heel length. When the ponderal index was used for classification, there were no statistically significant differences in mortality between the two groups. At present, however, actual mortality rates are difficult to assess, given that pregnancy termination is a frequent decision in severely malformed fetuses with harmonious IUGR diagnosed antenatally; the majority of fetuses with normal karyotype and harmonious IUGR are healthy infants. IUGR due to utero-placental insufficiency with adequate perinatal obstetric control should have mortality rates in such infants hardly higher than those of AGA infants.

In a study of 28-day survival rates of 6676 neonates with birth weights of 1250 g or less,[60] predictors of survival in descending order of significance in the multivariate analysis were gestational age and birth weight,[61,62] sex, race, single birth and SGA. In the study of Kilpatrick and colleagues,[63] singleton SGA neonates had a significantly greater perinatal mortality than twin SGA neonates matched for gestational age at delivery at 30 weeks or more. The effect of birth weight discordance in preterm twin gestations was studied in 122 live born twin sets delivered between 25 and 30 complete weeks' gestation.[64] Preterm twin gestations with > 30% birth weight discordance were associated with a higher incidence of infant death (25%), congenital anomalies (37.5%), SGA infants

Table 123.2 Biochemical and metabolic changes in small-for-gestational-age infants (modified from Babson and Kagas[50])

Carbohydrate and fat metabolism
Neonatal hypoglycemia
No changes in K_t (rate constant for glucose metabolism)
Decreased, increased or no change in insulin
Decreased, increased or no change in free fatty acids and glycerol[51,52]
Decreased or no change in *b*-hydroxybutyrate
Decreased hepatic gluconeogenesis
Decreased urinary epinephrine after hypoglycemia
Decreased levels of HDL-cholesterol, reduced activity of lecithin: cholesterol–acyl transferase[153]
Decreased insulin-like-growth factor-II (IGF-II)[53]
Increased lactate, pyruvate, alanine and glucagons
Increased or no change in ketone bodies
Increased levels of VLDL and lipoprotein lipid content[51]
Increased levels of IGF-I and IGF-binding protein-1[54,55]
Proteins and collagen
Decreased or no change in total protein and prealbumin
Decreased OH-proline turnover early and increased later
Decreased N-terminal propeptide of type III procollagen[56]
Increased ammonia, urea and uric acid
Increased uronic acid turnover
Immunocompetence[57]
Decreased IgG
Decreased humoral or cellular bactericidal capacity
Decreased phagocytic index
Decreased lysozyme
Decreased humoral and cellular immunocompetence
Increased IgM in some cases
Hematology
Increased hematocrit, erythroblast (H.I) count, erythrocytic volume and viscosity
Increased fetal hemoglobin
Increased erythropoietin
Increased, decreased or no change in prothrombin and partial thromboplastin time
Increased reticulocyte index but no change in reticulocyte count
Decreased platelets
Miscellaneous
Decreased serum ionic calcium
Decreased, increased or no change in amniotic fluid L/S ratio
Decreased, increased or no change in O_2 consumption
Increased cortisol or II-OH corticosteroids
Increased or no change in human growth hormone

(32%), Apgar score of < 7 at 5 min (33%) and periventricular leukomalacia (17%). The gestational age rather than the degree of discordance is a predicting factor for less favorable neonatal outcome.[65,66] Jacobs and colleagues,[67] using the 1995–97 Centers for Disease Control and Prevention's Matched Multiple Birth file, examined the association between increasing intratriplet birth weight discordance and risk of fetal death and smallness for gestational age and found also a positive association if the discordance was greater than 29%.

The main causes of death in full-term SGA infants included perinatal asphyxia, congenital anomalies

Table 123.3 Compositional changes in small-for-gestational-age infants (from Babson and Kagas[50])

Placenta
Decreased or no change in weight and DNA
Decreased, increased or no change in RNA
Decreased heat-stable alkaline phosphatase, glycogen, glucose and oxygen use
Decreased fibrinolysis (urokinase pathway)
No change in protein/DNA
Increased or no change in RNA/DNA, nitrogen or protein
Increased RNA polymerase, protein synthesis from proline and leucine and increased aromatization, glycogen use
Liver
Decreased weight and glycogen
No change in DNA and protein/DNA
Muscle
Decreased protein and fat
Decreased, increased or no change in total water and extracellular water
Decreased, increased or no change in DNA
Increased intracellular water
Decreased RNA, RNA/DNA, protein/DNA
Decreased zinc, potassium, magnesium and increased sodium
Brain
Decreased weight, especially cerebellar
Decreased cerebellar DNA, myelin lipid, galactolipid sulfotransferase and glucosaminoglycans
Heart
No change in DNA and protein/DNA
Decreased sarcoplasm and glycogen
Adrenals
Decreased fetal zone
Water
Increased total body water, extracellular water, intracellular water and plasma volume

and diseases related to poorly controlled metabolic problems, whereas in preterm SGA infants these were RDS, HIV infection and NEC.

Somatic growth disorders

Growth of SGA infants with chromosome abnormalities, multiple major birth defects or intrauterine symptomatic infections affecting the central nervous system is usually severely compromised, with overall and unequal degree of impairment of weight, height and head circumference. Results of different studies on postnatal somatic growth in SGA infants are inconsistent, probably owing to the heterogenicity of all newborn infants considered to be small for dates.

Type, severity and earliness of IUGR have been related to SGA features.[68–72] It has been shown that newborn infants were thinner and shorter than the general population when their IUGR began before 34 weeks' gestation, and that these characteristics persisted throughout the growth period. When IUGR began earlier, before 26 weeks' gestation, growth

Table 123.4 One-year catch-up growth (%) of small-for-gestational-age (SGA) infants with distinct anthropometric alterations at birth (from reference 18)

	Weight < 10th centile	Weight + height < 10th centile	Weight + HC < 10th centile	Weight + height + HC < 10th centile
Weight	79	62	65	38
Height		69		33
Head circumference			100	66
Ponderal index*	81	75	80	45

HC, head circumference. At birth: height < 10th centile, 53%; HC < 10th centile, 30%; ponderal index < 10th centile, 57%; *in 17.5% of SGA infants, when the ponderal index was > 10th centile at birth, it decreased to below the 10th centile by 1 year

impairment was still greater and may even have affected the head circumference. These infants were less susceptible to recuperation, and frequently suffered disorders associated with neurological development. IUGR of late onset was less severe and generalized, and showed a more rapid process of recuperation. However, considering IUGR as a whole, most studies indicated that intrauterine growth-restricted infants had a tendency to be thinner and shorter,[18,68,73–83] but others disagreed.[84–91] It is generally accepted that undernourished neonates (low ponderal index or disharmonious) recuperate sooner, whereas neonates apparently not undernourished (normal ponderal index or harmonious) remain thin, are of short stature and have a reduced cranial perimeter[18,92–95]; the more severe the malnutrition, the more time required for recuperation.[96] However, some authors consider that, although most infants with low ponderal index can grow faster during the first months of life, diminished height, weight and head circumference remain at the long-term follow-up.[97,98] Others consider that early nutrition of SGA infants is especially important,[99] as is catch-up growth during the first months of life, as predictors of recovery.Other authors, however, do not share this opinion.[77–79]

In full-term twins in which the weight of the smaller was < 2000 g and 25% less than that of the larger, Babson and Kagas[100] found that this difference persisted in relation to both physical development and intellectual capacity at the age of 8 years. On the other hand, Philip[101] showed that full-term twins with 20% discordant birth weights could attain the same height and head circumference at the age of 1 year, although remaining thinner. Differences by gender have been found in some studies. In a longitudinal follow-up of growth in 123 SGA children,[102] the boys showed an extremely fast weight catch-up, 85% of them reaching a weight greater than −2SD at the age of 3 months and all of them remaining above this level at 4 years of age. Such a fast catch-up growth was observed in only two-thirds of the girls, but at 4 years of age 85% of the girls were also above −2SD. Length catch-up was more gradual than weight catch-up. Acceleration of head growth may be more prominent in SGA males.[103] A recent longitudinal study about the outcomes of VLBW infants from birth to 20 years, found females having greater catch-up in growth than males. The negative effect of neonatal illness on 20 years' height attainment was greater among males.[104] According to some authors, head circumference may grow in parallel with, or faster than, weight or height.[71,104] Karlberg and Albertsson-Wikland[105] followed a singleton birth cohort ($n = 3650$) of full-term SGA infants from birth till they reached final height at about 18 years of age. SGA infants were found to have a sevenfold higher risk for short final stature in comparison with the non-SGA group. At 18 years of age, 22% of the total short population were short at birth, whereas when birth weight was used to define SGA, only 14% of the 18-year-old short population were light at birth. It is concluded that the vast majority (> 86%) will achieve catch-up in height during the first 6–12 months of life. Of the remaining non-catch-up infants, about 50% remain short in final height.

One-year catch-up growth of SGA infants with different anthropometric abnormalities at birth is shown in Table 123.4.

The role of preexisting or persistent hormonal defects in the postnatal growth processes of SGA infants is unclear.[50] Insulin plays a critical role in fetal growth. A significant correlation between linear growth velocity and insulin release after glucose overload has been reported.[106,107] In the study of Samaan and colleagues,[53] SGA infants had lower insulin-like growth factor-II (IGF-II) levels than AGA and large-for-gestational-age infants. These results suggest that IGF-II may play a major role in fetal growth. On the other hand, the mean serum IGF-I levels in SGA infants were significantly higher than in AGA infants, but not in their respective mothers. This indicates that the production of IGF-I in the maternal and fetal compartments is independent and that circulation of IGF-I across the placenta is unlikely. The concentration of IGF-I and insulin-like growth-factor-binding protein-1 (IGFBP-1) in the umbilical vessels at delivery showed an inverse correlation with birth weight, so that significantly higher values were found in SGA infants than in AGA neonates.[87] IGFBP-1 might inhibit the action of IGF-I in both the maternal and the fetal compartments, and the rise in IGFBP-1 could be a primary factor in retardation of fetal growth.[54,55] A positive correlation between C-peptide levels in cord blood and neonatal weight, ponderal index and maternal weight gain during gestation were also observed in SGA infants.[108] N-terminal propeptide of type III procollagen (PIIINP) concentration in cord serum of SGA infants was significantly lower than in AGA infants.[56] PIIINP assay may serve as a dynamic biochemical indicator of deviant fetal growth as the PIIINP results were also related to the severity or duration of IUGR. The lowest values were obtained in non-malformed SGA infants with small head circumference, known as an index for the chronicity of fetal nutritional deprivation.[90] Somatomedins seem to play a role in fetal growth.[109,110]

Some studies report the effects of growth hormone (GH) therapy in children with short stature secondary to IUGR,[110] showing significant results in patients with normal secretion of endogenous growth hormone when doses three times higher than in cases of growth hormone insufficiency were given.[111,112]

In July 2001, growth hormone GH was approved by the US Food and Drug Administration for the long-term treatment of growth failure in children who are born SGA and do not achieve catch-up growth by 2–3 years of age, at doses of 0.24–0.48 mg/kg/week.[113] The objectives of GH therapy in short SGA children are: catch-up in early childhood, maintenance of normal growth in childhood and achievement of normal adult height .Higher doses (up to 0.48 mg/kg/week) are more effective for the short term, but its advantages over lower doses on the long term is not yet know. Only adult height results of randomized dose–response studies will give a definite answer.

Whether measures of GH secretion provide clinically useful information for the routine treatment of short children who were born SGA is controversial. Arguments that favor evaluation for GH deficiency come from data suggesting that many short patients who were born SGA have diminished GH output, evidenced by low levels of spontaneous GH secretion, and depressed circulating concentrations of markers of GS secretion, such as IGF-I. Thus, the lack of catch-up growth in some cases might be attributable to reduced GH secretion.

However, standard laboratory GH stimulation tests do not predict growth response in most patients who are SGA. The present recommendation is that test of GH release only is performed when GH deficiency is suspected on clinical or biochemical backgrounds.

Neurological development and outcome: postnatal behavior

It has been widely recognized that SGA infants constitute a high-risk group for neonatal neurological problems, sensoral and neurodevelopmental sequelae and behavioral disturbances.[114–121] As early as in the neonatal period, deficits in muscular tone with decreased cephalic control, diminished spontaneous activity and poor and incomplete primary reflexes with a lower degree of impairment of tendon reflexes may be observed.[122] In a study in which the influence of IUGR on heart rate during sleep was assessed,[123] sympathetic and parasympathetic heart rate control was clearly different between SGA and AGA newborn infants, with a shorter RR interval and lower amplitude of heart rate variability in all bands of the polygraphic recordings. Circadian rhythmicity is established more slowly in growth restricted infants than in normal children.[124] Excretion of melatonin, also rhythmically and age related, is delayed in growth restricted infants.[125] During active and quiet sleep, Curzi-Dascalova and coworkers[126] and Riese[127,128] demonstrated significant modifications in the establishment of respiratory rhythm control (more central respiratory pauses, higher apnea index, and time spent with periodic breathing), dissimilar patterns for behavioral stability, reactivity and activity during sleep, significantly higher incidence of vigorous limb movements and right hand-to-mouth movements, more spontaneous smiles and a trend to more spontaneous startles. Abnormal responses in neurobehavioral performance at 40 weeks' conceptional age,[129] as well as two patterns of spontaneous general movements unique for the SGA infant might be used to discriminate between healthy and neurologically suspect newborn infants.[130]

When brainstem auditory evoked responses were examined in SGA children from birth to 6 years of age and compared with those of AGA children, Jiang and coworkers[131] demonstrated that I–V, I–III and III–V conduction intervals showed similar developmental trends. However, the III–V/I–III ratio followed a developmental course that differed markedly from that in AGA children. The ratio decreased slightly with age up to 2 years and was persistently smaller than in normal children after 1 year, indicating that the relative development of early and late brainstem conduction time deviates from normal.

Neurological development in SGA infants during the first years of life has been extensively studied. Fitzhardinge and Steven[114] considered that SGA infants constitute the second group in neurological sequelae following preterm infants with intraventricular hemorrhage (7% of neonates with a birth weight of < 3rd centile had neurological sequelae and up to 16% had mild deficits classified as minimal brain dysfunction). Preterm SGA neonates would be those at highest risk. In a neurological follow-up study of 37 SGA newborn infants,[132] 8% of the group had severe neurological sequelae at 1 year of corrected age. The statistical analysis showed a high correlation between subnormal weight gain and neurological and developmental abnormalities at 1 year. In a case–control study in which the risk of cerebral palsy in connection with

IUGR was analyzed,[133] the risk in SGA infants was significantly increased in term and moderately preterm infants. The most common abnormalities were tetraplegia, diplegia and dyskinetic cerebral palsy.[134] In full-term severely growth-retarded infants, a relationship was found between skull circumference < 3rd centile and the presence of minor neurological dysfunction at the age of 6 years, whereas body measurements, behavior at home and at school and school achievement were not related.[135]

In long-term follow-up studies, a higher prevalence of auditory problems in relation to IUGR has not been found, although speech disorders (delay in the onset of speech, poor and immature language, defects in articulation, etc.) have been documented by different authors.[53,136] With respect to visual defects, although 18% of male and 10% of female SGA infants in the study of Fitzhardinge and Steven[114] needed visual correction, these figures were similar to those found in the general population. According to the study of Getz and coworkers,[137] being SGA does not pose an additional risk for the development of grating acuity or binocular visual field size over the first 4 years of life in preterm children. Other studies[138,139] reported delayed visual directed prehension and abnormal visual brainstem evoked potentials.

Although minor motor dysfunctions, subtle neurodevelopmental and attention deficits, hyperactivity, failure at schools despite normal intelligence and increased fears have been reported,[80,140–142] it is difficult to ascertain whether these findings occur more frequently in SGA children.[115,143] The family environment may play an important role in the first developmental stages.

Recent studies point out the relation between reversal end-diastolic flow velocities (EDFVs) on antenatal assessment, with a wide range of problems at school age. Absence of EDFV is well recognized as a marker of fetal compromise which is associated with acute perinatal sequelae but not related with adverse neurodevelopmental outcome. This suggests that reversal EGFV could represent intrauterine decompensation which may have adverse effects on the developing brain.[144]

In a comparative study of the physical and developmental status of preschool SGA children, Pryor[145] found that mothers were less likely to have breastfed their babies and reported higher incidences of eating problems and visits to a general practitioner than those with AGA children. For all subjects, breast feeding was correlated with higher Stanford–Binet scores, and environmental factors appeared more salient for the progress of SGA children at this age than biological factors. At age 13, adolescents born SGA scored significantly lower than the AGA group on the WISC-R scales, and at the age of 15, they were rated by parents as having more behavioral problems.[146] Mothers' education has been associated with SGA infants' academic abilities,[147] and improper mothering behavior has also been postulated as a factor associated with behavioral disturbances in SGA children.[148,149]

It is generally considered that perinatal complications are important determinants of major neurological sequelae, whereas less severe behavioral problems in the long term would be more related to IUGR *per se*. The time of onset of IUGR (before 27 or before 34 weeks' gestation) has been associated with the degree of impairment of school performance; reading, writing and drawing abilities; creative and imaginative activities; and reasoning capacity.[150] More severe behavioral disturbances were observed in very early growth-retarded children and have been related to their short stature; boys were more irritable and anxious, and felt more unhappy and worried about their relationships with other children, whereas girls were more blubbering and irascible, and adopted defiant and intimidating attitudes against their schoolmates.

Smedler and colleagues[151] reported that healthy VLBW SGA infants aged 8–11 years scored significantly lower on measures of visuospatial ability, nonverbal reasoning, strategy formation and gross motor coordination, and they had also more behavioral and educational problems than control AGA infants matched for age, sex and socioeconomic background. These developmental deficits began to be increasingly evident at an early school age. Being born SGA at term is associated with poorer school performance at 12 and 18 years,[152] according to data obtained in a French regional cohort. Lagerstrom and coworkers[153] found that girls born SGA showed lack of school motivation and concentration difficulties both at age 10 and at age 13. These authors further observed that SGA children had lower scores than controls in WISC test performance and full scale scores at the age of 10 years; preterm SGA infants also had lower scores in the verbal scales.[154] Results from the British Birth Cohort in which school performance was assessed at 16 and 26 years were published recently.[155] At 16 years, those born SGA demonstrated small but significant deficits in academic achievement, and the teachers were less likely to rate those who were born SGA in the top 15th percentile of the class compared with those who were born AGA. At 26 years, the adults who were SGA did not demonstrate any differences in years of education, but they were less likely to have professional or managerial jobs and reported lower income than the AGA participants.

Adult conditions related to IUGR

Evidence that the quality of fetal growth and development has strong and, in widely varying populations, reproducible effects on susceptibility to many common adult human diseases has only been acquired relatively recently.

A further general point to be made in relation to studies in this area as they relate to human disease is the extremely crude nature and limited scope of the observations available reflecting the quality of human fetal growth and development at the present time. There is no such thing as a 'normal' birth weight. At the present, there is no way of knowing what the optimal fetal growth potential is of any particular child. The relationship of the prevalence of a disease to birth weight is often continuous throughout the range of birth weights. Studies in experimental animals have indeed shown that it is possible to expose pregnant women to particular insults, which do not change the birth weight of the offspring but yet do change their phenotype in other respects.[156]

Individuals who were born small-for-gestational age are a group of people who appear to be at increased risk of the detrimental consequences of obesity. In the cohort study of Ong and colleagues,[89] children who showed catch-up in weight or length between 0 and 2 years were heavier and taller than other children at 5 years, and had greater body mass index, percentage body fat, total fat mass, and central fat distribution, which are variables of childhood size linked to metabolic markers for risk of disease in adulthood and are predictive for adulthood obesity.

It appears that both poor fetal and early postnatal growth are separately linked to the risk of poor glucose tolerance as an adult.[156]

Adult hypertension and other cardiovascular disease, in people who were born small-for-gestational age, has been attributed to fetal adaptations to maternal undernutrition or placental dysfunction that permanently alters growth characteristics, postnatal metabolism and physiology.[157,158] The mechanisms underlying the programming of hypertension are likely to be multifactorial; however, a role for the kidney and the endotelium in the maintenance of raised blood pressure has been reported.[159] In some studies, postnatal physiological adaptation and maturation if IGUR infants is slower than normal and therefore they remain in a physiologically immature state for longer, the higher rates and greater cortisol excretion could be precursors to hypertension and cardiovascular disease seen in adult.[160]

The programming of the endocrine axes might occur during critical phases of fetal development and might thus be affected by intrauterine growth restriction. A northern Spanish group[161] has indicated associations between reduced fetal growth and the occurrence of precocious adrenarche, pubarche, hyperandrogenism, polycystic ovary syndrome and hyperinsulinism. However hyperandrogenism and precocious pubarche were not confirmed in a large Dutch study.[162] Both studies reported a lower number of follicles in the ovaries in girls born SGA. Most studies show that children born SGA start their puberty at a normal age but relatively early, within the normal range. Age at menarche seems comparable with controls.[163]

Intrauterine and early postnatal environments could have long-term consequences for infectious disease risk, as well as risk of other diseases with an immunologic component, including asthma and allergy, autoimmunity-related diseases and neoplasia. The success of immunization programs that target adolescent and young adults (e.g., tetanus and hepatitis B) could be affected.[164] A recent study of Hasselmar and colleagues[165] report a similar frequency of allergic diseases in SGA-born subjects as in controls deviating from the primary hypothesis of a protective effect on allergy development in the subgroup of IUGR subjects.

The underlying mechanisms explaining links between fetal growth and cancer are not clear but could well include permanent changes in growth factor expression and sensitivity.[156]

REFERENCES

1. Wilcox MA, Newton CS, Johnson IR. Paternal influences on birthweight. *Acta Obstet Gynecol Scand* 1995;74:5–8.
2. Drossou V, Diamantri E, Noutsia H, *et al.* Accuracy of anthropometric measurements in predicting symptomatic SGA and LGA neonates. *Acta Paediatr* 1995;84:1–5.
3. Baraibar R, Krauel J, Molina V, Sentis J. Cuantificación del grado y características del estado nutricional del recien nacido mediante la medida del espesor del pliegue cutáneo. *Clin Ginecol* 1981; 5:191–210.
4. Spinillo A, Capuzzo E, Stronati M, *et al.* Pregnancies complicated by idiopathic intrauterine growth retardation. Severity of growth failure, neonatal morbidity and two year infant neurodevelopmental outcome. *J Reprod Med* 1995;40:209–15.
5. Dubowitz V. Clinical assessment of gestional age in the newborn infant. *J Pediatr* 1970;77:1–7.
6. Lin YS, Chang FM, Chiu CH. Comparison of umbilical blood gas and acid–base status of small-for-date and normal Chinese newborns. *J Formos Med Assoc* 1992;91:396–9.
7. Thornberg E, Thiringer K, Odeback A, Milsom I. Birth asphyxia: Incidence, clinical course and outcome in a Swedish population. *Acta Paediatr* 1995;84:927–32.
8. Baraibar R. Neuroepidemiologia neonatal. *But Soc Cat Pediatr* 1982;42:235–88.
9. International Guidelines for Neonatal Resuscitation. An excerpt from the guidelines 2000 for cardiopulmonary resuscitation and emergency cardiovascular care: International Consensus on Science. *Pediatrics* 2000;106.c29.
10. Phillips B, Zideman D, Wyllie J, Richmond S, Van Reempts P. European Resuscitation Council Guidelines 2000 for Newly Born Life Support. A statement from the Pediatric Life Support Working Group and approved by the Executive Committee of the European Resuscitation Council. *Resucitation* 2001:48:235–9.
11. Spencer JA, Robson SC, Farkas A. Spontaneous recovery after severe metabolic acidaemia at birth. *Early Hum Dev* 1993;32:103–11.
12. Simmons RA, Gounis AS, Bangalore SA, Ogata ES. Intrauterine growth retardation: Fetal glucose transport is diminished in lung but spared in brain. *Pediatr Res* 1992;31:59–63.
13. Fredrick J, Butler NR. Certain causes of neonatal deaths. IV: Massive pulmonary haemorrhage. *Biol Neonate* 1971;18:243–6.
14. Lubchenco L. Incidence of hypoglycemia in newborn infants classified by birth weight and gestational age. *Pediatrics* 1971;47: 831–4.
15. Amiel-Tisson C. Hypotrophie foetale et hypoglicemie neonatal. *Arch Fr Pediatr* 1972;29:135–9.
16. Singhal PK, Singh M, Paul VK, *et al.* Neonatal hypoglycemia: Clinical profile and glucose requirements. *Indian Pediatr* 1992; 29:157–71.
17. Lucas A, Morley R, Cole TJ. Adverse neurodevelopmental outcome of moderate neonatal hypoglycemia. *Br Med J* 1988;297: 1304–8.

18. Baraibar R, Krauel J, Molina V. Aspectos neonatales del retraso de crecimiento intrauterino. In *IV Spanish Annual Meeting of AEP section of Perinatal Medicine, Libro de Ponencias*, Zaragoza, 1982:277–313.
19. Cowett RM. Hypoglycemia and hyperglycemia in the newborn. In Polin CA, Fox WW, eds. *Fetal and Neonatal Physiology*. Philadelphia, PA: WB Saunders, 1992:406–18.
20. Robertson NRC. Care of the normal small baby and the convalescing NICU graduate. In Roberston NRC, ed. *Textbook of Neonatology*, 3rd edn. Edinburgh: Churchill Livingstone, 1999: 389–99.
21. Hawdon JM, Ward Platt MP, Aynsley-Green A. Prevention and management of neonatal hypoglicemia. *Arch Dis Child* 1995; 73:60–5.
22. Hawdon JM, Ward Platt MP. Metbolic asaptation in small for gestational age infants. *Arch Dis Child* 1993;68:262–8.
23. Hawdon JM, Weddell A, Aynsley-Green A, Ward Platt MP. Hormonal and metabolic response to hypoglycaemia in small for gestational age infants. *Arch Dis Child* 1993;68:269–73.
24. Sparks JW, Cetin I. Intrauterine growth and nutrition. In Polin CA, Fox WW, eds. *Fetal and Neonatal Physiology*. Philadelphia, PA: WB Saunders, 1992:179–98.
25. Sann L, Ruitton A, Mathieu M, Lasne Y. Effect of intravenous hydrocortisone administration of glucose homeostasis of small for gestational age infants. *Acta Paediatr Scand* 1979;68:113–7.
26. Singhal PK, Singh M, Paul VK, *et al*. Prevention of hypoglycemia: A controlled evaluation of sugar fortified milk feeding in SGA infants. *Indian Pediatr* 1992;29:1365–9.
27. Sator-Kulic Z. Serum calcium in the early neonatal period in premature and small for gestational age infants. *Med Pregl* 1992;45:288–90.
28. Sinclair JC. Heat production and thermoregulation in the small for date infant. *Ped Clin North Am* 1970;14:47–57.
29. Malhotra AK, Deorari AK, Paul VK, *et al*. Gastric residuals in preterm babies. *J Trop Pediatr* 1992;38:262–4.
30. Simchen MJ, Beiner ME, Strauss-Liviathan N, *et al*. Neonatal outcome in growth-restricted versus appropriately grown preterm infants. *Am J Perinatol* 2000;17(4):187–92.
31. Zaw W, Gagnon R, da Silva O. The risk of adverse neonatal outcome among preterm small for gestational age infants according to neonatal versus fetal growth standards. *Pediatrics* 2003;111(6, Pt 1):1273–7.
32. Kurscheid T, Holschneider AM. Necrotizing enterocolitis (NEC). Mortality and long-term results. *Eur J Pediatr Surg* 1993;3:139–43.
33. Bernstein IM, Horbar JD, Badger GJ, Ohlsson A, Golan A. Morbidity and mortality among very-low-birth-weight neonates with intrauterine growth restriction. The Vermont Oxford Network. *Am J Obstet Gynecol* 2000;182(1, Pt 1):198–206.
34. Henderson G, Anthony MY, Mc Guire W. Formula milk versus preterm human milk for feeding preterm and low birth weight infants (Cochrane Review). *The Cochrane Library*, Issue 3. Chichester, UK; John Wiley and Sons, 2004.
35. Premji S, Chessell L. Continous nasogastric milk feeding versus intermittent bolus feeding for premature infants less than 1500 grams (Cochrane Review). *The Cochrane Library*, Issue 3. Chichester, UK; John Wiley and Sons, 2004.
36. Roberton NRC. Fetal growth, intrauterine growth retardations and small for gestational age babies. In Robertson NRC, ed. *Textbook of Neonatology*, 3rd edn. Philadelphia, PA: Churchill Livingstone, 1999:133–41.
37. Boehm G, Jakobsson I, Mansson M, Raiha NC. Macromolecular absorption in small for gestational age infants. *Acta Paediatr* 1992;81:864–7.
38. Olivares M, Llaguno S, Marin V, *et al*. Iron status in low birth weight infants, small and appropiate for gestational age. A follow-up study. *Acta Paediatr* 1992;81:824–8.
39. Bauer K, Cowett RM, Howard GM, *et al*. Effect of intrauterine growth retardation on postnatal weight change in preterm infants. *J Pediatr* 1993;123:301–6.
40. Amato M, Konrad D, Huppi P, Donati F. Impact of prematurity and intrauterine growth retardation on neonatal hemorrhagic and ischemic brain damage. *Eur J Neurol* 1993;33:299–303.
41. Procianoy RS, Garcia-Prats JA, Adams JM, *et al*. Hyaline membrane disease and intraventricular haemorrhage in small for gestational age babies. *Arch Dis Child* 1980;55:502–5.
42. Tyson JE, Kennedy K, Broyles S, Rosenfeldt CR. The small for gestational age infant: Accelerated or delayed pulmonary maturation? Increased or decreased survival? *Pediatrics* 1995;95:534–8.
43. Schiff E, Friedman SA, Mercer BM, Sibai BM. Fetal lung maturity is not accelerated in pre-eclamptic pregnancies. *Am J Obstet Gynecol* 1993;169:1096–101.
44. Thompson PJ, Greenough A, Gamsu HR, Nicolaides KH. Ventilatory requirements for respiratory distress syndrome in SGA infants. *Eur J Pediatr* 1992;151:528–31.
45. Ley D, Wide-Swanson D, Lindroth M, Sveningsen N, Marsal K. Respiratory distress syndrome in infants with impaired intrauterine growth. *Acta Paediatr* 1997;86:1090–6.
46. Snijders RJ, Abbas A, Melby O, *et al*. Fetal plasma erythropoietin concentrations in severe growth retardation. *Am J Obstet Gynecol* 1993;168:615–9.
47. Singh M, Singhal PK, Paul VK, *et al*. Polycythemia in the newborn: Do asymptomatic babies need exchange transfusion? *Indian Pediatr* 1990;27:61–5.
48. Pietersma AL, van der Stratten PJ, Van Haard PM, *et al*. Vitamin K_1 levels and K_1 dependent coagulation factors II and X in preterm and small for date neonates. *Eur J Pediatr* 1990;149:640–4.
49. Kupferminc MJ, Many A, Bar-Arm A, Lessing JB, Ascher-Landsberg J. Mid-trimester severe intrauterine growth restriction is associated with a high prevalence of trombophilia. *Br J Obstet Gynecol* 2002;109(12):1373–6.
50. Crouse DT, Cassady G. The small for gestational age infants. In Avery GB, Fletcher MA, McDonald MG, eds. *Neonatology*, 4th edn. Philadelphia, PA: JB Lippincott, 1994.
51. Morillas JM, Molto L, Robles R, *et al*. Lipoproteins in preterm and small-for-gestational-age infants during the first week of life. *Acta Paediatr* 1992;81:774–8.
52. Patel D, Kalhan S. Glycerol metabolism and triglyceride–fatty acid cycling in the human newborn: Effect of maternal diabetes and intrauterine growth retardation. *Pediatr Res* 1992;31:52–8.
53. Samaan NA, Schultz PN, Pham FK. Insulin growth factor II and nonsupressible insulin-like activity levels in newborns. *Am J Obstet Gynecol* 1990;163:1836–9.
54. Wang HS, Lim J, English J, *et al*. Serum levels of insulin-growth-factor-I and insulin-growth-factor-binding-protein-I in human umbilical cord serum at delivery: Relation to fetal weight. *J Endocrinol* 1991;129:459–64.
55. Verhaeghe J, Van Bree R, Van Herck E, *et al*. C-peptide, insulin-like growth factors I and II, and insulin-like growth factor binding protein-I in umbilical cord serum: Correlation with birth weight. *Am J Obstet Gynecol* 1993;169:89–97.
56. Vanhaesebrouck P, Kint J, Van Kets H, *et al*. Aminoterminal propeptide of type III procollagen in cord blood and amniotic fluid of high risk pregnancies: A biochemical approach to the dynamic assessment of deviant fetal growth. *Pediatr Res* 1994;36:71–6.
57. Chandra RK, Matsumura T. Ontogenic development of the immune system and effect of fetal growth retardation. *J Perinat Med* 1979;7:279–90.
58. Das US, Sysyn GD. Abnormal fetal growth: Intrauterine growth retardation, small for gestational age, large for gestational age. *Pediatr Clin North Am* 2004;51:639–54.
59. Balcazar H, Haas J. Classification schemes of small-for-gestational-age and type of intrauterine growth retardation and its implications to early neonatal mortality. *Early Hum Dev* 1990: 24:219–30.
60. Phelps DL, Brown DR, Tung B, *et al*. 28-day survival rates of 6676 neonates with birth weights of 1250 g or less. *Pediatrics* 1991; 87:7–17.
61. Piper JM, Xenakis EM, McFarland M, Elliott BD, Berkus MD, Langer O. Do growth-retarded premature infants have different rates of perinatal morbidity and mortality than appropriately grown premature infants? *Obstet Gynecol* 1996;87(2):169–74.
62. Bardin C, Zelkowith P, Papageorgiou A. Outcome of small-for-gestational age and appropriate-for-gestational age infants born before 27 weeks of gestation. *Pediatrics* 1997;100(2):E4.
63. Kilpatrick SJ, Jackson R, Croughan MS. Perinatal mortality in twins and singletons matched for gestational age and delivery at $\geq$ 30 weeks. *Am J Obstet Gynecol* 1996;174:66–71.
64. Cheung VY, Bocking AD, DaSilva OP. Preterm discordant twins: What birth weight difference is significant? *Am J Obstet Gynecol* 1995;1721:955–9.
65. Cohen SB, Elizur SE, Goldenberg M, *et al*. Outcome of twin pregnancies with extreme weight discordance. *Am J Perinatol* 2001;18(8):427–32.
66. Amaru RC, Bush MC, Berkowitz RL, Lapinski RH, Gaddipati S. Is discordant growth in twins an independent risk factor for adverse neonatal outcome?. *Obstet Gynecol* 2004;103(1):71–6.
67. Jacobs AR, Demissie K, Jain NJ, Kinzier WL. Birth weight discordance and adverse fetal and neonatal outcomes among triplets in the United States. *Obstet Gynecol* 2003;101(5, Pt 1):909–14.
68. Fithardinge PM, Steven EM. The small for date infant. I. Later growth patterns. *Pediatrics* 1972;49:671–5.

69. Farcourt R, Campbell S, Harvey D, Norman D. Follow-up study of small for date babies. *Br Med J* 1976;1:1421–84.
70. Wallis S, Harvey D. The consequences of being small for date at birth. *Ann Nestlé* 1982;40:30–42.
71. Davies PA, Davies JD. Very low birth weight and subsequent bad growth. *Lancet* 1970;2:1216–8.
72. Narbouton R. Lávenir des enfants atteints de RCIUR. *Med Infant* 1973;5:565–71.
73. Commey JOO, Fithardinge PM. Handicap in the preterm small-for-gestational-age infants. *J Pediatr* 1979;94:779–83.
74. Beck GJ, van den Berg BJ. The relationship of the rate of intrauterine growth of low birth weight infants to later growth. *J Pediatr* 1975;86:504–7.
75. Ounsted M. Postnatal growth of children who were SFD and LFD. *Dev Med Child Neurol* 1971;13:121–5.
76. Cruise MO. A longitudinal study of the growth of the low-birth-weight infants. I. Velocity and distance growth, birth to 3 years. *Pediatrics* 1973;511:620–8.
77. Beargie RA, James VL, Greene JW. Growth and development of small for date newborns. *Pediatr Clin North Am* 1970;17:159–70.
78. Wedgwood M, Holt KS. A longitudinal study of the dental and physical development of 2–3 year old children who were underweight at birth. *Biol Neonate* 1968;12:214–7.
79. Martell M, Falkner F, Bertolini LB. Early postnatal growth evaluation in full term, preterm and small for date infants. *Early Hum Dev* 1978;1:313–6.
80. Low JA, Galbraith RS, Muir D. Intrauterine growth retardation: A preliminary report of long term morbidity. *Am J Obstet Gynecol* 1978;130:534–7.
81. Piekkala P, Kero P, Sillanpää M, Erkkola R. The somatic growth of a regional birth cohort of 351 preterm infants during the first two years of life. *J Perinat Med* 1989;17:41–4.
82. Tenovuot A, Kero P, Piekkala P. Growth of 519 small for gestational age infants during the first two years of life. *Acta Paediatr Scand* 1987;76:636–40.
83. Lam B, Karlberg J, Yeungt CY. Incomplete catch-up growth in low birth weight Chinese infants in Hong Kong. *J Pediatr Child Health* 1995;31:428–34.
84. Chamberlain R, Davey A. Physical growth of twins, postmature and small for date children. *Arch Dis Child* 1975;50:437–10.
85. Davies DP, Beverley D. Changes in body proportions over the first year of life: Comparison between 'light for dates' and 'appropriate for dates' term infants. *Early Hum Dev* 1979;3:263–6.
86. Vohr BR, Oh W, Rosenfield AG. The preterm small for gestational age infants: A two year follow-up study. *Am J Obstet Gynecol* 1979;133:425–8.
87. Jaquet D, Lefer J, Tabone MD, *et al.* High serum leptin concentrations during catch-up growth of children born with intrauterine growth retardation. *J Clin Endocrinol Metab* 1999;84:1949–53.
88. Leger J, Limoni C, Collin D, *et al.* Prediction factors in the determination of final height in subjects born small for gestational age. *Pediatr Res* 1998;43:808–12.
89. Ong KL, Ahmed ML, Emmet PM, Preece MA, Dunger DB. Association between postnatal catch-up growth and obesity in childhood: Prospective cohort study. *Br Med J* 2000;320(7240):967–71.
90. Erikson J, Forsen T, Tuomilehto J, *et al.* Size at birth, childhood growth and obesity in adult life. *Int J Obes Relat Metab Disord* 2001;25:735–40.
91. Erikson J, Forsen T, Tuomilehto J, *et al.* Size at birth, fat-free mass and resting metabolic rate in adult life. *Horm Metab Res* 2002;34:72–6.
92. Walther FJ, Ramaekers LHJ. Growth in early childhood of newborns affected by disproportionate intrauterine growth retardation. *Acta Paediatr Scand* 1982;71:651–4.
93. Villar J, Belizan JM, Klein RE. Heterogeneous postnatal growth pattern of intrauterine growth retardation infants. *Am J Clin Nutr* 1982;35:860–5.
94. Villar J, Belizan JM, Spalding J, Klein RE. Postnatal growth of intrauterine growth retarded infants. *Early Hum Dev* 1982;6:265–8.
95. Smith DW, Tmog W, Dogers JE. Shifting linear growth during infancy: Illustration of generic factors in growth, fetal life through infancy. *J Pediatr* 1976;89:225–30.
96. Richter T, Lietz, R, Beyreiss K. Development of body weight and height of SGA infants to the degree of intrauterine retardation. *Kinderarztl Prax* 1991;59:341–5.
97. Ounsted M, Moar VA, Scott A. Proportionality of small for gestational age babies at birth, perinatal associations and postnatal sequelae. *Early Hum Dev* 1986;14:77–88.
98. Ounsted MK, Moar VA, Scott A. Children of deviant birthweight at the age of seven years: Health, handicap, size and developmental status. *Early Hum Dev* 1984;9:323–6.
99. Stanley OH, Spiedel BS. 'Catch-up' following severe intrauterine retardation of head growth. *Acta Pediatr Scand* 1985;13:583–6.
100. Babson SG, Kagas J. Preschool intelligence of undersized term infants. *Am J Dis Child* 1969;117:553–6.
101. Philip AGS. Term twins with discordant birth weights: Observations at birth and one year. *Acta Genet Med Gemellol* 1981;30:203–8.
102. Albersston-Wikland K, Wennergren G, Wennergren M, *et al.* Longitudinal follow-up of growth in children born SGA. *Acta Paediatr* 1993;82:438–43.
103. Ounsted M, Moar V, Scott A. Growth in the first year of life: Effects of sex and weight for gestational age at birth. *Dev Med Child Neurol* 1982;24:356–9.
104. Hack M, Schluchter M, Catar L, Rahman M, Cuttler L, Borawski E. Growth of very low weigth infant to age 20 years. *Pediatrics* 2003;(1, Pt 1):e30–8.
105. Karlberg J, Albertsson K. Growth in full-term SGA infants: From birth to final height. *Pediatr Res* 1995;381:733–9.
106. D'Ercole AJ, Underwood LE. Growth factors in fetal growth and development. In Novy MJ, Resjo JA, eds. *Fetal Endocrinology.* New York: Academic Press, 1981:155–65.
107. Colle E, Schiff D, Andrew J. Insulin responses during catch-up growth of infants who were small for gestational age. *Pediatrics* 1976;57:363–6.
108. Modesto Caballero C, Rodriguez Alarcon J, Aranguren G, *et al.* C-peptide in cord blood from macrosomatic and low birth weight for gestational age newborns. *Ann Esp Pediatr* 1993;39:29–32.
109. Marshall RN, Underwood, LE, Voina, SJ. Characterization of the insulin and somatomedin C-receptors in human placenta cell membranes. *J Clin Endocrinol Metabol* 1974;393:283–5.
110. Alberston-Wikland, K. Swedish Pediatric Study Group for Growth Hormone Therapy. Growth hormone secretion and growth hormone treatment in children with intrauterine growth retardation. *Acta Paediatr Scand* 1989;349:35–40.
111. Leger J, Czernichow P. Retard de croissance intraúterin. Pronostic statural et perspectives terapeutiques. *Presse Med* 1994;23:969–71.
112. de Zegher F, Albertsson-Wikland K, Wollmann HA, *et al.* Growth hormone treatment of short children born small for gestational age: Growth responses with continuous and discontinous regimens over 6 years. *J Clin Endocrinol Metab* 2000;85:2816–21.
113. Lee PA, Chernausek SD, Hokken-Koelega ACS, Czernichow P. International Small for Gestational Age Advisory Board Consensus Development Conference Statement: Management of short children born small for gestational age. *Pediatrics* 2003;111:1253–61.
114. Fitzhardinge PM, Steven EM. The small for date infant. II. Neurological and intellectual sequelae. *Pediatrics* 1972;50:50–4.
115. Allen MC. Developmental outcome and follow-up of the small-for-gestational-age infant. *Semin Perinatol* 1984;8:123–33.
116. Low JA, Galbraith RS, Muir D. Intrauterine growth retardation: A study of long term morbidity. *Am J Obstet Gynecol* 1982;142: 670–6.
117. Fitzhardinge PM, Inwood S. Long-term growth in small-for-dates children. *Acta Paediatr Scand* (Suppl) 1989;349:27–33.
118. Berg AT. Childhood neurological morbidity and its association with gestational age, intrauterine growth retardation and perinatal stress. *Pediatr Perinat Epidemiol* 1988;2:229–34.
119. Pena IC. The premature small-for-gestational-age infants during the first year of life: Comparison by birth weight and gestational age. *J Pediatr* 1988;113:1066–9.
120. Matalainen R. Neurodevelopmental screening of *in utero* growth retarded prematurely born children before school age. *Eur J Pediatr* 1987;146:453–5.
121. Vohr BR, Hack M. Developmental folow-up of low birth weight infants. *Pediatr Clin North Am,* 1982;29:1441–50.
122. Fredrikson WT, Brown JV. Gripping and Moro responses: Differences between small for gestational age and normal weight term newborns. *Early Hum Dev* 1980;4:69–72.
123. Spassov L, Curzi-Dascalova L, Clairambault J, *et al.* Heart rate and heart rate variability during sleep in SGA newborns. *Pediatr Res* 1994;35:500–5.
124. Kennaway DJ. Favtors influencing melatonin rhythmicity in humans. *J Clin Endocrinol Metab* 2000;81:1525–31.
125. Kennaway DJ, Flanagan DE, Moore VM, *et al.* The impact of fetal size and length of gestation on 6-sulphatoxymelatonin excretion in adult life. *J Pineal Res* 2001;30:188–92.
126. Curzi-Dascalova L, Peirano P, Christova E. Respiratory characteristics during sleep in healthy SGA newborns. *Pediatrics* 1996;97: 554–9.
127. Riese ML. Temperament prediction for neonate twins: Relation to size for gestational age in same-sex pairs. *Acta Genet Med Gemellol* 1992;41:123–35.

128. Riese ML. Size, gestational age and neonatal sleep variables: Behavioral indices of risk in full-term twins. *Acta Genet Med Gemellol* 1993;42:23–33.

129. Majnemer A, Rosenblatt B, Riley PS. Influence of gestational age, birth weight, and asphyxia on neonatal neurobehavioral performance. *Pediatr Neurol* 1993;9:181–6.

130. Van Kranen VH, Kingma H, Caberg HB, *et al.* Quality of spontaneous general movements in full term SGA and AGA newborn infants. *Neuropediatrics* 1994;25:145–53.

131. Jiang ZD, Wu YY, Zhen MS, *et al.* Development of early and late brainstem conduction time in normal and IUGR children. *Acta Pediatr Scand* 1991;80:494–9.

132. Gherpelli JL, Ferreira H, Costa HP. Neurological follow-up of SGA newborn infants. A study of risk factors related to prognosis at one year of age. *Arch Neuropsiquiatr* 1993;51:50–8.

133. Uvebrant P, Hagberg G. Intrauterine growth in children with cerebral palsy. *Acta Paediatr* 1992;81:407–12.

134. Pharoah POD, Cooke T, Rosembloom L, Cook RW. Effects of birth weight, gestational age, maternal obstetric history on birth prevalence of cerebral palsy. *Arch Dis Child* 1987;62:1035–40.

135. Hadders M, Touwen BC. Body measurements, neurological and behavioural development in six year old children born preterm and/or small for gestational age. *Early Hum Dev* 1990; 22:1–13.

136. Walther FJ, Ramaekers LHJ. Language development at the age of 3 years of infants malnourished *in utero*. *Neuropediatrics* 1982; 13:77–80.

137. Getz L, Dobson V, Luna B. Development of grating acuity, letter acuity and visual fields in SGA preterm infants. *Early Hum Dev* 1994:40:59–71.

138. Paine PA, Pasquali L, Spegiorin C. Appearance of visually directed prehensive related to gestational age and intrauterine growth. *J Genet Psychol* 1983;142:53–7.

139. Stanley OH, Fleming PJ, Morgant MH. Abnormal development of visual function following intrauterine growth retardation. *Early Hum Dev* 1989;19:87–91.

140. Als H, Tronick E, Adamson L, Brazelton TB. The behavior of the full term but underweight newborn infant. *Dev Med Child Neurol* 1976;18:590–5.

141. Michaelis R, Schulte FJ, Nolte R. Motor behavior of small-for-gestational-age newborn infants. *Pediatrics* 1970;76:208–13.

142. Low JA, Gallbraith RS, Muir D. Intrauterine growth retardation: A study of long-term morbidity. *Am J Obstet Gynecol* 1982;42: 670–3.

143. Walther FJ, Ramaekers LHJ. Developmental aspects of subacute fetal distress: Behavior problems and neurological dysfunction. *Early Hum Dev* 1982:6:1–8.

144. Schreuder AM, McDonnell M, Gaffney G, Johnson A, Hope PL Outcome at school age following antenatal detection of absent or reversed end diastolic flow velocity in the umbilical artery. *Arch Dis Child Fetal Neonatal* 2002;86:108–14.

145. Pryor JE. Physical and developmental status of preschool SGA children: A comparative study. *J Pediatr Child Health* 1992;28:162–7.

146. Pryor JE, Silva PA, Brooke M. Growth, development and behaviour in adolescents born SGA. *J Pediatr Child Health* 1995;31:403–7.

147. Roberton CMT, Etchest PC, Kyle JM. Eight-year school performance and growth of preterm, small-for-gestational-age infants: A comparative study with subjects matched for birth weight or for gestational age. *J Pediatr* 1990;116:19–23.

148. Leventhal JM, Berg A, Egerter SA. Is intrauterine growth retardation a risk factor for child abuse? *Pediatrics* 1987;79:515–8.

149. Miller HC, Hassanien K. Fetal malnutrition in white newborn infants: Maternal factors. *Pediatrics* 1973;52:5043–7.

150. Parkinson CE, Wallis S, Harvey D. School achievement and behaviour of children who were small for dates at birth. *Dev Med Child Neurol* 1981;23:41–50.

151. Smedler AC, Faxelius G, Bremme K, Lagerstrom M. Psychological development in children born with very low birth weight after severe intrauterine growth retardation: A 10 year follow-up study. *Acta Paediatr* 1991;81:197–203.

152. Larroque B, Bertrais S, Czernichow P, Léger J. School difficulties in 20-year-olds. Who were born small for gestational age at term in a regional cohort study. *Pediatrics* 2001;108(1):111–15.

153. Lagerstrom M, Bremme K, Eneroth P, Magnusson D. Behavior at 10 and 13 years of age for children with low birth weight. *Percept Mot Skills* 1990;71:579–94.

154. Lagerstrom M, Bremme K, Eneroth P, *et al.* WISC-test scores at the age of 10 for children born to women with risk pregnancies. *J Perinat Med* 1991;19:269–83.

155. Strauss RS. Adult functional outcome of those born small for gestational age. Twenty-six-year follow-up of the British Birth Cohort. *J Am Med Assoc* 2000;283:625–32.

156. Ozane SE, Fernandez-twinn D, Hales CN. Fetal growth and adult diseases. *Semin Perinatol* 2004;28(1):81–7.

157. Irving RJ, Belton NR, Elton RA, Walker BR. Adult cardiovascular risk factors in premature babies. *The Lancet* 2000;355:2135–6.

158. Eriksson JG, Forsen T, Tuomilehto J, Winter PD, Osmond C, Barker DJ. Catch-up growth in childhood and death from coronary hear disease: Longitudinal study. *Br Med J* 1999;318(7181):427–31.

159. Pinho Franco M, Nigro D, Fortes Zb, *et al.* Intrauterine undernutrition – renal and vascular origin of hypertension . *Cardiovasc Res* 2003;60(2):228–34.

160. Jackson JA, Wailoo MP, Thompson JR, Petersen SA. Early physiological development of infants with intrauterine growth retardation. *Arch Dis Child Fetal Neonatal* 2004;89:46–50.

161. Ibañez L, Ferrer A, Marcos MV, *et al.* Early puberty: Rapid progression and reduced final heigh in girls with low birth weight. *Pediatrics* 2000;106:1–3.

162. Sas T, se Waal W, Mulder P, *et al.* Growth hormone treatment in children with short stature born small for gestational age: Five years result of a randomized, double blind-response trial. *J Clin Endocrinol Metab* 1999;84:3064–70.

163. Anita CS, Hokken-Koèlega MD. *Best Pract Res Clin Endocrinol Metab* 2002;16(1):65–71.

164. McDade TW, Beck MA, Kuzawa C, Adair LS. Prenatal undernutrition, postnatal environments, and antibody response to vaccination in adolescence. *Am J Clin Nutr* 2001;74:543–8.

165. Hesselmar B, Dahlgren J, Wennergren G, Aberg N, Albertson-Wikland K. Born small for gestational age: Relation to future allergy and asthma. *Acta Paediatr* 2002;91:992–4.

124 Macrosomia: concept and epidemiology

E. Fabre, R. González de Agüero, J. L. de Agustín and A. Ezquerra

Introduction

The term macrosomia describes the condition of infants with birth weight of ≥4000 g, regardless of gestational age. Further subdivisions of macrosomia have been commonly used: mild macrosomia (4000–4499 g), very macrosomic (4500–4999 g) and extremely macrosomic (≥5000 g). However, other cutoff levels have also been used in the definition of the macrosomic fetus: birth weight of ≥4100 g[1], 4500 g[2] or 4536 g (10 lb).[3] Although weight is easy to determine, this criterion fails to reflect the influence of gestational age on birth weight.

Birth weight–gestational age tables are convenient methods to demonstrate the relationships between birth weight and perinatal outcome. The 10th and 90th percentiles of birth weight are common arbitrarily chosen limits of appropriate weight for gestational age (AGA). Large for gestational age (LGA) is defined as born with a weight ≥90th percentile for gestational age, and small-for-gestational age (SGA) as born with a weight < 10th percentile (Figure 124.1). However, because birth weights normal-for-gestational age may vary with geography and ethnicity, an infant that is LGA according to a set of normative data derived from one population may not meet the criteria derived from another population.

Although macrosomia has traditionally been defined on the basis of birth weight, not all macrosomic fetuses have the same anthropometric characteristics. It has long been recognized that the infant of a diabetic mother typically has a disproportionate increase in such insulin-sensitive tissues as adipose tissue, liver and muscle, but not in others such as bone, skull and brain, in which growth is relatively insulin insensitive.[4] In addition to differences in weight/length ratios, infants of diabetic mothers also differ in body composition and weight distribution from those of non-diabetic mothers. Fetal macrosomia in diabetes mellitus is characterized by organomegaly and increased adiposity and fetal muscle mass. Both fetuses and neonates of diabetic mothers have a significantly smaller head circumference than that of fetuses and neonates of gestational age-matched non-diabetic mothers,[5] but abdominal circumferences of LGA infants of diabetic mothers are significantly greater than those of LGA infants of non-diabetic mothers.[6] Among neonates weighing over 4000 g, the shoulder circumferences of infants of diabetic mothers were found to be significantly greater than those infants of non-diabetic mothers.[5] The disproportionate increase in the size of the abdomen and shoulders compared to the cranium contributes to the potential for traumatic vaginal delivery. The amount of subcutaneous fat present in the infant of a diabetic mother may be an indicator of the degree of glycemic control achieved during gestation.

Estimation of body composition, lean body mass and fat mass is a further anthropometric refinement in the assessment of growth. Lean body mass represents metabolically active tissue and is relatively stable *in utero* in relation to the alterations in the maternal metabolic milieu, while fetal fat mass accumulation may be more sensitive to factors that affect fetal growth.[7] In the normal-term neonate, lean body mass represents an average of 86% of total body weight and explains 83% of the variance in birth weight. In contrast, neonatal fat mass constitutes only 14% of birth weight but explains 46% of its variance.[8] Macrosomia in the fetus of a diabetic mother may represent the accumulation of excessive fetal fat as opposed to lean body mass.[9] Sparks[10] described a comparable rate of accretion of lean body mass in SGA, AGA and LGA fetuses but considerable variation in the accretion of fetal fat. Fat accretion in SGA fetuses is considerably less than in the AGA fetuses, which in turn is less than that of the LGA fetuses. Estimates of body composition, however, are rarely used to assess normal fetal growth, because of methodological difficulties. The ponderal index has been used as an estimate of the degree of obesity or thinness of an infant. Although birth weight is used in the derivation of the ponderal index, this explains only 22% of the variance in birth weight and correlates poorly with estimates of percentage body fat.[8]

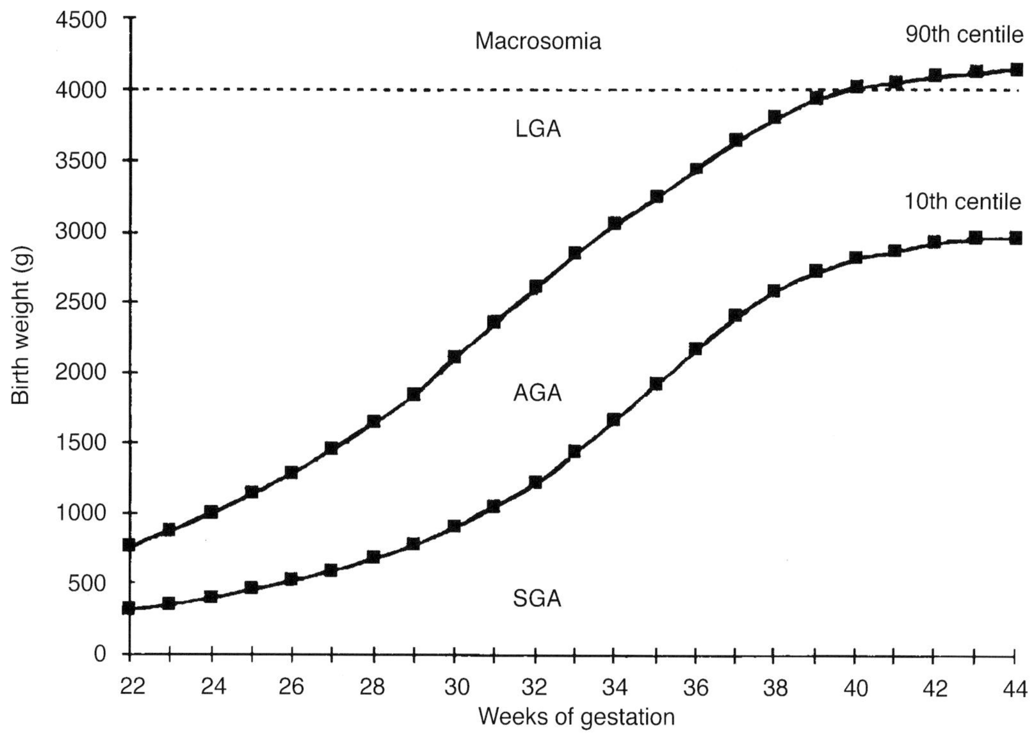

Figure 124.1 Increase in body weight of fetuses during the second half of gestation according to menstrual age. LGA, large; AGA, appropriate; and SGA, small-for-gestational age.

Epidemiology

Epidemiological factors

Women delivering macrosomic infants tend to be obese, tall, older and have increased parity.[11] It is also interesting that the macrosomic infant is more often male[12,13] (Table 124.1). Maternal factors that may predict macrosomia in the infant include previous history of macrosomia, obesity, prolonged pregnancy and diabetes mellitus.[2,13,14] Studies of pregestational and gestational diabetic women have demonstrated a similar relationship between macrosomic neonates and the aforementioned factors of risk.[15,16]

Fetal syndromes with genetics determination

There are different fetal syndromes which can determine a genetical growth acceleration. Their incidence is normally quite low. Most common ones are:

Beckwidth-Wiedemann syndrome, is characterized by a consistent set of symptoms including macroglossia, visceromegaly, macrosomia, umbilical hernia or omphalocele and neonatal hypoglycemia. Although most cases appear to be sporadic (85%), the etiology is generally accepted as genetic. Families with more than one affected relative have been reported, and linkage studies in these familial cases have located the gene on the short arm of chromosome 11 (11p15.5). This region contains the insulin-like growth factor, Type 2 (IGF2 gene), and the product of this gene is a major fetal growth factor.[17]

Nesiodioblastosis, autosomal recessive inheritance (11p15.1, 10q23.3, 7p15-p13), the main feature is a proliferation of beta pancreatic islets, producing hyperinsulinism and neonatal hypoglycemia.[18]

Sotos syndrome, in this syndrome, also called cerebral gigantism, babies are generally significantly larger and heavier than average, caused by excessive pre-natal and early post-natal growth. Characteristics include macrocephaly with accelerated bone maturation, delayed development and language problems, widely spaced eyes, prominent jaw, and high arched palate. Intelligence varies from normal to mild learning disability. Most cases are sporadic mutations. Once established, inheritance is autosomal dominant (5q35).[17]

Weaver syndrome, characterized by accelerated growth and advanced bone age (evident at birth), unusual craniofacial appearance, hoarse low-pitched cry, and hypertonia with camptodactyly, caused by mutations in a gene called NSD1 (5q35). The same gene is mutated in more than three-quarters of patients with another overgrowth disorder called Sotos syndrome.[17]

Nevo syndrome, Nevo syndrome is caused by mutation in the gene encoding lysyl hydroxylase and is therefore allelic with, or in the view of some, identical to, the kyphoscoliotic type of Ehlers Danlos

Table 124.1 Prevalence of macrosomia and odds ratios for selected factors (from Larsen *et al.*[13])

	Macrosomic infants (%)	Adjusted odds ratio (95% confidence interval)*
Body mass index		
≤25th	4.8	0.58 (0.55–0.62)
25th to <75th	8.1	l.00*
75th to <85th	10.8	1.34 (1.26–1.43)
85th to <95th	12.8	1.61 (l.52–170)
≥95th	17.0	2.15 (2.01–2.29)
Maternal height (quartiles)		
First	5.9	1.00*
Second	7.4	1.41 (1.32–1.52)
Third	9.3	1.93 (1.81–2.07)
Fourth	12.5	12.81 (2.63–3.01)
Maternal age (years)		
15–19	6.9	0.93 (0.88–0.99)
20–24	8.7	1.00*
25–29	10.3	1.09 (1.03–1.15)
≥30	13.5	1.33 (l.25–1.42)
Previous live births		
0	7.3	100*
1	8.8	1.25 (1.18–1.32)
2	10.3	1.41 (1.32–1.50)
≥3	12.0	1.54 (1.43–1.65)
Gestational age (weeks)		
37	3.9	0.38 (0.34–0.42)
38	5.1	0.49 (0.46–0.53)
39	7.1	0.69 (0.65–0.73)
40	10.1	1.00*
41	13.2	1.34 (1.26–1.41)
42	14.7	1.55 (1.45–1.66)
Sex of infant		
Male	11.2	1.00*
Female	6.7	0.52 (0.50–0.54)

*Multiple logistic regression with body mass index, height, ethnicity, smoking, maternal age, previous live births, gestational age and infant sex in the model

syndrome. Some of the characteristics are increased growth, kyphosis, prominent forehead, volar edema, spindle-shaped fingers, wrist drop, talipes, hyperbilirubinemia, generalized hypotonia and autosomal recessive inheritance (1p36.3–36.2).[17]

Congenital hyperinsulinism, is a clinically and genetically heterogeneous entity and causes severe hypoglycemia in neonates. The clinical heterogeneity is manifested by severity ranging from extremely severe, life-threatening disease to very mild clinical symptoms, which may even be difficult to identify. Most cases are caused by mutations in the cromosome 11p15 coding for either of the two subunits of the beta-cell. Recessive mutations of the beta-cell genes cause diffuse HI, whereas loss of heterozygosity together with inheritance of a paternal mutation causes focal adenomatous HI. Other cases are caused by mutations in gene coding for the beta-cell enzymes glucokinase (GK), glutamate dehydrogenase (GDH), and SCHAD.[19]

Maternal weight gain and prepregnancy weight

Maternal prepregnancy weight, as well as maternal weight gain during pregnancy, are directly related to birth weight. Underweight women tend to deliver infants with lower mean birth weights, and heavier women tend to deliver infants with higher mean birth weights.[20] A very important risk factor for macrosomic fetuses is maternal obesity.[3] Among women not selected on the basis of glucose intolerance, univariate analysis demonstrates a greater frequency of infant macrosomia among obese than among non-obese mothers.[21] After adjustment for factors known to be important predictors of birth weight, such as maternal age, smoking, race, height, parity, gestational age and infant gender, the odds of delivering a macrosomic infant are 2.2 times higher in severely overweight mothers than in those of normal weight[13] (Table 124.1). Among gestational diabetics, a positive association has also been demonstrated between birth weight and maternal prepregnancy body mass index, percentage ideal body weight and absolute weight.[22]

The evidence also indicates that women with large gestational weight gains are at increased risk for infants of high birth weight.[23] Low prenatal gain is associated with a more than doubled risk of SGA, and high prenatal gain gives a doubled risk of LGA.[24] Several studies have found a linear relationship between birth weight and maternal weight gain at all levels of prepregnancy weights,[25] whereas others have reported that, as prepregnancy weight increases, the importance of maternal weight gain diminishes.[26] Maternal weight gain significantly increases birth weight for women with body mass indices of ≤135% of the standard before pregnancy, with an equal effect in underweight and ideal-weight women and slightly less for moderately overweight women. However, weight gain during pregnancy has no significant effect on birth weight for very overweight women.[27] Compared to obese women who gained 7–11.5 kg, obese women who lose weight or do not gain weight are at higher risk for delivery of infants under 3000 g or SGA infants and those who gain more than 16 kg are at twice the risk for delivery of infants weighing 4000 g or more (Figure 124.2).[28] Nonetheless, obese women clearly have infants that are larger than those of non-obese women for the same weight gain.

Previous fetal macrosomia

The tendency to repeat increased birth weight in subsequent pregnancies is well accepted. Bakketeig and colleagues[29] found that the risk of an LGA infant was 48% in the second birth if the first was LGA, compared to a risk of 16% if the first birth was AGA. Infants with birth weight of ≥4500 g are 7.0 times more likely (95% confidence interval 5.4–9.1) to have a subsequent macrosomic sibling than are infants with smaller birth weight, after controlling for pregnancy smoking status, parity and gestational age. Race, maternal age or marital status and diabetes mellitus do not materially affect this relationship. The overall prevalence of macrosomic infants subsequent to previous macrosomic birth is 22%, a proportion that does not vary notably with parity, or when paternity changes between successive births. Mothers with one macrosomic infant are at marked risk for repeating macrosomic births.[30]

Post-term pregnancies

A recognized but often overlooked consequence of the prolonged pregnancy is fetal macrosomia. The post-date fetus should continue growing, although at a reduced rate, in the absence of uteroplacental insufficiency. Thus, an otherwise healthy fetus may become macrosomic with continuation of the pregnancy. Large, often macrosomic fetuses are more common in post-term pregnancies and predispose to dysfunctional labor, shoulder dystocia and operative deliveries. Boyd and coworkers[14] found a 16% incidence of macrosomic infants at 41 weeks' gestation and a 21% incidence at 42 weeks' gestation, both significantly increased when compared to the 8.2% incidence reported at less than 41 weeks' gestation. Similar results were reported by Arias,[31] who also found a 23.8% incidence of macrosomia in fetuses of more than 41 weeks' gestation. Figure 124.3 shows a continuous increase in the number of infants with birth weights of ≥4000 g for each week interval after 40 weeks' gestation. Usher and coworkers[32] reported that post-term fetuses are also more often macrosomic, with a birth weight of 4000 g or more in 23% of primiparas and 40% of multiparas at 42 weeks or later compared to 9% and 14%, respectively, at term. Chervenak and colleagues[33] reported an incidence of macrosomia at 42 weeks' gestation of 25.5%, significantly higher than 6% of macrosomic infants in the group of patients delivered between 38 and 40 weeks' gestation. In general, infants delivered at 42 weeks' gestation are three to seven times as likely to weigh more than 4000 g than those delivered before 41 complete weeks' gestation.

Diabetes mellitus

It is well known that infants born to diabetic mothers have an excessive size and weight at birth. Macrosomia has long been considered the hallmark of diabetic fetopathy. Maternal hyperglycemia induces fetal hyperglycemia, which in turn stimulates fetal endocrine pancreatic islets and insulin release; the persistent fetal hyperinsulinism promotes glucose uptake by fetal tissues and increases fetal growth, with resultant macrosomia.[34] The incidence of macrosomia in pregnancies complicated by diabetes is more than twice that for non-diabetic women.[14] Diabetes is more frequently

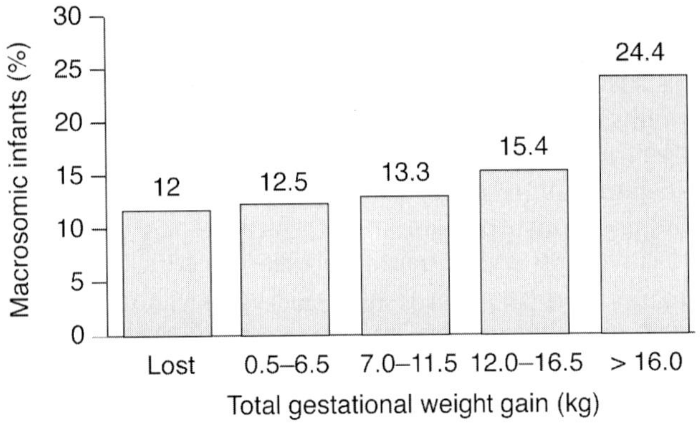

Figure 124.2 Incidence of macrosomia by total gestational weight gain in obese women. Data from Edwards *et al.*[28]

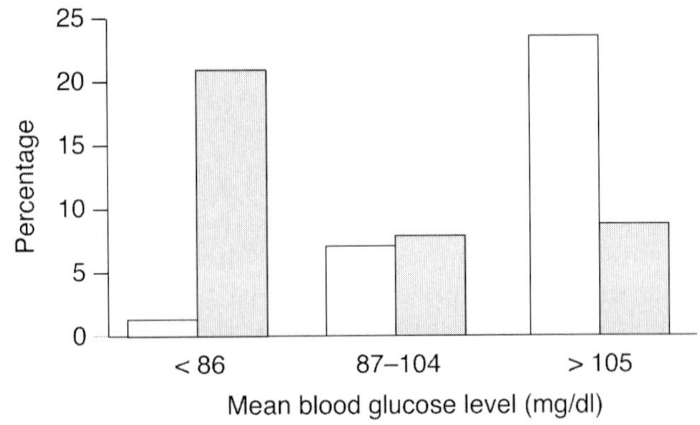

Figure 124.4 Association between neonatal size and level of glycemic control in gestational diabetes. Open bars, large; and shaded bars, small-for-gestational age. Modified from Langer *et al.*[39]

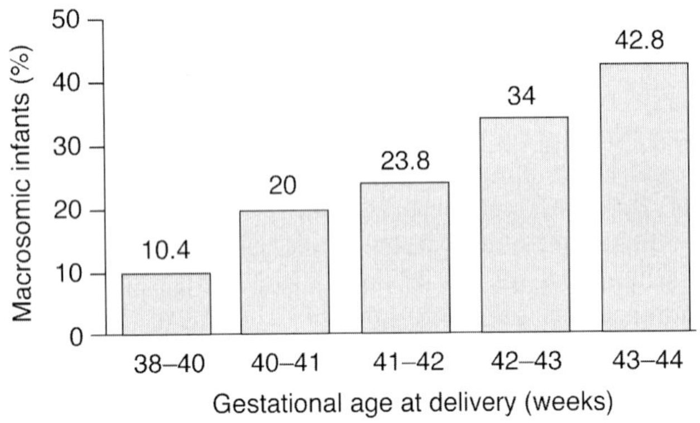

Figure 124.3 Incidence of macrosomia by gestational age at delivery. Data from Arias.[31]

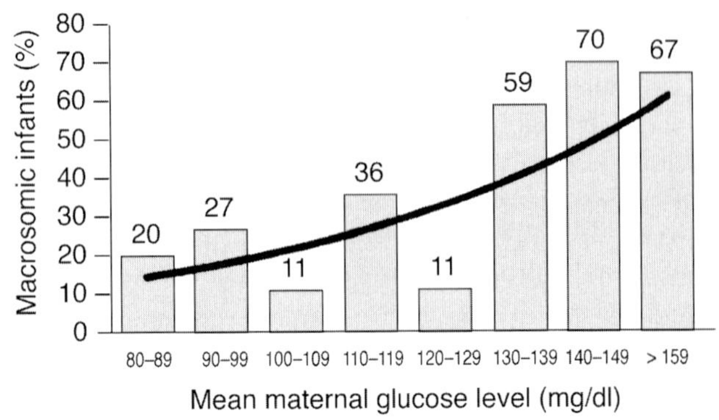

Figure 124.5 Incidence of macrosomia in relation to mean maternal glucose level. Data from Willman *et al.*[40]

present among mothers of infants whose birth weights exceed 4000 g than among those with lower birthweights.[3,14] However, when the gestational age is controlled, LGA infants are born with equal frequency to diabetic and non-diabetic mothers.[35] Inconsistencies in these findings may be explained by the influence of factors other than maternal diabetes on birth weight.[22]

In recent years tight glycemic control became a standard of care in the management of the pregnant diabetic in order to reduce perinatal mortality and morbidity. This resulted in the reduction of perinatal mortality to rates comparable to those observed in the normal population. In contrast, the incidence of perinatal morbidity as reflected by metabolic disorders and macrosomia remains relatively high. Although maternal hyperglycemia is clearly a factor implicated in the development of macrosomia, the evidence is often conflicting. Several investigators[36] have reported an association between maternal glucose control and macrosomia, but others have not been able to substantiate this finding.[37] Fetal growth appears to be affected by many factors in addition to maternal glucose levels. In non-diabetic women, maternal factors that have been shown to be related to macrosomia include parity, maternal size, weight gain and prolonged pregnancy.[14] Other determinants of birth weight that have been linked to excessive fetal size in non-diabetic women include fetal sex, history of a large infant and race.[38]

In a large study of patients with gestational diabetes, the relationship was examined between optimal levels of glycemic control and perinatal outcome (334 gestational diabetic women and 334 subjects matched for control obesity, race and parity).[39] Three groups were identified on the basis of mean glucose level throughout pregnancy. In the group with high levels (≥105 mg/dl) the incidence of LGA infants was approximately twofold higher than in the control group. Also, the incidence of LGA infants was 21-fold higher in the group with high mean blood glucose levels than in the group with low mean blood glucose levels (≤86 mg/dl), and fourfold higher than in the group with intermediate mean blood glucose levels (87–104 mg/d1). No significant difference was found between the control and the mean blood glucose category of 87–104 mg/dl in the incidence of SGA or LGA infants (Figure 124.4). Willman and colleagues[40] reported that there is a non-linear relationship between maternal glucose concentration and excessive fetal growth and that the incidence of macrosomia is not consistently increased until the mean glucose concentration is equal to or higher than 130 mg/dl (Figure 124.5). Also, the results of this study indicate that macrosomia among diabetic women is multifactorial in origin and not singularly the consequence of maternal hyperglycemia. Specifically, maternal obesity, maternal insulin requirements (which reflect greater insulin resistance and greater abnormality of fatty acid and lipid metabolism), maternal glucose level and history of a large infant are associated with fetal macrosomia. Therefore, factors known to be associated with excessive fetal size in non-diabetic women must also be considered when women with well-controlled diabetes inexplicably give birth to macrosomic infants.

In some studies of the relationship between maternal glucose concentrations and fetal macrosomia, there is an implicit assumption that the risk of the latter exists only for those who equal or exceed the threshold values defining gestational diabetes on a glucose tolerance test (GTT). However, this is probably not the case, as is suggested by a demonstrated risk of macrosomia among women exhibiting lesser degrees of glucose intolerance. In infants of women with diabetes, macrosomia is thought to occur because of fetal hyperinsulinemia due to maternal hyperglycemia. The same hypothesis has been used to explain the increase in neonatal birth weight found in studies of pregnant women with minor degrees of glucose intolerance. The exact degree of maternal glucose intolerance associated with fetal macrosomia is not well defined. As any criteria for the diagnosis of diabetes are arbitrary, their use lies in their clinical value. One may question whether the results of currently used screening tests accurately predict the patient's risk for fetal overgrowth.

The relationship between maternal glucose concentrations and fetal macrosomia has been explored in several publications. Some have failed to demonstrate any significant relationship. Others have found a positive relationship between maternal glucose levels and fetal macrosomia. One of these reports showed that patients who had elevated 1-h glucose screening test values and normal GTT (group study) results delivered macrosomic neonates (11.9%) significantly more often than those having normal glucose screens (6.4%). When the data were corrected for other macrosomia risk factors (advanced age, high parity, obesity, race and prolonged gestation) there was still a significantly higher frequency of macrosomia in the study group.[41] Another report demonstrated a trend of increasing birth weight with increasing 1-h glucose screening test values.[42] Women who have only one elevated value on a GTT have macrosomic neonates significantly more often (18.0%) than those having normal glucose screens (6.6%) (odds ratio 2.28; 95% CI 1.77–5.37), a relationship that persisted after controlling for risk factors.[43] The incidence of neonatal macrosomia in infants of mothers who had only one abnormal value in a 3-h GTT (20%) was greater than in those of normal values (12.4%); however, after adjustment for gestational age, there were no differences in birth weight and LGA percentage.[44]

Apart from glucose, many others factors are involved in fetal growth. Recently many studies have shown the correlation of blood cord levels of insulin-like growth factors (IGFs), IGF binding proteins (IGFBPs), leptin, and interleukin-6 (IL-6) with intrauterine growth.[45–47]

Incidence and perinatal mortality

In general, infants weighing more than 4000 g account for almost 10% of deliveries, while those of 4500 g or more account for about 1% of all deliveries.[3] The Spanish Perinatal Mortality Survey of the Perinatal Medicine Section of the Spanish Obstetrical and Gynecological Society recorded data of 597,585 births at hospital – with known birth weight and gestational age – in different Spanish regions from 1980 to 1992.[48] In the period surveyed, the incidence of infants weighing more than 4000 g was 6.7%, and 0.8% of infants weighed more than 4500 g. This is similar to the published rates of macrosomia. In a revision of 10 studies published from 1931 to 1980, the incidence of fetal macrosomia (≥4500 g) was between 0.6 and 1.9%.[3] Recent stastistics from the European Union show a significant variation in percentages of higher birth weights. In some countries like Denmark or Sweden, babies weighing more than 4500 g account for more than 4%, in others like France, Greece, Portugal or Luxembourg, the average is less than 1% of total live births.[49] Data obtained from the Center of Disease Control in the United States show a progressive decrease of the incidence of macrosomia, from 10.2% in 1996 to 9.2% in 2002 for babies over 4000g at birth (Tables 124.3 and 124.4).[49–51] Few epidemiological reports exist on the tendency over time regarding fetal macrosomia incidence. In the Spanish Perinatal Mortality Survey the macrosomic rate has decreased over recent years. From 1980 to 1992 the incidence of large infants (≥4000 g) diminished from 8.6% to 5.8%, and the incidence of infants weighing more than 4500 g decreased from 1.0% to 0.6% (Table 124.2). The incidence of infants weighing more than 5000 g remained stable, at round 0.1%.

The association of fetal growth abnormalities with perinatal morbidity and mortality is of interest to both obstetricians and neonatologists. The few studies of fetal overgrowth have shown that perinatal mortality plotted against birth weight follows a U-shaped distribution, even when controlled for the length of gestation. Perinatal mortality increases at the extremes of birth weight at each gestational age (Figure 124.6). Table 124.2 shows the mortality rates during the perinatal period in macrosomic fetuses. In the whole period surveyed, the fetal mortality rate in fetuses weighing more than 4000 g was very similar to that observed in fetuses weighing between 2500 and 3999 g (3.2 vs. 2.8/1000 births). A similar result was observed in the early neonatal mortality rate (1.5 vs. 1.6/1000 live births) and perinatal mortality rate (4.8 vs. 4.4/1000 births). However, when the mortality rates during the perinatal period between those born weighing over 4500 g and

Table 124.2 Trends in the incidence, fetal mortality, early neonatal mortality and perinatal* mortality rates in fetal macrosomia from 1980 to 1992 (Spanish Perinatal Mortality Survey of the Perinatal Medicine Section of the Spanish Obstetrical and Gynecological Society)

Birth weight (g) Incidence (%)	1980	1983	1986	1989	1992	Overall
≥4000	8.6	6.5	6.8	6.3	5.8	6.7
≥4500	1.0	0.8	0.8	0.7	0.6	0.8
Fetal mortality rate (%)						
2500–3999	3.1	3.0	2.8	2.7	2.3	2.8
≥4000	3.9	5.4	1.8	2.9	2.0	3.2
≥4500	9.2	8.2	8.1	7.4	6.6	7.8
Early neonatal mortality rate (%)						
2500–3999	2.4	1.5	1.7	1.4	1.4	1.6
≥4000	2.5	1.4	2.0	0.8	0.7	1.5
≥4500	6.2	5.5	5.6	4.7	3.9	5.1
Perinatal* mortality rate (%)						
2500–3999	5.5	4.5	4.5	4.1	3.6	4.4
≥4000	6.5	6.8	3.8	3.7	2.7	4.8
≥4500	15.4	13.6	13.6	12.0	10.4	12.9

*'Perinatal' includes fetal and early neonatal

Table 124.3 Live births > 4500 g in Europe from Simone Buitendijk *et al.*[49]

Member state	Data Source	> 4500gr (%)
Austria	A1- 2001	1.08
Belgium (Flanders)	B2- 2000	0.95
Belgium (French community)	B3- 2000	1.75
Denmark	DK1- 2000	4.20
Finland	FIN1- 2000	3.30
France (perinatal survey)	F1- 1998	0.81
Germany	D2- 1999	1.64
Greece (perinatal survey)	EL1- 1998	0.80
Ireland	IR1- 1999	3.00
Italy	I1- 1998	2.61
Luxemburg	L2- 2000	0.79
The Netherlands	NL1- 1999	2.31
Portugal	P1- 1999	0.74
Spain (Madrid, Valencia, País Vasco)	EL2- 2000	n/a
Sweden	S1- 2000	4.26
UK	UK1,6,7- 2000	1.75

Table 124.4 Prevalence of macrosomia in the United States (National Vital Statistics Report from Suneet *et al*.[50]

Variable	2002 (n)	2001 (n)	2000 (n)	1999 (n)	1998 (n)	1997 (n)	1996 (n)	P value
Total births	4,021,726	4,025,933	4,058,814	3,959,417	3,941,553	3,880,894	3,891,494	
Macrosomia	368,184 (9.2%)	378,976 (9.4%)	401,340 (9.9%)	392,683 (9.9%)	396,096 (10.1%)	390,071 (10.1%)	398,340 (10.2%)	<.0001
4000-4499 g	314,182 (7.8%)	322,346 (8.0%)	340,384 (8.4%)	332,863 (8.4%)	330,894 (8.5%)	330,894 (8.5%)	336,514 (8.6%)	< .0001
4500-4999 g	48,606 (1.2%)	51,132 (1.3%)	54,748 (1.3%)	53,751 (1.4%)	53,936 (1.4%)	53,936 (1.4%)	55,558 (1.4%)	<.0001
≥5000 g	5396 (0.1%)	5498 (0.1%)	6208 (0.2%)	6069 (0.2%)	5941 (0.2%)	5941 (0.2%)	6268 (0.2%)	< .0001

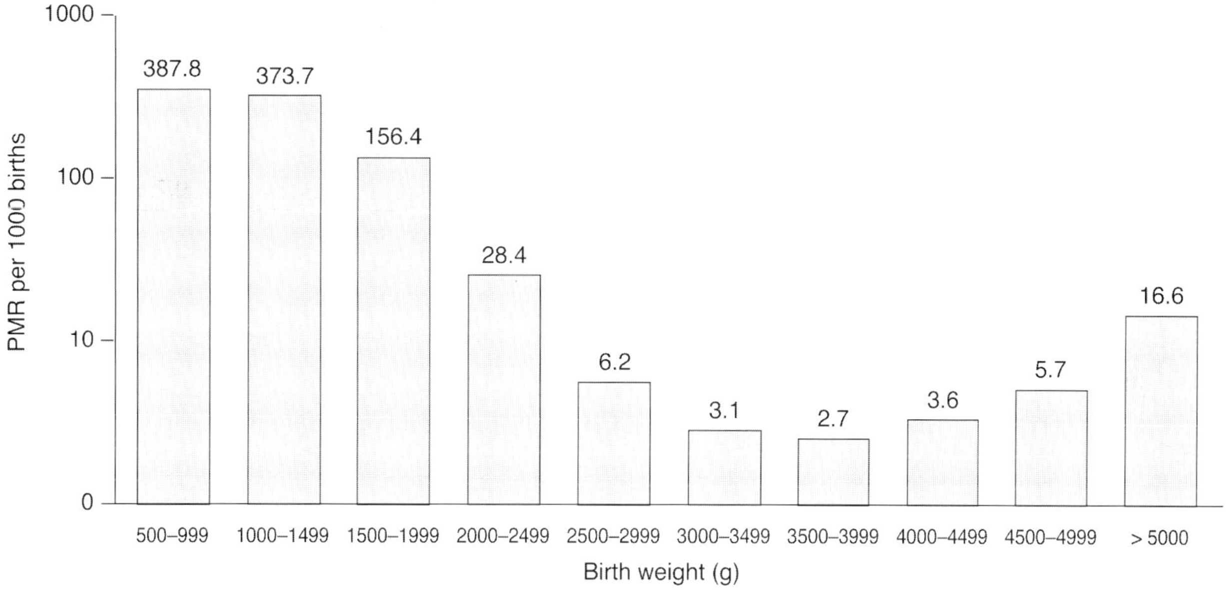

Figure 124.6 Perinatal mortality rate (PMR) for birth weight groups in those born at term (37–41 weeks' gestation) from the Spanish Perinatal Mortality Survey of the Perinatal Medicine Section of the Spanish Obstetrical and Gynecological Society from 1980 to 1992.

those born weighing in the range 2500–3999 g are compared, it is observed that fetal mortality rate is 2.8 times higher (7.8 vs. 2.8/1000 births), early neonatal mortality rate is 3.2 times higher (5.1 vs. 1.6/1000 live births) and perinatal mortality rate is 2.9 times higher (12.9 vs. 4.4/1000 births). The prognosis for the very large fetus, although substantially improved in recent years, remains less than desirable. From 1980 to 1992 in those born weighing more than 4500 g, the fetal mortality rate diminished from 9.2 to 6.6/1000 births, the early neonatal mortality rate from 6.2 to 3.9/1000 live births and the perinatal mortality rate from 15.4 to 10.4/1000 births. In other studies, a full-term infant weighing more than 4500 g was shown to have a risk of mortality three to four times higher than an infant of average birth weight.[52]

It is important to recognize the relatively high incidence of macrosomia, because of the complications associated with this condition. These include increased maternal and fetal trauma, shoulder dystocia resulting in Erb's palsy, perinatal asphyxia, meconium aspiration, increased rate of labor disorders, operative delivery and postpartum hemorrhage.[3] The incidence of shoulder dystocia directly relates to increasing fetal size. The overall incidence of shoulder dystocia varies between 8% and 10% with fetal weights of 4000–5000 g and is as high as 20–30% with fetal weights of more than 4500 g.[53] The risk of shoulder dystocia for LGA newborn (>4000 g) is 1.6% (OR = 22.3; 95% CI 16.7–29.8; P <0.001). The presence of maternal diabetes also increase the risk until 0.6% (OR = 2.8; 95% CI 2.0–4.0; P <0.001). Combining risk factors such as LGA, diabetes mellitus and vacuum delivery increased the risk for shoulder dystocia to 6.8% (OR = 32.6; 95% CI 10.1–105.8; P <0.001) (Figure 124.7).[54] Among infants of diabetic mothers, over two-thirds of shoulder dystocia cases occur in those weighing 4000 g or more.[55] Neonates experiencing shoulder dystocia have significantly greater shoulder-to-head and chest-to-head disproportions than do macrosomic neonates delivered without shoulder dystocia.[5] Fetal injuries, ranging from brachial plexus injuries to clavicular and humeral

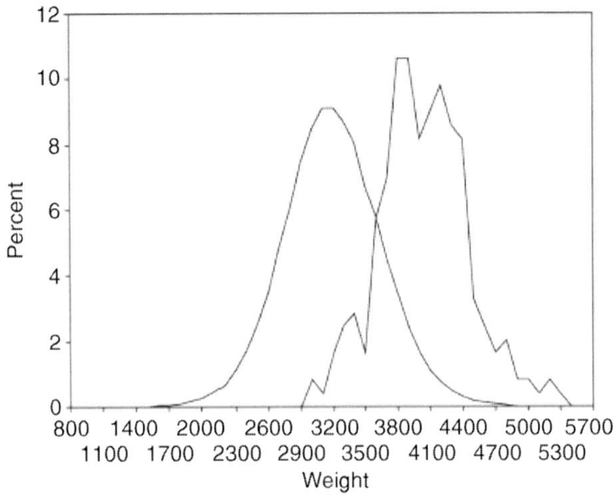

Figure 124.7 Birth-weight distribution among patients with shoulder dystocia (right curve; mean 4081.5 ± 416.1) and without shoulder dystocia (left curve; mean 3240.6 ± 449.2) from Sheiner *et al.*[54]

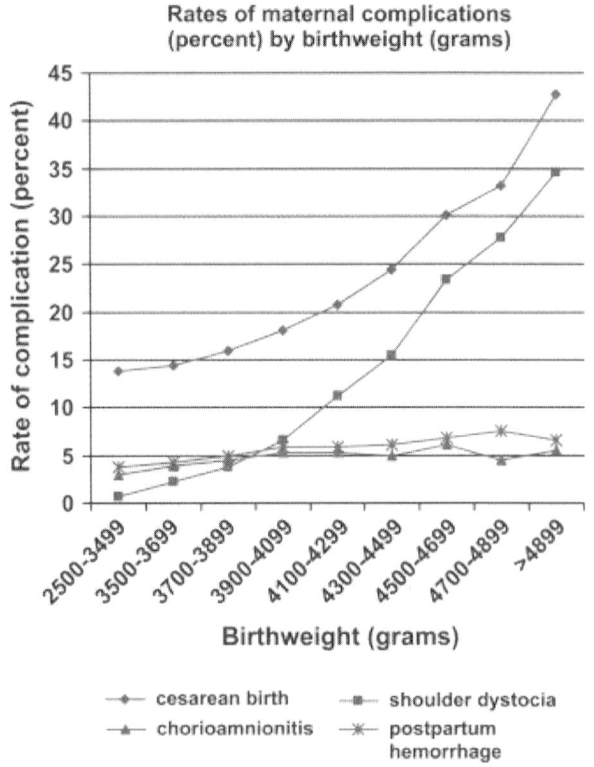

Figure 124.8 Rates of maternal complications (percent) by birth weight (g) from Stotland *et al.*[62]

fractures, are recognized complications of shoulder dystocia. However, most of these injuries appear to be transient, and permanent neurological injury or true asphyxia is uncommon. The management of large-for-date fetuses must be based not only on the estimated fetal weight, but also on functional criteria, and the mode of delivery will depend on a balance being struck between fetal and material risk, and the wishes of the parents.[56–61]

Several investigators have advocated for routine cesarean delivery when the fetus reaches a "macrosomic" weight, although there has been no consensus on what that weight should be. Benedetti and Gabbe[63], for example, considered an infant to be macrosomic when it was in excess of 4000 g, given the significantly increased risk of shoulder dystocia in this group. Alternatively, some investigators have suggested that the most appropriate fetal weight indication for cesarean delivery should be 4500 g, although others, such as ACOG (level C evidence), have recommended 5000 g.[64] But nowadays, among uncomplicated pregnancies, there is sufficient evidence that suspected macrosomia is not an indication for induction or for primary cesarean delivery. For pregnancies complicated by diabetes, with a prior cesarean delivery or shoulder dystocia, delivery of a macrosomic fetus increases the rate of complications, but there is insufficient evidence about the threshold of estimated fetal weight that should prompt cesarean delivery (Figure 124.8).[62–65]

REFERENCES

1. Golditch IM, Kirkman K. The large fetus: management and outcome. *Obstet Gynecol* 1978;52:26–30.
2. Spellacy WN, Miller S, Winegar A, Peterson PQ. Macrosomia – maternal characteristics and infant complications. *Obstet Gynecol* 1985;66:158–61.
3. Modanlou HD, Dorchester WI, Thorosian A, Freeman RK. Macrosomia – maternal, fetal and neonatal implications. *Obstet Gynecol* 1980;55:420–4.
4. Naeye RL. Infants of diabetic mothers: A quantitative, morphologic study. *Pediatrics* 1965;35:980–8.
5. Mondalou HD, Komatsu G, Dorchester W, *et al.* Large-for-gestational-age neonates: Anthropometric reasons for shoulder dystocia. *Obstet Gynecol* 1982;60:417–23.
6. Langer O, Koslowski S, Brustan L. Abnormal growth patterns in diabetes in pregnancy. *Isr J Med Sci* 1991;27:516–23.
7. Miller AT, Blyth CS. Lean body mass as a reference standard. *J Appl Physiol* 1953;5:311–16.
8. Catalano PM, Tyzbir ED, Allen SR, *et al.* Evaluation of fetal growth by estimation of neonatal body composition. *Obstet Gynecol* 1992;79:46–50.
9. Fee BA, Weil WB. Body composition of infants of diabetic mothers by direct analysis. *Ann N Y Acad Sci* 1963;110:869–97.
10. Sparks JW. Human intrauterine growth and accretion. *Semin Perinatol* 1984;8:74–93.
11. Carmona F, Cararach V. Concepto y etiopatogenia de la macrosomia fetal. In Carrera JM, ed. *Crecimiento fetal normal y patológico.* Barcelona: Masson SA, 1997:509–17.
12. Brunskill AJ, Rossing MA, Connell FA, Dalling J. Antecedents of macrosomia. *Pediatr Perinat Epidemiol* 1991;5:392–401.
13. Larsen CE, Serdula MK, Sullivan KM. Macrosomia: Influence of maternal overweight among a low-income population. *Am J Obstet Gynecol* 1990;162:490–4.
14. Boyd ME, Usher RH, McLean FH. Fetal macrosomia: Prediction, risks, proposed management. *Obstet Gynecol* 1983;61:715–22.
15. Fraser D, Weitzman S, Leiberman JR, Eschwege E. Factors influencing birth weight in newborns of diabetic and non-diabetic women. A population based study. *Eur J Epidemiol* 1990;6:427–31.
16. Phillipou G. Relationship between normal oral glucose tolerance test in women at risk for gestational diabetes and large for gestational age infants. *Diabetes Care* 1991;14:1092–7.

17. McKusick VA. Mendelian inheritance in man. Catalog of Autosomal Dominant, Autosomal Recesive and X-linked Phenotipes. 10ª ed. London: Johns Hopkins University; 1992.
18. Langer O. Macrosomía fetal: Factores causales. *Clínicas Obstet Ginecol* 2000; 2:263–75.
19. Fournet JC, Junien C. Genetics of congenital hyperinsulinism. *Endocr Pathol* 2004 Fall;15(3):233–40.
20. González de Agüero R, Fabre E, Sobreviela M. Efecto de la dieta materna sobre el crecimiento fetal. In Carrera JM, ed. *Crecimiento fetal normal y patólogico*. Barcelona: Masson SA, 1997:509–17.
21. Wolfe HM, Zador IE, Gross TL, *et al.* The clinical utility of maternal body mass index in pregnancy. *Am J Obstet Gynecol* 1991; 164:1306–10.
22. Sacks DA. Fetal macrosomia and gestational diabetes: what's the problem? *Obstet Gynecol* 1993;81:775–81
23. Ounsted M, Scott A. Associations between maternal weight, height, weight-for-height, weight-gain and birth weight. In Dobbing J, ed. *Maternal Nutrition in Pregnancy: Eating for Two?* London: Academic Press, 1981:113–29.
24. Parker JD, Abrams B. Prenatal weight gain advice: An examination of the recent prenatal weight gain recommendations of the Institute of Medicine. *Obstet Gynecol* 1992;79:664–9.
25. Luke B, Dickinson C, Petrie RH. Intrauterine growth: Correlations of maternal nutritional status and rate of gestational weight gain. *Eur J Obstet Gynecol Reprod Biol* 1981;12:113–21.
26. Winikoff B, Debrovner CH. Anthropometric determinants of birth weight. *Obstet Gynecol* 1981;58:678–84.
27. Abrams BF, Laros RK. Prepregnancy weight, weight gain, and birth weight. *Am J Obstet Gynecol* 1986;154:503–9.
28. Edwards LE, Hellerstedt WL, Alton IR, *et al.* Pregnancy complications and birth outcomes in obese and normal-weight women: Effects of gestational weight change. *Obstet Gynecol* 1996;87: 389–94.
29. Bakketeig LS, Hoffman HJ, Harley EE. The tendency to repeat gestational age and birth weight in successive births. *Am J Obstet Gynecol* 1979;135:1086–1103.
30. Davis R, Woelk G, Mueller BA, Daling J. The role of previous birthweight on risk for macrosomia in a subsequent birth. *Epidemiology* 1995;6:607–11.
31. Arias F. Predictability of complications associated with prolongation of pregnancy. *Obstet Gynecol* 1987;70:101–6.
32. Usher RH, Boyd ME, McLean FH, Kramer MS. Assessment of fetal risk in postdate pregnancies. *Am J Obstet Gynecol* 1988;158: 259 61.
33. Chervenak JL, Divon MY, Hirsch J, *et al.* Macrosomia in the postdate pregnancy: Is routine ultrasonographic screening indicated? *Am J Obstet Gynecol* 1989;161:753–6.
34. Perdersen J. Weight and length at birth of infants of diabetic mothers. *Acta Endocrinol* 1954;16:330–42.
35. Norlander E, Hanson U, Persson B. Factors influencing neonatal morbidity in gestational diabetic pregnancy. *Br J Obstet Gynaecol* 1989;96:671–8.
36. Jovanovic R, Jovanovic L. Obstetric management when normoglycemia is maintained in diabetic pregnant women with vascular compromise. *Am J Obstet Gynecol* 1984;149:617–23.
37. Miller JM. A reappraisal of 'tight control' in diabetic pregnancies. *Am J Obstet Gynecol* 1983;147:158–62.
38. Dougherty CRS, Jones AD. The determinants of birth weight. *Am J Obstet Gynecol* 1982;144:190–200.
39. Langer O, Levy J, Brustman L, *et al.* Glycemic control in gestational diabetes mellitus – how tight is tight enough: Small for gestational age versus large for gestational age? *Am J Obstet Gynecol* 1989;161:646–53.
40. Willman SP, Leveno KJ, Guzick DS, *et al.* Glucose threshold for macrosomia in pregnancy complicated by diabetes. *Am J Obstet Gynecol* 1986;154:470–5.
41. Leikin EL, Jenkins JM, Pomerantz GA, Klein L. Abnormal glucose screening test in pregnancy: A risk factor for fetal macrosomia. *Obstet Gynecol* 1987;69:570–3.
42. Green JR, Schumacher LB, Pawson IG, *et al.* Influence of maternal body habitus and glucose tolerance on birth weight. *Obstet Gynecol* 1991;78:235–40.
43. Lindsay MK, Graves W, Klein L. The relationship of one glucose tolerance test value and pregnancy complications. *Obstet Gynecol* 1989;73:103–6.
44. Kaufmann RC, McBride P, Amankwah KS, Huffman DG. The effect of minor degrees of glucose intolerance on the incidence of neonatal macrosomia. *Obstet Gynecol* 1992;80:97–101.
45. Lo HC, Tsao LY, Hsu WY, *et al.* Relation of cord serum levels of growth hormone, insulin-like growth factors, insulin-like growth factor binding proteins, leptin, and interleukin-6 with birth weight, birth length, and head circumference in term and preterm neonates. *Nutrition* 2002 Jul-Aug;18(7–8):604–8.
46. Vatten LJ, Nilsen ST, Odegard RA, *et al.* Insulin-like growth factor I and leptin in umbilical cord plasma and infant birth size at term. *Pediatrics* 2002 Jun;109(6):1131–5.
47. Ong KK, Ahmed ML, Sherriff A, *et al.* Cord blood leptin is associated with size at birth and predicts infancy weight gain in humans. ALSPAC Study Team. Avon Longitudinal Study of Pregnancy and Childhood. *J Clin Endocrinol Metab* 1999 Mar;84(3):1145–8.
48. Fabre E, González de Agüero, de Agustin JL, *et al.* Perinatal mortality in term and post-term births. *J Perinat Med* 1996;24:163–9.
49. Buitendijk S, Zeitlin J, Cuttini M, *et al.* Indicators of fetal and infant health outcomes. European Journal of Obstetrics & Gynecology and Reproductive Biology, Volume 111, Supplement 1, 28 November 2003, pp. S66–S77.
50. Chauhan SP, Grobman WA, Gherman RA, *et al.* Suspicion and treatment of the macrosomic fetus: A review. American Journal of Obstetrics and Gynecology. Volume 193, Issue 2, August 2005, pp. 332–46.
51. National Center for Health Statistics. *Advanced Report of Final Natality Statistics, 1992.* Monthly Vital Statistics Report, vol. 43, No. 5. Hyattsville, MD: Public Health Service, 1994.
52. Williams RL, Creasy RK, Cunningham GC, *et al.* Fetal growth and perinatal viability in California. *Obstet Gynecol* 1982;59:624–32.
53. Lipscomb KM, Gregory K, Shwan K. The outcome of macrosomic infants weighing at least ≥4500 grams: Los Angeles county + University of Southern California experience. *Obstet Gynecol* 1995; 85:558–64.
54. Sheiner E, Levy A, Hershkovitz R, *et al.* Determining factors associated with shoulder dystocia: a population-based study. European Journal of Obstetrics & Gynecology and Reproductive Biology, In Press, Corrected Proof, Available online 14 October 2004.
55. Langer O, Berkus MD, Huff RW, Samueloff A. Shoulder dystocia: Should the fetus weighing ≥4000 grams be delivered by Cesarean section? *Am J Obstet Gynecol* 1991;165:831–7.
56. Mulik V, Usha Kiran TS, Bethal J, *et al.* The outcome of macrosomic fetuses in a low risk primigravid population. *Int J Gynaecol Obstet* 2003 80:15–22
57. Sanchez-Ramos L, Bernstein S, Kaunitz AM. Expectant management versus labor induction for suspected fetal macrosomia: A systematic review. *Obstet Gynecol* 2002;100:997–1002.
58. Gilby JR, Williams MC, Spellacy WN. Fetal abdominal circumference measurements of 35 and 38 cm as predictors of macrosomia. A risk factor for shoulder dystocia. *J Reprod Med* 2000;45:936–8.
59. Wong SF, Chan FY, Cincotta RB, *et al.* Sonographic estimation of fetal weight in macrosomic fetuses: Diabetic versus non-diabetic pregnancies. *Aust NZ J Obstet Gynaecol* 2001;41:429–132.
60. Best G. Pressman, EK. Ultrasonographic prediction of birth weight in diabetic pregnancies. *Obstet Gynecol* 2002;99:740–4.
61. Conway DL. Delivery of macrosomic infant: Cesarean section versus vaginal delivery. *Semin Perinatol* 2002;26:225–31.
62. Stotland NE, Caughey AB, Breed EM, *et al.* Risk factors and obstetric complications associated with macrosomia. International Journal of Gynecology & Obstetrics, Volume 87, Issue 3, December 2004, pp. 220–6.
63. Benedetti TJ, Gabbe SG. Shoulder dystocia: a complication of fetal macrosomia and prolonged second stage of labor with midpelvic delivery. *Obstet Gynecol* 52 (1978), pp. 526–9
64. American College of Obstetricians and Gynecologists. Shoulder dystocia, The College, Washington (DC) (2002) Practice Bulletin No.: 40.
65. Irion O, Boulvain M. Induction of labour for suspected fetal macrosomia. From The Cochrane Library, Issue 1, 2006.

125 Etiology and pathogenesis of fetal macrosomia

F. Carmona and V. Cararach

Introduction

Macrosomia is the term used to define fetuses that present excessive weight at birth; however, there is no agreement on what is the maximum weight that can be considered normal at the moment of birth since the limits defined by different authors vary between 4000 and 4500 g.[1–3] The currently most widely accepted definition considers gestational age as well as weight; the the word macrosomia includes 'fetuses that are large for their gestational age' (birth weight above the 90th percentile of weight distribution for their gestational age).[4] However, with regard to the possible prevention of problems during delivery the limit is set at 4000 g.

Fetal development and growth are regulated by many factors, which include the fetus's own characteristics, the maternal environment, placental function, and the availability of nutrients for the fetus. There is a close correlation in normal pregnancies between fetal weight and gestational age, such that fetal growth may be considered as the result of the relationship between genetic potential for growth and external influences that may modulate it. During early pregnancy, fetal growth is due to an increase in the number of cells (hyperplasia), while in the third trimester it is principally a result of an increase in cell size (hypertrophy).

Since fetal needs in later pregnancy are greater, the external influences (particularly the placenta if its capacity is diminished) are more important and thus the rate of fetal growth tends to diminish after the 30th week in multiple pregnancies and after the 36th week in single pregnancies, making differences in fetal size during the third trimester more obvious than in earlier stages of the pregnancy.[5,6]

In this chapter, we review the main factors involved in the genesis of macrosomia.

Factors involved in fetal growth

Genetic factors

The basic determining factor for the size of different species is genetic in character. Nevertheless, the mechanisms that control growth, are not well known. In fact, birth weight varies widely: weight among percentiles 10 and 90 in the Hospital Clínic de Barcelona for 40-week newborns varies between 2900 and 3980 g; of this variation, 20% is believed to be attributable to the fetal genotype; maternal height and weight exert considerable influence on the final fetal weight.[7,8]

In only a small percentage of cases does macrosomia form a part of a genetically determined syndrome and there is no prenatal diagnostic test that can specifically identify this subgroup of patients. Although they are uncommon, we shall briefly describe the particular syndromes, which include macrosomia among their characteristics.

Beckwith–Wiedemann syndrome

Only 200 cases have been recorded in the literature since it was first described.[9] Newborns are characterized by excessive weight (mean birth weight 4000 g), macroglossia, linear creases in the outer ear, and, in a high percentage of cases, omphalocele. Hydramnios and prematurity are common and embryonal cancers of infancy and early childhood are also frequent. Macrosomia is mainly at the expense of the muscular and subcutaneous tissues, and in many cases there is hyperinsulinemia at birth; many cases (30–35%) show neonatal hypoglycemia. The majority of infants with hypoglycemia will be asymptomatic and have resolution of this condition within the first 3 days of life and less than 5% will have hypoglycemia beyond the neonatal period requiring either continuous feeding or a partial pancreatectomy.[10] It is also common to find an increase in the number of red blood cells, hyperviscosity, and dyspnea with, in some cases, slight to moderate mental retardation, which may improve if the condition is diagnosed and treated appropriately during the neonatal period. The neonatal complications are very similar to those presented by the offspring of diabetic mothers. There are descriptions of an increase in the number and affinity of erythrocyte insulin receptors and it has been suggested that the excessive growth is the consequence of an increased response to normal or slightly increased insulin concentrations,[11–13] resulting in hypoglycemia among newborns, which is often serious and produces convulsions. Treatment with hydrocortisone may improve the situation. Diagnosis must be regarded with suspicion until the birth, when macrosomia, omphalocele, and macroglossia can be diagnosed.[14]

Recent studies have identified the majority of genes associated with the Beckwith–Wiedemann syndrome in the 11p15 region and the genotype of persistent hyperinsulinemia–hypoglycemia of childhood also in the 11p15 region may provide a molecular basis for hypoglycemia in the Beckwith–Wiedemann syndrome involving abnormal methylation of either H19 or LIT1, which encodes unstralated RNAs on 11p15.[15] Prenatal diagnosis could be made in suspected cases studying by PCR the polymorphic loci on 11p 15.15 in the fetus, by amniocentesis or by chorionic villus sampling, or in both parents.[16]

Soto's syndrome

This occurs sporadically but familial cases with dominant autosomic heredity have been known with defects in the *NSD1* gene in nearly 60% of the patients.[17] The affected fetuses present macrocephaly, dolichocephaly, and prognathism with moderate to severe mental retardation in 83% of the cases. Fourteen percent of the affected newborns present abnormal glucose tolerance tests.[18] Prenatal echographic examination reveals the existence of a heavier-than-expected fetus with a cephalic perimeter/abdominal perimeter ratio that is greater than normal (similar to what happens in cases of asymmetric growth retardation).

Gillian Turner's syndrome

This is a recessive X-linked syndrome characterized by mental retardation, increase in genital size, and varying degrees of macrosomia. There may be cerebral gigantism

Weaver's syndrome

This is a rare syndrome characterized by accelerated skeletal maturation, unusual facies, and camptodactylia.[19]

Nesidioblastosis

This condition is characterized by the existence of a diffuse proliferation of the islets of Langerhans with a relative increase in beta cells. It has been suggested that the primary defect may be an alteration in the organization of the islets, which impedes the usual pancreatic regulation of insulin secretion, which is done by other hormones, such as somatostatin. The only efficient long-term treatment is the surgical resection of 95% of the pancreas. Although the etiology is unknown, it seems to be a recessive autosomic defect in pancreatic development. Newborns have a phenotype very similar to the offspring of diabetic mothers, with macrosomia due above all to hypertrophy of the muscular and subcutaneous tissue.

Other syndromes

Other genetic alterations have been related with fetal overgrowth. A recent report describes four children from two unrelated families presenting with macrosomia and a terminal duplication of the long arm of chromosome 15. In all cases, chromosome analysis of the parents showed a balanced translocation involving 15q26.1-qter.[20] Another report describes a case of non-diabetic macrosomia associated with Simpson–Golabi–Behmel syndrome.[21]

Fetal hormones

The genome controls fetal growth; the fetal hormones translate genetic information into real stimuli for growth. However, the exact mechanisms by means of which this control and regulation are carried out have not yet been established.

Insulin

This hormone plays a very important role in postnatal life, mainly in the metabolism of carbohydrates. During intrauterine life, however, insulin is the most important hormone in the regulation of fetal growth. Given that insulin cannot pass through the placental barrier, the only source of insulin found in the fetal plasma is its secretion by the fetal pancreas. Insulin is present in fetal plasma as early as 8–9 weeks' gestation, although it is relatively inactive until about the 20th week when fetal insulin response to glucose becomes evident;[22] the response to exogenous glucose depends on fetal glucose levels, which regulate the sensitivity of the beta cells of the pancreas.[23] Thus, chronic fetal hyperglycemia accelerates the development of insulin-secreting mechanisms in such a way that the offspring of diabetic mothers are predisposed to develop an insulin-secreting response similar to that of an adult.[24]

The insulin receptors in the fetal liver reach their maximum levels between weeks 19 and 25 of pregnancy; however, the maximum affinity of these receptors is reached later in pregnancy.[25]

Hyperinsulinemia induces the storage of glucose in the form of glycogen, lipogenesis, and the utilization of amino acids as an energy source. Experiments performed in rhesus monkeys on the effect of insulin on fetal growth have shown that this hormone produces organomegaly, increase in fetal and placental weight, and an increase in the crown–rump length (CRL).[26] In clinical practice, the importance of insulin in the control of fetal growth is better understood if it is kept in mind that in macrosomic syndromes, such as maternal diabetes, Beckwith–Wiedemann syndrome, and nesidioblastosis, hyperinsulinemia is very common.

Several human studies support the relationship between insulin and fetal macrosomia even in non-diabetic mothers. Akin *et al.* studied 20 non-diabetic mothers and their macrosomic infants with the appropriate-for-gestational age control group. Levels of hemoglobin A1c were similar in both the groups but the C peptide levels were significantly higher in macrosomic infants, suggesting that these infants were more likely to have hypersinsulinemia that were normal-sized infants and this hyperinsulinemia was not caused by the disregulation in glucose metabolism.[27] Valensise *et al.* determined the maternal plasma levels of C peptide in 206 consecutive patients submitted for an oral glucose tolerance test. They showed that a C peptide cutoff at 2.9 ng/ml resulted predictive for patients delivering large-for-gestational age newborns (OR=3.42; 95% CI=1.59–7.39).[28]

Insulin-like growth factors (IGFs)

This is a group of peptides with structural similarities to the proinsulin chain of amino acids.[29] They were previously known as somatomedins and may act through endocrine, paracrine, or autocrine mechanisms.[30] Their effect is to promote fetal growth though any of the following mechanisms: (a) stimulation of glucose metabolism; (b) DNA synthesis; and (c) cellular proliferation. There are two main IGFs: IGF I and IGF II, which can be detected from the 13th week of pregnancy and cannot cross the placenta; fetal and maternal IGF I levels increase as pregnancy advances and correlate with fetal and placental weight;[31] it is not possible to describe a similar relationship between IGF II and fetal weight, though it has been shown that the levels of this peptide in the amniotic fluid do not change during pregnancy.[32]

At the cell level also, two types of IGF receptors have been identified.[33] Type I receptors are very similar to insulin receptors, whereas type II receptors are IGF-specific. Two different transporting proteins have also been described, though the exact mechanism by which they act is not well known.

Animal models have shown that growth factors play an important role in the fetal growth. This role has been studied through transgenic animal models. Thus, growth hormone (GH)-deficient mice have been mated with IGF-I transgenic mice and their offspring have had normal body weight and linear growth, suggesting that IGF-I plays a larger role than GH in fetal growth.[34] Mice whose IGF-II gene has been eliminated are severely growth retarded *in utero* and have small placentas, but they survived and grew normally after birth. Mice with deleted IGF-I are also very small but have a normal placenta and they had severe postnatal arrest and neonatal death. This suggests that IGF-I plays a large role in prenatal as well in postnatal growth; however, IGF-II affects placental growth, and thus fetal size, but it is not essential for postnatal growth.[35]

Other hormones

The effect of the GH on fetal growth is minimal, since the liver is the only fetal tissue that expresses receptors for this hormone. Leptine is a hormone that plays an important role in the regulation of the fetal weight. The umbilical plasma levels of leptine are correlated with the birth weight and with the umbilical concentration of insulin, thus confirming that role.[36] The effect of other hormones on fetal growth is also minimal.

Maternal and environmental factors

There are certain factors that have been associated empirically with macrosomia. They include previous history of macrosomia, multiparity, maternal obesity, the mother's age, height, excessive weight gain during pregnancy, prolonged pregnancy, and prolonged labor.[37–40] Recently, a birth weight prediction equation based on maternal and pregnancy-specific characteristics, which achieved accuracy of prediction comparable to that obtained using ultrasonic fetal biometry, has been validated.[41] It has also been recently stressed that, in gestational diabetes pregnancies, the association of maternal glucose values and fetal macrosomia is limited to the fasting glucose levels between 32 and 35 weeks, while maternal obesity appears to be a strong risk factor of macrosomia throughout pregnancies with gestational diabetes.[42] In this sense, it has been described that the occurrence of obstetric complications, including macrosomia, parallels the level of obesity, but even moderate overweight amplifies the risk.[43]

To study the influence of these factors, we used a retrospective study of 22,745 births (of more than 20 weeks) in the Hospital Clínic de Barcelona between 1980 and 1992. To reduce difficulties of interpretation, we eliminated pregnancies in diabetic patients, which left 21,298 pregnancies, which we allocated as follows:

- *Group 1*: 500–2499 g (those with a low birth weight, totalling 1462 cases or 6.9%)
- *Group 2*: 2500–3999 g (those with normal weight, totalling 18,748 cases or 88%)
- *Group 3*: 4000–4249 g (first macrosome fraction, totalling 697 cases or 3.3%)
- *Group 4*: 4250–4449 g (intermediate macrosome fraction, totalling 275 cases or 1.3%)
- *Group 5*: over 4500 g (totalling 116 cases or 0.5%)

To describe and evaluate the distribution of the cases we used Habermann's contingency tables.

With regard to age there is a significant increase in cases of macrosomia (Table 125.1) after the age of 35, except in certain weight groups in ages above 40 in which, although there is a clear increase in frequency, it does not reach significant values due to the low number of cases in the group. Similar results are observed with parity. Beginning with the group with two or three previous pregnancies, there is a significant increase in frequency of macrosomes in all groups (Table 125.2). The same is found with maternal height when it is above 1.60 m and, especially when it is above 1.65 m (Table 125.3), with weight increase above 20% (Table 125.4), with a history of macrosomia (Table 125.5), and with fetal sex (Table 125.6). In the majority of cases, these factors increase the frequency

Table 125.1 Maternal age and birth weight

Maternal age	Birth weight (kg) 0.5–2.49	2.5–3.99	4–4.24	4.25–4.49	≥4.5	Total
≤16	59(10.7)*	472(86.1)	14(2.6)	3(0.5)		548
17–20	261(8.3)*	2,807(89)	59(1.9)**	17(0.5)**	11(0.3)	3,155
21–35	984(6.4)**	13,593(88.4)*	520(3.4)	204(1.3)	78(0.5)	15,379
36–40	87(6.3)	1,164(84.6)**	70(5.1)*	35(2.5)*	20(1.4)*	1,376
≥41	25(8.8)	238(83.5)**	13(4.6)	6(2.1)	3(1)	285
Not recorded	46	474	21	10	4	560
Total	1462	18,748	697	275	116	21,298

Results are expressed as *n* (%). Overall χ^2: 948.5; degrees of freedom: 16; $P < 0.0001$
*Higher than expected; **lower than expected

Table 125.2 Parity and birth weight

Number of previous births	Birth weight (kg) 0.5–2.49	2.5–3.99	4–4.24	4.25–4.49	≥4.5	Total
0	713(7.7)*	8243(88.7)*	240(2.5)**	64(.7)**	36(.4)**	9296
1	379(6.2)	5391(8805)	198(3.2)	86(1.5)	33(0.5)	6087
2–3	264(6.6)	3470(87)	161(4.0)*	74(1.8)*	23(0.6)	3992
4–5	65(6.0)	915(85)**	56(5.2)*	27(2.5)*	13(1.2)*	1076
6-7	27(4.4)**	526(85)**	36(5.8)*	21(3.4)*	9(1.4)*	619
Not recorded	14	203	6	3	2	228
Total	1462	18748	697	275	116	21298

Results are expressed as *n* (%). Overall χ^2: 160.5, degrees of freedom: 16; $P < 0.0001$
*Higher than expected; **lower than expected

Table 125.3 Maternal height and birth weight

Maternal height (m)	Birth weight (kg) 0.5–2.49	2.5–3.99	4–4.24	4.25–4.49	≥4.5	Total
≤1.44	14(6.1)	209(90.9)	3(1.3)	4(1.7)	0	230(1.3)
1.45–1.49	81(10)*	706(86.9)	14(1.7)**	10(1.2)	2(0.2)	813
1.5–1.54	165(6.1)	2,411(90.3)*	66(2.5)**	19(0.7)**	9(0.4)	2,685
1.55–1.59	201(5.3)**	3,363(89.3)*	130(3.4)	48(1.3)	24(0.6)	3,766
1.6–1.64	136(4.3)**	2,785(89.2)*	130(4.2)*	52(1.7)	18(0.6)	3,121(17.8)
≥1.65	65(4.0)**	1,436(87.9)	78(4.8)*	38(2.3)*	17(1.0)*	1,634(9.3)
Not recorded	800	7,838	276	104	46	9,064
Total	1462	18,748	697	275	116	21,298

Results are expressed as *n* (%). Overall χ^2: 1028.1; degrees of freedom: 20; $P < 0.0001$
*Higher than expected; **lower than expected

Table 125.4 Maternal weight gain and birth weight

Maternal weight gain > 20%	Birth weight (kg) 0.5–2.49	2.5–3.99	4–4.24	4.25–4.49	≥4.5	Total
No	1298(7.0)*	16,396(88.3)	564(3.0)**	218(1.2)**	92(0.5)**	18,568
Yes	51(3.1)**	1,420(87.3)	99(6.1)*	36(2.2)*	20(1.2)*	1,626
Not recorded	113	932	34	21	4	1,104
Total	1462	18,748	697	275	116	21,298

Results are expressed as *n* (%). Overall χ^2: 103.2; degrees of freedom: 4; $P < 0.0001$. χ^2 for trend: 93.7; $P < 0.0001$
*Higher than expected; **lower than expected

Table 125.5 Previous macrosomic fetus and birth weight

Previous macroscopic fetus	Birth weight (kg) 0.5–2.49	2.5–3.99	4–4.24	4.25–4.49	≥4.5	Total
No	1426(7.0)*	18,008(88.8)*	583(2.9)**	199(1.0)**	71(0.3)**	20,287(87.1)
Yes	21(2.5)**	590(70.1)**	113(13.4)*	74(8.8)*	43(5.1)*	841(7.6)
Not recorded	15	150	1	2	2	170
Total	1462	18,748	697	275	116	21,298

Results are expressed as *n* (%). Overall χ^2: 1051; degrees of freedom: 4; $P < 0.0001$. χ^2 for trend: 811.7; $P < 0.0001$
*Higher than expected; **lower than expected

Table 125.6 Fetal sex and birth weight

Fetal sex	Birth weight (kg) 0.5–2.49	2.5–3.99	4–4.24	4.25–4.49	4.5	Total
♂	686(6.2)**	9659(87.2)	54(4.1)*	190(1.7)*	75(0.7)	11,074(51.7)
♀	752(7.4)*	9014(88.9)	247(2.4)**	84(.8)**	40(.4)	10,140(47.3)

Results are expressed as *n* (%). Overall χ^2: 187.4; degrees of freedom: 4; $P < 0.0001$. χ^2 for trend: 9395; P=0.0016
*Higher than expected; **lower than expected

of macrosomia by two or three times, but the history of macrosomic previous fetuses increases macrosomia by nearly seven times.

Table 125.7 compares macrosomic newborns with newborns of normal weight, showing a statistically significant association between macrosomia and parity, maternal age, gestational age, maternal height and weight, and the maternal history of previous macrosomes. The implications of this and of other similar studies are that older women, obese women, multiparous women, and those with prolonged pregnancies each belong to a group with high risk of macrosomia, which is compounded when more than one is present at the same time. This is especially important in the selection of the group of pregnant women at risk of macrosomia, for whom we can consider adopting preventive attitudes toward the complications connected with this pathology.

The origin of macrosomia in diabetes

Since its description 150 years ago, macrosomia has been one of the main components of diabetic

Table 125.7 Epidemiology factors related with macrosomia in the Hospital Clínic de Barcelona (from Sack[1])

	Birth weight (kg)			
Factor	**< 2.5**	**2.5–4**	**> 4**	p^2
Parity				< 0.0001
Nuliparous	7.8	88.5	3.7	
Parous	6.2	87.5	6.2	
Maternal age				< 0.0001
< 20	8.6	88.5	2.8	
21–35	6.4	88.3	5.2	
< 36	6.7	84.4	8.8	
Maternal height				< 0.0001
< 1.5 m	8.6	88.3	3	
1.5–1.65 m	5.3	89.5	5,1	
> 1.65 m	3.9	87.8	8,2	
Maternal weight				< 0.0001
Non-obese	8	87.4	4.5	
Obese	3.4	89.4	7.1	
Gestational age				< 0.0001
< 36 weeks	46.4	52.7	0.8	
37–40 weeks	3.6	91.2	5.1	
> 41 weeks	1.4	87.5	11	
Previous macrosomic fetus				< 0.0001
No	7	88.7	4.2	
Yes	2.5	70.1	27.3	

Results are expressed as a percentage of each category. Chi-square test

fetopathy. It has been known for some time that the weight of the offspring of an untreated diabetic mother is 140% higher than that of the controls, but this increase is distributed asymmetrically in that CRL is increased by 112%, heart size by 175%, liver by 180%, lung and spleen by 130%, the adrenal glands by 160%, and the pancreas by 110%; the kidneys and the brain do not increase in size.[44] Moreover, the increase in weight is due to the increase in both the size and the number of cells.[44] In addition, the data from the Clinic Hospital of Barcelona mentioned above confirm that the distribution of macrosomes is significantly greater in diabetic compared with non-diabetic patients (data not shown).

The problem of excessive fetal growth in the diabetic pregnant woman is complex and may be the consequence of an abnormal supply of nutrients to the fetus. In the early 1950s Pedersen established the hypothesis that served for more than 30 years to explain fetal weight gain in diabetic mothers;[45] as a result of the characteristic hypoinsulinemia diabetic patients present hyperglycemia. The glucose easily crosses the placenta through a diffusion mechanism and reaches the fetus, 75% of the levels present in the mother's circulation. These high fetal blood glucose levels are an additional stimulus for the fetus, which responds by increasing insulin secretion, which causes fetal hyperinsulinemia, which in turn causes increases in hepatic glycogen and the synthesis of triglycerides in the adipocytes, all of which leads to increased weight and macrosomia.

This hypothesis was later extended by Freinkel and Metzger,[46] who examined the role played by other nutrients. In their model (Figure 125.1), reduction in maternal availability of insulin leads to an increase in maternal levels of glucose, which furthermore is underused. This produces changes in the levels of all maternal nutrients, with high plasmatic levels not only of glucose but also of lipids, some amino acids, and ketones. Placentary structure and function may be altered, allowing an abnormal mixture of nutrients to reach the fetus. This contributes to anabolism

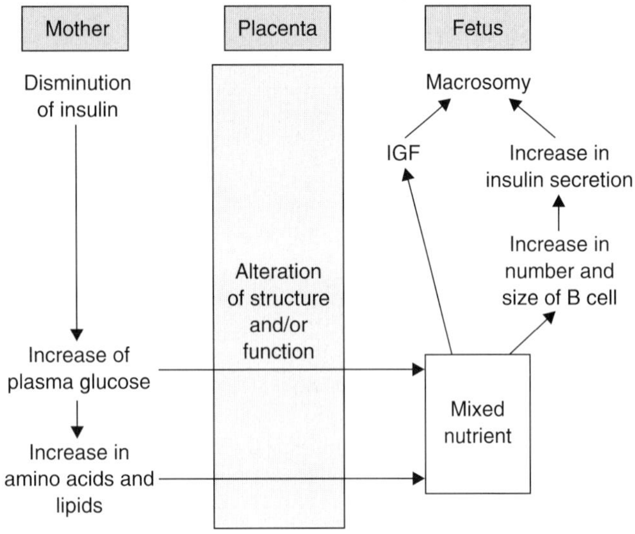

Figure 125.1

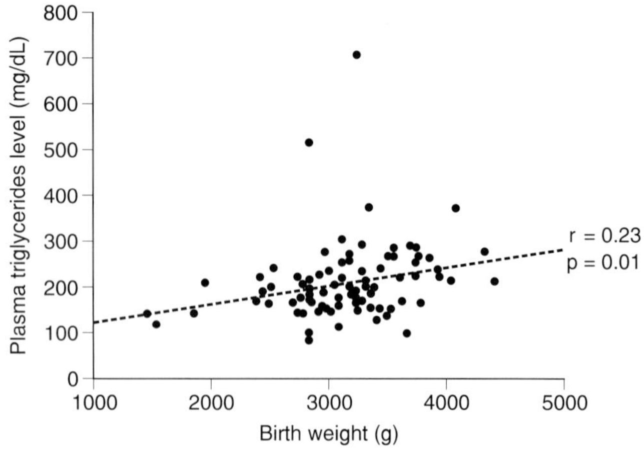

Figure 125.4 Correlation of neonatal weight and plasma triglycerides level in GDM patients.

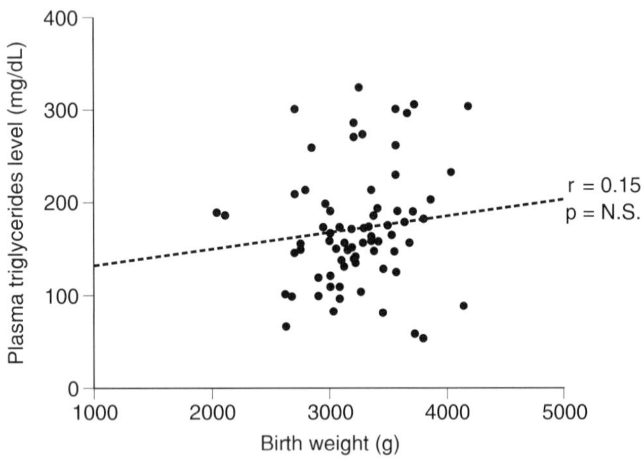

Figure 125.2 Correlation of neonatal weight and plasma triglycerides level in non-diabetic patients.

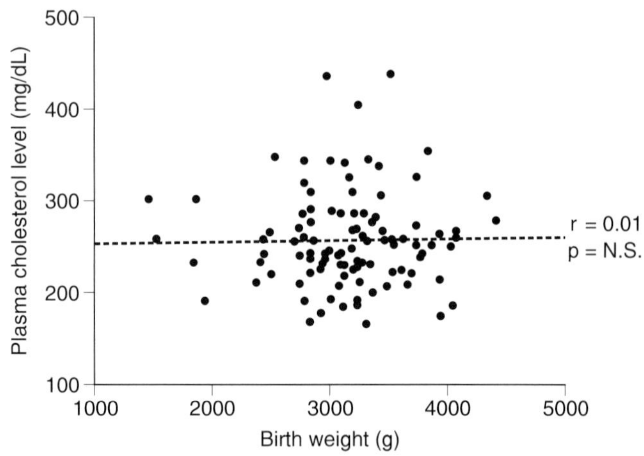

Figure 125.5 Correlation of neonatal weight and cholesterol level in GDM patients.

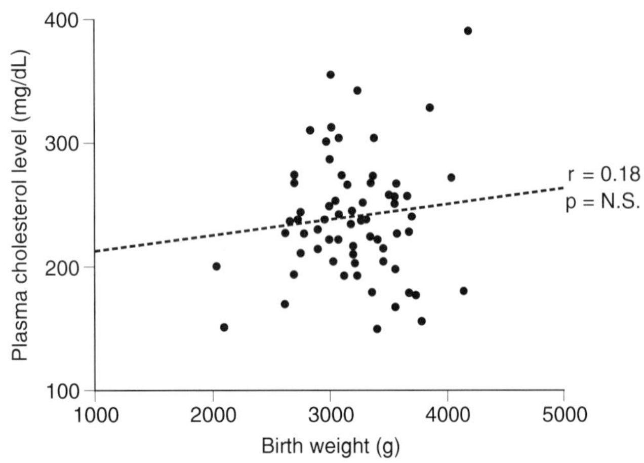

Figure 125.3 Correlation of neonatal weight and plasma cholesterol level in non-diabetic patients.

during the second half of pregnancy and produces excessive and premature insulin secretion, which leads to the growth in all the insulin-dependent organs.

We have recently investigated if there is any relationship between plasma lipid alterations and neonatal birth weight in pregnancies complicated with gestational diabetes mellitus (GDM). Between June 1994 and December 1995, 107 pregnancies complicated with GDM and 69 normal pregnancies were prospectively evaluated. The non-diabetic patients had normal O'Sullivan test during the early third trimester of their current pregnancy (26–29 weeks' gestation). GDM was diagnosed by a 3-h oral glucose tolerance test performed at 28–31 weeks' gestation. All women were studied after an overnight fast, between the 31st and the 34th gestational weeks. The levels of plasma cholesterol, triglycerides, high-density lipoproteins, and low-density lipoproteins were measured and their correlations with the birth

Table 125.8 Plasma lipid level in both groups studied

	Gamma	Control*	P**
Cholesterol (mg/dl)	256.5 ± 52.7	240.8 ± 47.6	0.04
Triglycerides (mg/dl)	208 ± 69.1	170 ± 64.4	0.001
Hypercholesterolemia	52 (48.6%)	30 (42.3%)	NS
Hypertriglyceridemia	86 (80.4%)	39 (54.9%)	< 0.01
Hyperlipemia	93 (86.9%)	47 (66.2%)	0.002

*Results are mean ± SD or *n* (%); **Student's test or chi-square test as appropriate

Table 125.9 Fetal birth weight in normal and GDM pregnancies by plasma level of cholesterol and triglycerides

	Plasma level*		
Parameter	**Normal**	**High**	***P*****
GDM group			
Cholesterol (mg/dl)	3099 ± 464	3190 ± 606	NS
Triglycerides (mg/dl)	2682 ± 697	3226 ± 470	0.01
Normal group			
Cholesterol (mg/dl)	3195 ± 437	3301 ± 362	NS
Triglycerides (mg/dl)	3154 ± 362	3248 ± 445	NS

*Results are mean ± SD; **Student's test

weight was determined in both the groups studied. The prevalence of hyperlipemia (hypertriglyceridemia and/or hypercholesterolemia) was greater among the GDM patients (Table 125.8), because a very high rate of hypertriglyceridemia is seen in these patients (85% vs. 56% in non-diabetic patients). The mean birth weight correlated positively with the plasma triglyceride level in the GDM patients but not in the non-diabetic group. The cholesterol did not correlate with the birth weight in the GDM group or in the normal patients group (Table 125.9 and Figures 125.2–125.5).

Clinical studies have shown that macrosomia may be associated with even minimal levels of hyperglycemia.[47,48] Freinkel and Metzger consider that other, as yet unidentified, defined growth factors may also contribute to excessive weight increase. The role of IGFs, among others, has been analyzed.[31,32]

The fetal pancreas is microscopically visible from the fourth week of embryonic life and insulin is detectable, as has been reported, from 7 to 10 weeks, albeit at levels much lower than those detectable in later stages of pregnancy. *In vitro* studies have shown that fetal pancreatic beta cells are functional from the 14th week of pregnancy, responding to amino acids, to ions such as Ca^{2+}, and to factors that increase intracellular cyclic adenosine monophosphate (cAMP), such as theophylline and glucagons.[49] Other studies have also shown that these cells release insulin in response to stimulation with glucose[50] in such a way that there is clear evidence to suggest that insulin may be a physiological regulator of glucose metabolism and fetal growth.[51]

Functional maturation of beta cells in fetuses of diabetic mothers is more premature than in fetuses of mothers with normal glycemia metabolism.[52] These studies emphasize the importance of understanding the physiological impact of early sensitivity to glucose: if this premature pancreatic maturation occurs, the onset of macrosomia may be much earlier than was previously believed.

Placental synthesis of substances such as human chorionic somatomamotrophin may influence nutrient availability. Likewise, decidual production of prolactin and lipotrophin, a precursor of the adrenocorticotropic hormone, and of endorphins may play a role in the modulation of fetal growth. Also, the hypothalamus–pituitary axis, which is well developed in the later part of pregnancy, may segregate peptides that promote fetal growth. Thus, fetal size at birth is a result of the integration of a system of three compartments: mother, placenta, and fetus. In a recent paper,[53] it has been hypothesized that fetal macrosomia could be the result of a placental defect because the placenta is interposed between both fetal and maternal compartments and it has its own glucose metabolism. One characteristic feature of the human placenta in diabetes is the increased deposition of glycogen. Neither hyperglycemia nor hyperinsulinemia increase the glycogen content in the trophoblast. Since the glycogen increments in diabetes are predominantly located around fetoplacental vessels, it is tempting to assume a fetal origin of glucose making up the glycogen deposits. In fat, glucose can be transported back from the fetus into the placenta and this reflux is increased in diabetes. Therefore, in conditions of fetal glucose levels exceeding the demand for sustaining fetal growth and metabolism, glucose can be stored in the liver and other fetal tissues. Once these stores are saturated, glucose is extracted from the fetal circulation by the glucose carriers GLUT1 and GLUT3 on cells surrounding the fetoplacental vasculature and stored therein, again in the form of glycogen. These processes might be under the control of fetal insulin, because insulin injected into the fetal circulation increases placental glycogen stores. Fetal macrosomia would then occur only when fetal hyperglycemia exceeds the placental capacity to store excess fetal glucose. Thus, according to this hypothesis, the placental failure to protect the fetus would cause the 'unexplained' phenotypic changes occasionally found in fetuses born to well-controlled diabetic women.[53]

Finally, the appearance of macrosomia is multifactorial and is probably due to an excessive supply of nutrients to the fetus, together with the action of other growth-promoting factors. However, the accumulated evidence suggests that fetal hyperglycemia may not be the only stimulus responsible for fetal hyperinsulinemia; in fact, in humans, glucose is just one of the substrates involved in the production of insulin and, although it is one of the most important, other nutrients seem to be also important.

REFERENCES

1. Sack RA. The large infant. *Am J Obstet Gynecol* 1969;104:195.
2. Golditch IM. The large fetus: Management and outcome. *Obstet Gynecol* 1978;52:26.
3. Modanlou HD, Dorchester WL, Thorosian A. Macrosomia. Maternal, fetal and neonatal implications. *Obstet Gynecol* 1980; 55:420.
4. Deter RL. Definition, epidemiology and classification of macrosomia. In Divon Y, ed. *Abnormal Fetal Growth.* Amsterdam: Elsevier Science Publishers, 1991.
5. McKeown T. Observations on fetal growth in multiple pregnancy in man. *J Endocrinol* 1952;8:388.
6. Fujikura T, Froehlich IA. Birthweight, gestational age, and renal glomerular development as indices of fetal maturity. *Am J Obstet Gynecol* 1972;113:627.
7. McKeown T, Marshall T. Influences on fetal growth. *J Reprod Med* 1976;47:167.
8. Kloosterman GJ. On intrauterine growth: The significance of prenatal care. *J Gynecol Obstet* 1970;8:895.
9. Jones KL. Beckwith–Wiedemann syndrome. In *Smith's Recognizable Patterns of Human Malformation,* 4th edn. Philadelphia: W. B. Saunders, 1988.
10. De Baun MR, King AA, White N. Hypoglycemia in Beckwith–Wiedemann syndrome. *Semin Perinatol* 2000;24:164.
11. Beckwith JB. Macroglossia, omphalocele, adrenal cytomegaly, gigantism, and hyperplastic visceromegaly. *Birth Defects* 1969;5:188.
12. Herzberg SA, Seyed S, Hill D. Possible etiological mechanisms for the overgrowth and hypoglycemia in patients with Beckwith–Wiedemann syndrome. *Clin Res* 1979;27:812.
13. Jones KL. Beckwith–Wiedemann syndrome. In *Smith's Recognizable Patterns of Human Malformation,* 4th edn. Philadelphia: W. B. Saunders, 1988.
14. Irving I. Exomphalos with macroglossia: A study of 11 cases. *J Pediatr Surg* 1967;2:499.
15. De Baun MR, Niemitz EL, McNeil DE, Brandenburg SA, Lee MP, Feinberg AP. Epigenetic alterations of H19 and LIT1 distinguish patients with Beckwith–Wiedemann syndrome with cancer and birth defects. *Am J Hum Genet* 2002;70:604.
16. Reish O, Lerer I, Amiel A, *et al.* Wiedemann–Beckwith syndrome: Further prenatal characterization of the condition. *Am J Genet* 2002;107:209–13.
17. Bajaut G, Rio M, Rossignol S, *et al.* Paradoxical mutations in Beckwith–Wiedemann syndrome and 11p15 anomalies in Sotos syndrome. *Am J Genet* 2004;74:715–20.
18. Jones KL. Soto's syndrome. In *Smith's Recognizable Patterns of Human Malformation,* 4th edn. Philadelphia: W. B. Saunders, 1988.
19. Weaver DD, Graham CB, Thomas IT, Smith DW. A new overgrowth syndrome with accelerated skeletal maturation, unusual faeces and camptodactylia. *J Pediatr* 1974;84:547.
20. Faivre L, Gosset P, Cormier-Daire V, *et al.* Overgrowth and trisomy 15q26.1-qter including the IGF1 receptor gene: Report of two families and review of the literature. *Eur J Hum Genet* 2002;10:699.
21. Yamashita H, Yashui I, Ishimaru T, Matsumoto T, Yamabe T. A case of non-diabetic macrosomia with Simpson–Golabi–Behmel syndrome: Antenatal sonographic findings. *Fetal Diagn Ther* 1995;10:134.
22. Adam PAJ, Teramo K, Raiha N. Human fetal insulin metabolism early in gestation. Responses to acute elevation of the fetal glucose concentration and placental transfer of human insulin-I-131. *Diabetes* 1969;18:409.
23. Fowden AL. Effects of arginine and glucose on the release of insulin in the sheep fetus. *J Endocrinol* 1980;87:113.
24. Oakley NW, Beard RW, Turner RC. Effect of sustained maternal hyperglycemia on the fetus in normal and diabetic pregnancies. *Br Med J* 1972;8:466.
25. Neufeld ND, Scott M, Kaplan SA. Ontogeny of the mammalian receptor. *Dev Biol* 1980;78:151.
26. Susa JB, Schwartz R. Effects of hyperinsulinemia in the primate fetus. *Diabetes* 1985;34:36.
27. Akin M, Ceran O, Atay E, Atay Z, Akin F, Akturk Z. Postpartum maternal levels of hemoglobin A1c and cord C-peptide in macrosomic infants of non-diabetic mothers. *J Maternal Fetal Neonatal Med* 2002;12:274.
28. Valensise H, Larciprete G, Vasapollo B, *et al.* C-peptide and insulin levels at 24–30 weeks' gestation: An increased risk of adverse pregnancy outcomes? *Eur J Obstet Gynecol Reprod Biol* 2002;103:130.
29. Daughaday WH, Heath E. Physiological and possible clinical significance of epidermal and nerve growth factors. *J Clin Endocrinol Metab* 1984;13:207.
30. D'Ercole AJ, Stiles AD, Underwood LE. Tissue concentrations of somatomedin C: Further evidence of multiple sites and paracrine/autocrine mechanisms of action. *Proc Natl Acad Sci USA* 1984;81:935.
31. Gluckman PD, Barret-Johnson JJ, Butler JH. Studies of insulin-like growth factors I and II by specific radioligand assays in umbilical cord blood. *Clin Endocrinol* 1983;19:405.
32. Ashton IK, Zapf J, Einschenk J. Insulin-like growth factors (IGF) I and II in human fetal plasma and relationship to gestational age and fetal size during mid-pregnancy. *Acta Endocrinol* 1985; 10:558.
33. Shigematsu K, Niwa M, Kurihara M. Receptor autoradiographic localization of insulin-like growth factor (IGF-I) binding sites in human fetal and adult adrenal glands. *Life Sci* 1985;45:383.

34. Behringer R, Lewin T, Quaife CJ, *et al.* Expression of insulin-like growth factor I stimulates normal somatic growth in growth hormone-deficient transgenic mice. *Endocrinology* 1990;127:1033.
35. Baker J, Liu JP, Robertson E, *et al.* Role of insulin-like growth factors in embryonic and postnatal growth. *Cell* 1993;75:73.
36. Silvan E, Lin WM, Homko CJ, Reece EA, Boden G. Leptin is present in human cord blood. *Diabetes* 1997;46:917.
37. Udall JN, Harrison GG, Vaucher Y. Interaction of maternal and neonatal obesity. *Pediatrics* 1978;62:17.
38. Hansen JP. Older maternal age and pregnancy outcome: A review of the literature. *Obstet Gynecol Surv* 1986;41:726.
39. Boyd ME, Usher RH, McLean FH, Kramer MS. Obstetric consequences of postmaturity. *Am J Obstet Gynecol* 1988;158:334.
40. O'Leary JA. Preconceptual risk factors. In O'Leary JA, ed. *Shoulder Dystocia and Birth Injury.* New York: McGraw-Hill, 1992.
41. Nahum GG, Stanislaw H. Validation of a birth weight prediction equation based on maternal characteristics. *J Reprod Med* 2002; 47:752.
42. Schaefer-Graf UM, Heuer R, Kilavuz O, Pandura A, Heinrich W, Vetter K. Maternal obesity not maternal glucose values correlates best with high rates of fetal macrosomia in pregnancies complicated by gestational diabetes. *J Perinatal Med* 2002;30:313.
43. Galtier-Dereure F, Bringer J. Obesity and pregnancy. *Ann Endocrinol* 2002;63:470.
44. Naeye RL. Infants of diabetic mothers: A quantitative morphologic study. *Pediatrics* 1965;35:980.
45. Pedersen J. *Diabetes and Pregnancy. Blood Sugar of Newborn Infants.* Copenhagen: Danish Science Press, 1952.
46. Freinkel N, Metzger BE. Pregnancy as a tissue-culture experience: The critical implications of maternal metabolism for fetal development. In *Pregnancy Metabolism, Diabetes and the Fetus.* CIBA Foundations Symposium 63 Amsterdam: Excerpta Medica, 1979.
47. Langer O, Brustman L, Anayegbunam A. The significance of one abnormal glucose tolerance test value on adverse outcome in pregnancy. *Am J Obstet Gynecol* 1987;157:758.
48. Langer O, Anayegbunam A, Brustman L, Divon M. A prospective randomized study: Management of women with one abnormal value (OGTT) reduces adverse outcome in pregnancy. *Am J Obstet Gynecol* 1989;161:593.
49. Hollingsworth DR. Infants of diabetic mothers. In Hollingsworth DR, ed. *Pregnancy, Diabetes and Birth,* 2nd edn. Baltimore: Williams and Wilkins, 1992.
50. Maitland JE, Parry DG, Turtle JR. Perfusion and culture of human fetal pancreas. *Diabetes* 1980;29:57–63.
51. Reddy S, Elliot RB. Reviews. Ontogenic development of peptide hormones in the mammalian fetal pancreas. *Experientia* 1988;44:1.
52. Otonkoski T, Andersson S, Knip M, Simell O. Maturation of insulin response to glucose during human fetal and neonatal development. Studies with perfusion of pancreatic islet-like cell clusters. *Diabetes* 1988;37:286.
53. Desoye G, Korgun ET, Ghaffari-Tabrizi N, Hahn T. Is fetal macrosomia in adequately controlled diabetic women the result of a placental defect? A hypothesis. *J Matern Fetal Neonatal Med* 2002; 11:258.

126 Macrosomia: obstetric management

B. Serra, J. M. Carrera and J. Mallafré

Introduction

As we have seen in an earlier chapter in this section, macrosomia is related to an increase in maternal and fetal complications. These include dystocia, prolonged birth, operative delivery, shoulder dystocia and postpartum hemorrhage. However, we must remember that a significant number of the mothers in these cases are diabetic, and this in itself increases fetal vulnerability.

It is also the case that the larger the fetus, the greater the duration of the birth, and the greater the risk of cephalopelvic disproportion and shoulder dystocia.

Management of the pregnancy

In our opinion there are three significant factors during pregnancy:

(1) *Prophylaxis of the macrosomia*, in particular the early detection and treatment of gestational diabetes (O'Sullivan's test, etc.). Appropriate advice on hygiene and diet should also be given to avoid obesity and a weight increase of over 20% during pregnancy. Finally, the remaining factors involving a risk of macrosomia must be evaluated thoroughly (age, parity, size, past history, prolonged gestation, etc.).

(2) *Evaluation of fetal weight*, bearing in mind not only the clinical evaluation of fetal size (uterine height over 34 cm at term or 32 cm in week 35), but more particularly the echographic estimate of fetal weight (biparietal diameter, head and abdominal circumferences). If the biometric values remain over the 90–95th percentiles, it is essential to establish the diagnosis of a probable macrosomia, but the following statements can be made regarding the accuracy of ultrasound in predicting fetal macrosomia:[1]

   (a) Independent of the formula used the relative accuracy of the estimated fetal weight decreases with increasing birth weight.
   (b) Ultrasound biometry, used to detect macrosomia, is characterized by low sensitivity, low positive predictive value and high negative predictive value. Thus, ultrasound's main value is to rule out the diagnosis.[2]
   (c) The positive predictive value can be increased making serial measurements.[3]
   (d) The measurement of fetal parts may not be very accurate in cases of combined maternal obesity, oligohydramnios and anterior placenta.
   (e) Every prenatal diagnosis center should use its own growth curves to select its particular cutoff value to predict macrosomia.
   (f) The time elapsed between the fetal weight estimation and delivery may influence the accuracy and precision of the estimate.
   (g) To date, none of the management algorithms based on ultrasonographically estimated fetal weight has shown any efficacy in reducing the incidence of shoulder dystocia or brachial plexus injury.

Although three-dimensional ultrasound and MR techniques have been used to assess fetal weight, they are still under investigation.

(3) *Prepartum obstetric strategy*, on which opinions are divided. While some authors[4] consider an induced birth inappropriate for avoiding any possible mechanical problems, since the risks can outweigh the benefits, others[2] favor induction from week 38 onwards if conditions are favorable (Bishop's test over 7). Their justification is that, if the birth is brought forward by 2 weeks, an increase in fetal weight of between 200 and 400 g may be avoided. In any case, the majority of authors agree that when the fetal weight is calculated as being over 4500 g, an elective cesarean section must be considered.[4–6]

Management of the birth

The decision regarding the route of delivery will depend on the estimated size of the fetus and the local conditions, as well as on whether the mother is diabetic.[2,7]

If the estimated fetal weight is over 4500 g, the cesarean option should be chosen, regardless of any other considerations, apart from cases of mothers admitted in labor.

If the mother is diabetic, a cesarean section should be indicated if the suspected fetal weight is 4000 g or more. According to Langer and colleagues,[8] 84% of shoulder dystocias are thus avoided. It must be borne in mind that a cesarean section for extracting a macrosomic fetus has associated risks, since the uterus may be torn if the uterine incision is insufficient.

If the fetal weight is under 4500 g, the mother is not diabetic and the local conditions are acceptable (cephalic presentation, multiple pregnancy, mature neck, etc.), a vaginal delivery should be attempted.

The intrapartum management depends on the evaluation of the dilatation and the expulsion. If the evolution is slow and there appears to be an intrapartum risk of shoulder dystocia, it is necessary to resort to a cesarean section. Extractions with forceps or vacuum must be avoided in all cases. The delivery of an apparently macrosomic fetus is considered as high risk, and it is essential that both an anesthesiologist and a neonatologist are in attendance in the delivery room. The staff present at the birth must be absolutely sure of what to do if a shoulder dystocia should suddenly appear.

Shoulder dystocia

A shoulder dystocia occurs when the bisacromial diameter of the fetus is too large for the maternal lower pelvic strait and the foremost shoulder of the fetus encounters the obstacle of the pubic bone once the head is already outside. Such a dystocia can occur in a birth that had been evolving normally up to that point, although it is usually preceded by a prolonged expulsive period. It seems that its incidence is higher in obese patients. The diagnosis can be suspected if the head, after being released, seems to go back in and wedge itself firmly against the perineum. If slight downward pressure does not succeed in dislodging the shoulder, then the diagnosis is confirmed. This is the cue for taking the following steps:[3]

(1) Forced flexion of the legs on the abdomen. The upward rotation of the symphysis can free the affected shoulder (McRoberts' maneuver). If this is unsuccessful:
(2) Wide half-lateral episiotomy. Begin or intensify anesthesia. Clean the fetal mouth and nose.
(3) Manual pressure on the suprapubic region to try to pass the shoulder under the pubic symphysis (Hibbard's maneuver), while the index finger of the other hand pulls away from the rear axilla to allow the rearmost shoulder to progress through the concavity.
(4) If the above maneuver is unsuccessful, apply pressure to the fetus' rear scapula and try to rotate it sideways and upward (Woods' maneuver). If this succeeds, then the rearmost shoulder will end up below the symphysis and will emerge first. In other words, the rearmost shoulder will become the foremost one.
(5) If this maneuver is fruitless, then the fetus' upper arm must be moved rapidly onto its thorax and brought out. The foremost shoulder will be then dislodged and lie below the symphysis.
(6) If this also fails, then a cleidotomy must be considered.

These maneuvers are easy to describe, but difficult to perform with dexterity.

Shoulder dystocia is associated with fetal asphyxia, death and residual complications, such as brachial plexus complications (Erb's paralysis), diaphragmatic paralysis and fractures in the humerus and clavicle. As for the mother, these cases usually give rise to hemorrhages in delivery, hematomas and vaginal tears and, in extreme cases, uterine rupture.

REFERENCES

1. Ben-Harough A, Yogev Y, Hod M. Fetal weight estimation in diabetic pregnancy and suspected fetal macrosomia. *J Perinat Med* 2004;32:113–21.
2. American College of Obstetrician and Gynecologists Practice Bulletin. *Fetal Macrosomia*, Number 22. Washington, DC: ACOG, 2000.
3. Hedriana HL, TR Moore. A comparison of single versus multiple growth ultrasonographic examinations in predicting birth weight. *Am J Obstet Gynecol* 1994;170:1600.
4. Fabre E, González de Agüero R. Parto distócico. In Cabero L, ed. *Riesgo Elevado Obstétrico*. Barcelona: Masson, 1996:473.
5. Cararach V, Carmona F, Palacio M, Cobo E. Conducta obstétrica ante un feto macrosoma. In Carrera JM, ed. *Crecimiento fetal*. Barcelona: Masson, 1997:527–35.
6. Carrera JM. *Protocolos de Obstetricia*, 3rd edn. Barcelona: Masson, 1996:353.
7. Conway DL. Choosing the route of delivery for macrosomic infant of a diabetic mother: Cesarean section versus vaginal delivery. *J Mater Fetal Neonat Med* 2002;12:442.
8. Langer O, Berkus MD, Huff RW, Samueloff A. Shoulder dystocia. *Am J Obstet Gynecol* 1991;165:831–7.

127 Macrosomia: neonatal aspects

E. Doménech and N. Marta Díaz-Gómez

Definition

Neonatal growth is assessed using anthropometric measures taken immediately after birth.[1,2] Newborns (NBs) with a birth weight between the 10th and 90th percentiles on the intrauterine growth curves are considered appropriate for gestational age (AGA) and those lower than the 10th percentile are small-for-gestational age (SGA).

An NB is considered large-for-gestational age (LGA) when its weight is greater than the 90th percentile for gestational age on intrauterine growth curves,[3] although some authors advocate two standard deviations above the mean of birth weight for gestational age. The term macrosomic is used when the birth weight exceeds 4000 g. Some authors[4] believe that the term macrosomic should refer to those whose weight is greater than or equal to 4500 g (1.7% of all NBs).

Certain infants are constitutionally large due to favorable combinations of genetic potential and maternal environment.[5] Normal intrauterine growth is affected by gender and race. Female neonates are smaller than males, and black neonates are smaller than whites, at each estimated gestational age. Thus, to classify a neonate as LGA we have to use intrauterine growth curves that are gender and race specific.[6] Altitude (> 4000 ft) may also negatively affect fetal growth.[6] Ouzilleau *et al.*,[7] using Canadian standards curves, have established the 90th percentile as 4200 g for boys and 4000 g for girls born at 40 weeks of gestational age.

In addition to weight, some have argued that neonatal body proportions have a role in defining macrosomia and predicting its complications. Fetuses with macrosomia of diabetic mothers have a greater shoulder to head circumference ratio, which increases the risk of shoulder dystocia. Disproportionate macrosomia (ponderal index exceeding the 90th percentile in relation to gestational age and sex of the reference population) has been associated with an increased likelihood of neonatal complications among infants of diabetic mothers,[8,9] and also with an increased likelihood of hypoglycemia in infants of non-diabetic mothers.[10]

Incidence

The overall incidence of macrosomia (≥4000 g) is 8% of all NBs and as much as 26% when they are infants of diabetic mothers (IDMs),[3] and appears to be increasing.[11] This increase is correlated with an increase in gestational diabetes, although a high percentage of infants with macrosomia are born to non-diabetic mothers.[8] In a study performed in Montreal, of 57,199 non-malformed singleton live births at or after term between 1978 and 1996, Kramer *et al.*[11] observed an increase in mean NB weight with a corresponding rise in the percentage of LGA. The increase was largely the result of a rise in prepregnancy body mass index, gestational weight gain and gestational diabetes, post-term deliveries as well as a substantial reduction in maternal cigarette smoking and changes in sociodemographic factors.

Endocrine factors that influence fetal growth

A brief review of fetal growth facilitates the understanding of some of the physiologic and pathologic events responsible for neonatal macrosomia.

Intrauterine growth depends on the interaction of maternal, placental and fetal endocrine factors. In normal placental function and a normal maternal environment, the fetal genome is the central controller of growth.

Several hormone and growth factors influence fetal growth. The more relevant are insulin, the insulin-like growth factor (IGF) system, adipocytokines, ghrelin, placental growth harmone (GH), placental lactogen and leptin.

Insulin-like growth factors

It is believed that IGF-1 is a major determinant of fetal growth and the role of the other possible endocrine regulators is likely to be mediated in part by the IGF system.

Table 127.1 Values of GH, IGF-1 in AGA, LGA or SGA full-term infants

	Cord blood			At first week of life		
	LGA	AGA	SGA	LGA	AGA	SGA
Weight (g)	4025 ± 223	3269 ± 376	2200 ± 2990	4011 ± 217	3270 ± 331	2179 ± 211
Seric GH (ng/ml)	16.8 ± 10.8	19.5 ± 20.1	24.0 ± 4.9	20.6 ± 9.3	40.9 ± 28.9	44.8 ± 22.0
Urine GH (ng/kg/day)	—	—	—	1.2 ± 2.7	2.9 ± 3.5	6.4 ± 4.5
Seric IGF-1 (ng/ml)	74.2 ± 29.3	63.5 ± 25.1	9.4 ± 5.8	37.9 ± 29.5	28.1 ± 28.0	20.3 ± 16.1

LGA, large-for-gestational age; AGA, appropriate-for-gestational age; SGA, small-for-gestational age; GH, growth hormone

IGF-1 circulates bound to one of six IGF-binding proteins (IGFBPs), which modulate IGF activity. IGF-1 and their binding proteins are synthesized in the liver and are also produced locally by most tissues, where they act in an autocrine or paracrine manner. The local IGF-1 production is very important for organ development during fetal life.

Han *et al.* have shown that IGFs, especially IGF-2, are present in placental trophoblasts and fetal membranes from as early as 6 weeks. Animal studies have demonstrated that IGF-2 is important in fetal growth during early gestation whereas IGF-1 is the predominant growth-promoting factor in late gestation.[12] IGFs lead to abnormal growth when genetic variation in expression is present.

The IGFBP-3 binds more than 95% of the IGF in serum. One of the main IGFBPs, IGFBP-1, is a potential inhibitor of IGF-1 action. The levels of IGFBP-1 vary in inverse proportion to insulin levels. The levels of IGF-1 and IGFBP-3 in the perinatal period are low and the levels of IGFBP-1 are high, compared with older children and adults.[13]

Whereas in the child and adult both GH and nutrition control the synthesis of IGF-1 and IGFBP-3, in the perinatal period the nutrition status is probably the main regulator of their secretion. This could be explained in part by the immaturity of the GH receptors during this period.[14,15]

IGFBP-1, an important IGF-binding protein in pregnancy, is the predominant IGFBP in decidual cells, amniotic fluid and fetal plasma. Its concentration in the maternal circulation increases during pregnancy. In the circulation IGFBP-1 normally exists in a highly phosphorylated (p) state; however, during pregnancy non-phosphorylated (np) isoforms of IGFBP-1 are found. Gibson *et al.*[16] have demonstrated that human decidualized endometrium produces both npIGFBP-1 and pIGFBP-1, and that in the presence of IGF-2, npIGFBP-1 was preferentially produced. Since npIGFBP-1 has decreased affinity for IGF-1, these effects should enhance IGF-1 bioavailability and are likely to represent an important mechanism for controlling fetal and maternal tissue growth.

We observed the highest levels of IGF-1 in LGA infants of non-diabetic mothers (Table 127.1), and the lowest in the SGA, and the reverse occurred with the levels of GH.[17–19] These findings coincide with those of other authors.[14,20]

Insulin

The role of insulin is thought to be permissive in fetal growth and is demonstrated by the phenotypes that characterize the extreme of insulin secretion. Neonates who are hyperinsulinemic have macrosomia, whereas severe growth restriction accompanies hypoinsulinemia. Hyperinsulinemia causes a decrease in IGFBP-1 levels, which increase IGF-1 bioavailability, and consequently accelerates fetal growth. Also, insulin itself may exert a direct mitogenic effect by binding to the IGF-1 receptors.[8]

Adipocytokines

Adipose tissue produces and secretes a number of hormones, collectively called adipocytokines. These include leptin and adiponectin, both of which are important in modulating metabolism and energy homeostasis.

Leptin, a hormone secreted by adipocytes and syncytiotrophoblast cells of the placenta, has been associated with intrauterine growth. This hormone is detectable in fetal umbilical cord blood at concentrations comparable with those found in adults. Plasma leptin levels in cord blood correlate with birth weight and their levels are significantly higher in LGA compared with AGA infants and are decreased by conditions that lead to low birth weight, such as maternal smoking and prematurity, although the mechanism by which it may by related to fetal growth remains unknown.[21] Christou *et al.*[22] found that the relationship between cord leptin levels and birth weight was independent of insulin and the IGF system.

Adiponectin is exclusively expressed and secreted from adipose tissue and is important in glucose and lipid metabolism. Plasma adiponectin levels decrease as adiposity increases in children and is inversely related to insulin, leptin and body weight. The role of adiponectin in fetal growth has not been clearly determined. Tsai *et al.*[23] have reported that high adiponectin levels are present in cord blood and are positively correlated with birth weight and adiposity. This suggests that adiponectin may be involved in regulating fetal growth.

Ghrelin

Ghrelin is secreted by the fundus of the stomach, the hypothalamus and the placenta. This peptide is closely associated with glucose metabolism and body mass. Hyperglycemia and insulin decrease plasma ghrelin. Fasting ghrelin concentration is decreased in patients with obesity. Insulin resistance and hyperinsulinism, commonly reported in obese subjects, have been proposed to explain part of this relationship.[24]

Farquhar *et al.*[25] have demonstrated the presence of ghrelin in cord plasma samples of NBs. They also found that its concentrations were inversely related to both birth weight *z*-score and glucose concentration. Plasma ghrelin levels in cord blood were 40% higher in SGA compared with AGA and LGA neonates, suggesting that ghrelin may play a physiological role in intrauterine malnutrition.

Placental lactogen and placental GH

Endocrine functions of the placenta include the synthesis of growth factors and hormones involved in cell reproduction and differentiation. Human placental lactogen, which is synthesized and secreted by the syncytiotrophoblast cells of the placenta, plays an important regulatory role in fetal growth, by stimulating the production of IGF-1 in the fetus and by increasing the availability of nutrients to fetal tissues.[26] On the other hand, placental GH has metabolic activities comparable to those of pituitary GH and is an important regulator of maternal IGF-1. Placental GH and maternal IGF-1 do not cross the placenta. Their effects on fetal growth are presumably mediated by effects on placental metabolism and substrate supply to the fetus.[27]

Causes of macrosomia

For proper management of macrosomia we should identify its possible cause. There are many possible causes for exaggerated fetal growth.

Congenital disorders

There are several congenital disorders associated with macrosomia, such as Sotos syndrome (cerebral gigantism), Carpenter syndrome, Weaver syndrome, Nevo syndrome, Nesidioblastosis, Beckwith–Wiedemann syndrome, Perlman syndrome, Marshall syndrome, Ruvalcaba–Mahre syndrome and some transpositions of the large arteries.

Hyperinsulinemia is a primary cause of macrosomia for many of these patients. Abnormalities in IGF secretion also have a significant role in many of these infants.

Nesidioblastosis (autosomal recessive disorder with hyperplasia of the β cells of the pancreas) is a life-threatening form of hypoglycemia that starts during the neonatal period in most cases and is caused by hyperinsulinism. Its diagnostic criteria are an extremely high demand for carbohydrates (> 15 g/kg/day), inadequately high plasma insulin level and an inhibited production of ketone bodies. The acute use of octreotide (somatostatin analog) produces prompt elevation of blood glucose, even in patients who fail to respond to diazoxide (5 mg/kg/dose, every 6 h) and hydrocortisone (25 mg/kg/day). In addition, it may be possible to avoid the need for partial or subtotal pancreatectomy by the long-term use of octreotide.[28]

Infants with Beckwith–Wiedemann syndrome (macrosomia and hyperinsulinism) may present (see Figure 127.1) typical phenotypic hyperinsulinemia features such as macroglosia, visceromegalia and omphalocele, as well as embryonic tumors and overproduction of IGF-2. These patients have anomalies in the short arm of chromosome 11 (replications, trisomies) where the insulin and IGF-2 genes are found, and in the neighboring genes including oncogene *H-ras* and the gene associated with Wilms tumor.

Other intrinsically fetal causes of accelerated growth are infrequent: twin receptors of a parabiotic pair are the most commonly cited. The NB with hydrops fetalis and with some fetal tumors (neuroblastoma, teratomas) also may have excessive weight for gestational age.

Diabetic pregnancy

The most common and best-known cause of LGA infants is the diabetic mother. In the USA, 0.2–0.3% of pregnancies are complicated by preexisting diabetes, and another 1–5% involve gestational diabetes.[29]

As a rule, the infant of a diabetic mother will be large for its gestational age, plump and born covered in an abundant layer of vernix caseosa, with a plethoric aspect, reddishness and cushingoid facial aspect, presenting limited motility and drowsiness during the first hours of life.

In the groups D, E and F of the White classification of diabetes with vasculopathy, there is often a placental insufficiency, which may give rise to children with normal or low birth weight.

The incidence of macrosomia in IDMs is approximately 25–30%, although we have found a decrease from 22.1% to 8.6% in recent years.[30] Fetal growth acceleration in LGA fetuses of diabetic mothers starts in the second trimester, from 18 weeks, and increases

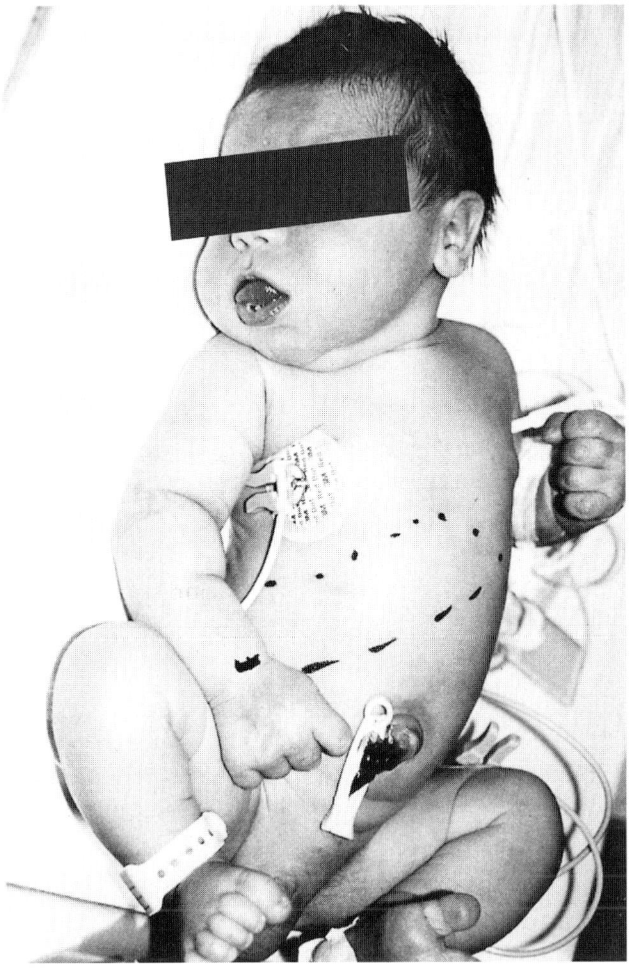

Figure 127.1 An infant with Beckwith–Wiedemann syndrome showing macroglosia, visceromegalia, macrosomia and umbilical hernia.

progressively as the gestation advances, reaching maximum differences in the third trimester.[31]

Macrosomia in these NBs could be attributed to the excessive transferral of glucose from the mother to the fetus inducing fetal hyperglycemia. The fetal pancreas responds with a hypertrophy of the cells of the pancreatic islets and hyperplasia of the β cells, which produce fetal hyperinsulinism, which is accepted as the principal mediator of macrosomia, neonatal hypoglycemia and other perinatal morbidities. Hyperaminoacidemia also has an intrauteral stimulating effect on the development of β cells and of the anabolic actions of the insulin, which could be mediated by the release of IGFs.[32] Fetal anabolism is facilitated in this way, with fatty expanses constituting most of the fetal mass increase.[33]

Organomegaly is selective, with the kidney, heart, suprarenal and bone length enlarged, which are increased in proportion to weight, but brain size does not increase (corresponding to its gestational age), so the head may seem disproportionately small.

Fetal hyperinsulinemia and excessive fetal growth are significantly associated with antepartum maternal hyperglycemia in diabetic pregnancy.[34] Gold *et al.*[35] have shown that first- and second-trimester HbA1 levels were associated with macrosomia and that periconceptional glucose control was most predictive of birth weight in type 1 diabetic pregnancy. A possible explanation could be that early programming of fetal growth by elevated maternal glucose levels during the periconceptional period may result in subsequent LGA babies.

A much improved quality of glycemic control in pregestational diabetic pregnancy has brought a marked improvement of perinatal outcome, with a reduction of premature deliveries and severe neonatal morbidity. However, the fact that fetal macrosomia remains five to six times higher than normal suggests that the glycemic threshold for enhanced fetal growth is closer to normal than it is for other fetal and neonatal complications.

Other causes of macrosomia

The birth of an infant of great weight increases the possibility of subsequent diabetes in the woman affecting future births. Many macrosomic infants have non-diabetic mothers.[3,36] Infants of large, tall and heavy mothers, of women who are obese prior to pregnancy or those who gain excessive weight during this period may be large. The rate of LGA infants is three times higher in multiparous than in primiparous mothers.[4,37]

In a retrospective study of 33,000 live NBs, 1.7% were considered macrosomics (neonatal weight of 4500 g or more).[4] Among the isolated high-risk factors for the existence of macrosomia were postmature pregnancy (15.4%), morbid obesity (10%), insulin-dependent diabetes (9.2%), gestational diabetes (6.4%) and obesity (5.6%).

Body composition

Different techniques have been used to assess body composition in neonates. It is possible to make a fair estimate of the body fat mass of the NB by using an anthropometric model that includes skin fold measure, by bioelectrical impedance analyses or by dual-energy x-ray absorptiometry. Using these techniques it has been shown that infants with macrosomia have a different body composition from that of the AGA infants at birth,[38] and others[39] have reported that LGA infants had significant higher total body fat, expressed as absolute amounts or as a proportion of body weight, and lower lean body mass. Maternal diabetes exaggerated these body composition changes (Table 127.2).

The effect of maternal diabetes on fetal bone mass is controversial. Hammami *et al.*[39] comparing 47 LGA neonates, 11 of them born to diabetic mothers, with 47 gestational age-matched AGA infants, found that LGA neonates have higher bone mineral content.

Table 127.2 Anthropometric measurements, body fat mass and body lean mass, estimated by bioelectrical impedance analyses, in term newborn infants from diabetic and non-diabetic mothers

	Infants of non-diabetic mothers			Infants of diabetic mothers	
	SGA ($n=21$)	AGA ($n=150$)	LGA ($n=29$)	AGA ($n=30$)	LGA ($n=20$)
Weight (g)	2162±199	3121±326	4030±338	3223±443	4093±420
Length (cm)	45.8±1.4	49.6±1.6	53.0±1.4	49.4±1.9	51.8±1.7
Head perimeter (cm)	32.3±0.7	34.1±1.1	35.9±0.6	34.2±1.6	35.4±0.8
Arm perimeter (cm)	8.2±0.5	9.9±0.8	11.0±1.0	10.3±0.8	11.8±0.9
Sum of four skin-folds (mm)	13.1±1.8	17.6±2.7	19.8±2.7	20.0±3.5	24.3±3.2
Total body lean mass (g)	2125±187	2636±291	3501±379	2693±293	3325±344
% body weight	97±1	85±7	87±6	85±9	82±8
Total body fat mass (g)	53±33	484±251	525±248	530±341	768±407
% body weight	3±1	15±7	13±6	15±9	18±8

LGA, large-for-gestational age; AGA, appropriate-for-gestational age; SGA, small-for-gestational age

Other authors found that infants of diabetic mothers have low bone mineral content (BMC) and high bone resumption marker at birth[40–42] and that infant BMC correlated inversely with poor control of diabetes in the mother, specifically first-trimester maternal mean capillary blood glucose concentration, suggesting that factors early in pregnancy might have an effect on fetal BMC.[42] Lower BMC and high bone resumption markers in infants of diabetic mothers could be related to the low vitamin D levels that have been found in NB of diabetic mothers than in control subjects.[43]

Neonatal complications

These apparently 'beautiful' NBs should be assessed by the neonatal specialist early on, as they may be more likely to present certain diseases, and should not be given an early discharge.

They should be screened for: glycemia, calcemia, hematocrits, bilirubin and, if they have respiratory distress, a gasometer and thoracic radiography scan should be carried out to detect cardiac or respiratory disorders. Other complications include increased risk of cesarean section, protracted labor, lacerations of the birth canal and hemorrhage in the mother, shoulder dystocia, brachial palsy, perinatal asphyxia and skeletal injuries in the infants.

Over the last 20 years significant reductions in complications have been achieved. However, recent reports have shown that even in Western countries, morbidity and mortality rates remain higher than in AGA infants.

The perinatal mortality rate is higher for infants weighing more than 4000 g, and this perinatal mortality is higher in the USA than in Norway;[44] however, we have not found this, except in IDMs.

Table 127.3 shows the morbidity and mortality rate in our environment (Canary Islands), based on a sample of 12,311 NBs, classified as AGA, LGA or SGA.

Obstetric trauma and perinatal asphyxia

Although NBs are getting bigger, the maternal pelvis has not been reported to do so. Macrosomia is associated with an increased rate of selective cesarean delivery (33.9%, almost three times that of control infants, obstetric trauma and perinatal asphyxia.[8]

In the macrosomic NB, except for infants of large mothers, obstetric trauma (clavicle fracture, Erb paralysis or paralysis of the frenic nerve) is common when they are born by vaginal route, as a consequence of the elevated presence of shoulder dystocia. Cesarean delivery is also more common in macrosomic than in normal birth weight.[8,45] Spontaneous rather than induced labor is associated with a lower chance of cesarean delivery among those fetuses with macrosomia. On the other hand, frequencies of shoulder dystocia, 1-min Apgar scores less than 7, and abnormal umbilical blood gas determinations are not different between vaginal and cesarean delivery.[46] Vaginal delivery seems a reasonable alternative to elective cesarean and a trial of labor can be offered.[47]

Sonographic methods for the diagnosis of macrosomia were developed in hopes of improving clinical estimates. However, the relative error associated with these methods limits their use in clinical practice. Serial sonographic measurements that are above the limits chosen to define macrosomia increase the likelihood that a birth weight will be macrosomic and could help to answer weight-related clinical questions such as mode and timing of delivery, especially for patients with diabetes.[48] Recently, Tisi *et al.*

Table 127.3 Morbidity and mortality of AGA, LGA and SGA newborns (1999–2003)

	AGA		LGA		SGA		Total	
	No.	NB %	No.	NB %	No.	NB %	No.	NB %
No. of NBs	11,182	90.8	743	6.1	386	3.1	12,311	100
Diabetic mothers (pre- or gestational)	421	3.7	123	16.3	5	1.3	549	4.5
Cesarean delivery	2,226	219.9	199	26.8	147	38.1	2,572	20.9
1-min Apgar < 7	722	6.5	69	9.3	50	12.9	841	6.8
Obstetric trauma	338	2.9	43	5.6	6	1.5	387*	3.1
Malformations	711	6.4	64	8.6	43	11.1	818**	6.6
Hypoglycemia (glycemia <40 mg/dl)	584	5.2	86	11.6	89	23.1	759	6.2
Hypocalcemia (Ca <7 mg/dl)	114	1.0	2	0.3	19	4.9	135	1.1
Hyperbilirubinemia (Br ≥ 13 mg/dl)	696	6.2	34	4.6	21	5.4	751	6.2
Respiratory distress (Silverman > 3)	207	1.8	8	1.1	8	2.1	223	1.8
Heart disease	82	0.7	4	0.5	9	2.3	95	0.9
Neonatal mortality	40	0.36	1	0.13	8	2.07	49	0.39

NB, newborn; AGA, appropriate-for-gestational age; LGA, large-for-gestational age; SGA, small-for-gestational age
*Including 238 cephalohematomas; **major and minor

demonstrated that mothers giving birth to LGA infants had a lower concentration of protein in amniotic fluid at 12–20 weeks' gestation compared with mothers of AGA infants, suggesting that amniotic fluid proteins might emerge as biomarkers of fetal growth.[49]

Hypoglycemia

Hypoglycemia is a very frequent complication in IDMs. Thirty to forty percent of IDMs present hypoglycemia after birth. The risk is higher in macrosomic infants of poorly controlled diabetic women and in cases of maternal hyperglycemia during delivery.[50]

Hypoglycemia in infants of diabetic mothers could be attributed to fetal hyperinsulinism, which is secondary to maternal hyperglycemia. After birth, with the source of glucose discontinued, this neonatal hyperinsulinism leads to hypoglycemia. In these infants a transitory intensified pancreatic response has been demonstrated, although temporarily, when using glucose solutions and intravenous arginine,[51] which suggests that the hypoglycemia is mainly due to neonatal hyperinsulinemia. After birth, there is a rapid drop in glycemia levels, with persistently low concentrations of free fatty acids, glycerol and hydroxybutyrate.[52]

Other endocrinological observations in IDMs are a reduction in the release of catecholamines and of the blood levels of glucagon after birth, which are less raised than in normal controls.[53]

Hypoglycemia most frequently occurs between 1 and 5 h of life, when the maternal glucose contribution has disappeared, but levels of circulating insulin remain raised.

IDMs that present hypoglycemia have raised C-peptide levels and free insulin at birth.[54] In infants of diabetic mothers, C-peptide should be determined in cord blood to define degree of hyperinsulinemia and glucose at birth (in cord blood or in plasma no later than 30 min after birth) and at regular intervals thereafter (before feeding at 1, 3, 6, 12, 24, 36 and 48 h of life) for detection of neonatal hypoglycemia. Monitoring may stop if normal plasma glucose levels are found on at least two consecutive measurements.

LGA NBs of non-diabetic mothers are also considered at increased risk for hypoglycemia. As happens with infants of diabetic mothers, chronic fetal hyperinsulinemia may be one of the causes of neonatal hypoglycemia in LGA infants of non-diabetic mothers. C-peptide concentrations in the cord blood of 29 macrosomic neonates born of non-diabetic mothers were higher than in 23 control infants whose birth weight was AGA, and there was a significant direct correlation between birth weight and C-peptide concentration. Six of the macrosomic infants studied (20%) had hypoglycemia in the first 24 h of life, compared with none of the infants born with appropriate weight.[10]

Because hypoglycemia in the immediate NB period is common in LGA infants, it has been recommended that these neonates should be routinely monitored for blood glucose levels. However, recently, Rooy *et al.*[55] have demonstrated that although low blood glucose levels did occur in LGA infants, this was offset by a normal ketone body response, equivalent to those observed in infants who were AGA. The authors argue that neonatal ketogenesis is a normal adaptive response that enables the transition from fetal to infant metabolism, and that LGA infants whose mothers did not have documented diabetes do not represent a high-risk group of abnormal neonatal adaptation. In view of this, routine blood glucose monitoring and routine formula milk supplementation for LGA infants are not recommended.

Under normal conditions at birth, the glucose levels in plasma of the umbilical cord correlate with the values of the mother. In nearly all cases, the levels of glycemia diminish in the first 2 h of life, and later increase and stabilize. It is not uncommon to observe an isolated value of hypoglycemia, and because of this, the diagnosis of this entity must be based on two consecutive low values on analysis made at an interval not greater than 30 min.

Hypoglycemia is defined by serum glucose values of less than 40 mg/dl (2.2 mmol/l) for full-term infants.[56]

In clinical practice, the primary detection of serum glucose is made with colorimetric strips impregnated with chromogen, but the blood sugar levels measured in this way are 10% less than those assessed by the current oxidase glucose method and they may overestimate the low glucose levels, and at times not identify the hypoglycemia.[45,57]

The diagnosis of hypoglycemia cannot be based on glucose measurement with reagent strips. Strip hypoglycemia (less than 40 mg/dl), should be verified in the laboratory.

In symptomatic hypoglycemia (defined as hypoglycemic signs and symptoms that disappear after glucose administration) we may find variable clinical manifestations: convulsions, apnea crises, hypotonia, lethargy, food rejection, wheezing and irregular breathing patterns, cyanosis, weak cry, etc.; it should be taken into account that at times intense hypoglycemia presents an asymptomatic course, with the possibility of causing irreparable cerebral damage.

We may differentiate between three situations requiring more control: asymptomatic IDM with normal glycemia, asymptomatic infants with hypoglycemia and symptomatic hypoglycemia:[30,52]

(1) In asymptomatic IDMs with normal glycemia in the first hour of life the early initiation of breast-feeding, in the first 30–60 min after delivery, can prevent hypoglycemia. Breast feeding should be frequent, at least 10–12 times per 24 h, and the infant should be put to the breast at the earliest signs of hunger (crying is a late sign of hunger).[58]

(2) In asymptomatic infants with risk factors,[56] continue breast feeding (every 1–2 h) or feed expressed breast milk or substitute (10–15 ml/kg). Recheck blood glucose concentration before subsequent feedings until the value is stable. If the plasma concentration is less than 2.0 mmol/l (36 mg/dl), a close surveillance should be maintained, an intervention is recommended if the neonate is unable to suck, does not tolerate the early and frequent feedings described above, common situations in IDMs, or if glucose is low despite feeding, or if abnormal clinical signs develop, the infant should be hospitalized. Begin intravenous glucose infusion of 4–8 mg/kg/min, according to the course of the glycemia. Repeat serum glucose within 30 min and serially thereafter until stable > 2.5 mmol/l (45 mg/dl). Then, continue breast feeding or bottle feeding and slowly reduce intravenous infusion.

(3) In cases of NBs with symptomatic hypoglycemia and/or weight < 2000 g, or respiratory difficulty, or glycemia < 20–25 mg/dl (1.1–1.4 mmol/l) or no increase 20–30 min after oral attempts, intravenous glucose (10%) should be administered, and one or more intravenous bolus of 200 mg/kg of 10% glucose should be administered, subsequently continuing with perfusion at a rate of 6–8 mg/kg/min and then adjusting infusion rate to maintain glycemia above 45 mg/dl. Encourage frequent breast feeding after relief of symptoms. As the amount of enteral feeding increases, the intravenous glucose supply is reduced progressively; avoid the sudden withdrawal of a significant parenteral contribution with a risk of reactive hypoglycemia developing.

The lack of hypoglycemic response to the intravenous glucose supply or its persistence over more than 48 h necessitates administration of 5 mg/kg/day of hydrocortisone, divided in three doses, and one should ascertain if there are other reasons to justify the prolonged hypoglycemia.

In these macrosomic NBs it is not easy to place the peripheral venoclysis. At times, it is interrupted by extravasation, producing a reactive hypoglycemia in hyperinsulinemic patients. Thus, central silastic catheters are commonly used, introduced through peripheral route. In the case of a symptomatic IDM on whom peripheral venoclysis cannot be performed because of lack of experience or means, 30–100 μg of glucagon/kg should be administered (to a maximum of 1 mg) by intramuscular or subcutaneous route. The increased glycemia that this provokes may last 2–3 h (or perhaps less, due to hyperinsulinemia reactive to postglucagon hyperglycemia), which permits the NB infant to be transferred to the appropriate center.

Congenital malformations

The association between isolated congenital anomalies and macrosomia has been evaluated in a retrospective study on 31,897 neonates with congenital anomalies, of whom 1800 were LGA (5.8%). Five anomalies were significantly associated with high birth weight: talipes calcaneovalgus, hydrocephaly, combined angiomatoses, hip subluxation, and non-brown-pigmented nevi.[59]

Table 127.4 Neonatal morbidity and mortality rates of infants of pre- or gestational diabetic mothers, related to the overall newborn population (1999–2003)

NBs	Total infants (%) (n=12,311)	Infants of diabetic mothers (%) (n=549)	Macrosomic infants ≥4000 g (%) (n=678)	Macrosomic infants of diabetic mothers (%) (n=47)
AGA	91.8	76.7		
LGA	6.1	22.4		
SGA	3.1	0.9		
Macrosomic	5.5	8.6		
Cesarean delivery	20.9	26.4	27.0	46.8
1-min Apgar < 7	6.8	6.4	8.7	12.7
Obstetric trauma (including cephalohematoma)	3.1	8.4	5.5	10.6
Hypoglycemia	6.2	35.9	26.7	42.8
Hypocalcemia	1.1	3.6	0.5	4.7
Hyperbilirubinemia	6.1	25.9	4.3	21.3
Respiratory distress	1.8	9.1	1.2	10.6
Heart disease	0.9	1.5	0.6	8.5
Malformations (including major and minor)	6.6	5.3	9.7	10.6
Neonatal mortality	0.39	0.55	0	0

NB, newborn; AGA, appropriate-for-gestational age; LGA, large-for-gestational age; SGA, small-for-gestational age

Diabetic pregnancies are associated with an increase in congenital anomalies. The rate of congenital malformations in IDMs is two to eight times higher than that of the general NB population.[8,29,60] However, the offspring of diabetic males have the same incidence of malformations as the general NB population and gestational diabetes does not represent a risk of congenital malformation.

Approximately, 40–50% of perinatal mortality in IDMs (it is increased two- to fivefold compared with the general population) is attributable to serious congenital malformations. The congenital anomalies seen in diabetes affect multiple organ systems. The most common abnormalities are seen in the cardiovascular system (6.1% live births) and in the central nervous system (2.5% live births).

Sacral agenesis and syndrome of caudal regression (agenesis or hypoplasia of the femora and sacral agenesis) seem to have a particularly strong association with diabetes. In the IDM there is an increase in the rate of anencephaly, meningomyelocele, holoprosencephalia[61] and congenital cardiac defects compared with the general population.[62]

Maintaining normal glycemic levels during organogenesis is accompanied by a significant reduction, but not total elimination, of congenital malformations in IDMs,[63,64] especially those in White's classes D, E and F with greater genetic predisposition to congenital defects. On the other hand, it is possible that in addition to sugars other metabolic fuels, from ketones to deranged lipid peroxidation, may be responsible for the path mechanisms of congenital malformations and the whole metabolic disturbance of the IDM and it is quite conceivable that besides the classical approach to strict glucose control, other dietary measures with supplementation or replacement of deficient substrates (arachidonic acid, myoinositol, antioxidants) may prove beneficial.[65]

Other neonatal complications in infants of diabetic mothers

Perinatal mortality in IDM diminished from 197 to 20 per 1000 NBs between 1967 and 1984,[29] but in our series neonatal mortality continued to be greater in infants of diabetic mothers (pre- or gestational) compared with the overall NB population (Tables 127.3 and 127.4). The rate of neonatal morbidity depends on the severity of the diabetes of the pregnant mother more than other factors. Taking morbidity as a reference for the IDMs in our environment (Table 127.3) and also the reported findings of other authors,[40,41] we may affirm that some of the clinical problems still affecting IDMs are fetal growth disorders (30–40%), hypoglycemia (20–30%), prematurity (10–15%), perinatal asphyxia (15–16%), respiratory distress syndrome (10–15%) and congenital malformations (4–8%).

These complications are seen especially in infants of uncontrolled diabetic mothers, although some of these morbidities are still more common in IDMs than the general population, in spite of good metabolic control, and, in general, these neonates still require a higher rate of admission to neonatal intensive care units.

Respiratory distress syndrome

Clinical investigations into the effects of gestation on the maturation of the fetal lung have generated contrasting data. In one series of 805 IDMs[66] the corrected risk of hyaline membrane disease was six times greater than in those of offspring of non-diabetic mothers, which was in relation to the premature birth and retarded maturation of the pulmonary surfactant. Coinciding with the best obstetric care during diabetic pregnancy, the incidence of hyaline membrane disease has decreased,[67] possibly because the child was born with greater gestational age, more commonly by vaginal route and with a lower degree of hyperinsulinism.

Insulin interferes with the maturation process of the lungs of the fetus, induced by glucocorticoids.[68] In a study of the components of pulmonary surfactant in the amniotic fluid of the diabetic pregnancy woman, a reduced concentration of some of its proteins has been detected (SP-A).[69]

IDMs may have a respiratory distress syndrome (RDS) even with a mature ratio of lecithin/sphingomyelin (L/S) in amniotic fluid (8% of the IDMs), with varying data regarding well-controlled diabetic pregnancies.[70]

Phosphatidylglycerol in amniotic fluid indicates that pulmonary maturation has been completed (is a marker of complete pulmonary maturation) and many obstetricians prefer to verify its presence before undertaking the planned delivery in diabetic women.[45,70]

Strict control of the diabetes, amniotic fluid analysis to evaluate pulmonary maturity, predelivery control of the biophysical parameters and avoiding of cesarean section or premature births should result in no more than 5% of hyaline membrane disease due to tensioactive deficiency and 5–10% additional cases of respiratory disorders from other causes (neonatal transitory tachypnea, hypertrophic cardiomyopathy, meconial aspiration and polycythemia).[45]

Hypertrophic myocardiopathy

In approximately 10–20% of IDMs, hypertrophic myocardiopathy is diagnosed by echocardiography showing asymmetrical septum hypertrophy, so that the hypertrophied septal muscles may bulge into the left ventricle, thereby narrowing the left ventricular outflow tract. The anterior wall of the right ventricle and the posterior of the left ventricle appear, at times, hypertrophied, though to a smaller degree than the interventricular septum.

The presence of this myocardial hypertrophy in some other patients with hyperinsulinemia, as in nesidioblastosis or in rhesus fetuses with primary fetal hyperinsulinemia, supports the hypothesis that high levels of insulin and an altered level in the uterus metabolic environment are responsible for an increase in the number of receptors and in the affinity for insulin.[71]

Approximately a third of these infants with hypertrophic myocardiopathy are asymptomatic. The clinical findings may be cardiomegalia, ejecting systolic breath, congestive cardiac insufficiency signs or low cardiac output. The resolution of the symptoms tends to occur between 2 and 4 weeks and echocardiography normalization in 2–12 months.[72] The use of digoxin is not recommended or any other inotropic that could increase obstruction of the exit tract of the left ventricle. The treatment of the most serious cases has been carried out with propranolol (0.01 mg/kg i.v. every 6 h in 10-min bolus, which may be increased to a maximum dose of 0.15 mg/kg every 6 h).

Hypocalcemia and hypomagnesemia

Approximately 25–50% of the infants of insulin-dependent diabetic mothers develop hypocalcemia (total calcium less than 7 mg/dl or ionic calcium less than 1 mmol/l).[73] The rate and severity of the hypocalcemia is directly related to the severity of the maternal diabetes. The incidence of hypocalcemia in the infants of mothers with gestational diabetes is not higher than in the control group.

Hypocalcemia generally manifests itself in the second or third day of postnatal life. It may present as convulsions, jitteriness, hyperexcitability, hyperreflex, hypertonia, apneas, cyanotic episodes, etc.

Among the factors involved in its etiology, the most accepted is the slowness in the elevation of parathyroid harmone (PTH) levels after birth, when the maternal supply of calcium disappears.[74] Some authors point out that sustained fetal hypomagnesemia, secondary to maternal hypomagnesemia (increased urinary loss of magnesium in serious diabetes) is responsible for the slow postnatal response of the PTH in IDMs to the low levels of calcium, as PTH secretion reduces, because magnesium is critical to normal PTH secretion. Other proposed mechanisms for explaining hypocalcemic episodes are the hyperphosphatemia produced by postnatal tissular catabolism, the abnormal metabolism of vitamin D (intestinal antagonism of raised levels of cortisol) and hypercalcitoninemia.

Generally, in apparently normal IDMs, hypocalcemia is resolved spontaneously without need of treatment. If there are symptoms suggestive of hypocalcemia or if the infant has disease and does not tolerate enteral feeding, 10% calcium gluconate by parenteral route should be administered (5 ml/kg/day). When symptomatic hypocalcemia does not respond to calcium therapy, the presence of associated hypomagnesemia should be investigated (levels less than 1.5 mg/dl), and corrected with magnesium sulfate at 50% (0.1–0.2 ml/kg i.m. or slow i.v.).

Hematological disorders. Polycythemia (venous hematocrit ≥65% or hemoglobin ≥20 g/100 ml) is detected in 20–40% of IDMs.[73]

Abundant nutrient supply and fetal hyperinsulinism produce an increase in metabolic rate and consumption of oxygen, which means oxygen demand may exceed availability. The final result of this sequence is relative fetal hypoxemia, which causes an increase in erythropoietin, erythropoiesis and polycythemia and, in general, hyperviscosity.[75] Also, it may contribute to the raised maternal levels of glycosylated hemoglobin, which involves a deviation to the left of the hemoglobin dissociation curve, eliminating less oxygen at the tissular level.

The risk for polycythemia is correlated with control of maternal diabetes and with the maternal total glycosylated hemoglobin level at delivery.[76]

In general, these NBs are plethoric, often with intense acrocyanosis and occasionally with central cyanosis. They may present cardiorespiratory symptoms, hyperexcitability or lethargy, priapism, testicular infarction, etc. Other complications of polycythemia, especially renal vein thrombosis, should be watched for in these infants. The time of cord clamping at delivery may significantly influence blood volume and the hematocrit value. Immediate clamping of the cord (within 20 s of delivery) should therefore be encouraged.[77]

Treatment of polycythemia involves an adequate supply of liquid and, at times (a partial exanguinotransfusion), an isovolemic exchange transfusion with albumin or saline to decrease the hematocrit value to the desired range.

With the hyperinsulinemia-induced expansion of the erythrocyte mass, an increase in fetal iron utilization occurs and the severely affected infants of diabetic mothers have reduced liver, heart and brain iron concentrations. The role of tissue iron deficiency in the genesis of the abnormal clinical findings in these infants deserves further consideration.[78]

There are higher percentages of total lymphocytes and lower percentages of activated T cells in children of diabetic mothers compared to children of the reference population between the age of 1–6 years. No significant differences in lymphocyte subpopulations between children of mothers with insulin-dependent diabetes mellitus (IDDM) and gestational diabetes have been detected. This may reflect a cellular immune reaction to the particular maternal environment, characterized by both an abnormal metabolic state and persisting autoimmunity in the affected mother.[79]

Hyperbilirubinemia

The incidence of hyperbilirubinemia (bilirubin ≥13 mg/dl) is greater in IDMs that in normal control groups of the same gestational age (Table 127.3). In well-controlled IDMs, with a longer pregnancy, hyperbilirubinemia is less frequent and significant.

A series of variables, frequent in IDMs, contributes to a greater or lesser degree of hyperbilirubinemia, that is, polycythemia (probably the most significant factor in absolute terms); turnover of increased hem (increased production of carboxyhemoglobin) due to the greater hemolysis of the red cells of the IDMs whose cellular membranes are less deformable because of their glycosylation; resorption of blood of cephalohematomas, equimosis or other hematic extravasations brought on by obstetric trauma; the postnatal fast that impedes the conjugation of bilirubin and increases enterohepatic circulation of the non-conjugated bilirubin and the functional immaturity of the required hepatic enzymes for the conjugation of the bilirubin.[8,9]

The treatment of hyperbilirubinemia involves phototherapy, proper hydration and exanguinotransfusion in exceptional cases.

Thrombosis

The incidence of thrombosis, particularly of the renal veins (which may develop intrauteral or postdelivery) in IDMs is higher than in the general population. In its development, hyperviscosity plays a significant role, along with low cardiac output (hypertrophic myocardiopathy, perinatal asphyxia, etc.) and coagulator disorders. Aortic thrombosis may be facilitated in IDMs with aortic catheters, introduced through the umbilical cord.

The postnatal presentation may be with hematuria, hypochondrial mass, signs of acute renal failure or embolic episodes. The diagnosis (also in the fetus) may be carried out by ultrasound. Most patients may be treated conservatively, which allows preservation of the renal tissue.

Long-term complications

High birth weight leads to greater adult obesity and chronic disease, and also increases the risk of cancer. In view of these observations, some authors suggest that adipose tissue may play a role in linking events in fetal growth to the subsequent development of adult disease.[80,81]

Neurodevelopment

Mild to moderate psychomotor and psychological disturbance has been reported in the offspring of diabetic mothers. Less optimal intellectual development is associated with reduced head circumference.

Different authors have found that ketonuria and glycohemoglobin of the pregnant woman bear a subsequent relation with low intellectual level of the IDMs.[82,83] In diabetic pregnancies with adequate metabolic control, these data were not detected.[2] Other authors have reported notably different results and it is not known for certain if the diabetic state causes subtle dysfunction of development.[84]

The presence of major congenital malformations has been associated with worse psychomotor development at 2 years.[85] The risk of malformations of the central nervous system (microcephalia, disorders of neuronal proliferation and migration) as well as sacral agenesia is well known, and there is evidence to suggest abnormal functional development of the nervous system.[86,87]

Cancer

Infants with macrosomia had increased risk of acute lymphocytic leukemia, Wilms tumor and neuroblastoma. A number of authors have postulated that a deregulation of growth factors may have a role in the development of soma childhood cancers. The association of Wilms tumor and Beckwith–Wiedemann syndrome suggests that overexpression of IGF-2 may have some role in both processes.

A questionnaire survey identified a possibly increased risk of malignancy for patients with Sotos syndrome.[88] The possible role of mutations at 3p21 in the etiology of Sotos syndrome and tumor development had been described.[89]

Obesity

In recent years, there has been accumulating evidence, from both animal studies and epidemiological data, to suggest that fetal β-cell hyperplasia and hyperinsulinism found in IDMs may induce irreversible changes leading to obesity and glucose intolerance.

At birth almost 50% of IDMs have corporal weight above the 90th percentile of the control, but at the end of the first year this difference is no longer noteworthy. Acceleration of the ponderal increase reappears at 5–8 years of life. By this time, half of the IDMs again exceed the 90th percentile of corporal weight and there is a higher probability of becoming obese adolescents than for those born with a normal birth weight,[90] but other authors have not confirmed these findings.

There is evidence that the offspring of insulin-dependent diabetic women are exposed to a greater risk of subsequently suffering diabetes (20 times more than children of non-diabetic mothers) and in a lower proportion than those of mothers with gestational diabetes.[45]

Care of the infants of the diabetic mothers should start well before conception, with preconceptional planning and strict glycemic control (HbA_{1c}=5–8%) throughout pregnancy to reduce the incidence of miscarriage, congenital malformations, macrosomia at birth and long-term complications.

Several studies have demonstrated that increased neonatal adiposity in LGA children born of non-diabetic mothers is also associated with obesity in later life. It has been suggested that there are three critical time periods for the development of adiposity during childhood: gestation and early infancy, a rebound period at 5–7 years and adolescence. Nutritional alterations that occur during these key ages may cause permanent physiologic alterations, placing the child at increased risk of adult obesity. Children born LGA, of diabetic and non-diabetic mothers, may be at risk for accumulating excess fat in early childhood and may be more likely to have an early adiposity rebound, increasing the risk for overweight in adulthood.[91]

The results of various studies[92,93] suggest that the positive association between high birth weight and later fatness is largely explained by prepregnancy maternal weight, which may be a more important risk factor for later obesity than birth weight.

A recent study on exclusively breast-fed infants demonstrates a slower growth rate from birth to 5 months of life in fatter NBs (larger arm fat area and higher weight-to-length ratio) than in thinner NBs. The authors hypothesize that the postuterine environment, particularly breast feeding, decelerates postnatal weight gain in fatter infants. Others factors, such as an increase in insulin sensitivity after birth or a higher free fatty acid (FFA) turnover due to higher fat mass may help explain this finding.[94]

Given all these considerations, the macrosomic infant requires specific follow-up to detect any possible complications. If the infant is of a diabetic mother, these risks may be increased and thus strict surveillance is necessary.

REFERENCES

1. Lubchenco LO, Hansman C, Boyd E. Intrauterine growth in length and head circumference as estimated from live births at gestational ages from 26 to 42 weeks. *Pediatrics* 1966;37:403–8.
2. Alexander GR, Himes JH, Kaufman RB, *et al.* A United States national reference for fetal growth. *Obstet Gynecol* 1996;87:163–8.
3. Chervenak JL. Macrosomia in the postdates pregnancy. *Clin Obstet Gynecol* 1992;35:151–5.
4. Spellacy WN, Miller S, Winegar A, Peterson PQ. Macrosomia-maternal characteristics and infant complications. *Obstet Gynecol* 1985;66:158–61.
5. Metcoff J. Clinical assessment of nutritional status at birth. Fetal malnutrition and SGA are not synonymous. *Pediatr Clin North Am* 1994;41:875–91.
6. Thomas P, Peabody J, Turnier V, Clark RH. A new look at intrauterine growth and the impact of race, altitude and gender. *Pediatrics* 2000;106:2,e21.
7. Ouzilleau C, Roy MA, Leblanc L, Carpentier A, Maheux P. An observational study comparing 2-hour 75-g oral glucose tolerance with fasting plasma glucose in pregnant women: Both poorly predictive of birth weight. *Can Med Assoc J* 2003;168:403–9.
8. Grassi AE, Giuliano MA. The neonate with macrosomia. *Clin Obstet Gynecol* 2000;43:340–8.
9. Ballard JL, Rosenn B, Khoury JC, Miodovnik M. Diabetic fetal macrosomia: Significance of disproportionate growth. *J Pediatr* 1993;122:115–9.
10. Balaguer JA, Garbayo J, Bofarull JM, Fernandez JD, Escribano J, Soler L. Hipoglucemias en recién nacidos a termino macrosomáticos no proporcionados. Valor del índice ponderal para predecir el riesgo de hipoglucemia neonatal. *An Esp Pediatr* 1995;43:124–7.
11. Kramer MS, Morin I, Yang H, *et al.* Why are babies getting bigger? Temporal trends in fetal growth and its determinants. *J Pediatr* 2002;141:538–42.

12. Baker J, Liu JP, Robertson EJ, Efstratiadis A. Role of insulin-like growth factors in embryonic and postnatal growth. *Cell* 1993;75:73–82.
13. Le Roith D. Insulin-like growth factors. *N Engl J Med* 1997;336: 633–40.
14. Salardi S, Orsini LF, Cacciari E, *et al.* Growth hormone, insulin-like growth factor I, insulin and C-peptide during human fetal life: In utero study. *Clin Endocrinol* 1991;34:187–90.
15. Gluckman PD, Breier BH, Oliver M, Harding J, Bassett N. Fetal growth in late gestation: A constrained pattern of growth. *Acta Paediatr Scand Suppl* 1990;367:105–10.
16. Gibson JM, Aplin JD, White A, Westwood M. Regulation of IGF bioavailability in pregnancy. *Mol Hum Reprod* 2001;7:79–87.
17. Doménech E, Díaz-Gómez NM, Barroso F, Cortabarria C. Endocrine factors related to perinatal period. *Prenat Neonat Med* 1998;3(Suppl 1):13.
18. Díaz Gómez NM, Doménech E, Barroso F, Cortabarria C, Rico J. Influencia de la GH y de la nutrición sobre el crecimiento en el periodo neonatal. *An Esp Pediatr* 1997;46:41–6.
19. Doménech E, Diaz-Gomez NM, Barroso F, Cortabarria C. Zinc and perinatal growth. Early Hum Dev 2001;65(Suppl):S111–7.
20. Quattrin T, Albini CH, Cara JF, Vandlen RL, Mills BJ, MacGillivray MH. Quantification of urinary somatomedin-C and growth hormone in preterm and full-term infants and normal children. *J Clin Endocrinol Metab* 1988;66:792–7.
21. Sivan E, Lin WM, Homko CJ, Reece A, Boden G. Leptin is present in human cord blood. *Diabetes* 1997;46:917–9.
22. Christou H, Connors JM, Ziotopoulou M, *et al.* Cord blood leptin and insuli-like growth factor levels are independent predictor of fetal growth. *J Clin Endocrinol Metab* 2001;86:935–8.
23. Tsai PJ, Yu CH, Hsu SP, *et al.* Cord plasma concentration of adiponectin and leptin in healthy term neonates: Positive correlation with birthweight and neonatal adiposity. *Clin Endocrinol* 2004;61:88–93.
24. Ikezaki A, Hosoda H, Ito K, *et al.* Fasting plasma ghrelin levels are negatively correlated with insulin resistance and PAI-1, but not with leptin, in obese children and adolescent. *Diabetes* 2002;51:3408–11.
25. Farquhar J, Mark H, Worg ACK, Wach R, Chessex P, Chanoine JP. Elevated umbilical cord ghrelin concentrations in small for gestational age neonates. *J Clin Endocrinol Metab* 2003;88:4324–7.
26. Hay WW, Catz ChS, Grave GD, Yaffe SJ. Workshop summary: Fetal growth: Its regulation and disorders. *Pediatrics* 1997;99: 585–91.
27. McIntyre HD, Serek R, Crane DI, *et al.* Placental growth hormone (GH), GH-binding protein, and insulin-like growth factor in normal, growth retarded, and diabetic pregnancies: Correlations with fetal growth. *J Clin Endocrinol Metab* 2000;85:1143–50.
28. Tauber MT, Harris AG, Rochiccioli P. Clinical use of the long acting somatostatin analogue octreotide in pediatrics. *Eur J Pediatr* 1994:153:304–10.
29. Centers for Disease Control. Perinatal mortality and congenital malformations in infants born to women with insulin-dependent diabetic mellitus – United States, Canada and Europe 1940–1988. *J Am Med Assoc* 1990;264:437–41.
30. Doménech E. Macrosomia: Neonatal aspects. In Kurjaj A, ed. *Textbook of Perinatal Medicine.* London: Parthenon Publishing Group, 1998;2:1296–306.
31. Wong SF, Oats JJN, Chan FY, McIntyre DH. Fetal growth spurt and pregestational diabetic pregnancy. *Diabetes Care* 2002;25: 1681–4.
32. Milner RDG. Endocrine control of fetal growth. In Linblad BS, ed. *Perinatal Nutrition.* New York: Academic Press. 1988:45–62.
33. Whitelaw A. Subcutaneous fat in newborn infants of diabetic mothers: An indication of quality of diabetic control. *Lancet* 1977;1:15–8.
34. Jang HC, Cho NH, Min YK, Han IK, Jung KB, Metzger BE. Increased macrosomia and perinatal morbidity independent of maternal obesity and advanced age in Korean women with GDM. *Diabetes Care* 1997;20:1582–8.
35. Gold AE, Reilly R, Little J, Walker JD. The effect of glycemic control in the pre-conception period and early pregnancy on birth weight in women with IDDM. *Diabetes Care* 1998;21:535–8.
36. Akinbi HT, Gerdes JS. Macrosomic infants of nondiabetic mothers and elevated C-peptide levels in cord blood. *J Pediatr* 1995; 127:481–4.
37. Chauhan SP, Sullivan CA, Lutton TC, Maganan EF, Morrison JC. Parous patient's estimate of birth weight in postterm infants. *J Perinatol* 1995;15:192–4.
38. Díaz-Gómez NM, Hernández MJ, González NL, Doménech E, Cortabarría C, Clemente I. Análisis de la composición corporal en el recién nacido de madre diabética. *An Esp Pediatr* 2000; 52(Suppl 4):209–10.
39. Hammami M, Walters JC, Hockman EM, Koo WWK. Disproportionate alterations in body composition of large for gestational age neonates. *J Pediatr* 2001;138:817–21.
40. Demarini S, Specker BL, Sierra IR, Miodovnik M, Tsang RC. Evidence of increased intrauterine bone resorption in term infants of mothers with insulin-dependent diabetes. *J Pediatr* 1995; 26:796–8.
41. Namgung R, Tsang RC. Bone in the pregnant mother and newborn at birth. *Clin Chim Acta* 2003;333:1–11.
42. Namgung R, Tsang RC. Factors affecting newborn bone mineral contents: In utero effects on newborn bone mineralization. *Proc Nutr Soc* 2000;59:55–63.
43. Clemente I, Díaz-Gómez NM, Barroso F, *et al.* Influences of diabetes on mother and fetal metabolism. *J Perinat Med* 2001; 29(Suppl 1):489.
44. Wilcox A, Skjaerven R, Buekens P, Kiely J. Birth weight and perinatal mortality: A comparison of the United States and Norway. *J Am Med Assoc* 1995;273:709–11.
45. Cordero L, Landon MB. Infant of the diabetic mother. *Clin Perinatol* 1993;20:635–48.
46. Friesen CD, Miller AM, Rayburn WF. Influence of spontaneous or induced labor on delivering the macrosomic fetus. *Am J Perinatol* 1995;12:63–6.
47. Lipscomb KR, Gregory K, Shaw K. The outcome of macrosomic infants weighing at least 4500 grams: Los Angeles County + University of Southern California experience. *Obstet Gynecol* 1995;85:558–64.
48. O'Reilly-Green C, Divon M. Sonographic and clinical methods in the diagnosis of macrosomia. *Clin Obstet Gynecol* 2000;43: 309–20.
49. Tisi DK, Emard JJ, Koski KG. Total protein concentration in human amniotic fluid is negatively associated with infants birth weight. *J Nutr* 2004;134:1754–8.
50. Anderson O, Hertel J, Schmolker L, Kuhl C. Influence of the maternal plasma glucose concentration at delivery on the risk of hypoglycaemia in infants of insulin-dependent diabetic mothers. *Acta Paediatr Scand* 1985;74:268–73.
51. Pilde RS, Lilien LD, Demarini S, Tsang RC, Morishima A, Danish RK. Metabolic and endocrino disorders. In Fanaroff AA, Martin RJ, eds. *Neonatal Perinatal Medicine.* St. Louis: Mosby Year Book, 1992:1152–292.
52. Aynsley-Green A, Soltesz G. The infant of a diabetic mother. In Roberton NCR, ed. *Textbook of Neonatology.* Edinburgh: Churchill Livingstone, 1992:333–8.
53. Bloom SR, Johnston DF. Failure of glucagon release in infants of diabetic mothers. *Br Med J* 1972;4:453–54.
54. Sosenko IR, Kitzmiller JL, Loo SW, Blix P, Rubenstein AH, Gabbay KH. The infant of the diabetic mother. Correlation of increased cord C-peptide levels with macrosomia and hypoglycemia. *N Engl J Med* 1979;301:859–62.
55. Rooy L, Hawdon J. Nutritional factors that affect the postnatal metabolic adaptation of full-term small- and large-for-gestational-age infants. *Pediatrics* 2002;109:3,e42.
56. Cornblath M, Hawdon JM, Williams AF, *et al.* Controversies regarding definition of neonatal hypoglycemia: Suggested operational thresholds. *Pediatrics* 2000;105:1141–5.
57. Holtrop PC, Madison KA, Kiechle FL, Karcher RE, Batton DG. A comparison of chromogen test strip (Chemstrip bG) and serum glucose values in newborns. *Am J Dis Child* 1990;144: 183–5.
58. The Academy of Breastfeeding Medicine. Clinical protocol number 1 – Guidelines for glucose monitoring and treatment of hypoglycemia in term breastfeeding neonates. The Academy of Breastfeeding Medicine, 1999:4. http://www.bfmed.org/
59. Lapunzina P, López Carmelo JS, Rittler M, Castilla EE. Risk of congenital anomalies in large for gestational age infants. *J Pediatr* 2002;140:200–4.
60. Becerra JE, Khoury MJ, Cordero JF, Erickson JD. Diabetes mellitus during pregnancy and the risks for specific birth defects: A population based case–control study. *Pediatrics* 1990;85:1–9.
61. Barr M, Hanson JW, Currey K, *et al.* Holoprosencephaly in infants of diabetic mothers. *J Pediatr* 1983;102:565–8.
62. Reece EA, Hobbins JC. Diabetic embryopathy: Pathogenesis, perinatal diagnosis and prevention. *Obstet Gynecol Surv* 1986;41: 325–35.

63. Goldman M, Kitzmiller JL, Abrams B, Cowan RM, Laros RK Jr. Obstetric complications with GDM. Effects of maternal weight. *Diabetes* 1991;40(Suppl 2):79–82.
64. Mills J, Knopp RH, Simpson JL. Lack of relation of increased malformation rates in infants of diabetic mothers to glycemic control during organogenesis. *N Engl J Med* 1988;318:671–6.
65. Carrapato MR. The infants of the diabetic mother: An overview. In Carrera JM, Cabero L, Baraibar R, eds. *The Perinatal Medicine of the New Millennium*. Bologna: Monduzzi Editore, 2001:469–74.
66. Robert M, Neff R, Hubbel J, Taeusch H, Avery M. Association between maternal diabetes and the respiratory distress syndrome in the newborn. *N Engl J Med* 1976;294:357–60.
67. Piper JM, Langer D. Does maternal diabetes delay fetal pulmonary maturity? *Am J Obstet Gynecol* 1993;168:783–6.
68. Carlson KS, Smith BT, Post M. Insulin acts on the fibroblast to inhibit glucocorticoid stimulation of lung maturation. *J Appl Physiol* 1984;57:1577–9.
69. Nogee L, McMahan M, Whitsett JA. Hyaline membrane disease and surfactant protein, SPA-35, in diabetes in pregnancy. *Am J Perinat* 1988;5:374–7.
70. Kjos SL, Walther FJ, Montoro M, Paul RH, Diaz F, Stabler M. Prevalence of etiology of respiratory distress in infants of diabetic mothers: Predictive value of fetal lung maturation tests. *Am J Obstet Gynecol* 1990;163:898–903.
71. Mehta S, Nuamah I, Kalhan S. Altered diastolic function in infants of mothers with gestational diabetes: No relation to macrosomia. *Pediatr Cardiol* 1995;1:24–7.
72. Trowitzsch E, Bigalke U, Gisbertz R, Kalifelz HC. Echocardiographic profile of infants of diabetic mothers. *Eur J Pediatr* 1983;140:311–5.
73. Mimouni F, Tsang RC, Hertzberg VS, Miodovnik M. Polycythemia, hypomagnesemia and hypocalcemia in infants of diabetic mothers. *Am J Dis Child* 1986;140:798–800.
74. Noguchi A, Eren M, Tsang RC. Parathyroid hormone in hypocalcemic and normocalcemic infants of diabetic mothers. *J Pediatr* 1980;97:112–4.
75. Widness JA, Susa JB, Garcia JF, *et al.* Increased erythropoiesis and elevated erytropoietin in infants born to diabetic mothers and in hyperinsulinemic rhesus fetuses. *J Clin Invest* 1981;67:637–42.
76. Green DW, Khoury J, Mimouni F. Neonatal haematocrit and maternal glycemic control in insulin-dependent diabetes. *J Pediatr* 1992;120:302–5.
77. Persson B, Hanson U. Neonatal morbidities in gestational diabetes mellitus. *Diabetes Care* 1998;21:B79–84.
78. Petry CD, Eaton MA, Wobken BS, Mills MM, Johnson DE, Georgieff MK. Iron deficiency of liver, heart, and brain in newborn infants of diabetic mothers. *J Pediatr* 1992;121:109–14.
79. Roll U, Scheeser J, Standl E, Ziegler AG. Alterations of lymphocyte subsets in children of diabetic mothers. *Diabetologia* 1994;37:1132–41.
80. Tsai PJ, Yu CH, Hsu SP, *et al.* Cord plasma concentrations of adiponectin and leptin in healthy term neonates: Positive correlation with birth weight and neonatal adiposity. *Clin Endocrinol* 2004;61:88–93.
81. Samaras TT, Elrick H, Storms LH. Birth weight, rapid growth, cancer, and longevity: A review. *J Natl Med Assoc* 2003;95:1170–83.
82. Stebhens JA, Baker GL, Kitchell M. Outcome at ages 1, 3 and 5 of children born to diabetic women. *Am J Obstet Gynecol* 1977;127:408–13.
83. Rizzo TA, Dooley SL, Metzger BE, Cho NH, Ogata ES, Silverman BL. Prenatal and perinatal influences on long-term psychomotor development in offspring of diabetic mothers. *Am J Obstet Gynecol* 1995;173:1753–8.
84. Goldstein E, Porter B, Galil A. Neurodevelopmental outcome of offspring of the diabetic mother: Need for further research. *Am J Dis Child* 1991;145:602–3.
85. Sells CJ, Robinson NM, Brown Z, Knopp RH. Long-term developmental follow-up of infants of diabetic mothers. *J Pediatr* 1994;125:S9–17.
86. Schulte FJ, Lassen U, Parl U, Nolte R, Jürgens U. Brain and behavioral maturation in newborn infants of diabetic mothers. Part II: Sleep cycles. *Neuropediatrie* 1992;1:36–43.
87. Castro JR, Gonzalez NL, Gonzalez-Campo C, Cortabarria C, Mendez A, Domenech E. Behavioral states in fetuses and newborn infants of diabetic women. *Prenat Neonat Med* 1996;1(Suppl 1):192A.
88. Hersh JH, Cole TR, Bloom AS, Bertolone SJ, Hughes HE. Risk of malignancy in Sotos syndrome. *J Pediatr* 1992;120:572–4.
89. Cole TR, Hughes HE, Jeffreys MJ, Williams GT, Arnold MM. Small cell lung carcinoma in a patient with Sotos syndrome: Are genes at 3p21 involved in both conditions? *J Med Genet* 1992;29:338–41.
90. Vohr BR, Lipsitt LP, Oh W. Somatic growth of children of diabetic mothers with reference to birth size. *J Pediatr* 1980;97:196–9.
91. Hediger ML, Overpeck MD, McGlynn A, Kuczmarski RJ, Maurer KR, Davis WW. Growth and fatness at three to six years of age of children born small- or large-for-gestational age. *Pediatrics* 1999;104:3,e33.
92. Parson TJ, Power C, Manor O. Fetal and early life growth and body mass index from birth to early adulthood in 1958 British cohort: Longitudinal study. *Br Med J* 2001;323:1331–5.
93. Vohr BR, McGarvey ST, Tucker R. Effects of maternal gestational diabetes on offspring adiposity at 4–7 years of age. *Diabetes Care* 1999;22:1284–91.
94. Sun M, Schutz Y, Grezzani A, Clementi M, Gaudino R, Maffeis C. Body size and early growth in appropriate- and large-for-gestational age infants. *Acta Paediatr* 2003;92:1127–32.

SECTION XIV

Preterm delivery

Section Editors: **G. C. di Renzo and R. Romero**

128 Mechanisms of the initiation of human parturition

L. F. Gonçalves, R. Romero, J. P. Kusanovic, E. Soto and J. Espinoza

Introduction

Parturition is the act of giving birth.[1] It is a complex process that includes the anatomical, physiological, biochemical and immunological events taking place in the maternal, placental and fetal compartments. These events are responsible for: (1) the preparation of the uterus for labor; (2) labor *per se*, leading to the delivery of the fetus and placenta; and (3) postpartum uterine involution, lactation and adaptation of maternal behavior.

The mechanisms responsible for labor resemble those involved in implantation. Both have been linked to carefully regulated inflammatory processes and, indeed, many of the molecular events associated with parturition have also been implicated in the process of implantation.

Abnormal parturition is a major cause of maternal and perinatal morbidity and mortality. The failure to initiate labor or prolonged pregnancy is associated with an increased risk of fetal death.[2] Preterm labor and delivery is the leading cause of perinatal morbidity and mortality worldwide.[3] Mothers also pay a price for labor abnormalities. For example, failure to progress in labor at term (often referred to as dystocia) is the most frequent indication for cesarean section.[4] Intrapartum infection (clinical chorioamnionitis) is a common complication that may result in maternal sepsis.[5] Inadequate hemostasis after delivery of the placenta (i.e., postpartum hemorrhage) is a leading cause of maternal death worldwide.[6] Hence, the importance of labor as a clinical entity. Yet, fundamental questions about the physiology and pathology of human parturition, a process that has played a key role in shaping the evolution of our species, remain unanswered at the beginning of the 21st century. In this chapter, we will review the mechanisms of parturition in normal pregnancies. Chapter 129 will address the mechanisms implicated in spontaneous preterm labor and preterm prelabor rupture of the membranes (PROM).

Normal duration of pregnancy

The mean duration of human pregnancy is 280 postmenstrual days or 40 weeks in women with a regular 28-day menstrual cycle (adjustments must be made for shorter or longer menstrual cycles). Studying 4000 women with reliable dates and regular menstrual cycles, Kloosterman[7] found that 4.5% of patients delivered on the expected date of confinement (also known as EDC, which corresponds to the expected date of delivery calculated from the Nägele rule), 29% at 40 weeks ± 3 days, and 80% between 38 and 42 weeks of gestation. Preterm delivery is defined as birth before 37 completed weeks. Post-term pregnancy is one in which the gestation extends beyond 42 weeks.

The duration of gestation varies remarkably among animal species.[8] A combination of fetal genetic and environmental factors appears to play a role in this variation, although the precise mechanisms are unknown. Conceptually, the duration of pregnancy should be linked to the time required for the birth of a developmentally mature fetus capable of surviving extrauterine life, and for the adaptations to be in place to react to changes in environmental conditions. Thus, mechanisms must exist to synchronize fetal growth and maturation with the maternal process of parturition. Evidence of a gene-environment interaction to determine the length of gestation derives from cross-breeding experiments. Allen *et al.*[9] transferred Thoroughbred embryos to the uteri of smaller Pony mares and Pony embryos to Thoroughbred mares in order to determine the effect of maternal size on placental and fetal size. These experiments also afforded an opportunity to examine the role of gene-environment interactions on the duration of gestation. A Thoroughbred in Thoroughbred group and a Pony in Pony group, established by artificial insemination, served as the control groups. The mean duration of gestation of the Thoroughbred in Thoroughbred pregnancy was 339 ± 3 days, while the Pony in Pony pregnancy was 325 ± 3 days. The duration of gestation in

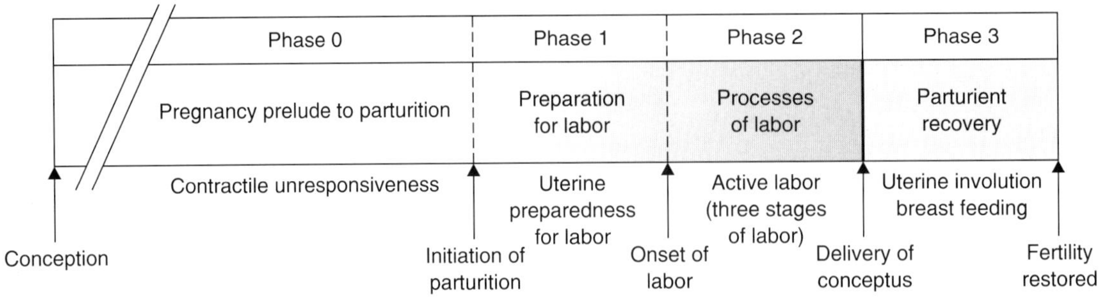

Figure 128.1 The initiation of parturition and the onset of labor. From: Cunningham *et al.*,[10] with permission

the experimental groups fell between these two. The Thoroughbred in Pony (also called 'deprived *in utero* environment') lasted 332 days ±2.8 days, while the Pony in Thoroughbred (also called 'luxurious *in utero* environment') lasted 331 days ±2.7 days. The authors concluded that the fetal and maternal genome, therefore, had an effect on the duration of pregnancy. A longer gestation was associated with a Thoroughbred genome, whether it was a mare or a foal. The longer gestation in the 'luxurious *in utero* environment' provided by the Thoroughbred mother gestating a Pony suggests that environmental factors operate to determine the duration of pregnancy. Otherwise, the fetus could have been born at the expected gestational age of the Pony. In contrast, the effect of the fetal genome is demonstrated in the Thoroughbred in Pony group in which gestational length was longer than that expected from the maternal genome alone in spite of a 'deprived *in utero* environment'. In conclusion, gestational length is likely a function of both genetic and environmental factors.

An overview of parturition and labor

The terms labor and parturition are often used interchangeably, although they are not synonymous. Labor is the acute process by which the fetus is expelled from the uterus, usually within 24 hours. Clinically, labor is defined as a state in which there is increased frequency and intensity of uterine contractions leading to progressive cervical effacement, dilatation and delivery. In contrast, parturition describes the changes that occur in preparation for, during and after labor. The process of parturition goes on for weeks, while labor lasts hours.

An integrated view of the relationship among implantation, pregnancy, labor and parturition was proposed by Paul MacDonald.[10] He suggested that this relationship could be represented to include four stages, which are described below (Figure 128.1).[10] We have slightly modified this insightful conceptual framework to take into account evidence gathered after MacDonald's initial proposal.

Phase 0 is characterized by myometrial tranquility, a state of cervical unripeness and intact membranes. A key feature of this phase of gestation is that the inherent propensity of the myometrium to contract is harnessed so that the uterine smooth muscle is refractory to natural stimulants such as oxytocin.[10] The chorioamniotic membranes remain intact. MacDonald proposed that this physiologic state lasts through 95% of pregnancy.[10]

Phase 1 of parturition is also called 'preparation for labor' and is characterized by the suspension of uterine tranquility and the development of myometrial responsiveness to agents that stimulate contractility (uterotonic agents). The initiation of parturition (not labor), considered as the switch from Phase 0 to Phase 1, is subclinical in nature. There is no current test that can identify this hypothetical switch with certainty. The traditional view has been that there is a progressive nature to the transition from Phase 0 to Phase 1, but this needs to be reconsidered based on clinical and experimental observations, including those demonstrating that parturition could have both a reversible and irreversible course. The irreversible course takes place when the switch from Phase 0 to Phase 1 is followed by Phase 2. For example, some maternal insults, such as pyelonephritis, can lead to increased uterine contractility and induce cervical changes.[11,12] Yet, early treatment of pyelonephritis can prevent preterm delivery.[12] Similarly, the administration of antiprogestins can induce a switch from Phase 0 to Phase 1 of parturition; although this is not always followed by progression to delivery (Phase 2).[13,14] Moreover, the administration of 17-α-hydroxyprogesterone or progesterone may prevent the transition from Phase 0 to Phase 1.[15–17]

Phase 2 corresponds to the process of labor and is clinically characterized by a dramatic increase in the intensity and frequency of uterine contractions (which become painful), progressive cervical effacement and dilatation, and membrane rupture. The term 'onset of labor' specifically refers to the transition from Phase 1 to Phase 2. Challis and Lye introduced the concept of 'activation' to refer to the changes in uterine function that take place between Phase 1 and Phase 2 of parturition.[18] From a clinical point of view,

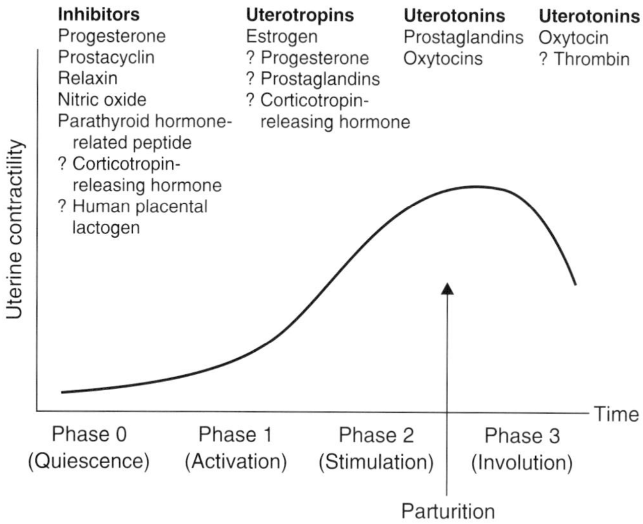

Figure 128.2 Biochemical mediators involved in the four phases of parturition. From: Norwitz *et al.*,[20] with permission.

some of the changes in Phase 2 can be objectively described with partograms, which display the relationship between cervical dilatation and the station of the presenting part as a function of time. The end of Phase 2 occurs at delivery of the conceptus. Clinicians often refer to the first stage of labor as the events taking place between the onset of clinical labor and complete dilatation of the cervix. The second stage is the period between full dilatation and delivery of the fetus. The third stage is the interval between delivery of the fetus and expulsion of the placenta. The first stage is clinically important because this is when most labor disorders are diagnosed (i.e., dysfunctional labor, dystocia, failure to progress in labor, etc.).

Phase 3 refers to the events that occur after delivery and are aimed at maternal recovery from childbirth, maternal contribution to survival of the infant (i.e., breast feeding) and restoration of the non-gestational state.

Challis and Lye proposed that a different set of biochemical mediators are involved in the four phases of parturition.[19] Candidate molecules are displayed in Figure 128.2.[20] For example, Phase 0 may be mediated by inhibitors of uterine contractility such as progesterone, prostacyclin, relaxin, and parathyroid hormone-related peptide (PTHrP).[19] Phase 1 is considered an active process involving fetal development and maturation. Specifically, the fetal hypothalamic–pituitary–adrenal (HPA) axis is hypothesized to increase the output of cortisol, which ultimately leads to upregulation of a group of genes that encode for contraction-associated proteins, including connexin-43 (the major protein of myometrial gap junctions) and oxytocin receptors, among others.[19] The role of the fetus and placenta in changing the concentrations of estrogen (uterotropin) and progesterone are considered central to this phase. Phase 2 of parturition refers to stimulation of a 'prepared' uterus by uterotonic agents, such as prostaglandins and oxytocin.[19] The latter hormone is also involved in uterine contractility after delivery of the placenta, breast milk ejection and maternal–fetal bonding.

The current descriptions of the mediators involved represent the contribution of many investigators using hypothesis-driven research strategies. The utilization of discovery techniques, such as genomics, proteomics and metabolomics (which allow a comprehensive description of the global changes in the transcriptome, proteome, and metabolome), are likely to yield new insights into the processes of normal and abnormal parturition, and allow integration of much of the research conducted to date.[21]

In broad terms, labor may begin because of: (1) removal of inhibitory actions of factors that promote uterine tranquility and a state of cervical unripeness during most of gestation; (2) the effect of stimulatory agents on the same target organs; or (3) a combination of both.

The common pathway of parturition: components

The common pathway of human parturition has been defined as the anatomic, biochemical, physiologic and clinical events that occur in the mother and/or fetus in both term and preterm labor. The intrauterine components of this pathway include increased uterine contractility, cervical ripening (dilatation and effacement) and decidual/fetal membrane activation (Figure 128.3). In addition, systemic processes (endocrinological, metabolic, etc.) are also part of the pathway. For example, term and preterm parturition are associated with an increase in the fetal and maternal plasma levels of corticotrophin-releasing hormone (CRH) and cortisol, as well as an increase in caloric metabolic expenditures.[22–31]

Increased uterine contractility

Although myometrial activity occurs throughout pregnancy, labor is characterized by a dramatic change in the pattern of uterine contractility that evolves from 'contractures' to 'contractions'. Nathanielsz and colleagues[32,33] defined contractures as epochs of myometrial activity that last several minutes and are associated with a modest increase in intrauterine pressure and very fragmented bursts of electrical activity on the electromyogram. In contrast, contractions are epochs of myometrial activity of short duration, associated with dramatic increases in intrauterine pressure and electromyographic activity. The switch from a contracture to a contraction pattern occurs during normal labor,[34] or can be induced by pathological events such as food withdrawal, infection or maternal intra-abdominal

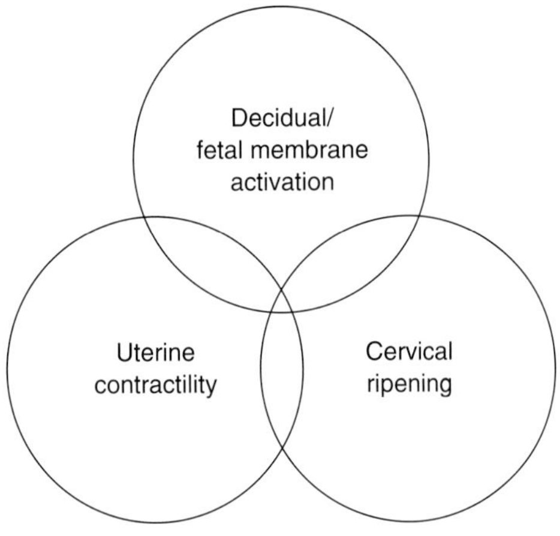

Figure 128.3 The common pathway of preterm and term parturition.

surgery.[35–37] The switch from a contracture to a contraction pattern is a potentially reversible phenomenon.[35,38–40] The increased birth rate observed immediately after a period of fasting suggests that a fasting-induced switch operates in humans.[39,40]

This change in pattern (from contracture to contraction) begins at night and labor is preceded by a progressive nocturnal increase in uterine activity of the contraction pattern.[41,42] The circadian nature of this rhythm suggests that uterine activity is under neural control. Plasma concentrations of oxytocin follow a circadian pattern similar to that of uterine contractility.[41] Oxytocin antagonists blunt the nocturnal increase in uterine activity that precedes the onset of parturition in monkeys,[41–45] suggesting that oxytocin may mediate the circadian rhythm in uterine contractility. Oxytocin is produced by human decidua and the paraventricular nuclei of the hypothalamus, while oxytocin receptors are present in myometrial cells and decidua.[46–52] This hormone, therefore, may play both an endocrine and a paracrine role in the control of parturition.[47,53–60]

Labor is characterized by a coordinated and effective generation of mechanical forces by the myometrium, which eventually lead to the expulsion of the conceptus. Increased cell-to-cell communication is thought to be responsible for the effectiveness of myometrial contractility during labor. Gap junctions develop in the myometrium just prior to labor and disappear shortly after delivery.[61–65] Gap junction formation and the expression of the gap junction protein connexin-43 in human myometrium is similar in term and preterm labor.[66–70] These findings suggest that the appearance of gap junctions and increased expression of connexin-43 may be part of the underlying molecular and cellular events responsible for the switch from contractures to contractions prior to the onset of parturition. Estrogen, progesterone and prostaglandins have been implicated in the regulation of gap junction formation, as well as in influencing the expression of connexin-43.[71–73] Lye *et al.*, for example, have referred to a set of distinct proteins called 'contraction-associated proteins' that are characteristic of this phase of parturition.[70,74,75]

Recently, Lye *et al.*[76] reported that the myometrium undergoes sequential phenotypic remodeling during pregnancy, specifically, that rat myometrium undergoes changes in the extracellular matrix (ECM). They also proposed that contractile proteins can be grouped into three phenotypes, including: (1) *Proliferative*, when the number of myocytes increase, as demonstrated by a higher proliferation cell nuclear antigen labelling and protein expression in early pregnancy. This phenotype coincides with a higher myometrial expression of anti-apoptotic proteins (BCl-2 and BCl-xL); (2) *Synthetic*, when the myometrial cells undergo hypertrophy, as demonstrated by a higher protein/DNA ratio in the second half of pregnancy and coincides with a higher secretion of ECM from the myocytes, in particular collagen I and collagen III, as well as with a high concentration of caldesmon (a marker of synthetic phenotype); and (3) *Contractile*, which occurs at the end of pregnancy and coincides with a low myometrial expression of interstitial matrix and high expression of components of the basement membrane (laminin and collagen IV). In addition, the authors reported a high protein expression of alpha actin in the myometrium in early pregnancy and a high protein expression in gamma actin associated with the contractile phenotype. The authors proposed that the switch from a proliferative to a synthetic phenotype may be regulated by caspase 3 and the switch from the synthetic to the contractile phenotype by a decrease in progesterone.[76] A concept of emerging importance is that mechanical factors, such as uterine stretch, can modify the uterine[76,77] and membrane[78] phenotype and play an important role in parturition.

Cervical ripening

The ability of the cervix to retain the conceptus during pregnancy is unlikely to depend on a traditional muscular sphincteric mechanism.[79,80] The normal function of the cervix during pregnancy depends on the regulation of the ECM. The major macromolecular components of the ECM are collagen, proteoaminoglycans, elastin and various glycoproteins such as fibronectins. Collagen is the most important component of the ECM and determines the tensile strength of fibrous connective tissue.[81] Changes in cervical characteristics during pregnancy have been attributed to modifications in collagen content and metabolism. Proteoaminoglycans have also been implicated in cervical physiology. The proteoaminogylcan decorin (PG-S2) has a high affinity for collagen and can cover the surface of the collagen fibrils, stabilize them, and promote the formation of thicker bundles of collagen fibers. In contrast, PG-S1 (biglycan) has no affinity for collagen and can therefore disorganize collagen fibrils. The predominant dermatan sulfate proteoglycan in the non-pregnant state is PG-S2 and in the term-pregnant state, PG-S1.[82]

The biochemical events that have been implicated in cervical ripening are: (1) a decrease in total collagen content; (2) an increase in collagen solubility (probably indicating degradation or newly synthesized weaker collagen); and (3) an increase in collagenolytic activity (both collagenase and leukocyte elastase).

Contrary to what is generally believed, ECM turnover in the cervix is high and, thus, the mechanical properties of the cervix can change rapidly. Uldbjerg *et al.*[81] demonstrated the importance of collagen content in cervical dilatation, reporting a strong correlation between the collagen content (measured by hydroxyproline determination) of cervical biopsies obtained after delivery and the time required for the cervix to dilate from 2 to 10 cm.

The changes in ECM components during cervical ripening have been likened to an inflammatory response.[83] Indeed, during cervical ripening there is an influx of inflammatory cells (macrophages, neutrophils, mast cell, eosinophyls, etc.) into the cervical stroma. It has been proposed that these cells produce cytokines (e.g., interleukin (IL)-8, IL-8) and other mediators (e.g., prostaglandins), both of which have an effect on ECM metabolism.[84–88]

The chain of events leading to physiological cervical ripening has not been defined. However, strong evidence supports a role for sex steroid hormones including: (1) intravenous administration of 17β-estradiol induces cervical ripening;[89] (2) estrogen stimulates collagen degradation *in vitro*;[90] (3) progesterone blocks estrogen-induced collagenolysis *in vitro*;[90] (4) administration of progesterone receptor (PR) antagonist induces cervical ripening in the first trimester of pregnancy;[91] and (5) IL-8 production by the uterine cervix is downregulated by progesterone.[92] A detailed review of the mechanisms responsible for the changes in cervical physiology during parturition has been recently published by Norman *et al.*[93] The reader is referred to this outstanding review for further details.

Prostaglandins have been widely used to ripen the cervix prior to the induction of labor or abortion. Within hours of administration, prostaglandin E_2 (PGE_2) produces clinical and histological cervical changes resembling physiological ripening that normally develops over several weeks of gestation. The mechanism of action of PGE_2 is thought to involve stimulation of collagenolytic activity and synthesis of PG-S1 by cervical tissue.[82]

Another mediator implicated in the mechanisms of cervical ripening is nitric oxide (NO),[94] which accumulates at sites of inflammation and can act as an inflammatory mediator at high concentration.[95–97] The expression of the inducible form of nitric oxide synthase (iNOS) and NO production in the cervix increase during labor in animals.[98] Moreover, the administration of L-nitro-arginine methylester (a non-specific inhibitor of iNOS) blocks cervical ripening,[98] whereas direct application of sodium nitroprusside (an NO donor) to the cervix can induce cervical ripening.[99] Similar results have been obtained in human clinical trials.[100–103]

Gene expression profiling has recently been used to identify molecular markers of physiological cervical ripening. Microarray analysis was used to compare the gene expression profile of cervical biopsy specimens obtained from 10 women undergoing spontaneous vaginal delivery and 10 women undergoing primary cesarean delivery at term. Messenger RNA expression of 40 genes increased more than 2.5-fold in patients with a ripe cervix. These genes mostly encoded cytokines, chemokines, growth factors, transcription factors and cell-matrix-associated proteins. Messenger RNA expression of 6 genes decreased to less than 0.5-fold in patients with a ripe cervix, including iNOS, FasL receptor, apoptosis regulator bclw, caspase-9 precursor and nucleobinding precursor. For a complete list of genes found to be differentially regulated in patients with a ripe cervix, the reader is referred to the original publication.[104]

Cervical changes precede the onset of labor, are gradual, and develop over several weeks.[105] Wood *et al.*[106] were the first to report that a short cervix was a risk factor for preterm labor and delivery. This observation has been subsequently confirmed by several investigators using both manual and sonographic examinations.[107–117]

Although cervical shortening is traditionally considered an irreversible change, anecdotal clinical observations indicate that some women can have a short cervix, remain pregnant for a long time, and even deliver at term. Reversibility of cervical ripening has been demonstrated with pharmacological intervention in the pregnant ewe. Dexamethasone administration induces cervical ripening and increases uterine contractility. These effects can be reversed with large doses of progesterone.[118]

Decidual/fetal membrane activation

The term 'decidual/fetal membrane activation' refers to a complex set of anatomical and biochemical events that result in the separation of the lower pole of the membranes from the decidua of the lower uterine segment, and eventually in spontaneous rupture of membranes. Untimely activation of this mechanism leads to preterm PROM, which accounts for 40% of all preterm deliveries. For a detailed description of the mechanisms involved in spontaneous rupture of the membranes in preterm PROM, the reader is referred to Chapter 129 (*Mechanisms of preterm labor and preterm premature rupture of the membranes*).

The role of progesterone

Estrogen and progesterone play a central role in the endocrinology and paracrinology of pregnancy.[119] Progesterone is thought to maintain myometrial quiescence, downregulate gap junction formation, and inhibit cervical ripening.[120–122] Estrogens have been

Table 128.1 Source of steroids and mechanism for progesterone withdrawal before parturition in several species (modified from Bernal,[123] with permission)

Species	Source of steroids in late pregnancy	Fall in maternal progesterone concentration	Mechanism
Mouse	Corpus luteum	Yes	Luteolysis
Rat	Corpus luteum	Yes	Luteolysis
Rabbit	Corpus luteum	Yes	Luteolysis
Goat	Corpus luteum	Yes	P450 c17/luteolysis
Cow	Placenta	Yes	P450 c17
Sheep	Placenta	Yes	P450 c17
Guinea pig	Placenta	No	?
Primates	Fetoplacental unit	No	?

P450 c17 enzymes (17-α-hydroxylase and C17-20 lyase activities) are induced in the placenta by an increase in fetal cortisol concentration. Luteolysis is provoked by prostaglandin F2α acting on FP receptor

implicated in increasing myometrial contractility and excitability, as well as in the induction of cervical ripening prior to the onset of labor.[121,122] However, the changes in sex steroid serum concentrations before spontaneous parturition are different among species (see Table 128.1).[123] In many species, a decrease in maternal serum progesterone concentration occurs prior to spontaneous parturition, but the mechanism for this 'progesterone withdrawal' depends, to a large extent, on whether or not the placenta or the corpus luteum is the major source of progesterone.[123]

Luteolysis is a crucial component of the mechanism for parturition in the rat, mouse and rabbit. In the sheep and goat, an increase in fetal plasma cortisol induces the placental production of P450 C17 enzymes (17-α-hydroxylase and C17-20 lyase) and these enzymes catalyze the conversion of progesterone to androstenedione (resulting in reduction of progesterone). Androstenedione would then be transformed by action of aromatases to estrogen.[123] The net effect is that parturition is preceded by a decrease in progesterone and an increase in estrogen concentration. In goats, however, the corpus luteum is responsible for most maternal progesterone production and luteal regression is still required before parturition. In contrast, in primates (including humans) and guinea pigs, there is no apparent change in circulating maternal progesterone concentration before parturition. The human placenta, contrary to the sheep's, lacks P450 C17 enzymes and, therefore, cannot synthesize estrogen and androstenedione (C-19 androgen) from C21-progestins. Consequently, progesterone is the final product of the human placenta. The principal precursor for estrogen synthesis in the human placenta is dehydroepiandrosterone sulfate (DHEA-S) from the fetal and maternal adrenal glands (for estradiol and estrone), as well as 16-OH-DHEA-S from the fetal liver (for estriol).[119] The reader is referred to an excellent review by Young for a comparative physiology of parturition in mammals.[124]

In both human and guinea pig pregnancies, a 'serum progesterone withdrawal' has not been demonstrated. Yet, this hormone is considered important in pregnancy maintenance because inhibition of progesterone action could result in parturition in these two species. For example, administration of antiprogestins [e.g., RU 486 (mifepristone) or ZK 98299 (onapristone)] to pregnant women,[125] primates[126] or guinea pigs[120] during pregnancy can induce abortion and/or labor.[119] Several investigators have proposed alternative mechanisms to explain a suspension of progesterone action without a serum progesterone withdrawal. These alternatives have included: (1) binding of progesterone to a high affinity protein and, thus, a reduced functional active form;[127,128] (2) increasing cortisol concentration in late pregnancy that can compete with progesterone for binding to the glucocorticoid receptors, resulting in functional progesterone withdrawal;[129] and (3) converting progesterone to an inactive form within the target cell before interacting with its receptor. Human amnion and chorion can convert progesterone to the inactive 20-α-dihydroxyprogesterone.[130,131] This metabolite has been observed to increase with advancing gestational age and around the time of parturition.[131] None of these hypotheses, however, have been proven.[132] Therefore, many investigators have shifted their attention to the abundance and modulation of estrogen–progesterone receptor expression, as well as progesterone binding capability to its nuclear response element.

Conflicting results have been reported for the role of the progesterone receptor (PR) in myometrium during human parturition. These discrepancies are probably due to the methods used to assess PR concentration (and binding) and the sampling site. Rezapour *et al.*[133] concluded that there was no relationship between human parturition and PRs in myometrium.[133] In contrast, How *et al.* examined estradiol and PR expression in the myometrium (lower uterine segment), from women undergoing cesarean deliveries at term in labor ($n=10$), term not in labor ($n=10$), preterm in labor ($n=9$) and preterm not in labor ($n=11$), by immunohistochemistry and Western immunoblot analysis.[134] The intensity of the immunostaining for PR was lower in patients in labor compared to those without labor (preterm and term gestations), indicating that a functional progesterone withdrawal might occur in human labor through a reduction in PR expression. Moreover, among patients without labor, the intensity of the immunostaining for PR was lower in patients at term compared to those of preterm pregnancies, suggesting that the preterm gestation may be more resistant to the effects of progesterone withdrawal than term pregnancies. In contrast, there was no obvious difference in estradiol receptor immunostaining among the four study groups.[134] In conclusion, this study supports the concept that functional progesterone withdrawal occurs in human pregnancy at both term and preterm parturition by reducing PRs in the myometrium.

Henderson and Wilson[135] measured the binding of PR to its nuclear response element in decidual tissue using gel shift assays, which measure progesterone receptor–progesterone responsive element binding, an essential step in progesterone transactivation.[135] The binding of the ligand causes the activation of the receptor through changes that include dimerization and shedding of a heat shock protein. The activated receptor then initiates transcription by binding to its specific DNA response element. A nine-fold decrease in PR binding to its response element was observed in tissues obtained after labor (in both term and preterm gestation) as compared to tissues obtained from women not in labor.[135] However, there was no significant difference in the binding of PR between preterm and term tissues.[135]

Progesterone receptor subtypes

The human PR exists as two major subtypes, PR-A (94 kDa) and PR-B (116 kDa), both encoded by a single gene independently regulated by separate promoters. PR-A is a truncated form of PR-B that lacks the first 164 N-terminal amino acids. In most human cells, type PR-B is the principal ligand-dependent transcriptional *activator* of progesterone-responsive genes, whereas PR-A is a ligand-activated *repressor* of the transcriptional activity mediated by PR-B. The human estrogen receptor (ER) also exists as two major subtypes: ERα and ERβ. Both are derived from separate genes, each having different ligand binding affinities and tissue distribution.[136] The selective actions of estrogens and various estrogen agonists and antagonists are thought to be to the result of differential expressions of ERα and ERβ.[137]

Using Western blot analysis, Pieber *et al.*[132] reported that PR-A protein was expressed in two out of three myometrial samples obtained from women at term after labor (delivered because of fetal distress). In contrast, PR-B protein was equally expressed in the myometrium of both women in labor and women not in labor.[132] Mesiano *et al.*, using quantitative RT-PCR, measured mRNAs encoding PR-A, PR-B, ERα, and ERβ expressions in myometrium from lower uterine segments of women at term with ($n=12$) and without labor ($n=12$).[138] The mRNA expression of PR-A, PR-B, PR-A/PR-B ratio, and ERα were significantly higher in the myometrium of women in labor than in those not in labor. ERβ mRNA expression was unchanged. The PR-A/PR-B ratio correlated with ERα mRNA expression in the myometrium of women not in labor. Furthermore, there was a relationship between ERα mRNA expression and the expression of cyclooxygenase type 2 (COX-2), as well as oxytocin receptor mRNA expression in non-laboring myometrium, indicating that the increase in ERα expression was directly associated with the activation of contraction-associated genes and estrogen responsiveness. These data suggest that in term human myometrium, a significant increase in the expression of PR-A relative to PR-B might be responsible for a functional progesterone withdrawal. Functional estrogen activation would occur because of an increased expression of ERα, resulting in a coordinated expression of a specific ER subtype and a functional progesterone withdrawal. Mesiano *et al.* suggested that the interaction between the PR and ER systems in the human myometrium may be critical for the control of parturition.[119,138]

In support of the interaction of the two isoforms of the PR, Pieber *et al.*[132] conducted a series of experiments in which myometrial cells obtained prior to the onset of labor were transiently transfected with expression vector for either the PR-A or PR-B. Only cells expressing the PR-B could significantly increase the expression of progesterone reporter activity when exposed to progesterone. When both isoforms (PR-A and PR-B) were co-transfected, PR-A exhibited a marked inhibitory effect on PR-B-mediated transcription. This repression was not simply due to an excess of PR-A, because significant repression of transcription was achieved even when a 5:1 ratio of PR-B and PR-A was used for transfection. The authors concluded that PR-A is, therefore, a dominant repressor of PR-B transactivation in myometrial and amnion cells and its increased expression at the onset of labor might cause a 'functional progesterone withdrawal'.[132,139]

An alternative mechanism explaining a 'functional progesterone withdrawal' has been advanced by Professor Phillip Bennett's laboratory.[140,141] The concept is that the activation of nuclear factor (NF)-kappa B in the amnion represses PR function. NF kappa B, a transcription factor in the cytoplasm, is bound by the inhibitor kappa B (IkB). NF-kappa B (activated by IL-1β and other cytokines) leads to phosphorylation and degradation of IkB protein, allowing NF-kappa B translocation to the nucleus, where it can bind to specific sites within the promoter sequence of target genes. Indeed, Belt *et al.*[142] demonstrated that stimulation of human myometrial cells with IL-1 could lead to rapid activation of NF-kappa B, inducing the increased expression of COX-2 mRNA, protein, and prostaglandin synthesis. The mutual negative interaction in which NF-kappa B represses PR function has been described in detail elsewhere.[143]

Using transient transfection followed by assays for transcriptional activation and promoter binding, Allport *et al.*[141] demonstrated constitutive activity of NF-kappa B in human amnion cells at the time of labor. The activation of NF-kappa B also induced COX-2 mRNA expression. In cells obtained before labor, when NF-kappa B was low, an increased progesterone concentration repressed NF-kappa B-dependent transcription, while the stimulation with IL-1β increased NF-kappa B activity and repressed progesterone activity. The investigators concluded that human labor is associated with the increased constitutive NF-kappa-B activity within the amnion, whose function is to increase mRNA expression of COX-2, while contributing to a 'functional progesterone withdrawal'.[141]

Collectively, there is substantial evidence supporting the view that a 'functional progesterone withdrawal' is present locally in intrauterine tissues during human parturition in both term and preterm gestation. The changes in estrogen and progesterone ratio activity could activate the three components of the common pathway of parturition, including myometrium, cervix and membranes, directly or indirectly through prostaglandins, or oxytocin and its receptor systems.[46] However, the signal eliciting the onset of these hormonal functional changes in human parturition remains to be determined.

The role of prostaglandins

Prostaglandins have been considered the key mediators for the onset of labor[144–159] since they can induce myometrial contractility,[146–159] changes in ECM metabolism associated with cervical ripening,[144,145,150–152] and decidual/membrane activation.[160]

The evidence traditionally invoked to support a role for prostaglandins in the initiation of human labor includes: (1) administration of prostaglandins can induce early or late termination of pregnancy (abortion or labor);[153,161–171] (2) treatment with indomethacin or aspirin can delay spontaneous onset of parturition in animals;[172–175] (3) concentrations of prostaglandins in plasma and amniotic fluid increase during labor;[14,176–185] (4) intra-amniotic injection of arachidonic acid, the precursor for prostaglandins, induces abortion;[155] (5) prostaglandin concentrations in amniotic fluid increase early during spontaneous labor at term.[184] These observations are consistent with those reported in PROM at term, and[185] similar findings have been described in longitudinal studies performed in non-human primates;[14] and (6) amniotic fluid prostaglandin concentrations increase before the onset of spontaneous labor in humans.[186] Therefore, most of the available evidence in humans, as well as in animals, suggests that prostaglandin concentrations increase prior to the onset of labor or during early labor.[14,184–191] Moreover, in all species examined thus far, including marsupials, prostaglandin secretion increases during labor.[8,192]

Prostaglandins are produced by intrauterine tissues including amnion,[193–195] chorion,[194] decidua,[196,197] myometrium,[198–201] and placenta.[191,194] Although there are many stimulants of prostaglandin biosynthesis, the precise signals responsible for their increase during the course of labor have not been determined. Candidates include cytokines (IL-1, tumor necrosis factor-α),[193,197,202] growth factors (i.e., epidermal growth factor),[203] cortisol,[204,205] and others.

Prostaglandin synthase (PGHS), also known as cyclo-oxygenase, is the enzyme responsible for the initial step in the production of prostaglandins. PGHS has two isozymes: PGHS1 and PGHS2. Recent reports indicate that there is a topographic variation in the distribution of PGHS2 during labor. Indeed, in pregnant baboons the mRNA expression of PGHS2 is higher in the lower uterine segment than in the fundus of the uterus. In contrast, the mRNA expression of 15-OH prostaglandin dehydrogenase (PGDH), the enzyme responsible for the prostaglandins' degradation, is reduced in the lower uterine segment compared to the expression in the fundus. It is possible that such topographic differences in the distribution of these enzymes may play a role in the physiologic control of parturition (see below).[206]

Prostaglandin receptors are classified based on the responses to various agonists and antagonists (IP, TP, DP, EP and FP).[192] The EP receptors are classified into four distinct subtypes, two of which stimulate contraction responses (EP_1 and EP_3) and two that induce a relaxation response (EP_2 and EP_4).[207] Recent studies have examined the expression of prostaglandin receptors in non-pregnant and pregnant human myometrium, as well as in several animal species.[206,208] Topographic differences in the expression of receptors that stimulate uterine contractility and those that inhibit uterine contractility have been found.[209–211] For example, Smith *et al.* reported an increased expression of the EP_2 receptor in the lower uterine segment (which induces relaxation) and increased expression of the EP_3 receptor mRNA in the uterine fundus, while both areas express FP and EP_4 in similar quantities.[212,213] These observations are important because PGE_2 elicits different contractile responses in myometrium, depending on the source of the myometrium. PGE_2 generally stimulates the fundus, but not the lower uterine segment. Collectively, these findings suggest that there may be functional regionalization of the uterus. On the other hand, a recent study examining *in vitro* contractile responses of the upper and lower segment has not produced findings consistent with those described by Smith *et al.*[212–214]

A role for the fetus in the timing of the onset of labor

A role for the fetus in the control of the timing of labor was demonstrated by the classic studies of Liggins *et al.*,[215,216] as well as by the cross-breeding experiments described at the beginning of this chapter (see Normal Duration of Pregnancy). The importance of the fetal brain has been shown, experimentally, because destruction of the paraventricular nucleus of the fetal hypothalamus results in prolongation of pregnancy in sheep.[217,218] The human counterpart to this animal experiment is anencephaly, which is also characterized by a tendency to have a prolonged pregnancy (if women with polyhydramnios are excluded).[219] However, the situation in human anencephaly is considerably more complicated than the one described in animal experiments. The discrepancy can be explained by the wide range of central nervous system and pituitary lesions found in human anencephaly.

Possible routes for the fetus to signal the onset of labor

The effector organs of labor are the myometrium, cervix and membranes. The fetus could signal the onset of parturition/labor by using a set of molecules which could be delivered to the effector organs using the following routes: (1) an endocrine pathway whereby the fetal circulation delivers the molecules to the placenta and reaches the uterus directly or through the maternal circulation; or (2) a paracrine pathway in which molecules produced by fetal organs, such as the lungs or kidneys, reach the amniotic cavity to exert an effect on the fetal membranes that transduce the signal to the myometrium and cervix (Figure 128.4).[220]

The current paradigm is that once maturity has been reached, the fetal brain, specifically the hypothalamus, increases corticotropin-releasing hormone (CRH) secretion, which in turn stimulates adrenocorticotrophic hormone (ACTH) and fetal cortisol production by the adrenals.[221–223] The increase in cortisol in sheep and DHEA-S in primates eventually leads to activation of the common pathway of parturition.[224,225] In the sheep, but not in the human, fetal cortisol induces expression of 17-α-hydroxylase, which catalyzes the conversion of progesterone to estrogen. Increasing concentrations of estrogen lead to the transcription of contraction-associated genes in the myometrium that favor the onset of labor. The experiments of Liggins *et al.*[215,216] demonstrated that damage to the fetal adrenal glands or pituitary glands would prolong pregnancy. The

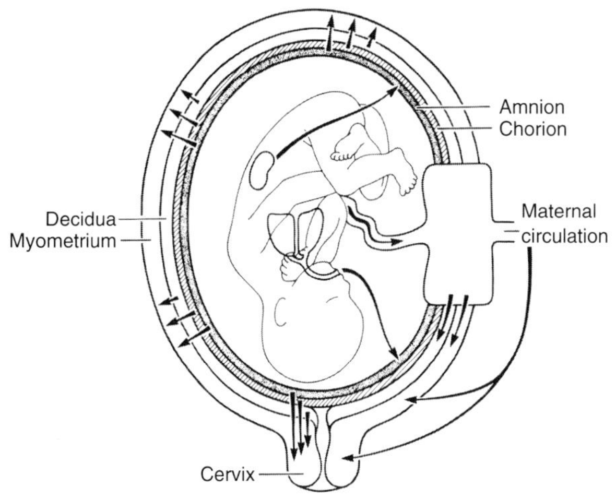

Figure 128.4 Possible routes of transmission of the signal for the initiation of labor from the conceptus to the mother. Note the large area of contact between the chorion and the decidua which makes the paracrine route an effective way of signal transmission from conceptus to mother. From: Schellenberg and Liggins,[220] with permission.

administration of a CRH-antagonist has a similar effect.[226] Nathanielsz has proposed that in non-human primates lacking 17-α-hydroxylase in the placenta, ACTH stimulates the production of androgens, which are converted into estrogens by the placenta and initiate the cascade of events responsible for parturition.[227]

Challis and Lye suggested that the apparent differences in the mechanisms of parturition between the sheep and human can be reconciled.[228] They propose that cortisol in primates has at least three important functions: (1) it increases prostaglandin production by intrauterine tissues directly or indirectly by stimulating the production of PGHS2; (2) it stimulates the production of CRH by the placenta; and (3) it inhibits the enzyme 15-OH prostaglandin dehydrogenase,[229] which catabolizes prostaglandins.[206,230]

CRH is a hormone that is largely produced by the placenta and can stimulate prostaglandin production and induce the fetal adrenal gland to secrete DHEA-S, a source of estrogens that drives the increased expression of oxytocin receptors, gap junctions, and prostaglandins.[231–233] It is important to note that while cortisol suppresses CRH production by the pituitary gland, this hormone stimulates CRH production by the placenta.[229] In support of the importance of cortisol in human parturition, we have reported that fetal plasma cortisol concentrations are elevated in the human fetus before the onset of labor in the context of preterm PROM, and that this elevation is associated with the fetal inflammatory response syndrome.[234]

Parturition as an inflammatory process

Liggins was the first to liken cervical ripening with an inflammatory response.[215] Since then, accumulating evidence supports that inflammation can be detected in the cervix, myometrium, chorioamniotic membranes, and the amniotic cavity in women in labor. Spontaneous labor at term is associated with infiltration of inflammatory cells in these tissues [235–237] and increased production of a wide range of pro-inflammatory cytokines (IL-1β, IL-6, TNF-α, IL-8)[238–240] and chemokines (GROα, MCP-1, ENA, GCSF, GMCSM, neutrophil attractant/activating peptide-1/IL-8, macrophage inflammatory protein-1α).[240–245] Stjernholm-Vladic *et al.*[245] have recently observed a decrease in glucocorticoid receptors (a mediator of glucocorticoid anti-inflammatory reactions) and a concomitant increase in the expression of NF-kappa-B (a key pro-inflammatory regulator) in cervical tissues obtained at the time of parturition, suggesting that these transcription factors are directly involved in the regulation of the inflammatory response associated with cervical ripening.

Recently, using a genome-wide screen, Haddad *et al.*[247] have been able to demonstrate that genes involved in the control of inflammation are upregulated in the chorioamniotic membranes after labor at term, even in the absence of histologic chorioamnionitis. Of interest is that an inflammatory signature was not observed in the maternal circulation in patients in spontaneous labor at term. This suggests that the inflammatory process is localized to the gestational tissues and specifically to the membranes. These observations are consistent with the findings of Kim *et al.* who reported upregulation of the Toll-like receptor (TLR)-2 and TLR-4 in normal spontaneous parturition.[248] This finding may reflect that spontaneous parturition is associated with increased pro-inflammatory cytokine and chemokine responses in gestational tissues.[240] Indeed, pro-inflammatory cytokines have been shown to upregulate the expression of TLR-2 and TLR-4.[249]

The role of the placenta

Sixty years ago, Van Wagenen and Newton[250] demonstrated that in pregnant primates, surgical removal of the fetus, but not of the placenta, does not affect the timing of labor, suggesting that the onset of labor is independent of the presence of the fetus. Similar results were reported by Albrecht *et al.*[251] However, Lanman *et al.*[252] and, more recently, Nathanielsz *et al.*[253] demonstrated that delivery of the placenta outlasts the normal duration of pregnancy in pregnant rhesus monkeys after fetectomy, indicating that the fetus plays an important role in the timing of delivery in primates, and that in the absence of the fetus, gestational length is significantly longer than in normal pregnancies.

A decade ago, McLean and Smith[22] proposed the existence of a 'placental clock' in human pregnancy, which is active at an early stage and determines the length of gestation and the timing of parturition. This proposal was based on the result of a large, longitudinal study in which women who delivered preterm had a significantly higher plasma concentration of CRH than those who delivered at term. In contrast, women who had prolonged pregnancies had a lower CRH concentration than those who delivered at term. Of note, these differences were already present at 16–18 weeks of gestation.[25] The association between a high maternal plasma concentration of CRH and preterm labor has been confirmed by other studies.[254–256] According to 'the placental clock hypothesis', the rate of increase in the maternal plasma concentration of CRH through pregnancy determines the timing of labor when saturation of the CRH binding protein is achieved and free CRH becomes available and triggers parturition.[22,257] High concentrations of CRH have been described in women with chronic stress and this condition has been associated with a high risk of preterm delivery.[256]

Conclusions

The common pathway of parturition is characterized by increased uterine contractility, cervical ripening and degradation of ECM, which predisposes to membrane rupture. There is growing evidence that parturition occurs over a period of weeks, rather than hours. The mechanisms responsible for the initiation of physiologic labor at term have not been determined in humans. Recent studies implicate the production of fetal or placental signals that would activate the common pathway, such as surfactant protein-A[258] and CRH/cortisol.[259]

This chapter serves as the basis for the understanding of mechanisms implicated in the extemporaneous activation of the common pathway of parturition leading to preterm delivery, which will be discussed in Chapter 129. The expanded utilization of discovery techniques, such as genomics, proteomics and metabolomics, which allow a comprehensive description of the global changes in the transcriptome, proteome, and metabolome, will continue to yield new insights into the processes of normal and abnormal parturition, allowing integration of much of the research conducted to date.[21,104,247]

REFERENCES

1. *Merriam-Webster's Collegiate Dictionary*. Springfield, MA: Merriam-Webster Inc., Publishers, 2003.
2. Yudkin PL, Wood L, Redman CWG. Risk of unexplained stillbirth at different gestational ages. *Lancet* 1987;1:1192–4.
3. Tucker J, McGuire W. ABC of preterm birth – Epidemiology of preterm birth. *Br Med J* 2004;329:675–8.
4. Porreco RP, Thorp JA. The cesarean birth epidemic: Trends, causes, and solutions. *Am J Obstet Gynecol* 1996;175:369–74.

5. Mabie WC, Barton JR, Sibai BM. Septic shock in pregnancy. *Obstet Gynecol* 1997;90:553–61.
6. Chang J, Elam-Evans LD, Berg CJ, *et al.* Pregnancy-related mortality surveillance – United States, 1991–1999. *MMWR Surveill Summ* 2003;52:1–8.
7. Kloosterman GJ. Prolonged pregnancy. *Gynaecologia* 1956;142: 372–88.
8. Jenkin G, Young IR. Mechanisms responsible for parturition; the use of experimental models. *Anim Reprod Sci* 2004;82–83:567–81.
9. Allen WR, Wilsher S, Turnbull C, *et al.* Influence of maternal size on placental, fetal and postnatal growth in the horse. I. Development in utero. *Reproduction* 2002;123:445–53.
10. Cunningham FG, Gant NF, Leveno KJ, Gilstrap LCI, Hauth JC, Wenstrom KD. Parturition. In Cunningham FG, Gant NF, Leveno KJ, Gilstrap LCI, Hauth JC, Wenstrom KD, eds. *Williams Obstetrics.* New York: McGraw-Hill; 2001:251–90.
11. Duff P. Pyelonephritis in pregnancy. *Clin Obstet Gynecol* 1984; 27:17–31.
12. Millar LK, DeBuque L, Wing DA. Uterine contraction frequency during treatment of pyelonephritis in pregnancy and subsequent risk of preterm birth. *J Perinat Med* 2003;31:41–6.
13. Chwalisz K, Fahrenholz F, Hackenberg M, Garfield R, Elger W. The progesterone antagonist onapristone increases the effectiveness of oxytocin to produce delivery without changing the myometrial oxytocin receptor concentrations. *Am J Obstet Gynecol* 1991;165:1760–70.
14. Haluska GJ, Stanczyk FZ, Cook MJ, Novy MJ. Temporal changes in uterine activity and prostaglandin response to RU486 in rhesus macaques in late gestation. *Am J Obstet Gynecol* 1987;157:1487–95.
15. da Fonseca EB, Bittar RE, Carvalho MH, Zugaib M. Prophylactic administration of progesterone by vaginal suppository to reduce the incidence of spontaneous preterm birth in women at increased risk: A randomized placebo-controlled double-blind study. *Am J Obstet Gynecol* 2003;188:419–24.
16. Keirse MJ. Progestogen administration in pregnancy may prevent preterm delivery. *Br J Obstet Gynaecol* 1990;97:149–54.
17. Meis PJ, Klebanoff M, Thom E, *et al.* Prevention of recurrent preterm delivery by 17 alpha-hydroxyprogesterone caproate. *N Engl J Med* 2003;348:2379–85.
18. Challis JRG, Gibb W. Control of parturition. *Prenat Neonat Med* 1996;1:283–91.
19. Challis JRG. Mechanism of parturition and preterm labor. *Obstet Gynecol Surv* 2000;55:650–60.
20. Norwitz ER, Robinson JN, Repke JT. Labor and delivery. In Gabbe SG, Niebyl JR, Simpson JL, eds. *Obstetrics: Normal and Problem Pregnancies.* New York: Churchill Livingstone; 2002:353–94.
21. Romero R, Kuivaniemi H, Tromp G. Functional genomics and proteomics in term and preterm parturition. *J Clin Endocrinol Metab* 2002;87:2431–4.
22. McLean M, Bisits A, Davies J, Woods R, Lowry P, Smith R. A placental clock controlling the length of human pregnancy. *Nat Med* 1995;1:460–3.
23. Ohrlander S, Gennser G, Eneroth P. Plasma cortisol levels in human fetus during parturition. *Obstet Gynecol* 1976;48:381–7.
24. Challis JR. CRH, a placental clock and preterm labour. *Nat Med* 1995;1:416.
25. Genazzani AR, Petraglia F, Facchinetti F, Galli PA, Volpe A. Lack of beta-endorphin plasma level rise in oxytocin-induced labor. *Gynecol Obstet Invest* 1985;19:130–4.
26. Korebrits C, Ramirez MM, Watson L, Brinkman E, Bocking AD, Challis JR. Maternal corticotropin-releasing hormone is increased with impending preterm birth. *J Clin Endocrinol Metab* 1998; 83:1585–91.
27. Petraglia F, Giardino L, Coukos G, Calza L, Vale W, Genazzani AR. Corticotropin-releasing factor and parturition: Plasma and amniotic fluid levels and placental binding sites. *Obstet Gynecol* 1990;75:784–9.
28. Randall NJ, Bond K, Macaulay J, Steer PJ. Measuring fetal and maternal temperature differentials: A probe for clinical use during labour. *J Biomed Eng* 1991;13:481–5.
29. Smith R. Alterations in the hypothalamic pituitary adrenal axis during pregnancy and the placental clock that determines the length of parturition. *J Reprod Immunol* 1998;39:215–20.
30. Leung TN, Chung TK, Madsen G, Lam PK, Sahota D, Smith R. Rate of rise in maternal plasma corticotrophin-releasing hormone and its relation to gestational length. *Br J Obstet Gynecol* 2001;108:527–32.
31. Florio P, Cobellis L, Woodman J, Severi FM, Linton EA, Petraglia F. Levels of maternal plasma corticotropin-releasing factor and urocortin during labor. *J Soc Gynecol Investig* 2002;9:233–7.
32. Nathanielsz P, Honnebier M. Myometrial function. In Drife J, Calder A, eds. *Prostaglandins and the Uterus.* London: Springer-Verlag; 1992:161.
33. Hsu HW, Figueroa JP, Honnebier MB, Wentworth R, Nathanielsz PW. Power spectrum analysis of myometrial electromyogram and intrauterine pressure changes in the pregnant rhesus monkey in late gestation. *Am J Obstet Gynecol* 1989;161:467–73.
34. Taylor NF, Martin MC, Nathanielsz PW, Seron-Ferre M. The fetus determines circadian oscillation of myometrial electromyographic activity in the pregnant rhesus monkey. *Am J Obstet Gynecol* 1983;146:557–67.
35. Binienda Z, Rosen ED, Kelleman A, Sadowsky DW, Nathanielsz PW, Mitchell MD. Maintaining fetal normoglycemia prevents the increase in myometrial activity and uterine 13,14-dihydro-15-keto-prostaglandin F2 alpha production during food withdrawal in late pregnancy in the ewe. *Endocrinology* 1990;127:3047–51.
36. Nathanielsz P, Poore E, Brodie A, *et al.* Update on molecular events of myometrial activity during pregnancy. In Nathanielsz P, Parer J, eds. *Research in Perinatal Medicine.* Ithaca, NY: Perinatology Press, 1987:111.
37. Romero R, Avila C, Sepulveda W, *et al.* The role of systemic and intrauterine infection in preterm labor. In Fuchs A, Fuchs F, Stubblefield P, eds. *Preterm Birth: Causes, Prevention, and Management.* New York: McGraw-Hill; 1993.
38. Fowden AL, Harding R, Ralph MM, Thorburn GD. The nutritional regulation of plasma prostaglandin E concentrations in the fetus and pregnant ewe during late gestation. *J Physiol* 1987;394:1–12.
39. Kaplan M, Eidelman AI, Aboulafia Y. Fasting and the precipitation of labor. The Yom Kippur effect. *J Am Med Assoc* 1983;250: 1317–8.
40. Maymon E, Mazor M, Romero R, *et al.* The Yom Kippur effect on human parturition. *Am J Obstet Gynecol* 1997;176:S115.
41. Honnebier MB, Jenkins SL, Wentworth RA, Figueroa JP, Nathanielsz PW. Temporal structuring of delivery in the absence of a photoperiod: preparturient myometrial activity of the rhesus monkey is related to maternal body temperature and depends on the maternal circadian system. *Biol Reprod* 1991;45:617–25.
42. Katz M, Newman RB, Gill PJ. Assessment of uterine activity in ambulatory patients at high risk of preterm labor and delivery. *Am J Obstet Gynecol* 1986;154:44–7.
43. Honnebier MB, Figueroa JP, Rivier J, Vale W, Nathanielsz PW. Studies on the role of oxytocin in late pregnancy in the pregnant rhesus monkey: Plasma concentrations of oxytocin in the maternal circulation throughout the 24-h day and the effect of the synthetic oxytocin antagonist [1-beta-Mpa(beta-(CH2)5)1, (Me(Tyr2, Orn8] oxytocin on spontaneous nocturnal myometrial contractions. *J Dev Physiol* 1989;12:225–32.
44. Owiny JR, Mitchell M, Nathanielsz PW. Effect of 48-hour infusion of the synthetic oxytocin antagonist, [1-beta-mercapto(beta-(CH2)5)1(OMe)Tyr2,Orn8]-oxytocin, on myometrial activity of pregnant sheep at 139–140 days of gestation. *Biol Reprod* 1992; 47:436–40.
45. Wilson L Jr, Parsons MT, Flouret G. Inhibition of spontaneous uterine contractions during the last trimester in pregnant baboons by an oxytocin antagonist. *Am J Obstet Gynecol* 1990;163:1875–82.
46. Blanks AM, Vatish M, Allen MJ, *et al.* Paracrine oxytocin and estradiol demonstrate a spatial increase in human intrauterine tissues with labor. *J Clin Endocrinol Metab* 2003;88:3392–400.
47. Blanks AM, Thornton S. The role of oxytocin in parturition. *Br J Obstet Gynecol* 2003;110(Suppl 20):46–51.
48. Chibbar R, Wong S, Miller FD, Mitchell BF. Estrogen stimulates oxytocin gene expression in human chorio-decidua. *J Clin Endocrinol Metab* 1995;80:567–72.
49. Mauri A, Argiolas A, Ticconi C, Piccione E. Oxytocin in human intrauterine tissues at parturition. *Reprod Fertil Dev* 1995;7: 1481–4.
50. Mitchell BF. Oxytocin synthesis and metabolism in human decidua. *Reprod Fertil Dev* 1995;7:319–21.
51. Mitchell BF, Chibbar R. Synthesis and metabolism of oxytocin in late gestation in human decidua. *Adv Exp Med Biol* 1995;395: 365–80.
52. Mitchell BF, Wong S. Metabolism of oxytocin in human decidua, chorion, and placenta. J *Clin Endocrinol Metab* 1995;80:2729–33.
53. Romero R, Sibai BM, Sanchez-Ramos L, *et al.* An oxytocin receptor antagonist (atosiban) in the treatment of preterm labor: a randomized, double-blind, placebo-controlled trial with tocolytic rescue. *Am J Obstet Gynecol* 2000;182:1173–83.
54. Moutquin JM, Sherman D, Cohen H, *et al.* Double-blind, randomized, controlled trial of atosiban and ritodrine in the treatment

of preterm labor: a multicenter effectiveness and safety study. *Am J Obstet Gynecol* 2000;182:1191–9.

55. The Worldwide Atosiban versus Beta-agonists Study Group. Effectiveness and safety of the oxytocin antagonist atosiban versus beta-adrenergic agonists in the treatment of preterm labour. *Br J Obstet Gynecol* 2001;108:133–42.
56. Coomarasamy A, Knox EM, Gee H, Khan KS. Oxytocin antagonists for tocolysis in preterm labour – a systematic review. *Med Sci.Monit* 2002;8:RA268–73.
57. Miller FD, Chibbar R, Mitchell BF. Synthesis of oxytocin in amnion, chorion and decidua: A potential paracrine role for oxytocin in the onset of human parturition. *Regul Pept* 1993;45:247–51.
58. Chibbar R, Miller FD, Mitchell BF. Synthesis of oxytocin in amnion, chorion, and decidua may influence the timing of human parturition. *J Clin Invest* 1993;91:185–92.
59. European Atosiban Study Group. The oxytocin antagonist atosiban versus the beta-agonist terbutaline in the treatment of preterm labor. A randomized, double-blind, controlled study. *Acta Obstet Gynecol Scand* 2001;80:413–22.
60. French/Australian Atosiban Investigators Group. Treatment of preterm labor with the oxytocin antagonist atosiban: A double-blind, randomized, controlled comparison with salbutamol. *Eur J Obstet Gynecol Reprod Biol* 2001;98:177–85.
61. Garfield RE, Hayashi RH. Appearance of gap junctions in the myometrium of women during labor. *Am J Obstet Gynecol* 1981;140:254–60.
62. Garfield RE, Puri CP, Csapo AI. Endocrine, structural, and functional changes in the uterus during premature labor. *Am J Obstet Gynecol* 1982;142:21–7.
63. Cole WC, Garfield RE, Kirkaldy JS. Gap junctions and direct intercellular communication between rat uterine smooth muscle cells. *Am J Physiol* 1985;249:C20–31.
64. Garfield RE, Sims S, Daniel EE. Gap junctions: their presence and necessity in myometrium during parturition. *Science* 1977;198: 958–60.
65. Garfield RE, Sims SM, Kannan MS, Daniel EE. Possible role of gap junctions in activation of myometrium during parturition. *Am J Physiol* 1978;235:C168–179.
66. Orsino A, Taylor CV, Lye SJ. Connexin-26 and connexin-43 are differentially expressed and regulated in the rat myometrium throughout late pregnancy and with the onset of labor. *Endocrinology* 1996;137:1545–53.
67. Ou CW, Orsino A, Lye SJ. Expression of connexin-43 and connexin-26 in the rat myometrium during pregnancy and labor is differentially regulated by mechanical and hormonal signals. *Endocrinology* 1997;138:5398–407.
68. Chow L, Lye SJ. Expression of the gap junction protein connexin-43 is increased in the human myometrium toward term and with the onset of labor. *Am J Obstet Gynecol* 1994;170:788–95.
69. Balducci J, Risek B, Gilula NB, Hand A, Egan JF, Vintzileos AM. Gap junction formation in human myometrium: A key to preterm labor? *Am J Obstet Gynecol* 1993;168:1609–15.
70. Lefebvre DL, Piersanti M, Bai XH, Chen ZQ, Lye SJ. Myometrial transcriptional regulation of the gap junction gene, connexin-43. *Reprod Fertil Dev* 1995;7:603–11.
71. Petrocelli T, Lye SJ. Regulation of transcripts encoding the myometrial gap junction protein, connexin-43, by estrogen and progesterone. *Endocrinology* 1993;133:284–90.
72. Lye SJ, Nicholson BJ, Mascarenhas M, MacKenzie L, Petrocelli T. Increased expression of connexin-43 in the rat myometrium during labor is associated with an increase in the plasma estrogen: progesterone ratio. *Endocrinology* 1993;132:2380–6.
73. Cook JL, Zaragoza DB, Sung DH, Olson DM. Expression of myometrial activation and stimulation genes in a mouse model of preterm labor: Myometrial activation, stimulation, and preterm labor. *Endocrinology* 2000;141:1718–28.
74. Lye SJ. The initiation and inhibition of labour: Towards a molecular understanding. *Semin Reprod Endocrinol* 1994;12:284–94.
75. Lye SJ, Mitchell J, Nashman N, *et al.* Role of mechanical signals in the onset of term and preterm labor. *Front Horm Res* 2001;27: 165–78.
76. Lye S, Tsui P, Dorogin A, *et al.* Myometrial programming: A new concept underlying the maintenance of pregnancy and the initiation of labor. *VII International Conference on the Extracellular Matrix of the Female Reproductive Tract and Simpson Symposia*, Centre for Reproductive Biology. University of Edinburgh, 2004.
77. Wen SW, Smith G, Yang Q, Walker M. Epidemiology of preterm birth and neonatal outcome. *Semin Fetal Neonat Med* 2004;9: 429–35.
78. Bryant-Greenwood GD, Millar LK. Human fetal membranes: their preterm premature rupture. *Biol Reprod* 2000;63:1575–9.
79. Schwahn H, Dubrausky V. The structure of the musculature of the human uterus-muscles and connective tissue. *Am J Obstet Gynecol* 1966;94:391.
80. Danforth D, Evanston I. The distribution and functional activity of the cervical musculature. *Am J Obstet Gynecol* 1954;68:1261.
81. Uldbjerg N, Ekman G, Malmstrom A. Ripening of the human uterine cervix related to changes in collagen, glycosaminoglycans and collagenolytic activity. *Am J Obstet Gynecol* 1982;147:662.
82. Uldbjerg N, Forman A, Peterson L, *et al.* Biomechanical and biochemical changes of the uterus and cervix during pregnancy. In Reece E, Hobbins J, Mahoney M, Petrie R, eds. *Medicine of the Fetus and Mother*. Philadelphia: JB Lippincott, 1992:849.
83. Liggins G. Cervical ripening as an inflammatory reaction. In Ellwood D, Anderson A, eds. *The Cervix in Pregnancy and Labour: Clinical and Biochemical Investigations*. Edinburgh: Churchill Livingstone, 1981.
84. Ito A, Hiro D, Ojima Y, Mori Y. Spontaneous production of interleukin-1-like factors from pregnant rabbit uterine cervix. *Am J Obstet Gynecol* 1988;159:261–5.
85. Ito A, Hiro D, Sakyo K, Mori Y. The role of leukocyte factors on uterine cervical ripening and dilation. *Biol Reprod* 1987;37: 511–7.
86. Ito A, Leppert PC, Mori Y. Human recombinant interleukin-1 alpha increases elastase-like enzyme in human uterine cervical fibroblasts. *Gynecol Obstet Invest* 1990;30:239–41.
87. Osmers RG, Blaser J, Kuhn W, Tschesche H. Interleukin-8 synthesis and the onset of labor. *Obstet Gynecol* 1995;86:223–9.
88. Maradny EE, Kanayama N, Halim A, Maehara K, Terao T. Stretching of fetal membranes increases the concentration of interleukin-8 and collagenase activity. *Am J Obstet Gynecol* 1996;174: 843–9.
89. Pinto R, Rabow W, Votta R. Uterine cervix ripening in term pregnancy due to the action of estradiol-17 beta. *Am J Obstet Gynecol* 1965;92:319.
90. Rajabi MR, Dodge GR, Solomon S, Poole AR. Immunochemical and immunohistochemical evidence of estrogen-mediated collagenolysis as a mechanism of cervical dilatation in the guinea pig at parturition. *Endocrinology* 1991;128:371–8.
91. Chwalisz K, Shi Shao O, Neff G, Elger J. The effect of antigestagen ZK 98, 199 on the uterine cervix. *Acta Endocrinol* 1987;283:113.
92. Ito A, Imada K, Sato T, Kubo T, Matsushima K, Mori Y. Suppression of interleukin 8 production by progesterone in rabbit uterine cervix. *Biochem J* 1994;301(Pt 1):183–6.
93. Norman JE, Thomson AJ, Osmers RG, Ledingham MA. Cervical physiology. In Critchley H, Bennett H, Thornton S, eds. *Preterm Birth*. London: RCOG Press, 2004:99–114.
94. Chwalisz K, Garfield RE. Role of nitric oxide in the uterus and cervix: implications for the management of labor. J Perinat Med 1998;26:448–57.
95. Chwalisz K, Buhimschi I, Garfield RE. The role of nitric oxide in obstetrics. *Prenat Neonat Med* 1996;4:292–328.
96. Evans CH, Stefanovic-Racic M, Lancaster J. Nitric oxide and its role in orthopaedic disease. *Clin Orthop* 1995;275–94.
97. Romero R. Clinical application of nitric oxide donors and blockers. *Hum Reprod* 1998;13:248–50.
98. Buhimschi I, Ali M, Jain V, Chwalisz K, Garfield RE. Differential regulation of nitric oxide in the rat uterus and cervix during pregnancy and labour. *Hum Reprod* 1996;11:1755–66.
99. Facchinetti F, Piccinini F, Volpe A. Chemical ripening of the cervix with intracervical application of sodium nitroprusside: A randomized controlled trial. *Hum Reprod* 2000;15:2224–7.
100. Thomson AJ, Lunan CB, Cameron AD, Cameron IT, Greer IA, Norman JE. Nitric oxide donors induce ripening of the human uterine cervix: A randomised controlled trial. *Br J Obstet Gynaecol* 1997;104:1054–7.
101. Tschugguel W, Schneeberger C, Lass H, *et al.* Human cervical ripening is associated with an increase in cervical inducible nitric oxide synthase expression. *Biol Reprod* 1999;60:1367–72.
102. Ekerhovd E, Weijdegard B, Brannstrom M, Mattsby-Baltzer I, Norstrom A. Nitric oxide induced cervical ripening in the human: involvement of cyclic guanosine monophosphate, prostaglandin F(2 alpha), and prostaglandin E(2). *Am J Obstet Gynecol* 2002; 186:745–50.
103. Ledingham MA, Thomson AJ, Young A, Macara LM, Greer IA, Norman JE. Changes in the expression of nitric oxide synthase in the human uterine cervix during pregnancy and parturition. *Mol Hum Reprod* 2000;6:1041–8.

104. Huber A, Hudelist G, Czerwenka K, Husslein P, Kubista E, Singer CF. Gene expression profiling of cervical tissue during physiological cervical effacement. *Obstet Gynecol* 2005;105:91–8.
105. Bishop E. Pelvic scoring for elective induction. *Obstet Gynecol* 1964;24:266.
106. Wood C, Bannerman R, Booth R, Pinkerton J. The prediction of premature labor by observation of the cervix and external tocography. *Am J Obstet Gynecol* 1965;91:396.
107. Catalano PM, Ashikaga T, Mann LI. Cervical change and uterine activity as predictors of preterm delivery. *Am J Perinatol* 1989;6:185–90.
108. Leveno KJ, Cox K, Roark ML. Cervical dilatation and prematurity revisited. *Obstet Gynecol* 1986;68:434–5.
109. Heath VC, Southall TR, Souka AP, Elisseou A, Nicolaides KH. Cervical length at 23 weeks of gestation: Prediction of spontaneous preterm delivery. *Ultrasound Obstet Gynecol* 1998;12:312–17.
110. Holbrook RH Jr, Falcon J, Herron M, Lirette M, Laros RK Jr, Creasy RK. Evaluation of the weekly cervical examination in a preterm birth prevention program. *Am J Perinatol* 1987;4:240–4.
111. Bouyer J, Papiernik E, Dreyfus J, Collin D, Winisdoerffer B, Gueguen S. Maturation signs of the cervix and prediction of preterm birth. *Obstet Gynecol* 1986;68:209–14.
112. Hassan SS, Romero R, Berry SM, *et al.* Patients with an ultrasonographic cervical length < or =15 mm have nearly a 50% risk of early spontaneous preterm delivery. *Am J Obstet Gynecol* 2000;182:1458–67.
113. Papiernik E, Bouyer J, Collin D, Winisdoerffer G, Dreyfus J. Precocious cervical ripening and preterm labor. *Obstet Gynecol* 1986;67:238–42.
114. Anderson AB, Turnbull AC. Relationship between length of gestation and cervical dilatation, uterine contractility, and other factors during pregnancy. *Am J Obstet Gynecol* 1969;105:1207–14.
115. Iams JD, Goldenberg RL, Meis PJ, *et al.* The length of the cervix and the risk of spontaneous premature delivery. National Institute of Child Health and Human Development Maternal Fetal Medicine Unit Network. *N Engl J Med* 1996;334:567–72.
116. Stubbs TM, Van Dorsten JP, Miller MC III. The preterm cervix and preterm labor: Relative risks, predictive values, and change over time. *Am J Obstet Gynecol* 1986;155:829–34.
117. Gomez R, Galasso M, Romero R, *et al.* Ultrasonographic examination of the uterine cervix is better than cervical digital examination as a predictor of the likelihood of premature delivery in patients with preterm labor and intact membranes. *Am J Obstet Gynecol* 1994;171:956–64.
118. Stys SJ, Clewell WH, Meschia G. Changes in cervical compliance at parturition independent of uterine activity. *Am J Obstet Gynecol* 1978;130:414–8.
119. Mesiano S. Roles of estrogen and progesterone in human parturition. *Front Horm Res* 2001;27:86–104.
120. Chwalisz K. The use of progesterone antagonists for cervical ripening and as an adjunct to labour and delivery. *Hum Reprod* 1994;9(Suppl 1):131–61.
121. Gorodeski IG, Geier A, Lunenfeld B, Beery R, Bahary CM. Progesterone (P) receptor dynamics in estrogen primed normal human cervix following P injection. *Fertil Steril* 1987;47:108–13.
122. Stjernholm Y, Sahlin L, Akerberg S, *et al.* Cervical ripening in humans: Potential roles of estrogen, progesterone, and insulin-like growth factor-I. *Am J Obstet Gynecol* 1996;174:1065–71.
123. Bernal AL. Overview of current research in parturition. *Exp Physiol* 2001;86:213–22.
124. Young IR. The comparative physiology of parturition in mammals. In Smith R, ed. *The Endocrinology of Parturition.* Basel: Reinhardt Druck, 2001:10–30.
125. Bygdeman M, Swahn ML, Gemzell-Danielsson K, Gottlieb C. The use of progesterone antagonists in combination with prostaglandin for termination of pregnancy. *Hum Reprod* 1994;9(Suppl 1):121–5.
126. Puri CP, Patil RK, Elger WA, Pongubala JM. Effects of progesterone antagonist ZK 98.299 on early pregnancy and foetal outcome in bonnet monkeys. *Contraception* 1990;41:197–205.
127. McGarrigle HH, Lachelin GC. Increasing saliva (free) oestriol to progesterone ratio in late pregnancy: A role for oestriol in initiating spontaneous labour in man? *Br Med J (Clin Res Ed)* 1984;289:457–9.
128. Westphal U, Stroupe SD, Cheng SL. Progesterone binding to serum proteins. *Ann N Y Acad Sci* 1977;286:10–28.
129. Karalis K, Goodwin G, Majzoub JA. Cortisol blockade of progesterone: A possible molecular mechanism involved in the initiation of human labor. *Nat Med* 1996;2:556–60.
130. Milewich L, Gant NF, Schwarz BE, Chen GT, MacDonald PC. Initiation of human parturition. VIII. Metabolism of progesterone by fetal membranes of early and late human gestation. *Obstet Gynecol* 1977;50:45–8.
131. Mitchell BF, Wong S. Changes in 17 beta,20 alpha-hydroxysteroid dehydrogenase activity supporting an increase in the estrogen/progesterone ratio of human fetal membranes at parturition. *Am J Obstet Gynecol* 1993;168:1377–85.
132. Pieber D, Allport VC, Hills F, Johnson M, Bennett PR. Interactions between progesterone receptor isoforms in myometrial cells in human labour. *Mol Hum Reprod* 2001;7:875–9.
133. Rezapour M, Backstrom T, Lindblom B, Ulmsten U. Sex steroid receptors and human parturition. *Obstet Gynecol* 1997;89:918–24.
134. How H, Huang ZH, Zuo J, Lei ZM, Spinnato JA, Rao CV. Myometrial estradiol and progesterone receptor changes in preterm and term pregnancies. *Obstet Gynecol* 1995;86:936–40.
135. Henderson D, Wilson T. Reduced binding of progesterone receptor to its nuclear response element after human labor onset. *Am J Obstet Gynecol* 2001;185:579–85.
136. Gustafsson JA. An update on estrogen receptors. *Semin Perinatol* 2000;24:66–9.
137. Warner M, Nilsson S, Gustafsson JA. The estrogen receptor family. *Curr Opin Obstet Gynecol* 1999;11:249–54.
138. Mesiano S, Chan EC, Fitter JT, Kwek K, Yeo G, Smith R. Progesterone withdrawal and estrogen activation in human parturition are coordinated by progesterone receptor A expression in the myometrium. *J Clin Endocrinol Metab* 2002;87:2924–30.
139. Pieber D, Allport VC, Bennett PR. Progesterone receptor isoform A inhibits isoform B-mediated transactivation in human amnion. *Eur J Pharmacol* 2001;427:7–11.
140. Bennett P, Allport V, Loudon J, Elliott C. Prostaglandins, the fetal membranes and the cervix. *Front Horm Res* 2001;27:147–64.
141. Allport VC, Pieber D, Slater DM, Newton R, White JO, Bennett PR. Human labour is associated with nuclear factor-kappaB activity which mediates cyclo-oxygenase-2 expression and is involved with the 'functional progesterone withdrawal'. *Mol Hum Reprod* 2001;7:581–6.
142. Belt AR, Baldassare JJ, Molnar M, Romero R, Hertelendy F. The nuclear transcription factor NF-kappaB mediates interleukin-1beta-induced expression of cyclooxygenase-2 in human myometrial cells. *Am J Obstet Gynecol* 1999;181:359–66.
143. Kalkhoven E, Wissink S, Van der Saag PT, van der BB. Negative interaction between the RelA(p65) subunit of NF-kappaB and the progesterone receptor. *J Biol Chem* 1996;271:6217–24.
144. Greer I. Cervical ripening. In Drife J, Calder A, eds. *Prostaglandins and the Uterus.* London: Springer-Verlag, 1992:191.
145. Calder A. Pharmacological management of the unripe cervix in the human. In Naftolin F, Stubblefield P, eds. *Dilatation of the Uterine Cervix.* New York: Raven Press, 1980:317.
146. Bennett PR, Elder MG, Myatt L. The effects of lipoxygenase metabolites of arachidonic acid on human myometrial contractility. *Prostaglandins* 1987;33:837–44.
147. Carraher R, Hahn DW, Ritchie DM, McGuire JL. Involvement of lipoxygenase products in myometrial contractions. *Prostaglandins* 1983;26:23–32.
148. Ritchie DM, Hahn DW, McGuire JL. Smooth muscle contraction as a model to study the mediator role of endogenous lipoxygenase products of arachidonic acid. *Life Sci* 1984;34:509–13.
149. Wiqvist N, Lindblom B, Wikland M, Wilhelmsson L. Prostaglandins and uterine contractility. *Acta Obstet Gynecol Scand Suppl* 1983;113:23–9.
150. Rajabi M, Solomon S, Poole AR. Hormonal regulation of interstitial collagenase in the uterine cervix of the pregnant guinea pig. *Endocrinology* 1991;128:863–71.
151. Ellwood DA, Mitchell MD, Anderson AB, Turnbull AC. The in vitro production of prostanoids by the human cervix during pregnancy: Preliminary observations. *Br J Obstet Gynaecol* 1980;87:210–14.
152. Calder AA, Greer IA. Pharmacological modulation of cervical compliance in the first and second trimesters of pregnancy. *Semin Perinatol* 1991;15:162–72.
153. Novy MJ, Liggins GC. Role of prostaglandins, prostacyclin, and thromboxanes in the physiologic control of the uterus and in parturition. *Semin Perinatol* 1980;4:45–66.
154. Mitchell MD. The mechanism(s) of human parturition. *J Dev Physiol* 1984;6:107–18.
155. MacDonald PC, Schultz FM, Duenhoelter JH, *et al.* Initiation of human parturition. I. Mechanism of action of arachidonic acid. *Obstet Gynecol* 1974;44:629–36.

156. Thorburn GD, Challis JR. Endocrine control of parturition. *Physiol Rev* 1979;59:863–918.
157. Challis JR, Olson D. Parturition. In Knobil E, Neill J, eds. *The Physiology of Reproduction*. New York: Raven Press, 1988:2177.
158. Bleasdale JE, Johnston JM. Prostaglandins and human parturition: Regulation of arachidonic acid mobilization. *Rev Perinat Med* 1985;5:151.
159. Challis JRG. Endocrine control of parturition. *Physiol Rev* 1979; 59:863.
160. Romero R, Mazor M, Munoz H, Gomez R, Galasso M, Sherer DM. The preterm labor syndrome. *Ann N Y Acad Sci* 1994;734:414–29.
161. Karim SM, Filshie GM. Therapeutic abortion using prostaglandin F2alpha. *Lancet* 1970;1:157–9.
162. Embrey MP. Induction of abortion by prostaglandins E1 and E2. *Br Med J* 1970;1:258–60.
163. Comparison of intra-amniotic prostaglandin F2 alpha and hypertonic saline for induction of second-trimester abortion. *Br Med J* 1976;1:1373–6.
164. Termination of second trimester pregnancy by intramuscular injection of 16-phenoxy-omega-17,18,19,20-tetranor-PGE2 methyl sulphonylamide. *Int J Gynaecol Obstet* 1982;20:383–6.
165. Husslein P. Use of prostaglandins for induction of labor. *Semin Perinatol* 1991;15:173–81.
166. Macer J, Buchanan D, Yonekura ML. Induction of labor with prostaglandin E2 vaginal suppositories. *Obstet Gynecol* 1984;63: 664–8.
167. MacKenzie IZ. Prostaglandins and midtrimester abortion. In Drife J, Calder A, eds. *Prostaglandins and the Uterus*. London: Springer-Verlag, 1992:119.
168. World Health Organization Task Force. Repeated vaginal administration of 15-methyl pgf2 alpha for termination of pregnancy in the 13th to 20th week of gestation. *Contraception* 1977;16:175.
169. Husslein P. Prostaglandins for induction of labour. In Drife J, Calder A, eds. *Prostaglandins and the Uterus*. London: Springer-Verlag, 1992.
170. Gordon-Wright AP, Elder MG. Prostaglandin E2 tablets used intravaginally for the induction of labour. *Br J Obstet Gynaecol* 1979;86:32–6.
171. Ekman G, Forman A, Marsal K, Ulmsten U. Intravaginal versus intracervical application of prostaglandin E2 in viscous gel for cervical priming and induction of labor at term in patients with an unfavorable cervical state. *Am J Obstet Gynecol* 1983;147: 657–61.
172. Skarnes RC, Harper MJ. Relationship between endotoxin-induced abortion and the synthesis of prostaglandin F. *Prostaglandins* 1972;1:191–203.
173. Harper MJ, Skarnes RC. Inhibition of abortion and fetal death produced by endotoxin or prostaglandin F2alpha. *Prostaglandins* 1972;2:295–309.
174. Giri SN, Stabenfeldt GH, Moseley TA, *et al*. Role of eicosanoids in abortion and its prevention by treatment with flunixin meglumine in cows during the first trimester of pregnancy. *Zentralbl Veterinarmed A* 1991;38:445–59.
175. Keirse MJ. Eicosanoids in human pregnancy and parturition. In Mitchell M, ed. *Eicosanoids in Reproduction*. Boca Raton, FL: CRC Press, 1990:199.
176. Sellers SM, Mitchell MD, Anderson AB, Turnbull AC. The relation between the release of prostaglandins at amniotomy and the subsequent onset of labour. *Br J Obstet Gynaecol* 1981;88:1211–6.
177. Romero R, Emamian M, Wan M, Grzyboski C, Hobbins JC, Mitchell MD. Increased concentrations of arachidonic acid lipoxygenase metabolites in amniotic fluid during parturition. *Obstet Gynecol* 1987;70:849–51.
178. Romero R, Wu YK, Mazor M, Hobbins JC, Mitchell MD. Increased amniotic fluid leukotriene C4 concentration in term human parturition. *Am J Obstet Gynecol* 1988;159:655–7.
179. Romero R, Emamian M, Quintero R, Wan M, Hobbins JC, Mitchell MD. Amniotic fluid prostaglandin levels and intra-amniotic infections. *Lancet* 1986;1:1380.
180. Romero R, Wu YK, Mazor M, Hobbins JC, Mitchell MD. Amniotic fluid prostaglandin E2 in preterm labor. *Prostaglandins Leukot Essent Fatty Acids* 1988;34:141–5.
181. Romero R, Emamian M, Wan M, Quintero R, Hobbins JC, Mitchell MD. Prostaglandin concentrations in amniotic fluid of women with intra-amniotic infection and preterm labor. *Am J Obstet Gynecol* 1987;157:1461–7.
182. Romero R, Wu YK, Sirtori M, *et al*. Amniotic fluid concentrations of prostaglandin F2 alpha, 13,14-dihydro-15-keto-prostaglandin F2 alpha (PGFM) and 11-deoxy-13,14-dihydro-15-keto-11, 16-cycloprostaglandin E2 (PGEM-LL) in preterm labor. *Prostaglandins* 1989; 37:149–61.
183. Keirse MJ. Endogenous prostaglandins in human parturition. In Keirse MA, Gravenhorst J, eds. *Human Parturition*. The Hague, Netherlands: Nijhoff Publishers, 1979:101.
184. Romero R, Baumann P, Gonzalez R, *et al*. Amniotic fluid prostanoid concentrations increase early during the course of spontaneous labor at term. *Am J Obstet Gynecol* 1994;171:1613–20.
185. Romero R, Baumann P, Gomez R, *et al*. The relationship between spontaneous rupture of membranes, labor, and microbial invasion of the amniotic cavity and amniotic fluid concentrations of prostaglandins and thromboxane B2 in term pregnancy. *Am J Obstet Gynecol* 1993;168:1654–64.
186. Romero R, Munoz H, Gomez R, *et al*. Increase in prostaglandin bioavailability precedes the onset of human parturition. *Prostaglandins Leukot Essent Fatty Acids* 1996;54:187–91.
187. Keirse MJ, Mitchell MD, Turnbull AC. Changes in prostaglandin F and 13,14-dihydro-15-keto-prostaglandin F concentrations in amniotic fluid at the onset of and during labour. *BrJ Obstet Gynaecol* 1977;84:743–46.
188. Keirse MJ, Turnbull AC. E prostaglandins in amniotic fluid during late pregnancy and labour. *J Obstet Gynaecol Br Commonw* 1973;80:970–3.
189. Dray F, Frydman R. Primary prostaglandins in amniotic fluid in pregnancy and spontaneous labor. *Am J Obstet Gynecol* 1976; 126:13–9.
190. Salmon JA, Amy JJ. Levels of prostaglandin F2 alpha in amniotic fluid during pregnancy and labour. *Prostaglandins* 1973;4:523.
191. Olson DM, Zakar T, Smieja Z, *et al*. A pathway for the regulation of prostaglandins and parturition. In Drife J, Calder A, eds. *Prostaglandins and the Uterus*. London: Springer-Verlag, 1992:149.
192. Myatt L, Lye SJ. Expression, localization and function of prostaglandin receptors in myometrium. *Prostaglandins Leukot Essent Fatty Acids* 2004;70:137–48.
193. Romero R, Durum S, Dinarello CA, Oyarzun E, Hobbins JC, Mitchell MD. Interleukin-1 stimulates prostaglandin biosynthesis by human amnion. *Prostaglandins* 1989;37:13–22.
194. Duchesne MJ, Thaler-Dao H, de Paulet AC. Prostaglandin synthesis in human placenta and fetal membranes. *Prostaglandins* 1978; 15:19–42.
195. Olson DM, Zakar T, Potestio FA, Smieja Z. Control of prostaglandin production in human amnion. *New Physiol Sci* 1990; 5:259.
196. Okazaki T, Casey ML, Okita JR, MacDonald PC, Johnston JM. Initiation of human parturition. XII. Biosynthesis and metabolism of prostaglandins in human fetal membranes and uterine decidua. *Am J Obstet Gynecol* 1981;139:373–81.
197. Romero R, Mazor M, Manogue K, Oyarzun E, Cerami A. Human decidua: A source of cachectin-tumor necrosis factor. *Eur J Obstet Gynecol Reprod Biol* 1991;41:123–7.
198. Hertelendy F, Zakar T. Prostaglandins and the myometrium and cervix. *Prostaglandins Leukot Essent Fatty Acids* 2004;70:207–22.
199. Molnar M, Hertelendy F. Signal-transduction in rat myometrial cells – comparison of the actions of endothelin-1, oxytocin and prostaglandin-F2-alpha. *Eur J Endocrinol* 1995;133:467–74.
200. Hertelendy F, Molnar M, Rigo J. Proposed signaling role of arachidonic-acid in human myometrium. *Mol Cell Endocrinol* 1995;110:113–8.
201. Molnar M, Romero R, Hertelendy F. Interleukin-1 and tumor-necrosis-factor stimulate arachidonic-acid release and phospholipid-metabolism in human myometrial cells. *Am J Obstet Gynecol* 1993;169:825–9.
202. Romero R, Manogue KR, Mitchell MD, *et al*. Infection and labor. IV. Cachectin-tumor necrosis factor in the amniotic fluid of women with intraamniotic infection and preterm labor. *Am J Obstet Gynecol* 1989;161:336–41.
203. Romero R, Wu YK, Oyarzun E, Hobbins JC, Mitchell MD. A potential role for epidermal growth factor/alpha-transforming growth factor in human parturition. *Eur J Obstet Gynecol Reprod Biol* 1989;33:55–60.
204. Novy MJ, Walsh SW. Dexamethasone and estradiol treatment in pregnant rhesus macaques: Effects on gestational length, maternal plasma hormones, and fetal growth. *Am J Obstet Gynecol* 1983; 145:920–31.
205. Potestio FA, Zakar T, Olson DM. Glucocorticoids stimulate prostaglandin synthesis in human amnion cells by a receptor-mediated mechanism. *J Clin Endocrinol Metab* 1988;67:1205–10.

206. Nathanielsz PW, Smith G, Wu W. Topographical specialization of prostaglandin function in late pregnancy and at parturition in the baboon. *Prostaglandins Leukot Essent Fatty Acids* 2004;70: 199–206.
207. Coleman RA, Kennedy I, Humphrey PP, Bunce K, Lumley P. In Hansch C, Sammes GTJB, eds. *Comprehensive Medicinal Chemistry*. Oxford: Pergamon Press, 1990:643–717.
208. Matsumoto T, Sagawa N, Yoshida M, *et al.* The prostaglandin E2 and F2 alpha receptor genes are expressed in human myometrium and are down-regulated during pregnancy. *Biochem Biophys Res Commun* 1997;238:838–41.
209. Wikland M, Lindblom B, Wiqvist N. Myometrial response to prostaglandins during labor. *Gynecol Obstet Invest* 1984;17:131–8.
210. Wiqvist N, Bryman I, Lindblom B, Norstrom A, Wikland M. The role of prostaglandins for the coordination of myometrial forces during labor. *Acta Physiol Hung* 1985;65:313–22.
211. Lye SJ, Ou CW, Tech TG, *et al.* The molecular basis of labour and tocolysis. *Fetal Matern Med Rev* 1998;10:121–36.
212. Smith GC, Wu WX, Nathanielsz PW. Effects of gestational age and labor on the expression of prostanoid receptor genes in pregnant baboon cervix. *Prostaglandins* 2001;63:153–63.
213. Smith GC, Baguma-Nibasheka M, Wu WX, Nathanielsz PW. Regional variations in contractile responses to prostaglandins and prostanoid receptor messenger ribonucleic acid in pregnant baboon uterus. *Am J Obstet Gynecol* 1998;179:1545–52.
214. Luckas MJM, Wray S. A comparison of the contractile properties of human myometrium obtained from the upper and lower uterine segments. *Br J Obstet Gynaecol* 2000;107:1309–11.
215. Liggins G, Fairclough RJ, Grieves SA, *et al.* Parturition in the sheep. In Knight J, O'Connor M, eds. *The Fetus and Birth*. Amsterdam: Elsevier, 1977.
216. Liggins GC, Fairclough RJ, Grieves SA, Kendall JZ, Knox BS. The mechanism of initiation of parturition in the ewe. *Recent Prog Horm Res* 1973;29:111–59.
217. McDonald TJ, Nathanielsz PW. Bilateral destruction of the fetal paraventricular nuclei prolongs gestation in sheep. *Am J Obstet Gynecol* 1991;165:764–70.
218. Gluckman PD, Mallard C, Boshier DP. The effect of hypothalamic lesions on the length of gestation in fetal sheep. *Am J Obstet Gynecol* 1991;165:1464–8.
219. Honnebier WJ, Swaab DF. The influence of anencephaly upon intrauterine growth of fetus and placenta and upon gestation length. *J Obstet Gynaecol Br Commonw* 1973;80:577–88.
220. Schellenberg JC, Liggins GC. Initiation of labour: uterine and cervical changes, endocrine changes. In Chard T, Grudzinskas JG, eds. *The Uterus*. Cambridge, UK: Cambridge University Press, 1994:308–35.
221. Kendall JZ, Challis JR, Hart IC, *et al.* Steroid and prostaglandin concentrations in the plasma of pregnant ewes during infusion of adrenocorticotrophin or dexamethasone to intact or hypophysectomized foetuses. *J Endocrinol* 1977;75:59–71.
222. Liggins G, Holm LW, Kennedy PC. Prolonged pregnancy following surgical lesions of the foetal lamb pituitary. *J Reprod Fertil* 1966;12:419.
223. Mecenas CA, Giussani DA, Owiny JR, *et al.* Production of premature delivery in pregnant rhesus monkeys by androstenedione infusion. *Nat Med* 1996;2:443–8.
224. Rees LH, Jack PM, Thomas AL, Nathanielsz PW. Role of foetal adrenocorticotrophin during parturition in sheep. *Nature* 1975;253:274–5.
225. Liggins GC. Premature parturition after infusion of corticotrophin or cortisol into foetal lambs. *J Endocrinol* 1968;42:323–9.
226. Chan EC, Falconer J, Madsen G, *et al.* A corticotropin-releasing hormone type I receptor antagonist delays parturition in sheep. *Endocrinology* 1998;139:3357–60.
227. Nathanielsz PW, Jenkins SL, Tame JD, Winter JA, Guller S, Giussani DA. Local paracrine effects of estradiol are central to parturition in the rhesus monkey. *Nat Med* 1998;4:456–9.
228. Whittle WL, Patel FA, Alfaidy N, *et al.* Glucocorticoid regulation of human and ovine parturition: the relationship between fetal hypothalamic–pituitary–adrenal axis activation and intrauterine prostaglandin production. *Biol Reprod* 2001;64:1019–32.
229. Challis JRG, Matthews SG, Gibb W, Lye SJ. Endocrine and paracrine regulation of birth at term and preterm. *Endocr Rev* 2000;21:514–50.
230. Tornblom SA, Patel FA, Bystrom B, *et al.* 15-hydroxyprostaglandin dehydrogenase and cyclooxygenase 2 messenger ribonucleic acid expression and immunohistochemical localization in human cervical tissue during term and preterm labor. *J Clin Endocrinol Metab* 2004;89:2909–15.
231. Grammatopoulos DK, Hillhouse EW. Role of corticotropin-releasing hormone in onset of labour. *Lancet* 1999;354:1546–9.
232. Quartero HW, Fry CH. Placental corticotrophin releasing factor may modulate human parturition. *Placenta* 1989;10:439–43.
233. Benedetto C, Petraglia F, Marozio L, *et al.* Corticotropin-releasing hormone increases prostaglandin F2 alpha activity on human myometrium in vitro. *Am J Obstet Gynecol* 1994;171:126–31.
234. Yoon BH, Romero R, Jun JK, *et al.* An increase in fetal plasma cortisol but not dehydroepiandrosterone sulfate is followed by the onset of preterm labor in patients with preterm premature rupture of the membranes. *Am J Obstet Gynecol* 1998;179:1107–14.
235. Osman I, Young A, Ledingham MA, *et al.* Leukocyte density and pro-inflammatory cytokine expression in human fetal membranes, decidua, cervix and myometrium before and during labour at term. *Mol Hum Reprod* 2003;9:41–5.
236. Thomson AJ, Telfer JF, Young A, *et al.* Leukocytes infiltrate the myometrium during human parturition: Further evidence that labour is an inflammatory process. *Hum Reprod* 1999;14:229–36.
237. Yellon SM, Mackler AM, Kirby MA. The role of leukocyte traffic and activation in parturition. *J Soc Gynecol Investig* 2003;10: 323–38.
238. Romero R, Brody DT, Oyarzun E, *et al.* Infection and labor. III. Interleukin-1: A signal for the onset of parturition. *Am J Obstet Gynecol* 1989;160:1117–23.
239. Romero R, Mazor M, Brandt F, *et al.* Interleukin-1 alpha and interleukin-1 beta in preterm and term human parturition. *Am J Reprod Immunol* 1992;27:117–23.
240. Keelan JA, Blumenstein M, Helliwell RJ, Sato TA, Marvin KW, Mitchell MD. Cytokines, prostaglandins and parturition – a review. *Placenta* 2003;24(Suppl A):S33–46.
241. Romero R, Gomez R, Galasso M, *et al.* Macrophage inflammatory protein-1 alpha in term and preterm parturition: Effect of microbial invasion of the amniotic cavity. *Am J Reprod Immunol* 1994;32:108–13.
242. Cohen J, Ghezzi F, Romero R, *et al.* GRO alpha in the fetomaternal and amniotic fluid compartments during pregnancy and parturition. *Am J Reprod Immunol* 1996;35:23–9.
243. Esplin MS, Romero R, Chaiworapongsa T, *et al.* Amniotic fluid levels of immunoreactive monocyte chemotactic protein-1 increase during term parturition. *J Matern Fetal Neonatal Med* 2003;14: 51–6.
244. Romero R, Ceska M, Avila C, Mazor M, Behnke E, Lindley I. Neutrophil attractant/activating peptide 1/interleukin-8 in term and preterm parturition. *Am J Obstet Gynecol* 1991;165:813–20.
245. Keelan JA, Yang J, Romero RJ, *et al.* Epithelial cell-derived neutrophil-activating peptide-78 is present in fetal membranes and amniotic fluid at increased concentrations with intra-amniotic infection and preterm delivery. *Biol Reprod* 2004;70:253–9.
246. Stjernholm-Vladic Y, Stygar D, Mansson C, *et al.* Factors involved in the inflammatory events of cervical ripening in humans. *Reprod Biol Endocrinol* 2004;2:74.
247. Haddad R, Tromp G, Kuivaniemi H, Chaiworapongsa T, Kim YM, Romero R. Spontaneous labor at term is characterized by a genomic signature of acute inflammation in the chorioamniotic membranes but not in the systemic circulation. *Am J Obstet Gynecol* 2004;191(6):S138.
248. Kim YM, Romero R, Chaiworapongsa T, *et al.* Toll-like receptor-2 and-4 in the chorioamniotic membranes in spontaneous labor at term and in preterm parturition that are associated with chorioamnionitis. *Am J Obstet Gynecol* 2004;191:1346–55.
249. Muzio M, Bosisio D, Polentarutti N, *et al.* Differential expression and regulation of toll-like receptors (TLR) in human leukocytes: Selective expression of TLR3 in dendritic cells. *J Immunol* 2000;164:5998–6004.
250. Van Wagenen G, Newton WH. Pregnancy in the monkey after removal of the fetus. *Surg Gynecol Obstet* 1943;77:539–43.
251. Albrecht ED, Crenshaw MC, Pepe GJ. The effect of estrogen on placental delivery after fetectomy in baboons. *Am J Obstet Gynecol* 1989;160:237–41.
252. Lanman JT, Mitsudo SM, Brinson AO, Thau RB. Fetectomy in monkeys (*Macaca mulatta*): Retention of the placenta past normal term. *Biol Reprod* 1975;12:522–5.
253. Nathanielsz PW, Figueroa JP, Honnebier MB. In the rhesus monkey placental retention after fetectomy at 121 to 130 days' gestation outlasts the normal duration of pregnancy. *Am J Obstet Gynecol* 1992;166:1529–35.

254. Wadhwa PD, Garite TJ, Porto M, *et al.* Placental corticotropin-releasing hormone (CRH), spontaneous preterm birth, and fetal growth restriction: a prospective investigation. *Am J Obstet Gynecol* 2004;191:1063–9.
255. Leung TN, Chung TKH, Madsen G, McLean M, Chang AMZ, Smith R. Elevated mid-trimester maternal corticotrophin-releasing hormone levels in pregnancies that delivered before 34 weeks. *Br J Obstet Gynaecol* 1999;106:1041–6.
256. Hobel CJ, Dunkel-Schetter C, Roesch SC, Castro LC, Arora CP. Maternal plasma corticotropin-releasing hormone associated with stress at 20 weeks' gestation in pregnancies ending in preterm delivery. *Am J Obstet Gynecol* 1999;180:S257–63.
257. McLean M, Smith R. Corticotrophin-releasing hormone and human parturition. *Reproduction* 2001;121:493–501.
258. Condon JC, Jeyasuria F, Faust JM, Mendelson CR. Surfactant protein secreted by the maturing mouse fetal lung acts as a hormone that signals the initiation of parturition. *Proc Natl Acad Sci USA* 2004;101:4978–83.
259. McKeown KJ, Challis JRG. Regulation of 15-hydroxy prostaglandin dehydrogenase by corticotrophin-releasing hormone through a calcium-dependent pathway in human chorion trophoblast cells. *J Clin Endocrinol Metab* 2003;88:1737–41.

The concepts described in this chapter, as well as some of the text, were originally published in the book *Preterm Birth*, published by the Royal College of Obstetricians and Gynaecologists in the United Kingdom (Edited by Professor Hilary Critchley, Professor Phillip Bennett and Professor Steven Thornton and published by the RCOG Press). That work, as well as the present work, has been produced by U.S. Government appointees and, therefore, is not subject to copyright. The editors, as well as the publisher, have been informed and agreed with this course of action and their position is gratefully acknowledged.

129 Mechanisms of preterm labor and preterm premature rupture of the membranes

R. Romero, L. F. Gonçalves, T. Chaiworapongsa, J. P. Kusanovic and J. Espinoza

Introduction

Preterm delivery, defined as delivery before 37 completed weeks of gestation, is the leading cause of perinatal morbidity and mortality worldwide.[1] Preterm delivery may result from: (1) spontaneous premature initiation of labor with intact membranes; (2) preterm prelabor rupture of membranes (PROM); or (3) medically indicated preterm delivery to protect the health of the mother and/or the fetus. In this chapter, we will review the mechanisms involved in the initiation of spontaneous preterm labor with or without preterm PROM, with emphasis on the preterm labor syndrome. Preterm birth is the major challenge to modern obstetrics in areas of the world where the problem of maternal mortality has been conquered.[2]

Premature parturition as a syndrome

The current taxonomy of disease in obstetrics is largely based on the clinical presentation of the mother and not the mechanism of disease responsible for the clinical manifestations. The term 'premature labor', for example, does not inform one as to whether the condition is caused by an infection, a vascular insult, uterine overdistension, abnormal allogeneic recognition, stress, or some other pathological process. The same applies to other obstetrical complications, such as pre-eclampsia, small-for-gestational age (SGA) fetal death, etc. The lack of recognition of the syndromic nature of obstetric diseases is responsible for the view that one diagnostic test will detect and one treatment will cure each of these conditions. The key features of obstetrical syndromes[3] are: (1) multiple etiologies; (2) chronicity; (3) fetal involvement; (4) clinical manifestations that are often adaptive in nature; and (5) susceptibility due to a gene–environment interaction.

We will review the available evidence to support the concept that premature labor has '*multiple etiologies*'. Clearly, women with a short cervix in the mid-trimester of pregnancy, with increased concentrations of fetal fibronectin in vaginal fluid, or the presence of bacterial vaginosis are at increased risk for preterm labor or preterm delivery,[4–7] demonstrating that the pathological disorder leading to these conditions is *chronic* in nature. For example, intrauterine infection can be detected at the time of routine mid-trimester amniocentesis for genetic indications and become clinically evident weeks later with either PROM or premature labor.[8–10] '*Fetal involvement*' has been demonstrated in women with microbial invasion of the amniotic cavity. Fetal bacteremia has been detected in 30% of patients with preterm PROM and a positive amniotic fluid culture for microorganisms.[11] Similarly, neonates born after spontaneous preterm labor or preterm PROM are more likely to be SGA, indicating a pre-existing problem with the supply line.[12–18] The *adaptive nature* of labor has been proposed in the context of intrauterine infection in which the onset of labor can be considered a mechanism of host defense against infection that enables the mother to eliminate an infected tissue and allows the fetus to exit from a hostile environment.[19,20] It is possible that other mechanisms of disease in premature labor may also threaten the maternal/fetal pair, and a key question is why some women develop fetal growth restriction

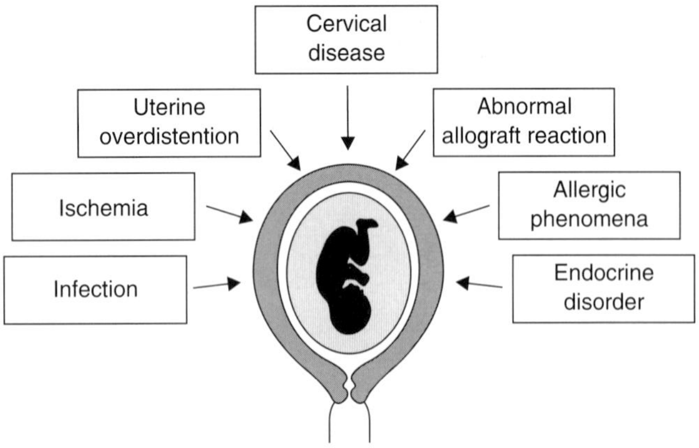

Figure 129.1 The pathological processes implicated in the preterm parturition syndrome From: Romero *et al.*,[21] with permission

and others pre-eclampsia, while yet another group resorts to the onset of preterm labor to deal with the threat. If the clinical manifestations are adaptive, then treatment of the components of the pathway (tocolysis, cerclage, etc.) could be considered symptomatic in nature and not aimed at the specific pathological processes that cause preterm labor. Finally, the predisposition to use a specific mechanism of host defense may be determined by *gene–environment interactions*, as in other disorders such as atherosclerosis and diabetes. However, complexity is added during pregnancy by the presence, and perhaps even the conflicting interests, of two genomes (maternal and fetal).

The pathological processes implicated in the preterm parturition syndrome include intrauterine infection, uterine ischemia, uterine overdistension, abnormal allograft reaction, allergy, cervical insufficiency and endocrine disorders (Figure 129.1). The following sections review the evidence for each of the potential mechanisms of disease.

Intrauterine infection and inflammation

Intrauterine infection has been recognized as a frequent and important mechanism of disease in preterm birth.[22–25] Indeed, it is the only pathological process for which a firm causal link with prematurity has been established with a defined molecular pathophysiology.[26] Moreover, fetal infection/inflammation has been implicated in the genesis of fetal or neonatal injury leading to cerebral palsy[27] and chronic lung disease.[28]

Evidence for a role of infection in the etiology of preterm birth includes: (1) intrauterine infection or systemic administration of microbial products to pregnant animals can result in preterm labor and delivery;[29–34] (2) systemic maternal infections, such as pyelonephritis, typhoid fever, malaria, and pneumonia, are frequently associated with the onset of premature labor in humans;[35–47] (3) subclinical intrauterine infections are associated with preterm birth;[48] (4) antibiotic treatment of ascending intrauterine infections can prevent prematurity in experimental models of chorioamnionitis;[31,49] and (5) treatment of asymptomatic bacteriuria prevents prematurity.[50]

Microbiological and histopathological studies suggest that infection/inflammation may account for 25–40% of cases of preterm delivery.[51] Since infection is frequently difficult to confirm, we often refer to women with histological evidence of acute chorioamnionitis/elevated proinflammatory cytokines in the amniotic fluid and documented microbial invasion of the amniotic cavity as belonging to the 'inflammatory cluster' associated with preterm PROM or preterm labor with intact membranes.

Frequency of intrauterine infection in spontaneous preterm birth

The prevalence of positive amniotic fluid cultures for microorganisms in women with preterm labor and intact membranes is approximately 13%.[52] The earlier the gestational age at preterm birth, the more likely that microbial invasion of the amniotic cavity will be present.[53] In preterm PROM, the prevalence of positive amniotic fluid cultures for microorganisms is approximately 32.4%.[22] Among women presenting with a dilated cervix in the mid-trimester, the prevalence of positive amniotic fluid cultures is 51%.[54] Microbial invasion of the amniotic cavity occurs in 11.9% of twin gestations presenting with preterm labor and delivering a preterm neonate and in 18.8% of patients in spontaneous labor at term.[55,56] The most common microorganisms found in the amniotic cavity are genital *Mycoplasmas*.

A higher prevalence of infection among pregnancies complicated by spontaneous preterm labor or preterm PROM has been identified with the use of molecular techniques.[57–66] Although amniotic fluid specimens were examined in most studies, a recent study examined amniotic fluid, gastric fluid and/or bronchoalveolar lavage fluid for bacterial 16s ribosomal RNA genes in a group of 36 pregnancies (41 neonates) delivered before 33 weeks of gestation.[66] The rationale for this approach is that amniotic fluid can be considered on a continuum with fetal lung and gastric fluids. Bacterial footprints were detected in at least one of the fluid compartments in 70% (7/10) of the pregnancies delivered after preterm PROM and 80% (8/10) of those delivered following spontaneous preterm labor. In contrast, bacterial 16s ribosomal RNA genes were only present in 9% (1/11) of the pregnancies that underwent preterm delivery for maternal or fetal indications and in none of the twin pregnancies delivered before 33 weeks ($n=5$). A strong association was observed between the detection of bacterial 16s ribosomal RNA genes in any fluid and elevated interleukin (IL)-6 and IL-8 in placental tissues, fetal membranes, and cord blood. Remarkably, only four pregnancies had positive cultures for microorganisms using conventional microbiology techniques.[66]

Intrauterine infection as a chronic process

Evidence in support of the chronicity of intrauterine inflammation/infection is derived from studies of the microbiological state of the amniotic fluid, as well as the concentration of inflammatory mediators at the time of genetic amniocentesis.

Cassell *et al.*[8] were the first to report the recovery of genital *Mycoplasmas* from 6.6% (4/61) of amniotic fluid samples collected by amniocentesis between 16 and 21 weeks of gestation. Two women had positive cultures for *Mycoplasma hominis* and two for *Ureaplasma urealyticum*. Women with *M. hominis* delivered at 34 and 40 weeks without neonatal complications, while those with *U. urealyticum* had premature delivery, neonatal sepsis, and neonatal death at 24 and 29 weeks. Subsequently, Gray *et al.*[9] reported a 0.37% prevalence (9/2461) of positive cultures for *U. urealyticum* in amniotic fluid samples obtained during second-trimester genetic amniocenteses. After exclusion of a therapeutic abortion case, all women (8/8) with positive amniotic fluid cultures had either a fetal loss within 4 weeks of amniocentesis ($n=6$) or preterm delivery ($n=2$). All had histological evidence of chorioamnionitis. These observations suggest that microbial invasion could be clinically silent in the mid-trimester of pregnancy and that pregnancy loss/preterm delivery could take weeks to occur. A similar finding was reported by Horowitz *et al.*,[10] who detected *U. urealyticum* in 2.8% (6/214) of amniotic fluid samples obtained between 16 and 20 weeks of gestation. The rate of adverse pregnancy outcome (fetal loss, preterm delivery and low birth weight) was significantly higher in women with a positive amniotic fluid culture than in those with a negative culture [3/6 (50%) vs. 15/123 (12%); $p=0.035$].

IL-6 concentrations in amniotic fluid are considered to be a marker of intra-amniotic inflammation frequently associated with microbiological infection in the amniotic fluid or the chorioamniotic space.[67–70] Romero *et al.*[71] reported the results of a case–control study in which IL-6 determinations were conducted in stored fluid of women who had a pregnancy loss after a mid-trimester amniocentesis and a control group who delivered at term. Women who had a pregnancy loss had a significantly higher median amniotic fluid IL-6 than those with a normal outcome. Similar findings were reported by Wenstrom *et al.*[72] Of note is that maternal plasma concentrations of IL-6 were not associated with adverse pregnancy outcomes.

The same approach was subsequently used to test the association between markers of inflammation in mid-trimester amniotic fluid of asymptomatic women and preterm delivery. The concentrations of matrix metalloproteinases (MMP)-8,[73] IL-6,[74] tumor necrosis factor-α (TNF-α),[75] and angiogenin[76] in amniotic fluid obtained at the time of mid-trimester amniocentesis were significantly higher in women who subsequently delivered preterm than in women who delivered at term.

Collectively, this evidence suggests that a chronic intra-amniotic inflammatory process may be present in early pregnancy and is associated with both miscarriage and spontaneous preterm delivery. Some indirect evidence suggests that such inflammatory processes may be detectable using maternal blood.[77]

Fetal involvement

The most advanced and serious stage of ascending intrauterine infection is fetal infection. The overall mortality rate of neonates with congenital neonatal sepsis ranges between 25% and 90%.[78–82] The wide range of results reflects the effect of gestational age on the likelihood of survival. One study,[78] which focused on infants born before 33 weeks of gestation, found that the mortality rate was 33% for those infected and 17% for non-infected fetuses. Carroll *et al.*[11] have reported that fetal bacteremia detected by cordocentesis is found in 33% of fetuses with positive amniotic fluid cultures and 4% of those with negative amniotic fluid cultures. Therefore, subclinical fetal infection is far more common than traditionally recognized.

Preterm labor and preterm PROM as 'adaptive responses'

We have proposed that the onset of preterm labor in the context of intrauterine infection is a host defense mechanism with survival value.[19,20] The hosts (mother and/or fetus) would signal the onset of labor for the mother to expel the infected tissue and maintain reproductive fitness. The molecular mediators involved in parturition are similar to those that have evolved to protect the host against infection (cytokines and other inflammatory mediators).

The current view is that during the course of an ascending intrauterine infection, microorganisms may reach the decidua where they can stimulate a local inflammatory reaction, as well as the production of proinflammatory cytokines, chemokines, and inflammatory mediators (platelet activating factor, prostaglandins, leukotrienes, reactive oxygen species, nitric oxide, etc.). If this inflammatory process is not sufficient to signal the onset of labor, microorganisms can then cross intact membranes into the amniotic cavity where they can also stimulate the production of inflammatory mediators by resident macrophages and other host cells within the amniotic cavity. Finally, microorganisms that gain access to the fetus may elicit a systemic inflammatory response syndrome, characterized by increased fetal plasma concentrations of IL-6[20] and other cytokines,[83–85] as well as cellular evidence of neutrophil and monocyte activation.[86]

Thus far, evidence for the participation of IL-1 and TNF-α in the mechanisms of preterm parturition is persuasive, although the precise role of other pro-inflammatory mediators remains to be elucidated. Evidence supporting a role for IL-1 and TNF-α in preterm parturition includes the following: (1) IL-1β[87–89] and TNF-α[90,91] stimulate prostaglandin production by amnion, decidua and myometrium; (2) human decidua can produce IL-1β and TNF-α in response to bacterial products;[88,89,92] (3) amniotic fluid IL-1β and TNF-α bioactivity and concentrations are elevated in women with preterm labor and intra-amniotic infection;[93–96] (4) in women with preterm PROM and intra-amniotic infection, IL-1β concentrations are higher in the presence of labor;[94,95] (5) IL-1β and TNF-α can induce preterm parturition when administered systemically to pregnant animals;[97,98] (6) fetal plasma IL-1β is dramatically elevated in the context of preterm labor with intrauterine infection;[99] and (7) placental tissue obtained from women in labor, particularly those with chorioamnionitis, produces larger amounts of IL-1β than that obtained from women not in labor.[100]

There is considerable redundancy in the cytokine network and, thus, it is not clear that a particular cytokine is required to signal the onset of labor. Results of knockout animal experiments suggest that infection-induced preterm labor and delivery occur in animals lacking the IL-1 type I receptor.[101] However, a recent observation with a double knockout system indicates that the IL-1 type I and the TNF-α type I receptors are essential mediators for bacterially-induced preterm birth (Hirsch E, personal communication).

Microbial invasion from the amniotic cavity to the fetus can lead to fetal infection and a systemic inflammatory response known as 'the fetal inflammatory response syndrome' (FIRS). FIRS is a subclinical condition originally described in fetuses of mothers presenting with preterm labor and intact membranes or preterm PROM and is operationally defined as a fetal plasma IL-6 concentration above 11 pg/ml.[20] IL-6 is a major mediator of the host response to infection and tissue damage that is capable of eliciting biochemical, physiological and immunological changes in the host, including stimulation of the production of C-reactive protein by liver cells, activation of T and natural killer cells, etc. Fetuses with FIRS have a higher rate of neonatal complications and are frequently born to mothers with subclinical microbial invasion of the amniotic cavity.[20] It is believed that fetal microbial invasion results in a systemic fetal inflammatory response that can progress towards multiple organ dysfunction,[102] septic shock, and death in the absence of timely delivery. Evidence of multisystemic involvement in cases of FIRS includes increased concentrations of fetal plasma MMP-9,[84] neutrophilia, a higher number of circulating nucleated red blood cells, and higher plasma concentrations of G-CSF.[83] The histological hallmark of FIRS is inflammation in the umbilical cord (funisitis) or chorionic vasculitis.[103] Preterm newborns with funisitis are at increased risk for neonatal sepsis[104], as well as long-term handicap, including bronchopulmonary dysplasia[105] and cerebral palsy.[106,107]

An important observation is that the fetuses with preterm PROM and FIRS are at risk for the impending onset of preterm labor regardless of the inflammatory state of the amniotic cavity.[19] This suggests that the human fetus plays a major role in the initiation of preterm labor. Nonetheless, systemic fetal inflammation and even fetal injury may occur in the absence of labor when the inflammatory process does not involve the chorioamniotic membranes and decidua. Examples of this are hematogenous viral infections of the fetus and/or alloimmunization.

Specific mechanisms involved in preterm PROM

Untimely decidua/membrane activation leads to preterm PROM, which accounts for 40% of all preterm deliveries.

Histological studies of the membranes in women with term PROM indicate that membranes ruptured prematurely have a decreased number of collagen fibers, disruption of the normal wavy patterns of these fibers, and a deposit of amorphous materials among them.[108] Similar changes have been observed in the membranes apposed to the cervix in women undergoing elective cesarean section at term with intact membranes.[109] The implication is that although spontaneous rupture of membranes normally occurs at the end of the first stage of labor, the process responsible for this phenomenon begins before the onset of labor.

Histological studies of the site of rupture have demonstrated a 'zone of altered morphology' (ZAM).[109,110] A significant decrease in the amount of collagen type I, III, or V and an increased expression of tenascin have been reported in the ZAM. Tenascin is an extracellular matrix that is characteristically expressed during tissue remodeling and wound healing. Its identification in the membranes thus intimates the presence of injury and a wound healing-like response. Observations by Bell and Mallak[111,112] propose that the changes in the ZAM are more extensive in the setting of preterm PROM. These morphological and biochemical observations are consistent with the results of biophysical studies suggesting that rupture of membranes results from the application of acute or chronic stress on localized areas of the membranes that are weaker.

Structural extracellular matrix proteins, such as collagens, have been implicated in the tensile strength of the membranes, while the viscoelastic properties were attributed to elastin.[113,114] Dissolution of extracellular cements (i.e., fibronectins) is thought to be responsible for the process that allows the membranes to separate from the decidua after the birth of the infant.

Fibronectins are a family of important extracellular cements. Oncofetal fibronectin can be found in the vagina during both term and preterm parturition.[115–118] Therefore, degradation of the extracellular matrix, assessed by the detection of oncofetal fibronectin, is part of the common pathway of parturition.

The precise mechanism of membrane/decidual activation remains to be elucidated. However, roles for matrix-degrading enzymes and apoptosis have been proposed. Several studies have demonstrated increased availability of MMP-1 (interstitial collagenase),[119] MMP-8 (neutrophil collagenase),[120] MMP-9 (gelatinase-B),[121] and neutrophil elastase[122] in the amniotic fluid of women with preterm PROM, compared with that of women in preterm labor with intact membranes. Plasmin has also been implicated in this process,[118] as this enzyme can degrade type III collagen, fibronectin and laminin.[123] Other MMPs are likely to be involved, but systematic studies have not been conducted to date.[124–126] A role for tissue inhibitors of MMPs (TIMPs) has also been postulated.[127]

Accumulating evidence suggests that apoptosis is important in the mechanisms of membrane rupture.[128,129] Rupture of membranes has been associated with overexpression of pro-apoptotic genes and decreased expression of anti-apoptotic genes.[130] Some MMPs, such as MMP-9, may induce apoptosis in amnion.[131–133] Bell and McParland have recently reviewed the subject in detail.[134]

Gene–environment interactions

Gene–environment interactions are important in the understanding of many complex disorders, such as atherosclerosis, obesity, hypertension, etc. A gene–environment interaction is said to be present when the risk of a disease (occurrence or severity) among individuals exposed to both a genotype and an environmental factor is greater or lower than that which is predicted from the presence of either the genotype or the environmental exposure alone.[135,136] There is now considerable evidence that the inflammatory response is under genetic control and, therefore, the interaction between the genotype of the host and microorganisms is important in determining the likelihood and course of some infectious diseases. An example of such an interaction has been reported for bacterial vaginosis, an allele for TNF-α and preterm delivery.[137]

Bacterial vaginosis is a risk factor for spontaneous preterm delivery.[7] However, randomized clinical trials with antibiotic administration to prevent preterm birth have yielded contradictory results.[138–150] Recently, Macones *et al.*[137] reported the results of a case–control study in which cases were defined as women who had a spontaneous preterm delivery and controls as women who delivered at term. The environmental exposure was symptomatic bacterial vaginosis. The allele of interest was TNF-α allele 2, given that its carriage had been demonstrated to be associated with spontaneous preterm birth.[151] The key observations were: (1) clinically diagnosed bacterial vaginosis was associated with an increased risk for preterm delivery [odds ratio (OR) 3.3; 95% CI 1.8–5.9]; (2) women who carried the TNF-α allele 2 were also at increased risk for preterm delivery (OR, 2.7; 95% CI 1.7–4.5); and (3) women with both bacterial vaginosis and the TNF-α allele 2 had an OR of 6.1 (95% CI 1.9–21) for spontaneous preterm delivery, suggesting that a gene–environment interaction predisposes to preterm birth. Other gene–environment interactions may determine the susceptibility to intrauterine infection, microbial invasion of the fetus, and the likelihood of perinatal injury.

Uteroplacental ischemia

Histologic studies of the placentas of patients with preterm labor and preterm PROM indicate that after infection, the most common type of lesions are vascular in nature and can involve the maternal and fetal circulations.[152] Maternal lesions include the failure of physiological transformation of the spiral arteries, atherosis, and thrombosis, while those observed in the fetal circulation include a decreased number of arterioles in the villi and fetal arterial thrombosis. The proposed mechanism linking vascular lesions and preterm labor/delivery is uteroplacental ischemia.

Evidence supporting a role for vascular disorders/uteroplacental ischemia as a mechanism of disease leading to preterm parturition includes the following: (1) experimental uterine ischemia in primates is associated with preterm labor and delivery;[153] (2) vascular lesions in decidual vessels attached to the placenta have been reported by Arias *et al.*[154] in 34% of women with spontaneous preterm labor and intact membranes and in 35% of those with preterm PROM, but only in 12% of women in the control group (term gestation without complications);[154] (3) placental abruption is more frequent in women who deliver preterm with intact membranes or rupture of membranes than in those who deliver at term;[154–159] (4) failure of physiologic transformation in the myometrial segment of the spiral arteries has been found in women with preterm labor and intact membranes and preterm PROM.[160,161] This developmental abnormality had been previously associated with pre-eclampsia and intrauterine growth restriction; (5) women presenting with preterm labor and intact membranes who have an abnormal uterine artery Doppler velocimetry (an index of increased impedance to flow in the uterine circulation) are more likely to deliver preterm than those with normal Doppler velocimetry;[162–165] and (6) the frequency of SGA neonates is increased in women delivering after preterm labor with intact membranes and preterm PROM.[12–18] Vascular lesions leading to compromise of the uterine supply line could account for both intrauterine growth restriction and preterm labor.

The molecular mechanisms responsible for the onset of preterm parturition in cases of ischemia have not been determined. A role for the renin–angiotensin system has been postulated, as the fetal membranes are endowed with a functional renin–angiotensin system[166] and uterine ischemia increases the production of uterine renin.[167,168] Angiotensin II can induce myometrial contractility either directly[169] or through the release of prostaglandins.[170]

When uteroplacental ischemia is severe enough to lead to decidual necrosis and hemorrhage, thrombin may activate the common pathway of parturition. Evidence in support of this includes: (1) decidua is a rich source of tissue factor, the primary initiator of coagulation and of thrombin activation;[171] (2) intrauterine administration of whole blood to pregnant rats stimulates myometrial contractility,[172] while heparinized blood does not (heparin blocks the generation of thrombin);[172] (3) fresh whole blood stimulates myometrial contractility *in vitro* and this effect is partially blunted by incubation with hirudin, a thrombin inhibitor;[172] (4) thrombin stimulates myometrial contractility in a dose-dependent manner;[172] (5) thrombin stimulates the production of MMP-1,[173] and urokinase type plasminogen activator (uPA), and tissue type plasminogen activator (tPA) by endometrial stromal cells in culture.[174] MMP-1 can digest collagen directly, while uPA and tPA catalyze the transformation of plasminogen into plasmin, that in turn can degrade type III collagen and fibronectin,[175] which are important components of the extracellular matrix in the chorioamniotic membranes;[176] (6) thrombin/antithrombin (TAT) complexes, markers of *in vivo* generation of thrombin, are increased in plasma[177] and amniotic fluid[178] of women with preterm labor and preterm PROM; and (7) an elevation of plasma TAT complex concentration in the second trimester is associated with subsequent preterm PROM.[179]

The recognition that thrombin may play an important role in uterine contractility can explain the clinical observations that retroplacental hematomas in early pregnancy are associated with preterm delivery.[180] Also, vaginal bleeding in the first or second trimester is a risk factor for preterm birth.[181–184]

Although some investigators proposed that fetal hypoxemia is a cause of preterm labor, studies with cordocentesis have indicated that fetal hypoxemia and metabolic acidemia are not more frequent in women with preterm labor and intact membranes who deliver preterm than in those who deliver at term.[185] Similarly, Carroll *et al.*[186] have demonstrated that hypoxemia is not more common in fetuses of women with preterm PROM. Therefore, uterine ischemia should not be equated with fetal hypoxemia, and no evidence currently supports fetal hypoxemia as a cause of preterm parturition.

Uterine overdistension

The mechanisms responsible for the increased frequency of preterm birth in multiple gestations and other disorders associated with uterine overdistension are unknown.[187–191]

The importance of stretch in the initiation of labor is supported by an experiment conducted in humans in which the uteri of pregnant women with a live term fetus or a dead fetus were distended with a balloon inflated with physiologic saline (up to 300 cm^3).[192] Regular uterine contractions occurred in all patients shortly after distension of the balloon, and all delivered within 21 h. This observation indicated that stretch can induce labor at term, regardless of whether the fetus is alive or dead. Moreover, amniotic fluid concentrations of prostaglandin F2α and its stable metabolite in plasma were increased in stretch-induced labor.[192] Recently, it has been reported that in women with twin pregnancies, the presence of polyhydramnios further increases the rate of preterm delivery.[193]

Central questions include how the uterus senses stretch and how these mechanical forces induce biochemical changes that lead to parturition. Lye *et al.* and other investigators have conducted several studies that explore the biochemical consequences of stretch on myometrium.[194–219]

Increased expression of oxytocin receptor,[207] connexin 43,[220] and the *c-fos* mRNA has been consistently demonstrated in the rat myometrium near term.[204–206,208,210] Using a model in which pregnancy was restricted to one of the two uterine horns (by unilateral tubal ligation), the expression of the same genes was substantially lower in the empty horn, but could be corrected by distending the uterus with a 3 mm tube and stretching the horn.[207,220] In another set of studies, progesterone was found to block stretch-induced gene expression in the myometrium.[221] Mitogen-activated protein kinases have been proposed to mediate stretch-induced *c-fos* mRNA expression in myometrial smooth muscle cells.[204–206,208,210]

In addition to the effects of stretch on myometrium, recent studies indicate that stretch can impact the chorioamniotic membranes.[222–236] For example, *in vitro* studies have demonstrated an increase in the production of collagenase, IL-8,[228,237] and prostaglandin E_2,[227] as well as the cytokine pre-B-cell colony-enhancing factor.[231] These observations provide a possible link between the mechanical forces operating in an overdistended uterus and rupture of membranes.

Abnormal allograft reaction

The fetoplacental unit has been considered nature's most successful semi-allograft, and abnormalities in the recognition and adaptation to fetal antigens has been proposed as a mechanism of disease in recurrent pregnancy loss, intrauterine growth restriction and pre-eclampsia.[238–240] Chronic villitis has been considered a lesion indicative of 'placental rejection' and such lesions have been found in the placentas of a subset of women who delivered after spontaneous preterm labor.[241] We have observed that some women with preterm labor, in the absence of demonstrable infection, have elevated concentrations of the IL-2 soluble receptor.[152] Such elevations are considered an early sign of rejection in non-pregnant patients with renal transplants.[242] Further studies are required to define the frequency and clinical significance of this pathological process in preterm labor. Recently, allorecognition, in which cytotoxicity and rejection reactions are not inevitable consequences of exposure to foreign antigens,[243] has been proposed as a more accurate means of describing the maternal–fetal relationship. This has implications for the concept of allograft rejection as a mechanism of disease in obstetrics. A role for complement and natural killer cells in adverse pregnancy outcome has been proposed,[244–254] but it is unclear whether these systems are disturbed in preterm parturition.

Allergy-induced preterm labor

The concept that an allergic-like mechanism (type I hypersensitivity reaction) may be one of the etiologies of preterm birth was proposed in the early 1990s based upon clinical observations and experimental studies.[255–257] Case reports documented that some women had preterm labor after exposure to an allergen, and that a subgroup of patients with preterm labor had eosinophils as the predominant cell type in amniotic fluid. Since the presence of eosinophils in body fluids is generally considered an indicator of an allergic reaction, patients with preterm labor and eosinophils as a predominant cell type in the amniotic fluid were proposed to represent a form of uterine allergy. Subsequent to this observation, a large body of experimental evidence has accumulated providing biological plausibility to this hypothesis. The key observations have been that mast cells are present in the uterus and their products of degranulation can stimulate uterine contractility. Observations supporting a role for a type I hypersensitivity reaction in preterm labor include the following:[258–269] (1) the human fetus is exposed to common allergens, such as house dust mite. The allergen Der p 1 has been detected in both amniotic fluid and fetal blood. Moreover, the concentrations of the allergen are higher in fetal blood than in maternal blood;[262] (2) allergen-specific reactivity has been demonstrated in umbilical cord blood at birth and as early as 23 weeks of gestation, indicating that the fetus can recognize the allergen and mount an immune response;[263] (3) pregnancy is considered a state in which there is a preponderance of a TH-2 cytokine response that favors the differentiation of naive $CD4^+$ T cells to the TH-2 phenotype and the production of IgE, the key immunoglobulin required for a type I hypersensitivity reaction; (4) the gravid uterus is a rich source of mast cells, the effector cells of allergic responses;[268] (5) several products of mast cell degranulation, such as histamine and prostaglandins, can induce myometrial contractility;[266,267] (6) pharmacological degranulation of mast cells with a compound called '48/80' induces myometrial contractility;[259,261] (7) incubation of myometrial strips from sensitized and non-sensitized animals with an anti-IgE antibody increases myometrial contractility;[261] (8) human myometrial strips obtained from women known to be allergic to ragweed demonstrate increased myometrial contractility when challenged *in vitro* by the allergen (Garfield RE, personal communication). Moreover, sensitivity of the myometrial strips of non-allergic women can be transferred passively by preincubation of the strips with human serum (Garfield RE, personal communication); and (9) premature labor and delivery can be induced by exposure to an allergen in sensitized animals and can be prevented by treatment with a histamine H1 receptor antagonist.[260]

In summary, there is clinical and experimental evidence that a type I hypersensitivity reaction can induce preterm parturition, although the frequency of this phenomenon in humans is still unknown.

Cervical insufficiency

Although cervical insufficiency (formerly known as cervical incompetence) is traditionally considered to be a cause of mid-trimester miscarriage, accumulating evidence suggests it can also be a cause of spontaneous preterm birth.[270] Cervical insufficiency may be the result of a congenital disorder (e.g., hypoplastic cervix or diethylstilboestrol exposure *in utero*), surgical trauma (e.g., conization resulting in substantial loss of connective tissue) or traumatic damage to the structural integrity of the cervix (e.g., repeated cervical dilatation associated with termination of pregnancy).[271] Some cases presenting with the clinical characteristics of cervical insufficiency may be due to infection. Indeed, intrauterine infection has been demonstrated in 50% of women presenting with acute cervical insufficiency.[54] A detailed review of this topic has been recently published by Romero *et al.*[272]

Progesterone deficiency as a potential mechanism of disease in preterm labor

The spectrum of reproductive abnormalities associated with progesterone deficiency is broad. For example, luteal phase deficiency (LPD) is widely believed to be a cause of infertility[273,274] and is commonly listed as a cause of recurrent spontaneous abortion.[275,276] This disorder has been defined as either a defect of progesterone secretion by the corpus luteum or a defect in the endometrial response to progesterone.[277,278] Thus, in LPD, the reproductive organ could function well enough to ovulate, but the function of corpus luteum and/or endometrium is below a physiologic threshold sufficient for conception or pregnancy maintenance. Since there is no general agreement on the criteria for the diagnosis of LPD,[273,274,279,200] its clinical significance and contribution to adverse pregnancy outcome remains uncertain. However, one retrospective study included 540 infertile patients with a diagnosis of luteal phase defect (endometrial biopsy was out of phase by 2 days in two consecutive cycles) and showed a high rate of preterm delivery [31.2% (169/540)] in patients who had not received progesterone treatment.[281] Interestingly, those patients who were treated with progesterone vaginal suppositories for at least 12 weeks demonstrated a significant reduction in the rate of preterm delivery at less than 32 weeks and less than 37 weeks of gestation [for 32 weeks, no progesterone: 12.5% (4/32) vs. progesterone 1.3% (6/469), $p < 0.01$; and for 37 weeks, no progesterone: 31.2% (10/32) vs. progesterone 13.7% (64/469), $p < 0.01$].[281]

Several pathophysiologic mechanisms have been proposed to explain LPD, though the precise etiology remains unclear.[282] Progesterone supplementation in patients with LPD has been reported to improve pregnancy outcomes (reduction in the rate of recurrent abortion)[283–285] and increase the rate of successful pregnancy[286,287] in some, but not all, studies.[288,289] Recently, the use of gonadotropin releasing hormone (GnRH) agonist to suppress a premature surge of luteinizing hormone during ovarian stimulation in *in vitro* fertilization (IVF) cycles has led to corpus luteum dysfunction and, subsequently, to abnormal progesterone and estrogen concentration/function in several infertile patients. A meta-analysis of randomized trials[290] showed that luteal phase supplementation with intramuscular progesterone injection significantly improved fertility outcomes (clinical pregnancy rates and the rate of pregnancies achieving 24 weeks of gestation). Thus, there is evidence suggesting that progesterone might be important in human pregnancy, especially in early gestation.

Other than a primary progesterone functional deficiency such as LPD, reduction of progesterone function could result from other pathologic mechanisms, such as, intrauterine infection. In animal models of ascending intrauterine infection, bacteria-induced and LPS-induced preterm birth is preceded by a significant fall in serum progesterone concentration,[291] and the mechanisms by which this occurs were attributed to: (1) LPS and pro-inflammatory cytokines induced prostaglandin synthesis and, subsequently, luteolysis; (2) a direct anti-gonadotropic effect of pro-inflammatory cytokines and, thus, the suppression of progesterone production; and (3) pro-inflammatory cytokines up-regulated an inducible form of nitric oxide synthase and, thus, inhibited steroidogenesis, including progesterone production. However, Hirsch and Muhle[292] have argued that the fall in serum progesterone concentration is unlikely to be a primary mechanism by which intrauterine inoculation with bacteria causes preterm parturition in mice, since the mean interval to delivery is shorter in animals with intrauterine infection than ovariectomized animals, despite a higher serum progesterone concentration in the former.[292]

Patients with preterm PROM who went into spontaneous labor and delivered within seven days of cordocentesis had a significantly higher median plasma concentration of fetal cortisol than those who delivered after seven days.[293] Fetal plasma cortisol concentration, but not maternal cortisol concentration, was an independent predictor of the duration of pregnancy after adjusting for gestational age and the results of amniotic fluid culture (hazards ratio 2.9, $p < 0.05$). There was a significant correlation between fetal plasma cortisol and fetal plasma IL-6 concentrations. This evidence suggests that the activation of the fetal hypothalamic–adrenal axis may be present and that it is associated with intrauterine infection.[293,294]

It is well known that intrauterine infection is associated with an increase in pro-inflammatory cytokines[295,296] (i.e., IL-1, TNF-α, etc.) in amniotic fluid,[93–96] fetal membranes,[297,298] decidua[88,89,92] and myometrium.[299–302] In the context of infection-related preterm birth, the increased concentration of IL-1β in gestational tissue could stimulate NF-kappa B.[303–305] The activation of NF-kappa B, other than increasing COX-2 (mRNA and protein expression) and prostaglandin production,[303] could repress progesterone activity, as proposed by Allport *et al.*,[306] resulting in 'functional progesterone withdrawal' and, thus, preterm parturition.

Conclusions

Term and preterm labor share a common pathway characterized by increased uterine contractility, cervical ripening and degradation of extracellular matrix, which predisposes to membrane rupture. The evidence presented in this chapter provides support for the concept that preterm parturition is a complex disorder, which is also syndromic in nature. The predominant clinical presentation of this syndrome (i.e., uterine contractility, preterm cervical ripening without significant clinical contractility, or PROM) will vary depending upon the type and timing of the insult. This conceptual framework has implications for the understanding of the mechanisms responsible for the initiation of preterm parturition, as well as the diagnosis, treatment, and prevention of preterm birth. Since preterm labor is a heterogeneous condition, it is unlikely that one diagnostic modality or one therapeutic intervention will prevent all preterm births. We believe that the way forward requires a systematic examination of the taxonomy of preterm labor, which is now possible using genomic, proteomic and metabolomic techniques.

REFERENCES

1. Tucker J, McGuire W. ABC of preterm birth – Epidemiology of preterm birth. *Br Med J* 2004;329:675–8.
2. Bryce J, Boschi-Pinto C, Shibuya K, Black RE. WHO estimates of the causes of death in children. *Lancet* 2005;365:1147–52.
3. Romero R. The child is the father of the man. *Prenat Neonat Med* 1996;1:8–11.
4. Iams JD, Goldenberg RL, Meis PJ, Mercer BM, Moawad A, Das A, Thom E, McNellis TE, Copper RL, Johnson F, Roberts JM. The length of cervix and the risk of spontaneous premature delivery. National Institute of Child Health and Human Development Maternal Fetal Medicine Unit Network. *N Engl J Med* 1996;334: 567–72.
5. Hassan SS, Romero R, Berry SM, Dang K, Blackwell SC, Treadwell MC, Wolfe HM. Patients with an ultrasonographic cervical length < or =15 mm have nearly a 50% risk of early spontaneous preterm delivery. *Am J Obstet Gynecol* 2000;182:1458–67.
6. Goldenberg RL, Mercer BM, Meis PJ, Copper RL, Das A, McNellis D. The preterm prediction study: fetal fibronectin testing and spontaneous preterm birth. NICHD Maternal Fetal Medicine Units Network. *Obstet Gynecol* 1996;87:643–8.
7. Meis PJ, Goldenberg RL, Mercer B, *et al.* The Preterm Prediction Study – Significance of vaginal infections. *Am J Obstet Gynecol* 1995;173:1231–5.
8. Cassell GH, Davis RO, Waites KB, *et al.* Isolation of *Mycoplasma hominis* and *Ureaplasma urealyticum* from amniotic fluid at 16–20 weeks of gestation: potential effect on outcome of pregnancy. *Sex Transm Dis* 1983;10:294–302.
9. Gray DJ, Robinson HB, Malone J, Thomson RB Jr. Adverse outcome in pregnancy following amniotic fluid isolation of *Ureaplasma urealyticum. Prenat Diagn* 1992;12:111–7.
10. Horowitz S, Mazor M, Romero R, Horowitz J, Glezerman M. Infection of the amniotic cavity with *Ureaplasma urealyticum* in the midtrimester of pregnancy. *J Reprod Med* 1995;40:375–9.
11. Carroll SG, Papaioannou S, Ntumazah IL, Philpott-Howard J, Nicolaides KH. Lower genital tract swabs in the prediction of intrauterine infection in preterm prelabour rupture of the membranes. *Br J Obstet Gynaecol* 1996;103:54–9.
12. Weiner CP, Sabbagha RE, Vaisrub N, Depp R. A hypothetical model suggesting suboptimal intrauterine growth in infants delivered preterm. *Obstet Gynecol* 1985;65:323–6.
13. MacGregor SN, Sabbagha RE, Tamura RK, Pielet BW, Feigenbaum SL. Differing fetal growth patterns in pregnancies complicated by preterm labor. *Obstet Gynecol* 1988;72:834–7.
14. Tamura RK, Sabbagha RE, Depp R, Vaisrub N, Dooley SL, Socol ML. Diminished growth in fetuses born preterm after spontaneous labor or rupture of membranes. *Am J Obstet Gynecol* 1984;148:1105–10.
15. Williams MC, O'Brien WF, Nelson RN, Spellacy WN. Histologic chorioamnionitis is associated with fetal growth restriction in term and preterm infants. *Am J Obstet Gynecol* 2000;183:1094–9.
16. Bukowski R, Gahn D, Denning J, Saade G. Impairment of growth in fetuses destined to deliver preterm. *Am J Obstet Gynecol* 2001; 185:463–7.
17. Ott WJ. Intrauterine growth retardation and preterm delivery. *Am J Obstet Gynecol* 1993;168:1710–15.
18. Zeitlin J, Ancel PY, Saurel-Cubizolles MJ, Papiernik E. The relationship between intrauterine growth restriction and preterm delivery: An empirical approach using data from a European case–control study. *Br J Obstet Gynecol* 2000;107:750–8.
19. Romero R, Gomez R, Ghezzi F, *et al.* A fetal systemic inflammatory response is followed by the spontaneous onset of preterm parturition. *Am J Obstet Gynecol* 1998;179:186–93.
20. Gomez R, Romero R, Ghezzi F, Yoon BH, Mazor M, Berry SM. The fetal inflammatory response syndrome. *Am J Obstet Gynecol* 1998;179:194–202.
21. Romero R, Espinoza J, Mazor M, Chaiworapongsa T. The preterm parturition syndrome. In: Preterm Birth. Critchley H, Bennett P, Thornton S (eds). RCOG Press, London; 2004; pp. 28–60.
22. Goncalves LF, Chaiworapongsa T, Romero R. Intrauterine infection and prematurity. *Ment Retard Dev Disabil Res Rev* 2002; 8:3–13.
23. Minkoff H. Prematurity: Infection as an etiologic factor. *Obstet Gynecol* 1983;62:137–44.
24. Romero R, Sirtori M, Oyarzun E, *et al.* Infection and labor. V. Prevalence, microbiology, and clinical significance of intraamniotic infection in women with preterm labor and intact membranes. *Am J Obstet Gynecol* 1989;161:817–24.
25. Romero R, Mazor M, Wu YK, *et al.* Infection in the pathogenesis of preterm labor. *Semin Perinatol* 1988;12:262–79.
26. Hirsch E, Wang H. The molecular pathophysiology of bacterially induced preterm labor: insights from the murine model. *J Soc Gynecol Investig* 2005;12:145–55.
27. Yoon BH, Jun JK, Romero R, Park KH, Gomez R, Choi HJ, Kim IO. Amniotic fluid inflammatory cytokines (interleukin-6, interleukin-1beta, and tumor necrosis factor-alpha), neonatal brain white matter lesions, and cerebral palsy. *Am J Obstet Gynecol* 1997;177:19–26.
28. Yoon BH, Romero R, Kim KS, Park JS, Ki SH, Kim BI, Jun JK. A systemic fetal inflammatory response and the development of bronchopulmonary dysplasia. *Am J Obstet Gynecol* 1999;181:773–9.
29. Fidel PL Jr, Romero R, Wolf N, *et al.* Systemic and local cytokine profiles in endotoxin-induced preterm parturition in mice. *Am J Obstet Gynecol* 1994;170:1467–75.
30. McDuffie RS Jr, Sherman MP, Gibbs RS. Amniotic fluid tumor necrosis factor-alpha and interleukin-1 in a rabbit model of bacterially induced preterm pregnancy loss. *Am J Obstet Gynecol* 1992;167:1583–8.
31. McKay DG, Wong TC. The effect of bacterial endotoxin on the placenta of the rat. *Am J Pathol* 1963;42:357–77.
32. Romero R, Munoz H, Gomez R, *et al.* Antibiotic therapy reduces the rate of infection-induced preterm delivery and perinatal mortality. *Am J Obstet Gynecol* 170;390:1994.
33. Takeda Y, Tsuchiya I. Studies on the pathological changes caused by the injection of the Shwartzman filtrate and the endotoxin into pregnant rabbits. *Jap J Exp Med* 1953;21:9–16.
34. Zahl PA, Bjerknes C. Induction of decidua-placental hemorrhage in mice by the endotoxins of certain gram-negative bacteria. *Proc Soc Exp Biol Med* 1943;54:329–32.
35. Benedetti TJ, Valle R, Ledger WJ. Antepartum pneumonia in pregnancy. *Am J Obstet Gynecol* 1982;144:413–17.
36. Cunningham FG, Morris GB, Mickal A. Acute pyelonephritis of pregnancy: A clinical review. *Obstet Gynecol* 1973;42:112–7.
37. Fan YD, Pastorek JG, Miller JM Jr, Mulvey J. Acute pyelonephritis in pregnancy. *Am J Perinatol* 1987;4:324–6.
38. Finland M, Dublin TD. Pneumococcic pneumonia complicating pregnancy and the puerperium. *J Am Med Assoc* 1939;112:1027–32.
39. Gilles HM, Lawson JB, Sibelas M, Voller A, Allan N. Malaria, anaemia and pregnancy. *Ann Trop Med Parasitol* 1969;63:245–63.
40. Herd N, Jordan T. An investigtion of malaria during pregnancy in Zimbabwe. *Afr J Med* 1981;27:62.
41. Hibbard L, Thrupp L, Summeril S, Smale M, Adams R. Treatment of pyelonephritis in pregnancy. *Am J Obstet Gynecol* 1967;98: 609–15.
42. Kass E. Maternal urinary tract infection. *N Y State J Med* 1962;1:2822–6.
43. Madinger NE, Greenspoon JS, Ellrodt AG. Pneumonia during pregnancy: Has modern technology improved maternal and fetal outcome? *Am J Obstet Gynecol* 1989;161:657–62.
44. McLane CM. Pyelitis of pregnancy: A five-year study. *Am J Obstet Gynecol* 1939;38:117.
45. Oxhorn H. The changing aspects of pneumonia complicating pregnancy. *Am J Obstet Gynecol* 1955;70:1057.
46. Stevenson CS, Glasko AJ, Gillespie EC. Treatment of typhoid in pregnancy with chloramphenicol (chloromycetin). *J Am Med Assoc* 1951;146:1190.
47. Wing ES, Troppoli DV. The intrauterine transmission of typhoid. *J Am Med Assoc* 1930;95:405.
48. Gomez R, Ghezzi F, Romero R, Munoz H, Tolosa JE, Rojas I. Premature labor and intra-amniotic infection. Clinical aspects and role of the cytokines in diagnosis and pathophysiology. *Clin Perinatol* 1995;22:281–342.
49. Fidel P, Ghezzi F, Romero R, *et al.* The effect of antibiotic therapy on intrauterine infection-induced preterm parturition in rabbits. *J Matern Fetal Neonatal Med* 2003;14:57–64.
50. Romero R, Oyarzun E, Mazor M, Sirtori M, Hobbins JC, Bracken M. Meta-analysis of the relationship between asymptomatic bacteriuria and preterm delivery/low birth weight. *Obstet Gynecol* 1989;73:576–82.
51. Romero R, Salafia CM, Athanassiadis AP, *et al.* The relationship between acute inflammatory lesions of the preterm placenta and amniotic fluid microbiology. *Am J Obstet Gynecol* 1992;166: 1382–8.
52. Romero R, Espinoza J, Chaiworapongsa T, Kalache K. Infection and prematurity and the role of preventive strategies. *Semin Neonatol* 2002;7:259–74.
53. Watts DH, Krohn MA, Hillier SL, Eschenbach DA. The association of occult amniotic fluid infection with gestational age and

neonatal outcome among women in preterm labor. *Obstet Gynecol* 1992;79:351–7.

54. Romero R, Gonzalez R, Sepulveda W, *et al.* Infection and labor. VIII. Microbial invasion of the amniotic cavity in patients with suspected cervical incompetence: Prevalence and clinical significance. *Am J Obstet Gynecol* 1992;167:1086–91.
55. Romero R, Shamma F, Avila C, *et al.* Infection and labor. VI. Prevalence, microbiology, and clinical significance of intraamniotic infection in twin gestations with preterm labor. *Am J Obstet Gynecol* 1990;163:757–61.
56. Romero R, Nores J, Mazor M, *et al.* Microbial invasion of the amniotic cavity during term labor. Prevalence and clinical significance. *J Reprod Med* 1993;38:543–8.
57. Blanchard A, Hamrick W, Duffy L, Baldus K, Cassell GH. Use of the polymerase chain reaction for detection of *Mycoplasma fermentans* and *Mycoplasma genitalium* in the urogenital tract and amniotic fluid. *Clin Infect Dis* 1993;17(Suppl 1):S272–9.
58. Jalava J, Mantymaa ML, Ekblad U, *et al.* Bacterial 16S rDNA polymerase chain reaction in the detection of intra-amniotic infection. *Br J Obstet Gynaecol* 1996;103:664–9.
59. Hitti J, Riley DE, Krohn MA, *et al.* Broad-spectrum bacterial rDNA polymerase chain reaction assay for detecting amniotic fluid infection among women in premature labor. *Clin Infect Dis* 1997;24:1228–32.
60. Markenson GR, Martin RK, Tillotson-Criss M, Foley KS, Stewart RS Jr, Yancey M. The use of the polymerase chain reaction to detect bacteria in amniotic fluid in pregnancies complicated by preterm labor. *Am J Obstet Gynecol* 1997;177:1471–7.
61. Oyarzun E, Yamamoto M, Kato S, Gomez R, Lizama L, Moenne A. Specific detection of 16 micro-organisms in amniotic fluid by polymerase chain reaction and its correlation with preterm delivery occurrence. *Am J Obstet Gynecol* 1998;179:1115–9.
62. Yoon BH, Romero R, Kim M, *et al.* Clinical implications of detection of *Ureaplasma urealyticum* in the amniotic cavity with the polymerase chain reaction. *Am J Obstet Gynecol* 2000;183:1130–7.
63. Gerber S, Vial Y, Hohlfeld P, Witkin SS. Detection of Ureaplasma urealyticum in second-trimester amniotic fluid by polymerase chain reaction correlates with subsequent preterm labor and delivery. *J Infect Dis* 2003;187:518–21.
64. Markenson GR, Adams LA, Hoffman DE, Reece MT. Prevalence of Mycoplasma bacteria in amniotic fluid at the time of genetic amniocentesis using the polymerase chain reaction. *J Reprod Med* 2003;48:775–9.
65. Yoon BH, Romero R, Lim JH, *et al.* The clinical significance of detecting *Ureaplasma urealyticum* by the polymerase chain reaction in the amniotic fluid of patients with preterm labor. *Am J Obstet Gynecol* 2003;189:919–24.
66. Miralles R, Hodge R, McParland PC, *et al.* Relationship between antenatal inflammation and antenatal infection identified by detection of microbial genes by polymerase chain reaction. *Pediatr Res* 2005;57:570–7.
67. Yoon BH, Romero R, Kim CJ, *et al.* Amniotic fluid interleukin-6: A sensitive test for antenatal diagnosis of acute inflammatory lesions of preterm placenta and prediction of perinatal morbidity. *Am J Obstet Gynecol* 1995;172:960–70.
68. Romero R, Avila C, Santhanam U, Sehgal PB. Amniotic fluid interleukin 6 in preterm labor. Association with infection. *J Clin Invest* 1990;85:1392–400.
69. Romero R, Sepulveda W, Kenney JS, Archer LE, Allison AC, Sehgal PB. Interleukin 6 determination in the detection of microbial invasion of the amniotic cavity. *Ciba Found Symp* 1992;167: 205–20.
70. Romero R, Yoon BH, Kenney JS, Gomez R, Allison AC, Sehgal PB. Amniotic fluid interleukin-6 determinations are of diagnostic and prognostic value in preterm labor. *Am J Reprod Immunol* 1993; 30:167–83.
71. Romero R, Munoz H, Gomez R, *et al.* Two thirds of spontaneous abortion/fetal deaths after genetic amniocentesis are the result of a pre-existing sub-clinical inflammatory process of the amniotic cavity. *Am J Obstet Gynecol* 1995;172:261.
72. Wenstrom KD, Andrews WW, Tamura T, DuBard MB, Johnston KE, Hemstreet GP. Elevated amniotic fluid interleukin-6 levels at genetic amniocentesis predict subsequent pregnancy loss. *Am J Obstet Gynecol* 1996;175:830–3.
73. Yoon BH, Oh SY, Romero R, *et al.* An elevated amniotic fluid matrix metalloproteinase-8 level at the time of mid-trimester genetic amniocentesis is a risk factor for spontaneous preterm delivery. *Am J Obstet Gynecol* 2001;185:1162–7.
74. Wenstrom KD, Andrews WW, Hauth JC, Goldenberg RL, DuBard MB, Cliver SP. Elevated second-trimester amniotic fluid interleukin-6 levels predict preterm delivery. *Am J Obstet Gynecol* 1998;178:546–50.
75. Ghidini A, Eglinton GS, Spong CY, *et al.* Elevated mid-trimester amniotic fluid tumor necrosis alpha levels: A predictor of preterm delivery. *Am J Obstet Gynecol* 1996;174:307.
76. Spong CY, Ghidini A, Sherer DM, Pezzullo JC, Ossandon M, Eglinton GS. Angiogenin: A marker for preterm delivery in mid-trimester amniotic fluid. *Am J Obstet Gynecol* 1997;176:415–8.
77. Goldenberg RL, Andrews WW, Mercer BM, *et al.* The preterm prediction study: Granulocyte colony-stimulating factor and spontaneous preterm birth. National Institute of Child Health and Human Development Maternal–Fetal Medicine Units Network. *Am J Obstet Gynecol* 2000;182:625–30.
78. Thompson PJ, Greenough A, Gamsu HR, Nicolaides KH, Philpott-Howard J. Congenital bacterial sepsis in very preterm infants. *J Med Microbiol* 1992;36:117–20.
79. Placzek MM, Whitelaw A. Early and late neonatal septicaemia. *Arch Dis Child* 1983;58:728–31.
80. Ohlsson A, Vearncombe M. Congenital and nosocomial sepsis in infants born in a regional perinatal unit: Cause, outcome, and white blood cell response. *Am J Obstet Gynecol* 1987;156:407–13.
81. Gerdes JS. Clinicopathologic approach to the diagnosis of neonatal sepsis. *Clin Perinatol* 1991;18:361–81.
82. Boyer KM, Gadzala CA, Kelly PD, Gotoff SP. Selective intrapartum chemoprophylaxis of neonatal group B streptococcal early-onset disease. III. Interruption of mother-to-infant transmission. *J Infect Dis* 1983;148:810–6.
83. Berry SM, Gomez R, Athayde N, *et al.* The role of granulocyte colony stimulating factor in the neutrophilia observed in the fetal inflammatory response syndrome. *Am J Obstet Gynecol* 1998;178:S202.
84. Romero R, Athayde N, Gomez R, *et al.* The fetal inflammatory response syndrome is characterized by the outpouring of a potent extracellular matrix degrading enzyme into the fetal circulation. *Am J Obstet Gynecol* 1998;178:S3.
85. Romero R, Maymon E, Pacora P, *et al.* Further observations on the fetal inflammatory response syndrome: A potential homeostatic role for the soluble receptors of tumor necrosis factor alpha. *Am J Obstet Gynecol* 2000;183:1070–7.
86. Berry SM, Romero R, Gomez R, *et al.* Premature parturition is characterized by in utero activation of the fetal immune system. *Am J Obstet Gynecol* 1995;173:1315–20.
87. Romero R, Durum S, Dinarello CA, Oyarzun E, Hobbins JC, Mitchell MD. Interleukin-1 stimulates prostaglandin biosynthesis by human amnion. *Prostaglandins* 1989;37:13–22.
88. Romero R, LaFreniere D, Duff G, *et al.* Human decidua: A potent source of interleukin-1 like activity. 32nd Annual Meeting for the Society for Gynecologic Investigation. Phoenix. Arizona. *J Soc Gynecol Investig* 1985.
89. Romero R, Durum SK, Dinarello CA, *et al.* Interleukin-1: A signal for the initiation of labor in chorioamnionitis. *33rd Annual Meeting for the Society for Gynecologic Investigation,* Toronto, Ontario, Canada, 1986.
90. Romero R, Mazor M, Manogue K, Oyarzun E, Cerami A. Human decidua: A source of cachectin-tumor necrosis factor. *Eur J Obstet Gynecol Reprod Biol* 1991;41:123–7.
91. Romero R, Mazor M, Wu YK, Avila C, Oyarzun E, Mitchell MD. Bacterial endotoxin and tumor necrosis factor stimulate prostaglandin production by human decidua. *Prostaglandins Leukot Essent Fatty Acids* 1989;37:183–6.
92. Casey ML, Cox SM, Beutler B, Milewich L, MacDonald PC. Cachectin/tumor necrosis factor-alpha formation in human decidua. Potential role of cytokines in infection-induced preterm labor. *J Clin Invest* 1989;83:430–6.
93. Romero R, Manogue KR, Mitchell MD, *et al.* Infection and labor. IV. Cachectin-tumor necrosis factor in the amniotic fluid of women with intraamniotic infection and preterm labor. *Am J Obstet Gynecol* 1989;161:336–41.
94. Romero R, Brody DT, Oyarzun E, *et al.* Infection and labor. III. Interleukin-1: A signal for the onset of parturition. *Am J Obstet Gynecol* 1989;160:1117–23.
95. Romero R, Mazor M, Brandt F, *et al.* Interleukin-1 alpha and interleukin-1 beta in preterm and term human parturition. *Am J Reprod Immunol* 1992;27:117–23.
96. Romero R, Mazor M, Sepulveda W, Avila C, Copeland D, Williams J. Tumor necrosis factor in preterm and term labor. *Am J Obstet Gynecol* 1992;166:1576–87.

97. Romero R, Mazor M, Tartakovsky B. Systemic administration of interleukin-1 induces preterm parturition in mice. *Am J Obstet Gynecol* 1991;165:969–71.
98. Silver RM, Lohner WS, Daynes RA, Mitchell MD, Branch DW. Lipopolysaccharide-induced fetal death: the role of tumor-necrosis factor alpha. *Biol Reprod* 1994;50:1108–12.
99. Gomez R, Ghezzi F, Romero R, *et al.* Two thirds of human fetuses with microbial invasion of the amniotic cavity have a detectable systemic cytokine response before birth. *Am J Obstet Gynecol* 1997;176:514.
100. Taniguchi T, Matsuzaki N, Kameda T, *et al.* The enhanced production of placental interleukin-1 during labor and intrauterine infection. *Am J Obstet Gynecol* 1991;165:131–37.
101. Hirsch E, Muhle RA, Mussalli GM, Blanchard R. Bacterially induced preterm labor in the mouse does not require maternal interleukin-1 signaling. *Am J Obstet Gynecol* 2002;186:523–30.
102. Romero R, Gomez R, Ghezzi F, *et al.* A novel form of fetal cardiac dysfunction in preterm premature rupture of membranes. *Am J Obstet Gynecol* 1999;180:S27.
103. Pacora P, Chaiworapongsa T, Maymon E, *et al.* Funisitis and chorionic vasculitis: The histological counterpart of the fetal inflammatory response syndrome. *J Matern Fetal Med* 2002;11:18–25.
104. Yoon BH, Romero R, Park JS, *et al.* The relationship among inflammatory lesions of the umbilical cord (funisitis), umbilical cord plasma interleukin 6 concentration, amniotic fluid infection, and neonatal sepsis. *Am J Obstet Gynecol* 2000;183:1124–9.
105. Yoon BH, Romero R, Kim KS, *et al.* A systemic fetal inflammatory response and the development of bronchopulmonary dysplasia. *Am J Obstet Gynecol* 1999;181:773–9.
106. Yoon BH, Romero R, Yang SH, *et al.* Interleukin-6 concentrations in umbilical cord plasma are elevated in neonates with white matter lesions associated with periventricular leukomalacia. *Am J Obstet Gynecol* 1996;174:1433–40.
107. Yoon BH, Romero R, Park JS, *et al.* Fetal exposure to an intra-amniotic inflammation and the development of cerebral palsy at the age of three years. *Am J Obstet Gynecol* 2000;182:675–81.
108. Skinner SJ, Liggins GC. Glycosaminoglycans and collagen in human amnion from pregnancies with and without premature rupture of the membranes. *J Dev Physiol* 1981;3:111–21.
109. McLaren J, Malak TM, Bell SC. Structural characteristics of term human fetal membranes prior to labour: Identification of an area of altered morphology overlying the cervix. *Hum Reprod* 1999; 14:237–41.
110. Malak TM, Bell SC. Structural characteristics of term human fetal membranes: A novel zone of extreme morphological alteration within the rupture site. *Br J Obstet Gynaecol* 1994;101:375–86.
111. Bell SC, Pringle JH, Taylor DJ, Malak TM. Alternatively spliced tenascin C mRNA isoforms in human fetal membranes. *Mol Hum Reprod* 1999;5:1066–76.
112. Malak TM, Mulholland G, Bell SC. Morphometric characteristics of the decidua, cytotrophoblast, and connective tissue of the prelabor ruptured fetal membranes. *Ann N Y Acad Sci* 1994; 734:430–2.
113. Hieber AD, Corcino D, Motosue J, *et al.* Detection of elastin in the human fetal membranes: Proposed molecular basis for elasticity. *Placenta* 1997;18:301–12.
114. Bryant-Greenwood GD. The extracellular matrix of the human fetal membranes: Structure and function. *Placenta* 1998;19:1–11.
115. Iams JD, Casal D, McGregor JA, *et al.* Fetal fibronectin improves the accuracy of diagnosis of preterm labor. *Am J Obstet Gynecol* 1995;173:141–5.
116. Lockwood CJ, Senyei AE, Dische MR, *et al.* Fetal fibronectin in cervical and vaginal secretions as a predictor of preterm delivery. *N Engl J Med* 1991;325:669–74.
117. Nageotte MP, Casal D, Senyei AE. Fetal fibronectin in patients at increased risk for premature birth. *Am J Obstet Gynecol* 1994; 170:20–5.
118. Oshiro B, Edwin S, Silver R. Human fibronectin and human tenascin production in human amnion cells. *J Soc Gynecol Invest* 1996;3:351A.
119. Maymon E, Romero R, Pacora P, *et al.* Evidence for the participation of interstitial collagenase (matrix metalloproteinase 1) in preterm premature rupture of membranes. *Am J Obstet Gynecol* 2000;183:914–20.
120. Maymon E, Romero R, Pacora P, *et al.* Human neutrophil collagenase (matrix metalloproteinase 8) in parturition, premature rupture of the membranes, and intrauterine infection. *Am J Obstet Gynecol* 2000;183:94–9.
121. Athayde N, Edwin SS, Romero R, Gomez R, Maymon E, Pacora P, Menon R. A role for matrix metalloproteinase-9 in spontaneous rupture of the fetal membranes. *Am J Obstet Gynecol* 1998;179: 1248–53.
122. Helmig BR, Romero R, Espinoza J, *et al.* Neutrophil elastase and secretory leukocyte protease inhibitor in prelabor rupture of membranes, parturition and intra-amniotic infection. *J Matern Fetal Neonatal Med* 2002;12:237–46.
123. Everts V, van der ZE, Creemers L, Beertsen W. Phagocytosis and intracellular digestion of collagen, its role in turnover and remodelling. *Histochem J* 1996;28:229–45.
124. Reboul P, Pelletier JP, Tardif G, Cloutier JM, Martel-Pelletier J. The new collagenase, collagenase-3, is expressed and synthesized by human chondrocytes but not by synoviocytes. A role in osteoarthritis. *J Clin Invest* 1996;97:2011–9.
125. Fortunato SJ, Menon R. Screening of novel matrix metalloproteinases (MMPs) in human fetal membranes. *J Assist Reprod Genet* 2002;19:483–6.
126. Velasco G, Pendas AM, Fueyo A, Knauper V, Murphy G, Lopez-Otin C. Cloning and characterization of human MMP-23, a new matrix metalloproteinase predominantly expressed in reproductive tissues and lacking conserved domains in other family members. *J Biol Chem* 1999;274:4570–6.
127. Maymon E, Romero R, Pacora P, *et al.* A role for the 72 kDa gelatinase (MMP-2) and its inhibitor (TIMP-2) in human parturition, premature rupture of membranes and intraamniotic infection. *J Perinat Med* 2001;29:308–16.
128. Lei H, Furth EE, Kalluri R, *et al.* A program of cell death and extracellular matrix degradation is activated in the amnion before the onset of labor. *J Clin Invest* 1996;98:1971–8.
129. Fortunato SJ, Menon R, Bryant C, Lombardi SJ. Programmed cell death (apoptosis) as a possible pathway to metalloproteinase activation and fetal membrane degradation in premature rupture of membranes. *Am J Obstet Gynecol* 2000;182:1468–76.
130. Fortunato SJ, Menon R, Lombardi SJ. Support for an infection-induced apoptotic pathway in human fetal membranes. *Am J Obstet Gynecol* 2001;184:1392–7.
131. Lei H, Kalluri R, Furth EE, Baker AH, Strauss JF III. Rat amnion type IV collagen composition and metabolism: implications for membrane breakdown. *Biol Reprod* 1999;60:176–82.
132. McLaren J, Taylor DJ, Bell SC. Increased incidence of apoptosis in non-labour-affected cytotrophoblast cells in term fetal membranes overlying the cervix. *Hum Reprod* 1999;14:2895–900.
133. McLaren J, Taylor DJ, Bell SC. Increased concentration of pro-matrix metalloproteinase 9 in term fetal membranes overlying the cervix before labor: Implications for membrane remodeling and rupture. *Am J Obstet Gynecol* 2000;182:409–16.
134. Bell SC, McParland PC. Fetal membrane rupture. In Critchley H, Bennett P, Thornton S, eds. *Preterm Birth.* London: RCOG Press, 2004:195–212.
135. Clayton D, McKeigue PM. Epidemiological methods for studying genes and environmental factors in complex diseases. *Lancet* 2001;358:1356–60.
136. Tiret L. Gene-environment interaction: a central concept in multifactorial diseases. *Proc Nutr Soc* 2002;61:457–63.
137. Macones G, Parry S, Elkousy M, Clothier B, Ural SH, Strauss JF III. A polymorphism in the promoter region of TNF and bacterial vaginosis: Preliminary evidence of gene–environment interaction in the etiology of spontaneous preterm birth. *Am J Obstet Gynecol* 2004;190:1509–19.
138. US Preventive Services Task Force. Screening for bacterial vaginosis in pregnancy. Recommendations and rationale. *Am J Prev Med* 2001;20:59–61.
139. Sexually transmitted diseases treatment guidelines 2002. Centers for Disease Control and Prevention. *MMWR Recomm Rep* 2002;51:1–78.
140. Carey JC, Klebanoff MA, Hauth JC, *et al.* Metronidazole to prevent preterm delivery in pregnant women with asymptomatic bacterial vaginosis. National Institute of Child Health and Human Development Network of Maternal–Fetal Medicine Units. *N Engl J Med* 2000;342:534–40.
141. Guise JM, Mahon SM, Aickin M, Helfand M, Peipert JF, Westhoff C. Screening for bacterial vaginosis in pregnancy. *Am J Prev Med* 2001;20:62–72.
142. Hauth JC, Goldenberg RL, Andrews WW, DuBard MB, Copper RL. Reduced incidence of preterm delivery with metronidazole and erythromycin in women with bacterial vaginosis. *N Engl J Med* 1995;333:1732–6.

143. Klebanoff MA, Guise JM, Carey JC. Treatment recommendations for bacterial vaginosis in pregnant women. *Clin Infect Dis* 2003; 36:1630–1.
144. Koumans EH, Markowitz LE, Hogan V. Indications for therapy and treatment recommendations for bacterial vaginosis in nonpregnant and pregnant women: A synthesis of data. *Clin Infect Dis* 2002;35:S152–72.
145. Lamont RF. Infection in the prediction and antibiotics in the prevention of spontaneous preterm labour and preterm birth. *Br J Obstet Gynecol* 2003;110(Suppl 20):71–5.
146. Leitich H, Brunbauer M, Bodner-Adler B, Kaider A, Egarter C, Husslein P. Antibiotic treatment of bacterial vaginosis in pregnancy: A meta-analysis. *Am J Obstet Gynecol* 2003;188:752–8.
147. McDonald H, Brocklehurst P, Parsons J, Vigneswaran R. Antibiotics for treating bacterial vaginosis in pregnancy. *Cochrane Database Syst Rev* 2003;CD000262.
148. McDonald HM, O'Loughlin JA, Vigneswaran R, *et al.* Impact of metronidazole therapy on preterm birth in women with bacterial vaginosis flora (*Gardnerella vaginalis*): A randomised, placebo controlled trial. *Br J Obstet Gynaecol* 1997;104:1391–7.
149. McGregor JA, French JI, Parker R, *et al.* Prevention of premature birth by screening and treatment for common genital tract infections: results of a prospective controlled evaluation. *Am J Obstet Gynecol* 1995;173:157–67.
150. Morales WJ, Schorr S, Albritton J. Effect of metronidazole in patients with preterm birth in preceding pregnancy and bacterial vaginosis: A placebo-controlled, double-blind study. *Am J Obstet Gynecol* 1994;171:345–7.
151. Roberts AK, Monzon-Bordonaba F, Van Deerlin PG, *et al.* Association of polymorphism within the promoter of the tumor necrosis factor alpha gene with increased risk of preterm premature rupture of the fetal membranes. *Am J Obstet Gynecol* 1999;180:1297–302.
152. Romero R, Sepulveda W, Baumann P, *et al.* The preterm labor syndrome: Biochemical, cytologic, immunologic, pathologic, microbiologic, and clinical evidence that preterm labor is a heterogeneous disease. *Am J Obstet Gynecol* 1993;168:288.
153. Combs CA, Katz MA, Kitzmiller JL, Brescia RJ. Experimental preeclampsia produced by chronic constriction of the lower aorta: Validation with longitudinal blood pressure measurements in conscious rhesus monkeys. *Am J Obstet Gynecol* 1993;169: 215–23.
154. Arias F, Rodriquez L, Rayne SC, Kraus FT. Maternal placental vasculopathy and infection: Two distinct subgroups among patients with preterm labor and preterm ruptured membranes. *Am J Obstet Gynecol* 1993;168:585–91.
155. Arias F. Placental insufficiency: an important cause of preterm labor and preterm premature ruptured membranes. Presented at the 10th Annual meeting of the Society for Perinatal Obstetricians, Jan. 23-27, 1990, Houston, TX.
156. Gonen R, Hannah ME, Milligan JE. Does prolonged preterm premature rupture of the membranes predispose to abruptio placentae? *Obstet Gynecol* 1989;74:347–50.
157. Major C, Nageotte M, Lewis D. Preterm premature rupture of membranes and placental abruption: Is there an association between these pregnancy complications? *Am J Obstet Gynecol* 1991;164:381.
158. Moretti M, Sibai BM. Maternal and perinatal outcome of expectant management of premature rupture of membranes in the midtrimester. *Am J Obstet Gynecol* 1988;159:390–6.
159. Vintzileos AM, Campbell WA, Nochimson DJ, Weinbaum PJ. Preterm premature rupture of the membranes: A risk factor for the development of abruptio placentae. *Am J Obstet Gynecol* 1987;156:1235–8.
160. Kim YM, Bujold E, Chaiworapongsa T, *et al.* Failure of physiologic transformation of the spiral arteries in patients with preterm labor and intact membranes. *Am J Obstet Gynecol* 2003;189: 1063–9.
161. Kim YM, Chaiworapongsa T, Gomez R, *et al.* Failure of physiologic transformation of the spiral arteries in the placental bed in preterm premature rupture of membranes. *Am J Obstet Gynecol* 2002;187:1137–42.
162. Brar HS, Medearis AL, De Vore GR, Platt LD. Maternal and fetal blood flow velocity waveforms in patients with preterm labor: Relationship to outcome. *Am J Obstet Gynecol* 1989;161:1519–22.
163. Brar HS, Medearis AL, DeVore GR, Platt LD. Maternal and fetal blood flow velocity waveforms in patients with preterm labor: Prediction of successful tocolysis. *Am J Obstet Gynecol* 1988; 159:947–50.
164. Strigini FA, Lencioni G, De Luca G, Lombardo M, Bianchi F, Genazzani AR. Uterine artery velocimetry and spontaneous preterm delivery. *Obstet Gynecol* 1995;85:374–7.
165. McMaster-Fay RA. Failure of physiologic transformation of the spiral arteries of the uteroplacental circulation in patients with preterm labor and intact membranes. *Am J Obstet Gynecol* 2004; 191:1837–8.
166. Poisner AM. The human placental renin–angiotensin system. *Front Neuroendocrinol* 1998;19:232–52.
167. Woods LL, Brooks VL. Role of the renin–angiotensin system in hypertension during reduced uteroplacental perfusion pressure. *Am J Physiol* 1989;257:R204–9.
168. Katz M, Shapiro WB, Porush JG, Chou SY, Israel V. Uterine and renal renin release after ligation of the uterine arteries in the pregnant rabbit. *Am J Obstet Gynecol* 1980;136:676–8.
169. Lalanne C, Mironneau C, Mironneau J, Savineau JP. Contractions of rat uterine smooth muscle induced by acetylcholine and angiotensin II in Ca^{2+}-free medium. *Br J Pharmacol* 1984;81:317–26.
170. Campos GA, Guerra FA, Israel EJ. Angiotensin II induced release of prostaglandins from rat uterus. *Arch Biol Med Exp (Santiago)* 1983;16:43–9.
171. Lockwood CJ, Krikun G, Papp C, *et al.* The role of progestationally regulated stromal cell tissue factor and type-1 plasminogen activator inhibitor (PAI-1) in endometrial hemostasis and menstruation. *Ann N Y Acad Sci* 1994;734:57–79.
172. Elovitz MA, Saunders T, Ascher-Landsberg J, Phillippe M. Effects of thrombin on myometrial contractions in vitro and in vivo. *Am J Obstet Gynecol* 2000;183:799–804.
173. Rosen T, Schatz F, Kuczynski E, Lam H, Koo AB, Lockwood CJ. Thrombin-enhanced matrix metalloproteinase-1 expression: A mechanism linking placental abruption with premature rupture of the membranes. *J Matern Fetal Neonatal Med* 2002;11:11–7.
174. Lockwood CJ, Krikun G, Aigner S, Schatz F. Effects of thrombin on steroid-modulated cultured endometrial stromal cell fibrinolytic potential. *J Clin Endocrinol Metab* 1996;81:107–12.
175. Lijnen HR. Matrix metalloproteinases and cellular fibrinolytic activity. *Biochemistry (Moscow)* 2002;67:92–8.
176. Aplin JD, Campbell S, Allen TD. The extracellular matrix of human amniotic epithelium: Ultrastructure, composition and deposition. *J Cell Sci* 1985;79:119–36.
177. Chaiworapongsa T, Espinoza J, Yoshimatsu J, *et al.* Activation of coagulation system in preterm labor and preterm premature rupture of membranes. *J Matern Fetal Neonatal Med* 2002;11:368–73.
178. Gomez R, Athayde N, Pacora P, Mazor M, Yoon BH, Romero R. Increased thrombin in intrauterine inflammation. *Am J Obstet Gynecol* 1998;178:S62.
179. Rosen T, Kuczynski E, O'Neill LM, Funai EF, Lockwood CJ. Plasma levels of thrombin–antithrombin complexes predict preterm premature rupture of the fetal membranes. *J Matern Fetal Med* 2001;10:297–300.
180. Nagy S, Bush M, Stone J, Lapinski RH, Gardo S. Clinical significance of subchorionic and retroplacental hematomas detected in the first trimester of pregnancy. *Obstet Gynecol* 2003;102: 94–100.
181. Funderburk SJ, Guthrie D, Meldrum D. Outcome of pregnancies complicated by early vaginal bleeding. *Br J Obstet Gynaecol* 1980;87:100–5.
182. Weiss JL, Malone FD, Vidaver J, Ball RH, Nyberg DA, Comstock CH, Hankins GD, Berkowitz RL, Gross SJ, Dugoff L, Timor-Tritsch IE, D'Alton ME; FASTER Consortium. Threatened abortion: A risk factor for poor pregnancy outcome, a population-based screening study. *Am J Obstet Gynecol* 2004;190:745–50.
183. Signore CC, Sood AK, Richards DS. Second-trimester vaginal bleeding: Correlation of ultrasonographic findings with perinatal outcome. *Am J Obstet Gynecol* 1998;178:336–40.
184. Williams MA, Mittendorf R, Lieberman E, Monson RR. Adverse infant outcomes associated with first-trimester vaginal bleeding. *Obstet Gynecol* 1991;78:14–8.
185. Gomez R, Romero R, Ghezzi F, *et al.* Are fetal hypoxia and acidemia causes of preterm labor and delivery? *Am J Obstet Gynecol* 1997;176:S115.
186. Carroll SG, Papaioannou S, Nicolaides KH. Assessment of fetal activity and amniotic fluid volume in the prediction of intrauterine infection in preterm prelabor amniorrhexis. *Am J Obstet Gynecol* 1995;172:1427–35.
187. Besinger R, Carlson N. The physiology of preterm labor. In Keith L, Papiernik E, Keith D, Luke B, eds. *Multiple Pregnancy: Epidemiology, Gestation and Perinatal Outcome.* London: Parthenon Publishing, 1995:415.

188. Hill LM, Breckle R, Thomas ML, Fries JK. Polyhydramnios: ultracsonically detected prevalence and neonatal outcome. *Obstet Gynecol* 1987;69:21–5.
189. Ludmir J, Samuels P, Brooks S, Mennuti MT. Pregnancy outcome of patients with uncorrected uterine anomalies managed in a high-risk obstetric setting. *Obstet Gynecol* 1990;75:906–10.
190. Phelan JP, Park YW, Ahn MO, Rutherford SE. Polyhydramnios and perinatal outcome. *J Perinatol* 1990;10:347–50.
191. Weiner CP, Heilskov J, Pelzer G, Grant S, Wenstrom K, Williamson RA. Normal values for human umbilical venous and amniotic fluid pressures and their alteration by fetal disease. *Am J Obstet Gynecol* 1989;161:714–7.
192. Manabe Y, Sagawa N, Mori T. Fetal viability does not affect the onset of stretch-induced labor and the increase in amniotic fluid prostaglandin F2 alpha and plasma prostaglandin F2 alpha metabolite levels. *Prostaglandins* 1992;44:119–28.
193. Orhan A, Kurzel RB, Istwan NB, Rhea D, Burgess E, Stanziano G. The impact of hydramnios on pregnancy outcome in twin gestations. *J Perinatol* 2005;25:8–10.
194. Barany K, Rokolya A, Barany M. Stretch activates myosin light chain kinase in arterial smooth muscle. *Biochem Biophys Res Commun* 1990;173:164–71.
195. Farrugia G, Holm AN, Rich A, Sarr MG, Szurszewski JH, Rae JL. A mechanosensitive calcium channel in human intestinal smooth muscle cells. *Gastroenterology* 1999;117:900–5.
196. Fisk NM, Ronderos-Dumit D, Tannirandorn Y, Nicolini U, Talbert D, Rodeck CH. Normal amniotic pressure throughout gestation. *Br J Obstet Gynaecol* 1992;99:18–22.
197. Fuchs AR, Periyasamy S, Alexandrova M, Soloff MS. Correlation between oxytocin receptor concentration and responsiveness to oxytocin in pregnant rat myometrium: Effects of ovarian steroids. *Endocrinology* 1983;113:742–9.
198. Holm AN, Rich A, Sarr MG, Farrugia G. Whole cell current and membrane potential regulation by a human smooth muscle mechanosensitive calcium channel. *Am J Physiol Gastrointest Liver Physiol* 2000;279:G1155–61.
199. Hu Y, Bock G, Wick G, Xu Q. Activation of PDGF receptor alpha in vascular smooth muscle cells by mechanical stress. *FASEB J* 1998;12:1135–42.
200. Kloeck FK, Jung H. In vitro release of prostaglandins from the human myometrium under the influence of stretching. *Am J Obstet Gynecol* 1973;115:1066–9.
201. Laudanski T, Rocki W. The effects on stretching and prostaglandin F2alpha on the contractile and bioelectric activity of the uterus in rat. *Acta Physiol Pol* 1975;26:385–93.
202. Lee HS, Millward-Sadler SJ, Wright MO, Nuki G, Al Jamal R, Salter DM. Activation of Integrin-RACK1/PKCalpha signalling in human articular chondrocyte mechanotransduction. *Osteoarthritis Cartilage* 2002,10:890–7.
203. Li C, Xu Q. Mechanical stress-initiated signal transductions in vascular smooth muscle cells. *Cell Signal* 2000;12:435–45.
204. Mitchell JA, Lye SJ. Regulation of connexin43 expression by c-fos and c-jun in myometrial cells. *Cell Commun Adhes* 2001;8: 299–302.
205. Mitchell JA, Lye SJ. Differential expression of activator protein-1 transcription factors in pregnant rat myometrium. *Biol Reprod* 2002;67:240–6.
206. Oldenhof AD, Shynlova OP, Liu M, Langille BL, Lye SJ. Mitogen-activated protein kinases mediate stretch-induced c-fos mRNA expression in myometrial smooth muscle cells. *Am J Physiol Cell Physiol* 2002;283:C1530–9.
207. Ou CW, Chen ZQ, Qi S, Lye SJ. Increased expression of the rat myometrial oxytocin receptor messenger ribonucleic acid during labor requires both mechanical and hormonal signals. *Biol Reprod* 1998;59:1055–61.
208. Piersanti M, Lye SJ. Increase in messenger ribonucleic acid encoding the myometrial gap junction protein, connexin-43, requires protein synthesis and is associated with increased expression of the activator protein-1, c-fos. *Endocrinology* 1995;136: 3571–8.
209. Ravens U. Mechano-electric feedback and arrhythmias. *Prog Biophys Mol Biol* 2003;82:255–66.
210. Shynlova OP, Oldenhof AD, Liu M, Langille L, Lye SJ. Regulation of c-fos expression by static stretch in rat myometrial smooth muscle cells. *Am J Obstet Gynecol* 2002;186:1358–65.
211. Shyy JY, Chien S. Role of integrins in endothelial mechanosensing of shear stress. *Circ Res* 2002;91:769–75.
212. Sideris IG, Nicolaides KH. Amniotic fluid pressure during pregnancy. *Fetal Diagn Ther* 1990;5:104–8.
213. Sladek SM, Westerhausen-Larson A, Roberts JM. Endogenous nitric oxide suppresses rat myometrial connexin 43 gap junction protein expression during pregnancy. *Biol Reprod* 1999;61:8–13.
214. Speroff L, Glass RH, Kase NG. The endocrinology of pregnancy. In Mitchell C, ed. *Clinical Gynecologic Endocrinology and Infertility*. Baltimore, MD: Williams & Wilkins, 1994:251–90.
215. Steers WD, Broder SR, Persson K, *et al.* Mechanical stretch increases secretion of parathyroid hormone-related protein by cultured bladder smooth muscle cells. *J Urol* 1998;160:908–12.
216. Ticconi C, Lye SJ. Placenta and fetal membranes in human parturition and preterm delivery – a workshop report. *Placenta* 2002;23(Suppl A):S149–52.
217. Tzima E, del Pozo MA, Shattil SJ, Chien S, Schwartz MA. Activation of integrins in endothelial cells by fluid shear stress mediates Rho-dependent cytoskeletal alignment. *EMBO J* 2001;20:4639–47.
218. Watson PA, Hannan R, Carl LL, Giger KE. Contractile activity and passive stretch regulate tubulin mRNA and protein content in cardiac myocytes. *Am J Physiol* 1996;271:C684–9.
219. Wu WX, Ma XH, Yoshizato T, Shinozuka N, Nathanielsz PW. Differential expression of myometrial oxytocin receptor and prostaglandin H synthase 2, but not estrogen receptor alpha and heat shock protein 90 messenger ribonucleic acid in the gravid horn and nongravid horn in sheep during betamethasone-induced labor. *Endocrinology* 1999;140:5712–8.
220. Ou CW, Orsino A, Lye SJ. Expression of connexin-43 and connexin-26 in the rat myometrium during pregnancy and labor is differentially regulated by mechanical and hormonal signals. *Endocrinology* 1997;138:5398–407.
221. Lye SJ, Mitchell J, Nashman N, *et al.* Role of mechanical signals in the onset of term and preterm labor. *Front Horm Res* 2001;27:165–78.
222. Barclay CG, Brennand JE, Kelly RW, Calder AA. Interleukin-8 production by the human cervix. *Am J Obstet Gynecol* 1993;169:625–32.
223. Calder AA. Prostaglandins and biological control of cervical function. *Aust N Z J Obstet Gynaecol* 1994;34:347–51.
224. Chwalisz K, Benson M, Scholz P, Daum J, Beier HM, Hegele-Hartung C. Cervical ripening with the cytokines interleukin 8, interleukin 1 beta and tumour necrosis factor alpha in guinea-pigs. *Hum Reprod* 1994;9:2173–81.
225. Denison FC, Calder AA, Kelly RW. The action of prostaglandin E2 on the human cervix: Stimulation of interleukin 8 and inhibition of secretory leukocyte protease inhibitor. *Am J Obstet Gynecol* 1999;180:614–20.
226. el Maradny E, Kanayama N, Halim A, Maehara K, Sumimoto K, Terao T. Interleukin-8 induces cervical ripening in rabbits. *Am J Obstet Gynecol* 1994;171:77–83.
227. Kanayama N, Fukamizu H. Mechanical stretching increases prostaglandin E2 in cultured human amnion cells. *Gynecol Obstet Invest* 1989;28:123–6.
228. Maehara K, Kanayama N, Maradny EE, Uezato T, Fujita M, Terao T. Mechanical stretching induces interleukin-8 gene expression in fetal membranes: A possible role for the initiation of human parturition. *Eur J Obstet Gynecol Reprod Biol* 1996;70:191–6.
229. Mazor M, Hershkovitz R, Ghezzi F, Maymon E, Horowitz S, Leiberman JR. Intraamniotic infection in patients with preterm labor and twin pregnancies. *Acta Obstet Gynecol Scand* 1996; 75:624–7.
230. Millar LK, Stollberg J, DeBuque L, Bryant-Greenwood G. Fetal membrane distention: Determination of the intrauterine surface area and distention of the fetal membranes preterm and at term. *Am J Obstet Gynecol* 2000;182:128–34.
231. Nemeth E, Tashima LS, Yu Z, Bryant-Greenwood GD. Fetal membrane distention: I. Differentially expressed genes regulated by acute distention in amniotic epithelial (WISH) cells. *Am J Obstet Gynecol* 2000;182:50–9.
232. Nemeth E, Millar LK, Bryant-Greenwood G. Fetal membrane distention: II. Differentially expressed genes regulated by acute distention in vitro. *Am J Obstet Gynecol* 2000;182:60–7.
233. Rajabi M, Solomon S, Poole AR. Hormonal regulation of interstitial collagenase in the uterine cervix of the pregnant guinea pig. *Endocrinology* 1991;128:863–71.
234. Sennstrom MK, Brauner A, Lu Y, Granstrom LM, Malmstrom AL, Ekman GE. Interleukin-8 is a mediator of the final cervical ripening in humans. *Eur J Obstet Gynecol Reprod Biol* 1997;74;89–92.
235. Stjernholm YM, Sahlin L, Eriksson HA, Bystrom BE, Stenlund PM, Ekman GE. Cervical ripening after treatment with prostaglandin E2 or antiprogestin (RU486). Possible mechanisms in relation to gonadal steroids. *Eur J Obstet Gynecol Reprod Biol* 1999;84; 83–8.

236. Yoon BH, Park KH, Koo JN, *et al.* Intra-amniotic infection of twin pregnancies with preterm labor. *Am J Obstet Gynecol* 1997; 176:535.
237. Maradny EE, Kanayama N, Halim A, Maehara K, Terao T. Stretching of fetal membranes increases the concentration of interleukin-8 and collagenase activity. *Am J Obstet Gynecol* 1996; 174:843–9.
238. Aksel S. Immunologic aspects of reproductive diseases. *J Am Med Assoc* 1992;268:2930–4.
239. Kilpatrick DC. Immune mechanisms and pre-eclampsia. *Lancet* 1987;2:1460–1.
240. McLean JM. Early embryo loss. *Lancet* 1987;1:1033–4.
241. Benirschke K, Kaufmann P. Villitis of unknown etiology. In Benirschke K, Kaufmann P, eds. *Pathology of the Human Placenta.* New York: Springer-Verlag, 1995:596.
242. Soulillou JP, Peyronnet P, Le Mauff B, *et al.* Prevention of rejection of kidney transplants by monoclonal antibody directed against interleukin 2. *Lancet* 1987;1:1339–42.
243. Loke YW, King A. Immunology of human implantation: An evolutionary perspective. *Hum Reprod* 1996;11:283–6.
244. Cunningham DS, Tichenor JR Jr. Decay-accelerating factor protects human trophoblast from complement-mediated attack. *Clin Immunol Immunopathol* 1995;74:156–61.
245. Girardi G, Berman J, Redecha P, *et al.* Complement C5a receptors and neutrophils mediate fetal injury in the antiphospholipid syndrome. *J Clin Invest* 2003;112:1644–54.
246. Gonzalez NC, Chairez JA, Cueto SM. Immunology of the fetal–maternal relationship. *Rev Alerg Mex* 1996;43:18–22.
247. Hagmann M. Embryos attacked by mom's natural defenses. *Science* 2000;287:408.
248. Holmes CH, Simpson KL, Okada H, *et al.* Complement regulatory proteins at the feto-maternal interface during human placental development: Distribution of CD59 by comparison with membrane cofactor protein (CD46) and decay accelerating factor (CD55). *Eur J Immunol* 1992;22:1579–85.
249. Holmes CH, Simpson KL. Complement and pregnancy: New insights into the immunobiology of the fetomaternal relationship. *Baillieres Clin Obstet Gynaecol* 1992;6:439–60.
250. Nishikori K, Noma J, Hirakawa S, Amano T, Kudo T. The change of membrane complement regulatory protein in chorion of early pregnancy. *Clin Immunol Immunopathol* 1993;69:167–74.
251. Pham TQ, Goluszko P, Popov V, Nowicki S, Nowicki BJ. Molecular cloning and characterization of Dr-II, a nonfimbrial adhesin-I-like adhesin isolated from gestational pyelonephritis-associated *Escherichia coli* that binds to decay-accelerating factor. *Infect Immun* 1997;65:4309–18.
252. Simpson KL, Jones A, Norman S, Holmes CH. Expression of the complement regulatory proteins decay accelerating factor (DAF, CD55), membrane cofactor protein (MCP, CD46) and CD59 in the normal human uterine cervix and in premalignant and malignant cervical disease. *Am J Pathol* 1997;151:1455–67.
253. Vanderpuye OA, Labarrere CA, McIntyre JA. The complement system in human reproduction. *Am J Reprod Immunol* 1992;27: 145–55.
254. Xu C, Mao D, Holers VM, Palanca B, Cheng AM, Molina H. A critical role for murine complement regulator crry in fetomaternal tolerance. *Science* 2000;287:498–501.
255. Corry DB, Kheradmand F. Induction and regulation of the IgE response. *Nature* 1999;402:B18–23.
256. Holgate ST. The epidemic of allergy and asthma. *Nature* 1999; 402:B2–4.
257. Romero R, Mazor M, Avila C, *et al.* Uterine "allergy": A novel mechanism for preterm labor. *Am J Obstet Gynecol* 1991;164:375.
258. Bulmer JN, Pace D, Ritson A. Immunoregulatory cells in human decidua: Morphology, immunohistochemistry and function. *Reprod Nutr Dev* 1988;28:1599–613.
259. Bytautiene E, Vedernikov YP, Saade GR, Romero R, Garfield RE. Endogenous mast cell degranulation modulates cervical contractility in the guinea pig. *Am J Obstet Gynecol* 2002;186:438–45.
260. Bytautiene E, Romero R, Vedernikov YP, El-Zeky F, Saade GR, Garfield RE. Induction of premature labor and delivery by allergic reaction and prevention by histamine H1 receptor antagonist. *Am J Obstet Gynecol* 2004;191(4):1356–61.
261. Garfield RE, Bytautiene E, Vedernikov YP, Marshall JS, Romero R. Modulation of rat uterine contractility by mast cells and their mediators. *Am J Obstet Gynecol* 2000;183:118–25.
262. Holloway JA, Warner JO, Vance GH, Diaper ND, Warner JA, Jones CA. Detection of house-dust-mite allergen in amniotic fluid and umbilical-cord blood. *Lancet* 2000;356:1900–2.
263. Jones AC, Miles EA, Warner JO, Colwell BM, Bryant TN, Warner JA. Fetal peripheral blood mononuclear cell proliferative responses to mitogenic and allergenic stimuli during gestation. *Pediatr Allergy Immunol* 1996;7:109–16.
264. Kammerer U, Schoppet M, McLellan AD, *et al.* Human decidua contains potent immunostimulatory CD83(+) dendritic cells. *Am J Pathol* 2000;157:159–69.
265. Lachapelle MH, Miron P, Hemmings R, Roy DC. Endometrial T, B, and NK cells in patients with recurrent spontaneous abortion. Altered profile and pregnancy outcome. *J Immunol* 1996;156: 4027–34.
266. Padilla L, Reinicke K, Montesino H, *et al.* Histamine content and mast cells distribution in mouse uterus: The effect of sexual hormones, gestation and labor. *Cell Mol Biol* 1990;36:93–100.
267. Rudolph MI, Bardisa L, Cruz MA, Reinicke K. Mast cells mediators evoke contractility and potentiate each other in mouse uterine horns. *Gen Pharmacol* 1992;23:833–6.
268. Rudolph MI, Reinicke K, Cruz MA, Gallardo V, Gonzalez C, Bardisa L. Distribution of mast cells and the effect of their mediators on contractility in human myometrium. *Br J Obstet Gynaecol* 1993;100:1125–30.
269. Shingai Y, Nakagawa K, Kato T, *et al.* Severe allergy in a pregnant woman after vaginal examination with a latex glove. *Gynecol Obstet Invest* 2002;54:183–4.
270. Iams JD, Johnson FF, Sonek J, Sachs L, Gebauer C, Samuels P. Cervical competence as a continuum: a study of ultrasonographic cervical length and obstetric performance. *Am J Obstet Gynecol* 1995;172:1097–103.
271. Romero R, Mazor M, Gomez R. Cervix, incompetence and premature labor. *Fetus* 1993;3:1.
272. Romero R, Espinoza J, Erez O, Hassan S. The role of cervical cerclage in obstetric practice: Can the patient who could benefit from this procedure be identified? *Am J Obstet Gynecol* 2006;194:1–9.
273. Balasch J, Vanrell JA, Marquez M, Rivera F, Gonzalez-Merlo J. Luteal phase in infertility: Problems of evaluation. *Int J Fertil* 1982;27:60–2.
274. Annos T, Thompson IE, Taymor ML. Luteal phase deficiency and infertility: Difficulties encountered in diagnosis and treatment. *Obstet Gynecol* 1980;55:705–10.
275. Stephenson MD. Frequency of factors associated with habitual abortion in 197 couples. *Fertil Steril* 1996;66:24–9.
276. Daya S. Issues in the etiology of recurrent spontaneous abortion. *Curr Opin Obstet Gynecol* 1994;6:153–9.
277. Jones GS. Luteal phase defect: A review of pathophysiology. *Curr Opin Obstet Gynecol* 1991;3:641–8.
278. Jones GS. The luteal phase defect. *Fertil Steril* 1976;27:351–6.
279. Balasch J, Fabregues F, Creus M, Vanrell JA. The usefulness of endometrial biopsy for luteal phase evaluation in infertility. *Hum Reprod* 1992;7:973–7.
280. Balasch J, Vanrell JA. Corpus luteum insufficiency and fertility: A matter of controversy. *Hum Reprod* 1987;2:557–67.
281. Check JH, Lee G, Epstein R, Vetter B. Increased rate of preterm deliveries in untreated women with luteal phase deficiencies. Preliminary report. *Gynecol Obstet Invest* 1992;33:183–4.
282. McNeely MJ, Soules MR. The diagnosis of luteal phase deficiency: A critical review. *Fertil Steril* 1988;50:1–15.
283. Daya S, Ward S, Burrows E. Progesterone profiles in luteal phase defect cycles and outcome of progesterone treatment in patients with recurrent spontaneous abortion. *Am J Obstet Gynecol* 1988; 158:225–32.
284. Wentz AC, Herbert CM, Maxson WS, Garner CH. Outcome of progesterone treatment of luteal phase inadequacy. *Fertil Steril* 1984;41:856–62.
285. Check JH, Chase JS, Wu CH, Adelson HG, Teichman M, Rankin A. The efficacy of progesterone in achieving successful pregnancy: I. Prophylactic use during luteal phase in anovulatory women. *Int J Fertil* 1987;32:135–8.
286. Rosenberg SM, Luciano AA, Riddick DH. The luteal phase defect: The relative frequency of, and encouraging response to, treatment with vaginal progesterone. *Fertil Steril* 1980;34:17–20.
287. Balasch J, Vanrell JA, Marquez M, Burzaco I, Gonzalez-Merlo J. Dehydrogesterone versus vaginal progesterone in the treatment of the endometrial luteal phase deficiency. *Fertil Steril* 1982;37:751–4.
288. Karamardian LM, Grimes DA. Luteal phase deficiency: Effect of treatment on pregnancy rates. *Am J Obstet Gynecol* 1992;167: 1391–8.
289. Daya S. Efficacy of progesterone support in the luteal phase following in-vitro fertilization and embryo transfer: meta-analysis of clinical trials. *Hum Reprod* 1988;3:731–4.

290. Pritts EA, Atwood AK. Luteal phase support in infertility treatment: a meta-analysis of the randomized trials. *Hum Reprod* 2002; 17:2287–99.
291. Fidel PI Jr, Romero R, Maymon E, Hertelendy F. Bacteria-induced or bacterial product-induced preterm parturition in mice and rabbits is preceded by a significant fall in serum progesterone concentrations. *J Matern Fetal Med* 1998;7:222–6.
292. Hirsch E, Muhle R. Intrauterine bacterial inoculation induces labor in the mouse by mechanisms other than progesterone withdrawal. *Biol Reprod* 2002;67:1337–41.
293. Yoon BH, Romero R, Jun JK, *et al.* An increase in fetal plasma cortisol but not dehydroepiandrosterone sulfate is followed by the onset of preterm labor in patients with preterm premature rupture of the membranes. *Am J Obstet Gynecol* 1998;179:1107–14.
294. Dudley DJ. Immunoendocrinology of preterm labor: the link between corticotropin-releasing hormone and inflammation. *Am J Obstet Gynecol* 1999;180:S251–6.
295. Keelan JA, Blumenstein M, Helliwell RJ, Sato TA, Marvin KW, Mitchell MD. Cytokines, prostaglandins and parturition – A review. *Placenta* 2003;24(Suppl A):S33–46.
296. Dudley DJ, Collmer D, Mitchell MD, Trautman MS. Inflammatory cytokine mRNA in human gestational tissues: Implications for term and preterm labor. *J Soc Gynecol Investig* 1996;3:328–35.
297. Menon R, Swan KF, Lyden TW, Rote NS, Fortunato SJ. Expression of inflammatory cytokines (interleukin-1 beta and interleukin-6) in amniochorionic membranes. *Am J Obstet Gynecol* 1995;172: 493–500.
298. Fortunato SJ, Menon R, Swan KF. Expression of TNF-alpha and TNFR p55 in cultured amniochorion. *Am J Reprod Immunol* 1994;32:188–93.
299. Sehringer B, Schafer WR, Wetzka B, *et al.* Formation of proinflammatory cytokines in human term myometrium is stimulated by lipopolysaccharide but not by corticotropin-releasing hormone. *J Clin Endocrinol Metab* 2000;85:4859–65.
300. Elliott CL, Slater DM, Dennes W, Poston L, Bennett PR. Interleukin 8 expression in human myometrium: Changes in relation to labor onset and with gestational age. *Am J Reprod Immunol* 2000;43:272–7.
301. Rauk PN, Chiao JP. Interleukin-1 stimulates human uterine prostaglandin production through induction of cyclooxygenase-2 expression. *Am J Reprod Immunol* 2000;43:152–9.
302. Todd HM, Dundoo VL, Gerber WR, Cwiak CA, Baldassare JJ, Hertelendy F. Effect of cytokines on prostaglandin E2 and prostacyclin production in primary cultures of human myometrial cells. *J Matern Fetal Med* 1996;5:161–7.
303. Belt AR, Baldassare JJ, Molnar M, Romero R, Hertelendy F. The nuclear transcription factor NF-kappa B mediates interleukin-1beta-induced expression of cyclooxygenase-2 in human myometrial cells. *Am J Obstet Gynecol* 1999;181:359–66.
304. Lappas M, Permezel M, Georgiou HM, Rice GE. Nuclear factor kappa B regulation of proinflammatory cytokines in human gestational tissues in vitro. *Biol Reprod* 2002;67:668–73.
305. Yan X, Sun M, Gibb W. Localization of nuclear factor-kappa B (NF kappa B) and inhibitory factor-kappa B (I kappa B) in human fetal membranes and decidua at term and preterm delivery. *Placenta* 2002;23:288–93.
306. Allport VC, Pieber D, Slater DM, Newton R, White JO, Bennett PR. Human labour is associated with nuclear factor-kappa B activity which mediates cyclo-oxygenase-2 expression and is involved with the 'functional progesterone withdrawal'. *Mol Hum Reprod* 2001;7:581–6.

The concepts described in this chapter, as well as some of the text, were originally published in the book *Preterm Birth*, published by the Royal College of Obstetricians and Gynaecologists in the United Kingdom (Edited by Professor Hilary Critchley, Professor Phillip Bennett and Professor Steven Thornton and published by the RCOG Press). That work, as well as the present work, has been produced by U.S. Government appointees and, therefore, is not subject to copyright. The editors, as well as the publisher, have been informed and agreed with this course of action and their position is gratefully acknowledged.

130 Management of preterm labor: pharmacological and non-pharmacological aspects

G. C. Di Renzo, A. Cutuli, L. Liotta, L. Burnelli and G. Luzi

Introduction

Tocolysis is the first therapeutic tool for treatment of threatened preterm labor allowing timely administration of corticosteroids, to induce lung maturation, and antibiotics when appropriate. However, before starting with tocolysis, careful diagnosis is needed, so as to detect manageable conditions and fetal and/or maternal contraindications. For pregnant woman with threatened preterm labor, bed rest is advisable, as well as monitoring by cardiotocography. If membranes are intact, cervical condition must be evaluated by means of digital and/or preferably sonography examinations. Relative and absolute contraindications related to tocolysis therapy are listed in Table 130.1.

As most contraindications are relative, tocolysis is preferable to the high risk of perinatal mortality or morbidity. Maternal medical conditions, such as diabetes mellitus, could be negatively influenced by administration of tocolytic agents like β-mimetics. Minor vaginal bleeding or spotting is often associated with preterm labor and cervical changes, but could be also due to abruptio placentae. If the cervix is dilated above 4–5 cm, tocolytic treatment can hardly be successful. If the pregnancy is between 22 and 26 weeks, prolongation of pregnancy by 1–2 weeks could positively affect the perinatal outcome, especially in multiple pregnancy.

Pharmacological treatment of preterm labor

The use of mild sedatives is sometimes advisable to reduce anxiety and fear. Bed rest and hydration do not have any significant effect on uterine contractions. Nevertheless, bed rest is usually recommended in the management of a patient with threatened preterm labor.

Tocolytic drugs currently used are:

(1) Magnesium sulfate
(2) Inhibitors of prostaglandin synthesis
(3) Calcium antagonists
(4) β-sympathomimetics
(5) Oxytocins antagonists
(6) Nitric oxide donors.

Magnesium sulfate

Magnesium sulfate has been widely used for the treatment of pre-eclampsia and as a tocolytic agent only over the last 20 years. Its inhibitory activity on the

Table 130.1 Absolute and relative contraindications to tocolysis

Absolute contraindications	Relative contraindications
Pregnancy induced hypertension	Mild chronic hypertension
Severe bleeding	Placenta previa
Chorioamnionitis	Maternal cardiac diseases
Fetal death	Hyperthyroidism
Fetal lethal anomalies	Uncontrolled diabetes mellitus
Severe IUGR	Fetal distress
	Fetal anomalies
	Mild IUGR
	Cervical dilation > 5 cm

smooth muscle is well known, but its mechanisms of action are still unexplored. A high concentration of magnesium has a central inhibitory effect, interfering with acetylcoline release and then with nervous conduction. Magnesium also suppresses the contractile activity of isolated myometrium. Furthermore, magnesium increases cyclic adenosine monophosphate and decreases intracellular calcium.

Myometrial contractility is inhibited by maternal serum levels of magnesium of 5–8 mg/dl. Concentrations of 9–13 mg/dl may provoke deep tendineal reflex and a level above 14 mg/dl may cause respiratory depression. Magnesium is excreted mainly by the kidneys, with at least 75% of the infused dose excreted during infusion and 90% during the subsequent 24 h. In two randomized and controlled studies, there were no advantages in using magnesium sulfate vs. placebo. A recent meta-analysis suggests that magnesium offers the slight advantage of delaying the time of delivery without affecting the newborn.

More than 45% of patients, especially during intravenous treatment, have hot flushes, headaches, nistagmus and lethargy. More than 75% of patients suffer from hypovisus or diplopy. Furthermore, a reduction of memory has been reported. Some cases have been published of transitory ischemia, maternal hypothermy, osteoporosis with spontaneous fractures from therapy over 60 days and neuromuscular block due to association with nifedipine.

In the presence of renal hypofunction, even a mild hypermagnesemia can lead to respiratory and cardiac dysfunction. Magnesium in patients with myasthenia gravis must be carefully administered. After infusion of magnesium, serum calcium decreases and is abundantly excreted by the urine. It also increases serum phosphorus and parathyroid hormone. These changes may involve a decrease of bone density during the first week after delivery, in case of prolonged magnesium therapy.

A study of 1000 patients treated with magnesium and terbutaline showed a relative low incidence of side effects. Other studies have demonstrated an increase in maternal side effects with combined use of ritodrine and magnesium.

In neonates with magnesium concentration ranging between 4 and 11 mg/dl in umbilical cord vessels, motor and respiratory depression has been noticed. In the newborns of mothers who underwent magnesium sulfate therapy with serum levels of 4–7 mg/dl, decrease of muscular tone and lethargy have been reported.

For plasmatic concentrations of 6–8 mg/dl per 24 h, 50% of fetuses show an unreactive cardiotocograph tracing and only 20% of breathing movements interfering with biophysical profile interpretation. The recommended starting dose is 4–6 g, administered intravenously for more than 20 min, followed by a maintenance dose of 1–4 g/h. The endovenous therapy must be continued for about 12 h, until the reduction of uterine contractions below four to six per hour has been reached.

As treatment with magnesium may lead to pulmonary edema, strict observation of intake and out-take is needed, daily decreasing the administration of fluids below 1500–2500 ml. It is recommended that constant examination of tendineal reflex and calcium and magnesium serum levels be done so as to avoid toxic effects. In case of toxic effects caused by hypermagnesemia, calcium gluconate should be promptly administered.

Inhibitors of prostaglandin synthesis

Several drugs such as indometacin, naproxen, ketoprofen and diclofenac interfere with the synthesis of prostaglandins, inhibiting both cyclooxygenases (COX), which catalyze the conversion of arachidonic acid into prostaglandins G, precursors of prostaglandins E and F.

Indometacin is a generic inhibitor of COX, after absorption by oral or rectal administration, which achieves the plasmatic peak in 1–2 h. The half-life is about 5 h. This drug binds largely to plasmatic proteins and is eliminated unmodified. Indometacin crosses the placenta and the concentration in the umbilical artery is similar to the maternal one 5 h after administration. In comparison with aspirin, indometacin binds reversibly to COX, having an inhibiting effect while the drug is in circulation. The half-life in the newborn is about 15 h. In the neonates, 90% of the drug binds to the proteins.

Several studies have shown tocolytic effects of this inhibitor of prostaglandin synthesis comparable to β-sympathomimetics and fewer maternal side effects. Tocolysis by indometacin may double the maternal bleeding time, although it does not influence the prothrombin levels or activate thromboplastin partial time. Prolonged administration may be associated with headache, dizziness and depression.

The inhibition of contractions by prostaglandin inhibitor synthesis can cause closure of the ductus arteriosus, neonatal pulmonary hypertension, ventricular hemorrhage and oligohydramnios, especially if the drug is administered after 30 weeks of pregnancy.

Studies on animals have shown that COX-1 is mainly responsible for patent ductus arteriosus. Indometacin inhibits both enzymes COX-1 and COX-2 and rapidly crosses the placenta. Serial fetal echocardiography has demonstrated that antenatal administration of indometacin may cause a narrowing of the ductus arteriosus, which can resolve within 24 h of drug interruption.

In other studies, of 53 fetuses exposed to indometacin, the narrowing of ductus appeared in 61% at 31–34 weeks, in 43% at 27–30 weeks and in none before 27 weeks. These findings suggest that limiting the use of indometacin to within 32 weeks of gestation and, furthermore, fetal echocardiography could help evaluate the narrowing of the ductus arteriosus in case of indometacin treatment for more than 48–72 h.

The etiology of neonatal primitive pulmonary hypertension could be the prolonged deviation of blood from the ductus arteriosus to the pulmonary vascular bed, probably with treatment lasting more than 48 h. Furthermore, antenatal exposure to indometacin seems to be associated with postnatal patent ductus arteriosus, and is refractory to medical therapy.

Fetal exposure to indometacin is correlated to a high incidence of intraventricular hemorrhage, when it is used after failure of other therapies or in combination with magnesium sulfate. Some authors did not confirm the increased risk of intraventricular hemorrhage associated with the use of indometacin. Indometacin can increase the risk of necrotizing enterocolitis. Its use in the last 5 weeks of pregnancy is associated with anuria, microcystic kidney lesions and increased neonatal mortality.

Treatment with indometacin is also associated with oligohydramnios due to decreased fetal urinary production. This effect is reversible with the interruption of the drug treatment. For this reason, some cases of polyhydramnios can be treated with indometacin.

Most studies used indometacin 50 or 100 mg suppository; alternatively, they used 50 mg per os, followed by 25–50 mg per os every 6 h, depending on the therapeutic effects. Tocolysis by indometacin must be limited for women before 32 weeks, without intrauterine growth restriction (IUGR) and normal amniotic fluid volume. The duration of administration should not exceed 48–72 h.

Calcium antagonists

Calcium antagonists are considered as tocolytic agents because of their important role in blocking cytoplasmatic free ion calcium into smooth muscular contractility. Nifedipine acts by inhibiting calcium passage through the plasmatic membrane, particularly interfering with voltage-dependent ion channels. Nifedipine reaches a plasmatic peak 30–60 min after oral administration, and more quickly by sublingual administration. The half-time is 1–2 h and it is excreted through the renal and intestinal system. The calcium channel block is reversible with interruption of therapy. Nifedipine crosses the placenta, yet its kinetics are not completely known.

In an observational study, nifedipine has been proved to abolish uterine activity and prevent delivery for 3 days in a significant percentage of cases vs. placebo. Some studies have demonstrated that nifedipine has a similar or better effect than ritodrine in the suppression of contraction and in delaying delivery for at least 48 h.

This substance causes vasodilation. Frequently, hyperemia is associated with headache and nausea, as well as transitory tachycardia and mild reduction of blood pressure. Occasionally, a significant hypotension may occur. The use of nifedipine in combination with magnesium may cause neuromuscular toxicity. In monkeys, after the administration of nifedipine, there may be a severe reduction of oxygen in the fetal circulation and a decrease of pH, probably due to a reduction of uterine blood flow.

Doppler investigations of pregnant women treated with nifedipine have shown changes in uteroplacental fetal circulation, with an increase of fetal cerebral flow, but no alteration in other districts.

The first dose is usually 10 mg of nifedipine per os, to be repeated after 20 min if the contractions persist. Sublingual administration must be avoided in patients at risk of hypotension. Oral therapy is to be carried out for 10–20 mg every 4–6 h. The duration of therapy has not been established.

β-sympathomimetics

Substances like ixosuprine, exoprenaline, fenoterol, ritodrine, salbutamol and terbutaline belong to this family. They have a $\beta 2$-adrenergic effect at the uterine level. Nevertheless, these drugs have a partial $\beta 1$-adrenergic activity. Their action is mediated by cyclic adenosine monophosphate, which inhibits the kinase of light chain of myosin, thus avoiding myometrial cell contraction. Most of these drugs are excreted unmodified or conjugated. Ritodrine and terbutaline cross the placenta, but fenoterol and exoprenaline cross the placenta in a lower concentration.

The maternal serum concentration of ritodrine rises with the increasing infusion dose, but it can vary more than 100% among patients at low doses. The half-time of ritodrine is about 2 h and about 3–4 h for terbutaline. Myometrial β-receptors decrease in the pregnant uterus treated with β-sympathomimetics. In sheep, continued exposure to β-adrenergic stimulation leads to a reduction of inhibition of the contractility induced by oxytocin, whereas intermittent administration of ritodrine does not show any changes in β-adrenergic receptor or adenyl cyclase activity, and maintains the inhibition of contractility induced by oxytocin.

There is no strong evidence about the better effect of one drug vs. another; these substances may delay delivery by 3–7 days, but the efficacy in decreasing preterm morbidity and the advantages for the newborn are still a matter of controversy. Oral administration is not useful, both for a long and for a short period, and meta-analysis does not show any advantage regarding the prevention of preterm delivery, the period of time until delivery as well as the recurrence of preterm delivery. Although these substances have a maximum effect on the uterus and a minimal effect at the extrauterine level, they may significantly influence the maternal cardiovascular physiology and metabolic system. Table 130.2 lists the changes in some maternal systems due to β-sympathomimetic administration.

Some effects are slight, but others may be dangerous for maternal life. The most important side effects are hypotension, cardiac arrhythmia, myocardial ischemia and pulmonary edema. The incidence in treated women is about 0.3–5%. Intravenous administration of ritodrine is associated with palpitations in about 30% of patients, hot flushes in 10–15% and

Table 130.2 β-Sympathomimetics responses of different body systems

Heart	↑Contractility
	↑Ejection volume
Smooth muscle	↓Vascular tone
	↓Uterine activity
	↓Bronchiolar tone
Bowel	↓Motility
Kidney	↑Renin
	↓Urinary output
Metabolism	↑Lipolysis
	↑Intracellular K^+
	↑Glucogenolysis
	↑Insulin release

chest pain in 8%. In 7–10% of patients, the therapy has to be interrupted. Maternal death has been observed in case of heart disease or unknown myocarditis.

The most frequent and severe effect is pulmonary edema. This complication rapidly regresses by interrupting the therapy and administrating diuretics. Predicting factors are twin pregnancies (about 50% of observed cases), persistent heart frequency higher than 130 bpm, anemia below 9 g/dl, maternal infection and iatrogenic fluid overload.

β-sympathomimetics stimulate the renin–aldosterone system, decrease urinary output and colloidal pressure by about 20% after 24 h of infusion. All these factors lead to an increase in fluids, especially if colloidal pressure decreases below 15 mmHg. Most cases of pulmonary edema have been reported 30–60 h after the beginning of treatment.

It has been reported that the incidence of pulmonary edema in patients treated with β-sympathomimetics and corticosteroids is similar to the incidence in patients treated only with corticosteroids. β-sympathomimetics increase glucogenolysis and maternal glycemia for 3–24 h from the beginning of therapy. In patients affected by insulin-dependent diabetes, there is an increased risk of ketoacidosis. Subsequent to hyperglycemia hypokalemia develops, although all parameters return to the normal range in 24–48 h. During treatment, nausea, vomiting, insomnia and agitation have often been reported, and also rarely paralytic ileus and dermatitis.

A low dose of infusion is not related to major changes in the fetal heart rate, whereas a high dose can provoke fetal tachycardia and reduction of variability. In a retrospective study on newborns from mothers delivering within 48 h of treatment with ixosuprine, it has been observed that the newborns may develop hypoglycemia, hypocalcemia, ileus and hypertension.

The incidence of intraventricular and periventricular hemorrhage is increased, according to two studies, in newborns exposed to β-sympathomimetics.

The follow-up of babies exposed to β-sympathomimetics in the uterus shows normal growth and development in the second year, with no alterations in anthropometric measurements, neurological tests and behavior in the sixth year. β-sympathomimetics may be administered intravenously, intramuscularly, subcutaneously or orally. The treatment with ritodrine or terbutaline can be started intravenously, using an infusion pump, intramuscularly with ritodrine or subcutaneously with terbutaline. Before treatment, the fluid balance needs to be recorded and fluid intake between 1500 and 2500 ml is recommended.

Initially, 0.005–0.10 mg/min of ritodrine is administered intravenously, with an increase of 0.05 mg/min every 10–30 min, up to a maximal dose of 0.350 mg/min. Terbutaline can also be administered endovenously, starting with 0.01 mg/min and increasing by 0.01 mg/min every 10–30 min, up to 0.08 mg/min. The infusion dose is adjusted according to the uterine activity or by considering the maternal side effects. However, the infusion must not cause an increase of maternal heart rate over 130 bpm or a decrease of blood pressure below 80–90 mmHg.

Some physicians continue infusion for 6–24 h after tocolysis, while others recommend a slow decrease to the lower tocolytic dose, protracting it for over 12 h.

Oxytocin antagonists

For several years research has been focused on molecules for specific uterine receptors, avoiding the influence on other tissues. Oxytocin antagonists tend to inhibit oxytocin receptors, inducing uterine contraction in human and animal models. Oxytocin antagonists inhibit the double oxytocin effect on myometrium, which activates channels and indirectly stimulates prostaglandin production by decidual and fetal membranes. The only commercially available oxytocin antagonist is atosiban, analog to oxytocin, which is able to block myometrium and decidual receptors of oxytocin competing specifically with the substance. It is a synthetic peptide characterized by fast action and dose-dependent effect. This was the first oxytocin antagonist used in clinical practice.

Atosiban is able to delay preterm delivery. It has a uterus-specific action and it is therefore safer than other tocolytics. Some studies show an affinity of atosiban for vasopressin receptors, but this is not a clinical problem, since during labor the oxytocin uterine receptors are more numerous than vasopressin receptors.

Therapeutic indications are:

(1) Gestational age at 24–33 weeks,
(2) Presence of four or more regular contractions for 30 min, lasting at least 30 s,

(3) Cervical dilation of 1–3 cm (0–3 for nulliparous) and cervical shortening ≥50% and
(4) Normal fetal cardiac activity.

The rare maternal side effects of atosiban are nausea, headache, dizziness, tachycardia, hypertension, hyperglycemia and allergic reactions. The effects on the fetus are not remarkable. The efficacy and safety of atosiban vs. β-sympathomimetics in the treatment of preterm labor have been studied in a randomized, multicentric, controlled, double-blind trial. A total of 742 women have been randomized, with a diagnosis of preterm labor and gestational age between 23 and 33 weeks; 733 underwent tocolytic therapy, 363 with atosiban and the other 379 with β-sympathomimetics, for at least 18 h and within a maximum of 48 h. No statistically significant difference was found between atosiban and β-sympathomimetics in delaying delivery, either for 48 h (88.1% vs. 88.9%) or for 7 days (79.7% vs. 77.6%).

The main gestational age at delivery was similar (35.8 vs. 35.5 weeks), as well as the birth weight. (2491 vs. 2461 g). Tolerability and efficacy were statistically different for pregnant women who delivered over 7 days, without requesting any alternative tocolytic drug (57.7% atosiban vs. 47.4% β-sympathomimetics; $P=0.0003$). There was no statistically relevant difference as far as the feto–neonatal outcome is concerned (bradicardia, tachycardia, fetal distress, neonatal morbidity and hospital stay in the neonatal intensive care unit).

Maternal side effects, especially cardiovascular, were observed more frequently in women treated with β-sympathomimetics than in those treated with atosiban (81.2% vs. 8.3%, respectively, 10 times less frequent), imposing the interruption of therapy in 15.4% vs. 1.1% of the cases, respectively. The modality of atosiban administration is indicated in Table 130.3.

Table 130.3 Modality of administration of atosiban

Stage	Regimen	Dosage	Modality	Time length
1	0.9 ml i.v.	6.75 mg	Bolo	1 min
2	e.v.	18 mg/h	24 ml/h	3 h
3	e.v.	6 mg/h	8 ml/h	Until 45 h

Nitric oxide

Nitric oxide (NO) is a myorelaxant gas that mainly acts on vessels, bowel and uterine muscle. Nitroglycerine is a NO donor. The application of nitroglycerine patches seems to be efficacious for treating preterm delivery, but it has some maternal hypotensive effects. NO is a lipophilic molecule with a low molecular weight, derived from arginine intake by diet. NO binds to cyclic guanosine monophosphate, causing relaxation of smooth muscle of vessels and inhibiting platelet aggregation and endothelial adhesion.

NO is synthesized by the endothelium, epatocytes, macrophages, platelets, human placenta (especially syncitiotrophoblast) and umbilical vessel. It is a vasodilator, neurotransmitter, cytotoxic and cytostatic agent. The maternal side effects are nausea, vomiting, tachycardia, orthostatic hypotension and cutaneous rash.

The fetal adverse effects are determined by variation of feto-placental flow, due to maternal vasodilation. Neonatal hypotension can be observed. The acute treatment of preterm delivery is represented by a transdermic patch of 10 mg, initially applied every 12 h, then every 6 h and finally replaced by another patch every 12 h. Conservative treatment is carried out by means of a transdermic patch of 5 mg, applied daily for 12 h.

Improving NO synthesis by increasing L-arginine synthesis could lead to a reduction of uterine contractility. Nevertheless, the findings from human studies are contradictory. *In vitro* studies show that NO donors do not have any significant effect on myometrial contractions; other studies show a decrease.

In conclusion, there is no evidence to support the routine administration of NO donors in the treatment of preterm delivery. It might be useful to combine them with other tocolytic drugs (atosiban and indometacin) for a synergistic effect, which may prevent the increase of maternal side effects.

Non-pharmacological aspects

Despite the high possibility of identifying the risk cases of preterm delivery, the range of prevention is still limited.

The chances that can currently be taken into consideration are listed:

(1) Identification of a risk subject by cervical sonography screening or by dosage of fetal fibronectin according to demographic factors (low social status), life habits (smoking and drugs use), working conditions (hard work), obstetric anamnesis (previous preterm deliveries, miscarriage due to cervical incompetence), gynecologic anamnesis (uterine malformations or cervical conization) or current pregnancy (multiple pregnancy, polyhydramnios and placenta previa). Some authors have proposed risk scoring systems depending on the presence or absence of the above risk factors. It is very important to detect high-risk subjects among the population, in order to identify the most appropriate diagnostic and therapeutic tool.
(2) Change in life habits. In risk subjects some working conditions need to be changed, and bed rest is advisable, as well as avoiding smoking and use of illicit drugs.
(3) Study of cervico-vaginal microbial flora and its correction. In about 15–20% of pregnant women, the vagina is colonized by microbic agents, such as gardnerella vaginalis and anaerobic bacteria (causing bacterial vaginosis). The association between bacterial vaginosis and preterm delivery

is particularly striking. Antibiotic treatment of bacterial vaginosis reduces the rate of preterm delivery only in high-risk patients, but not in the general population. It is useful to perform the cervico-vaginal culture specimen test in the second trimester, in order to detect and to treat bacterial vaginosis or infections by other microorganisms (chlamydia, ureaplasma or mycoplasma).

(4) Cervical cerclage. In the past it was widely used for all pregnancies considered at risk of preterm delivery. In a recent meta-analysis it has been shown to be efficacious only in cases at high risk. Recent evidence has shown that cervical cerclage on patients with cervical shortening, evaluated by transvaginal ultrasound, reduces the incidence of preterm delivery.

(5) Prophylactic therapies. There is no evidence that in high-risk patients (positive obstetric history, cervical shortening or positive fibronectin test) there is an advantage in the use of prophylactic tocolytic agents.

Role of progesterone

In the field of obstetric and gynecologic pharmacology no other drug has been so extensively studied as progesterone, since its synthesis in 1934. In particular, this hormone has been proposed and used in the treatment of different gynecological pathologies such as endometrial hyperplasia, dysfunctional uterine hemorrhage, amenorrhea, luteal phase deficiency, premenstrual syndrome, as well as being utilized as a contraceptive tool alone or in combination with estrogens and in assisted reproductive technologies and in the maintenance of pregnancy.

The mechanism of action of this hormone is mainly through specific cytoplasmatic receptors that are influenced by the concentrations of estradiol.

Preterm labor

The hypothesis of Csapo, 40 years ago, implicated progesterone in the mechanism of human parturition (at term and preterm) with alternative observation. Adequate progesterone levels in the myometrium have been shown to counteract prostaglandin stimulatory activity as well as oxytocin properties, enhancing the activity of β-mimetic agents. Moreover, progesterone decreases the concentration of myometrial oxytocin receptors, counteracting the effect of estrogens; the same is apparent in the number and properties of gap junctions. Progesterone also inhibits prostaglandin production by amnion–chorion–decidua and it has been shown that the increase in binding of progesterone at the level of fetal membranes at term gestation may justify the predominant effect of estrogen in promoting prostaglandin production and triggering labor.

A high dose of progesterone has been advocated as a possible tocolytic agent; however, its action is slow and its use has been abandoned in acute tocolysis except in conjunction with β-mimetics; in this regard the combination of the two drugs has shown a synergistic effect, reducing the need for high concentrations of β-mimetics with potential dangerous side effects (Tables 130.4 and 130.5).

Table 130.4 Efficacy of combined use of β-mimetics and progesterone (P4)

47 (only β-mimetics)	42 (β-mimetics + P4)
Mean gestational age: 30.5 (3.2)	Mean gestational age: 30.3 (2.7)
Ritodrine (100 mg in saline 0.1–0.3 mg/min)	Ritodrine (50 mg in saline 0.1–0.3 mg/min)$^{+}$ P4 (200 mg/day)
Delivery after 48 h: 87%	Delivery after 48 h: 85%
Delivery after 7 days: 65%	Delivery after 7 days: 68%

From: Di Renzo GC, A. Mattei, M. Gojnic, S. Gerli: Progesterone and Pregnancy. Current Opinion in Obstetrics and Gynecology, 2005 Dec; Vol 17 no 6 pp. 598–600.

Table 130.5 Side effects of combined use of β-mimetics and progesterone

β-mimetics	β-mimetics + P4
Maternal tachycardia (> 140 bpm): 97%	Maternal tachycardia: 52%
Nausea and vomiting: 28%	Nausea and vomiting: 16%
Trembling, dizziness: 26%	Trembling, dizziness: 12%
Palpitations: 32%	Palpitations: 32%
Chest pains: 15%	Chest pains: 10%
Hyperglycemia: 47%	Hypokalemia: 53%
Hypokalemia: 92%	

From: Di Renzo GC, A. Mattei, M. Gojnic, S. Gerli: Progesterone and Pregnancy. Current Opinion in Obstetrics and Gynecology, 2005 Dec; Vol 17 no 6 pp. 598–600.

Recently, the use of prophylactic progesterone in a high dose has been proposed in patients at high risk of preterm labor (one or more previous preterm deliveries before 32 weeks). An NIH randomized controlled trial has clearly shown that the weekly administration of 17-α-hydroxyprogesterone caproate at 300 mg intramuscularly is related to a decrease of almost 50% of the chances of having another preterm delivery before either 32 or 36 weeks, irrespective of the etiology.

This study has been reinforced by similar results obtained by De Fonseca *et al.*[12] with high-dose progesterone given vaginally.

In conclusion, progesterone may be utilized either in acute tocolysis in order to decrease the concentration of potentially harmful tocolytic drugs or as a preventive agent in a population at high risk for preterm delivery.

SUGGESTED READING

1. Althusius SM, Dekker GA, van Geijn HP, *et al*. Cervical incompetence prevention randomized cerclage trial (CIPRACT): Study design preliminary results. *Am J Obstet Gynecol* 2000;183:823.
2. American Academy of Pediatrics and American College of Obstetricians and Gynecologists. *Guidelines for Prenatal Care*, 5th edn. Washington, DC: American Academy of Pediatrics and American College of Obstetricians and Gynecologists, 2002:6.
3. Brocklehurst P, Hannah M, McDonald H. Interventions for treating bacterial vaginosis in pregnancy (Cochrane Review). In *The Cochrane Library*, Issue 4. Oxford: Update Software, 2002.
4. Caritis SN, Venkataramanan R, Darby MJ, *et al*. Pharmacokinetics of ritodrine administered intravenously: Recommendations for changes in the current regimen. *Am J Obstet Gynecol* 1990;162: 429.
5. Evidence Report/Technology Assessment No 18. *Management of Preterm Labor*. AHRQ Publication No 01-E021, October 2000. www.ahrq.gov.clinic/epix.htm.
6. Grether JK, Hoogstrate J, Selvin S, *et al*. Magnesium sulfate tocolysis and risk of spastic cerebral palsy in premature children born to women without pre-eclampsia. *Am J Obstet Gynecol* 2000; 183:717.
7. Keirse MJNC. Magnesium sulphate in preterm labor. In Keirse MJNC, Renfrew MJ, Neilson JP, *et al*. eds. *Pregnancy and Childbirth Module*. The Cochrane Collaboration. The Cochrane Pregnancy and Childbirth Database, Issue # 2. Oxford: Update Software, 1995.
8. Macones GA, Berlin M, Berlin JA. Efficacy of oral beta-antagonist maintenance therapy in preterm labor: A meta-analysis. *Obstet Gynecol* 1995;85:313.
9. Makrides M, Crowther CA. Magnesium supplementation in pregnancy. *Cochrane Database Syst Rev* 2001;4:CD000937.
10. Moutquin JM, Sherman D, Cohen H, *et al*. Double-blind, randomised, controlled trial of atosiban and ritodrine in the treatment of preterm labor: A multicenter effectiveness and safety study. *Am J Obstet Gynecol* 2000;182:1191.
11. Tsatsaris V, Papasonis D, Goffinet F, *et al*. Tocolysis with nifedipine or beta adrenergic agonists: A meta-analysis. *Obstet Gynecol* 2001;97:840.
12. De Fonseca EB, Bittar RE, Carvalho MH, Zugaib M. Prophylactic administration of progesterone by vaginal suppository to reduce the incidence of spontaneous preterm birth in women at increased risk: a randomized placebo-controlled double-blind study. *Am J Obstet Gynecol* 2003 Feb;188(2):419–24.

131 Efficient and simple program including community-based activities for prevention of very early premature birth

E. Saling, J. Lüthje and M. Schreiber*

Introduction

Overview

The rate of prematures (< 37 + 0 gestational weeks) in Germany is increasing, 9.4% in 2004, similar to other European countries and the USA. In the past, it was not possible to substantially reduce this rate.

One of the most urgent tasks for modern obstetrics is to reduce the rate of very early (< 32 + 0 gestational weeks) prematures, and those with a very low birth weight (< 1500 g). These infants form the group of newborns with the highest mortality and morbidity.

Mortality and morbidity

Although in industrial countries, neonatologists have achieved enormous success in keeping extremely premature infants alive, mortality increases rapidly with decreasing birth weight. The immediate and long-term sequelae of prematurity are also alarming – something that is sometimes neglected when just measuring the 'successes' of modern intensive care by mortality rates. Table 131.1 summarizes the complications caused by prematurity or low birth weight.

The psychological and physical burden, which often exists for the families concerned, is another important factor that underlines the urgent necessity for effective prematurity prevention activities.

Costs

The enormously high costs of intensive care and follow-up care should be an urgent inducement to make even

Table 131.1 Specific published complications caused by prematurity or low birth weight (from Berkowitz *et al.*,[1] Hack *et al.*,[2] Edwards *et al.*,[3] Saigal *et al.*,[4] Riegel *et al.*,[5] Monset-Couchard *et al.*[6] and Wolke *et al.*[7])

Perinatal morbidity and mortality
Respiratory distress syndrome
Intraventricular hemorrhage
Leucomalacia
Necrotizing enterocolitis
Infection
Long-term sequelae
Cerebral palsy
Hearing defects
Visual defects
Epilepsy
Lack of intelligence
Subnormal weight
Subnormal height
Poor gross-motor function
Poor adaptive functioning
Behavioral problems
Attention deficit
Schooling problems

*Coauthors of this chapter in the 1st edition of this book were T. Al-Taie, W. Masur and A. Placht

more efforts to reduce the number of very small prematures if possible.

After a calculation by Künzel,[8] based on the well-organized German perinatal studies, the costs of care of all prematures born at less than 32 gestational weeks (about 8000 per year) were about 300 million EUR, and the costs for those born between 32 and 36 gestational weeks (about 47,000 per year) were about 430 million EUR, amounting to 730 million EUR. Additionally, the costs of clinical management of mothers with threatened prematurity were about 360 million EUR, totalling more than 1 billion EUR per year. These calculations do not even include the costs of long-term care of children and adults who are impaired due to prematurity.

Lewit *et al.*[9] estimated that in the USA each year the costs of medical care, child care and education for 3.5–4 million children aged 0–15 years, who had been born with low birth weight, were between $5.5 billion and $6 billion more than they would have been if those children had been born with normal birth weight.

We want to emphasize that smoking and abuse of other drugs (especially alcohol) are important avoidable causes of prematurity and low birth weight. The physician should inform any pregnant woman about the risks of the above-mentioned and should encourage her to discontinue smoking, consuming alcohol or drug taking.

Causes of late abortions and prematurity

Overview

Late abortions and, in particular, very early prematurity should be considered together, because their etiology is often the same.

A number of reasons are known to cause late abortions and prematurity. Lockwood and Kuczynski[10] divided most of the known causes of prematurity into four pathogenetic processes:

- Activation of the maternal or fetal hypothalamic–pituitary–adrenal (HPA) axis
- Decidual chorioamniotic or systemic inflammation
- Decidual hemorrhage
- Pathological distension of the uterus.

The various pathomechanisms initially follow different pathways, merge later on and cause changes in the cervix, leading to premature contractions and/or premature rupture of the membranes and finally to premature birth.

As far as effective preventive measures are concerned, most of the avoidable causes, particularly before 32 gestational weeks, are to be found among patients with ascending genital infections, and the diagnostic and therapeutic strategies in this direction are of definitive importance.

As far as other less frequent causes are concerned, both the possibility of treatment being available and the chances of success are clearly lower than in the infection group. Furthermore, some problems are directly related to the causes resulting from genital infection.

Ascending infections

The first convincing and direct confirmation of the ascension infection genesis was found at the beginning of the 1980s when the operative early total cervix occlusion (ETCO) was introduced for patients with recurrent late abortions.[11] This creates a complete barrier within the ascension area and leads to remarkably good results.[†]

Profound biochemical studies later performed by Romero *et al.*[12] brought us immensely forward in understanding the mechanisms by which infections lead to premature birth. Another pioneering step that underlines how important it is to improve prevention of infections is the concept of the 'fetal inflammatory response syndrome'.[13] It explains that fetal inflammation is linked to the onset of labor, and that the multisystemic involvement in this condition can lead to fetal injury, such as brain damage, which predisposes the subsequent development of cerebral palsy.

In the meantime, association between infections and prematurity has been proved by many studies. If early diagnosed, infections can often be treated effectively. Besides ascending genital infections, for instance, due to *Chlamydia trachomatis*, other infections must be considered, especially urinary tract infections.

Infections with *Candida* alone do not normally increase the risk of prematurity. *Chlamydia* infections are associated with a risk of prematurity that is as high as the risk associated with bacterial vaginosis. Some authors also report a similarly high risk of infection with *Trichomonas*, but *Trichomonas* is often associated with bacterial vaginosis, although *Chlamydia* and *Trichomonas* infections are not as prevalent as bacterial vaginosis.

Table 131.2 shows several urogenital infections and their impact on pregnancy and morbidity of infants and mothers.

Stress and immune system

Concerning efforts to prevent prematurity, many publications and recommendations have been reviewed in the literature. Most of them, for example, by Papiernik,[15] are based on the fact that socioeconomical factors, such as low social status, psychological and physical stresses, are important reasons and causes for premature birth. Some successes have been achieved with programs based on these aspects, particularly in

[†]For details see our article 'Operative Early Total Cervix Occlusion for Prevention of Late Abortion and Early Prematurity'

Table 131.2 Urogenital infections and associated complications in pregnancy (from Martius *et al.*[14])

Infection	Increased rate of prematurity	Increased morbidity by infection of the mother	Increased morbidity by infection of the newborn
Bacterial vaginosis	Yes	Yes	Unknown
C. trachomatis	Yes	Yes	Yes
Streptococcus Group B	Unknown	Yes	Yes
N. gonorrhea	Yes	Yes	Yes
Trichomonas vaginalis	Unknown	Unknown	Seldom
Mycoplasma hominis	Unknown	Unknown	Unknown
Ureaplasma urealytikum	Unknown	Unknown	Unknown
Urinary tract infection	Yes	Yes	No
Candida species	No	Yes	Yes

model studies. However, the main obstacle preventing a consistent reduction in the number of very low birth weight infants on a broad scale concerns the amount of expense involved. Considerable organizational and personal expenses are necessary to realize such projects, and these resources are hardly available to such an extent in all countries.

Another interesting aspect is that, as far as the cellular and humoral parameters of the immune system are concerned, concrete signs of impairments of the immune status could be found in women with prematurity symptoms.[16] In pregnant women with symptoms of threatened prematurity, significantly lower levels of lymphocytes, T-lymphocytes and T-helper cells were measured than in women who had a normal course of pregnancy. The T_4/T_8 ratio was also clearly reduced in those cases where later preterm birth actually occurred; it was particularly low at 1.1 compared to 1.6 in cases with uncomplicated pregnancies. In the group of pregnant women with premature labor, the rate of those who found their situation 'very stressful' amounted to 65%, and in the group whose course of pregnancy was normal, the rate was 26%. We assume that ascending infections are probably enhanced by such impairments of the immune system. Furthermore, we conclude that those pregnant women living in critical socioeconomical environments and who, therefore, are more likely to have impaired immunity can be helped effectively through exposure to appropriate information and preventive medical measures initiated early in pregnancy.

Early intervention by the prematurity-prevention program (see below) is more realistic and, consequently, more successful in reducing prematurity than the complicated and necessarily expensive intensive measures given by social services or later in pregnancy when prematurity symptoms are evident.

The protective lactobacillus system

Role of lactobacilli

The human vagina possesses a biosystem that under normal conditions provides a balance between physiologic lactobacilli and pathogenic bacterial flora, and so ensures a good protection against the spreading of pathogens, including their ascension to the uterine cavity. The importance of lactobacilli for the normal vaginal milieu was first described by Döderlein.[17]

In an article of particular interest to us, Gregor Reid[18] describes the role of lactobacilli in the urogenital tract infections.

The following main functions of lactobacilli are known (Figure 131.1):

(1) They produce acids, mainly lactic acid.
(2) They produce hydrogene peroxide (H_2O_2), which releases oxygen and has a disinfecting effect. These factors, combined with
(3) Bacteriocines, inhibit the growth of pathogens, which are always present in the vagina.
(4) They produce biosurfactants, which cover the surface of the vaginal wall, thereby inhibiting the adhesion of pathogens.
(5) They produce coaggregation molecules, which block the spread of pathogens.

Not every lactobacillus strain produces all the factors mentioned above. That is the reason why some strains are more effective against specific infections than others. For instance, women with H_2O_2-producing lactobacilli have a lower risk of bacterial vaginosis than women whose lactobacilli do not produce H_2O_2.[19] Unfortunately, there are also some microorganisms, the growth of which is not or only marginally inhibited by lactobacilli (e.g. *Streptococci* and *Candida*).

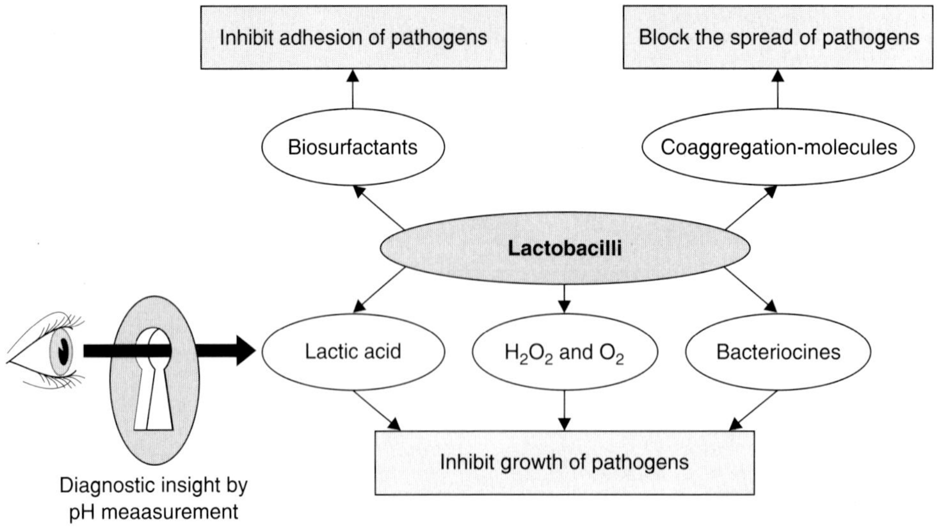

Figure 131.1

However, we can assume that lactobacilli are the main regulating factors of the vaginal milieu. Vaginal pH measurement gives us insight – like peering through a keyhole – into this protective biosystem. Vaginal pH measurement was already used by Döderlein, in order to distinguish pathological from normal vaginal fluid.[17]

Importance of pH measurement

The importance of lactobacilli and measurement of vaginal pH is illustrated, for instance, by the following facts:

Ernest *et al.*[20] found out that the risk of premature rupture of the membranes before 37+0 gestational weeks is three times higher when the vaginal pH is repeatedly above 4.5, compared to pregnant patients with pH $\leq$4.5.

A retrospective evaluation carried out by one of our coworkers reveals that: the earlier in pregnancy the examined children were born the more frequently the mothers had an increased vaginal pH when admitted to hospital. All 15 mothers (100%) of children with a gestational age lower than 32+0 gestational weeks had increased pH values; as far as prematures between 32+0 gestational weeks and 36+6 gestational weeks were concerned, the rate was still about 60%; when born mature only 43.5% were affected.[21] It follows, that ascending infections very frequently play a role concerning very early prematurity, and that in many of these cases threatening prematurity can be detected by measurement of increased pH values.

In a prospective study, Hengst[22] was able to show the practical importance of measuring the vaginal pH, which we recommend in routine prenatal care for the prevention of prematurity. In a cohort of pregnant women with a normal course of pregnancy until the study, who had an increased pH > 4.5 and who had received no therapy for acidification, the number of prematures amounted to 15.1%. On the other hand, the number was only 2.0% when an acidifying therapy with *Lactobacillus acidophilus* preparations had been applied.

In another earlier evaluation, we also found results concerning how many pregnant patients had normal vaginal pH values and how many had pathological ($\geq$4.7). In 67% of all the 695 evaluated cases, normal pH values were present; in 33%, the values were increased twice or more and 7% of these were permanently increased.[23]

It is of particular interest to examine the success rate in normalizing the pH, in cases with increased vaginal pH values, by using *L. acidophilus* therapy. Success was achieved in 83% of 75 such patients, and this is really an unexpectedly good result. The therapy was carried out for 5 ±3 days to achieve this success.[23]

Normal flora – disturbed milieu – infection

According to some published data, we assume that the main reason for the good results of our prematurity-prevention program (see below) is not the early detection of existing infections, but the early detection of their precursors, namely disturbances of the vaginal milieu.

- Hillier *et al.*[24] diagnosed an intermediate pattern between normal flora and bacterial vaginosis – see also Schröder[25] – in 16% of the pregnant women examined, while 22% of the women suffered from bacterial vaginosis, and 61% had a normal flora. Of the women with such a transitional stage in the second trimester, in the third trimester in about one-third the findings were the same, in about one-third the findings were normal, and about one-third developed a bacterial vaginosis.

- Hay *et al.* found in a study[26] an increased risk of loss of pregnancy, when just an intermediate pattern was present.
- Viehweg *et al.*[27] reported that an increasing pH value during the course of pregnancy leads to an increased risk of prematurity, even when the pH value stays within the normal range.

In the literature, there are controversial results concerning the success of treatment of bacterial vaginosis, and its effects on pregnancy outcome. However, there may have been little success, when screening, diagnosis and treatment took place rather late in the course of pregnancy, or when the diagnosis was incorrect, and there was probably a so-called 'aerobic vaginitis' (which is associated with aerobic microorganisms, mainly group B *Streptococci* and *Escherichia coli*) rather than bacterial vaginosis.[28]

We assume, that the main reason for those different results is that up to now no studies have been published where vaginal acidity was checked by pH measurement so early in pregnancy and at such short intervals (allowing early treatment), as is the case for the pregnant women who participate in our prenatal-care self-examination (see below).

We have first results that indicate that already disturbances of the vaginal milieu can be detected by pH measurement at regular intervals, before bacterial vaginosis develops.[29] In 24 pregnant patients who visited their doctor because they had themselves measured an increased vaginal pH value, 33 diagnoses were made:

- 46% of the patients were told that they only had a disturbance of the vaginal milieu, and not yet bacterial vaginosis.
- Bacterial vaginosis was diagnosed only in 4%.
- *Candida* were diagnosed in 33%, *Chlamydia* in 8% and other bacteria in 8%.

Although we received these data from the patients, and not directly from their physicians – and thus they should be interpreted with caution – there is no reason to question the results on principle.

Prematurity-prevention program

General aspects

We began our activities to reduce the rate of prematures in 1972,[30,31] but our successes[32] were only transiently satisfying. The program could not be maintained for long periods because it was too expensive for practical use. Fifteen years ago, we changed to another policy and developed a new prematurity-prevention program, which is based on the most frequent cause of prematurity, namely, as already mentioned above, the ascension infection genesis. Some reports on this program have already been published.[33–37] Its practical introduction into our clinical routine and later in general practitioners' offices by colleagues in the area has led to a considerable decrease in the number of very small, low birth weight infants. However, in spite of achieving a reduction rate of about 40% in our department and 50% in cooperation with practitioners, we had to admit that the practical employment of the program and the consequent application of preventive measures started at a relatively late stage in the entire prematurity pathogenetic process. Therefore, in 1993 we developed another supporting new concept, namely active cooperation of the pregnant patient herself.[38] Our present program is the combination of these two important parts. This solution appears to be quite different from conventional measures; it is a relatively simple, economical and more easily achieved way to attain considerable success in reducing the rate of very small and extremely small prematures.

Table 131.3 Risk factors for prematurity

Anamnestic risk factors
One or more premature births or stillbirths
Two or more pregnancy terminations
Prior cervical conization
Prior vaginal infections
After infertility treatment
In the present pregnancy
Low social status
Younger than 18 or older than 35 years
Multiples (twins, triplets, etc)
Polyhydramnios
Certain pressure situations (professional or private, physical or emotional)
Smoking, regular alcohol consumption, or use of other drugs

Diagnostic measures

Risk factors

Risk factors (Table 131.3) can be divided into anamnestic risk factors (mainly previous premature births or stillbirths) and events in the current pregnancy.

Screening for infections

Each time when a pregnant patient consults her physician, attention should also be paid to disturbances of the vaginal milieu or to manifest infections. Besides, medical history and physical examination (vaginal discharge, redness, etc.), especially measurement of the pH value should be performed. An increased pH value normally indicates a so-called 'dysbiosis', a bacterial vaginosis or – less frequently – another infection.

It is also important to note that some vaginal infections are normally not associated with increased pH values. This concerns *Candida* species, *C. trachomatis*, *Neisseria gonorrhoeae* and B-streptococci.

Systemic infections and urinary tract infections can also lead to prematurity. Therefore, we should always look for symptoms and signs of these infections (see also Ascending Infections and Table 131.2).

Measurement of pH value

The most important step during routine diagnosis in our prematurity-prevention program is to measure the pH value in the vagina. A high level of acidity in the vaginal milieu does not guarantee completely secure protection against ascending infections, but it is certainly very effective.

According to our investigations in an undisturbed course of pregnancy the pH-value at the introitus vaginae (at a depth of approximately 2–3 cm) is regarded as normal:

- ≤4.2 when measured with pH-meter
- ≤4.4 when measured with indicator paper.

In order to achieve uniformity, we recommend that measurements on principle be made in the lower area of the vagina. The higher in the vagina measured, that is, the nearer to the cervical canal, according to our examinations, the higher are the pH values.[39] In the cervical canal itself, for example, when measured in the external os, almost neutral pH conditions at 6.5 are to be found in women with an undisturbed course of pregnancy.

- A simple way of measuring the pH is to use a small portable pH-meter.
- If indicator strips are used, they have to be introduced into the area of the introitus vaginae with the finger either before or after the vaginal examination and compared with the corresponding color scale. We made by far the best measurements, when using Spezialindikator pH 4.0–7.0, art-no. 1.09542 by Merck, Darmstadt (Germany), because the reading is especially easy and reliable.
- In the meantime, special disposable gloves with the indicator paper from Merck fixed on the index finger are available for use by the physician. The gloves are almost identical to the ones that we recommend for the patients (see below). The only difference is that the paper in the version for the physician is attached to the *middle phalanx* of the index finger, so that during vaginal examination the pH value will be measured automatically at the introitus vaginae.

Stages and appropriate measures

The stages of threatened prematurity, prophylactic and therapeutic measures depending on diagnostic findings and/or the presence of symptoms as well as chances of success and efficiency of countermeasures are summarized in Table 131.4.

Stage 1: anamnestic risk

In the first, very early stage, a potentially increased risk is found in cases with poor medical history, such as one or more previous late spontaneous abortions or very premature labor. The best prophylactic countermeasure is to perform an operative ETCO at about 12 gestational weeks to create a barrier against ascension of organisms.[‡]

Stage 2: disturbance of vaginal milieu

The second early stage of increased risk is a disturbance of the vaginal milieu, which mostly can be detected by simple pH-measurement at the introitus. In such a case of so-called dysbiosis simple substitution with a *L. acidophilus* preparation for about 7 days is recommended. Especially effective are *Lactobacillus* strains that produce H_2O_2. For instance, the German preparation Gynoflor®[**] contains only H_2O_2-producing lactobacilli. Because *Lactobacillus* therapy normally takes 2–8 days, until the pH values normalize, additional local acidifying therapy might be indicated (e.g. lactic acid in the morning and *Lactobacillus* preparation in the evening). However, currently there is no scientific proof that this additional measure reduces the rate of prematurity.

Both stages 1 and 2 allow the best chances for success in prevention of prematurity.

Stage 3: infection

The third, also relatively early stage of increased risk includes cases without symptoms of premature labor, but in which vaginal infection has been confirmed, such as bacterial vaginosis, *Chlamydia* infection of the cervical canal or urethra, infections of the lower egg-pole (which can be detected by our egg-pole lavage[‡]) or significant bacteriuria. In such cases, we recommend:

- in case of bacterial vaginosis, local therapy with octenidine hydrochloride, metronidazole or clindamycin;
- when there is evidence of *Chlamydia* in the cervix or urethra, pregnant patients should get systemic therapy with erythromycine succinate;

[‡]For details see our article 'Operative Early Total Cervix Occlusion for Prevention of Late Abortion and Early Prematurity'

**Organon GmbH, personal communication, 25 August 2004

Table 131.4 Stages of threatened prematurity, prophylactic and therapeutic measures, and prognosis

Stage of endangerment	Symptoms and findings	Prophylactic and therapeutic measures			Chances of success
Anamnestic risk	Mean (one miscarriage or very small premature)	Small ETCO			
	High (≥two miscarriages or very small prematures)	Extensive ETCO			
Disturbance of vaginal milieu	pH ↑ and/or dysbiosis in native preparation, but No evidence of bacterial vaginosis No ascension of bacteria No increased contractions Normal cervical state	Only here treatment with *L. acidophilus* alone is recommended (maybe combined with acidifying therapy)			Best prognosis
Infection	Microscopically or culturally proved vaginal infection (such as bacterial vaginosis, *trichomoniasis, candidiasis*)	Local therapy Antiseptics Antibiotics Other chemotherapeutics (such as metronidazole)	Recommendation of rest and relaxing measures (among others, for improving immunological conditions)	After treatment with *lactobacillus* preparation in case pH ↑ (may be combined with acidifying therapy)	Still good prognosis
	Evidence of *Chlamydia* in cervix or urethra Evidence of bacteria at lower egg-pole Significant bacteriuria	Systemic antibiotic therapy + local acidifying therapy			
Symptoms of prematurity	Preterm labor and/or critical cervical state, and local infection in vagina, cervix or at lower egg-pole or signs of inflammation (e.g. CRP↑, leucocytosis)				Increasingly unsuccessful

- for other infections (including significant bacteriuria >100,000/ml), specific systemic antibiotic therapy.

In some countries, some colleagues are hesitant to apply antibiotics in pregnancy. Therefore, we want to stress that pregnancy is not an obstacle for a necessary local or systemic therapy against microorganisms.

The patients should have the recommended amount of physical rest, as well as use of psychological relaxing measures to try to improve their immunological status. The chances of success are still acceptable.

Stage 4: symptoms of threatened prematurity

This most advanced stage is found when symptoms of prematurity, such as apparent premature uterine contractions and/or critical cervical findings, are present. If organisms can be identified, or laboratory parameters, such as C-reactive protein (CRP), are positive, systemic antibiotic therapy (e.g. with clindamycin, or better according to the antibiogram, if available) is the method of choice. In most of these cases, admittance to hospital is recommended. In the last stage, the therapeutic measures are increasingly unsuccessful.

In both stages, an additional 'after treatment' with *L. acidophilus* preparations may be indicated because most of the therapeutic measures concerned also disturb the vaginal milieu, which can be confirmed by increased vaginal pH values.

In this context, it should be emphasized that our prematurity-prevention program contains, above all, measures most suitable for the prevention of premature rupture of the membranes, as ascending infection is the most frequent cause of this event.

Prenatal-care self-examination

The other, more important, part of our prevention program, is the so-called prenatal-care self-examination of the pregnant patient. The main points are given below.

pH self-measurement

Every pregnant woman is advised to measure the pH value in her vagina twice a week herself, by using a special indicator (see above). It can be used in the form of a test paper by itself, but in cooperation with us special disposable gloves with a piece of test paper fixed on the tip of the index finger have been developed (CarePlan VpH, made by Unipath). The majority

Table 131.5 Warning signs of a threatened premature birth (part of the patients brochure)

The patients are advised to get in touch with their doctor as soon as possible if any of these signs are present
Repeated measurement (with the test glove) of a vaginal pH value of 4.7 or higher. *Attention*: Particularly high values may be due to the loss of amniotic fluid (premature rupture of the membranes)
Vaginal bleeding or spotting
Bad smelling or highly increased discharge (a slight increase is normal during pregnancy)
Abnormally frequent urination (a slight increase is also normal) or a burning sensation when urinating
Itching or burning in the intimate region
Fever and/or diarrhea (these conditions are often associated with an increase in uterine activities)
Premature contractions:
Considerable pain similar to menstruation
Aching in the groin or in the sacral region
Temporary, repeated hardening of the uterus
Premature contractions should be regarded as critical to threatening, if they occur more than twice per hour, or more than 10 times during the whole day

of the women whom we consulted reported that it is much more comfortable to use the gloves, rather than the test paper alone.

The woman simply introduces the index finger into her vagina, withdraws it shortly afterward, and compares the color of the indicator paper with the enclosed special color scale, in order to read the pH value. When pH values are increased to 4.7 or higher, the patient should see her practitioner at once.

If her doctor confirms the reduced acidification, additional examinations should be performed, in order to find the cause of the acidity disturbance. The further procedure depends on the stage of threatened prematurity (see prematurity-prevention program above).

Self-observation of warning signs

Independent of the vaginal pH self-measurement, all expectant mothers should be made aware of the most important warning signs. They are listed in the information brochure (see Table 131.5). If anything unusual occurs, the patient should see her doctor.

Benefits of the self-care program

As the program is fundamentally based on a screening-principle, as many patients as possible should be motivated to take part, at best, every pregnant woman without exception. The reason for a recommendation such as this is that, during the course of even supposedly normal pregnancies, late abortions and preterm delivery can occur. It is very probable that a large number of these patients will have early symptoms that could have been detected but remained concealed.

The self-examination should be started very early on, to detect the threat of irregularities in good time, that is, at the earliest possible moment in the pregnancy. It would be even better, in cases with a poor history, to choose a preconceptional moment, that is, weeks or months before a planned pregnancy. For some women, it could be really important to detect potential risks themselves at such an early stage and to inform their practitioner even before the pregnancy has started or at least very early on in the pregnancy.

Recently, Hübner confirmed the importance of early onset of pH self-measurement in pregnancy. She evaluated questionnaires from 607 pregnant women, who participated in the Thuringia Prematurity Prevention Campaign 2000' (see below) (Hübner, in preparation).

Among women who started measurement before 15 + 0 gestational weeks, the total rate of prematures was 4.8%, and the rate of very early prematures was 0%. In contrast, when women started pH-measurement at 15 + 0 gestational weeks or later, there were 6.1% prematures and 0.9% very early prematures.

The main advantage achieved by the patient's active participation is that increases in vaginal pH or the manifestation of any other risk factors are identified very early and this leads to the detection of a considerable number of disturbances connected with spontaneous abortions and prematurity. This enables the practitioner to avoid longer, critical latency periods, sometimes of several weeks. In particular, without these new facilities, some symptoms remain concealed, although they are, in fact, easily recognizable. Furthermore, there is also a possibility of controlling the behavior of vaginal acidity at short intervals, for instance, to follow effects of therapeutic measures.

Hübner also confirmed that it is important to measure regularly at short intervals. Among patients who did not only start pH-measurement early in pregnancy, but also – according to our recommendations – measured twice a week, the total rate of prematures was 4.2%, and the rate of very early prematures was 0%. In contrast, in the group of women who started pH-measurement at 15 +0 gestational weeks or later, or measured less frequently than twice a week, there were 7.3% prematures, and 0.8% very early prematures. However, the differences between these rates are not statistically significant (Hübner, in preparation).

Now and then, some colleagues argue that self-measurement of vaginal pH would have no other effect than confusing the pregnant women. The opposite is true. In an inquiry, we asked the women who participated in our prenatal-care self-examination program regarding this point. The vast majority answered that they found it 'very good', 'reassuring' and had 'a good feeling' about it, etc. because they 'were able to do something themselves'. Although it might seem surprising, because of these simple regular self-examinations, most of the users have the feeling of not being a 'treated object' during pregnancy anymore but an 'active subject'.

Results of self-examination

The results evaluated up to now appear to justify the pH self-measurement by pregnant patients and demonstrate the efficiency of the prenatal-care self-examination program.

In a study by our department[39] of 100 women who had measured their vaginal pH themselves using indicator paper, 91% of the measurements corresponded with the results later measured by a physician with a pH-meter. In 9% of cases, the results were false-positive; this means that with the indicator paper an increased pH value was measured, but the value controlled by the pH-meter was normal. This is not a grave error, as there were no false-negative results, i.e. no pathological findings were overlooked.

Furthermore, we found that in about 70% of the patients who had increased pH values measured both by indicator paper and by the pH-meter, evidence of pathogenous organisms was found in the vagina and/or the cervix, whereas when the pH values were normal, the figure was only 8%.

The full prenatal-care self-examination program was started in September 1993. The program was advertised in publications that are frequently read by pregnant women.

To date, about 10,000 pregnant patients have participated or are still participating, and about 3000 returned the questionnaire to us. Of the 1715 women whose data have been evaluated so far, 595 were pregnant for the first time and 1120 had been pregnant before. The anamnestic information given by the group of women with previous pregnancies was particularly interesting. A high number of these women, namely 46.4%, had had miscarriages and about 18.3% had had underweight infants during the immediate previous pregnancies. To date, we are able to draw the conclusion that the participating women belong to a higher-risk group rather than to a lower-risk group. According to the returned records, 60.8% of the patients reported 'disturbed courses' in their present pregnancy.

Our evaluations have shown that the rate of underweight infants, in particular the very small ones (birth weight < 1500 g) in all pregnant patients who took part in this program is clearly lower at 1.3% than in previous pregnancies, when the rate was 7.8%. The rate of extremely small infants (< 1000 g) is 0.9% when the women participated in our program, compared with 3.9% in previous pregnancies.

Another evaluation shows comparisons between the results of the immediate previous pregnancies and the present pregnancies only of those women who had suffered a premature birth in the immediate previous pregnancy. Of the 111 women, only 20 (18%) again gave birth to a premature baby (< 37 +0 weeks of gestation). Of the 38 women who had given birth to a very early premature (< 32 +0 weeks' gestation) in the immediate previous pregnancy, only 3 (8%) suffered the same misfortune again, and, of the 22 who had given birth to an extremely early premature (< 28 +0 weeks of gestation), no recurrence occurred.

The effectiveness of our self-care program was also proved by two prospective campaigns.[40] The first was carried out in Erfurt (the capital of Thuringia, Germany), where pregnant women have been offered to perform self-measurements of their vaginal pH by means of test gloves. Patients who were not interested in participating served as a control group. In this study, the prematurity rate was 8.1% in the self-measurement/intervention group vs. 12.3% in the control group. Of the neonates 0.3% vs. 3.3% belonged to the group of very early prematures with a gestational age of < 32 +0. Premature rupture of membranes was registered in 22.8% vs. 30.8%, respectively.

Encouraged by these results, in 2000, a similar pH screening campaign was initiated in the whole state of Thuringia, in order to reduce prematurity. A significant reduction of early prematurity from 1.58% to 0.99%, and regarding low birth weights a significant reduction of cases in all groups, was achieved.

After this campaign had been finished, the prematurity rates monitored in 2002 were as high as they had been prior to the introduction of the activities.

That is why the new Thuringia prematurity prevention campaign 2004/2005 was started on September 1 2004.

Also, four major German health insurance companies currently offer our prenatal-care self-examination program as a pilot project to their pregnant members at no charge. This is especially important, because prematurity is most frequent in women with low social status. The companies started this project in December 2003, and after first internal evaluations, they have already saved a high amount of expenses.

Conclusion

Currently, our prematurity-prevention program, particularly with its self-care activities – as has been confirmed by our evaluation and afterward by two campaigns by Hoyme and coworkers – seems to be the most efficient, easily applicable and inexpensive program for prevention of very early prematurity. Thus, it has high importance in the field of health and social care, and has considerable value within our social community.

REFERENCES

1. Berkowitz GS, Papiernik E. Epidemiology of preterm birth. *Epidemiol Rev* 1993;15(2):414–43.
2. Hack M, Taylor HG, Klein N, Eiben R, Schatschneider Ch, Mercuri-Minich N. School-age outcomes in children with birth weights under 750 g. *N Engl J Med* 1994;331:753–9.
3. Edwards WH, Little GA. Outcomes of the very-low-birth-weight baby: An American experience. In Kurjak A, ed. *Textbook of Perinatal Medicine.* London: Parthenon Publishing Group, 1998: 141–52.
4. Saigal S, Rosenbaum P, Hattersley B, Milner R. Decreased disability rate among 3-year-old survivors weighing 501 to 1000 grams at birth and born to residents of a geographically defined region from 1981 to 1984 compared with 1977 to 1980. *J Pediatr* 1989; 114:839–46.
5. Riegel K, Ohrt B, Wolke D, Österlund K. *Die Entwicklung gefährdet geborener Kinder bis zum Fünften Lebensjahr.* Stuttgart: Enke, 1995.
6. Monset-Couchard M, de Bethmann O, Kastler B. Mid- and long-term outcome of 89 premature infants weighing less than 1000 g at birth, all appropriate for gestational age. *Biol Neonate* 1996; 70:328–38.
7. Wolke D. Psychological development of prematurely born children. *Arch Dis Child* 1998;78:567–570. (Free full-text article at http://adc.bmjjournals.com/cgi/content/full/78/6/567.)
8. Künzel W, Wulf KH, eds. *Frühgeburt.* Baltimore: Urban & Schwarzenberg, 1997:preface, p. V.
9. Lewit EM, Schuurmann Baker L, Corman H, Shiono PH. The direct cost of low birth weight. *Future Child* 1995;5(1): 35–56.
10. Lockwood CJ, Kuczynski E. Markers of risk for preterm delivery. *J Perinat Med* 1999;27:5–20.
11. Saling E. Der frühe totale Muttermundverschluß zur Vermeidung habitueller Aborte und Frühgeburten. *Z Geburtshilfe Perinatol* 1981;185:259–261.
12. Romero R, Gomez R, Baumann P, Mazor M, Cotton D. The role of the infection and cytokines in preterm parturition. In Chwalisz K, Garfield RE, eds. *Basic Mechanisms Controlling Term and Preterm Birth.* Ernst Schering Research Foundation, Workshop 7. New York: Springer, 1993:197–240.
13. Gomez R, Romero R, Ghezzi F, Yoon BH, Mazor M, Berry SM. The fetal inflammatory response syndrome. *Am J Obstet Gynecol* 1998;179:194–202.
14. Martius J. Infektionen. In Martius G, Rath W, eds. *Praxis der Frauenheilkunde, Band 3: Geburtshilfe und Perinatologie.* Stuttgart,: Thieme, 1998:304–39.
15. Papiernik E. Proposals for a programmed prevention policy of preterm birth. *Clin Obstet Gynecol* 1984;27:614–35.
16. Brandt-Niebelschütz S, Saling E, Uphoff A, *et al.* Untersuchungen zur Immunitätslage Schwangerer insbesondere beim Vorliegen einer Frühgeburtsymptomatik. *Geburtsh Frauenheilk* 1995;55: 456–63.
17. Döderlein A. *Das Scheidensekret und seine Bedeutung für das Puerperalfieber.* Leipzig: Eduard Besold, 1892.
18. Reid G. Probiotic agents to protect the urogenital tract against infection. *Am J Clin Nutr* 2001;73:437S–43S. (Free full-text article at http://www.ajcn.org/cgi/content/full/73/2/437S.)
19. Hillier SL, Krohn MA, Klebanoff SJ, Eschenbach DA. The relationship of hydrogen peroxide-producing lactobacilli to bacterial vaginosis and genital microflora in pregnant women. *Obstet Gynecol* 1992;79(3):369–73.
20. Ernest JM, Meis PJ, Moore ML, Swain M. Vaginal pH: A marker of preterm premature rupture of the membranes. *Obstet Gynecol* 1989;74:734–38.
21. Schumacher E. Infektionsbezogene diagnostische Parameter bei Patientinnen mit Frühgeburtsymptomatik. Doctoral thesis, Freie Universität Berlin, Germany, 1999.
22. Hengst P, Uhlig B, Bollmann R, Kokott Th. Nutzen der vaginalen pH-Messung zur Frühgeburtsvermeidung. *Z Geburtshilfe Perinatol* 1992;196:238–41.
23. Saling E, Fuhr N, Placht A, Schuhmacher E. Erste Ergebnisse der Selbst-Vorsorge-Aktion von Schwangeren zur Frühgeburtenvermeidung. *Arch Gynecol Obstet* 1995;257:178–85.
24. Hillier SL, Krohn MA, Nugent RP, Gibbs RS. Characteristics of three vaginal flora patterns assessed by Gram stain among pregnant women. *Am J Obstet Gynecol* 1992;166:938–44.
25. Schröder R. Zur Pathogenese und Klinik des vaginalen Fluors. *Zentralbl Gynakol* 1921;38:1350–61.
26. Hay PE, Lamont RF, Taylor-Robinson D, Morgan DJ, Ison C, Pearson J. Abnormal bacterial colonisation of the genital tract and subsequent preterm delivery and late miscarriage. *Br Med J* 1994;308:295–298. (Free full-text article at http://bmj.bmjjournals.com/cgi/content/full/308/6924/295.)
27. Viehweg B, Junghans U, Stepan H, Voigt T, Faber R. Der Nutzen vaginaler pH-Messungen für die Erkennung potentieller Frühgeburten. *Zentralbl Gynakol* 1997;119:33–7.
28. Donders GGG, Vereecken A, Bosmans E, Dekeersmaecker A, Salembier G, Spitz B. Definition of a type of abnormal vaginal flora that is distinct from bacterial vaginosis: Aerobic vaginitis. *Br J Obstet Gynecol* 2002;109:34–43.
29. Saling E, Schreiber M. Laktobazillen-Schutzsystem bei Schwangeren – effiziente Vermeidung von Frühgeburten durch Früherkennung von Störungen. *Z Geburtsh Neonatol* 2005; 209:128–34.
30. Saling E. Prämaturitäts- und Dysmaturitäts-Präventions-Programm (PDP-Programm). In Saling E, Dudenhausen JW, eds. *Perinatale Medizin III, 4. Deutscher Kongreß für Perinatale Medizin,* Berlin, 1971. Stuttgart: Thieme, 1972.
31. Saling E. Prämaturitäts- und Dysmaturitäts-Präventions-Programm (PDP-Programm). *Z Geburtshilfe Perinatol* 1972;176:70–81.
32. Giffei JM, Saling E. First results and experiences with our prematurity and dysmaturity prevention program (PDP-Program). *J Perinat Med* 1974;2:45–53.
33. Saling E. Program for the prevention of prematurity. In Hirsch HA, ed. *Infection and Preterm Labor.* Stuttgart: Thieme, 1991, 31–40.
34. Saling E, Brandt-Niebelschütz S, Schmitz C. Vermeidung von Spätaborten und risikoreichen Frühgeburten – für die Routine

geeignete Maßnahmen. *Z Geburtshilfe Perinatol* 1991;195: 209–221.

35. Saling E. Current measures to prevent late abortion or prematurity. In Saling E, ed. *Perinatology. Nestlé Nutrition Workshop Series.* New York: Raven Press, 1992;26:141–51.
36. Saling E. Effective prevention of premature birth – Some recent aspects and results. In Koppe JG, Eskes TKAB, van Geijn HP, Wiesenhaan PF, Ruys JH, eds. *Care, Concern and Cure in Perinatal Medicine.* New York: Parthenon Publishing Group, 1992:147–53.
37. Saling E. Infektiologische Spätabortursachen und operativer Muttermundverschluß. *Arch Gynecol Obstet* 1993;254:1265–71.
38. Saling E, Fuhr N, Placht A, Schumacher E. A new efficient strategy for prevention of prematurity. In Kurjak A, Latin V, Rippmann E, eds. *Advances on the Pathophysiology of Pregnancy.* Rome: CIC Edizioni Internationali, 1995:228–34.
39. Riedewald S, Hanifi-Afshar T, Saling E. pH-Selbstmessung in der Vagina durch die Schwangere (im Vergleich zu Kontrollmessungen durch den Arzt). *Z Geburtshilfe Perinatol* 1992;196:61–2.
40. Hoyme UB, Saling E. Efficient prematurity prevention is possible by pH-self measurement and immediate therapy of threatening ascending infection. *Eur J Obstet Gynecol Reprod Biol* 2004;115: 148–53.

132 Operative early total cervix occlusion for prevention of late abortion and early prematurity

E. Saling, M. Schreiber and J. Lüthje

Introduction

Recurrent late abortions and early prematurity continue to be two of the inadequately solved problems in modern obstetrics and perinatal medicine. The patients concerned often feel heavily burdened: On the one hand, they yearn for a child and on the other hand, they experience recurring losses, which are often accompanied by increasing psychological problems. To achieve a surviving infant is in such cases a particularly important medical and psychological task.

Several causes of late abortions and prematurity are known. Lockwood and Kuczinski[1] divided most of the known causes of prematurity into four pathogenetic processes. However, as far as the avoidable causes are concerned, infection, particularly ascending genital infection, is known to be the most common.*

The most efficient measure for preventing ascending genital infections in cases of recurrent late abortions and early prematurity is to establish a total barrier within the cervical canal by early total cervix occlusion (ETCO). We introduced this measure in 1981.[2,3]

Before that, there were only very few reports in the literature about operative cervix occlusion for treatment of imminent abortion, mainly in advanced stages. For instance, 40 years ago, Szendy published two articles on the topic 'Measures to Prevent the Birth of the Infant in Advanced Premature Labor' (translated from the German).[4,5] Thus, it was thought of as an emergency measure, to be taken mostly when prolapse of membranes had occurred.

We introduced the ETCO as an original early preventive measure for use when the cervix is still in an anatomically normal state and that should be performed early in pregnancy at about 12 gestational weeks (gw), and only in women with previous critical history. It is important to note that the ETCO is quite different from a cerclage (and in principle, also from the occasionally used pessary). The ETCO actually closes the cervical canal, thus preventing ascension of organisms, whereas the cerclage only tightens the canal (Figure 132.1) and has much poorer results (see below).

Definition

With regard to total cervix occlusion (TCO), we differentiate between 'early' and 'late' and between 'small' and 'extensive'.

- *ETCO* is performed at $< 16+0$ gw and with an almost normal state of the portio (sonographically measured† cervix length ≥ 30 mm or modified[6] Bishop score of ≤ 4).
- *Late TCO* is performed at $\geq 16+0$ gw or when the portio is in a critical state (cervix length < 30 mm or modified Bishop score of > 4).

Because the results (of preventing premature birth) are much better (see below), we recommend ETCO rather than late TCO.

- *Extensive TCO*: After removing both the glandular epithelium in the cervical canal and the epithelium of the portio surface, the cervix is closed by two to three circular internal sutures, followed by

*More details can be found in our article 'Efficient and Simple Program Including Community-Based Activities for Prevention of Very Early Premature Birth', Chapter 131.

†The sonographic measurement of the cervical length is more reliable than the assessment using the Bishop score and should therefore be preferred.

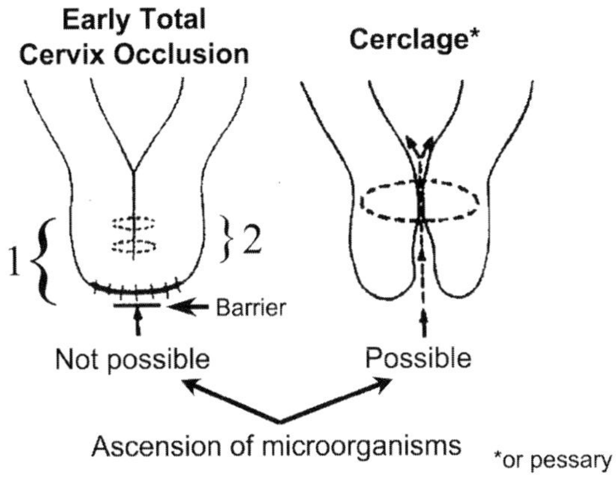

Figure 132.1 ETCO vs. cerclage or pessary: (1) 'extensive' ETCO and (2) 'small' ETCO.

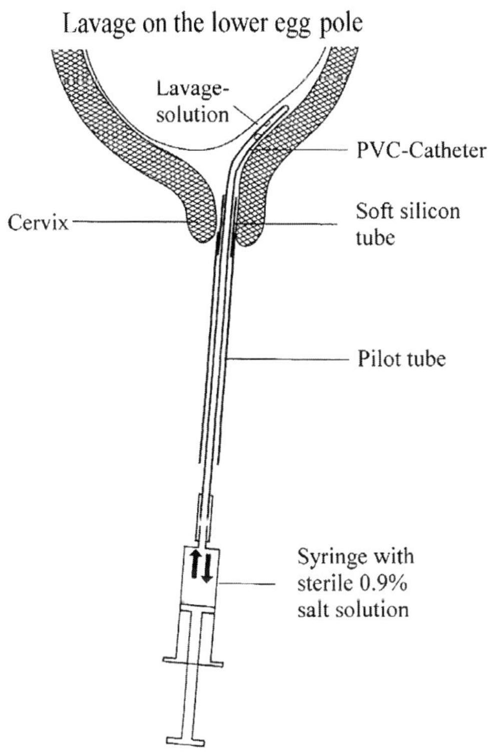

Figure 132.2 Lavage on the lower egg pole.

two transverse rows of knotted stitches to close the surface of the portio. See Figures 132.1(1) and 132.5(2)–(5). For most cases we recommend extensive TCO, preferably ETCO.

- *Small TCO*: Only the cervix canal is closed by two to three circular sutures after removing the glandular epithelium. See Figure 132.1(2).

Indications and contraindications

(1) *Indication* for ETCO is two or more

- late abortions (≥12 +0 gw) or
- early premature births (< 32 +0 gw) in the patient's history either
- with infection as the cause of these events or
- (in the absence of any other cause) when, for instance, premature rupture of the membrane (PROM) has occurred. Please note that the main reason for PROM is ascending vaginal infection.

(2) Up to now no study is available on whether in cases with only one previous late abortion or premature birth a consequent screening for vaginal infection (see Chapter 131, 'Efficient and Simple Program Including Community-Based Activities for Prevention of Very Early Premature Birth', in this section) will lead to similar good results as with ETCO. Therefore, one might consider an ETCO even after only *one* abortion or premature birth, particularly when additional risks exist, for instance, when the patient is older or when there have been problems with fertility. In these cases, a small occlusion of the cervix may be sufficient.

A *contraindication* is dilatation of the cervix with apparent signs of infection and labor activity, which cannot be inhibited.

Preoperative diagnostics and measures

Examinations for infections are compulsory, for example, vaginal and cervical smears with microscopic and/or bacteriologic examinations. Further, should pathological findings be present – such as bacterial vaginosis, candida, *Trichomonas* or *Chlamydia* infection – the patient should be given an appropriate local or systemic therapy.

After an ETCO has been performed, there is no further opportunity to examine whether organisms have already ascended to the intrauterine space. Therefore, we recommend performing a so-called egg-pole lavage (which we introduced in 1992) directly before the operative occlusion of the cervix.

Egg-pole lavage (Istmical lavage)

The use of this method is still not sufficiently widespread. In the beginning of the 1990s, we started to achieve direct access to the area of the lower uterine segment, namely, the egg pole, and have tried to obtain bacteriological information from this region.[7,8]

A pilot tube, the front part of which is made of silicone, is inserted into the cervical canal (see Figure 132.2). In this pilot tube a flexible 1.5-mm-diameter plastic (polyvinyl chloride) catheter is introduced and pushed further 2–6 cm forward, according to the state of separation of the membranes from the uterine wall. In this way, we can be sure that we have reached the area of the lower egg pole, and that the front end of the inner plastic catheter is in the uterus.

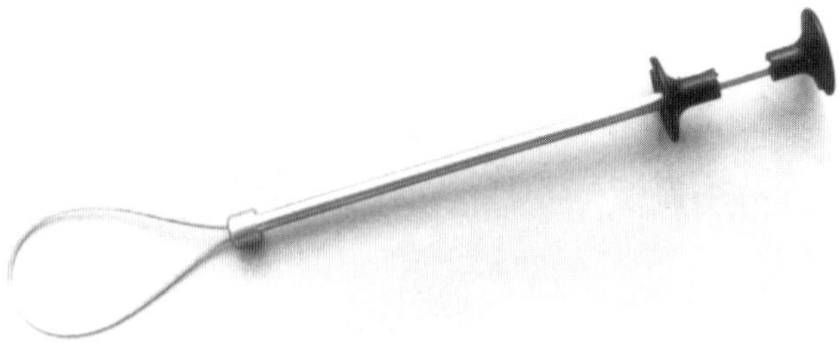

Figure 132.3 Ligature with the loop instrument:[9] There is a ratchet on the traction stick with a blocking spring. This allows the stainless steel plaited wire loop to be attached in a circle around the portio and to be fixed in a tightened state. We always try to clamp the loop so tight that there is minimal bleeding remaining. This is a sign that the tissue circulation is not completely interrupted. When the hemostasis has to be suspended at the end of the operation, the traction stick is turned about 90°. The blocking spring slides out of the traction and the loop is set free.

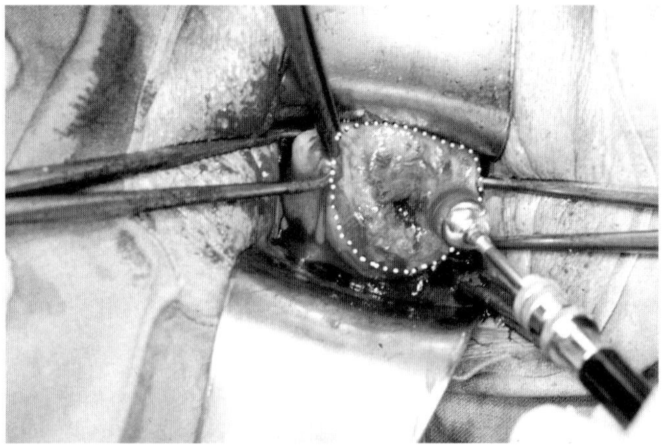

Figure 132.4 Removal of the portio epithelium with rotating wire brush. White points indicate the position of circular incision.

Then, using a syringe attached to the outer end of the catheter, 2 ml of sterile 0.9% physiological saline solution is slowly injected and, shortly afterwards, as much as possible of this solution is aspirated back. When we have reaspirated more than 0.3 ml (the dead space of the catheter), we can be certain that we have collected fluid that was in contact with the membranes or intrauterine wall at the lower egg pole.

The aspirated fluid undergoes bacteriological examination. If the laboratory is close enough, the syringe with the fluid at body temperature can be brought directly to the laboratory for all examinations. Otherwise, the fluid should be instilled into two blood culture bottles (one for aerobe and one for anaerobe examination). Additionally, special transport media provided by the laboratory should be used for other examinations, such as for *Chlamydia* and *Neisseria gonorrhoea*.

A disadvantage of the lavage method is that it is not yet possible to be certain of preventing some organisms from being carried up to the cervical canal. On the other hand, it must be assumed that organisms that have already reached the cervical canal will probably ascend further to the lower egg pole and can certainly develop pathogenicity there. Organisms from the vagina very probably are not transported, as the outer os uteri is treated with disinfectant before catheterization and the device is inserted under visual control directly into the cervical canal.

Operation technique

Before starting the actual operation, we recommend using a procedure and a device that we specially introduced to avoid considerable bleeding. This involves a tight circular ligation of the portio as high as possible, so that the circulation is almost cut off. This measure has two particular advantages: first, the blood loss, which can be considerable on account of the hypervascularization in pregnancy, is reduced to a minimum, and second, it is much easier to see and control the operation area. For a simple and successful ligature we have developed a special loop instrument[9] (see Figure 132.3).

In order to allow the os uteri to grow completely together, the upper surface of the portio has to be dissected, that is, the epithelium has to be almost completely removed. So as to clearly mark the surface to be removed, and also to find the exact positioning of the wounded area later for the row of stitches adapting the upper surface of the portio, we make a circular incision 1 mm deep with a radius of 10–15 mm around the external os uteri with a scalpel. Then, we remove the portio epithelium with a quick rotating wire brush or a special metal rasp in a similar way as is used in dermatology to smooth out scars (Figure 132.4). This method of removing the tissue is more effective and preserves the tissue better than the method we had previously used, when we removed the epithelium by sharp dissection using a scalpel.

Later, the glandular epithelium of the cervical canal is also removed, as far as possible to a depth of about 1–2 cm using the same rotating device, while the os uteri is spread out using mosquito clamps. Then, two to three circular inner stitches are made to close the cervical canal. Consequently, two rows of knotted stitches are made, which close the outer os uteri completely (Figure 132.5). For all the stitching we use synthetic monofile thread like PDS or braided thread, such as Vicryl. These threads, when compared to catgut, are much better for the healing process and are reabsorbed much more slowly.

Measures at the end of pregnancy

The scar should be opened:

- when labor starts spontaneously,
- when an induction of labor is planned or
- when 37 gw are completed.

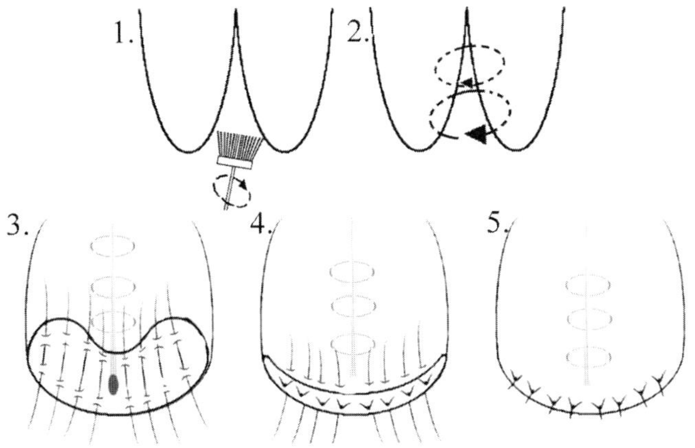

Figure 132.5 Operation technique of ETCO with the different sutures: (1) removal of the glandular epithelium, (2) two to three circular cervical sutures, (3) transverse stitching of the whole dissected area for deep adaptation, (4) second row of knotted stitches adapting the surface tissue and (5) situation after the operation.

We generally cut the portio scar with scissors under local anesthesia. Then, we penetrate with the finger to a depth of about 1–2 cm into the loose cervical tissue in the assumed direction of the cervical canal. If the patient wants to leave the hospital after the scar has been opened, to wait until labor starts spontaneously, we see no reason why she should not do so, provided there are no signs of any risk.

We do not think that a primary cesarean section is necessary at all. Quite the contrary: when recanalization of the cervix takes place during a vaginal delivery, it is in fact a good prerequisite for the reestablishment of normal anatomic conditions.

Results

To assess the results of ETCO, particularly in comparison with cerclage, one should look only at high-risk groups which match the above-mentioned indications for an ETCO (two or more late abortions or premature births). We have no knowledge of any randomized study on ETCO. On the basis of the results published so far we do not think that the operation can be withheld from any woman with such a critical history. A randomized study would not receive the approval of any ethic council – at least not in Germany – and no woman is likely to agree to being integrated into a control group anyway. Therefore, an acceptable solution is to compare the outcome of pregnancies after performing an ETCO with the outcome of former pregnancies of these patients.[3,6,10] We should also consider that the chances of giving birth to a surviving infant are reduced the more late abortions or premature births the woman has previously had.[11]

In 1990[12] we evaluated retrospectively the data from a group of 113 patients with previous recurrent abortions. From a total of 389 wanted pregnancies only 101 infants were born alive (26%). However, 35 of these infants died in the neonatal period. In total, 66 survived, which means that only 17% of all these pregnancies resulted in a surviving infant. Through the introduction of TCO (either early or late) the same patients achieved 132 pregnancies with 94 live and surviving infants (71%!). We could also show that the results in cases with an early TCO are twice as good as with a late TCO (80% vs. 40%).[12]

Similarly, good results have been obtained by other clinicians performing the TCO. In 1996 we reported the results of a multicenter evaluation, in which 11 German hospitals took part,[6] and the outcome of a total of 819 pregnancies with TCO was assessed. It emerged that the rate of surviving infants in the pregnancies before TCO had been performed was 21% compared to 74% in the pregnancies with TCO. Hormel and Künzel[10] reported similar good results.

As far as the mode of delivery is concerned, 71% of the patients with a cervical occlusion had a spontaneous delivery and 15% had an operative vaginal delivery. The rate of cesareans was 14% in comparison to 9% for the whole department at that time.[12]

In 1997 we reported the results of a follow-up examination carried out on 52 women who had previously had a TCO.[13] On the basis of these results, we can generally conclude that up to now no remarkable negative effects have been proven in connection with the operative TCO.

ETCO vs. cerclage

The cerclage is a widely used measure and there are numerous publications on it. Some authors report good results – but one should look at these reports very closely and verify whether or not cerclage had been performed on women at similar high risk (see above). But cerclage is hardly capable of preventing ascending infections because this method only tightens the cervical canal and does not close it (Figure 132.1). In our sample of women treated with ETCO, we found that in 51 previous pregnancies in which cerclage was performed, only 13 infants survived. This is a survival rate of only 26% (as compared to a survival rate of 80% with ETCO). These results underline how advisable it is to give the ETCO preference over cerclage in cases with such a critical history.

Conclusion

On the basis of previous experiences and available results, the TCO – in particular the early occlusion – is a convincingly efficient operative measure for the prevention of late abortions and early prematurity, particularly in cases where such events had previously occurred recurrently.

REFERENCES

1. Lockwood CJ, Kuczinski E. Markers of risk for preterm delivery. *J Perinat Med* 1999;27:5–20.
2. Saling E. Der frühe totale Muttermundverschluss zur Vermeidung habitueller Aborte und Frühgeburten. *Z Geburtshilfe Perinatol* 1981;185:259–61.
3. Saling E. Prevention of habitual abortion and prematurity by early total occlusion of the external os uteri. *Eur J Obstet Gynec Reprod Biol* 1984;17:165–70.
4. Szendi B. Verhinderung von fortgeschrittenen Fehl- und Frühgeburten durch vollkommenen Muttermundverschluss auf blutigem Weg. *Acta Chir II* 1961;413–8.
5. Szendi B. Vollständiges Zusammennähen des äußeren Muttermundes auf blutigem Wege zur Verhinderung von vorgeschrittenen Abortus und Frühgeburten. *Zentralbl Gynäk* 1961;83:1083–7.
6. Saling E, Schumacher E. Der operative Totale Muttermundverschluss (TMV). Erhebungen von Daten einiger Kliniken, die den TMV einsetzen. *Z Geburtshilfe Neonatol* 1996;200:82–7.
7. Saling E. Current measures to prevent late abortion or prematurity. In Saling E, ed. *Perinatology.* Nestlé Nutrition Workshop Series, vol. 26. New York: Raven Press, 1992.
8. Brandt-Niebelschütz S, Saling E, Küchler R. Weitere Erfahrungen mit der Eipol-Lavage (EPL) im Zusammenhang mit der Vermeidung von Frühgeburten. *Z Geburtshilfe Perinatol* 1992; 196:229–37.
9. Saling E, Lescinski R. Schlingeninstrument zur Blutstillung bei operativen Eingriffen an der Portio. *Z Geburtshilfe Perinatol* 1989;193: 213–20.
10. Hormel K, Künzel W. Der totale Muttermundverschluss. Prävention von Spätaborten und Frühgeburten. *Gynäkologe* 1995;28:181–6.
11. Künzel W. Epidemiologie der Frühgeburt. *Gynäkologe* 1995;28: 130–5.
12. Saling E. Infektiologische Spätabortursachen und operativer Muttermundverschluss. *Arch Gynecol Obstet* 1993;254:1265–71.
13. Saling E, Schumacher E. Ergebnisse einer Nachuntersuchung von Müttern nach vorausgegangenen operativen "Totalen Muttermund-Verschlüssen" (TMV) unter Berücksichtigung auch der Daten ihrer Kinder. *Z Geburtshilfe Neonatol* 1997;201:122–7.

133 Assessment of risk for preterm birth in asymptomatic patients and those with preterm labor

J. Espinoza, R. Romero, L. F. Gonçalves, J. P. Kusanovic and J. K. Nien

Introduction

Preterm delivery is the leading cause of neonatal mortality worldwide.[1] Several biochemical and biophysical markers have been proposed for the identification of patients at risk for preterm delivery, in both patients with threatened preterm labor and asymptomatic ones, with the hope that interventions could prevent preterm delivery. However, current interventions such as tocolysis, cerclage and antibiotic therapy have been ineffective in this regard. This may be due to the nature of these interventions, which are aimed at treating the symptoms, rather than the causes, of preterm labor or at modulating the mechanisms of disease involved in preterm parturition. Mechanisms of disease implicated in preterm labor include infection, vascular insults, stress, uterine overdistension, allergy, cervical insufficiency, hormonal disturbances and others (see Chapter 129). The clinical presentation of preterm labor may depend on (1) the intensity of the insult (i.e., microbial load or virulence), (2) the timing and duration of the insult (i.e. infection may cause abortion in the first trimester and preterm birth in the second or third trimester), and (3) the evolving nature of the host response.

This chapter will review the biophysical and biochemical markers that have been used to determine the risk of preterm birth among symptomatic and asymptomatic pregnant women.

Cervical ultrasonography to assess the risk for preterm delivery

Several investigators have examined the utility of cervical ultrasound to identify patients at risk for preterm delivery. In the early 1990s, Andersen *et al.*[2] examined the risk of preterm delivery by transabdominal and transvaginal ultrasonography, along with manual assessment of the cervix, in a group of 113 patients with singleton gestations and no cervical incompetence. Patients were examined once before 30 weeks of gestation. The patient population, with an overall prematurity rate of 15%, was not separated into low-risk and high-risk categories. Twenty-five percent of the patients with a cervical length <39 mm (50th percentile for gestational age) delivered preterm, compared to 6.7% of those with a cervical length ≥ 39 mm ($P=0.01$). When the cervical length was below 34 mm (25th percentile), 34.8% of the patients delivered prematurely, compared to 10.1% of those with a cervical length ≥ 34 mm ($P=0.003$). Using 34 mm as a cutoff point, the sensitivity and specificity of cervical length measurement by transvaginal ultrasound to identify patients at risk for preterm delivery were 47% and 84%, respectively, compared to 36% and 76% with manual assessment of the cervix.

Several studies have confirmed and extended the observations of Andersen *et al.* Details of studies performed on patients presenting with preterm labor,[3–12] asymptomatic patients at low risk for preterm delivery[2,13–17] and asymptomatic patients at high risk for preterm delivery[18–22] are presented in Tables 133.1–133.3. Only studies with adequate information to allow calculation of diagnostic indices and predictive values are included. Collectively, the information provided by these studies shows that cervical sonography is a powerful method to assess the risk of preterm delivery in patients presenting with preterm labor, low-risk asymptomatic patients, and patients at high risk for preterm delivery. Furthermore, in patients with a long cervical length, the likelihood of preterm delivery is low and, therefore,

Table 133.1 Measurement of cervical length by transvaginal ultrasound in women with symptoms of preterm labor and singleton pregnancies (adapted from Gomez *et al.*,[26] with permission)

Authors	*n*	Gestational age (weeks)	Cutoff (mm)	Definition of PTD (weeks)	Prevalence of PTD (%)	Sensitivity (%)	Specificity (%)	PPV (%)	NPV (%)
Murakawa *et al.*[3]	32	18–37	<20	<37	34	27	100	100	72
Iams *et al.*[4]	60	24–35	<30	<36	40	100	44	55	100
Gomez *et al.*[5]	59	20–35	≤18	<36	37	73	78	67	83
Rizzo *et al.*[6]	108	24–36	≤20	<37	43	68	79	71	76
Rozenberg *et al.*[7]	76	24–34	≤26	< 37	26	75	73	50	89
Cetin and Cetin[8]	65	26–35	<30	<37	74	100	46	58	100
Goffinet *et al.*[9]	108	24–34	≤27	<37	22	79	67	40	92
Hincz *et al.*[10]	82	24–34	≤31	≤28	17	100	47	28	100
Tsoi *et al.*[11]	216	24–36	≤15	Within 7 days	8	94	86	37	99
Tsoi *et al.*[12]	510	24–34	None	<35	7.1	76	OR: 0.92 (95% CI: 0.88–0.96)		

PTD, preterm delivery; PPV, positive predictive value; NPV, negative predictive value; OR, odds ratio

Table 133.2 Measurement of cervical length by ultrasound in low-risk asymptomatic pregnant women and preterm delivery rate according to different cutoff values (adapted from Chaiworapongsa *et al.*,[23] with permission)

Authors	*N*	Gestational age (weeks)	Cutoff (mm)	Definition of PTD (weeks)	Prevalence of PTD (%)	Sensitivity (%)	Specificity (%)	PPV (%)	NPV (%)
Andersen *et al.*[2]	113	<30	<39	<37	15	76	59	25	93
Tongsong *et al.*[13]	730	28–30	≤35	<37	12	66	62	20	93
Iams *et al.*[14]	2915	24	<20	<35	4	23	97	26	97
Taipale and Hiilesmaa[15]	3694	18–22	≤25	<37	2	6	100	39	99
Heath *et al.*[16]	2702	23	≤15	≤32	1.5	58	99	52	99
Hassan *et al.*[17]	6877	14–24	≤15	≤32	3.6	8	99	47	97

PTD, preterm delivery; PPV, positive predictive value; NPV, negative predictive value

avoiding aggressive intervention in the setting of premature labor may be justified.[23]

Some of the studies presented in Tables 133.1–133.3 represent significant contributions to understand the value of cervical sonography in screening for spontaneous preterm birth. These are described in greater detail below.

Cervical sonography in asymptomatic patients at low risk for preterm delivery

The Maternal–Fetal Medicine Units Network of the National Institute of Child Health and Human Development conducted a prospective cohort study entitled 'The Preterm Prediction Study'. This study evaluated the value of clinical, demographic, microbiological, biochemical and sonographic parameters in the prediction of preterm birth. Iams *et al.*[14] reported the cardinal observations of cervical sonography for the assessment of risk for preterm delivery. A total of 2915 low-risk asymptomatic patients were examined at 24 and 28 weeks of gestation by transvaginal sonography to evaluate the cervical length and calculate the risk of preterm birth. An exponential increase in the relative risk of delivering before 35 weeks was described. This large study confirmed the results of

Table 133.3 Measurement of cervical length by ultrasound in high-risk singleton gestations and preterm delivery rate according to different cutoff values

Authors	*n*	Gestational age (weeks)	Cutoff (mm)	Definition of PTD (weeks)	Prevalence of PTD (%)	Sensitivity (%)	Specificity (%)	PPV (%)	NPV (%)
Cook and	81	20	<30*	<34	20	50	89	56	86
Ellwood[18]	120	24				59	79	45	87
Andrews	53	20	≤25	<35	31	28	88	50	73
et al.[19]**	57	20–24			17	56	100	100	92
Owen *et al.*[20]	183	16–19	<25	<35	26	19	98	75	77
Guzman	469	15–24	<25	<34	11.8	76	68	20	96
et al.[21]			<15			81	72	29	96

PTD, preterm delivery; PPV, positive predictive value; NPV, negative predictive value
*Definition of abnormal in this study was a cervical length <30 mm plus dilation of the internal os of 5 mm or more; **high-risk factors: at least one prior spontaneous birth between 16 and 30 weeks

Andersen *et al.*,[2] which indicate that a short cervix increases the risk for preterm delivery, while a long cervix decreases such a risk. The study also extended the observations by allowing discernment of the comparative value of cervical length with other predictors of preterm delivery (i.e. demographic, biochemical, microbiological and clinical variables).[14]

An important series of studies reported by Heath *et al.*[16] and conducted at King's College Hospital in London examined the value of cervical sonography in screening for preterm birth. Cervical length was measured by transvaginal sonography in a low-risk population of 2702 patients. Patients with a history of preterm birth, of African-Caribbean origin, of low maternal age (< 20 years) and with a low body mass index had a shorter cervix than those without such risk factors. However, when logistic regression analysis was used to examine the contribution of all these parameters to the prediction of preterm birth (< 32 weeks), a short cervix was the only significant predictor.[24] These findings suggest that clinical and demographic risk factors associated with preterm birth operate through inducing cervical ripening. In this study, a cervix of 15 mm or less at 23 weeks of gestation in 1.7% of the population identified 60% of patients who subsequently had spontaneous preterm birth at less than 32 weeks and 80% of those who had spontaneous preterm birth at less than 28 weeks.

Hassan *et al.*[17] conducted a retrospective cohort study of 6877 women who had cervical sonography performed between 14 and 24 weeks. Examinations were conducted transabdominally and in cases of cervical length < 30 mm or suboptimal visualization, transvaginally. A cervical length of ≤15 mm had a positive predictive value of 48%, a negative predictive value of 97%, a sensitivity of 8% and a specificity of 99.7% for spontaneous preterm delivery at ≤32 weeks. A history of preterm delivery and African-American ethnicity were also associated with the occurrence of spontaneous preterm birth, although the odds ratio (OR) was considerably lower than that of a short cervix. The low sensitivity of a short cervix in this study is similar to that reported by Taipale *et al.*[15] in a large study conducted in Finland. The apparent discrepancy among the studies can be explained by the different gestational ages at which ultrasound examination was conducted. There is evidence that later scans are more predictive of preterm delivery than earlier ones. The study of Heath *et al.*[16] included exams conducted at 23 weeks, while the exams by both Hassan *et al.* and Taipale *et al.*[15] were performed at earlier gestational ages.

Cervical sonography in patients at high risk for preterm delivery

Cook *et al.*[18] conducted a prospective cohort study in 120 women considered to be at risk for preterm delivery. The patients at risk included those with a history of recurrent first-trimester loss, second-trimester loss, previous preterm delivery (< 34 weeks), previous cervical surgery and uterine anomalies. Initial cervical assessment was made between 9 and 29 weeks of gestation. Further assessments varied on weekly to monthly schedules, according to cervical findings and obstetric history. The parameters measured were cervical length, diameter and internal os dilatation. Twenty-four patients (20%) delivered before 34 weeks of gestation. Cervical length was the only significant factor found for the prediction of preterm delivery. A cervical length ≤20 mm before 20 weeks was associated with delivery before 34 weeks in 95% of the women studied.

Owen *et al.*[20] performed an observational study of 183 patients who had a history of spontaneous preterm birth before 32 weeks of gestation. The patients were enrolled between 16 and 19 weeks of gestation and were followed every 2 weeks until 24 weeks. Forty-eight (26%) women delivered before 35 weeks of gestation. A short cervix (< 25 mm) at the first scan was associated with a relative risk of 3.3 (95% CI: 2.1–5.0) for spontaneous preterm birth (< 35 weeks). The sensitivity, specificity and positive predictive values were 19%, 9% and 75%, respectively. After controlling for cervical length, neither funneling nor dynamic shortening was an independent contributor of spontaneous preterm birth. However, using the shortest cervical length on serial evaluations, after any dynamic shortening, the relative risk of a cervical length of less than 25 mm increased to 4.5 (95% CI: 2.7–7.6) with a sensitivity, specificity and positive predictive value of 69%, 80% and 55%, respectively. Therefore, based on these findings, a serial measurement through 24 weeks significantly improves the sensitivity but lowers the positive predictive value of the test.

Guzman *et al.*[25] enrolled 469 high-risk patients between 15 and 24 weeks of gestation. High risk was defined as the presence of a history of spontaneous preterm birth before 37 weeks of gestation, prior mid-trimester loss, more than two terminations of pregnancy, cone biopsy, uterine malformation, previous cerclage or diethylstilbestrol exposure. Transvaginal cervical sonography was performed and transfundal pressure was applied, and the shortest cervical length, funnel width, funnel length and cervical index were recorded serially. A cervical length of 25 mm or less had a sensitivity, specificity, positive predictive value and negative predictive value of 76%, 68%, 20% and 96%, respectively, to identify preterm birth at less than 34 weeks of gestation. Cervical length was the best parameter for the prediction of preterm birth in women with prior mid-trimester losses. The authors proposed that a cervical length of ≤ 15 mm had a sensitivity, specificity, positive predictive value and negative predictive value of 81%, 72%, 29% and 96%, respectively, in predicting spontaneous preterm delivery at less than 34 weeks. Cervical length was better at predicting earlier forms of prematurity (< 28 or < 30 weeks) than later forms (< 32 or < 34 weeks).

Odibo *et al.*[22] demonstrated the relationship between a short cervix and preterm premature rupture of membranes (PROM) leading to preterm birth in a high-risk population. They studied 69 women at high risk for preterm birth (by obstetric history and transvaginal cervical length < 25 mm) between 14 and 24 weeks of gestation. The incidence of preterm PROM was 39% (27/69). Cervical length of less than 10 mm had a sensitivity, specificity, positive predictive value and negative predictive value of 33%, 90%, 69% and 68%, respectively, in predicting preterm PROM at less than 35 weeks of gestation.

The evidence provided by these studies suggests that to prevent preterm delivery, patients with a previous history of preterm birth or mid-trimester pregnancy loss require a longer cervix than those without such a history.[23]

Cervical sonography in patients presenting with threatened preterm labor

There is now compelling evidence that examination of the cervix with ultrasound in patients presenting with preterm labor can assist in determining the risk for preterm delivery. Table 133.1 summarizes the results of some of the studies published to date. In general, the shorter the cervix, the higher the risk for preterm delivery and vice versa. Recently, Tsoi *et al.* analyzed the value of cervical length measurement for the prediction of preterm delivery at < 35 weeks among 510 pregnant women with singleton pregnancies who were admitted with symptoms of preterm labor between 24 and 34 completed weeks.[12] The authors reported that cervical length and vaginal bleeding were independent explanatory variables for the prediction of preterm delivery at < 35 weeks. However, among patients with threatened preterm labor, the inclusion of vaginal bleeding did not improve the performance of cervical length for the prediction of preterm delivery.[12]

In summary, cervical sonography is a powerful method to assess the risk of preterm delivery in asymptomatic patients and those presenting with preterm labor. In the latter group, avoiding aggressive intervention in patients who have a long cervix would probably be beneficial. In contrast, patients who have a short cervix would have a higher rate of preterm delivery and may benefit from targeted interventions (i.e. steroid administration and transfer to a center with a newborn special care unit).

Fetal fibronectin in vaginal fluid and preterm delivery

Fetal fibronectin in patients with preterm labor

Fetal fibronectin is a glycoprotein considered to be a major component of the extracellular matrix of the choriodecidual junction.[27] It has been proposed that a positive fetal fibronectin test in the second and third trimesters represents the separation of the chorion from the decidual layer of the uterus, with the release of intact or degraded chorionic components of the extracellular matrix into the cervical and vaginal secretions.[28] A growing body of evidence indicates that a positive fetal fibronectin test in cervical and/or vaginal fluid is associated with preterm delivery both in patients with threatened preterm labor[29–34] and in asymptomatic patients.[35–43] The conventional view is that the presence of fetal fibronectin in cervical and vaginal fluid before 20 weeks is due to the absence of complete fusion between the fetal membranes and the decidua.[27] However, it has recently been reported that a high concentration of fetal fibronectin in vaginal fluid between 13 and 20 weeks is also a risk factor for preterm delivery.[44] Honest *et al.* performed a systematic review that included 28 studies in asymptomatic pregnant women and 40 studies in women with threatened

Table 133.4 Likelihood ratios for positive fetal fibronectin test results of studies predicting spontaneous preterm birth before 34 weeks of gestation in asymptomatic women (adapted from Honest *et al.*,[45] with permission)

	Positive fetal fibronectin test result	Negative fetal fibronectin test result	LR(+) (95% CI)	LR(−) (95% CI)
Goldenberg *et al.*[37]	29/117	98/2812	7.27 (4.97–10.63)	0.80 (0.72–0.88)
Goldenberg *et al.*[37]	20/102	72/2329	6.20 (3.98–9.65)	0.81 (0.73–0.90)
Goldenberg *et al.*[37]	19/107	47/2403	8.00 (5.19–12.31)	0.74 (0.63–0.86)
Goldenberg *et al.*[37]	15/90	61/2222	5.88 (3.55–9.75)	0.83 (0.74–0.93)
Chang *et al.*[38]	3/5	3/229	57.0 (11.57–280.92)	0.50 (0.23–1.12)
Nageotte *et al.*[39]	12/42	1/45	2.28 (1.66–3.13)	0.13 (0.02–0.86)
Oliveira *et al.*[40]	8/34	2/18	1.29 (0.87–1.91)	0.52 (0.14–1.92)
Morrison *et al.*[41]	6/12	3/44	5.22 (2.17–12.57)	0.38 (0.15–0.97)
Morrison *et al.*[41]	4/9	2/10	1.73 (0.71–4.22)	0.54 (0.16–1.82)
Goldenberg *et al.*[44]	79/536	331/5972	2.57 (2.07–3.19)	0.87 (0.83–0.92)
Heath *et al.*[46]	15/182	30/4964	10.18 (6.56–15.80)	0.69 (0.56–0.85)
Tolino *et al.*[43]	14/32	1/36	2.75 (1.84–4.10)	0.10 (0.02–0.68)
Goldenberg *et al.*[47]	13/157	33/1713	3.58 (2.20–5.82)	0.78 (0.65–0.93)
Wennerholm *et al.*[42]	13/36	9/65	2.03 (1.24–3.31)	0.58 (0.34–0.97)
Goldenberg *et al.*[37]	11/25	36/122	1.67 (0.82–3.40)	0.89 (0.75–1.06)
Tolino *et al.*[43]	10/23	1/45	3.99 (2.39–6.66)	0.12 (0.02–0.77)
Wennerholm *et al.*[42]	7/13	12/75	4.24 (1.61–11.12)	0.69 (0.49–0.98)
Hux *et al.*[48]	3/8	1/46	7.50 (2.74–20.51)	0.28 (0.05–1.52)
Overall (95% CI)			4.01 (2.93–5.49)	0.78 (0.72–0.84)

*LR, likelihood ratio.

Table 133.5 Likelihood ratios for positive fetal fibronectin test results of studies predicting spontaneous preterm birth before 34 weeks of gestation in symptomatic women (adapted from Honest *et al.*,[45] with permission)

	Positive fetal fibronectin test result	Negative fetal fibronectin test result	LR(+) (95% CI)	LR(−) (95% CI)
Burrus *et al.*[29]	23/29	3/8	1.62 (0.93–2.83)	0.25 (0.07–0.88)
Malak *et al.*[33]	14/18	8/94	14.32 (5.22–39.26)	0.38 (0.22–0.66)
Lopez *et al.*[32]	11/20	4/65	5.70 (2.88–11.28)	0.31 (0.13–0.71)
Chuileannain *et al.*[30]	9/20	1/50	4.91 (2.77–8.70)	0.12 (0.02–0.79)
Goffeng *et al.*[31]	7/14	4/49	4.73 (2.08–10.75)	0.42 (0.19–0.93)
Parker *et al.*[34]	6/13	1/26	3.92 (1.90–8.06)	0.18 (0.03–1.13)
Cox *et al.*[49]	3/25	11/150	1.57 (0.53–4.60)	0.91 (0.69–1.20)
Nageotte *et al.*[50]	15/50	1/52	2.30 (1.73–3.06)	0.11 (0.02–0.71)
Overall (95% CI)			3.64 (2.32–5.73)	0.32 (0.16–0.66)

*LR, likelihood ratio.

preterm labor, and concluded that a positive fetal fibronectin test is a risk factor for delivery at < 34 weeks in both symptomatic and asymptomatic patients (Tables 133.4 and 133.5) and for delivery within 7–10 days in women with threatened preterm labor.[45] A negative fetal fibronectin test identifies patients at low risk for preterm delivery; however, a positive test has a limited positive predictive value.[27,45]

Table 133.6 Pooled estimates of likelihood ratios for bacterial vaginosis according to different diagnostic criteria in the prediction of spontaneous preterm birth in asymptomatic pregnant women and in those with threatened preterm labor (adapted from Honest *et al.*,[84] with permission)

Diagnostic criteria	Summary of likelihood ratio for a negative test (95% CI)	Summary of likelihood ratio for a positive test (95% CI)
Asymptomatic pregnant women		
Nugent's criteria (7 studies, n=13,729)	0.88 (0.84–0.92) (P=0.01)	1.64 (1.4–1.9) (P=0.01)
Spiegel's criteria (2 studies, n=927)	0.81 (0.64–1.0) (P=0.659)	2.4 (1.4–5.0) (P=0.498)
Clinical criteria (2 studies, n=3067)	1.00 (0.93–1.1) (P=0.49)	0.98 (0.59–1.6) (P=0.38)
Women with threatened preterm labor		
Spiegel's criteria (3 studies, n=575)	0.9 (0.73–1.00) (P=0.247)	1.3 (1.0–1.6) (P=0.04)

Bacterial vaginosis and the risk of preterm delivery

Bacterial vaginosis, a condition characterized by a change in the microbial ecosystem of the vagina,[51,52] is present in up to 15–20% of pregnant women[53–57] and is a risk factor for spontaneous preterm delivery[36,53,57–72] (Table 133.6), preterm PROM[73–76] and postpartum endometritis.[53,77] The change in the bacterial ecosystem is characterized by a decrease in the number of lactobacilli and an overgrowth of several anaerobic or facultative bacteria (such as *Mobiluncus* species, *Prevotella* species, *Gardnerella vaginalis* and genital Mycoplasmas – *Mycoplasma hominis* and *Ureaplasma urealyticum*).[52,78] Yet, despite the substantial microbial overgrowth, the conventional view has been that bacterial vaginosis is not associated with signs of inflammation (i.e. vaginal fluid leukocytes).[79–81] Hence, the condition is called vaginosis rather than vaginitis.[78,79] The reason for the absence of a local inflammatory response in most women with bacterial vaginosis, in spite of increased microbial load in the vaginal fluid, is yet to be determined. Clearly, the vaginal mucosa is capable of mounting an inflammatory response, as infections with *Trichomonas vaginalis* and *Candida* species can cause an intense inflammation that is clinically manifested as vaginitis.[82,83] Thus, it is noteworthy that bacterial vaginosis is asymptomatic in approximately 50% of patients.[51,83]

Although the cause of bacterial vaginosis is unknown, the condition can be considered as a microbial/mucosal immunity disorder. The clinical criteria for the diagnosis of bacterial vaginosis (Amsel's criteria) is based on the presence of at least three of the following findings: (1) a thin homogenous vaginal discharge; (2) vaginal pH > 4.5; (3) positive 'whiff' test (release of the amine odor with the addition of a base); and (4) clue cells on a saline wet mount.[85] However, the standard method for the diagnosis of bacterial vaginosis is a Gram stain examination of vaginal fluid.[86] Nugent *et al.* developed standardized criteria for the interpretation of the Gram stain based on the examination of four bacterial morphotypes.[87] A score of 7–10 is considered diagnostic of bacterial vaginosis. This method, both highly reproducible and reliable,[87–89] has been very helpful in advancing the state of knowledge of bacterial vaginosis. However, about 20% of women with bacterial vaginosis by Amsel's criteria have a Nugent score of 5 or 6.[90] Thus, it has been proposed that a score of 4–10, according to Nugent's criteria, should be considered to indicate 'abnormal vaginal flora'.[90]

Screening and treatment of bacterial vaginosis have been used to test whether antimicrobial agents can prevent preterm birth. The rationale behind this approach to prevent preterm parturition is that bacterial vaginosis is associated with intra-amniotic infection[57,58,70,71,91] and is a clear risk factor for preterm delivery[59,63,65,67,92,93] (Table 133.6). However, the results of randomized clinical trials have yielded conflicting results[94–107] (Table 133.7). The reader is referred to the original trials and systematic reviews for details of this controversy.[108–110]

The Centers for Disease Control, as well as some of the leaders in the field of infectious diseases in obstetrics and gynecology, have recommended that patients at high risk for preterm delivery (those with a previous history of a spontaneous preterm birth) should be screened and treated with prophylactic metronidazole or clindamycin.[108,110–116] However, a recent systematic review reported that antibiotic treatment of patients with a previous preterm birth and bacterial vaginosis in the index pregnancy does not reduce the rate of preterm birth regardless of the type of antibiotic used[116] (see Table 133.8).

Table 133.7 Treatment of bacterial vaginosis to prevent preterm birth (adapted from Riggs and Klebanoff,[116] with permission)

Study	Antibiotic	Placebo	Weight (%)	Odds ratio (95% CI)
Morales *et al.*[94]	8/44	16/36	5.93	0.28 (0.10–0.76)
McGregor *et al.*[95]	9/60	5/69	4.92	2.26 (0.71–7.16)
Hauth *et al.*[96]	54/172	42/86	11.49	0.48 (0.28–0.82)
Joesoef *et al.*[97]	51/340	46/341	13.11	1.13 (0.74–1.74)
McDonald *et al.*[105]	16/242	18/238	9.11	0.87 (0.43–1.74)
Carey *et al.*[98]	116/953	121/966	15.63	0.97 (0.74–1.27)
Gauschino *et al.*[99]	6/49	8/51	5.01	0.75 (0.24–2.34)
Kekki *et al.*[101]	9/187	7/188	5.93	1.31 (0.48–3.59)
Odendaal *et al.*[102]	42/136	25/133	10.94	1.93 (1.09–3.40)
Andrews *et al.*[103]	11/86	15/99	7.49	0.82 (0.36–1.90)
Ugwumadu *et al.*[104]	19/244	31/241	10.44	0.57 (0.31–1.04)
Overall (95% CI)	2513	2448	100.00	0.89 (0.66–1.20)

Bacterial vaginosis, tumor necrosis factor alpha (TNF-α) allele 2 and the risk of preterm birth

Macones *et al.*[117] reported the results of a case–control study in which cases were defined as patients who had a spontaneous preterm delivery (defined as < 37 weeks) and controls as women who delivered after 37 weeks. The environmental exposure was clinically diagnosed bacterial vaginosis (symptomatic vaginal discharge, a positive whiff test and clue cells on a wet preparation). The genotype of interest was TNF-α allele 2, given that carriage of this genotype had been demonstrated by the author to be associated with spontaneous preterm birth in previous studies.[118] The key observations were: (1) clinically diagnosed bacterial vaginosis associated with an increased risk for preterm delivery (OR: 3.3; 95% CI 1.8–5.9); (2) women who carried the TNF-α allele 2 were also at increased risk for preterm birth (OR: 2.7; 95% CI 1.7–4.5); and (3) patients with both bacterial vaginosis and the TNF-α allele 2 had an OR of 6.1 (95% CI 1.9–21) for spontaneous preterm delivery, suggesting that a gene–environmental interaction predisposes to preterm birth. These estimates were derived from logistic regression and are referred to Table 133.9.

The significance of this observation is that bacterial vaginosis, in a host defined by genotype analysis, substantially increases the risk for spontaneous preterm delivery. However, it is noteworthy that these patients had clinical symptoms requiring treatment with metronidazole and, thus, were different from those included in a large randomized clinical trial of bacterial vaginosis that included patients with an abnormal Gram stain of vaginal fluid, but excluded symptomatic women. It is possible that symptomatic women could have not only a change in the vaginal microflora (bacterial vaginosis), but also inflammatory changes and, hence, symptoms.

Table 133.8 Treatment of bacterial vaginosis to prevent preterm birth in women with a previous preterm birth (adapted from Riggs and Klebanoff,[116] with permission)

Study	Antibiotic	Odds ratio (95% CI)
Morales *et al.*[94]	Metronidazole	0.28 (0.10–0.76)
Hauth *et al.*[96]	Metronidazole + erythromycin	0.48 (0.25–0.91)
McDonald *et al.*[105]	Metronidazole	0.11 (0.01–1.09)
Carey *et al.*[98]	Metronidazole	1.35 (0.73–2.49)
Odendaal *et al.*[102]	Metronidazole	2.44 (1.09–5.43)
Ugwumadu *et al.*[104]	Clindamycin	0.33 (0.12–0.95)
Overall (95% CI)		0.61 (0.28–1.34)

Macones *et al.*[117] have called for additional studies that would allow confirmation of these findings. Such investigations are necessary in light of the recent history of conflicting results of genetic association studies.[117–122] However, if these observations are confirmed there may be substantial implications. For example, serious consideration would need to be given to the incorporation of genotype assessment in the design of clinical studies to reduce the rate of preterm birth. Assessment of the local host response (vaginal inflammation) and determination of the genotype may be required to identify patients who might benefit from intervention. Clearly, relying on the Gram stain for the diagnosis of bacterial vaginosis has not been sufficient.

Table 133.9 Contingency table to estimate genetic, environmental and gene–environment effects (adapted from Romero *et al.*,[122] with permission)

Environmental	Genotype	Cases	Controls	Odds ratio (95% CI)	Type
BV	TNF-α2				
–	–	57	171	1	
–	+	29	49	1.8 (1.0–3.1)	Genetic
+	–	12	22	1.6 (0.8–3.5)	Environmental
+	+	27	8	10.1 (4.4–23.5)	Interaction

BV = vacterial vaginosis; TNF-α 2 = tumor necrosis factor-alpha allele 2. Raw data provided by Macones *et al.*

Home uterine monitoring and the risk for preterm delivery

The assessment of the frequency of uterine contractions has been proposed to identify those at risk for preterm delivery in both asymptomatic[123,124] and symptomatic pregnant patients.[125] The rationale for this is that increased frequency of uterine contractions leads to preterm delivery. Thus, early detection and suppression of uterine contractions could potentially reduce the rate of preterm delivery. However, the results of randomized clinical trials have indicated that ambulatory uterine monitoring has not reduced the rate of preterm delivery.[126–130] For example, in 1995, the Collaborative Home Uterine Monitoring Study (CHUMS) group reported the results of a multicenter randomized controlled trial of home uterine monitoring.[126] The authors randomized 1292 pregnant women between 24 and 36 weeks of gestation at high risk of preterm labor or birth into home uterine activity monitoring with either active (data revealed) or sham (data concealed) devices. Seventy-two percent of these patients (n=842) completed the study. The data analysis was performed according to the intent to treat. The results of the study indicated that there were no differences in the rate of preterm birth, referral rates to the hospital, unscheduled emergency visits or antepartum admissions between the two arms of the study. Recently, Iams *et al.* demonstrated that the limited use of ambulatory uterine monitoring is due to its low sensitivity and a low positive predictive value of preterm delivery in both low- and high-risk patients[131] (Table 133.10).

Garfield *et al.*[132] proposed that more sensitive methods to measure uterine activity, such as uterine electromyography (a non-invasive assessment of uterine electrical signals) may allow for a more objective evaluation of uterine activity. The authors reported that the power spectrum peak frequency within the uterine electrical burst remained relatively low in patients with preterm labor, but increased dramatically 4 days prior to delivery. The authors proposed that uterine electromyography may predict preterm birth within 4 days of the evaluation.[133] The value of this technique to evaluate the risk of preterm delivery has not yet been determined.

Table 133.10 Diagnostic indices of ambulatory uterine monitoring for the prediction of delivery at < 35 weeks (adapted from Iams *et al.*,[131] with permission)

Test	Weeks of gestation at time of testing		
	22–24	27–28	31–32
Maximum nighttime contraction frequency ≥ 4/h			
Sensitivity	8.6	28.1	27.3
Specificity	96.4	88.7	82.0
Positive predictive value	25.0	23.1	11.3
Negative predictive value	88.3	91.1	93.0
Maximum daytime contraction frequency ≥ 4/h			
Sensitivity	0	12.9	13.6
Specificity	98.4	93.9	84.9
Positive predictive value	0	20.0	7.1
Negative predictive value	87.0	90.2	92.1

Values expressed as percentage

Corticotropin releasing hormone (CRH) and the risk of preterm delivery

A decade ago, McLean *et al.* proposed the existence of a 'placental clock' (which is active from an early stage in human pregnancy) that determines the length of gestation and the timing of parturition.[134] This proposal was based on the result of a large longitudinal study in which women who delivered preterm had a significantly higher plasma concentration of CRH than those who delivered at term. In contrast, women who had prolonged pregnancies had a lower CRH concentration than those who delivered at term. Of note, these differences were already present at 16–18 weeks of gestation.[134] The association between a high maternal plasma concentration of CRH and preterm labor has been confirmed by other studies.[135–137] Moreover, high plasma concentrations of CRH have been described in women with chronic stress, and this condition has been associated with a high risk for preterm delivery.[137] According to 'the placental clock hypothesis', the rate of increase in the maternal plasma CRH through pregnancy determines the timing of labor when saturation of the CRH binding protein is achieved and free CRH becomes available and triggers parturition.[134,138] However, Inder *et al.*[139] reported that a plasma concentration of CRH at 26 weeks of gestation of >90 pmol/l had a sensitivity of 45%, specificity of 94%, and positive predictive value of 46.7% for the prediction of preterm delivery. Based on these results, the authors suggested that maternal plasma CRH may identify patients at risk for preterm delivery, but it may not be a good screening method for preterm delivery.[139]

Salivary estriol and the risk of preterm delivery

McGregor *et al.*[140] performed a longitudinal study that included 241 singleton pregnancies with women at low [30% (72/241)] and high risk [70% (169/241)] for preterm labor. The authors measured salivary estriol concentration at least once a week from 22 weeks onward, and reported that patients who delivered at <37 weeks of gestation had a higher salivary estriol concentration than those who delivered at term. Moreover, a cutoff of 2.3 ng/ml had a sensitivity, specificity and false-positive rate of 71%, 77% and 23%, respectively, for the prediction of preterm delivery. The authors proposed that determination of salivary estriol concentration would be more accurate than clinical risk assessment in the prediction of preterm birth.[140] In a larger, more recent study, the same group of investigators reported that a cutoff of 2.1 ng/ml had a sensitivity, specificity, and positive and negative predictive values of 57%, 78%, 9% and 98%, respectively, for the prediction of preterm delivery.[141] Furthermore, the authors reported that the risk of preterm delivery was higher if a second salivary sample, collected within a week of the first sample, was also positive.[141,142] Collectively, this evidence indicates that a high concentration of salivary estriol is a risk factor for preterm birth, but it is unlikely to become a useful screening index because of the low positive predictive value.

Evidence of thrombin generation and the risk of preterm delivery

Thrombin is a multifunctional serine protease that results from the proteolysis of the prothrombin molecule into thrombin and prothrombin fragments 1 and 2. This protease plays a central role in the coagulation cascade by catalyzing the conversion of fibrinogen into fibrin and activating clotting factors (factors V and VIII).[143] Natural anticoagulant mechanisms limit thrombin action by binding antithrombin III to form a stable stoichiometric complex with thrombin, also known as the thrombin-antithrombin (TAT) complex.[144] TAT concentrations in plasma are widely considered to be an index of *in vivo* thrombin generation and, therefore, of activation of the coagulation cascade.

Normal pregnancy is a state in which there is excessive thrombin generation, as indicated by an increased concentration of fibrinopeptide A, prothrombin fragments 1 and 2, and TAT complexes.[144–146] Elovitz *et al.*[147] performed a case–control study of patients with preterm labor ($n=19$) and controls ($n=24$) between 24 and 32 completed weeks of gestation. The authors reported that the mean plasma TAT concentration was significantly higher in patients who delivered within 3 weeks (7.8 ± 2.86 ng/ml) of blood sampling than in those who delivered after 3 weeks (5.57 ± 1.69 ng/ml; $P<0.05$) and those in the control group (5.77 ± 1.43; $P<0.05$). A maternal plasma TAT cutoff of 6.8 ng/ml as determined by a receiver operating curve analysis, had a sensitivity of 80%, specificity of 71%, positive predictive value of 50%, and negative predictive value of 91% for the prediction of preterm delivery within 7 days. Similarly, a maternal plasma TAT concentration greater than 6.3 ng/ml had a sensitivity of 75%, specificity of 73%, positive predictive value of 67%, and negative predictive value of 73% for the prediction of preterm delivery within 3 weeks.[147] These observations are consistent with our previous report that women with preterm labor and intact membranes and preterm PROM had significantly higher median plasma TAT complex concentrations than normal pregnant women.[148] Collectively, these results indicate that preterm parturition is associated with an excess of thrombin generation, which may precede the clinical presentation of preterm labor.

Value of combining cervical ultrasonographic data and other biological markers of preterm delivery

Preterm delivery is a multifactorial condition and, therefore, individual screening tests are inherently limited in predicting all preterm births.[149] It has been recently suggested that to improve the sensitivity of cervical length assessment by ultrasound, new studies should focus on the development of scoring systems that combine ultrasound data with biochemical, hormonal and molecular diagnostic methods (e.g. fetal DNA assessment in maternal blood).[149,150]

Biomarkers in cervicovaginal secretions, cervical ultrasonography and the risk of preterm delivery

A positive fetal fibronectin test[6,7,10,26,46,93,151] or increased cytokine concentrations in cervicovaginal fluid[152] increase the predictive value of cervical ultrasonography to identify patients at risk for preterm delivery. Rizzo *et al.*[6] studied 180 patients with preterm labor and intact membranes and found that the combination of a cervical index $\geq$0.5 and a positive fibronectin test ($\geq$60 ng/mL) was more efficient than each test alone in the prediction of the admission-to-delivery interval. Similar findings were reported by Hincz *et al.*,[10] who proposed a two-step approach to the examination of patients with preterm labor. In their study, a positive fetal fibronectin test in patients with a cervical length between 21 and 30 mm was associated with a shorter admission-to-delivery interval (38.6 days, 95% CI: 26.7–50.4 vs. 109.2 days, 95% CI: 97.8–120.7; $P < 0.001$). More recently, Gomez *et al.*[26] measured cervical length and fibronectin concentrations in the vaginal fluid of 215 patients with preterm uterine contractions, intact membranes and cervical dilation $\leq$3 cm by digital examination. Although both tests had a comparable performance for the prediction of spontaneous preterm delivery, significant improvement was observed when fetal fibronectin results were added to those of cervical length.

Rizzo *et al.*[152] have also demonstrated that increased interleukin-8 concentrations in cervicovaginal fluid and a short cervix by ultrasonographic examination were independently associated with positive amniotic fluid cultures and histological chorioamnionitis. More recently, Kurkinen-Raty *et al.*,[153] using logistic regression analysis, proposed that a combination of interleukin-6 > 61 ng/l, interleukin-8 > 3739 ng/l and a cervical index > 0.36 improved the prediction of preterm delivery over that achieved with the use of each of these tests alone.

Collectively, the evidence reviewed in this chapter indicates that biophysical markers, biochemical markers, or a combination of both may identify patients at risk for preterm delivery. However, interventions aimed at modifying some of these markers have failed to prevent preterm delivery. This lack of effectiveness may be due to: (1) the limitations of the current tests, (2) inadequate interventions, (3) the timing of the interventions, and (4) an incorrect conceptual framework. We have proposed that preterm labor is one of the great obstetrical syndromes[154,155] together with SGA, preeclampsia, preterm PROM and fetal death. Thus, preterm labor has multiple etiologies, is chronic in nature and is frequently associated with fetal disease, and the clinical manifestations in both the mother and the fetus may be adaptive in nature (Chapter 129). Moreover, these manifestations may depend on the maternal and fetal gene–environment interaction. Therefore, it is not surprising that symptomatic treatment of preterm labor has been ineffective thus far.

Two main strategies have been used in the search for biomarkers for preterm delivery. The hypothesis-driven technique is a deductive scientific method used in most of the studies reviewed in this chapter. However, an alternative approach is provided by 'discovery science', an inductive scientific method that includes the so-called 'omics' sciences (genomics, transcriptomics, proteomics and metabolomics). These discovery techniques have been used to improve the taxonomy of the preterm labor syndrome.[156,157] Our group has recently reported that patients with preterm labor who delivered at term, those with infection/inflammation who delivered preterm and, more importantly, those without infection/inflammation who delivered preterm have a stereotypical metabolic profile. Indeed, unsupervised metabolomics analysis was able to discriminate these groups with 88.5% accuracy.[158] Discovery sciences hold the promise of accelerating the understanding of the mechanisms of disease of the great obstetrical syndromes, which may potentially provide better tools to identify women at risk for preterm delivery and guide the design of interventions aimed not at the symptoms but at the underlying causes of the disease or at modulating the mechanisms of disease (i.e. interleukin-10 or dexamethasone for modulation of intra-amniotic inflammation[159]). An intervention tailored to the mechanisms of disease and the genetic makeup of the mother/fetus is likely to be more effective in preventing preterm delivery than traditional interventions.

REFERENCES

1. Lawn JE, Cousens S, Zupan J. 4 million neonatal deaths: When? where? why? *Lancet* 2005;365:891–900.
2. Andersen HF, Nugent CE, Wanty SD, Hayashi RH. Prediction of risk for preterm delivery by ultrasonographic measurement of cervical length. *Am J Obstet Gynecol* 1990;163:859–67.
3. Murakawa H, Utumi T, Hasegawa I, Tanaka K, Fuzimori R. Evaluation of threatened preterm delivery by transvaginal ultrasonographic measurement of cervical length. *Obstet Gynecol* 1993;82:829–32.
4. Iams JD, Paraskos J, Landon MB, Teteris JN, Johnson FF. Cervical sonography in preterm labor. *Obstet Gynecol* 1994;84:40–6.
5. Gomez R, Galasso M, Romero R, *et al.* Ultrasonographic examination of the uterine cervix is better than cervical digital examination as a predictor of the likelihood of premature delivery in patients with preterm labor and intact membranes. *Am J Obstet Gynecol* 1994;171:956–64.
6. Rizzo G, Capponi A, Arduini D, Lorido C, Romanini C. The value of fetal fibronectin in cervical and vaginal secretions and of

ultrasonographic examination of the uterine cervix in predicting premature delivery for patients with preterm labor and intact membranes. *Am J Obstet Gynecol* 1996;175:1146–51.

7. Rozenberg P, Goffinet F, Malagrida L, *et al.* Evaluating the risk of preterm delivery: A comparison of fetal fibronectin and transvaginal ultrasonographic measurement of cervical length. *Am J Obstet Gynecol* 1997;176:196–9.
8. Cetin M, Cetin A. The role of transvaginal sonography in predicting recurrent preterm labour in patients with intact membranes. *Eur J Obstet Gynecol Reprod Biol* 1997;74:7–11.
9. Goffinet F, Rozenberg P, Kayem G, Perdu M, Philippe HJ, Nisand I. The value of intravaginal ultrasonography of the cervix uteri for evaluation of the risk of premature labor (in French). *J Gynecol Obstet Biol Reprod (Paris)* 1997;26:623–9.
10. Hincz P, Wilczynski J, Kozarzewski M, Szaflik K. Two-step test: The combined use of fetal fibronectin and sonographic examination of the uterine cervix for prediction of preterm delivery in symptomatic patients. *Acta Obstet Gynecol Scand* 2002;81: 58–63.
11. Tsoi E, Akmal S, Rane S, Otigbah C, Nicolaides KH. Ultrasound assessment of cervical length in threatened preterm labor. *Ultrasound Obstet Gynecol* 2003;21:552–5.
12. Tsoi E, Fuchs IB, Rane S, Geerts L, Nicolaides KH. Sonographic measurement of cervical length in threatened preterm labor in singleton pregnancies with intact membranes. *Ultrasound Obstet Gynecol* 2005;25:353–6.
13. Tongsong T, Kamprapanth P, Srisomboon J, Wanapirak C, Piyamongkol W, Sirichotiyakul S. Single transvaginal sonographic measurement of cervical length early in the third trimester as a predictor of preterm delivery. *Obstet Gynecol* 1995;86:184–7.
14. Iams JD, Goldenberg RL, Meis PJ, *et al.* The length of the cervix and the risk of spontaneous premature delivery. National Institute of Child Health and Human Development Maternal Fetal Medicine Unit Network. *New Engl J Med* 1996;334:567–72.
15. Taipale P, Hiilesmaa V. Sonographic measurement of uterine cervix at 18–22 weeks' gestation and the risk of preterm delivery. *Obstet Gynecol* 1998;92:902–7.
16. Heath VC, Southall TR, Souka AP, Elisseou A, Nicolaides KH. Cervical length at 23 weeks of gestation: Prediction of spontaneous preterm delivery. *Ultrasound Obstet Gynecol* 1998;12: 312–7.
17. Hassan SS, Romero R, Berry SM, *et al.* Patients with an ultrasonographic cervical length < or =15 mm have nearly a 50% risk of early spontaneous preterm delivery. *Am J Obstet Gynecol* 2000; 182:1458–67.
18. Cook CM, Ellwood DA. The cervix as a predictor of preterm delivery in 'at-risk' women. *Ultrasound Obstet Gynecol* 2000;15: 109–13.
19. Andrews WW, Copper R, Hauth JC, Goldenberg RL, Neely C, Dubard M. Second-trimester cervical ultrasound: Associations with increased risk for recurrent early spontaneous delivery. *Obstet Gynecol* 2000;95:222–6.
20. Owen J, Yost N, Berghella V, Thom E, *et al.* Mid-trimester endovaginal sonography in women at high risk for spontaneous preterm birth. *J Am Med Assoc* 2001;286:1340–8.
21. Guzman ER, Walters C, Ananth CV, *et al.* A comparison of sonographic cervical parameters in predicting spontaneous preterm birth in high-risk singleton gestations. *Ultrasound Obstet Gynecol* 2001;18:204–10.
22. Odibo AO, Berghella V, Reddy U, Tolosa JE, Wapner RJ. Does transvaginal ultrasound of the cervix predict preterm premature rupture of membranes in a high-risk population? *Ultrasound Obstet Gynecol* 2001;18:223–7.
23. Chaiworapongsa T, Espinoza J, Kalache K, Gervasi MT, Romero R. Sonographic examination of the uterine cervix. In Chervenak F, Kurjak A, Papp Z, eds. *The Fetus as a Patient: The Evolving Challenge.* New York: Parthenon Publishing, 2002:90–117.
24. Heath VC, Southall TR, Souka AP, Novakov A, Nicolaides KH. Cervical length at 23 weeks of gestation: Relation to demographic characteristics and previous obstetric history. *Ultrasound Obstet Gynecol* 1998;12:304–11.
25. Guzman ER, Mellon C, Vintzileos AM, Ananth CV, Walters C, Gipson K. Longitudinal assessment of endocervical canal length between 15 and 24 weeks' gestation in women at risk for pregnancy loss or preterm birth. *Obstet Gynecol* 1998;92:31–7.
26. Gomez R, Romero R, Medina L, *et al.* Cervicovaginal fibronectin improves the prediction of preterm delivery based on sonographic cervical length in patients with preterm uterine contractions and intact membranes. *Am J Obstet Gynecol* 2005;192:350–9.
27. Leitich H, Kaider A. Fetal fibronectin – How useful is it in the prediction of preterm birth? *Br J Obstet Gynaecol* 2003; 110(Suppl 20):66–70.
28. Lockwood CJ, Senyei AE, Dische MR, *et al.* Fetal fibronectin in cervical and vaginal secretions as a predictor of preterm delivery. *N Engl J Med* 1991;325:669–74.
29. Burrus DR, Ernest JM, Veille JC. Fetal fibronectin, interleukin-6, and C-reactive protein are useful in establishing prognostic subcategories of idiopathic preterm labor. *Am J Obstet Gynecol* 1995; 173:1258–62.
30. Chuileannain FN, Bell R, Brennecke S. Cervicovaginal fetal fibronectin testing in threatened preterm labour – Translating research findings into clinical practice. *Aust N Z J Obstet Gynaecol* 1998;38:399–402.
31. Goffeng AR, Holst E, Milsom I, Lindstedt G, Lundberg PA, Andersch B. Fetal fibronectin and microorganisms in vaginal fluid of women with complicated pregnancies. *Acta Obstet Gynecol Scand* 1997;76:521–7.
32. Lopez RL, Francis JA, Garite TJ, Dubyak JM. Fetal fibronectin detection as a predictor of preterm birth in actual clinical practice. *Am J Obstet Gynecol* 2000;182:1103–6.
33. Malak TM, Sizmur F, Bell SC, Taylor DJ. Fetal fibronectin in cervicovaginal secretions as a predictor of preterm birth. *Br J Obstet Gynaecol* 1996;103:648–53.
34. Parker J, Bell R, Brennecke S. Fetal fibronectin in the cervicovaginal fluid of women with threatened preterm labour as a predictor of delivery before 34 weeks' gestation. *Aust N Z J Obstet Gynaecol* 1995;35:257–61.
35. Goldenberg RL, Iams JD, Miodovnik M, *et al.* The preterm prediction study: Risk factors in twin gestations. National Institute of Child Health and Human Development Maternal–Fetal Medicine Units Network. *Am J Obstet Gynecol* 1996;175:1047–53.
36. Goldenberg RL, Thom E, Moawad AH, Johnson F, Roberts J, Caritis SN. The preterm prediction study: Fetal fibronectin, bacterial vaginosis, and peripartum infection. NICHD Maternal Fetal Medicine Units Network. *Obstet Gynecol* 1996;87:656–60.
37. Goldenberg RL, Mercer BM, Meis PJ, Copper RL, Das A, McNellis D. The preterm prediction study: Fetal fibronectin testing and spontaneous preterm birth. NICHD Maternal Fetal Medicine Units Network. *Obstet Gynecol* 1996;87:643–8.
38. Chang TC, Chew TS, Pang M, Tan AC, Yeo GS. Cervicovaginal foetal fibronectin in the prediction of preterm labour in a low-risk population. *Ann Acad Med Sing* 1997;26:776–80.
39. Nageotte MP, Casal D, Senyei AE. Fetal fibronectin in patients at increased risk for premature birth. *Am J Obstet Gynecol* 1994; 170:20–5.
40. Oliveira T, de Souza E, Mariani-Neto C, Camano L. Fetal fibronectin as a predictor of preterm delivery in twin gestations. *Int J Gynaecol Obstet* 1998;62:135–9.
41. Morrison JC, Naef RW III, Botti JJ, Katz M, Belluomini JM, McLaughlin BN. Prediction of spontaneous preterm birth by fetal fibronectin and uterine activity. *Obstet Gynecol* 1996;87:649–55.
42. Wennerholm UB, Holm B, Mattsby-Baltzer I, *et al.* Fetal fibronectin, endotoxin, bacterial vaginosis and cervical length as predictors of preterm birth and neonatal morbidity in twin pregnancies. *Br J Obstet Gynaecol* 1997;104:1398–404.
43. Tolino A, Ronsini S, Zullo F, Pellicano M, Regine V, Nappi C. Fetal fibronectin as a screening test for premature delivery in multiple pregnancies. *Int J Gynaecol Obstet* 1996;52:3–7.
44. Goldenberg RL, Klebanoff M, Carey JC, *et al.* Vaginal fetal fibronectin measurements from 8 to 22 weeks' gestation and subsequent spontaneous preterm birth. *Am J Obstet Gynecol* 2000;183:469–75.
45. Honest H, Bachmann LM, Gupta JK, Kleijnen J, Khan KS. Accuracy of cervicovaginal fetal fibronectin test in predicting risk of spontaneous preterm birth: Systematic review. *Br Med J* 2002;325:301–10.
46. Heath VC, Daskalakis G, Zagaliki A, Carvalho M, Nicolaides KH. Cervicovaginal fibronectin and cervical length at 23 weeks of gestation: Relative risk of early preterm delivery. *Br J Obstet Gynaecol* 2000;107:1276–81.
47. Goldenberg RL, Mercer BM, Iams JD, Moawad AH, Meis PJ, Das A, McNellis D, Miodovnik M, Menard MK, Caritis SN, Thurnau GR, Bottoms SF. The preterm prediction study: patterns of cervicovaginal fetal fibronectin as predictors of spontaneous preterm delivery. National Institute of Child Health and Human Development Maternal-Fetal Medicine Units Network. *Am J Obstet Gynecol* 1997;177(1):8–12.
48. Hux CH, Trolice MP, Kadar N. The value of a single fetal fibronectin assay as a screen for preterm labor and delivery. *J Matern Fetal Med* 1995;4:100–4.

49. Cox S, Little B, Dax J, Leveno K. Fetal fibronectin and preterm delivery. *Am J Obstet Gynecol* 1996;174:306. Abstract 9.
50. Nageotte MP, Hollenbach KA, Vanderwahl BA, Hutch KM. Oncofetal fibronectin in patients at increased risk for preterm delivery. *Am J Obstet Gynecol* 1992;166:274. Abstract 1.
51. Eschenbach DA, Hillier S, Critchlow C, Stevens C, DeRouen T, Holmes KK. Diagnosis and clinical manifestations of bacterial vaginosis. *Am J Obstet Gynecol* 1988;158:819–28.
52. Spiegel CA. Bacterial vaginosis. *Clin Microbiol Rev* 1991;4: 485–502.
53. Eschenbach DA, Gravett MG, Chen KC, Hoyme UB, Holmes KK. Bacterial vaginosis during pregnancy. An association with prematurity and postpartum complications. *Scand J Urol Nephrol Suppl* 1984;86:213–22.
54. McGregor JA, French JI. Bacterial vaginosis in pregnancy. *Obstet Gynecol Surv* 2000;55:S1–19.
55. Ugwumadu AH. Bacterial vaginosis in pregnancy. *Curr Opin Obstet Gynecol* 2002;14:115–8.
56. Sobel JD. Bacterial vaginosis. *Annu Rev Med* 2000;51:349–56.
57. Eschenbach DA. Bacterial vaginosis and anaerobes in obstetric-gynecologic infection. *Clin Infect Dis* 1993;16(Suppl 4): S282–7.
58. Gibbs RS. Chorioamnionitis and bacterial vaginosis. *Am J Obstet Gynecol* 1993;169:460–2.
59. Hillier SL, Nugent RP, Eschenbach DA, *et al.* Association between bacterial vaginosis and preterm delivery of a low-birth-weight infant. The Vaginal Infections and Prematurity Study Group. *N Engl J Med* 1995;333:1737–42.
60. Meis PJ, Goldenberg RL, Mercer B, *et al.* The preterm prediction study: Significance of vaginal infections. National Institute of Child Health and Human Development Maternal-Fetal Medicine Units Network. *Am J Obstet Gynecol* 1995;173:1231–5.
61. Goepfert AR, Goldenberg RL. Prediction of prematurity. *Curr Opin Obstet Gynecol* 1996;8:417–27.
62. Carey JC, Klebanoff MA. What have we learned about vaginal infections and preterm birth? *Semin Perinatol* 2003;27:212–6.
63. Flynn CA, Helwig AL, Meurer LN. Bacterial vaginosis in pregnancy and the risk of prematurity: A meta-analysis. *J Fam Pract* 1999;48:885–92.
64. Riduan JM, Hillier SL, Utomo B, Wiknjosastro G, Linnan M, Kandun N. Bacterial vaginosis and prematurity in Indonesia: Association in early and late pregnancy. *Am J Obstet Gynecol* 1993;169:175–8.
65. Kimberlin DF, Andrews WW. Bacterial vaginosis: Association with adverse pregnancy outcome. *Semin Perinatol* 1998;22: 242–50.
66. Paige DM, Augustyn M, Adih WK, Witter F, Chang J. Bacterial vaginosis and preterm birth: A comprehensive review of the literature. *J Nurse Midwifery* 1998;43:83–9.
67. Chaim W, Mazor M, Leiberman JR. The relationship between bacterial vaginosis and preterm birth. A review. *Arch Gynecol Obstet* 1997;259:51–8.
68. Subtil D, Denoit V, Le Goueff F, Husson MO, Trivier D, Puech F. The role of bacterial vaginosis in preterm labor and preterm birth: A case–control study. *Eur J Obstet Gynecol Reprod Biol* 2002; 101:41–6.
69. Newton ER, Piper J, Peairs W. Bacterial vaginosis and intraamniotic infection. *Am J Obstet Gynecol* 1997;176:672–7.
70. Martius J, Eschenbach DA. The role of bacterial vaginosis as a cause of amniotic fluid infection, chorioamnionitis and prematurity – A review. *Arch Gynecol Obstet* 1990;247:1–13.
71. Silver HM, Sperling RS, St Clair PJ, Gibbs RS. Evidence relating bacterial vaginosis to intraamniotic infection. *Am J Obstet Gynecol* 1989;161:808–12.
72. Hay PE, Lamont RF, Taylor-Robinson D, Morgan DJ, Ison C, Pearson J. Abnormal bacterial colonisation of the genital tract and subsequent preterm delivery and late miscarriage. *Br Med J* 1994; 308:295–8.
73. Gravett MG, Nelson HP, DeRouen T, Critchlow C, Eschenbach DA, Holmes KK. Independent associations of bacterial vaginosis and Chlamydia trachomatis infection with adverse pregnancy outcome. *J Am Med Assoc* 1986;256:1899–903.
74. Reynolds HD. Bacterial vaginosis and its implication in preterm labor and premature rupture of membranes. A review of the literature. *J Nurse Midwifery* 1991;36:289–96.
75. McGregor JA, French JI, Seo K. Premature rupture of membranes and bacterial vaginosis. *Am J Obstet Gynecol* 1993;169: 463–6.
76. Lamont RF. Recent evidence associated with the condition of preterm prelabour rupture of the membranes. *Curr Opin Obstet Gynecol* 2003;15:91–9.
77. Jacobsson B, Pernevi P, Chidekel L, Jorgen Platz-Christensen J. Bacterial vaginosis in early pregnancy may predispose for preterm birth and postpartum endometritis. *Acta Obstet Gynecol Scand* 2002;81:1006–10.
78. French JI, McGregor JA. Bacterial vaginosis. In Faro S, Soper DE, eds. *Infectious Diseases in Women.* Philadelphia: W. B. Saunders Company, 2001:221–39.
79. Donders GG, Bosmans E, Dekeersmaecker A, Vereecken A, Van Bulck B, Spitz B. Pathogenesis of abnormal vaginal bacterial flora. *Am J Obstet Gynecol* 2000;182:872–8.
80. Hill LV. Anaerobes and Gardnerella vaginalis in non-specific vaginitis. *Genitourin Med* 1985;61:114–9.
81. Blackwell A, Barlow D. Clinic diagnosis of anaerobic vaginosis (non-specific vaginitis). A practical guide. *Br J Vener Dis* 1982;58: 387–93.
82. Steele C, Fidel PL Jr. Cytokine and chemokine production by human oral and vaginal epithelial cells in response to Candida albicans. *Infect Immun* 2002;70:577–83.
83. Sobel JD. Vaginitis. *N Engl J Med* 1997;337:1896–903.
84. Honest H, Bachmann LM, Knox EM, Gupta JK, Kleijnen J, Khan KS. The accuracy of various tests for bacterial vaginosis in predicting preterm birth: A systematic review. *Br J Obstet Gynaecol* 2004;111:409–22.
85. Amsel R, Totten PA, Spiegel CA, Chen KC, Eschenbach D, Holmes KK. Nonspecific vaginitis. Diagnostic criteria and microbial and epidemiologic associations. *Am J Med* 1983;74:14–22.
86. Spiegel CA, Amsel R, Holmes KK. Diagnosis of bacterial vaginosis by direct gram stain of vaginal fluid. *J Clin Microbiol* 1983;18: 170–7.
87. Nugent RP, Krohn MA, Hillier SL. Reliability of diagnosing bacterial vaginosis is improved by a standardized method of gram stain interpretation. *J Clin Microbiol* 1991;29:297–301.
88. Schwebke JR, Hillier SL, Sobel JD, McGregor JA, Sweet RL. Validity of the vaginal gram stain for the diagnosis of bacterial vaginosis. *Obstet Gynecol* 1996;88:573–6.
89. Nelson DB, Macones G. Bacterial vaginosis in pregnancy: Current findings and future directions. *Epidemiol Rev* 2002;24: 102–8.
90. Cauci S. Biomarkers for adverse pregnancy outcome in vaginal fluid associated with altered vaginal flora. 2004.
91. Hillier SL, Martius J, Krohn M, Kiviat N, Holmes KK, Eschenbach DA. A case–control study of chorioamnionic infection and histologic chorioamnionitis in prematurity. *N Engl J Med* 1988;319:972–8.
92. Hill GB. Preterm birth: Associations with genital and possibly oral microflora. *Ann Periodontol* 1998;3:222–32.
93. Goldenberg RL, Iams JD, Mercer BM, *et al.* The preterm prediction study: The value of new vs standard risk factors in predicting early and all spontaneous preterm births. NICHD MFMU Network. *Am J Public Health* 1998;88:233–8.
94. Morales WJ, Schorr S, Albritton J. Effect of metronidazole in patients with preterm birth in preceding pregnancy and bacterial vaginosis: A placebo-controlled, double-blind study. *Am J Obstet Gynecol* 1994;171:345–7.
95. McGregor JA, French JI, Jones W, Milligan K, McKinney PJ, Patterson E, Parker R. Bacterial vaginosis is associated with prematurity and vaginal fluid mucinase and sialidase: results of a controlled trial of topical clindamycin cream. *Am J Obstet Gynecol* 1994;170(4):1048–60.
96. Hauth JC, Goldenberg RL, Andrews WW, DuBard MB, Copper RL. Reduced incidence of preterm delivery with metronidazole and erythromycin in women with bacterial vaginosis. *N Engl J Med* 1995;333:1732–6.
97. Joesoef MR, Hillier SL, Wiknjosastro G, Sumampouw H, Linnan M, Norojono W, Idajadi A, Utomo B. Intravaginal clindamycin treatment for bacterial vaginosis: effects on preterm delivery and low birth weight. *Am J Obstet Gynecol* 1995;173(5): 1527–31.
98. Carey JC, Klebanoff MA, Hauth JC, *et al.* Metronidazole to prevent preterm delivery in pregnant women with asymptomatic bacterial vaginosis. National Institute of Child Health and Human Development Network of Maternal–Fetal Medicine Units. *N Engl J Med* 2000;342:534–40.
99. Guaschino S, Ricci E, Franchi M, Frate GD, Tibaldi C, Santo DD, Ghezzi F, Benedetto C, Seta FD, Parazzini F. Treatment of asymptomatic bacterial vaginosis to prevent preterm delivery: a

randomized trial. *Eur J Obstet Gynecol Reprod Biol* 2003;110(2): 149–52.

100. Paavonen J, Mangioni C, Martin MA, Wajszczuk CP. Vaginal clindamycin and oral metronidazole for bacterial vaginosis: A randomized trial. *Obstet Gynecol* 2000;96:256–60.
101. Kekki M, Kurki T, Pelkonen J, Kurkinen-Raty M, Cacciatore B, Paavonen J. Vaginal clindamycin in preventing preterm birth and peripartal infections in asymptomatic women with bacterial vaginosis: A randomized, controlled trial. *Obstet Gynecol* 2001;97:643–8.
102. Odendaal HJ, Popov I, Schoeman J, Smith M, Grove D. Preterm labour–is bacterial vaginosis involved? *S Afr Med J* 2002;92(3): 231-4.
103. Andrews WW, Sibai BM, Thom EA, Dudley D, Ernest JM, McNellis D, Leveno KJ, Wapner R, Moawad A, O'Sullivan MJ, Caritis SN, Iams JD, Langer O, Miodovnik M, Dombrowski M. National Institute of Child Health and Human Development Maternal-Fetal Medicine Units Network. Randomized clinical trial of metronidazole plus erythromycin to prevent spontaneous preterm delivery in fetal fibronectin-positive women. *Obstet Gynecol* 2003;101(5 Pt 1):847–55.
104. Ugwumadu A, Manyonda I, Reid F, Hay P. Effect of early oral clindamycin on late miscarriage and preterm delivery in asymptomatic women with abnormal vaginal flora and bacterial vaginosis: A randomised controlled trial. *Lancet* 2003;361:983–8.
105. McDonald HM, O'Loughlin JA, Vigneswaran R, *et al.* Impact of metronidazole therapy on preterm birth in women with bacterial vaginosis flora (Gardnerella vaginalis): A randomised, placebo controlled trial. *Br J Obstet Gynaecol* 1997;104:1391–7.
106. Lamont DF. Changes in vaginal flora after 2% clindamycin vaginal cream in women at high risk of preterm birth. *Br J Obstet Gynaecol* 2003;110:788–9.
107. Rosenstein IJ, Morgan DJ, Lamont RF, *et al.* Effect of intravaginal clindamycin cream on pregnancy outcome and on abnormal vaginal microbial flora of pregnant women. *Infect Dis Obstet Gynecol* 2000;8:158–65.
108. Leitich H, Brunbauer M, Bodner-Adler B, Kaider A, Egarter C, Husslein P. Antibiotic treatment of bacterial vaginosis in pregnancy: A meta-analysis. *Am J Obstet Gynecol* 2003;188:752–8.
109. Brocklehurst P, Hannah M, McDonald H. Interventions for treating bacterial vaginosis in pregnancy. *Cochrane Database Syst Rev* 2000:CD000262.
110. Guise JM, Mahon SM, Aickin M, Helfand M, Peipert JF, Westhoff C. Screening for bacterial vaginosis in pregnancy. *Am J Prev Med* 2001;20:62–72.
111. Klebanoff MA, Guise JM, Carey JC. Treatment recommendations for bacterial vaginosis in pregnant women. *Clin Infect Dis* 2003;36:1630–1.
112. McDonald H, Brocklehurst P, Parsons J, Vigneswaran R. Antibiotics for treating bacterial vaginosis in pregnancy. *Cochrane Database Syst Rev* 2003:CD000262.
113. Koumans EH, Markowitz LE, Hogan V. Indications for therapy and treatment recommendations for bacterial vaginosis in nonpregnant and pregnant women: A synthesis of data. *Clin Infect Dis* 2002;35:S152–72.
114. US Preventive Services Task Force. Screening for bacterial vaginosis in pregnancy. Recommendations and rationale. *Am J Prev Med* 2001;20:59–61.
115. Centers for Disease Control and Prevention. Sexually transmitted diseases treatment guidelines 2002. *MMWR Recomm Rep* 2002;51:1–78.
116. Riggs MA, Klebanoff MA. Treatment of vaginal infections to prevent preterm birth: A meta-analysis. *Clin Obstet Gynecol* 2004;47:796–807.
117. Macones GA, Parry S, Elkousy M, Clothier B, Ural SH, Strauss JF III. A polymorphism in the promoter region of TNF and bacterial vaginosis: Preliminary evidence of gene–environment interaction in the etiology of spontaneous preterm birth. *Am J Obstet Gynecol* 2004;190:1504–8.
118. Roberts AK, Monzon-Bordonaba F, Van Deerlin PG, *et al.* Association of polymorphism within the promoter of the tumor necrosis factor alpha gene with increased risk of preterm premature rupture of the fetal membranes. *Am J Obstet Gynecol* 1999;180:1297–302.
119. Romero R, Kuivaniemi H, Tromp G, Olson J. The design, execution, and interpretation of genetic association studies to decipher complex diseases. *Am J Obstet Gynecol* 2002;187:1299–312.
120. Dizon-Townson DS, Major H, Varner M, Ward K. A promoter mutation that increases transcription of the tumor necrosis factor-alpha gene is not associated with preterm delivery. *Am J Obstet Gynecol* 1997;177:810–3.
121. Dahlman I, Eaves IA, Kosoy R, *et al.* Parameters for reliable results in genetic association studies in common disease. *Nat Genet* 2002;30:149–50.
122. Romero R, Chaiworapongsa T, Kuivaniemi H, Tromp G. Bacterial vaginosis, the inflammatory response and the risk of preterm birth: A role for genetic epidemiology in the prevention of preterm birth. *Am J Obstet Gynecol* 2004;190:1509–19.
123. Katz M, Newman RB, Gill PJ. Assessment of uterine activity in ambulatory patients at high risk of preterm labor and delivery. *Am J Obstet Gynecol* 1986;154:44–7.
124. Nageotte MP, Dorchester W, Porto M, Keegan KA Jr, Freeman RK. Quantitation of uterine activity preceding preterm, term, and postterm labor. *Am J Obstet Gynecol* 1988;158:1254–9.
125. Katz M, Gill PJ, Newman RB. Detection of preterm labor by ambulatory monitoring of uterine activity: A preliminary report. *Obstet Gynecol* 1986;68:773–8.
126. Multicenter randomized, controlled trial of a preterm birth prevention program. Collaborative Group on Preterm Birth Prevention. *Am J Obstet Gynecol* 1993;169:352–66.
127. Sachs BP, Hellerstein S, Freeman R, Frigoletto F, Hauth JC. Home monitoring of uterine activity. Does it prevent prematurity? *N Engl J Med* 1991;325:1374–7.
128. Grimes DA, Schulz KF. Randomized controlled trials of home uterine activity monitoring: A review and critique. *Obstet Gynecol* 1992;79:137–42.
129. US Preventive Services Task Force. Home uterine activity monitoring for preterm labor. Review article. US Preventive Services Task Force. *J Am Med Assoc* 1993;270:371–6.
130. Dyson DC, Danbe KH, Bamber JA, *et al.* Monitoring women at risk for preterm labor. *N Engl J Med* 1998;338:15–9.
131. Iams JD, Newman RB, Thom EA, *et al.* Frequency of uterine contractions and the risk of spontaneous preterm delivery. *N Engl J Med* 2002;346:250–5.
132. Garfield RE, Chwalisz K, Shi L, Olson G, Saade GR. Instrumentation for the diagnosis of term and preterm labour. *J Perinat Med* 1998;26:413–36.
133. Maner WL, Garfield RE, Maul H, Olson G, Saade G. Predicting term and preterm delivery with transabdominal uterine electromyography. *Obstet Gynecol* 2003;101:1254–60.
134. McLean M, Bisits A, Davies J, Woods R, Lowry P, Smith R. A placental clock controlling the length of human pregnancy. *Nat Med* 1995;1:460–3.
135. Wadhwa PD, Garite TJ, Porto M, *et al.* Placental corticotropin-releasing hormone (CRH), spontaneous preterm birth, and fetal growth restriction: A prospective investigation. *Am J Obstet Gynecol* 2004;191:1063–9.
136. Leung TN, Chung TK, Madsen G, McLean M, Chang AM, Smith R. Elevated mid-trimester maternal corticotrophin-releasing hormone levels in pregnancies that delivered before 34 weeks. *Br J Obstet Gynaecol* 1999;106:1041–6.
137. Hobel CJ, Dunkel-Schetter C, Roesch SC, Castro LC, Arora CP. Maternal plasma corticotropin-releasing hormone associated with stress at 20 weeks' gestation in pregnancies ending in preterm delivery. *Am J Obstet Gynecol* 1999;180:S257–63.
138. McLean M, Smith R. Corticotrophin-releasing hormone and human parturition. *Reproduction* 2001;121:493–501.
139. Inder WJ, Prickett TC, Ellis MJ, *et al.* The utility of plasma CRH as a predictor of preterm delivery. *J Clin Endocrinol Metab* 2001;86:5706–10.
140. McGregor JA, Jackson GM, Lachelin GC, *et al.* Salivary estriol as risk assessment for preterm labor: A prospective trial. *Am J Obstet Gynecol* 1995;173:1337–42.
141. McGregor JA, Hastings C, Dullien VV. A meta-analysis of salivary estriol (sE(3)) as a means to identify women at risk for preterm birth due to fetal-placental endocrine mechanisms. *Prim Care Update Ob Gyns* 1998;5:179.
142. Heine RP, McGregor JA, Goodwin TM, *et al.* Serial salivary estriol to detect an increased risk of preterm birth. *Obstet Gynecol* 2000;96:490–7.
143. Narayanan S. Multifunctional roles of thrombin. *Ann Clin Lab Sci* 1999;29:275–80.
144. Dati F, Pelzer H, Wagner C. Relevance of markers of hemostasis activation in obstetrics/gynecology and pediatrics. *Semin Thromb Hemost* 1998;24:443–8.
145. Romero R, Rickles FR, Matthews E, Scott D, Dinan C, Duffy T. Fibrinopeptide A during normal pregnancy. *Am J Perinatol* 1988;5:70–3.

146. Comeglio P, Fedi S, Liotta AA, *et al.* Blood clotting activation during normal pregnancy. *Thromb Res* 1996;84:199–202.
147. Elovitz MA, Baron J, Phillippe M. The role of thrombin in preterm parturition. *Am J Obstet Gynecol* 2001;185:1059–63.
148. Chaiworapongsa T, Espinoza J, Yoshimatsu J, *et al.* Activation of coagulation system in preterm labor and preterm premature rupture of membranes. *J Matern Fetal Neonatal Med* 2002;11:368–73.
149. Odibo AO, Ural SH, Macones GA. The prospects for multiple-marker screening for preterm delivery: Does transvaginal ultrasound of the cervix have a central role? *Ultrasound Obstet Gynecol* 2002;19:429–35.
150. Hoesli I, Tercanli S, Holzgreve W. Cervical length assessment by ultrasound as a predictor of preterm labour – is there a role for routine screening? *Br J Obstet Gynaecol* 2003;110(Suppl 20):61–5.
151. Gomez R, Romero R, Montiel C, *et al.* Cervicovaginal fetal fibronectin improves the prediction of preterm delivery estimated by sonographic cervical length in patients with preterm labor and intact membranes (Abstract # 66). *Am J Obstet Gynecol* 2002; 187:S80.
152. Rizzo G, Capponi A, Vlachopoulou A, Angelini E, Grassi C, Romanini C. Ultrasonographic assessment of the uterine cervix and interleukin-8 concentrations in cervical secretions predict intrauterine infection in patients with preterm labor and intact membranes. *Ultrasound Obstet Gynecol* 1998;12:86–92.
153. Kurkinen-Raty M, Ruokonen A, Vuopala S, *et al.* Combination of cervical interleukin-6 and -8, phosphorylated insulin-like growth factor-binding protein-1 and transvaginal cervical ultrasonography in assessment of the risk of preterm birth. *Br J Obstet Gynaecol* 2001;108:875–81.
154. Romero R, Sepulveda, W, Baumann, P, *et al.* The preterm labor syndrome: Biochemical, cytologic, immunologic, pathologic, microbiologic, and clinical evidence that preterm labor is a heterogeneous disease. *Am J Obstet Gynecol* 1993;168:288.
155. Romero R, Mazor M, Munoz H, Gomez R, Galasso M, Sherer DM. The preterm labor syndrome. *Ann N Y Acad Sci* 1994;734:414–29.
156. Gravett MG, Novy MJ, Rosenfeld RG, *et al.* Diagnosis of intra-amniotic infection by proteomic profiling and identification of novel biomarkers. *J Am Med Assoc* 2004;292:462–9.
157. Romero R, Kuivaniemi H, Tromp G. Functional genomics and proteomics in term and preterm parturition. *J Clin Endocrinol Metab* 2002;87:2431–4.
158. Romero R, Gomez, R, Nien, JK, *et al.* Metabolomics in premature labor: A novel approach to identify patients at risk for preterm delivery. *Am J Obstet Gynecol* 2004;191(6):S2.
159. Sadowsky DW, Novy MJ, Witkin SS, Gravett MG. Dexamethasone or interleukin-10 blocks interleukin-1beta-induced uterine contractions in pregnant rhesus monkeys. *Am J Obstet Gynecol* 2003;188:252–63.

134 Prevention of fetal and neonatal lung immaturity

M. M. Anceschi, L. Maranghi and E. V. Cosmi

Fetal lung immaturity is the principal contributor to neonatal mortality of preterm neonates; therefore, the lung has been the primary focus of strategies to improve the survival of newborn infants. If the lungs are immature, the infant will develop neonatal respiratory distress syndrome (NRDS), which still remains a leading cause of morbidity and death in preterm neonates. Untreated, around 25% of babies with NRDS born before 28 weeks of gestation will die within 28 days of birth, and another 25% will develop chronic lung disease, e.g. bronchopulmonary dysplasia (BPD), rendering affected babies dependent upon extra oxygen for long periods of time.

A deficit of pulmonary surfactant is known to be involved in the pathophysiology of NRDS; nevertheless, other factors may play an additional role, e.g. the immaturity of lung structure. Fetal lung maturity (FLM) is mainly the result of the enhancement (either quantitative or qualitative) of the synthesis and secretion of pulmonary surfactant and of structural changes of the lung parenchyma.[1] Factors that are known to be associated with increased or decreased risk of NRDS are summarized in Table 134.1.

The serendipitous findings by Liggins in 1969[2] that antenatal administration of glucocorticoids (GCs) prevented the development of NRDS in premature newborn lambs have stimulated a formidable deal of interest in the possibility of pharmacological enhancement of FLM. The effect of GCs on many parameters of FLM have been analyzed *in vitro* and *in vivo* in several mammalian species.[3]

Many clinical studies have confirmed the findings of the first trial by Liggins (1972)[4] that antenatal administration of GCs to the mother is associated with a statistically significant reduction in the incidence of NRDS. Over the past two decades, the strategy for the prevention and causal treatment of NRDS has been directed toward the acceleration of FLM *in utero* mainly by administering antenatal GCs (ANCs) to the mother and by intratracheal supplementation of surfactant to neonates for treatment of NRDS or to those at high risk for the disease.

Glucocorticoids

Betamethasone and dexamethasone are the preferred hormones used for antenatal corticosteroid therapy: both cross the placenta and are scarcely inactivated by placental enzymes, i.e. 11β-ol-dehydrogenase (11β-HSD), which convert active steroids into inactive 11-ketosteroids. Betamethasone crosses the placenta to the extent that fetal concentration is about 33% of those in maternal circulation.[5] Betamethasone and dexamethasone have a fluoride substituted in the steroid, greatly increasing GC potency and giving negligible mineralocorticoid effect. Both drugs are given intramuscularly (i.m.); this route is the most suited for clinical use, because of the rapid absorption of the drug, depending on its hydrosolubility. The most common hydrosoluble esters are 21-phosphate (dexamethasone and betamethasone) and 21-acetate. The use of 'Celestone Cronodose' (21-phosphate/21-acetate betamethasone) allows a continuous release with a prolonged therapeutic effect. Both drugs have a prolonged plasma half-life and a longer duration of biological action than cortisol and prednisolone.

Table 134.1 Risk factors for neonatal respiratory distress syndrome (NRDS)

Increased risk	Decreased risk
Low Apgar score	Labor before delivery
Male sex	Severe IUGR (< fifth percentile associated with ARED)
Genetic factors (SP)	Female sex
PIH	Smoking in pregnancy
Cesarean section	

SP, surfactant associated proteins; PIH, pregnancy-induced hypertension; IUGR, intrauterine growth retardation; ARED, absent/reverse end-diastolic flow

Cytoplasmatic receptors for GC are present in all fetal tissues, particularly in lung, liver, bowel, pancreas, stomach, skin, retina, brain, placenta, adrenal cortex and medulla and breast. In the fetal lung, the presence of these specific receptors and their progressive increase during gestation indicate that the maturing lung is a physiological target tissue for endogenous GCs.

The biological action of GCs depends on tissue distribution, metabolism, delivery to target cells and receptor affinity. The cellular mechanism underlying GC stimulation of pulmonary surfactant production and lung maturation is not completely understood. GCs are known to modulate the expression of several genes, by a mechanism that involves the binding of the activated receptor to specific DNA sequences. As a result, the transcription of specific messenger RNAs is then promoted and the synthesis of certain proteins activated. Because the receptors are saturated by physiological levels of GCs, their effect on FLM can be obtained with small doses. However, the ability of a particular tissue to respond to the hormone and the type of response depend on the degree of its cellular and biochemical differentiation and also upon the stage of fetal development.[6]

Aminophylline

Several studies indicate that aminophylline can stimulate fetal lung surfactant secretion, although it seems to exert only minor beneficial effects on FLM. Aminophylline is able to cross the human placenta (Cosmi and Condorelli, unpublished data) in significant amounts during late gestation and, through inhibition of phosphodiesterase, increases the levels of cyclic adenosine monophosphate (cAMP) in fetal lung tissue. Increased cAMP produces glycogen breakdown, contributing to surfactant synthesis and, above all, secretion. Studies on the efficacy of this drug to prevent NRDS are conflicting. Animal studies have shown that aminophylline administered to pregnant rabbits fails to accelerate the biochemical maturation of the fetal lung, but stimulates the synthesis and secretion of lung phospholipids that normally takes place at term. Animals treated with aminophylline had improved pressure–volume diagrams and increased amount of surface active phospholipids in lung lavage fluid; however, studies have shown that repeated antenatal administration of aminophylline to pregnant rabbits increases the survival rate and the respiratory frequency of preterm offspring, but other parameters of neonatal lung mechanics were unaffected.[7]

Among the proposed mechanisms of action in the perinatal lung adaptation, aminophylline may act as a central respiratory stimulant and also a smooth muscle relaxant (uterus, bronchi, vessels), promoting bronchodilatation in the premature lung. Aminophylline increases fetal breathing movements (FBM) in the human fetus and, therefore, may be useful in the prevention of fetal lung hypoplasia and in promoting the entry of supplementary surfactant following *in utero* administration, as it was recently shown by Ilia *et al.* in fetal rabbit[8] and for treatment of apnea of prematurity. Aminophylline remains a promising approach, but its use alone or in combination with other agents for the prevention of NRDS and other complications of prematurity needs further study.

Inositol

Inositol, a sugar alcohol, is a vitamin-like factor that is involved in growth and differentiation and is a precursor of cell membrane components responsible for signal transduction. Because of the effects of GCs on lung growth and body weight indexes, inositol has been given in association with GCs to pregnant animals counteracting their effects on growth parameters. Animal studies have shown that addition of inositol to the feeds of GC-treated pregnant rabbits increased surfactant in alveolar lavage from fetal lung. In rabbit fetuses prematurely delivered on day 28, inositol added to betamethasone on days 26 and 27 of gestation caused an increase in lung–thorax compliance and a decreased interstitium/air space, suggesting homogenous expansion of alveoli, not only with respect to controls, but also and, most importantly, with respect to animals treated with betamethasone alone. This finding was associated with an increase in lung weight, protein and DNA content. Furthermore, the association seemed to reverse the so-called male disadvantage in fetal lung maturation and the reported refractoriness to steroid treatment. Male neonates treated with betamethasone plus inositol had a mean lung–thorax compliance significantly higher than the corresponding males from the betamethasone-alone treated group.[9] These studies demonstrate that dietary inositol modifies the physiological and biochemical response of the immature lung to pharmacological doses of exogenous GCs.

A placebo-controlled randomized trial of inositol administration to preterm neonates with respiratory distress syndrome, who were receiving parenteral nutrition during the first week of life, showed that inositol supplementation was associated with increased survival without brochopulmonary dysplasia (BPD) and with a decreased incidence of retinopathy of prematurity.[10]

Betamimetics

Several studies have examined the outcome of premature infants delivered by mothers who received tocolytic therapy, and a positive effect on lung maturation in double-blind placebo-controlled studies has been observed. A decreased incidence of NRDS in babies born to mothers treated antenatally with ritrodine or isoxsuprine has been found by several authors, although others have reported no effect of the long-term administration of betamimetics on FLM.[11]

Currently beta-adrenergic agents are used as tocolytic drugs to prolong pregnancy in order to allow the administration of GCs.

Thyroid hormones

At least five trials on the effects of the combined use of antenatal thyrotropin releasing hormone (TRH) and GCs have shown a significant reduction in the risk of respiratory distress syndrome (RDS), the severity of RDS and the incidence of chronic lung disease, defined as dependency on oxygen at 28 days of life and/or oxygen dependency at 36 weeks post conception. The largest of such trials is by Ballard *et al.* published in 1992.[12] In humans, TRH associated with betamethasone at a dose of 400 μg intravenously every 8 h for 48 h determines a significant elevation in free and total thyroxine (T_4) and a depression of the TRH levels. Neonatal outcome showed that the combined use of GCs and TRH was more beneficial in preventing and ameliorating NRDS and its consequences than the use of GCs alone. Regarding fetal–neonatal side effects, transient elevations of fetal thyroid hormone levels have been found when TRH stimulation was performed during crucial periods of brain development. However, the results of the combination were challenged by a large Australian trial in 1234 women at 24–31 weeks' gestation, in which it was shown that the incidence of RDS and the need for assisted ventilation was not reduced following combined treatment involving up to four doses of 200 μg. In addition, the incidence of maternal symptoms (such as nausea, vomiting, lightheadedness) and hypertension (>140/90 mmHg) was significantly higher. Nonetheless, the results of the study have raised important questions that need to be clarified, e.g. the increased frequency of depressed 5-min Apgar scores and apparent protection against pulmonary hemorrhage.[13]

A recent meta-analysis including 13 trials on 4600 women at risk of very preterm birth who had received prenatal TRHs in addition to corticosteroids showed that the combination did not improve infant outcomes and could cause maternal side effects.[14]

Clinical studies

Among the hormones tested for the accelerating FLM, ANCs have proven effective in reducing the incidence of NRDS and of other complications, such as intraventricular hemorrhage (IVH), periventricular leukomalacia (PVL), retinopathy of prematurity (ROP), necrotizing enterocolitis (NEC), patent ductus arteriosus (PDA). A meta-analysis[15] comprising 18 trials including data on over 3700 babies showed that antenatal GC administration was associated with a 50% reduction of NRDS and that its effectiveness was more evident when delivery occurred after 24 h and within 7 days of drug administration (Table 134.2). For every 11 fetuses treated with ANC there will be one less case of NRDS and a similar reduced need for postnatal surfactant treatment. There will be also one less death in the neonatal period for every 23 treated fetuses and a similar reduction in IVH.[16] Since it is unlikely that further prospective controlled placebo trials on antenatal corticosteroids will ever be performed, the results of the meta-analysis by Crowley represent the definitive evidence-based proof of the effects of ANCs.

Table 134.2 The effects of antenatal glucocorticoid administration on neonatal outcome (from Crowley[15])

Effect on	Pooled odds ratio (95% CI)	*P*
NRDS (total)	0.55 (0.44–0.63)	0.001
NRDS (< 34 weeks)	0.36 (0.27–0.48)	0.001
NRDS (< 32 weeks)	0.33 (0.21–0.50)	0.001
NRDS (< 30 weeks)	0.48 (0.30–0.77)	0.001
NRDS (< 28 weeks)	0.64 (0.16–2.50)	NS
NRDS (< 48 h < 7 days after first dose)	0.38 (0.25–0.57)	0.001
NRDS (> 7 days after first dose)	0.41 (0.18–0.90)	0.04
NRDS (> 34 week)	0.65 (0.33–1.29)	0.20
Neonatal death	0.60 (0.48–0.75)	0.001
Intraventricular hemorrhage	0.29 (0.14–0.51)	0.001
NEC	0.59 (0.15–0.68)	0.09
Surfactant use at birth	0.41 (0.18–0.89)	0.02
Fetal and neonatal infection	0.82 (0.57–1.19)	0.30
Chronic lung disease	1.57 (0.87–2.84)	0.14

NRDS, neonatal respiratory distress syndrome, NS, not significant; NEC, necrotizing enterocolitis

There are, however, aspects that need to be further investigated. One relates to the type of GC to be administered to warrant optimal results. Kari *et al.*[17] in a randomized multicenter study on dexamethasone vs. placebo treatment in preterm pregnancies (< 32 weeks' gestation) showed that treated neonates had higher mean blood pressure during the first 3 days after birth. In the treated group, there was also a decreased incidence of IVH and PVL. The cerebral protection conferred by dexamethasone occurred in neonates born < 24 h after administration of GC, raising the possibility that prenatal steroids are beneficial even when delivery is imminent. These findings are suggestive of the fact that the protective effect of dexamethasone against cerebral complications is independent from the induction of FLM, possibly affecting the maturation of germinal matrix vessels and of the cardiovascular system, thus preventing neonatal hypotension that predisposes in turn to cerebral ischemia and hemorrhage.

To evaluate the effect on the occurrence of cystic PVL, a major cause of cerebral palsy, a cohort of 883 live-born infants, with gestational ages ranging from 24 to 31 weeks was retrospectively analyzed. The rate of cystic PVL was 4.4% among the infants whose mother received betamethasone, 11.0% among the infants whose mother received dexamethasone and 8.4% among the infants whose mother did not receive a GC. Antenatal exposure to betamethasone, but not dexamethasone, was associated with a decreased risk of cystic PVL among very premature infants.[18] In another retrospective cohort study including 1161 neonates with gestational age of 24–34 weeks and birth weights of 500–1750 g, ANCs were associated with significantly less PVL or IVH (23% vs. 31%), PVL with IVH (5% vs. 11%) and isolated PVL (3% vs. 7%). ANC treatment was associated with over 50% reduction in the incidence of PVL.[19] However, a recent study has challenged the conclusion, demonstrating that there are no advantages to maternal antenatal treatment with betamethasone compared with dexamethasone in reducing the risk of PVL in low birth weight ($\leq$1750 g) infants.[20]

In a recent review, Jobe and Soll have concluded that although these synthetic corticosteroids have almost identical structures, betamethasone is superior in preventing three major morbidities, i.e. NRDS, IVH and neonatal death.[21] The US National Institutes of Health Consensus Conference[22] has stated a general recommendation on the use of GC for the induction of FLM in fetuses at risk of preterm delivery. The optimal dose to administer has been fixed in two doses of 12 mg of betamethasone given i.m. 24 h apart or four doses of 6 mg of dexamethasone i.m. given every 12 h. These therapeutic regimens result in about 75% of corticosteroid receptor occupancy, providing a near maximal induction of antenatal corticosteroid receptor-mediated response in fetal tissues.

For infants born at 29–34 weeks' gestation, treatment with antenatal GC clearly reduces the incidence of NRDS and of overall mortality. While antenatal GCs do not clearly decrease the incidence of NRDS in infants born at 24–28 weeks' gestation, they reduce its severity. More important, antenatal GCs clearly reduce mortality and the incidence of IVH in this group.

All fetuses between 24 and 34 weeks' gestation should be considered candidates for this treatment, unless immediate delivery is imminent (< 24 h) or GC may have an adverse effect on the mother. The only absolute contraindications to the use of GC are: chorioamnionitis, peptic ulcer and tuberculosis. In infants born beyond 34 weeks' gestation the risk of neonatal mortality, NRDS and IVH is low. The use of GC in mothers expected to deliver at more than 34 weeks is therefore not recommended, unless there is evidence of pulmonary immaturity as assessed by amniotic fluid FLM tests.

Maternal side effects

Among maternal complications, pulmonary edema has been reported when GCs are used in combination with tocolytic agents. Since the mineralocorticoid action of beta- and dexamethasone is rather small, a potential role of GCs in sodium and water retention resulting in volume overload is considered rather negligible. Therefore, edema may develop as the consequence of the effects of betamimetic drugs, including: (1) increased electrolyte and water retention in the lung; (2) an increase in mean pulmonary arterial pressure; (3) a disturbance of membrane properties and (4) decreased blood vessel resistance. The potential of pulmonary edema seems to be particularly relevant in multifetal pregnancy or in severely infected women, or in any other circumstance in which fluids are administered injudiciously to the mother. Sporadic cases of maternal death have been reported in the 1980s following the combined treatment of betamimetics, especially fenoterol, with GCs. Overall, however, there is little evidence that one course of steroids alone causes major maternal side effects in healthy pregnant women. However, obstetricians should be cautious when steroids are administered to women with poorly compensated diabetes.

Fetal effects

GCs result in a variety of fetal effects that are unrelated to the process of acceleration of FLM. They affect fetal behavior; it is known that GC treatment abolishes diurnal rhythms in fetal hormones. Betamethasone produces a reduction of FBM, body movements and fetal heart rate (FHR) variability. Such effects are transient and return to normality occurs at discontinuation of therapy. Conversely, dexamethasone causes an increase in FHR variation.[23]

That these effects are gestational-age-dependent is shown by a study by Mulder *et al.* in fetuses exposed to betamethasone at 29–34 weeks' gestation, where a decrease in FHR on day 1 (indicative of baroreceptor reflex), and reduced breathing activity and prolonged episodes of quiescence with a concomitant decrease in body movements on days 1 and 2, was elicited. However, these changes were not observed if betamethasone administration occurred at 26–28 weeks' gestation. Betamethasone-induced reductions in FHR variability were similar in young and older fetuses. Age-related differential responsiveness to betamethasone was found for all the fetal processes studied (body and breathing movements, FHR and quiescence), except FHR variability, suggesting ontogenic changes in the mechanisms presumed to underlie these processes [GC receptor (GR) maturation, cardiovascular and neuroendocrine development].[24]

Table 134.3 Effects of corticosteroids on arterial Dopplers (from Visser[23])

Author	Population	Beta/Dex	Ut.art.	UA	MCA
Cohlen *et al.*[26]	High risk	B	—	—	—
Fallace *et al.*[27]	IUGR	B	—	↓	—
Wijnberger *et al.*[28,29]	IUGR	B	—	—	—
Rotmensch *et al.*[30]	High risk	B	—	—	—
Senat *et al.*[31]	IUGR	B/D	—	—	—
Chitrit *et al.*[32]	High risk	D	—	—	↓
Piazze *et al.*[33]	High risk	B	—	—	↓
Simchen[34]	IUGR/ARED	B	—	↓	—
Barkehall-Thomas[35]	High-risk twin	B	—	↓	—
Muller *et al.*[36]	High risk	B	—	—	↓

Ut.art., uterine artery; UA, umbilical artery; MCA, middle cerebral artery; B, betamethasone; D, dexamethasone; —, no change in waveform pattern; ↓, decrease in pulsatility index

The observed reductions in FHR variation and in body and breathing movements following betamethasone treatment might be interpreted as a sign of fetal hypoxemia. However, there are no striking changes in Doppler waveform patterns in uterine artery, umbilical artery or in various other fetal blood vessels in normally grown fetuses. Therefore, delivery on the basis of changes in biophysical variables 2 or 3 days after betamethasone administration should be considered with caution. If not, advantages of improved maturation might be offset by the risks of iatrogenic preterm delivery. It must be feared that in the past a number of fetuses has been unduly delivered as a result of suspected fetal distress following administration of betamethasone, which was given with the view to prevent the hazards of preterm delivery. In case of uncertainty about fetal condition, one may record Doppler waveform patterns of fetal vessels or monitor FHR with special emphasis to the occurrence of FHR decelerations.[23]

GCs exert a direct and potent vasodilatory effect on human umbilical artery resistance *in vitro*, thus providing an explanation for the previously unexplained vascular effects associated with antenatal administration of corticosteroids.[25] The effects of ANCs on the fetal vasculature and uterine vessels are summarized in Table 134.3. These effects are of considerable interest, especially in IUGR fetuses. As shown, these agents are known to have a vasodilatory effect on the human umbilical artery *in vitro* and to improve umbilical vascular dynamics transiently in many fetuses with absent end-diastolic flow.

Wallace and Baker[27] first found a temporary reduction in placental vascular resistance after betamethasone in fetuses with absent end-diastolic velocities in the umbilical artery. Simchen *et al.*[34] have recently identified a small subset of fetuses with intrauterine growth restriction who, rather than responding to steroids with a decrease in vascular resistance, actually increase resistance. This led to poor outcomes, presumably the result of an increase in systemic mean arterial pressure leading to an incremental increase in the after-load of very sick fetuses with impending cardiac failure.

Preterm premature rupture of the membranes

The use of antenatal GC to reduce infant morbidity in the presence of preterm premature rupture of membranes (pPROM) has been matter of controversy, particularly for the possible maternal and fetal adverse effects. According to the Crowley's meta-analysis,[15] it does not seem to be a significant increase in neonatal infection after GC treatment in pregnancies with pPROM. In pPROM at < 32 weeks, repeated administration of courses of steroids is not associated with an increase in the prevalence of clinical or histologic evidence in infectious outcome. However, Garite *et al.*[37] presenting combined data from seven randomized trials concerning GC and PROM, found that the risk of maternal infection after treatment with GC was increased by 70% over those women with pPROM who did not receive steroids.

In a recent meta-analysis, Harding *et al.*[38] combined data from 15 controlled trials involving more than 1400 women with pPROM and showed that GC reduces the risk of NRDS, IVH and NEC. Antenatal GC may also reduce the risk of neonatal death; they do not appear to increase the risk of infection in either mother or newborn infant. The duration of pPROM

Table 134.4 The effect of ANCs on neonatal outcomes in the setting of pPROM[38]

Effect on	Pooled odds ratio (95% CI)
NRDS	0.59 (0.48–0.71)
Intraventricular hemorrhage	0.47 (0.31–0.70)
NEC	0.21 (0.05–0.82)
Maternal infection	1.95 (0.83–4.59)
Fetal and neonatal infection	1.26 (0.55–2.86)
Neonatal death	0.68 (0.43–1.07)

NRDS, neonatal respiratory distress syndrome

did not alter these outcomes. The available data indicate that ANCs is beneficial in the setting of pPROM. In the opinion of the authors, further trials to address this question cannot be justified (Table 134.4).

The issue whether ANCs may affect the outcome of pregnancies complicated by chorioamnionitis was addressed by Elimian *et al.*[39] Among neonates exposed to antenatal steroids who had histologic chorioamnionitis, there was a significantly less incidence of low Apgar scores (18% vs. 33.5%), NRDS (39.6% vs. 55.9%), IVH and PVL (21.9% vs. 36.9%), major brain lesions (7.7% vs. 18.4%), PDA (14.8% vs. 23.7%) and neonatal death (8.3% vs. 16.2%), with no increase in rate of proven neonatal sepsis (18.3% vs. 14%). In the presence of histologic chorioamnionitis, antenatal steroids significantly decreased the incidence of RDS, IVH and PVL, major brain lesions and neonatal mortality, without increasing neonatal sepsis.

In a non-concurrent prospective analysis of women with singleton pregnancies who delivered between 24 and 32 weeks' gestation after pPROM, a single course of betamethasone administered antenatally to the mother with pPROM was associated with a decrease in the incidence of both NRDS and advanced grades of IVH without any increase in perinatal infections.[40]

Pregnancy-induced hypertension

A number of clinical evidences suggest that the administration of GC to induce FLM in patients with severe pregnancy-induced hypertension (PIH), who are carefully monitored, does not appear to be contraindicated.[41]

Contrary to the common perception of a decreased risk of NRDS as a result of increased fetal stress thereby resulting in acceleration of FLM, the risk of NRDS in fetuses < 32 weeks' gestational age born from pre-eclamptic patients is in fact increased (OR 1.35; 95% CI, 1.03–1.78).[42] As to the effect on FLM amniotic indexes, Piazze *et al.*[43] observed decreased FLM indexes in PIH, particularly evident between 24 and 33 weeks' gestation. GC treatment significantly improved FLM as judged from AF tests performed in the same gestational age, showing the greatest effectiveness between 29 and 33 weeks. No significant effect was observed in the period between 34 and 38 weeks, apart from increased lamellar bodies count.

The efficacy and side effects of corticosteroid therapy in pregnant women with severe pre-eclampsia at a gestational age between 26 and 34 weeks for the prevention of NRDS was studied in a prospective double-blind randomized trial. The incidence of the disease was significantly reduced in the corticosteroid group (23%) compared to the placebo group (43%). The relative risk of IVH, PDA and perinatal infection was also significantly decreased in the corticosteroid group: 0.35 (95% CI 0.15–0.86), 0.27 (95% CI 0.08–0.95) and 0.39 (95% CI 0.39–0.97), respectively. The study suggests that ANCs are a safe and efficient treatment in patients with severe preeclampsia at between 26 and 34 weeks' gestation.[44] ANCs also improve significantly the hematologic abnormalities associated with hemolysis, elevated liver enzymes and low platelet count (HELLP) syndrome. Two doses of betamethasone given 12 h apart was the most effective corticosteroid regimen.[45]

Twin pregnancy

The benefits of ANC on twin pregnancy are debated. Spinillo *et al.*,[46] in a retrospective study, showed a significant reduction in the incidence of NRDS in 21 pairs of twins treated with antenatal GC therapy. However, the reduction in NRDS may have been due to the significantly greater gestational age and birth weight, noted in the treated group compared to the non-treated group. Ardila *et al.*[47] reviewed 134 pairs of twins between 24 and 34 weeks' gestation and found a significant reduction in NRDS only at a gestational age of 28 and 32 weeks; no significant differences were found for the other gestational age group. Conversely, Turrentine *et al.*[48] did not find any difference in the incidence of NRDS in 21 pairs of twins, delivered between 24 and 34 weeks' gestation, compared to the controls. Interestingly, it has been suggested recently that administration of GC to enhance FLM in women with multiple pregnancy might predispose to earlier delivery.

The assumption that the maternal levels achieved with the current regimen of ANCs might not be high enough to reach both siblings resulting either from increased body mass of the pregnant women or from the increased mass of the placentas with their capacity for inactivating GC (*vide supra*) has prompted clinical studies. Mulder *et al.*[49] performed a prospective study to determine whether the effects of betamethasone on FHR and behavior in preterm twin pregnancy are similar to those observed in singleton pregnancies and whether the effects occur similarly in both twin members, in a group of 18 twin pregnancies receiving optimal corticosteroid treatment. Betamethasone administration was associated with significant transient decreases in basal FHR (day 1), FHR variability (days 2 and 3) and body and breathing movements (day 2). The overall changes in twins were similar to those previously found in singleton pregnancies. There was a high degree of association of response to betamethasone among individual members of twin pairs suggesting that the current regimen of antenatal corticosteroids used in preterm twin pregnancies results in achieving betamethasone levels high enough to reach the compartment of either twin member.

Repeated courses

Whether repeat doses should be given if delivery does not occur shortly after the initial course of GC is a matter of controversy. In women who remain undelivered but at continued risk of preterm birth, it is common practice to administer repeated doses of corticosteroids every 7–10 days. The practice has arisen because the evidence from randomized trials suggested that infants delivered after 7 days of maternal corticosteroid treatment did not have a lower incidence of NRDS, implying that the effect of treatment is short lived.

There exist some controversies about the disappearance of the beneficial effect of ANCs beyond 7 days from the initial administration. Animal experiments have shown that the induction of surfactant synthesis in the fetal lung is reversible and that betamethasone is cleared from the fetal circulation 48 h after maternal administration. More recent observations of preterm infants delivered over 7 days after maternal corticosteroid treatment showed that the efficacy of therapy was maintained,[50] though the effect of increasing gestational age is confounding. The finding does not seem to be operating in small fetuses. In infants who weighed 500–1500 g, the time interval between exposure to antenatal corticosteroids and delivery does not appear to affect neonatal outcome.[51]

A review on the effects of repeated doses of antenatal corticosteroids on lung and brain function and on growth restriction in animals has been recently published. Nineteen studies were included: the animals that were studied included sheep, monkeys, rabbits and mice. There were eight studies that assessed the effects of repeated doses of antenatal corticosteroids on lung function. All the studies reported improvement in lung function after repeated doses of antenatal corticosteroids. Seven studies investigated the effects of repeated doses of antenatal corticosteroids on brain or nervous system function or growth; all the studies found adverse effects with repeated doses of antenatal corticosteroids. Eleven studies looked at the effect of repeated doses of antenatal corticosteroids on fetal growth. Nine studies found evidence of fetal growth restriction with repeated doses of antenatal corticosteroids. One study assessed long-term behavioral outcomes in mice and found no effect. By reviewing all animal studies that these authors have collected, it is evident that repeated doses of antenatal corticosteroids may have beneficial effects in terms of lung function but may have adverse effects on brain function, i.e. delayed myelination and fetal growth. However, because of the differences between animals and humans, it is difficult to extrapolate directly the results of these studies to humans.[52]

The results of retrospective studies on repeated courses of ANCs are conflicting. In a study performed for 609 mothers and their 713 infants who were treated with 1–12 courses of ANCs, the incidence of NRDS was 45% for single-course and 35% for multiple-course groups (P=0.005; OR 0.44; 95% CI 0.25–0.79). The multiple-course group also had significantly less PDA (20% vs. 13%; P=0.016). The multiple-course group had a reduction of 0.46 ± 0.19 cm in head circumference at birth (P=0.013) when adjusted for gestational age and pre eclampsia. The authors concluded that the exposure to multiple courses of ANCs compared with a single course resulted in a significant reduction in the incidence of NRDS in singleton preterm infants delivered within a week of the last corticosteroid dose. This was associated with a reduction in the head circumference at birth and an increased incidence of maternal endometritis.[53]

In another study, Elimian *et al.*[54] have studied the effectiveness between single and multiple courses of ANCs in preterm infants who weighed 1750 g or less at birth. Infants exposed *in utero* to multiple courses had a significantly lower rate of NRDS (18% compared with 41%; $P \leq 0.001$) and surfactant use (43% vs. 57%; P=0.02) with no apparent increase in neonatal sepsis or disturbances in fetal growth.

In another study, the outcome for premature neonates after multiple courses of ANCs was examined through a *post hoc* non-randomized analysis on 710 neonates of 25–32 weeks' gestation and who received one, two, or three or more courses of ANCs. No detectable clinical difference in the incidence of NRDS, chronic lung disease and IVH related to courses of ANCs was observed, and outcome was similar for infants delivered at 7–13 days compared with those delivered at 1–6 days after receiving antenatal GC. Compared with those who received a single course, neonates who received two or more courses had significantly lower birth weights (−39 g), and those receiving three or more courses had increased risk of death (adjusted OR 2.8; 95% CI 1.3–5.9; P=0.01) and had lower levels of plasma cortisol at age 2 h. In this retrospective analysis, multiple courses of ANCs did not improve outcome and were associated with increased mortality, decreased fetal growth and prolonged adrenal suppression.[55]

When birth size, growth and development in preterm infants after repeated antenatal corticosteroids were analyzed, birth weight ratio decreased with increasing number of corticosteroid courses

($P=0.001$), and multivariate analyses confirmed a reduction in birth weight of as much as 9% ($P=0.014$) and a reduction in head circumference of as much as 4% ($P=0.0024$). There were no additional benefits in mortality or respiratory outcomes, and there was a trend toward more severe chronic lung disease. Repeated corticosteroids were associated with adverse effects on size at birth without apparent benefits. These changes have the potential to affect later development.[56]

A recent study on the effects of repetitive doses on lung mechanics at birth has shown that respiratory compliance was higher in the multiple-course group than in the remote single-course or untreated group; functional residual capacity (FRC) was higher in the multiple-course group than in the untreated group and similar to that of a single-course group, reflecting a maturation of the lung architecture independent of surfactant production.[57]

A National Institutes of Health (NIH) consensus conference[58] reaffirmed the practice of giving a single course of corticosteroids to pregnant women between 24 and 34 weeks' gestation who are at risk for preterm delivery, but underlined that there were insufficient evidence for giving repeat courses of the drugs.

The most important study addressing this issue has been published in 2001. This randomized, double-blind, placebo-controlled intention-to-treat trial was conducted in 13 academic centers in the USA from February 1996 through April 2000 on 502 pregnant women between 24 and 32 completed weeks' gestation at high risk of preterm delivery. All patients received a complete single course of antenatal corticosteroids (either betamethasone, 12 mg i.m. repeated once in 24 h for two doses, or dexamethasone, 6 mg i.m. repeated every 12 h for four doses). Participants who had not delivered 1 week after receipt of the single course were randomly assigned to receive either betamethasone, 12 mg i.m. repeated once in 24 h for 2 doses every week until 34 weeks' gestation or delivery, whichever came first ($n=256$), or a similarly administered placebo ($n=246$). Composite neonatal morbidity (including severe RDS, bronchopulmonary dysplasia, severe IVH, PVL, proven sepsis, NEC or perinatal death) occurred in 22.5% of the weekly-course group vs. 28.0% of the single-course group (unadjusted relative risk 0.80; 95% CI 0.59–1.10). Weekly courses of antenatal corticosteroids did not reduce composite neonatal morbidity compared with a single course of treatment. However, it must be noted that the incidence of severe RDS was significantly reduced in the repeated course group with respect to single course treatment.[59]

In order to evaluate the impact of repeated courses on neonatal lung function, pregnant women of 25–33 weeks' gestation, who remained undelivered 1 week after their first course of antenatal corticosteroids (two 12-mg doses of betamethasone) were randomized to weekly courses of corticosteroids vs. weekly placebo until delivery or 34 weeks' gestation. FRC was measured within 48 h of life. There was no significant difference in FRC (28.5 vs. 27.5 ml/kg) or respiratory compliance between the infants who received a single remote course of antenatal corticosteroids and those who received weekly courses of corticosteroids until delivery. There was no significant difference in admission head circumference or birth weights between the groups, demonstrating that weekly repetitive courses of AS do not significantly increase FRC or respiratory compliance in preterm infants when compared with a single remote course of steroids given at a mean gestational age of 29 weeks.[60]

To ascertain whether a repeated course may be of benefit in the setting of pPROM, the study by Yang *et al.* found that multiple courses of antenatal corticosteroid therapy were associated with an increased risk of clinical chorioamnionitis and seemed not to reduce the incidence of RDS and other neonatal morbidities in patients with pPROM.[61] In a companion prospective study on a group of 161 women with pPROM, half received weekly courses of steroids and half remained untreated following a single course. No significant differences in composite morbidity between the groups (34.2% vs. 41.8%; $P=0.41$) were observed. Chorioamnionitis was higher in patients who received weekly courses of antenatal steroids 49.4% vs. 31.7% ($P=0.04$). Repeated courses of ANCs in pPROM did not improve neonatal outcomes beyond that achieved with single-course therapy suggesting that ANCs should not repeated weekly in patients with pPROM.[62]

Incomplete courses

In everyday clinical practice, it is not uncommon that delivery occurs before the completion of the course of GC, i.e. two doses of 12 mg of betametasone 24 h apart. To find out whether beneficial effects may still ensue, an incomplete course of antenatal corticosteroids was associated with reduction in the need for vasopressors, the rate of IVH and neonatal death in preterm neonates in one study.[63] One dose of antenatal steroids given 4–24 h before delivery was clinically comparable in terms of reduction of IVH and mortality to the recommended schedule of the NIH in surfactant-treated preterm infants.[64]

Policies of administering antenatal GCs

In spite of guidelines on the use of ANCs issued twice by NIH over the last 10 years (1994 and 2000) and adopted by most of the National Societies of Maternal–Fetal Medicine and Perinatal Medicine, the policies of antenatal administration of corticosteroids may vary according to country, institutions and individuals. Several reports have addressed the issue.

A Canadian network study including 11,440 infants < 38 weeks' gestation admitted to the neonatal intensive care unit (NICU) from 1996 to October 1997 showed that the incidence of antenatal corticosteroid treatment was 42% for infants < 24 weeks' gestation, 59% for infants 24–34 weeks' gestation and 10% for infants > 34 weeks' gestation with wide institutional differences in the incidence of antenatal corticosteroid treatment for women. The authors concluded that increasing the use of antenatal corticosteroids for preterm deliveries could reduce neonatal mortality in Canada by up to 10%.[65]

The Europe Against Immature Lung (EURAIL) study group have investigated the practice of ANC administration in a survey of obstetric departments of 14 European countries: 11% of the respondents started ANCs from 23 to 24 weeks' gestation, 82% from 24 to 28 weeks and 7% from 28 to 36 weeks. The use of multiple ANC courses was observed in 85% of the units. After adjustment for country, number of infants delivered at 24–32 weeks' gestation annually in the NICU and maternal hypertension, maternal hypertension doubled the odds of using multiple courses of ANCs (OR 1.97; 95% CI 0.75–5.17), although the association was not significant ($P=0.17$). The survey's conclusion were that the high proportion of departments that initiated ANCs between 24 and 28 weeks of gestation is consistent with the high incidence of neonatal morbidity and mortality in that age range. Multiple courses are overwhelmingly prescribed in Europe; the practice appeared to be associated, albeit slightly, with maternal hypertension; this points out the importance of closely monitoring women at risk of premature delivery.[66] In a companion survey carried out in 1998 on all Fellows, Members and trainees of the Royal Australian College of Obstetricians and Gynaecologists, it was observed that 97% of obstetricians prescribe antenatal corticosteroids in the classical setting of uncomplicated early preterm labor and 85% prescribe repeated courses in those cases in which the risk of preterm birth persists or recurs; 50% of obstetricians prescribe this agent weekly in cases with persisting risk of preterm birth.[67]

In the UK, 98% of the obstetricians prescribed repeated courses, which shows that repeating courses is a common practice; the indications most commonly cited by units that prescribed steroids were prelabor spontaneous rupture of membranes (84.2%) and suspected preterm labor (81.8%).[68]

Follow-up studies

Concerns have been expressed for the potential short- and long-term adverse side effects on the fetus and the neonate of GC treatment. Follow-up studies of children exposed *in utero* to GC up to 12 years have shown that ANC treatment does not adversely affect physical growth or psychomotor development.[69] In order to study the late side effects of ANC on health and sexual development in subjects 20–22 years old, a follow-up study was conducted by Dessens *et al.*[70] No differences were found between corticosteroid-treated and placebo groups as to medical or psychological variables. In general, the subjects were healthy and had normal intellectual capacities. The 20-year follow-up study indicates that one course of ANC to prevent NRDS does not have adverse effects up to adulthood.

Higher blood pressure in adulthood has been described in several animal species after exposure to antenatal corticosteroids; however, reports in humans are scant. In a cohort study of 210 preterm survivors with birth weights of < 1500 g exposed to ANCs, blood pressure was measured at 14 years of age with a standard mercury sphygmomanometer. Children exposed to antenatal corticosteroids had higher systolic and diastolic blood pressures than those not exposed to corticosteroids. However, few had blood pressure in the hypertensive range.[71]

In animals, a dose-dependent decrease in birth weight after prenatal exposure to steroids has been found in rabbits[72] and in sheep.[73,74] Three courses of steroids given 1 week apart resulted in a 20–25% reduction in birth weight in sheep.[74]

In humans, a study of singleton preterm infants found an association between repeated antenatal administration of corticosteroids and reduced body weight and head circumference at birth;[75] reduction in growth of the head circumference in very low birth weight infants is known to be associated with poor neurodevelopmental outcome.[76] However, two out of four observational studies on repeated antenatal steroid courses report a decrease in birth weight.[77,78]

One recent study suggests that birth weight may already be reduced following one course of dexamethasone.[79] We have found a significant reduction of birth weight in pregnancies exposed to ANCs that eventually delivered at term (A. Ruozi, J. J. Piazze, M. M. Anceschi, unpublished).

In a follow-up study by Kumar *et al.*[80] of infants born between 24 and 34 weeks' gestational age exposed *in utero* to multiple courses of antenatal corticosteroids, it was found that treatment was not associated with increased incidence of abnormalities on subsequent neurodevelopmental outcome measures at 30 months of age.

To determine the effects of repeated courses of antenatal corticosteroids on childhood behavior and disabilities, including cognitive delay and cerebral palsy, French *et al.* have analyzed the physical, cognitive, and psychological assessments up to 6 years in infants who were exposed *in utero* to repeated courses of antenatal corticosteroids. Increasing numbers of antenatal corticosteroid courses were associated with a reduction in the rate of cerebral palsy. Three or more courses were also associated with increased rates of aggressive/destructive, distractible and hyperkinetic behavior and these effects were present at both ages 3 and 6 years. Measures of internalizing behavior and intelligence quotient were unaffected by antenatal corticosteroid use, suggesting that repeated antenatal courses of corticosteroids may protect against cerebral palsy but are associated with hyperactivity later in childhood.[81] Similarly, no difference was found with regard to head circumference, length of body and birth weight and at 4 years of age, as was the age at which the ability to sit and walk without assistance was attained in another follow-up study.[82]

In an elegant prospective observational study of 201 preterm singleton infants who received one or more courses of corticosteroids and were delivered between 24 and 34 weeks' gestation neurodevelopmental outcome was evaluated at 2 years corrected age. Two-thirds of infants were treated with betamethasone whereas the remaining third with dexamethasone. The prevalence of infant leukomalacia, including both prolonged echogenicity and cystic leukomalacia, was 25.9% after a complete corticosteroid course, 40% after one course, 42.3% after two courses and 44.4% after more than two additional courses, respectively (adjusted P for trend$=$0.011). In the same categories of steroid exposure, the corresponding prevalence of 2-year infant neurodevelopmental abnormalities were 18% (20/111), 21.4% (3/14), 29.2% (7/24) and 34.8% (8/23), respectively (adjusted P for trend$=$0.038). Compared with betamethasone, exposure to multiple doses of dexamethasone was associated with an increased risk of leukomalacia (OR$=$3.21, 95% CI$=$1.07–9.77) and overall 2-year infant neurodevelopmental abnormalities (OR$=$3.63, 95% CI$=$1.03–13.58).[83]

Future developments

Some questions still remain on the clinical use of antenatal GCs, i.e. the mode of administration, the minimum dose required, the minimum interval between their administration and delivery of the fetus, although the basic question revolves around the need to repeat courses in the circumstances under which the risk factors for preterm birth persist.

Regarding the mode of administration, animal studies has shown the feasibility of a direct fetal therapy (by intravascular or intramuscular injection of betamethasone). The minimum interval from fetal exposure to GCs to delivery for improving lung function was between 8 and 15 h, with an effect on pulmonary edema and blood pressure that was occurring within 8 h. Small observational series on direct intramuscular injection of betamethasone to the human fetus has been published showing effectiveness in prevention of RDS and no procedure-related complications, although no definitive conclusion can be drawn at the moment.[84,85]

The administration of supplementary surfactant directly to the fetus *in utero* via the amniotic fluid has been demonstrated either in the animal model,[86,87] and in humans either by intra-amniotic injection in the mouth area by Cosmi *et al.*[88,89] or directly into the mouth via endoscope through the vagina in the second stage of labor.[90] In the fetuses supplemented with surfactant *in utero* a decrease in the incidence of NRDS has been constantly observed, although the studies were observational or quasi-randomized.

This elegant approach may represent the true prophylactic antenatal treatment of NRDS. However, to the intriguing question whether the surfactant supplement injected into the amniotic fluid enters the trachea and eventually reaches the peripheral airways and lung tissue thereby altering the clinical course of lung development, no evidence is yet available in the human fetus. Although Hallman[91] has demonstrated in rabbit fetuses that only 6% of intra-amniotically injected surfactant was detected in the fetal lungs, with the majority entering into the gastrointestinal tract, in the same model Galan *et al.*[92] have shown that iron dextran (a substance mimicking the chemical–physical properties of surfactant) does enter the peripheral airways in unparalyzed rabbit fetuses and that is normal fetal breathing, not acute asphyxial gasping, that results in the movement of intra-amniotic iron dextran into the fetal lungs; further, the amount of substances that moves into the fetal lungs accumulated with time;[93] analogous conclusions have been reached by Illia *et al.* following intra-amniotic injection of natural bovine surfactant labelled with

Table 134.5 Summary of recommendations on the use of antenatal corticosteroids for the women at risk of preterm delivery (NIH and modified by EURAIL Study Group, from Visser and Anceschi[94])

- All pregnant women from 24 to 34 weeks' gestation who are at risk of preterm delivery within 7 days should be considered candidates for antenatal treatment with a single course of corticosteroids; pregnant women between 34 and 37 years of age are candidates as well in the presence of immature FLM tests
- Repeat courses of corticosteroids (i.e. more than one completed course), cannot be recommended at this time
- In IUGR fetuses, determination of fetal lung maturation may precede the use of corticosteroids
- Betamethasone seems to be a more effective drug than dexamethasone with respect to perinatal mortality and morbidity and might, therefore, be considered as the drug of choice, but be aware of the temporary effects that this drug has on FHR variation and on fetal movements

Tc-99 and with FBM stimulated by maternal injection of aminiphylline.[8]

At present one can only speculate that in the human fetus intra-amniotically administered surfactant may effectively achieve intrapulmonary distribution; reasons include: (1) injection in the mouth area; (2) FBM induced by administration of aminophylline to the mother and (3) possible bronchial smooth muscle relaxation induced by aminophylline facilitating entry.

Conclusions

Among the several methods proposed to accelerate FLM and to enhance lung adaptation in preterm neonates antenatal GC therapy remains one of the most striking successes in perinatal management of complicated pregnancies leading to premature birth. Despite this and the possibility of treatment with supplementary surfactant to neonates, NRDS still remains a major health problem, also as a result of the fact that not all fetuses delivered preterm have been exposed to therapeutic doses of GC and that NRDS is not solely the consequence of lack of surfactant. A summary of current recommendations on the use of antenatal GC is outlined in Table 134.5.

More recently, the possibility of surfactant administration directly to the fetus *in utero* may underscore a significant improvement in neonatal outcome, particularly for those fetuses necessitating immediate delivery.

REFERENCES

1. Gross I. Regulation of fetal lung maturation. *Am J Physiol* 1900; 259:337–44.
2. Liggins GC. Premature delivery of foetal lambs infused with glucocorticoids. *J Endocrinol* 1969;45:515–23.
3. Anceschi MM, Antsaklis A, Kurjak A, Pal A, Pereira Leite L. Beneficial effects of antepartum corticosteroids. *Prenat Neonatal Med* 2001;6(Suppl 2):31–41.
4. Liggins GC, Howie RN. A controlled trial of antepartum glucocorticoid treatment for prevention of the respiratory distress syndrome in premature infants. *Pediatrics* 1972;50:515–25.
5. Ballard PL, Ballard RA. Scientific bases and therapeutic regimens for use of antenatal glucocorticoids. *Am J Obstet Gynecol* 1995; 173:254–62.
6. Whitelaw A, Thoresen M. Antenatal steroids and the developing brain. *Arch Dis Fetal Neonatal Ed* 2000;83:F154–7.
7. Cosmi EV, Saitto C, Barbati A, *et al.* Effect of aminophylline on lung maturation in preterm rabbit fetuses. *Am J Obstet Gynecol* 1986;154:436–9.
8. Illia R, Solana C, Oliveri P, Toblli J, Imaz MU, Hablch D. Evidence of fetal pulmonary aspiration of intra-amniotic administered surfactant in animal experiment. *J Perinat Med* 2004;32(4):354–8.
9. Anceschi MM, Petrelli A, Zaccardo G, *et al.* Inositol and glucocorticoid in the development of lung stability in male and female rabbit fetuses. *Pediatr Res* 1988;24:617–21.
10. Hallman M, Bry K, Hoppu K, *et al.* Inositol supplementation in premature infants with respiratory distress syndrome. *N Engl J Med* 1992;326:1233–9.
11. Cosmi EV. Prenatal prevention of respiratory distress syndrome: New pharmacologic approaches. *Early Hum Dev* 1992;29: 283–6.
12. Ballard RA, Ballard PL, Creasy RK, *et al.* Respiratory disease in very-low-birth weight infants after prenatal thyrotropin-releasing hormone and glucocorticoid. TRH Study Group. *Lancet* 1992; 339(8792):510–5.
13. Australian collaborative trial of antenatal thyrotropin-releasing hormone (ACTOBAT) for prevention of neonatal respiratory disease. *Lancet* 1995;345(8954):877–82.
14. Crowther CA, Alfirevic Z, Haslam RR Thyrotropin-releasing hormone added to corticosteroids for women at risk of preterm birth for preventing neonatal respiratory disease. *Cochrane Database Syst Rev* 2004;2:CD000019.
15. Crowley P. Prophylactic corticosteroids for preterm birth (Cochrane Review). In *The Cochrane Library.* Chichester: Wiley, 2004;4.
16. Halliday H. Costs and benefits of perinatal corticosteroids. *Prenat Neonatal Med* 2000;5:201–3.
17. Kari MA, Hallman M, Eronen TK, Virtanen M, Koivisto M, Ikonen RS. Prenatal dexamethasone treatment in conjunction with rescue therapy of human surfactant: A randomised placebo controlled study. *Pediatrics* 1994;93:730–6.
18. Baud O, Foix-L'Helias L, Kaminski M, *et al.* Antenatal glucocorticoid treatment and cystic periventricular leukomalacia in very premature infants. *N Engl J Med* 1999;341:1190–6.
19. Canterino JC, Verma U, Visintainer PF, Elimian A, Klein SA, Tejani N. Antenatal steroids and neonatal periventricular leukomalacia. *Obstet Gynecol* 2001;97:135–9.
20. Bar-Lev MR, Maayan-Metzger A, Matok I, Heyman Z, Sivan E, Kuint J. Short-term outcomes in low birth weight infants following antenatal exposure to betamethasone versus dexamethasone. *Obstet Gynecol* 2004;104:484–8.
21. Jobe AH, Soll RF. Choice and dose of corticosteroid for antenatal treatments. *Am J Obstet Gynecol* 2004;190:878–81.
22. NIH Consensus Conference. Corticosteroids for fetal maturation on perinatal outcome. *J Am Med Assoc* 1995;275:413–7.
23. Visser GHA, Csermely T, Cosmi EV. Side effects of prenatal steroids. *Prenat Neonatal Med* 2001;6(Suppl 2):42–9.
24. Mulder EJ, Koenen SV, Blom I, Visser GH. The effects of antenatal betamethasone administration on fetal heart rate and behaviour depend on gestational age. *Early Hum Dev* 2004;76(1):65–77.
25. Potter SM, Dennedy MC, Morrison JJ.Corticosteroids and fetal vasculature: Effects of hydrocortisone, dexamethasone and betamethasone on human umbilical artery. *Br J Obstet Gynaecol* 2002;109(10):1126–31.
26. Cohlen BJ, Stigter RH, Derks JB, Mulder EJH, Visser GHA. Absence of significant haemodynamic changes in the uterus following maternal betamethasone administration. *Ultrasound Obstet Gynaecol* 1996;8:252–5.
27. Wallace EM, Baker LS. Effect of antenatal betamethasone administration on placental vascular resistance. *Lancet* 1999;353: 1404–07.
28. Wijnberger LDE, Bilardo CM, Hecher K, Stigter RH, Visser GHA. Antenatal betamethasone and fetoplacental blood flow. *Lancet* 1999;354:255–6.
29. Wijnberger LD, Bilardo CM, Hecher K, Stigter RH, Visser GH. Effect of antenatal glucocorticoid therapy on arterial and venous blood flow velocity waveforms in severely growth-restricted fetuses. *Ultrasound Obstet Gynecol* 2004;23(6):584–9.
30. Rotmensch S, Liberati M, Celentano C, *et al.* The effect of betamethasone on fetal biophysical activities and Doppler velocimetry of umbilical and middle cerebral arteries. *Acta Obstet Gynecol Scand* 1999;78:768–73.
31. Senat MV, Ville Y. Effect of steroids on arterial Doppler in intrauterine growth retarded fetuses. *Fetal Diagn Ther* 2000;15: 36–40.
32. Chitrit Y, Caubel P, Herrero R, Schwinte AL, Guillaumin D, Boulanger MCh. Effects of maternal dexamethasone administration on fetal Dopper flow velocity waveforms. *Br J Obstet Gynaecol* 2000;107:501–7.
33. Piazze JJ, Anceschi MM, La Torre R, Amici F, Maranghi L, Cosmi EV. Effect of antenatal betamethasone therapy on maternal–fetal Doppler velocimetry. *Early Hum Dev* 2001,60.225–32.
34. Simchen MJ, Adamson SL, Alkazaleh F, *et al.* The fetal cardiovascular response to antenatal steroids in severe early-onset intrauterine growth restriction. *Am J Obstet Gynecol* 2004;190:298–304.
35. Barkehall-Thomas A, Thompson M, Baker LS, Edwards A, Wallace EM. Betamethasone associated changes in umbilical artery flow

velocity waveforms in multiple pregnancies with umbilical artery absent end diastolic flow. *Aust N Z J Obstet Gynaecol* 2003; 43(5):360–3.

36. Muller T, Nanan R, Dietl J. Effect of antenatal corticosteroid administration on Doppler flow velocity parameters in pregnancies with absent or reverse end-diastolic flow in the umbilical artery. *Acta Obstet Gynecol Scand* 2003;82(9):794–6.
37. Garite TJ. The use of corticosteroids for acceleration of fetal pulmonary maturity in special clinical situations: Effect of corticosteroids for fetal maturation on perinatal outcomes. *NIH Consensus Conference*, National Institutes of Health, Bethesda, MD, March 1994.
38. Harding JE, Pang J, Knight DB, Liggins GC. Do antenatal corticosteroids help in the setting of preterm rupture of membranes? *Am J Obstet Gynecol* 2001;184:131–9.
39. Elimian A, Verma U, Beneck D, Cipriano R, Visintainer P, Tejani N. Histologic chorioamnionitis, antenatal steroids, and perinatal outcomes. *Obstet Gynecol* 2000;96:333–6.
40. Vermillion ST, Soper DE, Bland ML, Newman RB. Effectiveness of antenatal corticosteroid administration after preterm premature rupture of the membranes. *Am J Obstet Gynecol* 2000;183:925–9.
41. Ruvinsky ED, Douvas SG, Roberts WE, *et al.* Maternal administration of dexamethasone in severe pregnancy-induced hypertension. *Am J Obstet Gynecol* 1984;149:722–6.
42. Chang EY, Menard MK, Vermillion ST, Hulsey T, Ebeling M. The association between hyaline membrane disease and preeclampsia. *Am J Obstet Gynecol* 2004;191:1414–7.
43. Piazze JJ, Maranghi L, Nigro G, Rizzo G, Cosmi EV, Anceschi MM. The effect of glucocorticoid therapy on fetal lung maturity indices in hypertensive pregnancies. *Obstet Gynecol* 1998;92:220–5.
44. Amorim MM, Santos LC, Faundes A. Corticosteroid therapy for prevention of respiratory distress syndrome in severe preeclampsia. *Am J Obstet Gynecol* 1999;180:1283–8.
45. Tompkins MJ, Thiagarajah S. HELLP (hemolysis, elevated liver enzymes, and low platelet count) syndrome: The benefit of corticosteroids. *Am J Obstet Gynecol* 1999;181:304–9.
46. Spinillo A, Capuzzo E, Ometto A, *et al.* Value of antenatal corticosteroid therapy in preterm birth. *Early Human Dev* 1995;42: 37–47.
47. Ardila J, Le Guennec JC, Papageorgiou A. Influence of antenatal betamethasone and gender cohabitation in outcome of twin pregnancies 24 to 34 weeks of gestation. *Semin Perinatol* 1994;18:15–8.
48. Turrentine MA, Dupras-Wilson P, Wilkins IA. A retrospective analysis of the effect of antenatal steroid administration on the incidence of respiratory distress syndrome in preterm twin pregnancies. *Am J Perinat* 1996;13:351–4.
49. Mulder EJ, Derks JB, Visser GH. Effects of antenatal betamethasone administration on fetal heart rate and behavior in twin pregnancy. *Pediatr Res* 2004;56(1):35–9.
50. McNamara M, Bottoms S. The incidence of respiratory distress syndrome does not increase when preterm delivery occurs greater than 7 days after steroid administration. *Aust N Z J Obstet Gynaecol* 1998;38:8–10.
51. Sehdev HM, Abbasi S, Robertson P, *et al.* The effects of the time interval from antenatal corticosteroid exposure to delivery on neonatal outcome of very low birth weight infants. *Am J Obstet Gynecol* 2004;191:1409–13.
52. Aghajafari F, Murphy K, Matthews S, Ohlsson A, Amankwah K, Hannah M. Repeated doses of antenatal corticosteroids in animals: A systematic review. *Am J Obstet Gynecol* 2002;186(4): 843–9.
53. Abbasi S, Hirsch D, Davis J, *et al.* Effect of single versus multiple courses of antenatal corticosteroids on maternal and neonatal outcome. *Am J Obstet Gynecol* 2000;182:1243–9.
54. Elimian A, Verma U, Visintainer P, Tejani N. Effectiveness of multidose antenatal steroids. *Obstet Gynecol* 2000;95:34–6.
55. Banks BA, Cnaan A, Morgan MA, *et al.* Multiple courses of antenatal corticosteroids and outcome of premature neonates. North American Thyrotropin-Releasing Hormone Study Group. *Am J Obstet Gynecol* 1999;181:709–17.
56. French NP, Hagan R, Evans SF, Godfrey M, Newnham JP. Repeated antenatal corticosteroids: Size at birth and subsequent development. *Am J Obstet Gynecol* 1999;180:114–21.
57. McEvoy C, Bowling S, Williamson K, Collins J, Tolayamat L, Maher J. Timing of antenatal corticosteroids and neonatal pulmonary mechanics. *Am J Obstet Gynecol* 2000;183:895–9.
58. Antenatal corticosteroids revisited: Repeat courses. *NIH Consensus Statement* 2000;17(2):1–10.
59. Guinn DA, Atkinson MW, Sullivan L, *et al.* Single vs weekly courses of antenatal corticosteroids for women at risk of preterm delivery: A randomized controlled trial. *J Am Med Assoc* 2001; 286(13):1581–7.
60. McEvoy C, Bowling S, Williamson K, *et al.* The effect of a single remote course versus weekly courses of antenatal corticosteroids on functional residual capacity in preterm infants: A randomized trial. *Pediatrics* 2002;110:280–4.
61. Yang SH, Choi SJ, Roh CR, Kim JH. Multiple courses of antenatal corticosteroid therapy in patients with preterm premature rupture of membranes. *J Perinat Med* 2004;32(1):42–8.
62. Lee MJ, Davies J, Guinn D, *et al.* Single versus weekly courses of antenatal corticosteroids in preterm premature rupture of membranes. *Obstet Gynecol* 2004;103(2):274–81.
63. Elimian A, Figueroa R, Spitzer AR, Ogburn PL, Wiencek V, Quirk JG. Antenatal corticosteroids: Are incomplete courses beneficial? *Obstet Gynecol* 2003;102(2):352–5.
64. Sen S, Reghu A, Ferguson SD. Efficacy of a single dose of antenatal steroid in surfactant-treated babies under 31 weeks' gestation. *J Matern Fetal Neonatal Med* 2002;12(5):298–303.
65. Chien LY, Ohlsson A, Seshia MM, Boulton J, Sankaran K, Lee SK. The Canadian Neonatal Network. Variations in antenatal corticosteroid therapy: A persistent problem despite 30 years of evidence. *Obstet Gynecol* 2002;99(3):401–8.
66. Empana JP, Anceschi MM, Szabo I, *et al.* Antenatal corticosteroid policies in 14 European countries: Factors associated with multiple courses. The EURAIL survey. *Acta Paediatr* 2004;93(10): 1318–22.
67. Quinlivan JA, Evans SF, Dunlop SA, Beazley LD, Newnham JP. Use of corticosteroids by Australian obstetricians – A survey of clinical practice. *Aust N Z J Obstet Gynaecol* 1998;38(1):1–7.
68. Brocklehurst P, Gates S, McKenzie-McHarg K, Alfirevic Z, Chamberlain G. Are we prescribing multiple courses of antenatal corticosteroids? A survey of practice in the UK. *Br J Obstet Gynaecol* 1999;106:977–9.
69. Shmand B, Neuvel J, Smolders-De Haas, Hoeks J, Treffers PE, Koppe JG. Psychological development of children who were treated antenatally with corticosteroid to prevent respiratory distress syndrome. *Pediatrics* 1990;86:58–64.
70. Dessens AB, Haas HS, Koppe JG. Twenty-year follow-up of antenatal corticosteroid treatment. *Pediatrics* 2000;105:E77.
71. Doyle LW, Ford GW, Davis NM, Callanan C. Antenatal corticosteroid therapy and blood pressure at 14 years of age in preterm children. *Clin Sci* 2000;98:137–42.
72. Pratt L, Magness V, Phernetton T, *et al.* Repeated use of beamethasone in rabbits: Effects of treatment variation on adrenal suppression, pulmonary maturation and pregnancy outcome. *Am J Obstet Gynecol* 1999;180:995–1005.
73. Jobe AH, Wada N, Berry LM, Ikegami M, Ervin G. Single and repetitive maternal glucocorticoid exposures reduce fetal growth in sheep. *Am J Obstet Gynecol* 1998;178:880–5.
74. Huang WL, Brazly LD, Quinlivan JA, Evans SF, Newnham JP, Dunlop SA. Effects of corticosteroids on brain growth in fetal sheep. *Obstet Gynecol* 1999;94:213–8.
75. Shelton SD, Boggess KA, Murtha AP, Groff AO, Herbert WNP. Repeated fetal betamethasone treatment and birth weight and head circumference. *Obstet Gynecol* 2001;97:301–4.
76. French NP, Hagan R, Evans SF, Godfrey M, Newnham JP. Repeated antenatal corticosteroids: Size at birth and subsequent development. *Am J Obstet Gynecol* 1999;180:114–21.
77. Banks BA, Cnaan A, Morgan MA, *et al.* Multiple courses of antenatal corticosteroids and outcome of premature neonates. *Am J Obstet Gynecol* 1999;181:709–17.
78. Pratt L, Waschbusch L, Ladd W, Gagnon R, Hendricks SK. Multiple versus single betamethasone therapy: Neonatal and maternal effects. *J Reprod Med* 1999;44:257–64.
79. Bloom SL, Sheffield JS, McIntire DD, Leveno KJ. Antenatal dexamethasone and decreased birth weight. *Obstet Gynecol* 1991;97:485–90.
80. Kumar P, Seshadri R, Grobman WA. Neurodevelopmental outcome of very low birth weight infants after multiple courses of antenatal corticosteroids. *J Soc Gynecol Invest* 2004;11:483–7.
81. French NP, Hagan R, Evans SF, Mullan A, Newnham JP. Repeated antenatal corticosteroids: Effects on cerebral palsy and childhood behaviour. *Am J Obstet Gynecol* 2004;190:588–95.
82. Hasbargen U, Reber D, Versomld H, Schlze A. Growth and development of children to 4 years of age after repeated antenatal steroid administration. *Eur J Pediatr* 2001;160:552–5.

83. Spinillo A, Viazzo F, Colleoni R, Chiara A, Cerbo RM, Fazzi E. Two-year infant neurodevelopmental outcome after single or multiple antenatal courses of corticosteroids to prevent complications of prematurity. *Am J Obstet Gynecol* 2004;191:217–24.
84. Szabo I, Vizer M, Ertl T. Fetal betamethasone treatment and neonatal outcome in preeclampsia and intrauterine growth restriction. *Am J Obstet Gynecol* 2003;189(6):1812–3.
85. Ljubic A, Cvetkovic M, Sulovic V, *et al.* New technique for artificial lung maturation. Direct intramuscular fetal corticosteroid therapy. *Clin Exp Obstet Gynecol* 1999;26(1):16–9.
86. Galan HL, Cipriani C, Coalson JJ, Bean JD, Collier G, Kuehl TJ. Surfactant replacement therapy in utero for prevention of hyaline membrane disease in the preterm baboon. *Am J Obstet Gynecol* 1993;169:817–24.
87. Galan HL, Kuehl TJ. Effect of intra-amniotic administration of exosurf in preterm rabbit fetuses. *Obstet Gynecol* 1992;80(4):604–8.
88. Cosmi EV, La Torre R, Di Iorio R. Intraamniotic instillation of surfactant for prevention of neonatal respiratory distress syndrome (RDS): A preliminary report. *Appl Cardiopulm Pathophysiol* 1996;6:3–5.
89. Zhang JP, Wang YL, Wang YH, Zhamg R, Chen H, Su HB. Prophylaxis of neonatal respiratory distress syndrome by intra-amniotic administration of pulmonary surfactant. *Chin Med J (Engl)* 2004;117(1):120–4.
90. Petrikovsky BM, Lysikiewicz A, Markin LB, Slomko Z. In utero surfactant administration to preterm human fetuses using endoscopy. *Fetal Diagn Ther* 1995;10(2):127–30.
91. Hallman M, Lappalainen U, Bry K. Clearance of intra-amniotic lung surfactant: Uptake and utilization by the fetal rabbit lung. *Am J Physiol* 1997;273(1, Pt 1):L55–63.
92. Galan HL, Tennant LB, Marsh DR, Creasy RK. Paralysis of the preterm rabbit fetus inhibits the pulmonary uptake of intraamniotic iron dextran. *Am J Obstet Gynecol* 1997;177(1):42–9.
93. Pollack JA, Moise KJ Jr, Tyson WR, Galan HL. The role of fetal breathing motions compared with gasping motions in pulmonary airway uptake of intra-amniotic iron dextran. *Am J Obstet Gynecol* 2003;189(4):958–62.
94. Visser GHA, Anceschi MM. Guidelines on antepartum corticosteroids. *Prenat Neonatal Med* 2001;6:368–70.

135 Route of delivering and monitoring of the preterm fetus

R. Luzietti and G. C. Di Renzo

Introduction

The mode of delivery for the preterm fetus remains controversial, as incontrovertible data supporting either vaginal or abdominal delivery are not readily available. The mode of delivery for the preterm fetus is determined to some extent by the presentation (breech vs. cephalic), fetal weight and gestational age. The use of elective cesarean delivery has increased markedly over the last 20 years. The proportion of first-born singleton infants delivered by elective cesarean delivery between 20 and 27 weeks has increased from 5% in 1983–1985 to 13% in 1995–1997. For infants born between 28 and 31 weeks the increase has been from 21% to 36%; however, at 32–36 weeks the change was 12–16%, which is comparable to the 4–6% increase seen in term infants. The meta-analysis of the trials assessing the value of a policy of elective cesarean section vs. selective cesarean section for women in preterm labor at risk of delivering immature babies does not allow definitive conclusions. Controversy, therefore, still persists about the merits of vaginal vs. cesarean delivery, especially if the fetus is in a breech presentation. Controversy also exists as to whether forceps should be used to protect the more fragile preterm fetal head. Moreover, although it has long been thought that a use of generous episiotomy could reduce resistance to the preterm fetal head and minimize the risk of injury, data to support this theory have not been fully appreciated. As Stewart *et al.*[1] first showed a better prognosis for selected very low birth infants after cesarean section, subsequent investigators have also shown an improved long-term fetal outcome for preterm infants delivered by cesarean section. These reports turned attitudes in favor of abdominal delivery for selected preterm fetuses. Numerous authors subsequently reported on improved survival, reduction of hypoxia, and less intracranial trauma and intraventricular hemorrhage (IVH) after cesarean birth in subgroups of low birth weight neonates. During the last decade, however, many investigators have questioned the value of cesarean delivery for preterm fetuses. The reason for this shift is that many of the early investigations were retrospective, not well controlled, and biased in favor of heavier fetuses (> 1000 g). In many respects, obstetricians were biased against performing a cesarean unless the doctor reasonably believed that the fetus had a substantial chance of survival. In fact, more carefully controlled studies with adequate numbers have not found a neonatal benefit for routine cesarean birth. Thus, available information regarding the route of delivery of low birth weight infants is based primarily on retrospective investigations. Whether a randomized prospective study will be performed in the future to answer this important question is not known. In clinical practice preterm deliveries continue to increase, and survival rates of preterm infants have improved over the years. Elective delivery due to fetal and maternal complications have also increased among preterm deliveries. Most of these patients deliver abdominally because of an unfavorable cervix. In those cases, preterm infants may do better following abdominal delivery, although comparison of elective cesarean delivery to induction with careful fetal monitoring has not been adequately done. Moreover, studies on the application of prostaglandin E2 for cervical ripening in the preterm patients are limited and require further investigation. Regardless of the route of delivery, the goal is the avoidance of asphyxia and trauma to the preterm infant. This will necessarily include someone capable of neonatal resuscitation at the time of delivery.

It has also to be remembered that a cesarean section does not assure one of an easier delivery. Cesarean section in the preterm pregnancy can be complicated by an undeveloped lower uterine segment or an inadequate uterine incision. In the preterm pregnancy, the lower uterine segment is only 1.0 cm wide at 28 weeks and 4.0 cm at 34 weeks. With such a poorly developed and narrow lower uterine segment, a low transverse uterine incision may not be technically feasible. Moreover, an inadequate incision could lead to birth trauma or to lateral extension of the lower uterine segment incision, resulting in broad ligament lacerations and significant maternal morbidity. As a result, a higher rate of low vertical and classical uterine incisions is found in the preterm patient. The long-term impact of the classical incision will be less in patients available for a vaginal birth after cesarean in a subsequent pregnancy.

This does not mean a low transverse uterine incision cannot be made. Regardless of the type of incision, intraoperative complications including bladder injury, broad ligament lacerations and uterine artery laceration are more common at the time of preterm cesarean section than with delivery of term infants.

Preterm cephalic presentation

There is even less consensus for the optimal route of delivery in the preterm vertex presentation compared with the preterm breech. Cesarean section significantly improved the neonatal survival of the very low birth weight infants, but vaginal delivery also has advantages, such as the fetal chest compression facilitating lung expansion and the more complete placental transfusion to the fetus. Thus, it is evident that cesarean section should be more liberally used in the delivery of the preterm vertex. Nevertheless, cesarean section is probably more indicated in those below 30 weeks of gestation, while those infants greater than 32 weeks' gestation who carry a lower risk of immaturity may be delivered vaginally.

Although some reports have shown that cesarean delivery of the low birth weight fetus with a cephalic presentation may decrease trauma and the incidence of IVH, most investigations do not show a fetal or neonatal advantage or protective effect from cesarean delivery. Thus, cesarean delivery may not be the preferred route of delivery for a low birth weight infant presenting as a vertex over vaginal birth. Moreover, the incidence of germinal matrix bleeding that may extend to an IVH is probably unaffected by the route of delivery. Studies failed to show a difference in perinatal outcome between infants delivered by cesarean and those delivered vaginally. If, however, the case was complicated, cesarean appeared to improve perinatal outcome, but the use of cesarean delivery after the onset of labor does not prevent central nervous system (CNS) bleeding. According to some studies, cesarean delivery of very low birth weight infants reduces the incidence of IVH; however, Bejar and associates, using cranial ultrasound in the first 24 h of life, concluded that it was not the route of delivery but the presence of labor that was the critical factor in the development of IVH. Most studies, when corrected for gestational age, presentation and labor complications, fail to support these findings. Thus, we can identify situations requiring delivery in the face of a long-closed cervix that may tilt the analysis in these preterm fetuses away from a long and potentially morbid induction of labor toward elective cesarean birth; however, the studies to date have not provided sufficient evidence to recommend one route of delivery over another to prevent IVH. For example, there are many recognized conditions associated with IVH. These include prematurity, perinatal asphyxia, respiratory distress syndrome, neonatal trauma and the use of hyperosmolar solutions. It is unclear whether the route of delivery carries sufficient significance to be a factor when compared with these other known causes of IVH. Others have emphasized the complex basis for germinal matrix hemorrhage. Although immaturity does play a major role, additional factors also possibly play a role. Those suggested include intrapartum fetal distress and acidosis at birth, umbilical cord pH < 7.20, heparinization to avoid catheter-related thromboembolic events and vascular fluctuation in the velocity of cerebral blood flow. Attention to intrapartum events could help decrease the incidence of neonatal acidosis and may lessen the risk of IVH. There is, however, no evidence that routine cesarean delivery for the premature fetus presenting as a vertex will decrease the incidence of periventricular hemorrhage.

Notwithstanding, neonatal management of the preterm fetus can play a role in the subsequent development of IVH. In addition to the problems related to mechanical ventilation, medications such as muscle relaxants, phenobarbital, vitamin K and vitamin E appear to reduce the severity of IVH. Indometacin did not affect the incidence of hemorrhage.

Thus, there is no convincing evidence to support the concept that vaginal delivery should not be the mode of delivery when the fetus is in a vertex presentation, when the labor is progressing normally and when the fetal heart rate (FHR) pattern is within normal limits. While cesarean section may be indicated if there are reasons for urgent delivery on maternal or fetal grounds and/or vaginal birth is contraindicated, there is no good evidence to support its general use. The lower uterine segment may be poorly formed very early in pregnancy, making delivery difficult and the procedure poses significant risks to the woman, as well as consequences for her in any future pregnancies.

Until further information becomes available, use of cesarean section for preterm birth should only be undertaken if there is considerable clear benefit to the woman or her infant(s). The options should be discussed with her, including the need to extend the incision into the upper segment and the implications of that for future reproductive health.

Some other aspects should be considered like the routine use of forceps delivery and episiotomy. There are similarly few data to support these practices in preterm vertex births. Significant maternal morbidity occurs with both these procedures.

Episiotomy

A liberal episiotomy has been suggested for the vaginal delivery of the low birth weight infant to reduce resistance and shorten the second stage of labor. The theoretical basis for this recommendation is to protect the soft fetal head from injury; however, these forces are less than those generated by the cervix and muscles of the vagina through which the fetus has already passed. Thus, there are insufficient data to suggest that a liberal episiotomy will improve perinatal outcome in the low birth weight infant.

'Prophylactic' forceps

The National Collaborative Perinatal Project data found that premature infants (< 2500 g) delivered by low forceps had the best outcome. Recent studies, however, have not shown a benefit from the use of forceps. Moreover, there are studies that have suggested that the use of forceps in this circumstance may in fact be harmful to the fetus as several fetuses in their study had intracranial hemorrhages. Therefore, prophylactic use of forceps appears unnecessary when more than minimal traction is going to be required. The forceps are designed for infants weighing 1500–1900 g and appear to be too large for a fetus under 1000 g. Unlike the term fetus, midforceps should be avoided, where possible, because of the force required to pull the fetus through a resistant and unprepared vagina and firm perineum.

Preterm Breech

Breech presentation is more frequent in preterm labor with an incidence of 25% at 28 weeks' gestation compared with 2–3% at term. The optimum mode of delivery of women in preterm labor with a fetus presenting by the breech is controversial. Most of the published data are observational and retrospective and are prone to serious biases.

There is one study available that has tried to determine the optimum mode of delivery – vaginal vs. cesarean section – of the early preterm fetus in breech presentation. Four retrospective cohort studies, one incomplete randomized control trial and one comparative study indicated that the risk of neonatal death for infants with breech presentation born vaginally was significantly greater than for those born by cesarean section. Two retrospective cohort studies from Northern Nigeria and Jordan did not advocate the routine use of cesarean section for delivering preterm breech fetuses. Three retrospective cohort studies showed no difference in neonatal mortality between those born vaginally and those born by cesarean section. Nine of the 11 studies shared a similar outcome – neonatal mortality and morbidity. Of the remaining two studies, survival rates were examined at 2- and 5-year intervals.

Three of the studies detailed neonatal mortality according to weight and disease, two according to disease and weight alone, one by delivery and one by weight and gestational age. Seven of the studies obtained their data from the clinical environment while the remaining four studies extracted data from detailed births and deaths registries.

Retrospective cohort studies have yielded conflicting results regarding the appropriate delivery of the preterm breech infant. Jain *et al.*[2] and Sun Lee *et al.*[3] found that when comparing vaginal births with cesarean births, cesarean births had a lower neonatal (less than 28 days) mortality rate when ranked according to a birth weight group. In all birth weight groups, the difference in mortality between the vaginal births and the cesarean births was greater in the first hour of life. The difference decreased progressively throughout the day but remained significant in the first day of life. The least difference was noted in the period of 1–27 days. Gravenhorst *et al.*[4] and Kiely[5] also found a significantly lower neonatal mortality rate for breech presenting infants born by cesarean section compared with those delivered vaginally. They concede, however, that, because of the observational design and the fact that statistical analysis described only a trend, they were unable to conclusively state the appropriate mode of delivery. Supplementing the equivocal argument of Gravenhorst *et al.*[4] about the appropriateness of delivery were the studies undertaken by Gilady *et al.*[6], Kaplan *et al.*[7], Ziadeh *et al.*[8] and Wolf *et al.*[9] Both Gilady *et al.*[6] and Ziadeh *et al.*[8] reported no significant difference in the rate of neonatal mortality in the breech infants delivered by cesarean section and those delivered vaginally when compared by birth weight. Likewise, with Kaplan *et al.*[7] and Wolf *et al.*[9], a similar scenario was demonstrated only with a comparison made to the neonatal disease state. It was interesting to note, however, that Gilady *et al.*[6] proffered cautiously that breech infants weighing 1001–1600 g would benefit from a prophylactic cesarean section. This ran counter to the arguments put forward by Emembolu,[10] who claimed that a cesarean section would be an important morbidity consideration in his sample population. However, Gilady *et al.*[6] concedes that because of the potential limitations of such a study – problems of validity and reliability of medical record information, the duration of the study and its impact on treatment regimen and the challenges of the intention to treat analysis – only a mode of delivery trend has been identified. Thus, a prospective, randomized control trial would be essential.

Unfortunately, there was a paucity of prospective, randomized control data regarding the premature breech fetus and the appropriate mode of delivery. The incomplete study undertaken by Zlatnik[11] in the United States was able to recruit only 38 patients between 28 and 36 weeks' gestation from 1978 to 1983.

As a result of low patient recruitment, the authors terminated the study and lamented in their report the difficulties faced with randomization and the mode of delivery. In the second large non-randomized prospective evaluation, Malloy *et al.*[12] collected data on 437 very low birth weight breech infants admitted to seven intensive care units. After several neonatal variables were adjusted for by logistic regression, no significant difference was found in the rate of neonatal mortality in the breech infants delivered by cesarean section and those delivered vaginally, when compared by birth weight. However, Penn *et al.*,[13] like Zlatnik,[11] reported their experience in attempting to initiate a randomized controlled trial to compare elective cesarean delivery vs. a trial of vaginal delivery in the preterm breech infant. They surveyed 26 English hospitals to determine their willingness to participate. Unfortunately, only six hospitals were actively recruiting participants resulting in its termination by a governing body. They cite difficulty with obtaining consent, concern over the availability of skilled personnel, medicolegal issues and disagreement about the desirability of the trial as the cause of its demise.

In spite of the lack of clear scientific evidence that the mode of delivery of the breech presentation affects neonatal outcomes, the cesarean section rate for breech presentation continues to rise. In Australia, the cesarean section rate – as the preferred mode of delivery – has increased from 19.7% in 1996 to 21% in 1998.[14] In light of the medico-ethical dilemmas that may affect the clinician, it will be extremely difficult to launch any appropriately designed randomized controlled trial to answer this eluding question. We must therefore deal with non-selected and retrospective data to determine the course of clinical action.

Furthermore, bias existed in many of the studies available related to matching for gestational age and infant condition. Matching for gestational age at delivery may bias results against vaginal birth because a cesarean section will generally be performed earlier than a vaginal delivery. The difference in gestational age may be large, depending on the pressure to prevent vaginal delivery. This possible disadvantage of cesarean section might explain the increased need for artificial ventilation in those delivered by this method.

Regarding fetal condition it may be argued that for extremely low birth weight fetuses – 700 to 1000 g – the choice of the route of the delivery may in part reflect judgments on their viability. Specifically, it is possible that fetuses presumed to be less viable were selectively relegated to the vaginal mode of delivery. If true, such selection of high-risk patients for vaginal delivery may account for the survival advantage of the extremely low birth weight infants with breech presentation delivered by cesarean section.[16–25]

In conclusion the findings can be summarized as follows. Although the majority of obstetricians will use cesarean section for the uncomplicated preterm breech, only a minority believe that there is sufficient evidence to justify this policy. There is general acknowledgment that the numerous retrospective studies that suggest that cesarean section confers a better outcome in this situation have been subject to bias. This is acknowledged in some reports. The poor outcome for very low birth weight infants is mainly related to complications of prematurity and not the mode of delivery. Grant[15] has reviewed the controlled trials assessing the value of elective vs. selective cesarean delivery of the small baby. He felt that the data 'are not sufficient to justify a policy of elective caesarean section'. In the absence of good evidence that a preterm baby needs to be delivered by cesarean section, the decision about the mode of delivery should be made after close consultation with the laboring woman and her partner (Evidence Level III).[27–30]

Regarding twins, there is insufficient evidence to support cesarean section for the delivery of the first or second twin. The plan for delivery will need careful consideration and full discussion with the parents. Although many clinicians choose cesarean section when the first twin presents as a breech, because of concern about 'interlocking', this complication is extremely rare. Cohen *et al.* reported 'interlocking' occurring only once in 817 twin pregnancies. Oettinger *et al.* compared the outcome of breech presenting twins over two time periods where the cesarean section rate increased from 21% to almost 95%, and found no change in neonatal morbidity or mortality. They did, however, find an increase in maternal mortality in association with a cesarean section delivery. If the second twin is non-vertex (which occurs in about 40% of twins), vaginal delivery is considered safe. Rabinovici *et al.* carried out a randomized study of twin deliveries where the second twin presentation was non-vertex. Although the study included only 60 twins, the results showed no difference in 5-min Apgar scores or in any other indices in neonatal morbidity between the two groups.

There are other non-randomized reports on the safety of vaginal delivery for the non-vertex second twin. Laros had no fetal losses in either group of second twins with 74 being delivered by cesarean and 76 delivered vaginally.

Monitoring of the preterm fetus

During labor, the preterm fetus should be monitored with continuous fetal heart recording. It is noteworthy that the heart rate present in the preterm fetus has characteristics that are specific and different from that of the term fetus.[26] Cesarean section should be performed if there is any evidence of impending fetal hypoxia, which can contribute to the development of respiratory distress syndrome.

Cardiotocography (CTG) is the most widely used method for fetal monitoring. This technique provides

Table 135.1 Fetal development and cardiovascular response during 20–30 weeks' gestation
Immature parasympathetic system not fully developed (average baseline heart rate 150–155 bpm); variability within normal range of amplitude but with poorly defined cycles
Baroreceptor response present with frequent small baroreceptor response with movements (cord not protected by Wharton's jelly)
Peripheral chemoreceptors present and activated by decreased PO_2 and increased CO_2
Cerebral cortex immature, resulting in FHR accelerations, but with majority of them of less than 15-s duration
Constantly changing fetal state; REM state observed from 23 weeks

Table 135.2 Fetal development and cardiovascular response during 30–36 weeks' gestation
Maturing parasympathetic nervous system with decreased FHR baseline and increased cycles of variability
Baroreceptor response unexpected as cord is protected well (increased Wharton's jelly formation);
Chemoreceptors response: peripheral chemoreceptors present
Cerebral cortex maturing, resulting in FHR accelerations greater than 15 bpm lasting longer than 15 s
Quiet sleep (non-REM) emerging; longer time spent in specific states

useful information on fetal conditions but also presents well-recognized limitations. These limitations, in the term fetus, are mainly linked to the difficulty of interpretation of abnormal FHR patterns and to the poor specificity of the technique in identifying threatening hypoxia.

The normal FHR pattern is characterized by a baseline frequency between 110 and 150 bpm, the presence of periodic accelerations, a normal heart rate variability with a bandwidth between 5 and 25 bpm and the absence of decelerations.

The FHR pattern is abnormal when one or more of the following features are observed: a baseline frequency below 110 or above 150 bpm, the absence of accelerations for more than 45 min, decreased or absent FHR variability and the existence of repeated variable or late decelerations. Assessment of fetal well-being in the preterm fetus by analysis of FHR presents specific difficulties.

The antepartum non-stress test of recognized value in the term fetuses is of less well-defined value in the

Table 135.3 Fetal development and cardiovascular response during 36–40 weeks' gestation
Mature parasympathetic nervous system results in decreased baseline FHR with variability cycles well defined
Baroreceptor response unexpected (Wharton's jelly and amniotic fluid provide cushion)
Chemoreceptors response with both peripheral and central chemoreceptors able to function
FHR accelerations greater than 20 bpm lasting longer than 15–20 s, 90% correlated with fetal movements
Well-differentiated and extended behavioral states

preterm, due to more uncertainty in the relationship between baseline heart rate, reactivity and fetal conditions. During preterm labor the incidence of abnormal findings from intrapartum monitoring is higher as compared to term labor, when the same set of criteria for interpretation are used for both groups and, therefore, in preterm fetuses specific interpretative criteria considering the peculiar physiological aspects of the maturing fetus should be used. Together with 'extrinsic factors' (such as baseline maternal oxygen tension, maternal oxygen-carrying capacity, adequate blood flow to the uterus, uterine contractions, placental surface area and placental blood flow and umbilical cord occlusion or compression), the FHR is also influenced by 'intrinsic factors' such as the balance between the sympathetic and parasympathetic portions of the autonomic nervous system (constant interplay between the 'slowdown' influence of the parasympathetic system and the 'speed-up' influence of the sympathetic system), the CNS: medulla oblongata (integrative center for central and peripheral neural control of the cardiovascular system) and higher brain centers (responsible for variations in FHR in response to FBS); baroreceptors (homeostatic mechanism): pressure receptors located within the vessel walls of the aortic arch and carotid body; chemoreceptors (peripheral: aortic arch and carotid body, central: medulla): responsive to changes in the concentration of oxygen and CO_2 and hormonal influences, like, for example, catecholamine.

In the preterm fetus, the maturational process of the above-mentioned structures, influences the patterns of FHR, which results, with advancing gestation, in a progressive decrease in basal FHR, in a progressive increase in the amplitude of FHR accelerations and in a progressive increase in long-term FHR variability with advancing gestation (Tables 135.1–135.3).

The interpretation of FHR patterns of the preterm is not only more difficult because of the age of the fetus but also complicated by the impact on FHR of specific drugs, more frequently used in women with threatened or actual preterm labor (betamimetics, magnesium sulfate and steroids) or for other concomitant pathological conditions, for example, antihypertensives, that can influence FHR.

It is known, for example, that betamimetics increase the baseline FHR and are associated with a decrease in FHR variability, magnesium sulfate causes a decrease in FHR variability and antihypertensives may cause tachycardia, bradycardia, flattening of the accelerations or a decrease in variability. Betamethasone, contrary to dexamethasone, leads to a decrease in the incidence of fetal body and breathing movements and concomitantly a decrease in the number of accelerations and diminished variability.

Finally, the situation is also complicated by the fact that complementary techniques, like fetal electrocardiogram analysis, useful to improve the specificity of intrapartum fetal surveillance in the term fetuses, cannot be utilized in fetuses below 36 weeks of gestation.

In conclusion, interpretation of FHR changes in the preterm fetus presents specific difficulties in adjunction to the well-recognized limitation of CTG interpretation in term fetuses even if FHR nevertheless provide useful information about neurodevelopmental integration and the cardiovascular response to stress and hypoxia. FHR changes are the result of numerous intrinsic and extrinsic influences: interpretative criteria should consider the specific physiological aspects of the maturing fetus and in the interpretation of FHR patterns it is necessary to make adjustments for gestational age. It is important to underline that interpretation of FHR should not be separated by consideration of the complete clinical picture. Further studies are required to develop specific interpretative criteria considering the specific physiological aspects of the maturing fetus and to devise appropriate interpretative criteria for FHR monitoring of preterm fetuses.

REFERENCES

1. Stewart AL, Reynolds EO, Hope PL, Hamilton PA, Baudin J, Costello AM, Bradford BC, Wyatt JS. Probability of neurodevelopmental disorders estimated from ultrasound appearance of brains of very preterm infants. *Dev Med Child Neurol* 1987 Feb; 29(1):3–11.
2. Jain L, Ferre C, Vidyasagar D. Cesarean delivery of the breech very-low-birth-weight infant: Does it make a difference? *J Matern-Fetal Med* 1998;7:28–31.
3. Sun-Lee K, Khoshnood B, Sriram S, Hsieh HL, Singh J, Mittendorf R. Relationship of cesarean delivery to lower birth weight specific neonatal mortality in singleton breech infants in the United States. *Obstet Gynecol* 1998;92(5):769–74.
4. Gravenhorst J, Veen S, Brand R,Vanhorick SP, Verweij RA, Ens-Dokkum MH. Breech delivery in very preterm and very low birthweight infants in the Netherlands. *Br J Obstet Gynaecol* 1993; 100:411–5.
5. Kiely JL. Mode of delivery and neonatal death in 17,587 infants presenting by the breech. *Br J Obstet Gynaecol* 1991;98:898–904.
6. Gilady Y, Battino S, Reich D, Gilad G, Shalev E. Delivery of the very low birthweight breech: What is the best way for the baby? *Isr J Med Sci* 1996:32:116–20.
7. Kaplan B, Rabinerson D, Hirsch M, Mashiach R, Hod M, Neri A. Intrapartum management of the low-birth-weight breech fetus. *Clin Exp Obstet Gynaecol* 1995;22(4):307–11.
8. Ziadeh S, Abu-Heija AT, El-Sunna E, El-Jallad M, Shatnawi A, Obeidat A. Preterm singleton breech in North Jordan: Vaginal versus abdominal delivery. *Gynecol Obstet Invest* 1997;44:169–72.
9. Wolf H, Schaap AHP, Bruinse HW, Smolders-de Haas H, Ertbruggen I, Treffers PE. Vaginal delivery compared with caesarean section in early preterm breech delivery: A comparison of long term outcome. *Br J Obstet Gynaecol* 1999;106:486–91.
10. Emembolu J. The preterm breech delivery in Zaria, Northern Nigeria. *Int J Gynecol Obstet* 1992;38:287–91.
11. Zlatnik FJ. The Iowa premature breech trial. *Am J Perinatol* 1993; 10:60–3.
12. Malloy MH, Onstad L, Wright E. The effect of cesarean delivery on birth outcome in very low birth weight infants. National Institute of Child Health and Human Development Neonatal Research Network. *Obstet Gynecol* 1991;77:498–503.
13. Penn ZJ, Steer P, Grant A. A multicentre randomised controlled trial comparing elective and selective caesarean section for the delivery of the preterm breech infant. *Br J Obstet Gynaecol* 1996; 13:684–9.
14. Riley M, Halliday J. *Births in Victoria*. The Consultative Council on Obstetrics and Paediatric Mortality and Morbidity. Perinatal Data Collection Unit – Public Health and Development Division, 1999.
15. Grant A. Elective versus selective caesarean delivery of the small baby (revised July 24, 1995). In Keirse MJNC, Renfrew MJ, Neilson JP, Crowther C, eds. *Pregnancy and Childbirth Module*. The Cochrane Collaboration, Issue 2. Oxford: Update Software, 1995. (Available from BMJ Publishing Group, London.)
16. Acien P. A comparative study on breech deliveries attended in 1992: Hospital centers from Latin America versus Spain and Portugal. *Eur J Obstet Gynecol Reprod Biol* 1996;67:9–15.
17. Brown L, Karrison T, Cibils LA. Mode of delivery and perinatal results in breech presentation. *Am J Obstet Gynecol* 1994;171: 28–34.
18. Croughan-Minihane MS, Petitti D, Gordis L, Golditch I. Morbidity among breech infants according to method of delivery. *Obstet Gynecol* 1990;75:821–5.
19. Elective caesarean section versus expectant management for delivery of the small baby. Cochrane Review. From The Cochrane Library, Issue 4, 2005.
20. De Leeuw JP, de Haan J, Derom R, Thiery M, van Maele G, Martens G. Indications for caesarean section in breech presentation. *Eur J Obstet Gynecol Reprod Biol* 1998;79:131–7
21. Erkaya S, Tuncer RA, Kutlar I, Onat N, Ercakmak S. Outcome of 1040 consecutive breech deliveries: Clinical experience of a maternity hospital in Turkey. *Int J Gynecol Obstet* 1997;59:115–8.
22. FIGO Committee on Perinatal Health. Recommendations of the FIGO Committee on Perinatal Health on Guidelines for the Management of Breech Delivery. *Int J Gynecol Obstet* 1994;44: 297–300.
23. Gorbe, E, Chasen S, Harmath A, Patkos P, Papp Z. Very-low-birth-weight breech infants: Short term outcome by method of delivery. *J Matern Fetal Med* 1997;6:155–8.
24. Hennekens CH, Buring JE. *Epidemiology in Medicine*. Toronto: Little, Brown and Company, 1987.
25. Jonas, HA, Lumley JM. The effect of mode of delivery on neonatal mortality in very low birthweight infants born in Victoria, Australia: Caesarean section is associated with increased survival in breech-presenting, but not vertex-presenting, infants. *Paediatr Perinat Epidemiol* 1997;11:181–99.
26. Luzietti R, Clerici G, Taddei F, Liotta L, Di Renzo GC. Antepartum and intrapartum monitoring of the preterm fetus. *Prenat Neonat Med* 2001;6:47.
27. Morrison JJ, Rennie JM, Milton PJ. Neonatal respiratory morbidity and mode of delivery at term: Influence of timing of elective caesarean section. *Br J Obstet Gynaecol* 1995;102:101–6.
28. Pajntar M, Verdenik I, Pestevsek M. Cesarean section in breech by birth weight. *Eur J Obstet Gynecol Reprod Biol* 1994;54:181–4.
29. Penn ZJ, Steer PJ. How obstetricians manage the problem of preterm delivery with special reference to the preterm breech. *Br J Obstet Gynaecol* 1991;98:531–4.
30. RCOG Clinical Green Top Guidelines. *The Management of Breech Presentation*. London: RCOG, 2001:20.

136 Resuscitation of newborn infants

O. D. Saugstad

Introduction

It has been estimated that, of the 130 million infants born worldwide every year, approximately 3–5% (4–7 million) of newborns need some kind of resuscitation at birth, of these 4 million suffer from birth asphyxia. In turn 1 million of these will die and an equal number develop sequel. Further, approximately 1.6 million stillbirths occur annually due to intrauterine asphyxia. In low-income countries, it has been estimated that 30% of perinatal deaths are due to perinatal asphyxia. In the USA, it has been reported that 5% of all newborn infants require basic life support in the delivery room or nursery, constituting 200,000 newborn infants in the USA alone. In Western Europe there are similar figures, and in industrialized countries 2–6 per 1000 live births develop acute clinical sequel of intrauterine asphyxia, the so-called hypoxic-ischemic encephalopathy or neonatal encephalopathy. Of those who survive, 25% of moderate and 75–100% of severe cases seem to develop neurodevelopmental sequelae later. In low-income countries neonatal encephalopathy is more frequent, for instance, in Nepal it was observed in 6 per 1000 live births with birth weight > 2000 g, with a higher proportion of severe cases than, for instance, in Australia. Mortality of these children was three times higher in Nepal than in Australia. Due to the high mortality, few babies with neurodevelopmental handicap survive in such a low-income setting.

Some bodies do not recommend the term 'birth asphyxia' anymore. The American College of Obstetricians and Gynecologists, for instance, has abandoned both the terms 'fetal distress' and 'asphyxia'. 'Non-reassuring fetal status' is suggested instead of 'fetal distress'. In spite of this and different and sometimes rather vague definitions of birth asphyxia, the term is still in use and there is no doubt that a large number of newborn infants require resuscitation at birth both in industrialized and in low-income countries. It is very important, therefore, that existing resuscitation routines are based on scientific evidence. Furthermore, trained personnel and adequate equipment should be available at every delivery. As most deliveries throughout the world still occur at home, far away from a hospital and without authorized health personnel present, it is also important to develop simple resuscitation routines that can be handled by traditional birth attendants.

Birth asphyxia

As mentioned above, there is no uniform and clear definition of birth asphyxia. The term itself is Greek and means 'loss of pulse', but is often used synonymously with a condition where a combined respiratory and metabolic acidosis is found in the newborn infant. Today, the diagnosis of perinatal asphyxia is mainly based on its consequences and there is general agreement that the existence of multiple signs and symptoms are needed. Both intrapartum and neonatal distress combined with neurological symptoms in the newborn infant are usually required.

Intrapartum distress implies fetal bradycardia and hypoxemia resulting in a mixed acidosis. Intrapartum asphyxia can be diagnosed by measuring the heart rate and analyzing the heart-rate pattern by cardiotochography, as well as measuring pH in the scalp blood during delivery. Heart-rate abnormalities such as tachycardia and bradycardia are signs of intrapartum distress as in the so-called silent pattern, i.e. loss of heart-rate variability, and late or variable decelerations. Changes in the fetal QRS complex from the electrocardiogram (ECG) signal analyzed by computer-assisted electronic fetal monitoring have been recently obtained, and it seems to be an even more sensitive measure of *in utero* asphyxia. A clinical sign of fetal distress still in use is passage of meconium. A low cord blood pH is also a sign of intrapartum distress. A pH of < 7.05 or 7.00 and a base deficit (BD) > 12 mmol/l by many are held as evidence for intrauterine asphyxia.

Neonatal distress is most often diagnosed by using the Apgar scoring system. Low Apgar score, for instance < 4 for more than 5 or 10 min after birth, is often used as an indication of neonatal distress. Biochemical variables such as acid–base status, lactate, plasma and urinary hypoxanthine, erythropoietin, the number of nucleated erythrocytes in peripheral blood, brain-type creatine kinase isoenzyme, neuron-specific enolase and excitatory amino acid, as well as a number of other markers have been suggested and used to diagnose this condition. More sophisticated means such as magnetic resonance spectroscopy and positron emission tomography, as well as physiological indicators such as the electroencephalogram, evoked potential, cerebral blood flow, and oxygenation evaluated by near-infrared spectroscopy have also been used.

Apgar score is not a measure of asphyxia itself, but a low score still indicates the presence of neonatal distress. In a study from the USA, Apgar scores < 4 were found in 4.5% of newborn infants at 1 min and in 0.9% at 5 min of age. In Sweden, the incidence of infants with Apgar scores < 4 at 5 min was found to be 0.26%. In a Norwegian population with birth weight > 2500 g and no birth defects, a low Apgar score < 4 was found in only 0.7% at 1 min and 0.1% at 5 min.

Neurological symptoms and signs in the newborn following asphyxia vary depending also on when in the postpartum period the child is observed and include muscular hypotonia, feeding difficulties, and seizures. The term hypoxic-ischemic encephalopathy has been designed, a condition seen in term or near-term infants with onset within the first 24 h of life. Clinical scoring systems of this condition have been developed, classifying the condition according to its severity. Stage 1 usually has an excellent prognosis and stage 2 invariably results in sequelae, whereas stage 3, in most cases, leads to death or a severe injury of the child. In a recent survey of approximately 600 newly born infants mainly from low-income countries needing resuscitation, 30% developed hypoxic-ischemic encephalopathy; of these 45% had stage 3, 35% had stage 2 and 20% had stage 1 hypoxic-ischemic encephalopathy.

The term hypoxic-ischemic encephalopathy has by many authors been substituted by neonatal encephalopathy. This indicates that there are a number of other causes of newborn encephalopathy than asphyxia. In fact, one study from Australia indicates that the majority of newborn encephalopathy cases are due to factors other than asphyxia.

A practical definition of perinatal asphyxia given by the American College of Obstetricians and Gynecologist, where all four conditions must be fulfilled is:

(1) pH in umbilical cord blood < 7.0 and BD ≥12 mmol/l;
(2) Apgar scores < 4 more than 5 min;
(3) Multiple organ affection (brain, lung, myocardium, kidney, liver, and intestine);
(4) Evidence of neonatal neurologic sequelae.

From this definition it can also be appreciated that birth asphyxia is a retrospective diagnosis, which can be set not until some time has passed from birth. Resuscitation, which has to be initiated promptly, therefore, has to be carried out before a diagnosis of birth asphyxia is confirmed. In fact, BD > 12 mmol/l in umbilical arterial blood seems to represent a threshold value where cerebral and other organ injury may occur.

Guidelines for resuscitation of the newly born

There are several sets of international guidelines for newborn resuscitation. The World Health Organization published their guidelines for basic newborn resuscitation in 1998 applicable for most children around the world. The ILCOR guidelines from 1999 and the guidelines of the American Heart Association/American Academy of Pediatrics (AHA/AAP) from 2000 and 2005 are widely used internationally. A number of countries also have their own national guidelines. AHA/AAP has published an extensive textbook with CD-ROM demonstrations. These guidelines emphasize a practical approach and especially AHA/AAP has strived to be as evidence-based as possible.

Practical management

Selection of risk cases

It is important to anticipate those infants at risk: the antepartum and intrapartum history can often be of help in predicting which infants will need resuscitation. Some risk factors are listed in Table 136.1.

Fetal-movement counting, non-stress testing, fetal biophysical profile, electronic fetal monitoring, and scalp pH measurement all contribute to an identification of infants at risk for low Apgar scores and need for resuscitation. Electronic fetal-heart monitoring combined with scalp pH determinations improves the specificity; however, sensitivity is low. In spite of these measures, the need for resuscitation often cannot be foreseen and 20–50% of the infants requiring resuscitation have no identifiable risk factors; therefore, at every delivery, the caregiver should be prepared for a possible need of intervention.

Preparation for birth, personnel, and equipment

Most deliveries are uneventful and the adaptation to extrauterine life occurs smoothly. Only in some infants should more vigorous resuscitation procedures be carried out. Most of these can be performed with a bag and a face mask, but in some newborn infants, endotracheal intubation and more sophisticated treatment and observation are needed.

Resuscitation is team work, and at least one person skilled in resuscitation and one assistant should attend to the delivery. Optimally, two trained persons

Table 136.1 Factors indicating increased risk of need for resuscitation of newborn infants

Abnormal presentations
Congenital malformations
Decreased fetal activity
Fetal bradycardia or distress
Maternal age >35 years
Maternal illness
Anemia or isoimmunization
Cardiovascular disease
Chronic or pregnancy-induced hypertension
Diabetes mellitus
Drug therapy
Hemorrhage
Infection
Renal failure
Substance abuse
Maternal sedation
Meconium-stained amniotic fluid
Multifetal gestation
No prenatal care
Premature rupture of membranes
Preterm
Previous fetal or perinatal death
Prolapsed cord
Prolonged labor
Post-term
Small fetus for maternal dates

Table 136.2 Equipment needed for newborn resuscitation

Adhesive tape
Bulb syringe
Clock
Disinfectant
ECG monitoring if available
Endotracheal tubes and connectors (2.5, 3.0, 3.5, and 4.0 mm internal diameter)
Endotracheal tube introducers
Face masks, newborn, and premature sizes
Feeding tube 8F
Gloves, sterile
Laryngoscopes (at least two), straight bladed Nos. 0 (preterm) and 1 (term)
Magill forceps for nasal endotracheal intubation
Meconium aspirator
Medications
Epinephrine (1:10,000)
Naloxone hydrochloride (1 or 0.4 mg/ml)
Sodium bicarbonate (0.5 mmol/ml)
Volume expander (normal saline or Ringer's lactate)
Mucus extractor
Nasogastric tubes
Neonatal resuscitation bags
Oropharyngeal airways 0, 00, and 000 sizes or 30, 40, and 50 mm lengths)
Pulse oximeter if available
Radiant warmer
Scalpel
Scissors
Stethoscope
Suction catheters 5F or 6F, 8F, 10F, and 12F
Suction with manometers
Syringes 1, 3, 5, 10, 20, and 50 ml, needles (25, 21, and 18 gauge), intravenous cannulae and specimen bottles
Three-way stopcock
Umbilical catheters 3.5F and 5F
Umbilical vessel catheterization tray
Warmed linens

should actually perform the resuscitation and one should assist. All equipment should be at hand and functioning. Table 136.2 lists equipment needed for optimal resuscitation, which should be available in the delivery room. It is important to have specific daily routines, checking that the necessary equipment and drugs are present and that the equipment is functioning. The care provider should check, before the infant is born, the oxygen supply and equipment for intubation and that the bag, mask, and suction are functioning. Each team member should identify himself/herself, and it should be clear who the team leader is. Each order should be stated clearly and repeated by the recipient.

Most deliveries worldwide occur in the community outside hospitals and, if any, only basic equipment is at hand, such as a warm and clean bed, stethoscope, bag and face mask, and suction apparatus. A sterile scalpel to cut the cord should be used at every delivery.

Indication for resuscitation

The decision to resuscitate or not is a purely clinical one. The most important indication of the need for resuscitation is failure to breathe after birth. If the

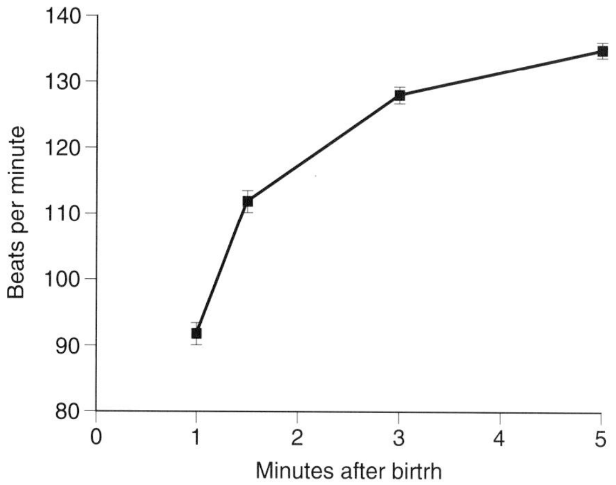

Figure 136.1 Heart rate in the first 5 min of life of approximately 600 newborn infants from the Resair 2 study resuscitated due to bradycardia (heart rate < 80 bpm) and or apnea or insufficient respirations. Values are expressed as mean and SEM.

newborn does not cry or breathe, or is only gasping after the initial quick suctioning, drying, and tactile stimulation, resuscitation should be started. Apneic infants with heart rate > 100 per minute probably represent those with primary apnea, and the infants often require tactile stimulation and a few inflations with a bag and mask only. Apnea and heart rate < 100 per minute may represent secondary apnea, and ventilation should be initiated. In most of these cases, the heart rate improves and spontaneous ventilation quickly develops (Figure 136.1).

Resuscitation, when needed, should start as soon as possible, not later than 30 s after birth. By observing breathing movements, tone, color, and, not the least, heart rate indications, it may be decided whether the infant is in need of resuscitation or not. According to AHA/AAP, every time a child is delivered, the following four questions should be answered:

- Is amniotic fluid clear of meconium?
- Is the baby breathing or crying?
- Is there a good muscle tone?
- Was the baby born at term?

If the answer is 'no' to any of these questions, resuscitation should be considered. Clinical judgment should be based on heart rate, breathing, color, and tone. If the child has apnea or insufficient breathing movements and/or heart rate < 100 bpm, and is blue or pale, resuscitation should be started.

ABC of resuscitation

The ABC of resuscitation is the same whatever the size of the patient: A, airways should be cleared and the infant positioned correctly; B, breathing should be stimulated or performed; and C, circulation should be assessed by heart rate and skin color.

The AHA/AAP guidelines have divided resuscitation into five major steps:

(1) Assess babies' response to birth.
(2) Keep the baby warm and position the baby correctly and keep airways clear. Stimulate to breathe by drying or giving oxygen (if necessary), suctioning.
(3) Establish effective ventilation by bag and mask or in some intubate endotracheally.
(4) Provide chest compression.
(5) Administer medications.

Every newborn goes through the first two; however, only a few go through the last steps. A few – approximately 5% – need the third: bag and mask resuscitation. The fourth step, chest compression, is needed in approximately 1–3% of those needing bag and mask, that is, 1–2 per 1000 deliveries. The fifth and final stage, medication, is very rare.

Evaluation

The sequence of events following asphyxia has been studied in animals. Immediately after asphyxia, there is a period of regular small-volume breaths followed by a fall in heart rate and cessation of breathing. This is the so-called primary apnea. This might last for a minute or so, and is followed by spontaneous gasping for 4–5 min before the secondary apnea develops. If resuscitation is not carried out at this stage, the infant will die.

As soon as the infant is delivered, a clock is started and, during the transport to the resuscitation table, the personnel should form a preliminary opinion regarding the seriousness of the situation, do an eval uation that is performed continuously during the resuscitation process. For instance, a completely lifeless and pale infant probably needs a more aggressive approach than a blue infant with some movements and perhaps also a feeble cry.

During the short period of the initial stabilization, the respiratory efforts are assessed, the heart rate recorded, and color noticed. Heart rate should, after the short initial stabilization, be monitored more precisely. Bradycardia combined with no respiratory efforts or gasping are warnings of immediate intervention. Central cyanosis indicates insufficient oxygenation, whereas acrocyanosis is common even in vigorous newborn infants. Pallor may be sign of reduced cardiac output, anemia, hypovolemi, hypothermia, or acidosis. Apgar scoring in itself should never be used as a criterion for resuscitation because Apgar scoring is not performed before 1 min of life and, in addition, it takes some time. It requires experience to determine Apgar scores correctly, and they are dependent on a number of factors other than the severity of asphyxia, such as drugs given to the mother and the degree of prematurity. It is clinical judgment, therefore, that should be used in deciding when and what kind of resuscitation should be initiated.

Step 1: assess babies' response

Most infants require only to be delivered into a warm room where they can be dried immediately. Their cord should be cut with sterile equipment and their breathing pattern should be observed. The mother herself is most often the best caregiver and provider of warmth, food, and protection from infections. Occasionally, the heart rate of the infant should be monitored preferably by auscultation of the left side of the thorax or alternatively by palpating the pulse for instance at the base of the umbilical cord.

Step 2: warmth, position, and suctioning

Newborn infants and especially asphyxiated ones have an unstable thermoregulation. Hypothermia is an important risk factor, possibly inducing hypotension and delaying the recovery from acidosis. Also, a healthy newborn infant, when exposed to a relatively cold delivery room, may experience a significant decrease in body temperature. Heat loss should be prevented and this is one important reason why deliveries should be performed in a warm delivery room. The newborn should be quickly dried with towels, with particular attention to the drying of the head, and swept into preferably prewarmed towels or other linens. It is recommended that the infant be placed under a prewarmed radiant heater on a table designed for resuscitation.

Some recommend that the nose and mouth should be suctioned with a bulb syringe after delivery of the shoulders but before the thorax has been delivered. However, as this may delay initiation of the resuscitation, this should be considered carefully in each individual case. The infant should be carried to the resuscitation table and placed in a supine position with the head toward the care provider. The neck should be in a neutral position, as both overextension and flexion may cause obstruction of the airways.

At the resuscitation table, the heart rate is quickly recorded by auscultation. An experienced person needs to listen for only a few seconds to obtain an impression of the degree of bradycardia. Count ten s and multiply by six. The nose and mouth should then be suctioned thoroughly but quickly, and for not more than 5–15 s. A bulb syringe or a mechanical suction apparatus attached to an 8F or 10F suction catheter should be used, and the negative pressure should not exceed 136 cmH_2O (100 mmHg). Suction can induce bradycardia and even heart arrest via vagal reflexes, especially when deep suctioning in the oropharynx is performed. Laryngospasm and pulmonary artery vasospasm have also been reported after suctioning. Suction bulb is less likely than suction catheters to induce cardiac arrhythmias but they are probably not as efficient. There is no justification for the practice of routine gastric suctioning not even after cesarean section and such suctioning might even be harmful.

Simultaneously, the other member(s) of the resuscitation team should continue drying the infant with warm and clean towels and changing the initial linens, which are usually wet. This also provides tactile stimulation. which may help initiate breathing in mildly depressed infants. No further stimulation is appropriate. This initial stabilization should be finished within 30 s.

Step 3: establish effective ventilation

After initial correct stabilization, positioning, suctioning, and drying, the infants who fulfill the criteria for further resuscitation, that is those having apnea or heart rate < 100 bpm, should be given ventilatory support. In the majority of these, a bag and face mask is adequate. Various bags and masks are available, but a bag with a reservoir and a 'pop-off' valve that automatically opens if the inflation pressure exceeds a certain figure, usually between 30 and 40 CmH_2O, is recommended, especially in preterm infants. A self-inflating bag is often preferable, as it is independent of gas supply, and ambient air can be used. Bags used for newborns should have a volume of 200–750 ml. Only a soft mask provides a tight seal where the mask is applied to the newborn's face to achieve adequate pressures. A soft-rimmed mask with a small dead space gives the best face seal.

The first breath of the newborn often generates a negative pressure, sometimes of the magnitude of 70 cmH_2O and even more, although in most infants the negative pressure generated by the first breath is < 10 cmH_2O. The first artificial breath given to the infant, therefore, requires a high pressure for term infants, perhaps in the range of 30–40 cmH_2O or even greater, but lower in preterm infants. The succeeding inflations usually require less pressure, around 15–20 cmH_2O. It is preferable to have a manometer coupled to the bag, so that peak inflation pressures can be recorded. The recommended rate of ventilation according to the AHA/AAP is 40–60 breaths per minute. The best way to monitor successful ventilation is to observe movements of the chest wall and follow the heart rate. The pulse picks up very quickly during a successful resuscitation procedure (Figure 136.1). At least three-quarters of asphyxiated infants have spontaneous breathing after establishing these initial steps.

The effects of bag and mask ventilation has been investigated in some studies. In unexpanded lungs, a satisfactory tidal volume is not achieved, and bag and mask ventilation on apneic newborn infants is probably futile. It has been suggested that the most important contribution by using bag and mask ventilation is that the Head's paradoxical reflex is elicited. This means that newborn infants in primary apnea often respond to rapid lung inflation by gasping instead of apnea. This makes the child inflate the lungs. The effect of bag and mask ventilation is therefore less efficient in babies in secondary apnea, since reflexes are not released in such babies. In aerated lungs, correct

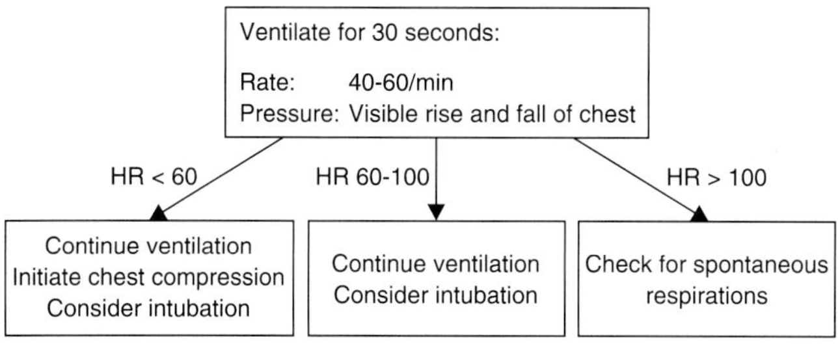

Figure 136.2 Flow chart for ventilation, chest compression and/or endotracheal intubation.

bag and mask ventilation provides tidal volumes of 5–15 ml.

After adequate ventilation has been established for 15–30 s, the heart rate should be recorded for 10 s. If the heart rate is at least 100 per minute and spontaneous respirations are established, positive pressure ventilation may be discontinued. If the heart rate is between 60 and 100 per minute and improving, ventilation should continue. If the heart rate is less than 60 per minute and not improving, assisted ventilation is continued and external heart massage is started (Figure 136.2).

Endotracheal intubation. Endotracheal intubation is necessary when bag–mask ventilation is not efficient enough to normalize the heart rate and establish spontaneous respiration. If chest compression does not quickly improve heart rate or prolonged assisted ventilation is anticipated, endotracheal intubation should also be carried out. A newborn infant without any heart beat or respiratory movement should also be promptly intubated, as bag and mask ventilation probably is not very efficient (see above).

Endotracheal intubation is rare in term infants. The indications are mainly tracheal plugging, for instance, by meconium. Some infants in secondary apnea need intubation and also the most immature infants who often do not have enough muscle strength for their respiratory drive to be sufficient. It has been estimated that 5–6% of all newborn infants need bag and mask ventilation. Of these, 4–20% according to different authors would need endotracheal intubation, approximately 2–10 per 1000. Recent studies indicate that the need for endotracheal intubation is even lower both in term and preterm infants.

The equipment for endotracheal intubation should be ready at hand. Equipment needed in addition to suction devices includes a laryngoscope(s) and blades, straight No. 01; a Magill forceps for nasal endotracheal tubes; endotracheal tubes of 2.5-, 3.0-, 3.5- and 4.0-mm inner diameter; and endotracheal tube stylets. Illumination of the laryngoscopes should be checked before the infant is born. Extra batteries and bulbs should be available. The length of the tube can be calculated in several ways. When nasal intubation is used, the length of the tube can be estimated to be 1.5 times the distance from the anterior part of the tragus to the lateral and caudal part of the ipsilateral ala nasi. The length of the tube from the tube tip to the lips, when oral intubation is performed, can be estimated in centimeters to be (6 + the weight in kg). An infant weighing 3 kg, therefore, needs an oral tube of 6 + 3 = 9 cm. Whether one should intubate orally or nasally is a matter of experience. If the tube is cut remember to add 1–2 cm for taping the tube.

After intubation, the position of the tube should be checked by listening to equal breath sounds, especially in the axillae, and for absence of breath sound in the stomach. Symmetrical movements of the chest wall are also an indication of proper placement of the tip of the tube. However, primarily, improvement in heart rate and color and activity of the infant are indications of adequate ventilation and oxygenation. An infant with open eyes and adequate movements is not a severely depressed infant. The position of the tube can also be checked by repeated visualization of the larynx and in the case of a prolonged intubation by chest x-ray. Some centers are using pneumotachographs or color methods to detect CO_2 in the expired air to assure the tube is correctly placed.

Oxygen supplementation. A high concentration of supplemental oxygen (80–100%) has usually been recommended in most textbooks and guidelines dealing with newborn resuscitation. There is, however, no scientific basis for such recommendations. The Resair 2 study has shown that most newborn infants can be resuscitated as efficiently with room air as with 100% oxygen. Even the most depressed newborn infants seem to be adequately resuscitated with room air when assessed by response in the neonatal period. A meta-analysis of five studies including more than 1700 newly born infants in need of resuscitation has shown that early recovery is faster if resuscitation is carried out with ambient air instead of 100% O_2. Time to first breath was registered earlier, heart rate at 90 s, and 5-min Apgar scores were higher. More importantly perhaps, the neonatal mortality is significantly reduced in room-air resuscitated babies. For this reason 100% oxygen should be avoided as a routine for newborn resuscitation. New recommendations seem to favor the use of room air to start out with having oxygen available as back up. The reasons for the toxic effects of oxygen are not fully understood. However, it has been shown in animal studies that resuscitation with oxygen triggers inflammation in the lung, heart, and brain and also seems to exaggerate brain injury. In humans it has been demonstrated that an increased oxidative stress lasting at least 4 weeks is triggered by resuscitation with pure oxygen. The use of oxygen consumes antioxidants and it may take a long time till these are restored, hence a long-lasting increased oxidative stress is induced, although the exposure to oxygen in most cases is very brief, a few minutes.

If room-air resuscitation is not successful within 90 s, we have supplemented it with oxygen. In such a case, it is probably optimal to monitor the arterial oxygen saturation by pulse oximetry. The oxygen supply in all delivery units should have a blender, so that the oxygen concentration can be adjusted to the requirement. If giving supplemental oxygen is justified, for instance, if central cyanosis or bradycardia persists for more than 90 s, it is recommended to start with 40–60% oxygen and adjust according to the clinical response and, if possible, oxygen saturation measured by pulse oximetry.

Step 4: chest compression

Chest compression is rarely needed and not recommended for basic newborn resuscitation. If bradycardia persists with a heart rate of less than 60 per minute and no signs of improvement after 30 s, adequate ventilation and chest compressions should be carried out. In the Resair 2 study, only 1.7% had a heart rate of 60 or less after 180 s and 1.2% after 300 s. Still almost 20% received chest compression.

AHA/APA recommends that chest compression should be performed by placing the two thumbs on the middle third of the sternum with the fingers encircling the chest and supporting the back. The thumbs should be placed side by side on the sternum just below an imaginary line drawn between the nipples. In small, premature infants the two thumbs may have to be superimposed instead of being placed side by side. The tips of the middle finger and either the index or ring finger of one hand positioned directly above the chest can also be used for chest compression. The sternum is compressed to a depth of 1/3 of its anterior–posterior diameter with a somewhat longer time for the relaxation phase. Chest compression should always be carried out simultaneously with adequate ventilation. A synchronized chest compression and ventilatory rate of 3:1 giving 90 compressions and 30 breaths per minute is recommended. An adequately performed resuscitation with chest compressions obviously requires at least two trained persons.

Heart rate should be assessed after 30 s of well-coordinated chest compressions and ventilation. When the spontaneous pulse rate has reached 60 per minute, chest compression should be discontinued and positive pressure ventilation is continued at a rate of 40–60 breaths per minute (Figure 136.2).

Step 5: medications

When oxygenation is established through adequate ventilation of the asphyxiated infant, it is extremely rare that drugs are needed. Epinephrine (Adrenalin) is indicated in asystole or in sustained bradycardia (heart rate < 60 bpm) in spite of a minimum of 30 s of adequate ventilation and oxygenation and another 30 s of coordinated chest compressions and ventilations. Epinephrine (1:10,000 solution – 0.1 mg/ml) is given as a bolus as rapidly as possible intravenously or intratracheally in a dose of 0.01–0.03 mg/kg (0.1–0.3 ml/kg) – a higher range of dose if endotracheal administration is chosen. The dose may be repeated every 3–5 min if needed. Bradycardia due to insufficient ventilation technique should be corrected by adequate ventilation before administration of epinephrine. Higher doses to premature infants should be avoided.

Naloxone hydrochloride is a narcotic antagonist; however, few studies have documented any benefit of this drug given during resuscitation. The potential negative effects are of concern, as it increases metabolic requirements and redistributes blood flow. Naloxone administration should be restricted, therefore, only to infants who are considered depressed from narcotics administrated to the mother during labor, within 4 h of the delivery, and who require active resuscitation in the immediate postnatal period. Adequate positive pressure ventilation that restores normal heart rate and color should always be established before administration of Naloxone. The appropriate dose is debated, but AHA/AAP recommends an initial dose, given intravenously or intratracheally, of 0.1 mg/kg of a 1- or 0.4-mg/ml solution, which can be repeated every 2–3 min as needed. Naloxone should not be given to newly born infants whose mothers are suspected of having recently abused narcotic drugs, because it may precipitate abrupt withdrawal signs.

The optimal treatment of hypovolemia and shock seems to be unclear; however, shock may be treated with repeated transfusions of volume expanders, usually 10 ml/kg. As volume expanders, normal saline or Ringer's lactate are recommended. The volume expander may be given over 5–10 min and repeated. Albumin or other plasma substitutes are not recommended. Blood volume expanders during acute resuscitation are only indicated when there are unmistakable signs of shock with evidence of acute blood loss, including feto-maternal hemorrhage. In case of blood loss, O-negative blood cross-matched with the mother's blood is given.

Sodium bicarbonate or Tribonat has no routine place in newborn resuscitation. No randomized studies have shown beneficial effects of these drugs. In fact, sodium bicarbonate may be counterproductive by decreasing intracellular pH. Only in prolonged cardiac arrest not responding to other therapy, administration of sodium bicarbonate, in a dose of 2 mmol/kg infused slowly, could be used. Sodium bicarbonate should be given only after all other steps of resuscitation described above have been taken and if ventilation is established. This drug is very caustic and if given should not be given endotracheally but in a large vein.

There is no evidence that atropine or calcium has any beneficial effect during the acute phase of resuscitation of the newborn infant.

In the Resair 2 study, a large trial comprising approximately 600 infants in need of resuscitation, 15% were given one or more drugs. Seven percent were given epinephrine, 6% were given sodium bicarbonate, 1% received Naloxone, and only 0.6% was infused with albumin or underwent blood transfusion.

Meconium aspiration

Meconium aspiration syndrome significantly increases morbidity and mortality. Meconium in the amniotic fluid is present in 10–12% of deliveries. However, only approximately 5% of these develop the meconium aspiration syndrome. In the Resair 2 study, approximately 40% had meconium-stained amniotic fluid.

If the amniotic fluid is meconium-stained, there is no evidence that suctioning the oropharynx before the thorax is delivered has any beneficial effects. As this is not harmful, this procedure is still often recommended. There are, today, no indications that an infant with thick meconium-stained amniotic fluid benefits from routine intubation and suctioning. It is therefore not recommended any more that suctioning of the nose, mouth, and posterior pharynx should be carried out thoroughly before delivery of the shoulder and thorax. A bulb syringe may also be adequate. Routine endotracheal intubation and suctioning of every infant born with meconium-stained amniotic fluid is not justified. However, it is recommended to intubate and suction, through the endotracheal tube with a bore suction catheter larger than 10F, all meconium-stained infants who are not vigorous. It has also been recommended previously to intubate and suction the infant if the meconium is thick or particulate. However, any positive effects of this procedure have not been demonstrated.

Preterm infants

Recent studies have shown that cardiorespiratory resuscitation of extremely low birth weight infants in the delivery room is not futile and a more active approach therefore seems to be established. In fact, studies show that intact survival of delivery room cardiopulmonary resuscitation of infants with birth weight < 750 g is identical to age and gender-matched controls not in need of resuscitation. Advanced cardiopulmonary resuscitation, therefore, is justified also in extremely low birth weight infants.

There are no or very few studies on optimal resuscitation of premature infants. This means that even the extremely low gestational age newborn infants are mainly resuscitated according to the guidelines and principles established for term and near-term infants. Obviously there is an urgent need for separate guidelines for the most immature ones. The following is, however, especially important for the preterm and is more important, the more immature the infant is:

- These infants have a relatively large surface area and a thin skin, therefore losing heat quickly.
- They have low tidal volume, for instance, only 5–10 ml or even lower. Just a few blows with large tidal volumes may ruin their lungs. On the other hand their lungs may be stiffer due to surfactant deficiency. Those with gestational age < 28 weeks are, therefore, often intubated by giving surfactant and in some centers they are immediately extubated.
- Premature infants have a fragile germinal matrix in their brain. Rapid changes in blood pressure or vascular volume in addition to hypoxia may be associated with germinal matrix hemorrhage. These infants should be handled as gently as possible. Rapid boluses of fluid and quick changes in body positions should be avoided.

According to one study, premature infants also have higher neonatal mortality if resuscitated with 100% oxygen compared with room air. There are no data for infants with birth weight < 1000 g but there are reasons to believe these are even more vulnerable to high oxygen exposures.

Response to resuscitation

In the Resair 2 study, the heart rate rose from a mean of 92 per minute at 1 min of age to 112 per minute at 90 s, and 128 at 3 min (Figure 136.1); only 8% and 5% of the infants had a heart rate of < 100 per minute at 3 and 5 min of age, respectively. Apgar scores were (median) 4 at 1 min and increased to 7 at 5 min, and 8 at 10 min of age. The median duration of ventilation was 2 min; 3/4 required less than 4 min, 1/10 required 10 min or more, with approximately 1/20 being ventilated for more than 30 min. Mean BD and pH in umbilical cord were 14.3 mmol/l and 7.11, respectively. After 10 min, arterial values did not show much difference with a BD of 14.1 mmol/l and a pH of 7.16, respectively. However, at 30 min of age, BD was (mean) 11.7 mmol/l and pH was 7.26. This means that heart rate is a much more sensitive indicator of the success of resuscitation than acid–base status, which normalizes very slowly. BD seems to fall 6–7 mmol/l/h during adequate ventilation and oxygenation.

To withdraw or withhold resuscitation

From the large Collaborative Perinatal Project of the National Institute of Neurological and Communicative Disorders and Stroke in the USA, it is known that very low Apgar scores for 15 min or more substantially increase the risk for severe sequel. In this study, in surviving infants with birth weight more than 2500 g, an Apgar score < 4 after 15 min or more substantially increased the risk of cerebral palsy. If the duration of very low Apgar scores was 5 min, the rate of cerebral palsy was found to be approximately 1%; however, after 20 min, the rate had increased to 57%. As it is often problematic to estimate the duration of prenatal asphyxia, resuscitation should consequently always be carried out for a minimum of 15–20 min without response, before withdrawal. Animal studies have shown, however, that the more immature the fetus, the longer is the period of hypoxia tolerated. A preterm infant, therefore, probably tolerates a substantially longer period of hypoxia than a term infant before severe hypoxic-ischemic encephalopathy develops. On the other hand, the preterm infant has an increased risk of developing intracranial hemorrhage.

In some cases, resuscitation should be withheld. Infants with malformations incompatible with life should not be resuscitated. Many centers do not resuscitate newborn infants with gestational age of less than 23 weeks. According to the author's opinion, the following conditions represent contraindications to newborn resuscitation: anencephaly, bilateral renal agenesis, spinal muscular atrophy type I (Werdnig–Hoffmann disease) with neonatal onset, trisomy 13, trisomy 18, and other diseases/conditions not compatible with survival beyond the neonatal period or infancy. The author resuscitates and tries to stabilize all infants with a gestational age of 23 weeks or more. Often, neither the exact diagnosis nor the gestational age is known at birth. A liberal policy of resuscitation is recommended whenever doubt about the care of the individual infant exists. This allows the doctor to collect more information about the clinical status and prognosis of the child. This also allows one to inform the parents, so that they can be prepared and perhaps participate in the discussion and decisions about subsequent therapy. How much the parents should participate in the decision is debatable. Active participation in the decision process requires a thorough understanding of the prognosis of the individual child. The final formal decision, therefore, belongs to the doctor. However, each institution needs a clear policy and guidelines in these matters, so that these difficult decisions are not left to individuals.

Postresuscitation care

After a successful resuscitation, heat loss should be prevented by drying the child with dry towels. The child should be labeled and frequently checked with regard to breathing efforts, respiratory rate, color, heart rate, signs of birth injury, or malformations. If the resuscitation was brief and the situation was not too dramatic, the newborn could be monitored in the nursery, provided an adequate respiration is established. The child could be placed with the mother so that skin-to-skin contact with the mother is obtained. However, this depends on the local conditions and the possibilities for adequate observation by a trained observer.

Even if the infant is not in need of artificial ventilation following resuscitation, the child is often brought to the intensive care unit for further close follow-up, which includes monitoring of the heart rate, ventilation, and determination of arterial pH, blood gases, and electrolytes. Any hypotension should be treated with volume expanders or pressors, appropriate fluid therapy, and seizures treated according to standard guidelines. During the first hours following the resuscitation, the newborn infant should be regularly screened for any hypoglycemia or hypocalcemia. Breast-feeding should be encouraged, if possible, as soon as 1 h after birth. If the resuscitation was unsuccessful and the child died, the parents need a close follow-up.

Documentation

It is useful if only one attending person observes and immediately writes down the procedures followed. A thorough documentation in the medical record of all observations and actions is required before the resuscitation is complete. Each institution should keep records documenting the condition and procedures carried out at birth. The important details of resuscitation to be recorded are identification of the newborn, the condition at birth (Apgar scores, etc.), procedures undertaken to initiate respiration (suctioning, stimulation, bag–mask ventilation, intubation, chest compression, oxygen, drugs, etc.), clinical observations during and after resuscitation, and identification of the resuscitation team.

Training programs in neonatal resuscitation

Birth asphyxia requires immediate availability and recognition of qualified personnel. A training program is necessary, at least at the local level. Some countries have implemented national training programs as, for instance, the successful program in India: 'Give a breath, save a life'. In the USA, AHA/AAP, through the National Resuscitation Program (NRP), provides teaching programs and courses and it is recommended that renewal take place every second year. This means continuous education for doctors, nurses, and midwives should be organized in each region/country.

Every institution that provides deliveries must develop its own standards for newborn resuscitation, and a plan of action should exist. The personnel should gain and maintain skills in newborn resuscitation by training using manikins, and an evaluation of the training is necessary.

Summary of practice and guidelines

- Approximately 3–5% of all newborn infants require resuscitation immediately after birth, which represents 4–7 million newborns worldwide every year. Resuscitation of the newly born infant, therefore, is one of the most frequent procedures carried out in medicine. Simple and clear guidelines for this procedure should exist. Training programs, identification of risk cases, and preparation for the resuscitation procedures should be part of the routine. The resuscitation itself can be divided into five steps. Not all infants requiring resuscitation go through all these steps, but the different steps of resuscitation should be clearly identified and be based on scientific evidence. Today, this is not the case, and there is obviously a need for more research in this field.
- Optimal resuscitation is a team effort. Every birth should be prepared so that adequate personnel skilled in resuscitation are present and adequate equipment is at hand. It is important that newborn infants in need of resuscitation are immediately identified and that trained personnel perform the procedures adequately.
- The asphyxiated newborn infant should be quickly evaluated and initially stabilized by drying and stimulation, proper suctioning, and positioning. Ventilation with a soft face mask and a self-inflating bag, in most cases, establishes spontaneous breathing. A small fraction of resuscitated infants only need endotracheal intubation, and data indicate that ambient air is at least as efficient as 100% oxygen for newborn resuscitation. If supplementary oxygen is used, it should be given with care and preferably simultaneously with continuous recording of arterial oxygen saturation by pulse oximetry. External heart massage and drugs are rarely needed. If there is no adequate response to the resuscitation procedure, ventilation is stopped after approximately 20 min.
- A liberal policy for initiation of newborn resuscitation is recommended. Preterm babies and those with meconium aspiration need specific guidelines. Resuscitation should be withheld in newborn infants with conditions incompatible with life; however, each institution should have its own guidelines concerning when resuscitation should be withheld or withdrawn.
- Postresuscitation care includes both the care of the newborn and the communication with the parents. Documentation of all observations and actions, as well as an adequate training program, is required in a proper resuscitation program for newborn infants.

REFERENCES

1. American College of Obstetrician and Gynecologists. Inappropriate use of the terms fetal distress and birth asphyxia. *Obstet Gynecol* 2004;104:903–4.
2. American Heart Association/American Academy of Pediatrics. Neonatal resuscitation. In Kattwinkel J, ed. *Textbook*, 4th edn. American Heart Association, American Academy of Pediatrics, 2000.
3. Badawi N, Kurinczuk JJ, Keogh JM, *et al.* Antepartum risk factors for newborn encephalopathy: The Western Australia case–control study *Br Med J* 1998;317:1549–53.
4. Badawi N, Kurinczuk JJ, Keogh JM, *et al.* Intrapartum risk factors for newborn encephalopathy: The Western Australia case–control study. *Br Med J* 1998;317:1554–8.
5. David R. Closed chest cardiac massage in the newborn infant. *Pediatrics* 1988;81:552–4.
6. Dawes G. *Fetal and Neonatal Physiology.* Chicago: Year Book, 1968.
7. Ellis M, Manandhar N, Manandhar DS, deL Costello AM. Risk factors for neonatal encephalopathy in Kathmandu, Nepal, a developing country: Unmatched case–control study. *Br Med J* 2000;32:1229–36.
8. Finer NN, Tarin T, Vaucher YE, Barrington K, Bejar R. Intact survival in extremely low birth weight infants after delivery room resuscitation. *Pediatrics* 1999;104:e40.
9. Guha DK. *Neonatal Resuscitation and Beyond.* New Delhi: Jaypee Brothers Medical Publishers, 1996.
10. Kumar R. Effect of training on the resuscitation practice of traditional birth attendants. *Trans R Soc Trop Med Hyg* 1994;88:459–60.
11. Low JA. Intrapartum fetal asphyxia: Definition, diagnosis, and classification. *Am J Obstet Gynecol* 1997;176:957–9.
12. Milner AD, Vyas H, Hopkin IE. Efficacy of facemask resuscitation at birth. *Br Med J Clin Res Ed* 1984;289:1563–5.
13. Moster D, Lie RT, Irgens LM, Bjerkedal T, Markestad T. The association of Apgar score with subsequent death and cerebral palsy: A population-based study in term infants. *J Pediatr* 2001;138: 798–803.
14. Nelson KB, Ellenberg JH. Apgar scores as predictors of chronic neurologic disability. *Pediatrics* 1981;68:36–44.
15. Palme C, Nystrom B, Thunell R. An evaluation of the efficiency of face masks in the resuscitation of newborn infants. *Lancet* 1985;2:207–10.
16. Palme-Kilander C. Methods of resuscitation in low-Apgar score newborn infants – A national survey. *Acta Paediatr* 1992;81:739–44
17. Palme-Kilander C, Thunell R. Pulmonary gas exchange during face mask ventilation immediately after birth. *Arch Dis Child* 1992;68:11–16.
18. Paul VK. Newborn care in India: A perspective. *Regional Health Forum* 1996;1:23–31.
19. Ramji S, Ahuja S, Thirupuram S, Rootwelt T, Rooth G, Saugstad OD. Resuscitation of asphyxic newborn infants with room air or 100% oxygen. *Pediatr Res* 1993;34:809–12.
20. Roberton NRC. Resuscitation of the newborn. In Rennie JM, Roberton NRC, eds. *Textbook of Neonatology,* 3rd edn. Edinburgh: Churchill Livingstone, 1999:241–65.
21. Sarnat HB, Sarnat MS. Neonatal encephalopathy following fetal distress. A clinical and electroencephalographic study. *Arch Neurol* 1976;33:696–705.
22. Saugstad OD, Ramji S, Irani SF, *et al.* Resuscitation of newborn infants with 21% or 100% oxygen: Follow-up at 18 to 24 months. *Pediatrics* 2003;112:296–300.
23. Saugstad OD, Ramji S, Rootwelt T, Vento M. Response to resuscitation of the newborn: Early prognostic variables. *Acta Paediatr,* 2005;94:1535–7.
24. Saugstad OD, Ramji S, Vento M. Resuscitation of depressed newborn infants with ambient air or pure oxygen: A meta-analysis. *Biol Neonate* 2005;87:27–34.
25. Saugstad OD, Rootwelt T, Aalen OO. Resuscitation of asphyxiated newborn infants with room air or oxygen: An international randomised trial. The Resair 2 study. *Pediatrics* 1998;102:e1.
26. Tyson JE. Immediate care of the newborn infant. In Sinclair JC, Bracken MB, eds. *Effective Care of the Newborn Infant.* Oxford: Oxford University Press, 1992:21–39.

27. Vain NE, Szyld EG, Prudent LM, Wiswell TE, Aguilar AM, Vivas NI. Oropharyngeal and nasopharyngeal suctioning of meconium-stained neonates before delivery of their shoulders: Multicentre, randomised controlled trial. *Lancet* 2004;364: 597–602.
28. Vento M, Asensi M, Sastre J, Garcia-Sala F, Pallardo FV, Vina J. Resuscitation with room air instead of 100% oxygen prevents oxidative stress in moderately asphyxiated term neonates. *Pediatrics* 2001;107:642–7.
29. Vyas H, Milner AD, Hopkins IE. Intrathoracic pressure and volume changes during the spontaneous onset of respiration in babies born by caesarean section and by delivery. *J Pediatr* 1981;99:787–91.
30. Vyas H, Milner AD, Hopkins IE, *et al.* Physiologic response to prolonged and slow-rise inflation in the resuscitation of the asphyxiated newborn infant. *J Pediatr* 1981;99:635–9.
31. Wiswell TE, Gannon CM, Jacob J, *et al.* Delivery room management of the apparently vigorous meconium-stained neonate: Results of the multicenter, international collaborative trial. *Pediatrics* 2000;105:1–7.
32. World Health Organization. *Basic Newborn Resuscitation: A Practical Guide.* Geneva: WHO. http://www.who.int/reproductive-health/publications/MSM 98 1/MSM 98 1 table of contents. en.html.
33. International Liason Committee on Resuscitation: Neonatal resuscitation. *Resuscitation* 2005;67:293–303.

SECTION XV

Fetal monitoring

Section Editors: **K. Maeda and H. P. van Geijn**

137 Intrapartum fetal asphyxia: prediction and diagnosis

J. A. Low

Controversy is currently centered on the benefits, risks and costs of intrapartum fetal surveillance. This is appropriate, recognizing the effort that has been committed to the development and application of methods for this purpose.

These questions will not be answered until the objectives of intrapartum fetal surveillance are clearly defined. Epidemiological studies indicate that a small component of long-term morbidity, such as cerebral palsy, can be attributed to intrapartum fetal asphyxia.[1,2] It is not realistic to anticipate that intrapartum fetal surveillance and management will have a major effect on long-term morbidity.

A realistic goal of intrapartum fetal surveillance is the diagnosis of fetal exposure to asphyxia and the prevention of morbidity and mortality due to this process. Thus the outcome measure for intrapartum fetal surveillance should be metabolic acidosis in the fetus and related morbidity in the newborn in the neonatal period.

This review will discuss outcome criteria and define the magnitude of the problem in the intrapartum period. The status of technology used in clinical practice or under development to predict this outcome will be examined.

Significance of fetal asphyxia

Exposure of the fetus to asphyxia has been a concern since the first report of an association between perinatal events and the mental and physical condition of the child.[3] The need for an animal model to systematically examine the effect of asphyxia and ischemia on the fetus was recognized in the late 1940s.[4] Since that time, research studies in the fetal monkey and lamb have advanced our understanding of the significance of asphyxia to the fetus.

Fetal asphyxia of a particular degree and duration may cause brain damage. Studies of the association between fetal asphyxia and brain damage in the fetal monkey and lamb have examined the effect of anoxia,[5,6] hypoxia[7–10] and ischemia.[11] Brain damage may occur in each model. However, in every instance, brain damage did not occur until the asphyxia was severe and hypotension with cerebral ischemia was present.

The studies of hypoxia in particular have demonstrated that the majority of fetuses who experience an asphyxial exposure do not have evidence of brain damage. This is due in part to the cardiovascular response of the fetus. The concept of fetal compensation has been established on the basis of studies in the fetal lamb. The effect of fetal asphyxia due to maternal hypoxemia,[12,13] reduced uteroplacental blood flow[14,15] and cord occlusion[16,17] on fetal cardiovascular function have been examined. There is a centralization of the fetal circulation with increased blood flow to the brain, heart and adrenal glands.

This cardiovascular response with increased cerebral blood flow is important to the integrity of the central nervous system during the compensatory phase. Cerebral oxygen metabolism is maintained because of the combination of increased cerebral blood flow and oxygen extraction and decreased oxygen requirements.[18] However, if the asphyxial exposure continues, decompensation with a progressive metabolic acidosis and a fall in arterial pressure will occur. The combination of hypoxemia and cerebral ischemia due to hypotension results in a marked reduction of cerebral oxygen metabolism, leading to cerebral dysfunction and brain damage.

This pathophysiological sequence of events is summarized in Figure 137.1. The important feature of anoxia is the short duration of the sequence of events with limited compensation prior to the threshold of brain damage. On the contrary with hypoxia, compensation may continue for variable periods (hours) before the threshold of decompensation leading to brain damage is reached.

Diagnosis of fetal asphyxia

A Task Force set up by the World Federation of Neurology Group defined asphyxia as a condition of

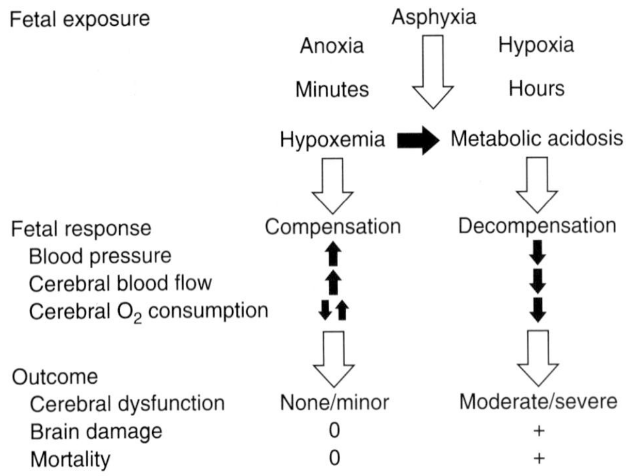

Figure 137.1 The pathophysiological sequence of events after exposure to asphyxia.

impaired blood gas exchange, leading, if it persists, to progressive hypoxemia and hypercapnia.[19] This is a good definition of asphyxia as it may affect the fetus and newborn. However, this may occur in a transient fashion which, although of physiological interest, has no pathological significance. Additionally, hypercapnia and respiratory acidosis alone do not account for organ system dysfunction or damage.[20] Significant fetal asphyxial exposure, leading to tissue oxygen debt with accumulation of fixed acids, results in a metabolic acidosis. Thus, for intrapartum fetal asphyxia, the following addition is proposed for this definition:

> Fetal asphyxia is a condition of impaired blood gas exchange leading to progressive hypoxemia and hypercapnia with a significant metabolic acidosis.

The diagnosis of intrapartum fetal asphyxia requires a blood gas and acid–base assessment. The important question is the threshold of a metabolic acidosis beyond which fetal morbidity or mortality may occur.

Umbilical vein and artery blood gas and acid–base measures at delivery represent valuable reference points of asphyxial exposure during labor. The umbilical vein reflects the effectiveness of maternal fetal blood gas exchange while the umbilical artery reflects the acid–base status of the fetus. The introduction of microelectrode blood gas systems has provided the opportunity to examine these measures in all pregnancies at delivery without risk to the fetus and newborn. Reference data for these measures in the umbilical vein and artery for 21,744 deliveries in our center are presented in Table 137.1.

Umbilical vein and artery acid–base status, and in particular the assessment of umbilical artery metabolic acidosis, is the most valuable indicator of fetal exposure to asphyxia during labor. Recognizing the importance of this measure, the Plymouth group was the first to emphasize the need for quality data to provide the basis for interpretation.[21] Several procedural and technical errors may occur during umbilical cord blood sampling and subsequent blood gas analysis.

Table 137.1 Mean blood gas and acid–base measures for 21,744 deliveries

	Umbilical vein		Umbilical artery	
	Mean	SD	Mean	SD
pH	7.340	0.07	7.248	0.069
pco_2	40.4	7.7	54.5	9.7
po_2	27.2	6.1	15.1	5.1
Base deficit	3.0	2.7	6.8	3.2

Table 137.2 Quality assessment of umbilical cord blood gas and acid–base data

	n	%
Single umbilical vein sample		
Single sample	1671	7.7
Two samples, single vessel	290	1.3
Paired samples, pco_2 error		
pco_2 outside physiological range	32	0.1
Artery–vein $pco_2 \leq 0$ mmHg	165	0.7
Artery–vein pco_2 1–3 mmHg	255	1.2
Paired samples, satisfactory criteria	19,931	89

Optimal interpretation requires a paired sample from both umbilical vein and artery. A single sample from the umbilical vein will define venous metabolic state but cannot rule out an arterial metabolic acidosis. During sampling, two aliquots may be drawn from the umbilical vein. Such a procedural error is implied when the vein–artery pH difference is less than 0.02. The accuracy of the calculated measures of metabolic acidosis is dependent upon the quality of the pH and pco_2 estimations. The accuracy of the pco_2 estimation should be questioned when the pco_2 value is outside the physiological range or the pco_2 artery–vein difference is a negative value or less than 4 mgHg. In these circumstances, the interpretation should be limited to pH alone. A review of our data in Table 137.1 indicated possible procedural or technical errors in 11% of the samples examined (Table 137.2).

Because of the lability of pco_2, pH is not a satisfactory proxy for metabolic acidosis.[22] Thus, an umbilical artery blood measure of metabolic acidosis is the best indicator of tissue oxygen debt experienced by the fetus. Lactate is the principal fixed acid contributing to this metabolic acidosis. However, an increase of lactate may be due to an increase of pyruvate as well as hypoxia.[23] We established an umbilical artery base deficit > 12 mmol/l as a criterion of fetal asphyxia. This represented 2 standard deviations below the mean adjusted for the component attributable to tissue oxygen debt. Whether this criterion reflects the threshold for

Table 137.3 Prevalence of significant intrapartum fetal asphyxia

	Per 1000 births
Metabolic acidosis	
UABD > 12 mmol/l	20
UABD > 16 mmol/l	5
Metabolic acidosis = cerebral dysfunction	3
Metabolic acidosis = brain damage	1–2

UABD, umbilical artery base deficit

morbidity in the fetus and newborn has been examined in recent studies.

Fifty-nine term fetuses with a metabolic acidosis, i.e. an umbilical artery base deficit > 16 mmol/l, were matched with 59 fetuses with normal blood gas measures at delivery. Forty percent of the newborns with an umbilical artery base deficit > 16 mmol/l had moderate or severe complications in one or more of the central nervous system, cardiovascular system, respiratory system or kidney.[20] A similar association was demonstrated in a matched case–control study of preterm newborns between 32 and 36 weeks of gestational age.[24]

In view of these findings, a study was conducted to determine the threshold of metabolic acidosis. This was a matched case–control study of three groups of term fetuses based on umbilical artery base deficit at birth. The three groups were umbilical artery base deficit 12–16 mmol/l ($n=58$), umbilical artery base deficit 8–12 mmol/l ($n=58$) and umbilical artery base deficit 4–8 mmol/l ($n=58$). Moderate and severe newborn complications occurred only in the fetuses with an umbilical artery base deficit > 12 mmol/l. The incidence of moderate and severe complications with an umbilical artery base deficit 12–16 mmol/l was 10%.[25] There is a progression of frequency of such complications with increasing metabolic acidosis, as noted in the study reported above, with a 40% incidence of moderate and severe complications when the umbilical artery base deficit was > 16 mmol/l.

These studies would support the contention that the threshold of fetal metabolic acidosis beyond which moderate or severe newborn complications *may* occur is an umbilical artery base deficit > 12 mmol/l.

The magnitude of the clinical problem is determined by the prevalence of a significant metabolic acidosis (Table 137.3). Approximately 20 fetuses per 1000 births will have a metabolic acidosis at delivery which exceeds the threshold for morbidity. The probability is greater in five fetuses per 1000 deliveries who have a metabolic acidosis with a base deficit > 16 mmol/l. The best measure of morbidity after intrapartum fetal asphyxial exposure is newborn cerebral dysfunction, expressed by moderate or severe newborn encephalopathy. Based upon our experience, the prevalence of

Table 137.4 Predictive value of antepartum risk factors (group 1) and antepartum plus intrapartum risk factors (group 2) for intrapartum fetal asphyxia

	Group 1		Group 2	
	Asphyxia present*	Asphyxia absent	Asphyxia present*	Asphyxia absent
Risk present	22	663	34	1081
Risk absent	22	1202	10	784
Sensitivity (%)	50		77	
Specificity (%)	64	42		
Positive predictive value (%)	3		3	
Negative predictive value (%)	98		99	

*Umbilical artery buffer base deficit > 12 mmol/l

intrapartum fetal asphyxia with a significant metabolic acidosis and moderate or severe newborn encephalopathy is of the order of three per 1000 births. Cerebral dysfunction does not necessarily imply brain damage with subsequent major handicap. A meta-analysis of the best available studies indicates that deficits due to brain damage occur in 20% after moderate newborn encephalopathy and 80% after severe newborn encephalopathy.[26] This implies a prevalence of intrapartum fetal asphyxia with brain damage in approximately one to two per 1000 births.

Prediction of intrapartum fetal asphyxia

The clinical paradigm which has been widely used combines clinical risk scoring with fetal heart rate surveillance to identify the fetus at risk of asphyxial exposure. The diagnosis can be confirmed or ruled out by a caput sample with a fetal blood gas and acid–base assessment. This has not resolved the problem due to shortfalls of each element of the paradigm which have become evident with increasing clinical experience.

Clinical risk scoring

The limitations of clinical risk scoring have been demonstrated in two studies. The predictive value of selected clinical risk factors was examined in 1909 consecutive pregnancies (Table 137.4) and in a second population of 100 consecutive pregnancies with biochemically determined intrapartum fetal asphyxia.[27] A second study examined the association between clinical risk factors and pregnancies resulting in a perinatal death with evidence of brain damage due to fetal asphyxia on postmortem examination.[28] These studies highlighted two points.

Fetal exposure to asphyxia occurs in pregnancies with no clinical risk factors. This occurred in 23% of the pregnancies studied to assess the predictive value of risk factors and in 35 of the 100 consecutive pregnancies with biochemically determined intrapartum fetal asphyxia. In the review of the perinatal mortality with postmortem evidence of brain damage due to antepartum or intrapartum fetal asphyxia, approximately 40% of the pregnancies had no clinical risk factors.

In those cases in which clinical risk factors were present, risk was determined by a wide range of clinical complications, with no single risk factor demonstrating a strong association with intrapartum fetal asphyxia. The positive predictive value for both antepartum and intrapartum risk factors for intrapartum fetal asphyxia was 3%. This low predictive value was true for all risk factors. Thus clinical risk scoring has a major problem with false-positive prediction of intrapartum fetal asphyxia.

Thus, the first step in the fetal assessment paradigm has not been validated. All pregnancies are at risk for this complication. The term 'low risk' based on clinical markers cannot be applied in regard to fetal exposure to asphyxia during labor. A number of clinical markers, such as antepartum hemorrhage, pregnancy-induced hypertension, fetal growth retardation and meconium in the amniotic fluid, are associated with a modest increased risk. However, in each case, the positive predictive value is low.

Fetal heart rate surveillance

Fetal heart rate observations began early in the 19th century with intermittent auscultation. Subsequently, continuous electronic fetal heart rate monitoring has been developed during the 20th century.[29] It has been difficult to determine if this surveillance has contributed to a decrease of fetal mortality or morbidity due to asphyxia.

Evidence has been presented to indicate that the introduction of electronic fetal heart rate monitoring has been associated with a reduction in the number of intrapartum fetal deaths.[30,31] However, mortality has not been resolved. Intrapartum fetal deaths continue to be reported in randomized clinical trials and in studies of perinatal mortality of stillbirths and early neonatal deaths after fetal asphyxia. In the last UK Confidential Enquiry into stillbirths and death in infancy, 9% of all deaths between 20 and 44 weeks of gestation were related to labor and, of the normally formed babies weighing at least 2500 g, 4.3% could be linked to intrapartum events.[32]

There is no evidence that fetal heart rate surveillance has been associated with a decrease in long-term morbidity as expressed by brain damage and cerebral palsy. The evidence of an association between abnormal fetal heart rate patterns and subsequent neurological abnormality has been limited.[33,34] A matched case–control study in our center examined the heart rate of fetuses with no metabolic acidosis at delivery who had a motor and cognitive assessment at 1 year. There was no difference in the fetal heart rate characteristics during the last 2–4 h of labor between the children with and without motor and cognitive disability at 1 year (unpublished data). Rosen and Dickinson[35] failed to find consistent fetal heart rate patterns that would predict brain injury. The authors concluded that these findings should not be surprising because the majority of brain damage occurs outside the intrapartum period.

A role for fetal heart rate surveillance to predict fetal metabolic acidosis holds greater promise. Laboratory studies in the fetal lamb and monkey have demonstrated a relationship between fetal heart rate behavior and fetal hypoxemia and metabolic acidosis. Late decelerations have been shown to occur when fetal oxygen tension decreases below a critical level. The interval between the onset of the contraction and the onset of the deceleration reflects the time necessary for fetal oxygen tension to fall below this threshold.[36–38] Late decelerations due to fetal hypoxemia in a previously normoxic fetus are due to chemoreceptor initiated reflex bradycardia which can be blocked by atropine, while in previously hypoxic fetuses the bradycardia is presumably due to a direct effect upon the myocardium.[39,40] The interpretation of heart rate variability by studies in the fetal lamb has been confounded by an apparent species difference. The late gestation sheep fetus consistently and reliably experiences an increase of heart rate variability with acute hypoxemia with or without acidosis.[41] In contrast, the hypoxemic human fetus generally exhibits a decrease of fetal heart rate variability.[42,43]

Two clinical studies have demonstrated an association between decreased baseline variability and late and prolonged decelerations and fetal metabolic acidosis at delivery.[44,45] An algorithm of three fetal heart rate patterns were defined on the basis of the presence of these fetal heart rate variables in six 10-min cycles in 1 h (Table 137.5). The sensitivity of this algorithm was good identifying 75% of fetal asphyxia and 96% of moderate and severe fetal asphyxia. The positive predictive value of the predictive fetal heart rate pattern was 90%. However, the positive predictive value of potentially predictive patterns ranged from 5% to 10%. The striking number of false positives for potentially predictive patterns represents the outstanding problem in the use of fetal heart rate surveillance as a screening test for intrapartum fetal asphyxia.

Well-designed, randomized, controlled trials are proposed as a means of minimizing selection bias and providing a measure of the true risks and benefits of a medical intervention. There have been no randomized clinical trials to compare fetal heart rate surveillance with intermittent fetal heart rate auscultation. The randomized clinical trials comparing intermittent auscultation and continuous electronic fetal heart rate

Table 137.5 Predictive and potentially predictive fetal heart rate patterns for intrapartum fetal asphyxia

	Baseline variability (cycles/h)		Decelerations late/prolonged (cycles/h)
Predictive	Absent ≥1	+	≥2
Potentially predictive	Minimal ≥2	+	≥2
	Minimal ≥2	or	≥2

monitoring have not demonstrated that continuous electronic fetal heart rate monitoring was associated with a decrease of fetal and newborn morbidity. Two factors have confounded these studies. The prevalence of intrapartum fetal asphyxia with cerebral dysfunction or brain damage is low. The magnitude of the randomized trials to date has not been sufficient to discriminate this infrequent outcome. The largest trial reported a decrease of newborn encephalopathy but not cerebral palsy.[46] The study protocols in these trials have modified clinical management by providing one-to-one support of care, assuring continuous surveillance during labor, a circumstance which, although widely advocated, is rarely achieved in clinical practice.

The randomized clinical trials have made an important contribution, confirming the occurrence of false-positive interpretation of electronic fetal heart rate recording, with unnecessary interventions. Nine randomized clinical trials, three with electronic fetal monitoring alone and six with electronic fetal monitoring with scalp sampling, have been analyzed in the Cochrane Pregnancy and Child Birth Database.[47,48] These studies have demonstrated that electronic fetal heart rate monitoring in relation to intermittent auscultation has been associated with increased incidence of cesarean section for fetal distress and dystocia, increased operative delivery and general anesthesia. It must be recognized that these outcomes are not due to the method of fetal heart rate surveillance but are a result of inappropriate interpretation of the fetal heart rate data.

The continuing use of fetal heart rate surveillance must recognize these limitations, i.e. some cases of asphyxial exposure will be missed and a large number of false positives must be clarified in order to avoid unnecessary intervention. Additionally, it is important that the quality of the fetal heart rate data be adequate for interpretation. This requires an optimal signal, recognition of interpretation problems and a satisfactory assessment protocol.

The data provided for interpretation by continuously recorded electronic fetal heart rate are superior to intermittent auscultation.[49] Interpretation of baseline variability can only be achieved from continuously recorded data interpreted either visually or by computer. The quality of the data must be adequate for interpretation. The ultrasound fetal heart rate signal and the tocodynometer have provided an attractive non-invasive option. These methods provide a good signal but not necessarily consistently. This is particularly true for the tocodynometer. A scalp electrode and an intrauterine catheter should be used in such circumstances.

Differences of classification criteria, decelerations in particular, remain. Classifications of late decelerations have, on the one hand, given first priority to the timing of the nadir of the deceleration, while others have emphasized the waveform. Interpretation of the waveform has focused on the onset to the nadir[50] or examined the residual component of the waveform.[51,52] Efforts to quantify decelerations are continuing.[53,54] Until a consensus is developed, criteria used in clinical practice should be clearly defined and consistently applied.

Encouraging progress has been made on computer-based programs for the interpretation of fetal heart rate patterns. However, the vast majority of clinical records are read visually. The limited interobserver reliability for the visual interpretation of fetal heart rate patterns has been well documented.[55] A study has been recently completed in our program. The interobserver reliability *k* values were: baseline fetal heart rate 0.70, baseline variability 0.55, accelerations 0.56, variable decelerations 0.46 and late decelerations 0.57. However, the interobserver reliability for an abnormal fetal heart pattern over 1 h of recording, based upon the presence of decreased baseline variability and/or late decelerations, was good. This experience supports the practice of defining patterns rather than assessing individual fetal heart rate variables.

There is no consensus in regard to the protocol for fetal heart rate assessment. Since low-risk and high-risk pregnancies for fetal asphyxia cannot be defined, fetal heart rate screening must be available for all patients. Since the objective of fetal heart rate screening is the prediction of asphyxial exposure, surveillance should begin early in labor with continuous recording of reasonable duration to permit interpretation. Visual interpretation requires that the fetal heart rate be carefully scored to establish the presence of abnormal patterns over a period of time.

Two clinical interventions have been advocated as options to improve the specificity of abnormal fetal heart rate patterns. Vibroacoustic stimulation with an acceleration response has been proposed as a sign of fetal reactivity and as a means of ruling out fetal acidosis in the presence of fetal heart rate patterns with decreased baseline variability and late decelerations with no accelerations.[56] However, subsequent reports of the predictive value of vibroacoustic stimulation have been equivocal.[57–59] A number of trials of amnioinfusion, particularly in the presence of oligohydramnios, have demonstrated a beneficial effect, relieving variable decelerations and reducing the rate of cesarean section for fetal distress.[60–64] These clinical interventions require further investigation.

Complementary technologies

The assessment of the fetal electrocardiographic (ECG) waveform is an attractive option since the signal can be obtained from the same fetal scalp electrode used for recording the fetal heart rate. It is possible to study the waveform in detail with appropriate filter characteristics and signal processing.[65] The time segments of ECG waveforms studied have included the ST segment and the PR interval.

Laboratory studies have examined the effect of hypoxemia and acidosis on the ST segment. In studies of acute hypoxemia, the ratio of the T-wave height to QRS height increased.[66–69] However, the results have not been consistent. ST segment depression with negative T-waves has been observed in experimentally growth-retarded guinea-pigs.[70] Slowly developed acidemia in fetal lambs was not detected by ST waveform analysis.[71]

Preliminary clinical observations suggested caution in the interpretation of ST waveforms.[72] Newborns with acidosis have had T/QRS ratios in the normal range.[73] Weak relationships have been reported between T/QRS ratios and fetal academia.[74,75] The recent development of higher-order FHR analysis has provided monitoring systems that can add automated fetal ECG ST segment analysis to the standard FHR and uterine contraction information which have been applied in a number of clinical trials. The result of the first trial was a 46% reduction of operative deliveries for fetal distress without change in newborn outcome.[76] Meta-analysis of two large randomized clinical trials of fetal heart rate assessment with the support of ST waveform analysis have shown that the number of babies born with metabolic acidosis at delivery could be reduced in conjunction with a reduction of operative deliveries for fetal distress.[77]

Laboratory studies of acute hypoxemia and fetal acidemia have demonstrated a conversion from negative relationships between the PR interval and the fetal heart rate to a positive relationship.[69,78] Preliminary observational studies and a randomized clinical trial suggest that this observation may be of value in the assessment of the human fetus during labor.[79,80]

Pulse oximetry provides a non-invasive measure of oxygen saturation which has proven of great value in patient surveillance in anesthesia and critical care. Fetal pulse oximetry is being developed for intrapartum assessment.[81,82]

Fetal pulse oximetry must have an acceptable level of precision and accuracy in measuring oxygen saturation. There have been technical problems unique to the fetus. The fetal signal is much smaller. The light-emitting diodes are placed in reflective rather than transmission mode. The sensor contact with the skin must be a good site free of hair. Progress has been made and the precision of newer prototypes has been encouraging.[83] The validation of the accuracy of pulsatile oxygen saturation measures in the human fetus is difficult. An encouraging correlation has been reported between pulse oximetry oxygen saturation and scalp blood oxygen saturation with cord vein oxygen saturation.[84,85]

Prospective clinical trials of pulse oximetry require a critical threshold of oxygen saturation. Chronic hypoxemia studies in fetal lambs have demonstrated that normal acid–base status in terms of pH and base deficit is maintained until oxygen saturation approaches 30%.[86,87] Data from the human fetus are limited. There is a decrease of fetal oxygen saturation during labor.[82,88] An examination of the relationship of a 30% threshold with pH in umbilical cord blood reported an encouraging sensitivity but poor specificity.[89] Carefully controlled clinical trials are required before this promising technology can be used as an adjunct to electronic fetal heart rate monitoring in intrapartum fetal assessment.

Near infrared spectroscopy has been used to provide quantitative data of cerebral oxygenation and hemodynamics in the newborn infant.[90] Near infrared spectroscopy is being developed as a means of continuous, non-invasive real-time measurement of change in fetal cerebral oxygenation and hemodynamics during labor. Preliminary reports of the application of this technology for fetal assessment during labor have been published.[91,92] There is some evidence of a correlation with pulse oximetry oxygen saturation during labor[91] and with acid–base status at delivery.[93] However, much research remains to be done before this technology can be considered for intrapartum fetal assessment. The outstanding issues have been reviewed recently.[94] These include the satisfactory maintenance of fetal contact of the sensor, confounding factors affecting the measurements and normative data during labor.

Fetal blood gas and acid–base assessment

The diagnosis of fetal asphyxia requires a blood gas and an acid–base assessment with evidence of a significant metabolic acidosis. An assessment can be carried out on fetal capillary blood obtained by scalp sampling during labor or in umbilical vein and artery blood at delivery. Such an assessment can confirm or rule out a metabolic acidosis.

The limitations of fetal sampling and blood gas and acid–base assessment are well known. This assessment provides a measure at one point in the continuum of labor and delivery. Continuous rather than intermittent assessment of acid–base status would be an optimal method of fetal surveillance. However, pH electrodes tested in recent years have had to contend with technical difficulties and artifacts.[95,96] Thus, this option is not available for clinical practice at the present time. The second problem is that fetal scalp sampling may not be technically feasible in early labor, while later in labor the procedure is invasive with a small but significant risk. This is a constraint in regard to repeated sampling in a fetus with a developing metabolic acidosis during labor and the frequent sampling required to clarify false-positive abnormal fetal heart rate patterns.

Discussion

Intrapartum fetal asphyxia is important to the fetus and newborn. Laboratory studies in the fetal monkey and lamb have established that a single severe episode of asphyxia accompanied by cardiovascular decompensation with cerebral ischemia can cause brain damage.

The responsibility of the obstetrician is early recognition to prevent morbidity and mortality. Clinical studies have established that asphyxial exposure with a significant metabolic acidosis occurs in approximately 20 per 1000 births. The key to understanding the significance of an asphyxial exposure is expressed by the equation:

$$\text{Fetal asphyxial exposure} + \text{fetal response} = \text{outcome}$$

The majority of fetuses are not compromised because of the fetal compensatory response to the asphyxial exposure. This fact provides the window of opportunity for the obstetrician to make a precise diagnosis of fetal exposure with a developing metabolic acidosis and to intervene before fetal compromise has occurred. Based on the animal studies, this window ranges from minutes to hours subject to the severity and nature of the asphyxial exposure. There is reason to speculate that, during labor, in most cases the asphyxial exposure is relative in degree and intermittent in nature. Thus, the window of opportunity to predict and diagnose asphyxial exposure tends to be longer rather than shorter.

Fetal exposure with fetal decompensation does occur. Clinical studies indicate that morbidity after fetal asphyxia is uncommon with cerebral dysfunction in three per 1000 births and brain damage in one to two per 1000 births. The responsibility of the neonatologist is early diagnosis, continuing assessment, and management of the newborns to minimize morbidity. Within the foreseeable future, medical interventions may be available to interrupt the cascade of biochemical events leading to neuronal death in order to minimize brain damage.

An appropriate objective for intrapartum fetal asphyxia would be to reduce the incidence of fetal exposure from 20 to 10 per 1000 births and prevent asphyxial exposure with cerebral dysfunction and brain damage. There is little evidence that intrapartum fetal surveillance has achieved such a goal, while the modest specificity of current methods has led to an increase of unnecessary interventions. This can be attributed to the limitations of current assessment protocols and technology.

Clinical risk scoring of pregnancies for intrapartum asphyxia has not proven to be of benefit. Asphyxial exposure occurs in pregnancies without clinical risk factors, while relevant risk factors have limited predictive value. Thus fetal heart rate assessment has become the primary method of screening for intrapartum asphyxia. Fetal heart rate patterns of decreased baseline variability and late decelerations have predictive value. However, the sensitivity is modest with 25% of fetal exposures not identified, while specificity is poor with a large number of false-positive fetal heart rate patterns requiring clarification. Fetal acid–base assessment will provide a definitive diagnosis. However, these measures provide a measure at one point in the continuum of labor and delivery.

The significance of fetal asphyxia justifies continuing efforts to improve the predictive sensitivity and specificity of intrapartum fetal surveillance protocols. Fetal heart rate surveillance has predictive value and should continue. However, the limitations must be recognized. In order to be a useful predictor, quality data beginning early in labor and of sufficient duration to permit interpretation are required. Satisfactory interpretation requires standardized criteria with well designed assessment protocols which can serve as a basis of ongoing evaluation of this method. It is widely acknowledged that fetal heart rate surveillance will require supplementary assessment methods to improve sensitivity and specificity of prediction. The role of fetal ECG waveform analysis and pulse oximetry is being examined. Near infrared spectroscopy is at a much earlier stage in development. These complementary measures are not yet ready for use in clinical practice.

The liberal use of fetal blood gas and acid–base assessment must be entertained until the predictive characteristics of current screening modalities have improved. Routine umbilical vein and artery blood gas assessments at delivery ensure that all asphyxial exposures during labor are identified. This is a valuable outcome measure for intrapartum fetal assessment and ensures that the neonatologist is forewarned of all newborns that have experienced an asphyxial exposure during labor. Periodic fetal scalp sampling and acid–base assessment during labor represent the only definitive methods to confirm that a suspected fetal exposure is occurring or to establish that an abnormal fetal heart rate pattern represents a false-positive prediction.

REFERENCES

1. Blair E, Stanley FJ. Intrapartum asphyxia: A rare cause of cerebral palsy. *J Pediatr* 1988;112:515–19.
2. Gaffney G, Sellers S, Flavell V, *et al.* Case–control study of intrapartum care, cerebral palsy and perinatal death. *Br Med J* 1994; 308:743–50.
3. Little WJ. On the influence of abnormal parturition, difficult labor, premature birth and asphyxia neunatorum on the mental and physical condition of the child, especially in relation to deformities. *Trans London Obstet Soc* 1862;3:293–325.
4. Windle WF. Neurological and psychological deficits of asphyxia neonatorum: With consideration of the use of primates for experimental investigations. By twenty-eight contributors. *Symposium in Neurology*. Springfield, IL: Charles C. Thomas, 1958.
5. Ranck JB, Windle WF. Brain damage in the monkey, *Macacca mulatta*, by asphyxia neonatorum. *Exp Neurol* 1959;1:130–54.
6. Mallard EC, Gunn AJ, Williams CE, *et al.* Transient umbilical cord occlusion causes hippocampal damage in the fetal sheep. *Am J Obstet Gynecol* 1992;167:1423–30.
7. Myers RE. Two patterns of perinatal brain damage and their conditions of occurrence. *Am J Obstet Gynecol* 1972;112: 246–76.
8. Ting P, Yamaguchi S, Bacher JD, *et al.* Hypoxic–ischemic cerebral necrosis in mid-gestational sheep fetuses: Physiopathologic correlations. *Exp Neurol* 1983;80:227–45.
9. Gunn AJ, Parer JT, Mallard EC, *et al.* Cerebral histologic and electrocorticographic changes after asphyxia in fetal sheep. *Pediatr Res* 1992;31:486–91.
10. deHaan HH, vanReempts JLH, Vles JSH, *et al.* Effects of asphyxia on the fetal lamb brain. *Am J Obstet Gynecol* 1993;169:1493–1501.
11. Williams CE, Gunn AJ, Mallard C, Gluckman PD. Outcome after ischemia in the developing sheep brain; an electro-encephalographic and histological study. *Ann Neurol* 1992;31:14–21.
12. Cohn HE, Sacks EJ, Heymann MA, Rudolph AM. Cardiovascular responses to hypoxemia and acidemia in fetal lambs. *Am J Obstet Gynecol* 1974;120:817–24.
13. Peeters LL, Sheldon RE, Jones MD, *et al.* Blood flow to fetal organs as a function of arterial oxygen content. *Am J Obstet Gynecol* 1979;135:637–46.
14. Jensen A, Roman C, Rudolph AM. Effects of reducing uterine blood flow on fetal blood flow distribution and oxygen delivery. *J Dev Physiol* 1991;15:309–23.
15. Ball RH, Espinoza MI, Parer JT, *et al.* Regional blood flow in asphyxiated fetuses with seizures. *Am J Obstet Gynecol* 1994; 170:156–61.
16. Itskovitz J, LaGamma EF, Rudolph AM. Effects of cord compression on fetal blood flow distribution and O_2 delivery. *Am J Physiol* 1987;252:H100–9.
17. Ball RH, Parer JT, Caldwell LE, Johnson J. Regional blood flow and metabolism in ovine fetuses during severe cord occlusion. *Am J Obstet Gynecol* 1994;171:1549–55.
18. Richardson BS, Rurak D, Patrick JE, *et al.* Cerebral oxidative metabolism during sustained hypoxemia in fetal sheep. *J Dev Physiol* 1989;11:37–43.
19. Bax M, Nelson KB. Birth asphyxia: A statement. World Federation of Neurology Group. *Dev Med Child Neurol* 1993;35:1002–24.
20. Low JA, Panagiotopoulos C, Derrick EJ. Newborn complications after intrapartum asphyxia with metabolic acidosis in the term fetus. *Am J Obstet Gynecol* 1994;170:1081–7.
21. Westgate J, Garibaldi JM, Greene KR. Umbilical cord blood gas analysis at delivery: A time for quality data. *Br J Obstet Gynaecol* 1994;101:1054–63.
22. Low JA. Fetal asphyxia and brain damage. *Curr Obstet Gynaecol* 1993;3:213–28.
23. Low JA, Pancham SR, Piercy NW, *et al.* Maternal and fetal lactate characteristics during labor and delivery. *Lactate in Acute Conditions. Proceedings of an International Symposium.* Basel: Karger, 1979:29–47.
24. Low JA, Panagiotopoulos C, Derrick EJ. Newborn complications after intrapartum asphyxia with metabolic acidosis in the preterm fetus. *Am J Obstet Gynecol* 1995;172:805–10.
25. Low JA, Lindsay BG, Derrick EJ. Threshold of metabolic acidosis associated with newborn complications. *Am J Obstet Gynecol* 1997;177:1391–4.
26. Pelowski A, Finer NN. Birth asphyxia in the term infant. In Sinclair J, Lucey J, eds. *Effective Care of the Newborn Infant.* London: Oxford University Press, 1992:363–6.
27. Low JA, Simpson LL, Tonni G, Chamberlain S. Limitations in the clinical prediction of intrapartum fetal asphyxia. *Am J Obstet Gynecol* 1995;172:801–4.
28. Low JA, Simpson LL, Ramsey DA. The clinical diagnosis of asphyxia responsible for brain damage in the human fetus. *Am J Obstet Gynecol* 1992;167:11–15.
29. Sureau C. Historical perspectives: Forgotten past, unpredictable future. *Baillieres Clin Obstet Gynecol* 1996;10:167–84.
30. Quilligan EJ, Paul RH. Fetal monitoring: Is it worth it? *Obstet Gynecol* 1975;45:96–100.
31. Vintzoleos AM, Nochimson DJ, Guzman ER, *et al.* Intrapartum electronic fetal heart rate monitoring versus intermittent auscultation: A meta-analysis. *Obstet Gynecol* 1995;85: 149–55.
32. Gardosi J. Monitoring technology and the clinical perspective. *Baillieres Clin Obstet Gynecol* 1996;10:325–39.
33. Holmquist P, Svenningsen NW, Ingermarsson I. Neurodevelopmental outcome and electronic fetal heart rate monitoring in a neonatal intensive care population. *Acta Obstet Gynecol Scand* 1984;63:527–32.
34. Painter MJ, Scott M, Hirsch RP, *et al.* Fetal heart rate patterns during labor: Neurologic and cognitive development at six to nine years of age. *Am J Obstet Gynecol* 1988;159:854–8.
35. Rosen MG, Dickinson JC. The paradox of electronic fetal monitoring: More data may not enable us to predict or prevent infant neurologic morbidity. *Am J Obstet Gynecol* 1993;168: 745–51.
36. James LS, Morishimo HO, Daniel SS, *et al.* Mechanism of late decelerations of the fetal heart rate. *Am J Obstet Gynecol* 1972; 113:578.
37. Mueller-Heubach E, Myers RE, Adamson K. Fetal heart rate and blood pressure during prolonged partial asphyxia in the rhesus monkey. *Am J Obstet Gynecol* 1980;137:48–52.
38. Murata Y, Martin CB, Ikenoue T, *et al.* Fetal heart rate accelerations and late decelerations during the course of intrauterine death in chronically catheterized rhesus monkeys. *Am J Obstet Gynecol* 1982;144:218–23.
39. Martin CB. Regulation of the fetal heart rate and genesis of fetal heart rate patterns. *Semin Perinatol* 1978;2:131–46.
40. Parer JT, Krueger TR, Harris JL. Fetal oxygen consumption and mechanisms of heart rate response during artificially produced late decelerations of fetal heart rate in sheep. *Am J Obstet Gynecol* 1980;136:478–82.
41. Bocking AD. The relationship between heart rate and asphyxia in the animal fetus. *Clin Invest Med* 1993;16:166–75.
42. Ribbert LSM, Snijders RJM, Nicolaides KH, Visser GHA. Relation of fetal blood gases and data from computer assisted analysis of fetal heart rate patterns in small for gestation fetuses. *Br J Obstet Gynaecol* 1991;98:820–3.
43. Dawes GS, Moulden M, Redman CWG. Short term fetal heart rate variation, decelerations and umbilical flow velocity waveforms before labor. *Obstet Gynecol* 1992;80:673–8.
44. Low JA, Cox MJ, Karchmar EJ, *et al.* The prediction of intrapartum fetal metabolic acidosis by fetal heart rate monitoring. *Am J Obstet Gynecol* 1981;139:299–305.
45. Low JA, Victory R, Derrick EJ. Predictive value of electronic fetal monitoring for intrapartum fetal asphyxia with metabolic acidosis. *Obstet Gynecol* 1999;93:285–91.
46. MacDonald D, Grant A, Sheridan-Perreira M, *et al.* The Dublin randomized controlled trial of intrapartum fetal heart rate monitoring. *Am J Obstet Gynecol* 1985;152:524–39.
47. Neilson JP. EFM alone vs. intermittent auscultation in labor (revised 04 May 1994). In Keirse MJNC, Renfrew MJ, Neilson JP, Crowther C, eds. Pregnancy and Childbirth Module. In *The Cochrane Pregnancy and Childbirth Database. The Cochrane Collaborative Issue 2.* Oxford: Update Software, 1995.
48. Neilson JP. EFM + scalp sampling vs. intermittent auscultation in labor (revised 04 May 1994). In Keirse MJNC, Renfrew MJ, Neilson JP, Crowther C, eds. Pregnancy and Childbirth Module. In *The Cochrane Pregnancy and Childbirth Database. The Cochrane Collaboration Issue 2.* Oxford: Update Software, 1995.
49. Hon EH. The electronic evaluation of the fetal heart rate. Preliminary report. *Am J Obstet Gynecol* 1958;75:1215–30.
50. Hon EH, Quilligan EJ. Electronic evaluation of fetal heart rate. Further observations on pathologic fetal bradycardia. *Clin Obstet Gynecol* 1968;11:145–67.

51. Sureau C, Charmine J, Michelon B. Le probleme du rhythme cardiaque foetal. Difficulties d'interpretation, solutions techniques. *Gynecol Obstet Paris* 1970;69:259–86.
52. Uzan S, Fouillot JP, Sureau C. Computer analysis of FHR patterns in labour. In Spencer JAD, ed. *Fetal Monitoring*. Tunbridge Wells: CHP, 1989:159–64.
53. VanGeijn H, Dekker G, deVries J, Van Vugt J. Fetal heart rate patterns during labor. In VanGeijn JP, Copray FJA, eds. *A Critical Appraisal of Fetal Surveillance*. Amsterdam: Elsevier, 1994: 238–70.
54. Chang A, Sahota DS, Reed NN, *et al.* Computerized fetal heart rate analysis in labor – Effect of sampling rate. *Eur J Obstet Gynecol Reprod Biol* 1995;59:125–9.
55. Paneth N, Bommaritom, Stricker J. Electronic fetal monitoring and later outcome. *Clin Invest Med* 1993;16:159–65.
56. Smith CV, Nguyen HN, Phelan JP, Paul RH. Intrapartum assessment of fetal well being. A comparison of fetal acoustic stimulation with acid–base determinations. *Am J Obstet Gynecol* 1986;155:726–8.
57. Richards DS, Cefalo RC, Thorpe JM, *et al.* Determinants of fetal heart rate response to vibroacoustic stimulation in labor. *Obstet Gynecol* 1988;71:535–40.
58. Umstad M, Bailey C, Permezel M. Intrapartum fetal stimulation testing. *Aust N Z J Obstet Gynaecol* 1992;32:222–4.
59. Anyaegbunam AM, Ditchik A, Stoessel R, Mikhail MS. Vibroacoustic stimulation of the fetus entering the second stage of labor. *Obstet Gynecol* 1994;83:963–6.
60. Miyazaki FS, Nevarez F. Saline amnioinfusion for relief of repetitive variable decelerations: A prospective randomized study. *Am J Obstet Gynecol* 1985;153:301–6.
61. Owen J, Hensen BV, Hauth JC. A prospective randomized study of saline solution amnioinfusion. *Am J Obstet Gynecol* 1990; 162:1146–9.
62. MacGregor SN, Banzhaf WC, Silver RK, Depp R. A prospective randomized evaluation of intrapartum amnioinfusion. Fetal acid–base status and cesarean delivery. *J Reprod Med* 1991;36: 69–73.
63. Strong TH, Hetzler G, Sarno AP, Paul RH. Prophylactic intrapartum amnioinfusion: A randomized clinical trial. *Am J Obstet Gynecol* 1990;162:1370–5.
64. Schrimmer DB, Macri CJ, Paul RH. Prophylactic amnioinfusion as a treatment of oligohydramnios in laboring patients: A perspective randomized trial. *Am J Obstet Gynecol* 1991;165:972–5.
65. Greene KR. The ECG waveform. *Baillieres Clin Obstet Gynecol* 1987;1:131–55.
66. Rosen KG, Hrbek A, Karlsson K, *et al.* Changes in the ECG and somatosensory evoked EEG responses (SER) during intrauterine asphyxia in the sheep. *Biol Neonate* 1976,30.95–101.
67. Greene KR, Dawes GS, Lilja H, Rosen KG. Changes in the ST waveform of the fetal lamb electrocardiogram with hypoxemia. *Am J Obstet Gynecol* 1982;144:950–8.
68. Widmark C, Hokegard KH, Lagercrantz H, *et al.* Electrocardiographic waveform changes and catecholamine responses during acute hypoxia in the immature and mature fetal lamb. *Am J Obstet Gynecol* 1989;160:1245–50.
69. Widmark C, Lindecrantz K, Murray H, Rosen KG. Changes in the PR, RR intervals and the ST waveforms of the fetal lamb electrocardiogram with acute hypoxemia. *J Dev Physiol* 1992; 18:99–103.
70. Widmark C, Jansson T, Lindecrantz K, Rosen KG. ECG waveform, short term heart rate variability and plasma catecholamine concentrations in response to hypoxia in intrauterine growth retarded guinea-pig fetuses. *J Dev Physiol* 1991;15:161–8.
71. deHaan HH, Ijzermans ACM, deHaan J, Hasaart THM. The T/QRS ratio of the electrocardiogram does not reliably reflect well being in fetal lambs. *Am J Obstet Gynecol* 1995;172:35–43.
72. Westgate J, Harris M, Curnow JSH, Greene KR. Plymouth randomized trial of cardiotocogram only versus ST waveforms plus cardiotocogram for intrapartum monitoring in 2400 cases. *Am J Obstet Gynecol* 1993;169:1151–60.
73. Newbold S, Wheeler T, Clewlow F. Comparison of the T/QRS ratio of the fetal electrocardiogram and the fetal heart rate during labour and the relation of these variables to condition at delivery. *Br J Obstet Gynaecol* 1991;98:173–8.
74. MacLachlan NA, Spencer JAD, Harding K, Arulkumaran S. Fetal acidemia, the cardiotocograph and the T/QRS ratio of the fetal ECG in labour. *Br J Obstet Gynaecol* 1992;99:26–31.
75. Murphy KW, Russell V, Johnson P, Valente J. Clinical assessment of fetal electrocardiogram monitoring in labour. *Br J Obstet Gynaecol* 1992;99:32–7.
76. Amer-Wahlin I, Hellsten C, Noren H, et al. Cardiotocography only versus cardiotocography plus ST analysis of fetal electrocardiogram for intrapartum fetal monitoring: A Swedish randomized controlled trial. *Lancet* 2001;358:534–8.
77. Amer-Wahlin I, Bordahl P, Eikeland T, *et al.* ST analysis of fetal electrocardiogram during labor: Nordic observational multicenter study. *J Matern Fetal Neonatal Med* 2002;12:260–6.
78. vanWijngaarden WJ, deHaan HH, Sahota DS, *et al.* Changes in the PR interval – Fetal heart rate relationship of the electrocardiogram during fetal compromise in chronically instrumented sheep. *Am J Obstet Gynecol* 1996;175:548–54.
79. Mohajer MP, Sahota DS, Reed NN, *et al.* Cumulative changes in the fetal electrocardiogram and biochemical indices of fetal hypoxia. *Eur J Obstet Gynecol Reprod Med* 1994;55:63–70.
80. vanWijngaarden WJ, Sahota DS, James DK, *et al.* Improved intrapartum surveillance with PR interval analysis of the fetal electrocardiogram: A randomized trial showing a reduction in fetal blood sampling. *Am J Obstet Gynecol* 1996;174:1295–9.
81. Gardosi JO, Schram CM, Symonds EM. Adaptation of pulse oximetry for fetal monitoring during labour. *Lancet* 1991;1:1265–7.
82. Johnson N, Johnson VA, Fischer J, *et al.* Fetal monitoring with pulse oximetry. *Br J Obstet Gynaecol* 1991;98:36–41.
83. Nijland R, Jongsma HW, Nijhuis JG. Reflectance pulse oximetry (RPOX): Two sensors compared in piglets (abstract). *Am J Obstet Gynecol* 1995;172:365.
84. Luttkus A, Fengler TW, Friedmann W, Dudenhausen JW. Continuous monitoring of fetal oxygen saturation by pulse oximetry. *Obstet Gynecol* 1995;85:183–6.
85. McNamara H, Chung DC, Lilford R, Johnson N. Do fetal pulse oximetry readings at delivery correlate with cord blood oxygenation and acidemia. *Br J Obstet Gynaecol* 1992;99:735–8.
86. Richardson BS, Carmichael L, Homan J, Patrick JE. Electrocortical activity, electro-ocular activity and breathing movements in fetal sheep with prolonged and graded hypoxemia. *Am J Obstet Gynecol* 1992;167:553–8.
87. Nijland R, Jongsma HW, Nijhius JG, *et al.* Arterial oxygen saturation in relation to metabolic acidosis in fetal lambs. *Am J Obstet Gynecol* 1995;172:810–19.
88. Dildy GA, van den Berg PP, Katz M, *et al.* Intrapartum fetal pulse oximetry. Fetal oxygen saturation trends during labor and relation to delivery outcome. *Am J Obstet Gynecol* 1994;171:679–84.
89. Dildy GA, Thorp JA, Yeast JD, Clark SL. The relationship between oxygen saturation and pH in umbilical blood. Implications for intrapartum fetal oxygen saturation monitoring. *Am J Obstet Gynecol* 1996;175:682–7.
90. Wyatt JS, Cope M, Delpy DT, *et al.* Quantitation of cerebral blood volume in newborn human infants by near infrared spectroscopy. *J Appl Physiol* 1990;68:1086–91.
91. Peebles DM, Edwards AD, Wyatt JS. Changes in human fetal cerebral hemoglobin concentration and oxygenation during labor measured by near-infrared spectroscopy. *Am J Obstet Gynecol* 1992;166:1369–73.
92. O'Brien PMS, Doyle PM, Rolfe P. Near infrared spectroscopy in fetal monitoring. *Br J Hosp Med* 1993;49:483–7.
93. Aldrich CJ, D'Antona D, Wyatt JS, *et al.* Fetal cerebral oxygenation measured by near infrared spectroscopy shortly before birth and acid-base status at birth. *Obstet Gynecol* 1994;84:861–6.
94. Hamilton RJ, Hodgett SG, O'Brien PMS. Near infrared spectroscopy applied to intrapartum fetal monitoring. *Baillieres Clin Obstet Gynaecol* 1996;10:307–24.
95. Lauersen NH, Miller FC, Paul RH. Continuous intrapartum monitoring of fetal scalp pH. *Am J Obstet Gynecol* 1979;133:44–50.
96. Small ML, Beall M, Platt LD, *et al.* Continuous tissue pH monitoring in the term fetus. *Am J Obstet Gynecol* 1989;161:323–9.

138 Cardiotocography

H. P. van Geijn

Introduction

Until the second half of the 20th century, assessment of the fetal condition depended on very limited information: the growth of the uterus and its contents, the movements of the fetus perceived by the mother and listening to the fetal heart beat with a mono- or biauricular stethoscope.[1] Sudden absence of fetal movements in the second half of pregnancy was, at that time, not only a very emotional but also a serious diagnostic problem. Usually one had to wait for some weeks in order to observe any growth of the uterus before the decision could be reached to induce labor. The Spalding's sign at x-ray examination, showing overlapping of the fetal skull bones like roof tiles as a result of advanced maceration of the fetal tissues, was one of the few helpful objective diagnostic signs of fetal demise.

This recurrent dilemma of whether or not the fetus had died *in utero* formed the major impulse for the development of cardiotocography.[2] Initially, fetal abdominal electrocardiography and phonocardiotocography were experimented with, but failed, primarily due to technical problems.

It was only when the fetal heart beat was found to be detected easily by means of ultrasound (the Doppler-shift) or through the application of direct electrocardiography that cardiotocography became popular as the method for monitoring the condition of the fetus. Currently, the majority of obstetric decisions to assist delivery of the baby by artificial means (cesarean section, forceps or vacuum extraction) for reasons of suspected fetal distress rely on information gathered through the application of cardiotocography.

It is the confirmation that the fetal heart rate (FHR) pattern is normal and, therefore, the near 100% certainty that the fetus is in a good condition, which have made cardiotocography so attractive and have encouraged its widespread use. This development is very understandable considering the dependence on indirect signals from the fetus and the problems mentioned above concerning the very limited means of monitoring the condition of the fetus prior to the introduction of cardiotocography. However, now cardiotocography has been in use for some decades, criticism of the method itself and objections to its widespread application are increasing (Table 138.1). These criticisms and objections will be discussed in more detail and an attempt made to reach a more meaningful conclusion.

The normal and abnormal fetal heart rate pattern

The normal FHR pattern is characterized by a baseline frequency of between 110 and 150 beats/min, presence of periodic accelerations, a normal heart rate variability with a bandwidth of between 5 and 25 beats/min and the absence of decelerations.[3] In this regard, the importance placed on the 120 and 160 frequencies is misleading. It originates from the second half of the 19th century when the normal frequencies were stated by Von Winckel to be between 120 and 160 beats/min.

The FHR pattern is abnormal when one or more of the following features are observed: a baseline

Table 138.1 Criticisms of cardiotocography

Insufficient understanding of the (patho)physiological background
Too indirect a signal of the fetal condition
Number of technical pitfalls
Differences in recording techniques
Primarily qualitative information (pattern recognition)
Lack of uniform classification systems
Confusion due to the many influences on the fetal heart rhythm
Substantial intra- and interobserver variation regarding the interpretation
Low validity, high incidence of false-positive findings
Primarily screening method, too often applied as a diagnostic
Leads to an increase in artificial deliveries
Lack of agreement on how, when and whom to monitor
Contributes to medico-legal vulnerability

frequency of below 110 or above 150 beats/min, absence of accelerations for more than 45 min, decreased or absent FHR variability and the existence of repeated variable or late decelerations. A baseline frequency between 100 and 110 can be considered as normal when the duration of pregnancy has exceeded 41 weeks.

Are the criticisms of cardiotocography justified?

In recent years cardiotocography has been criticized for a number of reasons. A far from complete summary is given in Table 138.1. The criticisms have a very diverging character. Each of them will be commented on in the following sections.

The FHR pattern is too indirect as a signal of the fetal condition

The (patho)physiological background of the fetal heart rhythm is extremely complex.[4] Blood pressure, cardiovascular regulation, the condition of the autonomic and voluntary central and peripheral nervous system, respiration, temperature regulation, the renin–angiotensin system, the functioning of the adrenals, endocrine mechanisms, the cardiac conduction systems, the condition of the vessel walls and cellular processes all contribute to the shape of the heart rate pattern recorded on paper or a visual screen. Under normal circumstances the FHR pattern primarily represents the state of the central nervous system, i.e. the 24-h (circadian) rhythms and the cycling of behavioral states (ultradian rhythms). When the condition of the fetus is being threatened there is a shift to a more likely representation of disturbances in the regulation of the blood pressure and the cardiac performance, and ultimately a direct influence on the fetal heart.

Artificial occlusions of the umbilical cord circulation and the uterine circulation in animal experiments have contributed to a better understanding of the various aspects of the FHR pattern under pathological circumstances. The human situation is far more complex however: successive uterine contractions vary in duration and intensity; the position of the human fetus may change; the amount of amniotic fluid varies from fetus to fetus; occlusions of the uterine circulation, umbilical vessels and/or placental circulation can be absent, be partial or even be total; and the circulation in the umbilical vein and/or one or both umbilical arteries can be affected. These are just a few of the many combinations on the circulatory level that may occur when the fetal condition is threatened. Next there are the many complex variations regarding the biochemical status of the fetus, in particular the state of the acid–base balance. It should be remembered that depth, duration and shape of variable decelerations have no direct relation to the acid–base balance of the fetus at a particular moment.[5]

Differences in technique

For a correct understanding of the FHR pattern as recorded on paper or a screen, it is essential to understand the technical procedures involved with the acquisition and processing of the heart beat signal obtained through ultrasound or direct electrocardiography.[6] The cardiotocographic equipment has been improved markedly since the introduction of cardiotocography. Nevertheless, some technical problems have never been fully resolved: some artificial FHR variability, halving and doubling of heart rate frequencies, no recording made of cardiac arrhythmias with Doppler ultrasound and recording of the maternal instead of the FHR frequency. The major problems, however, occur in clinical practice. There is no uniform opinion regarding the preferred paper speed. Recording speeds vary from 1 to 2 to 3 cm/min, depending on the obstetric unit. A low paper speed facilitates the overview of a recording but has definite disadvantages: 'long-term' FHR variability is artificially accentuated, 'short-term' variability is hardly recognizable and the time-relation between uterine contractions and decelerations is more difficult to assess.

The many influences of the FHR pattern

The healthy near-term fetus demonstrates a characteristic FHR pattern with continuous cycling of a 'reactive' and a 'non-reactive' FHR pattern representing the cycling of the sleep states 2F [rapid eye movement (REM)-sleep, active sleep] and 1F (non-REM-sleep, quiet sleep).[7] This cycling is interspersed, in particular around midnight, with periods of fetal activity (jogging) accompanied by recurrent accelerations sometimes mimicking fetal tachycardia. The maximum duration of a 1F state is 45 min in a healthy fetus.

When pregnancy advances, accelerations increase in number, duration and amplitude. Variability increases during the 2F states, but is nearly constant after 26 weeks of gestational age in 1F states.[8] The variability in the 1F states primarily relates to the absence or presence of clusters of regular mouthing movements (associated with oscillations!) or breathing movements (associated with short-term variability!).[9] FHR variability may vary from day to day and week to week in the individual fetus.[8]

Interpretation of a cardiotographic tracing is particularly difficult early preterm. In general, the decision to start cardiotocography is determined by a serious obstetric problem such as the presence of intrauterine growth restriction, rupture of membranes, vaginal blood loss or pregnancy-induced hypertension.

Interpretation then is not only more difficult because of the age of the fetus and the presenting obstetric problem, but also because of the use of maternally administered medication. Betamimetics increase the baseline FHR and are associated with a decrease in FHR variability. Magnesium sulfate causes a decrease in FHR variability. Antihypertensives may cause tachycardia, bradycardia, flattening of the accelerations or a decrease in variability. Bethamethasone, contrary to dexamethasone, leads to a decrease in the incidence of fetal body and breathing movements and concomitantly a decrease in the number of accelerations and diminished variability.[10]

High intra- and interobserver variability

Reading, classification and interpretation should be the successive steps in the assessment of cardiotocographic tracings. Often, too easily a conclusion is reached in (vague) terms of a suspicious, pathological, ominous or terminal FHR pattern.

The high intra- and interobserver variability concerning the classification and interpretation of FHR patterns has been substantiated in a large number of publications. Assessment of the baseline frequency and the presence or absence of accelerations and decelerations is rather uniform, but lacks any uniformity when FHR variability and deceleration types are concerned.[11] Easy, exact guidelines as to how to determine and interpret FHR variability are lacking. It appears that in daily obstetric practice variable decelerations far too often are classified as early or late decelerations, merely on the basis of the time-relation between the associated uterine contraction and the deceleration. The typical characteristics of the variable decelerations are that they vary in shape, duration and depth and, on this basis, nearly all decelerations occurring during labor should be classified as being of the variable type.[12] The 'shouldering', i.e. the increase in FHR prior to and following a variable deceleration, can incorrectly be interpreted as an acceleration. Their monotonous and recurrent character is, however, very different from the irregularly spaced accelerations occurring in association with fetal body movements. Recurrent increases in the FHR during uterine contractions should raise suspicion that the (umbilical) venous circulation is being obstructed.

The low validity, high false-positive rate

The low validity of cardiotocography has been concluded from a very limited number of earlier performed randomized studies, in which cardiotocography was compared with intermittent auscultation. These studies suffer from a number of serious drawbacks and inadequacies concerning patient selection, sample size, randomization procedures, in- and exclusion criteria, the knowledge of the responsible obstetricians as to how to classify and interpret cardiotocographic tracings and the comparability of the applied intermittent auscultation with daily obstetric practice (dedicated nurses participated in the auscultation groups).

A major problem with these and other studies aiming to assess the validity of cardiotocography and related procedures is the lack of solid endpoints concerning the fetal condition. One of the few hard endpoints is the status of the acid–base balance in arterial and venous cord blood, often applied to assess justification of artificial deliveries for reasons of suspected fetal distress. The primary aim of obstetric interventions in this regard is, however, to prevent fetal distress and as such these measures are not very helpful in assessing the adequacy of obstetric management in individual cases.

Cardiotocography increases medico-legal vulnerability

Ultrasonography and cardiotocography have been named as the 'minefields of obstetrics'. In contrast to antepartum monitoring, it is the intrapartum application of cardiotocography which may lead to litigation. The knowledge that their baby was in a good condition at the start of the birthing process is for parents an unbearable thought when the baby suffers from handicaps in later life which may possibly relate to the occurrence of fetal distress during the process of labor and delivery. The consumers, supported by legal experts, expect from the obstetrician not so much that she/he diagnoses fetal distress, but that a serious threat to the fetal condition is being avoided, certainly if it concerns a child with full potential for later life. The layman wonders why obstetricians do not all apply the same monitoring techniques and cannot understand why FHR patterns cannot be classified and interpreted uniformly.

The medico-legal vulnerability associated with the application of cardiotocography and other monitoring techniques is a very complex area.[13] Many aspects are involved, such as the time path followed, the standard of care at a certain moment, the preceding training experienced, the chain of command at a certain moment, the limitations of indirect information, uncertainty when damage to the infant occurred, the confusing nomenclature in use and the lack of exact definitions and guidelines. Nearly all cases are discussed 'in retrospect' knowing the fatal result of a particular case. Laymen have little understanding of peak loads in clinical care, the time span necessary before conclusions can reasonably be reached and the intensity of communication prior to a secondary cesarean section. The consumers demand optimal care at each moment in order to maximize future potentials for their child. They exert more and more pressure on decision making and easily push for a cesarean section when the condition of their child might be endangered.

Cardiotocography leads to an increase in obstetric interventions

One of the objections toward electronic fetal monitoring is that the widespread application has induced an increase in the number of obstetric interventions, in particular the incidence of cesarean sections. Randomized studies in the 1970s and early 1980s have demonstrated a higher incidence of artificial deliveries when cardiotocography was compared with (dedicated) intermittent auscultation. This was especially apparent when FHR monitoring was applied in low-risk pregnancies. The adding of microblood sampling as a second mode of fetal surveillance, to assess the fetal acid–base status in case of suspicious or abnormal FHR patterns, clearly reduces the number of obstetric interventions if compared with the application of cardiotocography alone.

Following the introduction of cardiotocography, however, obstetrics and maternal–fetal medicine have developed in different directions. Certain changes in attitudes of the profession and the public have favored obstetric intervention: a shift toward a far lower gestational age at which all is done to increase chances for fetal survival and diminished neonatal morbidity, another approach toward the fetus in breech position both preterm and term, an increase in the maternal age for the first pregnancy, an increase in the number of twins and triplets, another look at the pain experienced by the mother during labor and delivery, other criteria for the duration of the birthing process, etc. The main line in obstetric policies has moved toward prevention of serious maternal and fetal risks in whatever circumstances. Large randomized studies in high-risk populations and a recent meta-analysis provide evidence of an approximate 60% reduction in perinatal mortality due to fetal distress when electronic fetal monitoring is applied as a routine in high-risk groups.[14] These and other studies support earlier recommendations to apply cardiotocography in risk groups. Risks with a potential impact on the condition of the fetus may be identified before pregnancy (hypertension, diabetes), may show up during the course of pregnancy (vaginal blood loss, early preterm rupture of membranes) or may occur during the process of labor and delivery (meconium staining, FHR decelerations). An anticipative attitude by the obstetrician taking care of the pregnant mother should always be warranted.

The future of cardiotocography

Cardiotocography was initially introduced merely on an empirical basis. At the start little was understood of the (patho)physiology at the basis of the FHR pattern, the many factors influencing the shape of the FHR pattern and the clinical implications to be drawn from 'abnormal' FHR patterns. A classic example is the pseudosinusoidal pattern related to fetal sucking which for a long time was not distinguished from the truly sinusoidal pattern associated with serious fetal anemia or severe fetal acidosis. The simultaneous introduction of guidelines for classifying and interpreting FHR patterns by outstanding obstetricians living on different continents (Caldeyro-Barcia, Hammacher, Hon, Maeda, Wood) has further contributed to the confusion in nomenclature and definitions, a problem which has not been resolved in mondial terms until today.

In spite of many efforts, improvements in the quality of the instrumentation, better understanding of the FHR patterns and improved recognition of the position of cardiotocography among the full arsenal of fetal surveillance techniques, the current status of cardiotocography is still at the awkward age. It certainly has not reached full maturity yet. Major weaknesses are found in its application. Differences in paper speed, lack of uniform and exact definitions, uncertainties regarding how, when and whom to monitor, problems with storage of cardiotocographic tracings, uncertainty if and when fetal microblood sampling should be applied, the generally very limited training of those who are directly involved with fetal monitoring and the lack of guidelines on how to handle the great variety of (often complex) clinical circumstances are just a few of the problems which have weakened the position of cardiotocography as a monitoring technique. Another aspect is the department's organization regarding responsibilities at various locations, i.e. the outpatient clinics, the antenatal clinics and the labor and delivery unit. Are

Table 138.2 Improvements in cardiotocography

Improvements in cardiotocography
Further understanding of (patho)physiology
Knowledge of technical pitfalls
Uniform paper speed, vertical scaling
Knowledge of the many factors influencing fetal heart rate (FHR) patterns
Knowledge of all relevant clinical data
Discipline in reading, classification and interpretation of FHR patterns
Recognition that cardiotocography is an indirect parameter of fetal condition
Recognition that cardiotocography is only one parameter of fetal condition
Recognition that cardiotocography is only a screening technique
Disposition of maximal possible information (microblood sampling)
Availability of protocols how, when and whom to monitor
Availability of quantitative, objective FHR analyses
Digital storage of fetal heart rate data
Systematic pre- and postgraduate training

there solid and uniform arrangements and can one trust that they are continuously followed by each and every member of the department? Ways in which cardiotocography could be improved are shown in Table 138.2.

A computerized system permitting digital processing and storage of all FHR data has a number of potential advantages: the availability of quantitative information including analysis of trends, easy retrieval of relevant cardiotocographic traces for education purposes, decreased medico-legal vulnerability concerning lost cardiocographic traces, etc. The currently available integration of a number of fetal (heart rhythm, oxygen saturation) and maternal (heart rhythm, electrocardiogram, oxygen saturation, blood pressure) variables in one monitor offers more possibilities for fetal monitoring in future, in particular studies of the effects of changes in the maternal cardiovascular status on the condition of the fetus. There have been some initial experiences with management supporting systems in which clinical, biophysical and biochemical data of the mother and the fetus are integrated. These systems still have a long way to go, but certainly deserve further study.

Cardiotocography in itself is a useful and indispensable adjunct for monitoring the condition of the (endangered) fetus. In this regard, the continuous debate concerning its usefulness compared with intermittent auscultation is meaningless. Both methods, in principle, provide similar information. However, cardiotocography in comparison with intermittent auscultation results in continuous vs. spot-like, and objective vs. subjective, data.

REFERENCES

1. De Snoo K. *Leerboek der Verloskunde*. Groningen: Wolters Uitgeversmaatschappij, 1946.
2. Sureau C. The history of fetal surveillance. In Van Geijn HP, Copray FJA, eds. *A Critical Appraisal of Fetal Surveillance*. Amsterdam: Elsevier, Excerpta Medica, 1994:3–10.
3. Rooth G, Huch A, Huch R. Guidelines for the use of fetal monitoring. *Int J Gynecol Obstet* 1987;25:159–67.
4. Van Ravenswaay-Arts CMA, Kollee LAA, Hopman JCW, Stoelinga GBA, Van Geijn HP. Heart rate variability; clinical applicability in adults. *Ann Intern Med* 1993;118:436–47.
5. De Haan HH, Gunn AJ, Gluckman PD. Fetal heart rate changes do not reflect cardiovascular deterioration during brief repeated umbilical cord occlusions in near-term fetal lambs. *Am J Obstet Gynecol* 1997;176:8–17.
6. Van Geijn HP. Developments in CTG analysis. *Baillières Clin Obstet Gynecol; Intrapartum Surveill* 1996;10:185–209.
7. Nijhuis JG. *Fetal Behaviour: Development and Perinatal Aspects*. Oxford: Oxford University Press, 1992.
8. Mantel R, Van Geijn HP, Ververs IAP, Colenbrander GJ, Kostense PJ. Automated analysis of antepartum fetal heart rate in relation to fetal rest–activity states: A longitudinal study of uncomplicated pregnancies using the Sonicaid System 8000. *Eur J Obstet Gynecol Reprod Biol* 1996;71:41–51.
9. Van Woerden EE, Van Geijn HP, Swartjes JM, Caron FYM, Brons JTY, Arts NFTh. Fetal heart rhythms during behavioural state 1F. *Eur J Obstet Gynecol Reprod Biol* 1988;28:29–38.
10. Mulder EJH, Derks JB, Zonneveld MF, Bruinse HW, Visser GHA. Transient reduction in fetal activity and heart rate variation after maternal betamethasone administration. *Early Hum Dev* 1994; 36:49–60.
11. Donker DK, Hasman A, Van Geijn HP. Interobserver variation in the assessment of fetal heart rate recordings. *Eur J Obstet Gynecol Reprod Biol* 1993;52:21–8.
12. Van Geijn HP, Dekker GA, De Vries JIP, Van Vugt JMG. Fetal heart rate patterns during labour. In Van Geijn HP, Copray FJA, eds. *A Critical Appraisal of Fetal Surveillance*. Amsterdam: Elsevier, Excerpta Medica, 1994:238–70.
13. Van Geijn HP. Some reflections on fetal surveillance. In Van Geijn HP, Copray FJA, eds. *A Critical Appraisal of Fetal Surveillance*. Amsterdam: Elsevier, Excerpta Medica, 1994:659–74.
14. Gardosi J. Monitoring technology and the clinical perspective. *Baillières Clin Obstet Gynecol; Intrapartum Surveill* 1996;10:325–40.

139 Intrapartum fetal heart rate monitoring

T. Ikeda, H. Sameshima, M. Kaneko, Y. Kodama and T. Ikenoue

Introduction

In developed countries, fetal heart rate (FHR) monitoring is widely used to survey fetal well-being in the intrapartum period. In the early stage of introduction of FHR monitoring by Hon,[1] Caldeyro-Barcia *et al.*,[2] and Hammacher and Werners,[3] it seemed that FHR monitoring could contribute to a decrease in perinatal mortality and morbidity and to a decrease in incidence of perinatal brain damage, including cerebral palsy and mental retardation.[4] Despite early enthusiasm, subsequent randomized controlled trials comparing FHR monitoring with intermittent auscultation did not support the efficacy of FHR monitoring in preventing adverse fetal outcomes.[5–7] These trials unexpectedly showed higher rates of cesarean section and operative delivery in FHR monitoring groups than in auscultation groups, without exception. A meta-analysis of 58,855 pregnant women from 12 studies confirmed these observations.[8] Low specificity of FHR monitoring to detect fetal asphyxia is a partial explanation for increased cesarean section and operative delivery rates.

Concurrently, epidemiologists used advanced statistical techniques to analyze the real origin of cerebral palsy in large cohort[9] and population-based studies,[10] and concluded that intrapartum asphyxia causes no more than 10% of cerebral palsy cases, significantly less than had previously been thought. Intrapartum FHR monitoring seemed to lose its role in preventing the majority of cerebral palsy and major mental retardation cases, playing a preventive role in just 10% of cerebral palsy and minor mental retardation cases.

However, there is a discrepancy between the statistical evidence against intrapartum FHR monitoring and good clinical acceptance by caregivers.[11] There was a need to reevaluate the effectiveness and safety of FHR monitoring, following agreement on definitions and nomenclature of FHR patterns, and the establishment of management algorisms in hospitals. Guidelines published in 1997 for interpreting electronic FHR monitoring[12] fitted the first need exactly.

Here, we first explain FHR patterns of classification according to the National Institute of Child Health and Human Development (NICHD) guidelines, and physiological and pathological meanings underlying these FHR patterns. Secondly, we discuss several issues important to the successful application of this new research guideline to clinical practice. Finally, we emphasize the need to urgently establish a standard clinical management algorism and discuss the clinical endpoints we should reach.

NICHD Research Planning Workshops and research guidelines for interpreting electronic FHR

NICHD research planning workshops were held between May 1995 and November 1996 in Bethesda, MD, and Chicago, IL. Eighteen specialists in the field attended, mainly from North America, with various educational and research backgrounds. The guidelines developed at the workshops only include definitions and classifications of FHR patterns that most members agreed on. Therefore, it is important to note that these guidelines constitute an inadequate basis for decision making by caregivers; other classifications and nomenclatures are needed, as we discuss later. There are four basic components of FHR to read and understand: (1) baseline rate, (2) baseline FHR variability, (3) acceleration, and (4) deceleration.

Baseline rate

The baseline FHR is the approximate mean FHR rounded to 5 beats/min during a 10-min segment, excluding (Figure 139.1):

- Periodic or episodic changes
- Periods of marked FHR variability
- Segments of the baseline which differ by more than 25 beats/min.

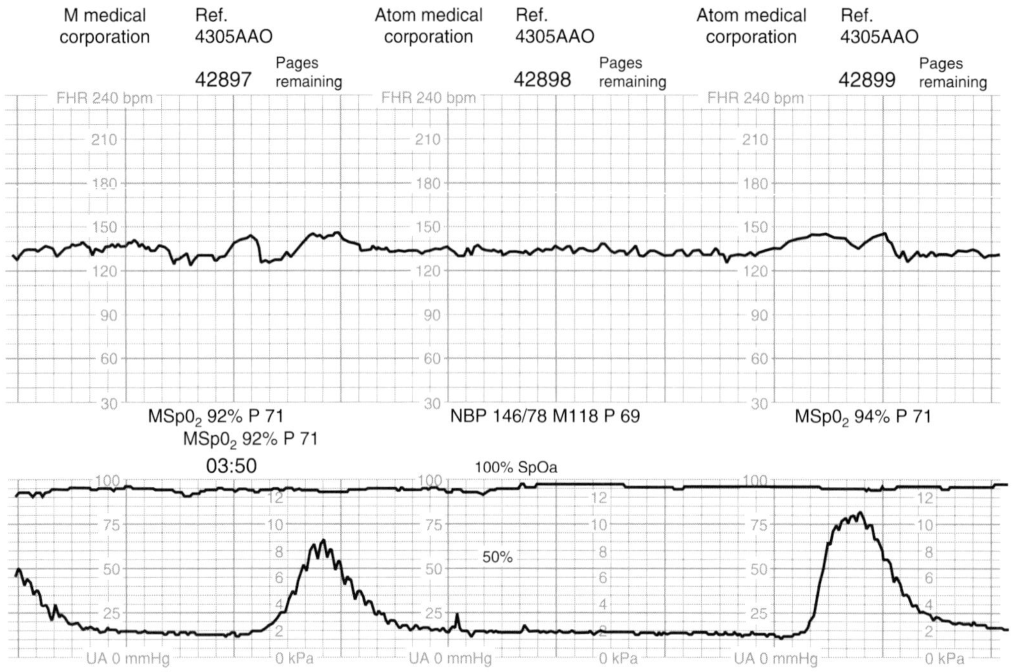

Figure 139.1 The baseline fetal heart rate (FHR) is the approximate mean FHR rounded to 5 beats/min during a 10-min segment. The baseline FHR in this case is 135 beats/min.

In any 10-min window, the minimum baseline duration must be at least 2 min, otherwise the baseline for that period is indeterminate, in which case one may need to refer to the previous 10-min segment(s) for determination of the baseline. The normal baseline FHR is regarded as between 110 and 160 beats/min. Values below 110 beats/min are regarded as bradycardia and those above 160 beats/min are regarded as tachycardia.

The baseline rate is determined by two autonomic nervous systems, sympathetic and parasympathetic, with the latter system being the more important contributor.

Baseline FHR variability

Baseline FHR variability is deemed as fluctuations in the baseline FHR of 2 cycles/min or greater. These fluctuations are irregular in amplitude and frequency and are visually quantified as the amplitude of the peak-to-trough in beats per minute as follows:

- Amplitude range undetectable = *absent* FHR variability
- Amplitude range detectable but ≤5 beats/min = *minimal* FHR variability
- Amplitude range 6–25 beats/min = *moderate* FHR variability
- Amplitude range > 25 beats/min = *marked* FHR variability

These grades of fluctuation are illustrated in Figure 139.2, together with a sinusoidal pattern. The sinusoidal pattern differs from variability in that it has a smooth, sine wave-like pattern of regular frequency and amplitude and is excluded in the definition of FHR variability.

Baseline variability has been thought to be a product of a 'push-and-pull' relationship between sympathetic and parasympathetic systems. However, the degree of each contribution is not the same; the parasympathetic system is more dominant than the sympathetic system. This is evidenced by the fact that atropine, a parasympathetic blocker, completely diminishes variability, whereas propranorol, a beta-sympathetic blocker, does not.[13] The presence of normal variability guarantees that perfusion and oxygenation to the cerebral cortex, mid-brain, heart and connections between these organs is well maintained.[14] Therefore, baseline variability is the most important parameter to ensure fetal well-being.

Baseline variability can be evaluated by eye, because it is well correlated with computer-calculated values.[15] In clinical practice, the observer does not need to differentiate short-term and long-term variability, as they almost always change concurrently and separate evaluation of the two kinds of variability is not helpful in clinical decision making.

Accelerations

An acceleration is a visually apparent abrupt increase (defined as onset of acceleration to peak in less than 30 s) in FHR above the baseline. The increase is calculated from the most recently determined portion of the baseline. The acme is more than 15 beats/min

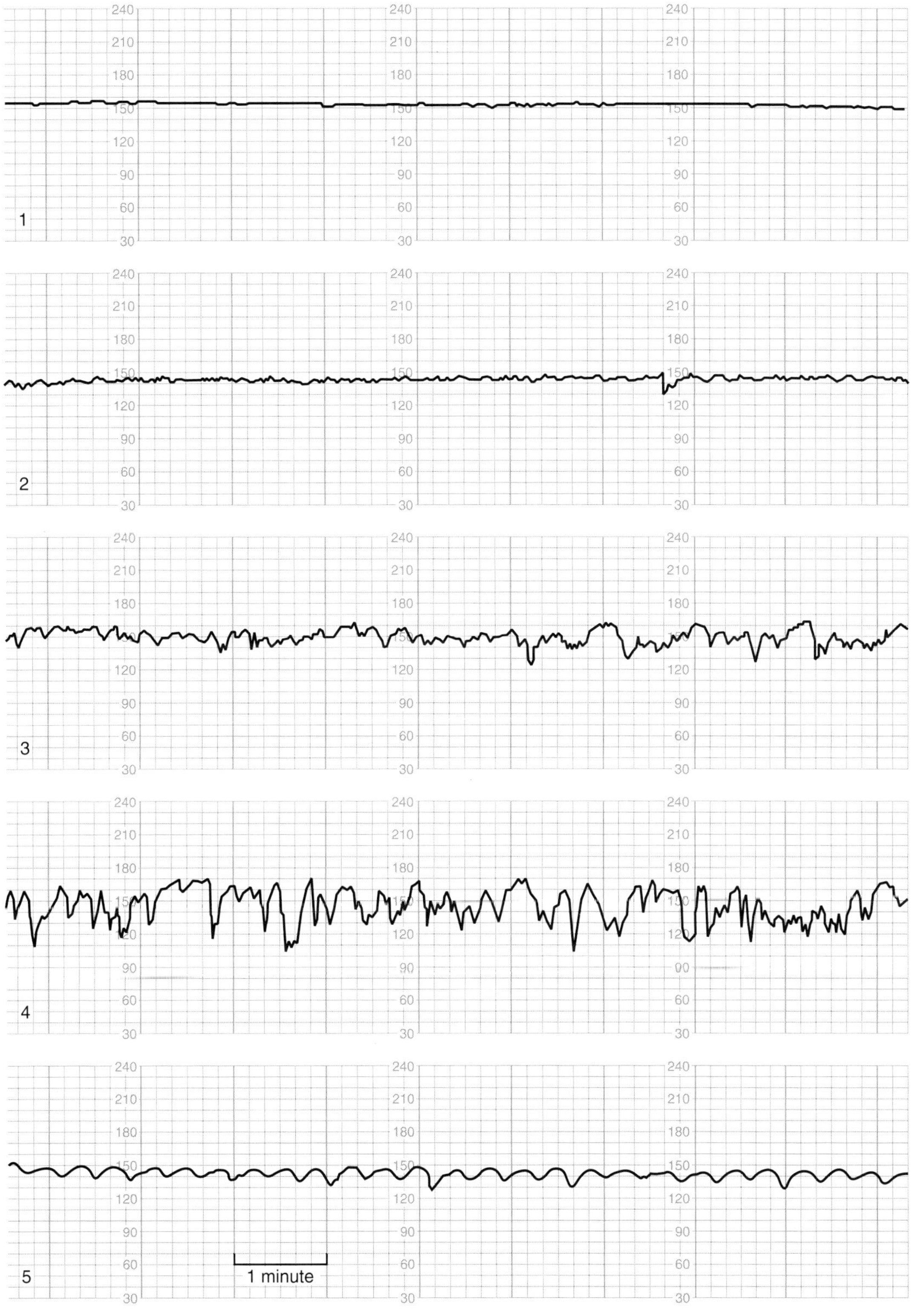

Figure 139.2 Varying degrees of FHR variability. 1, Undetectable; 2, minimal; 3, moderate; 4, marked; 5, sinusoidal pattern. Original scaling, 30 beats/min per centimeter vertical axis, and paper speed 3 cm/min horizontal axis. From National Institute of Child Health and Human Development Research Planning Workshop.[12]

above the baseline, and the acceleration lasts more than 15 s but less than 2 min from the onset to return to baseline. Before 32 weeks of gestation, accelerations are defined as having an acme of more than 10 beats/min above the baseline and duration of more than 10 s. A prolonged acceleration is between 2 and 10 min in duration. There is a close association between the presence of accelerations and normal FHR variability, and both accelerations and normal variability have the same positive prognostic

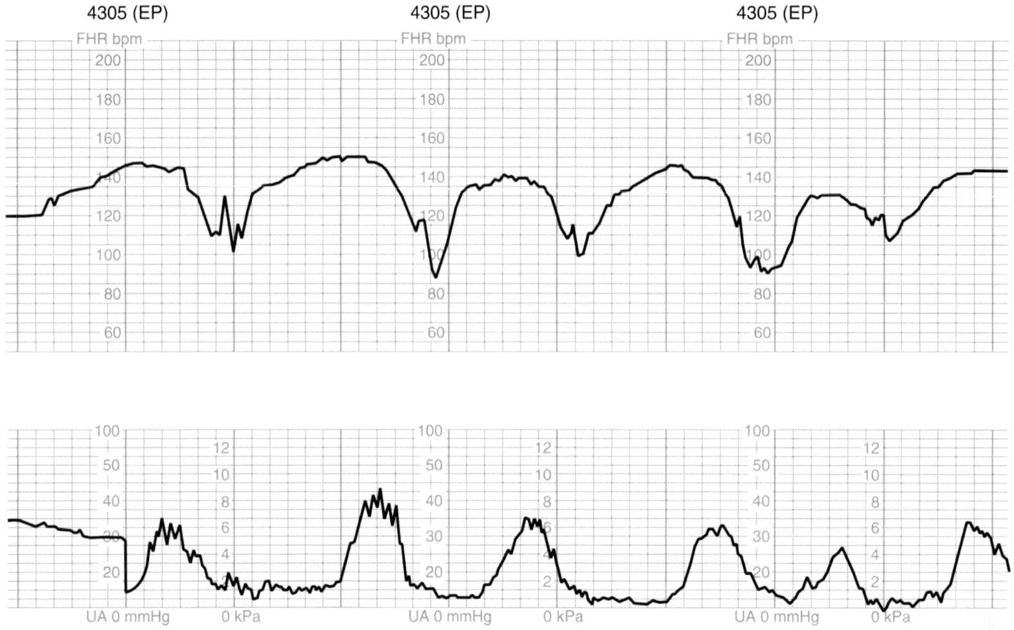

Figure 139.3 'Non-reflex late deceleration'. Primiparous 31-year-old woman was received cesarean section for fetal asphyxia and placental abruption was confirmed. The gas analysis of umbilical arterial blood showed severe metabolic acidosis: pH, 6.982; pco_2, 43.0 mmHg; po_2, 19.2 mmHg; base excess −21 mEq/l. Apgar score is 5 and 6 at 1 and 5 min after birth, respectively. Newborn elicited convulsion at her first day.

significance of normal fetal oxygenation.[14] In the dying monkey fetus, loss of acceleration is always preceded by the appearance of late deceleration.[16]

Decelerations

Periodic patterns are the alterations in FHR associated with uterine contractions. The three characteristic periodic patterns seen are late decelerations, early decelerations, and variable decelerations. Prolonged decelerations are a subcategory of variable or late decelerations. Episodic decelerations are similar to periodic patterns, but do not have the same constant association with contractions.

Late deceleration of the FHR is a visually apparent gradual decrease (defined as onset of deceleration to nadir more than 30 s) and return to baseline FHR associated with a uterine contraction. In most cases, the onset, nadir, and recovery are all late in relation to the beginning, peak, and ending of the contraction, respectively.

There are two types of late deceleration in terms of mechanisms to appear. One type is related to chemoreceptor and baroreceptor reflex to fetal hypoxemia,[17] and is sometimes called 'reflex late deceleration'. The other type is related to myocardial depression and is called 'non-reflex late deceleration' (Figure 139.3). Reflex late deceleration usually accompanies baseline variability and normal acid–base status, but with non-reflex late deceleration, baseline variability shows a minimal or undetectable fall in fetus acidosis. It is clinically important to differentiate these two types of late deceleration.

Early deceleration of the FHR is a visually apparent gradual decrease (defined as onset of deceleration to nadir longer than 30 s) and return to baseline FHR associated with a uterine contraction. The nadir of the deceleration coincides with the peak of the contraction. In most cases, the onset, nadir, and recovery all coincide with the beginning, peak, and ending of the contraction, respectively.

Variable decelerations are visually apparent abrupt decreases (defined as onset of deceleration to beginning of nadir less than 30 s) in FHR from the baseline. The decrease in FHR below the baseline is at least 15 beats/min, lasting (from baseline to baseline) at least 15 s, but less than 2 min. When variable decelerations are associated with uterine contractions, their onset, depth, and duration commonly vary with successive contractions (Figure 139.4).

Until now, two mechanisms have been thought to produce variable deceleration: umbilical cord compression and head compression. Both mechanisms require the presence of vagal reflex. It is important to note that a severe degree of variable deceleration with deep and long heart rate can cause a fetus to decompensate and suffer acidosis.[14] Therefore, to rule out acidosis in clinical practice, it is critical to keep track of the presence of baseline variability.

Prolonged deceleration is a subcategory of variable deceleration. The decrease in FHR below the baseline is at least 15 beats/min, lasting between 2 and 10 min. The definition changes to a change in baseline rate (e.g. bradycardia) if the prolonged deceleration is longer than 10 min.

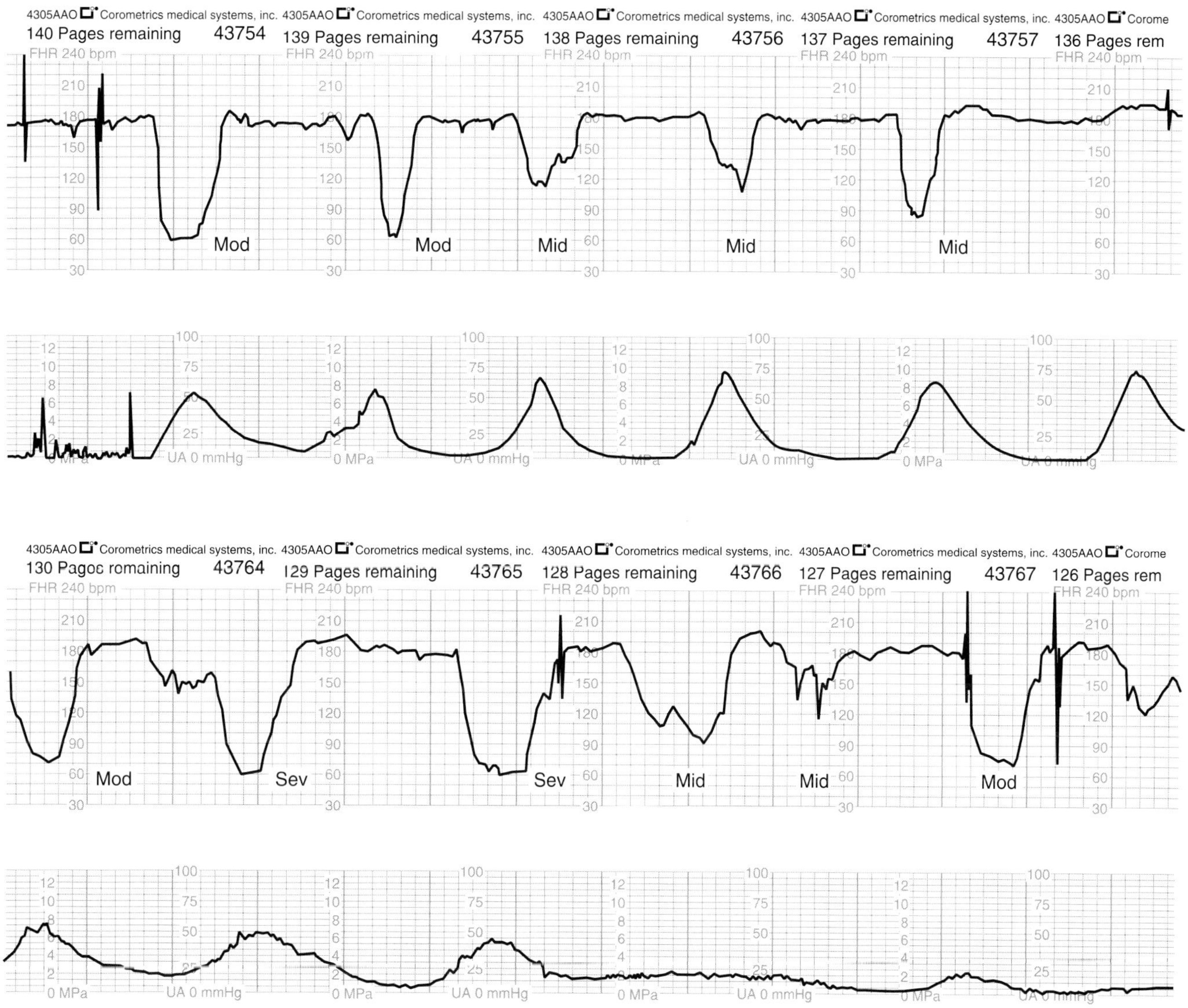

Figure 139.4 Variable decelerations. According to Kubli *et al.*'s classification, mild (Mid), moderate (Mod), and severe (Sev) variable decelerations are classified based on the nadir and duration of the deceleration.

Application of NICHD guidelines to intrapartum clinical management

As stated earlier, because the NICHD guidelines derive from the consensus of only 18 experts, other considerations about FHR patterns are needed in clinical decision making.

Consideration of clinical background

It is important to consider the clinical background, because different fetuses with different characteristic backgrounds show the same FHR pattern, and such patterns have a different clinical effect on each fetus. With intrapartum FHR decelerations, intrauterine growth restriction fetuses had a significantly higher lactate level than that appropriate for gestational age fetuses.[18] When an FHR pattern signifying hypoxia or asphyxia is observed in fetuses suspected antenatally to have intrauterine growth restriction, intervention should be considered earlier than appropriate-for-gestational-age fetuses.

Gestational age should be taken into account whenever FHR patterns are assessed. Premature fetuses have a propensity to higher basal FHR rates, lower amplitude of acceleration, and lower baseline variability compared with mature fetuses. In addition, the higher variability (active) phase and the lower variability (resting) phase can be differentiated after 28 weeks of gestational age in human fetuses.[19]

Maternal medication is another important factor affecting FHR patterns. Drugs known to decrease baseline variability include narcotics (e.g. morphine, meperidine), tranquilizers (e.g. diazepam), magnesium sulfate, and vagal blockade drugs (e.g. atropine, scopolamine). There have been few studies on causal

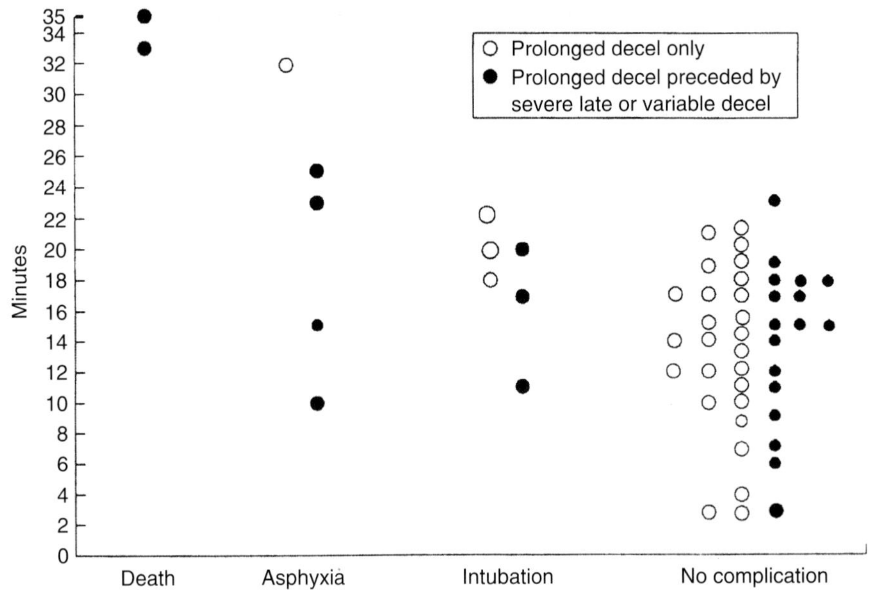

Figure 139.5 Prenatal outcome as related to time of delivery from onset of prolonged decelerations. From Leung *et al.*[20] When the prolonged deceleration or bradycardia followed the normal FHR pattern, no newborns showed umbilical cord artery pH < 7.0 and/or organ damage if they were born in less than 17 min of prolonged deceleration or bradycardia. In contrast, when prolonged deceleration or bradycardia was preceded by severe late or variable deceleration, no newborn showed asphyxic status in less than 9 min of prolonged deceleration or bradycardia.

relationships between given FHR patterns and outcomes in patients with disorders such as intrauterine infection, pre-eclampsia, diabetes mellitus, overterm, and congenital malformation.

Considering evolution of FHR patterns

Leung *et al.*[20] correlated the duration from onset of prolonged deceleration or bradycardia to delivery in 56 women with uterine rupture. When the prolonged deceleration or bradycardia followed the normal FHR pattern, no newborns showed umbilical cord artery pH < 7.0 and/or organ damage if they were born in less than 17 min of prolonged deceleration or bradycardia (Figure 139.5). In contrast, when prolonged deceleration or bradycardia was preceded by severe late or variable deceleration, no newborn showed asphyxic status in less than 9 min of prolonged deceleration or bradycardia. It is very important for the observer to take into consideration the evolution of FHR patterns.

It is important to understand the worsening pattern of deceleration. Late deceleration changes to have greater depth, with lower baseline rate or with higher baseline rate than normal range, and baseline variability becoming minimal or undetectable. Variable deceleration changes to an atypical variable pattern as described by Krebs *et al.*,[21] in addition to the changing pattern of late deceleration.

In a study by Fleischer *et al.*,[22] the average time duration from appearance of late decelerations to the time umbilical arterial pH reached 7.25 was 115 min; for variable decelerations, 145 min, and for flat line tracings, 185 min.

Baseline variability, the most important parameter indicating acidosis

Loss of variability, especially in the presence of other periodic patterns during labor, is the most sensitive indicator of metabolic acidemia in a fetus.[14] The factors of minimal or undetectable baseline variability are divided into asphyxic and non-asphyxic causes. Non-asphyxic causes include prematurity, tachycardia, drugs (such as narcotics, anesthetics, and parasympathomimetics), non-rapid eye movement sleep, and cardiac arrhythmia (such as atrioventricular block). Clinically, it is important to differentiate asphyxia-induced decreased variability from non-asphyxia-induced variability. One indication is that if the decreased variability is not accompanied by decelerations, it is likely to be non-asphyxial.[14] As reported by Samueloff *et al.*,[23] decreased baseline variability does not correctly predict umbilical arterial acidosis (defined as pH < 2.0) or a low Apgar score (< 7 at 5 min of life), if not accompanied by decelerations.

On the contrary, when decreased variability was accompanied by decelerations, predictability for acidosis (umbilical arterial blood pH < 7.1) was higher than when we did not take the presence of deceleration into account. In our recent study of 5522 low-risk pregnancies, the positive predictive value of umbilical artery pH < 7.1 increased exponentially from 0% in no deceleration, to 1% in occasional late decelerations, and 6–12% in recurrent late decelerations with moderate variability regardless acceleration present or not. In comparison, the positive predictive value was 54% in recurrent late

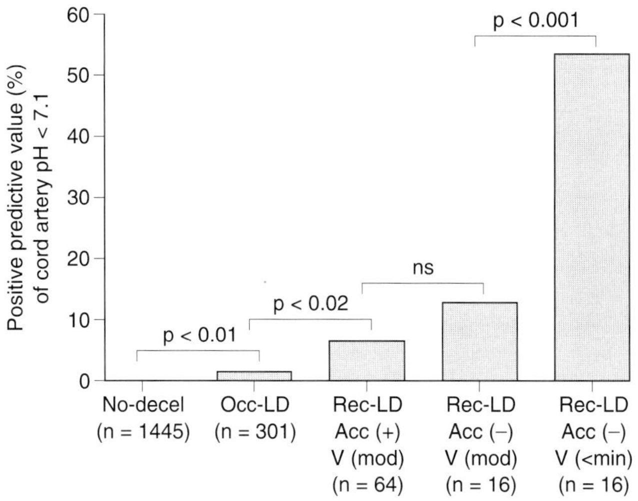

Figure 139.6 Predictive value of umbilical artery pH < 7.1 was increased as the FHR patterns were deteriorated from no-decel (no decelerations), occ-LD (occasional late decelerations), rec-LD (recurrent late decelerations) with accelerations present [Acc(+)] and variability moderate [V(mod)], to rec-LD with accelerations absent [Acc(−)] and variability minimal/absent [V(min)]. From Sameshima and Iknenoue.[24]

decelerations with acceleration absent and variability minimal/absent (Figure 139.6).[24]

Severity of decelerations

Paul *et al.*[25] correlated severity of late deceleration to fetal scalp blood pH (Figure 139.7a and b). They categorized cases into three subgroups according to the decrease in deceleration: mild late deceleration, less than 15 beats/min; moderate late deceleration, between 15 and 40 beats/min; severe late deceleration, more than 40 beats/min; and each subgroup was divided into two according to presence or decrease of baseline variability. The severity was significantly correlated with fetal acid–base status as well as the presence of variability.

Kubli *et al.*[26] also correlated severity of variable deceleration to fetal scalp blood pH in 85 cases. Their categorization was based on two parameters: nadir and duration of the deceleration. The average scalp blood pH in the severe variable deceleration group was 7.15 ± 0.069, significantly lower than in the mild and the moderate variable deceleration groups (7.29 ± 0.046 and 7.26 ± 0.044, respectively). In their study, they did not mention the variable deceleration with or without baseline variability, as Paul *et al.*[25] did. One drawback of using Kubli *et al.*'s categorization for variable deceleration is difficulty in recall, whereas Chao[27] created a mnemonic scale (Figure 139.8).

Regarding prolonged deceleration, Gull *et al.*[28] studied 27 prolonged decelerations just before vaginal delivery, and found a strong relationship between the length of loss of short-term variability and base deficit. They also noted that base deficit is significantly correlated with the duration and depth of prolonged decelerations, although these correlations were not as strong as the relationship to loss of variability.

Ancillary methods assuring fetal non-acidemia

To improve the specificity of FHR monitoring, two ancillary methods of assessing fetal acidemia are useful: fetal scalp blood sampling and fetal scalp stimulation. Fetal scalp blood sampling was developed as a method to assess intrapartum fetal well-being at almost the same time as FHR monitoring.[29] Clark *et al.*[30] subsequently showed that no fetus responding to scalp blood sampling with an acceleration of heart rate of 15 beats/min for 15 s had a scalp pH < 7.21. Since then, the fetal scalp stimulation test has replaced scalp blood sampling because it is simpler and less invasive.

The presence of an accelerated FHR in response to tactile or atraumatic clamp stimulation virtually assures a fetal blood pH above 7.2.[31] Almost one-third of fetuses who did not show accelerations revealed fetal acidosis. Scalp stimulation can be a useful adjunct when delivery is remote and the FHR tracing is non-reassuring but not clearly indicative of fetal acidemia.

Utility of FHR monitoring in intrapartum management

To develop a strategy to establish a management algorithm, we should clarify the surrogate endpoint of FHR monitoring. *Fetal acidosis* is defined as < 7.1 or < 7.0 in umbilical artery or fetal sampled blood pH, the incidences of which are about 3% and 0.3%, respectively.[14] The incidence of organ damage is significantly increased when pH is less than 7.0.[32,33] *Base deficit or excess*, representing metabolic acidosis, is a more important surrogate because metabolic acidosis is a more critical factor in organ damage than respiratory acidosis. The threshold is usually 12 or 16 mEq/l.[34]

In comparison with blood acid–base status, a depression index of a newly born infant, such as low *Apgar score* and *time duration of initial spontaneous respiration*, could be affected by observer bias.

Neonatal seizure, one of the most important signs of neonatal encephalopathy, is another surrogate endpoint for efficacy of FHR monitoring, which occurs in 0.3% of cases.[14] One case-controlled study showed that 29% of neonatal encephalopathy was caused by intrapartum factors or antepartum plus intrapartum factors.[35] The meta-analysis by Thacker *et al.*[8] showed that the incidence of neonatal seizures in FHR monitoring cases were decreased to half of that in the cases managed with intermittent auscultation. This result is staggering, because 0.09%

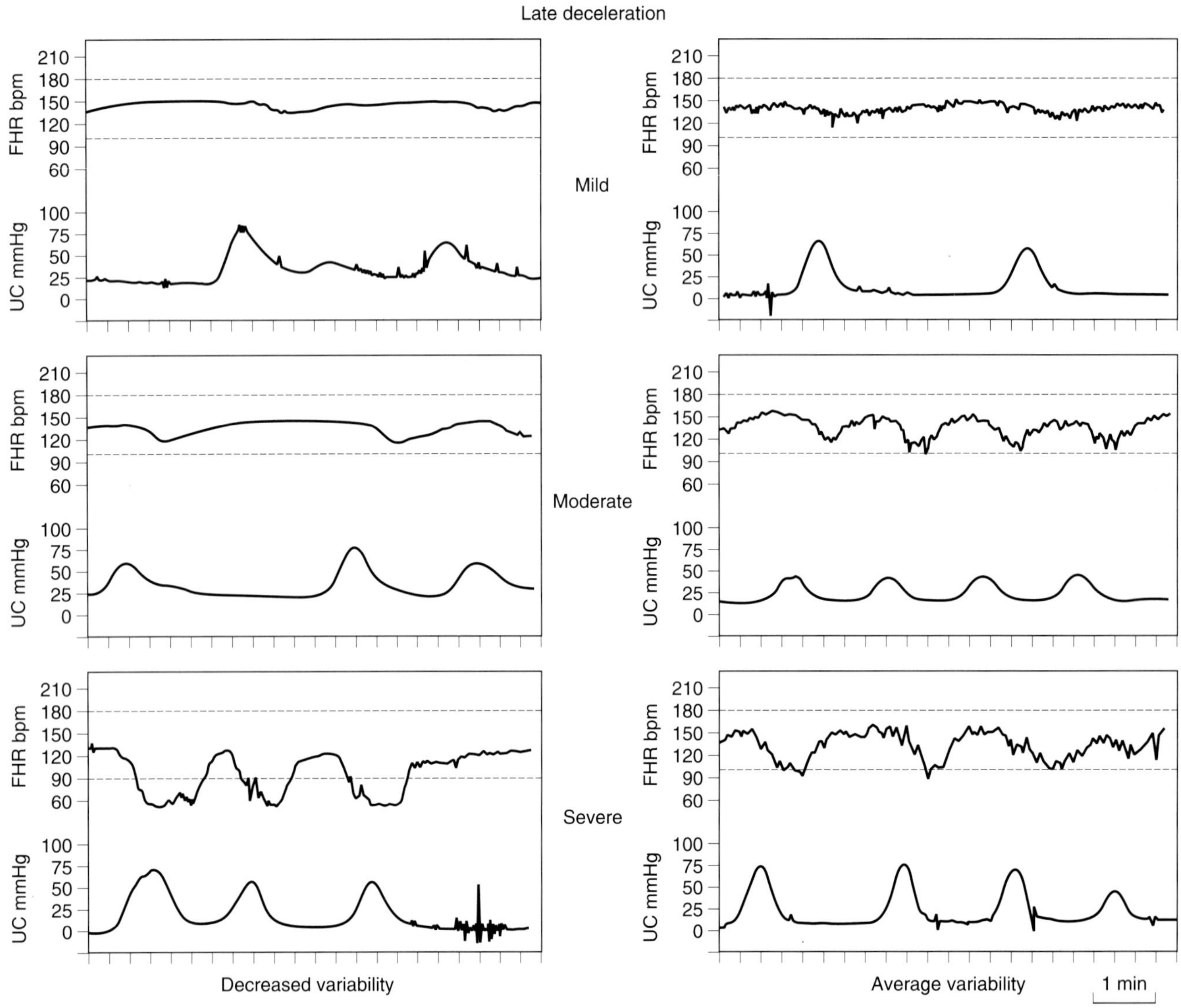

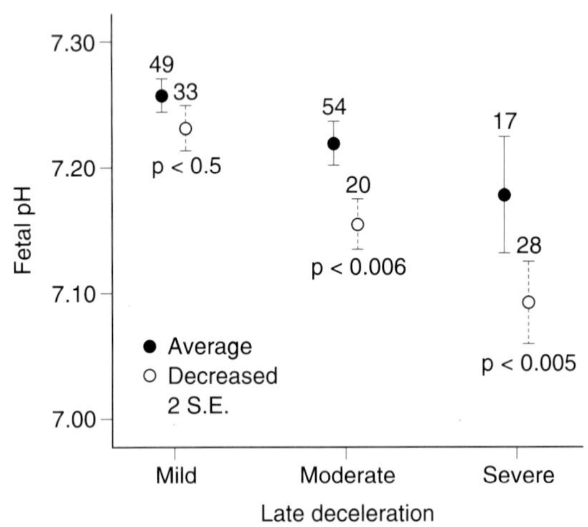

Figure 139.7 (a) Late deceleration FHR patterns are separated into mild (< 15 beats/min), moderate (15–40 beats/min), and severe (> 40 beats/min) groups. Examples associated with decreased variability, on the left, can be contrasted with those showing average or greater variability on the right. (b) As late deceleration patterns become more marked, the mean pH value falls. However, when FHR variability is present in association with late deceleration patterns, the mean pH is consistently higher than when it is decreased. From Paul *et al.*[25]

(0.3% × 0.29) is the incidence rate for neonatal encephalopathy in all pregnancies that is a target one hopes to avoid through use of intrapartum FHR monitoring.

Because the incidence of cerebral palsy is 0.2–0.3%, and less than 10% of all cerebral palsy cases are caused by intrapartum asphyxia, intrapartum FHR monitoring is of benefit in less than 0.03% of cases. Furthermore, it takes more than 12 months to make a diagnosis of cerebral palsy. Because of the problems of follow up and rarity of its incidence, cerebral palsy does not seem to be a

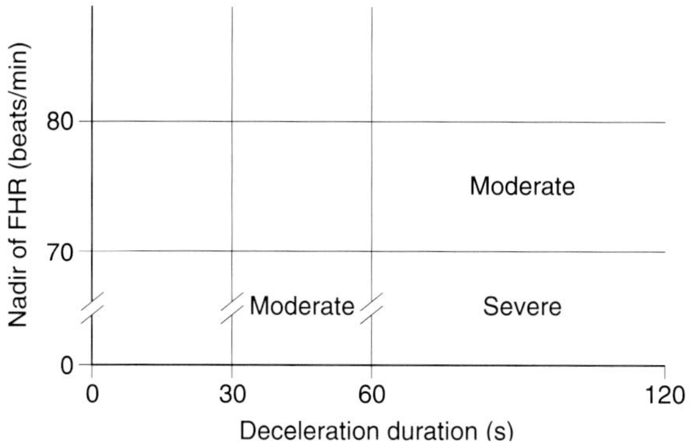

Figure 139.8 Chao's mnemonic for severity of variable deceleration.

feasible outcome measure for intrapartum FHR monitoring.

Another endpoint for intrapartum FHR monitoring is rates of cesarean section and operative vaginal delivery. It has been well known that cases managed with continuous FHR monitoring in labor and delivery tend to have an operative delivery. However, in a recent study using the cumulative meta-analysis of nine studies from 1976 to 1993, with more than 18,000 patients, the FHR group showed a relative risk of cesarean section of 1.21 compared with the intermittent auscultation group; for combined cesarean section and operative vaginal deliveries, the relative risk in the FHR group was 1.23.[8]

In conclusion, we recommend three major parameters as surrogate endpoints for efficacy of intrapartum FHR monitoring:

- umbilical arterial pH and base excess (or deficit);
- incidence of neonatal encephalopathy, especially neonatal seizure; and
- rate of operative delivery.

REFERENCES

1. Hon EH. The electronic evaluation of the fetal heart rate; preliminary report. *Am J Obstet Gynecol* 1958;75:1215–30.
2. Caldeyro-Barcia R, Poseiro JJ, Pantle G, Negreiros C, Gomez-Rogers C, Faunders AEA. Effects of uterine contractions on the heart rate of the human fetus. *Digest of the Fourth International Conference on Medical Electronics*, New York, 1961.
3. Hammacher K, Werners PH. On the evaluation and documentation of CTG (cardiotocographic) results. *Gynaecologia* 1968;166:410–23.
4. Quilligan EJ, Paul RH. Fetal monitoring. Is it worth it? *Obstet Gynecol* 1975;45:96–100.
5. Haverkamp AD, Thompson HE, McFee JG, Cetrulo C. The evaluation of continuous fetal heart rate monitoring in high-risk pregnancy. *Am J Obstet Gynecol* 1976;125:310–20.
6. Haverkamp AD, Orleans M, Langendoerfer S, McFee J, Murphy J, Thompson HE. A controlled trial of the differential effects of intrapartum fetal monitoring. *Am J Obstet Gynecol* 1979;134: 399–412.
7. MacDonald D, Grant A, Sheridan-Pereira M, Boylan P, Chalmers I. The Dublin randomized controlled trial of intrapartum fetal heart rate monitoring. *Am J Obstet Gynecol* 1985;152:524–39.
8. Thacker SB, Stroup DF, Peterson HB. Efficacy and safety of intrapartum electronic fetal monitoring: An update. *Obstet Gynecol* 1995;86:613–20.
9. Nelson KB, Ellenberg JH. Antecedents of cerebral palsy. Multivariate analysis of risk. *N Engl J Med* 1986;315:81–6.
10. Blair E, Stanley FJ. Intrapartum asphyxia: A rare cause of cerebral palsy. *J Pediatr* 1988;112:515–19.
11. Parer JT. Obstetric technologies: What determines clinical acceptance or rejection of results of randomized controlled trials? *Am J Obstet Gynecol* 2003;188:1622–5; discussion 1625–8.
12. National Institute of Child Health and Human Development Research Planning Workshop. Electronic fetal heart rate monitoring: Research guidelines for interpretation. *Am J Obstet Gynecol* 1997;177:1385–90.
13. Dalton KJ, Dawes GS, Patrick JE. The autonomic nervous system and fetal heart rate variability. *Am J Obstet Gynecol* 1983;146: 456–62.
14. Parer JT, Nageotte, MP. Intrapartum fetal surveillance. In Creasy RK, Resnik R, eds. *Maternal–Fetal Medicine*, 4th edn. Philadelphia: W.B. Saunders Company, 2004.
15. Knopf K, Parer JT, Espinoza MI, *et al.* Comparison of mathematical indices of fetal heart rate variability with visual assessment in the human and sheep. *J Dev Physiol* 1991;16:367–72.
16. Murata Y, Martin CB Jr, Ikenoue T, *et al.* Fetal heart rate accelerations and late decelerations during the course of intrauterine death in chronically catheterized rhesus monkeys. *Am J Obstet Gynecol* 1982;144:218–23.
17. Martin CB Jr, de Haan J, van der Wildt B, Jongsma HW, Dieleman A, Arts TH. Mechanisms of late decelerations in the fetal heart rate. A study with autonomic blocking agents in fetal lambs. *Eur J Obstet Gynecol Reprod Biol* 1979;9:361–73.
18. Lin CC, Moawad AH, Rosenow PJ, River P. Acid–base characteristics of fetuses with intrauterine growth retardation during labor and delivery. *Am J Obstet Gynecol* 1980;137:553–9.
19. Dawes GS, Houghton CR, Redman CW, Visser GH. Pattern of the normal human fetal heart rate. *Br J Obstet Gynaecol* 1982;89: 276–84.
20. Leung AS, Leung EK, Paul RH. Uterine rupture after previous cesarean delivery: Maternal and fetal consequences. *Am J Obstet Gynecol* 1993;169:945–50.
21. Krebs HB, Petres RE, Dunn LJ. Intrapartum fetal heart rate monitoring. VIII. Atypical variable decelerations. *Am J Obstet Gynecol* 1983;145:297–305.
22. Fleischer A, Schulman H, Jagani N, Mitchell J, Randolph G. The development of fetal acidosis in the presence of an abnormal fetal heart rate tracing. I. The average for gestational age fetus. *Am J Obstet Gynecol* 1982;144:55–60.
23. Samueloff A, Langer O, Berkus M, Field N, Xenakis E, Ridgway L. Is fetal heart rate variability a good predictor of fetal outcome? *Acta Obstet Gynecol Scand* 1994;73:39–44.
24. Sameshima H, Iknenoue T. Predictive value of late decelerations for fetal acidemia in unselected low risk pregnancies. *Am J Perinatol*, in press.
25. Paul RH, Suidan AK, Yeh S, Schifrin BS, Hon EH. Clinical fetal monitoring. VII. The evaluation and significance of intrapartum baseline FHR variability. *Am J Obstet Gynecol* 1975;123:206–10.
26. Kubli FW, Hon EH, Khazin AF, Takemura H. Observations on heart rate and pH in the human fetus during labor. *Am J Obstet Gynecol* 1969;104:1190–206.
27. Chao A. Graphic mnemonic for variable decelerations. *Am J Obstet Gynecol* 1990;163:1098.
28. Gull I, Jaffa AJ, Oren M, Grisaru D, Peyser MR, Lessing JB. Acid accumulation during end-stage bradycardia in term fetuses: How long is too long? *Br J Obstet Gynaecol* 1996;103:1096–101.
29. Saling E, Schneider D. Biochemical supervision of the foetus during labour. *J Obstet Gynaecol Br Commonw* 1967;74: 799–811.

30. Clark SL, Gimovsky ML, Miller FC. Fetal heart rate response to scalp blood sampling. *Am J Obstet Gynecol* 1982;144:706–8.
31. Clark SL, Gimovsky ML, Miller FC. The scalp stimulation test: A clinical alternative to fetal scalp blood sampling. *Am J Obstet Gynecol* 1984;148:274–7.
32. Gilstrap LC 3rd, Leveno KJ, Burris J, Williams ML, Little BB. Diagnosis of birth asphyxia on the basis of fetal pH, Apgar score, and newborn cerebral dysfunction. *Am J Obstet Gynecol* 1989;161:825–30.
33. Goldaber KG, Gilstrap LC 3rd, Leveno KJ, Dax JS, McIntire DD. Pathologic fetal acidemia. *Obstet Gynecol* 1991;78:1103–7.
34. Low JA, Lindsay BG, Derrick EJ. Threshold of metabolic acidosis associated with newborn complications. *Am J Obstet Gynecol* 1997;177:1391–4.
35. Badawi N, Kurinczuk JJ, Keogh JM, *et al.* Intrapartum risk factors for newborn encephalopathy: The Western Australian case–control study. *Br Med J* 1998;317:1554–8.

140 Quantitative fetal heart rate evaluation without pattern classification: FHR score and artificial neural network analysis

K. Maeda, Y. Noguchi, F. Matumoto and T. Nagasawa

Introduction

Fetal heart rate (FHR) monitoring, used by us in Kyushu University in the 1960s,[1] led to a reduction in the incidence of severe neonatal asphyxia, which in turn unmasked underlying neonatal intrinsic disorders, and facilitated the studies on congenital diseases. In the 1970s, in a controlled study at Tottori University, perinatal deaths were reduced by the use of fetal monitoring.[2] In addition, in the 1970–1980s, the use of full intrapartum monitoring resulted in the reduction of neonatal asphyxia, perinatal deaths and cerebral palsy at Yohka General Hospital, where the cesarean section rate was only 10%.[3] Pediatric neurologists have noted the reduction of cerebral palsy in whole births after the introduction of widespread fetal monitoring in the Tottori area in the 1980s.[4] Although it has been reported that monitoring with an internal fetal scalp electrode after rupture of the membranes does not improve outcome,[5] real improvements in outcome were achieved through external monitoring throughout pregnancy and labor.[2–4] Full intrapartum monitoring was not easy because all labors are monitored continuously by cardiotocography (CTG) watching and detailed FHR pattern classification.[2,3] It was thought that computerized FHR analysis and diagnosis would solve these problems.

Although FHR patterns are the main criteria in visual CTG diagnosis, it has been controversial even in modern classification. Therefore, quantitative analysis was required in precise studies and in clinical diagnosis. The more simple measurements of FHR tracing, based on manual analysis of FHR score, were adopted instead of pattern classification in the 1960s[1,6] and we introduced conventional computer diagnosis in the 1970s.[7,8] Recently, neural network computer assessment was introduced,[9,10] where the purpose is highly objective and easy FHR evaluation which cannot be carried out either with CTG observation or FHR pattern classification.*

FHR score in conventional computer systems

The conventional program was characterized by quantitative FHR evaluation without pattern classification from early studies on automated diagnosis.[7,8]

FHR score

FHR score was the first quantitative measure reported early in 1969. Although there were pattern classifications by Caldeyro-Barcia *et al.*[11] and Hon,[12] no criteria were present in the quantitative FHR measurement in the 1960s. We simply measured baseline heart rate, number of decelerations, its duration, nadir heart rate (dip HR), recovery time from the dip HR to the baseline, lag time of dip HR from the peak of the contraction, in 5 min of fetal monitoring (Figure 140.1).[1] No labor was intervened by rapid delivery because, in the trial, we did not know what the warning quantitative FHR signs were. The parameters of frequent changes

*Author contributions: KM worked on medical data and postprocessing, YN and FM dealt with the neural network computer, and TN performed the Fast Fourier Transform (FFT) analysis of FHR

were detected and each abnormality score was established according to the percentages of fetal death and neonatal depression (Table 140.1). Abnormality scores were accumulated to establish the FHR score repeatedly every 5 min and the highest FHR score in the labor was evaluated.[1]

The FHR score is easily compared to other numeric phenomena because it is a single quantitative value. The score correlated with the neonatal Apgar score, where the FHR score was 10 or more when the Apgar score was six or less (Figure 140.2). It also correlated with umbilical arterial blood pH and base excess (BE), where pH was lower than 7.20 when the FHR score was 10 or more (Figure 140.3).[1,6] The correlation was studied by meta-analysis of the results from the 1960–1970s, where an adverse outcome was suggested when the FHR score was higher than 10. The score also correlated with fetal scalp blood pH (Figure 140.4).[1] The correlation coefficient was 0.85 and subsequently scalp blood sampling was not considered to be indispensable during clinical monitoring. The technique was so easy that the FHR score was manually determined even before computer processing.[1,6]

After Dr Hon criticized the FHR scoring technique as there was no inclusion of FHR-baseline variability, new parameters were added to the new fetal distress (FD) index (Table 140.2). When umbilical arterial pH was higher than 7.25, FD index is 2 or less while when pH was 7.25 or less, FD index is 3 or more (Table 140.3).[13] Therefore, fetal blood pH may be assessed by FHR score as well as by FD index. The score and index flag fetal abnormalities during fetal monitoring with the conventional computer program.[7,8] We recognized the usefulness of quantitative FHR evaluation in studies on FHR score and FD index.

Conventional computer program for FHR analysis and diagnosis

An external fetal monitor is composed of a fetal heart beat detector, a fetal heart rate meter and a tocodynamometer.[14] The electrical output of FHR and contractions are each converted into 150 digital data in 5 min, saved in computer memory and analyzed. The program is divided into two parts: analysis and diagnosis.[7,8] The analytic computer detects FHR

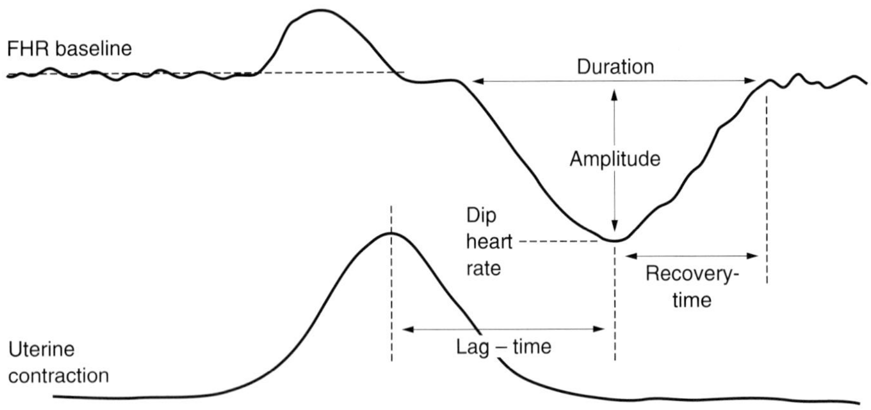

Figure 140.1 The FHR tracing has been quantitatively analyzed with simple measurement for the determination of FHR score since the 1960s.[1]

Table 140.1 Abnormality scores for the calculation of FHR score[1]

Signs	Apgar score (1 min) lower than 7 (%)	Abnormality score
FHR baseline		
110–130 or 160–180 bpm	27.5	1
< 110 or > 180 bpm	75.0	3
Deceleration		
Duration > 60 s	71.4	3
Dip heart rate < 100 bpm	37.1	2
Amplitude > 50 bpm	50.0	2
Recovery time > 40 s	63.2	3
Lag time > 40 s	71.4	3
No accompanied acceleration	44.7	2
W-shaped deceleration	100.0	4

FHR score = Total sum of abnormality scores detected in 5 min. FHR score is abnormally high when it is 10 or more, and severely abnormal when it is 20 or more

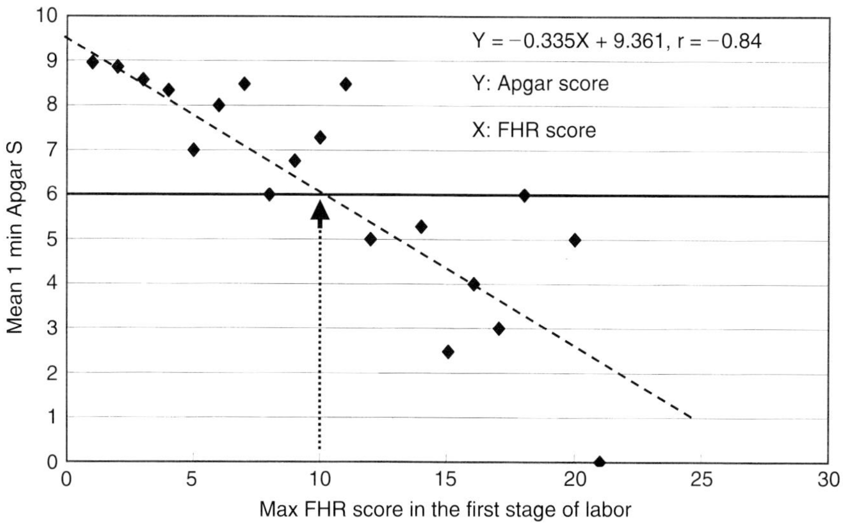

Figure 140.2 Maximum FHR score, even in the first stage of labor, correlates with the Apgar score at 1 min. Meta-analysis of original data, all obtained in the 1960s,[1] are presented in Figures 140.2 and 140.3 of the present study.

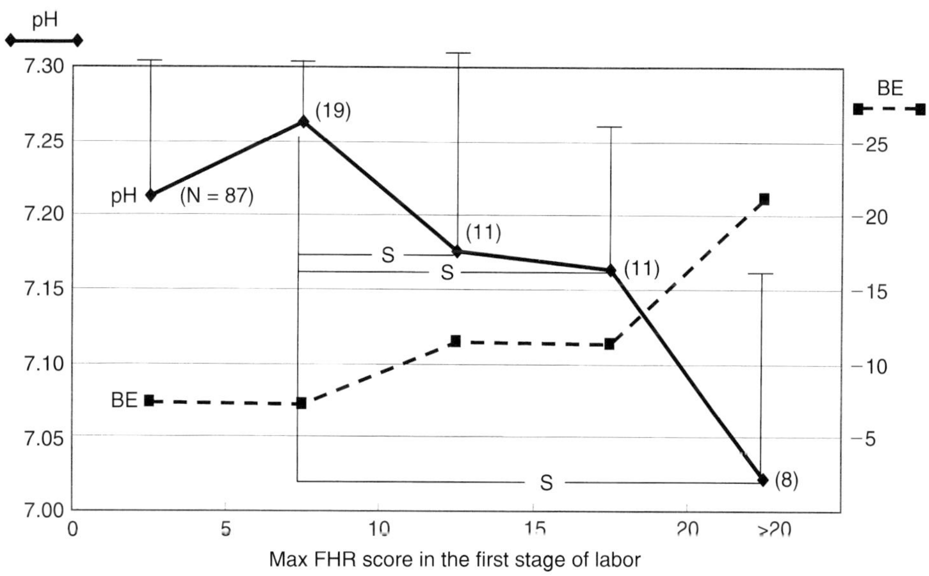

Figure 140.3 The maximum FHR score, even in the first stage of labor, correlates with umbilical arterial blood pH and BE at delivery. The pH is lower at 0–5 points of FHR score than at 5–10 points, while BE is equal in corresponding BE. It may show the metabolic nature of BE and the influence of respiratory acidosis on the pH. The figure is the meta-analysis of the data obtained in the 1960s.[1]

parameters, which are used in the FHR score and also in the artificial neural network in the recent studies.[9]

FHR data are divided into 20 steps in the analytic part. Data are averaged in the step where there are more and the result is the FHR baseline during 5 min. The average of all downslope variations is added to the baseline to form the upper reference line to detect the acceleration. The averaged variation is subtracted from the baseline to determine the deceleration below the lower reference line. Baseline variability is determined by excluding the acceleration and deceleration. The duration, dip HR, recovery time from the nadir to the baseline, lag time from the nadir to the contraction peak are measured in a deceleration.[7,8]

The dip area of a deceleration, which is the area surrounded by the baseline and deceleration, is divided by the product of duration and amplitude of the deceleration, to determine 'dip shape value'. Cord compression is suggested when the dip shape value is large and periodic deceleration is defined when the dip shape is small.[15] Late deceleration is determined in 15 min if all dip shape values are small, lag time is greater than 20 s and deceleration number is almost the same as the contractions. Non-reactive FHR is suggested if there is no acceleration in 20 min. An excessively large area under the contraction suggests uterine hyperactivity. Abnormal FHR is detected and fetal non-reassuring status is diagnosed by the high FHR score and index, as well as by baseline abnormality, loss of variability and abnormal decelerations in the diagnostic part of the computer. The study started in 1974 and was completed in 1980.[7,8] The program has been incorporated in various monitoring devices (TOITU[†], Tokyo, Japan) and has been used by obstetricians for more than 20 years without major problems. The value and usefulness of quantitative FHR evaluation is confirmed in the conventional program.

[†] http://www.toitu.co.jp/e

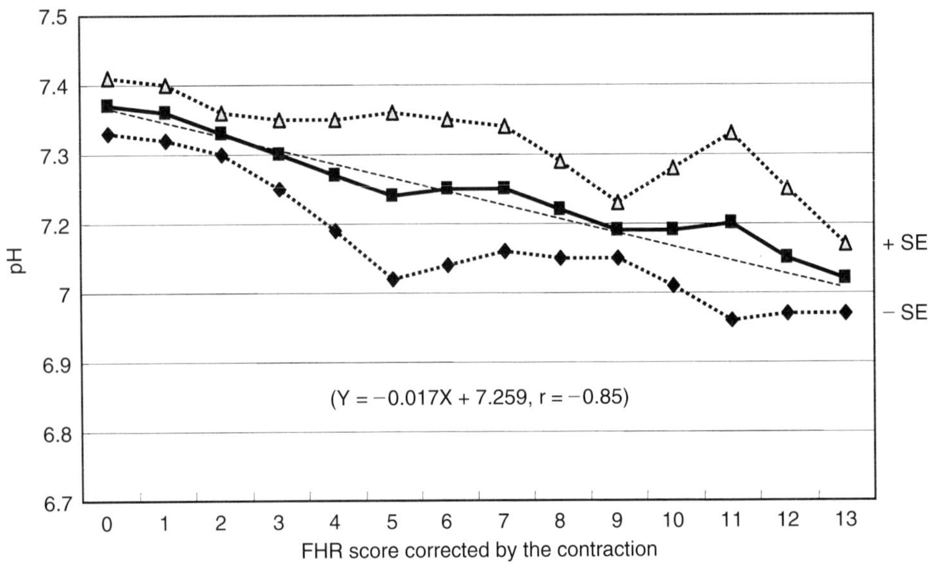

Figure 140.4 FHR score correlated with fetal scalp blood pH. The score was corrected by the state of uterine contraction, and the score was determined 20 min before blood sampling.[1]

Table 140.2 Calculation of FD index

Add 1 point
FHR score: 10–19
Loss of variability: the variability is less than 5 during 20 or more minutes
Late decelerations: quantitatively determined by 'dip-shape' and lag time
Bradycardia (100–110 bpm) lasted for 10–30 min
Tachycardia (>160 bpm) lasted for more than 30 min

Add 2 points
FHR score: 20 or more
Bradycardia (100–110 bpm) lasted for more than 30 min

Add 3 points
Bradycardia (<100 bpm) lasted for 5 min

The value 3 or more of total FD index suggests fetal distress[13]

Table 140.3 Umbilical arterial pH (UApH) is low if FD index is 3 or more at 30 min before the birth[13]

FD index	UApH is 7.25 or less	UApH is higher than 7.25	Total
3	19	4	23
<3	3	39	42
Total	22	43	65

Sensitivity: 86.64%, specificity: 90.70%, Fisher's exact test: P=0.00000; positive predictive value: 82.61%, negative predictive value: 92.86%

Artificial neural network computer analysis

Further highly objective evaluation is intended by the introduction of artificial neural network analysis under the collaboration of computer specialist Noguchi and colleagues. The computer is not programmed by experts' knowledge, instead it is educated by repeated training with eight FHR data of typical outcome cases. The FHR data are detected in 5 min and includes baseline heart rate, variability, sinusoidal heart rate, number of decelerations, and their duration, nadir heart rate, recovery time and lag time, by the analytic conventional computer from database, and sometimes by visual CTG analysis. Fifteen minutes of 24 parameters of 20 cases of known outcome are digitized and are manually input into the computer, instead of the full CTG data, which require enormous input units and long processing time, i.e. we selected a hybrid neural network system. The intermediate layer is composed of 30 units and the output layer is 3 units (Figure 140.5).[9,10] The computer is a common Dell PC that is automatically educated 10,000 times repeatedly by using a back propagation system to obtain the most effective neural network construction for outcome prediction. The computer education was successful and the internal check perfect. The network output is for probabilities to be normal, pathologic or suspicious outcomes. Output evaluation is easy because the probability is shown in percentages. We tentatively educated the computer with 50 min of data, and its accuracy was 86% in 50 min of 29 other cases.[9] Educated and completed neural network software can be transferred into any other computer with uniform diagnostic accuracy. No hardware board is used because it is educated in each computer, where no uniformity is expected in its diagnostic accuracy.

Computerized detection of fetal sinusoidal heart rate

Seven of the eight components are baseline and deceleration data detected by the conventional analyzing computer. However, when using the educated neural network computer for diagnosis, fetal sinusoidal heart rate (FSHR) becomes a complex problem in diagnosis with an educated neural network computer.

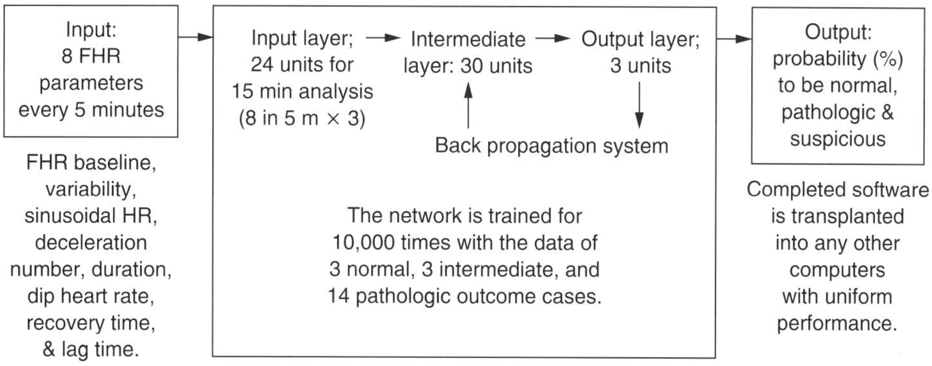

Figure 140.5 The artificial neural network computer is constructed of three layers and a back propagation system. It is repeatedly educated for 10,000 times using eight FHR parameters. The software of the completed neural network can be transplanted into any other computer.[9]

Table 140.4 Pathologic FSHR is diagnosed, when the ratio of La/Ta is 39% or greater and is combined with a PPSD value of 300 or more. If these criteria are fulfilled, the true positive rate is 100% and false-positive and false-negative rate are 0%[17]

La/Ta ratio 39% and PPSD 300	FSHR Pathologic	FSHR Physiologic*	Total
Yes	9	0	9
No	0	12	12
Total	9	12	21

*Physiologic FSHR and normal FHR

FSHR should be able to be automatically diagnosed before input into the neural network computer. Physiologic and pathologic FSHRs, however, cannot be differentiated by simple CTG observation. An actocardiogram can detect physiologic FSHR,[16] but it is a visual diagnosis and it is not compatible with computer processing. We have to use FHR alone for the automatic detection of pathologic FSHR.

Therefore, the following data were collected, scanned, digitized and studied by FFT frequency analysis: nine FHR tracings of pathologic FSHR caused by fetal anemia or hypoxia, which resulted in unfavorable outcome, fetal therapy or cesarean section; seven physiologic FSHR including periodic fetal movements detected by actocardiogram in those who had normal vaginal delivery and normal outcome; five normal FHR. The area under the power spectrum between 0.031 and 0.1 Hz (2–6 cycles/min) is La and the area under the whole power spectrum is Ta; the La/Ta ratio is studied. Peak power spectrum density (PPSD) is another FSHR parameter. La/Ta ratio and PPSD are both large in pathologic FSHR, whereas physiologic FSHR shows small La/Ta ratio or small PPSD. Therefore, the combination of large La/Ta and PPSD is suitable to separate pathologic FSHR from normal physiologic FSHR (Table 140.4).[17] The algorithm will be installed into actual neural network systems for FHR diagnosis.

Outcome probability trend gram

We also studied the trend gram of the probabilities obtained in the neural analysis; i.e. the time train of outcome probability, which is obtained every 5 min by analysis of 15 min of data. Upward bars show normal outcome probability while pathologic and suspicious probability are shown by reverse downward bars (Figure 140.6).[9] A trend gram of such short duration as 1 h is easily evaluated, whereas prolonged trend gram, for example of 4 h duration, is difficult to evaluate by visual examination. No outcome is expected even by the line graph connecting pathologic probabilities in 4 h of monitoring. KM's trial was a manual averaging of all past pathologic probabilities every 5 min and formation of a line graph of averaged pathologic probabilities. Evaluation is still difficult by the pathologic probability curve.[10]

Neural index obtained by averaged outcome probability

The next trial is the comparison of averaged normal probability curves to pathologic probability. The final average of normal probability is higher than an averaged pathologic one immediately before delivery. The technique is useful in outcome prediction because the neonate is normal in the case. However, the method is not used because it is still a visual evaluation (Figure 140.7). In further progress in the development of this technique, averaged pathologic probability is subtracted from averaged normal probability every 5 min. After processing, a final single curve and a single value are obtained. We have named this value ‘neural index’ (Figure 140.8). The final stage of the neural index immediately before the birth is greater than zero and the neonatal state is normal in the case. Results show possible FHR evaluation even after very prolonged monitoring.

Nine trend grams were evaluated by the neural index. In four cases where all of the neonates were normal and showed no asphyxia, the neural index was greater than zero. However, in another five cases, neural index was below zero before delivery and the neonates were all depressed and showed various grades of neonatal asphyxia (Table 140.5). Case no. 3 shows the lowest index; it was continuously −100%,

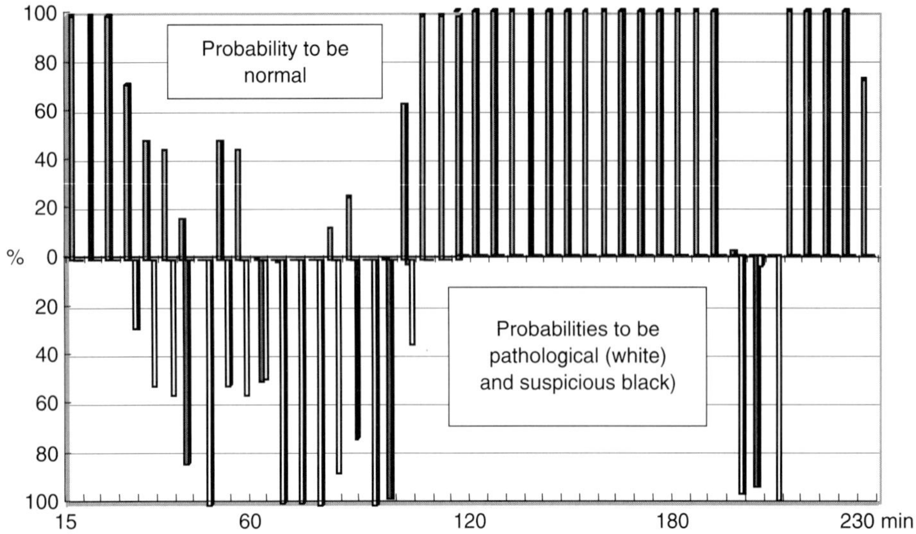

Figure 140.6 The trend gram bars show outcome probabilities obtained by the artificial neural network computer in case 1, who was monitored for 3 h and 50 min. Upward bar indicates the probability for normality, while reverse bars indicate probabilities for pathology (white) or suspicious (black).[9]

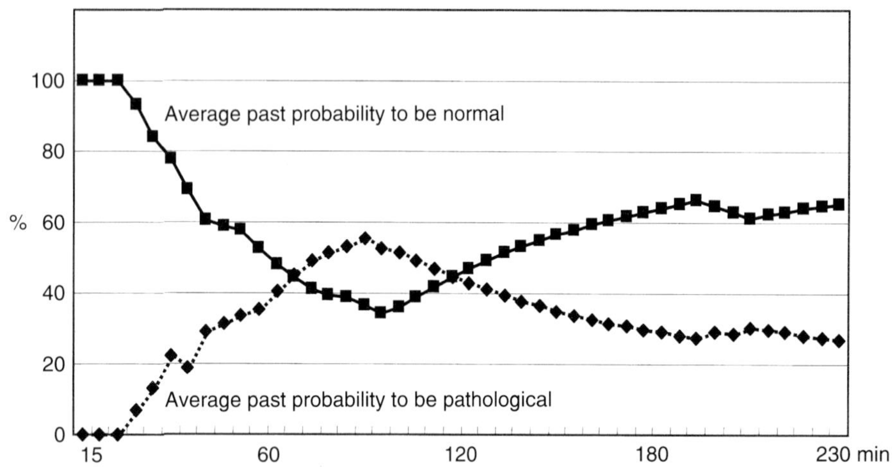

Figure 140.7 Past normal and pathologic outcome probabilities are averaged every 5 min and expressed as two line graphs in case 1.[10] Averaged normal probability is higher than the pathologic one. Neonatal condition is normal.

Apgar score was 3, and the infant expired 3 months later due to brain hemorrhage. Case no. 10, who was pathologic in the trend gram and in negative neural index, had an asphyxiated neonate.[10]

Using Fisher's exact test for statistical analysis, the neural index shows significant differences of neonatal states. The sensitivity, specificity, positive and negative predictive values are 100%. Therefore, the internal check of the neural index is perfect and a value lower than zero will inform of the danger of an intrapartum fetus during the monitoring process.

The place and role of neural index

The neural index can be used either in a personal computer connected to the fetal monitor, an intelligent individual monitor, or any other system where accurate and easy FHR evaluation is requested. We plan to carry out an external check of the neural system in a central monitor (TOITU MF-7400) after the installation of completed neural computer software. The system will be composed of a conventional program and a trained neural network. Both computers will analyze FHR and contractions. The central system monitors multiple pregnant women. The person responsible for the system studies the CTG and automatic diagnosis only after the system beeps when it alarms an irregular FHR, abnormal scores or abnormal indices. The display shows not only the neural index, but also outcome probability, CTG, alarming signs, FHR score, FHR findings in 5 min, and the contraction area that warns of uterine hyperactivity. The computer displays past CTG and its analysis on demand by the playback of computer memory. There is neither a CTG recorder nor a chart, but the CTG can be printed on demand. Original signals are stored in a large computer memory.

Monitoring by a central system is easy because computers monitor continuously without being subjected to sleepiness or fatigue, continuous CTG watching is not required and CTG display and automatic diagnosis are studied only after the alarm is sounded. There is no difficult pattern classification, but

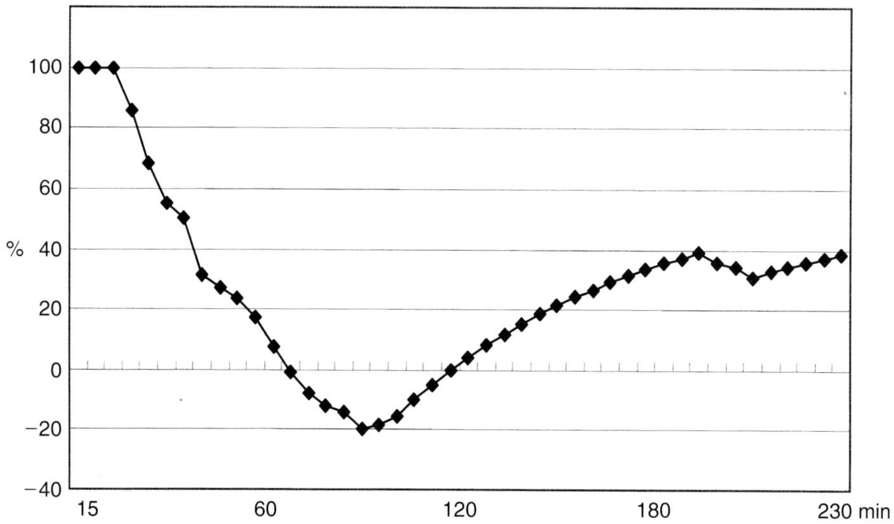

Figure 140.8 Averaged past pathologic outcome probabilities are subtracted from the averaged normal probabilities every 5 min in case 1, and the 'neural index' formed a single line graph. The final neural index is greater than zero and neonatal condition is normal in case 1.[10]

Table 140.5 Neural index correlates with neonatal condition[10]

Final neural index	Neonatal depression Present	Neonatal depression Absent	Total
<0	5	0	5
>0	0	4	4
Total	5	4	9

Sensitivity: 100%, specificity: 100%, Fisher's exact test: $P = 0.008$, positive predictive value: 100%, negative predictive value: 100%

instead, the pathologic outcome is shown by objective numeric values. Full monitoring of all births can be achieved. In a Seirei hospital where a central monitoring system was introduced without a neural network since 1996, the number of monitored cases increased 10-fold in 2 years. Objective and easy diagnosis will be further promoted by the neural network analysis.

Discussion

Quantitative FHR measurement made it possible to simply analyze FHR tracing and to express FHR condition with a continuous value. FHR score is quite different from FHR pattern classification, which has been commonly used and is helpful in fetal diagnosis. The method of pattern classification is to overlap an FHR change on typical templates proposed by the originators. The technique was generally accepted because it was similar to the diagnosis of a syndrome, i.e. the disease is diagnosed if the symptom complex coincides with the template of a syndrome. FHR pattern is classified when the FHR change overlaps clearly on a template. However, it is difficult to determine when the FHR change is far from any pattern in the classification. Although pattern classification has been accepted and is useful in fetal surveillance, FHR analysis is controversial and only its originator may be able to classify a difficult pattern. This may be the reason for various modifications which have been proposed by multiple originators.

As the pattern classification is of binary character, it evaluates FHR only by two categories. The pattern classification has been rarely studied by common scientific methods of regression and correlation with other biological phenomena. For example, its correlation with fetal blood acid–base or gas status has hardly ever been analyzed. Therefore, it was necessary to combine fetal scalp blood pH with CTG and was another reason of our quantitative FHR analysis.

FHR pattern classification needs multiple procedures. The first step is the study of FHR patterns to gain correct knowledge. Secondly, the FHR tracing is analyzed and patterns are classified. Thirdly, fetal pathophysiology has to be evaluated in the patterns. Finally, fetal status and prospective outcome are diagnosed by the observation of whole tracing. Obstetric and maternal conditions are simultaneously analyzed to plan any intervention. The presence of multiple steps may increase the risk of incorrect interpretation of the classification. Quantitative FHR score skips many analyzing steps in pattern classification to reach the score for which a certain outcome is expected. Neural analysis further indicates normal and pathologic probabilities using percentages. Finally, of these different methods, the neural index most clearly shows the outcome, economizing several steps which may present in pattern diagnosis.

Although pattern classification was useful in the initial stage of FHR diagnosis and its strict application promoted improved outcome in common obstetrics and in our past clinical studies,[1–4] its scientific analysis is difficult and it has a subjective nature. For example, the delay time of late deceleration was undetermined and later Chik *et al.*[18] measured typical late decelerations and determined the delay time as 20 or more seconds. Modern classification does not define the delay time yet. The shape difference of periodic and variable changes has not been scientifically studied, while quantified technique made the separation possible with 'dip-shape value' in our study.[15]

The visual FHR evaluation with pattern classification is standardized at present only by the consensus of authorities, not on the scientific basis of objective measurement. The subjectivity and vague definition of FHR pattern might cause false-positive FHR diagnosis, although 50–70% of false-positive cases was reduced by the introduction of actocardiogram.[19,20] The FHR should be analyzed by scientific procedures to improve outcomes because, at present, continuous and non-invasive fetal surveillance through pregnancy and labor is achieved only by FHR monitoring. Obstetric care and patient management should not be hampered by complicated visual CTG classification. Similar to the automatic diagnosis of adult electrocardiogram, the analysis should be left to computer processing where fetal abnormalities are diagnosed and outcome is predicted automatically by an informed advanced computer. Time can be economized by the computer for the management of increased jobs to save the mother and child in modern obstetrics.

Apart from the complex pattern classification, simple measurement of FHR tracing is useful for the objective description. Regression and correlation analyses with other phenomena are easy in quantitative FHR analysis, e.g. FHR score and FD index were easily compared to Apgar score and fetal blood pH. The benefits are confirmed in this paper. Fetal blood Po_2, Pco_2 or SPO_2, can be also analyzed with numeric scores and indices. Artificial neural network is introduced in our FHR studies on the basis of past beneficial evaluation of quantitative FHR analysis.

Artificial neural network analysis has been studied in various definitive purposes – the traveling salesman problem,[21] various business areas and widely in medicine, including EEG,[22] histology,[23] brain function,[24] brain tumor,[25] smear categorization,[26] visual field determination,[27] respirator fault detection,[28] coronary artery SPECT,[29] and HIV protein structure.[30] In our field, it has been used in ultrasonic fetal weight estimation,[31] estimation of the duration of the first-stage labor,[32] CTG feature extraction[33] and diagnosis of fetal hypoxia with FHR variability and pulse oximetry.[34] The aim of using a neural network in the present study is the highly objective FHR analysis, which is acceptable to general physicians.

In the past, conventional systems were mainly the experts' knowledge system, which was sometimes unacceptable to other scientists. In the artificial neural network, we used eight simplified FHR data obtained from normal and abnormal outcome cases. Data acquisition and its processing are totally objective and includes no opinion of experts. The outcome is shown by outcome probability and neural index. Details of FHR tracing are known by the conventional analyzing computer, if it is requested.

Although it is ideal to use all FHR data in the neural network processing, the data of FHR and the contraction will be 1500 in 15 min when the sampling interval is 2 s. A large number of units are required for input, and analysis time will be prolonged. For these cases, only off-line processing is suitable. We wanted real-time on-line processing in clinical monitoring and therefore, we selected a hybrid-type artificial neural network. The results are promising, and the completed neural network soft ware can be installed into clinical systems to achieve correct and easy fetal monitoring. All child births can be monitored by its application in the central system.

An artificial neural network will be useful not only in FHR analysis, but also in various other fields of medicine. An idea on the neural network is automatic diagnosis of ultrasound images. There are many tissue characterization reports in ultrasound images. Maeda *et al.*[35–37] reported a tissue evaluation by the gray-level histogram width, which was successful and clinical studies are promising. It will be also successful, if large sequential gray-scale data of typical diagnosis are input into a neural computer, which is completed by repeated education and used in actual diagnosis. The large volume of pixel data can be analyzed by off-line processing. Automatic diagnosis of malignancy, for example, will greatly contribute clinical medicine. The progress of computer technology is likely to make the author's ideas real in the future.

Conclusion

The FHR tracing is successfully evaluated by quantitative analysis of parameters including FHR score, FD index and artificial neural index without FHR pattern classification. The correlation and regression of quantitative FHR analyses to fetal blood pH and BE are successful, but not in pattern classification. The outcome of prolonged FHR monitoring is successful by the neural index obtained by the artificial neural network. Pathologic sinusoidal heart rate is diagnosed by a computerized frequency analysis. A high-grade CTG recorder and chart are not required in quantitative FHR evaluation. Difficult interpretation and study of pattern classification is of no use in quantitative evaluation, while late and variable decelerations are detected by the quantified computer analysis of FHR. Details of FHR tracing are displayed by the conventional analytic computer.

REFERENCES

1. Maeda K, Kimura S, Fukui Y, *et al. Pathophysiology of Fetus.* Fukuoka: Fukuoka Printing, 1969.
2. Maeda K. Healthy baby and reduced fetal death by improved obstetric management. In Karim SMM, Tan KI, eds. *Problems in Perinatology.* Singapore: Singapore University, 1979:525–9.
3. Tsuzaki T, Sekijima A, Morishita K, *et al.* The survey on the perinatal variables and the incidence of cerebral palsy for 12 years before and after the application of the fetal monitoring system. *Nippn Sanka Fujinka Gakkai Zasshi* 1990;42:99–105.
4. Takeshita K, Ando Y, Ohtani K, Takashima S. Cerebral palsy in Tottori, Japan. *Neuroepidemiology* 1989;8:184–92.
5. MacDonald D, Grant A, Sheridan-Perenia M, Boyland P, Charmers I. The Dublin randomized controlled trial of intrapartum fetal heart rate monitoring. *Am J Obstet Gynecol* 1985;152:524–39.
6. Endo S. Studies on the changes of fetal heart rate score along with the progress of labor. *Yonago Igaku Zasshi* 1972;23:266–85.
7. Maeda K, Arima T, Tatsumura M, Nagasawa T. Computer-aided fetal heart rate analysis and automatic fetal-distress diagnosis during labor and pregnancy utilizing external technique in fetal monitoring. *MEDINFO* 1980;80:1214–19.
8. Maeda K. Computerized automatic diagnosis of fetal distress with the use of external monitoring technique. In Krause W, ed. *Computerdiagnostik in der Geburtsmedizin.* Jena: Friedrich-Sciller-Universität, 1981:28–49.
9. Maeda K, Utsu M, Makio A, *et al.* Neural network computer analysis of fetal heart rate. *J Matern Fetal Invest* 1998;8:163–71.
10. Maeda K, Noguchi Y, Matsumoto F. Evaluation of prolonged fetal monitoring with normal and pathologic outcome probabilities determined by artificial neural network. *Fetal Diagn Ther* 2003;18:370–5.
11. Caldeyro-Barcia R A, Poseiro JJ, Gulin LO. Effects of abnormal uterine contractions on fetal heart rate during labor. *The 5th World Congress on Gynaecology and Obstetrics*, Sydney, 1967:9–29.
12. Hon EH. *An Atlas of Fetal Heart Rate Patterns.* New Haven: Harty Press, 1968.
13. Irie, T. Automated fetal heart rate analysis and its trend gram in relation to the gas analysis and acid-base balance of umbilical arterial blood. *Nippon Sanka Fujinka Gakkai Zasshi* 1986;38:1623–31.
14. FIGO News, Maeda K, *et al.* Evaluation and standardization of fetal monitoring. *Int J Gynecol Obstet* 1997;59:169–73.
15. Mizu M. Fundamental studies on the automatic analysis in fetal heart rate. *Nippon Sanka Fujinka Gakkai Zasshi* 1976;28:1383–92.
16. Ito T, Maeda K, Takahashi H, Nagata N, Nakajima K, Terakawa N. Differentiation between physiologic and pathologic sinusoidal FHR pattern by fetal actocardiogram. *J Perinat Med* 1994;22:39–43.
17. Meda K, Nagasawa T. Automatic computerized diagnosis of fetal sinusoidal heart rate. *Fetal Diagn Ther* 2005;20:328–34.
18. Chik L, Rosen MG, Hirsch VJ. An analysis of lag time and variability of fetal heart rate measurements. *Am J Obstet Gynecol* 1974;118:237–42.
19. Stanco LM, Rabello Y, Medearis AL, Paul RH. Does Doppler-detected fetal movement decrease the incidence of nonreactive nonstress test? *Obstet Gynecol* 1993;82:999–1003.
20. Teshima N. Non-reactive pattern diagnosed by ultrasonic Doppler fetal actocardiogram and outcome of the fetuses with non-reactive pattern. *Nippon Sanka Fujinka Gakkai Zasshi* 1993;45:423–30.
21. Tokuda I, Nagashima T, Aihara K. Global bifurcation structure of chaotic neural networks and its application to traveling salesman problems. *Neural Netw* 1997;10:1673–90.
22. Weng W, Khorasani K. An adaptive structure neural networks application to EEG automatic seizure detection. *Neural Netw* 1996;9:1223–40.
23. Moul JW, Snow PB, Fernandez EB, Maher PD, Sesterhenn IA. Neural network analysis of quantitative histological factors to predict pathological stage in clinical stage I nonseminomatous testicular cancer. *J Urol* 1995;153:1674–7.
24. Ruppin E, Reggia JA. A neural model of memory impairment in diffuse cerebral atrophy. *Br J Psychiatry* 1995;166:19–28.
25. Arle JE, Morriss C, Wang ZJ, Zimmerman RA, Philipps PG, Sutton LN. Prediction of posterior fossa tumor type in children by means of magnetic resonance image properties, spectroscopy, and neural networks. *J Neurosurg* 1997;86:755–61.
26. Brickley MR, Cowpe JG, Shepherd JP. Performance of a computer-simulated neural network trained to categorize normal, pre-malignant and malignant oral smears. *J Oral Pathol Med* 1996;25:424–8.
27. Mutlukan E, Keating D. Visual field interpretation with a personal computer-based neural network. *Eye* 1994;8:321–3.
28. Westenskow DR, Orr JA, Simon FH, Bender HJ, Frankenberger H. Intelligent alarms reduce anesthesiologist's response time to critical faults. *Anesthesiology* 1992;77:1074–9.
29. Fujita H, Katafuchi T, Uehara T, Nishimura T. Application of artificial neural network to computer-aided diagnosis of coronary artery disease in myocardial SPECT bull's-eye images. *J Nucl Med* 1992;33:272–6.
30. Andreassen H, Bohr H, Bohr J, Brunak S, Bugge T. Analysis of the secondary structure of the human immunodeficiency virus (HIV) proteins p17, gp120, and gp41 by computer modeling based on neural network methods. *J Acquir Immune Defic Syndr* 1990;3:615–22.
31. Farmer RM, Medearis AL, Hirata GI, Platt LD. The use of a neural network for the ultrasonic estimation of fetal weight in the macrosomic fetus. *Am J Obstet Gynecol* 1992;166:1467–72.
32. DeVoe LD, Samuel S, Prescott P, Work BA. Predicting the duration of the first stage of spontaneous labor using a neural network. *J Matern Fetal Neonatal Med* 1996;5:256–61.
33. Keith RD, Westgate J, Ifeachor EC, Greene KR. Suitability of artificial neural networks for feature extraction from cardiotocogram during labour. *Med Biol Eng Comput* 1994;32(Suppl 4):51–7.
34. Salamalekis E, Thomopoulos P, Giannaris D, *et al.* Computerized intrapartum diagnosis of fetal hypoxia based on fetal heart rate monitoring and fetal pulse oximetry recordings utilizing wavelet analysis and neural networks. *BJOG* 2002;109:1137–42.
35. Maeda K, Utsu M Kihaile PE. Quantification of sonographic echogenicity with grey-level histogram width: A clinical tissue characterization. *Ultrasound Med Biol* 1998;24:225–34.
36. Maeda K, Utsu M, Yamamoto N, Serizawa M. Echogenicity of fetal lung and liver quantified by the grey-level histogram width. *Ultrasound Med Biol* 1999;25:201–8.
37. Maeda K, Utsu M, Yamamoto N, Serizawa M, Ito T. Clinical tissue characterization with gray level histogram width in obstetrics and gynecology. *Ultrasound Rev Obstet Gynecol* 2002;2:124–8.

141 The fetal electrocardiogram

W. J. van Wijngaarden

Introduction

Electronic fetal monitoring (EFM), based on the recording and interpretation of the fetal heart rate (FHR), is practiced routinely in antenatal and intrapartum care throughout the world. This is analogous to diagnosing ischemic heart disease in adult medicine by recording an adult's pulse rate over a period of time. By only measuring the RR interval of the fetal electrocardiogram (FECG), as is done in EFM, a potential wealth of information on a fetus's well-being is discarded. During labor, the FECG is continuously available for analysis and reflects the cellular metabolic condition of the myometrium and the cardiac conduction system. FECG analysis in the detection of fetal compromise has been the focus of research of a relatively small number of groups for many years and has, in some instances, now reached the stage of clinical trials. Based on these, commercial enterprise is already advocating its implementation into clinical practice and is marketing specially devised monitoring systems.

The first FECG was recorded by Cremer in 1906[1] through silver electrodes attached to the abdominal wall and inserted into the vagina, with a simple string galvanometer used to display the very small signal. As concern over the maternal condition outweighed interest in fetal well-being, its clinical potential was not considered until many years later. However, already in 1930 it was recognized that for any analysis of the FECG to be made possible, the small FECG signal had to be amplified.[2] The potential of the FECG to aid diagnosis and management in certain conditions (drug effects on the fetal heart, congenital heart disease, umbilical cord problems, multiple pregnancies and abnormal labor) was suggested as early as in 1936.[3]

Signal processing

Technical difficulties with the small, trans-abdominally derived signal and background noise were first seriously addressed in the early 1950s with the introduction of bandpass filters, allowing only frequencies between 30 and 100 Hz to be amplified.[4] Thus QRS complexes were isolated and analyses of the FECG over longer periods were made possible. The first reports on changes in the FECG waveform during fetal hypoxemia were published in the 1950s.[5]

A major change in FECG research came with the introduction of the fetal scalp electrode in the early 1960s and as a result the main problems in obtaining transabdominal recordings (signal amplitude, signal identification and isolation) could be addressed. The ability to make accurate RR distance measurements led to the introduction of FHR analysis. However, low amplitude P and T waves were still often buried in background noise or filtered out when reducing the baseline drift of the signal which would otherwise interfere with signal detection. As a result, accurate, often manual, measurements were difficult to obtain and resulted in many inconsistencies in the earlier FECG waveform analysis studies. To amplify the FECG, so that the low amplitude waves could be identified and measured both automatically and accurately, a number of signal filtering and enhancement techniques have been developed.

The signal must be 'cleaned' from high and low frequency noise (such as baseline drift) by appropriate filters, leaving the frequency of the FECG waveform intact. In FECG recordings, a high pass cut-off of 0.16 Hz at −3 dB has been found to be adequate because of the shorter time intervals and higher heart rate than in adults where 0.05 Hz is a more appropriate high pass cut-off.[6]

Group averaging techniques were introduced by Hon and Lee[7] using a so-called 'CAT system'. This 'block averaging' technique meant stopping and resetting the system after each calculated averaged complex, which in the 1960s was an off-line and time-consuming procedure. An improvement on this was the development of 'sliding window' or 'running' averaging techniques, in which a new enhanced (averaged) complex is recalculated each time a new waveform is added to the calculation and the oldest is removed. Weighting of this running average was introduced later to allow for more transient changes to be detected. With this technique, all complexes are given a certain weight, with the latest the highest weighting factor or impact in the calculation of the enhanced waveform. With each new incoming

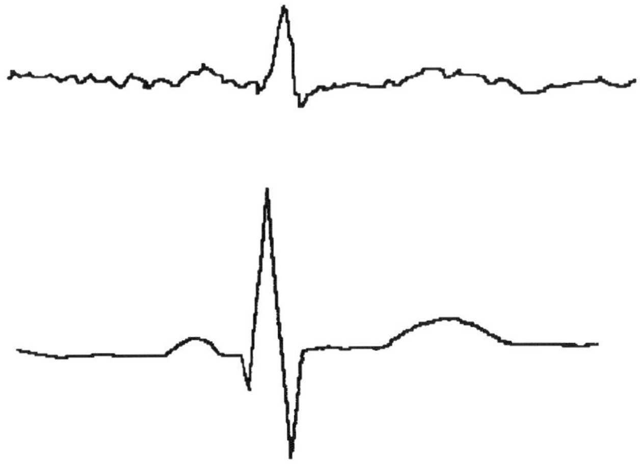

Figure 141.1 A raw fetal electrocardiogram (FECG) waveform (top) and enhanced FECG waveform after averaging (bottom).

complex, all the previous weighting factors are changed and a new enhanced waveform is calculated.[8] The number of raw complexes and their respective input into the resultant averaged and enhanced signal can be varied. The result of this averaging or enhancement routine is the attenuation of electrical noise and other non-repetitive features such as movements, leaving the FECG waves recognizable and analyzable (Figure 141.1).

After having obtained an enhanced FECG waveform, several techniques can be applied to perform measurements. The Nottingham FECG analyzer measures the components of the enhanced FECG waveform by identifying the segments of the averaged complex using a 'line-fit routine'.[9] The location of the start, peak and end of each wave is calculated from the intersections of straight lines which are fitted by a linear regression technique to represent the incline and decline of each wave (Figure 141.2). The STAN 21 system (Neoventa) uses a set number of complexes for its block averaging technique. In exactly which way the changes in the ST segment are recognized and monitored is not public domain.

The developments of the above described techniques, aided by rapid developments in microprocessing technology, have made it possible to automatically and accurately identify the FECG waveform, reduce waveform distortion (fetal and maternal movements and electrical signals, 50 Hz interference) and to perform continuous on-line FECG analysis on small personal computer-based systems usable in a clinical setting. Furthermore, large amounts of generated data can now be handled easily and transformed into clinically interpretable patterns.

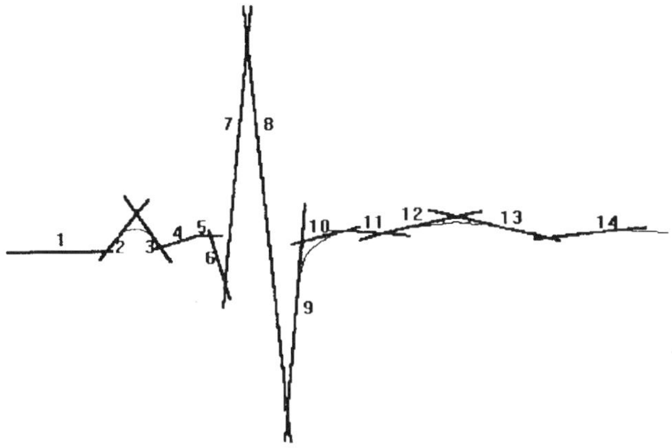

Point	Intersection
P onset	1 – 2
P peak	2 – 3
P end	3 – 4
Q onset	5 6
Q peak	6 – 7
R peak	7 – 8
S peak	8 – 9
S end	9 – 10
T onset	11 – 12
T peak	12 – 13
T end	13 – 14

Figure 141.2 Regression line-fit routine of the average fetal electrocardiogram (FECG) waveform.

Signal acquisition

In human fetuses during labor, the FECG signal is obtained through a fetal scalp electrode. Single spiral scalp electrodes (Corometrics Medical Systems, Connecticut, USA and Cetro AB, Sweden) have a superior frequency response and a high signal amplitude with a low signal-to-noise ratio.[10] Although this may be of importance in morphological FECG analysis, the frequency response and signal-to-noise ratio of the Copeland electrode (Surgicraft Ltd, Redditch, UK) allows for adequate detection of the time intervals within the FECG. Therefore, both systems have been found to function satisfactorily in FECG time interval analysis but caution needs to be expressed when comparing FECG morphology measurements using different fetal scalp electrodes.

In FECG morphology analysis, changes in the various amplitudes are recorded within a certain cardiac vector. The direction of this vector is determined by the location of the reference electrode in relation to the exploring electrode attached to the fetal skin. In the fetal lamb, the changes in the T wave after an isoprenaline challenge were seen to be mainly in the YZ plane, whereas the routinely used bipolar lead system would only be optimal in identifying T-wave changes in the XZ axis of the fetal body.[11] In the standard bipolar configuration of a spiral fetal scalp electrode, the distance between the electrodes is small and has been suggested to be a cause for baseline drift, noise and fluctuating vector directions which may result in alterations in FECG waveform morphology.[12]

The Copeland fetal scalp electrode (also a bipolar configuration) has a long reference electrode which is less likely to cause vector fluctuations. It has been proposed that a unipolar configuration, with one electrode on the fetal scalp and one on the maternal thigh, would be more stable and better to detect changes in the longitudinal axis of the fetus (e.g. wave changes). Experience with the Nottingham FECG analyzer, however, would suggest a satisfactory detection of T-wave changes using a bipolar lead system and we have not found any benefit from using a unipolar system, nor were there any changes in the FECG waveform configuration seen when such a lead configuration was used. In humans, bipolar lead systems would appear as sensitive as unipolar systems to detect changes in the Y axis of the fetus. For obvious reasons, FECG time interval analysis is not influenced by potential errors due to different vector configurations.

Antenatal signal acquisition is usually performed transabdominally with Ag/AgCl skin electrodes. Signals can also be obtained by the detection of changes in the magnetic field caused by electrical fluctuations of the fetal heart[13] or directly during intra-amniotic procedures such as fetal cord blood sampling *in utero*.[14]

Other means of obtaining a fetal ECG signal include the placement of wire electrodes under the skin, which requires operative techniques and is commonly used in obtaining data in animal rather than in human studies.

FECG analyzers

A number of FECG analyzers have been used in direct signal sampling research over the past 10 years. Of these, the Nottingham FECG analyzer (University of Nottingham) and the STAN S21 analyzer (Neoventa Medical, Gothenburg, Sweden) are the only FECG analyzers used in an on-line real-time trial setting on the labor ward. The STAN S21 analyzer filters the incoming signal with a bandwidth of 0.05–100 Hz and digitizes it with a sampling rate of 500 Hz. A block averaging technique is applied to create an enhanced waveform using 10 accepted complexes.[15] The system is specifically designed to measure ST waveform changes but can also calculate the PR time interval. The waves are recognized by an amplitude search for the points of maximum deviation within a fixed time zone. For quality control, every 2 min the current average T/QRS ratio and averaged FECG complex are printed alongside a cardiotocographic (CTG) record.[16]

The Nottingham FECG analyzer filters the raw signal with a bandwidth of 0.16–150 Hz and digitizes the analog FECG signal at a sampling rate of 500 Hz. A matched filter is used to recognize the QRS complex by comparing of frequency spectrum characteristics. The averaged or enhanced FECG complex is created by using a 'time coherent' approach. This is established by correlating each new incoming raw complex, consisting of a total of 256 data points, with the enhanced waveform. Proper alignment of the new incoming and the enhanced FECG complex is ensured by cross-correlating 15 points around the R peak of the enhanced waveform with the R peak of the new ECG complex. In other words, the identified R peak becomes the fixed point around which raw FECG complexes are superimposed. The enhanced waveform is calculated after 'weighting' the complexes with the most recent signals having the most input. After this, a line-fit routine (see above) is applied to identify the individual waves. The capability of this time coherent weighted averaging routine to accurately isolate rapid changes of the unprocessed or raw FECG signal has clinically been validated by comparing fast changes in the raw signal with those detected in the averaged signal.[17] The Nottingham FECG analyzer measures 18 FECG waveform parameters (morphology as well as time interval) and calculates four more simultaneously at 2 s intervals including signal-to-noise ratio estimation for signal quality control. Only waveforms with a ratio exceeding 3:1 are included in the resultant waveform calculation. For quality control, the desired measurements are displayed in real time on a VDU screen along with the raw waveform and the averaged waveform (Figure 141.3). All 22 parameter measurements and calculations are stored in the system's memory for retrospective analysis.

The system used in Southampton in off-line intrapartum recordings used a band pass filter of 0.1–40 Hz and sampling rate of 1000 Hz. The system was designed to measure the T/QRS ratio. Measurements were performed on every second of four incoming raw complexes, thus at best, T/QRS ratios of only 25% of all incoming complexes were available.[18] Averaging of the T/QRS ratios was performed after the actual waveform measurements.

Cardiac electrophysiology

The electrocardiogram is a record of myocardial action potential fluctuations during the cardiac cycle. The electrical discharge of each cycle starts in the sinoatrial (SA) node. The membrane potential of the pacemaker cells of the SA node is unstable and declines continuously until a trigger level is reached. At this stage there is a dramatic increase of Na^{+} ion influx and K^{+} ion efflux, resulting in the depolarization of the SA node. This is accompanied by an increase in membrane permeability to Ca^{2+} ions and results in 'slow' inward current of Ca^{2+} ions which is responsible for the upstroke of the action potential in the SA node and, consequently, its frequency of reaching firing threshold levels or heart rate. This slow inward current of Ca^{2+} ions consists of three components. The main component responsible

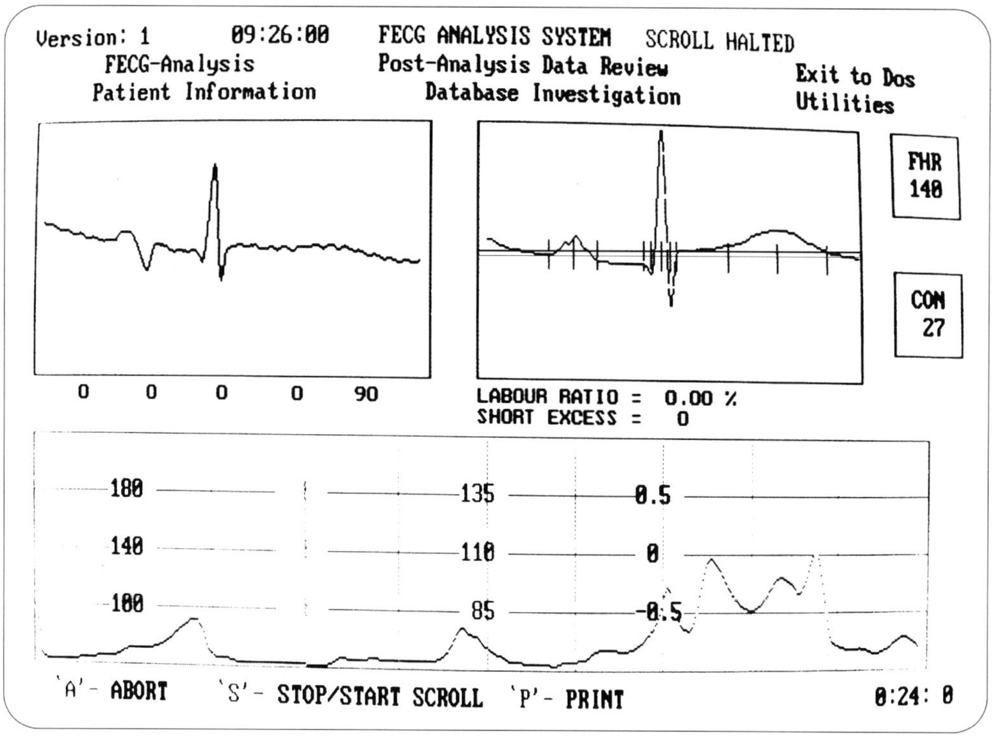

Figure 141.3 VDU display of the Nottingham analyzer: the raw waveform is displayed in the top left window, the averaged waveform in the top right window and the conduction index is displayed as a moving window at the bottom. The ratio index is displayed as a number next to 'labor ratio'.

for SA node repolarization is influenced by both adenosine triphosphate (ATP) and epinephrine which increase its conductance. As a result, during hypoxemia which is accompanied by reduced levels of ATP, the conductance is reduced. The atrioventricular (AV) node contains, in addition to 'slow' oxygen-sensitive Ca^{2+} channels, also fast Na^{+} channels which are less sensitive to oxygen.[19,20] Changes in oxygenation will therefore have less effect on the upstroke of the action potentials in the AV node than in the SA node.

Following the electrical discharge of the SA node, depolarization spreads through the atrial muscles. In the ECG this is represented by the P wave. Before the action potential is further propagated to the ventricles, it is delayed in the AV node. After the AV node, conduction is very rapid through the special conduction tissue of the bundle of His, which separates into the left and right bundle branches and the Purkinje fibers within the ventricular muscle mass. As the QRS complex is caused by ventricular depolarization, most of the PR interval reflects the conduction time (depolarization) of the AV node. Atrial repolarization is usually submerged in the QRS complex and ventricular repolarization is reflected by the T wave. The Na^{+}/K^{+} pump fuelled by ATP and activated by intracellular Ca^{2+} plays a central role in all these processes. The Na^{+}/K^{+} pump maintains the ion gradient across the cell membrane by Na^{+} ion efflux and K^{+} ion influx, with a resultant net positive extracellular charge. An increase in heart rate is a result of an increase in Na^{+}/K^{+} pump activity, which results in an increase in the outward current. This leads to a shorter repolarization time and therefore a shortening of the time to reach the following trigger level for depolarization. Under normoxemic conditions, this will not lead to any major changes in the morphology of the FECG waveform and the time intervals will shorten simultaneously.

The control of the FHR and the conduction of action potentials in the heart is complex. Spontaneous firing of the pacemaker cells of the SA node, the effect of baro- and chemoreceptor stimulation, autonomic nervous system reflexes and tone all directly or indirectly influence the SA and the AV node. Hypoxemia may not only induce an adrenal catecholamine release but also directly slow the conduction of action potentials in the myocardium[21] and the AV node.[22]

Normal values for the FECG waveform

Ranges for the normal values of FECG parameters using an old model of the STAN system and the Nottingham system have been reported for both acidotic and non-acidotic human fetuses during labor. Using the STAN-alyser system, a mean T/QRS ratio during labor has been quoted as 0.148, with an SD of 0.048.[23] A list of normal values for FECG waveform

Table 141.1 Normal values for fetal electrocardiogram (FECG) time interval and morphology parameters as measured with the Nottingham FECG analyzer during the first 20 min of recording time in the first stage of labor; time intervals in ms (from Mohajer[30] with permission)

Parameter	Mean values (SD)
Fetal heart rate	134.38 (13.3)
PR (interval)	102.72 (12.5)
P (duration)	63.34 (12.2)
QRS (duration)	43.61 (5.4)
R/S (ratio)	2.89 (0.6)
PRe (segment elevation)	97.49 (4.0)
STe (segment elevation)	102.86 (6.4)
RT (interval)	147.77 (21.3)
T (duration)	127.75 (24.1)
P (height)	9.44 (4.2)
Q (height)	10.77 (9.2)
R (height)	70.94 (15.2)
S (height)	24.58 (19.3)
T (height)	7.79 (6.7)
S/N ratio	9.39 (5.9)
P (area)	6.08 (3.5)
T (area)	10.63 (6.2)

measurements performed by the Nottingham FECG analyzer during the first 20 min of recording in first-stage labor of term pregnancies with uncompromised infants at delivery [umbilical artery pH > 7.20, base excess (BE) > −8 mmol/l] weighing over 2500 g is given in Table 141.1.

The FECG and changes during fetal compromise

All aspects of the FECG waveform have been analyzed and related to changes in biochemical markers or CTG patterns. The earlier studies in particular need to be interpreted with caution because of potential errors due to noise, inappropriate filter settings and manual measurement techniques. Furthermore, caution needs to be exerted when changes are reported in cross-sectional data sets, as individual trends may be of greater importance and more informative. The use of means and standard deviations in not normally distributed populations (such as the T/QRS ratio) should be avoided as it may lead to wrongly assumed definitions of abnormality.[24]

The P wave

The aspects of the P wave which have been studied are changes in its duration, height and area. P-wave duration increases progressively from the 17th week of gestation with increasing cardiac mass.[25] Changes in P-wave morphology (i.e. notching, inversion, biphasic), as well as its (sometimes transient) complete disappearance, have all been reported to occur in association with decelerations but not necessarily with an abnormal acid–base balance.[7,17,26–29] Care needs to be exerted when interpreting changes in the P-wave height using averaging techniques. It was found on examination of the raw FECG complexes that the P wave could be dislocated from its normal position during bradycardia beyond the FECG analyzer's ability of detection and consequently lead to a false apparent reduction in its height.[30]

The duration of the P wave may change during fetal respiratory acidemia[31] and was noted to be loosely related to umbilical vein norepinephrine levels.[17,28] The significant correlation between umbilical artery blood gases and change in P-wave duration during the last hour of labor was found to be too low (r_{pH}=0.13) for clinical use.[17] No significant difference was found between the duration, the height and the area of the P wave of non-compromised term fetuses, acidemic fetuses (umbilical artery pH < 7.16, BE < −10 mmol/l) regardless of gestational age and small-for-gestational-age fetuses (birth weight < 2500 g). Nor was any significant difference found when the first 20 min of these labors was compared to the last 20 min of labor of each group individually.[30]

The P-wave area has been seen to increase with fetal acidemia,[31] to decrease with fetal distress[27] and to be unrelated to fetal acid–base balance apart from a clinically impractical but significant correlation (r_{pco_2}=−0.15) with umbilical artery pco_2 levels over the last hour of labor.[17]

The PR segment

Changes in the height of the PR segment are common but have not been found to be related to any biochemical changes.[17,28] In FECG morphology measurements, the height of the PR segment is important when it is used as the isoelectric line, as is done by the STAN system. It may be a source of discrepancies when identical recordings are analyzed by different systems, as the Nottingham FECG analyzer and the system used in Southampton both use the pre-P segment as the isoelectric line.[32] No significant difference in the height of the PR segment was found when cross-sectional intrapartum measurements were compared between uncompromised term fetuses, compromised fetuses and small-for-gestational-age fetuses. Nor were there any significant differences between the first and last 20 min of labor in each of these groups.[30]

The PQ and PR intervals

In animals, manual measurements of the FECG waveform showed both a prolongation of the PQ interval during hypoxemia in lambs[33] and a lengthening of the PR interval after cord occlusion in baboons.[34] More recently, the changes in the PR interval seen during hypoxemia in fetal lamb experiments have been clearly documented. Acute maternal aortic occlusion was seen to be followed immediately by an initial prolongation of the PR interval simultaneous to RR interval lengthening (vagal reflex) and superseded by a shortening of the PR interval. This was reverted to a lengthening of the PR interval after release of the occluder.[35] The shortening of the PR interval following the vagal reflex is thought to be secondary to an increased adrenergic activity and the lengthening after release of the occluder as a result of baroreceptor stimulation. Murray[17] showed that the initial vagal reflex could be abolished with atropine premedication. In the same study, isoprenaline was shown to decrease both the PR and the RR intervals during normoxemia. Baro- and chemoreceptor reflexes probably do not have a great influence on this as the same changes were seen in experiments on very premature fetal lambs in which these reflexes are not yet fully developed (H. Murray, personal communication).

In humans, large changes in the FHR have been found to coincide with changes in the PR interval.[17] Table 141.2 displays the observations from various studies of changes in the PR interval in relation to periodic changes of the FHR.

In a study of 40 normal labors, the PR interval was noted to shorten significantly during contractions, whether induced by syntocinon infusion or not, without any significant change in coincident FHR pattern.[36] In one study, a significant difference in PR interval was reported when comparing male to female fetuses in labor.[37] Possible explanations for this phenomenon are the slightly higher heart rate and/or the higher sympathetic tone in males and exaggerated reaction to stress when compared with females.[38]

Earlier work suggested that the overall trend for the PR interval to shorten during normal labor did not have a relationship with biochemical compromise.[6,31] In a study comprising 309 labors, the mean PR interval duration was found to change little until the last hour of labor.[17] In 59% of labors, a significant shortening in the mean duration was noted during the last hour, although this was within the standard error of measurement in 13% of these. During this time, changes in the mean PR interval duration were significantly correlated ($r=0.2$) to umbilical artery cord gas measurements, but were too weak for clinical use. This was supported by a later study which did not find a change in the PR interval between the first and last 20 min of labors in uncompromised fetuses but noted a shortening of 10% in the group with evidence of fetal compromise, which was statistically not significant.[30] Importantly, Murray[17] found the average PR interval duration over the last 15 min of labor to be inversely related to epinephrine ($r_{epi}=-0.47$, $P<0.001$) and norepinephrine ($r_{norepi}=-0.26$, $P<0.001$) levels in arterial cord blood. As catecholamine levels increase during the second stage of labor and even more so in the compromised fetus, a strong adrenergic influence on the AV node and therefore PR interval duration could be an explanation for the changes in the PR interval seen during labor.

Table 141.2 The relationship between the PR interval and periodic changes in the fetal heart rate

	Study	PR interval
Accelerations	Murray[17]	↓
	Mohajer[30]	↓
Decelerations		
Early	Lee and Blackwell[26]	↓
	Murray[17]	↓↑ *
	Mohajer[30]	↑
Variable	Roemer *et al.*[65]	↓
	Pardi *et al.*[27]	↓
	Murray[17]	↓ **
	Mohajer[30]	↓
Late	Pardi *et al.*[27]	↓↑ ***
	Murray[17]	↓
	Mohajer[30]	↓

↑ Lengthening; ↓ shortening; *shortens in 50%, lengthens in 50%; **shortens after an initial lengthening; ***lengthens during 'mild' and shortens during 'moderate' and 'severe' late decelerations

The R/S ratio

The direction of spread of depolarization through the ventricles is called the cardiac axis and is represented by the R/S ratio. Right axis deviation occurs in congenital heart disorders and in conditions where there is a strain on the right side of the heart leading to right ventricle hypertrophy. Left axis deviation can occur with hypertrophy of the left ventricle but is commonly due to conduction defects.

Mohajer[30] found a reduction trend in the R/S ratio when cross-sectionally comparing the first 20 min with the last 20 min of labor in both non-compromised and compromised fetuses, indicating a right axis shift. The opposite was seen in small-for-gestational-age fetuses. In addition, small-for-gestational-age fetuses were observed to start labor with a non-significant but substantially higher ratio than non-compromised fetuses.

No change in the R/S ratio was seen during or between contractions.[37] Symonds[39] observed acidosis and hypokalemia in the umbilical vein to be accompanied by a left shift of the cardiac axis during labor. This was also seen to accompany late decelerations and bradycardia. However, with increasing acidosis as measured by fetal scalp blood sampling, there was a tendency toward right axis deviation. This right axis deviation during labor was also noted to be associated with umbilical cord entanglement and hypoxemia at birth.[40] The association between a right axis deviation and acidemia was also seen by Strachan *et al.*[41] who found a significant correlation between a decreasing R/S ratio during the last half-hour of labor and an umbilical artery pH and BE of less than 7.15 and –8 mmol/l, respectively. Acute pressure changes in the umbilical cord vessels may lead to intracardiac pressure changes which can result in cardiac axis deviations. Chronic hypoxia, on the contrary, may cause left ventricular strain and result in left axis deviation.[42] The tendency for left axis deviation in small-for-gestational-age fetuses seen in other studies would support this.[30]

The QRS duration

The QRS duration represents the time for the action potential to spread through the ventricles. It is significantly longer in males than in females[37] and is, as in adults,[43] directly related to myocardial mass.[44] This would be in keeping with anatomical studies showing the male fetal heart to be heavier than the female fetal heart.[45] The relationship between the QRS duration and birth weight is highly significant (r=0.38, P=0.001)[37] and should be borne in mind when quoting and reporting normal values. Although early and variable decelerations have been seen to be associated with a shortening of the QRS duration,[26] no relationship between QRS duration and fetal compromise during labor has been found.[5,17,46] Contractions do not influence QRS duration.[37]

The observation that chronic impaired oxygenation may lead to an increase in QRS duration[47] is supported by the clear correlation found between ventricular depolarization time and hemoglobin levels in pregnancies complicated by rhesus isoimmunization.[48] Reactive myocardial hypertrophy, resulting in a larger QRS duration, appears a logical explanation for this. Therefore, it has been suggested that serial antenatal QRS duration measurements may improve the detection of fetal growth retardation. One report quotes a sensitivity of 82% and specificity of 93%.[49]

The QT and RT intervals

The QT and RT intervals are closely related to the FHR and, if corrected for this, little significance in the relationship with clinical features has been found.[28,30,42] The QT interval during episodes of hypoxia has been seen to decrease in rabbit experiments,[50] not to change after placental separation[46] and to increase significantly during acidosis in human fetuses.[42] A shortening has been observed during early and variable decelerations.[26] Although this was also observed in a recent study on 68 fetuses with metabolic acidemia at birth, a significant shortening rather than a lengthening of the QT interval was found at the end of the recording when compared with the beginning which was independent of heart rate.[51] Further work is awaited to clarify the potential of the QT interval in fetal monitoring.

The ST interval and T-wave duration

As in all the low-frequency waves, the setting of the filter characteristics is essential in the ability to identify the beginning and end accurately. If too high, the onset of the ST segment will smoothen and continue indistinguishable into the T wave. If too low, noise will swamp the signal, rendering it unidentifiable. Group averaging techniques and, to a lesser degree, moving windows weighted averaging techniques will artefactually lengthen the T wave as a result of changes in the RT interval, secondary to normal RR duration variation. Mohajer[30] observed a trend of shortening of the T-wave duration during labor which was not significant. Changes in the T-wave duration have not been found to be related to fetal intrapartum compromise.[52]

The ST segment and T-wave height

In adults, ST waveform changes occur during episodes of myocardial hypoxemia and infarction. These include ST segment height changes and both an increase and inversion of the T-wave height. The observation of similar changes in compromised fetuses forms the background of ST waveform analysis in the detection of fetal hypoxemia. Repolarization of the cardiac ventricles, as opposed to depolarization, is an active and energy-requiring process. Therefore, the morphology of the ST waveform is dependent on the sequence of ventricular depolarization, functional hemodynamic changes, the local metabolic status and substances influencing the Na^+/K^+ pump and, importantly, the vector of the leads used.[53] Reduced efficiency of the Na^+/K^+ pump, regardless of the cause, leads to potassium release, a change in membrane potential and consequently an elevation of the T wave. Quantitative measurements of the T wave are commonly expressed as the T/QRS ratio to eliminate changing amplification factors.

Controlled animal experiments have clearly demonstrated the presence of ST waveform changes during episodes of fetal hypoxemia.[33,54] In myocardial metabolism studies in fetal lambs, the decrease in high-energy substances during hypoxia was accompanied by a decrease in the T-wave amplitude when

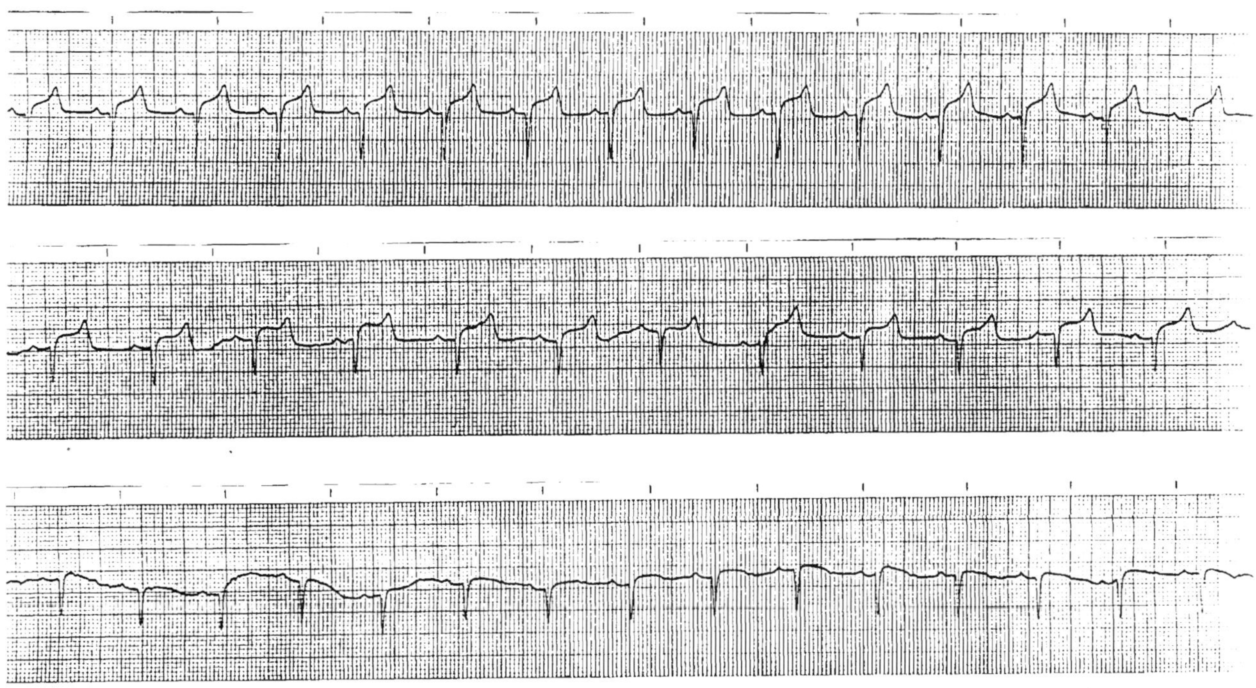

Figure 141.4 Reversion to normal of an elevated T/QRS ratio and ST segment elevation in a fetal lamb with a pH between 7.01 and 7.03 and a base excess between –14.8 and –17.8 mmol/l in fetal sheep experiments conducted by Drs H de Haan and THM Hasaart, Maastricht.

signs of failing cardiovascular functions occurred.[55] The decrease in amplitude of a previously elevated T wave during severe fetal compromise was also observed in another fetal sheep experiment and should caution against reassurance of a sound fetal condition with normal T/QRS ratios alone (Figure 141.4; van Wijngaarden, De Haan and Hasaart, unpublished data).

The rate of glycogenolysis has been found to be significantly correlated ($r=0.73$, $P=0.001$) with an increase in T-wave amplitude, indicating a relationship between myocardial glycogen utilization and T-wave amplitude.[55] Given the glycogenolytic effect of catecholamines, this is in keeping with the ST waveform changes seen with the administration of β-sympathicomimetics, epinephrine surges during hypoxia and the strong correlation between plasma epinephrine levels and the T/QRS ratio in mature fetal sheep.[35,56,57] The lack of this correlation in immature fetal sheep could be due to a different adrenergic response to hypoxia as a result of an immature neuroendocrine development.[35] A change in the normal adrenergic response to hypoxia may also be accountable for the different ST waveform changes seen in growth-retarded guinea-pig fetuses as compared to fully grown guinea-pig fetuses.[58] Perhaps a different setting of the basal sympathetic tone as a result of chronic stimulation, leaving little room for response to further excitation, may be responsible for this. However, as propranolol (a β-adrenoreceptor blocker) was seen to inhibit ST waveform changes during moderate but not during marked hypoxia, catecholamines alone may not be solely responsible for the observed changes.[57]

In studies on chronically instrumented fetal sheep, the T/QRS ratio was seen to have a linear relationship with hypoxemia and to be significantly correlated to acidemia, lactate and (nor)epinephrine levels and blood pressure.[59–61] As the acidemia was mainly due to increasing levels of lactate, increasing T/QRS ratios were suggested to indicate anaerobic metabolism.[59] T-wave changes have been observed to occur during normoxemia in combination with increased myocardial performance, indicating simultaneous epinephrine release. On the contrary, hypoxic episodes, with a decrease in oxygen content down to 64% without an increase in epinephrine levels, were not accompanied by ST waveform changes.[60,62] It has been suggested, therefore, that an increase in T-wave amplitude could serve as an index of myocardial energy balance which becomes negative when glycogenolysis sets in.[62] These findings and the correlation with lactate levels suggest that ST waveform changes occur when the fetal myocardium switches to an anerobic metabolism and the elevation of the T wave occurs when fetal adaptation to hypoxemia with an increased coronary blood flow is no longer sufficient.[63]

In a large study of 47 chronically cannulated lambs subjected to profound levels of hypoxia, the large changes seen in the T/QRS ratio and fetal biochemical status did not appear to be very well correlated.[64] The clinically important conclusion from this report was that the T/QRS ratio is a poor predictor of fetal compromise.

Observational ST waveform studies in human fetuses during hypoxemia are more equivocal than those in animals. In early work, using manual measurement techniques, hypoxia was seen to be accompanied by ST segment depression and T-wave inversion,[42,65] but no relationship was found between ST waveform changes during late decelerations and fetal scalp blood pH.[27] Using the STAN-alyser (Cinventa, Sweden), Lilja *et al.*[66] found an increased T/QRS ratio in half of the fetuses with an abnormal FHR pattern. In another study, low Apgar scores were associated with an increased T/QRS ratio.[67] Using the Nottingham FECG analyzer, ST waveform changes were seen to accompany low arterial cord pH values.[28,68] The average increase in the T/QRS ratio of 1.02% (range –3.07% to 10.0%, $P < 0.004$) seen during contractions may be explained by catecholamine surges and transient hypoxemia.[69] It is of note that this increase in T/QRS ratio was significantly higher in pre-edited raw complexes, which emphasizes the potential inaccuracy of FECG waveform morphology measurements from noisy data.

Other studies, however, could not confirm a relationship between birth asphyxia and the T/QRS ratio.[18,70,71] One report found a raised T/QRS ratio to have a considerably lower detection rate for fetal acidemia during labor at term than a pathological CTG.[72] During normal labor, T/QRS ratios appear to wander greatly[18,24,73] and the average T/QRS ratio in normal labor varies substantially: 10%,[18] 15%,[23] 18–26%[73] and 20%.[64] The setting of the isoelectric line may be responsible for differences when different systems are used.[18,32,70] A study which compared electrical signal conduction of different fetal scalp electrodes using the STAN-alyser, suggested the T/QRS ratio to have a linear relationship with the amplitude of the QRS complex.[74] Although this could not be confirmed on the Nottingham FECG database using the Nottingham FECG analyzer (W.J. van Wijngaarden and B.K. Strachan, unpublished data), further studies are required.

As the T/QRS ratio is not normally distributed and varies greatly between cases, it may be better to perform analyses using individually calculated criteria for abnormality rather than cross-sectionally acquired derived cut-off levels.[24] In a retrospective analysis of 20 intrapartum fetal electrocardiogram recordings, only two were found to have a T/QRS ratio which was normally distributed.[75] An increase in the T/QRS ratio over the 97.5th and 99.5th centile for 2 consecutive minutes, with the centiles calculated on an individual basis, would appear to discriminate best between biochemically compromised and non-compromised fetuses. However, the effect on the intervention rate remains to be established. In no case the T/QRS ratio was seen to exceed 0.25 for periods previously described to be related to poor outcome. It was concluded that the use of an absolute threshold for T/QRS ratio abnormality based on the assumption of a normal distribution needs to be viewed with caution.

The first randomized controlled trial (RCT) on the clinical value of ST segment and T/QRS ratio changes in intrapartum fetal surveillance reported in 1993 and included over 2400 labors.[76] Intrapartum monitoring was performed by conventional CTG or by ST waveform analysis in conjunction with CTG. The results of this trial[76] suggest the STAN-alyser safe to use in conjunction with conventional CTG and may reduce the number of fetal blood samples (FBS) carried out (but not the number of patients having a FBS carried out). The numbers of operative deliveries for an abnormal FBS were similar in both groups, indicating similar sensitivities to detect an abnormal scalp pH. The operative intervention rate for presumed fetal distress was significantly higher in the control group but as both groups had a similar incidence of abnormal FBS results, this appeared to be based on CTG interpretation only. There was no difference in intervention rate with normal cord gas measurements between both groups. Although there were fewer cases with metabolic acidosis in the ST analysis arm of the trial, it was not clear whether these were actually identified by ST analysis, as the incidence of mild acidosis was almost identical in the two groups.

Another clinical analysis of the application of T/QRS ratio changes in the detection of fetal compromise during labor showed that, when using the T/QRS ratio only, with values over 0.25 for depicting abnormality, over 75% of abnormal FBS results would have been missed.[77] Although the first intrapartum trial suggests that during labor a normal ST waveform reassures the birth attendants of a sound fetal condition, the latter study emphasizes that a normal ST waveform should not be regarded to be reassuring in the presence of CTG abnormalities.

A new model of the STAN system was introduced in the late 1990s (STAN S21) by Neoventa Medical, Gothenburg, Sweden, which not only calculates the T/QRS ratio, but also reports on ST segment changes. A number of retrospective and prospective observational studies and one RCT have since been reported, most by or in association with the same research group in Sweden. The final report of a large Swedish-based European multicenter implementation study is awaited. In a prospective observational study on 573 labors in 12 Nordic centers, of a total of 15 neonates with neurological symptoms and/or acidemia (cord artery $pH < 7.05$ and base deficit > 12.0 mmol/l), five neonates had neurological symptoms and ST abnormalities during the first stage and eight showed ST changes during pushing.[78] Of the eight cases that had acidemia and a normal neonatal outcome, seven had CTG + ST abnormalities.

In another prospective observational study, of the 637 labors which were monitored using a STAN S21 system, only 70.5% was, for various reasons, available for outcome analysis.[79] Eighteen (4.0%) of the 22 of the neonates with metabolic acidosis (same definition as above) were in this group. Fetal scalp blood samples (total 192) with a pH < 7.20 were associated with ST changes in 67%, whereas this occurred in 11% of cases with a pH ≥ 7.20. In all five cases with an umbilical cord artery pH < 7.00, significant changes occurred in the ST segment 18–31 min before birth, whereas these were not present in seven of the 13 neonates with a pH between 7.00 and 7.04. In 57% of the 61 cases with ST segment changes > 10 min before birth the umbilical artery blood pH was < 7.15. Of note is that in the severe acidemia group of five cases, no neonatal sequelae were reported. Although it was concluded that CTG plus ST analysis was more specific in detecting fetal acidemia than CTG alone, it would appear from this study that a normal ST analysis result is not highly predictive for a normal scalp blood pH (89%) and a normal ST waveform should not lull one into complacency and CTG changes must be taken serious as always. It would appear from this study that the timing of ST changes before delivery of (severe) acidemic neonates warrants further efficacy studies.

In a recent retrospective study on 143 labors in a setting which relies on CTG interpretation without the routine use of fetal scalp blood sampling as a second-line screening tool for fetal well-being, a sensitivity of 43%, specificity of 74%, negative predictive value of 96%, and a positive predictive value of 8% for metabolic acidemia at birth (umbilical cord artery pH < 7.15 and base deficit ≥ 12 mmol/l) using the STAN clinical guidelines was found.[80] In this study, problems with good-quality FECG signals occurred in 11% of the recording time. Although the authors concluded that the STAN system has a poor predictive value sensitivity for metabolic acidosis, it should be emphasized that their definition of metabolic acidosis at birth is debatable.

In 2001, a Swedish multicenter trial was reported in which a total of 4966 term labors were recruited in three centers.[81,82] Significantly lower rates of metabolic acidosis (umbilical artery pH < 7.05 and base deficit > 12 mmol/l) and operative delivery for presumed fetal distress were found in the ST analysis group with a risk ratio (RR) = 0.47 (95% CI: 0.25–0.86) and with an RR = 0.83 (95% CI: 0.69–0.99) respectively. Of the nine cases with HIE grade II and III, eight occurred in the CTG-only group and one in the ST analysis group, a significant difference. It was concluded that CTG plus ST analysis may prevent intrapartum asphyxia and neonatal encephalopathy. Since then, a Swedish-based EU project to introduce ST analysis into clinical practice entailing 7823 term singleton labors monitored with ST waveform analysis clinical guidelines, was completed.[83] At the time of writing the final analysis of this study is awaited.

Although human observational studies and controlled animal experiments on the benefits of ST waveform analysis during labor are inconclusive, the Swedish RCT appears to indicate a positive role in the reduction of adverse neonatal outcome. It must be emphasized however, that at the basis of the ST waveform analysis algorithm of the STAN S21 system is the ability of proper interpretation of conventional CTG recordings. This is of concern as misinterpretation of the CTG and suboptimal response to CTG abnormalities are still major factors in case of perinatal death and cerebral palsy.[84,85]

A number of issues regarding the ST waveform analysis remain to be addressed. For instance, the non-Gaussian distribution and the large 'normal' range of the T/QRS ratio during labor. In the commercially available algorithm, the cut-off for normal is calculated on the false assumption that there is a normal distribution. Furthermore, the impact of ST waveform abnormalities during the second stage on the time to delivery and outcome is not clear. The potential for ST waveform analysis to be used as a substitute for fetal scalp blood analysis needs further work as is indicated by the results of a large observational study.[79]

Clearly, with perinatal death and cerebral damage, undisputedly as the most important outcome measures, being relatively rare, and in the interest of evidence-based medicine, larger RCTs in other populations are required to confirm the conclusions of the Swedish studies before establishing ST waveform analysis as a diagnostic tool in fetal monitoring as was already proposed by the Swedish study group.[86]

The PR–FHR relationship

Under normal conditions, normoxemic fetuses, healthy children and exercising adults all exhibit an inverse relationship between the PR interval and the heart rate.[28,87,88] During mild hypoxemia in fetal sheep, a brief vagally mediated lengthening of the PR interval was seen to be followed by a simultaneous increase in the FHR and a shortening of the PR interval and to be accompanied by an increase in epinephrine levels.[35] Further hypoxemia resulted in a slowing of the FHR but did not affect the reduction of the PR interval. The same reversal of the normally inverse relationship between the PR interval and FHR was observed in hypoxemic fetal sheep with and without blocking vagal influences with atropine.[17] This changing relationship was confirmed in the analysis of fetal sheep experiments, in which profound and prolonged hypoxemia and acidemia were induced comparable to levels in compromised human fetuses during labor[89] (Figure 141.5). In fetal sheep this changing relationship occurred simultaneously to the accumulation of serum lactate at a rate of at least 5 mmol/l per 30 min, indicating anerobic metabolic

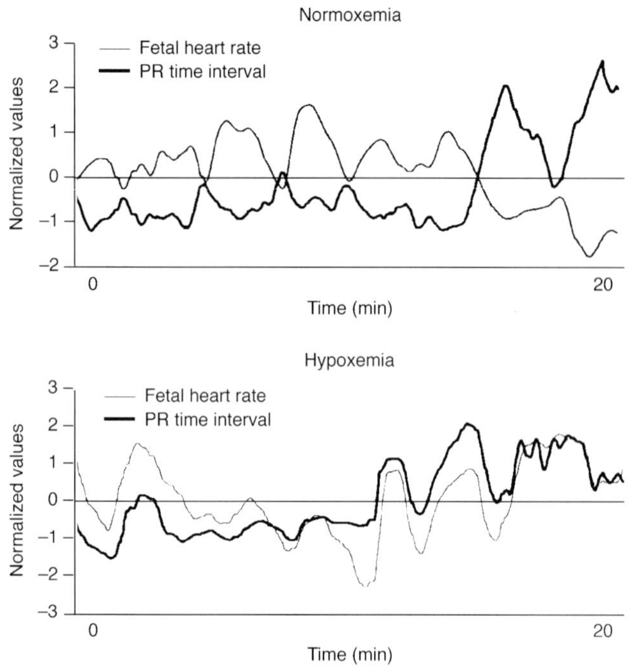

Figure 141.5 Two-second fetal heart rate (FHR) and PR interval measurement during normoxemia (top) and hypoxemia (bottom) in fetal sheep. Reprinted with permission from Bailliere Tindal.

circumstances.[17] Clinical observational studies indicated that a change of the fetal PR interval–FHR correlation during labor from negative to positive was associated with acidemia at birth, and in particular if sustained for 20 min or longer.[17,28]

An explanation for this reversal is the different response of the SA node and the AV node to hypoxemia.[17] The observed shortening of the PR interval during vagally mediated decelerations is contrary to how the AV node responds to parasympathetic stimuli and is more likely due to an increase in catecholamine levels associated with hypoxemia or stress.[17,90] Catecholamine levels rise during mild hypoxemia. This will increase the FHR and shorten the PR interval and sustain their negative relationship. Increasing hypoxemia will reduce ATP levels and affect the slow oxygen-dependent calcium channels of the SA node: the FHR will drop. The reduction in available oxygen does not yet affect the fast sodium channels of the AV node at this stage and the rising levels of epinephrine will continue to shorten the PR interval. Consequently, the PR–FHR relationship will change from negative to positive.[17]

The clinical application of this phenomenon in intrapartum surveillance has taken shape in two calculations to assess normality. The conduction index (CI) is a PR interval–FHR Pearson's correlation coefficient which is calculated by the Nottingham FECG analyzer every 2 s and, if it is positive for longer than 20 min, is thought to be an indication of recent fetal deterioration.[17] The ratio index (RI) is the product of the standard deviation values of the FHR and PR interval exceeding two positive standard deviations, expressed as a percentage of total recording (labor) time. It was found to be significantly related to umbilical artery pH, lactate, norepinephrine and hypoxanthine at birth, with a predictive accuracy of 89.4% when using 4% as a cut-off.[91] As this calculation incorporates data from the whole labor, it is thought to be an indicator of more chronic rather than acute fetal deterioration. A retrospective study of 250 high-risk labors indicated that the use of these two FECG parameters, in conjunction with CTG interpretation, could have resulted in an almost 50% reduction of unsuspected acidemia at birth and a reduction in unnecessary fetal blood sampling from 85.6% to 26.8%, without an increase in the assisted delivery rate.[92]

These findings prompted a randomized prospective trial which initially reported a significant reduction in fetal blood sampling of over 70%, with those taken more likely to be abnormal when FECG analysis was used in conjunction with EFM (RR=1.61, 95% CI: 0.91–2.84).[93] The final report in 2000, including a total of 1038 labors, showed a trend toward fewer operative interventions for presumed fetal distress in the PR analysis plus CTG group (RR=0.80, 95% CI: 0.59–1.08).[94] No significant difference between the groups was found in the number of cases with a cord artery pH ≤7.15 (RR=1.01, 95% CI: 0.7–1.47), or in the frequency of unsuspected acidemia (RR=1.17, 95% CI: 0.76–1.79). It was concluded that although there was a trend in decreasing operative intervention there was no significant benefit in the addition of PR time interval analysis to conventional CTG in neonatal outcome.

The effects of epidural analgesia on the FHR in relation to the PR interval have been studied in women in labor and the results suggest the possibility of a transient local anesthetic-induced effect on the fetal cardiac conduction system.[95,96] Further studies are required to assess the impact of repeated epidural 'top-ups' on the FECG during labor.

Combining FECG time interval and morphology analysis

Recent work suggests that the addition of the T/QRS ratio (with individualized cut-offs for abnormality) to the combination of EFM, RI and CI may reduce the number of unsuspected fetal acidemia at birth further but will simultaneously increase the number of unnecessary interventions.[24] This study showed further that the RI appears to be the most sensitive FECG parameter in detecting fetal compromise and the first to become abnormal during adverse situations. It was concluded that in future work more emphasis should be placed on this calculation of the PR–FHR relationship. It is clear that more research in combining FECG time intervals and morphology changes in the detection of fetal compromise is required.

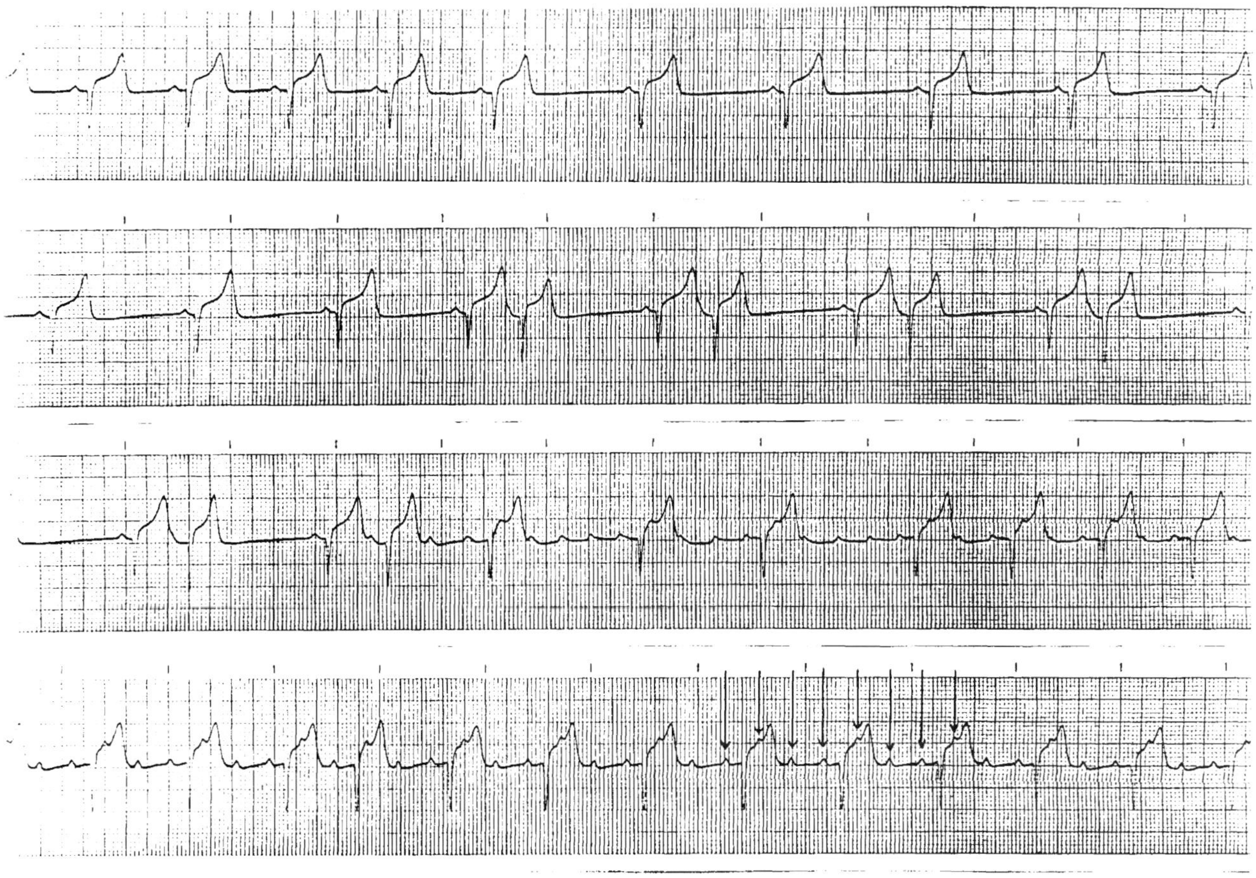

Figure 141.6 Conduction defects (bigeminy and second-degree AV block) at a pH between 7.06 and 7.10 and a base excess between –11.6 and –13.6 mmol/l in fetal sheep experiments conducted by Drs H de Haan and THM Hasaart, Maastricht.

Cardiac conduction defects

Cardiac conduction defects have been well described in adults suffering from coronary artery disease, myocardial ischemia, digitalis toxicity and electrolyte imbalances. In animal experiments, AV blocks have been induced by head compression and cord occlusion but not after vagotomy.[97,98] Yeh *et al.*[34] showed that in baboon fetuses myocardial conduction defects during vagal stimulation secondary to cord occlusion could be prevented by atropine. However, it was suggested that, apart from parasympathetic stimulation, these conduction defects could also be due to an increased sensitivity of the fetal myocardium to acetylcholine under hypoxic conditions. Pardi *et al.*[27] observed a prolongation of the PQ interval during 'mild late decelerations' and suggested that this was caused by mild vagal stimulation, resulting in a depression of the AV conduction system. Such a prolongation could continue to become the dislocation of the P wave from its normal position, as seen during bradycardia,[91] indicating a first-degree AV block. The third-degree AV block observed during severe variable decelerations indicates a complete disruption of conduction between the SA node and the AV node and may suggest hypoxic rather than vagal influences as a cause for this.[29] In controlled fetal sheep experiments, cardiac conduction defects in the form of second-degree heartblock and bigeminy were observed during profound hypoxemia and acidemia (Figure 141.6; van Wijngaarden, De Haan and Hasaart, unpublished data). These observations would confirm the potential of cardiac conduction defects in the detection of fetal compromise during labor. Although many decelerations are vagally mediated, those accompanied by a second- or third-degree AV heartblock may indicate a direct effect of hypoxemia on the myocardium or conductive tissues. The occurrence of such AV blocks during decelerations may therefore be an aid to distinguish between vagally induced decelerations and those associated with fetal compromise.[29] To detect these in real time, however, analysis of raw complexes is required. To achieve this, background noise and signal quality need to be addressed further to allow direct measurements of the filtered unenhanced FECG complex.

Fetal systolic time interval measurements

The pre-ejection period (PEP), the isovolumetric contraction time (IVC) and the ventricular ejection time (VET) are considered to be the most important fetal systolic time interval measurements.[99] Although not absolutely required for the latter two, these are best measured by simultaneous FECG and Doppler ultrasound recordings. The PEP is measured from the onset of the Q wave to the opening of the aortic valve. The IVC is measured from the closure of the mitral valve to the opening of the aortic valve and the VET is measured from aortic valve opening to aortic valve closure. The PEP of the fetal heart reflects the inotropic and loading state of the heart and has the potential of an index for fetal hypoxemia and cord compression. The PEP has been reported to become prolonged during both cord compression without a change in the FHR and variable decelerations. During late decelerations, however, the PEP tends to shorten.[99] More recent animal and human studies suggest that the PEP and PEP/VET ratio in particular, are good predictors of fetal acid–base status.[100] Simultaneous measurement of the PR interval may have some benefit in clarifying the influence of the autonomic nervous system on myocardial contractility. However, the value of PEP measurements in intrapartum monitoring is yet to be established by further studies. In theory, it might be expected to be of more value antepartum in assessing cardiac function.

Transabdominal FECG recordings

Transabdominal FECG analysis has a number of potential benefits. The relationship between cardiac size and the QRS ratio have been well described and could be used as an aid in predicting fetal weight and intrauterine growth retardation.[49] Antenatal FECG analysis could be employed to detect congenital conduction defects such as prolonged QT syndrome and heartblock. Furthermore, it could be used as an adjunct to other methods in the assessment of fetal well-being, especially in circumstances where cardiac failure can occur. FECG time interval and morphology changes and the length of the PEP (time between the QRS complex and opening of the aortic valve) could be informative regarding the health of the conduction system and myocardium, fetal compromise and changes in (para-) sympathic tone.

Intrapartum transabdominal FECG analysis has the potential of being able to record the FHR simultaneously with the uterine myogram, producing a completely electronically derived 'cardiotocogram'. It is easy to apply, with less discomfort to the mother than when using conventional belts. The main problem, however, is the inconsistency and uncertainty in obtaining an analyzable signal.

Transabdominal signal acquisition of the very small amplitude FECG (usually $< 30\,\mu$V) with adult ECG surface electrodes is greatly hindered by noise generated by maternal muscular activity, maternal and fetal movements, maternal ECG signals and most of all by the enormous variation with which the electrical signals are propagated from the fetal heart to the maternal abdominal surface. Interference by maternal ECG complexes is not a problem since the introduction of a range of software routines successfully addressing this. It is still unclear how many electrodes should be used, which configuration of electrode positioning is optimal and during which fetal state the best recordings can be expected. From 20 weeks onward, the signal strength increases until 28 weeks, after which it decreases to a minimum at about 30 weeks. Following this, it increases again until delivery. The reasons for this have been suggested to be the formation of vernix caseosa with a 62-times decrease in electrical conductivity, and fetal fat formation with a 30-times decrease in electrical conductivity.[101] Oostendorp *et al.*[102] found that a multilead system of 32 electrodes which used vectors within a fetal reference frame could remove inter- and intra-individual variation of signal acquisition, but only before a gestational age of 28 weeks. The absence of vernix caseosa before 28 weeks, allowing for homogeneous conduction, has been suggested as a cause for this. The occurrence of gaps in the skin-covering vernix after 32 weeks could be responsible for the improvement in signal acquisition after this gestational age but, by its random nature, will result in a great variation in conduction and therefore optimal electrode positioning.[103] It is our experience that the best recordings are obtained with a simple two-lead system in a vertical midline configuration with one electrode at the fundus, one suprapubically and one ground lead on the arm or leg. This is supported by the observation that the maximum FECG amplitude is sometimes obtained between electrodes placed outside or at the edge of the maternal abdomen.[104] Ciccinelli *et al.*[105] reported signal acquisition rates as high as 93.6% in gestations from 29 to 42 weeks, with reliable P- and T-wave identification in 72.8%. These QRS detection rates have not been confirmed by other studies which quote maximum success rates ranging between 63% and 77%.[101,106,107]

A recent prospective cross-sectional observational study on 241 singleton, 58 twin and five triplets pregnancies with a gestational age ranging from 15 to 41 weeks of gestation, reported a significant reduction in signal separation success rate between 27 and 36 weeks of gestation.[108] A 12-lead system was used for all singleton pregnancies and a 16-lead system was used for all multiple pregnancies. Recordings took 15–20 min, typically providing approximately 5 min of data from which a 60-s sample with all the R waves available was selected visually for further processing. In singletons, the success rate of signal separation was 85%. T waves could be obtained in 78% with most failures before 24 weeks (63%). In twins and triplets, separate signals were obtained in 78% and 93%, respectively. Although P, Q, R, S waves were seen in all averaged FECG complexes, T waves could not be identified in 41% and 43% of recordings, respectively. Normal pregnancy FECG time interval reference ranges with gestation are reported.

Fetal magnetocardiography (FMCG) offers the potential of signal acquisition under circumstances with reduced electrical conductivity. As no electrodes are placed on the maternal abdomen, it is not influenced by interference of maternal ECG complexes and abdominal muscle action. Furthermore, the (hypothetical) insulating effect of vernix caseosa hindering successful acquisition of an electrode-derived transabdominal FECG as seen during late, mid and early third-trimester gestation, is negated.[109] A superconducting quantum interference device (SQUID), placed just above the abdominal skin without touching it, detects changes in the magnetic field created by changes in the intracellular current density of the fetal heart. Quinn *et al.*[13] obtained a 67% success rate in detecting the QRS complex. P waves and T waves were detectable in 75% and 72% of these, respectively. Horigome *et al.* reported a success rate of 68% and 43% for the detection of these waves, respectively.[110] More recently, much higher success rates were obtained by Lowery *et al.*[111] using a newly developed 151-channel magnetic sensor array. In 102 recordings between 27.5 to 39.5 weeks of gestation, they identified 100% of QRS complexes, 95.1% of P waves and 87.3% of T waves. Crowe *et al.*[112] showed the potential for FMCG to produce recordings of similar amplitude and quality to the FECG derived with abdominal electrodes. The main disadvantages of the system are the high cost of the superconductor, the prerequisite of a magnetically shielded environment to reduce interference and the specially purpose-built magnetically inert chair. In a series of 253 FMCG recordings (gestational age 15–42 weeks), Van Leeuwen *et al.*[113] showed that the antenatal determination of cardiac time intervals can be accurate and reproducible as long as signal-to-noise ratio and fetal maturation (signal amplitude) are taken into account.

The Enschede group in The Netherlands have developed a large FMCG database with time interval reference values on which they reported on in 2002.[114] It is based on FMCG recordings of a total of 582 uncomplicated pregnancies. The results compared to the time intervals found with transabdominal electrode recordings and in neonates. Although the scatter of measurements was wide (probably due to physiological variation, measuring system, signal processing and interobserver variation), fetuses with cardiac conduction disorders may be diagnosed with the help of this database.

With the development of new multichannel SQUID systems with a very high success rate of detecting all the waves of the FECG, it would appear that it is only the costs involved that would make one pursue further development of electrode-derived transabdominal FECG recordings. It is of great importance to note that the multichannel SQUID system can also be used to record auditory and visual evoked responses and brain activity antenatally. This opens the way to multimodal testing of fetal well being with a direct method of fetal neurological assessment.

REFERENCES

1. Cremer M. Ueber die direkte Ableitung der Aktionsstrome des menschlichens Herzens vom Oesophagus und ueber das Electrokardiogram des Foetus. *Muench Med Wschr* 1906;53:811–13.
2. Maekawa M, Toyoshima J. The fetal electrocardiogram of the human subject. *Acta Sch Med Univ Kyoto* 1930;12:519–21.
3. Strassmann EO. The fetal electrocardiogram in late pregnancy. *Proc Staff Meetings Mayo Clinic* 1936;11:778–82.
4. Smyth CN. Experimental electrocardiography of the foetus. *Lancet* 1953;1:1124–6.
5. Southern EM. Fetal anoxia and its possible relation to changes in the prenatal electrocardiogram. *Am J Obstet Gynecol* 1957;73: 233–47.
6. Marvell CJ, Kirk DL, Jenkins HML, Symonds EM. The normal condition of the fetal electrocardiogram during labour. *Br J Obstet Gynaecol* 1980;87:786–96.
7. Hon EH, Lee ST. Noise reduction in fetal electrocardiography (II). Averaging techniques. *Am J Obstet Gynecol* 1963;87:1086–96.
8. Rhyne VT. Digital signal enhancement of the fetal electrocardiogram. *Am J Obstet Gynecol* 1968;102:549–55.
9. Marvell CJ, Kirk DL. A simple software routine for the reproducible processing of the electrocardiogram. *J Biomed Eng* 1980; 2:216–20.
10. Westgate J, Keith RD, Curnow JS, *et al.* Suitability of fetal scalp electrodes for monitoring the fetal electrocardiogram during labour. *Clin Phys Physiol Meas* 1990;11:297–306.
11. Lindecrantz K, Lilja H, Widmark C, Rosen KG. Fetal ECG during labour: A suggested standard. *J Biomed Eng* 1988;10:351–3.
12. Lindecrantz K, Widmark C. The fetal scalp lead ECG. In Gennser G, Marsal K, Svenningsen N, Lindstom K, eds. *Fetal and Neonatal Physiological Measurements. III. Proceedings of the Third International Conference on Fetal and Neonatal Measurements,* Malmo-Ronneby, Sweden, 1988:125–31.
13. Quinn A, Weir A, Shahani U, *et al.* Antenatal magnetography: A new method for fetal surveillance? *Br J Obstet Gynaecol* 1994; 101:866–70.
14. Arulkumaran S, Nicolini U, Fisk NM, Tannirandorn Y, Rosen KG, Rodeck CH. Direct antenatal fetal electrocardiographic waveform analysis. *Br J Obstet Gynaecol* 1991;98:829–31.
15. Lindecrantz K, Lilja H. New software QRS detector algorithm suitable for real time applications with low signal-to-noise ratios. *J Biomed Eng* 1988;10:280–4.
16. Rosen KG, Lindecrantz K. STAN – the Gothenburg model for fetal surveillance during labour by ST analysis of the fetal electrocardiogram. *Clin Phys Physiol Meas* 1989;10(Suppl B): 51–6.
17. Murray HG. Evaluation of the fetal electrocardiogram (ECG). M.D. thesis, University of Nottingham, Nottingham, 1992.
18. Newbold S, Wheeler T, Clewlow F, Soul F. Variation in the T/QRS ratio of fetal electrocardiograms recorded during labour in normal subjects. *Br J Obstet Gynaecol* 1989;96:144–50.
19. Noble D. The surprising heart: Review of recent progress in cardiac electrophysiology. *J Physiol* 1984;353:1–50.
20. Hart G. Physiology of cardiac conduction. *Br J Hosp Med* 1985; 33:128–35.
21. Fishmann EJ, Reid PR, Varghese PJ. Transition from theory to clinical application. In Nelson CV, Geselowitz DB, eds. *The Theoretical Basis of Electrocardiography.* Oxford: Clarendon Press, 1976:499–540.
22. Senges J, Mizutani T, Pelzer D, *et al.* Effect of hypoxia on the sinoatrial node, atrium and atrioventricular node in the rabbit heart. *Circ Res* 1979;44:856–63.
23. Lilja H, Arulkumaran S, Lindecrantz K, Ratnam SS, Rosen KG. Fetal ECG during labour: A presentation of a microprocessor system. *J Biomed Eng* 1988;10:348–50.

24. Van Wÿngaarden WJ. The fetal electrocardiogram in the detection of intrapartum compromise. D.M. thesis, University of Nottingham, Nottingham, 1977:170–96.
25. Polvani F, Brambati B, Pardi G. Analysis of the fetal ECG during pregnancy and labour. In Crosignani PG, Pardi G, eds. *Fetal Evaluation during Pregnancy and Labour.* London: Academic Press, 1971:221.
26. Lee KH, Blackwell R. Observations on the configuration of the fetal electrocardiogram before and during labor. *J Obstet Gynaecol Br Commonw* 1974;81:61–9.
27. Pardi G, Tucci B, Uderzo A, Zanini D. Fetal electrocardiogram changes in relation to fetal heart rate patterns during labor. *Am J Obstet Gynecol* 1974;118:243–50.
28. Murray HG. The fetal electrocardiogram: Current clinical developments in Nottingham. *J Perinat Med* 1986;14:399–404.
29. Mohajer MP, Sahota DS, Reed NN, James DK. Atrio-ventricular block during fetal heart rate decelerations. *Arch Dis Child* 1995;72:F51–3.
30. Mohajer MP. The fetal electrocardiogram and intrapartum asphyxia. D.M. thesis, University of Nottingham, Nottingham, 1994.
31. Jenkins HML. A study of the intrapartum electrocardiogram using a real-time computer. M.D. thesis, University of Nottingham, Nottingham, 1984.
32. Skillern L, Cockburn J, Benjamin M, *et al.* A comparative study of the fetal electrocardiogram recorded by the STAN and Nottingham systems. *Br J Obstet Gynaecol* 1994;101:582–6.
33. Pardi G, Uderzo A, Tucci E, Arato GD. Electrocardiographic patterns and cardiovascular performance of the sheep fetus during hypoxia. In Crosignani PG, Pardi G, eds. *Fetal Evaluation during Pregnancy and Labour.* London: Academic Press, 1971:157–74.
34. Yeh MN, Morishima HO, Niemann WH, James LS. Myocardial conduction defects in association with compression of the umbilical cord. *Am J Obstet Gynecol* 1975;121:951–7.
35. Widmark C, Lindecrantz K, Murray H, Rosen K-G. Changes in the PR, RR intervals and the ST waveform of the fetal lamb electrocardiogram with acute hypoxemia. *J Dev Physiol* 1992;18:99–103.
36. Morgan M. Conduction times in the human fetal heart during parturition. D.M. thesis, University of Nottingham, Nottingham, 1989.
37. Morgan M, Symonds EM. Natural history determinants of the time constants of the fetal electrocardiogram. *Eur J Obstet Gynecol Reprod Biol* 1991;42:s9–13.
38. Brown HF, Noble SJ. Effects of adrenaline on membrane currents underlying pacemaker activity in frog atrial muscle. *J Physiol* 1974;238:51–3.
39. Symonds EM. Vectorcardiography and acid–base balance in the human fetus. *J Obstet Gynaecol Br Commonw* 1972;79:416–23.
40. Larks SD, Larks GG. The electrical axis of the fetal heart: A new criterion for fetal well being or distress. *Am J Obstet Gynecol* 1965;93:975–83.
41. Strachan BK, Sahota DS, Chang AZM, Van Wijngaarden WJ, James DK. Computerised intrapartum fetal heart rate and fetal electrocardiogram interpretation. Book of Abstracts, 2nd Annual Conference British Maternal and Fetal Medicine Society, Warwick, UK, March 20–21, 1997. *J Obstet Gynaecol* 1997; 17(Suppl 1):S18.
42. Symonds EM. Configuration of the fetal electrocardiogram in relation to fetal acid–base balance and plasma electrodes. *J Obstet Gynaecol Br Commonw* 1971;78:957–70.
43. Wilson FN, Herrmann GR. Relation of QRS interval to ventricular weight. *Heart* 1929;15:135–40.
44. Brambati B, Pardi G. The intraventricular conduction time of the fetal heart in uncomplicated pregnancies. *Br J Obstet Gynaecol* 1980;87:941–8.
45. Schulz DL, Giordano DA. Hearts of infants and children. *Arch Pathol* 1962;74:464–71.
46. Gennser G, Johansson BW, Kullander S. Electrocardiographic and tissue lactate changes in the human fetus in mid pregnancy. *J Obstet Gynaecol Br Commonw* 1968;75:941–8.
47. Larks SD, Longo LD. Electrocardiographic studies of the fetal heart during delivery. *Obstet Gynaecol* 1962;19:740–7.
48. Brambati B, Pardi G. The intraventricular conduction time of the fetal heart in pregnancies complicated by rhesus haemolytic disease. *Br J Obstet Gynaecol* 1981;88:1233–40.
49. Pardi G, Ferazzi E, Cetin I, *et al.* The clinical relevance of the abdominal fetal electrocardiogram. *J Perinat Med* 1986;14:371–8.
50. Gelli MG, Gyulai F. Effect of glucose infusion in the mother before delivery on the ECG of rabbit foetuses under anoxia. *Acta Obstet Gynaecol Scand* 1969;48:56–63.
51. Oudijk MA, Kwee A, Visser GH, Blad S, Meijboom EJ, Rosen KG. The effects of intrapartum hypoxia on the fetal QT interval. *BJOG* 2004;111:656–60.
52. Murray HG. The intrapartum fetal electrocardiogram – A study of time intervals. In Gennser G, Marsal K, Svenningsen N, Lindstom K, eds. *Fetal and Neonatal Physiological Measurements III. Proceedings of the Third International Conference on Fetal and Neonatal Measurements,* Malmo-Ronneby, Sweden, 1989:133–48.
53. Noble D, Cohen I. The interpretation of the T wave of the electrocardiogram. *Cardiovasc Res* 1978;12:13–27.
54. Rosen KG, Kjellmer I. Changes in the fetal heart rate and ECG during hypoxia. *Acta Physiol Scand* 1975;93:59–66.
55. Hokegard KH, Eriksson BO, Kjellmer I, *et al.* Myocardiac metabolism in relation to electrocardiographic changes and cardiovascular function during graded hypoxia in the fetal lamb. *Acta Physiol Scand* 1981;113:1–7.
56. Rosen KG, Isaakson O. Alterations in the fetal heart rate and the ECG correlated to glycogen, creatine phosphate and ATP levels during graded hypoxia. *Biol Neonate* 1976;30:17–22.
57. Hokegard KH, Karlsson K, Kjellmer I, Rosen KG. ECG changes in the fetal lamb during asphyxia in relation to beta-adrenoceptor stimulation and blockade. *Acta Physiol Scand* 1979;105:195–303.
58. Widmark C, Jansson T, Lindecrantz K, Rosen KG. ECG waveform, short term heart rate variability and plasma catecholamine concentrations in response to hypoxia in intrauterine growth retarded guinea-pig fetuses. *J Dev Physiol* 1991;15:161–8.
59. Rosen KG, Hokegard KH, Kjellmer I. A study of the relationship between the electrocardiogram and haemodynamics in the fetal lamb during asphyxia. *Acta Physiol Scand* 1976;98:275–84.
60. Rosen KG, Dagbjartson A, Henrikson BA, *et al.* The relationship between circulating catecholamines and ST waveform in the fetal lamb electrocardiogram during asphyxia. *Am J Obstet Gynecol* 1984;149:190–5.
61. Watanabe T, Okamura K, Tanigawara S, *et al.* Change in electrocardiogram T-wave amplitude during umbilical cord compression is predictive of fetal condition in sheep. *Am J Obstet Gynecol* 1992;166:246–55.
62. Rosen KG. Alterations in the fetal electrocardiogram as a sign of fetal asphyxia – Experimental data with a clinical implication. *J Perinat Med* 1986;14:355–63.
63. Greene KR, Dawes GS, Lilja H, Rosen KG. Changes in the ST waveform of fetal lamb electrocardiogram with hypoxia. *Am J Obstet Gynecol* 1982;144:950–7.
64. De Haan HH, Ijzermans ACM, De Haan J, Hasaart THM. The T/QRS ratio of the electrocardiogram does not reliably reflect well-being in fetal lambs. *Am J Obstet Gynecol* 1995;172:35–43.
65. Roemer VM, Ruppin E, Bartschi R. Direct fetal electrocardiography in management of high risk pregnancies. *Proceedings of the International Symposium on the Treatment of Foetal Risks,* Baden, Austria, 1972:135–59.
66. Lilja H, Green KR, Karlsson K, Rosen KG. ST waveform changes of the fetal electrocardiogram during labour – A clinical study. *Br J Obstet Gynaecol* 1985;92:611–17.
67. Hokegaard KH, Karlsson K, Lilja H, Rosen KG. Neonatal electrocardiographic changes in relation to cardiotocographic changes. *Br J Obstet Gynaecol* 1978;85:165–70.
68. Jenkins HML, Symonds EM, Kirk DL, Smith PR. Can fetal electrocardiography improve the prediction of intrapartum acidosis? *Br J Obstet Gynaecol* 1986;93:6–12.
69. Newbold S, Wheeler T, Clewlow F. The effect of uterine contractions on the T/QRS ratio of the fetal ECG. *Proceedings of the 4th International Conference on Fetal and Neonatal Physiological Measurements,* Noordwijkerhout, The Netherlands. Rotterdam: Hoboken Congress Organisation, Erasmus Universiteit, 1991:96.
70. Newbold S, Wheeler T, Clewlow F. Comparison of the T/QRS ratio of the fetal electrocardiogram and the fetal heart rate during labour and the relation of these variables to condition at delivery. *Br J Obstet Gynaecol* 1991;98:173–8.
71. Murphy KW, Russell V, Johnson P. Clinical assessment of fetal electrocardiogram monitoring in labour. *Br J Obstet Gynaecol* 1992;99:32–7.
72. Maclachlan NA, Spencer JAD, Harding K, Arulkumaran S. Fetal acidaemia, the cardiotocograph and the T/QRS ratio of the fetal ECG in labour. *Br J Obstet Gynaecol* 1992;99:26–31.
73. Thaler I, Timor IE, Rotem S. Interpretation of the fetal ECG during labor. The effect of uterine contractions. *J Perinat Med* 1987;15(Suppl 1):35.
74. Deans A, Genevier E, Steer P. A comparative study of the FECG signal obtained from simultaneously applied single spiral and

Copeland fetal scalp electrodes. *Proceedings from the 3rd International Symposium on Intrapartum Surveillance*, Berkeley Court, Dublin, 1995.

75. van Wijngaarden WJ, Strachan BK, Sahota DS, James DK. Improving intrapartum surveillance: An individualised T/QRS ratio? *Eur J Obstet Gynecol Reprod Biol* 2000;88:43–8.
76. Westgate J, Harris M, Curnow JSH, Greene KR. Plymouth randomised trial of CTG only versus ST waveform plus CTG intrapartum monitoring in 2400 cases. *Am J Obstet Gynecol* 1993;169:1151–60.
77. O'Brien PMS, Warwick K. Can fetal T/QRS ratio replace fetal blood sampling. *Proceedings from the 3rd International Symposium on Intrapartum Surveillance*, Berkeley Court, Dublin, 1995.
78. Amer-Wahlin I, Bordahl P, Eikeland T, *et al.* ST analysis of the fetal electrocardiogram during labor: Nordic observational multicenter study. *J Matern Fetal Neonatal Med* 2002;12:260–6.
79. Kwee A, van der Hoorn-van den Beld CW, Veerman J, Dekkers AH, Visser GH. STAN S21 fetal heart monitor for fetal surveillance during labor: An observational study in 637 patients. *J Matern Fetal Neonatal Med* 2004;15:400–7.
80. Dervaitis KL, Poole M, Schmidt G, Penava D, Natale R, Gagnon R. ST segment analysis of the fetal electrocardiogram plus electronic fetal heart rate monitoring in labor and its relationship to umbilical cord arterial blood gases. *Am J Obstet Gynecol* 2004;191:879–84.
81. Amer-Wahlin I, Hellsten C, Noren H, *et al.* Cardiotocography only versus cardiotocography plus ST analysis of fetal electrocardiogram for intrapartum fetal monitoring: A Swedish randomised controlled trial. *Lancet* 2001;358:534–8.
82. Noren H, Amer-Wahlin I, Hagberg H, *et al.* Fetal electrocardiography in labor and neonatal outcome: Data from the Swedish randomized controlled trial on intrapartum fetal monitoring. *Am J Obstet Gynecol* 2003;188:183–92.
83. Rosen KG, Amer-Wahlin I, Luzietti R, Noren H. Fetal ECG waveform analysis. *Best Pract Res Clin Obstet Gynaecol* 2004;18:485–514.
84. CESDI (Confidential Enquiry into Stillbirths and Deaths in Infancy) (1997) *Annual Report*. London: HMSO.
85. Gaffney G, Sellers, Flavell V, Johnson A. Case–control study of intrapartum care, cerebral palsy and perinatal death. *Br Med J* 1994;308:743–50.
86. Rosen KG, Amer-Wahlin I, Luzietti R, Noren H. Fetal ECG waveform analysis. *Best Pract Res Clin Obstet Gynaecol* 2004; 18:485–514.
87. Atterhog JH, Loogna E. PR interval in relation to heart rate during exercise and the influence of posture and autonomic tone. *J Electrocardiol* 1977;10:331–6.
88. Donnerstein RL, Scott WA, Thomas TR. Spontaneous beat to beat variation of PR interval in normal children. *Am J Cardiol* 1990; 66:753–4.
89. Van Wijngaarden WJ, De Haan HH, Sahota DS, James DK, Symonds EM, Hasaart THM. Changes in the PR time interval – fetal heart rate relationship of the ECG during fetal compromise in chronically instrumented sheep. *Am J Obstet Gynecol* 1996;175: 548–54.
90. Myers RE. Two patterns of perinatal brain damage and their conditions of occurrence. *Am J Obstet Gynecol* 1972;112: 246–76.
91. Mohajer MP, Sahota DS, Reed NN, *et al.* Cumulative changes in the fetal electrocardiogram and biochemical indices of fetal hypoxia. *Eur J Obstet Gynecol Reprod Biol* 1994;55:63–70.
92. Reed NN, Mohajer MP, Sahota DS, James DK, Symonds EM. The potential of PR interval analysis of the fetal electrocardiogram (FECG) on intrapartum fetal monitoring. *Eur J Obstet Gynecol Reprod Biol* 1996;86:87–92.
93. Van Wijngaarden WJ, Sahota DS, James DK, *et al.* Improved intrapartum surveillance with PR interval analysis of the fetal electrocardiogram (FECG): A randomised trial showing a reduction in fetal blood sampling. *Am J Obstet Gynecol* 1996; 174:1295–9.
94. Strachan BK, van Wijngaarden WJ, Sahota D, Chang A, James DK. Cardiotocography only versus cardiotocography plus PR-interval analysis in intrapartum surveillance: A randomised, multicentre trial. FECG Study Group. *Lancet* 2000;355:456–9.
95. Ramasubramanian R, Murray H, Dannels L, *et al.* Fetal electrocardiographic changes following lumbar analgesia in labor. *Anesth Analg* 1987;66:S145.
96. Morgan M, Ramasubramanian R, Murray HG, *et al.* Monitoring fetal cardiac conduction during epidural analgesia in labour. *Anaesthesiology* 1989;71:A851.
97. Harned HS, Wolkoff AS, Pickrell J, MacKinney LG. Hemodynamic observations during birth of the lamb. Studies on the unanesthetized full-term animal. *Am J Dis Child* 1961;102:180–9.
98. Reeves JT, Daoud FS, Eastin C. Effects of vagotomy on arterial pressure and blood gases in the fetal calf. *Am J Physiol* 1971; 221:349–55.
99. Fleming JEE, Raymond SPW, Smith GCS, Whitfield CR. The measurement of systolic time intervals: Lessons from ultrasound. *Eur J Obstet Gynecol Reprod Biol* 1986;23:289–94.
100. Lewinsky RM. Cardiac systolic time intervals and other parameters of myocardial contractility as indices of fetal acid–base status. *Ballières Clin Obstet Gynaecol* 1994;8:663–81.
101. Caughey AF, Krohn MS. Variation in the fetal electrocardiogram with period of gestation. *Am J Obstet Gynecol* 1963;87:525–8.
102. Oostendorp TF, Van Oosterom A, Jongsma HW. The fetal ECG throughout the second half of gestation. *Clin Phys Physiol Meas* 1989;10(Suppl B):147–60.
103. Oostendorp TF, Van Oosterom A, Jongsma HW. The effect of changes in the conductive medium on the fetal ECG throughout gestation. *Clin Phys Physiol Meas* 1989;10(Suppl. B):11–20.
104. Oostendorp TF, Van Oosterom A, Jongsma HW, Van Dongen PWJ. The potential distribution generated by the fetal heart at the maternal abdomen. *J Perinat Med* 1986;14:435–44.
105. Ciccinelli E, Bortone A, Carbonara I, *et al.* Improved equipment for abdominal fetal electrocardiogram recording: Description and clinical evaluation. *Int J Biomed Comput* 1994;35:193–205.
106. Carter MC, Gunn P, Beard RW. Fetal heart rate monitoring using the abdominal fetal electrocardiogram. *Br J Obstet Gynaecol* 1980;87:396–401.
107. Herbert JM, Huang XB, Crowe JA, *et al.* Antepartum fetal ECG extraction and analysis. In *Proceedings: Computers in Cardiology*. Los Alimatos, CA: IEEE Computer Society Press, 1993:875–7.
108. Taylor MJ, Smith MJ, Thomas M, *et al.* Non-invasive fetal electrocardiography in singleton and multiple pregnancies. *BJOG* 2003;110:668–78.
109. Wakai RT, Lengle JM, Leuthold AC. Transmission of electric and magnetic foetal cardiac signals in a case of ectopia cordis: The dominant role of the vernix caseosa. *Phys Med Biol* 2000;45:1989–95.
110. Horigome H, Takahashi MI, Asaka M, Shigemitsu S, Kandori A, Tsukada K. Magnetocardiographic determination of the developmental changes in PQ, QRS and QT intervals in the foetus. *Acta Paediatr* 2000;89:64–7.
111. Lowery CL, Campbell JQ, Wilson JD, *et al.* Noninvasive antepartum recording of fetal S-T segment with a newly developed 151-channel magnetic sensor system. *Am J Obstet Gynecol* 2003;188:1491–6.
112. Crowe JA, Herbert JM, Huang XB, *et al.* Sequential recording of the abdominal fetal electrocardiogram and magnetogram. *Physiol Meas* 1995;16:43–7.
113. Van Leeuwen P, Lange S, Klein A, *et al.* Reproducibility and reliability of fetal cardiac time intervals using magnetocardiography. *Physiol Meas* 2004;25:539–52.
114. Stinstra J, Golbach E, van Leeuwen P, *et al.* Multicentre study of fetal cardiac time intervals using magnetocardiography. *BJOG* 2002;109:1235–43.

142 Fetal magnetocardiography and fetal magnetoencephalography

T. Hosono and Y. Chiba

Fetal magnetocardiography

Introduction

Electrical activity of the heart and brain can be recorded on the body surface of a living body by a form of electrocardiogram and electroencephalogram, respectively. These electrical recording methods are widely used in clinical practice for newborns, infants, children and adults. Electrical activities of the heart and brain cause weak changes of the magnetic field. Since magnetic lines of force can pass through internal organs and skin without attenuation, magnetic activity of the heart and brain can be recorded without skin contact. Tracings of the magnetic activity of the heart and brain are magnetocardiogram and magnetoencephalogram, respectively.

Cardiac magnetic activity is measured in the order of 50 picotesla (pT) in adults and less than 10 pT in fetuses. These values are about one million times smaller than the static magnetic field of the earth. The first adult magnetocardiogram was recorded using induction coils.[1] However, since magnetic field strength caused by the fetal heart and brain are too small to record using induction coils, devices to measure fetal magnetocardiogram and magnetoencephalogram were anticipated, and as superconductor technology progressed, a superconducting quantum interference device (SQUID) was developed.

Fetal magnetocardiogram was first recorded about three decades ago using SQUID technology.[2] The amplitude of fetal QRS complex exceeded 5 pT and could be clearly distinguished from the maternal magnetocardiogram. Fetal QRS was more successfully recorded between 30 and 40 weeks of gestation when the fetus was in cephalic presentation with the left side facing the detector than when the right side faced the detector. The shorter the distance between the fetal heart and the detector, the weaker the fetal magnetocardiographic signals. The consecutive application of fetal magnetocardiogram to fetal heart rate monitoring was also reported.[3] Fetal heart rates were simultaneously calculated from fetal magnetocardiogram and electrocardiogram, and both tracings thoroughly coincided. However, after the initial development, fetal magnetocardiography has not progressed for nearly two decades. The improvement and advantage of fetal echocardiography and Doppler ultrasound technology for fetal heart rate monitoring also surpassed relatively primitive biomagnetism technology.[4] In the early 1990s, the usefulness of magnetocardiography has received more attention. The spread of fetal magnetocardiography is due to advances in several aspects of biomagnetism technology; a highly efficient magnetically shielded room and multichannel SQUID sensors of very high sensitivity.

Fetal magnetocardiogram provides clinicians with similar information to a fetal electrocardiogram. However, it is still difficult to record electrocardiograms because the surface of the fetal body is covered with caseous vernix in the latter half of the second trimester and the first half of the third trimester of pregnancy. The caseous vernix mainly consists of fat, which has low electrical conductivity. Thus, a fetal electrocardiogram is hard to record from the maternal abdominal surface. Direct fetal electrocardiogram, which attaches the leads of the fetal electrocardiogram to the fetal shoulder and buttocks by inserting needle electrodes via the maternal abdomen under ultrasonography guiding, is one solution of the problem, but is invasive.[5] Magnetic flux can pass through the caseous vernix and magnetocardiography is a non-invasive method to measure the electrical activity of the fetal heart.

Data processing of magnetocardiography

Multichannel system

Figure 142.1 shows a multichannel SQUID system (MC6400; Hitachi Hi-technologies Ltd, Tokyo, Japan) installed in the National Cardiovascular Center in Osaka, Japan. The system is placed in an active

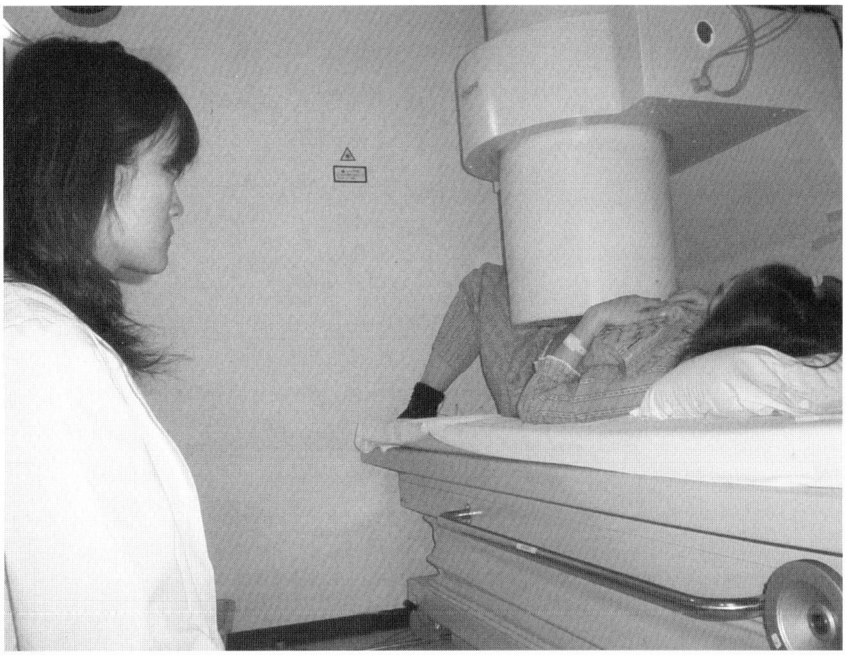

Figure 142.1 Magnetocardiography system using multichannel SQUID sensors (MC6400; Hitachi Hi-technologies Ltd). The dewar, including SQUID sensors, is positioned above the abdomen of a pregnant patient lying on a bed.

magnetically shielded cabin in a non-magnetically shielded room in a hospital building. The active magnetic shield system produces compensating magnetic fields, which negate the magnetic fields of earth. The system is composed of 64-channel SQUID sensors with a sensitivity of less than 20 femtotesla (fT)/Hz. The gradiometer array is 8 × 8 matrix distributed and its sensor pitch is 25 mm. The array is installed in a dewar stored in liquid helium. The bed is positioned under the dewar and the patient lies on the bed usually after verifying the fetal heart position by ultrasonography. In other centers, a multichannel system such as a 37-channel system[6] and 67-channel system[7] have been used recently.

Data processing

The recorded magnetocardiographic signals are digitized and stored in a computer at a sampling frequency of 1 kHz. After passing through a low-pass filter, signals are processed several times. The removal of the maternal magnetocardiogram is indispensable for further signal processing. The maternal electrocardiogram is simultaneously recorded to aid the removal of the maternal magnetocardiogram. We calculated the average maternal magnetocardiogram by triggering R peaks of the maternal electrocardiogram. The averaged maternal magnetocardiogram is subtracted from the raw recordings at the time of each maternal heartbeat. Typical signal processing is the average triggered at R waves of the fetal magnetocardiogram. Since the P wave and T wave stay in the range of noises in the raw magnetocardiogram even when QRS complexes exceed the noise levels, averaging is required for a better signal-to-noise ratio to reveal the P wave and T wave. Our group adopted 100-times averaging from 2-min raw magnetocardiograms.

RR intervals in fetal magnetocardiogram are also often measured. The RR intervals are usually changed to the fetal heart rate, which is widely used in obstetrical practice.

Mapping

Although a multichannel system for magnetocardiogram has recently been commonly employed, only a few mapping techniques are available. The geometrical distribution of magnetocardiogram tracing is often used to display multichannel results.[4] The demonstration of all magnetocardiograms, usually averaged magnetocardiograms, at each of the used multichannels in one plane aligned along the baseline is designated 'butterfly plotting'.

The current-arrow map is a unique mapping technique showing the magnetic field and hypothetic current vectors in one plane.[8] The current arrows (I_x, I_y) are obtained from derivatives of the normal vertical component (B_z) of the fetal magnetocardiogram from the following equations:

$$I_x = +\mathrm{d}B_z/\mathrm{d}y$$
$$I_y = -\mathrm{d}B_z/\mathrm{d}x$$

Contour lines showing the strength of current arrows $[(I_x^{\,2}+I_y^{\,2})^{-1/2}]$ also visualize the current-arrow distributions. The current-arrow map is designed for obstetricians to better understand the current distribution although the current-arrow map is not the

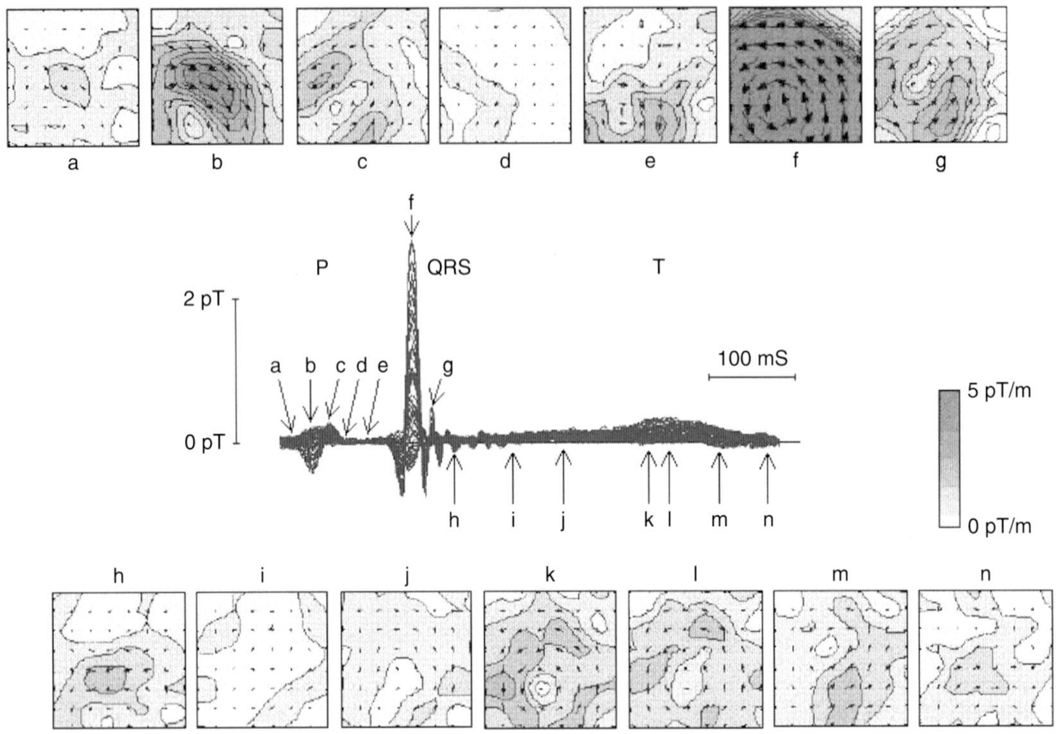

Figure 142.2 An example of an averaged fetal magnetocardiogram (center). P, QRS, T indicates the P wave, QRS complex and T wave, respectively. Figures with subscripts a–n are current-arrow maps calculated at the timing indicated in the averaged fetal magnetocardiogram.

complete solution of the so-called inverse problem. Figure 142.2 shows an example of a current-arrow map. Note that current-arrow maps at the R wave and T wave are in a circular pattern although the current-arrow map at the P wave is in a pattern aimed in one direction.

Standards of fetal magnetocardiogram

The peaks in the magnetocardiogram are called P, QRS and R similar to the electrocardiogram. The P wave indicates atrial depolarization preceding atrial contractions, the QRS complex indicates ventricular depolarization preceding ventricular contractions, and the T wave indicates ventricular repolarization preceding ventricular diastole. Indeed, the consistency of the fetal electrocardiogram and fetal magnetocardiogram is demonstrated by simultaneously recording the cardiograms.[4] Waveforms of the fetal magnetocardiogram, i.e. amplitudes, polarities and phases, vary depending on the spatial mutual relation between the fetal heart and detectors similar to waveforms of the electrocardiogram vary depending on the leads. Each component of the magnetocardiogram even in normal fetuses appears in a biphasic or negative pattern, but the causes of such patterns have not been clarified yet.

The amplitudes of the QRS complex, P wave and T wave increases with gestational age. However, the amplitudes of the P wave and T wave are often in noise levels, thus it is difficult to detect P and T waves in raw magnetocardiograms. Averaging the magnetocardiographic signals is the usual method to improve the signal-to-noise ratio and to analyze the waveforms of fetal magnetocardiograms,[9] but signal processing by averaging inevitably misses small beat-to-beat variations. Fetal heart position is also an important factor to improve the detectable limit of fetal signals. QRS complex can be detected by magnetocardiogram even at 17 weeks of gestation with a favorable fetal presentation. Kandori *et al.*[10] revealed by theoretical calculations that the depth between the sensor and fetal ventricular muscles is the most important factor for detection and that the fetal magnetocardiogram can be detected after 22 weeks of gestation if the depth between the sensor and the fetal ventricular muscle is 50 mm. The result of the theoretical analysis coincides well with practical data from 35 normal fetuses. If the distance between the fetal heart and the detector is 80 mm, the magnitude of the fetal magnetocardiogram stays at approximately 1 pT. If the detection limit of the fetal magnetocardiogram is as low as 1 pT, the minimum distance between the fetal heart and the detector is approximately 50 mm at 25 weeks of gestation, and is 80 mm at 35 weeks of gestation. Note that the distance between the fetal heart and the detector is approximately equal to the distance between the fetal heart and mother's abdominal surface. In clinical practice, the detection rate of the QRS complex is 67% by raw signals and the detection

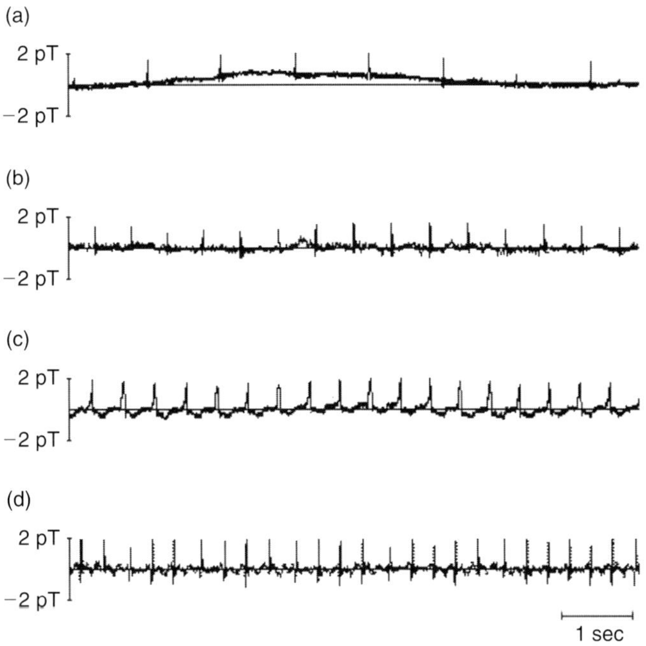

Figure 142.3 Examples of fetal arrhythmia: (a) complete atrioventricular block; (b) long QT syndrome; (c) WPW syndrome; (d) atrial flutter.

rates of the P wave and T wave in averaged fetal magnetocardiogram are 75% and 72%, respectively.[11]

The normal values for the components of fetal magnetocardiogram have also been studied. Horigome *et al.*[12] reported normal values of each component of magnetocardiogram for normal fetuses. The detected rates of P and T waves in averaged magnetocardiograms were 68% and 43%, respectively, although the detected rate of the QRS complex was 85% in raw magnetocardiograms. For a total of 150 magnetoencephalograms of normal fetuses of between 20 and 41 weeks of gestation, RR, PQ, QRS, QT intervals (durations) were 421 ± 27 (ms; mean $\pm$ SD), 100 ± 16, 49 ± 8, 223 ± 39, respectively. QT_c (corrected QT interval; QT interval divided by the square root of the RR interval) was 378 ± 52. Although QT and PQ intervals were constant between 20 and 41 weeks of gestation, the QRS interval increased as the gestational weeks increased. A similar gestational increase of QRS interval was also reported by Leuthold *et al.*[9]

Fetal arrhythmia

The diagnosis of arrhythmia has attracted a great deal of attention in fetal magnetocardiogram. Recently, prenatal diagnoses of fetal arrhythmias have been accumulated.

Bradyarrhythmia

One of the most life-threatening pathological bradyarrhythmias is atrioventricular block. Figure 142.3(a) shows a case of complete atrioventricular block. Magnetocardiographic observations of complete atrioventricular block coincide well with the findings by echocardiography, direct fetal electrocardiogram and neonatal electrocardiogram.[5] It is important to record completely independent P waves and QRS complexes in the diagnosis. Averaged fetal magnetocardiogram is also useful for the diagnosis because P waves are never detected in the averaged magnetocardiogram. Wakai *et al.*[13] reported an interesting case of complete atrioventricular block in which ventricular rates increase in association with the increase of atrial beats. Hosono *et al.*[14] reported a case of complete atrioventricular block with alternating ventricular pacemakers, which were revealed by the alternating amplitude of R wave recorded by magnetocardiography.

The diagnosis of QT prolongation is a good application of fetal magnetocardiography. QT prolongation, often by heredity, is rather hard to diagnose by echocardiography.[15] Hamada *et al.*[16] reported the first case of prenatal diagnosis of familial long QT syndrome by magnetocardiography. In this case, the mother was complicated with long QT syndrome and had a history of syncope at 10 years old. The nonstress test of the fetus at late gestation demonstrated a non-reactive pattern of fetal mild bradycardia of 110 bpm with decreased fetal heart rate variability. The QT interval was 410 ms, which is beyond the upper limit of 300 ms,[12] by averaged fetal magnetocardiography. The neonatal electrocardiogram coincided well with the fetal magnetocardiogram. Menéndez *et al.*[17] reported two additional cases, one of which was familial and the other was sporadic. Hosono *et al.*[15] also reported a case of familial long QT syndrome, which was suspected of sustained mild fetal bradyarrhythmia of about 110 bpm with decreased variability and maternal QT prolongation. Figure 142.3(b) shows a case of long QT syndrome. Kandori *et al.*[18] described two cases of long QT syndrome in which detailed diagnoses were achieved by current-arrow maps. The accuracy of magnetocardiogram in time domain exceeds further than that of echocardiography, and thus magnetocardiography enables the prenatal diagnosis of long QT syndrome, which requires precise determination of the QT interval.

Tachyarrhythmia

Fetal tachyarrhythmia often causes fetal heart failure and induces general hydrops fetalis. Supraventricular tachycardia and atrial flutter are the most common causes of fetal tachyarrhythmia. Atrial fibrillation is generally considered rare.

Wolff–Parkinson–White (WPW) syndrome was first successfully diagnosed by magnetocardiography (Figure 142.3c). Hosono *et al.*[19] reported the prenatal diagnosis of fetal WPW syndrome by magnetocardiography. In a case of fetal paroxysmal supraventricular tachyarrhythmia, a typical delta wave, short PR interval and wide QRS duration were revealed by averaged fetal magnetocardiography. The averaged magnetocardiogram during the attack of supraventricular tachyarrhythmia showed normal QRS complex with normal duration and normal PR interval. In this case, cardioversion was obtained by prescribing oral propranolol to the mother. Fetal hydrops disappeared soon after sufficient dose administration. Another case of fetal WPW syndrome was described by Kähler *et al.*[20] The fetus exhibited intermittent tachyarrhythmia and hydrops fetalis after the administration of tocolytic agents. The magnetocardiogram at 33 weeks of gestation showed a delta wave. Oral flecainide, not digoxin, was prescribed and cardioversion was achieved within a few days. Digoxin is contraindicated in WPW syndrome due to the adverse effect of the atrioventricular conduction mechanism. Although digoxin has been widely used in therapy for fetal tachyarrhythmia, the prenatal diagnosis of fetal WPW syndrome by magnetocardiography may change the prescription of fetal therapy. The tachyarrhythmia and retrograde conduction of the P wave were also reported by Menéndez *et al.*[21] Wakai *et al.*[6] analyzed the initiation and termination of 13 cases of supraventricular tachyarrhythmia and revealed the mechanism of attack of tachyarrhythmias. The most common cause of fetal supraventricular tachycardia was revealed to be re-entrant premature atrial contractions. Kandori *et al.*[22] succeeded in the identification of accessory pathways in fetal WPW syndrome using current-arrow maps. The current-arrow maps at the time of the delta wave and the R peak of two cases of fetal WPW syndrome were produced and the vector sums of the current arrows were calculated. When the vector sum of the current arrows at the R peak was fitted to the position of the ventricular septum, the vector sum of the current arrows at the delta waves was revealed to be positioned at the left ventricle, indicating that an accessory pathway exists in the left heart. The WPW syndrome, which has an accessory pathway in the left heart, is type A, which shows a typical electrocardiogram with a high-voltage positive delta wave in the T1 lead. The neonatal electrocardiogram of each case exhibited a high-voltage positive delta wave in the T1 lead of the electrocardiogram.

Cases of atrial flutter have also been reported by several authors (Figure 142.3d).[21,23] Hosono *et al.*[24] also reported a case of fetal atrial flutter. The F wave, which represents fast atrial reciprocal excitation, appeared in a form of fluctuation of the baseline, similar to the teeth of a saw. The averaged fetal magnetocardiogram showed two P waves preceding the QRS complex, indicating 2:1 atrioventricular conduction. In another case, atrial flutter with 3:1 atrioventricular conduction was also demonstrated by magnetocardiography.[25] Kandori *et al.*[26] successfully made a differential diagnosis between atrial flutter and atrial fibrillation by evacuating QRS complexes from raw magnetocardiogram and by spectral analysis of atrial beats by fast-Fourier-transform processing. The spectrum of atrial flutter had a sharp peak at around 7 Hz, whereas the spectrum of atrial fibrillation was distributed diffusely in the range of 2–8 Hz. Since atrial flutter is caused by reciprocal pulse conductions of a certain frequency in the atrium, the spectrum showed a sharp peak at this frequency. However, since atrial fibrillation is generated by multiple independent pulse generators in the atrium, the spectrum might have a diffusely distributed pattern.

Ventricular tachycardia is rare in fetal arrhythmia. Menéndez *et al.*[21] succeeded in recoding *tosades de poites* of the fetus at 32 weeks of gestation.

Extrasystoles

Since extrasystoles are the most common fetal arrhythmia, extrasystoles have been reported since the pioneer period of fetal magnetocardiogram.[3] Van Leeuwen *et al.*[27] reported a variety of fetal extrasystoles such as ventricular extrasystoles, supraventricular extrasystoles, and sinoatrial block. Wakai *et al.*[28] reported a case of fetal complicated heart malformation that exhibited a fetal heart rhythm alternating between the period of normal sinus rhythm and the period of junctional rhythm associated with respiratory sinus arrhythmia. Single-channel magnetocardiography revealed the increase of fetal arrhythmia during ritodrine treatment for threatened premature delivery.[29]

Fetal heart rate monitoring

Magnetocardiography has been applied for fetal heart rate monitoring since the genesis era of fetal magnetocardiogram.[3,30] Since magnetocardiogram has a high resolution in the time domain, beat-to-beat variability of the fetal heart rate can be measured. The commonly used Doppler technique of ultrasound needs data processing of autocorrelation, and thus subtle beat-to-beat variability is essentially non-recordable.

Spectral analysis of fetal heart rate variability has been reported by several groups. Wakai *et al.*[31] analyzed fetal heart rate patterns from magnetocardiograms of 10 healthy fetuses and revealed a frequency distributed in a lower frequency range of less than 0.2 Hz in a fetal resting state but the spectrum is distributed in a wide range of less than 1.0 Hz during fetal respiratory arrhythmia. Rassi and Lewis[32] also performed spectrum analysis of the fetal heart rate and observed that the power spectral density at a high frequency of nearly 3 Hz increased as the gestational age increased, and thus variability of fetal heart rate increased in late gestation. Van Leeuwen and colleagues[7,33] calculated several statistical parameters from fetal heart rate tracings measured by magnetocardiography. They concluded that the significance of statistical parameters representing fetal heart variability and complexity reflects fetal development.

The monitoring of fetal heart rate using magnetocardiography is still in a pilot study and is beyond clinical application.

Instruments for fetal heart monitoring in recent clinical practice have employed the Doppler technology of ultrasound because of its convenience. Magnetocardiographic instruments generally require a magnetically shielded room. Baffa *et al.*[34] attempted to record magnetocardiograms using a single-channel SQUID system in an unmagnetically shielded environment and successfully detected the QRS complex. Spectral analysis of the fetal heart rate revealed that the spectrum of variability was distributed from 0.5 to 1.0 Hz.

Applications of magnetocardiography for other fetal heart diseases

Kähler *et al.*[35] reported an application of fetal magnetocardiography in congenital heart disease. Using the magnetocardiogram of a case of slight hypoplasia of the right ventricle with a small right ventricular outflow tract, prolonged duration of the QRS complex was revealed, suggesting morphological abnormalities of the pulse conduction system in the fetal heart. The magnetocardiographic findings were well coincided with the electrocardiographic findings of the neonate.

Horigome *et al.*[36] estimated the magnitude of the single current dipole of fetal heart by fetal magnetocardiography. The magnitude of current dipole was well correlated with gestational age in normal fetuses, indicating an increased amount of currents in myocardial muscles. However, in cases of cardiomegaly with myocardial abnormalities such as twin-to-twin transfusion, malformation of the Galen vein and endocardial cushion defects, the magnitude of dipole current exceeded the normal range, indicating excess increase of the cardiomuscular mass.

Hosono *et al.*[37] revealed that QT prolonged fetuses with severe congenital structural anomalies such as mitral atresia, transposition of the great arteries and so on, had poor neonatal prognosis of death within 28 days after birth in spite of specialist neonatal intensive care.

Magnetoencephalography

The strength of the magnetic field by the brain is far weaker than that by the heart. The range of magnetoencephalogram in fetuses is in the order of femtotesla whereas that of adults is in the order of picotesla.

Magnetoencephalography was first reported about a decade after the first fetal magnetocardiography.[38] When the fetal face is almost parallel to the mother's abdominal surface, verified using high-resolution ultrasonography, a total of 300 acoustic stimulus with a frequency of 1 kHz and a duration of 100 ms was applied through the maternal abdomen. The stimuli evoked magnetical responses of the fetal brain. Although the number of fetuses with complete recording was small, typical auditory responses were successfully revealed by averaging.

Wakai *et al.*[39] reported the success of fetal magnetoencephalogram nearly a decade after the pioneering work. A seven-channel SQUID detector was placed on the maternal abdomen located near the fetal auditory canal and external canthus. A total of 100 trials of auditory stimulus applied to a brief tone burst of 1.5 kHz frequency, 20 ms duration and 100 dB amplitude from the speaker placed about 1.5 m from the mother evoked distinct auditory responses with latencies of approximately 200 ms. The amplitude of auditory brain response was 100 fT. Evoked fetal auditory magnetoencephalographic signals were well coincided with the neonatal auditory magnetoencephalographic responses evoked by similar auditory stimuli.

Eswaran *et al.*[40] recorded fetal magnetoencephalographic-evoked auditory responses using a 100-ms tone burst of 120 dB intensity using 151-channel magnetoencephalography system specially designed for pregnant women. By consecutive trials of fetal magnetoencephalographic responses, they succeeded in recording at least one of several trial sessions. Eswaran *et al.*[41] also succeeded in recording visually evoked brain activity in fetuses using magnetoencephalography. Light pulses of 8800 lux, 33 ms duration and an approximately 2 s ± 50 ms randomized interval were applied for 6 min (180 flushes). They succeeded in recording visually evoked electroencephalographic responses in four of 10 healthy fetuses. The amplitude of the magnetoencephalogram was about 30 femtotesla at maximum.

Conclusion

Fetal magnetocardiography has been shown as suitable to reveal a variety of fetal heart diseases during the second and the third trimesters of gestation. In particular, fetal arrhythmia is a good indication of fetal magnetocardiography. Magnetocardiographic analysis revealed detailed cardiac activity of the fetal heart, which has not been detected by fetal echocardiography. However, the number of reports on the application of fetal magnetocardiography in other fetal heart diseases such as structural heart diseases and fetal heart hypertrophy is still small. Fetal heart rate monitoring by fetal magnetocardiography is attractive because magnetocardiography can estimate beat-to-beat variability, but it has not been used in routine clinical practice.

Fetal magnetoencephalograms are still a significant area of study. Evoked auditory responses have been successfully measured in healthy fetuses, but evoked visual responses were recorded by only a few groups.

The amplitudes of fetal magnetocardiogram and magnetoencephalogram are in the order of picotesla and femtotesla. The SQUID system requires superconducting substances of low transition temperature, which inevitably requires liquid helium. A more portable SQUID system which clinicians can use at the bedside without a magnetically shielded room is anticipated.

REFERENCES

1. Baule G, McFee R. Detection of the magnetic field of the heart. *Am Heart J* 1963;55:95–6.
2. Kariniemi V, Ahopelto J, Karp PJ, Katila TE. The fetal magnetocardiogram. *J Perinat Med* 1974;2:214–15.
3. Hukkinen K, Kariniemi V, Katila TE, Laine H, Lukander R, Mäkipää P. Instantaneous fetal heart rate monitoring by electromagnetic methods. *Am J Obstet Gynecol* 1976;125:1115–20.
4. Wakai RT, Wang MH, Martin CB. Spatiotemporal properties of the fetal magnetocardiogram. *Am J Obstet Gynecol* 1994;170:770–9.
5. Hosono T, Chiba Y, Shinto M, *et al.* A case of fetal complete heart block recorded by magnetocardiography, ultrasonography and direct fetal electrocardiography. *Fetal Diagn Ther* 2001;16:38–41.
6. Wakai RT, Strasburger JF, Li Z, Deal BJ, Gotteiner NL. Magnetocardiographic rhythm patterns at initiation and termination of fetal supraventricular tachycardia. *Circulation* 2003;107:307–12.
7. Van Leeuwen P, Lange S, Bettermann H, Grönemeyer D, Hatzmann W. Fetal heart rate variability and complexity in the course of pregnancy. *Early Hum Dev* 1999;54:259–69.
8. Tsukada K, Mitsui T, Terada Y, Horigome H, Yamaguchi I. Noninvasive visualization of multiple simultaneously activated regions on torso magnetocardiographic maps during ventricular depolarization. *J Electrocardiol* 1999;32:305–13.
9. Leuthold A, Wakai RT, Martin CB. Noninvasive in utero assessment of PR and QRS intervals from the fetal magnetocardiogram. *Early Hum Dev* 1999;54:235–43.
10. Kandori A, Miyashita T, Tsukada K, *et al.* Sensitivity of foetal magnetocardiograms versus gestation week. *Med Biol Eng Comput* 1997;37:5454–8.
11. Quinn A, Weir A, Bain R, Maas P, Donaldson G. Antenatal fetal magnetocardiography: A new method for fetal surveillance? *Br J Obstet Gynaecol* 1994;101:866–70.
12. Horigome H, Takahashi MI, Asaka M, Shigemitsu S, Kandori A, Tsukada K. Magnetocardiographic determination of the developmental changes PQ, QRS and QT intervals in the foetus. *Acta Paediatr* 2000;89:1–5.
13. Wakai RT, Leuthold AC, Martin CB. Atrial and ventricular fetal heart rate patterns in isolated congenital complete heart block detected by magnetocardiography. *Am J Obstet Gynecol* 1998;179:258–60.
14. Hosono T, Shinto M, Chiba Y, Kandori A, Tsukada K. Prenatal diagnosis of fetal complete atrioventricular block with QT prolongation and alternating ventricular pacemakers using multichannel magnetocardiography and current arrow maps. *Fetal Diagn Ther* 2002;17:173–6.
15. Hosono T, Kawamata K, Chiba Y, Kandori A, Tsukada K. Prenatal diagnosis of long QT syndrome using magnetocardiography: A case report and review of the literature. *Prenat Diagn* 2002;22:198–200.
16. Hamada H, Horigome H, Asuka M, *et al.* Prenatal diagnosis of long QT syndrome using fetal magnetocardiography. *Prenat Diagn* 1999;19:677–80.
17. Menéndez T, Achenbach S, Beinder E, *et al.* Prenatal diagnosis of QT prolongation by magnetocardiography. *PACE* 2000;23:1305–7.
18. Kandori A, Miyashita T, Tsukada K, *et al.* Prenatal diagnosis of QT prolongation by fetal magnetocardiogram – Use of QRS and T-wave current-arrow maps. *Physiol Meas* 2001;22:377–87.
19. Hosono T, Chiba Y, Shinto M, Kandori A, Tsukada K. A fetal Wolff–Parkinson–White syndrome diagnosed prenatally by magnetocardiography. *Fetal Diagn Ther* 2001;16:215–7.
20. Kähler C, Schleussner E, Schneider U, Seewald HJ. Prenatal diagnosis of the Wolf-Parkinson–White syndrome by fetal magnetocardiography. *Br J Obstet Gynaecol* 2001;108:335–6.
21. Menéndez T, Achenbach S, Beinder E, *et al.* Usefulness of magnetocardiography for the investigation of fetal arrhythmia. *Am J Cardiol* 2001;88:334–6.
22. Kandori A, Hosono T, Chiba Y, *et al.* Classifying cases of fetal Wolf–Parkinson–White syndrome by estimating the accessory pathway from fetal magnetocardiograms. *Med Biol Eng Comput* 2003;41:33–9.
23. Quartero HWP, Stinstra JG, Golbach EGM, Meiboom EJ, Peters MJ. Clinical implications of fetal magnetocardiography. *Ultrasound Obstet Gynecol* 2002:20;142–53.
24. Hosono T, Kanagawa T, Chiba Y, Neki R, Kandori A, Tsukada K. Fetal atrial flutter recorded prenatally by magnetocardiography. *Fetal Diagn Ther* 2002;17:75–7.
25. Hosono T, Kanagawa T, Chiba Y, Kandori A, Tsukada K. The coincidence of fetal magnetocardiography and direct electrocardiography in a case of fetal atrial flutter due to intracardiac tumor. *Fetal Diagn Ther* 2002;17:331–3.
26. Kandori A, Hosono T, Kanagawa T, *et al.* Detection of atrial-flutter and atrial-fibrillation waveforms by fetal magnetocardiogram. *Med Biol Eng Comput* 2002;40:213–7.
27. Van Leeuwen P, Hailer B, Bader W, Geissler J, Trowitzsch E. Magnetocardiography in the diagnosis of fetal arrhythmia. *Br J Obstet Gynaecol* 1999;106:1200–8.
28. Wakai RT, Leuthold AC, Wilson AD, Martin CB. Association of fetal junctional rhythm and respiratory arrhythmia detected by magnetocardiography. *Pediatr Cardiol* 1997;18:201–3.
29. Anastasiadis PG, Anninos P, Assimakoppoulas E, Koutlaki N, Kotini A, Glazios G. Fetal heart rate patterns in normal and ritodrine-treated pregnancies detected by magnetocardiography. *J Matern Fetal Med* 2001;10:250–4.
30. Kariniemi V, Hukkinen K. Quantification of fetal heart rate variability by magnetocardiography and direct electrocardiography. *Am J Obstet Gynecol* 1977;128:526–9.
31. Wakai RT, Wang M, Pedron SL, Reid DL, Martin CB Jr. Spectral analysis of antepartum fetal heart rate variability from fetal magnetocardiogram recordings. *Early Hum Dev* 1993;35:15–24.
32. Rassi D, Lewis MJ. Power spectral analysis of the foetal magnetocardiogram *Physiol Meas* 1995;16:111–20.
33. Cysarz D, Van Leeuwen P, Bettermann H. Irregularities and nonlinearities in fetal heart rate period time series on the course of pregnancy. *Herzschr Elektrophys* 2000;11:179–83.
34. Baffa O, Wakai RT, Sousa PL, Verzola RMM. Fetal heart rate monitoring by magnetocardiograms. *Braz J Med Biol Res* 1995;28:1333–7.
35. Kähler C, Grimm B, Schleussner E, *et al.* The application of fetal magnetocardiography (FMCG) to investigate fetal arrhythmias and congenital heart defects (CHD). *Prenat Diagn* 2001;21:176–82.
36. Horigome H, Shiono J, Shigemitsu S, *et al.* Detection of cardiac hypertrophy in the fetus by approximation of the current dipole using magnetocardiography. *Pediatr Res* 2001;50:242–5.
37. Hosono T, Kandori A, Chiba Y, *et al.* Magnetocardiography in fetuses with congenital structural heart diseases. In Halgren E, Ahlfors S, Hämäläinen M, Cohen D, eds. *BIOMAG2004, Proceedings of the 14th International Conference on Biomagnetism*, Boston, MA, USA, 2004:319–20.
38. Blum T, Saling E, Bauer R. First magnetoencephalographic recordings of the brain activity of a human fetus. *Br J Obstet Gynaecol* 1985;92:1224–9.
39. Wakai RT, Leuthold AC, Martin CB. Fetal auditory responses detected by magnetoencephalography. *Am J Obstet Gynecol* 1996;174:1484–6.
40. Eswaran H, Preissl H, Wilson JD, *et al.* Short-term serial magnetoencephalography recordings of fetal auditory evoked responses. *Neurosci Lett* 2002;331:128–32.
41. Eswaran H, Wilson JD, Preissl H, *et al.* Magnetographic recordings of visual evoked brain activity in the human fetus. *Lancet* 2002;360:779–80.

143 Fetal pulse oximetry

P. P. van den Berg and H. W. Jongsma

Introduction

Accurate assessment of the fetal condition during labor is a major problem in clinical obstetric practice. Electronic fetal monitoring (EFM) was introduced into clinical practice in the 1960s without proper validation. Subsequent performed randomized trials failed to show the real benefit of EFM compared with intermittent auscultation.[1–4] No clear differences were found in direct neonatal course or long-term follow-up between the two groups.[5,6] There was, however, an increase in obstetric interventions in the EFM group. When EFM and fetal scalp blood sampling (FBS) are combined, the efficacy of fetal surveillance improves.[7] Although this concept has gained worldwide recognition, in the majority of obstetric units FBS is not consistently used.[8,9] One of the reasons may be that blood sampling requires a blood gas analyzer which needs maintenance and frequent calibration. Others objected to the method being invasive, cumbersome and disliked by the patients.[9,10] It is also a disadvantage that the information is only available at the time of sampling and further samples are needed to determine a trend. This has led to the situation that EFM is still used in most labor rooms as the single diagnostic tool to assess the fetal condition instead of EFM being used as a screening method and FBS as the method to verify the fetal oxygenation.

Pulse oximetry, which measures the arterial oxygen saturation (SaO_2) continuously, has become a standard monitoring technique in anesthesia, intensive care and neonatal care, and may become equally helpful for the obstetrician in monitoring the fetal condition during labor. It is minimally invasive and easy to use. Moreover, the SaO_2 is an adequate parameter to measure oxygen supply, because 99% of the oxygen in the blood is bound to hemoglobin.[11] Fetal SaO_2 values (range 30–80%) are on the steep part of the oxygen dissociation curve, due to a relatively low fetal partial pressure of oxygen. Consequently, minor reduction in oxygen supply will lead to a detectable decrease in fetal SaO_2 (Figure 143.1). Optimism about pulse oximetry, as an alternative technique for assessing the fetal intrapartum condition, rose when it appeared possible to obtain signals from the fetal scalp during labor for prolonged periods.[12–14]

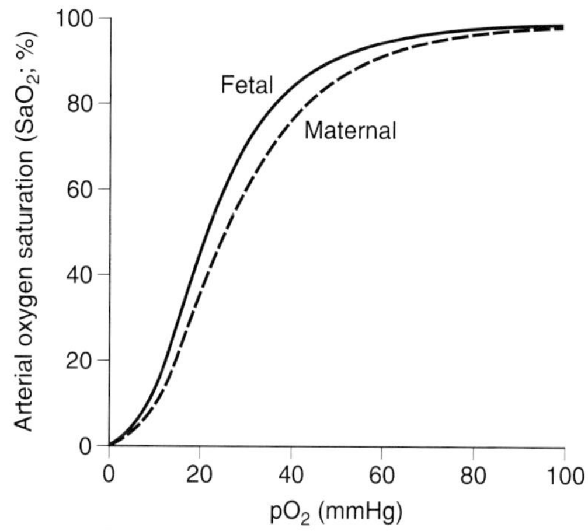

Figure 143.1 Maternal and fetal oxygen dissociation curve.

Principles of the measurement

Basic principles of pulse oximetry

The oxygen saturation of hemoglobin is expressed as a percentage ratio of the concentration of oxyhemoglobin (HbO_2) to the sum of the concentrations of oxyhemoglobin and deoxyhemoglobin (Hb). The measurement of oxygen saturation in arterial blood with pulse oximetry is based on two principles.

The first is that oxyhemoglobin and deoxyhemoglobin differ in their absorption spectrum. Figure 143.2 shows the absorbance spectra of HbO_2 and Hb.[15] Pulse oximetry uses two wavelengths in the red and infrared region of the light spectrum. In the red region (around 660 nm), deoxyhemoglobin absorbs much more light than oxyhemoglobin, while in the infrared region of the spectrum (890–940 nm) this is vice versa. These absorption differences of oxyhemoglobin and deoxyhemoglobin lead to the visible difference between well oxygenated arterial blood, which looks bright red, and less oxygenated venous blood, which appears more brown-violet.[16]

The second principle is that cyclic changes of the blood volume in tissue, caused by arterial blood, result in detectable pulsatile changes in the absorption of red and infrared light. During systole the blood volume in

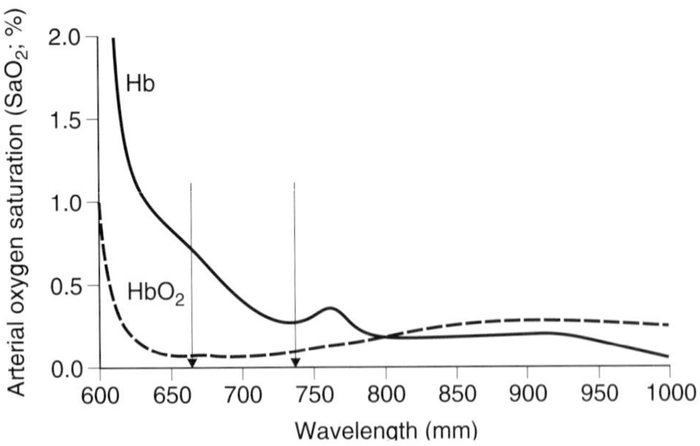

Figure 143.2 Absorbance spectrum of oxyhemoglobin (HbO_2) and deoxyhemoglobin (Hb). Arrows indicate 660 and 735 nm wavelengths.

the tissue increases, which causes an increase in the absorption of both red and infrared light. During diastole the blood volume in the tissue, and correspondingly the absorption of light, decrease.

The absorption of red and infrared light, which is caused by the skin, subcutaneous tissue, venous blood, non-pulsatile arterial blood and other absorbers in the light paths, leads to an additional, non-pulsatile component in the total absorption. The pulsatile or alternating component (ac) and the non-pulsatile or direct component (dc) of both red and infrared (IR) light are used to calculate a red to infrared ratio $[(ac_{red}/dc_{red})/(ac_{IR}/dc_{IR})]$. This ratio is assumed to be dependent only on changes in absorption in the arterial vascular tissue. In the pulse oximeter, the measured red/infrared ratio is converted into an oxygen saturation value, usually denoted by SpO_2, which is displayed. As the pulse oximetry principle assumes that pulsatile signals are caused by pulsations of arterial origin, other pulsatile signals (such as venous pulsations or rhythmic motion artifacts) may cause false SpO_2 readings.

Adaptations for fetal use

Reflectance sensor

To adapt this technique for fetal application, changes were made. In transmission sensors, which are commonly used for monitoring anesthetic patients and neonates, the light emitting diode (LED) and the photodetector are placed on opposite sides of the tissue. Light absorption is measured across the vascular bed. These sensors are placed on fingers or earlobes and are not suitable for application on the fetus during labor, as the presenting part is usually the fetal head. Reflectance sensors were designed, where LED and photodetector are placed on the same side of the tissue and light absorption is determined from light that scatters back to the surface. This made fetal utilization possible.

Plethysmographic signals from the fetal scalp can also be obtained by the transmission principle by using a hollow spiral scalp electrode containing an optical fiber; light is transmitted through the vascular bed from the spiral tip to the surface of the skin.[17]

Application of the reflectance sensor

In early studies, the sensor was applied to the fetal scalp using suction, gluing, clipping or using an incorporated spiral electrode[18] for fixation.

After the early results,[12–14] it became obvious that the fetal scalp is not the ideal area for measurement. Reduced peripheral perfusion, due to caput succedaneum, as well as hair, may lead to signal attenuation or erroneous measurements. When caput succedaneum is present, significant optical shunting may occur via the edematous area. In this case, light reaches the photodetector without passing through vascularized tissue. Dark hair absorbs a significant amount of light, particularly red light, and this reduces the signal amplitude. To avoid this, Nellcor Puritan Bennett and also Gardosi *et al.*[19] developed a reflectance sensor which is placed at the side of the fetal face (temple or cheek area) and held in place by means of the pressure of the uterine wall (Figure 143.3a). However, with this approach the sensor cannot be seen during application and monitoring, which is a potential problem. Incorrect apposition of the sensor may lead to false readings.[20,21] Therefore, the sensor should incorporate a means of assessing the correct placement on the fetal skin. In the sensor developed by Nellcor Puritan Bennett, this was realized by impedance measurement across contact points in the sensor as an indication of adequate sensor to skin contact (Figure 143.3b).

Side-effects

Thermal safety has been investigated in non-perfused tissue in an *in vitro* model. Under these conditions, the temperature increase is less than or equal to 3.0 °C. In well perfused tissue like the fetal face, the temperature increase is expected to be smaller because of the cooling effect of the blood flow. Sensors of this design have been extensively used in different centers worldwide in over 10,000 patients; complications such as uterine wall perforation, umbilical cord trauma, eye or ear injury, were not reported.[22] No significant difference in estimated blood loss and maximum recorded postpartum temperatures was found.[23]

Problems specific for fetal pulse oximetry

Calibration

The calibration of reflectance pulse oximetry for fetal use is more complicated than the calibration of transmission pulse oximetry for adult or neonatal use,

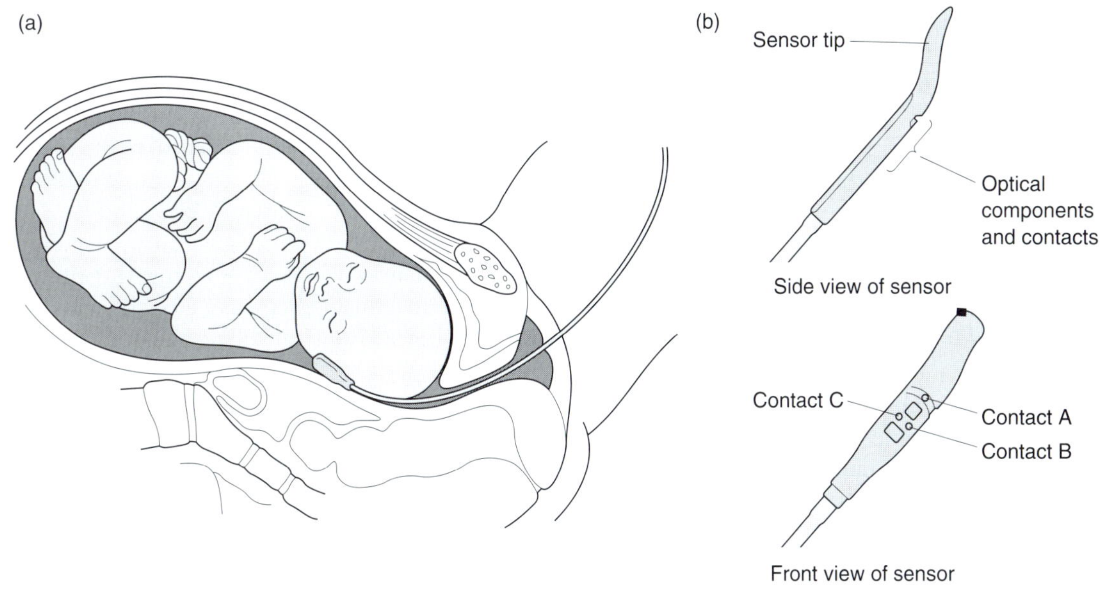

Figure 143.3 (a) Sensor positioned between the temple or cheek area of the fetal face and the uterine wall; (b) FS-14 sensor: the fetal oximeter and the sensor used in most studies reported were developed by Nellcor Puritan Bennett. The sensor consists of a flexible silicone tip curved toward the uterine wall. After insertion, the sensor is gently pulled back and wedged between the fetal face and the uterine wall. The sensor is supplied sterilized and meant for single use only. Dimensions of the sensor head are 3 × 1 cm. All surfaces are smooth, and the materials of the sensor have been tested for sensitization, pyrogenicity and irritation on different body regions. Adequate contact between the sensor and the fetal skin is verified by measuring the impedance between conductive contacts on the sensor. Low impedance values indicate that the contacts are immersed in amniotic fluid and that there is no adequate fetal skin–sensor contact. In this case the fetal oximeter will not accept data. After confirmation that the sensor is contacting tissue, the oximeter must determine whether the obtained pulsatile signals (plethysmograms) originate from fetal arterial blood.

as sample SaO_2 values cannot be obtained in the human fetus. Normal values of SaO_2 in the human fetus range from 30% to 80%.[24] The human adult is not a suitable subject because normal fetal SaO_2 values are mainly below 70% and it is unsafe to subject adults to such low saturation levels. In critically ill neonates, SaO_2 values may become as low as 60%,[25] an SaO_2 value still not low enough for a fetal calibration. Therefore, animal models are used to calibrate reflectance pulse oximetry against blood sample SaO_2 measurements.

For the comparison of two methods measuring the same quantity, i.e. SaO_2, it is recommended that the mean difference and standard deviation of differences is calculated.[26] The mean difference is called the bias and may show a systematic over- or underestimation of a method relative to the standard method. The standard deviation of differences is called the precision and represents the random 'variability' of the system. Another measure for the random 'variability' of the system can be obtained by calculating the standard deviation of residuals with linear regression analysis. The standard deviation of residuals and the precision will be equal if the bias is zero. The correlation coefficient is not a sufficient measure of accuracy. If the accuracy of a reflectance pulse oximeter is evaluated in the same study in which the reflectance sensor is calibrated, the bias will be zero and will give no additional information.

The accuracy of various reflectance pulse oximetry systems has been reported in animal models. Initial reports indicated a precision of 2.5–6.6% for sensors with 660 nm red wavelength and 890, 925 or 940 nm for the infrared LED.[27–31] Subsequent studies with a greater number of animals showed a much lower precision between 7.3% and 12.9%.[32,33]

Alternative approaches in sensor design

From the reviewed studies, it is clear that reflectance pulse oximetry is much more sensitive for all kinds of physiological variables in the fetal SaO_2 range of 10–80% than transmission pulse oximetry in an SaO_2 range of 70–100%. Alternative approaches in sensor design must therefore be considered for intrapartum use. One theoretical suggestion is using three photodetectors at different distances of the LEDs.[34]

Changing the red wavelength from 660 to 735 nm (Figure 143.2) leads to less attenuation of the red light at low SaO_2 levels. In a theoretical Monte Carlo model based on both absorption and scattering of light, Mannheimer *et al.*[35] predicted a significantly better similarity of light propagation for a 735/890 nm combination of LED than for a 660/890 nm combination of LED. A prototype reflectance sensor with a combination of 735 and 890 nm LEDs, and with a photodetector at a distance of 10 mm from both LEDs, developed by Nellcor Puritan Bennett, yielded much better results in six piglets compared with the

660/890 nm sensor[33]; the precision was 5.4%. A new version of this prototype sensor developed for intrapartum use, in which the LED–photodetector distance was changed from 10 to 14 mm, was evaluated in two independent laboratories.[36] The precision was around 5% with a small bias of 1.6% between the laboratories. Measurements were made over an SaO_2 range of 17–100%, with various sensors at several positions on each animal.[36]

Hemoglobin

Differences in the light absorption characteristics of hemoglobin of other species in the spectral range might lead to a different calibration line for the human fetus, although no differences were found at 660 and 940 nm for dogs and rabbits.[37,38] Presumably, hemoglobin light absorption characteristics of other mammals will not differ substantially from humans.

Being a two-wavelength device, a pulse oximeter can only measure the ratio of concentrations of HbO_2 and Hb, which makes it specifically sensitive to changes in SaO_2. However, other hemoglobin derivatives, like carboxyhemoglobin (COHb) and methemoglobin (MetHb) also absorb light in the visible range and might therefore lead to errors in the SpO_2. The error caused by the presence of 10% COHb appeared to be insubstantial over the whole SaO_2 range, for the wavelengths 660 and 940 nm.[15,39] In the presence of 10% MetHb, the pulse oximeter will underestimate the SaO_2 above 70% and overestimate below 70% SaO_2.[15,39–41] However, concentrations of 10% COHb and 10% MetHb are not expected in the human fetus during labor. In non-smoking pregnant women and their newborns, COHb concentrations are reported to be $< 0.5\%$. COHb concentrations in blood of newborns of cigarette smoking mothers were 1.9% (SD 1.2%).[42]

Human fetal (HbF) and human adult hemoglobin (HbA) differ slightly in their spectra in the visible range.[15] Commercial pulse oximeters programmed with a calibration curve derived from studies in healthy adults will not be affected by high concentrations of HbF in the neonatal SaO_2 range of 70–100%.[43] However, at an SaO_2 level of 25%, such commercial pulse oximeters will underestimate the SaO_2 by 5%.

Composition of the tissue compartment

The attenuation of the light received at the photodetector is not only caused by absorption, but also by scattering of light in tissue. The scattering of light by erythrocytes (e.g. velocity, size and shape) is of special importance, because it causes most of the fundamental problems in pulse oximetry at low saturation values. The scattering is largely determined by the hematocrit, blood flow conditions and blood volume changes. Erythrocyte differences between human subjects and between animals might have an effect on the accuracy of pulse oximetry but this factor has not been studied yet.

The effect of hematocrit, blood flow and blood volume fraction have been studied in *in vitro* models and animal models. In general, variation of these factors has hardly any effect above 70% SaO_2.[44] However, at SaO_2 values of 25%, a substantial bias can be observed.[45] Also varying the pressure on the sensor can cause bias, probably by variations in the venous blood fraction in the tissue.[46]

Sensor–skin interface

Scattering of light occurs in all situations where there are variations of the refractive index, i.e. at cross-sections of different tissue layers, at the boundaries of blood vessels and even within the cells themselves (e.g. by the mitochondria). It is therefore likely that differences in skin structure between animals and humans will influence the calibration of reflectance pulse oximetry. For none of the animal models is the magnitude of this effect known.

All intravascular dyes or pigments on the skin, which cause an unequal absorption of red and infrared light, may also cause an inaccurate reading. For example, meconium-stained skin caused an inaccurate oxygen saturation reading in a neonate because red light is more readily absorbed by meconium than infrared light.[47]

Optical shunting through hair is also mentioned as a possible cause for inaccuracy. However, differences between measurements on wet hair or shaved skin were not observed in fetal lambs.[32] Improper contact of the sensor to the skin can lead to erroneous pulse oximeter readings, if the light is directly shunted toward the photodetector.[21]

Technical problems

Certain technical situations may interfere with a reliable estimation of the SaO_2. Some problems related to the use of fetal reflectance pulse oximetry will be discussed in this paragraph, i.e. small pulses and signal analysis, and the choice of the LED wavelengths.

Small pulses

The fetal plethysmographic signals obtained with reflectance pulse oximetry are typically one-tenth of the adult transmission pulse oximetry signals. The amplitude of the pulsatile component of the signal is often below 0.2% of the total signal, which is at the lower limit of signal acceptance for some commercial transmission pulse oximeters.[48,49] These small pulses lead to a lower signal-to-noise ratio and, as a consequence, a less accurate device. To optimize signal quality, fetal plethysmographic signals should be maximized while the noise is minimized. Pulse oximeters use several ways to enhance the signal processing. The fetal electrocardiogram can be used to cardiosynchronize the red and infrared pulses. A high-pass filter is used to detect the red and infrared peak and trough and the pulse oximeter verifies if the red and infrared peak and trough are in phase with each other. A weighted moving average of red to infrared ratios is calculated over several heart beats[22] and the average value is converted into an SpO_2 value. If the red and infrared pulses are not properly synchronized to the fetal electrocardiogram or not in phase with each other, inaccurate SaO_2 estimations may be the result.[50] Such phase shifts of the red and infrared pulses with the heart rate were observed by placing a 660/940 sensor on a caput succedaneum.[50]

Wavelength accuracy

The LEDs used in commercial transmission sensors are not ideal light sources. The LEDs emit light in a narrow spectral range. However, the center wavelength of the emitted light varies between diodes of the same type of sensor, by up to 15 nm.[16] A shift in the wavelength results in a different extinction coefficient (Figure 143.2) and hence in an error in the estimated SaO_2. The effect of variation in the center wavelength will be greater for the red (660 nm) than for the infrared wavelength because its absorption spectrum shows a steeper slope. This problem can be solved in two ways. First, LEDs with center wavelengths which fall outside a specified range may be rejected. Second, the pulse oximeter may be programmed to accept several ranges of LED center wavelength for both the red and infrared, and to correct for these different wavelengths internally.[49]

Another problem related to the 660 nm LED is that a small amount of light in the infrared region is often emitted in addition to the center wavelength.[16] Although this so-called 'secondary emission' does not influence the accuracy at high SaO_2 values, it might influence the accuracy at low fetal SaO_2 values.

Clinical studies

In the first reports of this technique used in the human fetus, the investigators used equipment that was designed for adults, without suitable calibration curves and using sensors of their own design. This may explain the wide range in mean values that were reported during normal labor.

Clinical studies published since 1996 were performed with the improved 735/890 nm sensor. These studies are reported in a separate paragraph. Studies published before 1996 were performed with older type sensors that are less reliable.

Normal values

The first studies reported a mean SpO_2 value of 68% (range 11–81%) in the early part of the first stage of labor, which decreased to 58% (range 29–81%) at the end of dilation,[51] a mean SpO_2 value of 82% (range 50–95%),[20] and a median value of 60% (range 10–95%).[52]

Dildy *et al.*[53] were the first to report normal values using an oximeter and sensor (660 nm red wavelength) especially designed for fetal use, and validated in adult volunteers and fetal sheep. He reported adequate signals during 40–60% of the time. The mean SpO_2 was 58% (range between 45% and 59%).

Breech presentation

In the fetal lamb, the difference in oxygen saturation across the ductus arteriosus is 4–5% and remains the same even during hypoxia, when redistribution of the blood flow occurs to protect the vital organs.[54] In a clinical study, saturations of 27–32% lower than vertex presentation were reported,[20] probably because these breeches indeed had lower saturation values.

Relationship with scalp blood

Correlations between oxygen saturation and pH in fetal scalp blood and SpO_2 values have been investigated by several groups.[55,56] Correlation coefficients were low ($r^2 < 0.5$) in all cases, as might have been expected.

Maternal oxygen therapy

The effect of maternal oxygen therapy was studied by McNamara *et al.*[57] and Dildy *et al.*,[58] both using validated equipment (Nellcor Puritan Bennett). In these studies, a significant increase in SpO_2 values was found, when 100% oxygen was given to the mother. McNamara *et al.* found an increase of 11%, Dildy *et al.* reported an increase of 14%. When lower concentrations of oxygen were given to the mothers, inconsistent results were obtained. McNamara *et al.*[57] observed an increase in fetal SpO_2 of 7.5% when 27% oxygen was administered to the mother. However, Dildy *et al.*[58] found no increase in SpO_2 after supplying 40% oxygen to the mother. This discrepancy in results was the reason for the re-evaluation of the data reported by Dildy *et al.*[58] by van den Berg and Jongsma.[59] They found that maternal oxygen administration with both high (100%) and moderate (40%) inspired oxygen concentrations was beneficial to those fetuses whose oxygen saturation is near a critical lower limit (40%).

Correlations with neonatal outcome

Pulse oximetry readings were compared with SaO_2 measurements in the umbilical cord blood at delivery. McNamara *et al.*[60] and Langer *et al.*,[55] both using validated equipment (Nellcor Puritan Bennett), observed a significant correlation with the venous oxygen saturation, arterial pH and venous pH, but not with SpO_2. McNamara *et al.* analyzed the data only when there was an acceptable signal within the 30 min before the birth of the child. Langer *et al.* analyzed the data when the oximetry signal was obtained within 15 min of birth.

Studies for the validation of this method in the human fetus have limitations. During the period between the last obtained SpO_2 values and umbilical cord blood sampling, large differences in placenta perfusion and thus in fetal arterial po_2 may occur. As fetal oxygen saturation values are on the steep part of the oxygen dissociation curve, a small difference in po_2 will result in large differences in arterial oxygen saturation.

Carbonne *et al.*[61] defined a desaturation index as the difference between the mean SpO_2 of the last hour of stage 1, and the mean SpO_2 of the last 5 min of available recordings (interval between last SpO_2 measurement and birth < 10 min). This index correlated with the umbilical vein pH ($r=0.62$) and the 1-min Apgar score ($r=0.71$).[61]

Seelbach-Göbel *et al.*[62] correlated the duration of time below an SpO_2 level of 30%, between 30–60% and above 60% and the umbilical artery pH. The duration of low SpO_2 values was significantly longer in neonates with an umbilical artery pH < 7.15 compared to neonates with an pH ≤ 7.15. Another approach to address the efficacy of fetal pulse oximetry is to investigate the potential effect of adding fetal pulse oximetry to fetal heart rate (FHR) monitoring. In that study,[63] four expert obstetricians retrospectively evaluated intrapartum FHR tracings initially without and then with SpO_2 values obtained with an 660/890 nm reflectance sensor. They were requested to indicate if they felt there was a need for intervention. They were also requested to estimate the umbilical artery pH. In the 119 patients evaluated in the study, the clinicians managing labor were blinded to SpO_2 values obtained with fetal pulse oximeters. Acidosis and fetal compromise was defined as an umbilical artery pH < 7.15. Sensitivity and specificity for fetal compromise was determined for each referee. With the SpO_2 information, all of the referees would have intervened less often and in most of the cases predicted a higher pH value. The authors state that fetal pulse oximetry would not only lead to less unnecessary interventions but may also lead to undetected fetal acidosis. They raise the concern that SpO_2 may be falsely reassuring. One of the reasons for this might be the amount of signal loss (mean percentage of adequate signal was 65%).

Studies with the 735/890 nm sensor

Several groups have used the Nellcor 735/890 nm reflectance sensor (FS 14) during labor. The mean percentage of time with adequate signal during measurement ranged from 65% to 80%.[64–67] The reproducibility of two double-sensor studies showed a mean absolute saturation difference between two sensors on the same fetus of −0.7% and 6.3%, and with a standard deviation of a single sensor of 5.3% and 6.3%, respectively.[65,68]

Normal values are reported in several studies, i.e. in which the neonatal outcome showed an umbilical artery pH > 7.15 and Apgar score at 5 min ≥ 7.[65–69] Mean values of SpO_2 during labor ranged between 42% and 50%. No significant difference was seen during phase I (dilatation phase) and phase II (pushing phase). All individual SpO_2 values ranged between 30% and 70% for fetuses with a normal outcome.[65–69] Occasionally, an SpO_2 of below 30% was seen, but always with a quick return to values above 30%.[69] These values agree with blood sample values in the awake fetal lamb in which the SaO_2 could be decreased to 30% before metabolic acidosis became apparent.[70,71] Weak but significant correlations were found between the mean fetal SpO_2 during the last 30 min before birth and the umbilical artery and vein SaO_2, as with the umbilical artery pH and base excess.[66]

The 735/890 nm sensors were further used to study SpO_2 in cases with meconium aspiration,[72] and in cases of severe FHR abnormalities.[64,73] In both situations, SpO_2 values were significantly lower compared to normal situations, i.e. with normal FHR patterns and without meconium aspiration.[64,72,73] However, more studies are needed of these specific situations before definite conclusions can be drawn.

In two studies, intrapartum monitoring of fetal SpO_2 was used as a diagnostic test to predict acidosis at birth.[66,74] Alshimmiri *et al.*[66] concluded that fetal SpO_2 was of limited use in predicting acidosis at birth, regardless of the SpO_2 cut-off value used. For predicting acidosis at birth, Carbonne *et al.*[74] concluded that the predictive value of intrapartum fetal SpO_2 with a cut-off value of 30% was as equally predictive as fetal scalp blood analysis with a cut-off value of pH ≤ 7.20. Fetal pulse oximetry became superior at higher threshold levels.[74]

A multicenter randomized trial to study the efficacy of fetal pulse oximetry was published in 2000.[75] The primary hypothesis was that the cesarean delivery rate for non-reassuring FHR patterns would be halved if SpO_2 was used as an adjunct to EFM.

However although this rate was reduced by more than 50%, the overall cesarean rate was unchanged between the control and the study group. This was due to an increased percentage of cesareans for dystocia in the study group. Further analysis could not explain the reason for this increase. A follow-up study found that women with more clinically worrisome FHR patterns had a significantly higher incidence of cesarean for dystocia although co-monitored with SpO_2.[76] In a randomized trial in 146 patients with term pregnancies, in labor and abnormal FHR patterns, the hypothesis was tested if pulse oximetry in addition to EFM and FBS reduces operative deliveries performed because of non-reassuring fetal status. A reduction of 50% in operative deliveries and FBS was achieved without an increase in cesarean section for dystocia.[77]

Current status

The aim of fetal surveillance during labor is straightforward: to identify fetal distress which may, if uncorrected, cause short-term morbidity, death, or possibly long-term morbidity. Undeniably, improved obstetric care, together with cardiotocography, has led to a decrease in perinatal mortality in Western countries since 1960. The expected decrease in perinatal and long-term morbidity, however, was not observed and, due to a poor predictive value of cardiotocography, operative interventions during labor increased dramatically. In an effort to improve this unfortunate clinical situation new techniques which supply objective parameter about the fetal status are warranted.

Fetal monitoring with SpO_2 with the Nellcor device was approved by the FDA in May 2000 for clinical use in the USA and became commercially available. In Europe, fetal pulse oximetry is available from Nellcor (Pleasanton, CA, USA) and OB Scientific (Germantown, WI, USA).

In September 2001, the American College of Obstetricians and Gynecologists (ACOG) released a Committee Opinion on fetal pulse oximetry (no. 258). There were three main concerns: signal registration time, possible false-negative readings and lack of proven cost benefit. The committee recommended that new prospective randomized clinical studies are needed to establish the role of fetal pulse oximetry during labor.[78]

In March 2002, the Society of Obstetricians and Gynaecologists of Canada published guidelines for fetal surveillance during labor. It stated that fetal pulse oximetry as an adjunct to EFM in patients with non-reassuring fetal status, should not be considered a standard of practice.[79]

In early 2003, FDA labeling for the Nellcor monitor was revised. This was based on postapproval surveillance of over 12,000 cases. The conclusion was that FPO is meant as an adjunct to EFM, not as a replacement.

The future of fetal pulse oximetry as an adjunct to EFM is still uncertain and its value can only be established by further clinical research.

REFERENCES

1. Kelso IM, Parsons RJ, Lawrence GF, *et al.* An assessment of continuous fetal heart rate monitoring in labor – A randomized trial. *Am J Obstet Gynecol* 1978;131:526–32.
2. Haverkamp AD, Orleans M, Langendorfer M, *et al.* A controlled trial of the differential effects of intrapartum fetal monitoring. *Am J Obstet Gynecol* 1979;134:399–412.
3. Luthy DA, Shy KK, van Belle G, *et al.* A randomized trial of electronic fetal monitoring in preterm labor. *Obstet Gynecol* 1987;69:687–95.
4. MacDonald D, Grant A, Sheridan-Pereira M, *et al.* The Dublin randomized controlled trial of intrapartum fetal heart rate monitoring. *Am J Obstet Gynecol* 1985;152:524–39.
5. Grant A, O'Brian N, Joy M, *et al.* Cerebral palsy among children born during the Dublin randomized trial of intrapartum monitoring. *Lancet* 1989;2:1233–6.
6. Shy KK, Luthy DA, Bennett FC, *et al.* Effects of electronic fetal heart rate monitoring, as compared with periodic auscultation, on the neurologic development of premature infants. *N Engl J Med* 1990;322:588–93.
7. van den Berg PP, Schmidt S, Gesche J, Saling E. Fetal distress and the condition of the newborn using cardiotocography and fetal blood analysis during labour. *Br J Obstet Gynaecol* 1987;94:72–5.
8. Wheble AM, Gillmer MDG, Spencer JAD, Sykes GS. Changes in fetal monitoring practice in the UK: 1977–1984. *Br J Obstet Gynaecol* 1984;96:1140–7.
9. Clark SL, Paul RH. Intrapartum fetal surveillance: The role of fetal scalp blood sampling. *Am J Obstet Gynecol* 1985;153:717–20.
10. Nickelsen C, Thomsen SG, Weber T. Continuous acid–base assessment of the human fetus during labour by tissue-pH and transcutaneous carbon dioxide monitoring. *Br J Obstet Gynaecol* 1985;92:220–5.
11. Tremper KK, Barker SJ. Pulse oximetry and oxygen transport. In Payne JP, Severinghaus JW, eds. *Pulse Oximetry.* Berlin, New York: Springer, 1986:19–30.
12. Peat S, Booker M, Lanigan C, Ponte J. Continuous intra partum measurement of fetal oxygen saturation. *Lancet* 1988;2:213.
13. Johnson N, Lilford RJ. Continuous intrapartum measurement of fetal oxygen saturation. *Lancet* 1988;2:517.
14. Gardosi J, Carter M, Becket T. Continuous intrapartum monitoring of fetal oxygen saturation. *Lancet* 1989;2:692–3.
15. Zijlstra WG, Buursma A, Meeuwsen-van der Roest WP. Absorption spectra of human fetal and adult oxyhemoglobin, de-oxyhemoglobin, carboxyhemoglobin, and methemoglobin. *Clin Chem* 1991;37:1633–8.
16. Pologe JA. Pulse oximetry; technical aspects of machine design. *Int Anesthesiol Clin* 1987;25:137–3.
17. Buschmann J, Rall G, Knitza R. Fetal oxygen saturation measurement by transmission pulse oximetry. *Lancet* 1992; 339:615.
18. Knitza R, Rall G, Mainz S, *et al.* Fetale Geburtsüberwachung durch Oxykardiotokographie (OCTG). *Geburtsh Frauenheilk* 1993;53: 849–53.
19. Gardosi J, Reed N, Sahota B. Fetal pulse oximetry with the balloon probe. In Knitza R, ed. *Hypoxische Gefährdung des Fetus Sub Partu.* Darmstadt: Steinkopff, 1994:179–83.
20. Gardosi JO, Schram CM, Symonds EM. Adaptation of pulse oximetry for fetal monitoring during labour. *Lancet* 1991;1:1265–7.
21. Gardosi JO, Damianou D, Schram CMH. Artifacts in fetal pulse oximetry: Incomplete sensor-to-skin contact. *Am J Obstet Gynecol* 1994;170:1169–73.
22. Nellcor Puritan Bennett. *Technical Issues of Noninvasive Fetal Oxygen Saturation Monitoring using the Nellcor N-400.* Pleasanton, CA: Nellcor Puritan Bennett, 1995:1–13.
23. Johnson N, Baker M, McNamara H. The effect of monitoring the fetus with a pulse oximeter on the puerperal morbidity. *Br J Obstet Gynaecol* 1994;14:11–13.
24. Dildy GA, van den Berg PP, Katz M, *et al.* Intrapartum fetal pulse oximetry: Fetal oxygen saturation trends during labor in relation to delivery outcome. *Am J Obstet Gynecol* 1994;171:679–84.
25. Boxer RA, Gottesfeld L, Singh S, *et al.* Noninvasive pulse oximetry in children with cyanotic congenital heart disease. *Crit Care Med* 1987;15:1062–4.
26. Bland JM, Altman DG. Statistical methods for assessing agreement between two methods of clinical measurement. *Lancet* 1986;i: 307–10.
27. Jongsma HW, Crevels J, Menssen JJM, *et al.* Application of transmission and reflection pulse oximetry in fetal lambs. In Lafeber HN, Aarnoudse JG, Jongsma HW, eds. *Fetal and Neonatal Physiological Measurements.* Amsterdam: Elsevier, 1991:123–8.

28. Mendelson Y, Yocum BL. Noninvasive measurement of arterial oxyhemoglobin saturation with a heated and non-heated skin reflectance pulse oximeter sensor. *Biomed Instrum Technol* 1991;25:472–80.
29. Dassel AC, Graaff R, Aarnoudse JG, *et al.* Reflectance pulse oximetry in fetal lambs. *Pediatr Res* 1992;31:266–9.
30. Takatani S, Davies C, Sakakibara N, *et al.* Experimental and clinical evaluation of a noninvasive reflectance pulse oximeter sensor. *J Clin Monit* 1992;8:257–66.
31. Harris AP, Sendak MJ, Chung DC, Richardson CA. Validation of arterial oxygen saturation measurements *in utero* using pulse oximetry. *Am J Perinatol* 1993;10:250–4.
32. Nijland R, Jongsma HW, Menssen JJM, *et al.* Reflectance pulse oximetry: Accuracy of measurements from the neck of fetal lambs. In Ince C, Kesecioglu J, Telci L, Apkir K, eds. *Oxygen Transport to Tissue XVII.* New York: Plenum Press, *Adv Exp Med Biol* 1996;388:69–75.
33. Nijland R, Jongsma HW, Nijhuis JG. Is reflectance pulse oximetry reliable for fetal monitoring? Two sensors validated in piglets. *J Matern Fetal Invest* 1997;7:68–71.
34. Graaff R. Tissue optics applied to reflectance pulse oximetry. Ph.D. thesis, Groningen, The Netherlands, 1993.
35. Mannheimer PD, Casciani JR, Fein ME, Nierlich SL. Wavelength selection for low-saturation pulse oximetry. *IEEE Trans Biomed Eng* 1997;44:148–58.
36. Nijland R, Nierlich S, Jongsma HW, *et al.* Validation of reflectance pulse oximetry: An evaluation of a new sensor in piglets. *J Clin Monit* 1997;13:43–9.
37. Sendak MJ, Harris AP, Donham RT. Accuracy of pulse oximetry during arterial oxyhemoglobin desaturation in dogs. *Anesthesiology* 1988;68:111–14.
38. Vegfors M, Sjöberg F, Linberg L-G, *et al.* Basic studies of pulse oximetry in a rabbit model. *Acta Anaesthesiol* 1991;35:596–9.
39. Nijland R, Jongsma HW, Nijhuis JG, *et al.* Notes on the apparent discordance of pulse oximetry and multiwavelength hemoglobin photometry. *Acta Anaesthesiol Scand* 1995;39(Suppl 107):49–52.
40. Barker SJ, Tremper KK, Hyatt J. Effect of methemo-globinemia on pulse oximetry and mixed venous oximetry. *Anesthesiology* 1989;70:112–17.
41. Reynolds KJ, Palayiwa E, Moyle JTB, *et al.* The effect of dyshemoglobins on pulse oximetry: Part I, theoretical approach and part II, experimental results using an *in vitro* test system. *J Clin Monit* 1993;9:81–90.
42. Fogh-Andersen N, Sindberg Eriksen P, Grinsted J, Siggaard-Andersen O. HbCO in mothers and newborns. *Scand J Clin Lab Invest* 1988;48(Suppl 189):27–32.
43. Rajadurai VS, Walker AM, Yu VYH, Oates A. Effect of fetal haemoglobin on the accuracy of pulse oximetry in preterm infants. *J Paediatr Child Health* 1992;47:1084–5.
44. De Kock JP, Tarassenko L. *In vitro* investigation of the factors affecting pulse oximetry. *J Biomed Eng* 1991;13:61–6.
45. Nijland R, Jongsma HW, Verbruggen IM, Nijhuis JG. Reflectance pulse oximetry in fetal lambs: Subcutaneous vessels and vasoconstriction affects its reliability. *J Clin Monit* 1996;12:225–30.
46. Dassel ACM, Graaff R, Sikkema M, *et al.* Reflectance pulse oximetry at the forehead improves by pressure on the probe. *J Clin Monit* 1995;11:237–44.
47. Johnson N, Johnson VA, Bannister J, McNamara H. The effect of meconium on neonatal and fetal reflectance pulse oximetry. *J Perinat Med* 1990;18:351–5.
48. Wukitsch MW, Petterson MT, Tobler DR, Pologe JA. Pulse oximetry: Analysis of theory, technology, and practice. *J Clin Monit* 1988;4:290–301.
49. Tremper KK, Barker SJ. Pulse oximetry. *Anesthesiology* 1989;70: 98–108.
50. Schram CMH, Gardosi JO. Artifacts in fetal pulse oximetry: Nonarterial pulsatile signals. *Am J Obstet Gynecol* 1994;170: 1174–7.
51. Johnson N, Johnson VA, Fisher J, *et al.* Fetal monitoring with pulse oximetry. *Br J Obstet Gynaecol* 1991;98:36–41.
52. Knitza R. Erfahrungen und Ergebnisse mit der Oxykardiotokographie. In Knitza R, ed. *Hypoxische Gefährdung des Fetus Sub Partu.* Darmstadt: Steinkopff, 1994:211–18.
53. Dildy GA, Clark SL, Loucks CA. Preliminary experience with intrapartum fetal pulse oximetry in humans. *Obstet Gynecol* 1993;81:630–5.
54. Nijland R, Jongsma HW, Crevels J, *et al.* The ductus arteriosus, pre- and postductal oxygen saturation measurements in fetal lambs. *Eur J Obstet Gynecol Reprod Biol* 1994;55:135–40.
55. Langer B, Boudier E, Haddad J, *et al.* Fetal pulse oximetry during labor and at birth. In Knitza R, ed. *Hypoxische Gefährdung des Fetus Sub Partu.* Darmstadt: Steinkopff, 1994:139–44.
56. Luttkus A, Fengler TW, Friedmann W, Dudenhausen JW. Continuous monitoring of fetal oxygen saturation by pulse oximetry. *Obstet Gynecol* 1995;85:183–6.
57. McNamara H, Johnson N, Lilford R. The effect on fetal arteriolar oxygen saturation resulting from giving oxygen to the mother measured by pulse oximetry. *Br J Obstet Gynaecol* 1993;100:446–9.
58. Dildy GA, Clark SL, Loucks CA. Intrapartum fetal pulse oximetry: The effects of maternal hyperoxia on fetal arterial oxygen saturation. *Am J Obstet Gynecol* 1994;171:1120–4.
59. van den Berg PP, Jongsma HW. Effects of maternal inhalation of 40% oxygen on fetal oxygen saturation. *Am J Obstet Gynecol* [Letter] 1995;172:1940.
60. McNamara H, Chung C, Lilford R, Johnson N. Do fetal pulse oximetry readings at delivery correlate with cord blood oxygenation and acidaemia? *Br J Obstet Gynaecol* 1992;99:735–8.
61. Carbonne B, Audibert F, Segard L, *et al.* Fetal pulse oximetry: Correlation between changes in oxygen saturation and neonatal outcome. Preliminary report on 39 cases. *Eur J Obstet Gynecol Reprod Biol* 1994;57:73–7.
62. Seelbach-Gobel B, Huepel M, Kuhnert M, *et al.* The prediction of fetal acidosis by means of intrapartum fetal pulse oximetry. *Am J Obstet Gynaecol* 1999;180:73–81.
63. van den Berg PP, Dildy GA, Luttkus A, *et al.* The efficacy of intrapartum fetal surveillance when fetal pulse oximetry is added to cardiotocography. *Eur J Obstet Gynecol Reprod Biol* 1997;72(Suppl 1):S67–71.
64. Butterwegge M. Fetal pulse oximetry and non-reassuring heart rate. *Eur J Obstet Gynecol Reprod Biol* 1997;72(Suppl 1):S63–6.
65. East CE, Colditz PB, Phil D, *et al.* Human fetal intrapartum oxygen saturation monitoring: Agreement between readings from two sensors on the same fetus. *Am J Obstet Gynecol* 1996;174: 1594–8.
66. Alshimmiri M, Bocking AD, Gagnon R, Natale R, Richardson BS. Prediction of umbilical artery base excess by intrapartum fetal oxygen saturation monitoring. *Am J Obstet Gynecol* 1997;177:775–9.
67. Goffinet F, Langer B, Carbonne B, *et al.* Multicenter study on the clinical value of fetal pulse oximetry. I. Methodologic evaluation. *Am J Obstet Gynecol* 1997;177:1238–46.
68. Davies MG, Greene KR. Fetal pulse oximetry – A preliminary report on sensor precision determined by dual sensor studies. *Eur J Obstet Gynecol Reprod Biol* 1997;72(Suppl 1):S35–41.
69. Chua S, Yeong SM, Razvi K, Arulkumaran S. Fetal oxygen saturation during labour. *Br J Obstet Gynaecol* 1997;104:1080–3.
70. Richardson B, Carmichael L, Homan J, Patrick J. Electrocortical activity, electroocular activity, and breathing movements in fetal sheep with prolonged and graded hypoxemia. *Am J Obstet Gynecol* 1992;167:553–8.
71. Nijland R, Jongsma HW, Nijhuis J, van den Berg PP, Oeseburg B. Arterial oxygen saturation in relation to metabolic acidosis in fetal lambs. *Am J Obstet Gynecol* 1995;172:810–19.
72. Carbonne B, Cudevile C, Sivan H, *et al.* Fetal oxygen saturation measured by pulse oximetry during labour with clear or meconium-stained amniotic fluid. *Eur J Obstet Gynecol Reprod Biol* 1997;72(Suppl 1):S51–5.
73. Langer B, Carbonne B, Goffinet F, *et al.* Fetal pulse oximetry and fetal heart rate monitoring during stage II of labour. *Eur J Obstet Gynecol Reprod Biol* 1997;72(Suppl 1):S57–61.
74. Carbonne B, Langer B, Goffinet F, *et al.* Multicenter study on the clinical value of fetal pulse oximetry. II. Compared predictive values of pulse oximetry and fetal blood analysis. *Am J Obstet Gynecol* 1997;177:593–8.
75. Garite TJ, Dildy GA, McNamara H, *et al.* A multicenter controlled trial of fetal pulse oximetry in the intrapartum management of nonreassuring fetal heart rate patterns. *Am J Obstet Gynecol* 2000;183:1049–58.
76. Porecco RP, Boehm FH, Dildy GA, *et al.* Dystocia in nulliparous patients monitored with fetal pulse oximetry. *Am J Obstet Gynecol* 2004;190:113–7.
77. Kuhnert M, Schmidt S. Intrapartum management of nonreassuring fetal heart rate patterns: A randomized controlled trial of fetal pulse oximetry. *Am J Obstet Gynaecol* 2004;191(6):189–95.
78. ACOG Committee opinion, no. 258, 2001. Fetal pulse oximetry. *Obstet Gynaecol* 2001;98:523–4.
79. Liston R, Crane J, Hughes O, *et al.* Fetal health surveillance in labour. *J Obstet Gynaecol Can* 2002;24:342–55.

144 Intrapartum fetal monitoring – objective and subjective assessment of the main methods

E. Saling and S. Schmidt

Introduction

Fetal blood analysis (FBA) was first performed in June 1960 and published in 1961.[1] It was the first method which allowed the human fetus to be directly examined by sampling its blood.[2] Fetal blood analysis was one of the four essential clinical methods with which Prenatal Medicine or so-called Fetal Medicine started.[3]

The first continuous cardiotocogram conducted from an anencephalic fetus was described by Caldeyro-Barcia in 1958.[4] In 1966, with his CLIP-electrode that could be inserted vaginally after the membranes were ruptured, Hon introduced direct fetal electrocardiotocography during labor.[5] Widespread clinical utilization of cardiotocography (CTG), particularly in cases with intact membranes, could not start earlier than 1968 because of the lack of suitable equipment, which has been developed by Hammacher in co-operation with Hewlett Packard. We reported on these and other historic landmarks in 1988.[6] The combined intrapartum electronic–biochemical supervision by CTG and FBA was introduced by us in 1968[7] shortly after the first cardiotocographs became available for widespread clinical application. Since then, this combination continues to provide the safest supervision of the fetus during labor to prevent serious hypoxia and to minimize unnecessary operative interventions.[8–13]

The purposes of both methods are:

(1) Cardiotocography as a way of continuous electronic monitoring should enable the obstetrician:

 (a) To confirm the undisturbed condition of the fetus in all cases with normal cardiotocogram (CTGm); and

 (b) To select all fetuses with abnormal CTGm. Less than half of them are really threatened by hypoxia, but the majority of the fetuses in this group is not endangered.

(2) Fetal blood analysis from the presenting part, as a biochemical method, should only be employed as a complementary measure in cases of abnormal CTGm:

 (a) To clarify whether or not biochemical changes confirm imminent fetal hypoxia and/or acidosis which has been indicated by CTG; and

 (b) To help in deciding whether further important clinical consequences like tocolysis for inhibition of uterine contractions and conservative improvement of fetal supply or termination of labor by operation are necessary.

In this way, by using both CTG and FBA if necessary, it is possible to achieve a minimum of operative deliveries, which is of advantage to the mothers (cesarean) and to the fetuses (difficult vaginal intervention), with an optimal safety for the fetuses (low incidence of hypoxic morbidity).

One of the main disadvantages of using electronic fetal heart rate monitoring – this means CTG on its own – is a high rate of erroneously diagnosed cases of fetal hypoxia and consequently a relatively high number of unnecessary cesarean sections and of avoidable difficult vaginal deliveries, the latter in cases of abnormal CTGm early in the second stage when the presenting part is still high.

So, for instance, after an evaluation together with Goeschen *et al.*[14] in our department we found in cases with abnormal CTGm that an operative termination of

Table 144.1 Fetal blood analysis (FBA) is indicated when the heart rate patterns shown in the table are present

Heart rate pattern	Time	Precondition
Acute bradycardia	Immediately	Presenting part not yet on the pelvic floor or in the pelvic outlet, as then a vaginal operation to terminate labor should be performed without FBA
Late decelerations Variable decelerations if ≥30 bpm Early decelerations if ≥60 bpm	After three decelerations or at the latest after 10 min	
Variable decelerations if < 30 bpm	After six decelerations or at the latest after 20 min	

labor was indicated when using the Hammacher score in 73% of women, but when pH values were used simultaneously termination was indicated in only 14% of women. This means that when CTG is used on its own, about 60% unnecessary operations would have been performed.

How very subjective the interpretation of CTGm can also be from highly experienced colleagues has been impressively studied and published, particularly by Donker *et al.*[15] from the research group of van Geijn *et al.*[16] Logically, CTG can only be used as a method of selection of suspicious cases and not as a method for diagnosis of fetal hypoxia in all its stages. Therefore, the best way to solve this problem is the use of an additional biochemical method in all cases with abnormal fetal heart rate patterns.

Suitable blood parameters

For clinical routine, the actual pH values are the most suitable parameters to differentiate whether imminent or progressive fetal hypoxia is present or not. In each stage of intrauterine hypoxia, namely in the early mainly respiratory complication, and later in the stage of anaerobic glycolysis, the pH values are decreasing. Additional use of blood gases can certainly be of help in the differentiation of the character of the disturbance but is not essential for clinical decisions. So, for instance, $p\text{CO}_2$ values can help to differentiate the degree to which respiratory disturbances are also present – mostly in acute complications – or whether metabolic disturbances predominate when the $p\text{CO}_2$ values are not increased so much. The use of oxygen saturation values in the form of fetal pulse oximetry has in the meantime reached clinical usable state[17] but it has not found a wide acceptance in routine work up to now.

Indications for FBA

Fetal blood analysis is indicated in all cases when the CTGm shows patterns which lead to suspicion of hypoxia. For about 36 years, after CTG became available for clinical use in 1968, the schematic, but practicable, indication scheme shown in Table 144.1 has been used in routine practice in our department with success.

Repetition of FBA and clinical consequences

Fetal blood analysis should be repeated, depending on the character of the disturbance. When an acute complication (occurrence of acute bradycardia) is suspected, it is recommended to take a blood sample as quickly as possible, then immediately a second one and if necessary a third.

In order not to lose any time in cases with hypoxia, two other measures should be taken at the same time:

(1) Inhibition of the contractions through tocolysis; and
(2) Warning should be given for the operative team to be ready in case an emergency cesarean section should be necessary.

If further FBA do not show a critical fall in pH, then one should wait. Usually the fetal heart rate pattern recovers within a short time. If, however, the pH values decrease in spite of preventive measures, a cesarean section should be performed immediately or, if the labor is so far advanced, a vaginal operation should be performed to deliver the baby.

All other suspicious heart rate patterns indicate a complication advancing relatively slowly. The first FBA should be made after about 10 min. When decelerations are persistent, particularly if the pattern becomes more marked, and the first pH value was not suspicious, further blood samples should be taken at intervals of about 15 min. If the pH values remain suspicious after two or three samples have been taken, and if the heart rate pattern concerned does not occur again in a stronger or more marked form, then further FBA can be made at longer intervals or dispensed with.

If a normal pH value (such as 7.3) was measured from the first blood sample after suspicious decelerations have occurred, then the blood analysis should be repeated at short intervals of 5-10 min in order to establish the trend of the blood acidity if there is a further fall in pH values.

When the intensity remains the same or when the suspicious heart rate patterns disappear, the intervals between the blood sampling can be gradually lengthened and finally further blood analysis can be dispensed with if the pH values increase again. Should the pH values continue to decrease to prepathologic (pH 7.20–7.24) or even to pathologic values ($pH < 7.2$) in spite of tocolytic therapy, an operation to terminate the labor should be performed.

There is one possibility which leads to slightly different consequences, namely the so-called maternogenic increase of fetal acidity. This situation is caused by overflow of lactic acid from the mother to the fetus. Maternogenic acidity increase is not as dangerous as acidosis caused by fetal hypoxia. Therefore, it is not necessary to terminate the labor immediately by operation. To rule out such cases with maternogenic origin of acidity increase, we recommend measuring maternal and fetal acidity simultaneously. If the difference between mother and fetus is less than 0.15 pH units, maternogenic acidity increase is confirmed.[18] The incidence of cases with maternogenic acidity increase is relatively low. Out of all cases with acidosis ($pH < 7.2$), it occurs in about 9% and of cases with progressed acidosis ($pH < 7.1$), it occurs in 1%.[19]

The aim of modern supervision of the fetus during labor

The combined use of electronic and biochemical monitoring of the fetus should enable an obstetrician to detect all fetuses endangered by hypoxia during labor. While intrapartum mortality was mainly used as an important factor of quality control in the past, recent studies have focused more on the morbidity of the newborn. In this context the neurologic outcome is a decisive parameter for judging the validity of fetal monitoring methods.

The one measure of neonatal outcome which has shown significant results by more intensive intrapartum monitoring have been neonatal seizures. Due to the result of randomized trials this effect seems to be restricted to electronic fetal monitoring backed by fetal pH measurement.[20]

A 50% reduction in the risk of neonatal seizures, associated with continuous monitoring of the fetal heart and fetal acid–base analyses, is potentially very important. Indeed, between a quarter and a third of babies who suffer neonatal seizures die, and a further quarter to a third are seriously impaired in childhood.

But such considerations of the neurologic status should not ignore the other pathophysiological events caused by longer-lasting intrauterine hypoxia. The fetus consists of many organs, not only the brain, even though many authors focus their investigations on the central nervous system. If the certainly important central system is less endangered during labor than otherwise assumed, a variety of other organs and functions still exist which may very well suffer from hypoxia and acidosis.

As we demonstrated, there is a close connection between manifest acidosis and the overall well-being of the infant. In the literature several authors report about the dangers of severe hypoxia, e.g. Shankaran *et al.*[21] and Low *et al.*[22]

According to these considerations fetuses at hypoxic risk should therefore be identified as early as possible for instance shortly after abnormal CTG appears and long before a dangerous chock syndrome with all its pathological consequences can develop in fetal organ systems.

Intermittent character of FBA

This so-called disadvantageous property of FBA is compensated to a certain degree by the fact that most intrauterine complications – more than 90% – progress so slowly[23] that there is enough time to detect the disturbance also under such conditions of intermittent diagnostic insight and to react properly in the clinical routine, i.e. if one consequently follows the CTG, and, if abnormal patterns occur, the obstetrician starts early enough with fetal blood sampling.

Methods for continuous measurement of pH, PO_2 and PCO_2 (sometimes simultaneously) have been under development for more than 20 years. These measurements have mainly contributed to the understanding of the physiologic status of the fetus.[24] No method has up to now been convincingly reliable or suitable for use in routine practice. The electrodes commonly used for continuous tissue pH measurements have been unsatisfactory for a number of reasons.

They are large, fragile and tend to become detached. Continuous transcutaneous PO_2 monitoring is still unsatisfactory.[25] The occurrence of caput succedaneum and compression of the electrode influence the reliability of these measurements. Transcutaneous PCO_2 monitoring looked the most promising from a theoretical and technical point of view, but the problems common to all methods of continuous biochemical monitoring still have to be solved.[26] None of these new techniques has been tried in more than a relatively small group of fetuses.

The newly available sensor for spectroscopy (NIR) (modified laser spectroscopy) for fetal physiologic measurements provides information about biochemical parameters and is potentially an additional technique for fetal surveillance.[27] Using laser spectroscopy, it was possible to trace changes in absorbances at four different wavelengths and to calculate relative changes of HbO_2, desaturated hemoglobin, total hemoglobin, and cytochrome aa_3. NIR has been used as a research tool and holds the promise of a non-invasive surveillance providing continues monitoring. Up to now NIR is not clinically accessible with an adequate monitor and sensor.[20]

Pulse oximetry allows measurements of oxygen saturation. It is based on the premise that light transmission by blood varies with the change in blood volume in a tissue with each pulse of a fetal sensor (SpO_2). The sensor is placed against the fetal cheek. Studies indicate that results may be obtained from 2 cm dilation in between 45% and 60% of cases.[29] Although results vary between studies, a SaO_2 of more than 30% is indicative of fetal well-being as this is the level below which anaerobic respiration begins.[30,31]

More recently this borderline has been validated further by the demonstration that SaO_2 of less than 30% for longer than 10 min correlated well with low scalp pH if the signal loss is limited.[32] A prospective randomized trial implicates a reduction in cesarean section rates in cases with pathologic heart rate pattern.[33] A further improvement of the sensor for routine application seems essential, since a reliable SpO_2 signal is precondition. The reliability during clinical applications to detect disturbances early enough has been questioned.[34,35]

Frequency of false-positive findings with fetal monitoring during labor

It is the aim of clinical obstetrical care to perform an operative delivery in those cases where the risk is adequately identified. Due to the large number of false-positive heart rate patterns the considerable increase of unnecessary interventions during continuous electronic monitoring is a logical consequence. FBA as additional biochemical method is particularly suitable to resolve this problem. Van den Berg *et al.*[36] showed how convincingly the rate of cases with false-positive findings can be reduced by means of combined supervision with FBA.

A misleading clinical conclusion is to consider infants who were born in a good condition after intrapartum pathology as diagnostically false-positive cases, as has for instance been described by Sykes *et al.*[37] The inevitable confusion resulting from this has led to some scientifically untenable conclusions. The aim of supervising the fetus during labor is to recognize threatening, real fetal distress situations, namely falling pH values, and to draw the correct clinical conclusions before the infant has gone into a state of depression due to hypoxia or has become severely acidotic. From the special study which we performed, the frequency of correct positive findings was 94% out of 110 controlled cases using additional fetal blood sampling.[13]

Critical appraisal of prospective studies on fetal monitoring during labor

In spite of the evidence of the benefit of the additional use of the FBA during fetal monitoring in prospective randomized trials its clinical use is not generally accepted.[38] This obvious discrepancy between scientific findings and clinical acceptance has been discussed in recent publications.[39]

Perhaps, it can be explained by the characteristics of the papers mentioned on prospective randomized trials concerning fetal monitoring. Sometimes one gets the impression that it would be more worthwhile to examine what went wrong in the application, or in the performance of such prospective studies. It seems that a number of researchers prefer to use highly sophisticated statistical rather than established clinical methods. For our critical appraisal we have chosen two studies particularly often cited in the past. In the study by Haverkamp *et al.*[40] the groups were small. The termination of labor in cases of fetal distress was performed late, namely when fetal acidosis was already present. Consequently, the overall number of acidotic and depressed newborns was high. The important finding in Haverkamp *et al.*'s study was the reduction of operative deliveries using FBA, compared with the use of CTG without FBA.

In the frequently cited largest prospective Dublin study,[41] only umbilical vein blood samples were used. However, it is well known that such samples are not representative for the fetal condition compared with umbilical artery blood. Blood in the umbilical vein has passed the placenta and has accordingly been changed in its composition. Thus it cannot reflect the situation in fetal tissues as umbilical artery blood can after it has passed parts of the fetal body. Moreover, the pH measurement in umbilical blood was performed in only 500 of the 6500 cases. If one projects the differences found between the examined groups to all the cases in this study, then an apparently significant difference can be established, i.e. not only a significantly higher incidence of seizures of newborns was found in the Dublin study in the auscultation group, but also a significantly higher number of acidotic newborn (pH $<$ 7.1) must have been present. These important results have, as far as we know neither been stated in the publication concerned nor recognized by any other author who has cited this study.

How do the results of prospective randomized trials correlate with large databases?

The evaluation of a perinatal survey in Germany that included a large number ($>$ 500,000) of cases focused on death rate of mature infants in the intrapartum and perinatal period as well as during the first days of life. The authors found that structural problems in small obstetrical units ($<$ 500 deliveries per year) were the major cause of perinatal death.[42] Furthermore, the data of this survey indicate an improved perinatal outcome in the cases with pathologic heart rate pattern and additional use of FBA in regionalized obstetrical care.

Direct comparisons of electronic fetal monitoring, with and without additional FBA, show that access to scalp sampling reduces the number of cesareans due to fetal distress, with no clear differences in neonatal outcome. Data from indirect comparisons point both to better maternal and better neonatal outcome if FBA is used.

Subjective considerations of FBA

Fetal blood analysis is sometimes exposed to subjective considerations such as 'it is labor intensive' or 'it is inconvenient for the mother'. But in view of the incomparable higher expenses caused by unnecessary caesarean sections, which can be prevented by FBA, such opinions must be seen as subordinate and objectively as untenable.

The interpretation of the results and drawing the consequences – clinical measures after FBA – are relatively simple. Thus the use of FBA might be enhanced when the given evidence of benefit is adequately addressed.

Future prospects

In the future, we will probably discontinue the subjective visual interpretation of fetal heart rate patterns. More and more a computer-assisted evaluation will take place which allows a more objective assessment. For the antepartum supervision such a Sonicaid system, developed by Dawes and Redman at Oxford University has been available since 1977. In the meantime, Sonicaid also prepared a version available for intrapartum use.

Later in 1980, Maeda created a computer software for an automatic fetal heart rate analysis during labor with warning system in case abnormal heart rate patterns occur. Apart from this, a so-called QCTG-program system is available developed by Roemer[*] in Detmold (Germany) and a Trium CTG-Online System developed by M. Daumer[†] in Munich (Germany).

But even with computer assistance, we should be aware that CTG is in principle an indirect biophysical 'detour-method' which we clinicians try to use for the diagnosis of biochemical problems as hypoxia. Therefore the same reliability as can be achieved by FBA, which is a direct biochemical method, cannot be expected from CTG.

This means that the number of false-positive findings by use of computer-assisted CTG will apparently be reduced, but not definitely eliminated. Thus, for an expert FBA will maintain its clinical value.

Summary

Combined intrapartum electronic–biochemical supervision of the fetus during labor by CTG and FBA was introduced by us in 1968, shortly after the first cardiotocographs became available for widespread clinical application. By using both CTG and, if necessary, additional FBA, it is possible to achieve a minimum of operative deliveries (cesarean sections and difficult vaginal interventions), which is of advantage for both mother and fetus, with an optimum safety for the fetus by minimizing the incidence of hypoxic morbidity. The best suitable blood parameter of FBA is the actual pH value because it reflects the biochemical situation of the fetus in each stage of intrauterine hypoxia. FBA is indicated in all cases when abnormal CTGm shows patterns suspicious of hypoxia. Repetition of FBA depends on the character of the assumed intrauterine disturbance. In acute cases (bradycardia), FBA should be repeated as quickly as possible. All other suspicious heart rate patterns indicate a slower advancing complication. FBA should be repeated depending on the severity of the CTGm pattern within 5–10–15 min. In cases with slow progressive decrease of fetal blood pH, maternogenic acidity increase should be diagnosed and clinically interpreted accordingly.

The aim of modern supervision of the fetus during labor is primarily to minimize short-term morbidity of the fetus and the newborn and secondarily to prevent cerebral palsy and other organ injuries. The intermittent character of FBA can be compensated to a high degree by the fact that most intrauterine complications during labor progress rather slowly and there is generally enough time to detect the disturbance and to react properly within the clinical routine. The frequency of false-positive findings with FBA is much less than erroneously described. Some of the frequently cited prospective studies concerning fetal monitoring during labor have supported the additional use of FBA in cases with pathologic heart rate pattern.

Direct comparisons of electronic fetal monitoring, with and without additional FBA, show that access to scalp sampling reduces the number of cesareans due to fetal distress. Data from indirect comparisons including postnatal morbidity point to both better maternal and better neonatal outcome if FBA is used.

Due to the evidence of the benefit of the additional use of the FBA during fetal monitoring in prospective randomized trials, its clinical value should generally be accepted. The interpretation of the results and drawing the consequences – clinical measures after FBA – are relatively simple. Thus the use of FBA will be enhanced when the given evidence of benefit is adequately addressed. Alternative methods for continuous biochemical monitoring of the fetus such as $tcPO_2$, $tcPCO_2$, pH and NIRS are at this stage not accessible for clinical use.

Pulse oximetry, which has been in discussion during the last few years, could be useful in

*Michael.Roemer@Klinikum-lippe.de

†Trium CTG Online is a class IIb CE-marked product, see <http://www.trium.de>

combination with FBA, in spite of all reservations, provided that SpO_2 sensors could be improved to better prevent registration gaps. Of all the investigated techniques for continuous biochemical monitoring of the fetus, SpO_2 is the only one that proved beneficial during a prospective randomized trail.

In the future, computer-assisted evaluation of heart rate patterns will very probably find more acceptance for a better objective assessment of cardiotocograms in clinical routine. The number of false-positive findings will be reduced, but not definitely eliminated. Thus FBA will maintain its clinical value.

REFERENCES

1. Saling E. Neue Untersuchungsmöglichkeiten des Kindes unter der Geburt. *Zbl Gyn* 1961;83:1906–7.
2. Saling E. Neues Vorgehen zur Untersuchung des Kindes unter der Geburt (Einführung, Technik, Grundlagen). *Arch Gynäkol* 1962;197:108–22.
3. Dobbs RH, Gairdner D. Editorial: Foetal medicine – who is to practise it? *Arch Dis Child* 1966;41:453.
4. Caldeyro-Barcia R. Estudio de la anoxial fetal intrauterina mediante el ECG fetal y el registro continuo de la frecuencia cardiaca fetal. *Proceedings of III Cong Latinoamerican Obstetrics Gynecology*, Mexico, 1958;2:383.
5. Hon EH. A fetal electrographic electrode. *Yale J Biol Med* 1966; 39:54.
6. Saling E, Arabin B. Historic landmarks of perinatal medicine in obstetrics. *J Perinat Med* 1988;16:5–21.
7. Saling E. Elektronische und biochemische Überwachung des Feten unter der Geburt. *Bull Soc R Belge Gynecol Obstet* 1968; 38:289–99.
8. Saling E, Dudenhausen JW. The present situation of clinical monitoring of the fetus during labor. *J Perinat Med* 1973;1:75–103.
9. Saling E. Fetal scalp blood analysis. *J Perinat Med* 1981;9:165–77.
10. Saling E. Introduction and clinical aspects of biochemical monitoring of the fetus. *J Perinat Med* 1988;16(Suppl 1):23–47.
11. Saling E, Langner K. Fetal acid-base measurement in labor. In Spencer John AD, ed. *Fetal Monitoring.* Tunbridge Wells: Castle House Publications Ltd, 1989.
12. Saling E, Bartnicki J. Clinical importance of biochemical monitoring of the fetus during labor with demonstration of typical cases. In Chatterjee MS, ed. *Biochemical Monitoring of the Fetus.* New York, Berlin: Springer, 1993:1–12.
13. Brandt-Niebelschütz S, Saling E. Indications for operative termination of labor on cardiotocography and fetal blood analysis: The reliability of these methods. *J Perinat Med* 1994;22:19–27.
14. Goeschen K, Gruner T, Saling E. Stellenwert des Hammacher-Scores und der Fetalblutanalyse bei der subpartualen Überwachung des Kindes. *Z Geburtsh Perinat* 1984;188:12–20.
15. Donker DK, van Geijn HP, Hasmann A. Interobserver variation in the assessment of fetal heart rate recordings. *Eur J Obstet Gynecol Reprod Biol* 1993;52:21–8.
16. van Geijn HP, Donker DK, Hasmann A, for Nestec Ltd, Switzerland. How objective is visual evaluation of antepartum and intrapartum cardiotocograms? In Saling E, ed. *Perinatology, Nestlé Nutrition Workshop Series*, Vol. 26. New York: Raven Press Ltd, 1992:67–77.
17. Saling E. Combined intrapartum fetal supervision if the fetus by heart rate monitoring and biochemical control, including pulse oximetry. In Kurjak A, ed. *Textbook of Perinatal Medicine – A Comprehensive Guide to Modern Clinical Perinatology.* London, New York: The Parthenon Publishing Group, 1998.
18. Rooth G, McBride R, Ivy BJ. Fetal and maternal pH measurements. *Acta Obstet Gynecol Scand* 1973;52:47–50.
19. Goeschen K, Höhn R, Dudenhausen JW, Saling E. Ansäuerung des Feten durch die Mutter sub partu und klinische Konsequenzen. *Z Geburtsh Perinat* 1984;188:68–73.
20. Grant A. Monitoring the fetus during labour. In Chalmers I, Enkin M, eds. *Effective Care in Pregnancy and Childbirth*, Vol. 2. Oxford New York, Toronto: Marc J.N.C. Kreirse Archie Cochrane, 1991.
21. Shankaran S, Woldt E, Koepke T, *et al.* Acute neonatal morbidity and long-term central nervous system sequelae of perinatal asphyxia in term infants. *Early Hum Dev* 1991;25:135–48.
22. Low JA, Panagiotopolous C, Derrick EJ. Newborn complications after intrapartum asphyxia with metabolic acidosis in the term fetus. *Am J Obstet Gynecol* 1994;170:1081–7.
23. Saling E, Schneider D. Biochemical supervision of the foetus during labor. *J Obstet Gynaecol Br Commonw* 1967;74:799–811.
24. Braun T, Sierra F, Seiler D, Schmidt S. Continuous telemetric monitoring of fetal oxygen partial pressure during labor. *Arch Gynecol Obstet* 2004;270:40–5.
25. Huch A, Huch R, Schneider H, Rooth G. Continuous transcutaneous monitoring of fetal oxygen tension during labor. *Br J Obstet Gynecol* 1984;84:4–39.
26. Schmidt S, Saling E. The continuous measurement of transcutaneous carbon dioxide tension (TcPCOs), an atraumatic tool to verify fetal acidosis? *Br J Obstet Gynecol* 1987;94:963–6.
27. Schmidt S. Laser spectroscopy in the fetus during labor. *Eur J Obstet Gynecol* 2003;110:127–31.
28. Aldrichs Ch, Wyatt JS, Spencer JAD, Reynolds EOR, Delepy DT. The effect of maternal oxygen administration on human fetal cerebral oxygenation measured during labour by near infrared spectroscopy. *Br J Obstet Gynecol* 1994;101:509–13.
29. Dildy G, Thop J, Yeast J, Clark S. The relationship between oxygen saturation and pH in umbilical blood: Implications for intrapartum fetal oxygen saturation monitoring. *Am J Obstet Gynecol* 1996; 175:682–7.
30. Seelbach-Göbel B, Butterwegge M, Kühnert M, Heupel M. Fetale Reflektionspulsoxymetrie sub partu, Erfahrungen – Prognostische Bedeutung und Konsequenz – Ziele. Z Geburtsh Perinat 1994; 198:67–71.
31. Seelbach-Göbel B. Beurteilung der cerebralen Sauert-stoffversorgung des Feten sub partu durch Pulsoxymetrie und Nahinfrarotspektroskopie. In Butterwegge M, ed. Fetale Pulsoxymetrie sub partu. Stuttgart: Enke, 1996:62–78.
32. Kühnert M, Seelbach-Göbel B, Butterwegge M. Predictive agreement between the fetal arterial oxygen saturation and fetal scalp-pH: Results of the German multicenter study. *Am J Obstet Gynecol* 1998;178:330–5.
33. Garite TJ, Dildy GA, McNamara H. A multicenter controlled trial of fetal pulse oximetry in the intrapartum management of non reassuring fetal heart rate patterns. *Am J Obstet Gynecol* 2000; 183:1049–1058.
34. Schmidt S, Koslowski S, Sierra F, Meyer-Wittkopf M, Heller G. Clinical usefulness of pulse oximetry in the fetus with non-reassuring heart rate patterns? *J Perinat Med* 2000;28:298–305.
35. Luttkus AK, Callsen TA, Stupin JH, Dudenhausen JW. Pulse oximetry during labour does it give rise to hope? Value of saturation monitoring in comparison to fetal blood gas status. *Eur J Obstet Gynecol* 2003;110:132–8.
36. van den Berg P, Schmidt S, Gesche J, Saling E. Fetal distress and the condition of the newborn using cardiotocography and fetal blood analysis during labour. *Br J Obstet Gynaecol* 1987;94:72–5.
37. Sykes GS, Molloy PM, Johnson P, *et al.* Fetal distress and the condition of the newborn infant. *Br Med J* 1983;287:943-5.
38. Goodwin TM, Milner-Masterson L, Paul PH. Elimination of fetal scalp blood sampling on a large clinical service. *Obstet Gynecol* 1994;83:971–4.
39. Parer JT. Obstetric technologies: What determines clinical acceptance or rejection of results of randomized controlled trials? *Am J Obstet Gynecol* 2003;188(6):1622–8.
40. Haverkamp D, Orleans M, Langendoerfer S, *et al.* A controlled trial of the differential effects of intrapartum fetal monitoring. *Am J Obstet Gynecol* 1979;134:399–408.
41. Donald DM, Grand A, Sheridan-Pereira M, Boylan P, Chalmers I. The Dublin randomized controlled trial of intrapartum fetal heart rate monitoring. *Am J Obstet Gynecol* 1985;152:524–39.
42. Heller G, Misselwitz B, Schmidt S. Early neonatal mortality, asphyxia-related deaths and timing of low risk births in Hesse, Germany, 1990–1998. *Br Med J* 2000;321:274–5.

SECTION XVI

Multiple pregnancy and delivery

Section Editors: **J. W. Dudenhausen and I. Blickstein**

145 The epidemiology of multiple births

R. Derom, J. Orlebeke and A. Eriksson

Secular trends

The number of twins born per 1000 pregnancies differs considerably between different parts of the world as well as between different periods of time. In Europe and North America, for example, the twinning rate averaged between 12 and 14 per 1000 maternities during the first seven decades of the 20th century. In contrast, it was only about six per 1000 in Japan[1] and about 40 per 1000 in Nigeria[2,3] during these same years. In addition, the twinning rate has varied widely over the past three centuries in those countries where twin births were registered. In Scandinavian countries, epidemiologists have at their disposal registers of births that are kept for centuries by the churches. From these old data sets, it appears that, prior to 1900, several albeit unknown conditions led to considerably higher twinning rates than have been recorded in the 20th century. In the Scandinavian countries, for example, the frequency of twin births was about 17 per 1000 maternities during the second part of the 18th century and even higher (more than 20 per 1000) in areas with a low migration rate, such as the islands in the Baltic Sea.[4] The fluctuations in twinning rate over the last 250 years in Sweden are illustrated in Figure 145.1.

Since 1900, the twinning rate in most European countries has stabilized at around 11–13 per 1000. Official figures for the Netherlands, kept by the governmental Central Bureau of Statistics since 1907, are presented in Figure 145.2, and exemplify the general Western European trend from the 19th to 20th century.

The decreasing twinning rate from the previous to the current century has presumably to be ascribed to the disappearance of isolated societies within nations and the concomitant process of industrialization and urbanization.[5] An even more important reason for the gradual decline in the number of multiple pregnancies could be the lowering of mean maternal age and the smaller total number of maternities per woman (parity). When twinning rates in different countries and different years are corrected for differences in maternal age and parity, temporal and regional variations in the twinning rate can still be observed.[5–7] This has been convincingly documented for Sweden during the period 1870–1970[8,9] (Figure 145.3), a 100-year period uncontaminated by modern obstetric techniques for the improvement of fertility.

After about 1960, a sudden rapid decline in the twinning rate was observed in most European countries. The nadir of this decline occurred in the middle of the 1970s when twinning rates fell to between nine and 10 per 1000 maternities. Beyond that point, an equally rapid recovery to the pre-1960 figures, or even to the high values of the 19th century in recent years, took place. The U-shape of these shifts between 1960 and 1990 in six representative countries can be seen in Figure 145.4.

Such a remarkable and fast change in an otherwise rather stable biological phenomenon, presenting itself in nearly the same manner in several countries, is challenging. There is strong evidence that the decline in twinning rate between 1960 and 1975 can be predominantly ascribed to a parallel drop in maternal

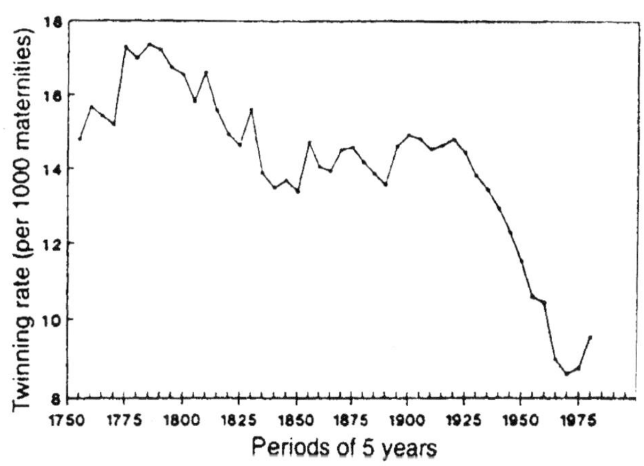

Figure 145.1 Secular variations in twinning rate in Sweden between 1756 and 1990; data are averaged per 5-year period.

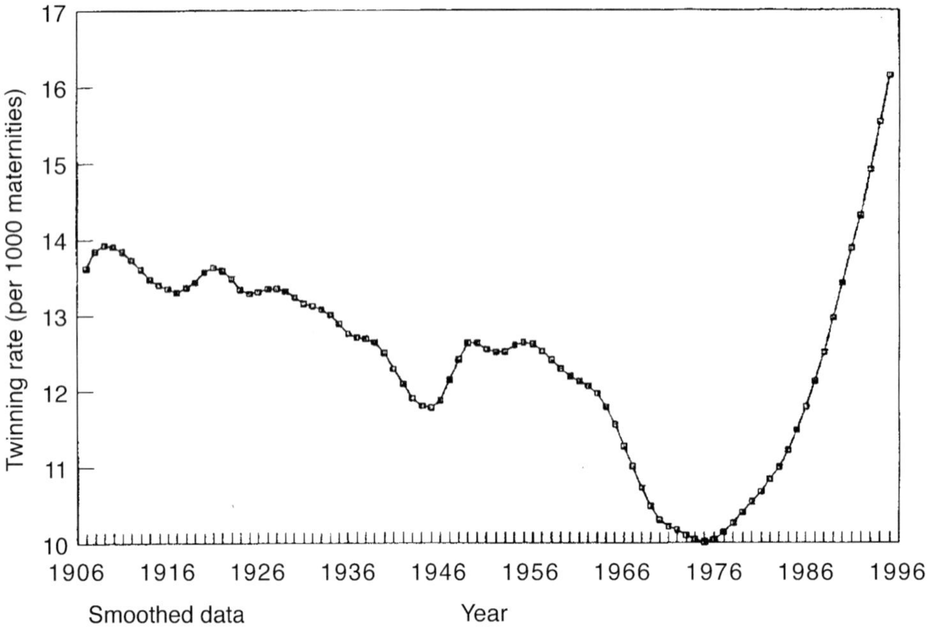

Figure 145.2 Total twinning rate in the Netherlands during 1907–1995.

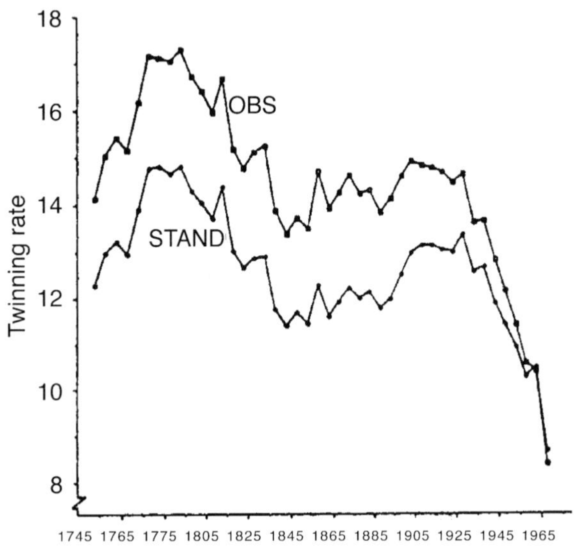

Figure 145.3 Secular variations in twinning rate in Sweden between 1751 and 1970: upper curve gives observed values (corresponding to those in Figure 145.1); lower curve represents same data, corrected for effect on twinning rate of changes in the maternal age. OBS, observed; STAND, standardized.

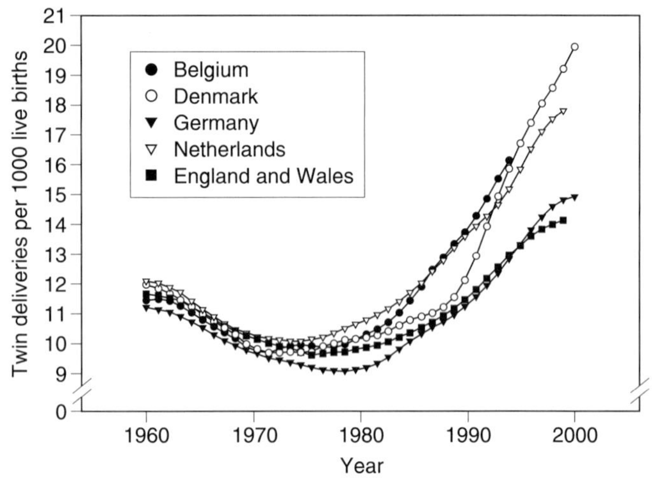

Figure 145.4 Twinning rates between 1960 and 2002 for six European countries.

age at delivery. We have tested this for the Netherlands. Several investigators[10,11] have shown that the probability of a dizygotic (DZ) twin pregnancy doubles in mothers between 35 and 40 years of age compared with mothers below 25. In the Netherlands, the 1960–1975 fall in the total twinning rate was accompanied by a parallel decline in maternal age at delivery. Figure 145.5 shows both the maternal age and the twinning rate changes over time.

As can be seen in Figure 145.5, the increase in the twinning rate after about 1984 is stronger than might be expected from the continuing increase in general maternal age. This 'additional' growth is very likely due to the increasing influence of modern obstetric technology. The excess number of twin pairs (i.e. more than may be expected from the quantitative relationship between the twinning rate and the proportion of deliveries by mothers $\geq$30 years) was about 300 in 1990, or about 10% of all twin pairs born in that year. This number equals the outcome of an independent calculation carried out by Merkus (personal communication) based on the number of women treated with hormones, in most cases clomiphene citrate (Clomid®). Or, to put it another way, the left

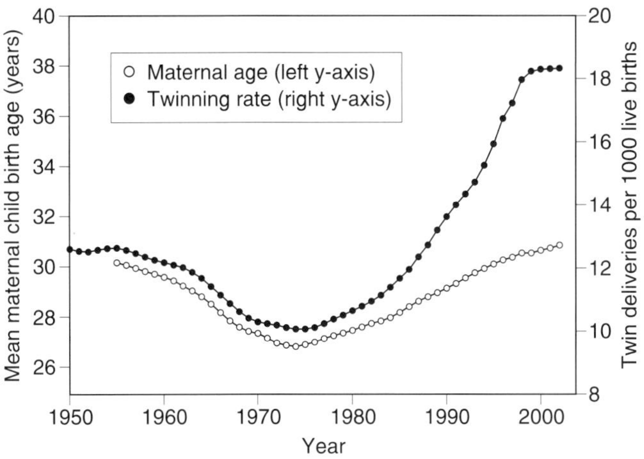

Figure 145.5 Correspondence in the Netherlands between changes in twinning rate and changes in maternal age (operational as percentage of maternities from mothers of 30 years and over). Recent years show disproportional growth in twinning rate relative to increase in maternal age.

sides of the U-shaped curves in Figures 145.4 and 145.5 very likely reflect only the influence of a rapid change in the mean age at which women become pregnant (an interesting societal phenomenon, manifest in most European countries: mean maternal age in the Netherlands, for example, was 30.2 years in 1995; maternal age at first pregnancy was 28.6 years on average; both these figures were never so high during the 20th century). In contrast, the right sides of the Us are produced by a combination of the increase in maternal age and the application of fertility-improving techniques. The relative contribution of these two factors (from the mid-1970s until the present) obviously varies between countries.

Zygosity

Figures 145.4 and 145.5 present data on all twin maternities. The question of to what degree the epidemiological changes in twin prevalence cited above are related to the occurrence of DZ twins, monozygotic (MZ) twins or both cannot be answered unequivocally. Zygosity of a twin can be ascertained with reasonable reliability with the aid of testing for blood groups or DNA. For epidemiological purposes, these methods, however, cannot be used for both practical and budget reasons. A classic method used frequently to estimate the relative contribution of MZ and DZ twin maternities to the total twinning rate was proposed by Weinberg[12,13] and applied many times since. According to this Weinberg rule, the number of MZ twin births equals the difference between all twin births and twice the number of twin births of unlike-sexed twin pairs. This method assumes that the number of unlike-sexed DZ twin pairs equals that of like-sexed twin pairs. Applying this method to a year-to-year time series of twin maternities in a given country consistently demonstrates that the changes in total twinning rate can predominantly be ascribed to changes in DZ twinning rate. In contrast, the MZ rate varies much less and hovers around 4 per 1000 maternities. Figure 145.6 gives the results of the application of Weinberg's rule to recent twin prevalence figures in England and Wales, and in the Netherlands.

Figure 145.6 also shows that the MZ twinning rate increased slightly after 1975. This trend has been recorded in several countries.[14] The hypothesis that the use of oral contraceptives is responsible for this phenomenon[15] appears to be untenable because, in several countries, the increase in the MZ rate began before the (widespread) use of oral contraceptives, whereas in others it started later. A different explanation was proposed by Orlebeke and colleagues,[16] who contend that the rise in the MZ twinning rate is the artificial consequence of another phenomenon, that is, the decrease in twin maternities of unlike sex relative to the number of DZ like-sexed twin maternities. If the latter hypothesis is true, then Weinberg's differential rule loses its basic assumption, that is, the equality of DZ like-sex and DZ unlike-sex prevalence. A relatively low number of DZ unlike-sexed twin pairs automatically leads the Weinberg method to overestimation of the MZ rate.[16] Several other authors have also expressed doubt about the DZ like-sex/DZ unlike-sex equality assumption,[17–20] but still others[21,22] opine that the assumption underlying Weinberg's rule is correct, at least in some countries. The discussion is not purely academic because the Weinberg rule is the major tool available for the study of trends in MZ and DZ twinning rates. A lively debate exists, which we will try to summarize in the following paragraphs.

A number of authors[16–20] adhere for several reasons to the hypothesis of a change in the proportion of like/unlike-sex DZ twinning, a change leading to a flaw of the Weinberg rule. First, if one considers the Weinberg-based year-to-year time series of DZ and MZ twinning rates, then a basic prerequisite for the justification of the use of the Weinberg rule is the absence of a correlation between the two series. This is so because the underlying mechanisms of MZ and DZ twinning are unrelated. Only if some common external factor would influence the frequency of MZ and DZ twinning or if the assumption about equality of DZ like-sex and DZ unlike-sex frequencies is incorrect could a correlation between the two time series be expected. Orlebeke and colleagues[16] calculated this correlation for the Netherlands (period 1904–1989), Denmark (1910–1985), Sweden (1961–1985) and Norway (1931–1985). The Pearson correlations for each country were $r=-0.69$, $r=-0.42$, $r=-0.56$ and $r=-0.12$, respectively. A closer look at the data additionally reveals that the calculated MZ twinning rate has increased very slowly from the beginning of the 20th century until the present decade. Stated

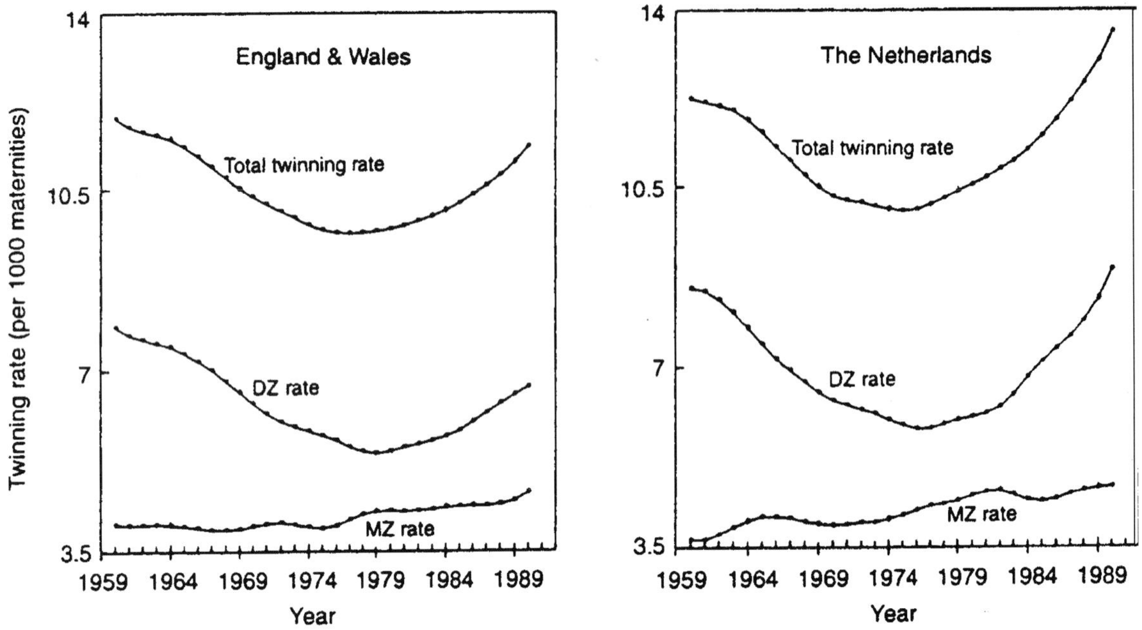

Figure 145.6 Application of Weinberg's differential rule to twin prevalence figures in England and Wales and in the Netherlands, 1959–1989, DZ, dizygotic; MZ, monozygotic.

another way, the increase in 'Weinberg-estimated' MZ frequency is not a recent phenomenon (although it has gone up during the past decade), but rather seems to have been present since the beginning of the 20th century. In Germany, for example, the MZ twinning rate was about 3.25 per 1000 during the second decade of the 20th century, 3.70 during the 1960s and about 4.4 during the past few years. A comparable trend is present in the Netherlands: 3.50 per 1000 around 1915, 3.90 in the 1960s and 4.60 during the past few years. In Denmark, these figures are 3.67, 4.40 and 4.60, respectively, and for England and Wales 3.38 during the early 1940s (we did not analyze older data), 3.55 during the 1960s and 4.50 in recent years. These arbitrarily selected examples make plausible the concept that a gradual shift in the Weinberg estimations of MZ twinning rate is not a phenomenon of the past one or two decades, but rather one that was present long before the introduction of oral contraceptives and ovulation-inducing drugs, although the latter might be held responsible for the very fast changes in MZ rate during the past decade.

Second, analysis of secular variations in sex combinations of twins in the Åland and the Åboland archipelagos (of Finland) demonstrate that the estimated rate of MZ twin maternities increased consistently during the six 50-year periods between 1650 and 1949.[23] It remains possible that this observation is the result of incompleteness of registrations. Mistakes and omissions in the registrations may diminish the proportion of MZ twins, because the frequency of stillbirths is higher among MZ than among DZ twins.

The above-mentioned negative correlation between the DZ and MZ time series, combined with the observations of James[20] and others, strongly suggests that the observed MZ twinning rate increase can be ascribed to a gradual shift in the DZ unlike/like-sex ratio from about unity (or maybe even higher) during roughly the first half of the 20th century to less than unity in later years. Another indication that the number of unlike-sex twin pairs is decreasing comes from the following observation. In all countries from which the total twinning rate is presented in Figure 145.4 the proportion of unlike-sexed pairs, relative to all twin pairs, is consistently higher (about 30.5%) during the period of a decreasing total twinning rate between about 1965 and 1975 relative to the comparable right part of the curve (about 29%). In other words, when the total twinning rate is the same, then DZ unlike-sex twinning rate declines nevertheless. This trend is summarized in Table 145.1. It is possible that this observation reflects an increasing MZ rate. Figures from the Dutch Twin Register, however, support the former interpretation. Of 4186 twin pairs in the register (all children below the age of 6), zygosity was assessed with the help of a questionnaire filled out by the parents. The parents of 392 twin pairs did not answer the questions (mostly because they were too uncertain). From the remaining 4186 pairs, 986 were classified as MZ, 1740 as DZ like-sex and 1460 as DZ unlike-sex. Application of the Weinberg rule would lead to an estimated number of MZ twins of 1266 (instead of 986) and a number of DZ twins of 2920 (instead of 3200).

Table 145.1 Mean proportion of dizygotic (DZ) unlike-sex twin pairs relative to all twin pairs

Country	Period 1	Period 2
Belgium	29.9%	27.8%
Denmark	30.4%	28.6%
England and Wales	30.4%	28.6%
Netherlands	30.9%	29.4%
West Germany	31.0%	28.9%

Period 1: period of decreasing total twinning rate; period 2: comparable subsequent period of increasing total twinning rate

The first group of authors[16–20] conclude that there must be some mechanism that has led to a decrease of the number of DZ unlike-sex twin pairs relative to the number of DZ like-sex pairs. The nature of that mechanism is still unclear; it has produced an artificial enhancement in the Weinberg-based estimations of MZ twinning rate during the past 10–20 years compared with earlier years. It is possible that the assumption of a constant MZ rate is better for the calculation of zygosity proportions than Weinberg's assumption that DZ unlike-and like-sex numbers are equal.

An opposite view has been put forward by a second group of authors who do not consider the presence of a correlation between the MZ and DZ twinning rates as a reason to invalidate the Weinberg rule. Bulmer,[24] writing in 1970, stated: 'It should be observed that *m* (the MZ rate) and *d* (the DZ rate) are negatively correlated since the number of unlike-sexed twins occurs in the formulas for both of them but with a different sign. This negative correlation means that *m* is likely to be an overestimate of the true value when *d* is an underestimate, and vice versa', Moreover, in a large population-based registry of multiple births, the East Flanders Prospective Twin Survey (EFPTS),[22] no reason was found to invalidate Weinberg's rule. This survey is characterized by accurate zygosity determinations. A total of 2589 twin pairs were investigated, of which 2577 were of known zygosity and placentation. The estimates of Weinberg's rule agreed well with the results of the direct zygosity determination. As pointed out by James,[25] in the East Flanders study, the area of uncertainty could be reduced in the group in which zygosity diagnosis is most difficult, that is, the group of same-sexed dichorionic pairs. In such pairs, monozygosity cannot be diagnosed with certainty. In each pair, according to the number of similar markers, a probability of monozygosity should be computed, which should reach at least 0.95 and, ideally, more than 0.99. In the EFPTS study, about one-half of the 401 same-sex dichorionic pairs classified as monozygotic had probabilities of monozygosity of less than 0.95. Husby and coworkers[26] describing a Danish series of 352 consecutive pairs in which direct determination of zygosity was performed, also came to the conclusion that their data were consistent with Weinberg's formulation. James[25] concludes his critical analysis by stating, 'The conclusion of both sets of authors that their data at present are consistent with Weinberg's rule is true but they are also consistent with the hypothesis that the rule is appreciably flawed'.

As suggested by James,[25] one way to solve the controversy would be to retest/those pairs (or those who survive), especially those with lower probabilities of monozygosity. The uncertain pairs would then be rediagnosed as DZ or reassigned a higher probability of monozygosity. Another way would be to perform population-based studies of placentation. Two-thirds of MZ twins are monochorionic. It follows that the number of MZ twins can be calculated by multiplying the number of monochorionic twins by 1.5.

Recent data of EFPTS[1] on a greater number of twin pairs ($n=5703$) and a lower number of uncertain zygosity pairs ($n=117$) confirmed the former results. In addition, the spontaneous twins and the iatrogenic twins were considered separately. The results in both groups validated Weinberg's rule. So, the second group of authors firmly recommends the use of the rule in population-based studies, at least in Caucasian populations. They also doubt that, in recent decades, the proportion of DZ-unlike sex and DZ-like sex differs from unity.

Prevalence of triplets

Compared to the change in twinning rates during the past 20 years (about 30–50% produced by an increasing maternal age and by use of fertility-enhancing techniques), the increase in triplet deliveries has been much more dramatic. In England and Wales and in West Germany, the triplet rate increased about 170% between 1975 and 1990. In the Netherlands, the increase was more than 300% and in Belgium (figures only available until 1988), the increase was still higher. Figure 145.7 depicts the triplet rates between 1971 and 1990 for the countries mentioned above.

Without doubt, ovulation induction and *in vitro* fertilization (IVF) are the principal causes of this change. Data on the etiology of triplet maternities were collected for 112 triplet sets born between the end of 1986 and the summer of 1991. All sets were part of the Dutch Twin Register. Only 30 sets were spontaneous; 39 were induced and 39 the result of IVF. Four sets were of unknown etiology. Most of the excess triplet sets are trizygotic (TZ). The epidemiological counterpart of the Weinberg rule for the estimation of zygosity proportions among triplets was proposed by Allen in 1960:[28]

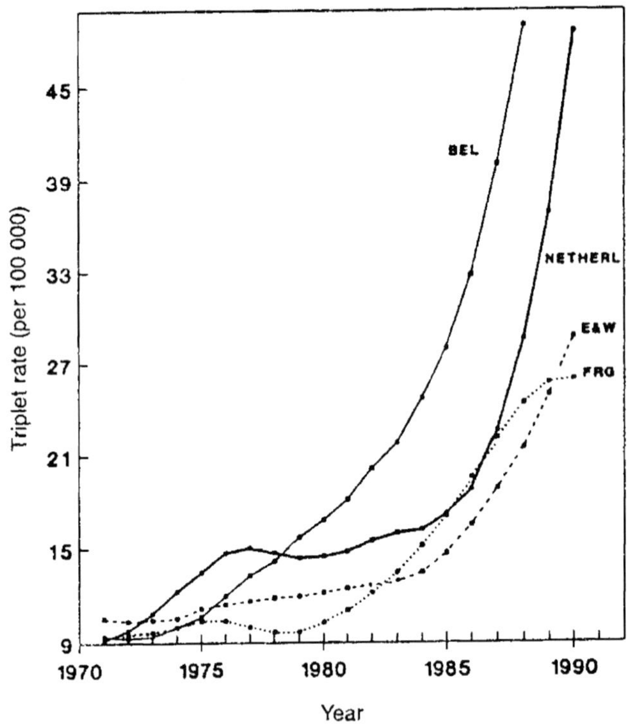

Figure 145.7 Changes in triplet rate during 1971–1990 in four European countries. BEL, Belgium; NETHERL, the Netherlands; E&W, England and Wales; FRG, Germany.

$$\text{Number of MZ triplets} = L - \frac{1}{2}D - \frac{1}{4}T$$

$$\text{Number of DZ triplets} = D = 2\ (\text{MZ twinning rate} \times \text{DZ twinning rate})N$$

$$\text{Number of TZ triplets} = T = (U - \frac{1}{2}D)\ 1/3$$

In these formulas, L is the number of like-sex triplets, U is the number of unlike-sex triplets and N is the total number of maternities. Application of the Allen formula to all triplets born in about the same period as the 112 registered triplet sets leads to estimated proportions of 4.5% MZ, 20.3% DZ and 75.2% TZ. This corresponds rather well with the empirical proportions among the registered 112 triplets: 6.3%, 21.4% and 72.3%, respectively. The Allen method, thus, seems to be a useful approximation for the estimation of zygosity rates in triplets. If we apply the method to triplet prevalence figures from before 1970 (i.e. when ovulation induction and IVF were still unknown or at least not widely used), zygosity proportions appear to be rather different from those of today, roughly about 20% of all triplets estimated to be MZ, 40% DZ and 40% TZ.[28] In other words, modern obstetrical technology has not only increased the triplet rate in general, but has also changed the proportional contributions of zygosity types to the total number of triplets.

Factors determining rates

Twinning rates are influenced by genetic and environmental factors. Some of the latter are undoubtedly related, a circumstance that increases the difficulty of assessing the importance of each factor on its own. Moreover, the actions of genes and the environment are interrelated in some instances. Finally, highly significant temporal fluctuations also impact on many of these environmental variables. As a result, great caution is required before assigning a significant role to any of the environmental variables discussed below.

In addition, at least in most industrialized countries, as will be discussed later in this chapter, iatrogenic twinning rates have reached such proportions that sensible studies can no longer be performed on a number of factors such as maternal age, parity, geographical variation, seasonality and genetics. Vital statistics, for instance, will be strongly biased unless the spontaneous and the induced sets of multiplets can be distinguished. Except in East Flanders, Belgium[30] such data are not available.

Maternal age

Duncan,[31] the famous Scottish obstetrician, was clearly aware of the relationship between maternal age and twinning frequency. In 1865, he stated, 'From the earliest childbearing period till the age of 40 is reached, that is till a period when fecundity has become extraordinarily diminished the fertility of mothers in twins gradually increases'.

Waterhouse[32] analyzed the total births in England and Wales for the 10-year period 1938–1948 in an attempt to understand how the twinning rate varies with maternal age and parity (Figure 145.8). Clearly, increased maternal age and increasing parity exert separate and independent positive influences on the twinning rates. However, recent data from the USA do not corroborate the British findings (Figure 145.9). According to data from Taffel,[33] only in first US births does the twinning rate increase with maternal age. In subsequent live births, the rates either remain approximately at the same level or fall. This contrast is of interest and obviously must be explained. To begin with the respective periods of observation differ by almost 40–50 years (between 1938–1948 and 1987). During this time, essentially the second half of the 20th century, the entire way of life has changed dramatically. Of all possible changes, the status of women and their reproductive behavior has been modified in ways that could hardly have been conceived in the first part of the century. Much of this change relates to availability of contraception, age at first pregnancy, abortion on demand, smaller family size, infertility treatment and probably also other factors. Further studies clearly are needed to track down the reasons behind this remarkable new phenomenon in the epidemiology of twinning.

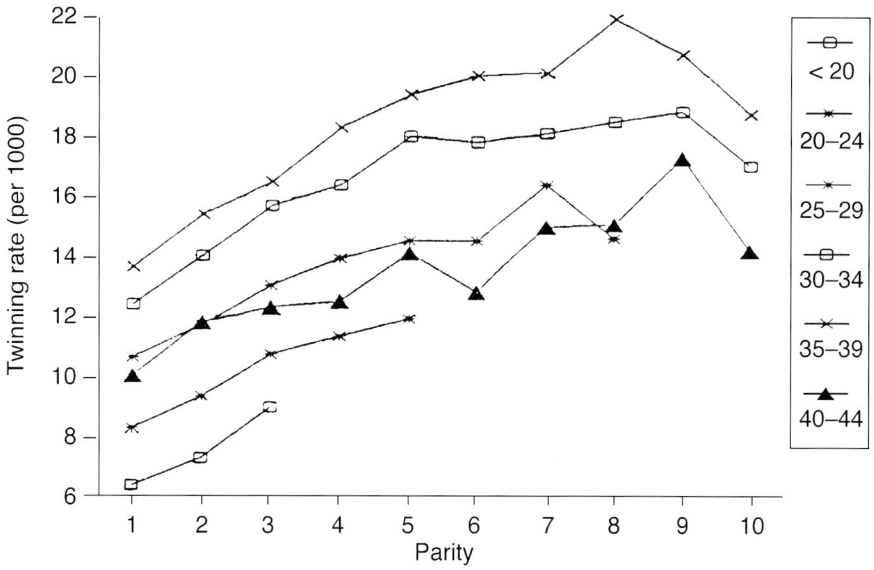

Figure 145.8 Twinning frequency according to maternal age and parity. England and Wales 1938 1948. Drawn from data of Waterhouse.[32]

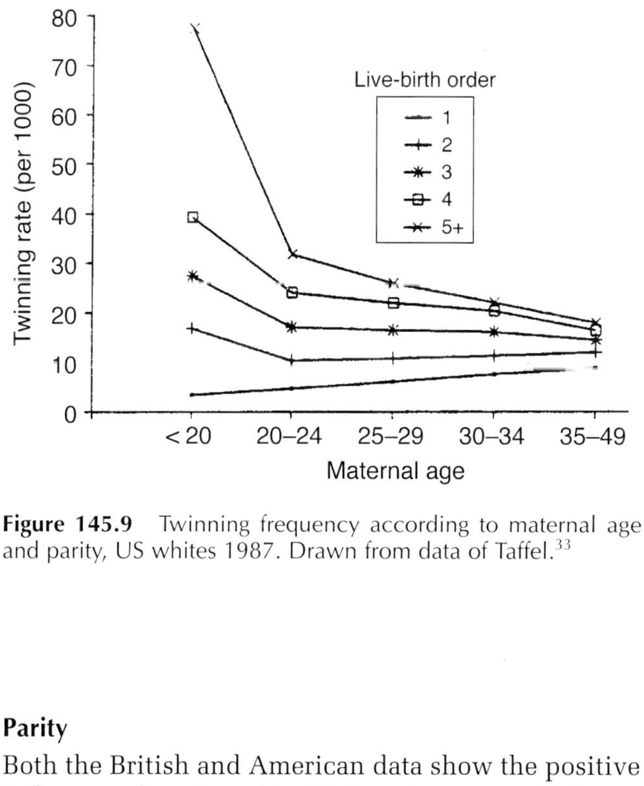

Figure 145.9 Twinning frequency according to maternal age and parity, US whites 1987. Drawn from data of Taffel.[33]

Parity

Both the British and American data show the positive influence of parity or live-birth order, respectively, on the twinning rate. There are no directional changes in these trends, as is the case with maternal age, but substantial changes in magnitude are present. Note, for instance, that in the age bracket of 25–29 years, the rates in 1938–1948 increased by 37% from parity 1 to 4 (Figure 145.8) but this increase amounted to 129% in 1987 (Figure 145.9). This almost three-fold difference will also require explanation by epidemiologists in the future.

It is not possible to determine the exact influence of parity derived from US live-birth certificates, because each live-born twin in a twin delivery is assigned a different, adjacent live-birth order. For example, in a parity 2 twin delivery, the first-born child is assigned live-birth order 2 while the second will be assigned live-birth order 3. Clearly, despite this shortcoming, one may safely surmise that higher parity is associated with increasing prevalence rates of twinning.

Height

As early as 1877, Tchouriloff[34] suggested that an association was present between height and the rate of twinning in a population. He observed that men rejected for military service because of small stature came from various parts of Europe in which the rate of twinning was known to be low. Studies of the height of mothers of MZ and DZ twins, performed in Oxford, England, and Aberdeen, Scotland, respectively, support the hypothesis that mothers of DZ twins are taller than those of MZ twins. In reality, the mean difference between the two groups is estimated at 1.03 ± 0.74 cm: mothers of MZ twins resemble mothers of singletons.[35]

Geographical variation

Studies indicate that the further north, the higher the twinning rate: the relationship, though, is far from close and is limited to DZ twinning. According to James,[36] the correlation coefficient between latitude and age-standardized DZ twinning rates in Europe in the late 1950s and the early 1960s reached a value of $+0.68$ ($P < 0.01$). This trend seems consistent with time, because similar findings had been reported by Davenport[37] in 1930 for the total twinning rate. For US whites, the correlation is +0.54 ($P < 0.001$); for US blacks it is positive (+0.31) but not significant. Bulmer[24] speculated that geographical variations in DZ twinning rates in Europe might have some genetic basis. James[36] observed that there is no reason to suppose that genetic clones in the Old World are duplicated by latitude in the New World. Indeed, the fact that the latitudinal variations in DZ twinning are similar in Europe and the USA suggests an environmental rather than genetic cause.

Superimposed on latitude variations are differences between countries and regions. It is not meaningful to report on all or even most national and/or regional figures. Only some examples of differences not fitting the latitude differences will be mentioned. Earlier in this chapter, Finnish and Swedish twinning rates were noted to vary between the mainland and islands or groups of islands in which endogamy was important.[4,5,23] Data from France, collected between the years 1858 and 1865, show regional variations ranging from 8.1 per 1000 in the southwest to 11.8 per 1000 in Alsace/Lorraine in the north.[38] In Italy, between 1892 and 1904, not only was there a decrease from north to south, which fits the latitudinal model, but also higher frequency of twins was noted in the east than the west, at least in the upper part of the country.[39] Finally, the twinning rate in the Irish Republic is higher than that in the UK. In 1968, it was 13.6 per 1000 vs. 10.8 per 1000 in Northern Ireland and 10.0 per 1000 in England and Wales, respectively. Only part of the difference is accounted for by the higher age and, to a very small extent, the higher parity of the mothers of the Irish Republic, indicating that the standardized twinning rate is higher in Ireland.[42]

Seasonality

Seasonality in the birth rates has been demonstrated in a number of European countries. The peak rate occurs, in April–May and the troughs appear in November–December.[41] The question arises whether twinning rates show similar variation. It could even be surmised that, during the more fertile months of the year the twinning rate would rise as well. According to James,[42] there is good evidence that, at least in England and Wales, the incidence of opposite-sexed (and by inference, DZ) twin births is seasonal, being about 5% higher in December than in June. Triplet births also show a similar seasonal variation but with double the magnitude. Evidence with regard to seasonal variation in MZ twinning rates is equivocal. Richter and coworkers[43] evaluated twinning rates over a period of 250 years (1611–1860) in Görlitz, Germany. The rates were relatively stable in spring and fall, but varied greatly in winter and summer. In contrast, analysis of data from the Aberdeen City District (1969–1983) showed little variation in either DZ or MZ twinning by month of last menstrual period.[11] These are but three reports from a voluminous literature, which have been critically analyzed by MacGillivray and coworkers.[11] Unfortunately, in many studies, clear-cut conclusions cannot be drawn, because of methodological problems, e.g. the use of improper statistical analysis, and the possibility that artifacts in the seasonal patterns are caused by the determination of zygosity by the use of an indirect technique such as the Weinberg formula.

According to MacGillivray and coworkers,[11] and this is also our view, the seasonal evidence has been inconclusive until the middle of the present century. However, circumstances have changed during the past decade or, possibly, since the 1970s. Figure 145.10 shows the seasonal variations in singleton and twin births in the Netherlands from 1987 to 1991. Peaks and troughs for twins are relatively higher and lower than for singletons. Considering the fact that as many as 50% of these pregnancies were planned in Western Europe during these years, one may speculate that these variations are the results of the parents' choice as to the best period of the year to have a baby. Since 1988, the seasonal variations are clearly more pronounced with the twin deliveries. Dionne and colleagues[44] compared birth dates of all twins that were born between 1984 and 1990 in the state of Washington, USA, with birth dates of singleton brothers and sisters from the same families. Thus, only families with both a twin pair and a singleton sib could enter the sample of 1168 families. It appeared that especially DZ opposite-sex twins (thus, presumably all DZ twins) were procreated significantly more than their singleton siblings during summer periods. The authors consider this finding as support for their view that the longer periods of sunlight increase the probability of multiovulation, mediated by the pineal gland.

Genetics

Twins undoubtedly run in families. The mode of inheritance, however, is not clear. Most authors agree that MZ and DZ twinning must be considered separately, and that the evidence for inheritance is much stronger in the latter. Although only a few studies have examined the heredity of MZ twinning, the strong similarity in their results is remarkable: on the one hand, there is a low increase in the probability of repeat MZ twinning among the relatives of MZ pairs; on the other, there are a small number of case studies of families with more than one pair of MZ twins among the first three degrees relationship.[45] The best hypothesis seems to be that of monogenic, dominant inheritance with a low penetrance. However, the inheritance seems to be restricted to only a small fraction of the MZ twin families.

Weinberg[12] was the first to investigate the heredity of DZ twinning. He discovered that, in Stuttgart and the

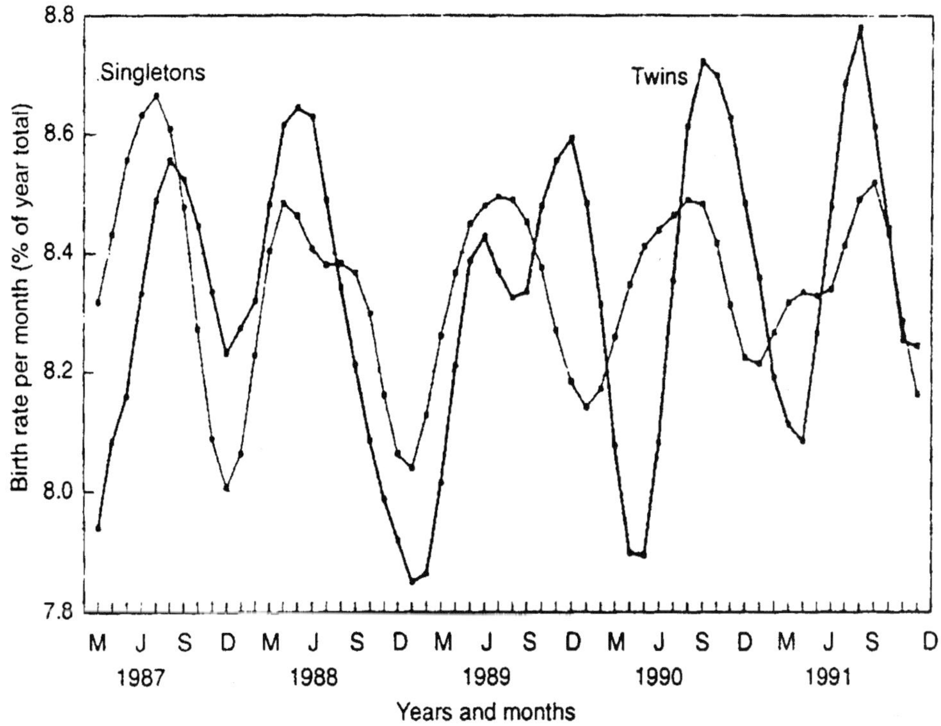

Figure 145.10 Seasonal variation of singleton and twin birth in the Netherlands, 1987–1991.

areas surrounding Würtenberg, Germany, the twinning frequency was increased by almost 54% among mothers of twins and the sisters and daughters of the mothers, but was not elevated or was even lower among the relatives of fathers of twins. He concluded that the inheritance of DZ twinning is restricted to the female line. A similar study was conducted in the Orkla valley in Norway.[46] Wyshak and White[47] analyzed the offspring of unlike-sexed twin pairs using the archives of the Genealogical Society of the Church of Jesus Christ of Latter Day Saints in Utah, USA. The DZ twinning frequency computed by the Weinberg method among the offspring of the female twins and their sisters amounted to 14.45 and 16.52, respectively, per 1000 maternities compared with 6.86 per 1000 maternities among the offspring of the male co-twins. These findings led Wyshak and White to accept the theory of a maternal autosomal recessive mode of inheritance. Although this point of view is supported by earlier studies,[12,46] questions about this type of research remain. As the hereditary factor interferes with normal ovulation by causing the production of two or more ova, phenotypic proof of the presence of the gene or genes fails on the paternal side. The unobserved transmission in a pedigree through the males may mislead scientists. Indeed, instead of investigating the offspring of the male twin or his male sibs, scanning the offspring of the daughters of the male DZ twin and of his male sibs should reveal comparable results. This observation underlines once more the important problem of the sex-limited expression. No doubt, rather large samples are needed to detect effects that are diluted 50% by additional segregation.

Starting from a working hypothesis, Bulmer[24] approached the problem in the same manner as Wyshak and White,[47] evaluating recessiveness and dominance, but based on a theoretical background rather than on empirical data. He assumed that DZ twinning is controlled by a pair of genes, *T* and *t*, and that women with either of the genotypes *TT* or *Tt* have a twinning rate p_1, while the twinning frequency among *tt* women amounts to p_2, Supposing that both genes, the dominant *T* and the recessive *t*, appear at the same frequency, this results in phenotypic frequencies of 3/4 and 1/4 for p_1 and p_2, respectively, given random mating and a Hardy–Weinberg equilibrium. This allowed the calculation of the gene frequencies using the twin-bearing probability, which can be regarded as a random variable with its own probability density function and mean. Bulmer rejected the dominant-gene hypothesis but adopted recessiveness as the mode of inheritance. Limiting himself to this single hypothesis, he could not find the reason why the twinning rate among mothers of TZ triplets was double the rate among the DZ twin mothers, although both had the same *tt* genotype. Referring to the long tail in the graph of the distribution of twinning rate *p*, the possibility of another group of women with a higher predisposition for DZ twinning seems to be the most logical explanation. Polygenic models are not rejected by these data.

Eriksson and Fellman[23,48,49] conducted extensive studies on the secular changes of the DZ twinning rates in Finland and Sweden. These two countries possess the oldest population statistics in the world for a whole nation. In the Åland archipelago in the Northern Baltic Sea, for example, as well as in Sweden, the DZ twinning rate has decreased, particularly in the past half century. Until recently, these island populations, particularly the outer parishes, had DZ twinning rates that were significantly higher than on the mainlands of Sweden and Finland. The higher frequencies of multiple maternities in these insular populations may well reflect the effect of inbreeding and endogamy. Indeed, these populations, which have descended from a relatively small group of founding settlers, have a more markedly decreasing trend of twinning, especially DZ twinning, compared with the mainland populations. This steep decline in twinning cannot be explained simply by a lower maternal age and parity. The decrease may be partly a consequence of the changes in matrimonial migration patterns, by breaking up of the isolation and by reducing the endogamy. In this case, the high twinning frequencies of previous centuries on these islands are consistent with a recessive mode of inheritance for the DZ twinning process.

In the recent analysis of multiple births by Eriksson and colleagues,[50] high frequencies of multiple maternities were found on the maternal side of families with triplets. The twinning rate among mothers with triplets was four times that of normal mothers. According to the senior author of this investigation, a simple genetic model is not sufficient to explain this high frequency. Eriksson's hypothesis is that this higher propensity for twinning, particularly on the maternal side, is caused by multifactorial inheritance.

To conclude, in the majority of instances, the inheritance of DZ twinning possibly results from a recessive character caused by an unknown number of genes. However, recessiveness does not seem to be the only potential mode of inheritance. Indeed, several authors[24,46,51] have already suggested that other modes of inheritance must also be investigated for a dimensionally undefined group of twin mothers. Besides the genetic propensity, environmental factors, such as maternal age, parity and race, increase the individual probability of twin bearing.

Considering the variety of models that have been suggested to date, and especially the necessity to investigate more fully the hereditary transmission through the female as well as the male line, our group has teamed up with the Genetic Epidemiology Division, Department of Medical Informatics, University of Utah, to conduct a large-scale study of the genetics of twinning in Belgian and Dutch population-based samples. The inheritance of spontaneous DZ twinning was investigated in 1422 three-generation pedigrees of mothers of spontaneous DZ proband twins. DZ twinning was modeled as a trait of the mother and defined as a dichotomous phenotype. Complex segregation analysis showed that the trait of 'having DZ twins' was inherited by an autosomal monogenic dominant model with a gene frequency of 0.035 and a female-specific penetrance of 0.10.[52]

The same model applies to DZ twinning among relatives of induced DZ twins, i.e. twins born of artificial induction of ovulation, one of the many modes of treatment of infertility. It seems, therefore, that women over-reacting to the administration of ovulation-inducing drugs are those carrying the twinning gene.[53]

The hereditary transmission through the female as well as the male must be investigated. Confusion with the sex-limited expression of the factor not only pushed scientists to come to the wrong conclusions but also obscures the transmission along the male side. Generally, one can consider female as well as male carriers. Future research should focus on the hereditary paradox: male vs. female inheritance, recessiveness vs. other manners of transmission and environmental vs. genetic twinning.

Infertility treatment

Recent data pertaining to twin- and triplet-delivery rates in six European nations have been analyzed in the first part of this chapter. Part of the increase has resulted from treatment of infertility. In all six countries, the rates are soaring, but in different degrees. As already stated, part of the increase is associated with the new methods of infertility treatment. In the East Flanders Prospective Twin Survey (EFPTS), the origin of the pregnancy has been recorded since 1976. From January 1, 1976, to 31 December 31, 1991, a total of 437 multiple births that resulted from artificial induction of ovulation (AIO) and Artificial Reproduction Technology (ART) were recorded. Only the pregnancies in which one of the children weighed more than 500 g or, if birth weight was unknown, the gestational age was greater than or equal to 22 weeks, have been considered for the present discussion. The zygosities of these pregnancies were compared with the zygosities of spontaneously occurring multiple pregnancies in terms of their relative frequency. All dichorionic MZ twins and trichorionic DZ triplets born after AIO had a probability of monozygosity and dizygosity, respectively, of at least 0.95.

Figure 145.11 shows the yearly numbers of spontaneous and induced twin births registered by EFPTS between 1976 and 2002.[30] In 1976, the total number of registered twin births approached 140 per year, whereas since 1991, the total has numbered more than 200. Figure 145.1 clearly documents that the increase in the total number of twins is entirely due to the use of fertility-enhancing agents, because the number of spontaneous twin births did not rise appreciably during these years. Between 1976 and 1985, the number of induced twin births increased slowly but substantially whereas after 1985, it was more dramatic. To be exact, AIO and ART pregnancies accounted for more than one-third of all twin births in 1991 and 1992 and almost one-half in 1996. The

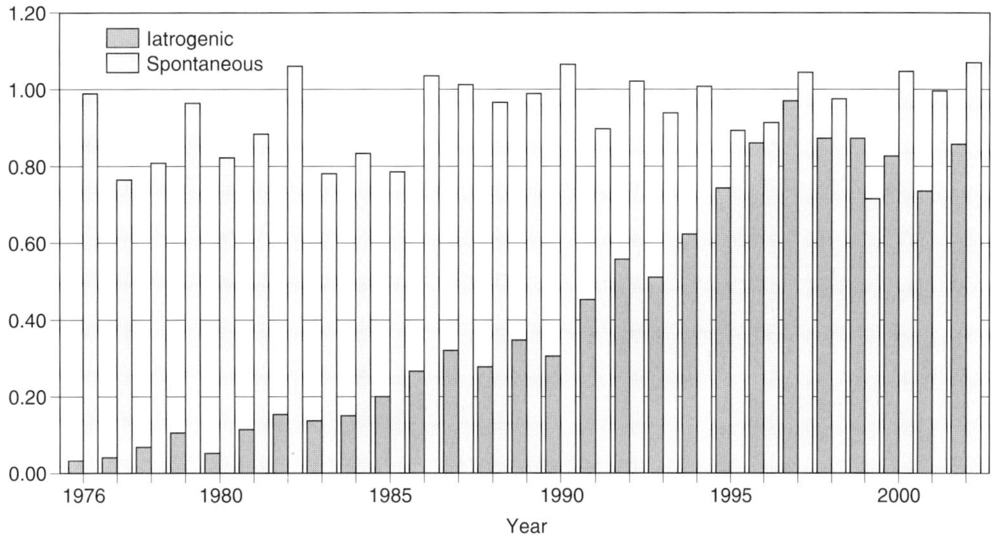

Figure 145.11 East Flanders Prospective Twin Survey, 1976–2002: yearly numbers of spontaneous and iatrogenic twins and iatrogenic twin maternities.

decline in the number of spontaneous twin births during the years 1983–1985 was due to a decrease in the total number of births. Figure 145.12 extends the analysis by showing the relative frequency of twins and triplets born after AIO and ART (1%) between 1976 and 1996. As was the case in the other countries cited above, the increase in the number of triplet births far outweighed the concomitant increase in the number of twin births.

Pooling the data over the years, Figure 145.13 shows that most of the induced multiple gestations in Figures 145.11 and 145.12 do not result from the advanced technologies of assisted reproduction such as IVF and embryo transfer (IVF–ET), gamete intrafallopian transfer (GIFT) and zygote intrafallopian transfer (ZIFT). Rather, they result from the use of fertility-enhancing drugs alone. In 80% of the iatrogenic twin pregnancies and 78% of the iatrogenic triplet pregnancies, AIO was the only treatment. Clomiphene and the sequential use of human menopausal and human chorionic gonadotropin were the regimens most commonly used in the mothers of these multiplets. Before 1986, the use of IVF–ET, GIFT and ZIFT was limited in East Flanders. In the past 4 years, however, the number of pregnancies resulting from these procedures represented more than 35% of all induced twin pregnancies, so their contribution to the increase in multiple births can no longer be neglected or denied.

In contrast with common expectation, all induced twin and triplet pregnancies were not DZ or TZ (Table 145.2). As reported earlier,[54] the frequency of zygotic splitting after AIO (1.0%) is higher than that observed after spontaneous ovulation (0.45%). There is no significant difference in the rate of zygotic division between the pregnancies that resulted from AIO only and those that occurred after IVF–ET, GIFT or ZIFT, or between the pregnancies induced by clomiphene and those induced by gonadotropins.

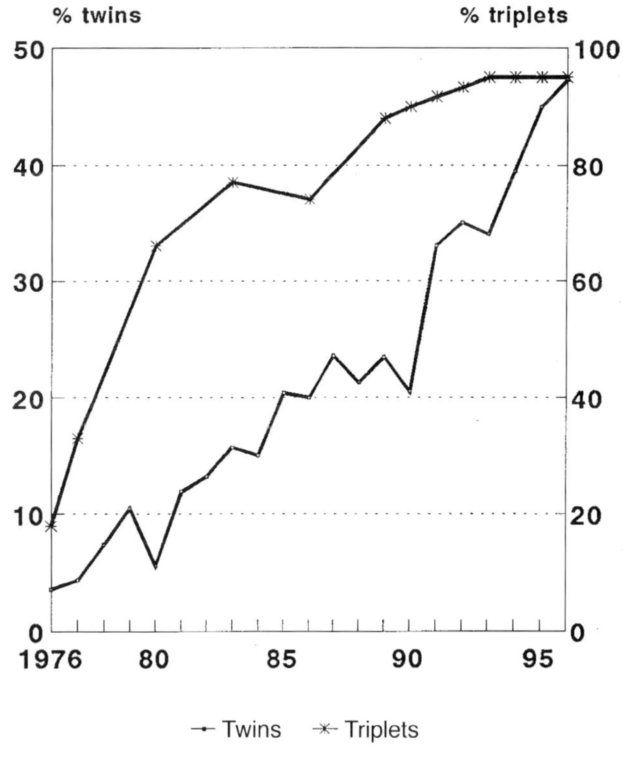

Figure 145.12 East Flanders Prospective Twin Survey, 1976–1996: relative frequencies of induced twin and triplet maternities. Twin maternities are shown on 50% scale, triplet maternities are shown on 100% scale; frequencies refer to the total number of twin and triplet maternities.

The increase in the rate of multiple pregnancies represents an important public health problem. If this trend continues, the rates of very preterm births and very low birth weight infants will undoubtedly rise, as in multiple, compared to singleton, pregnancies, the trend toward infants whose birth weight is less than 1500 g is dramatic. Because very low birth weight

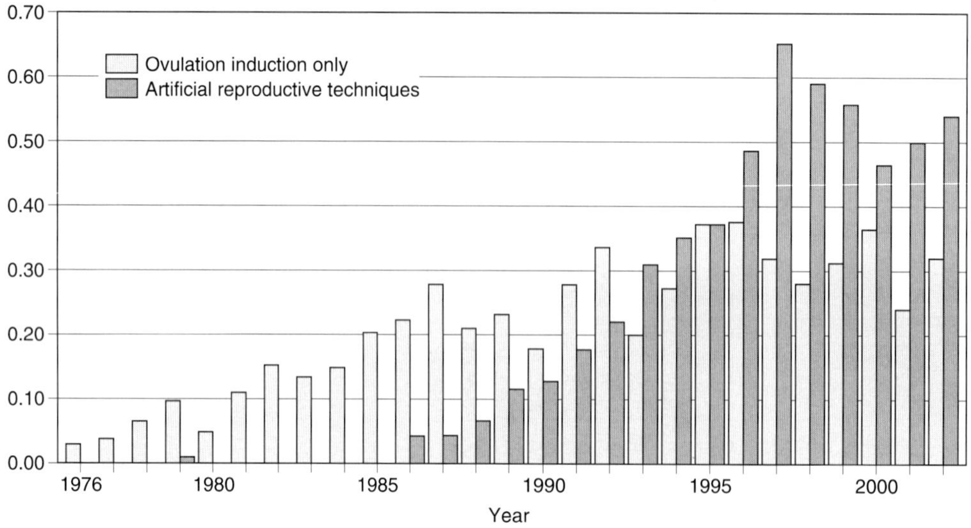

Figure 145.13 East Flanders Prospective Twin Survey, 1976–2002: yearly numbers of iatrogenic twin deliveries according to type of treatment, ovulation induction only and artificial reproduction techniques (ART).

Table 145.2 East Flanders Prospective Twin Survey: 1976–2000. Zygosity of twins and triplets born after artificial induction of ovulation

	Twins	Triplets
Monozygotic (MZ)	74	0
Dizygotic (DZ)	1442	16
Trizygotic (TZ)	—	112
Unknown	12	0
Total	1528	128

Frequency of zygotic splitting in iatrogenic DZ twinning:

$$\frac{\text{number of DZ triplets}}{2\times\text{number of (DZ twins + DZ triplets)}} = \frac{7}{2\times(1442+7)} = 0.0055$$

infants have high perinatal mortality and morbidity rates, they represent a high cost to the community in terms of an increased patient load to the neonatal intensive care units and an increased number of lifelong physical and mental handicaps.[55–57]

The fact that a number of MZ twins are born after AIO and ART and that the frequency of zygotic division after AIO and ART is higher than after naturally occurring ovulation is of fundamental biological importance. It is clear that hormonal induction of ovulation acts not only on the ovary but also on the zygote in as much as it stimulates division. To date, no conditions were known that could influence the MZ twinning rate. Treatment with clomiphene and/or gonadotropins is the first exception.

The spectacular iatrogenic increase of the rates of multiple maternities upsets the epidemiology of twinning and higher-order multiple births. When comparing population data from countries or regions where ART and ovulation induction are commonplace, the proportion of MZ/DZ twinning should be duly considered. The number of unlike-sex pairs should be mentioned and the Weinberg rule applied. Appropriate statistics can be applied if there are significant differences. By the way, the same procedure allows valid comparison between ethnicities with high and low DZ rates.

Perinatal and infant mortality

Innumerable studies on perinatal mortality of multiple births have been published worldwide. The major specific variables considered were, and still are, birth order, placentation, zygosity, maternal age, parity, height, social class, birth weight, mode of delivery, differences in rates in like- vs. unlike-sex pairs, etc. Many of these studies, however, are only of historical importance, mainly because of the changes in the definitions of stillbirth and live birth. Recently, excellent recent studies have been performed on US multiple[58] and Scottish[59] twin births.

Two population-based studies will be considered in this chapter: they are based on data from the US vital statistics and the East Flanders Prospective Twin Survey (EFPTS).

United States National Natality files[60] have been used to generate intrauterine growth curves for twins, and the linked Birth/Infant Death files to analyze the risk of neonatal and infant death for US black and white twins. As demonstrated in Figures 145.14 and 145.15 twins have a survival advantage over singletons at certain ranges of both birth weight and gestational age. Despite this, the overall risk of infant death among twins continues to be four to six times greater than that of singletons. Optimal duration of twin gestation and birth weight are 39 weeks for whites and 37–38 weeks for blacks, and range from 2750 to 3500 g for whites and from 3250 to 3500 g for blacks.

In the EFPTS, the structure of the fetal membranes and the zygosity have been determined at the time of

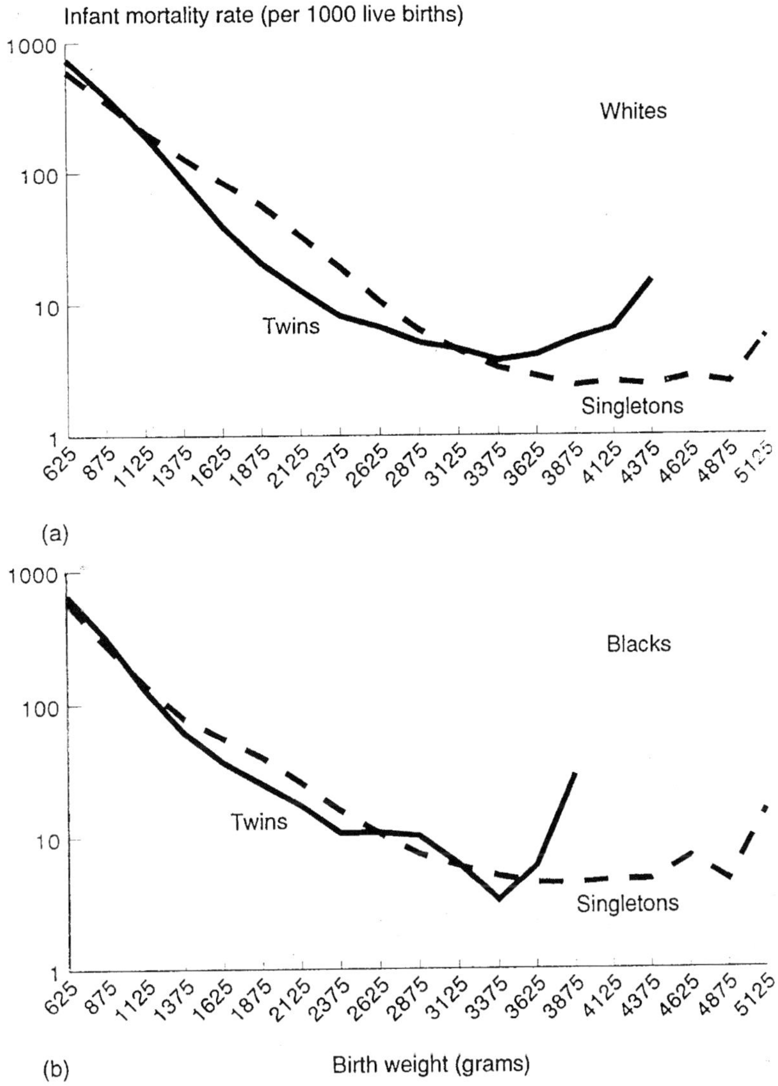

Figure 145.14 Birth weight-specific infant mortality for US white (a) and black (b) singletons and twins, calculated from linked Birth/Infant Death files for 1983–1985.[60]

birth.[61] These data allow differentiation of the perinatal mortality rates according to zygosity and chorion type. In MZ dichorionic twins (Table 145.3), the rate is not increased compared with that of DZ twins (data not given). In monochorionic twins (which are MZ), the rates are clearly increased, less so in the diamniotic than in the monoamniotic subgroups. Cord entanglement and conjoined twins are responsible for the very high rate in the latter subgroup.

As shown in Table 145.4 the second twin is, independently of the chorion type, at greater risk of mortality than the first twin, but much less so in the 1980s and 1990s than in the two preceding decades.

Congenital anomalies

If there is an epidemiological domain that is bedeviled by ascertainment biases, it is most probably that of congenital anomalies. Besides the usual biases, e.g. definitions, diagnostic criteria, extent of investigation to ascertain the presence of malformation and length of time that a population is followed, there are biases specific to twin studies: accurate zygosity diagnosis, calculation of concordance rates, sample size (small number of twins with malformations), etc. The reader is referred to several reviews[62–64] for detailed discussions of these problems.

Studies of congenital anomalies in twins are of major interest because they allow differentation of genetic from antenatal environmental influences in their origin (nature vs. nurture). However, except for occasional case reports in which concordant or discordant malformations were found in MZ twins, only a handful of studies of sufficient size meet the criteria mentioned above.

Major findings in the numerous studies of congenital anomalies in twins are summarized below:

(1) Although few studies have compared singletons and twins with adequate methods, overall, the prevalence rates are higher in twins.[64]
(2) The higher prevalence is probably greatly or entirely to be attributed to MZ twins.[64,65] Indirect

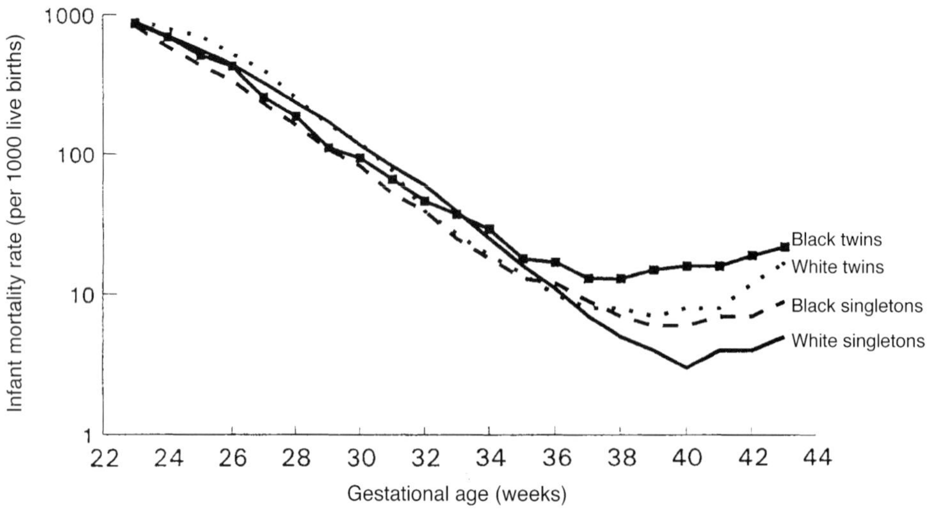

Figure 145.15 Gestation-specific infant mortality rates for US singletons and twins, calculated from linked Birth/Infant Death files for 1983–1985.[60]

Table 145.3 East Flanders Prospective Twin Survey (EFPTS): 1964–1989. Monozygotic twins: perinatal mortality according to placentation[61]

Placentation	Number of pairs	Perinatal mortality, *n* (%)	
		Twin 1	Twin 2
Dichorionic (PMZ ≥95%)	438	14 (3.2)	26 (5.9)
Monochorionic–diamniotic	871	65 (7.5)	84 (9.6)
Monochorionic–monoamniotic	30	9 (30)	7 (23)

PMZ, probability of monozygosity

Table 145.4 East Flanders Prospective Twin Survey (EFPTS): 1964–1989. Perinatal mortality rates (%) according to chorion type and birth order, twin 1 vs. twin 2

Time Period	Number of pairs	Chorion type	Twin 1	Twin 2
1964–1979	1852	MC	10.3	13.1
		DC	5.0	8.0
1980–1996	2766	MC	7.5	8.5
		DC	2.5	3.5

MC, monochorionic; DC, dichorionic

evidence is provided by many studies in which the frequency of anomalies among like-sex twins has been higher than that among unlike-sex twins. Few studies have been reported in which zygosity has been determined by a direct method.[64]

(3) In MZ twins, the prevalence varies according to placentation: lowest (possibly not increased) in the dichorionic, highest in the monochorionic–monoamniotic and intermediate in the monochorionic–diamniotic subgroups.[65]

(4) Specific to twinning are acardia and conjoined twinning (which occur only in monochorionic–monoamniotic pairs), and fetus *in fetu*.[64]

(5) In MZ pairs, most anomalies are discordant. Clearly, antenatal environmental factors must play an important role in their origin.[65]

(6) Cardiac anomalies are a good example to illustrate what we have discussed in the preceding paragraphs. Preliminary results show that they are more frequent in monochorionic pairs, pointing to the role played by the twin-to-twin vascular anastomoses as a possible causal mechanism.[66]

(7) A large majority of conjoined twins are of the female sex. This is probably not related to the malformation itself but to the placental structure: the overall proportion of males/females of monoamniotic pairs is very low.[66]

Table 145.5 Relative number of male infants born per 1000 females in US births (1915–1948)[72]

Total born living	1055
Twins	1043
Triplets	1007
Quadruplets	940
Quintuplets	935

Table 145.6 Sex proportion of spontaneous twins in EFPTS (1970–2000) according to zygosity and placentation

Zygosity and chorionicity	Sex proportion
Dizygotic	0.514
Monozygotic–dichorionic	0.501
Monochorionic–diamnionic	0.499
Monochorionic–monoamnionic	0.212
All monozygotic	0.494
All (n=3765 pairs)	0.506

(8) Whether ART or AIO increases the risk of congenital anomalies makes doctors and patients uneasy. Only four methodologically valid studies have been devoted to this disquieting question.[67–70] They conclude that the outcome of twin pregnancies obtained with ART is comparable with that of normally conceived twins. The number of cases is limited and does not allow ruling out any teratogenic action. Hypothetically, such action should be considered because in ISCI natural selection of the fertilizing sperm is surpassed, a potential risk of facilitating congenital anomalies. No data are available on the outcome of twin pregnancies following induction or enhancing of ovulation. A warning, therefore, is mandatory and additional research is needed.[71]

Sex proportions at birth

The proportion of males in multiple births has been and still is a matter of lively debate. Clearly, there are differences between singletons and multiplets. The question remains, however, of the explanation for these differences and whether the differences could throw some light on the mechanisms of the human sex proportions at birth.

The proportion of males in the human species decreases with each increase in the number of fetuses per pregnancy. An overview in the white population of the United States is given in Table 145.5.

Twins

In twins, the lower male/female proportion is for the greater part due to the MZ twins (Table 145.6). In the EFPTS series, the sex proportions of the DZ pairs and the singletons did not differ significantly. To our knowledge, no other studies comparing the sex proportions between MZ and DZ twins and singletons have been published. James has studied the sex proportions extensively, and has reviewed the literature on MZ twins whose sex was ascertained at birth.[73–75]

Adding the data from nine studies on Caucasian samples with known placentation, the male/female proportions were as follows: overall 0.499, monochorionic pairs 0.492 (in five of the nine reports, monoamniotic twins have been omitted) and dichorionic twins 0.571 (only three of the nine authors reported data on these twins). The ratio of 0.499 is lower, but not significantly lower, than that estimated for all Caucasian pairs, 0.5047±0.001, by Bulmer.[24] James concludes that there is direct (although admittedly inconclusive) evidence here that MZ twins have a lower male/female proportion than DZ twins.

According to our data from East Flanders and those of the literature, it may be concluded that the male/female proportion in MZ twins with monochorionic placentas is lowered, albeit to a smaller extent in the diamniotic and a much greater extent in the monoamniotic variety. One can only speculate about the reasons for this remarkable biological phenomenon. Various hypotheses have been put forward. James[76] and Guerrero[77] independently suggest that the sex of a human zygote is influenced by the time of its formation within the menstrual cycle, with more male zygotes being formed, on average, both early and very late in the cycle, whereas more female zygotes are formed during the middle of the cycle. Experiments in lower vertebrates such as fish, amphibians and chickens have led to MZ twins by retarding the development of the fertilized ova, depriving them of oxygen or maintaining them at a lower temperature. Delayed ovulation seems to induce MZ twinning in rabbits.[78] As suggested by James, it seems possible that the delay hypothesized as being associated with the formation of female zygotes runs parallel with the delay associated with the splitting of the ovum. If this is the case, then MZ twins could be composed of a higher proportion of females.

One or two percent of MZ pairs of twins share the chorion and the amnion at birth. They represent twinning that occurred after the differentiation of the amnion (on about day 7). Fusion of the embryos[79] gives rise to conjoined twins and could occur even later, after the second week of development. Because of the rarity of conjoined twins, it is as yet unknown whether further subdivision of the monoamniotic twins into unjoined and conjoined pairs will clarify the enigma of their very low male/female proportion. As only three conjoined pairs (all of them female) emerged in our relatively large series, only a registry of almost continental scale could provide the amount of data needed to answer this question. It is well documented that conjoined twins include a high proportion of girls.[80]

It is useful to enquire whether female embryos are more likely to undergo delayed splitting than male embryos, or if embryonal or fetal mortality in the late-splitting group predominantly affects the male embryos. In their series of spontaneously aborted twins, Uchida and colleagues[81] found two male conjoined pairs with normal chromosomes, the result of consecutive abortions in the same mother. Because both conjoined twins and male monoamniotic twins are rare, this single finding could suggest a predominantly male early fetal mortality in monoamniotic twins. With regard to the first question, Burn and associates[82] hypothesized that unequal lyonization may represent a cause of late twinning unique to female embryos. If this is true, analysis of the DNA methylation patterns of the X chromosome[83] of monoamniotic twins should throw more light on the question. We have performed such an analysis.[84] It shows that the earlier the splitting, the more unequal lyonisation, invalidating the hypothesis of Burn and associates. The sex proportions discussed so far deal with spontaneous twinning, rather than iatrogenic twins. A series of studies have addressed this question, but the results are not in agreement. No large-scale population-based inquiries have been performed. Hence, one can question whether the samples are representative. In the EFPTS, the sex proportions of the iatrogenic and the spontaneous DZ twins do not differ significantly.

Triplets

One finding of the increase in triplet rates (especially TZ) is a decreasing male/female sex proportion. In the population in general, about 1000 girls are born per 1045 boys: a ratio of 1.045. Among the 336 triplet individuals from the Dutch Twin Register there were 157 boys and 179 girls: a sex ratio of 0.88. The Dutch population triplet male/female ratio (i.e. triplets born during about the same period as the sample studied) is 0.87. A closer look at the triplet sets from a different etiology reveals that only among the induced triplets does the ratio deviate significantly from unity: 50 boys and 67 girls. This supports James' hypothesis[85–87] that hormonal induction of ovulation increases the mother's gonadotropin levels at the time of conception and that this, in turn, increases the probability of female offspring. In the EFPTS, however, opposite results are found: 47 girls and 66 boys.

Whether the decreasing male/female ratio in triplets is unevenly distributed among the three zygosity groups is unknown. Very few population-based studies of zygosity in triplets have been published. In all of these, the number of cases is too small to enable a firm conclusion to be made.

Acknowledgments

This work was aided by grant Nos. 3.0038.02 of the Fund for Medical Scientific Research (Belgium), 002818470 of the Prae-ventiefonds (Netherlands), 86/0823 of NATO, and by the Association for Scientific Research in Multiple Births (Belgium). This chapter has been adapted and revised from Derom *et al.*[88]

REFERENCES

1. Imaizumi Y, Inouye E. Analysis of multiple birth rates in Japan. I. Secular trend, maternal age effect, and geographical variation in twinning rates. *Acta Genet Med Gemellol (Roma)* 1979;28:107.
2. Nylander PPS. Ethnic differences in twinning rates in Nigeria. *J Biosoc Sci* 1971;3:151.
3. Rehan N, Tafida DS. Multiple births in Hausa women. *Br J Obstet Gynaecol* 1980;87:997.
4. Eriksson AW, Eskola MR, Fellman JO. Retrospective studies on the twinning rate in Scandinavia. *Acta Genet Med Gemellol (Roma)* 1976;25:29.
5. Eriksson AW, Fellman JO. Differences in the twinning trends between Finns and Swedes. *Am J Hum Genet* 1973;25:141.
6. James WH. Second survey of secular trends in twinning rates. *J Biosoc Sci* 1982;14:481.
7. Parisi P, Caperna G. The changing incidence of twinning: One century of Italian statistics. In Gedda L, Parisi P, Nance WE, eds. *Twin Research 3, Part A, Twin Biology and Multiple Pregnancy.* New York: Alan R. Liss, 1981:35–48.
8. Fellman JO, Eriksson AW. Statistical models for the twinning rate. *Acta Genett Med Gemellol (Roma)* 1987;36:297.
9. Fellman JO, Eriksson AW. Standardization of the twinning rate. *Hum Biol* 1990;62:803.
10. Bulmer MG. Is Weinberg's method valid. *Acta Genet Med Gemellol (Roma)* 1976;25:25.
11. MacGillivray I, Samphier M, Little J. Factors affecting twinning. In MacGillivray I, Campbell DM, Thompson B, eds. *Twinning and Twins.* Chichester: Wiley, 1988:67–97.
12. Weinberg W. Beiträge zur Physiologie und Pathologie der Mehrlinggeburten beim Menschen. *Arch Gesamte Physiol* 1901; 88:346.
13. Weinberg W. Differenzmethode und Geburtenfolge bei Zwillingen. *Genetica* 1934;16:282.
14. Bressers WMA, Eriksson AW, Kostense PJ, *et al.* Increasing trend in monozygotic twinning rate. *Acta Genet Med Gemellol (Roma)* 1987;36:397.
15. Emery AEH. Identical twinning and oral contraception. *Biol Soc* 1986;3:23.
16. Orlebeke JF, Eriksson AW, Boomsa DI, *et al.* Changes in the DZ unlike/like sex ratio in the Netherlands. *Acta Genet Med Gemellol (Roma)* 1991;40:319.
17. Renkonen KO. Is Weinberg's rule defective? *Ann Hum Genet* 1967;30:277.
18. Nylander PPS, Corney G. Placentation and zygoticity of twins in Ibadan, Nigena. *Ann Hum Genet* 1969;33:31.
19. James WH. Excess of like sexed pairs of dizygotic twins. *Nature (Lond)* 1971;232:277.
20. James WH. Is Weinberg's differential rule valid? *Acta Genet Med Gemellol (Roma)* 1979;28:69.
21. Bulmer MG. The effect of parental age, parity and duration of marriage on the twinning rate. *Ann Hum Genet* 1959;23:454.
22. Vlietinck R, Derom C, Derom R, *et al.* The validity of Weinberg's rule in the East Flanders Prospective Twin Survey (EFPTS). *Acta Genet Med Gemellol (Roma)* 1988;37:137.
23. Eriksson AW. *Human Twinning in and around the Åland Islands.* Helsinki: Societas Scientiarum Fennica, 1973.
24. Bulmer MG. *The Biology of Twinning in Man.* Oxford: Clarendon Press, 1970.
25. James WH. The current status of Weinberg's differential rule. *Acta Genet Med Gemellol (Roma)* 1992:41:33.
26. Husby H, Holm NV, Gernow A, *et al.* Zygosity, placental membranes and Weinberg's rule in a Danish consecutive twin series. *Acta Genet Med Gemellol (Roma)* 1991;40:147.
27. Derom C, Vlietinck R, Thiery E, *et al.* The East Flanders Prospective Twin Survey (EFPTS). *Twin Res* 2002;5:337–41.
28. Allen G. A differential method for estimation of type frequencies in triplets and quadruplets. *Am J Hum Genet* 1960;12:210.
29. Allen G. Frequency of triplets and triplet zygoticity types among US births, 1964. *Acta Genet Med Gemellol (Roma)* 1988;37:299.
30. Derom C, Derom R, Vlietinck R, *et al.* Iatrogenic multiple pregnancies in East Flanders, Belgium. *Fertil Steril* 1993;60:493.

31. Duncan JM. *Fecundity, Fertility, Sterility and Allied Topics.* Edinburgh: A & C Black, 1986.
32. Waterhouse JA. Twinning in twin pedigrees. *Br J Soc Med* 1950; 4:197.
33. Taffel SM. Demographic trends in twin births: USA. In Keith LG, Papiernik E, Keith DM, *et al.*, eds. *Multiple Pregnancy, Epidemiology, Gestation and Perinatal Outcome.* Carnforth, UK: Parthenon Publishing, 1995:145–62.
34. Tchouriloff M. Sur la statistique des naissances gémellaires et leur rapport avec la taille. *Bull Soc Anthropol Paris* 1877:12:440.
35. Corney G, Seedburgh D, Thompson B, *et al.* Maternal height and twinning. *Ann Hum Genet (Lond)* 1979;43:55.
36. James WH. Dizygotic twinning, birth weight and latitude. *Ann Hum Biol* 1985;5:441.
37. Davenport CB. Litter size and latitude. *Arch Rassen Ges Biol* 1930:24:87.
38. Puechs A. Des accouchements multiples en France et dans les principales contrées de l'Europe. *Ann Hyg Pub II* 1874;Ser 41:197.
39. Prinzing F. Die örtlichen Verschiedenheiten der Zwillinghäufgkeit und deren Ursachen. *Z Geburtsh Gynäkol* 1907;60:420.
40. Dean G, Keane T. An investigation of the high twinning rate in the Republic of Ireland. *Br J Prev Soc Med* 1972;26:186.
41. Huntington E. *Season of Birth: Its Relation to Human Abilities.* New York: Wiley, 1938.
42. James WH. Seasonably in twin and triplet births. *Ann Hum Biol* 1980;7:163.
43. Richter J, Miura T, Nakamura I, *et al.* Twinning rates and seasonal changes in Görlitz, Germany, from 1611 to 1860. *Acta Genet Med Gemellol (Roma)* 1984;33:121.
44. Dionne CE, Soderstrom M, Schwartz SM. Seasonal variation in twin births in Washington state. *Am J Med Genet* 1993;42:41.
45. Harvey MA, Huntley RMC, Smith DW. Familial monozygotic twinning. *J Pediatr* 1977;90:246.
46. Bonnevie K, Sverdrup A. Hereditary disposition to dizygotic twin births in Norwegian peasant families. *J Genet* 1926:16:125.
47. Wyshak G, White C. Genealogical study of human twinning. *Am J publ Health* 1965;55:1586.
48. Eriksson AW. Variations in the human twinning rate. *Acta Genet Med Gemellol (Roma)* 1962:12:242.
49. Eriksson AW, Fellman G. Ethnological differences in twinning trends. *Scand J Clin Lab Invest* 1967;19(Suppl 95):73.
50. Eriksson AW, Bressers WMA, Kostense PJ, *et al.* Twinning rate in Scandinavia, Germany and the Netherlands during years of starvation. *Acta Genet Med Gemellol (Roma)* 1988:37:277.
51. Eriksson AW. Genetic epidemiological aspects on variation in human twinning in Sweden. Presented at the *VIIth Congress of the European Anthropological Association,* 1990.
52. Meulemans WJ, Lewis CM, Boomsma DI, *et al.* Genetic modelling of dizygotic twinning among relatives of sponteous dizygotic twins. *Am J Med Genet* 1996;61:258.
53. Meulemans WJ, Lewis CM, Boomsma DI, *et al.* Segregation analysis of dizygotic twinning in pedigrees of dizygotic proband twins conceived after artificial induction of ovulation. *Am J Hum Genet* 1994;55(Suppl); Abstract 913.
54. Derom C, Derom R, Vlietinck R, *et al.* Increased monozygotic twinning rate after ovulation induction. *Lancet* 1987;1:1236.
55. Keith L, Papiernik E, Luke B. The cost of multiple pregnancy. *Int J Gynaecol Obstet* 1991;36:109–14.
56. Luke B, Keith L. The contribution of singletons, twins and triplets to low birthweight, infant mortality and handicaps in the United States. *J Reprod Med* 1992;36:661.
57. Luke B, Minogue J, Witter FR. The role of fetal growth restriction and gestation age on length of hospital stay in twin infants. *Obstet Gynecol* 1993;81:949.
58. Kiely JL. The epidemiology of perinatal mortality in multiple births. *Bull N Y Acad Med* 1990;66:618.
59. Campbell DM, MacGillivray I. Outcome of twin pregnancies. In MacGillivray I, Campbell DM, Thompson B, eds. *Twinning and Twins.* Chichester: Wiley, 1988:179–202.
60. Powers WF, Kiely JL, Fowler MG. The role of birth weight, gestational age, face and other infant characteristics in twin intrauterine and infant mortality. In Keith LG, Papiernik E, Keith DM, *et al.*, eds. *Multiple Pregnancy, Epidemiology, Gestation and Perinatal Outcome.* Carnforth, UK; Parthenon Publishing, 1995: 163–74.
61. Derom R, Vlietinck R, Derom C, *et al.* Perinatal mortality in the East Flanders Prospective Twin Survey (preliminary results). *Eur J Obstet Gynecol Reprod Biol* 1991;41:25–6.
62. Myers C, Elias S, Arrabal P. Congenital anomalies and pregnancy loss. In Keith LG, Papiernik DM, *et al*, eds. *Multiple Pregnancy, Epidemiology, Gestation and Perinatal Outcome.* Carnforth, UK: Parthenon Publishing, 1995:73–92.
63. Little J, Carr-Hill RA. Problems of ascertainment of congenital anomalies. *Acta Genet Med Gemellol (Roma)* 1984;33:97.
64. Little J, Bryan EM. Congenital anomalies. In MacGillivray I, Campbell DM, Thompson B, eds. *Twinning and Twins.* Chichester: Wiley 1988;20–40.
65. Cameron AH, Edwards JH, Derom R, *et al.* The value of twin surveys in the study of malformations. *Eur J Obstet Gynecol Reprod Biol* 1983;14:34–56.
66. Derom C, Vlietinck R, Derom R, *et al.* Population-based study of sex-proportion in monoamniotic twins. *N Engl J Med* 1988;319: 119–20.
67. Dhont M, De Zutter P, Ruyssinck G, *et al.* Perinatal outcome of pregnancies after assisted procreation. *AM J Obstet Gynecol* 1999;181:688–95.
68. Koudstaal J, Bruinse HW, Helmerhorst FM, *et al.* Obstetric outcome of twin pregnancies after in-vitro fertilization: A matched control study in four Dutch University hospitals. *Hum Reprod* 2000;15:935–40.
69. Lambalk CB, van Hoof M. Natural versus induced twinning and pregnancy outcome: A Dutch nationwide survey of primiparous dizygotic twin deliveries. *Fertil Steril* 2001;75:731–6.
70. Pinborg A, Loft A, Rasmussen S, *et al.* Neonatal outcome in a Danish national cohort of 3438 IVF/ICSI and 10,362 non-IVF/ICSI twins born between 1995 and 2000. *Hum Reprod* 2004;14: 435–41.
71. Novak K. Reason to keep an eye on ICSI. *Nature Med* 1999;5: 1133.
72. Strandskov HH, Siemens GJ. An analysis of the sex ratios among single and plural births in the total, the 'white' and the 'colored' populations. *Am J Physiol Anthrop* 1946;4:49l–501.
73. Nichols JB. Statistics of births in the United States (sex ratio). *Am J Obstet Gynecol* 1952;64:376.
74. James WH. Sex ratio in twin births. *Ann Hum Biol* 1975;2:365.
75. James WH. The sex proportion of monoamnionic twin pairs. *Ann Hum Biol* 1977;4:143.
76. James WH. Sex ratio and placentation in twins. *Ann Hum Biol* 1980;7:273.
77. Guerrero R. Sex ratio: A statistical association with the type and time of insemination in the menstrual cycle. *Int J Fertil* 1970; 15:221.
78. James WH. Cycle day of insemination, coitus rate and sex proportion. *Lancet* 1971;1:112.
79. Spencer R. *Conjoined Twins.* Baltimore & London: The Johns Hopkins University Press, 2003.
80. Zake EZ. Case reports of 16 sets of conjoined twins from a Uganda hospital. *Acta Genet Med Gemellol (Roma)* 1984;33:75–80.
81. Uchida IA, Freeman VCP, Gedeon M, *et al.* Twinning rate in spontaneous abortion. *Am J Hum Genet* 1983;35:987.
82. Burn J, Povey S, Boyd Y, *et al.* Duchenne muscular dystrophy in one of monozygotic twin girls. *J Med Genet* 1986;23:494.
83. Fearon ER, Winkelstein JA, Civin CL, *el al.* Carrier detection in X-linked agammaglobulinemia by analysis of X-chromosome inactivation. *N Engl J Med* 1987;316:427.
84. Chitis S, Derom C, Vlietinck R, Derom R, Monterio J, Gregerson PK. X Chromosome inactivation patterns confirm the late splitting of monoamniotic-MZ twining. *Am J Hum* Genet 1999;65: 570–1.
85. James WH. The sex ratio of infants born after hormonal induction of ovulation. *Br J Obslet Gynaecol* 1985;92:299.
86. James WH. Sex ratio, dominance status and maternal hormone levels at the time of conception. *J Theor Biol* 1985;114:505.
87. James WH. Hormonal control of sex ratio. *J Theor Biol* 1986; 118:427.
88. Derom R, Orlebeke J, Eriksson A. The epidemiology of multiple births in Europe. In Keith LG, Papiernik E, Keith DM, Luke B, eds. *Multiple Pregnancy, Epidemiology, Gestation and Perinatal Outcome.* Carnforth, UK: Parthenon Publishing, 1995:145–62.
89. Pinborg A, Loft A, Schmidt L, *et al.* Neurological sequelae in twins born after assisted conception: Controlled national cohort study. *B Med J* 2004;329:311–29.
90. Pinborg A, Loft A, Schmidt L, *et al.* Maternal risk and perinatal outcome in a Danish National cohort of 1005 twin pregnancies: The role of in vitro fertilisation (IVF). *Acta Gynecol Obstet Scand* 2004, In press.

146 Monozygosity

I. Blickstein

Zygosity of multiple pregnancies

The human female is programmed to ovulate once in every menstrual cycle, and if ovulation results in fertilization, a single zygote will develop, i.e. a monozygotic (MZ) pregnancy. This is the case in 99.2% of pregnancies following spontaneous conceptions. In the remaining 0.8%, more than one oocyte is ovulated, resulting in polyzygotic pregnancies [i.e. dizygotic (DZ) twins, trizygotic triplets, etc]. Such polyzygotic pregnancies seem to have a phenotypic and genetic background as they occur more often in tall, heavily built, older, parous, and black women. Moreover, a genetic trait is strongly supported by the fact that DZ pregnancies have clear racial differences and occur more frequently in women who have 'twins in the family'.[1] On the whole, polyzygosity represents a reproductive anomaly whereby more than the usual single zygote is formed during a single ovulatory cycle.

This situation, however, changed profoundly with the implementation of assisted reproductive technologies, which share a common denominator – creating a higher number of oocytes available for fertilization, irrespective of whether fertilization occurs *in vivo* or *in vitro*. Current data indicate that where assisted conceptions are widely available, the frequency of DZ twins increases from 66% to 95%.[2]

Whereas polyzygotic multiples are common in many species, the human female is among the unique species (the other is the nine-banded armadillo) in which the product of conception – the zygote – is able to undergo splitting into MZ twins. This is a rare phenomenon observed in about 0.4% (4/1000) of births following spontaneous conceptions. As will be discussed below, and as is the case with DZ twins, all methods of assisted conceptions are associated with increased splitting rates of the zygote.[3]

Placentation

Each fetus comes along with a set of placenta and placental membranes. This design, obvious in singletons, is also true for DZ twins. However, because the uterine cavity is of limited space, placentas may develop very near to each other and eventually become fused. It follows that DZ twins have dichorionic–diamniotic (DC–DA) fused or separate placentas. In MZ twins, on the other hand, the type of placenta depends on the time of splitting. According to the current theory, the twin placenta resembles the (double) singleton placenta in early (< 3 days after fertilization) splitting. It follows that some (about one-third) of MZ twins may have a DC placenta, indistinguishable from that in DZ twins. The bad news is that DZ twins who have the same gender (comprising 50% of the cases) cannot be distinguished from MZ twins with a DC placenta, unless sophisticated genetic analysis is performed to establish zygosity.

When the split occurs after the chorion has already been developed, the remaining MZ twins (about two-thirds) must have one chorion and are termed monochorionic (MC) twins. The vast majority of these splits occur within 1 week when the amnion is not yet differentiated, and the MC twins have two amniotic sacs (MC–DA). However, in cases when the split occurs even later, the amnion is also differentiated, and the resulting pairs are nested within a single amniotic cavity – monoamniotic (MA) twins. MA twins (essentially MC–MA) are very rare and comprise less than 1% of all twins.

One may wonder what causes a zygote to undergo division. In the absence of a clear explanation, and in the presence of a much-increased frequency of anomalies, it is assumed that the mechanism(s) involved in zygotic splitting is/are also involved in the generation of anomalies. The most bizarre anomaly emerges when the zygote is split at a very advanced age after fertilization, after the amnion is already formed (i.e. MA twins) and the only remaining structure to be divided is the fetus itself. In this case, conjoined twins are formed. Figure 146.1 is a schematic presentation of the relationship between chorionicity and amnionicity.

Antenatal and postnatal diagnosis of zygosity/chorionicity

From the previous section it is clear that zygosity can be determined with certainty only if the twins are of unlike sex (in this case they must be DZ) and when an

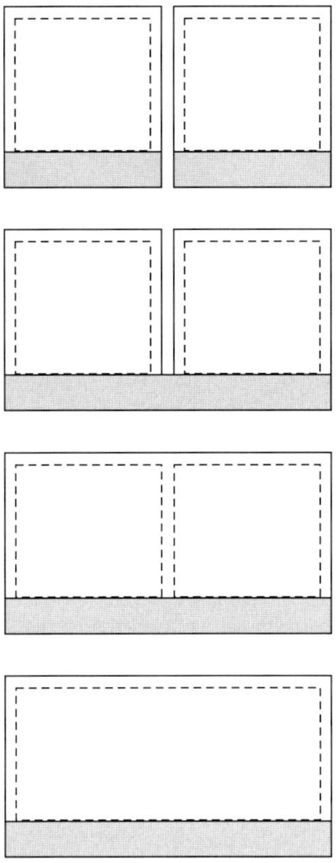

Figure 146.1 Schematic presentation of the relationship between chorionicity and amnionicity.

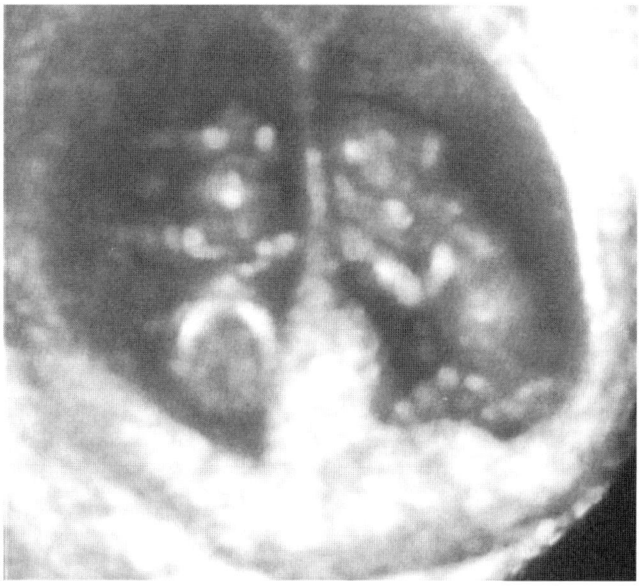

Figure 146.2 3D image of the twin peak (lambda) sign in dichorionic placentas.

MC placenta is found (in this case they must be MZ). It follows that we are blind to zygosity in as many as half of the DZ twins who are of the same sex and in one-third of the MZ twins who have a DC placenta. Altogether, these amount to 4/9 of the twins (44%).[3] An interesting approach to improve the detection of MZ conceptions comes from the Australian study of the number of corpora lutea in the ovary in a twin gestation.[4] According to this innovation, if there are two corpora lutea, it is likely that there were two ovulations, and the twins are likely to be DZ. Conversely, if there is only one corpus luteum, the twins are likely to be MZ. Although this method is by no means practical, it still represents the urge of clinicians to improve the antenatal (in this case, postconceptional) prediction of zygosity.

Irrespective of the above-mentioned difficulties to ascertain zygosity, the important clinical information is not zygosity but chorionicity. As it appears, the most complex pathology involves an MC placenta. Hence, it is imperative to establish the presence of MC twins as early as possible.[5] The fact is, however, that it is much easier to exclude MC placentation than to prove it. As early as 1992, the presence of a triangular decidual projection between the double bilayer of the intertwin membrane was described in practically all DC placentas.[6] This so-called 'twin peak' or lambda sign (Figure 146.2) is easily seen in first-trimester ultrasound but may diminish by the mid-pregnancy increase in the volumes of the amniotic sacs.

In the absence of the lambda sign, the clinician should look for signs of MC placentation. In most cases, a simple reflection of a rather thin intertwin membrane – the tau sign – can be visualized (Figure 146.3). Admittedly, the thin intertwin membrane might be elusive at first scan leading to an erroneous impression of MA twins. The diagnosis of chorionicity is relatively easy during the first trimester and becomes increasingly difficult when looked for after 20 weeks' gestation. At this stage, one may rely on ancillary sonographic signs such as number of layers (Figure 146.3) membrane thickness, same-sex twins, and single placenta.

It goes without saying that zygosity cannot be determined from postpartum examination of the placenta. At the same time, however, every effort to establish chorionicity should be done after each twin delivery. The placenta should be delivered with minimal trauma. Two separate or a single fused placenta is easily discerned and differentiated from the single placenta. At the fetal side, the insertion of the umbilical cords is noted. Very adjacent cords are commonly seen in MA twins (Figure 146.4). Velamentous insertion of umbilical cord found by ultrasound and/or placental examination is quite common in MC placentas and should alert the clinician to that possibility. Machin[7] reported on 45% of MC having velamentous cord insertion, and that the combination of one twin with centrally inserted cord and one with a velamentous cord was found in 53% of pairs. Moreover, this combination constitutes a subgroup at risk because such setting was associated with highest rates of growth discordance > 20%, unequal placental parenchymal sharing, uncompensated anastomoses and perinatal demise.[7,8]

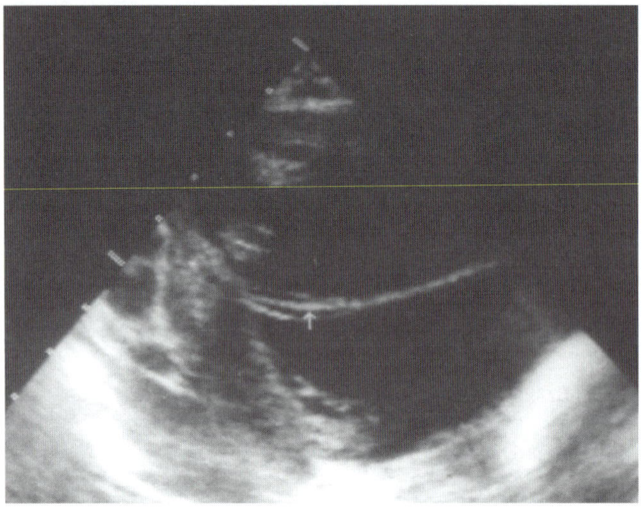

Figure 146.3 Intertwin membrane comprising a double amniotic layer. The reflection of the membrane from the placenta is referred to as the tau sign.

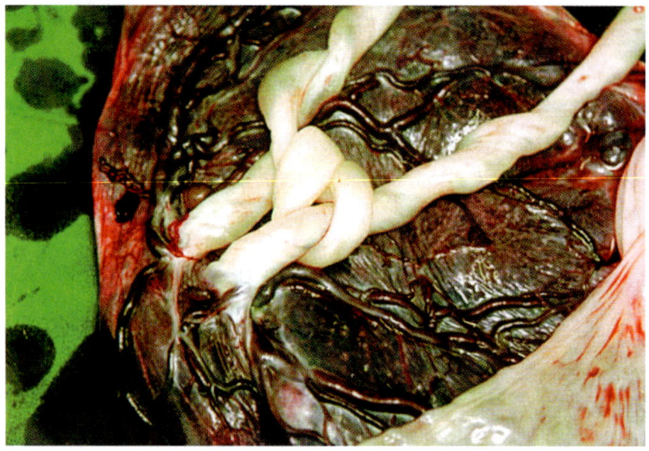

Figure 146.4 Close insertions of entangled umbilical cords of an MA placenta.

The 'gold standard' of monochorionicity is by counting the number of layers in the intertwin membrane. Careful peeling of the layers can do this; however, when the membrane is disrupted, histological examination may distinguish between the two-layer and the four-layer membranes in MC and DC placentas, respectively. Importantly, the number of the layers can sometimes be counted by ultrasound (Figure 146.3).

One of the most important observations in the MC placenta is the presence of intertwin, transplacental anastomoses. In fact, practically all MC placentas show intertwin connecting vessels, which might be arterio-arterial, veno-venous, and arterio-venous. The latter form is the putative anastomosis active in the twin–twin transfusion syndrome (TTTS), but the other types are probably involved in compensating mechanisms that reduce or balance the unidirectional shunt.[9]

Zygosity can be estimated in populations of spontaneous pregnancies by using the Hardy–Weinberg rule. The basic assumption behind this rule is that like- and unlike-sex pairs occur at the same frequency in DZ twins, and therefore, the number of DZ twins is twice the number of unlike-sex pairs in a population. The difference between the total number of twins and the number of DZ twins is the number of MZ twins. It should be remembered that there are reservations about the Hardy–Weinberg rule in general and in particular in a population of mixed spontaneous and iatrogenic twins.[3]

Etiology of MZ twinning

The reason why a single zygote splits to form MZ twins is unknown. For certain, this phenomenon is obviously abnormal and, therefore, it is not surprising that MZ twinning is associated with so many pathologies. Hall proposed the first of the current two hypotheses for MZ twinning in the mid-1990.[10] Normally, the cells of the zygote-blastocyst – the blastomeres – undergo condensation to form the inner cell mass. Hall suggested that different cells of the early embryo might develop differently during the same period and that this developmental discordance between adjacent cells might cause repulsion (rather than condensation) and splitting of the early embryo.

The second, and more widely cited hypothesis, describes the splitting event as the division of the early embryo during hatching. The mechanism responsible for the division presumably causes a breach in the integrity of the zona pellucida, herniation of blastomeres, and splitting of the embryo.[3] This hypothesis is based on the reported increased frequencies of MZ twins after all methods of zona manipulation used in assisted reproduction. However, observations from conceptions following ovulation induction also show increased MZ rates.[2] The latter observations suggest that the trigger for zygotic splitting might be at the stage of ovulation induction (the common denominator of all assisted pregnancies) rather than tampering the zona pelucida.[3]

Regardless of the etiology, the most comprehensive population-based analysis of twins – the East Flanders Prospective Twin Survey – where all like-sex dichorionic twins undergo genetic evaluation of zygosity, recently showed that spontaneous MZ twin comprise about 0.45%, MZ births after ovulation induction occur in 6.3% (16-fold increased rate), and those after *in vitro* fertilization (IVF) techniques occur in 2.6% (sixfold increased rate). The latter finding is in full accord with the estimation of the frequency of MZ twins after IVF procedures based on single embryo transfers.[11] This method assumes that if multiples occur following single embryo transfer in an IVF procedure, they must be MZ.

Chromosomal anomalies

It is assumed that because the two fetuses are derived from the same zygote, they must be genetically identical. However, a plethora of evidence suggest that postzygotic events exist and lead to discordant genetic anomalies as well as to the more puzzling phenomenon of heterokaryotypic MZ twins. As mentioned above, a potential reason for repulsion of the blastomeres – the basis for the cell-repulsion theory for MZ twinning[10] is genetic differences in these cells, including aneuploidy, X-inactivation, and imprinting. The literature cites many cases of XY or XYY/XO, male/female, 'identical twins', and randomization of X-inactivation may result in MZ twin girls who are different in respect to X-linked diseases such as muscular dystrophy, color blindness, Hunter disease, etc. Moreover, the pattern of X-inactivation confirms the timing of late splitting events.[12] Uniparental disomy – when a cell has both chromosomes from the same parent – may also occur after zygotic division. For example, imprinting of the gene responsible for the Wiedemann–Beckwith syndrome usually manifests in only one of the MZ twins.

A subset of genetically discordant MZ twins is the case of polar body fertilization, whereby one spermatozoon fertilizes the oocytes and another fertilizes the polar body (containing the same haplotype set of chromosomes as the oocytes) derived from the first meiotic division. In the human, this phenomenon was implicated in the pathogenesis of an acardiac (twin reversed perfusion – TRAP sequence) twin of a normal co-twin.[13]

Despite the potential genetic differences between MZ twins, the majority is concordant in terms of the usually obtained genetic karyotype. Because the risk of double sampling during genetic amniocentesis outweighs the risk of heterokaryotypic twins, most clinicians would sample one of the two sacs in cases that are definitely MZ, i.e. in MC twins.

Structural anomalies

Twins have more structural anomalies compared to singletons and most texts cite a two- to threefold increased risk. It is currently believed that the excess of malformations is limited to MZ pairs. Anomalies in twins are categorized under four subheadings[14] (Table 146.1). The first category includes malformations that are more frequently seen among multiples. The second type involves malformations found in MZ twins only such as TRAP sequence and the various manifestations of conjoined twins. The third category relates to consequences of placental malformations, in particular the MC placenta, resulting in the TTTS and higher frequency of velamentous cord insertion. The last type involves postural abnormalities such as clubfoot that are caused by intrauterine crowding.

Table 146.1 Categories of structural defects in twins

Category of malformation	Defect
More common in twins than in singleton	Neural tube defects Hydrocephaly Congenital heart disease Esophageal and anorectal atresia Intersex Genitourinary tract anomalies
Unique to monozygotic twins	Amniotic band syndrome TRAP sequence Conjoined twins Twin embolization syndrome
Placental malformations	Single umbilical artery Twin–twin transfusion syndrome Velamentous cord insertion
Intrauterine crowding	Skeletal malformations

Importantly, some of the malformations may impact on the non-malformed twin. For example, in the TRAP sequence, the circulation of the severely anomalous acardiac–acephalic twin is entirely supported by the normal (the so-called 'pump') twin. Without intervention, this cardiac overload may eventually lead to cardiac insufficiency of the 'pump' twin. In TTTS, where both twins are completely normal, the transplacental shunt of blood may cause serious morbidity in both twins. The most striking example is the case of single fetal demise in MC twins, whereby the live fetus may die *in utero* soon after the death of its co-twin, or – if it survives – serious end-organ damage is reported in as many as 30%.

Growth

Compared with the recognized adverse outcomes among MC twins (increased early pregnancy loss, perinatal mortality and morbidity, congenital anomalies, and long-term sequelae), the relation between MC twinning and growth aberrations is less clear. Most authors agree that MC twins are more likely to exhibit absolute growth restriction and low birth weight.

Similarity between MC twins, arising from a single zygote, is intuitively assumed to be greater than that between DC twins, comprising DZ as well as MZ sets. The alleged similarity between MC twins is therefore assumed to be associated with fewer or similar, but no more, growth discordance compared with DC sets. Counterintuitively, however, there were conflicting views regarding the frequency of discordance among MC twins, with reports showing a doubled risk of severe discordance,[15–17] and, on the other hand, reports that find similar discordance frequencies in the MC compared with DC twins.[18–21] Figure 146.5 shows the comparison between 939 DC and 216 MC

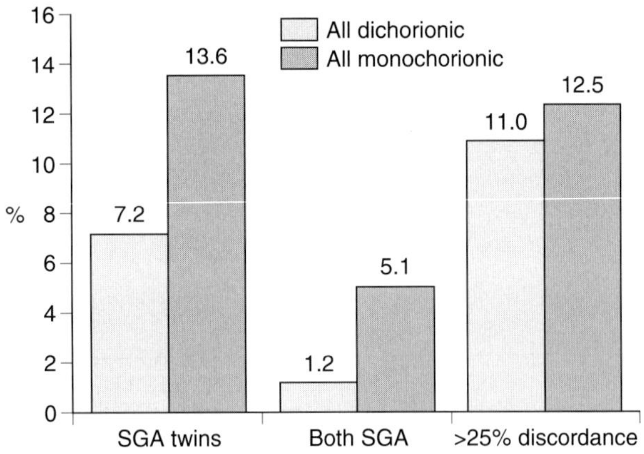

Figure 146.5 Frequency of small-for-gestational-age infants and severely (> 25%) discordant pairs by chorionicity. Data from the Northwestern Twin Chorionicity Study.

twin pregnancies from the Northwestern Twin Chorionicity Study (Blickstein *et al.*, unpublished observation) showing that small for gestational age (SGA) infants are less frequent among DC twins [odds ratio (OR) 0.4], fewer sets with two SGA infants exist among DC than among MC pairs (OR 0.3), but twins of all placental types have similar gestational ages (not shown) and frequencies of discordance > 25%.

Single fetal demise

Single fetal death has an entirely different connotation in MC twins compared with DC twins. In DC twins, unless the reason for fetal death endangers the entire pregnancy (i.e. chorioamnionitis), the survivor is generally unaffected. This is not the case in MC sets, where the co-twin frequently dies soon after the first demise, and, if not dead, the survivor quite often suffers from end-organ damage (brain, kidneys, etc.). In the past, products of fetal decay (the so-called thromboplastin-like material) were believed to embolize via the intertwin anastomosis and cause damage in the survivor – the so-called fetal embolization syndrome. Postmortem studies in the early 1990s, however, did not find any embolus in the brains of survivors that succumbed during early infancy. Subsequently, the 'embolic' theory was replaced by the 'ischemic' theory, whereby acute shunting of blood from the survivor to the low-resistant circulation of the demised twin causes acute hypertension, ischemia, and damage. Importantly, ischemic injury via acute shift of blood can occur during pregnancy even without fetal death and cause end-organ injury in one of the twins.[22]

Because the actual timing of fetal death is rarely known, any form of intervention, especially preterm, should be balanced against the risks of prematurity to the survivor. The idea behind treatment, beside prompt delivery, is that if acute feto-fetal hemorrhage occurs at the time of death, an immediate intrauterine transfusion may save the anemic survivor. This management includes proof of anemia in the survivor (either by cordocentesis or by measuring the peak systolic velocity of middle cerebral artery) followed by rescue therapy in the form of blood transfusion to the umbilical vein.[23–25] The reported outcomes, however, are less than optimistic.

To date, when fetal death is diagnosed before term, and the surviving fetus seems to be intact, most clinicians will not intervene, as the real risk of preterm birth is greater than the potential risk from the fetal embolization syndrome. Imaging is necessary to exclude visible end-organ lesions. At near-term, especially when the etiology of fetal demise is unknown, immediate delivery instead of continued close monitoring of the pregnancy might be a valid option.

Twin–twin transfusion

An unbalanced, deep, arterio-venous anastomosis, probably existing in MC placentas only, is necessary for the development of the TTTS. TTTS has been known for centuries, but only in the last two decades a significant change occurred in understanding the underlying process. As late as the mid-1980s, the diagnosis of TTTS was usually made postpartum, when weight and hemoglobin discordant pair was born. By the end of the 1980s and with the advent of ultrasound, a conceptual change has been introduced and TTTS became an antenatal diagnosis. At the same time, innovative and exciting methods to treat TTTS were proposed.[26]

Due to blood shunting, one twin – the so-called 'donor' twin – becomes anemic and hypovolemic. The co-twin – the so-called 'recipient' twin – becomes plethoric and hypervolemic. The discordant cardiac load soon results in discordant urinary output and the oligo-polyhydramnios sequence. Eventually, the small donor might be 'entrapped' within its amnion and pushed to the side of the uterus by the polyhydramnios surrounding the larger recipient, giving rise to the sonographic image of the 'stuck' twin. These findings constitute the first degree of TTTS of what is currently known as the Quintero criteria[27] (Table 146.2). In the next stage, the urinary bladder of the donor is no longer visible. In the third Quintero stage, abnormal Doppler findings are seen, representing an advanced decompensation of the cardiovascular systems of the twins. The ongoing cardiac overload in the recipient may lead to hydrops fetalis – which constitutes Quintero stage IV. Finally, at the last stage, either twin may die *in utero*.

TTTS may occur as early as the beginning of the second trimester and, rarely, intrapartum. When TTTS occurs late in pregnancy, most clinicians will opt for delivery because the fetal condition can be better managed in the neonatal intensive care unit. It

Table 146.2 Quintero's criteria for severity of TTTS

Stage	TOPS (O < 2 cm, P > 8 cm)	Absent bladder in donor	CADs (A/REDV, Rev DV, Puls UV)	Hydrops	Demise
I	+	–	–	–	–
II	+	+	–	–	–
III	+	+	+	–	–
IV	+	+	+	+	–
IV	+	+	+	–	+

TOPS, twin oligo (O) poly (P) sequence. Numbers relate to amniotic fluid index. CAD, critical abnormal Doppler measurements; A/REDV, absent/reversed end-diastolic velocity; Rev DV, reversed flow in ductus venosus; Puls UA, pulsatility in umbilical vein

follows that the earlier TTTS occurs the greater the risk for the twins. Consequently, clinicians tend to buy time by some form of intervention,[28] and currently – by stage tailored therapy.[29,30] At this stage, the three most common interventions are amnio-reduction (removal of a large quantity of amniotic fluid) with or without septostomy (puncturing the intertwin membrane), fetoscopic laser ablation of the putative anastomoses, and fetocide (by cord occlusion). The latter method is reserved for Quintero stage III–IV cases[31] and it is currently not yet established whether to terminate the donor or the recipient.

Although amnioreduction and endoscopic laser surgery differ conceptually as well as in the technology and expertise involved, they yielded similar outcomes. However, a recent randomized trial comparing laser surgery with amnioreduction showed that the laser group had a higher likelihood of survival of at least one twin to 28 days of age (76% vs. 56%) and 6 months of age. Infants in the laser group also had a lower incidence of brain injury (6% vs. 14%) and a lower incidence of neurological complications at 6 months of age (52% vs. 31%).[32]

Twin reversed arterial perfusion sequence

TRAP sequence is a condition whereby one twin transfuses its co-twin via an arterio-arterial anastomosis. Hence, the transfused twin receives blood by an artery instead of a vein – giving rise to reversed perfusion clearly seen on Doppler studies. The recipient in such cases is usually extremely malformed – the so-called acephalic–acardiac twin (Figure 146.6). The main clinical problem comes from the total dependence of the acardiac twin on the circulation of the 'pump' twin. Sooner or later, the 'pump' twin may develop cardiac insufficiency, and, as a result, the cardiac condition determines the time of delivery. A proxy to impending cardiac insufficiency is the relative size of the acardiac twin compared with the pump twin.

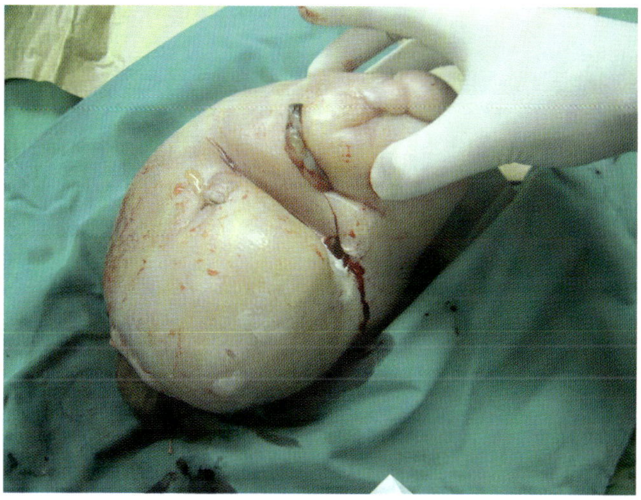

Figure 146.6 The acardiac–acephalic twin in the TRAP sequence.

TRAP sequence is easily diagnosed in the second trimester, when the typical ovoid mass, lacking the usual fetal structure, is visualized. When the diagnosis is made early enough, selective reduction of the acardiac twin by cord occlusion is recommended. However, in more advanced gestations, the cord might be too thick for bipolar coagulation and more invasive, intrahepatic coagulation might be necessary.[33]

Monoamniotic pregnancies

MA twinning is rare, occurring in less than 1% of all spontaneous twins. Before the availability of ultrasound, the diagnosis was made postpartum, when two dead fetuses with entangled cords were born. Indeed, cord entanglement is the rule rather than the exception in MA twins (Figure 146.4), and can be found as early as the beginning of the second trimester by dedicated Doppler ultrasound visualizing the characteristic braid of umbilical cords. With modern sonographic equipment, it should not be difficult to exclude MA placentation, especially if chorionicity/amnionicity is assessed in the first trimester. In that case, counting the number of yolk sacs may be misleading and repeated sonography, with different angles of scanning is recommended.

In addition to all the problems associated with an MC twinning (except for a lower probability to develop TTTS), the MA pair is at increased risk for cord entanglement and for the consequent morbidity and mortality of one or both twins. This risky situation is usually unexpected, and demands intensive monitoring. Many clinicians would feel more comfortable to hospitalize the patient for twice or thrice daily monitoring, starting at 28–29 weeks. Lung maturity is usually enhanced by antenatal corticosteroids. Delivery, usually by cesarean section, is performed at 32–33 weeks' gestation. A more conservative approach is based on the assumption that with advanced gestation, the potential space for fetal movements as well as the risk of tightening the cords is reduced. Consequently, it was proposed that if nothing happened until 32 weeks, the likelihood for tight entanglement is low. This policy should be carried by those who are able to assess the tightness of the cord by Doppler velocimetry.[34]

Conjoined twins

Conjoined twins are very rare, and the average obstetrician is not likely to see more than one or two cases in his lifetime. Obviously, the mechanism of conjoining is by itself a formidable malformation. If the parents want to continue the pregnancy, the most important clinical problem of the attending obstetrician is to estimate the feasibility of postpartum separation surgery.

Currently, 2D and 3D ultrasound, combined with Doppler assessment and supplement with magnetic resonance imaging, provide excellent visualization of the conjoined structures and the level of risk to the twins after separation. Because separation of conjoined twins is rare, it is advisable to consult with centers that gained experience in such difficult procedures.

Cerebral palsy

It is not clear whether cerebral palsy (CP) is more common in MC twins without TTTS or in the absence of fetal death.[35] This ambiguity is a result of the lack of series with established chorionicity/zygosity and adequate neurodevelopmental follow-up. Moreover, failure to register vanishing twins or fetal deaths may lead to a significant underestimate of the risk of CP in multiple gestations and an overestimate of the risk in apparently singleton infants.[22] To circumvent this difficulty, researchers compared the prevalence of CP in like-sex vs. unlike-sex pairs. In a recent review, Pharoah[22] commented that a greatly increased risk of CP among multiples is associated with MC placentation. This risk is particularly notable in the surviving twin with fetal or early infant death of the co-twin. Pharoah proposed, in addition to the above-mentioned theories for damage in the fetal embolization syndrome, that hemodynamic instability during pregnancy may cause bidirectional shunting of blood between the two fetuses. This may have caused lethal damage in one twin and CP in the other, and would explain the finding of increased prevalence of CP among survivors in twin pairs in which one of the twins died in the neonatal period.

It is currently believed that funisitis – inflammation of the umbilical cord – is a very sensitive marker for CP. The Northwestern Twin Chorionicity Study[36] examined the question whether discordant inflammation depends on chorionicity. In a retrospective analysis of 1156 twin placentas, the authors evaluated the association between chorionicity and discordant chorioamnionitis and funisitis in twin gestations. This study found that in the case of chorioamnionitis in DC twins (with either separate or fused placentas), the non-presenting twin is less frequently affected than the presenting twin. Such discordant inflammation is not apparent in MC twins. The results were somewhat accentuated in the case of funisitis – a more advanced state of inflammation (including inflammatory evidence within the walls of umbilical vessels or in Wharton's jelly). Whereas the difference between DC and MC twins persists, discordant funisitis was greatest among separate DC twins, less so among fused DC twins, and was absent among MC twins. The interpretation of these results was that DC placentas confer significant protection against the spread of chorioamnionitis from the presenting to the non-presenting sac. The difference between the separate and fused dichorionic twins implies that the paranchymal separation between these placentas and not the DC septum might be responsible for the protection. In simple terms, the different morphologic features of a four-layer intertwin membrane and the separate placentas may restrict the spread of inflammation. These findings might be relevant in the discussion of the presumable increased risk of CP among MC twins.

As attractive as these theories are, the excess risk of CP in MZ twinning in general and in the subset of MC twins in particular has to be established.

Summary

Monozygosity is a mysterious phenomenon in human conceptions. Splitting of the zygote destined to become a singleton is by itself an abnormal event, and it is not surprising that such pregnancies are associated with increased morbidity and mortality. Most of our knowledge about MZ twinning comes from the subset of MC twins because we are unable to differentiate the MZ–DC from the like-sex DZ–DC twins. This problem seems negligible because most of the pathology associated with MZ seems to be associated with MC twins. Modern diagnostics – mainly ultrasound and Doppler – are able to diagnose most of the associated pathologies quite early in pregnancy and help clinicians in counseling, planning appropriate follow-up, and tailoring treatment when necessary.

REFERENCES

1. Meulemans WJ, Lewis CM, Boomsma DI, *et al.* Genetic modelling of dizygotic twinning in pedigrees of spontaneous dizygotic twins. *Am J Med Genet* 1996;61:258–63.
2. Derom C, Derom R. The East Flanders Prospective Twin Survey. In Blickstein I, Keith LG, eds. *Multiple Pregnancy*, 2nd edn. London: Taylor & Francis, 2004:39–47.
3. Blickstein I. Estimation of iatrogenic monozygotic twinning rate following assisted reproduction: Pitfalls and caveats. *Am J Obstet Gynecol* 2005;192(2):365–8.
4. Tong S, Vollenhoven B, Meagher S. Determining zygosity in early pregnancy by ultrasound. *Ultrasound Obstet Gynecol* 2004;23: 36–7.
5. Machin GA. Why is it important to diagnose chorionicity and how do we do it? *Best Pract Res Clin Obstet Gynaecol* 2004;18: 515–30.
6. Finberg HJ. The "twin peak" sign: Reliable evidence of dichorionic twinning. *J Ultrasound Med* 1992;11:571–7.
7. Machin GA. Velamentous cord insertion in monochorionic twin gestation. An added risk factor. *J Reprod Med* 1997;42:785–9.
8. Loos RJ, Derom C, Derom R, Vlietinck R. Birthweight in liveborn twins: The influence of the umbilical cord insertion and fusion of placentas. *Br J Obstet Gynaecol* 2001;108:943–8.
9. Machin GA. Vascular anatomy of monochorionic twin placentas. In Blickstein I, Keith LG, eds. *Multiple Pregnancy*, 2nd edn. London: Taylor & Francis, 2004:193–200.
10. Hall JG. Twinning. *Lancet* 2003;362:735–43.
11. Blickstein I, Jones C, Keith LG. Zygotic splitting rates following single embryo transfers in in-vitro fertilization: A population-based study. *New Engl J Med* 2003;348:2366–7.
12. Chitnis S, Derom C, Vlietinck R, Derom R, Monteiro J, Gregersen PK. X chromosome-inactivation patterns confirm the late timing of monoamniotic–MZ twinning. *Am J Hum Genet* 1999;65:570–1.
13. Bieber FR, Nance MM, Morton CC, *et al.* Genetic studies of an acardiac monster: Evidence for polar body twinning in man. *Science* 1981;213:775–77.
14. Blickstein I, Smith-Levitin M. Multifetal pregnancy. In Petrikovsky BM, ed. *Fetal Disorders: Diagnosis and Management.* New York: Wiley, 1998:223.
15. Hatkar PA, Bhide AG. Perinatal outcome of twins in relation to chorionicity. *J Postgrad Med* 1999;45:33–7.
16. Victoria A, Mora G, Arias F. Perinatal outcome, placental pathology, and severity of discordance in monochorionic and dichorionic twins. *Obstet Gynecol* 2001;97:310–5.
17. Gonzalez-Quintero VH, Luke B, O'Sullivan MJ, *et al.* Antenatal factors associated with significant birth weight discordancy in twin gestations. *Am J Obstet Gynecol* 2003;189:813–7.
18. Dube J, Dodds L, Armson BA. Does chorionicity or zygosity predict adverse perinatal outcomes in twins? *Am J Obstet Gynecol* 2002;186:579–83.
19. Snijder MJ, Wladimiroff JW. Fetal biometry and outcome in monochorionic vs. dichorionic twin pregnancies; a retrospective cross-sectional matched-control study. *Ultrasound Med Biol* 1998;24:197–201.
20. Sebire NJ, D'Ercole C, Soares W, Nayar R, Nicolaides KH. Intertwin disparity in fetal size in monochorionic and dichorionic pregnancies. *Obstet Gynecol* 1998;91:82–5.
21. Hanley ML, Ananth CV, Shen-Schwarz S, Smulian JC, Lai YL, Vintzileos AM. Placental cord insertion and birth weight discordancy in twin gestations. *Obstet Gynecol* 2002;99:477–82.
22. Pharoah PO. Risk of cerebral palsy in multiple pregnancies. *Obstet Gynecol Clinic North Am* 2005;32(1):55–67.
23. Senat MV, Bernard JP, Loizeau S, Ville Y. Management of single fetal death in twin-to-twin transfusion syndrome: A role for fetal blood sampling. *Ultrasound Obstet Gynecol* 2002;20:360–3.
24. Tanawattanacharoen S, Taylor MJ, Letsky EA, Cox PM, Cowan FM, Fisk NM. Intrauterine rescue transfusion in monochorionic multiple pregnancies with recent single intrauterine death. *Prenat Diagn* 2001;21:274–8.
25. Senat MV, Loizeau S, Couderc S, Bernard JP, Ville Y. The value of middle cerebral artery peak systolic velocity in the diagnosis of fetal anemia after intrauterine death of one monochorionic twin. *Am J Obstet Gynecol* 2003;189:1320–4.
26. Blickstein I. The twin–twin transfusion syndrome. *Obstet Gynecol* 1990;76:714–22.
27. Quintero RA, Morales WJ, Allen MH, Bornick PW, Johnson PK, Kruger M. Staging of twin–twin transfusion syndrome. *J Perinatol* 1999;19:550–5.
28. Ropacka M, Markwitz W, Blickstein I. Treatment options for the twin–twin transfusion syndrome: A review. *Twin Res* 2002;5: 507–14.
29. Taylor MJ, Govender L, Jolly M, Wee L, Fisk NM. Validation of the Quintero staging system for twin–twin transfusion syndrome. *Obstet Gynecol* 2002;100(6):1257–65.
30. Quintero RA, Dickinson JE, Morales WJ, *et al.* Stage-based treatment of twin–twin transfusion syndrome. *Am J Obstet Gynecol* 2003;188:1333–40.
31. Nakata M, Chmait RH, Quintero RA. Umbilical cord occlusion of the donor versus recipient fetus in twin–twin transfusion syndrome. *Ultrasound Obstet Gynecol* 2004;23:446–50.
32. Senat MV, Deprest J, Boulvain M, Paupe A, Winer N, Ville Y. Endoscopic laser surgery versus serial amnioreduction for severe twin-to-twin transfusion syndrome. *N Engl J Med* 2004;351: 136–44.
33. Weisz B, Peltz R, Chayen B, *et al.* Tailored management of twin reversed arterial perfusion (TRAP) sequence. *Ultrasound Obstet Gynecol* 2004;23:451–5.
34. Bilardo CM, Arabin B. Monoamniotic twins. In Blickstein I, Keith LG, eds. *Multiple Pregnancy*, 2nd edn. London: Taylor & Francis, 2004:574–82.
35. Blickstein I. Cerebral palsy in multifoetal pregnancies. *Dev Med Child Neurol* 2002;44:352–5.
36. Phung DT, Blickstein I, Goldman RD, Machin GA, LoSasso RD, Keith LG. The Northwestern Twin Chorionicity Study: I. Discordant inflammatory findings that are related to chorionicity in presenting versus nonpresenting twins. *Am J Obstet Gynecol* 2002;186:1041–5.

147 Population-based risk of perinatal mortality and morbidity among multiple births

M. S. Wingate, G. R. Alexander, S. Boulet, R. Kirby and H. Salihu

Introduction

Over the past two decades, infant mortality (death of a liveborn up to 1 year of life) has declined significantly. From 1980 to 2001, infant mortality rates have decreased 46% (12.6 to 6.8 per 1000 live births, respectively). Neonatal death (death less than 28 days after birth), has dropped from 8.5 to 4.5 per 1000 live births, a decline of 47%. Though less marked, the rate of fetal death (death occurring at 20 weeks' gestation or greater per 1000 live births plus fetal deaths) has declined as well, from 9.1 fetal deaths to 6.5 per 1000 live births plus fetal deaths, from 1980 to 2001.[1] This overall improvement in perinatal survival appears to be due in large part to decreasing risks of birth weight and gestational age-specific mortality.[2,3] These improvements can likely be attributed to the technological and medical advances in high-risk obstetric and neonatal care, including antenatal steroids, ultrasound, high-frequency ventilation, and exogenous surfactant.[4–16] Also, regionalization of perinatal services and an increase in early entry into prenatal care seem to have increased the utilization of these services among high-risk populations.[17–19]

While these advances have influenced the health and well-being of many children, there are still many challenges in the perinatal field. The risk of morbidities associated with low birth weight (LBW) (less than 2500 g) and preterm birth (delivery prior to 37 weeks' gestation) has increased as the number of babies born too small and too soon has risen steadily over the past two decades. LBW rates climbed from 7.0 to 7.8 per 1000 live births from 1990 to 2002. Preterm birth rates increased 13%, from 10.6 per 1000 live births in 1990 to 12.0 per 1000 live births in 2002.[1,20] The rise in LBW and preterm birth has numerous causes. One of the most often cited contributions to this increase is the dramatic rise in multiple births over the past 20 years.[20] Multiple births, having higher mortality rates compared to singleton deliveries, are at an increased risk of preterm birth and LBW.[21,22] At least one-half of twins and almost 90% of triplets and higher-order multiples are LBW and/or preterm.[23] From 1980 to 2002, the number of twins in the USA rose by 65%, from 68,339 to 125,134. In 2002, the rate of triplets or higher-order multiple births continued to decline after an increase of nearly 400% between 1980 and 1998.

Several factors have been suggested for this rising incidence of multiple births in the USA. A frequently cited factor of this trend is the development and use of assisted reproductive technologies (ART).[22,24,25] The explosive increase in triplets and quadruplets due to ART has led to a call by obstetric and gynecologic organizations to actively reduce the multiple birth delivery associated with ART.[26–28] Those infants who are products of higher-order multiple pregnancies are at increased risk of complications, such as ventricular hemorrhages, cerebral palsy, and other conditions that can lead to morbidities in later life.[29]

Simultaneous to the rise in ART is the shift in the age demographics of mothers in the USA. Over the past two decades, the average age of the mother at the time of delivery has risen markedly.[20] In most developed nations, the rise in the rates of multiple births, particularly twins and triplets, can also be attributed to the increase in maternal age, as older mothers have an increased likelihood of spontaneous multiple births. In addition, an association has been shown between advancing maternal age and the use of ART as the conditions that influence infertility increase with age.[22–24] Previous studies indicate that

Table 147.1 Trends in mortality rates among multiple births

	Singletons			Twins			Triplets or higher		
	White	Black	Ratio	White	Black	Ratio	White	Black	Ratio
Fetal Mortality									
1985–88	6.0	12.0	1.99	24.6	28.3	1.15	36.3	43.6	1.20
1995–98	5.5	12.0	2.19	18.3	27.6	1.51	25.5	60.4	2.37
% change	−9.6	−0.5	10.07	−25.7	−2.4	31.40	−29.8	38.6	97.38
Hebdomadal Mortality									
1985–88	3.7	8.6	2.31	29.4	52.3	1.78	93.8	127.9	1.36
1995–98	2.6	6.6	2.58	18.9	36.4	1.93	50.0	88.1	1.76
% change	−31.1	−23.3	11.33	−35.9	−30.5	8.40	−46.7	−31.1	29.26
Neonatal Mortality									
1985–88	4.6	10.2	2.23	33.9	57.6	1.70	106.5	138.6	1.30
1995–98	3.3	8.0	2.45	21.9	41.2	1.88	57.3	95.5	1.67
% change	−28.4	−21.5	9.68	−35.5	−28.5	10.78	−46.2	−31.1	27.96
Infant Mortality									
1985–88	7.5	16.0	2.2	40.9	72.9	1.78	118.9	153.1	1.29
1995–98	5.2	12.3	2.4	26.0	51.6	1.98	63.1	114.8	1.82
% change	−29.8	−23.3	9.2	−36.4	−29.2	11.27	−47.0	−25.0	41.35

'White' and 'Black' may include persons of Hispanic ethnicity because of the change in birth certificate reporting of race/ethnicity in 1989
Fetal mortality rate: death in utero 20 weeks' gestation or greater per 1000 live births plus fetal deaths
Hebdomadal mortality rate: death less than 7 days after live birth per 1000 live births
Neonatal mortality rate: death less than 28 days after live birth per 1000 live births
Infant mortality rate: death less than 1 year after live birth per 1000 live births
Ratio: Black/White rate ratio

between one-fourth and one-third of the increase in the twin and triplet rates can be attributed to the increase in maternal ages without the influence of fertility treatment.[21]

While the rise in multiple births is of great concern, another important issue related to perinatal health pertains to racial disparities, particularly between blacks and whites. While infant mortality among blacks and whites has declined since 1980, the black/white infant mortality rate ratio has increased from 2.0 to 2.5.[1,30] This disparity is apparent across all measures of mortality including fetal, neonatal, postneonatal, and perinatal mortality. While the disparity between blacks and whites continues to exist for outcomes such as LMW and preterm birth, rates of both LBW and preterm birth for blacks have declined since 1990 in contrast to observed increases among whites. The proportion of preterm deliveries decreased for blacks, while it increased for whites over the past decade.[31] However, in 2002, 17.5% of black infants were born prior to 37 weeks' gestation, compared to 11.0% of white infants.[1] For multiple gestations, as expected, the rate of preterm birth increased among whites and blacks, but the relative increase was larger among whites. While there has been an overall increase in multiple births, the increase among whites was almost twice that of blacks from 1989 to 1997.[32] As the USA has one of the most diverse populations in the world, it is imperative to examine these trends by specific population; however, few studies have examined the racial disparities in outcomes of multiple births.[32]

This chapter describes the population-based risk of perinatal mortality and morbidity among multiples with a particular focus on racial disparities. First, we describe the trends in mortality rates for singletons and multiple births by racial/ethnic groups between 1985–1988 and 1995–1998. Next, we examine the mortality rates by gestational age, plurality, and race. Finally, we examine the risks of mortality and morbidity among multiple births and specific racial/ethnic populations. We compare and contrast rates and risks to evaluate patterns involved in morbidities and mortalities among multiple births by racial and ethnic group classifications. For these analyses, we use the U.S. National Center for Health Statistics 1985–88 and 1995–98 Linked Live Birth/Infant Death Cohort files and the Fetal Death files from the U.S. Perinatal Mortality data file, as well as the 1995-98 Matched Multiple Linked files.[33–41]

Results

Trends in mortality

Table 147.1 presents the trends in mortality among multiple births by race and plurality. This table presents mortality rates from 1985–1988 and 1995–1998, along with the percent change for each race and the race rate ratio. Fetal mortality rates decreased for whites in all plurality groups. As the plurality increases, that is, from singleton to twin, the negative percent change reveals improvement

Table 147.2 Gestational age-specific perinatal mortality rates by race

	Singletons			Twins			Triplets or higher-order multiples		
	Perinatal mortality rate			Perinatal mortality rate			Perinatal mortality rate		
Gestational age (weeks)	Whites	Blacks	Black/white rate ratio	Whites	Blacks	Black/white rate ratio	Whites	Blacks	Black/white rate ratio
20–21	948.9	904.1	0.95	945.1	902.2	0.95	948.6	975.9	1.03
22–23	871.6	786.2	0.9	867.7	775.8	0.89	849.9	802.8	0.94
24–25	570.9	451.7	0.79	512.4	410.8	0.8	404.7	463.2	1.14
26–27	313.4	266.6	0.85	238.2	197.7	0.83	139.6	262.8	1.88
28–29	190.5	153.8	0.81	113.7	110.4	0.97	61.4	63.2	1.03
30–31	104.6	82.5	0.79	53.2	56.5	1.06	19.0	57.8	3.04
32–33	53.9	46.0	0.85	25.7	31.7	1.23	14.0	24.5	1.75
34–35	23.1	23.0	1	12.3	15.7	1.27	8.9	11.1	1.24
36–37	9.0	11.7	1.3	7.5	11.3	1.52			
38–39	3.8	6.1	1.6	6.1	9.8	1.6			
40–41	3.1	5.2	1.71	8.4	10.3	1.23			
>=42	4.1	6.6	1.63	9.4	10.4	1.1			
Total	9.2	20.9	2.27	36.8	66.7	1.81	71.3	288.4	4.05

Singletons: 1995–98 Linked Live birth-Infant death cohort files
Multiples: 1995–98 Multiple birth files
'White' and 'Black' indicate Non-Hispanic White and Black; Missing cells indicate small numbers
Perinatal mortality rate: fetal deaths plus infant deaths per 1000 live births plus fetal deaths

in the fetal mortality rate. The fetal mortality rate among white singleton infants decreased from 6.04 in 1985–1988 to 5.46 per 1000 live births plus fetal deaths in 1995–1998, an overall decrease of 9.60%. The percent change for twins and triplets or higher-order multiples is 25.70% and 29.78%, respectively. Among black infants, variations in fetal mortality rates among singleton twins were less apparent. Compared to white twins with a percent decrease of 25.70, the fetal mortality rate of black twins decreases from 28.26 per 1000 live births plus fetal deaths in 1985–1988 to 27.59 in 1995–1998, a 2.37% decrease. Among black triplets, there is an almost 39% increase in fetal mortality rate from 1985–1988 to 1995–1998.

While the data suggest that there has been some improvement in fetal mortality among whites and blacks, it should be noted that there is an increase in the percent change of the race rate ratios for each plurality group. For example, among twins, the race rate ratios increase from 1.15 in 1985–1988 to 1.51 in 1995–1998, a 31.40% increase. Hebdomadal mortality rates (death less than 7 days after birth per 1000 live births) had a similar pattern, but the percent change among blacks is similar to that of whites, contrary to the fetal mortality data. While an increase in the percent change of the race rate ratios is apparent, the increase is not as marked among multiples for hebdomadal mortality as for fetal mortality.

Similar patterns are also noted for neonatal and infant mortality. As plurality increases, the percent change for race rate ratios for neonatal mortality (death less than 28 days after birth) also increases. In addition, the rate ratio percent change among singletons is 9.7% and 28.0% among triplets or higher order multiples. Considering infant mortality, there was a moderate increase in the race rate ratio among singletons and twins from 1985–1988 to 1995–1998, but for triplets and higher-order multiples, the increase was almost 48%. Overall, for all mortality classifications, the percent change from 1985–1988 to 1995–1998 in mortality rates were less marked among blacks compared to whites, particularly among multiple births.

Gestational age-specific perinatal mortality

Table 147.2 provides the gestational age-specific perinatal mortality (fetal death plus infant deaths) for blacks and whites as well as the race rate ratio. Figure 147.1 illustrates the gestational age-specific perinatal mortality race rate ratios for singletons and twins using 1995–98 data. For singletons, blacks have a lower perinatal mortality rate compared to whites, until roughly 34 weeks' gestation, at which the rates are roughly equal. At approximately 36 weeks' gestation, a crossover is observed in which the perinatal mortality rate of blacks begins to exceed that of whites and the disparity continues to grow.

Among twins, a crossover occurs at 30 weeks' gestation, where white perinatal mortality rate (53.16 per 1000 live births) is less than that of blacks (56.57 per 1000 live births). As seen among singletons, the

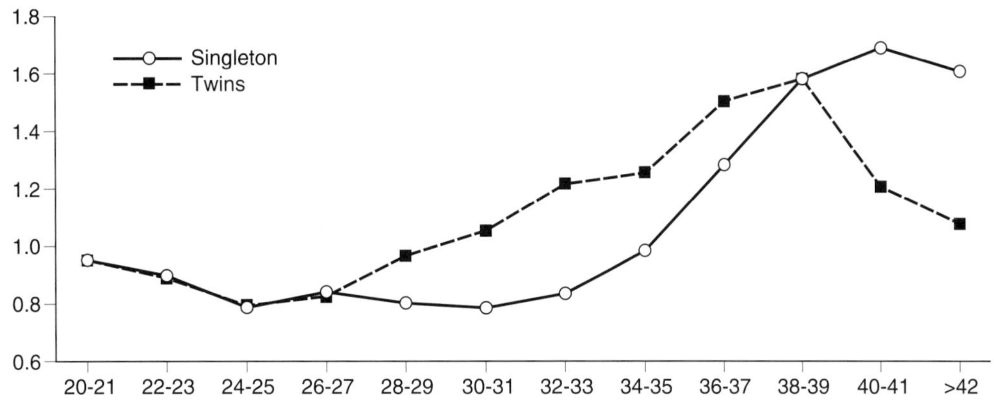

Figure 147.1 1995–98 Gestational age-specific perinatal mortality race rate ratios (Black/White).

disparity between blacks and whites grows, but the overall race rate ratio is less compared to that of singletons. Interestingly, at 38 weeks, the perinatal mortality rate for black singletons is equivalent to that of white twins at 38 weeks' gestation. Among triplets or higher-order multiples, the pattern is less delineated and, for the most part, whites exhibit better survival than blacks. The racial disparity exists but, unlike among singletons and twins, there is no distinct crossover for an improvement in the white mortality. The greatest rate ratio occurs at 26 weeks (1.88). Due to the small number of triplets or higher-order multiples among blacks, it is not possible to calculate the race rate ratio for all gestational ages.

Mortality rates for selected maternal characteristics

Tables 147.3 and 147.4 provide mortality rates for selected maternal characteristics by race. Table 147.3 provides fetal and hebdomadal mortality rates. Table 147.4 provides neonatal and infant mortality rates. The mortality rates differ slightly from Table 147.1 because the data in Tables 147.3 and 147.4 are for non-Hispanic whites and blacks, whereas the rates found in Table 147.1 are those of blacks and whites. Prior to the 1989 change of the birth certificate, the reporting related to ethnicity was poor.

In Tables 147.3 and 147.4, high and low education for age is defined according to an algorithm referenced in Petersen and Alexander, 1992.[44] High education for age is defined as 2 or more years above grade level appropriate for age. Low education for age is defined as 2 or more years below grade level appropriate for age. High gravidity for age defined as having had more than 6 pregnancies at any age; more than 2 pregnancies less than age 18; 3 pregnancies less than age 22; 4 pregnancies less than age 25; and 5 pregnancies less than age 30. The prenatal care utilization index (R-GINDEX) is defined further in Alexander and Cornely, 1987.[45]

Fetal mortality

Among singletons, white fetal mortality rates were lower than those of blacks for all selected maternal characteristics. For older mothers ($\geq$35 years), higher education for age, primigravid, previous pregnancy loss (PPL), hypertension, diabetes, incompetent cervix, and adequate and inadequate prenatal care utilization, the difference in mortality rates was greater than twofold. Among twins, fetal mortality rates were lower among unmarried and teenage black mothers than among whites. The rates were two times higher for blacks compared to whites among mothers with hypertension and diabetes. For triplets, unmarried black mothers had much lower fetal mortality rates (84.46 per 1000 live births plus fetal deaths) compared to white mothers (152.53 per 1000 live births plus fetal deaths), but the mortality rate was much lower for older (35 years) white mothers (14.99 per 1000 live births plus fetal deaths) compared to older black mothers (47.62 per 1000 live births plus fetal deaths).

Hebdomadal mortality

Among singleton births, black infants have a hebdomadal mortality rate that is 2.64 times greater than that of whites. While there is a disparity among twins and triplets or higher-order multiples, the relative differences in mortality rates are not as apparent. Among singletons, there is a threefold difference between black and white mothers with high education for age and PPL. For twins, the overall mortality rate for whites is 17.46 per 1000 live births and for blacks it is 32.82 per 1000 live births, a rate ratio of 1.88. For all selected maternal characteristics, blacks have an increased mortality rate, particularly among those with PPL. For triplets, blacks have a decreased mortality rate among women with low education for age and for PPL compared to whites, but the hebdomadal mortality rate among blacks is almost five times higher compared to whites among women with hypertension.

Neonatal mortality

Overall, black mothers have higher neonatal mortality rates compared to whites. Specifically among singletons, the race rate ratio is 2.5, thereby indicating

Table 147.3 Fetal and hebdomadal mortality rates for selected maternal characteristics by race

	Fetal Mortality (rate per 1000 live births plus fetal deaths)									Hebdomadal Mortality(rate per 1000 live births)								
	Singletons			Twins			Triplets or higher			Singletons			Twins			Triplets or higher		
	White	Black	B/W Ratio	White	Black	B/W Ratio	White	Black	B/W Ratio	White	Black	B/W Ratio	White	Black	B/W Ratio	White	Black	B/W Ratio
Overall	**4.9**	**10.9**	**2.21**	**16.8**	**24.9**	**1.48**	**21.9**	**54.2**	**2.48**	**2.5**	**6.6**	**2.64**	**17.5**	**32.8**	**1.88**	**42.4**	**77.7**	**1.83**
Unmarried	11.1	12.7	1.15	44.7	28.9	0.65	152.5	84.5	0.55	3.7	6.8	1.87	23.6	35.0	1.49	55.1	92.3	1.67
<18 years	6.5	10.8	1.65	35.3	32.3	0.92	78.6	103.5	1.32	3.8	6.1	1.61	35.0	49.0	1.4	108.5	123.1	1.13
>=35 years	6.3	15.3	2.41	13.0	25.5	1.96	15.0	47.6	3.18	2.8	8.1	2.96	12.1	22.4	1.85	30.9	38.9	1.26
High ed for age	3.7	8.2	2.22	13.5	19.0	1.41	19.2	45.0	2.34	1.9	5.9	3.08	14.9	27.5	1.85	39.7	51.7	1.3
Low ed for age	5.5	8.4	1.52	20.0	20.8	1.04	19.9	51.9	2.6	3.4	5.8	1.74	23.7	34.6	1.46	85.8	74.6	0.87
Primigravid	4.6	10.2	2.19	22.5	37.0	1.64	28.3	74.1	2.62	2.6	6.3	2.42	22.4	38.3	1.71	47.7	95.0	1.99
High gravidity for age	9.8	17.3	1.76	18.7	23.7	1.27	33.8	37.0	1.1	4.2	9.9	2.34	17.1	32.5	1.9	44.2	76.9	1.74
Previous pregnancy loss	21.5	45.1	2.1	59.5	82.5	1.39	106.7	189.2	1.77	4.7	14.6	3.12	22.8	53.2	2.34	53.1	41.7	0.79
Smoking	6.7	13.3	1.98	19.6	22.6	1.16	47.9	87.0	1.82	3.4	8.1	2.41	19.7	31.9	1.62	60.7	133.3	2.2
C-section	2.7	3.5	1.33	0.3	0.4	1.4				3.7	5.8	1.59	10.9	13.8	1.26			
Hypertension	6.1	20.1	3.28	8.7	20.7	2.39	13.1	18.0	1.37	2.4	5.0	2.11	6.3	11.6	1.82	8.7	42.7	4.91
Diabetes	5.8	16.9	2.93	10.5	24.0	2.29	7.3	19.2	2.64	2.2	5.2	2.37	9.7	14.8	1.52			
Incompetent Cervix	46.0	98.8	2.15	81.5	107.7	1.32	49.0	87.0	1.77	51.3	107.2	2.09	138.9	220.9	1.59	95.3	190.5	2
Prenatal Care Utilization (R-GINDEX)																		
Intensive	2.8	4.8	1.73	7.4	8.0	1.09	9.6	17.9	1.86	2.3	4.1	1.78	9.0	11.9	1.31	20.3	21.3	1.05
Adequate	5.1	10.4	2.06	14.3	20.8	1.46	20.6	49.3	2.4	2.8	7.6	2.69	17.8	34.2	1.92	50.6	85.4	1.69
Intermediate	2.5	5.7	2.34	12.2	19.4	1.59	9.5	48.0	5.08	1.3	3.0	2.42	13.6	23.3	1.71	53.7	41.3	0.77
Inadequate	3.6	5.5	1.51	11.3	8.1	0.72				1.7	2.5	1.44	9.7	9.6	0.99			
No Care	30.8	39.8	1.29	42.7	70.2	1.64	27.5	90.9	3.3	18.8	30.1	1.6	91.1	111.2	1.22	198.1	233.3	1.18
Missing	24.7	36.6	1.48	84.0	76.4	0.91	78.8	167.4	2.12	9.1	18.6	2.04	52.7	73.1	1.39	89.6	190.2	2.12

Singletons: 1995–98 Linked Live birth-Infant death cohort files
Multiples: 1995-98 Multiple birth files
'White' and 'Black' indicate Non-Hispanic White and Black
Missing cells indicate that numbers were too small to calculate rates

Table 147.4 Neonatal and infant mortality rates for selected maternal characteristics by race

	Neonatal Mortality (rate per 1000 live births)									Infant Mortality(rate per 1000 live births)								
	Singletons			Twins			Triplets or higher			Singletons			Twins			Triplets or higher		
	White	Black	B/W Ratio	White	Black	B/W Ratio	White	Black	B/W Ratio	White	Black	B/W Ratio	White	Black	B/W Ratio	White	Black	B/W Ratio
Overall	**3.2**	**8.0**	**2.5**	**20.4**	**37.8**	**1.86**	**49.7**	**85.3**	**1.72**	**5.2**	**12.4**	**2.38**	**24.4**	**48.4**	**1.99**	**55.4**	**105.6**	**1.91**
Unmarried	4.6	8.3	1.79	26.6	40.3	1.51	56.2	99.1	1.76	8.1	13.2	1.64	34.7	51.9	1.5	62.9	121.6	1.93
<18 years	4.9	7.6	1.54	40.5	54.2	1.34	114.3	137.9	1.21	8.8	12.7	1.44	53.0	67.7	1.28	114.3	158.1	1.38
>=35 years	3.5	9.8	2.83	14.2	27.0	1.91	35.0	42.3	1.21	5.0	13.9	2.8	17.0	34.7	2.04	38.6	68.8	1.78
High ed for age	2.4	7.2	2.94	17.4	32.1	1.85	47.1	57.0	1.21	3.7	10.1	2.73	20.0	40.5	2.03	52.0	75.7	1.45
Low ed for age	4.5	7.4	1.65	27.9	41.6	1.49	88.5	75.5	0.85	9.0	13.9	1.55	37.6	55.6	1.48	106.2	103.8	0.98
Primigravid	3.3	7.7	2.31	25.8	43.6	1.69	51.7	106.5	2.06	5.1	11.2	2.21	29.6	51.5	1.74	57.4	120.4	2.1
High gravidity for age	5.3	11.8	2.23	19.8	38.5	1.94	47.1	80.3	1.7	8.2	18.7	2.28	24.5	51.4	2.1	52.2	92.6	1.77
Previous pregnancy loss	5.6	16.3	2.91	24.8	55.6	2.25	53.8	33.8	0.63	8.1	21.1	2.61	28.7	67.5	2.35	58.3	40.5	0.69
Smoking	4.4	9.9	2.23	23.5	39.4	1.68	77.6	139.1	1.79	8.6	18.4	2.14	31.4	54.9	1.75	90.8	147.8	1.63
C-section	5.1	8.4	1.65	14.6	19.6	1.35				7.9	14.2	1.8	19.0	31.0	1.63			
Hypertension	3.5	7.1	2.01	8.2	14.7	1.79	13.5	47.9	3.55	5.8	12.2	2.1	11.8	23.3	1.98	16.8	71.9	4.29
Diabetes	3.1	6.7	2.15	11.7	22.4	1.92	17.8			5.3	10.5	1.99	15.3	32.6	2.13	20.3	19.2	0.95
Incompetent Cervix	53.9	105.5	1.96	140.0	210.1	1.5	102.4	202.9	1.98	58.1	115.3	1.99	145.5	229.6	1.58	111.9	275.4	2.46
Prenatal Care Utilization (R-GINDEX)																		
Intensive	3.3	5.7	1.72	11.2	16.5	1.47	27.0	34.0	1.26	5.5	9.5	1.74	14.7	26.8	1.82	31.6	51.9	1.64
Adequate	3.6	9.3	2.58	21.0	40.3	1.92	58.0	95.9	1.65	5.4	13.3	2.46	24.8	50.3	2.03	65.2	110.5	1.7
Intermediate	1.8	4.0	2.3	16.3	27.3	1.68	66.2	65.5	0.99	3.5	7.7	2.19	20.7	37.9	1.83	72.1	91.7	1.27
Inadequate	2.4	3.5	1.44	11.8	13.1	1.1				5.8	8.7	1.49	19.3	22.8	1.18			
No Care	21.0	32.6	1.56	94.4	114.3	1.21	211.0	212.1	1.01	27.8	43.9	1.38	105.8	135.7	1.28	220.2	242.4	1.1
Missing	10.2	20.2	1.99	53.5	73.6	1.38	93.6	162.9	1.74	12.9	25.3	1.96	58.7	84.8	1.44	97.2	199.1	2.05

Singletons: 1995-98 Linked Live birth-Infant death cohort files
Multiples: 1995-98 Multiple birth files
'White' and 'Black' indicate Non-Hispanic White and Black
Missing cells indicate that numbers were too small to calculate rates

Table 147.5 Mortality rates of selected infant characteristics by race and plurality

	Singleton			Twins			Triplets or higher		
	White	Black	B/W Rate Ratio	White	Black	B/W Rate Ratio	White	Black	B/W Rate Ratio
				Fetal Mortality[†]					
LBW	63.7	67.4	1.06	27.5	33.7	1.23	20.9	47.9	2.29
VLBW	242.2	203.5	0.84	119.2	105.7	0.89	49.1	89.5	1.82
Preterm	36.8	47.1	1.28	22.4	32.7	1.46	17.7	45.2	2.55
Very Preterm	155.9	136.8	0.88	72.3	75.2	1.04	30.9	69.8	2.26
SGA	20.8	22.6	1.09	19.2	23.0	1.2	23.6	44.5	1.89
				Hebdomadal Mortality[‡]					
LBW	39.1	50.7	1.3	34.5	55.1	1.6	49.3	84.7	1.72
VLBW	192.2	203.7	1.06	182.8	204.4	1.12	125.9	168.8	1.34
Preterm	21.6	32.7	1.51	30.0	51.7	1.73	44.4	77.7	1.75
Very Preterm	112.5	117.8	1.05	113.3	136.0	1.2	85.7	128.7	1.5
SGA	8.3	10.0	1.2	14.9	22.4	1.51	31.6	45.2	1.43
				Neonatal Mortality[‡]					
LBW	43.5	55.7	1.28	39.3	62.0	1.58	57.0	93.1	1.63
VLBW	168.4	187.3	1.11	185.9	210.7	1.13	140.1	177.9	1.27
Preterm	25.0	37.2	1.49	34.5	59.2	1.71	52.3	87.5	1.68
Very Preterm	111.2	119.5	1.07	122.7	147.5	1.2	98.9	141.4	1.43
SGA	10.5	12.2	1.17	17.6	25.9	1.47	36.1	58.9	1.63
				Infant Mortality[‡]					
LBW	53.8	70.2	1.3	45.6	76.1	1.67	63.0	113.3	1.8
VLBW	189.2	216.1	1.14	202.8	240.0	1.18	152.7	209.5	1.37
Preterm	31.2	48.0	1.54	40.3	73.7	1.83	58.5	109.0	1.86
Very Preterm	127.6	142.0	1.11	135.9	172.8	1.27	109.2	171.5	1.57
SGA	16.1	19.5	1.21	22.5	35.3	1.57	40.9	78.5	1.92

'White' and 'Black' indicate Non-Hispanic White and Black
1995–98 Cohort files
1995–98 Multiple birth files
[†]Rate per 1000 live births plus fetal deaths
[‡]Rate per 1000 live births
Fetal mortality rates: per 1000 live birthplus fetal deaths
Hebdomadal, neonatal, and infant mortality rates: per 1000 live births

that the neonatal mortality rate among blacks is 2.5 times greater compared to whites. For all of the selected outcomes, black mothers have higher neonatal mortality rates than whites, with particular differences noted for older mothers, mothers with high education for age, and PPL. Among twins, neonatal mortality rates are higher for black mothers in all the selected characteristics. However, the race rate ratios for most characteristics were lower compared to those of singletons. For triplets or higher-order multiples, a similar pattern is seen as compared to twins; however, the mortality rate of black mothers with low education for age and PPL is less than that of white mothers.

Infant mortality

As seen for all other mortality classifications, infant mortality rates among blacks are higher compared to whites. Among singletons, the race rate ratios indicate that among older mothers, mothers with higher education, and those with PPL, black mothers have much higher infant mortality rates, 2.80, 2.73, and 2.61 per 1000 live births, respectively. Among twins, a similar pattern is seen. For triplets, black women who have low education for age and PPL have lower mortality rates compared to whites.

Mortality rates of selected infant characteristics

Table 147.5 provides the mortality rates of selected infant characteristics by race and plurality. Fetal mortality rates are lower for whites and blacks among twins and triplets compared to singletons with adverse infant outcomes of LBW, very LBW, preterm, and very preterm. For hebdomadal mortality, a similar pattern is seen among some outcomes, but for LBW and preterm infants, the mortality rates increase for triplets or higher-order multiples. Among black infants, hebdomadal mortality rates increase among very LBW infants, while for whites, there is a decrease. For neonatal mortality, the mortality rates of twins with certain outcomes are higher compared to those of triplets or higher-order multiples. While the pattern for infant mortality is less clear, there do appear to be differences in the changes in rates for blacks and whites.

Table 147.6 Adjusted odds ratio for mortality risks by race and plurality

	Blacks		
Mortality	**Singletons**	**Twins**	**Triplet or higher order multiples**
Fetal mortality	1.28 (1.25–1.30)	0.78 (0.74–0.84)	0.72 (0.55–0.94)
Hebdomadal mortality	2.23 (2.18–2.29)	1.60 (1.50–1.69)	1.58 (1.27–1.96)
Neonatal mortality	2.13 (2.09–2.18)	1.60 (1.51–1.69)	1.54 (1.26–1.89)
Infant mortality	1.95 (1.92–1.98)	1.66 (1.58–1.74)	1.75 (1.45–2.11)

Reference group, white non-Hispanic; controlling for marital status, age, education, gravidity, female sex, PPL, and smoking

Among singletons, while there is evidence of disparity among blacks and whites for some infant outcomes, the differences are not as pronounced as previously noted. Very low birth weight black infants have a lower fetal mortality rate (203.46 per 1000 live births plus fetal deaths) compared to white infants (242.17 per 1000 live births plus fetal deaths). A similar pattern is seen for very preterm infants and for very LBW twins. For triplets or higher-order multiples, the race rate ratios indicate greater differences for selected infant outcomes. For example, the hebdomadal mortality rate among black VLBW infants was only slightly higher than that of white VLBW infants. For neonatal and infant mortality, a similar pattern is seen, with the race rate ratios being lower for very LBW and very preterm infants.

Adjusted odds ratios

Table 147.6 shows the mortality risks of black singleton, twins, and triplets or higher-order multiples compared to whites. After controlling for marital status, age, education, gravidity, female sex, PPL, and smoking, these data suggest that among singletons, black infants are at an increased risk of all mortality outcomes compared to whites.

Among twins, blacks are 22% less likely to experience fetal mortality, yet they are roughly 60% more likely to experience hebdomadal, neonatal, and infant mortality. A similar pattern is noted among triplets and higher-order multiples with a protective effect (28% decreased risk) of fetal death among blacks compared to whites.

Comments

Overall, this study indicates that the racial disparities in mortality noted among singleton births persist in multiple births. The data indicate that there has been improvement in the mortality rates over the last decade and the decline is more notable in multiple births compared to singletons. However, a less-marked decline has been noted among blacks. While it is beyond the scope of this study and ability of the data to tease out the underlying factors of the decrease in mortality, these findings do suggest an improvement in clinical management of multiple births. While the advances have lessened the overall impact of the dramatic rise in multiple births on perinatal indicators, there is some indication in these findings that there may be disparities in the access to and utilization of these advances. Discussion of these potential disparities has been noted elsewhere.[43]

It should be noted that the same pattern of improved survival observed among black singleton infants is seen among twin births, with the crossover point at an earlier gestational age. Fetal, hebdomadal, and neonatal mortality rates among very preterm and VLBW black infants are roughly equivalent to or lower compared to whites for singletons and twins, again indicating an increased survival at lower gestational ages and birth weights.

The information presented in this chapter has important clinical and public health implications. It is noteworthy that certain maternal and infant characteristics, while eliciting higher mortality rates among black singletons, may actually be protective in multiples. For example, fetal mortality rates among black infants are lower among those who are unmarried than among those who are married. This information could be useful in further classification for treatment and interventions.

Acknowledgment

This work was supported in part by DHHS, HRSA, MCHB grant 6T76MC00008.

REFERENCES

1. Arias E, MacDorman MF, Strobino DM, Guyer B. Annual summary of vital statistics – 2002. *Pediatrics* 2003;112(6): 1215–30.
2. Allen MC, Alexander GR, Tompkins ME, *et al.* Racial differences in temporal changes in newborn viability and survival by gestational age. *Paediatr Perinat Epidemiol* 2000;14:152–8.
3. Alexander GR, Tompkins ME, Allen MC, *et al.* Trends and racial differences in birth weight and related survival. *Matern Child Health J* 1999;3(1):71–9.
4. Goldenberg RL, Rouse DJ. Prevention of premature birth. *N Engl J Med* 1998;339(5):313–20.
5. Goldenberg RL. The prevention of low birth weight and its sequela. *Prevent Med* 1994;23:627–31.
6. Ballard PL. Scientific rationale for the use of antenatal glucocorticoids to promote fetal development. *Pediatr Rev* 2000; 1(5):E83–90.
7. Thorp JM, Hartmann KE, Berkman ND, *et al.* Antibiotic therapy for the treatment of preterm labor: A review of the evidence. *Am J Obstet Gynecol* 2002;186:587–92.
8. Curley AE, Halliday HL. The present status of exogenous surfactant for the newborn. *Early Hum Dev* 2001;61(2):67–83.
9. Eichenwald EC, Stark AR. High-frequency ventilation: Current status. *Pediatr Rev* 1999;20(12):e127–33.
10. Horbar JD, Lucey JF. Evaluation of neonatal intensive care technologies. *Future Child* 1995;5(1):139–61.
11. Reger R, Dolfin T, Ben-Nun Y, *et al.* Survival rate and 2-year outcome in very low birth weight infants. *Isr J Med Sci* 1995; 31(5):309–13.
12. Schwartz RM, Luby AM, Scanlon JW, *et al.* Effects of surfactant on morbidity, mortality, and resource use in newborn infants weighing 500 to 1500 g. *N Engl J Med* 1994;330(21):1476–80.
13. Avery ME, Tooley WH, Keller JB, *et al.* Is chronic lung disease in low birth weight infants preventable? A survey of eight centers. *Pediatrics* 1987;79(1):26–30.
14. Copper RL, Goldenberg RL, Creasy RK, *et al.* A multicenter study of preterm birth weight and gestational age-specific neonatal mortality. *Am J Obstet Gynecol* 1993;168(1):78–84.
15. Howell EM, Vert P. Neonatal intensive care and birth weight-specific perinatal mortality in Michigan and Lorraine. *Pediatrics* 1993;91(2):464–70.
16. Philip, AGS. Neonatal mortality rate: Is further improvement possible? *J Pediatr* 1995;126(3):427–32.
17. Hulsey TC, Heins HC, Marshall TA, *et al.* Regionalized perinatal care in South Carolina. *J SC Med Assoc* 1989;85(8):357–84.
18. Alexander GR, Kogan MD, Nabukera S. Racial differences in prenatal care use in the United States: Are the disparities decreasing? *Am J Public Health* 2002;92(12):1970–5.
19. Kogan MD, Martin J, Alexander GR, *et al.* The changing pattern of prenatal care utilization in the U.S., 1981–1995: Using different prenatal care indices. *J Am Med Assoc* 1998;279(20):1623–8.
20. Martin JA, Hamilton BE, Sutton PD, Ventura SJ, Menacker F, Munson ML. *Births: Final Data for 2002.* National Vital Statistics Reports, vol. 52, No. 10. Hyattsville, MD: National Center for Health Statistics, 2003.
21. Blondel B, Kaminski M. Trends in the occurrence, determinants, and consequences of multiple births. *Semin Perinatol* 2002; 26(4):239–49.
22. Reynolds MA, Shieve LA, Martin JA, Jeng G, Macaluso M. Trends in multiple births conceived using assisted reproductive technology, United States, 1997–2000. *Pediatrics* 2003;111(5, Pt 2): 1159–62.
23. Russell RB, Petrini JR, Damus K, Mattison DR, Schwarz RH. The changing epidemiology of multiple births in the United States. *Obstet Gynecol* 2003;101(1):129–35.
24. Jewell SE, Yip R. Increasing trends in plural births in the United States. *Obstet Gynecol* 1995;85:229–32.
25. Misra DP, Ananth CV. Infant mortality among singletons and twins in the United States during 2 decades: Effects of maternal age. *Pediatrics* 2002;110(6):1163–8.
26. Templeton A. Avoiding multiple pregnancies in ART. Replace as many embryos as you like – one at a time. *Hum Reprod* 2000; 15:1662.
27. Olivennes F. Double trouble: Yes a twin pregnancy is an adverse outcome. *Hum Reprod* 2000;15:1663–5.
28. ESHRE Campus Course Report. Prevention of twin pregnancies after IVF/ICSI by single embryo transfer. *Hum Reprod* 2001;16:790–800.
29. Polin JI, Frangipane WL. Current concepts in management of obstetric problems for pediatricians. II. Modern concepts in the management of multiple gestations. *Pediatr Clin North Am* 1986; 33:649–61.
30. Centers for Disease Control and Prevention. Infant mortality and low birth weight among black and white infants – United States, 1980–2000. *Morb Mortal Wkly Rep* 2002;51:589–92.
31. Demissie K, Rhoads GG, Ananth CV, *et al.* Trends in preterm birth and neonatal mortality among blacks and whites in the United States from 1989 to 1997. *Am J Epidemiol* 2001;154(4):307–15.
32. Salihu HM, Kinniburgh BA, Aliyu MH, Kirby RS, Alexander GR. Racial disparity in stillbirth among singleton, twin, and triplet gestations in the United States. *Obstet Gynecol* 2004;104(4):734–40.
33. National Center for Health Statistics. *1995–1998 Matched Multiple Birth Data Set.* CD-ROM Series 21, No. 13a. Hyattsville, MD: Public Health Service, January 2003.
34. National Center for Health Statistics. *1998 Birth Cohort Linked Birth/Infant Death Data Set.* CD-ROM Series 20, No. 16a. Hyattsville, MD: Public Health Service, October 2002.
35. National Center for Health Statistics. *1997 Birth Cohort Linked Birth/Infant Death Data Set.* CD-ROM Series 20, No. 15a. Hyattsville, MD: Public Health Service, October 2002.
36. National Center for Health Statistics. *1996 Birth Cohort Linked Birth/Infant Death Data Set.* CD-ROM Series 20, No. 14a. Hyattsville, MD: Public Health Service, October 2002.
37. National Center for Health Statistics. *1995 Birth Cohort Linked Birth/Infant Death Data Set.* CD-ROM Series 20, No. 12a. Hyattsville, MD: Public Health Service, October 2002.
38. National Center for Health Statistics. *1998 Perinatal Mortality Data File.* CD-ROM Series 20, No. 18. Hyattsville, MD: Public Health Service, December 2000.
39. National Center for Health Statistics. *1997 Perinatal Mortality Data File.* CD-ROM Series 20, No. 15. Hyattsville, MD: Public Health Service, September 1999.
40. National Center for Health Statistics. *1996 Perinatal Mortality Data File.* CD-ROM Series 20, No. 14. Hyattsville, MD: Public Health Service, November 1998.
41. National Center for Health Statistics. *1995 Perinatal Mortality Data File.* CD-ROM Series 20, No. 12. Hyattsville, MD: Public Health Service, April 1998.
42. Kessel SS, Kleinman JC, Koontz AM, Hogue CJ, Berendes HW. Racial differences in pregnancy outcomes. *Clin Perinatol* 1988;15(4):745–54.
43. Ranganathan D, Wall S, Khoshnood B, Singh JK, Lee KS. Racial differences in respiratory-related neonatal mortality among very low birth weight infants. *J Pediatr* 2000;136(4):454–9.
44. Petersen DJ, Alexander GR. Seasonal variation in adolescent conceptions, induced abortions, and late initiation of prenatal care. *Public Health Rep* 1992;107(6):701–6.
45. Alexander GR, Cornely DA. Prenatal care utilization: Its measurement and relationship to pregnancy outcome. *Am J Prev Med* 1987;3(5):243–53.

148 Prevention of preterm birth in single and multiple pregnancies

E. Papiernik

We will describe in this chapter how the policy for prevention of preterm birth was successful in France from 1972 to 1988, and how the recent increase in preterm births can be explained. The results are very different for single pregnancies for which prevention did work; the reduction of spontaneous preterm births was clearly found in singleton pregnancies,[1] while an increase was observed for indicated preterm (by medical decision) in single pregnancies.[2] The global increase of preterm births since 1988 was not observed for single pregnancies, whose rates remained stable or with a non significant increase in national representative samples in 1995 and 1998.[3] But for twin and triplet pregnancies no comparable reduction in preterm birth has been measured; on the contrary, a significant rise in preterm births was demonstrated for two associated reasons: first, an increase in the rate of twin pregnancies and second, an increase of the rate of preterm births in twin pregnancies.

Prevention in this chapter will be understood as primary prevention, before the beginning of the disease, before any sign of preterm labor, and will not address the treatment of preterm labor and the treatment given to the mother for an advanced maturity of the newborn.

The task of preventing preterm delivery is very different if the risk is obvious, for women with a previous preterm birth or a previous second-trimester spontaneous abortion, or in the absence of such a previous history. The risk is very different in single pregnancies and in twins or triplet pregnancies. We will first address the situation of single pregnancies with an obvious risk factor, and then those without a risk factor, and address later the problem of prevention of preterm births in twin and triplet pregnancies.

In spite of remarkable progress in the efficacy of neonatal care, prevention remains an important aim, especially the prevention of very early preterm births, as the risk related to preterm birth for the newborn exponentially decreases with each week of gestational age, measured in deaths, severe disease, and hospital neonatal costs[4] as well as by risk of development delay and of cerebral palsy.[5]

Single pregnancies with an obvious risk factor

The major predictor of risk of preterm delivery is the outcome of the previous pregnancy, as established by all scoring systems;[6] the risk is important if the previous pregnancy ended in a preterm birth, and even more important if the mother had two preterm births or one preterm and one second-trimester spontaneous abortion. The risk of a second preterm is 15% if the mother had a first preterm delivery and 32% if she had two previous preterm deliveries.[7,8]

Cervical incompetence is difficult to define but is described by McDonald[9,10] as 'the history of one or two mid-trimester abortions, with early rupture of the membranes, usually before onset of labor. The labor is short and relatively pain-free'. Repeated middle-term abortions at the same time of gestation are significant.

For women with two previous losses as preterm births or late spontaneous abortions, controlled trials have shown that a cerclage has a measured efficacy for the reduction of the recurrence rate of preterm birth. The most important is the trial of the MRC/RCOG Working Party on Cervical Cerclage,[11] which compared 454 cases and 451 controls, and showed that in this high-risk group defined by two losses (either previous second-trimester miscarriage or preterm delivery), cerclage did reduce the risk of delivery before 33 weeks (odds ratio: 0.61, 95% CI: 0.40–0.93) and reduced the risk of miscarriage, stillbirth, or neonatal death (odds ratio: 0.54, 95% CI: 0.33–0.90). But no efficacy was shown for women in lower level risk groups, in the MRC/RCOG trial and by Lazar *et al.*[12]

For women with a history of one previous preterm delivery, cerclage does not help to reduce the risk of a preterm birth in the next pregnancy. But treatment with progestins had been demonstrated to be effective in reducing the occurrence of a second preterm birth in women with a previous spontaneous preterm birth.[13–17]

Single pregnancies without an obvious risk factor

For the majority of women without any obvious risk factor known before or at the beginning of pregnancy, the reasons for preterm birth are more difficult to understand and the task of prevention is not easy.

In 1895, Adolphe Pinard was the first to propose that preterm delivery could be the effect of exposure of poor single mothers to excessive workload; this hypothesis resulted from an observation.[18]

These women, most often young, unmarried, and without social support, worked in a standing position for many hours, 6 days a week. His intervention was simple, by removing these women from their normal working environment to 'rest homes', a simple lodging, kept clean by themselves, with proper meals and adequate sleeping accommodation. His experiment was successful, as the women included in the program had more often deliveries at term, with normal-weight babies, in striking contrast to the frequent preterm deliveries in women not included in this program. The principle that heavy work could be the cause of preterm births became the basis for the medical program adopted for pregnant women as part of the health policy advocated by the League of Nations in 1932.[19]

At the end of World War II, in 1945, all European countries voted for laws for the protection of mothers and children, including several weeks of work leave before the expected date of delivery and after birth, with financial compensation of the salary.

The early focus on reduction of physically arduous work as a preventive measure for reducing preterm births has had an important impact on French perinatal health policy, which was put into place in the 1970s. The proposal that reduction of physical effort was a key intervention during pregnancy for the prevention of preterm birth formed the basis of the national prevention policy proposed in 1972,[20] for women for whom a risk factor would be recognized by a systematic screening, using a risk scoring system,[6] or for those for whom exposition to hard working conditions had been identified. For those women with identified risk factors, a reduction of physical effort or a medically prescribed work leave for employed women would be recommended. This policy remains an active part of the French policy. This intervention on physical effort was part of a global improvement of prenatal care, which will be presented. At present, hard work is no longer a risk factor for the majority of pregnant women in France.

The policy for prevention of preterm births, effective in France since 1972, was designed with several components: (1) early and equal access to prenatal care for all women; (2) provision of information that would convince women to change their lifestyles; (3) recognition, during prenatal care, of warning signs increasing the risk of preterm birth; and (4) appropriate use of maternity work leave and reduction of physical activity.

The French prevention programs target all women and not only high-risk cases. Initial studies on the impact of the prevention program were tested on a demonstration intervention including all women who were delivered in a region of eastern France, in Alsace, in the city of Haguenau on 16,000 women from 1971 to 1982. The reduction of preterm births was demonstrated with the progressive acceptance of the new policy.[21] In this program, it was clear that the reduction of preterm births was not observed for women with high-risk predictors; this is shown in Table 148.1. No reduction of preterm birth could be measured for women with a previous preterm birth, for those with a history of stillbirth, or for those with an episode of bleeding in the second or third trimester.

However, a statistically significant reduction was observed in the middle-risk women, those with 'soft' risk predictors,[22] those in their first pregnancy, those less than 21 years of age, or 36 years or older, those with a low or average level of education measured by the number of years of school attendance. Not surprisingly, the program was not efficient for women in the low-risk groups, such as those with the highest level of education or those in their second or third pregnancy.

This finding was incorporated into policy: prevention efforts to be comprehensive and applied to every pregnant woman. In this regard, the French policy for the prevention of preterm delivery follows the public health approach to the prevention of cardiovascular diseases, which does not target only 50-year-old men who are sedentary, obese, with high cholesterol and high blood pressure, but is directed to the entire population, before risk factors are obvious.

These programs were also focused on those risk factors that could be modified during the present pregnancy, such as information to the woman on her pregnancy, quality of care, or physical effort during pregnancy. It was obvious that the major risk factors, which are important for their predictive value,[6,23,24] could not be used for prevention as they could not be modified during the actual pregnancy. This is true for age, low level of education, low income, or single status, or with a previous adverse history of preterm birth, second-trimester fetal loss, or stillbirth, or for women with an episode of bleeding during the second or the third trimester, with a low-lying placenta, or if the pregnancy is of twins or triplets.

Early and equal access to prenatal care is the basic condition for reaching every pregnant woman and convincing her to be followed and to accept some of

Table 148.1 The rate of preterm births among women delivered at the maternity in the city of Haguenau, in the 'Perinatal Study at Haguenau', for whom a prevention program was proposed, for three successive time periods of observation (1971–1974, 1975–1978, 1979–1982), and the progressive acceptance of the program

Period of observation		1971–1974	1975–1978	1979–1982	P
Prior PTD parous woman	Yes	52/408 (12.7%)	31/248 (12.5%)	33/269 (12.3%)	n.s.
	No	124/2868 (4.3%)	71/2247 (3.2%)	68/3008 (2.9%)	<0.01
Prior SB parous woman	Yes	7/65 (10.8%)	7/53 (13.2%)	7/79 (8.9%)	n.s.
	No	169/3211 (5.3%)	95/2442 (3.9%)	114/3198 (3.6%)	<0.001
Parity	0	152/2343 (6.7%)	108/2325 (4.8%)	115/2574 (4.6%)	<0.01
	1–2	105/2275 (4.6%)	76/2023 (3.8%)	103/2740 (3.8%)	n.s.
	3+	71/1002 (7.1%)	26/472 (5.5%)	18/537 (3.4%)	<0.01
Age	<21	70/961 (73%)	52/801 (6.5%)	49/806 (6.0%)	n.s.
	21–35	227/417 (25.4%)	146/3770 (3.9%)	177/485 (13.6%)	<0.001
	36+	31/461 (6.7%)	10/181 (5.5%)	10/180 (5.6%)	n.s.
Years/school	8	200/3125 (6.4%)	143/2837 (5.0%)	168/3701 (4.5%)	<0.001
	9–12	118/2194 (5.4%)	57/1612 (3.5%)	57/1717 (3.3%)	<0.01
	13+	10/300 (3.3%)	10/371 (2.7%)	11/433 (2.5%)	n.s.
Bleeding in the second trimester	Yes	27/148 (18.2%)	20/97 (20.6%)	18/126 (14.3%)	n.s.
	No	120/1931 (6.2%)	108/2804 (3.9%)	164/4371 (3.8%)	<0.001
Bleeding in the third trimester	Yes	24/140 (17.1%)	8/68 (11.8%)	20/87 (23.0%)	n.s.
	No	179/3392 (5.3%)	159/3967 (4.0%)	194/5429 (3.6%)	<0.001

The reduction in preterm births was observed only in women without major risk factors, but no reduction of preterm birth rates was observed in women with an obvious risk factor, such as previous preterm birth (among parous women), a previous history of stillbirth (among parous women), age below 21 years, or 36 years and above, 8 years of education or 9–12 years of school attendance, an episode of bleeding during the second or third trimester. (Trimester measured among those women who were followed at the prenatal clinic of the Haguenau maternity during the second or the third trimester of pregnancy.) PTD, preterm birth; SB, stillbirth

the proposals for prevention. Free prenatal care in France is a reality and has been so since 1945. All women, regardless of income, educational accomplishments, or legal or alien civil status have access to this as a right. Although the cost of care is variably addressed either privately or in public hospital systems, significant effort has been devoted to convince pregnant women to be included early in basic prenatal care. The choice of the team for antenatal care and the choice of the site of delivery are the patient's decision, and the decision to deliver at a level III institution may be made early on the basis of patient preference or later on the basis of physician referral.

The French national perinatal surveys show that this principle of providing early and adequate care for pregnant women has been successfully implemented, for instance, by the proportion of pregnant women with seven or more prenatal visits measured on representative samples of all French births:[25] 22.2% in 1972, 33.9% in 1976, 54.9% in 1981, 90.5% in 1995; the proportion of pregnant women without any prenatal visit during the first trimester was at 3.6% in 1976 and 2.4% in 1981. A comparison with other European countries shows that France is one of the more successful among its European neighbors in ensuring timely access to medical care during pregnancy.[26]

This effective outreach for most pregnant women is only limited by recent immigration, for women less used to utilizing the facilities offered free to them; this has been measured in a recent study on all women delivered in Seine-Saint-Denis, a poor district northeast of Paris, on more than 40,000 women in 1998/1999,[27] as shown in Table 148.2. For this population, even if a larger proportion among the new immigrants (not born in France) than among women born in France did not have the national social security coverage, the complementary system proposed to all pregnant women by the local district authority, called Protection Maternelle et Infantile (PMI), allows a high proportion of pregnant women to be included early in prenatal care, measured by the proportion with no visits in the first trimester or the proportion of women with

Table 148.2 National insurance coverage, trimester of first prenatal visit, by country of birth, district of Seine-Saint-Denis, October 1998–December 2000, 48,746 singleton live births (after Zeitlin *et al.*[27])

Country of birth of the mother	Continental France ($n = 22,875$)	French Caribbean & Indian Ocean ($n = 1752$)	Southern Europe ($n = 3266$)	Northern Africa ($n = 7602$)	Sub-Saharan Africa ($n = 5803$)	Southeast Asia ($n = 2778$)
National health insurance						
No coverage	1.0	2,2	6.3	5.7	18.7	10.7
Coverage	99.0	97.8	93.7	94.3	81.3	89.3
(% Missing)	(4.1)	(6.9)	(6.7)	(6.9)	(8.8)	(10.2)
First antenatal visit:						
First trimester	94.1	89.8	89.2	90.2	84.4	86.6
Second trimester	4.9	8.5	7.8	7.4	11.2	10.3
Third trimester	1.1	1.7	3.0	2.4	4.4	3.0
(% Missing)	(0.2)	(0.2)	(0.2)	(0.3)	(0.5)	(0.6)
Less than four antenatal visits	3.5	5.6	5.9	6.5	9.2	6.0
No. of antenatal visits (mean)	8.3	8.2	8.0	8.0	7.2	7.8
(% missing)	(9.0)	(10.7)	(10.2)	(9.4)	(11.8)	(11.2)

This table shows that the coverage by national health insurance varies with the site of birth of the mother, in reality with the proportion of recent immigration, with two categories of non-covered, from southern Europe or North Africa, or from sub-Saharan Africa or Southeast Asia. The absence of health insurance coverage is reflected by the proportion of women without a first prenatal visit during the first trimester, but few women have their first prenatal visit during the third trimester, and few have less than four prenatal visits

less than four antenatal visits, or the mean number of antenatal visits.

Here also, collective social agreement reached in France did participate in supporting 'lifestyle changes' during the pregnancy that recognize two facts. The first is that this social agreement accepts that the 9-month period is the only chance the mother will ever have to 'gestate' her baby and help ensure its future as much as possible. The second is the disastrous consequences of preterm delivery in terms of morbidity, mortality, and immediate and long-term familial and societal costs.

French women are informed by articles in the lay press and television networks about the need for lifestyle change and the benefits that can derive from this measure. This is particularly true for the need to obtain work leave and the reduction of physical effort. This is also true but more difficult to implement for women not working outside their home, for whom the rate of preterm birth remains higher than for those employed.

The proposal was to collect two major clinical signs during every routine antenatal care visit following a risk scoring.[6] The first is uterine contractions, the second is the clinical measure of cervical length.

To help the mother to be able to recognize a uterine contraction by herself, obstetricians, midwives, and nurses must take the time to explain what are uterine pains to women who have had no previous pregnancy and are not able to recognize the symptoms. The most common expression for this abnormal feeling is the description of low abdominal 'pressure'. The prenatal attendants should question this woman to discern what circumstances precede the onset of contractions. When questioned carefully, pregnant women describe precisely the circumstances in their daily life that induce uterine contractions. For some women, it is a fast walk; for some, it is carrying an older child; and for others, it is bearing heavy loads at work or working in an imposed rhythm. For still others, it is working in a standing position for hours and for the rest, it is the stressful events in professional or private life.

The second clinical sign is a repetitive quantification of the length and opening of the uterine cervix, which is measured by digital vaginal examination. The efficacy of this proposal for risk screening was confirmed by a prospective study of 8303 pregnant women, which clearly demonstrated the value of these clinical signs in measuring the risk of preterm delivery.[28] The predictive value for the risk of preterm birth of the precocious opening or shortening of the cervix has been documented by the presence of fetal fibronectin in cervical secretions[29] and/or by the shortening of the cervix by vaginal ultrasound measure of cervical length.[30,31] The fibronectin measure or the ultrasound measure of the length of the cervix has not been accepted as routine in France; this corresponds to the available meta-analysis showing no effect in the reduction of preterm births, in spite of their good predictive value.[32]

In France, the local tradition from the end of the 19th century is to use a clinical measure of the length of the cervix at every prenatal visit, even though the efficacy of this practice was not evident. The only available controlled trial on the use of the clinical measure of cervix length did confirm its predictive value,[33] but did not test its usefulness for prevention of preterm birth. No specific intervention was proposed to those women with a short cervix. The statement of this study on the non-usefulness of cervical examination as one of the steps included in the policy of prevention of preterm birth could be a misleading inference[34] as the only action was on the diagnosis side, without any specific action to prevent preterm deliveries for women with a short cervix. This is not different from the statements of Iams[35] or Faron[32] that the diagnostic tools of ultrasound or fetal fibronecin do not by themselves help to reduce preterm births.

In the years following the demonstration of the value of documenting cervical change, physiologic studies have shown that cervix distensibility is a good predictor for preterm labor, because a distended cervix prematurely reaches the low resistance normally observed at term.[36] The mechanism of premature start of labor for women with a short cervix shows that infection or vaginal colonization is a major mechanism of secondary trigger, as infection or vaginal colonization by itself does not increase the risk of prematurity, but the same vaginal infection or colonization is a risk factor for those women with a short or open cervix.[37]

Swedish politicians decided in 1935 to grant for all pregnant women maternity leave during the last weeks of pregnancy for the prevention of preterm birth (and a work leave for several months after delivery to improve breast-feeding), and other Scandinavian countries soon followed suit. Of equal importance, women who went on leave received financial compensation and job protection. Finally, maternity leave became mandatory by law for all women and, along with free prenatal care, was an important part of the European 'System for Protection of Mothers and Children'.

During the year 1945, immediately after the end of World War II, all countries from West as well as East Europe decided to provide all women with maternity leave with financial compensation of the salary for the specific purpose of preventing preterm birth. Leave begins during the last 6–8 weeks of pregnancy in Belgium, France, Germany, Ireland, Italy, and The Netherlands; 10 weeks prenatally in Sweden; and 12 weeks before the expected date of delivery in Norway and the United Kingdom. In France, Belgium, Bulgaria, Germany, The Netherlands, and Poland, salaries are compensated at 100%, up to a stated limit, during maternity leave. In Czechoslovakia, Denmark, and Sweden, salaries are compensated at 90%. In Italy and Greece, the compensation rate is about two-thirds.

All countries also provide a possible addition of sick leave to maternity leave, for as long as necessary during pregnancy, although the proportion of salary compensation for sick leave is less than that given for maternity leave.

During the 1960s, it became obvious that the French policy since 1945, with a maternity prenatal leave for the 6 last weeks, beginning at 35 weeks of pregnancy, was not more adapted to the present needs, not at all adapted to the improvement of survival of those preterm infants born much earlier than 35 weeks. This maternity leave was adapted only to the women in the labor force, and did not target the unemployed women. Thus, a means for earlier intervention had to be proposed, and this was accomplished by proposing to reduce the pregnant woman's workload.[6] This proposal was based on the knowledge available at that time.

It was known that nurses who worked in standing positions were more prone to preterm births, particularly if they worked in very demanding jobs such as in a neonatal intensive care. This information was confirmed by other studies showing that hard work was a risk factor during pregnancy,[23,38–42] even before the start of maternity work leave.

However, such a major intervention as workload reduction could not be proposed for all women, because the cost would be enormous and many women would not accept it. It was therefore necessary to define an intervention and a specific group of women for whom it would be effective and acceptable.

A decision was made to propose the intervention of reduction of physical effort in daily life for those women who had some risk factors identified at the prenatal visit, the risk factors being either a complaint of uterine contractions or evidence of uterine cervix shortening, softening, or opening.

In some cases, the reduction of physical effort could be achieved by a simple change in behavior, with slower walking, not carrying an older child, not shopping for a period, or avoiding long-distance travel by car. If uterine contractions were related to work, however, such as to long hours in a standing position, bearing heavy weights, or commuting 2 h or more every day, then simply changing habits would not effectively reduce physical exertion. In these situations, the only way to modify the physical load was to propose leave from work. At that time, French law did not permit maternity leave to begin earlier than 35 weeks. (The law was changed in 1976 to permit 2 weeks of maternity leave before 35 weeks if medically needed). Under these circumstances, the only solution was sickness leave, and we were able to convince the physicians in the social security system responsible for approving sickness leave that during pregnancy this should be considered as a preventive intervention.

The use of sickness leave was monitored on representative samples of all French women delivering in

Table 148.3 Proportion of employed women with a medical prescription of work leave since the first year of the French national perinatal program in 1972, in which a medical prescription of work leave for prevention of preterm births was provided (after Saurel-Cubizolles and Kaminiski[43])

Percentage of employed women with a prescription of work leave by trimester of pregnancy	1972	1976	1981
French national representative samples *N* women	5727	2463	2955
First trimester	12.5	18.2	23.2
Second trimester	18.4	26.6	33.3
Third trimester	24.0	36.4	40.8

The proportion of employed women with a medical prescription of work leave did increase progressively; in 1995, less than a third of employed women did work during the third trimester

1972, 1976, and 1981,[43] as shown in Table 148.3. The main fact is that the proportion of employed women effectively working in the third trimester of pregnancy was remarkably reduced.

Hard work and work in a standing position were also monitored. The hardness of work decreased over the years for reasons unrelated to the prevention program, but to evolution of the working conditions in all industrial sectors ($P < 0.001$, comparing 1972 with 1976 with 1981).[43]

Leave prescribed by medical doctors, general practitioners, or obstetricians was carefully analyzed, as was the distribution of this intervention by trimester of pregnancy.[43] The proportion of employed women on work leave in the third trimester in 1995 reached 68.5%.[3] These changes represented a major change in the working habits of pregnant women in France.

In France, the prescription of work leave for prevention of preterm labor was accepted by the national insurance system, in addition to the work leave given to all women at 35 weeks, keeping in mind that this prescription was used to reduce the difference with the systematic maternity work leave proposed to all pregnant women in the United Kingdom at 28 weeks or in Sweden at 30 weeks.

The reason for prescription was not directly measured; it could be the presence of a warning sign observed during prenatal care, or just the patient's request, without direct relationship with the presence of a warning sign. At present, less than one-third of employed women work during the third trimester.

Evaluation of this intervention is not easy, as it was not constructed on an experimental basis, as all pregnant women in France were exposed to the intervention without a possible control population.

One of the only possible evaluation tools was to determine that the risk factor of hard work did lose its predictive value for the risk of preterm birth. In fact, the predictive value of hard work disappeared in France, but this was not the case in other European countries in which the prescription of work leave was not as commonly accepted as in France. This differential evolution was measured in a multicenter European study called EUROPOP (for European Study on Preterm Delivery Related to Work) (Table 148.4). This study compared global policies by countries with different practices of frequent or infrequent work leave prescriptions. This was a case–control study in 17 maternities (one per country) between 1994 and 1997, including all consecutive preterm births in the participating clinics (5145 preterm births from 22 to 36 weeks) and a control group including every 10th consecutive term birth (7911 births at or after 37 weeks[44] of which 2369 preterm and 4098 term births were to women employed during pregnancy, as shown in Table 148.4. The two risk factors related to work condition are the number of working hours per week, comparing 30/39 to 40/42 and 43+, and the number of hours of work in a standing position, comparing < 2, 2–6, and > 6 h/day. Three groups of countries were compared, the first group with low figures of infant mortality (below 8 per 1000 births) and frequent prenatal work leave (France, Germany, Italy, Slovenia, Czech Republic); a second group of countries with low infant mortality and infrequent prenatal work leave (Finland, Greece, Ireland, Scotland, Spain, Sweden, The Netherlands); and the third group of countries with infant mortality figures of 10 per 1000 or more and infrequent prenatal work leave (Hungary, Poland, Romania, Russia).

The high number of working hours per week is not predictive of preterm birth in the first group, but is predictive of the risk of preterm birth in the second and the third groups. The same is true for more than 6 h of work in a standing position (Table 148.4). The predictive value of hard work is not more observed in countries with frequent prescriptions of work leave in Europe, but remains as a risk factor for preterm birth in those European countries with infrequent prescriptions of work leave during pregnancy.

Table 148.4 Preterm births related to working conditions (after Saurel-Cubizolles *et al.*[44]) by working hours per week, by group of countries with different policies of prenatal work leave. The predictive value of long working hours per week is not more statistically significant in the group of countries with the practice of long prenatal work leave in group A1, but remains predictive in countries of group A2 without the practice of long prenatal leaves, and is predictive of preterm in countries with less developed perinatal care

Adjusted* odds-ratio of preterm birth related to working conditions	A1 (infant mortality < 8/1000; frequent long prenatal work leave)	A2 (infant mortality < 8/1000; infrequent long prenatal work leave)	B (infant mortality > 10/1000)
Number of employed women after the third month of pregnancy	1833 term births, 936 preterm births	1600 term births, 853 preterm births	616 term births, 534 preterm births
Working hours per week			
30–39	1	1	1
40–42	0.85 (0.4–1.1)	1.20 (0.9–1.5)	1.43 (1.0–2.1)
43+	1.12 (0.8–1.5)	1.40 (1.0–1.9)	1.65 (1.0–2.7)
Standing position hours per day			
Less than 2	1	1	1
2–6	0.98 (0.8–1.3)	1.09 (0.9–1.4)	1.15 (1.1–2.3)
More than 6	1.06 (0.8–1.3)	1.38 (1.1–1.7)	1.55 (1.1–2.3)

Preterm birth related to working conditions, more than 6 h/day, is not more predictive of the risk of preterm birth in the group of countries with the practice of long prenatal leaves (A1), but remains strongly predictive of premature birth in the group of countries with no practice of long prenatal leaves (A2), and in the countries with less developed perinatal care. A1: France, Germany, Italy, Slovenia, the Czech Republic; A2: Finland, Greece, Ireland, Scotland, Spain, Sweden, The Netherlands; B: Hungary, Poland, Romania, Russia

*Adjusted for age, educational level, marital status, obstetrical history, and country. One model was calculated for each of the variables describing working conditions

France is one of the few countries in which a decrease in the preterm birth rate has been documented over the past 30 years. In other European countries with low rates of preterm births, the trends have not been measured; no information is available on the effect of the program for protection of pregnant mothers and children effective since 1935 in Sweden; no estimate before the program can be compared to the low figures observed; and in the same way, no information is available on the effect of 12 weeks of work leave before the expected due date in use since 1945 in the United Kingdom.

In France, the proportion of deliveries before 37 weeks for singleton pregnancies decreased from 8.2% in 1972 to 6.8% in 1976, 5.6% in 1982, and 4.9% in 1988.[1] This reduction was more marked for early preterm births and in the number of very low birth weight babies. The most important results were in deliveries at less than 34 weeks: these decreased in national representative samples from 2.4% of deliveries in 1972 to 1.7% in 1976, 1.2% in 1981, and 0.9% in 1988.[1] In addition, the incidence of very low birth weight babies (less than 1500 g) decreased from 0.8% in 1972 to 0.7% in 1976 and 0.4% in 1981; it remained stable or increased to 0.5% in 1988.

The decrease was observed for all singleton deliveries, but should be described separately for spontaneous or indicated preterm births, as these two components show a different evolution. A significant decrease in spontaneous preterm deliveries was observed. On the other hand, indicated preterm births (after induction of labor or after scheduled cesarean section before spontaneous onset of labor) did increase during these years, as shown in Table 148.5, with a change in the proportion of indicated preterm vs. spontaneous preterm births.[1]

This decrease could not be explained by the technique to measure the duration of gestation, as ultrasound scans were used since 1972, and as the mean birth weight of premature born babies decreased after introduction of first-trimester ultrasound scans.[1]

While data exist to prove that preterm birth rates have declined in France and data also exist to show that policy goals were achieved – a high proportion of women receive timely care and there is a clear reduction in physical activity and workload during

Table 148.5 Preterm births among all live births in the national French representative randomized samples, for singleton and multiple births (after Bréart *et al.*[1] for 1972, 1981, 1988 and Blondel *et al.*[3] 2001 for 1995 and 1998). The preterm birth rate did decrease significantly from 1972 to 1988 ($P<0.001$); after this year, the rate of preterm birth increased

Year	1972	1981	1988	1995	1998
< 37 weeks (%)	6.89	5.39	3.80	5.43	6.27
Spontaneous	6.38	4.66	2.80	3.51	3.86
Induced	0.51	0.73	1.00	1.92	2.31
% Induced	7.3	13.5	26.5	35.4	36.0

The rate of spontaneous preterm births was reduced from 1972 to 1988 by 45%, but began to increase after that year, but remaining at a rate under 4% of all births, much less than the rate at 6% before the preventive intervention. The rate of induced preterm, either after induction of labor or after scheduled section before spontaneous labor, shows a progressive and significant increase, with a rising proportion of induced vs. spontaneous preterm births, describing a major change in obstetrical practice

pregnancy – it is much more difficult to show that these links are causal.

Experimental evaluation of public health policies is very difficult because for interventions proposed to all women in the population, no possible controls exist, if in reality all women were included. This is the case in France, since this policy was directed at the entire population and not just a subgroup of women. This is why we used historical trends, using the fact that for any intervention, there is a gradient in the acceptance of the new policy, and this gradient could be monitored and used for evaluation, for instance, in the Perinatal Study of Haguenau,[45] or for the national data in France.[1]

But this trend for less premature births has changed since 1988, with a progressive increase in the incidence of preterm births (for all births) observed in national figures for 1995 and 1998 (Table 148.6).[3] There are several causes for this increase: the first is the change in medical attitude when a fetal growth restriction is recognized by an ultrasound scan, the second is the progressive rise in the number of multiple births and the rise in preterm deliveries among multiples.

The proportion of medically decided preterm births has increased in 1995 and even more in 1998 in French national samples of all births (Table 148.5). The evolution is in relation with the technical progress allowing a better recognition of fetal growth restriction; this was monitored on a population basis in the district of Seine-Saint-Denis.[46] This study has shown how obstetrical practice did change,[47] with more medical decisions, before 37 weeks, to induce labor or to decide a scheduled cesarean section before spontaneous onset of labor.

On this total population basis was measured the rate of preterm birth for singleton live births, for the years 1998/1999, for women born in France or for new immigrant women born in southern Europe, North Africa, south and east Asia. The rates were low for all these groups, in spite of recent immigration and important differences in income and education among groups. These groups do not show differences in the rates of severe preterm births, and no difference in the proportion of spontaneous and induced preterm births (Table 148.7). Two groups of women were measured with higher rates, women born in the French Caribbean Islands or in the Island of Reunion in the Indian Ocean, and women born in sub-Saharan Africa. These two groups are different by education and income, which are lower in the new immigrants from sub-Saharan Africa, but they share the same African ethnic origin. In these two groups, the rate of spontaneous preterm is significantly higher, as is the rate of severe preterm birth before 33 weeks; the rates are higher for spontaneous preterm births, and the relative risk is higher for induced preterm births when compared to the group of women born in France, southern Europe, North Africa, or south and east Asia. This study also showed that both groups of women with African roots share higher rates of high blood pressure and pregnancy complications related to this high blood pressure.

This prevention policy would not have been successful had our program targeted only high-risk women. Indeed, we have been unable to reduce the risk of preterm delivery in women with a major risk factor, such as previous preterm birth or bleeding in the second or third trimester, or teenagers not included in a shelter program, or women over 35 years of age.[22] Clearly, preventive effort is not effective if applied to high-risk women. This is not surprising, as primary prevention works only before the disease occurs, and before the highly effective risk predictors are present. This concept has been well established in the management of other health problems, including coronary heart disease. Confusion develops because the same word 'prevention' is used to refer to secondary prevention, which is the reduction of disease incidence in people with high-risk factors (obesity, hypertension, high cholesterol), and primary prevention, which is the reduction of disease incidence in people without high-risk factors. Whereas secondary prevention is addressed to individuals, primary prevention must be addressed to all people in a given population.

Our program for prevention of preterm birth did exactly what it was supposed to do. It achieved a risk reduction. Obvious risk factors were reduced in the population, such as a history of a previous preterm birth or the incidence of bleeding during the second or the third trimester (Table 148.8), as demonstrated in the perinatal study of Haguenau,[22] resulting in fewer spontaneous preterm births. Several European countries proposed the same policy for the prevention of preterm

Table 148.6 Preterm births in the French randomized representative samples among all births in 1995 and 1998 (Blondel *et al.*[3])

Preterm births <37 weeks	1995			1998			
	No. of births	No. of pretem births	%	No. of births	No. of preterm births	%	*P*
All live births	13,105	710	5.4	13,358	837	6.2	0.008
All single live births	12,777	577	4.5	13,073	613	4.7	n.s.
All twin live births	316	124	39.2	453	212	46.8	0.04

The increase in the rate of preterm birth is mostly related to twin pregnancies, with an increase in their incidence (from 2.41% in 1995 to 3.35% in 1998), and an increase in the proportion of preterm births among multiples. The rate of preterm births among singleton pregnancies did not show a significant small increase from 1995 to 1998

Table 148.7 Preterm births by country of birth of the mother (percentage and odds-ratio compared to the results for women born in continental France) for singleton pregnancies for all pregnant women delivered in the district of Seine-Saint-Denis, northeast of Paris in the years 1998–1999, with rates of births before 33 weeks, from 33 to 36 weeks, for spontaneous and indicated preterm births, with rates and odds ratio for the comparison of the groups to the results for women born in France, adjusted for age and parity (after Zeitlin *et al.*[27])

Country of birth	Timing of preterm birth			
	< 33 weeks GA (%)	Adjusted OR* (CI)	33–36 weeks GA (%)	Adjusted OR* (CI)
Continental France	0.9	1	3.7	1
French Caribbean/ Indian Ocean	2.3	2.67 (1.91–3.78)	5.5	1.52 (1.22–1.88)
Southern Europe	1.0	1.15 (0.77–1.71)	4.0	1.07 (0.88–1.32)
Northern Africa	1.0	1.12 (0.86–1.46)	3.7	0.99 (0.87–1.14)
Sub-Saharan Africa	2.1	2.43 (1.93–3.05)	5.1	1.39 (1.21–1.59)
Southeast Asia	0.8	0.94 (0.61–1.44)	4.3	1.16 (0.95–1.41)
Test of equality between coefficients			*P*=0.0003	
	Onset of preterm birth			
	Spontaneous GA (%)	**Adjusted OR* (CI)**	**Indicated GA%**	**Adjusted OR* (CI)**
Continental France	3.5	1	1.0	1
French Caribbean/ Indian Ocean	4.6	1.34 (0.91–1.38)	2.9	2.91 (2.14–3.95)
Southern Europe	3.9	1.12 (0.91–1.38)	1.1	1.06 (0.73–1.56)
Northern Africa	3.3	0.96 (0.83–1.11)	1.2	1.15 (0.90–1.47)
Sub-Saharan Africa	4.7	1.38 (1.19–1.58)	2.3	2.26 (1.82–2.80)
Southeast Asia	3.8	1.09 (0.89–1.35)	1.1	0.99 (0.67–1.46)
Test of equality between coefficients			*P*=0.0003	

CI, confidence interval; GA, gestational age; OR, odds ratio
The rates of preterm birth for immigrants from southern Europe, northern Africa, and Southeast Asia are not different from those observed for women born in continental France, but rates for women born in the French Caribbean or Indian Ocean French possessions or those born in sub Saharan Africa are significantly higher

Table 148.8 Evolution of the frequency of risk factors after the acceptance of the prevention policy in the Perinatal Study of Haguenau, during three observation periods, for the risk factors of previous preterm birth among parous women, bleeding during the second trimester, and bleeding during the third trimester (after Bouyer *et al.*[22])

Study period	1971–1974	1975–1978	1979–1982	*P*
Births/period	5622	4824	5852	
Previous preterm parous week	428/3418 (12.5%)	259/2604 (10.0%)	280/3357 (8.3%)	< 0.001
Bleeding in the second trimester	151/2134 (7.1%)	99/2961 (3.3%)	187/5948 (2.8%)	< 0.001
Bleeding in the third trimester	143/3630 (3.9%)	71/4122 (1.7%)	88/5572 (1.6%)	< 0.001

A prevention policy achieved what was expected, a reduction in the proportion of pregnant women with a major risk factor, either from their previous pregnancy (fewer parous women with a previous preterm birth) or during that index pregnancy (fewer women with an episode of bleeding, during either the second or the third trimester)

births, as was determined by the EUROPOP study, and show similar results as those observed in France. In countries without any policy for work leave during pregnancy, such as the United States, the proportion of births prior to 37 weeks has increased from 9.4% in 1981 to 12.1% in 2002.[48]

Prevention of preterm births in multiple pregnancies

As shown in all population based registers, the rate of preterm birth among twins has increased; the question then is to ask if prevention of preterm birth is at all possible, and if yes, to define the goals that could be reached by a prevention policy of preterm birth for twin pregnancies. The question of prevention of preterm births is even more important in twin pregnancies than for single pregnancies, as the risk of cerebral palsy is higher for twin-born infants than for singletons, and even higher for triplets,[49] with the rate for infants with cerebral palsy being 2.3 per 1000 survivors in singletons, 12.6 per 1000 survivors in twins, and 44.8 per 1000 survivors in triplets. Confirmation of these facts was given by the meta-analysis of Stanley *et al.*[5] showing a higher risk of cerebral palsy with an odds ratio of 5.5 (95% CI: 4.34–12.06); this difference is even higher for triplets with an odds ratio of 18.21 (95% CI: 8.74–31.15); the major risk factor is to be born too early or to be born too small.

No program was able to show a reduction in the rate of preterm births in twins and triplets. This chapter will show that many programs were able to reduce the rate of very early preterm births in twins, with a subsequent reduction in neonatal deaths. A program for prevention of preterm births in twin pregnancies should focus on the extreme preterm births.[50]

By comparison with the problem of prevention of preterm delivery in single pregnancies, the problem to address in twin or triplet preterm birth prevention is very different as the risk for preterm birth in twin pregnancies is 50% and for triplet pregnancies, 90%. This means that the risk of severe preterm birth before 32 weeks of gestation is eight times higher for twins than for singletons in the United States, according to the CDC/NHCHS data collection,[51] and the risk of birth before 32 weeks for triplets is 26 times higher than for singletons in the same study.

Prevention should be an important point of discussion as the rate of twin pregnancies continues to rise in the USA[52] and Europe,[53] and the rate of preterm births among twins also continues to rise. Prevention should be an important focus of prenatal care as the consequences of preterm births from multiple pregnancies are better measured on familial impact.[54]

The rate of preterm birth in twins has increased since 20 years, due to more medical interventions aiming at preventing fetal death or fetal disease related to fetal growth retardation.

The rate of preterm births among twins in the United States[55] increased from 40.9% in 1981 to 55.0% in 1997. Twin births account for an ever-increasing percentage of all preterm births from 8.3% in 1981 to 13.0% in 1997. The spontaneous preterm birth rate among twins did not change for US twin births from 1989 to 1997; the proportion of twin births after induction of preterm delivery showed a small change, but an increase has been measured for preterm twin births after scheduled cesarean section for 1995/1997 by comparison with the figures for 1989/1991 and those for 1992/1994.

During these years, the increase of preterm deliveries in twins was contemporary to a remarkable improvement in infant mortality rates[55] for all twin births, for all durations of gestation. Newborn twins have benefited from the transformation of neonatal intensive care, and also from the improvement of obstetrical practice.

The same observation was made in other developed countries;[53] the French national figures show an increase in preterm births among twins,[53] and at the same time an increase of twin births.

In France, this evolution of medical practice toward more medically decided preterm births in twin and triplet pregnancies can be measured on the register (FIVNAT) of all pregnancies following *in vitro* fertilization (IVF) and related assisted reproduction techniques (ART).[56] In this register, we studied the reasons for preterm deliveries and the relationship with fetal growth retardation.

The FIVNAT register shows the differences in the rates of preterm births, comparing single to twin and triple pregnancies. The major difference is in the rate of early preterm births, here defined as births at less than 33 weeks, with 2.3% in singletons, 8.4% in twins, and 30.4% in triplets.

This register collected information about the spontaneous beginning of preterm birth, or after induction of labor or scheduled cesarean section before onset of labor. In single, twin, or triplet pregnancies, there is a clear relationship between fetal growth restriction and medically decided preterm birth.

The proportion of scheduled cesarean sections is not different for single, twin, and triplet pregnancies in the 22–27-week period; between single, twin, and triplet pregnancies at weeks 28–32; and for twin and singleton pregnancies at weeks 32–35. But it is higher for triplet pregnancies, $P < 0.0001$, at weeks 32–35, much higher for twins compared to singletons at week 36, and weeks 37 and above, and even higher in triplets.

This description of the progressive rise of twin births and of prematurity among twins does not mean that nothing can be done; the possible action varies with gestation duration.

It is useful to distinguish three periods within the large proportion of preterm births among twins, with different risk status for the infants born from twin pregnancies, with the inclusion of new knowledge about the risk of cerebral palsy among twin infants.

The risk of cerebral palsy is not the same for different periods of gestation among preterm twins; this gives a strong argument for distinguishing three different periods in the description of preterm births in twin pregnancies, in relation to differences in the risk of cerebral palsy risk among twin infants.

For twins as well as singletons, the risk of neonatal death, severe neonatal disease, long-term developmental handicap, and, specifically, cerebral palsy depends first on the severity of prematurity, measured by the shortness of gestation duration, but the risk might be higher for twin-born infants compared to singletons of the same gestational age,[57,5] with three periods with varying relative risk.

In the period from 22 to 27 weeks, the risk of cerebral palsy is higher for twin infants compared to singletons of the same gestational age, with an odds ratio of 1.94 (95% CI: 1.16–3.24).[5] My proposed interpretation of this higher rate in twins compared to singletons is the specific contribution of monochorial twin pregnancies with the adverse effect of twin–twin transfusion syndrome. The aim of prevention would be to reduce the occurrence of extreme preterm births for cases not related to a twin–twin transfusion syndrome. Strong arguments are in favor of effective prevention of these very early births in twins.

In the period from 28 to 32 weeks, the risk of cerebral palsy is the same for twin and singletons infants, with an odds ratio in the meta-analysis of 1.03 (95% CI: 0.65–1.62). This period is the most important for the prevention program, as it is not in competition with the need to consider fetal growth retardation, as in the next period.

In the period of late preterm births, from 33 to 36 weeks, the risk of cerebral palsy is higher in twins than in singleton infants, with an odds-ratio of 2.25 (95% CI: 1.35–3.74). My interpretation of this fact is based on the different proportion of fetal growth restriction, much higher in twins than in singletons.[5,57] During this period from 32 to 36 weeks, the aim of prevention of preterm births is in opposition to the action adopted in relation to possible fetal growth restriction and the aim to reduce the potential danger to the fetus as a consequence of fetal growth restriction. This risk could be a good reason for termination of pregnancy by induction of labor or by scheduled cesarean section before the spontaneous onset of labor. The prevention policy is only aimed at twin pregnancies without fetal growth restriction of one or both fetuses.

The risk of preterm birth is high for twin pregnancies and is acknowledged as soon as the diagnosis of twinning is made; prevention can be proposed as soon as the first ultrasound scan is performed, and as the mean gestation duration for twin births is 36 weeks, it means that about 50% of all twin pregnancies will end before 37 weeks. But the real problem is to be able to recognize those women at risk of extreme preterm (22–27 weeks) births and early (28–32) preterm births.

The late recognition of twin or multiple gestation is an important risk factor for preterm delivery and perinatal deaths, as shown by the results of a controlled trial with or without a systematic ultrasound scan in the first trimester;[58] the rate of preterm birth is higher in the absence of early diagnosis. The observed difference was for extreme preterm births, with a higher rate for the control group without scan. This difference had an impact on the final result, with neonatal deaths at 27.8 per 1000 births for twin babies born to women with the systematic scan, compared to a neonatal mortality rate of 105.8 per 1000 twin births for the group of women without the systematic scan.

It is also of importance to recognize chorionicity, as monochorionic twin pregnancies show specific complications and a higher rate of extreme preterm births before 28 weeks, in relation to twin–twin transfusion syndrome.[59] This was measured in a population-based study including all twins delivered in a study of perinatal deaths among 67,819 births in the district of Seine-Saint-Denis,[60] where 551 twin deliveries were included beginning at 22 weeks up to the first month of live birth (28 days). Monochorionic twin pregnancy complications explained 50% of all fetal and neonatal deaths, when the proportion of monochorionic pregnancies was not different from the rate of 30% commonly recorded. Complications of extreme preterm births before 28 weeks occur more frequently in monochorionic pregnancies, mostly with the loss of both twins, often with a direct relationship to a twin–twin transfusion syndrome.

Nuchal translucency thickness at 10–14 weeks of gestation is a predictor of severe twin–twin transfusion syndrome.[61] Twin–twin transfusion syndrome can be a specific cause of neurological damage of the fetus and the developing child.[62] In twins resulting from ART, these complications are not observed, as most of the twin pregnancies from ART are dichorionic.

Lack of prenatal care always was and still remains a major risk factor, measured in all twin births in the United States for the years 1998–2000, with a significant difference in the rate of preterm births, before 37 weeks, for twin pregnant women: 57.2% without and 51.2% with prenatal care for Caucasian women, 70.3% vs. 61.6% for African-american women.[63] Women with intensive use of prenatal care for twin pregnancies show the lowest infant mortality rates, compared to those with inadequate prenatal care.[55]

To belong to a high-level social group with good access to information and the capacity to choose the obstetrical team best qualified to follow a twin pregnancy has been shown as a predictor for a better outcome as measured by the study of perinatal deaths for all twin infants born from 1989 to 1991 in the district of Hauts de Seine southwest of Paris, France.[64]

The social status of the mother measured in years of education and level of income is related to important differences in the perception of risk related to a twin pregnancy, and to the choice by the mother of the prenatal outpatient clinic and the maternity.[65] This study was population based and included all twin deliveries in this district of 2,000,000 inhabitants, and between 250 and 300 twin pregnancies per year, in 541 mothers delivered from October 1, 1989, to September 30, 1991, with a direct questionnaire the day of delivery or during the next 2 days, in the 22 maternities of this district where the delivery took place. There were questions on the level of education measured by years of school attendance, income from herself and her husband or companion, the perception of specific risks for the children related to the twin pregnancy, or for the mother herself, the reason for the choice of the maternity. Data were collected on gestation duration, beginning at 26 weeks (and 500 g or more of birth weight), including fetal deaths, and neonatal outcome up to 28 days for all infants, back at home or admitted in a pediatric department. The perception of specific risk for the children or the mother in relation to the twin pregnancy is described in different terms and is less for women of low socioeconomic level; the more educated women have a higher degree of concern ($P < 0.01$). The difference of attitude is also measured by the choice of the maternity in which they decide to be followed; women belonging to the higher socioeconomic level show a more frequent choice of a level 3 maternity, in a perinatal center with on-site availability of neonatal intensive care.

An important progress in the risk assessment has been made by the measure of cervix length by transvaginal scans. A prospective study showed that twin mothers whose cervical length at 24 weeks was 35 mm or more were at low risk of spontaneous delivery before 34 weeks.[66] A meta-analysis of 46 studies including 31,577 women confirms the importance of this technique; cervical length shortening and cervical funneling, alone or in combination, appear to be useful in predicting spontaneous preterm birth in asymptomatic women.[67] The change of cervical length in repeated systematic transvaginal ultrasound scans shows that shortening of the cervix and change of the shape of the inner os, opening with tunneling, can be recognized early in those women who deliver early, before 34 weeks. The median shortening rate was 2.9 mm (0.8–5.2) per week in women who gave birth preterm and 1.2 mm (0.8–2.4) per week in those who gave birth at term.[68]

While the predictive value of cervical length measurement is well established, there are no intervention studies that have evaluated the importance of this measurement in the prevention of preterm birth.

Among the clinical signs collected at the prenatal clinic, the length and orientation of the cervix, the height of the presenting part remain good predictors for the risk of early preterm birth in twins. In spite of the lack of precision, clinical cervical assessment appears to be safe and may be effective in monitoring twin gestation, if transvaginal ultrasound is not available or is too expensive; clinical examination is more subjective and less reproductible.[69–71]

Home uterine activity monitoring can be helpful in identifying women at increased risk of preterm labor before cervical dilation occurs; this information has not resulted in a reduction in the incidence of preterm labor, of advanced cervical dilatation at presentation or preterm birth in controlled trials.[72–75]

The classical risk factors are of interest, such as height and prepregnancy short stature of the mother, limited weight gain[76,77] with a protective value of higher body mass index and of significant weight gain.[78]

Most of the techniques used for the reduction of prematurity in twin or triplet pregnancies have not proven their effectiveness in controlled trials.

Bed rest is the oldest proposed method for the prevention of preterm deliveries in multiple pregnancies. A meta-analysis of six controlled trials[79] involved 600 women and 1400 babies. Systematic bed rest in hospital did not reduce the risk of preterm birth or perinatal mortality. There is a trend to decrease the number of low birth weight babies, with an odds ratio of 0.79 (95% CI: 0.63–0.99), but there is no difference in the number of very low birth weight infants or in neonatal outcome. On the other hand, bed rest in hospital for women with an uncomplicated pregnancy did increase the rate of very preterm births, below 34 weeks, with an odds ratio of 1.84 (95% CI: 1.01–3.34). The only positive outcome related to bed rest is the reduced risk of pregnancy hypertension, with an odds ratio of 0.55 (95% CI: 0.32–0.97).

Prophylactic cerclage has not been shown to be effective in twins,[80] through a meta-analysis of six randomized controlled trials comparing cervical cerclage in low- and moderate-risk women for second-trimester pregnancy loss with expectant management during pregnancy, describing a total of 2175 women. Four trials compared prophylactic cerclage with no cerclage and two examined the therapeutic role of cerclage when ultrasound examination revealed a short cervix. Pooled results failed to show a significant reduction in pregnancy loss and preterm delivery, although a small reduction of births at less than 33 weeks was seen in the largest trial. Cerclage was associated with mild pyrexia, increased use of tocolytic therapy, and more hospital admissions, but no serious morbidity. The conclusion of this meta-analysis was to propose that the effectiveness of prophylactic cerclage in preventing preterm deliveries in mothers with a low or medium risk of second-trimester pregnancy loss was not proven.

Prophylactic betamimetics have not been shown to be effective in twin pregnancies,[81–85] but progestins have been proven as of interest for high-risk single or twin pregnancies, as shown by a meta-analysis by Keirse[86] with the use of 17 alpha hydroxyprogesterone caproate, with an odds ratio of 0.50 (95% CI: 0.30–0.85), with a major confirmation for women with a single pregnancy but at very high risk of recurrent preterm births.[87] But the only specific controlled trial on twin pregnancies has shown a negative result.[88]

Treatment of the mother with systematically prescribed antenatal corticosteroids was not effective for improvement of neonatal outcome for twin neonates,[89] with no reduction of respiratory distress syndrome, with an odds ratio of 0.7 (95% CI: 0.2–2.0), but with a reduction in mean birth weight in term babies of 129 g (95% CI: –218 to 33).

Weight gain during pregnancy might be a protective factor against preterm birth in twin pregnancies. No controlled trial is available to measure the possible effectiveness of recommending high weight gain for mothers of twins, but this question is of interest as mothers with a significant weight gain early in pregnancy, before 24 weeks, are less at risk of preterm births and low birth weight babies.[90,91] The Higgins Nutritional Program in Canada[92] recommended a 1000-cal regimen over recommendations for singleton pregnancies, which resulted in an 80-g increase in twin birth weight and a 15% reduction in preterm birth below 37 weeks. The specialized care described by Luke *et al.*[93] includes a nutritional intervention on the amount of calories and vitamins as well as calcium, magnesium, and zinc, and claims for this non-random study a significant benefit in reduction of early preterm deliveries, a significant difference in birth weight of twin babies, a significant difference in neonatal hospitalization days, and better results at 3 years of age. But it is difficult in this multiproposal intervention to decide whether this was the effect of nutritional intervention or the effect of other proposals for better prenatal care, or the effect of the personal choice of the women in the program compared to those not included in the program.

Work leave prescription on medical advice and life style modifications by information given to the mother are the basic techniques of a policy for prevention of preterm deliveries addressed to all French women,[94] and have been effective for the reduction of spontaneous preterm births in singleton pregnancies. For twin pregnancies the same program has been proposed, but has to be set in action early in pregnancy, as the major goal is the prevention of extreme preterm births. The proposal is a prescription of work leave for employed twin pregnant women between 22 and 24 weeks. No controlled trial is available to test the potential effectiveness of this policy.

The evaluation of this policy was to measure if its application for all twin pregnant women of a given population would reduce the commonly observed social differences in preterm deliveries and in perinatal mortality figures.

A specific study has measured the results of such a policy proposed for all pregnant women with twins in the population of a French district (Hauts de Seine) in the years 1989–1991, 546 women for whom the mean gestation duration at prescription of work leave was 22.6 weeks.[64] The goal of the prevention policy was that this proposal should be available for every pregnant woman, regardless of her social level. The effective action was measured by the mean gestation duration at the first prenatal visit, the mean gestation duration at the first ultrasound scan, the number of prenatal visits, the number of ultrasound scans, the gestation duration at prescription of work leave. It was not the aim to measure the effect of work leave itself, as this specific proposal was included in a much larger prevention policy.

The reality of equal access for all women, regardless of their social level, to the prenatal care proposal was measured by the fact that no difference was observed for time at the first prenatal visit, time at first ultrasound, time for prescription of work leave by socioeconomic level. The observation of results by socioeconomic level showed no difference in the distribution of gestation duration, but there was a higher but not significant difference in births before 28 weeks for the lowest socio-economic group. The only difference between socioeconomic groups of women was in the choice of the maternity,[65] the the best-informed chose more often a level 3 maternity unit, with intensive neonatal care available on site.

The major outcome measure was the rate of preterm births from 26 to 32 weeks, which was 6%, when available comparisons on populations show higher figures, such as 11% before 32 weeks for all US twin births.[95]

This low rate of early and extreme preterm birth seems to explain the low rate of perinatal deaths at 22 per 1000, with a fetal death rate at 8 per 1000 (8/1082) and a low neonatal mortality rate at 15 per 1000 (16/1074) live births, with no significant difference by socioeconomic group. These figures are lower than the perinatal mortality rates for all twin births in United States in 1989/1991 of 28.7 per 1000.[51]

The twin clinic

Several programs have described special sessions in the outpatient department devoted to mothers with multiple pregnancies, conducted by a trained team of doctors and midwifes or nurses offering specific attention to these mothers, specific education on the risk factors, on the importance of limitation of physical activity and avoidance of heavy work, nutritional advice, and specific educative sessions. Such a specialized outpatient twin clinic also gives an opportunity for twin mothers and fathers to meet and provide mutual support. The first description of such a proposal and of effective results was given in Germany.[96]

The first historical comparison with a demonstration of the positive effect of a twin clinic for all twin pregnant women of a region was given in Scotland.[97] In this setting, there was a reduction of extreme preterm births below 28 weeks, and of babies of less than 1500-g weight, in the two last historical periods, 1976/1980 and 1981/1983, compared to the four previous historical periods from 1956 to 1975. The improvement is in the number of neonatal deaths, from a mean level of 60 neonatal deaths per 1000 twin live births to figures of 18.4 per 1000 and 16.2 per 1000, since the twin clinic was made available for all twin pregnant women in Dundee, Scotland.

This type of care has been proposed in many other settings.[98] The specialized prenatal care proposed by Luke *et al.*[93] is another example of a twin clinic with several proposals, including early work leave, information about reduction in physical effort, more visits with a well-informed member of the team, and specific nutritional advice; this intervention claims a significant reduction in the rate of preterm births and a better outcome for twin newborns and twin infants followed at 3 years of age.

A preventive proposal should be proposed not only at the outpatient clinic of the department, but also to all women in the population with a twin pregnancy.

The difficult task of preventing preterm birth in twin pregnancies and the impossibility of prevention of preterm births in triple pregnancies is a strong argument for the prevention of multiple pregnancies in IVF and related techniques, up to the point of preventing twins, by the transfer of a single embryo.[99–102]

In triplet pregnancies, no improvement of gestation duration can be seen comparing earlier and present publications. The mean gestation duration remains in all publications at about 33 weeks, even if there has been a remarkable improvement in the rates of perinatal deaths (PND) from the earlier series to recent ones, from Itzkovic[103] on 59 mothers in 1946/1976 with 132 PND/1000 and Holcberg *et al.*[104] on 78 mothers in 1975/1988 with 312 PND/1000, to better results reported by Lipitz *et al.*[105] on 78 mothers in 1975/1988 with 93 PND/1000, Newman *et al.*[106] on 198 mothers in 1985/1988 with 66 PND/1000, Pons *et al.*[107] on 91 mothers in 1975/1993 with 80 PND/1000, to the more recent period with Ballabh *et al.*[108] in 1993/2000 on 116 mothers with 47 PND/1000 and Barr *et al.*[109] on 51 mothers in 1993/2002 with 40 PND/1000.

The rate of preterm birth in triplets is very different from the rate in twins or singletons, as given, for example, in the French register of all births following IVF or related techniques,[56] in the FIVNAT register for the years 1986/1999. The rate of extreme preterm births below 28 weeks is 3.3%, 1.9 times more than for twins and 5.5 times more than for singletons. The rate of severe preterm births at 28–32 weeks is 27.1% of all triplet births, 3.9 times more than for a twin pregnancy and 15.9 times more than for a singleton pregnancy in the same register. But an improvement in gestation distribution would have been difficult to measure because for triplets, as for twins, a significant proportion of preterm deliveries result from a medical decision, after a better recognition of growth retardation of one, two, or three fetuses with the decision to induce labor or to go in for a scheduled cesarean section. The register FIVNAT gives a comparative description of the decision of elective cesarean section for triplet pregnancies, by duration of pregnancy in six gestation periods. At 28–32 weeks, the proportion of births following elective caesarean section is 57% in singletons, 49% in twins, and 58% in triplet pregnancies, with no significant difference between single, twin, or triplet pregnancies. A difference was measured for the next period, 33–35 weeks, with 48% in single or twin pregnancies and 82% in triplet pregnancies ($P < 0.001$).

Few techniques used for prevention of spontaneous preterm births were tested by controlled trials, none of them with proven efficacy in triplet pregnancies.

Bed rest was tested by a controlled trial,[110] comparing bed rest beginning at 28 weeks with conventional care and normal physical activity at home, with a not significant longer gestation duration for the group at bed rest, a higher birth weight of the newborn babies, and a shorter stay in the neonatal unit, but the meta-analysis did not confirm this difference.[111] The study of Skrablin *et al.*[112] comparing hospital bed rest since the beginning of the second trimester with hospital bed rest at 28 weeks, by choice of the mother herself, shows a benefit for the group of women accepting early bed rest, for gestation duration at delivery, mean birth weight, and perinatal mortality rates. But this is not a controlled study, and the results of the 'normal care' group were very bad, with a mean gestation duration at 30.0 weeks, a mean birth weight at 1228 g, and a perinatal mortality rate of 430 per 1000 births, opening a real question on the negative consequences of the personal choice of the mothers who did not accept the hospital bed rest proposal in this non-randomized study. Adams *et al.*[113] claims a better birth weight of the newborn in a historical comparison of women with or without hospital bed rest; for women offered bed rest at hospital, less intraventricular bleeding was observed in the newborn babies, but no difference in gestation duration and no difference in perinatal mortality rates.

Cerclage with a stitch on the uterine cervix, proposed systematically and not for specific indications for a previous second-trimester pregnancy loss, has not proven its efficacy for triplets,[105,114,115] with an improvement in gestation duration but no difference in neonatal mortality rates.[116]

Systematic prescription of betamimetics has not been proven to improve the results for triplet pregnancies, but has proven that accidents related to utilization of betamimetics perfusion were possible, even early in gestation.[117]

The only proven technique to reduce preterm births related to triplet pregnancies or twin pregnancies is to avoid multiple gestations by a better use of ART and the transfer of only two embryos at routine[99,102] and even only one embryo at a time.[100,101]

REFERENCES

1. Bréart G, Blondel B, Tuppin P, Grandjean H, Kaminsky M. Did preterm deliveries continue to decrease in France in the 1980s. *Paediatr Perinatol Epidemiol* 1995;9:296–356.
2. Papiernik E, Zeitlin J, Rivera L, Bucourt M, Topuz B. Preterm birth in a French population: The importance of births by medical decision. *Br J Obstet Gynaecol* 2003;110:430–2.
3. Blondel B, Norton J, du Mazubrun C, Bréart G. Pour la Coordination des enquêtes nationales périnatales. Evolution des principaux indicateurs de santé périnatale en France métropolitaine entre 1995 et 1998. *J Gynecol Obstet Biol Reprod* 2001;30: 552–64.
4. Gilbert WM, Nesbitt TS, Danielsen B. The cost of prematurity: Quantification by gestational age and weight. *Obstet Gynecol* 2003;102:488–92.
5. Stanley F, Blair E, Alberman E. (eds) The special case of multiple pregnancy. In *Cerebral Palsies: Epidemiology and Causal Pathways*. London: Mac Keith Press, distributed by Cambridge University Press, 2000;109–23.
6. Papiernik E. Le coefficient de risque d'accouchement premature. *La Presse Médicale* 1969;77:793–4.
7. Bakketeg LS, Hoffman HJ, Harley EE. The tendency to repeat gestational age and birthweight in succesive pregnancies. *Am J Obstet Gynecol* 1979;135:1086–106.
8. Carr-Hill RA, Hall MH. The repetition of spontaneous preterm labour. *Br J Obstet Gynaecol* 1985;92:921–8.
9. McDonald IA. Suture of the cervix for inevitable miscarriage. *J Obstet Gynecol Br Empire* 1957;64:346–50.
10. McDonald IA. Cervical cerclage. *Clin J Obstet Gynecol* 1980; 7:461–79.
11. MRC/RCOG Working Party on Cervical Cerclage. Interim report of the Medical Research Council Royal College of Obstetricians and Gynecologists multicentre randomized trial of cervical cerclage. *Br J Obstet Gynaecol* 1988;95:437–45.
12. Lazar P, Gueguen S, Dreyfus J, Renaud R, Pontonnier G, Papiernik E. Multicentred controlled trial of cervical cerclage in women at moderate risk of preterm delivery. *Br J Obstet Gynaecol* 1984;91:731–5.
13. Goldstein PA, Sacks HS, Chalmers TS. Hormone administration for the maintenance of pregnancy. In Chalmers I, Marc ME, Keirse JNC, eds. *Effective Care in Pregnancy and Childbirth*. London: Oxford University Press, 1989:612–23.
14. De Fonseca EB, Bittar RE, Carvalho MHB, Zugaib M. Prophylactic administration of progesterone by vaginal suppository to reduce the incidence of spontaneous preterm birth in women at increased risk: A randomized placebo-controlled double-blind trial. *Am J Obstet Gynecol* 2003;188:419–24.
15. Meis PJ, Klebanoff M, Thom E, *et al.* Prevention of recurrent preterm delivery by 17 alpha hydroxyprogesterone caproate. *N Engl J Med* 2003;348:2379–85.
16. Petrini JR, Callaghan WM, Klebanoff M, Green NS, Lackritz EM, Howse JL, Schwarz RH, Damus K. Estimated effect of 17 alpha-hydroxyprogesterone caproate on preterm birth in the United States. *Obstet Gynecol* 2005;105:267–72.
17. Papiernik E. Double blind study of an agent to prevent preterm delivery among women at increased risk. *Shering ed Ser 4* 1970:65–8.
18. Pinard A. Prévention des accouchements prématurés par les Refuges et Asiles des femmes enceintes. *Bull Soc Med Pub Hyg Prof Paris* 1895;XVIII:326–32.
19. Debré R, Jouannon P, Cremieu-Alcan MT. *La Mortalité Infantile et la mortinatalité. Résultats de l'enquête poursuivie en France et dans cinq pays d'Europe sous les auspices du Comité d'Hygiène de la Société des Nations*. Paris: Masson, 1933;1:464.
20. Ministere de la santé publique et de la sécurité sociale. Le plan périnatalité. In *Pour une politique de la santé*. Paris: La Documentation Française, 1971:50–107.
21. Papiernik E, Bouyer J, Dreyfus J *et al.* Prevention of preterm births: A perinatal study in Hagueneau, France. *Pediatrics* 1985;76:154–8.
22. Bouyer J, Papiernik E, Gueguen S. Changes in the frequency of risk factors for preterm delivery and their predictive value over time. In Papiernik E, Keith LG, Bouyer J, Dreyfus J, Lazar P, eds. *Effective Prevention of Preterm Birth: French Experience Measured at Haguenau*. Preventing Birth Defects, Original Articles Series, vol. 25. March of Dimes, 1989;1:115–22.
23. Kaminski M, Goujard J, Rumeau-Rouquette C. Prediction of low birthweight and prematurity by a multiple regression analysis with maternal characteristics known since the begining of pregnancy. *Am J Epidemiol* 1973;2:195–204.
24. Berkowirtz GS, Papiernik E. The epidemiology of preterm births. *Epidemiol Rev* 1994;15:414–43.
25. Blondel B, Breat G, Du Mazubrun C, *et al.* La situation périnatale en France, evolution entre 1981 et 1995 (The perinatal situation in France, trends between 1981 and 1995). *J Gynecol Obstet Biol Reprod* 1997;26:770–80.
26. Wildman K, Blondel B, Nijhuis J, Defoot P, Bakoula C. European indicators of health care during pregnancy, delivery and the postpartum period. *Eur J Obstet Gynecol Reprod Biol* 2003;111: S53–65.
27. Zeitlin J, Bucourt M, Rivera L, Topuz B, Papiernik E. Preterm birth and maternal country of birth in a french district with a multiethnic population. *Br J Obstet Gynaecol* 2004;111:1–7.
28. Papiernik E, Bouyer J, Gueguen S. Precocious cervical reopening and preterm labour. *Obstet Gynecol* 1986;67:238–42.
29. Lockwood CJ, Senyi AE, Distre MR. Fetal fibronectin in cervical and vaginal secretions as a predictor for preterm delivery. *N Engl J Med* 1991;325:669–74.
30. Anderson HF, Nugent CE, Wanty SD, Hayashi RH. Prediction of risk for preterm delivery by ultrasonographic measurement of cervical length. *Am J Obstet Gynecol* 1990;163:859–67.

31. Iams JD, Goldenberg RC, Meis PJ, Mercer BM, Moawad A, Das A. The length of the cervix and the risk of spontaneous preterm delivery. *N Engl J Med* 1996;334:567–72.
32. Faron G, Boulvain M, Irion O, Bernard PM, Frazer WD. Prediction of preterm delivery by fetal fibronectine: A meta-analysis. *Obstet Gynecol* 1998:92;153–8.
33. Buekens P. Alexander S, Boutsen M, Blondel B, Kaminski M, Reid M. Randomised control trial of routine cervical examination in pregnancy European Community Collaborative Study Group on Prenatal Screening. *Lancet* 1994:344;841–4.
34. Khan S. Khan SN, Woqu C, Arnott N, Chien P. Misleading authors' inferences in obstetric diagnostic test literature. *Am J Obstet Gynecol* 1999;181:112–5.
35. Iams JD. Prediction and early detection of preterm labor. *Obstet Gynecol* 2003;101:402–12.
36. Cabrol D, Jannet D, Lehouezec R. Mechanical properties of the pregnant human uterus cervix, use of an instrument to measure the index of distensibility. *Gynecol Obstet Invest* 1990;29:32–6.
37. Chambers S, Pons JC, Richard A,Chiesa M, Bouyer J, Papiernik E. Vaginal infections, cervical ripening and preterm delivery. *Eur J Obstet Gynecol Reprod Biol* 1990;38:103–8.
38. Mamelle N, Laumon B, Lazar P. Prematurity and occupational activity during pregnancy. *Am J Epidemiol* 1984,119:309–22.
39. Ahlborg G Jr, Bodin L, Hogstedt C. Heavy lifting during pregnancy. A hazard to the fetus? A prospective study. *Int J Epidemiol* 1990; 19:90–7.
40. Homer CJ, James SA, Siegel E. Work related psychosocial stress and risk of preterm low birth weight delivery. *Am J Public Health* 1990;80:173–7.
41. Saurel-Cubizolles MJ, Kaminski M. Is preterm delivery still related to physical condition in pregnancy. *J Epidemiol Community Health* 1991;45:29–4.
42. Klebanoff MA, Shono PH, Rhoads GC. Outcomes of pregnancy in a national sample of resident physicians. *N Engl J Med* 1990;323:1040–5.
43. Saurel-Cubizolles MJ., Kaminski M. Activité professionnelle pendant la grossesse. In Rumeau-Rouquette C, Du Mazubrun C, Rabarison Y, eds. *Naitre en France, 10 ans d'évolution.* Paris: Inserm-Doin, 1984;1:139–47.
44. Saurel-Cubizolles MJ, Zeitlin J, Lelong N, *et al.* Employment, working condition and preterm birth: Results from the European case–control survey. *J Epidemiol Community Health* 2004;58: 395–401.
45. Papiernik E, Bouyer J, Collin G, Winisdoerffer G, Dreyfus J. Precocious cervical ripening and preterm labor. *Obstet Gynecol* 1986;67:238–42.
46. Zeitlin J, Ancel PY, Saurel-Cubizolles MJ, Papiernik E. The relationship between intrauterine growth restriction and preterm delivery: An empirical approach using data from the EUROPOP case–control study. *Br J Obstet Gynaecol* 2000;107:750–8.
47. Papiernik E, Zeitlin J, Rivera L, Bucourt M, Topuz B. Preterm birth in a French population: The importance of births by medical decision. *Br J Obstet Gynaecol* 2003;110:430–2.
48. Martin JA, Kochanek KD, Strobino DM, Guyer B, MacDorman MF. Annual summary of vital statistics—2003. *Pediatrics* 2005;115: 619–34.
49. Pharoah PO, Cooke T. Cerebral palsy and multiple births. *Arch Dis Child Fetal Neonatal Ed* 1996;75:174–7.
50. Papiernik E. The rate of preterm twin births (22–27 weeks) as a criterion for measuring the quality of prenatal care. *Twin Res* 2001; 4:426–30.
51. Kiely JL. What is the population based risk of preterm births among twins and other multiples. *Clinical Obstet Gynecol* 1998; 41:3–11.
52. Martin JA, Hamilton BE, Ventura SJ, Menacker F, Park MM, Sutt PD. Births: Final data for 2001. *Natl Vital Stat Rep.* 2002;51:1–102.
53. Blondel B, Kogan MD, Alexander GR, *et al.* The impact of increasing number of multiple births on the rates of preterm births and low birth weight: An international study. *Am J Public Health* 2002; 8:1323–30.
54. Bryan E. The impact of multiple preterm births on the family. *Br J Obstet Gynaecol* 2003;110(Suppl 20):24–8.
55. Kogan MD, Alexander GR, Kotelchuck M, *et al.* Trends in twin birth outcomes and prenatal care utilization in the United States, 1981–1997. *J Am Med Assoc* 2000;284:335–41.
56. Papiernik E, De Mouzon J. Triplet pregnancies from French IVF centers: 1968–98. In Keith JG, Blickstein I, eds. *Triplet Pregnancies and Their Consequences.* London: Parthenon Publishing Group, 2002: 45–54.
57. Williams K, Hennessy E, Alberman E. Cerebral palsy: Effect of twinning, birthweight, and gestational age. *Arch Dis Child Fetal Neonatal Ed* 1996;75:F178–82.
58. Saari-Kemppainen A, Karjalainen O, Ylöselo P, Heinonen OP. Ultrasound screening and perinatal mortality: Controlled trial of systematic one stage screening in pregnancy. *Lancet* 1990;336: 387–91.
59. Blickstein I. The twin–twin transfusion syndrome. *Obstet Gynecol* 1990;76:714–22.
60. Chitrit Y, Filidori M, Pons JC, Duyme M, Papiernik E. Perinatal mortality in twin pregnancies: A three years analysis in Seine-Saint-Denis (France). *Eur J Obstet Gynecol Reprod Biol* 1999; 86:23–8.
61. Sebire F, D'Ercole C, Hughes K, Carvalho M, Nicolaides KH. Increased nuchal translucency thickness at 10–14 weeks as a predictor of severe twin–twin transfusion syndrome. *Ultrasound Obstet Gynecol* 1997;10:86–9.
62. Larroche JC, Girard N, Nancy F, Fallet C. Abnormal cortical plate (polymicrogyria), heterotopias and brain damage in monozygotous twins. *Biol Neonate* 1994;65:343–52.
63. Vintzileos AM, Ananth CV, Simulian JC, Scorza WE. The impact of prenatal care on preterm births among twin gestations in the United States, 1989–2000. *Am J Obstet Gynecol* 203;189:818–23.
64. Papiernik E, Richard A, Tafforeau J, Keith LG. Social groups and prevention of preterm births in a population of twin mothers. *J Perinat Med* 1996;24:669–76.
65. Papiernik E, Richard A, Tafforeau J, Keith LG. Perception of risk, choice of maternity site, and socio economic level of twin mothers *J Perinat Med* 1997;25:139–45.
66. Imseis HM, Albert TA, Iams JD. Identifying twin gestations at low risk for preterm birth with transvaginal ultrasonographic cervical measurement at 24 weeks gestation. *Am J Obstet Gynecol* 1997; 177:1149–55.
67. Honest H, Bachman LM, Coomarasamy A, Gupka JK, Kleijnen J, Khan KS. Accuracy of cervical transvaginal sonography in predictiong preterm birth: A systematic review. *Ultrasound Obstet Gynecol* 2003;22:305–22.
68. Bergelin I, Valentin L. Cervical changes in twin pregnancies during the latter half of pregnancy: A longitudinal observation study. *Ultrasound Obstet Gynecol* 2003;21:556–63.
69. Bivins HA, Newman RB, Ellings JM. Risk of antepartum cervical examination in multifetal gestations. *Am J Obstet Gynecol* 1991; 169:22–5.
70. Newman RB, Godsey RK, Ellings JM, Campbell BA, Eller DP, Miller MC. Quantification of cervical change: Relationship to preterm delivery in the multifetal gestation. *Am J Obstet Gynecol* 1991;165:264–9.
71. Gomez R, Galasso M. Romero R. Ultrasonic examination of the uterine cervix is better than cervical digital examination as a predictor of likelihood of premature delivery in patients with preterm labor and intact membranes. *Obstet Gynecol* 1994;171: 956–64.
72. Knuppel RA, Lake MF, Watson DL, *et al.* Preventing preterm birth in twin gestation: Home uterine activity monitoring and perinatal nursing support. *Am J Obstet Gynecol* 1990;76:24S–27S.
73. Collaborative Home Uterine Monitoring Study (CUHMS) Group. A multicenter randomised controlled trial of home uterine monitoring: Active versus sham device. *Am J Obstet Gynecol* 1995;173:1120–7.
74. Colton T, Kayne HL, Zhang Y, Heeren TA. A meta-analysis of home uterine monitoring. *Am J Obstet Gynecol* 1995;173:1499–505.
75. Rust OA, Perry KG, Andrew ME, Roberts WE, Martin RW, Morrison JC. Twins and preterm labor. *J Reprod Med* 1997;42: 229–34.
76. Pederson AL, Worthington-Roberts B, Hickok DE. Weight gain patterns during twin gestation. *Am J Diet Assoc* 1989;89:642–6.
77. Luke B. Maternal weight gain in ideal twin pregnancies. *Am J Diet Assoc* 1996;96:178–81.
78. Riese ML, Swift HM, Barnes SL. Newborn twin outcome predicted by maternal variables: Differentiation by term and sex. *Twin Res* 2003;6:12–8.
79. Crowther CA. Hospitalisation and bed rest for multiple pregnancy. *Cochrane Database Syst Rev* 2000;2:CD000110.
80. Drakeley AJ, Roberts D, Alfirevic Z. Cervical stich (cerclage) for preventing pregnancy loss in women (Cochrane Review). In *Cochrane Library,* issue 4. Chichester, UK: Wiley, 2003.
81. Cetrullo CL, Freeman RK. Ritodrine HCl for the prevention of preterm labor in twin pregnancies. *Acta Genet Med Gemellol* 1976;321–5.

82. Marivate M, De Villers KQ, Fairbrother P. Effect of prophylactic outpatient administration of fenoterol on the time of onset of spontaneous labor and fetal growth in twin pregnancy. *Am J Obstet Gynecol* 1977;128:707–9.
83. O'Connor MC, Murphy H, Darymple IJ. Double blind trial of ritodrine and placebo in twin pregnancy. *Br J Obstet Gynaecol* 1979;86:706–9.
84. Gummerus M. Halonen O. Prophylactic long term oral tocolysis of multiple pregnancies. *Br J Obstet Gynaecol* 1987;94:249–51.
85. Ashworth MF, Spooner SF, Verkuyl DA, Waterman R, Ashurt HM. Failure to prevent preterm labour and delivery in twin pregnancy using oral salbutamol. *Br J Obstet Gynaecol* 1990;97:878–82.
86. Keirse M. Progestogen administration in pregnancy may prevent preterm delivery. *Br J Obstet Gynaecol* 1991;97:149–52.
87. Meis PJ, Klebanoff M, Thom E, *et al.* Prevention of recurrent preterm delivery by 17 alpha hydroxy progesterone caproate. *N Eng J Med* 2003;348:2379–85.
88. Hartikainen-Sorri AL, Kauppila A, Tuimala R. Inefficacy of 17 alpha hydroxyprogesterone caproate in the prevention of prematurity in twin pregancy. *Obstet Gynecol* 1980;56:692–5.
89. Murphy DJ. Caukwell S, Joels LA, Wardle P. Cohort study of the neonatal outcome of twin pregnancies treated with prophylactic or rescue antenatal corticosteroids. *Am J Obstet Gynecol* 2002;187:483–8.
90. Luke B, Minogue J, Witter FR. The ideal twin pregnancy; patterns of weight gain, discordancy and length of gestation. *Am J Obstet Gynecol* 1993;169:588–97.
91. Lantz ME, Chez RA, Rodriguez A, Porter KB. Maternal weight gain patterns and birth weight outcome in twin gestation. *Obstet Gynecol* 1996;87:551–6.
92. Dubois S, Dougherty C, Duquette MP, Hanley JA, Moutquin JM. Twin pregnancu: The impact of the Higgins Nutrition Intervention Program on maternal and neonatal outcomes. *Am J Clin Nutr* 1991;53:1397–1403.
93. Luke B, Brown MB, Misiunas R, *et al.* Specialized prenatal care and maternal and infant outcomes in twin pregnancy. *Am J Obstet Gynecol* 2003;189:934.
94. Papiernik E, Bouyer J, Dreyfus J, *et al.* A perinatal study in Haguenau, France. *Pediatrics* 1985;76:154–8.
95. Taffel SM. Demographic trends in twin births: USA. In Elder MG. Romero R, Lamont RF, eds. *Preterm Labor.* New York: Churchill Livingstone, 1997:127–52.
96. SholtesG. Uberwachung und betrevung des mehrlins schwangershahten gebursthilfe. *Frauenheilkd* 1977;37:747–55.
97. Osborne CK, Patel NH. An assessment of perinatal mortality in twin pregnancies. *Acta Genet Med Gemellol* 1985;34:193–9.
98. Ellings JM. Newman RB, Hulsey TC, Bivins HA, Keenan A. Reduction in very low birth weight deliveries and perinatal mortality in a specialized multidisciplinary twin clinic. *Obstet Gynecol* 1993;81:1057–8.
99. Hazekamp J, Bergh C, Wennerholm UB, Hovatta O, Karlsröm PO, Selbing A. Avoiding multiple pregnancies in ART. *Hum Reprod* 2000;15:1217–9.
100. Olivennes O, Avoiding multiple pregnancies in ART/double trouble: Yes a twin pregnancy is an adverse outcome. *Hum Reprod* 2000;15:1663–5.
101. Gerris J, Van Royen E, Avoiding multiple pregnancy in ART: Replace as many embryos as you like-one at a time. *Hum Reprod* 2000;15:1662–2.
102. ESHRE Campus course report. Prevention of twin pregnancies by single embryo transfer. *Hum Reprod* 2001;16:790–800.
103. Itzkovic D. A survey of 59 triplet pregnancies. *Br J Obstet Gynaecol* 1979;86:23–8.
104. Holcberg G, Biale Y, Lewenthal H, Insler V. Outcome of pregnancy in 31 triplet gestations. *Obstet Gynecol* 1982;59:505–9.
105. Lipitz S, Reichman B, Paret G, *et al.* The improving outcome of triplet pregnancies. *Am J Obstet Gynecol* 1989;161:1279–84.
106. Newman RB, Hamer C, Miller C. Outpatient triplet management. A contemporary view. *Am J Obstet Gynecol* 1989;161: 547–55.
107. Pons JC, Charlemaine C, Dubreuil E, Papiernil E, Frydman R. Outcome of 91 triplet pregnancies. *Eur J Obstet Gynecol Biol Reprod* 1998;76:131–9.
108. Ballabh P, Kumari J, Alkouatly HB, *et al.* Neonatal outcome of triplet versus twin and singleton pregnancies: A matched case control study. *Eur J Obstet Gynecol Biol Reprod* 2003;100:28–36.
109. Barr S, Poggi S, Keszler M. Triplet morbidity and mortality in a large case series. *J Perinatol* 2003;23:368–71.
110. Crowther CA, Verkuyl DAA, Ashworth MF, Bannerman C, Ashurst HM. The effects of hospitalisation for bed rest on duration of gestation, fetal growth and neonatal morbidity in triplet pregnancy. *Acta Genet Med Gemellol* 1991;40:63–8.
111. Crowther CA, Hospitalisation and bed rest for multiple pregnancy. *Cochrane Database Syst Rev* 2001;1:CD000110.
112. Skrablin S, Kuvacic I, Jukic P, Kalafatic B. Hospitalization versus outpatient care in the management of triplet gestations. *Int J Obstet Gynecol* 2002;77:223–9.
113. Adams D, Sholl JS, Haney EI, *et al.* Perinatal outcome associated with outpatient management of triplet pregnancy. *Am J Obstet Gynecol* 1998;178:848–57.
114. Elimian A, Figueroa R, Nigam S, Verma U, Tejani N, Kirchenbaum N. Perinatal outcome of triplet gestation: Does prophylactic cerclage make a difference. *J Matern Fetal Med* 1998;8:119–22.
115. Strauss A, Heer IM, Janben U, Dannecker C, Hillemanns P, Muller-Egloff S. Routine cervical cerclage in higher order multiple gestation, does It prolong pregnancy. *Twin Res* 2002;5: 67–70.
116. Mordel N, Zajicek G, Benshushan A, Schencker JG, *et al.* Elective suture of uterine cervix in triplets. *Am J Perinatol* 1993; 10:63–8.
117. Boulot P, Hedon B, Pellicia G, *et al.* Favorable outcome in 33 triplet pregnancies managed between 1985 and 1990. *Eur J Obstet Gynecol Biol Reprod* 1992;43:123–9.

149 The vanishing fetus in multiple pregnancy

H. J. Landy and L. G. Keith

Introduction

The 'vanishing twin' phenomenon has been well described over the past two decades. Ultrasound scans performed during early pregnancy have demonstrated that the number of conceived multiple pregnancies exceeds the multiple birth rate. Spontaneous first-trimester fetal loss of multifetal gestations occurs relatively frequently.[1,2] Over the years, spontaneous pregnancy loss in multiple gestations has been confirmed in both animals and humans, especially after technological advancement in sonographic techniques and the introduction of assisted reproductive technologies (ARTs).[1]

Diagnosis and frequency

Early pregnancy fetal disappearance likely involves resorption and/or formation of blighted ova, though the precise mechanisms of this phenomenon have yet to be elucidated. Reports of the vanishing twin from the 1970s and 1980s inaccurately suggested a wide range of occurrence; however, technological progress has helped to refine these numbers.[1,2] In the past, reports of high rates of multiple gestation likely resulted from sonographic error in the misinterpretation of normal early embryonic structures or of other conditions (e.g. subchorionic hematomas or collections of subchorionic fluid).[1–3] Sonographically defined characteristics were first proposed by Blumenfeld *et al.* in 1992 in order to better recognize a true intrauterine gestational sac and minimize interpretive error.[4] These characteristics include: (1) a double contour; (2) identification of a yolk sac within the gestational sac; and (3) recognition of an embryonic heart beat after 6 weeks of gestation.[4]

Transvaginal sonography, available since the late 1980s, provides detailed visual information regarding early pregnancy. Early resorption in multiple gestations has been well described over the last 20 years. The figures included demonstrate the sonographic images of pregnancies in which the vanishing twin phenomenon has been documented (Figures 149.1–149.3).

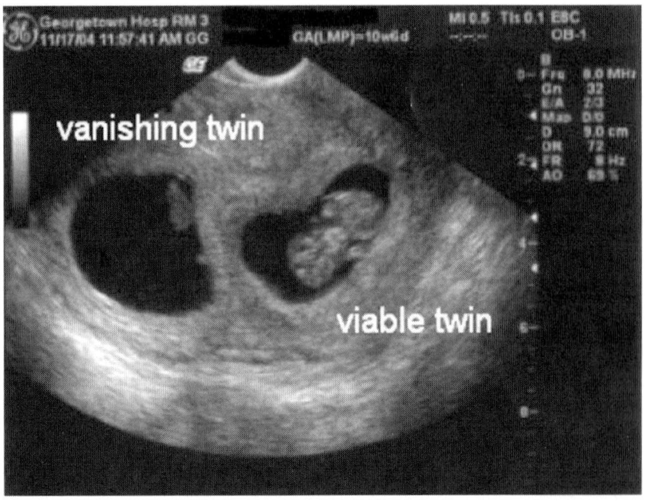

Figure 149.1 Sonogram demonstrating one viable twin in the right sac and a non-viable twin in the left sac. One week earlier, two viable twins were seen.

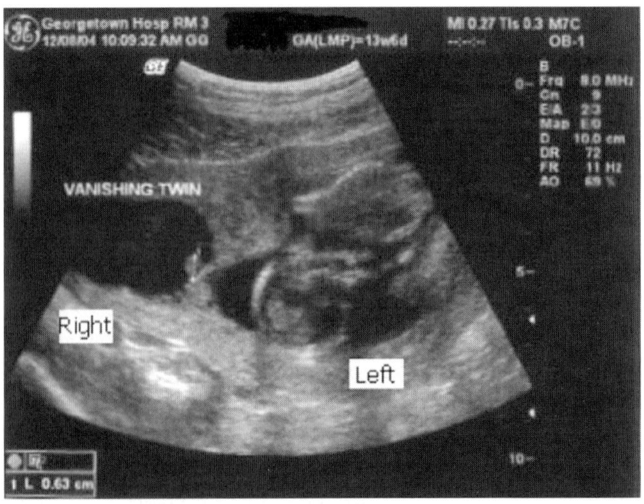

Figure 149.2 Sonogram of the same patient as in Figure 149.1 4 weeks later demonstrating one viable twin in the left sac and the resorbing, vanishing twin in the right sac.

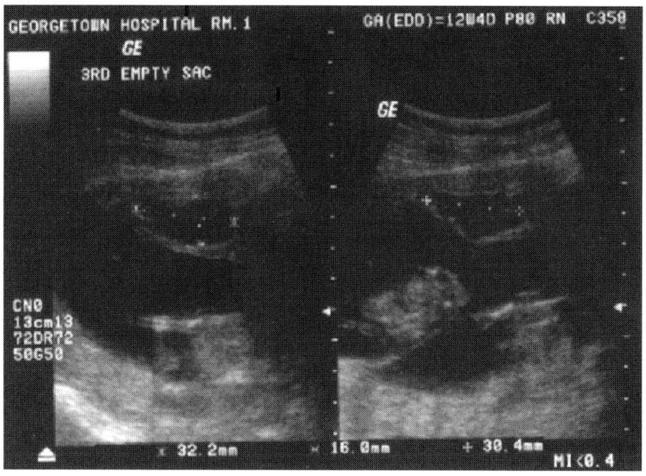

Figure 149.3 Sonogram demonstrating a third empty sac (measuring 32.2 × 16.0 × 34.4 mm) in a previously viable triplet gestation.

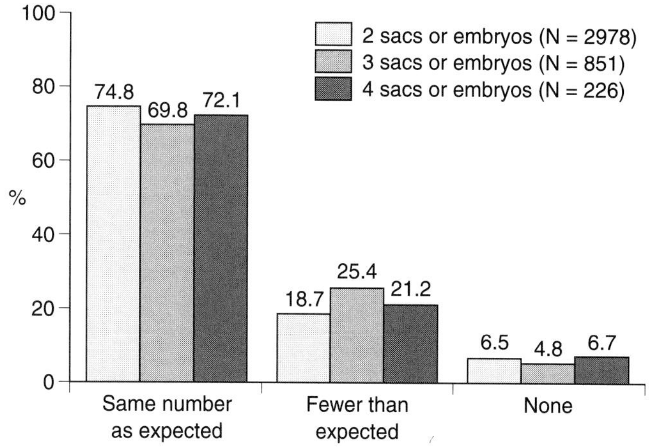

Figure 149.4 Outcome beyond the first trimester after the sonographic diagnosis of 2–4 gestational sacs and/or embryos: Number of fetuses after the sonographic diagnosis of 2 sacs or embryos, 3 sacs or embryos, and 4 sacs or embryos.[4–15]

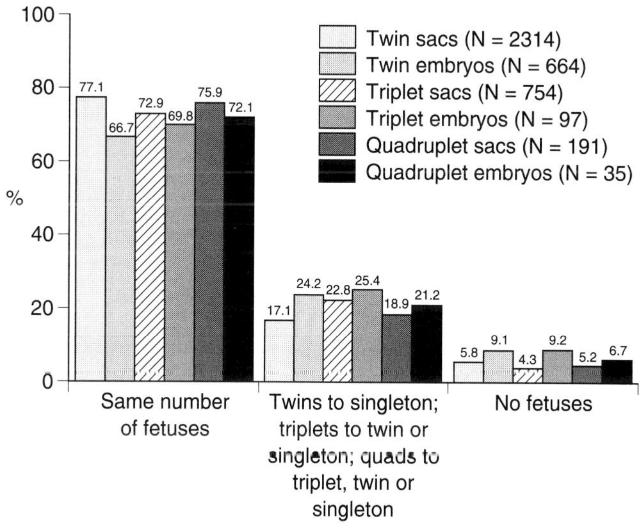

Figure 149.5 Outcome beyond the first trimester after the early sonographic diagnosis of multiple sacs or embryos: Pregnancy outcome after the sonographic diagnosis of twins (N = 2978), triplets (N = 851), or quadruplets (N = 226).[4–15]

Until recently, most published data described pregnancies with two or three gestational sacs or embryos.[4–14] One of our earlier papers cited information based on the few quadruplet pregnancies reported by the 1998 publication date.[1] In 2003 and 2004, however, several papers included sizable numbers for pregnancies with four sacs and/or embryos.[15–17] Despite this, there is little information available for pregnancies of higher order. Combining current data suggest that approximately 70% of pregnancies with multiple sacs or embryos continue with the same number of fetuses as expected (Figure 149.4). This 70% maintenance rate appears to be constant for pregnancies that began with two, three, or four sacs or embryos. Spontaneous resorption occurred in 18.7% of twins, 25.4% of triplets, and 21.2% of quadruplet gestations (Figure 149.4).[4–15] Further stratification of these data is seen in Figure 149.5. The growing body of literature confirms that the prevalence of fetal disappearance in multiple gestations is fairly constant.

Are there differences in the vanishing twin rate in different populations? One questions the impact of ART on this area. Answering this question is confounded by the fact that most published data on early pregnancy loss in multiple gestations describe ART pregnancies rather than spontaneous conceptions. Figures 149.6 and 149.7 demonstrate available data comparing spontaneous pregnancies and those conceived using ART (*in vitro* fertilization, IVF; intracytoplasmic sperm injection, ICSI; and ovulation induction), evaluating loss rates after the sonographic diagnosis of two sacs (Figure 149.6) and two embryos (Figure 149.7). Higher loss rates are seen when only gestational sacs are demonstrated sonographically rather than when embryos are visualized. Data obtained for Figures 149.6 and 149.7 have been compiled from different studies where very few patients with spontaneous conceptions are reported compared to those conceived with ART.[4,5,8–13,15–18] Moreover, many patients with spontaneous conceptions underwent ultrasonography because of pregnancy complications such as vaginal bleeding. These data, especially for those spontaneously conceived, therefore, should not be extrapolated to the general population. With the ultrasound identification of viable twins, loss of one twin occurs in 29.7% of IVF/ICSI conceptions, 32.5% of pregnancies conceived with ovulation induction, and 10.2% of spontaneous conceptions (Figure 149.7).

Disappearance of gestational sacs or embryos has been described throughout the first trimester, although unconfirmed beyond 13 weeks.[4,5] Spontaneous reduction rates are higher earlier in gestation, though precise frequencies per given gestational week cannot be extrapolated.[4–6,18]

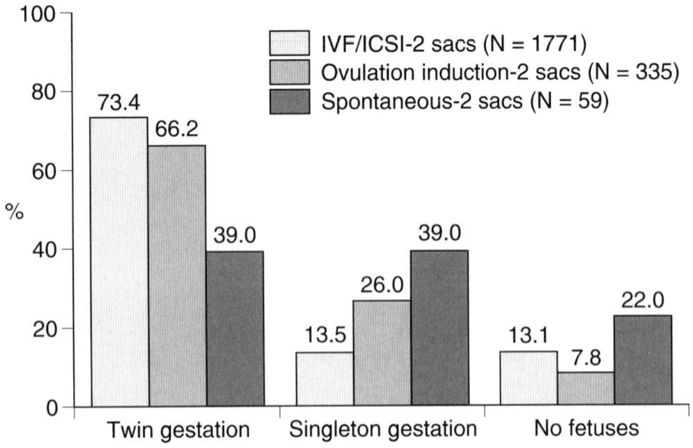

Figure 149.6 Outcome beyond the first trimester in assisted vs. spontaneous conceptions after the early sonographic diagnosis of two sacs (N=2135): Comparison of IVF/ICSI, ovulation induction, and spontaneous conceptions.[8,9,11,12,16,17]

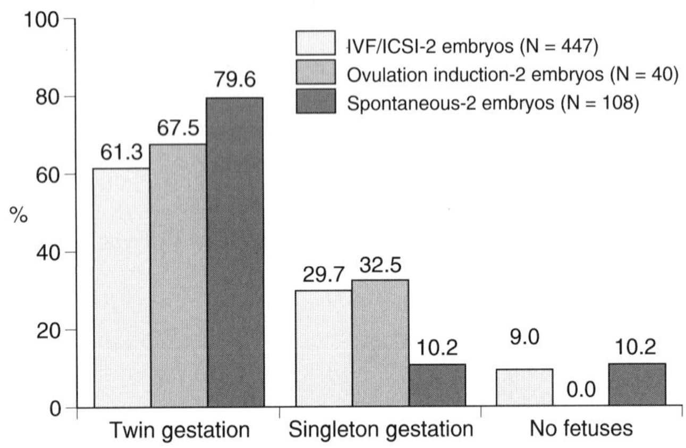

Figure 149.7 Outcome beyond the first trimester in assisted vs. spontaneous conception after sonographic diagnosis of 2 embryos (N=595): Comparison of IVF/ICSI, ovulation induction, and spontaneous conceptions.[4,5,10,13,15,18]

Complications and prognosis

Vaginal bleeding

Vaginal bleeding or spotting, commonly reported in the first trimester by all pregnant women, appears to be the only apparent complication associated with disappearance of an embryo or a gestational sac. Rates as high as 76.5% have been reported, varying with study and patient populations.[1] The finding of clinical bleeding seems to coincide with the vanishing process. Regardless of chorionicity, the prognosis for continuing a pregnancy associated with spontaneous resorption is good.[1,18]

Continued viability

Predicting continued fetal viability among sonographically identified twin gestations early in pregnancy may be challenging. More reliable prognoses can be made at later gestational ages and in the absence of abnormal sonographic findings (e.g. subchorionic hemorrhage). Disappearance rates occur more than twice as often in monochorionic compared to dichorionic twin gestations (50% compared to 21%).[18] Increasing maternal age is associated with higher spontaneous resorption rates in some studies,[8,17] though results are conflicting.[7,15] In one study, no association was seen between twin resorption and maternal age, spontaneous vs. induced conception, or indication for sonography.[7] Further, La Sala *et al.* did not discern a correlation between early spontaneous loss of multiple gestations and the starting number of embryos transferred in IVF patients.[15]

Though identification of an embryonic heartbeat confirms a viable pregnancy, its initial presence cannot guarantee continued fetal viability in multiple gestations. Kelly *et al.* found a more reliable predictor of ongoing viability to be the rate of increase of serum human chorionic gonadotropin levels rather than the presence of embryonic cardiac activity.[10] Differences in crown–rump length measurements between embryos may be associated with fetal aneuploidy or congenital anomalies[19] as well as a vanishing twin.[13]

Cerebral palsy

Worldwide data demonstrate that the prevalence of cerebral palsy increases with plurality, being more common with a higher number of fetuses.[20] Higher cerebral palsy rates are seen with preterm and low birth weight infants.[20] Though studies describe higher risks of cerebral palsy in children resulting from ART,[21,22] confounding issues include high frequency of multiple gestations, low birth weight and premature deliveries.[20] Higher rates of cerebral palsy are described in monochorionic twin survivors after demise of a co-twin and in cases of the twin transfusion syndrome.[23,24]

In 1997, Pharoah and Cooke hypothesized that cerebral palsy of unknown etiology in singletons could be attributable to the early loss of a previously unrecognized monochorionic twin.[25] They theorized that the survivor's antenatal neurological development would be impaired, resulting in the clinical manifestation of spastic cerebral palsy.[25] A similar line of thought was proposed in a Norwegian study in 2000.[26] Though intriguing, a follow-up report from this same group of authors was not supportive of their original hypothesis.[27] Further, this concept is not supported by tangential evidence, given the lack of reported cases of cerebral palsy following multifetal pregnancy reduction, a procedure that is not unlike the vanishing twin phenomenon.[20]

Miscellaneous

Though surviving co-twins in multiple gestations associated with a vanished twin have not been found to have an increase in congenital anomalies, the case series by Casale *et al.* proposes that blighted conjoined twinning may result in cloacal exstrophy variants.[28] The vanishing twin phenomenon perhaps may explain some isoimmunization cases that develop during gestation in which a Rh-positive twin disappears in a previously unsensitized Rh-negative mother.[1,2] The emotional needs of the mother who has experienced a vanished twin requires sensitivity and humanistic communication.[29]

Pathological considerations

Pathological documentation of the resorption process can be confirmed by histological findings from the fetal surface of the placenta. Such findings include sacs or cysts; placental nodules or plaques; areas of degenerated chorionic villi; fibrin deposition or fibrinoid degeneration; embryonic remnants; and macerated embryos.[1,2,30,31] The vanishing twin phenomenon has been used to explain discordant chromosome results, including various trisomies, triploidy, tetraploidy, and sex chromosome discrepancies.[1,2,31–33]

Conclusions

In summary, the 'vanishing twin' phenomenon is a common sonographic finding among multiple pregnancies. The risk of resorption appears to be relatively constant at approximately 20% of conceptions, whether the pregnancy begins with two, three, or four sacs or embryos. Disappearance is more frequently described earlier in the first trimester. Higher resorption rates are reported in pregnancies conceived using ART though the numbers of spontaneously conceived multiple gestation are lacking. Better outcomes are seen with dichorionic rather than monochorionic twin gestations. The main complication associated with embryonic or fetal resorption is vaginal bleeding. Detailed sonographic evaluation is recommended to follow the progression of the resorption process as well as to assess viability and evaluate growth in the remaining fetus(es). Though conflicting data exist regarding risks of cerebral palsy to the surviving infants, the association does not seem likely. Close inspection of the placenta and membranes after delivery may confirm earlier sonographic findings.

With continued technological advances, sonography of early pregnancy will continue to provide a thorough understanding of embryonic development and the relationship of early pregnancy loss in multiple gestations.

REFERENCES

1. Landy HJ, Keith LG. The vanishing twin: A review. *Hum Reprod Update* 1998;4:177–83.
2. Landy HJ, Weiner S, Corson SL, Batzer FR, Bolonese FJ. The "vanishing twin": Ultrasonographic assessment of fetal disappearance in the first trimester. *Am J Obstet Gynecol* 1986;155: 14–19.
3. Dickey RP, Olar TT, Taylor SN, *et al.* Incidence and significance of unequal gestational sac diameter or embryo crown–rump length in twin pregnancy. *Hum Reprod* 1992;7:1170–2.
4. Blumenfeld Z, Dirnfeld M, Abramovici H, Amit A, Bronshtein M, Brandes JM. Spontaneous fetal reduction in multiple gestations assessed by transvaginal ultrasound. *Br J Obstet Gynaecol* 1992;99:333–7.
5. Sampson A, de Crespigny LCh. Vanishing twins: The frequency of spontaneous fetal reduction of a twin pregnancy. *Ultrasound Obstet Gynecol* 1993;2:107–9.
6. Benson CB, Doubilet PM, David V. Prognosis of first-trimester twin pregnancies: Polychromotous logistic regression analysis. *Radiology* 1994;192;765–8.
7. Manzur A, Goldsman MP, Stone SC, Frederick JL, Balmaceda JP, Asch RH. Outcome of triplet pregnancies after assisted reproductive techniques: How frequent are the vanishing embryos? *Fertil Steril* 1995;63:252–7.
8. Dickey RP, Taylor SN, Lu PY, *et al.* Spontaneous reduction of multiple pregnancy: Incidence and effect of outcome. *Am J Obstet Gynecol* 2002;186:77–83.
9. Bateman BG, Nunley WC, Kolp LA, Kitchen JD, Felder R. Vaginal sonography findings and hCG dynamics of early intrauterine and tubal pregnancies. *Obstet Gynecol* 1990;75:421–7.
10. Kelly MP, Binor Z, Molo MW, Rawlins RG, Maclin VM, Radwanska E. Human chorionic gonadotropin rise in normal and vanishing twin pregnancies. *Fertil Steril* 1991;56:221–4.
11. Seoud MA-F, Toner JP, Kruithoff C, Muasher SJ. Outcome of twin, triplet, and quadruplet *in vitro* fertilization pregnancies: The Norfolk experience. *Fertil Steril* 1002;57:825–34.
12. Botchan A, Yaron Y, Lessing JB, *et al.* When multiple gestational sacs are seen on ultrasound, 'take-home baby' rate improves with *in-vitro* fertilization. *Hum Reprod* 1993;8:710–3.
13. Kol S, Drugan A, Levron J, Itskovitz-Eldor J, Lewit N. The natural history of multiple pregnancies after assisted reproduction: Is spontaneous fetal demise a clinically significant phenomenon? *Fertil Steril* 1993;60:127–30.
14. Rodriguez-Gonzalez M, Serra V, Garcia-Velasco JA, Pellicer A, Remohi J. The 'vanishing embryo' phenomenon in an oocyte donation programme. *Hum Reprod* 2002;17:798–802.
15. La Sala GB, Nucera G, Gallinelli A, Nicoli A, Villani MT, Blickstein I. Spontaneous embryonic loss following in vitro fertilization: Incidence and effect on outcomes. *Am J Obstet Gynecol* 2004;181:741–6.
16. Tummers P, De Sutter P, Dhont M. Risk of spontaneous abortion in singleton and twin pregnancies after IVF/ICSI. *Hum Reprod* 2003;18:1720–3.
17. Ulug U, Jozwiak EA, Mesut A, Berksoy MM, Bahceci M. Survival rates during the first trimester of multiple gestations achieved by ICSI: A report of 1448 consecutive multiples. *Hum Reprod* 2004; 19:360–4.
18. Benson CB, Doubilet PM, Laks MP. Outcome of twin gestations following sonographic demonstration of two heart beats in the first trimester. *Ultrasound Obstet Gynecol* 1993;3:343–5.
19. Weissman A, Achiron R, Lipitz S, Blickstein I, Mashiach S. The first-trimester growth-discordant twin: An ominous prenatal finding. *Obstet Gynecol* 1994;84:110–4.
20. Blickstein I. Do multiple gestations raise the risk of cerebral palsy? *Clin Perinatol* 2004;31:395–408.
21. Schieve LA, Meikle SF, Ferre C, Peterson HB, Jeng G, Wilcox LS. Low and very low birth weight in infants conceived with use of assisted reproductive technology. *N Engl J Med* 2002;346: 731–7.
22. Stromberg B, Dahlquist G, Ericson A, Finnstrom O, Koster M, Stjernqvist K. Neurological sequelae in children born after in-vitro fertilization: A population-based study. *Lancet* 2002;359:461–5.
23. Pharoah PO. Cerebral palsy in the surviving twin associated with infant death of the co-twin. *Arch Dis Child Fetal Neonatal Ed* 2001;84:F111–6.
24. Reisner DP, Mahony BS, Petty CN, *et al.* Stuck twin syndrome: Outcome in thirty-seven consecutive cases. *Am J Obstet Gynecol* 1993;169:991–5.
25. Pharoah PO, Cooke RW. A hypothesis for the aetiology of spastic cerebral palsy – The vanishing twin. *Dev Med Child Neurol* 1997; 39:292–6.

26. Brodtkorb E, Myhr G, Gimse R. Is monochorionic twinning a risk factor for focal cortical dysgenesis? *Acta Neurol Scand* 2000; 102:53–9.
27. Newton R, Casabonne D, Johnson A, Pharoah PO. A case–control study of vanishing twin as a risk factor for cerebral palsy. *Twin Res* 2003;6:83–4.
28. Casale P, Grady RW, Waldhausen JH, Joyner BD, Wright J, Mitchell M. *J Urol* 2004;173:1103–6.
29. Briscoe L, Street C. "Vanished twin": An exploration of women's experiences. *Birth* 2003;30:47–53.
30. Sulak LE, Dodson MG. The vanishing twin: Pathologic confirmation of an ultrasonographic phenomenon. *Obstet Gynecol* 1986; 68:811–5.
31. Rudnicki M, Vejerslev LO, Junge J. The vanishing twin: Morphologic and cytogenetic evaluation of an ultrasonographic phenomenon. *Gynecol Obstet Invest* 1991;31:141–5.
32. Cytogenetic analysis of chorionic villi for prenatal diagnosis: An ACC collaborative study of U.K. data. Association of Clinical Cytogeneticists Working Party on Chorionic Villi in Prenatal Diagnosis. *Prenat Diagn* 1994;14:363–79.
33. Lloveras E, Lecumberri JM, Perez C, *et al.* A female infant with a 46,XX/48,XY,+8,+10 karyotype in prenatal diagnosis: A 'vanishing twin' phenomenon? *Prenat Diagn* 2001;21:896–7.

150 Sonographic evaluation of multiple pregnancies

A. Matias, N. Montenegro and I. Blickstein

... The day will come soon
when a routine ultrasound examination
will be offered to every pregnant women ...

Ian Donald, 1974

Over the last decade, perinatal mortality and morbidity in multiple pregnancies have fallen due to advances in fetal medicine and improvement in perinatal care. One of the most decisive contributing factors was the widespread use of ultrasound evaluation in early pregnancy, defining the number of fetuses, assigning chorionicity and screening for major aneuploidies and malformations.

Diagnosis of chorionicity and amnionicity

Clearly, it is chorionicity rather than zygosity that determines several aspects of antenatal management and perinatal outcome. Thus, the routine assignment of chorionicity and the earliest possible diagnosis of monochorionic twinning are highly desirable, though seldom achieved in practice.

Zygosity refers to the type of conception whereas chorionicity denotes the type of placentation. The type of placentation depends on the time of splitting of the fertilized ova: if it occurs too early, two placentas will be found and a dichorionic diamniotic twin pregnancy will be identified; if it occurs after the third day, a single placenta, that is, a monochorionic twin pregnancy will be established.

Caution should be taken when using the number of chorionic sacs (Figure 150.1) and the number of yolk sacs alone to determine the number of embryos. Shortly after the sixth postmenstrual week, embryonic heartbeats are visible and one can confidently count the number of embryos by the number of beating hearts.

By that time, to determine the number of amnions in a monochorionic twin pregnancy, in which two embryos are seen within the chorionic sac, it is wise to wait until the eighth postmenstrual week to ascertain amnionicity. The amniotic membrane is so thin that it may remain inconspicuous until 8–9 weeks, leading to the incorrect consideration of a monochorionic–monoamniotic gestation. After that gestational age, it is clear that no amniotic membrane is present

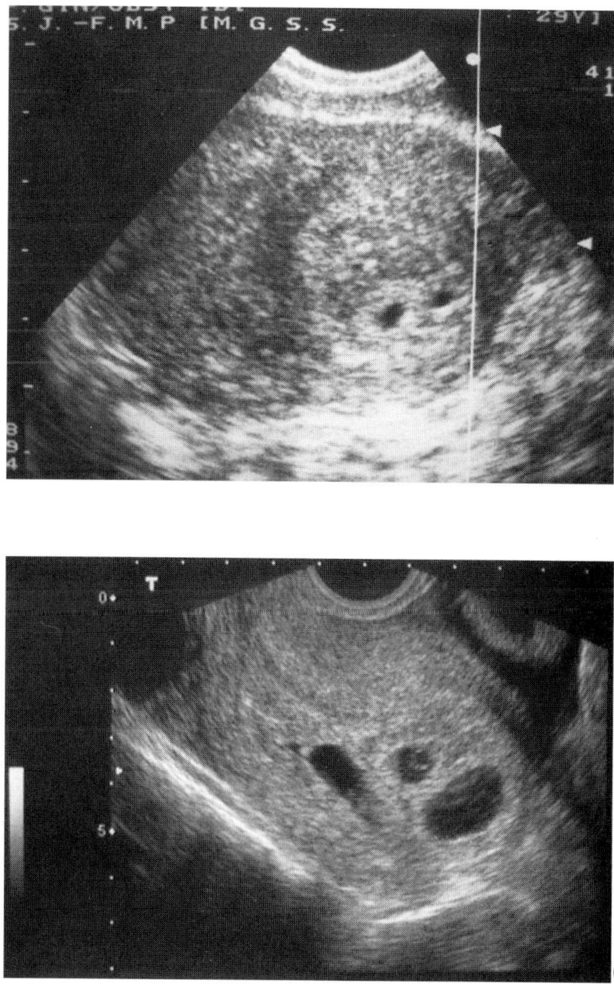

(a)

(b)

Figure 150.1 (a) Early scan at 5 weeks of gestation showing a dichorionic twin pregnancy with two chorionic sacs. (b) Early scan at 6 weeks of gestation showing three chorionic sacs and defining a trichorionic triamniotic twin pregnancy.

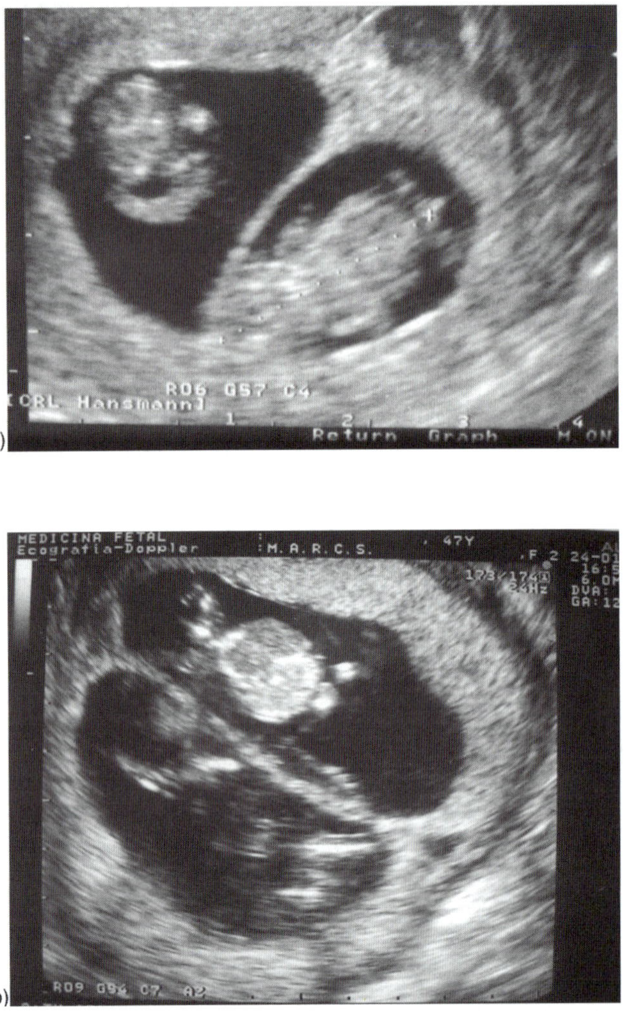

Figure 150.2 (a) Lambda sign at 11 weeks of gestation, depicting a thick layer of chorion between the two layers of amnion, and defining a dichorionic dimaniotic twin pregnancy. (b) Example of a dichorionic diamniotic twin pregnancy with two differently located placentas.

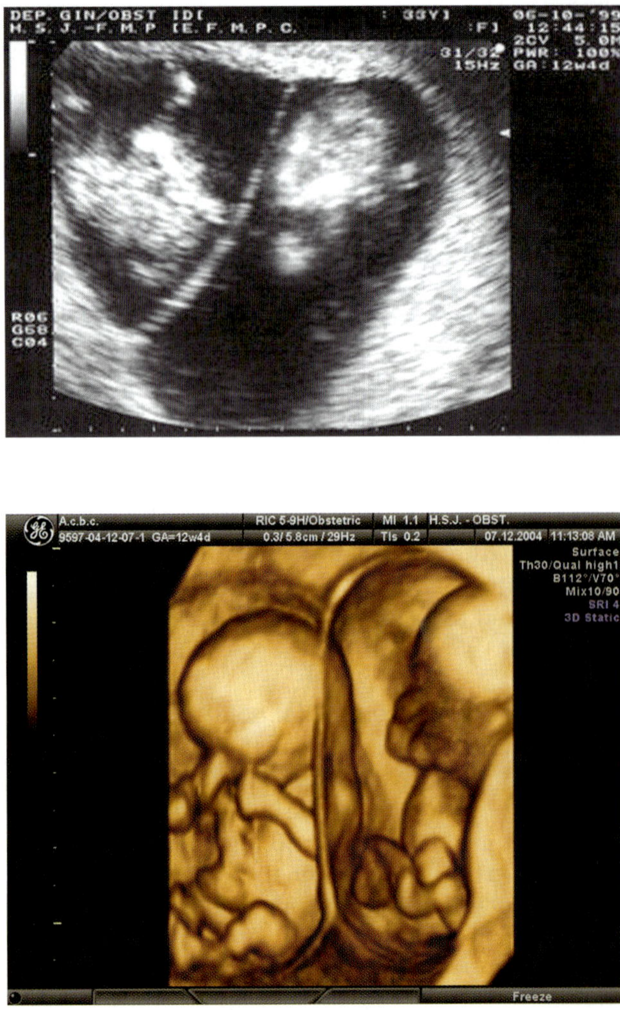

Figure 150.3 (a) Example of a monochorionic twin pregnancy at 11 weeks of gestation showing a thin dividing membrane without chorion between the amnion layers. (b) 3D imaging of a monochorionic diamniotic twin pregnancy at 11 weeks showing the thin intertwin membrane with two layers of amnion.

between the embryos and only one yolk sac is visualized. From then on it is important to look for sonographic signs of cord entanglement, potentially depicted as early as 12 weeks, with the help of color Doppler.

When two embryos or fetuses assume a parallel, head-to-head position, conjoined twins should be suspected. A jerk with the probe should be inflicted to induce movement between the two fetuses, away from each other or close together when conjoined twins are in question.

At 10–14 weeks, the gold standard 'window' for chorionicity definition, the chorion frondosum is sufficiently thick to be identified between the two layers of amnion as a wedge-shaped structure in a dichorionic twin pregnancy (not obligatory dizygotic twin pregnancy), yielding the fully diagnostic 'twin peak' or 'lambda' or 'delta' sign (Figure 150.2a and b).[1,2] However, the number of 'twin-peak' signs is no secure indication of how many chorionic sacs exist within a given pregnancy. If two fused layers of amnion, without any chorion interposed, are found in the scan creating a T-shaped 'take-off' (T sign), showing a very thin membrane with strictly two layers (Figure 150.3a and b), a monochorionic twin pregnancy can be diagnosed with 100% certainty.[3]

After 16 weeks, physiologically the chorion frondosum regresses and chorionicity becomes a more confounding issue. The delta sign disappears[4] and, if sexes are alike, monochorionicity can be wrongly inferred. It is the conjugation of several sonographic criteria that approaches the correct diagnosis of chorionicity, the most and ultimate determinant of perinatal prognosis. Therefore, an adequate first-trimester scan of a multifetal pregnancy makes the subsequent second- and third-trimester evaluation much more meaningful, simpler and faster.

Identifying a single placenta with a paper-thin, reflective hair-like septum without chorion between the two amnions, with a very thin septum with less

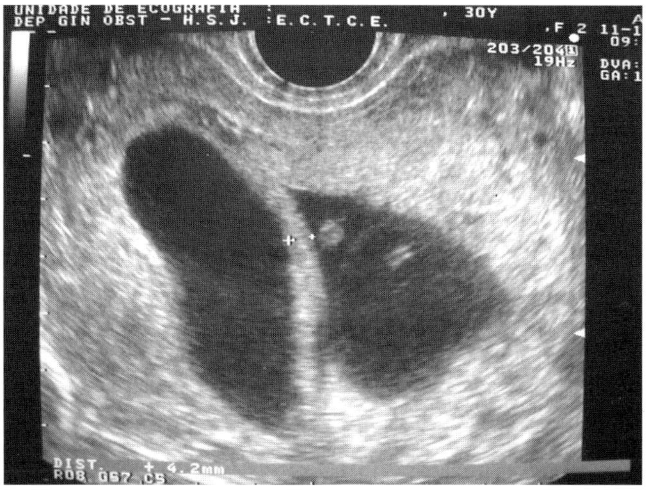

Figure 150.4 Thick intertwin membrane with chorion interposed in a dichorionic diamniotic twin pregnancy at 11 weeks of gestation.

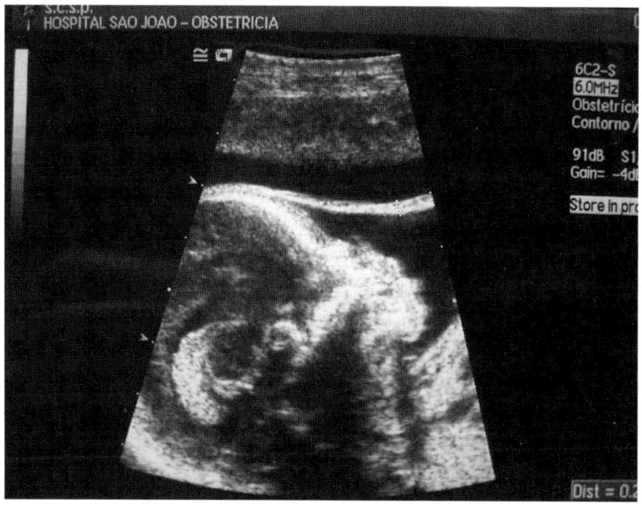

Figure 150.5 Thin intertwin membrane with two layers of amnion without chorion interposed in a monochorionic diamniotic twin pregnancy at 11 weeks of gestation, better imaged by zooming in.

than 2 mm and like-sex twins, placentation will most probably be monochorionic. If contrarily one finds two separate placentas of different location, or two fetuses of a different sex or a thick membrane >2 mm with more than two layers (Figure 150.4), dichorionicity is strongly suggested. Note that to identify the interfetal membranes, a right-angled orientation of the probe in relation to the membranes should be obtained to take advantage of the axial over the lateral resolution. In order to count the number of layers one must 'zoom in' (Figure 150.5). In contrast, a membrane placed parallel to the ultrasonic beam will appear thinner and poorly imaged, rendering it impossible to be sure about the number of layers of the intertwin membrane.

Down's syndrome screening in multiple pregnancies

Down's syndrome is the most prevalent autosomic chromosomal abnormality in the human race (birth prevalence of about 1 in 800) and accounts for almost 50% of all aneuploidies.

Maternal age has been a widely accepted screening method since it is cheap, universally available, has no intra- or interobserver variation, is non-invasive and is understandable by the women screened, but yields a sensitivity dependent on the prevalence of women with maternal age over 35 years (50% sensitivity for a 15% prevalence of women older than 35 years). In the late 1980s, the quantification of various fetoplacental products in the maternal circulation (*biochemical screening*) was introduced.

In the 1990s, screening by a combination of maternal age and fetal *nuchal translucency* thickness (NT) at 11–14 weeks for a given crown–rump length was introduced, identifying about 75% of trisomy-21-affected fetuses for a screen-positive rate of about 5%.[5] More recently, combining NT and nasal bone[6] with two biochemical markers between 11 and 14 weeks of gestation [free β-human chorionic gonadotropin (β-hCG) and pregnancy-associated plasma protein-A (PAPP-A)],[7,8] provided a detection rate of 95% for a screen-positive rate of 2%.

Screening for chromosomal abnormalities in twin pregnancies implies, however, a different reasoning.[9,10] The overall probability that a multiple gestation contains an aneuploid fetus is directly related to its zygosity. In *dizygotic* pregnancies, each fetus has an independent risk of aneuploidy; thus, the risk for chromosomal abnormalities for each twin may be the same as in singleton pregnancies, but the chance that at least one fetus is affected by a chromosomal defect is twice as high as in singleton pregnancies. This means that for dizygotic twin pregnancies, the pregnancy-specific risk is calculated by summing the individual risk estimates for each fetus.

In *monozygotic* twins, the risk of an affected fetus approximates the risk of a singleton pregnancy and, in the vast majority of cases, the risk for one fetus is, in expectation, the same as the risk for the other.

If zygosity is unknown, the risk of at least one aneuploid fetus can be approximated as five-thirds (1.667) that of the singleton risk. This is based on the assumption that a third of all twin pairs are monozygotic.[11]

Counseling based on chorionicity, clinically more feasible than zygosity, results that in monochorionic twins both fetuses can be affected equally. If the pregnancy is dichorionic, the parents should be counseled that the risk of discordance for a chromosomal abnormality is about twice that in singleton pregnancies, whereas the risk that both fetuses would be affected is a much rarer event, corresponding to the singleton

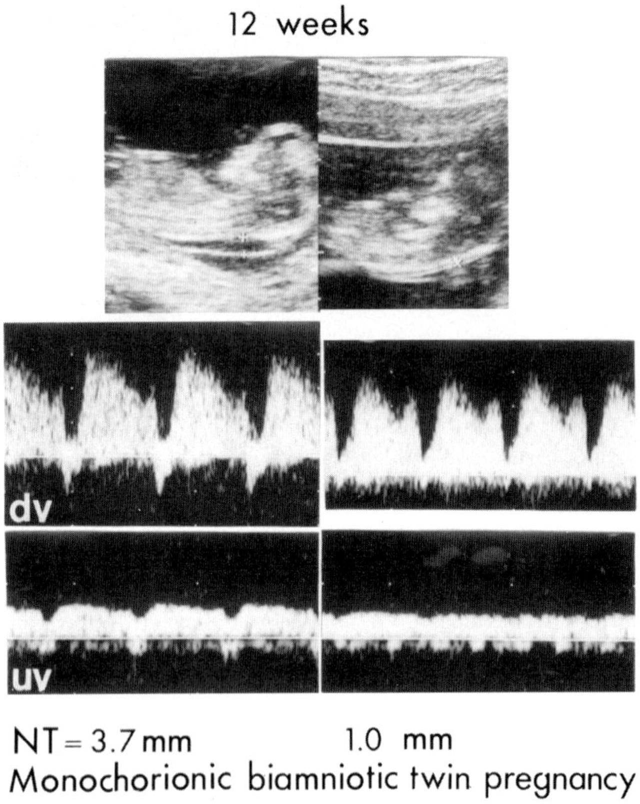

Figure 150.6 A monochorionic diamniotic twin pregnancy was established at 12 weeks of gestation. Doppler blood flow waveforms in both fetuses were obtained in the umbilical vein (UV) and ductus venosus (DV) in the same scan. A nuchal translucency (NT) discrepancy was noted (NT=3.7/1.0 mm). The fetus with increased nuchal translucency shows an inverted A-wave in the DV and dicrote pulsatile flow in the UV. TTTS developed at 17 weeks and the patient was referred for laser ablation of anastomosis.

risk squared. For example, in a 40-year-old pregnant woman with a risk for trisomy of about 1 in 100 based on maternal age, in a dizygotic twin pregnancy the risk that one fetus would be affected would be 1 in 50 (1 in 100 plus 1 in 100), whereas the risk that both fetuses would be affected is 1 in 10,000 (1 in 100 × 1 in 100). Unlike all monochorionic pregnancies that are always monozygotic, only about 90% of dichorionic pregnancies are dizygotic, so these calculations are slightly inaccurate.

When calculating the risk of higher order multiples, estimates can be made multiplying the singleton risk by the number of fetuses.[12] This method assumes unique chorionicity for each fetus, though monozygosity can occur more frequently than usually thought at higher rates in multiple gestations through assisted reproductive techniques (Wenstrom *et al.*, 1993; Blickstein *et al.*, 1999).[13]

In twin pregnancies, interpretation of biochemical screening is clearly more problematic since each serum marker necessarily relates to the pregnancy and is not specific to the fetus, deriving solely a pregnancy- and not a fetus-specific risk. As biochemical screening in twins is still investigational and far less powerful than in singletons, it should not be recommended in general practice. Even if prospective studies demonstrate that biochemical screening in twins is effective, there is a 10% lower detection rate for an acceptable high false-positive rate and if screening is positive there is no distinctive feature to identify which of the fetuses is affected.

In contrast, the availability of a more credible sonographic parameter for trisomy 21 risk assessment in the first trimester of pregnancy shifted the consideration of a *pregnancy-specific risk* to a *fetus-specific risk*. If it is proved that the distribution of NT measurements in twin fetuses with trisomy 21 is similar to that in singletons,[13–16] NT can be considered the gold standard of screening in twins.

In a monochorionic twin pregnancy, presumably, both fetuses will be affected or both will be unaffected. It is therefore appropriate to take the average of the two NT measurements, so that a single risk estimate can be calculated (*averaging method*). Prevalence of increased NT was found twice as much as in monochorionic than in singleton pregnancies, but concomitantly the likelihood ratio of developing twin-to-twin transfusion syndrome (TTTS) in those twins with increased NT was higher (3.5 times).[17,18] In those cases, our group has demonstrated that the combined evaluation of NT and ductus venosus (DV) at 11–14 weeks could anticipate which of them would develop TTTS. In those cases presenting both increased NT and abnormal flow in the DV, TTTS eventually developed (Figure 150.6). In contrast, whenever NTs were discrepant but with normal flow in the DV, no cases of TTTS were found (Figure 150.7).[19,20]

In a dichorionic twin pregnancy, the twins are dizygotic in about 90% of the cases, which means that one of the fetuses, or both fetuses could be affected. As each fetus has an independent risk, the risks derived from NT measurements should be summed (*summing method*) (Figure 150.8). The 10% of dichorionic twin pregnancies that are monozygotic will incorrectly have their risks calculated by the summing rather than the averaging method, but the effect on screening performance will be a negligible one.

For higher-order multiples more credible data have been obtained using NT alone to assess risk in triplets or more.[20] Not only was it feasible and reproducible, but also mean NT was similar for both groups.[21]

Considering that biochemical screening alone cannot specifically identify the fetus at risk in the presence of twins discrepant for Down's syndrome, it seems reasonable to combine NT and maternal biochemical markers, as suggested by Spencer.[22] In this modeled study, it was demonstrated that biochemical screening would add a further 5% to the detection rate obtained by using NT alone and thus offering a detection rate for Down's syndrome of about 80% compared to the 90% in singleton pregnancies, which could be a worthwhile addition. Interestingly, the combined test is more discriminative in monochorionic than

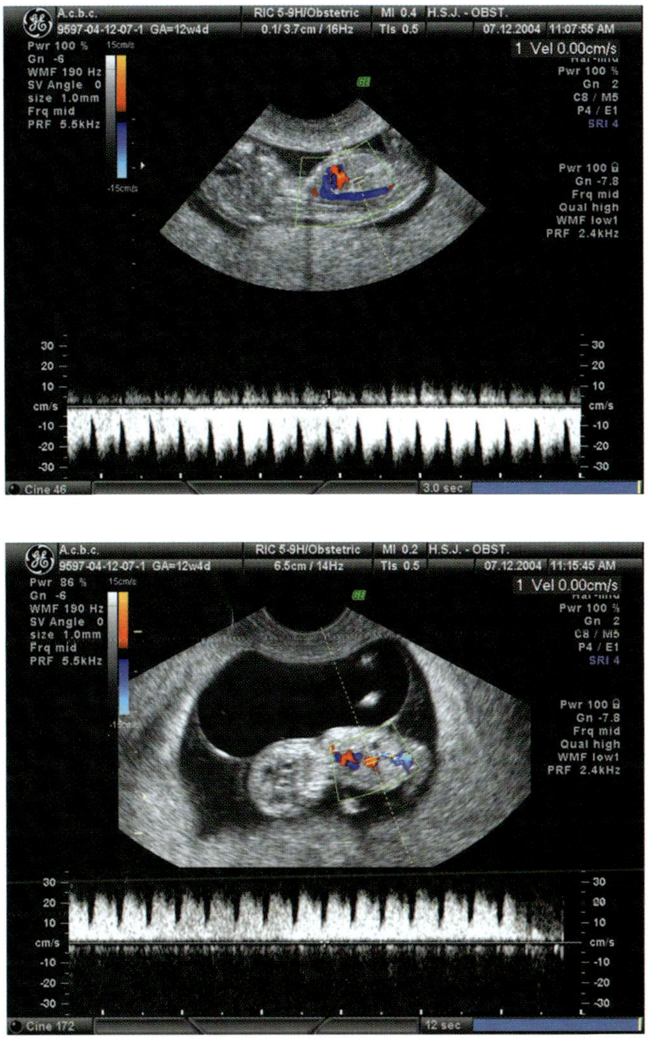

Figure 150.7 Doppler blood flow waveforms in the ductus venosus (DV) obtained in a monochorionic twin pregnancy at 11 weeks of gestation. Both DV waveforms were normal and NT were within normal range and non-discrepant. The pregnancy was uneventful and no TTTS developed.

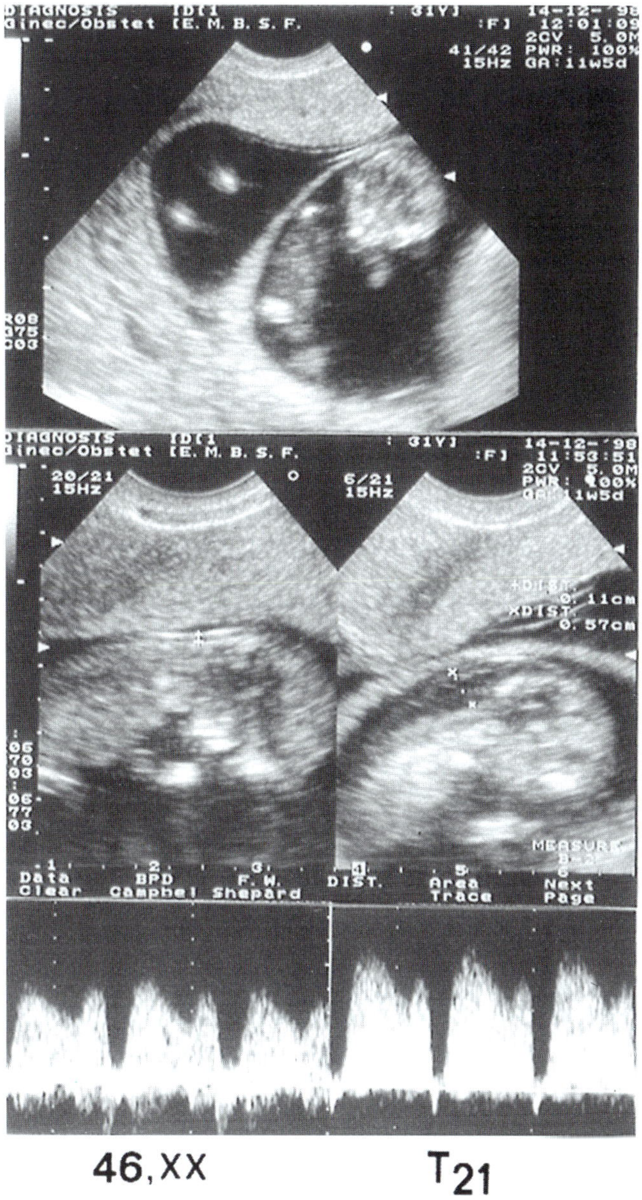

Figure 150.8 A dichorionic diamniotic twin pregnancy was established at 11 weeks +5 days. The measurements of nuchal translucency (NT) were discrepant (1.1/5.7 mm) and ductus venosus (DV) blood flow was reversed in the fetus with increased nuchal translucency. Amniocentesis revealed a normal karyotype (46,XX) for the fetus with normal NT and DV blood flow; a trisomy 21 was identified in the fetus with increased NT and abnormal flow in the DV.

dichorionic twin pregnancies, since in dichorionic pregnancies the median serum marker level in affected pregnancies will be artificially lowered by the unaffected twin, whereas in monochorionic pregnancies no dilution of the serum markers is expected from an unaffected pregnancy.

Until more data are available from larger studies on the distribution of markers in concordant or discordant twins, NT estimated for each fetuses should be the predominant factor by which women presenting with increased risk should be counseled regarding invasive testing.

Screening and diagnosis of TTTS

TTTS affects about 15% of monochorionic twin pregnancies (1:400 pregnancies) and it accounts for 17% of perinatal mortality. Though clinically identifiable and with expected ominous prognosis, this condition is still far from being effectively anticipated and treated. By definition, it affects *structurally* normal babies, it is a *placenta-based disease*, it is associated with *important perinatal morbidity and mortality* but still is amenable to *curative* therapy.

TTTS reflects primarily a pathological form of circulatory imbalance that develops chronically between hemodynamically connected monochorionic twin fetuses. A vicious cycle of hypervolemia–polyuria–hyperosmolality is established and results in a mid-trimester discordance in amniotic fluid volume and fetal growth, with signs of hypovolemia and uteroplacental insufficiency in the donor twin and hypervolemia and cardiac dysfunction in the recipient twin.

In the past, diagnosis of the syndrome was made only after delivery of the affected twin pair and careful examination of the placenta. A difference in cord hemoglobin concentrations of 5 g/dl or more and a difference in birth weights of 20% or more established the diagnosis, but both criteria were later found to be inaccurate and non-specific.

Considering the inadequacy of neonatal findings in the diagnosis of TTTS and the more consistent sonographic antenatal criteria,[23–26] ultrasound revealed to be crucial in screening and diagnosing TTTS.

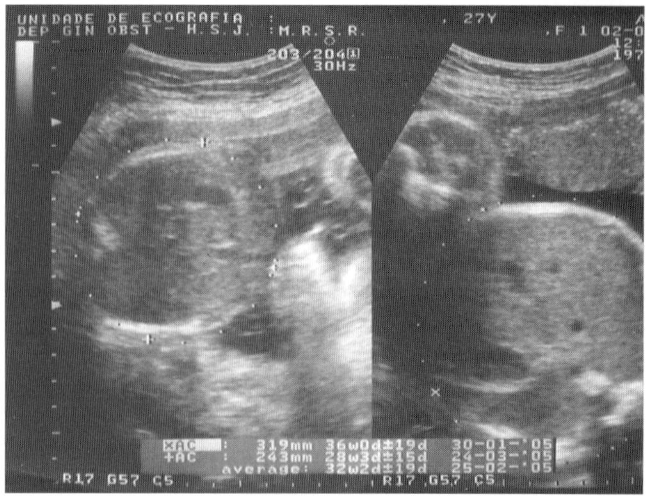

Figure 150.9 Scan performed at 35 weeks in a dichorionic diamniotic twin pregnancy showing discrepancy > 25% in the abdominal circumference.

Determination of monochorionicity

TTTS is a syndrome expected to develop in monochorionic pregnancies. Only in the first trimester of pregnancy (10–14 weeks of gestation), type of placentation can be assigned with a 100% certainty. The definition of monochorionicity is based on the presence of the T sign (one placenta with a paper-thin, reflective hair-like septum without chorion between the two amnion) (Figure 150.3a and b).

Discordance in size

In TTTS, the recipient fetus tends to be a bigger and more plethoric baby in contrast with the donor, defined as a smaller and leaner fetus (Figure 150.9). A cut-off value of 20 mm for the difference in abdominal circumference between twins indicated growth discordance of more than 20%.

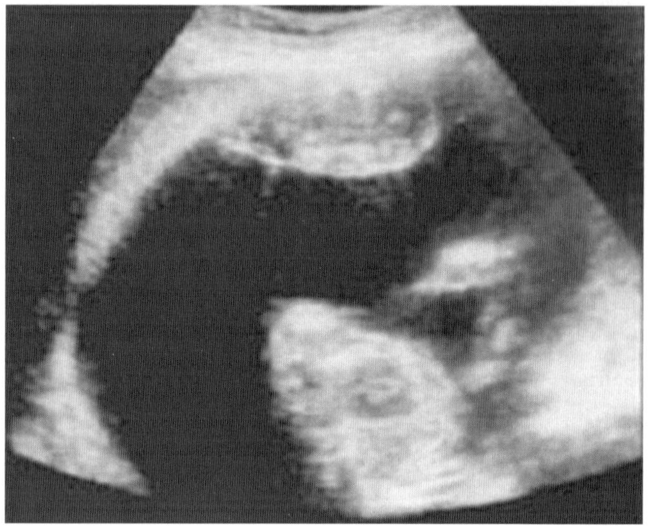

Figure 150.10 Image of a stuck twin in a monochorionic twin pregnancy at 20 weeks with TTTS showing a fetus with severe polyhydramnios and the other one shrouded with a thin membrane, with anhydramnios and pushed against the uterine wall.

Discordance in amniotic fluid volume (oligohydramnios sequence)

We understand TTTS as a manifestation of hemodynamic imbalance. Fetal renal perfusion is asymmetric: the congestive heart failure in the recipient will overperfuse the kidneys with consequent polyuria and excess of amniotic fluid; hypovolemia in the donor causes inadequate perfusion of the kidneys with decrease in urinary output and oligohydramnios.

Consequently, differences in the amniotic fluid volume are expected: oligohydramnios if the deepest vertical pool in the donor sac is < 2 cm and polyhydramnios if the deepest vertical pool is >8 cm in the recipient's sac. Not infrequently anhydramnios in the donor sac results in its becoming 'stuck', shrouded by the intertwin membrane, while the recipient's sac becomes severely polyhydramniotic (Figure 150.10). The presence of discordant anomalies in twins that imply differences in amniotic fluid volume, such as one twin with esophageal atresia and consequent polyhydramnios, or with renal agenesis, with consequent oligohydramnios/anhydramnios, is confounding.

Further confirmatory features include a small or nonvisible bladder in the donor, along with a distended urinary bladder with resulting excessive micturition in the recipient.

Abnormal Doppler findings

Alterations in cardiac hemodynamics are indirectly put on evidence by alterations in venous blood flow waveforms. The most striking feature is the reduced or reversed flow during atrial contraction in the DV commonly found in fetuses with congenital heart defects,[27,28] growth retardation (Hecher 1995) and TTTS.[19,20] (Figure 150.6). Hecher and coworkers[29] found umbilical vein pulsations and absent or reversed flow during atrial contraction in the DV in the recipient with fully established TTTS. Zosmer *et al.*[30] showed that some surviving twins of TTTS had a persistent right ventricular hypertrophic cardiomiopathy with right ventricular tract obstruction (functional pulmonary stenosis) and pulmonary hypertension in the neonatal period.

Recently, diastolic abnormalities were described in the right ventricle, with abnormal filling patterns, prolonged isovolumic relaxation time and abnormal flow patterns in the inferior vena cava and ductus venosus. In addition to hemodynamic remodeling, the role of increased endothelin-1 in the recipient, mainly in the hydropic recipient, as a mitogenic factor to smooth muscle cell in systemic and pulmonary vasculature and for ventricular myocyte proliferation is well recognized.

Abnormalities of vascular distensibility were also described in survivors of TTTS in infancy.[31] The donor fetus shows evidence of chronic hypovolemia causing the activation of the renin–angiotensin system and transfusion of increased concentrations of angiotensin II with increased vascular stiffness in the surviving donor in childhood.

Other ultrasonographic findings

Identification of cord insertion: Velamentous insertion of the cord is more frequent in monochorionic twins.

Funipuncture: Theoretically, it may allow the antenatal evaluation of intertwin hemoglobin difference, the degree of fetal anemia in the donor twin and the twin zygosity through blood group studies. However, middle cerebral artery Doppler studies seem promising in identifying anemia in the surviving twin of a TTTS pair.[32]

Signs of hydrops in the recipient twin: In an advanced stage of TTTS, the recipient twin affected by congestive heart failure may present signs of serosa effusions, such as ascites, pleural effusion and subcutaneous edema.

Difference in color of the placentas: Due to hyperperfusion, the placenta of the recipient tends to be denser in color while the donor tends to show a paler placenta (Figure 150.11).

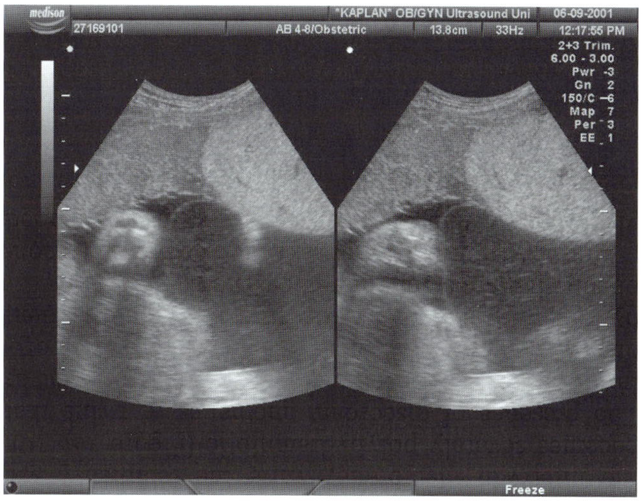

Figure 150.11 Example of a monochorionic twin pregnancy at 32 weeks with TTTS showing a clear difference in echogenecity between the two parts of the placenta. The placenta from the recipient is more echogenic due to congestion and the one from the donor is less echogenic due to blood depletion. Image courtesy of B. Caspi and I. Blickstein, Kaplan Medical Center.

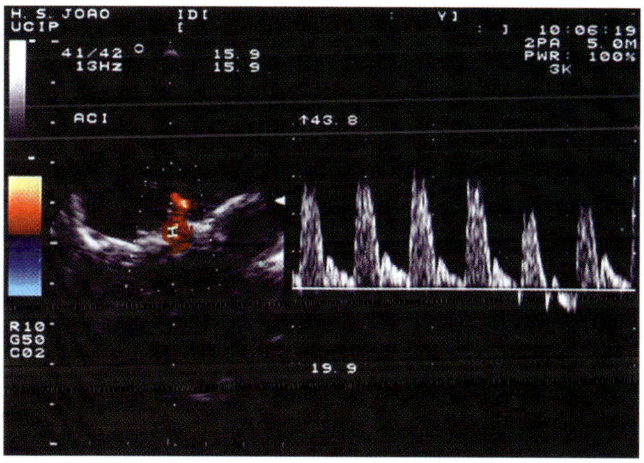

Figure 150.12 Doppler blood flow waveform obtained in the middle cerebral artery. Peak systolic velocity is measured to non-invasively assess the degree of fetal anemia.

Monitoring of anemia in the surviving twin

Intrauterine fetal demise of one fetus in a multiple gestation is a rare event, complicating approximately 0.5–6.8% of twin pregnancies during the second and third trimesters.[33] Demise of both twins has been reported rather infrequently. In higher-order multiples, demise of a single fetus could be more common, ranging from 4.3% to 17% in triplet pregnancies.[34]

The incidence of ominous outcome is dramatically increased in monochorionic twins due to vascular anastomosis. When the death of a co-twin happens, acute hypotension most frequently occurs in the surviving twin with the expected ischemic changes in the spleen, kidney, gastrointestinal tract and skin.[35] More dramatic are the ischemic lesions in the brain of the co-twin, resulting in permanent adverse neurological sequelae (multicystic encephalomalacia, porencephalic cysts).[36,37]

In order to evaluate fetal anemia, invasive techniques such as amniocentesis and cordocentesis are currently used. More recently an alternative noninvasive method, the measurement of middle cerebral artery peak systolic velocity (MCA-PSV), has been proposed to evaluate the level of fetal anemia, namely in pregnancies complicated by rhesus isoimmunization (Figure 150.12).[38] In a study in which a comparison between MCA-PSV and amniotic fluid optical density at 450 nm was performed, both were useful and reliable in the prediction of fetal anemia, with the former having the advantage of being non-invasive.[39]

In the case of intrauterine death of one twin, in which the surviving twin will endure profound exsanguinations with consequent acute and severe anemia, the measurement of MCA-PSV has been used as a simple and reliable diagnostic tool and may be helpful in counseling and planning invasive assessment.[31] Besides, Senat and coworkers demonstrated that after the correction of the anemia by intrauterine transfusion, MCA-PSV decreased with good correlation between MCA-PSV and hemoglobin concentration.[32,40]

Growth discrepancy in multiple pregnancies: distinguishing between adaptation, promotion and restriction

Discordant growth is a common finding/complication of twin pregnancies. It is commonly accepted regarding this controversial issue that (a) not all discordant pairs are similar; (b) discordant growth does not necessarily represent growth restriction; (c) a discordance level may have a different clinical implication in different gestational ages; (d) the larger the discordance level the greater is the risk for an adverse outcome and (e) the smaller fetuses in severely discordant pairs are at disproportionate risk for perinatal mortality and morbidity.

Intertwin growth discordance may represent a normal variation between sibs working as an adaptive measure to promote gestational age at the same uterine size. Nature seems to favor maturity rather than size: data from large twin and triplet series suggest that significant birth weight discordance result from the inability of the uterine milieu to equally nurture twins.[43] In order to promote maturity – gestational age – mild compensation in the form of size discordance begins after mid-gestation. When the uterine environment competently nurtures multiples, total birth weight increases and discordance decreases. In fact, the entire 'fetal mass' of a multiple pregnancy can exceed the 90th birth weight percentile of a singleton of the same gestational age and the individual fetuses may exhibit growth patterns compatible with adaptation to the limited uterine environment rather than pathological restriction.[41] Adaptation can take the form of relative growth restriction (i.e. discordance in weight or abdominal circumference), whereby not all fetuses show a decelerating growth pattern or hemodynamic compromise.[43]

Further away in this process, when adaptation fails, severely discordant pairs often exhibit patterns of growth restriction. However, even in cases with significant discordance, about 40% of the smaller twins, weigh above the 10th birth weight percentile. Clinically relevant is the fact that recognizing the transition from the physiologic adaptation into the pathologic process of growth restriction. Therefore, the smallest fetus should be evaluated to perceive whether its growth is being promoted (abdominal circumference >P50), adapted (abdominal circumference P5–50) or restricted (abdominal circumference <P5) in conjunction with Doppler blood flow evaluation. From the large series it is recognized that about 75% of twins exhibit <15% discordance (designated concordant), 20% are 15–25% (mildly) discordant, and about 5% are more than 25% (severely) discordant (Figure 150.9).[42,43] Higher frequencies and increased severity are observed among triplets.[44]

Growth curves of twins and triplets do not support the growth restriction pattern seen in singletons. At the same time that individual members of a twin or a triplet set may be smaller than singletons of the same gestational age, only a minority are indeed growth-restricted by singleton standards.[45]

The evaluation of fetal growth depends on stricter sonographic criteria to define normal or abnormal growth. Abdominal circumference rather than head measurements of twins was proposed as the most reproducible and meaningful one. Besides, considering that fetal weight estimations based on singleton growth charts may be inadequate for twins, the abdominal circumference criterion should be definitely used for the sonographic diagnosis of divergent twin growth. A cutoff value of 20 mm for the difference in abdominal circumference between twins indicated growth discordance of more than 25%.

Identification of the genuinely growth-restricted fetuses is an imperative step in the management of birth weight discordance in twin gestations as it has dramatic implications on perinatal morbidity and mortality. Neonatal mortality rates among discordant twins were compared among three groups of discordant twins (> 25%), distinguished by the birth weight of the smaller twin being < 10th, 10th to 50th or > 50th percentile.[45] Among the 10,683 pairs of twins who were studied, the respective proportions of the three groups were 62.4%, 32.9% and 4.7%. The neonatal mortality rate was significantly higher among pairs in which the smaller twin weighed < 10th birth weight percentile (29 vs. 11.1 and 11 per 1000; odds ratio, 2.7; 95% CI, 1.3–5.7). This difference results from the higher mortality rates among the smaller but not among the larger twins. Severely discordant twin pairs in whom the smaller twin is also small for gestational age are at an increased risk of neonatal death.[46]

In order to identify the groups at risk, complimentary to abdominal circumference measurements (Figure 150.9), Doppler blood flow evaluation of the arterial (umbilical artery, middle cerebral artery) and venous (umbilical vein and ductus venosus) compartments should be the next step. Whenever end-diastolic blood flow is absent or reversed in the

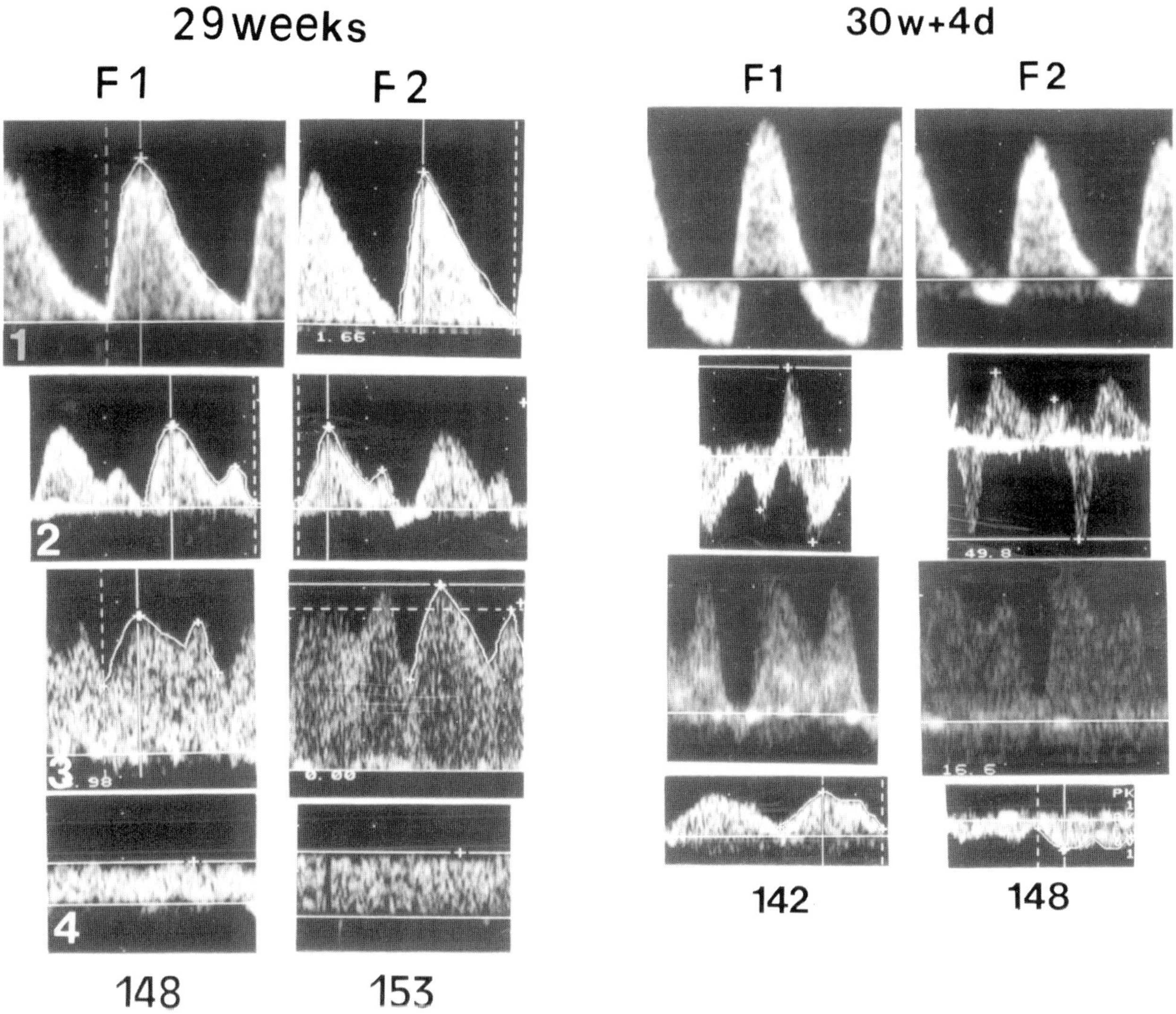

Figure 150.13 Doppler blood flow waveforms from umbilical artery (1), inferior vena cava (2), ductus venosus (3) and umbilical vein (4) obtained in fetuses F1 and F2 of a dichorionic diamniotic twin pregnancy. The first examination was performed at 29 weeks with present end-diastolic flow in the umbilical artery and normal venous flow. The scan performed at 30 weeks +4 days, on the day of the elective delivery, shows reverse end-diastolic flow in the umbilical artery, with a high velocity A-wave in the inferior vena cava, absent flow during the atrial contraction in the ductus venosus and dicrote pulsatile flow in the umbilical vein in both fetuses. Both babies are alive and well, but were born growth-restricted. Reproduced with permission from *Journal of Perinatal Medicine*.

umbilical artery, blood flow in the middle cerebral artery should be assessed looking for adaptive centralization. Venous Doppler waveforms are affected slightly later and depict confidently hemodynamic deterioration and correctly predict acid–base status, mainly when absent or reversed flow appears in the ductus venosus (Figure 150.13).[47–50] The evaluation of amniotic fluid volume as a chronic marker of intrauterine hypoxia may constitute a further differentiating parameter between an adapted or genetically small baby, and a restricted and suffering baby. This hemodynamic deterioration is sequential and can be monitored longitudinally. The timing of delivery has most of its clues in the Doppler flowmetry sequential evaluation both for singletons and multiples, bearing in mind that previously known chorionicity makes a difference when talking about growth discrepancy.

Malformations in multiple gestations

Acardiac twin/TRAP sequence

Acardiac twins were first documented in 1533 and were first diagnosed by ultrasound in 1978.[51] This is a unique complication to monochorionic twinning. Due to a paradoxical retrograde perfusion by a structurally normal 'pump' twin there is a disruption of development of the cardiovascular system and a cascade of disruption of organ development in the perfused twin (TRAP sequence – twin reversed arterial perfusion).[52] However, the anomalous twin may have an underlying cytogenetic anomaly or a primary malformed cardiovascular system prior to anastomosis development.

It is a rare condition, occurring with a reported incidence of 1 in 35,000 deliveries, 1% of monozygotic twins and 1 in 30 monozygotic triplets.[53] The

(a)

(b)

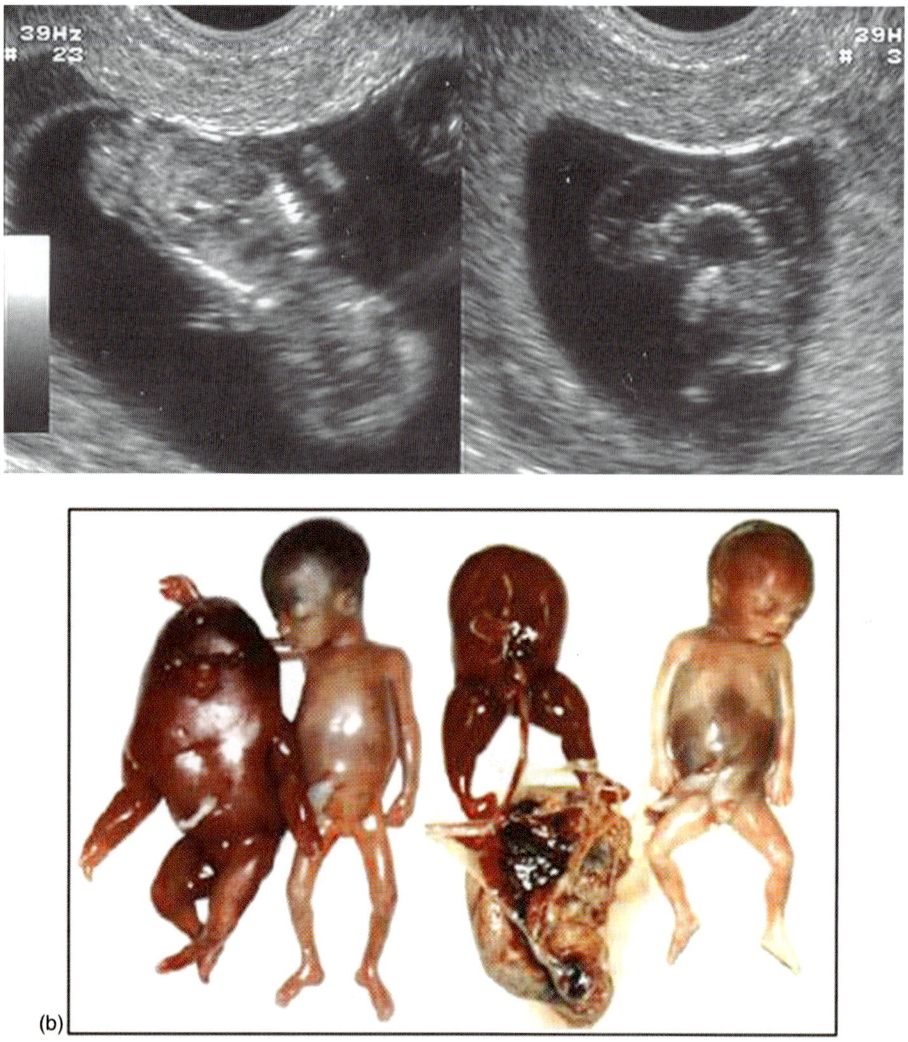

Figure 150.14 (a) Image of an acardiac twin showing a malformed head and trunk and the normal co-twin in the first trimester of pregnancy. (b) Two necropsic specimens of an acardiac twin and the normal co-twin. The one on the right has a rudimentary head ('anceps acardia') and the one on the left represents the most common form of acardiac twin, without head and trunk, with a plethoric appearance. Courtesy of C. Comas.

hemodynamically advantaged or pumping structurally normal twin is at risk for *in utero* cardiac failure and without treatment dies in more than 75% of cases. This risk has three causes: the high cardiovascular demands of the parasitic twin on the pump twin will cause high-output heart failure; an important increase in uterine volume will be caused by the continuing excessive growth of the acardiac twin; and the deoxygenated blood from the pump twin, that will be further deoxygenated by the acardiac twin, will circulate back to the pump twin with a low content of oxygen and will provoke chronic hypoxia and growth restriction.

Acardiac twins can be diagnosed antenatally on the ultrasound by the absence of identifiable cardiac motion. In some cases, due to a rudimentary heart or transmitted pulsation from the pump twin, cardiac pulsation may be suspected. In addition, there is poor definition of the head, trunk and upper extremities, deformed lower extremities, which may show some movements, and usually conspicuous subcutaneous edema and abnormal cystic areas in the upper part of the body of the affected twin[54] (Figure 150.14a and b). In about 70% of the acardiac fetuses, there is polyhydramnios with a functional urinary tract. However, the main clue to the diagnosis seems to be the continued growth of a 'presumed dead' twin on subsequent scans in a monochorionic twin pregnancy.

Color Doppler ultrasound, first used in the prenatal detection as well as documentation of the reversed arterial perfusion, reported by Pretorious *et al.*,[55] is a very useful tool in the definitive diagnosis of an acardiac twin. Those acardiac twins missed in an early pregnancy were those in which color Doppler was not used, namely to put in evidence the two vessel cord (in more than two-thirds of the cases) and the paradoxical direction of arterial blood flow toward rather than away from the acardiac twin, and from caudal to cranial in this twin's abdominal aorta.

Intrauterine diagnosis of acardiac twin has been achieved in some cases in the first trimester of pregnancy,[56,57] suggesting that the pathogenesis in acardia is cardiac dysmorphogenesis secondary to reversal of blood flow rather than cardiac agenesis, since cardiac beats in the malformed twin were seen until the seventh week and stopped thereafter, along with reversed flow through the umbilical cord into the recipient twin via arterioarterial anastomosis of placental vessels.

Essentially, every single organ system is affected, but the most commonly associated anomalies are cardiac defects: the heart may be completely absent, reduced to tubular or a two-chamber heart. A single umbilical artery is the rule. The lower extremities are usually spared because the femoral arteries contain the most oxygen and nutrients. The abdominal viscera are hardly discernible. The external genitalia may be normal, deficient or absent. The thoracic structures may be present, rudimentary, severely dysplastic or absent. Marked edema and cystic hygroma may be massive. They are typically acephalic with absent upper extremities. When cranial structures are present ('acardius anceps'), or in the rarest form when there are cranial elements but no body structure ('acardius acormus'), anencephaly, holoprosencephaly or facial clefts may be present.

Poor prognostic factors for the pump twin can be assessed by ultrasound: acardiac-to-pump twin weight ratio of > 70%, hydrops in the pump twin, polyhydramnios, acardiac twin with presence of arms or an anceps acardia, a small resistance index < 0.20 in the umbilical artery of both the acardiac and pump twins.[58] Fetal demise will occur unless salvage invasive procedure is performed by disconnecting intertwin blood circulation. Therefore, TRAP sequence should be monitored on a weekly basis by ultrasound, including size estimation, Doppler flowmetry and echocardiography.

Conjoined twins

Conjoined twins are defined as monochorionic and monoamniotic twins, originating from a single fertilized ovum, fused at any portion of their body as a result of an incomplete division of the embryonic disk, which occurs after the 13th day of conception. The term 'conjoined' is actually a misnomer, since this malformation results from failure of complete separation and not from inadequate fusion. Conjoined twins occur as often as 1 in every 40,000 births but only 1 in every 200,000 live births. The overall survival rate for conjoined twins is between 5% and 25%. Conjoined twins are more likely to be female (70–75%). There are no documented cases of conjoined triplets or quadruplets.

Conjoined twins are usually classified by the point at which they are joined (the Greek word *pagos*, meaning 'that which is fixed'). There have been as many as three-dozen separate types identified in the last century. The most frequent varieties are thoracopagus (40%), omphalopagus (33%), pygopagus (18%), ischiopagus (6%) and craniopagus (2%). The fact of sharing the heart or not makes an important prognostic difference.

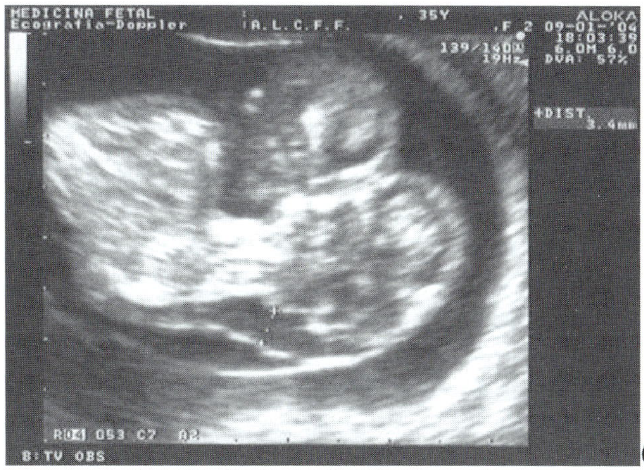

(a)

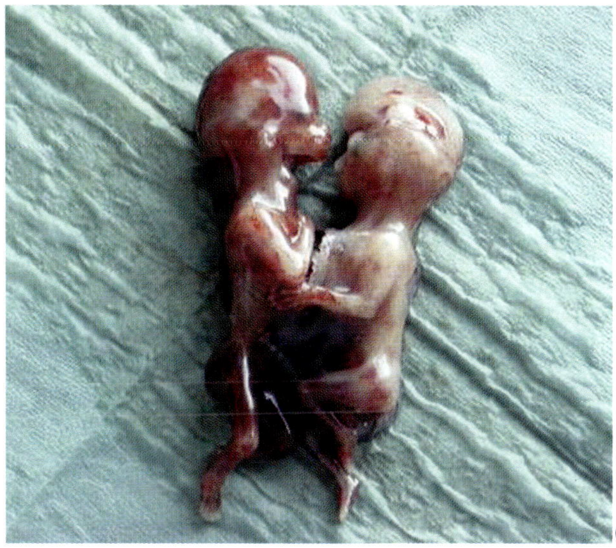
(b)

Figure 150.15 (a) Scan of thoracopagus conjoined twins at 12 weeks of gestation. Note the parallel, mirror image, head-to-head position of both fetuses, with a shared single heart. (b) Necropsic specimen of the same case, confirming the thoracopagus type of conjoined twins with a single heart.

The first-trimester scan can be very useful to detect and to define the type of conjoined twins.[59] This situation must always be considered whenever a monochorionic monoamniotic twin pregnancy is suspected. Discordant presentation does not exclude conjoined twins.

Basically, the scan must demonstrate fused portion of the bodies of monozygotic–monoamniotic twins (Figure 150.15a and b). Several other sonographic signs can be looked for to avoid misdiagnosis:

- Bifid appearance of the first-trimester fetal pole ('V'- or 'Y'-shaped twin pregnancy)
- Absence of interamniotic membrane between the twins
- Inability to separate fetal bodies and permanent position of the fetus relative to the other, even after maternal abdomen stimulation
- Abnormal number of vessels (more than three) in the umbilical cord

- The heads and bodies of both twins are seen at the same level and a mirror-image can occasionally be seen
- Unusual proximity of the extremities
- Unusual hyperextension of the spines
- Single heart
- Presence of other fetal anomalies.

The timely recognition of this condition enables the parents to consider the possibility of terminating the pregnancy. If not, one should bear in mind that conjoined twins present a higher prevalence of congenital anomalies other than the shared organs of about 50%. Cardiac defects are the most common association (20–30%), and thus echocardiography is recommended in all cases. Neural tube defects and midline fusion defects, orofacial clefts, imperforate anus and diaphragmatic hernia are also frequently seen. Polyhydramnios is observed in more than half of the cases.

Major malformations

It is well established that congenital anomalies are found more frequently in monozygotic twinning than in singleton pregnancies.[60] These anomalies are of different types: some are related to the twinning process itself, others are due to vascular factors, and a few are structural malformations not exclusively found in twins but observed more frequently in monozygotic twinning.[61] The largest study, combining data from nine registries based in European and Latin American countries, analyzed 260,865 twins and 5572 malformations were reported.[61] An expected excess of malformations in twins compared with singletons was found, and all anatomical sites were involved.

Here again, ultrasound has an irreplaceable role in experienced hands and with high-quality equipments in the screening and diagnosis of fetal malformations as early as the first trimester of pregnancy.

REFERENCES

1. Sepulveda W, Sebire N, Hughes K, Odibo A, Nicolaides KH. The lambda sign at 10–14 weeks of gestation as a predictor of chorionicity in twin pregnancies. *Ultrasound Obstet Gynecol* 1996;7:421–3.
2. Wood SL, St Onge R, Connors G, Elliot PD. Evaluation of the twin peak sign in determining chorionicity in multiple pregnancy. *Obstet Gynecol* 1996;88:6–9.
3. Fisk NM, Bennett PR. Prenatal determination of chorionicity and zygosity. In Ward RH, Whittle W, eds. *Multiple Pregnancy*. London: RCOG Press, 1995:56–66.
4. Sepulveda W, Sebire N, Hughes K, Kalogeropoulos A, Nicolaides KH. Evolution of the lambda or twin-chorionic peak sign in dichorionic twin pregnancies. *Obstet Gynecol* 1997;89:439–41.
5. Snijders RJM, Noble P, Sebire JN, Souka A, Nicolaides KH. UK multicentre project on assessment of risk of trisomy 21 by maternal age and fetal nuchal translucency thickness at 10–14 weeks of gestation. *Lancet* 1998;351:343–6.
6. Cicero S, Curcio P, Papageorghiou A, Sonek J, Nicolaides KH. Absence of nasal bone in fetuses with trisomy 21 at 11–14 weeks of gestation: An observational study. *Lancet* 2001;358:1665–7.
7. Bindra R, Heath V, Liao A, Spencer K, Nicolaides KH. One-stop clinic for assessment of risk of trisomy 21 at 11–14 weeks: A prospective study of 15,030 pregnancies. *Ultrasound Obstet Gynecol* 2002;20:219–25.
8. Spencer K, Souter V, Tul N, Snijders RJM, Nicolaides KH. A screening program for trisomy 21 at 10–14 weeks using fetal nuchal translucency, maternal serum free β-human chorionic gonadotropin and pregnancy-associated plasma protein-A. *Ultrasound Obstet Gynecol* 1999;13:231–7.
9. Spencer K, Salonen R, Muller F. Down's syndrome screening in multiple pregnancies using alpha-fetoprotein and free beta hCG. *Prenat Diagn* 1994;18:537–42.
10. Cuckle H. Down's syndrome screening in twins. *J Med Screen* 1998;5:3–4.
11. Rodis JF, Egan JF, Craffey A, Ciarleglio L, Greenstein RM, Scozza WE. Calculated risk of chromosomal abnormalities in twin gestations. *Obstet Gynecol* 1990;76:1037–41.
12. Jenkins TM, Wapner RJ. The challenge of prenatal diagnosis in twin pregnancies. *Curr Opin Obstet Gynecol* 2000;12:87–92.
13. Blickstein I, Verhoeven HC, Keith LG. Zygotic splitting after assisted reproduction. *N Engl J Med* 1999;340(9):738–9.
14. Pandya PP, Hilber F, Snijders RJM, *et al.* Nuchal translucency thickness, crown–rump length in twin pregnancies with chromosomally normal fetuses. *J Ultrasound Med* 1995;14:565–8.
15. Sebire NJ, Snijders RJM, Hughes K, Sepulveda W, Nicolaides KH. Screening for trisomy 21 in twin pregnancies by maternal age and fetal nuchal translucency thickness at 10–14 weeks of gestation. *Br J Obstet Gynaecol* 1996;103:999–1003.
16. Sebire NJ, Noble PL, Psarra A, Papapanagioutou G, Nicolaifdes KH. Fetal karyotyping in twin pregnancies: Selection of technique by measurement of fetal nuchal translucency. *Br J Obstet Gynaecol* 1996;103:887–90.
17. Sebire NJ, D'Ercole C, Hughes K, Carvalho M, Nicolaides KH. Increased nuchal translucency thickness at 10–14 weeks of gestation as a predictor of severe twin-to-twin transfusion syndrome. *Ultrasound Obstet Gynecol* 1997;10:86–9.
18. Sebire NJ, Souka A, Skentou H, Geerts L, Nicolaides KH. Early prediction of severe twin–twin transfusion syndrome. *Hum Reprod* 2000;15:2008–10.
19. Matias A, Montenegro N, Areias JC. Anticipating twin–twin transfusion syndrome in monochorionic twin pregnancy. Is there a role for nuchal translucency and ductus venosus blood flow evaluation at 11–14 weeks? *Twin Res* 2000;3:65–70.
20. Matias A, Ramalho C, Montenegro N. Search for hemodynamic compromise at 11–14 weeks in monochorionic twin pregnancy: Is abnormal flow in the ductus venosus predictive of twin-to-twin transfusion syndrome? *J Matern Fetal Neonatal Med* 2005;18(2): 79–86.
21. Maymon R, Dreazen E, Rozinsky S, *et al.* The feasibility of nuchal translucency measurement in higher order multiple gestation achieved by assisted reproduction. *Hum Reprod* 1999;14:2102–5.
22. Spencer K. Screening for trisomy 21 in twin pregnancies in the first trimester using free β-hCG and PAPP-A, combined with fetal nuchal translucency thickness. *Prenat Diagn* 2000;20: 91–5.
23. Wittmann BK, Baldwin VJ, Nichol B. Antenatal diagnosis of twin-to-twin transfusion syndrome by ultrasound. *Obstet Gynecol* 1981;58:123–6.
24. Brennan JN, Diwan RV, Rosen MG, Bellon EM. Fetofetal transfusion syndrome: Prenatal ultrasonographic diagnosis. *Radiology* 1982;143:535–6.
25. Brown DL, Benson CB, Driscoll SG, Doubilet PM. Twin–twin transfusion syndrome: Sonographic findings. *Radiology* 1989;170:61–3.
26. Blickstein I. The twin–twin transfusion syndrome. *Obstet Gynecol* 1990;76(4):714–22.
27. Montenegro N, Matias A, Areias JC, Castedo S, Barros H. Increased nuchal translucency: Possible involvement of early cardiac failure. *Ultrasound Obstet Gynecol* 1997;10:265–8.
28. Matias A, Gomes C, Flack N, Montenegro N, Nicolaides KH. Screening for chromosomal defects at 11–14 weeks: The role of ductus venosus blood flow. *Ultrasound Obstet Gynecol* 1998; 12:380–4.

29. Hecher K, Ville Y, Snijders R, Nicolaides KH. Doppler studies of the fetal circulation in twin-to-twin transfusion syndrome. *Ultrasound Obstet Gynecol* 1995;5:318–24.
30. Zosmer N, Bajoria R, Weiner E, Rigby M, Vaughan J, Fisk N. Clinical and echographic features of in utero cardiac dysfunction in the recipient twin-to-twin transfusion syndrome. *Br Heart J* 1994;72:74–9.
31. Gardiner HM; Taylor M, Karatza A, *et al.* Twin–twin transfusion syndrome: The influence of intrauterine laser photocoagulation on arterial distensibility in childhood. *Circulation* 2003;107:1–6.
32. Senat MV, Loizeau S, Coouderc S, Bernard JP, Ville Y. The value of the middle cerebral artery peak systolic velocity in the diagnosis of fetal anemia after intrauterine death of one monochorionic twin. *Am J Obstet Gynecol* 2003;189:1319–23.
33. Johnson CD, Zhang J. Survival of other fetuses after a fetal death in twin and triplet pregnancies. *Obstet Gynecol* 2002;99:698–703.
34. Gonen R, Heyman E, Asztalos E, *et al.* The outcome of triplet gestations complicated by fetal death. *Obstet Gynecol* 1990;75:175–8.
35. Bulla M, von Lilien T, Goecke H, *et al.* Renal and cerebral necrosis in survivor after in utero death of co-twin. *Arch Gynecol* 1987; 240:119–24.
36. D'Alton ME, Newton ER, Cetrulo CL. Intrauterine fetal demise in multiple gestation. *Acta Genet Med Gemellol* 1984;33:43–9.
37. Weiss JL, Cleary-Goldman J, Tanji K, Budorick N, D'alton ME. Multicystic encephalomalacia after first-trimester intrauterine fetal death in monochorionic twins. *Am J Obstet Gynecol* 2004;190: 563–5.
38. Alshimmiri MM, Hamoud MS, Al-Saleh EA, Mujaibel KY, Al-Harmi JA, Thalib L. Prediction of fetal anemia by middle cerebral artery peak systolic velocity in pregnancies complicated by rhesus isoimmunization. *Perinatology* 2003;23:536–40.
39. Nishie EN, Brizot ML, Liao AW, Carvalho MH, Toma O, Zugaib M. A comparison between middle cerebral artery peak systolic velocity and amniotic fluid optical density at 450 nm in the prediction of fetal anemia. *Am J Obstet Gynecol* 2003;188:214–9.
40. Mari G, Rahman F, Olofsson P, Ozcan T, Copel JA. Increase of fetal hematocrit decreases the middle cerebral artery peak systolic velocity in pregnancies complicated by rhesus isoimmunization. *J Matern Fetal Med* 1997;6:206–8.
41. Blickstein I. Is it normal for multiples to be smaller than singletons? *Best Pract Res Clin Obstet Gynecol* 2004;18:613–23.
42. Blickstein I. Normal and abnormal growth of multiples. *Semin Neonatol* 2002;7:177–85.
43. Blickstein I, Goldman RD. Intertwin birth weight discordance as a potential adaptive measure to promote gestational age. *J Reprod Med* 2003;48:449–54.
44. Blickstein I, Kalish RB. Birthweight discordance in multiple pregnancy. *Twin Res* 2003;6:526–31.
45. Blickstein I, Kalish RB, Sharma G, Rhea DJ, Keith LG. The ponderal index in triplets: Relationship to small for gestational age neonates. *J Perinat Med* 2004;32:62–5.
46. Blickstein I, Keith LG. Neonatal mortality rates among growth-discordant twins, classified according to the birthweight of the smaller twin. *Am J Obstet Gynecol* 2004;190:170–4.
47. Montenegro N, Matias A, Areias JC, Castedo S, Barros H. Increased nuchal translucency: Possible involvement of early cardiac failure. *Ultrasound Obstet Gynecol* 1997;10:265–8.
48. Areias JC, Matias A, Montenegro N. Venous return and right ventricular diastolic function in ARED flow fetuses. *J Perinat Med* 1998;26:157–67.
49. Baschat AA. Pathophysiology of fetal growth restriction: Implications for diagnosis and surveillance. *Obstet Gynecol Surv* 2004;59:617–27.
50. Baschat AA, Guclu S, Kush ML, Gembruch U, Weiner CP, Harman CR. Venous Doppler in the prediction of acid–base status of growth-restricted fetuses with elevated placental blood flow resistance. *Am J Obstet Gynecol* 2004;191:277–84.
51. Lehr C, DiRe J. Rare occurrence of a holocardius acephalic monster: A sonographic and pathologic findings. *J Clin Ultrasound* 1978;6:259–61.
52. van Allen MI, Smith DW, Shepard TH. Twin reversed arterial perfusion (TRAP) sequence: A study of 14 twin pregnancies with acardius. *Semin Perinatol* 1983;7:285–93.
53. James WH. A note on the epidemiology of acardiac monsters. *Teratology* 1977;16:211–6.
54. Sebire NJ, Sepulveda W, Jeanty P, Nyberg DA, Nicolaides KH. Multiple gestations. In Nyberg DA, McGahan JP, Pretorious DH, Pilu G, eds. *Diagnostic Imaging of Fetal Anomalies.* Philadelphia, PA: Lippincott Williams & Wilkins, 2003:777–813.
55. Pretorious DH, Leoplold GR, Moore TR, Benirschke K, Sivo JJ. Acardiac twin. Report of Doppler sonography. *J Ultrasound Med* 1988;7:413–6.
56. Coulam CB, Wright G. First trimester diagnosis of acardiac twins. *Early Pregnancy* 2000;4:261–70.
57. Kamitomo M, Kouno S Ibuka K, *et al.* First-trimester findings associated with twin reversed arterial perfusion sequence. *Fetal Diagn Ther* 2004;19:187–90.
58. Dashe JS, Fernandez CO, Twickler DM. Utility of Doppler velocimetry in predicting outcome in twin reversed arterial perfusion sequence. *Am J Obstet Gynecol* 2001;185:135–9.
59. Lam YH, Sin SY, Lam C, Lee CP, Tang MH, Tse HY. Prenatal sonographic diagnosis of conjoined twins in the first trimester: Two case reports. *Ultrasound Obstet Gynecol* 1998;11:289–91.
60. Myrianthopoulos NC. Congenital malformations: The contribution of twin studies. *Birth Defects Orig Artic Ser* 1978;14:151–65.
61. Baldwin VJ. Anomalous development of twins. In Baldwin VJ, ed. *Pathology of Multiple Pregnancy.* New York: Springer-Verlag, 1994:169–97.
62. Mastroiacovo P, Castilla EE, Arpino C, *et al.* Congenital malformations in twins: An international study. *Am J Med Genet* 1999; 12:117–24.

151 Genetic diagnosis in multiple pregnancies

Z. Appelman and B. Furman

Introduction

The likelihood of finding chromosomal anomalies and Mendelian diseases is increased in multiple gestations compared to singletons. Prenatal diagnosis may therefore be indicated in multiple pregnancies to a no lesser extent than in the singleton. The most common situations discussed in the context of multiple pregnancies are screening and diagnostic measures to detect aneuploidy, genetic counseling when a structural anomaly is detected and in circumstances with increased risk of specific inherited conditions. The basic rules of genetic counseling in singletons are applicable also in multiples; however, there are specific facets in multiple gestations that need special attention, which makes counseling more complex. Indeed, it is the combination of medical and ethical aspects that makes it so complicated. The basic difference between counseling singletons and multiples is the fact that, as opposed to singletons, any decision in multiples should take into consideration the implication of that decision for the other sib(s). This includes both diagnostic and therapeutic measures. However, genetic counseling is often provided by a general obstetrician, who may benefit from a simplified approach. This chapter describes specific medical situations that require the attention of a genetic counselor.

Prenatal genetic diagnosis – an overview

The incidence of multifetal pregnancies has increased exponentially during the past two decades mostly because of assisted reproduction technologies (ART).[1] Typically, pregnant women after ART are older. Hence, the age-related risk of aneuploidy is often significant. The likelihood of at least one twin having a chromosomal abnormality is five-third times higher than in singleton pregnancy.[2] The decision to undergo prenatal diagnosis in multiple gestations is complex and must take into consideration not only the risk of aneuploidy, but also the procedure-related complications. In addition, abnormal results sometimes require selective termination of an affected sib, a procedure entailing moral, ethical and medical implications. Invasive prenatal diagnosis techniques include chorionic villus sampling (CVS), amniocentesis (AC), cordocentesis, fetal tissue sampling, embrioscopy and fetoscopy (Table 151.1). The indications for prenatal diagnostic genetic testing determined as routine and applicable for singleton and twin gestations are advanced maternal age, familial history of chromosomal abnormalities, previous children with a chromosomal abnormality or neural tube defects (NTDs) and suspected abnormalities identified during sonographic examination.

Advanced maternal age was defined as any expectant mother who will be 35 years old by the time of

Table 151.1 Characteristics of AC and CVS

	AC	CVS
Timing	16–18 weeks	10–12 weeks
Placement	TA	TA and TC
Risk of miscarriage	0.5–1%	TA – 1–2%; TC – 2–6%
Sampling success	99%	99%
Time to diagnosis	3 weeks (FISH available)	2–3 weeks (rapid direct technique may be considered)
Accuracy	High	High
Mosaicism	Rare	Confined placental 1–2%
Open NTD	AFP in amniotic fluid detects 95% of NTDs	Other test required

FISH, fluorescence *in situ* hybridization; TA, transabdominal; TC, transcervical birth. Nowadays, the age of 35 years still stands as a turning point in prenatal supervision and is recommended as the age at which aggressive screening should be done using AC or CVS. Not everyone accepts categorical age of 35 or even 37 years as an absolute indication for invasive genetic diagnosis. Some would prefer to adjust the risk individually according to the maternal age and some non-invasive risk assessment. In multiple pregnancies, the logical approach would be the combination of maternal age and nuchal translucency (NT) measurement. It is also possible to add to the risk assessment the presence or absence of 'soft' sonographic signs of aneuploidy. It makes sense since chromosomal aneuploidy increases with advanced maternal age. The risk of Down's syndrome in 35-year-old women is 1:365[3] and increases to 1:109 at 40 years and even 1:12 at 49 years. The overall probability that a multiple gestation contains an aneuploid fetus is directly related to zygosity. The risk of both twins being simultaneously abnormal in monozygotic (MZ) twins is the same as the age-related risk in singletons, since one oocyte was fertilized. In contrast, for dizygotic (DZ) twins, each of the fetuses has an independent risk of abnormal chromosomal composition, because at least two different ova were fertilized. Clinically, the risk of only one affected fetus in a dizygotic pregnancy is approximately two times the age-related risk of a singleton. Since the risk of only one affected fetus in MZ twins is basically zero,[4] the overall birth prevalence of Down's syndrome is only 3% greater in twin pregnancies than in singletons.[5] The risk of both the fetuses having a chromosomal abnormality is small. If zygosity is unknown, the risk of one aneuploid fetus can be approximated as five-thirds that of a singleton.[6] This is based on the principle that one-third of twins are MZ. However, this is only an unfulfilled approach because rates of MZ and DZ twins are dependent on maternal age, ethnicity and mainly on the mode of conception.

MZ (twinning from a single egg) twins happen once in 250 pregnancies. This is unaffected by age, race or any other factors except mode of conception. In DZ, or 'fraternal', twins not only maternal age, but also the parity increases the chances of twins. The frequency of twins is three times higher in women over 35 years with at least four other children than in nulliparas under 20 years of age. When parity is considered alone, the chance of twins doubles from the first pregnancy to the fourth pregnancy. African-American women have a 1:79 probability for twins, Caucasians 1:100 and Oriental women 1:155.

Spontaneous twins occur in 1 in 80 births, but in the era of ART and the trend toward delayed childbirth increased dramatically and the incidence of twins is now 1 in 40 births. The increasing use of ART procedures (defined as any procedure that entails the handling of both eggs and sperm or of embryos for the purpose of establishing a pregnancy) and other non-ART fertility treatments (i.e. intrauterine insemination and ovulation-inducing drugs) in the past two decades increased the multiple birth rates.[7,8]

Another factor that increases the twinning rate is the concurrent shift in maternal age distribution as more women delay childbearing into their late 30s and 40s. The extraordinary rise in high-order multiple births over the past two decades, especially in triplet births, has also been associated with the above-mentioned trends: advances in and greater access to ovulation-inducing drugs and ART, and older age at childbirth.[9] Since 1990, the twin birth rate rose 80% among women 40–44 years of age (from 24.7 to 44.5 per 1000), and almost 600% among women aged 45–49 years (from 23.8 to 155.7 per 1000), compared to only a 6% rise for women under age 20 years (14.3–15.2 per 1000). Data are not available, however, for women aged 50–54 years, but in 1999 more than one-third of births (34%) to women in the oldest age group were twin deliveries.[9]

Determination of chorionicity

Determination of chorionicity is crucial in assessing the perinatal risk as well as the risk of aneuploidity and is probably the most important factor in genetic counseling in multiples.[10] In addition, it helps in perinatal risk assessment.[11] The probability of both the DZ twins being chromosomally abnormal is the product of their separate probabilities. For example, the age-related risk for Down's syndrome in a woman is 1:100 for singletons as well as for each twin, thus the probability of having the syndrome for both is $1{:}100 \times 1{:}100 = 1{:}10{,}000$.

First-trimester ultrasound is now accepted as the most accurate for determination of chorionicity (Figure 151.1). Identification of the twin-peak sign in the first trimester provides 100% accuracy for the diagnosis of dichorionic (DC) twins.[12] However, accuracy is reduced when chorionicity assessment is performed later in pregnancy. In midtrimester, after the fusion between the chorion and the amnion, the accuracy of chorionicity determination is about 90%.[13] Other techniques for chorionicity determination like septal thickness measurements and counting the number of intertwin membranes are less popular and seem to depend on the operator's skills and the transducer in use.[14,15] It should be stressed that one-third of MZ twins are DC. However, at present, it is impossible to differentiate DC MZ from DC-like-sex DZ twins on clinical grounds. It follows that assessment of both the twins is inevitable in all DC twins irrespectively of zygosity.

From the genetic point of view, monochorionic (MC) twins imply monozygosity and high genetic resemblance. On the other hand, only unlike-sexed DC twins are 100% DZ, and zygosity is unknown in all like-sexed DC twins. This uncertainty is even greater in iatrogenic conceptions, because the proportion of DZ to MZ twins (about 10:1), as well as the proportion of DC to MC in the subpopulation of MZ twins (proportion

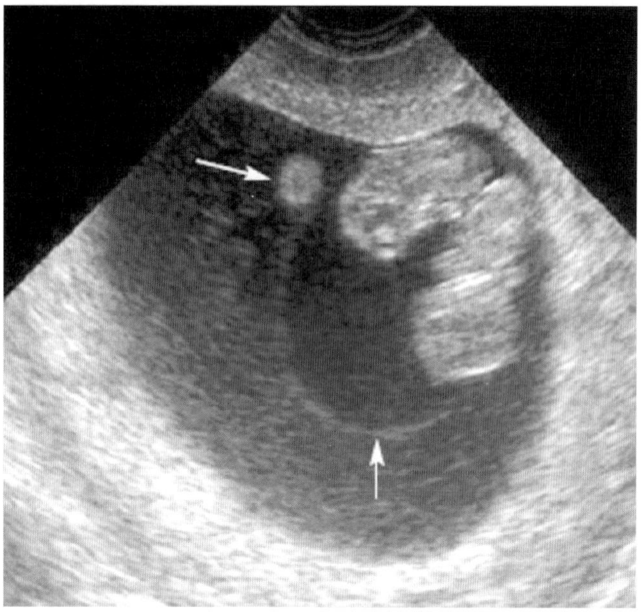

Figure 151.1 A single yolk sac (upper arrow) and two fetuses were observed within a single amniotic sac (lower arrow). This sonographic scan at 9 weeks led to the diagnosis of monoamniotic twins. Image courtesy of B. Caspi, MD, Kaplan Medical Center.

unknown), is different from that of spontaneous conceptions. When chorionicity is unclear and management decisions might be altered by determination of zygosity, prenatal DNA studies should be considered. An example of the difficulty arising from inconclusive chorionicity determination in the later parts of pregnancy is presented in a case of twin pregnancy discordant for hydrocephaly and oligohydramnios in which sonographic evaluation could not exclude MC twinning. Before considering selective feticide, blood samples from both the fetuses were examined by DNA 'fingerprint' analysis. The different banding patterns of the blood samples established dizygosity.[16] Similarly, DNA zygosity studies were performed on amniocytes to guide the management of four such pregnancies.[17] In this series, DNA zygosity analyses provided >99% likelihood of MZ twins in two cases, a fact that altered counseling regarding selective termination options.[17] In the other two cases, DNA studies were used to assess risk to the normal twin in the event of the co-twin's demise, based on the differentiation of twin–twin transfusion syndrome (TTTS) from discordant severe intrauterine growth restriction (IUGR) and oligohydramnios.[17]

Should all MC twin gestations receive genetic counseling?

MZ twins have a two- to threefold increased risk of structural anomalies. When an MC gestation comes to the attention of the genetic counselor, the patient should be informed about this risk, and should be referred for a comprehensive sonographic scan, including detailed echocardiography. When a discordant structural anomaly is found, discussion of management options should consider the vascular anastomoses between the circulations of the twins. This circumstance precludes termination of the anomalous twin by intracardiac KCl injection, which may lead to the so-called 'embolization' syndrome. Selective termination of the malformed twin can be carried out by one of the cord occlusion techniques. Similarly, single fetal demise of a MC twin may indicate appropriate counseling regarding the potential damage to the survivor. When a case of MC twins is referred early enough, there seems to be a clear benefit of NT measurement. Although NT assessment may be indicated in all twins in order to detect chromosomal aberrations and cardiac anomalies, an increased NT in MC twins may also be an early sign of TTTS. It should be noted, however, that the risk of TTTS is mainly associated with MC–diamniotic twins and is rarely seen in MC–monoamniotic twins.

The fact that utility of biochemical screening in twins is limited and practically not available in higher-order multiples only underscores the importance of performing NT measurements in all multiples (Figure 151.2a and b). Sebire *et al.*[18] prospectively screened 448 twins at 10–14 weeks of gestation. Fetal NT thickness was measured by ultrasound examination at 10–14 weeks. Sensitivity and false-positive rates of screening for trisomy 21 by a combination of fetal NT thickness and maternal age were calculated. In the 448 twin pregnancies, the NT thickness was above the 95th centile of the normal range (for crown–rump length in singletons) in 65/896 fetuses (7.3%), including 7/8 (88%) with trisomy 21. Increased translucency was also present in four fetuses with other chromosomal abnormalities. In the chromosomally normal twin pregnancies, the prevalence of increased NT was higher in fetuses from MC (8.4%, 16/190) than in those with DC pregnancies (5.4%, 37/688). The minimum estimated risk of trisomy 21, based on maternal age and fetal NT thickness, was 1 in 300 in 19.5% (175/896) of the twins including all eight of those with trisomy 21. They concluded that in twin pregnancies, the sensitivity of fetal NT thickness in screening for trisomy 21 is similar to that in singleton pregnancies, but the specificity is lower because translucency is also increased in chromosomally normal MC twin pregnancies. In another study,[19] 67 twin pregnancies were identified at the time of an ultrasound scan for determination of fetal NT thickness, where the parents requested karyotyping. The risk of chromosomal defects in each fetus was calculated from the maternal age and the fetal NT thickness at 10–14 weeks of gestation. If the estimated risk of either fetus was 1 in 50 or greater, CVS was the method of choice, whereas if the risk was less than 1 in 50, second-trimester AC was performed. The estimated risk of trisomies was more than 1 in

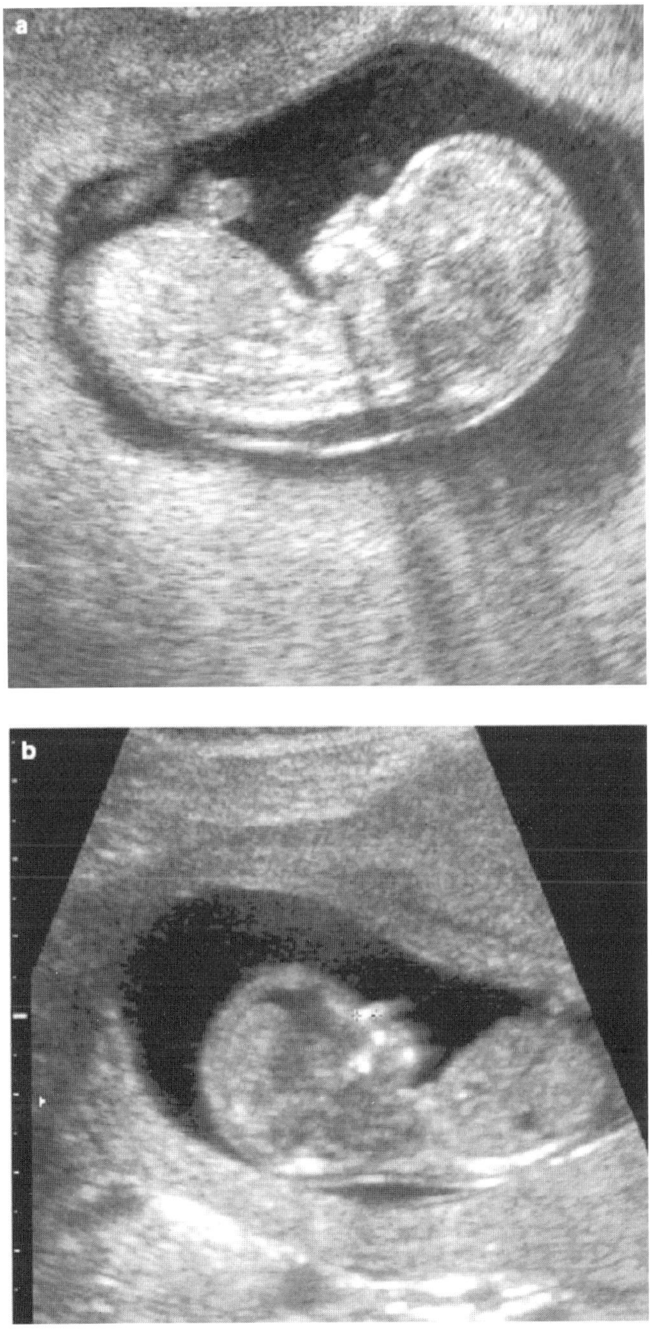

Figure 151.2 Twins screened for NT and the absence of a NB. (a) Image showing an increased NT and absent NB. (b) Image showing a normal NT and presence of a NB (calipers). Images courtesy of B. Caspi, MD, Kaplan Medical Center.

50 in 34 pregnancies and 23.5% of these fetuses were found to be chromosomally abnormal. In contrast, in the 33 low-risk pregnancies, chromosomal abnormalities were found in only 1.5% of the fetuses. The conclusion was that in twin pregnancies, the technique for fetal karyotyping may be selected by calculating the risk of chromosomal abnormality based on maternal age and fetal NT thickness.

The evaluation of screening for fetal trisomy 21 in the first trimester of twin pregnancies by a combination of maternal serum biochemistry and ultrasonography was presented by Spencer *et al.*[20] The population included 230 twin pregnancies in women of all ages presenting with pregnancies between 10 weeks 3 days and 13 weeks 6 days of gestation. Screening using a combination of maternal serum free β-human chorionic gonadotropin (hCG) and pregnancy-associated plasma protein-A (PAPP-A) and fetal NT thickness was offered. Women at increased risk of carrying a fetus with trisomy 21 or trisomy 13/18 ($\geq$1 in 300 at sampling) were offered counseling and an invasive diagnostic procedure. For women who on examination were at 14 weeks of gestation or greater, screening was performed in the same time frame using only maternal serum free β-hCG and alpha fetoprotein (AFP). Overall, 97.4% of the women with twins (224/230) accepted first-trimester screening. The rate of detection of trisomy 21 was 75% (3/4). A risk of trisomy 21 was calculated for each fetus based on the individual fetal NT thickness and the maternal biochemistry. The false-positive rate among those eligible for first-trimester screening was 9.0% (19/206) of pregnancies and 6.9% of fetuses (28/412). Uptake of invasive testing was 59% (10/17) with CVS in eight cases and AC in two. One case of trisomy 21 was identified for every three invasive procedures. First-trimester screening for trisomy 21 in twin pregnancies was both theoretically possible and practically achievable using a combination of NT thickness and maternal serum biochemistry. However, dilemmas for the mother and health professionals when both NT thickness measurements are normal might suggest that greater reliance be placed on the NT thickness risk alone when counseling women about invasive testing.

In a study of 180 twin pregnancies, Spencer[21] has examined the distribution of maternal serum free-βhCG and PAPP-A, in addition to fetal NT thickness, in twins classified as MC or DC, based on ultrasound appearance at 10–14 weeks of gestation. In 45 MC and 135 DC twin pregnancies the multiple of the median (MoM) of free βhCG was not significantly different (1.00 vs. 1.01), while that for PAPP-A was lower (0.89 vs. 1.01), but with no statistical significance. Previous reports of an increased fetal NT in MC twin pregnancies were not confirmed (1.03 vs. 1.00). It was concluded that the existing pseudorisk twin correction algorithm is appropriate for both MC and DC twins in providing accurate first-trimester risks of trisomy 21.

It is currently not definite whether the absence of the fetal nasal bone (NB) (sign for trisomy 21) during NT measurements will significantly increase the screening efficacy of ultrasound in twin pregnancies (Figure 151.2). The absence of NB has been noted in trisomy 21 fetuses at first-trimester ultrasound. In the study of Zoppi *et al.*,[22] the NB was evaluated in relation to fetal karyotype in unselected pregnancies. The fetal facial profile was examined at the 11–14 weeks' scan for screening by NT. NT screening was performed in 5532 fetuses from 5425 pregnancies (85 twins, 8 triplets,

2 quadruplets). The visualization of fetal profile was obtained in 5525 fetuses (99.8%), and in 5491 fetuses (99.4%) the NB was present and in 34 cases (0.6%) it was absent. Fetal karyotype and pregnancy outcome were available in 3503 pregnancies, and 40 chromosomal abnormalities were diagnosed (27 trisomies 21, 5 trisomies 18, 2 trisomies 13, 3 Turner syndromes, 1 partial trisomy 9 and 2 others). The NB was absent in 19 (70%) trisomies 21, 4 trisomies 18 (80%), 2 Turner syndromes (66%), in the partial trisomy 9, in 7 normal karyotype fetuses (0.2%) and in a case with spontaneous first-trimester abortion before prenatal diagnosis. A significant difference was found between NT thickness, expressed as an MoM, in trisomy 21 fetuses with NB present and absent.

Invasive diagnostic procedures

When considering an invasive diagnostic procedure, complications, such as procedure-related fetal loss, are weighed against the probability of an abnormal result. The accuracy of the procedure is of importance as well. The conventional approaches include second-trimester AC or first-trimester CVS. The gestational age at which the procedure is performed should be considered because most patients favor an early diagnosis. Moreover, early diagnosis in multiple pregnancies enables early decision making concerning selective termination of an affected fetus or termination of the entire pregnancy.

AC was first described by Elias *et al.*[23] The procedure is routinely performed between 16 and 20 weeks' gestation. Ultrasound is performed for appropriate fetal measurements, number and location of each placenta and location and characteristics of the dividing membrane. A 22-gauge needle is inserted under continuous ultrasound guidance into one sac and fluid is retrieved, 1–2 ml of inert dye (indigo carmine) is injected and the needle is removed. In the same fashion, a second needle is inserted into the second twin sac under ultrasound guidance and clear, dye-free fluid is retrieved.

With improvement of ultrasound technology and diagnostic skills, another technique for AC sampling was proposed without using the dye.[24,25] In this technique, the initial ultrasound examination visualizes both sacs and the dividing membrane in the same plane. The needle is inserted into the first sac, fluid is retrieved and under direct visualization the needle is pushed through the dividing membrane into the second sac. Using this technique, misdiagnosis may occur due to possible sampling twice the same sac or due to possible cell contamination.

Sampling in MC pregnancy is an additional challenge. Because the fetuses develop from the same zygote, the karyotypes should be exactly the same, and, therefore, sampling of both sacs is not recommended. There are rare cases in which MC twins have discordant chromosomal results. Given that the diagnosis of monochorionicity was accurate, postzygotic non-disjunction can lead to such discordant karyotypes. Because of the rarity of these events, most authors do not recommend sampling of both sacs in cases with characteristic signs of monochorionicity.

Late karyotyping

Karyotyping is possible not only in the first trimester (by CVS) but also in the third trimester by late AC.[26] Late karyotyping after viability carries certain advantages in extremely high-risk pregnancies by avoiding the risk of miscarriage following second-trimester AC. Criteria for late AC include women over 41 years, conception after prolonged infertility and systemic diseases during the period of second-trimester AC.[27] Undoubtedly, this practice is applicable only in countries where the law permits termination of pregnancy after viability. This approach is based on studies of third-trimester AC showing that fetal karyotyping in late gestation provides accurate results with a better fetal outcome in terms of deliveries beyond 30 weeks of gestation.[28] In addition to medicolegal considerations, this practice raises significant ethical dilemmas: which pregnancies are of 'extremely high-risk', should one perform late AC for all pregnant women and avoid procedure-related term birth, should one perform late AC 'per request'.

The loss rates following AC in multiple gestations

There are no randomized control trials documenting the safety of AC in multiple gestations. Figure 151.3 shows the pregnancy loss rates before 20 and 28 weeks in various studies.[25,29–36] Pregnancy loss rates in these studies ranged from 0% to 6% until 20 weeks and from 0% to 8% until 28 weeks. Overall, the mean pregnancy loss until 20 weeks is 1.9% and 3.5% until 28 weeks. The risk of pregnancy loss before 28 weeks in unsampled twins after a normal second-trimester ultrasound is 4.5%–7.2%.[28] Ghidini *et al.*[34] reported similar pregnancy loss rates between twins and their gestational age-matched unsampled controls, (3.0% vs. 2.8%, respectively). The rate of procedure-related pregnancy loss after AC in twin pregnancies is not different from that of singletons and is empirically estimated to be approximately 1%. However, Yukobowich *et al.*[38] in a retrospective study comparing 476 women with DC twins undergoing AC and 477 sampled twin pregnancies found a statistically significant difference between pregnancy loss rates at 4 weeks after AC (2.7% vs. 0.6%, respectively; $P=0.01$). A recent study of Toth-Pal *et al.*[39] compared spontaneous pregnancy losses between 175 women with twins after AC and 300 twin pairs as controls. The authors found that spontaneous losses in multiple pregnancies between 18 and 24 weeks occurred in 2.39%, whereas if AC was performed, the loss rate before the 24th week was 3.87%. Despite the non-significant statistical difference, the investigators

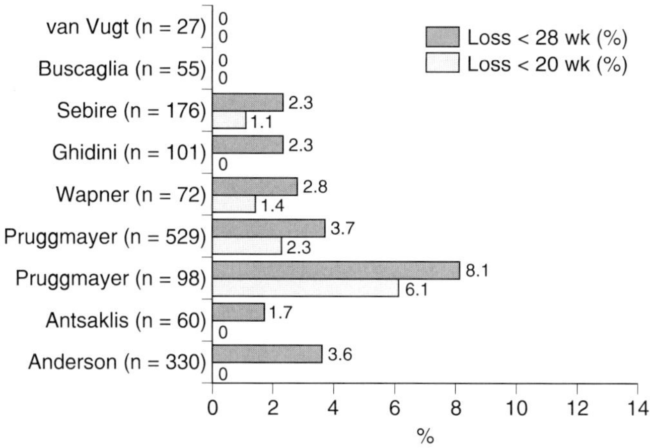

Figure 151.3 Pregnancy loss rates after AC in twins.

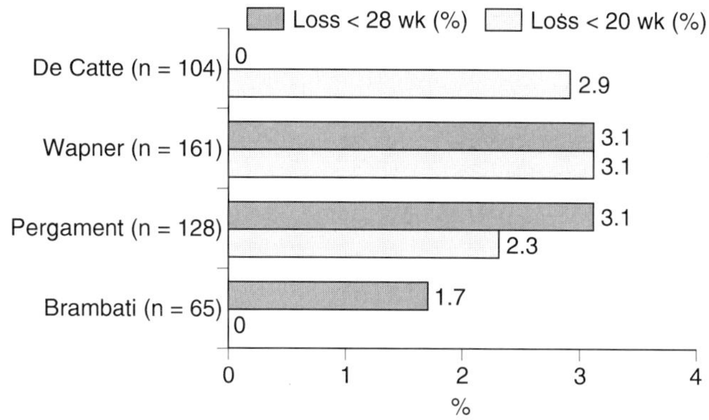

Figure 151.4 Pregnancy loss rates after CVS in twins.

concluded that genetic AC in multiple pregnancies slightly increases the fetal loss rate until the 24th week. Moreover, patients undergoing AC for twins should be informed that there is a greater risk of pregnancy loss than in singletons, although most cases are not related to the procedure.

CVS in twins

CVS has emerged as a safe and efficacious alternative to AC for the identification of genetic abnormalities. The standard of care is to perform CVS after 10 gestational weeks in order to avoid limb reduction defects. A detailed ultrasound examination should be undertaken to determine fetal age, chorionicity, placental location and the presence of major malformation. Performance of CVS in multiple pregnancies demands an accurate assessment of the site of placental implantation for each fetus and zygosity determination. Both transcervical and transabdominal approaches are used for carrying out this procedure.[40] Some pitfalls exist when performing CVS because there is no apparent way to ensure sampling of each frondosum site. Therefore, the same fetus can be inadvertently sampled twice. In some studies, the intertwin villi contamination and sampling errors occurred in about 4% of the samples.[41] Another study compared the diagnostic accuracy of second-trimester AC (n=297) and CVS (n=163) in twins and triplets.[42] Successful sampling using the two-pass approach was achieved in 99.3% vs. 99.7%, respectively. Uncertain results were present in seven CVS cases (five with placental mosaicism). No uncertain results were found in the AC group. Four of the 15 triplet sets were sampled by CVS and 11 underwent AC; however, one from each group required further AC due to abnormal results. The authors conclude that fetal cell contamination and confined placental mosaicism can be kept to a minimum with CVS and do not lead to critical mistakes.

Loss rates following CVS in multiple gestations

First-trimester CVS in multiple gestations appears to have pregnancy loss rates comparable to that of AC. Figure 151.4 represents pregnancy loss rates after CVS in twins. According to these,[33,40,41,43] the rate of pregnancy loss until 20 weeks following CVS is 2.3–3.1%, and 1.7–3.1% until 28 weeks. In 458 twin pairs, the overall pregnancy loss rates before 20 as well as before 28 weeks were similar (2.8%). Wapner *et al.*[33] compared the procedure-related loss rates between first-trimester CVS and second-trimester AC. Fetal loss rate following the procedure until 28 weeks' gestation was 2.9% following AC and 3.2% following CVS. Altogether, the total fetal loss (corrected for anomalies) was 9.3% following AC and only 4.9% following CVS. It was therefore concluded that CVS is at least as safe and as reliable as AC for prenatal diagnosis of twin pregnancies.

Figure 151.5 shows the reported outcomes of CVS in twin pregnancies by pregnancy losses before 22 weeks of gestation and by total fetal loss.[33,40,41,43] In 614 twin pregnancies, the mean rate of pregnancy loss before 22 weeks was 3.1%, and the mean total pregnancy loss was 4.6%.[44]

Counseling of the older patient

The increased maternal age in multiple pregnancies observed worldwide has led to adapted approaches to these patients. On the one hand, the risk of aneuploidy is age dependent, placing the older mother at increased risk. On the other hand, every invasive diagnostic test entails risks of miscarriage, and very rarely infection and fetal injury. Many of these pregnancies are considered 'premium' because of adverse prior maternal reproductive history; the reluctance for invasive testing in the older patients seems understandable.

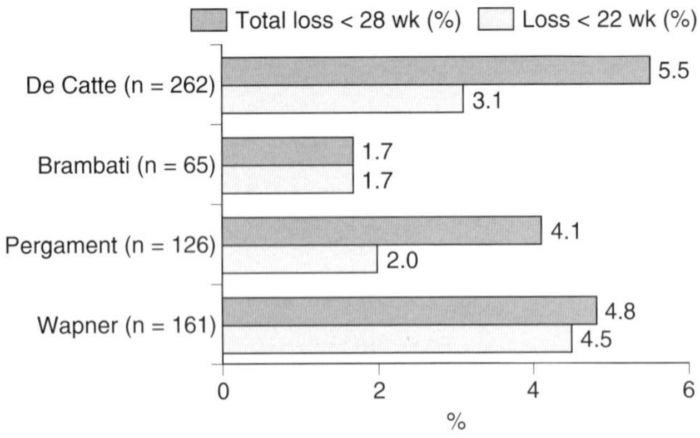

Figure 151.5 Outcome of CVS in twins.

Calculations suggest that the risk of aneuploidy (mainly trisomy 21) in one of the fetuses in DZ twins should lower the maternal age at which AC is recommended in singletons (from 35 to about 32 years). Meyers *et al.*[45] tried to determine the maternal age at which twin gestations have a risk of fetal aneuploidy comparable to that of singleton pregnancies at maternal age 35 years, accounting for variation in DZ twinning rates by maternal age and race. Known aneuploidy risks and rates of DZ twinning by maternal age and race were used to calculate the risk of fetal aneuploidy at term and in the second trimester by maternal age and race in twin gestations. The risk of at least one aneuploid twin at term was 1/193 at maternal age of 31 years for both white and African-American women, which is comparable to the risk of 1/192 for an aneuploid singleton-term pregnancy at maternal age 35 years. The risk of at least one aneuploid twin at AC at maternal age 31 was 1/190 for Caucasian and 1/187 for African-American women, which is slightly lower than the rate in singletons of 1/135. They concluded that invasive prenatal diagnosis for detection of fetal aneuploidy should be offered to all women with twin gestations at age 31, regardless of race. This risk, however, has not been accepted as an indication for invasive genetic testing. A Belgian group recently collected 512 prenatal diagnoses (AC or CVS) from 278 twin pregnancies.[46] The most frequent indications were maternal age ≥35 years (38.8%), assisted reproduction (12.3%) and suspicious ultrasound findings (7.2%). Autosomal chromosome aberrations were found in eight twin sets (2.9%): four inherited balanced rearrangements (two Robertsonian translocations and two paracentric inversions of chromosome 11) and four cases of trisomy 18. Surprisingly, the authors did not detect any trisomy 21 in this population.

A remarkable issue is the case of pregnancies following the use of donor oocytes. Naturally, one may think that the donor's age should be used for aneuploidy risk assessment. However, the donor's age may not always be known or reliable. For example, in a series of established pregnancies from oocyte donation in women aged ≥50 years, the authors found one case of Down's sydrome in 23 infants.[47] Although this single case does not imply an increased risk in pregnancies following oocyte donation, it demands the same attention as all other multiples to markers of aneuploidy.

'Reversed' cytogenetics

Reversed cytogenetics refers to an indication for cytogenetic analysis following a suspected or a pathognomonic ultrasonographic finding. The literature is replete with such signs in singletons, but, regrettably, does not discuss extensively the value of these signs in multiples. It should be remembered that some findings, which indicate further assessment in singletons, are seen more frequently in twins (i.e. major anomalies, such as cardiac malformations, or minor anomalies, such as a single umbilical artery, IUGR, polyhydramnios, oligohydramnios, etc.). Regardless, the approach in such cases should be the same as in singletons with the same presentation.

Ethical consideration

Genetic counseling frequently involves tough ethical issues. In the antepartum period, a conflict may arise in the case of discordant anomalies, when any form of treatment of the anomalous twin may endanger the co-twin. For instance, consider the possibility of a DC twin pregnancy with a suspected discordant chromosomal anomaly. Would it be ethical to perform an invasive procedure to reach the diagnosis, and, at the same time, put the co-twin at risk for potential adverse outcome? Moreover, in the context of multiple pregnancies, these issues are not restricted to prenatal diagnosis only. It may start postpartum with parental requests for zygosity diagnosis of their infants. In the absence of a medical indication, would it be ethical to perform any procedure to satisfy the curiosity of the parents to know if their twins are 'identical'? This may go on to adulthood, when one twin of an MZ set is diagnosed with a late-onset genetic disease. Is there an ethical obligation to reveal the patient's disease state to his/her co-MZ twin? Finally, consider the situation when one twin wishes to know the results of her deceased mother's tests for *BRCA1* mutations (increased risk of breast cancer) and the second twin objects to researchers making this information available.[48] Who is in a position to decide? Obviously, answers are not at hand, and for many cases called into question, the lines of ethic certainty become less clear. Unfortunately, is seems that technical advances will always precede ethical dilemmas, and in this respect, especially in multiple pregnancies, the future does not seem to facilitate the ethical conflicts in genetic counseling.

REFERENCES

1. Evans MI, Littmann L, St Louis L, *et al.* Evolving patterns of iatrogenic multifetal pregnancy generation: Implications for aggressiveness of infertility treatments. *Am J Obstet Gynecol* 1995;172:1750–3.
2. Rodis JF, Egan JF, Craffey A, Ciarleglio L, Greenstein RM, Scorza WE. Calculated risk of chromosomal abnormalities in twin gestations. *Obstet Gynecol* 1990;76:1037–41.
3. Carothers AD, Hecht CA, Hook EB. International variation in reported livebirth prevalence rates of Down syndrome, adjusted for maternal age. *J Med Genet* 1999;36:386–93.
4. Pergament E. Diagnostic genetic testing in multiple pregnancies. In Blickstein I, Keith LG, eds. *Multiple Pregnancy: Epidemiology, Gestation and Perinatal Outcome*, 2nd edn, Taylor and Francis Group, London, 2005, pp. 393–402.
5. Cuckle H. Down's syndrome screening in twins. *J Med Screen* 1998;5:3–4.
6. Jenkins TM, Wapner RJ. The challenge of prenatal diagnosis in twin pregnancies. *Curr Opin Obstet Gynecol* 2000;12:87–92.
7. Schieve LA, Peterson HB, Meikle SF, *et al.* Live-birth rates and multiple-birth risk using in vitro fertilization. *J Am Med Assoc* 1999;282:1832–8.
8. Reynolds MA, Schieve LA, Jeng G, Peterson HB, Wilcox LS. Risk of multiple birth associated with in vitro fertilization using donor eggs. *Am J Epidemiol* 2001;154:1043–50.
9. Ventura SJ, Martin JA, Curtin SC, Menacker F, Hamilton BE. *Births: Final Data for 1999.* National Vital Statistics Report. Maryland: National Center for Health Statistics 2001;49:1–99.
10. Fisk MN, Bryan E. Routine prenatal determination of chorionicity in multiple gestation: A plea to the obstetrician. *Br J Obstet Gynaecol* 1993;100:975–7.
11. Sebire NJ, Snijders RJM, Hughes K, Sepulveda W, Nicolaides KH. The hidden mortality of monochorionic twin pregnancies. *Br J Obstet Gynecol* 1997;104:1203–7.
12. Sepulveda W, Sebine NJ, Hughes K, Kalogeropoulos A, Nicolaides KH. Evolution of the lambda or twin-chorionic peak sign in dichorionic twin pregnancies. *Obstet Gynecol* 1997;89:439–41.
13. Wood SL, St Orange R, Connors G, Elliot PD. Evaluation of the twin peak or lambda sign in determining chorionicity in multiple pregnancy. *Obstet Gynecol* 1996;88:6–9.
14. Stagiannis KD, Sepulveda W, Southwell D, *et al.* Ultrasonographic measurements of the dividing membrane in twin pregnancy during the second and third trimesters: A reproducibility study. *Am J Obstet Gynecol* 1995;173:1546–50.
15. Vayssiere CF, Heim N, Camus EP, *et al.* Determination of chorionicity in twin gestations by high frequency abdominal ultrasonography: Counting the layers of the dividing membrane. *Am J Obstet Gynecol* 1996;175:1529–33.
16. Appelman Z, Manor M, Magal N, *et al.* Prenatal diagnosis of twin zygosity by DNA "fingerprint" analysis. *Prenat Diagn* 1994;14: 307–9.
17. Norton ME, D'Alton ME, Bianchi DW. Molecular zygosity studies aid in the management of discordant multiple gestations. *J Perinatol* 1997;17:202–7.
18. Sebire NJ, Snijders RJ, Hughes K, *et al.* Screening for trisomy 21 in twin pregnancies by maternal age and fetal nuchal translucency thickness at 10–14 weeks of gestation. *Br J Obstet Gynaecol* 1996;103:999–1003.
19. Sebire NJ, Noble PL, Psarra A, *et al.* Fetal karyotyping in twin pregnancies: Selection of technique by measurement of fetal nuchal translucency. *Br J Obstet Gynaecol* 1996;103:887–90.
20. Spencer K, Nikolaides KH. Screening for trisomy 21 in twins using first-trimester ultrasound and maternal serum biochemistry in a one-stop clinic: A review of three years experience. *Br J Obstet Gynecol* 2003;110:276–80.
21. Spencer K. Screening for trisomy 21 in twin pregnancies in the first trimester: Does chorionicity impact on maternal serum free beta-hCG or PAPP-A levels? *Prenat Diagn* 2001;21:715–7.
22. Zoppi MA, Ibba RM, Axiana C, *et al.* Absence of fetal nasal bone and aneuploidies at first-trimester nuchal translucency screening in unselected pregnancies. *Prenat Diagn* 2003;23: 496–500.
23. Elias S, Gerbie A, Simpson JL, Nadler HL, Sabbagha KE, Shkolnik A. Genetic amniocentesis in twin gestations. *Am J Obstet Gynecol* 1980;138:169–74.
24. Jeanty P, Shah D, Roussis P. Single-needle insertion in twin amniocentesis. *J Ultrasound Med* 1990;9:511–7.
25. Sebire MJ, Noble PL, Odibo A, Malligiannis P, Nicolaides KH. Single uterine entry for genetic amniocentesis in twin pregnancies. *Lancet* 1996;47:26–31.
26. Fisk NM, Fordham K, Abramsky L. Elective late fetal kariotyping. *Br J Obstet Gynecol* 1996;103:468–70.
27. Shalev J, Meizner I, Rabinerson D, *et al.* Elective cytogenetic amniocentesis in the third trimester for pregnancies with high-risk factors. *Prenat Diagn* 1999;19:749–52.
28. Lipitz S, Shalev E, Meizner I, *et al.* Late selective termination of fetal abnormalities in twin pregnancies: A multicenter report. *Br J Obstet Gynecol* 1996;103:1212–6.
29. Anderson RL, Goldenberg JD, Golbus MS. Prenatal diagnosis in multiple gestation: 20 years' experience with amniocentesis. *Prenat Diagn* 1991;11:263–70.
30. Antsaklis A, Gougoulakis A, Mesogitis S, *et al.* Invasive techniques for fetal diagnosis in multiple pregnancy. *Int J Gynecol Obstet* 1991;34:309–14.
31. Pruggmayer M, Baumann P, Schutte H, *et al.* Incidence of abortion after genetic amniocentesis in twin pregnancies. *Prenat Diagn* 1991;11:637–40.
32. Pruggmayer MRK, Jahoda MGJ, Van der Pol JG, *et al.* Genetic amniocentesis in twin pregnancies: Results of a multicenter study of 529 cases. *Ultrasound Obstet Gynecol* 1992;2:6–10.
33. Wapner RJ, Jonhson A, Davis G. Prenatal diagnosis in twin gestation: A comparison between second trimester amniocentesis and first trimester chorionic villus sampling. *Obstet Gynecol* 1993;82: 49–56.
34. Ghidini A, Lynch L, Hicks C, *et al.* The risk of second-trimester amniocentesis in twin gestations: A case–control study. *Am J Obstet Gynecol* 1993;169:1013–6.
35. Buscaglia M, Chisoni L, Bellotti M, *et al.* Genetic amniocentesis in biamniotic twin pregnancies by a single transabdominal insertion of the needle. *Prenat Diagn* 1995;15:17–9.
36. Van Vugt M, Nieuwint A, van Geijn HP. Single-needle insertion: An alternative technique for early second-trimester genetic twin amniocentesis. *Fetal Diagn Ther* 1995;10:178–81.
37. Pretorious D, Budorick N, Sciossia A, Krabbe JK, Ko S, Myhre CM. Twin pregnancies in the second trimester in an a-fetoprotein screening program. Sonographic evaluation and outcome. *Am J Roentgenol* 1993;161:1007–13.
38. Yukobowich E, Anteby EY, Cohen SM, Lavy Y, Granat M, Yagel S. Risk of fetal loss in twin pregnancies undergoing second trimester amniocentesis. *Obstet Gynecol* 2001;98:231–4.
39. Toth-Pal E, Papp C, Beke A, Ban Z, Papp Z. Genetic amniocentesis in multiple pregnancies. *Fetal Diagn Ther* 2004;19:138–44.
40. Brambati B, Tului L, Lanzana A, Simoni G, Travi M. First trimester genetic diagnosis in multiple pregnancies: Principals and potential pitfalls. *Prenat Diagn* 1991;11:767–74.
41. Pergament E, Schulman J, Copeland K, *et al.* The risk of and efficacy of chorionic villus sampling in multiple gestation. *Prenat Diagn* 1992;12:377–84.
42. Van den Berg C, Braat APG, Van Opstal D, *et al.* Amniocentesis or chorionic villus sampling in multiple gestations? Experience with 500 cases. *Prenat Diagn* 1999;19:234–44.
43. De Catte L, Liebaers I, Foulon W, *et al.* First trimester chorionic villus sampling in twin gestations. *Am J Perinatol* 1996;13:413–7.
44. De Catte L, Liebaers I, Foulon W. Outcome of twin gestations after first trimester chorionic villus sampling. *Obstet Gynecol* 2000; 95:714–20.
45. Meyers C, Adam R, Dungan J, Prenger V. Aneuploidy in twin gestations: When is maternal age advanced? *Obstet Gynecol* 1997; 89:248–51.
46. Jamar M, Lemarchal C, Lemaire V, *et al.* A low rate of trisomy 21 in twin-pregnancies: A cytogenetics retrospective study of 278 cases. *J Genet Couns* 2003;14:395–400.
47. Sauer MV, Paulson RJ, Lobo RA. Pregnancy in women 50 or more years of age: Outcomes of 22 consecutively established pregnancies from oocyte donation. *Fertil Steril* 1995;64:111–5.
48. Green RM, Thomas AM. Whose gene is it? A case discussion about familial conflict over genetic testing for breast cancer. *J Genet Couns* 1997;6:245–54.

152 Intrauterine behavior of multiples

B. Arabin and J. van Eyck

Introduction

The phenomenon that two or more children simultaneously grow *in utero*, are borne by the same mother and are characterized by specific similarities in features, behavioral expression and interaction has inspired mythological and religious stories, artists, writers and finally also researchers since ancient times. Hippocrates as well as further Greek and Roman scholars discussed the twinning phenomenon.[1] Prenatal activity and communication of twins was already anticipated in the Bible: Esau and Jacob were supposed to struggle in the womb for the right to breath, to cry or to be welcomed *ex utero* as the first.[2]

In his classical paper *The History of Twins as a Criterion of the Relative Powers of Nature and Nurture* dated 1876 Sir Francis Galton was the first to argue that twins could be of value in the study of the effects of hereditary and environmental influences.[3] Still, not until the 1920s did it become obvious that there are different kinds of twins. The breakthrough of the 'twin method' relating to either mono- or dizygocity being an 'experiment of nature' and a challenge for scientific exploration, dates back to observations of the American psychologist Curtis Merriman and the German dermatologist Hermann Siemens in 1924.[4]

The classic twin method is based on some assumptions: monozygotic (MZ) twins or higher order multiples originate from splitting of the same zygote into two or more embryos during the first 14 days after fertilization and subsequent separate development. Any difference recognized between the MZ co-multiples necessarily is supposed to originate from environmental – which means other than genetic factors – influences. The other mechanism is polyovulation and consequent multiple fertilization resulting in the simultaneous development of dizygotic (DZ) or polyzgotic (PZ) siblings. Both, MZ and DZ twins are of the same age and share prenatally and usually to a large extent also postnatally the same environment. It is assumed that the extent of any characteristics exhibiting a higher within-pair similarity in MZ compared to DZ co-twins reflects the genetic control of a specific variable.

There have been doubts about how far results based on the twin method represent a general population. Bias can arise from antenatal (e.g., different forms of twinning or specific risks of multiple pregnancy) and postnatal (e.g., varieties in the common environment) conditions. Also, the last decades have witnessed tremendous progress in cytogenetics, molecular genetics and chronogenetics. Still, the study of twins remains a precious tool in behavioral genetics, developmental studies, matched-pair designs and epidemiology.

Focusing on prenatal twins and multiples[5,6] and using more sophisticated techniques of supervision and statistical analysis it might be possible to observe still unknown phenomena and achieve new perspectives of human development under normal and pathological conditions.

Methods to describe prenatal behavior of multiples

Brief summary of methods used in singleton pregnancies

Despite over 100 years of interest in prenatal behavior in the medical literature[7] and over 20 years of systematic research initiated by the Prechtl's group,[8–10] the examination of prenatal behavior is still not widely accepted as a potential tool for researchers and clinicians. Difficulties start from its definition, which may be characterized by 'any observable action/reaction towards stimuli'.[11]

Embryonic and fetal movements emerge during the first trimester with 'just discernible movements' at around 7 completed weeks. Subsequently, more complex movement patterns emerge, many of them remaining recognizable throughout life. Prenatal motility is considered to reflect the developing nervous system and involves functional and maturational properties of hemodynamics, muscle or organ tissue.

For the investigation of prenatal behavior various methods have been applied: Fetal body movements *in utero* were first recorded objectively with a kymograph by Haled in 1905 using the displacement of an inverted glass funnel by the distortions of the maternal abdominal wall resulting from movements of the underlying fetus.[12] In 1944 Hooker observed movements and reflexes after cutaneous stimulation of embryos after therapeutic terminations of pregnancy by hysterotomy maintaining them at body temperature in an isotonic fluid bath.[13]

With the introduction of real-time ultrasound, it became possible to observe prenatal motility *in utero*. Reinhold was one of the first to describe fetal activity stressing the spontaneous character of early prenatal movements.[14] Better resolution of ultrasound equipment made it possible to identify qualities of prenatal activity.[9] Cyclic changes of fetal activity accompanied by fetal heart rate (FHR) variability were described at the end of the 1970s[15,16] but were still not linked with sleep–wake states in neonates.[17] By combining FHR-patterns with presence or absence of fetal movements (FMs), it became evident that bandwidth, amplitude and accelerations of FHR are related to the type of FM. FHR and FM patterns were used to classify behavioral states before 36 gestational weeks.[18] Subsequently, Nijhuis *et al.*[10] took advantage of the first prenatal descriptions of fetal eye movements (FEM).[19,20] Thus they were able to detect four behavioral states during the last weeks comparable to those described by Prechtl in neonates.[17] The implication of Doppler velocimetry in addition allowed consumptions that under normal conditions fetal hemodynamics are related to behavioral states.[21]

Independently, prenatal reactions evoked by external stimuli such as sound and vibration,[22] touch,[23] light[24] or merely maternal noise[25] have been investigated.

All methods have meanwhile been integrated into a cohesive whole to describe prenatal behavior in singleton pregnancies.

In twins and higher-order multiples, the same techniques can be applied in principle, though this demands more sophisticated methodological and statistical efforts because of the following reasons:

- two or more different individuals have to be observed simultaneously,
- there might be inter-twin or inter-multiple influences.

Specific conditions of multiple pregnancy such as zygosity, chorionicity, sex and position as well as pathological conditions have to be systematically defined and considered for interpretations.

Methods to document prenatal multiple behavior at early gestation

All types of movements that develop in singleton pregnancies seem to be present up to 15 weeks. This is why we regard the interval between 8 and 16 gestational weeks as an appropriate interval for the study of early twin behavior. In addition, this has a pragmatic background: from 16 weeks onwards it becomes more difficult to visualize both twins completely on one ultrasound monitor.

Though the pioneering work describing the emergence of qualitative movement patterns in singletons was performed with the aid of transabdominal sonography,[9] transvaginal sonography (TVS) has developed as the method of choice during the first 12 weeks of gestation.

Considering individual differences of compliance and abdominal wall thickness of the mothers we switch to transabdominal ultrasound observations from around 12 completed weeks. The type and position of the transducers are selected to optimize accurate simultaneous visualization.

As a compromise between maternal compliance or possible side effects and scientific curiosity our protocol has included weekly ultrasound examinations until at least 30 min of good quality are documented by video registration. Sometimes it might be difficult to visualize two or three members of the multiple pregnancy simultaneously in their full length. Under such conditions it is advisable to change either the position of the mother towards the transducer or to move the transducer to an oblique position.

Selection of study groups

Parents with early diagnosed twin or triplet pregnancy have taken part in our studies of early behavior of multiples. A high percentage of twin and higher-order multiple pregnancies results from fertility treatment such as *in vitro* fertilization, artificial induction of ovulation or artificial insemination. The criteria should be documented and gestational age adapted.

Parents who volunteer to take part in the study, have to be informed that there are still no follow-up studies about bioeffects of long-term ultrasound observations. Our own research protocol had been submitted to the local research ethics committee and approval had been granted. Parents are also informed about possible advantages of the study, such as a more careful evaluation of the development, exclusion of early markers for chromosomal defects between 10 and 14 weeks and the possibility to witness the development of their children. All specific variables which might have an effect on prenatal behavior such as maternal risks, medication or abnormal ultrasound findings have to be documented.

Sonographic determination of placentation and position

Precise analysis of the membranes is of primary importance not only for the classification but also for later management decisions. Already from 5 to 6 weeks onwards chorionicity can be defined by the number of chorionic sacs. In dichorionic (DC) placentation the

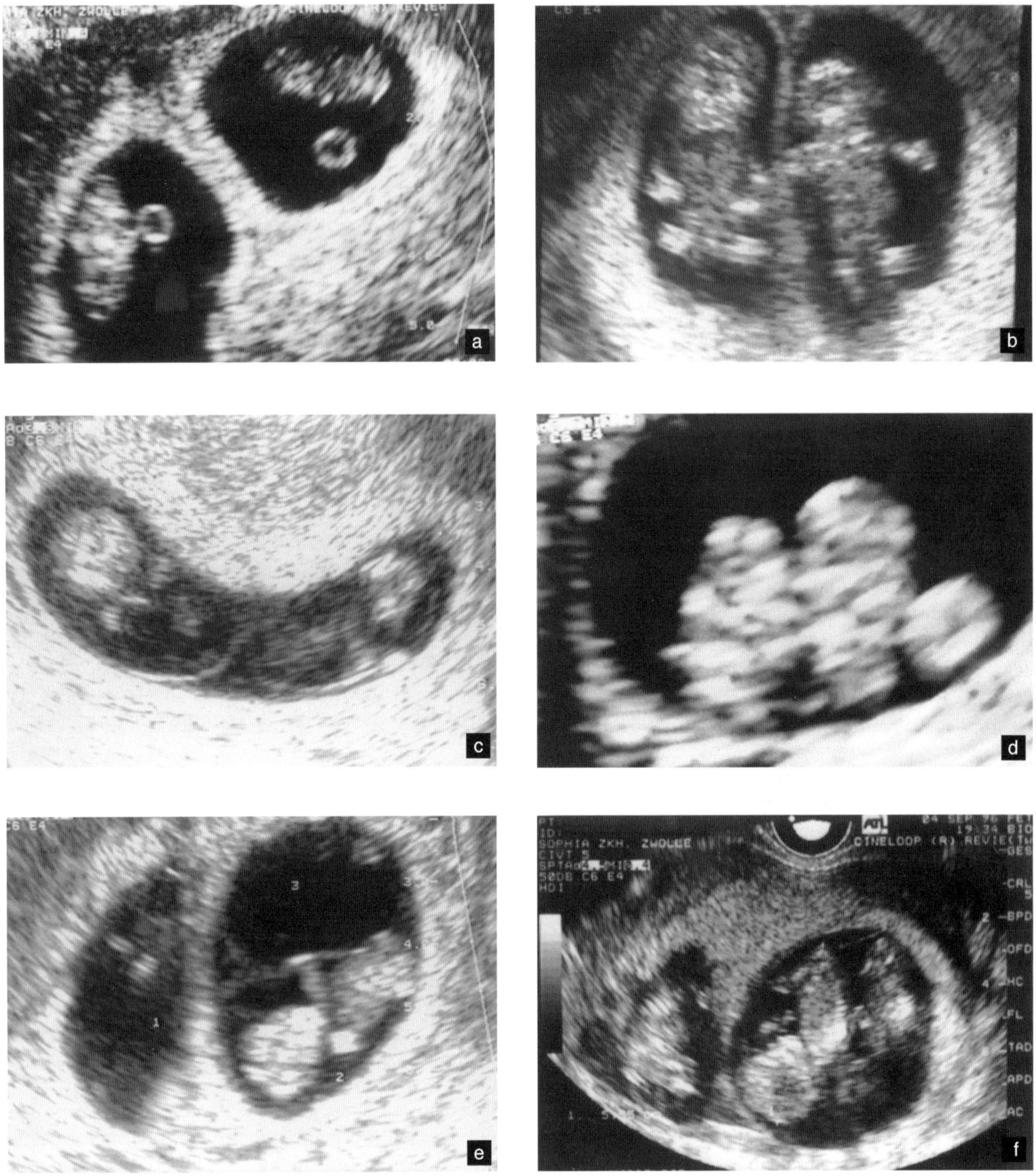

Figure 152.1 Sonographic illustration of chorionicity, impact for inter-twin contact. (a) DC twin pregnancy at 8 weeks still with surrounding villi: no contact possible. (b) DC twin pregnancy at 12 weeks with thick dividing membrane and lambda sign: moment of first inter-twin reaction towards touch. (c) MC DA twin pregnancy at 10 weeks with a single placenta and separate amnions: moment of first inter-twin reaction towards touch. (d) MC MA twin pregnancy at 9 weeks illustrating two adjoining embryos in a single sac: moment of first inter-twin reaction towards touch. (e) DC TA triplet pregnancy at 10 weeks illustrating simultaneous differences of dividing membranes: chorion laeve (left) and thin inter-triplet amnion (right): the two right triplets demonstrated with earlier reactions towards touch. (f) CD DA triplet pregnancy at 10 weeks with one thick inter-triplet membrane (left) and two triplets within one amniotic cavity (right): the two right triplets demonstrated with earlier and more frequent reactions towards touch.

villous stems surround the amniotic cavity (Figure 152.1a) until chorion frondosum and chorion laeve are further differentiated. As in singletons amnion and chorion remain separated by the coelom cavity up to around 12 weeks. The developing dividing membrane consists of two chorions and two amnions and appears echogenic. From around 12 weeks the presence of lambda-shaped structures at the attachment to the placenta is indicative of the dichorial nature (Figure 152.1b).[26] In monochorionic (MC) placentation it is recommended to evaluate whether each multiple is surrounded by an amniotic membrane, so that the

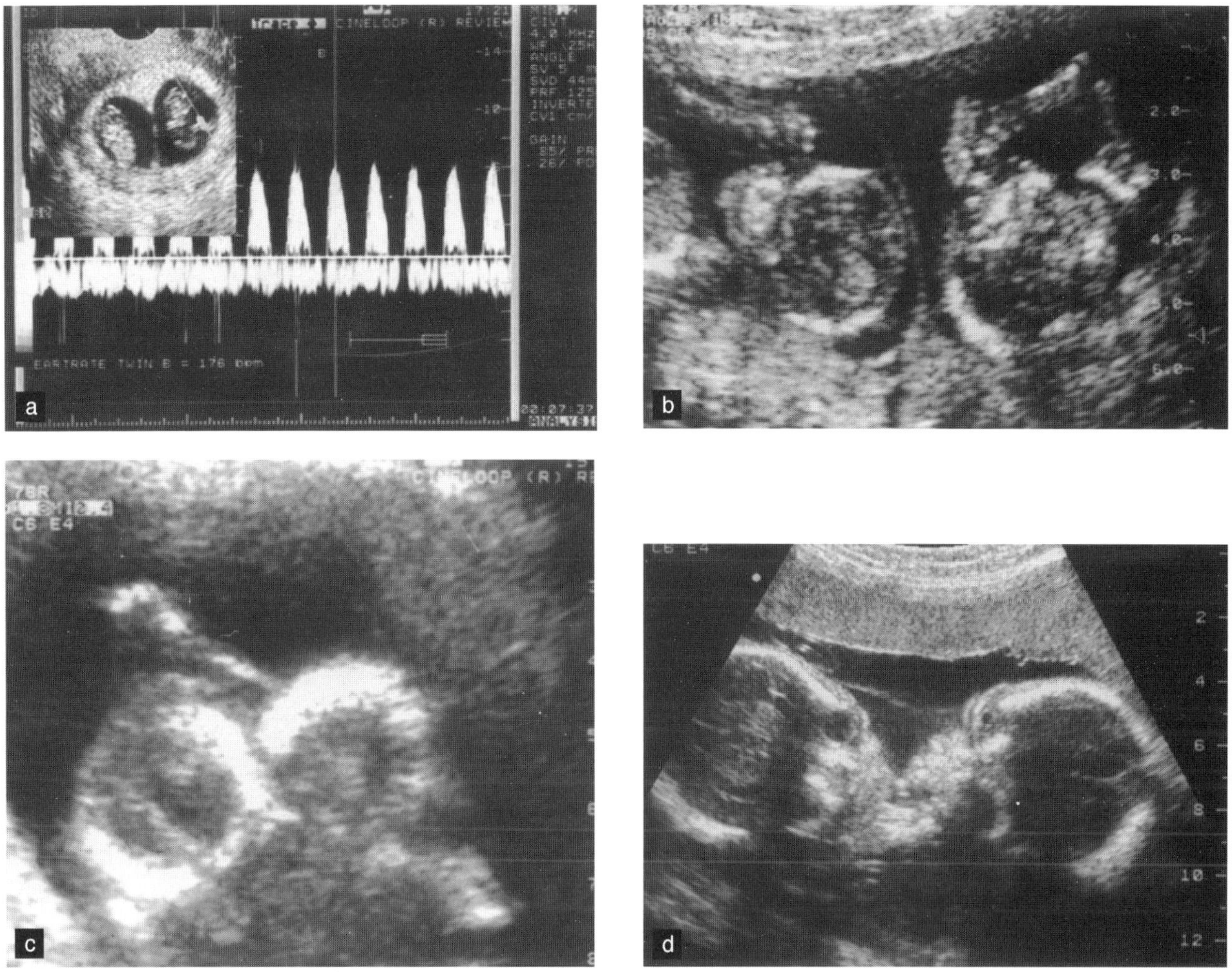

Figure 152.2 Hemodynamics and behavioral patterns at early gestation. (a) Doppler velocity wave forms of umbilical vessels at 10 weeks illustrating pulsatile arterial and venous flow (probe directed on umbilical cord). (b) Simultaneous activities (hand–face contacts) of twins at 12 weeks. (c) Complex contact ('embracement') at 14 weeks. (d) Mouth contact ('kiss') at 16 weeks.

dividing membrane consists of two amnions (Figure 152.1c) or whether there is only one amniotic cavity containing both twins without any dividing membrane (Figure 152.1d). Accordingly, there are six different types of chorionicity in triplet pregnancies, e.g., DC triplets can be triamniotic (TA) (Figure 152.1e) or diamniotic (DA) (Figure 152.1f). All ultrasound findings should be registered.

In utero twins and triplets can also be characterized by their position. Therefore it is important to compare carefully whether transvaginal and transabdominal definitions are in agreement.

In DC twin pregnancies with different sex we have followed the position of twins from 16 weeks onwards and have up to now not recognized a change of position from the primary definitions. We admit that in monoamniotic (MA) twins identification may be a problem.

Longitudinal examination of growth, structure and hemodynamics

It is recommended to document biometry and presentation *in utero* (e.g., vertex/breech) during each session and to notify early growth differences.[27] We have designed early growth charts specific for multiples.[28]

The prevalence of multiple pregnancy, which is related to maternal age and assisted reproduction techniques, has increased and accordingly the number of multiple pregnancies at risk for chromosomal abnormalities. Early ultrasound diagnosis of fetal nuchal translucency thickness, which has been proven to be as sensitive as in singletons in DC multiples, though with a lower specificity in screening for trisomy 21 in MC twins,[29] is recommendable to help the parents to decide for or avoid further invasive techniques. Serial ultrasound examinations of early behavior have the advantage of allowing a careful evaluation of nuchal translucency without further efforts and should therefore be included in all early behavioral studies.

Doppler velocimetry of the umbilical vessels can be theoretically registered from 8 weeks onwards and may allow to detect early heart rate (Figure 152.2a). Subsequently, Doppler velocimetry may be performed in several vessels such as the ductus venosus, the aorta or cerebral vessels.

Longitudinal examination of early activity

Using video documentation of early twin behavior we have defined first qualities of activities of twins which are analyzed separately for each multiple most of them are comparable to the definitions found by abdominal ultrasound in singletons.[9]

First discernible movements are defined according to their name. Startles are abrupt generalized movements, starting in the limbs and spreading to the trunk and neck including flexion and extension of both arms and legs at the same time. Hiccups are jerky contractions of the diaphragm followed by an abrupt displacement of thorax and abdomen. Hiccups are frequently seen at regular intervals of 2–3 s. Hand–face contacts are characterized by a touch between hands and face (Figure 152.2b). Movements of single fingers and touch of the mouth just with the thumb may be differentiated. Mouth openings without swallowing are differentiated from swallowing movements, which are accompanied by a displacement of the tongue and are often initiated by sucking. During swallowing, fetuses are able to 'drink' amniotic fluid which can be visualized by color imaging and Doppler velocimetry. Breathing movements are paradoxical in nature, accompanied by slow simultaneous movements of the diaphragm (downwards), thorax movements (inwards) and abdominal movements (outwards). They may occur at regular or irregular intervals and may also be accompanied by aspiration and expiration of fluid.

Head movements include retroflexion, anteflexion or rotation of the head. Extremity movements may involve extension, flexion, external or internal rotation or abduction and adduction of arms and/or legs. Jumping appears as a consequence of pushing off the uterine wall with the legs and may occur incidentally and repetitively. Twisting may be defined when the body leans to the left and the right side repetitively. The 'turning point' of the movement may be neck and/or rump. It may appear as 'dancing' and may even initiate a somersault.

Stretching is a complex motor pattern consisting of an extreme extension of the spine, retroflexion of the head, abduction, external rotation and elevation of the arms. The movement may last several seconds. Prenatal yawning is comparable to yawning after birth. Yawning is often accompanied by a retroflexion of the head. After a slow opening, the mouth remains open for several seconds and then quickly closes. Like stretching this movement pattern is nonrepetitive.

In all multiples it is interesting to compare whether the described activities occur independently, 'in turn' or simultaneously (Figure 152.2b).

Longitudinal examination of early contacts

Using video documentation of early twin behavior we have defined first qualities of contacts. 'First reach and touch' is classified when multiples touch without giving evidence of reactions. 'First reaction' was defined as the first movement of the co-twin within 1 s of a touch (Figure 152.1b–d). Thereafter, the part of the body initiating the contact and the speed of the primary contact are classified as 'slow' or 'fast' arm, leg, head or body contact. All short contacts following an action/reaction model are called primary contacts. With advancing gestational age and smaller distance from each other, more complex contacts are observed lasting more than 5 s. Action and reaction might be repetitive so that initiatives cannot be exclusively correlated to only one twin. Thereby both bodies and extremities may be involved (Figure 152.2c). Twins may even touch the head or mouth of the co-twin with the lips followed by a reaction of the co-twin which we classify as 'mouth contact' (Figure 152.2d). Parents often interpreted these contacts as 'embraces' and 'kisses'. With advancing gestation, diffuse interactions, characterized by initiations or reactions, which are difficult to distinguish, are observed.

Using only the speed of initiations and reactions other classifications of contacts can be used such as contacts characterized by slow initiations with a slow reaction, a fast initiative with a slow reaction, a slow initiative followed by a fast reaction and a fast initiative followed by a fast reaction. It is interesting to compare whether contacts are preferably initiated by one of the multiples or whether there are differences in the frequency and sensitivity to react towards touch.

Analysis

Video tapes are retrospectively analyzed documenting gestational age in days, time of the day and meal intake. After a training period we recommend to determine the intra- and interobserver variability of observed qualities. For the observed activities and contacts we have found an interobserver variation coefficient between 88% and 100%. For all activities and contacts the gestational age of the first observation are documented.

The activities can be analyzed separately for each twin or multiple, the contacts can be classified according to described criteria. Throughout the observation period it is possible to calculate the occurrence of activity and contact patterns. In addition, inter-twin variance of activities and dominance can be evaluated. Using a short (1 min) window, rest–activity cycles are analyzed. In our studies all data were coded, collected and analyzed by computer programs.

Methods to document prenatal multiple behavior at advanced gestation

Although fetal activity of twins in the third trimester has been analyzed,[30–32] there are confusing methodological differences relating to whether FM were recorded by mother's perception, real-time ultrasound or electromagnetic devices. Ultrasound observations of fetal activity allow the most precise analysis of the quality of FM. In advanced pregnancy two ultrasound equipments are necessary to document all movements of head, body and extremities of only one child, which then is unrealistic for twins or higher order multiples.

In singleton pregnancy, a Doppler device for simultaneous recording of FM and FHR (actocardiograph MT 320[33]) registers slow and fast FM with a high sensitivity and specificity.[34–36] We have used a similar equipment designed for multiple pregnancies (actocardiograph MT 430). This portable device captures the signals of FHR and FM with one external Doppler transducer for each twin, the signals are simultaneously recorded on separate channels and designed on one tracing. Thus, FM and FHR patterns can be easily correlated with each other. The simultaneous recording of both FM patterns in combination with FHR patterns on one tracing is the method of choice for acute supervision of advanced multiple pregnancies also in clinical routine. We have published that this method is also a useful tool for research purposes[5,6] and proposed several qualitative criteria to classify prenatal behavior in twin pregnancies roughly summarized as 'concordant' or 'discordant' behavior. The same equipment is useful for simultaneous FHR monitoring of triplets during vaginal delivery.[37]

Selection of study groups

We have performed systematic studies of spontaneous and reactive FHR–FM patterns in normal twin pregnancies from 24 weeks onwards. Mothers who volunteered to take part in the study, were informed about the protocol. For inclusion into the study protocol early ultrasound examinations to confirm gestational age and define chorionicity was a prerequisite. Data from risk pregnancies such as premature labor, pre-eclampsia, diabetes or growth retardation have to be excluded for definition of normal values or analyzed separately.

Sonographic determination of the position, growth and hemodynamics

At the beginning of each session the position of the placenta, presentation (e.g., vertex/breech) and the size of the twins including their estimated weight have to be registered. Using FHR monitoring identification on the tracing is facilitated by different thickness of the FHR-tracings and different height of the FM tracings for each twin. Doppler flow measurements of the umbilical artery (at least) should be performed and the amount of amniotic fluid should be estimated.

Longitudinal examination of spontaneous FHR combined with FM patterns

Usually we have registered behavior of twins over a period of at least 1 h combining spontaneous behavior during the first 30 min and the registration of reactive behavior during the consecutive 30 min. We have used a paper speed of 2 cm/min. It has to be considered that there is no signal loss or disturbances caused by maternal movements. An example of an actocardiographic tracings of spontaneous FHR/FM patterns is presented in Figure 152.3(a).

Longitudinal examination of reactive FHR combined with FM patterns

Studies to examine answers of peripheral sensory receptors face the problem in how far the occurrence of a response is causally related to the stimulus, whether it is accurately measured and reproducible and in how far the present behavioral state has an influence on the occurrence, magnitude and course of the response. Prechtl has described various patterns of responses to external stimuli in relation to different neonatal states.[17]

In contrast to the neonate, the human fetus is surrounded by amniotic fluid, which diminishes technical feasibility to objectify and quantify stimuli as well as responses.

Still various kinds of external stimulations to provoke reactions of a single fetus have been reported and are summarized in detail.[38,39] For all methods of prenatal external stimulation problems have to be overcome due to attenuation and uncertainties of transmission through the maternal abdomen of either touch, sound or light. The possible effect of the attachment alone has to be excluded by touching the abdomen with the instrument without stimulation ('sham stimulation'[40]).

Methodological problems in multiple pregnancies are as follows. Stimulations by light or touch have to be performed for each multiple and still the stimulus might vary dependent on the position of the fetus towards the stimulus (front or back side). The first reaction to light stimulation is often just a short movement of the bulbi, which can only be observed by ultrasound if the fetal face is visualized.

Vibroacoustic stimulations (VAS) using an electronic artificial larynx (EAL) producing a broadband noise at a fundamental frequency of 87 Hz with multiple harmonics up to 15,000 Hz was used in singleton pregnancies.[41] Coupling between the vibrating surface of the instrument and the maternal tissue provides optimal transmission of frequencies of up to 20,000 Hz.[42] When placed between the twins it can be suggested that the stimulus reaches both members in a comparable way. It has been proven that the position of the EAL in relation to the fetus is without influence on the kind of reaction[43] because it is transmitted via the amniotic fluid and the intensity of the sound *in utero* does not vary.[44] It was demonstrated that a stimulus with EAL of 3 s is sufficient to cause a reaction even from quietness to an active state.[45] In our studies we tried to perform a stimulus of around 2 s.

A further problem arises if twins do not demonstrate the same rest-activity state before stimulation. We have only started with sham/final stimulations till at least 10 min of quiet behavior was recorded. Waiting for this condition can extend the duration of the session. An example of an actocardiographic tracing after VAS with various FHR/FM responses is presented in Figure 152.3(b).

Analysis of polygraphic tracings

From each session the tracings are analyzed documenting gestational age in days, time of the day and meal intake. After a training period we recommend

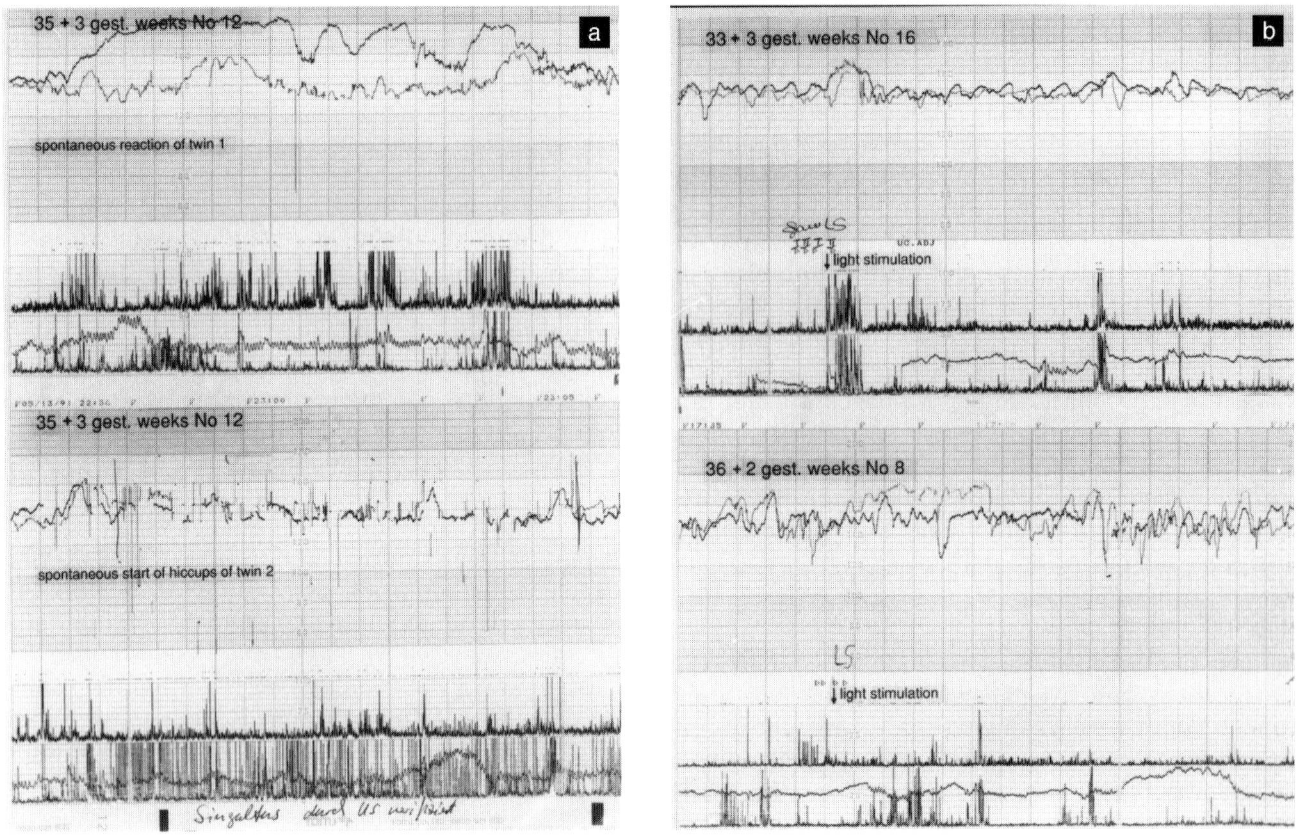

Figure 152.3 Hemodynamics and behavioral patterns at advanced gestation. (a) Actocardiographic patterns demonstrating spontaneous 'discordant'. FHR-FM patterns: spontaneous increase of FHR of twin A (above), spontaneous onset of hiccup of twin B (below). (b) Actocardiographic patterns demonstrating reactive 'concordant' and 'discordant' FHR-FM patterns: both twins react with a FHR-acceleration combined with FM (above), only one twin reacts with a short FM and an increase of FHR-baseline (below).

the determination of the intra- and interobserver variability. For the actocardiographic tracings we have found an interobserver variation coefficient between 80% and 90%. For all reactions towards external stimuli gestational age of the first occurrence can be documented.

For systematic studies we have meanwhile classified FHR/FM patterns according to possible combinations of variability, accelerations and FM (Table 152.1). To classify these periods 3 min consistency is required in a tracing of at least 30 min of good quality. The longest and shortest periods as well as the total distribution as percentage of the registration time can be calculated for the whole study group, subgroups and for each twin pair throughout the observation interval.

FHR/FM patterns after VAS were classified according to possible combinations of FHR accelerations in combination with FM, the duration of the reaction and the change of states. For direct comparison of twin pairs all described criteria can be used. The described parameters can also be combined by semi-quantitative scoring systems.[3] Thereby the degree of difference in FHR-variability, baseline, number and synchronicity of FHR accelerations and FM can be compared. The latter are classified as simultaneous if there are less than 10 s difference.[46]

Postnatal assessment

Postnatal assessment of placenta and zygosity

Placentation of multiple pregnancies is influenced by the number of zygotes, blastocysts and the division of the inner cell mass. When two placentas are present, they are always DC, most are dizygotic (DZ), but some are monozygotic (MZ), when division occurs before implantation. Single placentas can be present in DC and MC as well as in DZ and MZ pregnancies.

A proper examination of the membranes allows definite statements concerning the zygosity, which are summarized for twins and triplets.[47]

(1) DZ twins are DC; (2) MZ twins are either DC or MC; (3) MC placenta proves MZ twins

(1) TZ triplets are TC; (2) DZ triplets are either DC or TC; (3) MZ triplets are either TC, DC or MC; (4) DC triplets are MZ or DZ; (5) MC triplets are MZ.

The following placental features should be examined still in the delivery room and used for protocols[47]: the structure of fetal membranes, the unity of the placenta, the site of umbilical cord insertions and the extent of vascular anastomoses in MC placentas. Placental weight, surface area, insertion of the umbilical cord, disturbances of maturation or circulation and signs of infection should be examined.

Table 152.1 Classification of fetal heart rate (FHR) and fetal movement (FM) patterns in twins obtained by the Actocardiograph MT 420

FHR-FM pattern	Variability (amplitude/bpm)	Fetal movements	Accelerations
I	< 10 bpm	NO	NO
II	< 10 bpm	YES	NO
III	> 10 bpm	NO	NO
IV	> 10 bpm	NO	YES
V	> 10 bpm	YES	NO
VI	> 10 bpm	YES	YES

Examination of placentation and gender determines zygosity in around 50% of cases.[48] This ratio varies worldwide. Zygosity remains unclear in cases with the same sex and DC/TC placentation. In these cases sequential blood group testing can be performed considering ABO, Rh, MNSs, Kell and Duffy subgroups. DC twins can be correctly identified if only one (or more) of the subgroups vary. If all subgroups are identical, the probability of MZ twins is around 97%, still 3% are DZ.[49] In uncertain cases, the use of DNA methods to analyze variable numbers of 'tandem' repeat sequences dispersed in the human genome has become the most powerful tool for accurate diagnosis of zygosity. DNA fingerprint can be performed of each twin's leukocytes, umbilical cord tissue or even placental tissue even after being frozen at −20°C.[50,51]

Statistical methods

All data of subgroups of MC vs. DC twin pregnancy or of different gender combinations can be calculated. Our datasets are shown as box–whisker plots using SPSS (Statistical Package for Social Sciences). Thereby the mean, the 75th and 25th centile and the limits of extreme values are plotted so that 50% of the values are collected within the 'box'; the 'whisker' represents all values up to the 1.5-fold distance of the given centiles. Significant differences can be calculated for two or three variables by the Mann–Whitney–Wilcoxon and the Kruskal–Wallis test or by chi-square tests. Multivariate analysis can be used to find parameters with an impact on behavior of multiples.

Possible discussions relating towards long time ultrasonography

Bioeffects of ultrasound have been studied for sixty years now and can be classified as nonthermal and thermal effects. Nonthermal processes are enhanced by gas-body activation occurring when gas filled structures become biologically active when exposed to megahertz frequencies.[52] The 'spatial peak pulse average' (SPPA) represents the average intensity of a pulse. At SPPA values of 10–100 W/cm^2 signs of cavitations were never seen.[53]

Thermal effects of ultrasound depend on the intensity of the ultrasound waves, the duration of exposition and the absorption coefficient of the tissue. Ultrasound waves cause oscillation and heat production. Temperature elevation of less than 1°C is considered to be without any effect for the fetus;[54,55] thermal effects have not been reported in mammals below 39°C.[56] The critical temperature for fetal tissue is 41°C and its exposition limit at this temperature is 16 min.[54] However, in animal experiments a temperature of 41°C is only reached with intensities of > 300 mW/cm^2 and an exposure duration of > 60 min.[57] The SPTA (spatial peak temporal average) values have to be considered.

Mutagenic effects of ultrasound are only described in *in vitro* cell lines.[58,59] Epidemiological research has been performed in children, who were exposed to ultrasound during pregnancy and no increased risk for malignancy was found.[60,61]

Recently, it has been suggested that there is an association between routine ultrasonography and subsequent non-right-handedness[62] and growth restriction if ultrasound is performed frequently.[63] However, no other differences in intelligence, neuromuscular or psychological development were found. However, there were critics on methodological aspects of these studies.[64] Side-effects of long-term ultrasound have not yet been noticed. In any case, it is important to discuss these subjects with parents openly and not to use ultrasound in an unreflected way.

Development of activities, hemodynamics, reactions towards touch and external stimuli

Onset of twin activities

The first increase in axodendritic and axosomatic synapses occurs between 8 and 10 weeks.[65] In this period movement patterns differentiate rapidly. Another striking increase in the number of axosomatic synapses is described between 12 and 15 weeks.[66] In these weeks simple general movements of body, head and extremities as well as more complex activity patterns such as swallowing, stretching and yawning emerge. Besides the study of Samueloff *et al.*[67] and our own reports, prenatal twin behavior has not been studied in early pregnancy.

First appearance of the described activities can be correlated to the gestational age; however, it has to be considered that all phenomena could have emerged already during the interval of the sessions. During the first weeks of gestation movements become more frequent and appear faster. The cascade of developing activities in twins is demonstrated in Figure 152.4(a).

The clinical importance of qualitative observations was stressed from replays of video recordings of neonatal movements. It was possible to distinguish between

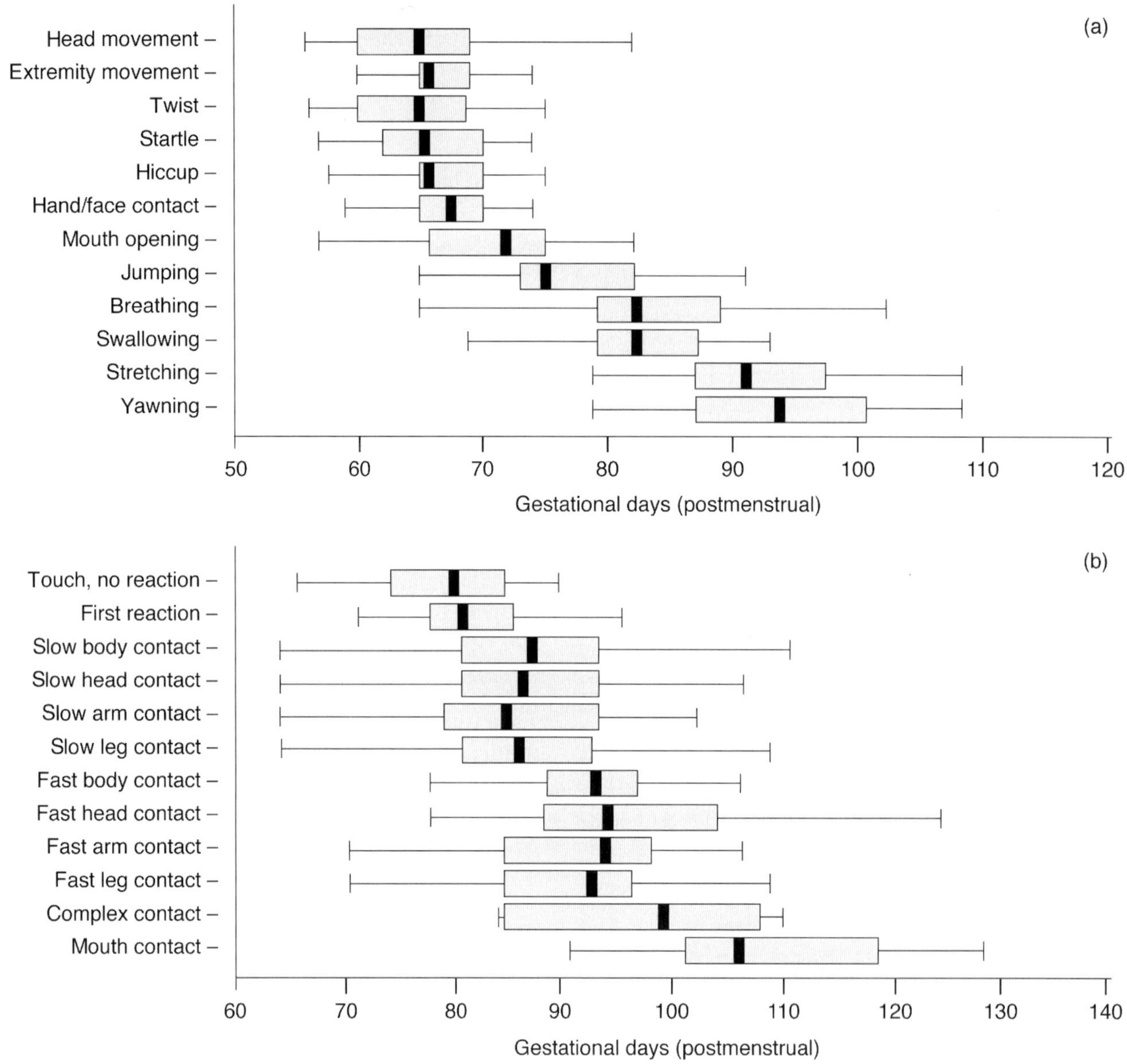

Figure 152.4 Onset of behavioral patterns in box–whisker plots, ultrasound observations at 1-week intervals, $n=25$ (20 DC and 5 MC) twin pairs. (a) Onset of activities. (b) Onset of inter-twin contacts.

infants with intact nervous system and brain lesions, though there was no difference in the quantity of movements. Neonates with brain lesions seemed to demonstrate with abnormal movements lacking elegance, fluency and rotations superimposed to limb movements.[68] These 'subjective' observations had a high interobserver agreement of around 90%,[69] which is comparable to our own correlation coefficients.

Onset of intertwin contacts

To study reactions of singletons towards touch *in utero* would be combined with ethical and practical restraints. However, twins are naturally exposed to sensory stimulations of the co-twin and thus ideal models to study the onset of reactions towards touch *in vivo*. As it was supposed for motor activities of singletons[70] the primacy of contact patterns may also indicate that contacts develop before being 'useful' responses to biological or psychological relevant sensory input.

Studying movements in twins in the last trimester Sadovsky stated[31]: 'The possibility that movements of one twin stimulate the other to move was rejected by the fact that in no instant did one fetus move immediately after the second started to move'. Looking at our video tapes we arrived at different conclusions.[71] Similarly, inter-twin contacts have been supposed to cause increased rates of simultaneous twin activities in early pregnancy.[68]

As described for activities, primary contacts can be correlated to the gestational age, still it has to be considered, that all phenomena could have emerged during the interval before the session. Both, the first interhuman contacts without and with reaction were primarily observed in a MC MA twin pair of two boys at 57 and 65 postmenstrual days, respectively. The cascade of developing contacts from simple to more complicated patterns in twins is demonstrated in Figure 152.4(b).

Prenatal contacts start with slow initiatives followed by slow reactions, giving the appearance of a 'tender' contact. This may be due to the still poorly developed muscular and sensory system. As described *in vitro*[3] we found *in vivo* that embryos respond to tactile stimulation as early as at 8–9 weeks. Yet at this age the receptors to perceive tactile stimuli have not yet penetrated the basement layer of the skin.[72] It is speculated that the developing neural system is responsive prior to the formation of specific receptor cells.[73] In MC twins contacts occur earlier, which might be interpreted with the smaller distance and the thinner intertwin membranes.

Continuity of early twin activities

A change in motility has been reported from 'rather jerky' around 12 weeks to 'slow and harmonious' at 16 weeks[74] for singletons. Interindividual differences in the quantity of FM have been described for singletons.[75] In twin pregnancies the question is whether they depend on systematic variables such as gender, zygosity, position *in utero* or possibly on 'early individuality', so that activity *in utero* might already be an early expression of temperament. Particular movements, for example, twisting and jumping, showing large ranges and unsystematic differences might be representative of individual differences. In contrast, some movements might be considered merely as reflexes (startles, hiccups) or seem to be essential for fetal development of organs (breathing movements and swallowing). These activity patterns show smaller inter-twin differences.

The number of most exhibited patterns increases throughout early gestation, except for twisting, which seems to be an early pattern that disappears after 13 weeks. Startles and hiccups decline after 13 weeks. Breathing and swallowing display a constant rise up to 16 weeks. Frequencies of hand–face contacts remain stable throughout. In Figure 152.5(a), the course of breathing movements, given as number per hour is plotted separately for twin A and B. In Figure 152.5(b), the course of twisting is demonstrated. There are large unsystematic differences between the two twins reflecting the incidental and possibly individual character, after 14 weeks twisting movements seem to disappear.

Continuity of early inter-twin contacts

The described change from 'rather jerky' activity around 12 weeks to 'slow and harmonious' activity at 16 weeks[74] correlates with our observations of the development of diffuse contact patterns during these weeks. Contacts may be explained by the onset of movements whereby incidental touches cannot be avoided *in utero* or are responded by early reflexes. Both, the part of the body that initiates the contacts as well as the reacting part may be randomly involved. Some reactions may be just incidental endogenously evoked movements or passive answers towards touch. Early contacts of MC twins are also more in number. Our classification of early contacts might be a subjective one. We tried to establish 'normal values' of the described qualities which cannot be demonstrated in detail. We just show two examples of our normal values classified according to the speed of either initiative or reaction (Figure 152.5c and d).

Hemodynamics during early multiple gestation

It is well known that normal values of FHR fall during the first 10 weeks of pregnancy.[76,77] This also holds true for twins and triplets. Due to the decrease of vascular resistance within the placental bed there is also a fall in pulsatility index (PI) of the umbilical artery in twins and triplets.

As an example we demonstrate our normal PI values and the FHR of twins in Figure 152.6(a) and (b) possibly of use for further research of the influence between early activity and hemodynamics.

Spontaneous FHR/FM patterns after 26 weeks

Observations of spontaneous FHR–FM patterns have been published in twin pregnancies before,[30,31,32,46,78] however, no normal values were established which is a prerequisite for further scientific and clinical evaluation.

As described we have tried to classify periods according to FM and FHR patterns (Table 152.1). If a 3 min window was used, the distribution of all periods varied per week, but there were no systematic changes throughout the observation period of 26–36 weeks. The distribution of periods with or without FM demonstrates the high percentage of active periods (mean around 80%) compared with singletons,[6] which might be caused by intertwin stimulations. Accordingly periods with a variability of >10 bpm were present in around 80% of the registration time (Figure 152.7a).

The question of whether or how often spontaneous FHR–FM patterns of co-twins are comparable, has been investigated in small samples. Sadovsky observed 10 normal twin pregnancies between 33 and 39 weeks looking whether the twins moved simultaneously or independently. Of all observed fetal movements around 75% were independent of the movements of the co-twin.[31] Similarly completely similar patterns were found in 26% of the observation time.[32] Still it could be demonstrated that FHR accelerations are more often associated (in 57%) than

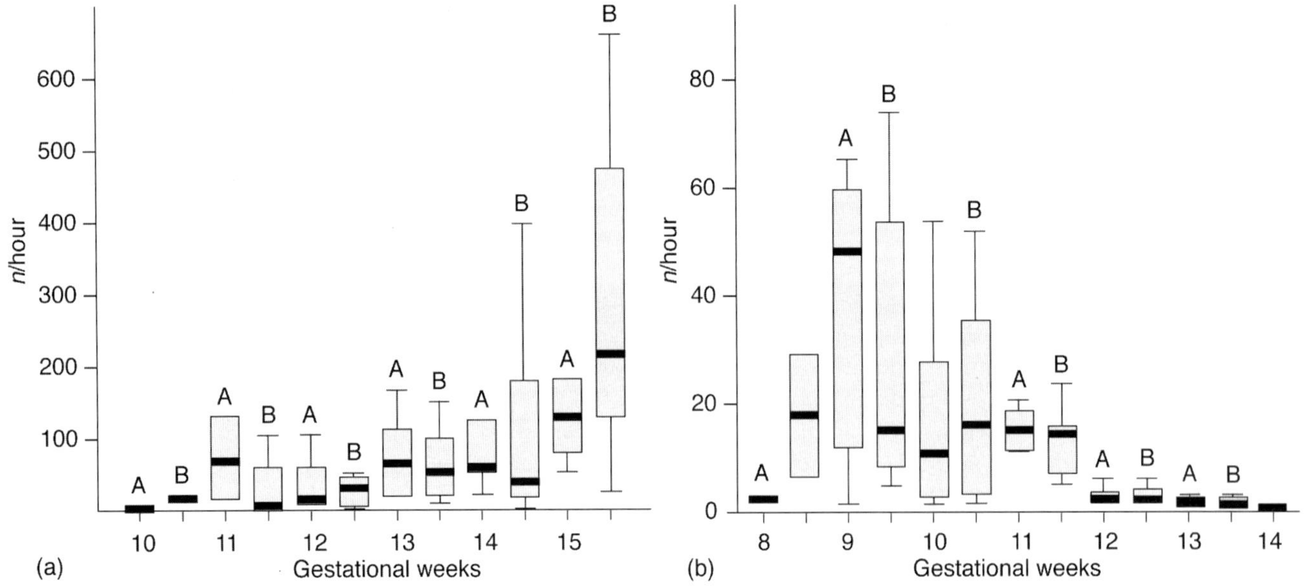

Figure 152.5 Continuity of early behavioral patterns in box–whisker plots, ultrasound observations at 1-week intervals, $n=25$ (20 DC and 5 MC) twin pairs. (a) Breathing movements (number per hour) separate for twin A and B. (b) Twisting movements (number per hour) separate for twin A and B. (c) Slow initiations with slow reactions between corresponding twins. (d) Fast initiations with fast reactions between corresponding twins.

statistically expected within the members of a twin pair.[78] Whether this proves the similarity of endogeneous behavioral patterns or just 'inter-twin stimulations' must remain open.

In our group of longitudinally investigated twins we have analyzed how far oscillation amplitude and fetal activity can be compared. Two members of a twin pair showed the same pattern of either FHR-variability < 10 bpm (patterns I and II), respectively, > 10 bpm (pattern III–IV) in around 50%. Similarly two members of a twin pair demonstrated simultaneously with an inactive pattern (I, II, IV) in 49% and with comparable active patterns in 43%.

Onset of reactions towards external stimuli

A measurable response of the fetus towards external stimuli depends on developmental differentiation of sensory receptors, adequate stimulation and fetal state. Emphasis in this section is put on two further sensory routes through which the fetus may be stimulated: vision and hearing.

Vision

After 18 weeks synapses appear on the eye rods. Between 20 and 24 weeks fetal eyelids may open, later followed by the development of the maculae

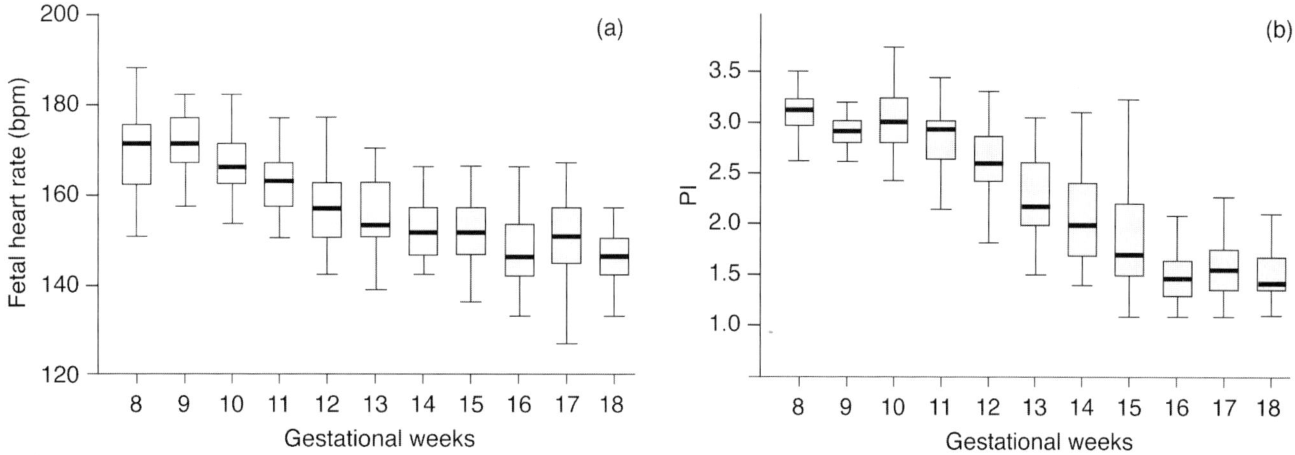

Figure 152.6 Development of early hemodynamics (box–whisker plots, ultrasound observations at 1-week intervals, $n = 31$ twin pairs). (a) Course of fetal heart rate ($p < 0.001$, Kruskal–Wallis test). (b) Course of pulsatility index in the umbilical artery ($p < 0.001$, Kruskal–Wallis test).

and photoreceptors.[38] There are only few studies of stimulations in singletons and up to now none in multiples.

As explained we have incidentally observed movements of the bulbi ('twinkling') by ultrasound towards stimulation with flash light from 28 weeks onwards. Reactions of FHR and FM in twins were observed by our team from 28 weeks onwards, at 30 weeks we even observed simultaneous reactions of two twins. However, probably due to the described methodological problems reactions of FHR–FM patterns were only registered in 29/390 light stimulations (around 8%) in our series. Therefore, we did not collect further systematic data for normal values or inter-twin comparison.

Audition

In the 4–5-week-old embryo the otocyst divides into two parts for cochlea and labyrinth. At 6 months, peripheral vibration-sensitive endings include Meissner's and Pacinian corpuscles, which transmit vibrotactile stimuli. The cochlea and peripheral sensory end organs have reached normal development at around 24–25 weeks.[39] Still, auditory brain stem response in the premature newborn have not been registered before 26 completed weeks.[79]

Auditory stimuli are the most documented and are even used clinically. External stimuli have to overrule intrauterine background noise *in utero* as well as attenuation by the maternal tissue. After the first suggestion to use FHR-monitoring in combination with external pure tone stimulation[80] a wide variety of acoustic stimuli have been introduced. The most 'reliable' responses were registered after stimulation with the EAL.[39]

Whether the FHR-response is a direct one or concomitant with muscular activity cannot always be differentiated. In singletons, first reactions to acoustic stimulations were observed as a 'aurepalpebral reflex' at 28 weeks[81] on a regular basis. Using FHR–FM monitoring responses in the form of FM and/or FHR-accelerations, reactions were observed as early as from 26 gestational weeks.[82,83]

Up to now, there are only a few studies on reactive behavioral patterns in multiples.[6,31,84,85] We have studied reactions of twins, though we still withheld it from clinical routine. Only by using the actocardiograph, we could observe a first fetal reaction in twins at a gestational age of 26 weeks +4 days characterized by a short FM in combination with a change from FHR–FM pattern I to II. First simultaneous reactions of two members of a twin pair were observed at 27 weeks and 2 days.

Reactive FHR/FM patterns after 26 weeks

After stimulation with the EAL we have investigated twin reactions throughout pregnancy. The distribution of the number and type of reactions changes significantly during the observation period.

After VAS short reactions describing a rapid FM possibly combined with FHR accelerations and reactions with a longer duration of more than 60 s can be differentiated in singletons and twins. Throughout the observation period we have observed significant increases of short reactions consisting predominantly of FM and FHR-accelerations (Figure 152.7b) as well as in the number of reactions of longer durations of more than 60 s characterized by changes of the baseline and/or FHR-variability (Figure 152.7c). In addition, we have investigated changes of the described FHR–FM patterns after VAS.

Before 30 weeks, the mean duration of a long reaction of twins is 184 (1–990) s and after 34 weeks it is 237 (3–690) s. Before 30 weeks the mean increase of the baseline after VAS is 3.5 bpm, after 34 weeks the mean increase is 11.9 bpm, the mean increase of the oscillation amplitude is 1.3 and 2.4 bpm, respectively, in a group of 32 longitudinally investigated twins.

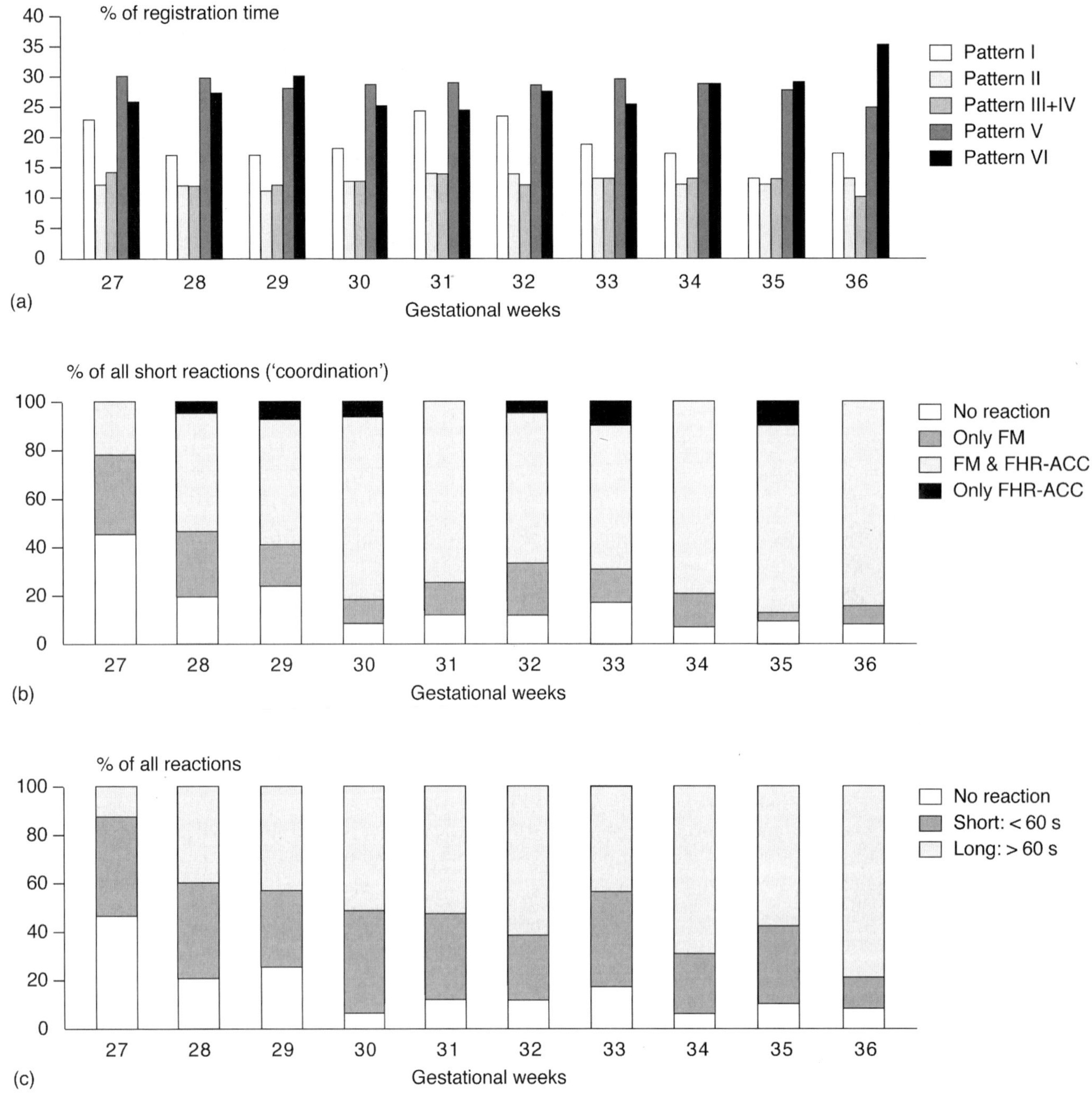

Figure 152.7 Continuity of behavioral patterns at advanced gestation (actocardiographic monitoring, $n=32$ twin pairs). (a) Distribution of spontaneous FHR-FM patterns (mean, $n=320$ tracings, ns). (b) Distribution of combinations of short reactive FHR-FM patterns (mean, $n=320$ tracings, $p<0.001$, Kruskal–Wallis test). (c) Distribution of combinations of short reactive FHR-FM patterns (mean, $n=320$ tracings, $p<0.001$, Kruskal–Wallis test).

Multivariate analysis demonstrates that the influence of gestational age on both variables is significant with even a higher impact on the baseline in all twins independent of their sex, zygosity or position. Stimulations without any alteration of either baseline or oscillation amplitude decrease in the group of twins from 98% at 27 weeks to around 55% at 36 gestational weeks. The described phenomena were observed in all twin groups independent of their zygosity, their sex and their presentation, though the degree of alterations shows significant differences.

Simultaneous FHR and FM-alterations after VAS were already described.[81] Investigating variables such as the duration of the reaction, the kind of the combined reaction and change of combined FHR–FM pattern synchronous reactions are demonstrated in around 70–80% of 'normal' co-twins. This again is a model for proving the effect of a stimulus.

Table 152.2 Comparison of the onset of contacts 8–16 weeks: Male vs. female vs. mixed pairs and monochorionic (MC) vs. dichorionic (DC) pairs: earlier onset in male and MC pairs (n=340 video tracings/25 twin pairs, Kruskal-Wallis & Mann-Whitney test)

First contact	Different gender (male vs. female vs. mixed)	Different chorionicity (MC vs. DC)
First reaction	p=0.29 (NS)	p=0.005
Slow body contact	p=0.29 (NS)	p=0.001
Fast body contact	p=79 (NS)	p=0.02
Complex contacts	p=0.01	p=0.009
Mouth contact	p=0.46 (NS)	p=0.79 (NS)

Influences on prenatal behavior under normal conditions

Prenatal twin studies offer the opportunity to observe two fetuses developing in the same environment. Apart from spontaneous activities and functions, inter-twin reactions towards touch as well as reactions towards external stimuli have a developmental aspect. One of the challenges is to examine inter-twin differences in specific subgroups relating to onset, qualities and quantities of behavioral variables.

Some simple questions are: Is there a difference in subgroups with different zygosity, gender, chorionicity and position? What is the influence of gestational age? Is there a dominant twin *in utero*? If the hypothesis holds true, that the character and incidence of activities, contacts and reactions is determined by individual genetics or by gender-specific variances, intermultiple differences are expected to be smaller within MZ or sex-alike compared to DZ or sex-unlike multiples. If the hypothesis holds true, that activities, reactions towards touch or external stimuli are determined by what we call 'environmental influences *in utero*', behavioral differences would be smaller in MC compared to DC multiples or in multiples lying in the same position.

It has to be considered that all these models are simplifications since there are interactions between intrinsic and extrinsic variables.

Influences on behavioral variables in early multiple pregnancy

From adult life we know that there are individual characteristics of behavioral patterns – also in the way how people move and communicate. In our series we up to now found a trend that the onset of activities is more similar between MZ than between DZ twins. The frequency of activities did not reveal significant inter-twin differences with a few exceptions: MZ and MC twins demonstrate with a higher incidence of 'jumping' compared to DZ or DC twins. No significant differences were found between pairs with different gender combinations except for yawning and mouth opening; however, the results may be biased by the low incidence of these patterns.

Contact patterns offer more obvious differences in their onset and incidence depending on chorionicity, zygosity and sex.

Analyzing the onset of early contacts we found that in the total group of MC twins ($n=5$), including one MC MA twin, mean and minimum of nearly all forms of contacts are observed significantly earlier than in the 20 DC twins (Table 152.2). This might be interpreted with the smaller distance and the thinner inter-twin membranes.

Analyzing the subgroups according to different gender combinations we did not yet detect systematic differences in the onset of primary contacts except for complex contacts which seem to occur significantly earlier in the group of only female twins (Table 152.2).

Analyzing the course of early contacts we found that within the first 16 gestational weeks all contacts in MC twins are more numerous (Table 152.3). It is not surprising and even known from adult life, that long interhuman distances and interhuman 'walls' make physical contacts impossible. The question of how far the observed contacts only occur because – here the multiples – are forced to move in a limited space remains open.

Surprisingly, we found significant differences in the speed of initiatives and reactions within subgroups of different gender combination as early as during the observation period of 8–16 weeks. In the group of only male twins, fast initiatives combined with fast or slow reactions were significantly increased compared to only female or mixed twin pairs (Table 152.3). Also the number of complex contacts within same-sex male pairs were significantly increased. It is suggested from animal experiments that differences of testosterone levels, being recognizable from around 12–14 weeks might even have an impact on early development *in utero*. Sex differences in adult human behavior have been reported for a

Table 152.3 Comparison of the number of contacts 8-16 weeks: Male vs. female vs. mixed pairs and monochorionic (MC) vs. dichorionic (DC) pairs: higher incidence in male and MC pairs (n=340 video tracings/25 twin pairs, Kruskal–Wallis & Mann–Whitney test)

First contact	Different gender (male vs. female vs. mixed)	Different chorionicity (MC vs. DC)
Extremity contact	p=0.01	p=0.00001
Fast initiative/slow reaction	p=0.0007	p=0.00001
Fast initiative/fast reaction	p=0.0058	p=0.00001
Complex contact	p=0.01	p=0.0014
Mouth contact	p=0.45 (NS)	p=0.001

number of dimensions of cognition, aggression, sensation seeking, affiliation and sociability and biological explanations have focused on the organizational or sensitizing influences of pre- and perinatal exposure to steroid hormones as well as neuroanatomic differences. The fact that hormones may have an impact on the anatomical development *in utero* leaves us with the following question. How far either females or males will be influenced by their opposite-sex co-twin?

Influences on behavioral variables in advanced normal pregnancy

Investigation of spontaneous FHR–FM patterns up to now have not shown a 'dominant' twin.[78] Gallagher *et al.* compared FHR patterns of five MC pairs with 10 DC pairs and found that simultaneous patterns occurred in 100% of all MC but only 92% of all DC pairs. The group found a 98% vs. 92% rate of simultaneous patterns in twin pairs with the same sex compared to twin pairs of different sex.[46] The differences were calculated as significant. As opposed to these results, Zimmer *et al.* did not find an influence of gender on FHR patterns of twins, however he could prove that twins who were lying on the right side of the uterus were significantly more active.[32]

In twin pairs with a DC fused placenta it was described that the rate of similar FHR-patterns regarding the amplitude of accelerations or the baseline was significantly higher (70%) as compared to twins with DC-separate placenta (30%).[86]

Accordingly, we have used the described distribution of active and passive periods as well as periods with variability of above or below 10 bpm to investigate whether different subgroups of twins demonstrate with more or less comparable patterns. Using chi-square tests, we could prove that female twin pairs demonstrate significantly more often with periods of the same variability (60%) as compared to mixed and male groups (50% and 38%, respectively). No influence could be proven by zygosity or position. MZ twins demonstrated more often with active periods compared to DZ twins, which might be attributed to the thinner inter-twin membrane.

FHR–FM patterns after VAS were examined between different subgroups. The mean increase of the baseline was found to be higher in twin pairs with vertex compared to breech position ($p < 0.01$, Kruskal–Wallis test). Multivariate analysis demonstrated a dominant influence of the gestational age, the presentation, and gender. Before 30 weeks, the state before VAS had an influence. An increase of the oscillation amplitude was more frequent in male as compared to female or mixed pairs ($p < 0.01$, Kruskal–Wallis test) and in pairs with both in vertex position ($p < 0.05$, Kruskal–Wallis test). No differences were found in MZ vs. DZ or left compared to right twins. Multivariate analysis demonstrated a significant influence of the state before the stimulation, presentation, gender and gestational age on the oscillation amplitude.

The kind of the first short reaction characterized by either no reaction, only FM or FM with FHR-accelerations is more frequently comparable among twins of the same sex (79% vs. 61%, $p < 0.05$, chi-square test), multivariate analysis demonstrates in addition a significant influence of zygosity after 30 weeks and of the presentation before 34 weeks.

The distribution of reactions of either short or long duration mainly depends, as expected, on the gestational age, the state before VAS and the chorionicity. The presentation only had an influence after 33 weeks. No differences could be found between right and left twins by multivariate analysis. By direct combination, 81% of twins with the same sex demonstrated with reactions of the same duration compared to only 68% of twins with different sex ($p < 0.05$, chi-square test).

The degree of changes of FHR–FM patterns is significantly more similar in MZ than in DZ twin couples (72% vs. 59%, $p < 0.05$, chi-square test). Multivariate analysis demonstrates that the state before VAS, gestational age, presentation and zygosity have significant influences on the degree of state changes between 26 and 36 weeks.

Also, the score by which we considered several FHR–FM variables was significantly more 'similar' in twins with the same presentation, with the same sex and between 31 and 33 weeks in MZ twins.

Table 152.4 Comparison of possibilities to describe fetal reactions towards vibroacoustic stimulation (left column): The parameters listed according to gestational age groups have a significant influence on the corresponding reactive behavioral pattern (n = 390 video tracings/32 twin pairs, multivariate analysis)

Kind of reaction	< 30 weeks	30–33 weeks	33–36 weeks
First reaction		state/zygosity	position
Change of state	state	state/sex	state
Kind of reaction	state	state/sex/position	state/position
Duration of reaction	state	position	position
Score of concordance	position	zygosity	sex

To summarize results from multivariate analysis we list the significant variables according to tracings of age intervals (Table 152.4). With more sophisticated variables and advancing gestational age the influence of gender, zygosity and position increases.

Influences on prenatal behavior under pathologic conditions

The rate of malformations is increased in MZ twins, concordance of malformations is only seen in around 10–20% even within MZ twin pairs.[87] Postulated theories explaining the increased rate of malformations are 'crowding' causing mostly concordant musculoskeletal malformations, early defects in the splitting process with the ultimate example of conjoined twins and vascular compromise secondary to a shared placenta leading to early organ embolization (e.g., disruption).[88]

Differences in the location of the nidation, connective mechanisms between embryonic and trophoblast circulation resulting in variances of umbilical insertion and differences in vasculatory support from the uterine vessels may be a reason for the development of circulative inter-twin differences and A–B asymmetry. Twins represent a unique model to study adaptive changes resulting from unequal placental nourishment. Hereditary difference in growth potential for each infant could be proposed as an alternative mechanism in DZ but not in MZ twins. Differences of fetal behavior in cases with A–B asymmetry – mainly if also detected by Doppler examinations – might be classified as 'environmental' ('nurture').

It is interesting that twins exposed *in utero* to the same 'environmental' influences may react with different degree of abnormality. This indicates that differences in fetal susceptibility or in the speed of their development may be of importance for the expression of syndromes caused by 'environmental' or teratogenic influences ('nature and nurture').

Influences on behavioral variables in early gestation

Individual growth of multiples is comparable with growth of singletons during the first and second trimester. Early growth differences between twins demand further evaluation. Weissman *et al.* reported retrospectively on five cases with discordant growth of > 5 days' difference during the first trimester. In all cases major anomalies were identified.[89]

Up to now in 3/80 multiple pregnancies with intermultiple growth differences of > 7days between 8 and 10 gestational weeks we prospectively performed early behavioral studies including Doppler examinations at 1-week intervals. Behavioral parameters were analyzed from the video tapes and karyotyping was performed.

In the first case (Figure 152.8a), a DC twin pregnancy, a triploidy xxx was diagnosed in the smaller twin next to a healthy boy. The sick twin demonstrated a significantly later onset of activities and contact initiations; some complex patterns such as swallowing and yawning were not observed at all. This twin died *in utero* at a gestational age of 26 weeks. Pregnancy continued until 35 weeks.

In the second case, a TC TA triplet pregnancy, one embryo appeared as a 'vanishing triplet' at 11 weeks. The most striking behavioral difference was a reduced number of movements and lower heart rate until intrauterine death.

In the third case, a TC TA triplet pregnancy after ovulation stimulation, a normal karyotype in all triplets (3x xy) was diagnosed and superfecundation was suspected. Behavioral patterns did not differ throughout the observation period. The mother developed premature rupture of membranes (PROM) 1 week after amniocentesis. All triplets died due to amnioninfection and prematurity.

The analysis of these cases might suggest that detailed analysis of early behavioral patterns including early Doppler parameters as suggested recently[90] might improve non-invasive diagnosis mainly in cases when other symptoms of risk are present.

Twin-to-twin transfusion syndrome (TTTS) may also develop as early as from 10 weeks onwards. The earliest case we have observed presented with extreme hydops of the recipient with tricuspid and mitral valve regurgitation of the recipient at 16 weeks. Laser treatment was performed at Kings College Hospital in London.[91] Though the condition of the twins stayed

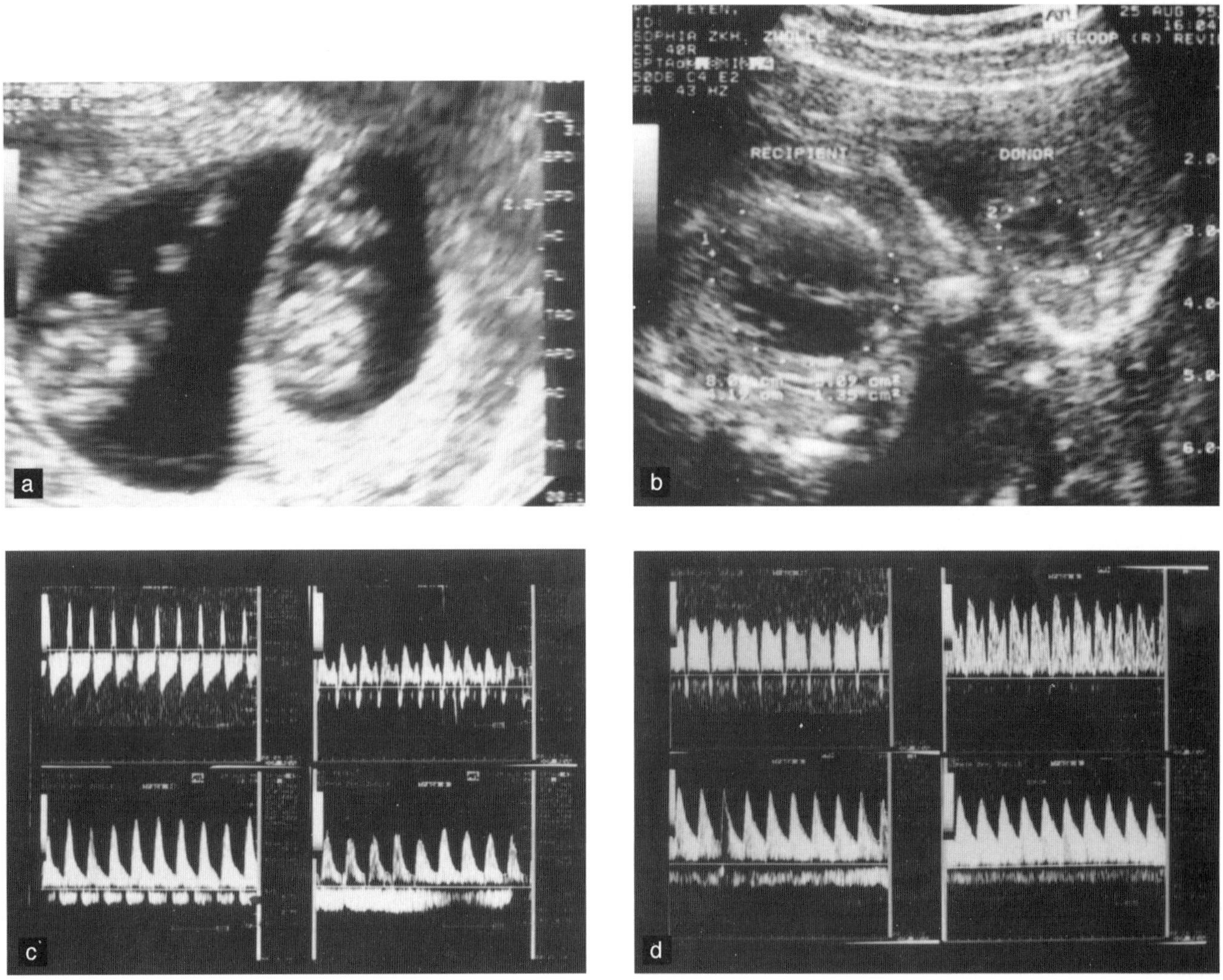

Figure 152.8 Ultrasound pictures of pathologic early twin gestation. (a) Early growth difference in a dichorionic twin pregnancy at 10 weeks (triploidy xxx). (b) Early TTTS at 16 weeks with hydrops of the recipient twin (left), there is evident inter-twin difference in cardiac dilatation. (c) Doppler flow velocity wave forms of the ductus venosus (above) and the umbilical vessels (below) of recipient (left) and donor twin (right) before treatment. (d) Doppler flow velocity wave forms of the ductus venosus (above) and the umbilical vessels (below) of recipient (left) and donor twin (right) after treatment.

stable, the hydrops did not disappear until we started with digitalization of the mother. Before treatment the ductus venosus velocity waveforms of the recipient showed a significant reverse flow as described[92] and umbilical flow demonstrated with venous pulsations (Figure 152.8c, left). Only some days after digitalization the hydrops disappeared and behavioral patterns of both twins switched towards more active periods (Figure 152.9a). The donor twin presented with increased activity (Figure 152.9b). Doppler velocity waveforms improved (Figure 152.8d, left). Placental evaluation by computer-angiography revealed that there were no communications between the two placental parts.

Doppler examination is regarded as an important tool in the diagnosis of MA twinning visualizing common tangle at the cord insertion[93] or later in gestation the occurrence of notches.[94] In the two cases with MC MA placentations (Figure 152.1c and f) that we have followed up to now we observed two arterial patterns with different heart rhythm reflected from the entangled umbilical cords already at 10 weeks. Though we were skeptical about the prognosis we could continue even the DC DA triplet pregnancy until lung maturity was proven at 34 weeks. Growth and FHR–FM patterns were not at all affected during the whole course of pregnancy, though excessive entanglement was diagnosed during caesarean section. Close monitoring including behavioral patterns and circulation helps clinical decision making, but can also give confidence to parents and doctors in charge.

Influences on behavioral variables in advanced gestation

Interesting aspects of behavioral studies can be drawn from twin gestations discordant for fetal anomalies also in advanced gestation. In a case report of a DC

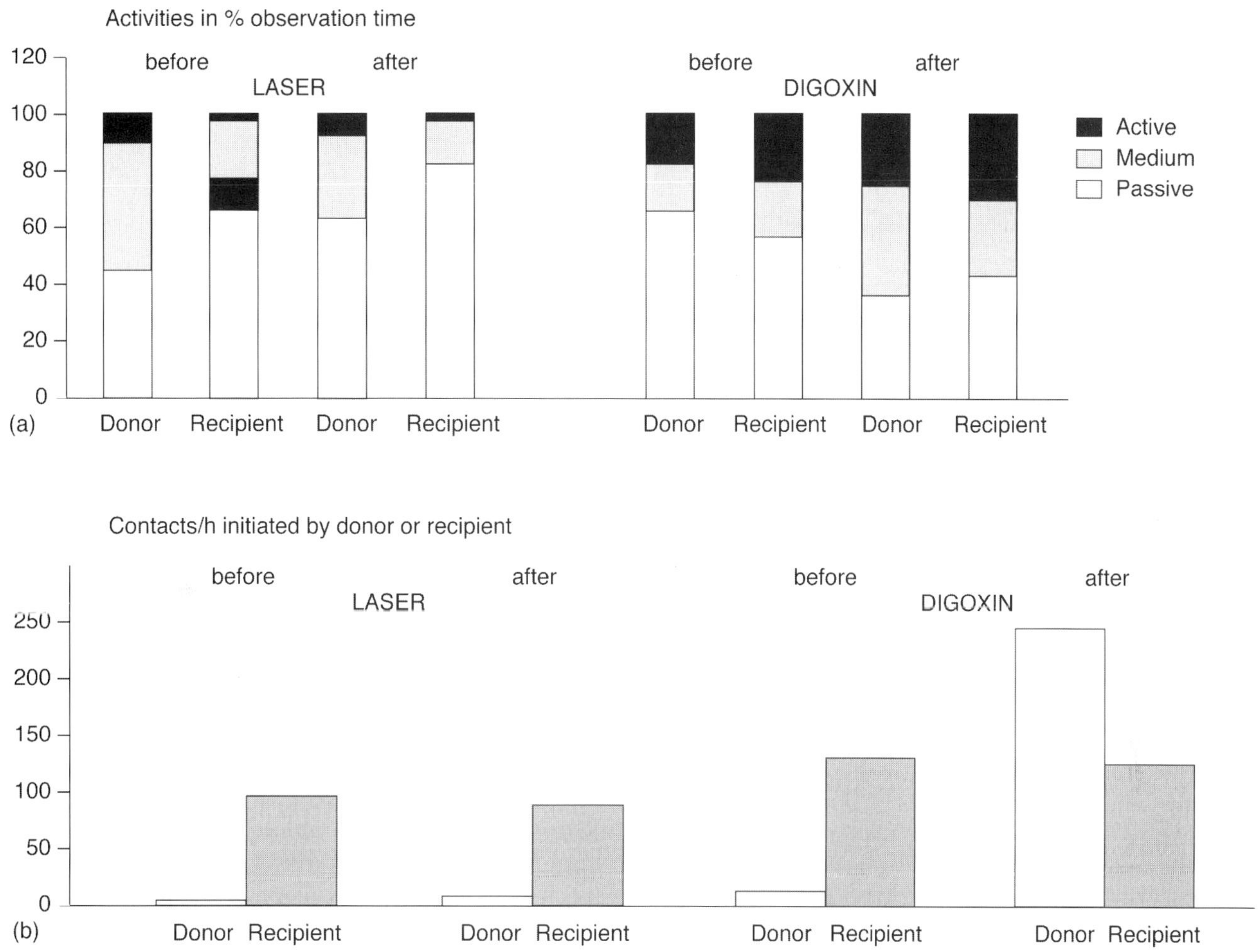

Figure 152.9 Behavioral patterns before and after treatment of early TTTS between 16 and 20 gestational weeks. (a) Activities given as active (fast FM), medium (slow FM) and passive (no FM). (b) Contacts with reactions of the co-twin.

twin pregnancy discordant for anencephaly significant inter-twin differences could be found.[95] Data analysis of ultrasound observations revealed that the incidence of startles and jumping, decreasing in the normal fetus, remained high in the anencephalic one. It is suggested that these movements are due to spinal cord stimulations and their elimination is usually controlled by the brain above the medulla oblongata. In contrast, breathing movements and hiccups were limited or nearly absent in the anencephalic twin indicating that at least an intact medulla oblongata and pons are required for preparatory movements.

In a similar case that we have documented from 30 to 34 weeks of gestation, we have additionally observed that FHR-variability was significantly decreased in the anencephalic fetus whereas FMs were increased, maybe due to the polyhydramnios. Reactions towards VAS did not occur in the anecaphalic fetus (unpublished).

The clinical significance of FHR–FM patterns in advanced pregnancy of twins or higher-order multiples, in general, does not differ significantly from those in singleton pregnancy. Still, probably due to inter-twin stimulation or difficulties in interpretations of two simultaneous FHR tracings, FHR–FM patterns might not be as an early indicator of threatening fetal hypoxia as in singletons.

As already known from singleton pregnancy, Doppler flow velocity wave forms of umbilical, arterial cerebral and venous vessels are now prerequisite for the control of pathologic multiple pregnancies to differentiate the underlying pathologic processes. In TTTS umbilical arterial Doppler is of no obvious value and is meanwhile replaced by venous Doppler measurements[92] as already described at early gestation. Predictive sensitivity of Doppler examination in the internal carotid and the umbilical artery preceded diagnosis of growth retardation in twins by a mean of 3.7 weeks, combining ultrasound improves the sensitivity to 84%[96] and interpair differences also improve prediction of discordant growth of twins[96] and triplets.[97] It would be interesting to examine, whether intrauterine stress may cause accelerated maturation measurable by behavioral variables.

It has to be considered that with advancing gestational age behavioral states might have an influence

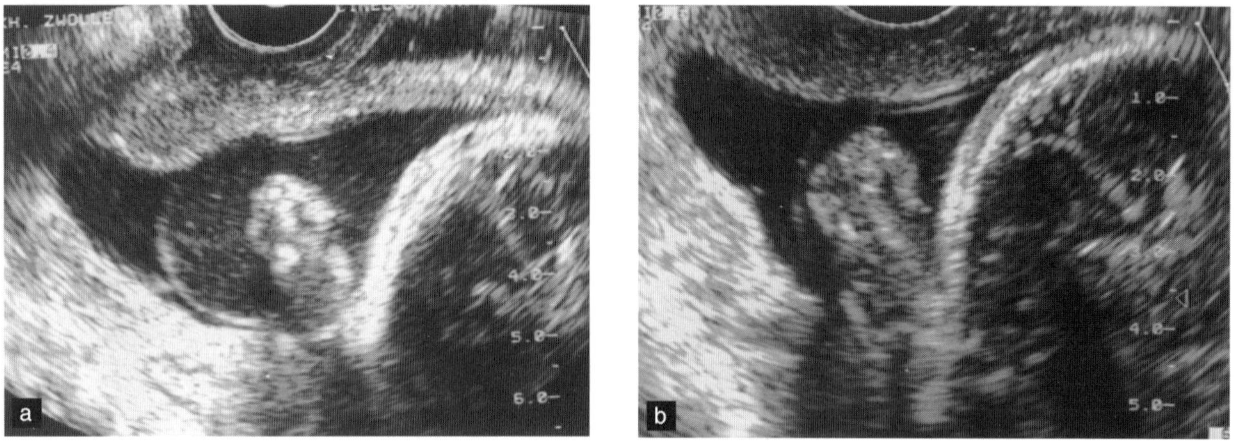

Figure 152.10 Future aspects of twin behavior: 'the self examining twin'. (a) Funneling with spiriting amnion and chorion. (b) Examining hand of the first twin.

on Doppler velocity waveforms as proven for singletons.[21,98,99] We have up to now not yet repeated these studies for twins, since the simultaneous registration of FEM would demand to use two Doppler equipments and separate ultrasound equipments. To investigate multiple behavior during advanced gestation under pathologic conditions is awaited for, but would definitely imply, that all data from Doppler examinations have to be included in the protocols.

Though we have used VAS as a tool for research under described conditions, we have up to now consciously withheld it from clinical routine and therefore no experience with systematic clinical testing besides from controlled trials. Warning hints from the literature not to use VAS in cases with low variability and possible hypoxia to avoid unnecessary stresses for the fetus[100] may be taken even more seriously in twins.

An interesting aspect of multiple gestation are pregnancies in which both twins are exposed to the same pathologic influences such as drugs, alcohol or nicotine. In a set of DC twins of a frankly alcoholic mother, one twin presented with the stigmata of fetal alcohol syndrome, whereas the other just displayed mild fetal alcohol effects.[101] Whether different susceptibility to ethanol dysmorphogenesis or exposure to different concentrations due to different circulation of the corresponding placenta is of primary etiology remains an open question. At present we are investigating the influence of nicotine and caffeine on behavior and hemodynamics of multiples.

Implications for future research

Methodological improvements

Realizing that skepticism often arises toward pioneering work, we are aware that many readers will have doubts on the described phenomena at early gestational age. This might hopefully stimulate them to improve the methods by more intense research efforts.

Methodological self-criticism is realized: Proposing time-intervals and durations of ultrasound sessions we have to compromise with the patients compliance, e.g., discomfort when proposing longer or more frequent ultrasound sessions or anxieties about bioeffects of serial ultrasound studies. Still we realize that within 30–60 min of documentation the whole pattern of possible contacts may not be reflected and that within a week new contacts may emerge without being realized. We still do not know the impact of the time of the day, health or emotion of the mother, food intake or even of ethnic differences on the onset and early development of activities and contacts. Though we have documented these data, larger series are needed.

Methodological criticism also relates to the present form of presentation of this article. Books are being replaced or accompanied by database systems combined with addresses of researchers in charge of the most recent information or meta-analysis.[102] Processes by which moving images are predominant can be presented on CD-ROM and thus improve our understanding tremendously.[103] For several ultrasound features including behavioral patterns and hemodynamics, as well as for delivery management, 'multimedia documentations' would be of enormous advantage.

Computer analysis of behavioral FHR and FM patterns has been described, mostly for singleton pregnancies.[104] In twins, the advantage is that the high number of data can be compromised. There are still a lot of disadvantages: most computer programs only concentrate on just one of two parameters such as FHR-variability and incidence of movements. The tremendous advantage of behavioral observations are, however, primarily to describe and analyze qualities of activities or phenomena that have to be carefully described in order not to lose precious information.

Reaction of the family toward ultrasound visualization of multiples' 'bonding'

The first steps *in utero* are observed with enthusiasm by parents and siblings. Visualization of prenatal twin life seems to evoke even more surprising reactions than in singletons. The existence of inter-twin contacts *in utero* is perceived with great amazement. The early tender touches are moving, the more forceful hitting and kicking at a later stage may sometimes cause laughter. It is impressive that the fetuses are touching and reacting without seeing each other. Following the expression of parents, they 'embrace' and 'kiss' without having had teachers. Questions arise about the inborn aspect of contacts in humans.

Parent–infant bonding is defined as a one-way concern and affection of adults towards children they care for during the first days of life was systematically described only as late as 1972.[105] As soon as the contact is reciprocal, even if it is only by crying or smiling, we speak of attachment. In mothers who experience extra contact with their infants at the time of delivery and during the first days of life, maternal–infant bonding is facilitated.[106] It is also suggested that emotional attachment to the fetus starts shortly after conception and deepens as pregnancy progresses. This is also true in high-risk pregnancies[106] – as multiple pregnancies often are. Early affectionate relationships may also develop towards two newborns[107] though initial bonding difficulties were seen more frequently due to medical problems, prematurity and maternal feelings of inadequacy. Early ultrasound examination might prepare parents of their future task and allow space for talks and dreams.

The impact of ultrasound on expectant parents in singletons has been found to be a reassuring experience[107] inducing a positive attitude towards the growing baby.[108] After a single ultrasound examination between 12 and 20 weeks[109] the baby was perceived as being more active, more beautiful and familiar as well as the woman's own body as more pleasant, relaxed and less fearful. Integrating other family members might facilitate that all members of the new family will be welcomed more easily. We always ask that besides the husbands, older young brothers and sisters also take part in the ultrasound sessions and stimulate them to paint the future family in order to avoid later jealousy.

Prospective studies of the effect of frequent and early ultrasound examinations on bonding or attachment in multiple pregnancy have not yet been performed. Unfortunately, it is only recently that we became increasingly aware of the impact of our examinations on bonding and on the doctor–patient relationship and therefore have only performed retrospective questionnaires. Prospective research and sampling procedures might demand professional efforts of psychologists and large sample sizes.

Follow-up

Follow-up examinations are the best control – yet this is far from reality. Many perinatologiosts only hear incidentally of the further development of their prenatal patients and are sometimes surprised to hear of either positive or negative outcomes. Unfortunately, health systems do not care sufficiently to promote direct 'bonding' between pediatricians and perinatologists which makes it difficult to get systematic data on specific risk groups. This also holds true for twins and higher-order multiples and even more, if comparison of prenatal and postnatal behavior is concerned. We admit that prospective studies would be time-consuming for both sides.

Activity itself promotes growth and dendritic branching of individual neurons. Sensation from receptor cells promotes the development of the neural system.[110] The fact that twins experience more tactile stimuli than singletons might improve their development. This was speculated by early follow-up examinations,[111] showing accelerated functional maturation in multiples born between 32 and 37 weeks[112] and by long-term follow-up studies at the age of 6 where multiples scored better than singletons.[113] It can be speculated that intrauterine neurological development is accelerated by increased rates of intrauterine stress of multiples as proven for lung maturation processes.[114] Simultaneous assessment of functional and metabolic maturation of the central nervous system and the lungs at birth of growth-discordant MZ (ideally DC) multiples not due to TTTS or of MZ multiples discordant for PROM would be an interesting topic for a multicenter trial.

Prenatal learning, habituation or adaptation toward touch of the co-twin, as described for repetitive auditory stimuli,[110,115,116] deserves further evaluation. Yet in early gestation nothing is known about the phenomenon of habituation. Again, twin pregnancies would be a perfect model to study eventual 'learning' which is defined as any change resulting from past experience.[117]

Follow-up studies in opposite-sex twins are fascinating: We found a study[118] based on the findings of Zuckerman *et al.*[119] that aspects of sensation seeking are consistently increased in males relative to females. In comparing age-adjusted data for opposite- and same-sex twins, it was shown that there is a predicted increase of sensation seeking in female members of opposite-sex pairs. Though psychosocial explanations cannot be excluded, the findings are consistent with hypothesized *in utero* hormonal influences of prenatal androgen exposure on later behavioral development of females. Influences of estrogen in opposite-sex males could not be proved. This might suggest that it is not sufficient to just analyze all females or all males of all twin pregnancies, but to differentiate as it was performed in our studies, between mixed or pure male and pure female twin pairs. Further comparisons of prenatal and postnatal series are required.

Similarly surprising are follow-up studies in MZ DC vs. MZ MC twins. Intrapair differences in personality and cognitive ability among MZ distinguished by MC or DC placentation were calculated. Absolute differences of individualized personality inventory scores for children between MC MZ co-twins were smaller than between DC MZ twins.[120] The findings are interpreted as follows. Variation in timing of embryological division and possible effects on MZ twins' placental vasculature may have consequences for some dimensions of their behavioral development as well.

Controlled follow-up studies concentrating on side effects of frequent early ultrasound examinations should be recommended. These studies could be combined with other study proposals and be collected in an international 'behavioral register'. Still, manpower, limited international communication and statistical evaluation play a limiting role.

How far increased intelligence scoring of postnatal twins as compared to singletons,[113] matched for gestational age and birth weight, suits the intrauterine multiples is an open question. In a prospective study to detect the diagnostic value to predict prematurity, we could describe that separation of amnion and chorion included in funneling of the cervix was diagnosed as a new risk factor (Figure 152.10a and b).[121]

Conclusions

Multiple pregnancies do not only represent sorrows and problems as indicated in the obstetric literature. They also represent challenges mainly for their parents and perinatologists. Therefore, we would like to add the statement supported by more than 1000 publications during the last decade: 'It is tough to be a twin: The risk of disorder, disease and death are greater for all members of a plural set from the moment of conception to the end of their life span and encompass physical, psychological and social threats'[122] ...by a new statement: 'It is also great to be a twin: The stimulating pleasure of close company, contact, competitive challenges and interaction are unique for all members of a plural set from the moment of conception to the end of their life span and encompass physical, psychological and research chances'. Do not forget: No pleasure without risk!

Acknowledgments

We thank Brigitte Güner, Renske Rijlaarsdam, Rinske Bos and Hubertus Adt, Axel Mohnhaupt for help with data analysis and preparation.

REFERENCES

1. Gedda L. *Twins in the History of Science*. Springfield, IL: C.C. Thomas, 1961:21–4.
2. Bible, *Genesis* 25, 22.
3. Galton F. The history on twins as a criterion of the relative powers of nature and nurture. *J Anthropol Inst Great Britain Ireland* 1875;5:391–406.
4. Rende RD, Plomin R, Vandenberg SG. Who discovered the twin method? *Behav Genet* 1990;20:227–35.
5. Arabin B, van Eyck J, Wisser J, Versmold H, Weitzel HK. Fetales Verhalten bei Mehrlings-gravidität: methodische, klinische und wissenschaftliche Aspekte. *Geburtsh Frauenheilk* 1991;51:869–75.
6. Arabin B, Gembruch U, van Eyck J. Fetal behavior in multiple pregnancies. *J Perinat Med* 1993;21:285–94.
7. Preyer W. Spezielle Physiologie des Embryo. Untersuchungen über die Lebenserscheinungen vor der Geburt. Leipzig: Grieben Verl, 1885.
8. Prechtl HFR, Beintema DJ. The neurological examination of the full term newborn infant. *Clinics in Developmental Medicine*. Vol. 12. London: Heinemann, 1964.
9. De Vries JIP, Visser GHA, Prechtl HFR. The emergence of fetal behaviour I, qualitative aspects. *Early Hum Dev* 1982;7:301–22.
10. Nijhuis JG, Prechtl HFR, Martin CB Jr. Are there behavioural states in the human fetus? *Early Hum Dev* 1982;6:177–95.
11. Hepper PG. Fetal behavior: Why so special? *Ultrasound Obstet Gynecol* 1996;8:145–8.
12. Ahlfeld F. Die intrauterine Tätigkeit der Thorax-und Zwerchfell-muskulatur, intrauterine Atmung. *Mon Geburtsh Gynäk Berlin* 1905;21:143–63.
13. Hooker D. *The Prenatal Origin of Behavior*. Kansas: University of Kansas Press, 1952.
14. Reinold E. Clinical value of fetal spontaneous movements in early pregnancy. *J Perinat Med* 1973;1:65–72.
15. Timor-Tritsch IE, Dierker LJ, Hertz LH, Deagan NC, Rosen MG. Studies of antepartum behavioural state in the human fetus at term. *Am J Obstet Gynecol* 1978;132:524–8.
16. Junge HD. Behavioral state and state related heart rate and motor activity patterns in the newborn and the fetys ante partum. A comparative study. *J Perinat Med* 1979;7:85–107.
17. Prechtl HFR. The behavioural states of the newborn infant. *Brain Res* 1974;76:185–212.
18. Arduini D, Rizzo G, Giolandino C, Valensise H, Dell'Aqua S, Romanini C. The development of behavioural states. A longitudinal study. *Prenat Diagn* 1985;5:269–76.
19. Birnholz JC, Stephens JC, Faria M. Fetal movement patterns: a possible means of defining neurologic milestones in utero. *AJR Am J Roentgenol* 1978;130:537–40.
20. Bots RSGM, Nijhuis JG, Martin CB Jr, Prechtl HFR. Human fetal eye movements: Detection in utero by ultrasonography. *Early Hum Dev* 1981;5:87–94.
21. Van Eyck J, Wladimiroff JW, Noordam MJ, Tongue HM, Prechtl HFR. The blood flow velocity waveform in the fetal descending aorta; its relationship to fetal behavioural states in normal pregnancy at 37–38 weeks of gestation. *Early Hum Dev* 1985;14: 99–107.
22. Grimwade J, Walker DW, Bartlett M. Human fetal heart rate change and movement in response to sound and vibration. *Am J Obstet Gynec* 1971;109:86–90.
23. Ron M, Yaffe H, Sadovsky E. Fetal heart response to amniocentesis in cases of decreased fetal movements. *Obstet Gynecol N Y* 1976;48:456–9.
24. Polishuk WZ, Laufer N, Sadovsky E. Fetal response to external light stimulus. *Harefuah* 1975;89:395–6.
25. Walker D, Grimwade J, Wood C. Intrauterine noise: a component of fetal environment. *Am J Obstet Gynecol* 1971;109:91–5.
26. Chitkara U, Berkowitz R.. Assessment of multiple pregnancy. In Chervenak FA, Isaacson GC, Campbell S, eds. *Ultrasound in Obstetrics and Gynecology*. Boston, MA: Little, Brown, 1993: 413–20.
27. Rijlaarsdam R, Bos R, van Eyck J, Arabin B. Comparison of biometry, circulation and behaviour in multiple pregnancies with early growth differences. *Ultrasound Obstet Gynecol* 1996; 8(Suppl 1):118.
28. Bos R, Rijlaarsdam R, Van Eyck J, Arabin B. Longitudinal analysis of growth, fetal heart rate and umbilical artery Doppler values in early multiple pregnancies. *Ultrasound Obstet Gynecol* 1996; 8(Suppl 1):117.
29. Sebire NJ, Snijders RJM, Hughes K, Sepullveda W, Nicolaides KH. Screening for trisomy 21 in twin pregnancies by maternal age and fetal translucency thickness at 10–14 weeks of gestation. *Br J Obstet Gynaecol* 1996;103:999–1003.
30. Ohel G, Samueloff A, Navot D, Sadovsky E. Fetal heart rate accelerations and fetal movements in twin pregnancies. *Am J Obstet Gynecol* 1985;152:686–7.
31. Sadovsky E, Ohel G, Simon A. Ultrasonographical evaluation of the incidence of simultaneous and independent movements in twin fetuses. *Gynecol Obstet Invest* 1987;23:5–9.

32. Zimmer EZ, Goldstein I, Alglay S. Simultaneous recording of fetal breathing movements and body movements in twin pregnancy. *J Perinat Med* 1988;16:109–12.
33. Maeda K. Studies on new ultrasonic fetal actograph and continous recording of fetal movement. *Acta Obstet Gynaecol* 1984;36: 280–8.
34. Arabin B, Riedewald S, Zacharias C, Saling E. Quantitative analysis of fetal behavioural patterns. *Gynaecol Obstet Invest* 1988;26:211–18.
35. Schwöbel E, Fallenstein F, Huch R, Huch A. Combined electronic FHR and FM monitor – a preliminary report. *J Perinat Med* 1987; 15:179–84.
36. Besinger RE, Johnson TRB. Doppler recording of fetal movement: clinical correlation with real-time ultrasound. *Obstet Gynecol* 1989;74:277–80.
37. Van Eyck J, Arabin B. Actocardiographic monitoring of triplets during vaginal delivery. *Am J Obstet Gynecol* 1992;166:1293–5.
38. Timor- Tritsch IE. The effect of external stimuli on fetal behaviour. *Eur J Obstet Gynecol Reprod Biol* 1986;21:321–9.
39. Gagnon R. Fetal behaviour in relation to stimulation. In Nijhuis JG, ed. *Fetal Behaviour Developmental and Perinatal Aspects*. Oxford: Oxford Medical Publications, 1992:209–26.
40. Schmidt W, Boos R, Gnirs J, Auer L, Schulze S. Fetal behavioral states and sound stimulation. *Early Hum Dev* 1985;12:145–53.
41. Gagnon R, Hunse C, Foreman J. Human fetal behavioural states after vibratory stimulation. *Am J Obstet Gynecol* 1989;161:1470–6.
42. Gagnon R, Foreman J, Hunse C, Patrick J. Effects of low-frequency vibration on human term fetuses. *Am J Obstet Gynecol* 1989;161: 1479–85.
43. Eller DP, Robinson LJ, Newman RB. Position of the vibroacoustic vibrator does not effect the response. *Am J Obstet Gynecol* 1992; 167:1137–9.
44. Nyman M, Arulkumaran SM, Hsu TS, Ratnam SS, Till O, Westgreen M. Vibroacoustic stimulation and intrauterine sound pressure levels. *Obstet Gynecol* 1991;78:803–6.
45. Pietrantoni M, Angel JL, Parsons MT, Mc Clain L, Arango HA, Spellacy WN. Human fetal response to vibroacoustic stimulation as a function of stimulus duration. *Obstet Gynecol* 1991;78: 807–11.
46. Gallagher MW, Costigan K, Johnson TRB. Fetal heart rate accelerations, fetal movement and fetal behaviour patterns in twin gestation. *Am J Obstet Gynecol* 1992;167:1140–4.
47. Derom R, Derom C, Vlietink R. Placentation. In Keith LG, Papiernik E, Keith DM, Luke B, eds. *Multiple Pregnancy – Epidemiology, Gestation & Perinatal Outcome*. New York: Parthenon, 1995:331–49.
48. Vlietinck R. Determination of the zygosity of twins. Thesis, Leuven, 1986.
49. Juel Nielsen N, Hauge M. On the diagnosis of zygosity in twins and the value of blood groups. *Acta Genet* 1958;8:256–60.
50. Jeffreys AJ, Brookfiel JFY, Semeonoff R. Positive identification of an immigration test case using human DNA fingerprints. *Nature* 1985;317:818–19.
51. Derom C, Vlietinck R, Derom R, Boklage C, Thiery M, Pearson P. Genotyping macerated stillborn fetuses. *Am J Obstet Gynecol* 1991;164:797–800.
52. Miller DL. A review of the ultrasonic bioeffects of microsonation, gas-body activation and related cavitation-like phenomena. *Ultrasound Med Biol* 1987;13:443.
53. Rott HD. Zur Frage der Schädigungsmöglichkeit diagnostischen Ultraschalls. *Ultraschall* 1981;2:56–64.
54. Kaufman GE. Mutagenicity of ultrasound in cultured mammalian cells. *Ultrasound Med Biol* 1985;11:497–501.
55. Doida Y, Miller MW, Cox C, Church CC. Confirmation of an ultrasound-induced mutation in two in-vitro mammalian cell lines. *Ultrasound Med Biol* 1990;16:699–705.
56. National Council on Radiation Protection. Biological effects of ultrasound: Mechanisms and clinical implications. Report no. 74, Bethesda, 1983.
57. American Institute of Ultrasound in Medicine. Bioeffects considerations for the safety of diagnostic ultrasound. *Ultrasound Med Biol* 1988;7:1.
58. Miller MW, Ziskin MC. Biological consequences of hyperthermia. *Ultrasound Med Biol* 1989;15:707–22.
59. Lele PP. Safety and potential hazards in the current applications of ultrasound in obstetrics and gynecology. *Ultrasound Med Biol* 1979;5:307–20.
60. Kinnier Wilson LM, Waterhouse JAH. Obstetric ultrasound and childhood malignancies. *Lancet* 1984;2:997–8.
61. Cartwright RA, McKinney PA, Hopton PA, *et al*. Ultrasound examinations in pregnancy and childhood cancer. *Lancet* 1984;2: 999–1000.
62. Salvesen KA, Vatten LJ, Eik-Nes SH, Hughdahl K, Bakketeig LS. Routine ultra-sonography in utero and subsequent handedness and neurological development. *Br Med J* 1993;307:159–64.
63. Newnham JP, Evans SF, Michael CA, Stanley FJ, Landau LI. Effects of frequent ultrasound during pregnancy: A randomised controlled trial. *Lancet* 1993;342:887–91.
64. Keirse MJNC. Frequent prenatal ultrasound: Time to think again. *Lancet* 1993:342.
65. Okado N. Development of the human cervical spinal cord with reference to synapse formation in the motor nucleus. *J Comp Neurol* 1980;191:495–513.
66. Okado N, Kojima T. Ontogeny of the central nervous system: neurogenesis, fibre connection, synaptogenesis and myelination in the spinal cord. In Prechtl HFR, ed. *Continuity of Neural Functions from Prenatal to Postnatal Life*. Oxford: Blackwell Scientific 1984: 46–64.
67. Samueloff A, Younis JS, Strauss N, Baras M, Sadovsky E. Incidence of spontaneous and evoked fetal movements in the first half of twin pregnancy. *Gynecol Obstet Invest* 1991;31:200–3.
68. Ferrari F, Cioni G, Prechtl HFR. Qualitative changes of general movements in preterm infants with brain lesions. *Early Hum Dev* 1990;23:193–231.
69. Prechtl HFR. Qualitative changes of spontaneous movements in fetus and preterm infant are a marker of neurological dysfunction. *Early Hum Dev* 1990;23:151–8.
70. Prechtl HFR. Continuity and change in early neural development. In Prechtl HFR, ed. *Continuity of Neural Functions from Prenatal to Postnatal Life. Clinics in Developmental Medicine*. Oxford: Blackwell Scientific, 1984;94:1–15.
71. Arabin B, Bos R, Rijlarsdam R, van Eyck J. The onset of inter-human contacts. Longitudinal ultrasound observations in twin pregnancies. *Ultrasound Obstet Gynecol* 1996;8(3):166–73.
72. Humphrey T. The development of trigeminal nerve fibres to the oral mucosa compared to with their development to cutaneous surfaces. *J Comp Neurol* 1966;126:91–108.
73. Hepper PG. Fetal psychology: an embryonic science. In Nijhuis JG, ed. *Fetal Behaviour. Developmental and Perinatal Aspects*. Oxford: Oxford University Press, 1992:130–56.
74. Boué J, Vignal P, Aubry JP, Aubry MC, Aleese JM. Ultrasound movement patterns of fetuses with chromosome anomalies. *Prenat Diagn* 1982;2:1–65.
75. De Vries JIP, Visser GHA, Prechtl HFR. The emergence of fetal behaviour III. Individual differences and consistencies. *Early Hum Dev* 1988;16:85–103.
76. Schats R, Jansen CAM, Wladimiroff JW. Embryonic heart activity: appearance and development in early human pregnancy. *Br J Obstet Gynaecol* 1990;97:989–94.
77. Wisser J, Dirschede P. Embryonic heart rate in dated human embryos. *Early Hum Dev* 1994;37:107–15.
78. Sherer DM, Nawricki MN, Peco NE, Metalay LA, Woods JR. The occurrence of simultaneous fetal heart rate accelerations in twins during non stress-testing. *Obstet Gynecol* 1990;76:817–21.
79. Despland PA, Galambos R. The auditory brain stem response (ABR): A useful diagnostic tool in the intensive care nursery. *Pediatr Res* 1980;15:154–8.
80. Read JA, Miller FC. Fetal heart rate acceleration in response to acoustic stimulation as a measure of fetal well-being. *Am J Obstet Gynecol* 1977;129:512–17.
81. Birnholz J, Benacerraf B. The development of fetal hearing. *Science* 1983;222:516–18.
82. Druzin ML, Edersheim TG, Hutson JM, Bond AL. The effect of vibroacooustic stimulation on the nonstress test at gestational ages of thirty-two weeks or less. *Am J Obstet Gynecol* 1989;161:1476–8.
83. Arabin B, Zacharias C, Riedewald S, Blucher U, Saling E. Analyse fetaler Reaktionen auf akustische Reize mit unterschiedlicher Registriertechnik. *Geburtsh Frauenheilk* 1980;49:653–7.
84. Sherer DM, Abramowicz JS, D'Amico ML, Caverly CB, Woods JR. Fetal vibratory acoustic stimulation in twin gestations with simultaneous fetal heart rate monitoring. *Am J Obstet Gynecol* 1991; 164:1104–6.
85. Arabin B, Gembruch U, van Eyck J. Intrauterine behavior. In Keith LG, Papiernik E, Keith DM, Luke B, eds. *Multiple Pregnancy – Epidemiology, Gestation & Perinatal Outcome*. New York: Parthenon, 1995:331–49.
86. Devoe LD. Simultaneous antepartum testing of twin fetal heart rates. *Southern Med J* 1985;78(4):380–3.

87. Wigglesworth JS, Singer DB, eds. *Textbook of Fetal and Perinatal Pathology*. Cambridge, MA: Blackwell Scientific Publications, 1991:221–62.
88. Rumack CM, Wilson SR, Charboneau JW, eds. *Diagnostic Ultrasound*. St. Louis, MO: Mosby Year Book, 1991:746–8.
89. Weissman A, Achiron R, Lipitz S. The first trimester growth-discordant twin: an ominous prenatal finding. *Obstet Gynecol* 1994;84:110–14.
90. Montenegro N, Matias A, Areias JC, Barros H, Nicolaides KH. Early cardiac failure as a putative pathogenic mechanism for increased nuchal translucency. *Ultrasound Obstet Gynecol* 1996;8(Suppl 1):111.
91. VilleY, Hyett J, Hecher K, Nicolaides KH. Preliminary experience with endoscopic laser surgery for severe twin–twin transfusion syndrome. *N Engl J Med* 1995;332:224–7.
92. Hecher K, Ville Y, Nicolaides KH. Doppler studies of the fetal circulation in twin–twin transfusion syndrome. *Ultrasound Obstet Gynecol* 1995;4:318–24.
93. Filly RA, Goldstein RB, Callen PW. Monochorionic twinning: sonographic assessment. *AJR Am J Roentgenol* 1990;154:459–69.
94. Abuhamad AZ, Mari G, Copel JA, Cantwell CJ, Evans AT. Umbilical artery flow velocity waveforms in monoamniotic twins with cord entanglement. *Obstet Gynecol* 1995;86:674–7.
95. Kuraucji O, Ohno Y, Mizutani S, Tomoda Y. Longitudinal monitoring of fetal behaviour in twins when one is anencephalic. *Obstet Gynecol* 1995;86:672–4.
96. Degani S, Gonen R, Shapiro I. Doppler flow velocity waveforms in fetal surveillance of twins: A prospective longitudinal study. *J Ultrasound Med* 1992;11:537–41.
97. Giles WB, Trudinger BJ, Cook CM. Umbilical artery waveforms in triplet pregnancy. *Obstet Gynecol* 1990;75:813–16.
98. Van Eyck J, Wladimiroff JW, van den Wijngaard JAGW, Noordam MJ, Prechtl HFR. The blood flow velocity waveform in the fetal internal carotid and umbilical artery. ist relationship to fetal heart rate pattern, eye and body movements in normal pregnancy. *Br J Obstet Gynecol* 1987;94:734–41.
99. Van Eyck J, Stewart PA, Wladimiroff JW. Human fetal foramen ovale flow velocity wave forms relative to behavioral state in normal term pregnancy. *Am J Obstet Gynecol* 1990;163:1239–42.
100. Romero R, Mazor M, Hobbins JC. A critical appraisal of fetal acoustic stimulation as an antenatal test for fetal well-being. *Obstet Gynecol* 1988:781–3.
101. Chasnoff I. Fetal alcohol syndrome in twin pregnancy. *Acta Genet Med Gamellol* 1985;34:229–32.
102. Cochrane Database, e-mail: update@cochrane.co.uk (Europe); tstarr@powergrid.electriciti.com (USA). Update Software, PO Box 696/Oxford OX2 7YX England.
103. de Vore GR. Internet Fetal Echocardiography, CD ROM, http://www.fetalecho.com; e-mail: fetalecho@ fetalecho.com, 1996.
104. Maeda K, Tatsumura M, Nakajima K, Ida T, Nagata N, Minagawa I. The ultrasonic Doppler fetal actocardiogram and its computer processing. *J Perinat Med* 1988;16:327–31.
105. Klaus M, Jeraululd R, Kreger N, *et al*. Maternal attachment: importance of the first postpartum days. *N Engl J Med* 1972;286:460–3.
106. Kemp VH, Page CK. Maternal prenatal attachment in normal and high risk pregnancies. *J Obstet Gynecol Neonat Nurs* 1987;16:179–84.
107. Villeneuve C, Laroche C, Lippman A, Marrache M. Psychological aspects of ultrasound imaging during pregnancy. *Can J Psychiatry* 1988;33:530–5.
108. Campbell S, Reading AE, Cox DN. Ultrasound scanning in pregnancy: the short-term psychological effects of early real time scans. *J Psychosom Obstet Gynaecol* 1982;1:57–60.
109. Langer M, Ringler M, Reinold E. Psychological effects of ultrasound examinations: Changes of body perception and child image in pregnancy. *J Psychosom Obstet Gynaecol* 1988;8:199–208.
110. Hepper PG. Fetal psychology: an embryonic science. In Nijhuis JG, ed. *Fetal Behaviour: Developmental and Perinatal Aspects*. Oxford: Oxford University Press, 1992;:130–56.
111. De Man K, Samson JF, Lafeber HN. Morbidity and mortality of neonatal intensive care unit admitted preterm infants born from multiple pregnancies, influence of in vitro fertilisation techniques. In *Course Book Genetic Epidemiology of Twins and Twinning*. Amsterdam: PAOG Amsterdam, 1994:22–3.
112. Amiel-Tison C, Maillard F, Lebrun F, *et al*. Acceleration of neurologic and physical maturity in multiple pregnancies. Presented at the *European Congress of Perinatal Medicine*, Helsinki, June 4–7, 1994.
113. Meyer R, Wolke D, Riegel K. Bedeuten Mehrlinge mehr Entwicklungsprobleme bei sehr kleinen Frühgeborenen – eine Längsschnittstudie. Presented at the *50th Congress of the German Society of Obstetrics and Gynaecology*, Munich, August 23–27, 1994.
114. Kulocvich MV, Gluck L. The lung profile II - complicated pregnancy. *Am J Obstet Gynecol* 1979;135:71–8.
115. Thomson RF, Spencer WA. Habituation: a model for the study of neuronal substrates of behavior. *Psychol Rev* 1966;73:16–43.
116. Bornstein MH. Stability in early mental development: from attention and information processing in infancy to learning and cognition in childhood. In Bornstein MH, ed. *Stability and Continuity in Mental Development*. New Jersey: Lawrence Erlbaum, 1989: 147–70.
117. Bernstein DA, Roy EJ, Wickens CD, Srull TK. *Psychology*. Boston, MA: Houghton Mifflin, 1988.
118. Resnick SM, Gottesman II, McGue MM. Sensation seeking in opposite-sex twins: An effect of prenatal hormones? *Behav Genet* 1993;23(4):323–9.
119. Zuckerman M, EyseneckS BG, Eyseneck HJ. Sensation seeking in England and America: Cross-cultural, age and sex comparisons. *J Consult Clin Psychol* 1978;46:139–49.
120. Sokol DK, Moore CA, Rose RJ, Williams CJ, Reed T, Christian JC. Intrapair differences in personality and cognitive ability among young monozygotic twins distinguished by chorion type. *Behav Genet* 1995;25(5):457–66.
121. Aardenburg R, van Eyck J, Arabin B. Systematic antenatal functional evaluation (SAFE) for prematurity in multiple pregnancies: Comparison of predictive values of biophysical, clinical and biochemical parameters. *Ultrasound Obstet Gynecol* 1996; 8(Suppl 1):120.
122. Farr V. Prognosis for the babies, early and late. In McGillary I, Nylander PPS, Corney G, eds. *Human Multiple Reproduction*. Philadelphia, PA: W.B. Saunders, 1975:188–211.

153 Invasive antenatal interventions in complicated multiple pregnancies

L. Lewi, E. Gratacos and J. Deprest

Abstract

Multiple pregnancies still pose challenging problems in modern obstetrics. Monochorionic (MC) multiple pregnancies have received much interest recently as they indeed are at much higher risk than dichorionic multiplets. Some complications can be treated today by sonoendoscopic interventions on the placenta and umbilical cord. Fetoscopic laser coagulation of vascular anastomoses has recently been shown to be the best first-line treatment for severe twin-to-twin transfusion syndrome. In selected indications, fetoscopic or ultrasound-guided cord coagulation can be offered and is an effective technique for selective feticide in MC twins, albeit with still considerably higher fetal loss rates as compared to selective feticide by KCl injection in dichorionic twins. Long-term outcome of these procedures seems good. The place of surgical interventions for other indications, such as some forms of selective intrauterine growth restrictions in MC twins, has not been established yet.

Twins have a more complicated *in utero* stay than singletons. Also, management is complicated by the fact that more than one fetus has to be taken into account and varies according to chorionicity. About 30% of twins are monozygotic and 70% dizygotic. Dizygotic twins result from the fertilization of two different eggs. By definition, dizygotic twins are therefore dichorionic and diamniotic (Figure 153.1). Monozygotic twins result from the fertilization of a single egg followed by early division into two cell masses, which further develop separately. In 30%, cleavage occurs prior to the third day postfertilization resulting in dichorionic diamniotic twins, whereas in 70% splitting takes place after the third day, resulting in MC twins in its different manifestations.

Correct and timely determination of chorionicity is paramount to appreciate the risks and correctly manage multiple pregnancies. Ultrasound is highly accurate when performed in the first trimester (Figure 153.2).[1] MC multiplets run the highest risk of complications and the well-being of one fetus crucially depends on that of the other(s) because of the almost ever-present vascular anastomoses in the common placenta (Figure 153.3).[2] These vascular anastomoses can cause significant blood volume shifts between the fetuses, leading to complications such as twin-to-twin transfusion syndrome (TTTS), acute exsanguination of the survivor in the fetoplacental unit at the time of demise of its co-twin, as well as in the presence of large intertwin arterio-arterial (AA) anastomoses, for instance, in case of selective intrauterine growth restriction (sIUGR), or in its extreme form, the twin reversed arterial perfusion (TRAP). Sonoendoscopic surgery on the placenta and the umbilical cord today plays an important role in the treatment of certain complicated MC multiple pregnancies and has acquired an established place in modern fetal medicine.[3] TTTS affects about 10–15% of MC twins and fetoscopic laser treatment of the vascular anastomoses is currently the best treatment available.[4] For selective feticide in MC multiple pregnancies, the conventional method of potassium chloride injection into the target fetus' circulation is unsuitable because the toxic drug may embolize to the healthy fetus(es). Furthermore, patent anastomoses can trigger acute exsanguination of the surviving fetus into the demised fetus' circulation[5] Therefore, minimally invasive techniques have been developed to separate and occlude the sacrificed fetus' circulation completely and permanently.[6] The presence of vascular anastomoses in the single placenta seems to be the basis of many complications, and it seems logical to apply experience with the above techniques in other complicated MC twins. At this moment, however, such therapies remain experimental and should be restricted to expert centers and within strict protocols.

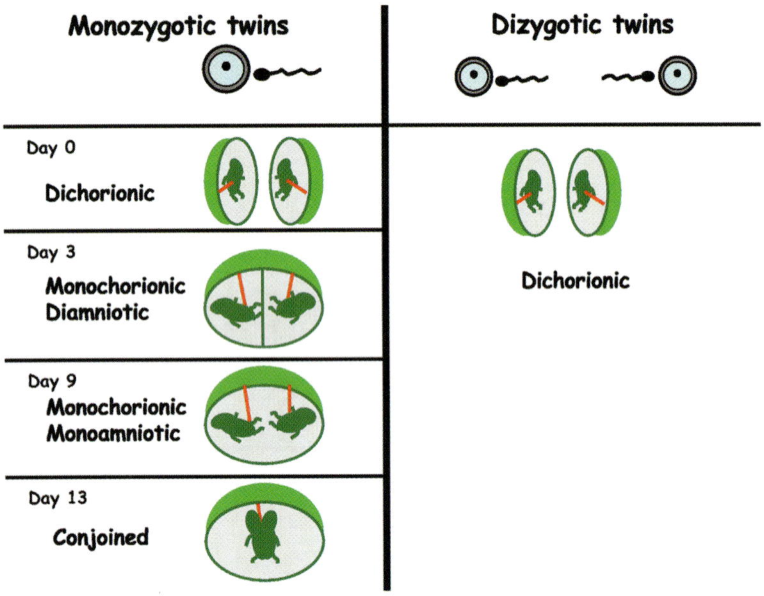

Figure 153.1 Zygosity and chorionicity in twin pregnancies.

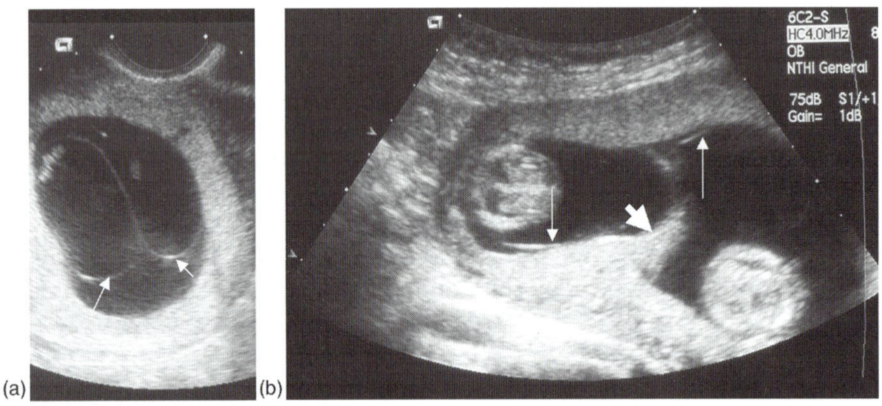

Figure 153.2 Chorionicity determination in the first-trimester ultrasound scan. (a) Monochorionic diamniotic twins: only two thin amniotic membranes (arrows) separate the two fetuses. (b) Dichorionic diamniotic twins: the fetuses are separated by three layers (amnion, chorion–chorion, amnion; arrows).

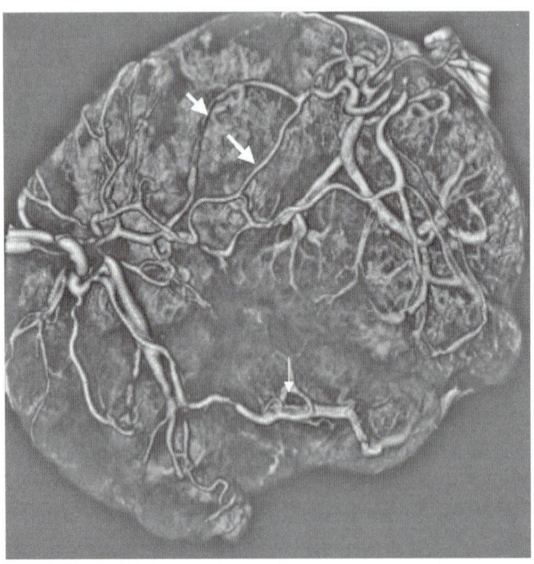

Figure 153.3 3D reconstruction of a CT angiogram of a monochorionic placenta at term, showing an equal distribution of the injected placental mass and a large arterio-arterial and veno-venous superficial anastomosis (arrows). Photo in collaboration with the Department of Radiology, M. Cannie, UZ Leuven, Belgium.

Fetoscopic laser treatment for twin-to-twin transfusion syndrome

Introduction

In most MC multiple pregnancies, interfetal transfusion is a constant but usually balanced phenomenon. However, in about 10–15%, a chronic imbalance in net flow develops, resulting in TTTS. The donor twin becomes hypovolemic, resulting in oliguria and oligohydramnios, which leads to the typical 'stuck twin' sequence on ultrasound. Hypervolemia, polyuria and polyhydramnios evolve in the recipient twin, who can develop circulatory overload and hydrops. TTTS typically occurs between 15 and 26 weeks and is a sonographic diagnosis based on the following criteria (www.eurofoetus.org):

- Polyhydramnios in the sac of the recipient twin (defined as the deepest vertical pocket of ≥ 8 cm prior to 20 weeks and ≥ 10 cm between 20 and 26 weeks) with signs of polyuria (distended bladder).

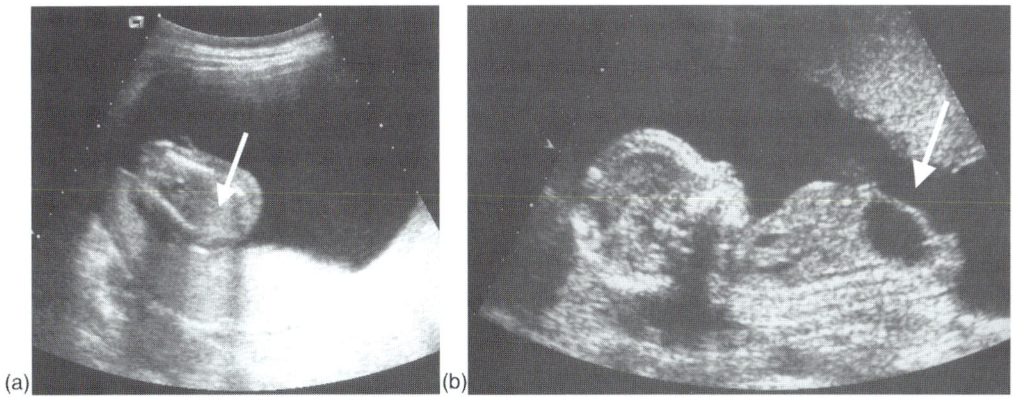

Figure 153.4 Ultrasound image of TTTS. (a) The donor is stuck to the uterine wall without bladder filling. (b) There is polyhydramnios in the sac of the recipient, who has a distended bladder.

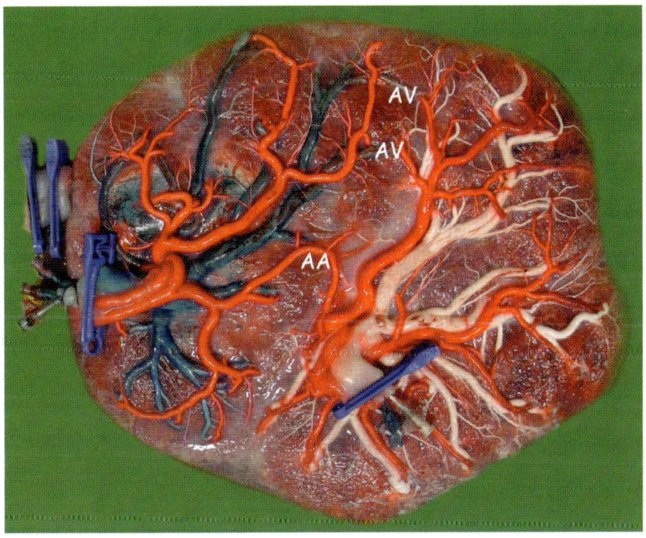

Figure 153.5 Macroscopic image after dye injection of a monochorionic placenta. (a) Superficial AA and deep AV anastomosis. (b) AV and oppositely directed VA anastomosis.

- Oligohydramnios in the donor's sac (the deepest vertical pocket ≤2 cm) with signs of oliguria (small or empty bladder) (Figure 153.4).

The diagnosis is made by ultrasound only; discordant growth may be present, but is not a prerequisite.

The pathophysiology of TTTS is usually explained on an angioarchitectural basis. Placental anastomoses can be AA, arterio-venous (AV or VA) and veno-venous (VV) or a combination of these types.[7] AA and VV anastomoses are typically superficial, bidirectional anastomoses on the surface of the chorionic plate, forming direct communications between the arteries and veins of the two fetal circulations. AV anastomoses occur at the capillary level, deep within a shared cotyledon, receiving arterial supply from one twin and providing venous drainage to the other twin. The supplying artery and draining vein of the AV anastomosis can be visualized on the placental surface, piercing the chorionic plate at close proximity to each other to supply the shared cotyledon, which may receive other vessels too (Figure 153.5). AV anastomoses allow flow in one direction only, and hence can create an imbalance in the interfetal transfusion leading to TTTS, unless balanced by an oppositely directed transfusion through other (superficial or deep) anastomoses.

Untreated, severe mid-gestational TTTS has a mortality rate of nearly 100%. Polyhydramnios may lead to spontaneous abortion, rupture of the membranes and/or extreme preterm delivery. It may also have a direct effect on fetal hemodynamics and placental function. *In utero* fetal death (IUFD) may result from cardiac failure in the recipient or poor perfusion in the donor, which may lead to acute, agonal or postmorten intertwin transfusion into the dead fetus. Additionally, there are substantial risks of cerebral and cardiac sequelae in survivors due to the chronic or acute hemodynamic imbalance. Initially, only serial amnioreduction was available as a treatment option to reduce the polyhydramnios and intrauterine pressure, thus alleviating symptoms and prolonging pregnancy. Repeated amnioreduction is a simple and widely available technique, but it does not address the vascular basis of TTTS. The anastomoses remain patent maintaining the pathologic chronic transfusion process or, in the event of single IUFD, allow acute interfetal transfusion, putting the surviving twin at high risk of IUFD, anemia and neurological damage. Vascular anastomoses can in most cases be visualized on the chorionic surface during fetoscopy, and their coagulation would therefore be a causative treatment. A recent randomized trial set up by the Eurofoetus research consortium comparing serial amnioreduction vs. laser coagulation for severe TTTS prior to 26 weeks showed that laser had significantly better outcome in terms of survival of at least one twin (76% vs. 51%), gestational age (GA) at delivery (33.3 vs. 29.0 weeks) and neurological damage (6% vs. 14%),).[4] Laser, therefore, appears to be a better first-line treatment than amnioreduction.

Technique of laser coagulation

Hardware

Today good-quality videoendoscopic hardware is a given, including a high-quality light fountain, lightweight video camera and monitor. For fetoscopic operations, some extra investments are needed, such as a range of purpose-designed fetoscopes and adapted sheaths, long light cables and a twin camera system mixing ultrasound and endoscopic images may be helpful. Further, appropriate energy sources are needed to coagulate the vessels of interest. Laser energy sources with specific absorbance in the red are preferred, such as Nd:YAG (minimal power requirements 60–100 W) or diode (minimal power requirements 30–60 W), which typically comes with bare fibers of 400–600 μm. For intrafetal or cord electro-coagulation, a conventional electrosurgical generator can be used.

Fetoscopic endoscopes differ from their hysteroscopic or laparoscopic counterparts but are delivered by the same suppliers. At present, there is no evidence that one particular brand or even type of endoscope performs better than another. Intuitively, one strives for a combination of minimal diameter, appropriate length and maximal light transmission and resolution. Personal preference, local factors such as after sales-service and compatibility with other operation room equipment will influence the choice of the manufacturer. In Europe, considerable investments have been made by the European Commission in its 'Biomed 2 Programme' for instrument development by a partner of the Eurofoetus research consortium (Karl Storz Endoskope).[8] Thanks to this project, a range of 20–30 cm fetoscopes with diameters of 1.0–2.3 mm are now available (Figure 153.6).[9] The majority are semiflexible 0° fiberoptic scopes, which can be curved, e.g. to direct the scope toward an anterior located placenta.[10] Rod lens telescopes have also been fabricated, with angles of inclination up to 30°, with an associated deflecting mechanism for the laser fiber. Steerable fiberscopes have also been used for an anterior placenta;[11,12] however, image quality is not optimal because of poor light transmission (unpublished observations). A double-access method with side firing fibers has also been reported in that case. All scopes are used within a sheath, housing the endoscope and any additional instrument such as a laser fiber or other. Fibers are usually inserted through an additional working channel, which keep the fiber in a stable position. Luer lock connections allow irrigation or drainage of fluid.

To gain entry, the sheath can either be introduced directly or through a cannula. For direct introduction, the sheath is loaded with its accompanying trocar. The sheath is inserted into the amniotic cavity under ultrasound guidance and once inside, the trocar is removed and replaced by the fetoscope. During the procedure, the sheath can be moved back and forward – causing friction at the membrane–myometrium interface, but cannot be withdrawn without losing access to the amniotic cavity. The use of formal cannulas obviates this problem, as the port remains during the entire procedure and instruments and scopes can be interchanged numerous times. We ourselves use teflon cannulas, which are thin-walled and therefore add only 0.3 mm to the external diameter of the sheath, are semiflexible to accommodate curved instruments and come in a variety of diameters with purpose-developed fitting trocars.[9] There are currently no data available to support either the direct or cannula access method to the amniotic cavity. Further technical details on endoscopes and ancillary equipment are available in more recent handbooks on fetal therapy.[13–15]

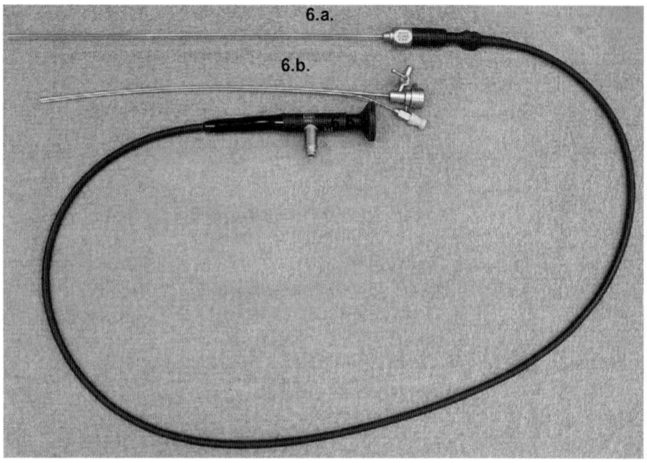

Figure 153.6 Example of fetoscopic instruments as used for laser coagulation of the vascular anastomoses in TTTS. (a) Straight forward telescope, diameter 2 mm, length 30 cm, with remote eyepiece (Karl Storz, Tuttlingen, Germany). (b) Fetoscopic sheath with channel for laser fibers up to 600 μm with one stopcock and one luer-lock adaptor (Karl Storz).

Procedure

Preoperatively, in our institution, all patients receive 2 g cefazolin i.v. and 20 mg slow release nifedipin postoperatively (PO), which will be continued for 48 h. Laser coagulation is performed by percutaneous approach (Figure 153.7) through a 3-mm incision under local or locoregional anesthesia and under strict aseptic conditions. The position of the fetuses, umbilical cord insertions and placenta is mapped by ultrasound scan. A skin incision is made the size of the sheath, and under ultrasound guidance the cannula or fetoscopic sheath is inserted into the hydramniotic sac (Figure 153.8). At all times, the placenta, fetal parts, maternal vessels and bowel are avoided. We personally use, in addition, transplacental sedation of the fetus while administering remifentanyl to the mother, which is a short-acting agent.[16]

In TTTS, fetoscopic detection of the anastomoses is improved by the presence of polyhydramnios. The amniotic fluid is normally clear by dilution and its volume flattens the placenta. Occasionally though vision may be hampered by blood (from previous procedures or bleeding) or debris. In these instances, amnioexchange with warmed Hartmann's solution heated by a blood warmer or a special amnioirrigator[17] can improve visibility. Three fixed landmarks are used to identify any anastomosing vessels: the intertwin membrane, the recipient's and the donor's cord insertion. The intertwin septum and its placental insertion are easily identified as a white line (Figure 153.9). From there, blood vessels leaving the donor usually cross under the septum in the direction of the recipient. These blood vessels are followed to identify any anastomosing vessels. Importantly, the vascular equator does usually not coincide with the intertwin septum and cannot be predicted by simple determination of the cord insertions. Alternatively, vessels can also be followed starting from the recipient's or donor's cord insertion. The purpose of the procedure is to visualize the entire vascular equator and to coagulate *all* anastomoses. A 'hyperselective' approach, as discussed by Machin *et al.*[18] – coagulating only the causative AV anastomosis – is probably wishful thinking and not at all used in the European centers practicing laser coagulation. Any residual anastomoses put the remaining fetuses at risk of hypovolemic events in case of single IUFD and may even lead to persistence or reversal of transfusion. Arteries are distinguishable from veins, as they have a darker color due to the deoxygenated blood. Also, arteries usually cross over the veins.

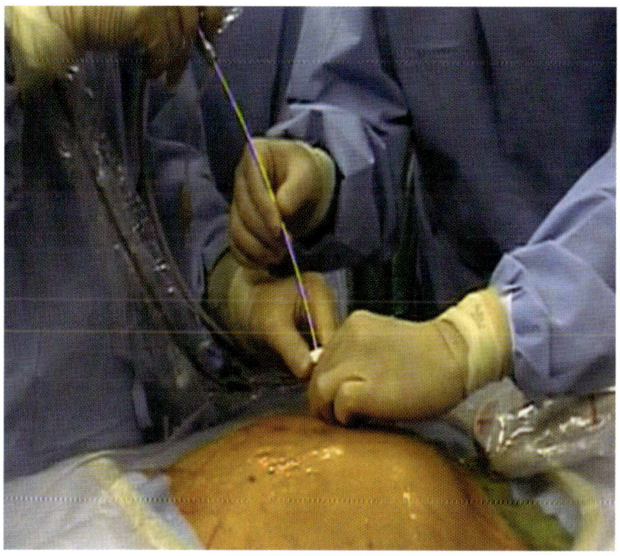

Figure 153.7 Image of the operative setup and percutaneous access used for fetoscopic interventions.

Occasionally, it may be impossible to determine whether vessels anastomose or not, due to the position of the intertwin septum, placenta, fetus or other physical limitations. In these instances, the vessels with uncertain course are coagulated as well. Also, with an anterior placenta, the amniotic sac as well as the vessels on the placenta may be more difficult to access. As mentioned above, instruments for anterior placentas have been purpose-developed, but it is yet unclear whether this improves performance. So far, similar outcomes have been reported for anterior and posterior located placentas.

Coagulation is performed at a distance of approximately 1 cm and ideally at a 90° angle, using a non-touch technique (Figure 153.10). Sections of about 1 cm are coagulated with shots of about 3–4 s, according to tissue response. Laser energy is adapted to the source used, the diameter of the vessels and the tissue response. Typically, a Nd:YAG laser is set at 50–70 W

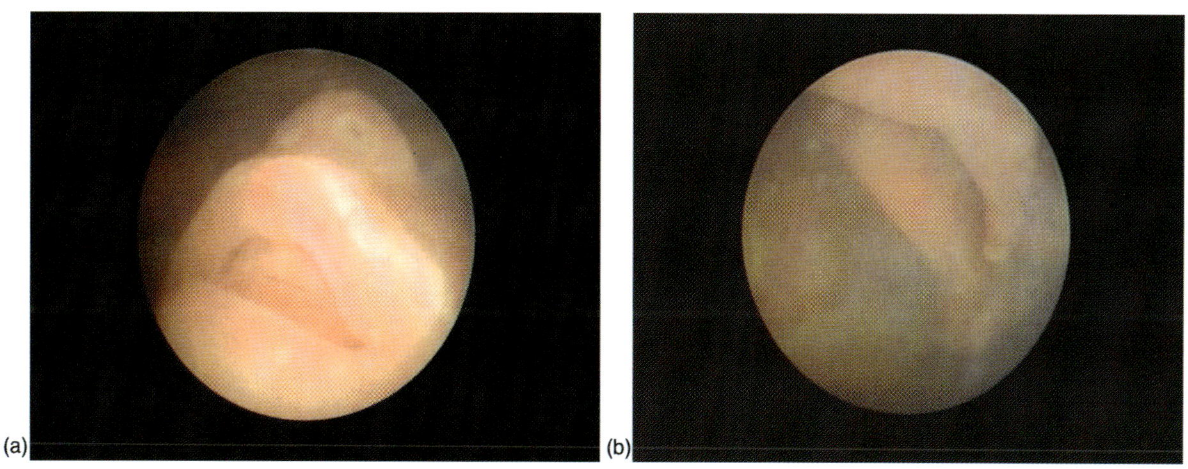

Figure 153.8 (a) Fetoscopic image of the face of the recipient, who moves freely in the hydramniotic sac. (b) Fetoscopic image of the feet of the donor, who is stuck behind the intertwin septum.

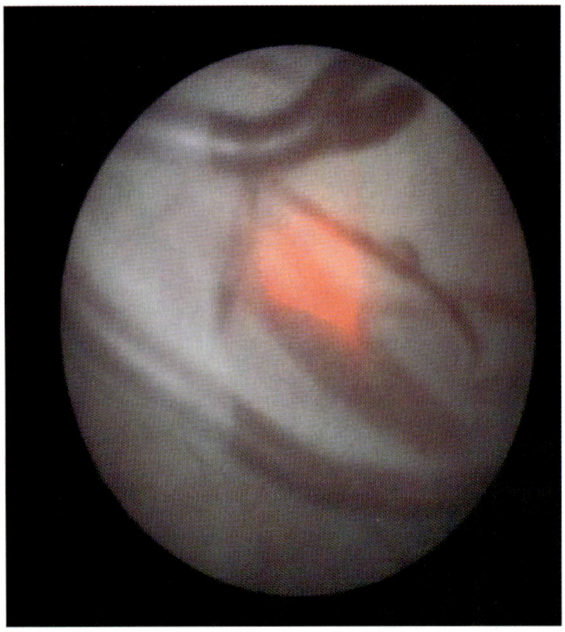

Figure 153.9 Fetoscopic image of the intertwin septum inserting on the chorionic surface with the donor's vessels crossing underneath.

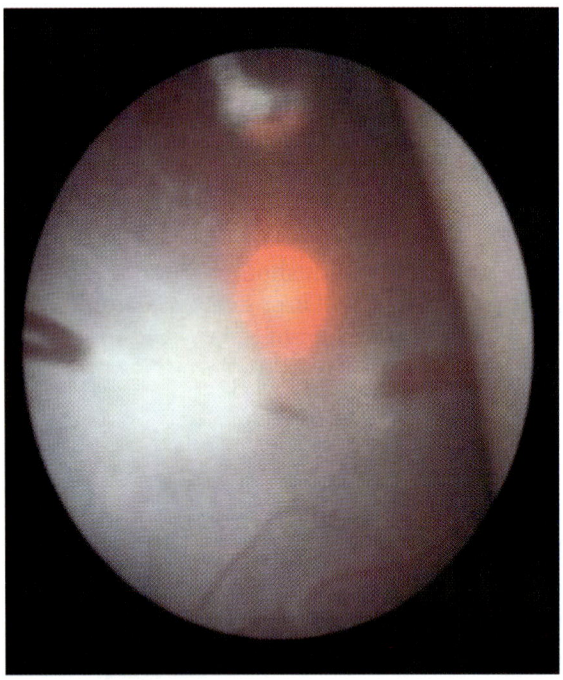

Figure 153.10 (a) Fetoscopic image of a coagulated AV anastosomosis.

and a diode laser at 30–40 W. Large vessels can be coagulated from various angles to obtain progressive narrowing and eventual coagulation. The use of excessive laser power levels should be avoided, as this may cause vessel perforation and fetal hemorrhage. Once all vessels are coagulated, the vascular equator is followed once more to ascertain that all anastomoses have indeed been fully coagulated and that flow has not resumed.

The procedure is completed by amnioreduction until normal amniotic fluid pockets are seen on ultrasound scan. The cannula or sheath is removed under ultrasound guidance to detect any significant bleeding from the uterine wall. In continental Europe, the patient remains as an in-patient for 48 h. Blood pressure, pulse, temperature and fluid balance are monitored. Ultrasound scan is repeated the first and second days to document fetal viability, Dopplers, amniotic fluid volume and bladder filling. Cefazolin is repeated every 8 h for 24 h and the patient stays on nifedepin PO 12-hourly for 48 h.

Hecher *et al.* demonstrated a learning curve, with improving results in terms of survival as well as neurologic outcome over time. We have seen the number of patients developing preterm prelabor rupture of the membranes (PPROM), a strong predictor of preterm delivery, and hence morbidity, dropping with experience. This argues against scattering the experience over too many centers.[19]

Risks and outcome of the procedure

In contrast to amnioreduction, where IUFD of one or both fetuses often occurs remotely from the procedure, most IUFD with laser are diagnosed within 48 h. In our experience with our first 100 cases, this happens in 18% and affects the donor as often as the recipient. The cause of these deaths remains largely unexplained, although it is generally assumed that too little placental mass may remain after laser for both fetuses to survive.[20] However, preliminary data suggest that preoperative MRI accurately predicts placental distribution in TTTS and that postoperative IUFD is not restricted to the fetus with the smallest placental mass.[21] Further research is therefore needed into the exact cause of these losses yet attempting to prevent these. Nonetheless, the surviving twin appears far less likely to be anemic after laser[22] or to sustain neurological sequelae[23,24] compared to survivors after amnioreduction where the anastomoses remain patent.

Another important fetal risk is preterm delivery. In the Eurofoetus research consortium trial (RCT), median GA at delivery was higher in the laser than in the amnioreduction group (33.3 vs. 29.0 weeks' gestation), with 42% and 69% women, respectively, delivering prior to 32 weeks. However, PPROM remains the most important complication of invasive antenatal procedures, accounting for a high morbidity and mortality if the membranes rupture prior to viability. In our own experience of the first 100 cases, PPROM within 5 weeks of the procedure occurred in 16%. The overall incidence of PPROM (<37 weeks) was 45% with median GA at delivery of 30 weeks in cases with PPROM as compared to 35 weeks in those without PPROM group. Amniotic fluid volume drained, cervical shortening or prior procedures may be contributing to that risk. The intra-amniotic injection of platelets and clotting factors may be a successful technique to treat cases of early postoperative PPROM.[25,26] Other rare fetal complications include congenital skin loss, gangrenous limb lesions, microphthalmia and intestinal atresia.[27,28] These anomalies have been described in TTTS not treated by laser[29] and can therefore also originate from the disease process itself.

The neurological infant outcome in laser for TTTS may be determined by the severity of the disease, the GA at delivery and the procedure. In the Eurofoetus RCT, infants in the amnioreduction group had higher incidences of cystic periventricular leukomalacia (laser: 6% vs. amniodrainage: 14%), in particular the recipients. Presently, the children are being followed until 2 years of age and these results are eagerly awaited. A recent long-term follow-up study of children surviving an uncontrolled series managed by laser (age between 14 and 44 months of age) observed major neurological problems in 11% of survivors.[30]

Maternal safety remains a priority, and serious maternal complications should be registered carefully in a registry, such as the one set up by Eurofoetus.[3] Transient maternal mirror or Ballantyne syndrome with pulmonary edema, placental abruption, chorioamnionitis and bleeding requiring transfusion are reported, but none yet leading to maternal death. In the Eurofoetus RCT, there was no severe maternal morbidity (no woman required ICU admission or blood transfusion), although three placental abruptions occurred at the end of the amnioreduction (two in the drainage and one in the laser group); all requiring immediate delivery. Infection is another potential problem. In our study on fertility and pregnancy outcome in a consecutive series of 100 patients, fetoscopic interventions did not appear to influence future fertility and pregnancy outcome.[31]

Selective feticide in multiple pregnancies

Introduction

The indications, technique and outcome of selective feticide in complicated multiple pregnancies crucially depend on an exact chorionicity determination in the first trimester. In MC multiple pregnancies, selective feticide may be contemplated for several indications: (1) a severe discordant structural or chromosomal anomaly, (2) severe discordant growth with high risk of IUFD, (3) TRAP and (4) severe TTTS with associated discordant anomaly or where inspection of the chorionic plate was precluded by the position of the fetus and placenta. In contrast, in dichorionic twins, selective feticide is restricted to the management of discordant structural or chromosomal anomalies.

Structural anomalies are more common in twins. Unfortunately, most studies have not related their incidence to zygosity or chorionicity. Nonetheless, it seems that in dizygotic twins the rate per fetus is the same as in singletons, whereas in the monozygotic twins the rate is two to three times higher.[32] Even in MC twins, in more than 80% of cases, only one fetus is affected.[33] The exact mechanism of this increased prevalence remains unknown.

In dizygotic twins, the age-related risk of chromosomal abnormalities for one twin is independent of the risk for the other and should be the same as in singletons. Therefore, the risk of at least one fetus, e.g. having Down's syndrome should theoretically be double that in singletons. In contrast, all MC twins are monozygotic and the risk for chromosomal abnormalities should therefore be the same as for singletons and in the vast majority both fetuses are equally affected. Nonetheless, discordance in MC twins for nearly all common human aneuploidies (trisomy 13,[34] trisomy 21,[35] monosomy 45,X[35]) has been reported, most cases involving one twin with Turner syndrome and the other with either a female or male phenotype but usually a mozaic karyotype. This rare phenomenon is called heterokaryotypic monozygotism; going into its exact genetics mechanisms would lead us to far. Our series of selective feticide includes five such cases of discordant chromosomes in MC twins (46,XY/47,XY,+21; 46,XX/47,XX,+13; 46,XY/45,X; two cases of 46,XX/45,X).[36] Heterokaryotic MC twins can only be diagnosed prenatally if an amniocentesis is performed of both amniotic sacs, which is recommended in the event of discordant anomalies in MC twins.[35]

There are essentially three management options for discordant structural and chromosomal anomalies: conservative management, selective feticide or termination of the entire pregnancy. For anomalies that are non-lethal but may well result in serious handicap, parents must thus decide whether the burden of a handicapped child is enough to risk the loss of the healthy twin from feticide-related complications. For lethal anomalies in dichorionic twins, it may be best to avoid such risk and conservative management is preferable, unless the condition threatens the well-being of the healthy co-twin. Such a dilemma is illustrated by twins discordant for anencephaly, which is always lethal but due to associated polyhydramnios places the healthy co-twin at risk of severe preterm delivery. While in dichorionic twins expectant management may be preferable for anomalies with a high risk of *in utero* demise, in MC twins this specifically warrants selective feticide. In dichorionic twins, single IUFD is associated with perinatal death or handicap of the surviving twin in 5–10%, and that is largely due to extreme preterm delivery. In contrast, single IUFD in MC twins has a co-twin IUFD rate of 10–25% and antenatal cerebral lesions in 25–45% of surviving twins, due to acute exsanguination in the fetoplacental unit of the dead twin, which adds to the effects of extreme preterm delivery.[37,38]

An extreme manifestation of TTTS is TRAP, which complicates about 1% of MC twin pregnancies. In TRAP, blood flows from an umbilical artery of the pump twin in a reverse direction into the umbilical artery of the perfused twin, via an AA anastomosis. The perfused twin's blood supply is by definition deoxygenated and results in variable degrees of deficient development of the head, heart and upper limb structures. Two criteria seem to be necessary for the development of a TRAP sequence. The first is an AA anastomosis and the second a discordant development[39] or an IUFD[40] in one of the MC twins, allowing for reversal of blood flow. The increased burden to perfuse the parasitic twin puts the pump twin at risk for congestive heart failure and hydrops.[41] Because of the rarity of the disorder, the natural history of antenatally diagnosed cases is still poorly documented with reported survival rates for the pump twin varying between 14%[42] and 90%.[43] Data on long-term outcome are not available, although the risk of cardiac and neurodevelopmental sequelae may be high due to hemodynamic imbalances *in utero*.[44,45] Prediction of outcome of TRAP diagnosed is challenging, particularly early in pregnancy. Several parameters have been suggested to indicate poor prognosis such as a high acardiac/pump weight ratio,[46] a rapid increase in the acardiac mass[47] and small differences in the umbilical artery Doppler values.[48,49] These parameters were mostly studied in late second and third trimesters, and do not necessary apply in the early second trimester, where spontaneous resolution as well as sudden, yet unpredictable death of the pump twin have been observed. Early intervention is an issue, as the diagnosis is now usually made at an early stage in pregnancy and the techniques are available. Early prophylactic intervention may preclude the technical difficulties of achieving arrest of flow in larger and often hydropic acardiac masses, as well as cardiac failure. Some may therefore prefer to offer prophylactic, minimally invasive intervention if no spontaneous arrest of flow has occurred by 16 weeks, recognizing the pump twin may survive without any intervention in at least half of cases. It is unlikely whether a more expectant rather than an aggressive prophylactic attitude will ever be shown to be superior, given the rarity of the condition.

For the treatment of TTTS, selective feticide has been proposed, merely to try to salvage one twin.[50,51] The rationale is that laser coagulation has such a high risk of IUFD of one twin that it acts as a selective feticide. Therefore, cord occlusion may appear an alternative, as it is technically easier to perform and may better protect the surviving twin. This approach is at least open for debate, as this will by definition at best yield a 50% survival rate, given no complications occur. It necessarily leads to some difficult decisions. Not only does it pose a tremendous strain on the parents to give up a structurally normal fetus, but also it may not always be easy to determine which fetus will have the worst prognosis. Initially, it was thought to be the donor, especially if abnormal umbilical artery Dopplers were present, but these can normalize after occlusion of the recipient's cord. Access to the donor is also technically more challenging and recipients appear to be at higher risk of neurological[4] and cardiac sequelae.[52] As laser can salvage fetuses at all stages of the disease, advanced disease is not an indication.[20] In our opinion therefore, fetoscopic laser coagulation remains the preferred first-line treatment available in Europe, and selective feticide should be restricted to highly selected and exceptional cases. The place of selective feticide in sIUGR will be discussed further on.

Technique and outcome of selective feticide in dichorionic twins

Selective feticide in dichorionic twins is performed by intracardiac or intrafunicular injection of potassium chloride under ultrasound guidance. It is of utmost importance to ascertain that the correct fetus is terminated by identification of gender differences, obvious structural anomalies, placental localizations and cord insertions. The risks of selective termination are loss of the entire pregnancy and premature delivery. The overall loss rate reported by the international selective feticide registry of 402 multiple pregnancies including some higher-order multiple pregnancies is 7.5%. Preterm delivery before 33 weeks occurred in 22%, with 6% delivering between 25 and 28 weeks.[53] One center with 200 selective feticides reported an overall loss rate of only 4%, with 16% of patients delivering before 32 weeks.[54] This underscores the importance of the procedure being performed by experienced hands, just as for any other invasive procedure. In order to reduce loss rates, it has also been proposed to defer selective feticide to 28–32 weeks, which is obviously only an option in countries where late termination is legal and may be emotionally more difficult to accept for both parents and doctors. In a series on 23 dichorionic twins with non-lethal anomaly, there were no fetal losses and all patients delivered beyond 35 weeks.[55]

Technique and outcome of selective feticide in MC twins

As mentioned above, for selective feticide in MC multiple pregnancies, the conventional techniques of potassium chloride injection cannot be used. Therefore, minimally invasive techniques have been proposed to arrest and isolate the target twin's circulation completely and permanently,[6] although all have considerably higher risks for fetal loss as compared to the injection of potassium chloride.

Currently, the preferred method for selective feticide in MC multiple pregnancies is cord occlusion by either laser/bipolar coagulation. The initially reported method of umbilical cord embolization using a variety of agents is no longer recommended because of failure rates of > 60%,[6,56] probably due to incomplete vascular obliteration or migration of the toxic products to the co-twin. Fetoscopic cord ligation is already a historical technique, although it does cause immediate, complete and permanent interruption of both arterial and venous flow. Despite the fact that co-twin survival rates are over 70% when done fetoscopically, it is a quite cumbersome technique with a high risk for PPROM.[57] In contrast, fetoscopic laser coagulation of the umbilical cord is a simple technique, which is similar to fetoscopic coagulation of the vascular anastomoses in TTTS. It has been performed as early as 16 weeks, using a double-needle loaded with a 1 millimeter fetoscope and a 400 μm laser fiber.[58] The procedure allows optimal visual control but may fail beyond 20 weeks because of increasing size of the umbilical cord vessels.[59] Ultrasound-guided bipolar cord coagulation was therefore introduced for selective feticide at later gestational ages. In our institution, we primarily use laser coagulation prior to 21 weeks GA. Later on, we may attempt laser coagulation, but in over 75% of bipolar cases will be needed between 21 and 26 weeks, which can be used even later on.[60]

The pre- and postoperative care and access method are similar to those described for laser coagulation of the vascular anastomoses in TTTS. At all times, a double setup for fetoscopic laser and ultrasound-guided bipolar coagulation is prepared. The site of port insertion is chosen according to the position of the placenta, the amniotic sac of the target fetus and its umbilical cord. Preferentially, entry is in the sac of the target fetus to avoid direct interference with the other sac in case of PPROM. Whenever necessary, amniodrainage or amnioinfusion with warmed Hartmann's solution at 38°C is performed to reduce or expand the working space around the target cord and/or to improve endoscopic vision.

Laser coagulation is performed by an Nd:YAG laser or diode laser with bare fibers of 600 μm. The cord is coagulated over a distance of 5–10 cm, using a non-touch technique in continuous mode (Figure 153.11). Absence of flow is interrogated by color Doppler. Septostomy can be performed by laser when direct access to the target sac is not possible and laser coagulation through the intertwin septum fails (Figure 153.12). Bipolar coagulation is performed with a 3.0 or 2.4 mm forceps, according to the cord diameter (Karl Storz). Under ultrasound guidance, a portion of the umbilical cord is grasped at the abdominal wall, at its placental insertion or any other appropriate place

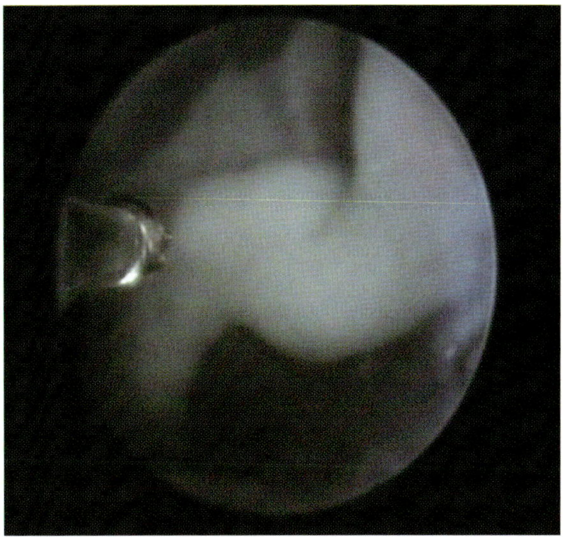

Figure 153.11 Fetoscopic image of laser cord coagulation.

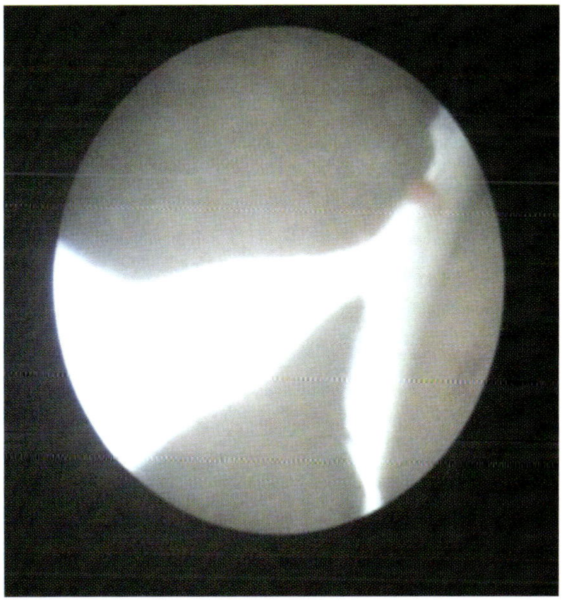

Figure 153.12 Fetoscopic image of the hole in the intertwin septum after septostomy by laser.

as to ensure correct identification and enhance stability (Figure 153.13). Direct contact with the placenta, fetus or membranes is avoided. To improve visual control, a new 'optical' forceps is being evaluated within the Eurofoetus project that combines the advantages of bipolar coagulation and fetoscopy. Coagulation starts at power settings of 15 W applied for approximately 15 s with progressive increments of 2–5 W until the appearance of turbulence and steam bubbles indicative of local heat production and hence eventual tissue coagulation between the forceps' blades (usually between 25 and 45 W). Higher initial energy settings are avoided to prevent tissue

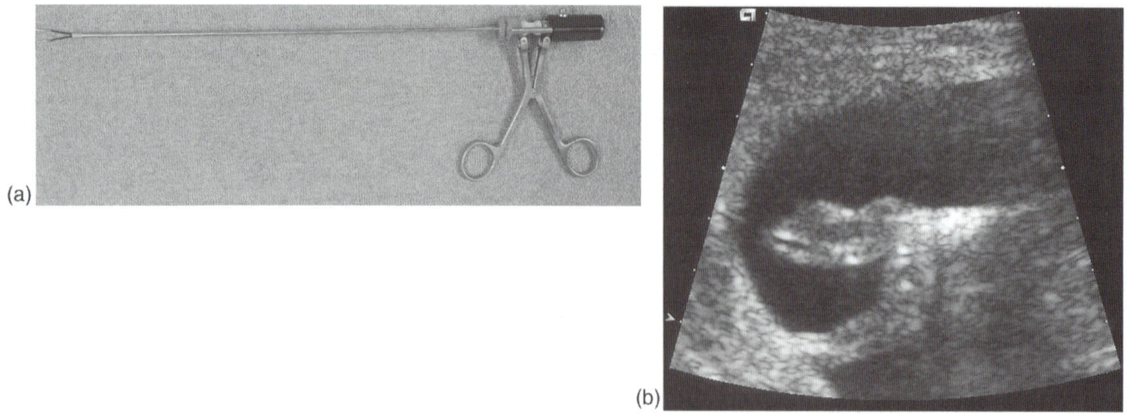

Figure 153.13 (a) Reusable 2.4-mm bipolar forceps (Karl Storz). (b) Ultrasound image of the bipolar forceps grasping the umbilical cord at its placental inertion.

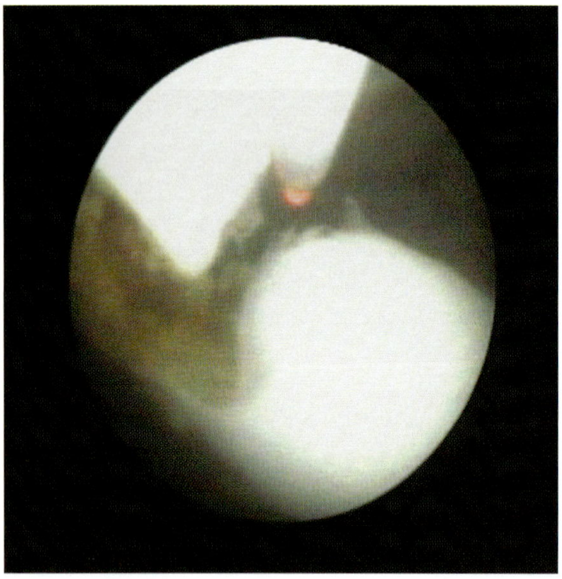

Figure 153.14 Fetoscopic image of a cord transection by laser in contact mode after selective feticide in monoamniotic twins.

carbonization, which may lead to the cord becoming stuck to the forceps' blades and eventual cord perforation. Confirmation of arrest of flow is performed after the forceps is freed from the umbilical cord by gentle manipulation. Even if there is no longer any visible flow, two additional cord segments (preferentially at a site more proximal toward the target fetus) are coagulated. This is an additional safety precaution, because absence of Doppler flow may be caused by temporary vasospasm rather than by true vascular obliteration. In monoamniotic twins, to avoid later cord entanglement, the cord is first coagulated and then transected with laser in contact mode (Figure 153.14). After completion of the procedure, amniodrainage of excessive fluid is carried out before removal of the cannula. Middle cerebral artery Dopplers are performed postoperatively to detect fetal anemia.

In our initial 10 cases, two patients had PPROM and underwent a termination. The other eight patients delivered at a mean gestation age of 35 weeks, i.e. more than 15 weeks after the procedure.[56] Later Nicolini *et al.* reported their experience with 17 cases.[61] The survival rate was 81% (13/16 survivors; one patient had TOP because of an abnormality diagnosed later on). There was one fetal hemorrhage caused by cord perforation, which may be avoided by not applying too much energy. We reported the outcome of 50 consecutive cord coagulations in complicated MC multiplets (including four triplets) by laser and/or bipolar coagulation performed between 16 and 28 weeks (mean 21 weeks).[62] Indications were TRAP (38%), discordant anomaly (38%), severe TTTS (20%) and selective IUGR (4%). In 75%, laser was used as the primary energy, but additional bipolar was necessary in about half of the cases. Overall survival was 75% with normal outcome (range: 1–36 months, 63% follow-up), except for one child with mild developmental delay born after PPROM < 28 weeks GA. Persistent PPROM < 30 weeks occurred in 25%, and if < 25 weeks, was associated with a mortality of 80%. There were no serious maternal complications, except for one mild transient mirror or Ballantyne syndrome. To avoid the risks of early PPROM for the healthy co-twin, there is a strong argument to defer selective feticide until after 24 weeks in highly selected cases of discordant anomaly where the risk of IUFD is small (such as in severe discordant central nervous system, genitourinary, skeletal anomaly), at least in countries where this is legally possible, and when ethically acceptable. Bipolar coagulation can then be performed using the 3.0-mm forceps by overstretching the blades whereupon the forceps opens more widely to accommodate for the larger cord diameter, as we showed in a consecutive series of five cases performed between 26 and 30 weeks

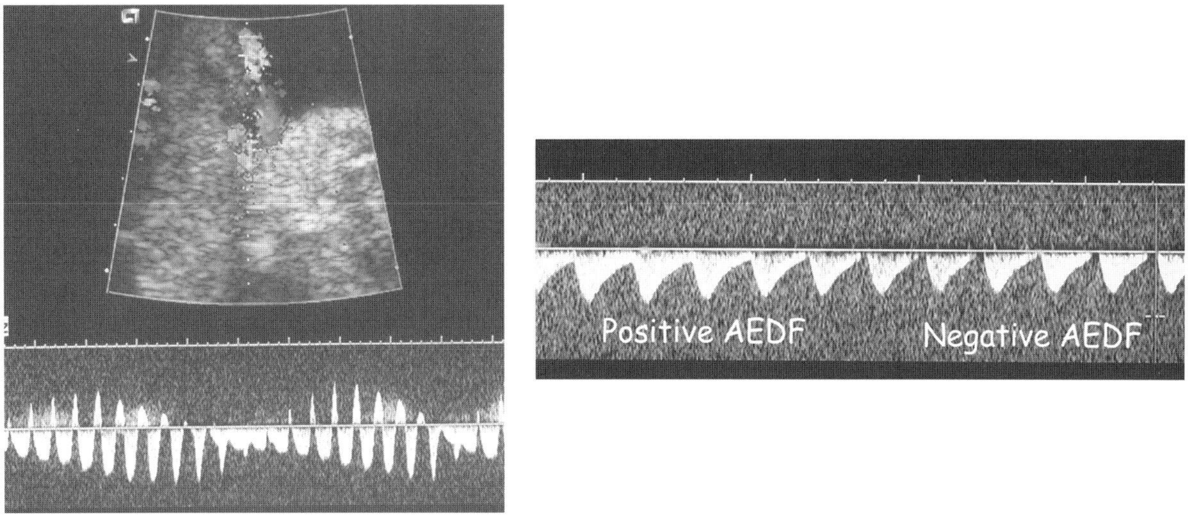

Figure 153.15 iA/REDF: Abnormal Doppler findings in umbilical artery with intermittently a positive, and negative flow (right) and reversed flow (left), a sign of retrograde transmission of an AA wave from in the umbilical artery.

GA. All deliveries occurred beyond 31 weeks (range: 31–37 weeks). All infants survived, except for one unrelated neonatal death of a child born at 36 weeks due to a complication of balloon dilatation for pulmonary stenosis.[63]

Selective growth retardation in MC twins

sIUGR complicates approximately 7% of all MC twin pregnancies.[64] sIUGR is usually defined as fetal growth below the P_{10} for GA together with an intertwin weight discordance of >25%, calculated as [(larger twin – smaller twin)/larger twin]. It is usually associated with an unequal distribution of the placental vascular territory. While the incidence is similar in dichorionic and MC twins, the nature and incidence of risks is not. Neurological damage is much more frequent in MC with sIUGR, mainly due to the existence of intertwin placental anastomoses.[65] Intrauterine demise of the IUGR twin may result in agonal postmortem acute feto-fetal transfusion, with concomitant death of the larger twin (occurring in 25–30% of cases) and neurological damage in 30% of survivors.[66] Recent clinical studies indicate a substantial risk for neurological damage in the absence of single IUFD of the small twin.[67,68] In one series ($n=13$),[67] abnormal neurodevelopment was observed in 42% of children and cerebral palsy rates were 19%. There were four instances of IUFD; three children survived and all had cerebral palsy. The other series ($n=42$)[68†] showed an IUFD rate of 10% with 12% parenchymal brain damage in surviving infants. This clearly demonstrates that MC twins with discordant growth are at especially high risk of adverse outcome.

Up to 50% of MC twins with sIUGR present with a pattern of intermittent absent or reversed end-diastolic flow (iA/REDF) on umbilical artery Doppler velocimetry.[66,69] iA/REDF, a sign unique to MC twins, is characterized by the presence of absent and/or reversed end-diastolic flow in the umbilical artery, alternating over seconds or minutes with positive diastolic flow (Figure 153.15). This pattern reflects retrograde transmission of an AA waveform in the umbilical artery. It is strongly associated with sIUGR coexisting with the presence of large-diameter intertwin placental AA anastomoses.[70] The presence or absence of this sign predisposes to a different pregnancy course and outcome, and therefore the clinical management will be discussed separately.

MC twins with sIUGR and iA/REDF in the umbilical artery

Twins with iA/REDF have an atypical clinical course and do not show the Doppler and biophysical profile changes observed in most fetuses with severe IUGR secondary to placental restriction. Umbilical artery waveform patterns indeed reflect downstream vascular resistance, but in MC twins this is determined not only by the adequacy of spiral artery invasion but also by the direction and degree of shunting across the anastomoses. This makes interpretation of Doppler findings problematic, since absent end-diastolic flow and reversed flow in the sIUGR twin, a sign known to

† Small, but important case series on the finding of cyclic changes in umbilical artery waveforms in the smaller of growth discordant MC twins

be associated with fetal distress in singletons, may rather indicate the presence of (a) large AA anastomose(s). Despite the apparently benign nature of this situation, sudden intrauterine death in the small twin occurs in up to 25% of the cases[66] and neurological damage of the appropriately grown twin may develop in up to 30% of the cases.[71] This clinical course is thought to be caused by acute intertwin blood transfer episodes through the large AA anastomoses, necessary to allow this pattern and which might interfere with the natural history of the growth-retarded twin.

The clinical management of these cases constitutes at present a dilemma. The smaller twin will not show any sign of fetal deterioration, but conservative management may result in serious complications as discussed above, without typical alarm signs. In theory, laser coagulation of placental anastomoses, including the predisposing AA anastomosis, would be a potential and causative therapy. Delinking the two fetal circulations would protect the appropriately grown fetus in the event of IUFD of the growth-retarded fetus and may render the use of Doppler for fetal well-being theoretically more reliable. Quintero *et al.*[71] reported his early experience in a small and more heterogeneous series and compared it to 17 cases managed expectantly. However, there was no significant difference in survival or neurological morbidity[70] between treated and expectantly managed patients. In our own experience in a small clinical series of MC with growth discrepancy and iA/REDF in the umbilical artery, we observed more and different technical limitations as compared to laser therapy for TTTS (unpublished data).

Selective termination does not appear as an immediate option, as it implies selective termination of a fetus, which in up to 75% of cases would survive in good conditions. Finally, considering that in our clinical series neurological damage occurred in most pregnancies beyond 32 weeks, a policy of elective delivery at 30–31 weeks could reduce, in part, the incidence of complications. The best management option for sIUGR with iA/REDF remains to be formally evaluated in future clinical trials, their nature and design still being undefined.

MC twins with IUGR and without iA/REDF

In these cases, the IUGR twin may have a normal or pathologic umbilical blood flow pattern, but it is 'constant' or unchanged during the course of the Doppler interrogation. As opposite to those with iA/REDF, MC sIUGR fetuses with absent or reverse 'constant' diastolic flow will show a clinical evolution similar to what has been described for single fetuses or dichorionic twins with growth restriction, and the typical cascade of fetal hypoxic deterioration can be assessed by means of Doppler and/or fetal heart rate patterns.[4] The observation of significant fetal deterioration indicating a high risk of intrauterine demise of the IUGR twin is a clear indication for active management in order to prevent the typical risks of monochorionicity to the normally grown fetus. Selective termination is considered as a first option in previable cases. Later in pregnancy, and particularly before 32 weeks, the decision whether to perform selective termination vs. elective delivery must be carefully discussed with parents, certainly between 24 and 28 weeks, where complications of cord occlusion, such as PPROM, may compromise the outcome of the appropriately grown twin.[62] This is ethically a very challenging dilemma.[72]

Conclusion

Complications unique to MC twins and the shared circulation have stimulated a revival of fetoscopy as a means to operate on the placenta and umbilical cord. At present, fetoscopic laser coagulation of the vascular anastomoses is the preferred first-line treatment for TTTS, complicating 10–15% of MC multiple pregnancies. Minimally invasive cord coagulation appears to be an effective technique for selective feticide in MC twins complicated with discordant anomaly, severe early discordant growth, TRAP and selected cases of TTTS. However, these procedures still have considerably higher fetal loss rates (20%) as compared to selective feticide in dichorionic twins (7.5%).

Acknowledgments

Dr L. Lewi is a beneficiary from a grant of the European Commission in its 5th Framework Programme (#QLG1-CT-2002-01632 EuroTwin2Twin). The other members of the EuroTwin2Twin Consortium are thanked for setting up the group: Y. Ville (Poissy), K. Hecher (Hamburg), E. Gratacos (Barcelona), R. Vlietinck (Leuven), M. van Gemert (Amsterdam), G. Barki (Tuttlingen), K. Nicolaides (London), R. Denk (Munich) and C. Jackson (London).

REFERENCES

1. Caroll SGM, Soothill PW, Abdel-Fattah SA, *et al.* Prediction of chorionicity in twin pregnancies at 10–14 weeks of gestation. *Br J Obstet Gynaecol* 2002;109:182–6.
2. Denbow ML, Cox P, Taylor M, *et al.* Placental angioarchitecture in monochorionic twin pregnancies: Relationship to fetal growth, fetofetal transfusion syndrome, and pregnancy outcome. *Am J Obstet Gynecol* 2000;182:417–26.
3. Gratacós E, Deprest J. Current experience with fetoscopy and the Eurofoetus registry for fetoscopic procedures. *Eur J Obstet Gynecol Reprod Biol* 2000;92:151–60.

4. Senat MV, Deprest J, Boulvain M, Paupe A, Winer N, Ville Y. Endoscopic laser surgery versus serial amnioreduction for severe twin-to-twin transfusion syndrome. *N Engl J Med* 2004;8,351(2): 136–44.
5. Lewi L, Van Schoubroeck D, Gratacos E, Witters I, Timmerman D, Deprest J. Monochorionic diamniotic twins: Complications and management options. *Curr Opin Obstet Gynecol* 2003;15:177–94.
6. Challis D, Gratacós E, Deprest J. Selective termination in monochorionic twins. *J Perinat Med* 1999;27:327–38.
7. Campbell S. Opinion: Twin-to-twin transfusion syndrome-debates on the etiology, natural history and management. *Ultrasound Obstet Gynecol* 2000;16:220–13.
8. Eurofoetus. Endoscopic feto-placental surgery: From animal experimentation to early human experimentation. Programme funded by the European Commission, within the Biomed 2 Programme, BMH CT 4 97 2382.
9. The Eurofoetus Group: Deprest J, Ville Y, Barki G, *et al.*, eds. *Manual of Fetoscopes: Endoscopy in Fetal Medicine.* Tuttlingen, Germany: Endopress, ISBN 3-89756-427-0, 2004:1–58.
10. Deprest J, Van Schoubroeck D, Van Ballaer P, *et al.* Alternative access for fetoscopic Nd:YAG laser in TTS with anterior placenta. *Ultrasound Obstet Gynecol* 1998;12:347–52.
11. Luks FI, Deprest JA, Vandenberghe K, *et al.* Fetoscopy-guided fetal endoscopy in a sheep model. *J Am Coll Surg* 1994;178:609–12.
12. Quintero RA, Bornick PW, Allen MH, Johnson PK. Selective photocoagulation of communicating vessels in severe twin–twin transfusion syndrome in women with an anterior placenta. *Obstet Gynecol* 2001;97:477–81.
13. Deprest J, Ville Y. Obstetric endoscopy. In Harrison M, Evans M, Adzick NS, Holzgreve W, eds. *The Unborn Patient: The Art and Science of Fetal Therapy.* Philadelphia: W. B. Saunders, 2000:213–32.
14. Deprest J, Van Schoubroeck D, Carreras E, *et al.* Operative fetoscopy. In Evans M, Johnson M, Wapner R, eds. *Prenatal Diagnosis.* New York: McGraw-Hill, 2006.
15. Quintero RA, ed. Diagnostic and operative fetoscopy: Technical issues. In *Diagnostic and Operative Fetoscopy.* New York: Parthenon Publishing, 2002:7–20.
16. Vandevelde M, Van Schoubroeck D, Lewi L, *et al.* Randomized double blind comparison of remifentanil and diazepam for fetal immobilization and maternal sedation during fetoscopic surgery. *Anesth Analg* 2005;101(1):251–8.
17. Bonati F, Perales A, Novak P, *et al.* Ex vivo testing of a temperature and pressure controlled amnio-irrigator for fetoscopic surgery. *J Pediatr Surg* 2002;37:18–24.
18. Feldstein VA, Machin GA, Albanese CT, *et al.* Twin–twin transfusion syndrome: The 'select' procedure. *Fetal Diagn Ther* 2000;15: 257–61.
19. Hecher K, Diehl W, Zikulnig L, Vetter M, Hackeloer BJ. Endoscopic laser coagulation of placental anastomoses in 200 pregnancies with severe mid-trimester twin-to-twin transfusion syndrome. *Eur J Obstet Gynecol Reprod Biol* 2000;92(1):135–40.
20. Quintero RA, Comas C, Bornick PW, Allen MH, Kruger M. Selective versus non-selective laser photocoagulation of placental vessels in twin-to-twin transfusion syndrome. *Ultrasound Obstet Gynecol* 2000;16(3):230–6.
21. Lewi L, Cannie M, Vandecaveye V, Jani J, Dymarkowski S, Deprest J. A pilot study to assess the role of placental MR imaging to predict placental distribution and the position of the vascular equator in twin-to-twin transfusion syndrome. *Ultrasound Obstet Gynecol* 2004;24(3):OC118, 248.
22. Senat MV, Loizeau S, Couderc S, Bernard JP, Ville Y. The value of middle cerebral artery peak systolic velocity in the diagnosis of fetal anemia after intrauterine death of one monochorionic twin. *Am J Obstet Gynecol* 2003;189(5):1320.
23. Sutcliff AG, Sebire NJ, Pigott AJ, Taylor B, Edwards PR, Nicolaides KH. Outcome of children born after in utero laser ablation therapy for severe twin-to-twin transfusion syndrome. *Br J Obstet Gynaecol* 2001;108:1246–50.
24. Lopriore E, Nagel HT, Vandenbussche FP, Walther FJ. Long-term neurodevelopmental outcome in twin-to-twin transfusion syndrome. *Am J Obstet Gynecol* 2003;189(5):1314–9.
25. Quintero RA, Morales WJ, Allen M, Bornick PW, Arroyo J, LeParc G. Treatment of iatrogenic previable premature rupture of membranes with intra-amniotic injection of platelets and cryoprecipitate (amniopatch): Preliminary experience. *Am J Obstet Gynecol* 1999;181(3):744–9.
26. Lewi L, Van Schoubroeck D, Van Ranst M, *et al.* Successful patching of iatrogenic rupture of the fetal membranes. *Placenta* 2004; 25(4):352–6.
27. Stone CA, Quinn MW, Saxby PJ. Congenital skin loss following Nd:YAG placental coagulation. *Burns* 1998;24:275–7.
28. Luks F, Carr S, Tracy T. Intestinal complications associated with twin twin transfusion syndrome after antenatal laser treatment: Report of 2 cases (replying letter). *J Pediatr Surg* 2001;36:1105–6.
29. Scott F, Evans N. Distal gangrene in a polycythemic recipient fetus in twin–twin transfusion. *Obstet Gynecol* 1995;86:677–9.
30. Banek CS, Hecher K, Hackeloer BJ, Bartmann P. Long-term neurodevelopmental outcome after intrauterine laser treatment for severe twin–twin transfusion syndrome. *Am J Obstet Gynecol* 2003;188(4):876–80.
31. Lewi L, Vandenberghe G, Deprest J. Fertility and pregnancy outcome after fetoscopic surgery. *Am J Obstet Gynecol* 2003;6: S189,S597.
32. Baldwin VJ. Anomalous development in twins. In *Pathology of Multiple Pregnancies.* New York: Springer-Verlag, 1994:169–197.
33. Bryan E, Little J, Burn J. Congenital anomalies in twins. *Baillieres Clin Obstet Gynaecol* 1987;1:697–721.
34. Heydanus R, Santema JG, Steward PA, *et al.* Preterm delivery rate and fetal outcome in structurally affected twin pregnancies: A retrospective matched control study. *Prenat Diagn* 1993;13(3):155–62.
35. Nieuwint A, Van Zalen-Sprock R, Hummel P, *et al.* 'Identical' twins with normal karyotypes. *Prenat Diagn* 1999;19(1):72–6.
36. Lewi L, Blickstein I, van Schoubroeck D, Gloning KP, Casteels M, Brandenburg H, Fryns JP, Deprest J. Diagnosis and management of heterokaryotypic monochorinic twins. *Am J Med Genet* 2005; 140A:272–5.
37. Bajoria R, Wee LY, Anwar S, Ward S. Outcome of twin pregnancies complicated by single intrauterine death in relation to vascular anatomy of the monochorionic placenta. *Hum Reprod* 1999;14(8):2124–30.
38. Nicolini U, Poblete A. Single intrauterine death in monochorionic twin pregnancies. *Ultrasound Obstet Gynecol* 1999;14:297–301.
39. Van Allen MI, Smith DW, Shephard TH. Twin reversed arterial perfusion (TRAP) sequence: A study of 14 twin pregnancies with acardiacus. *Semin Perinatol* 1983;7:285–93.
40. Gembruch U, Viski S, Bagamery K, *et al.* Twin reversed arterial perfusion sequence in twin-to-twin transfusion syndrome after the death of the donor co-twin in the second trimester. *Ultrasound Obstet Gynecol* 2001;17:153–6.
41. Gilliam DL, Hendricks CH. Holoacardius: Review of literature and case report. *Obstet Gynecol* 1953;2:647–53.
42. Sogaard K, Skibsted L, Brocks V. Acardiac twins: Pathophysiology, diagnosis, outcome and treatment. Six cases and review of the literature. *Fetal Diagn Ther* 1999;14(1):53–9.
43. Sullivan AE, Varner MW, Ball RH, Jackson M, Silver RM. The management of acardiac twins: A conservative approach. *Am J Obstet Gynecol* 2003;189(5):1310–3.
44. Chandra S, Crane JM, Young DC, Shah S. Acardiac twin pregnancy with neonatal resolution of donor twin cardiomyopathy. *Obstet Gynecol* 2000;96(5, Pt 2):820–1.
45. Kosno-Kruszewska E, Deregowski K, Schmidt-Sidor B, *et al.* Neuropathological and anatomopathological analyses of acardiac and "normal" siblings in an acardiac-twin pregnancy. *Folia Neuropathol* 2003;41(2):103–9.
46. Moore TR, Gale S, Benirschke K. Perinatal outcome of forty-nine pregnancies complicated by acardiac twinning. *Am J Obstet Gynecol* 1990;163(3):907–12.
47. Brassard M, Fouron JC, Leduc L, Grignon A, Proulx F. Prognostic markers in twin pregnancies with an acardiac fetus. *Obstet Gynecol* 1999;94(3):409–14.
48. Sherer DM, Armstrong B, Shah YG, Metlay LA, Woods JR Jr. Prenatal sonographic diagnosis, Doppler velocimetric umbilical cord studies, and subsequent management of an acardiac twin pregnancy. *Obstet Gynecol* 1989;74:472–5.
49. Dashe JS, Fernandez CO, Twickler DM. Utility of Doppler velocimetry in predicting outcome in twin reversed-arterial perfusion sequence. *Am J Obstet Gynecol* 2001;185(1):135–9.
50. Mahone PR, Sherer DM, Abramowicz JS, Woods JR. Twin transfusion syndrome: Rapid development of severe hydrops of the donor following selective fetocide of the recipient. *Am J Obstet Gynecol* 1993;169:166–8.
51. Taylor MJ, Shalev E, Tanawattanacharoen S, *et al.* Ultrasound-guided umbilical cord occlusion using bipolar diathermy for stage III/IV twin–twin transfusion syndrome. *Prenat Diagn* 2002;22(1): 70–6.
52. Zosmer N, Bajoria R, Weiner E, *et al.* Clinical and echocardiographic features of in utero cardiac dysfunction in the recipient twin in twin-twin transfusion syndrome. *Br Heart J* 1994;72: 74–9.

53. Evans MI, Goldberg JD, Horenstein J, *et al.* Selective termination for structural, chromosomal, and mendelian anomalies: International experience. *Am J Obstet Gynecol* 1999;181(4):893–7.
54. Eddleman KA, Stone JL, Lynch L, Berkowitz RL. Selective termination of anomalous fetuses in multifetal pregnancies: Two hundred cases at a single center. *Am J Obstet Gynecol* 2002;187(5):1168–72.
55. Shalev J, Meizner I, Rabinerson D, *et al.* Improving pregnancy outcome in twin gestations with one malformed fetus by postponing selective feticide in the third trimester. *Fertil Steril* 1999; 72(2):257–60.
56. Denbow ML, Overton TG, Duncan KR, Cox PM, Fisk NM. High failure rate of umbilical vessel occlusion by ultrasound guided injection of absolute alcohol or enbucrilate gel. *Prenat Diagn* 1999;19:527–32.
57. Deprest JA, Evrard VA, Van Ballaer PP, *et al.* Experience with fetoscopic cord ligation. *Eur J Obstet Gynecol Reprod Biol* 1998;81:157–64.
58. Hecher K, Hackeloer BJ, Ville Y. Umbilical cord coagulation by operative microendoscopy at 16 weeks' gestation in an acardiac twin. *Ultrasound Obstet Gynecol* 1997;10(2):130–2.
59. Ville Y, Hyett JA, Vandenbussche FP, Nicolaides KH. Endoscopic laser coagulation of umbilical cord vessels in twin reversed arterial perfusion sequence. *Ultrasound Obstet Gynecol* 1994; 4(5):396–8.
60. Ville Y. Selective feticide in monochorionic pregnancies: Toys for the boys or standard of care? *Ultrasound Obstet Gynecol* 2003; 22(5):448–50.
61. Nicolini U, Poblete A, Boschetto C, *et al.* Complicated monochorionic twin pregnancies: Experience with bipolar cord coagulation. *Am J Obstet Gynecol* 2000;185:703–7.
62. Lewi L, Gratacos E, Ortibus E, Van Schoubroeck D, Carreras E, Higueras T, Perapoch J, Deprest J. Pregnancy and infant outcome of 80 consecutive cord coagulations in complicated monochorionic multiple pregnancies. *Am J Obstet Gynecol* 2005, 193, in press.
63. Deprest J, Van Schoubroeck D, Senat M-V, *et al.* Cord coagulation in monochorionic multiplets late in gestation. *Am J Obstet Gynecol* 2003;6:S189,S612.
64. Sebire NJ, Snijders RJ, Hughes K, Sepulveda W, Nicolaides KH. The hidden mortality of monochorionic twin pregnancies. *Br J Obstet Gynaecol* 1997;104:1203–7.
65. Bejar R, Vigliocco G, Gramajo H, *et al.* Antenatal origin of neurologic damage in newborn infants. II. Multiple gestations. *Am J Obstet Gynecol* 1990;162:1230–6.
66. Gratacós E, Lewi L, Carreras E, *et al.* Incidence and characteristics of umbilical intermittent absent and/or reversed diastolic flow in complicated and uncomplicated monochorionic twin pregnancy. *Ultrasound Obstet Gynecol* 2004;23:456–60.
67. Adegbite AL, Castille S, Ward S, Bajoria R. Neuromorbidity in preterm twins in relation to chorionicity and discordant birth weight. *Am J Obstet Gynecol* 2004;190(1):156–63.
68. Gratacós E, Carreras E, Becker J, *et al.* Prevalence of neurological damage in monochorionic twins with selective intrauterine growth retardation and intermittent absent or reversed end diastolic umbilical artery flow. *Ultrasound Obstet Gynecol* 2004;24: 159–63.
69. Nakai Y, Ishoko O, Nishio J, *et al.* Cyclic changes in the umbilical arterial flow in monochorionic diamniotic twin pregnancy. *Eur J Obstet Gynecol Reprod Biol* 2002;101:135–8.
70. Myers SA, Bennett TL. Selective photocoagulation of monochorionic twin pregnancy (letter). *Am J Obstet Gynecol* 2002;187(1).
71. Quintero RA, Bornick PW, Morales WJ, *et al.* Selective photocoagulation of the communicating vessels in the treatment of monochorionic twins with selective growth retardation. *Am J Obstet Gynecol* 2001;185:689–96.
72. Deprest J, Van Schoubroeck D, Senat MV, *et al.* Cord coagulation in monochorionic multiplets late in gestation (abstract 612). *Am J Obstet Gynecol* 2003;S226.

154 Route of delivery

J. W. Dudenhausen and J. A. S. Dimer

The principal issues for neonatal morbidity and mortality in multiples are intrauterine growth restriction and prematurity.[1] Nevertheless, the route of delivery of multiples affects the perinatal morbidity and mortality rates.[2] There is no general consensus regarding the optimal route of delivery in multiple gestations. We must clearly separate the mode of delivery of higher-order gestations and triplets from that of twins.

Triplets and higher-order pregnancies

The route of delivery of triplets and higher-order gestations is widely variable and is controversial. In North America, the planned cesarean section is widely accepted as standard care; in South Africa, on the other hand, a cesarean section rate of 14% was reported by Pheiffer and Golan in 1979[3] as well as by Deale and Cronje in 1984.[4] In the African experience, the majority of cases that were described are those where a higher-order gestation was first discovered during the birth. Thus, few conclusions should be made from isolated birth statistics without regard to the obstetrical environment in which those statistics were gleaned.

In 1989, Lipitz *et al.*[5] reported the outcome of 78 sets of triplets; the cesarean section rate was 78% in this collective. Triplets born vaginally had a higher rate of low Apgar scores and respiratory distress. In 1988, Feingold *et al.*[6] published their experience with a group of 15 triplet pregnancies undergoing vaginal birth; the mortality and morbidity of the initial infant was 21%, of the second infant 31% and of the third infant 43%. These observations were not seen by Ron-El *et al.*[7] In comparison, in 1990, Olofsson[8] reported the experience of 14 triplets and quadruplets. In this group, vaginal birth was initiated in the 34th week of gestation, even when the presenting fetus was breech. In three cases, the vaginal birth was interrupted and an emergency cesarean section was performed for intrapartum fetal indications. During 1989, the obstetrical experience in a large group of 198 triplet pregnancies delivered at 24 different hospitals was reported by Newman *et al.*,[9] where 94% of the infants were delivered abdominally and 12% were delivered solely vaginally. In 2004, Alran *et al.*[10] investigated a series of 93 triplet pregnancies in a single perinatal department. Of these, 66 (84%) had a successful vaginal delivery, 12 delivered by emergency cesarean section and 15 by elective cesarean section. The perinatal mortality was 48/1000.

In a review of the literature in 1989, Petrikovsky and Vintzileos[11] evaluated the route of delivery of higher-order gestations. Although malpresentations were common, a broad spectrum of complications were seen such as placental abruption, intrauterine oxygen deprivation, umbilical cord prolapse and vaginal bleeding. An elective cesarean section avoided the majority of these complications and allowed for the antepartum organization of the obstetric and neonatology personnel. The importance of this interdisciplinary cooperation and the availability of neonatal beds should not be underestimated. When the decision has been made to proceed with a vaginal trial of labor, the attending obstetrician should plan to have the assistance of another well-trained obstetrician who is capable of diagnosing an anomalous fetal presentation with ultrasound, and who is able to be a competent operative assistant if a malpresentation is seen. Furthermore, during the second stage of labor, there must be adequate obstetric personnel at hand, who are able to monitor the fetal movement ultrasonographically.

The potential safety of the vaginal delivery of triplets has been studied in recent years in a few European centers. In 1995, Dommergues *et al.*[12] reported for a group in Paris about a case–control study of 69 consecutive triplet pregnancies delivered at the same institution. He found the neonatal mortality was not significantly increased by vaginal birth and concluded that vaginal delivery of triplets may be safe in carefully selected cases. Also, in 1995, Wildschut *et al.*[13] in the Netherlands reported the results of a retrospective study comparing planned abdominal with planned vaginal birth in triplet pregnancies. He found two centers in the Netherlands with two distinctly different primary modes of delivery: in Leiden 80% of women were delivered by cesarean section and in Amsterdam 87% favored vaginal birth. Similar reports of planned vaginal delivery of triplets have emphasized that the greater maturity of the infants delivered vaginally

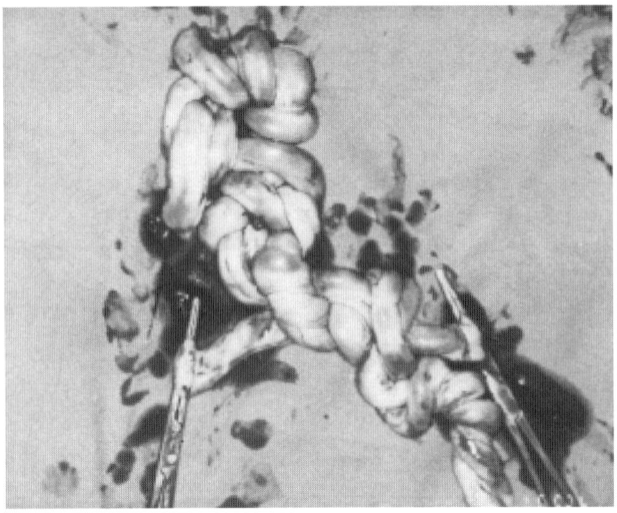

Figure 154.1 Complex umbilical cord knot from monoamniotic twins. Courtesy of Dr D. Berg, Amberg/Germany.

appeared to be the major factor for the lower neonatal morbidity and mortality seen in such a review.[14]

Multifetal reduction of triplets to twins yields an improved perinatal outcome compared with non-reduced triplets and a similar outcome compared with non-reduced twins.[15] Probably, the best means of reducing the perinatal morbidity of higher-order multiple gestations is to prevent multiple pregnancies in *in vitro* fertilization programs by reducing the number of embryos transferred per cycle.[16]

As a rule, today, obstetricians choose to deliver triplets and higher-order multiples with a planned cesarean section. This operative procedure should be performed by obstetricians who are experienced in the delivery of multiple gestations from malpresentations and who are also experienced in the treatment of intractable postpartum hemorrhage and possible hysterectomy. A comparison of the maternal and neonatal outcomes in patients following transverse and longitudinal uterine incisions has concluded that a transverse lower segment uterine incision should be used to increase the chances of a normal vaginal delivery in the future.[17] The anesthesia team should also be well experienced and prepared to manage a potentially life-threatening circulatory collapse. It deserves to be emphasized that a generous dose of oxytocin should be given following the delivery of the infants to prevent the development of uterine atony.

In a study from the USA in 1995, the total cost involved in the delivery, prenatal and neonatal care for triplet pregnancies was estimated to be $64,347 per family. Neonates averaged 13.7 hospital days and mothers averaged 16.7 in-patient hospital days.[18] Improvement in the neonatal resuscitation and care as well as delivery by cesarean section are felt to be responsible for lower mortality rates and overall better outcomes.[19]

Antepartum intrauterine death of one fetus in a multiple gestation may be associated with significant morbidity and mortality in the surviving infants, and it may be a factor in deciding the time and route of delivery. Neurological damage is recognized to be higher in the surviving infants, especially when intrauterine fetal death is associated with monochorionic placentation.[20]

Delayed interval delivery in triplet pregnancies has been reported in the literature.[21,22] In the rare circumstance that the presenting fetus is expelled, conservative management of the remaining viable fetuses has resulted in 34 and 49 days of interval time before the birth of the remaining three or two infants, respectively.

Twins

The prerequisites involved in the decision of the optimal mode of delivery in twins are manifold because one must always consider the different fetal presentation constellations. Chervenak[23] reported the following fetal presentations: vertex/vertex 42.5%, vertex/non-vertex 38.4%, non-vertex/vertex or non-vertex 19.1%. These findings take into consideration the clinically important factors necessary to make a decision regarding mode of delivery.

In the case of monoamniotic twins, regardless of fetal lie and presentation, the literature frequently recommends primary cesarean section to reduce the risks of umbilical cord complications and locked fetal heads[24] (Figure 154.1). Umbilical cord entanglement is the most common complication and often results in intrauterine fetal demise. These umbilical cord complications may be seen when one twin suddenly descends in labor.

Locked twins is a rare intrapartum complication; it is seen once in 1000 twins births.[25] The risk of locked twins is clearly higher in monochorionic–monoamniotic twins than in dichorionic–diamniotic twins. Both oligohydramnios and low birth weight increase the risk of locked twins.

Conjoined twins are a uniquely demanding situation for the obstetrician. The twins should be systematically evaluated ultrasonographically antepartum to determine if the anatomical findings are compatible with extrauterine life. To avoid the maternal risks resulting from an obstruction of labor, an elective cesarean section should be recommended.

Vertex/vertex

Vaginal delivery is appropriate for vertex/vertex twins. A thorough review of the literature on this constellation supports an attempt at vaginal birth.[26] Some authoritative sources have reported that 75% of all vertex/vertex twins may be delivered vaginally without difficulty.[27] On the other hand, other authors propose that cesarean delivery should be indicated for preterm birth or estimated fetal weight under a given value.[28] The weight cutoff and gestational age restriction are variable. In a consensus article,[29] this estimated fetal weight cutoff was recommended to be 1800 g.

There are exceptions to this rule that only vertex/vertex twins estimated to weigh over 1800 g should be encouraged to attempt a vaginal trial of labor. If there is an estimated fetal weight on ultrasound indicating that the weight of the second twin is 15–25% higher[30] than the first, an elective cesarean section is indicated to avoid complications during the birth of the second twin.

Course of labor following the birth of the first vertex twin

Following the birth of the first twin, a brief physiologic pause between uterine contractions usually ensues. An intravenous oxytocin infusion is appropriate to shorten this pause. Before initiating the oxytocin infusion, ultrasound and/or external abdominal palpation to discern the fetal lie should be performed. Furthermore, the heart rate of the second twin (just as was indicated before the birth of the presenting twin) should be continuously monitored. A vaginal examination will determine if the amniotic membranes are intact and what fetal part is presenting. Following the return of uterine contractions and the descent of the fetal presenting part, an amniotomy may be performed and the fetal heart rate can be obtained via the direct mode.[31] The fetal heart pattern should remain reassuring throughout this procedure. In the presence of a non-reassuring fetal heart rate tracing, an operative delivery is indicated.

The time interval between deliveries has been a topic of discussion in the literature for decades. During the 1960s in Europe, the approach was rather conservative and non-interventional for adopting strict norms regarding this time interval. In comparison, the Anglo-Saxon language literature of the times seemed to support a 30-min cutoff to avoid the risk of intrapartum hypoxia of the second twin that could result from umbilical cord prolapse, placental abruption and the clamping down of the cervix. There was no controversy, however, on the fact that there is a clear correlation between the difference in the umbilical artery pH values (twin I minus twin II) and the time interval between deliveries regardless of the fetal heart tracings.[32] Current obstetrical practice mandates that the fetal heart rate be continuously monitored and taken into consideration in the management scheme. A relationship exists between the frequency of fetal hypoxia in the second twin and the time interval between deliveries, especially in those where a fetal heart rate pattern is non-reassuring. In these cases, it is recommended that a timely completion of the delivery be accomplished; this frequently requires an operative delivery of the second twin.

When the fetal heart pattern of the second twin is within normal limits following the birth of the first twin, this correlation with time interval between deliveries does not apply. Although expectant management in view of reassuring fetal heart pattern may be indicated, this should not imply that the attending obstetrician should wait until the cervix has clamped down.[33]

There are three modes of delivery of twins: both are delivered by cesarean section (C–C), both are delivered vaginally (V–V) and the first twin is delivered vaginally but the second one is delivered by cesarean section (V–C). The higher neonatal morbidity of the V–C-mode is caused by labor and delivery complications after the delivery of the first twin.[34,35] The increase of neonatal morbidity and mortality in the second twin is more evident in term births than in preterm births.[36]

Vertex/non-vertex

Intrapartum management of vertex/non-vertex and vertex/transverse twins has been debated in the literature. In the American literature, support can be found for a general indication for elective cesarean section in such cases.[37] This opinion is not generally seen by European authors and practicing obstetricians.[38]

In the case of a malpresentation of the second twin, intrapartum management includes an attempt at external cephalic version of the second twin. An internal version combined with extraction from a non-vertex presentation should be handled the same way as a vaginal breech delivery.

External version of the second twin

Reports of external version of the second twin conflict markedly. Although a few authors recommend the external cephalic version of the second twin and have analyzed their own extensive experience,[39] other authors criticize this maneuver because it increases the risk of umbilical cord compromise and wastes time.

Alternatively, the breech presentation of the second twin is less controversial. There is no increased rate of neonatal compromise following the unremarkable vaginal breech birth.[40,41] One report presented experience with 39 vertex/breech twins following vaginal birth. The author found no difference in the outcome of the study and control groups when the second twin had converted to a vertex presentation. Another prospective study compared elective cesarean section, external version and breech extraction.[42] This study included only fetuses with an ultrasound estimating fetal weight over 1500 g. The best outcome was present following vaginal delivery; there was no increased neonatal or maternal morbidity. An external version was successful in 20 of 41 cases. An emergency cesarean section was necessary in a single case. Manual breech extraction of the second twin is a rather uncomplicated procedure, as cited in the literature on twins over 1800 g in weight. The combination of the version of a second twin in transverse lie to breech and delivery via total breech extraction is usually possible for the experienced obstetrician. With certain risk factors such as oligohydramnios, dorsoposterior transverse lie and macrosomia, this version–extraction combination may be difficult. In these cases, a cesarean section may be indicated instead of the difficult operative vaginal manipulations.

Non-vertex/vertex or non-vertex/non-vertex

It is generally accepted that an elective cesarean section is indicated in these cases.[43] The locking of the fetal heads is a potentially lethal complication of the vaginal birth when the first twin is breech. It must be said that these statements have not been extensively validated by clinical studies in this area.

REFERENCES

1. Garite TJ, *et al.* Twins and triplets: The effect of plurality and growth on neonatal outcome compared with singleton infants. *Am J Obstet Gynecol* 2004;191:700–7.
2. Koutopoulos EL, *et al.* The impact of route of delivery and presentation on twin neonatal and infant mortality: A population-based study in the USA, 1995–1997. *J Matern Fetal Neonatal Med* 2004;15:219–24.
3. Pheiffer EL, Golan A. Priplet pregnancy. A 10-year review of cases at Baragwanath Hospital. *S Afr Med J* 1979;55:843–6.
4. Deale CJ, Cronje HS. A review of 367 triplet pregnancies. *S Afr Med J* 1984;66:92–4.
5. Lipitz S, Rechman B, Paret G, *et al.* The improving outcome of triplet pregnancies. *Am J Obstet Gynecol* 1989;161:1279.
6. Feingold M, Cetrulo C, Peters M, Chaudhury A, Schuroys S, Geifman O. Mode of delivery in multiple birth of higher order. *Acta Genet Med Gemellol Roma* 1988;37:105.
7. Ron-El R, Mor Z, Weinraut Z, *et al.* Triplet, quadruplet and quintuplet pregnancies-management and outcome. *Acta Obstet Gynaecol Scand* 1992;71:347.
8. Olofsson P. Triplet and quadruplet pregnancies – A forthcoming challenge also for the 'general' obstetrician. *Eur J Obstet Gynecol Reprod Biol* 1990;35:159.
9. Newman RB, Hamer C, Miller MC. Outpatient triplet management: A contemporary review. *Am J Obstet Gynecol* 1989;161:547.
10. Alran S, *et al.* Maternal and neonatal outcome of 93 consecutive triplet pregnancies with 71% vaginal delivery. *Acta Obstet Gynecol Scand* 2004;83:554–9.
11. Petrikovsky BM, Vintzileos AM. Management and outcome of multiple pregnancy of high fetal order: Literature review. *Obstet Gynecol Surv* 1989;44:578.
12. Dommergues M, Mahieu-Caputo D, Mandelbrot L, Huon C, Moriette G, Dumaz Y. Delivery of uncomplicated triplet pregnancies: Is the vaginal route safer? A case–control study. *Am J Obstet Gynecol* 1995;172:513–7.
13. Wildschut HI, van Roosmalen J, van Leeuwen E, Keirse MJ. Planned abdominal compared with planned vaginal birth in triplet pregnancies. *Br J Obstet Gynaecol* 1995;102:292–6.
14. Clarke JP, Roman JD. *Aust N Z J Obstet Gnaecol* 1994;34: 50–3.
15. Macones GA, Schemmer G, Pritts E, Weinblatt V, Wapner RJ. Multifetal reduction of triplets to twins improves perinatal outcome. *Am J Obstet Gynecol* 1993;169:982–6.
16. Nijs M, Geerts L, van Roosendaal E, Segal-Bertin G, Vanderwalmen P, Schoysman R. Prevention of multiple pregnancies in an in vitro fertilization program. *Fertil Steril* 1993;59:1245–50.
17. Mordel N, Ezra Y, Benshushan A, Dorembus D, Schenker JG, Sadovsky E. Transverse versus longitudinal uterine incision in cesarean delivery of triplets. *J Reprod Med* 1993;38:695–6.
18. Chelmow D, Penzia AS, Kaufman G, Cetrulo C. Costs of triplet pregnancy. *Am J Obstet Gynecol* 1995;172:677–82.
19. Creinin M, Katz M, Lros R. Triplet pregnancy: Changes in morbidity and mortality. *J Perinatol* 1991;11:207–12.
20. Lui S, Venirschke K, Scioscia AL, Mannino FL. Intrauterine death in multiple gestation. *Acta Genet Med Gamellol Roma* 1992; 41:5–26.
21. van Heusden AM, Bots RS. Delayed interval delivery in a triplet pregnancy: A case report. *Eur J Obstet Gynecol Reprod Biol* 1991;38:75–8.
22. Chua EK, Tsakok FH. *Ann Acad Med Singapore* 1996;25:279–80.
23. Chervenak FA. The controversy of mode of delivery in twins: The intrapartum management of twin gestation (part II). *Semin Perinatol* 1986;10:44–9.
24. Nissen ED. Twins: Collision, impaction, compaction and interlocking. *Obstet Gynecol* 1958;11:514–26.
25. Bryan E. *Twins and Higher Multiple Births: A Guide to Their Nature and Nurture.* London: Edward Arnold, 1992.
26. Keith L, Hughey MJ. In Gerbie AB, Sciarra JJ, eds. *Gynecology and Obstetrics*, 2nd edn. New York: Harper & Row, 1981:1–10.
27. Chervenak FA, Johnson RE, Youcha S, *et al.* Intrapartum management of twin gestation. *Obstet Gynecol* 1985;65:119–24.
28. Barrett JM, Staggs SM, van Mooydonk JE, *et al.* The effect of type of delivery upon neonatal outcome in premature twins. *Am J Obstet Gynecol* 1982;143:360–7.
29. Dudenhausen JW. Care of the twin pregnancy and the twin delivery. *Perinat Med* 1990;2:1.
30. Blickstein I, *et al.* The growth discordant twin. *Obstet Gynecol Surv* 1988;43:509.
31. Bakker PC, *et al.* Quality of intrapartum cardiotokography in twin deliveries. *Am J Obstet Gynecol* 2004;191:2114–9.
32. Müller-Holve W, Saling E, Schwarz M. The significance of the time interval in twin delivery. *J Perinat Med* 1976;4:100.
33. Stucki D. Various aspects of the management of twin pregnancy and delivery. *Gynakol Rundsch* 1984;24(Suppl 1):108–15.
34. Smith GC, *et al.* Birth order, gestational age, and risk of delivery related perinatal death in twins: Retrospective cohort study. *Br Med J* 2002;325:1004–9.
35. Shi WW, *et al.* Neonatal morbidity in second twin according to gestational age at birth and mode of delivery. *Am J Obstet Gynecol* 2004;191:773–7.
36. Shi WW, *et al.* Neonatal mortality in secon twin according to cause of death, gestational age, and mode of delivery. *Am J Obstet Gynecol* 2004;191:778–83.
37. Cetrulo C. The controversy of mode of delivery in twins: The intrapartum management of twin gestation. *Semin Perinatol* 1986;23: 533–48.
38. Wolff K. Excessive use of cesarean section for the second twin. *Gynecol Obstet Invest* 2000;50:25–32.
39. Chervenak FA, Johnson RE, Berkowitz RL, *et al.* Intrapartum external version of the second twin. *Obstet Gynecol* 1983;62:160–5.
40. Blickstein I, Schwarz-Schamon Z, Lancet MD, Borenstein R. Vaginal delivery of the second twin in breech presentation. *Obstet Gynecol* 1987;69:774–6.
41. Acker D, Leberman M, Holbrook H, *et al.* Delivery of the second twin. *Obstet Gynecol* 1982;59:710–11.
42. Goecke SE, Nageotte MP, Garite T, Towers CV, Dorcester W. Management of the nonvertex second twin: Primary cesarean section, external version, or primary breech extraction. *Am J Obstet Gynecol* 1989;162:111–14.
43. Nassar AH, *et al.* Breech presenting twin A: Is vaginal delivery safe? *J Perinat Med* 2004;32:470–4.

155 Delayed interval delivery in multiple pregnancy

J. van Eyck, B. Arabin and R. A. van Lingen

Introduction

In the recent decades, the number of multiple pregnancies has increased rapidly, primarily due to the use of assisted reproduction techniques (ART) and increased maternal age. Multiple pregnancy is frequently complicated by premature delivery, which is a major cause of perinatal mortality and morbidity. Luke *et al.* reported relative risks of mortality in twin pregnancies and triplet pregnancies of 6.6 and 19.4, respectively, whereas among survivors the relative risks of severe handicap were 1.7 for twins and 2.9 for triplets.[1] After premature vaginal delivery of the first baby of a multiple pregnancy, arrest of labor may occur. Traditionally, only a few attempts were undertaken to postpone delivery of the remaining fetus(es), and thus increase their chance of survival. Since 1957, several case reports and small series have been published reporting on delayed interval delivery in multiple pregnancies. In 1998, we published the largest series ($n=17$) of that moment on delayed interval delivery in twins originating from one single center.[2] In our series, a fixed treatment protocol was used and the 'success rate' was 53%. This was in contrast to a review of the literature, which showed a large variation in the treatment protocols and a very high success rate (93%), suggesting that mainly cases with successful outcomes were reported. Because of this selection bias, it was only possible to speculate on both prognosis and recommendations concerning treatment protocols. In this chapter, we report on data from our department, which provides again the largest series of delayed interval deliveries in twins and triplets originating from one single center, including neonatal follow-up.

In our chapter published in 1998, we reviewed the literature between 1957 and 1996.[2] In this chapter, a review of the literature between 1996 and 2004 is performed and compared with the former review.

Population and techniques

Between 1991 and 2004, a total of 78 twin pregnancies and 21 triplet pregnancies were complicated by vaginal delivery of the first fetus between 16 and 31 weeks of gestation. After exclusion of pregnancies in which a cesarean section had to be performed for the second twin, labor progressed or patients with specific contraindications to postpone delivery, such as ongoing infection, 33 women with twin pregnancy and 8 women with triplet pregnancy could be included in our final study. Mean maternal age in the group with twins was 30.8 years (range: 23–39 years) and in the group with triplets 33 years (range: 25–41 years). In twin pregnancies, 67% of women conceived spontaneously, whereas all women with triplets conceived after ART. When preterm delivery was anticipated, women were asked to give informed consent and were treated according to a fixed protocol, in which four phases can be distinguished: phase 1: preparation, phase 2: delivery of the first baby, phase 3: period between the birth of the first and the remaining fetus(es) and phase 4: delivery of the last multiple including the evaluation of the placenta. Each phase is characterized by specific measures that have to be taken.

Phase 1

The procedure starts with ruling out contraindications and obtaining informed consent. Contraindications include fetal distress or severe congenital abnormalities of the remaining fetus, chorioamnionitis, severe vaginal blood loss and other situations in which the maternal condition is compromised (e.g. preeclampsia, suspicion of placental abruption, infection). Membranes of the remaining fetus(es) must be intact, since early-onset long-term oligohydramnios is associated with pulmonary hypoplasia.[3] Considering the potential risks of the procedure vs. the risks of perinatal mortality and morbidity, it is not appropriate to pursue delayed interval delivery after 31 weeks of gestation, especially when corticosteroids have been administered to stimulate fetal lung maturation.

Informed consent consists of thorough explanation of the procedure to both future parents, its limited success rate and the potential risks for mother and her unborn child(ren), such as chorioamnionitis, placental abruption and, although rare, maternal coagulation disorder. Side effects of anticipated medication, such as tocolytics, should also be discussed.

In the Netherlands, immature delivery before 25 weeks is practically always associated with neonatal death. However, parents should be made aware that if delivery of the remaining fetus takes place between 25 and 28 weeks, neonatal mortality may be reduced, but neonatal morbidity remains high. The latter may be considered an even greater and costly burden for the future parents and society. Motivation of the parents is an absolute prerequisite for starting a delayed interval delivery procedure.

For tocolytic treatment, we administered ritodrine and more recently atosiban intravenously or nifedipine orally and, if necessary, indometacin suppositories. Fetal lung maturation is stimulated by giving two doses of 12 mg betametasone intramuscularly with an interval of 24 h to the patient between 25 and 32 weeks of gestation. After cervical and urinary culture was obtained, antibiotics are administered intravenously for at least 1 week.

Phase 2

The birth of the first baby deserves special consideration. Expulsion forces should be kept limited. During delivery of the first baby, administration of tocolytics and antibiotics are usually continued. As episiotomy is a source of infection; it should be avoided mainly since there is no proof of better outcome after episiotomy. After delivery of the first baby, no efforts should be undertaken to deliver the placenta. A culture is taken from the cervix and the vagina is intensively disinfected. The umbilical cord has to be ligated as high as possible near the cervix. We do not recommend cervical cerclage. In rhesus-negative women, 1000 IU of anti-D globulin is injected intramuscularly immediately after the first delivery.

Phase 3

After delivery of the first baby, digital examination is avoided. Cervical length, dilatation and funneling are monitored, preferably by transvaginal sonography, applying the transducer only into the proximal part of the vagina. Monitoring the maternal condition focuses on (early) detection of chorioamnionitis, recurrent preterm labor, placental abruption and coagulation disorders. Body temperature is measured four times daily. Cervical cultures are taken weekly and antibiotics are administered according to their results. Laboratory tests (infection and coagulation) are performed periodically. Fetal monitoring consisted of very frequent biophysical assessment, including cardiotocography, Doppler flow velocimetry and real-time ultrasound. Fetal biometry and the amount of amniotic fluid are examined by ultrasound at regular intervals. The patient remains hospitalized as long as contractions and/or cervical dilatations are present. Peridural analgesia is frequently given during the first three phases of the procedure and offers good relief of pain and discomfort.

Phase 4

After delivery of the remaining fetus(es), the placenta must be carefully examined in order to prevent retention of the placenta, and also of the first baby. All placentas were histologically examined for signs of infection and chorionicity. During the whole procedure, parents are counseled regularly by our social worker and special attention is paid to their emotional state, which is frequently ambiguous in the situation when one baby is dead and the other may survive.

Results

Within our series of 99 multiple pregnancies with vaginal delivery of the first baby before 32 gestational weeks, we have treated 33 twin and 8 triplet pregnancies according to our protocol.

Data of all 33 twin pregnancies are shown in Table 155.1. The mean gestational age at delivery of the first baby was 24.8 weeks (range: 16–31 weeks). The mean birth weight was 751 g (range: 140–1660 g). Perinatal mortality of all first-born twins was 70%. All 18 first babies born before 26 weeks died and had a mean birth weight of 481 g (range 140–1000 g). Survival rate of 10 first-born babies, born between 26 and 29 weeks, was 50%. From 29 weeks onward, all five first-born babies survived, but needed artificial ventilation in contrast to their later-born sibs. On average, delivery of the remaining fetus could be postponed for 20.6 days (range: 0.5–106 days). Mean birth weight of the 33 remaining second-born fetuses was 1163 g (range: 250–2995 g). Perinatal mortality of these children was 30%. Six of the remaining fetuses were delivered by cesarean section because of partial placental abruption ($n=1$), cord prolaps ($n=1$), fetal distress ($n=1$) and in three women because of chorioamnionitis, in one case associated with prolapse of the umbilical cord. One woman had a relaparotomy because of a postoperative intra-abdominal hemorrhage. This woman developed pulmonary embolism postpartum despite prophylactic use of anticoagulants. In 18 twin pregnancies, in which the first baby was born before 26 weeks, it was possible to delay the second delivery until at least 26 weeks in 9 of 18 cases (50%), resulting in a perinatal mortality of the second baby of only one of nine cases (13%). In 80% of all women, it was possible to administer complete betamethasone treatment. Histological examination of the placenta showed 29 dichorionic (DC) and

Table 155.1 Twin pregnancies ($N=33$): maternal age, gestational age at delivery, interval, birth weight and sex, mode of delivery, outcome, placenta and mode of conception

N	Maternal age (years)	Delivery		Interval (days)	Weight and sex		Mode of delivery	Outcome	Placenta	Mode of conception
		1	2		1	2				
1	25	16+2	20+2	28	140 m	490 m	V/V	D/D	DC	Spontaneous
2	26	19+0	19+5	5	250 f	300 f	V/V	SB/D	DC	ICSI
3	33	19+1	20+4	10	235 m	250 f	V/V	D/D	DC	Spontaneous
4	31	20+1	20+2	1	320 f	360 m	V/V	D/D	DC	Spontaneous
5	37	20+1	21+6	12	300 m	390 m	V/V	D/D	DC	IVF
6	34	20+1	27+4	52	330 m	1000 f	V/CS	D/A	DC	Spontaneous
7	32	21+1	31+4	73	350 f	1890 m	V/V	D/A	DC	IVF
8	31	22+0	37+1	106	465 f	2995 f	V/V	D/A	DC	ICSI
9	36	22+4	26+6	30	410 f	795 f	V/CS	SB/A	DC	Spontaneous
10	29	22+5	24+3	12	550 f	620 f	V/V	D/D	MC/DA	IVF
11	27	22+5	26+3	25	310 f	710 m	V/V	D/D	DC	Stimulation
12	31	23+1	25+6	19	550 f	740 m	V/V	D/SB	DC	IVF
13	39	24+0	26+2	16	795 m	860 m	V/V	D/A	MC/DA	ICSI
14	23	24+2	26+2	14	615 f	805 f	V/V	D/SB	DC	Spontaneous
15	27	24+4	25+1	4	680 m	765 m	V/V	D/A	DC	ICSI
16	26	24+6	25+4	5	670 m	750 f	V/V	D/A	DC	IVF
17	28	24+6	27+3	18	690 m	1250 m	V/V	D/A	DC	Spontaneous
18	29	24+6	30+0	36	1000 m	1530 f	V/V	D/A	DC	Spontaneous
19	29	26+1	26+4	3	875 m	715 m	V/V	D/D	MCDA	Spontaneous
20	29	26+2	26+5	3	780 f	870 f	V/V	D/A	DC	Stimulation
21	35	26+2	29+6	25	940 f	1470 f	V/CS	D/A	DC	IVF
22	35	26+3	26+4	1	850 f	855 m	V/V	A/A	DC	Spontaneous
23	39	26+3	28+1	12	835 f	1340 f	V/CS	A/A	DC	Spontaneous
24	33	26+3	32+3	42	850 m	1690 m	V/CS	A/A	DC	Spontaneous
25	32	26+3	34+0	53	840 m	2310 f	V/V	A/A	DC	Stimulation
26	28	28+1	30+3	16	865 m	1470 m	V/V	D/A	DC	Spontaneous
27	35	28+5	31+3	19	1220 m	1645 m	V/CS	SB/A	DC	ICSI
28	32	28+6	29+1	2	1150 f	1040 f	V/V	A/A	DC	Spontaneous
29	31	29+3	29+3	0.5	1305 m	1580 m	V/V	A/A	DC	Spontaneous
30	26	30+1	32+1	14	1450 m	1550 f	V/V	A/A	DC	Spontaneous
31	34	30+2	31+4	9	1220 m	1945 m	V/V	A/A	DC	Spontaneous
32	26	30+5	31+2	4	1660 m	1770 m	V/V	A/A	MCDA	Spontaneous
33	28	31+0	32+2	9	1271 f	1625 m	V/V	A/A	DC	Stimulation

m, male; f, female; V, vaginal; CS, cesarean section; D, perinatal death; SB, stillborn; A, alive; MC, monochorionic; DA, diamniotic; DC, dichorionic

4 monochorionic–diamniotic (MC–DA) placentas. Twenty placentas (5%) showed histological signs of chorioamnionitis. In eight women, the placenta had to be removed manually. Four of these women had a postpartum hemorrhage of more than 1 L. Nine women had clinical signs of chorioamnionitis. In three women, cesarean section had to be performed. Prolapse of the umbilical cord occurred in 4 out of 33 pregnancies and in two of them it was necessary to perform a cesarean section. In the other two, a breech

Table 155.2 Triplet pregnancies ($N=8$): maternal age, gestational age at delivery, interval, birth weight and sex, mode of delivery, outcome, placenta and mode of conception

	Maternal age	Delivery			Interval days		Weight and sex						
N	(years)	1	2	3	1–2	2–3	1	2	3	Mode of delivery	Outcome	Placenta	Mode of conception
1	33	18+6	19+0	19+1	1	1	250 m	250 m	280 m	V/V/V	D/D/D	TC	ICSI
2	34	18+6	23+5	23+5	34	0	220 m	520 f	580 m	V/V/V	D/D/D	TC	Stimulation
3	35	24+4	25+3	25+3	6	1	332 f	570 f	670 m	V/V/V	SB/D/D	TC	Stimulation
4	31	24+5	25+2	25+2	4	0	329 f	660 m	580 f	V/V/V	D/D/D	TC	IVF
5	34	25+4	27+1	27+3	11	2	645 m	900 m	810 m	V/V/CS	D/D/D	TC	Stimulation
6	25	26+0	26+6	26+6	6	0	830 f	900 f	850 f	V/V/V	A/A/A	TC	IVF
7	33	26+0	27+6	27+6	13	0	820 f	1000 m	1200 m	V/CS/CS	A/A/D	TC	ICSI
8	34	26+1	26+3	26+3	2	0	675 m	870 f	900 f	V/V/V	D/D/D	TC	IVF

M, male; f, female; V, vaginal; CS, cesarean section; D, perinatal death; SB, stillborn; A, alive; TC, trichorionic

extraction was performed because there was full dilatation and gestational age was below 25 weeks. Two women had a partial placental abruption, one of them delivered by breech extraction because there was fully dilatation. One woman had an isolated transient elevation of liver enzymes, but serological tests for viral infections were negative. One woman had a transient atrium fibrillation, which was successfully treated with digitalis and heparin. In one woman, appendectomy was performed in the puerperium.

Data of all eight triplet pregnancies are shown in Table 155.2. The mean gestational age at delivery of the first baby was 23.8 weeks (range: 18–26 weeks). The mean birth weight was 513 g (range: 220–830 g). Perinatal mortality of all first-born triplets was 75%. All five first-born babies born before 26 weeks died and had a mean birth weight of 355 g (range: 220–645 g). Mean interval between delivery of the first baby and the second baby was 9.6 days (range: 1–34 days). Three women delivered on three separate days. Mean interval between the second and the third delivery was 1.3 days (range: 1–2 days). Perinatal mortality of all 16 remaining fetuses was 81%. Perinatal mortality of the eight remaining fetuses that were delivered after 26 weeks was 63%. In two women a cesarean section was performed on a remaining multiplet because of fetal distress and chorioamnionitis, respectively. The latter had a relaparotomy because of a hemorrhage in the abdominal wall and she also developed urosepsis. She recovered completely. In one woman, the placenta that had to be removed manually, postpartum hemorrhage was more than 1 L. Two women developed clinical signs of chorioamnionitis. Histological examination of the placenta showed that all placentas were trichorionic. Four placentas showed histological signs of chorioamnionitis.

Short- and long-term neonatal follow-up was evaluated in our series.[4] Long-term follow-up at the corrected age of 1 and/or 2 years is not yet known in children born after 2002 and was not available for those born before 1997, and was therefore only analyzed in 17 sets of twins and 3 sets of triplets. As expected, mean birth weight and gestational age was significantly higher in the second born infants. Nine of 11 surviving first-born infants and 16 of 23 second-born infants needed assisted ventilation for an average period of 17 days and 14 days, respectively. This difference in the need for and duration of assisted ventilation was not significantly different. Idiopathic respiratory distress syndrome (RDS) and patent ductus arteriosus were more prevalent in first-borns, whereas second-born infants developed sepsis and bronchopulmonary disease more often. However, these differences are not significant either. For long-term outcome, we evaluated neuromotor development at the corrected age of 9 months, the developmental outcome at the ages of 1 and 2 years post-term using a Bayley score and adverse outcomes, defined as either mortality or a suspect (score between –1 SD and –2 SD) or an abnormal Bayley test (score < -2SD), at the corrected age of 2 years. At the corrected age of 9 months, neuromotor development of seven first-borns was normal in 71%, suspect in 14% and abnormal in 14%. In the group of infants ($n=17$) born after delayed interval delivery, neuromotor development was normal in 76%, suspect in 18% and abnormal in 6%, which was comparable to a reference group. One first-born and four children who were born later were lost to long-term follow-up. We obtained a Bayley score on four first-borns (group 1) and nine infants (group 2) who were born after delayed interval delivery. The differences were not statistically significant. In group 1, the results after 1 year were that two children had normal developmental outcome, whereas one child was scored abnormal. At the age of 2 years, the score of these children had not changed. In group 2, after 1 year there were three children with normal developmental outcome, whereas two children were scored as having a suspect developmental outcome. At the age of 2 years, of the latter two children, one appeared to have a normal developmental outcome and the other an abnormal outcome. Adverse outcome was 74% in group 1 and 30% in group 2.

Review of the literature

In 1957, Abrams was the first to report on a woman with uterus simplex and twin pregnancy, who gave birth to two children with an interval of 35 days between the deliveries and were both alive at time of birth.[5] At 23.3 weeks of gestation, the mother delivered a girl of 396 g, who died 3 h after birth at home. Five weeks later, she delivered a living boy weighing 1033 g. Unfortunately, neonatal outcome and further development were not stated. Since 1957, several well-documented case reports were published on delayed interval delivery from women, in which the first baby was born before 32 weeks of gestation. In 1998, we reviewed data published between 1957 and 1996, consisting of 21 small series including 30 cases with delayed interval deliveries in twins, 11 single case reports in triplets and 3 single case reports in quadruplets.[2] At that moment, there were only two larger series: Arias *et al.* had presented a series of delayed interval procedures in eight twin and three triplet pregnancies,[6] whereas Van Eyck *et al.* had reported a series of 13 twin and 4 triplet pregnancies.[2] As already mentioned, the success rate of the smaller series was almost twice as high as in the two larger series, suggesting that in the smaller series mainly cases with successful outcomes were reported. Furthermore, in the smaller series and case reports there was a great variety in the treatment protocols and a lack of neonatal follow-up.

Since 1996, several small studies have been published on delayed interval delivery in twins (12), triplets (10), two studies on quadruplets and quintuplets and one study on very high-order multiplets (more than five fetuses). Furthermore, three larger series of more than six cases were published originating from a single center and three studies reporting on results of multicenter databases.

Small series (six or fewer cases) on twin pregnancies originating from a single center

Table 155.3 shows 12 studies including 30 cases of delayed interval delivery in twins published in the period between 1996 and 2004.[7–18] The most important variation in treatment protocols implied the use of cervical cerclage, which was performed in 53% of the cases. Tocolytics were administered in 93%, antibiotics in 100%, whereas corticosteroids were administered in 100% of the cases when a gestational age of more than 24 weeks was reached. Mean gestational age at delivery of the first-born baby was 22 weeks (range: 15–27 weeks). Mean interval between the two deliveries was 55 days (range: 1–153 days). The survival rate of the first-borns was 23%. Survival rate of the second twins was 87%. Neonatal follow-up was reported in six studies. Maternal complications consisted of placental abruptions ($n=2$), sepsis ($n=2$), chorioamnionitis ($n=7$) and thrombophlebitis of the left ovarian vein ($n=1$).

Small series (six or fewer cases) on triplet pregnancies originating from a single center

Table 155.4 summarizes 10 studies reporting on 12 cases of delayed interval delivery in triplets, which were published in the period between 1996 and 2004.[8,9,11,14,16,19,20–23] Besides the use of antibiotics (100%), treatment protocols varied largely with respect to the use of cervical cerclage (25%) and administration of tocolytics (58%). Corticosteroids were given in 75% of pregnancies in which a gestational age of more than 24 weeks was reached.

Mean gestational age at delivery of the first-born was 22 weeks (range: 17–31 weeks). Mean interval between the birth of the first and the remaining fetuses was 30 days (range: 3–70 days). Only one delivery took place on three separate days. The survival rate for 12 first-borns was 25% and that of the 24 remaining fetuses was 67%. Neonatal follow-up was reported in one study. Maternal complications consisted of placental abruption ($n=1$), chorioamnionitis ($n=2$) and sepsis with multiorgan failure ($n=1$).

Quadruplet pregnancies originating from a single center

Table 155.5 shows two studies reporting on two cases of delayed interval delivery in quadruplets, which were published in the period between 1996 and 2004.[24,25] In both series, tocolytics, antibiotics and corticosteroids were given and no cervical cerclage was performed. Gestational age at delivery of the first-born was 19 and 26 weeks, respectively. The interval between the birth of the first and the remaining fetuses was 92 and 12 days. Only one of the two first-borns survived, whereas five out of six (=83%) of the remaining fetuses survived. In both series deliveries took place on two separate dates.

Quintuplet pregnancies originating from a single center

Table 155.6 shows two studies reporting on two cases of delayed interval delivery in quintuplets, which

Table 155.3 Twin pregnancies, smaller series ($N=12$): reference, year of publication, gestational age at delivery, interval, birth weight and sex, mode of delivery, outcome, placenta and treatment

Reference	Year	Delivery		Interval (days)	Weight and sex		Mode of delivery	Outcome	Placenta	Treatment			
		1	2		1	2				T	A	C	Cortico
Chang et al.[7]	1996	18	28 + 2	72	n.s.	1232 m	V/V	SB/A	DADC	+	+	+	–
Antsaklis et al.[8]	1996	20	34	98	n.s.	2100 m	V/V	SB/A	DADC	+	+	–	–
		15	28	85	n.s.	1270 f	V/V	SB/A	DADC	+	+	–	–
Kalchbrenner et al.[9]	1998	23 + 1	27 + 1	28	685 n.s.	1095 n.s.	V/CS	D/A	n.s.	+	+	+	+
		24 + 3	25 + 3	7	660 n.s.	690 n.s.	V/V	A/A	n.s.	+	+	+	+
		24 + 3	25 + 1	5	720 n.s.	740 n.s.	V/CS	A/A	n.s.	+	+	+	+
		24 + 5	37 + 6	92	610 n.s.	2750 n.s.	V/CS	A/A	n.s.	+	+	+	+
		24	30	42	650 n.s.	1665 n.s.	V/V	A/A	n.s.	+	+	+	+
Watson et al.[10]	1998	23 + 6	36 + 3	88	510 f	3510 f	V/CS	A/A	n.s.	+	+	+	–
Platt and Rosa[11]	1999	21 + 1	21 + 6	5	n.s.	n.s.	V/V	D/D	n.s.	–	+	–	–
Song et al.[12]	2000	24 + 6	33 + 1	58	260 n.s.	2110 f	V/V	SB/A	n.s.	+	+	–	–
		27 + 6	33 + 6	42	60 n.s.	2430 f	V/V	SB/A	MCDA	+	+	–	+
Clerici et al.[13]	2001	22 + 6	25 + 3	18	520 f	775 f	V/CS	A/A	DADC	+	+	–	+
Van der Straeten et al.[14]	2001	19 + 3	36 + 2	117	259 n.s.	2800 n.s.	V/V	D/A	n.s.	+	+	–	+
		24 + 6	27 + 4	19	n.s.	999 n.s.	V/V	SB/A	n.s.	+	+	–	+
		25 + 4	28 + 1	18	690 n.s.	1240 n.s.	V/V	D/A	n.s.	+	+	–	+
		24 + 1	26 + 1	14	495 n.s.	900 n.s.	V/V	D/A	n.s.	+	+	–	+
		20 + 5	27 + 4	48	335 n.s.	1020 n.s.	V/V	D/A	n.s.	+	+	–	+
Platt and Rosa[15]	2001	18	25	49	n.s.	704 m	V/CS	D/A	DADC	–	+	+	+
Weemhoff et al.[16]	2001	19 + 4	37 + 6	136	255 m	3480 f	V/V	D/A	DADC	+	+	+	+
		18 + 1	19 + 3	9	160 m	270 m	V/V	SB/D	DADC	+	+	+	–
		26 + 6	28 + 6	14	980	1260 m	V/V	A/A	DADC	+	+	–	+
		24 + 3	24 + 4	1	586 n.s.	575 f	V/V	D/D	DADC	+	+	–	+
Benden et al.[17]	2001	24 + 2	29	33	410 f	1320 m	V/V	SB/A	DADC	+	+	–	+
Hamersley et al.[18]	2002	24 + 5	36 + 3	82	n.s.	2806 n.s.	V/V	D/A	DADC	+	+	+	+
		20 + 1	36 + 1	112	n.s.	2240 n.s.	V/CS	D/A	DADC	+	+	+	+
		15 + 3	37 + 2	153	n.s.	2863 n.s.	V/CS	D/A	DADC	+	+	+	–
		18 + 6	22 + 1	23	n.s.	n.s.	V/V	D/D	DADC	+	+	+	–
		19 + 6	34 + 5	104	n.s.	2325 n.s.	V/V	D/A	DADC	+	+	+	–
		21 + 6	30 + 6	62	n.s.	1332 n.s.	V/CS	D/A	DADC	+	+	+	+

m, male; f, female; V, vaginal; CS, cesarean section; D, perinatal death; SB, stillborn; A, alive; MC, monochorionic; DA, diamniotic; DC, dichorionic; T, tocolysis; A, antibiotics; C, cerclage; cortico, corticosteroids; n.s., not stated

Table 155.4 Triplet pregnancies, smaller series ($N=10$): reference, year of publication, gestational age at delivery, interval, birth weight and sex, mode of delivery, outcome, placenta and treatment

		Delivery			Interval (days)		Weight and sex						Treatment			
Reference	Year	1	2	3	1–2	2–3	1	2	3	Mode of delivery	Outcome	Placenta	T	A	C	Cortico
Chua and Tsakok[19]	1996	24	29	29	35	0	295 n.s.	1155 f	1025 F	V/CS/CS	SB/A/A	n.s.	+	+	–	+
Antsaklis *et al.*[8]	1996	17	27	27	70	0	n.s. n.s.	670 m	1040 F	V/CS/CS	SB/SB/A	TC	–	+	–	–
Matalliotakis *et al.*[20]	1998	24	32	32	56	0	n.s. n.s.	1790 m	1610 F	V/CS/CS	D/A/A	TC	–	+	–	+
Kalchbrenner *et al.*[9]	1998	18+6	26+5	26+5	55	0	220 n.s	1150 n.s.	1110 n.s.	V/V/V	D/A/A	n.s.	+	+	+	+
		19	19+3	19+3	3	0	142 n.s.	275 n.s.	270 n.s.	V/V/V	D/D/D	n.s.	+	+	+	–
Giannacopoulou *et al.*[21]	1998	23	32	32	56	0	n.s. n.s.	1790 m	1610 F	V/CS/CS	D/A/A	TC	–	+	–	–
		26	26+6	26+6	6	0	850 m	1030 m	950 M	V/CS/CS	A/A/A	TC	–	+	–	–
Flatt and Rosa[11]	1999	21+1	21+6	21+6	5	0	n.s. n.s.	n.s. n.s.	n.s. n.s.	V/V/V	SB/D/D	TC	–	+	–	–
Van der Straeten *et al.*[14]	2000	26+4	27	29+4	3	18	970 n.s.	860 n.s.	1395 n.s.	V/V/V	A/A/D	n.s.	+	+	–	+
Weemhoff *et al.*[16]	2001	31+4	32	32	3	0	1530 m	1860 m	1258 F	V/V/V	A/A/A	n.s.	+	+	–	+
Kursun *et al.*[22]	2002	21	27	27	42	0	n.s. n.s.	978 f	925 F	V/CS/CS	SB/A/A	n.s.	+	+	–	+
Hoffman and Sciscione[23]	2004	21	22	22	7	0	445 n.s.	n.s. n.s.	n.s. n.s.	V/V/V	D/D/D	n.s.	+	+	+	–

m, male; f, female; V, vaginal; CS, cesarean section; D, perinatal death; SB, sti lborn; A, alive; TC, trichorionic; T, tocolysis; A, antibiotics; C, cerclage; cortico, corticosteroids; n.s., not stated

Table 155.5 Quadruplet pregnancies smaller series ($N=2$): reference, year of publication, gestational age at delivery, interval, birth weight and sex, mode of delivery, outcome, placenta, treatment and neonatal follow-up

Reference	Year	Neonate	Gestational age at delivery	Interval (days)	Birth weight and sex	Mode of delivery	Outcome	Placenta	Treatment T	Treatment A	Treatment C	Treatment Cortico	Neonatal follow-up
Marinoff *et al.*[24]	1998	1	19 + 5	0	260 f	V	SB	n.s.	+	+	–	–	–
		2	32 + 6	92	n.s.	V	SB	=	+	+	–	+	–
		3	32 + 6	=	1470 f	V	A	=	+	+	–	+	28 days
		4	32 + 6	=	1700 f	V	A	=	+	+	–	+	28 days
Kirshon[25]	2002	1	26 + 6	0	780 m	V	A	QC/QA	+	+	–	+	1 year
		2	28 + 4	12	990 m	V	A	=	+	+	–	+	1 year
		3	28 + 4	=	1040 m	CS	A	=	+	+	–	+	1 year
		4	28 + 4	=	860 f	CS	A	=	+	+	–	+	1 year

m, male; f, female; V, vaginal; CS, cesarean section; SB, stillborn; A, alive; QC, quadrochorionic; QA, quadroamnionic; T, tocolysis; A, antibiotics; C, cerclage; cortico, corticosteroids; n.s., not stated

Table 155.6 Quintuplet pregnancies ($N=2$): reference, year of publication, gestational age at delivery, interval, birth weight and sex, mode of delivery, outcome, placenta, treatment and neonatal follow-up

Reference	Year	Neonate	Gestational age at delivery	Interval (days)	Birth weight and sex	Mode of delivery	Outcome	Placenta	Treatment T	A	C	Cortico	Neonatal follow-up
Rosa *et al.*[26]	1995	1	19+2	0	n.s.	V	D	n.s.	–	+	–	–	–
		2	19+2	0	n.s.	V	D	n.s.	–	+	–	–	–
		3	19+3	1	n.s.	V	D	n.s.	–	+	–	–	–
		4	21+3	14	n.s.	V	D	n.s.	–	–	–	–	–
		5	21+3	=	n.s.	V	D	n.s.	–	–	–	–	–
Elias *et al.*[27]	1998	1	24	0	400 f	V	D	QC/QA	+	+	–	–	–
		2	26	21	700 m	V	D	=	+	+	–	–	–
		3	27	23	700 m	V	D	=	+	+	–	–	–
		4	32	61	1000 m	CS	A	=	+	+	–	+	1 year
		5	32	=	850 f	CS	D	=	+	+	–	+	–

m, male; f, female; V, vaginal; CS, cesarean section; D, perinatal death; A, alive; QC, quinchorionic; QA, quinamnionic; T, tocolysis; A, antibiotics; C, cerclage; cortico, corticosteroids; n.s., not stated

were published in the period between 1996 and 2004.[26,27] In both studies, no cervical cerclage was performed. In both studies antibiotics were given. When a gestational age of 24 weeks was reached tocolytics and corticosteroids were administered. Gestational age at delivery of the first-born was 19 and 24 weeks. The interval between the birth of the first fetus and the last fetuses was 14 and 61 days. No first-borns and only one of the remaining fetuses survived. This infant had normal development after 1 year. No maternal complications were reported.

Very high-order (more than five fetuses) multiple pregnancies originating from a single center

Table 155.7 shows one study of two cases of delayed interval delivery in very high-order (more than five fetuses) multiple pregnancies.[25] Kirshon reported on delayed interval delivery in a woman with a sextuplet pregnancy, who already had a cerclage placed at the end of the first trimester.[25] Despite tocolytics, the first baby was born at 22 weeks and 4 days through the anterior cervix. At 26 weeks, she had vaginal blood loss and full dilatation. A cesarean section was performed. Five neonates were born with birth weights between 580 and 760 g. One of the five surviving infants had intraventricular hemorrhage grade III, with resultant hydrocephalus. The other four had no significant long-term sequelae. Kirshon also reported on delayed interval delivery in a woman with octuplet pregnancy. Despite tocolytics, the first baby was born at 25 weeks after removal of the cervical cerclage. A girl of 690-g weight was born and developed uneventfully. At 26 weeks and 5 days a cesarean section was performed because of fetal distress of one multiplet. Seven neonates were born with birth weights between 320 and 810 g. Postoperative course was complicated by intra-abdominal bleeding, relaparotomy and the necessity to apply a large amount of blood products. At the age of 1 year, all seven surviving infants were neurologically intact and met all their milestones.

Larger series (more than six cases) originating from a single center

Since 1996, a total of three larger series originating from a single center were reported. In 1998, Porreco *et al.* reported on nine cases (six twin and three triplet pregnancies).[28] Monochorionicity was considered as an exclusion criterion. The treatment protocol consisted of cervical cerclage and administration of tocolytics and antibiotics. Mean gestational age at delivery of the first baby was 23.9 weeks (range: 19.4–27.9 weeks). Mean latency interval was 34 days (range: 3–76 days). Perinatal mortality was 70% for first-borns and 18% for the neonates born after delayed interval. No information is given on birth weights, neonatal follow-up or maternal complications.

Van Doorn *et al.* reported in 1999 on 15 cases (10 twins and 5 triplets).[29] The treatment protocol

Table 155.7 Very high-order (> 5 fetuses) pregnancies ($N=1$): reference, year of publication, gestational age at delivery, interval, birth weight and sex, mode of delivery, outcome, placenta, treatment and neonatal follow-up

Reference	Year	Neonate	Gestational age at delivery	Interval (days)	Birth weight and sex	Mode of delivery	Outcome	Placenta	Treatment				Neonatal follow-up
									T	A	C	Cortico	
Kirshon[25]	2002	1	22+4	0	340 m	V	SB	SC/SA	+	+	–	–	–
		2	26+0	24	650 m	CS	A	=	+	+	–	–	1 year
		3	26+0	=	590 f	CS	A	=	+	+	–	–	1 year
		4	26+0	=	760 m	CS	A	=	+	+	–	–	1 year
		5	26+0	=	740 f	CS	A	=	+	+	–	–	1 year
		6	26+0	=	580 f	CS	A	=	+	+	–	–	1 year
		1	25	0	690 f	V	A	OC/OA	+	+	–	+	1 year
		2	26+5	12	760 f	CS	A	=	+	+	–	+	1 year
		3	26+5	=	800 f	CS	A	=	+	+	–	+	1 year
		4	26+5	=	730 f	CS	A	=	+	+	–	+	1 year
		5	26+5	=	320 f	CS	D	=	+	+	–	+	–
		6	26+5	=	500 m	CS	A	=	+	+	–	+	1 year
		7	26+5	=	810 m	CS	A	=	+	+	–	+	1 year
		8	26+5	=	520 f	CS	A	=	+	+	–	+	1 year

m, male; f, female; V, vaginal; CS, cesarean section; D, perinatal death; SB, stillborn; A, alive; SC, sexchorionic; SA, sexamnionic; OC, octachorionic; OA, octa-amniotic; T, tocolysis; A, antibiotics; C, cerclage; cortico, corticosteroids; n.s., not stated

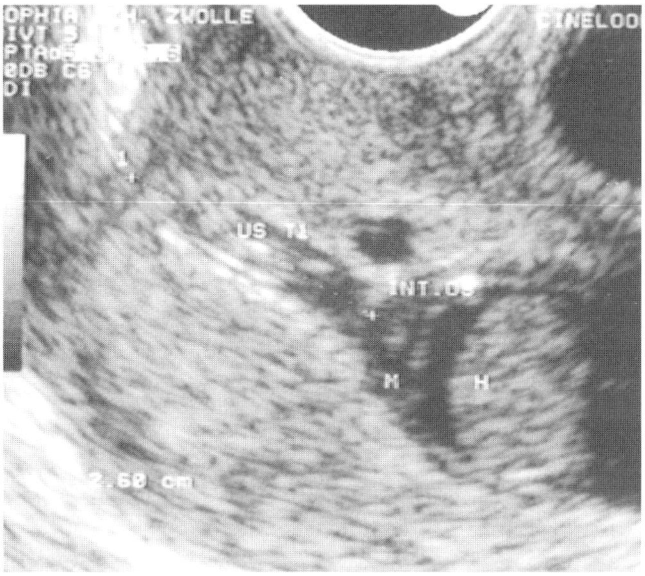

Figure 155.1 Ultrasonic image of a cervix 2 days after delivery of the first baby, showing the umbilical cord of the first baby in the cervical canal, which regained a length of 2.6 cm.

consisted of administration of tocolytics and antibiotics. In one case, a cervical cerclage was performed. Mean gestational age at delivery of the first baby was 26 weeks (range: 19.7–30.4 weeks). In five women, the attempted interval delivery resulted in a delay of less than 3 h between separate deliveries. The mean latency interval within the 10 remaining pregnancies was 12 days (range: 1–53 days). Five of 15 first-borns survived. Survival rate of the 20 neonates born after delayed interval was 50%. In all triplet pregnancies, the second and the third child were born on the same day. Long-term follow-up revealed one child with axial hypotonia and strabismus and one child with rachitis. Maternal morbidity consisted of chorioamnionitis in three women and one woman with postpartum hemorrhage necessitating blood cell transfusion.

Farkouh *et al.* reported in 2000 on 24 cases (20 twin and 4 triplet pregnancies).[30] The treatment protocol consisted of cerclage and administration of tocolytics and antibiotics. Administration of corticosteroids was not mentioned. Mean gestational age at delivery of the first baby was 22.7 weeks (range: 16.4–28.6 weeks). Mean latency interval was 36 days (range: 3–123 days). Patients with a previous cervical cerclage during the index pregnancy had significantly shorter mean latency intervals than patients without previous cerclage. There were no survivors among first-born infants when the gestational age at presentation was 24 weeks or less. Perinatal mortality of the first-born infants was 84%, whereas perinatal mortality of the infants who were retained after the birth of the first-borns was 37%. The duration of hospital stay of the survivors was used to express the short-term neonatal morbidity. Hospitalization of the surviving first-born infants ($n=4$) lasted on average 86 days (range: 72–106 days). In the surviving siblings who were retained after delayed interval delivery ($n=17$), hospitalization lasted on average 47 days (range: 2–126 days). The duration of hospitalization was significantly shorter for the 'retained' group. Long-term neonatal morbidity was not studied. Seven women developed postpartum endometritis and one woman, septic pelvic endometritis.

Multicenter studies

Three larger series originating from a multicenter database were published.[31–33] Zhang *et al.* studied the US 1995–1998 Matched Multiple Birth File.[31] Two hundred twin pregnancies were identified in which the first twin was delivered between 17 and 29 weeks and the second twin two ore more days later. These 200 delayed interval deliveries were individually matched with 347 twin pregnancies in which the second twin was delivered on the same or the next calendar day. Among the 200 pregnancies with delayed delivery, the mean gestational age at first delivery was 23 weeks and the median duration of delay was 6 days (range: 2–107 days). One week of delay in delivery was associated with a mean increase in infant birth weight of 131 g. Furthermore, 56% of the delayed second twins survived to 1 year of age, whereas only 24% of the non-delayed second twins survived to 1 year of age ($P<0.001$). However, 11% of the second twins in delayed delivery (95% CI: 6–16%) experienced fetal death before 24 weeks. There was no information on treatment protocols, maternal and neonatal morbidity.

Fayad *et al.* published a series of 35 cases (28 twin and 7 triplet pregnancies) of delayed interval delivery originating from 12 tertiary care centers over 10 years.[32] Treatment protocols varied and consisted of a high ligation of the cord (in 78%), cervical cerclage (in 32%), administration of antibiotics (in 100%), tocolytics (in 82%) and hospitalization (in 93%). In relation to the 'success' expressed by the duration of the interval, there was no statistical difference whether or not a cerclage was performed; antibiotics or tocolytics were administered or whether the patient was admitted or not. Mean gestational age of the first twin deliveries was 20.8 ± 5.5 weeks and the mean birth weight of first twins was 497 ± 239 g. Only 7% of the first-borns survived. The mean interval between deliveries was 47 days (range: 3–140 days). The mean birth weight of the second twin was 1217 ± 602 g. The survival rate of these second twins was 79%. In each of the seven triplet pregnancies, only one delayed interval delivery procedure was performed. The mean interval between deliveries was 23 days. Survival rate of the first, second and third triplets was 9.5%, 19% and 14.2%, respectively. No data were presented with respect to maternal and neonatal morbidity or neonatal follow-up.

Livingston *et al.* published a series of 14 cases (nine twin and five triplet pregnancies) of delayed interval delivery originating from two tertiary care centers over 12 years.[33] The mean gestational age of delivery of the first multiplets was 21 weeks. All women received tocolytics and intravenous antibiotics. Two of three attempts to place a cerclage were successful. The mean latency was 2 days (range: 1–70 days). There was one survival of a first-born multiplet. Of the 19 retained fetuses, 2 died *in utero*, 10 died between birth and day 57 of life and 7 (37%) survived until hospital discharge. Six of he seven survivors had major sequelae from prematurity. One of 19 fetuses (5%) was discharged without major sequelae. Maternal morbidity included two pregnancies with placental abruption and eight pregnancies with infectious morbidity including one septic shock.

Discussion

Even the review of the recent literature shows a large variety of treatment protocols and relatively higher success rates in smaller compared to larger series. However, compared to our review of the literature, which was published in 1998,[2] a larger number of studies were published reporting also on procedures that were not favorable. Only few studies include long-term neonatal follow-up. With respect to treatment protocols, the use of cervical cerclage for delayed interval delivery is still controversial. In the smaller series, there is no consistency with respect to performing a cervical cerclage. Even if this were the case, it would be impossible to draw conclusions because of the selection bias. Retrospective multicenter studies report on large series, but have the disadvantage that there is a large variety in treatment protocols, especially with respect to the use of cervical cerclage. Zhang *et al.* examined whether cervical cerclage after the first delivery prolonged the interdelivery interval in reports on delayed interval delivery published between 1880 and 2002.[34] Seven larger series (81 cases) were selected that identified all cases of delayed interval delivery in their institutions during a specified period. Studies in which a cerclage was infrequently used reported a shorter interdelivery interval compared to studies where cerclage was used (median: 9 vs. 26 days, respectively, $P < 0.001$) despite similar gestational age at the first delivery, similar use of antibiotics, tocolytics and incidence of infection. After controlling for other factors, the use of cerclage did not significantly increase the risk of intrauterine infection. Zhang *et al.* suggest that cervical cerclage after the first delivery is associated with a longer interdelivery interval without increasing the risk of intrauterine infection. In contrast, we never performed cervical cerclage in our series of 41 cases, which resulted in a mean interval of 21 days (range: 0.5–106 days) in twin and 10 days (range: 1–34 days) in triplet pregnancies. There is still a debate not only on whether to perform but also on when to perform a cerclage. Some authors perform a cervical cerclage immediately after delivery of the first twin,[6,35–37] and others perform a cerclage only if cervical dilatation persists.[32,38,39]

There is meanwhile more information on maternal complications and morbidity in relation to cervical cerclage.[9,23,30,33,34] Hoffman *et al.*[23] reported on a procedure in a triplet pregnancy, resulting in chorioamnionitis, septic shock, multiorgan failure and artificial ventilation because of RDS and even dialysis for the treatment of acute renal tubular necrosis. Kalchbrenner *et al.*[9] reported on four cases of chorioamnionitis, including two cases of sepsis and one of placental abruption. In a series of 24 cases, Farkouh *et al.*[30] observed eight cases of endometritis, including one case of septic pelvic thrombophlebitis. In a series of 14 cases, Livingston *et al.*[33] reported on two pregnancies with placental abruption, eight cases of infectious morbidity, including one case of septic shock. In a review of 66 case reports and case series published between 1880 and 2002, Zhang *et al.*[34] stated that despite prophylactic routine use of broad-spectrum antibiotics, the average incidence of clinical intrauterine infection after the first delivery was 36% and the incidence of maternal sepsis was 4.9%. A remarkable complication in a special kind of interval delivery was reported by Porreco *et al.*[40] At 28 weeks and 4 days of gestation a cesarean section was performed in a woman with twin pregnancy because of growth retardation of one fetus. A neonate of 619 g was born and the other fetus was kept *in utero*, which was closed in two layers with fibrin glue interposed. The woman was discharged on home uterine activity monitoring and modified bed rest. The mother complained of left lower uterine pain and increasing uterine activity at 31 weeks and 6 days of gestation. Ultrasonic evaluation showed anhydramnios and the fetal heart tracing showed variable and prolonged decelerations. The retained sibling (a boy of 1738 g) was delivered by laparotomy and had normal Apgar scores and umbilical cord blood gases. A complete uterine scar dehiscence was noted with prolapse of a loop of umbilical cord into the peritoneal cavity. The infant was delivered through the dehiscence, the edges were debrided and the uterus was closed in layers. The mother was discharged on her fourth postoperative day.

Our study describes a large series originating from a single center. In this series, the survival rate of at least one remaining baby is comparable with other large series.[28–30] In contrast to these series, we never performed cervical cerclage. Success rate depends on numerous criteria, including the length of postponement or merely whether time was obtained to give corticosteroids for lung maturation of the remaining fetus or whether there was a reduction of mortality or morbidity. With respect to viability of the remaining baby, the goal of our series was to postpone the second delivery until a gestational age of at least 26 weeks, resulting in a reduction of perinatal mortality to 13%. All remaining babies born after at least 29 weeks survived. Due to the small number of infants available for follow-up, we could not find a significant difference between the two groups. If, however, we bear in mind that the reason for postponing the delivery of the second sib is the birth of a viable baby and adverse outcome is defined as death or abnormal development, there was a significant difference. Nonetheless, it is important to recognize that delayed interval delivery may be associated with a relatively high degree of maternal morbidity. Besides the technical aspects of this procedure, it is important to consider psychosocial and emotional support to the patient and her partner.

Conclusion

If twin pregnancies are complicated by immature or very premature delivery of the first baby, delayed interval delivery results in a significant reduction of perinatal mortality of the second infant. Single case reports and small series have a higher success rate than larger series, suggesting selection bias, based on the fact that only successful results were published. The significant reduction of adverse neonatal outcome has to be considered in relation to the degree of complications and maternal morbidity. For further recommendations, randomized studies performed for all multiple pregnancies with a vaginal delivery of the first multiplet before 26 weeks might be an option to differentiate whether a cervical cerclage improves the outcome. In any case, for an adequate counseling of future parents about the described procedure including pros and cons, it is important to document protocols and outcome of all cases (also the failures) of each single center.

REFERENCES

1. Luke B, Keith LG. The contribution of singletons, twins and triplets to low birth weight, infant mortality and handicap in the United States. *J Reprod Med* 1992;37:661–6.
2. Van Eyck J, Risseeuw JJ, Arabin B. Delayed interval delivery in multiple pregnancy: Techniques and results. In Kurjak A, ed. *Textbook of Perinatal Medicine*. New York: The Parthenon Publishing Group, 1998:1542–9.
3. McIntosh N, Harrison A. Prolonged premature rupture of membranes in the preterm infant: A 7 year study. *Eur J Obstet Gynecol Reprod Biol* 1994;57:1–6.
4. Rosbergen HMF, Vogt HP, Baerts W, *et al.* Long and short term outcome after delayed-interval delivery in multi-fetal pregnancies. *Eur J Obstet Gynecol* 2005;122:66–72.
5. Abrams RH. Double pregnancy. Report of a case with thirty-five days between deliveries. *Obstet Gynecol* 1957;9:435–8.
6. Arias F. Delayed delivery of multifetal pregnancies with premature rupture of membranes in the second trimester. *Am J Obstet Gynecol* 1994;170:1233–7.
7. Chang HC, Wu MY, Ho HN, Yang YS. Delayed delivery of surviving triplet after fetal reduction and spontaneous abortion. *J Formos Med Assoc* 1996;95(11):881–4.
8. Antsaklis A, Daskalakis G, Papageorgiou I, Aravantinos D. Conservative treatment after miscarriage of one fetus in multifetal pregnancies. Report of three cases and review of the literature. *Fetal Diagn Ther* 1996;11(5):366–72.
9. Kalchbrenner MA, Weisenborn EJ, Chyu JK, Kaufman HK, Losure TA. Delayed delivery of multiple gestations: Maternal and neonatal outcome. *Am J Obstet Gynecol* 1998;179:1145–9.
10. Watson WJ, McNelis T. Delayed interval delivery: Infection is not an absolute contraindication. *Am J Perinatol* 1998;15(6):387–8.
11. Platt JS, Rosa C. Delayed interval delivery in multiple gestations. *Obstet Gynecol Surv* 1999;54(5):343–8.
12. Song TB, Jeong J, Kim YH, Kim EK. Delayed interval delivery in multiple gestations. *Arch Gynecol Obstet* 2000;263(4):185–7.
13. Clerici G, Cutuli A, Renzo GC. Delayed interval delivery of a second twin. *Eur J Obstet Gynecol Reprod Biol* 2001;96(1):121–2.
14. Van der Straeten FM, De Ketelaere K, Temmerman M. Delayed interval delivery in multiple pregnancies. *Eur J Obstet Gynecol Reprod Biol* 2001;99(1):85–9.
15. Platt JS, Rosa C. Delayed interval delivery military style. *Mil Med* 2001;166(3):278–80.
16. Weemhoff M, van Meir CA, Walther FJ, Twaalfhoven FC, van Roosmalen J. Delayed birth of the second child in multiple gestation. *Ned Tijdschr Geneeskd* 2001;145(29):1377 80.
17. Benden D, Miller M, Hatoum N. 39-day delay in delivery of twins. A case report. *J Reprod Med* 2001;46(12):1071–7.
18. Hamersley SL, Coleman SK, Bergauer NK, Bartholomew LM, Pinckert TL. Delayed-interval delivery in twin pregnancies. *J Reprod Med* 2002;47(2):125–30.
19. Chua EK, Tsakok FH. Delayed interval delivery in a triplet pregnancy: A case report. *Ann Acad Med Singapore* 1996;25(2):279–80.
20. Matalliotakis IM, Makrigiannakis AS, Giannakopoulou CC, Neonaki MA, Goumenou AG, Koumantakis EE. Delayed interval delivery and survival of the two fetuses after second trimester loss of one triplet. *Eur J Obstet Gynecol Reprod Biol* 1998;80(2):159–60.
21. Giannacopoulou C, Matalliotakis I, Hatzidaki E, *et al.* Conservative treatment of multiple pregnancies after delivery and a fetal miscarriage: Two case reports. *Clin Exp Obstet Gynecol* 1998;25(1–2):54–5.
22. Kursun S, Simsek M, Trak B, Boneval C, Melikoglu M, Taskin O. Delayed-interval delivery of triplet pregnancy following preterm labor. A case report. *Fetal Diagn Ther* 2002;17(5):293–4.
23. Hoffman MK, Sciscione AC. Sepsis and multisystem organ failure in a woman attempting interval delivery in a triplet pregnancy: A case report. *J Reprod Med* 2004;49(5):387–8.
24. Marinoff DN, Spitzberg EH, Chueh JT, Goldman JM, Downs T. Delayed-interval delivery in a quadruplet pregnancy after intrauterine death of a partial molar pregnancy and preterm delivery. A case report. *J Reprod Med* 1998;43(12):1051–4.
25. Kirshon B. Interval delivery and aggressive tocolysis in high-order multiple gestation. A report of three cases. *J Reprod Med* 2002;47(10):867–70.
26. Rosa C, Fontenot JP, Harlass FE. Clomiphene-induced quintuplets with a failed attempt at delayed-interval delivery. *Mil Med* 1995;160(12):646–7.s
27. Elias M, Heimrath J, Zimmer M, Woyton J, Goluda M. Delayed interval delivery in a quintuplet pregnancy. *Hum Reprod* 1998;13(1):224–6.
28. Porreco RP, Sabin ED, Heyborne KD, Lindsay LG. Delayed-interval delivery in multifetal pregnancy. *Am J Obstet Gynecol* 1998;178(1 Pt 1):20–3.

29. Van Doorn HC, van Wezel-Meijler G, van Geijn HP, Dekker GA. Delayed interval delivery in multiple pregnancies. Is optimism justified? *Acta Obstet Gynecol Scand* 1999;78(8):710–5.
30. Farkouh LJ, Sabin ED, Heyborne KD, *et al.* Delayed-interval delivery: Extended series from a single maternal-fetal medicine department. *Am J Obstet Gynecol* 2000;183:1499–1503.
31. Zhang J, Hamilton B, Martin J, Trumble A. Delayed interval delivery and infant survival: A population-based study. *Am J Obstet Gynecol* 2004;191(2):470–6.
32. Fayad S, Bongain A, Holhfeld P, *et al.* Delayed delivery of second twin: A multicentre study of 35 cases. *Eur J Obstet Gynecol Reprod Biol* 2003;109(1):16–20.
33. Livingston JC, Livingston LW, Ramsey R, Sibai BM. Second trimester asynchronous multifetal delivery results in poor perinatal outcome. *Obstet Gynecol* 2004;103:77–81.
34. Zhang J, Johnson CD, Hoffman M. Cervical cerclage in delayed interval delivery in a multifetal pregnancy: A review of seven case series. *Eur J Obstet Gynecol Reprod Biol* 2003;108(2): 126–30.
35. Abifadel W, Afif N, Azouri J. Delayed interval delivery: Case report and review of the literature. *J Gynecol Obstet Biol Reprod* 1997;26:711–4.
36. Laverty JP, Austin RJ, Schaefer DS, Aladjem S. Asynchronous multiple birth: A report of five cases. *J Reprod Med* 1994;39: 55–60.
37. Cardwell MS, Caple P, Baker CL. Triplet pregnancy with delivery on three separate days. *Obstet Gynecol* 1988;71:448–9.
38. Wittman BK, Farquharson D, Wong GP. Delayed delivery of second twin: A case report. *Obstet Gynecol* 1992;79:260–3.
39. Woolfson J, Fay F, Bates A. Twins with 54 days between deliveries: Case report. *Br J Obstet Gynaecol* 1983;90:685–6.
40. Porreco RP, Diss Sabin E, Heyborne KD, Lingle JR. Selective delivery in a twin gestation. *Am J Obstet Gynecol* 1998;179: 264–5.

156 Cerebral palsy in multiple pregnancy

P. O. D. Pharoah

Introduction

Cerebral palsy (CP) is not a single disease entity, rather it is a syndrome, the manifestations of which vary in severity and topographical involvement of the extremities and the site, type and timing of cerebral impairment.

The earliest clinical description is usually attributed to Little and the syndrome eponymously bears his name.[1] Inherent in the title of Little's paper is that difficulties in labor, preterm delivery and neonatal asphyxia placed the child at risk for cerebral impairment.

Variation in the manner by which CP is manifested and the overlap of presenting symptoms and signs with many other conditions has promulgated several attempts to classify and to formulate a definition of the syndrome. Suggested classifications have been based on timing of the impairment (intrauterine, birth or intrapartum palsies and postnatal or acquired palsies),[2] limb topography (hemiplegia, paraplegia – now regarded as diplegia to distinguish it from a paralysis attributable to a spinal cord lesion that is not considered to be CP, quadriplegia and disordered movements without rigidity),[1,3] muscle tonicity and clinical features (spasticity, hypotonia, dystonia, ataxia choreoathetosis and mixed forms).[4] Epidemiological description demands a definition of the syndrome that is being studied and there have been several definitions of CP.[4–10] Such plurality of definition is testament to the variability of what is or is not CP. Common to these definitions is that CP is a disorder of movement or posture due to a cerebral impairment that is non-progressive though not unchanging, i.e. it is not due to progressive lesions such as cerebral tumors or the lipoidoses but the symptoms and signs may alter as the child develops. It is also mentioned in the definition that the timing of the impairment is during early development although this begs the question as to what is meant by 'early' development.

Epidemiology of CP

The descriptive epidemiology of CP has been dependent on special surveys or on specific CP disease registers. Early studies reported population prevalence rates that ranged from 0.76 to 5.8 per 1000.[11] The development of specific CP disease registers, with an emphasis on the definition of the syndrome and efforts to ensure complete ascertainment of cases, has narrowed the range of CP prevalence to 2–2.5 per 1000 live births.[12–14]

It has been customary in the past to distinguish CP as those that are 'congenital', i.e. infants whose cerebral impairment occurred before birth, and those that are 'acquired', i.e. cerebral impairment that occurred postnatally. However, this distinction is unsatisfactory because of the difficulty, particularly in very preterm infants, of determining the precise timing of the cerebral insult. The alternative classification of 'early' impairment that has been sustained during fetal development or in the perinatal period and 'late' impairment sustained after the seventh postnatal day has been suggested.[15,16]

Late impairment (acquired) CP

Late impairment CP is usually attributable to head injury, both accidental and non-accidental and infections of the central nervous system such as encephalitis and meningitis.[17] These contribute about 10% of all CP,[11] are of marginal relevance to perinatal medicine and will not be considered further.

Early impairment (congenital) CP

Two risk factors dominate the epidemiology of early impairment CP. These are preterm delivery or low birth weight and multiple births. There is also the confounding of these risk factors in that an inverse association exists between the degree of plurality at birth and birth weight.

Prevalence and incidence in CP

It is essential, when examining the epidemiology of CP, to acknowledge the difference between incidence and prevalence of the condition. The incidence is a measure of the number of new cases entering a population and a changing incidence is primarily a pointer to what may be of etiological significance. The point

Table 156.1 Birth weight specific prevalence of CP

<table>
<tr><th>Birth weight group</th><th>Sweden* 1991–1994[13]</th><th>Western Australia** 1990–1994[18]</th><th>Oxford* 1984–1997[17]</th><th>Mersey** 1984–1989[19]</th></tr>
<tr><td>< 1000 g</td><td>48.5</td><td>92.5</td><td rowspan="2">48.2</td><td>87.3</td></tr>
<tr><td>1000–1499 g</td><td>81.0</td><td>48.3</td><td>86.2</td></tr>
<tr><td>1500–2499 g</td><td>11.4</td><td>7.9</td><td>9.4</td><td>11.8</td></tr>
<tr><td>≥2500 g</td><td>1.3</td><td>1.6</td><td>1.2</td><td>1.4</td></tr>
<tr><td>All birth weights</td><td>2.1</td><td>2.3</td><td>2.1</td><td>2.6</td></tr>
</table>

*Prevalence per 1000 live births
**Prevalence per 1000 neonatal survivors

prevalence is a measure of the number of cases in a population at a point in time and is affected by both the incidence and the duration of the disease. The arithmetic relationship is:

$$\text{Prevalence} \propto \text{Incidence} \times \text{Duration}$$

and, at a given point in time, Prevalence = Incidence × Duration, if the incidence and the mean duration of the disease are unchanging. This relationship merits emphasis in perinatal medicine and, in particular, in conditions such as CP and the congenital anomalies when the impairment may occur prepartum. There are two caveats that must be borne in mind when examining population prevalence of CP:

(1) It is unusual to make a firm diagnosis of CP before the age of 3 months and often it is not made until much later. In early impairment CP, the impairment may be of such severity that the child succumbs before a diagnosis can be made. The true incidence cannot be established and only the prevalence at a point in time is possible. If the cerebral impairment occurs during fetal development, contrary to expectation, improvements in fetal and neonatal medicine will lead to an *increasing* prevalence of CP. The impaired infant that would otherwise have died now survives with an increase in duration leading to an increase in prevalence. The corollary to this is that, when the impairment occurs during the perinatal period as may occur with hypoxic-ischemic injury in very preterm infants, improvements in medical management thereby preventing such injury will be associated with a *decrease* in the prevalence of CP.

(2) The population denominator for the prevalence must be stated. This assumes significance when birth weight specific prevalence of CP is considered. Very low birth weight infants have a much-increased neonatal mortality and the denominator used in calculating the CP prevalence will reflect this. The CP prevalence per 1000 live births may differ significantly from that per 1000 neonatal survivors.

Risk factors in CP

Birth weight and gestational age show a strong inverse association with the prevalence of CP. Indeed, Little's seminal description of CP in 1862 noted the relevance of prematurity.[1] Table 156.1, compiled from different population registers of CP, illustrates the inverse association of birth weight with CP prevalence.

Birth asphyxia and CP

Birth or perinatal asphyxia is usually taken to mean asphyxia sustained intrapartum or in the immediate postpartum period. Particularly in very preterm infants, the difficulty in maintaining normality of physiological variables, with the attendant risks of hypoxic-ischemic cerebral impairment manifest as periventricular leucomalacia or hemorrhage, is well recognized. Undoubtedly, peripartum asphyxia may lead to CP, usually of the dyskinetic hypertonic type. Also, CP in some very preterm infants, irrespective of whether they are multiple or singleton births, is attributable to hypoxic-ischemic damage sustained soon after birth, i.e. postnatal asphyxial damage.

Particularly in very preterm infants, distinguishing between intrapartum and immediate postpartum asphyxial damage is fraught with uncertainty. Abnormal ultrasound appearances, not present at birth but appearing shortly thereafter, are discriminant for CP.[20] Nevertheless, there is an increasingly prevalent view that this is less of a problem than had been previously assumed.[21] White matter damage in preterm infants shown by neonatal echoencephalography, even in those of birth weight < 1000 g, was more likely to have been sustained antenatally.[22]

The contribution of intrapartum asphyxia to the genesis of CP has also been downgraded in importance.[23] In a case–control study, although an association was observed between clinical signs of birth asphyxia and subsequent CP, it was estimated that in only about 8% was intrapartum asphyxia the possible cause of the brain damage.[24] In one cohort study, the proportion of CP in infants with complicated deliveries,

Table 156.2 Birth weight specific cerebral palsy prevalence in singleton and multiple births (from the National Perinatal Epidemiology Unit[17], Williams *et al.*[31] and Pharoah and Cooke[33])

BW	Singletons		Twins		Triplets	
	No. CP/neonatal survivors	CP prev per1000 survivors	No. CP/neonatal survivors	CP prev per 1000 survivors	No. CP/neonatal survivors	CP prev per 1000 survivors
< 1500 g	379/5,533	68.4	84/1,388	60.5	13/276	47.1
1500–2499 g	441/42,414	10.4	92/9,714	9.5	6/582	10.3
≥2500 g	1227/905,347	1.4	38/11,074	3.4	0/61	0
All BW	2047/953,294	2.1	214/22,176	9.7	19/919	20.7

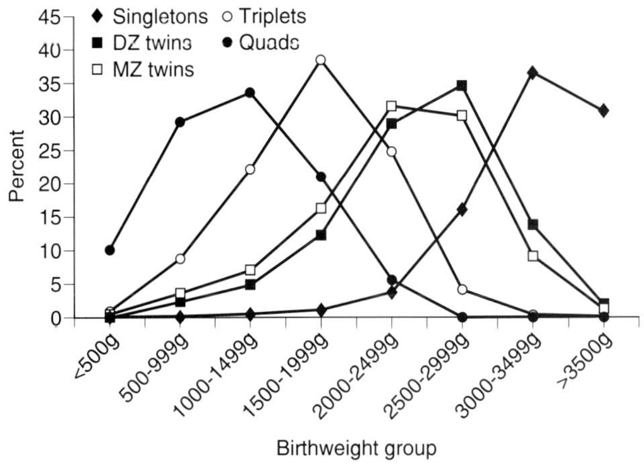

Figure 156.1 BW frequency distribution of singletons and multiples. Reprinted from Pharoah POD. *Obstet Gynecol Clin North Am* 2005;32(1):55–67 with permission from Elsevier.

low Apgar scores and neonatal hypoxemic-ischemic encephalopathy was only 13%.[25,26] In another cohort study, 10% of CP was attributable to birth asphyxia.[27]

Thus, CP of perinatal or postperinatal origin accounts for about 20% of all CP, and the remaining 80% is considered attributable to an insult occurring during fetal development.

Multiple births and CP

Over a century ago, Freud recognized that multiple births are at increased risk of CP compared with singleton births.[3] Several studies have confirmed this observation[28–34] with twins having about a fivefold increase in risk compared to singletons. Table 156.2, compiled from two population-based CP registers, shows birth weight specific CP prevalence per 1000 neonatal survivors.[18,33] From Table 156.2, compared with singletons, the relative risk for twins is 5.2 and for triplet and higher-order multiple births it is 12.6. Both values are highly statistically significant.

However, the inverse association of birth weight and CP prevalence means that birth weight is an important confounding variable when comparing crude relative risks. In Table 156.2, the prevalence of CP in twins and higher-order multiple births compared to singletons is not significantly different for the birth weight groups < 1500 and 1500–2499 g. Therefore, there are two components to the increased crude relative risk of CP associated with multiple births. One component is attributable to the high proportion of very low birth weight infants. The second component, evident as a striking feature of Table 156.2, is that for normal birth weight infants, i.e. ≥2500 g, the relative risk for twins compared to singletons is 2.5 (95% confidence interval 2.2–4.8; $P < 0.00001$). The increased risk in normal birth weight infants must be attributable to something other than problems of neonatal management of very immature infants. (The number of triplet and higher-order multiple births weighing ≥2500 g is too small for a meaningful estimation of relative risk.)

The higher the order of multiplicity at birth, the greater is the proportion that is preterm or of low birth weight. The birth weight frequency distributions for singleton and multiple births shown in Figure 156.1, have been compiled from the national birth registration statistics for England and Wales, 1993–2000. Applying Weinberg's rule to the data, the birth weight frequency distribution of twins was subdivided into dizygous (DZ) and monozygous (MZ) components.[35] The rule assumes that opposite-sex twins are DZ and that an equal number of same-sex twins are DZ. The remainder, obtained by subtracting twice the number of opposite-sex from the total, gives the number of MZ twins.

Of particular note, the birth weight frequency distribution of MZ is shifted to the left of DZ twins. The lower the birth weight of twins, the greater is the likelihood that they are MZ. Among Caucasian populations, MZ comprise about one-third of all twins. However, among twins of birth weight < 1000 g, 40%

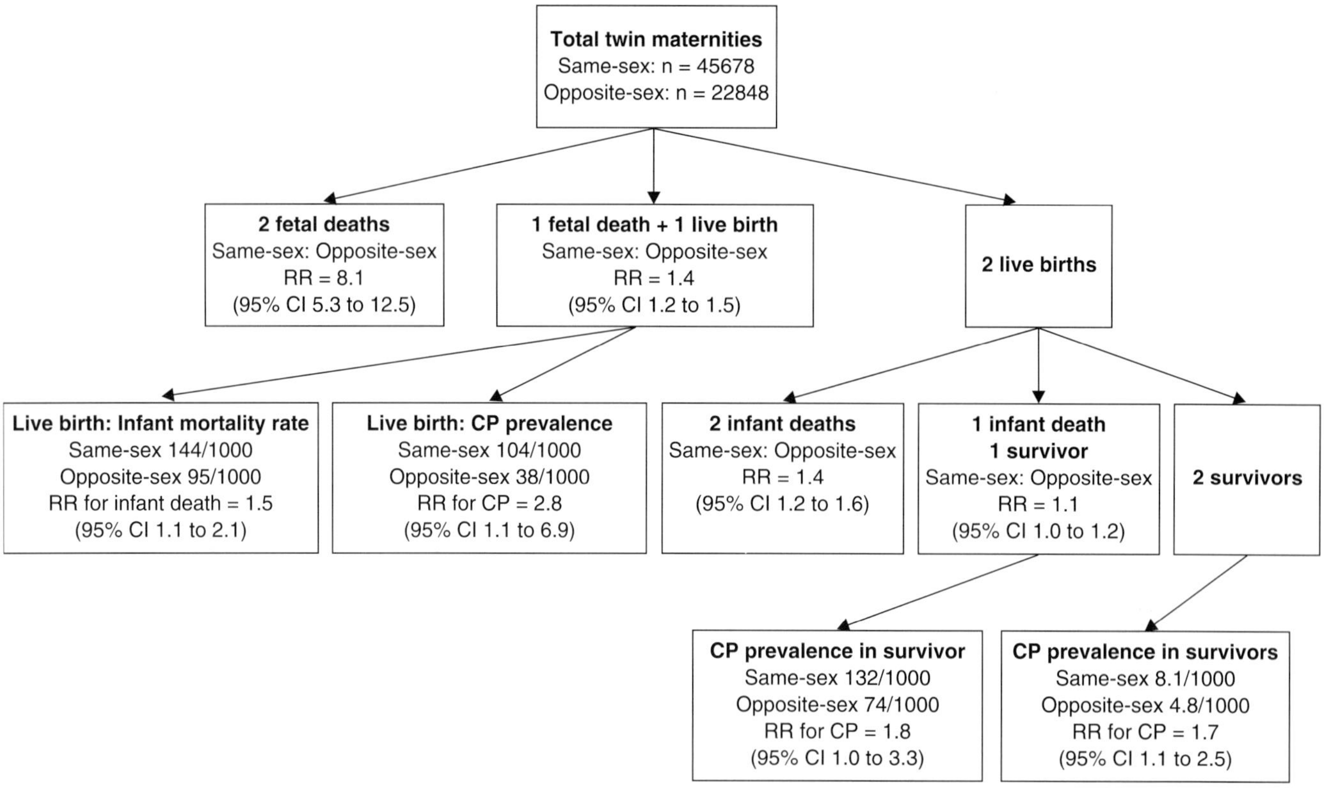

Figure 156.2 Mortality and CP risks in same- and opposite-sex twins.

are MZ, but in those of birth weight ≥3000 g, about 25% are MZ. This difference in birth weight distribution will place MZ at greater risk of CP than DZ twins.

Mortality and CP risk associated with zygosity

CP, whether in singleton or multiple births, needs to be considered as part of a spectrum of severity of cerebral impairment. This spectrum may range from early or late fetal death through a live birth that results in death in infancy to a survivor that presents with CP. The severity of the disabilities that comprise CP also varies extensively from a child with severe motor, cognitive and sensory abnormalities to one having minimal cerebral dysfunction.

In the context of multiple births, zygosity is a major determinant of fetal death and subsequent morbidity, particularly CP. In national birth and death registrations, zygosity in multiple gestations is not recorded, nevertheless, as a partial substitute, same-sex and opposite-sex comparisons may be used as an indicator for DZ and MZ risks.

There is a significantly greater risk for same-sex compared with opposite-sex at all points of the spectrum of severity as shown in Figure 156.2.

When both twins suffer fetal death, the same-sex:opposite-sex relative risk is 8.1. When one twin dies *in utero*, infant mortality in the surviving co-twin is very high irrespective of zygosity, but within this group, it is significantly higher at 144 per 1000 in same-sex compared with 96 per 1000 live births in opposite-sex twins. An analysis of multiple births in the United States found that same-sex twins were two times more likely than opposite-sex twins to die after intrauterine demise of one fetus at 25–32 weeks and more than three times more likely to die after a death at 33 + weeks.[36]

When both twins are live births, same-sex compared with opposite-sex twins are at a 40% increased risk for both to die in infancy. There is a high preponderance of very preterm infants when both twins die in infancy. Therefore, in part the excess risk is attributable to the shift to the left in the birth weight frequency distribution of same-sex twins. However, even after adjusting for birth weight in 500 g groups, the same-sex:opposite-sex relative risk is 1.21 (95% CI 1.12–1.32; $P < 0.00001$). The excess fetal and infant mortality in same-sex compared with opposite-sex twins is associated with the zygosity of the pregnancy.

Further along the spectrum of severity, not only is there an increased risk of fetal and infant death in same-sex compared with opposite-sex twins, but there is also a significantly increased risk of CP in a survivor whose co-twin died *in utero* (Figure 156.2). There are numerous case reports of a variety of congenital anomalies in the surviving co-twin. Predominantly, cerebral impairments such as multicystic encephalopathy, ventriculomegaly, porencephaly, polymicrogyria, cerebral atrophy and hydranencephaly have been described. These impairments are frequently, though

Table 156.3 Birth weight specific cerebral palsy prevalence in twins (from Pharoah and Adi[45], Pharoah[46,48] and Glinianaia *et al.*[47]) (reprinted from *Multiple Pregnancy*)

Birth weight	Same-sex		Opposite-sex	
	Cerebral palsy/number responders	Cerebral palsy prevalence/1000 infant survivors	Cerebral palsy/number responders	Cerebral palsy prevalence/1000 infant survivors
(a) Cerebral palsy in surviving twin of co-twin fetal death*				
< 1500 g	15/91	164.8	3/29	103.4
≥1500 g	20/246	81.3	2/104	19.2
All	35/337	103.9	5/133	37.6
(b) Cerebral palsy in surviving twin of co-twin infant death**				
< 1500 g	44/207	212.6	12/87	137.9
≥1500 g	8/187	42.8	0/75	0
All	52/394	132.0	12/162	74.1
(c) Cerebral palsy: both twins survive infancy***				
< 1500 g	52/984	52.8	17/393	43.3
≥1500 g	54/12037	4.5	13/5841	2.2
All	106/13021	8.1	30/6234	4.8
(a+b+c) Combined cerebral palsy birth-weight-specific prevalence****				
< 1500 g	111/1282	86.6	32/509	62.9
≥1500 g	82/12470	4.5	15/6020	2.5
All	193/13752	14.0	47/6529	7.2

*Same-sex vs. opposite-sex, Mantel–Haenszel weighted relative risk 2.60 (95% CI 1.06–6.39); **same-sex vs. opposite-sex, Mantel–Haenszel weighted relative risk 1.77 (95% CI 1.01–3.25); ***same-sex vs. opposite-sex, Mantel–Haenszel weighted relative risk 1.29 (95% CI 0.71–2.21); ****same-sex vs. opposite-sex, Mantel–Haenszel weighted relative risk 1.76 (95% CI 1.29–2.41)

not necessarily, clinically manifest as CP, and almost invariably with MZ and, specifically, monochorionic twinning.[37–43] Population registers of CP confirm the high risk associated with fetal demise of a co-twin. The Californian Registry noted that, in children who survived fetal death of a co-twin, CP was 108 times more prevalent than in singletons and 13 times more prevalent than in twins whose co-twin was born alive.[44] The Mersey registry observed a 1 in 10 probability of CP in the surviving twin whose co-twin died *in utero*.[33] Further evidence of the vulnerability of the surviving co-twin to serious morbidity has been reported in cohort studies. The CP prevalence data shown in Figure 156.2 are from a national[45,46] and a regional[47] survey and confirms the very high risk of CP in the surviving co-twin of a fetal death. The risk is significantly greater in same-sex than in opposite-sex twins. However, it is pertinent that, when both twins are live born and one dies in infancy, the risk of CP in the surviving twin also is extremely high with the risk being greater in same-sex compared with opposite-sex twins.

Because birth weight is an important confounding variable, birth weight specific comparison of CP prevalence between same- and opposite-sex twins should be examined (Table 156.3).

The weighted relative risk of CP in same-sex compared with opposite-sex twins is significant for the surviving twin whose co-twin either died *in utero* or was liveborn but died in infancy (Table 156.3a and b). This observation is confirmed in a collaborative study combining the data from five population-based registers and the difference in the prevalence of CP persists after adjusting for birth weight and gestational age.[49]

When both twins survive infancy (Table 156.3c), the relative risk, though not statistically significant, is nevertheless greater in same-sex than in opposite-sex twins. In the collaborative study, only a marginal difference in CP prevalence was observed between same- and opposite-sex twins.

Problems associated with birth registration in multiple births

When determining the prevalence of CP, population denominators are obtained from birth registrations. The very high prevalence of CP associated with fetal or infant death of a co-twin emphasizes the importance that should be given to ensure that birth registrations in multiple gestations, particularly of fetal deaths, are complete and, for the purpose of comparison of same- with opposite-sex, the correct sex of the fetus is registered.

The World Health Organization defines a fetal death for registration purposes as 'death prior to the complete expulsion or extraction from its mother of a product of conception, irrespective of the duration of the pregnancy'. It is inherent in this definition that it is the gestational age at expulsion or extraction from the mother and not the gestational age at death of the fetus that determines whether such a fetus from a multiple pregnancy is registered. This applies particularly to a fetal death in the midtrimester that is clinically manifest as a fetus papyraceous at birth. Usually, it is the legal requirement of the parents to register a birth. However, obstetricians differ as to whether or not the parents should be informed that a fetus papyraceous has been delivered or, if the parents are informed, that the fetus should be registered.[50] Furthermore, the sex of a fetus papyraceous is not usually known but, in England and Wales, the parents who register the fetus papyraceous may be allowed the choice as to whether the fetus is registered as male or female. As fetal death is more common in MZ gestations, arbitrary allocation of sex to a fetal death, comparisons of same- and opposite-sex will underestimate the contribution of monozygosity to the prevalence of CP.

In the United States, the 1992 Revision of the Model State Vital Statistics Act and Regulations recommends reporting of fetal deaths of 350 g or more, or if the weight is unknown, of 20 completed weeks gestation or more. However, there are regional variations, some using birth weight or gestational age as the primary determinant, while others require all fetal deaths to be reported. There is, therefore, variation in the registration of those fetal deaths weighing less than 350 g or of gestational age less than 20 weeks.

In an analysis of 18 cases of CP in the twin survivor of a fetal death and where the fetal death had been recorded in the obstetric case records, in only 12 instances had both twins been registered and six cases of CP had been registered as singletons.[51] This accentuates the importance of completeness of registration of all births not only for elucidating the pathogenesis of CP but also in counseling and advising parents who have suffered fetal loss in a multiple pregnancy.

Initially, it was considered that only late fetal death was associated with neurological impairment in the surviving co-twin.[52–54] Subsequently, second-trimester demise of one fetus was also reported to have neurological consequences for the survivor.[40,55]

Since the initial report of the loss of one fetus early in a multiple gestation,[56] the phenomenon of the 'vanishing' twin is now well recognized.[57] Such first-trimester loss of a twin has been reported in association with neurological polymicrogyria in the surviving co-twin[37] and report of a further four cases of CP in the surviving co-twin led to the hypothesis that CP in an apparently singleton child may be attributable to first-trimester loss of a fetus as the vanishing twin.[58] Fetal death of one twin may be associated with cerebral impairment in the surviving co-twin irrespective of the gestational age at which the fetal death occurs.

Mechanisms of neurological impairment in multiple births

Hypoxic-ischemic impairment sustained peripartum in a vulnerable preterm infant may occur irrespective of the multiplicity or zygosity of the gestation. In addition to the increased risk associated with preterm delivery of multiple gestations, there is the risk associated with monozygosity and, specifically, monochorionicity. While MZ gestations are of the same genotype, they may differ significantly in their phenotype and these differences hinge predominantly on the placentation that the fetuses share and the vascular anastomoses within the placenta. The chorionicity of MZ gestations is dependent on the stage of splitting of the fertilized ovum as depicted in Figure 156.3. Fertilization of two ova produces dichorionic, dizygotic twins with either separate placentas or a fused placenta but without vascular anastomoses. Early splitting of a single fertilized ovum may also lead to dichorionic placentation without vascular anastomoses. Later splitting produces monochorionic MZ twins with intraplacental anastomoses and late incomplete splitting presents as conjoint twins.

Case reports that have observed cerebral impairment in association with fetal death of a co-twin note that monochorionicity is invariably present. The crucial role of monochorionicity lies in the vascular anastomoses within the placenta that provide a shared circulation between the fetuses.

Initially, it was hypothesized that thromboplastin or thromboemboli from the dead fetus passing to the co-twin led to cerebral damage from disseminated intravascular coagulation or embolization.[42,59–61] This proposed mechanism considered the dead fetus to be the donor and the surviving fetus to be the receptor. However, in the majority of cases neither disseminated intravascular coagulation nor thromboli has been demonstrated in the surviving twin.

Subsequently an alternative explanation proposed that the dead fetus acted as the receptor with the surviving fetus as the donor. Ischemic damage to the surviving fetus was attributed to an acute twin–twin transfusion with exsanguination into the dead fetus that acted as a low-resistance vascular sump.[41,62]

In both mechanisms the dead fetus, either the donor or the receptor, is the cause of the cerebral impairment in the surviving co-twin. However, fetal death of a twin is not a necessary component as the prevalence of CP is significantly in excess among same-sex compared with opposite-sex twin when both twins are live births and one dies in infancy or when both survive (Table 156.3).

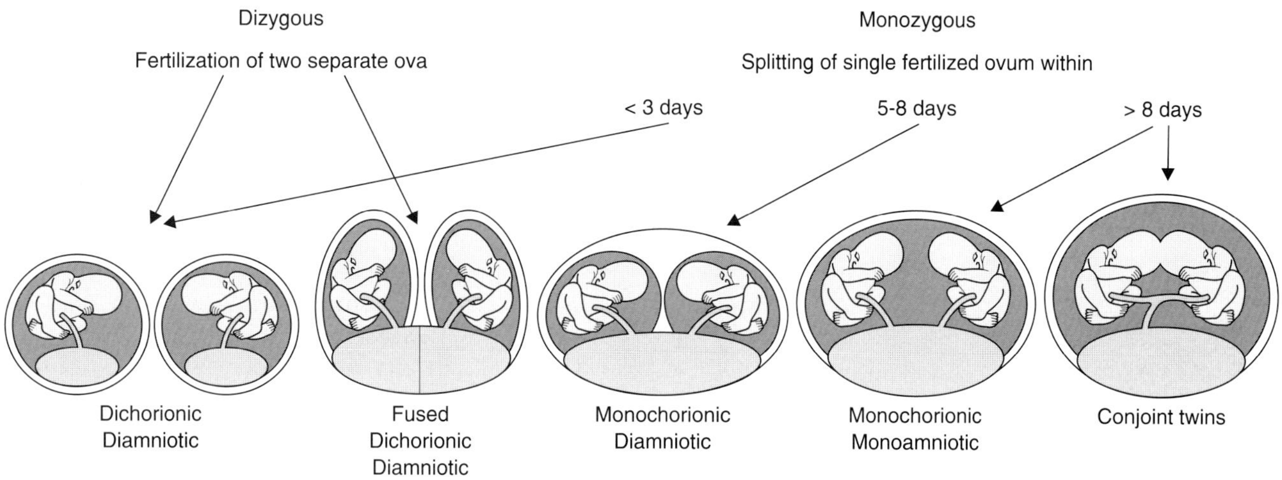

Figure 156.3 Zygosity and chorionicity in twin gestations. Reprinted from: Pharoah POD. *Semin Neonatol* 2002;7:223–30 with permission from Elsevier.

A third proposed mechanism is that the fetal death of one twin and the cerebral impairment in the co-twin are both the result of vascular instability with acute episodes of bidirectional shunting and that either twin may be donor or receptor.[63–66] This mechanism is sufficient to account for the extreme range of mortality and morbidity that may be observed in both fetuses of a monochorionic gestation. Early fetal death of both fetuses will present as a spontaneous abortion, an outcome recognized as being more common in monochorionic than dichorionic gestations.[67,68] Later fetal death will present as two stillbirths also significantly more common in monochorionic than dichorionic gestations (Figure 156.2). When both twins are live births, same-sex compared with opposite-sex twins are at greater risk of infant death and CP (Figure 156.2 and Table 156.3).

If monochorionicity with acute episodes of feto-fetal transfusion leading to cerebral impairment is an important cause of CP of antenatal origin, explanation is needed for those cases of CP observed in the twins of opposite sex. The hypothesis that CP in a singleton infant may be attributable to loss of a twin, either as a 'vanishing' twin or as a recognized but non-registered twin such as a fetus papyraceus[58] is applicable to higher-order multiple gestations. Loss of one of an MZ pair within a triplet gestation may result in twin births of opposite sex. Therefore, it cannot be assumed that twin births of opposite sex are *both* from a DZ gestation. Also, placental vascular communications, albeit rarely, have been observed in dichorionic placentas.[69,70] Additionally, the arbitrary allocation of gender to a fetus papyraceus at the time of registration of the births will introduce further misclassification over whether twins are of the same or opposite sex.

Assisted reproductive technology (ART) and CP

The increased prevalence of CP among multiple gestations has inevitably posed questions over the possible effect of ART on CP prevalence. Over the past quarter century, there has been a striking increase in rates of multiple births, predominantly as a result of ART.[71–73] The possible effect of this increase in multiple births on the prevalence of CP needs to consider the two major components that affect CP prevalence, low birth weight or immaturity and chorionicity.

Multiple births, whether spontaneously conceived or by ART, are at increased risk of low birth weight. However, cohort and matched control studies have shown that ART singleton births are at increased risk of being born preterm or of very low birth weight.[74,75] An adverse birth weight distribution will predispose to a higher prevalence of CP in ART conceptions. Based on published data, CP prevalence was estimated at 2.7, 8.8, 10.3 and 16.9 per 1000 neonates in spontaneous conceptions, two transferred embryos, three transferred embryos reduced to twins and three transferred embryos, respectively.[76] The estimates suggest that iatrogenic reduction from three to two embryos can be expected to decrease the prevalence of CP. In a study of trichorionic triplet pregnancies, iatrogenic reduction to twins increased the gestational age at delivery and there were three cases of CP among 183 survivors, a prevalence of 16.4 per 1000. As the gestations were trichorionic, monochorionicity was not a risk factor and all three cases of CP were of birth weight < 1500 g.[77]

The increased risk of CP attributable to monochorionicity may be relevant because MZ division occurs more commonly in ART than in spontaneous conceptions.[78,79] About 1 in 10–15 ART gestations undergo MZ division.[80] It is not known why MZ division is more frequent than expected in ART conceptions but the specific method of assisted reproduction may be important. Embryos from intracytoplasmic sperm injection were found to be at lesser risk of MZ division than those from other techniques of *in vitro* fertilization[81] and there was no difference in neurodevelopmental scores in children conceived following *in vitro* fertilization by intracytoplasmic sperm injection and their matched controls.[82] The extent to which ART gestations may be at risk of CP will depend on the proportion that are of very low birth weight, the proportion that undergo MZ division and within the latter group, the number that are monochorionic.

Summary

CP is 5–10 times more common in multiple compared with singleton gestations. There are two components to this increased risk. The shift to the left in the birthweight-frequency distribution of multiple compared with singleton births places them at risk of cerebral impairment of peripartum origin. The second component is MC placentation when the risk of CP is very high in a surviving twin if the co-twin dies *in utero* or is a liveborn who dies in infancy.

The increased risk associated with MC placentation has been variously ascribed to transfer of thromboplastin or thromboemboli from the dead to the surviving fetus, exsanguination of the surviving fetus into the low-pressure reservoir of the dead fetus or hemodynamic instability with bidirectional shunting of blood between the two fetuses.

The risk of CP in multiple gestations may be considerably underestimated owing to failure to register or record early loss of a vanishing twin or later fetal demise as a fetus papyraceus.

An increase in risk of CP in ART gestations is likely because of the higher proportion of very preterm births. Because ART gestations are predominantly DZ, the risk of CP attributable to MC placentation will be limited to the minority that undergoes MZ division.

REFERENCES

1. Little WJ. On the incidence of abnormal parturition, difficult labour, premature birth and asphyxia neonatorum of the mental and physical condition of the child, especially in relation to deformities. *Trans Obstet Soc Lond* 1892;3:293–344.
2. Sachs B, Peterson F. A study of the cerebral palsies of early life. *J Nervous Mental Dis* 1890;17:295–332.
3. Freud S. Infantile Cerebrallähumung. In Nothnagel, ed. *Specielle Pathologie und Therapie*. Wien: A Holder, 1897. (Infantile cerebral paralysis. Translation by Russin LA, University of Miami Press, Florida, 1968.)
4. Little Club. Memorandum on terminology and classification of cerebral palsy. *Cereb Palsy Bull* 1959;1:27–35.
5. Evans PR. Antecedents of cerebral palsy. *Arch Dis Child* 1948; 23:213–9.
6. Crothers B, Paine RS. *The Natural History of Cerebral Palsy*. Cambridge, MA: Harvard University Press, 1959.
7. Ingram TTS. A study of cerebral palsy in the childhood population of Edinburgh. *Arch Dis Child* 1955;30:244–50.
8. Kurland LT. Definitions of cerebral palsy and their role in epidemiological research. *Neurology* 1957;7:641–54.
9. Nelson KB, Ellenberg. Neonatal status as predictors of cerebral palsy. *Pediatrics* 1979;64:225–32.
10. Mutch L, Alberman E, Hagberg B, Kodama K, Perat MV. Cerebral palsy epidemiology: Where are we now and where are we going. *Dev Med Child Neurol* 1992;34:547–51.
11. Paneth N, Kiely J. The frequency of cerebral palsy: A review of population studies in industrialised nations since 1950. In Stanley F, Alberman E, eds. *The Epidemiology of the Cerebral Palsies*. Clinics in Developmental Medicine. Oxford: Blackwell, 1984;87:46–56.
12. Stanley FJ, Watson L. Trends in perinatal mortality and cerebral palsy in Western Australia, 1967 to 1985. *Br Med J* 1992;304: 1658–63.
13. Hagberg B, Hagberg G, Beckung E, Uvebrant P. Changing panorama of cerebral palsy in Sweden. VIII. Prevalence and origin in the birth year period 1991–94. *Acta Paediatr* 2001;90: 271–7.
14. Pharoah POD, Cooke T, Johnson MA, King R, Mutch L. Epidemiology of cerebral palsy in England and Scotland. *Arch Dis Child Neonatal Ed* 1998;79:F21–5.
15. Maudsley G, Hutton JL, Pharoah POD. Cause of death in cerebral palsy: A descriptive study. *Arch Dis Child* 1999;81:390–4.
16. Pharoah POD, Cooke T, Rosenbloom L. Acquired cerebral palsy. *Arch Dis Child* 1989;64:1013–6.
17. National Perinatal Epidemiology Unit. *Oxford Register of Early Childhood Impairments*. Annual Report, 2002.
18. Watson L, Stanley F, Blair E. *Report of the Western Australia Cerebral Palsy Register. To Birth Year 1994*. Western Australia: TVW Telethon Institute for Child Health Research, 1999.
19. Pharoah POD, Cooke T, Cooke RWI, Rosenbloom L. Birthweight specific trends in cerebral palsy. *Arch Dis Child* 1990;65:602–6.
20. Cooke RWI. Cerebral palsy in very low birthweight infants. *Arch Dis Child* 1990;65:201–6.
21. Stanley FJ. Survival and cerebral palsy in low birthweight infants: Implications for perinatal care. *Paediatr Perinat Epidemiol* 1992; 6:298–310.
22. Bejar R, Wozniac P, Allard M, *et al.* Antenatal origin of neurologic damage to newborn infants. *Am J Obstet Gynecol* 1988;159:357–63.
23. Bedrick AI. Perinatal asphyxia and cerebral palsy. *Am J Dis Child* 1989;143:1139–40.
24. Blair E, Stanley FJ. Intrapartum asphyxia: A rare cause of cerebral palsy. *J Pediatr* 1988;112:515–9.
25. Nelson KB, Ellenberg JH. Antecedents of cerebral palsy. Multivariate analysis of risk. *N Engl J Med* 1986;315:81–6.
26. Nelson KB. What proportion of cerebral palsy is related to birth asphyxia. *J Pediatr* 1988;112:572–4.
27. Yudkin PL, Johnson A, Clover LM, Murphy KW. Assessing the contribution of birth asphyxia to cerebral palsy in term singletons. *Paediatr Perinat Epidemiol* 1995;9:156–70.
28. Alberman ED. Cerebral palsy in twins. *Guys Hosp Rep* 1964;113: 285–95.
29. Illingworth RS, Woods GE. The incidence of twins in cerebral palsy and mental retardation. *Arch Dis Child* 1960;35:333–5.
30. Russell EM. Cerebral palsied twins. *Arch Dis Child* 1961;36: 328–36.
31. Williams K, Hennessy E, Alberman E. Cerebral palsy: Effects of twinning, birthweight, and gestational age. *Arch Dis Child Fetal Neonatal Ed* 1996;75:F178–82.
32. Patterson B, Nelson KB, Watson L, Stanley F. Twins, triplets, and cerebral palsy in births in Western Australia in the 1980s. *Br Med J* 1993;307:1239–43.
33. Pharoah POD, Cooke T. Cerebral palsy and multiple births. *Arch Dis Child Fetal Neonatal Ed* 1996;75:F174–7.
34. Scher AI, Petterson B, Blair E, *et al.* The risk of mortality or cerebral palsy in twins: A collaborative population-based study. *Pediatr Res* 2002;52:671–81.
35. Johnson CD, Zhang J. Survival of other fetuses after a fetal death in twin or triplet pregnancies. *Obstet Gynecol* 2002;99:698–703.
36. Weinberg W. Beiträge zur physiologie und pathologie der mehrlingsgeburten beim menschen. *Archiv für die gesamte Physiologie des Menschen und der Tiere* 1902;88:346–430.
37. Baker EM, Khorasgani MG, Gardner-Medwin D, Gholkar A, Griffiths PD. Arthrogryposis multiplex congenita and bilateral parietal polymicrogyria in association with the intrauterine death of a twin. *Neuropediatrics* 1996;27:54–6.
38. Bordarier C, Robain O. Microgyric and necrotic cortical lesions in twin fetuses: Original cerebral damage consecutive to twinning? *Brain Dev* 1992;14:174–8.
39. Larroche JCl, Girard N, Narcy F, Fallet C. Abnormal cortical plate(polymicrogyria), heterotopias and brain damage in monozygous twins. *Biol Neonate* 1994;65:343–52.

40. Anderson RL, Golbus MS, Curry CJR, Callen PW, Hastrup WH. Central nervous system damage and other anomalies in surviving fetus following second trimester antenatal death of co-twin. *Prenat Diagn* 1990;10:513–8.
41. Fusi L, Gordon H. Twin pregnancy complicated by single intrauterine death. Problems and outcome with conservative management. *Br J Obstet Gynaecol* 1990;97:511–6.
42. Hoyme EH, Higginbottom MC, Jones KL. Vascular etiology of disruptive structural defects in monozygotic twins. *Pediatrics* 1981; 67:288–91.
43. Jung JH, Graham JM, Schultz N, Smith DW. Congenital hydranencephaly/porencephaly due to vascular disruption in monozygotic twins. *Pediatrics* 1984;73:467–9.
44. Grether JK, Nelson KB, Cummins CK. Twinning and cerebral palsy: Experience in four Northern Californian counties, births 1983 through 1985. *Pediatrics* 1993;92:854–8.
45. Pharoah POD, Adi Y. Consequences of in-utero death in a twin pregnancy. *Lancet* 2000;355:1597–602.
46. Pharoah POD. Cerebral palsy in the surviving twin associated with infant death of the co-twin. *Arch Dis Child Fetal Neonatal Ed* 2001;84:F111–6.
47. Glinianaia SV, Pharoah POD, Wright C, Rankin JM. Fetal or infant death in twin pregnancy: Neurodevelopmental consequence for the survivor. *Arch Dis Child Fetal Neonatal Ed* 2002;86:F9–F15.
48. Pharoah POD, Price TS, Plomin R. Cerebral palsy in twins: A national study. *Arch Dis Child Fetal Neonatal Ed* 2002;87:F122–4.
49. Scher AI, Petterson B, Blair E, *et al.* The risk of mortality or cerebral palsy in twins: A collaborative population-based study. *Pediatr Res* 2002;52:671–81.
50. Heys RF. Selective abortion. *Br Med J* 1996;313:1004.
51. Pharoah POD, Cooke RWI. Registering a fetus papyraceus. *Br Med J* 1997;314:441–2.
52. Yoshida K, Soma H. Outcome of the surviving co-twin of a fetus papyreceus or a dead fetus. *Acta Genet Med gemellol* 1986;35: 91–8.
53. Carlson Nj, Towers CV. Multiple gestation complicated by the death of one fetus. *Obstet Gynecol* 1989;73:685–9.
54. Prompeler HJ, Madjar H, Klosa W, *et al.* Twin pregnancies with single fetal death. *Acta Obstet Gynecol Scand* 1994;73:205–8.
55. Van Bogaert P, Donner C, David P, Rodesch F, Avni EF, Szliwowski HB. Congenital bilateral perisylvian syndrome in a monozygotic twin with intra-uterine death of the co-twin. *Dev Med Child Neurol* 1996;38:166–71.
56. Hellman LM, Kobayashi M, Cromb E. Ultrasonic diagnosis of embryonic malformations. *Am J Obstet Gynecol* 1973;115:615–23.
57. Landy HJ, Keith LG. The vanishing twin: A review. *Hum Reprod Updat* 1998;4:177–83.
58. Pharoah POD, Cooke RWI. A hypothesis for the aetiology of spastic cerebral palsy – the vanishing twin. *Dev Med Child Neurol* 1997;39:292–6.
59. Benirschke K. Twin placenta in perinatal mortality. *N Y State J Med* 1961;61:1499–508.
60. Moore CM, McAdams AJ, Sutherland J. Intrauterine disseminated intravascular coagulation: A syndrome of multiple pregnancy with a dead twin fetus. *J Pediatr* 1969;74:523–8.
61. Durkin MV, Kaveggia EG, Pendleton E, Neuhäuser G, Opitz JM. Analysis of etiologic factors in cerebral palsy with severe mental retardation. I. Analysis of gestational, parturitional and neonatal data. *Eur J Pediatr* 1976;123:67–81.
62. Fusi L, McParland P, Fisk N, Nicolini U, Wigglesworth J. Acute twin–twin transfusion: A possible mechanism for brain-damaged survivors after intrauterine death of a monochorionic twin. *Obstet Gynecol* 1991;78:517–20.
63. Larroche J Cl, Droulle P, Delezoide AL, Narcy F, Nessmann C. Brain damage in monozygous twins. *Biol Neonate* 1990;57:261–78.
64. Bejar R, Vigliocco G, Gramajo H, *et al.* Antenatal origin of neurologic damage in newborn infants. II. Multiple gestations. *Am J Obstet Gynecol* 1990;162:1230–6.
65. Gonen R. The origin of brain lesions in survivors of twin gestations complicated by fetal death. *Am J Obstet Gynecol* 1991;161: 1897–8.
66. Grafe MR. Antenatal cerebral necrosis in monochorionic twins. *Pediatr Pathol* 1993;13:15–9.
67. Sebire NJ, Snijders RJM, Hughes K, Sepulveda W, Nicolaides KH. The hidden mortality of monochorionic twin pregnancies. *Br J Obstet Gynaecol* 1997;104:1203–7.
68. Benson CB, Doubilet PM, Laks MP. Outcome of twin gestations following sonographic demonstration of two heart beats in the first trimester. *Ultrasound Obstet Gynecol* 1993;3:343–5.
69. Robertson EG, Neer KJ. Placental injection studies in twin gestation. *Am J Obstet Gynecol* 1983;147:170–3.
70. Hagihara S, Matsubara S, Kuwata T, *et al.* Discordant twin: Marked vascular communication between separated dichorionic diamniotic placentas. *Twin Res* 2003;6:267–9.
71. Imaizumi Y. A comparative study of twinning and triplet rates in 17 countries. *Acta Genet Med Gemellol* 1998,47.101–14.
72. Kiely JL, Kiely M. Epidemiological trends in multiple births in the United States, 1971–1998. *Twin Res* 2001;4:131–3.
73. Platt MJ, Marshall A, Pharoah POD. The effects of assisted reproduction on the trends and zygosity of multiple births in England and Wales 1974–99. *Twin Res* 2001;4:417–21.
74. Bergh T, Ericson A, Hillensjö T, Nygren K-G, Wennerholm U-B. Deliveries and children born after in-vitro fertilisation in Sweden 1982–95: A retrospective cohort study. *Lancet* 1999;354:1579–85.
75. Helmerhorst FM, Perquin DAM, Donker D, Keirse MJNC. Perinatal outcome of singletons and twins after assisted conception: A systematic review of controlled studies. *Br Med J* 2004;328:261–4.
76. Blickstein I, Weissman A. Estimating the risk of cerebral palsy after assisted conceptions. *N Engl J Med* 1999;341:1313–4.
77. Dimitriou G, Pharoah POD, Nicolaides KH, Greenough A. Cerebral palsy in triplet pregnancies with and without iatrogenic reduction. *Eur J Pediatr* 2004;163:449–51.
78. Derom C, Derom R, Vlietinck R, Van Den Berghe H, Thiery M. Increased monozygotic twinning rates after ovulation induction. *Lancet* 1987;i:1236–8.
79. Wenstrom KD, Syrop CH, Hammitt EG, Van Voorhis BJ. Increased risk of monochorionic twinning associated with assisted reproduction. *Fertil Steril* 1993;60:510–3.
80. Blickstein I, Keith LG. The spectrum of iatrogenic multiple pregnancy. In Blickstein I, Keith LG, eds. *Iatrogenic Multiple Pregnancy: Clinical Implications*. London: Parthenon Publishing, 2001:1–7.
81. Blickstein I, Verhoeven HC, Keith LG. Zygotic splitting after assisted reproduction. *N Eng J Med* 1999;340:738–9.
82. Sutcliffe AG, Taylor B, Saunders K, Thornton S, Lieberman BA, Grudzinskas JG. Outcome in the second year of life after in-vitro fertilisation by intracytoplasmic sperm injection: A UK case–control study. *Lancet* 2001;357:2080–4.

SECTION XVII

Infectious disease

Section Editors: **J. Schenker and C. Sen**

157 Infectious disease in pregnancy

J. G. Schenker

Introduction

Infection may be defined as multiplication of microbes (viruses, bacteria, fungi and protozoa) or multicellular parasites in the tissue. The host may or may not be symptomatic. In the evolution of any infectious disease, the virulence of the organism, the susceptibility of the host as well as the inoculums of the infectious agent are determinants of the clinical course. Infection during pregnancy poses a unique situation, since two patients become potentially involved – the mother and the fetus. Fetal and neonatal infections can occur at different stages of gestation from conception to birth. The mother is at risk because of certain changes induced by pregnancy, such as depression of immunity, urinary tract infection, genital tract infection due to premature rupture of membranes or prolonged labor, injuries to the genital tract during birth or retained products of conception.

Infections that occur at fertilization or during the early stages of conception often destroy the zygote or pre-embryo, and only rarely leave definite evidence. The inability of most agents to infect the pre-embryo probably depends largely on the local barriers to the infectious agent. Some viruses can infect only embryos of certain developmental stages. After implantation, most infectious agents reach the fetus hematogenously by transplacental infection. The fetus is at risk as a result of ascending infection from the birth canal or during passage down the birth canal. Viruses can infect the embryo and the fetus, and this kind of infection, which is often trivial in the adult, can be devastating to the newborn. Fetal infections during the organogenetic period can cause major malformations, and the most serious are those affecting the central nervous system. Bacterial infections increase perinatal wastage, mainly due to premature labor. Postnatal infections may be acquired from the mother via secretions, blood, milk or from attending medical personnel or the hospital environment.

Major advances have been made in the later part of the present century in the development of new antibiotic preparations. In spite of this, infections continue to be of great concern in obstetric practice.

We have tried in this section on infectious diseases to introduce the various clinical aspects of infections that affect the mother and her fetus. Sexually transmitted diseases (STD) are a special threat to population. They may adversely affect pregnancy, causing pregnancy losses, and the disease may be transmitted to the offspring *in utero* or during delivery. Because STD in women is often asymptomatic, screening for the most common infections is an important component of prenatal care, particularly in highly predisposed women. Although more than 20 infectious diseases may be sexually acquired, the chapter on STD deals with syphilis, gonorrhea, chlamydia, herpes, trichomoniasis, human papilloma virus, chancroid and donovanosis. Since human immunodeficiency virus (HIV) infection is a global threat in the developed and developing world, and poses a special threat to pregnant women and their fetuses, special attention is given to acquired immunodeficiency syndrome (AIDS).

The traditional bacterial infection by Group A β-hemolytic streptococcus is at present a minor clinical problem, but infections by β-hemolytic streptococcus can cause a serious or even fatal infection in the newborn infant.

Group B streptococcus (GBS) is an extremely important human pathogen causing thousands of maternal and neonatal infections yearly. In the last 5 years clinical research has put much effort into understanding the risk factors for GBS and strategies for its early detection and prevention. Future studies will determine whether GBS infections can be prevented by administration of vaccine in high-risk women. Pregnant women who are in an immunodeficient state are at risk for pneumonia infection due to agents such as *Pneumocystis carinii*, *Mycobacterium avium* and *Mycobacterium tuberculosis*. Recently, pneumococcal infections have become partly or completely resistant to penicillin or its synthetic components. Varicella pneumonia requires special attention in pregnant women.

Obstetrical interventions are associated with increased incidence of infectious morbidity, especially the common procedure of cesarean section. The prevention of infection may be accomplished by applying aseptic techniques, but is mainly achieved today by prophylactic antibiotics.

Septicemia and septic shock are dramatic clinical syndromes that result from acute invasion of the bloodstream by certain microorganisms or their toxic products. Even with the appropriate antimicrobial and supportive care, many patients die of septic shock, making strategies for prevention and more effective treatment of this critical condition of primary importance.

Infections of the gastrointestinal tract may have an impact on the course of pregnancy and its outcome. Several pathogens such as *Salmonella* and *Campylobacter* cause bacteremia with secondary infection of the placenta and the fetus. Other microorganisms cause severe circulatory compromise due to dehydration and electrolyte imbalance, and may bring about fetal hypoxia. Several aspects of gastrointestinal infections during pregnancy and the neonatal period are discussed.

Central nervous system (CNS) infections in pregnant women are divided into different clinical syndromes according to the principle site of the infection within the CNS (meningitis, encephalitis and myelitis). CNS infections may be caused by a wide variety of infectious agents: bacteria (including rickettiae, spirochets and mycobacteria), viruses, fungi and protozoa. The clinical course of CNS systemic infections in pregnancy, the diagnostic tools and the effects of the disease and the therapy on the fetus and the newborn are reported.

Puerperal pelvic infections are usually caused by anaerobic flora resistant to common antibacterial drugs. There is increasing evidence that infections ascending from the lower genital tract, which may be caused by an anaerobic organism, are risk factors for chorioamnionitis, postabortion septicemia, and septic shock and postcesarean infection. The treatment of anaerobic infections in pregnancy follows the usual rule of antimicrobial treatment, which includes the following agents: metronidazole, clindamycin, some penicillins, chloramphenicol and impipenem–cilistatin. By applying these treatment modalities one should balance the benefits of the treatment with their potential side effects.

Parasitic infections are common throughout the world, but most clinicians have no experience in the diagnosis and treatment of these diseases. Clinicians are increasingly confronted with parasitic infections such as malaria, schistosomiasis and leishmaniasis because of the increase in international travel and emigrations. Malaria is one of the most prevalent and serious infectious disease problems throughout the tropical and subtropical areas of the world. Intrauterine transmission of malaria from mother to fetus frequently occurs, although the mechanism of transplacental passage of the parasite is unknown. In the endemic areas, prophylaxis for pregnant women is recommended.

Pregnant women are more prone than non-pregnant women to have vaginal colonization with fungal infectious agents such as candida. Rarely, the infection can ascend and involve the uterine content, producing chorioamnionitis and congenital candidiasis. Viral infections can cause damage to the fetus through passage across the placenta. Approximately 5% of pregnancies will be complicated by one or more viral infections, excluding the common cold. Vaccines are at present being successfully developed in order to prevent these viral infections. Measles can be severe during pregnancy and has been associated with spontaneous abortion and premature delivery. However, in contrast to rubella, the measles virus is not known to cause congenital anomalies of the fetus. Mumps is generally a benign condition during pregnancy, but it affects the fetus by increasing the rate of abortion, prematurity and congenital malformations. Vaccination against mumps is available, but it should not be administered to pregnant women. The treatment of the disease is only symptomatic, and there is no antiviral agent available yet.

Only a few antimicrobial agents have been shown to be completely non-toxic when given to pregnant women, and some of them have teratogenic potential. Thus, the administration of an antimicrobial drug during pregnancy should always be a carefully considered action in which a balance between the need of the mother and the possible adverse effect of the drug on the fetus should be taken into consideration. The Food and Drug Administration of the United States has established a fetal risk summary, which divides drugs into categories, based on accumulated safety data from animal and human studies. Therefore, a physician, when administering any antimicrobial or antiviral agent, should find out to which category the drug belongs.

158 Sexually transmitted infections in women with special reference to pregnancy

M. Dan

Introduction

Sexually transmitted infections (STIs) represent a special threat to the feminine population. Many STIs are transmitted more efficiently from men to women than from women to men. STIs are often asymptomatic in women; thus, treatment is not sought, and the disease remains uncontrolled, often leading to pelvic inflammatory disease, which in turn can damage the fallopian tubes irreversibly. Tubal scarring is a major cause of mechanical sterility and ectopic pregnancy. STIs may adversely affect pregnancy, causing spontaneous abortion, stillbirth and premature delivery. The infected pregnant women can transmit the disease to her offspring *in utero* or at delivery. Venereal infection present on delivery can be responsible for postpartum endometritis. Risk factors identified for most STIs include young age, multiple sex partners, early onset of sexual activity, being single, substance abuse and Black race. Consequently, when all STIs are considered together, they may represent one of the most common medical complications in pregnancy, especially in high-risk groups, such as indigent urban populations plagued with drug abuse and promiscuity. Because STIs in women are often asymptomatic, screening for the most common infections is considered by some authors as an important component of prenatal care, particularly in highly predisposed women. Although more than 20 infectious diseases may be sexually acquired, only those transmitted primarily by sexual contact and causing genital disease will be discussed in this chapter.

Syphilis

Syphilis is a chronic spirochetal infection with many diverse clinical manifestations that occur in distinct stages. It holds a special place in the history of medicine as the 'great imitator' or 'great imposter'.

The Pathogen

Treponema pallidum subspecies *pallidum*, the causative agent of syphilis, is a slender, tightly coiled, motile organism. Belonging to the family Sperochaetaceae, the genus *Treponema* includes several other members, some of which are human pathogens; *T. pallidum* subsp. *pallidum* is the only one that can be transmitted by sexual contact. The pathogenic troponomes cannot be cultivated *in vitro*, and the distinction between them is based primarily on the clinical presentation.

Pathogenesis

Syphilis is most often acquired through sexual contact. Venereal transmission of *T. pallidum* is possible only when mucocutaneous syphilitic lesions are present. Immediately after *T. pallidum* penetrates the intact mucosa or gains access through disrupted skin, it enters the lymphatic and blood stream and disseminates throughout the body. Virtually any organ can be invaded including the central nervous system. Once established, the natural history of the disease is divided into several stages: primary, secondary, latent and tertiary (late) syphilis. The primary stage is characterized by the development of a chancre at the site of inoculation, which consists of an intense infiltration of plasma cells, scattered histocytes and the typical obliterative endarteritis. The secondary stage reflects the dissemination of the infection to the entire body and is characterized by a variety of diffuse mucocutaneous lesions and constitutional symptoms. Secondary syphilis can recur up to 4 years after acquisition of infection in about 25% of the patients, the risk of recurrence being higher in patients with suppressed cellular immunity, e.g., third-trimester pregnancy; most relapses (90%) occur within the first year. During the latent period, the only evidence for the presence of infection is the positive serologic response after the lesions of primary and secondary disease have vanished. The Centers for Disease Control and Prevention (CDC) define an infection of less than 1 year as early latent syphilis (recurrence of secondary disease possible, high infectivity), and infection of more than 1 year as late latent syphilis (recurrence unlikely). Tertiary syphilis develops in about one-third of untreated patients after a variable interval of latency. Two types of lesions can develop during this stage of the disease: the most common variety is the obliterative endarteritis of the vasa vasorum of the aorta and the arteries of the central nervous system as seen in cardiovascular syphilis and meningovascular neurosyphilis and where *T. pallidum* can be demonstrated by appropriate staining. The other type is the gumma which is a granulomatous-like lesion consisting of a necrotic, coagulated center surrounded by an inflammatory zone and fibrosis. The lesions, which may contain spirochetes, can be found anywhere in the body, most often in the liver, skin, bones and spleen.[1]

In the infected woman, syphilis is not associated with impairment of subsequent ability to conceive.[1] The pathologic consequences of *T. pallidum* infection are less prominent during pregnancy.[2] Since many of the manifestations of adult and congenital syphilis are thought to have an immunologic basis, the milder form of syphilis in the pregnant female is consistent with the relative state of immunosuppression which accompanies pregnancy. At least two-thirds of fetuses of women with early (infectious) syphilis during pregnancy are affected. Once the infection reaches the placenta during maternal spirochetemia, fetal infection usually follows. The infected placenta becomes large and pale. Microscopically, the villi appear to have lost their characteristic arborescent appearance and to have become thicker and club shaped. The blood vessels may decrease in number or almost disappear as a result of endarteritis. Vascular resistance in uterine and umbilical arteries may be increased.[3] Evidence of fetal involvement is more likely to be documented after the 18th gestational week, although spirochetes were detected as early as 9 weeks' gestation.[2] Thus, syphilis is not associated with early abortion. It has been proposed that the lesions of congenital syphilis do not become evident until the fetus becomes immunologically competent at about the 16th gestational week.[2] The consequences of congenital syphilis depend on the severity of the infection: late abortion, stillbirth, neonatal death, premature labor, delayed intrauterine growth, neonatal disease, or latent infection may be seen. These appear to be largely due to the dysfunction of the maternal–fetal endocrine axis, resulting from decreased levels of dehydroepiandrosterone produced by the fetal adrenal glands.[4]

Epidemiology

Although the vast majority of cases of syphilis result from transmission by sexual intercourse, the infection can also be acquired by passage of the organism through the placenta (congenital syphilis), by kissing or touching a person who has active lesions, by transfusion of fresh blood (*T. pallidum* cannot survive longer than 24–48 h in stored blood units), or by accidental direct inoculation (syphilis of the fingers in medical personnel). Sexual transmission is highest during the primary and secondary stages: one-third of contacts will acquire the infection.

In the United States, the incidence of syphilis declined sharply after the introduction of penicillin therapy and broad based public health programs, attaining its lowest levels in the 1950s (annual rate of primary and secondary syphilis, ~5 cases per 100,000 population).[5] An increase in the rate of primary and secondary syphilis was observed during the late 1980s with an incidence of 20 cases per 100,000 population in 1990. More recently, the rate decreased again, and in 2000 it was the lowest (2.1 cases per 100,000) since reporting began, although a slight increase was observed thereafter (2.5 cases per 100,000 in 2003). This increase was due to the rise of the rate of primary and secondary syphilis among men (4.2 cases per 100,000 in 2003), while in women the incidence continued to decline (0.8 cases per 100,000 in 2003).[6] In 2003, almost 40% of cases of primary and secondary syphilis reported to the CDC occurred among African-Americans, with a rate 5.2 times higher than the rate among Whites.[6]

Women usually have had lower rates of disease than men although most recently the male-to-female rate ration in White Americans was 1.0. Women cycled at low levels until the epidemic of the 1980s, when rates, primarily in Black women, increased rapidly (Figure 158.1), a trend that also led to a dramatic increase in congenital syphilis. This change is probably related to the development of a new highly promiscuous life style which is marked by exchange of sexual favors for drugs, especially crack cocaine.[7] A sharp decrease of primary and secondary syphilis among women was observed during the 1990s and the early 2000s, with an incidence of 0.8 case per 100,000 in 2003.[6] The vast majority of cases occur as expected in the most sexually active age group (15–29-year-olds).

In other industrialized countries, the incidence of syphilis has generally been lower than in the United States even before the recent epidemic. In Western Europe and Canada, a sharp decline in the rates had been observed after the advent of penicillin. A further decrease in incidence has occurred in the 1980s with rates of ≤2 cases per 100,000 since 1983, probably as a consequence of changes in sexual behavior imposed by the AIDS epidemic.[5] During the 1990s, until 1998, the number of cases of infectious syphilis diagnosed in England remained stable among both sexes, but then more than doubled between 1998 and 2000 in

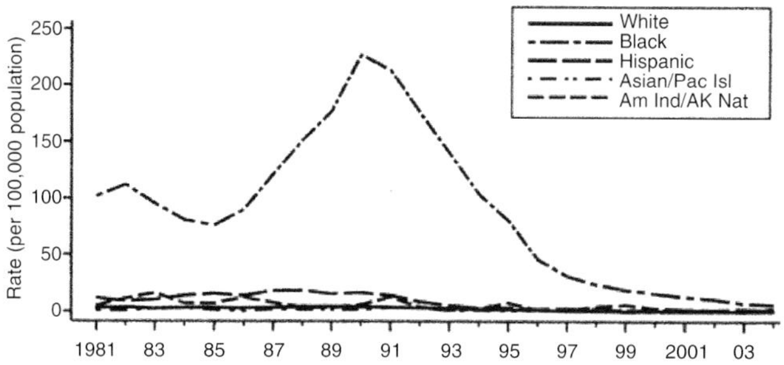

Figure 158.1 Primary and secondary syphilis. Rates among 15- to 19-year-old females by race and ethnicity: United States, 1981–2004 (from Centers for Disease Control and Prevention[6]).

men and rose by 53% in women. In 2000, 48% of syphilis infections in men were homosexually acquired, rates being highest in London (men 2.9/100,000; women 0.8/100,000) and in northwest England (men 2.0/100,000; women 0.2/100,000) regions.[8] A similar trend has been observed in Israel with a significant decline in the incidence of syphilis since the 1970s (less than 0.5 per 100,000 in 1990). Since the mid-1990s, however, an increase in the incidence was documented (3 cases of primary and secondary syphilis per 100,000 in 2001), mostly due to morbidity among newly arrived immigrants.[9] In Eastern Europe, on the other hand, a brisk increase in the incidence of primary and secondary syphilis was observed in countries formerly belonging to the USSR (32 cases per 100,000 in Russia).[10] Very limited information is available on the prevalence of syphilis in non-industrialized countries. The estimates for parts of Africa are 360 cases per 100,000 in 1990.[11]

In pregnant women, the prevalence of positive serologic tests for syphilis in the penicillin era in Northern Europe and the United States has been roughly 0.1–0.6%.[1] More recently, 1.5% of women who delivered in a large tertiary care urban hospital in Detroit, Michigan, USA, had reactive serologic tests. Seropositive mothers were primarily Black, multigravida with a mean age of 25 years and had a history of crack heroine use.[12] Women with untreated syphilis apparently may remain infectious to their fetuses for many years, although the proportion of affected fetuses and the severity of fetal disease decrease with longer duration of untreated maternal infection. According to World Health Organization (WHO) estimates, a million pregnancies each year are adversely affected by syphilis due to maternal infection, and about 270,000 infants are born with congenital diseases. Primary or secondary syphilis during pregnancy affects virtually 100% of fetuses with 50% of such pregnancies resulting in premature delivery or perinatal death. Pregnancy during early latent syphilis results in a 40% rate of prematurity or perinatal death, whereas late syphilis causes congenital infection in 10% of infants and 10-fold risk of perinatal death.[2] According to the 1988 Centers of Disease Control Surveillance case definition, a presumptive case of congenital syphilis includes any infant whose mother had untreated of inadequately treated syphilis at delivery, regardless of findings in the infant, as well as symptomatic infants.[13] Trends in congenital syphilis occurrence closely parallel trends in rates of primary and secondary syphilis in women in the peak childbearing age group (15–29 years) which is also the peak age group in which early syphilis occurs. Peaks in congenital syphilis usually occur 1 year after peaks in primary and secondary syphilis among women. At present, syphilis is an uncommon cause of stillbirth in industrialized countries: the incidence of congenital syphilis has steadily declined in recent decades reaching an all time low of 2–3 cases per 100,000 births in the late 1970s.[1] However, since the early 1980s, an increase in congenital syphilis was noted in the United States.[1,6] In 1987, the incidence of reported congenital syphilis in infants less than 1 year of age was about 12 cases per 100,000 live births, and it continued to increase steeply until 1991 when 107 cases per 100,000 live births were reported. A sharp decline was observed thereafter with 10.3 cases per 100,000 live births in 2003.[6] In 2003, Blacks accounted for the majority of congenital syphilis cases with a rate of 33.9 cases per 100,000 live births, followed by Hispanics (18.1 per 100,000 live births) and non-Hispanic Whites (1.3 cases per 100,000 live births).[6] In the United Kingdom, each year around two infants are born with congenital syphilis. Similar low rates are reported in other West European countries such as France and Switzerland.[14] In Israel, congenital syphilis is also rare: during the period 1991–2000, a mean of 2.4 cases were reported annually to the Ministry of Health (range, 0–4 cases per year). The annual incidence during this period was ≤0.08 cases per 100,000 live births.[9] On the other hand, a 50-fold increase in the incidence of congenital syphilis was documented in the former Soviet Union during the decade 1990–1999.[14]

Maternal and congenital syphilis still remain a major problem in developing countries, especially in sub-Saharan Africa. Prevalences of syphilis seropositivity in pregnant women attending antenatal clinics in Africa range from 10% to 15% in most reports.[1] In Zambia, congenital syphilis was documented in 1% of the babies delivered at a Lusaka hospital, and seropositivity rates ranging from 2.9% to 6.5% was noted among infants under 6 months of age.[1] In another study from Zambia, serologic tests for syphilis were positive in 43% of women who delivered stillborn babies, 19% of those who aborted and in 13% of women attending their first antenatal visit; 19% of miscarriages in this country were attributed to syphilis.[1] In Durban, South Africa, congenital syphilis is the fourth, and in Addis Ababa, Ethiopia, the fifth leading cause of perinatal death.[2] Also, in the latter city, syphilis is responsible for as many as 10% of all perinatal deaths.[15] According to other sources the impact of congenital syphilis on perinatal mortality in sub-Saharan Africa is even higher.[14] In most of the North African, Latin American and Asian countries the rates of syphilis among pregnant women range between 2% and 5%.[14]

Clinical manifestations

Treponema pallidum infection may remain asymptomatic in many cases: 11% of infected women develop signs of primary syphilis, 41% develop signs of secondary disease, and 48% remain asymptomatic. The classical primary chancre appears at the site of inoculation (labia, the posterior fourchette, cervix, vagina, anus, etc.) as a single painless papule after an average 21-day incubation period (range, 3–90 days). It quickly erodes to form an indurated ulcer with a smooth, clean base, and firm, raised borders. Multiple chancres can occur, however, especially in the person infected with HIV. Other variations in presentation are possible; thus any genital lesion should raise the suspicion of syphilis ('any anogenital ulcer is syphilis until proven otherwise'). The cervical location is more common in pregnant women, probably because of inoculation of the friable cervix.[3] In some instances, the lesion may be somewhat larger than usual, presumably because of increased genital vascularity. On other occasions, it may be of such a small size or be located as to go unnoticed.[3] The chancre is often accompanies by non-tender, non-suppurative enlarged inguinal lymph nodes. Primary syphilis must be differentiated principally from herpes virus infections, chancroid and traumatic superinfected genital lesions. The chancre heals spontaneously within 3–6 weeks (range, 1–12 weeks), while the lymphadenopathy usually persists for a longer duration.

Secondary syphilis usually appears approximately 6 weeks (range, 2–8 weeks) after the appearance of the chancre, and up to 6 months after exposure, in the form of highly variable mucocutaneous lesions and constitutional symptoms. In about 15% of women, the chancre may still be present. Skin lesions occur in 80% of patients in form of macular, papular, maculpapular and/or pustular rash that may persist from a few days to 8 weeks. Any surface area of the body can be affected with all of the different rashes being present at one time; the involvement of palms and soles strongly suggests the diagnosis. Temporary patchy alopecia and loss of eyebrow may be seen. In warm, moist intertriginous areas (perianal area, vulva, etc.) highly infectious plaques, called condyloma lata, may develop. Mucous patches, in form of silvery gray superficial erosions, may also be noted on the mucous membranes of the vagina, cervix, mouth, pharynx, etc. The constitutional symptoms include low-grade fever, malaise, anorexia, weight loss and generalized painless lymphadenopathy. The cerebrospinal fluid may be inflamed in up to 40% of the patients, but most of them do not develop neurosyphilis after treatment with one of the currently recommended regimens. Virtually any organ can be affected: kidney (glomerulonephritis, nephrotic syndrome), liver (high serum alkaline phosphatase levels), spleen (splenomegaly), eyes (iritis, uveitis), the osteoarticular system (synovitis, osteitis) and cranial nerves (palsies).

Tertiary syphilis is a slowly progressive inflammatory disease that can touch any organ in the body and can produce clinical illness years after the initial infection. It is generally referred to as cardiovascular syphilis (syphilitic aortitis), gummatous syphilis (can affect any organ), or neurosyphilis (asymptomatic, meningovascular or parenchymatous). Neurosyphilis encompasses a heterogeneous collection of neurologic syndromes and psychiatric manifestations with tabes dorsalis and Argyll Robertson pupil being the most specific for syphilis. The parenchymatous neurologic lesions are usually irreversible and respond only slightly to therapy.

Most syphilitic infants lack manifestations at birth.[1] Neonates who are born with manifest syphilis are usually severely affected and carry a worse prognosis. In symptomatic patients the earliest sign (appearing usually on the third to eighth week of life) is a rhinitis (snuffles) followed by a diffuse maculopapular desquamative rash with skin sloughing particularly on the palms, soles and about the anus and mouth. In contrast to acquired syphilis, a vesicular rash and bullae may be seen. Necrotizing funisitis (swollen and discolored umbilical cord) is pathognomonic. Osteochondritis and perichondritis can affect all bones of the osteoarticular system, most prominently the nose (saddle nose) and the metaphyses of the lower extremities ('saber shin'). The liver is often heavily involved with accompanying splenomegaly, anemia, thrombocytopenia and jaundice. Immune-complex glomerulonephritis can develop at about the fourth month of life. Neonatal congenital syphilis must be differentiated from other generalized congenital infections (TORCH). Late congenital syphilis (beyond 24 months of life) is characterized by the frequency of interstitial keratitis and neurosyphilis, while cardiovascular syphilis is rare. Other typical lesions include recurrent arthropathy, deformed upper central incisors (Hutchinson's teeth), frontal bossing and other craniofacial malformations.[1]

Laboratory diagnosis

Demonstration of the pathogen

Since *T. pallidum* is not culturable on artificial medium, the organism can be diagnosed only by direct demonstration in an appropriate specimen. Dark-field examination of a serous exudate from a moist lesion is the quickest and most productive technique. *Treponema pallidum* will have a corkscrew appearance and will move in a characteristic spiraling motion which is not seen in non-pathogenic treponemes. An alternative technique, which can be used also in biopsy specimens, is the direct or indirect immunofluorescence or immunoperoxydase staining.[16] Promising results were recently obtained with the polymerase chain reaction (PCR) technique which can be applied also on paraffin-embedded tissue. The PCR technique could be extremely valuable in diagnosing infection in congenital syphilis (in amniotic fluid, neonate's serum and cerebrospinal fluid, CSF) and neurosyphilis.[17]

Serologic tests

Serology remains the most useful diagnostic tool in women. These tests cannot distinguish, however, between syphilis and other treponemal infections. Hence, the interpretation of reactive serologic tests can be difficult in patients who live in or come from areas where non-venereal treponematoses are common. Two different types of tests are used in concert.[1] *The non-treponemal tests:* inexpensive, rapid and convenient means for screening large numbers of sera, and when used quantitatively, can give an indication of disease activity. Limitations of the non-treponemal tests include their lack of sensitivity in early primary cases (less than 5 weeks) and in late syphilis (negative in up to 30% of cases); the possibility of *prozone reaction* (false-negative reaction in undiluted serum because of antibody excess); or false-positive results which can occur in association with advanced age, pregnancy, drug addiction, connective tissue diseases, chronic liver disease, cancer, multiple myeloma and a variety of infectious diseases including early HIV infection.[11] These tests detect antibodies directed against a lipoidal antigen that is the result of the interaction of host tissue with *T. pallidum*. The standard antitreponemal test is the VDRL (Venereal Diseases Research Laboratory). The rapid plasma reagin (RPR) card test and the automated reagin test (ART) are two modifications of the standard test used for routine screening. A positive screening test should be further evaluated with a confirmatory treponemal test and a non-treponemal quantitative test. Following adequate therapy early syphilis, the titers of the quantitative test should decline until little or no reaction is detected after the first year.[18] A persisting positive test with insufficient decline of the titer in a treated patient suggests: (a) persistent infection, (b) reinfection, or (c) biologically false-positive reaction. However, after an appropriate clinical response to treatment, non-treponemal titers persist at low levels in some individuals for a long time (sometimes for life), a response referred to as a 'serofast' state. Up to 15% of HIV-negative patients with early syphilis who received therapy at recommended or greater dosages do not demonstrate a 2-dilution decline in RPR/VDRL titers at 12 months following therapy, without evidence of clinically defined treatment failure. No further therapy is required in serofast states if titers are not increasing, clinical disease resolves (primary and secondary syphilis), clinical disease does not recur (primary and secondary disease) or develop (early latent syphilis), and the patient is HIV-negative. HIV-positive patients with a serofast reaction to treatment of latent syphilis may need a lumbar puncture for further evaluation.[19]

Treponemal tests

Treponemal tests are used primarily to verify the reactivity of the non-treponemal tests. In primary syphilis, they may become reactive before the non-treponemal tests.[17] Three tests are currently considered the standard: the fluorescent traponemal antibody absorption test (FTA-ABS), the *T. pallidum* hemagglutination (TPHA), and the microhemagglutination assay for antibodies to *T. pallidum* (MHA-TP). All these tests use *T. pallidum* as the antigen to detect antibodies. The treponemal tests are technically more difficult and costly to perform than the non-treponemal tests and cannot be used to monitor therapy. For most infected persons, test results may remain positive for life-time even after successful therapy. About 1% of the general population have false-positive results: these are also associated with systemic lupus erythematosus and some other spirochetal and non-spirochetal infections.[2,11] A reactive treponemal test result on a sample that is also reactive in a non-treponemal test is, however, highly specific.[17] If late latent syphilis is suspected, serologic testing of the CSF should be considered to rule out neurosyphilis. A definitive diagnosis is made on the basis of a reactive VDRL-CSF test[17] or the intrathecal *T. pallidum* antibody (ITPA) index.[16] All patients with diagnosed syphilis should be tested for HIV.

Treatment

Experience has shown that a single benzathine penicillin G dose had a success of 95% or higher in early syphilis in patients with intact immune system. In late syphilis, because spirochetes are thought to divide more slowly, the suggested duration of therapy is longer.[11] Recommended choice and dosages of antimicrobial agents for the various clinical forms of syphilis are shown in Table 158.1. During pregnancy, syphilis therapy must be guided not only by its ability to cure the mother, but also by its ability to prevent or cure fetal infection. Treatment in the pregnant woman is generally the same as that of the non-pregnant patient and depends on the duration of infection, the presence or absence of central nervous system involvement and the competence of the patient's immune system. Some experts recommend, however, additional therapy (e.g., a second dose of benzathine penicillin G 2.4 million units IM) 1 week after the initial dose, particularly for those women in the third

Table 158.1 Recommended therapeutic regimens for syphilis[20]

Stage	Treatment of choice	Alternative regimens*
Primary, secondary early latent (≤1 year)	Benzathine penicillin G, 2.4 million units IM in a single dose	Doxycycline 100 mg po bid ×14 days
		or
		Tetracycline 500 mg po qid ×14 days
		or
		Erythromycin 500 mg po qid ×14 days
		or
		Cefriaxone (dosage not established; see Schafer *et al.*[22])
Late (or of unknown duration) latent tertiary (cardiovascular, gummatous)	Benzathine penicillin G, 3 doses of 2.4 million units, IM each at 1 week intervals	Doxycycline 100 mg po bid ×14 days
		or
		Tetracycline 500 mg po qid ×14 days
Neurosyphilis	Aqueous crystalline penicillin G, 2–4 million units IV every 4 h for 10–14 days	
	or	
	Procaine penicillin 2.4 million units IM daily, plus probenecid 500 mg po qid, both for 10–14 days	
Congenital	Aqueous crystalline penicillin G, 50,000 units/kg IV every 12 h during the first 7 days, and every 8 h thereafter, for 10–14 days	
	or	
	Procaine penicillin G, 50,000 units/kg IM daily for 10–14 days	

*For patients allergic to penicillin; not recommended for use in pregnant women

trimester and for women who have secondary syphilis during pregnancy.

In patients with a history of penicillin allergy, skin testing with penicillin G minor determinant mixture and penicylloyl polylysine is recommended. If skin tests are reactive, penicillin desensitization should be performed using the technique described by Wendel *et al.*[20] Alternative therapy during pregnancy with one of the non-penicillin regimens is discouraged by the CDC because of reported treatment failures in preventing congenital syphilis, especially with erythromycin, and potential adverse effects on the mother and the fetus.[16] Initial reports on treatment of early syphilis with cefriaxone are promising.[21,22]

The Jarisch–Herxheimer reaction is a well described phenomenon often occurring in pregnant patients treated for primary or (more particularly) secondary syphilis. Symptoms usually occur within 24 h after any therapy for syphilis. Approximately 1–2 h after therapy has been initiated, systemic manifestations of fever, rigors, tachycardia, hyperventilation, vasodilatation, hypotension, profuse sweating headache, myalgia and arthralgia. Uterine contractions frequently develop during the reaction, and they may be followed by evidence for fetal distress manifested as late fetal heart decelerations.[3] The reaction is self limited and can be treated with aspirin or prednisone if manifestations are severe.

All patients treated for early syphilis should have repeat quantitative non-treponemal tests at 3, 6 and 12 months post-therapy. In pregnant women, serologic tests should be performed monthly until adequacy of treatment has been assured. All patients with syphilis of more than 1 year duration should also be tested 24 months after treatment. Patients with documented neurosyphilis should be carefully followed serologically and have a CSF examination for at least 5 years unless all abnormal parameters normalize before.

The risk of infection for the infant is minimal (less than 2%) if the mother has received adequate penicillin therapy during pregnancy. However, the child must be examined monthly after delivery and until the non-treponemal test or PCR analysis become negative. Treatment of the infant should be considered in the following circumstances: (a) mother had received inadequate penicillin therapy or was treated with antibiotics other than penicillin, (b) the treatment status of the mother is not well documented, (c) the mother was treated appropriately, but a significant decrease in non-treponemal antibody (≥fourfold) has not been achieved or documented after therapy to indicate adequate response, and (d) the infant could be difficult to follow. Additionally, any infant with physical, radiologic or serologic (quantitative titer ≥fourfold greater than the mother's titer) evidence of active diseases should be fully treated.[23] Since neurosyphilis is difficult to exclude in newborns, treatment regimens similar to those recommended for neurosyphilis should be used in infants. If the mother was appropriately treated *during* pregnancy (more than 4 weeks before delivery), mother's titers decreased fourfold, and the infant was normal on physical exam and serologically (titers <fourfold the maternal's), no evaluation is required; yet, it is recommended to give the infant a single dose of IM benzathine penicillin G 50,000 units/kg.[23]

Syphilis in HIV-infected patients often presents with a more protracted and malignant course, greater constitutional symptoms, organ involvement, atypical and florid skin rashes and a significant predisposition to develop neurosyphilis.[16] HIV-infected patients are more likely to show an aberrant serologic response.[16] Therapeutic recommendations vary: some authors recommend more vigorous and prolonged regimens, while others suggest that regimens used for non-HIV patients are satisfactory.[23] Failure of even high dose intravenous therapy to cure symptomatic neurosyphilis in HIV infected patient has been reported.[24] Penicillin should always be administered and careful follow-up is essential. Since syphilis increases the risk for the acquisition and transmission of HIV,[11] testing for HIV is recommended for all persons in whom syphilis is diagnosed.[23]

Case detection and prevention

Any person sexually exposed to a patient with syphilis in any stage should be evaluated clinically and serologically.[23]

Congenital syphilis is entirely preventable in an appropriate case detection program. Most congenital syphilis today is the result of failure to detect and treat syphilis in pregnant women. In the recent epidemic of congenital syphilis in the United States, half of the infected infants were born to women who received prenatal care, but in whom serological screening was not done and thus maternal syphilis was not treated.

Prenatal first-trimester serologic screen is cost-beneficial even in countries with prevalence of maternal syphilis as low as 1:20,000.[2,14] The CDC recommend serologic testing at the beginning of prenatal care and, for high-risk women, at the beginning of the third trimester and at delivery. Any woman who delivers a stillborn infant after 20 weeks' gestation should also be tested.[23] To improve early detection in pregnant women, particularly in developing countries and in poor and minority women in industrialized countries, the following practical measures are suggested: on-site pregnancy testing of women in STI clinics and drug addiction programs whose menstrual periods are late; routine PRP testing whenever a positive pregnancy test is reported in all pregnancy testing programs; and early testing by prenatal programs before the regularly scheduled prenatal visit when the waiting time for their first scheduled visit is long.[2] No infant or mother should leave the hospital unless the maternal serologic status has been documented at least once during pregnancy and preferably again at delivery.[23] All infants born to mothers seropositive to syphilis should have a quantitative non-treponemal serologic test performed on infant serum (treponemal tests are not necessary). These infants should also be examined for signs of congenital syphilis: non-immune hydrops, jaundice, hepatosplenomegaly, rhinitis, skin rash and/or pseudoparalysis of an extremity. Pathologic examination of the placenta or the umbilical cord is suggested, and microscopic examination of suspicious lesions or body fluids for tremonema is recommended. Laboratory tests should include CSF analysis for VDRL, cell count and protein, complete blood count and differential, platelet count. Other tests if clinically indicated: radiographs, liver function tests, ophthalmologic examination, etc.[23]

Gonorrhea

Gonorrhea may present as a localized infection of the lower genital tract, an invasive infection of the upper genital tract or disseminated disease with systemic manifestations. Ascending genital infection in women is responsible for salpingitis, one of the leading causes of infertility in the world.

The Pathogen and pathogenesis

Neisseria gonorrhoeae is a non-motile, non spore-forming, gram-negative coccus that typically grows in pairs (diplococci). The bacterial cell surface is an important determinant in the pathogenesis of the gonococcal infection, and specific surface components have been related to adhesion, tissue and intracellular penetration, cytotoxicity and invasion of host defenses both systemically and at the mucosal level. These include protein structures such as pili, porins and opacity proteins, lipoligosaccharids and phospholipids. Some of the gonococcal serovars are associated with resistance to the bactericidal effect of normal human serum and with enhanced propensity to cause bacteremia.[25]

Gonococci primarily infect columnar and cuboidal epithelium. Attachment to mucosal epithelium, mediated in part by pili and opacity proteins, is followed within 24–48 h by penetration of the bacterium into the submucosal tissue.[25] The primary site of gonococcal infection in women is the endocervix, although the organism can also invade the urethra and occasionally the periurethral and Bartholin's glands. In 10–20% of women with gonorrhea, the infection can extend to the upper genital organs and involve the endometrium, fallopian tubes and the ovaries. *Neisseria gonorrhoeae* can invade the upper genital tract as a solitary pathogen or as part of a polymicrobial infection. From the fallopian tubes the infection can extend further to the liver capsule and the overlying peritoneum to give acute perihepatitis. However, the most serious complications of pelvic inflammatory disease (PID) are infertility and ectopic pregnancy due to fallopian tube scarring.[26] Infertility occurs in 15–20% of women after a single episode and up to 80% of those with three or more episodes. Evidence for prior salpingitis can be found in 50–80% of women with ectopic pregnancies.[27]

Extragenital sites of infection include the rectum, the pharynx (following anogenital and orogenital sexual exposure, respectively), the conjunctiva (resulting from autoinoculation in the adult, or acquired through contact with the infected birth canal in the newborn), or disseminated gonococcal infection. Gonococcal dissemination is associated with some host factors, such as complement deficiency, female sex, menstruation and perhaps pharyngeal gonococcal infection and pregnancy.[25] Disseminated gonococcal infection, occurring in 0.5–3% of patients with gonorrhea, results from bacteremic spread of *N. gonorrhoeae* to the skin and articular or periarticular tissues; various immunologic mechanisms are also involved in some cases.[25]

In most pregnant women, gonococcal infection is limited to the lower genital tract. Acute salpingitis is rare, but can develop if cervical infection ascends before obliteration of uterine cavity through fusion of the chorion and decidua at 12 weeks. Rarely, preexisting infection can cause a tubo-ovarian abscess. Local cervical factors also decrease the risk for ascending gonococcal infection. Serum progesterone concentrations are greatly increased in pregnancy; high concentrations of this hormone are known to inhibit the growth of *N. gonorrhoeae in vitro*. Cervical mucus becomes impermeable to motile sperm and perhaps to microorganisms under the influence of progesterone.[2] Although PID during pregnancy is quite rare, it can be particularly virulent resulting in severe morbidity and in higher rates of pregnancy loss. The prevalence of pharyngitis as the sole gonococcal infection may be higher during pregnancy (15–30% of infected women) reflecting perhaps an increase in the frequency of fellatio as pregnancy progresses.[2] There are conflicting reports as to whether pregnancy is a risk factor for disseminated gonococcal infection.[25]

Gonococcal infection may have a deleterious effect on the pregnancy outcome at any stage, although the consequences on late pregnancy have been better studied. Antenatal gonorrhea is associated with increased risks of chorioamnionitis, spontaneous abortions, premature labor, early rupture of membranes, perinatal infant mortality and postpartum upper genital tract infections.[28–35] It is not clear, however, whether gonococcal infection is always directly responsible for all of these complications or is merely a marker for high risk due to concomitant pathogens. A threefold increased relative risk for endometritis was observed in patients who had untreated gonococcal infection when compared with uninfected control subjects.[31] Elliot *et al.* found that the attributable risk for preterm birth was 14%.[33] Stoll and colleagues showed that treatment of gonococcal carriage reduced the increased risk for adverse pregnancy outcome.[34] Infected mothers can transmit *N. gonorrhoeae* to the newborn *in utero*, during delivery or in the postpartum period.[25] Conjunctivitis (ophthalmia neonatarum) is the most common postnatal complication, occurring in 30–42% of infants born to infected women,[35] although septicemia and arthritis can also be rarely seen. Gonococcal conjunctivitis of the newborn is still a common cause of blindness in some developing countries.

Epidemiology

The risk of transmission of gonorrhea from an infected male to a female partner is approximately 50% per contact. The risk of female to male transmission is approximately 20% per intercourse.[25,36] Transmission by rectal intercourse appears to be similarly efficient, while spread by oral–genital contact is believed to be lower.[25] Gonorrhea is usually a short-lived infection, even when not treated. Therefore, high rates of partner change are required to maintain the spread of infection. Individuals at high risk of acquiring and transmitting gonorrhea – the core transmitters – are characterized by young age (20–24 years), low educational and socioeconomic level, urban residence, being single, prostitution activity, illicit drug use and reduced access to health care.[25,36] The role of anovulary contraceptives as a predisposing factor for contracting gonorrhea has remained controversial. High rates of gonorrhea have recently been observed also in rural communities in the southeastern United States, surpassing those in urban counties.[37] Risk factors are generally similar in pregnancy as in the non-pregnant state. More cases of gonorrhea are reported in men than in women, reflecting a greater ease of diagnosis in men; in the United States the male:female case ratio was 1.3:1 in 1992.[25]

Gonorrhea is most common in developing countries. In a survey conducted by the WHO in Senegal and Uganda in 1990–1991, the prevalence of gonorrhea was 0.6% among military men and 13.1% among commercial sex workers.[38] The prevalence of gonorrhea in unselected populations of pregnant women has been estimated to be 10% in Africa, 5% in Latin America and 4% in Asia.[39] Gonococcal conjunctivitis of the newborn was diagnosed in about 4% of all live births in Kenya in 1987.[39] According to a survey performed in 1990–1991[38] the prevalence of gonorrhea among pregnant women in Senegal and Uganda was 1.4%. The prevalence rates in the United States have been generally higher than those in other industrialized countries. The annual incidence in the United States had reached a peak in 1975 with 468 cases per 100,000. It declined thereafter, attaining a rate of 116 cases per 100,000 in 2003.[6] Since 1997, the rates of gonorrhea among men and women are almost identical. The highest rates of gonorrhea among women in the United States are in the age group of 15–29 years. When analyzed by ethnic groups, incidence rates (in 2003) were highest among the Black population (655.8 per 100,000), followed by Native Americans and Hispanics (103.5 and 71.7 cases per 100,000, respectively), and was lowest in the White population (32.7 cases per 100,000).[6] Not unexpectedly, the difference between the Black and White populations in the prevalence of gonorrhea was also documented among pregnant women.[40] The incidence of gonorrhea has been substantially lower in most European countries, and indigenous gonorrhea was virtually eliminated in Sweden. More recently, however, a trend toward the resurgence of gonorrhea is being observed in several West European countries, such as Sweden, Denmark, United Kingdom and France.[41] In Israel, following a period very low reported rates during most of the 1990s (0.7 cases per 100,000 in 1994–1995),[9,42,43] a sharp increase in the incidence of the disease was documented in the late 1990s and early 2000s (13.8 cases per 100,000 in 2001).[44] The reasons for this change in the epidemiology of gonorrhea are not evident, however, the role of sex tourism and immigration of sex workers originating from countries with high gonorrhea prevalence (eastern Europe) was evoked.[11,44] After attaining a peak incidence of 16/100,000 in 2002, a trend toward a decrease in the incidence was observed more recently (8.5/100,000 in 2004) (Department of Epidemiology, Ministry of Health, Israel; unpublished data). In a survey conducted among young female soldiers, gonococcal infection was detected by PCR in 1.0%.[45]

Risk factors for PID include teenage, use of intrauterine device, prior PID and vaginal douching.[25] In the United States 20–40% of PID in most urban areas were associated in the 1980s with *N. gonorrhoeae*, whereas in Sweden and Israel, where gonorrhea has become very rare, the organism is seldom isolated from patients with PID.[43] It has been estimated that in a cohort of 100 women with gonorrhea, of whom 25 were pregnant, effective treatment would prevent 25 cases of PID, one of ectopic pregnancy, six instances of infertility, and seven cases of neonatal ophthalmia.

Clinical manifestations

Many infected women remain asymptomatic or develop only minor symptoms. In surveys in which infections are detected through screening, up to 90% of women with gonorrhea may be asymptomatic. The incubation period is variable: symptoms appear within 10 days in most cases. The dominant symptoms of lower genital tract infection include increased vaginal discharge, dysuria, usually without urgency or frequency, and intermenstrual bleeding.[25] Abdominal pain usually indicates infection of the upper genital tract. On examination, purulent or mucopurulent cervical exudate, cervical edema and bleeding, and purulent urethritis can be seen. Gonococcal Bartholin's abscesses associated with gonorrhea most often are unilateral, acutely suppurative and painful.

Rectal infection, seen in up to 40% of women with gonorrhea, is most often asymptomatic, although acute proctitis can develop in some patients, manifested by anal pruritus, tenesmus, purulent discharge or rectal bleeding.[25] Pharyngeal gonorrhea can be found in 10–25% of heterosexual women with genital infection. The infection is most often asymptomatic and resolves spontaneously.[25]

Gonococcal PID often follows the onset of menses by a few days. It usually presents acutely: abdominal pain usually bilateral and often associated with manifestations of cervicitis, is the most common symptom. High fever, chills, nausea and vomiting can be seen in a minority of the patients.[25] On examination, pelvic adnexal and uterine fundal tenderness is often noted and pain can be produced on moving the cervix; mucopurulent cervicitis is usually present. The lower abdomen is tender on palpation and signs of peritoneal inflammation are common in severe cases. Abscess formation is uncommon. Leukocytosis, accelerated erythrocyte sedimentation and elevated C-reactive protein levels are present in about two-thirds of patients with PID. The minimal criteria for diagnosis of PID include uterine-adnexal tenderness or cervical-motion tenderness.[23] The differential diagnosis includes appendicitis, septic abortion, adnexal torsion, and ectopic pregnancy. Chronic pelvic pain that may be very disabling can be a complication in up to 20% of women with PID and is often difficult to distinguish from recurrent PID. Perihepatitis (Fitz–Hugh–Curtis syndrome) manifests with abdominal pain and hepatic tenderness; in many cases pelvic symptoms and signs are lacking. The definitive diagnosis is made by laporoscopy which can visualize the 'violin string' adhesions between the liver capsule and the parietal peritoneum.[25]

Disseminated gonococcal infection is characterized by the 'arthritis–dermatitis syndrome'. The initial manifestations consist of additive and sometimes migratory polyarthritis; physical signs of arthritis and synovitis are present.[25] Typically, a few joints are involved in an asymmetric manner. A characteristic dermatitis can be seen in about 75% of patients and consists of lightly scattered discrete papular and pustular lesions (occasionally hemorrhagic, bullous or necrotic), localized predominantly on the extremities. Subsequently, septic arthritis develops in one or two joints and can occasionally be the sole manifestation of disseminated gonococcal infection. Fever, systemic toxicity and leukocytosis are usually mild when present. Infective endocarditis, meningitis, osteomyelitis and fulminant septicemia are rare yet severe manifestations of disseminated gonococcal infection.[3]

Gonococcal conjunctivitis in the adult is usually severe and can be complicated by corneal ulcerations. In the newborn, purulent conjunctivitis develops within 1 week of delivery. It can result in perforation of the globe and blindness if inadequately treated.

Laboratory diagnosis

Isolation of *N. gonorrhoeae* by culture is the preferred method for diagnosing gonococcal infection. Endocervical specimens are obtained after wiping exudate from the endocervix, while avoiding contact with the vaginal mucosa or secretions.[25] Rectal specimens are best obtained by collecting purulent secretions or swabbing in an inflamed area under direct visualization by anoscopy.

For direct identification of diplococci with their typical morphology, smears of discharge are stained with Gram stain or methylene blue. This technique is very specific (95–100%) when performed by highly trained personnel, although its sensitivity is low when used for endocervical or rectal specimens (40–60%).[25] A definitively positive urethral or cervical smear (showing intracellular gram-negative of blue stained diplococci within neutrophils) is diagnostic.

Specimens should be transferred to the laboratory in a non-nutrient transport medium without refrigeration and inoculated onto growth medium within 6 h.[25] Immediate inoculation onto growth medium (e.g., Thayer–Martin medium or New York City medium) at room temperature with prompt incubation is preferable.

All gonococcal isolates should undergo antimicrobial susceptibility testing and be tested for β-lactamase (penicillinase) production. Penicillinase producing strains were first discovered almost simultaneously in 1975–1976 in the United States, western Europe, The Philippines and western Africa.[25] In 1990, penicillinase producing strains accounted for about 10% of isolates in the United States and western Europe and 30–60% in most developing countries. More recently, strains of *N. gonorrhoeae* with high level resistance to tetracycline have been detected and increasingly noted, particularly in Africa.[46] Resistance to quinolones is now being reported from several areas around the world.[47] Resistance to third generation cephalosporins has been rarely reported.

Nucleic acid amplification tests (NAATs) such as polymerase chain reaction (PCR) or ligase chain reaction (LCR), are highly specific and sensitive techniques,[25] and often perform better than culture. These tests, which are designed to amplify nucleic acid sequences that are specific for the pathogen being detected, do not require viable organisms. Another advantage consists of the possibility to use urine samples for the testing. On the other hand, if diagnosis is based on these tests solely, antimicrobial susceptibility tests cannot be done. All other non-culture tests are less sensitive than culture, especially for endocervical specimens, and are little better than Gram stain.

The possibility of concurrent sexually transmitted infections should be taken into consideration when diagnosing and treating gonorrhea. Up to 35–50% of women with gonorrhea are also infected with *C. trachomatis*.[25]

Treatment

Because of public health implications, an acceptable regimen for the treatment of gonorrhea should have efficacies that approach 100% and not less than 95%. Antibiotic treatment of gonorrhea is most often empiric, and should follow local guidelines which take into consideration the local antimicrobial resistance patterns. Thus, penicillin and tetracyclines should not be used any more in most cases for the empiric treatment of gonococcal infections. More recently, resistance to fluroquinolones has emerged and is spreading worldwide, particularly in the Far East, Australia, Hawaii, California, Israel, and in some countries in Europe.[47] Fluoroquinolones should not be used empirically anymore in patients infected in these areas.

Uncomplicated gonorrhea in adults

The regimens recommended by the U.S. Public Health Services[23] are presented in Table 158.2. Ceftriaxone cures genital, pharyngeal, rectal and conjunctival gonococcal infection, probably aborts incubatory syphilis, and is safe and effective in pregnant women. Ceftriaxone in a single dose of 125–150 mg IM is in fact the only regimen recommended for pregnant women. However, in areas where penicillin resistant strains represent less than 1% of all isolates, an acceptable alternative is aqueous procaine penicillin 2.8 million units injected IM at two sites with 1.0 g probenecid given by mouth. The efficacy of cefixime against incubating syphilis is uncertain. Quinolones should be avoided in pregnant women, and they will not abort incubatory syphilis. Spectinomycin 2 g IM is highly effective for genital and rectal, but not for pharyngeal gonorrhea, and it does not affect *T. pallidum*. Its main indication is the treatment of pregnant women with history of immediate allergy to penicillin or documented cephalosporin allergy. Cephalosporins can be given to patients with history of delayed reaction to penicillins.

The treatment of gonorrhea should be accompanied with a regimen active against *C. trachomatis* if co-infection by this organism has not been ruled out, and serologic testing for HIV and syphilis should be done. Since tetracyclines are contraindicated during pregnancy, most authorities recommend following ceftriaxone administration with 7–10-day course of erythromycin.[23,25] Azithromycin, 1 g orally, single dose is an acceptable alternative to erythromycin, although

Table 158.2 Recommended regimens for the empiric treatment of uncomplicated gonococcal urethritis/cervicitis/proctitis (from Centers for Disease Control and Prevention[23])

Target	Agent	Dosage
Gonorrhea	Cefixime	400 mg orally, single dose
	or	
	Ceftriaxone	125–250 mg intramuscularly, single dose
	or	
	Ciprofloxacin*	500 mg orally, single dose
	or	
	Ofloxacin*	400 mg orally, single dose
	or	
	Levofloxacin*	250 mg orally, single dose
	or	
	Spectinomycin	2.0 g intramuscularly, single dose
	plus	
Chlamydia**	Azithromycin	1.0 g orally, single dose
	or	
	Doxycycline	100 mg orally twice a day for 7 days

*Quinolones should not be used for infections acquired in areas with increased prevalence of quinolone resitance
**If chlamydia infection is not ruled out

it should be used with caution in pregnant women. HIV carriers with gonococcal infection should receive the same treatment as patients not carrying the virus.[23] Retesting to document cure is not recommended by most authorities if one of the suggested treatment regimens is used, unless therapeutic compliance is in question or symptoms persist.[23,25]

Disseminated gonococcal infection

Hospitalization is recommended for initial therapy which consists of ceftriaxone 1.0 g once daily IM or IV. Other third generation cephalosporins and spectinomycin 2.0 g IM twice daily are probably as effective. After clinical improvement, and in absence of complications, such as septic arthritis, treatment may be switched to oral cefixime 400 mg twice daily (or a quinolone in a non-pregnant patient) to complete 7–10 days of total therapy.[23] Meningitis should be treated with a 10–14-day course of ceftriaxone 1–2 g IV every 12 h, and patients with gonococcal endocarditis should receive at least 4 weeks of parenteral therapy.

Neonates and children

The advised regimen for neonates and children, weighing 45 kg or less, is ceftriaxone 25–30 mg per kg body weight, not to exceed 125 mg. It should be given as single dose for uncomplicated gonorrhea and conjunctivitis, or as a daily dose for 7 days in disseminated infection, and for 10–14 days if meningitis is documented. For conjunctivitis, topical antibiotic therapy alone is inadequate and is unnecessary if systemic treatment is administered; local care of the eyes by an expert is also important. Test for chlamydial infection should be done, and specific therapy should be withheld unless infection is diagnosed.[23]

PID

Close observation and aggressive antibiotic therapy are advised. Therapeutic regimens must provide empiric, broad spectrum coverage of likely pathogens because the specific organisms responsible for the infection usually are not known. Antimicrobial coverage should include *N. gonorrhoeae*, *C. trachomatis*, gram-negative facultative bacteria, anaerobes and streptococci.[23] For outpatients, the recommended regimen consists of ofloxacin, 400 mg orally twice a day for 14 days, or levofloxacin, once a day for 14 days, with or without metronidazole, 500 mg orally twice a day for 14 days; this regimen is not suitable for infections caused by quinolone-resistant gonococci. An alternative regimen, effective against quinolone-resistant gonococci, consists of ceftriaxone 250 mg intramuscularly as a single dose, or cefoxitin 2 g intramuscularly as a single dose, plus probenecid, 1 g orally, plus doxycycline, 100 mg twice a day for 14 days, with or without metronidazole, 500 mg twice a day for 14 days. The inpatient regimen includes cefotetan, 2 g intravenously every 12 h, or cefoxitin, 2 g intravenously every 6 h, plus doxycycline 100 mg orally or intravenously every 12 h. An alternative inpatient regimen includes clindamycin, 900 mg intravenously every 8 h, plus gentamicin 2 mg per kg of body weight (loading dose), followed by 1.5 mg per kg every 8 h (this regimen is less suitable for gonococcal infections). The parenteral therapy for PID should be continued for 24–48 h after clinical improvement occurs and should be followed by oral therapy with doxycycline, 100 mg twice a day, or clindamycin, 450 mg four times a day, for a total of 14 days.[23] For the management of PID during pregnancy the recommendations of the CDC are very brief and consist of the suggestion that 'pregnant women with suspected PID should be hospitalized and treated with parenteral antibiotics'.[23] Some of the regimens recommended for the treatment of PID in non-pregnant women include agents such as doxycycline, ofloxacin, levofloxacin or gentamicin, which should be avoided during pregnancy (these agents belong to categories C and D of the Food and Drug Administration Fetal Risk Drug Classification[48]). The following empirical regimens probably provide an effective and safe coverage of salpingitis in pregnant women: cefoxitin 1–2 g IV every 6 h or cefotetan 1–2 g IV every 12 h, plus erythromycin 500 mg IV or orally every 6 h. Ceftriaxone 1 g IV or IM every 24 h is probably also effective, although it is less active than the former cephalosporins against anaerobic bacteria. The alternative regimen recommended by the CDC for non-pregnant patients, clindamycin 900 mg IV every 8 h, plus gentamicin 1.5 mg/kg every 8 h (following a loading dose of 2 mg/kg), should be avoided in pregnancy because of the aminoglycoside component, and should be used only when essential. Therapy should continue for a total of 14 days. Recommendations for continued oral therapy are difficult to formulate, particularly for an adequate coverage of gram-negative facultative bacteria.

Prevention and control

Use of a condom provides a high degree of protection for the non-infected partner. Because gonococcal infection, which is often subclinical in women, may have deleterious effects on pregnancy outcome, a screening cervical culture is recommended by most authorities at the first prenatal visit or prior to an induced abortion. In high-risk populations (young, non-White, single, primigravada, low socioeconomic status, IV drug use, current or past STI), some authorities recommend that a repeat culture be obtained during the third trimester.[23] Sexual partners of infected patients and parents of infected infants should be examined and treated for *N. gonorrhoeae* and *C. trachomatis* infection regardless of whether clinical evidence of gonorrhea is found. Patients should be instructed to avoid intercourse until patient and partner(s) are cured.

An endocervical swab for Gram stain and culture for *N. gonorrhoeae* should also be obtained in women with premature rupture of membranes, intrapartum fever or septic abortion.[2]

Treatment of gonococcal and chlamydial infection in pregnant women is the method for preventing neonatal infection. However, ocular prophylaxis in newborn infants is useful in areas where the prevalence of maternal gonococcal infection is greater than 1% and is required by law in many countries. Infants should receive ocular prophylaxis as soon as possible after delivery whether delivery is vaginal or cesarean. The preparations recommended by the CDC are: silver nitrate (1%) aqueous solution in a single application; or erythromycin (0.5%) ophthalmic ointment in a single application; or tetracycline ophthalmic ointment (1%) in a single application.[23] Silver nitrate aqueous solution and tetracycline ointment were found equally efficient in reducing the incidence of gonococcal conjunctivitis when compared with a historical control group who did not receive prophylaxis.[2] It should be noted that prophylaxis with 1% silver nitrate is not effective against *C. trachomatis*. Recently, povidone-iodine administered as a 2.5% solution was found to be as effective as silver nitrate or erythromycin against *N. gonorrhoeae* and more effective than the two other agents against *C. trachomatis*[49]; its use has not been approved yet by the CDC. Some authorities recommend that neonates born to mothers with documented untreated antepartum or intrapartum gonococcal infection should receive parenteral antibiotics in the standard curative dosage in addition to topical ocular prophylaxis.[2]

Chlamydial infections

Chlamydia trachomatis is responsible for two distinct genital infections which are caused by different serovars and differ in their clinical presentation and potential sequelae: the urethritis–cervicitis entity which is by far the most common form, especially in developed countries, and lymphogranuloma venereum which is endemic in the tropics and will be discussed separately. The most important impact of genital chlamydial infection concerns the reproductive health sequelae of upper genital tract infections in women: ectopic pregnancy and tubal infertility.[50]

The Pathogen

Chlamydia trachomatis is a true parasite closely resembling gram-negative bacteria with a biphasic life cycle. The extracellular infectious form, the elementary body, attaches to a susceptible epithelial cell, penetrates it by endocytosis and transforms to a reticulate body which is the replicative form. The reticulate body uses the host cell energy resources and amino acids to replicate and retransform to elementary bodies which are released to reinfect new cells. Of the 15 serovars, serovars A–C are associated with ocular trachoma, D–K with genital tract infection and inclusion conjunctivitis, and serovars L_1–L_3 cause lymphogranuloma venereum.[51]

Pathogenesis

The genital serovars of *C. trachomatis* (D–K) attack the squamocolumnar epithelial cells of the endocervix and upper genital tract in women, and the urethra, rectum and conjunctiva in both men and women. In infants, the pathogen can infect the columnar epithelium of the respiratory tract.[51] The acute inflammatory stage is succeeded by formation of lymphoid follicles which consist of aggregates of lymphocytes and macrophages in the submucosa, seen in both ocular and genital disease.[51] Papillae can form as result of epithelial proliferation. Finally, fibrosis and scarring occur as inflammation resolves. The inflammatory and fibrotic process intensifies with each additional episode of recurrent infection, leading to the development of substantial scarring and deformation of the fallopian tubes when the upper genital tract is involved. It has been suggested that the pathogenesis of chlamydial disease is due at least partly to the host immune response to a chlamydial sensitizing antigen (the 60-kDa heat shock protein). The presence of serum antibodies reactive with the chlamydial heat-shock protein was associated with ectopic pregnancy and infertility.[51]

The immune response to chlamydial genital infection is only partially protective. Although recurrent chlamydial infections are quite common in sexually active individuals with genital tract infections, patients with a prior history of a sexually transmitted disease are at lower risk for acquiring a new chlamydial infection than those without such history.[51]

Little is known about the natural history of endocervical infection with *C. trachomatis*. Some data suggest that chlamydial can persist for a prolonged period of time in the female genital tract.[51] Thus, untreated infections among women often persist for months; during this period complications may develop and infection transmitted to others.

Chlamydia trachomatis is an important cause of PID with sequelae including infertility, ectopic pregnancy and chronic pelvic pain. Up to two-thirds of cases of tubal infertility and one-third of cases of ectopic pregnancy have been attributed to *C. trachomatis* infection. These conclusions derive mainly from studies that have demonstrated higher rates of antibodies to *C. trachomatis* in women with the above complications than in normally pregnant women.[2,52,53] Moreover, colonization of the fallopian tubes by *C. trachomatis* has been demonstrated in infertile women without symptoms and in the absence of laparoscopic signs of active pelvic infection.[50] The mechanism that accounts for tubal occlusion after chlamydial infection is not fully known, although an immune-mediated process might be involved. Chlamydia apparently causes more severe subclinical tubal inflammation and tubal damage than other pathogens despite its more benign appearing symptomatology.[52]

It has been suggested that pregnancy may influence shedding of *C. trachomatis* from the cervix since the rate of isolation of the organism was found to be higher during the third than the first or second trimester.[2] Shedding of chlamydia in pregnancy may be influenced by the development of ectopy which is positively correlated with *C. trachomatis* isolation and/or by the depressed cellular immunity observed during pregnancy.

Endocrinologic changes associated with pregnancy may increase the virulence of both symptomatic and asymptomatic chlamydial infection. Animal studies have demonstrated that treatment with estradiol resulted in florid endometritis, salpingitis and cystitis while in control animals infection was limited to vagina and the cervix. Moreover, direct *C. trachomatis* infection may occur more commonly in trophoblastic tissue and the conceptus than is generally recognized.[54]

Chlamydial infection during pregnancy has been incriminated in causing ectopic pregnancy, pregnancy loss, inadequate fetal development, bleeding, premature labor or premature rupture of membranes. Whether *C. trachomatis* infection can cause abortion is unknown. It is though, however, that chlamydial infection of endometrial or decidual cells or fetal trophoblast cells may alter maternal–fetal tolerance mechanisms that are integral to successful pregnancy. The increased local production of cytokines caused by chlamydial infection may decrease cell-mediated tolerance at maternal fetus interfaces.[54]

Studies on the role of genital *C. trachomatis* infection in prematurity and perinatal mortality have given conflicting results. While a series of studies have all shown a correlation of antenatal chlamydial infection with prematurity, no such association could be found by others.[54] Some of the 'negative' studies have suggested, however, that women with either recent or more extensive and invasive chlamydial infection (associated with the presence of IgM antibodies) are at increased risk for premature rupture of membranes, premature birth and low birth weight.[54] In two studies, but not in a third, women successfully treated for chlamydial infection and uninfected control women had significantly less adverse pregnancy outcomes compared with untreated women.[55] Correlation of antenatal *C. trachomatis* infection with perinatal mortality was observed in only one study and has not been confirmed in others.[2] Antepartum chlamydial infection may also have a role in amnionitis and postpartum infection. Studies have found that intrapartum fever and/or postpartum endometritis were significantly associated with antepartum *C. trachomatis* infection. Other studies, however, have failed to document a significant association between cervical chlamydial infection and postpartum or postcesarean endometritis.[2,54] A delayed postpartum uterine infection with *C. trachomatis* 2–3 weeks after delivery, causing vaginal bleeding or discharge, low-grade fever, lower abdominal pain and uterine tenderness, has been described.[3] An excess rate of postabortal PID has been observed among women with chlamydial infection at the time of the procedure.[55]

Vertical transmission of *C. trachomatis* during vaginal delivery occurs in about two-thirds of infants born to infected women[54]; however, not all infected infants develop clinically overt disease. Colonization or infection may take weeks to months to become detectable and can involve multiple sites including the conjunctiva, nasopharynx, rectum and vagina. The nasopharynx is the most common site of organism recovery after birth.[54] Although chlamydial pneumonia is usually not progressive, affected infants may be subjected to a prolonged respiratory disease, with impaired lung function tests later in childhood and perhaps chronic lung disease.[50] Perinatally acquired *C. trachomatis* infection may persist in the nasopharynx, urogenital tract or rectum for more than 2 years.[51]

Epidemiology

Chlamydia seems to be more difficult to transmit than *N. gonorrhoeae*. Among couples, men apparently transmit the organism to their female partners 40% of the time, while women transmit the infection to their male partners, 32% of the time.[50] Transmission during

Table 158.3 Risk factors for chlamydial genital infection (from Cates and Wasserheit[52] and Centers for Disease Control and Prevention[55])

Less than 20 years of age
Intercourse at an early age
Unmarried status
Lower socioeconomic status
Living in the inner-city
Nulliparity
Black race
Cervical ectopy
Multiple sexual partners/more than one sexual partner
New sexual partner
Concomitant or past other STIs
Oral contraception
Inconsistent use of barrier contraception

a single coitus is probably much lower. Symptomatic individuals are more infectious than asymptomatic carriers of the pathogen.[51] Among the risk markers for chlamydial genital infection (Table 158.3), young age (less than 25 years and, in particular less than 20 years) has been the factor most strongly and consistently associated with the infection. This association is largely due to the more intense sexual activity among younger women, and the larger area of ectopic columnar epithelium surrounding the ectocervix; this ectopy provides a larger target area for chlamydial infection than is present in older women. Although barrier contraception (condom, diaphragm) protects from chlamydial infection, evidence that oral contraception increases the risk for infection is inconsistent.[46,50]

Genital chlamydial infection is not a reportable disease in most countries, and the actual incidence of the entity is not known. However, a large number of studies have examined its prevalence. In the United States, surveys published in the 1980s and 1990s have reported a prevalence of 6–13% among sexually active women attending family planning clinics, 15–19% among female patients of STI clinics, 5–10% among women attending university clinics and 2–4% among female patients seen in private clinics.[50] In North America, genital infections caused by *C. trachomatis* were probably three times more frequent than those caused by *N. gonorrhoeae* during the same period.[52] Chlamydia infection is more common than gonorrhea among Whites, pregnant women, oral contraceptive users and asymptomatic individuals.[52] Recently, a decline in the prevalence of chlamydial infection has been noted among girls (age 13–19 years) attending adolescent health clinics in Indianapolis, Indiana, between 1985 (rate 25.9%) and 1994 (rate 9.7%). Behavioral data showed decreases in the frequency of sexual intercourse and in lifetime years of sexual activity, as well as an increase in condom use.[56] Reporting of chlamydia infection became mandatory in all U.S. states in 2000. In 2003, the incidence of reported infections was 304.3 cases per 100,000 population, which constitutes a slight increase compared with the preceding year. The incidence in women (466.9/100,000) was over three times higher than the rate among men, and seven times higher among African-American women (1633.1/100,000) than among White females.[6]

In Sweden (Uppsala county), the prevalence of genital chlamydial infection among women had been 6% in the 1980s, and it has declined to 3.2% in the early 1990s.[57] However, an increase in the incidence of the infection was noted in the Nordic countries in the second half of the 1990s.[58] In the United Kingdom, recent data suggest that the rate of infection among young women exceeds 10%. In a survey conducted in Israel in 1995, endocervical cultures yielded *C. trachomatis* in 2.0% of sexually active women presenting to a gynecologic clinic; none had evidence of mucopurulent cervicitis.[59] More recently *C. trachomatis* infection was detected by PCR in urine samples of 3.2% of young Israeli female soldiers.[45] These rates are markedly lower from those reported by surveys conducted in the 1970s and 1980s.[60]

In contrast with other STIs, chlamydial infection rates in developing countries often have been comparable to or even lower than rates in Western countries. Prevalence of chlamydial antigen has been reported to be between 8% and 14% in most studies conducted in Africa.[61–65] It has been suggested that the low rates of chlamydial infection among highly exposed women in Africa may be caused by relative immunity, although other factors such as technical diagnostic problems or indiscriminate use of tetracycline cannot be excluded.[46]

The prevalence of genital chlamydial infections in pregnant women is generally similar to that of non-pregnant women with comparable demographic and epidemiologic characteristics. *Chlamydia trachomatis* was isolated or its antigen detected in genital specimens in 5–10% of low income Hispanic and White women in the United States,[66,67] 15% of unmarried and 5.6% married women in Japan,[68] 15–24% of young inner-city women attending public clinics in the United States[23,67] and 26.7% of pregnant women in Martinique.[69] In Africa, on the other hand, the prevalence of genital chlamydial infection among pregnant women varies between 2% and 15% in most studies.[46,62,70]

It is estimated that about 8% of women with endocervical *C. trachomatis* infection develop acute salpingitis.[52] The proportion of women with PID from whom chlamydia can be isolated from the urogenital tract ranges between 5% and 51% depending on the population studied and the techniques of detection used.[44,52] Up to two-thirds of cases of tubal-factor infertility and one-third of cases of ectopic pregnancy may be attributable to *C. trachomatis* infection.[71] Among pregnant women, endometritis may develop during late postpartum period in 19–34% of infected women who deliver vaginally and at term.[2] Similarly, endometritis, and possibly salpingitis, developed among 10–28% of pregnant women who underwent induced abortion.[55]

Approximately two-thirds of infants born to infected women have serologic evidence of chlamydial infection.[54,55] *Chlamydia trachomatis* is the most common cause of neonatal conjunctivitis and is one of the most common causes of pneumonia during the first few months of life.[48] Chlamydial conjunctivitis is seen in 22–44% of infants born to women with infected cervix, while 11–22% of such infants develop chlamydial pneumonia.[55]

Clinical manifestations

The vast majority of chlamydial genital infections in women (and men) do not cause symptoms: as many as 85–90% of women harboring *C. trachomatis* are symptomless, and asymptomatic infections can persist for several months.[50,71] The spectrum of clinical manifestations of *C. trachomatis* infections includes cervicitis, urethritis, bartholinitis, endometritis, salpingo-oophoritis, PID, perihepatitis and reactive arthritis. The endocervix is the organ most often infected. Infection of the cervix and urethra may cause dysuria, abnormal vaginal discharge, and postcoital bleeding. The most frequent symptoms are vaginal discharge and dysuria. Despite the frequent absence of symptoms, at least one-third of infected women have local signs of infection.[71] On examination, the cervix may appear normal or exhibit signs of mucopurulent cervicitis: edema, erythema and hypertrophy with mucopurulent discharge. The presence of green or yellow mucus in the cervical os, or cervical friability (bleeding upon introduction of a cotton swab), or ≥ 10 polymorphonuclear leukocytes per oil immersion field of a gram-stained smear of cervical secretions, have been strongly associated with chlamydial infection.[50] The specificity and sensitivity of these parameters are, however, poor in predicting *C. trachomatis* infection in pregnant women.[72] Chlamydial urethritis should be considered in women with acute urethral syndrome and 'culture negative' pyuria.[72] *Chlamydia trachomatis* has been isolated from the Bartholin's gland in women with bartholinitis.

Endometritis and salpinigitis may cause lower abdominal pain, which may be constant or intermittent, irregular uterine bleeding and menstrual abnormalities. Increased vaginal discharge or fever may or may not be present. Commonly symptoms begin at the time of menstruation. On examination, uterine tenderness or cervical pain on motion can be noted. Women with chlamydial salpingitis are more likely to experience a chronic, subacute course with longer duration of abdominal pain insidious onset and prolonged course than those with gonocococcal PID. Yet they have as much or more tubal inflammation at laparoscopy.[49]

Rectal infection with the genital serovars of *C. trachomatis*, resulting usually from anal intercourse, generally produces a mild disease ranging from asymptomatic carriage to variable degree of acute proctitis with rectal pain, mucopurulent discharge, abdominal pain, diarrhea and rectal bleeding.[49]

Inclusion conjunctivitis in the adult results from autoinoculation with infected genital secretions or direct inoculation from an infected partner during oral–genital sexual contact. The presentation is that of an acute follicular conjunctivitis often with a foreign body sensation in the eye. Untreated the condition can persist for many months and scarring may occur. Chlamydial infection appears to be the most common triggering event for sexually reactive arthritis, which is seen less often in women than in men.[49]

An infant born to a mother with active chlamydial infection has a risk of acquiring infection at any anatomical site of 50–75%. Approximately 30–50% of infants born to chlamydia-positive mothers will have conjunctivitis, and at least 50% of infants with chlamydial conjunctivitis will also have nasopharyngeal infection. Chlamydia pneumonia develops in about 30% of infants with nasopharyngeal infection.[71] Neonatal chlamydial conjunctivitis usually develops within 5–14 days of delivery and presents with ocular discharge, swollen eyelids and erythematous conjunctiva.[2] Significant corneal scarring develops in a minority of cases. A mucopurulent rhinitis and vulvovaginitis are often associated with conjunctivitis.[51] Infant chlamydial pneumonia usually develops 4–17 weeks following delivery. Onset is usually mild and subacute, although the initial respiratory manifestations may, especially in very young infants, be more severe and include prolonged spells of apnea or respiratory failure. Physical findings are often nonspecific, and the infant is often afebrile. The chest radiograph shows diffuse interstitial or patchy alveolar infiltrates with hyperinflation. Peripheral eosinophilia, arterial hypoxemia and elevated serum immunoglobulins are characteristic. Untreated, the course is prolonged, lasting weeks to months.[51]

Laboratory diagnosis

Because most genital chlamydial infections are asymptomatic or have mild and non-specific presentation, they require laboratory confirmation for definitive diagnosis. Although typical intracytoplasmic inclusion can be identified in conjunctival or endocervical scrapings, this finding is not sensitive enough for diagnostic purposes, especially in adult infection.

Isolation of the pathogen

Cell culture has remained the gold standard for the diagnosis of chlamydial infection. It is particularly preferred for specimens with low numbers of organisms which is often the case in low-prevalence population and asymptomatic infection. Although *C. trachomatis* grows well in a variety of cell lines, the most commonly used are the cycloheximide-treated McCoy cells. Three to seven days are required to obtain a result. The sensitivity of culture is between 70% and 90%, while the specificity is 100%.[51] For best results the specimen should contain columnar epithelial cells from the endocervix or the urethra. Culturing both the endocervix and the urethra can increase the rate of positive culture by 23%.[51] Secretions and discharge should be removed from the cervical os before obtaining a specimen. The swab should be inserted 1–2 cm into the endocervical canal and rotated against its wall for 10–30 s. The swab should then be withdrawn without touching any vaginal surface and be placed in an appropriate transport medium. Urethral swabs should be obtained 2 h after the patient has voided. The swab should be inserted 1–2 cm into the urethra and rotated for 5 s.[55] Swabs used for specimen collection (Dacron or rayon material is preferred) should be free from substances that may be toxic to the organism; wooden shafts should not be used. The specimen must be kept refrigerated, but for no longer than 24 h before inoculation. Alternatively, the sample can be stored at –80°C until it is processed at a later date, but this may result in loss of some organisms. Specimens should never be stored at –20°C.

Non-culture tests

These tests are based on the detection of the chlamydial antigen or its nucleic acids. In general, non-culture tests are more reliable in symptomatic patients who shed large numbers of organisms, than in asymptomatic individuals who usually shed fewer organisms.[55] The presence of the chlamydial antigen in the clinical specimen can be demonstrated by direct fluorescent antibody (DFA) staining which detects the elementary bodies using a fluorescent-labeled monoclonal antibody. This test allows also assessment of the quality of the specimen, but requires a highly skilled microscopist for proper interpretation.[51] Another technique, the enzyme-linked immunosorbent assay (EIA), employs polyclonal or monoclonal antibodies conjugated with an enzyme that reacts with the substrate which produces a colored product if chlamydial organisms are present. The EIA requires less skilled personnel but generally takes longer to perform. Nucleic and hybridization tests use a chemiluminescent-type DNA probe that is complementary to a sequence of ribosomal RNA in the chlamydial genome of the patient's sample. The assay is relatively easy to perform and interpret, is species specific for *C. trachomatis* and does not cross-react with other bacteria. Specimens can be stored at room temperature in a special transport material up to 7 days before being processed. The accuracy of the three diagnostic techniques is similar, with sensitivities greater than 70% and specificities of 97–99% in populations of men and women with a prevalence of infection of ≥5%.[55] In low-prevalence populations (< 5%), a significant proportion of positive test will be falsely positive. Verification of a positive test is therefore desirable by culture (which should be preferred in medicolegal situations) or a second non-culture test targeting a different antigen or nucleic acid.[55] The most newly developed nucleic acid assays are the amplification tests based on the detection of chlamydial DNA using polymerase or ligase chain reactions. These tests are species specific and appear to be more sensitive and as specific as cultures.[51,73] Moreover, they can be performed on urine specimens from both symptomatic and asymptomatic men and women; however, their sensitivity is slightly lower compared with endocervical specimens.[51,73] Recently, specimens obtained form the vaginal introitus were found highly effective for *C. trachomatis* testing by polymerase chain reaction.[74,75]

Serology

Serologic tests have little value in routine clinical evaluation of patients suspected of having chlamydial genital infection.[55] The specificity of serology is low because antibodies generated against chlamydiae can persist for years. The microimmunofluorescence test is highly sensitive and detects antichlamydial IgG in ≥99% of women with cervicitis, adults with inclusion conjunctivitis and infants with pneumonia. Antichlamydial IgM is present in 100% of infants with pneumonia, but is uncommon in adults with genital tract infection.[51] The complement fixation test measures antibodies against genus-specific antigens. It is less specific and less sensitive than the microimmunofluorescence test.

Treatment

The main purpose of treating chlamydial infection would be to decrease the likelihood of sequelae in women with cervical infection, to prevent transmission to infants during delivery, and to prevent transmission to sexual partners. Several studies have provided evidence that treatment of *C. trachomatis* in the antenatal period decreases the incidence of poor pregnancy.[76] The active antichlamydial agents are tetracyclines, macrolides, rifampin and some fluoroquinolones. Penicillin has limited activity because its intracellular concentration is low and chlamydiae lack peptidoglycan.

Doxycycline, 100 mg orally, twice daily for 7 days, has been the standard regimen used for the treatment of uncomplicated urethral, cervical or rectal *C. trachomatis* infections in non-pregnant women.[55] Failure rates have ranged from 0% to 8% among women with cervicitis.[50] However, tetracyclines, including doxycycline, are contraindicated in pregnant women because of possible adverse effects on the

Table 158.4 Regimens recommended by Centers for Disease Control and Prevention[55] for the treatment of chlamydial infections during pregnancy

Regimen	Options
First choice	Erythromycin base, 500 mg orally 4 times a day for 7 days
	or
	Amoxicillin, 500 mg orally 3 times a day for 7–10 days
Alternatives	Erythromycin base, 250 mg orally 4 times a day for 14 days
	or
	Erythromycin ethylsuccinate, 800 mg orally 4 times a day for 7 days
	or
	Erythromycin ethylsuccinate, 400 mg orally 4 times a day for 14 days
	or
	Azithromycin, 1 g orally, single dose

fetus such as discoloration of deciduous teeth. Erythromycin base, 500 mg orally four times a day for 7 days, has been the first alternative and the drug of choice in pregnant women and infants (Table 158.4). Women unable to tolerate erythromycin at the standard dose can be treated with 250 mg four times a day for 14 days. Erythromycin estolate should be avoided in pregnant women since 10% of those receiving the drug develop liver enzyme impairment. Other alternative regimens include amoxycillin and clindamycin. Eradication rates of 86–98% were reported in studies of amoxycillin treatment for *C. trachomatis* infection in pregnant women.[77] Clindamycin appears to be as efficacious as erythromycin in both pregnant (92.7% vs. 83.8% cure rate) and non-pregnant women.[78] It is recommended by the American College of Obstetricians and gynecologists, but not by the CDC, as an alternative regimen in pregnancy.[76] However, caution is advised because of the possible occurrence of pseudomembranous celitis. Recently, azithromycin given as a single 1 g dose has been found to be as effective as a seven day course of doxycycline.[79] This is the only antimicrobial agent effective against *C. trachomatis* infection as a single dose therapy. Moreover, azithromycin is well tolerated and is associated with significantly lower rate of gastrointestinal adverse effects than erythromycin. It is now considered by the CDC as an equivalent regimen to doxycycline for the treatment of chlamydial infections in non-pregnant women.[55] In pregnant women the success rates with the same regimen of azithromycin were between 91% and 100%.[80,81] Azithromycin is classified as a pregnancy category B agent, and its use in pregnancy is indicated only if clearly needed.[78] Although comparable to doxycycline in the treatment of uncomplicated chlamydial genital tract infection, ofloxacin at a dose of 300 mg twice daily for 7–10 days, offers no advantage over the standard regimen and is contraindicated in patients under the age of 18 years, pregnant women and lactating mothers.[50] Retesting for chlamydia may be considered 3 weeks after completion of treatment with erythromycin (because of low compliance), amoxycillin or clindamycin (because of limited clinical experience). This is usually unnecessary if the patient was treated with doxycycline, azithromycin or ofloxacin, unless symptoms persist or reinfection is suspected.[55]

Because of the risks of infertility and other sequelae of PID, clinicians should have a low threshold for the prompt institution of treatment in women who are at risk for chlamydial infection. The delay of antibiotic therapy is associated with an increased risk of adverse outcome (The regimens recommended for the therapy of PID are detailed in the section on gonorrhea.)

The timely treatment of the patient's sexual partner is also essential in order to reduce the risk of reinfection. The sexual partners should be evaluated, tested, and treated if they have had sexual contact with the patient during the 60 days preceding the diagnosis.[71]

For the treatment of infant chlamydial infection, oral erythromycin 50 mg/kg of body weight per day in four divided doses for 10–14 days, is the treatment of choice for both inclusion conjunctivitis and pneumonia. The efficacy of this regimen in both indications is approximately 80%, and a second course may be required.[23] Topical treatment of inclusion conjunctivitis is not recommended. Mothers of infants with chlamydial infection should be evaluated and treated.

Case detection and prevention

The main objective of chlamydial prevention strategies is to prevent chlamydial salpingitis and its sequelae, as well as perinatal and postpartum infection. For this purpose, both primary and secondary prevention strategies should be applied.[55]

Primary prevention of chlamydial infection consists of two approaches: (1) behavioral changes that reduce the risk of acquiring or transmitting chlamydial infection as well as other STDs: delaying age at first intercourse, decreasing the number of sex partners, partner selection and use of barrier contraception; and (2) identifying and treating persons with genital chlamydial infection before they infect their sex partners, and for pregnant women, before they infect their babies. Because chlamydial infections are usually asymptomatic, active screening and referral of sex partners of infected persons are required. A recent study that sought to identify criteria for selective screening concluded that a combination of young age and attending an urban clinic was highly predictive of chlamydial infection and identified a minimum of 85% of infected women in all public clinic settings.[82] In countries where an extensive educational and control program has been applied, there has been a dramatic decline in chlamydial infection over the last decade.[58,79]

Secondary prevalence strategies include efforts to prevent complications (such as salpingitis and its sequelae) among persons infected with chlamydial: (1) screening women, mainly sexually active adolescent and young females, to identify and treat asymptomatic infections; (2) treating sex partners of infected men; and (3) recognizing clinical conditions, such as mucopurulent cervicitis or urethral syndrome, which are often caused by chlamydia and applying appropriate diagnostic tests and treatment.[55] In a large randomized trial of screening and treatment of women at high risk of chlamydial infection, the incidence of PID was significantly lower in the screened group compared with the usual care group.[83] However, it is not clear yet who should be screened and how often. Screening on the basis of age (less than 25 years) appears to be effective in areas where the prevalence of chlamydial infection is low to moderate (3–6%); women with other risk factors for chlamydial infection (Table 158.3) should also be considered for screening. In high-risk women screening should be done every 6 months; otherwise, annual screening is reasonable.[71]

There is some evidence that screening high-risk women for *C. trachomatis* during pregnancy can reduce the rate of adverse outcomes of pregnancy.[71] The American College of Obstetricians and Gynecologists recommends screening high risk pregnant women in their first prenatal visit and again in the third trimester. The CDC recommends screening high-risk pregnant women preferably during the third trimester.[55] High-risk factors for chlamydial infection in pregnant women are the same as in non-pregnant women (Table 158.3).

Prevention of neonatal *C. trachomatis* infection should consist of detection and treatment of chlamydial infection during pregnancy together with ocular prophylaxis. Recently, povidone-iodine administered as a 2.5% solution was found more effective than silver nitrate solution or erythromycin ointment in preventing ocular *C. trachomatis* infection.[49] It should be borne in mind that topical prophylaxis of conjunctivitis does not prevent pneumonia.

Lymphogranuloma venereum

Lymphogranuloma venereum (LGV) is a sexually transmitted disease caused by L_1, L_2 and L_3, serovars of *C. trachomatis* and characterized by acute inguinal lymphadenitis (bubo) and other local and systemic manifestations. We are not aware of any report on the adverse effect of LGV on pregnancy or the newborn.

The LVG strains are more virulent and more invasive than the A–K serovars, and may cause disseminated infection. The pathogen gains entrance into the body through breaks in the skin or infects epithelial cells of the genital tract and rectal mucosa.[84] It is then carried by lymphatic drainage to the regional lymph nodes where it multiplies inside mononuclear phagocytes. Histologically, granuloma are formed, and small abscesses develop that may coalesce to form diamond-shaped suppurative foci which are progressively replaced by fibrosis. This histopathologic picture is suggestive although not specific to LGV.

The infection is endemic in tropical and subtropical countries: areas of Africa (Ethiopia, Nigeria, Swaziland), India, Southeast Asia, South America and the Caribbean.[85] Clinic-based series of patients with genital ulcers suggest that LVG is an uncommon cause of genital ulceration in Africa.[86] It occurs only sporadically in developed countries, where it is usually found in promiscuous persons (homosexual men and prostitutes) and individuals returning from endemic areas (sailors, travelers, military personnel). Clinical disease is sixfold more common in men than in women.

The clinical course of LGV can be divided into three stages: the primary stage involves the site of inoculation; the secondary stage involves the regional lymph nodes and sometimes the anorectum; the tertiary stage consists of late sequelae affecting the genitals and/or the rectum. A total of 3–30 days after infection occurs, a primary lesion appears in the form of a small papule, vesicle or ulcer on the genital mucosa or the adjacent skin.[51] The lesion may not always occur, and when present it is often not noticed because symptoms are few or absent and healing is rapid without leaving a scar. Symptomatic urethritis can occur if the lesion develops in the urethra. Days to weeks later and up to 6 months after exposure, regional lymphadenopathy and systemic symptoms develop. Inguinal lymphadenopathy is less common in women than in men, since lymphatic drainage of the vagina and the cervix is to the retroperitoneal rather than the inguinal lymph nodes. Lymphadenopathy is initially discrete and tender, and is unilateral in two-thirds of the cases.[84] The localization of enlarged lymph nodes above and below the groin gives a groove appearance ('groove sign') which is regarded as pathognomonic for LGV although it is seen in only 10–20% of cases. The inflammatory process spreads from the affected lymph nodes into the surrounding tissue forming an inflammatory mass consisting of abscesses that coalesce to give a bubo. The bubo can rupture spontaneously in one-third of the cases, with development of fistulae or a sinus tract. Otherwise the bubo hardens and forms an inguinal mass which gradually evolves over time. The untreated lesion may, however, persist in an active form for years.[87] Proctitis, characterized by a bloody mucopurulent anal discharge and tenesmus, is seen mainly in women and homosexual men, and is often accompanied by pronounced systemic symptoms. Cervical lymphadenopathy has been reported following inoculation during oral sex, while ocular inoculation can give rise to follicular conjunctivitis accompanied by preauricular lymphadenopathy.[86] Systemic symptoms, noted during the acute stage of lymphadenitis, include fever, chills, sweats, malaise, headache, myalgia, anorexia, nausea and vomiting. A variety of skin manifestations, such as erythema nodosum and erythema multiforme, can be seen. Other rare manifestations include conjunctivitis, arthritis, hepatitis and meningitis. Lymphatic obstruction, secondary to fibrotic changes, may lead to elephantiasis of the genitalia. Other local complications consist of fistulae formation involving the rectum, perineum, vulva and vagina; esthiomene, a chronic, granulomatous enlargement with ulcerations of the external genitalia; and rectal strictures resulting from the replacement of inflamed muscle layer by fibrous tissue.[51] Mild leukocytosis with an increase in monocyte and eosinophil counts is frequent in the early bubonic stage.

Diagnosis is based on serology or isolation of the pathogen. Complement fixing antibodies usually appear within 4 weeks after infection starts. The test is genus specific, and therefore does not distinguish between infections with different chlamydiae (trachomatis, psittaci, pneumoniae). Because of its increased invasiveness, LGV is associated with higher serum antibody titers than is *C. trachomatis* infection.[86] Virtually 100% of individuals with LGV will have complement fixing antibody titers greater than 1:16.[51] In an appropriate clinical setting a complement fixation titer of $\geq$1:256 is strongly supportive of a diagnosis of LGV, although confirmation requires a fourfold titer rise between acute and convalescent sera.[51] The micro-immunofluorescence test is invariably positive, the titer being usually higher than 1:512 during the acute phase. The test can distinguish between infections with different chlamydial species, but its use in clinical practice has been limited because it requires a fluorescent microscope and a skilled technologist.[86] Isolation of *C. trachomatis* from bubo aspirates, genital or rectal tissue is possible in only about one-third of cases.[84] The organism can also be identified by direct fluorescent microscope using a commercially available conjugated monoclonal antibody on a smear of bubo or ulcer material. Histopathology, although non-specific, can lead to a presumptive diagnosis when combined with serologic tests in an appropriate clinical setting. A skin test (Frei test) has been used in the past, but is not currently available. The differential diagnosis includes genital herpes, chancroid, donovanosis, syphilis and occasionally, lymphoma.

Treatment of LVG consists of doxycycline, 100 mg twice daily for 14–21 days. Alternatively, erythromycin, 500 mg four times daily, or sulfisoxazole can be used.[23] Fluctuant bubos should be aspirated to prevent rupture, using a lateral approach through normal skin. Antibiotic therapy results in rapid decline of systemic symptoms, but has limited effect on bubo resolution. The general rules of STI prevention are also applicable to the management of LGV patients.

Herpes simplex infections

Herpes simplex infection is life long and is characterized by recurrences that are either symptomatic or not. Genital herpes is caused by herpes simplex virus type 1 (HSV-1) or herpes simplex virus type 2 (HSV-2). While usually annoying and troublesome for the infected woman,[88] the virus can have devastating effect on the newborn.[89] Women with genital herpes who are pregnant should be identified so that preventive measures can be applied.

The pathogen

Herpes simplex virus (HSV) has an internal core containing double-stranded DNA, an icosahedral capsid composed of 162 polypeptide capsomers and a lipid containing envelope. HSV can be distinguished from other members of the herpes virus group by its cytopathogenic affects and by its antigenic and DNA base composition. The two subtypes of HSV differ primarily by their clinical and epidemiologic characteristics and can also be separated by a variety of biochemical and biologic properties. HSV type 1 is transmitted essentially by a non-genital route and causes mainly non-genital infections, such as labial blisters, keratitis and adult encephalitis; however, in many developed countries it has become the leading cause of genital herpes. HSV type 2 is transmitted by genital contact and is responsible for most of the herpetic genital and neonatal infections.[88]

Pathogenesis

Inoculation occurs following exposure of mucosal surfaces or abraded skin to secretions or mucosa containing the virus. After penetration, HSV replicates locally in parabasal and intermediate epithelial cells. Virus replication results in lysis of infected cells and development of local inflammatory reaction. In individuals with depressed immune mechanisms (particularly cell-mediated immunity), infection can disseminate resulting in viremia and visceral involvement (liver, lungs, central nervous system). From the primary site of infection, HSV is transported along the axon to the nerve cell bodies in the sensory and autonomic ganglia, where the virus becomes latent. During latency, viral replication almost ceases, and the viral genome is maintained in a repressed state. Several non-specific stimuli, e.g., bacterial or other viral infection, ultraviolet radiation, nervous stimuli, or hormonal changes can trigger reactivation of HSV. Reactivation and replication of the virus in the ganglia does not result in cell lysis. The virus then migrates back to the skin by peripheral sensory nerve fibers that share the infected ganglia. Viral reactivations occur periodically, characterized by viral shedding that may be symptomatic or subclinical. The vast majority of recurrent episodes are due to viral reactivation not reinfection.[90] Most recurrences of genital herpes infection are caused by HSV-2 which readily establishes latency in the sacral ganglia, while HSV-1 is less prone to do so. Autoinoculation from genital areas to other sites, including hands, thighs and buttocks, is not uncommon.

A complex immune response is involved in the natural history of HSV infection. Cell-mediated immunity is essential for recovery from both primary infection and recurrences. The presence of high titers of neutralizing HSV antibodies may limit recurrences. High levels of antibodies transferred by the mother to the fetus may have a protective effect on the neonate from contracting the virus during passage through an infected birth canal.

Primary genital herpes infection occurring in a pregnant woman before 20–23 weeks of gestation may cause spontaneous abortion in up to a half of the cases and low birth weight in one-third.[91,92] Primary infection during pregnancy may also lead to premature labor and congenital infection causing microencephaly, chorioretinitis and large skin scars.[92,93] Infection of the neonate during passage through the birth canal is common and can have devastating effects including encephalitis with high rates of mortality and residual morbidity.[88] On the other hand, recurrent episodes of genital herpes during pregnancy are no worse than recurrences in non-pregnant women, and they are not associated with prematurity or other obstetrical adverse events. Neonatal infection is uncommon and less devastating, not only because of the protective effect of transplacentally acquired maternal antibodies, but also due to a smaller viral inoculum and lower rates of cervical virus shedding associated with recurrent infection.[94,95] The increased neonatal susceptibility to HSV infection which persists for several months following delivery is presumably related to the poor cellular immune response during this period of life.[2]

Genital ulcer disease, including that caused by HSV-2, is a well-recognized risk factor for the transmission of human immunodeficiency virus (HIV). High titers of HIV are found in genital herpes ulcerations, and the plasma HIV viral load increases when HSV-2 infection is reactivated in HIV-infected persons.[96]

Epidemiology

Humans appear to be the only natural reservoir of HSV.[88] Direct contact, most often sexual, with infected genital secretions or mucosa is the principal mode of transmission of HSV. Direct contact other than sexual intercourse can result in viral spread if an area of viral shedding comes into contact with the skin or mucous membranes of a susceptible person. Because of virus fragility, transmission by fomites is rare. HSV can be acquired both from persons with symptomatic infection and from asymptomatic excretors, although transmissibility is greater from the former. However, asymptomatic viral shedding accounts for much of the transmission of HSV. Herpes simplex virus DNA can be detected by PCR in genital specimens from HSV-2-seropositive women on 28% of days, and the virus may be transmitted to a sexual partner during such periods of subclinical shedding. Although the risk of transmission of HSV-2 from an infected person to a susceptible sexual partner is higher when genital lesions are present, because individuals with symptomatic genital herpes usually abstain from sexual activity during this period of time and asymptomatic shedding occurs much more frequently than symptomatic disease, most experts believe that transmission results from asymptomatic shedding in most cases.[97] The risk of heterosexual acquisition of HSV is greater in women than in men.[88,98] In a study of HSV-2 transmission between monogamous couples in which only one member of each couple had a history of genital herpes, the annual rate of acquisition was 9.7%, being higher in women and in those who lacked HSV-1 antibodies.[98] Infection with HSV-2 occurs mainly following puberty and corresponds to the period of intense sexual activity between 14 and 44 years. Rates of infection with HSV-2 are higher in unmarried individuals, in females, in those with increased numbers of sexual partners, in individuals with history of STI and in those of lower socioeconomic status,[90,99,100] although the association with the last factor has been inconsistent[90,99]; in the United States the infection is more common among Blacks and Hispanics. Recurrences are less common in women than in men; overall, approximately 60–90% of those with an initial episode will have recurrences.[88]

The prevalence of genital HSV-1 infection, which is usually acquired through oral–genital contact, has also increased dramatically and has replaced HSV-2 as the principal causative pathogen of genital herpes in several developed countries.[101] In Israel, for example, a retrospective analysis of positive herpes isolates found that HSV-1 accounted for 66% of isolates.[102]

In neonates, most infections result from the retrograde spread of HSV-2 secondary to maternal genital infection or via passage of the infant through an infected birth canal. The risk of transmission of HSV to the neonate is 10 times greater if delivery occurs during an episode of primary genital infection (33–50%) than if it occurs during a recurrence (~3%).[88,90,95] Up to one-half of neonates acquiring HSV infection have been exposed to mothers with primary disease occurring in late pregnancy.[2] In most of the remaining cases, the newborn is infected from an asymptomatic mother shedding the virus.[103] The risk of neonatal infection correlates directly with the amount of virus present in the birth canal at delivery, and with the duration of ruptured membranes. Cesarean section significantly reduces this risk if performed within 4 h of rupture of membranes; whereas if membranes are ruptured for more than 4 h, infants acquire the infection irrespective of the route of delivery.[92] Use of fetal scalp electrodes also predisposes for neonatal infection.[104] Transplacental transmission can also occur, although rarely: a recent study has documented congenital infection in 9 out of 192 (4.7%) cases of neonatal HSV.[93] Also rarely, neonatal herpes can be acquired postnatally from an infected family member. The occurrence of neonatal HSV-1 associated genital herpes (including fatal cases) after Jewish ritual circumcision has been reported.[105]

Herpes simplex virus has a global distribution. The worldwide prevalence of genital herpes infection continues to increase despite the increased public awareness of STIs, and seroprevalence of HSV-2 has reached unprecedented rates.[98] Much of this may be related to the chronicity of the infection and the high rate of unrecognized cases. In Western countries HSV is by far the most prevalent genital ulcer disease, well ahead of syphilis and chancroid.[98] The estimated annual incidence of clinically apparent infection in the United States is 50 cases per 100,000 adults, and this rate has been increasing constantly. The highest annual incidence among women occurs at 20–24 years of age and is estimated to be 210 per 100,000.[83] Using HSV-2 specific antibody assays, it was estimated that 16–33% of the general population in the United States have antibodies to this HSV type.[90] Up to 46% of women attending a STD clinic and 9% of college students were reported to have serologic evidence of genital herpes. In adults $\geq$30 years of age, HSV-2 antibody was found in approximately 25% of White women and over 60% of Black women; seropositivity rate was associated with increasing age.[100] Similar rates of seroprevalence (10–40%) were found in other Western countries.[98]

In developing countries, the serologic prevalence of HSV-2 is generally higher, ranging from 40% to 80%. In Kinshasa, the seroprevalence was found to be higher among HIV positive prostitutes (95%) than among HIV negative prostitutes (75%).[98]

The prevalence of genital herpes in pregnant women depends on the population studies. In an inner city cohort, serologic evidence of HSV-2 infection was detected in 36% of women attending an obstetric clinic in the 1970s.[91] More recently, 32% of pregnant women followed by private obstetricians in Stanford, California, were seropositive.[99] In three studies of asymptomatic pregnant women, cervical isolation rates of 0.2–0.65% were reported.[91,100,104] Pregnancy had no influence on the frequency of asymptomatic virus shedding.[100]

The increasing incidence of genital HSV infection in women has been accompanied by an increase in neonatal HSV in some areas of the United States. In King County, Washington, the incidence increased from 1.6 to 11.9 cases per 1,000,000 live births.[100] More recently, the incidence of neonatal HSV has been estimated to be between 1 in 2000 to 1 in 10,000 live births and was higher in premature than in full-term infants.[92,93,104]

Clinical manifestations

The manifestations of genital herpes vary widely, not only among individuals, but also between episodes of the same patient. It has been estimated that at least two-thirds (and up to 90%) of HSV-2 seropositive women did not have histories compatible with genital herpes – they were infected asymptomatically.[92,100] Corey has suggested that asymptomatic genital herpes often is unrecognized symptomatic infection.[98]

The clinical episodes are classified as follows: genital herpes in the absence of antibodies to HSV-1 and HSV-2 is called primary infection; a first episode infection in the presence of antibodies to either HSV-1 or HSV-2 is termed first episode non-primary infection; and a recurrent infection is one caused by the same virus (usually HSV-2) that previously infected the patient and has reactivated after a latent period.

Primary herpes genitalis

The average incubation period after the genital acquisition of HSV-1 or HSV-2 is approximately 4 days (range 2–12), although the incubation period can reach 20 days. Local and systemic symptoms associated with primary HSV-1 infection are generally of the same intensity as those associated with primary HSV-2 infection. Local prodromal symptoms, including itching, erythema, paresthesia, burning sensation and pain, usually precede genital lesions by 1–2 days. Vulvar involvement is common, and the cervix is affected in almost 90% of the patients, while vaginal lesions are present in less than 5% of infected women. The initial lesions are small painful vesicles or pustules; the mean duration of local pain and virus shedding is 12 days. Vaginal discharge is present in approximately 75%. The cervix is friable, a mucopurulent discharge is often noted. In general, new lesions continue to appear over 4–10 days. After a few days, the individual lesions coalesce into large wet ulcers that persist for 1–2 weeks, and eventually heal without scars, usually within 3 weeks of onset of lesions. Tender inguinal adenopathy appears in most patients and is the last sign to resolve. Dysuria is present in most cases.

Systemic symptoms occur in more than two-thirds of women with primary infection and usually last for 3–7 days. They include fever, malaise, myalgia, headache, abdominal pain and backache. Self-limited neurologic signs, such as stiff neck, photophobia, and inflammatory cerebrospinal fluid, can be seen. Approximately one-third of women and 10% of men with primary infection have meningeal signs, whereas such signs are rare among patients with non-primary infection. Autonomic nervous system dysfunction can also occur, manifesting as urinary retention, constipation, lower extremity weakness, due to sacral radiculopathy or transverse myelitis. Benign recurrent lymphocytic meningitis (Mollaret's meningitis) can also complicate genital herpes. Herpetic encephalitis with poor prognosis can rarely complicate primary infection. Viral dissemination to the lungs, liver and kidneys is rare in the normal host.

Pharyngitis can accompany primary genital herpes in approximately 10% of cases. Primary infection of the perianal and anal area may be responsible for severe rectal pain, discharge and tenesmus. Systemic symptoms are prominent in patients with herpatic proctitis.

First episode non-primary infection

About one-half of all patients with first attack genital herpes have preexisting antibodies to HSV-1 or HSV-2. Compared with primary infection, women with non-primary first episode have less often (~16%) and fewer systemic symptoms, fewer lesions and shorter duration of pain (~9 days) and shedding of virus (~7 days). The lesions heal within a mean of 16 days. Extragenital manifestations and complications are uncommon.[98]

Recurrent infection

The clinical course is usually mild. At least one-half of the patients have prodromal symptoms ranging from mild tingling sensations occurring 0.5–48 h before the eruption, to shooting pains in the buttocks, legs or hips occurring as long as 5 days before the eruption. Uncommonly, systemic symptoms can occur. Genital lesions involve mainly the labia and perineum; the cervix is affected in only 12% of the episodes. There are fewer lesions present than in primary infection; they shed the virus during approximately 5 days and heal completely within 7–10 days. Other manifestations, such as dysuria, vaginal discharge and tender lymphadenopathy, occur less often and extragenital lesions and systemic complications are very rare. Most patients (90%) with a documented first episode of genital HSV-2 infection have at least one recurrence within 12 months after diagnosis, 38% have six or more recurrences, and 20% have 10 or more recurrences. Genital HSV-1 infections recur less frequently than do genital HSV-2 infections, explaining why most cases of symptomatic HSV-1 genital disease are primary cases. Irrespective of viral type and whether or not suppressive therapy is used, recurrence rates decrease over time.

Pregnancy does not appear to modify the clinical course of primary or recurrent infection, although cases of severe gestational primary infection with dissemination and high death rate have been reported.[91,106] Among young women with recently acquired genital herpes infection, approximately 80% will have an average of two to four symptomatic recurrences during pregnancy.[107,109] Concomitant cervical shedding is identified in 15–30% of women with symptomatic vulvar recurrences.[107] The prevalence of positive cultures at any time during pregnancy or delivery is 1–2%.

Congenital infection may be recognized at birth along with jaundice, hepatosplenomegaly, a bleeding diathesis, microcephaly, microphthalmia, seizures, chorioretinitis and skin vesicles. In the newborn clinical presentation can range from a mild localized infection to a fatal disseminated one. Onset of disease usually occurs in the first week after birth, but it has been described up to one month after delivery. The herpetic lesions can involve the central nervous system (cranial nerve palsy, seizures, coma), the skin, and less often, the eye. If the central nervous system is affected the mortality is high, and survivors usually suffer from profound neurologic dysfunction. Disseminated infection, with or without central nervous system involvement, can affect the liver, the lungs or the hematopoietic system, leading to respiratory failure and disseminated intravascular coagulation.[110]

In order to avoid unnecessary tension in couples, it should be explained that many first clinical episodes of symptomatic genital herpes may represent infection that was acquired years before, and that a new diagnosis of genital herpes in a member of a monogamous couple does not necessarily imply recent acquisition of infection from another partner.

Diagnosis

The clinical spectrum of genital herpes being diverse, the clinical diagnosis has reasonable specificity but poor sensitivity[113]; it is prudent to seek laboratory confirmation of the diagnosis. The Tzanck smear and the Papanicolaou smear may detect cellular changes suggestive of HSV infection, but both tests have low sensitivity.

Culture

Viral culture represents the most sensitive method for diagnosing HSV infection.[90] Vesicles should be unroofed with sterile needle, and the base of the lesion should be rubbed vigorously with a cotton or a Dacron-tipped swab (calcium alginate swabs may inactivate herpes virus). The swab should be placed immediately into a suitable transport medium and maintained at 4°C, where it can stay no longer than 3 days before being processed. Samples can be stored for longer periods of time at –70°C, but should not be kept at –20°C because the virus will be destroyed immediately. The older the lesion the lower the chance to detect the virus: it can be isolated from 90% of vesicles, from 70% of ulcerative lesions, and from only 30% of crusted lesions. The yield of virus recovery is also low (~50%) in lesions of recurrent episodes because recurrent disease is associated with a lower viral load than primary infection.[100] Cultures of amniotic fluid for HSV have given both false-positive and false-negative results for congenital infection, making such tests of questionable usefulness.[112] Cytopathic effects appear rapidly, usually within 24–48 h if the virus inoculum is high.

Rapid diagnostic tests

The most sensitive tests for antigen detection use labeled monoclonal antibodies that bind to HSV proteins. The sensitivity of these tests for specimens obtained from visible lesions ranges between 65% and 90% compared with virus isolation, and the results are available within 1–2 h. These methods should not be used to detect viral shedding in asymptomatic women because of the low virus titers.

Serology

Serology may be helpful in diagnosing primary HSV infection by demonstration of seroconvertions or a fourfold rise in antibody titers. Detection of IgM is less accurate by the presently available methods; however, it can be used in infants for the diagnosis of neonatal infection.[88] Such antibodies usually appear within the first 4 weeks of life and may persist for many months. Recently, type-specific serologic testing for HSV, using enzyme-linked immunosorbent assays or immunoblot tests based on HSV-specific glycoproteins G1 and G2, have been commercially available for clinical use. Type-specific serologic tests may be useful for diagnosis in patients with symptomatic genital disease who have healing lesions (in whom culture is likely to be negative). Testing should be performed at the time of an initial episode and, if negative, repeated 3 months later. Because almost all HSV-2 infections are sexually acquired, type-specific HSV-2 antibody indicates anogenital infection, but the presence of HSV-1 antibody does not distinguish anogenital from orolabial infection.[23] Type-specific serologic analysis can aid in the classification of infection as primary, non-primary, or recurrent, and thus may guide counseling. It may help to manage sex partners of persons with genital herpes, and may also be used in screening.

The differential diagnosis of labial ulcerations seen in genital herpes includes primary syphilis (one or more painless, indurated ulcers occurring at the site of inoculation), and chancroid (painful, tender, non-indurated ulcerationss characterized by a serpiginous border surrounding a friable base covered with gray or yellow, necrotic, purulent exudates). Noninfectious conditions that can mimic genital herpes include Crohn's disease, Behçet's syndrome, trauma, contact dermatitis, erythema multiforme, Reiter's syndrome, psoriasis, and lichen planus.

Treatment

Although herpes infections enjoy the most efficacious antiviral therapy, the available agents neither eradicate latent virus nor affect subsequent risk, frequency or severity of recurrences after administration of the drug is discontinued. The mainstay of herpes antiviral therapy is acyclovir. It has demonstrated the ability to alleviate symptoms of both primary and recurrent herpes infection. Acyclovir is available in both oral and intravenous forms for systemic treatment and in ointment for topical use. Recently, two new derivatives, famcyclovir and valacyclovir (an acyclovir prodrug) have been approved for the treatment of herpes infections. Their main advantage resides in their favorable pharmacokinetic profile, allowing administration of fewer doses per day compared to acyclovir. HSV infections that are resistant to acyclovir, valacyclovir, or famciclovir are rare, and when they occur, they are usually in immunocompromised persons.

The CDC recommendations for the use of acyclovir, valacyclovir and famciclovir in sexually acquired herpes infections are listed in Table 158.5. Systemic acyclovir provides partial control of the symptoms and signs when given to patients with first clinical episode or when used as suppressive therapy. Topical acyclovir provides no benefit in the episodic treatment of genital herpes and is not recommended.[23] In recurrent episodes the effect of acyclovir therapy can be achieved only if the treatment is instituted during the prodrom or at the first sign of a recurrence; even then the benefit of the treatment is quite limited, and the impact on pain and itching is minimal.[88] Consequently, its use in immunocompetent patients with recurrent disease is not generally recommended.[23]

Daily suppressive therapy with oral acyclovir in patients with frequent recurrences of HSV (i.e., six or more episodes per year), reduces the frequency of episodes by at least 75%. Suppressive treatment will also significantly reduce although not totally eliminate viral shedding and the potential for its transmission.[91,113] Safety and efficacy have been documented for as long as 5 years of daily administration. Patients should be advised yearly to discontinue the suppressive therapy; since frequency of genital recurrences decreases over time for both patients who receive suppressive therapy and those who do not, withholding the drug periodically allows for reassessment of whether suppression is still needed.

Symptomatic sex partners should be managed in the same manner as any patient with genital lesions.

The safety of systemic acyclovir therapy among pregnant women has not been established, although current registry data do not indicate an increase in the number of birth defects.[114] There is no information on the effectiveness of preterm acyclovir treatment of mothers with recurrence of genital herpes at time of delivery. Acyclovir administration to pregnant women is indicated only for life-threatening maternal HSV infection. All infants with evidence of neonatal herpes should be treated with systemic acyclovir.[115]

Case detection and prevention

During symptomatic episodes of genital herpes, patients should abstain from sexual contact until the lesions are healed completely. Because most instances of transmission result from exposure to an asymptomatic carrier, the use of a condom is recommended for any person who has evidence of prior HSV-2 infection. When condoms are used during more than 70% of sexual encounters between an HSV-2-positive man and an HSV-2–negative woman, the risk of transmission is reduced by more than 60%. Another approach is the use of antiviral suppressive therapy in the seropositive partner. Neither approach, however, completely eliminates the risk of transmission.[97]

During the initial antenatal visit, the pregnant women should be questioned carefully about a history of genital herpes in herself or her partner. The development of signs and symptoms of genital herpes at any time during pregnancy requires that samples from

Table 158.5 Centers for Disease Control and Prevention recommended regimens for treatment of sexually acquired herpes infection[23]

Condition	Regimen
First clinical episode	
Genital herpes	Acyclovir 200 mg orally 5 times a day for 7–10 days
	or
	Acyclovir 400 mg orally 3 times a day for 7–10 days
	or
	Valacyclovir 1 g orally twice a day for 7–10 days
	or
	Famciclovir 250 mg orally 3 times a day for 7–10 days
Herpes proctitis	Acyclovir 400 mg orally 5 times a day for 10 days
Recurrent episodes	Acyclovir 200 mg orally 5 times a day for 5 days
	or
	Acyclovir 800 mg orally 2 times a day for 5 days*
	or
	Valacyclovir 500 mg orally 2 times a day for 3–5 days
	or
	Valacyclovir 1.0 g orally once a day for 5 days
	or
	Famciclovir 125 mg orally 2 times a day for 5 days
Suppressive therapy	Acyclovir 400 mg orally 2 times a day
	or
	Valacyclovir 500 mg orally once a day
	or
	Valacyclovir 1.0 g orally once a day
	or
	Famciclovir 250 mg orally 2 times a day
Severe disease	Acyclovir 5–10 mg/kg body weight IV every 8 h for 5–7 days or until clinical resolution is attained
Perinatal infection	Acyclovir 30 mg/kg body weight IV per day for 10–14 days

*An even shorter regimen of acyclovir for the treatment of recurrent episodes (800 mg orally 3 times a day for 2 days) was found to be significantly superior to placebo (Wald A, *et al. Clin Infect Dis* 2002;34:944)

the patient be cultured to confirm the diagnosis. Weekly cultures should be obtained if a positive culture is documented and should be repeated until a negative result is obtained.[23] Although primary genital HSV in early pregnancy may cause spontaneous abortion, congenital infection is uncommon. Hence, therapeutic abortion is not recommended for pregnancies complicated by primary infection.[2] Because primary genital herpes contracted late in pregnancy usually is associated with prolonged shedding and frequent reactivation, it has been suggested that weekly viral cultures should be obtained from these women.[90] If viral shedding ceases before labor ensues and there is no clinical evidence of disease activity, vaginal delivery should be permitted. However, if viral shedding continues until delivery, a cesarean section is recommended.[90] Since infants born vaginally to mothers with primary infection are at particular risk of invasive disease, consideration should be given to the early empiric use of acyclovir in this circumstance.[2]

Although many infants with perinatal HSV infection are born to mothers with asymptomatic genital infection, the risk of transmission of the virus to the newborn remains very low (1/5000 live births to mothers with history of recurrent genital herpes). Weekly surveillance for asymptomatic HSV shedding in mothers near term is extremely expensive.[2] Moreover, asymptomatic intrapartum shedding of HSV is not predictable from antepartum cultures for HSV.[2] Based on these considerations, the following approach is now recommended by most authorities.[112] Any woman with a history or recurrent genital herpes should have a careful genital examination conducted during admission for delivery. If lesions consistent with herpes are present, abdominal delivery should be undertaken. Cesarean section should be done ideally before membranes rupture or as soon thereafter as possible; however, abdominal delivery does not prevent all cases of neonatal herpes, even when done before the membranes rupture. In a recent surveillance study, 10 of 184 infants with neonatal herpes were delivered by cesarean section before the membranes ruptured.[116] If no maternal lesions are present at delivery, vaginal delivery is recommended.

Several small randomized studies have suggested that suppressive acyclovir therapy during the last four weeks or so of pregnancy in women with a history of genital herpes decreases the occurrence of clinically apparent genital HSV disease at the time of delivery, with an associated decrease in the rate of cesarean sections performed because of genital HSV. However, because viral shedding still occurs (albeit with reduced frequency), neonatal infection is still possible. There are currently insufficient data to justify the routine use of suppressive therapy in pregnant women who have had genital herpes.[97]

The infected mother and any other infected family members must be instructed in proper hygienic techniques to prevent postnatal transmission of infection to the newborn. Breast feeding is allowed unless lesions of the breast are present.

An HSV-2 glycoprotein-D-subunit vaccine was recently demonstrated to be safe and, in women who were seronegative for HSV-1 and HSV-2 before vaccination, reasonably effective in preventing clinically apparent HSV-1 or HSV-2 genital herpes disease (efficacy, 75%).[57] The vaccine was neither effective in men, nor in women with preexisting anti–HSV-1 antibodies.[117] Further study of this vaccine in women who are seronegative for HSV-1 and HSV-2 is under way.

Trichomoniasis

Trichomoniasis is one of the most common sexually transmitted diseases, affecting millions of people worldwide.[118] It represents a vexing health problem especially for women in whom it can cause a persistent discomfort if untreated. More recently, trachomonal infection has been incriminated as a significant risk factor for premature rupture of membranes, preterm birth and posthysterectomy vaginal cuff cellulitis.[119] The association of trichomoniasis with HIV acquisition seems to be clear.[120]

The pathogen and pathogenesis

Trichomonas vaginalis is a motile, ovoid, flagellated anaerobic protozoan. *T. vaginalis* lives only in the genitourinary tract, and human beings are its only natural hosts. This extracellular parasite has four anterior flagella and a fifth posterior flagellum which extends along its body and is embedded in an undulating membrane. The presence of hormonal receptors has been demonstrated on the protozoan's cell surface. The parasite is actively mobile and is easily identified by its characteristic twitching motility. *T. vaginalis* can survive only on squamous epithelial cells lining the anterior fornix of the vagina, Skene glands and urethra in women and in the urethra, the prostate and the foreskin of uncircumcised men.[121]

Trichomonas vaginalis attaches to mucosal cells via specific adhesions. It can damage epithelial cells by releasing a cell-detaching factor[122] and cause microulcerations; there is no invasion of the mucosa.[118] *T. vaginalis* produces phospholipases and proteases,[122] and activates the alternative complement pathway. The parasite attracts polymorphonuclear neutrophils which can kill the organism. On the other hand, it can sense and move away from toxic materials such as products of polymorphonuclear oxidative metabolites and metronidazole.[119,121] Protective immunity does not occur with trichomoniasis. The antigenic diversity, which is displayed on the parasite's external membrane and subject to regulation, may also contribute to the pathogenicity.[122] Trichomoniasis is often associated with a change of the normal vaginal environment consisting of an overgrowth of facultative and anaerobic bacteria and reduction of lactobacilli.

Evidence regarding the association between *T. vaginalis* infection and adverse pregnancy outcome has been conflicting.[118,121–125] Trichomoniasis during pregnancy has been associated with premature rupture of membranes, preterm birth, low birth weight, postpartum fever and postabortal infection. It has been suggested that the role of trichomonal infection is rather indirect, acting via the associated overgrowth of anaerobic bacteria.[121] In a large multicenter study, after adjusting for demographic, behavioral, and microbiological variables, trichomonas was significantly associated with low birth weight, premature rupture of membranes, and preterm delivery.[123] However, pregnant women with asymptomatic trichomoniasis who were treated with metronidazole had higher rates of preterm delivery than those who received placebo.[126]

Epidemiology

Trichomoniasis is transmitted almost exclusively by sexual contact. The parasite is more readily transmitted to women (85% infectivity after exposure) than to men (70% infectivity).[122] Perinatal acquisition has also been documented with transmission rates of 2–17% of female offspring of infected women.[127] Because the organism can survive for hours on moist objects and clothing used by infected women, nonsexual transmission by fomites is theoretically possible although it should be extremely rare, and no well-documented cases were reported.[121] Yet, high prevalence of trichomoniasis was found in some institutionalized populations.[118] The incidence of trichomoniasis is highest among Black women, women with multiple sexual partners and in those with history of STI.[119] Unlike other STIs, trichomonal infection is more evenly distributed among sexually active women of all age groups, with a mean age of 35 years; Reproductive hormone levels may be partly responsible for higher prevalence of trichomoniasis in older women. Trichomoniasis is frequently seen with other STIs, particularly chlamydial infection (15–28% co-infection rate) and gonorrhea (10%), and may be a sensitive marker of high-risk sexual behavior. It is also often seen in association with bacterial vaginosis.[120] Hence, women with trichomonal infection should be evaluated for the presence of other STIs. The infection is less common among women using oral contraceptives than in women using no form of birth control.[119] Estrogens may act by changing the vaginal environment or directly on the pathogen itself.[128]

Acquisition of HIV has been associated with trichomoniasis in several studies conducted in Africa, possibly as the result of local inflammation often caused by the protozoan.[120]

Trichomoniasis is the most prevalent non-viral STI. It has been diagnosed in about 5% of US women in family planning clinics compared with 13–25% of women attending gynecology clinics, up to 40% of women attending STD clinics and 50–75% of prostitutes.[118,122] The incidence of trichomonal infections appears to be declining during the last decade in the US and Western Europe. A Swedish STD clinic reported a prevalence of 5.4% in 1980, while in 1987, it was only 0.7%.[129] A decline by 30% in the incidence of trichomoniasis was observed in genitourinary medicine clinics in England and Wales between 1976 and 1986.[130] In Israel in the early 1990s, trichomonal infection was diagnosed in 7% of women attending a gynecology clinic for vaginal symptoms and in 2% of asymptomatic women seen in the same clinic (author's unpublished data). In a study conducted recently in Burkina Faso, trichomononiasis was diagnosed in 27.8% of women with genitourinary complaints.[131]

In pregnant women, the prevalence of trichomoniasis is generally similar to that in the general feminine population. In a multicenter survey between 1984 and 1989 among pregnant American women from urban clinics, the prevalence of trichomoniasis at mid-pregnancy was 12.6% (range 8.5–21.8%). The infection rate was 6.2% among White women, 6.6% among Hispanic and 22.8% in Black women.[132] Women colonized with *T. vaginalis* were significantly more likely to be Black, cigarette smokers, unmarried, less educated, had greater number of sexual partners and a history of gonorrhea.[123] A study from Britain reported a 4% infection rate among third-trimester women.[127] In Africa the prevalence rate of trichomoniasis in pregnant women has ranged from 10% to 30%, and it often did not differ significantly from that among prostitutes.

Clinical manifestations

Between 10% and 50% of women attending an STD clinic who carry *T. vaginalis* are asymptomatic, while most (90%) infected men appear to be asymptomatic.[119] The incubation period in women ranges from 5 to 28 days.[133] Symptoms are nonspecific and cannot be used to differentiate trichomoniasis from other genital infections. They begin or exacerbate during or immediately following the menstrual period. Vaginal discharge is noted by 50–75% of infected women. About 10% of the women describe the discharge as malodorous. One-fourth to one-half of the symptomatic women complain of pruritus which is often severe. Up to one-half of patients report a dyspareunia; the same proportion of women may note dysuria. Urinary tract infection may be common; thus consideration should be given to the presence of trichomoniasis for women with dysuria as a sole complaint. Lower abdominal pain, possibly resulting from pelvic lymphadenitis, has been described by 5–12% of the patients; salpingitis caused by other sexually transmitted organisms should be ruled out. Physical examination reveals a diffusely erythematous vulva in up to one-third of the patients; edema may be noted with more severe infection. Excessive, rather loose discharge, which pools in the posterior vaginal fornix, is noted in most infected women. The typical yellow-green and frothy discharge is seen in less than a half of the patients. Although yellow secretions are suggestive of trichomoniasis, they can also be seen in mucopurulent cervicitis and desquamative inflammatory vaginitis; a frothy discharge is also found in bacterial vaginosis. The vaginal walls are erythematous in up to 75% of patients with trichomoniasis. The exocervix is often inflamed; punctate hemorrhages (colpitis macularis) with strawberry appearance are observed with a naked eye in about 1–2% of cases, but in 45% when colposcopy is used. The presence of this finding strongly suggests trichomoniasis.[118]

The vaginal discharge has a high pH (> 4.5) in up to 90% of cases. A positive whiff test (malodor produced by application of 10% KOH on a sample of the vaginal discharge) and the presence of excessive numbers of polymorphonuclear leukocytes on a wet mount preparation are noted in about 75% of patients.[118]

If untreated, trichomonal infection in women can last for months and even 3–5 years. Symptoms and signs of chronic infection do not vary much from those of acute infection.[134] Trichomoniasis can be rarely complicated by vaginitis emphysematosa in which gas filled blebs occur in the vaginal wall. The condition will resolve when infection is eradicated.[135] Women with trichomoniasis are more likely to develop vaginal cuff cellulitis after abdominal hysterectomy.[136] This complication, like the obstetrical ones, probably results from the changes in the bacterial flora that accompany the protozoan infection.

Laboratory diagnosis

The accurate diagnosis of trichomoniasis cannot relay on clinical findings and depends on demonstrating the pathogen in the vaginal discharge.[133]

Microscopic examination

Trichomonads can be identified in vaginal secretions using the wet mount technique. A sample of vaginal fluid is mixed with a drop of saline on a slide. The preparation is covered with a cover slip and viewed under a phase contrast microscope at medium magnification. *T. vaginalis* is easily recognized by its characteristic movements. This technique detects 60–80% of cases and is less sensitive in asymptomatic patients.[108] In the majority of cases (50–75%) large numbers of white blood cells (> 1 per epithelial cell) are also seen. The epithelial cells appear normal; in florid infection epithelial cell turnover may be rapid and increased numbers of parabasal cells (small and ovid) can be observed. The bacterial flora consists of either rods or coccobacilli.[118]

The Gram, Giemsa and acridine orange stains and Papanicolaou smear are less useful than the wet mount. Direct fluorescent antibody staining, latex agglutination, enzyme linked immunosorbent assay and oligonucleotide probe techniques are more sensitive than the wet mount (80–90%) but less so than culture.[119,137,138] The PCR techniques show high sensitivity (~95%) and specificity (~98%) when performed on vaginal specimens,[139] although results may vary, especially in women and with urine samples.[120] As of 2005 these tests are not yet approved for diagnostic purposes.

Culture

This remains the most sensitive (≥ 95%) technique for the diagnosis of trichomoniasis. Culture should preferably be inoculated anaerobically; most isolates show growth within 48 h. The modified Diamond's medium is considered the 'gold standard'[122]; however, a modified thioglycolate medium was recently found to be as reliable and readily available.[140] The combination of culture and wet mount examination will give a sensitivity close to 100% and remains the standard approach for detecting *T. vaginalis* in patient samples.

Treatment

CDC-recommended treatment regimen is 2 g of metronidazole as a single oral dose for both females and males.[23] Cure rates range from 82–88%, with concurrent treatment of partners improving efficacy to more than 95%.[122] Alternative regimens consist of metronidazole 500 mg orally twice daily or 250 mg orally three times daily for 7 days. The advantage of the extended course therapy over the single dose treatment, is its higher efficacy in men and its improved tolerance.[122] On the other hand, the prolonged administration may decrease compliance. Because of the gastrointestinal side effects of systemic metronidazole (nausea, bad taste, Antabuse-like effects), one is tempted to use the drug intravaginally; however, only systemic therapy is capable of eradicating trichomonads from extravaginal sites. The major concern with metronidazole administration is its potential carcinogenicity and teratogenicity. Although the available literature[141,142] does not support the association between the drug and these risks, metronidazole remains relatively contraindicated during the first trimester of pregnancy. Symptomatic pregnant women may initially be treated with clotrimazole, 100 mg vaginal tablet at bedtime for 1–2 weeks, which will cure the infection in some and relieve symptoms in most cases. After the first trimester, the CDC recommends the single 2 g regimen for infected pregnant women.[23]

In case of metronidazole treatment failure, one should consider: (a) reinfection from an untreated sexual partner; (b) noncompliance; (c) increased hepatic inactivation of the drug (e.g., when coadministered with phenobarbital); and (d) true drug resistance. Metronidazole resistance remains rare and can be overcome with higher and more prolonged regimens: 2 g daily for 3–14 days, with or without intravaginal metronidazole tablets, 500 mg twice daily. Some resistant cases have been cured with intravenous metronidazole, up to 2 g every 6–8 h for 3 days or more.[119] Successful therapy with tinidazole (another 5-nitromidazole derivative) 2 g daily for 2 days or more, has been reported in a number of metronidazole resistant cases.[134]

Prevention

Asymptomatic infected women should be treated because they represent an important reservoir of the pathogen; moreover, about one-third of these women will become symptomatic during the following few months. Sex partners should be treated. Infected male sex partners are usually asymptomatic. Patients should be instructed to avoid sex until patient and partner are cured. Screening for *T. vaginalis* of high-risk pregnant women on entry into prenatal care and of those undergoing high risk obstetrical or gynecological procedures has been advised.[122]

Genital warts (human papillomavirus infection)

Human papillomavirus (HPV) attacks the squamous epithelium and causes lesions ranging from benign genital warts (condyloma acuminatum) to dysplasia and invasive squamous carcinoma of the lower genital tract. In pregnant women, genital warts may rapidly enlarge with advancing gestation and mechanically obstruct labor. Perinatal exposure may result in the development of laryngeal papillomatosis in the infant. Only the clinical aspects of genital warts will be discussed herein, the carcinogenic effects of HPV being beyond the scope of this chapter.

The pathogen and pathogenesis

Human papillomaviruses are highly species-specific, and cross-species infections do not occur. The virus, which is non-enveloped, has an icosahedral capsid containing a double-stranded circular DNA genome. Over 70 types of HPV have been identified based on DNA homology, approximately one-third of which infect the genital tract.[143] Each type is associated with a distinct histopathologic process: benign exophytic and flat genital warts are most commonly caused by HPV types 6 and 11 and less often by types 42–45.[144,145] The types that are strongly associated with dysplasia and carcinoma (e.g., 16, 18, 31, 33 and 35) usually cause subclinical infection, although occasionally are found in exophytic warts.

It is assumed that the virus replicative cycle begins with the entry of particles into the basal epithelial cells. Some infected cells undergo the characteristic transformation of koilocytosis consisting of large, polygonal squamous cells with a shrunken nucleus lodged inside a large cytoplasmic vacuole.[144] It is speculated that HPV infection may persist throughout life in a dormant state and become infectious intermittently. Exophytic genital warts may rarely transform into squamous cell carcinoma.[144] Women with a history of anogenital warts have a 30-fold increased risk of anal cancer.[146]

Anti-HPV antibodies, which tend to disappear with disease resolution, probably contribute to virus neutralization.[144] The importance of the cellular immune system in the resolution of HPV disease is suggested by the observation that the regression of one wart is frequently followed by disappearance of others.[144] The decrease of HPV prevalence in older women may suggest an increase in immunity to HPV with age.[147] HPV infection occurs frequently and is often more severe in patients with both primary and secondary immune deficiencies. Genital warts are particularly persistent in patients with diabetes mellitus, organ transplantation, corticosteroid therapy, lymphoma or HIV infection.[144]

The suppressed cellular immunity may probably explain the increased incidence and severity of HPV disease in pregnancy.[144] It has been suggested that hormonal changes during pregnancy may also play a role in the enhancement of viral infection or expression.[143,148] Transmission during delivery can result in the development of juvenile laryngeal papillomatosis which is most commonly associated with types 6 and 11. Rarely the disease can spread to the trachea and bronchi.[145]

Epidemiology

About two-thirds of sexual contacts of patients with anogenital warts subsequently develop the disease.[144] The risk of acquiring condyloma acuminatum is strongly associated with increased number of sexual partners and younger age.[147,149,150] Whether patients with subclinical HPV infection are as contagious as patients with warts is unknown. In children, anogenital warts should raise the suspicion of sexual abuse; however, about one-fifth of prepubertal children with condyloma acuminatum have 'non-genital' types of HPV.[144] Infants can acquire the virus during passage through an infected birth canal.[151] Many children with respiratory papillomatosis are first-born infants who were delivered vaginally to young mothers.[151] Acquisition of the virus *in utero* is also possible, probably by ascending infection from the mother's genital tract, as suggested by cases in which the disease was documented at birth even after cesarean delivery.[144,152,153] The role of fomites in the transmission of HPV if not clear, although theoretically possible since HPV is resistant to heat.

It is estimated that genital HPV causes approximately 30 million new infections annually.[149] Anogenital warts are the most common viral sexually transmitted in the United States and United Kingdom.[149] Several studies conducted in these countries have shown that the incidence of the disease has continued to increase rapidly in the 1980s.[144,149] A comparative analysis of women attending a STD clinic and college women showed that 11% of the patients with an STD but only 2% of the college students presented with visible genital warts. However, when cervical specimens from women without visible lesions were analyzed, 10% of the patients with an STD and 11% of the students were positive for HPV DNA or antigen.[154] In a recent investigation among an ethnically diverse group of urban adolescent females, genital HPV infection was documented in 24%, while genital warts were observed in 3.5% of women. There was a strong association with number of lifetime sexual partners; no ethnic difference in prevalence was noted.[150] A similar prevalence of genital HPV DNA (29%) was documented among women attending a STD clinic in Jamaica.[147] In Sweden, one-third of women 25 years of age and younger who visited a contraception clinic reported a history of condyloma.[149]

Clinically apparent HPV infection of the female genital tract seems to occur more frequently during pregnancy and regresses rapidly after delivery.[155,156] Schneider *et al.*[157] reported detection of HPV DNA in exfoliated cervical cells of 28% of pregnant women compared with 12.5% in non-pregnant women control women. In their longitudinal study, Rando *et al.*[148] have observed a dramatic increase in the percentage of pregnant women harboring HPV DNA in exfoliated cervical cells from the first (21%) to the third trimester (46%), with a sharp decrease in the postpartum examination (17.5%). This association between pregnancy and increased prevalence of HPV infection was not reconfirmed in a recent cross-sectional study.[158] Transmission of HPV from infected mothers to their newborns is rare and does not appear to be associated with persistent infection. Transmission rates are similar for newborns born vaginally and those delivered by cesarean section.[159]

Laryngeal papillomatosis has a bimodal age distribution with peaks in children 2–5 years of age and young adults. It is estimated that the incidence of juvenile respiratory papillomatosis is similar to that of neonatal HSV infection: 1/2500 to 1/10,000 cases per year.[143]

Clinical manifestations

Wives of American soldiers returning from the Korean war with penile warts developed genital warts after an incubation period of 4–6 weeks after exposure.[144] The majority of lesions are located in the posterior introitus and to a lesser degree in the labia majora and minora and the clitoris. Other sites that may be involved are the perineum, vagina, anus and urethra.[144] Only rarely do condylomata develop in the cervix.[143] The warts appear as flesh- to gray-colored exophytic papules, either sessile or, more frequently, attached by a short, broad peduncle. Their size ranges from less than a millimeter in diameter to several square centimeters when they merge into plaques. Flat condyloma can be demonstrated on the uterus cervix by colposcopy after soaking with 3% acetic acid. Typically these lesions are shiny, white patches with poorly defined borders and an irregular surface containing characteristic capillary loops.[144] In the vagina, in addition to the flat condylomas, small white nodosities, called spiked condylomas, have been described.[144]

About one-fourth of patients with anogenital warts are symptomatic.[144] Itching, burning, tenderness and pain are common complaints. Not less important are the psychological consequences of the disease that may be severe.[144] Spontaneous remission of lesions may occur: this has been noted in 10–20% of untreated patients over a few months' period.[144]

During pregnancy condylomas may become so large as to impair normal delivery mechanically.[144] The lesions often regress spontaneously after delivery.

Patients with laryngeal warts present with hoarseness or, in infants, with an altered cry; respiratory distress may follow. Rapid growth of lesions in young children often threatens the patency of the upper respiratory tract and may require repeat surgical excision to prevent suffocation. If spread to the lower respiratory tract occurs, lesions can lead to obstruction, infection and respiratory failure.[144]

Diagnosis

Because of their distinctive appearance genital warts are usually diagnosed by physical examination. Condyloma acuminatum should rarely be confused with other STDs, although it may be difficult to distinguish from molluscum contagiosum, particularly in its more atypical form. Molluscum contagiosum is a benign human disease caused by a pox virus. Of worldwide occurrence, it spreads by close contact, including sexual intercourse. The typical lesions are in the form of small firm umbilicated papules which resolve spontaneously. In contrast to condyloma acuminatum, the lesions of malluscum contagiosum tend to predominate over the pubis and are rarely pedunculated, but rather appear to be very smooth sessile domes from which cheesy material can be expressed.[160]

The use of colposcope with prior application of an acetic acid solution is an important diagnostic tool for HPV infection. To confirm diagnosis, careful colposcopic examination of the genital area should be done after application for 3–5 min of a 3% acetic acid solution; the white epithelium should be noted and biopsied. Koilocytes on histology or cytologic smear are the hallmark of HPV infection. Depending on the patient's age, the location and the nature of the HPV infection, the sensitivity of Pap's smear in detecting the infection ranges from 30% to 90%.[144] Dysplasia and malignant changes should be ruled out.

Diagnosis of HPV infection by DNA detection is currently possible, but no consensus exists as to the indication for such testing in clinical practice. No clear management strategy has been established for patients who test positive for HPV DNA but who have no detectable high-grade dysplasia.

Treatment

With the currently available therapeutic arsenal, the only clear indication for treatment of HPV infection is alleviation of symptoms and restoration of normal anatomy when large lesions obstruct the birth canal.[23] Most therapeutic means consist of physical and chemical destruction of macroscopic lesions; no therapy has been shown to eradicate HPV and recurrence rates are high with all modalities.[143] No studies have assessed whether treatment of warts reduces transmission of HPV.

Treatment of genital warts should be guided by the preference of the patient, while taking care to avoid expensive, toxic and scar-forming modalities. For women with cervical warts, dysplasia must be excluded before therapy is started.

For the treatment of extensive warts, carbon dioxide laser and surgery are most useful. Laser is expensive and requires general anesthesia; its efficacy is 43%, with recurrence rate of 5–50%. Surgical excision is effective in 35–70% of cases with 29% recurrence rate[23]; scarring is common.

Interferon therapy is not recommended by the CDC because of its cost, frequency of side effects and an efficacy that is not greater than that of other methods.[23]

Imiquimod 5% cream is a topical cell-mediated immune response modifier. The efficacy of imiquimod ranges between 30% and 50%, with a relatively low recurrence rate of 15%. Local inflammatory reactions are common (70%). Imiquimod can weaken condoms and diaphragms, and sexual contact is not recommended while the cream is on the skin.

5-Fluorouracil cream frequently causes local irritation. Controlled experience with this method is limited, and it is not recommended by the CDC for treatment of genital warts. The use of 5-fluorouracil in pregnancy is contraindicated.[23]

Cryotherapy with liquid nitrogen or cryoprobe is relatively inexpensive, does not require anesthesia and can be used in all localizations. It does not result in scarring if performed properly and is safe in pregnancy. The efficacy of cryotherapy ranges between 63% and 88%, with a relatively low recurrence rate of 21–39%.[23]

Podophyllin is a resin extract of the mayapple plant. It is simple to use: a 10–25% solution is applied directly on the wart once weekly and should thoroughly be washed-off in 1–4 h. Efficacy rate: 32–79%, recurrences are seen in 5–30% of cases. Local irritation or pain can occur after treatment. Severe systemic complications can develop if the solution is applied on a large area (application should be limited to a volume not exceeding 1 ml/day). Use of podophyllin is contraindicated in pregnancy. Podofilox (0.5% solution) is a purified derivative of podophyllin. It is less toxic than podophyllin and can be self-applied by the patient at home. Efficacy is 45–88%; recurrence, 33–60%. It is contraindicated during pregnancy.

Trichloroacetic acid, 80–90%, has a limited controlled experience. It should be applied only on warts, and unreacted acid should be removed with talcum powder. Application is painful and can cause ulcers. Trichloroacetic acid can be useful for vaginal lesions. Efficacy is 81% and recurrence rate is 36%. It is safe in pregnancy.

Few data are available on efficacy of electrodesiccation or electrocautery. In a single randomized trial, electrodessiccation was effective in 94% of cases, with a recurrence rate of 22%. Local anesthesia is required, and it can cause moderate discomfort and leave scarring.

Removal of genital warts is recommended prior to delivery. The preferred modalities in pregnancy include electrocautery, electrodiseccation and cryotherapy. Podophyllin, podofilox and 5-fluorouracil are contraindicated.[144]

Prevention

After warts have been removed, follow-up is not necessary. However, annual cytologic screening is recommended for women with or without warts. Examination of sex partners is not necessary for management because the role of reinfection is probably minimal. The use of condom may reduce transmission to uninfected sex partners. Cesarean delivery is not justified solely to prevent transmission of HPV to the newborn. However, cesarean section may be indicated in rare cases in which warts may be so extensive as to cause pelvic outlet obstruction, or if vaginal delivery would result in excessive bleeding.[23] Anti-HPV vaccines against oncogenic strains are currently under development.

Chancroid

While considered a rare disease in industrialized countries, chancroid is the most common cause of genital ulcer disease in many parts of the world, particularly in the developing countries of Africa and Asia. The disease is characterized by necrotizing genital ulceration which may be accompanied by inguinal lymphadenitis and bubo formation. The most important public health problem associated with *Haemophilus ducreyi* infection is its role as cofactor in transmission of HIV.

The pathogen and pathogenesis

Haemophilus ducreyi is a small pleomorphic gram-negative coccobacillus with fastidious growth requirements.[161] It is believed that *H. ducreyi* initiates an infective process within the genital skin after the formation of epidermal microabrasions during sexual intercourse. The pathogenesis of *H. ducreyi* infection is still poorly understood. Most wild-type isolates express pilli. The role of *H. ducreyi* surface lipooligosaccharide and cytotoxin in producing chancroid lesions is being investigated. Recent data have linked genital ulcer disease, especially chancroid, to an increase in heterosexual transmission of HIV infection.[161] No adverse effects of chancroid or pregnancy outcome or on the fetus have been reported.

Epidemiology

Transmission of the infection from an infected individual to a sex partner has been well documented. A study in Kenya has revealed that 59% of secondary female contacts of males with chancroid have also developed *H. ducreyi* ulcers; only one contact (3%) carried the organism in the cervix without evidence of ulcer formation.[162] The infection is associated with low socioeconomic status and poor hygienic conditions.[163] Chancroid is most often seen in non-White, uncircumcised men.[163] In North America, only 10% of the reported cases are in women, an observation that might be due to clinically unapparent carrier state and/or infected prostitutes with large numbers of male contacts.[164,165]

Chancroid is worldwide in distribution. The infection is endemic in the tropics, where it is the most common cause of genital ulcer disease. In sub-Saharan Africa and Southeast Asia, *H. ducreyi* can be isolated from 20–60% of patients with genital ulcerations.[166]

Although long considered of rare occurrence in developed countries, the incidence of chancroid began to rise in 1986 in the United States and peaked in 1989 when 5191 cases were reported.[164,167] Major outbreaks of chancroid have recently occurred in Canada and the United States,[164,165] related to prostitution and other forms of promiscuous sexual behavior associated with the use of crack cocaine.[167] A high rate of HIV infection among patients with chancroid has been reported in the tropics as well as in the United States. HIV seropositive patients have increased numbers of genital ulcers which may heal at lower rates.[168] As many as 10% of patients with chancroid may be coinfected with *T. pallidum* or HSV.[23]

Clinical manifestations

The incubation period of chancroid is usually between 3 and 10 days, although it can extend to several weeks. The lesion begins as a tender papule surrounded with erythema. The papule ulcerates within 1–2 days to form the typical chancroid ulcer which is painful, minimally indurated and has undermined ragged edges. The base is covered with a purulent exudate and bleeds easily during swabbing. Individual ulcers vary from 1 to 20 mm in diameter. Adjacent lesions may merge and form confluent giant or serpiginous ulcerations. Multiple ulcers (up to 10 or more have been reported) are seen more often in women; they are frequently due to auto-inoculation ('kissing ulcers'). Superinfeciton of ulcers may occur and lead to rapid and extensive destruction of external genitalia (phagedenic chancroid). In women, lesions are most often located at the entrance of the vagina, particularly on the fourchette, and can also be found on the labia, clitoris, cervix and anus.[161] In approximately half of the cases painful inguinal lymphadenopathy appears within a week after the initial lesion. It is usually unilateral and may become fluctuant (bubo). Therapeutically undrained buboes may rupture spontaneously to form chronic draining sinuses or extensive ulceration of surrounding tissue. Extragenital cases of chancroid with lesions on inner thighs, breasts, and fingers have been reported but are rarely seen in clinical practice.[168] Untreated, the mean duration of lesions is approximately 60 days.[161,166]

Diagnosis

Clinical diagnosis of chancroid is inaccurate because genital ulcers of other etiologies may appear similar and may occur concomitantly. A gram-stained smear of material from the ulcer may be difficult to interpret because of the possible presence of various other bacteria. Smears of bubo aspirate are more specific when typical gram-negative coccobacilli are demonstrated, although the diagnostic sensitivity of the procedure is low. Diagnosis of chancroid should be confirmed by isolation of *H. ducreyi* from a lesion.[161] However, *H. ducreyi* is an extremely difficult organism to culture from clinical specimens in the hands of inexperienced laboratory staff, and conventional culture facilities are often not available. Even if culture facilities are available, it often takes several days for the organism to grow. The sensitivity of culture relative to the multiplex PCR is approximately 75%.[168]

The multiplex PCR technique offers a highly sensitive and specific way to detect *H. ducreyi*. However, this is an expensive tool which is mostly used in research and outbreak investigation.[168] Other diagnostic techniques, such as detection of *H. ducreyi* in ulcer material by immunofluorescence, oligonucleotide probes and serologic assays, have been reported.[161] Their usefulness in the diagnosis of chancroid remains to be established.

Because similarity in presentation and possible coexistence, it is important to exclude syphilis and HIV infection in every case of suspected chancroid. Patients should be tested for HIV and syphilis at the time of diagnosis and 3 months later if initial results are negative.

Treatment

The classical drugs used to treat chancroid, i.e., tetracycline and sulfamethoxazole-trimethoprim, are no longer appropriate because of high rates of resistance to these agents.[161] In addition, most isolates of *H. ducreyi* in recent years have been shown to produce β-lactamases.[167]

The therapeutic regimens proposed by the CDC[23] are shown in Table 158.6. Of the recommended regimens, azithromycin and ceftriaxone offer the advantage of single dose therapy,[170,171] which is an important factor in controlling STDs.

In addition to antibiotic therapy, drainage of buboes by needle aspiration through normal skin, or incision and drainage, is required to avoid spontaneous rupture which may result in chronic draining sinuses or extensive ulcerations.

Patients with HIV coinfection may need longer courses of therapy; healing in these patient may be slower and treatment failures do occur.

If treatment is effective, improvement occurs within seven days of its initiation. If no improvement is observed, the following possibilities should be considered: incorrect diagnosis; coinfection with another STDs agent; HIV coinfection; lack of compliance; or isolate is resistant to the administered agent.

Table 158.6 Regimen proposed by the Centers for Disease Control and Prevention for the treatment of chanroid[23]

Recommended regimens
Azithromycin,* 1 g orally in a single dose
or
Ceftrioxone, 250 mg intramuscularly in a single dose
or
Erythromycin, 500 mg orally 4 times a day for 7 days
Alternative regimens
Amoxicillin, 500 mg, plus clavulanic acid, 125 mg orally 3 times a day for 7 days
or
Ciprofloxacin,** 500 mg orally 2 times a day for 3 days†

*Safety for pregnant and lactating women has not been established
**Contraindicated in pregnant and lactating women and in individuals < 17 years of age
†A single dose appears to be as effective (recommended by WHO)[168]

Prevention

Symptoms in individuals who had sexual contact with a patient within the 10 days preceding onset should be examined and treated. Eradication of infection in human reservoirs of *H. ducreyi*, such as prostitutes, is imperative in controlling outbreaks of chancroid[161,164] and may have contributed to the decrease in the incidence of the disease in the United States since 1989. As for any STD, properly used condom may be useful in preventing transmission of chancroid.

Donovanosis

Donovanosis (formerly called granuloma inguinale) is characterized by slowly progressive hypertrophic ulceration with tissue destruction of the lower genital tract.

The pathogen and pathogenesis

Calymmatobacterium granulomatis, the causative organism of donovanosis was discovered by Donovan in 1905. The encapsulated, pleomorphic gram-negative bacilli with bipolar densities ('Donovan bodies') can be found in the cytoplasma of large mononuclear cells. After intracellular multiplication, the organisms are released from the ruptured intracytoplasmic vacuoles to infect other cells. *C. granulomatis* shares antigenic and morphologic characteristics with *Klebsiella* species. The organism is otherwise poorly characterized because it is difficult to culture *in vitro* or to propagate in laboratory animals.[166,172]

Epidemiology

Several arguments such as the age distribution of patients, the frequent coexistence of other STDs and the predominance of the genital involvement, advocate for the sexual transmission of the infection. However, the possibility of additional mechanisms of spread is suggested by the existence of extragenital lesions and by the occurrence in young children. The infection affects predominantly the lower socioeconomic classes and is characterized by low infectivity.[172]

Donovanosis is endemic in parts of Africa, Southeast Asia, southern India, South America, the Caribbean Islands and among the indigenous populations of Australia. The disease is rare in Europe and North America, with less than 100 cases reported annually in the United States.[172]

Donovanosis is frequently diagnosed during pregnancy, and it has been suggested that pregnancy may exacerbate the disease.[173] However, it is also possible that the routine examination during pregnancy is associated with increased detection rate of asymptomatic lesions.[172]

Clinical manifestations

The incubation period of donovanosis is 8–80 days, but may extend up to 6 months.[172] The initial small painless papule ulcerates and progresses over a course of days to weeks into an exuberant beefy-red granulomatous ulcer that bleeds easily. New lesions may form by auto-inoculation, and multiple lesions may coalesce into large destructive ulcers. Spontaneous healing results in scar formation and secondary deformities. When the scar tissue blocks the lymphatics, lymphedema develops that may lead to elephantiasis of external genitalia. In women, the labia and the fourchette are most often involved, but lesions can also be seen in the vagina and cervix. The infection can spread to the inguinal region causing groin swelling that involves the soft tissues, but not the lymph nodes ('pseudobuboes').[172]

Systemic spread is rare but can occur more often in women with cervical lesions. Hematogenous spread can result in pelvic granulomas and bone and joint lesions, while lymphatic spread can lead to lymphadenitis in rare cases.[172] Constitutional symptoms should suggest secondary bacterial infection or another concomitant STD.

Diagnosis

The clinical diagnosis of donovanosis, based on the identification of characteristic lesions, should be confirmed by the demonstration of intracytoplasmic encapsulated Donovan bodies in macrophages. A specimen of tissue is obtained by curettage or punch biopsy from the edge of an active lesion and crushed between two glass slides to prepare an impression smear which is stained with Giemsa, Wright or Leishman stain.[174] Under the microscope the organisms appear in clusters of blue or black with the characteristic safety-pin configuration. In cases where malignancy has to be ruled out, biopsy specimens are mandatory. If the diagnosis of donovanosis cannot be confirmed by microscopy, the genital ulcer should be cultured for *H. ducreyi*.[166]

Treatment

Most information on therapeutic efficacy of various antibiotic regimens derives from open, non-comparative trials. Tetracyclines, in a standard dosage, are considered the drug of choice. Trimethoprin-sulfamethoxazole, administered for at least 2 weeks, has also been reported to be effective. Comparable results were obtained with erythromycin, 500 mg four times daily, which has been used mainly in pregnant women.[173] Other useful antibiotics are the quinolones, chloramphenicol and aminoglycosides.[172] With successful therapy lesions begin to heal from the edges toward the center. Treatment should be continued until complete epithelialization occurs.[172]

REFERENCES

1. Radolf JD, SanchezPJ, Schultz KF, Murphy FK. Congenital syphilis. In Holmes KK, Sparling PF, Mardh PA, *et al*, eds. *Sexually Transmitted Diseases*, 3rd edn. New York: McGraw-Hill, 1999:1165.
2. Watts DH, Brunham RC. Sexually transmitted diseases including HIV infection in pregnancy. In Holmes KK, Sparling PF, Mardh PA, *et al*, eds. Sexually *Transmitted Diseases*, 3rd edn. New York: McGraw-Hill, 1999:1089.
3. Cunningham FG, MacDonald PC, Leveno KJ, Gant NF. Sexually transmitted diseases. In Cunningham FG, MacDonald PC, Levens KJ, *et al*, eds. *Williams Obstetrics*, 19th edn. Englewood Cliffs, NJ: Prentice-Hall International, 1993:1299.
4. Parker CR, Wendel GD. The effects of syphilis on endocrine function of the fetoplacental unit. *Am J Obstet Gynecol* 1988; 159:1327.
5. Nakashima AK, Ralfs RT, Flock ML, Kilmar P, Greenspan JR. Epidemiology of syphilis in the United States, 1941–1993. *Sex Transm Dis* 1995;23:16.
6. Centers for Disease Control and Prevention. Sexually Transmitted Disease Surveillance, 2003. Atlanta, GA: U.S. Department of Health and Human Services, September 2004.
7. Finelli L, Budd J, Spitalny KC. Relationship to sex, drugs and changes in high risk behavior from 1987–1990. *Sex Transm Dis* 1993;20:89.
8. Doherty L, Fenton KA, Jones J, *et al*. Syphilis: old problem, new strategy. *Brit Med J* 2002;325:153.
9. Israel Center for Disease Control. Notifiable Infectious Diseases in Israel. 50 Years of Surveillance, 1951–2001. Ministry of Health, State of Israel. Publication No 224, July 2003.

10. Linglof T. Rapid increase of syphilis and gonorrhea in parts of the former USSR. *Sex Transm Dis* 1995;22:160.
11. Hook EW, Maria CM. Acquired syphilis in adults. *N Eng J Med* 1992;326:1060.
12. Reyes MP, Hunt N, Ostrea EM, George D. Maternal/congenital syphilis in a large tertiary-care urban hospital. *Clin Infect Dis* 1993;17:1041.
13. Centers for Disease Control. Guidelines for the prevention and control of congenital syphilis. *MMWR Morb Mortal Wkly Rep* 1988;37(Suppl 1):1.
14. Walker DG, Walker GJA. Forgotten but not gone: The continuing scourge of congenital syphilis. *Lancet Infect Dis* 2002;2:432.
15. Naeye RL, Tafari N, Marboe CC, Judge DM. Causes of perinatal mortality in an African city. *Bull WHO* 1977;55:63.
16. Tramont EC. Treponema pallidum (syphilis). In Mandell GL, Bennett JE, Dolin R, eds. *Principles and Practice of Infectious Diseases*, 5th edn. New York: Churchill Livingstone, 2000:2474.
17. Larsen SA, Steiner BM, Rudolph AH. Laboratory diagnosis and interpretation of tests for syphilis. *Clin Microbiol Rev* 1995;8:1.
18. Romanowski B, Sutherland R, Fick GH, Mooney D, Love EJ. Serologic response to treatment of infections syphilis. *Ann Intern Med* 1991;114:1005.
19. Rolfs RT, Joesoef MR, Hendershot EF, *et al.* A randomized trial of enhanced therapy for early syphilis in patients with and without human immunodeficiency virus infection. The Syphilis and HIV Study Group. *N Engl J Med* 1997;337:307.
20. Wendel GD, Stark RJ, Jamison RR, Molina RD, Sullivan TJ. Penicillin allergy and desensitization in serious infections during pregnancy. *N Eng J Med* 1985;312:1229.
21. Hook EW, Roddy RE, Hansfield HH. Ceftriaxone therapy for incubating and early syphilis. *J Infect Dis* 1988;158:88.
22. Schafer H, Vogt HJ, Milbradt R. Ceftariaxone for treatment of primary and secondary neurosyphilis. *Chemotherapy* 1989; 95:140.
23. Centers for Disease Control and Prevention. Sexually transmitted diseases treatment guidelines 2002. *MMWR Morb Mortal Wkly Rep* 2002;51(RR-6):1.
24. Malone JC, Wallace MR, Hendrick BB, *et al.* Syphilis and neurosyphilis in a human immunodeficiency virus type-1 seropositive population: Evidence for frequent serologic relapse after therapy. *Am J Med* 1995;99:55.
25. Sparling PF, Handsfield HH. *Neisseria gonorrhoeae*. In Mandell GC, Bennett JE, Dolin R, eds. *Principles and Practice of Infectious Diseases*, 5th edn. New York: Churchill Livingstone, 2000:2242.
26. World Health Organization Task Force on the Prevention and Management of Infertility. Tubal infertility: Serologic relationship to past chlamydial and gonococcal infection. *Sex Transm Dis* 1995;22:71.
27. Doyle MB, DeCherney AH, Diamond MP. Epidemiology and etiology of ectopic pregnancy. *Obstet Gynecol Clin North Am* 1991;18:1.
28. Edwards LE, Barrada MMI, Hermann AA, *et al.* Gonorrhea in pregnancy. *Am J Obstet Gynecol* 1978;132:637.
29. Schultz KF, Cates W Jr, O'Mara PR. Pregnancy loss, infant death, and suffering: Legacy of syphilis and gonorrhea in Africa. *Genitourin Med* 1987;63:320.
30. Handsfield HH, Hodson WA, Holmes KK. Neonatal gonococcal infection: I. Orogastric contamination with *Neisseria gonorrhoeae*. *J Am Med Assoc* 1973;225:697.
31. Burkman RT, Tonascia JA, Atienza MF, King TM. Untreated endocervical gonorrhea and endometritis following elective abortion. *Am J Obstet Gynecol* 1976;126:648.
32. Alger LS, Lovchik JC, Hebel JR, Blackman LR, Crenshaw MC. The association of *Chlamydia trachomatis, Neisseria gonorrhoeae,* and group B streptococci with preterm rupture of the membranes and pregnancy outcome. *Am J Obstet Gynecol* 1988;159:397.
33. Elliot D, Brunham RC, Loga M, *et al.* Maternal gonococcal infection as a preventable risk factor for low birth weight. *J Infect Dis* 1990;161:531.
34. Stoll BJ, Kanto WP, Glass RI, Pushkin J. Treated maternal gonorrhea without adverse effect on outcome of pregnancy. *South Med J* 1982;75:1236.
35. de Toledo AR, Chandler JW. Conjunctivitis in the newborn. *Infect Dis Clin North Am* 1992;6:807.
36. Jolly AM, Orr PH, Hammond G, Young TK. Risk factors for infection in women undergoing testing for *Chlamydia trachomatis* and *Neisseria gonorrhoeae* in Manitoba, Canada. *Sex Transm Dis* 1995;22:289.
37. Thomas JC, Schoenbach VJ, Weiner DM, Parker EA, Earp JA. Rural gonorrhea in the southeastern United States: A neglected epidemic? *Am J Epidemiol* 1996;143:269.
38. Roseberry WL, Heymann DL, Ndoye I, Nsubuga PS. Rapid sexually transmitted disease assessment in two developing countries. *Sex Transm Dis* 1994;21(Suppl):S84.
39. Brunham PC, Enbree JE. Sexually transmitted diseases: current and future dimensions of the problem in the Third World. In Germain A, Holmes KK, Piot P, *et al*, eds. *Reproductive Tract Infections: Global Impact and Priorities for Women: Reproductive Health.* New York: Plenum Press, 1992:35.
40. Goldenberg RL, Klebanoff MA, Nugent R, *et al.* Bacterial colonization of the vagina during pregnancy in four ethnic groups. *Am J Obstet Gynecol* 1996;174:1618.
41. Dan M. The return of gonorrhea. *Isr Med Assoc J* 2004;6:164–6.
42. Samra Z, Dan M, Segev S, *et al.* Prevalence of sexually transmitted pathogens among women attending a methadone clinic in Israel. *Genitourin Med* 1991;67:133.
43. Dan M, Samra Z, Katz A, Debby A, Gutman R, Zakut H. Etiology of laparoscopy proven acute pelvic inflammatory disease. *Sex Transm Dis* 1993;20:158.
44. Green MS, Anis E, Gandacu D, Grotto I. The fall and rise of gonorrhoea incidence in Israel: An international phenomenon? *Sex Transm Infect* 2003;79:116.
45. Bamberger ES, Siegler E, Makler-Shiran E, *et al.* Chlamydia trachomatis infections in female soldiers, Israel. *Emerg Infect Dis* 2003;10:1344–6
46. Laga M. Epidemiology and control of sexually transmitted disease in developing countries. *Sex Transm Dis* 1994;21(Suppl 2):S45.
47. Dan M. The use of fluoroquinolones in gonorrhea: The increasing problem of resistance. *Expert Opin Pharmacother* 2004;5:829.
48. Hedstrom S, Martens MG. Antibiotics in pregnancy. *Clin Obstet Gynecol* 1993;36:886.
49. Isenberg SJ, Apt L, Wood M. A controlled trial of povidone-iodine in prophylaxis against ophthalmia neonatrum. *N Engl J Med* 1995;332:562.
50. Weinstock H, Dean D, Bolan G. *Chlamydia trachomatis* infections. *Infect Dis Clin North Am* 1994;8:797.
51. Jones RB, Batteiger BE. Chlamydia trachomatis. In Mandel GL, Bennett JE, Dolin R, eds. *Principles and Practice of Infectious Diseases*, 5th edn. New York: Churchill Livingstone, 2000:1989.
52. Cates W, Wasserheit JN. Genital chlamydial infections: Epidemiology and reproductive sequelae. *Am J Obstet Gynecol* 1991;164:1771.
53. Mehanna MTR, Rizk MA, Eweiss NYM, *et al.* Chlamydial serology among patients with tubal factor infertility and ectopic pregnancy in Alexandria, Egypt. *Sex Transm Dis* 1995;22:317.
54. McGregor JA, French JI. *Chlamydia trachomatis* infection during pregnancy. *Am J Obstet Gynecol* 1991;164:1782.
55. Centers for Disease Control and Prevention. Recommendations for the prevention and management of *Chlamydia trachomatis* infections, 1993. *MMWR Morb Mortal Wkly Rep* 1993;42:1.
56. Katz BP, Blythe NJ, Van Der Pol B, Jones RB. Declining prevalence of chlamydial infection among adolescent girls. *Sex Transm Dis* 1996;23:226.
57. Herrmann B, Egger M. Genital *Chlamydia trachomatis* infections in Uppsala County, Sweden, 1985–1993: Declining rates for how much longer? *Sex Transm Dis* 1995;22:253.
58. Hitunen-Back E, Haikala O, Kautiainen H, Ruutu P, Paavonen J, Reunala T. Nationwide increase of *Chlamydia trachomatis* infection in Finland. Highest rise among adolescent women and men. *Sex Transm Dis* 2003;30:737–41.
59. Dan M, Kaneti N, Levin D, Poch F, Samra Z. Vaginitis in a gynecological practice in Israel: causes and risk factors. *Isr Med Assoc J* 2003;5:629–32.
60. Herman A, Roach Z, Samra Z, *et al.* Prevalence of low genital tract infectious agents in young Israeli women. *Isr J Med Sci* 1985;21:346.
61. Duncan ME, Jamil Y, Tibaux G, Pelzer A, Mehari L, Darougar S. Seroepidemiological and socioeconomic studies of genital chlamydial infection in Ethiopian women. *Genitourin Med* 1992;68:221.
62. Mabey DC, Whittle HC. Genital and neonatal chlamydial infection in a trachoma endemic area. *Lancet* 1982;2:300.
63. Kaptue L, Zekeng L, Djoumessi S, Monny-Lobe M, Nichols D, Debuysschar R. HIV and chlamydial infection among prostitutes in Yaounde, Cameroun. *Genitourin Med* 1991;67:143.
64. Mason PR, Gwanzura L, Latif AS, Marowa E. Genital infections in women attending a genito-urinary clinic in Harare, Zimbabwe. *Genitourin Med* 1990;66:178.

65. Ismail SO, Ahmed HJ, Jama MA, *et al.* Syphilis, gonorrhoea and genital chlamydial infeciton in a Somali village. *Genitourin Med* 1990;66:70.
66. Campos-Outcalt S, Ryan K. Prevalence of sexually transmitted diseases in Mexican-American pregnant women by country of birth and length of time in the United States. *Sex Transm Dis* 1995;22:78.
67. Goldenberg RL, Klebanoff MA, Nugent R, *et al.* Bacterial colonization of the vagina during pregnancy in four ethnic groups. *Am J Obstet Gynecol* 1996;174:1618.
68. Korokin M, Kumamoto Y, Hirose T, *et al.* Epidemiologic study of *Chlamydia trachomatis* in pregnant women. *Sex Transm Dis* 1994;21:329.
69. Chout RT, Vaton S, Duval-Violton D, Leguyader-Despres P, Orfila J. Screening for *Chlamydia trachomatis* infection in pregnant women in Martinique. *Sex Transm Dis* 1995;22:221.
70. Roseberry WL, Heymann DL, Ndoye I, Nsubuga PS. Rapid sexually transmitted disease assessment in two developing countries. *Sex Trans Dis* 1994;21(Suppl 2):S84.
71. Peipert JF. Genital chlamydial infections. *N Engl J Med* 2003; 349:2424.
72. Nugent RP, Hillier, SL. Mucopurulent cervicitis as a predictor of chlamydial infection and adverse pregnancy outcome. *Sex Transm Dis* 1992;19:198.
73. Lee HH, Chernesky MA, Schachler J, *et al.* Diagnosis of *Chlamydia trachomatis* genitourinary infection in women by ligase chain reaction assay of urine. *Lancet* 1995;345:213.
74. Wiesenfeld HC, Heini RP, Rideout A, *et al.* The vaginal introitus: A novel site for *Chlamydia trachomatis* testing in women. *Am J Obstet Gynecol* 1996;174:1542.
75. Witkin SS, Inglis SR, Polanecaky M. Detectino of *Chlamydia trachomatis* and *Trichomonas vaginalis* by polymerase chain reaction in introital specimens from pregnant women. *Am J Obstet Gynecol* 1996;175:165.
76. Allaire A, Naton L, Martens MG. *Chlamydia trachomatis*: Management in pregnancy. *Infect Dis Obstet Gynecol* 1995;3:82.
77. Alary M, Joly JR, Moutquin J-M, *et al.* Randomized comparison of amoxycillin in treatment of genital chlamydial infection in pregnancy. *Lancet* 1994;344:1461.
78. Weber JT, Johnson RE. New treatment for *Chlamydia trachomatis* genital infection. *Clin Infect Dis* 1995;20(Suppl 1):S66.
79. Martin DH, Mroczkowski TF, Dalu AZ, *et al.* A controlled trial of a single dose of azithromycin for the treatment of chlamydial urethritis and xervicitis. *N Eng J Med* 1992;327:921.
80. Miller JM. Efficacy and tolerance of single-dose azithromycin for treatment of chlamydial cervicitis during pregnancy. *Infect Dis Obstet Gynecol* 1995;3:189.
81. Rosen MF, Macones GA, Silverman NJ. Randomized trial of erythromycin and azithromycin for treatment of chlamydial infection in pregnancy. *Infect Dis Obstet Gynecol* 1995;3:241.
82. Finelli L, Nakashima AK, Hillis S, Crayne E, Spitalny KC. Selective screening versus presumptive treatment criteria for identification of women with chlamydial infection in public clinics: New Jersey. *Am J Obstet Gynecol* 1996;174:1527–33.
83. Scholes D, Stergachis A, Heidrich FE, *et al.* Prevention of pelvic inflammatory disease by screening for cervical chlamydial infection. *N Engl J Med* 1996;334:1362.
84. Perine PL, Osoba AO. Lymphogranuloma venereum. In Holmes KK, Mardh P-A, Sparling PF, eds. *Sexually Transmitted Diseases*, 2nd edn. New York: McGraw-Hill, 1990:195.
85. Kuo C-C, Grayston JT. Chlamydia: In Warren KS, Mahmond AAF, eds. *Tropical and Geographical Medicine*, 2nd edn. New York: McGraw-Hill, 1990:644.
86. Mabey D, Peeling RW. Lymphogranuloma venereum. *Sex Transm Infect* 2002;78:90–2.
87. Dan M, Rotmensch HM, Eylan E, *et al.* A case of lymphogranuloma venereum of 20 years' duration. *Br J Vener Dis* 1980;56:344.
88. Corey L. Herpes simplex virus. In Mandell GL, Bennett JE, Dolin R, eds. *Principles and Practice of Infectious Diseases*, 5th edn. New York: Churchill Livingstone, 2000:1564.
89. Corey L, Spear PG. Infections with herpes simplex virus. *N Engl J Med* 1986;314:686–691, 749.
90. Prober CG. Herpetic vaginitis in 1993. *Clin Obstet Gynecol* 1993;36:177.
91. Maccato M. Herpes in pregnancy. *Clin Obstet Gynecol* 1993;36:869.
92. Brown ZA, Vontver LA, Benedetti J, *et al.* Effects on infants of a first epidose of genital herpes during pregnancy. *N Engl J Med* 1987;317:1246.
93. Hutto C, Arvin A, Jacobs R, *et al.* Intrauterine herpes simplex virus infection. *J Pediatr* 1987;110:97.
94. Prober CG, Sullander WM, Yasukawa LL, Au DS, Yeager AS, Arvin AM. Low risk of herpes simplex virus infections in neonates exposed to the virus at the time of vaginal delivery to mothers with recurrent genital herpes simplex virus infections. *N Engl J Med* 1987;316:240.
95. Yeager AS, Arvin AM. Reasons for the absence of a history of recurrent genital infections in mothers of neonates infected with herpes simplex virus. *Pediatrics* 1984;73:188.
96. Corey L, Handsfield HH. Genital herpes and public health: addressing a global problem. *J Am Med Assoc* 2000;283:791.
97. Kimberlin DW, Rouse DJ. Genital herpes. *N Engl J Med* 2004;350:1970–7.
98. Corey L. The current trend in genital herpes. Progress in prevention. *Sex Trans Dis* 1994;21(Suppl):S38.
99. Kulhanjian JA, Soroush V, Au DS, *et al.* Identification of women at unsuspected risk of contracting primary herpes simplex type 2 infecions during pregancy. *N Engl J Med* 1992;326:916.
100. Mertz GJ. Epidemiology of genital herpes infections. *Infect Dis Clin North Am* 1993;7:825.
101. Cherpes TL, Meyn LA, Hillier SL. Cunnilingus and vaginal intercourse are risk factors for herpes simplex virus type 1 acquisition in women. *Sex Transm Dis* 2005;32:84.
102. Samra Z, Scherf E, Dan M. Herpes simplex virus type 1 is the prevailing cause of genital herpes in the Tel Aviv area, Israel. *Sex Transm Dis* 2003;30:794.
103. Whitley RJ, Nahmias AJ, Visintine AM, *et al.* The natural history of herpes simplex virus infection of mother and newborn. *Pediatrics* 1980;66:489.
104. Brown ZA, Benedetti J, Ashley R, *et al.* Neonatal herpes simplex virus infection in relation to asymptomatic maternal infection at the time of labor. *N Engl J Med* 1991;324:1247.
105. Gesundheit B, Grisaru-Soen G, Greenberg D, *et al.* Neonatal genital herpes simplex virus type 1 infection after Jewish ritual circumcision: modern medicine and religious tradition. *Pediatrics* 2004;114:e259.
106. Peacock JE Jr, Sarubbi FA. Disseminated herpes simplex virus infection during pregnancy. *Obstet Gynecol* 1983; 61(Suppl 3):135.
107. Brown ZA, Vontver CA, Benedetti J, *et al.* Genital herpes in pregnancy. Risk factors associated with recurrences and asymptomatic viral shedding. *Am J Obstet Gynecol* 1958;153:24.
108. Vontver LA, Hicock DE, Brown Z, Reid C, Corey L. Recurrent genital herpes simplex virus infections in pregnancy. Infant outcome and frequency of asymptomatic recurrences. *Am J Obstet Gynecol* 1982;143:75.
109. Harger JH, Amortegui AJ, Meyer MP, Pazin GJ. Characteristics of recurrent genital herpes simplex infections in pregnant women. *Obstet Gynecol* 1989;73:367.
110. Whitley R, Arvin A, Prober C, *et al.* Predictors of morbidity and mortality in neonates with herpes simplex virus infection. *N Engl J Med* 1991;324:450.
111. Koutsky LA, Stevens CE, Holmes KK, *et al.* Underdiagnosis of genital herpes by current clinical and viral isolation procedures. *N Engl J Med* 1992;326:1533.
112. The American College of Obstetricians and Gynecologists. Perinatal herpes simplex virus infections.: Technical Bulletin. Washington, DC: ACOG.
113. Wald A, Zeh J, Barnum G, Davis LG, Corey L. Suppression of subclinical shedding of herpes simplex virus type 2 with acyclovir. *Ann Intern Med* 1996;124:8.
114. Andrews EB, Yankaskas BC, Cordero JF, Schoeffer K, Hampp S, The Acyclovir in Pregnancy Registry Advisory Committee. Acyclovir in pregnancy registry: six years' experience. *Obstet Gynecol* 1992;79:7.
115. Committee on Infectious Diseases, American Academy of Pediatrics. *Report of the Committee on Infectious Diseases*, 22nd edn, 1991.
116. Stone KM, Brooks CA, Guinan ME, Alexander ER. National surveillance for neonatal herpes simplex virus infection. *Sex Transm Dis* 1989;16:152.
117. Stanberry LR, Spruance SL, Cunningham AL, *et al.* Glycoprotein-D-adjuvant vaccine to prevent genital herpes. *N Engl J Med* 2002;347:1652.

118. Rein MF, Muller M. *Trichomonas vaginalis* and trichomoniasis. In Holmes KK, Mardh P-A, Sparling AF, *et al*, eds. *Sexually Transmitted Diseases*, 2nd edn. New York: McGraw-Hill, 1990:481.
119. Rein MF. Trichomonas vaginalis. In Mandell GL, Bennett JE, Dolin R, eds. *Principles and Practice of Infectious Diseases*, 5th edn. New York: Churchill Livingstone, 2000; :2894.
120. Schwabke JR. Update on trichomoniasis. *Sex Transm Infect* 2002;78:378.
121. Thomason JL, Gelbart SM. *Trichomonas vaginalis. Obstet Gynecol* 1989;74536.
122. Heine P, McGregor JA. *Trichomonas vaginalis*: A reemerging pathogen. *Clin Obstet Gynecol* 1993;36:137.
123. Cotch MF, Pastorek JG, Nugent RP, *et al. Trichomonas vaginalis* associated with low birth weight and preterm delivery. *Sex Transm Dis* 1997;24:341.
124. Meis PJ, Goldenberg RL, Mercer B, *et al.* The preterm prediction study: significance of vaginal infections. Nation Institute of Child Health and Human Development Maternal-Fetal Medicine Units Network. *Am J Obstet Gynecol* 1985;173:1231.
125. Germain M, Krohn MA, Hillier SL, Eschenbach DA. Genital flora in pregnancy and its association with intrauterine growth retardation. *J Clin Microbiol* 1994;32:2162.
126. Klebanoff M, Carey J, Hauth JC, *et al.* Failure of metronidazole to prevent preterm delivery among pregnant women with asymptomatic *Trichomonas vaginalis* infection. *N Engl J Med* 2001;345:487.
127. Bramley M. Study of female babies of women entering confinement with vaginal trichomoniasis. *Br J Vener Dis* 1976;25:58.
128. Garber GE, Lemchuck-Favel CT, Rousseau G. Effect of beta-estradiol on production of the cell detaching factor of *Trichomoniasis vaginalis. J Clin Microbiol* 1991;29:1847.
129. Schou M, *et al. Trichomoniasis vaginalis* is now a very rare disease in Sweden. Scandinavian Society for Genitourinary Medicine, Vth Meeting, 1988, p37.
130. Summary information from Form KC60 (SM 12 B). New cases seen at National Health Service Genitourinary Medicine Clinics in England. 1990 Annual Figures. London: Department of Health, 1993.
131. Ledru S, Nicolas M, Mohamed F, *et al.* Etiologic study of genitourinary infections in childbearing age in Bobo-Dioulasso, Burkina Faso, 1996. *Sex Transm Dis* 1996;23:151.
132. Goldenberg RL, Klebanoff MA, Nugent R, *et al.* Bacterial colonization of the vagina during pregnancy in four ethnic groups. *Am J Obstet Gynecol* 1996;174:1618.
133. Wolner-Hanssen P, Krieger JN, Stevens CE, *et al.* Clinical manifestation of vaginal trichomoniasis. *J Am Med Assoc* 1989;264:571.
134. Dan M, Sobel JD. Trichomoniasis as seen in a chronic vaginitis clinic. *Infect Dis Obstet Gynecol* 1996;4:77.
135. Josey WE, Campbell WG Jr. Vaginitis emphysematosa. A report of four cases. *J Reprod Med* 1990;35:974.
136. Soper DE, Bump RC, Hurt WG. Bacterial vaginosis and trichomoniasis vaginitis are risk factors for cuff cellulitis after abdominal hysterectomy. *Am J Obstet Gynecol* 1990;163:1016.
137. Krieger NJ, Tam MR, Stevens CE, *et al.* Diagnosis of trichomoniasis: Comparison of conventional wet mount examination with cytologic studies, cultures, and monoclonal antibody staining of direct specimen. *J Am Med Assoc* 1988;259:1223.
138. DeMeo LR, Draper DL, McGregor JA, *et al.* Evaluation of deoxyribonucleic acid probe for the detection of *Trichomoniasis vaginalis* in vaginal secretions. *Am J Obstet Gynecol* 1996;174:1339.
139. Patel SR, Wiese W, Patel SC, Ohl C, Byrd JC, Estrada CA. Systematic review of diagnostic tests for vaginal trichomoniasis. *Infect Dis Obstet Gynecol* 2000;8:248.
140. Poch F, Levin D, Levin S, Dan M. Modified thioglycolate medium: A simple reliable means for detection of *Trichomoniasis vaginalis. J Clin Microbiol* 1996;34:2630.
141. Burtin P, Taddis A, Ariburner J, Einasson TR, Koren G. Safety of metronidazole in pregnancy: a meta-analysis. *Am J Obstet Gynecol* 1995;172:525.
142. Falayas ME, Walker AM, Jick H, Ruthazer R, Griffith J, Snydham DR. Cancer incidence after metronidazole use: A matched metronidazole user/non-user study of 60,054 subjects. *Presented at the 36th Conference on Antimicrobial Agents and Chemotherapy*, New Orleans, LA, 1996. Abstract K41:September.
143. Phelps WC, Alexander KA. Antiviral therapy for human papillomavirus: Rationale and prospects. *Ann Intern Med* 1995;123:368.
144. Bonnez W, Reichman RC. Papillomaviruses. In Mandell GL, Bennett JE, Dolin R, eds. *Principles and Practice of Infectious Diseases*, 5th edn. New York: Churchill Livingstone, 2000:1630.
145. Smotkin D. Human papillomavirus infection of the vagina. *Clin Obstet Gynecol* 1933;36:188.
146. Daling JR, Weiss NS, Hislop TG, *et al.* Sexual practices, sexually transmitted diseases and the incidence of anal cancer. *N Engl J Med* 1987;317:973.
147. Figueroa JP, Ward E, Luthi TE, Vermund SH, Brathwaite AR, Burk RD. Prevalence of human papillomavirus among STD clinic attendees in Jamaica: Association of younger age and increased sexual activity. *Sex Transm Dis* 1995;22:114.
148. Rando RF, Lindheim S, Hasty L, Sedlacek V, Woodland M, Eder C. Increased frequency of detection of huma papillomavirus deoxyribonucleic acid in exfoliated cervical cells during pregnancy. *Am J Obstet Gynecol* 1989;161:50.
149. Karlsson R, Jonsson M, Edlund K, *et al.* Lifetime number of partners as the only independent risk factor for human papillomavirus infection: a population-based study. *Sex Transm Dis* 1995;22:119.
150. Jamison JH, Kaplan DW, Hammon R, Eagar R, Beach R, Douglas JM. Spectrum of genital human papillomavirus infection in a female adolescent population. *Sex Transm Dis* 1995;22:236.
151. Puranen M, Yliskoski M, Saarikoski S, Syrjanen K, Syrjanen S. Vertical transmission of human papillomavirus from infected mother to their newborn babies and persistence of the virus in childhood. *Am J Obstet Gynecol* 1996;174:694.
152. Tseng C-J, Lin C-Y, Wang R-L, *et al.* Possible transplacental transmission of human papillomavirus. *Am J Obstet Gynecol* 1992;166:35.
153. Steinberg BM. Papillomavirus: effects upon mother and child. *Ann N Y Acad Sci* 1988;549:118.
154. Kiviat NB, Koutsky LA, Paavonen JA, *et al.* Prevalence of genital papillomavirus infection among women attending a college student health clinic or sexually transmitted disease clinic. *J Infect Dis* 1989;159:293.
155. Gary R, Jones R. Relationship between cervical condylomata, pregnancy and subclinical papillomavirus infection. *J Reprod Med* 1985;30:393.
156. Fife KH, Rogers RE, Zwicki BW. Symptomatic and asymptomatic cervical infections with human papillomavirus during pregnancy. *J Infect Dis* 1987;156:904.
157. Schneider A, Hotz M, Gissmann L. Increased prevalence of human papillomavirus in the lower genital tract of pregnant women. *Int J Cancer* 1987;40:198.
158. Kemp EA, Hakenewerth AM, Laurent SL, Gravitt PE, Stoerker J. Human papillomavirus prevalence in pregnancy. *Obstet Gynecol* 1992;79:649.
159. Smith EM, Ritchie JM, Yankowitz J, *et al.* Human papillomavirus prevalence and types in newborns and parents: Concordance and modes of transmission. *Sex Transm Dis* 2004;31:57.
160. Neff JM. Parapoxoviruses and molluscum contagiosum and tanopox viruses. In Mandell GC, Bennett JE, Dolin R, eds. *Principles and Practice of Infectious Diseases*, 5th edn. New York: Churchill Livingstone, 2000:1556.
161. Hand WC. Haemophilus species (including chanroid). In Mandell GL, Bennett JE, Dalin R, eds. *Principles and Practice of Infectious Diseases*, 5th edn. New York: Churchill Livingstone, 2000:2378.
162. Plummer FA, D'Costa LJ, Nsanze H, *et al.* Epidemiology of chanroid and *Haemophilus ducreyi* in Nairobi, Kenya. *Lancet* 1983;2:1293.
163. Nsanze H, Fast M, D'Costa CJ, *et al.* Genital ulcer in Kenya: A clinical and laboratory study of 100 patients. *Br J Vener Dis* 1981;57:371.
164. Schmid GP, Sanders LL Jr, Blount JM, *et al.* Chanroid in the United States: reestablishment of an old disease. *J Am Med Assoc* 1987;258:3265.
165. Flood JM, Sarafian SK, Bolan GA, *et al.* Multistrain outbreak of chanroid in San Francisco, 1989–1991. *J Infect Dis* 1993;167:1106.
166. Piot P, Holmes KK. Sexually transmitted diseases. In Warren KS, Mahmoud AAF, eds. *Tropical and Geographical Medicine*, 2nd edn. New York, McGraw-Hill, 1990:894.
167. Centers for Disease Control and Prevention, Division of STD/412 Prevention. *Sexually Transmitted Disease Surveillance 1992.* Atlanta, GA: Center for Disease Control, 1992.
168. Lewis DA. Chancroid: Clinical manifestations, diagnosis, and management. *Sex Transm Infect* 2003;79:68.

169. DiCarlo RP, Armentor BS, Martin DM. Chanroid epidemiology in New Orleans men. *J Infect Dis* 1995;172:446.
170. Tyndall MW, Agoki E, Plummer FA, Malisa W, Ndinya-Achola JO, Ronald AR. Single dose azithromycin for the treatment of chanroid: a randomized comparison with erythromycin. *Sex Transm Dis* 1994;21:231–4.
171. Martin DH, Sergent SJ, Wendel GD, McCormack WM, Spier NA, Johnson RB. Comparison of azithromycin and ceftriaxone for the treatment of chanroid. *Clin Infect Dis* 1995;21:409–19.
172. Ballard RC. Calymmatobacterium granulomatis (donovanosis, granuloma inguinale). In Mandell GL, Bennett JE, Dolin R, eds. *Principles and Practice of Infectious Diseases*, 5th edn. New York, Churchill Livingstone, 2000:2457.
173. O'Farrell N. Donovanosis (granuloma inguinale) in pregnancy. *Int J STD AIDS* 1991;2:447.
174. Richens J. The diagnosis and treatment of donovanosis (granuloma inguinale). *Genitourin Med* 1991;67:441.

159 Human immunodeficiency virus/AIDS in pregnancy and delivery

K. Olshtain-Pops and S. Maayan

Epidemiology

In the latter part of the 1990s, human immunodeficiency virus (HIV) infection spread to all continents, infecting some 30,000,000 individuals.[1] The greatest burden of the infection was felt in the developing world, where an estimated 90% of infected individuals resided. The World Health Organization has estimated that by the year 2000 a total of 40,000,000 individuals will have been infected by the AIDS virus since the start of the epidemic in 1981.[2] Four different patterns of spread of HIV have been described.[3] Pattern 1 is seen mainly in the developing world; HIV infection spreads mainly as a sexually transmitted disease (STD), about 50% of those affected being women. Pattern 2 is seen mainly in the developed world; the virus spreads mainly among homosexuals, drug abusers and persons receiving contaminated blood transfusions. Heterosexual spread is the exception rather than the rule and thus only 20% of HIV seropositives are women, and most are intravenous drug abusers. Although the rate of heterosexually acquired HIV infection among females in pattern 2 countries has been increasing steadily, it is not expected to reach the rates in the developing world.[4] Pattern 3 spread has been described in Southeast Asia and India,[5,6] and is characterized by a late introduction of HIV infection (in the early 1990s) and a rapid spread among heterosexuals. Male-to-female ratios reach African proportions of roughly 1:1. Pattern 4 spread has been seen in the Middle East, with a slow spread of the epidemic, mainly among established groups with risky behavior.[7,8]

The AIDS virus, target cells for the virus and molecular epidemiology of HIV1

The AIDS virus, human immunodeficiency virus 1 (HIV1), is a member of the retrovirus family to which three other human viruses [HIV2, human T-cell lymphoma virus 1 (HTLV1) and HTLV2] and several other primate viruses (SIV in monkeys, FELV in cats) belong. Only HIV1 and HIV2 cause immunodeficiency, but HIV2, a less pathogenic virus than HIV1, is endemic only in West Africa.[9] HIV1 has spread worldwide. Like other retroviruses, HIV1 is characterized by the retroversion of its genetic material, from RNA to DNA, upon penetration to target cells. This retroversion is done by the viral enzyme, reverse transcriptase, in the cytoplasm of target cells. The AIDS virus uses two major receptors on target cells for anchoring and penetration: CD4 and CCR5/CXCR2.[10–12] Research on CD4 receptors detected their abundance on T-helper cells, macrophages, Langerhans and glia cells. All these cells are thus targets for HIV1. Although no CD4 receptors were detected on spermatozoites, HIV1 was detected,[13] the idea being that CD4 receptor is present but not expressed on spermatozoites.[9] The CCR5/CXCR2 receptors were shown in 1996 to be second and indispensable receptors for HIV to penetrate target cells.[10] It was also shown that macrophages and Langerhans tropical strains of HIV uses the CCR5 receptor, while lymphocyte tropical strains use the CXCR2 receptor.[12] As was recently shown, the lack of this second receptor confers natural resistance to HIV infection.[11]

HIV subtypes and their importance

HIV1 is constantly mutagenic in its component (envelope, core and enzymes). The rate of mutations, however, is not constant.[12] Mutations in the envelope region tend to cluster in several patterns, giving rise to different viral clades (quasispecies, subtypes). Eight HIV subtypes (A–F) were thus described. All were found to circulate in equatorial Africa. Only the B subtype is endemic in North America, Europe and Australia, while in Southeast Asia, the B, C and E sub types predominate.[15,16] Some studies have recently suggested that different viral strains have different tropism to target cells in the immune system: E and C HIV subtypes replicate better in Langerhans cells, which are abundant in the sexual organs, while B subtypes replicate better in peripheral blood lymphocytes derived from the circulation.[17,18] The suggestion was made that this different pattern of replication may account in part for the difference in the prevailing mode of transmission of HIV in the different continents. Thus, in areas where non-B subtypes prevail (Africa and Asia), heterosexual transmissions of the virus prevail. In areas where the B subtype prevails, contact with contaminated blood plays a significant role in HIV transmission. Recently, a preferential expression of the CCR5 receptor on Langerhans cells was proposed as accounting for the preferential heterosexual transmission of macrophage tropical HIV strains.[18,19]

Diagnosis of HIV1 infection

The mainstay of diagnosis of HIV1 is antibody tests (AIDS tests).[19] Two types of tests are being used: ELISA tests for screening and western blot tests for confirmation. Screening tests, very sensitive and somewhat less specific, employ selected recombinant HIV proteins as antigens. Confirmatory (western blot) tests employ all HIV proteins as antigens. Since confirmatory tests are more specific than the screening tests, all positive screening tests need to be confirmed. Diagnostic pitfalls of HIV infection arise mainly in two situations:

(1) The initial 3 months following seroconversion ('window period'). In this period antibody levels are too low to be detected with the current HIV screening tests, giving false-negative results.
(2) During the perinatal period and up to 18 months of age in infants born to HIV seropositive mothers. Due to passive transfer of HIV antibodies through the placenta, HIV antibody tests in these infants will invariably be positive even if perinatal transmission of HIV did not occur. Since the current rate of HIV transmission in zidovudine-treated women is about 8%, most perinatal HIV antibody tests give false-positive results[21] (discussed elsewhere in this book). All infants seropositive due to passive transfer will serorevert by 18 months.[22]

To overcome the diagnostic difficulties during these periods, HIV(P24) antigen tests can be used. The presence of HIV antigen in the serum points to active replication of HIV (established infection). A positive test in the window period or during the perinatal period confirms the presence of true HIV infection. Clinical data suggest, however, that the sensitivity of the antigen test may not be higher than the current antibody tests.[23]

Other potentially useful tests in this category employ virologic tests: the polymerase chain reaction technique for detection of HIV DNA sequences in lymphocytes and for measuring HIV viral load. Negative tests by 6 months of age exclude perinatal HIV transmission.[22]

Natural history of HIV infection: viral dynamics

During the initial 2–10 weeks following seroconversion, acute HIV syndrome, with a pattern resembling infectious mononucleosis, may appear in 50–80% of individuals.[24] The main symptoms of fever, maculopapular rash and lymphadenopathy are at times accompanied by meningoencephalitic features. Viral load during this phase is very high, with millions of copies of HIV RNA/ml. The syndrome usually resolves spontaneously, viral load decreases to lower levels and the infected person enters the asymptomatic clinical phase, lasting an average of 2–8 years. During this period, massive viral replication and destruction of target cells continues relentlessly, mainly in the lymph glands. On average, some 2 billion CD4+ cells are eliminated by the virus every 24 h with partial replenishment from preexisting pools.[24–26] This gradual elimination of CD4+ cells leads to the gradual loss of almost all cell-mediated immunity, which, in turn, results in the development of full-blown AIDS (the reactivation of opportunistic infections) and death, usually by 8–10 years following infection.

Drug therapy for HIV infection

The late 1990s have witnessed significant breakthroughs in the field of antiretroviral treatment.[27] The combination of two, three or four drugs highly active antiretroviral (HAART) of the reverse transcriptase and protease inhibitors has shown promise in arresting HIV replication over long periods and lowering HIV load in plasma to undetectable levels. In addition, these 'cocktail' HAART combinations prevented the emergence of resistant HIV mutants over periods of over 2 years.[28,29] The clinical effectiveness of these combinations was soon to be manifested in the form of lowering hospitalization and death rates of AIDS patients.[30] The 'cocktail' combinations are available only in the West. Their cost prohibits their present and future usage in the developing world, where most HIV infections occur. Although very effective, the long-term side effects and effectiveness of these combinations are still unknown.

Three types of antiretroviral agents form the current 'cocktail' combinations:

(1) *Reverse transcriptase inhibitors*: These drugs, nucleic acid analogs, cause chain termination in the process of transcribing HIV RNA to DNA by the viral enzyme reverse transcriptase in the cytoplasm.

The currently approved drugs are zidovudine, zalcitabine, didanosine, 3TC and D4T. When given as monotherapy, these drugs lose their effectiveness after a few months due to the rapid emergence of resistant mutations of the reverse transcriptase enzyme. The drug should be administered in combination with other drugs, non-reverse-transcriptase inhibitors, in order to lower the rate of emergence of resistant viral mutants.

(2) *Non-nucleoside reverse transcriptase inhibitors*: These block reverse transcription by mechanisms other than being nucleoside analogs. These drugs should always be given in combination with other drugs. The available drugs are nevirapine, atevridine and delavridine.

(3) *Protease inhibitors*: These drugs block HIV protease activity during proteolitic cleavage of viral proteins following transcription. Despite their great *in vitro* effectiveness, rapid emergence of resistance follows their use as monotherapy. The available drugs are indinavir, ritonavir, saquinavir and nelfimaviz.

Natural history of HIV infection in women and during pregnancy

In controlled studies, no appreciable gender differences in the rate of acceleration of established HIV infection were observed.[31,32] Detection of HIV infection among women was sometimes delayed due to a lack of awareness of the importance of vaginal candidiasis as a presenting sign of HIV infection. An increased incidence of cervical dysplasia was found among HIV seropositive women[33,34] and cervical neoplasia has been clearly associated with human papilloma virus infection.[35] Pregnancy does not seem to affect the natural course of HIV infection.[36] Congenital anomalies due to HIV infection in the first trimester were described, although their occurrence is rare.[36]

HIV transmission through the female genital tract

The presence of concomitant STD and bacterial vaginosis was found to play a critical role in easing HIV transmission.[37–39] Treatment of STD, as seen in the African setting, was shown to reduce HIV transmission rates. An association between HIV load in vaginal secretions and the presence of vaginal inflammation was also demonstrated. Other biochemical and physical factors, e.g. the use of contraceptive pills, the lack of male circumcision, vitamin A deficiency, the presence of bacterial vaginosis and trichomonas vaginalis, were also associated with increased rates of acquisition of HIV in the African setting.[38–45]

Perinatal transmission of HIV

Multiple factors probably play a role in aiding perinatal HIV transmission. Detailed studies recently demonstrated a direct correlation between high HIV viral load in the plasma of pregnant women and the increased rate of HIV transmission to the newborn.[42,43] However, in the landmark placebo-controlled zidovudine intervention study of over 800 pregnant women followed to term in the USA, Europe and Australia, HIV transmission occurred at all levels of HIV viral load.[46] A low CD4 level during pregnancy was also associated with increased rates of HIV transmission, as well as low vitamin A levels (in African women).[44] The most important obstetrical factor associated with increased HIV transmission was found in a large prospective US study to be the premature rupture of membranes of over 4 h in HIV seropositive women.[47]

Timing of HIV transmission

Despite the findings of placentitis in placentas of seropositive mothers,[38] studies have indicated that most HIV transmission to the newborn occurs during delivery and the perinatal period, rather than in the first trimester of pregnancy.[48,49] Supporting evidence for this comes from the rarity of congenital HIV syndrome and from analysis of twins born to HIV seropositive mothers: statistically, more first- than second-borns are found to be infected by HIV, suggesting transmission during passage in the birth canal.[50,51]

The importance of breast feeding in HIV transmission during the perinatal period has been demonstrated since early on in the epidemic in studies carried out in Australia and Africa.[52,53] It is estimated that 15–20% of perinatal HIV transmission in Africa occurs as a result of breast feeding. However, since the alternative, bottle feeding, carries a far greater danger to infant health in the form of gastroenteritis and dehydration, UNESCO has ruled that breast feeding should continue to be the practice of choice in infant nutrition during the AIDS era in underdeveloped countries.[54,55]

Drug therapy with zidovudine to reduce perinatal transmission of HIV

A pivotal study, completed in 1994 and updated in 1996, has demonstrated conclusively that zidovudine, given in the second and third trimesters as well as during delivery and for 6 weeks to the newborn infant, reduces HIV transmission to the newborn by approximately 66% (from 22.6% to 7.6%).[46,48] This cornerstone, placebo-controlled study, has changed the practice of obstetrics in pregnant HIV seropositive women in the West. The exact factors that determine the lowering of HIV transmission in zidovudine-treated women are still poorly understood. In many of the study participants receiving zidovudine, HIV transmission did not occur despite a meager degree of reduction in plasma viral HIV load. Other factors, such as the zidovudine level in the newborn tissues, may account for the apparent protection. The success of this intervention study has prompted modifications aimed at making zidovudine treatment accessible to pregnant women in the developing world. Newer protocols such as a single dose of zidovudine given during delivery or parenteral zidovudine given only during active delivery are being studied in Africa and Thailand. Other protocols with combination antiretrovirals aimed at lowering perinatal transmission of HIV even further.[56–58]

Other interventions

No conclusive evidence for the protective role of cesarean section has yet surfaced, although two meta-analyses addressing this issue have demonstrated the existence of clear benefit of this procedure in reducing HIV transmission to the newborn compared to vaginal delivery.[59,60] The analyses were carried out prior to the introduction of zidovudine to the routine care of pregnant women. Other procedures, such as cleansing of the vaginal canal with chlorhexidine prior to delivery were not shown to reduce the rate of HIV transmission.[61]

Recommended zidovudine protocol for the prevention of HIV transmission during delivery

To the expectant mother, zidovudine 500 mg is given daily in the second and third trimesters. During delivery, a loading dose of intravenous zidovudine 2 mg/kg is given over 1 h. Maintenance intravenous zidovudine is administered, 1 mg/kg/h until half an hour after termination of delivery. Within 8–12 h following delivery, administration of zidovudine syrup to the newborn is started, 2 mg/kg/dose every 6 h for 6 weeks.[54]

Additional recommendations

Cesarean section should be considered if the delivering women are at advanced stages of HIV infection, will not receive intravenous zidovudine and have had over 4 h of premature rupture of membranes.[47]

Breast feeding should be discouraged for all infants born to HIV seropositive mothers in developed countries.[54] All killed vaccines (e.g. pneumococcal, hepatitis B) as well as Hib and influenza virus should be given to the pregnant woman. They should also receive the same prophylactic regimens as non-pregnant women. Trimethoprim sulfamethoxazole appears safe as prophylaxis against pneumocystic pneumonia during pregnancy. Dapsone is also safe and should be used in cases of allergy to trimethoprim sulfamethoxazole.

Conclusion

HIV among women continues to spread unabated worldwide, especially in sub-Saharan Africa and Southeast Asia. In recent years, important biological factors have been defined as cofactors in HIV transmission to women and during delivery. The lack of access to medical care in many parts of the world delays effective therapy. However, no biological differences in disease progression or response to antiretroviral drugs, when available, can be detected among women.

REFERENCES

1. Global HIV/Aids Surveillance. *Weekly Epidemiological Records* 1997;72:365–72.
2. UNAIDS/WHO. Report on the global HIV/AIDS epidemic. *Lancet* 1997;350:1683.
3. Mertens TE, Burton A. Estimates and trends of the HIV/AIDS epidemic. *AIDS* 1996;10(Suppl):S221–8.
4. Stein Z, Susser M. AIDS – An update on the global dynamics. *Am J Public Health* 1997;87:901.
5. Richner B, Laurent D, Sunnarat, *et al.* Spread of HIV1 to children in Cambodia. *Lancet* 1997;349:1451–2.
6. Muller O, Ungchusak K, Leng HB, Chung A, Tadiar F. HIV and AIDS in Southeast Asia. *Lancet* 1997;350:288.
7. Quinn TC. The global burden of the HIV pandemic. *Lancet* 1997;348:99–105.
8. Weniger BG, Brown T. The march of AIDS through Asia. *Lancet* 1996;335:343–4.
9. Travers K, Mboup S, Marlink R, *et al.* Natural protection against HIV1 infection provided by HIV2. *Science* 1995;268:1612–5.
10. Huang Y, Paxton WA, Wolinsky SM, *et al.* The role of mutant CCR5 allele in HIV1 transmission and disease progression. *Nat Med* 1996;2:1240–3.
11. Liu R, Paxton WA, Choe S. Homozygous defect in HIV1 coreceptor accounts for resistance of multiple exposed individuals to HIV1 infection. *Cell* 1996;86:367–77.
12. Berger EA. HIV entry and tropism. The chemokine receptor connection. *AIDS* 1997;11(Suppl A):S3–16.
13. Basarga O, Farzadegan H, Seshamma T, Oakes JW, Saah A, Pomerantz RJ. Detection of HIV1 proviral DNA in sperm from HIV1 infected men. *AIDS* 1994;8:1669–74.
14. UNAIDS. HIV1 subtypes – Implication for epidemiololgy, pathogenicity, vaccine and diagnosis. *AIDS* 1997;11:S17–36.
15. Gehring S, Maayan S, Ruppach H, *et al.* Molecular epidemiology of HIV in Israel. *J AIDS* 1997;15:296–303.
16. Ou CY, Takebe Y, Lou CC, *et al.* The epidemiology of HIV infection and AIDS in Thailand. *AIDS Res Hum Retroviruses* 1992; 8:1471–2.

17. Fowke KR, Nagelkerthe NJD, Kimani J, *et al.* Resistance to HIV1 infection among persistently seronegative prostitutes in Nairobi, Kenya. *Lancet* 1996;348:1347–51.
18. Soto Ramirez LE, Rengifo B, McLane M, *et al.* HIV1 LC tropism associated with heterosexual transmission of HIV. *Science* 1996;271:1291–3.
19. Graziosi C, Pantaleo G. The multifaceted personality of HIV. *Nat Med* 1997;3:1318–20.
20. Zaitseva A, Blauvelt A, Lee S, *et al.* Expression and function of CCR5 and CXCR4 on human LC's and macrophages: Implications for HIV primary infection. *Nat Med* 1997;3:1369–75.
21. CDC. Serologic testing for antibody against HIV1. *Morbid Mortal Weekly Rep* 1988;36:833–45.
22. CDC-USPHS. Recommendations for HIV counseling and voluntary testing for pregnant women. *Morbid Mortal Weekly Rep* 1995;44:1–14.
23. Chaisson ME, Volberding PA. Clinical manifestations of HIV infection. In Mandell, Douglas, Bennett, eds. *Principles and Practice of Infectious Diseases,* 4th edn. 1995:1217–47.
24. Pantaleo G, Graziosi C, Demarest JF, *et al.* HIV infection is active and progressive in lymphoid tissue during the clinically latent stage of disease. *Nature (Lond)* 1993;362:355–8.
25. Ho DD, Neuman AU, Perelson AS, Chan W, Leonard JM, Markovitz M. Rapid turnover of plasma virions and CD4 lymphocytes in HIV infection. *Nature (Lond)* 1995;373:123–6.
26. Wolthers KC, Bea G, Wisman A, *et al.* T cell telomere length in HIV1 infection: No evidence for increased CD4 T cell turnover. *Science* 1996;274:1543–7.
27. Cameron B, Heath-Chiozzi M, Kravcik S, *et al.* Prolongation of life and prevention of AIDS in advanced HIV immunodeficiency with ritonavir. Presented at the *Third Conference on Retrovinises,* Washington, DC, 1996: Abstract LB6a.
28. Hammer SM, Katzenstein DA, Hughes MD, *et al.* A trial comparing nucleoside monotherapy with combination therapy in HIV infected adults with CD4 counts 200–500/ml (the 75 trial). *N Engl J Med* 1996;335:1081–90.
29. Carpenter CC, Fischl MA, Hammer SM, *et al.* Antiretroviral therapy for HIV infection in 1997. *J Am Med Assoc* 1997;277:1962–9.
30. Staszewski S, Bartlet J, Hill AM, Katlama C, Johnson J. Reduction in HIV1 disease progression for zidovudine–ramivudine relative to control treatments. *AIDS* 1997;11:474–83.
31. Johnson MA, Johnstone F, eds. *HIV Infection and Women.* London: Churchill Livingstone, 1993.
32. Cotton DJ. Aids in women. In Pizzo, Wilfert, eds. *Pediatric Aids, the Challenge of HIV Infection in Infants, Children and Adolescents,* 2nd edn. Baltimore: Williams & Wilkins, 1994:161–8.
33. Henry M, Stanley M, Cruishank S, Carson L. Association of HIV, HPV and cervical intraepithelial neoplasia. *Am J Obstet Gynecol* 1989;160:52–3.
34. Schrager L, Friedland GH, Maud D, *et al.* Cervical and vaginal squamous cell abnormalities in women infected by HIV1. *J AIDS* 1989;2:570–5.
35. Munoz N, Bosch FX, Jensen OM. *Epidemiology of Cervical Cancer.* WHO Agency for Research on Cancer: Scientific Publications, 1989:9–39.
36. Koonin LM, Elklerbrook TV, Atrawsh HK, *et al.* Pregnancy associated death due to AIDS in the US. *J Am Med Assoc* 1989;3:1306–9.
37. Selwyn PA, Schoenbaum EE, Davenny K, *et al.* Prospective study of HIV infection and pregnancy outcome in intravenous drug users. *J Am Med Assoc* 1989;261:1289–94.
38. Plummer FA, Simonsen JN, Cameron DW, *et al.* Cofactors in male–female sexual transmission of HIV1. *J Infect Dis* 1991;163:233–9.
39. Laga M, Alary M, Nzila N, *et al.* Condom promotion, sexually transmitted diseases treatment, and declining incidence of HIV1 in female Zairian sex workers. *Lancet* 1994;344:246–8.
40. Grosskurth H, Mosha F, Todd J, *et al.* Impact of improved treatment of sexually transmitted diseases on HIV infection in rural Tanzania. *Lancet* 1995:346:530–6.
41. Sewenkamblo N, Gray RH, Wawer M, *et al.* HIV1 infection associated with abnormal vaginal flora morphology and bacterial vaginosis. *Lancet* 1997;350:546–50.
42. Moss GB, Overbaugh J, Welch M, *et al.* HIV1 DNA in urethral secretions in men: Association with gonococcal urethritis and CD4 depletion. *J Infect Dis* 1995;172:1469–75.
43. Eron JJ, Gilliam B, Fiscus S, Dyer J, Cohen MS. HIV1 shedding and chlamydia urethritis. *J Am Med Assoc* 1996;275:36.
44. Mostad SB, Overbangh J, Devange DM. Hormonal contraception, vit A deficiency and other risk factors for shedding of HIV 1 infected cells from the cervix and vagina. *Lancet* 1997;350:992–7.
45. Moses S, Bradley JE, Nagalkerke NJ, Ronald AR, Njinya JO, Plummer FA. Geographical patterns of male circumcision practices in Africa: Association with HIV prevalance. *Int J Epidemiol* 1990;19:693–7.
46. Sperling RS, Shapiro DE, Coomby RW, *et al.* Maternal viral load, zidovudine treatment and the risk of transmission of HIV1 from mother to infant. *N Engl J Med* 1996;335:1621–9.
47. Landesman SH, Kalish LH, Burns DN, *et al.* Obstetrical factors and the transmission of HIV1 from mother to child. *N Engl J Med* 1996;334:1617–23.
48. Connor EM, Sperling RS, Gelber R, *et al.* Reduction of maternal infant transmission of HIV1 with Zidovudine (the 076 study). *N Engl J Med* 1994;331:1173–80.
49. Goedert JJ, Duliege AM, Amos CI, Felton S, Biggar RJ. High risk of HIV1 infection for first born twins. *Lancet* 1991;338:1471–5.
50. Ehrnst A, Lindgren A, Dicor M, *et al.* HIV in pregnant women and their offsprings: Evidence for late transmission. *Lancet* 1991; 338:203–7.
51. Rogers MF, Ou CY, Kilbornne B, Schochetman G. Advances and problems in the diagnosis of HIV infection in infants. *Pediatr Inf Dis J* 1991;10:523–31.
52. Ziegler JB. Breast feeding and HIV. *Lancet* 1993;342:1437–8.
53. Ekpini ER, Wiktor SZ, Satten GA. Late postnatal mother to child transmission of HIV1 in Abidjan, Cote d'Ivoire. *Lancet* 1997;349:1054–9.
54. WHO/UNICEF. Statement on breast feeding and HIV. WHO/ UNICEF consultative meeting. *Weekly Epidemiol Rec* 1992;67:177–84.
55. European Collaborative Study. Risk factor for mother to child transmission of HIV1. *Lancet* 1992;339:1007–12.
56. Cohen J. Bringing AZT to poor countries. *Science* 1995;269:624–5.
57. Wiznia AA, Crane A, Lambert G, Sansary J, Harris A, Solomon L. Zidovudine use to reduce perinatal HIV1 transmission in an urban medical center. *J Am Med Assoc* 1996;275:1504–6.
58. Fiscus SA, Adimora AA, Schonbach UJ, *et al.* Prenatal HIV infection and the effect of zidovudine therapy on transmission in rural and urban counties. *J Am Med Assoc* 1996;275:1483–8.
59. European Collaborative Study. Caesarian section and risk of vertical transmission of HIV1 infection. *Lancet* 1994;343:1464–7.
60. Villari P, Spino C, Chalmers TC, Sacks HS. Caesarian section to reduce perinatal transmission of HIV1. A meta-analysis. *On-line J Curr Clin Trials* 1993:Document 74.
61. Biggar RJ, Miotti PF, Taha TE, *et al.* Perinatal intervention trial in Africa: Effect of a birth canal cleansing intervention to prevent HIV transmission. *Lancet* 1996;347;1647–50.
62. Zidovudine for the prevention of HIV transmission from mother to infant. *Morbid Mortal Weekly Rep* 1994;43:286–9.

160 Pneumonia in pregnancy

D. Miron and R. Raz

Introduction

The prevalence of antepartum pneumonia is 1 in 350 to 2300 deliveries. Maternal conditions associated with increased risk for the infection are immunodeficiency state (e.g. HIV/AIDS, malignancy and chemotherapy), chronic cardiopulmonary disease, diabetes mellitus, poor nutrition, cocaine use, smoking and anemia. Such risk factors were found in up to 45% of pregnant women who presented with pneumonia.[1–5]

Etiology

The agents associated with pneumonia in a pregnant woman are those that most commonly cause pneumonia in non-pregnant women. Currently, in 40–60% of patients, no agents can be found despite improved laboratory diagnosis (see below).[1,5]

The most frequent organism causing community-acquired pneumonia is *Streptococcus pneumoniae.* Other less common agents are *Haemophilus influenzae* and β-hemolytic streptococcus. A large section of pregnant women with pneumonia is made up of those with atypical pneumonia. Common etiologic agents include *Mycoplasma pneumonia*, *Legionella pneumophilia*, *Chlamydia pneumonia* and viruses.[1,2,6,7] Infection with *Coxiella burneti* (Q-fever) can occur in endemic areas (including Israel) with frequent contact with domestic animals or unpasteurized milk.[7] The bacteria can infect the placenta, resulting in prematurity, low birth weight or fetal death. Chicken pox during pregnancy is associated with pneumonitis in 10–20% of patients, which may be life-threatening. In endemic areas, yeast infections such as *Coccidioides immitis* or *Histoplasma capsultum* may be life-threatening. Nosocomial pneumonia is usually caused by gram-negative bacteria (e.g. *Klebsiella pneumonia*, *Pseudomonas* spp.) or anaerobic bacteria.[1,2,5]

More women with primary or secondary immunodeficiency are now surviving through their reproductive years and attempting pregnancy. In these women, unusual agents have been associated with pneumonia, including *Pneumocystis carinii*, *Mycobacterium avium* complex (mostly in women with AIDS) and *Mycobacterium tuberculosis* (MTB). In areas endemic for tuberculosis, infection of pregnant women with MTB can be associated with either congenital tuberculosis or infection of young infants by untreated mothers.[2,4,5]

Diagnosis

In about 40–60% of women with pneumonia a specific agent can be found. The most helpful tests are sputum for gram stain and culture, sputum and urine for antigen detection, blood culture and serology. Specific diagnostic measures for the main causes of pneumonia are presented in Table 160.1.

An adequate sputum test is defined as > 25 neutrophils and < 10 epithelial cells per low-powered microscopic field. Sputum can be obtained either by induction or by bronchoalveolar lavage (BAL). Gram stain of the sputum remains the commonest way for rapid identification of causative agents. For example, predominance of gram-positive diplococci is highly suggestive of pneumococcal pneumonia.[1,2]

Several rapid, highly sensitive and specific diagnostic methods have recently been developed using sputum. Direct fluorescent assays for *Legionella* and *Pneumocystis carinii* antigens have 50–80% sensitivity and > 95% specificity. DNA hybridization tests for ribosomal RNA and polymerase chain reaction (PCR) amplification are also highly sensitive, specific and rapid tests that are commercially available for identification of *Legionella* and MTB. These tests can profoundly shorten the time of identification of the agent and initiation of effective therapy. In 5–20% of patients with bacterial pneumonia, blood cultures are positive. Most of the available serology tests are of enzyme-linked immunosorbent assay (ELISA). These tests are highly sensitive and specific. A radioimmunoassay test for identifying *Legionella pneumophilia* serogroup I antigen in the urine is a new method with comparable sensitivity to other methodologies, and is much easier to perform.[1,2,5]

Clinical manifestations

Signs and symptoms of pneumonia vary, depending on the agent causing the disease and the patient's

Table 160.1 Laboratory diagnosis of pneumonia

Agent	Sputum	Blood culture	Serology	Others
Bacterial pneumonia	Gram stain, culture of pleural	Positive		Fluid
S. pneumoniae				
H. influenzae				
Group A streptococci				
β-hemolytic streptococcus				
Atypical pneumonia				
L. pneumophilia	Direct fluorescent assay, DNA tests	Positive		Urine antigen
M. pneumonia	Probe, culture		Positive	
C. pneumonia			Positive	
Viral	Culture		Positive	
M. tuberculosis	Acid fast stain, Gastric lavage Culture Pleural biopsy DNA probe, PCR		Mantoux	Test
P. carinii	Direct fluorescent assay Bronchoalveolar Giemsa stain Lavage or lung biopsy			
Fungal pneumonia biopsy	Gram stain, culture			Lung

PCR, polymerase chain reaction

underlying immune status. Generally, most pneumonia occurs during fall and winter. Pneumococcal pneumonia presents with high fever, productive cough, chills and pleuritic chest pains. These patients may develop a stormy disease with sepsis syndrome, hypoxemia and adult respiratory distress syndrome (ARDS). The chest x-ray shows involvement of one or more lobes, or bronchopneumonia. In patients with involvement of the pleural membranes, fluid collection within the pleural cavity can be demonstrated. In such patients the disease may have a range from pleural effusion to emphysema, necessitating invasive drainage procedures and prolonged antibiotic therapy. Chest ultrasound and/or computed tomography are helpful for evaluation of the fluid volume viscosity, for the development of intrapleural cavity septa and for drainage procedures. Atypical pneumonia is more insidious in onset, with moderate fever, non-productive and sometimes prolonged cough, headache and myalgias. The disease may occasionally progress to a more advanced level. In many patients, history of a similar infection can be elicited in other family members. Chest x-ray usually demonstrates broncho- or interstitial pneumonia. Patients with *Legionella* pneumonia may present with abdominal pains (10–20%), diarrhea (25–50%), hepatitis and neuralgic symptoms ranging from lethargy to encephalopathy.[1–3,6] Contact with domestic animals (such as goats or sheep), or unpasteurized milk, could raise the possibility of Q-fever in an endemic area.[7] In patients with tuberculosis there is usually a history of exposure to an infected person. The typical presentation is of prolonged fever and cough with persistent pulmonary infiltrate (with or without pleural effusion), or cavity on the chest x-ray. These women, if not aggressively diagnosed and treated, may be highly infectious to the fetus and close contacts. In every HIV/AIDS patient with a history of prolonged cough and dyspnea, with or without fever, *Pneumocystis carinii* pneumonia must be considered. Chest x-ray shows an interstitial pattern of pneumonia, although rarely lobar involvement and abscess-like formation have been reported. Involvement of the lungs in *Mycobacterium avium* complex infection is part of multiorgan involvement in a patient with advanced AIDS or other immunocompromised conditions. *Varicella zoster* pneumonia should be suspected in every woman with chicken pox who develops dyspnea. Chest x-ray demonstrates interstitial pneumonitis. These women may deteriorate rapidly to ARDS. Chicken pox during the first half of pregnancy may be associated with a congenital varicella syndrome in 3–5% of fetuses.[2,4,5]

Prognosis

The prognosis for pregnant women with pneumonia has improved markedly since the introduction of antibiotics. Important added factors include the availability of ventilatory aids and more precise technology to monitor fluid requirements and vital signs. These advances have resulted in a reduction of maternal death from about one-third of cases to 4%. Clinical features that are associated with significant morbidity include: (1) more than one lobe involved; (2) respiratory rate greater than 30 breaths/min; (3) severe hypoxemia, hypoalbuminemia and septicemia; (4) chronic underlying disease such as immunodeficiency syndrome, diabetes mellitus or chronic pulmonary disease and poor nutrition and (5) maternal smoking.[2,3]

However, obstetric complications have not been altered, with a rate of preterm delivery of 15–43%, and perinatal death rate of 4–11%. Several factors are associated with poor outcome of the fetus. In pregnancy there is a mild increase in the alveolar–capillary difference because of an increased oxygen consumption and peripheral extraction by mother and fetus. As early as 4 weeks' gestation, progesterone effects occur, resulting in maternal hyperventilation and respiratory alkalosis.[3,4,8]

This hyperventilation of pregnancy decreases fetal oxygen tension, so that any disease such as pneumonia that causes hypoxia and dyspnea will increase the respiratory rate and have adverse effects. These include a decrease in uterine blood flow with vasoconstriction, a decrease in maternal venous return and a decrease in umbilical blood flow. Hyperventilation and hypocapnia shift the oxygen–hemoglobin dissociation curve to the left for both mother and fetus, resulting in increased hemoglobin affinity for oxygen. A dangerous situation exists if the blood pH exceeds 7.6 or the PaO_2 falls below 55 mmHg. In addition to the above effects, the increased effort from the work of breathing may result in further extraction of oxygen from the fetus and organs such as the placenta, uterus and kidneys. The uteroplacental circulation is a low-pressure, highly vascularized system, well developed by the 12th gestational week. Its blood flow is 20% of the cardiac output by the 26th gestational week. Any maternal oxygen debt will harm the fetus.[3,4,8]

It is apparent that oxygen consumed for the work of breathing has a proportionately small and smooth increase during gestation. If the mother has dyspnea and hypoxia from pulmonary disease, the oxygen required for the work of breathing may be taken from the fetus and organs such as the placenta, uterus or kidneys.[3,6,8]

Immunologic changes in the mother and fetus may contribute to the adverse outcome of pneumonia in pregnancy. The fetus has a decreased immunologic defense since only immunoglobulin G can cross the placenta, so any infection of the mother can be disastrous for the fetus. There is an increase in the normal number of T-suppressive cells formed to protect against the rejection of the fetus as a foreign body, and this may explain the reduced immune response to infections.[3]

The precise reasons for the high rate of preterm labor despite effective antimicrobial therapy are not fully explained. One postulated mechanism is a production of prostaglandins, either locally in the cervicovaginal area, or as part of the inflammation in the lungs. These agents could circulate to the uterus and produce preterm labor.

Perinatal death associated with pneumonia in pregnancy could be due to either maternal hypoxemia or premature delivery.[5,6,8]

Therapy

The key to the care of a pregnant woman with pneumonia is early diagnosis. Patients with respiratory symptoms should immediately be evaluated for the possibility of lower respiratory infection, including chest x-ray when needed. In such women with pneumonia, the etiology must be elicited by using blood cultures, sputum Gram stain and culture and other diagnostic tests as necessary. In addition, careful monitoring of arterial PO_2 and appropriate oxygenation should be performed. A healthy fetus depends on the mother keeping oxygen debt to a minimum, and supplementing oxygen is vital whenever hypoxia is manifested. A warning sign of dyspnea in pregnancy is a respiratory rate > 18 breaths/min. Premature labor can present difficulties, necessitating adequate hydration and close monitoring of uterine activity.[1,2]

Antimicrobial therapy is limited because of known or possible adverse effects on the fetus (Table 160.2). Most patients with community-acquired pneumonia can be treated as outpatients unless they are dehydrated, clinically ill or immunocompromised. For patients with typical pneumococcal pneumonia penicillin should be started, either orally or intravenously. For patients allergic to penicillin, erythromycin is the drug of choice.[1,2,5]

Recently, pneumococci that are either partially or completely resistant to penicillin have been reported from different areas in the world to cause pneumonia and other invasive diseases. In areas with a high frequency of such pneumococci, either second- or third-generation cephalosporins should be empirically initiated until sensitivity studies are available. The drug of choice for atypical pneumonia is erythromycin. Recently, new second-generation macrolides and azoles derivatives (e.g. azithromycin) have been approved for use for such infections. They have equal activity, but less adverse effects on the mother. In many cases of pneumonia, the exact causative agent cannot be

Table 160.2 Antimicrobial agents for pneumonia

Agent	Indication route	FDA pregnancy categories*
Penicillin	Typical pneumonia PO, IV, IM	B
Ampicillin or amoxicillin+BLI	Typical pneumonia PO, IV**	B
Cephalosporins	Typical pneumonia PO, IV, IM***	B
Gentamicin	Nosocomial pneumonia IV, IM	C
Amikacin	Nosocomial pneumonia IV	D
Erythromycin estolate	Bacterial and atypical pneumonia IV, PO	B
Clanthromycin	Bacterial and atypical pneumonia PO	C
Azithromycin	Atypical pneumonia PO	B
Amphotericin B	Fungal pneumonia IV	B
Fluconazole	Fungal pneumonia PO	C
Itraconazole	Fungal pneumonia PO	C
Isoniazide	Tuberculosis PO	C
Rifampin	Tuberculosis PO	C
Sulfonamides	PCP PO, IV	C
Pyrazinamide	Tuberculosis PO	–
Ethambutol	Tuberculosis PO	–
Acyclovir	Varicella pneumonia IV, PO	C

FDA, Food and Drug Administration; BLI, β-lactamase inhibitors; PCP, *Pneumocystis carinii* pneumonia; PO, oral; IV, intravenous; IM, intramuscular
*FDA pregnancy categories: A, adequate studies in pregnant women, no risk; B, animal studies show no risk but human studies not adequate, or animal toxicity but human studies show no risk; C, animal studies show toxicity, and human studies inadequate, but benefit of use may exceed risk; D, evidence of human risk, but benefits may outweigh risk; **for ampicillin sulbactan no oral drug is available; ***only third-generation cephalosporins should be used by intravenous route

determined. In these patients, therapy should be directed against the most likely organisms, which are pneumococci, *Mycoplasma* and *Legionella*. Erythromycin or second-generation macrolides have been found to be active against all and should be given empirically.[1,5]

Varicella zoster pneumonia requires special attention in pregnant women. In general, patients who are not immunocompromised are at high risk for ARDS when infected with varicella viruses, and in these cases acyclovir should be started. If a patient complains of dyspnea or tachypnea, then admission should be considered and acyclovir should be given intravenously. While in hospital, appropriate isolation measures should be taken.[2,5]

REFERENCES

1. Donowitz GR, Mandell GL. Acute pneumonia. In Mandell GL, Bennet JE, Dolin R, eds. *Principles and Practice of Infectious Diseases.* New York: Churchill Livingstone, 1995:619–37.
2. Nolan TE, Hankins GDV. Acute pulmonary dysfunction and distress. *Obstet Gynecol Clin N Am* 1995;22(1):39–54.
3. Tenholder MF, South-Paul JE. Dyspnea in pregnancy. *Chest* 1989; 96(2):381–9.
4. Berkowitz K, LaSala A. Risk factors associated with the increasing prevalence of pneumonia during pregnancy. *Am J Obstet Gynecol* 1990;163:981–5.
5. Ledger W. Respiratory tract infection. In Reece EA, Hobbins JC, Mahoney MJ, Petrie RA, eds. *Medicine of the Fetus and Mother,* 1st edn. Philadelphia: JB Lippincott Co., 1992:1187–8
6. Richey SD, Roberts SW, Ramin KD, *et al.* Pneumonia complicating pregnancy. *Obstet Gynecol* 1994;64:525–8.
7. Rault D, Stein A. Q fever during pregnancy – A risk factor for women, fetuses and obstetrician. *New Engl J Med* 1995;330:371.
8. Madinger NE, Greenspoon JF, Elrodt AG. Pneumonia during pregnancy: Has modern technology improved maternal and fetal outcome? *Am J Obstet Gynecol* 1989;61:657–62.

161 Prevention of infection in cesarean section

A. Dražančić

Introduction

The rate of cesarean sections has increased to more than 10% of all deliveries, predominantly because of fetal indications. Without an elevated incidence of cesarean section rate it is impossible to achieve low perinatal mortality and to avoid the early and late neonatal sequelae. Numerous complications are possible during and after the operation. Immediate complications, anesthesiologic and surgical, are not frequent. Early postoperative complications are more frequent, predominantly due to infection: puerperal fever, endomyometritis and suppuration of the abdominal wall, paralytic ileus, pelveoperitonitis and diffuse peritonitis and/or sepsis.

The frequency of infectious complications is variously quoted in the literature.[1–5] This is because of the difference of interpretation of the symptoms, the variety of surgical aseptic approaches and the differences in pharmacological prophylaxis and treatment. By analysis of 15 publications[2] the range of complications was established: the average for puerperal fever was 19%, endomyometritis 4.4%, pelveoperitonitis 1.2% and wound infection 1.5% (Table 161.1).

Maternal infections follow cesarean section in spite of the usual surgical aseptic measures, which include washing and cleaning of the lower abdominal wall skin and the use of sterile instruments and other operative materials. In fact, during operation the uterine cavity has to be opened, in which the aerobic and anaerobic gram-positive and -negative bacteria can be found.[6,7]

Bacteria are always present in the uterine-amniotic cavity when more than 6 h has elapsed since the rupture of the membranes.[7,8] Even when the amniotic membranes persist during labor, pathogenic bacteria have been established by amniocentesis in the amniotic fluid in 8 out of 78[9] and in 18 out of 31[10] deliveries. Among the isolated bacteria the most frequent are the gram-negative aerobes and anaerobes; among the aerobes the most frequent are *Escherichia coli* and *Enterococcus*, and among the anaerobes, *Peptostreptococcus*.[6–12] The same bacteria have been isolated from the surgeon's gloves and thereafter from the wound suppuration[6] and from the peritoneal cavity, amniotic fluid and wound suppuration.[8] There is a relationship between the colonization of the amniotic fluid and the time elapsed from membrane rupture.[13] The bacteria detected during postcesarean infection may be regularly isolated from the vagina.[14] The clinical manifestation of infection is related to the number of vaginal examinations and to the invasive monitoring during delivery,[15] to the time elapsed since the rupture of the membranes and to the existence of the signs of infection before the operative procedure. In our analysis in 1981, the relationship of puerperal fever and wound infection to the duration of time since membrane rupture was established (Table 161.2).

The presence of bacterial agents in the amniotic fluid and uterine cavity, and the possibility of propagation of the infection during cesarean section to the endometrium, myometrium, peritoneum and even the blood circulation,[16] has stimulated clinicians to start antibiotic prophylaxis of infection during and following cesarean section. The various antibiotics are given alone or in combination, during the operative procedure or following it, in a single or repeated dose.

The first report was published by Miller and Crichton in 1968.[17] By the application of penicillin during the 5 days following cesarean section, puerperal morbidity has been reduced by 50%. In Table 161.3 the type of antibiotic prophylaxis, i.e. the antibiotic used, the time and duration of application and their effect upon the puerperal postcesarean endometritis and wound infection are presented. From the table, the favorable effect of antibiotic prophylaxis can be seen. Until 1980, the penicillins, and thereafter the cephalosporins, have been used predominantly. The cephalosporins have an advantage in relation to the penicillins due to their broader spectrum of activity, especially on the gram-negative agents (*E. coli*).

Table 161.1 Reported rates of puerperal fever, endomyometritis, pelveoperitonitis and wound infection in women following cesarean section (data from Dražančić and Orešković[2])

	Mean incidence (%)	Range (%)
Puerperal fever	19.0	7.3–48.0
Endomyometritis	4.4	1.0–7.3
Pelveoperitonitis	1.2	0.2–4.7
Wound infection	5.4	1.6–7.5

Table 161.2 Puerperal fever and wound infection in relation to the duration of membrane rupture in 263 cesarean sections without pharmacological prophylaxis performed by Zagreb in 1981

Time from membrane rupture	Puerperal fever	Wound infection
Existing membranes ($n=106$)	12 (11.3%)	1 (0.9%)
1–6 h ($n=58$)	13 (22.4%)	2 (3.5%)
7–12 h ($n=42$)	14 (33.3%)	6 (14.3%)
> 13 h ($n=57$)	18 (31.6%)	12 (21.0%)
Total ($n=263$)	57 (21.7%)	21 (8.0%)

Since there is no difference between the effect of a single intraoperative dose and a multiple postoperative application (Table 161.4), the trend today is to apply a single intraoperative dose immediately after cord clamping.

Nevertheless, pharmacological prophylaxis does not seem to be sufficient. We would like to present our results of 13 years' follow-up of cesarean section deliveries, grouped into five periods, according to the pharmacological and surgical proceedings.

Materials and methods

Our approach to the prevention of infection in cesarean deliveries has changed during the past 13 years; we can distinguish five periods, which followed one after another. For each period the results with regard to puerperal morbidity, i.e. fever and the wound infection, will be presented.

First period, 1981–1982

Antibiotic prophylaxis was not performed. The antibiotics were applied after operation, depending on the clinical behavior of the patient, the temperature, bowel function and leukocyte count. The surgical procedure was 'usual': the laparotomy was by transverse incision; after the opening of the abdomen the uterus was wrapped in gauze; following extraction of the child and the placenta, and the removal of the gauze, the uterus was sutured by two rows of single catgut sutures, or one row of single and another of continued catgut sutures.

Second period, 1983–1986

Antibiotic prophylaxis was by cefuroxim for 3–5 days, 3 × 1.5 g daily starting after the operation. The surgical procedure was as before.

Third period, 1987–1989

Antibiotic prophylaxis was as before. After opening of the uterus, suction of the amniotic fluid and blood was carried out. After removing the gauze, wiping and washing out of the peritoneal cavity was performed with isotonic solution.

Fourth period, 1990–1992

Pharmacological prophylaxis was administered only in cases with membrane rupture over 6 h, and after cord clamping cefuroxim 1.5 g was given intravenously. The surgical procedure was as before, with suture of the uterus incision by one row of interrupted single Dexon sutures; before closing the abdominal wall there was a change of sheets, instruments and surgical gloves.

Fifth period, 1993–1994

Pharmacological prophylaxis was administered in all cases after cord clamping, with cefuroxim 1.5 g intravenously. The surgical procedure was as before.

In all cases puerperal fever and wound infection were evaluated. For puerperal fever, all cases with temperature more than 38°C, starting from the second day of puerperium were registered. For wound infection, all cases of suppuration, irrespective of the involved layer of the abdominal wall, were declared.

The first 12 months of each period were included in the analysis, except the fourth period, for which two complete years were analyzed.

In the first period, 263 cases were analyzed, 99 (37.6%) of them with a rupture of membranes (ROM) of more than 6 h; in the second period 237 cases, 105 (44.3%) of them with ROM > 6 h; in the third period 428 cases, 180 (42.1%) of them with ROM > 6 h; in the fourth period 1153 cases, 332 (28.8%) of them with ROM > 6 h and in the fifth period 333 cases were analyzed, 74 (22.2%) of them with ROM > 6 h.

Results and discussion

The results are presented in Table 161.5. In the first period, without pharmacologic or extended surgical

Table 161.3 Review of the antibiotic prophylaxis of infection following cesarean section

	Antibiotic	Effect: Endometritis*	Effect: Wound infection (%)
Miller and Crichton[17]	Ampicillin 5 days postoperatively	Reduction for 50%	
Weissberg *et al.*[18] (*n*=40)	Penicillin+kanamycin 5 days	Reduction from 35 to 10% postoperatively	
Gibbs *et al.*[19] (*n*=67)	Ampicillin+kanamycin	45–19%	16–0
D'Angelo and Sokol[20] (*n*=49)	Cefalexin 1 day, 4×1.0 g	65–29%	
	Cefalexin 5 days, 4×0.5 g	65–20%	
Dillon *et al.*[21] (*n*=31)	Cefoxitin 5 days, 4×1.0 g	Infection reduced	
Harger and English[22] (*n*=196)	Cefoxitin 1 day, 3×2.0 g	20–10%	7.4–1.0
Gonik[23] (*n*=50)	Cefoxitin 1 day, 3×1.0 g	14%	
Von Mandach *et al.*[24]			
(*n*=76)	Ceftriaxon intraoperatively, 1.0 g	12.0%	
(*n*=75)	Cefoxitin 1 day, 3×1.0 g	13.2%	
McGregor *et al.*[25]			
(*n*=195)	Cefamycin intraoperatively, 1×2.0 g	4.1%	2.5
(*n*=91)	Cefoxitin 1 day, 3×2.0 g	9.9%	3.3
Kristensen *et al.*[26] (*n*=102)	Cefuroxim intraoperatively, 1.5 g	10–1%	1.0–0
Neuman *et al.*[27]			
(*n*=87)	Penicillin 10 million+1 day tetracycline 2×250 mg	7.3%	5.2
(*n*=96)	Penicillin 10 million+3 days ampicillin 3×2.0 g and tetracycline 3×0.5 g	4.8%	6.9
Ehrenkranz *et al.*[20] (*n*=906)	Intraoperatively**	2.1 to 0.7%	2.0–0.2
Faro *et al.*[29]			
(*n*=161)	Cefazolin 1 day, 3×1.0 g	22.5%	
(*n*=148)	Cefazolin intraoperatively, 2.0 g	10.6%	
(*n*=141)	Ampicillin intraoperatively, 2.0 g	12.8%	
Carlson and Duff[30]			
(*n*=192)	Cefazolin intraoperatively, 2.0 g	19.3%	1.6
(*n*=185)	Cefamycin intraoperatively, 2.0 g	21.1%	1.6
Watts *et al.*[31]			
(*n*=50)	Cefamycin intraoperatively, 2.0 g	18.0%	4.0
(*n*=52)	Cefoxitin 1 day, 3×2.0 g	13.5%	3.9

*Endometritis and/or puerperal fever; **type of antibiotic not specified

prophylaxis, there is an evident increase of puerperal fever after ROM, especially after 6 h. Wound infection increased continuously from 0.9% to 21.0% (see Table 161.1).

In the second period the pharmacologic postoperative prophylaxis does not reduce the incidence of puerperal fever (44.3%) and wound infection (10.5%).

In the third period, with the same pharmacologic prophylaxis and with surgical prophylaxis, there is a slight decrease of febrile puerperiums (10.2%) and wound infection (6.1%).

In the fourth period, with intraoperative single-dose antibiotic prophylaxis only in cases of ROM more than 6 h, and with systematically performed

Table 161.4 The intraoperative and postoperative antibiotic prophylaxis of wound infection

	Antibiotic	Incidence of wound infection (%)	
		Postoperative prophylaxis	Intraoperative prophylaxis
McGregor *et al.*[25]	Cefamycin or cefoxitin	3.3	2.5
Neuman *et al.*[27]	Penicillin+tetracyclin	6.9	5.2
Watts *et al.*[31]	Cefoxitin or cefuroxim	3.9	4.0
Dražančić and Orešković[2]	Cefuroxim	6.1	1.6

Table 161.5 Puerperal fever and wound infection in relation to the type of pharmacologic and surgical prophylaxis

Type of prophylaxis	*N*	Puerperal fever	Wound infection
Antibiotics postoperatively and selectively (1981)	263	57 (21.6%)	21 (8.0%)
Cefuroxim postoperatively 3–5 days (1983)	237	105 (44.3%)	25 (10.5%)
Cefuroxim 3–5 days, surgical prophylaxis partial (1987–1988)	428	44 (10.2%)	26 (6.1%)
Cefuroxim intraoperatively when membrane rupture > 6 h, surgical prophylaxis extended (1990–1991)	1153	129 (11.2%)	18 (1.6%)
Cefuroxim intraoperatively in all cases, surgical prophylaxis extended (1993–94)	333	13 (3.9%)	2 (0.6%)

surgical prophylaxis, there is no change in the rate of febrile puerperium (11.2%), and there is a decrease in wound infection to 1.6%.

Only in the fifth period with extended surgical prophylaxis and pharmacological prophylaxis in all cases, irrespective of ROM, is the evident decrease of puerperal fever (3.9%) and wound infection (0.6%) established.

The more detailed analysis of 1153 cases during the fourth period (Table 161.6), with systematically extended surgical prophylaxis, revealed the importance of combined pharmacological and surgical prophylaxis. There are no significant differences between the cases with and without antibiotic application within the separate groups. Puerperal fever was established by persistent membranes in 10.2% vs. 7.9%, by ROM 0–3 h in 7.7% vs. 10.3% and by ROM 4–6 h in 12.9% vs. 11.5% of the cases, respectively. Among 81 cases without ROM or with ROM less than 6 h, which manifested puerperal fever, 45 (55.6%) were without membrane rupture and without antibiotic prophylaxis. Wound infection, which is more specific and indicative of puerperal infection, appeared in 10 cases with persistent membranes without antibiotic prophylaxis, that is, 55.6% of the 18 cases with wound infection. The above data influenced us to introduce the regime of extended surgical plus pharmacological prophylaxis in all cases, irrespective of membrane rupture. In this way, out of 333 cases of cesarean section during the period July 1993 to March 1994 only 13 cases (3.9%) of febrile puerperium and only two cases (0.6%) of wound infection were registered (Table 161. 5). The causes of febrility over 38°C were two cases of wound infection, three cases of endomyometritis, one case of pelveoperitonitis (cured conservatively), one case with pyelonephritis and six cases without established origin of febrility.

Since 1993 we have introduced general pharmacological and surgical prophylaxis in all cases of cesarean section. The pharmacological prophylaxis includes all cases, irrespective of rupture of the membranes. As a routine, 1.5 g of cefuroxim is administered intravenously immediately after the cord clamping. The surgical prophylaxis comprises the wrapping of the uterus with gauze, suction of the blood and amniotic fluid that flows out from the uterine incision, one row of interrupted suture of the uterine incision, wiping and washing of the peritoneal cavity and – at the end – a change of the sheets, surgical gloves and instruments before the suturing of the abdominal wall.

The surgical prophylaxis seems to be of special importance. After 6 h following ROM, all the uterine cavities are infected[7,8] and even with persisting membranes the amniotic fluid may be infected.[9,10] The suction of the blood and amniotic fluid during uterotomy and the wiping and washing of the peritoneal cavity hinders the dissemination of (infected) uterine contents

Table 161.6 Peurperal fever and wound infection in relation to the rupture of membranes and to antibiotic prophylaxis (Zagreb 1990–1991)

		n	Fever >38°C	Wound infection
Membranes persistent	A	443	45 (10.2%)	10 (2.3%)
	B	89	7 (7.9%)	0
Membranes ruptured 0–3 h	A	91	7 (7.7%)	3 (3.3%)
	B	58	6 (10.3%)	0
Membranes ruptured 4–6 h	A	62	8 (12.9%)	4 (6.4%)
	B	78	8 (11.5%)	0
Membranes ruptured >6 h	B	332	47 (14.2%)	1 (0.3%)
Total		1153	129 (11.2%)	18 (1.6%)

A, without antibiotic prophylaxis; B, antibiotic prophylaxis, one dose intraoperatively

to the peritoneum. The exchange of sheets, instruments and gloves prevents the implantation of infectious material to the abdominal wall. The one-row uterine suture should prevent myometritis, because it hinders the formation of uterine wall pockets with retention of the potentially infected material; during the one-row suturing the possibility of a hematoma forming at the edges of the uterine incision is reduced.

The selective antibiotic prophylaxis in the cases with membrane rupture of more than 6-h duration is, without doubt, beneficial. However, with this type of antibiotic prophylaxis about 20% of infected cases are missed in the deliveries with persistent membranes or with membrane rupture of less than 3-h duration.

The one-dose antibiotic application intraoperatively is not less effective than several days' postoperative treatment,[23–27,29] but it is less expensive.[32] We used cefuroxim, but other cephalosporins of the third generation resistant to β-lactamase and first-generation cephalosporins are also efficient. The single-dose application is efficient as a prophylactic measure. It does not suffice when the cesarean section is performed during delivery with evident intrauterine infection: fever during delivery, tachycardia, uterine tenderness, pus discharge from the uterus and excessive leukocytosis with a shift to the left. In such cases, intensive antibiotic treatment with a combination of penicillins, aminoglycosides and metranidazol, or cephalosporins and clindamycin, before operation and for some days after operation are necessary.

The prophylaxis of infection after cesarean section has to start during pregnancy and continue during labor and after delivery. During pregnancy the treatment of vaginitis and bacterial vaginosis will be beneficial. During labor all procedures that propagate ascending infection should be avoided: superfluous vaginal examinations, invasive fetal monitoring and prolonged labor.

Pharmacological prophylaxis should be selective or total. If it is selective, it is administered in cases with a higher risk of infection: membrane rupture over 6 h, maternal age over 35 years, obesity, diabetes or persistent or previous uroinfection. We incline to total prophylaxis, i.e. for all women undergoing cesarean section. Pharmacologic prophylaxis has to be in parallel with extended surgical prophylaxis.

Conclusion

Careful and extended surgical prophylaxis combined with pharmacological antibiotic prophylaxis decreases the incidence of infectious complications after cesarean section to the minimum: less than 5% for puerperal fever (endomyometritis) and less than 1% for wound infection.

Cefuroxim or other cephalosporins in a single intraoperative intravenous dose successfully reduce the rate of endomyometritis and wound infection and several days of postoperative prophylaxis is not more effective.

REFERENCES

1. Cunningham FC, Hauth JC, Strong JP, Kappus SS. Infectious morbidity following cesarean section. *Obstet Gynecol* 1978;52:456–61.
2. Dražančić A, Orešković S. Prevention of infection by cesarean section. *Gynecol Perinatol* 1994;(Suppl 3):83–7.
3. Henriksen HM. Maternal complications after delivery by cesarean section. *Z Geburtsh Perinatol* 1981;183:351–3.
4. Nielsen TF, Hokegard KH. Post operative cesarean section morbidity: A prospective study. *Am J Obstet Gynecol* 1983;146:911–6.

5. Tissot-Guerraz F, Moussy I, Agniel F, *et al.* Infection hospitaliere en maternite. *J Gynecol Obstet Biol Reprod* 1990;19:19–24.
6. Cooperman NR, Kasim M, Rajashekaraih KR. Clinical significance of amniotic fluid, amniotic membranes and endometrial biopsy cultures at the time of cesarean section. *Am J Obstet Gynecol* 1980;137:536–42.
7. Yoder PR, Gibbs RS, Blanco JD, Castaneda YS, Clair PJ. A prospective, controlled study of maternal and perinatal outcome after intra-amniotic infection at term. *Am J Obstet Gynecol* 1983;145: 695–701.
8. Gilstrap LC III, Cunningham FG. The bacterial pathogenesis of infection following cesarean section. *Obstet Gynecol* 1979;53: 545–9.
9. Prevedourakis G, Papadimitriou G, Ioannidou A. Isolation of pathogenic bacteria in the amniotic fluid during pregnancy and labor. *Am J Obstet Gynecol* 1970;106:400–2.
10. Miller JM, Pupkin MJ, Hill GB. Bacterial colonization of amniotic fluid from intact fetal membranes. *Am J Obstet Gynecol* 1980; 136;796–804.
11. Middleton JR, Apuzzio J, Lange M, Sen P, Bonamo J, Louria DB. Post cesarean section endometritis: Causative organisms and risk factors. *Am J Obstet Gynecol* 1980;137:144–5.
12. Berenson AB, Hammill HA, Martens MG, Faro S. Bacteriologic findings of post cesarean endometritis in adolescents. *Obstet Gynecol* 1990;75:627–9.
13. Bobitt JR, Ledger WJ. Amniotic fluid analysis. Its role in maternal–neonatal infection. *Obstet Gynecol* 1978;51:56–62.
14. Ledger WJ. A historical review of pelvic infections. *Am J Obstet Gynecol* 1988;158:687–93.
15. Ledger WJ. Premature rupture of membranes and the influence of invasive monitoring techniques upon fetal and newborn infection. *Semin Perinatol* 1977;1:79–87.
16. Dizerega GS, Yonekura ML, Keegan K, Roy S, Nakamura R. Bacteremia in post cesarean section endometritis: Differential response to therapy. *Obstet Gynecol* 1980;55:587–90.
17. Miller RD, Crichton D. Ampicillin prophylactic antibiotics in cesarean section. *Obstet Gynecol* 1971;38:290–3.
18. Weissberg SM, Edwards NL, O'Leary JA. Prophylactic antibiotics in cesarean section. *Obstet Gynecol* 1971;38:290–3.
19. Gibbs RS, Hunt JE, Schwarz RH. A follow-up study on prophylactic antibiotics in cesarean section. *Am J Obstet Gynecol* 1973; 117:419–22.
20. D'Angelo I, Sokol RJ. Short versus long-course antibiotic prophylactic treatment in cesarean section. *Obstet Gynecol* 1980;55: 583–6.
21. Dillon WP, Seigel MS, Amol S, O'Leary JL. Evaluation of cefoxitin prophylaxis in cesarean section. *Int J Obstet Gynecol* 1981; 19:133–7.
22. Harger JH, English DH. Selection of patients for antibiotic prophylaxis in cesarean section. *Am J Obstet Gynecol* 1981;141: 752–8.
23. Gonik P. Single-versus three-dose cefotaxime prophylaxis for cesarean section. *Obstet Gynecol* 1985;65:189–92.
24. Von Mandach U, Fiedler R, Huch R, Huch A. Ceftriaxon versus cefoxitin in der antibiotischen. Prophylaxe bei Kaiserschnitt mit erhohtem Infektrisiko. *Gynaek Rsch* 1987;27:22–9.
25. McGregor JA, Gordon SF, Krotec, J, Pointexter A. Results of a randomized, multicenter comparative trial of a single dose of cefotetan versus multiple doses of cefoxitin as prophylaxis in cesarean section. *Am J Obstet Gynecol* 1988;158:701–6.
26. Kristensen GB, Beiter EC, Mather O. Single dose cefuroxim prophylaxis in non-elective cesarean section. *Acta Obstet Gynecol Scand* 1990;69:497–500.
27. Neuman M, Langer R, Rachar R, Golan A, Bukovsky I, Caspi E. Penicillin-tetracycline prophylaxis in cesarean delivery: Prospective and randomized comparison of short- and long-term therapy. *J Perinat Med* 1990;18:145–8.
28. Ehrenkranz NJ, Blackwelder BC, Pfaaff SJ, Poppe D, Yerg DE, Kaslow RA. Infections complicating low-risk cesarean sections in community hospitals: Efficacy of antibiotic prophylaxis. *Am J Obstet Gynecol* 1990;162:337–43.
29. Faro S, Martens MG, Hammill HA, Riddle G, Tortolero G. Antibiotic prophylaxis: Is there a difference? *Am J Obstet Gynecol* 1990;162:900–7.
30. Carlson C, Duff P. Antibiotic prophylaxis for cesarean delivery: Is an extendent spectrum agent necessary? *Obstet Gynecol* 1990; 76:343–6.
31. Watts DH, Hillier SL, Eschenbach DA. Upper genital tract isolates at delivery as predictors of post cesarean infections among women receiving antibiotic prophylaxis. *Obstet Gynecol* 1991; 77:287–92.
32. Duff P. Prophylactic antibiotics for cesarean delivery: A simple cost-effective strategy for prevention of post operative morbidity. *Am J Obstet Gynecol* 1987;157:794–8.

162 Septicemia and septic shock

S. J. Fasouliotis and J. G. Schenker

Definition

Septicemia and septic shock are dramatic clinical syndromes that result from acute invasion of the bloodstream by certain microorganisms or their toxic products. Fever, chills, tachycardia, tachypnea and altered mentation are common acute manifestations of septicemia. When hypotension and signs of inadequate organ perfusion develop, the condition is termed septic shock. The circulatory insufficiency is characterized by a lowered systemic vascular resistance, decreased myocardial contractile function and pooling and altered distribution of blood in the microcirculation. Diffuse cell and tissue injury and, ultimately, widespread organ failure develop. Even with appropriate antimicrobial and supportive care many patients die of septic shock, making strategies for prevention and more effective treatment of critical importance.

Etiology

Septicemia can be caused by all classes of organisms; however, septic shock is most commonly caused by gram-negative bacteria (60–70% of cases).[1] Gram-positive organisms and especially staphylococci, pneumococci and streptococci are less frequent causes (20–40% of cases), as are opportunistic fungi (2–3%) and, rarely, mycobacteria or certain viruses or protozoans. *Escherichia coli, Klebsiella, Enterobacter, Proteus, Pseudomonas* and *Serratia* are the most frequent blood culture isolates in septic shock, followed by *Staphylococci* and *Pneumococci*. Gram-negative bacteremia is complicated by shock in about 40% of patients; shock is seen in 5–15% of patients with acute bacteremias caused by pneumococci or staphylococci. The incidence of suppurative complications (metastatic seeding to bones, joints and viscera), on the other hand, is much higher with gram-positive microorganisms. Gram-positive bacteria have the capability of adhering to endothelial cells and subendothelial matrix substances (such as fibronectin, laminin, fibrinogen and endothelial cell proteins) to a much greater degree than do gram-negative organisms, so that seeding to heart valves, to other organs and especially to foci of trauma and/or preexisting inflammation is much more common.

Epidemiology

Infections most commonly occur in the hospital setting. Many infected patients become bacteremic. It is estimated that of 100 randomly chosen patients who appear to be infected (septic) in a hospital setting, approximately 90% are actually infected. Of these, about 20% develop some evidence of hemodynamic instability and appear, at least temporarily, to have shock. About half of shock patients (or about 10% of all septic-appearing patients) go on to real septic shock and/or manifest serious end-organ malfunction related to the septic episode, such as adult respiratory distress syndrome (ARDS), renal failure or disseminated intravascular coagulation (DIC). Since about 5% of all hospital patients are either admitted with or develop an infection during hospitalization, the number of patients at risk of developing septic shock is large. Despite the introduction of new antimicrobial agents, the overall mortality from gram-negative bacteremia has averaged about 25% over the past two decades, and is highest in patients who have major associated diseases or shock. Predisposing factors include diabetes mellitus, cirrhosis, alcoholism, leukemia, lymphoma or disseminated carcinoma, cytotoxic chemotherapy and immunosuppressive drugs that cause neutropenia, total parenteral nutrition, a variety of surgical procedures, and infections arising from the urinary, biliary or gastrointestinal tracts. Gram-positive bacteremias are more often community acquired, except staphylococcal sepsis from indwelling intravenous catheters. Opportunistic fungal sepsis is most often seen in immunosuppressed patients with severe neutropenia, or in postoperative patients with intravenous catheters, and usually follows prolonged antibiotic therapy.

Pathogenesis and pathology

Most of the bacteria causing gram-negative sepsis are normal commensals in the gastrointestinal tract. From

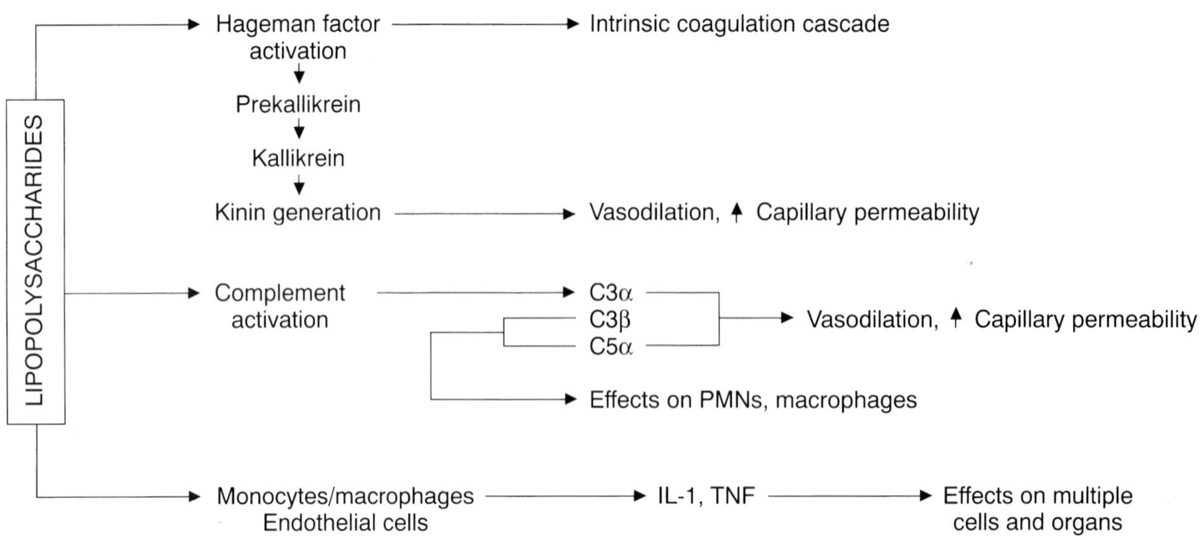

Figure 162.1 Schematized interactions between gram-negative lipopolysaccharides (LPS) and host humoral and cellular mediator systems in sepsis. PMNs, polymorphonuclear leukocytes; IL-1, interleukin 1; TNF, tumor necrosis factor-α.

there they may spread to contiguous structures, as in peritonitis after appendiceal perforation, or they may migrate from the perineum into the urethra or bladder. The genitourinary, gastrointestinal and biliary tracts or the lungs, are usually the primary sites from where gram-negative bacteremia starts, and less commonly from the skin, bones and joints. On the other hand, gram-positive bacteremias usually arise from the skin or respiratory tract. Bacteremia, mainly caused by gram-positive or anaerobic organisms, may be complicated by the formation of metastatic abscess.[2]

Pathophysiology

The classic clinical picture of septicemia and septic shock is a result of the interactions between microbial substances and host mediator systems. A vicious circle is established regarding vascular perfusion and organ function, which result in altered blood flow in the microcirculation and progressive injury to the capillary endothelium and tissues. Unless this circle is interrupted by control of the infection and correction of the hemodynamic and metabolic alterations, death usually results.

Microbial factors that are most important include gram-negative lipopolysaccharides (LPS), especially the lipid A component, peptidoglycans from gram-positive organisms, or mannan from fungal cell walls, certain polysaccharides and extracellular enzymes (e.g. streptokinase) or toxins (e.g. toxic shock enterotoxins of staphylococci). LPS, which has been studied thoroughly, seems to activate directly humoral or cellular systems, which in turn promote the development of the septicemic and shock syndromes, whereas other microbial products, although not as well defined, seem to affect the same systems in varying degrees.

Host mediators that have been associated with the pathogenesis of septic shock include active metabolites of the complement kinin, and coagulation systems as well as factors released from stimulated cells, in particular the cytokines, tumor necrosis factor-a (TNF) and interleukin-1, enzymes and oxidants from polymorphonuclear leukocytes (PMN), vasoactive peptides and products of the metabolism of arachidonic acid. In addition, the secretion and action of counterregulatory vasoactive catecholamines, angiotensin, pituitary hormones, insulin and glucagon all contribute to the clinical laboratory events in sepsis.

One of the proposed mechanisms involves the direct activation of both the coagulation and kinin systems by LPS through its effect on Hageman factor (Figure 162.1). The intrinsic coagulation cascade is activated, and increased amounts of factors XII, VIII and V, and fibrinogen are found. Plasmin is also generated by activated Hageman factor. Cleavage of prekallikrein to kallikrein by the activated Hageman factor leads to the production of bradykinin and related kinins, which are potent vasodilators, increase capillary permeability, and increase gastrointestinal motility. The complement system can also be activated by LPS and other microbial products and the generation of the anaphylatoxins C3α and C5α contributes to the vasodilation and increased capillary permeability. A reduction of C3 levels in septic shock has been associated with a fatal outcome. Effects on PMN include aggregation, increased adhesion to endothelial cells, promotion of lysosomal enzyme release and activation of the superoxide generating system. The activated PMN has enhanced bactericidal capabilities, and also the capability of damaging host tissues. The activated PMN possesses increased amounts of lysosomal enzymes and a variety of toxic metabolites of molecular oxygen, all of which are both bactericidal and cytocidal. Also, the activated PMN produces both inflammatory prostaglandins and several products of the lipoxygenase system, many of which enhance inflammation by also producing vasodilation, capillary leakage and chemotaxis and PMN activation. The activated PMN adhere to each other (the leukopenic phase of sepsis during which PMN aggregates in capillaries) and to endothelial cells to cause severe damage and capillary leakage.

The production of TNF and interleukin-1 by macrophages, endothelial cells and perhaps other cells plays a central role in the multiple actions of LPS and other microbial products in sepsis.[3] Large doses of TNF in experimental animals produce all the systemic and pathologic features of LPS- or bacteria-induced septic shock, including hypotension, pulmonary injury with platelet and leukocyte thrombi and hemorrhagic necrosis of the intestine, acute renal failure, severe metabolic acidosis and death. Classic symptoms appearing in sepsis, such as fever, myalgia and somnolence follow administration of small amounts of recombinant TNF or interleukin-1 to human beings. Experimental studies have shown that these two cytokines act synergistically, contributing to many of the characteristic hormonal and metabolic changes seen in sepsis in human beings [hypoalbuminemia, hyperlipidemia and elevations in plasma adrenocorticotropic hormone, arginine vasopressin (AVP), growth hormone, cortisol, catecholamines, glucagons and insulin].[4]

Arachidonate metabolites also seem to participate in this complex process. Thromboxanes produced by activated platelets and PMN are platelet aggregating agents and induce pulmonary arterioral constriction. On the other hand, prostacyclins, which are formed by endothelial cells, are potent vasodilators and increase capillary permeability. Interleukin-1, TNF and LPS induce the production of these factors as well as of the classic prostaglandins. LPS can also cause the production, by various cells, of leukotrienes (which can induce asthma and pulmonary edema) and of the platelet activating factor, which is a vasodilator, increases capillary permeability and also has effects on PMN that duplicate those of the leukotrienes.[5]

After the initiation of this cascade process, the interactions between these varying contributing mediators become very complex. Endothelial cells and the microcirculation are major sites of reaction. There is evidence of cytotoxicity, precapillary shunting, the plugging of postcapillary venules, with PMN and platelet thrombi, and fibrin deposition. A generalized capillary leak syndrome appearing as pulmonary edema is a common event. Kinins, C3a, C5a, histamine released by mast cells, arachidonate metabolites, proteases and oxygen products released by activated neutrophils, monocytes and macrophages can all contribute to the vasomotor alterations characteristic of sepsis, and can participate in capillary damage. Tissue hypoxia and eventual cell death result from the disordered microcirculation.

Severe sepsis produces hemodynamic changes in two phases. Septic patients initially have hemodynamic changes primarily reflecting vasodilatation. Systemic vascular resistance is decreased, the pulse rate increases to compensate and cardiac output is dramatically increased. A state of cardiodepression exists during severe sepsis, and a circulating myocardial depressant factor (MDF) has recently been discovered. This MDF seems to be TNF. Septic patients develop a fall in cardiac ejection fractions to 20–25%, despite the markedly increased cardiac output. As this hyperdynamic state develops, complement-mediated leukoagglutination combines with other inflammatory mediators to cause a severe capillary leak, the intravascular volume decreases, the blood pressure falls and the cardiac output now further declines. Several additional factors contribute to the decline in cardiac output. Peripheral resistance increases in late septic shock, and other cardiodepressants participate, such as vasopressin and encephalin. Hyperventilation is a characteristic early response to sepsis, leading to varying degrees of respiratory alkalosis. Blood lactate concentrations rise early in sepsis, and in the late stages marked metabolic acidosis usually predominates.[6]

Individual organs may be damaged independently of the hypotensive events. Sepsis is the leading cause of ARDS. A progressively widening alveolar–arterial oxygen gradient and the appearance of diffuse pulmonary infiltrates on chest x-ray are characteristic features. ARDS develops in 20–45% of patients with severe sepsis, and it is associated with an 80–90% mortality rate, with complicating secondary pneumonias responsible for many of the deaths that occur late in the course.

Evidence of renal hypoperfusion or renal injury including oliguria, azotemia, proteinuria and the appearance of tubular and epithelial cells and coarse granular casts in the urine will be detected in the majority of patients. Late complications include acute tubular necrosis or, rarely, renal cortical necrosis as part of a generalized Shwartzman reaction.

The direct action of LPS as well as activation of platelet aggregation by multiple mechanisms seem to be responsible for the thrombocytopenia that is seen in up to 70% of patients with septicemia. Platelet counts below 50,000 μl are usually associated with evidence of DIC. Activation of Hageman factor and release of plasminogen activator from macrophages and endothelial cells also contribute to the appearance of this syndrome.

The syndrome of multiple organ failure has a central role in evaluating the damage that occurs during sepsis. Septicemia is the most important of a number of precipitating causes. Other causes include severe trauma, burns, pancreatitis and all other causes of shock. Once the syndrome is initiated, the patient becomes febrile and hypermetabolic, exhibits hyperactive hemodynamic measurements and develops progressive failure of one or more organs. Mortality approaches 90% despite all modern therapeutic measures.

Clinical manifestations

Early phase

The abrupt onset of sepsis is characterized by fever and chills. However, up to 13% of patients may be hypothermic, with rectal temperature $< 36.5°C$ at the onset of sepsis, and an additional 5% of patients who are not initially hypothermic may fail to mount a febrile response above 37.5°C. The absence of fever is seen primarily in the elderly and in those with underlying diseases such as alcoholism and uremia, and has been associated with a poor prognosis. The skin is warm and dry and a redness of the facial skin is usually observed. In the initial stages of sepsis, alterations in mental status may be subtle, with disorientation or personality change as the only manifestation. During this phase, which is called 'hyperdynamic' or 'warm', increased cardiac output and decreased peripheral resistance are observed due to the peripheral vasodilatation that afterward leads to hypotension and in general to a hyperdynamic circulation. Tachypnea follows, which results in respiratory alkalosis. The duration of this phase varies from 30 min to 16 h and the response to treatment may be satisfactory.

Late phase

A hypodynamic circulation ('hypodynamic' or 'cold' phase) characterizes this phase as a result of the hypotension and the hypovolemia due to the capillary leakage of fluids. Peripheral vasoconstriction follows, whereas the skin becomes cold, dry and cyanotic. Respiratory alkalosis is followed by metabolic acidosis. While increased lactate production by poorly perfused tissues may be a factor, reduced removal of lactate by the liver and kidneys appears to play a major role. In the late stages of septic shock, generalized hypoperfusion and the use of vasoconstricting pressors also aggravate the acidosis. Gastrointestinal manifestations are seen in approximately one-third of patients. They include nausea, vomiting, diarrhea or ileus. Upper gastrointestinal bleeding may occur, and rarely hemorrhagic necrosis of the bowel, which may be exacerbated by preexisting atherosclerotic disease. Mild to moderate jaundice may be present related to a sepsis-induced defect in bile secretion. Less frequently, shock-induced hepatic necrosis occurs. Also, later in the disease, more obvious changes of obtundation and coma may be present. Death is associated with refractory hypotension and persistently low systemic vascular resistance, progressive lactic acidosis and evidence of multiple organ failure (ARDS, DIC, acute renal failure and hepatic failure) despite administration of fluids, pressors and antibiotics.[7]

Laboratory findings

Several laboratory tests are often helpful in the evaluation of a potentially septic patient. There is usually leukocytosis with a left shift, but normal white blood cell counts and even leukopenia can occur. As white cells aggregate, platelets become caught up in the process. Thrombocytopenia is common, and when severe it is usually a sign of concomitant DIC, and is associated with a prolonged thrombin time, decreased fibrinogen level and elevated fibrin degradation products. Abnormalities in serum electrolytes can include an elevated anion gap with reduction of the bicarbonate concentration and metabolic acidosis. Liver function test abnormalities include modest hyperbilirubinemia and elevations of the transaminases that may be pronounced in severe shock. Hypoalbuminemia, mild at first, may progress as sepsis continues and malnutrition supervenes. Serum lipids are often elevated. Rarely, changes in serum calcium and phosphorus levels are seen. On urinalysis, mild abnormalities are seen, such as proteinuria, whereas with shock, acute tubular necrosis may develop with oliguria, azotemia and cellular or granular casts. In the initial stages of sepsis there is respiratory alkalosis and arterial blood gases reveal an elevated pH and decreased pCO_2. Serum lactate elevation is highly predictive of deterioration, leading to septic shock, and the blood may show hypoxemia and a metabolic acidosis. Chest x-ray abnormalities may include an underlying pneumonia as the source of sepsis, congestive heart failure as a result of myocardial depression and volume resuscitation or the diffuse infiltrates of ARDS. The electrocardiogram often shows non-specific ST–T wave abnormalities.

Diagnosis

The presumptive diagnosis of sepsis must be made when the setting and attendant clinical signs are suggestive. In general, patients with fever should be considered septic until proven otherwise. Therapy should always be initiated for high-risk febrile patients in advance before microbiologic confirmation of sepsis. The setting in which the episode is occurring should be evaluated promptly. Crucial to appropriate initial decision-making are the background history, which may help to define the type of host–defense defect present, and prior culture data, which might predict the infecting organism. The physical examination should be directed at quickly but thoroughly searching for the septic source as well as signs of end-organ failure that might indicate progression to shock, such as altered mental status, progressive edema and hypotension. All potentially infected foci should be appropriately sampled, and the material obtained should be gram-stained and cultured. The diagnosis and etiology of sepsis is confirmed by finding pathogenic organisms in the blood or at other sites of infection. Other entities often confused with septic shock include myocardial infarction, pulmonary embolus, drug overdose, occult hemorrhage, cardiac tamponade, rupture of aortic aneurysm and aortic dissection.

Treatment

Management of the septic patient involves several stages. Determination and withdrawal of the source of bacteremia is essential, as removal or drainage of the source can turn a potentially fatal disease into an easily treatable one. Intravenous, Foley and drainage catheters should be checked and replaced if necessary.

The severity of the underlying disease influences the outcome of sepsis. Measures, according to the disease, should be undertaken in order to improve this outcome. For example, patients who are immunosuppressed by virtue of drugs or a disease will have an improved outcome if the immunosuppressive medication can be decreased or discontinued, or if the underlying disease can be effectively treated.

Support of respiration is necessary. Arterial oxygen should be monitored by pulse oximetry or by direct measurement. Oxygen should be provided nasally or by mask, sufficient to maintain arterial oxygen saturations in excess of 95%. If respiratory failure develops, intubation with mechanical ventilation should be employed.

Hemodynamic support should also be provided. Fluids should be administered as a measure against hypotension. It is not clear whether colloids or crystalloids are superior. Blood transfusions may be needed in cases of severe anemia. The pulmonary capillary wedge pressure should be maintained between 15 and 20 mmHg or the central venous pressure between 10 and 12 cm H_2O. Urine output should be kept above 20 ml/h. Mean arterial pressures > 60 mmHg are considered satisfactory in previously normotensive patients. About a third of patients will respond to fluid administration alone, with reversal of the hypotension; if volume resuscitation fails to increase blood pressure, pressor drugs should be given. Dopamine, dobutamine and norepinephrine are the agents most frequently used.[8]

Therapy of acidosis and DIC is required. Acidosis often resolves with therapy of the underlying infection and correction of hypoperfusion. If the pH falls below 7.20, sodium bicarbonate should be given. Treatment of the underlying infection is of critical importance in the management of DIC. Asymptomatic DIC (laboratory abnormalities only) or mild manifestations, such as ecchymoses or oozing at venipuncture sites, do not require specific therapy. If major bleeding is detected, replacement of clotting factors and platelets is essential.

Broad antibiotic coverage is required in patients with severe sepsis. Prior to the institution of antibiotics, blood cultures as well as cultures of relevant body fluids and exudates should be obtained. Identification of a portal of entry or localized site of infection can guide initial antibiotic therapy. When considering the choice of antibiotics prior to the availability of culture results, an antibiotic or combination of antibiotics should be chosen with activity against both gram-positive and gram-negative organisms. Once the results of the culture are known, therapy can be more specific.

Recently, two multicenter studies prospectively compared high doses of methylprednisolone sodium succinate (MPSS) with placebo in a blinded protocol in over 600 severely septic patients. Glucocorticoids were administered within 4 h of recognition of the septic event. Both studies showed no efficacy of MPSS and one study showed increased mortality in patients who had mild degrees of renal malfunction or who developed ARDS. Thus, glucocorticoid therapy has no proven role in the treatment of human sepsis.[9,10]

The use of anti-inflammatory drugs such as the antiprostaglandins is under active investigation. These agents may selectively suppress inflammatory damage caused by the activated PMN, without interfering with the antibacterial capabilities of these important host defense cells.

Naloxone, an opiate antagonist, has been used by several clinicians in the treatment of septic shock on the basis of the contribution of the endorphin system to hemodynamic instability. However, in primate models naloxone appears to increase blood pressure without leading to improved tissue perfusion. Also, data from small controlled trials in human sepsis have not documented any long-term benefits from naloxone administration.[11]

Administration of polyclonal antibodies directed at common core LPS antigens of the J5 mutants of *E. coli* has been shown to decrease mortality in patients with gram-negative bacteremia and septic shock and to prevent the development of shock when given prophylactically to high-risk patients. Immunotherapy for gram-negative sepsis is under investigation using monoclonal antibodies to core components of LPS and to TNF. Results are not yet available, but both techniques hold promise as a possible novel approach to therapy.[12]

Prognosis

Most febrile patients lacking other signs of severe sepsis will usually do well even when bacteremic. Such patients usually respond quickly to fluid administration, antibacterial therapy and drainage of the primary focus of infection. However, the presence of shock and/or progressive dysfunction in any organ system significantly increases morbidity and mortality. Even when the inciting infection is localized, shock is associated with a 30–50% mortality rate. Full-blown bacteremia-associated septic shock has a greater than 50% mortality rate. Early diagnosis and treatment of severely septic patients decrease morbidity and mortality.

Prevention

Prevention of infection, especially in the hospital, is the key to reducing morbidity and mortality associated with septic shock. This fact emphasizes the need to limit invasive procedures, limit the use of intravenous lines, avoid Foley catheterization and practice good infection control at all times in an attempt to prevent the occurrence of these infections. The use of active and passive immunization against cell wall components of gram-negative organisms holds promise as a preventive measure in the future.

Bacteremia and septic shock in obstetric and gynecological patients

Infections that most commonly cause bacteremia and septic shock in obstetric patients are septic abortion, antepartum pyelonephritis and puerperal sepsis. Septic abortion most commonly refers to an infected, incomplete abortion, although some patients present prior to the passage of any products of conception. Therefore, any threatened, inevitable, or incomplete abortion associated with elevated temperature should be considered a septic abortion. Incomplete passage of the products of conception may follow spontaneous abortion, legal abortion or illegal abortion. The pathophysiology includes the ascending spread of microorganisms that are normally found in the upper vagina and cervix. Retained products of conception act as a nidus for the development of local infection, which can then lead to a more generalized sepsis. Bacteria migrating through the uterine wall via venous and lymphatic channels may produce cellulitis and abscesses in the broad ligaments and retroperitoneal space of the pelvic floor. Tubo-ovarian abscesses may occur as direct extensions of intrauterine infection. In severe cases, septic pelvic thrombophlebitis may result in multiple, small septic pulmonary emboli, bacteremia and metastatic infection to other organs.

The most common microorganisms isolated from both the blood and the uterine cavity are anaerobes and microaerophilic bacteria. Anaerobic gram-positive cocci are the most common isolates, but *Bacteroides* species and *Clostrodium* species can also play a major role in the pathogenesis of septic abortion. The most common aerobic isolates include *E. coli* and group B streptococci. Treatment involves the use of broad-spectrum antibiotics, uterine curettage and supportive therapy in severe cases. Hysterectomy is seldom indicated unless the uterus has been lacerated or is obviously intensely infected.

Acute pyelonephritis is the most common serious medical complication of pregnancy, occurring in 1–2% of pregnant women. In most women, renal parenchymal infection is caused by bacteria that ascend from the lower tract. Between 75% and 90% of renal infections are caused by bacteria that have P-fimbrial adhesions. The most common isolates include *E. coli*, *Klebsiella pneumoniae* and *Enterobacter* or *Proteus*. About 15% of women with acute pyelonephritis also have bacteremia. For women with pyelonephritis, continuing sepsis is usually from urinary obstruction caused by calculi or a perinephric abscess or phlegmon. Ureteral catheterization or percutaneous nephrotomy may be life-saving, and if this fails, surgical exploration may be indicated. In some cases end-stage pyelonephritis is found as a source of continuing sepsis and nephrectomy must be performed.

Puerperal sepsis may be caused by infection in the genital tract, by infection of the respiratory tract, pyelonephritis, thrombophlebitis and in cases of laparotomy by incisional wound abscess. Postpartum uterine infection, also called endometritis, is relatively common following uncomplicated vaginal delivery, but still continues to be a major problem in women delivered by cesarean section. In the majority of cases, bacteria responsible for pelvic infection are those that normally reside in the bowel and also colonize the perineum, vagina and cervix. Complications of uterine infections include wound infections, necrotizing fasciitis, peritonitis and septic pelvic thrombophlebitis. Treatment includes broad-spectrum antibiotics, and in cases where it is indicated, surgical intervention should be applied.

Among infections that most commonly cause bacteremia and septic shock in gynecological patients are pelvic inflammatory disease and postoperative infections. Pelvic inflammatory disease affects thousands of women every year. Microorganisms most commonly causally related to inflammatory disease include *Neisseria gonorrhoeae*, *Chlamydia trachomatis*, *Hemophilus influenzae*, *E. coli*, group B streptococci, anaerobes (*Peptostreptococcus* species, *Peptococcus*, *Bacteroides* species), *Mycoplasma hominis*, *Ureoplasma urealyticum* and *Actinomyces israelii*. Most cases are caused by an ascending infection. Usually, an endocervical infection exists and the microorganisms gain entrance to the endometrial cavity when the cervical mucus barrier to infection alters, either in conjunction with menstruation or through changes in the hormonal milieu. In the endometrium, the microorganism stimulates an inflammatory response. With continued canilicular spread, with help from a vehicle such as a sperm or by reflux of menstrual blood into the fallopian tubes, the gonococcus reaches the tubes and peritoneal surface, stimulating inflammatory reactions. Pelvic inflammatory disease comprises cervicitis–endometritis–salpingitis–peritonitis and, in some cases, oophoritis with abscess formation occurs. Ambulatory management with antibiotics is applied in mild cases, and in-patient intravenous antibiotic treatment in severe cases.

Postoperative infections that may lead to sepsis include incisional infection, pelvic cellulitis, vaginal cuff abscess, pneumonia, pelvic abscess, septic thrombophlebitis, urinary tract infection and catheter sepsis. In wound infections the most common isolates include *Staphylococcus*, *E. coli*, *Proteus*, *Pseudomonas*, non-hemolytic *Streptococcus* and *Klebsiella*. Management includes opening of the incision, removal of all necrotic tissue and debris and frequent dressing drainages. Antibiotics are indicated when there is evidence of significant cellulitis, systemic signs suggesting bacteremia or signs suggestive of a necrotizing infection, or in high-risk patients (diabetes, patients under steroid treatment). Necrotizing wound infections are uncommon, but of life-threatening potential, demand prompt recognition and accurate therapy and do not resolve without surgical intervention. The incidence of soft tissue pelvic infections has decreased over recent years with the advent of prophylactic antibiotics; however, pelvic cellulitis remains a significant problem in gynecological surgery. Treatment includes antibiotics, and in cases where abdominal or pelvic abscess is suspected, drainage of the abscess, either percutaneously or through open laparotomy, is mandatory.

REFERENCES

1. Kreger BS, Craven DE, Carling PC, *et al*. Gram-negative rod bacteremia III: Reassessment of etiology, epidemiology, and ecology in 612 patients. *Am J Med* 1980;68:332–43.
2. Root RK, Jacobs R. Septicemia and septic shock. In Wilson JD, *et al*., eds. *Harrisson's Principles of Internal Medicine*, 12th edn. 1992:502.
3. Beutler B, Cerami A. Cachectin: More than a tumor necrosis factor. *N Engl J Med* 1987;316:379–85.
4. Michie HR, Monogue KR, Spriggs DR, *et al*. Detection of circulating tumor necrosis factor after endotoxin administration. *N Engl J Med* 1988;318:1481–6.
5. Ball HA, Cook JA, Wise WC, *et al*. Role of thromboxane, prostaglandins, and leukotrienes in endotoxic and septic shock. *Intensive Care Med* 1986;12:116–26.
6. Parillo JE, Parker MM, Natanson C, *et al*. Septic shock in humans. Advances in the understanding of pathogenesis, cardiovascular dysfunction and therapy. *Ann Intern Med* 1990;113:227–42.
7. Harris RL, Musher DM, Bloom K, *et al*. Manifestations of sepsis. *Arch Intern Med* 1987;147:1895–906.
8. Higgins TL, Chenow B. Pharmacotherapy of circulatory shock. *Dis Mon* 1987;33:309–61.
9. Bone RC, Fisher CJ, Clemmer TP, *et al*. A controlled clinical trial of high dose methylprednisolone in the treatment of severe sepsis and septic shock. *N Engl J Med* 1987;317:653–8.
10. The Veterans Administration Study Group. Effects of high-dose glucocorticoid therapy in patients with clinical signs of systemic sepsis. *N Engl J Med* 1987;317:659–65.
11. Faden AL, Holaday JW. Experimetal endotoxin shock: The pathophysiologic function of endorphins and treatment with opiate antagonists. *J Infect Dis* 1980;142:229–38.
12. Ziegler EJ, McCutchan JA, Fierer J, *et al*. Treatment of gram-negative bacteremia and shock with antiserum to a mutant *E. coli*. *N Engl J Med* 1982;303:1225–30.

163 Gastrointestinal infections in pregnancy and neonates

I. Krause and S. Ashkenazi

Infectious gastrointestinal disease may have an impact on the course of pregnancy and its outcome. Several pathogens such as *Salmonella* and *Campylobacter* may cause bacteremia with secondary infection of the placenta and the fetus. Other microorganisms cause severe circulatory compromise due to dehydration and electrolyte imbalance, and may bring about fetal hypoxia.

Some infections in mothers can be transmitted during delivery, and later on by the fecal–oral route, to the neonate. Neonatal infections often have atypical presentation, with a more serious course. Breast feeding is of great importance as a preventive measure against many gastrointestinal infections. Special considerations should be made regarding antimicrobial therapy during pregnancy.

This chapter deals with several aspects of gastrointestinal infections during pregnancy and the neonatal period.

Salmonella species

Salmonellae are motile, gram-negative, non-capsulated, non-sporulating rods that belong to the family Enterobacteriaceae. The large number of different serotypes makes the classification of salmonellae somewhat confusing; therefore different systems have been suggested. There are three main groups of salmonellae, named by the species *Salmonella enteritidis*, *S. typhi*, and *S. cholerasuis*. These species are further divided into serogroups and serotypes according to principal antigens: flagellae (H) antigens, the cell wall (O) lipopolysaccharide antigen, and the envelope virulence (Vi) heat-labile antigens.[1]

Salmonellae are resistant to many physical agents, but can be killed by heating to 54.4°C for 1 h or 60°C for 15 min. They may remain viable for days and even weeks in sewage, dried food and fecal material.

The precise mechanisms of salmonellae virulence are not completely understood. Two-thirds of *Salmonella* strains produce enterotoxin immunologically related to cholera toxin, and this may explain the watery diarrhea often seen in *Salmonella* gastroenteritis. Salmonellae secrete several protein synthesis-inhibiting cytotoxines that are not immunologically related to the cytoxines produced by *Shigella dysenteriae* or *Escherichia coli* (mainly serotype O157:H7). The pathogenic role of these cytotoxins is unclear. The ability of salmonellae to survive inside the phagolyposomes of phagocytic cells due to the properties of their lipopolysaccharides has major clinical significance. It may explain treatment failure with antibiotics, which do not penetrate the phagolyposomes, prolonged fever even with adequate therapy, and relapses of the disease after apparent recovery.

Both humoral immunity and cell-mediated immunity are activated during *Salmonella* infection; it is thought that cellular immunity plays a more important role in eradication of the microorganism, because macrophages activated by T cells have the ability to kill intracellular bacteria.

Non-typhoid salmonellosis

Epidemiology

Salmonellosis is one of the most common gastrointestinal infections in humans worldwide. Salmonellae cause disease in animals as well, although most of the infections are asymptomatic. More than 500,000 culture-proven cases of salmonellosis are reported annually in the United States, and the actual estimated number is up to 4,000,000. The highest isolation rate is reported among infants less than 1 year of age. The incidence of *Salmonella* infection during the first year of life is about 75 cases per 100,000 infants. Meat, milk, poultry, and eggs are the main sources of *Salmonella*. Up to 50% of poultry, 5% of beef, 16% of pork, and 40% of frozen egg products contain *Salmonella*. Reptiles, particularly pet turtles, may serve as a source of the infection. In hospitals, *Salmonella* infection may be transmitted by contaminated food, personnel, inadequately sterilized equipment, and administration of animal extracts (pituitary, liver, pancreas, etc.). The occurrence of nursery outbreaks and intrafamilial infection suggests person-to-person spread.

Salmonella is rarely acquired by the neonate from the mother during delivery, but it can easily be transmitted to the neonate by infected mothers after delivery. The mother may be symptomatic or asymptomatic. Contaminated human milk, raw milk, formula, fomites such as delivery room resuscitators, rectal thermometers, oropharyngeal suction devices, and air condition filters may serve as reservoirs of *Salmonella*.[2] Once having entered a nursery, *Salmonella* is difficult to eradicate. Epidemics lasting for up to 30 months have been reported. The risk of the newborn becoming infected once *Salmonella* is introduced into a nursery may be as high as 20–27%.[2] The incubation period varies from 6 h to several days.

Outbreaks of salmonellosis may be widespread, and it is important to find the source of the infection. Outbreak tracing has improved with the development of molecular epidemiology techniques such as plasmid analysis and endonuclease digestion of chromosomal genes. After infection, non-typhoidal *Salmonella* are excreted in feces for a median of 5 weeks. Chronic carrier state is rare in non-typhoidal salmonellosis (< 1%) in healthy individuals, but occurs with higher frequency in young children and in patients with biliary disease or immune deficiency.

Pathogenesis

Ingested salmonellae enter the stomach. Gastric acidity provides the first protective barrier, as most organisms are killed at a pH of 2.0. Several factors may interfere with this protective effect: achlorhydria, buffering medications, and rapid gastric emptying. Neonates and infants have hypochlorhydria and rapid gastric emptying, and are therefore more susceptible to symptomatic salmonellosis.[3] Premature and low birth weight infants appear to be at higher risk of acquiring *Salmonella* infection than full-term infants.[4] Bacterial flora of the small and large intestines, which may be affected by antibiotic therapy, serve as an additional barrier to *Salmonella*. Decreased intestinal motility due to anatomic causes or medications prolongs the contact time of salmonellae with the mucosa and increases its pathogenicity.[1]

The organisms multiply within the lumen and then penetrate the mucosa, usually at the distal part of the ileum and the proximal part of the colon. Afterward, salmonellae enter the Peyer patches. Most non-typhoidal salmonellae remain within the lamina propriae and the local lymph nodes. *S. dublin* and *S. choleraesuis* may rapidly invade the blood stream with little intestinal damage. The ability to cause bacteremia is related to specific virulent genes, which are found in strains of *S. typhimurium*, although any *Salmonella* strain may produce bacteremia. Patients with impaired reticuloendothelial or cellular immune response such as chronic granulomatous disease and acquired immune deficiency syndrome (AIDS) are prone to *Salmonella* infections. Sickle cell anemia predisposes to *Salmonella* septicemia and osteomyelitis, probably due to multiple infarcts in the gastrointestinal tract, bones, and reticuloendothelial system. Chronic infections are more common in the presence of cholelithiasis and hepatosplenic disease caused by *Schistosoma mansoni*.

Pathology

Pathologic findings are consistent with enterocolitis and include diffuse mucosal inflammation, edema, erosions, and microabscesses. Penetration of mucosa by salmonellae does not usually cause destruction of epithelial cells, hence mucosal ulcers are not found. Polymorphonuclear cells and macrophages infiltrate the lamina propria. Enlargement of intestinal lymphoid tissue is seen; the reticuloendothelial system in the liver and spleen may undergo hyperplasia.

Clinical manifestations

Several clinical syndromes occur with non-typhoidal *Salmonella* infection.

Acute gastroenteritis

This is the most common presentation of non-typhoidal salmonellosis. In neonates and young infants there is an abrupt onset of nausea, vomiting, and crampy abdominal pain, followed by diarrhea, which may be watery or dysenteric – green, mucous- and sometimes blood-containing stools. Fever of 38.5–39°C is found in about 70% of patients. Abdominal examination may reveal tenderness, and mild leukocytosis can be detected. There are some differences in presentation of the disease depending on the *Salmonella* serotype. A few infants with *Salmonella* gastroenteritis develop necrotizing enterocolitis, although it is not clear whether *Salmonella* is the causative agent.[5]

The duration of symptoms is 2–7 days in healthy individuals. In neonates, young infants, and patients with immune deficiency, the disease may last for several weeks. In patients with AIDS, the infection may cause multisystem involvement, septic shock, and death.

Gastrointestinal complications of *Salmonella* infection include protracted diarrhea due to secondary carbohydrate intolerance, and non-specific chronic diarrhea associated with prolonged excretion of *Salmonella*.

Bacteremia

The precise incidence of bacteremia is unknown, and differs according to the age of the patient and the presence of risk factors. Prospective studies of infants in the first year of life suggest a risk of bacteremia of 1.8–6%.[6] Several retrospective studies have reported the risk to be as high as 30–50% during the first month of life.

Extraintestinal spread may occur in infants who initially present with diarrhea and in those without gastrointestinal tract symptoms. Some serotypes of *Salmonella* are more invasive in the first 2 months of life than in older patients, for example, *S. newport*, *S. enteritidis*, *S. infantis* and *S. typhimurium*, but virtually any *Salmonella* serotype can cause bacteremia in neonates.

The spectrum of clinical signs and symptoms in patients with *Salmonella* bacteremia ranges from toxic appearance with high-grade fever and chills to good general condition and absence of fever;[7] enlarged liver and spleen are common. Certain underlying conditions put the patient in a high-risk group for bacteremia: neonates and infants (aged less than 3 months), AIDS and other immune deficiency states, malignancies, immunosuppressive or steroid therapy, hemolytic anemias, including malaria and bartonellosis, collagent vascular disease, inflammatory bowel disease, gastrectomy, achlorhydria or antacid medications, schistosomiasis, and malnutrition. Although infants with bacteremia may have spontaneous resolution without therapy, a sufficient number develop complications. The complications are most common during the first month of life.

In pregnancy, *Salmonella* septicemia may cause sepsis and fetal loss.[8] Two cases of *Salmonella* urinary tract infection during pregnancy have been reported.[9]

Extraintestinal focal infection

Salmonella may cause suppurative infection of almost any organ. The most common focal infections involve the skeletal system, meninges, and the endocardium. Endophthalmitis, hepatic abscesses, intra-abdominal abscesses, mastitis, pericarditis, peritonitis, pleuropneumonia, soft tissue abscesses, splenic abscesses and genitourinary tract infection, otitis media, cholecystitis, and infected cephalhemotoma have all been reported to be caused by *Salmonella*.[10] Endocarditis has rarely been reported in neonates. Meningitis is the most frightening complication. Of all cases of non-typhoidal *Salmonella* meningitis, 50–75% occur during the first 4 months of life.[11] The serotypes associated with neonatal meningitis are *S. typhimurium*, *S. heidelberg*, *S. enteritidis*, *S. sant-paul*, *S. Newport*, and *S. panama*. The presenting symptoms are vague: little or no fever, bulging fontanelle, and decreased appetite. Rapid deterioration and a high mortality rate (30–60%) occur despite appropriate antibiotic therapy. Relapse has been reported in up to 64% of cases. The survivors suffer from early and late neurologic sequelae including hydrocephalus, seizures, ventriculitis, abscess formation, subdural empyema, mental retardation, hemiparesis, visual impairment, and athetosis.

Asymptomatic infection

After clinical recovery from *Salmonella* gastroenteritis, asymptomatic fecal excretion of the organism occurs for several weeks. A chronic carrier state is defined as asymptomatic excretion of *Salmonella* species for more than 1 year. The precise incidence is not known, but the condition seems to be rare. Patients with biliary tract disease are prone to become carriers.

Diagnosis

Diagnosis is based on culturing the organism from stools, blood, cerebrospinal fluid, or aspirated specimens from sites of local suppuration. Selective media such as MacConkey, xylose-lysine decarboxylase (XLD), bismuth sulfite, or Salmonella–Shigella agar should be used for specimens normally containing bacterial flora. Two tests, based on latex agglutination and fluorescence, are commercially available for the rapid diagnosis of *Salmonella* colonies growing in stool culture.[1] Clinical experience is limited. An experimental method for rapid detection of *Salmonella* using chromosomal fragments, which are unique to the genus, as DNA probes, is under evaluation.[1] Serologic assays for detecting antibodies against *S. typhimurium* and *S. enteritidis* are available, although their clinical relevance is unclear. Because of the potential complications of *Salmonella* infection during pregnancy, bacteremia, fetal loss, and urinary tract infection, diarrheal disease during pregnancy should be evaluated for a possibility of *Salmonella* infection.

Prevention

Adequate food hygiene practices, chlorination of water, and hand washing are important for preventing salmonellosis. Hospitalized patients should be isolated. Proper sterilization of medical equipment should be performed.

Individuals with symptomatic or asymptomatic excretion of *Salmonella* need to be excluded from handling food and taking care of children until repeated stool cultures are negative. Control of the spread of *Salmonella* in humans requires control of the infection in animal reservoirs and use of appropriate food processing.

Breast feeding may prevent *Salmonella* infection by reducing the risk of contamination relative to other foods, especially in developing countries, and by class-specific antibodies against *Salmonella*.[12]

Treatment

The most important aspect of treating *Salmonella* gastroenteritis is supportive care, i.e. correction of dehydration and electrolyte and acid–base imbalances. Antimotility agents should be avoided because they prolong intestinal transit time and may increase the risk of invasion. Antimicrobial therapy is not routinely recommended in patients with uncomplicated *Salmonella* gastroenteritis, because it does not shorten the clinical course, or eliminate fecal excretion of *Salmonella*.

Antibiotics may suppress normal intestinal flora, prolong the excretion of *Salmonella*, and increase the risk for chronic carrier state. Antibiotic therapy is indicated in infants of less than 3 months because of a high rate of extraintestinal complications, in patients with underlying conditions that increase the risk of a disseminated disease, and in those with a severe or protracted course of the disease. Patients with bacteremia or extraintestinal focal *Salmonella* infections should always receive antimicrobial therapy.

The choice of the antibiotic drug depends on the epidemiologic data, because antibiotic susceptibility of *Salmonella* differs significantly from region to region. In areas where *Salmonella* is susceptible to ampicillin, it is an effective agent (200 mg/kg/24 h in four divided doses, adults 2–12 g/24 h). Trimethoprim–sulfamethoxazole (TMP–SMX) is not recommended for use in neonates and pregnant women because of the risk of kernicterus. If chloramphenicol is used, serum levels must be closely monitored to avoid toxicity.

Increasing resistance of *Salmonella* to these three agents is reported from all over the world. For this reason, third-generation cephalosporins are used with increasing frequency. Cefotaxime 100–200 mg/kg/24 h in three to four divided doses (in adults 2–12 g/24 h) or ceftriaxone 50–100 mg/kg (in adults 1–4 g/24 h) in one or two divided doses are effective.

Quinolones, although effective, are not approved for use in children and in pregnant women because of the potential damage to growing cartilage. The dosage, route of application, and duration of therapy depend on the site and severity of the infection.

Acute gastroenteritis may be treated for 3–5 days by antibiotics given orally. Ceftriaxone may be given intramuscularly on an ambulatory basis. Patients with bacteremia are treated for 10–14 days intravenously, acute osteomyelitis warrants 4–6 weeks of therapy, and meningitis should be treated for 4 weeks intravenously with the highest recommended dosage.

Enteric fever

Enteric fever is a clinical syndrome produced by *S. typhi* (typhoid fever) and occasionally by other serotypes of *Salmonella*.

Epidemiology

The incidence of enteric fever has decreased in developed countries. In the United States, 400 cases of enteric fever are reported each year (incidence of less than 0.2:100,000). The incidence is similar in Western Europe and Japan. In southern Europe, the annual incidence is estimated to be 4.3–14.5 per 100,000. In developing countries, the incidence may be as high as 500:100,000. Every year 12.5 million cases occur worldwide according to the estimation of the World Health Organization. The disease is not common in neonates. Humans are the only natural reservoir of *S. typhi*. The most common mode of transmission is ingestion of food or water contaminated with human feces. Congenital transmission of the disease can occur by transplacental infection from a bacteremic mother to the fetus, while intrapartum transmission may occur by the fecal–oral route.[2]

Pathogenesis

The inoculum size required to cause disease is 10^5–10^9 for *S. typhi* organisms. Ingested organisms adhere to the microvilli of the ileal brush border, invade the epithelial cells, enter the intestinal lymph node follicles, and reach the mesenteric lymph nodes. Organisms enter the blood stream through the thoracic duct. Reticuloendothelial cells in the liver, spleen, and bone marrow are infected with circulating bacteria. Following proliferation in the reticuloendothelial system, the bacteremia recurs. The gallbladder is especially prone to infection.

Clinical manifestations

The incubation period is usually 7–14 days, but may be as short as 3 days and as long as 30 days.

Neonatal infection

Neonatal disease may begin within 3 days of delivery, with vomiting, diarrhea, and abdominal distension. Fever as high as 40.5°C may be present. Seizures, jaundice, anorexia, and weight loss may be seen. Hepatosplenomegaly can be found. Laboratory findings include low blood leukocyte counts, thrombocytopenia, disturbed liver function test results, and proteinuria. Fecal leukocytes or blood are common.

Complications include intestinal perforation and hemorrhage, myocarditis, central nervous system manifestations, hepatitis, cholecystitis, osteomyelitis, and arthritis. Pneumonia or bronchitis may occur.[13]

Infection during pregnancy

Enteric fever during pregnancy puts women at risk of aborting the fetus. In 1930, 64 pregnant women with typhoid fever were reported.[14] Fetal and maternal mortality rates of 26% and 60%, respectively, were noted. The rate of premature delivery was 25%. With prompt diagnosis and appropriate antibiotic therapy, pregnancy does not appear to put the woman at increased risk of death from enteric fever.[15] Premature labor and fetal death are reported occasionally, despite adequate antimicrobial therapy.[16,17] In one case of spontaneous abortion due to typhoid fever, extensive fetal necrosis was found.[15] Typhoid fever must be considered in the differential diagnosis of pelvic pain, urinary symptoms, and fever in pregnant patients. One case of typhoid cholecystitis, which required surgical intervention, has been reported.[18]

Diagnosis

Diagnosis is based on culturing. Blood cultures are positive in 40–60% of patients early in the course of the disease.[1] Repeated blood cultures are recommended. Stool and urine cultures may become positive after the first week. Late in the course of the disease, when blood cultures are sterile, *Salmonella* may be found in bone marrow. Bone marrow culture is the most sensitive test (positive in 85–90%). *Salmonella* may be cultured in amniotic fluid, cervical swabs, and placenta in cases of premature labor due to enteric fever.[16,17]

New methods for rapid diagnosis include direct detection of *S. typhi*-specific antigens in the serum or urine by monoclonal antibodies and polymerase chain reaction (PCR).[1] Serologic tests are of little clinical value. The Widal test, which measures antibody titer against O- and H-antigens of *S. typhi*, is not sensitive or specific.

Prevention

Appropriate sanitation, hand washing, control of food production, and eradication of *S. typhi* from carriers are needed. Several vaccines (parenteral and oral) against *S. typhi* are available.[19] Parenteral heat-phenol-inactivated vaccine provides only limited protection (51–70%) and is associated with a high rate of adverse effects such as fever, headache, and local reactions. The most effective vaccine that is currently in use is an oral live-attenuated preparation of the Ty21a strain of *S. typhi*. The efficacy is 67–82%, and no significant adverse effects have been reported. This vaccine should not be used in immunocompromised patients, and is not recommended for children under 6 years because of limited experience. Infants do not seem to develop immune response with this preparation.

Treatment

Antibiotic therapy should be given to all patients with suspected enteric fever. Prompt antimicrobial treatment is of great importance during pregnancy, since it may prevent fetal loss and maternal morbidity. High resistance rates to many antibiotic drugs, including ampicillin, chloramphenicol, and TMP–SMX, are currently common worldwide. Resistant strains are usually susceptible to third-generation cephalosporins. Cefotaxime 200mg/kg/24 h (maximal dose 12g/24 h) intravenously, divided in three to four doses, and ceftriaxone (100 mg/kg/24 h, maximal dose 4 g/24 h) intravenously in one or two doses are effective in treating enteric fever. Ceftriaxone is used in pregnancy, although its safety has not been established. Fluoroquinolones are efficacious but currently not approved for use in children and pregnant women, although several authors recommend ciprofloxacin as a drug of choice for treatment of ampicillin-resistant typhoid fever during pregnancy.[20] Given orally, ciprofloxacin produces more rapid resolution of fever than parenteral ceftriaxone. A short course of dexamethasone, 3 mg/kg for the initial dose, followed by 1 mg/kg every 6 h for 48 h, has been shown to improve the survival rate of patients with shock. Supportive treatment is needed to correct fluid and electrolyte imbalance. Attempts to eradicate chronic carriage of *S. typhi* are recommended. A course of 4–6 weeks of high-dose ampicillin or amoxycillin with probenecid results in an 80% cure rate. In the presence of biliary disease, the eradication is difficult and sometimes cholecystectomy is recommended.

Shigella species

Shigellosis is the clinical illness caused by bacteria of the genus *Shigella*, which belong to the family Enterobacteriaceae.[21] Shigellae are gram-negative rods that are non-motile and do not ferment lactose or do so slowly. They are divided into four species or serogroups: *Shigella dysenteriae*, serogroup A; *Shigella flexneri*, serogroup B; *Shigella boydii*, serogroup C; and *Shigella sonnei*, serogroup D. The species differ in their geographic distribution. *S. sonnei* is the most common species in developed countries, where its relative prevalence is increasing.[21] In developing countries, *S. flexneri* is most frequent, with outbreaks that are often caused by *S. dysenteriae.*

Shigellosis has worldwide distribution, and the organisms spread through the fecal–oral route. Because of the low infectious dose – 10–200 organisms can transmit the disease – person-to-person transmission of shigellosis is common. However, transmission by contaminated food, drinking water, swimming pools, and flies has been documented.[21] Seasonality in the incidence of *Shigella* infections is well documented. In temperate climates, including the United States, the peak incidence of shigellosis is during summer and early fall; in the tropics the disease peaks in the rainy season.

The major virulence trait of shigellae is their ability to invade mammalian cells. This ability depends on a 120–140-MDa plasmid, which encodes the synthesis of several polypeptides that are necessary for invasion.[21] Several chromosomal loci are needed to regulate the invasion polypeptides and for complementary virulence traits. Of particular importance are loci encoding the synthesis of bacterial lipopolysaccharide, which is mandatory for full virulence and determines the serotype of *Shigella*.

Shigella strains excrete several toxins. Best known is Shiga toxin, which is produced mainly by *S. dysenteriae* serotype 1 and plays a major role in the complications of shigellosis.[22] Shiga toxin is capable of damaging mammalian cells by inhibiting protein synthesis. Two *Shigella* enterotoxins have recently been identified, cloned, and sequenced; additional toxins are probably produced.

Clinical manifestations

Shigellosis is characterized by acute diarrhea, which develops after an incubation period of 1–2 days. The illness often starts as watery diarrhea and in about half of the patients then progresses to bloody or mucous stools. Diarrhea is usually accompanied by high fever, generalized toxicity, anorexia, and vomiting. Defecation is painful, with urgency. When untreated, diarrhea usually lasts about 1 week. More prolonged diarrhea and even chronicity have been described in immunocompromised patients, especially those with AIDS and malnourished infants. The disease caused by *S. dysenteriae* type 1 is usually more severe. Physical examination during the acute disease may show abdominal distention, tenderness, and hyperactive bowel sounds.

Although usually self-limited, several complications of shigellosis may develop. Intra-abdominal complications include ileus, toxic megacolon, pseudomembranous colitis, perforation with local abscesses, and cholestatic hepatitis.

Neurologic symptoms are among the most frequent extraintestinal manifestations of shigellosis, mainly in children. Of these, convulsions are the best documented, developing in 12–45% of hospitalized children with culture-proven shigellosis.[21] Seizures are usually benign, self-limited, and have no neurologic sequelae. Other neurologic symptoms include lethargy, confusion, severe headache, and hallucinations, and are often referred to as encephalopathy. Fatal outcome can occur. The pathogenesis of *Shigella*-associated neurologic symptoms is not clear.

Septicemia is occasionally seen in patients with shigellosis. A study in Bangladesh found *Shigella* bacteremia in 4% of patients. Septicemia with other enteric bacteria is also found during shigellosis, probably secondary to the damaged gut and loss of the intestinal barrier function. Focal extraintestinal infections of *Shigella* include vaginitis, cystitis, conjunctivitis, iritis, arthritis, and pneumonia. Reactive arthritis and Reiter syndrome may develop.

Especially with *S. dysenteriae* type 1 infection, hemolysis, hemolytic uremic syndrome, and thrombotic thrombocytopenic purpura may develop. It is thought that damage to endothelial cells by Shiga toxin is the initial event in pathogenesis.[22]

Shigellosis in pregnancy and neonates

Shigellosis is relatively rare in neonates and young infants. This is related, at least in part, to protecting maternal antibodies that are transferred through the placenta and by breast feeding.[21] According to published series, less than 4% of *Shigella* cases occur during the first 3 months of life and less than 2% in the neonatal period.[23,24] Of the neonatal *Shigella* cases, more than half occur within 3 days of birth, suggesting fecal–oral transmission during parturition. Haltalin found that in 11 of 16 neonates with shigellosis, the mothers or other family members had clinical diarrhea, sometimes with isolation of *Shigella* species from their stools.[24] Infection from asymptomatic mothers can sometimes occur. Intrauterine infection with *Shigella* is rare; Armor described chorioamnionitis caused by *S. sonnei*, with transmission of the infection to the neonate as pneumonia.[25]

Shigellosis in the neonatal period has distinct clinical characteristics. As compared to older children and adults, neonates with shigellosis usually have low-grade (< 39°C) fever or are afebrile, a lower rate of typical bloody diarrhea, and often abdominal distention.[23,24,26] Lethargy, general toxicity, and feeding difficulties are more frequent in neonates.[24]

Complications are relatively frequent in neonatal shigellosis. Hypothermia, electrolyte imbalance, especially hypernatremia, acidemia, and dehydration are seen.[23] Toxic megacolon, necrotizing enterocolitis, and perforation may develop.[26–28] Chronic diarrhea leading to malnutrition may be seen.[27]

Development of septicemia is of particular importance. *Shigella* bacteremia has been reported to occur in 12% of infants younger than 3 months who had shigellosis,[23] with the rate in neonates even higher.[24,29] Bloodstream invasion with *Shigella* has been reported in an asymptomatic newborn infant.[29] Two neonates have been reported with *Shigella* meningitis.[23,30]

Data on age-related mortality during *Shigella* infections show a particularly high fatality rate during the neonatal period. In the series of Huskins and colleagues, five of 24 (21%) neonates with shigellosis died, and in infants younger than 3 months the mortality rate was over 16%.[23] It has been estimated that in developing countries the mortality rate of neonatal shigellosis is over 50%.[24]

Diagnosis

Culturing is the cornerstone in the diagnosis of neonatal shigellosis, particularly because of the atypical presentation of the disease in this age group. Shigellosis should be suspected not only in neonates with diarrhea, but also in those who look septic and in those presenting with shock and abdominal symptoms suggesting necrotizing enterocolitis, midgut volvulus, and intussusception. A history of diarrhea in the mother or other family members is important.

Stool, but also blood and when relevant cerebrospinal fluid, specimens should be obtained for culture. Culture media should include MacConkey agar as well as selective media such as xylose-lysine decarboxylase (XLD) and Salmonella–Shigella agars. After growth, the species (serogroups) are identified by agglutination. Identification of *Shigella* by culture takes at least 2–3 days, and the yield of stool specimens is relatively low. New techniques for more rapid and possibly more sensitive diagnosis include DNA probes, PCR, and antigen detection methods. These, however, are still being developed.

Treatment

Correction of fluid and electrolyte disturbances is always the mainstay in treating patients with diarrhea. Particular attention should be given to neonates with shigellosis who are more likely to develop dehydration, hypernatremia, hypoglycemia, and acidemia.

Appropriate antibiotic therapy has been shown to be efficacious in shigellosis. Clinically, it shortens the duration of fever, diarrhea, and general toxicity; bacteriologically, fecal excretion of shigellae is stopped in a few days. Complications are probably decreased by antibiotics.

The major problem is the increasing antimicrobial resistance of *Shigella* species worldwide. Oral TMP–SMX, in daily doses of 10 mg/kg of trimethoprim and 50 mg/kg of sulfamethoxazole, divided into two doses, is the usual recommended therapy.[21] TMP-SMX is not recommended in young infants because of the potential risk of kernicterus, nor is it recommended during pregnancy. In addition, in certain geographic locations, high rates of TMP–SMX resistance of shigellae have been reported.

When epidemiologic or laboratory data suggest susceptibility to ampicillin, it can be used orally or parenterally, according to the condition of the patient. The daily dose is 100 mg/kg divided into four doses. Chloramphenicol treatment, with careful monitoring of blood levels, may be considered. Third-generation cephalosporins, and especially ceftriaxone (50 mg/kg/day in a single dose), are adequate alternatives, especially for the more severe cases. Although efficacious, quinolones are not approved for use in children (< 17 years) because of potential damage to the growing cartilage.

Antimotility agents, such as diphenoxylate and atropine, can prolong the duration of fever, diarrhea, and fecal excretion of the pathogen in patients with shigellosis, and should therefore not be used when shigellosis is suspected. Intestinal motility with constant fluid flow may actually be an important host defense mechanism for rapid clearance of the infection.

Prevention

Breast feeding can reduce the risk of *Shigella* infection in early infancy or lessen its severity. It should be especially recommended in developing countries, where *Shigella* infections are more frequent and have a significant impact on nutrition and growth.[21] Because person-to-person transmission of shigellosis is common, strict personal hygiene, and especially hand washing after defecation or diaper changing, and before food preparation and consumption, is mandatory. In developing countries, running water and closed sewage systems are important. Several approaches to the development of *Shigella* vaccines are currently under investigation.

Yersinia enterocolitica

Yersinia are gram-negative bacilli of the family Enterobacteriaceae. Adherence to the intestinal epithelial cells and production of heat-stable enterotoxin produce watery diarrhea. Cytotoxin secreted by *Yersinia* causes ulcerative ileocolitis with mesenteric adenitis. Pathogenic strains require iron and survive only in red-blood-cell-containing products. Patients with hemochromatosis or after accidental overdose of iron are susceptible to septicemia with *Yersinia*.[31]

Epidemiology

Animals, food, and water are the major reservoirs of *Yersinia enterocolitica*. Swine, cattle, goats, dogs, and cats are the most common carriers of this organism. Transfusion-transmitted *Y. enterocolitica* infection has been reported. The risk of transfusion-associated disease increases with blood stored for over 2 weeks. Person-to-person transmission may occur by the oral–fecal route. Infection occurs primarily in children and young adults.

Clinical manifestations

Infection with *Y. enterocolitica* has not been reported in association with complications during pregnancy. Neonatal infection with *Y. enterocolitica* is rare.[32] Infants present either with watery diarrhea or with stools containing mucus and blood. Bacteremia and sepsis are common (20–30%) in infants younger than 3 months,[33] and meningitis is rare. Complications include erythema nodosum, hemolytic anemia, thrombocytopenia, and reactive arthritis.

Diagnosis

Diagnosis is based on culturing the organism. *Y. enterocolitica* can be recovered from stool, throat swabs, peritoneal fluid, blood, and mesenteric lymph nodes. Stool culture should be performed on *Yersinia*-selective agar and incubated at reduced temperatures. It is worthwhile to keep the culture for longer periods. Isolation from body fluids that do not normally contain bacteria (blood, cerebrospinal fluid) may be made on routine media.

Distinction between pathogenic stool strains and nonpathogenic ones may be made by Congo red–magnesium oxalate agar and certain biochemical tests. Antibody titers against *Y. enterocolitica* can be measured but are useful for epidemiologic purposes only.

Prevention

Appropriate means of preparing food, especially meat, pasteurization of milk, and hand washing, may prevent transmission of *Y. enterocolitica*. Human milk might inhibit adhesion of *Y. enterocolitica*.[34]

Treatment

Antibiotic therapy is indicated in culture-proven septicemia, in patients less than 3 months with gastroenteritis, who have a high rate of septicemia. Otherwise, uncomplicated enterocolitis due to *Y. enterocolitica* in previously healthy patients is a self-limited disease and the benefit of antimicrobial treatment has not been established. Aminoglycosides in combination with third-generation cephalosporins, or TMP–SMX, are effective against *Y. enterocolitica* infections.

Vibrio cholerae

Vibrio cholerae are gram-negative, non-spore-forming, curved, motile rods with a polar flagellum. There are many serotypes of *V. cholerae*, but only *V. cholerae* 01 and 0139 (Bengal) cause epidemics. *V. cholerae* 01 is divided into two serotypes, Inaba and Ogawa, and two biotypes, classical and E1 Tor.[35]

Epidemiology

V. cholerae is found in warm, salty water, roots of plants, and shellfish. Person-to-person transmission is rare. Epidemics of cholera still occur worldwide. In 1991, epidemic of cholera appeared in South and Central America. In 1992, strains of a new serotype 0139 caused an outbreak in Madras (now called Chennai), India.

Pathophysiology

In order to cause disease, vibrios, which are acid-sensitive, must overcome the stomach barrier and reach the small bowel. Vibrios adhere to the mucous layer and produce proteolytic enzymes. Virulence of *V. cholerae* is mainly due to production of enterotoxins. The most important of these toxins is cholera toxin, a large heat-labile protein containing a single A subunit and five B subunits. B subunits are responsible for toxin binding to the enterocyte membrane ganglioside GM1, and the A subunit is an adenosine diphosphate (ADP)-ribosyltransferase, which causes elevation of cyclic adenosine monophosphate (cAMP) levels. cAMP decreases the active absorption of sodium and chloride by villous cells and increases active secretion of chloride by crypt cells. Another toxin produced by *V. cholerae* alters the intracellular tight junctions and increases the permeability of intestinal mucosa to water and electrolytes. A third enterotoxin is an ion-transporting ATPase. These three enterotoxins are coded by chromosomal genes.

Clinical manifestations

The most common clinical presentation is watery diarrhea and vomiting. The incubation period varies from 6 h to 5 days. Fever may be present. In severe cases, there is profuse diarrhea with 'rice water' consistency and fishy odor. Dehydration may cause circulatory collapse, acidosis, impaired consciousness, electrolyte imbalance, and renal failure.

Pregnancy

Cholera during pregnancy, especially in the third trimester, is associated with a high incidence of fetal death.[36] Bacteremia is unusual with cholera, and it has not been found in cultures of placenta and aborted fetuses. Miscarriage is probably attributed to fetal acidosis and hypoxemia resulting from the marked metabolic and circulatory changes in the sick mother. Risk of stillbirth is correlated with the severity of maternal disease.[2]

Neonatal cholera

Neonatal cholera is rare. Even infants born to mothers with active diarrheal disease may not be infected.[37] Several factors may contribute to the low rate of infection in newborn infants. Breast feeding provides effective protection due to the existence of specific antibodies against *V. cholerae*,[38] receptor-like glycoprotein that inhibits adherence of the bacteria,[39] and gangliosides that bind cholera toxin.[40] The limited exposure to contaminated food and water further reduces the neonatal risk of acquiring cholera.

Diagnosis

Two selective media are used to culture *V. cholerae*: thiosulfate–citrate–bile–sucrose (TCBS) and tellwrite–taurocholate–gelatin agar (TTGA). Specific antibody tests and DNA probe methods for direct detection in stool samples are available. Vibriocidal, agglutinating, and toxin-neutralizing antibodies may be found 7–14 days after the onset of illness, though providing only retrospective diagnosis.

Prevention

Breast feeding is the most practical method of prevention in infants. Proper handling of food and water are needed to prevent epidemics. A vaccine composed of killed bacteriae given parenterally is currently available.[1] The efficacy of this vaccine is about 50% by 3–6 months after vaccination. It has a high frequency of adverse reactions (pain, erythema, local induration, fever, headaches). The vaccine is not recommended for children under 6 months of age. New vaccines using combinations of killed whole cells with cholera toxin B subunit, live recombinant organisms, or synthetic peptides are under investigation.

Treatment

The most important purpose in treating cholera is correction of fluid and electrolyte imbalance. Oral rehydration solution (ORS), recommended by the World Health Organization and containing 90 mmol/l Na^+, 20 mmol/l K^+, 80 mmol/l ClV^-, 111 mmol/l glucose, and 30 mmol/l bicarbonate, has been shown to be highly effective. When fluids cannot be given orally, parenteral fluid and electrolyte replacement should be provided.

Antibiotics, although of secondary importance in treating cholera, shorten the duration of the illness. TMP–SMX and tetracycline are effective, but these agents are not recommended for use in pregnancy and the neonatal period. Alternative therapy may consist of ampicillin.

Campylobacter species

Etiology

Campylobacter is a curved gram-negative rod. The genus *Campylobacter* includes 15 species, and 8 of them are considered pathogenic for humans: *C. jejuni*, *C. fetus*, *C. coli*, *C. hypointestinalis*, *C. laridis*, *C. cinaedi*, *C. fennelliae*, and *C. upsaliensis*. *Campylobacter* organisms are microaerophilic, with optimal growth at 5–6% oxygen. The growth in blood culture may take as long as 5–14 days after the initial inoculation.[41]

Epidemiology

Campylobacter is one of the most common causes of bacterial gastroenteritis worldwide. In the United States, isolation rates of this organism range from 28 to 71 per 100,000 annually. The most common pathogen of gastroenteritis is *C. jejuni*. *C. coli* and *C. laridis* cause gastrointestinal infections as well. Extraintestinal and systemic infections are associated with *C. fetus*. *Campylobacter* gastroenteritis is more common in children under 17 years of age, with the highest incidence in the first year of life. The second peak occurs in adolescents and young adults. Infection may be asymptomatic. The mode of transmission is zoonosis. The gastrointestinal tract of many domestic and wild animals such as chickens, turkeys, young dogs and cats, and waterfowl serve as the main resevoir of infection. *Campylobacter* is transmitted from animals to persons by the fecal–oral route, by ingestion of contaminated meat, milk, or water. The inoculum needed to cause disease is between 2×10^2 and 10^4 organisms.

Perinatal and person-to-person transmission may occur, although it is much less common. Communicability is greatest during the acute phase of the illness, and may last as long as 2–3 weeks. Chronic carriage is uncommon. Homosexual men are at increased risk for *C. cinaedi* and *C. fennelliae* infections.[2]

The organism is often carried asymptomatically in the intestinal or biliary tract of sheep and cattle. It has a high affinity for placental tissue, and during bacteremia in pregnancy it may invade the uterus and multiply in the fetus. The infected fetuses are usually aborted. It is not clear whether humans acquire *C. fetus* only from animals or from asymptomatic human carriers who transmit it venereally. *C. fetus* infections predominantly occur in older men with a history of animal exposure, and in pregnant women during the third trimester.[42]

Pathogenesis

Mucosal invasion is mediated by bacterial surface proteins. *Campylobacter* produces cytotoxins, and some strains of *C. jejuni* secrete cholera-like enterotoxin. *C. fetus* contains a surface protein capsule that inhibits opsonophagocytosis and enables the pathogen to reach the reticuloendothelial system and bloodstream.

Clinical manifestations

Pregnancy

Infection with *Campylobacter* is an uncommon cause of abortion and premature labor.[42] Although *C. fetus* is most frequently implicated as a pathogen in cases of septic abortion,[43] invasion of the amniotic cavity causing abortion by other strains of *Campylobacter*, such as *C. coli*, *C. upsaliensis*, and *C. jejuni*, has also been reported.[44–47]

Infection with *C. fetus* is usually associated with mild or no symptoms during pregnancy, but often leads to premature labor[43] and may cause recurrent abortions. Cervical cultures remain positive in women who have recurrent abortions and whose husbands have a high titer of antibodies to *C. fetus*.[48] Prolonged febrile illness with bacteremia and pneumonitis in the third trimester of pregnancy has been reported.[2] Unless appropriately treated, symptoms usually resolve only after abortion or delivery of an infected fetus.[42]

Campylobacter infection should be actively sought for in pregnant women with suspected infectious diarrhea, because it may lead to stillbirth and perinatal infection.[47,49] Diarrhea caused by *C. jejuni* consists of loose, watery stools or blood and mucus-containing stools. Fever, vomiting, abdominal pain, malaise, and myalgia are common. The incubation period is 1–7 days. Most patients recover in less than 1 week, but illness may last longer in immunocompromised hosts. Fecal excretion of the organisms in untreated patients usually lasts for 2–3 weeks, but may last as long as several months. Young children tend to shed the organisms for longer periods.

Perinatal infection

Maternal *C. fetus* and *C. jejuni* infections may cause neonatal sepsis and meningitis.[50] The infected neonates, who are often premature, develop signs suggesting sepsis, including fever, cough, respiratory distress, vomiting, diarrhea, cyanosis, convulsions, and jaundice. Newborn infection with *C. jejuni* is associated with diarrhea that may be bloody.[51] Focal infections caused by *C. jejuni*, such as pancreatitis, cholecystitis, urinary tract infection, arthritis, and peritonitis, may occur in neonates.

Late complications

Guillain–Barré syndrome has been reported 1–3 weeks after culture-proven *C. jejuni* gastroenteritis. Serologic studies suggest that 20–40% of patients with Guillain–Barré syndrome have evidence of recent infection with *C. jejuni*.[41] Other late immunoreactive complications include arthritis, erythema nodosum, hemolytic anemia, and immune complex glomerulonephritis.

Diagnosis

The diagnosis is based on identification of *Campylobacter* in cultures. Selective media such as Skorrow's or Batzler's media are used. Rapid diagnosis of *Campylobacter* enteritis may be made by direct carbolfuchsin stain of fecal smear, indirect fluorescence antibody test, dark field microscopy, or latex agglutination. Diagnosis with species-specific DNA probes and gene amplification by PCR have been described.

Prevention

Proper food handling and hand washing after contact with animals decrease the risk of infection with *Campylobacter*.

Breast feeding protects against infectious diarrhea caused by *C. jejuni*. Specific immunoglobulin A antibodies have been found in human milk.[52]

Treatment

Erythromycin (50 mg/kg/24 h, maximal dose 500 mg × 4/day for 5 days) is the drug of choice for treatment of *C. jejuni* and *C. coli* infections. Antibiotic therapy significantly shortens fecal excretion of *Campylobacter*. Erythromycin resistance has been reported. Antibiotic treatment should be given to patients with the dysenteric form of the disease, high-grade fever, pregnant women and immunocompromised hosts. Infections with *C. fetus* require parenteral antibiotic therapy for 3–4 weeks. Gentamicin is the recommended drug until antibiotic susceptibility is proven.

Parasitic infections: *Entamoeba histolytica*

Etiology

Infection is caused by ingestion of parasite cysts that exist in the small intestine to form trophozoites. Trophozoites colonize the lumen of the large intestine and may invade the mucosa.

Epidemiology

Humans are the major reservoir. It is estimated that 12% of the population worldwide is infected with *E. histolytica;* symptomatic disease occurs in 1–17% of infected subjects. Chronically institutionalized persons, homosexual men, and lower socioeconomic groups are at increased risk of acquiring *E. histolytica*. The most common modes of transmission are consumption of food or water contaminated with cysts, and direct fecal–oral contact.

Clinical manifestations

Intestinal amebiasis is the most common form of the disease. The presentation may be with gradual onset of bloody mucous diarrhea and abdominal pain. Fever is found in one-third of patients and constitutional symptoms are usually absent. Complications include extraintestinal spread, local perforation, and peritonitis.

Hepatic amebiasis occurs in 1% of infected individuals, usually in patients with amebic colitis, although it may appear in patients with no clear history of intestinal disease. Hepatic amebiasis presents with fever, abdominal pain, and enlarged, tender liver. Elevation of the diaphragm may be seen on chest x-ray examination. Leukocytosis, anemia, and elevation of liver enzymes may be present.

Pregnancy

Amebiasis is known to be more severe and even fatal in pregnant women.[53] This is thought to be due to several factors, including high progesterone levels[54] and failure of immunoglobulin levels to rise during infection.[55] Pregnant women are more susceptible to hepatic amebiasis as well. Several cases of rupture of amebic liver abscesses and peritonitis during pregnancy and puerperium have been reported.[56] Hepatic amebiasis may cause premature delivery,[56] but early diagnosis and adequate treatment results in successful outcome of the pregnancy. Vertical transmission of *E. histolytica* has not been reported. Infection in neonates probably results from ingestion of fecal material at birth, from oral fluids given as a supplement to breast feeding, or from close contact with infected mothers. The disease in newborns may be severe.[57]

Diagnosis

This is based on detecting the organisms in stool samples, tissue biopsy samples, and aspirates of a liver abscess. At least three stool samples should be examined, within 30 min of passage. In patients with hepatic amebiasis, stool cultures are negative in 50% of the cases. Indirect hemagglutination test is used to detect antibody titer.

Treatment

Intestinal amebiasis may be treated with iodoquinol, which is a luminal amebicide and has been used in pregnancy, apparently without causing fetal harm.[58] Invasive amebiasis of the intestine, liver, or other organs should be treated with metronidazole, a tissue-amebicidal drug. The use of metronidazole in the first trimester of pregnancy is controversial, although several studies have described the safe use of metronidazole in pregnancy.[58] Since invasive amebiasis is a life-threatening disease, particularly in pregnancy, and metronidazole is the drug of choice for this condition, the benefit of use outweighs the risk.

Small hepatic abscesses may be treated with metronidazole alone, but larger abscesses should be treated with transabdominal aspiration. If rupture is suspected, laparotomy is essential and life-saving.

Other parasitic infections

Infections with several protozoa including *Giardia lamblia*, *Cryptosporidium* and *Isospora belli* may cause diarrheal disease in neonates. Adverse effects in pregnancy have not been reported. Breast feeding is believed to protect against symptomatic infection.[2]

REFERENCES

1. Ashkenazi S, Cleary TG. Salmonella infections. In Behrman YS, Kliegman RM, Arvin AM, eds. *Textbook of Pediatrics*. Philadelphia: W. B. Saunders, 1996:784–90.
2. Pickering LK, Guerrant RL, Cleary TG. Microorganisms responsible for neonatal diarrhea. In Remingron JS, Klein JO, eds. *Infectious Diseases of the Fetus and Newborn Infant*. Philadelphia: W. B. Saunders, 1995:1142–222.
3. Silverio B. Gastric emptying time in the newborn and the nursling. *Am J Med Sci* 1964;247:732–4.
4. Sasidharan CK, Rajagopal KC, Panicker CK. *S. typhimurium* epidemic in newborn nursery. *Indian J Pediatr* 1983;50:599–605.
5. Puri V, Thirupuram S, Khalil A, Vergheese A, Gupta S. Nosocomial *S. typhimurium* epidemic in a neonatal special care unit. *Indian J Pediatr* 1980;17:233–9.
6. Torrey S, Fleisher G, Jaffe D. Incidence of *Salmonella* bacteremia in infants with *Salmonella* gastroenteritis. *J Pediatr* 1986;108: 718–21.
7. Meadow WL, Schneider H, Beem MO. *Salmonella enteritidis* bacteremia in childhood. *J Infect Dis* 1985;152:185–9.
8. Revhaug A, Berdal B. Septic abortion caused by *Salmonella enteritidis*. *Acta Obstet Gynecol Scand* 1988;67:185–6.
9. Tettmar RE, Faithfull-Davies DN. Salmonella urinary tract infection in pregnancy. *J Hosp Infect* 1985;6:227–9.
10. Goldberg MB, Rubin RH. The spectrum of *Salmonella* infection. *Infect Dis Clin North Am* 1988;2:571–98.
11. Cohen JI, Bartlett JA, Corey GR. Extraintestinal manifestations of *Salmonella* infections. *Medicine* 1987;66:349–88.
12. Achi R, Dac-Cam P, Forsum U, *et al*. Titers of class-specific antibodies against *Shigella* and *Salmonella* lipopolysaccharide antigens in colostrum and breast milk of Costa Rican, Swedish and Vietnamese mothers. *J Infect* 1992;2–5:89–105.
13. Mahle WT, Levine MM. *Salmonella typhi* infection in children younger than 5 years of age. *Pediatr Infect Dis J* 1993;12:627–31.
14. Villarma A, Galang YS. Typhoid fever in pregnancy. *Phillipine Med Assoc* 1930;10:311–5.
15. Riggal F, Salkind G, Spellacy W. Typhoid fever complicating pregnancy. *Obstet Gynecol* 1974;44:117–21.
16. Amster R, Lessing JB, Jaffa AJ, Peyser MR. Typhoid fever complicating pregnancy. *Acta Obstet Gynecol Scand* 1985;64:685–6.
17. Awadalla SG, Mercer LY, Brown LG. Pregnancy complicated by intraamniotic infection by *Salmonella typhi*. *Obstet Gynecol* 1983;65:30S–1S.
18. Lewis GJ. A rare cause of cholecystitis in pregnancy. *Int J Gynaecol Obstet* 1983;21:175–7.
19. Centers for Disease Control and Prevention. Typhoid immunization: Recommendations of the Immunization Practices Advisory Committee. *Morbid Mortal Weekly Rep* 1990;39:1.
20. Leung D, Venkatesan P, Bosewell T, Innes JA, Wood MJ. Treatment of typhoid in pregnancy (letter). *Lancet* 1995;34:648.
21. Ashkenazi S, Cleary TG. Shigella infections. In Feigin RD, Cherry JD, eds. *Textbook of Pediatric Infectious Diseases*. Philadelphia: W. B. Saunders, 1992:637–46.
22. Ashkenazi S. Role of bacterial cytotoxins in hemolytic uremic syndrome and thrombotic thrombocytopenic purpura. *Ann Rev Med* 1993;44:11–8.
23. Huskins WC, Griffiths JK, Faruque ASB, Bennish ML. Shigellosis in neonates and young infants. *J Pediatr* 1994;125:14–22.
24. Haltalin KC. Neonatal shigellosis. *Am J Dis Child* 1967;117:142.
25. Armor SA. Periparturitional shigellosis. *Nebr Med J* 1990;75: 239–41.
26. Lett DW, Marsh TD. Shigellosis in a newborn. *Am J Perinatol* 1993;10:58–9.
27. Kraybill EN, Controni G. Septicemia and enterocolitis due to *S. sonnei* in a newborn infant. *Pediatrics* 1968;42:529.
28. Starke JR, Baker CJ. Neonatal shigellosis with bowel perforation. *Pediatr Infect Dis J* 1985;4:405.
29. Raderman JW, Stoller KP, Pomerance JJ. Bloodstream invasion with *S. sonnei* in an asymptomatic newborn infant. *Pediatr Infect Dis J* 1986;4:405.
30. Whitefield C, Humphries JM. Meningitis and septicemia due to *Shigella* in a newborn infant. *J Pediatr* 1967;70:805.
31. Ashkenazi S, Cleary TG. Yersinia. In Oski FA, De Angelis CD, Feigin, RD, McMillan, JA, Warshaw JB, eds. *Principles and Practice of Pediatrics*. Philadelphia: J. B. Lippincott Company, 1993: 1259–63.
32. Paisley JW, Lauer BA. Neonatal *Yersinia enterocolitica* enteritis. *Pediatr Infect Dis J* 1992;11:331–2.
33. Challapalli M, Cunningham DG. *Yersinia enterocolitica* septicemia in infants younger than 3 months of age. *Pediatr Infect Dis J* 1993;12:168–9.
34. Jensen OM, Paerregaard A. Inhibition of plasmid-encoded adhesion of *Yersinia enterocolitica* by non-immunoglobulin fraction of human milk. *Acta Pathol Microbiol Immunol Scand* 1991;99:657–60.
35. Glass RI, Libel M, Brandling AD. Epidemic cholera in the Americas. *Science* 1992;256:1524–6.
36. Hirschhorn N, Chowdhury AK, Lindenbaum J. Cholera in pregnant women. *Lancet* 1969;1:1230–2.
37. Lindenbaum J, Akbar R, Gordon RS Jr. Cholera in children. *Lancet* 1966;1:1066–8.
38. Glass RI, Svennerholm AM, Stoll BJ, *et al*. Protection against cholera in breast-fed children by antibodies in breastmilk. *N Engl J Med* 1983;308:1389–92.
39. Holmgren J, Svennerholm AM, Lindblad M. Receptor-like glycocompounds in human milk that inhibit classical and El Tor Vibro choleral cell adherence (hemagglutination). *Infect Immun* 1983;39:147–54.
40. Laegreid A, Otnaess AB, Fugleslang J. Human and bovine milk. Comparison of ganglioside composition and enterotoxin inhibitory activity. *Pediatr Res* 1986;20:416–21.
41. Ashkenazi S, Cleary TG. Campylobacter. In Behrman RE, Kliegman RM, Arvin AM, eds. *Textbook of Pediatrics*. Philadelphia: W. B. Saunders, 1996:800–2.
42. Eden AN. Perinatal mortality caused by *Vibrio fetus*: Review and analysis. *J Pediatr* 1966;68:297–9.
43. Sauerwein RW, Bisseling J, Horrevorts AM. Septic abortion associated with *Campylobacter fetus* subspecies *fetus* infection: Case report and review of the literature. *Infection* 1993;21:331–3.
44. Mazor M, Chaim W, Bar-David J, *et al*. Prenatal diagnosis of microbial invasion of the amniotic cavity with *Campylobacter coli* in preterm labor. *Br J Obstet Gynaecol* 1995;102:71–2.
45. Gurgan T, Diker KS. Abortion associated with *Campylobacter upsaliensis*. *J Clin Microbiol* 1994;32:3093–4.
46. Quentin R, Chevrier D, Guesdon JL, Martin C, Pierre F, Goudeau A. Use of nonradioactive DNA probes to identify *Campylobacter jejuni* strain causing abortion. *Eur J Clin Microbiol Infect Dis* 1993;12:627–30.
47. Goh J, Flynn M. *Campylobacter jejuni* in pregnancy. *Aust N Z J Obstet Gynaecol* 1992;32:246–8.
48. Hood M, Todd JM. *Vibrio fetus* – A cause of human abortion. *Am J Obstet Gynecol* 1960;80:506–7.
49. Denton KJ, Clarke T. Role of *Campylobacter jejuni* as a placental pathogen. *J Clin Pathol* 1992;45:171–2.
50. Torphy DE, Bond WW. *Campylobacter fetus* infections in children. *Pediatrics* 1979;64:898–900.

51. Reina J, Borrell N, Fial M. Rectal bleeding caused by *Campylobacter jejuni* in a neonate. *Pediatr Infect Dis J* 1992;11:500–1.
52. Torres O, Cruz, JR. Protection against *Campylobacter* diarrhea: Role of milk IgA antibodies. *Acta Paediatr* 1993;82:835–8.
53. Abioye AA. Fatal amoebic colitis in pregnancy and the puerperium. *J Trop Med Hyg* 1973;76:97–100.
54. Biagi FF, Beltram MF. The challenge of amoebiasis: Understanding pathogenic mechanisms. *Int Rev Trop Med* 1969;3:219–39.
55. Abioye AA, Lewis EA, McFarlane H. Clinical evaluation of serum immunoglobulins in amoebiasis. *Immunology* 1972;23:937–46.
56. Constantine G, Menon V, Luesley D. Amoebic peritonitis in pregnancy in the United Kingdom. *Postgrad Med J* 1987;63: 495–6.
57. Dykes AC, Ruebush TK, Gorelkin L, Lushbaugh WB, Upshur JK, Cherry JD. Extraintestinal amebiasis in infancy: Report of three patients and epidemiologic investigations of their families. *Pediatrics* 1980;65:799–803.
58. Briggs GG, Freeman RK, Yaffe SJ. *Drugs in Pregnancy and Lactation*, 4th edn. Baltimore: Williams & Wilkins, 1994:455,585.

164 Central nervous system infections in pregnancy

E. Rubinstein and B. Rubinovitch

Introduction

Central nervous system (CNS) infection in a pregnant woman is the result of the same expected epidemiological and predisposing factors that operate in CNS infections in non-pregnant adults. Chances for CNS invasion and disease are generally very low, even for a pathogenic microorganism that is more likely to colonize and infect women during pregnancy and/or the puerperium (e.g. *Listeria monocytogenes*, streptococcus group B).

Infections of the CNS are divided into different clinical syndromes according to the principal site of the infection within the CNS (meningitis, encephalitis and myelitis) and with regard to the time course of the disease (acute or chronic). The distinction between syndromes is clinically useful in guiding management, but is artificial in terms of etiology and pathology.

In this chapter are discussed the principal CNS infectious syndromes, with emphasis on aspects unique to pregnancy, mainly the impact of infection, disease and therapy on the fetus and the newborn.

Meningitis

Meningitis is an inflammation of the subarachnoid space and is identified by an abnormal number of white blood cells in the cerebrospinal fluid (CSF). The acute meningitis syndrome is characterized clinically by the sudden onset of symptoms (high fever, headache, photophobia, stiff neck and altered mental status) over a course of hours or days. It may be caused by a wide variety of infectious agents: bacteria (including rickettsiae, spirochetes and mycobacteria), viruses, fungi and protozoa, and may also be a manifestation of non-infectious diseases. Most commonly, it is caused by viruses (aseptic meningitis) or bacteria. Chronic meningitis typically has a gradual onset of symptoms and signs (over weeks to months) and the patient is more likely to present a picture of chronic general debility, as well as having symptoms referable to the CNS.[1]

Acute bacterial meningitis

Epidemiology and microbiology

Bacterial meningitis remains an important disease worldwide. Despite the development of new and more effective antimicrobial agents, the overall case fatality rate remains about 25%. Nowadays, the three most common meningeal pathogens in adults with community-acquired meningitis are *Streptococcus pneumoniae, Neisseria meningitidis* and *L. monocytogenes*, with pneumococci and meningococci accounting for half of the cases. Uncommon pathogens are *Staphylococcus aureus*, streptococci (groups A, B, D), *Haemophilus influenzae* and gram-negative bacilli.[1,2]

Pathogenesis

Nasopharyngeal colonization of a typical meningeal pathogen *(S. pneumoniae, N. meningitidis, H. influenzae)*, which is asymptomatic, usually precedes meningitis. Mucosal invasion and bacteremia follow colonization, depending on the interplay between specific virulence factors and host defense mechanisms. Meningeal invasion occurs due to unknown mechanism(s). Bacterial replication in the subarachnoid space and release of bacterial components initiate subarachnoid space inflammation (i.e. meningitis).[1]

Clinical presentation

Two-thirds of the patients have the classical triad of fever, nuchal rigidity and change in mental status, ranging from confusion to lethargy and coma. Ninety percent have headache. Seizures (occurring in 30% of patients), and focal cerebral signs (10–20%) are the result of inflammation and thrombosis of subarachnoid blood vessels, causing cortical and subcortical ischemia. Cranial nerve palsies, especially those involving cranial nerves III, IV, VI and VII (10–20%), develop as the nerve becomes enveloped by exudate in the arachnoid sheath surrounding it. Isolated palsy of cranial nerve VI may be a sign of increased intracranial pressure. Other signs of elevated intracranial

Table 164.1 Normal CSF composition, and composition with bacterial meningitis

CSF parameter	Normal value	Typical value in bacterial meningitis
Opening pressure (mmH_2O)	50–180	> 180
White blood cell count	< 4/mm^3	1000–5000/mm^3
Neutrophilic percentage	1%	> 80%
Protein level (mg/dl)	20–45	100–500
Glucose level (mg/dl)	40–70	< 40
Lactate level (mg/dl)	10–20	> 35

CSF, cerebrospinal fluid

pressure are coma, hypertension and bradycardia. Papiledema is seen in 1% of cases. Unilateral pupil dilatation, due to involvement of the parasympathetic fibers of cranial nerve III, heralds transtentorial brain herniation.

Accompanying signs and symptoms may suggest a specific etiologic diagnosis. Rash is noted on admission in 10% of patients, of whom two-thirds have meningococcal meningitis.

An obvious primary focus of bacteremia is found in more than half of the adults with community-acquired meningitis, and the most common are pneumonia, acute otitis media and sinusitis.[1]

Characteristics of CSF

Diagnosis of bacterial meningitis rests on examination of the CSF by lumbar puncture. Typical findings are elevated opening pressure, neutrophilic pleocytosis, elevated protein level, hypoglychorrachia and elevated lactate level.[1] Pregnancy by itself does not alter normal CSF composition and pressure. Typical CSF findings are presented in Table 164.1.

Many patients with bacterial meningitis have atypical CSF findings (e.g. lymphocytic predominance, normal glucose value, slightly elevated protein level, very low CSF white blood cell count), therefore a Gram stain and cultures should be performed on all spinal fluid specimens regardless of the composition.

Microbiological evaluation

Gram stain examination of CSF identifies accurately the causative microorganism in 60–90% of all cases. It is less sensitive for meningitis caused by gram-negative bacilli or *L. monocytogenes*. In addition, sensitivities of Gram stain and culture are reduced by prior antibiotic use. Latex agglutination assays for detection of bacterial antigens in CSF currently detect the antigens of *S. pnuemoniae, H. influenzae, N. meningitidis*, streptococcus group B and *Escherichia coli* K1. Sensitivity ranges from 50–90%, depending on the kit used.[1]

Initial management of a patient suspected to have bacterial meningitis

Bacterial meningitis should be considered in the differential diagnosis of a febrile patient with any of the following: meningeal signs, change in mental status, headache, photophobia, convulsions and/or focal neurological signs, petechial rash or close contact with patients with meningitis. In suspected bacterial meningitis, performance of lumbar puncture is mandatory.

The timing of performance of lumbar puncture, head and brain computed tomography scan and initiation of antibiotic therapy depend on the following factors:

Pattern of onset: In approximately 20% of cases, patients become critically ill within hours. Others develop meningeal symptoms over several days. In critically ill patients, and whenever results of lumbar puncture cannot be obtained in 30 min, empirical antimicrobial therapy may precede lumbar puncture and should be given immediately after obtaining blood cultures. Whenever possible, consultation with an infectious diseases expert, an internist or an intensivist should be sought.

Presence of papilledema or other signs of elevated intracranial pressure: A simple method to reduce intracranial pressure is elevation of the head of the bed to 30°, to maximize venous drainage with minimal compromise to cerebral perfusion. Hyperventilation and use of manitol should be performed by experienced personnel.

Presence of focal neurologic signs or seizures: More than 50% of patients with focal findings (excluding ophthal-moplegia) or seizures have evidence on computed tomography scan of an intracranial abnormality (i.e. cerebral edema, hydrocephalus, subdural effusion or empyema, cavernous sinus thrombosis, abscesses). Because of the potential risk of brain herniation, computed tomography scan of the head should be performed prior to lumbar puncture if the above signs are present.[1,3]

Table 164.2 Specific antimicrobial therapy of bacterial meningitis in adults

Microorganism	Standard therapy	Dosage per 24 h
Streptococcus pneumoniae		
Penicillin MIC < 0.1 mg/ml	Penicillin G	4×10^6 U × 6
Penicillin MIC 0.1–1.0 mg/ml	Ceftriaxone or	2 g × 2
	Cefotaxime	2 g × 4–6
Penicillin MIC ≥ 2.0 mg/ml	Vancomycin plus	1 g × 2–3
	ceftriaxone or cefotaxime	As above
	±rifampicin	600 mg × 1
Neisseria meningitidis	Penicillin G	4×10^6 U × 6
Haemophilus influenzae		
β-Lactamase negative	Ampicillin	2 g × 6
β-L actamase positive	Ceftriaxone or cefotaxime	As above
Listeria monocytogenes	Ampicillin or penicillin G	As above
	±gentamicin	3–5 mg/kg
Streptococcus agalactiae	Ampicillin or penicillin G	As above
	±gentamicin	3–5 mg/kg

MIC, minimal inhibitory concentration

Recommended empirical therapy is aimed against the most common pathogens (i.e. *S. pneumoniae, N. meningitidis*). Currently, the drug of choice is a parenteral third-generation cephalosporin.[1,3] Penicillin should be added whenever certain risk factors for *L. monocytogenes* meningitis exist. Specific recommendations are given in relevant sections and are summarized in Table 164.2.

Adjunctive corticosteroid therapy

As described earlier, subarachnoid space inflammatory response is a major factor contributing to morbidity and mortality. Recent evidence has indicated that antibacterial agents initially potentiate cerebral inflammation, by causing bacterial lysis and discharging bacterial components that accelerate release of cytokines. This has renewed interest in adjunctive therapies such as corticosteroids. Ample data support the routine use of dexamethasone in infants and children with bacterial meningitis. In adults, the benefits of steroids are currently less certain. However, adults with severely impaired mental status, documented cerebral edema or markedly elevated intracranial pressure, as well as patients with a high CSF bacterial concentration, may benefit from adjunctive dexamethasone. For optimal effect, the first dose of dexamethasone should be administered shortly before or concomitantly with the first dose of antibiotics. Recommended dosage is 0.15 mg/kg intravenously every 6 h for 4 days or 0.4 mg/kg every 12 h for 2 days.[1,3]

S. pneumoniae meningitis

Pneumococci are encapsulated gram-positive, lancet-shaped diplococci. This is a major respiratory pathogen, frequently colonizing the nasopharynx of normal adults and healthy children. *S. pneumoniae* is the most common etiologic agent of bacterial meningitis in adults, accounting for a third of cases.[1] Specific immunodeficiencies and chronic diseases predispose to severe pneumococcal infections. The most relevant for women of childbearing age are absent or hypofunctioning spleen and acquired immunodeficiency syndrome (AIDS). In addition, patients with previous head trauma, CSF leak, or a break in the integrity of the dura, have a unique predisposition to recurrent meningitis caused by pneumococci.[1,2] Africans seem to have a peculiar susceptibility to severe pneumococcal infections, including pneumococcal meningitis. An unexplained association of pneumococcal meningitis with pregnancy and the puerperium was recorded in Nigeria in the early 1960s.[4]

Clinical manifestations

Pneumococcal meningitis in pregnancy has no distinctive clinical or laboratory features. Fever, headache, nuchal rigidity and altered mental status are common. One-third of patients have seizures. Most cases occur in late pregnancy and the first week of the puerperium. Apparent sources of infection are pneumonia and purulent otitis media or sinusitis as expected, but a high percentage have primary bacteremia. Although *S. pneumoniae* is only occasionally isolated in puerperal or postabortal sepsis,[5] ascending infection of the female genital tract may be relevant as a source of bacteremia and meningitis in some cases of puerperal and postabortal meningitis. The fatality rate for maternal pneumococcal meningitis is 27%, and is correlated with obtunded mental status. In Nigeria, hyperthermia (body temperature above 41°C) was found to be a bad prognostic sign. About half of the survivors have neurologic sequelae (i.e. deafness, hemiparesis and cranial nerve palsies and cognitive impairment).[4] Rates of mortality and neurological morbidity in adults with pneumococcal meningitis have not decreased much in the last 30 years,[1,2] reflecting the severe damage caused by the subarachnoid inflammatory process. In severe maternal pneumococcal disease, overall fetal loss is 45% (abortion, stillbirth and early neonatal death).[4,5] Whenever pregnancy continues to term, newborns survive. Neonates of mothers with puerperal pneumococcal meningitis may also develop pneumococcal meningitis, pneumonia and/or sepsis.[6] Mode of transmission is either transplacental (hematogenous spread) or through a colonized birth canal. Neonatal pneumoccocal disease has an early onset and carries a grave prognosis.[5] The mortality rate is 48% and of the survivors 13% are left with neurologic sequelae. Fatal maternal meningitis may spare the newborn, as seen in a rare case of successful postmortem cesarean section in fulminant pneumococcal meningitis.[7]

Diagnosis

Examination of a gram-stained specimen of CSF provides the correct diagnosis unless antibiotic has already been administered. In the latter case latex agglutination assay for detection of pneumococcal capsular antigen is useful. Cultures of CSF specimens, blood and any other relevant material (e.g. from the genital tract) should always be performed.

Treatment

Penicillin can no longer be recommended as empirical therapy in suspected pneumococcal meningitis due to an increasing frequency of penicillin resistance in pneumococci. A parenteral third-generation cephalosporin is recommended pending results of susceptibility tests (see Table 164.2). Optimal therapy for meningitis caused by pneumococci highly resistant to penicillin [i.e. minimal inhibitory concentration (MIC) greater than 1 mg/ml] is a subject of debate. Currently, vancomycin and a third-generation cephalosporin are recommended. Some authorities advise the addition of rifampicin (RMP).[1,3] Penicillin G and the cephalosporins (first, second and third generation) are considered safe in pregnancy. Data on the use of vancomycin in pregnancy are limited; however, no toxicity was demonstrated in a small controlled study of infants exposed in the second and third trimesters. RMP has caused teratogenic effects in rodents treated with high doses, and is probably best avoided during pregnancy.[1,8] The duration of antimicrobial therapy is 10–14 days.[1,9]

N. meningitidis meningitis

Meningococci are gram-negative encapsulated diplococci. Strain serogrouping is based on capsular polysaccharides. Serogroups A, B and C are the most important clinically, while current commercial vaccines contain polysaccharides of groups A, C, Y, and W-135, and are effective in 90% of recipients 2 years of age or older. *N. meningitidis* is the second most common cause of community-acquired bacterial meningitis, accounting for 13–20% of cases. In epidemics, meningococci are more likely to be implicated than pneumoccoci as a cause of meningitis. Patients with deficiencies in the terminal complement components have a markedly increased incidence of meningococcal diseases. However, the vast majority of patients with meningococcemia and/or meningitis have an intact complement system.[1]

Clinical manifestations

Meningococcal infections are capable of diverse presentations, which range from transient fever and bacteremia to fulminant disease with circulatory collapse and death ensuing within hours of the onset of clinical symptoms. Meningeal or neurological signs do not distinguish meningitis caused by meningococci from meningitis caused by other etiologies. The most important clinical finding is the rash, which is typically petechial, but can be purpuric or sometimes maculopapular. The presence of petechiae in conjugation with purulent meningitis has a very high sensitivity and specificity rate for *N. meningitidis* meningitis. Lesions are found on the trunk, lower portions of the body, the face and mucous membranes, and new petechiae may appear during the physical examination.

Shock, heart failure and disseminated intravascular coagulation are complications of overwhelming meningococcemia and are associated with poor prognosis.[1]

Meningococcal meningitis in pregnancy is apparently uncommon.[10] In one study, meningitis occurred in late pregnancy, and the newborns were delivered while the mothers were acutely ill. One newborn died immediately, although there was no evidence of infection; the mothers survived.

Diagnosis

CSF examination provides the diagnosis in 50–90% of cases. Blood cultures are positive in 50% of cases. Latex agglutination assays are useful when prior antibiotic has been administered. Bacterial antigens can be detected longer in the urine than in other body fluids, and concentrated urine specimens, in addition to CSF, should be studied for antigen in such patients.[1]

Treatment

Penicillin G is the treatment of choice for meningococcal meningitis.[1,3] Strains of meningococci that are relatively resistant to penicillin have emerged, but their clinical significance is unclear. For penicillin-allergic patients a third-generation cephalosporin is an alternative. Duration of therapy is 7 days.[9]

Antibacterial prophylaxis

Therapy to eliminate asymptomatic nasopharyngeal colonization is recommended for all intimate contacts of the index case (household and nursery-school contacts). The index case should also receive therapy to eradicate nasopharyngeal carriage (after completion of therapy for meningitis), unless treated with a cephalosporin.[1] RMP, 600 mg for adults or 10 mg/kg for children, 12 hourly for 2 days, is used as prophylaxis. An alternative for pregnant women is a single dose of intramuscular ceftriaxone 250 mg.

Vaccination

Vaccination with the quadrivalent meningococcal vaccine is recommended during outbreaks of disease caused by the serogroups represented in the vaccine preparation. Vaccination is not contraindicated in pregnancy.[1]

L. monocytogenes meningitis

L. monocytogenes is a gram-positive bacillus that is widespread in nature. Outbreaks are associated with consumption of contaminated food, but most cases are sporadic. *L. monocytogenes* is the third most common cause of community-acquired bacterial meningitis in adults, accounting for 10% of cases.[1,2] Patients susceptible to listeriosis are those with suppressed T-cell-mediated immunity, serious underlying diseases, the elderly, and pregnant women and their offspring.[1,11]

Clinical manifestations

Listeria infection of the CNS manifests either as fulminant bacterial meningitis or as subacute meningoencephalitis. Meningitis in pregnancy occurs rarely, although listeriosis associated with pregnancy accounts for a third of all cases. It is not known why CNS invasion occurs very rarely in pregnant women, but does occur in half of the cases not associated with pregnancy.[1,11–13] *Listeria* meningitis in immunocompromised hosts has a mortality rate of 20–40%; in previously healthy adults the risk of mortality is very low. All pregnant women reported with *Listeria* meningitis have survived. While serious illness in the mother is rare, transmission to the fetus and neonate causes serious diseases with high mortality rates. Fetal loss is high with early intrauterine infection, and perinatal mortality rates are 20–50% for the 'late' form. The devastating illness granulomatosis infantisepticum is almost always fatal.[1,11,13]

Diagnosis

CSF findings do not distinguish between *Listeria* and other bacterial etiologies of meningitis. CSF Gram stain for detection of *L. monocytogenes* has a low sensitivity, but the organism will usually grow on appropriate culture media.[1]

Treatment

The treatment of choice for *Listeria* meningitis is either penicillin or ampicillin in sufficient dosages[1] (see Table 164.2). The addition of gentamicin is based on laboratory data only. Duration of therapy should be 14–21 days.[9] For penicillin-allergic patients, trimetoprim–sulfamethoxazole is an alternative. Sulfonamides should not be administered during the last month of pregnancy due to increased risk of kernicterus in the newborn. The teratogenicity of trimetoprim is not clearly defined.[1,8]

Standard empirical therapy for bacterial meningitis in the adult would be a third-generation cephalosporin (see above), an antimicrobial agent to which *Listeria* is inherently resistant. Taking into account the rarity of *Listeria* meningitis in pregnancy, it is suggested that penicillin need not be added routinely to the standard empirical treatment of bacterial meningitis in the otherwise healthy young pregnant woman.

Streptococcus agalactiae meningitis

S. agalactiae [group B streptococcus (GBS)] is a gram-positive coccus, which frequently colonizes the genitourinary tract and lower gastrointestinal tract of pregnant women. GBS is an important cause of maternal postpartum infections, as well as bacteremia and meningitis, in the neonate.[1] It is a rare cause of meningitis in adults, representing < 1% of etiologic agents, with most affected patients having severe underlying diseases.[14]

Clinical manifestations

The presentation is similar to that of other types of acute bacterial meningitis, with a high incidence of neurological dysfunction. Cases of postpartum GBS meningitis are reported rarely,[14] occurring during the first 2 days postpartum. In contrast with an overall mortality rate of 27% for GBS meningitis in adults, all parturient women recovered. Mortality rates of neonatal GBS infections have decreased to 2–8% in term infants, but a significant number of the neonates surviving GBS meningitis will suffer neurologic sequelae.[1,14]

Diagnosis

CSF Gram stain and culture provide the diagnosis in 90% of cases. Concomitant bacteremia is frequent.

Treatment

High-dose penicillin G is the drug of choice for GBS meningitis in adults; addition of gentamicin is based on *in vitro* synergy. Duration of therapy is 14–21 days.[1,14]

Acute viral meningitis

Enteroviruses (echoviruses and coxackieviruses)

Echoviruses and coxackieviruses group B are currently the leading recognizable causes of the acute aseptic meningitis syndrome.[1] These are RNA viruses, members of the Picornaviridae family, with a worldwide distribution.

Epidemiology

Most cases occur in children and young adults. There is a marked summer/fall seasonality, but infection may occur at any time.

Clinical manifestations

Fever, headache, meningismus, nausea, vomiting and photophobia are common. There may be accompanying non-specific signs and symptoms such as rash, diarrhea, upper respiratory findings and myalgia. Illness is sometimes biphasic, with fever and myalgia present for a few days, followed by defervescence and absence of symptoms for 2–10 days before the sudden reappearance of fever and headache signaling the onset of meningitis. Duration of illness is usually less than 1 week, and most children and adults recover uneventfully without sequelae. Seizures, lethargy and coma or full-blown encephalitis occur in less than 5% of cases. A more severe meningoencephalitis may be seen in neonates (and in individuals with deficient humoral immunity that impairs clearance of enteroviruses). In such cases morbidity and mortality are considerable.[1]

Enteroviral meningitis complicating pregnancy is a rare occurrence.[15] Specific echovirus and coxackievirus serotypes are usually responsible for severe, frequently fatal disease in the perinatally infected neonate.[1] Ample experimental evidence indicates that the fetus is relatively protected during maternal infection by the placenta, but the newborn has the highest risk of infection. Thus, the most critical factor determining the outcome of neonatal enterovirus infection is the timing of maternal infection in relation to the development of maternal virus-specific immunoglobulin G antibodies and delivery of the infant.

Diagnosis

CSF parameters are aseptic meningitis with lymphocytic pleocytosis (10–1000 cells/mm^3), mildly elevated CSF protein and usually normal glucose level. Early in the course there may be polymorphonuclear neutrophil predominance and it may be difficult to exclude bacterial meningitis on the basis of CSF analysis alone. Diagnosis is based on enterovirus isolation from stools, nasopharyngeal swabs and CSF. Serology is useful only to confirm diagnosis for specific type.

Treatment

No specific antiviral therapy exists. In cases of severe neonatal disease (as in the rare cases of chronic enterovirus meningoencephalitis in agammaglobulinemic patients), high doses of intravenous immunoglobulin have been reported to improve outcome.[1]

Human immunodeficiency virus

Human immunodeficiency virus (HIV) causes acute aseptic meningitis syndrome associated with the acute retroviral syndrome in 5–10% of cases. Onset of illness ranges from 1 to 6 weeks after exposure to the virus. Clinical manifestations are non-specific, with fever, headache, photophobia and meningismus. Typical CSF findings show mild lymphocytic pleocytosis (20–300/mm^3), mildly elevated protein and normal or slightly decreased glucose.

Diagnosis is based on detection of HIV p24 core antigen in serum and CSF, since the enzyme-linked immunosorbent assay (ELISA) for HIV antibodies remains negative for an average of 2–3 months.[1]

For management strategies regarding HIV-infected pregnant women, the reader should consult HIV authorities.

Acute viral encephalitis

Enecephalitis is an inflammation of the brain. Acute encephalitis associated with viral infections includes two distinct clinico-pathological diseases: acute viral encephalitis of which the most important etiologies are herpes simplex virus type 1 (HSV-1), and the arthropod-borne viruses (arboviruses), and postinfectious encephalomyelitis, with the number of cases decreasing greatly since the institution of immunization against measles, mumps and rubella.[16] Important issues in the differential diagnosis of encephalitis are to rule out non-viral diseases (which may require urgent treatment) and to properly identify cases due to HSV-1, where morbidity and mortality can be greatly reduced with specific antiviral therapy.

Herpes simplex encephalitis

HSV-1, a member of the Herpesviridae family, is the commonest cause of localized sporadic encephalitis in otherwise healthy adults and children

Clinical manifestations

The distinctive pathology, localization of inflammation and necrosis to the temporal and frontal lobes, determines the clinical manifestations. Signs that suggest a localized lesion in one or both temporal lobes are present in 90% of patients.[16] This may manifest itself as personality changes, bizarre behavior and hallucinations, which can dominate the clinical picture for a few days before other signs evolve. Onset may be abrupt or insidious. Fever, headache and altered consciousness are very common. Other focal findings (seizures, dysphasia, hemiparesis, autonomic dysfunction, ataxia and cranial nerve palsies) occur in 30–80% of the cases The course in untreated patients is usually one of rapid deterioration, over several days, to coma and death. Therapy reduces the mortality rate from 70% to 19%, but patients may suffer severe neurological sequelae, even with early specific treatment.[1,16]

HSV encephalitis in pregnancy is rare, but carries significant morbidity and mortality for the mother and fetus. Only a few cases that were treated with acyclovir have been reported, and most had a favorable outcome, for both the mother and the fetus.[17]

Diagnosis

CSF findings are abnormal in more than 95% of patients. Typical findings are mildly elevated protein level, lymphocytic pleocytosis and normal glucose level. Red blood cells are found in 20–50% of cases.[16] Computed tomography scan may show a low-density abnormality in one or both temporal lobes, but is less sensitive than magnetic resonance imaging (MRI) for detecting focal findings, especially early in the course of the disease. The electroencephalogram is always abnormal but its specificity is low.

The 'gold standard' for diagnosis is brain biopsy, with appropriate histologic and cultural techniques. Non-invasive diagnostic tests such as viral culture of CSF, and CSF and serum serology have unacceptably low sensitivity and/or specificity regarding therapeutic decisions. Newer diagnostic tests [e.g. ELISA for CSF antigen detection and polymerase chain reaction (PCR) assay of CSF] appear to be highly sensitive and specific but are not widely available.[16]

It is generally accepted that even with extensive clinical experience, the accuracy of the diagnosis of HSV encephalitis is only 50% by using clinical judgment, spinal fluid examination and imaging. Should all patients with suspected HSV encephalitis be biopsied? In view of the disastrous nature of the disease, the effectiveness of the available treatment and its low toxicity (see below), empirical acyclovir treatment is justified in most cases of acute sporadic encephalitis in the normal host.[1,16]

Treatment

Acyclovir is currently the drug of choice for HSV encephalitis.[1] Dosage is 10 mg/kg intravenously every 8 h for 14 days. Dosage should be modified with renal function impairment. Use of acyclovir during pregnancy was not found to be teratogenic in animal studies.[1] Human experience with high intravenous dosages during the first trimester is lacking. No adverse reactions for the fetus have been reported when the drug has been used during the third trimester.[17]

Arbovirus encephalitis

The term arbovirus refers to viral pathogens transmitted by arthropod vectors (mosquito or tick). More than 20 arboviruses cause human encephalitis. Each has a specific geographic distribution, is associated with a different ratio of inapparent to clinical infections and causes encephalitis of variable severity.[16]

Japanese encephalitis virus is the causative agent of the most important arbovirus encephalitis worldwide. The virus is a member of the Flaviviridae family and is widely distributed in Asia. Most human infections are asymptomatic, with only 1 in 300 infections resulting in typical encephalitis.[16]

Clinical manifestations

Illness begins with non-specific febrile prodrome lasting several days, followed by abrupt onset of encephalitis with focal spastic paralysis, most commonly of the upper extremities, cranial nerve palsies and extrapyramidal signs. After 2–4 days, patients begin to improve or deteriorate rapidly. The case-fatality rate is 25% and neurological sequelae occur in up to 70% of the survivors.[1,16] In pregnant women infected during the first or second trimester, spontaneous abortion and fetal death have been documented, and the virus has been isolated from the conceptus. The risk of transmission during the third trimester is not known.[1,18]

Diagnosis

Typical CSF findings are lymphocytic pleocytosis, mildly elevated protein level and normal glucose level. Imaging studies of the brain (MRI and to a lesser degree computed tomography) may show abnormalities in basal ganglia and the brain stem. Specific diagnosis is serologic, by means of virus-specific immunoglobulin M ELISA, performed on CSF or on paired (acute and convalescent) sera.

Treatment and vaccination

No specific antiviral treatment exists. However, an inactivated whole virus vaccine is available and is indicated for travelers to endemic or epidemic areas. The vaccine is 90% effective and is not contraindicated in pregnancy.[1]

Tuberculous meningitis

Tuberculosis is caused by *Mycobacterium tuberculosis*, an acid-fast bacillus, for which humans are the only reservoir. In developed countries tuberculosis has emerged as an important problem since 1985, due to a combination of interrelated factors, namely illicit drug abuse, urban homelessness and the AIDS epidemic.[1] Tuberculosis in pregnancy has been a topic of concern and controversy for many decades.[1,19] Currently, it seems that the impact of pregnancy on tuberculosis is minimal, except for potentially obscuring the diagnosis and possibly increasing the risk of disease activation during the postpartum period. Tuberculous meningitis in adults is usually caused by rupture of a quiescent subependimal tubercle into the subarachnoid space. Less often, it is a complication of milliary tuberculosis (i.e. hematogenous spread).

Clinical manifestations

Usually, illness is subacute in presentation, and begins with a prodrome of malaise, intermittent headache and low-grade fever, followed within 2–3 weeks by protracted headache, vomiting, confusion, meningismus and focal neurologic signs.

The clinical spectrum is broad, ranging from chronic headache or subtle mental status alteration to sudden and severe meningitis progressing to coma.[1] Tuberculous meningitis in pregnancy tends to occur during the postpartum period or late pregnancy. The clinical presentation is often of chronic meningitis. Mortality and neurological morbidity are correlated with delay in diagnosis and initiation of appropriate therapy.[20] There is no evidence that tuberculosis affects the course of pregnancy. Intrauterine transmission of tuberculosis is very rare.[19] The neonate is at risk of acquiring tuberculosis postpartum if born to a mother with open pulmonary tuberculosis.[1,19]

Diagnosis

Findings on physical examination, chest x-ray films and extraneural cultures are often not helpful. The initial tuberculin skin test is negative in more than half of the patients.

The cornerstone of diagnosis is examination of the CSF. Characteristic findings are lymphocytic pleocytosis (occurring in three-quarters of patients), hypoglycorrhachia (with initially normal glucose value in many patients) and elevated protein level. CSF smears are positive for acid-fast bacilli in a minority of cases on initial examination, but when four consecutive smears from lumbar punctures are examined, the sensitivity approaches 90%. Cultures are positive in the majority of cases, but growth takes 10–21 days. Newer rapid diagnostic tests include various antibody and antigen detection assays, but these are currently not widely available. The PCR to detect mycobacterial DNA in CSF has limitations due to the high rates of false-positive results.[1]

Treatment

Modern therapy for tuberculous meningitis consists of isoniazide (INH, oral 300 mg daily), RMP (oral 600 mg daily) and pyrazinamide (PZA, oral 20–35 mg/kg daily) plus initially either ethanbutol (EMB, oral 15–25 mg/kg) or streptomycin (STM, intramuscularly 0.5–1 g daily), if drug resistance is suspected. Duration of therapy is 6–12 months, depending on the protocol used. The adjunctive use of corticosteroid (prednisone 60–80 mg daily for 1–2 weeks, with gradual decrease) is advised in patients with altered mental status or other neurologic findings.[1] In a large epidemiologic study of antituberculous drugs in pregnancy, RMP was associated with fetal abnormalities in 3% of exposed fetuses, compared to 2% for EMB and 1% for INH. STM should not be used during pregnancy due to the risk of nerve toxicity in the fetus. The risk of teratogenicity for PZA has not been determined.[8]

Neurosyphilis

Syphilis is a complex systemic disease with protean clinical manifestations, caused by the spirochete *Treponema pallidum*. The pathogen cannot be cultivated *in vitro*.

Clinical manifestations

There are numerous presentations of neurosyphilis. Syphilitic meningitis as a complication of secondary syphilis is often asymptomatic, and its diagnosis is based on CSF abnormalities (lymphocytic pleocytosis, elevated protein level, decreased glucose concentration) and/or positive Venereal Disease Research Laboratory test response. Symptomatic secondary syphilitic meningitis usually presents similarly as other forms of aseptic meningitis with headache, nausea and vomiting. Meningeal signs occur in 60% of patients and fever in less than half. Cranial nerve palsies are relatively common (45%). Other focal abnormalities or mental status changes are not common. Late (tertiary) symptomatic neurosyphilis is divided into two major clinical categories that are correlated with pathologic findings: meningovascular neurosyphilis, usually starting 5 years after acquisition of syphilis, and parenchymatous neurosyphilis (general paresis and tabes dorsais), appearing 10–25 years after primary syphilis.[1] Although syphilis occurs in a relatively small percentage of the population, data support the widespread screening of obstetric patients for syphilis. Among pregnant women found to have latent syphilis, a fifth of patients have evidence of asymptomatic neurosyphilis following examination of spinal fluid.[21] Despite maternal therapy, 11% of the infants born to mothers with syphilis have reactive serum and CSF involvement.

Diagnosis

Whenever a positive serum treponemal test (fluorescent treponemal absorption test or *T. pallidum* hemagglutination assay) is detected, the clinical staging of syphilis must be accomplished by examination of the CSF. Abnormal CSF findings (even a few cells), a positive CSF non-treponemal test and/or a positive treponemal test establish the diagnosis of neurosyphilis.

Treatment

Only penicillin reliably treats the infant, therefore the treatment of choice for pregnant women with neurosyphilis is penicillin G 2–4 million units intravenously every 4 h for 10 days. An alternative for the penicillin-allergic patient is ceftriaxone 1 g intravenously or intramuscularly for 2 weeks.[1]

CNS toxoplasmosis

Toxoplasmosis is a worldwide zoonosis, caused by *Toxoplasma gondii*, an intracellular protozoan parasite. In humans, toxoplasma infection is acquired either orally (through the ingestion of undercooked meat containing tissue cysts or water and food contaminated by oocysts) or congenitally. Acute toxoplasma infection in an immunocompetent host, including pregnant women, goes unrecognized in ~90% of cases, but may result in a tragic outcome for the offspring (discussed elsewhere in this book). Chronic (latent) infection ensues in all infected patients, due to persistence of *T. gondii* in the cyst form. Reactivation, with resultant life-threatening (mostly CNS) toxoplasmosis, occurs exclusively in patients who are severely immunocompromised.[1] In women receiving chronic immunosuppression after organ transplantation, not a single case of CNS toxoplasmosis was observed during pregnancy.[22] In pregnant women who are infected with HIV, the incidence of CNS toxoplasmosis is very low,[1,22,23] is correlated with HIV immunosuppression (CD4 cell count $< 100\ mm^3$) and is not influenced by pregnancy. At present, data are insufficient to define the risk of congenital transmission of *T. gondii* by HIV-infected mothers who have chronic toxoplasma infection.[1]

Clinical manifestations

A wide range of clinical signs and symptoms are seen with CNS toxoplasmosis. Characteristically, there is a subacute onset of encephalitis with focal neurologic signs. CSF is normal or may show a non-specific mild 'viral' inflammatory response.

Diagnosis

Brain biopsy with appropriate cultural and histologic techniques is the gold standard for diagnosis of CNS toxoplasmosis. Serological tests (serum and CSF) are not helpful. Brain imaging studies (MRI and to a lesser degree computed tomography scan) show characteristic multiple lesions, which tend to occur at the corticomedullary junction and involve the basal ganglia. In AIDS patients, such focal CNS lesions suggest the diagnosis.[1]

Treatment

For the immunodeficient patient with CNS toxoplasmosis, standard therapy is a combination of pyrimethamine (oral 200 mg loading dose, then 50–75 mg daily) and sulfadiazine (oral 1–1.5 g every 6 h) or clindamycin (oral or intravenously 600–1200 mg every 6 h). Addition of folinic acid (oral, intravenously or intramuscularly 10–20 mg daily) minimizes pyrimethamine-associated myelotoxicity.

Duration of treatment is 4–6 weeks, followed by lifelong maintenance treatment.[1] For the HIV-infected woman the reader is advised to consult HIV authorities.

REFERENCES

1. Mandell GL, Bennett JE, Dolin R, eds. *Principles and Practice of Infectious Diseases*, 4th edn. New York: Churchill Livingstone, 1995.
2. Durand ML, Calderwood SB, Weber DJ, *et al.* Acute bacterial meningitis in adults. A review of 493 episodes. *N Engl J Med* 1993;328:21–8.
3. Tunkel AR, Scheld WM. Acute bacterial meningitis. *Lancet* 1995; 346:1675–80.
4. Lucas AO. Pneumococcal meningitis in pregnancy and the puerperium. *Br Med J* 1964;1:92–5.
5. Westh H, Skibsted L, Korner B. Streptococcus pneumonia infections of the female genital tract and in the newborn child. *Rev Infect Dis* 1990;12:416–22.
6. Tempest B. Pneumococcal meningitis in mother and neonate. *Pediatrics* 1974;53:759–60.
7. Stiener ZP, Manor Y, Smorjik J, *et al.* Successful postmortem cesarean section in a case of fulminant pneumococcal meningitis. *Isr J Med Sci* 1978;14:287–8.
8. Korzeniowski OM. Antibacterial agents in pregnancy. *Infect Dis Clin North Am* 1995;9:639–51.
9. O'Neill P. How long to treat bacterial meningitis. *Lancet* 1993; 341:530.
10. Finan MA, Smith SG, Sinnott JT, *et al.* An interesting case presentation: Peripartum meningococcal meningitis. *J Perinatol* 1992; 12:78–80.
11. McLauchlin J. Human listeriosis in Britain, 1967–85, a summary of 722 cases. *Epidemiol Infect* 1990;104:181–9.
12. Boucher M, Yonekura ML. Listeria meningitis during pregnancy. *Am J Perinatol* 1984;1:312–8.
13. Sirry HW, George RH, Whittle MJ. Meningoencephalitis due to *Listeria monocytogenes* in pregnancy. *Br J Obstet Gynaecol* 1994;101:1083–4.
14. Dunne DW, Quagliarello V. Group B streptococcal meningitis in adults. *Medicine* 1993;72:1–9.
15. Johnson RT. Acute encephalitis. *Clin Infect Dis* 1996;23:219–26.
16. Frieden EJ, Ordorica SA, Goodgold AL, *et al.* Successful pregnancy with isolated herpes simplex virus encephalitis: Case report and review of the literature. *Obstet Gynecol* 1990;75:511–3.
17. McKernan PD, Schare MB. Type B-2 coxaxievirus meningitis in pregnancy. A case report. *J Reprod Med* 1988;33:667–70.
18. Chaturvedi UC, Mathur A, Chandra A, *et al.* Transplacental infection with Japanese encephalitis virus. *J Infect Dis* 1980;141:712–5.
19. Hamadeh MA, Glassroth J. Tuberculosis and pregnancy. *Chest* 1992;101:1114–20.
20. Kingdom JC, Kennedy DH. Tuberculous meningitis in pregnancy. *Br J Obstet Gynaecol* 1989;96:233–5.
21. Jones JE, Harris RE. Diagnostic evaluation of syphilis during pregnancy. *Obstet Gynecol* 1979;54:611–4.
22. Biederman K, Flepp M, Fierz W, *et al.* Pregnancy, immunosuppression and reactivation of latent toxoplasmosis. *J Perinat Med* 1995;23:191–203.
23. Hedriana HL, Mitchell JL, Brown GM, *et al.* Normal fetal outcome in a pregnancy with CNS toxoplasmosis and HIV infection. A case report. *J Reprod Med* 1993;38:747–50.

165 Anaerobic infections in pregnancy

Y. Schlesinger

Introduction

The role of anaerobic organisms as a cause of infections of the female genital tract is well established. Anaerobic bacteria, among others, can be cultured from virtually all specimens from women with clinically important gynecological infections. Anaerobic infections in pregnancy are particularly important due to the impact of the infection on both the pregnant mother and the developing fetus. There is increasing evidence that ascending infection from the lower genital tract is an important cause of preterm delivery and low birth weight infants. Similarly, bacterial vaginosis has been linked to a number of complications of pregnancy, including preterm labor and delivery, chorioamnionitis, postcesarean amnionitis, and postabortion septic thrombophlebitis. This chapter will attempt to summarize the impact of and the approach to anaerobic infections in the pregnant woman.

The pathogens

The classification of anaerobic bacteria has changed dramatically over the last decade, due to the introduction of molecular biology techniques in this field. A detailed description of the new nomenclature of anaerobic bacteria is beyond the scope of this chapter, and the interested reader is referred to recent comprehensive reviews.[1–3]

The normal flora of the vagina has been the subject of several studies in both healthy women and those with pathologic conditions.[4–6] The microbial environment of the vagina is very delicately balanced and can be altered by many factors. These include hormonal changes from aging, pregnancy and oral contraceptives. Also, in certain conditions such as antibiotic therapy and uncontrolled diabetes mellitus, the normal vaginal flora is altered. Local factors such as malformation and anatomic deformities after surgery, vaginal douching and foreign material such as contraceptives (intrautorinc device, diaphragm and spermicides) and tampons also play an important role. In the healthy woman, the vaginal flora is dominated by lactobacilli. In contrast, in the vaginal flora of women with bacterial vaginosis, the predominance of lactobacilli is replaced by a combination of aerobic, facultatively anaerobic and strictly anaerobic bacteria. The most important pathogens include *Gardnerella vaginalis* (the 'clue' cell organism), *Bacteroides* species, *Prevotella (Bacteroides) melaninogenicus*, *Mycoplasma hominis* and *Mobiluncus* species. The importance of bacterial vaginosis in pregnancy will be discussed later in detail.

Numerous anaerobic bacteria are encountered in obstetric and gynecological infections. Most of these infections are of polymicrobial nature and include both aerobic and anaerobic bacteria. In a large-scale survey by Brook and colleagues,[5] anaerobic pathogens were recovered from 714 out of a total of 736 patients sampled. These specimens included 53 from infected Fallopian tubes, 470 from infected endomotrium, 94 from infected amniotic fluid, 57 aspirates of cul-de-sacs in instances of pelvic inflammatory disease, 14 labial and vaginal abscesses and 26 of Bartholin's cyst abscess. A total of 2052 isolates were recovered, out of which 1139 were anaerobes (1.6 per specimen). The most commonly isolated anaerobic bacteria were *Bacteroides* species (566 isolates), anaerobic gram-positive cocci (391), *Clostridium* species (48) and *Fusobacterium* species (36).

The most important anaerobic infection of the genital tract during pregnancy is bacterial vaginosis, due to the possible effect on the outcome of pregnancy. Therefore, most of the rest of this chapter will be devoted to the diagnosis and treatment of bacterial vaginosis. Other forms of anaerobic infections in pregnancy are clinically less significant and will be mentioned only briefly.

Bacterial vaginosis

Bacterial vaginosis is not an infection in the ordinary sense. In contrast to vaginitis, in which there is an inflammatory response of the vaginal wall, bacterial vaginosis is not associated with such inflammation.

The manifestations of bacterial vaginosis are an increased homogenous vaginal discharge that has an elevated pH, a characteristic odor after addition of potassium hydroxide and a microscopical appearance characterized by epithelial cells with adherence of bacteria (mostly *G. vaginalis*) to the cell margins (the so-called 'clue cell'). In bacterial vaginosis the normal lactobacillus-dominated vaginal flora is replaced with anaerobic bacteria, *Mobiluncus* species, *G. vaginalis* and *M. hominis*. A standard method for the diagnosis of bacterial vaginosis has been described by Spiegel and colleagues[7] and Nugent and associates.[8]

The normal vaginal flora of 171 pregnant women in labor at term was studied by Hillier and colleagues.[6] A score of 0–10 was assigned in light of the relative proportions of large gram-positive rods (lactobacilli), small gram-negative or gram-variable rods (*Bacteroides* or *Gardnerella*) and curved gram-variable rods (*Mobiluncus*). The flora was categorized as normal (a score of 0–3, *Lactobacillus*-predominant), intermediate (a score of 4–6) or representative of bacterial vaginosis (a score of 7–10). Bacterial vaginosis was diagnosed in 39 women (23%); the vaginal flora was diagnosed as normal in 50% of cases and as intermediate in 27%. The microorganisms most frequently recovered from women with bacterial vaginosis were *G. vaginalis*, anaerobic bacteria (*Prevotella* species, *Bacteroides* species, *Fusobacterium, Peptostreptococcus*), *Mobiluncus* species, viridance streptococci, *Ureaplasma urealiticum*, and *M. hominis*. The presence of H_2O_2-producing lactobacilli was inversely associated with the presence of bacterial vaginosis.

The effect of bacterial vaginosis on the outcome of pregnancy has been the subject of several studies in the last decade.[9–18] Most investigators agree that there is an association between bacterial vaginosis and premature delivery, premature rupture of membranes (PROM), infection of the chorion and amnion,[15,16] histologic chorio-amnionitis,[16] and infection of amniotic fluid. In a recent multicenter comprehensive study by Hillier and colleagues,[13] a cohort of 10,397 pregnant women was followed. The study end point was a preterm (< 37 weeks) or a low birth weight (< 2500 g) delivery. In 16% of all the women, bacterial vaginosis was detected at 23–26 weeks of gestation, based on vaginal pH and Gram stain. In a multivariant analysis, bacterial vaginosis was found to be associated with preterm delivery or low birth weight (odds ratio 1.4, 95% confidence interval 1.1–1.8). Among women with bacterial vaginosis, the highest risk of preterm delivery or a low birth weight infant was found among those with both vaginal *Bacteroides* and *M. hominis* (odds ratio 2.1, 95% confidence interval 1.5–3.0). In contrast to these and other findings, Hillu and associates[14] found no evidence that bacterial vaginosis is associated with prematurity or adverse pregnancy outcome. The authors suggest that the characteristics of their study population, i.e. differences in normal vaginal flora due to different antibiotic usage habits, may account for the conflicting results. Kurki and colleagues also found conflicting results[11] in an assessment of the association between bacterial vaginosis early in pregnancy and adverse pregnancy outcome. Bacterial vaginosis in this particular study was diagnosed by Gram stain, bacterial culture and Papanicolaou stain, performed between 8 and 17 weeks of gestation. Bacterial vaginosis was diagnosed in 169 of 790 women (21.4%), and associated with a 2.6-fold risk (95% confidence interval 1.3–4.9) for preterm labor (premature contractions), a 6.9-fold risk (2.5–18.8) for preterm birth, and a 7.3-fold risk (1.8–29.4) for PROM. However, the authors indicate that due to the high rate of false-positive findings, the positive predictive value of bacterial vaginosis for pregnancy outcome is only 4–11%. Hence, the role of treatment of bacterial vaginosis in the prevention of adverse pregnancy outcome remains unclear.

The mechanism by which bacterial vaginosis causes premature delivery is not completely clear. It may involve prostaglandins, endotoxins, mucinase, salicidase, interleukin-1 and other mediators derived from fetal membranes or decidua, as well as these and other agents released from the bacteria themselves. The role of chorioamniotic infection and histologic chorioamnionitis in prematurity was the subject of a study by Hillier and colleagues.[16] Microorganisms were recovered from the chorioamnion in 23 of 38 placentas (61%) from women with premature labor (< 37 weeks of gestation) and in 12 of 56 placentas (21%) from women who delivered at term (odds ratio 5.6, 95% confidence interval 2.1–15.6). The most frequent isolates from the placentas of those whose infants were delivered prematurely were *U. urealiticum* and *G. vaginalis*. The recovery of any organism from the chorioamnion was strongly associated with histologic chorioamnionitis and bacterial vaginosis. Silver and colleagues[15] also found that bacterial vaginosis organisms (*M. hominis*, anaerobes and *G. vaginalis*) were associated with each other in 408 cases of intra-amniotic infection, and that women with bacterial vaginosis were most likely to have *M. hominis* and *G. vaginalis* in their amniotic fluids. These and other studies suggest that the mechanism of premature labor in patients with bacterial vaginosis, especially early in pregnancy, is amniotic fluid infection and chorioamnionitis.

The timing of bacterial vaginosis in relation to prematurity has also been investigated. Riduan and colleagues[17] examined the association between preterm delivery and bacterial vaginosis in early and late pregnancy. A total of 490 pregnant women were evaluated for the presence of bacterial vaginosis at 16–20 weeks and 28–32 weeks of gestation, and subsequently followed to delivery. A significant association was found between preterm delivery (< 37 weeks of gestation) and bacterial vaginosis diagnosed at 16–20 weeks of gestation (odds ratio 2.0, 95% confidence interval 1.0–3.9). In contrast, no significant correlation was found with bacterial vaginosis diagnosed at 28–32 weeks of gestation. The authors suggest that these findings are in accordance with the assumption that bacterial vaginosis causes an ascending infection resulting in chorioamnionitis, which in turn is the cause of prematurity, since chorioamnionitis is likely to occur at an earlier stage. Russel[19] found that the incidence of chorioamnionitis declined as gestational age increased, from 94.4% for women who delivered at a gestational age of 21–24 weeks, to 39.6% at 25–28 weeks, 35.4% at 29–32 weeks and 10.7% at 33–36 weeks. A reasonable conclusion from these findings is that early detection and treatment of bacterial vaginosis may reduce the rate of prematurity and low-birthweight deliveries. In contrast, other studies do not confirm these results.[14] Four hundred women from the north of Israel were followed up to delivery. The presence of bacterial vaginosis was evaluated twice: at 15–20 weeks and 27–32 weeks of gestation. Bacterial vaginosis was found in 15% of the women at 15–20 weeks and in 12.5% of the women at 27–32 weeks of gestation. However, no association was found between bacterial vaginosis in either stage of pregnancy and premature delivery. As mentioned before, these conflicting results may be explained in part by differences in normal vaginal flora due to different antibiotic usage habits between the study populations.

Given this information, should bacterial vaginosis be screened for and treated during pregnancy with the aim of reducing premature delivery, low birth weight infants and PROM? This issue is still debated, due to the marginal efficacy and the microbiological and financial cost of unnecessary mass antimicrobial usage. In a randomized, double-blinded controlled study, Hauth and colleagues[20] found that compared to placebo, treatment of women with bacterial vaginosis with metronidazole and erythromycin lowered the rate of prematurity (31% vs. 49%, $P=0.006$). This effect was not found in women at high risk for premature delivery who did not have bacterial vaginosis.[20] These findings are in accordance with those of McGregor and associates,[21] who found in a prospective study that screening for bacterial vaginosis in pregnancy and treatment with oral clindamycin 300 mg twice daily for 7 days resulted in approximately 50% reduction in preterm birth and/or rupture of membranes. Similarly, Morales and coworkers[22] compared treatment of asymptomatic women with both a history of preterm birth and findings of bacterial vaginosis with oral metronidazole or placebo. They obtained nearly 70% reduction in prematurity, low-birthweight and PROM in the clindamycin-treated women.[22] In contrast, based on data derived from several studies, Joesoef and Schmid concluded that treatment of bacterial vaginosis should be reserved only for symptomatic patients.[23] In their review, the authors suggest that treatment of asymptomatic patients with the rationale of preventing adverse pregnancy outcome should be deferred until further data are available. Hence, no firm recommendations about the routine screening for and treatment of bacterial vaginosis in pregnancy can be given at the current time. However, due to substantial evidence that bacterial vaginosis, at least in the second trimester, is associated with adverse pregnancy outcome, and the relative low cost and simplicity of oral or topical antibiotics for the treatment of bacterial vaginosis, it is probably reasonable to offer such therapy in this subset of patients.[18,24]

Other forms of anaerobic infections in pregnancy

All the anaerobic bacteria mentioned previously can contribute to virtually every type of obstetric infection,[5] varying in severity from minor to life-threatening infections. These infections commonly include abscess of the perianal soft tissue or glands, endometritis, salpingitis, tubo-ovarian abscess, septic abortions and postoperative infections. Clues to the presence of anaerobes in these infections include a foul-smelling discharge, presence of gas in tissue, abscess formation and pelvic thrombophlebitis.

Clostridia species are isolated from 5–10% of normal vaginal flora, and up to 19–29% of women in the postabortion period. Hence, their presence does not necessarily indicate the presence of infection. An important exception in which *Clostridia* clearly play a major role is uterine gas gangrene, now a rare complication that was previously seen in the setting of septic abortion. Rarely, uterine gas gangrene has followed amniocentesis,[25] or a cesarean section. It is debatable whether or not hysterectomy should always be performed in cases of uterine gas gangrene.

Treatment

The treatment of anaerobic infections in pregnancy follows the usual rules of antimicrobial treatment of anaerobic infections. The primary agents that are effective against most anaerobic bacteria include metronidazole, clindamycin, some penicillins, chloramphenicol and imipenem–cilistatin. Among the penicillins, those that are combined with beta-lactamase inhibitors, i.e. amoxicillin–clavulanate, piperacillin–tazobactam, ticarcillin–clavulanate and others, are particularly effective. Various treatment regimens can be offered. The decisions regarding the specific agent, the dose, the route of administration (parenteral, oral or topical) and the length of therapy are dictated by the type and severity of the particular infection being treated. Antibiograms, derived from *in vitro* susceptibility testing, are very difficult to perform and interpret for anaerobic bacteria and should not be used routinely in the selection of the antimicrobial agent. Bacterial vaginosis can be treated with oral metronidazole 500 mg twice daily for 1 week, or just as effectively by metronidazole or clindamycin gel.[24,26] Treatment of the male sex partner is controversial, but may be recommended in cases of recurrent bacterial vaginosis.[23,24] Treatment of bacterial vaginosis prior to surgical abortion with the aim of preventing postabortion pelvic inflammatory disease is recommended by some authors.[23] The use of metronidazole in pregnancy has traditionally been avoided due to a fear of teratogenicity. However, in a meta-analysis by Burtin and colleagues[27] it was shown that metronidazole is safe for use in pregnancy and lactation and therefore need not be avoided. Other forms of therapy include surgical debridement and hyperbaric oxygen, but these are reserved for invasive infections in severe cases.

REFERENCES

1. Summanem P. Microbiology terminology update: Clinically significant anaerobic gram-positive and gram-negative bacteria (excluding spirochetes). Summary of current nomenclature, taxonomy and classification of various microbial agents. *Clin Infect Dis* 1993;16:606–9.
2. Summanem P. Recent taxonomic changes for anaerobic gram-positive and selected gram-negative organisms. *Clin Infect Dis* 1993;16(Suppl 4):S168–74.
3. Shah NH, Gharbia SE. Ecophysiology and taxonomy of *Bacteroides* and related taxa. *Clin Infect Dis* 1993;16(Suppl 4)160–7.
4. Mardh PA. The vaginal ecosystem. *Am J Obstet Gynecol* 1991; 165:1163–8.
5. Brook I, Frazier EH, Thomas RL. Aerobic and anaerobic microbiological factors and recovery of beta-lactamase-producing bacteria from obstetric and gynecological infection. *Surg Gynecol Obstet* 1991;172:138–44.
6. Hillier SL, Krohn MA, Rabe LK, Klebanoff SJ, Eschenbach DA. The normal vaginal flora, H_2O_2-producing *Lactobacilli*, and bacterial vaginosis in pregnant women. *Clin Infect Dis* 1993; 16(Suppl 4):S273–81.
7. Spiegel CA, Amsel R, Holmes KK. Diagnosis of bacterial vaginosis by gram stain of vaginal fluid. *J Clin Microbiol* 1983;18:170–7.
8. Nugent RP, Krohn MA, Hillier SL. Reliability of diagnosing bacterial vaginosis is improved by a standardized method of gram stain interpretation. *J Clin Microbiol* 1991;29:297–301.
9. Minkoff H, Grunebaum AN, Schwartz RH, *et al.* Risk factors for prematurity and premature rupture of membranes: A prospective study of the vaginal flora in pregnancy. *Am J Obstet Gynecol* 1984;165:965–72.
10. Martius J, Krohn MA, Hillier SL, Stamn WE, Holmes KK, Eschenbach DA. Relationship of vaginal *Lactobacillus* species, cervical *Chlamydia trachomatis*, and bacterial vaginosis to preterm birth. *Obstet Gynecol* 1988;71:89–95.
11. Kurki T, Sivonen A, Renkonen OV, Savia E, Ylikorkala O. Bacterial vaginosis in early pregnancy outcome. *Obstet Gynecol* 1992;80: 173–7.
12. Hay PH, Lamont RF, Taylor-Robinson D, Morgan DJ, Ison C, Pearson J. Abnormal bacterial colonization of the genital tract and subsequent preterm delivery and late miscarriage. *Br Med J* 1994; 308:295–8.
13. Hillier SL, Nugent RP, Eschenbach DA, *et al.* Association between bacterial vaginosis and preterm delivery of a low-birthweight infant. *N Engl J Med* 1995;333:1737–42.
14. Hillu J, Kenes J, Shalev E. Bacterial vaginosis in pregnancy and the association to preterm delivery (in Hebrew). *Harefuah* 1996; 131:83–5.
15. Silver HM, Sperling RS, St Clair PJ, Gibbs R. Evidence relating bacterial vaginosis to intra-amniotic infection. *Am J Obstet Gynecol* 1989;161:808–12.
16. Hillier SL, Martius J, Krohn M, Kiviat N, Holmes KK, Eschenbach DA. A case-control study of chorioamnionitic infection and histologic chorioamnionitis in prematurity. *N Engl J Med* 1988;319: 972–8.
17. Riduan JM, Hillier SA, Utomo B, Wiknjosastro G, Linnan M, Kandum N. Bacterial vaginosis and prematurity in Indonesia: Association in early and late pregnancy. *Am J Obstet Gynecol* 1993;169:175–8.
18. McGregor JA, French JI. Bacterial vaginosis and preterm birth (letter). *N Engl J Med* 1996;334:1337–8.
19. Russel P. Inflammatory lesions of the human placenta. I. Clinical significance of the acute chorioamnionitis. *Am J Diagn Gynecol Obstet* 1979;1:127–37.
20. Hauth JC, Goldenberg RL, Andrews WW, DuBard MB, Cooper RL. Reduced incidence of preterm delivery with metronidazole and erythromycin in women with bacterial vaginosis. *N Engl J Med* 1995;333:1732–6.
21. McGregor JA, French JI, Parker R, *et al.* Prevention of premature birth by screening and treatment for common genital tract infections: Results of a prospective controlled evaluation. *Am J Obstet Gynecol* 1995;173:157–67.
22. Morales WJ, Schorr S, Albritton J. Effect of metronidazole in patients with preterm birth in preceding pregnancy and bacterial vaginosis: A placebo-controlled, double blind study. *Am J Obstet Gynecol* 1994;171:345–9.
23. Joesoef MR, Schmid GP. Bacterial vaginosis: Review of treatment options and potential clinical indications for therapy. *Clin Infect Dis* 1995;20(Suppl 1):S72–9.
24. Eschenbach DA. Pelvic infections and sexually transmitted diseases. In Scott JR, Disaria PJ, Hammond CB, Spellacy NS, eds. *Danforth's Obstetrics and Gynecology*, 7th edn. Philadelphia: J. B. Lippincott Company, 1994:641–4.
25. Hovav Y, Hornstein E, Pollack RN, Yaffe C. Sepsis due to *Clostridium perfringens* after second-trimester amniocentesis (letter). *Clin Infect Dis* 1995;21:235–6.
26. Ferris GD, Litaker MS, Woodward L, Mathis MT, Hendrich J. Treatment of bacterial vaginosis: A comparison of oral metronidazole, metronidazole vaginal gel, and clindamycin vaginal cream. *J Fam Pract* 1995;41:443–9.
27. Burtin P, Taddio A, Ariburnu O, Einarson TR, Koren G. Safety of metronidazole in pregnancy: A meta-analysis. *Am J Obstet Gynecol* 1995;172:525–9.

166 Malaria in pregnancy

I. Kassis, M. Giladi and M. Efrat

Introduction

Malaria, the most important of the human parasitic protozoa, is endemic in many parts of the world, mainly in the tropical and subtropical areas. An annual incidence of > 300 million new cases and 2–3 million deaths is almost undoubtedly an underestimation. Mortality and morbidity are greatest in children and pregnant women, especially in sub-Saharan Africa, as well as in non-immune travelers. In the latter, disease may develop months to years after leaving an endemic area, and thus the diagnosis can be easily delayed and possibly missed. Delay in diagnosis can lead to significant morbidity and even death.

Globally, *Plasmodium vivax* accounts for 80% of cases, and *Plasmodium falciparum* for 10–15%. The remaining cases are caused by *Plasmodium ovale* or *Plasmodium malariae*. Occasionally, mixed infections can occur. The epidemiology of human malaria varies, and different species may predominate in different areas. Severe complications and mortality are almost always due to falciparum malaria.

The parasite and life cycle

Malaria is acquired when the female anopheline mosquito bites for a blood meal. Sporozoites travel via the blood stream to the liver. They invade hepatocytes and develop into mature tissue schizonts. Within 1–2 weeks, infected hepatocytes rupture and thousands of merozoites are released from each tissue schizont into the bloodstream. Each merozoite may invade a human erythrocyte. Each parasite replicates asexually every 48–72 h and releases 8–32 merozoites during rupture of infected erythrocytes. Some erythrocytic parasites develop into sexual forms (gametocytes). These forms are ingested by the feeding *Anopheles*. After completing the stages of sexual reproduction in the mosquito, sporozoites develop and migrate to the mosquito's salivary gland. They will be injected into, and will potentially infect, the next human bitten. Alternatively, erythrocytic forms may infect humans by blood or by maternal–fetal transfusion.

In the liver, *P. vivax* and *P. ovale* may exist as dormant forms (hypnozoites). These forms may cause relapse (in almost a third of cases), even years after the primary infection. *P. falciparum* has no dormant form and there is no true relapse. Deterioration after a period of clinical improvement may occur, but not due to liver hypnozoites, and is termed recrudescence.

P. malariae is the rarest cause of human disease. It may exist in peripheral blood for years, causing low-grade parasitemia, often asymptomatic.

Clinical manifestations

The clinical picture is highly variable. Some infected people may have few symptoms and others may develop a rapidly fatal course. The pattern of fever and other symptoms in primary infection is not typical and may imitate many other febrile diseases. Furthermore, the state of host immunity plays a major role, thus a high level of suspicion is required. Malaria should be suspected in every patient in the proper epidemiological setting.

During the initial period of symptomatic malaria, patients may not exhibit the typical cyclical fever classically attributed to malaria. They may have low-grade fever with random peaks. After several days, synchronous febrile peaks may occur. One to 2 h of feeling cold with rigors are followed by 4–6 h of high fever, which is then followed by an often massive diaphoresis and a concomitant reduction of temperature, and exhaustion. These paroxysms are coincident with the rupture of erythrocytes and release of parasites into the circulation. This pattern occurs roughly every 72 h in *P. malariae* infection and every 48 h in the others (*P. falciparum*, *P. vivax* and *P. ovale*). Other symptoms may occur including lethargy, anorexia, nausea, vomiting, diarrhea, headache and low back pain. Malaria may mimic many other febrile illnesses prevalent in both endemic and non-endemic regions.

Untreated patients with malaria due to *P. vivax* and *P. ovale* may have attacks for weeks. Spontaneous recovery after several attacks is the rule. Clinical symptoms due to *P. falciparum* may begin as early as 8–12 days after infection. If untreated, paroxysms may continue for 3 weeks. Recrudescence may occur. In some instances, the clinical course of disease may progress with severity and rapidity and lead to complications and death. This is determined, in part, due to factors, such as age (children are more susceptible), general medical and nutritional status, degree of immunity to malaria, virulence of the parasite, pregnancy and time of onset of effective treatment. Life-threatening severe and complicated malaria develops almost exclusively with *P. falciparum* infection, although the majority of falciparum infections do not progress to this extreme form, even if not treated. In those who develop complications, the variable spectrum of manifestations may include anemia with or without hyperparasitemia, pulmonary edema, renal failure, acidosis, shock, cerebral involvement, disseminated intravascular coagulation and death.

Central nervous system (CNS) involvement (cerebral malaria) with confusion, obtundation, seizures, coma and death may occur. It is of supreme importance to note that patients with malaria and CNS symptoms may have other reasons for these symptoms. Bacterial meningitis should be excluded by lumbar puncture. Encephalitis and various causes of encephalopathy should be considered. Hypoglycemia, another potential cause of CNS symptomatology, may complicate malaria, especially during pregnancy and childhood, and is further augmented by treatment with quinine or quinidine.

Hypovolemia, renal microvascular sequestration of erythrocytes and hemoglobinuria may act together to cause renal failure, which is more common in non-immune patients and is usually non-oliguric. Hemodialysis or hemofiltration may be required. Pulmonary edema is uncommon in developing countries. It may be precipitated by iatrogenic fluid overload. This complication occurs mainly in adults and is usually associated with high-grade parasitemia (> 250,000/ml, > 5%).

Patients with specific organ complications usually die if not appropriately treated with both antimalarials and supportive therapy. Patients who survive cerebral malaria may be left with varying degrees of neurological sequelae.

Pathogenesis

P. falciparum is the most severe form of disease. This species invades erythrocytes of all ages. Parasitized red blood cells adhere to endothelial cells in capillaries and postcapillary venules of the brain, kidneys, lungs and other organs. Mature asexual forms of the parasite disappear from peripheral blood and sequester in the microcirculation. The adherence of parasitized erythrocytes to endothelial cells in the postcapillary venules is considered the main mechanism of pathogenesis. Uninfected circulating erythrocytes bind to infected erythrocytes with mature parasites (rosetting). Microvascular obstruction facilitates tissue hypoxia, hypoglycemia and the production of lactate. In addition, tumor necrosis factor-α (TNF-α) and other cytokines, nitrous oxide and free oxygen radicals, contribute to the pathogenetic sequence of events at the tissue level. The resultant severe metabolic dysfunction is manifested by specific organ complications. With the institution of appropriate therapy, most of these effects are abolished, largely without permanent damage. The absence of neurological sequelae in the majority of cases (but not all) implies that reversible metabolic mechanisms, e.g. synaptic dysregulation by tissue mediators, are responsible for cerebral malfunction. Anemia occurs frequently in malaria. Its etiology is multifactorial. Infected erythrocytes rupture with the release of parasites. This is associated with the release of cytokines, such as TNF-α, which has a suppressive effect on erythropoiesis (dyserythropoiesis). Activated reticuloendothelial cells, mainly in the spleen, destroy defective erythrocytes as well as uninfected erythrocytes that are coated with malaria antigens. In developing countries, underlying anemia is common (malnutrition, intestinal parasites, physiological effects of pregnancy, etc.).

P. vivax and *P. ovale* infect mainly reticulocytes and young erythrocytes (1–2% of erythrocytes) and microvascular sequestration does not occur. Tissue involvement is not present and hemolysis is usually mild.

P. malariae invades primarily senescent erythrocytes. Low-grade parasitemia may continue even asymptomatically for years. Immune complex glomerulonephritis and hypersplenism may develop.

Diagnosis

Malaria is a life-threatening disease. It should always be suspected in the appropriate epidemiological setting. Clinical symptoms and signs may be misleading, therefore clues, such as living in or traveling to endemic areas even years before, a history of previous malaria, previous prophylaxis for malaria or blood transfusions, may help. Blood smear is still the cornerstone of diagnosis. Trained personnel should prepare thick and thin peripheral blood smears, which are best stained with Giemsa. Smears should be examined at length before they are declared negative. In order to confirm or exclude the diagnosis of malaria by classical methods, smears should be examined every 6–8 h for up to 3 days. The degree of parasitemia should be assessed. To exclude the possibility of drug resistance, follow-up smears are required after the institution of therapy.

Falciparum malaria must be differentiated from the other forms. When initial speciation cannot be determined, treatment must be for *P. falciparum*. When chloroquine-resistant *P. falciparum* is a possibility, initial treatment must reflect this possibility. Other diagnostic methods such as serology are available, but have limited value in practice. Sensitive staining techniques (acridine orange) and antigen detection (by specific antibodies) are being increasingly used, especially in non-endemic countries. In the future, field-adapted molecular diagnostic tests may become available for diagnosis and for the identification of drug-resistant parasites.

Malaria in pregnancy

Malaria has a special impact on pregnant women, the placenta, the fetus and the newborn infant. In endemic areas, the frequency and severity of falciparum malaria and its complications are greater during pregnancy. The impact of non-falciparum malaria on the materal–fetal unit has yet to be accurately defined. Almost 500 million women live in endemic areas; in some regions more than 50% of the pregnant women may be parasitemic and have clinical manifestations of variable severity, or may be asymptomatic.

Parasitemia and malaria attacks are 4–12 times more common during pregnancy. The susceptibility to infection and severity of disease are determined in part by the prepregnancy immune status. In areas where transmission of malaria is low or seasonal, acquired antimalarial immunity is poor. Pregnancy alone downregulates immune responses, thus pregnant women may suffer more from malaria and its complications. In endemic areas where the transmission of malaria occurs year-round, protective immunity may develop and disease tends to be less severe, albeit more prevalent. In non-immune women, the susceptibility to infection with malaria is similar in all parities. In endemic areas with intense transmission, primigravidara are more often infected, and the severity of the disease is greater. In areas with seasonal or low-level transmission, the effects of malaria are felt in subsequent pregnancies as well. Interestingly, for grand multipara, the effect of protective immunity wanes. Some specific features and complications of malaria during pregnancy deserve special mention. Other than anemia, the following complications occur uniquely with *P. falciparum*.

Anemia

Anemia is very common in pregnancy, especially in developing countries. It usually develops during the second trimester. Anemia is usually normochromic and normocytic, and hemoglobin levels of < 7 g/dl are not uncommon. In the anemia associated with malaria, factors like hemolysis, activation of the macrophage–monocyte system, hypersplenism, suppression of bone marrow by TNF-α and peripheral sequestration may act together. Regardless of endemicity or the level of immunity, anemia contributes significantly to maternal and fetal morbidity. Prophylactic iron supplementation is advised during pregnancy, including in malaria-endemic areas. It has a positive effect on mothers and newborn infants.

Iron overload may increase host susceptibility to malaria. Iron supplementation may be detrimental to women with sickle cell trait. In this group, low antimalarial antibody levels and iron overload may act in concert to make women more susceptible to malaria during pregnancy. In fact, the advantages of some hemoglobinopathies (i.e. sickle cell anemia) in protection against malaria have not been clearly proven in pregnancy.

Blood transfusions may be required to correct severe anemia. The risk of transmission of malaria and other infectious agents (i.e. hepatitis B, hepatitis C, HIV), mainly in areas with poor medical facilities, should be weighed against the risk of heart failure and hypovolemic and hemorrhagic shock. Anemia may be chronic and its rapid correction may induce acute heart failure and pulmonary edema. In all instances, blood should be given with strict monitoring. Blood is usually transfused when the hematocrit is below 20%. Antimalarial therapy may be indicated for all pregnant women with severe anemia since placental malaria with negative blood smears can occur, especially in semi-immunes. In areas where transfusion practices involve an increased risk of acquiring blood-borne infections, a more conservative approach is indicated as long as there are no signs of maternal and/or fetal distress.

Liver problems

Mild hepatomegaly may be found in about half of cases of falciparum malaria. Hyperbilirubinemia with clinical jaundice due to hepatic damage with elevated hepatocellular enzymes may be seen in severe malaria, and rarely, malaria-associated severe hepatic necrosis may lead to death. It is important to remember that acute liver failure may complicate pregnancy without malaria.

Spleen problems

Early in the course of malaria, splenic macrophages are activated. Thrombocytopenia and leukopenia occur early in the course of infection, while splenomegaly is rarely seen at this stage. In endemic areas where recurrent or chronic infections are the rule, splenomegaly may be pronounced, sometimes in the form of hyperreactive malarial splenomegaly or tropical splenomegaly syndrome. Rarely, splenic rupture occurs and may cause death.

Cerebral malaria

Cerebral malaria is particularly common in pregnant women and in children. Altered consciousness, confusion, seizures, behavioral disturbances, focal neurologic findings, ataxia and coma are the main features. Patients may deteriorate rapidly, within a few hours. Untreated, this situation may lead to death within a few days. Recurrent convulsions and coma are poor prognostic signs. Supportive treatment includes preventing aspiration, treating hyperpyrexia and administering anticonvulsants. The mortality rate of cerebral malaria during pregnancy is considerably higher than in general. It is not clear if malaria predisposes to pre-eclampsia or eclampsia. In cerebral malaria, hypertension is very unusual, thus distinguishing it from eclampsia. Fever is also not typical of eclampsia.

Hypoglycemia

Hypoglycemia is very common in pregnant women with severe falciparum malaria. Predisposing factors include reduced glycogen stores due to starvation and vomiting, increased metabolic demands during febrile episodes, tissue hypoxia, quinine and quinidine stimulation of islet cells inducing hyperinsulinism, glucose consumption by large numbers of parasites, the hypoglycemic effect of TNF-α and possibly the toxic effect of iron or parasite-specific factors.

Hypoglycemia should be suspected and aggressively treated in any patient, in particular those with abnormal CNS symptoms. Abnormal behavior, sweating, convulsions or sudden loss of consciousness should be considered to be due to hypoglycemia. Correcting hypoglycemia results in their rapid reversal and should be tried immediately without awaiting the results of blood tests. The rapid assessment of blood glucose by a standard finger-prick method is useful.

Glucose solution may be administered orally or, when necessary, by nasogastric tube. The intravenous infusion of 10% dextrose or a therapeutic trial of 25–50 ml of 50% dextrose will rapidly abolish signs of hypoglycemia. Hypoglycemia may be prevented by the infusion of 5–10% dextrose (mainly when quinine is being given). Glucose overload may lead to fluid overload, rebound hyperinsulinism, hypokalemia and metabolic acidosis. Even subclinical maternal hypoglycemia may affect fetal growth and the development of the fetal CNS.

Pulmonary edema

Pregnancy is associated with an increased blood volume. Fluid overload, hyperparasitemia, renal failure and blood transfusions all increase the risk of developing pulmonary edema. The basic pathogenetic mechanism is capillary leak. Iatrogenic fluid overload by infusions, especially during labor, greatly increases the risk of pulmonary edema. After the initial treatment of dehydration when indicated, central venous pressure should be maintained at 0–5 cmH_2O. Pulmonary edema may develop even several days after institution of antimalarial drugs. Respiratory status should be monitored adequately. Treatment is supportive and may include oxygen, diuretics, fluid restriction and even mechanical ventilation.

Bacterial infections

Bacterial infections are not uncommon during pregnancy and the immediate postpartum period. Meningitis and encephalitis are endemic in most malaria zones and may be confused with cerebral malaria and may even occur concomitantly. Pneumococcal infections, gram-negative sepsis, typhoid fever, urinary tract infections and endometritis should also be considered. Immediate diagnosis and treatment according to local epidemiological data are needed. Aspiration pneumonia and sepsis may occur in the severely ill, comatose patient. In summary, bacterial infections mimic as well as complicate malaria.

Renal involvement

Proteinuria is common in pregnancy and malaria. Renal failure is rare. In most cases, urinary output is restored with adequate hydration. The combination of cerebral and renal malaria in pregnancy may mimic eclampsia.

Blackwater fever

This severe form of hemolysis is associated with falciparum malaria and is rare during pregnancy. Large numbers of non-parasitized red blood cells are destroyed, possibly due to antigen–antibody complex formation. Quinine may aggravate this phenomenon. Severe anemia, prostration, chills, vomiting, jaundice and bloody-black urine result in renal failure and even death.

The effect of malaria on labor

Malaria, especially *P. falciparum* malaria in the non-immune host, may induce preterm labor. Fetal distress and prematurity may add substantially to the neonatal morbidity and mortality. Ante- as well as postpartum fever may be the first manifestation of malaria.

The effect of malaria on the placenta

By the fourth month of pregnancy, the placenta becomes a highly vascularized organ. The intervillous spaces serve as preferential sites for parasite development, because they are, in part, sequestered from the immune system. Also, blood flow is sluggish and macrophages are scarce.

In endemic areas, placentas from primigravida are highly parasitized. Even in women living in areas of high endemicity, where immunity to malaria in adulthood is said to be the rule, high-grade placental parasitemia may be found. Parasites may be seen in placental blood smears even when they are absent in peripheral blood. Thus, in some areas, negative blood films cannot exclude the diagnosis of malaria in a pregnant woman.

P. falciparum parasites bind to placental ligands (e.g. chondroitin sulfate A) and selectively sequester in the placenta. Pathological changes include the presence of parasites in erythrocytes, malarial pigment deposits in intervillous spaces, monocytes, trophoblasts and mesenchymal stroma. There is trophoblastic damage with focal necrosis, loss of microvilli, irregular thickening of the trophoblastic basement membrane and protrusion of syncytiotrophoblastic projections into the basement membrane. The severity of these changes is correlated with the level of maternal and placental parasitemia. Histochemical stains may demonstrate deposits of immunoglobulins G and E, C3 and malarial antigens in the trophoblastic cytoplasm and basement membrane. Clinical manifestations of these pathological changes may include reduced placental weight, decreased nutrient and oxygen exchange between the mother and the fetus and reduced hormone secretion by the placenta.

High-level parasitemia may lead to intrauterine growth retardation, preterm delivery, low birth weight and, possibly, stillbirth. On the other hand, the placenta may serve as a barrier sequestering parasites selectively on the maternal side, thus preventing invasion of the fetal circulation and the resultant possibility of disease in the newborn infant. Parasites are seldom seen in the fetal circulation and in placental fetal blood smears. They are, however, seen much more frequently than the incidence of clinical congenital malaria. The incidence of congenital malaria is very low when compared with the large numbers of women who have malaria during pregnancy.

The effect of malaria on the fetus

Malaria is an important cause of low birth weight in the tropics. Low birth weight is more frequent in primigravidas in areas with intense malaria transmission. In areas where transmission is seasonal or sporadic, the effect of malaria on the fetus is extended to subsequent pregnancies. Growth is adversely affected by the degree of placental parasitemia, maternal nutrition and anemia. Effective antimalarial prophylaxis and iron supplementation during pregnancy have been shown to increase birth weight. Maternal hypoglycemia may cause fetal brain damage. The chronic inflammation of placental malaria may increase the probability of mother-to-child transmission of HIV.

Malaria-associated fever, dehydration, acidosis and placental insufficiency may cause fetal distress and induce premature labor. Prematurity, especially in the malaria-endemic areas of the world, has a great impact, since the medical facilities equipped for treating premature infants are inadequate or non-existent. The association of malaria and abortion or stillbirth is not clear-cut.

Drug therapy of malaria during pregnancy and lactation

Two major issues in drug therapy are addressed: the treatment of disease and the prophylaxis against the acquisition of malaria for both residents of endemic areas as well as traveling women. Data from studies in endemic areas show that malaria prophylaxis during pregnancy is beneficial to the fetomaternal unit. The once unequivocal benefit of large scale prophylaxis is now problematic, especially in the context of increasing parasite drug resistance and the lack of financial resources in many endemic areas. In areas where antimalarial prophylaxis is effective and financially feasible, this practice should be continued. In all endemic areas, chemical and physical barriers (e.g. mosquito repellents, insecticide-impregnated bed nets, etc.) should be used. Intermittent presumptive therapy is another potential strategy. Close obstetrical follow-up including the frequent measurement of hematocrit and blood smears for malaria detection should be routine.

Recommendations for the treatment of malaria vary in different areas of the world. The changing patterns of drug resistance, mainly in falciparum malaria, necessitate constant review. Treatment is best tailored by specialists who are familiar with the disease and the continually evolving epidemiology of drug resistance. In pregnancy, full doses of antimalarial therapy should be given. The utility of early cesarean section in malaria has not been proven.

Chloroquine is the cornerstone of malaria treatment and prophylaxis. Today, its use in falciparum malaria is limited due to the widespread resistance of *P. falciparum* to this drug. It remains central to the prophylaxis and treatment of *P. vivax*, *P. ovale* and *P. malariae* malaria. Chloroquine has been used for many years during pregnancy and is safe. It crosses the placenta readily. In rats, very high doses are teratogenic, and rare cases of teratogenicity have been described in patients with collagen vascular diseases treated with high doses of chloroquine for years. Doses used for the treatment and prophylaxis of malaria are not teratogenic. In some circumstances, amodiaquine might be considered during pregnancy.

Fansidar is a combination of sulfadoxine and pyrimethamine. It has been used safely during pregnancy without severe adverse effects, although large doses of pyrimethamine in animals may induce folic acid deficiency. The addition of folinic acid may reverse this effect. Sulfa-containing drugs are not considered teratogenic in humans. In rats and mice, cleft palate and thyroid tumors have been described. Theoretically, sulfa-containing drugs may cause neonatal hyperbilirubinemia and kernicterus when used within 2 weeks prior to delivery. The combination of pyrimethamine and sulfa was used for treatment and prophylaxis of malaria until its use was discontinued due to adverse cutaneous reactions and increasing parasite resistance. The drug combination is also used to treat toxoplasmosis during pregnancy.

Mefloquine is considered safe during the second and third trimesters and some will use this drug during the first as well. Safety during the first trimester has yet to be determined. Data on teratogenicity are lacking.

Information regarding the safety of halofantrine during pregnancy is lacking, thus it should not be used.

Quinine is the drug of choice for treating falciparum malaria where the possibility of chloroquine resistance exists (in most areas of the world). It is usually used in combination with another drug (i.e. tetracycline, clindamycin). High doses of quinine may stimulate the uterus, but at therapeutic doses it can be administered safely, even during the third trimester, with no oxytocic effect. Its hypoglycemic effect is prominent during pregnancy. When given in high doses, quinine is teratogenic in guinea pigs, but not in monkeys. Its possible association with human congenital anomalies (X rating by FDA) has rarely been mentioned in most major reviews on the subject.

Quinidine can be used alternatively when quinine is unavailable. Other than its excellent antimalarial activity, it has a similar hypoglycemic effect. Teratogenicity and oxytocic effects have not been reported in humans. Neonatal thrombocytopenia has been reported.

Tetracyclines are used in combination with quinine for treatment of resistant falciparum malaria. Their administration is contraindicated during pregnancy. Tetracyclines cause fetal bone and enamel abnormalities as well as potentially fatal fatty hepatic degeneration in the pregnant woman. An acceptable alternative is quinine and clindamycin.

Primaquine is used to eradicate the liver hypnozoite stage in *P. vivax* and *P. ovale* malaria, and is usually given for 2 weeks, commencing after the completion of chloroquine treatment. It is given in order to reduce the risk of relapse. It is contraindicated in glucose-6-phosphate dehydrogenase (G6PD) deficiency and may induce hemolysis *in utero* if the fetus is G6PD deficient. Fetal hemoglobin is even more sensitive to its deleterious effects. Primaquine is contraindicated before delivery. Instead, prophylaxis with weekly chloroquine should suppress relapse until after delivery when primaquine can be given to the mother.

Artemesinin derivatives are increasingly given during pregnancy, especially after the first trimester, though data about safety and possible teratogenic effects are lacking. They should be used in combination with drugs such as mefloquine and lumefantrine. To date, however, there is insufficient data about the use of these combinations during pregnancy, especially during the first trimester.

Proguanil has been used along with chloroquine for prophylaxis during pregnancy. It is considered safe for the fetus. Malarone (aotvaquone-proguanil) cannot yet be recommended for the treatment of pregnant women. Proguanil-dapsone is another potential candidate for treating malaria during pregnancy.

The concentration of antimalarial drugs in breast milk is minimal. Lactation is possible while on antimalarials. When indicated, the infant should be given prophylaxis since the concentration of antimalarial drugs in breast milk is not protective. Prolonged administration of tetracyclines to lactating mothers should be avoided. Given that hemolysis in G6PD deficiency is not necessarily dose dependent, primaquine should be avoided while breast feeding infants with this disorder.

Congenital malaria

The incidence of malaria during pregnancy in endemic areas can be high. Placental involvement is found in more than 30% of the pregnancies in endemic areas. The incidence of congenital malaria in infants of immune mothers is estimated to be 0.1–0.3%, but is as high as 10% in non-immune mothers. In endemic areas, malaria parasites have been found in almost 10% of cord blood samples when prospectively studied. Interestingly, congenital malaria is considered a rare disease. The mother does not always have clinical disease. Furthermore, a transient febrile episode during pregnancy due to malaria may go unnoticed. Only a few hundred cases have been described, mainly from non-endemic areas. This is in part due to under-reporting. In non-endemic areas, congenital malaria is seen mainly in infants of travelers to endemic areas and of refugees.

Parasites may infect the fetus *in utero* (congenital acquisition) or may be acquired as a result of the admixture of maternal and fetal blood during delivery (perinatal acquisition). Both these processes may cause malaria in the newborn. Transfer of antimalarial immunoglobulin G during the third trimester may have some protective effect on the fetus as well as on the newborn for the first few months after delivery. In true congenital malaria, the infant is born ill, although this condition is exceedingly rare. Perinatally acquired malaria is much more common, but is difficult to distinguish from vector-transmitted malaria in endemic areas.

The onset of symptoms usually occurs 3–8 weeks after birth, but may occasionally begin within a few hours after delivery and up to 15 months later. When disease starts later than 1 week of age in endemic areas, it is impossible to discriminate between congenital and early perinatally acquired infection.

Symptoms include fever, irritability, lethargy, poor feeding, diarrhea, jaundice, hepatosplenomegaly, anemia, leukopenia, thrombocytopenia and elevated levels of liver enzymes. Complications include coma and seizures, disseminated intravascular coagulopathy (*P. falciparum*), hypersplenism, splenic rupture, autoimmune phenomena, gastrointestinal symptoms with malabsorption, electrolyte imbalance and nephrotic syndrome. Untreated infants may progress to a state of wasting, malnutrition, secondary infection and even death. Manifestations of congenital malaria are not specific and may suggest many other diseases of the newborn. A high index of suspicion is needed in the appropriate epidemiological setting (maternal and travel history).

The early diagnosis of this potentially lethal disease is crucial. Treatment of congenital malaria is with chloroquine except for the resistant falciparum malaria. Primaquine is not required for treating congenital malaria since there is no liver hypnozoite stage.

Traveling during pregnancy

Women who are pregnant or likely to become pregnant should avoid travel to malaria-endemic areas. The impact of disease on the non-immune pregnant female is great. Other than areas without chloroquine-resistant *P. falciparum*, no chemoprophylactic regimen is likely to be completely effective.

When traveling is unavoidable, women may take chloroquine during pregnancy. Proguanil is used in some areas together with chloroquine for prophylaxis, though the combined use of these two individually safe drugs during pregnancy has not been studied rigorously.

Mefloquine is used as a prophylactic agent in chloroquine-resistant falciparum areas. It may be used during the second and third trimesters of pregnancy, and during the first trimester if intense exposure to chloroquine-resistant *P. falciparum* is unavoidable. In areas of mefloquine resistance (i.e. parts of Thailand) doxycycline is usually used for prophylaxis, but this drug is contraindicated in pregnancy. Women should avoid traveling to these areas during pregnancy. In addition to prophylaxis with antimalarial drugs, other methods for malaria prevention should be stressed (avoidance of being outside in rural areas during the evening and night hours, use of mosquito repellents, bed nets, etc.).

SUGGESTED READING

1. Baird JK. Effectiveness of antimalarial drugs. *N Engl J Med* 2005;352:1565–77.
2. Bergstrom S, Fernandes A, Schwalbach J, Perez O, Miyar R. Materno-fetal transmission or malaria in pregnancy: An immunoparasitological study in 202 parturients in Maputo. *Gynecol Obstet Invest* 1993;35:103–7.
3. CDC. Malaria. In *Health Information for International Travel 2005–2006*. Atlanta: US Department of Health and Human Services. Public Health Service, 2005.
4. Fairhurst RM and Wellems TE. Plasmodium species (malaria). In Mandell GL, Bennett JE, Dolin R, eds. *Principles and Practice of Infectious Diseases*, 6th edn. Phildelphia: Elsevier Churchill Livingstone, 2005:3121–3144.
5. Garcia LS, Suizer AJ, Healy GR, Grady KK, Bruckner DA. Malaria (in blood and tissue protozoa). In Balows A, Hausler WT Jr, Herrmann KL, *et al.*, eds. *Manual of Clinical Microbiology*, 6th edn. Washington, DC: American Society for Microbiology Press, 1995:1171–9
6. Hoffman SL, Campbell CC, White NJ. Malaria. In *Tropical Infectious Diseases, Principles, Pathogens & Practice*, 2nd edn. Philadelphia: Elsevier Churchill Livingstone, 2006:1024–62.
7. Joffe A, Tadavji T. Congenital malaria: A case report of a preventable disease. *Pediatr Infect Dis J* 1990;9:522–3.
8. MacLeod CL, Whiteside ME. Malaria. In MacLeod CL, ed. *Parasitic Infections in Pregnancy and the Newborn*. Oxford: Oxford University Press, 1988:8–42.
9. McGready R, Ashley EA, Moo E, Cho T, Barends M, Hutagalung R, Looareesuwan S, White NJ, Nosten F. A randomized comparison of artesunate-atovaquone-proguanil versus quinine in treatment for uncomplicated falciparum malaria during pregnancy. *J Infect Dis* 2005;192:846–53.
10. Nosten F, Rogerson SJ, Beeson JG, McGready R, Mutabingwa TK, Brabin B. Malaria in pregnancy and the endemicity spectrum: what can we learn? *Trends in Parasitol* 2004;20:425–32.
11. Okoko BJ, Enwere G, Ota MOC. The epidemiology and consequences of maternal malaria: a review of immunological basis. *Acta Tropica* 2003;87:193–205.
11. Taylor WRJ, White NJ. Antimalarial drug toxicity: a review. *Drug Safety* 2004;27:25–61.
12. Whitty CJ, Edmonds S, Mutabingwa TK. Malaria in pregnancy. *Br J Obstet Gynaecol* 2005;112:1189 95.
13. WHO guidelines for the treatment of malaria. World Health Organization, 2006.

167 Toxoplasmosis: pregnancy, delivery and the effect on the fetus and the newborn

D. T. Spira

Etiology

Toxoplasmosis is caused by the protozoan *Toxoplasma gondii*, an intestinal coccidian parasite of cats and other felines. The parasite was first described at the beginning of the century by Nicolle and Manceau,[1] isolated from the North African rodent *Ctenodactylus gundi*. Thirty years later in 1939, Wolf and Cowen[2] reported the first congenital transmission in man. The importance of the disease was immediately recognized and a large volume of data on epidemiology, serology, clinical picture and experimental systems were available. It took another 30 years for the whole life cycle of the parasite to be elucidated.[3]

Life cycle

The cycle of reproduction of *Toxoplasma gondii*, including the asexual schizogony and sexual gametogony, occurs in the intestinal epithelium of felines. Cats and all the other felines are therefore considered the definitive host of this parasite. Kittens get infected by oocysts excreted in large numbers (up to 10^7/cat/day) in infected cat feces, or later in life by tissue cysts in the prey. The ingested cysts release, in the small intestine, comma-shaped (2–6 mm) parasites, with a single nucleus and the rhoptrie apparatus necessary to penetrate into host cells, in this case the cat enterocytes. Cat enterocytes can be infected either by the eight sporozoites released from oocysts in cat feces, or by thousands of bradyzoites released from tissue cysts found in the organs or muscles of the prey. Both sources of infection initiate in the cat an enteric infection, with the production of micro- and macrogametes, fertilization and development of oocysts discharged in the feces. Considering that the primary infection renders the cat immune, young kittens should be considered the main source of environmental dissemination of the disease. The oocysts are about 9–15 mm in size, extremely resistant, and may remain infective for years.

In the intermediate host, *T. gondii* does not infect intestinal epithelium, rather it penetrates it and is hematogenously disseminated through the body. Parasites enter cells, preferentially phagocytes, although they can infect any mammalian cell except erythrocytes. In the cells, the parasites divide in a unique way known as endodyogony (division within the membrane of the mother cell) and are released when the host cell is destroyed by multiplication of the parasite. The early, fast-dividing stage in the life cycle of *T. gondii* is known as tachyzoite. After a few cycles of division and cell destruction, and concurrent with the development of a specific immune reaction in the intermediate host, *T. gondii* enters a different phase of its life cycle. The parasite now called bradyzoite divides slowly, preserving the host cell and creating a cyst wall within the host cell. The cyst finally outgrows the cell, which at this time disappears, leaving a 100–200-mm large round cyst filled with thousands of dormant bradyzoites. The three parasite stages, sporozoites in the oocyst, tachyzoites in host cells and bradyzoites in tissue cysts, are morphologically and structurally similar and all have the same infectious capabilities. The inactive tissue cysts persist in the mammalian host for many years, either till consumed by a predator or by man in insufficiently cooked meat or till the immune system of the host is compromised, the cysts break down and the dormant bradyzoites are reactivated.[4]

Epidemiology

Distribution of *T. gondii* is worldwide, and the parasite has been found in sheep even in cat-free areas of Australia. From epidemiological studies and comparisons, one can assume that man is infected both by oocysts from infected cat feces, which have contaminated food or water, and by tissue cysts in undercooked meat. The prevalent source of infection in each country depends on hygiene of food handling and on cooking habits (raw or 'rare' meat). Sheep, pork, cattle and horse meat, and apparently even poultry, have been found as potential sources of infection to man, if consumed insufficiently cooked. High infection rates have been found in most countries surveyed: thus, in Europe 45–80% of women of childbearing age have anti-*T. gondii* antibody; in the US and Canada 10–40%; and in Israel about 30% of adults. In some developing countries up to 90% of the adult populations have been exposed to the parasite. It can be assumed that in countries with lower standards of hygiene, the main source of infection originates from oocysts in cat feces, which contaminate food or water, whereas in developed countries undercooked meat is the main source. The importance to public health of *T. gondii* depends therefore on the method of transmission and the age of primary contact with the parasite.

Immune response

The immune response to *T. gondii* infection in man and in laboratory models is primarily cell-mediated. Both CD-4 and CD-8 lymphocytes as well as natural killer cells are active in the process. Primary *T. gondii* infection induces profound cytokine production, mainly of γ-interferon, tumor necrosis factor-α, interleukin-2 and interleukin-12, and thus stimulation of various immune mechanisms. A 65-kDa heat shock protein expressed on infected macrophages seems to act as a very strong antigen stimulating the responses. It is as if the parasite, instead of using ways to impair immunological recognition and thus to diminish the immune reaction of the intermediate host, advertises its presence inviting a fast and profound reaction, without achieving sterile immunity, thus guiding the life cycle toward bradyzoites and permanent tissue cysts.[5]

Clinical picture

Immunocompetent adult

Toxoplasma gondii in man can be considered the ultimate opportunistic parasite. Infection of the immunocompetent adult is subclinical as a rule, initiating an effective immune response, which abolishes the active stage of infection and causes the appearance of the inactive tissue cyst. Infection during pregnancy of immunocompetent mothers can, in the majority of cases, be considered in this category, as there is no difference in the clinical picture in the pregnant or non-pregnant female.

Immunocompromised host

In AIDS patients, as the paradigm of immunocompromised hosts, toxoplasmosis is severe, and in the great majority of cases considered to be the result of reactivated cysts in the central nervous system. Toxoplasmic encephalitis is the major expression, with lesions, in nearly all cases, in the cerebral hemispheres, but in about 50% also in the cerebellum and in 6% in the spinal cord. Toxoplasmic lesions have also been found in the lungs, kidneys and muscles including the myocardium. The dispersion is evidently hematogenic as parasites have been cultured from blood. *T. gondii* infections have been induced by organ transplantation into non-immune immunosupressed recipients.

Children infected after birth

Of the few newborns and children that develop clinical toxoplasmosis, the majority (about 90%) present with lymphadenitis, mainly of the deep cervical nodes, about 5% with chorioretinitis or cerebral lesions and 1.5% with myocarditis. These cases usually resolve even without treatment, when the parasites transform into the latent tissue cysts.

Congenital toxoplasmosis

This is the most severe presentation of the disease, and has a pathology quite distinct from the other types. There is a profusion of surveys and estimates on the number of infections during pregnancy and the percentage of transplacental infections of the fetus. The latest surveys estimate that only 10% of primary infections acquired during pregnancy are transmitted to the fetus. Of these, 75% induce a subclinical infection, and 15% present with mild and 10% with grave symptoms. In general, the earlier the infection occurs during pregnancy, the lower the chances of transmission, but the higher the probability of serious consequences. Infections acquired later in pregnancy tend to cross the placenta more often, but with a lower chance of inducing pathological changes in the child.

As stated, pathological signs in the pregnant woman are quite infrequent. Posterior cervical lymphadenopathy, fever, sometimes splenomegaly, all disappear after a few days to a week. After 10–14 days the parasite might traverse the placenta and appear in the fetus. *T. gondii* may be found in the cord and membranes, but only infrequently in the villi of the placenta. In the developing fetus, tachyzoites multiply in phagocytic cells, causing local inflammation and necrosis, but the proven neurotropy of the parasite soon concentrates the major damage in the neural tissue of the brain and eyes.

Brain pathology usually appears as glial nodules, microinfarctions and necrosis leading to calcifications. Yellowish necrotic nodules can be observed on the brain surface or in the brain substance. *T. gondii* multiplies in the ependymal cells lining the ventricles. The subependymal area is usually inflamed. The outlet of the ventricular system (aqueduct of Sylvius) is blocked by granulation tissue and by necrotic debris causing fluid accumulation and hydrocephalus. In the eye, chorioretinitis appears first as small hemorrhages gradually enlarging, bordered by black pigment. The lesions have a predilection for the macular region.

Clinically, chorioretinitis is the most common sign, often causing only minor problems. Punctate lesions in the eye may be harmless unless in the macular region, but some may flare up much later in adolescence and even adulthood. Other symptoms observed at birth that correlate with the acute infection of the fetus, mainly as a result of infections in the third trimester, are fever, jaundice, lymphadenopathy and sometimes dermal lesions. The most severe expression of congenital toxoplasmosis is the so-called 'tetrad of signs': chorioretinitis, micro- or hydrocephalus, cerebral calcifications and convulsions as a result of cerebral damage. Hydrocephalus is the most dramatic but least common of the clinical signs.

In cases of intense damage to the fetus one can expect abortion, fetal death *in utero* or preterm birth. In cases with less intense damage there may be neonatal or infant death, or the infant may survive with defects.

Diagnosis

Direct evidence

Parasitological diagnosis of *T. gondii* is limited, and gives false-negative results. Parasites might be found in amniotic fluid by tissue culture or by mouse inoculation. Both tests are difficult, take a long time and are expensive. Attempts to find circulating *T. gondii* antigen do not succeed in all cases of clinically proven infections. Polymerase chain reaction (PCR)-based discovery of *T. gondii* DNA in blood or amniotic fluid is slowly gaining acceptance, but is still not fully reliable.

Serology

Diagnosis of *T. gondii* in man is indirect, based on the presence of specific antibody, seroconversion or relative titers of different immunoglobulin classes. Diagnosis of fetal infection is therefore doubly indirect, as it relies on serology of the mother. Considering that only a small percentage of infected mothers transmit the infection to the fetus, sometimes with grave or even fatal consequences, the reliability of serologic diagnosis and its interpretation are of prime importance.

Different serologic techniques have been employed in the measurement of the various immunoglobulin classes. Each has its advantages and drawbacks, and this is not the place to deal with them. It is sufficient to explain the kinetics of antibody appearance and fading, and the relative sensitivities of the various tests. In general, all antibody classes rise during the second and third weeks postinfection. Immunoglobulin G is the most persistent, with significant titers for years. Considering the ease and reliability of tests based on immunoglobulin G or total immunoglobulins, it is the best way to diagnose 'old' infections at the beginning of pregnancy, thus marking pregnancies with no danger to the offspring.

Immunoglobulins M and A, rising rapidly and fading after 6 months, are the most reliable for establishing and following infection during pregnancy. Considering that as a rule they do not pass through the placenta, positive immunoglobulin M or A in the newborn is diagnostic for *T. gondii* infection. According to accepted algorithms, women negative for antitoxoplasma antibody or with a high titer, pointing to a recent infection in early pregnancy, should be followed during pregnancy and any rise in titer of immunoglobulin M or A antibodies should be carefully evaluated. When there is suspicion of infection, chemotherapy or abortion, depending on the history and stage of pregnancy, diagnostic imaging of the fetus and clinical examinations, should be considered. All cases of positive serology in the newborn, with or without clinical signs, should also receive chemotherapy to prevent late sequelae of the infection.

Treatment

Fortunately, *T. gondii* readily responds to treatment, and the problems are only in the clinical evaluation of whether the parasite has passed through the placenta.

Treatment of the mother

It has been verified that treatment, even of an asymptomatic mother who has acquired infection during pregnancy, greatly reduces the danger of fetal infection and sequelae. In all cases of *T. gondii* infection, a combination of spiramycin and sulfa plus pyrimethamine is recommended. One of the protocols states that if no overt infection of the fetus can be recognized, spiramycin 100 mg/kg/day and 25 mg pyrimethamine and 500 mg sulfadoxine twice weekly should be administered from 16 weeks of pregnancy. If the fetus is presumed to be infected, spiramycin plus 50 mg pyrimethamine and 3.0 g sulfadiazine daily should be given. As the combination of sulfa plus pyrimethamine inhibits folic acid synthesis, it should always be accompanied by 15 mg/day of leucovorin to prevent megaloblastic anemia.

Treatment of the neonate

In cases of an infected child with symptoms, spiramycin 100 mg/kg/day for 2 weeks, followed by alternating 1 month of pyrimethamine 1 mg/kg/day and sulfadiazine 100 mg/kg/day, and 1 month of spiramycin 100 mg/kg/day is recommended. This regimen should continue for 1 year.

Asymptomatic neonates with serologically proven infection should also be treated in the first 2 weeks with spiramycin and then by sulfadoxine–pyrimethamine 1 + 20 mg/kg/week in the first year of life. In all cases close clinical observation is suggested.

Other drugs and drug combinations are certainly possible, thus trimetoprim–sulfamethoxazole and clindamycin can be used. A novel antimalarial drug, Atovaquone, seems to be very effective against *T. gondii*, but large-scale clinical tests in pregnancy and on neonates have yet to be performed.[6]

Prevention

Many European countries have instituted compulsory testing for anti-*T. gondii* antibody during pregnancy, and others are preparing their legislatures for such tests. This approach seems the most promising in the prevention of *T. gondii* damage to the fetus or the neonate. On the personal hygiene basis, avoidance of contact with cat feces and consumption of only cooked or pickled meat and careful handling of raw meat and meat products should be part of health education preceding pregnancy.

REFERENCES

1. Nicolle C, Manceaux L. Sur une infection a corps de Leishman (ou organismes voisins) du gondi. *C R Acad Sci* 1908;147:763–6.
2. Wolf A, Cowen D, Paige BH. Toxoplasmic encephalo-myelitis. *Trans Am Neurol Assoc* 1939;65:76–9.
3. Hutchinson WM, Dunachie JF, Slim JC, Work K. Life cycle of *Toxoplasma gondii. Br Med J* 1969;4:806.
4. Dubey JP. *Toxoplasma, Hammondia, Besnoitia, Sarcocystis,* and other tissue cyst-forming coccidia of man and animals. In Kreier JP, ed. *Parasitic Protozoa.* New York: Academic Press, 1977: 101–238.
5. Subauste CS, Remington JS. Immunity to *Toxoplasma gondii. Curr Opin Immunol* 1993;5:532–7.
6. Vaudaux B, Rudin Ch, Kind C, *et al.* Toxoplasmose congenitale: Pris en charge pediatrique. *Schweiz Med Wochenschr* 1955; 125:(Suppl 65)70S–81S.

168 Fungal infections presenting particular features during pregnancy

M. Dan

Introduction

Among more than 50,000 known species of fungi, only about 200–300 are pathogenic to humans in varying degrees. The clinical manifestations of fungal infections range from bothersome cutaneous or mucosal lesions to invasive disease associated with severe morbidity and high mortality rates, particularly in immunosuppressed patients.

Fungal infections are classified according to the initial site of infection. The superficial mycoses are usually mild infections and are limited to the epidermis, the nails and hair and the mucosal surfaces. The principal pathogens in this group are the dermatophytes and *Candida* species. The subcutaneous mycoses involve the dermis, subcutaneous tissues and bone. They are usually acquired by traumatic inoculation of organisms of environmental origin. The systemic mycoses usually occur following inhalation of spores from the environment. The infection often disseminates from the lungs to various other organs. They can be caused by true pathogens, such as *Histoplasma capsulatum* and *Coccidioides immitis*, that invade the tissues and survive in the normal host, producing mild infection of short duration. In the immunosuppressed host, however, the same pathogens can be responsible for life-threatening infections. Alternatively, opportunistic fungi, such as *Aspergillus fumigatus*, mucor and *Cryptococcus neoformans*, are able to invade tissues only in immunocompromised patients. In addition, the commensal *Candida* can disseminate in debilitated patients and cause severe bloodstream infection or invade internal organs, such as the liver and the spleen.[1]

This chapter will discuss only fungal infections that present particular aspects in pregnancy.

Candida infections

Organisms belonging to the genus *Candida* are commensals of the gastrointestinal and genital tracts. *Candida* species usually cause superficial infections of the mucosa, skin and nails. In debilitated individuals, however, the fungus may invade the bloodstream and internal organs. Pregnant women are more prone than non-pregnant women to vaginal colonization and clinical infection with *Candida*. Rarely, the infection can ascend and involve the uterine content, producing chorioamnionitis and congenital candidiasis.

The pathogen and pathogenesis

Candidal organisms are dimorphic fungi, growing as ovoid yeast cells or as pseudomycelium. Blastospores represent the phenotypic form responsible for transmission or spread, and they are often associated with asymptomatic vaginal colonization. Germinated yeasts, on the other hand, produce mycelia, which can invade tissues and are associated with symptomatic disease. Although *Candida albicans* is the species most commonly isolated from the vagina, at least eight other members of the genus are recognized as human pathogens (*Torulopsis glabrata*, *Candida tropicalis*, *Candida parapsilosis*, etc.).

Candida organisms reach the vagina from the perianal area. In order to colonize the vaginal mucosa, the yeast must first adhere to the vaginal epithelial cells. It has been shown that fucose disaccharides serve as receptors for *Candida* ligands.[2] *C. albicans* adheres more avidly to the vaginal epithelium than do non-albicans species. Although there is a considerable interperson variation with regard to vaginal cell receptivity to *Candida* adherence, vaginal cells from women with recurrent vulvovaginal candidiasis do not show increased cell affinity for *Candida*, and all *C. albicans* strains appear to adhere equally well to epithelial cells.[3] In many women *Candida* inhabits the vagina in low numbers without causing symptoms. The transition from a vaginal commensal to a pathogen that causes symptoms probably depends on factors related to the organism and to the vaginal environment. Germination of the yeast enhances colonization, facilitates tissue invasion and precipitates symptomatic vaginitis. Epithelial cell damage and mucosal inflammation can result from direct hyphal invasion of tissues or hypersensitivity reaction.[3,4] *Candida* elaborates proteolytic enzymes, toxins and phospholipases that may be associated with virulence.[3] Candidal vaginitis occurs predominantly in women of child-bearing age, suggesting that gonadal hormones may play a major role in the pathogenesis of this entity. Indeed, during pregnancy the vagina is more susceptible to candidal infection, resulting in a higher incidence of colonization and symptomatic vaginitis, particularly in the third trimester. Symptomatic recurrences are more common, and cure rates are significantly lower during pregnancy.[5–7] However, other studies have suggested that the risk of *Candida* vulvovaginitis in pregnant women does not differ significantly from that in other gynecological patients.[8,9] Estrogens provide a carbon source for *Candida* growth and germination by increasing the glycogen content in the vaginal mucosa. These hormones also enhance vaginal epithelial cell avidity to *Candida* adherence, and facilitate yeast mycelial formation. It has been reported that peripheral blood lymphocyte responses are depressed during pregnancy and oral contraceptive use.[10–12] Cytoplasmic receptors for female reproductive hormones have been documented in yeast cells.[10,13] Data on the risk of *Candida* vulvovaginitis in women on oral contraceptives are conflicting; increased vaginal colonization rates have been documented mostly with high-estrogen oral contraceptive use, while studies on low-estrogen pills have not found an increase in occurrence of *Candida* vaginitis.[3,14]

The natural vaginal flora is thought to provide a colonization resistance barrier and prevent candidal germination and mucosal invasion. It has been suggested that lactobacilli compete with *Candida* for nutrients and interfere with candidal adherence to vaginal epithelial cells. Lactobacilli also elaborate bacteriocins that inhibit yeast proliferation and germination. Reduced numbers of lactobacilli were found in vaginal cultures obtained from women with symptomatic *Candida* vaginitis. The association between antibiotic use, increased colonization rates and precipitation of symptomatic *Candida* vaginitis is explained by the suppressive effect of antibiotics on the normal protective bacterial flora of the vagina.[3]

Other host factors that may contribute to the increased incidence of candidal vaginitis include (1) uncontrolled diabetes mellitus;[15] (2) increased local perineal moisture and temperature resulting from the use of tight, poorly ventilated nylon underclothing and (3) a high-carbohydrate diet.[14]

Cell-mediated immunity is considered to be the most important defense system in preventing mucosal invasion by *Candida* species. It has been demonstrated that cytokines can reduce hyphal formation.[16] Polymorphonuclear leukocytes and monocytes play an important role in limiting systemic candidal infection and deep tissue invasion, while humoral immunity is only marginally involved, if at all, in protecting against vaginal yeast infection.

Recurrent vaginitis is not usually associated with any precipitating or causal event. Three possible mechanisms have been proposed to explain recurrent candidal infections. First, repeated fungal reinoculation of the vagina from the intestinal reservoir is possible. Isolates from the vagina and the rectum are often of the same biotype. However, recurrences of candidal vaginitis have been demonstrated in the absence of *Candida* growth in rectal cultures,[17] and reduction of intestinal yeast carriage by nystatin treatment did not prevent recurrences of vaginal candidiasis. Second, sexual transmission may also be suggested due to the increased penile colonization by identical strains of *Candida* in male partners of women with recurrent vulvovaginal candidiasis. However, treatment of sexual partners does not prevent recurrences in women.[3] A third recurrence mechanism is relapse of persisting carriage in the vagina: following effective antimycotic treatment with mycologic eradication, an identical strain may be recultured in a quarter of the women within 4–6 weeks of therapy. Hence, recurrence is rather due to relapse than to reinfection. More recently, it has been suggested that idiopathic recurrent vulvovaginal candidiasis may result from a local dysfunction of cell-mediated immune mechanisms in the vaginal mucosa.[18]

Although *Candida* colonization of the vagina is common in pregnant women, ascending infection resulting in chorioamnionitis rarely occurs. *Candida* can cross intact membranes, and ruptured membranes are not a prerequisite for intrauterine invasion by *Candida*. Several reports have suggested, however, an association between intrauterine infection and the presence of a retained intrauterine device (IUD) or other foreign materials, such as cerclage sutures.[19–24] Mothers with *Candida* chorioamnioitis and premature labor have delivered at an earlier date when an IUD was present (mean gestational age, 25 weeks) than in its absence (mean, 31.5 weeks).[25] Very rarely *Candida* infection can further disseminate in the pregnant woman and become systemic, even in the absence of a particular predisposing factor other than the pregnancy state.[26]

Epidemiology

In most patients *Candida* infections are caused by organisms from the individual's own endogenous flora in the gastrointestinal and genital tracts. The pathogen may, however, be transmitted from person to person: neonatal oral candidiasis is more common in infants born to mothers with candidal vaginitis, suggesting that the infection may be acquired during passage through the birth canal.

About 75% of women will have at least one episode of vulvovaginal candidiasis during their child-bearing years, and approximately 40–50% of these will experience a second attack.[27] Some 5% of adult women suffer from recurrent, often intractable, episodes of candidal vaginitis.[3] Approximately 20% (range, 10–55%) of healthy, asymptomatic women of reproductive age harbor *Candida* in their genital tract at any point in time. A total of 25–40% of women with positive vaginal cultures for *Candida* are free of complaints. Asymptomatic vaginal colonization with *Candida* is increased in pregnancy: 30–40% of pregnant women carry the yeast in their lower genital tract. The incidence of symptomatic vulvovaginal candidiasis has been reported to be 2–20-fold higher during pregnancy than in non-pregnant women.[28] Other factors associated with increased carriage rate include estrogen-containing oral contraceptives, uncontrolled diabetes mellitus, corticosteroid therapy, antimicrobial therapy and tight-fitting synthetic underclothing.[14]

Candida is the most common cause of vaginal infection in Europe, while in North America it is the second most common (after bacterial vaginosis). In both areas the incidence of candidiasis has shown a sharp increase in the last decade.[3]

Candida species were found in 10% of positive amniotic fluid cultures in women with preterm labor.[24] In a study of 3500 placentas from high-risk pregnant women, *Candida* chorioamnionitis and funisitis were found in 18 (0.5%) cases. In eight (45%) of these patients, an IUD was present *in utero*.[21] In another report of six cases of *Candida* chorioamnionitis, a retained IUD was noted in three (50%) of the patients.[22]

Clinical manifestations

Characteristically, symptoms of vulvovaginal candidiasis are exacerbated in the week preceding the onset of menses. Vulvar pruritus is the most frequent symptom; vulvar burning, dyspareunia and external dysuria commonly occur. Vaginal discharge is often minimal and typically cottage cheese-like, although it can vary from watery to homogenously thick. On examination, the labia and vulva are erythematous and edematous; the vaginal mucosa is also erythematous and an adherent white discharge is typically noted. Symptoms are usually milder when infection is caused by *T. glabrata*.

Candida chorioamnionitis often presents with premature labor. The fetus is often affected: congenital candidiasis characteristically presents with skin lesions or erythematous rash seen at birth. *Candida* can be cultured from specimens of amniotic fluid, placenta and lesions of the newborn. Infection is often mild in term neonates: systemic disease is rare and the cutaneous rash often clears spontaneously. In preterm infants, on the other hand, disseminated disease frequently develops, and mortality is high. Early initiation of systemic antifungal therapy can improve survival rates.[29]

Laboratory diagnosis

Symptoms and signs of *Candida* vulvovaginitis are often non-specific and should not be used for establishing the diagnosis. Culture of vaginal discharge cannot distinguish between colonization, however the presence of large numbers of organisms is characteristic of symptomatic vaginitis.

The diagnosis of vulvovaginal candidiasis should be based on the microscopic examination of vaginal secretions. A saline preparation (wet mount) will often identify yeast or mycelia and will allow the consideration of other causes of vaginitis, such as trichomoniasis and bacterial vaginosis (presence of clue cells). The 10% potassium hydroxide preparation is more sensitive than the wet mount in identifying yeasts. Alternatively, the organisms can be easily seen on a gram-stained smear. The pH of vaginal secretions is usually normal (<4.5) in *Candida* vaginitis, and a finding of a higher pH indicates an alternative or concomitant condition. Culture of vaginal secretions should be considered in the presence of high clinical suspicion of candidal infection and negative microscopic results.[3]

Diagnostic amniocentesis for microbiologic evaluation of the amniotic fluid should be considered for all pregnant women with retained IUD and preterm labor with or without intact membranes.

Treatment

Vaginal fungal infections are easy to treat, but may be difficult to cure. This is at least partially due to the fact that the presently available antimycotic drugs are rather fungistatic than fungicidal. There is no indication that formulation influences therapeutic efficacy; the patient's preference should dictate which formulation is used to deliver the medication. However, relief of symptoms is achieved earlier with topical drugs than with those administered systemically. Among the available agents (Table 1), nystatin is the only polyene derivative, while the rest belong to the azole group. The average mycologic cure rate with

Table 168.1 Drugs recommended for the treatment of *Candida* vaginitis

Drug	Formulation	Dosage	Category*
Clotrimazole	Cream 1%	5 g × 7–14 days	B
	Vaginal tablet		
	100 mg	100 mg × 7 days	
	200 mg	200 mg × 3 days	
	500 mg	500 mg single dose	
Miconazole	Cream 2%	5 g × 7 days	B
	Vaginal suppository		
	100 mg	100 mg × 7 days	
	200 mg	200 mg × 3 days	
	1200 mg	1200 mg single dose	
Econazole	Vaginal tablet 150 mg	150 mg × 3 days	
Ticonazole	Cream	5 g × 3 days	
	2%	5 g single dose	
	6.5%		
Terconazole	Cream	5 g × 7 days	B
	0.4%	5 g × 8 days	
	0.8%		
	Vaginal suppository 80 mg	80 mg × 3 days	
Nystatin	Vaginal tablet 100,000 U	100,000 U × 14 days	B
Fluconazole	Oral tablet 150 mg	150 mg single dose	C
Ketoconazole	Oral tablet 200 mg	400 mg × 5 days	C
Itraconazole	Oral tablet 100 mg	200 mg × 3 days	C
		400 mg single dose	

*Food and Drug Administration Fetal Risk Drug category[32]

nystatin is 75–80%. There is no evidence of increased congenital anomalies when used during pregnancy:[30] it is classified in the B category of the Food and Drug Administration Fetal Risk Drug Summary. The various azole agents are of comparable efficacy, although they achieve slightly higher clinical and mycologic cure rates (85–90%) than does nystatin. In two studies miconazole was more efficacious than nystatin in treating vulvovaginal candidiasis during pregnancy.[28,31]

Clinical trials have shown that short courses and single-dose regimens of most azole agents are as effective as longer courses.[3] It seems reasonable, however, to use short regimens only in patients with infrequent episodes of mild to moderate severity.[3] During pregnancy, clinical response tends to be slower and recurrences are more frequent. Although single high-dose therapy with clotrimazole has been efficacious in pregnant women, it is generally recommended to prescribe topical antifungal agents for longer periods of 1–2 weeks. Side effects are minimal and consist most often of local burning and discomfort. Although azoles may inhibit estrogen and testosterone biosynthesis in animals and are embryotoxic in high doses in rodents, there is no evidence for an increase in human teratogenesis, including after first-trimester topical exposure. Most authorities believe that topical azoles are safe to use after the first trimester of pregnancy and that treatment during the first trimester should be reserved only for severe infections.[30] Clotrimazole and miconazole are category B drugs.[32]

The oral antimycotic agents – ketoconazole, fluconazole and itraconazole – are highly effective in achieving clinical and mycologic cures in acute candidiasis. Clinical results are similar or minimally superior to those obtained with topical agents. Most women consider oral therapy more convenient. However, oral therapy is more expensive and might be associated with higher rates of side effects, toxicity and teratogenicity. Ketoconazole therapy is accompanied by gastrointestinal upset in 10% of the cases. Of more concern is the risk of hepatotoxicity, which although rare (1/10,000–150,000 women treated) can be fatal.[3] Similar side effects are much less frequent with fluconazole and itraconazole. Ketoconazole also has antiandrogenic properties in humans. High doses of the drug are teratogenic in rats (cleft palate and patent incisive foramena) and embryotoxic in rabbits.[30] Animal embryotoxicity consistent with inhibition of estrogen synthesis was also documented with high dosages of fluconazole (cleft palate, abnormal craniofacial ossification).[33] A follow-up study conducted among 289 women who had taken fluconazole at some time during the months before or during pregnancy, did not reveal any harmful effects.[34] Nevertheless, oral azoles should be avoided in pregnancy (category C drugs).

Treatment of recurrent and chronic vulvovaginal candidiasis remains unsatisfactory. First, the diagnosis of *Candida* infection should be confirmed and the *Candida* species identified. Possible underlying conditions, such as uncontrolled diabetes mellitus, use of corticosteroids and other hormones, should be recognized and treated. Although most episodes of vulvovaginal candidiasis will respond to standard therapy, definitive eradication of the organism is often impossible and most women require long-term suppressive drug administration. Good results are obtained with intravaginal clotrimazole 500 mg weekly or oral fluconazole 150 mg weekly. Discontinuation of maintenance therapy usually results in resurgence of symptomatic infection in more than half the patients.

Vaginal infections caused by uncommon *Candida* species, such as *T. glabrata*, *C. tropicalis* and *Saccharomyces ceréviceae*, may not respond to conventional therapy. *T. glabrata* is inherently resistant to fluconazole. Its response to therapy with other drugs is quite unpredictable. Cases not responding to clotrimazole may still be cured by intravaginal nystatin, flucytosin or boric acid 600 mg twice daily for 2 weeks. The latter two agents should not be used in pregnant women.[3]

A number of other therapeutic approaches of unproven value have been recommended for prevention of recurrence of vulvovaginal candidiasis: oral nystatin to eradicate the gastrointestinal reservoir, treatment of male sexual partner, ingestion or local application of yoghurt, and use of *Lactobacillus acidophilus* capsules.

The optimal management of *Candida* amnionitis has not been established yet. Indications for and against the use of oxytocin to effect delivery rather than the continuation of tocolysis and systemic antifungal therapy are unclear, and no conclusions can be drawn from the insufficient data currently available. Amphotericin B has traditionally been the standard of treatment for systemic fungal infections; however, experience with the use of this agent in pregnancy is limited.[35] The pharmacokinetics of amphotericin B during pregnancy seem to be similar to those in non-pregnant women.[36] Intravenously delivered amphotericin B crosses the placenta and achieves effective concentrations in placental tissues and cord serum.[35] In most reported cases (~80%), the mother and infant tolerated therapy well, and there are no reports of teratogenesis.[37] However, toxicity in the form of renal function impairment and hypokalemia can occur in both in the same manner as described in non-pregnant patients, and appropriate monitoring is mandatory. Amphotericin B is a category B drug according to the classification of the Food and Drug Administration Fetal Risk Drug Summary,[32] and its use is usually indicated in serious fungal infections. Fluconazole has been demonstrated to be of comparable efficacy to amphotericin B in immunocompetent patients with systemic *Candida* infections.[38] It has the advantage of being markedly less toxic and showing good gastrointestinal absorption and cerebrospinal fluid penetration. However, because the drug has been shown to be embryotoxic in animal models,[33] its use in pregnancy should be avoided (category C drug).

There is no consensus about whether *Candida* colonization during pregnancy should be looked for and treated to prevent intrauterine infection. Vaginal antifungal prophylaxis should probably be considered for pregnant women with *Candida* colonization and risk factors, such as retained IUD and previous preterm delivery with no other identifiable causes.

Coccidioidomycosis

Coccidioidomycosis is most often a mild respiratory disease, occurring predominantly in endemic areas; only a minority of symptomatic patients experience a severe course. Pregnant women with coccidioidomycosis are at higher risk for dissemination and mortality than non-pregnant women.

The pathogen

C. immitis is a dimorphic fungus that exists in the soil in the mycelial phase. The mycelial growth results from apical elongation into branching, septate hyphae. With maturity, alternating compartments lose their cytoplasm. The walls of these degenerating cells are easily fractured and the infectious spores, the arthroconidia, can be released. The arthrospores are dispersed in dust in the air to infect new sites in the soil (saprophytic cycle). If inhaled by an animal host, the spores become spherical and develop a thick wall. These spherules reproduce by formation of internal spores (endospores). A single spherule may produce as many as 800 endospores. When the spherule ruptures, the endospores are released and each in turn can transform into a new spherule (parasitic cycle). If returned to the soil, the endospore develops into hyphae.[39]

Pathogenesis

Inhalation of the arthrospores into the lower airway triggers a complex immunologic response involving macrophage-mononuclear cells, neutrophils, complement activation and stimulation of T-lymphocytes.[40] Spherules and endospores are quite resistant to killing by neutrophils or products of oxidative metabolism. Spherule-produced substances can have a suppressive effect on cell-mediated immune reactions. Overall, T-lymphocytes play a major role in anticoccidioidal immunity. Monocytes recruited to the site of inflammation process the fungal antigens. This is followed by clonal expression of T-lymphocytes bearing receptors to coccidioidal antigens. The development of the specific cell-mediated immune response is essential for resistance to reinfection.[41]

The pathologic findings in coccidioidomycosis resemble those seen in tuberculosis, with granulomatous reaction, caseation and fibrosis. Although endosporulating spherules are the characteristic tissue form of the fungus, hyphae can be found in most pulmonary cavities. If the initial infection in the lung is not contained by the host defenses, progressive pulmonary disease or dissemination can occur. Conditions that predispose to expansion of the infectious process include large fungal inoculum and an immunosuppressive state of the patient. It is possible that T-suppressive cells and/or macrophage suppressors play a role in the fungal-specific immune suppression that is seen in severe forms of coccidioidal disease. Dissemination may involve almost any organ of the body at one or more sites, although the heart and gastrointestinal tract are rarely affected.[40]

The increased rate of dissemination in pregnant women is attributed to the relative immunosuppression associated with pregnancy and an agonist effect of 17β-estradiol and progesterone on the growth of *C. immitis*. A specific binding site for progesterone has been identified on the fungal cell wall.[42,43] Coccidioidal disease during pregnancy is associated with the tendency for spontaneous abortion in the first trimester and for premature labor in later gestation.[44] Rates of fetal loss as high as 43% and prematurity rates of 29% have been reported.[45] Although dissemination of infection during pregnancy can involve the placenta, there is no evidence for transplacental spread of the fungus.[46] It is postulated that the large size of the spherules and the acute thrombotic and chronic granulomatous reactions in the placenta protect villous capillaries from transplacental spread.[46] Neonatal infection is probably acquired following aspiration of infected decidua or postnatal inhalation.[46]

Epidemiology

Coccidioidomycosis is endemic in areas characterized by arid to semiarid climates, alkaline soil and sparse flora. The short rainfall season favors mycelial proliferation in the soil, and the long summer period allows the production of large numbers of arthrospores and their dispersion in the air. The majority of infections occur in seven southwestern states of the USA and in certain areas of Central and South America (Mexico, Guatemala, Honduras, Venezuela, Paraguay and Argentina).[47] Cases can occur, however, outside these endemic areas in individuals who have visited endemic regions (exposure of only a few hours may suffice), or as reactivation of infection in former residents of endemic areas, or as infection acquired from fomites originating in endemic areas (e.g. fruit, cotton).[48] About 20% of coccidioidomycosis cases are seen by physicians outside endemic zones.[49]

Infection is almost always acquired by inhalation of soil dust contaminated with arthrospores. Person-to-person transmission can occur only in special circumstances when the fungus reverts to its airborne form in contaminated secretions.[50]

In parts of the endemic regions more than 90% of inhabitants have had the infection. In the USA about 20,000 cases of mild coccidioidomycosis and 200 cases of severe disease occur each year, with nearly 60 deaths.[51] In southwestern USA the average annual incidence among young adults is 0.4% of the susceptible (i.e. skin-test negative) population.[52]

In endemic areas, 1 in 1000 (in the 1940s) to 1 in 5000 (in the 1980s) pregnant women have had coccidioidomycosis.[44,53] The dissemination rate during pregnancy is 40–100 times that in the general population. The dissemination and mortality rates increase as pregnancy advances: the estimated first-trimester dissemination rate is 23%, second trimester, 59% and third trimester, 68%.[54] The risk of death is nearly 100% in untreated pregnant women as compared to 50% in non-pregnant patients.[45]

Clinical manifestations

About 40% of those infected develop symptoms, the incubation period being 1–4 weeks.[40] The most common symptoms are fever and pleuritic chest pain mimicking a flu-like self-limited illness. Cough, headache, myalgia, arthralgia, malaise, night sweats and loss of appetite are often present. A mild diffuse erythematous or maculopapular rash (toxic erythema) can develop in about one-half of patients, while one-third of infected individuals suffer from erythema nodosum (2–11 times more common in women) or erythema multiforme. Segmental lung infiltrate is the most common radiologic finding, although other abnormalities, such as hilar lymphadenopathy, pleural effusion, nodules or cavities can be seen; these usually last a couple of weeks. Eosinophilia in the range of 5–10% of the peripheral white cell count is often noted in primary infection. Marked elevation of the peripheral eosinophilic count has been proposed as an indicator of non-meningeal dissemination.[55]

In about 5% of infected patients a nodule or cavity can persist for as long as 2 years. Most of these patients are asymptomatic, although hemoptysis can occur. Some patients do not follow such a benign course, but rather develop an acute progressive pneumonia that can be fatal. In other patients, in particular diabetics and immunosuppressed individuals, the lung infection progresses to a chronic pulmonary disease mimicking tuberculosis. Cavities are commonly seen, but bronchiectasis, emphysema or bronchopleural fistula can also develop. The disease may wax and wane over many years with fever, cough, chest pain and weight loss.

About 0.5% of infected individuals develop extrapulmonary disseminated disease. Dissemination occurs more often in men (who are five times more predisposed than women), immunocompromised hosts (with AIDS, malignancy, immunosuppressive or corticosteroid therapy), pregnant women and dark-skinned races. Dissemination can occur within a few weeks of initial infection or as reactivation of a previous quiescent infection in individuals who later become immunosuppressed. The clinical manifestations of disseminated disease range from an indolent chronic illness that persists for months or years to a fulminant illness that is often fatal within weeks if untreated. The organs most often involved are the skin and soft tissues, bone, joints and meninges; one or more sites may be affected. Cutaneous and soft tissue involvement is common and of varied presentations: verrucous papules, ulcers, erythematous plaques and nodules. Osteomyelitis occurs in about 40% of patients with disseminated disease. Most cases are asymptomatic or there are complaints of a dull pain. On radiography the bony lesions may be lytic or sclerotic. The infection may spread into contiguous joints or adjacent soft tissues causing subcutaneous abscesses, which often drain through spontaneously formed sinuses. Meningitis is the most serious manifestation of disseminated coccidioidomycosis, often complicated by hydrocephalus. Central nervous system involvement occurs in approximately one-third of pregnant women with disseminated disease. Although the onset is often insidious and fever is minimal or absent, the disease is fatal if left untreated. Other possible sites of infection include lymph nodes, liver, spleen, adrenal glands, eye and peritoneum.[40]

Women with a history of antecedent infection are not usually considered to be predisposed to relapse during pregnancy if they have a positive skin test before conception. Some authors recommend that patients with prior disseminated disease be considered at risk for relapse during pregnancy.[54]

Neonatal infection is characterized by gradual and non-specific onset of symptoms. Gastrointestinal manifestations may predominate over the classic fever and respiratory symptoms. Consequently, there is usually a low degree of clinical suspicion, as shown by the fact that more than half of the reported cases are diagnosed only at postmortem examination.[50]

Laboratory diagnosis

Mycological diagnosis

Microscopic examination of a standard 10% potassium hydroxide preparation or a wet mount preparation of clinical material can be diagnostic if the characteristic large thick-walled endospore-containing spherules are seen. Immature spherules can, however, be confused with other yeasts and some pollens. Visualization of the organism in cerebrospinal fluid is extremely rare. *C. immitis* can be isolated from various clinical specimens, although spinal fluid culture is positive only in about one-third of the cases. Several saprophytic fungi resemble *C. immitis* on ordinary media and a special medium containing cycloheximide should be used to inhibit the saprophytes. Identification of the organism by its morphologic characteristics is difficult even in the most experienced hands and confirmation can be achieved by using special media and incubation conditions, injection of a suspension of sporulating cultures into rodents or testing with reference antisera. Cultures of *C. immitis* represent a severe biologic hazard, and specimens and cultures should be handled only by experienced laboratories using appropriate safety equipment and procedures.[40]

Serology

Serum immunoglobulin M antibodies to the mycelial antigen coccidioidin can be demonstrated by several methods, 1–3 weeks after the onset of symptoms of primary infection in 75% of patients, and disappear within 4 months. Serum immunoglobulin G antibodies appear 4–12 weeks after onset of infection and may last for 6–8 months. Immunoglobulin G titers correlate with disease progression or recovery. Elevated titers of complement-fixing immunoglobulin G antibodies (CFA) are the hallmark of disseminated disease: 60% of patients have titers of ≥1:32, and in 40% the titers are ≥1:64. Titration can also be carried out with the immunodiffusion test, which is sensitive and simple to perform. In meningeal disease, serum titers remain low or absent, while in the cerebrospinal fluid, CFA are initially present in 70% of patients and in almost all of them as the disease progresses. The CFA titers in the spinal fluid parallel the course of the meningeal disease. Occasional cross-reaction can occur in patients with histoplasmosis or blastomycosis.[56]

Skin tests

Skin tests for coccidioidal antigens (coccidioidin, spherulin) give positive results (> 5 mm induration) 10–45 days after infection, usually before the first serologic reactions are detectable. By 1 month after onset, almost every symptomatic patient has a positive skin test. Anergy is common in disseminated disease. Skin testing can be useful if a conversion from a negative to a positive result is documented, or as a preliminary indication of infection while awaiting serologic results.[40]

Treatment

Although most patients with symptomatic primary infection recover without treatment, chemotherapy is indicated in some circumstances. These include severe disease, symptoms persisting for more than 6 weeks, rising or elevated titers of immunoglobulin G > 1:64, immunosuppression, presence of concurrent disease (diabetes mellitus, chronic lung disease) likely to be adversely affected by the infection, pregnant women, infants, and dark-skinned persons. Treatment is almost always indicated in extrapulmonary disease.

Amphotericin B given intravenously in doses of 1–1.5 mg/kg/day to a total dose of 1–2.5 g is the standard regimen in disseminated coccidioidomycosis. Smaller doses, 0.6 mg/kg/day (0.5–1.0 g total dose), may suffice in primary infection. Some authors recommend addition of local administration of the drug (irrigation of sinuses, instillation of abscesses or intra-articular therapy). Intrathecal therapy with amphotericin B is the traditional treatment modality in coccidioidal meningitis. The daily dose should be gradually increased as tolerated to 0.5–1.0 mg. Intrathecal administration of amphotericin B is associated with neurotoxicity and local reactions that can be reduced by concomitant intrathecal administration of hydrocortisone. Treatment should continue until 3 months after the spinal fluid CFA has disappeared, with follow-up of spinal fluid serology for at least 2 years.[57]

If active infection is present during pregnancy, some authors recommend considering abortion or early delivery (depending on the stage of pregnancy).[40] Good maternal and neonatal results have been obtained, however, with amphotericin B therapy of disseminated fungal infection during pregnancy. Aggressive use of the drug has significantly improved the previously often fatal maternal outcome.[46]

Alternative regimens for the treatment of coccidioidomycosis include the azole drugs, which have the advantage of good intestinal absorption and a low toxicity profile. They are, however, contraindicated in pregnancy (see section on candidiasis). Most experience has been acquired with ketoconazole (400 mg once daily) and itraconazole (200 mg twice daily) in non-meningeal coccidioidomycosis. Relapse rates of 25–30% even after 12 months of treatment have been reported. The best results have been obtained in patients with cutaneous or joint involvement. Similarly, good results have been obtained with fluconazole (400–600 mg once daily). Duration of azole therapy should probably be 6 months after disease activity has become undetectable or 12 months in total.[40]

Chemotherapy should often be supplemented with surgical measures: removal of pulmonary cavities is indicated if persistence, enlargement, recurrence or hemoptysis occurs. In musculoskeletal involvement, infected bone or synovium should be resected, and adjacent soft tissue pus drained. Immobilization is an important part of the treatment.[40]

REFERENCES

1. Richardson MD, Warnock DW. *Fungal Infection: Diagnosis and Management.* London: Blackwell Scientific Publications, 1992.
2. Douglas LJ. Mannoprotein adhesins of *Candida albicans.* In Bennett JE, Hay RJ, Peterson PK, eds. *New Strategies in Fungal Disease.* Edinburgh: Churchill Livingstone, 1992:34–9.
3. Sobel J. Candidal vulvovaginitis. *Clin Obstet Gynecol* 1993;36: 153–65.
4. Witkin SS. IgE antibodies to *Candida albicans* in vaginal fluids of women with recurrent vaginitis. Presented at the *Annual Meeting of the American Society of Microbiology,* Palm Springs, CA, March 1987.
5. Carroll CT, Hurley R, Stanley VD. Criteria for diagnosis of *Candida* vulvovaginitis in pregnant women. *J Obstet Gynecol* 1973;80:258–63.
6. Gillespie HL, Inman WB, Slater V. Incidence of *Candida* in the vagina during pregnancy. *Obstet Gynecol* 1960;16:185–8.
7. Gugnani HC, Nzelibe FK, Gini PC, *et al.* Incidence of yeasts in pregnant and non-pregnant women in Nigeria. *Mycosen* 1989; 32:131–5.
8. Hopsu-Havu VK, Gronroos M, Punnonen R. Vaginal yeasts in parturients and infestation of the newborns. *Acta Obstet Gynecol Scand* 1980;59:73–7.
9. Reed BD, Huck W, Zavove P. Differentiation of *Gardnerella vaginalis, Candida albicans* and *Trichomonas vaginalis* infections of the vagina. *J Fam Pract* 1989;28:673–80.
10. Powell BL, Frey CC, Drutz DJ. Identification of a 17-estradiol-binding protein in *Candida albicans* and *Candida (torulopsis) globrata. Exp Mycol* 1984;8:304–6.
11. Mazumder DN, Ghose N, Mirta J, Dutta G, Santra A. Immunological status of women with prolonged oral contraceptives and occurrence of giardiasis. *J Indian Med Assoc* 1990;88:129–31.
12. Brunham RC, Martin DH, Hubbard TW, *et al.* Depression of the lymphocyte transformation response to microbial antigens and to phytohemagglutinin during pregnancy. *J Clin Invest* 1983;72: 1629–38.
13. Kinsman OS, Collard AE. Hormonal factors in vaginal candidiasis in rats. *Infect Immun* 1986;53:498–504.
14. Reed BD. Risk factors for *Candida* vulvovaginitis. *Obstet Gynecol Surv* 1992;47:551–60.
15. Sobel JD. Epidemiology and pathogenesis of recurrent vulvovaginal candidiasis. *Am J Obstet Gynecol* 1985;152:924–35.
16. Kalo-Klein A, Witkin SS. Prostaglandin E_2 enhances and γ-interferon inhibits germ-tube formation in *Candida albicans. Infect Immun* 1990;58:260–2.
17. O'Conner MI, Sobel JD. Epidemiology of recurrent vaginal candidiasis: Identification and strain differentiation of *Candida albicans. J Infect Dis* 1986;154:358–63.
18. Fidel PL, Sobel JD. Immunopathogenesis of recurrent vulvovaginal candidiasis. *Clin Microbiol Rev* 1996;9:335–48.
19. Schweid AI, Hopkins GB. Monilia chorionitis associated with an intrauterine contraceptive device. *Obstet Gynecol* 1968;31: 719–21.
20. Ho CY, Aterman K. Infection of the fetus by *Candida* in a spontaneous abortion. *Am J Obstet Gynecol* 1970;106:705–10.
21. Whyte RK, Hussein Z, de Sa D. Antenatal infection with *Candida* species. *Arch Dis Child* 1982;57:528–35.
22. Bruner JP, Elliott SP, Kilbride HW, *et al. Candida* chonoamnionitis diagnosed at amniocentesis with subsequent fetal infection. *Am J Perinatol* 1986;3:213–18.
23. Smith CV, Horenstein J, Platt CD. Intra-amniotic infection with *Candida albicans* associated with a retained intrauterine contraceptive device: A case report. *Am J Obstet Gynecol* 1988;159: 123–4.
24. Mazor M, Chaim W, Pak I, Goldstein D. Intra-amniotic infection with *Candida albicans* associated with a retained intrauterine device. *J Reprod Med* 1992;37:950–2.
25. Delprado WJ, Baird PJ, Russell P. Placental candidiasis: Report of three cases with a review of the literature. *Pathology* 1982; 14:191–5.
26. Potasman I, Leibovitz Z, Sharf M. *Candida* sepsis in pregnancy and the postpartum period. *Rev Infect Dis* 1991;13:146–9.
27. Hurley R. Recurrent *Candida* infection. *Clin Obstet Gynecol* 1981;8:209–14.
28. McNellis D, Mcleod M, Lawson J, Posquale S. Treatment of vulvovaginal candidiasis in pregnancy: A comparative study. *Obstet Gynecol* 1977;50:674–8.
29. Van Winter JT, Ney JA, Ogburn PL, Johnson RN. Preterm labor and congenital candidiasis. *J Reprod Med* 1994;39:987–90.
30. Sullivan C, Smith LG. Management of vulvovaginitis in pregnancy. *Clin Obstet Gynecol* 1993;36:195–205.
31. Wallenburg HC, Wladimirnoff JW. Recurrence of vulvovaginal candidiasis during pregnancy: Comparison of miconazole versus nystatin treatment. *Obstet Gynecol* 1976;48:491–6.
32. Hedstrom S, Martens MG. Antibiotics in pregnancy. *Clin Obstet Gynecol* 1993;36:886–92.
33. Lee BE, Feinberg M, Abraham JJ, Murthy AR. Congenital malformations in an infant born to a woman treated with fluconazole. *Pediatr Infect Dis J* 1992;11:1062–4.

34. Inman W, Pearce G, Wilton L. Safety of fluconazole in the treatment of vaginal candidiasis. A prescription-event monitoring study, with special reference to the outcome of pregnancy. *Eur J Clin Pharmacol* 1994;46:115–18.
35. Dean JL, Wolf JE, Ranzini AC, Laughlin MA. Use of amphotericin B in pregnancy: Case report and review. *Clin Infect Dis* 1994; 18:364–8.
36. McCoy MJ, Ellenberg JF, Killam AP. Coccidioidomycosis complicating pregnancy. *Am J Obstet Gynecol* 1980;137:739–40.
37. Cohen I. Absence of congenital infection and teratogenesis in three children born to mothers with blastomycosis and treated with amphotericin B during pregnancy. *Pediatr Infect Dis* 1987; 6:76–7.
38. Rex JH, Bennett J, Sugar AM *et al.* A randomized trial comparing fluconazole with amphotericin B for the treatment of candidemie in patients without neutropenia. *N Engl J Med* 1994;331:1325–30.
39. Huppert M, Sun SH. Overview of mycology, and the mycology of *Coccidioides immitis.* In Stevens DA, ed. *Coccidioidomycosis: A Text.* New York: Plenum Medical, 1980:21–32.
40. Stevens DA. *Coccidioides immitis.* In Mandell GL, Bennett JE, Dolan R, eds. *Principles and Practice of Infectious Diseases,* 4th edn. New York: Churchill Livingstone, 1995:2365–75.
41. Beaman L, Pappagianis D, Benjamini E. Mechanisms of resistance to infection with *Coccidioides immitis* in mice. *Infect Immun* 1979;23:681–5.
42. Drutz DJ, Huppert M, Sun SH, *et al.* Human sex hormones stimulate the growth and maturation of *Coccidioides immitis. Infect Immun* 1981;32:897–907.
43. Powell BL, Drutz DJ, Huppert M, *et al.* Relationship of progesterone and estradiol-binding proteins in *Coccidioides immitis* to coccidioidal dissemination in pregnancy. *Infect Immun* 1983; 40:478–85.
44. Vaughan JE, Ramirez H. Coccidioidomycosis as a complication of pregnancy. *Calif Med* 1951;74:121–5.
45. Smale LE, Waechter KG. Dissemination of coccidioidomycosis in pregnancy. *Am J Obstet* 1970;107:356–61.
46. Spark RP. Does transplacental spread of coccidioidomycosis occur? *Arch Pathol Lab Med* 1981;105:347–50.
47. Papagianis D. Epidemiology of coccidioidomycosis. In McGinnis MR, ed. *Current Topics in Medical Mycology.* New York: Springer-Verlag, 1988;2:199–238.
48. Rothman PE, Graw RG, Harris JC. Coccidioidomycosis: Possible fomite transmission: A review and report of a case. *Am J Dis Child* 1969;118:792–801.
49. Salkin D, Evans BH. Coccidioidomycosis. In Steele JD, ed. *The Treatment of Mycotic and Parasitic Disease of the Chest.* Springfield, IL: Thomas Publishing, 1964:55–61.
50. Eckmann BH, Schaefer GL, Huppert M. Bedside interhuman transmission of coccidioidomycosis via growth on fomites: An epidemic involving six persons. *Am Rev Respir Dis* 1964;89:175–9.
51. Egeberg RO. Socioeconomic impact of coccidioidomycosis. In Einstein HE, Catanzaro A, eds. *The Fourth International Congress on Coccidioidomycosis.* Washington, DC: Foundation for Infectious Disease, 1985:27.
52. Kerrick SS, Lundergan LL, Galgiani JN. Coccidioidomycosis at a university health service. *Am Rev Respir Dis* 1985;131:100–2.
53. Wack EE, Ampel NM, Galgiani JN, Bronnimann DA. Coccidioidomycosis during pregnancy. An analysis of ten cases among 47,120 pregnancies. *Chest* 1988;94:376–9.
54. Peterson CM, Schuppert K, Kelly PL, Pappagianis D. Coccidioidomycosis in pregnancy. *Obstet Gynecol Rev* 1993;48: 149–56.
55. Harley WB, Blaser MJ. Disseminated coccidioidomycosis associated with extreme eosinophilia. *Clin Infect Dis* 1994;1:627–9.
56. Pappagianis D, Zimmer BL. Serology of coccidioidomycosis. *Clin Microbiol Rev* 1990;3:247–68.
57. Drutz D. Amphotericin B in the treatment of coccidioidomycosis. *Drugs* 1983;26:337–48.

169 Mumps in pregnancy

A. Morag

Introduction

The word 'mumps' probably derives from the British word 'to mump', which means to grimace or grin. Thus, the name of the disease likely refers to the marked parotid swelling, which is the most common manifestation of infection with this virus.

Mumps is an acute generalized viral infection that occurs primarily in school-age children and adolescents. The disease caused by this virus is usually benign and self-limited, with about 30% of those infected not showing any clinical manifestations.

The agent

Mumps virus is an RNA virus, a member of the Paramyxoviridae family, which also includes some of the other common causes of childhood infections, such as parainfluenza, measles and respiratory syncitial viruses.

The complete mumps virion has an irregular spherical shape with a diameter averaging 200 nm. The external surface is regularly studded with glycoproteins possessing hemagglutinin, neuraminadase and cell-fusion activity. Mumps virus has a lipid envelope, is ether-sensitive and is stable at 4°C for several days and at −70°C for years. The virus can be propagated in various tissue cultures (see diagnosis), and causes cytopathic effects, with eosinophilic cytoplasmic inclusions.

Epidemiology and clinical manifestations

During mumps infection the virus is shed heavily in respiratory secretions. Transmission, therefore, is by droplet infection or fomites, and the virus enters through the nose or mouth.[1] Mumps virus has also been recovered from the urine of infected individuals.[2]

Mumps is endemic throughout the world. There are no known immunologic differences among the various strains of mumps virus, and natural infection with wild-type virus or immunization with live-attenuated mumps virus vaccine, provides long-lasting immunity.[3] In the United States, before the introduction of vaccine in 1967, epidemics occurred every 2–5 years, with peak incidence between January and May.

Man is the only known host for the mumps virus in nature. The virus is uncommonly observed in infants less than 1 year of age, and primarily infects young children during their early school years.[4] Due to mass immunization programs the occurrence of mumps has shifted from younger to older children and adolescents. In recent years, only 25% of cases have occurred in the 5- to 9-year age group, and more than 50% have occurred in the teenage group. In Western countries, about 10–20% of the adult populations have no demonstrable antibodies against the mumps virus. This susceptible postpubescent population is at risk of the increased severity and higher complication rate seen in mumps infection within this age group.[5]

With a 10–20% susceptibility in this population, mumps infection can occur during pregnancy. The incidence of mumps infection during pregnancy in the United States is estimated to be between 1 in 1000 and 1 in 3000.[1]

The incubation period of mumps averages 14–18 days. Following a short prodromal period, which comprises non-specific complaints such as fever, anorexia, myalgia and malaise, the parotitis becomes evident in about 60–70% of infected individuals. The parotid and sometimes other salivary glands are swollen and tender, with symptoms lasting about 1 week.[3] The patient may have difficulty with pronunciation, and mastication and ingestion of citrus juices typically exacerbates the pain. Fever up to 40°C is often observed during the phase of parotitis.

Involvement of other organs is sometimes observed in addition to the salivary glands. Epididymo-orchititis is observed in 25% of cases in postpubertal men[6] and oophoritis in 5% of infected postpubertal women. Orchitis is usually unilateral and very rarely causes sterility. Oophoritis is manifested with fever, nausea, vomiting and lower abdominal pain. Impaired fertility and premature menopause have been reported as a consequence of ovarian involvement, but this is very rare.[7]

Involvement of the central nervous system is quite common in mumps. Cerebrospinal fluid pleocytosis is observed in about half of the cases. Clinical meningitis occurs in 1–10% of individuals with mumps parotitis; on the other hand only 40–50% of patients with mumps meningitis have parotitis.[8] Mumps encephalitis is rare, and occurs in about 0.1% of mumps cases.

Mumps-associated pancreatitis is a late effect of mumps infection. It is usually diagnosed on the basis of mild clinical symptoms, but can be manifested by severe epigastric pain and tenderness accompanied by fever, nausea and vomiting. There is still controversy concerning the possible association of mumps and the development of diabetes mellitus.[9]

Deafness secondary to mumps labyrinthitis is a rare complication of mumps virus infection.[10] This hearing loss is severe and of sudden onset.

Other mumps-associated complications may include thyroiditis, myocarditis, arthritis and renal involvement.[10]

Mumps in pregnancy

When mumps occurs in pregnant women, the illness is generally benign and not more severe than it is in other adult women.[11] In pregnant women as well as in the population as a whole, deaths from mumps are exceedingly rare.

Effects of gestational mumps on the fetus

Abortion

Gestational viral infections have been extensively investigated by Siegel and associates.[12] They observed excessive fetal deaths when mumps developed during the first trimester but not during the second and third trimesters.[12] Many other reports describe isolated cases of abortion associated with gestational mumps, nearly all of these occurring in the first 4 months of pregnancy.[13] In one instance, mumps virus was isolated from a 10-week-old fetus spontaneously aborted 4 days after the mother developed clinical mumps.[14]

Prematurity

In the only prospective study of low birth weight in relation to maternal mumps infection, no significant association was found. However, analysis of data showed that the effect was greatest when mumps occurred in the first trimester.[15]

Congenital malformations

Evidence in experimentally infected animals suggests that mumps virus can cross the placenta, infect the fetus and induce congenital malformations.[16]

Definitive evidence of a teratogenic potential for mumps virus in humans is yet unclear. Many reports describe the occurrence of congenital malformations after gestational mumps, but no data are available concerning the occurrence of similar anomalies in matched controls. Malformations described as associated with gestational mumps include chorioretinitis and optic atrophy, intestinal atresia, corneal cataracts, urogenital anomalies, hydrocephalus and others.[17]

Endocardial fibroelastosis

In the 1960s, St. Geme and colleagues suggested an association between endocardial fibroelastosis and mumps virus infection.[18] They reported that a high proportion of children with primary endocardial fibroelastosis exhibit cutaneous delayed hypersensitivity to mumps virus antigens and that their mothers often had mumps or exposure to mumps during gestation. An experimental model in the chicken supports a possible association between mumps and the occurrence of cardiac lesions in the developing fetus. Definite evidence for such an association does not exist.

Laboratory diagnosis

Isolation of mumps virus from clinical specimens

Mumps virus is readily isolated in various tissue culture cell lines. The most commonly used are Vero, human embryonic kidney and chick embryo fibroblasts.[1] The virus can be isolated from urine during the period from 6 days before to 15 days after the onset of parotitis, and from saliva from 7 days before until 9 days after the onset of salivary gland enlargement.

Serological diagnosis

The most commonly used serological test today is an enzyme linked immunosorbent assay detecting specific immunoglobulin G or M antibodies to mumps virus. Serological diagnosis can also be made by determination of neutralizing and other types of specific antibodies.[4]

Prevention and treatment

Active immunization with the Jeryl Lynn strain of attenuated mumps virus vaccine has been available in the United States since 1967. A single subcutaneous immunization produces protective levels of mumps-neutralizing antibodies in more than 95% of vaccines, and adequate titers are maintained for more than 10 years.[19]

All children over 12 months of age should be immunized. Vaccination should take place at 12–15 months of age and again at 5–12 years of age, as a part of combined measles–mumps–rubella viruses' vaccine (MMR). As with other live virus vaccines, mumps vaccine should not be administered to pregnant women and immunocompromised patients. Treatment for mumps patients is only symptomatic, as there is as yet no antiviral agent efficiently active against the mumps virus.

REFERENCES

1. Gershon AA. Chickenpox, measles and mumps. In Remington JS, Klein JO, eds. *Infectious Diseases of the Fetus and Newborn Infant,* 44th edn. Philadelphia: W. B. Saunders Company, 1995:565–658.
2. Utz JL. Viruria in man: An update. *Prog Med Viral* 1974;17:77–90
3. Klein JO. Mumps. In Klein JO, ed. *Report of the Committee on Infectious Diseases,* 19th edn. Elk Grove Village, IL: American Academy of Pediatrics, 1982:142–5.
4. The Immunization Practices Advisory Committee (ACIP). Mumps vaccine. *MMWR Morb Mortal Wkly Rep* 1980;29:87–94.
5. Meyer HM Jr, Hopps HE, Parkman PD. Appraisal and re-appraisal of viral vaccines. *Adv Intern Med* 1980;25:533–600.
6. Laubert B. The incidence of mumps and mumps orchitis. *Acta Genet Stat Med* 1951;2(Suppl 1):1.
7. Morrison JC, Givens JR, Wider WL. Mumps oophiritis: A cause for premature menopause. *Fertil Steril* 1975;26:655.
8. Johnstone JA, Ross CAC, Dunn M. Meningitis and encephalitis associated with mumps infection. *Arch Dis Child* 1972;47:647.
9. Craighead JE. The role of viruses in the pathogenesis of pancreatic disease and diabetes mellitus. *Prog Med Virol* 1975;19:161–214.
10. The Association for the Study of Infectious Diseases. A retrospective survey of the complications of mumps. *J R Coll Gen Pract* 1974;24:552–6.
11. Harsdy JB. Viral infection in pregnancy. A review. *Am J Obstet Gynecol* 1965;93:1052.
12. Siegel M, Fuerst HT, Peress NS. Comparative fetal mortality in maternal virus diseases: A prospective study on rubella, measles, mumps, chickenpox and hepatitis. *N Engl J Med* 1966; 274:768.
13. Ylinen O, Jervinen PA. Parotitis during pregnancy. *Acta Obstet Gynecol Scand* 1953;32:121.
14. Kurtz J, Tomlinson A, Pearson J. Mumps virus isolated from a fetus. *Br Med J* 1982;248:471.
15. Siegel M, Fuerst HT. Low birth weight and maternal virus disease: A prospective study of rubella, measles, mumps, chickenpox and hepatitis, *J Am Med Assoc* 1966;197:88.
16. Robertson GG, Williamson AP, Blattner RJ. Origin and development of lens cataracts in mumps-infected chick embryos. *Am J Anat* 1964;115:473.
17. Grenvall H, Selander P. Some virus diseases during pregnancy and their effect on the fetus. *Nord Med* 1948;37:409.
18. St Geme JW Jr, Noren FR, Adams P. Proposed embryopathic relation between mumps virus and primary endocardial fibroelastosis. *N Engl J Med* 1966;275:339.
19. Weibel RE, Buynak EB, Mclean AA, *et al.* Persistence of antibody in human subjects following administration of combined live attenuated measles, mumps and rubella vaccines. *Proc Soc Exp Biol Mcd* 1980;165:260.

170 Measles in pregnancy

A. Morag

Introduction

Measles virus is a member of the family Paramyxoviridae and the genus *Morbillivirus*. This virus has a single-stranded RNA genome and a lipoprotein envelope that contains proteins associated with hemaglutinating, hemolyzing and membrane fusion properties of measles viruses.[1]

Epidemiology and clinical manifestations

Man is the natural host for measles virus, although other primates are susceptible to naturally transmitted measles infection. Measles occur in all parts of the world inhabited by man. Climate and natural boundaries influence the occurrence of measles only to the extent that they limit contact between susceptible and contagious individuals.

From 1912 to 1959, 200,000–600,000 cases of measles were reported annually in the United States, and the morbidity rate remained relatively constant at 200–500 cases per 100,000 per year.[2] With the introduction of the measles vaccine in 1963, the annual number of reported cases fell rapidly. With the improvement of vaccination programs in the early 1980s the annual rate of reported cases reached less than 2 cases per 100,000.[3] Within more than 30 years of the introduction of the measles vaccine, the age-specific incidence of measles shifted upward as the overall incidence of measles declined. Measles today occurs primarily in preschool children, and to a lesser extent in school children, probably due to primary vaccine failures. Measles occurs less frequently during pregnancy than mumps or chickenpox.[4] Measles is the most communicable of the childhood exanthems.[5] Transmission is by infected droplets entering the respiratory system of a susceptible individual through the nose or oropharynx, and probably also through the conjuctival mucosa. A person with measles is capable of transmitting infection from as early as 3 days prior to the onset of symptoms, and until the rash desquamates.[6] Infectivity is maximal during the prodrome.

The incubation period of measles is 10–14 days. A prodromal phase lasting several days is manifested by fever, malaise, anorexia, conjunctivitis and respiratory symptoms such as coryza and cough. Shortly before the appearance of systemic skin rash, a pathognomonic sign of measles, Koplik's spots appear as lesions resembling grains of salt or sand, on the inflamed, reddish, buccal mucosa. The skin rash is systemic and is erythematous and maculopapular.[7] At that time the patient is very sick. The appearance of the rash coincides with the appearance of serum antibody and the termination of communicability of the disease. Although measles virus has been isolated from the skin lesions in the early stage of the rash, it has been postulated that the rash might be a reaction of hypersensitivity of the host to the virus. The rash lasts for about 5 days, and a few days later the fever goes down and the patient feels better.

Complications of measles are often in the respiratory tract or the central nervous system, manifesting as pneumonia (measles virus or bacterial) and as encephalitis.

Modifications of the clinical presentation of measles have been observed in various forms:

(1) Modified measles, which is very mild measles occurring in individuals with some degree of passive immunity to the virus.
(2) Atypical measles, which is a phenomenon believed to be a result of hypersensitivity to measles virus in a partially immune host.[8] It has been described in individuals who are exposed to the live measles virus (wild or attenuated) some years following immunization with killed measles vaccine. The clinical syndrome may be very severe with hemorrhagic phenomena, pneumonia, hepatic involvement and high fever.
(3) Measles in the altered host often occurs as a very severe disease with increased risk of mortality. This has been observed in immunocompromised patients (either due to underlying disease or chemotherapy[9]) and in malnourished children, mainly in Africa.[10]

Diagnosis

Clinical diagnosis is often achieved in a patient with severe respiratory tract illness, conjunctivitis, Koplik's spots and rash.

Laboratory diagnosis is more often made by serology, demonstrating specific antibodies of the M and G classes of immunoglobulin, most commonly by enzyme linked immunosorbent assay. Virus isolation is also possible, but it is more difficult to perform, and is less often used as a routine diagnostic approach.

Measles in pregnancy

When measles occurs in adults, it is often a more severe illness than in children. In patients with measles reported to the Centers for Disease Control and Prevention in 1991, the incidence of complications was higher in those over 20 years of age than in children.[11] Measles can be severe during pregnancy and has been associated with spontaneous abortions and premature delivery. However, in contrast to rubella, measles virus is not known to cause congenital anomalies of the fetus.[12] Measles in the newborns of mothers with measles may be severe, and it is therefore recommended that such newborns be passively immunized with human immunoglobulin at birth.[13]

Treatment and prevention

There is no specific antiviral therapy against measles virus infection. The patient should be given supportive therapy, such as antipyretic and fluids, as indicated. Bacterial superinfection should be treated promptly, directed against the causative bacterial agent.

Prevention can be accomplished by passive or active immunization. Measles virus infection can be very effectively prevented or modified to a less severe illness by early postexposure administration of human gamma-globulins.

Immunoglobulins should be administered to individuals at risk of developing severe or fatal measles, such as children receiving chemotherapy or radiotherapy, or children with deficits in cell-mediated immunity for various reasons. Also at increased risk are babies younger than 1 year of age, including newborns whose mothers have measles.

Passive immunization should be given within 6 days after exposure. Later administration is usually without any beneficial effect. Infants younger than 1 year of age who receive human immunoglobulin (dosage 0.25 ml/kg intramuscularly) should be given active immunization at 15 months of age.[14] Active immunization is by live attenuated measles virus vaccine, incorporated into the combined mumps–measles–rubella vaccine (MMR). The current recommendation is the administration of two doses of MMR, the first at 12–15 months of age and the second in childhood.[15] Live measles vaccine is contraindicated in persons with deficits in cell-mediated immunity and in pregnant women. It is currently recommended that children with HIV infection should be vaccinated with measles vaccine at the age of 15 months.[14]

REFERENCES

1. Waterson AP. Measles virus. *Arch Gestamte Virusforsch* 1965;16:57.
2. Laigmnr AD. Medical importance of measles. *Am J Dis Child* 1962;103:224.
3. Centers for Disease Control and Prevention. Measles – United States, 1981. *MMWR Morb Mortal Wkly Rep* 1982;31:37.
4. Sever J, White LR. Intrauterine viral infections. *Ann Rev Med* 1968;19:471.
5. Hope-Simpson RE. Infectiveness of communicable diseases in the household (measles, mumps and chickenpox). *Lancet* 1952;2:549.
6. Gordon JE, Ingalls TH. Modern measles. *Am J Med Sci* 1954;228:334.
7. Suring DWR, Bank LJ, Ackerman AB. Role of measles virus in skin lesions and Koplik's spots. *New Engl J Med* 1970;283:1139.
8. Fulginiti VA, Eller JJ, Downie AW, *et al.* Altered reactivity to measles virus. *J Am Med Assoc* 1967;202:1075.
9. Siegal MM, Walker TK, Ablin AR. Measles pneumonia in childhood leukemia. *Pediatrics* 1977;60:38.
10. Hayden RJ. The epidemiology and nature of measles in Nairobi before the impact of measles immunization. *East Afr Med J* 1974;51:199.
11. Centers for Disease Control and Prevention. Public sector vaccination efforts. *MMWR Morb Mortal Wkly Rep* 1992;41:522.
12. Gershon A. Chickenpox, measles and mumps. In Remington J, Klein J, eds. *Infectious Diseases of the Fetus and Newborn Infant.* Philadelphia: W. B. Saunders, 1995:565.
13. Gazala E, Karplus M, Liberman JR *et al.* The effect of maternal measles on the fetus. *Pediatr Infect Dis J* 1985;4:203.
14. American Academy of Pediatrics. *Report of the Committee on Infectious Diseases,* 22nd edn. Evanston, IL: American Academy of Pediatrics, 1991.
15. Chui L, Marusyk RG, Pabst HF. Measles virus-specific antibody in infants in a highly vaccinated society. *J Med Virol* 1991;33:204.

171 Antimicrobial drugs in obstetrics and gynecology

M. Shapiro

Introduction

Since only a few antimicrobial drugs have been shown to be completely non-toxic when given to pregnant women, and the teratogenic potential of the majority of antimicrobial agents is unknown, these drugs should generally be avoided during pregnancy. On the other hand, the patient's best interest may require that an antimicrobial drug be administered. Studies in animal models offer some information but may be unreliable in predicting human teratogenicity. Thus, the administration of an antimicrobial drug should always be a carefully considered action in which a balance is struck between the needs of the mother and the possible adverse effects of the drug. Most drug-associated congenital abnormalities are produced during the first trimester while differentiation of the embryo is occurring. There is a smaller risk during the second and third trimesters because most organ systems are developed by this time, and it is the metabolic processes that are at most risk. Almost all antimicrobial agents administered to the lactating mother can be detected in her milk. Although detrimental effects to the newborn have only occasionally been encountered, there are possible dangers, especially when large doses of antimicrobial agents are given to premature infants or to those with impaired drug elimination pathways.[1]

The Food and Drug Administration (FDA) has established a Fetal Risk Summary, which divides drugs into categories based on accumulated safety data from animal and human studies (Table 171.1). Category A drugs represent no fetal risk. Currently, there are no antimicrobial agents that fall into this category. Category B drugs are relatively safe to use during pregnancy. If possible, agents should be selected from this category. A designation of category C means that the fetal risk is unknown. These agents should be used only when there is no safer alternative, or when the benefit outweighs the risk. Although there is some evidence of fetal risk in category D, it may be necessary to use these drugs for life-threatening or serious infections for which safer drugs cannot be used or prove ineffective. Drugs listed as category X cause abnormalities and are contraindicated for use in pregnancy. The risk of using these antimicrobial agents in pregnant women clearly outweighs any possible benefit. A

Table 171.1 Pregnancy categories for drugs (Food and Drug Administration)

Category	Description
A	Controlled studies fail to demonstrate a risk to the fetus in the first trimester (and there is no evidence for risk in later trimesters); the possibility of fetal harm appears remote
B	Fetal risk not demonstrated in animal studies, but there are no controlled studies in pregnant women or animal reproduction studies have shown an adverse effect that was not confirmed in controlled studies in women during the first trimester (and there is no evidence of risk in later trimesters)
C	Either animal studies have revealed adverse effects on the fetus (teratogenic, embryocidal or other) and there are no controlled human studies or studies in animals and women are not available
D	There is positive evidence of human fetal risk, but the benefits from use in pregnant women may be acceptable despite the risk (e.g. if the drug is needed in a life-threatening situation or for a serious disease for which safer drugs cannot be used or are ineffective)
X	Studies in animals or humans have demonstrated fetal abnormalities or there is evidence for fetal risk based on human experience or both, and the risk of the use of the drug in pregnant women clearly outweighs any possible benefit. The drug is contraindicated in women who are or may become pregnant

Table 171.2 Antimicrobial agents in pregnancy

Generally contraindicated:
flucytosine, ganciclovir, griseofulvin, nalidixic acid, nitrofurantoin,* primaquine, quinine, quinolones, streptomycin, tetracyclines

Try to avoid, use only if essential:
acyclovir, albendazole, amikacin, amphotericin B, chloramphenicol*, cotrimoxazole, erythromycin estolate, ethionamide, fluconazole, gentamicin, itraconazole, ketoconazole, metronidazole, pentamidine, pyrimethamine, trimethoprim/sulfamethoxazole,* vancomycin, zidovudine

Probably safe, use when clearly indicated:
cephalosporins, clindamycin, erythromycin, ethambutol, imipenem, isoniazid, methenamine mandelate, nystatin, penicillin, pyrazinamide, rifampicin

*Contraindicated at term

summary of the use of antimicrobial drugs in pregnancy is given in Table 171.2.

Selecting an antimicrobial drug

The selection of agents for therapy is determined by many factors, including the suspected site(s) of infection (e.g. urinary tract or pelvic infection), the efficacy of the specific antibiotic at the target site (e.g. renal parenchyma, intracellular or extracellular bacterium, vegetation of endocarditis), the severity of illness (e.g. presence of renal function impairment), putative adverse effects of the agent on the mother and fetus and on the environment, and the cost of administering the drug. Whenever possible, a narrow-spectrum drug is to be preferred to a broad-spectrum agent, and single therapy in most instances is preferable to multiple drug use. Pollution of the environment with antibiotics can only lead to a vicious circle involving emergence of increasingly resistant endemic flora that require ever more esoteric and expensive antibiotics for adequate treatment.

Empiric therapy must often be administered before the specific infecting microorganism has been isolated, or before its sensitivity to various antibiotics has been established. In most instances, knowledge of the anatomic site(s) of infection will be apparent (e.g. pneumonia, peritonitis, endometritis, pelvic inflammation). This, together with the circumstances under which the infection developed (e.g. community- or hospital-acquired, immunosuppressed host, postoperative) will provide a reasonable indication of the putative pathogen(s) involved. Antimicrobial drugs can then be administered in accordance with their activity against the suspected microorganisms. Consequently, the physician should be aware of the organisms that are currently the endemic nosocomial pathogens in the hospital milieu, and know their common sensitivity patterns, since these frequently differ among institutions and change over time within the confines of a particular hospital.

The penicillins

Penicillins kill bacteria by attaching to enzymes (penicillin-binding proteins) that are involved in the normal process of synthesizing the cell wall in growing bacteria.[2] In general, these antibiotics are well distributed throughout the tissues of the body, although high doses are needed to achieve bactericidal concentrations in the cerebrospinal fluid (CSF). They are relatively non-toxic, although about 10% of patients will develop an allergic reaction, which is the main adverse effect of all penicillins.[3] A report of penicillin allergy in the past is often misleading and incorrect, and a careful history will often elicit data that will make this highly unlikely, e.g. the patient has since received other penicillin preparations without any adverse reaction. However, patients who are allergic to one penicillin must be regarded as being allergic to all the penicillins.

Penicillin G (benzyl penicillin)

Benzyl penicillin, discovered by Fleming in 1928, was originally active against a wide variety of organisms including gram-positive cocci (streptococci, staphylococci), gram-negative cocci (gonococci, meningococci), gram-negative anaerobic rods belonging to the normal mouth flora and gram-positive anaerobic rods (e.g. *Clostridium* species). In addition, penicillin is also active against many anaerobic, non-spore-forming bacilli (e.g. *Actinomyces*, *Propionibacterium*). However, over the years many bacteria have developed resistance, particularly by acquiring the ability to secrete enzymes (β-lactamases) that destroy the β-lactam ring of the penicillin nucleus,[4] such as staphylococci or *Escherichia coli*, or anaerobic flora of the mouth (*Bacteroides melaninogenicus*). Another important mechanism of resistance is achieved by the bacteria being able to alter the penicillin-binding proteins so that they no longer bind the penicillins well.[5] The most important organisms that have become relatively resistant to penicillin by this mechanism include the pneumococci and some of the viridans streptococci of the oral cavity. Consequently, community-acquired aspiration pneumonia will no longer always respond to penicillin G.[6] On the other hand, β-hemolytic streptococci such as *Streptococcus pyogenes* or group B β-hemolytic streptococci have remained exquisitely sensitive to penicillin G, as have most viridans streptococci and pneumococci. Invasive pneumococcal infections with organisms that are relatively resistant to penicillin G are becoming more common.[7] These organisms respond only to high doses of penicillin G, except in sanctuaries such as the CSF where sufficiently high concentrations of the antibiotic cannot be obtained to eradicate the infection, necessitating the use of other drugs such as the third-generation cephalosporins.

Treponema pallidum remains sensitive to penicillin, as are most strains of *Neisseria meningitidis*, although the gonococcus has acquired β-lactamases that render it resistant in many areas of the world.

Phenoxymethyl penicillin (penicillin V)

These penicillins have a similar spectrum of activity as the benzyl penicillins, but are less active against the *Neisseria* species. They are administered orally instead of intravenously.

Metabolism, dosage and routes for benzyl and phenoxymethyl penicillins

Benzyl penicillin and phenoxymethyl penicillins are excreted mainly in the urine, and, to a much lesser extent, in the bile. Crystalline benzyl penicillin is administered by intravenous injection, in doses that may range from 1,000,000 units every 6 h, to much higher doses, in the case of pneumonia caused by relatively resistant pneumococci, for example, when 12,000,000 units may be administered daily in six divided doses. In the case of meningitis caused by a sensitive organism, the drug may be administered every 2 h.

Sustained-release intramuscular preparations are also available, and may be used in the case of infection due to a known sensitive organism such as *Streptococcus pneumoniae*. In this case procaine penicillin G may be used in the dose of 600,000–1,200,000 units every 12 h. Benzathine penicillin G results in a very slow release of penicillin from the intramuscular compartment. The usual dose is 2.4 million units of benzathine penicillin at intervals that depend on the indication (mainly syphilis and prevention of rheumatic fever).

Indications in obstetrics and gynecology

Benzyl penicillin is the drug of choice for β-hemolytic streptococcal infections, for the treatment of actinomycosis, which may occur in association with intrauterine device (IUD) usage, and for clostridial infections.

Use in pregnancy

The benzyl penicillins and phenoxymethyl penicillins have been used extensively in pregnancy and are considered safe for the fetus.

Penicillinase-resistant antistaphylococcal penicillins (methicillin, oxacillin, cloxacillin, dicloxacillin, flucloxacillin and nafcillin)

These semisynthetic penicillins, which are resistant to the penicillinases, are used mainly for the treatment of staphylococcal infections. They have a much narrower spectrum of activity than benzyl penicillin. Streptococci are more sensitive to penicillin G, but, except for enterococci which are resistant, will usually respond to therapy with one of the antistaphylococcal penicillins. Although the incidence of interstitial nephritis seems to be more common with methicillin there is no clinical evidence that justifies favoring one of these agents over the others.

In infections suspected to be caused by gram-positive cocci, one of this group of drugs should be used before final identification and sensitivity results are available. Such a situation might include postoperative wound infection, line sepsis, or presence of gram-positive cocci in grape-like clusters in secretions or pus. Staphylococci develop resistance to these drugs as a result of alterations in their penicillin-binding proteins that result in a lower affinity of these enzymes for the antibiotics.[8] If the prevalence of resistant staphylococci is high, then vancomycin should be the drug of choice when gram-positive infection is suspected.

Metabolism, dosage and route

These drugs are excreted in the urine by both glomerular filtration and tubular secretion, and a small proportion is excreted in the bile. Nafcillin reaches high concentrations in the CSF of patients with normal meninges and in those with meningitis.

Methicillin and nafcillin are administered by the intravenous route only, whereas cloxacillin, dicloxacillin and flucloxacillin can be given by the oral route as well. The doses of these drugs vary between 4.0 and 12.0 g/day depending on how serious an infection is being treated.

Indications in obstetrics and gynecology

These drugs are indicated almost exclusively for the treatment of infections due to *Staphylococcus aureus*, including the toxic shock syndrome.

Use in pregnancy

All these drugs cross the placenta, and are not known to cause any fetal damage.

Aminopenicillins (ampicillin and amoxycillin)[9]

Ampicillin and amoxycillin have the same antibacterial spectrum. The only real clinical difference between them is the much increased absorption of amoxycillin from the gastrointestinal tract, so that amoxycillin should be used for oral therapy and ampicillin for intravenous administration when necessary. The aminopenicillins are clinically effective against the same organisms as penicillin G. In addition, they are highly active against gram-negative organisms such as *E. coli*, *Salmonella* spp., *Shigella* spp. (for which amoxycillin should not be used) and *Hemophilus influenzae*. However, the proportion of these organisms in the community, which have acquired resistance to these drugs, is such that ampicillin can no longer be regarded as an adequate empiric choice for the treatment of severe infections, including urinary tract or pelvic infection, or meningitis, in which these organisms are suspected of being the causative agents. Ampicillin is still the treatment of choice for infections caused by *Enterococcus faecalis* and *Listeria monocytogenes*. Although aminoglycosides are synergistic with ampicillin against the enterococci, this combination is not usually necessary except in situations such as endocarditis where bactericidal activity against the organisms is essential to obtain a cure.

Association with β-lactamase inhibitors (amoxycillin/clavulanic acid, ampicillin/clavulanic acid)

These antibiotics are becoming increasingly popular in clinical practice. The β-lactamase inhibitor potassium clavulanate irreversibly binds and inhibits many bacterial β-lactamase enzymes that are coded for by plasmids, but not by chromosomes. Thus, the addition of the inhibitor to amoxycillin effectively broadens the spectrum of this antibiotic (Augmentin) to β-lactamase-producing organisms such as *H. influenzae*, *E. coli*, most *Bacteroides fragilis* and staphylococci that are not resistant to methicillin. Augmentin plus doxycycline is an excellent oral regimen for the treatment of pelvic inflammatory disease.

Sulbactam is a penicillanic acid sulfone β-lactamase inhibitor, which, in a similar manner to clavulanic acid, extends the effective antibacterial spectrum of this drug when combined with ampicillin (Unasyn). Unasyn has been shown to be effective in soft tissue pelvic infections and in polymicrobial infections.

Metabolism, dosage and route

The aminopenicillins are excreted mainly in the urine, and to a small extent in the bile. The usual oral dose of amoxycillin is 250–500 mg three times a day, and the intravenous dose is 1.0 g three times per day. The usual intravenous dose of ampicillin is 1–2 g every 4–6 h, depending on the severity of the disease. Ampicillin/sulbactam (Unasyn) is available as 1.0 g of sulbactam to every 2.0 g of ampicillin. The usual dosage is 0.5 to 1.0 g sulbactam plus 1–2 g of ampicillin every 6 h.

Indications in obstetrics and gynecology

Ampicillin can be used in the treatment of cystitis in those areas where *E. coli* resistance is rare, but should no longer be used for the initial treatment of pyelonephritis, although its use should be encouraged in urinary tract infections where the organism is known to be sensitive to ampicillin. It is still the drug of choice in infections caused by the enterococcus, and may be used in serious pelvic infections in association with other drugs that are effective against anaerobes and have a wider spectrum of activity against the Enterobacteriaceae.

Use in pregnancy

Ampicillin has been used extensively in pregnancy and is regarded as safe in pregnancy. The β-lactamase inhibitors have been used less frequently in pregnancy, but there is no evidence for their causing fetal abnormalities, and they can be used when indicated.

Carboxypenicillins (carbenicillin and ticarcillin)

These antibiotics are similar to ampicillin but extend the spectrum to indole-positive *Proteus* spp., *Enterobacter* spp. and especially *Pseudomonas aeruginosa*. They have been replaced generally by the ureidopenicillins (see below).

Combination with β-lactamase inhibitors (timentin)

Ticarcillin plus clavulanate extends the spectrum of ticarcillin greatly against β-lactamase-producing strains of *H. influenzae*, *Staphylococcus* coagulase-positive, *B. fragilis*, Enterobacteriaceae and other organisms. Timentin is a reasonable choice for the treatment of soft tissue pelvic infections and polymicrobial infections.

Ureidopenicillins (mezlocillin, azlocillin and piperacillin)

These drugs extend the range of activity of penicillin and ampicillin, and have a similar spectrum of antibacterial activity to the carboxypenicillins (see above), but their range is somewhat wider. Their activity against *Klebsiella pneumoniae* and *P. aeruginosa* is notable. There is no clinical evidence that differences between these antibiotics have any clinical relevance. They have a lower sodium content (1.85–2.17 meq/g) than the carboxypenicillins, and thus have a lesser tendency to produce hypokalemia. Single agent therapy with the ureidopenicillins has been shown to be effective in a wide range of serious infections, including pneumonia, bacteremia, soft tissue infections and intra-abdominal infections. In many hospitals the proportion of Enterobacteriaceae and *P. aeruginosa* that are resistant to these antibiotics may well preclude their use as single drugs in serious infections. In all patients with granulocytopenia and fever of unknown origin, they need to be administered with another drug, such as an aminoglycoside, but care must be taken to ensure that these two drug groups are not mixed in solution before administration.

Combination with β-lactamase inhibitors (piperacillin/tazobactam)

Tazobactam is another irreversible β-lactam inhibitor, which has been combined with piperacillin to increase its antimicrobial spectrum to include Enterobacteriaceae, *B. fragilis* and Staphylococci, and has been successfully used in the treatment of pelvic infections. This drug is especially useful in nosocomially acquired infections, and has been successfully used as a single agent in fever of unknown origin in patients with granulocytopenia.

Metabolism, dosage and route

The ureidopenicillins are excreted primarily by the kidneys, by means of glomerular filtration and tubular secretion. The dose of mezlocillin is 200–300 mg/kg/day; usually 5.0 g four times daily given intravenously. Piperacillin is given intravenously in a dose of 4 g every 4–6 h. Piperacillin/tazobactam is given in the dose of 3 g piperacillin with 0.375 g tazobactam every 6 h.

Indications in obstetrics and gynecology

Clinical investigations have confirmed the efficacy of mezlocillin or piperacillin as single agents for the treatment of mixed aerobic–anaerobic soft tissue pelvic infection, although one study has found the combination of clindamycin and gentamicin to be superior to mezlocillin. However, in another study, piperacillin was approximately equivalent.

Adverse effects of all penicillins

Allergic reactions are the commonest adverse effects encountered with all the penicillins, and may be present in 3–5% of the population and up to 10% of those who have previously received penicillin. Local application of the penicillins should never be used because of the high risk of producing sensitization. It cannot be emphasized strongly enough that cross-allergenicity exists among all the penicillins, and if a true allergic reaction has occurred to any one of the penicillins it must be assumed that the patient is allergic to all penicillins.

Drug fever and various skin rashes are common. Drug fever can be especially difficult to interpret in a patient who is being treated for serious infection, since the clinical picture may be indistinguishable, and a high index of suspicion is essential to make the correct diagnosis. Severe reactions that occur include drug rashes, angioneurotic edema, serum sickness and anaphylaxis. About 5% of patients will show cross-allergenicity with the cephalosporins, which can be useful alternatives in the penicillin-allergic patient, but they should be avoided if there is a history of a type I allergic reaction. Less common adverse effects include hemolytic anemia, granulocytopenia and interstitial nephritis (especially with methicillin). Massive doses, especially in renal failure, may produce neurological symptoms and signs, including hallucinations and generalized convulsions. Electrolyte disturbances may be produced by the high sodium load of the carboxypenicillins and the relatively high potassium load (1.6 meq/1 million units) that can occur with the administration of potassium penicillin G in patients with impaired renal function.

Cephalosporins

These are synthetic β-lactam antibiotics that, like penicillin, interfere with construction of the bacterial cell wall. They have a broad spectrum of activity including an extremely wide range of microorganisms, but the enterococcus is resistant. Resistance among gram-negative bacteria is almost always the result of inactivation by β-lactamases. Classically, these agents have been divided into first-, second- and third-generation cephalosporins, based on their activity and not the chronology of their marketing.

First-generation cephalosporins (the parenteral drugs: cephalothin, cefazolin, cephradine and the oral drugs: cephapirin, cephalexin, cefaclor and cefadroxil)

The antibacterial activity of first-generation cephalosporins is interchangeable practically among the different preparations. The antibacterial spectrum is roughly that of the antistaphylococcal penicillins plus ampicillin, although *H. influenzae*, *E. faecalis* and *L. monocytogenes*, which are resistant to all the cephalosporins, are very important exceptions. They are active against the streptococci (except enterococci) and methicillin-sensitive staphylococci. The cephalosporins must not be used to treat methicillin-resistant staphylococci that may be reported by the laboratory as being sensitive to first-generation cephalosporins since clinical failure is likely. The first-generation cephalosporins are also active against *E. coli*, *Klebsiella* spp. and non-indole-positive *Proteus* spp., whereas *Enterobacter* spp., *S. marcescens*, *Citrobacter*, other Enterobacteriaceae and *P. aeruginosa* are resistant, as are *Chlamydia trachomatis* and mycoplasmas. These drugs are not active against *B. fragilis*, and do not cross the blood–brain barrier in high enough concentrations to be useful in the treatment of meningitis.

Metabolism, dosage and route

All the first-generation cephalosporins are excreted via the renal route, but some (cephalothin, cephradine and cephapirin) are also excreted via the liver, and must thus be given at more frequent dosage intervals. In renal failure, dosage adjustments are necessary. Cephalothin is administered intravenously in doses that vary from 4.0 to 12.0 g/day, depending on the severity of the infection. Since cefazolin is excreted only via the kidneys and thus has a half-life of 1.8 h, it can be given 8-hourly. Cephalexin and cephradine are administered in the dose of 250 mg every 6 h, cefadroxil 1.0 g every 12 h and cefaclor 250 mg daily.

Indications in obstetrics and gynecology

The first-generation cephalosporins are the drugs of choice for prophylaxis in obstetric and gynecological procedures.[10] Although these drugs are not the drugs of choice for many infections, they are extremely useful in patients with delayed-type hypersensitivity to the penicillins, since there is little cross-reaction between the drug groups. However, if there has been a severe reaction to any penicillin in the past (e.g. anaphylaxis) the cephalosporins should be avoided unless there is no alternative. The first-generation cephalosporins are also useful in the treatment of mild to moderate pyelonephritis, which is caused by organisms resistant to ampicillin and cotrimoxazole, and may be used in other infections that are caused by an organism of known sensitivity, e.g. *K. pneumoniae* pneumonia.

Use in pregnancy

These drugs are considered safe in pregnancy.

Second-generation cephalosporins (cefamandole, cefoxitin, cefuroxime,[11] cefonicid, cefotetan, ceforanide and cefmetazole)

These drugs retain sufficient activity to be effective against gram-positive cocci. Thus, they are indicated when the infecting organisms have not yet been identified and a mixed infection including gram-positive cocci is suspected or has been proven. All drugs of this group (except cefoxitin) show excellent activity against all *H. influenzae*. Cefuroxime should not be used for meningitis, nor should other members of this group. Good activity against *B. fragilis* is shown by cefoxitin, which is thus a useful drug in the treatment of mixed infections with anaerobes, gram-negative aerobes and gram-positive cocci such as occurs in the infected diabetic foot.[12] Cefotetan is also active against *B. fragilis* and has a half-life of up to 4.5 h, so that it need be administered only every 12 h. Penicillinase-producing *N. gonorrhea* are sensitive to cefoxitin and cefotetan. The antimicrobial spectra of cefuroxime, cefonicid and ceforanide are very similar. They do not include *B. fragilis*, and these drugs are not usually used in pelvic infections. *C. trachomatis* and the genital mycoplasmas are resistant to the second-generation cephalosporins.

Metabolism, dosage and route

Most of these drugs are excreted mainly in the urine, and thus need a dose adjustment in patients with renal impairment. For initial treatment of infections with cefoxitin the dosage is 1–2 g intravenously every 6 h, for cefamandole 2–3 g every 6 h and for cefotetan 1–2 g every 8–12 h.

Indications in obstetrics and gynecology

Cefoxitin and cefotetan have been used successfully as single drugs in pelvic infections.

Use in pregnancy

Cefoxitin, cefotetan and cefamandole have been widely used in pregnancy and are considered safe.

Third-generation cephalosporins (cefotaxime, ceftizoxime, ceftriaxone, moxalactam, cefoperazone, ceftazidime, cefsulodin, cefixime and cefpodoxime)

Some of these drugs broaden the spectrum of activity of the cephalosporins against the Enterobacteriaceae, and others against *P. aeruginosa*, but they all show decreased activity against the gram-positive cocci and (except for moxalactam and ceftizoxime) they have no activity against β-lactamase-producing anaerobes such as *B. fragilis*. The third-generation cephalosporins are the drugs of choice in gram-negative bacillary meningitis in adults.[13] Cefotaxime still retains useful, although inferior, activity against the gram-positive cocci and is ineffective against *P. aeruginosa*. Ceftriaxone is almost identical in its antibacterial activity to cefotaxime, having little antipseudomonas activity, but because of its extraordinary half-life (nearly 6 h) it need be given only once daily. On the other hand, ceftazidime has almost no activity against staphylococci, but is as active as cefotaxime against the Enterobacteriaceae and, in addition, is particularly active against *P. aeruginosa*. Ceftazidime has been used successfully as a single drug in the treatment of infections caused by *P. aeruginosa*, including meningitis.[14] Ceftizoxime is similar to cefotaxime in its antibacterial activity, but also has a useful effect on *B. fragilis*.[15] Cefsulodin is used clinically only against *P. aeruginosa*. Against *N. gonorrhea*, activity of cefotaxime, ceftazidime cefoperazone, moxalactam and especially ceftriaxone is excellent.

Metabolism, dosage and route

These drugs differ in their metabolism. Cefotaxime has a short half-life since it is excreted both in the urine and via the bile, and should be administered every 6 h at a dose of 1–2 g per dose. Cefoperazone and ceftazidime are administered at a dose of 2.0 g every 8–12 h. Ceftriaxone, which has the longest half-life of all, is administered at a dose of 2.0 g every 24 h. Cefotetan is given every 12 h at a dose of 2.0 g.

Indications in obstetrics and gynecology

Although some of these drugs have been used as single agents in pelvic infections, the lack of coverage against *B. fragilis* and *C. trachomatis* makes them poor choices in serious infections. Cefoxitin, ceftizoxime and cefotetan do have reasonable coverage against *B. fragilis*. Ceftriaxone is the drug of choice for anorectal gonorrhea.

Use in pregnancy

A suitable choice of a cephalosporin may be confusing. It is most appropriate to use an older or earlier-generation cephalosporin whenever possible, in order to decrease as far as possible the emergence of resistant bacteria. When treating infections where gram-positive cocci are the putative pathogens, such as cellulitis, or in patients with proven staphylococcal or streptococcal (not enterococcal) infections who have a history of penicillin allergy (not type I) cefazolin is probably the drug of choice. It is also the commonest cephalosporin used for surgical prophylaxis. In community-acquired pneumonias, especially in patients with chronic obstructive pulmonary disease or in young children

Table 171.3 Recommended dosages for some parenterally administered cephalosporin antibiotics in adults with normal renal function

Antibiotic	Daily dose (g)	Time between doses (h)	Maximal dose (g/day)
First-generation			
Cefazolin	1	8	4
Second-generation			
Cefoxitin	2	4–6	12
Cefuroxime	1.5	6–8	9
Cefonicid	1	12	2
Cefotetan	2	12	6
Third-generation			
Cefotaxime	2	6	12
Ceftizoxime	2	8	12
Ceftriaxone	1	12	2
Cefoperazone	2	8	8
Ceftazidime	2	8	6

where *H. influenzae* may be the offending pathogen, cefuroxime is preferred. The widespread use of cephalosporins has led to the emergence of the enterococci as nosocomial pathogens. Enterobacteriaceae that are resistant to multiple antibiotics should be treated with cefotaxime, ceftriaxone or ceftizoxime. When *P. aeruginosa* is the offending pathogen, or when a gram-negative hospital-acquired pathogen is suspected, ceftazidime would be the appropriate cephalosporin to choose for initial therapy. Under these circumstances, many infectious disease experts would prefer an aminoglycoside with a ureidopenicillin (e.g. gentamicin or amikacin plus mezlocillin or piperacillin).

Adverse effects of all cephalosporins

The cephalosporins are relatively non-toxic when compared to other antimicrobial drugs. The main adverse effects, as with other β-lactams, are allergic or hypersensitivity reactions that occur in 1–5% of patients, but anaphylaxis is rare.[16] On the other hand, the cephalosporins are a common cause of drug fever, and isolated eosinophilia has been noted in 7% of patients receiving cefoperazone or ceftazidime. Cross-reactions between penicillins and cephalosporins occur in about 5% of cases. Cephalosporins can usually be administered safely to patients who have not had an immediate-type reaction to the penicillins, but should be avoided in patients who have had such a reaction. A positive Coomb's reaction occurs frequently, but is usually not associated with hemolysis. Bleeding due to the inhibition of vitamin K synthesis in the liver has been a problem particularly with moxalactam, but can potentially occur with cefoperazone, cefamandole, cefmenoxime and cefotetan, which also bear the methylthiotetrazole (MTT) group side-chain. This same substitution can also produce a disulfiram-like reaction due to inhibition of the hepatic acetyldehydrogenase enzyme. Ceftriaxone has been associated with the formation of biliary sludge, which may lead to symptoms and signs of cholecystitis, but this phenomenon is reversible on withdrawal of the drug.[17] Rare complications include neutropenia, thrombocytopenia and hepatic dysfunction. Renal failure is highly unlikely, although the combination of gentamicin with cephalothin is probably more nephrotoxic than gentamicin alone.[18]

Superinfections frequently occur, and the wide use of cephalosporins has also resulted in the emergence of *E. faecalis* as a nosocomial pathogen. Candida infections may occur, and are particularly troublesome in severely compromised patients who have received intravenous therapy with broad-spectrum antibiotics for prolonged periods. Dosages for several cephalosporin drugs in severe infections are shown in Table 171.3.

Other β-lactam antibiotics (imipenem and azthreonam)

Imipenem consists of the active principle thienamycin, which is a carbapenem, combined with cilastatin, which has no antibacterial activity but inhibits the enzymatic destruction of thienamycin by the dipeptidase enzymes of the renal tubular brush border and prevents renal toxicity. Imipenem has the widest spectrum of all antimicrobial drugs, including gram-positive cocci and gram-negative bacilli, penicillinase-resistant staphylococci, *P. aeruginosa*, *Acinetobacter* spp. and β-lactamase-producing anaerobes (including *B. fragilis*). The one organism that is consistently resistant is *Stenotrophomonas* (*Pseudomonas*) *maltophilia*. Imipenem has proven very useful in the treatment of hospital-acquired infections, especially when caused by Enterobacteriaceae. When used as a single drug against *P. aeruginosa*, resistant organisms have emerged. This drug should be reserved for serious hospital-acquired infections, both because of its cost and the need to minimize the emergence of resistant bacteria.

The main adverse effects of imipenem are those of all β-lactams, with perhaps a greater tendency to produce neurological adverse effects such as seizures. Rapid infusion may produce nausea and emesis.

Aztreonam is a monobactam, i.e. its basic structure consists of only a single β-lactam ring. This antibiotic is a narrow-spectrum antimicrobial drug, which is very active against gram-negative organisms only, and has no effect on *E. faecalis* or the anaerobes.[19] It has been used as a single drug in severe infections (septicemia, pneumonia, skin and soft tissue) caused by sensitive gram-negative organisms, including *P. aeruginosa*. It has no activity against *C. trachomatis*. The usual dose of aztreonam is 1.0–2.0 g given every 8 h intravenously. Aztreonam accumulates in renal failure in the presence of which the dose should be modified. Aztreonam has been used in combination with other antibiotics such as clindamycin in the treatment of severe pelvic infections, since it can replace the aminoglycosides for community and (most) nosocomial infections. The chemical structure of aztreonam apparently results in an absence of allergic cross-reactions between this drug and the penicillins or cephalosporins.

Vancomycin[20]

Vancomycin is a narrow-spectrum, complex glycopolypeptide antibiotic, which acts by inhibiting synthesis of bacterial cell-wall peptidoglycan. Its main indication is for therapy of methicillin-resistant staphylococcal infections (both coagulase-positive and-negative), and for treatment of serious methicillin-sensitive staphylococcal infections when the patient is intolerant to the penicillins and cephalosporins. In addition, this antibiotic can be used to treat enterococcal endocarditis in patients who have serious penicillin allergy and cannot be desensitized. Since vancomycin is bacteriostatic to streptococci, it should be combined with an aminoglycoside (streptomycin or gentamicin) with which it is synergistic and bactericidal. Vancomycin is also the drug of choice in resistant *Corynebacterium* spp. infections. It is poorly absorbed when given by mouth, and pseudomembranous enterocolitis caused by *Clostridium difficile* can be treated with vancomycin given orally, in a dose of 125 mg four times daily for 7–10 days, although this should be avoided if at all possible in order to minimize the emergence of vancomycin-resistant enterococci (VREF).

Besides the emergence of resistance among enterococci the main adverse effects of vancomycin include local irritation, so the drug must be given intravenously. If infused rapidly the so-called 'red man' syndrome may be produced, including an erythematous or maculopapular rash involving the upper portion of the body, with or without hypotension and/or syncope. This is not a true allergic reaction, and is probably due to a non-immunologically mediated release of histamine. If this occurs, the drug may be re-administered, provided it is infused slowly. Vancomycin is excreted solely via the kidneys, and the dose must be modified in patients with renal dysfunction, as auditory (and rarely vestibular) damage may be produced. Rarely, drug fever or leukopenia occurs.

Tetracyclines (tetracycline hydrochloride, minocycline and doxycycline)

These antibiotics have similar antibacterial spectra, and exert their antibacterial activity by binding to the 30 S ribosomes where they inhibit protein synthesis. The tetracyclines penetrate well into the body tissues and fluids. They are active against gram-positive cocci including pneumococci and streptococci, gram-negative Enterobacteriaceae including *E. coli*, *H. influenzae* and *K. pneumoniae* and anaerobic bacteria (*Propionibacterium acnes*, *Bacteroides* spp.). However, many of these organisms have developed resistance to the tetracyclines, and these drugs are no longer used as a first-line treatment when serious infections caused by these organisms occur. Chlamydia, mycoplasmas, rickettsiae and some protozoa (including *Plasmodium falciparum*) remain sensitive to these drugs, which are now most frequently indicated for ambulatory infections such as sexually transmitted diseases. Approximately 50% of penicillin-resistant gonococci are also resistant to tetracyclines. The main indications for use of tetracyclines in serious disease are for infections caused by rickettsia (e.g. Rocky Mountain spotted fever, or Q-fever endocarditis), and for brucellosis, relapsing fever (*Borrelia recurrentis*), tularemia, cholera and plague (*Yersinia pestis*).

Metabolism, dosage and route

All tetracyclines are excreted by the kidneys via glomerular filtration. Although they are excreted in the bile, a large proportion is reabsorbed by the gastrointestinal tract. The dose of tetracycline is 500 mg every 6 h, and of minocycline and doxycycline 100 mg every 12 h on the first day, followed by 100 mg every 24 h.

Indications in obstetrics and gynecology

In gynecology, the main indication of tetracyclines is for the treatment of *C. trachomatis*, *M. hominis* and ureaplasma infections.

Use in pregnancy

Tetracyclines cross the placenta readily and are in category D because they are known teratogens. They should be avoided in pregnancy unless absolutely essential (see below).

Adverse effects

The major adverse effects are gastrointestinal intolerance, skin rashes and secondary infections of the mucous membranes with *Candida albicans* (vaginal candidiasis). Fatty necrosis of the liver may be caused by intravenous tetracycline, especially if more than 2 g per day is administered, especially during pregnancy.[21] Minocycline tends to produce dose-related vestibular toxicity, with dizziness, ataxia, nausea and vomiting. Phenytoin and barbiturates may shorten the half-life of doxycycline by increasing hepatic metabolism of the drug. Except for doxycycline, the tetracyclines aggravate renal failure by inhibiting protein synthesis. Because of dose-related yellow mottling, hypoplasia and enamel defects[22] of developing teeth and deposition in growing bones of infants where they may disturb longitudinal growth,[23] these drugs should not be given to pregnant or lactating women or to children under 8 years of age, unless under very special circumstances, e.g. a short course in Rocky Mountain spotted fever.[24]

Chloramphenicol

Chloramphenicol inhibits synthesis of bacterial protein by binding to the 50 S ribosomal subunit. It is very well absorbed from the gastrointestinal tract even in the presence of food, and is widely distributed throughout the body tissues and fluids. This antibiotic is inactivated in the liver, and may reach toxic levels when the glucuronyltransferase activity is low, as occurs in liver disease or in the immature neonate. Chloramphenicol is excreted rapidly and does not accumulate in renal failure. It is a very wide-spectrum antibiotic, which is effective against most Enterobacteriaceae, and has excellent activity against *B. fragilis*. Chloramphenicol is effective in brain abscesses caused by susceptible organisms. It is an important drug in the treatment of typhoid fever and severe rickettsial infections in patients who cannot receive tetracyclines (e.g. during pregnancy).

The major adverse effect of chloramphenicol is an idiosyncratic aplastic anemia that occurs in 1/40,000 to 1/100,000 courses of therapy, and is almost always fatal. A dose-related bone suppression that reverses when chloramphenicol is discontinued also occurs. In liver disease and neonates chloramphenicol is better avoided, but if it has to be given, serum levels must be measured. Chloramphenicol inhibits the hepatic microsomal enzymes so that the half-life of drugs that are metabolized by this system (e.g. dicumarol, phenytoin, chlorpropamide and tolbutamide) may be prolonged.

Macrolides (erythromycin, roxithromycin, clarithromycin and azithromycin)

These antimicrobial drugs are all macrolides, and have a similar, although not quite identical spectrum (see below). In general, if an organism is resistant to one member of this group, it is with some exceptions resistant to all other members.

Erythromycin

This macrolide antibiotic acts by binding to the 50 S ribosomal subunit, where it inhibits protein synthesis. It is well distributed throughout the body except in the CSF and brain. It is active against most bacteria that are sensitive to penicillin G, and also against staphylococci, although the latter often become resistant when the use of erythromycin is widespread. It is the drug of choice for the treatment of *M. pneumoniae* and *Legionella*,[25] *Hemophilus ducreyi* and *Corynebacterium diphtheriae* infections. Erythromycin is also active against *C. trachomatis*, *M. hominis* and *U. urealyticum*. It can be used in penicillin-allergic patients against *T. pallidum*. *S. aureus* is generally sensitive to erythromycin but resistance does develop during treatment, and while superficial infections caused by staphylococci may be treated with this drug, in severe or deep-seated infections (intra-abdominal abscess) the organism tends to develop resistance, and the macrolides should not be used.

Adverse effects

This is a very safe antibiotic, the most common problem being severe gastrointestinal disturbances. In addition, reversible hepatitis may be produced, particularly, but not exclusively, by the oral estolate. Reversible deafness may be produced by high dosages, especially when renal function is impaired. Erythromycin may increase the serum concentration of cyclosporine because of competition for protein-binding sites. All the macrolides including erythromycin, clarithromycin and azithromycin (see below) interact with terfenadine and astemizole, to produce a prolonged Q–T interval and life-threatening arrhythmias.

Metabolism, dosage and route

Erythromycin can be administered via the oral or intravenous route. Oral preparations include erythromycin base, which requires enteric coating to make it palatable, stearate, which hydrolyzes to the base in the duodenum, estolate and ethylsuccinate, which are acid-stable. Erythromycin is excreted primarily in the bile. The dose of oral erythromycin is 250–500 mg every 6 h. The intravenous form is administered in high doses (0.9 g every 6 h) for *Legionella* infections.

Indications in obstetrics and gynecology

Erythromycin may be used for staphylococcal or streptococcal infections in penicillin-allergic patients (see above). It is especially useful for the treatment of *C. trachomatis* infection in pregnancy when tetracycline is contraindicated.

Use in pregnancy

Erythromycin has been extensively used and is safe in pregnancy.

Clarithromycin

Except for enhanced activity against *H. influenzae* and Mycobacterium–avium complex, the spectrum of activity of this drug is similar to that of erythromycin. The dose varies from 250 to 500 mg every 12 h. The most common side effect is gastrointestinal disturbance, but this is less frequent than with erythromycin. Clarithromycin should only be used during pregnancy when definitely indicated (e.g. infection with Mycobacterium–avium complex).

Azithromycin

Azithromycin has the same general spectrum of activity as erythromycin, although it is slightly less active against the gram-positive cocci, but more active against *H. influenzae*.

Metabolism, dosage and route

Azithromycin is better absorbed than erythromycin. Blood levels of the antibiotic are low, but the levels in the polymorphonuclear leukocytes and in the tissues at the site of infection are 10- to 100-fold higher than serum levels. Moreover, the half-life in the tissues is 2–4 days, thus allowing earlier cessation of therapy while the antibiotic remains active at the site of infection for several more days. The dose is 1.0 g as a single dose for chlamydial cervicitis, and 2.0 g as a single dose for uncomplicated gonococcal infections. For lower respiratory tract infections the dose is 500 mg as a single dose on day 1, followed by 250 mg once daily on days 2–5 for a total dose of 1.5 g.

Use in pregnancy

Currently this drug is not recommended in pregnancy since no data are available regarding its safety.

Rifampicin

Rifampicin, a rifamycin compound, exerts its action by inhibition of DNA-dependent RNA polymerase. This antibiotic has an extremely wide antibacterial spectrum, but is used primarily for the treatment of tuberculosis. In addition, it is remarkably active against both coagulase-positive and coagulase-negative staphylococci. Thus, it is often recommended in infections caused by these organisms that are not responding well to therapy, or that are expected to be difficult to eradicate, e.g. meningitis in the presence of an artificial device, or endocarditis on an artificial valve.[26]

Because of its marked *in vitro* activity against *Legionella* spp. it is also sometimes recommended for treating pneumonia caused by this organism, which does not respond to erythromycin therapy. Among its other indications is prophylaxis of meningococcal meningitis in close contacts of infected patients. The rapid emergence of resistance when rifampicin alone is given is notable. Consequently, rifampicin is usually administered with another antibiotic.

Adverse effects

A red-orange staining of urine, tears and soft contact lenses may occur with short courses of therapy. Gastrointestinal and cutaneous manifestations may occur. Intermittent therapy and administration of doses larger than 1200 mg/day have been associated with an increased incidence of severe side effects, including a flu-like syndrome, hemolysis, renal failure and even shock. Rifampicin is one of the most active inducers of the hepatic microsomal enzymes, and results in decreased efficacy of many compounds, including barbiturates, cimetidine, oral contraceptives, cyclosporine, digoxin, ketoconazole, β-blockers, sulfonylureas, theophyline, thyroxin and warfarin.

Use in pregnancy

Rifampicin may be used for the treatment of tuberculosis in pregnancy.

Clindamycin

Clindamycin is bacteriostatic and acts by attaching to the ribosome where it inhibits protein synthesis. It has a similar antimicrobial spectrum of activity to erythromycin, except that it is much more active against *B. fragilis* and other β-lactamase-producing anaerobes. It is thus indicated in aspiration pneumonia where it may be used as a single drug, although some authorities might still try penicillin G in this situation when the circumstances are not critical. Clindamycin can be used in association with an aminoglycoside in intra-abdominal infections, and also in penicillin- and cephalosporin-allergic patients for streptococcal and staphylococcal infection (but not for endocarditis).[27] It reaches high concentrations in bone, and is useful as a second-line drug in osteomyelitis. Recently, clindamycin has been used as an adjunct therapy in resistant *P. falciparum* malaria.

Adverse reactions

The major serious adverse reaction to clindamycin is the occurrence of pseudomembranous enterocolitis,[28] the result of a toxin produced by a colonic overgrowth of *C. difficile*. The incidence of this complication varies geographically and the onset may occur several weeks after the administration of clindamycin has been stopped. It is not dose-related and may occur after oral or intravenous administration. The patient suffers from diarrhea that may be bloody, abdominal cramps and fever, and the disease may be fatal. Yellow-white plaques on the colonic mucosa may be seen by proctoscopy. The toxin of *C. difficile* can be detected in nearly all patients with this complication. The treatment includes prompt cessation of clindamycin administration, and either metronidazole (250 mg every 8 h) or vancomycin (125 mg every 6 h) should be given orally as therapy against the toxin-producing organism.

Metabolism, dosage and route

Clindamycin is metabolized by the liver, and excreted in an inactive form in the urine. Reduction in dose should be made for patients with liver impairment or severe renal impairment. The dose ranges from 600 mg every 8 h intravenously, to 150–300 mg orally every 6 h. The dose recommended for *C. trachomatis* infection is 450 mg every 6 h.

Indications in obstetrics and gynecology

Clindamycin is indicated in polymicrobial infections of the pelvis including pelvic abscess, tubo-ovarian abscess, endometritis and infection following hysterectomy. In these cases, it should be combined with an aminoglycoside. *C. trachomatis* can be treated with clindamycin, which can also be used for susceptible gram-positive infections including non-enterococcal streptococci and staphylococci. Clindamycin 300 mg every 12 h for 7 days, or clindamycin cream 2% intravaginally twice daily for 5 days are effective in the treatment of bacterial vaginosis.

Use in pregnancy

Clindamycin is probably safe in pregnancy, and if necessary can be used. However, there are no specific infections requiring clindamycin during pregnancy.

Aminoglycosides (streptomycin, kanamycin, gentamicin, tobramycin, netilmicin, amikacin and neomycin)

These antibiotics act by binding to the 30 S bacterial ribosome whereby they disrupt protein synthesis, but are nevertheless bactericidal. They have an extremely wide spectrum of activity, especially on the gram-negative Enterobacteriaceae and *P. aeruginosa*, and are also active against staphylococci. Even though *Salmonella* spp. may be sensitive *in vitro* to the aminoglycosides, they are not effective *in vivo* in the treatment of infections produced by this group of organisms. On the other hand, although aminoglycosides are ineffective against streptococci, they are synergistic with penicillin or vancomycin against these organisms. Uptake of the aminoglycosides by bacteria is oxygen-dependent, so that these drugs do not inhibit anaerobic bacteria. Since these drugs are not metabolized and are rapidly excreted via the renal route only, the half-life increases markedly with declining renal function. In renal failure, it is prudent to avoid the use of aminoglycosides. Serum trough levels should be monitored to prevent accumulation of the drug in the case of poor renal function or in the elderly. On the other hand, the dose may need to be greatly increased if the patient does not respond and the serum levels remain below the maximum peak recommended concentrations.

Streptomycin

Since most Enterobacteriaceae have acquired resistance, this drug is used almost exclusively with other drugs to treat: (1) endocarditis caused by *S. viridans* or susceptible enterococci, together with penicillin or vancomycin (in penicillin-allergic patients);[29] (2) brucellosis, together with tetracycline; (3) tularemia and the plague (as a single drug) and (4) occasionally as one of a combination of drugs in tuberculosis. Streptomycin toxicity is mainly vestibular and auditory and it is the least nephrotoxic of the aminoglycosides.

Gentamicin and tobramycin

These two drugs are very similar with regard to their antibacterial spectrum and pharmacodynamics. They show no clinically important differences, and continue to be the aminoglycosides of choice for serious bacterial infections. Many community-acquired gram-negative infections are now caused by organisms that are relatively resistant, and the use of these drugs in seriously ill patients on admission to hospital (e.g. pyelonephritis with suspected septicemia) is appropriate. Gentamicin or tobramycin are also the aminoglycosides of choice for severe hospital-acquired infections caused by most Enterobacteriaceae and *P. aeruginosa* (e.g. pneumonia, urinary tract infection, septicemia). They are indicated in endocarditis caused by viridans streptococci and enterococci that display high-level resistance to streptomycin. In febrile neutropenic patients, it is appropriate to administer gentamicin or tobramycin in combination with other drugs (e.g. ureidopenicillins or third-generation cephalosporins) that have a better gram-positive spectrum and that can be synergistic against gram-negative organisms such as *P. aeruginosa*. Netilmicin is similar to gentamicin and tobramicin in activity and dosage.

Amikacin

This is the aminoglycoside that is most resistant to the aminoglycoside-modifying enzymes, and should be used empirically when gentamicin resistance is prevalent.

Adverse reactions of aminoglycosides

Adverse reactions include dose-related ototoxicity and vestibular damage[30,31] and renal toxicity. The therapeutic–toxic ratio of all these drugs is low, so that serum levels have to be monitored in these patients who are usually seriously ill, since their renal function often fluctuates and is not reflected immediately by the serum creatinine or blood urea nitrogen. Another important, though rare, event is the production of neuromuscular paralysis, which is enhanced by the presence of curare-like drugs and in patients with myasthenia gravis when very high concentrations of the aminoglycoside are present at the neuromuscular junction.[32] This should be avoided by not giving intravenous bolus injections or introducing large quantities of aminoglycosides into the pleural or peritoneal cavities.

Metabolism, dosage and routes for aminoglycosides

These drugs are administered intramuscularly or intravenously as a single dose or in three divided doses (see Table 171.4). Recently, emphasis has been

Table 171.4 Aminoglycoside doses and recommended serum levels in adults with normal renal function

Antibiotic	Standard dose (mg/kg/day)	Serum concentration (mg/l)	
		Peak	Trough
Streptomycin	15	20–30	<5
Gentamicin	3–5	<10	<2
Tobramycin	3–5	<10	<2
Netilmicin	3–5	<10	<2
Amikacin	15	20–30	5–10

placed on the administration of aminoglycosides as a single daily dose. This is possible because of the prolonged postantibiotic effect of these drugs, of the apparent lower renal and auditory toxicity with this form of administration, and the greater efficacy of aminoglycosides with high peak concentrations. There is great variation in the individual response to aminoglycoside administration, so that serum levels should be monitored, especially in the obese, during the puerperium, and in the presence of renal impairment. The dose has to be modified in accordance with renal function, response to treatment and serum antibiotic levels. Aminoglycosides should not be mixed with β-lactams in the same solution since chelation inactivates the aminoglycoside.

Indications in obstetrics and gynecology

These drugs are used in particular for severe urinary tract infections, and, in combination with clindamycin, for serious soft tissue pelvic infections. Their use is often limited to the initial therapy until culture results are available, after which less toxic drugs may be used in their stead.

Use of aminoglycosides in pregnancy

Streptomycin is known to cause eighth nerve damage *in utero*. Although pregnancy should not be considered an absolute contraindication to the other aminoglycosides, these drugs should be avoided if possible.[33] Only gentamicin is listed in category C. The serum levels attained in pregnancy are lower than expected, because of the increased volume of distribution, and must be carefully monitored. Aminoglycoside doses and recommended serum levels in adults with normal renal function are shown in Table 171.4.

Metronidazole[34]

Metronidazole has been used for many years for the treatment of parasitic infections caused by *Giardia lamblia*, *Entamoeba histolytica* and *Trichomonas vaginalis*, but is now the major drug for the treatment of infections caused by anaerobic bacteria.[35] Its mode of action is not clear, but is thought to be bactericidal via the toxic effect of reductive activation of the compound within the bacterial cell in which there is an interaction with DNA. Metronidazole is most active against the gram-negative anaerobic bacteria, including those that produce β-lactamase, and less active against the anaerobic gram-positive cocci such as peptostreptococci. It is, however, bactericidal against *Clostridium perfringens* and *B. fragilis*, and is thus indicated in the rare instances of meningitis or endocarditis produced by this organism. Metronidazole also has activity against *Helicobacter pylori* and *Gardnerella vaginalis*. Its main indication is in the treatment of deep-seated anaerobic infections, such as in the diabetic foot, intra-abdominal surgical infections and aspiration pneumonia. In all these infections, it should be administered together with a drug that is active against the accompanying aerobic flora that is almost invariably present. Metronidazole is as useful as vancomycin in antibiotic-associated pseudomembranous enterocolitis produced by *C. difficile*.

Metabolism, dosage and route

Metronidazole is very well absorbed, and diffuses well into nearly all tissues. It is eliminated primarily via the liver. Oral doses vary between 2 and 4 g as a single dose (for trichomoniasis) or 250–750 mg every 8 h. Giardiasis is treated with 250 mg tid for 7 days, non-dysenteric amebiasis with 500 mg tid for 10 days, and severe amebic disease with 750 mg tid for 10 days. In bacterial vaginosis, the dose is 500 mg bid for 7 days. For pseudomembranous enterocolitis, the recommended dose is 500 mg tid for 7–10 days.

Indications in obstetrics and gynecology

Metronidazole is the drug of choice in bacterial vaginosis caused by *G. vaginalis*, in association with other anaerobic organisms. Metronidazole gel 0.75% is available for this indication. Since it should not be used in lactating women, it is not used as first-line therapy in deep-seated pelvic infections following labor.

Use in pregnancy

Metronidazole has been used extensively during pregnancy without any apparent problem, but it is recommended that it be avoided during the first trimester of pregnancy. Lactating women should not receive metronidazole, or breast feeding should be discontinued for 24 h following the administration of a single dose of metronidazole.

Adverse effects

Serious adverse effects are rare. The major toxic reactions are nausea and other gastrointestinal disturbances, an unpleasant metallic taste and peripheral neuropathy following prolonged therapy with high doses in patients with renal insufficiency. An antabuse-like reaction may be seen.

Cotrimoxazole[36]

This drug consists of a combination of sulfamethoxazole (a sulfonamide) and trimethoprim (a diaminopyrimidine), which are sequential inhibitors in the bacterial synthetic chain of folinic acid. Cotrimoxazole is well distributed in the body tissues and fluids, including the CSF. The antibiotic is excreted in the urine and bile, and when the creatinine clearance decreases below 30 ml/min the dosage should be adjusted.

Cotrimoxazole has a very wide spectrum of activity against both gram-positive and gram-negative organisms, but anaerobic organisms are resistant. Its main use is in the outpatient setting for urinary tract infections. The recommended dose is one double-strength tablet (trimethoprim 160 mg, sulfamethoxazole 800 mg) every 12 h. It may also be used in other infections if the organism that is isolated is sensitive *in vitro*. Cotrimoxazole is the treatment of choice for pneumocystis pneumonia infections in patients with AIDS. In this condition, the maximum dose (20 mg/kg/day trimethoprim and 100 mg/day sulfamethoxazole) should be administered orally or intravenously for at least 3 weeks, after which a prophylactic dose should be continued. Another important indication for cotrimoxazole is in patients with infections caused by *Nocardia asteroides*, an important pulmonary and intracerebral pathogen in immunocompromised hosts.

Use in pregnancy

Trimethoprim is in category C and is generally avoided because it inhibits folic acid metabolism. However, cotrimoxazole may be used in pregnancy when indicated and other agents are not available. Sulfonamides are in category B but should be avoided near the end of gestation (third trimester) because of the increased risk of kernicterus in the infant. Kernicterus occurs when the sulfonamide competes with bilirubin for albumin binding, thus causing hyperbilirubinemia. The placenta can clear unconjugated bilirubin, but once the infant is born, it has no elimination mechanism. Infants with glucose-6-phosphate deficiency can develop hemolytic anemia if the mother takes sulfonamides late in pregnancy.[37] At high doses, gross fetal malformations have been reported in animals,[38] but in humans only two studies suggest an association between these drugs and birth defects.[39,40]

Adverse effects

Major adverse effects are rare, but include anaphylaxis, severe cutaneous eruptions, Steven's Johnson syndrome and leukopenia, thrombocytopenia and hemolytic anemia (especially in patients with glucose- 6-phosphate dehydrogenase deficiency). In patients with AIDS, the skin rashes and other toxicities seem to be more frequent. Of special note in these patients is the bone marrow suppression that is engendered by the combination of cotrimoxazole prophylaxis (or therapy) and zidovudine therapy for the underlying AIDS condition.

Nitrofurantoin

Nitrofurantoin is an FDA category B agent. Nitrofurantoin is often an alternative to trimethoprim/sulfamethoxazole for the prophylaxis and treatment of lower urinary tract infections during pregnancy. It has low serum concentrations and, to a very small extent, crosses the placenta.

Use in pregnancy

Teratogenicity or fetal adverse effects have not been observed in animal studies. Several clinical reports support the safety of nitrofurantoin use during pregnancy.[41,42]

Adverse effects

Nitrofurantoin can induce acute hemolytic anemia in patients with glucose-6-phosphate dehydrogenase deficiency or with glutathione-deficient red blood cells. No instances of hemolytic anemia have been reported in newborns. However, the manufacturer cautions the use of nitrofurantoin in pregnant women at term and in infants less than 1 month of age.

Quinolones (norfloxacin, ciprofloxacin, ofloxacin and lomefloxacin)

All the quinolones have a similar structure, are bactericidal and act by inhibiting the enzyme topoisomerase (gyrase) that is required for the supercoiling of DNA strands within the bacterial cell.

The quinolones have a wide spectrum of activity and are particularly effective against the Enterobacteriaceae, including the common urinary pathogens (*E. coli*, *Proteus* spp. and *K. pneumoniae*), *Salmonella typhi* and *S. paratyphi*, and *Shigella* spp. They are also effective against *P. aeruginosa*, even when given orally. With regard to the gram-positive cocci, activity is shown against *S. aureus* and epidermidis, but against streptococci and anaerobes, activity is borderline to poor, and failures are not infrequent. Consequently, these drugs should not be used in community-acquired and aspiration pneumonias, although they have been very successful in hospital-acquired pneumonia, and urinary activity against *E. faecalis* is often sufficient. The quinolones also have activity against *Legionella pneumophila*, *M. hominis*, *M. pneumoniae* and atypical mycobacteria. Ofloxacin is also recommended for the treatment of infections caused by *C. trachomatis*, and all the quinolones are active against *Neisseria gonorrhea* and *Hemophilus ducreyi*.

Nalidixic acid was the original quinolone, but, because of rapid emergence of resistance, it is used today only for urinary tract infection either as prophylaxis for recurrent acute cystitis, or for therapy. It can also be used as therapy for *Shigella* and other gastrointestinal infections. Norfloxacin is used almost exclusively for infections of the urinary tract, whereas ciprofloxacin, ofloxacin and pefloxacin achieve sufficiently high concentrations within the body fluids and organs to be useful when administered orally. Ciprofloxacin and ofloxacin achieve high concentrations within the macrophages and leukocytes. These drugs can also be administered intravenously in serious infections when oral therapy is contraindicated.

Metabolism, dosage and route

Norfloxacin and ciprofloxacin are excreted by the liver and kidney, whereas ofloxacin and lemefloxacin are excreted mainly by the kidneys. A major advantage of all the quinolones is that they are generally well absorbed following oral administration. Antacids reduce the absorption of quinolones and should not be taken until at least 2 h after taking quinolones. Sucralfate should be administered at least 6 h before any quinolone.

The serum half-lives are prolonged, so they need only be administered twice daily in most instances.

Indications in obstetrics and gynecology

In the community, the quinolones are used for first-line therapy of more serious and complicated urinary tract infections such as pyelonephritis and in patients with kidney stones. The quinolones are also extremely useful in treating uncomplicated gonorrhea, urinary tract infections, diarrheal diseases (including traveller's diarrhea) and chlamydial infections for which ofloxacin has been approved. In the treatment of pelvic inflammatory disease the quinolones need to be combined with an antianaerobic agent such as clindamycin or metronidazole.

These drugs should be used for the oral therapy of infections that would otherwise require intravenous administration of antibiotics. This allows for continuation of therapy of serious infections on an outpatient basis, after they have been controlled during hospitalization, e.g. pseudomonas osteomyelitis. They are generally not used as first-line drugs for the treatment of serious infections within the hospital, although they have proven to be effective in serious infections within intensive care units, in respiratory tract infections, osteomyelitis, infections of the skin and soft tissues, and in intra-abdominal infections when combined with antianaerobic therapy.[43] Although they cross into the CSF, their use in meningitis is anecdotal.

Use in pregnancy

These drugs are deposited in cartilage and result in irreversible arthropathy in animal studies, so that their use in pregnancy is contraindicated.

Adverse effects

The main adverse effects are gastrointestinal, rashes (including photosensitivity) and rarely neurological, including sleep disturbances, acute reversible toxic psychosis and grand malseizures. Because articular damage has been shown in juvenile animals these drugs are presently not approved for use in children under 18 years of age. They are also contraindicated in patients with glucose-6-phosphate dehydrogenase deficiency, in whom they may produce hemolysis.

Antituberculous drugs

Although safety in pregnancy of the drugs commonly used to treat tuberculosis is unknown or poor (Table 171.5), and only ethambutol is in category B, they are not contraindicated during pregnancy because of the risks to the pregnant woman resulting from untreated tuberculosis.[44]

For active tuberculosis, isoniazid and rifampicin are recommended as the initial treatment regimen.[45] Ethambutol should be added unless primary isoniazid resistance is unlikely. Pyrazinamide should probably not be used because of the lack of teratogenic data. Pyridoxine should be added to the regimen to protect against isoniazid neurotoxicity. Isoniazid crosses the placenta, but it appears to be well tolerated. The risk of hepatotoxicity to the mother from this drug may be increased during pregnancy. Neurologic abnormalities have been reported in one small study.[46] Streptomycin (category B) should not be used during pregnancy since it can cause eighth cranial nerve damage and deafness in children born to mothers receiving this drug during pregnancy.

Antifungal agents

Amphotericin B

Amphotericin B (category B) is the treatment of choice for systemic fungal infections, despite the availability of the azole antifungal agents – ketoconazole, fluconazole and itraconazole. Nephrotoxicity and electrolyte wasting are the most significant toxic effects of amphotericin B but they do not occur any more

Table 171.5 Antituberculous agents during pregnancy

Antituberculous agent	Category	Maternal toxicities	Fetal/neonatal toxicities
Isoniazid	C	Hepatotoxicity	Possible neurologic symptoms
Rifampicin	C	Hepatotoxicity, hypoprothrombinemia, bleeding	No known teratogenicity in humans
Ethambutol	B	Optic neuritis	None known
Pyrazinamide	C	Hepatotoxicity	Limited data
Streptomycin	D	Ototoxicity, nephrotoxicity	Ototoxicity

frequently in pregnant women than in non-pregnant women. Teratogenesis or persistent toxic effects have not been found.[47]

Azole antifungals (ketoconazole, fluconazole and itraconazole)

Safety in pregnancy has not been established. Flucytosine is contraindicated during pregnancy because of teratogenic effects observed in rats.[48] Although the manufacturer does not recommend breast-feeding by women using fluconazole, some commentators have concluded that the use of fluconazole is 'probably safe' during lactation.[49]

Antiviral agents

Acyclovir is used in the treatment of herpes simplex virus (HSV) and varicella zoster virus (VZV) infections.[50] Although its safety in pregnancy has not been formally established, in animals it has not caused toxicity or teratogenicity and numerous case reports have been published describing its use in pregnant women with disseminated HSV infections or VZV pneumonia.[51] Of 312 pregnancies followed prospectively, there was no consistent pattern of fetal abnormality or adverse outcome.[52]

Valaciclovir (category C), an acyclovir analog, is rapidly converted to acyclovir in the intestine and liver. It is better absorbed than acyclovir, thus producing higher plasma concentrations of acyclovir. Consequently, the effect on mother and fetus should be similar to that of acyclovir, but this has not been well studied.

Famciclovir (category B), a prodrug of penciclovir, is similar in activity to acyclovir. Its safety during pregnancy is unknown. Ganciclovir and foscarnet (both category C) have activity against cytomegalovirus (CMV). Because of their severe toxicity and the lack of studies of their use in pregnant women, there are no current indications for either agent. The only case in which the benefit of either drug may outweigh the risk is in severe, sight-threatening CMV retinitis.

Anti-human immunodeficiency virus drugs

There are numerous approved agents for use against the human immunodeficiency virus (HIV). Zidovudine (AZT), didanosine (ddI), zalcitabine (ddC), stavudine (d4T) and lamivudine (3TC) all work by inhibiting the reverse transcriptase enzyme produced by the virus. Saquinavir inhibits the activity of the HIV protease enzyme and prevents cleavage of viral protein precursors.

Zidovudine has not been associated with premature births, malformations or fetal distress.[53] It reduces significantly the risk of HIV transmission from mother to infant by 67.5%.[54] Women with CD4+ cell counts above 200 cells/mm^3 and no clinical indications for antepartum zidovudine therapy took the drug from weeks 14–34 of gestation and continuing throughout pregnancy. The infants were then continued on therapy from 8 to 12 h after birth for a 6-week duration.

Didanosine and saquinavir are in category B. Saquinavir has not shown teratogenicity at plasma concentrations in animals up to five times those achieved in humans at the recommended doses.[55] Zalcitabine, stavudine and lamivudine are all category C drugs since at very high doses in some animals they have been shown to be teratogenic or toxic, or to cause early fetal death. Zalcitabine has been found to be teratogenic.

REFERENCES

1. Chow AW, Jewesson PJ. Pharmacokinetics and safety of antimicrobial agents during pregnancy. *Rev Infect Dis* 1985;7:287–313.
2. Tomasz A. The mechanism of the irreversible antimicrobial effects of penicillins; how the beta-lactam antibiotics kill and lyse bacteria. *Annu Rev Microbiol* 1979;33:113–37.
3. Saxon A. Immediate hypersensitivity reaction to β-lactam antibiotics. *Rev Infect Dis* 1983;5(Suppl 2):368–79.
4. Sykes RB, Matthew M. The beta-lactamases of gram-negative bacteria and their role in resistance to β-lactam antibiotics. *Antimicrob Agents Chemother* 1976;2:115–57.

5. Malouin F, Bryan LE. Modification of penicillin-binding proteins as mechanisms of beta-lactam resistance. *J Antimicrob Chemother* 1986;30:1–5.
6. Levison ME, Mangura CT, Lorber B, *et al.* Clindamycin compared with penicillin for the treatment of anaerobic lung abscess. *Ann Intern Med* 1983;98:466–71.
7. Applebaum PC. World-wide development of antibiotic resistance in pneumococci. *Eur J Clin Microbiol* 1987;6:367–77.
8. Hartman BM, Tomasz A. Low-affinity penicillin-binding protein associated with beta-lactam resistance in *Staphylococcus aureus*. *J Bacteriol* 1984;158:513–6.
9. Neu HC. Aminopenicillins: Clinical pharmacology and use in disease states. *Int J Clin Pharmacol Biopharm* 1975;11:132–44.
10. Hemsell DL. Prophylactic antibiotics in gynecologic and obstetric surgery. *Rev Infect Dis* 1991;13(Suppl):S821–41.
11. Smith BR, LeFrock JL. Cefuroxime: Antimicrobial activity, pharmacology, and clinical efficacy. *Ther Drug Monit* 1983;5:149–60.
12. Lefrock JL, Blais F, Schell RD, *et al.* Cefoxitin in the treatment of diabetic patients with lower extremity infections. *Infect Surg* 1983;23:61–74.
13. Lecour H, Seara A, Miranda AM, *et al.* Treatment of 160 cases of acute bacterial meningitis with cefotaxime. *J Antimicrob Chemother* 1984;14(Suppl B):195–202.
14. Fong IW, Tompkins KB. Review of *Pseudomonas aeruginosa* meningitis with special emphasis on treatment with ceftazidime. *Rev Infect Dis* 1985;7:604–12.
15. Fu KP, Neu HC. Antibacterial activity of ceftizoxime, a beta-lactamase stable cephalosporin. *Antimicrob Agents Chemother* 1980;17:583–90.
16. Petz LD. Immunologic cross-reactivity between penicillins and cephalosporins: A review. *J Infect Dis* 1978;137(Suppl):S74–9.
17. Schaad UB, Tschappeler H, Lentze MJ. Transient formation of precipitations in the gallbladder associated with ceftriaxone therapy. *Pediatr Infect Dis J* 1986;5:708–10.
18. Wade JC, Petty BG, Conrad G, *et al.* Cephalothin plus an aminoglycoside is more nephrotoxic than methicillin plus an aminoglycoside. *Lancet* 1978;2:604–6.
19. Sykes RB, Bonner DP, Bush K, *et al.* Aztreonam (SQ 26776), a synthetic monobactam specifically active against aerobic gram-negative bacteria. *Antimicrob Agents Chemother* 1982;21:85–92.
20. Alexander MR. Review of vancomycin after 15 years of use. *Drug Intell Clin Pharm* 1974;8:520.
21. Whalley PJ, Adams RH, Combes B. Tetracycline toxicity in pregnancy: Liver and pancreatic dysfunction. *J Am Med Assoc* 1964; 189:357–62.
22. Knothe H, Dette GA. Antibiotics in pregnancy: Toxicity and teratogenicity. *Infection* 1985;13:49–51.
23. Cohlan SQ, Bevelander G, Tiamsci T. Growth inhibition of prematures receiving tetracycline. *Am J Dis Child* 1963;105:453–61.
24. Grossman ER, Walcheck A, Freedman H. Tetracycline and permanent teeth: The relationship between doses and tooth color. *Pediatrics* 1971;47:567–70.
25. Kirby BD, Snyder KM, Meyer RD, Finegold SM. Legionnaires' disease: Report of 65 nosocomially-acquired cases and review of the literature. *Medicine* 1980;59:188–205.
26. Archer GL, Tenenbaum MJ, Haywood HB III. Rifampin therapy of *S. epidermidis*: Use in infection of indwelling artificial devices. *J Am Med Assoc* 1978;240:751–3.
27. Watanakunakorn C. Clindamycin therapy of *Staphylococcus aureus* endocarditis. Clinical relapse and development of resistance to clindamycin, lincomycin and erythromycin. *Am J Med* 1976;60:419–25.
28. Tedesco FJ. Clindamycin and colitis: A review. *J Infect Dis* 1977; 135(Suppl):S95–8.
29. Moellering RC Jr, Wennersten C, Weinberg AN. Studies in antibiotic synergism against enterococci. I. Bacteriologic studies. *J Clin Lab Med* 1971;77:821–8.
30. Moore RD, Smith CR, Lietman PS. Risk factors for the development of auditory toxicity in patients receiving aminoglycosides. *J Infect Dis* 1984;149:23–30.
31. Lerner SA, Matz GJ, Hawkins JE, eds. *Aminoglycoside Ototoxicity*. Boston: Little, Brown and Company, 1981.
32. Wright JM, Collier B. The effects of neomycin upon transmitter release and action. *J Pharmacol Exp Ther* 1977;200:576–87.
33. Mollering RC Jr. Special consideration of the use of antimicrobial agents during pregnancy, post partum, and in the newborn. *Clin Obstet Gynecol* 1979;22:373–8.
34. Rosenblatt JE, Edson RS. Metronidazole. *Mayo Clin Proc* 1987; 62:1013–7.
35. Nastro LJ, Finegold SM. Bactericidal activity of five antimicrobial agents against *Bacteroides fragilis*. *J Infect Dis* 1972;126:104–7.
36. Reeves D. Sulphonamides and trimethoprim. *Lancet* 1982;2: 370–3.
37. Hawkins DF. Teratogenesis and other adverse effects on the fetus of antimicrobial drugs used in pregnancy. *Clin Exp Obstet Gynecol* 1986;13:113–24.
38. Kato T, Kitagawa S. Production of congenital abnormalities in fetuses of rats and mice with various sulphonamides. *Congenit Abnorm* 1973;13:7–15.
39. Nelson MM, Forfar JO. Associations between drugs administered during pregnancy and congenital abnormalities of the fetus. *Br Med J* 1971;1:523–7.
40. Saxen I. Associations between oral clefts and drugs taken during pregnancy. *Int J Epidemiol* 1975;4:37–44.
41. Hailey FJ, Fort H, Williams JC. Fetal safety of nitrofurantoin macrocrystals therapy during pregnancy: A retrospective analysis. *J Int Med Res* 1993;11:364–9.
42. Lenke RR, VanDorsten JP, Schitrin BS. Pyelonephritis in pregnancy: A prospective randomized trial to prevent recurrent disease: Evaluating suppressive therapy with nitrofurantoin and close surveillance. *Am J Obstet Gynecol* 1983;146:953–7.
43. Webster A, Gaya H. Quinolones in the treatment of serious infections. *Rev Infect Dis* 1988;10(Suppl):225–33.
44. Snider DE, Layde RM, Johnson MW, *et al.* Treatment of tuberculosis during pregnancy. *Am Rev Respir Dis* 1980;122:65–79.
45. American Thoracic Society. Treatment of tuberculosis and tuberculous infection in adults and children. *Am J Respir Crit Care Med* 1994;149:1359–74.
46. Monnet P, Kalb JC, Pujol M. Harmful effects of isoniazid on the fetus and infants. *Lyon Med* 1967;217:431–55.
47. Dean JL, Wolf JE, Ranzini AC, *et al.* Use of amphotericin B during pregnancy: Case report and review. *Clin Infect Dis* 1994;18: 364–8.
48. Chow AW, Jewesson PJ. Use and safety of antimicrobial agents during pregnancy. *West J Med* 1987;146:761–4.
49. Briggs GG, Freeman RK, Yaffe SJ. *Drugs in Pregnancy and Lactation*, 4th edn. Baltimore, MD: Williams and Wilkins, 1994:370–1.
50. Tucker WE. Preclinical toxicology profile of acyclovir: An overview. *Am J Med* 1982;73(Suppl):S27–30.
51. Watts DH. Antiviral agents. *Obstet Gynecol Clin North Am* 1992;19:563–85.
52. Andrews EB, Uankaskas BC, Cordero JF, *et al.* Acyclovir in pregnancy registry: Six years' experience. *Obstet Gynecol* 1992;79:7–13.
53. Sperling RS, Stratton P, O'Sullivan MJ, *et al.* A survey of zidovudine use in pregnant women with human immunodeficiency virus infection. *N Engl J Med* 1992;326:857–61.
54. Centers for Disease Control and Prevention. Recommendations of the US Public Health Service task force on the use of zidovudine to reduce perinatal transmission of human immunodeficiency virus. *Morb Mortal Wkly Rep* 1994;43:1–19.
55. Package insert. Invirase (saquinavir mesylate). Roche Laboratories, Nutley, NJ, December 1995.

172 Preterm delivery and infections

Y. Baytur and C. Şen

Birth before 37 weeks' gestational age or before 259 days is defined as preterm birth according to the World Health Organization.[1] Preterm birth is the major clinical problem associated with perinatal mortality, serious neonatal morbidity and moderate to severe childhood disability in both developed and underdeveloped countries and its prevention is the major aim of modern obstetrics. At present, there are no effective diagnostic tests for preterm birth and there are no effective treatments for this condition. Preterm birth could be qualified according to its clinical presentation: medically induced, preterm premature rupture of membranes (PPROM) and spontaneous preterm labor leading to preterm delivery. We need to be aware that preterm labor is not a disease, but an event that may result from single or multiple, independent or interdependent pathways. The etiology of spontaneous preterm labor is multifactorial, but there is overhelming evidence to implicate infection as a possible cause in up to 40% of cases.[2,3] Systemic maternal infection (e.g. pneumonia, influenza) may cause preterm delivery. However, the frequency in developed countries is low.[4,5] No large clinical or epidemiologic study has implicated viral diseases in the etiology of preterm delivery; however, both cytomegalovirus and herpes simplex virus infections may cause preterm delivery. Both urinary tract infection and periodontal disease may induce labor.[6,7] In a high proportion of pregnancies complicated by preterm labor and preterm prelabor amniorrhexis, the underlying cause may be ascending infection from the lower genital tract. Abnormal colonization of the lower genital tract with microorganisms, such as *Mycoplasma hominis, Ureaplasma urelayticum*, Group B hemolytic streptococci, *Chlamydia trachomatis, Gardnerella vaginalis*, is associated with intrauterine infection, preterm labor and also neonatal adverse outcome, such as cerebral palsy, chronic lung disease of prematurity and fetal inflammatory response syndrome (FIRS).[5,8] Positive amniotic fluid cultures, with organisms commonly found in the vagina, are present in about one-tenth of pregnancies in preterm labor with intact membranes and in more than one-third of cases with preterm prelabor amniorrhexis.[2] Vaginal organism first ascends into the choriodecidual space and stimulates an inflammatory reaction in the placenta, membranes and decidua. Preterm labor and delivery are then caused by a maternal and fetal response to this inflammatory reaction with increased prostaglandins secretion.[8–21]

This chapter will focus on the evidence that infection is causally associated with spontaneous preterm birth and the interactions between microorganisms, cytokines and prostaglandins and also adverse neonatal outcome.

The causes and mechanism of intrauterine infection

In patients with preterm labor and intact membranes, the amniotic fluid concentration of prostaglandins, leukotrienes and cytokines is higher in those with positive amniotic fluid cultures; in this group, tocolytics are less successful in arresting labor than in those with no infection.[2] The most common pathway of intrauterine infection is the ascending route, although transplacental infections, accidental introduction of pathogens into the cavity at the time of invasive procedures and invasion of systemic maternal infections may be involved.[5] According to Romero *et al.*,[22] ascending intrauterine infection is considered to have four stages. Stage 1 consists of a change in the vaginal/cervical microbial flora or the presence of pathologic organisms in the cervix. Some forms of bacterial vaginosis may be an early manifestation of this initial stage. In stage 2 microorganisms enter the cavity and then reside in the decidua. After microorganisms create an inflammatory response in the decidua, they invade the fetal vessels (choriovasculitis) or membranes (amnionitis), leading to intra-amniotic infection (stage 3). Once in the amniotic cavity, the bacteria may gain access to the fetus through various ports of entry (Stage 4). Intrauterine infection is often chronic and asymptomatic until labor or membrane rupture, without fever, abdominal pain, leucocytosis or fetal tachycardia.[23]

It is necessary to define abnormal genital tract colonization. Lamont[3] defined a classification of abnormal genital flora. He divided abnormal genital tract flora into four groups: (1) pathogens (*Neisseria gonorrhoeae*, *C. trachomatis*, *Trichomonas vaginalis*), (2) Group B hemolytic streptococci, (3) enteropharyngeal organism (*Escherichia coli*, *Enterococcus faecalis*) and (4) bacterial vaginosis-related organisms (anaerobes, *M. hominis* and *G. vaginalis*). A number of studies have shown that abnormal genital tract flora, either in the form of bacterial vaginosis or as bacterial vaginosis-related organisms, such as anaerobes, *Ureaplasma urealyticum*, *M. hominis* or *G. vaginalis*, is associated with preterm birth.[24–26] However, it has also been suggested that lower genital tract colonization with *U. urealyticum*, *M. hominis* or *G. vaginalis* is not associated with preterm birth.[27–29] On the other hand, these microorganisms are frequently found in the amniotic fluid of the women with premature labor and PPROM.[30,31] In a recent clinical trial, Gerber *et al.*[32] found that polymerase chain reaction testing of second-trimester amniotic fluid for *U. urealyticum* can identify women at risk of subsequent preterm labor and delivery. *U. urealyticum* has been identified in 11% of asymptomatic women who underwent transabdominal amniocentesis at 15–17 weeks' gestation. A subsequent preterm labor occurred in 58% of urealyticum-positive women, compared with 4% urealyticum-negative women.

A case-controlled study showed that cervical infection with *C. trachomatis* at 24 weeks' gestation increases by two to three times the risk of preterm delivery.[33] But the results of studies have been conflicting.[34–36] Romero *et al.*[5] stated that the association with prematurity in women with genital colonization of *C. trachomatis* is unclear, but the treatment is indicated because of serious neonatal adverse outcome, such as pneumonia and ophthalmia neonatarum, in case of vertical neonatal transmission. The presence of *T. vaginalis* in pregnant women was associated with an increased risk of preterm delivery, but the treatment of trichomoniasis with metronidazole (two 2 g doses) in asymptomatic women did not prevent the rate of preterm delivery. Another microorganism that may be related to preterm delivery and prematurity is *N. gonorrhoeae*.[37] It has been recommended to culture samples from high-risk women during pregnancy and to treat with antimicrobial agents. Amoxicillin plus probenecid, ceftriaxone or cefixime may be used as a treatment agent and have similar cure rates.

Group B hemolytic streprococci are worthwhile considering in a class of their own because of the devastating effects that these organisms can have on low birth weight or preterm infants.[37,38] Although asymptomatic bacteriuria with Group B hemolytic streprococci is a risk factor of preterm delivery and its treatment is associated with a reduction in the rate of preterm delivery, colonization of the lower genital tract with Group B streprococci is not a risk factor for preterm delivery.[5]

Asymptomatic bacteriuria is strongly associated with preterm delivery, pyelonephritis and also mental retardation and developmental delay in the fetus.[39–42] Antibiotic administration to patients with asymptomatic bacteriuria is associated with a significant reduction in the rate of preterm birth.[40] The incidence of asymptomatic bacteriuria is reported as 2–14% during pregnancy.[41] Considering the relatively high incidence of asymptomatic bacteriuria during pregnancy and its dangerous results, it has been recommended to screen and treat asymptomatic bacteriuria routinely in all pregnant women.[41–43] Not enough evidence was found to support one approach over the other for the screening and treatment. The gold standard for screening asymptomatic bacteriuria is urine culture and it was recommended by the U.S. Preventive Services Task Force that all pregnant women be screened by urine culture at their initial prenatal visit.[39] However, it was suggested that the routine use of urine cultures in the assessment of preterm labor is costly and adds little value to obtaining a diagnosis except in the presence of specific complaints.[44] The microscopic urinalysis and dipstick urine tests may be used as effective and cheaper alternative methods for detecting asymptomatic bacteriuria.[6,39] The treatment alternatives are single-dose phosphomycin 3 g, one of the β-lactams (amoxicillin, cefalexin, etc.) or nitrofurantoin for 3–7 days.[39]

Screening and treatment of bacterial vaginosis to prevent preterm delivery

According to review articles and meta-analysis, bacterial vaginosis increases the risk of preterm delivery by approximately 40–60%.[3–5,25,45,46] By the time a woman is admitted with preterm labor, there may be irreversible changes in the cervix, which render attempts to inhibit the process unsuccessful. It is important to diagnose and treat abnormal genital tract flora in early pregnancy before the symptoms of preterm delivery. First, it should be defined as abnormal colonization and classification of abnormal genital tract flora in pregnancy. Bacterial vaginosis is a condition in which there is a change in the microbial flora of the vagina characterized by replacement of the lactobacilli by other organisms, such as anaerobic bacteria, genital mycoplasmas, *G. vaginalis*, etc. In most cases, the condition is asymptomatic. The standard method for the diagnosis of this condition is a Gram stain examination of vaginal fluid. However, the studies in the literature that investigated the relationship between bacterial vaginosis and preterm birth have used different criteria and assessment methods based on either clinical finding or Gram staining. Recently, Honest *et al.*[17] have investigated the accuracy of various types of tests for bacterial vaginosis to predict spontaneous preterm birth in pregnant women. In this study, there were four different bacterial vaginosis testing methods: gram-staining tests using either Nugent's or Spiegel's criteria, gas liquid chromatography and clinical (Amsel's) criteria. They did not find any difference in the accuracy of the various bacterial vaginosis tests for predicting preterm birth in both asymptomatic and symptomatic women with threatened preterm labor. It was suggested that the presence of coccobacilli in Pap smears within 4 weeks before delivery was associated with a more than fourfold increase in the risk of very preterm delivery (≤31 weeks) and the authors concluded that if coccobacilli are detected in Pap smears during the second trimester, antibacterial treatment may lower the risk of very preterm delivery.[48] The detection of fetal fibronectin in cervical/vaginal secretion has been proposed as a marker for clinically silent upper genital tract microbial infections. The relationship between bacterial vaginosis/fetal fibronectin and preterm labor/birth has been investigated.[49] The time interval from gestational age at testing until delivery was significantly shorter for +bacterial vaginosis/+fetal fibronectin and −bacterial vaginosis/+fetal fibronectin groups than for the groups with negative results of fetal fibronectin and bacterial vaginosis. However, it was recommended that the use of the fetal fibronectin test should be limited to its negative predictive value and the use of antibiotics for preventing preterm birth according to positive fetal fibronectin results should be discouraged.[50]

Intrauterine infection may result from a chronic infection early in pregnancy that eventually becomes symptomatic with contractions and leads to spontaneous abortion or preterm labor and birth. Bacterial vaginosis in early pregnancy may be a stronger risk factor of preterm delivery than bacterial vaginosis later in pregnancy. In a meta-analysis that consists of 20,232 women, bacterial vaginosis increased the risk of preterm delivery greater than twofold. Higher risks were found in women who were screened for bacterial vaginosis at <16 weeks of gestation (odds ratio, 7.55; 95% CI, 1.80–31.65) or at <20 weeks of gestation (odds ratio 9.91; 95% CI, 1.99–49.34).[25] Screening after 26 weeks' gestation was associated with 1.4- to 1.9-fold increased risk, whereas screening in the second trimester was associated with a 2- to 6.9-fold increased risk of preterm birth.[45]

Although the results of studies support the theory of a chronic infection starting early in pregnancy, strategies to screen for and treat bacterial vaginosis in pregnancy remain controversial. Screening and treating bacterial vaginosis in low-risk asymptomatic pregnant women are not recommended.[51,52] Tebes *et al.*[53] reviewed the studies on effect of treatment on preterm birth with levels of evidence ranging from I to II between 1994 and 2001. They found that several trials reported a decrease in the incidence of preterm labor when bacterial vaginosis was treated, but most of those trials were performed on women with a history of preterm labor. Therefore, based on these studies and the current guidelines of the Centers for Disease Control and Prevention (CDC), they concluded that treating pregnant women in high-risk populations, who are diagnosed with bacterial vaginosis, provides the clinician with an opportunity to possibly prevent preterm labor in this population. In nulliparous women without a history of preterm birth, treatment is recommended if other risk factors are present (e.g. gonorrhea or chlamidia). But in the general low-risk populations, routine screening is not indicated. The largest trial reported today is the ORACLE II. In this study, 6295 women in spontaneous preterm labor with intact membranes and without evidence of clinical infection were randomly allocated to receive erythromycin, co-amoxiclav, both, or placebo. Antibiotic administration prolonged pregnancy and was associated with a significant reduction in the rate of maternal infection. Unfortunately, antibiotic administration had no significant effect on the primary neonatal outcome, which included neonatal death, chronic lung disease or major cerebral abnormality on ultrasonography before discharge.[54]

Lamont *et al.*[3] criticized the ORACLE study and emphasized three points in this investigation. First, the women were not screened for infection. The etiology of preterm birth is multifactorial and infection is responsible for only 40% of preterm birth. It is logical that antibiotics would not have any beneficial effect on spontaneous preterm labor without infectious etiology. Second, the antibiotics that were used in the study (erythromycin and co-amoxiclav) are not useful in bacterial vaginosis. Finally, one of the study groups received a combination of erythromycin and co-amoxiclav. Since one antibiotic is bactericidal and the other bacteriostatic, the actions are cancelled out. They suggested that the wrong antibiotics were used in the wrong patients too late in pregnancy.

Recently, a meta-analysis including 11 trials with ORACLE study and 7428 women shows a reduction in maternal infection with the use of prophylactic antibiotics but fails to demonstrate a benefit or harm for any of the neonatal outcomes. The authors concluded that antibiotic treatments cannot be currently recommended for routine practice.[55]

However, Lamont *et al.*[45] has used 2% clindamycin vaginal cream for women with abnormal genital tract flora before 20 weeks' gestation and they reported 60% reduced incidence of preterm birth and the need for neonatal intensive care when compared with the placebo. Once the inflammatory mediators, such as cytokines, have increased in fetomaternal tissues, it may be too late or harmful to try and stop labor. Antibiotics alone are unlikely to be helpful at that stage. It is logical that antibiotics used to prevent preterm birth should be given early in pregnancy in high-risk and symptomatic patients with bacterial vaginosis. Although intravaginal treatment may be effective on infections localized to the vagina, in late stages, systemic rather than local vaginal antibiotic regimens should be used.

Role of cytokines and other inflammatory mediators in preterm birth

Patterns of expression of cytokines in the fetal membranes and decidua suggest that inflammatory activation occurs modestly with term labor, but much more robustly in preterm delivery, particularly in the presence of intrauterine infection. The placenta and extraplacental membranes are sources of a large number of cytokines, chemokines and related factors.[11] In addition, infiltrating inflammatory cells, especially monocytes/macrophages, produce these cytokines in intrauterine tissues as the host reaction to infections.[10] Therefore, microorganisms that gain access to the fetus may elicit a systemic inflammatory response syndrome, which is characterized by the increased concentration of interleukin-6 (IL-6) and other cytokines, as well as cellular evidence of neutrophil and monocyte activation.

Recent studies with complimentary DNA (cDNA) array identified a cluster of inflammation-associated genes upregulated with labor both at term and preterm with infection and without infection.[56] Normal-term labor is associated with only a modest upregulation of these chemokines and cytokines. In contrast, preterm deliveries complicated with chorioamnionitis are associated with a dramatically elevated expression of a number of genes and proteins, particularly those of the chemokine class. However, chemokine expression is also elevated in gestational tissues with preterm labor that have no evidence of infection. It was suggested that an incidental exposure of infection may elicit an inappropriately robust immune response in some women, which fails to resolve and commences a feed-forward inflammatory loop, triggering parturition.[11]

Major attention has been focused on the role of proinflammatory cytokines, such as IL-1β, TNF-α and IL-8. However, other proinflammatory and anti-inflammatory cytokines together with chemokines increase with preterm labor; examples include IL-6, IL-10, granulocyte macrophage-colony stimulating factor (GM-CSF), G-CSF, leukemia inhibitory factor, platelet-activating factor (PAF), macrophage inflammatory protein (MIP)-1α, RANTES (regulated on activation, T-cell expressed and secreted) and growth-related oncogene-α.[5,8,10,11] Human decidua produces IL-1 and TNF-α in response to bacterial products, such as lipopolysaccharides (LPS).[57] Human amnion and chorion also have the ability to produce cytokines on stimulation with either LPS or IL-1 and TNF-α.[58] Several cytokines and chemokines in cervicovaginal and amniotic fluids, such as IL-1β, TNF-α, IL-6, IL-8 and monocyte chemotactic protein-1 can be detected before labor onset, particularly in women who deliver preterm with associated intra-amniotic infection.[2,8,11,21,59]

Chemokines play a crucial role in the process by regulating the leukocyte traffic. Leukocytes that are abundant in the majority of tissues from microbiologically confirmed infection-positive pregnancies have been shown to be activated in infection-associated preterm deliveries. The primary cellular source of cytokine production in the presence of intrauterine infection is, therefore, likely to be leukocytes that are recruited into the gestational membranes to fight the pathogen.[11] Recently, intra-amniotic secretion and abundance of epithelial cell-derived neutrophil-activating peptide (ENA-78), a potent chemoattractant and activator of neutrophils, has been studied in term and preterm parturition. It was found that ENA-78 was expressed immunohistochemically in chorionic trophoblasts and amniotic epithelium in term and preterm gestational membranes. ENA-78 increased more in preterm labor than term labor in amniotic membrane and showed a positive correlation with the leukocyte infiltration. More interestingly, in amniotic fluid, ENA-78 levels from pregnancies with preterm labor with intra-amniotic infection were significantly higher than those from pregnancies with preterm deliveries without infection.[60] Neutrophil defensins (HNP 1-3), bactericidal/permeability-increasing protein and calprotectin (MRP8/14) are antimicrobial peptides stored in the leukocytes that act as effector molecules of the innate immune response. The association between the amniotic fluid concentration of these peptides and the microbial invasion of amniotic cavity, PROM and parturition, was investigated. Microbial invasion of amniotic cavity, PROM and preterm parturition, was found to be associated with the increased amniotic fluid concentration of these peptides. Moreover, elevated amniotic fluid levels of these peptides were associated with intra-amniotic inflammation, histological chorioamnionitis and shorter amniocentesis-to-delivery interval in patients with preterm labor and intact membranes.[17]

In contrast to the increase in cytokine production observed in the fetal membranes and decidua during labor, the placenta involves less in the cytokine production. Studies of placental cells and tissue *in vitro* have demonstrated their ability to respond to inflammatory stimuli, such as pathogenic bacteria, LPS or IL-1β, with increased production of cytokines (IL-1β, IL-6, IL-10), chemokines (macrophage chemotactic protein-1, IL-8) and prostanoids.[11] However, the response of the placenta to the stimuli of TNF-α is very weak. The placenta might play a more important role in cytokine signaling in the process of labor and this process may be controlled by suppressors of cytokine-signaling proteins.[11]

The suggested mechanism for the association between intrauterine infection and labor is infection-mediated release of cytokines, which stimulate production of prostaglandins that induce myometrial contraction, cervical ripening and membrane rupture. IL-1β and TNF-α are known to stimulate prostaglandin biosynthesis in amnion, chorion, decidua and myometrium cells through an increase in cyclo-oxygenase (COX)-2 synthesis and activity.[10] These cytokines also increase the expression of prostaglandin H synthase (PGHS)-2 and decrease the activity of 15-hydroxyprostaglandin dehydrogenase within the fetal membrane, which is one of the key enzymes for prostaglandin degradation. PGHS-2 can be increased rapidly up to 80-fold in response to cytokines and bacterial endotoxins.[12] IL-1β induces PGHS-2 mRNA expression and prostaglandin E_2 (PGE_2) production in primary human amnion cells, chorion and deciduas. IL-6 has also been shown to stimulate prostaglandin production by the amnion and deciduas.[11] Protein levels of microsomal PGE_2 synthase and COX-2 are stimulated by cytokines (IL-1β and TNF-α) in human placenta and villous trophoblast cultures.[61] Dexamethasone and IL-10 reverse these effects of IL-1β in cultured villous and chorion trophoblast cells.[20,62,63]

Another possible mechanism for preterm labor may be PAF-mediated uterine contractions. IL-1β and TNF-α enhance PAF activity by suppressing the secretion of PAF-acetylhydrolase (inactivating enzyme for PAF). PAF stimulates PGE_2 production by the chorion decidua before labor and it may act synergistically with other stimulatory cytokines in the fetal membranes during labor.[10]

Cytokines increase the level of matrix metalloproteinase (MMP) expression and activity. The concentration of MMP-9 in chorion increases in term and preterm labor. Since this gelatinase enzyme contributes to the controlled degradation of collagen within the fetal membranes, and MMP-9 activity is increased by PGE_2, MMP-9 may be responsible for the PPROM.[11,12] Furthermore, intrauterine infection has been associated with higher MMP-9 concentrations in amniotic fluid, whether or nor membrane rupture occurred. TNF-α also stimulates MMP-1 and MMP-3.[11] Treatment with amniochorion explants with LPS also results in an increase in MMP-2 secretion and release.[64] This effect of LPS on MMP-2 and MMP-9 is inhibited by IL-10. MMP-3 is significantly increased in amniotic fluid of women with term and preterm parturition, but not in those with PROM.[18] Cytokines and prostaglandins may produce apoptotic effect on the membranes and lead to membrane rupture.[65] Expression of proapoptotic genes *bax* and *p53* is increased in the amniochorion of women with preterm PROM, while expression of the antiapoptotic gene *bcl-2* is decreased.[66] It has been suggested that Fas/CD95, a member of the TNF receptor superfamily, which is expressed in the fetal membranes, might play a key role in triggering the apoptosis, particularly in the presence of infection. These cytokine-induced and metalloproteinase-associated pathways may also play a role in cervical ripening. The increase in IL-8 during cervical ripening correlates with increases in leukocyte infiltration and concentrations of MMPs in the tissue.[11] Concentrations of IL-1β, TNF-α and IL-6 in the lower uterine segment also increase with cervical dilatation. IL-1β and TNF-α induce an increased expression of endothelial adhesion molecules with subsequent extravasation of granulocytes in the cervical stroma. The chemotaxis and degranulation of these cells in the stroma are triggered by IL-8. Concentrations of inflammatory cytokines, especially IL-8, in cervicovaginal secretion increases during labor and may be responsible for cervical ripening.[9,11] IL-8 production is activated by fibroblasts and macrophages. It plays a key role in cervical ripening, since this cytokine induces chemotaxis, activation and degranulation of neutrophilic granulocytes with the consequent release of various proteases, including collagenase.

Detection of intrauterine infection and predicting preterm delivery

It is well known that the admission-to-delivery interval is significantly shorter than in those cases with intrauterine infection compared to those without infection in preterm delivery. Attempts at prevention of preterm delivery in those with intrauterine infection have generally been unsuccessful. For avoiding unnecessary use of tocolytics, it is important to define women with intrauterine infection. The diagnosis of intrauterine infection is made by culture of amniotic fluid and fetal blood in PPROM or preterm labor with intact membranes. However, it takes at least 2 days before the results of culture are available and consequently, a series of rapid tests, such as Gram stain of the amniotic fluid, leukocyte count and glucose concentration, have been developed to predict the presence of infection.[2] The detection of proinflammatory cytokines in the amniotic fluid has also been proposed as a rapid test to predict preterm delivery.[67] High concentrations of IL-6, IL-18, monocyte chemotactic protein-1 in amniotic fluid were associated with microbial invasion of the amniotic fluid, intra-amniotic infection and prompt delivery.[8,21] However, these tests are required an invasive procedure and it is logical to use a less invasive test for predicting the possibility of preterm delivery.

The concentration of cytokines in the cervicovaginal secretions, maternal and fetal plasma as well as amniotic fluid increases with microbial invasion of the membranes in the preterm labor and PPROM cases. The cytokines and chemokines involved in the infection-induced preterm labor have also been studied for predicting preterm delivery. Cervicovaginal IL-6 demonstrated the ability to predict delivery between 2 and 7 days. Using 35 pg/ml as a cutoff, IL-6 had a sensitivity and specificity of 60% and 77% for predicting delivery within 2 days, and 62% and 80% within 7 days.[68] High concentration of IL-18 in cervical mucus in contrast to amniotic fluid was not found useful for predicting intra-amniotic infection and prompt delivery.[21] Monocyte chemotactic protein-1 in cervical secretions is elevated in preterm labor and PPROM and correlates to intra-amniotic infection/ inflammation.[8] Another potential marker in cervicovaginal fluid is intercellular adhesion molecule-1 (ICAM-1) in women presenting with preterm labor. Elevated ICAM-1 concentrations in cervical secretions have been shown to predict short intervals to delivery with high specificity. It has been found that, sensitivity, specificity, positive and negative predictive value were 33%, 98%, 75% and 93%, respectively, for predicting delivery within 3 days at 3-ng/ml threshold.[69] However, maternal serum levels of IL-6, IL-8 and TNF-α are not increased in preterm labor patients and the usefulness of maternal serum measurement of cytokines for detecting early fetal infection in preterm labor is doubtful and needs further evaluation.[70]

Although there is an association between infection, cytokine production and preterm delivery, it is not clear that a particular cytokine is required to signal the onset of labor. Studies with the animals showed that infection-induced preterm delivery does not require a specific cytokine.[71,72] However, tocolytics may prevent preterm delivery through the modulation of cytokines. Formoterol, a β2-adrenoreceptor agonist, has potent tocolytic effects in the rats. It is blocked $PGF_{2\alpha}$, IL-1α and IL-6, but not IL-10 in LPS-induced preterm delivery in rats.[73] Intrauterine inflammation is associated with decreased serum progesterone levels and decreased transcription of progesterone receptor-B in animals. It has shown that medroxyprogesterone acetate (MPA) suppressed the activation of contraction-associated genes and inflammatory mediators and prevented cervical ripening in response to intrauterine inflammation. LPS-induced preterm delivery rates in rats reduced from 100% to 63% and 0% with treatment with progesterone and MPA, respectively.[74] It has also been suggested that treatment with IL-10 prevents LPS-induced preterm delivery in the rats.[75]

Neonatal consequences of intrauterine infection

Intrauterine infection causes several acute or chronic adverse events in the newborn, such as increased incidence of neonatal infections, brain injury, cerebral palsy and chronic lung disease.[76,77] Neonatal sepsis in patients with PPROM is probably acquired *in utero* rather than during delivery. Supporting evidence is provided by the finding that the incidence of neonatal sepsis in pregnancies with positive amniotic fluid cultures is much higher than in the general population. Moreover, the causative organisms in neonatal infections are similar to those in vaginal infections.

It is believed that fetal microbial invasion results in a systemic fetal inflammatory response and this reaction may progress towards serious complications such as cerebral palsy, multiple organ dysfunction and septic shock, if the fetus remains undelivered.[5,13] This condition is named as the FIRS and generally occurs in fetuses of women with subclinical infection. The level of inflammatory cytokines (IL-6) often elevates in fetuses affected by this syndrome. Elevated cytokine levels induce the infiltration of inflammatory cells into the amnion and activate MMP in the fetus. As a result, preterm birth occurs.[5] The high levels of inflammatory cytokines in the fetus are associated with the development of bronchopulmonary dysplasia and periventricular leukomalacia in the newborn.[13,76] Except for the elevation of fetal IL-6 levels, there is still no specific clinical or laboratory sign of the FIRS. Umbilical cord plasma IL-6 concentrations were higher in the neonates born with funisitis than in those without this lesion. Funisitis is associated with amniotic fluid infection, congenital neonatal sepsis and the FIRS.[78] Increased IL-6 levels in the fetal plasma and the presence of the funisitis are used for the diagnosis of the FIRS and histologic findings of funisitis are better specificity and positive predictive value for predicting impaired neurological outcome.[79] Although the FIRS seems crucial to the association between intrauterine infection and white matter disease in human preterm infants, the underlying mechanisms remain unclear. In a rabbit model of intrauterine infection, it has been shown that in the fetuses with both diffuse cell death and focal periventricular white matter cysts mimicking cystic periventricular leukomalacia, a strong rabbit macrophage and inducible nitric oxide synthase immunostaining was observed at the border of these cystic lesions. In contrast, in the fetuses with only diffuse and significant cell death, no inflammatory or astroglial responses were detected in the white matter or hippocampus. In this model, focal white matter cysts are accompanied by a robust inflammatory response, and diffused cell death, which may mimic the white matter and hippocampal damage seen in very and extremely preterm infants, occurs in the absence of a detectable brain inflammatory response.[80] Proinflammatory cytokines, such as IL-6, have been implicated in the mechanisms that are responsible for brain injury in cases of intrauterine infection. IL-6 is a major mediator of the host response to infection and tissue damage and may play a role in the brain injury.

Fetal inflammation has been linked to the onset of labor in association with ascending infection. However, systemic fetal inflammation may occur in the absence of labor when the inflammatory process is secondary to a systemic maternal infection. In the presence of intrauterine infection, for preventing FIRS sequence, the fetus should be delivered timely, but the problems related to prematurity should be considered. The use of antibiotics seems to be not useful because the FIRS sequence has already been started before antibiotic administration. Agents such as anti-inflammatory cytokines may play a role in interrupting this sequence but this should be investigated more.

REFERENCES

1. World Health Organisation. *The Prevention of Perinatal Mortality and Morbidity*. WHO Technical Report Series, Report 457. Geneva: World Health Organization, 1970.
2. Carroll SG, Sebire NJ, Nicolaides KH. Infection: Amniorrhexis, preterm delivery, neonatal sepsis. In Nicolaides KH, ed. *Preterm Prelabour Amniorrhexis*. New York: The Parthenon Publishing Group, 1996:51–74.
3. Lamont RF. Infection in the prediction and antibiotics in the prevention of spontaneous preterm labor and preterm birth. *Br J Obstet Gynecol* 2003;110(Suppl 20):71–5.
4. Haram K, Mortensen JH, Wollen AL. Preterm delivery: An overview. *Acta Obstet Gynecol Scand* 2003;82:687–704.
5. Romero R, Espinoza J, Chaiworapongsa T, Kalache K. Infection and prematurity and the role of preventive strategies. *Semin Neonatal* 2002;7:259–74.
6. Kutlay S, Kutlay B, Karaahmetoglu O, Ak C, Erkaya S. Prevalance, detection and treatment of asymptomatic bacteriuria in a Turkish obstetric population. *J Reprod Med* 2003;48(8):627–30.
7. Jeffcoat MK, Hauth JC, Geurs NC, *et al.* Periodontal disease and preterm birth: Results of a pilot intervention study. *J Periodontal* 2003;74(8):1214–8.
8. Jacobsson B. Infectious and inflammatory mechanism in preterm birth and cerebral palsy. *Eur J Obstet Gynecol Reprod Biol* 2004; 115(2):159–60.
9. Jacobsson B, Holst RM, Wennerholm UB, Andersson B, Lilja H, Hagberg H. Monocyte chemotactic protein-1 in cervical and amniotic fluid: Relationship to microbial invasion of the amniotic cavity, intra-amniotic inflammation, and preterm delivery. *Am J Obstet Gynecol* 2003;189:1161–7.
10. Winkler M. Role of cytokines and other inflammatory mediators. *Br J Obstet Gynecol* 2003;110(Suppl 20):118–23.
11. Saji F, Samejima Y, Kamiura S, Sawai K, Shimoya K, Kimura T. Cytokine production in chorioamnionitis. *J Reprod Immunol* 2000;47:185–96.
12. Keelan JA, Blumenstein M, Helliwell RJA, Sato TA, Marwin KW, Mitchell MD. Cytokines, prostoglandins and parturition – A review. *Placenta* 2003;17:33–46.
13. Challis JR, Sloboda DM, Alfaidy N, *et al.* Prostoglandins and mechanism of preterm birth. *Reproduction* 2002;124:1–17.
14. Goldenberg RL, Culhane JF. Infection as a cause of preterm birth. *Clin Perinatol* 2003;30(4):677–700.
15. Premyslova M, Li W, Alfaidy N, *et al.* Differential expression and regulation of microsomal prostaglandin E(2) synthase in human fetal membranes and placenta with infection and in cultured trophoblast cells. *J Clin Endocrinol Metab* 2003;88(12):6040–7.
16. Friese K. The role of infection in preterm labour. *Br J Obstet Gynecol* 2003;110(Suppl 20):52–4.
17. Espinoza J, Chaiworapongsa T, Romero R, *et al.* Antimicrobial peptides in amniotic fluid: Defensins, calprotectin and bacterial/permeability-increasing protein in patients with microbial invasion of the amniotic cavity, intra-amniotic inflammation, preterm labor and premature rupture of membranes. *J Matern Fetal Neonatal Med* 2003;13(1):2–21.
18. Park KH, Chaiworapongsa C, Kim YM, *et al.* Matrix metalloproteinase 3 in parturition, premature rupture of the membranes, and microbial invasion of the amniotic cavity. *J Perinat Med* 2003; 31(1):12–22.
19. Rhone SA, Magee F, Remple V, Money D. The association of placental abnormalities with maternal and neonatal clinical findings: A retrospective cohort study. *J Obstet Gynaecol Can* 2003; 25(2):123–8.
20. Sato TA, Keelan JA, Mitchell MD. Critical paracrine interactions between TNF-alpha and IL-10 regulate lipopolysaccharide – Stimulated human choriodecidual cytokine and prostaglandin E2 production. *J Immunol* 2003;170(1):158–66.
21. Jacobsson B, Holst RM, Mattsby-Baltzer I, Nikolaitchouk N, Wennerholm UB, Hagberg H. Interleukin-18 in cervical mucus and amniotic fluid: Relationship to microbial invasion of the amniotic fluid, intra-amniotic inflammation and preterm delivery. *Br J Obstet Gynecol* 2003;110:598–603.
22. Romero R, Mazor M. Infection and preterm labor. *Clin Obstet Gynecol* 1988;31:553–84.
23. Goldenberg RL, Hauth JC, Andrews WW. Intrauterine infection and preterm delivery. *N Engl J Med* 2000;342:1500–7.
24. Chin BM, Lamont RF. The microbiology of preterm labor and delivery. *Contemp Rev Obstet Gynaecol* 1997;9:285–96.
25. Leitich H, Bodler-Adler B, Brunbauer M, Kaider A, Egarter C, Husslein P. Bacterial vaginosis as a risk factor for preterm delivery: A meta-analysis. *Am J Obstet Gynecol* 2003;189:139–47.
26. Gibbs RS. The relationship between infections and adverse pregnancy outcomes: An overview. *Ann Periodontol* 2001;6:153–63.
27. Romero R, Mazor M, Oyarzun E, Sirtori M, Wu YK, Hobbins JC. Is genital colonization with Mycoplasma hominis or Ureaplasma urealyticum associated with prematurity/low birth weight? *Obstet Gynecol* 1989;73:532–6.
28. Carey JC, Blackwelder WC, Nugent RP, *et al.* Antepartum cultures for ureaplasma urealyticum are not useful in predicting pregnancy outcome. The vaginal infections and prematurity study group. *Am J Obstet Gynecol* 1991;164:728–33.
29. Harrison HR. Cervical colonization with Ureaplasma urealyticum and pregnancy outcome: Prospective studies. *Pediatr Infect Dis* 1986;5:266–9.
30. Vintzileos AM, Campbell WA, Nochimson DJ, Weinbaum PJ, Escoto DT, Mirochnick MH. Qualitative amniotic fluid volume versus amniocentesis in predicting infection in preterm premature rupture of the membranes. *Obstet Gynecol* 1986;67:579–83.
31. Gauthier DW, Meyer WJ, Bieniarz A. Biophysical profile as a predictor of amniotic fluid culture results. *Obstet Gynecol* 1992; 80:102–5.
32. Gerber S, Vial Y, Hohlfeld P, Witkin SS. Detection of Ureaplasma urealyticum in second-trimester amniotic fluid by polymerase chain reaction correlates with subsequent preterm labor and delivery. *J Infect Dis* 2003;187(3):518–21.
33. Andrews WW, Goldenberg RL, Mercer B, *et al.* The preterm prediction study: Association of second-trimester genitourinary Chlamydia infection with subsequent spontaneous preterm birth. *Am J Obstet Gynecol* 2000;183:662–8.
34. Gravett MG, Nelson HP, DeRouen T, Critchlow C, Eschenbach DA, Holmes KK. Independent associations of bacterial vaginosis ND Chlamydia trachomatis infection with adverse pregnancy outcome. *J Am Med Assoc* 1986;256:1899–903.
35. Brocklehurst P, Rooney G. Interventions for treating genital Chlamydia trachomatis infection in pregnancy. *Cochrane Database Syst Rev* 2000:CD000054.
36. Sweet RL, Landers DV, Walker C, Schachter J. Chlamydia trachomatis infection and pregnancy outcome. *Am J Obstet Gynecol* 1987;156:824–33.
37. Kaufman D, Fairchild KD. Clinical microbiology of bacterial and fungal sepsis in very low birth weight infants. *Clin Microbiol Rev* 2004;17(3):638–80.
38. Lin FY, Weisman LE, Troendle J, Adams K. Prematurity is the major risk factor for late-onset group B streptococcus disease. *J Infect Dis* 2003;188(2):267–71.
39. Cram LF, Zapata MI, Toy EC, Baker B III. Genitourinary infections and their association with preterm labor. *Am Fam Physician* 2002;65(2):241–8.
40. Goncalves LF, Chaiworapongsa C, Romero R. Intrauterine infection and prematurity. *Ment Retard Dev Disabil Res Rev* 2002;8(1):3–13.
41. Uncu Y, Uncu G, Esmer A, Bilgel N. Should asymptomatic bacteriuria be screened in pregnancy? *Clin Exp Obstet Gynecol* 2002;28(4):281–5.
42. McDermott S, Callaghan W, Szwejbka L, Mann H, Daguise V. Urinary tract infections during pregnancy and mental retardation and developmental delay. *Obstet Gynecol* 2000;96:113–9.
43. Kremery S, Hromec J, Demesova D. Treatment of lower urinary tract infection in pregnancy. *Int J Antimicrob Agents* 2001;17:279–82.
44. Hundley AF, Onderdonk AB, Greenberg JA. Value of routine urine culture in the assessment of preterm labor. *J Reprod Med* 2003; 48(11):853–7.
45. Lamont RF, Duncan SL, Mandal D, Bassett P. Intravaginal clindamycin to reduce preterm birth in women with abnormal genital tract flora. *Obstet Gynecol* 2003;101:516–22.
46. Klein LL, Gibbs RS. Use of microbial cultures and antibiotics in the prevention of infection-associated preterm birth. *Am J Obstet Gynecol* 2004;190(6):1493–502.
47. Honest H, Bachmann LM, Knox EM, Gupta JK, Kleijnen J, Khan KS. The accuracy of various tests for bacterial vaginosis in

predicting preterm birth: A systematic review. *Br J Obstet Gynecol* 2004;111(5):409–22.

48. Buchmayer S, Sparen P, Cnattingius S. Signs of infection in Pap smears and risk of adverse pregnancy outcome. *Paediatr Perinat Epidemiol* 2003;17(4):340–6.
49. Stevens AO, Chauhan SP, Magann EF, *et al.* Fetal fibronectin and bacterial vaginosis are associated with preterm birth in women who are symptomatic for preterm labor. *Am J Obstet Gynecol* 2004;190(6):1582–7.
50. Andrews WW, Goldenberg RL, National Institute of Child Health and Development Maternal-Fetal Medicine Units Network. What we have learned from an antibiotic trial in fetal fibronectin positive women. *Semin Perinatol* 2003;27(3):231–8.
51. Kekki M, Kurki T, Kotomaki T, Sintonen H, Paavonen J. Cost-effectiveness of screening and treatment for bacterial vaginosis in early pregnancy among women at low risk for preterm birth. *Acta Obstet Gynecol Scand* 2004;83(1):2–3.
52. Carey JC, Klebanoff MA, National Institute of Child Health and Human Development Maternal-Fetal Medicine Units Network. What have we learned about vaginal infections and preterm birth? *Semin Perinatol* 2003;27(3):212–6.
53. Tebes CC, Lynch C, Sinnott J. The effect of treating bacterial vaginosis on preterm labor. *Infect Dis Obstet Gynecol* 2003;11(2): 123–9.
54. Kenyon SL, Taylor DJ, Tarnow –Mordi W. Broad spectrum antibiotics for spontaneous preterm labor, the ORACLE II randomized trial. ORACLE Collaborative Group. *Lancet* 2001;357:989–94.
55. King J, Flenady V. Prophylactic antibiotics for inhibiting preterm labor with intact membranes. *Cochrane Database Syst Rev* 2002;4:CD000246.
56. Marvin KW, Keelan JA, Eykholt RL, Sato TA, Mitchell MD. Use of cDNA arrays to generate differential expression profiles for inflammatory genes in human gestational membranes delivered at term and preterm. *Mol Hum Reprod* 2002;8:399–408.
57. Romero R, Wu YK, Mazor M, *et al.* Human decidua: A source of interleukin-1. *Obstet Gynecol* 1989;73:31–4.
58. Bowen JM, Chamley L, Mitchell MD, Keelan JA. Cytokines of the placenta and extra-placental membranes: Biosynthesis secretion and roles in establishment of pregnancy in women. *Placenta* 2002;23:239–56.
59. Kayem G, Maillard F, Batteux F, Weill B, Cabrol D, Goffinet F. Interleukin-8 mRNA in vaginal secretions: A prenatal marker of congenital infection in case of preterm labor with intact membranes. *Prenatal Diagn* 2004;24(1):58–62.
60. Keelan JA, Yang J, Romero RJ, *et al.* Epithelial cell-derived neutrophil-activating peptide 78 is present in fetal membranes and amniotic fluid at increased concentrations with intra-amniotic infection and preterm delivery. *Biol Reprod* 2004;70(1):253–9.
61. Premyslova M, Li W, Alfaidy N, *et al.* Differential expression and regulation of microsomal prostaglandin E(2) synthase in human fetal membranes and placenta with infection and in cultured trophoblast cells. *J Clin Endocrinol Metab* 2003;88(12):6040–7.
62. Xue S, Slater DM, Bennett PR, Myatt L. Induction of both cytosolic phospholipase A2 and prostoglandin H synthase-2 by interleukin -1ß in WISH cells is inhibited by dexamethasone. *Prostoglandins* 1996;51:107–24.
63. Pomini F, Caruso A, Challis JRG. Interleukin-10 modifies the effects of interleukin-1 and tumor necrosis factor-α on the activity and expression of prostaglandin H synthase-2 and the NAD$^+$ dependent 15-hydroxyprostaglandin dehydrogenase in cultured term human villous trophoblast and chorion trophoblast cells. *J Clin Endocrinol Metab* 1999;84:4645–51.
64. Fortunato SJ, Menon R, Lombardi SJ. Amniochorion gelatinase-gelatinase inhibitor imbalance in vitro: A possible infectious pathway to rupture. *Obstet Gynecol* 2000;95:240–4.
65. Lonergan M, Aponso D, Marvin KW, *et al.* Tumor necrosis factor-related apoptosis-inducing ligand (TRIAL), TRIAL receptors, and the soluble receptor osteoprotegerin in human gestational membranes and amniotic fluid during pregnancy and labor at term and preterm. *J Clin Endocrinol Metab* 2003;88:3835–44.
66. Fortunato SJ, Menon R, Bryant C, Lombardi SJ. Programmed cell death (apoptosis) as a possible pathway to metalloproteinase activation and fetal membrane degradation in premature rupture of membranes. *Am J Obstet Gynecol* 2000;182:1468–76.
67. Romero R, Yoon BH, Mazor M, *et al.* A comparative study of the diagnostic performance of amniotic fluid glucose, white blood cell count, interleukin-6, and Gram stain in the detection of microbial invasion in patients with premature rupture of membranes. *Am J Obstet Gynecol* 1993;169:1099–114.
68. Coleman MA, Keelan JA, McCowan LM, Townend KM, Mitchell MD. Predicting preterm delivery: Comparison of cervicovaginal interleukin (IL)-1, IL-6 and IL-8 with fetal fibronectin and cervical dilatation. *Obstet Gynecol* 2001;95:154–8.
69. Marvin KW, Keelan JA, Coleman MA, McCowan LM, Zhou RL, Mitchell MD. Intercellular adhesion molecule-1 (ICAM-1) in cervicovaginal fluid of women presenting with preterm labor: Predictive value for preterm delivery. *Am J Reprod Immunol* 2000;43:264–71.
70. Bahar AM, Ghalib HW, Moosa RA, Zaki ZM, Thomas C, Nabri OA. Maternal serum interleukin-6, interleukin-8, tumor necrosis factor-alpha and interferon-gamma in preterm labor. *Acta Obstet Gynecol Scand* 2003;82(6):543–9.
71. Hirsch E, Muhle RA, Mussalli GM, Blanchard R. Bacterially induced preterm labor in the mouse does not require maternal interleukin-1 signaling. *Am J Obstet Gynecol* 2002;186: 523–30.
72. Yoshimura K, Hirsch E. Interleukin-6 is neither necessary nor sufficient for preterm labor in a murine infection model. *J Soc Gynecol Invest* 2003;10(7):423–7.
73. Shinkai N, Takasuna K, Takayama S. Inhibitory effects of formoterol on lipopolysaccharide-induced premature delivery through modulation of proinflammatory cytokine production in mice. *Reproduction* 2003;125(2):199–203.
74. Elovitz M, Wang Z. Medroxyprogesterone acetate, but not progesterone, protects against inflammation induced parturition and intrauterine fetal demise. *Am J Obstet Gynecol* 2004;190(3): 693–701.
75. Terrone DA, Rinehart BK, Granger JP, Barrilleaux PS, Martin JN, Bennet WA. Interleukin-10 administration and bacterial endotoxin-induced preterm birth in a rat model. *Obstet Gynecol* 2001;98:476–80.
76. Lyon A. Chronic lung disease of prematurity. The role of intrauterine infection. *Eur J Pediatr* 2000;159:798–802.
77. Sullivan MH, Steel J, Kennea N, Feldman RG, Edwards AD. The role of intrauterine bacteria in brain injury. *Acta Pediatr Suppl* 2004;93(444):4–5.
78. Yoon BH, Romero R, Park JS, *et al.* The relationship among inflammatory lesions of the umbilical cord (funisitis), umbilical cord plasma interleukin 6 concentration, amniotic fluid infection, and neonatal sepsis. *Am J Obstet Gynecol* 2000;183(5):1124–9.
79. Mittendorf R, Montag AG, MacMillan W, *et al.* Components of the systemic fetal inflammatory response syndrome as predictors of impaired neurologic outcomes in children. *Am J Obstet Gynecol* 2003;188(6):1438–44.
80. Debillon T, Gras-Leguen C, Leroy S, Caillon J, Roze JC, Gressens P. Patterns of cerebral inflammatory response in a rabbit model of intrauterine infection-mediated brain lesion. *Brain Res Dev Brain Res* 2003;145(1):39–48.

173 Perinatal infectious morbidity in multiple pregnancies

I. Blickstein and E. L. Yashphe

Introduction

Multiple pregnancies seem to be more prone to perinatal infectious morbidity compared with singleton gestations. Two explanations may support this statement. First, preterm premature rupture of the membranes (PPROM) is more frequent among multiples and, second, the uterine cavity is more likely to be accessed for diagnostic and therapeutic procedures during a multiple gestation. In addition, multiples are exposed to infections via the hematogenic route to the same extent as singletons. Figure 173.1 is a schematic depiction of the possible routes of infection in multiple pregnancies.

In contrast to singletons, the unique situation of discordant fetal infection may be seen in twins and higher-order multiples, whereby only the presenting gestational sac is exposed to ascending infection. In this circumstance, it is possible that the presenting twin somehow protects its non-presenting sib.

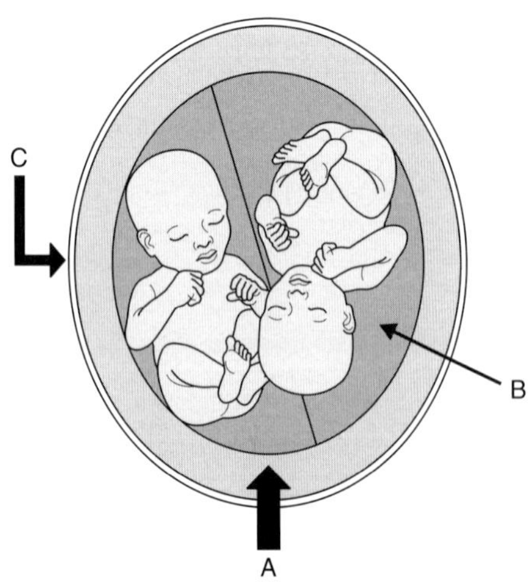

Figure 173.1 Potential routes of infection in multiple pregnancies: (A) ascending infection, (B) infection due to invasive procedures, and (C) hematogenic infections.

In this chapter, we shall discuss several issues related to perinatal infectious morbidity among multiples.

Preterm premature rupture of membranes

A multiple gestation, within an overdistended uterus, is an important risk factor for PPROM, leading to a number of maternal and fetal/neonatal complications. The mother is at a greater risk for developing chorioamnionitis, endometritis, and bacteremia. For the fetus/neonate, the risk for PPROM-related morbidity and mortality are even greater, resulting in premature labor and preterm birth associated with respiratory distress syndrome (RDS), intraventricular hemorrhage (IVH), septic morbidity, and necrotizing enterocolitis (NEC).

The incidence of PPROM is higher and occurs earlier in multiple pregnancies.[1] Mercer *et al.* compared 99 twin with 99 well-matched singleton pregnancies complicated by preterm rupture of the membranes. The authors found that PPROM occurs more frequently in twin than in singleton gestations (odds ratio, OR 2.1) and that PPROM at < 26 weeks' gestation complicated 1.4% of twin gestations (18.2% of those with PPROM) compared with 0.52% of singleton gestations (OR 2.71). Despite these differences, the etiology of PPROM in twins seems similar to that in singleton pregnancies with the main identifiable cause being maternal genital tract infection. Uterine overdistention, however, may also play a role in multiple pregnancies. Not surprisingly, membrane rupture usually occurs in the presenting sac, but may develop in the non-presenting sac following invasive procedures. Management of PPROM in twins depends on the presence or absence of clinical maternal infection, labor, gestational age, and fetal well-being. The management algorithm includes administration of antibiotics and steroids, whereas immediate delivery is usually reserved for cases with clinical evidence of intra-amniotic infection, fetal distress, established lung maturity, or more advanced gestational ages.

Several studies examined the perinatal outcome after PPROM in twin compared with singleton gestations. Mercer *et al.*[1] found no significant differences in infectious morbidity in terms of chorioamnionitis and postpartum fever between twin and singleton gestations despite the presence of an intact amniotic sac in the second twin. In contrast, Myles *et al.*[2] observed a somewhat higher incidence of chorioamnionitis in singleton pregnancies and explained this finding by the longer latency period among singletons – as was also observed by Bianco *et al.*[3] and Mizrahi *et al.*[4] The latter group compared perinatal outcomes in spontaneously conceived 435 sets of twins and 4754 singletons born preterm. Twin gestation had significantly lower rates of PPROM and clinical chorioamnionitis (12.2% vs.17.3%, and 1.8% vs. 5.2%, respectively).

In the case of multiple gestations, which are at a greater risk of very preterm birth, the management of extremely PPROM (EPPROM, < 25 weeks' gestation) seems to be more pertinent. In a recent series of 47 pregnancies including 10 twin and 2 triplet gestations, the comparison of multiple with singleton pregnancies with EPPROM at the same median gestational age (22 weeks) revealed that fewer infants of a multiple pregnancy were considered viable and admitted to the neonatal intensive care unit (NICU).[5] Among those who were admitted, mortality rate was almost twice higher despite a similar incidence of serious sequelae.[5]

Finally, it should be remembered that multiple pregnancies are the best example of how imaginative diagnostic as well as therapeutic methods are implemented in modern perinatology. The invasive nature of most of them undoubtedly increases the risk of PPROM and infection. For example, laser treatment of twin–twin transfusion needs several ports of entry, amniocentesis for dizygotic twins usually needs two punctures, and even simple lung maturity testing needs needle insertion into both sacs.

Endometritis

Women with multiple gestations are at an increased risk for several maternal complications compared to women carrying singletons. Endometritis, an infection of the endometrium or decidua, with and without extension to the myometrium and parametrium, is the most common cause of postpartum fever. Risk factors for this condition include prolonged rupture of membranes and labor with multiple vaginal examinations, both of which may be more prevalent in multiple pregnancies and births. One might therefore expect to find more cases of endometritis following multiple pregnancies.

One large historical cohort study, addressing maternal complications, evaluated 885,338 gestations, of which 15,484 were twin gestations, delivered in Latin America.[6] A significant association between multiple pregnancies and puerperal endometritis was found, with a higher risk among nulliparous mothers. The larger placental bed in multiple pregnancies and the higher cesarean section rate (2.5 higher compared with singleton pregnancies) were the explanation for these findings.

As noted above, prolonged rupture of membranes is a significant risk factor for both maternal and neonatal infections. Indeed, the higher incidence of PPROM in multiple pregnancies increases the risk for endometritis, and this risk correlates with the latency period between membrane rupture and delivery. The question whether the mode of delivery affects the risk of maternal infections is particularly pertinent because many clinicians suggest a cesarean birth in the majority of twin pregnancies and in practically all triplet pregnancies.[7] This question was studied by Suonio and Huttunen,[8] who prospectively compared the infectious complications of 122 consecutive abdominal twin deliveries with 761 singleton abdominal births. The incidence of endometritis was nearly threefold after twin deliveries and the incidence of abdominal wound infections nearly twofold compared with singleton abdominal pregnancies. The risk of amnionitis was increased 10-fold when 6 h elapsed after rupture of the membranes in abdominal twin delivery, but no such connection was found between amnionitis and endometritis in singleton abdominal deliveries. The authors performed a multiple regression analysis and found only two risk factors for puerperal endometritis after abdominal twin delivery: age under 25 years and an interval of more than 6 h from rupture of membranes to delivery. In contrast, a retrospective study of 93 consecutive triplet pregnancies with 71% vaginal delivery found that vaginal delivery had no deleterious effect on neonatal and maternal outcomes; however, endometritis was slightly more frequent in the group undergoing trial of labor as compared with the group delivering by planned cesarean section.[9]

A study examining 718 twin births found that the endometritis rate was higher in the cesarean group than in the vaginal group.[10] In the subgroup of vaginal births, the incidence of endometritis was similar in those deliveries with and without manipulations. The length of time between delivery of twin A and twin B did not affect the endometritis rate.

Discordant infection/inflammation by chorion type

A unique situation exists in multiple pregnancies whereby an ascending genital infection may not affect both gestational sacs, resulting in discordant infection or inflammation. Mazor and coworkers[11] evaluated microbial invasion of the amniotic cavity by transabdominal amniocentesis under sonographic guidance in multiple pregnancies. Amniotic fluid from both sacs was cultured for aerobic and anaerobic microorganisms

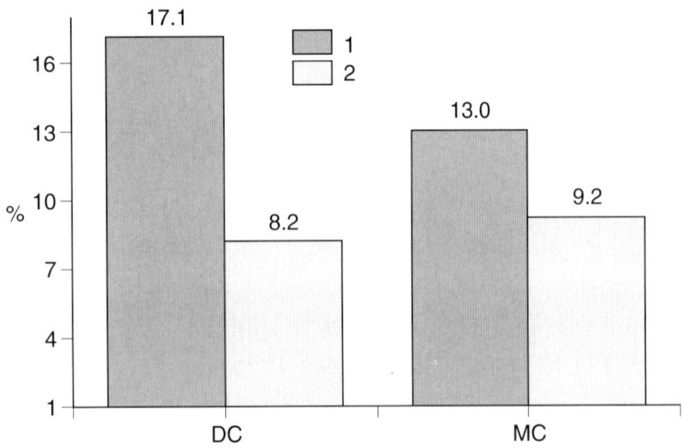

Figure 173.2 Frequency (%) of chorioamnionitis by chorionicity and presentation. 1, Presenting twin; 2, non-presenting twin. DC, dichorionic; MC, monochorionic. Adapted from Phung *et al.*[12]

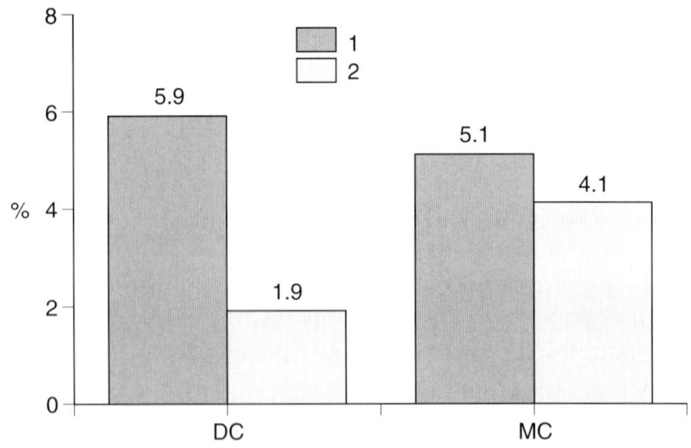

Figure 173.3 Frequency (%) of chorioamnionitis and funisits by chorionicity and presentation. 1, Presenting twin; 2, non-presenting twin; DC, dichorionic, MC, monochorionic. Adapted from Phung *et al.*[12]

as well as for *Mycoplasma* species. Amniotic fluid was obtained from 74 patients. Sixty-eight women delivered prematurely (91.9%). Amniotic fluid culture results were positive for microorganisms in nine cases of the 74 patients in the study cohort, including five isolated from the presenting sac (55.6%), three from both sacs (33.3%), and one from the upper sac (11.1%). Patients with a positive culture had a higher incidence of clinical chorioamnionitis than those with a negative culture.

The so-called Northwestern Twin Chorionicity Study[12] examined the question whether discordant inflammation depends on chorionicity. The authors retrospectively analyzed 1156 twin placentas to evaluate the association between chorionicity and discordant chorioamnionitis and funisitis in twin gestations. This study found that in the case of chorioamnionitis in dichorionic twins (with either separate or fused placentas), the non-presenting twin was less frequently affected than the presenting twin. Such discordant inflammation was not apparent in monochorionic twins (Figure 173.2). The results were somewhat accentuated in the case of funisitis – a more advanced state of inflammation (including inflammatory evidence within the walls of umbilical vessels or in Wharton's jelly) (Figure 173.3). Whereas the difference between dichorionic and monochorionic twins persists, discordant funisitis was greatest among separate dichorionic twins, less so among fused dichorionic twins, and absent among monochorionic twins. The interpretation of these results was that the dichorionic placentas confer significant protection against the spread of chorioamnionitis from the presenting to the non-presenting sac. The difference between the separate and fused dichorionic twins implies that the paranchymal separation between these placentas and not the dichorionic septum might be responsible for the protection. In simple terms, the different morphologic features of a four-layer intertwin membrane and the separate placentas may restrict the spread of inflammation.

More intriguing and somewhat puzzling is the finding of twins discordant for infections with a presumably hematogenic spread.[13–16] For example, Vogler and coworkers[13] described a stillborn male twin from a diamniotic–dichorionic pregnancy with disseminated cytomegalovirus (CMV) identified morphologically and the other was liveborn without clinical or laboratory evidence of CMV infection. The placenta of the affected twin had chronic villitis but that of the liveborn was normal. The authors suggested that dissimilar immune responses between the affected and unaffected twin and direct extension of uterine CMV infection to only one twin might be responsible for the discordant infection. Similarly, Barlow and Mok[14] described twin girls born at 37 weeks' gestation to a mother infected by human immunodeficiency virus (HIV) and hepatitis C virus. Twin A had symptomatic HIV infection by 9 months but was negative for hepatitis C virus antibody and RNA whereas twin B became HIV antibody negative by 15 months but was positive for anti-hepatitis C virus and RNA.

The discordant infection with HIV is particularly important (see below).[15,16] For example, the acquired immunodeficiency syndrome-related complex was identified in a mother and one of her dizygotic twins. Generalized lymphadenopathy was first noted in the infant at age 17 months. Both parents and the patient had hypergammaglobulinemia, low T-helper-to-suppressor-cell ratio, and positive serum antibody to HIV. The twin brother was in good health with a normal immunologic profile and negative antibody to HIV.[13]

Infection and delayed interval delivery

When a multifetal pregnancy is complicated by PPROM and premature labor, in particular at a previable stage, it may be possible to deliver the presenting fetus and to salvage, by delayed interval delivery, the second twin (or more fetuses in higher-order pregnancies). In this circumstance, precious time may be gained, thus reducing the risks of prematurity for the undelivered fetus(es). Because of the rarity of this situation, the literature on the subject comprises case reports and relatively small series. In addition, a publication bias may exist, whereby successful cases are reported whereas complicated cases are not published. In order to consider delayed interval delivery after PPROM of one gestational sac, a number of conditions must be met: most important, intra-amniotic infection should be excluded. If the situation is appropriate, management comprises high ligature of the first twins' cord, strict bed rest, aggressive tocolysis, prophylactic antibiotics, and steroids. The use of cervical cerclage is controversial, and the use of anticoagulation may be considered in some cases.[17] A recent retrospective cohort study matched delayed deliveries with twin pairs that were delivered without delay and compared the perinatal outcomes and infant survival.[18] The mean duration of delay was 6 days. The authors found that 56% of the delayed second twins survived to 1 year of age compared with 24% of second twins born immediately.

Conceptually, one should assume that the birth of the presenting fetus was a result of an infectious or inflammatory process. Therefore, with the success rates in mind on the one hand, and the alternative of delivering multiples before or at the limit of viability on the other, it is important to consider the risk of chorioamnionitis in such cases.

Chorioamnionitis seems to be a universally accepted contraindication to attempting delayed interval birth in a multiple gestation. However, Watson and McNelis[19] maintained that infection is not an absolute contraindication for such a heroic procedure, and present a delay of 00 days between the birth of the two infants, in which chorioamnionitis was observed immediately after the delivery of twin A and successfully treated with antibiotics. On the other side of the scale, Hoffman and Sciscione[20] reported on a woman attempting interval delivery of triplets at 21 weeks who developed severe septic complications including chorioamnionitis, acute RDS, and tubular necrosis 7 days after delivery of the first fetus.

Delayed interval delivery is discussed in length elsewhere in this book. However, it is our personal view that the risk of intrauterine infection (up to 30%) and maternal sepsis (about 5%)[21] should deter both clinicians and patients from attempting this kind of formidable birth when chorioamnionitis is not categorically excluded. Having said this, it seems that delayed delivery remains a therapeutic option in selected cases for improving the survival rates of the remaining fetuses in correlation to the latency period achieved.[21]

HIV in twins

There are two pertinent questions related to the occurrence of congenital HIV infections: when does transmission of infection occur during the peripartum period and what role does the mode of delivery play in determining the risk of infections? Because twins share the same uterine environment as well as genetic similarities, the evaluation of outcomes in twins delivered to HIV carriers may lead to better understanding of the transmission of different infectious agents, including HIV.

Several studies indicate that the majority of infections occur during labor or delivery and not antepartum. In this scenario, despite cases of intrauterine infection, transmission occurs mainly due to exposure of the newborn to blood, mucus, and other secretions during the passage through the birth canal. Therefore, one would expect to find a higher transmission rate among first-born twins (similar to that found in singletons) compared with second-born twins. The results of some studies concur with this hypothesis; however, other studies found that infections were more concordant than would be expected by chance.

In an international study, 66 sets of twins were evaluated. This registry found HIV-1 infections to be more common in first-born than in second-born twins.[22] A higher concordance was found in monozygotic than dizygotic twins, implying that infection *in utero* may exist at least in some cases. Another study of 115 pairs confirmed these results and concluded that HIV infection of second twins occurs predominantly *in utero*, whereas the infection of the first twins occurs mainly intrapartum.[23]

In contrast to the above-mentioned findings, more recently, a large study that examined 315 twin pairs in Africa found different results.[24] This group found that birth order has no effect on the infection rate, either *in utero* or perinatally in vaginal deliveries. Others found similar results, albeit in a much smaller sample.[25] If indeed the major mode of transmission is the passage of the neonates through the birth canal, cleansing of the birth canal with virucidal agents or a cesarean delivery could reduce the risk of transmission. In Africa, cleansing the birth canal during labor did not seem to reduce the risk of infection, but these results should be interpreted with caution because the prevalent breast-feeding among the HIV-infected women and the potential transmission during lactation cannot be excluded. Elective cesarean birth, on the other hand, can minimize the risk of transmission by reducing the newborn's contact with maternal infective secretions and the potential exposure to contractions associated with labor and 'micro' maternal–fetal blood transfusions during contractions. Many studies found a reduction in transmissions when a cesarean section was performed – up to 81% reduction in one study.[24] This is especially true after decreasing the viral load pharmacologically, although a substantial proportion of first- and second-born twins delivered in this way were found to be infected. Indeed, several researchers[25] believe that viral load reduction may have a greater implication on infection rate than the change in the mode of delivery. Several studies found discordant HIV infection in twins, but also found different quasispecies of the virus in the two sibs,[26] as well as a different immune response to the virus in the years following birth.[27]

These conflicting findings in twins highlight the controversial nature of this issue. Because of the rare occurrence of the combination of HIV and twins, better understanding is expected only with a large sample of cases.

Summary

Multiple pregnancies are associated with increased risk of infectious perinatal morbidity such as chorioamnionitis and endometritis, mainly as a result of more frequent PPROM and higher cesarean section rate. In addition, the uterine cavity is more likely to be accessed for diagnostic and therapeutic procedures during a multiple gestation. Finally, multiples are exposed to infections via the hematogenic route to the same extent as singletons. In contrast to singletons, a unique situation of discordant fetal infection may be seen in twins and higher-order multiples, whereby only the presenting gestational sac is exposed to ascending infection. This circumstance is an excellent opportunity to study the relative role of hematogenic and contact disease transmission during parturition in cases of blood-borne infections such as HIV.

REFERENCES

1. Mercer BM, Crocker LG, Pierce F, Sibai BM. Clinical characteristics and outcome of twin gestation complicated by preterm premature rupture of the membranes. *Am J Obstet Gynecol* 1993;168:1467–73.
2. Myles TD, Espinoza R, Meyer W, Bieniarz A. Preterm premature rupture of membranes: Comparison between twin and singleton gestations. *J Matern Fetal Med* 1997;6:159–63.
3. Bianco AT, Stone J, Lapinski R, Lockwood C, Lynch L, Berkowitz RL. The clinical outcome of preterm premature rupture of me branes in twin versus singleton pregnancies. *Am J Perinatol* 1996;13:135–8.
4. Mizrahi M, Furman B, Shoham-Vardi I, Vardi H, Maymon E, Mazor M. Perinatal outcome and peripartum complications in preterm singleton and twins deliveries: A comparative study. *Eur J Obstet Gynecol Reprod Biol* 1999;87:55–61.
5. Dinsmoor MJ, Bachman R, Haney EI, Goldstein M, Mackendrick W. Outcomes after expectant management of extremely preterm premature rupture of the membranes. *Am J Obstet Gynecol* 2004;190:183–7.
6. Conde-Agudelo A, Belizan JM, Lindmark G. Maternal morbidity and mortality associated with multiple gestations. *Obstet Gynecol* 2000;95:899–904.
7. Blickstein I. Cesarean section for all twins? *J Perinat Med* 2000; 28:169–74.
8. Suonio S, Huttunen M. Puerperal endometritis after abdominal twin delivery. *Acta Obstet Gynecol Scand* 1994;73:313–5.
9. Alran S, Sibony O, Luton D, *et al.* Maternal and neonatal outcome of 93 consecutive triplet pregnancies with 71% vaginal delivery. *Acta Obstet Gynecol Scand* 2004;83:554–9.
10. Alexander JM, Gilstrap LC, Cox SM, Ramin SM. The relationship of infection to method of delivery in twin pregnancy. *Am J Obstet Gynecol* 1997;177(5):1063–6.
11. Mazor M, Hershkovitz R, Ghezzi F, Maymon E, Horowitz S, Leiberman JR. Intraamniotic infection in patients with preterm labor and twin pregnancies. *Acta Obstet Gynecol Scand* 1996;75:624–7.
12. Phung DT, Blickstein I, Goldman RD, Machin GA, LoSasso RD, Keith LG. The Northwestern Twin Chorionicity Study: I. Discordant inflammatory findings that are related to chorionicity in presenting versus nonpresenting twins. *Am J Obstet Gynecol* 2002;186:1041–5.
13. Vogler C, Kohl S, Rosenberg HS. Cytomegalovirus infection and fetal death in a twin. A case report. *J Reprod Med* 1986;31:207–10.
14. Barlow KM, Mok JY. Dizygotic twins discordant for HIV and hepatitis C virus. *Arch Dis Child* 1993;68:507.
15. Park CL, Streicher H, Rothberg R. Transmission of human immunodeficiency virus from parents to only one dizygotic twin. *J Clin Microbiol* 1987;25:1119–21.
16. Young KK, Nelson RP, Good RA. Discordant human immunodeficiency virus infection in dizygotic twins detected by polymerase chain reaction. *Pediatr Infect Dis J* 1990;9:454–6.
17. Van der Straeten FMA, De Ketelaere K, Temmerman M. Delayed interval delivery in multiple pregnancies. *Eur J Obstet Gynecol Reprod Biol* 2001;99:85–9.
18. Zhang J, Hamilton B, Martin J, Trumble A. Delayed interval delivery and infant survival: A population based study. *Am J Obstet Gynecol* 2004;191:470–6.
19. Watson WJ, McNelis T. Delayed interval delivery: Infection is not an absolute contraindication. *Am J Perinatol* 1998;15:387–8.
20. Hoffman MK, Sciscione AC. Sepsis and multisystem organ failure in a woman attempting interval delivery in a triplet pregnancy: A case report. *J Reprod Med* 2004;49:387–8.
21. Fayad S, Bongain A, Holhfeld P, *et al.* Delayed delivery of second twin: A multicenter study of 35 cases. *Eur J Obstet Gynecol Reprod Biol* 2003;109:16–20.
22. Goedert JJ, Duliege AM, Amos CI, Felton S, Biggar RJ. High risk of HIV 1 infection for first born twins. The international registry of HIV exposed twins. *Lancet* 1991;338:1471–5.
23. Duliege AM, Amos CI, Felton S, Biggar RJ, Goedert JJ. Birth order, delivery route and concordance in the transmission of HIV 1 from mothers to twins. International registry of HIV exposed twins. *J Pediatr* 1995;126:625–32.
24. Biggar RJ, Cassol S, Kumwenda N, *et al.* The risk of HIV 1 infection in twin pairs born to infected mothers in Africa. *J Infect Dis* 2003;188:850–5.
25. Krasinski K, Turner BJ, Hauck WW, Fanning TR. HIV infection in a population based twin sample. *Pediatr AIDS HIV Infect* 1997;8:114–9.
26. Goedert JJ. Vertical transmission of HIV 1. Insights from studies of multiple pregnancies. *Acta Paediatr Suppl* 1997;421:56–9.
27. Gaggero A, Escanilla D, Larranaga C, Uribe P, Espejo R. Progression of viral infection in twins born from a mother infected with HIV. *Rev Med Child* 1995;123:1189–98.

SECTION XVIII

Labor and delivery

Section Editors: **W. Cohen and D. Weinstein**

174 The assessment of labor

W. R. Cohen and E. A. Friedman

Assisting women during their labor and delivery is a remarkable privilege and a weighty responsibility. To do it well requires a clear and comprehensive understanding of the physiology of labor and delivery, sensitivity to the emotional and physical needs of the parturient, fine clinical judgment, and good dexterity. The oversight of labor and delivery is among the most challenging and important endeavors undertaken by obstetricians and midwives. That oversight is important to all pregnancies; it takes on special importance when the prenatal course has been complicated by maternal or fetal compromise or when certain risk factors for adverse outcome are present. The management of labor often requires complex decision making, and combines the need for skillful physical examination and the interpretation of high technology data in a serial fashion. Although most labors will progress normally, the sapient observer will be able to distinguish those that can benefit from some medical intervention.

From the perspective of the obstetrician, a finite number of clinical features of labor are readily determinable that can potentially help establish whether a labor is normal. These are the frequency, intensity, and duration of uterine contractions, the effacement and degree of dilatation of the cervix, and the descent of the fetus through the birth canal. In addition, related details about pelvic architecture, fetal position, attitude, and cranial molding can be ascertained, and assessment of fetal oxygenation and the presence of infection carried out. Information about all of these factors must be integrated and interpreted periodically during labor to assess the probability that a safe vaginal delivery can occur. When that probability is low, the obstetric attendant will opt for cesarean delivery as the best alternative for mother and fetus.

While uterine contractions are of obvious importance in labor, information about the contractile pattern of the uterus is relatively little information as to whether the labor is normal or not.[1,2] We recognize, of course, that neither cervical dilatation nor fetal descent is possible without a sequence of strong coordinated uterine contractions. Nevertheless, because we are unable to utilize specific information about the nature of the contractility pattern to assess the labor clinically, we must focus on other features to help determine whether or not the labor is normal. In this regard, two features of labor, cervical dilatation and fetal descent, constitute the essential functional components of the work necessary for the pregnant woman and her uterus to achieve in order for delivery to occur.

During normal labor rather characteristic, reproducible patterns in the course of progressive cervical dilatation and fetal descent occur.[3–5] These characteristics have allowed the development of a practical tool for following the course of an individual parturient's labor and thus provide objective evidence for determining if her labor is normal. Furthermore, this approach has permitted analysis of labor data derived from large numbers of patients to help elucidate the types and causes of abnormalities that arise, the efficacy of various therapies for each of them, and the prognosis for mother and fetus according to the type of labor pattern and treatment given.[3] This information in turn can be used by obstetric attendants to help manage individual patients optimally.

The labor graph

A pictorial representation of the labor process can be obtained by using a simple square-ruled graphic template (Figure 174.1). The horizontal axis of the graph represents time elapsed during the patient's labor, in hours. The origin is the onset of labor, although this is not always precisely determinable. To avoid confusion or difficulty in this regard, use the pragmatic criterion of the time when the patient perceived the onset of regular uterine contractions. Defining the onset of labor in this way avoids the dilemma of having to identify labor more arbitrarily on the basis of the cervix having achieved a certain degree of effacement or dilatation.

The vertical axis of the graph is divided into 10 equal segments. Two scales are designated, cervical dilatation and fetal station. Each division on the dilatation scale represents a centimeter of dilatation,

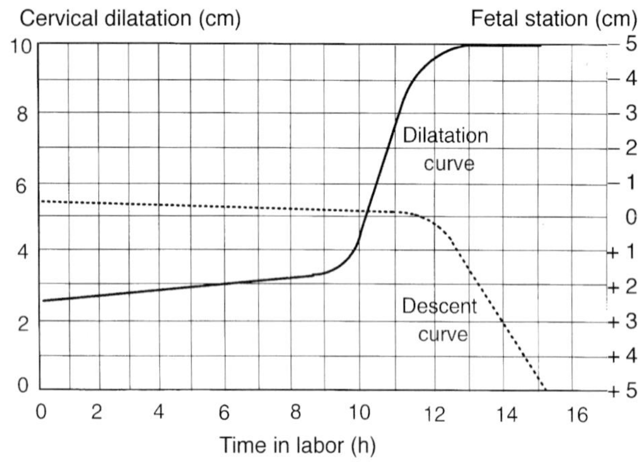

Figure 174.1 Characteristic patterns of normal cervical dilatation and fetal descent as depicted graphically against elapsed time.

ranging from 0 (closed cervix) to 10 cm (full cervical dilatation). The choice of 10 cm for full cervical dilatation is a practical approximation because the cervix will only dilate sufficiently to permit the fetal presenting part to traverse it. Since most term-sized fetal heads are approximately 9.5 cm in diameter this number would be more accurate, but in most cases it makes little practical importance. However, for preterm or very large fetuses upward or downward scales of adjustment would represent the true measure of cervical dilatation needed to accommodate passage of an individual fetal head.

Each division of the fetal station scale depicts a centimeter of station, defined as the level of the forward leading edge of the fetal presenting part with reference to the plane of the ischial spines. The range extends from –5 (5 cm above the referent plane, or about the level of the true inlet of the maternal pelvis) through station 0 (the referent plane of the ischial spines) to station +5 (5 cm caudad to the plane of the ischial spines, or the station at which crowning of the fetal head occurs at the vaginal outlet). The use of this system provides an accurate means to assess the rate of descent of the fetus through the birth canal.

One constructs the patterns of cervical dilatation and fetal descent by simply entering each clinical observation at the appropriate place on the graph (Figure 174.1). As additional data are collected from the sequential examinations done during labor, each dilatation and station observation is entered at its appropriate position. In this way the patterns of dilatation and descent are traced and observed prospectively while the patient's labor is evolving, providing a simple, utilitarian, visual tool to evaluate labor progress in real time. The addition of other pertinent information to the labor graph can also be helpful. Thus, the relationship of dilatation and descent to events such as rupture of fetal membranes, analgesic or anesthetic administration, or the effects of oxytocin can be visualized readily.

The graphic method of labor analysis should be mastered and employed by all who care for women during labor. This recommendation notwithstanding, it is obvious that labor curves cannot be used in a clinical vacuum. They provide information vital to clinical decision making, but which must be integrated with other obstetric data. For example, information obtained from the labor curves must be assessed in the context of that derived concerning cephalopelvic relationships, pelvic architecture, effects of medications, state of fetal oxygenation and maternal condition in order to make the most enlightened clinical judgments.

Normal labor pattern

While labor may be properly considered to begin with the onset of regular uterine contractions that lead ultimately to cervical dilatation and descent of the fetus through the birth canal, biochemical and biophysical preparation of the cervix and uterus begin well in advance of that time. These changes are most evident clinically in the maturation (ripening) of the cervix and the development of the lower uterine segment, as well as the increasing frequency and intensity of Braxton–Hicks contractions.[6,7] These events are, to a variable degree, completed before the onset of labor. The extent of this prelabor maturation governs the duration of the *latent phase* of labor. The latent phase, which commences with the onset of labor, is characterized by little or no cervical dilatation for some time despite the presence of uterine contractions that may be quite strong. Notwithstanding the absence of dramatic changes in dilatation, many important events are taking place in the cervix during this portion of labor. Biochemical modifications of the connective tissue and ground substance occur, extensions of the process of cervical maturation or ripening that, as noted, often has begun prior to the onset of labor. This breakdown of dense connective tissue within the cervix results in a clinically palpable softening and an increase in compliance that are necessary preliminaries to the more active dilatation that will occur later.

The latent phase is followed in due course under normal circumstances by an *active phase*. Together, latent and active phases comprise the *first stage* of labor. The active phase is characterized normally by rapid and progressive change in cervical dilatation, continuing in a linear fashion without interruption until it ends at the onset of the second stage, when the cervix has retracted around the maximum diameter of the presenting part and is said to be fully or completely dilated. The beginning of the active phase can be identified on the graphic pattern by the upswing of the dilatation curve. Interestingly, this generally occurs without any discernible objective change in the uterine contractile pattern and often without a subjective change in the parturient's perception of her contractions.

It is during the active phase that most of the cervical dilatation is achieved. Although on average the active phase begins when the cervix has reached about 4 cm dilatation, it often starts with a smaller or larger dilatation; the degree of dilatation cannot, therefore, be used as the sole indicator that the labor is in the active phase.[3,4,8] Some demonstration that the rate of dilatation has accelerated is necessary.

The active phase is divisible into three recognizable components. It starts with an initial acceleration phase, followed by a central linear phase of maximum slope, and is concluded by a terminal deceleration phase. The acceleration phase represents the transition from the nearly flat slope of the latent phase to the rapid dilatation of the phase of maximum slope. The latter typically traces a straight line in the labor graph proceeding quickly to about 8–9 cm when, at the onset of the deceleration phase, the curve appears to slow down. There is no true slowing as the name implies, but rather an artifactual appearance of slowing of cervical dilatation just prior to the second stage. The cervix continues in fact to dilate at the same rate, but as it retracts around the presenting part the edges of the cervix are moving more cephalad than laterally; hence the lateral change in dilatation measured clinically and plotted on the curve slows. Uterine contractions often increase in frequency, intensity and duration at about this time, and simultaneously the patient's perception of discomfort from the contractions is often markedly enhanced. This portion of labor has sometimes been called transition.

The curve of fetal descent is likewise divisible into phases similar to, but not completely congruent with those of the dilatation curve. It also begins with a latent phase starting at the onset of labor, but the latent phase of the descent pattern does not end at the same time as the beginning of the active phase of dilatation. It continues thereafter, not concluding until the dilatation curve has completed almost all of its active phase. The active portion of the descent curve generally begins somewhere at or beyond the midpoint of the phase of maximum slope of dilatation; it ordinarily reaches its own maximum slope at the onset of the deceleration phase of dilatation and no later than the beginning of the second stage.

Once the active phase of descent begins, one can expect fetal descent to continue without interruption until the presenting part encounters the pelvic floor. While the descent pattern is usually represented as hyperbolic in shape, it does have a deceleration phase – more correctly, a perineal phase-which is too short in the usual clinical situation to be apparent in the graphic pattern. The constant interrelationship between the dilatation curve and the descent curve is an important clinical diagnostic feature to aid in disclosing the presence of labor abnormalities.

Abnormal labor patterns

The analysis of cervical dilatation and fetal descent patterns in large numbers of cases allowed a detailed analysis that provided information about the statistical distributions of various aspects of the cervical dilatation or fetal descent vs. time relationships. Thus, the mean, central tendency, the 5th and 95th percentile confidence intervals, and the range of each measured duration and slope could be determined. Limits of normal for each of the definable components were determined based on these confidence intervals (Table 174.1).[3–5,9]

Table 174.1 Limits of normal labor pattern components

Component	Nulliparas*	Multiparas
Latent phase duration (h)	20	14
Maximum slope of dilatation (cm/h)	1.2	1.5
Deceleration phase duration (h)	3	1
Maximum slope of descent (cm/h)	1.0	2.0

*Includes parous women who have never had a vaginal delivery[46]

Labor disorders may be categorized into three groups, based on similarities in their attributes and prognostic implications: prolonged latent phase; protraction disorders (of dilatation and descent); and arrest disorders (arrest of dilatation or descent, prolonged deceleration phase, and failure of descent) (Table 174.2; Figure 174.2).

A *prolonged latent phase*, which often reflects inadequate prelabor cervical ripening or some other factor inhibiting progression into the active phase, is diagnosed when the duration of the latent phase exceeds 20 h in the nullipara and 14 h in the multipara.[10,11] A *protracted active phase* of dilatation and *protracted descent* are diagnosed when dilatation or descent occur in a linear progressive manner during their active phase, but at a rate below the critical limit of normal (the 5th percentile derived from a series of labors uninfluenced by medical intervention).[10,12,13] An *arrest of dilatation* is identified when, having entered the active phase, dilatation ceases for a period of at least 2 h.[10,14] (Although this is the standard definition, some data indicate that 1 h of arrest of dilatation is sufficient to make a diagnosis.)[15] The analogous disorder of descent, *arrest of descent*, can be diagnosed when active descent has ceased for a period of 1 h.[10,16]

A special kind of dilatation abnormality, a *prolonged deceleration phase*, reflects a delay in the terminal portion of dilatation and is diagnosed when the duration of deceleration of the dilatation curve exceeds 3 h in nulliparas or 1 h in multiparas. If expected descent does not begin when normally anticipated, i.e. during the later portion of dilatation or by the onset of the second stage, a *failure of descent* can be said to exist.[3]

Table 174.2 Abnormal labor patterns as defined by dilatation and descent curves

Dysfunction	Nulliparas	Multiparas
Prolonged latent phase	>20 h duration	>14 h duration
Arrest of dilatation	2 h without progress in active phase	2 h without progress in active phase
Arrest of descent	1 h without progress after active descent has begun	1 h without progress after active descent has begun
Prolonged deceleration phase	>3 h duration	>1 h duration
Failure of descent	No descent by deceleration phase or second stage onset	No descent by deceleration phase or second stage onset
Protracted dilatation	< 1.2 cm/h slope	< 1.5 cm/h slope
Protracted descent	< 1.0 cm/h slope	< 2.0 cm/h slope

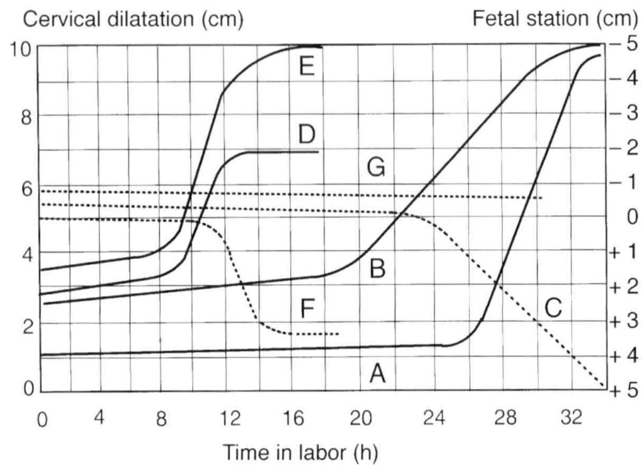

Figure 174.2 Labor disorders that can be identified on the basis of deviations from the expected normal durations, slopes, and patterns of the dilatation and descent curves are illustrated graphically: (A) prolonged latent phase; (B) protracted dilatation; (C) protracted descent; (D) arrest of dilatation; (E) prolonged deceleration phase; (F) arrest of descent; (G) failure of descent.

Prolonged latent phase

Labors with the descriptively named prolonged latent phase are characterized by little or no change in cervical dilatation despite many hours of regular uterine contractions. The differentiation between a prolonged latent phase and false labor (which underlies about 10% of diagnoses of prolonged latent phase) can seldom be made with any degree of certainty, except in hindsight. The latent phase can be prolonged by the administration of narcotics or sedative agents for pain relief. Peridural anesthesia has the capacity to prolong the latent phase considerably, probably because uterine contractility is more easily inhibited by analgesia and anesthesia during this time of labor. Frequently (nearly 20% of those with this labor disorder) the cervix has failed to achieve the essential prelabor maturation and preparation expected. That is, the cervix is long, closed and resistant, rather than more favorably soft, effaced and partially dilated. In such cases, one can expect the latent phase will take a long time to modify the cervix in anticipation of later active dilatation.

While the diagnosis of prolonged latent phase sometimes lacks precision because of the difficulty of ascertaining the exact time of labor onset, the simple recognition of the fact that the latent phase may be normally quite long is of considerable importance in the management of labor. Prolonged latent phase *per se* does not appear to confer an increased need for operative delivery and is not a predictor of more serious active phase disorders strongly associated with the need for cesarean delivery. Moreover, its presence does not appear to increase perinatal morbidity.[17–19] Ignorance about the normal course of the latent phase sometimes leads nevertheless to unnecessary cesarean section under the erroneous assumption that continuous progress should be expected in all phases of labor, or that very long labors are always abnormal. Concern is sometimes raised during the latent phase about the station of the fetal head. A fetal head floating above the pelvic brim in early labor is a risk factor for cesarean delivery later in labor[20]; but this is true whether or not the latent phase is prolonged.

Treatment of a prolonged latent phase may consist of active efforts to stimulate uterine contractility or heavy maternal sedation (Figure 174.3). Both are equally effective. The conversion to active phase labor generally occurs within 3 h. The choice between uterine stimulation and therapeutic rest for treatment of prolonged latent phase depends on the clinical situation. Concerns exist about transient fetal deoxygenation occurring with some kinds of narcotic drugs,[21] but no adverse outcomes after this kind of treatment for prolonged latent phase have been recognized. The approach does not seem to be associated with an increased rate of newborn depression, although if the mother delivers unexpectedly early a narcotic antagonist should be available for

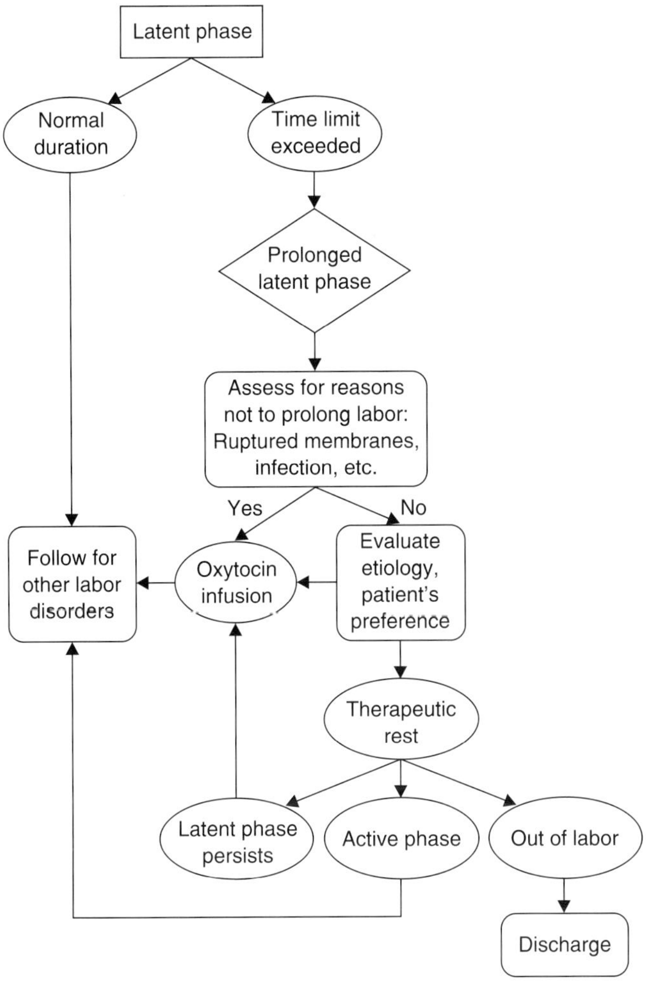

Figure 174.3 Management of the latent phase of labor. Prolonged latent phase is diagnosed when more than 20 h in a nullipara or more than 14 h in a multipara have elapsed. Oxytocin stimulation and narcotic sedation are equally effective treatments, and are chosen according to patient preference and the presence of factors that militate against prolonging the labor.

administration to the newborn. Whenever a fetal or maternal condition exists that could be worsened by prolonging labor, active intervention should be used, unless there is a contraindication to the administration of oxytocin. Similarly, when there is a reason to minimize the duration of labor (e.g. infection, pre-eclampsia) it is reasonable to intervene in the latent phase even before it reaches the limit of normal. The presence of prolonged ruptured membranes, preeclampsia, early intrauterine infection or certain acute maternal diseases thus favor an approach of active stimulation of labor. The mother's wishes should be taken into consideration as well. Some prefer oxytocin stimulation; others welcome the interposition of some rest into an arduous and stressful experience.

Prolonged latent phase is almost always innocuous with regard to its potential impact on mother and fetus. It responds to treatment in most cases (about 85%), and affected patients have no increased disposition to develop more serious labor aberrations. The fetuses of women whose labor is complicated by prolonged latent phase generally do well and can be expected to suffer no adverse consequences.[11,17–19]

Protraction and arrest disorders

The obstetric conditions associated with protraction and arrest disorders are similar but the therapeutic approaches to them differ (Figure 174.4).[10,13,14] Both dysfunctions are observed in association with cephalopelvic disproportion, malpositions, excessive sedation or anesthesia, and uterine infection.[3,22,23] Myometrial contractile dysfunction, which may be primary or a consequence of the preceding factors, may also cause or contribute to active phase dysfunction. Evaluation of a parturient with an active phase labor abnormality requires a search for associated, etiologic, or predisposing conditions. Careful clinical cephalopelvimetry is useful to determine the likelihood of disproportion. Assessment of factors such as pelvic architecture, fetal position and attitude, the degree of molding of cranial bones, and of dynamic aspects of cephalopelvic relationships allows a reasonable judgment to be made about the probability of disproportion. In addition, vaginal examination during the peak of a contraction in advanced cervical dilatation with gentle fundal pressure applied (the Müller–Hillis maneuver) provides useful assessment of the degree of descent, rotational tendencies, and attitudinal changes likely to occur with subsequent contractions.[24] Malpositions occur commonly, and can probably cause or, at times be a consequence of, active phase disorders. Labors affected by a protraction disorder tend to be sensitive to the inhibitory effects of sedation and anesthesia; thus, these factors may aggravate an already existing functional abnormality, rather than cause it.

If cephalopelvic disproportion seems unlikely and position of the fetal head is normal, assessment of uterine contractility, a search for chorioamnionitis, and evaluation for the presence of drugs or other factors that might inhibit labor are necessary. The risk of dysfunctional active phase labor may be increased in older mothers,[3,25] but diagnosis and therapy should not be influenced by maternal age.

No form of therapy has been shown effective in correcting the slow rates of dilatation and descent in protraction disorders that arise *de novo*. No matter how much one may attempt to encourage contractility with oxytocin, it does not appear to alter the dilatory course of labor significantly. Amniotomy, though it may be advisable in order to provide access for direct fetal heart rate monitoring to assess fetal oxygenation optimally in the presence of a protraction disorder, may actually result in superimposition of an arrest disorder.

Given the absence of benefit from ecbolic agents and their potential harm, they are best avoided for treating patients with a protraction disorder. This leaves very little in our therapeutic armamentarium.

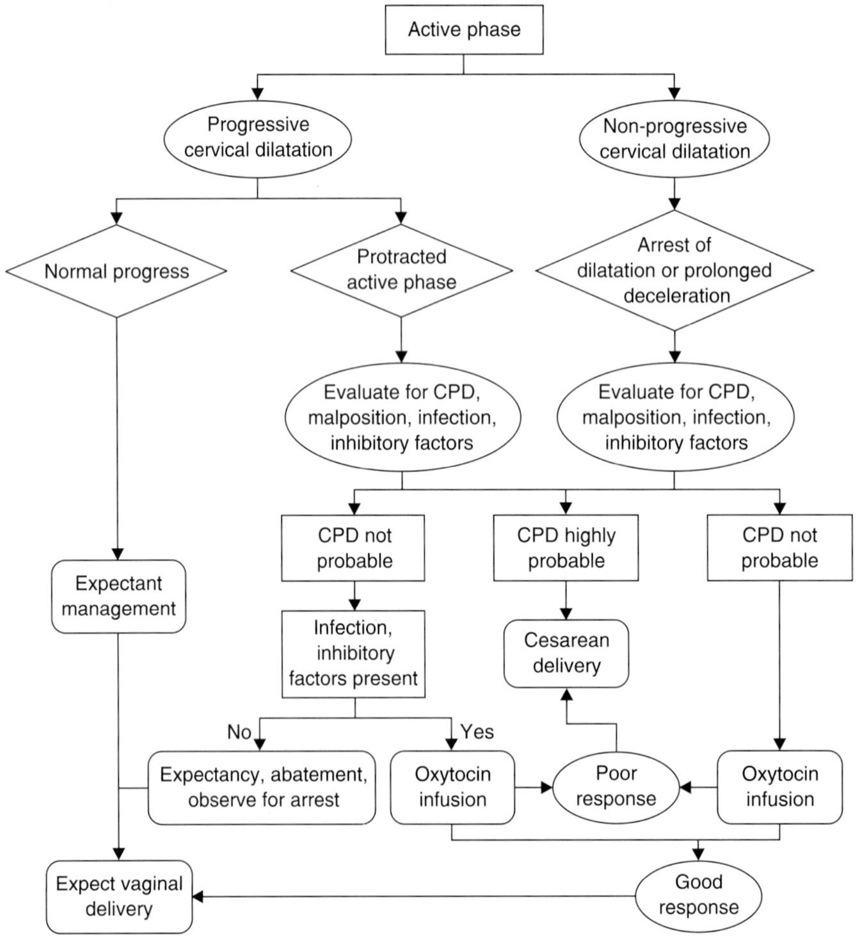

Figure 174.4 Management of the active phase of labor. Active phase abnormalities are frequently associated with cephalopelvic disproportion (CPD), and thorough clinical cephalopelvimetry is therefore important. A good response to oxytocin in an arrest disorder is defined as one in which the postarrest slope is equal to or greater than the prearrest slope. In protraction disorders it is when the rate of dilatation or descent becomes normal.

We recommend that, once the condition is diagnosed (and cephalopelvic determined to be unlikely), the patient be advised of the nature of her condition and the fact that the labor is likely to be quite prolonged and uncomfortable. Women with a protraction disorder need intense psychologic and social support coupled, when possible, with the avoidance of medications likely to retard progress further. Thus, expectancy and careful observation for adverse maternal or fetal development are essential. Oxytocin may be of therapeutic value if the protraction disorder appears to have resulted from some inhibitory influence. For example, if the protraction dysfunction was provoked by conduction anesthesia or by drugs that have the potential to suppress contractility, oxytocin may override these inhibitory influences and restore normal dilatation. One randomized trial suggested that oxytocin stimulation increased the rate of dilatation in what was termed 'primary dysfunctional labor', a diagnosis that probably included protraction disorders; but the degree of enhancement was not documented, and many patients responded to placebo infusion.[26] The role of epidural anesthesia in altering the course of labor is controversial. The best information supports the idea that a properly administered epidural (i.e. one using proper anesthetic or analgesic drugs in appropriate concentrations and achieving an optimal level of sensory block) probably has little or no influence on the first stage of labor.[27,28] It may, however, lengthen the second stage because the sensation of the urge to push is blunted and bearing-down may be less effective because of motor blockade.

The maternal and fetal outcome after protraction disorders is not optimal. A substantial number, at least 25–30%, will require cesarean delivery because of presumed cephalopelvic disproportion. Cesarean section should also be considered whenever there is any evidence of irremediable fetal distress or when signs of chorioamnionitis develop at a time when vaginal delivery is not likely to occur soon. If an arrest disorder should supervene, the prognosis for vaginal delivery worsens because disproportion becomes increasingly likely.

Fetal prognosis depends principally on the method of delivery that follows the protracted labor. If delivery can be achieved spontaneously by the vaginal route or by cesarean section, there is no discernible difference in outcome from that of infants born after normal labor patterns, provided there is no intervening factor placing the fetus in jeopardy. Operative vaginal delivery, however, carries a worse prognosis for the fetus. There is a threefold or greater increase in perinatal mortality associated with both low forceps and midforceps delivery.[17] A long-term deleterious impact on speech, language, hearing, and I.Q. also occur with increased frequency.[18,19]

Arrest disorders are arguably the most important labor aberrations because of their very common association with cephalopelvic disproportion.[14–16,22,29] When one or more of these abnormalities occurs, there is at least a 40–50% likelihood that cesarean delivery will be necessary because of disproportion. The treatment of arrest disorders is uterotonic stimulation, unless there is evidence of abnormal fetal heart rate patterns or compelling indications of disproportion. It is important to remember that progress can be achieved by oxytocin even in the face of major degrees of disproportion. This means that one cannot use oxytocin infusion as a clinically reliable 'test of labor' to demonstrate the presence or absence of disproportion. It becomes essential, therefore to ensure that disproportion is ruled out as best as possible by evaluating the maternal pelvic architecture and capacity, the fetal head dimensions, molding, cranial bone overlapping, and the aggregate of cephalopelvic relationships. When using the Müller–Hillis maneuver, if the head is felt to advance 1–2 cm, often in association with appropriate rotation and flexion, one can be confidently assured that no disproportion exists at that level of the pelvis. If the head is fixed instead, with no compensatory room palpable around it to permit additional descent without extreme molding, this represents clinically evident cephalopelvic disproportion. In that case, cesarean delivery would be acceptable with no further trial of labor. When disproportion has been reasonably excluded, oxytocin stimulation can be expected to correct the arrest and result in vaginal delivery in due course. If an error has been made – that is, if one has failed to detect disproportion that actually does exist – the subsequent pattern of dilatation and descent will usually serve as a telltale indicator. The postarrest slope of the curve (the measurements of the rate of progress achieved after oxytocin is begun) should be at least as great as the prearrest slope; if not, special care must be taken to reevaluate the maternal pelvis and its relation to the fetal head before allowing labor to proceed.

Patients treated with oxytocin who have normal postarrest slopes can be expected to deliver spontaneously without further complication. Instrumental delivery is best avoided in these cases because of the adverse impact it may have on the fetus. Overall, fetal prognosis is poorer after labor complicated by an arrest disorder. Although this can probably be minimized by adequate fetal surveillance, careful assessment for cephalopelvic disproportion, and use of the postarrest slope for verification of adequate pelvic capacity, results are still not quite optimal. Outcomes are worsened when the delivery procedure that follows the arrest disorder is low forceps or midforceps. Comparably adverse long-term results are also seen with increased frequencies of abnormal cognitive test results and lowered intelligence quotients. These data suggest that there may be an intrinsic adverse impact from the labor abnormalities that constitute the arrest disorders, and that this deleterious influence is enhanced by attempts to effect delivery by the vaginal route.[17–19]

When oxytocin is given for the treatment of an arrest disorder, about 85% of those patients who respond with dilatation that resumes at or above the prearrest rate of dilatation will have done so within about 3 h of having the infusion initiated.[3] Most such patients will eventually deliver vaginally without complication. If there has been no progress, or the new slope of dilatation is lower than the prearrest slope, it may generally be assumed that cesarean delivery is necessary. More prolonged oxytocin administration should be used only when the clinical situation suggests a high likelihood of a safe vaginal delivery. In some women arrest disorders resolve without the need for oxytocin. This may occur spontaneously, or as a result of awaiting abatement of inhibitory factors such as excess anesthesia or infection.

The goal of oxytocin infusion should be individualized, but should generally be the achievement of firm contractions (about 50 mmHg in amplitude) that occur every 2–3 min. Use of a quantitative measure of contractility, such as Montivideo Units is sometimes helpful; but the relation between contractility assessed in this way and the likelihood of change in cervical dilatation and descent has not been defined clearly.

Many obstetricians use artificial rupture of the fetal membranes as a means to accelerate labor and, specifically, to treat arrest disorders. This is based on the widely held notion that rupture of the membranes stimulates labor progress. The evidence for the latter is controversial. While rupture of membranes can certainly induce labor in some women, it is less clear that the progress of an already-established active phase can be augmented by rupturing membranes. Such an effect, if it exists, must be modest.[30–32] There are probably some situations in which rupture of membranes in an arrest disorder can effect change. The few patients who do respond do so promptly. There is, nevertheless, a virtue of ruptured membranes in the presence of an arrest disorder. It allows direct fetal heart rate monitoring, providing the most precise data for heart rate pattern interpretation. This is of importance because of evidence that dysfunctional labors may predispose to abnormal fetal heart rate patterns.[33]

Also of potential use in the presence of arrest or protraction disorders is changing maternal position.

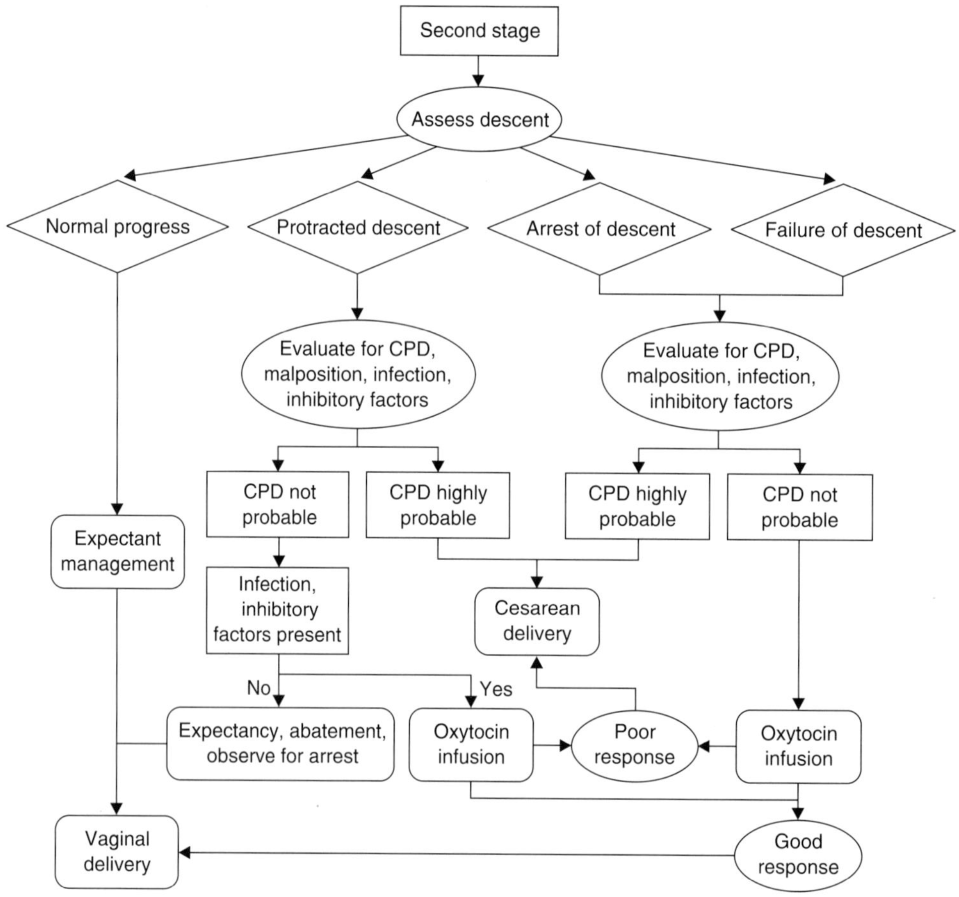

Figure 174.5 Management of the second stage of labor. Progress is measured by the rate of descent rather than by elapsed time. Fetal position, station, attitude and cranial molding should be assessed at each examination. A good response to oxytocin in an arrest of descent is defined as a postarrest slope equal to or greater than the prearrest slope of descent. In protracted descent it is when the rate of descent is normalized. CPD, cephalopelvic disproportion.

Using upright postures (squatting, standing, etc.) may benefit some labors by altering pelvic diameters or increasing uterine contractility.[34–38] While convincing objective proof of the efficacy of position changes is lacking, they can cause no harm, and may do some good. They should be tried.

A prolonged deceleration phase has the same associations and etiologies as arrest disorders, and should be assessed and treated in much the same manner. It is of particular importance because of its strong association with disproportion,[3] as well as with an increased risk of shoulder dystocia if vaginal delivery occurs.[39] It is frequently accompanied or followed by failure of descent, and the combination of these disorders makes safe vaginal delivery unlikely.

The second stage

The *second stage* of labor, which extends from complete cervical dilatation to delivery of the fetus, involves the major portion of fetal descent and rotational movements (Figure 174.5). The efficiency of the descent mechanism is assessed by measuring the rate of descent of the presenting part through the birth canal. This is preferable to judging the second stage solely by its length. In fact, second stage duration has little significant influence on neonatal or maternal morbidity or mortality,[40–43] except when it is exceptionally long (more than 3 h).[42] In that case the very high frequency of cesarean delivery has an effect on maternal outcome.

The rate at which active descent occurs is governed by several factors, including uterine contractile force; voluntary maternal expulsive efforts; fetal size, position and attitude; the deformability of the fetal head; pelvic architecture; and the characteristics of the pelvic of pelvic floor. Each should be assessed clinically to help judge the likelihood of vaginal delivery. In this regard, all obstetricians should be capable of performing a thorough and systematic examination of the pelvis and the cephalopelvic relationships. Information from such an evaluation is necessary to make informed judgments about delivery.[40] For example, an arrest of descent often occurs in the midpelvis with a posterior position of the occiput. This may be an entirely appropriate position in a large pelvis with anthropoid features. In such a case, if the sacrum is inclined posteriorly and the sidewalls parallel and minimal fetal cranial molding, the arrest may be due to factors other than disproportion. Continuing a trial of labor might be appropriate. If, however, the arrest occurs in a pelvis with a flattened sacral curve (preventing further descent as a posterior) and a narrow interspinous dimension or convergent sidewalls (resisting anterior rotation), with considerable overlapping of the cranial plates evident, safe vaginal delivery may be far less likely and cesarean section a reasonable option without further labor.

Precipitate labor

While most concerns about dysfunctional labor have focused on abnormally slow or arrested parturition, excessively rapid labor may also have important consequences. *Precipitate labor* has been defined in two ways: labors that are exceptionally short (usually < 3 h); labors in which there is abnormally rapid cervical dilatation or fetal descent. There is greater virtue in the latter approach because it excludes labors that are short simply because the latent phase is short (usually related to advanced cervical ripening prior to labor onset). There is evidence that the excess morbidity that can accrue to fetuses exposed to very short labors (meconium passage, abnormal heart rate patterns and low Apgar scores) affects predominantly those with precipitate dilatation or descent.[44] These are defined by rates greater than 5 cm/h in nulliparas and 10 cm/h in multiparas.[3] Of course, spontaneous precipitate labor can generally be neither predicted nor prevented. When oxytocin is being used to stimulate contractility, however, it is important to avoid provoking excessive uterine contractility forces leading to high rates of dilatation and descent.

Conclusion

The approach to the assessment of labor outlined above requires a disciplined style of evaluation and treatment. This allows a considerable degree of evidence-based clinical objectivity to be combined with clinical art to yield optimal results for both mother and fetus. If we aspire to a uniform standard of nomenclature, we will enhance communication, permit objective study of labor, and maximize outcomes.[45]

Oxytocin or therapeutic rest may be used with equivalent benefit for prolonged latent phase. Expectancy and support are most appropriate for protraction disorders and oxytocin stimulation is best for arrest disorders, provided that cephalopelvic relationships have been judged adequate. If there is a high likelihood of disproportion based on clinical examination associated with either a protraction or arrest disorder, cesarean section is recommended as the option most compatible with safety. Such decisions must always be made in the context of assessing all available pertinent clinical data, with the parturient's full understanding of the situation, and with her participation in decision making when appropriate. The obstetrician cannot always guarantee a good outcome for every labor; but through application of the principles of assessment outlined in this chapter, one can maximize diagnostic accuracy and patient safety in the context of a satisfying and emotionally enriching birth experience.

REFERENCES

1. Seitchik J, Chatkoff ML. Intrauterine pressure wave form characteristics in hypocontractile labor before and after oxytocin administration. *Am J Obstet Gynecol* 1975;123:426–34.
2. Shulman J, Romney S. Variability of uterine contractions in normal human parturition. *Obstet Gynecol* 1970;36:215–21.
3. Friedman EA. *Labor: Clinical Evaluation and Management*, 2nd edn. New York: Appleton-Century-Crofts, 1978.
4. Friedman EA. Graphic analysis of labor. *Am J Obstet Gynecol* 1954;68:1568–75.
5. Friedman EA. Primigravid labor: A graphicostatistical analysis. *Obstet Gynecol* 1956;8:691–703.
6. Ekman G, Malmström A, Uldbjerg N, Ulmsten U. Cervical collagen: An important regulator of cervical function in term labor. *Obstet Gynecol* 1986;67:633–6.
7. Osmers RGW, Andelmann-Grill BC, Rath W, Stuhlsatz HW, Tschesche H. Biochemical events in cervical ripening dilatation during pregnancy and parturition. *J Obstet Gynecol* 1995;21:185–94.
8. Peisner DB, Rosen MG. Transition from latent to active labor. *Obstet Gynecol* 1985;68:448–51.
9. Friedman EA, Sachtleben MR. Dysfunctional labor: VII. A comprehensive program for diagnosis, evaluation, and management. *Obstet Gynecol* 1965;25:844–7.
10. Friedman EA, Sachtleben MR. Dysfunctional labor: VI. Abnormal progress in the multipara. *Obstet Gynecol* 1963;22:478–94.
11. Friedman EA, Sachtleben MR. Dysfunctional labor: I. Prolonged latent phase in the nullipara. *Obstet Gynecol* 1961;17:135–48.
12. Friedman EA, Sachtleben MR. Dysfunctional labor: II. Protracted active phase dilatation in the nullipara. *Obstet Gynecol* 1961;17:566–78.
13. Friedman EA, Sachtleben MR. Station of the fetal presenting part: V. Protracted descent patterns. *Obstet Gynecol* 1970;36:558–67.
14. Friedman EA, Sachtleben MR. Dysfunctional labor: III. Secondary arrest of dilatation in the nullipara. *Obstet Gynecol* 1962;19:576–91.
15. Bottoms SF, Sokol RJ, Rosen MG. Short arrest of cervical dilatation: A risk for maternal/fetal/infant morbidity. *Am J Obstet Gynecol* 1981;140:108–16.
16. Friedman EA, Sachtleben MR. Station of the fetal presenting part: VI. Arrest of descent in nulliparas. *Obstet Gynecol* 1976;47:129–32.
17. Friedman EA, Sachtleben MR. High risk labor. *J Reprod Med* 1971;7:52–6.
18. Friedman EA, Sachtleben MR, Bresky PA. Dysfunctional labor: XII. Long-term effects on infant. *Am J Obstet Gynecol* 1977;127:779–83.
19. Friedman EA, Neff RK. *Labor and Delivery. Impact on Offspring.* Littleton, MA: PSG Publishing Co., 1987:65–145.
20. Murphy K, Shah L, Cohen WR. Labor and delivery in nulliparas who present with an unengaged fetal head. *J Perinatol* 1998;18:122–25.
21. Baxi L, Petrie RH, James LS. Human fetal oxygenation ($tcPO_2$), heart rate variability, and uterine activity following maternal administration of meperidine. *J Perinat Med* 1988;16:23–30.
22. Handa VL, Laros RK. Active-phase arrest in labor: Predictors of cesarean delivery in a nulliparous population. *Obstet Gynecol* 1993;81:758–63.
23. Satin AJ, Maberry MC, Leveno KJ, Sherman ML, Kline DM. Chorioamnionitis: A harbinger of dystocia. *Obstet Gynecol* 1992;79:913–15.
24. Hillis DS. Diagnosis of contracted pelvis. *Illinois Med J* 1938;74:131–4.
25. Cohen WR, Newman L, Friedman EA. Frequency of labor disorders with advancing maternal age. *Obstet Gynecol* 1980;55:414–16.
26. Cardozo L, Pearce JM. Oxytocin in active phase abnormalities of labor: A randomized study. *Obstet Gynecol* 1990;75:152–7.
27. Zhang J, Yancey MK, Klebanoff MA, Schwarz J, Schweitzer D. Does epidural analgesia prolong labor and increase the risk of

cesarean delivery? A natural experiment. *Am J Obstet Gynecol* 2001;185:128–34.
28. Studd JWW, Crawford JS, Duignan NM, Rowbotham CJF, Hughes AO. The effect of lumbar epidural analgesia on the rate of cervical dilatation and the outcome of labour of spontaneous onset. *Br J Obstet Gynaecol* 1980;87:1015–21.
29. Friedman EA. Trial of labor: Formulation, application, and retrospective clinical evaluation. *Obstet Gynecol* 1957;10:1–9.
30. Laros RK, Work BA, Witting WC. Amniotomy during the active phase of labor. *Obstet Gynecol* 1972;39:702–4.
31. Friedman EA, Sachtleben MR. Amniotomy and the course of labor. *Obstet Gynecol* 1963;22:755–70.
32. Van Praagh I, Hendricks CH. The effect of amniotomy during labor in multiparas. *Obstet Gynecol* 1964;24:258–65.
33. Porreco RP, Boehm FH, Dildy GA, *et al.* Dystocia in nulliparous patients monitored with fetal pulse oximetry. *Am J Obstet Gynecol* 2004;190:113–17.
34. McKay SR. Maternal position during labor and birth. *J Obstet Gynecol Neonat Nurs* 1980;9:288–91.
35. McManus TJ, Calder AA. Upright positions and the efficiency of labor. *Lancet* 1978;1:72–4.
36. Russell JGB. Moulding of the pelvic outlet. *J Obstet Gynaecol Br Commonw* 1969;76:817–20.
37. Downe S, Gerrett D, Renfrew MJ. A prospective randomized trial of the effect of position in the passive second stage of labour on birth outcome in nulliparous women using epidural analgesia. *Midwifery* 2004;20:157–64.
38. Bodner-Adler,B, Bodner K, Kimberger O, Lazanov P, Husslein P, Mayerhofer K. Women's position during labour: Influence on maternal and neonatal outcome. *Wien Klin Wochenschr* 2003;115:720–3.
39. Hopwood HG. Shoulder dystocia: Fifteen years' experience in a community hospital. *Am J Obstet Gynecol* 1982;144:162–6.
40. Cohen WR. The pelvic division of labor. In Cohen WR, Acker DB, Friedman EA, eds. *Management of Labor,* 2nd edn. Rockville, MD: Aspen Publishers, Inc., 1989:19–60.
41. Cohen WR. Influence of the duration of second stage labor on perinatal outcome and puerperal morbidity. *Obstet Gynecol* 1977;49:266–9.
42. Cohen WR, Mahon T, Chazotte C. *The Very Long Second Stage of Labor. Proceedings of the Third World Congress on Labor and Delivery.* New York: Parthenon Publishing, 1998:348–51.
43. Roemer VM, Buess H, Harms K. Zum problem der leitung der austreibungs-und pre-periode. *Arch Gynaekol* 1977;222:29–43.
44. Mahon T, Chazotte C, Cohen WR. Short labor: Characteristics and outcome. *Obstet Gynecol* 1994;84:47–51.
45. Schifrin BS, Cohen WR. Labor's dysfunctional lexicon. *Obstet Gynecol* 1989;74:121–4.
46. Chazotte C, Madden R, Cohen WR. Labor patterns in women with previous cesareans. *Obstet Gynecol* 1990;75:350–5.

175 Induction of labor

I. Z. MacKenzie and K. Duckitt

Introduction

The need to time delivery has been recognized and practiced for centuries. Although the indications have doubtless changed during the past 200 years, with the emphasis on fetal rather than maternal health in recent times, effective and safe methods of achieving delivery must always have been the primary objectives. Most methods of inducing labor employed before the 20th century involved mechanical manipulations, including Galvinism, repeated pressurized douches, extra-amniotic aqua picea, tents, bougies and catheters. The use of threats, incantations and chants was doubtless popular when nothing else was to hand, while the administration of potions and latterly castor oil, quinine, and posterior pituitary extract was also utilized. During the past 50 years, labor induction has mostly involved combining the recognized advantages of physical stimulation with a pharmacologic myometrial stimulant.

During the 1980s and 1990s, patients' acceptance of when and how delivery was achieved became a significant and sometimes overpowering consideration; this has not necessarily always been in the long-term best interests of mother or baby. In some countries, the fear of legal redress if the pregnancy outcome is not entirely favorable has become of such concern that patient demands are frequently acquiesced to, and in many cases requests for delivery by cesarean section are agreed to even without a clear medical indication. This chapter appraises the indications for and methods of labor induction and augmentation. It reviews their virtues and risks, together with an assessment of the views of the women whose labor has been induced and a consideration of the economics of such intervention.

Definition and rates of labor induction

It is difficult to compare the rates of induction between obstetric units, states or countries because of variations in the definition of induced or augmented labor. Examples of the differences that exist and which will influence calculations of induction rates include the following:

(1) When the membranes have spontaneously ruptured at term but labor has not established, to stimulate labor is variably called induction or augmentation;
(2) When efforts are made to ripen the unfavorable cervix and labor commences, is variably listed as induced or spontaneous labor; and
(3) There may be ready resort to elective prelabor cesarean, particularly if the cervix is unfavorable: should such cases be included with the statistics for labor induction?

The first two examples should logically be included in labor induction statistics. The concept of 'cervical ripening' was widely acknowledged and introduced into clinical practice by the late 1970s with the adoption of local prostaglandin administration. The changes that occur in cervical form during the latter weeks of pregnancy are accelerated as labor establishes and are thus not physiologically separable. It seems inappropriate therefore to consider therapeutically-induced cervical ripening and labor induction as two distinct entities. Elective prelabor cesarean section should be included with inductions under the all-encompassing title of 'timed' deliveries.

In England and Wales between 1980 and 1995 the induction rate varied between 16.8% and 20.6% (Figure 175.1).[1] This trend continued with just over 20% of births being induced in 2002–2003.[2] The equivalent rate for induction of labor in the USA in 2002 was 20.5%.[3]

Indications for labor induction

The indications for labor induction may be subdivided into maternal, fetal, or social, or a combination of these, and such indications may either be indicated or anticipated. Table 175.1 illustrates many of the indications that are widely acknowledged. An example of the relative frequency with which the indications occur is shown in Table 175.2 of data derived

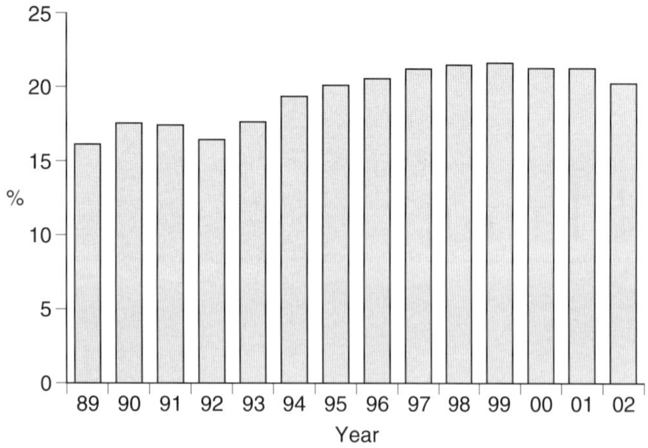

Figure 175.1 Induction rates for England and Wales, 1989–2002.

from the Obstetrics Department in Oxford for 5980 labor inductions during 2000–2004.

Specific definitions and the relative importance of the various indications for labor induction vary among obstetricians and countries. 'Post-term pregnancy' leading to induction is probably the commonest indication in many units, but definitions may include any gestation beyond 40 completed weeks; cephalopelvic disproportion may be managed by early induction at 38 weeks of gestation or ignored in the belief that spontaneous labor is to be preferred and results in a more favorable outcome. Some obstetricians consider that cervical state should determine the timing of delivery, particularly when 'post-term pregnancy' is the indication for induction; it should, however, be recognized that there is often a poor relationship between cervical favorability and gestational age.

Hypertensive states constitute the second most common primary indication for labor induction in many obstetric units, generally because of anticipated fetal or maternal problems rather than because of evidence of deteriorating ill health for mother or baby. The remaining unspecified indications are varied, some probably universally accepted, such as recent or current antepartum hemorrhage, diabetes mellitus, red cell isoimmunization, demonstrable placental failure and previous unexplained post-term stillbirth, and others with little logic, such as fetal macrosomia and suspected cephalopelvic disproportion.

Labor induction performed for maternal request or convenience at term is widely frowned upon. However,

Table 175.1 Common indications for induction of labor

	Fetal	Maternal	Social
Clinical evidence	Growth retardation Antepartum hemorrhage Polyhydramnios Red-cell alloimmunization Diabetes mellitus Unstable lie Fetal infection Macrosomia	Deteriorating health Renal Hypertension Psychological Malignancy Autoimmune Diabetic fragility Intrauterine infection Coagulopathy Abruptio placentae Polyhydramnios Discomfort	Specialist services availability X-matched blood Anesthesia Fetal surgery NICU/SCBU cot Partner availability
Prophylactic indications	Prolonged pregnancy Growth retardation Previous obstetric history Ruptured membranes Diabetes mellitus Antepartum hemorrhage Multiple pregnancy Red-cell alloimmunization	Hypertension Fetopelvic disproportion Intrauterine fetal death Previous section Ruptured membranes	

Table 175.2 Indications for labor induction for 5980 patients in the John Radcliffe Hospital, Oxford, 2000–2004

Indication for induction	2001	2002	2003	2004	Total
Prolonged pregnancy (%)	31.5	28.2	26.6	23.1	27.2
Hypertensive disorders (%)	16.4	16.3	15	14.8	15.6
SROM without labor (%)	18.6	19.8	21.9	23.3	21
Fetal death *in utero* (%)	1.2	1.6	0.9	1.3	1.2
Term and social (%)	0.3	0.3	0.5	0.4	0.4
Other (%)	49.6	33.7	35	37.1	38.6
Total number of inductions	1363	1466	1577	1594	5980

SROM, spontaneous rupture of membranes

Table 175.3 Components of Bishop's pelvic scoring system[4]

	Score			
	0	1	2	3
Station of presenting part	−3	−2	−1.0	+1
Cervical dilatation (cm)	Closed	1–2	3–4	5+
Cervical effacement (%)	0–39	40–59	60–79	80+
Cervical consistency	Firm	Medium	Soft	
Cervical position in pelvis	Posterior	Mid	Anterior	

the reluctance to accommodate such requests, believing that it is not in the best interests of mother or baby, is at variance with the willingness to allow patients to opt for delivery by elective cesarean section, usually performed before full term, particularly in cases such as breech presentation or previous delivery by section. Such reluctance is not logical. As demonstrated later, the rates of failed induction should be very low if the induction is managed correctly, and the fear of this should thus be limited.

Methods of induction

Cervical condition exerts a significant influence upon induced labor outcome, and in consequence the decision about how to induce labor must take account of the favorability of the cervix. To assist the obstetrician in deciding how to induce labor, a cervical scoring system is used. More than 12 different pelvic or cervical scoring schemes have been described during the past several decades, but that described by Bishop[4] is the one most widely employed (Table 175.3). An objective cervical scoring system is also essential as a research tool to enable comparisons of different induction methods and protocols to be made and to allow new methods to be developed and introduced.

Two different approaches to induction are employed: one relies on mechanical stimulation to provoke cervical effacement, dilatation and ultimately uterine contractions; the other uses pharmacologic agents to modify cervical form, with or without stimulating uterine contractions. Frequently, a combination of both approaches is used. As a general principle, the simplest inductions, those which probably precede the spontaneous onset of labor by a few hours to a day or two, rely upon mechanical techniques alone, while the most difficult inductions are often managed with pharmacologic agents, frequently involving more than one drug and often combined subsequently with a mechanical stimulus. Figure 175.2 lists the various techniques or agents used with reference to cervical condition.

Prior to the induction being started, a final check should be made to ensure that the indication to induce still pertains, and any specific labor management that may be required as a consequence of the indication should be reaffirmed. Palpation of the abdomen should confirm that the fetal lie is longitudinal and the presentation is as anticipated; the fetal heart beat should be present and healthy unless fetal death is the indication for the induction. Induction should not proceed if the fetal lie is not longitudinal; manipulation of the fetus to a longitudinal lie followed by management to ensure that the lie remains stable during the induction process can be employed.

The place for the routine use of continuous electronic fetal heart rate monitoring and intrauterine pressure measurement has still not been proven. The reliance on continuous electronic heart monitoring has unfortunately led to less clinical attention being paid to the duration and intensity of uterine contractions; this should be discouraged since valuable information about labor progress is often overlooked. A return to more clinical vigilance of uterine contractility, which remains an important part of the management of labor, is to be encouraged. Adequate analgesia should be available, as for spontaneous labor, and ideally should include the simple approaches such as, inhalational gases, parenteral narcotics and regional amnesia: some of the newer approaches including transcutaneous electrical nerve stimulation, massage techniques, aromatherapy and use of a birthing pool, although claimed to be beneficial, have not yet been shown objectively to offer any advantage.

Induction when the cervix is favorable (Bishop score > 6)

With a ripe or favorable cervix, mechanical methods of induction, which probably act by stimulating release of endogenous prostaglandins, and thereby promote uterine contractions, are frequently all that is required to achieve established progressive labor.

Membrane sweep and cervical stretch

When the cervix is particularly ripe, simple cervical examination and stretching of the membranes off the lower uterine segment can be very effective. Performed using a sterile glove, introducing one or two fingers through the cervix and stretching the os, this produces further dilatation; in addition, one of the fingers is swept around the internal surface of the cervix, dislodging the membranes from the cervical surface. When performed daily over 3 days, labor is induced in 69% of cases, depending upon the degree of cervical favorability at the time of the initial examination.[5]

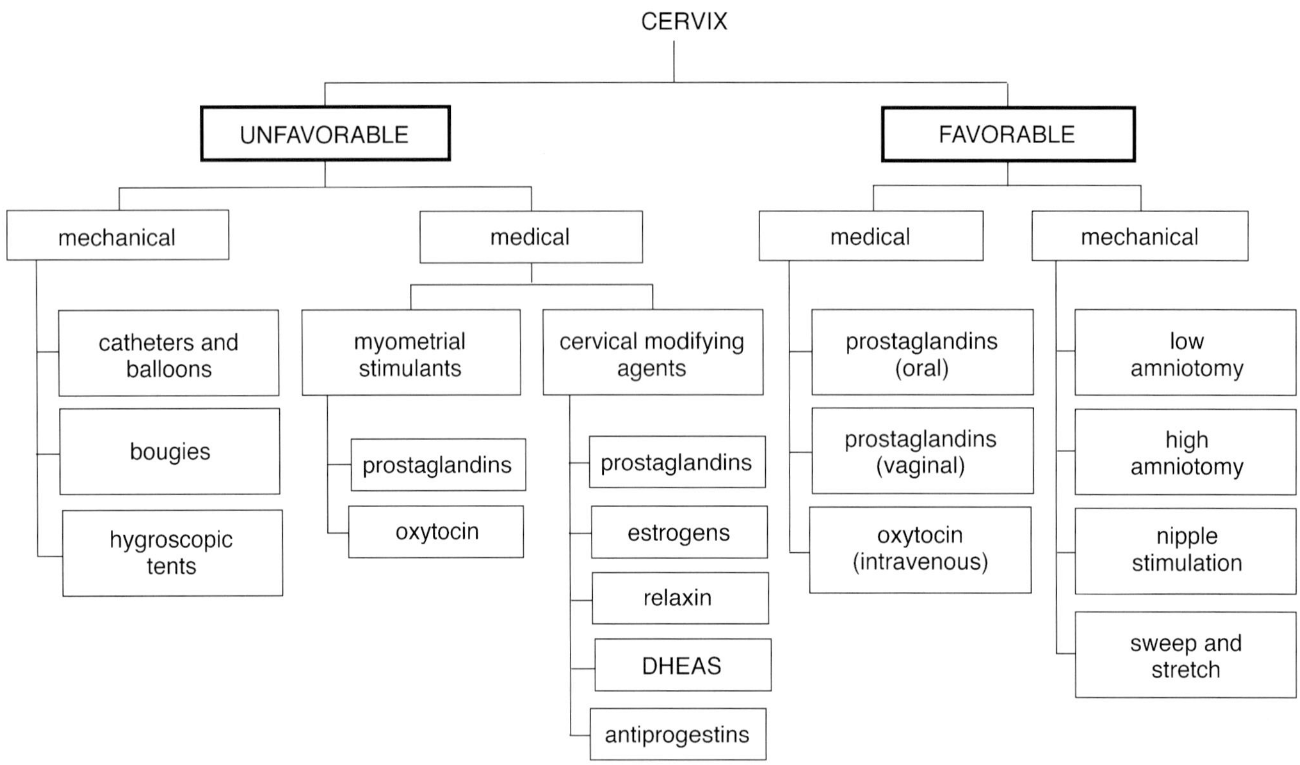

Figure 175.2 Therapeutic agents and devices that have been used for the induction of labor, according to the state of the cervix. When indicated, either low amniotomy is performed after the administration of the oxytocic agent when contractions are occurring, or an oxytocic is given, once the mechanical effect upon the cervix has been achieved. The timing for these additional therapies will depend upon circumstances and obstetrician preferences. DHEAS, dehydroepiandrosterone sulfate.

Sweeping of the membranes, performed routinely in women at term, is associated with a reduced duration of pregnancy and a reduced frequency of pregnancy continuing beyond 41 weeks [relative risk (RR) 0.62, 95% confidence interval (CI) 0.49–0.79] and 42 weeks (RR 0.28, 95% CI 0.15–0.50). To avoid one additional formal induction of labor, a stretch and sweep must be performed in seven women (number needed to treat (NNT = 7)). Maternal or neonatal infection does not seem to be increased.[6]

Low or forewater amniotomy

Abdominal palpation must confirm that the presenting part, head or breech, is either engaged or apparently securely settled in the pelvic brim; previous placental localization should have been performed in whom placenta praevia had previously been suspected. Amniotomy is usually performed in the labor suite. The maternal bladder should be emptied by spontaneous voiding immediately before the procedure, and ideally the rectum should be empty, if necessary following the prior administration of a suppository or enema. The dorsal or lithotomy position with some mild degree of left lateral tilt is used to reduce the chances of supine hypotension occurring, causing a decrease in placental bed blood flow.

The size and shape of the mid-cavity and outlet of the pelvis are assessed, and stretching of the cervix and sweeping the membranes off the lower uterine segment as described above is performed, at which time it is necessary to ensure the cord is not presenting. The membranes are then ruptured using a pair of toothed forceps, or a purpose-designed instrument such as an amniotomy hook. Amniotic fluid is released, encouraged by controlled elevation of the presenting part. A further check is made to ensure that the presentation is unchanged and the cord is not palpable, and the station and position of the presenting part are noted. The condition of the amniotic fluid is also noted and the fetal heart rate pattern checked to ensure that it is satisfactory. If continuous electronic monitoring is indicated, the preferred electrode can be attached to the most appropriate area of the presenting part before completing the procedure, unless an external ultrasound recording is to be used. Labor is then awaited.

The interval between amniotomy and any pharmacologic augmentation, if required, is variable, ranging from immediately after amniotomy to a delay of up to 24 h. Approximately 98% of women with a high Bishop score will labor after amniotomy alone.[7] Amniotomy with early intravenous oxytocin infusion, however, produces a significant reduction in women undelivered after 24 h compared with those managed by amniotomy alone.[8,9]

Hindwater amniotomy

There are few indications nowadays for using this method of labor induction unless ecbolic drugs are not available. It is usually reserved for inductions when the presenting part is high in relation to the pelvic cavity and associated with polyhydramnios. The objective is to achieve a controlled release of amniotic fluid from a puncture in the membranes above the level of the presenting part, so reducing the chances of subsequent malpresentation, compound or funic presentation, and placental abruption.

Preparation for the procedure is the same as that described for low amniotomy; every attempt should be made using ultrasound to exclude a posterior placenta implanted low on the uterine wall. A sterilized Drew-Smythe catheter[10] is guided through the vagina and cervix alongside two examining fingers in the vagina, directing the leading end behind the presenting part. With an assistant stabilizing the longitudinal lie of the fetus by continuous pressure against the long axis of the uterus by abdominal palpation, the stylet of the catheter is advanced to puncture the membranes, and the amniotic fluid is allowed to drain through the lumen of the catheter until a sufficient amount has been released and the presenting part has descended and stabilized at or below the pelvic brim, when the catheter is withdrawn. Postamniotomy observations should be performed as for low amniotomy, but with particular attention to the possibility of placental abruption occurring in cases of polyhydramnios. An intravenous infusion of oxytocin may be given prior to the amniotomy or immediately afterwards, to try to ensure that uterine contractility is soon established to help retain the longitudinal lie and the presenting part fixed in the pelvis. Until then, careful repeated palpations are necessary to prevent the lie changing or to identify as soon as possible any deviation from this situation.

Oxytocin

Buccal oxytocin citrate 100–400 units[11] or demoxytocin 50 units[12] given at 30-min intervals as tablets held under the tongue to allow the oxytocin to be absorbed across the buccal mucous membrane is not widely used because of fears of uncertain absorption and unpredictable uterine response, and has thus largely been abandoned.

Protocols using intravenous infusions of oxytocin that are used these days are largely based on the work of Turnbull and Anderson.[13] Although originally given at a constant low dose infusion at less than 10 mU/min, this has been replaced by titrated doses, determined by the intensity and frequency of the uterine contractions. The rate is controlled using either basic clinical observations of contraction rate, duration and intensity, assessed by staff who alter the infusion rate using mechanical pumps and electronic drip counters, or by automatic infusion pumps governed by feedback from intrauterine contraction pressure using solid-state pressure transducers. Concentrations of oxytocin infusates range between 5 and 20 units oxytocin in 1000 ml solution of saline, N/5 dextrose-saline, or 5% dextrose solution. Infusion rates normally start at 1–4 mU/min and increase variably,[14] arithmetically[15] or logarithmically[16] at 15–30-min intervals, often to a maximum of around 32 mU/min, or until satisfactory labor has been established; occasionally higher rates may be required.[16] Most workers consider that the rate required to establish labor should be maintained into the second stage, and increased once the third stage of labor is reached, being maintained for approximately 1 h following delivery of the placenta and membranes. A modification has been suggested, giving 1-min infusions every 10 min,[17] to reduce the chances of unnecessarily overdosing the patient; this approach has not been widely adopted.

Automatically-controlled infusion systems were devised to eliminate the imprecision of clinical assessment of uterine contractions by repeated fundal palpation. The infusion rate is adjusted using a continuous measure of intrauterine pressure obtained with a transcervical intrauterine pressure catheter and either an open-loop infusion system, which requires the rate to be controlled manually once contractions are adequate,[18] or a closed-loop feedback system which allows an automatic decrease in infusion rate and theoretical avoidance of overdosage. Small studies, either randomized[19] or uncontrolled,[20] have produced conflicting results, suggesting that there is probably little advantage from such technology. As a consequence, despite the apparent enhanced safety features, these automated feedback systems have not found wide acceptance.

The place of amniotomy in inductions using intravenous oxytocin continues to be debated. Most obstetricians combine the two, with low amniotomy followed by intravenous oxytocin titration immediately or within 1 h, while some advocate a delay of 4–6 h. Alternatively, a titrated infusion of oxytocin can be started and amniotomy delayed until contractility is established in cases where the presenting part is very mobile at or above the pelvic brim; such a method should reduce the chances of compound presentation and cord prolapse or malpresentation occurring at amniotomy.

Prostaglandins

Potent ecbolics at all gestational ages, the prostaglandins have become the mainstay of labor induction in many countries. They may be administered in a variety of ways (Figure 175.3), the route being influenced by the indication for labor induction and the state of the cervix. The oral administration of prostaglandin E_2 (PGE_2) 0.5 mg tablets taken hourly with an incremental increase of 0.5 mg every 2 h to a maximum of 2.0 mg per hour should establish labor in most cases[21]; some advocate half-hourly medication.[22] Treatment may be continued for a maximum of 6 h or maintained as long as necessary to establish labor. Amniotomy may be performed before prostaglandin treatment, when cervical dilatation starts to occur, when labor begins to establish, or after 6 h. Some clinicians favor leaving the membranes intact unless rupturing them is indicated for other reasons.

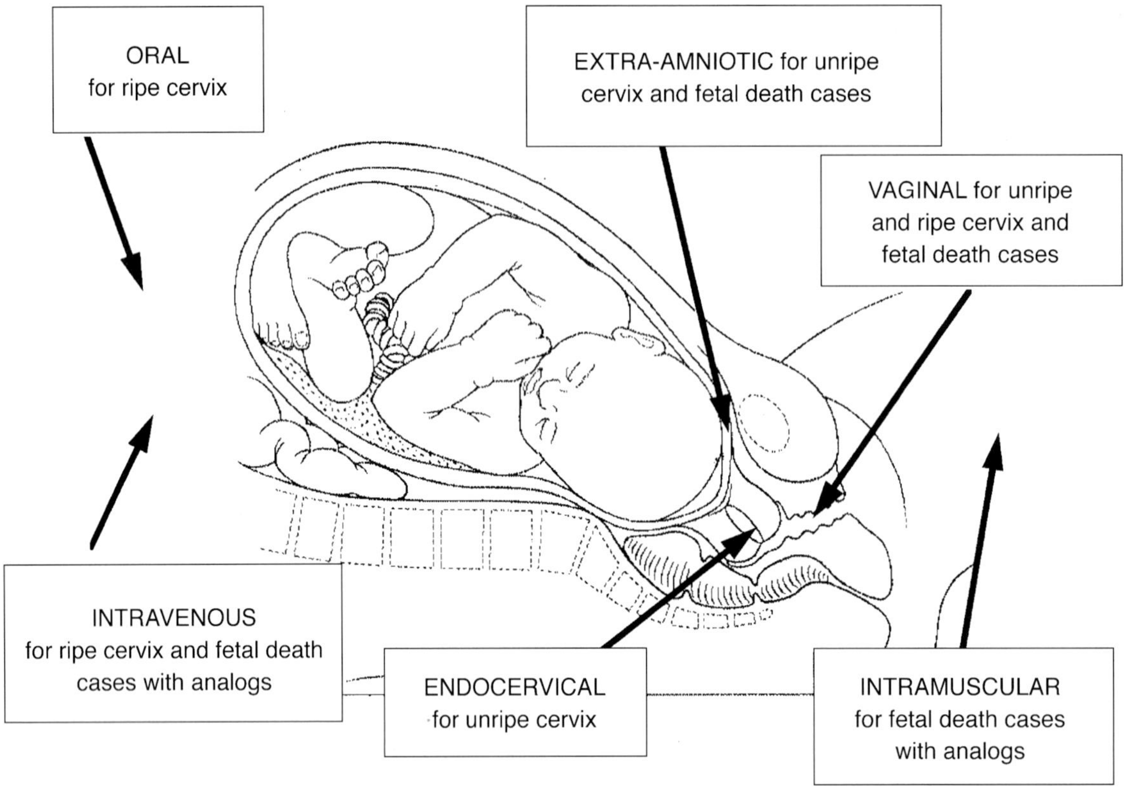

Figure 175.3 Routes of prostaglandin administration for the induction of labor.

Intravenous infusions are not widely used because of the gastrointestinal side-effects and local erythema at the infusion site associated with their use. Infusion rates usually start at PGE_2 0.1–0.5 µg/min or prostaglandin $F_{2\alpha}$ ($PGF_{2\alpha}$) 3–5 µg/min and either remain constant or increase arithmetically or logarithmically at 30-min intervals as necessary to a maximum of PGE_2 2–4 µg/min or $PGF_{2\alpha}$ 18–30 µg/min.[23,24] As with oxytocin, the infusion rate may be adjusted using routine clinical criteria, a peristaltic drip counter or an automatic feedback loop system. The place of amniotomy when using intravenous prostaglandins is similar to that described for intravenous infusions of oxytocin.

A single PGE_2 1–3 µg dose administered into the posterior vaginal fornix as a dry tablet, viscous gel or wax pessary, followed by low amniotomy after 3 h will induce labor in approximately 60% of primiparas and 80% of multiparas.[25–27] Augmentation can be provided with intravenous oxytocin, or repeated prostaglandin treatments at 6 h intervals. Timing of the amniotomy and further oxytocic augmentation is debatable, but most consider that oxytocin should not be administered for at least 3 h after any prostaglandin treatment.

Nipple stimulation

Uterine contractions can be induced by mechanical stimulation of the nipples, even to the extent of apparently causing uterine hypertonus.[28] A systematic review suggests that there is a significant reduction in the number of women not in labor after 72 h, when breast stimulation is compared with no treatment (RR 0.67, 95% CI 0.60–0.70),[29] but this technique has not found a role in common practice.

Sexual intercourse

Sexual intercourse is sometimes advised at term to encourage the onset of labor, with the premise that the high concentrations of prostaglandins in semen, the physical stimulation of the cervix and lower uterine segment leading to endogenous prostaglandin release, or orgasm may encourage uterine contractions. However, evidence to substantiate this advice is lacking. One small randomized clinical trial compared women having sexual intercourse with semen deposit, but no nipple stimulation, for three nights in a row at term, with women who abstained from this activity. There was no change in the Bishop score between the two groups and there was no difference in the number of women who delivered within 3 days of the intervention (46% vs. 47%, RR 0.99, 95% CI 0.45–2.20).[30]

Induction when the cervix is unripe (Bishop score < 7)

The unripe cervix can present a major problem when delivery is necessary and labor induction is indicated; rarely is it a problem for multiparas, except occasionally for those women previously delivered by cesarean section. The concept of cervical ripening or priming involves treatment to render the cervix more favorable, followed by a formal induction method, unless labor supervenes with the 'ripening' procedure. The distinction between ripening and labor induction is artificial;

a subdivision between the latent prelabor phase and the active acceleratory phase is unphysiologic. Such a subdivision may encourage the idea of abandoning the attempt to induce labor if cervical ripening is not easily achieved: when this approach is adopted there must be a question about the wisdom of the initial indication to induce labor.

Ripening may be achieved either medically or mechanically. Two principles of management have been explored using pharmacologic agents in this situation: those that modify the cervix and stimulate uterine contractions (oxytocin and prostaglandins), and those that influence cervical form and consistency, by modifying the cervical ground-substance without seemingly provoking any change in myometrial contractility (estrogens, antiprogestins, relaxin, dehydroepiandrosterone sulfate). Both groups of substances may be used in isolation, or in combination with other modalities of treatment.

Prostaglandins

Both PGE_2 and $PGF_{2\alpha}$ have been used, although there is much less experience reported using $PGF_{2\alpha}$. Various synthetic prostaglandin analogs have been explored for pregnancy termination and in cases of fetal death; there is increasing experience with misoprostol, the PGE_1 analog, for term labor induction with a viable fetus. When the cervix is unripe, local administration routes are most applicable. Oral and intravenous administration of PGE_2 and $PGF_{2\alpha}$ usually result in high rates of side-effects with the doses required to achieve clinical benefit, and are thus not generally used. Although misoprostol can be administered orally and even bucally and sublingually, these routes do not seem as effective as vaginally administered misoprostol.[31–33]

Extra-amniotic infusion or instillation. With prior vulvar and vaginal toilet, and using aseptic techniques, a catheter is guided through the cervical canal with the tip placed in the extra-amniotic space, either by the vaginal examining fingers or under direct vision using a speculum. Once introduced, the catheter can be left in place by distending a self-retaining balloon with 20–50 ml sterile isotonic saline and the catheter connected to an infusion pump, or it can be removed once a single bolus of prostaglandins has been given. If using an infusion the rate commences at PGE_2 20 μg/h, with 10 μg incremental increases at 15-min intervals as necessary using a solution concentration of 1.5–5 μg/ml[34,35] or $PGF_{2\alpha}$ 180–600 μg/ml with similar proportional incremental dose increases; the infusion is maintained until the catheter is expelled into the vagina. Bolus doses of PGE_2 (300–500 μg) or $PGF_{2\alpha}$ (5 mg in 10 ml volumes of viscous gel) can be given as a single instillation, and this is a simpler and equally efficacious method.[36] Amniotomy may be performed once labor is established, and oxytocin augmentation started thereafter. Inadvertent perforation of the fetal membranes is a disadvantage and disturbance of a previously unsuspected placenta previa may provoke excessive hemorrhage, requiring immediate cesarean section.

Endocervical instillation. A catheter is passed into the cervical canal as described above and PGE_2 500–1000 μg in 2–4 ml viscous gel is discharged into the endocervical canal.[37] Subsequent management is as described for the extra-amniotic instillation approach. There must be doubt about the precise location of the gel after initial injection, some probably reaching the extra-amniotic space and some leaking into the vagina. Attempts have been made to confine the drug to the cervical canal using a system of balloons, but the benefits of the system have yet to be demonstrated.[38] Some of the disadvantages of the extra-amniotic approach should be avoided with endocervical instillation, but there must be uncertainties over the duration of the gel being retained in the canal; the method is not particularly suitable for a patient with an uneffaced cervix that admits an examining finger, as occasionally occurs. Endocervical placement may be the most logical, with the prostaglandins being adjacent against the end organ concerned, although studies comparing endocervical extra-amniotic and vaginal protocols suggest the clinical responses are very similar.

Vaginal instillation. Many different vehicles including dry tablets,[24] wax pessaries,[25] viscous gels,[39] non-biodegradable hydrogel polymers,[40] and water-soluble polymers,[41] incorporating many different doses have been tried. There is no clearly established most appropriate protocol to recommend. Published results suggest that PGE_2 (2–5 mg) in biodegradable pessaries and gels and PGE_2 (5–10 mg) in the non-biodegradable formulations as a single instillation are appropriate; the lower doses are probably as effective as the higher ones. A latent period of 12 h is necessary before formal induction is performed in many cases to achieve the desired clinical effect on the cervix. Some protocols use repeated prostaglandin treatments at 6-hourly intervals for three or more doses, and others describe amniotomy and oxytocin titration 15 h after a single prostaglandin treatment unless labor has already supervened. Repeated small doses of PGE_2 0.5 mg at 2–3-hourly intervals have been used,[42,43] but have not been widely adopted. A prospective randomized study examining a single vs. repeat dose after 6 h reports that no advantage is obtained by repeating the dose of prostaglandins, suggesting that the initial exposure to prostaglandins is sufficient to achieve the desired effect on cervical function[44]; it appears that tachyphylaxis may occur in those women with a resistant cervix, and repeated dosing will probably not improve outcome. The controlled release hydrogel pessary,[40] with its maximum release rate of prostaglandins of less than 1 mg/h from a 10 mg reservoir, providing a prolonged source of prostaglandins over many hours, offers potential advantages; in particular, it may be removed from the

Table 175.4 Labor outcome using local prostaglandin E_2 protocols with an unripe cervix

Protocol	n	Maximum cervical score	Labor length (h)	Additional oxytocic (%)	Cesarean section (%)	Failed induction (%)
Extra-amniotic 240–480 μg[36]	121	3	10.7	80	14	0.8
Endocervical 500 μg[106]	27	5	10.7	34	7	3.7
Vaginal 3 mg wax pessaries[107]	110	4	16.0	20	21	5.5
Vaginal 2 mg gel[39]	102	3	10.5	76	13	3.0
Vaginal 10 mg hydrogel pessaries[108]	32	3	10.6	72	12	

Table 175.5 Use of misoprostol in pregnancy*

May be considered for cervical ripening or labor induction in hospitalized patients
The dose is 25 μg intravaginally every 3–6 h
A dose of 50 μg every 6 h may be considered in some situations, but is associated with uterine tachysystole and possibly hyperstimulation, and meconium in amniotic fluid
Oxytocin should not be given within 4 h of the last misoprostol dose
Fetal heart rate and uterine activity should be continuously monitored
Misoprostol should not be administered to women with a previous hysterotomy (cesarean delivery or major uterine surgery)

*Adapted from American College of Obstetricians and Gynecologists. ACOG Committee Opinion No. 283. *Obstet Gynecol* 2003;101:1049.

vagina if indicated.[45] Prospective comparative trials are needed to assess the pessary against the alternatives. Table 175.4 summarizes the results from the published literature obtained for nulliparas with an unfavorable cervix undergoing induction using local PGE_2. Prostaglandin $F_{2\alpha}$ 25–50 mg in viscous gel has also been studied, but the objective evidence available suggests that it is less efficient than PGE_2, although it has demonstrable benefits over placebo.[58,59]

Misoprostol is licensed for the treatment and prevention of gastroduodenal ulcers. Its use for induction of labor remains an off-label unlicensed use.[46,47] It is available as 100 and 200 μg tablets that have to be broken to provide 25 or 50 μg doses. It is inexpensive, can be stored at room temperature and is rapidly absorbed from both the oral and vaginal route. Misprostol, administered vaginally, improves cervical ripening compared with placebo.[48] Experience with misoprostol is changing rapidly. Currently the evidence suggests that when compared with vaginal or intracervical PGE_2 or oxytocin, its use at doses of 25 μg every 3 h or more is associated with less epidural analgesia use, fewer failures to achieve vaginal delivery within 24 h but more uterine hyperstimulation. Compared with vaginal or intracervical PGE_2, oxytocin augmentation was less common with misoprostol but meconium-stained amniotic fluid was more common. This may be due to a direct effect on fetal bowel activity. Cesarean section rates did not differ between groups. The optimal dose and timing interval of intravaginally applied misoprostol are unknown. However, there was less uterine hyperstimulation with lower doses (25 μg every 4 h or less) as opposed to higher doses of misoprostol. More limited information on these lower doses suggest equivalent efficacy to conventional methods of induction.[48] More comparisons between different doses of oral misoprostol and vaginal misoprostol are required. Reports of uterine rupture following labor induction with misoprostol, even in unscarred uteri, are a cause for concern.[49–52] The use of misoprostol has been endorsed by ACOG[53–55] (Table 175.5) but the professional bodies in the UK and Canada remain cautious about its use outside randomized controlled trials.[56,57]

Oxytocin

Intravenous infusions, intramuscular injections, buccal tablets and even nasal sprays of forms of oxytocin have all been used, but in general all have been abandoned in favor of alternatives, if available. Controlled studies have indicated that oxytocin is not very effective when the cervix is unfavorable, especially when compared with local prostaglandins. Prior to the introduction of prostaglandins, inductions were managed by repeated infusions or buccal courses of oxytocin over 8–15-h periods, with breaks overnight and repeated the next day and as often as necessary until labor was induced, or the attempt at induction abandoned.

Estrogens

Estradiol 150–300 mg in viscous gel extra-amniotically, endocervically or vaginally, or estradiol 10 mg intramuscularly and estriol 150–250 mg in viscous gel extra-amniotically, can produce improvement in cervical scores with minimal myometrial stimulation.[60,61] When formal induction is performed 12–24 h later, there appears to be little improvement in the outcome of labor. However, since estradiol has a 10-fold higher estrogenic potency than estriol, and there was a considerable dosage range in these studies, the true value of estrogens for cervical ripening remains uncertain, but present evidence suggests that their role is probably very limited.

Dehydroepiandrosterone sulfate

Intravenous dehydroepiandrosterone sulfate (DHEAS), which is transformed into estrogens in the fetoplacental unit, has been explored as a possible cervical ripening agent, achieving effacement without inducing uterine contractions. The results were not encouraging when DHEAS 100 mg injected intravenously twice a week from 38 weeks of gestation was compared with placebo,[62] and the concept has received little further attention.

Relaxin

Like DHEAS, this has been studied in the human, using purified porcine relaxin 1–4 mg in viscous gel vaginally or endocervically, in the hope that it would have the same properties as exhibited in certain animal species. To date, there have been no well-conducted trials to determine its value for ripening the unfavorable cervix and enhancing the outcome of induced labor without stimulating uterine activity, and more studies enabling a critical scientific assessment to be made are required before considering it to be of any clinical value. With the production of recombinant human relaxin, interest was renewed in studying this polypeptide for induction. Trials to date exploring different dosages, given vaginally, suggest that there is no evidence that 1, 2 or 4 mg cause any maternal or fetal toxicity,[63] but unfortunately there appears to be little evidence of any therapeutic effect.[64] Further studies with larger doses and alternative administration methods are required before large clinical trials can be mounted. Enthusiasm for this agent for labor induction must at present be muted.

Antiprogestins

Epostane, the 3β-hydroxysteroid dehydrogenase inhibitor, and more recently mifepristone, the progesterone receptor blocker, have been shown to have a dramatic effect on reducing the induction-to-abortion intervals during second-trimester therapeutic pregnancy termination.[65,66] Similar benefits might be expected for labor induction at term, but experience reported to date is limited. Labor may be induced following exposure to mifepristone, and cervical condition can be improved; the need for delivery by cesarean section has not been found to be reduced compared with placebo.[67] It had been thought that mifepristone might revolutionize labor induction but experience is still limited and there are no trials that compare mifepristone with alternative methods of inducing labor, e.g. prostaglandins.

Mechanical dilators

Dilatation, and to a lesser extent effacement, can be produced by the introduction of catheters, balloons, bougies and tents into the cervical canal. The devices are introduced most easily using the lithotomy position, taking aseptic precautions; after a variable period the device is either spontaneously expelled or removed. Thereafter, the induction can be advanced either by low amniotomy or administration of an oxytocic. However, results are unpredictable and when assessed objectively such devices probably offer little, if any, benefit.[68] Since intrauterine infection is a theoretical risk, which probably increases with prolonged retention of the foreign body, a careful watch needs be kept on maternal pulse and temperature. The advantages of these methods are their wide availability and the low cost, especially balloon catheters. Storage and preservation of mechanical devices is less problematic than PGE_2, which should be kept at low temperature. There seems little place for this method if prostaglandins are available. However, when compared with prostaglandins and misoprostol their use is associated with significantly less risk of hyperstimulation and fetal heart rate changes, advantages that may be important in high risk cases.[68]

Homeopathy

Homeopathy involves the use, in dilution, of substances that cause symptoms in their undiluted form. A type of herb *Caulophyllum thalictroides* is a homeopathic therapy used to induce labor. Although two small randomized clinical trials have looked at this method of inducing labor there was not enough detail presented to draw any firm conclusions about its effectiveness.[69]

Acupuncture

Although observational studies suggest that acupuncture may stimulate the onset of labor[70–72] and ripen the cervix,[73,74] the only clinical trial to compare acupuncture with no acupuncture in women who were post-term included only 56 subjects and did not lead to any convincing conclusions because of its large loss to follow-up and significant post-randomization exclusions.[75]

Labor induction in specific situations

Post-term pregnancy

The most frequent indication for labor induction in most units is prolonged pregnancy, an indication that stems from the findings of the 1958 Perinatal Mortality Survey of England and Wales[76]; many studies examining this area define post-term pregnancy as one undelivered by the 41st week of gestation determined by menstrual calculation or ultrasound assessment. It is thus performed for anticipated problems derived from statistical analyses, although the principle has been challenged in recent years, with alternative management strategies advocated which involve repeated frequent fetal surveillance methods using a combination of various cardiotocographic and ultrasound monitoring procedures. The end result, if assessed by need for delivery by cesarean section, suggests that there is no obvious benefit from avoiding induction. A meta-analysis of 19 randomized trials showed that routine induction of labor reduced perinatal mortality (OR 0.20, 95% CI 0.06–0.70) with the benefit being due to the effect of induction of labor after 41 weeks. Routine induction of labor in post-term pregnancies was not associated with an increased risk of cesarean section overall or in any subgroup of women, regardless of parity, state of the cervix or method of induction.[77]

Once the expected date of confinement has passed, and delivery is still awaited, many women are keen to be delivered. In addition, the incidence of meconium staining of the amniotic fluid increases with advancing gestation, and this often influences the care that is provided during labor and the handling of the newborn. It is unlikely that there will be a dramatic change in the incidence of induction for post-term women unless obstetricians are prepared, at the start of pregnancy, to recalculate the expected date of delivery as 42 completed weeks rather than 40 weeks: such a change could reduce patients' demands for induction because of prolonged pregnancy.

Previous cesarean section

Opinions vary over the wisdom of inducing labor in women previously delivered by lower-segment cesarean section; the majority considers that a previous classical section and previous repeated lower-segment sections should usually be considered as contraindications to attempting labor. For those who favor allowing labor induction, the most appropriate method to use is debated. Some believe it only appropriate to induce labor by low amniotomy, others to limit the ecbolic agent to low doses of oxytocin, while there are those who do not restrict the method to be used. There is widespread agreement that a patient should not labor if obvious fetopelvic disproportion is present, if she has delivered previously by cesarean section.

Management of the induction should be little different from other inductions, but perhaps conducted with greater caution. Continuous electronic monitoring of the fetal heart rate is advocated by many, and continuous intrauterine pressure recording by a smaller number.[78] Although logical as a way of anticipating or avoiding scar rupture, the major concern in this situation, experience has not confirmed the benefits of either form of continuous monitoring. It is difficult, therefore, to argue that either should be provided as routine.

A scarred uterus is a stated contraindication for the use of prostaglandins by the pharmaceutical companies marketing PGE_2. Despite this, a survey of 230 consultant obstetric units in the UK found that 78% used prostaglandins in such patients.[79] It has been argued, contrary to the recommendations of the pharmaceutical industry, that PGE_2 might have advantages in patients previously delivered by lower-segment cesarean section, because it produces more physiologic contractions than oxytocin and improves cervical compliance, theoretically reducing the intensity of myometrial contractions necessary to achieve full cervical dilatation. In consequence, there should be less risk of compromise to the scar.[39] Work in recent years has substantiated that view, comparing pressures generated by prostaglandins and oxytocin in spontaneous and induced labor.[13] Personal experience suggests, however, that full dilatation may be achieved too readily in the presence of cephalopelvic disproportion if prostaglandins are used, and thus the obstetrician needs to be particularly aware of this possibility.

Controversy also exists about the extent to which the use of prostaglandins and oxytocin to induce or augment labor increase the risk of scar rupture in women with a previous cesarean. A meta-anaylsis[80] found that oxytocin use was associated with a two- to fourfold increased risk of uterine rupture in two case–control studies; but this finding was not confirmed in cohort studies or controlled trials. In prospective cohort studies, the use of oxytocin (five trials) or prostaglandin (two trials) was not associated with a higher risk of uterine rupture. A large prospective study published subsequently[81] indicated that augmentation of labor with oxytocin and induction of labor, regardless of method, were associated with a two- to fourfold increased risk of uterine rupture compared with spontaneous labor without the use of oxytocin. However, the absolute risk was still very low, with only an 8% prospect of serious perinatal morbidity of death occurring when uterine rupture occurs.

Multiple pregnancy

When multiple pregnancies are considered in texts or monographs, little attention is paid to the place or method of inducing labor. There is thus little information about the experiences of induction using various methods. In a series of 656 twin pregnancies managed in Oxford, labor started spontaneously in 52%, was induced in 35% and elective cesarean section was performed in 13%. Of those in whom labor was induced, prostaglandins were used in 137 and amniotomy and oxytocin without prostaglandins in 91 cases. There appeared to be little difference in the outcomes, although prostaglandins were generally given when the cervix was less favorable and thus any conclusions that may be drawn must be guarded (I. Z. MacKenzie and N. C. Watson, 1996, unpublished data).

The methods described earlier for labor induction are equally applicable to twin pregnancies, and as with other complicated pregnancy situations, continuous electronic fetal monitoring of both babies is considered by some to be essential, but has not been shown objectively to be of any advantage and thus this recommendation has not been substantiated. Since postpartum hemorrhage due to uterine hypotonia is a recognized added risk of labor for twin pregnancies, it has been suggested that the prostaglandins might be particularly appropriate; this potential advantage has not been proven.

Intrauterine fetal death

When fetal death occurs, spontaneous expulsion will occur in the majority of cases within a few days. Once the diagnosis has been confirmed, evacuation can be arranged at the request of the woman to relieve emotional distress. If the fetal membranes have ruptured, prolonged retention may result in intrauterine infection, and if the dead fetus is retained for longer than 4 weeks, a consumptive coagulopathy may develop.[82] The methods of achieving evacuation are either surgical or pharmacologic, depending on gestational stage and uterine size.

Up to 14 weeks of gestational size, evacuation by cervical dilatation and aspiration under general or local anesthetic is the most expedient management. At later gestations, with the uterus at least equivalent to a 14-week gestation, prostaglandins have revolutionized management. Administration routes appropriate in this situation are illustrated in Figure 175.3 and include intravenous, extra-amniotic, intramuscular and vaginal. In this situation, some of the analogs of the prostaglandins have been used with great success, the fear of ill-effects upon the fetus not being a restricting factor. The oral route is not appropriate with the natural prostaglandins, since the doses required cause very high rates of side-effects. The intra-amniotic route has been used but may be unwise for two reasons: (1) puncturing the fetal membranes by amniocentesis may enhance the possibility of amniotic fluid embolism, a hazard thought to be more common in cases of fetal death *in utero*, and (2) the risk of intrauterine infection may be increased. The few reports of this method for managing such cases have not, however, observed these problems.

Clinical management is essentially the same whichever protocol is used. A check of the clotting status should be made if fetal death is thought to have occurred at least 3 weeks previously, and appropriate investigations should be initiated to assist in determining the etiology for those cases in which death was unexpected. Progress once treatment has started is assessed by vaginal examinations as indicated, and adequate analgesia is provided according to needs. Delivery of the dead fetus and placenta are similar to when the fetus is liveborn, although attempts are made to avoid perineal damage if possible. Administration of ergometrine or a prostaglandin analog should be done to enhance uterine contractility following delivery, thus reducing the chances of excessive hemorrhage occurring from uterine atonia.

The antiprogestins might be helpful in this situation, but physiologically there is little reason to anticipate this with the recognized low levels of progesterone already present in cases of fetal death.[83]

Complications of induction

There are a number of potential hazards for both mother and fetus or neonate from induction of labor, either as a result of initiating labor before spontaneous onset, or as a consequence of the method of induction used. There has been, however, a surprising lack of information about infant development after induced, compared with spontaneous, labor onset. Two small studies that examined babies up to 12 months[84] and 3 years of age[85] suggested there is probably no reason to anticipate any disturbance to development as a consequence of a labor induction with oxytocin or prostaglandins when compared with spontaneous labor or elective cesarean. Some specific complications are, nevertheless, recognized as a consequence of labor induction.

Uterine hyperstimulation

Hypersystole and hypertonia occur during both spontaneous and induced labors. The true incidences are unclear, but hypertonus occurs in about 1 in 500 labors, whether induced or spontaneous.[86] The prostaglandins classically provoke low-amplitude contractions at 1–2-min intervals which are often subclinical and generally do not cause fetal or maternal disturbance. If hypertonus occurs, it can be counteracted by the administration of a tocolytic agent. Subcutaneous and intravenous injections as well as inhalation have been used,[87] although the benefit of the latter route is uncertain. This management strategy can be used either to treat an acute episode and allow labor to continue if the fetus is not distressed and normal uterine contractility is restored, or as a first aid measure while preparing for emergency cesarean section.

Fetal distress

Fetal distress should be expected to occur more frequently during induced than spontaneous labor, since some induction indications, such as those for intrauterine growth retardation, are associated with intrapartum fetal distress. When diagnosed, management will depend upon circumstances at the time, including the degree of cervical dilatation and the suspected cause of the distress, such as abruptio placentae, cord prolapse, hyperstimulation, and previously suspected placental insufficiency; tocolytic therapy may be given prior to emergency cesarean section.[88] The concept of concomitant tocolytic therapy with the administration of prostaglandins for cervical ripening has been examined to try to achieve ripening without myometrial contractions, thus reducing the chances of fetal distress being provoked. It was concluded, unfortunately, that the tocolysis could reduce uterine activity, but it also reduced the influence of the prostaglandins upon cervical ripening, and thus was considered counterproductive.[89]

Failed induction

There is no universally accepted definition for 'failed' induction. It should perhaps be reserved for those cases in which the cervix does not dilate beyond 3 cm despite adequate and appropriate oxytocic stimulation of good-quality uterine contractions for 8 h in a nullipara and 4 h in a multipara; there should be no fetopelvic disproportion. It is generally confined to nulliparas with an unfavorable cervix at the time of induction, and is a rare complication in multiparas, except those whose only previous delivery was by cesarean section. In the high risk group of nulliparas with an unfavorable cervix, failed induction rates have been reported in 15–35% of cases induced with intravenous oxytocin, and should be no greater than 3–5% of nulliparas induced with local prostaglandins.

Cord prolapse

When the membranes rupture spontaneously during stimulation with an oxytocic, cord prolapse may result. This occurs most commonly with a high presenting part in patients with polyhydramnios and when there is a flexed breech presentation. An urgent operative vaginal delivery may be appropriate if at full dilatation; otherwise delivery is by emergency cesarean section, with measures taken to prevent pressure on the cord at the pelvic brim using the knee–chest position, or the vaginal examining fingers exerting counter pressure against the presenting part. It also occurs with spontaneous labor, when the outcome may be less favorable because of some inevitable delay in diagnosis, the cord prolapse occurring when the membranes rupture spontaneously and staff are not immediately available.

Abruptio placentae

This may occur during the first or second stage of labor, but is most likely to occur when the membranes rupture either spontaneously or at amniotomy, especially in cases of polyhydramnios. In theory, the use of hindwater membrane rupture reduces the chances of this happening. There has been a suggestion that the prostaglandins may predispose to this complication when used for labor induction, but there has been only one report[90] to suggest the relationship, and at present the evidence for such an association is therefore unconfirmed. The lack of such a complication being reported in many large series of labor inductions with prostaglandins suggests that there is unlikely to be any direct relationship.

Uterine rupture

Extremely uncommon in nulliparas, this complication may occur in any labor at risk, whether induced or spontaneous. It is a particular risk in multiparas of high parity and those previously delivered by cesarean section. Clearly this hazard should be recognized in the patient, with staff mindful of the possibility, with facilities available for emergency management when indicated.

Inadvertent preterm delivery

This is a risk with any term induction, whichever method is used. With the widespread use of ultrasound examinations in early pregnancy, there is a belief that this hazard can be eliminated. Cases still occur, however, especially when gestation has been inappropriately reassigned to an earlier expected delivery date by 2–3 weeks using the ultrasound measurements. There is little substantiated evidence of reduced rates of labor induction or of unplanned preterm delivery as a consequence of routine ultrasound dating scans, although routine early pregnancy ultrasound does reduce the incidence of post-term pregnancy (OR 0.68, 95% CI 0.57–0.82).[77]

Hyponatremia

Prolonged infusions of relatively high doses of oxytocin in dilute solutions of saline may lead to severe maternal electrolyte disturbance due to maternal fluid retention. Coma and death have been recorded.[91] Similar derangements in neonatal biochemistry leading to neonatal seizures in severely disturbed cases have also been reported.[92] Caution is therefore essential in those cases when the induction process is prolonged. Close attention should be continuously paid to maternal fluid balance, restricting intravenous fluid intake whenever possible.

Hyperbilirubinemia

The incidence of neonatal hyperbilirubinemia is increased following induction with intravenous oxytocin compared with prostaglandin inductions and spontaneous labor.[93,94] Prostaglandins have been associated with reduced rates of hyperbilirubinemia, possibly because of their apparent steroidogenic properties.[95]

Hypotonic uterine postpartum hemorrhage

Postpartum hemorrhage is more commonly encountered following induced labor than spontaneous labor[96]; the frequency is possibly lower following prostaglandin- than oxytocin-induced labors, but this has yet to be established for certain. The mechanism for this difference in effect is not entirely clear.

Augmentation of labor

For the purposes of this chapter, augmentation of labor refers to stimulating uterine contractions in those women whose membranes have ruptured but labor has not followed. The decision to intervene in this situation is strongly influenced by gestational age, which in turn is influenced by the facilities available to support the very preterm neonate. Apart from the statistical arguments relating to survival chances for the baby, intervention may be precipitated by clinical suspicion of developing intrauterine infection. There would, however, appear to be a lack of logic in waiting until there are clinical signs indicative of sepsis and thus potentially fatal infection: action is then possibly being taken too late.

There have been many studies examining the outcome of 'uncomplicated' cases of ruptured membranes without ensuing labor at full term, and the debate will not be rehearsed here. However, once the decision has been reached to augment labor, the most appropriate way of 'inducing' labor in this situation then needs to be addressed.

Each of the oxytocic protocols described for routine labor induction is potentially appropriate, but it is wise before commencing oxytocic treatment to examine the patient vaginally to assess the state of the cervix and determine whether the forewaters are intact and whether leakage is the consequence of a forewater or hindwater rupture; a forewater amniotomy may then be indicated.

A titrated intravenous infusion of oxytocin, repeated oral prostaglandins or vaginal prostaglandin protocols are widely used. There are theoretical concerns about sepsis with vaginal instillation protocols, and the extra-amniotic and endocervical methods do not seem appropriate, carrying an even greater risk of introducing infection. However, published series have not identified sepsis as a problem using these methods. There have been a number of prospective studies comparing oxytocin with various prostaglandin protocols. It appears fairly certain that PGE_2 offers no advantage over oxytocin for inducing labor in this situation,[97] whether given orally[98] or vaginally.[99,100] The current enthusiasm to explore misoprostol for this purpose[101] needs to be tempered with caution; experience is limited, but the early impression is that that this agent probably offers no advantage over PGE_2 other than economic, but has the disadvantage of a lack of information about fetal toxicology.

Maternal views on induction

Consumer opinion has gained considerable importance, and is now, in the views of some, the only opinion to be considered. Although it is widely suggested that women are against obstetric intervention, surveys of patients' attitudes have produced conflicting results.[102,103] A prospective survey of 352 women conducted in Oxford in 1989, by staff not involved in the decision to advise labor induction, found that 36% of nulliparas and 57% of multiparas wanted to have their labor induced. As expected, a large proportion of women expressed a wish to avoid labor induction in their next pregnancy, an observation that was more frequent among mothers who had just delivered their first baby (62%) compared with multiparas (47%). It would have been surprising if the reverse result had been obtained. Interestingly, patients' understanding of the indication for induction was frequently at variance with that recorded by the obstetric staff who gave the recommendation for labor induction: 276 of the 352 women (78%) gave the same indication for the induction as recorded by the obstetric staff, and the others either did not know why the induction was advised (9%), or gave a different reason (13%) (J. Boland, E. McKinlay and I. Z. MacKenzie, 1990, unpublished data).

Assessing patient's opinion about the way the induction was performed is extremely difficult. Prospective randomization with subsequent questionnaire completion unfortunately will not provide much worthwhile information, since nulliparas will have nothing with which to compare the experience; for multiparas, second labors are known to be associated with more favorable outcomes with regard to labor duration, discomfort, need for assisted delivery and perineal suturing compared with first confinements, and there is a risk that patients' previous experiences would compromise any analyses, potentially rendering the results meaningless. Acknowledging this, Kennedy *et al.*[25] found that induction with prostaglandins was more acceptable than intravenous oxytocin. Among the 352 patients surveyed in Oxford, six of 298 (2%) with an unfavorable cervix who received vaginal prostaglandins were unhappy about the method of induction compared with two of 54 (4%) with a favorable cervix who did not receive any prostaglandins; the other patients in both groups expressed satisfaction with the method of induction used. Four of these eight patients complained that the induction was too rushed or too uncomfortable. Women's views on induction with misoprostol have not yet been published.

Economics of induction

In the UK, and probably in many other countries, financial calculations about patient management have become a major consideration when deciding what medical facilities and treatments should be provided. Cost–benefit analyses have not featured prominently in discussions about the appropriateness of labor induction or the methods used to the present time. The cost of an induction depends on how it is managed and the outcome achieved. A prospective analysis of

Table 175.6 Workload on delivery unit related to spontaneous labor and labor induced with vaginal prostaglandin E_2 (P. Young, M. Vicaretti and I. Z. MacKenzie, 1989, unpublished data)

	Spontaneous labor	Induced labor	*P*-value
n	184	79	
Nulliparae (%)	49	49	NS
Gestation (weeks)	39.7 ± 1.8	39.9 ± 1.4	NS
Oxytocin infusion (%)	29	67	
Duration of infusion (min)	312 ± 216	453 ± 289	0.005
No. of medical visits in labor	1.3 ± 2.1	3.0 ± 2.9	NS
No. of VEs in labor	2.1 ± 1.2	3.1 ± 2.9	NS
Length of labor (min)	378 ± 219	292 ± 204	< 0.003
Time on labor ward (h)	6.8 ± 7.5	9.9 ± 7.8	NS
1-min Apgar < 8 (%)	22	27	NS
5-min Apgar < 8 (%)	2	0	NS
Resuscitation at birth (%)	15	15	NS

Data given as percentages or mean ±SD. VE, vaginal examination; NS, not significant

the workload associated with induction using prostaglandins compared with spontaneous labor was performed in Oxford in 1989 (Table 175.6). These data were not matched and are thus of limited value, but the impression was that labor induction was probably more costly than managing spontaneous labor, although the differences should be small, providing an efficient approach to induction is used. A similar analysis is probably worth performing prospectively, and ideally using random assignment, for women having a labor induction for social reasons at term compared with a conservative non-induction approach. It is possible that patient choice will need to be restricted if induction is confirmed to be more costly than spontaneous labor and resources are limited as in the UK.

Personal experience of costing an induction has been discouraging. The Canadian experience, however, has suggested induction is marginally cheaper than conservative management of post-term pregnancy.[104] In the UK it appears that hospital units are very uncertain of the costs of most procedures; many procedure costings need to be calculated using first principles, but the results cannot be readily confirmed. An analysis of the costs incurred using one or two doses of prostaglandins for labor induction found that the most expensive item is the midwife attending the patient during labor, with cesarean section being the next major factor, largely due to the more protracted hospitalization following delivery.[105] Thus protocols that can reduce the amount of time parturients spend on the labor ward and the need for cesarean section will prove very attractive to those who pay for the care: it is possible that a prelabor cesarean section is economically more attractive than inducing labor in those women with an unripe cervix.

Conclusions

There can be little doubt that the widespread acceptance of locally administered prostaglandins for induction of labor has had a dramatic impact upon the outcome of labor, reducing maternal and fetal morbidity and improving the relationship between doctor, midwife and patient. There are prospects that further improvements may well be achieved, with yet further reductions in failed inductions and the unwanted side-effects that are occasionally seen with prostaglandins. The convenience of misoprostol combined with its low cost makes its use for induction very attractive, particularly in low resource settings, but concerns still exist about its safety and optimal dosing regimen. The goal remains to induce cervical effacement and dilatation with little uterine contractility and thus risk of fetal compromise, followed by a short period of labor and uncomplicated delivery. Whether such a goal can be achieved in the near future remains to be seen.

Not only must efforts continue to be made to develop methods of labor induction that are effective and safe, but these methods must also be shown to be acceptable to women. Additionally, far greater attention will need to be paid to an analysis of the cost–benefit equation. While such considerations are entirely reasonable, we must ensure that safety and acceptability are not demoted in importance at the expense of financial efficiency.

REFERENCES

1. Macfarlane A, Mugford M. *Care of Mothers and Babies. Birth Counts: Statistics of Pregnancy and Childbirth.* London: The Stationary Office, 2000:191–242.
2. NHS Maternity Statistics England 2002–03, March 2004. Statistical Bulletin 2004/10 downloadable from www.dh.gov.uk ISBN 1 841828416.
3. Martin JA, Hamilton BE, Sutton PD, Ventura SJ, Menacker F, Munson ML. *Births: Final Data for 2002. National Vital Statistics Reports,* Vol. 52, no. 10. Hyattsville, MD: National Center for Health Statistics, 2003.
4. Bishop EH. Pelvic scoring for elective induction. *Obstet Gynecol* 1964;24:266–8.
5. Swann RO. Induction of labor by stripping membranes. *Obstet Gynecol* 1958;11:74–8.
6. Boulvain M, Stan C, Irion O. Membrane sweeping for induction of labour. *The Cochrane Database of Systematic Reviews,* 2001, Issue 2. Art. No.: CD000451. DOI: 10.1002/14651858.CD000451.
7. Booth JH, Kurdizak VB. Elective induction of labor: A controlled study. *Can Med Assoc J* 1970;103:245.
8. Patterson WM. Amniotomy with or without simultaneous oxytocin infusion. A prospective survey. *J Obstet Gynaecol Br Commonw* 1971;78:310–16.
9. Saleh YZ. Surgical induction of labour with and without oxytocin infusion. A prospective study. *Aust N Z J Obstet Gynaecol* 1975; 15:8033.
10. Drew-Smythe HJ. Indications for the induction of premature labour. *Br Med J* 1931;1:1018–20.
11. Pentecost AF. The effect of buccal Pitocin on the unripe cervix. *Curr Med Opin* 1973;482–4.
12. Sorensen SS, Brocks V, Lenstru C. Induction of labor and cervical ripening with intracervical prostaglandin E_2. *Obstet Gynecol* 1985;65:110–14.
13. Turnbull AC, Anderson AB. Induction of labour. 3. Results with amniotomy and oxytocin 'titration'. *J Obstet Gynaecol Br Commonw* 1968;75:32–41.
14. Lamont RF, Neave S, Baker AC, Steer PJ. Intrauterine pressures in labours induced by amniotomy and oxytocin or vaginal prostaglandin gel compared with spontaneous labour. *Br J Obstet Gynaecol* 1991;98:441–7.
15. Kurup A, Chua S, Arulkumaran S, Tham KF, Tay D, Ratnam SS. Induction of labour in nulliparas with poor cervical score: Oxytocin or prostaglandin vaginal pessaries? *Aust N Z J Obstet Gynaecol* 1991;31:223–6.
16. Toaff ME, Hezroni J, Toaff R. Induction of labour by pharmacological and physiological doses of intravenous oxytocin. *Br J Obstet Gynaecol* 1978;85:101–8.
17. Pavlou C, Barker GH, Roberts A, Chamberlain GVP. Pulsed oxytocin infusion in the induction of labour. *Br J Obstet Gynaecol* 1978;85:96–100.
18. Francis JG, Turnbull AC, Thomas FF. Automatic oxytocin infusion equipment for induction of labour. *J Obstet Gynaecol Br Commonw* 1970;77:594–602.
19. Steer PJ, Carter MC, Choong K, Hanson M, Gordon AJ, Pradhan P. A multicentre prospective randomized controlled trial of induction of labour with an automatic closed-loop feedback controlled oxytocin infusion system. *Br J Obstet Gynaecol* 1985;92:1127–33.
20. Gibb DM, Arulkumaran S, Ratnam SS. A comparative study of methods of oxytocin administration for induction of labour. *Br J Obstet Gynaecol* 1985;92:688–92.
21. Yip SK, Ma MK, Ng KH. Induction of labour with oral prostaglandin E_2. *J Obstet Gynaecol Br Commonw* 1973;88:442–5.
22. Miller JF, Welpy GA, Elstein M. Prostaglandin E_2 tablets compared with intravenous oxytocin in induction of labour. *Br Med J* 1975; 1:14–16.
23. Calder AA, Embrey MP. Comparison of intravenous oxytocin and prostaglandin E_2 for induction of labour using automatic and non-automatic infusion techniques. *Br J Obstet Gynaecol* 1975;82: 728–33.
24. Thiery M, Vroman S, de Hemptinne D, *et al.* Elective induction of labor conducted under lumbar epidural block. II. Labor induction by amniotomy and intravenous prostaglandin. *Eur J Obstet Gynecol Reprod Biol* 1977;7:181–200.
25. Kennedy JH, Stewart P, Barlow DH, Hillan E, Calder AA. Induction of labour: A comparison of a single prostaglandin E_2 vaginal tablet with amniotomy and intravenous oxytocin. *Br J Obstet Gynaecol* 1982:89:704–7.
26. Shepherd JH, Bennett MJ, Laurence D, Moore F, Sims CD. Prostaglandin vaginal suppositories; a simple and safe approach to the induction of labor. *Obstet Gynecol* 1981;58:596–600.
27. MacKenzie IZ, Bradley SG, Embrey MP. A simpler approach to labor induction using a lipid-based prostaglandin E_2 vaginal suppository. *Am J Obstet Gynecol* 1981;141:158–62.
28. Viegas OA, Arulkumaran S, Gibb DM, Ratnam SS. Nipple stimulation in late pregnancy causing uterine hyperstimulation and profound fetal bradycardia. *Br J Obstet Gynaecol* 1984;91:364–6.
29. Kavanagh J, Kelly AJ, Thomas J. Breast stimulation for cervical ripening and induction of labour. *The Cochrane Database of Systematic Reviews,* 2001, Issue 4. Art. No.: CD003392. DOI: 10.1002/14651858.CD003392.
30. Bendvold E. Coitus and induction of labour [Samleie og induksjon av fodsel]. Tidsskr Jordmodre 1990;96:6–8.
31. Alfirevic Z. Oral misoprostol for induction of labour. *The Cochrane Database of Systematic Reviews,* 2001, Issue 2. Art. No.: CD001338. DOI: 10.1002/14651858.CD001338.
32. Muzonzini G, Hofmeyr GJ. Buccal or sublingual misoprostol for cervical ripening and induction of labour. *The Cochrane Database of Systematic Reviews,* 2004, Issue 2. Art. No.: CD004221.pub2. DOI: 10.1002/14651858.CD004221.pub2.
33. Hofmeyr GJ, Gülmezoglu AM. Vaginal misoprostol for cervical ripening and induction of labour. *The Cochrane Database of Systematic Reviews,* 2002, Issue 4. Art. No.: CD000941. DOI: 10.1002/14651858.CD000941.
34. Calder AA, Embrey MP, Hillier K. Extra-amniotic prostaglandin E_2 for induction of labour at term. *Br J Obstet Gynaecol* 1974;81: 39–46.
35. Miller AWF, Mack DS. Induction by extra-amniotic prostaglandins. *Br J Obstet Gynaecol* 1974;81:706–8.
36. Calder AA, Embrey MP, Tait T. Ripening of the cervix with extra-amniotic prostaglandin E_2 in viscous gel before induction of labour. *Br J Obstet Gynaecol* 1977;84:264–8.
37. Wingerup L, Anderson K-E, Ulmsten U. Ripening of the cervix and induction of labor in patients at term by single intracervical application of prostaglandin E_2 in viscous gel. *Acta Obstet Gynecol Scand* 1979;84:11–14.
38. Atad J, Bornstein J, Petrikovsky B, Calderon I, Sorokin Y, Abramovici H. A non-pharmaceutical ripening of the unfavorable cervix and induction of labor by a novel double balloon device. *Obstet Gynecol* 1990;77:146–52.
39. MacKenzie IZ, Embrey MP. Cervical ripening with intravaginal prostaglandin E_2 gel. *Br Med J* 1977;2:1381–4.
40. Embrey MP, Graham NB, McNeill ME. Induction of labour with a sustained-release prostaglandin E_2 vaginal pessary. *Br Med J* 1980;281:901–2.
41. Arulkumaran S, Adaikan PG, Anandakumar C, Viegas OA, Singh P, Ratnam SS. Comparative study of a two-dose schedule of PGE_2 3 mg pessary and 1700-μg film for induction of labour in nulliparae with poor cervical score. *Prostaglandins Leukot Essent Fatty Acids* 1989;38:37–41.
42. Liggins GC. Controlled trial of induction of labour by vaginal suppositories containing prostaglandin E_2. *Prostaglandins* 1979; 18:167–72.
43. Hunter IWE, Cato E, Ritchie J. Induction of labor using high-dose or low-dose prostaglandin vaginal pessaries. *Obstet Gynecol* 1984;63:418–20.
44. MacKenzie IZ, Burns E. Randomised trial of one versus two PGE_2 doses for labour induction. I: clinical outcome. *Br J Obstet Gynaecol* 1997;104:1062–7.
45. Westgate J, Williams JA. Evaluation of a controlled release vaginal prostaglandin E_2 pessary with a retrieval system for the induction of labour. *J Obstet Gynaecol* 1994;14:146–50.
46. Wagner M. Off-label use of misoprostol in obstetrics: A cautionary tale. *BJOG* 2005;112:266.
47. Weeks AD, Fiala C, Safar P. Misoprostol and the debate over off-label drug use. *BJOG* 2005;112:269.

48. Hofmeyr GJ, Gülmezoglu AM. Vaginal misoprostol for cervical ripening and induction of labour. *The Cochrane Database of Systematic Reviews*, 2002, Issue 4. Art. No.: CD000941. DOI: 10.1002/14651858.CD000941.
49. Gherman RB, McBrayer S, Browning J. Uterine rupture associated with vaginal birth after cesarean section: A complication of intravaginal misoprostol? *Gynecol Obstet Invest* 2000;50:212–13.
50. Hill DA, Chez RA, Quinlan J, Fuentes A, LaCombe J. Uterine rupture and dehiscence associated with intravaginal misoprostol cervical ripening. *J Reprod Med* 2000;45:823–6.
51. Majoko F, Magwali T, Zwizwai M. Uterine rupture associated with the use of misoprostol for induction of labor. *Int J Gynecol Obstet* 2002;76:77–8.
52. Daisley H. Maternal mortality following the use of misoprostol. *Med Sci Law* 2000;40(1):78–82.
53. American College of Obstetricians and Gynecologists. *Induction of Labor with Misoprostol*. ACOG Committee Opinion No. 228. Washington, DC: American College of Obstetricians and Gynecologists, 1999.
54. American College of Obstetricians and Gynecologists. *Response to Searle's Drug Warning on Misoprostol*. ACOG Committee Opinion No. 248. Washington, DC: American College of Obstetricians and Gynecologists, 2000.
55. American College of Obstetricians and Gynecologists. *Induction of Labor*. Practice Bulletin No. 10. Washington, DC: American College of Obstetricians and Gynecologists, 1999.
56. *Induction of Labour, RCOG Clinical Guideline*. Available: http://www.rcog.org.
57. Available: http://www.sogc.org.
58. MacKenzie IZ, Embrey MP. A comparison of PGE_2 and $PGF_{2\alpha}$ vaginal gel for ripening the cervix before induction of labour. *Br J Obstet Gynaecol* 1979;86:167–70.
59. Neilson DR, Prins RP, Bolton RN, Mark C, Watson P. A comparison of prostaglandin E_2 gel and prostaglandin F gel for pre-induction cervical ripening. *Am J Obstet Gynecol* 1983;146:526–30.
60. Magnani M, Cabrol D. Declenchement artificel du travail par la prostaglandine E_2 apres maturation du col par l'estradiol. *Inserm* 1986;51:109–18.
61. Thiery M, De Grezelle H, Van Ketz H, *et al.* The effect of locally administered estrogen on the human cervix. *Z Geburtsh Perinatol* 1979;183:445–8.
62. Sasaki K, Nakano R, Kadoya Y, Iwao M, Shima K, Sowa M. Cervical ripening with dehydroepiandrosterone sulphate. *Br J Obstet Gynaecol* 1982;89:195–8.
63. Bell RJ, Permezel M, MacLennan A, Hughes C, Healy D, Brennecke S. A randomized, double-blind, placebo-controlled trial of the safety of vaginal recombinant human relaxin for cervical ripening. *Obstet Gynecol* 1993;82:328–33.
64. Brennand JE, Calder AA, Leitch CR, Greer IA, Chou MM, MacKenzie IZ. Recombinant human relaxin as a cervical ripening agent. *Prog Relaxin Res* 1995;26:380–8.
65. Selinger M, MacKenzie IZ, Gillmer MDG, Phipps SL, Ferguson J. Progesterone inhibition in midtrimester termination of pregnancy: Physiological and clinical effects. *Br J Obstet Gynaecol* 1987;94: 1218–22.
66. Hill NCW, Selinger M, Ferguson J, Lopez-Bernal A, MacKenzie IZ. The physiological and clinical effects of progesterone inhibition with RU486 (mifepristone) in the second trimester. *Br J Obstet Gynaecol* 1990;97:487–92.
67. Frydman R, Lelaidier C, Baton-Saint-Mleux C, Fernandez H, Vial M, Bourget P. Labor induction in women at term with mifepristone (RU486): A double-blind, randomized, placebo-controlled study. *Obstet Gynecol* 1992;80:972–5.
68. Boulvain M, Kelly A, Lohse C, Stan C, Irion O. Mechanical methods for induction of labour. *The Cochrane Database of Systematic Reviews*, 2001, Issue 4. Art. No. CD001233. DOI: 10.1002/14651858.CD001233.
69. Smith CA. Homoeopathy for induction of labour. *The Cochrane Database of Systematic Reviews*, 2003, Issue 4. Art. No. CD003399. DOI: 10.1002/14651858.CD003399.
70. Theobald GW. *The Electrical Induction of Labour*. New York: Appleton-Century-Crofts, 1973.
71. Kubista E, Kucera H, Muller-Tyl E. Initiating contractions of the gravid uterus through electro-acupuncture. *Am J Chinese Med* 1975;3:343–6.
72. Dunn PA, Rogers D, Halford K. Transcutaneous electrical nerve stimulation at acupuncture points in the induction of uterine contractions. *Obstet Gynecol* 1989;73:286–90.
73. Tremeau ML, Fontanie-Ravier P, Teurnier F, Demouzon J. Protocol for cervical maturation by acupuncture [Protocole de maturation cervicale par acupuncture]. *J Gynecol Obstet Biol Reprod (Paris)* 1992;21:375–80.
74. Romer A, Weigel M, Zieger W, Melchart F. Prenatal acupuncture: Effects on cervical maturation and duration of labour. *Geburtshilfe Frauenheilkunde* 2000;60:513–18.
75. Rabl M, Ahner R, Bitschnau, Zaisler H, Husslein P. Acupuncture for cervical ripening and induction of labour at term: A randomised controlled trial. *Wien Klin Wochenschr* 2001;113(23/24):942–6.
76. Butler NR, Bonham DG. *Perinatal Mortality*. Edinburgh: E. and S. Livingstone Ltd, 1963.
77. Crowley P. Interventions for preventing or improving the outcome of delivery at or beyond term. *The Cochrane Database of Systematic Reviews*, 1997, Issue 1. Art. No.: CD000170. DOI: 10.1002/14651858.CD00017.
78. Flamm BL, Dunnett C, Fischermann E, Quilligan EJ. Vaginal delivery following Cesarean section: Use of oxytocin augmentation and epidural anesthesia with internal tocodynamic and fetal monitoring. *Am J Obstet Gynecol* 1984;148:759–63.
79. MacKenzie IZ, Boland J. Current therapeutic uses of prostaglandins in obstetrics in the United Kingdom. *Contemp Rev Obstet Gynaecol* 1993;5:9–14.
80. Guise JM, McDonagh MS, Osterweil P, Nygren P, Chan BK, Helfand M. Systematic review of the incidence and consequences of uterine rupture in women with previous caesarean section. *BMJ* 2004;329:19–25.
81. Landon MB, Hauth JC, Leveno KJ, *et al.*; National Institute of Child Health and Human Development Maternal-Fetal Medicine Units Network. Maternal and perinatal outcomes associated with a trial of labor after prior cesarean delivery. *N Engl J Med* 2004; 351:2581–9.
82. Pritchard JA. Fetal death in utero. *Obstet Gynecol* 1959;14: 573–80.
83. Selinger M. Progesterone inhibition in mid-pregnancy with Epostane. *Contemp Rev Obstet Gynaecol* 1988;94:67–79.
84. Van Pelt C, De Coster W, Thiery M. Preinduction cervical ripening with prostaglandin E_2: Influence on psychomotor evolution in the first year. *Eur J Obstet Gynecol Reprod Biol* 1984;18:299–301.
85. MacKenzie IZ, McKinlay E. Paediatric follow-up study: Follow-up of infants delivered by spontaneous vaginal delivery, following PGE_2 or oxytocin induction, or by cesarean section. In Calder AA, Keirse MJNC, MacKenzie IZ, eds. *Propan RS – A Clinical Review*. Hastenove: Euromed, 1995:37–9.
86. MacKenzie IZ. Clinical studies on cervical ripening. In Ellwood DA, Anderson ABM, eds. *The Cervix in Pregnancy and Labour*. London: Churchill Livingstone, 1981:161–86.
87. Kurup A, Arulkumaran S, Tay D, Ingemarsson I, Ratnam SS. Can terbutaline be used as a nebuliser instead of intravenous injection for inhibition of uterine activity? *Gynecol Obstet Invest* 1991;32:84–7.
88. Ingemarsson I, Arulkumaran S, Ratnam SS. Single injection of terbutaline in term labor. II. Effect on uterine activity. *Am J Obstet Gynecol* 1985;153:865–9.
89. Taylor AV, Boland JC, MacKenzie IZ. Prostaglandin-induced cervical ripening under tocolytic cover in primiparae: Results of a double-blind placebo-controlled trial. *Br J Obstet Gynaecol* 1990;97:827–31.
90. Leung A, Kwok P, Chang A. Association between prostaglandin E_2 and placental abruption. *Br J Obstet Gynaecol* 1987;94:1001–2.
91. Hatch MC. Maternal deaths associated with induction of labor. *N Y State J Med* 1969;69:599–602.
92. Schwartz RH, Jones RWA. Transplacental hyponatraemia due to oxytocin. *Br Med J* 1978;1:152–3.
93. Beazley JM, Weekes ARL. Neonatal hyperbilirubinaemia following the use of prostaglandin E_2 in labour. *Br J Obstet Gynaecol* 1976;83:62–7.
94. Conway DI, Read MD, Baver C, Martin RH. Neonatal jaundice – A comparison between intravenous oxytocin and oral prostaglandin E_2. *J Int Med Res* 1976;4:241–6.
95. Saruta T, Kaplan NM. Adrenocortical steroidogenesis: The effects of prostaglandins. *J Clin Invest* 1972;51:2246–51.
96. Brinsden RS, Clark AD. Postpartum haemorrhage after induced and spontaneous labour. *Br Med J* 1978;2:855–6.
97. Hannah ME, Ohlsson A, Farine D, *et al.* Induction of labor compared with expectant management for prelabor rupture of the membranes at term. TERMPROM Study Group. *N Engl J Med* 1996;334:1005–10.

98. Lange AP, Secher NJ, Nielsen FH, Pedersen GT. Stimulation of labor in cases of premature rupture of the membranes at or near term. A consecutive randomized study of prostaglandin E_2 tablets and intravenous oxytocin. *Acta Obstet Gynecol Scand* 1981; 60:207–10.
99. McQueen D, Neilson JP, Whittle MJ. Prelabour rupture of membranes with an unripe cervix: A random trial of management. *J Obstet Gynaecol* 1990;10:495–8.
100. Ray DA, Garite TJ. Prostaglandin E_2 for induction of labor in patients with premature rupture of membranes at term. *Am J Obstet Gynecol* 1992;166:836–43.
101. Ngai SW, To WK, Lao T, Ho PC. Cervical priming with oral misprostol in pre-labor rupture of membranes at term. *Obstet Gynecol* 1996;87:923–6.
102. Stewart P. Patients' attitudes to induction and labour. *Br Med J* 1977;2:749–52.
103. Cartwright A. Mothers' experiences of induction. *Br Med J* 1977; 2:745–9.
104. Goevee R, Hannah M, Hewson S. Cost-effectiveness of induction of labour versus serial antenatal monitoring in the Canadian Multicentre Post-term Pregnancy Trial. *Can Med Assoc J* 1995; 152:1145–50.
105. MacKenzie IZ, Magill P, Burns E. Randomised trial of one versus two PGE_2 doses for labour induction: Cost–benefit analyses. *Br J Obstet Gynaecol* 1997;104:1068–72.
106. Ekman G, Perssen PH, Ulmsten U, Wingerup L. The impact on labour induction of intracervically applied PGE_2 gel, related to gestational age in patients with an unripe cervix. *Acta Obstet Gynecol Scand* 1983;113:173–5.
107. Shepherd JH, Pearce JMF, Sims CD. Induction of labour using prostaglandin E_2 pessaries. *Br Med J* 1979;2:108–10.
108. Embrey MP, MacKenzie IZ. Labour induction with a sustained-release prostaglandin E_2 polymer vaginal pessary. *J Obstet Gynaecol* 1985;6:38–41.

176 Electronic fetal monitoring

B. S. Schifrin, S. Myers, W. R. Cohen and R. Kates

Understanding fetal heart rate patterns

Introduction

The introduction of electronic fetal heart rate monitoring (EFM) more than 30 years ago was accompanied by extraordinary expectations. It was expected that by timely detecting, then intervening in the presence of certain fetal heart rate (FHR) features, EFM would reduce the intrapartum stillbirth rate, enhance neonatal condition, diminish the risk of long-term disability and reduce the cesarean section rate for fetal distress.[1] While indeed the fetal and neonatal death rates have fallen considerably since the introduction of EFM, the risk and severity of neurologic handicap have not.[2,3] Moreover, the rise in the cesarean section rate over the past 30 years has been attributed at least in part to the use of EFM.[4] Clearly, the benefits of EFM, as envisioned by its early enthusiasts, have not been realized.[5,6]

Reservations about the value of EFM prompted a number of randomized controlled trials (RCTs) comparing it with auscultation.[7–9] The nomenclature of FHR patterns, experimental design and indeed the results of these studies diverge widely and permit almost any conclusion about the benefit or lack thereof of EFM or auscultation.[10,11] One may thus conclude from available studies that EFM reduces the risk of neonatal seizures, or increases the risk of cerebral palsy in prematures, or that it is of no benefit at the expense of an increased, presumably unnecessary, risk of cesarean section or that the failure to demonstrate benefit is related to selection bias or other methodological flaws. Furthermore, marked differences exist in the interpretation of FHR patterns even among experts, even when the nosology is agreed upon.[12] Indeed, the trials were premature, not reproducible, beset by technical and statistical difficulties. It is reasonable to argue that the benefits of EFM remain unsatisfactorily tested and that RCTs confuse the issue. Nevertheless, the recommendations by the American College of Obstetricians and Gynecologists, the International Federation of Obstetricians and Gynecologists, the Society of Obstetricians and Gynecologists of Canada, and the Royal College of Obstetricians and Gynecologists, based on the results of these RCTs, all assert that auscultation is equivalent to EFM, that EFM is not required on admission to labor and delivery, that intermittent auscultation is relevant as a primary or indeed the only necessary method of surveillance.[13] While the basis of these guidelines rests with the presumed equivalence of outcome between auscultation and EFM in the RCTs, there is no contemporary study comparing auscultation against no FHR surveillance at all, or any explanation as to why, if FHR is a reflection of fetal health, a technique that inarguably provides more accurate and complete information about it would not be better than one less effective in that regard. Customary auscultation (not part of a controlled study) appears less reliable than structured auscultation with a Doppler device.[10] Others, conceding the extraordinary specificity of the 'reassuring' FHR pattern, advocate alternative strategies for the evaluation of the abnormal tracing including fetal scalp blood sampling, fetal pulse oximetry and computerized evaluation of the fetal ECG.[14–17] Despite the lingering uncertainties about the relevance of EFM, the reproducibility and meaning of FHR patterns and some articles calling for its outright abandonment, there remains virtually universal application of this technique during labor.[6,18]

Pathophysiology

Before discussing the interpretation and management of individual EFM tracings, it is necessary to point out certain physiologic principles of FHR monitoring along with the technical and logistic pitfalls that impede the ability to realize the objectives originally vouchsafed for EFM.

FHR patterns during labor and before are influenced by numerous factors including gestational age and the behavioral state of the fetus (activity level, breathing movements, electroencephalographic pattern, etc.), as well as medications, infection, anomalies, arrhythmias and maternal disease.[19] Beyond these, FHR patterns during labor are also influenced to a considerable degree by uterine contractions and expulsive efforts of

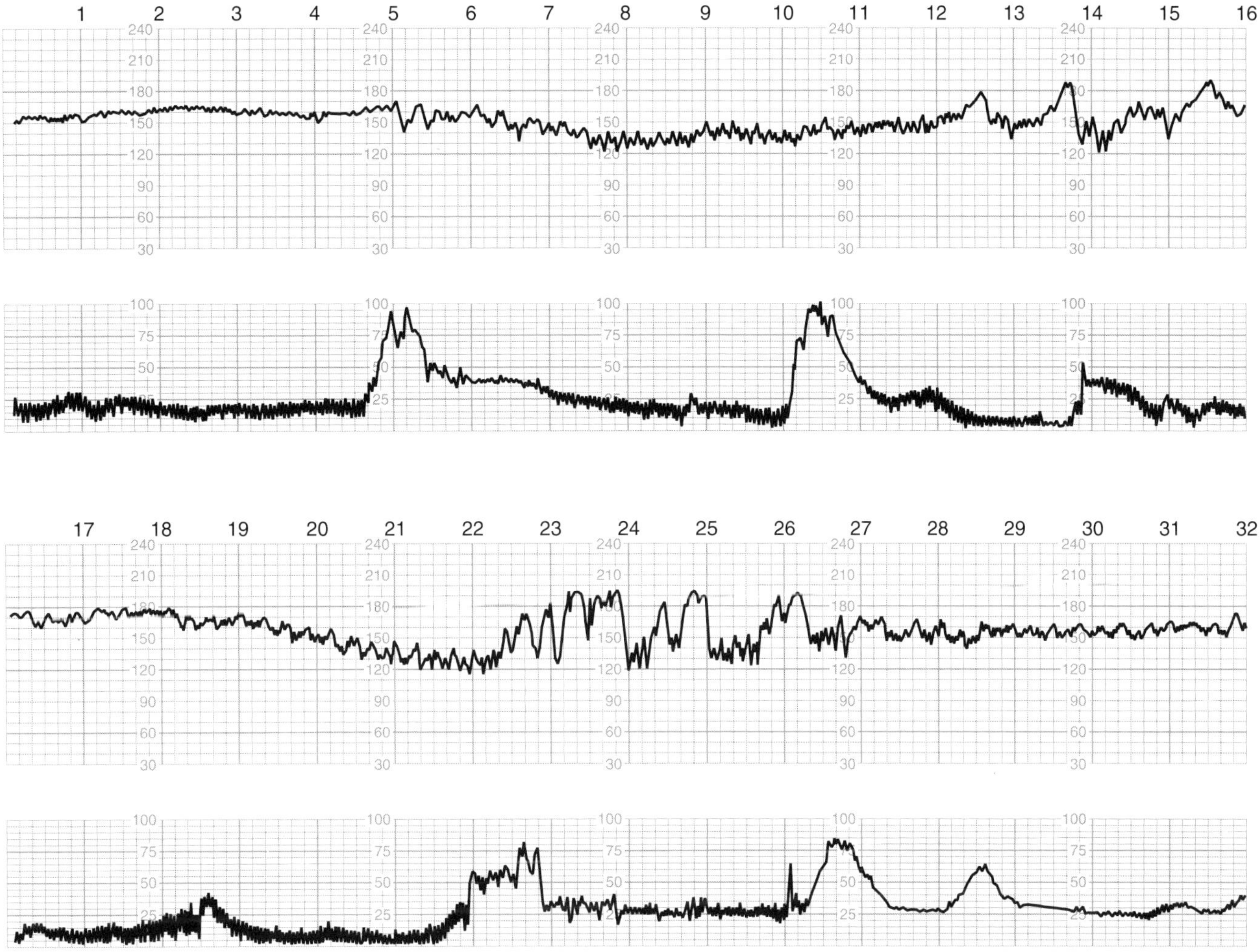

Figure 176.1 Non-decelerative pattern. Reactive tracing. Normal variations in FHR pattern produced by changes in fetal behavioral state. Note the three obvious epochs in top half of the tracing which begins with absent variability and no accelerations. The rate then decreases somewhat with an obvious increase in the variability. The third epoch shows obvious accelerations and variability, but different from that in the previous epoch.

the mother as well as the station, position, attitude and molding of the fetal head, fetal temperature, the presence of infection, and perhaps by dysfunctional labor.[20,21]

The normal-term FHR pattern has identifiable features corresponding to various behavioral states (Figure 176.1). These include a stable baseline rate and absent decelerations and alternating epochs of (a) decreased variability and absent accelerations (sleep/rest) and (b) average variability and accelerations associated with fetal movement (awake/active).[22–29] When present, these features, particularly including the cyclic activity, permit the inference of both normal fetal behavior (neurologic integrity) and absent hypoxia. They represent the fundamental properties of the FHR pattern of the normally oxygenated and neurologically responsive fetus, who will not likely deteriorate from hypoxia, sepsis, or trauma without changes in baseline rate and variability.

As will be discussed below, not all changes in rate and variability represent deterioration, and if only brief segments of the tracing are analyzed some of the normal features of the rest cycle (for example, reduced variability and absence of accelerations) carry the potential for adverse interpretation.[19] Thus, brief periods of absent variability (fetal sleep) and sinusoidal heart rate pattern (fetal sucking), even certain 'late' decelerations (with stable baseline rate and maintained variability) that correspond to periods of active fetal breathing should not be confused with fetal abnormality.[24–26] The evolution of these episodic changes is best evaluated during antepartum heart rate testing in both normal and pathologic pregnancies.[23,27–31] Absent decelerations during labor, these patterns may be observed for reasonable lengths of time before consideration is given to intervention.

The normal baseline FHR is defined as the persistently stable rate in the absence of (or between) contractions or provocations.[32] The baseline rate can be characterized in a very narrow range, perhaps 5–10 bpm at best, and is usually described according to the rate, the stability of the rate and the presence of short- and long-term variability in the intervals between contractions. Short-term variability represents the abrupt and seemingly random changes between consecutive heart beats (usually only about 1–2 bpm) giving rise to a rather unpredictable, somewhat chaotic pattern of changes. Long-term variability represents the more predictable changes in the oscillations in the rate over many beats, is usually classified according to the range (peak to trough) of heart rates over about 1 min and normally averages about 5–15 bpm. Changes in long- and short-term variability tend to correspond. When only short-term variability is present, however, the tracing is usually considered acceptable. When the long-term oscillations are regular (sinusoidal) with a frequency of about 2–6 cpm and an amplitude of 5–15 bpm it is often referred to as *sinusoidal* if reactivity elsewhere in the tracing is absent. Whether the pattern is intermittent or persistent and reactivity elsewhere is absent, it likely represents an ominous situation in the fetus such as severe anemia, neurologic injury or anomaly.[33–39] However, the most typically encountered sinusoidal pattern is either a variant of normal or the result of narcotic administration and correctable by nalorphine.[40] While most attention has been paid to the abnormalities associated with decreased (< 5 bpm) or absent (< 2 bpm) long-term variability, it is important to emphasize that increased variability, either long- or short-term (> 15 bpm), is no more 'normal' than is decreased variability. Indeed, increased variability may be a harbinger of impending or early hypoxia secondary to alpha-adrenergic activity.[41]

Baseline tachycardia and bradycardia are frequently defined as heart rates outside the range of 'normal' (e.g. 110–160 bpm) for at least 10–15 min.[32] (Indeed the definitions of the various 'guidelines' differ.) Defining fetal bradycardia and tachycardia by some 'normal range' based on cross-sectional studies, however, seems to violate a more physiologic approach of using the fetus as its own control. For example, a fetal baseline rate that rises from 155 to 165 bpm (tachycardia by the above definition) represents much less of a problem than a rise to 155 bpm from a baseline of 110 bpm, even though both of the latter values are in the normal range for the population. The baseline heart rate established on admission should be used as the reference point for subsequent changes. Thus, if the FHR on admission were about 130 bpm, a rise to a persistent 150 bpm should be considered a relative tachycardia while a fall in heart rate to a persistent 115 bpm, even with normal or increased variability would represent relative bradycardia. Neither should be considered part of the normal range of this particular fetus. A number of factors, many of which do not represent hypoxia, may increase the heart rate including fever, cardioactive drugs, maternal dehydration, arrhythmia and hypoxia (with decelerations).

Thus in a review of any tracing, it is important to look at the beginning of the pattern to establish the baseline and ask if the fetal behavior was ever demonstrably normal. As the fetus deteriorates before the onset of labor, behavioral cycles become disrupted with lengthening sleep cycles, disappearance of variability, and sometimes a rise in the baseline. Only then do accelerations disappear, decelerations appear with contractions, the baseline becomes unstable, it falls, and the fetus dies.[42,43] If the fetus enters labor with persistently absent variability, it cannot be defined as having normal neurologic potential. If there has been no preceding testing to help ascertain the acuity of these findings, then the differential diagnosis is broad and includes: drug effect, placental insufficiency, infection, genetic disorders, anemia, neurologic injury (infarction, hemorrhage, asphyxia), congenital anomaly, and tumor.

It is critical to the understanding of FHR patterns to recognize that in the presence of uterine contractions, acute fetal hypoxemia will be reflected by the appearance of decelerations before any rise in the baseline rate or decrease in variability.[43,44] With continued mild to moderate oxygen deprivation, the decelerations persist, accompanied by a rising baseline heart rate and a diminution in baseline variability (and developing acidosis) eventually leading to a fixed elevated rate (rarely above 160 bpm). As the fetus approaches death the baseline falls and becomes unstable; decelerations may be less obvious and less easily separable into type – i.e. late or variable. With severe or profound hypoxemia the initial response may be a prolonged deceleration or bradycardia, which requires immediate attention if not relieved or improving after about 4 min.

To connote significant fetal hypoxemia, therefore, transient decelerations must provoke a rise in a previously normal baseline rate. If the fetal baseline rate is already increased over the initial normal baseline, then no apparent change in baseline will necessarily occur. Irrespective of the deceleration pattern (late, variable, or prolonged), transient decelerations unaccompanied by a rise in heart rate cannot represent developing tissue hypoxia or troublesome ischemia. Similarly, elevations of the heart rate or loss of variability without decelerations during labor also cannot represent ongoing tissue oxygen deprivation. Thus, in the absence of changes in baseline rate and variability there is no meaningful distinction among , late, variable, even prolonged decelerations. Prolonged decelerations (usually in the second stage of labor) arising from a previously normal FHR patterns are rarely of (acid–base) consequence if the deceleration stabilizes at 80 bpm or above, and especially if variability is maintained (*vide infra*).[45,46] If the prolonged deceleration continues to fall below 80 bpm and loses

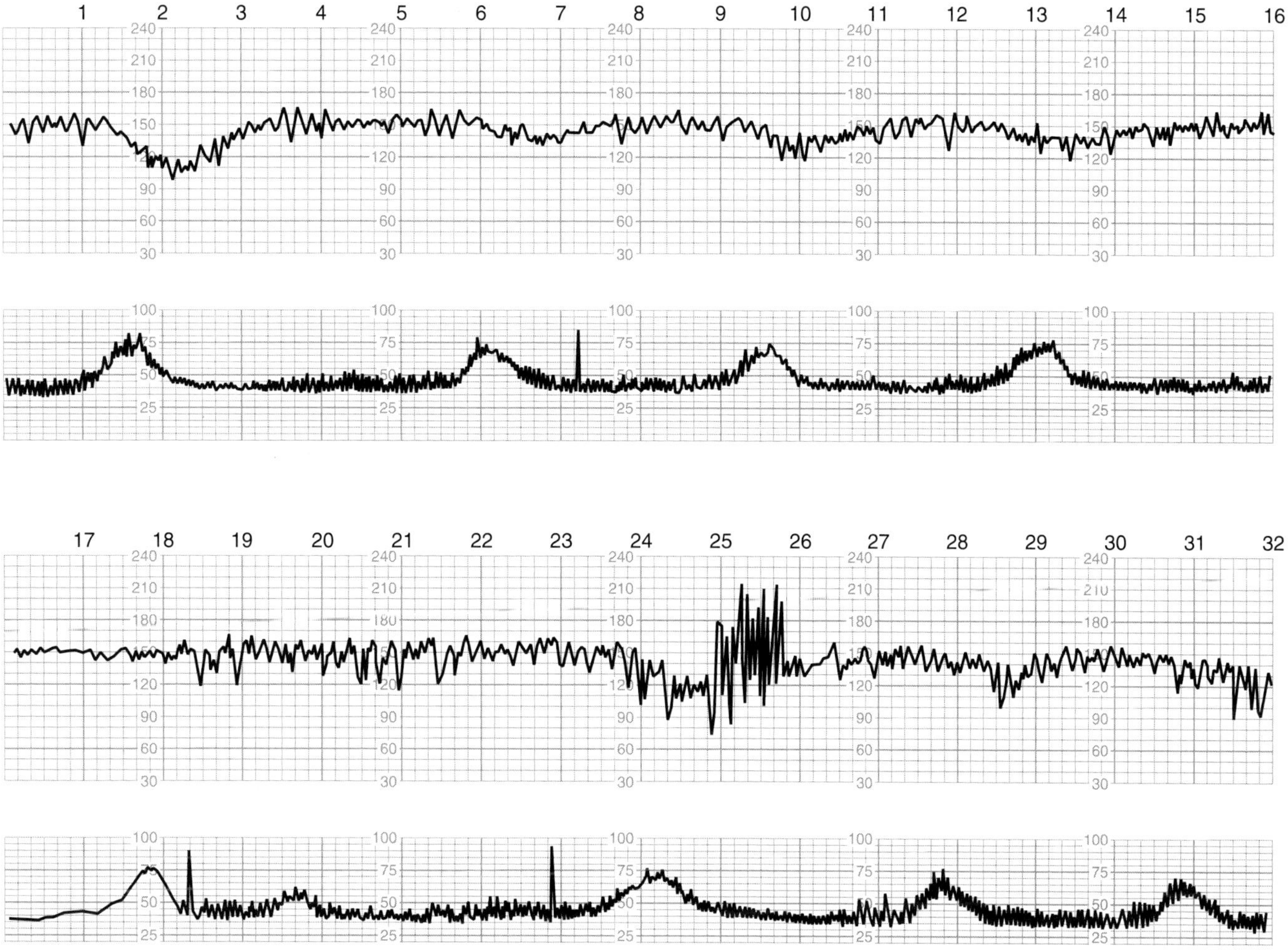

Figure 176.2 Late deceleration pattern in association with fetal breathing movements (FBM). The upper portion of the panel has what appear to be late decelerations. They are not related to hypoxemia; rather, they represent a response to active FBM which, when picked up by the tocodynamometer, are seen as high-frequency low-amplitude spikes. When FBM abate (16–20 min) the decelerations disappear without residual tachycardia or decrease in variability.

variability, the prognosis is much more ominous. Whether or not the deceleration is agonal or not, the first response is to attempt to ameliorate it by position change, the elimination of contractions and, as a minimum, refraining from pushing.

The pattern of decelerations provides important insights into the mechanism of hypoxia: The fetus may suffer hypoxia related either to (1) a decreased availability of oxygen to the fetus (hypoxemic hypoxia) or (2) interference with blood flow to the brain or placenta (ischemic hypoxia). We consider those changes associated with late decelerations *hypoxemic* while those associated with variable or prolonged decelerations of sudden onset *ischemic.* The bases for this distinction derive from the clinical and experimental work of several authors.[44,47–56] The difference is important because of the markedly different ways the fetus responds to such limitations of oxygen, in the speed of deterioration and in the relationship to subsequent injury. Hypoxemia may occur without ischemia, and in this context is rarely associated with organ damage unless there has been considerable neglect. Tissue ischemia, however, may occur in the absence of systemic hypoxemia and cause end-organ injury – sometimes rapidly.[57]

Late decelerations represent an early response to fetal hypoxemia, even before the development of changes in baseline rate and variability.[43,58,59] They may also represent a benign response to a behavioral pattern of normal fetal breathing episodes (Figure 176.2).[26] When associated with a rising baseline rate and decreasing variability, they are accompanied by transient hypotension during the deceleration and a slow decrease in oxygen availability and cerebral blood flow (CBF) and may be tolerated for many hours while the fetus accumulates a metabolic acidosis.[43,58,59] As the hypoxia and acidosis increase, the FHR becomes fixed (absent variability) usually with a relative tachycardia and continuing decelerations. The decelerations at this time might be quite minimal in amplitude, but

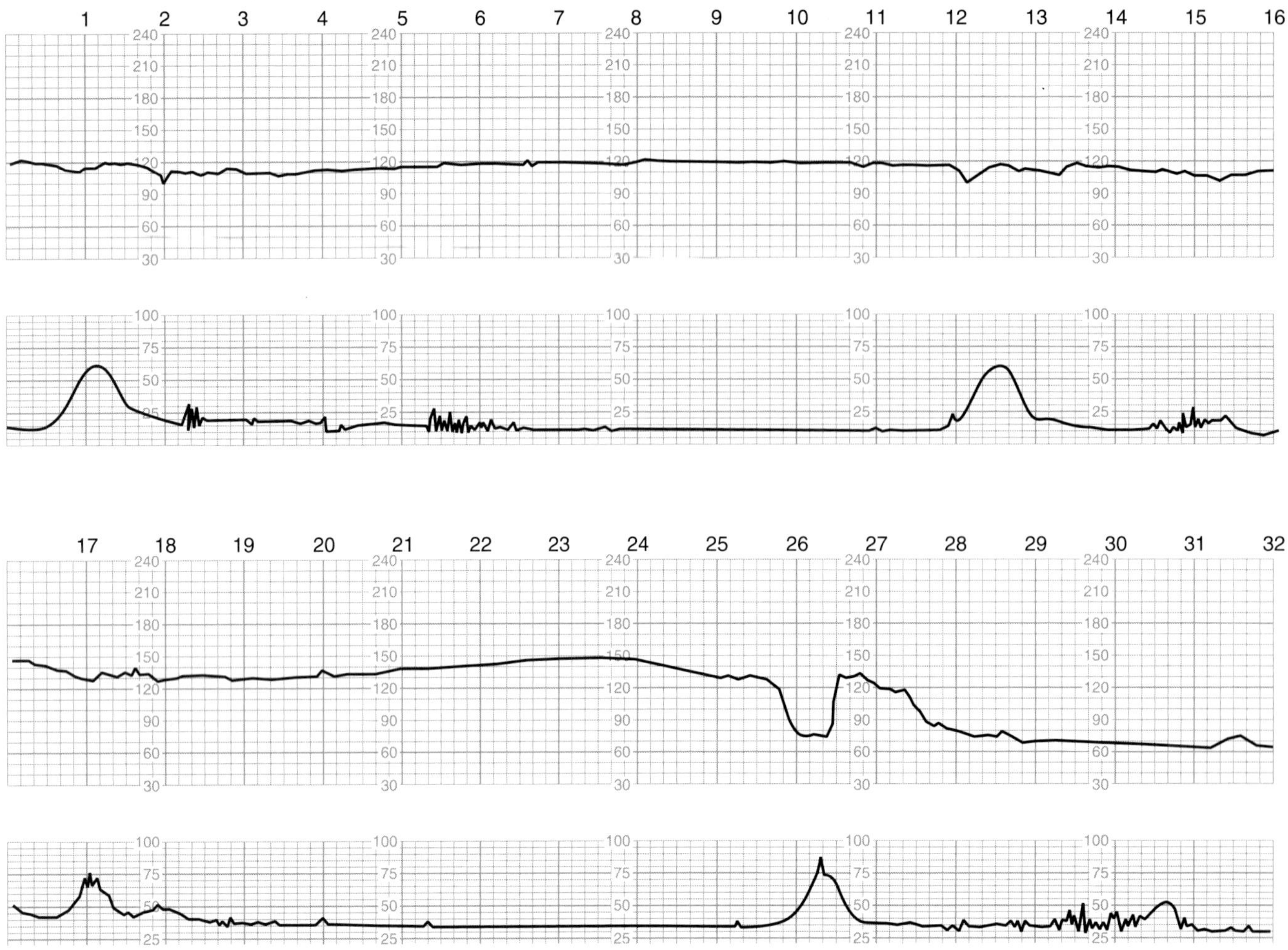

Figure 176.3 In this agonal pattern, death (attributed to a tight knot in the cord) was preceded by absent variability, an unstable baseline, and a terminal bradycardia.

are usually discernible because of the marked reduction in the amount of both long- and short-term variability.

Late in the course of continuing and progressive hypoxia, there eventually comes a point when the severity of the oxygen deprivation and the resulting acidosis and loss of energy substrate conspire so that the fetus is no longer be able to maintain cardiac output to even priority organs. Blood flow to the brain will then diminish and injury will supervene as the fetus approaches death. On the monitor this is revealed as an unstable, slowly oscillating, diminishing heart rate, less obvious decelerations with absent variability, and, eventually, asystole (Figure 176.3).[36,60] As mentioned above, the fetus with this agonal pattern is unlikely to survive or to survive intact after delivery. This is the 'pure' sequence of changes that most likely results in severe acidosis at birth, prolonged, low Apgar scores and severe neonatal hypoxic–ischemic encephalopathy in the immediate neonatal period.[61–64] This agonal pattern requires intervention as rapidly as can be performed with reasonable safety for mother and fetus. While failing to intervene will surely result in fetal death, it must be understood, nevertheless, that this fetus may die or already be seriously handicapped irrespective of the speed of intervention.

It is important here to distinguish between the features of the sudden bradycardia or prolonged deceleration (Figure 176.4) seen commonly at the very end of labor and the 'agonal' pattern (seen at any time) (Figure 176.3). In the prolonged deceleration pattern, the preceding FHR pattern has been normal or contained minimal decelerations unassociated with a rising baseline rate or decreased variability. While the appearance of the sudden prolonged deceleration suggests an acute, ischemic stress, it may not be used to infer injury. At least as importantly, prompt intervention may produce a neurologically intact child. In the terminal decelerative pattern, in which one may often anticipate injury if the infant survives, the preceding pattern reveals absent variability, an unstable baseline rate and nondescript decelerations. Death or injury is probably inevitable and not preventable.

As noted, the initial appearance of late decelerations represents an early marker of hypoxemia, even before the appearance of acidosis. As such it will be, early in

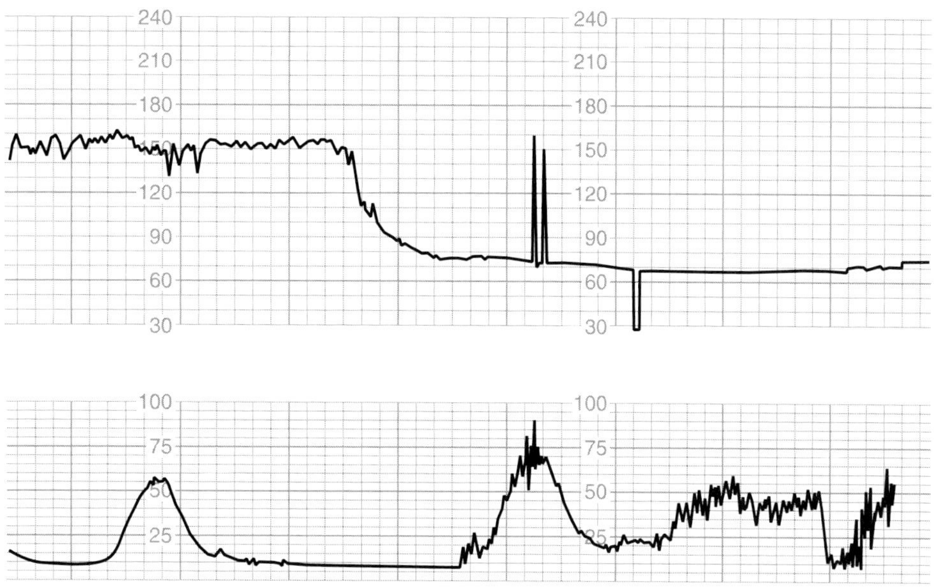

Figure 176.4 A sudden prolonged deceleration preceded by a normal pattern. The presumptive cause was placental abruption and prompt delivery resulted in a good outcome.

the course, a poor predictor of subsequent poor outcome at delivery or long-term outcome.[65] Those factors associated with the early appearance of late decelerations include: fever, frequent or prolonged uterine contractions, maternal hypotension, placental disease, and fetal anemia. We emphasize here that if the mother is febrile, the fetus and placenta are also febrile – at an even higher temperature – with increased metabolic demands.[66,67]

Variable and prolonged decelerations may be considered acute, responses to any diminution in cerebral or umbilical blood flow (ischemia).[19,40,50,68–71] When the cord is compressed, the rapidity of the onset and the depth of the deceleration result from an exuberant increase in fetal peripheral resistance and blood pressure. Head compression causes variable decelerations by a different mechanism, but they are morphologically indistinguishable clinically from those produced by cord compression. When hypoxemia ensues from any cause there may be redistribution of blood flow within the fetus so that flow to the vital structures in the organism, i.e. the brain, the adrenals, the heart and the placenta are maintained and flow to less critical areas (the gut, skin, muscles, etc.) is sacrificed. This is referred to as the 'dive reflex' and is similar to that found in the diving mammal, including the human.[72,73] Under these manifold responses and redirection of blood flow, specific areas of the fetus from which blood has been shunted or where flow has been inadequate may suffer injury in a short period of time, even without ongoing, systemic hypoxia.[57,74] Variable decelerations deteriorate with much the same changes as described for late decelerations above, but the course may be considerably shorter. It is axiomatic therefore, that for this reflex to indeed protect the brain for example, it must overcome any meaningful obstruction to blood flow to the brain.[75,76] Sometimes, as the result of expulsive efforts, malposition of the fetal head and non-progressive labor, cerebral blood flow (CBF) may not be maintained. It is likely that most variable decelerations, especially in the second stage of labor and especially in the OP position, are related to head compression.

This approach to the evaluation of decelerations prompts here a definition of the term 'recovery' from a deceleration. In this context 'total' recovery from a deceleration sequence means a return to the previously normal baseline rate and variability. When the fetus recovers from even significant hypoxia or ischemia, first the decelerations diminish in amplitude and disappear; then the baseline rate and variability return to normal. The disappearance of decelerations alone is insufficient to declare the fetus 'recovered'. Irrespective of the type or duration of the deceleration, recovery as defined here, appears to preclude injury during the episode. On the contrary, abnormalities in the recovery of variable decelerations sometimes called 'atypical' variables, or those with 'slow return', represent the yet unrecovered responses to the hemodynamic changes reflected in the variable deceleration.[70,71] They require no increased attention – provided that the baseline rate and variability recover to their previously normal state before the next contraction.[77]

While many classify the severity of decelerations based on the duration and the amplitude, these factors have not been shown to be predictive of adverse outcome.[78–81] Paul *et al.* showed that the severity of the acidosis accompanying late decelerations was a

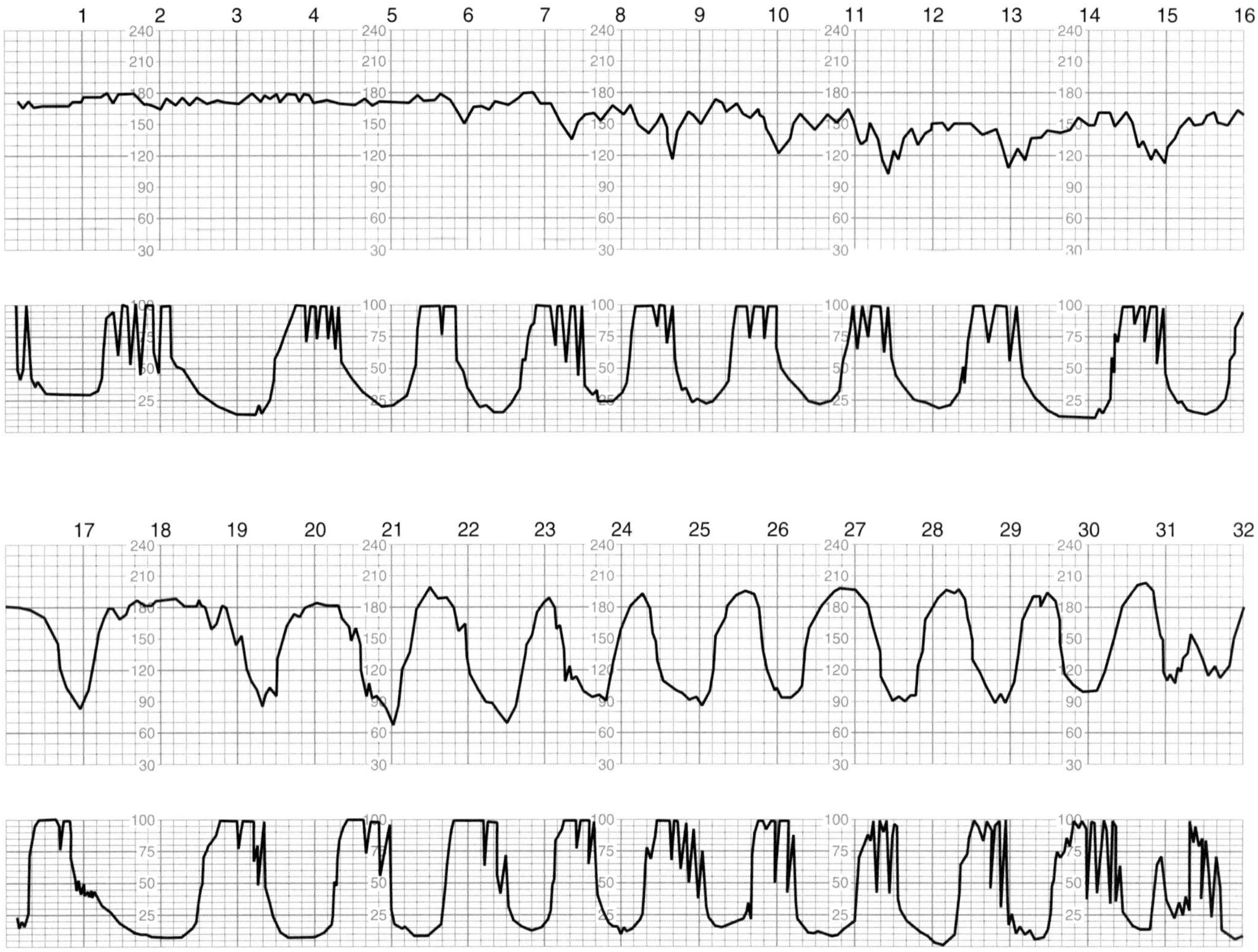

Figure 176.5 Progressive decelerative pattern (variable decelerations). At the start of the second stage of labor the fetal heart rate patterns is normal with absent decelerations. With the onset of pushing the fetus develops a series of variable decelerations with progressively decreasing variability. This represent recurrent ischemic events but the pattern in itself does not permit the diagnosis of injury. The frequency of contractions should be diminished and the patients expulsive efforts moderated.

function of the amount of variability in the baseline and not of the amplitude or the duration of the deceleration.[82] Zalar and Quilligan[83] and Visser *et al.*[42] showed that pH was almost invariably normal in fetuses with poor variability provided there were no decelerations. A similar dichotomous division of pH results was demonstrated with fetal tachycardia.[84] Those fetuses with tachycardia and no late decelerations had normal pH values, while those with late decelerations were more likely to be acidotic. Fetuses with persistent bradycardia during the second stage of labor are frequently, but not invariably, normal.[45,46,85] Here again, other features of the tracing need to be considered.

The most telling parameter in attempting to determine hypoxia is the impact of the deceleration on the subsequent baseline rate and variability. According to this notion, most decelerations developing during labor either represent no significant difficulty for the fetus, or are remediable with conservative care. Thus, careful control of contraction frequency, whether or not oxytocin or prostaglandins are used, minimizing supine hypotension associated with maternal position or epidural anesthesia, and observing the fetal response to maternal pushing in the second stage of labor can forestall decelerations from appearing in the first place. Even when decelerations are progressive, the change from a developing to persistent hypoxia is more or less gradual, in part related to the strength and frequency of contractions and the amount of head or umbilical cord compression due to descent and maternal expulsive efforts (Figure 176.5). Thus in the majority of instances decelerations are correctable, or failing that, permit timely intervention. Occasionally, most especially in the second stage with frequent contractions and unrestrained pushing, the transition from early to advanced hypoxia and ischemia can be abrupt (Figure 176.6).

The second stage of labor

The second stage of labor begins with the completion of cervical dilatation. The frequency of decelerations

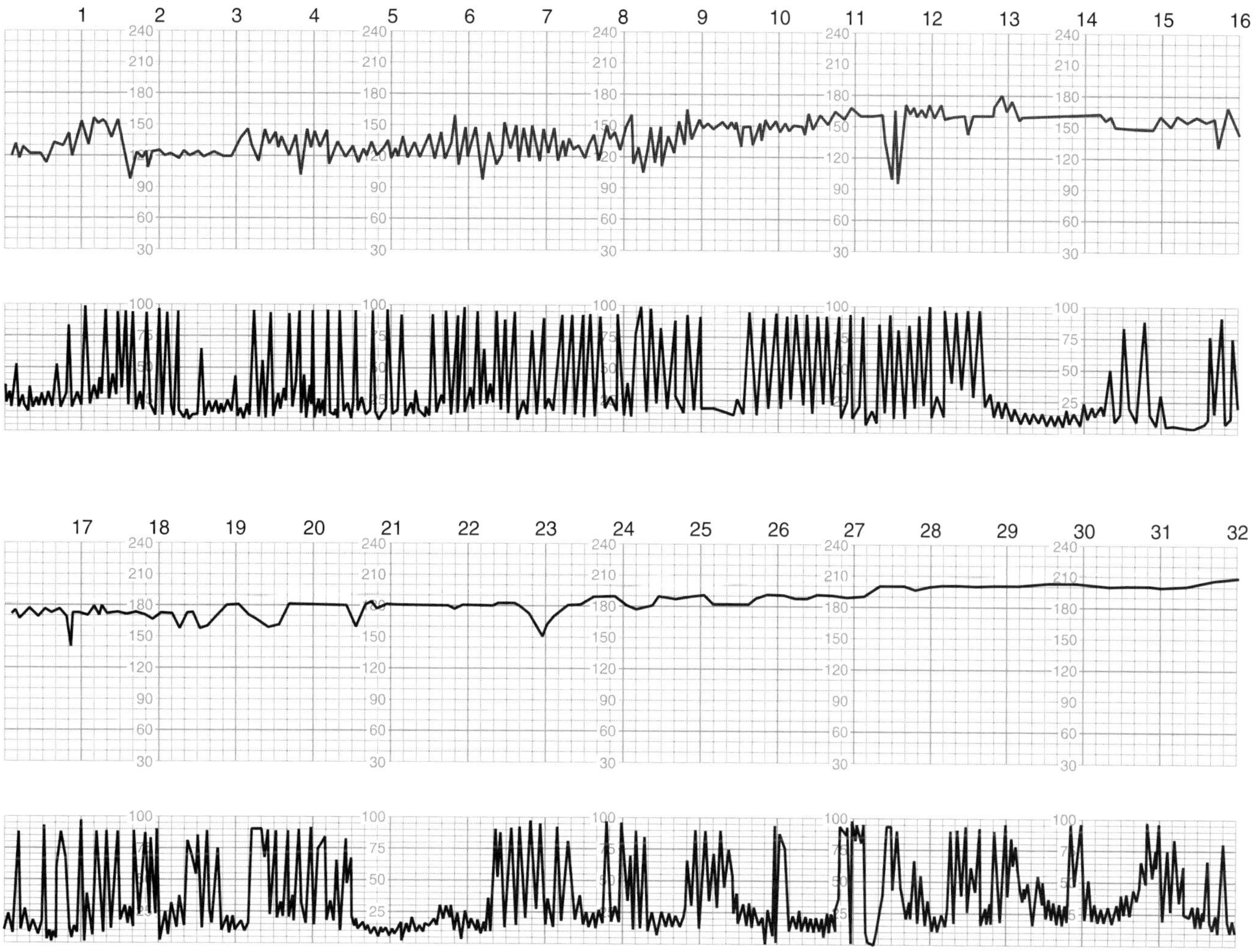

Figure 176.6 Progression of normal decelerative pattern to injury during the second stage of labor in a fetus in occiput posterior position and relentless pushing.[103] The tracing reveals a diminution in baseline rate to 120 bpm from the normal fetal baseline of 135 bpm accompanied by an increase in baseline variability. It is important to emphasize that increased variability is no more normal than is decreased variability. At 18 min the fetus develops a sudden tachycardia and absent variability. Notice also the disappearance of the decelerations. The infant was born with massive intracranial hemorrhage but normal acid–base balance.

usually increases dramatically in the second stage of labor, probably due to the effects of frequent uterine contractions along with the effect of maternal expulsive forces on the fetal head and the cord. While no pattern is unique to the second stage, increased variability, prolonged decelerations and rising baseline are especially common, as are variable decelerations.[19,86] Alterations of the baseline, especially tachycardia, are often associated with acidosis, an effect confirmed in the bovine model.[87] Baseline bradycardia is not uncommon; it is frequently related to the pushing strategy (see below) and only infrequently associated with adverse outcome or acidosis, especially if variability is maintained.[86]

It is widely believed, however, that patterns during the second stage are different and may even require their own classification.[20,46,88] The enormous potential variation in second-stage decelerations makes understandable why so many patterns are other than 'normal' and why in the largest RCT of monitoring, 40% of second stage patterns could not even be classified.[7,88] We emphasize, however, that the principles of interpretation of FHR patterns apply irrespective of the timing of the tracing (antepartum, first stage of labor, second stage of labor).[20]

We believe that decelerations during the second stage are made more difficult to classify not because of inherent changes in their appearance but because of the frequency of contractions and the conduct of maternal pushing. In the first stage of labor decelerations usually induce treatment to diminish the frequency of contractions and avoid additional stresses. In the second stage of labor, maternal pushing is often sustained and encouraged in spite of decelerations. In this situation there may be no opportunity for the fetus to recover from one contraction before the next one begins. Under these circumstances it may not be possible even to determine the fetal baseline rate between contractions.

Table 176.1 Principles of EFM interpretation

- Cyclic activity with accelerations, normal baseline variability and a stable baseline heart rate alternating with epochs of decreased variability and absent accelerations are hallmarks of fetal health
- Accelerations arise out of normal variability during cyclic variation in the baseline heart rate. Accelerations without baseline variability should be considered suspicious. In the second stage of labor, they may represent the maternal heart rate pattern
- Abnormal patterns may represent the effects of drugs, fetal anomaly, fetal injury or infection – not only hypoxia
- Significant hypoxia will not occur without changes in baseline rate and variability. When contractions are present, decelerations appear before changes in rate and variability
- Periods of decreased variability and stable baseline heart rate in the normal range without decelerations may represent quiet fetal sleep. During labor, they are unlikely to represent hypoxia
- Before labor, hypoxic fetuses may have a normal baseline FHR of 110–150 bpm with no accelerations and baseline variability of < 5 bpm for < 40 min. During labor the additional presence of decelerations is required for the presumptive diagnosis of hypoxia
- With diminished baseline variability < 5 bpm even shallow late decelerations < 15 bpm are ominous in a non-reactive trace
- During labor, too frequent contractions represent a threat to the fetus irrespective of the presence of abnormal heart rate patterns
- Abruption, cord prolapse, and scar rupture can cause acute hypoxia and should be suspected clinically. (May give rise to prolonged decelerations/bradycardia)
- Fetal hypoxia and acidosis may develop faster with an abnormal trace when there is scanty, thick meconium, intrauterine growth retardation, intrauterine infection with pyrexia and/or pre-or post-term labor
- In preterm fetuses (especially < 34 weeks), signs of hypoxia and acidosis (the presence of an abnormal trace) [increase the likelihood of respiratory distress syndrome and may contribute to intraventricular hemorrhage] warrant earlier intervention than in the term fetus
- Hypoxia can be aggravated by excessive uterine activity (e.g. oxytocin), maternal hypotension (epidural analgesia) and by mechanical/traumatic stresses (difficult operative delivery)

As a result, decelerations may pile one on top of the other, creating virtually any type or duration of deceleration pattern, including prolonged deceleration.

Focusing specifically on the second stage draws attention to the role of head position, compression and reduction in brain blood flow in the etiology of fetal cardiac decelerations during this period. Fetuses in the occiput posterior position, for example, demonstrate an increased likelihood of decelerations and adverse outcomes.[89,90]

Many of the cases in which the FHR pattern deteriorates during the second stage are related to excessive frequency of contractions and unrestrained maternal bearing down.[19,91,92] Safety requires that contractions appear no more often than every 2 min or more preferably, no more than 7 in 15 min, and that pushing with the contraction be resumed only if the baseline heart rate and variability have recovered to their previously normal levels (see definition of recovery above). Determining the significance of second stage decelerations is best approached by analyzing them in the absence of pushing. This requires both diminishing the frequency of contractions when necessary (by reducing the oxytocin infusion rate) and curtailing the mother's pushing. Thus, if the deceleration is prolonged beyond the contraction or the baseline rate is rising between contractions the expulsive efforts of the mother must be temporarily modified. This may require some effort and discipline, especially if the mother is not receiving analgesia or epidural anesthesia. Failing this, the practitioner exhorts the patient to push exuberantly in an attempt to 'outrun the fetal distress', but succeeds only in precipitating an unremitting, prolonged deceleration. Alternatively, he or she may be tempted to undertake a potentially difficult operative delivery that is often unsuccessful. It must be remembered that the first objective of fetal surveillance is to keep the fetus out of harm's way; that is a more effective approach than rescue. Principles of interpretation are summarized in Table 176.1.

Pitfalls

Given all the insights that fetal monitoring provides about the condition of the fetus, it is necessary to explore why it is subjected to so much criticism and skepticism about its value. We will not deal further with the several randomized clinical trials relating to the subject, whose merits and limitations have been discussed elsewhere.[93–96] Rather, we will focus on those relevant technical and philosophical issues that have not received broad discussion in the literature.

Nomenclature

While several attempts have been made to standardize nomenclature,[88,97–100] it is clear that diverse systems of limited compatibility are in vogue throughout the world and receive inconsistent interpretation.[101] It is also clear that these classifications function primarily to direct attention to phenomena within the tracing (decelerations, variability, tachycardia, etc.); they do little to explain the source of the heart rate pattern abnormalities or the probability that they arise from clinically important pathology. Moreover, in each case, the classification is deemed relevant only to the detection of hypoxia and acidosis and not in relationship to neurologic integrity and behavior.[102–105]

These drawbacks have doubtless contributed to the current official disparagement of the term 'fetal distress', and to general skepticism about EFM. As the term is commonly employed, "fetal distress" refers to an abnormal heart rate pattern thought to represent oxygen deprivation. The distress is seldom qualified further or quantified at all. In addition, there are clearly other kinds of stress, some potentially as devastating to the fetus as systemic hypoxia. These include infection, anemia, arrhythmia, anomaly, and localized ischemia of the brain or other organs related to perfusion or mechanical trauma. The more in-vogue but vague and imprecise terms 'fetal intolerance to labor' and 'non-reassuring fetal status' however, surely underscore the failure of current classifications to provide insight into the mechanism(s) of the problem, the likelihood of recovery, the interaction among various heart rate patterns or a basis upon which to relate the events of labor to subsequent outcome. This helps us understand why there are no useful computerized models for the interpretation of intrapartum FHR patterns and even why 'alarm' systems are so readily abandoned.[106]

The problem of nomenclature is best illustrated by a brief discussion of the requirements for a 'reactive NST'.[107] In designating an NST tracing as 'reactive' we do not mention the specific baseline rate if it is in the normal range, or the amount of variability, or the fact that there are periods of time when the baseline variability is poor or absent (Figure 176.1). The entire pattern has a name – the reactive NST.

Technical issues

Technical issues must be understood as well. Abnormalities of the tracing are found predominantly during the expulsive phase of labor when technical difficulties are most likely to interfere with proper registration. The source of the FHR and uterine contraction signals (internal or external) will influence both the accuracy of the interpretation and the potential for misrepresentation of the baseline rate and the variability. Indeed, the monitor may mistake the maternal heart rate pattern for the fetal pattern with sometimes catastrophic results.[108,109] Under these circumstances, the 'baby has been lost' on the monitor and deterioration has not been appreciated. This situation has become commonplace in medical malpractice cases.

Correlation with outcome

The correlation of FHR patterns with outcome was originally confined to measures of immediate neonatal condition based on the potential effects of oxygen deprivation: neonatal death, pH of umbilical cord blood, Apgar scores, or need for neonatal intensive care.[84,110–114] While a normal intrapartum FHR pattern virtually excludes the presence of acute fetal hypoxia, and while abnormal patterns show an increased likelihood of acidosis and neonatal depression, most abnormal patterns fail to show any correlation with hypoxia or adverse outcome. The presence of a normal pattern, especially one with evidence of normal fetal behavioral states, correlates strongly with normal long-term neurologic outcome.[115–117] Abnormal FHR patterns, both before and during labor, are indeed associated with abnormal neurologic activity, including subsequent cerebral palsy.[65,102,118,119–123] Nevertheless, most abnormal patterns, when defined traditionally based on presumptions about the presence of hypoxia, show only a poor correlation with adverse outcome.[65,119] These generalizations apply despite differences in classification of FHR pattern.

As originally conceived, EFM was predicated on the benefits of the early detection of and timely intervention for fetal hypoxia. The test of hypoxia was the presence of certain specific decelerations. So unique were the *individual* decelerations thought to be in 1967[124] that they were named according to the presumed mechanism. Thus, late decelerations were thought to represent 'uteroplacental insufficiency', variable decelerations to 'cord compression', and early decelerations to 'head compression'. It is now clear that this represents a simplistic view of FHR patterns. Variable decelerations, for example, are caused by both umbilical cord compression and (probably more commonly) by fetal head compression. Early decelerations are pathophysiologically probably the same as variable decelerations. Late decelerations may occur other than in the context of hypoxia.

Figure 176.7 (bottom half) illustrates the importance of understanding the provenance of the patterns. It illustrates a series of combined variable and late decelerations and absent variability. There is a very high likelihood of a poor outcome associated with such a pattern. If the FHR recording preceding this

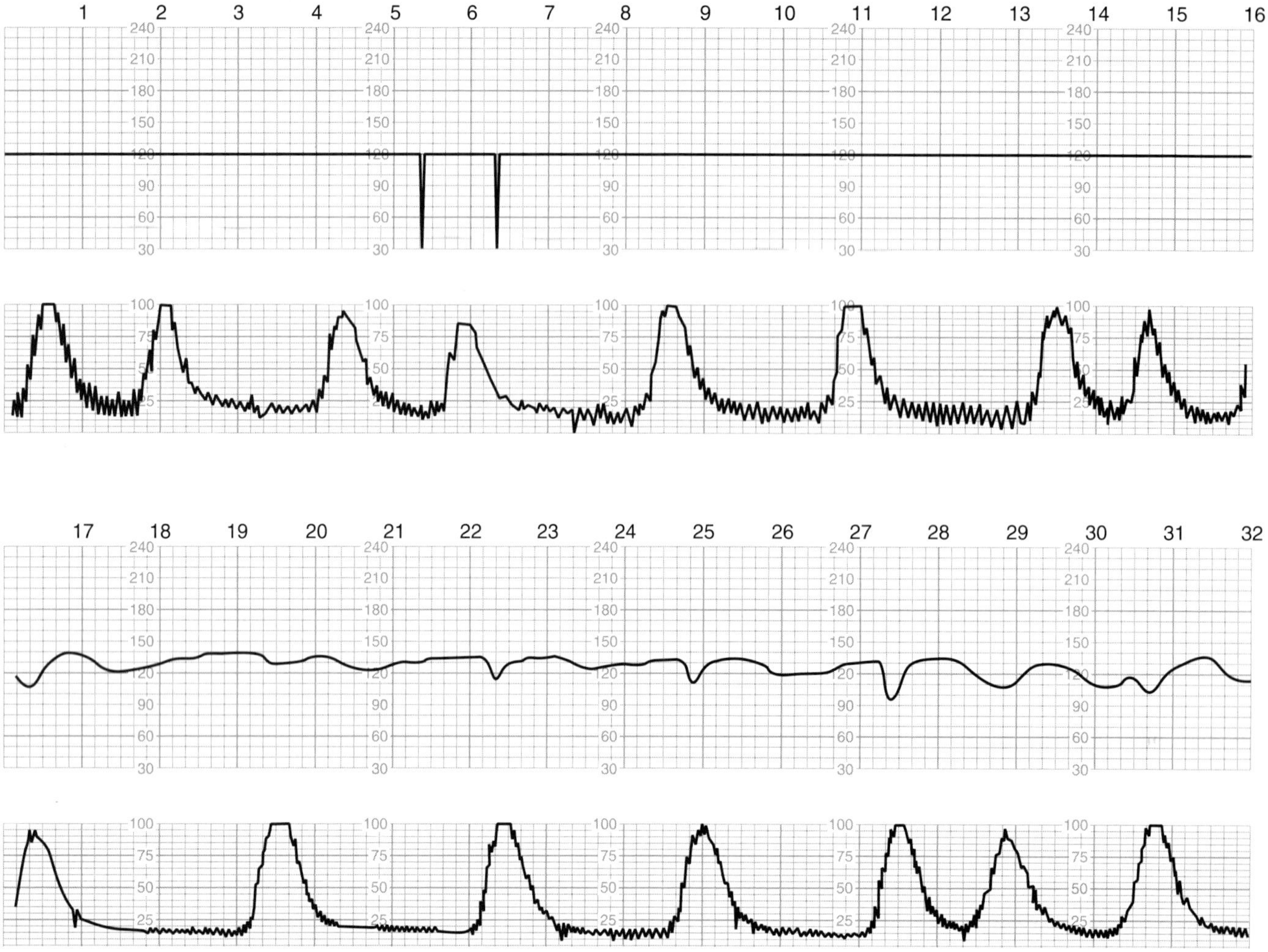

Figure 176.7 Pattern of injury. Note the persistent absence of baseline variability as well as the absence of decelerations in the top panel. In the bottom panel, several hours later, we find the combination of absent variability and small variable decelerations with overshoot and late decelerations in the presence of a stable baseline rate. This sequence and the absence of any normal tracing suggest that that threshold of injury had been crossed by the time monitoring was initiated. The infant was found to have low Apgar scores at birth but normal cord blood gases. The infant subsequently developed cerebral palsy.

tracing was normal then the progression of the pattern from normal to ominous suggests an acute and ongoing problem that could (and may already have) progressed to brain injury. If, however, the fetus was admitted with diminished variability, even absent decelerations (as in this case – top figure), then it is likely that the fetus was already injured at the time of admission.

FHR patterns and the diagnosis of neurologic injury

To understand the potential for using FHR patterns to detect neurologic injury, consider a principle widely used for the neurologic evaluation and prognosis of a person after a near-drowning accident. Irrespective of the severity of immediate asphyxia and neurologic manifestations thereof, the diagnosis of permanent neurologic injury must await the resolution of acidosis, hypoxia, and cerebral edema. Only then does a neurologic prognosis become reasonable. In the studies of Ikeda *et al.* on fetal lambs, the umbilical cord circulation was interrupted completely to a level of profound hypoxia and acidosis (pH < 6.9, and base deficit > 20 mmol/l).[35,125] The occlusion was then relieved, and the lambs were allowed to recover. Their brains were later examined for the severity of injury. The authors found no correlation between the duration of the fetal bradycardia or the severity of the hypoxia or acidosis and the severity of brain injury. Several features of this study appear to have critical relevance to the analysis of intrapartum events and their relationship to injury. The mechanism of injury in the animal studies was an acute abrupt and profound ischemic assault reaching extraordinary levels of hypoxia and acidosis. But, although the FHR responded to this oxygen deprivation and severe acidosis, the duration of the bradycardia was not directly related to the severity of the neurologic injury. The factors that did correlate to the severity of injury were the (1) duration of the diminished perfusion of the brain (the ischemia), which could be measured in the experiment, but cannot be measured directly in the human fetus and (2) the appearance of the FHR pattern *after the event*. Of clinical importance was the observation that, despite the duration and the severity of the assault, when the obstruction to blood flow in the umbilical cord was removed, the pH and the base deficit returned to normal, but the injury remained. These experiments revealed the potential for acid–base (but not histologic) recovery of an obvious and severe asphyxial insult, the variability of neurologic injury among fetuses exposed to the same severe insult and extreme values of acidosis, and the potential relevance of the FHR pattern that occurs in the wake of a severe ischemic insult. No estimate of severity could be gleaned from the type or duration of the FHR pattern during the acute episode. Similar conclusions can be drawn from other experimental data.[126]

These findings contradict the prevailing opinion that for acute intrapartum asphyxia to be diagnosed, there must be evidence of abnormalities in Apgar score and pH at birth.[61,64] That may be reasonable for a model of injury that is one of progressive systemic hypoxia with relentless deterioration of the pH, and severe systemic manifestations of hypoxia at the end of labor. It makes, however, no concession for injury by any other mechanism (e.g. mechanical trauma, pure ischemia), or for the likelihood that host or environmental factors influence the vulnerability of individual fetuses to injury, even when exposed to the same degree of oxygen deprivation. It also makes no accommodation for a profound hypoxic event from which the fetus has recovered metabolically but not neurologically, and gives no consideration to the baseline condition of the fetus at the time the acute insult occurred. The issue is complex, and too poorly understood at this time to allow such definitive requirements.[102,127]

Clinical FHR tracings illustrate that the fetus may be injured during an hypoxic/ischemic episode from which it recovers from the hemodynamic and metabolic standpoints, but not from a neurologic one.[102,103,105,128] Decelerations need not be present to consider the potential for adverse neurologic consequences on the basis of the tracing. In this respect the diagnosis is a neurologic one, not a hypoxic one. When adverse features including persistently absent short-term variability and small variable decelerations with overshoot or intermittent sinusoidal pattern (Figure 176.6 – bottom half) are associated with absence of accelerations the potential for adverse neurologic outcome increases considerably, especially if the preceding antepartum or intrapartum tracing was reactive.[102,120,122,129] This 'pattern of injury' may be recoverable under certain circumstances, e.g. when there is severe metabolic ketoacidosis in the mother.[130,131] The pattern of injury appears in about 0.2% of all patients undergoing monitoring, but in about 50% of fetuses who subsequently develop neurologic disability in the form of cerebral palsy.[120,122,123] The overwhelming majority of patients with this pattern will have normal pH values. Only those whose patterns show obvious decelerations also show acidosis.[123] Thus, when one encounters this pattern under the circumstances described above it seems reasonable to anticipate a significant problem with the baby and to understand that even the most aggressive and timely management may not change the outcome.

In other, rare circumstances, the decelerations disappear and the baseline rate returns to normal, but the variability remains persistently exaggerated as the marker of the neurological injury; but normal behavioral cycles are usually not maintained.[132]

On occasion the transition from a normal to a pathologic pattern is obvious and dramatic, as in the sudden development of ischemic or hemorrhagic injury – a pattern we have referred to as the 'conversion pattern'.[102,103] Figure 176.6 illustrates the dramatic conversion of a previously normal tracing to one of absent variability in a fetus who suffered a stroke during labor. These events, which may be far more common than realized, are compatible only with a regional, ischemic event, not one of progressive, systemic asphyxia. The appearance of such tracings further underscores the limitations of trying to identify neurologic problems in the fetus using a nosology of decelerations designed only to demonstrate systemic hypoxia.

While the 'conversion' pattern shows an extraordinary correlation with subsequent adverse neurologic outcome, it cannot be used in any way to ascertain the severity of that involvement[122] or that its continuation necessarily represents ongoing deterioration of the fetal condition. It is important to emphasize the determination of injury is not based solely on the presence of a tracing with absent variability and other features. To define injury or the potential for it, one must either demonstrate or have reason to believe that the pattern of injury represents the conversion from a previously normal FHR pattern.[122,128] This distinction is important because this pattern of injury may be emulated in all respects by the administration of atropine to the mother or fetus.[51,133,134] It may also appear in the non-injured fetus as a result of prematurity, extreme tachycardia from any cause, and in anomalous fetuses.[135] Abnormalities of variability in the heart rate pattern may also be seen in older children with cerebral palsy and brain damaged adults.[136–138]

Effects on the cesarean rate

Most studies suggest that the use of EFM, because of the high incidence of abnormal FHR patterns that do not reflect severe asphyxia, increases the cesarean section rate, without apparent benefit for fetal outcome. As a result, there has been considerable interest in techniques that will increase the sensitivity of the 'non-reassuring' pattern for identifying significant oxygen deprivation or acidosis. Fetal capillary blood sampling has some potential benefits in this regard, but is no longer widely used, owing primarily to its technical challenges and intrinsic measurement errors.[139,140]

The U.S. Food and Drug Administration recently approved the marketing of the Nellcor N-400 fetal pulse oximeter to be used as an adjunct to FHR monitoring to monitor fetal intrapartum oxygen saturation continuously in a singleton vertex fetus with a gestational age of at least 36 weeks in the presence of a non-reassuring heart rate pattern after fetal membranes have ruptured. The stated and the implied benefits of the technique include: (1) reduced cesarean section rate for so-called 'non-reassuring FHR patterns' (NRFHRP); (2) simplicity – ostensibly only a single reading of more than 30% between contractions is assurance that the fetus is adequately oxygenated.[15,141] This notion eliminates the requirement for understanding the periodic changes in fetal oxygen saturation associated with contractions and prevents any misunderstanding about the meaning of various FHR decelerations and their impact on the baseline heart rate and variability. It would also seem to attenuate the risk of any medicolegal challenge relative to the interpretation of FHR patterns.[142]

When the device was used in conjunction with FHR monitoring in a randomized clinical trial there was indeed a reduction in cesarean delivery rates for 'non-reassuring FHR patterns'; but there was no difference in the immediate neonatal outcomes or the overall cesarean delivery rates (the latter as a result of an increase in abdominal delivery for dystocia in the pulse oximetry group).[15] Given these data, along with data suggesting that the correlation with scalp or umbilical pH is poor and that pulse oximetry may fail to recognize FHR changes associated with neurologic injury, the net value of the device for its stated purpose is unobvious.[142–144]

According to the rationale for using adjunctive techniques such as capillary pH measurements or pulse oximetry, overreaction to abnormalities in the FHR tracing will prompt unnecessary intervention if the FHR monitor is used alone, while intervention, if ultimately necessary, can be safely delayed as long as the oxygen saturation or pH is normal.[15] There would seem to be no obvious advantage for pulse oximetry to reduce somewhat the cesarean section rate, but increase the risk of urgent interventions or more difficult operative deliveries.

Precepts of monitoring

Perhaps a broader perspective is necessary. The original incentive for implementing fetal monitoring was the notion that the unique decelerations produced in relationship to contractions would allow early detection of fetal hypoxia and early intervention, in other words, *rescue* the fetus from impending decompensation. This oft repeated precept of EFM about intervention may indeed be the major impediment to realizing its benefits. To optimize the timing of intervention, there must be knowledge about the types of FHR patterns and mechanisms that produce injury, the speed of deterioration and the options for recoverability. Clearly some patterns develop slowly with ample, non-critical, opportunities for intervention with the expectation of normal outcome. Other patterns progress more rapidly and the timing of intervention becomes critical if the fetus is to be rescued. Still other patterns develop so rapidly and unpredictably that timely intervention is improbable and, irrespective of the speed of intervention, the fetus may not escape injury or death. In other circumstances, the opportunity for timely intervention has long passed and intervention, required by the standard of care, may not change the inevitable handicap or death. There has been little meaningful discussion of these issues.

Perhaps a better understanding of the benefits of EFM will be realized if the perspective of its role is changed from rescue to prevention. To begin to realize this role for EFM requires that the medical personnel attending the parturient continuously answer three questions: 'Does anything have to be done for the mother?' 'Does anything have to be done for the fetus?' And thirdly, 'What is the feasibility of safe vaginal delivery, given the circumstances of the labor, the fetal condition and the maternal condition?' Focusing on the FHR pattern for a moment, it seems axiomatic that irrespective of any abnormality of the FHR pattern, labor can only be permitted as long as there is reasonable expectation of the feasibility of safe vaginal delivery. That is, the decelerations that can be tolerated at full dilatation of the cervix with a head ready to deliver would not reasonably be tolerated in early labor before descent of the head, rupture of the membranes and the potential for cord compression, factors likely to further increase the severity of decelerations. Indeed, the lower the feasibility of safe vaginal delivery, the lower should be the threshold for intervention for abnormal FHR patterns irrespective of the severity of the FHR pattern, or the amount of acidosis.

For example, in the patient with an arrest of dilatation with the FHR demonstrating a rising baseline with decreasing variability and recurrent decelerations, what can be the benefit of waiting for an abnormal fetal oxygen saturation or critically low pH? Abnormal FHR patterns, in fact, anticipate difficulty in labor and the need for cesarean section for dystocia.[21] Perhaps, decelerations occur for a reason. The increased frequency of decelerations, operative intervention, and subsequent adverse neurologic outcome with fetuses in occiput posterior positions have been known for some time.[89,145–148] It stands to reason that the longer and more difficult the labor the greater are the options for decelerations from fetal head or cord compression and for subsequent harm and the less likely is safe vaginal delivery from the OP position.[103,146–149]

Continued, unproductive labor may be associated with increased cranial molding and deeper lodgement of the fetal head into the pelvis. It may provoke protracted fetal bradycardia or make ultimate operative delivery by either vaginal or abdominal routes that much more difficult. The question then arises, what is the value of delaying delivery in the face of progressive abnormalities in the FHR pattern, even if one knew the scalp blood pH or transcutaneous oxygen saturation were normal? Delaying intervention – waiting until the fetal condition deteriorates or becomes critical before intervention – seems to be a violation of one of the fundamental tenets of obstetric care – keeping the mother and fetus out of harm's way.

When the FHR pattern is reactive, there is reasonable diagnostic certainty that there is no *fetal* indication for intervention. It does not exclude intervention on the basis of fetal size or presentation or position, pelvic size or a maternal condition. Thus, the determination of the timing of intervention will depend as much on the heart rate pattern as it does on the estimated feasibility and timing of safe vaginal delivery. The strength of such evaluations is modified by the reliability and predictability of the information, the skill of the interpreter, and the clinical context. The approach we have recommended here emphasizes the need to examine and codify trends in FHR patterns in an effort to identify the boundaries that separate the normally oxygenated and normally behaving fetus from the hypoxemic one and to distinguish pure hypoxia from that likely to be associated with ischemia.

We have tried to avoid here discussing tracings as a 'snapshot' of various patterns without discussion of their evolution.[150] Such limited perspective cannot permit an accurate assessment of the fetal condition or thoughtful deliberation about the urgency and route of delivery. Assessing 'non-reassuring patterns' would seem to require less attention to specific features of the types and timing of decelerations or variability, than to changes in these values over time – we need to use the fetus as its own control. The normal tracing with a stable baseline, cyclic accelerations and variability, and absent decelerations defines absent hypoxia and normal fetal behavior. Fetuses appear not to deteriorate without first modifying their FHR baseline and variability, even in the presence of decelerations. If patterns thought to represent fetal compromise were present at the outset of labor, then any adverse outcome likely represents antepartum insult. If such patterns evolve over time during labor after an initially normal FHR, however, then less severe signs of 'distress' were likely present. Irrespective, 'rescue' at this time may not allow a normal outcome.

We believe that much more is known about the determinants of FHR patterns than is currently used clinically in their analysis or classification. Perinatal asphyxia does not mean that the fetus was injured. Perinatal injury does not mean that the fetus was asphyxiated or that it was preventable. The evaluation of these tracings, therefore, requires that testing must be performed properly and in a timely way; the results must be interpreted and communicated correctly using an agreed upon, widely understood classification, and the interpretation must provoke an appropriate response in the larger clinical context relating to the condition of the mother and the feasibility of safe vaginal delivery. To a greater or lesser extent all these components must be included in any evaluation of the reproducibility of EFM, to its comparison with alternatives, and finally to the evaluation of its role in the allegation of obstetric negligence.

As much insight as tracings are able to provide, however, they cannot be used to explain all adverse outcomes. Indeed, they provide limited affirmative evidence of adverse outcomes associated with maladroit resuscitation, congenital anomaly, traumatic or difficult delivery, sepsis, or medication. The majority of infants depressed at birth have a normal blood pH and the majority of infants with low pH have normal outcome. There is, however, no reported example of sudden, unexpected fetal death on a monitor.

Thus, all of these modalities (EFM, fetal pulse oximetry, pH) should at least anticipate, if not prevent, fetal death in labor because this outcome, unlike neurologic injury, is universally associated with either progressive hypoxia and acidosis or an acute, catastrophic event, e.g. massive abruption. But whether any of these techniques, by a single value or feature or even a combination thereof, can dictate the critical time for delivery of the fetus with a problematic FHR pattern and a abnormal labor, is unresolved. There yet seems to be a place for skilled interpretation of FHR patterns, for understanding the expected course of labor and for the Art of Obstetrics in dealing with the parturient in labor. Rescuing the fetus is not good obstetrics; preventing injury is. It should not be concluded that universal cesarean would be the obvious solution to preventing all hypoxic and ischemic injury; rather, informed and insightful management of labor, including intelligent fetal surveillance would seem to be the best route to that end. For the acceptance and benefit of monitoring to improve, we will have to learn from the mistakes of the past and learn to ask the right questions about both immediate and long-term outcomes. We will have to broaden the understanding of both fetal and physician behavior and let the fetus act as its own control. We need to pay more attention to understanding the mechanism of fetal injury while abandoning the myths and fear of malpractice. We will need to value more both the responses of the fetus before and during labor and the potential benefits of skilled human intervention.

REFERENCES

1. Paul RH, Gauthier RJ, Quilligan EJ. Clinical fetal monitoring. The usage and relationship to trends in cesarean delivery and perinatal mortality. *Acta Obstet Gynecol Scand* 1980;59:289–95.
2. Visser G, Narayan H. The problem of increasing severe neurological morbidity in newborn infants: Where should the focus be? *Pernat Neonatal Med* 1996;1:12–15.
3. Stanley FJ. Cerebral palsy trends. Implications for perinatal care. *Acta Obstet Gynecol Scand* 1994;73:5–9.
4. McCusker J, Harris DR, Hosmer DW Jr. Association of electronic fetal monitoring during labor with cesarean section rate and with neonatal morbidity and mortality. *Am J Public Health* 1988;78:1170–4.
5. Freeman R. Intrapartum fetal monitoring – a disappointing story. *N Engl J Med* 1990;322:624–6.
6. Natale R, Dodman N. Birth can be a hazardous journey: Electronic fetal monitoring does not help. *J Obstet Gynaecol Can* 2003;25:1007–9.
7. MacDonald D, Grant A, Sheridan-Pereira M, Boylan P, Chalmers I. The Dublin randomized controlled trial of intrapartum fetal heart rate monitoring. *Am J Obstet Gynecol* 1985;152: 524–39.
8. Vintzileos AM, Nochimson DJ, Guzman ER, Knuppel RA, Lake M, Schifrin BS. Intrapartum electronic fetal heart rate monitoring versus intermittent auscultation: A meta-analysis. *Obstet Gynecol* 1995;85:149–55.
9. Shy KK, Luthy DA, Bennett FC, *et al.* Effects of electronic fetal-heart-rate monitoring, as compared with periodic auscultation, on the neurologic development of premature infants. *N Engl J Med* 1990;322:588–93.
10. Mahomed K, Nyoni R, Mulambo T, Kasule J, Jacobus E. Randomised controlled trial of intrapartum fetal heart rate monitoring. *BMJ* 1994;308:497–500.
11. Mahomed K, Nyoni R, Mlambo T, Jacobus E, Kasule J. Intrapartum foetal heart rate monitoring – continuous electronic versus intermittent Doppler – a randomised controlled trial. *Cent Afr J Med* 1992;38:458–62.
12. Donker DK, van Geijn HP, Hasman A. Interobserver variation in the assessment of fetal heart rate recordings. *Eur J Obstet Gynecol Reprod Biol* 1993;52:21–8.
13. Liston R, Crane J, Hughes O, *et al.* Fetal health surveillance in labour. *J Obstet Gynaecol Can* 2002;24:342–55.
14. Rosen KG, Amer-Wahlin I, Luzietti R, Noren H. Fetal ECG waveform analysis. *Best Pract Res Clin Obstet Gynaecol* 2004; 18:485–514.
15. Garite TJ, Dildy GA, McNamara H, *et al.* A multicenter controlled trial of fetal pulse oximetry in the intrapartum management of nonreassuring fetal heart rate patterns. *Am J Obstet Gynecol* 2000;183:1049–58.
16. Ayres-de-Campos D, Costa-Santos C, Bernardes J. Prediction of neonatal state by computer analysis of fetal heart rate tracings: The antepartum arm of the SisPorto((R)) multicentre validation study. *Eur J Obstet Gynecol Reprod Biol* 2005;118: 52–60.
17. Luttkus AK, Noren H, Stupin JH, *et al.* Fetal scalp pH and ST analysis of the fetal ECG as an adjunct to CTG. A multi-center, observational study. *J Perinat Med* 2004;32:486–94.
18. Lent M. The medical and legal risks of the electronic fetal monitor. *Stanford Law Rev* 1999;51:807–37.
19. van Geijn HP, Copray FJ, Donkers DK, Bos MH. Diagnosis and management of intrapartum fetal distress. *Eur J Obstet Gynecol Reprod Biol* 1991;42(Suppl):S63–72.
20. Piquard F, Hsiung R, Mettauer M, Schaefer A, Haberey P, Dellenbach P. The validity of fetal heart rate monitoring during the second stage of labor. *Obstet Gynecol* 1988;72:746–51.
21. Porreco RP, Boehm FH, Dildy GA, *et al.* Dystocia in nulliparous patients monitored with fetal pulse oximetry. *Am J Obstet Gynecol* 2004;190:113–17.
22. Spencer JA, Johnson P. Fetal heart rate variability changes and fetal behavioural cycles during labour. *Br J Obstet Gynaecol* 1986;93:314–21.
23. Nijhuis JG. Fetal behavior. *Neurobiol Aging* 2003;24(Suppl 1): S41–6; discussion S7–9, S51–2.
24. van Woerden EE, van Geijn HP, Swartjes JM, Caron FJ, Brons JT, Arts NF. Fetal heart rhythms during behavioural state 1F. *Eur J Obstet Gynecol Reprod Biol* 1988;28:29–38.
25. van Woerden EE, van Geijn HP, Caron FJ, van der Valk AW, Swartjes JM, Arts NF. Fetal mouth movements during behavioural states 1F and 2F. *Eur J Obstet Gynecol Reprod Biol* 1988;29: 97–105.
26. Schifrin BS, Artenos J, Lyseight N. Late-onset fetal cardiac decelerations associated with fetal breathing movements. *J Matern Fetal Neonatal Med* 2002;12:253–9.
27. Nijhuis IJ, ten Hof J, Mulder EJ, *et al.* Fetal heart rate in relation to its variation in normal and growth retarded fetuses. *Eur J Obstet Gynecol Reprod Biol* 2000;89:27–33.
28. Nijhuis IJ, ten Hof J, Nijhuis JG, *et al.* Temporal organization of fetal behavior from 24-weeks gestation onwards in normal and complicated pregnancies. *Dev Psychobiol* 1999;34:257–68.
29. Gagnon R, Hunse C, Fellows F, Carmichael L, Patrick J. Fetal heart rate and activity patterns in growth-retarded fetuses: Changes after vibratory acoustic stimulation. *Am J Obstet Gynecol* 1988;158: 265–71.
30. Gagnon R, Hunse C, Carmichael L, Fellows F, Patrick J. Human fetal responses to vibratory acoustic stimulation from twenty-six weeks to term. *Am J Obstet Gynecol* 1987;157:1375–81.
31. Patrick J, Campbell K, Carmichael L, Probert C. Influence of maternal heart rate and gross fetal body movements on the daily pattern of fetal heart rate near term. *Am J Obstet Gynecol* 1982; 144:533–8.
32. National Institute of Child Health and Human Development Research Planning Workshop. Electronic fetal heart rate monitoring: Research guidelines for interpretation. *Am J Obstet Gynecol* 1997;177:1385–90.
33. Kang AH, Boehm FH. The clinical significance of intermittent sinusoidal fetal heart rate. *Am J Obstet Gynecol* 1999;180(1 Pt 1): 151–2.
34. Krebs HB. Definition of sinusoidal fetal heart rate. *Am J Obstet Gynecol* 1980;138:1231–3.
35. Ikeda T, Murata Y, Quilligan EJ, *et al.* Fetal heart rate patterns in postasphyxiated fetal lambs with brain damage. *Am J Obstet Gynecol* 1998;179:1329–37.
36. Cetrulo CL, Schifrin BS. Fetal heart rate patterns preceding death in utero. *Obstet Gynecol* 1976;48:521–7.
37. Gleicher N, Runowicz CD, Brown BL. Sinusoidal fetal heart rate pattern in association with amnionitis. *Obstet Gynecol* 1980; 56:109–12.
38. Cotton DB, Rivera-Alsina M, Palma PA, Schifrin BS. Sinusoidal fetal heart rate pattern in hydranencephaly. A case report. *J Reprod Med* 1983;28:631–3.
39. Sacks DA, Bell KE, Schwimmer WB, Schifrin BS. Sinusoidal fetal heart rate pattern with intrapartum fetal death. *J Reprod Med* 1980;24:171–3.
40. Murphy KW, Russell V, Collins A, Johnson P. The prevalence, aetiology and clinical significance of pseudo-sinusoidal fetal heart rate patterns in labour. *Br J Obstet Gynaecol* 1991;98: 1093–101.
41. Parer JT, Dijkstra HR, Vredebregt PP, Harris JL, Krueger TR, Reuss ML. Increased fetal heart rate variability with acute hypoxia in

chronically instrumented sheep. *Eur J Obstet Gynecol Reprod Biol* 1980;10:393–9.

42. Visser GH, Bekedam DJ, Ribbert LS. Changes in antepartum heart rate patterns with progressive deterioration of the fetal condition. *Int J Biomed Comput* 1990;25:239–46.
43. Murata Y, Martin CB Jr, Ikenoue T, *et al.* Fetal heart rate accelerations and late decelerations during the course of intrauterine death in chronically catheterized rhesus monkeys. *Am J Obstet Gynecol* 1982;144:218–23.
44. Itskovitz J, Goetzman BW, Rudolph AM. The mechanism of late deceleration of the heart rate and its relationship to oxygenation in normoxemic and chronically hypoxemic fetal lambs. *Am J Obstet Gynecol* 1982;142:66–73.
45. Herbert CM, Boehm FH. Prolonged end-stage fetal heart rate deceleration: A reanalysis. *Obstet Gynecol* 1981;57:589–93.
46. Krebs HB, Petres RE, Dunn LJ. Intrapartum fetal heart rate monitoring. V. Fetal heart rate patterns in the second stage of labor. *Am J Obstet Gynecol* 1981;140:435–9.
47. Ball RH, Espinoza MI, Parer JT, Alon E, Vertommen J, Johnson J. Regional blood flow in asphyxiated fetuses with seizures. *Am J Obstet Gynecol* 1994;170(1 Pt 1):156–61.
48. Ball RH, Parer JT. The physiologic mechanisms of variable decelerations. *Am J Obstet Gynecol* 1992;166(6 Pt 1):1683–8; discussion 8–9.
49. Harris JL, Krueger TR, Parer JT. Mechanisms of late decelerations of the fetal heart rate during hypoxia. *Am J Obstet Gynecol* 1982; 144:491–6.
50. Itskovitz J, LaGamma EF, Rudolph AM. Heart rate and blood pressure responses to umbilical cord compression in fetal lambs with special reference to the mechanism of variable deceleration. *Am J Obstet Gynecol* 1983;147:451–7.
51. Parer JT, Krueger TR, Harris JL. Fetal oxygen consumption and mechanisms of heart rate response during artificially produced late decelerations of fetal heart rate in sheep. *Am J Obstet Gynecol* 1980;136:478–82.
52. Yagel S, Anteby E, Lavy Y, *et al.* Fetal middle cerebral artery blood flow during normal active labour and in labour with variable decelerations. *Br J Obstet Gynaecol* 1992;99:483–5.
53. Mueller-Heubach E, Battelli AF. Variable heart rate decelerations and transcutaneous PO_2 during umbilical cord occlusion in fetal monkeys. *Am J Obstet Gynecol* 1982;144:796–802.
54. Murata Y, Quilligan EJ, Ninomiya Y, *et al.* Variable fetal heart rate decelerations and electrocortical activities. *Am J Obstet Gynecol* 1994;170:689–92.
55. Ozden S, Demirci F. Significance for fetal outcome of poor prognostic features in fetal heart rate traces with variable decelerations. *Arch Gynecol Obstet* 1999;262:141–9.
56. Richardson BS, Carmichael L, Homan J, Johnston L, Gagnon R. Fetal cerebral, circulatory, and metabolic responses during heart rate decelerations with umbilical cord compression. *Am J Obstet Gynecol* 1996;175(4 Pt 1):929–36.
57. Clapp JF, Peress NS, Wesley M, Mann LI. Brain damage after intermittent partial cord occlusion in the chronically instrumented fetal lamb. *Am J Obstet Gynecol* 1988;159:504–9.
58. Aldrich CJ, D'Antona D, Spencer JA, *et al.* Late fetal heart decelerations and changes in cerebral oxygenation during the first stage of labour. *Br J Obstet Gynaecol* 1995;102:9–13.
59. Fleischer A, Schulman H, Jagani N, Mitchell J, Randolph G. The development of fetal acidosis in the presence of an abnormal fetal heart rate tracing. I. The average for gestational age fetus. *Am J Obstet Gynecol* 1982;144:55–60.
60. Lewinsky RM, Oppenheimer LW, Morrow RJ, Adamson SL, Farine D, Ritchie JW. Cardiac electromechanical dissociation in the hypoxic fetal sheep may have clinical implications. *Am J Obstet Gynecol* 1992;167:246–9.
61. ACOG. *Neonatal Encephalopathy and Cerebral Palsy: Defining the Pathogenesis and Pathophysiology.* Washington, DC: ACOG, 2003.
62. Hankins GD, Speer M. Defining the pathogenesis and pathophysiology of neonatal encephalopathy and cerebral palsy. *Obstet Gynecol* 2003;102:628–36.
63. MacLennan A. A template for defining a causal relation between acute intrapartum events and cerebral palsy: International consensus statement. *BMJ* 1999;319:1054–9.
64. MacLennan A. A template for defining a causal relationship between acute intrapartum events and cerebral palsy: International consensus statement. International Cerebral Palsy Task Force. *Aust N Z J Obstet Gynaecol* 2000;40:13–21.
65. Nelson KB, Dambrosia JM, Ting TY, Grether JK. Uncertain value of electronic fetal monitoring in predicting cerebral palsy. *N Engl J Med* 1996;334:613–18.
66. Morishima HO, Glaser B, Niemann WH, James LS. Increased uterine activity and fetal deterioration during maternal hyperthermia. *Am J Obstet Gynecol* 1975;121:531–8.
67. Impey L, Greenwood C, MacQuillan K, Reynolds M, Sheil O. Fever in labour and neonatal encephalopathy: A prospective cohort study. *BJOG* 2001;108:594–7.
68. Kates RB, Schifrin BS. Fetal cardiac asystole during labor. *Obstet Gynecol* 1986;67:549–55.
69. Cibils LA. Clinical significance of fetal heart rate patterns during labor. V. Variable decelerations. *Am J Obstet Gynecol* 1978;132: 791–805.
70. Kazandi M, Sendag F, Akercan F, Terek MC, Gundem G. Different types of variable decelerations and their effects to neonatal outcome. *Singapore Med J* 2003;44:243–7.
71. Krebs HB, Petres RE, Dunn LJ. Intrapartum fetal heart rate monitoring. VIII. Atypical variable decelerations. *Am J Obstet Gynecol* 1983;145:297–305.
72. Houk PG, Smith V, Wolf SG. Brain mechanisms in fatal cardiac arrhythmia. *Integr Physiol Behav Sci* 1999;34:3–9.
73. Quigley KS, Shair HN, Myers MM. Parasympathetic control of heart period during early postnatal development in the rat. *J Auton Nerv Syst* 1996;59:75–82.
74. Mallard EC, Williams CE, Johnston BM, Gunning MI, Davis S, Gluckman PD. Repeated episodes of umbilical cord occlusion in fetal sheep lead to preferential damage to the striatum and sensitize the heart to further insults. *Pediatr Res* 1995;37: 707–13.
75. O'Brien WF, Davis SE, Grissom MP, Eng RR, Golden SM. Effect of cephalic pressure on fetal cerebral blood flow. *Am J Perinatol* 1984;1:223–6.
76. Amiel-Tison C, Sureau C, Shnider SM. Cerebral handicap in full-term neonates related to the mechanical forces of labour. *Baillieres Clin Obstet Gynaecol* 1988;2:145–65.
77. Dellinger EH, Boehm FH, Crane MM. Electronic fetal heart rate monitoring: Early neonatal outcomes associated with normal rate, fetal stress, and fetal distress. *Am J Obstet Gynecol* 2000;182: 214–20.
78. Chen SZ, Koike S, Mizutani K, Teshima H, Mori H, Kigawa T. Semi-quantitative evaluation of the intrapartum variable deceleration of the FHR pattern and its association with umbilical cord blood gas analysis. *Nippon Sanka Fujinka Gakkai Zasshi* 1987;39:411–19.
79. Tortosa MN, Acien P. Evaluation of variable decelerations of fetal heart rate with the deceleration index: Influence of associated abnormal parameters and their relation to the state and evolution of the newborn. *Eur J Obstet Gynecol Reprod Biol* 1990;34: 235–45.
80. Tournaire M, Sturbois G, Ripoche A, *et al.* Evaluation of the fetal state by automatic analysis of the heart rate. 2. Deceleration areas and umbilical artery blood pH. *J Perinat Med* 1976;4: 118–30.
81. Albrecht H, Bokelmann J, Morgenstern J, Schmidt H. Some remarks concerning the fetal heart rate total dip areas. *J Perinat Med* 1975;3:226–30.
82. Paul RH, Suidan AK, Yeh S, Schifrin BS, Hon EH. Clinical fetal monitoring. VII. The evaluation and significance of intrapartum baseline FHR variability. *Am J Obstet Gynecol* 1975;123:206–10.
83. Zalar RW Jr, Quilligan EJ. The influence of scalp sampling on the cesarean section rate for fetal distress. *Am J Obstet Gynecol* 1979;135:239–46.
84. Kubli FW, Hon EH, Khazin AF, Takemura H. Observations on heart rate and pH in the human fetus during labor. *Am J Obstet Gynecol* 1969;104:1190–206.
85. Katz M, Shani N, Meizner I, Insler V. Is end-stage deceleration of the fetal heart ominous? *Br J Obstet Gynaecol* 1982;89:186–9.
86. Roemer VM, Fritz U. Fetal bradycardia in labor. *J Perinat Med* 1989;17:237–43.
87. Jonker FH, Van Geijn HP, Chan WW, Rausch WD, Van der Weijden GC, Taverne MA. Characteristics of fetal heart rate changes during the expulsive stage of bovine parturition in relation to fetal outcome. *Am J Vet Res* 1996;57:1373–81.
88. Melchior J, Bernard N. Second-stage fetal heart rate patterns. In Jad S, ed. *Fetal Monitoring, Physiology and Techniques of Antenatal and Intrapartum Assessment.* Turnbridge Wells: Castle House Publications, Ltd, 1989.

89. Ingemarsson E, Ingemarsson I, Solum T, Westgren M. Influence of occiput posterior position on the fetal heart rate pattern. *Obstet Gynecol* 1980;55:301–4.
90. Badawi N, Kurinczuk JJ, Keogh JM, *et al.* Intrapartum risk factors for newborn encephalopathy: The Western Australian case–control study. *BMJ* 1998;317:1554–8.
91. Thomson AM. Pushing techniques in the second stage of labour. *J Adv Nurs* 1993;18:171–7.
92. Aldrich CJ, D'Antona D, Spencer JA, *et al.* The effect of maternal pushing on fetal cerebral oxygenation and blood volume during the second stage of labour. *Br J Obstet Gynaecol* 1995;102:448–53
93. Vintzileos AM. Electronic monitoring: Who needs a Trojan horse? *Birth* 1994;21:235–6.
94. Thompson MS. Decision-analytic determination of study size. The case of electronic fetal monitoring. *Med Decis Making* 1981;xx: 165–79.
95. Thacker SB, Stroup DF. Revisiting the use of the electronic fetal monitor. *Lancet* 2003;361:445–6.
96. Simkin P. Is anyone listening? The lack of clinical impact of randomized controlled trials of electronic fetal monitoring. *Birth* 1986;13:219–20.
97. Hammacher K, Brun del Re R, Gaudenz R, De Grandi P, Richter R. Cardiotocographic diagnosis of fetal hazard using a CTG-score. *Gynakol Rundsch* 1974;14(Suppl 1):61–3.
98. Hon EH. The classification of fetal heart rate. I. A working classification. *Obstet Gynecol* 1963;22:137–46.
99. Rooth G, Huch A, Huch R. Guidelines for the use of fetal monitoring. *Int J Gynaecol Obstet* 1987;25:159067.
100. The National Institute of Child Health and Human Development Research Planning Workshop. Electronic fetal heart rate monitoring: Research guidelines for interpretation. *J Obstet Gynecol Neonatal Nurs* 1997;26:635–40.
101. Ayres-de-Campos D, Bernardes J, Costa-Pereira A, Pereira-Leite L. Inconsistencies in classification by experts of cardiotocograms and subsequent clinical decision. *Br J Obstet Gynaecol* 1999;106:1307–10.
102. Schifrin BS. The CTG and the timing and mechanism of fetal neurological injuries. *Best Pract Res Clin Obstet Gynaecol* 2004; 18:437–56.
103. Asakura H, Schifrin BS, Myers SA. Intrapartum, atraumatic, non-asphyxial intracranial hemorrhage in a full-term infant. *Obstet Gynecol* 1994;84:680–3.
104. Freeman JM, Nelson KB. Intrapartum asphyxia and cerebral palsy. *Pediatrics* 1988;82:240–9.
105. Freeman RK. Problems with intrapartum fetal heart rate monitoring interpretation and patient management. *Obstet Gynecol* 2002;100:813–26.
106. van Woerden E, van Geijn H. Factors influencing the fetal heart rate. In Copray HvGaF, ed. *A Critical Appraisal of Fetal Surveillance.* Amsterdam: Elsevier, Exerpta Medica, 1994: 211–20.
107. Schifrin BS, Harwell R. FHR terminology. *J Obstet Gynecol Neonatal Nurs* 1999;28:123.
108. Murray ML. Maternal or fetal heart rate? Avoiding intrapartum misidentification. *J Obstet Gynecol Neonatal Nurs* 2004;33:93–104.
109. Sherman DJ, Frenkel E, Kurzweil Y, Padua A, Arieli S, Bahar M. Characteristics of maternal heart rate patterns during labor and delivery. *Obstet Gynecol* 2002;99:542–7.
110. Ruth VJ, Raivio KO. Perinatal brain damage: Predictive value of metabolic acidosis and the Apgar score. *BMJ* 1988;297:24–7.
111. Hon EH, Khazin AF, Paul RH. Biochemical studies of the fetus. II. Fetal pH and Apgar scores. *Obstet Gynecol* 1969;33:237–55.
112. Low JA, Victory R, Derrick EJ. Predictive value of electronic fetal monitoring for intrapartum fetal asphyxia with metabolic acidosis. *Obstet Gynecol* 1999;93:285–91.
113. Low JA, Panagiotopoulos C, Derrick EJ. Newborn complications after intrapartum asphyxia with metabolic acidosis in the term fetus. *Am J Obstet Gynecol* 1994;170:1081–7.
114. Westgate JA, Gunn AJ, Gunn TR. Antecedents of neonatal encephalopathy with fetal acidaemia at term. *Br J Obstet Gynaecol* 1999;106:774–82.
115. Painter MJ, Depp R, O'Donoghue PD. Fetal heart rate patterns and development in the first year of life. *Am J Obstet Gynecol* 1978; 132:271–7.
116. Keegan KA Jr, Waffarn F, Quilligan EJ. Obstetric characteristics and fetal heart rate patterns of infants who convulse during the newborn period. *Am J Obstet Gynecol* 1985;153:732–7.
117. Horimoto N, Koyanagi T, Nakano H, Ueda K. The in utero determination of lesion site affecting the central nervous system assessed by abnormal behavioral patterns in the human fetus. *No To Hattatsu* 1992;2:147–51.
118. Gaffney G, Sellers S, Flavell V, Squier M, Johnson A. Case–control study of intrapartum care, cerebral palsy, and perinatal death. *BMJ* 1994;308:743–50.
119. Spencer JA, Badawi N, Burton P, Keogh J, Pemberton P, Stanley F. The intrapartum CTG prior to neonatal encephalopathy at term: A case–control study. *Br J Obstet Gynaecol* 1997;104:25–8.
120. Phelan JP, Ahn MO. Perinatal observations in forty-eight neurologically impaired term infants. *Am J Obstet Gynecol* 1994; 171:424–31.
121. Phelan JP, Kim JO. Fetal heart rate observations in the brain-damaged infant. *Semin Perinatol* 2000;24:221–9.
122. Schifrin BS, Hamilton-Rubinstein T, Shields JR. Fetal heart rate patterns and the timing of fetal injury. *J Perinatol* 1994;14:174–81.
123. Shields JR, Schifrin BS. Perinatal antecedents of cerebral palsy. *Obstet Gynecol* 1988;71:899–905.
124. Hon EH, Quilligan EJ. The classification of fetal heart rate. II. A revised working classification. *Conn Med* 1967;31:779–84.
125. Ikeda T, Murata Y, Quilligan EJ, *et al.* Physiologic and histologic changes in near-term fetal lambs exposed to asphyxia by partial umbilical cord occlusion. *Am J Obstet Gynecol* 1998;178:24–32.
126. George S, Gunn AJ, Westgate JA, Brabyn C, Guan J, Bennet L. Fetal heart rate variability and brain stem injury after asphyxia in preterm fetal sheep. *Am J Physiol Regul Integr Comp Physiol* 2004;287:R925–33.
127. Dear P, Newell S. Establishing probable cause in cerebral palsy. How much certainty is enough? *BMJ* 2000;320:1075–6.
128. van der Moer PE, Gerretsen G, Visser GH. Fixed fetal heart rate pattern after intrauterine accidental decerebration. *Obstet Gynecol* 1985;65:125–7.
129. Visser GH. Abnormal antepartum fetal heart rate patterns and subsequent handicap. *Baillieres Clin Obstet Gynaecol* 1988;2: 117–24.
130. Hagay ZJ, Weissman A, Lurie S, Insler V. Reversal of fetal distress following intensive treatment of maternal diabetic ketoacidosis. *Am J Perinatol* 1994;11:430–2.
131. Gimovsky ML, Eichenlaub J, Keroack E. Fetal heart rate monitoring casebook. Fetal heart rate monitoring in diabetic ketoacidosis. *J Perinatol* 1993;13:79–82.
132. Patrick JE, Dalton KJ, Dawes GS. Breathing patterns before death in fetal lambs. *Am J Obstet Gynecol* 1976;125:73–8.
133. Ikenoue T, Quilligan EJ, Murata Y. Circulatory response to atropine in sheep fetus. *Am J Obstet Gynecol* 1976;126:253–60.
134. Renou P, Newman W, Wood C. Autonomic control of fetal heart rate. *Am J Obstet Gynecol* 1969;105:949–53.
135. Garite TJ, Linzey EM, Freeman RK, Dorchester W. Fetal heart rate patterns and fetal distress in fetuses with congenital anomalies. *Obstet Gynecol* 1979;53:716–20.
136. Lowensohn RI, Weiss M, Hon EH. Heart-rate variability in brain-damaged adults. *Lancet* 1977;1:626–8.
137. MacCulloch MJ, Williams C, Davies P. Heart-rate variability in a group of cerebral palsied children. *Dev Med Child Neurol* 1971;13:645–50.
138. van Ravenswaaij-Arts CM, Kollee LA, Hopman JC, Stoelinga GB, van Geijn HP. Heart rate variability. *Ann Intern Med* 1993;118: 436–47.
139. Goodwin TM, Milner-Masterson L, Paul RH. Elimination of fetal scalp blood sampling on a large clinical service. *Obstet Gynecol* 1994;83:971–4.
140. Perkins RP. Requiem for a heavyweight: The demise of scalp blood pH sampling. *J Matern Fetal Med* 1997;6:298–300.
141. Dildy GA 3rd. Fetal pulse oximetry: A critical appraisal. *Best Pract Res Clin Obstet Gynaecol* 2004;18:477–84.
142. Schifrin BS. Is fetal pulse oximetry ready for clinical practice? Writing for the CON position. *MCN Am J Matern Child Nurs* 2003;28:65.
143. Rijnders RJ, Mol BW, Reuwer PJ, Drogtrop AP, Vernooij MM, Visser GH. Is the correlation between fetal oxygen saturation and blood pH sufficient for the use of fetal pulse oximetry? *J Matern Fetal Neonatal Med* 2002;11:80–3.
144. Kirkendall C, Phelan J. Ischemic fetal brain injury and normal fetal pulse oximetry. *Obstet Gynecol* 2002;99:628.
145. Sokol RJ. Occiput posterior position and FHR patterns. *Obstet Gynecol* 1981;57:266–7.

146. Pearl ML, Roberts JM, Laros RK, Hurd WW. Vaginal delivery from the persistent occiput posterior position. Influence on maternal and neonatal morbidity. *J Reprod Med* 1993;38:955–61.
147. Ponkey SE, Cohen AP, Heffner LJ, Lieberman E. Persistent fetal occiput posterior position: Obstetric outcomes. *Obstet Gynecol* 2003;101:915–20.
148. Fitzpatrick M, McQuillan K, O'Herlihy C. Influence of persistent occiput posterior position on delivery outcome. *Obstet Gynecol* 2001;98:1027–31.
149. Akmal S, Kametas N, Tsoi E, Howard R, Nicolaides KH. Ultrasonographic occiput position in early labour in the prediction of caesarean section. *BJOG* 2004;111:532–6.
150. Quintero R, Meyers S, Schifrin B. Problems with intrapartum fetal heart rate monitoring interpretation and patient management. *Obstet Gynecol* 2003;101:617; author reply 618.

177 Pain relief during labor

D. J. Birnbach and E. M. Davidson

Introduction

The numerous challenges presented by the parturient requesting analgesia makes the job of the anesthesiologist working in labor and delivery both demanding and rewarding. Those providing analgesia to the obstetric patient must be familiar with the unique physiology of the parturient and the effects of many medications and techniques on the parturient and fetus, and on the labor.

Continuous improvements in drugs and techniques have led to a significant decrease in anesthetic-related deaths in the delivery suite.[1] The maternal mortality rate in the United States is estimated at 7.5 per 100,000 live births[2]; however, under-reporting makes this probably a minimum estimate.[3] A recent retrospective analysis of maternal mortality during hospital admission by Panchal *et al.* indicated that anesthesia-related complications accounted for 5.2% of maternal deaths.[4]

The American College of Obstetricians and Gynecologists (ACOG) and the American Academy of Pediatrics (AAP) have made several recommendations concerning anesthetic management in the labor and delivery suite. These include the availability of 24-h coverage in larger facilities with complicated patients, the ability to perform an emergency cesarean section within all facilities with delivery suites, and the availability of properly trained personnel to manage anesthetic complications. They further suggest that, in the event of fetal compromise, the team should be capable of starting an operative delivery within 30 min.[5] Immediate availability of anesthesiologists remains a major problem in many parts of the world, and even when available, communication between the obstetrician and anesthesiologist may be suboptimal. To provide optimal better care for the pregnant patient, obstetricians and anesthesiologists must understand the physiologic changes that exist in these patients. Maternal changes in pregnancy occur as a result of hormonal alterations, mechanical effects of the gravid uterus, increased metabolic and oxygen requirements, metabolic demands of the fetoplacental unit, and hemodynamic alterations associated with the placental circulation. Such changes become more significant as pregnancy progresses and have major implications for anesthetic management. In the section on deaths related to anesthesia in a most recent triennial report of the United Kingdom, it was noted that poor communication between obstetric and anesthetic teams remained a problem, with anesthesiologists often being presented with difficult cases as emergencies, with no prior warning.[6]

Appreciation of the roles of the obstetrician, anesthesiologist, pediatrician, and other personnel in the care of the mother and child will facilitate the highest level of care. This chapter will provide an overview of the principles and techniques utilized by the anesthesiologist in the labor and delivery suite.

Physiologic changes of pregnancy

The cardiovascular system is impacted by pregnancy and may place the parturient with preexisting cardiac disease at great risk of morbidity and mortality.[7,8] Cardiovascular changes throughout pregnancy (Table 177.1) include an increased total blood volume of up to 40%, the consequence of increases in both plasma volume and red blood cell mass, the latter increasing relatively less than the plasma. This leads to 'physiologic anemia' of pregnancy with average hemoglobin and hemocrit of 11.6 g/dl and 35.5%, respectively.[9] Increased cardiac output (30–50%) due to increased heart rate, increased stroke volume and decreased systemic vascular resistance is also present.[10] Obstruction of the inferior vena cava occurs in many term parturients in the supine position and may produce hypotension in at least 5% of patients near term.[11] Kerr *et al.* reported that 10 out of 12 pregnant patients whom they studied had signs of complete obstruction of the inferior vena cava.[12] Aortocaval compression causes an obstruction to venous return and also an increased uterine venous pressure, thus further decreasing uterine blood flow (Figure 177.1).[13] Drugs causing vasodilatation or regional anesthetic techniques causing a sympathetic blockade may further decrease venous return and worsen this supine hypotension. Left uterine displacement has been found to reverse some of these effects and to improve cardiac output.[14]

Table 177.1 Cardiovascular changes in pregnancy

Parameter	Change	Amount
Heart rate	Increased	20–30%
Stroke volume	Increased	20–50%
Cardiac output	Increased	30–50%
Contractility	Variable	~10%
Central venous pressure	Unchanged	—
Pulmonary capillary wedge pressure	Unchanged	—
Systemic vascular resistance	Decreased	20%
Systemic blood pressure	Slight decrease	Mid-trimester 10–15 mmHg, then rises
Pulmonary vascular resistance	Decreased	30%
Pulmonary artery pressure	Slight decrease	—

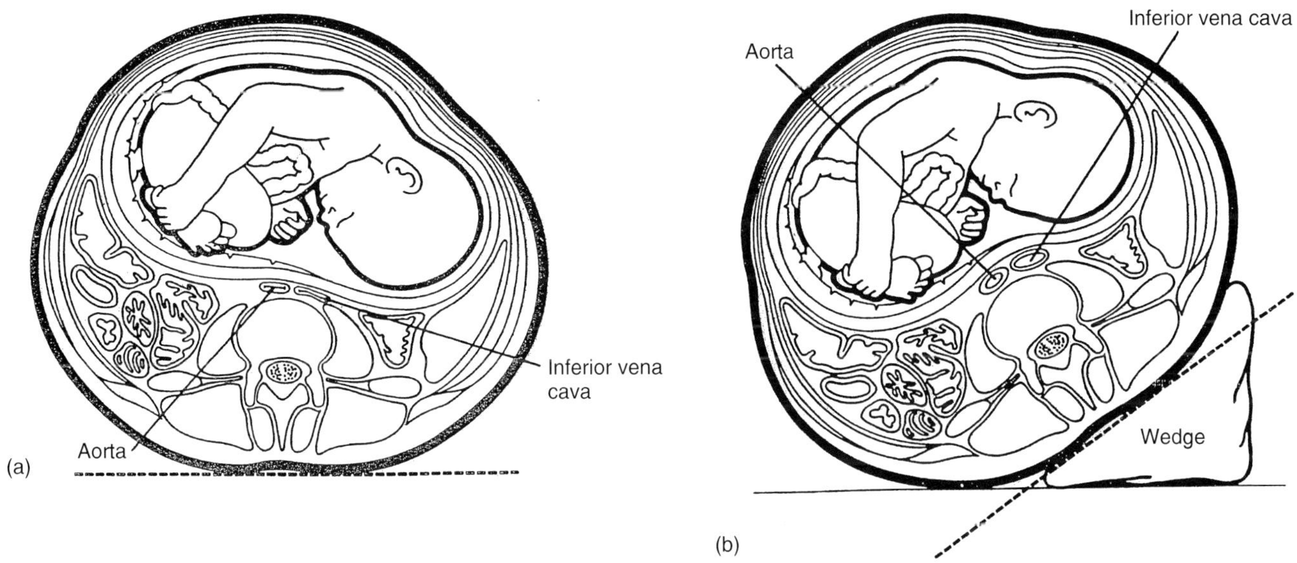

Figure 177.1 In (a) the patient is in the supine position, and the uterus compresses the aorta and inferior vena cava. A wedge under the hip (b) displaces the uterus and relieves aortocaval compression. From Fisher S, Ostheimer G, Warren TM. Obstetric analgesia and anesthesia. In Cohen WR, Acker DB, Friedman EA, eds. *Management of Labor*, 2nd edn. Rockville, MD: Aspen Publishers, 1989:80–81, with permission.

A state of hypercoaguability, which is thought to be a protective adaptation to lessen the risks of acute hemorrhage, exists in pregnancy with increased levels of most coagulation factors (Table 177.2). This hypercoaguable state may, however, lead to thromboembolism, one of the leading causes of maternal mortality.

Respiratory changes (Tables 177.3 and 177.4) include increased oxygen consumption, decreased functional residual capacity, increased minute and alveolar ventilation, increased tidal volume, and a decreased arterial carbon dioxide pressure.[15,16] The decreased functional residual capacity, in combination with the increased minute ventilation, causes lowered oxygen reserve and a risk of hypoxia developing more rapidly during attempted intubation as part of general endotracheal anesthesia.[17]

Other pregnancy-related changes of the respiratory tract and oropharynx may have important anesthetic implications. Capillary engorgement of the mucosa and edema of the oropharynx, larynx, and trachea may result in difficult intubation. Any manipulation of the upper airway such as suctioning, insertion of airways, or laryngoscopy may cause edema, bleeding, and upper airway trauma. Because of the particularly friable mucosa of the nasopharynx, instrumentation of the nose should be avoided. When performing intubation of the pregnant patient, a smaller endotracheal tube (size 6.0–7.0) should be used, and repeated attempts at laryngoscopy minimized. Every member of the medical team taking care of the parturient should be able to assess the patient's airway[18] (Mallampati classification), and should be able to recognize features that may cause difficulty in managing the airway.

Table 177.2 Coagulation factors in pregnancy

Factor	Change
II	Unchanged
VII	Increased+++
VIII, IX, X, XII	Increased
XI	Reduced
Fibrinogen	Increased+++
Platelets	Unchanged

Table 177.3 Changes in respiratory physiology at term gestation

Parameter	Change
Lung volumes	
Inspiratory reserve volume	+5%
Tidal volume	+45%
Expiratory reserve volume	−25%
Residual volume	−15%
Lung capacities	
Inspiratory capacity	+15%
Functional residual capacity	−20%
Vital capacity	No change
Total lung capacity	−5%
Dead space	+45%
Respiratory rate	*No change*
Ventilation	
Minute ventilation	+45%
Alveolar ventilation	+45%

Table 177.4 Effects of pregnancy on respiratory mechanics (adapted from Conklin[9])

Parameter	Change*
Diaphragm excursion	Increased
Chest wall excursion	Decreased
Pulmonary resistance	Decreased 50%
FEV_1	No change
FEV_1/FVC	No change
Flow volume loop	No change
Closing capacity	No change

FEV_1: Forced expiratory volume in 1 s
*Relative to non-pregnant women

Gastrointestinal changes in the pregnant patient increase the risk associated with the administration of anesthesia, by increasing the aspiration risk. The stomach and intestines are displaced in pregnancy, gastrointestinal motility is decreased, gastric acid secretion is increased, gastric volume is increased, and pH is decreased.[19,20] Because of these physiologic changes, many authors have suggested the routine administration of an antacid prior to initiation of anesthesia in the pregnant patient.[21] The use of a non-particulate antacid, such as sodium citrate, has many advantages, no major disadvantages and has become standard practice in the United States prior to cesarean delivery.[22]

The renal system undergoes major changes in the pregnant patient, mainly because of the effects of progesterone and the mechanical effects of compression by the enlarging uterus. Urea, creatinine, and uric acid clearance all rise in pregnancy. The renal plasma flow and glomerular filtration rate (GFR) increase rapidly and relate to the increase in cardiac output. GFR rises by almost 50%; this, accompanied by the dilutional effect of plasma volume expansion, accounts for the fall in plasma creatinine and urea. Hence, 'normal' renal indices in pregnancy are lower than in the non-pregnant state. Therefore, BUN and creatinine levels that would be considered marginally elevated in the non-pregnant patient are usually indicative of severe renal impairment in the parturient. The increase in GFR usually precedes the expansion of blood volume and is generally considered to be a marker of pregnancy-induced vasodilation.[23] Glycosuria is a common finding due to the increase in GFR and reduced renal tubular resorption capacity.

Analgesia for labor

Before deciding on one of the various analgesic options available to the parturient, it is important to understand the mechanisms and pain pathways of labor. Pain perception by the parturient is a dynamic process that involves both peripheral and central mechanisms.

Many factors impact on the degree of pain experienced by a woman during labor. These include psychological preparation, quality of emotional support during labor, previous experiences, patient's expectations regarding the birthing process, and whether or not the labor is augmented. An abnormal fetal presentation (such as occiput posterior) may also cause labor pain to be more intense. For most women childbirth is associated with very severe pain, which often exceeds expectations.[24] In fact, as reported on the McGill pain questionnaire, labor pain is one of the most intense pains a woman can experience, and it is typically worse than a toothache, back pain, and pain associated with deep laceration.[25] A study of women in the first stage of labor reported that 60% of primiparous women described the pain of uterine contractions as being 'unbearable, intolerable, extremely severe, or excruciating'.[25]

During the first stage of labor, pain impulses arise primarily from the uterus. Uterine contractions may result in myometrial ischemia, which ultimately causes the release of bradykinin, histamine, and serotonin. In addition, stretching and distension of the lower uterine segment and cervix may stimulate mechanoreceptors. These noxious impulses follow sensory nerve fibers that accompany sympathetic nerve endings; they travel through the paracervical region and the hypogastric plexus to enter the lumbar sympathetic chain.[26] These stimuli enter the spinal cord at the T10, 11, 12, and L1 spinal segments. Parturients describe this pain as dull in nature and often poorly localized. With the onset of the second stage of labor and stretching of the perineum, somatic afferent nerve fibers transmit impulses via the pudendal nerve to the spinal cord at S2, 3, and 4 levels.

Labor causes increased maternal levels of adrenocorticotropic hormone (ACTH) and cortisol, epinephrine, norepinephrine and β-endorphins.[27,28] Animal studies suggest that these substances may decrease uterine blood flow and cause fetal hypoxia.[29] In addition to the obvious immediate problems associated with pain, it has also been reported that increased pain in labor was associated with a higher incidence of postpartum depression.[30]

Pain impulses may be blocked at the level of the peripheral nerves (local anesthetic, peripheral nerve blocks), the spinal cord (spinal, epidural, or combined spinal–epidural anesthesia) or centrally (systemic medications, such as opioids, general anesthesia).

The following section of this chapter will give an overview of the various methods and techniques of analgesia currently utilized.

Systemic medication

When systemic medications are chosen for labor analgesia, opioids are the most commonly used class of drugs. All opioids are associated with certain side effects including respiratory depression, nausea and vomiting, and mental status changes (ranging from euphoria to excessive sedation). All opioids cross the placenta because of their physicochemical characteristics, and they may cause respiratory depression in the newborn. However, when used in appropriate doses, systemic narcotics can be somewhat effective in alleviating labor pain for short periods of time. Other systemic drugs used in the treatment of labor pain include sedative tranquilizers and ketamine.

Meperidine (demerol, pethidine)

Meperidine is the most commonly used parenteral opioid for labor analgesia. A recent American survey examined the use of parenteral opioids in obstetric units and reported their use at 39–56%. In units with over 1500 deliveries per year, parenteral opioids were administered to 39% of women; that percentage increased as the number of deliveries decreased.[31] The intramuscular dose ranges from 50 to 100 mg, with peak effect at 40–50 min; intravenous doses of 25–50 mg act within 5–10 min. The analgesic effect lasts approximately 3–4 h. This drug may cause loss of beat-to-beat variability in fetal heart rate (FHR) tracings. Fetal exposure to meperidine is highest between 2 and 3 h following maternal administration.[32] Meperidine is felt to cause less respiratory depression in the neonate than morphine; therefore, it is more commonly used.[33]

Despite the known problems associated with meperidine, a recent meta-analysis suggested that other opioids (tramadol, meptazinol, diamorphine, pentazocine, nalbuphine, and butanorphanol) were not superior to meperidine for labor analgesia.[34] Several authors, however, have proposed that fentanyl and remifentanil are better choices.[35,36]

Fentanyl

Intravenous fentanyl is an alternative analgesic option for patients in whom regional anesthesia is contraindicated. Its short half-life makes it suitable for prolonged use in labor, either as an IV bolus or administered using a patient-controlled analgesia delivery system.[37] It provides adequate analgesia with minimal neonatal depression.[38] Although it provides strong analgesia, its use in labor has been limited by side effects and short duration of action. One study that evaluated intravenous fentanyl for labor reported that 4 of the 11 newborns whose mothers received fentanyl for analgesia during labor required naloxone treatment.[39] The usual dose of IV fentanyl for labor analgesia is 25–50 μg when given as a bolus. The peak effect occurs within 3–5 min and it has a duration of 30–60 min. A prospective evaluation of fentanyl for labor concluded that an intravenous dose during early labor was associated with temporary depressant effects on fetal biophysical parameters without apparent harm noted at time of delivery.[40] A study evaluating intravenous fentanyl in labor reported that mild sedation and a transient decrease in FHR variability were also noted.[41] Several investigators, however, have determined that intravenous fentanyl is preferable to meperidine as a labor analgesic.[42] Fentanyl offers another advantage in that it can be administered in non-parenteral modalities including orally and via a patch. These uses, however, have not been evaluated for use in the laboring patient.

Remifentanil

Remifentanil is a potent, short-acting mu-opioid receptor agonist which has been approved for clinical use. It is a piperidine derivative with a normal opioid configuration, but it contains an ester linkage that allows metabolism by non-specific esterases throughout the plasma and muscle tissue. This gives it a unique pharmacologic profile in comparison to other opioids. Remifentanil has an extremely rapid plasma clearance and offset of action. Its estimated half-life is 1.3 min and prolonged administration does not appear to cause accumulation of this drug. Studies have demonstrated an umbilical vein-to-maternal artery ratio of 0.88.[35] Thus, fetal exposure to the drug is minimized due to its rapid metabolism or redistribution. These properties make it an attractive alternative systemic analgesic in those parturients in whom regional anesthesia is contraindicated. There are growing data in the literature regarding the use of this drug for labor analgesia.[36,43] Dose–response studies using intravenous remifentanil in patient-controlled analgesia suggest a median effective bolus dose of 0.4 μg/kg with a lockout time of 1 min[44] or a continuous infusion of remifentanil at 0.05 μg/kg/min and a bolus of 25 μg with a lockout time of 5 min provides satisfactory analgesia.[36] There is also a report of its prolonged use for 34 h in a complex parturient in whom regional techniques were contraindicated; there were no adverse effects.[45] Studies using remifentanil in labor have not fully answered whether or not it is a superior systemic opioid analgesic for parturients.[46] While preliminary reports have been promising, it is still somewhat premature to advocate the use of remifentanil until larger studies have fully evaluated its use.

Butorphanol and nalbuphine

Butophanol and nalbuphine are opioid agonist-antagonists that are structurally related to oxymorphone and naloxone. They have the potential advantages of producing less nausea and vomiting as compared with other opioids. Butorphanol is a kappa-agonist, a mu-antagonist, and has minimal affinity for sigma-receptors. Its dose is 1–2 mg IM or IV, and it has a duration of action up to 4 h. Nalbuphine is a partial kappa-agonist and a potent mu-antagonist with minimal sigma-receptor activity. A dose of 10 mg IV or IM is equivalent to 10 mg morphine with an onset of 2–3 min for IV or 10–15 min for the IM route. It provides analgesia for up to 6 h.

One advantage of these agents as compared to mu-agonists is that they demonstrate a 'ceiling effect' so that increasing doses do not produce further respiratory depression.[47] Unfortunately, the use of these drugs is limited in clinical practice because they are rapidly transferred across the placenta and have produced sinusoidal FHR patterns.[48,49] While it appears that this FHR pattern is benign and does not signify life-threatening fetal jeopardy as usually associated with such a pattern, many obstetricians do not wish to administer a drug that might mimic this ominous FHR tracing. In addition, the use of antagonists or agonist–antagonists may precipitate acute withdrawal syndrome in the mother and the newborn of an opioid-dependent parturient. This has been reported following both parenteral and neuraxial administration.[50]

Sedative tranquilizers

Sedative tranquilizers, including barbiturates, phenothiazines, hydroxyzine, and benzodiazepines, have been used during labor. While barbiturates such as secobarbitol were once popular, especially during early labor, they are currently unfashionable due to potential anti-analgesic effects in the mother and prolonged depressant effects on the neonate. Even with small doses of barbiturates that result in no depression of the Apgar score, the newborn's attention span may be depressed for upwards of 4 days.[51]

Promethazine is a phenothiazine occasionally used in the obstetric patient. Administered together with meperidine, it can be given in doses of 25–50 mg to reduce the risk of emesis. Its ability to potentiate the analgesic effects of opioids, however, has been challenged.[52] Promethazine appears in the fetal blood within 1–2 min following intravenous injection in the mother and reaches equilibrium within 15 min.[53]

Ketamine is an *N*-methyl D-aspartate (NMDA) receptor antagonist that produces dissociative anesthesia and has been used in pregnant patients. As a phenylcyclidine derivative, its mechanism of action may be mediated by an interaction with phencyclidine receptors located in the limbic and corticothalamic areas of the brain. There is evidence, however, suggesting that NMDA antagonism is central to the effects of ketamine. Ketamine has been used in subanesthetic doses (0.5–1 mg/kg or 10 mg every 2–5 min to a total of 1 mg/kg over 30 min) during labor.[54] Its main disadvantages are the potential for hypertension and emergence reactions. High doses (greater than 2 mg/kg) can cause psychomimetic effects and increased uterine tone; causing lower Apgar scores and abnormalities in neonatal muscle tone.[55]

Benzodiazepines such as diazepam (valium), lorazepam (ativan), and midazolam (versed) can be used as sedatives and anxiolytics in labor. When administered intravenously, these drugs readily cross the placenta with elimination half-lives as long as 48 h for diazepam and upwards of 120 h for its main metabolite *N*-desmethyldiazepam.[56] There is anecdotal evidence suggesting that exposure to the benzodiazepines (valium) early *in utero* may result in malformations such as cleft lip.[57] Closer analysis involving first trimester administration of benzodiazepines, however, demonstrates that the majority of infants were normal at birth and had normal postnatal development.[56] The use of these drugs during labor will obviously have no effect on fetal malformations, but they may be associated with other problems in the neonate including sedation, hypotonia, cyanosis, and impaired metabolic responses to stress. In addition, since these drugs are potent amnestic agents, a parturient may not be able to remember her birthing experience.[58] Many of the adverse effects can be reversed by the administration of flumazenil, which is a competitive benzodiazepine-receptor antagonist.

Recently, a study evaluating the use of intrathecal midazolam has suggested that this may be advantageous. This study, however, which was performed in Australia, used a non-preservative-containing formulation of midazolam which is not available in the United States and many other countries.[59]

Inhalation analgesia

Inhalation analgesia consists of the administration of subanesthetic concentrations of inhalational anesthetic agents to relieve pain during labor. This pain relief technique should not be confused with inhalation anesthesia (during general anesthesia), which produces unconsciousness and loss of protective laryngeal reflexes. Although inhalation analgesia provides some degree of pain relief, it is not associated with an adequate level of analgesia to provide sufficient pain relief for most mothers. It may, however, have a place as an adjunct to neuraxial techniques or in parturients for whom regional anesthesia is contraindicated. Inhaled analgesics can be administered either intermittently (e.g., during contractions) or continuously. They can be self-administered, but the patient should have a healthcare provider present in order to ensure an adequate level of consciousness and proper use of the equipment. Although inhalational agents continue to be used in parts of Europe as well as in some developing countries, they are seldom used for labor analgesia in the United States.

Entonox (50:50 N_2O/O_2 mixture) has been used for many years both as a sole analgesic and adjuvant to systemic and regional techniques for labor. Associated side effects include dizziness, nausea, dysphoria, and inability of the parturient to cooperate. The maximum analgesic effect occurs after 45–60 s of inhalation, and it is therefore important that the parturient uses entonox at the early onset of her contractions and discontinues its use after the peak of the contraction. The lack of scavenging systems in labor rooms may theoretically put staff at risk of exposure to excessive levels of this agent over a prolonged period. The administration of nitrous oxide and oxygen in a 50:50 combination appears to have no effect on hepatic, renal, cardiac, or pulmonary functions. While safe and economic, it is unfortunate that analgesia with 50% nitrous oxide has not been demonstrated to be reliable.[60]

Desflurane (0.2%), enflurane, and isoflurane (0.2–0.25%) have also been used successfully to provide labor analgesia, but their effectiveness appears to be comparable to nitrous oxide. While Abboud and coworkers found that enflurane and nitrous oxide were equipotent, others have found that enflurane 1% provided better pain relief.[61–63] The use of these volatile agents, however, is limited by drowsiness, an unpleasant smell, and high cost. The major risk when using volatile agents is accidental overdose resulting in unconsciousness and loss of protective reflexes. In addition, proper scavenging of gases in a labor room remains problematic.

Local and regional anesthesia for labor

Local anesthesia can provide differing degrees of sensory and motor block over specific regions of the body. Advantages over intravenous analgesia include lack of maternal central nervous system depression and low maternal-to-fetal transfer of drugs. It may be produced with peripheral nerve blocks (pudendal and paracervical blocks) or central nerve blocks at the level of the spinal cord or spinal nerve roots (caudal, epidural, spinal, combined spinal–epidural). Currently, the most commonly performed regional techniques for labor are epidural, and combined spinal–epidural. Less frequently, lumbar sympathetic blocks are performed.[64] Paracervical, pudendal, and local perineal infiltration are occasionally used by the obstetrician, but use is limited by side effects.

Patient evaluation and preparation

It is important to evaluate all patients prior to placement of a regional block by obtaining a focused medical and obstetric history, performing a clinical examination, and an airway evaluation. Use of herbal medications by the general population is gaining in popularity,[65] and obstetric patients are no different. It has recently been reported that there is a 7.1% incidence of herbal remedy use by parturients after 20 weeks' gestation.[66] Preparations containing garlic, ginkgo, ginseng, ginger, and feverfew may have anesthetic implications.

The obstetric plan and fetal well-being should be noted during this preoperative assessment. Patients should be evaluated and screened for contraindications for neuraxial blocks. Certain medical conditions require lab testing prior to performance of a neuraxial blockade. Informed consent must be obtained, and the anesthesiologist should explain the procedure and the potential complications of the technique. A retrospective study of patients' attitudes toward labor analgesia satisfaction and the consent process revealed that pain and distress during labor did not interfere with the women's ability to understand the information associated with the consent process prior to epidural placement. Furthermore, patients felt that the most valuable information received was either from the anesthesiologist who placed the epidural or from an antenatal course. A full check of emergency equipment must be performed to ensure the immediate availability of resuscitative drugs and equipment. In addition, an intravenous infusion should be started and appropriate maternal and fetal monitoring should in place before starting the procedure.

Epidural analgesia

The epidural space is a potential space containing blood vessels, fat, and lymphatics. This space extends from the end of the sacrum to the foramen ovale. For analgesia during labor it is usually entered via the lumbar intervertebral space (usually L3–L4 or L4–L5). There is no physical end-point to guide epidural catheter placement, such as free-flow of cerebrospinal fluid (CSF) when initiating spinal anesthesia. Therefore, identification of the epidural space is made using either the 'loss of resistance' or 'hanging drop' techniques to allow verification of needle placement. The epidural needle is relatively large (usually 17 or 18 gauge) so as to allow passage of a 19- or 20-gauge catheter, which is threaded into the epidural space.

Before dosing with local anesthetic, proper placement of the epidural catheter should be assured. Accidental intravenous or subarachnoid placement may prove disastrous if unrecognized. The volume of local anesthetics necessary to achieve anesthesia are much larger than the required spinal doses, and if an epidural volume is injected into the spinal space it may cause a 'total spinal' with resultant hypotension, respiratory paralysis, and unconsciousness. Epidural doses of local anesthetics given intravascularly may cause symptoms ranging from mild central nervous system effects (tinnitus, lightheadedness) to total circulatory collapse, depending on agent, dose and rate of injection. For this reason a 'test dose', often consisting of a local anesthetic with a small amount of epinephrine, is sometimes given, especially before the use of the catheter for cesarean delivery. Evidence of significant sensory and/or motor block indicates an intrathecal placement of the catheter, while a sudden increase in heart rate shortly after injection may indicate intravascular placement of the epidural catheter. Intravascular infusions of ultradilute local anesthetics (e.g., 0.0625% bupivacaine) do not pose a serious threat unless given for prolonged periods. However, if the concentrated local anesthetic is administered for operative delivery, intravascular injection remains a real hazard.

Once the proper placement of the epidural catheter is assured, a dilute solution of local anesthetic may be given to provide labor analgesia. To achieve analgesia during the first and second stages of labor, a segmental block from the lower thoracic to the sacral dermatomes is needed. The dermatomal segments blocked depend on the location of the catheter as well as the dose, concentration and volume of the anesthetic agent used.

It has been suggested that epidural analgesia for labor may influence the outcome of labor.[67] Studies that have examined the effect of an epidural on the length of labor, incidence of malposition, and incidence of operative delivery, however, have been conflicting in their conclusions, with some finding no effect.[68–70] and others finding an increased risk of operative delivery.[71,72] Unfortunately, the majority of studies which have attempted to answer this question have been non-blinded, non-randomized, or retrospective. More recent studies suggest that there is no increased risk for cesarean delivery with epidurals as currently administered[73] although there is still controversy as to the possible increase of instrumental deliveries and possible prolongation of labor that may occur. Despite the controversy surrounding the influence of epidural analgesia on labor progress, this technique remains the most effective method of providing pain relief during parturition.[71]

Bupivacaine, in concentrations ranging from 0.0625% to 0.125%, is often used to provide epidural analgesia in the laboring patient. Initially, 8–12 ml of local anesthetic is administered via the epidural catheter (often in divided doses) to initiate analgesia. The dilute local anesthetic concentrations provide a solid sensory block with only minimal motor block. Because hypotension may occur, ephedrine and phenylephrine should be available to treat hypotension if it occurs.

Because of concerns about cardiotoxicity with inadvertent intravascular injection of bupivacaine,[74] levo isomers, thought to be less cardiotoxic, are being used by some anesthesiologists. Ropivacaine, with a similar phamacodynamic profile as bupivacaine but with less cardiotoxicity,[75] may replace bupivacaine as the local anesthetic of choice for epidural anesthesia. Santos *et al.*[76] reported that intravenous ropivacaine did not lead to any decrease in uterine artery blood flow in pregnant sheep. Levobupivacaine is also being studied and may provide an improved safety profile as compared with racemic bupivacaine.

Continuous epidural infusions

Most obstetric anesthesiologists now advocate the use of continuous infusions of dilute local anesthetic solutions for labor. Local anesthetics are used either alone or, more commonly, in combination with an opioid. The addition of epinephrine may enhance the quality of the analgesia by reducing vascular uptake, systemic absorption of local anesthetic, and by a direct agonist effect on alpha-2 spinal receptors.[77,78] From a parturient's perspective, a continuous infusion offers numerous benefits because it allows for a continuous level of comfort rather than waiting for intermittent epidural top-ups, but may be associated with higher incidence of anesthetic interventions as compared to patient-controlled techniques.[79]

Patient-controlled epidural analgesia

Patient-controlled epidural analgesia (PCEA) is a safe and effective technique.[80] This method of delivery offers effective labor analgesia and excellent patient satisfaction. It reduces the total amount of local anesthetic used; consequently, it lessens unwanted effects such as motor block. It also reduces the demands on the labor floor staff, and it gives many patients a feeling of self-control. Typically, after analgesia is established (either via spinal or epidural) the catheter is connected to the PCEA device, and the patient can then self-administer further boluses as required. Some authors advocate a continuous infusion with patient controlled top-ups; others suggest only boluses be used.[81]

Spinal analgesia

Opioids with or without small doses of local anesthetics introduced into the intrathecal space may be used to provide analgesia for labor vaginal delivery. The block produced by spinal agents may produce anything from a little to complete sensory and motor block, depending on the agent used and its concentration. Intrathecal opioids have the advantage of providing satisfactory analgesia without causing a motor block. Commonly used intrathecal opioids which may provide labor analgesia include sufentanil and fentanyl. While meperidine and morphine have been used, they have side effect profiles that make them suboptimal as sole agents.[82,83] Combinations of opioids plus local anesthetics have also been described.[84] The addition of 2.5 mg bupivacaine to a spinal opioid has been shown to prolong the sensory block without significantly increasing motor block.[85]

A sensory block to T10 is considered adequate for controlling the pain of the first stage of labor. In situations where analgesia or anesthesia is only needed in the sacral dermatomes (as in the provision of anesthesia for a forceps delivery), a 'saddle block' may be performed. With this technique, spinal anesthesia is performed using small amounts of hyperbaric local anesthetics with the patient in the sitting position. Because the solution given is heavier than cerebrospinal fluid and the patient is sitting while the local anesthetic is administered, only the lowest dermatomes are blocked.[86]

Spinal blocks for labor may be associated with the complications that may occur with any central nerve block, including hypotension and dural puncture. The risk of postdural puncture headache can be greatly reduced, however, through the use of atraumatic spinal needles. These newer needles (including Sprotte, Gertie Marx, Whitacre, and Pencan needles) are pencil-point in shape and do not cut the dural fibers to the same extent as conventional (Quincke) spinal needles.[87]

A major disadvantage of single-injection spinal analgesia for labor is the inability to administer more medication should labor last longer than the duration of the spinal medication, or should cesarean section become necessary. Continuous spinal analgesia via a spinal microcatheter is no longer used in the United States due to Food and Drug Administration (FDA) sanctions, which arose as a result of several reports of cauda equina syndrome after use of intrathecal microcatheters.[88] The use of macrocatheters (placing an epidural needle subarachnoid and advancing a standard epidural catheter into the spinal space) has been advocated, especially in very high risk parturients or following accidental dural puncture ('wet-tap').

Combined spinal–epidural analgesia

The combined spinal–epidural (CSE) technique is widely used in obstetric practice to provide analgesia for parturients. It offers effective, rapid onset of spinal analgesia along with the ability to prolong the duration of analgesia, as required, via an epidural catheter. In addition, should an operative delivery become necessary, that same catheter can be used to provide operative anesthesia. Onset of spinal analgesia is almost immediate, and the duration is between 2 and 3 h depending on whether fentanyl or sufentanil is chosen.

In addition to the advantage of the rapid onset of pain relief, the CSE technique may reduce the incidence of several potential problems associated with the conventional epidural, including incomplete blockade, motor block, and poor sacral spread. Another potential advantage of the CSE technique is that some preliminary evidence suggests that it may be associated with a significantly reduced duration of the first stage of labor in nulliparous parturients.[89]

Side effects of intrathecal opioids include pruritis, nausea and vomiting, and urinary retention. Respiratory depression (due to cephalad spread of opioid) is rare when using lipid soluble opioids.

Use of a dilute concentration of a continuous epidural infusion (0.0625–0.1% bupivacaine) provides sensory analgesia without motor block; consequently, it permits many parturients to ambulate during labor. Prior to ambulation, however, women should be observed for approximately 30 min to ensure maternal and fetal well-being, and be assessed for adequate motor function.

Paracervical block

The paracervical block utilizes local anesthetic placed via transvaginal injection in the lateral fornix on each side of the cervix. This produces anesthesia to the nerves of the uterus (T10–L1), which is helpful in relieving pain of the first-stage labor. Currently, this block is infrequently used because of a high incidence of potentially severe and life-threatening complications. These include the possibility of local anesthetic-induced maternal seizures from intravascular injection, hematoma formation, and a high incidence of fetal bradycardia, which has been reported in 10–70% of patients who receive these blocks. Fishburne *et al.*[90] suggested that the fetal bradycardia results from decreased placental perfusion due to drug-induced uterine artery vasoconstriction, although other theories include high blood concentrations of local anesthetic in the fetus, and an increase in uterine activity.[91] Because of these risks, paracervical block is considered to be a suboptimal choice when fetal compromise exists or is anticipated.[92]

Pudendal block

A pudendal block may be performed to reduce the pain of the second stage of labor, facilitate forceps delivery, or allow the performance of a painless episiotomy. The pudendal nerve (S2–S4) innervates the vagina and the perineum, but does not affect the pain felt from uterine contractions, so its block is ineffective for the first stage of labor. In addition, perineal analgesia is incomplete, so discomfort may be felt if the episiotomy is extended or the vaginal delivery is difficult. This block is performed by anesthetizing the pudendal nerves as they travel just posterior to the junction of the ischial spine and the sacrospinous ligament. Aspiration prior to injection of the local anesthetic is essential in order to decrease the risks associated with paracervical block. This block has a low incidence of maternal hypotension and fetal bradycardia when properly performed. Rare complications of paracervical block, however, include infection, puncture of the rectum, hematoma formation, toxic reactions of the local anesthetic, and sciatic nerve block if the needle is inserted too deeply.[93]

Lumbar sympathetic blocks

Another nerve block that can be considered an alternative to central neuraxial block is the paravertebral lumbar sympathetic technique. This block can be used to block transmission of pain from the uterus during the first stage of labor.[94] Although it is a technically difficult block to perform, it appears to be associated with far fewer complications when compared to paracervical blockade.

Local anesthetic agents

Bupivacaine

Bupivacaine is an amide local anesthetic commonly used for spinal and epidural anesthesia and analgesia in obstetric practice. Its long duration of action, differential sensory to motor block,[95] and relative lack of tachyphylaxis makes it a popular choice.

The placental transfer of bupivacaine, as with other amide local anesthetics, is governed by two factors: the degree of ionization at physiologic pH, and the extent of protein binding. Bupivacaine has a pK_a of 8.05 (highly ionized at physiologic pH) and is 95% protein-bound; thus, it has limited transfer to the placenta when compared to other local anesthetics. In the 1980s, safety concerns were raised following reports of several deaths related to cardiovascular or cardiac toxicity of bupivacaine.[96,97] Following these reports, the FDA prohibited the use of 0.75% concentration epidural solution in obstetric practice. Bupivacaine consists of two stereoisomers *S*(–) and *R*(+) and is marketed as a racemic mixture of these. When separated, the R component was found to predominantly contribute to bupivacaine's toxicity.[98,99] This led researchers to develop the use of *S*(–) isomers for clinical practice, and it resulted in the introduction of ropivacaine (the *S*-isomer of the propyl homologue of bupivacaine) and levobupivacaine (the *S*-isomer of bupivacaine).

Lidocaine

Lidocaine has been used for many years in obstetric anesthesia. It has a quick onset with an intermediate duration of action. Umbilical venous/maternal venous ratios reported in the literature are approximately 0.4–0.6.[100] Although lidocaine is very popular for use as an epidural local anesthetic for operative delivery (especially 2% with epinephrine), it is not popular for providing labor analgesia. While early reports suggested that lidocaine compromised neonatal neurobehavioral function,[101] numerous follow-up studies have not confirmed this.[102] Controversy has developed regarding the use of 5% hyperbaric lidocaine for spinal anesthesia because of reports of transient neurologic symptoms. In 1994, the FDA issued a letter concerning 5% hyperbaric lidocaine; it urged physicians to dilute the lidocaine with saline or CSF prior to injection. These precautions were subsequently incorporated into the package insert for this drug. More recent data indicate, however, that the 2.5% and 2% solutions may still cause transient radicular irritation (TRI).[103] As a result, and despite many years of use without clinical evidence of neurotoxicity, many anesthesiologists have abandoned the use of 5% hyperbaric lidocaine for cesarean section.

2-Chloroprocaine

2-Chloroprocaine is an ester local anesthetic with a rapid onset time and short-lived duration of action. Its rapid metabolism by ester hydrolysis ($t_{1/2}=45$ s) makes it a very safe agent for use in obstetrics since almost no drug crosses the placenta.[104] Because of this and its speed of onset, its primary role in obstetric anesthesia is for establishment of epidural anesthesia for emergency cesarean (when an epidural catheter is already in place). In addition to its short duration of action, a potential disadvantage of chloroprocaine is that it may interfere with the action of epidurally administered opioids.[105] This interaction may be due to antagonism at the mu and kappa receptors.[106] Furthermore, it has been reported that chloroprocaine may also interfere with the action of epidurally administered bupivacaine.[107] Previous preparations of 2-chloroprocaine were considered to be potentially neurotoxic because of reports of arachnoiditis following unintentional subarachnoid injection of this anesthetic.[108] Subsequent reports incriminated the low pH of the anesthetic along with the preservatives used for stabilization.[109] Removal of metabisulfite and methylparaben have decreased the risk of neurotoxicity. However, caution is advised because despite the availability of preservative-free preparations (marketed as MPF or methylparaben free), older formulations containing preservatives are still commercially available.[110]

Levobupivacaine

Based on the evidence that the cardiotoxicity of bupivacaine was more pronounced with the *R*(+) enantiomer, the *S*(–) enantiomer of bupivacaine (levobupivacaine), was developed for clinical use. Levobupivacaine is a long-acting local anesthetic with a similar clinical profile to bupivacaine. Both animal and human volunteer studies have demonstrated its greater safety profile compared to racemic bupivacaine.

Assessment of sensory block between 0.5% bupivacaine and 0.5% levobupivacaine demonstrated no difference in adequacy of block or time taken to reach a surgically adequate block. Similarly, other authors have recently reported that there was no difference with regard to onset or duration of sensory block when patients received either levobupivacaine 0.5% or bupivacaine 0.5% for cesarean section. In addition, the onset and regression of sensory and motor blockade, quality of anesthesia, and muscle relaxation were comparable between the two groups.[111] Levobupivacaine has also been used to provide epidural analgesia for labor. A recent multicenter study comparing levobupivacaine and bupivacaine reported these drugs have equivalent analgesic efficacy. In addition, motor blockade was similar between the groups.[112] As with other local anesthetics, recent evidence suggests that fentanyl significantly reduces levobupivacaine requirements for epidural analgesia in labor.[113]

Ropivacaine

Ropivacaine is a homolog of mepivacaine and bupivacaine, and was the first *S*-levo isomer local anesthetic to be marketed. Ropivacaine is less soluble than bupivacaine and therefore may be less potent. While clinical evidence suggests that the two drugs might be similar in potency,[114] Minimum Local Anesthetic Concentration (MLAC) studies have suggested that the analgesic potency of ropivacaine was 0.60 (0.47–0.75) relative to bupivacaine. Claims for reduced toxicity and motor block must be considered with differences in analgesic potency kept in mind,[115] because, in theory, more drug would need to be administered and any safety advantage might be minimized.

Psychoprophylaxis – non-pharmacological methods

'Natural childbirth' stems from a phrase coined by Grantley Dick-Read in 1933; he believed that childbirth was a painless process that did not need medical intervention if the mother was adequately prepared.[116] The Pavlovian methods of controlling childbirth pain used in Russia were adapted by the French obstetrician Fernand Lamaze in the late 1950s, and his work popularized natural childbirth as an option for parturients. This method focuses on teaching the mother conditioned reflexes to overcome the pain as well as the fear of childbirth. It also employs an education program, human support during labor, breathing techniques, relaxation techniques, a strong focus of attention, and specific activities to assist concentrate during contractions. Indeed, even the effect of the presence of another woman during labor to support the expectant mother has been shown to have a positive effect on outcomes, including duration of labor.[117]

Transcutanaeous electrical nerve stimulation

Transcutanaeous electrical nerve stimulation (TENS) is thought to reduce pain by nociceptive inhibition at a presynaptic level in the dorsal horn by limiting central transmission. Electrical stimulation preferentially activates low threshold myelinated nerves. Afferent inhibition effects inhibit propagation of nociception along unmyelinated small 'c' fibers by blocking impulses to target cells in the substantia gelatinosa of the dorsal horn. TENS is also thought to enhance release of endorphins and dynorphins centrally.[118] Placement of electrode pads over the lower back in the distribution of T10–L1 has been shown to provide some degree of analgesia for some patients in early labor.[119] However, other reports have failed to demonstrate its effectiveness for labor analgesia or as an adjunct to epidural analgesia.[120,121]

Anesthetic drugs and the fetus

After drug uptake into the maternal circulation, a portion of the drug will cross the placenta and enter the fetal circulation. The amount of drug that ultimately is delivered to the fetus will depend on numerous factors, including uterine blood flow, the characteristics of the drug itself, and the characteristics of the placenta.

Placental transfer of drugs

Since the placenta has the properties of a lipid membrane, the physiochemical factors related to transfer may be described by the Fick law, which states that:

$$Q/T = KA\,(C_m - C_f)/D$$

where Q/T is the rate of diffusion, A is area of placenta involved in diffusion, C_m is the maternal blood concentration, C_f is the fetal blood concentration, D is the thickness of the membrane, and K is the diffusion constant which is unique to each drug and is dependent on the properties of the drug itself including its degree of ionization, lipid solubility, protein binding, and molecular weight.

Factors that favor transfer across the placenta include low molecular weight, low degree of ionization, high lipid solubility, and low protein binding.[122] Since most anesthetic drugs are weak bases, a decrease in pH of the blood (acidemia) will increase the percentage of drug that will be in the ionized form. This will decrease the amount of drug transferred across the placenta.

The increasing ionization of most drugs with decreasing pH may cause high levels of drugs to accumulate in the fetus. For example, if lidocaine is transferred from the blood of the mother to an acidemic fetus, the lower pH of the fetal blood will increase ionization of the lidocaine. This additional ionization may make the lidocaine less able to diffuse back across the placental membrane to the mother. Thus, the ratio of lidocaine level in the fetus compared to the lidocaine level in the mother's blood will be higher. This phenomenon is known as *fetal ion trapping*, and explains why increased blood levels of anesthetic drugs may be seen in the compromised (acidemic) fetus.[123]

Fetal circulation and anesthetic drugs

During general anesthesia for cesarean section, the mother is unconscious and her muscles paralyzed. The newborn child, however, is removed from the uterus fully awake and moving. This is explained by maternal circulation and the physiochemical processes of drug transfer across the placenta from mother to fetus.[124] An additional factor is the unique physiology of the fetal circulation.[125] The lack of muscle paralysis in the newborn is explained by the highly ionized nature of muscle relaxants, which permits minimal drug to cross the placental membrane to enter the fetal circulation. However, induction drugs (such as thiopental) freely pass through the placental membrane. The lack of rapid fetal effect of these drugs is explained by the fetal circulation. Drugs crossing the placenta are directed to the liver which will act as a reservoir for a portion of the drug. Some of the drug reaching the fetal circulation, however, will bypass the liver via the ductus venosus and proceed to the right atrium via the inferior vena cava. From the right atrium, a portion of the drug will be shunted via the foramen ovale to the left-sided circulation from which eventually it will reach the fetal brain, where the greatest effect will occur. However, a majority of the drug that enters the right ventricle passes through the ductus arteriosus into the lower systemic circulation, with very little drug reaching the brain.

Regional anesthesia and drug effects in the newborn

A well-conducted regional anesthetic given for pain control in labor will have no long-term neurobehavioral effects in the newborn. Local anesthetics injected into the intrathecal or epidural space have very limited uptake into the maternal circulation. Opioids injected into the intrathecal space for labor require only small doses compared to those needed for analgesia via the intravenous route. This results in low maternal blood levels and distribution to the fetus. The acid–base status of infants whose mothers receive epidural anesthesia during the first stage of labor is more favorable than when mothers do not receive regional anesthesia. Apgar scores are not affected in mothers receiving epidural analgesia, even when continuous epidural infusions of low-dose bupivacaine and fentanyl are maintained for many hours.[126]

Uterine activity and anesthesia

In the uterus there are α_1- and β_2-adrenergic receptors. Stimulation of α-receptors increases uterine tone, while β-stimulation produces uterine relaxation. The pain and stress of labor causes the adrenal gland to release epinephrine, which has primarily β_2-stimulating properties. This may reduce uterine contractility and slow the progress of labor. However, labor analgesia and anesthesia, because they decrease maternal pain and the stress response, may decrease adrenal epinephrine secretion.

The effect of neuraxial anesthesia on the progress of labor depends on when it is administered. If given during the active phase of labor, epidural analgesia will have little effect on the progress of labor and may even increase uterine activity. This is presumed to be due to a decreased release of epinephrine from the maternal adrenal gland in response to a decrease in pain. Systemic narcotics may also have a negative impact on labor. When given during the latent phase of labor they generally reduce uterine contractility, but when given after labor is well established they generally have no effect or increase uterine contractility.

Uterine blood flow and anesthesia

Uterine blood flow is directly proportional to uterine perfusion pressure and inversely proportional to uterine vascular resistance. Uterine perfusion pressure is the difference between uterine arterial pressure and uterine venous pressure. Since uterine arterial pressure is proportional to maternal mean blood pressure, anything that decreases maternal blood pressure will ultimately decrease transfer of respiratory gases across the placenta. This may result in a compromised, acidotic fetus. Anything that increases uterine vascular resistance may also have a negative effect on the fetus because it decreases uterine blood flow.

Anesthetic agents may both directly and indirectly change uterine blood flow. Regional anesthesia may decrease maternal blood pressure and thus indirectly impact on uterine blood flow. This may be due to the sympathectomy caused by local anesthetics, particularly if the patient is hypovolemic. Deep general anesthesia with volatile agents may also decrease maternal blood pressure due to decreases in systemic venous resistance and/or cardiac output. These unwanted effects of both regional and general anesthesia may be exaggerated if aortocaval compression is present.

Very high concentrations of local anesthetics in the uterine circulation may cause an increase in uterine vascular resistance. This may occur when large doses of local anesthetics are accidentally given intravenously. In animal studies, vasopressor agents that directly stimulate α_1-adrenergic receptors, such as phenylephrine, norepinephrine and epinephrine, have been associated with increased intrinsic vascular resistance in the uterine vasculature. Ephedrine has been considered the vasopressor of choice in obstetric anesthesia because it does not decrease uterine blood flow. This is because ephedrine has primarily direct β_1-adrenergic agonist activity. It has some α-stimulating effects, but this is by an indirect mechanism (release of catecholamines from sympathetic terminals instead of directly stimulating the α_1-receptors). Recently, many anesthesiologists have begun using phenylephrine or a combination of phenylephrine and ephedrine to treat hypotension in the parturient following administration of neuraxial analgesia or anesthesia.[127]

Increased uterine tone may also decrease uterine vascular resistance. This occurs with physiologic contractions associated with labor and may be especially pronounced with oxytocin infusions, resulting in tetanic contractions. Accidental intravascular injections of large amounts of local anesthetics can also cause increased uterine tone, which may result in fetal compromise.

Anesthesia for cesarean section

Cesarean birth has become the most common hospital-based operative procedure in the United States and accounts for more than 25% of all live births.[128] The increased use of the procedure has been attributed to the liberalization of indications for fetal 'distress' as well as elective repeat cesarean sections.[129] The most common indications for cesarean delivery include 'failure to progress', non-reassuring fetal status, cephalopelvic disproportion, malpresentation, prematurity, and prior uterine surgery. The choice of anesthesia for cesarean section depends on the indications for the surgery, degree of urgency, maternal status, and the desires of the patient.

Regional anesthesia for cesarean section

The use of regional anesthesia has dramatically increased, and since 1997 that of general anesthesia for cesarean section has been steadily decreasing in the United States.[130] Regional anesthesia techniques have several advantages, including a decreased risk of failed intubation, and aspiration of gastric contents, avoidance of depressant agents, and the ability of the mother to remain awake and participate in the birthing experience. In addition, it has been suggested that blood loss is reduced under regional anesthesia for cesarean delivery.[131]

Although epidural, spinal, continuous spinal, and CSE techniques have all been advocated, most straightforward cesarean sections are now performed under single-shot spinal anesthesia which has been found to be faster, provide a superior block, and is more cost effective than alternative techniques.[132]

Spinal anesthesia

Spinal anesthesia offers many advantages for cesarean delivery. It has a rapid onset and provides a dense sensory block. Because of the small doses used, there is little risk of local anesthetic toxicity, and there is minimal transfer of drug to the fetus. In addition, failure rates including incomplete or patchy blocks are very infrequent with spinal anesthesia. Disadvantages of this technique include the finite duration of anesthesia and a higher incidence of hypotension, associated with the very fast onset and associated sympathetic blockade.

Spinal anesthesia can be initiated with the patient either in the sitting or the lateral position and using either plain or hyperbaric solutions. Each method has its advantages and disadvantages. The sitting position, however, appears to be optimal for placement of a neuraxial block in the obese parturient.[133] Hyperbaric solutions have an advantage of greater predictability of block height than plain solutions, and they allow the anesthesiologist the ability to adjust block height by adjusting table position.[134]

Despite achieving an adequate (T4) block, some women under spinal anesthesia will experience some degree of visceral discomfort during cesarean section. This is particularly true in situations in which the obstetrician exteriorizes the uterus. Quality of the spinal anesthesia has been reported to be improved by the addition of epinephrine,[135] morphine,[136] fentanyl,[137] or sufentanil.[138]

Epidural anesthesia

When flexibility is necessary (e.g., for a potentially prolonged cesarean section or need to bring up a block slowly), a catheter technique is optimal, and an epidural approach is often chosen. In addition, women with an indwelling epidural catheter for labor who require cesarean section usually receive medication via that catheter. In high-risk parturients, such as women with 'difficult airways', epidurals are often placed early so they will be available in the event that emergency cesarean section becomes necessary. This illustrates the importance of continuous assessment of epidural catheters and their effectiveness during labor.

The ideal local anesthetic agent for cesarean section should provide rapid onset of dense sensory or motor block with an appropriate duration of action. Commonly used agents include 2-chloroprocaine, lidocaine, and bupivacaine. As compared to spinal anesthesia, very large doses of local anesthetic are used to achieve adequate levels for cesarean section. Epidural catheters can migrate and even a negative aspiration of the catheter does not absolutely rule out intrathecal or intravascular placement. Since large volumes of potentially toxic local anesthetics are administered via an epidural catheter, several measures can be utilized to reduce the risks of local anesthetic toxicity. First, the catheter should be aspirated before use and an appropriate test dose administered. Second, the anesthetic should be administered in fractionated doses. Last, safer drugs (such as chloroprocaine and lidocaine) or the newer amide local anesthetics (such as ropivacaine and levobupivacaine) should be considered.

Intraoperative analgesia under epidural anesthesia may be improved if fentanyl (50–100 μg)[139] or sufentanil (10–20 μg)[141] are added to the local anesthetic. Clonidine has also been used as an additive to epidural local anesthetics, but it has been associated with sedation, bradycardia, and hypotension.[141]

Combined spinal–epidural technique

The combined spinal–epidural (CSE) technique has recently increased in popularity.[143] The advantage of this technique is that it provides rapid onset of dense surgical anesthesia while allowing the ability to prolong the block with an epidural catheter. In addition, because the block can be supplemented at any time, the CSE technique allows the use of smaller doses of spinal local anesthetics which may, in turn, reduce the incidence of high spinal block and hypotension.[143]

Continuous spinal anesthesia

Continuous spinal anesthesia has many potential advantages as compared to single-shot spinal or continuous epidural techniques. The classic technique required the use of large bore epidural needles or a 32-gauge microcatheter inserted through a 26-gauge spinal needle.[144] The technique rapidly gained in popularity despite technical difficulties, but, as previously described, it was abandoned following withdrawal of these catheters by the FDA. The advantages of continuous spinal anesthesia, however, remain and macrocatheters (e.g., placing an epidural catheter intrathecally) can still be used in high-risk parturients. In order to perform a continuous spinal anesthetic, the anesthesiologist intentionally pierces the dura with an epidural needle and then threads the epidural catheter 3 cm within the intrathecal space. Catheter placement can be tested by aspiration of CSF. Since a catheter is being used, smaller doses can be given in an incremental fashion. This is particularly advantageous in high-risk parturients such as those with cardiac disease, respiratory disease, morbid obesity, and those with neuromuscular disease. In order to reduce the risk of headache following this technique, the epidural needle should be turned so that it is parallel to the dural fibers at the time of insertion. In addition, to reduce further the risk of headache, it has been suggested that several steps be taken, including leaving the epidural catheter *in situ* for more than 12 h and injecting a bolus of preservative-free normal saline prior to its removal.[145]

General anesthesia

Although the use of general anesthesia for cesarean delivery has dramatically declined during recent decades, it is still necessary for the management of several situations, including maternal hemorrhage, overt coagulopathy, life-threatening fetal compromise, or in cases in which patients refuse regional anesthesia. A recent study found that anesthesia-related maternal mortality associated with regional anesthesia has declined, but the number of deaths involving general anesthesia has remained relatively constant. This has led to an increase in the relative risk of fatality during general anesthesia to more than 16 times that for regional.[146] Despite these problems, general anesthesia has the advantages of speed of induction, control of the airway, and superior hemodynamics. The frequency of the use of general anesthesia is dependant on many factors including the number of patients at that institution who receive epidural analgesia for labor, the percentage of high-risk parturients, and the skills of the anesthesiologist. Although there are no absolute contraindications to general anesthesia, certain conditions such as malignant hyperthermia or the patient with a difficult airway may require a modified anesthetic technique. Potential problems associated with general anesthesia for cesarean section include failed intubation, pulmonary aspiration of gastric contents, neonatal depression, and maternal awareness.

Steps to provide anesthesia in the healthy parturient for cesarean section include the following:

(1) Administer a non-particulate antacid. Additional agents such as metoclopramide or an H2-blocker should be considered in the patient at high risk for aspiration or failed intubation.
(2) Apply routine monitors including EKG, pulse oximetry, and capnography. Ensure that suction is functioning and that failed intubation equipment is readily available.
(3) Position patient with left uterine displacement and optimize airway position.
(4) Denitrogenate with high flow of oxygen for 3–5 minutes or four vital capacity breaths.
(5) After the drapes are applied and the surgeon is ready, initiate a rapid sequence induction. Apply cricoid pressure and continue this pressure until correct position of the endotracheal tube is verified and cuff is inflated. In hypotensive crises, ketamine 1–1.5 mg/kg should be substituted for thiopenthal. A defasiculating dose of muscle relaxant is not necessary.
(6) Ventilate with 50% oxygen and 50% nitrous oxide and volatile agent as necessary. Maintain normocarbia and use muscle relaxation as necessary with either a non-depolarizing muscle relaxant or succinylcholine infusion. Administer 0.5–0.75 MAC of volatile agent until delivery.
(7) After delivery, increase nitrous oxide to 70%, discontinue or reduce volatile agent, administer opioid and benzodiazepine. Add oxytocin to intravenous fluids.
(8) Insert orogastric tube prior to completion of surgery.
(9) Reverse neuromuscular blockade, as necessary, at completion of surgery.
(10) Extubate when patient is awake, adequately reversed, and following commands.

Failed endotracheal intubation

A study of anesthesia-related deaths in the United States between 1979 and 1990 revealed that the case fatality rate with general anesthesia was 16.7 times greater than with regional anesthesia.[146] Most anesthesia-related deaths were due to hypoxemia when difficulties securing the airway were encountered. The most commonly occurring adverse respiratory events have been failure to intubate, failure to recognize esophageal intubation, and failure to ventilate. It has been recently reported that airway evaluation can often identify the parturient with a difficult airway, but it was not performed in upwards of 10% of cases in which maternal mortality occurred.[147] Others have evaluated the risk factors associated with difficult intubation, and it appears that the greatest risks are associated with a Mallampatti 4 airway, short neck, protruding maxillary incisors, and mandibular recession.[148] From these data, an estimated prediction of a difficult airway has been calculated. Regardless of the initial assessment, all patients must have a repeat airway examination performed before initiation of anesthesia for cesarean section because it has been demonstrated that pregnancy and labor may be associated with changes in the maternal airway.[149,150]

Complications of regional anesthesia in the pregnant patient

Hypotension

Hypotension is defined as a fall of systolic blood pressure to less than 100 mmHg or > 20% from baseline values. The reported incidence of hypotension in the parturient receiving a conduction anesthetic varies depending on the type of anesthetic, the extent of the block, the type of prophylaxis, the site and frequency of blood pressure monitoring, and the definition of hypotension.[151] Ralston and Shnider[152] reported that the incidence of hypotension was reduced from 82% to 14% by conservative measures, including administration of lactated Ringer's solution and left uterine displacement. Hypotension following induction or regional anesthesia occurs primarily as a result of the sympathetic blockade, since a block of sympathetic fibers will alter the blood vessel tone and cause vasodilatation. When hypotension is recognized and immediately treated, no negative sequelae occur. However, if hypotension is not adequately treated, it may have profound effects on fetal well-being.[153] These fetal effects are primarily due to a decrease in uterine blood flow. If maternal hypotension is not treated, the uterine blood flow may decrease to the point where fetal hypoxia and acidosis occur. This is because, at term, the placental vasculature is usually completely dilated. Any untoward fetal effects of regional anesthesia are due to the ensuing hypotension and are not secondary to the anesthesia *per se*.

Treatment of hypotension should start in the preanesthetic period with appropriate prophylaxis. An intravenous catheter must be inserted prior to initiation of the block and 500–1000 ml crystalloid should be administered in order to avoid hypotension associated with vasodilatation.[154] Since glucose easily crosses the placenta, the rapid administration of glucose-containing solutions may actually cause newborn hypoglycemia and are generally best avoided.[155] Left uterine displacement is also vital in order to avoid hypotension due to compression of the aorta and inferior vena cava.

If recognized and treated promptly, transient maternal hypotension should not be associated with maternal or neonatal morbidity.[156] As previously discussed, while intravenous ephedrine in 5–10 mg increments remains a first-line treatment, recent evidence supports the use of phenylephrine.[157] There appears to be no benefit in the prophylactic administration of commonly used doses of ephedrine.[158,159]

Accidental dural puncture

A relatively common and problematic complication of epidural placement is accidental puncture of the dura ('wet tap'), with an incidence of up to 3%.[160] This complication can lead to the development of a postdural puncture headache (PDPH) in the majority of cases.[161] The traditional management of accidental dural puncture has been to remove the epidural needle and reinsert it at a different interspace. In more recent years, however, many anesthesiologists have advocated that the epidural catheter should be placed into the CSF, providing intrathecal delivery of local anesthetic as a continuous spinal technique. This establishes rapid and effective pain relief that can be very carefully titrated. In addition, analysis of aggregate data from limited retrospective trials demonstrated a significant reduction in the incidence of PDPH and the need for epidural blood patch in those patients who received continuous spinal analgesia after unintentional dural puncture.[162] In addition, the catheter provides excellent labor analgesia and a route toward almost instant onset of blockade for cesarean section. Furthermore, a recent review suggested that spinal headache could be reduced if five steps were followed. They include: (1) injection of the cerebrospinal fluid from the epidural syringe back into the subarachnoid space through the epidural needle; (2) insertion of an epidural catheter into the subarachnoid space; (3) injection of preservative-free normal saline through the intrathecal catheter before its removal; (4) administration of continuous intrathecal labor analgesia; and (5) leaving the intrathecal catheter in-situ for a total of 12–20 h.[163]

Not all postpartum headaches occur as a result of a dural puncture. A large analysis reported that headaches occurred in 15% of parturients who did not receive an epidural, and 12% of parturients who had an epidural but did not show evidence of dural puncture.[164] Other causes of headache in the postpartum period include non-specific headache, migraine, hypertension, pneumocephalus, infection including sinusitis and meningitis, cortical vein thrombosis, and intracerebral pathology. A recent report also suggested that neurocysticercosis should be considered in the differential.[165] In addition, since coffee and tea intake is so prevalent, one should also consider caffeine withdrawal in the differential diagnosis. A PDPH has a typical presentation of a postural headache that is worsened by standing or straining and relieved by lying down. Generally, PDPH is initially treated conservatively with increased intake of both oral and intravenous fluid administration of caffeine and analgesics. There is no evidence, however, that increasing the fluid intake will cause a greater production of CSF; recently, the use of intravenous fluid has been questioned.

Drugs that have been used to treat PDPH include caffeine, vasopressin, theophyline, sumatriptan, and ACTH. Caffeine, a cerebral vasoconstrictor, has been successfully used, but the effects appear to be transient.[166] Caffeine treatment is more effective when headaches are the result of smaller rather than larger needles. A negative aspect of the caffeine treatment is that patients may feel anxious and unable to sleep. In addition, there are reports of seizures and cardiac arrhythmias following caffeine administration.[167] While some of the caffeine is present in breast milk, it has not been shown to have a deleterious effect on the newborn.[168]

If symptoms are severe enough to limit a mother's activity, or if evidence of cranial nerve involvement appears, an epidural blood patch (EBP) should be considered. The epidural blood patch was first described more than 40 years ago and it still appears to be the most effective treatment for PDPH. Although early reports suggested immediate and permanent cure of PDPH, it has recently been suggested that complete success rates are approximately 75% and that the effectiveness of EBP is decreased if the dural puncture is caused by a large-bore needle.[169] One study reported that although immediate relief occurred in almost all patients, a permanent cure following EBP was achieved in only 61%.[170] The success of an epidural blood patch is probably not as simple as the clotted blood obstructing the dural tear. CSF volume replacement is not rapid, yet the symptoms resolve almost immediately. Other explanations for the effectiveness of EBP include the increase in CSF pressure and cerebral vasoconstriction.[171] There is some controversy regarding the optimal volume of blood to be injected; however, most practitioners use 15–25 ml and stop injection of the blood if severe pain occurs. While the incidence of complications (especially back pain) increases with increased volume of blood injected, it appears that increased volume also increases the success rate.[172]

Total spinal

This rare complication occurs when the level of anesthesia rises higher than C4 and thus prevents movement of the diaphragm and effective spontaneous ventilation. It may occur from an excessive spread of local anesthesia after intrathecal injection of a correct dose, from injection of a miscalculated dose of a spinal drug, or more commonly, from an inadvertent intrathecal injection of an epidural dose. This complication may occur initially or during the course of a previously uneventful epidural anesthetic.[173] Treatment consists of immediate establishment of an airway and initiation of adequate ventilation. Since these patients cannot protect their airway, endotracheal intubation will allow for ventilation while providing protection against aspiration. Severe bradycardia progressing to cardiac asystole has been reported and therefore bradycardia should be treated early.[174] If cardiac arrest occurs, a full resuscitation dose of epinephrine should be immediately administered.[175]

Table 177.5 Maximum recommended doses of local anesthetics commonly used in obstetrics*

	Dosage (mg/kg) LA without epinephrine	LA with epinephrine
Lidocaine	4–5	7
Mepivacaine	5–6	8–9
Bupivacaine, ropivacaine	2.5–3	2.5–3
Chloroprocaine	8–10	15

*Caution note – the recommended maximum safe dose is influenced by many factors and should be adjusted to the site of injection

Local anesthetic toxicity

Local anesthetic toxicity occurs when high blood concentrations of local anesthetics occur. This can occur following accidental intravascular injection of therapeutic amounts of epidural local anesthetic or by administration of massive doses of local anesthetic into the proper space. Accidental intravascular injection can occur with any regional anesthetic technique. Table 177.5 lists the maximal recommended doses of the local anesthetics commonly used in obstetrics.

Local anesthetic toxicity is usually recognizable by prodromal symptoms of central nervous system toxicity, including ringing in the ears, perioral numbness, disorientation, and excitation. These symptoms, if unchecked, may progress to frank convulsions. Cardiovascular toxicity often begins with hypertension but quickly progresses to hypotension, arrhythmias, and cardiac arrest. Because it generally takes a higher blood level of local anesthetic to induce cardiovascular symptoms, the central nervous system and cardiovascular reactions may be usually temporally separated. Of all the local anesthetics commonly used in obstetrics, bupivacaine represents the greatest

Table 177.6 Resuscitative equipment and medications that should be immediately available*

Emergency medications	Hemodynamic support – atropine, ephedrine, phenylephrine, epinephrine Muscle relaxation – succinylcholine Hypnotics – propofol, thiopental, brevital
Equipment for emergency airway management	Laryngoscope and assorted blades Endotracheal tubes, with stylets Laryngeal mask airways of assorted sizes Device for emergency non-surgical airway ventilation-jet ventilator, combitube Device for emergency surgical airway Oxygen source Self-inflating bag and mask for positive pressure ventilation Suction source with tubing and catheters

*The items listed represent suggestions and should be customized to preferences and skills of the practitioner and health care facility

risk due to its potential for cardiotoxicity and the difficulty associated with resuscitation of these patients.[176] Morishima *et al.* demonstrated that bupivacaine is more cardiotoxic than other local anesthetics.[177] Because of these risks, the manufacturers of bupivacaine have suggested that 0.75% bupivacaine not be used for obstetric patients. To minimize the risks associated with this drug, it has become standard practice to administer local anesthetics by incremental injection. As noted previously, newer local anesthetics, including levobupivacaine and ropivacaine, may prove to offer improved qualities while being less cardiotoxic.[178–180]

Treatment of local anesthetic toxicity involves preventive measures (such as aspiration of the catheter and fractionated doses), early recognition and prompt response. Adequate oxygenation is of paramount importance and endotracheal intubation usually needs to be immediately performed. Benzodiazepines may be used to stop the convulsions. If cardiac arrest occurs, the patient should be treated with cardiac massage, defibrillation and cardiotonic drugs, as necessary. Emergency cesarean delivery should be considered, as early delivery following cardiac arrest has been demonstrated to increase the chances of maternal as well as infant survival.[181] Table 177.6 outlines the resuscitative medications and equipment that should be immediately available.

Allergic reactions to local anesthetics

True allergy to local anesthetics is rare.[182] Currently used local anesthetics are either amino esters or amides. Allergic reactions to amide local anesthetics (e.g., lidocaine, bupivacaine) are extremely rare. However, allergic reactions to esters (procaine, tetracaine) occur more commonly. Since allergy to *p*-aminobenzoic acid might suggest a potential for allergic reaction to an ester (which gets broken down to PABA), patients with a possible history of local anesthetic allergy should be asked about allergies to cosmetics and sunscreens. If a patient states that she has had an allergic reaction to a local anesthetic, she should be referred for an antepartum evaluation. Should a patient arrive on labor and delivery with a question of local anesthetic allergy, a thorough and detailed clinical history (including the exact symptoms and timing of the supposed allergic reaction) may reveal a history of 'adverse reaction' and exclude true hypersensitivity.[183] Recent evidence suggests that latex allergy is increasing and may be the cause of anaphylaxis in the parturient. Physicians should be aware of this growing problem and be prepared to manage the patient with a known or suspected latex allergy.[184] Management of an allergic reaction to a local anesthetic will depend on the severity of reaction. Despite the potential for alterations of uterine blood flow, epinephrine is the drug of choice in severe reactions.

Neurological complications

Direct nerve injury from spinal or epidural needles is extremely rare. Pressure on the cord or intraneural injection causes severe pain. While neuraxial blockade may cause neurologic sequelae, it is important to note that not all neurologic complications after labor and delivery are due to administration of a regional anesthetic. The process of childbirth may itself cause neurologic sympotoms. In fact, the first documented case of maternal postpartum palsy was reported in 1838, prior to the introduction of either regional or general anesthesia.[185] Obstetric causes for neurologic injury include poor patient positioning, incorrectly positioned stirrups, prolonged application of retractors and difficult forceps application.[186] Potential neurologic complications of spinal and epidural anesthesia include epidural hematoma, epidural abscess, or meningitis. Chemical contaminants have also been reported as a cause of neurologic injury, but with the use of disposable epidural and spinal kits and commercially prepared drug ampoules, chemical meningitis is exceedingly rare. Unfortunately, there continue to be case reports describing the neurologic sequelae of accidental administration of intravenous drugs into an epidural catheter.[187–189] These accidents can be prevented by vigilance, careful handling, and inspection of drug ampoules, and the use of portless epidural tubing.

Compression of the spinal cord by a spinal or epidural hematoma is a potentially devastating complication which, if diagnosed early, does not necessarily cause permanent neurologic sequelae. The incidence of neurologic injury resulting from hematoma associated with neuraxial anesthesia is very low, with estimates of 1 in 150,000 and 1 in 220,000 for epidural and spinal anesthesia, respectively.[190] A review of 61 cases of spinal hematoma associated with spinal or epidural anesthesia reported evidence of hemostatic abnormality in 68% of patients and difficult or bloody placements of needles and catheters in 25% of cases. A new risk factor for development of spinal hematoma is the high-risk parturient who is receiving low molecular weight heparin (LMWH). Recent guidelines by the American Society of Regional Anesthesia (ASRA) suggest that neuraxial techniques should be deferred for 10–12 h in the parturient who has received preoperative LMWH or 24 h for those parturients on higher doses of LMWH (e.g., enoxaparin 1 mg/kg twice daily).[192]

Backache

Low back pain is common following delivery. Many patients believe that back pain is linked in some way to epidural analgesia administered for labor; and the alleged relationship between labor epidurals and postpartum backache has been suggested by several retrospective studies.[192,193] Recently, however, prospective studies evaluating labor epidural analgesia and postpartum back pain failed to find a significant link between epidural placement and pain. One study reported that the incidence of postpartum backache in women who received epidural anesthesia was equivalent to those who did not (44% vs. 45%).[194] Further data analysis in that study demonstrated an association between new-onset postpartum back pain with greater weight and shorter stature; postpartum back pain was also associated with a previous history of back pain, greater weight, and younger age. Similarly, another recent study found no difference in the incidence of long-term low back pain in patients who received epidurals for labor compared to controls.[195]

Anesthesia for the high-risk parturient

Parturients are considered to be 'high risk' from an anesthesiology perspective if they have a preexisting medical condition, obstetric complication, a problem that can potentially necessitate an emergency cesarean section, or a potential uncertainty regarding anesthetic management.

Pre-eclampsia–eclampsia

Analgesia for vaginal delivery

Although in the past it had been suggested that epidural analgesia should not be performed in the pre-eclamptic patient, there is a growing body of opinion among anesthesiologists and obstetricians that epidural analgesia (if there is no coagulation abnormality) is the preferred method of providing analgesia to the pre-eclamptic.[196] Epidural analgesia offers several advantages, including:

(1) It may facilitate blood pressure management;
(2) It potentially increases uteroplacental perfusion by decreasing endogenous catecholamines;
(3) It allows a fast route for cesarean section, if necessary, without the use of general anesthesia.

Anesthesia for cesarean section

General anesthesia. If general anesthesia is necessary, one should consider the following:

(1) Laryngeal edema and other airway changes may make endotracheal intubation difficult.
(2) Hypertension may be worsened by laryngoscopy and therefore elevated blood pressure should be treated prior to induction of anesthesia. Drugs that have been suggested include: labetalol, hydralazine, nitroglycerin, trimethophan and nitroprusside.
(3) Magnesium sulfate may potentiate the effects of neuromuscular blocking agents.

Regional anesthesia. Although spinal anesthesia has recently been advocated by some authors,[197,198] others suggest that epidural anesthesia causes fewer changes in blood pressure and should be used when regional anesthesia is chosen for severely pre-eclamptic women undergoing cesarean section. Points to consider include:

(1) Epinephrine-containing local anesthetics[199] may exacerbate hypertension.
(2) Consider central venous line, or pulmonary artery catheter prior to initiation of epidural, if volume status is in question.
(3) Ephedrine (and phenylephrine) should be used in small incremental doses to treat hypotension.

Assessment of platelet function in pre-eclamptic women

It is generally accepted that if the platelet count in pre-eclampsia is greater than 100,000/mm^3, it is likely that the other indices of coagulation will be normal.

However, rarely, pre-eclamptic women may have a normal platelet count with abnormal platelet function. While in the past the bleeding time had been suggested as a good test to determine platelet function, it is no longer performed by most obstetric anesthesiologists since it has not been shown to predict the risk of hematoma formation. Rogers and Levin[200] stated that 'our analysis of bleeding time data from 640 publications reveals that the value of the test in diagnosis remains unclear'. Thromboelastography can be used as a bedside measure of viscoelastic changes but has not yet been shown to be predictive in pre-eclamptic women.

Regional anesthesia can be safely performed on the pre-eclamptic patient if:

(1) A recent platelet count is normal;
(2) The recent platelet count is not dramatically lower than the previous value;
(3) There is no clinical evidence of coagulopathy.

Antepartum hemorrhage

Placenta previa

Actively bleeding/major blood loss (general endotracheal anesthesia). The following steps should be taken:

(1) Get help; second intravenous placement;
(2) Intravenous fluid administration (via rapid infusion device with warmer, if available); and
(3) Rapid sequence induction; consider ketamine 1 mg/kg.

No active hemorrhage; hemodynamic stability. If there is no hypovolemia, epidural or spinal anesthesia may be used.

Placenta accreta

Since placenta previa in a patient for a repeat cesarean delivery may be associated with placenta accreta,[201] these patients should be treated as though major blood loss will occur. Two intravenous lines should be inserted, blood should be available, and the patient should be made aware that a cesarean hysterectomy may become necessary and that general anesthesia may be required to provide appropriate operating conditions and to protect her airway in the event of massive hemorrhage and cesarean hysterectomy. In an elective repeat cesarean delivery in a patient with a placenta previa, regional anesthesia may be used and if hemodynamics remain stable, and may be continued even if a hysterectomy following delivery is performed. In a recent multi-institutional study, 12 patients received epidural anesthesia for elective or emergency cesarean hysterectomy and none required intraoperative induction of general anesthesia.[202] Should the patient become unstable, however, general anesthesia should be considered.

Fetal distress

The American College of Obstetricians and Gynecologists has issued a Committee Opinion entitled *Anesthesia for Emergency Deliveries*.[203] They suggest:

(1) Failed intubation and pulmonary aspiration remain prominent causes of maternal morbidity and mortality from anesthesia.
(2) The obstetric care team should be alert to the presence of risk factors that place the parturient at increased risk for complications from emergency general or regional anesthesia.
(3) When risk factors are identified, the obstetrician should obtain an antepartum anesthesia consultation.
(4) Strategies should be developed to help minimize the need for emergency induction of general anesthesia. Such strategies might include early placement of an epidural or spinal catheter.

Regional anesthesia for fetal distress

(1) Consider placement of epidural catheters in patients who are at increased risk for operative delivery [non-reassuring fetal heart rate tracing, intrauterine growth restriction, pre-eclampsia, preterm labor, vaginal birth after cesarean section (VBAC), multiple gestations, breech presentation, diabetes].
(2) If an epidural is functioning at the time of cesarean section, administer 15–20 ml of 3% chloroprocaine in 5 ml increments. Onset of block is within 3–5 min. Chloroprocaine is rapidly metabolized in the mother and fetus and placental transfer is not increased in the presence of fetal acidosis.
(3) The use of spinal anesthesia for emergency cesarean section remains controversial, but is routinely practiced at many institutions. Several authors have reported excellent results with spinal anesthesia in the presence of fetal distress. If the patient is not hypovolemic or acutely bleeding and if anesthesia can be achieved quickly (i.e., the patient is not morbidly obese), spinal anesthesia is an attractive alternative to general anesthesia for emergency cesarean section. If early attempts at dural puncture are unsuccessful, the anesthesiologist must have the discipline to abandon further attempts and proceed with an alternative plan (such as general anesthesia).
(4) Intravenous fluid should be administered prior to initiation of a spinal anesthetic, but there is evidence that the anesthetic need not be delayed until the total amount of fluid is administered. Consider having pressure infusion bags available so that fluid can be administered quickly in the scenario in which a patient without prior intravenous fluid administration needs an emergency cesarean section.

(5) If possible, continue to monitor the fetal heart rate in the operating room while placing the regional anesthetic.
(6) In the absence of an ongoing epidural or continuous spinal anesthetic in a case of profound 'fetal distress' (e.g., profound acidosis or fetal bradycardia, not resolving) in a patient with a normal airway, general anesthesia (with a rapid sequence induction) should be considered.
(7) In the event of a history of a failed or difficult intubation, the anesthesiologist should consider an awake fiberoptic intubation or regional anesthetic.
(8) A large bore atraumatic needle (such as a 22-gauge Sprotte needle) may speed the initiation of a spinal while still minimizing the risk of postdural puncture headache.

Summary

Obstetric anesthesia and the anesthesiologist play an important role on the labor and delivery suite. To optimize patient care and to offer the best care to our patients, cooperation and open lines of communication between all health care personnel are required.

REFERENCES

1. Hawkins JL, Koonin LM, Palmer SK, Gibbs CP. Anesthesia-related deaths during obstetric delivery in the United States, 1979–1990. *Anesthesiology* 1997;86:277–8.
2. The Centers for Disease Control and Prevention. Maternal mortality: United States, 1982–1996. *Morb Mortal Wkly Rep* 1998;47:705–7.
3. Berg CJ, Atrash HK, Koonin LM, *et al.* Pregnancy related mortality in the United States, 1987–1990. *Am J Obstet Gynecol* 1996;88: 161–7.
4. Panchal S, Arria AM, Labhsetwar SA. Maternal mortality during hospital admission for delivery: a retrospective analysis using a state-maintained database. *Anesth Analg* 2001;93:134–41.
5. American Academy of Pediatrics and American College of Obstetricians and Gynecologists. *Guidelines for Perinatal Care*, 3rd edn. Washington, DC: ACOG, 1992.
6. *Report on Confidential Enquiries into Maternal Deaths in England and Wales*. London: Her Majesty's Statistics Office, 1989.
7. Clark SL, Cotton DB, Lee W, *et al.* Central hemodynamic assessment of normal term pregnancy. *Am J Obstet Gynecol* 1989;161:1439–42.
8. Metcalfe J, Ueland K. Maternal cardiovascular adjustments to pregnancy. *Prog Cardiovasc Dis* 1974;16:363–74.
9. Conklin KA. Maternal physiological adaptations during gestation, labor and the puerperium. *Semin Anesth* 1991;10:221–234.
10. Skerman JH, Birnbach DJ, Swayze CR. Effects of anesthesia on maternal/fetal circulation. *Semin Anesth* 1991;10:235–46.
11. Holmes F. Incidence of the supine hypotensive syndrome in late pregnancy. *J Obstet Gynaecol Br Emp* 1960;67:254–8.
12. Kerr MG. The mechanical effects of the gravid uterus in late pregnancy. *J Obstet Gynaecol Br Commonw* 1965;72:513–29.
13. Marx GF. Aortocaval compression: incidence and prevention. *Bull N Y Acad Med* 1974;50:443–6.
14. Newman B, Derrington C, Dore C. Cardiac output and the recumbent position in late pregnancy. *Anaesthesia* 1983;38:332–5.
15. Gee JB, Packer BS, Millen JE. Pulmonary mechanics during pregnancy. *J Clin Invest* 1967;46:945–52.
16. Prowse CM, Gaensler EA. Respiratory and acid base changes during pregnancy. *Anesthesiology* 1965;26:381–92.
17. Archer GW Jr, Marx GF. Arterial oxygen tension during apnoea in parturient women. *Br J Anaesth* 1974;46:358–60.
18. Gaiser RR, McGonigal ET, Litts P, Cheek TG, Gutsche BB. Obstetricians' ability to assess the airway. *Obstet Gynecol* 1999;93(5, Pt 1):648–52.
19. Gryboski WA, Spiro HM. The effect of pregnancy on gastric secretion. *N Engl J Med* 1956;255:1131–4.
20 Sandhar BK, Elliot RH, Windram I, *et al.* Peripartum changes in gastric emptying. *Anaesthesia* 1992;47:196–8.
21. Dewan DM, Floyd HM, Thistlewood JM, *et al.* Sodium citrate pretreatment in elective Cesarean section. *Anesth Analg* 1985;64:34–7.
22. Dewan DM, Floyd HM, Thistlewood JM, Bogard TD, Spielman FJ. Sodium citrate pretreatment in elective cesarean section patients. *Anesth Analg* 1985;64(1):34–7.
23. Sibai BM, Frangieh A. Maternal adaptation to pregnancy. *Curr Opin Obstet Gynecol* 1995;7:420.
24. Stolte K. A comparison of women's expectations of labor with the actual event. *Birth* 1987;14:99–103.
25. Melzack R. The myth of painless childbirth. The John J. Bonica Lecture. *Pain* 1984;19(4):321–37.
26. Eltzchig HK, Lieberman ES, Camann WR. Regional anesthesia and analgesia for labor and delivery. *N Engl J Med* 2003;348:319.
27. Lederman RP, McCann DS, Work B. Endogenous plasma epinephrine and norepinephrine in last trimester pregnancy and labor. *Am J Obstet Gynecol* 1977;129:5–8.
28. Fletcher JE, Thomas TA, Hill RG. Beta endorphin and parturition. *Lancet* 1980;1:310.
29. Rosenfeld CR, Barton MD, Meschia G. Effects of epinephrine on distribution of blood flow in the pregnant ewe. *Am J Obstet Gynecol* 1976;124:156–63.
30. Hiltunen P, Raudaskoski T, Ebeling H, Moilanen I. Does pain relief during delivery decrease the risk of postnatal depression? *Acta Obstet Gynecol Scand* 2004;83(3):257–61.
31. Hawkins JL, Beaty BR. Update on obstetric anesthesia practices in the United States (abstract). *Anesthesiology* 1999;91:A1060.
32. Kuhnert BR, Kuhnert BM, Tu ASI, *et al.* Meperidine and normeperidine levels following meperidine adminisration during labor. Fetus and neonate. *Am J Obstet Gynecol* 1979;133:909–14.
33. Way WL, Costley EC, Way EL. Respiratory sensitivity of the newborn infant to meperidine and morphine. *Clin Pharmacol Ther* 1965;6:454–461.
34. Bricker L, Lavender T. Parenteral opioids for labor pain relief: a systematic review. *Am J Obstet Gynecol* 2002;186(5 Suppl Nature):S94–109.
35. Kan RE, Hughes SC, Rosen MA, *et al.* Intravenous remifentanil: placental transfer, maternal and neonatal effects. *Anesthesiology* 1998;88:1167–74.
36. Roelants F, De Franceschi E, Veyckemans F, *et al.* Patient-controlled intravenous analgesia using remifentanil in the parturient. *Can J Anaesth* 2001;48:175–8.
37. Nikkola EM, Ekblad UU, Kero PO, *et al.* Intravenous fentanyl PCA during labour. *Can J Anaesth* 1997;44:1248–55.
38. Craft JB, Coaldrake LA, Bolan JC, *et al.* Placental passage and uterine effects of fentanyl. *Anaesth Analg* 1983;62:894.
39. Morley-Forster PK, Reid DW, Vandeberghe H. A comparison of patient controlled analgesia; fentanyl and alfentanil for labour analgesia. *Can J Anaesth* 2000;47:113–19.
40. Smith CV, Rayburn WF, Allen KV, Bane TM, Livezey GT. Influence of intravenous fentanyl on fetal biophysical parameters during labor. *J Matern Fetal Med* 1996;5(2):89–92.
41. Rayburn W, Rathke A, Leuschen P, *et al.* Fentanyl citrate analgesia during labor. *Am J Obstet Gynecol* 1989;161:202.
42. Rayburn WF, Smith CV, Parriott JE, *et al.* Randominzed comparison of meperidine and fentanyl during labor. *Obstet Gynecol* 1989;4:604–6.
43. Volikas I, Male D. A comparison of pethedine and remifentanil patient-controlled analgesia in labour. *Int J Obstet Anesth* 2001; 10:86–90.
44. Volmanen P, Akural EI, Raudaskoski T, *et al.* Remifentanil in obstetric analgesia: a dose-finding study. *Anesth Analg* 2002;94: 913–17.

45. Owen MD, Poss MJ, Dean LS, *et al.* Prolonged intravenous remifentanil infusion for labor analgesia. *Anesth Analg* 2002;94: 918–19.
46. Saunders TA, Glass PSA. A Trial of labor for remifentanil. *Anesth Analg* 2002;94:771–3.
47. Gal TJ. Analgesia and respiratory depressant activity of nalbuphine: A comparison with morphine. *Anesthesiology* 1982;55:367.
48. Hatjis CG, Meis PJ. Sinusoidal fetal heart rate pattern associated with butanorphal administration. *Anesthesiology* 1986; 67:377.
49. Feinstein SJ, Lodeiro JG, Vintzileos M. Sinusoidal fetal heart rate pattern after administration of nalbuphine hydrochloride: A case report. *Am J Obstet Gynecol* 1986;154:159.
50. Weintraub SJ, Naulty JS. Acute abstinence syndrome after epidural injection of butorphanol. *Anesth Analg* 1985;64:452–3.
51. Irving FC. Advantages and disadvantages of barbiturates in obstetrics. *R I Med J* 1945;28:493.
52. McQuitty FM. Relief of pain in labour: a controlled double-blind trial comparing pethedine and various phenothiazine derivatives. *J Obstet Gynaecol Br Commonw* 1967;74:925–928.
53. Eisenstein JI, Rubin EJ, Arnold M, *et al.* Propiomazine hydrochloride in obstetrics. *Am J Obstet Gynecol* 1964;88:606–11.
54. Mercier F, Benhamou D. Promising non-narcotic analgesic techniques for labour. *Baillieres Clin Obstet Gynaecol* 1998;12: 397–407.
55. Akamatu TJ, Bonica JJ, Rehmet R, *et al.* Experiences with the use of ketamine for parturition. I. Primary anesthesia for vaginal delivery. *Anesth Analg* 1974;53:284–7.
56. McElhatton PR. The effects of benzodiazepine use during pregnancy and lactation. *Reprod Toxicol* 1994;8:461–75.
57. Shiono PH, Mills JL. Oral clefts and diazepam use during pregnancy. *N Engl J Med* 1984;311:919–20.
58. Seideman SF, Marx GF. Midazolam in obstetric anesthesia. *Anesthesiology* 1987;67:443–44.
59. Tucker AP, Mezzatesta J, Nadeson R, Goodchild CS. Intrathecal midazolam II: Combination with intrathecal fentanyl for labor pain. *Anesth Analg* 2004;98(6):1521–7.
60. Irestedt L. Current status of nitrous oxide for obstetric pain relief. *Acta Anaesthesiol Scand* 1994;38:771.
61. Abboud TK, Swart F, Shu J, *et al.* Desflurane analgesia for vaginal delivery. *Acta Anaestheisol Scand* 1996;39:259–61.
62. Wee MY, Hasan MA, Thomas TA. Isoflurane in labour. *Anaesthesia* 1993;48:369–72.
63. Ross JA, Tunstall ME, Campbell DM, *et al.* The use of 0.25% isoflurane premixed in 50% nitrous oxide and oxygen for pain relief in labour. *Anaesthesia* 1999;54;1166–72.
64. Suelto MD, Shaw DB. Labor analgesia with paravertebral lumbar sympathetic block. *Reg Anesth Pain Med* 1999;24:179–181.
65. Eisenberg DM, Davies RB, Ettner SL, *et al.* Trends in alternative medicine use in the USA 1990–97. Results of a follow-up national survey. *J Am Med Assoc* 1998;280:1569–75.
66. Hepner DL, Hartnett M, Segal S, *et al.* Herbal medicine use in parturients. *Anesth Analg* 2002;94:690–3.
67. Ramin SM, Gambling DR, Lucas MJ, *et al.* Randomized trial of epidural versus intravenous analgesia during labor. *Obstet Gynecol* 1995;86:783–9.
68. Chestnut DH, Vanderwalker GE, Owen CL, *et al.* The influence of continuous epidural bupivacaine analgesia on the second stage of labor and method of delivery in nulliparous women. *Anesthesiology* 1987;66:774–80.
69. Chestnut DH, McGrath JM, Vincent RD, *et al.* Does early administration of epidural analgesia affect obstetric outcome in nulliparous women who are in spontaneous labor? *Anesthesiology* 1994;80:1201–8.
70. Phillips KC, Thomas TA. Second stage of labor with or without extradural analgesia. *Anaesthesia* 1983;38:972–6.
71. Howell CJ. Epidural versus non-epidural analgesia for pain relief in labour. *Cochrane Database Syst Rev* 2000;(2):CD000331.
72. Lieberman E, Lang JM, Cohen A, *et al.* Association of epidural analgesia with Cesarean delivery in nulliparas. *Obstet Gynecol* 1996;88:993–1000.
73. Zhang J, Yancey MK, Klebanoff MA, Schwartz J, Schweitzer D. Does epidural analgesia prolong labor and increase risk of cesarean delivery? A natural experiment. *Am J Obstet Gynecol* 2001;185(1):128–34.
74. Albright GA. Cardiac arrest following regional anesthesia with etidocaine or bupivacaine. *Anesthesiology* 1979;51:285–7.
75. Scott DB, Lee A, Fagan D. Acute toxicity of ropivacaine compared with that of bupivacaine. *Anesth Analg* 1989;69:563–9.
76. Santos AC, Arthur GR, Roberts DJ, *et al.* Effect of ropivacaine and bupivacaine on uterine blood flow in pregnant ewes. *Anesth Analg* 1992;74:62–7.
77. Priddle HD, Andros GJ. Primary spinal anesthetic effects of epinephrine. *Anesth Analg* 1950;29:156–62.
78. Curatalo M, Petersen-Felix S, Arendt-Nielson L, *et al.* Epidural epinephrine and clonidine, segmental analgesia and effects on different pain modalities. *Anesthesiology* 1997;87:785–94.
79. van der Vyver M, Halpern S, Joseph G. Patient-controlled epidural analgesia versus continuous infusion for labour analgesia: A meta-analysis. *Br J Anaesth* 2002;89(3):459–65.
80. Viscomi C, Eisanach JC. Patient controlled epidural analgesia during labor. *Obstet Gynecol* 1991;77:348.
81. Paech MJ. Patient controlled epidural analgesia in obstetrics. *Int J Obstet Anesth* 1996;5:115–25.
82. Scott PV, Bowen FE, Cartwright P, *et al.* Intrathecal morphine as a sole analgesic during labor. *Br Med J* 1980;281:351–5.
83. Honet JE, Arkoosh VA, Norris MC, *et al.* Comparison among intrathecal fentanyl, meperidine, and sufentanil for labor analgesia. *Anesth Analg* 1992;75:734–9.
84. Leighton BL, DeSimone CA, Norris MC, Ben-David B. Intrathecal narcotics for labor revisited: the combination of fentanyl and morphine intrathecally provides rapid onset of profound, prolonged analgesia. *Anesth Analg* 1989;69:122–5.
85. Campbell DC, Camann WR, Datta S. The addition of bupivacaine to intrathecal sufentanil for labor analgesia. *Anesth Analg* 1995; 81:305–9.
86. Green NM. Distribution of local anesthetic solutions within the subarachnoid space. *Anesth Analg* 1985;64:715–30.
87. Cesarini M, Torielli R, Lahaye F, *et al.* Sprotte needle for intrathecal anesthesia for Caesarean section. *Anaesthesia* 1990;45: 656–8.
88. Rigler ML, Drasner K, Krejcie T, *et al.* Cauda equina syndrome after continuous spinal anesthesia. *Anesth Analg* 1991;72:275–81.
89. Tsen L, Thue B, Datta S, *et al.* Is combined spinal–epidural analgesia associated with more rapid cervical dilation in nulliparous patients when compared with conventional epidural analgesia? *Anesthesiology* 1999;91:920–5.
90. Fishburne JI, Griess FC Jr, Hopkinson R, *et al.* Response of the gravid uterine vasculature to arterial levels of local anesthetic agents. *Am J Obstet Gynecol* 1979;133:753–61.
91. Shnider SM, Asling JH, Holl JW, Margolis AJ. Paracervical block anesthesia in obstetrics. I. Fetal complications and neonatal morbidity. *Am J Obstet Gynecol* 1970;107:619–25.
92. Carrlson BM, Johansson M, Westin B. Fetal heart rate pattern before and after paracervical anesthesia. A prospective study. *Acta Obstet Gynecol Scand* 1987;66:391–5.
93. Qvigstad E, Jerne F. Severe infection following pudendal anesthesia. *Int J Gynecol Obstet* 1980;18:385–6.
94. Leighton BL, Halpern SH, Wilson DB. Lumbar sympathetic blocks speed early and second stage induced labor in nulliparous women. *Anesthesiology* 1999;90:1039–46.
95. Albaladejo P, Bouaziz H, Benhamou D. Epidural analgesics: How can safety and efficacy be improved? *CNS Drugs* 1998;10:91–104.
96. Albright G. Cardiac arrest following regional anesthesia with etidocaine or bupivacaine. *Anesthesiolgy* 1979;51:285–7.
97. Heath ML. Deaths after intravenous regional anaesthesia. *Br Med J* 1982;285:913–14.
98. Aberg G. Toxicological and local anaesthetic effects of optically active isomers of 2 local anaesthetic compounds. *Acta Pharmacol Toxicol* 1972;31:273–86.
99. Luduena FP, Bogado EF, Tullar BF. Optical isomers of mepivacaine and bupivacaine. *Arch Int Pharmacodyn* 1972;200:359–69.
100. Brown WU, Bell GC, Lurie AL, *et al.* Newborn blood levels of lidocaine and mepivacaine in the first postnatal day following maternal epidural anesthesia. *Anesthesiology* 1975;42:698–707.
101. Scanlon JW, Brown WJ Jr, Weiss JB, *et al.* Neurobehavioral responses of newborn infants after maternal epidural anaesthesia. *Anesthesiology* 1974;40:121.
102. Kuhnert BR, Harrison MJ, Linn PL, *et al.* Effects of maternal epidural anesthesia on neonatal behavior. *Anesth Analg* 1984;63:301.
103. Pollock JE, Neal JM, Stephenson CA, *et al.* Prospective study of the incidence of transient radicular irritation in patients undergoing spinal anesthesia. *Anesthesiology* 1996;84:1361–7.
104. Kuhnert BR, Kuhnert PM, Philipson EH, *et al.* The half life of 2-chloroprocaine. *Anesth Analg* 1986;65:273.
105. Karembelkar DJ, Ramanathan S. 2-Chloroprocaine antagonism of epidural morphine analgesia. *Acta Anaesthesiol Scand* 1997;41: 774–8.

106. Coda B, Bausch S, Haas M, *et al.* The hypothesis that antagonism of fentanyl analgesia by 2-chloroprocaine is mediated by direct action on opioid receptors. *Reg Anesth* 1997;22:43–52.
107. Corke BC, Carlson CG, Dettbarn W. The influence of 2-chloroprocaine on the subsequent analgesic potency of bupivacaine. *Anesthesiology* 1984;60:25–7.
108. Reisner LS, Hochman BN, Plumer MH. Persistent neurologic deficit and adhesive arachnoiditis following intrathecal 2-chloroprocaine injection. *Anesth Analg* 1980;59:452.
109. Gissen AJ, Datta S, Lambert D. The chloroprocaine controversy. I. A hypothesis to explain the neural complications of chloroprocaine epidural. *Reg Anesth* 1984;9:124.
110. Winnie AP, Nader AM. Santayana's prophecy fulfilled. *Reg Anesth Pain Med* 2001;26:558–64.
111. Cheng CR, Su TH, Hung YC, *et al.* A comparative study of the safety and efficacy of 0.5% levobupivacaine and 0.5% bupivacaine for epidural anesthesia in subjects undergoing elective caesarean section. *Acta Anaesthesiol Sin* 2002;40:13–20.
112. Burke D, Henderson DJ, Simpson A, *et al.* Comparison of 0.25% *S*(–) bupivacaine with 0.25% *R–S* bupivacaine for epidural analgesia in labour. *Br J Anaesth* 1999;83:750–5.
113. Robinson AP, Lyons GR, Wilson RC, *et al.* Levobupivacaine for epidural analgesia in labor: The sparing effect of epidural fentanyl. *Anesth Analg* 2001;92:410–14.
114. Stienstra R, Tonker TV, Bourdez P. Ropivacaine 0.25% versus bupivacaine 0.25% for continuous epidural analgesia in labor: A double-blind comparison. *Anesth Analg* 1995;80:285–9.
115. Capogna G, Celleno D, Fusco P, *et al.* Relative potencies of bupivacaine and ropivacaine for analgesia in labour. *Br J Anaesth* 1999;82:371–3.
116. Read GD. *Natural Childbirth.* London: Heinemann, 1933.
117. Kennell J, Klaus M, McGrath S, *et al.* Continuous emotional support during labor in a US hospital. *J Am Med Assoc* 1991;265:2197–201.
118. Han JS, Chen XH, Sun SL, *et al.* Effect of low-and high-frequency transcutaneous electrical nerve stimulation on Met-enkephalin-Arg-phe and dynorphin A immunoreactivity in human lumbar CSF. *Pain* 1991;47:295–8.
119. Kaplan B, Rabinerson D, Lurie S, *et al* Transcutaneous electrical nerve stimulation for adjunct pain relief during labor and delivery. *Int J Gynaecol Obstet* 1998;60:251–5.
120. Van der Ploeg JM, Vervest HA, Liem AL, *et al.* Transcutaneous electrical nerve stimulation for adjunct pain relief during the first stage of labour: A randomized controlled trial. *Pain* 1996; 68:75–8.
121. Tsen L, Thomas J, Segal S, *et al.* Transcutaneous electrical nerve stimulation does not augment epidural labor analgesia. *J Clin Anesth* 2001;13:571–5.
122. Finster M, Pedersen H, Santos AC. Placental transfer of drugs. In Van Zundert A, Ostheimer GW, eds. *Pain Relief and Anesthesia in Obstetrics.* New York: Churchill Livingstone, 1996:149.
123. Brown WU Jr, Bell GC, Alper MH. Acidosis, local anes-thetics and the newborn. *Obstet Gynecol* 1976;48:27–30.
124. Morgan DJ, Blackman GL, Paul JD, *et al.* Pharmacokinetics and plasma binding of thiopental. II. Studies at Cesarean section. *Anesthesiology* 1981;54:468–74.
125. Rudolph AM, Heyman MA. Fetal and neonatal circulation and respiration. *Annu Rev Physiol* 1974;36:187.
126. Bader AM, Fragneto R, Terui K, *et al.* Maternal and neonatal fentanyl and bupivacaine concentrations after epidural infusion during labor. *Anesth Analg* 1995;81:829–32.
127. Mercier FJ, Riley ET, Frederickson WL, Roger-Christoph S, Benhamou, Cohen SE. Phenylephrine added to prophylactic ephedrine infusion during spinal anesthesia for elective cesarean section. *Anesthesiology* 2001;95(3):668–74.
128. Curtin SC, Park MN. Trends in the attendant, place, and timing of births, and in the use of obstetric interventions: United States, 1989–97. *Natl Vital Stat Rep* 1999;47(21):1–12.
129. Depp R. Cesarean delivery and other surgical procedures. In Gabbe SG, Niebyl JR, Simpson JL, eds. *Obstetrics. Normal and Problem Pregnancies.* New York: Churchill Livingstone, 1991:635.
130. Hawkins JL, Giffs CP, Orleans M, *et al.* Obstetric anesthesia work force survey, 1981 versus 1992. *Anesthesiology* 1997;87:135–43.
131. Andrews WW, Ramin SM, Maberry MC, *et al.* Effect of type of anesthesia on blood loss at elective repeat cesarean section. *Am J Perinatol* 1992;9:197–200.
132. Riley ET, Cohen SE, Macario A, *et al.* Spinal versus epidural anesthesia for cesaresan section: A comparison of time efficiency, costs, charges, and complications. *Anesth Analg* 1995;80:709–12.
133. Hamza J, Mohammed S, Benhamou D, *et al.* Parturient's posture during epidural puncture affects the distance from the skin to epidural space. *J Clin Anesth* 1995;7:1–4.
134. Russell IF. Spinal anaesthesia for caesarean section: The use of 0.5% bupivacaine. *Br J Anaesth* 1983;55:309–14.
135. Abouelish EI. Epinephrine improves the quality of spinal hyperbaric bupivacaine for cesarean section. *Anesth Analg* 1987;66:395.
136. Abouelish EI, Rawal N, Fallon K, *et al.* Combined intrathecal morphine and bupivacaine for cesarean section. *Anesth Analg* 1988;67:370.
137. Hunt CO, Nolte S, Bader AM, *et al.* Perioperative analgesia with subarachnoid fentanyl–bupivacaine for cesarean delivery. *Anesthesiology* 1989;71:535.
138. Courtney MA, Bader AM, Hartwell B, *et al.* Perioperative analgesia with subarachnoid sufentanil administration. *Reg Anesth* 1992;17:274.
139. Preston PG, Rosen MA, Hughes SC, *et al.* Epidural anesthesia with fentanyl and lidocaine for cesaresan section: Maternal effects and neonatal outcome. *Anesthesiology* 1988;68:938.
140. Vertommen JD, Van Aken H, Vandermeulen E, *et al.* Maternal and neonatal effects of adding epidural sufentanil to 0.5% bupivacaine for cesarean delivery. *J Clin Anesth* 1991;3:371–6.
141. Eisanach J, Detweiler D, Hood D. Hemodynamic and analgesic actions of epidurally administered clonidine. *Anesthesiology* 1993; 78:277–87.
142. Carrie LES, O'Sullivan GM. Subarachnoid bupivacaine 0.5% for cesarean section. *Eur J Anaesthesiol* 1984;1:275–83.
143. Crowhurst J, Birnbach DJ. Low dose neuraxial block. Heading towards the new millennium. *Anesth Analg* 2000;90:241–2.
144. Hurley RJ, Lambert DH. Continuous spinal anesthesia with a microcatheter technique. Preliminary experience. *Anesth Analg* 1990;70:97–102.
145. Kuczkowski KM, Benumof JL. Decrease in the incidence of post-dural puncture headache: Maintaining CSF volume. *Acta Anaesthesiol Scand* 2003;47:98–100.
146. Hawkins JL, Koonin LM, Palmer SK, *et al.* Anesthesia-related deaths during obstetric delivery in the United States, 1979–1990. *Anesthesiology* 1999;86:277–84.
147. Morgan M. Anaesthetic contribution to maternal mortality. *Br J Anaesth* 1987;59:842–55.
148. Rocke DA, Murray WB, Rout CC, *et al.* Relative risk analysis of factors associated with difficult intubation in obstetric anesthesia. *Anesthesiology* 1992;77:67.
149. Pilkington S, Carli F, Dakin MJ, *et al.* Increase in Mallampati score during pregnancy. *Br J Anaesth* 1995;74:638–42.
150. Farcon EL, Kim MH, Marx GF. Changing Mallampatti score during labor. *Can J Anaesth* 1994;41:50–1.
151. Birnbach DJ, Datta S, Ostheimer GW. Maternal hypotension during regional anaesthesia for Caesarean section. *Curr Opin Anaesthesiol* 1988;1:151–6.
152. Ralston DH, Shnider SM. The fetal and neonatal effects of regional anesthesia in obstetrics. *Anesthesiology* 1978;48:34–64.
153. Brizgys RV, Dailey PA, Shnider SM, *et al.* The incidence and neonatal effects of maternal hypotension during epidural anesthesia for Cesarean section. *Anesthesiology* 1987;67:782–6.
154. Clark RB. Prevention of spinal hypotension associated with Cesarean section. *Anesthesiology* 1976;45:670–4.
155. Kenepp NB, Kumar S, Shelley WC, *et al.* Fetal and neonatal hazards of maternal hydration with 5% dextrose before Cesarean section. *Lancet* 1982;1:1150–2.
156. Norris MC. Hypotension during spinal anesthesia for cesarean section: Does it affect neonatal outcome? *Reg Anesth* 1987; 12:191.
157. Mercier FJ, Riley ET, Frederickson WL, *et al.* Phenylephrine added to prophylactic ephedrine infusion during spinal anesthesia for elective cesarean section. *Anesthesiology* 2001;95:668–74.
158. Tsen LC, Boosalis P, Segal S, *et al.* Hemodynamic effects of simultaneous administration of intravenous ephedrine and spinal anesthesia for cesarean delivery. *J Clin Anesth* 2000;12:378–82.
159. Ngan Kee WD, Khaw K, Lee BB, *et al.* A dose–response study of prophylactic intravenous ephedrine for the prevention of hypotension during spinal anesthesia for cesarean delivery. *Anesth Analg* 2000;90:1390–5.
160. Norris MC, Leighton BL, DeSimone CA. Needle bevel orientation and headache after inadvertent dural puncture. *Anesthesiology* 1989;70:729–31.
161. Reynolds F. Dural puncture and headache. *Br Med J* 1993;306: 874–5.

162. Russell I. In the event of accidentla dural puncture by an epidural needle in labour, the catheter should be passed into the subarachnoid space. *Int J Obstet Anesth* 2002;11:23–7.
163. Kuczkowski KM, Benumof JL. Decrease in the incidence of post-dural puncture headache: maintaining CSF volume. *Acta Anaesthes Scand* 2003;47:98–100.
164. Benhamou D, Hamza J, Ducot B. Postpartum headache after epidural analgesia without dural puncture. *Int J Obstet Anesth* 1995;4:17–20.
165. Browne IM, Birnbach DJ. Neurocysticercosis: A new differential in the diagnosis of postdural puncture headach. *Anesth Analg* 2003;97:580–2.
166. Camann WR, Murray RS, Mushlin PS, *et al.* Effects of oral caffeine on postdural puncture headache: A double-blind placebo-controlled rial. *Anesth Analg* 1990;70:181–4.
167. Bolton VE, Leicht CH, Scanlon TS. Postpartum seizure after epidural blood patch and intravenous caffeine sodium benzoate. *Anesthesiology* 1989;70:146–9.
168. Ryu JE. Effect of maternal caffeine consumption on heart rate and sleep time of breast fed infants. *Dev Pharmacol Ther* 1985;8: 353–63.
169. Safa-Tisseront V, Thormann F, Malassine P, *et al.* Effectiveness of epidural blood patch in the management of post-dural puncture headache. *Anesthesiology* 2001;95:334–9.
170. Taivaninen I, Pitkanen M, Touminen M, *et al.* Efficacy of eidural blood patch for postdural puncture headache. *Acta Anaesthesiol Scand* 1993;37:702–5.
171. Coombs DW, Hooper D. Subarachnoid pressure with epidural blood patch. *Reg Anesth* 1979;4:3–6.
172. Szeinfeld M, Ihmeidan IH, Moser MM, *et al.* Epidural blood patch: Evaluation of the volume and spresad of flood injected into the epidural space. *Anesthesiology* 1986;64:820–2.
173. Abouleish E, Goldstein M. Migration of an extradural catheter into the subdural space. *Br J Anaesth* 1986;58:1194–7.
174. Wetstone DL, Wong KC. Sinus bradycardia and asystole during spinal anesthesia. *Anesthesiology* 1974;41:87–9.
175. Caplan RA, Ward RJ, Posner K, Cheny FW. Unexpected cardiac arrest during spinal anesthesia: A closed claims analysis of predisposing factors. *Anesthesiology* 1988;68:5–11.
176. Clarkson CW, Hondeghem LM. Mechanism for bupivacaine depression of cardiac conduction: Fast block of sodium channels during the action potential with slow recovery from block during diastole. *Anesthesiology* 1985;62:396–405.
177. Morishima HO, Pedersen H, Finster M, *et al.* Bupivacaine toxicity in pregnant and nonpregnant ewes. *Anesthesiology* 1985;63:134–9.
178. Scott DB, Lee A, Fagan D, *et al.* Acute toxicity of ropivacaine compared with that of bupivacaine. *Anesth Analg* 1989;69:563–9.
179. Santos AC, Pedersen H, Sallustro JA, *et al.* Pharmaco-kinetics of ropivacaine in nonpregnant and pregnant ewes. *Anesth Analg* 1990;70:262–6.
180. Groen K, Mantel M, *et al.* Pharmacokinetics of the enantiomers of bupivacaine and mepivacaine after epidural administration of the racemates. *Anesth Analg* 1998;86:361–6.
181. American Heart Association. Guidelines for cardio-pulmonary resuscitation and emergency cardiac care. *J Am Med Assoc* 1992; 268:2289–95.
182. Giovannitti JA, Bennett CR. Assessment of allergy to local anesthetics. *J Am Dental Assoc* 1979;98:701–6.
183. Incaudo G, Shatz M, Patterson R. Administration of local anesthetics to patients with a history of prior adverse reaction. *J Allergy Clin Immunol* 1978;61:339–45.
184. Stewart PD, Bogod D. Latex anaphylaxis during late pregnancy. *Int J Obstet Anesth* 1995;4:48–51.
185. Beatty TE. Second report of the new Lying-In Hospital, Dublin. *Dublin J Med Sci* 1938;12:273.
186. Cole JT. Maternal obstetric paralysis. *Am J Obstet Gynecol* 1946; 52:372–86.
187. Shanke KB, Palkar NV, Nishkala R. Paraplegia following epidural potassium chloride. *Anaesthesia* 1985;40:45–7.
188. Bickler P, Spear R, McKay W. Intralipid solution mistakenly infused into epidural space. *Anesth Analg* 1990;71:712–13.
189. Dror A, Henriksen E. Accidental epidural magnesium sulfate injection. *Anesth Analg* 1987;66:1020–1.
190. Tryba M. Epidural regional anesthesia and low molecular weight heparin: Pro [in German]. *Anasthsiol Intensivmed Notfallmed Schmerzther* 1993;28:179–81.
191. Regional anesthesia in the anticoagulated patient – Defining the risks. American Society of Regional Anesthesia Consensus Statement 2002, www.asra.com
192. Macarthur C, Lewis M, Knox FG, *et al.* Epidural anaesthesia and longterm backache after childbirth. *Br Med J* 1990;301:9–12.
193. Russell R, Groves P, Taub N, *et al.* Assessing longterm backache after childbirth. *Br Med J* 1993;306:1299–303.
194. Breen TW, Ransil BJ, Groves PA, *et al.* Factors associated with back pain after childbirth. *Anesthesiology* 1994;81:29–34.
195. Howell CJ, Dean T, Lucking L, *et al.* Randomised study of longterm outcome after epidural versus non-epidural analgesia during labour. *Br Med J* 2002;325:357–61.
196. Newsome LR, Bramwell RS, Curling PE. Severe preeclampsia: hemodynamic effects of lumbar epidural anesthesia. *Anesth Analg* 1986;65:31–6.
197. Aya AG, Mangin R, Vialles N, *et al.* Patients with severe preeclampsia experience less hypotension during spinal anesthesia for elective cesarean delivery than healthy parturients: A prospective cohort comparison. *Anesth Analg* 2003;97:867–72.
198. Hood DD. Spinal anesthesia is the preferred technique for cesarean section severe preeclampsia: proponent position. *Acta Anaesthesiol Belg* 2002;53:305–10.
199. Hadzic A, Vloka J, Patel N, Birnbach DJ. Hypertensive crisis after successful placement of an epidural anesthetic in a hypertensive parturient. *Reg Anesth* 1995;20:156–8.
200. Rogers RPC, Levin J. A critical reappraisal of the bleeding time. *Semin Thromb Hemost* 1990;16:1–20.
201. Clark SL, Koonings PPP, Phelan JP. Placenta previa/accreta and prior Cesarean section. *Obstet Gynecol* 1985;66:89–92.
202. Chestnut DH, Dewan DM, Redick LF, *et al.* Anesthetic management for obstetric hysterectomy. A multi-institutional study. *Anesthesiology* 1989;70:607–10.
203. American College of Obstetricians and Gynecologists Committee on Obstetrics: Maternal and Fetal Medicine. *ACOG Committee Opinion No. 104.* Washington, DC: ACOG, 1992.

178 Instrumental delivery

H. Hopp and P. Husslein

Vaginal operative delivery involves the extraction of the fetus by traction on its head. In some cases, this may also involve correcting the fetal attitude and position. Whether an operative delivery is appropriate depends on the circumstances of the labor, the informed consent of the mother, and the relevant experience and ability of the obstetrician. Because vaginal operative births can cause severe trauma to mother and child, it is generally accepted that they should be avoided when possible. The option of completely eliminating assisted vaginal delivery is, however, unreasonable, as there are situations in obstetrics in which such deliveries would be less traumatic and safer for a mother and child than a cesarean section or allowing the labor to continue.

In general, the degree of risk that accrues to mother and child is directly proportional to how high the head of the fetus lies in the birth canal when the delivery has begun, and to how much the sagittal suture deviates from the antero-posterior axis of the pelvis at that time. Operative delivery should be resorted to only when necessary, and midcavity deliveries should be carried out only by qualified and experienced obstetricians.

Frequency and indications

In the state of Berlin, the number of vaginal operative births decreased from 10% to 8.6% during the 1990s and has been 8.1% since 2000. The proportion of forceps deliveries, in comparison to vacuum extraction, is about 20%. In Austria, the figure for vacuum extraction deliveries during the 1990s was just below 4%, and forceps deliveries just over 1%; in 2003, the frequencies of these were 4.7% and only 0.3%, respectively (Figure 178.1). In the United States, approximately 9% of births are assisted vaginal births, of which 3% are forceps and 6% vacuum assisted deliveries, with the proportion clearly shifting toward vacuum extraction in recent years.[1]

Vaginal operative delivery can be indicated for maternal or fetal reasons. Sometimes emergencies arise in response to evidence of fetal oxygen deprivation derived from fetal heart rate monitoring or blood gas analysis. In these urgent situations,

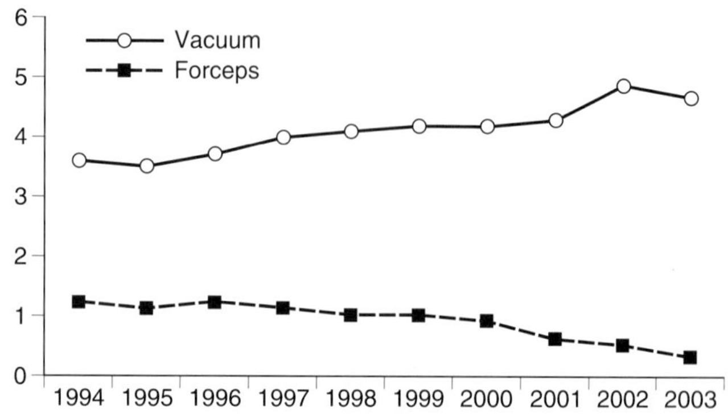

Figure 178.1 Instrumental delivery in Austria, 1994–2003.

judgment is required to determine what the safest and most expeditious mode of delivery should be.

In the event of contraction-induced acute fetal endangerment, intrauterine resuscitation measures should be used, including tocolysis when necessary, even if operative delivery is planned. This can serve to minimize further deterioration, and reduce the need for unnecessary emergency operations. If the infant's head is positioned suitably for forceps and there is a highly abnormal fetal heart rate pattern, the shortening of the bearing-down period in the second stage by operative delivery can reduce the risk of severe fetal acidosis. The heart rate pattern alone is not always adequate to make a reliable prediction of the fetal blood gas status; fetal capillary blood sampling can be an important correlative technique.

Maternal indications (sometimes combined with those related to the fetus) occur. An example would be severe pre-eclampsia, or abnormalities of fetal descent, particularly arrest of descent. If the fetus is in good health and the mother has sufficient energy reserves, the American College of Obstetricians and Gynecologists (2000) set the following maximum time limits for the expulsion phase of labor:[2] for nulliparas, 3 h with and 2 h without regional anesthesia; for multiparas, 2 h with and 1 h without regional anesthesia.

It is not uncommon for the birth to be delayed due to abnormalities of fetal position (e.g. occiput posterior) and attitude (e.g. marked deflexion). In such cases, the circumference of the head that must be accommodated by the birth canal is larger than if the head were well flexed and anterior. Exhaustion of the mother can sometimes be an indication for operative delivery, as can the existence of various maternal diseases that would mitigate against excessive bearing-down efforts (e.g. cardiopulmonary and cerebrovascular diseases). For psychological reasons, vaginal operative deliveries should be subject to relatively strict indications and should not be carried out as prophylactic measures, which were, at one time, promoted.[3]

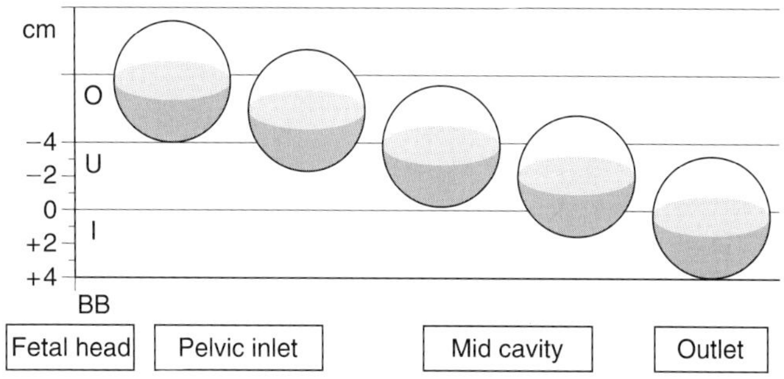

Figure 178.2 The determination of station of the presenting part and plane of passage, according to Hodge – parallel levels and according to De Lee – zero plane. BE Beckeneingang (Pelvic inlet), BM Beckenmitte (Mid cavity), BB Beckenboden (Pelvic floor), O Obere Schossfugenrandebene (Superior edge of the symphysis), U Untere Schossfugenrandebene (Inferior edge of the symphysis) I Interspinalebene (Level of the ischial spines), BB Beckenbodenebene (Pelvic floor plane)

Conditions for operative delivery

A skillful operator working in the context of an appropriate indication ensures that the operative procedure will be as gentle as possible for the mother and fetus. Prior to the operation an accurate diagnosis must be established and documented in the record. This should include assessment or assurance of the following:

- The cervix is completely dilated
- Station of the fetal head
- Fetal presentation, position, and attitude
- Membranes must have ruptured
- Description of fetal pelvic relationships, and comment on the likelihood of disproportion
- Fetal condition
- Maternal condition.

Station of the fetal head

The precise determination of fetal station and the assessment of whether operative correction of any positional abnormalities is appropriate or possible are of utmost importance for the assisted vaginal delivery. The determination of station is based on the definition of the pelvic planes. In order to understand this concept, the pelvic inlet, the narrowest region of the pelvis, should be considered as one plane. The midpelvic region consists of a large curved cavity with anterior and posterior walls of different lengths; it reaches from the terminal plane of the pelvic inlet to the pelvic outlet plane.[4] The pelvic floor is anatomically equivalent to the pelvic diaphragm, which restricts the pelvic outlet surrounded by the bony pelvis. While the plane of passage cannot be determined accurately by vaginal examination, the level of the presenting part within the birth canal can be situated by indicating the number of centimeters below (negative values) or above (positive values) the midcavity plane. This division, according to DeLee,[3] considers the midcavity at the level of the ischial spines as the zero plane and allows the station of the presenting part to be determined in relation to it. Thus, the assessment of fetal descent is based on the station of the presenting part in relation to the station of the plane of passage at the pelvic inlet or midcavity (Figure 178.2). The exact station of the fetal head is assessed by clinical examination and must be documented prior to the operative procedure. The vaginal operative delivery should be carried out only if the station has been documented as being in the midcavity region or, preferably, on the pelvic floor.

With a vertex presentation, the midcavity position is reached when the occiput has completely engaged into the pelvis. The head has passed the pelvic inlet with its narrowest part at the level of the ischial spines and extends approximately 4 cm above the midcavity line. The leading edge of the head in the axis of the birth canal has reached the midcavity plane (station 0). The midpelvic position ends as soon as the presenting part has descended to the pelvic floor (+4). It follows that the fetal head, in a flexed position and with a palpable bony presenting part at 0 to +3 is in the midcavity.

When the station is in the midpelvic cavity, rotation has generally not been completed and instrumental deliveries from this area require a great deal of operative expertise. The degree of difficulty and danger for the operative delivery increases if the presenting part is at a station above +2, or if the sagittal suture deviates from the antero-posterior position by more than 45 degrees. If the obstetrician does not have the necessary expertise to perform such deliveries, cesarean section is generally preferred.

Operative delivery from the midcavity generally requires stricter indications than those done when the head has reached the pelvic floor, and should be carried out only in exceptional circumstances. Due to the fact that in most departments of obstetrics (at least in German-speaking countries) the proportion of births per trainee and junior level physicians has decreased quite considerably over recent years, it has become increasingly difficult to teach assisted vaginal deliveries. It is therefore anticipated that cesarean section will largely replace midpelvic operative deliveries in the near future.

When the presenting part has reached the pelvic floor (+4) the plane of passage (the biparietal

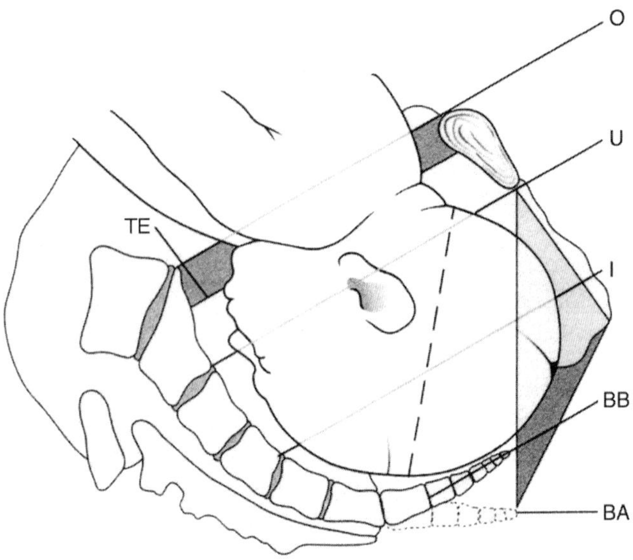

Figure 178.3 Head on the pelvic floor O Obere Schossfugenrandebene (Superior edge of the symphysis), U Untere Schossfugenrandebene (Inferior edge of the symphysis) I Interspinalebene (Level of the ischial spines), BB Beckenbodenebene (Pelvic floor plane), BA Beckenausgangsebene (Pelvic outlet level)

diameter of the head in a vertex presentation) is located parallel to the pelvic floor at the level of the ischial spines (Figure 178.3). At this time the spines and the sacral hollow are no longer readily palpable on vaginal examination. The head is visible in the vagina, and the sagittal suture has completed internal rotation, or deviates only slightly from the antero-posterior diameter of the pelvis (exceptions occur depending on the architecture of the pelvis). The majority of instrumental deliveries are performed with the presenting part at the pelvic floor. If the fetal head has descended to the introitus and remains visible between contractions, the plane of passage reaches the final phase of the birth mechanism and soon crowns at the pelvic outlet. If the baby's head does not progress naturally in this situation, operative delivery is referred to as outlet forceps or outlet vacuum extraction. In most situations, operative delivery in this situation serves primarily in a supporting role to help the mother cope with her physical exhaustion.

Contraindications

Assisted vaginal delivery of a flexed vertex presentation with the presenting part above 0 station is contraindicated; with a deflexed head the station must be at least +2. Because of the considerable distance between the plane of passage and the leading edge of the presenting part, when the head is deflexed it has generally not passed the pelvic inlet, despite the fact that the presenting part can be palpated at station 0. Operative vaginal delivery should never be attempted without clear evidence that the head has engaged.

With the station of the presenting part at or below +2, operative delivery should generally be attempted only when the sagittal suture is within 45 degrees of the antero-posterior position. Even so, it should be performed only by an experienced and qualified obstetrician. With a marked delay in progress during the second stage and clinical or sonographic evidence of fetal macrosomia, the decision to perform vaginal operative delivery is problematic, even if the fetal head has already reached the midcavity. If in doubt, a cesarean section is generally preferred. Incorrect assessments that disregard deflexed attitudes or marked molding that deforms the head are the most common contributors to failed vaginal operative delivery.

The above considerations must be taken into account independent of the choice of delivery instrument. The fact that a vacuum cup can be easily placed does not justify its use in an unengaged head. It is particularly important in situations in which there are alternative treatment methods being considered (vaginal operative delivery or cesarean delivery) to inform the patient of these options and to explain the relevant benefits and risks. In most situations, it is necessary to respect the mother's wishes. It cannot be stressed enough that these discussions should be started at the first sign of abnormalities during the pregnancy or labor that could necessitate vaginal operative delivery. That is the best way to guarantee that the mother has had sufficient opportunity to participate in the decision-making process.

Contraindications for vaginal operative delivery may be summarized as follows:

- Station of the presenting part above 0 with well-flexed vertex presentation
- Presenting part above +2 with a diagonal or transverse sagittal suture
- Station above +2 with deflexion of the head
- Cephalopelvic disproportion
- Abnormal progress in descent with fetal macrosomia

Forceps delivery technique

Instruments

Forceps consist of two blades, which are locked together in a crossed (e.g. Naegele, Simpson, Kielland) or in a parallel fashion (e.g. Shute, Bamberger Divergence forceps). Each blade consists of the headpiece, the shank, and the handle. The headpiece is curved to secure an application to the curvature of the contour of the fetal head. The conformation of the forceps to the axis of the pelvis is accomplished by the pelvic curvature of the shank, one of the factors that differentiate each forceps model.

Procedure

After it has been determined that forceps delivery will be done, the patient is placed in the dorsal lithotomy

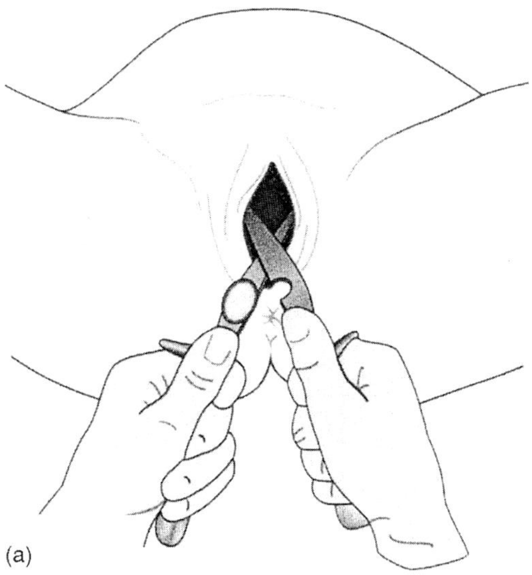

(a)

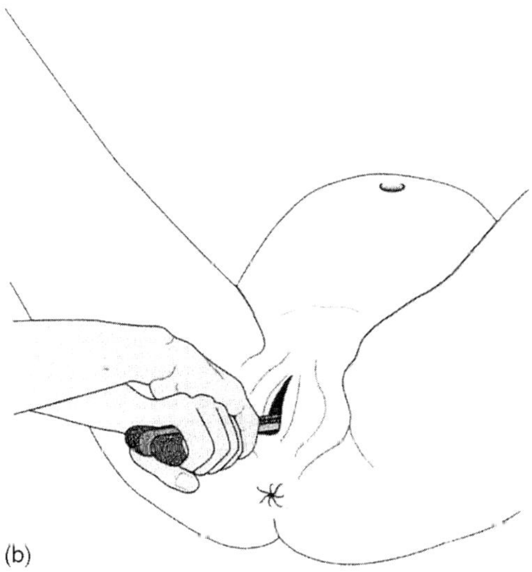

(b)

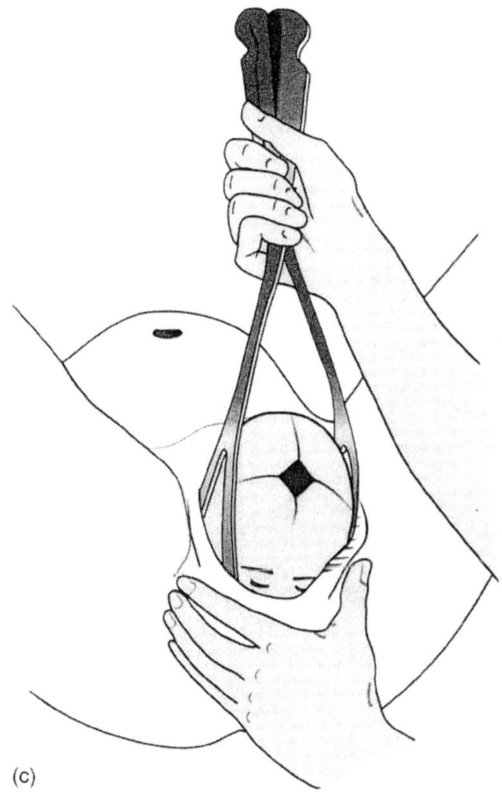

(c)

Figure 178.4 Forceps delivery procedure
(a) Closing of forceps
(b) Traction toward the forceps handles
(c) Vertical traction and perineum support with the free hand

position. It is useful to hold the closed forceps in front of the introitus in what will be their final orientation once they are inserted. It is helpful to judge the correctness of placement by observing the orientation of the handles after insertion. In order to achieve a biparietal application to a head in an anterior position using forceps with a crossed lock, the left hand takes the handle of the left blade, the convex side of the headpiece of which is on the left of the mother. The left hand positions the left blade so that it is initially vertical and hanging in front of the vulva. After the index and middle finger of the right hand have been placed between the vaginal wall and the fetal head, the blade should initially slide toward the sacrum and then, after lowering the handle along the inserted fingers, should slide into the birth canal. The right blade should be held with the right hand in the same manner, and must slide along the inserted fingers of the left hand between the vaginal wall and the fetal head after lowering the handle. If the head has not internally rotated completely, one blade must be made to wander, i.e. it must be guided gently from its initial position at insertion across the head toward the symphysis in order to be able to position the inserted blades biparietally in the first or second diameter of the lesser pelvis. The blades of the instrument can be locked by appropriate action of the relevant hand (Figure 178.4a).

The obstetrician's hand is placed in the vagina to ensure that the forceps are correctly positioned on the baby's head and that no soft tissue is trapped between them. A trial of traction is then carried out by the left hand, which grasps the lock of the upper handle and carries out a short tentative traction. The right hand checks the progression of the head during this maneuver. The progression of the head during the contraction combined with the trial of traction ensures that a gentle and successful delivery is likely to occur.

Both hands are then used to hold the handles of the forceps. The right hand grasps the instrument from above at the level of the lock. The left hand has a firm grip on the handles and controls the instrument. With classical types of forceps, the right hand is clasped over the Busch–Drawhook. Never use excessive traction and ensure that the direction of traction is only in the midline of the pelvis and not laterally.

With an occiput anterior vertex presentation from low in the pelvis, the extraction from the curved position is slowly corrected into a flexion. Following the biparietal application, the forceps are pulled initially horizontally (toward the handles) until the hypomochlion (hairline at the nape of the neck) has reached the lower border of the symphysis pubis (Figure 178.4b). The deeper the head descends into the pelvis, the higher the handles of the forceps should be held. The delivery of the head is completed with the forceps handles being almost vertical. The obstetrician then turns either to the left or right side of the patient (to the side of the hand that is clasping the forceps above the lock) and, ideally, supports the perineum with his or her free hand (Figure 178.4c).

If the head has not internally rotated completely, the forceps extraction requires that flexion and rotation of the head be completed before traction is applied. The forceps blades are placed in a biparietal application. This requires the drifting of the anterior blade across the face of the fetus toward the symphysis. With the first attempt at traction, flexion is completed and the head is carefully rotated into the occiput anterior position. The minimum necessary force should be applied to ensure gentle progression of the fetus down the birth canal.

The forceps delivery of occiput posterior presentations must be appropriate to the relevant mechanical birthing procedures. The traction vector is more downward (posterior) than with an anterior vertex presentation; the head is flexed by raising the forceps handles after the fetal brow has stemmed under the symphysis. In other words, the exit mechanism of a fetal attitude abnormality is to be emulated during the extraction. Due to the risk of severe trauma to the fetus, vaginal operative delivery should not be carried out if the brow or face is presenting.

Vacuum extraction

To achieve sufficient traction with the vacuum cup, designed initially by Mälmstrom in 1954 (Figure 178.5), the area of the cup above the opening is expanded.[5] The various modifications of the original metal cup have retained this basic principle, which, with increasing vacuum, allows the soft tissues of the fetal scalp to be drawn into the cup. The artificially created caput succedaneum helps fix the cup to the fetal head, which allows the extraction. In addition to the metal cup, silicone vacuum cups have been developed that attach to the head by adhesion and do not cause the caput succedaneum (Figure 178.6). The advantage of this cup is the rapid accumulation of pressure. The vacuum strength, however, is relatively less, so this tool is recommended primarily for outlet deliveries.

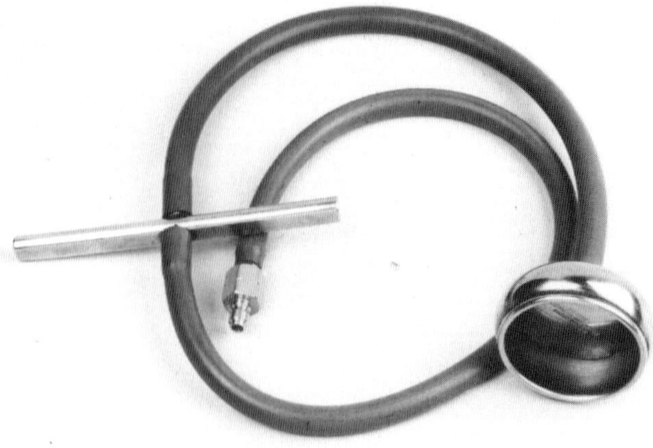

Figure 178.5

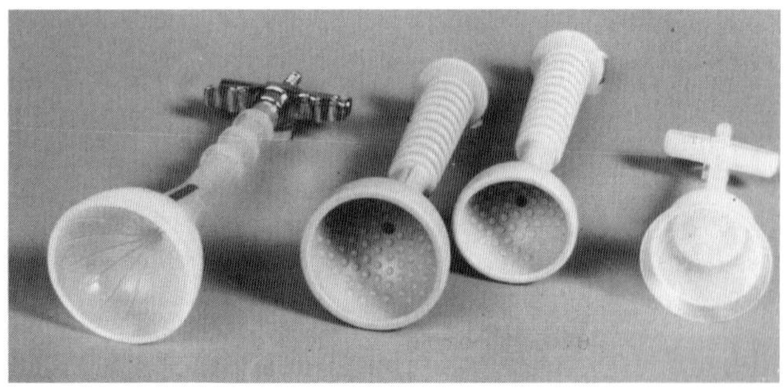

Figure 178.6

In a 2001 review of nine studies on the effect of soft and rigid vacuum extractor cups, Johanson and Menon concluded that metal cups are more suitable for occiput posterior, transverse, and difficult occiput anterior positions.[7] The success rate of soft cups for vaginal deliveries is lower, but their use is associated with fewer scalp injuries to the baby. The technique of application involves choosing the largest cup possible that will fit in the available space. The cup is placed in the vagina, rotated 90 degrees, and placed on the fetal scalp. The cup is placed on the presenting part of an occiput anterior vertex presentation over the small (posterior) fontanel. With occiput posterior presentations it is placed over the anterior fontanel. The development of the vacuum should occur in several steps over a period of about 2 min. After the first step,

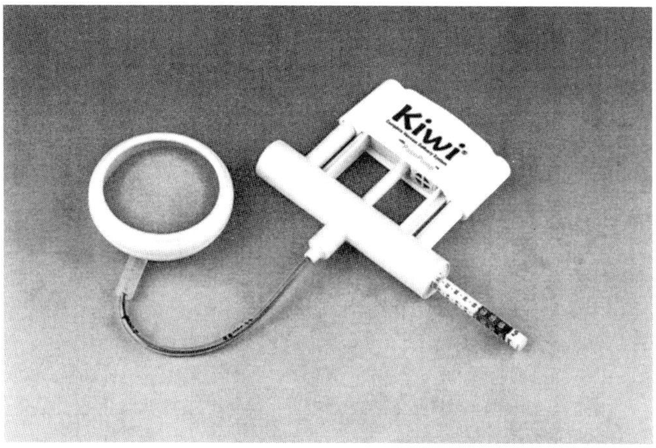

Figure 178.7

the position of the cup is rechecked to ensure that there is no maternal tissue between the fetal head and the vacuum cup. After the cup has been attached with low pressure of about 0.8 kg/cm^2 (600 mmHg) the trial traction confirms whether the head is descending appropriately during traction. Various manufacturers recommend different optimal vacuum pressures for their instrument, and physicians who use vacuum extraction instruments should be familiar with the recommendations and the specifications of the particular unit they employ.

In recent years, easy to use disposable rigid plastic vacuum cups (e.g. the Kiwi Omnicup) have been developed.[8] They allow the buildup of adequate pressure through an attachable hand pump (Figure 178.7). Maximum strength of the suction is more likely to be severely restricted by this method; however, the preparation for this form of operative delivery is much less complicated, which can have a positive psychological effect on the parents.

Traction on the vacuum device should occur coincident with maternal contractions, with increasing and decreasing traction forces paralleling those of the contraction. Using Kristeller pressure on the fundus can be helpful for the extraction if done gently.

When the fetus presents as occiput, anterior traction should occur in the axis of the birth canal and change according to the anatomic curve of the canal. The right hand is placed on the cross-handle of the cup; the left hand, or contact hand, confirms whether the fetal head is descending and whether its attitude is being maintained and rotation is proceeding as anticipated. As the head crowns, the perineum is supported to control the speed of the delivery. The obstetrician can step to the patient's left and support the perineum with the right hand. An episiotomy is not necessarily required, but can sometimes make it easier for the head to pass the terminal portions of the birth canal. After the head has been delivered, the vacuum pump is switched off. Following depressurization, the cup can be lifted easily from the head as soon as the shoulders and trunk are visible. The caput will usually resolve spontaneously after 12–24 h. The risk of cephalohematoma depends on the duration of traction, which should therefore be minimized.[9] Severe abrasions of fetal skin related to long periods of extraction, excessive pulling, and popping off of the metal or even the silicone vacuum cup can occur.

If fetal attitude is abnormal or internal rotation has not been completed, the vacuum cup should be placed over the portion of the head that will need to be flexed and rotated. Following careful reexamination of the situation, the eccentric application of the vacuum cup and the required direction of travel are established. With this kind of application, correction of fetal attitude can be attained. In most cases, the outstanding rotation is achieved by correction of the attitude and descent of the head.

Choice of instrument

Whether the attendant chooses to use obstetric forceps or the vacuum extractor depends on several factors. These include the condition of the fetus prior to attempts at delivery, and, of utmost importance, the expertise of the obstetrician with a particular instrument. Although in German-speaking countries the vacuum cup is the dominant instrument, for most of the last century forceps delivery was favored in the United States. Recently, however, increasing numbers of obstetric centers there have changed, and now emphasize vacuum extraction as the preferred approach in most situations. Although the American College of Obstetricians and Gynecologists recommended in 2000[2] that an experienced obstetrician should master both methods and use them depending on the given situation, this seems unrealistic, especially because the number of operative deliveries has been decreasing over recent decades, and as a consequence the opportunity to achieve and maintain expertise with two instruments is diminished.

With regard to the risk of trauma for full-term babies, there is no documented difference between the two methods. The listed advantages and disadvantages take into account the results of prospective studies[10–12] and were included in the recommendations of the German Institute for Gynecology and Obstetrics regarding vaginal operative delivery from the midcavity.[13]

Decisions favoring vacuum over forceps may have been influenced by the recent technical advances in vacuum cups ('soft cups', 'M-cup') and higher rate of injuries to the mother caused by forceps, with their potential for long-term effects on pelvic floor function. As a consequence, the frequency of vacuum extractions has been increasing progressively, even in countries that previously preferred the use of forceps.[14,15]

The conclusion of a *Cochrane Review* of the issue is that vacuum extraction is the preferred instrument to minimize maternal morbidity. There is a counter-balancing benefit of forceps delivery, in the reduction of cephalohematomas and retinal hemorrhage.[16]

Midcavity delivery

Instrumental delivery from the midcavity is indicated to manage acute fetal distress or arrest of descent during the expulsion phase of labor. When there is a persistent fetal bradycardia during the terminal portion of labor, an experienced obstetrician will usually prefer vaginal operative delivery to cesarean section because of the ability to deliver the baby more expeditiously. Complex midcavity deliveries should, however, be avoided. Forced vacuum extractions should under no circumstances be carried out because of the risk of injury to the fetus. A rapid buildup of pressure, followed by popping off of the cup and related intracranial pressure fluctuations can contribute to a high risk of intracranial hemorrhage. The general guideline to initially attempt vaginal operative delivery rather than opting directly for cesarean section is no longer accepted universally. Under the premise that severe trauma for mother and child cannot always be avoided following vaginal operative deliveries and because of the increased danger of floor damage and permanent impairment of urinary and anal incontinence, instrumental delivery is questionable.

The significance of the patient's psychological well-being associated with the delivery experience has been highlighted as an important consideration in obstetric decision making. Recently, vaginal operative delivery was shown to be undesirable in this regard.[17] However, after long second stages of labor, cesarean section may be considered equally undesirable.[18] Certain changes in the anterior pelvic floor compartment (paravaginal defect) have already occurred in a high proportion of cases and the morbidity and mortality during a secondary cesarean section as compared to vaginal birth is still significantly increased. With a vaginal operative delivery, the risk of injury to mother and child is greater the higher the head lies and the more the sagittal suture deviates from the antero-posterior dimension of the pelvis. This type of operation should, therefore, be kept to a minimum or, preferably, avoided altogether. The midcavity delivery, especially with the station of the presenting part above +2, should be carried out by an experienced and qualified obstetrician. The decision to opt for an instrumental midcavity delivery is greatly influenced by the personal experience of the physician. In borderline situations, such as the station of a presenting part above +2 or a deviation of the sagittal suture more than 45° from the vertical with acute fetal distress, a cesarean section must be carried out immediately, especially in the presence of fetal growth restriction.

If it becomes apparent during the operation that the assessment of the station or the position of the head was incorrect, or if excessive force appears to be required, vaginal operative delivery must be abandoned. Therefore, the preparations for a possible emergency cesarean section must be made as soon as the decision for a vaginal operative delivery has been made. In some cases, the trial of forceps or vacuum extraction may require the presence of an anesthesiologist and surgical staff in the operating room. However, due to the severe psychological stress it creates for the mother a trial of operative delivery should remain an exception. The exceptional circumstances of these situations should always be discussed clearly with the patient and her partner. The neonatal morbidity associated with these deliveries should be stressed. The risk of intracranial bleeding in newborns is highest if cesarean section must be carried out after the failure of instrumental vaginal delivery.[19] This high risk of injury applies as well when delivery is attempted with both instruments in sequence, most commonly vacuum followed by forceps. We may conclude that a vaginal operative delivery should not generally be attempted if the success rate is considered to be low. Moreover, persistent attempts to complete the delivery vaginally when difficulties are encountered are fraught with danger. Keen judgment is necessary to avoid trauma in these situations, and abandoning attempts at forceps or vacuum in favor of cesarean should by no means be considered a failure; in fact it may signal good medical judgment.

Outlet instrumental delivery

Vaginal operative delivery when the head has reached the pelvic floor is considered safe and presents minimal risk to mother and fetus when performed properly. This is true when the head is in a direct anterior position, or with the sagittal suture no more than 45 degrees from the midline. When the head has assumed a transverse position the risks of forceps delivery are considerably greater, and the obstetrician must have expert knowledge of the mechanisms of labor and of the expertise required to correct abnormalities in fetal position and attitude. Often a persistent transverse position with the head relatively low in the pelvis results from the head failing to flex. The fontanelles are consequently palpated at the same level of the pelvis. Flexion of the head with the forceps or vacuum is necessary in order to allow internal rotation, descent, and delivery.

To accomplish this flexion using the vacuum extractor, the vacuum cup is positioned eccentrically over the small fontanelle, primary traction to the opposite side and dorsally is carried out until the head is in a direct anterior position. The increasing flexion of the head produces the passive rotation and

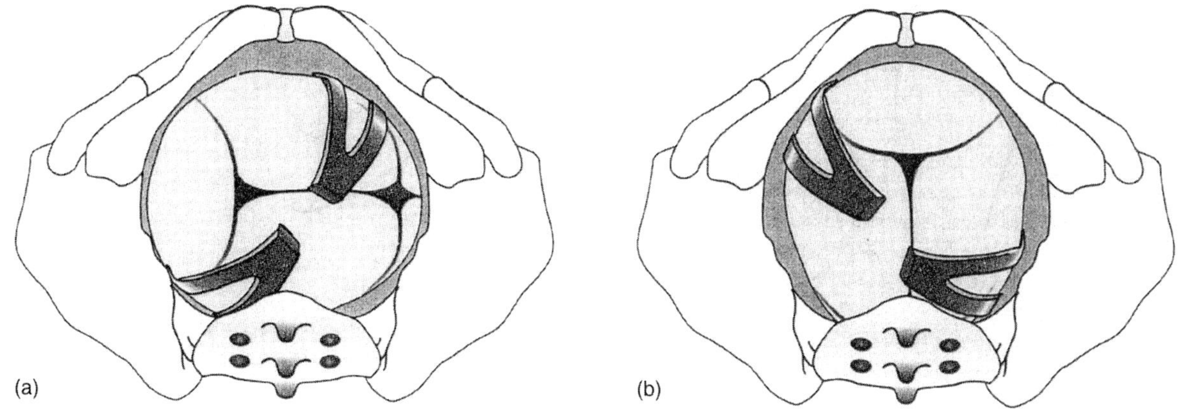

Figure 178.8 Forceps delivery of a fetus in low transverse position
a. With right low transverse position the forceps are positioned in the first diameter of the lesser pelvis
b. After rotation into vertical position, the progression of the occiput anterior vertex presentation follows

no further assistance is required in this regard. The subsequent traction follows the axis of the birth canal with appropriate changes in the direction.

Forceps may also be used to effect delivery of a fetus in a low transverse position. In a right occiput transverse, the left blade of the forceps is inserted first between the head and the sacrum. It is then moved carefully across the fetal face to achieve a diagonal application. The right blade is then inserted in the first diameter of the lesser pelvis (Figure 178.8a). During the extraction, the forceps must be initially rotated so that the small fontanelle is directed underneath the symphysis pubis. The resulting occiput anterior vertex presentation thereby progresses along the axis of the birth canal with no need to alter the application of the forceps before applying traction (Figure 178.8b).

Kielland forceps, a special instrument that lacks a pelvic curve, were designed especially for the rotation of the head in a transverse or posterior position. Some operators remove them after the rotation and apply classical forceps for the traction.

Complications

The risk of fetal and maternal injury related to forceps or vacuum use is increased in proportion to the complexity of the vaginal operative delivery. With fetal stations above +2, correct positioning of the forceps is difficult to achieve and often results in hematomas and abrasions of the fetal skin. When instrumental rotation of the head is necessary, rotational shearing forces can cause severe maternal injuries.

Technical conditions concerning vacuum extraction influence risk. Proper application of the cup is important, as is applying sufficient traction in the correct direction. The potentially lower tractive force generated when the cup is positioned eccentrically and the prolonged extraction time when it is necessary to correct fetal attitude and position increase the danger of the cup popping off, which can cause intracranial pressure fluctuations of up to 50 mmHg as well as injury to the scalp. Subgaleal hemorrhage may occur and be severe enough to be life-threatening. Excessive force or inappropriately long durations of traction should be avoided irrespective of the choice of instrument. The easy placement of the vacuum cup cannot *per se* justify attempting delivery from above the midpelvis.

Fetal injuries

Excessive force should under no circumstances be used during vacuum extraction because of substantial risks of injury to the fetus. The rapid development of pressure from excessively forceful traction followed by popping off of the cup can lead to considerable intracranial pressure fluctuations and a risk of intracranial hemorrhage.[20]

The most common external fetal trauma from vaginal operative delivery is cephalohematoma, which occurred in 3% of 1672 forceps deliveries and in 12% of 371 vacuum extractions.[21] The indication 'impending asphyxia' during vacuum extractions resulted in the frequency of cephalohematomas increasing 10-fold, presumably related to the perceived need for rapid development of the vacuum. In a review of 10 randomized studies of instrumental delivery, Johanson and Menon[16] concluded that cephalohematomas and retinal bleeding occurred more often during vacuum extractions than forceps delivery. The pathogenesis of retinal bleeding that is the consequence of instrumental delivery is uncertain, as are its long-term effects.

Skin injuries from the vacuum extractor can result in long-term alopecia, caused by scarring. Fetal injuries following forceps deliveries include abrasions of the skin, hematomas, and transient (rarely, permanent) paresis of the facial nerves. Skull fractures and intracranial bleeding occur rarely with both methods if the operative technique is applied correctly.

Neonatal morbidity (5-min Apgar score less than 7 and umbilical artery pH below 7.20) following vaginal operative deliveries from the midcavity did not differ from instrumental delivery from the pelvic floor, despite the higher operative pressure and manipulation suffered by a head that has not yet descended or completed its flexion and rotation.[21] In comparing the results of midcavity forceps to cesarean delivery, one study showed no difference regarding the neonatal adjustment responses for the frequency of linguistic and neuromotor development delays.[22] There is, however, controversy about this area (see Chapter 187).

Maternal injuries

Maternal injuries, such as lacerations of the perineum, vagina, or cervix, are a function of the choice of instrument as well as the degree of expertise of the obstetrician. There is evidence[16] that vacuum extraction causes significantly fewer maternal injuries than does forceps delivery. Vacuum delivery is also associated with less use of regional and general anesthesia and less pain during delivery and in the 24 h after birth.

Cheong *et al.*[23] demonstrated that an approach to teaching precision in vaginal operative delivery did not necessarily increase the success rate but clearly reduced the number of complications to mother and child. Weitzel and Hopp[21] found little difference between instruments in the frequency of vaginal lacerations (25% during forceps deliveries and 23% during vacuum extractions). However, forceps deliveries resulted in significantly more third- and fourth-degree perineal tears than vacuum extraction (7.4% vs. 1.7%), particularly when performed from the midcavity. Similar results were found by Johanson *et al.*[11] and Sultan *et al.*[24] who reported that the number of hidden anal sphincter injuries (35% with spontaneous births) doubled following forceps deliveries. In a recent inquiry, their group[25] discovered that vaginal delivery, particularly after forceps or vacuum, was associated with a reduction of anal pressure and increase in sphincter trauma, independent of the choice of instrument.

The risk of injury to the mother and child is greater the higher the head lies and the more the sagittal suture deviates from the antero-posterior diameter of the pelvis at the time the instrumental delivery is begun.[2] Because injuries are relatively frequent, it is necessary to inspect the vagina and cervix thoroughly after each vaginal operative delivery to make an early diagnosis of these injuries and to repair them surgically.

Questionnaires received from patients showed that 18% of mothers who had vacuum deliveries and 27% who had forceps delivery reported unbearable pain during the delivery, and 7% and 18%, respectively, reported similarly of severe pain in the perineal region on the fourth day after delivery.[11,14] Garcia *et al.*[26] made the following statement: 'Compared to forceps delivery, women who deliver by vacuum extraction suffer less pain, but have more trouble with their babies'. This was confirmed in a study[27] in which a total of 31,000 vacuum and 19,000 forceps deliveries between 1991 and 1996 were examined. It was established that there was a relative risk of 0.48 of perineal trauma during vacuum extraction. The risk of subarachnoid bleeding was, however, 5.4 times greater and the risk of cephalohematoma was twofold higher compared to that of a forceps delivery.

For vaginal operative delivery, in addition to the benefit of pain relief, relaxation of the pelvic muscles by pudendal block analgesia (when the head is at the pelvic floor) or epidural anesthesia (when the head is in the midcavity) is beneficial. Pudendal block analgesia is easy to carry out transvaginally. It allows the active participation of the parturient during the delivery process. Vacuum delivery from the pelvic floor, however, is often carried out relatively easily and does not always require anesthesia.

Guidelines for operative vaginal delivery

Guidelines for the physician regarding the indications and contraindications for vaginal operative delivery are based on clinical experience as well as on recommendations of expert committees.[2,13,28] In terms of choice of instrument, convincing evidence is available based on meta-analyses.[7,16] These indicate that both forceps and the vacuum extractor are acceptable and safe instruments for vaginal operative delivery. The expertise of the operator is imperative for the choice of instrument in a particular situation. The meta-analyses indicate that vacuum extraction is associated with a higher rate of failed operations as well as more cephalohematomas, retinal bleeding, and neonatal jaundice. Forceps are associated with higher associated rates of regional or general anesthesia and maternal trauma. There is no apparent difference between the two instrument types with regard to cesarean section rates, Apgar scores, and 5-year follow-up of maternal and child condition. With regard to the choice of cup material, metal cups have a higher rate of scalp injuries than do silicone cups. The latter, however, are associated with more failed operations, especially with malpositions of the occiput and delivery from the midcavity.

Other recommendations are based on more limited or inconsistent scientific evidence.[10,19,29] It can be concluded that vaginal operative delivery from the midcavity with a station of +2 should be carried out if the clinically estimated likelihood of success is high and if the obstetrician is qualified and trained in the method. The length of the vacuum application is related to the frequency of cephalohematoma formation and other forms of head trauma; therefore, this time should be minimized. The incidence of intracranial bleeding is highest in newborns delivered by cesarean section following a failed operative delivery. This risk is high as well when the combination of vacuum extraction and forceps is used. One can conclude that vaginal operative delivery should not be attempted if the *a priori* success rate is considered to be low.

Forensic viewpoint

The law in many countries is becoming increasingly strict with regard to the physician's requirement to inform the patient of the risks, benefits, and alternatives of medical procedures. As soon as there is any indication that the birth may require an operative procedure, the obstetrician must discuss this with the patient and request her authorization. The earlier this is carried out the more likely is the patient to be still fit enough to agree, i.e. still able to follow the conversation and weigh the advantages and risks of the recommended procedure.

If treatment alternatives can result in different levels of pain and suffering for the mother or fetus, or have different success rates, the doctor is required to inform the patient of these. It is important, especially with midcavity positioning of the baby's head, that the patient be aware of the different delivery options: vacuum extraction, forceps, and cesarean. Because the dangers to the mother and fetus are different in each of these methods, according to German and Austrian law, the mother has the option of either making her own interests a priority or choosing according to the best interests of her baby. There is great discrepancy between the legal requirement and the reality of birth, however, which results in the patient sometimes being completely overwhelmed with the decision process. Moreover, the need to process objectively information that may be complex and unfamiliar during a time of great stress is at best challenging, and at worst impossible. It is the physician's duty to respect the patient's autonomy and to assist her as best as possible to comprehend the situation and its potential harm and benefits.

This basic principle applies: the more urgent the situation, the shorter the time to inform the patient. If adequate information can still be conveyed in an emergency, but would delay an urgent operation, the doctor will be held liable in the case of damage.[11] With expected complications during a vaginal operative delivery (delivery with a possible requirement for a cesarean section), the patient must be informed of the increased fetal risk. The patient should ideally have already received basic information about vaginal and abdominal surgical procedures during her prenatal care, so that further information can be given in abbreviated form during an emergency.

REFERENCES

1. Wegner EK, Bernstein IM. Operative vaginal delivery. *UpToDate* Online 12.3, 2004.
2. American College of Obstetricians and Gynecologists. Practice Bulletin number 17 (2000). Operative vaginal delivery. *Int J Gynecol Obstet* 2001;74:69–76.
3. DeLee JB. The prophylactic forceps operation. *Am J Obstet Gynecol* 1921;1:34–7.
4. Weitzel HK, Hopp H. Wann steht der Kopf zangengerecht-vakuumgerecht? *Gynäkologe* 1998;31:742–50.
5. Malmstrom T. The vacuum extractor. Indications and results. *Acta Obstet Gynecol Scand* 1954;43(Suppl 1):42.
6. Huikeshoven FJ. Venthouse delivery. In Kurjak A, ed. *Textbook of Perinatal Medicine*. London: Parthenon Publishing Group, 1998:1811–22.
7. Johanson RB, Menon BKV. Soft versus rigid vacuum extractor cups for assisted vaginal delivery. *Cochrane* 2001;4:1–8.
8. Vacca A. *Handbook of Vacuum Delivery in Obstetric Practice*. Australia: Vacca Research, 2003.
9. Bofill JA, Rust OA, Devidas M, Roberts WE, Morrison JC, Martin JN Jr. Neonatal cephalohematoma from vacuum extraction. *J Reprod Med* 1997;42:565–9.
10. Bofill JA, Rust OA, Schorr SJ, *et al.* A randomized prospective trial of the obstetric forceps versus the M-cup vacuum extractor. *Am J Obstet Gynecol* 1996;175:1325–30.
11. Johanson RB, Rice C, Doyle M, *et al.* A randomized prospective study comparing the new vacuum extractor policy with forceps delivery. *Br J Obstet Gynaecol* 1993;100:524–530.
12. Williams MC, Knuppel RA, Weiss A, Kanarek N, O'Brien WF. A prospective randomized comparison of forceps and vacuum-assisted delivery. *Am J Obstet Gynecol* 1991;164: 323–8.
13. Hopp H, Dudenhausen JW, Martius G, *et al.* Vaginal-operative Entbindungen aus Beckenmitte. Deutsche Gessellschaft für Gynäkol. *Geburt Frauenarzt* 1999;40:1471–3.
14. Drife JO. Choice and instrumental delivery. *Br J Obstet Gynaecol* 1996;103:608–11.
15. Meniru GI. An analysis of recent trends in vacuum extraction and forceps delivery in the United Kingdom. *Br J Obstet Gynaecol* 1996;103:168–70.
16. Johanson RB, Menon BKV. Vacuum extraction versus forceps for assisted vaginal delivery. *Cochrane Library* 2000;2:1–7.
17. Husslein P. Perspektiven in der Geburtshilfe. *Geburtsh Frauenheilk* 1998;58:M50–4.
18. Schindl M, Birner P, Reingrabner M, Joura EA, Husslein P, Langer M. Elective cesarean section versus spontaneous delivery: A comparative study of birth experience. *Acta Obstet Gynecol Scand* 2003;82:834–40.
19. Towner D, Castro MA, Eby-Wilkens E, Gilbert WM. Effect of mode of delivery in nulliparous women on neonatal injury. *N Engl J Med* 1999;341:1709–14.
20. Castillo M, Fordham LA. MR of neurologically symptomatic newborns after vacuum extraction delivery. *AJNR Am J Neuroradiol* 1995;16:816–8.
21. Weitzel HK, Hopp H. Zangen- versus Vakuumextraktion. In Künzel W, Kirschbaum M, eds. *Giessener Gynakologische Fortbildung 1995*. Berlin: Springer, 1996:219–27.
22. Dierker LJ, Rosen MG, Thompson K, Lynn P. Midforceps deliveries: Long-term outcome of infants. *Am J Obstet Gynecol* 1986;154:764–8.
23. Cheong YC, Abdullahi H, Lashen H, Fairlie FM. Can formal education and training improve the outcome of instrumental delivery? *Eur J Obstet Gynecol* 2004;113:139–44.

24. Sultan AH, Kamm MA, Hudson CN, Thomas JM, Bartram CI. Anal sphincter disruption during vaginal delivery. *N Engl J Med* 1999;341:1709–14.
25. Chaliha CH, Sultan AH, Bland JM, Monga AK, Stanton SL. Anal function: Effect of pregnancy and delivery. *Am J Obstet Gynecol* 2001;185:427–32.
26. Garcia J, Anderson J, Vacca A, Elbourne D, Grant A, Chalmers I. Views of women and their medical and midwifery attendants about instrumental delivery using vacuum extraction and forceps. *J Psychosom Obstet Gynaecol* 1985;4:1–9.
27. Wen SW, Liu S, Kramer MS, *et al.* Comparison of maternal and infant outcomes between vacuum extraction and forceps deliveries. *Am J Epidemiol* 2001;153:103–7.
28. Johanson RB. Instrumental vaginal delivery. *RCOG Clinical Green Top Guideline.* London: Royal College of Obstetricians and Gynaecologists, 2000.
29. Bashore RA, Phillips WH Jr, Brinkman CR III. A comparison of the morbidity of midforceps and cesarean delivery. *Am J Obstet Gynecol* 1990;162:1428–34.

179 Cesarean delivery

M. Pajntar

Cesarean delivery is defined as the delivery of the fetus through an incision in the abdominal wall (laparotomy) and the uterine wall (hysterotomy). This definition does not include the removal of the fetus from the abdominal cavity in the case of a rupture of the uterus or an abdominal pregnancy.[1]

Frequency

Monitoring of cesarean delivery rates is one way to take the pulse of obstetric practice and is a key factor in any form of obstetric audit and in international comparisons.[2] Over the last three to four decades, a substantial increase in cesarean delivery rates has been registered almost everywhere in the developed world. The incidence of cesarean delivery has increased from 4–5% to 15–25% on average; however, some countries report much higher rates (e.g. 40% in South Korea in 2000,[3] 52% in Italy, especially in Campania[4] in 2000, and in some hospitals in Brazil as high as 72%[5]). This increasing incidence has been observed despite the recommendation of the World Health Organization to keep it below 10–15%.[6]

Comparative studies of cesarean delivery rates in industrialized countries in the mid- to late 1980s showed a wide variation.[7–9] Almost a quarter of births in the USA and one-fifth in Canada were by cesarean delivery, compared with 6–7% in the Netherlands, Japan, Slovenia, and the former Czech Republic. The rates for other developed countries, for which data are available, ranged from 10% to 15%.[2] A further increase in almost all countries has been observed since the late 1990s: in 2002 it was 26.1% in the USA[10] and 13% in Slovenia.

Fear of litigation is widely held to have played a key part in the rise in the cesarean delivery rates in the USA and the UK.[11–13] In Canada, however, where litigation is not nearly so widespread as in the USA, the rate is nearly as high and well above that for most European countries.[12,13] One factor may be that doctors rather than midwives supervise most of the deliveries in the USA, and the countries in which midwife deliveries predominate generally have lower cesarean rates. Methods of payment may also be important: high rates have been observed among private patients, in private hospitals and in other settings where fee-for-service payments are involved.[14,15] In Sao Paolo, Brazil, the cesarean section rate in the private sector is 80%, and in the public health system, 32.1%.[16] Although the evidence that an elective operative delivery leads to a better outcome for term breeches[2,17,18] or for very small babies[17] is controversial, cesarean rates for these indications have also increased considerably in developed countries.[2]

Fetal distress and a previous cesarean delivery were important contributors to the growth of cesarean delivery rates in Scotland, Norway and Sweden in recent decades. Cesarean deliveries for a previous cesarean delivery and dystocia are the primary contributors to a substantially higher cesarean delivery rate in the USA.[19]

In the Netherlands, the largest increase in the cesarean delivery rate was found within the medium-risk group (singleton, at term, vertex presentation, normal birth weight, mothers aged 20–35 years and with a normal diastolic blood pressure). Although no evident pathology can be found in the data, these women no longer belonged to the low-risk group, because they had been referred to an obstetrician.[20]

Increasing cesarean delivery rates coincided with several changes in obstetric practice, including the introduction and dissemination of technology (ultrasound, cardiotocography); women becoming pregnant and delivering despite severe diseases; improved safety for women undergoing operative delivery;[9] the increased inclination of obstetricians to operative delivery, uncritically transferring the experiences of others to their own institution; and ever-less obstetrical experience in maternity hospitals with a decreasing number of deliveries, resulting in obstetricians being no longer skilled in various operative deliveries (e.g., breech delivery). Numerous articles have been published on the effects of vaginal delivery on the pelvic floor, urinary incontinence, pelvic organ prolapse, and, especially, fecal incontinence. All these publications conclude that cesarean section has a protective effect.[21] An association exists between pelvic floor damage and childbirth, but this cannot be attributed entirely to vaginal delivery and occurs after a cesarean delivery as well.[22]

The incidence of cesarean delivery performed on request without a medical indication is rising too. The reasons for this are not only a perceived medical benefit but also social, cultural, and psychological factors. The legal and ethical issues of cesarean deliveries on request are complex. In dealing with requests for a cesarean section, obstetricians should establish the reasons for the request and provide clear, unbiased information based on the best available evidence.[22]

Although some claim that over the last 20 years the decrease in the perinatal mortality rate from 20–30 per 1000 to 10 per 1000 is mainly due to the increased cesarean delivery rate, there are others who disagree this. For example, while data show a close relationship between mortality and cesarean rate in the USA, the same fall in mortality was observed in Ireland without a significant change in its cesarean rate.[23] The decrease in perinatal mortality has occurred for various reasons, such as higher patient educational and socioeconomic levels and generally improved perinatal care, but primarily, it has been due to better neonatal intensive care and therapy.

Many studies have found no relationship between the frequency of cesarean delivery and the level of perinatal mortality. The comparison among different countries has also shown that in some populations, low levels of early infant mortality can be achieved despite a low cesarean delivery rate.[17,24] On the contrary, it has been found that in many instances, cesarean delivery increases the risk to the mother, fetus, and neonate. Different authors have demonstrated that the overall cesarean delivery rate can be safely lowered without increasing the maternal, fetal, or neonatal morbidity and mortality (from 17.5% to 7.8% and from 31.1% to 15.4%).[26–28]

A stated USA national goal by the year 2000 was to reduce the cesarean delivery rate from 25% to 15%. It was estimated that this 10% reduction in the national cesarean rate could save more than 1 billion US health care expenditure dollars annually.[29] This goal was, however, not achieved.

In our opinion, and that of many others,[20,30,31] the cesarean delivery rate could be decreased by decreasing the number of repeat cesareans, active management of dystocia, efforts to increase the vaginal breech delivery rate, improving methods of diagnosing fetal distress, and preventive and timely active management of labor (timely termination of pregnancy, augmentation of weak contractions, external cephalic version for a transverse lie and breech presentation, etc.).

Indications

There are various indications for cesarean delivery. Generally, they can be divided into fetal, maternal, and fetomaternal indications. However, they are greatly affected by the different policies of individual maternity hospitals, and by individuals; this has also been reported in a study performed in five maternity hospitals.[32] It was found that the clinical and nonclinical factors that influence the cesarean delivery rate are highly site-dependent. This implies that physicians practicing at different sites are influenced by different criteria when deciding whether a cesarean delivery should be performed.

The majority of cesareans are performed for fetal indications; a few are done solely for maternal reasons, and some for the benefit of both the fetus and the mother. The most frequent indications for a cesarean delivery found in the literature are the following: arrest of progress of labor (dystocia), fetal distress, breech presentation, and repeat cesarean delivery with various possible combinations. In different countries, the cesarean delivery rate by indications may be quite disparate.

In the early 1990s, the cesarean delivery rate was three times higher in the USA than in Slovenia, which was then known for a relatively low operative delivery rate (12% of deliveries were done by cesarean, vacuum extraction, or forceps).[24] The cesarean delivery rate for various indications in Slovenia was quite different. The relative share of repeat deliveries and dystocia was smaller, whereas for all other indications it was larger. The absolute rate for all other indications was 2.14% in Slovenia, even lower than in the USA (3.3%) (Table 179.1).

In Slovenia, with 19,108 deliveries in 1995, and an overall early neonatal mortality (over 500 g) of 2.4 per 1000 live births, the cesarean delivery rate was 9.2% in 1994 and 1995. The comparison between the time periods 1988–1991 and 1992–1995 (Table 179.1) shows an increase in cesarean deliveries with all indications, the highest being for breech presentation and the lowest for dystocia. Despite these good results, the cesarean delivery rate in Slovenia increased to 13% in 2002, while the early neonatal mortality rate remained the same (2.4 per 1000 live births).

Over the last few years, the number of cesarean deliveries done in response to patient request has been increasing. While for many women the experience of vaginal delivery is among the most fulfilling of their entire life, comparable only to sexuality-related moments of ecstasy, there are women who regard delivery as the worst thing ever to have happened to them, an experience attended by pain, fear, loneliness, and

Table 179.1 Cesarean delivery rates (per 100 deliveries) for selected indications in the United States and in Slovenia (the data for USA are adapted from Cunningham *et al.*[1])

	Rate (%)		
Indication	**USA, 1985**	**Slovenia 1988–1991**	**Slovenia 1992–1995**
Repeat section	9.0 (36)	1.25 (17.0)	1.55 (17.9)
Dystocia	7.6 (31)	1.41 (19.2)	1.56 (18.0)
Fetal distress	2.3 (9)	1.30 (17.7)	1.52 (17.6)
Breech	2.5 (10)	1.25 (17.0)	1.58 (18.3)
All others	3.3 (13)	2.14 (29.1)	2.44 (28.2)
Total	24.7 (100)	7.35 (100)	8.65 (100)

perhaps long-lasting negative consequences.[33] In some countries, the indication 'cesarean delivery on request' has been accepted and is documented in records; thus, in Norway the rate of cesarean delivery on request is known to have been 7.6% in recent years.[34] In most countries, this indication is not officially recognized. However, many believe[35] that a woman can always find an obstetrician willing to perform a cesarean section for non-medical reasons. Of course, the indications for these sections are hidden, mostly under the diagnosis of dystocia.

Many distinguish between absolute indications for a cesarean delivery, and clinical situations in which a cesarean delivery may be indicated (relative indications). However, there are many different opinions, especially concerning the clinical situations in which a cesarean delivery may be performed.

The absolute indications include the following.

(1) Placenta previa totalis (centralis)
(2) Placental abruption (with fetal distress, jeopardized mother)
(3) Cephalopelvic disproportion (evident)
(4) Umbilical cord prolapse (with incomplete cervical dilatation)
(5) Transverse lie
(6) Proven (pH) fetal distress (with incomplete cervical dilatation)
(7) Active genital herpes infection
(8) Obstructive benign and malignant tumors
(9) Impending maternal death.

The relative indications include the following.

(1) Previous classical cesarean delivery
(2) Previous uterine surgery
(3) Arrest of progress of labor (dystocia)
(4) Abnormal presentation
(5) Fetal anomalies
(6) Suspected fetal distress [fetal heart rate (FHR)]
(7) Multiple pregnancy (triplet or higher).

Decisions for cesarean for fetal distress must include thorough analysis, an interpretation of FHR pattern abnormalities, with consideration of the stage and progress of labor, and the presence of factors such as intrauterine growth restriction, thick meconium, and oligohydramnios.

Various maternal diseases are classified among the relative indications, i.e. cases in which the physician treating the basic disease fears an increased risk to the parturient, especially with prolonged and difficult labor. The risks to the fetus for various diseases, such as rhesus isoimmunization should also be taken into account.

Each relative indication provokes a higher risk if combined with another. All decisions for intrapartum cesarean should be strongly influenced by assessment of the progress of labor. The decision making process should be influenced by evidence-based considerations when possible; but often there will be no good quality studies to bear on specific situations, and the obstetrician must use his or her own clinical wisdom and experience.

Contraindications

In modern obstetrics, with a good anesthesiology service, there are no absolute contraindications for a cesarean delivery, but there exist several relative contraindications.

The most common inappropriate reasons for cesarean include the following.

(1) Diagnosis of failed induction when the labor is still in a normal latent phase
(2) Diagnosis of inadequate uterine contractions when oxytocin stimulation has not been properly applied, or there has been exceedingly heavy sedation
(3) Diagnosis of abnormal fetal descent before complete cervical dilatation
(4) Breech presentation as the only indication
(5) Transverse lie without a previous attempt at external cephalic version
(6) Fetal distress (without a reliable cardiotocographic evaluation or pH measurement)
(7) One previous cesarean delivery
(8) Single or combined indications, such as advanced maternal age in a nullipara, infertility, high-risk pregnancy, etc.
(9) Intrauterine fetal demise.

Repeat cesarean

The attitude toward the management of labor after a previous cesarean has greatly changed over the last two decades. The policy of many maternity hospitals followed the principle of 'once a cesarean, always a cesarean' for many years. However, with the recognition that vaginal delivery can be effected safely after a cesarean, this policy has changed.

The main concerns about laboring after a prior cesarean delivery relate to the risk of uterine rupture and its consequences. These were most frequent when the cesarean was done through a vertical incision in the uterine fundus (now referred to a as a 'classical' cesarean), which was commonly performed in the past. Repeat cesarean delivery remains the leading indication in many maternity hospitals. In the USA in 1978 repeat cesarean deliveries were performed in 98.0% of cases, and represented 30% of all the indications for a cesarean delivery.[35] Repeat cesarean delivery was thus one of the main reasons for the increased cesarean delivery rate in the USA.

Once obstetricians began to do most cesareans using a low transverse uterine incision, the occurrence of uterine rupture decreased considerably, thus making the possibility of a vaginal delivery following a cesarean section more feasible. There is evidence that the mother with a previous low-segment vertical cesarean delivery can undertake a trial of labor with relative maternal and perinatal safety. The likelihood of a successful outcome and the incidence of complications are comparable with those published for trials of labor after a previous low-segment transverse incision.[36]

A substantial reduction in the cesarean rate can be achieved safely and efficiently by using a trial of labor for appropriate cases with prior cesareans. In a study of 17,322 patients with a previous cesarean delivery, a trial of labor was used in 80% of women with one previous cesarean, 54% with two, and 30% with three and more. The success rate was significantly higher with one previous cesarean delivery (83%) than with two or more (75.3%).[37] Others report 75–81% success rates with trial of labor.[38–40] In a large retrospective analysis of trials of labor, the variables that significantly predicted success were prior vaginal delivery, malpresentation, pregnancy-induced hypertension, and Bishop score ≥ 4.[38]

The indications for a previous cesarean delivery, such as cephalopelvic disproportion or arrest in the progress of labor, are not absolute contraindications for trial of labor in a subsequent pregnancy. With these indications for a previous cesarean section, a trial of vaginal delivery was successful in 50–75% of women.[35–38] Multiple previous cesarean deliveries are not an absolute contraindication either. Comparative studies report results almost as favorable for trials of labor after two previous cesarean deliveries as after a single previous cesarean.[35] The maternal and perinatal mortality rates were not increased, but there were slightly more uterine dehiscences and lacerations of a minor degree (up to 3.8%).[35] A trial of labor for patients with more than one previous cesarean delivery is allowed under the conditions that permit prompt recognition and treatment of emergencies.

Thus, the results of many studies show the beneficial effect of trial of labor after a previous cesarean delivery, especially if there are no strict contraindications. The repeat cesarean delivery is done only if new indications for a cesarean occur.

A vertical lower uterine segment incision has been reintroduced in some maternity hospitals for preterm cesarean deliveries, because a thick undeveloped lower uterine segment may not safely accommodate a standard transverse incision. This seems to have resulted in more reports of uterine rupture. It has been found,[35] however, that they are not as frequent as with classical incisions, probably due to the preterm cesarean incision being made in the lower segment rather than in the fundus. The difference between uterine rupture following a lower transverse incision and that following a vertical incision on the uterine corpus is that the latter frequently occurs suddenly and unpredictably in pregnancy, and is thus more dangerous. According to our experience, there is usually no proper indication for a vertical incision in preterm labor. With an unripe lower uterine segment, we recommended making a transverse incision somewhat higher than in normal conditions.

Procedures with a trial of labor

The use of oxytocin for either induction or augmentation of labor in women with a prior cesarean had long been controversial. The overview of various reports shows that the use of oxytocin does not increase the incidence of rupture; therefore, it can be used for induction and augmentation of labor under the same conditions as in labor in an unscarred uterus.[42] In most Slovenian maternity hospitals, oxytocin has been successfully used in induction and augmentation of a trial of labor after a previous cesarean delivery for many years.

The use of analgesia and regional and epidural anesthesia has also been greatly discussed. In the opinion of some, analgesia could mask the pain and uterine sensitivity at the site of the scar, thus delaying identification of a rupture; others claim that the use of analgesia does not increase the risk of trial of labor after a previous cesarean delivery.[35]

In 1970, Greenhill[43] recommended that the uterus be digitally examined after every vaginal delivery. In some maternity hospitals, this recommendation is still being followed. Enkin[35] considers the question of the thinning or laceration of the uterus to be of a purely academic nature. If there is no bleeding, repair of injuries to the uterus is not necessary. Besides, no beneficial effect of a digital examination of the uterus following delivery has been reported so far. There is always a possibility of infection, or of enlarging a simple dehiscence into a greater rupture. Some recommend digital examination of the uterus only if significant bleeding persists more than 1 h after delivery. Improved techniques of cesarean delivery have almost abolished severe ruptures, and only one-half of uterine dehiscences are due to a previous cesarean delivery.

Conclusion

In the absence of an absolute contraindication to vaginal delivery, based on history and the situation in the current pregnancy, a trial of labor is highly recommended. The management of this labor follows the same principles as that of labor without a previous cesarean delivery, except that more careful monitoring is required for the development of risk factors, signs, or symptoms of uterine rupture. Should there be a threatened rupture of the uterus, the decision for cesarean delivery is made earlier than it might be in a labor without a uterine scar.

Cesarean delivery for breech presentation

Over recent decades, cesarean delivery rates for breech presentation have increased in most developed countries, thus contributing to the overall rise in the incidence of cesarean delivery (see Chapter 181). This approach is based on the experience of some obstetricians who have attempted to prevent the poor outcomes of vaginal breech delivery by recourse to cesarean section, beginning especially after publication of the studies of Kubli and colleagues and Ingemarsson and associates pointing towards acidemia and adverse long-term sequelae for the newborn after vaginal breech delivery.[44] The rates of cesarean delivery thereafter continued to rise; thus, in many European and North American maternity hospitals, especially in small ones, breech presentation *per se* is an accepted indication for a cesarean delivery. Over the last two decades, the management of breech delivery has changed from mainly vaginal to principally abdominal delivery[45] in some maternity units, while in some others this policy has never been accepted.[46–48] In maternity units with moderate policy, the cesarean delivery rate in mature breech deliveries has in many European countries increased to 30–40%.[46,48]

Authors of numerous studies propose a policy of either routine cesarean or selective vaginal breech delivery. Some claim that the registered data on singleton-term breech deliveries imply that vaginal delivery is associated with increased morbidity and mortality.[49] The results of many other studies suggest that a routine cesarean delivery does not in itself guarantee a reduction in neonatal morbidity and mortality, and should not be promoted at the expense of maternal health.[48,50,51] Poor perinatal outcomes of breech deliveries are primarily related to factors other than breech presentation; moreover, the route of delivery in infants weighing more than 1500 g does not influence neonatal outcome.[52] Cesarean delivery solely for breech presentation in birth weights of more than 1500 g does not appear to be justified.[53] Observational data, based on the Slovenian perinatal database, suggested better outcomes in 5012 singleton breeches delivered vaginally than in those delivered by cesarean.[54]

The increased cesarean delivery rate in breech presentation has resulted in a 5- to 25-fold higher maternal mortality rate[53] and up to a 38-fold increase in maternal morbidity.[54,55] Cesarean delivery can reduce the risk of adverse childhood neurologic outcomes for those born with myelomeningocele and may reduce the rate of brachial plexus palsies, neonatal herpes virus and human immunodeficiency virus (HIV) infections. However, children born by cesarean have no reduced risk of childhood neurologic problems or cerebral palsy that can be documented.[56]

While some[57] report better outcomes of cesarean deliveries in babies weighing between 1000 and 1500 g, others are of the opinion that there are no differences between the respective modes of delivery in this weight group. In a prospective study, Weisbach *et al.*[58] found no differences in the outcome of delivery of babies of less than 1500 g according to the route of delivery. Among breeches, the route of delivery does not significantly influence the outcome among complete and frank presentations; abdominal delivery may offer some benefit for footling breeches.

An observational study using the Slovenian database[59] showed that the outcomes of 6020 singletons in breech presentation weighing more than 1000 g (excluding the babies with lethal malformations and stillbirths) delivered vaginally using the Bracht or Covianov maneuver were most favorable in terms of early neonatal mortality and some signs of neonatal morbidity. Less-favorable outcomes were achieved with abdominal deliveries, and the poorest by all kinds of vaginal extraction.

Conclusions

On the basis of recommendations by the International Federation of Gynecology and Obstetrics Committee on Perinatal Health, Eskes and Wallenburg[44] proposed a solution to the problem, i.e. external cephalic version at term, as well as the use of physicians well trained and experienced in handling vaginal breech delivery.

Complications of cesarean delivery

Maternal morbidity and mortality

Maternal morbidity following a cesarean is much higher than following a vaginal delivery, the main causes being infections, hemorrhage and injuries to the urinary tract. Infections are very common; 10–80% of women have elevated body temperature, usually due to endometritis.[60] Dehiscences and wound infections are less frequent. Infections are often associated with low socioeconomic status of the mother, frequent vaginal examinations, long duration of labor, and a long interval from rupture of membranes to cesarean delivery. In long labor, in which delivery starts more than 6 h after the rupture of the membranes, endometritis occurs in up to 85% of cases.[7]

In a meta-analysis of several prospective studies, Enkin[35] found that febrile morbidity was significantly less frequent in the vaginal (2.4–23.1%) than in the cesarean delivery group (9.8–37.7%). In addition, blood transfusion, infection of the abdominal wound, thromboembolic complications, anesthesia-associated complications, pyelonephritis, pneumonia, and septicemia were also less frequent in the vaginal delivery group. Between the two groups, no significant differences in perinatal morbidity and mortality were found.

In many cesarean deliveries blood loss is great, especially with placenta previa, placental abruption, pre-eclampsia, and multiple pregnancy. It depends on the surgical technique used; it is greater if a classical longitudinal incision is made into the uterine corpus. It is less when a transverse or a small longitudinal incision in the lower uterine segment is made. If a transverse incision is made too low in the lower uterine segment of an unripe uterus, uterine arteries may often be injured.

The incidence of injuries to the urinary bladder in a cesarean delivery is 0.3%. The incidence may be higher in a repeat cesarean.[9] Injuries to the urinary bladder are more frequent in the presence of adhesions between the bladder and the anterior abdominal wall. Injuries to the ureter occur less frequently, mainly when attempts are made to stop the bleeding from major uterine vessels.

Late complications of cesarean delivery include intestinal obstruction from adhesions, dehiscence of the uterine scar in subsequent pregnancies, and incisional hernia in a longitudinal skin incision (laparotomia mediana inferioris). Multiple cesarean deliveries pose little risk to the mother, but may be associated with an increased neonatal risk, attributed mainly to a preterm non-elective cesarean delivery.[57]

In developed countries, maternal mortality related to cesarean delivery has decreased over the last two decades. In the USA and Great Britain, maternal mortality is less than 1 per 1000 cesarean deliveries. In other parts of the world, maternal mortality resulting from cesarean delivery is markedly higher.[61] Generally, it is 2–4 times higher than with vaginal delivery.[61] The main causes of death following a cesarean delivery are infections, hemorrhage, pulmonary embolism, and anesthesia-associated complications, the most frequent being aspiration pneumonia and cardiopulmonary arrest. Cesarean delivery was an important underlying cause of death in Norway and contributed to the increased maternal death ratio in the last decade.[62]

Neonatal morbidity

Cesarean delivery is not always atraumatic to the fetus. Although injuries are fewer than with vaginal delivery, they are also relatively frequent during cesarean section, especially in premature babies and in forceful deliveries or extractions. The fetal head in the vertex presentation is sometimes injured when the head is low in the birth canal or the operative incision is too small, resulting in difficulty extracting it. Fractures of long bones may also occur. All these injuries are more frequent with extraction by the feet. In breech deliveries, the soft tissues, bones and fetal head are most exposed to injuries.

In babies delivered by cesarean, the incidence of respiratory distress is higher, and so is the neonatal mortality due to hyaline membrane disease. The lecithin/sphyngomyelin ratio is poorer after elective cesarean than after induced labor. In babies delivered by an elective cesarean, the volume of the lungs is smaller, and the resistance of the respiratory tract is increased compared to babies delivered vaginally. The outcome of babies delivered by an emergency cesarean delivery is ranked somewhere in between.[63]

Cesarean delivery is associated with an increased risk of disorders of placentation in subsequent pregnancies. Delivery by cesarean delivery in the first pregnancy could increase the risk of an unexplained stillbirth in the second. The risk of unexplained antepartum stillbirth at or after 39 weeks' gestation is about double the risk of stillbirth or neonatal death from intrapartum uterine rupture.[64]

Unfortunately, there are few data to suggest that the liberalized indications for a cesarean delivery have reduced the incidence of cerebral palsy and other long-term disabilities. This is probably because most perinatal morbidity and mortality is caused by premature births, fetal anomalies, or antepartum events.[65,66]

Elective and emergency cesarean delivery

A delivery is designated an elective cesarean delivery when the obstetrician decides on a cesarean delivery prior to labor, for various indications. To facilitate the elective cesarean delivery, some induce labor for an hour or two before the procedure in order to achieve the thinning of the lower uterine segment and better uterine contractility, which may result in reduced blood loss and improved adaptation of the newborn to extrauterine life. Although the onset of labor is induced, the delivery is still referred to as an elective cesarean. Emergency cesarean delivery occurs when indications for delivery arise during labor, which require a cesarean.

In developed countries, the rates of elective cesarean delivery are increasing, especially in cases where cesarean is commonly performed on patient request, for breech presentation and for twins. In the USA, the cesarean delivery rate for the second twin after vaginal delivery of the first twin is approximately 9.5%.[54]

Technique of cesarean delivery

Preparation of the parturient

At emergency cesarean delivery, the preparation of the parturient is short, especially when done in haste. The parturient should be given an explanation of the procedure, of the risks involved, and she should be given the reason why the procedure is necessary. The appropriate informed consent form(s) should be signed by the woman, stating the type of procedure, the type of anesthesia, potential complications necessitating further procedures (blood transfusion, hysterectomy, if necessary), and any special requests of the parturient. The blood group should be verified and pubic hair shaved.

Prior to elective cesarean delivery there is enough time to discuss the reasons for the procedure, the procedure itself, and the postoperative course with the woman in greater detail. The obstetrician enquires about the possibility of sterilization. The woman is advised to do respiratory exercises, and if a smoker, she is advised not to smoke for some time before the procedure. She has to have her blood group determined, if this has not been already done, and some basic blood tests are performed as well. The woman is examined by an anesthesiologist, and additional tests are carried out if she suffers from any disease (heart or kidney diseases, diabetes mellitus, etc.).

Prophylactic amnioinfusion in women with thick meconium decreases the incidence of meconium below the fetal vocal cords and the impact on the incidence of meconium aspiration syndrome may be apparent in future in larger series.[67]

Anesthesia

Considerable data support the presumption that the fetal condition worsens as the time of exposure to general anesthesia lengthens. Progressive fetal depression as the induction-to-delivery time is prolonged makes it important to avoid unnecessary delay during the operative procedure. The abdomen should be fully prepared, draped, and ready for the incision before general anesthesia is induced.[40]

Just before surgery, the woman should be given antacid to neutralize the acids in the stomach contents to prevent pulmonary complications in case of vomiting and aspiration. It is not yet clear which agent best achieves this effect.

In Slovenia, a cesarean delivery is performed under general endotracheal anesthesia. In some countries, regional anesthesia is increasing in popularity as the mother feels more involved in the birth of her baby and there is less likelihood of neonatal respiratory depression.[68] The procedure of anesthesia is described in detail elsewhere.

Usually 1–2 l of fluid containing electrolytes is infused during and immediately after the operation. Throughout the procedure, and subsequently while in the recovery area, the blood pressure and urine flow are monitored closely to ascertain that the perfusion of vital organs is satisfactory.

Position of the patient and immediate preparation

At a cesarean delivery, the woman is at high risk of developing thrombophlebitis and thromboembolism. Therefore, proper care of the parturient's legs in the operating room is important, and spontaneous movements of the legs and early ambulation after a cesarean delivery are strongly recommended.

In Slovenia, a cesarean delivery is usually performed with the parturient on the gynecologic operating table and her legs spread on the leg supports (Figure 179.1). Thus, vaginal interventions are made possible, if necessary (e.g. pushing up the head). Immediately before the procedure, the urinary bladder is catheterized, and methylene blue injected, so that an incision of the bladder is quickly recognized.

The most convenient position for the parturient is slightly lateral (15°) and light Trendelenburg position (15°).

Skin incision

Two skin incisions are commonly used: transverse, the incisio secundum Pfannenstiel being more common, and vertical (laparotomia mediana inferior). Advocates of the former claim that the incision leaves a better cosmetic effect, as the scar is smaller, and is usually covered with pubic hair, and that incisional hernia is a less frequent consequence. The advocates of the latter consider the vertical incision to offer more rapid access and better visibility of the whole abdomen. In general, the transverse incision is reproached for slower access, especially in the case of a repeated incision, and the vertical incision for a less cosmetically desirable scar, and more frequent incisional hernias.[69]

In agreement with the enumerated advantages of the transverse incision, we are of the opinion that it should be used in the majority of the cases. The vertical incision should only be used in exceptional cases when good visibility of the upper abdominal cavity is required.

Uterine incision

Two uterine incisions are mainly used: transverse in the lower uterine segment, and a vertical incision. Some distinguish between the vertical incision of the lower uterine segment and the high vertical incision of the uterine corpus, although a combination of both is most commonly used. Frequent occurrence of serious uterine ruptures during subsequent pregnancies following a high vertical approach has made this incision nearly obsolete. In the opinion of some,[68] it is appropriate with a neglected transverse lie, when the approach to the lower uterine segment is not easy (congenital anomalies, severe adhesions following inflammations and surgeries, tumors of the lower uterine segment – primarily leiomyomas – and severe kyphoscoliosis of the parturient), and with the preterm uterus with an undeveloped lower segment. A skilled surgeon has to revert to the vertical uterine incision only rarely.

Recommended technique

We recommend a technique that, in our experience, provides relatively quick access to the uterus and results in little blood loss, minimal lacerations of the uterus and major uterine vessels, infrequent postoperative complications, and a favorable cosmetic effect.

Incision of the abdominal wall

The surgeon stands to the left of the parturient, the first assistant to the right. The second assistant, if required for expected operative complications (multifetal pregnancy, etc.), stands between the patient's legs. The skin incision (Pfannenstiel) should be made with a determined move transversely in a slightly curvilinear direction, approximately 2 cm above the symphysis pubis, preferably in the skin fold (Figure 179.2a) at the level of the pubic hairline. An incision of 12 cm is sufficient. A subcutaneous tissue incision is made somewhat higher than the skin incision, but only in the middle to provide access to the fascia. Minor bleeding veins are ignored; arterial bleeding, which occurs uncommonly with such a small incision, is managed with a small clamp, which is left in place.

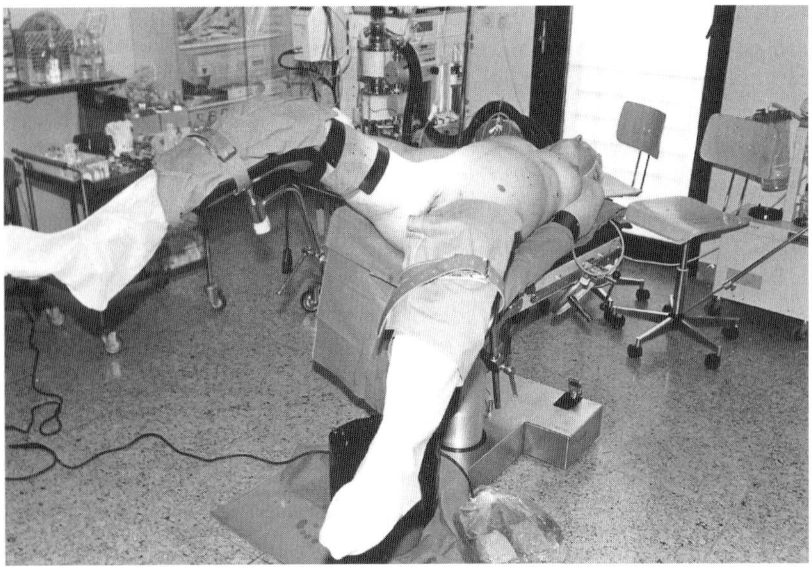

Figure 179.1 Position of the patient for cesarean delivery (slightly lateral and light Trendelenburg position, legs spread on the leg supports).

A short median transverse incision in the anterior rectus fascia is made with a scalpel (Figure 179.2b). The fascia is separated from the underlying muscle with closed scissors in the direction of the intended incision; then, pushing the half-open scissors laterally, the fascia is incised curvilinearly on either side for 7–8 cm (Figure 179.2c). The surgeon and the assistant grasp the superior edges of the fascia and elevate them with strong forceps. The surgeon and the assistant hold the upper incised edge of the fascia approximately 2 cm from the midline on each side, and separate the fascial sheath from the underlying rectus muscles with the index finger (Figure 179.2d) for 2 cm on either side of the intact midline and upward almost to the umbilicus. They should be careful not to rupture the blood vessels coursing between the muscles and the fascia. Ruptures occur only rarely if we take care not to separate the fascial sheath from the muscles too laterally from the midline. In case of a rupture, the blood vessel is clamped and ligated. With semicurved scissors, the midline of the fascia is then sharply separated from the rectal muscles to near the umbilicus (Figure 179.2e).

The rectus muscles are separated with the index fingers or with the tip of the closed forceps and the separation is stretched in the direction symphysis–umbilicus; the pyramidalis muscles are detached in the midline with the scissors.

The surgeon and the assistant grasp the parietal peritoneum and incise as far cephalad as possible to avoid damage to the bladder. This incision of the peritoneum is then lengthened, first upward, and then downward. Some surgeons prefer simply to perforate the peritoneum, after which the two sides are stretched with the index fingers. This may reduce the risk of bladder injury.

The laparotomy wound may be covered with soft gauze. Only a sufficiently wide anterior hook is inserted into the abdominal cavity in a downward direction to uncover the site of the uterine incision.

Uterine incision

With smooth forceps, the surgeon grasps and lifts the serosa in the midline, approximately 1 cm above the bladder and incises with the scissors (Figure 179.2f). The scissors are inserted between the serosa and myometrium, which are then separated laterally and incised. The incision, made curvilinearly somewhat in a cranial direction, is approximately 5 cm long on either side. Varices, if any, should be avoided. Extremely unripe cervices in low gestational age or extremely dilated cervices demand the incision to be made 1 cm or more higher. It is not necessary to separate the bladder from the myometrium. The small low transverse uterine incision is begun in the middle (Figure 179.2g). To avoid incising the fetus, it is safer to perforate a thin posterior layer of the uterine wall with a finger or a handle of the scalpel. With the two index fingers the incision is extended by spreading the incision to achieve the required size of the opening. The initial incision needs only rarely to be lengthened using the scalpel or scissors. This may, however, be the case with an unripe uterus, when the uterine wall is thick and the incision is made too low. The incision should be made carefully, curving it laterally cephalad, to avoid injuries to the major uterine vessels. If the membranes are still intact, they should be ruptured, and the amniotic fluid suctioned. If the placenta is encountered in the line of incision, it must be incised. When the placenta is incised, the cord should be clamped as soon as possible to prevent fetal hemorrhage. The anterior hook is removed to enlarge the opening.

Delivery of the baby

Delivery of the fetus in the vertex presentation. The surgeon's left hand gently slips behind the symphysis and between the lower uterine wall and the head, attempting to reach as far below the fetal head as possible. The head should then be flexed gently and elevated into the incision. When the fetal head is rather tightly wedged into the birth canal, a careful

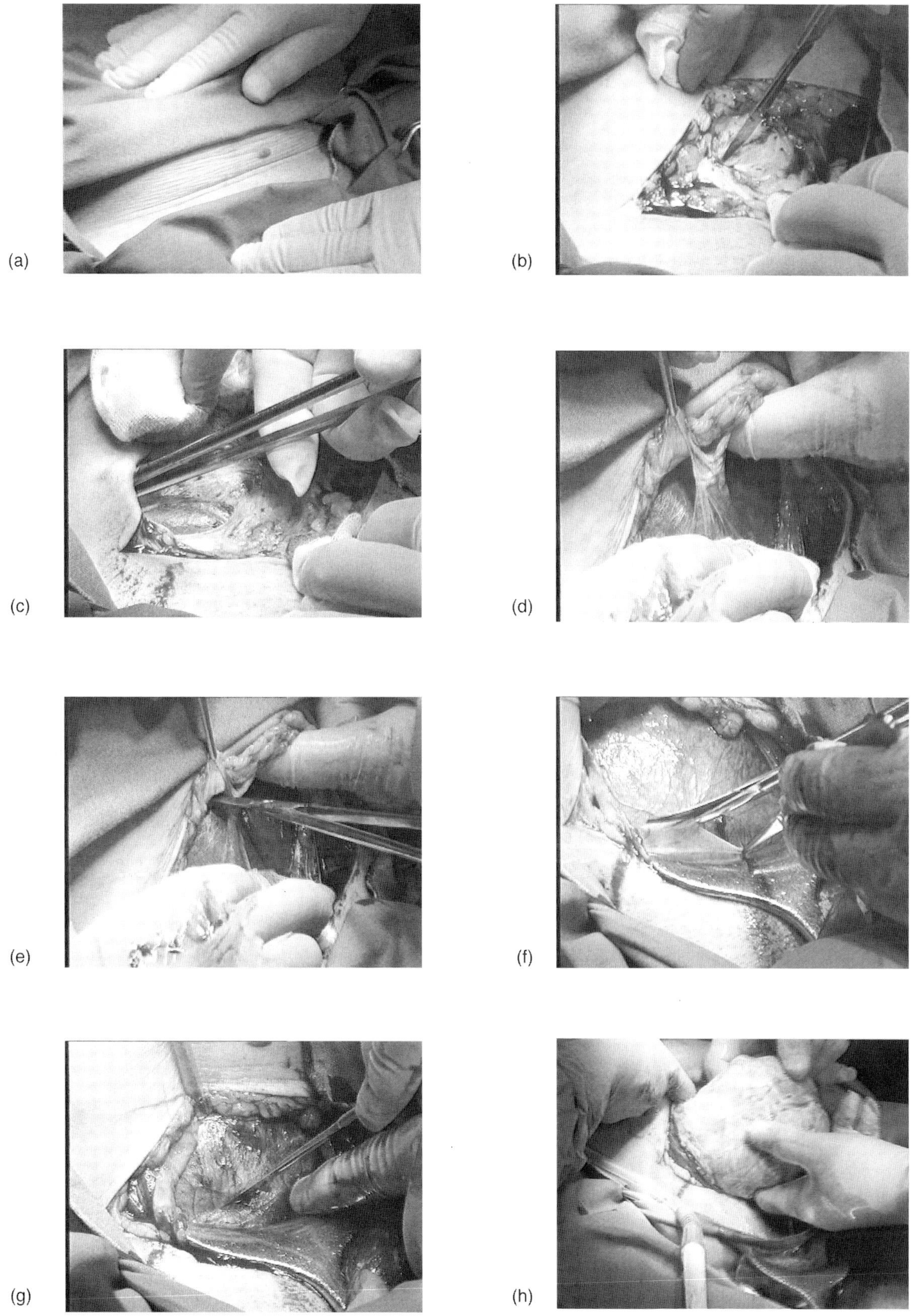

Figure 179.2 (a) Skin incision in skin fold; (b) small incision of the fascia with scalpel; (c) incision of the fascia with scissors; (d) separation of the fascia with index finger; (e) sharp separation of the fascia from rectal muscles; (f) incision of visceral peritoneum; (g) incision of the uterine wall; (h) delivery of fetal breech;

(i) 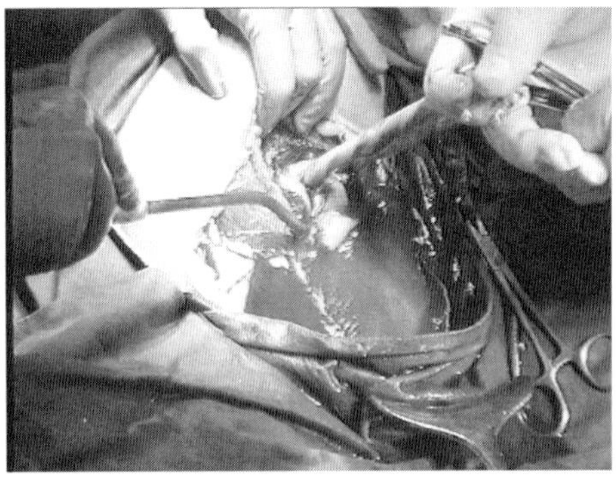 (j) 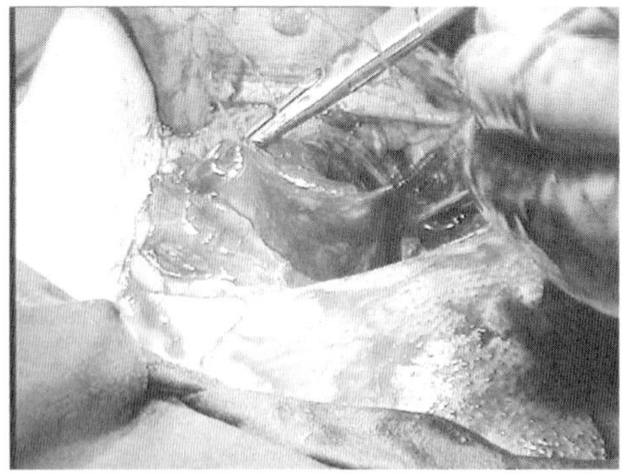

(k) 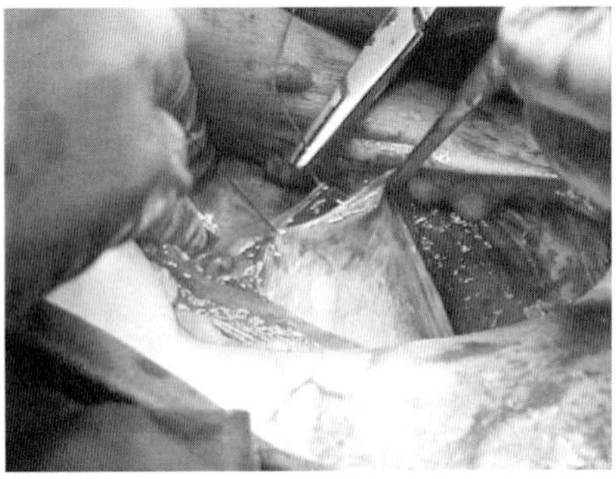 (l) 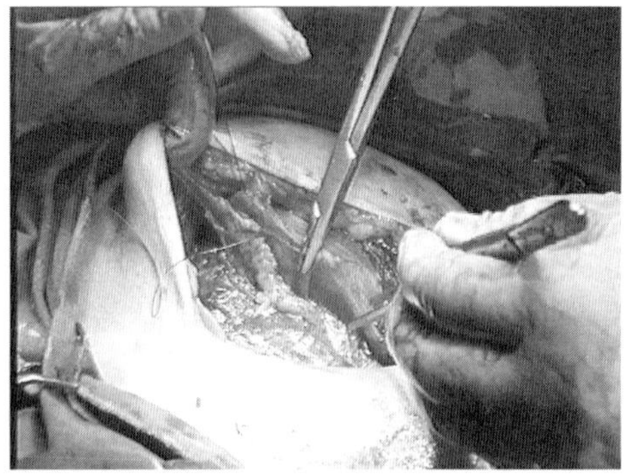

(m) 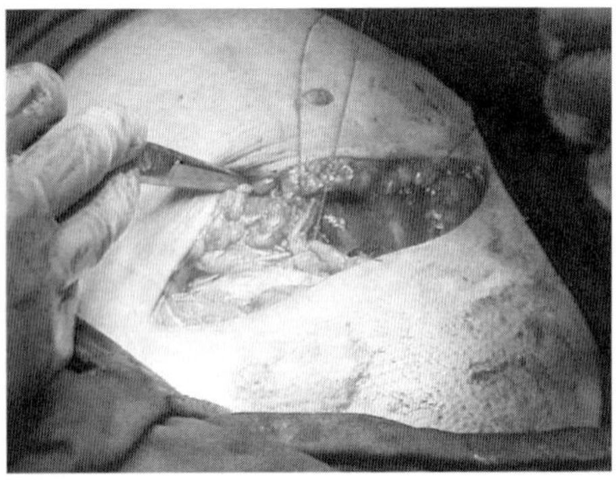 (n) 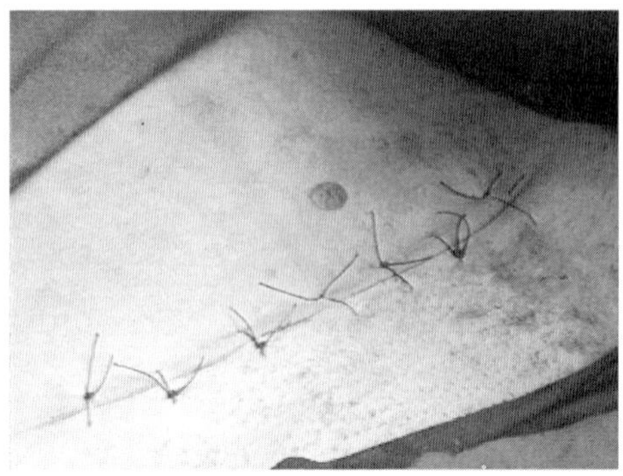

Figure 179.2 (i) delivery of placenta with cords traction; (j) continuous suturing of the uterine wall; (k) continuous suturing of the visceral peritoneum; (l) continuous suturing of the parietal peritoneum; (m) continuous suturing of the fascia; and (n) interrupted sutures of the skin.

upward pressure exerted through the vagina by an assistant will help to dislodge the head. It is of the utmost importance that the surgeon's right hand presses the uterine fundus, retaining it and preventing it from moving upward. When pressing the fetal head upward, especially if it is already deep in the birth canal and thus more force is required, the surgeon may, especially if too forceful, push the entire uterus upward, resulting in an unwanted extension of the initial incision. If the fetal head and the surgeon's hand are both large, the use of the right blade of the forceps may prove helpful in flexing and directing the fetal head. Once the fetal head is directed toward the incision, the assistant helps deliver the head by pressing the uterine fundus through the abdominal wall. If necessary, the surgeon simultaneously retracts the uterine wall over the head with the fingers of his or her right hand. When the head is delivered, and the baby's mouth and nose are wiped, the head is held with both the surgeon's hands in an attempt to deliver the trunk, in similar manner to vaginal delivery. If the baby is large, the shoulders are usually delivered by pressing the baby's head toward the umbilicus. First, the inferior shoulder is delivered; then, by pressing the head against the symphysis, the superior one. The baby should not be held above the level of the uterus until the cord is clamped, otherwise the blood will tend to drain from the fetus to the placenta.

After the baby is born, the umbilical cord is clamped at three sites to obtain blood for pH measurement, which is important for evaluation of the baby's condition at birth.

Breech delivery. At a frank breech presentation, the buttocks are directed toward the incision by the surgeon's left hand in a similar manner to the fetal head at a vertex delivery. If this manipulation fails, the surgeon attempts to deliver the buttocks by hooking the fetal inguinal regions with both index fingers (Figure 179.2h). With various types of footling presentations, or with transverse and oblique lies, the delivery is started by delivering a foot, or feet, if possible. By the traction on a foot or feet, the fetal trunk is delivered. Traction limited to one foot only should be performed carefully to avoid fracturing the femur, especially when rotating the foot. At delivery of the aftercoming head, a spasm of the uterine muscles around the fetal neck sometimes occurs, especially when the traction has been hasty, or when the fetus is smaller with a relatively larger head. In the rare instance in which the extraction of the fetal head by a modified Mauriceau–Smellie–Veit maneuver fails, the uterine incision should be extended, usually by T-incision.

In either mode of delivery, an ecbolic agent (ergometrine 0.25 mg or oxytocin 5 units) is administered intravenously after the fetal head is delivered. By gentle traction on the umbilical cord, the placenta is delivered (Figure 179.2i). To avoid heavier bleeding, manual removal of the placenta is not recommended. The edges of the uterine incision should be grasped with ring forceps, first at the angles, and then in the middle of the lower edge. If heavy bleeding occurs at other sites, they are also clamped with ring forceps. When the delivered placenta is incomplete, or the membranes have been retained, the uterine cavity is explored and wiped using a swab on a stick. Manual exploration should be avoided, especially with preterm rupture of the membranes and with suspected chorionitis. Should manual exploration be absolutely necessary, surgical gloves should be changed after suturing the uterine wall.

The hysterotomy incision is then reapproximated with either continuous or interrupted sutures (Figure 179.2j), usually in one layer when the uterine wall is thin, and in two layers when the uterine wall is thick. The endometrium should be directed toward the uterine cavity. Sutures are applied as far apart as possible (1.5–2 cm), not tightly tied, or not sutured with a running-lock, to avoid ischemia.

When the second layer is being sutured, the stitches are put between the stitches of the first layer. After each layer has been sutured, massage of the uterus is necessary. If after the suturing there is still bleeding, additional hemostatic sutures are introduced.

Serosal edges are usually approximated with continuous sutures (Figure 179.2k). Many do not close the visceral peritoneum. Nagele *et al.*[70] reported that nonclosure of the visceral peritoneum was associated with lower febrile and infectious morbidity.

After the suturing, the uterus is massaged again, the adnexa are examined, and the abdominal cavity above the uterus manually explored to verify the possible presence of adhesions. Blood is also removed, usually by hand. If a gauze pack is used for the purpose, forceful wiping should be avoided, as it may cause postoperative atony of the bowels or lead to injuries of the serosa. The injured serosa presents a higher risk of subsequent adhesion formation than the retained blood.

Continuous sutures, avoiding forceful traction of the suture, can be used to close the parietal peritoneum (Figure 179.2l). Some do not approximate the peritoneum; its non-closure does not cause increased postoperative complications.[71,72]

After delivery, the suturing of the rectus abdominus muscles is not necessary, or just one suture is made at the top of the pyramidalis muscles.

The fascial edges may be reapproximated with either a continuous suture (Figure 179.2m) or interrupted sutures about 1 cm apart, mostly with synthetic resorbable sutures. Care must be taken not to wipe off the blood clots, which are hemostatic; therefore, only gentle blotting is applied. The clamps, if used, are removed, and ligation is used only if bleeding occurs. A few interrupted sutures may be made to obliterate the dead space and reduce the tension on the skin edges. If there is abundant adipose tissue, these sutures should not be too tightly tied either. The skin is usually sutured with interrupted sutures (Figure 179.2n), which should not be too close together or tied too tightly. Alternatively, we can use staples.

Cesarean delivery performed in the manner described usually takes 15–17 min. The most common operative errors are the following.

(1) Making the skin incision too long
(2) Making the transverse skin incision too high
(3) Excessive coagulation or ligation of the bleeding sites, leading to necrosis and development of favorable conditions for infections
(4) Making the rectus fascia incision shorter than the skin incision
(5) Separating the anterior rectus fascia from the rectal muscles too laterally
(6) Not separating the fascia from the rectal muscles up to the umbilicus
(7) Separation of the bladder from the myometrium in the case of a low transverse uterine incision
(8) Making a transverse uterine incision too low, especially when the cervix is unripe or fully dilated
(9) Failing to curve the lateral portions of the uterine incision upward, with consequent rupture of uterine vessels
(10) Forceful extraction of the fetus, leading to risks of uterine laceration and damage to the fetus
(11) Tying the sutures too closely and too tightly, resulting in ischemia and greater risk of infections
(12) Forceful wiping of the uterus and abdominal cavity

(13) Suture of the anterior fascia too laterally, resulting in the entrapment of the cutaneous nerves (genitofemoralis) consequent pain after the operation.

Hemorrhage

Parturients undergoing a cesarean delivery, in whom factors for an increased risk of hemorrhage exist, can be identified prospectively. These women will benefit greatly from extended preoperative counseling when possible, effective utilization of blood bank technology through the type and cross-match requests, and preventive measures during abdominal delivery to minimize blood loss.[73]

The woman of average size with a hematocrit of 30% or more, and a normally expanded blood volume and extracellular fluid volume, most often tolerates blood loss up to 1500 ml without difficulty.[1,5] The average reported blood loss during a cesarean delivery is 800–1100 ml.[74] In the Ljubljana maternity hospital, the mean blood loss is 500 ml. In only 5% of women is the blood loss greater than 1000 ml.

Antibiotic prophylaxis

The advantages and disadvantages of antibiotic prophylaxis of the parturient at a cesarean delivery have been discussed for years. In our opinion, antibiotic prophylaxis (treatment) should be used at every cesarean delivery after a preterm rupture of the membranes, with suspected chorioamnionitis, with prolonged labor and thus numerous vaginal examinations, and in maternity hospitals with frequent postpartum infections. In all such cases, after the umbilical cord is clamped, intravenous antibiotic (ampicillin or preferably a cephalosporin) should be injected. The administration is usually repeated twice.

Postoperative procedure

The basics of the postoperative course are the following.

(1) Regular monitoring of uterine contraction and hemorrhage (at least twice on the day of surgery, and once daily afterward)
(2) Monitoring of the operative wound (once daily)
(3) Infusion: 1500–2000 ml of fluid, usually Ringer lactate in a 5% glucose solution, on the day of surgery and the following day
(4) Analgesia: intravenously when access is available; afterward oral or intramuscularly, if required
(5) Getting up: 3–6 h after surgery
(6) Breast-feeding: almost immediately after recovery from anesthesia
(7) Nutrition: fluids and light food as soon as bowel sounds reappear and nausea disappears
(8) Active physical exercises immediately after surgery: arms, legs, breathing, pelvic floor
(9) Removal of sutures: 4–6 days after surgery

Discharge from hospital is becoming dictated by the economic and insurance conditions, rather than an ideal management. In the opinion of some authors, the mother may be safely discharged from hospital on the third or fourth postpartum day, unless there are complications in the puerperium.[1] In Slovenia, the mother is usually discharged from hospital on the seventh or eighth day.

REFERENCES

1. Cunningham FG, MacDonald PC, Gant NF, Leveno KJ, Gilstrap LC III. *Williams Obstetrics*, 19th edn. Norwalk: Appleton & Lange, 1993:591–613.
2. Macfarlane A, Chamberlain G. What is happening to caesarean section rates? *Lancet* 1993;342:1005–6.
3. Lee SI, Khang YH, Lee MS. Women's attitudes toward mode of delivery in South Korea – A society with high cesarean section rates. *Birth* 2004;31:108–16.
4. Saporito M, Arsieri R, Pugliese A, Formisano V, Triassi M. Increase of births by cesarean section in Campania in 2000. *Epidemiol Prev* 2003;27:291–6.
5. Guzman Ibarra Mde L, Ablanedo Augirre J, Basvilvazo Rodriguez MA, Martinez Rodriguez OA, Ahumada Aramirez E. Is the high frequency of caesarean sections in a higly specialized gyneco-obstetric hospital justifiable? *Gynecol Obstet Mex* 2003;71: 291–6.
6. Rozenberg P. Evaluation of cesarean rate: A necessary progress in modern obstetrics. *J Gynecol Obstet Biol Reprod (Paris)* 2004; 33:79–83.
7. De Palma RT, Cunningham FG, Leveno KG, Roark ML. Continuing investigation of women at high risk for infection following cesarean delivery. *Obstet Gynecol* 1982;60:53–9.
8. Duff P. Antibiotic prophylaxis for a cesarean section: A review of the American literature since 1970. *Sex Med Today* 1985;9: 18–22.
9. Duff P. Cesarean delivery and cesarean hysterectomy. In Pauerstein CJ, ed. *Clinical Obstetrics.* New York: Churchill Livingstone, 1987:883–921.
10. Martin JA, Hamilton BE, Sutton PD, Ventura SJ, Menacker F, Munson ML. Births: Final data for 2002. *Natl Vital Stat Rep* 2003;52:1–113.
11. Savage W, Francome C, Lewison H, Churchill H. *Caesarean Birth in Britain.* London: Middlesex University Press, 1983.
12. Notzon FC. International differences in the use of obstetric interventions. *J Am Med Assoc* 1990;263:3286–91.
13. Nair C. Trends in cesarean section deliveries in Canada. *Health Rep* 1991;3:203–19.
14. Macfarlane AJ. Holding back the tide of caesareans. *Br Med J* 1988;297:852.
15. Stafford RS. Cesarean section use and source of payment: An analysis of Canadian hospital discharge abstracts. *Am J Publ Health* 1990;80:313–5.
16. Yazlle ME, Rocha JS, Mendes MC, Patta MC, Marcolin AC, de Azevedo GD. Incidence of cesarean section regarding the financial support source for delivery care. *Rev Saude Publica* 2001;35:202–6.
17. Enkin MW, Keirse MJNC, Renfrew MJ, Neilson JP, eds. Pregnancy and childbirth module. *Cochrane Database Systemic Reviews Published through Cochrane Updates on Disk.* Oxford: Update Software, 1993.
18. Pajntar M, Verdenik I, Pestevsek M. Cesarean section in breech by birth weight. *Eur J Obstet Gynecol Reprod Biol* 1994;54:181–4.
19. Notzon FC, Cnattingius S, Bergsjo P, *et al.* Cesarean section delivery in the 1980s: International comparison by indication. *Am J Obstet Gynecol* 1994;170:495–504.

20. Elferink-Stinkens PM, Brand R, Van Hemel OJ. Trends in cesarean section rates among high- and medium-risk pregnancies in the Nederlands 1983–1992. *Eur J Obstet Gynecol Reprod Biol* 1995;59:159–67.
21. Rozenberg P. Evaluation of cesarean rate: A necessary progress in modern obstetrics. *J Gynecol Obstet Biol Reprod (Paris)* 2004; 33:279–89.
22. Devendra K, Arulkumararan S. Should doctor perform elective cesarean section on request. *Ann Acad Med Singapore* 2003; 32:577–81.
23. O'Driscoll K, Foley M. Correlation of decrease in perinatal mortality and increase in cesarean section rates. *Obstet Gynecol* 1983;61:1–5.
24. Verdenik I, Pajntar M. *Perinatologia Slovenica 1995.* Ljubljana: University Medical Centre Ljubljana, 1996.
25. Stembera Z. Development of indications for cesarean section in the Czech Republic and certain developed countries. *Cas Lek Cesk* 1992;131:225–30.
26. Lagrew DC Jr, Morgan MA. Decreasing the cesarean section rate in a private hospital: Success without mandated clinical changes. *Am J Obstet Gynecol* 1996;174:184–91.
27. Myers SA, Gleicher N. A successful program to lower cesarean section rates. *N Engl J Med* 1988;319:1511–6.
28. Ziadeh SM, Sunna EI. Decreased cesarean birth rates and improved perinatal outcome: A seven-year study. *Birth* 1995;*22*: 144–7.
29. Raul RH, Miller DA. Cesarean birth: How to reduce the rate. *Obstet Gynecol* 1995;172:1903–11.
30. Finkler MD, Wirtschafter DD. Why pay extra for cesarean section deliveries? *Inquiry* 1993;30:208–15.
31. Soliman SRH, Burrows RF. Cesarean section: Analysis of the experience before and after the national consensus conference on aspects of cesarean birth. *Can Med Assoc J* 1993;148: 1315–20.
32. Hueston WJ. Site-to-site variation in the factors affecting cesarean section rates. *Arch Fam Med* 1995;4:346–51.
33. Husslein P. Elective caesarean section versus vaginal delivery. *Arch Gynecol Obstet* 2001:265–74.
34. Kwee A, Kohlen BJ, Kanhai HH, Visser GH. Cesarean section on request: A survey in the Netherlands. *Eur J Obstet Gynecol Reprod Biol* 2004;113(2):186–90.
35. Enkin M. Labour and delivery following previous cesarean section. In Chalmers I, Enkin M, Keirse MINC, eds *Effective Care in Pregnancy and Childbirth.* New York: Oxford University Press, 1989:1198–215.
36. Naef RW III, Ray MA, Chauhan SP, Roach H, Blake PG, Martin JN Jr Trial of labor after cesarean delivery with lower-segment, vertical uterine incision: Is it safe? *Am J Obstet Gynecol* 1995;172: 1666–74.
37. Miller DA, Diaz FG, Paul RH. Vaginal birth after cesarean: A 10-year experience. *Obstet Gynecol* 1994;84:255–8.
38. Weinstein D, Benshushan A, Tanos V, Zilberstein R, Rojansky N. Predictive score for vaginal birth after cesarean section. *Am J Obstet Gynecol* 1996;174:192–8.
39. Flam BL, Goings JR, Liu Y, Wolde-Tsadik G. Elective repeat cesarean delivery versus trial of labor: A prospective multicenter study. *Obstet Gynecol* 1994;83:927–32.
40. Cowan RK, Kinch RAH, Ellis B, Anderson R. Trial of labor following cesarean delivery. *Obstet Gynecol* 1994;83:933–6.
41. Rosen MG, Dickinson JC, Westhoff CL. Vaginal birth after cesarean: A meta-analysis of morbidity and mortality. *Obstet Gynecol* 1991;77(3):465–70.
42. Sakala EP, Kaye S, Murray RD, Munson LJ. Oxytocin use after previous cesarean: Why a higher rate of failed labor trial? *Obstet Gynecol* 1990;75:356–9.
43. Greenhill JP. Editorial. *Year Book of Obstetrics and Gynecology.* Chicago: Year Book Publishers, 1970:202–3.
44. Eskes TKAB, Wallenburg HCS. How to handle breech presentation and delivery? *Eur J Obstet Gynecol Reprod Biol* 1995;61:83.
45. Notzon FC, Placek PJ, Taffel SM. Comparisons of national cesarean section rates. *N Engl J Med* 1987;316:386–9.
46. Cruikshank DP. Breech presentation. *Clin Obstet Gynecol* 1986; 29:255–63.
47. Hofmeyr GJ. Effect of external cephalic version in late pregnancy on breech presentation and cesrean section rate: A controlled trial. *Br J Obstet Gynaecol* 1983;90:392–9.
48. Pajntar M, Verdenik I, Pestevšek M. Cesarean section in breech by birth weight. *Eur J Obstet Gynaecol Reprod Biol* 1994;54:181–4.
49. Nielsen TF, Hokegard KH. Postoperative cesarean section morbidity: A prospective study. *Am J Obstet Gynecol* 1983; 146:911–5.
50. DeLeeuw JP. Management of breech presentation in two university hospitals: Preliminary results of a prospective comparative study. *Eur J Obstet Gynecol Reprod Biol* 1987;24:94–6.
51. Bingham P, Lilford R. Outcome of breech delivery at term. *Br Med J* 1992;305:500.
52. Smith GC, Pell JP, Dobbie R. Cesarean section and risk of unexplained stillbirth in subsequent pregnancy. *Lancet* 2003; 362(9398):1779–84.
53. De Crespigny LJ, Pepperell RJ. Perinatal mortality and morbidity in breech presentation. *Obstet Gynecol* 1979;53(2):141–5.
54. Confino E, Gleicher N, Elrad H, Ismajovich B, David MP. The breech dilemma. A review. *Obstet Gynecol Surv* 1985;40:330–7.
55. Odibo AO, Macones GA. Current concepts regarding vaginal birth after cesarean delivery. *Curr Opin Obstet Gynecol* 2003; 15:479–82.
56. Falconer AD, Poyser LM. Fetal sympatho-adrenal mediated metabolic responses to parturition. *Br J Obstet Gynaecol* 1986;93: 747–53.
57. Seidman DS, Paz I, Nadu A, *et al.* Are multiple cesarean sections safe? *Eur J Obstet Gynecol Reprod Biol* 1994;57:7–12.
58. Weisbach W, Menzel K, Wagner F, Bratanoff E, Jager KH. Zur Morbiditat und Mortalitet in den Jahren 1984-1985 aus Beckendlage geborener Prematurer mit einem Geburtsgewicht < 1500 g. Eine Prospectivstudie zur Fragestellung vaginaler oder abdominaler Endbindugsweg. *Zentralbl Gynakol* 1985;108: 424–34.
59. Pajntar M, Verdenik I. Vaginal breech delivery. *Sing J Obstet Gynaecol* 1996;27:75–9.
60. Wirakusumah FF. Maternal and perinatal mortality/morbidity associated with cesarean section in Indonesia. *J Obstet Gynaecol* 1995;21:475–81.
61. Miller JM Jr. Maternal and neonatal morbidity and mortality in cesarean section. *Obstet Gynecol Clin North Am* 1988;15: 629–38.
62. Vangen S, Bergsjo P. Do woman die from pregnancy these days? *Tidsskr Nor Laegeforen* 2003;123:3544–5.
63. Fortney JA, Higgins JE, Kennedy KI. Delivery type and neonatal mortality among 10749 breeches. *Am J Public Health* 1986;76: 980–5.
64. Brown L, Karrison T, Cibils LA. Mode of delivery and perinatal results in breech presentation. *Am J Obstet Gynecol* 1994; 171:28–34.
65. Scott JR. Cesarean delivery. In Scott JR, Disaia PJ, Hammon CB, Spellacy WN, eds. *Danforth's Obstetrics and Gynecology*, 7th edn. Philadelphia: J.B. Lippincott Company, 1994:563–76.
66. Scheller JM, Nelson KB. Does cesarean delivery prevent cerebral palsy or other neurologic problems of childhood? *Obstet Gynecol* 1994;83:624–30.
67. Eriksen NL, Hostetter M, Parisi VM. Prophylactic amnioinfusion in pregnancies complicated by thick meconium. *Am J Obstet Gynecol* 1994;171:1026–30.
68. Hibbard BM. *Principles of Obstetrics.* London: Butterworths & Co, 1988:500–37.
69. Lindholt JS, Möller-Christensen T, Steele RE. The cosmetic outcome of the scar formation after cesarean section: Percutaneous or intracutaneous suture? *Acta Obstet Gynecol Scand* 1994; 73:832–5.
70. Nagele F, Karas H, Spitzer D, *et al.* Closure or nonclosure of the visceral peritoneum at cesarean delivery. *Am J Obstet Gynecol* 1996;174:1366–70.
71. Hull DB, Varner MW. A randomized study of closure of the peritoneum at cesarean delivery. *Obstet Gynecol* 1991;77: 818–21.
72. Pietrantoni M, Parsons MT, O'Brien WF, Collins E, Knuppel RA, Spellacy WN. Peritoneal closure or non-closure at cesarean. *Obstet Gynecol* 1991;77:293–6.
73. Naef RW III, Chauhan SP, Chevalier SP, Roberts WE, Meydrech EF, Morrison JC. Prediction of hemorrhage at cesarean delivery. *Obstet Gynecol* 1994;83:923–6.
74. Gilson GJ, Kephart WH, Izquierdo LA, Joffe GM, Qualls CR, Curet LB. Comparison of absorbable uterine staples and traditional hysterotomy during cesarean delivery. *Obstet Gynecol* 1996;87:384–8.

180 Transverse lie, brow and face presentations

Ž. Novak-Antolic

The lie and presentation assumed by the fetus have considerable influence on perinatal and maternal morbidity and mortality. These influences relate in part to the factors that cause abnormal lies or presentations and in larger measure to the complications that accrue to pregnancies with these abnormalities during the process of labor and delivery. In this regard, abnormal lies and presentations have an increased risk of cesarean delivery (CD), as well as of fetal injury during labor and vaginal birth. The early diagnosis of these abnormalities is important for optimal management.

Maternal and fetal factors are involved in the term fetus assuming the most commonly encountered longitudinal cephalic–occiput presentation. At the end of gestation the fetus probably adjusts to the position in which it best fits: generally its podalic pole is where there is more space and, because of the piriform shape of the uterus, the fundus is more spacious. When the normal tonus of the uterus, the abdominal wall or the fetus is absent or other factors are present, an abnormal lie or presentation ensues. Other factors are fetal and uterine anomalies, polyhydramnios, uterine leiomyomas or other pelvic tumors, and placenta previa. Hydrocephalic and anencephalic fetuses are often in breech presentations; those with nuchal teratomas or goiter are likely to be in face presentation.

Transverse lie

Face and brow presentations

Definition

The lie of the fetus is determined with regard to the relation between the longitudinal axis of the fetal spine and that of the maternal spine. Longitudinal axes are usually parallel; when they are not, the lie is transverse or oblique. The latter is sometimes referred to as an unstable or transitory lie. When labor starts, most transverse lies change into longitudinal ones. We do not know when or whether this is about to occur, and at the end of pregnancy, interventions to convert the fetus to a more favorable lie before labor starts may prevent complications and perinatal and maternal morbidity and mortality.[1]

Diagnosis

The diagnosis can sometimes be made solely by inspection, and suspected with palpation and vaginal examination. Ultrasound should be used to confirm the lie and to rule out placenta previa. With early diagnosis, complications can be reduced.[2]

Labor and delivery

The presenting part is the fetal shoulder. The fetal back can be superiorly, inferiorly, anteriorly, or posteriorly positioned. A full-term fetus in a transverse lie cannot be delivered without serious injury. (If, however, the fetus is previable or dead it can be delivered.) If the regular strong contractions have fixed the fetus in the transverse lie, a CD should be performed immediately. The technique of CD itself may need to be modified, because the lower uterine segment has not generally softened and thinned. Sometimes the vertical cervico-isthmic incision is the proper solution. When possible, intraoperative version just before the uterus is incised may be performed.

If the labor proceeds, the most serious complication, the so-called neglected transverse lie, results: after rupture of the membranes and when uterine contractions push a fetal shoulder into the pelvis, the lower uterine segment becomes very thin. A fetal arm may prolapse through the cervix (Figure 180.1). With further contractions, the risk of uterine rupture is substantial. It can occur spontaneously, or be provoked by any vaginal manipulation at this stage.

Epidemiology and predisposing factors

Among more than 52,000 deliveries in 3 years (1997–1999) in Slovenia, the overall occurrence of transverse lie was 0.24%. With placenta previa, transverse lie occurred in 13.6%; in babies weighing less than 1500 g, in 3.3%; and with uterine anomalies, in 4.5%. The percentages are quite similar to those in the period from 1987 to 1995, calculated for more than 204,000 deliveries.[3] The percentage was the

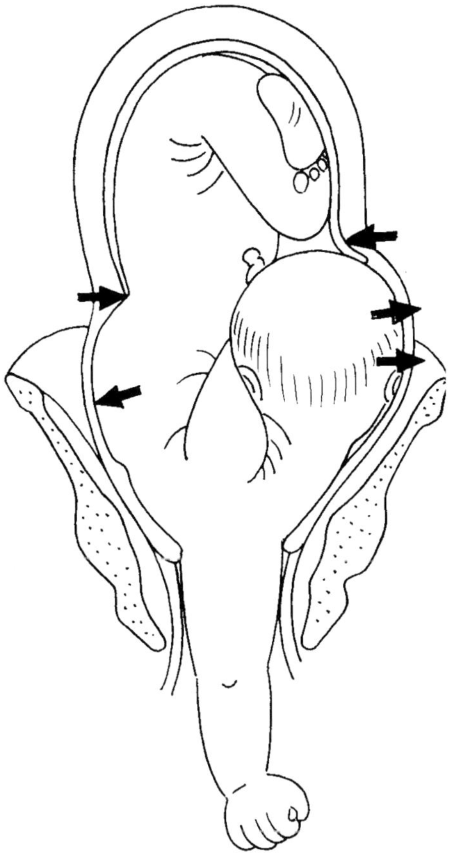

Figure 180.1 Neglected transverse lie.

highest at 27 weeks (11.5%), and dropped to 0.1% at term. With polyhydramnios there were 1.7%, with a lethal malformation 1.4%, and with myomas present there were 1.2% of transverse lies. The occurrence of transverse lie was 0.5% if the maternal age was over 35 years. Transverse lie occurred in 0.13% of nulliparas and in 0.9% of those with a parity of four or more, which is significantly different from brow, breech, and vertex presentations.

Therefore, the factors predisposing to transverse lie are as follows: placenta previa, uterine anomalies, low birth weight, prematurity, polyhydramnios, lethal malformations, myomas, maternal age over 35 years, and multiparity.

Complications

The complications of transverse lie are cord prolapse, obstructed labor, rupture of the uterus, and infection. As these complications are rare, the numbers calculated for the larger of the above-mentioned populations[3] are presented: in the transverse lie, cord prolapse occurred 17 times more often (1.7% vs. 0.1%), perinatal mortality was 12 times higher (8.4% vs. 0.7%), and rupture of the uterus occurred 10 times more often (0.3% vs. 0.03%) than in cephalic presentations. Also, blood transfusion was given six times more often, as placenta previa is a frequent cause of transverse lie. Postpartum infections were four times more common.

Conclusions

Whenever the presenting part cannot be felt in the pelvic inlet in late pregnancy, ultrasound should be performed to diagnose a possible transverse lie and also to rule out placenta previa, pelvic tumors, and fetal anomalies. When fetal maturity is reached, the cervix is ripe, and there are no contraindications, external cephalic version (ECV) could be performed, followed by amniotomy and oxytocin infusion. In a randomized trial, ECV with epidural analgesia was more successful[4] than without. ECV was also described in a woman with ruptured membranes; however, prolapse of the cord ensued.[5] It should be noted that pregnancies after successful version should not be considered the same as normal pregnancies.[6] For breech presentation at term it appears that ECV reduces the chance of non-cephalic birth and cesarean section; there is not enough evidence to quantify most risks of ECV at term.[7] There are no useful data for other malpresentations. During labor, or when the membranes have ruptured, one cannot wait and a CD should be performed as promptly as possible. Internal podalic version (IPV) is contraindicated because of its associated high perinatal mortality.[8] Even in resource-poor countries, safe cesarean section is regarded as a technology that should be employed to help reduce maternal mortality.[9]

Transverse lie of the second twin

Epidemiology

Among 2226 pairs of twins (Slovenia, 1987–1995),[3] 55.2% were both in cephalic presentation, and the CD rate was 16.8%. There were 17.2% of cases that presented as cephalic (first twin)/breech (second twin), of which 24.3% were delivered by cesarean; 10.8% were breech/breech (CD 63%); and 7.5% were breech/cephalic (CD 58.5%). Transverse lies were not uncommon: 4.7% presented as cephalic/transverse (CD 55.9%), 3.3% as breech/transverse (CD 91.7%), and in 0.7% both were in a transverse lie (CD 100.0%); 0.3% were transverse/breech and the same percentage were transverse/cephalic. The percentages of various combinations were similar for the population of 780 pairs of twins born during 1997–1999; the CD rate, however, being higher for all combinations in the more recent period. In roughly 1% of cases, CD was performed for the second twin only.

Combined delivery

The indications for the so-called combined delivery, in which the first twin is delivered vaginally and the second by cesarean, are most often prolapse of the cord, transverse lie, brow, face and compound presentations, cephalopelvic disproportion, fetal distress, placental abruption, contracted cervix, extreme discordance, and failed versions.[10–12] The setting must be such that the interval between births

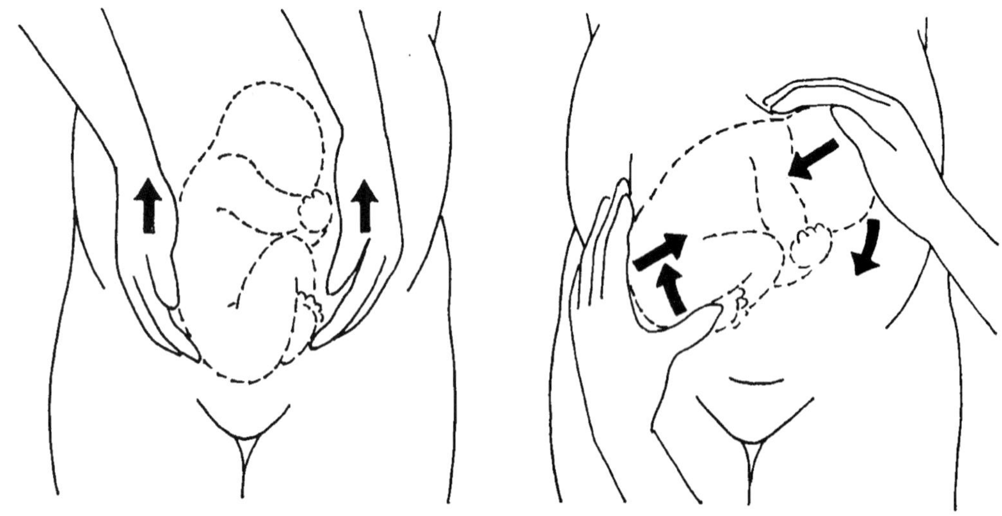

Figure 180.2 Intrapartum external cephalic version.

is not too long; otherwise, the outcomes are not good.[13] A Cochrane review indicated that caesarean section for the birth of a second twin not presenting cephalically is associated with increased maternal febrile morbidity with, as yet, no identified improvement in neonatal outcome; this policy should not be adopted except within the context of further controlled trials.[14] The occurrence of combined deliveries is directly proportional to the increased use of CD for twin pregnancy.[11] One of the causes of an increasing occurrence of cesarean births in twins is the fact that obstetric experience in the cases of vaginal delivery in these circumstances is not easily acquired; the other is the threat of litigation.

External cephalic version

Intrapartum ECV (Figure 180.2) of the second twin, whether in transverse lie or breech presentation, is most successful in gestations over 35 weeks, with intact membranes of the second diamniotic twin, no oligohydramnios, and no nuchal cord.[15]

The complication rate of ECV (cord prolapse, persistent abnormal fetal heart rate tracings, abruptio placentae, and compound presentation) is 10 times higher[16] for the second twin compared to ECV in singletons before labor. Possible explanations for the high complication rate are more premature deliveries, advanced cervical dilatation, and less experience of the operator in twin deliveries, in which ECV occurs in the context of labor, whereas in singletons it is planned.

Internal podalic version

IPV with unruptured membranes using nitroglycerin as a uterine relaxant was performed under epidural anesthesia successfully in 20 of 22 second twins found in transverse lie.[17] In their report, the authors stated that IPV is superior to ECV.[18,19] The numbers reported in most studies were small, and the studies were neither prospective nor randomized.

The attitude of a group of doctors toward the mode of delivery of twins was surveyed; it is interesting to note that 64% of respondents on twin births were interested in a randomized controlled trial to compare planned caesarean section with planned vaginal birth for twin pregnancies.[20] In a cohort study it was found that, at comparable gestational ages, the neonatal morbidity of second twins was comparable to that of a low-risk population. It should be remembered that because immediate management of the vaginally delivered second twins often needs to be more intensive than that of vaginally delivered singletons in the cephalic presentation, appropriate obstetric and neonatal care must be available to ensure optimal outcome.[21]

Deflexion attitudes

Brow presentation

Definition

The fetal head is extended more in the face presentation and less in the brow presentation (Figure 180.3), the presenting part being the part of the fetal head from the anterior fontanelle to the root of the nose (Figure 180.4). Reported incidences differ because of the different times when the diagnosis was made.

Diagnosis

Twenty-four percent are not diagnosed before the second stage.[22] The root of the nose, the upper part of the orbits, frontal sutures, and the anterior fontanelle

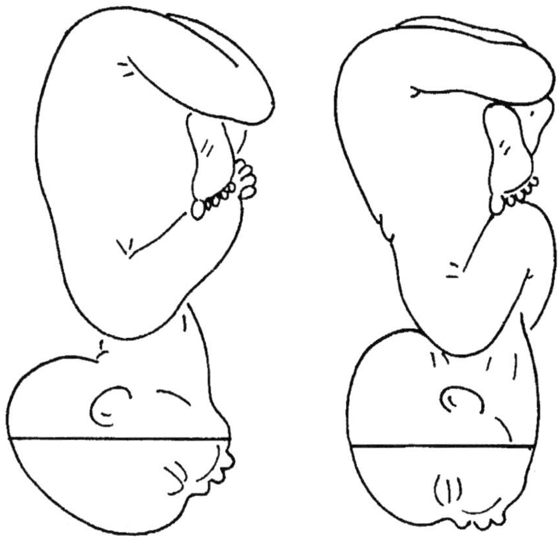

Figure 180.3 Brow (left) and face (right) presentation.

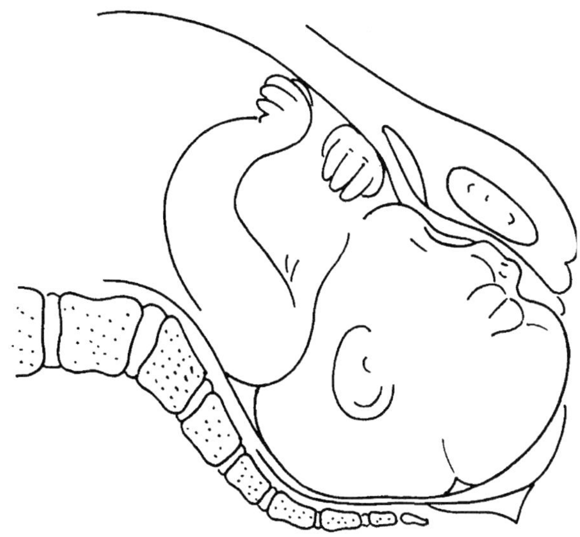

Figure 180.4 Brow presentation. Small fetus.

are felt on vaginal examination. The anterior fontanelle is the point of orientation.

Labor and delivery

Brow presentation is transient in most cases: it is delivered as a vertex if the head flexes, or as a face presentation if the head further extends. As long as labor progresses without signs of fetal distress, one can wait. Very small babies can be delivered vaginally even without further flexion or extension.

With the electrodes for internal fetal heart rate monitoring, damage may be done to the fetus if the electrode is attached to the face or over the anterior fontanelle; therefore, the external mode is preferred. Likewise, one must be very careful with the sites chosen for fetal blood sampling.

In persistent brow presentation, delivery is only possible with a very small baby when the fetal back is posterior or when the pelvis is extremely large. Extensive molding of the head occurs so that the occipitomental diameter is diminished, and usually there is a large caput succedaneum over the forehead. Swelling might be such that it feels to the examiner as if the head is descending. Delivering over the perineum, the fetal head first flexes so that the brow, the sinciput, and the occiput are delivered, and then it extends so that the face is delivered. In most cases, when brow persists and the labor is dysfunctional, a CD should be performed, as vaginal manipulations increase perinatal mortality dramatically.

Epidemiology and predisposing factors

At the time of delivery, brow presentations were present in 0.09% of more than 204,000 deliveries over 9 years (1987–1995) in Slovenia.[3] During the second period analyzed (1997–1999) there were also 0.096% of brow presentations. With polyhydramnios, the occurrence of brow presentation was 0.4%, and in babies weighing less than 1500 g it was 0.19%. The percentage was the highest before 34 weeks (0.16%), dropped to 0.08% at term, and rose slightly after 42 weeks to 0.10%. Brow presentation occurred in 0.1% of nulliparas, and in 0.04% of those whose parity was four or more, which is significantly different from the face presentation and transverse lie. The predisposing factors, listed in decreasing order of appearance, were polyhydramnios, low birth weight, prematurity, and postmaturity. Uterine leiomyomas were not predisposing factors, nor were uterine anomalies, lethal malformations, maternal age over 35 years, or birth weight over 4000 g.

Mode of delivery and complications

In the above-mentioned population of brow presentations,[3] 69% were delivered by cesarean and 5.9% by vacuum extraction. Compared to vertex presentations, cord prolapse occurred five times more often, and rupture of the uterus 17 times more often (0.5% vs. 0.03%); blood transfusion was three times more likely, and postpartum infections occurred four to five times more often than in vertex presentations. The perinatal mortality was 1.6% compared to 0.7% in vertex presentations.

Conclusions

When a brow presentation is diagnosed early in labor, a policy of watchful waiting is usually appropriate. Oxytocin should be used cautiously if uterine contractions are weak, but should be avoided when the descent is absent, or abnormal, or cephalopelvic disproportion is suspected. If a brow presentation persists, a full-term fetus should be delivered by cesarean.

Face presentation

Definition

The fetal head is completely extended. The position during labor is designated by the mentum, which can be on the left or on the right and anterior or posterior, as felt on vaginal examination.

Diagnosis

Forty-nine percent are not diagnosed before the second stage.[22] Sometimes, by abdominal palpation, parts of the fetal head are palpated better on the side of the fetal back. The nose, eyes, mouth, and chin are felt on vaginal examination. The chin is the point of orientation. If the face is swollen, which is common, it can be mistaken for a breech.

Labor and delivery

A direct electrode should not be applied (or, if absolutely necessary, with extreme caution on the fetal chin; it must be removed carefully to avoid injury to the skin), but external fetal heart rate monitoring should be used. For the same reason, fetal blood sampling cannot be performed. Stimulation of the face is sometimes used as an indicator of good fetal condition. Very careful oxytocin stimulation may be used. Labor should proceed as in vertex presentation: arrest of labor and fetal distress are indications for CD.

The mentum anterior position with the fetal back posterior may be delivered vaginally (Figure 180.5). The neck is relatively short and can flex around the pubic symphysis; but because it cannot flex around the sacrum, term fetuses in the mentum posterior position cannot safely deliver vaginally. A persistent mentoposterior (Figure 180.6) is therefore accepted as an absolute indication for CD. In the anterior position, the head delivers by flexing, so first the face emerges, then the brow, the sinciput, and the occiput. An episiotomy should be performed.

The mento-occipital diameter might be somewhat elongated because of molding. The baby's face is often quite swollen, and difficulties may sometimes arise because of laryngeal edema.

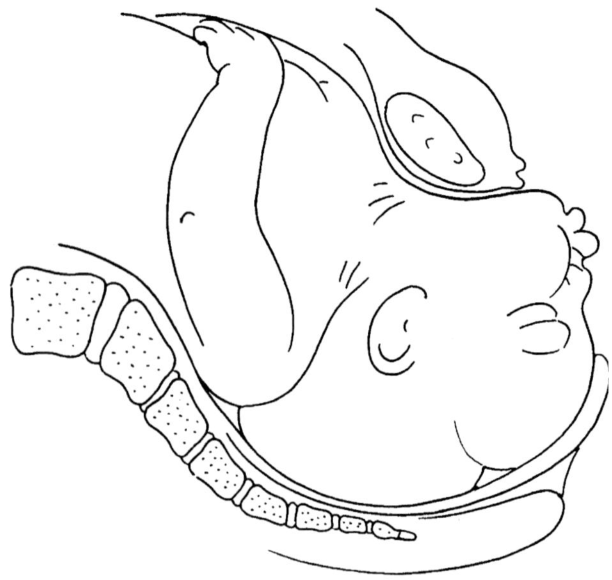

Figure 180.5 Face presentation, mentum anterior.

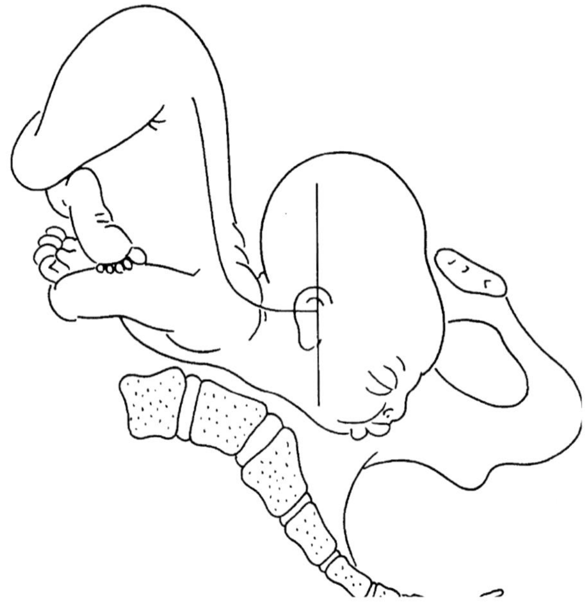

Figure 180.6 Face presentation, mentum posterior: indication for cesarean delivery.

Epidemiology and predisposing factors

Face presentations constituted 0.11% among more than 204,000 deliveries over 9 years in Slovenia,[3] an incidence similar to that reported by other authors.[22] Face presentation occurred in 0.9% of babies with a lethal malformation; in babies weighing less than 1500 g, 0.71% were face presentations. In association with polyhydramnios, 0.63% of the presentations were face, and with placenta previa, 0.46%. The percentage was the highest before 34 weeks (0.51%), dropped to 0.09% at term, and rose after 42 weeks to 0.18%. In primiparas there were 0.08%, in secundiparas 0.12%, in terciparas 0.16% and in those who delivered for the fourth time or more 0.18%, which is significantly different from brow presentation. The predisposing factors, listed in decreasing order of appearance, were the following: lethal malformations, low birth weight, polyhydramnios, prematurity, postmaturity, multiparity.

Myomas were not predisposing factors, nor were uterine anomalies, maternal age over 35 years, or birth weight over 4000 g.

Mode of delivery and complications

In the above-mentioned Slovenian sample, cesarean deliveries were performed in 44% of cases. Cord prolapse occurred nine times more often, rupture of the uterus 30 times more often (0.9% vs. 0.03%), and blood transfusion was given twice as often as in vertex presentations. The perinatal mortality was 5.8% compared to 0.7% in vertex presentations.

Conclusions

When labor starts, one can wait as long as there is no fetal distress and labor proceeds normally. Fetal anomalies should be ruled out. Very often, the face presentation does not undergo internal rotation until the face has encountered the pelvic floor. A persistent mentum posterior position is indication for a CD.

Figures by Bojan Pecar, reprinted with permission from Pajntar M, Novak-Antolic Z (eds): Pregnancy, labour and delivery management, Second edition, Slovenia, CZ 2004

REFERENCES

1. Chhabra S, Bhagwat N, Chakravorty A. Reduction in the occurrence of uterine rupture in Central India. *J Obstet Gynaecol* 2002;22:39–42.
2. Seffah JD. Maternal and perinatal mortality and morbidity associated with transverse lie. *Int J Gynaecol Obstet* 1999;65:1–5.
3. Verdenik I, Pajntar M. Perinatologia Slovenica 1995. Ljubljana: Reseach Unit, Department of Obstetrics and Gynecology, University Medical Centre, 1996:1–60.
4. Mancuso KM, Yancey MK, Murphy JA, Markenson GR. Epidural analgesia for cephalic version: A randomized trial. *Obstet Gynecol* 2000;95:648–51.
5. Berghella V. Prolapsed cord after external cephalic version in a patient with premature rupture of membranes and transverse lie. *Eur J Obstet Gynecol Reprod Biol* 2001;99:274–5.
6. Chan LY, Tang JL, Tsoi KF, Fok WY, Chan LW, Lau TK. Intrapartum cesarean delivery after successful external cephalic version: A meta-analysis. *Obstet Gynecol* 2004;104:155–60.
7. Hofmeyr GJ, Kulier R. External Cephalic Version for Breech Presentation at Term (Cochrane Review). The Cochrane Library, Issue 2, 2004.
8. Chauhan AR, Singhal TT, Raut VS. Is internal podalic version a lost art? Optimum mode of delivery in transverse lie. *J Postgrad Med* 2001;47:15–18.
9. Hofmeyr GJ. Obstructed labor: Using better technologies to reduce mortality. *Int J Gynecol Obstet* 2004;85(Suppl 1):S62–S72.
10. Bider D, Korach J, Hourvitz A, Dulitzky M, Goldenberg M, Mashiach S. Combined vaginal–abdominal delivery of twins. *J Reprod Med* 1995;40:131–4.
11. Blickstein I, Zalel Y, Weissman A. Cesarean delivery of the second twin after the vaginal birth of the first twin. Misfortune or mismanagement? *Acta Genet Med Gemellol* 1991;40:389–94.
12. Samra JS, Spillane H, Mukoyoko J, Tang L, Obhrai MS. Cesarean section for the birth of the second twin. *Br J Obstet Gynaecol* 1990;97:234–6.
13. Roopnarinesingh AJ. Abdominal delivery of the second twin. *J Obstet Gynaecol* 2002;22:379–80.
14. Crowther CA. Caesarean Delivery for the Second Twin (Cochrane Review). The Cochrane Library, Issue 2, 2004.
15. Tchabo J-G, Tomai T. Selected intrapartum external cephalic version of the second twin. *Obstet Gynecol* 1992;79:421–3.
16. Chauhan SP, Roberts WE, McLaren RA, Roach H, Morrison JC, Martin JN Jr. Delivery of the nonvertex second twin: Breech extraction versus external cephalic version. *Am J Obstet Gynecol* 1995;173:1015–20.
17. Dufour P, Vinatier D, Vanderstichele S, Ducloy AS, Depret S, Monnier JC. Intravenous nitroglycerin for internal podalic version of the second twin in transverse lie. *Obstet Gynecol* 1998;92:416–9.
18. Cristalli B, Stella V, Heid M, Izard V, Levardon M. La grande extraction du deuxième jumeau avec ou sans version par manoeuvres internes. *J Gynecol Obstet Biol Reprod* 1992; 21:705–7.
19. Gocke SE, Nageotte MP, Garite T, Craig VT, Dorcester W. Management of the non vertex second twin: Primary cesarean section, external version, or primary breech extraction. *Am J Obstet Gynecol* 1989;161:111–14.
20. Hutton EK, Hannah ME, Barrett J. Use of external cephalic version for breech pregnancy and mode of delivery for breech and twin pregnancy: A survey of Canadian practitioners. *J Obstet Gynaecol Can* 2002;24:804–10.
21. Sibony O, Touitou S, Luton D, Oury JF, Blot PH. A comparison of the neonatal morbidity of second twins to that of a low-risk population. *Eur J Obstet Gynecol Reprod Biol* 2003;108:157–63.
22. Lenehan PM, MacDonald D, Turner MJ. Face and brow presentation. *J Obstet Gynecol* 1986;7:102–6.

181 Breech presentation

M. Foley and M. Alarab

Introduction

The incidence of breech presentation is relatively low at term, but because cesarean birth is the mode of delivery in at least 50% of cases, maternal mortality and morbidity are increased. Perinatal mortality and morbidity rates are increased for a number of reasons, of which prematurity is the most significant. The incidence of breech presentation is about 20% at 28 weeks' gestation and 3% at term, indicating that most fetuses that are in a breech presentation early in gestation undergo spontaneous cephalic version. In countries with high rates of premature birth, the incidence of breech delivery is therefore proportionately higher.

The major controversy regarding the management of breech presentation concerns the question of what method should be used for delivery at term: is a trial of labor and vaginal delivery in selected cases as safe as universal cesarean section? This question took on particular importance following publication of the Term Breech Trial in 2000,[1] which concluded that elective cesarean birth was best for breech presentations at term. Interestingly, at the same time this approach was being recommended as the standard of care, individual centers were reporting the safety of vaginal breech birth.[2–4] Of great concern with regard to setting policy is that vaginal breech delivery requires a degree of skill acquired by practice and experience. Even if vaginal delivery by an experienced attendant were appropriate, one may reasonably ask how today's obstetricians in training can acquire that skill in the context of shorter work hours and fewer vaginal breech deliveries available to allow the requisite acquisition of skill and clinical judgment? Of course, those skills will be necessary under any circumstances because a proportion of planned cesarean births will labor and may present in advanced labor when the expertise for a safe vaginal delivery is needed; also, some mothers may opt to have a trial of vaginal breech birth.

External cephalic version (ECV) would seem an obvious answer for the breech problem, but suffers from variable popularity in different countries and within institutions, possibly because the procedure is not without risk (albeit small), requires a measure of skill and experience, and has a relatively high failure rate – an unpopular combination with many obstetricians. There is a danger that this expertise may also be lost as part of the breech controversy, because some obstetricians now feel that cesarean section is the only solution for breech presentation in general. Moreover, a greater proportion of women are declining the offer of ECV than in the past and are opting for cesarean birth. Perhaps, critical to the current controversies is the question of informed consent based on objective evidence for both trial of vaginal breech delivery and ECV, balancing short- and long-term risks of cesarean delivery for the mother and baby.

Cesarean delivery for breech birth has been shown to increase both short- and long-term maternal morbidity and mortality in both observational and randomized controlled studies,[5–8] not least because it predisposes to further cesareans in subsequent pregnancies. A change to cesarean delivery for all breech presentations in institutions currently offering a trial of vaginal delivery (with a 50% vaginal delivery rate) would double the cesarean rate attributable to breech presentation from 2% to 4% of all term deliveries, with an inevitable incremental effect on the repeat cesarean rate.

Etiology

Premature delivery is the commonest reason for breech presentation, just because there will have been insufficient opportunity for spontaneous version. The fetus may be a factor: the majority of breech presentations at term have extended legs, suggesting that this posture prevents spontaneous version. Version is less likely to occur spontaneously in nulliparas compared with multiparas, probably because of increased uterine tone or abdominal wall tone or both and is also less likely to occur in a patient who has had a previous breech delivery, presumably because of some uterine factor[9] (Table 181.1; Figure 181.1). A fetal malformation may be a factor. For example, hydrocephalus may prevent version, as may a neurologic deficit in which poor muscular activity does not promote spontaneous version. Seemingly high rates of long-term handicap have been reported

Table 181.1 Likelihood of spontaneous turning during pregnancy in two groups of mothers (from Westgren *et al.*,[9] with permission)

Ultrasound findings	Persistent breech ($n=133$)	Spontaneous cephalic version ($n=177$)
Fetal size		
Biparietal diameter, mm (SD)	82.2 (4.4)	82.6 (3.9)
Abdominal diameter,* mm (SD)	90.4 (5.6)	91.2 (5.4)
Femur length, mm (SD)	62.3 (2.8)	(2.9)
Fetal posture		
Legs flexed at knees, *n* (%)	27 (20)	92 (52)**
Legs extended, *n* (%)	106 (80)	85 (48)
Placenta location		
Fundal, *n* (%)	49 (37)	65 (37)
Anterior, *n* (%)	53 (40)	91 (51)
Posterior, *n* (%)	31 (23)	21 (12)

*Mean of anterior–posterior and transverse diameters; **significant difference between the two groups, $P<0.001$

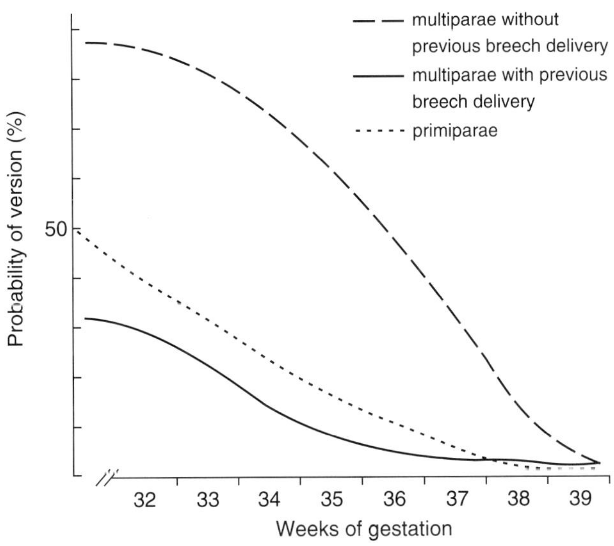

Figure 181.1 Probability of spontaneous version of breech to cephalic presentation according to parity, gestational age, and prior breech delivery

in term breech fetuses independent of the method of delivery – cesarean or vaginal – but data on outcome of cephalic births were not always available for comparison.[10] While there has always been the anecdotal suggestion of an 'inherent' breech problem, this may not be true when corrected for prematurity and intrauterine growth restriction.[11] Excessive or reduced amniotic fluid volume are risk factors, as is placenta previa, the management of which takes priority over the presentation. Uterine malformations are obvious causes, and occasionally a pelvic tumor, e.g. a leiomyoma or ovarian cyst, may prevent spontaneous cephalic version.

Techniques of breech delivery and their attendant risks are related in part to the type of breech presentation that exists (Figure 181.2). The commonest type of breech presentation is the extended or frank breech, in which both legs are extended at the knee (60%). The flexed or complete breech (15%) has both legs flexed at the knee. The footling breech (25 %) has one or both feet presenting.

Perinatal mortality and morbidity

Prematurity and its consequences are the major contributors to mortality and morbidity: extreme prematurity incompatible with survival, intraventricular hemorrhage, respiratory distress syndrome, infection, necrotizing enterocolitis, jaundice, feeding difficulties, and the psychosocial effects of being in a neonatal intensive care unit all affect outcome. Neonatal respiratory morbidity is also increased up to fivefold following elective cesarean delivery,[12] and while delaying delivery until after 39 weeks' gestation can minimize this, the chance of having to deal with a breech in spontaneous labor increases.

Perinatal mortality specific to vaginal breech delivery includes cord prolapse, anoxia caused by delay in the actual delivery of the breech, and traumatic intracranial hemorrhage. The latter can be related to difficulty delivering the head, or in the opposite case, to a rapid uncontrolled delivery associated with sudden compression and then decompression of the unmolded head. Both situations can result in tearing of the falx cerebri and associated catastrophic intracranial hemorrhage. Intrapartum and early neonatal hypoxic deaths are highest when intrauterine growth restriction has been undiagnosed[13], and when there exist fetal heart rate abnormalities in labor.[14] Skeletal trauma can include fracture of the femur during vaginal delivery and can also be a problem at cesarean delivery when the legs are extended. The clavicle or humerus may be fractured during delivery of the shoulders. Skeletal injuries generally heal quickly with no long-term sequelae. Cranial nerve or nerve root injury can occur but seem to be less common than with shoulder dystocia;[1] recovery depends on the degree of the initial trauma.

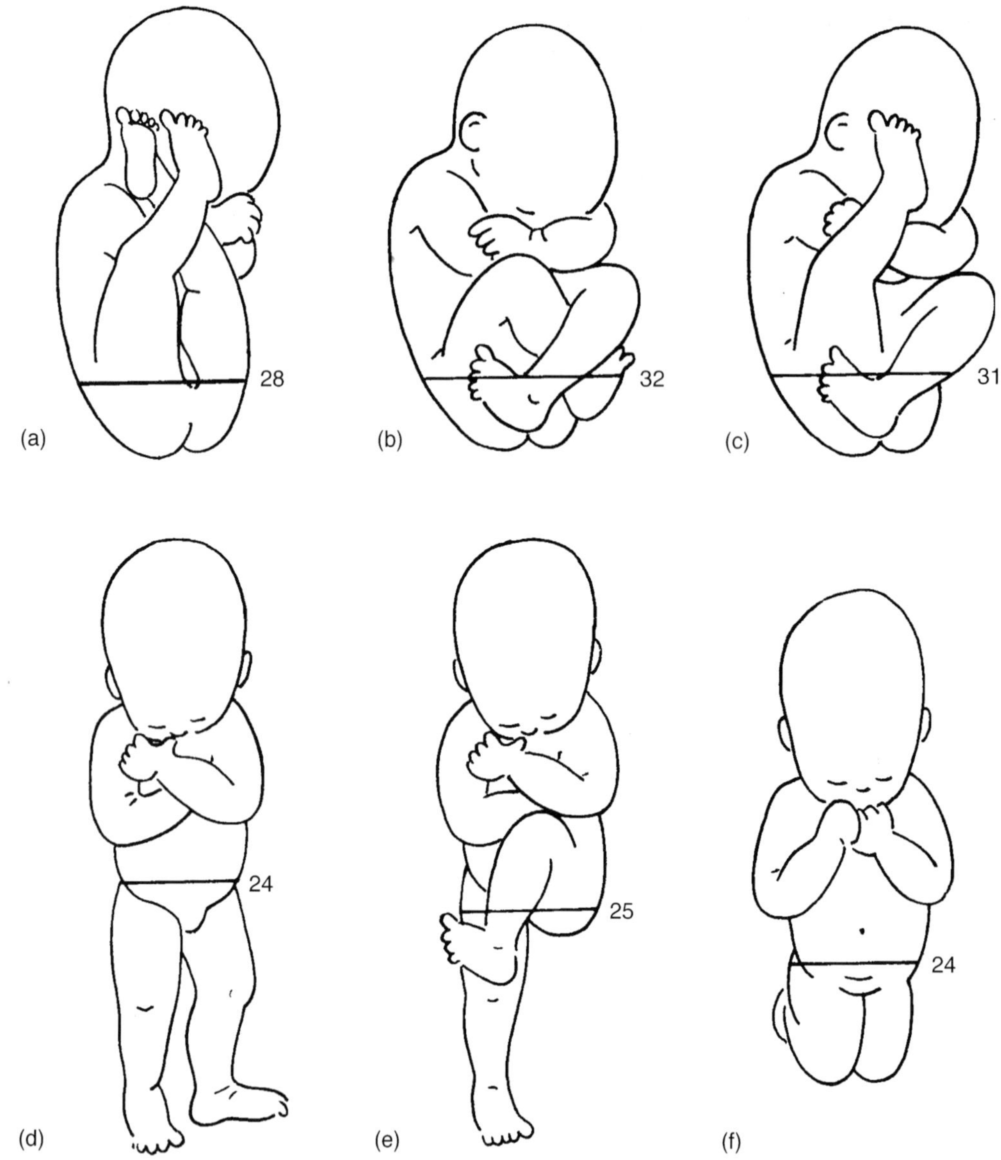

Figure 181.2 Types of breech presentations: (a) frank breech; (b) complete breech/footling; (c) incomplete breech/footling; (d) complete footling; (e) incomplete footling; (f) knee. Numbers indicate largest circumference of the presenting part (cm) in an average size fetus. From Pajntar, M. Breech presentation. In Kurjak A. *Textbook of Perinatal Medicine*, 1st edn. London: Parthenon Publishing, 1998.

The genitalia, facial structures, and even intra-abdominal viscera may be injured, but these injuries area not exclusive to vaginal breech delivery; they can also occur at cesarean section. The 2-year neurologic follow-up of babies in the Term Breech Trial[15] showed no differences between the planned vaginal breech delivery and the planned cesarean section groups, and similar results have been reported at 7 years comparing breech and cephalic deliveries.[16]

Diagnosis

The diagnosis is made by abdominal palpation, and while not really relevant until 34 weeks' gestation, it is worth noting at earlier visits to serve as an *aide memoire* for 34 weeks when the option of ECV should first be considered. Difficulty palpating a fetal head above the pelvic brim, or the sense that there is a deeply engaged head should raise the possibility of malpresentation. With increasing use of imaging in antenatal care, the incidence of undiagnosed breech presentation should be minimal, and while a cephalic presentation can revert to a breech at any time in multiparas, this probably almost never happens in late pregnancy in nulliparas.

Occasionally, a patient will present in labor with an indeterminable presentation on vaginal examination. The differential diagnosis generally includes breech presentation, face presentation, compound presentation, shoulder presentation, fetal malformation (e.g. anencephaly), and, rarely, a pelvic tumor (e.g. a cervical fibroid or an ovarian cyst in the Pouch of Douglas), or even a congenital uterine abnormality (e.g. a prolapsed uterine horn). The diagnosis is made by palpation but should be confirmed by ultrasound. The management of most of these cases, with the exception of anencephaly, often is cesarean section. A plain film of the abdomen might be helpful in some circumstances when neither palpation nor ultrasound can confirm the diagnosis.

External cephalic version

With the decline in enthusiasm for vaginal breech delivery the main opportunity for reducing the rate of cesarean section for breech presentation is to increase the use of ECV, and the availability of this procedure to all patients is recommended by both the American and the Royal Colleges of Obstetricians and Gynecologists.[17,18] Since the Term Breech Trial, however, there has been a decline in enthusiasm for ECV as well as for vaginal breech delivery.[19]

There is good evidence that ECV reduces the incidence of non-cephalic births by nearly 60%,[20] although the risk of intrapartum cesarean is still higher after successful ECV than for spontaneous cephalic presentations.[21] One study calculated that four attempted version procedures were required to prevent one cesarean section, reducing to two attempts if applying current practice of cesarean section for all term breech presentations.[22] Despite this, the technique is not part of routine clinical service in many centers;[23,24] and in general the uptake of ECV is low, partly because of patient refusal.[22,25] The success rate is greater in multiparas (60%) compared with nulliparas (40%), presumably because uterine and abdominal wall tone is greater in nulliparas, which is a strong argument for analyzing all data separately by parity. A disproportionately higher number of nulliparas presented in our series[4] with a breech presentation, which may have reflected the higher success rate of ECV in multiparas. Although the success rate of ECV declines with advancing gestational age, it is generally recommended that it be carried out at 37 weeks' gestation, to allow for spontaneous version in some cases, reduce the incidence of spontaneous reversion of the fetus, and minimize potential neonatal problems in the event of an emergency delivery being required.

Comparing ECV at 34–36 weeks' gestation with 37–38 weeks' gestation, the rates of breech presentation at birth were lower in the early ECV group, but not significantly so,[26] and a recent Cochrane review[27] concluded that early ECV was not effective in lowering non-cephalic presentation or the rate of cesarean section. A survey of practice in Australia and New Zealand[24] (74% response rate) found, nevertheless, that almost 40% of obstetricians attempted ECV before 37 weeks. While neither of the authors of this chapter has experience in the use of tocolytics to facilitate ECV, analysis of a variety of interventions, including use of tocolytics, fetal acoustic stimulation, epidural or spinal regional analgesia vs. none, showed that only the use of routine tocolysis with beta-stimulants was associated with fewer failures of ECV.[28]

Therefore, the major decisions concerning the use of ECV relate to the gestational age at which the procedure is attempted, particularly in relation to parity, and the use of tocolytic drugs. Despite all the evidence, our experience is that the best chance of ECV in nulliparas is between 34 and 36 weeks. It is extremely rare for a cephalic presentation to convert to breech in nulliparas and for this to occur after a 'successful' ECV would suggest that the ECV was not successful in the first place. The same is not true of multiparas and for them ECV at 37–38 weeks is reasonable, but has to be balanced against parity. A multipara with one previous pregnancy is not the same as one with five, who might almost be regarded as having an unstable lie. On this basis, if tocolytics are to be used they should certainly be offered to nulliparas. It is our understanding that many of these questions will be answered by ongoing randomized trials.

Complications of ECV are well documented. Antepartum hemorrhage complicating the procedure must be interpreted as being due to placental separation and therefore requiring delivery, usually by cesarean. Factors predisposing to placental separation (hypertension, a previous antepartum hemorrhage) are therefore relative contraindications to ECV. Fetomaternal transfusion is an issue in two respects: in the rhesus-negative patient immunoprophylaxis is recommended, which may deter patients from undergoing ECV; also, a major fatal fetomaternal transfusion may rarely occur during the procedure. The potential complication of cord entanglement unfortunately captures the imagination (particularly of the patient), but should not be any more common than with spontaneous version. Certainly, the fetal heart slows down if pressure is applied to the fetal head and a bradycardia is common after an attempted or successful ECV. The wise option is to perform fetal heart rate monitoring as well as an ultrasound scan prior to the procedure, because in some cases breech presentation is associated with preexisting fetal compromise (abnormal fetal heart rate pattern, fetal growth restriction, reduced amniotic fluid) and this should be excluded as far as possible before embarking on ECV. The fetal heart rate should be monitored after the procedure, but it must be borne in mind that temporary fetal heart rate abnormalities are common after ECV and should be anticipated. The risk of emergency cesarean section for fetal distress following ECV is small, at less than 1%.[29,30] Both Royal and American Colleges recommend that the procedure be performed in a hospital setting with emergency facilities available; whether it should be performed in the operating theatre with the patient fasting is questionable. Relative contraindications to ECV include previous cesarean section and other previous uterine surgery (e.g. myomectomy) and an estimated birth weight at term of greater than 3800 g, as the failure rate is higher with larger babies.

The management of ECV

Ideally, cases should be referred to a dedicated breech clinic. The question of consent, balancing the risks of ECV, vaginal breech delivery, and cesarean birth should be initiated by the referring doctor; but if presented in a negative fashion it is probably not worth referring the patient. A good service, well organized and with good results, would obviously help to dispel any negative preconceptions. Every attempt should be made to diagnose breech presentation at 34 weeks' gestation, to allow plenty of time to formulate a plan of management. The initial assessment includes a structured ultrasound examination documenting placental site, estimated fetal weight, amniotic fluid estimation, type of breech, fetal attitude, and fetal morphology. ECV is offered with informed consent if the estimated fetal weight, amniotic fluid volume, placental site, and fetal morphology are normal. A non-stress test is performed before and after the procedure.

A useful technique is as follows: The presenting breech is first disengaged from the pelvis and directed laterally at least 90 degrees; generally, the head would have passed 90° in the other direction. Then, both poles can be manipulated in tandem to complete the ECV. Manipulation of the head as a first step is less likely to be successful except perhaps in a multiparous patient. When a tocolytic is to be prescribed, and provided there are no medical contraindications, the drug is administered 30 min before the procedure. Most recommend no more than two attempts at ECV in any one session, but ECV can be repeated later in the pregnancy; this decision is determined by how early the initial attempt is made.

The premature breech

The management of the premature breech in labor has clearer established guidelines, mainly favoring cesarean delivery, although this approach has not been subjected to large clinical trials. The evidence suggests that cesarean birth reduces neonatal mortality in babies less than 32 weeks and weighing less than 1500 g,[31,32] with no differences in the incidence of handicap between the two methods of delivery.

Condition at birth is a major determinant of early neonatal progress, and while neonatologists would probably favor cesarean delivery for the premature baby, abdominal delivery does not guarantee an easy birth. When the lower uterine segment is poorly developed, a high transverse incision is preferable to an inadequate low incision, which may necessitate extending the incision into the upper uterine segment or making a T-incision in order to deliver the baby. Anecdotal evidence suggests that a high transverse incision through the upper segment of the uterus is less likely to rupture in a subsequent pregnancy than a vertical incision in that area. Prior preterm cesarean section is, however, a risk factor for uterine rupture in a subsequent labor[33] and this should be a consideration when deciding to perform a preterm cesarean delivery, particularly if subsequent deliveries are likely to be poorly supervised. When the birth weight is between 1500 and 2500 g the concern is that the cervix may entrap the aftercoming head and for that reason cesarean section is recommended. This is an unpredictable and unpreventable emergency and the treatment options include using traction and making relieving incisions in the cervix. The main complications are trauma and asphyxia secondary to delayed delivery, often with a catastrophic outcome for the neonate.

Vaginal breech delivery at term

Case selection and management in labor are most important when considering a trial of vaginal delivery, and the old maxim of 'breech and any other problem – cesarean section' still holds true. General non-specific obstetric indications for elective prelabor cesarean delivery include maternal age, infertility, maternal disease likely to put the fetus at risk (e.g. diabetes), and significant preeclampsia. In our center, prelabor cesarean delivery is offered at 41 weeks as an alternative to induction because oxytocin to induce or augment labor is more likely to be required following induction of labor and for prolonged pregnancy, particularly in nulliparas; oxytocin is not used either to augment or to induce labor with a breech presentation.

It is generally felt that an estimated birth weight of 3800 g at term should be the cutoff for a trial of vaginal delivery, but there are difficulties in predicting birth weight on palpation and by ultrasound. To be a candidate for a vaginal delivery, the fetus should be in the extended or flexed position, i.e. not footling. Hyperextension of the fetal head – an angle of extension of greater than 90° – is rare, but must be excluded because hyperextension makes vaginal delivery of the head very difficult. If the problem is not recognized in labor until delivery of the head, it may be, unfortunately, too late to prevent spinal cord injury. Any evidence of fetal compromise such as suspected intrauterine growth restriction or oligohydramnios is an indication for cesarean section.

Although the selection criteria for elective cesarean section from various centers are similar, the reported percentage considered suitable for a trial of vaginal delivery varies from less than 20% in some hospitals

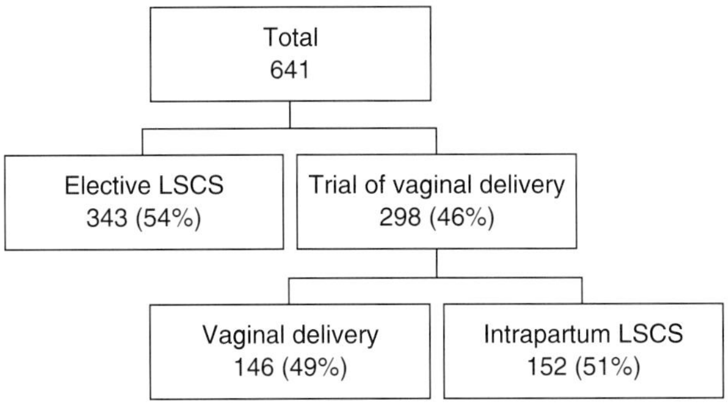

Figure 181.3 Obstetric outcome in 641 consecutive vaginal breech presentations at term, analyzed according to intended and actual route of delivery. Adapted from Alarab *et al.*,[4] with permission.

in the USA[34,35] to around 70% in some European centers;[3,36] 56% were considered suitable for a trial of labor in the Term Breech Trial. Less clearly defined in most series are the criteria for management of breech labor, particularly in relation to the timing of the onset of labor, and hence the diagnosis of prolonged labor, time limits for the duration of the first and second stages of labor both for nulliparas and multiparas, the use of oxytocin to augment labor, the question of induction of labor, and the expertise of the obstetrician conducting or supervising a vaginal breech delivery.

In our unit, patients are offered a trial of vaginal delivery if the following criteria are fulfilled: (1) estimated fetal weight 2500–3800 g; (2) deepest amniotic fluid pool 30 mm or more; (3) normal fetal morphology and normal placental location; (4) absence of hyperextension of the fetal head (an angle exceeding 90°); and (5) flexed (complete) or extended (frank) breech presentation. Management of fetal anomalies depends on the type of malformation identified. Elective prelabor cesarean section is advised based on the following indications: estimated fetal weight more than 3800 g, footling breech, hyperextension of the fetal head, or when fetal compromise is suspected. Maternal indications for elective cesarean section include maternal preference, previous cesarean section, significant preeclampsia, and placenta previa. Induction of labor is not practiced with breech presentation. Elective prelabor cesareans are scheduled for 39 weeks' gestation or, if a trial of labor has been planned, at 41 weeks if labor has not ensued.

On admission in spontaneous labor, a vaginal examination is carried out early in labor to confirm the type of presentation, to exclude cord presentation, and to rupture the membranes in order to inspect the amniotic fluid. Oxytocin is not used to augment labor in the first or second stage. Time constraints for the first and second stages are based on the average duration of the first and second stages of labor in this hospital for nulliparas and multiparas.[37] The average first-stage durations are 6 and 2 h, and the active second stages 1 h and 30 min, respectively; up to 1 h may be allowed for descent of the presenting part at full dilatation but not associated with active pushing. We have a very low threshold for intervention and cesarean section in both the first and second stages of labor if there is delay or if fetal distress is noted. The presence of meconium with a breech presentation does not necessarily indicate fetal distress; nevertheless, its presence should not be altogether ignored if detected in early labor. All should have continuous external monitoring in labor, and cesarean section should be performed for suspected fetal distress with a breech presentation. Epidural administration is based on maternal request. An experienced obstetrician (senior resident with at least 4 years' experience or a consultant) conducts all vaginal breech deliveries, and a pediatrician is also in attendance.

In our institution, during a 42-month study period[4] up to the year 2000, 641 patients presented with singleton breech presentation at term, of whom 374 (58%) were nulliparas and 267 (42%) were multiparas. They were managed according to the guidelines outlined above. Applying our selection criteria, 343 patients (54%) underwent elective prelabor cesarean section, and 298 (46%) progressed to a trial of vaginal delivery (Figure 181.3). Specific obstetric indications for elective prelabor cesarean delivery were present in 56% of cases; these included birth weight more than 3800 g, gestation more than 41 weeks, previous cesarean section, pre-eclampsia, oligohydramnios, suspected intrauterine growth restriction, hemolytic disease, and placenta prevail. Non-specific indications, such as maternal or obstetrician's preference pertained in 151 cases (44%).

Of 298 patients who progressed to a trial of vaginal delivery, 146 (49% of the total) delivered vaginally and 152 (51%) were delivered by intrapartum cesarean section (Figure 181.2); 13 (8.6%) intrapartum cesareans were performed in the second stage of labor. One hundred and forty-three of the intrapartum cesarean sections (94%) were performed for failure to progress in labor and seven (4.6%) for suspected fetal distress; all seven babies had Apgar scores of 9 at 1 min. The vaginal delivery rate in multiparas (63%) was significantly higher than the rate in nulliparas (37%) ($P < 0.001$) (Figures 181.4 and 181.5). Nine patients (6%), two nulliparas and seven multiparas, were ready to deliver on admission to the delivery ward. There were two intrapartum cesarean sections for cord prolapse: one was detected on admission in labor and one 2 h after admission. Epidural analgesia was used in 53% of labors (nulliparas 61% and multiparas 45%); 82 (56%) women with epidural analgesia delivered vaginally.

Mean birth weight and the frequency of birth weight exceeding 3800 g were significantly greater in

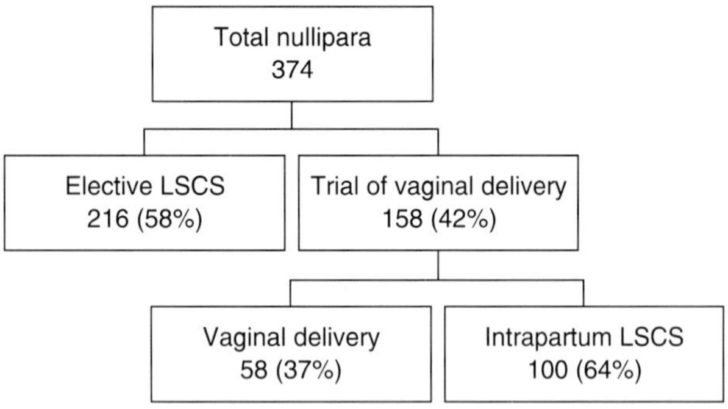

Figure 181.4 Outcome of labor in nulliparas. Adapted from Alarab *et al.*[4] with permission.

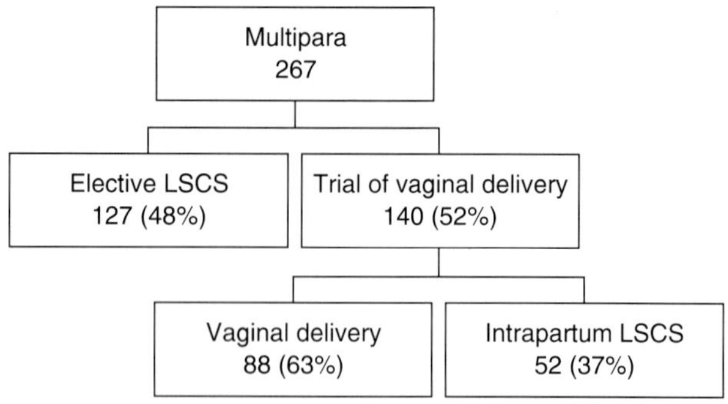

Figure 181.5 Outcome of labor in multiparas. Adapted from Alarab *et al.*[4] with permission.

women delivered by elective or intrapartum cesarean section compared with those delivered vaginally, particularly among nulliparas. The mean durations of the first and second stages of labor for nulliparas who delivered vaginally were 4.4 h (range 0.5–11), and 24 min (5–75), respectively, and for multiparas they were 3.0 h (0.2–11), and 13 min (10–45), respectively, indicating that our criteria for management of labor, including avoiding oxytocin and applying strict time limits for the first and second stages of labor, select out the larger babies for cesarean delivery. There was no significant neonatal morbidity and no intrapartum or neonatal deaths in normally formed infants in either the vaginally or cesarean delivered cohorts.

This study, in keeping with other well-organized retrospective studies[2,3,34,38,39] showed that vaginal delivery is still a safe option provided strict criteria for selection for a trial of labor and for the management of labor are applied, with a low threshold for cesarean delivery in either the first or the second stage of labor, and an experienced obstetrician to conduct the delivery.

The Term Breech Trial showed that cesarean delivery was safer than vaginal delivery for a breech birth and that perinatal morbidity and mortality were increased by a factor of 3 in the planned vaginal breech delivery group. These findings have been criticized for a number of reasons.[34,40] Intrauterine growth restriction, one of the exclusion criteria for vaginal breech delivery, was underdiagnosed; fetal monitoring in labor was inadequate; induction and oxytocin augmentation of labor were freely used; the definitions of prolonged first and second stages of labor would be questionable in most centers with a cephalic presentation; the study was conducted in 26 different centers with a range of approaches and possibly experience, and some of the centers had very few vaginal breech deliveries. An unexpected finding was that a composite of adverse perinatal outcomes was worse in countries with low background perinatal mortality rates; but analysis of perinatal deaths only showed no difference and revealed that some were unrelated to the method of delivery. The definition of perinatal morbidity used in the study has been questioned, and the normal outcome at 2 years for both arms of the trial supports that criticism.[15]

The study was, however, unique because of its size and organization and will probably never be repeated. While the Term Breech Trial was randomized and prospective, a large retrospective study[36] of over 33,000 breech deliveries from the Netherlands in Northern Europe reported results similar to those of the Term Breech Trial. This report from a country in which practices have been fairly standard and stable over years, and where vaginal breech delivery is widely practiced, probably carries more weight on this side of the Atlantic, because of their strong background experience of vaginal breech delivery and also because of a presumption in that country that vaginal breech delivery was perfectly safe with careful selection (at least until the publication of their recent trends[19]). The Dutch study also addressed one important question by showing that cesarean section was safer even in a group managed without induction or augmentation of labor with oxytocin, thus addressing a potential weakness in the interpretation of the Term Breech Trial. They did report that the highest neonatal morbidity and mortality occurred with delivery of the aftercoming head and was related to the duration of the second stage (a 20% complication rate with the aftercoming head after 90 min in the second stage).[36] This is a complication that we advise could be minimized with stricter guidelines for the duration of the second stage for nulliparas and multiparas. Although the question of the presence of an experienced obstetrician for the delivery was not addressed, we would assume that this was the case in the Netherlands. The authors suggested that obstetricians had rushed with 'unseemly haste' (*Macbeth*) to abandon vaginal breech delivery and perhaps should show more consideration for the long-term consequences of cesarean delivery.[36]

A study from Finland that compared breech cesarean delivery, breech vaginal delivery, and vertex vaginal delivery interestingly found no significant differences in perinatal mortality between the vertex and breech vaginal deliveries and less trauma in the vaginal breech delivery group, although the Apgar scores were lower in the breech vaginal group. All adverse events were lowest in the planned cesarean section group. The breech vaginal group required fewer admissions to the outpatient department and the cumulative incidence of long-term morbidity in the breech vaginal delivery group was smaller to the age of 7 years than in the breech planned cesarean group. Age at going to school and school performance showed no dependence on the mode of delivery. They asked the question, 'Are our expectations of term breech infants unrealistically high?'.[16] A neonatal follow-up of babies born in the Term Breech Trial showed no significant differences at 2 years between the various groups.[15] Our study showed that with careful selection, careful management in labor, and the mandatory presence of an experienced obstetrician (arguably the most important factor), safe vaginal delivery could be achieved. With fewer vaginal breech deliveries, and shorter working hours for physicians (at least in Europe), the need for an experienced attendant at a breech delivery is fast becoming the weak link in the chain.

Studies[1,8] comparing morbidity in elective vs. emergency cesarean section for breech presentation showed no difference, although it has been argued[41] that the increased morbidity associated with emergency cesarean section in general outweighs the gain in vaginal breech delivery once the number of vaginal breech deliveries falls below a critical level. With our criteria for the management of breech labor, emergency cesareans are performed relatively early in labor (average 3.8 h, range 0.5–9 h in nulliparas and 2.4 h, range 0.5–8 h in multiparas) and because the lower segment has thinned out and the breech is usually not deeply engaged in the pelvis they are arguably the easiest cesareans from a technical point of view. Emergency cesareans after prolonged labor with a cephalic presentation are as difficult as an elective cesarean section with a poorly formed vascular lower segment, whatever be the presentation. We are not recommending a trial of vaginal breech delivery to facilitate a subsequent cesarean section, but feel strongly that the argument regarding an increased morbidity with emergency cesarean section is irrelevant within the guidelines for the duration of labor in our reported series.

Conduct of vaginal breech delivery

The breech is allowed to descend spontaneously to the maternal perineum; the fetal anus should be visible with a contraction. When delivery appears imminent, timing is critical to ensure that the delivery commences at the start of a contraction, holding back the presenting part if necessary. As the contraction begins, an episiotomy is timed to coincide with a concentrated maternal effort, the objective being to deliver the trunk of the baby with a single contraction. If the trunk delivers only up to halfway, we do not advise delivering the legs at this stage because the extended legs of the frank breech act as a splint to protect the cord, and may also provide a better stimulus for the next contraction than the soft fetal abdomen. If difficulty is experienced with delivery of the shoulders with the next contraction, traction should be applied to the fetal pelvis, keeping in mind the potential risk of damaging intra-abdominal viscera. Lovsett's maneuver should be used to deliver the shoulders. In general, traction should only be required as a last resort and the breech should be allowed to deliver by maternal effort. The breech should now be suspended from the mother, as this facilitates passage of the fetal head into the pelvis. Delivery of the head is controlled by either the Mauriceau–Smellie–Veit maneuver or with obstetric forceps. Some obstetricians find it easier to control the descent and delivery of the head using forceps and employ them routinely; in this case, the forceps are not used for traction. The most important principle is to deliver the head slowly, as rapid compression and decompression of a fetal head that has not undergone gradual molding can result in a tentorial tear or other injury. The same principles hold for cesarean breech delivery.

If the head does not descend into the pelvis on its own and delivery is not imminent with the next contraction, either of the above procedures can be used to deliver the head into the pelvis. In most centers, operative deliveries are performed in the lithotomy position, but delivery in the left lateral position should be considered because access is easier, and the baby can be suspended over the side of the bed when the trunk has been delivered.

Alternative approaches

Alternative methods to encouraging cephalic version and for vaginal breech delivery are described as part of an excellent and balanced review of the whole question of breech birth[42] but we have no personal experience with these.

The aftermath of the Term Breech Trial

The experience in the aftermath of publication of the Term Breech Trial was an almost immediate, dramatic change in practice, amplifying an already existing trend of rising cesarean sections rates for term singleton breech presentation. This trend had been first reported from the Netherlands,[18] with similar experience in the USA,[43] Canada,[44] and Australia/New Zealand.[19,45] The incidence of term breech has increased significantly in the periods studied, which may reflect a degree of indifference to the practice of ECV, which has been proposed as a viable solution for the rising cesarean section rate for breech presentation.[23] What was most surprising in some of the centers was the rapidity with which vaginal breech delivery was dropped in favor of cesarean section. It seemed almost as if a generation of obstetricians, secretly terrified of vaginal breech delivery, could hardly wait for the 'permission' to abandon the practice that the Trial seemed to provide.[19] Nevertheless, the experience from the randomized trial (10%) and from our study (6%) showed that a proportion of women scheduled for planned cesarean breech delivery presented in an advanced stage of labor and required a vaginal delivery. In some cases, the diagnosis of a breech presentation will first be made in labor; in a comparison of such cases with antenatally diagnosed breeches, a higher vaginal delivery rate with no increase in neonatal morbidity among the cases diagnosed in labor was reported.[46]

In an editorial[43] titled 'Teaching Infrequently Used Skills: Vaginal Breech Delivery', the editor of the *American Journal of Obstetrics and Gynecology* argued that given two opposing views (vaginal vs. cesarean breech delivery), the one appearing to minimize professional liability risk will prevail in this litigious age. This view makes more compelling the question: How will we teach vaginal breech delivery? Perhaps we need to learn from educational approaches used for other infrequently used skills such as cardiopulmonary resuscitation (CPR) and management of shoulder dystocia. Teaching films, hands-on sessions, and mannequins have been shown to be of value in teaching CPR. Such approaches should be brought to bear for breech delivery. It is also important to remember that the technique of breech delivery during a cesarean section is similar to a vaginal breech delivery. All the common maneuvers – Lovsett, Mauriceau–Smellie–Veit, and application of forceps to the aftercoming head – are routinely employed, and a formal teaching approach could be used at this time.

In conclusion, the evidence suggests that most obstetricians feel that cesarean section is the preferred method of delivery for breech presentation, and this is already the prevalent approach in the developed world. There is evidence that ECV can reduce the incidence of breech presentation at term. Numerous studies from individual institutions have reported the safety of vaginal breech delivery at term, but whether this expertise can be maintained with fewer vaginal breech deliveries requires careful monitoring. Developing countries will have to balance a practice of prelabor cesarean for breech presentation against the long-term maternal risk of cesarean delivery, particularly where subsequent labor is likely to be poorly supervised, and also with the immediate complications and cost implications. It is an interesting irony that when the expertise for vaginal breech delivery exists and where vaginal breech delivery is widely practiced, there are arguably better results for this presentation compared with the developed world.[1]

REFERENCES

1. Hannah ME, Hannah WJ, Hewson SA, Hodnett ED, Saigai S, Willan AR. Planned caesarean section versus planned vaginal birth for breech presentation at term: A randomised multicentre trial. *Lancet* 2000;356:1375–83.
2. De Leeuw JP, De Hann J, Derom R, Thiery M, Martens G, Van Maele G. Mortality and early neonatal morbidity in vaginal and abdominal deliveries in breech presentation. *J Obstet Gynaecol* 2002;22:127–39.
3. Giuliani A, Scholl W, Basver A, Tamussino K. Mode of delivery and outcome of 699 term singleton breech deliveries at a single center. *Am J Obstet Gynecol* 2002;187:1694–8.
4. Alarab M, Regan C, O'Connell MP, Keane DP, O'Herlihy C, Foley ME. Singleton vaginal breech delivery at term: Still a safe option. *Am J Obstet Gynecol* 2004;103:407–12.
5. Schuitemaker N, van Roosmalen J, Dekker G, van Donegen P, van Geijn H, Bennebroek GJ. Maternal mortality after cesarean section in the Netherlands. *Acta Obstet Gynecol Scand* 1997;75: 332–4.
6. Green R, Gardeil F, Turner MJ. Long-term implications of cesarean section. *Am J Obstet Gynecol* 1997;176:254–5.
7. Hemminiki E, Merilainen J. Long-term effects of cesarean sections: Ectopic pregnancies and placental problems. *Am J Obstet Gynecol* 1996;174:1569–74.
8. Sanchez-Ramos L, Wells TL, Adair CD, Arcelin G, Kaunitz AM, Wells DS. Route of breech delivery and maternal and neonatal outcomes. *Int J Gynecol Obstet* 2001;73:7–14.
9. Westgren M, Edvall H, Nordstrom L, Svalenius E, Ranstam J. Spontaneous cephalic version of breech presentation in the last trimester. *Br J Obstet Gynaecol* 1985;92:19–22.
10. Danielian PJ, Wang J, Hall MH. Long-term outcome by method of delivery of fetuses in breech presentation at term: Population based follow up. *Br Med J* 1996;312:1451–3.
11. Haheim LL, Albrechtsen S, Berge LN, *et al.* Breech birth at term: Vaginal delivery or elective cesarean section? A systemic review of the literature by a Norwegian review team. *Acta Obstet Gynecol Scand* 2004;83:126–36.
12. Levine EM, Ghai V, Barton JJ, Strom CM. Mode of delivery and risk of respiratory diseases in newborns. *Obstet Gynecol* 2001;97: 439–42.
13. Krebs L, Langenhoff-Roos J, Weber T. Breech at term: Mode of delivery? *Acta Obstet Gynecol Scand* 1995;74:702–6.
14. Eilen B, Fleisher A, Schulman H, Jagani N. Fetal acidosis and abnormal fetal heart rate tracing: The term breech fetus. *Obstet Gynecol* 1984;63:233–6.
15. Whyte H, Hannah M, Saigal S. Outcomes of children at 2 years of age in the Term Breech Trial. *Am J Obstet Gynecol (Suppl)* 2003; 189:S57.
16. Ulander VM, Gissler M, Nuutila M, Ylikorkala O. Are health expectations of term breech infants unrealistically high? *Acta Obstet Gynecol Scand* 2004;83:180–6.
17. American College of Obstetricians and Gynecologists. ACOG practice patterns: External cephalic version. Number 4, July 1997. *Int J Gynecol Obstet* 1997;59:73–80.
18. Royal College of Obstetricians and Gynaecologists. The management of breech presentation. In *Clinical Green Top Guidelines 2001*. London: RCOG, 2001.
19. Molkenboer JF, Bouckaert PJ, Roumen FJ. Recent trends in breech delivery in the Netherlands. *Br J Obstet Gynecol* 2003;110:948–51.
20. Hofmeyr GJ. External cephalic version facilitation for breech presentation at term. *Cochrane Database Syst Rev* 2000;2: CD000184.
21. Lau TK, Kit KW, Rogers M. Pregnancy outcome after successful external cephalic external version for breech presentation at term. *Am J Obstet Gynecol* 1997;176:218–23.
22. Varma R, Horwell D. External cephalic version should be routine clinical practice in the UK. *Br Med J* 2002;321:19.
23. Shennan A, Bewley S. How to manage term breech deliveries. Avoid vaginal breech deliveries but offer external cephalic version. *Br Med J* 2001;323:244–7.
24. Phipps H, Roberts CL, Nasser N, Raynes-Greenow CH, Peat B, Hutton EK. The management of breech presentation in Australia and New Zealand. *Aust N Z J Obstet Gynaecol* 2003;43:294–7.

25. Yogev Y, Horowitz E, Ben-Haroush B, Chen R, Kaplan B. Changing attitudes towards mode of delivery and external cephalic version in breech presentation. *Int J Gynecol Obstet* 2002;79:221–4.
26. Hutton EK, Kaufman K, Hodnett E, *et al.* External cephalic version beginning at 34 weeks' gestation versus 37 weeks gestation: A randomized trial. *Am J Obstet Gynecol* 2003;189:245.
27. Hofmeyr G. External cephalic version for breech presentation before term (Cochrane Review) 2003. In *The Cochrane Library*, Issue 1. Oxford: Update Software.
28. Hofmeyr G. Intervention to help external cephalic version for breech presentation at term (Cochrane Review) 2002. In *The Cochrane Library*, Issue 3.Oxford: Update Software.
29. Impey L, Lissoni D. Outcome of external cephalic version after 36 weeks gestation without tocolysis. *J Matern Fetal Med* 1999: 8:203–7.
30. Johnson R. External cephalic version. The Diplomate. *R Coll Obstet Gynaecol* 1999;5:178–82.
31. Gravenhorst JB, Schreuder AM, Veen S, *et al.* Breech delivery in very preterm and very low birth weight infants in the Netherlands. *Br J Obstet Gynaecol* 1993;100:411–5.
32. Lee KS, Khoshnood BK, Spiram S, Hsieh H, Singh J, Mittendorf R. Relationship of cesarean delivery to lower birth weight-specific neonatal mortality in singleton breech infants in the United States. *Obstet Gynecol* 1998:92;769–74.
33. Rochelson B, Pagano M, Conetta L, Goldman B, Frey M, Day C. Previous preterm cesarean section: Identification of a new risk factor for uterine rupture. *Am J Obstet Gynecol (Suppl)* 2004; 189:S138.
34. Hauth J, Cunningham FG. Vaginal breech delivery is still justified. *Obstet Gynecol* 2002;99:1115–6.
35. Diro M, Puangsricharern A, Royer L, O'Sullivan MJ, Burkett G. Singleton term breech deliveries in nulliparous and multiparous women. A 5-year experience. The University of Miami/Jackson Memorial Hospital. *Am J Obstet Gynecol* 1999;181:247–52.
36. Rietberg CC, Elferink-Stinkens PM, Brand R, vanLoon AJ, Van Hemel OJS, Visser GHA. Term breech presentation in the Netherlands from 1995 to 1999: Mortality and morbidity in relation to the mode of delivery of 33,824 infants. *Br J Obstet Gynaecol* 2003;110:604–9.
37. O'Driscoll K, Foley M, MacDonald D. Active management of labor as an alternative to cesarean section for dystocia. *Obstet Gynecol* 1984;63:485–90.
38. Irion O, Hirsbrunner-Almagbaly P, Morabia A. Planned vaginal delivery versus elective cesarean section: A study of 705 singleton term breech presentations. *Br J Obstet Gynaecol* 1998;105:710–7.
39. Roman J, Bakos O, Cnattingius S. Pregnancy outcomes by mode of delivery among term breech births: Swedish experience 1987–1993. *Obstet Gynaecol* 1998;92:945–50.
40. van Roosmalen J, Rosendaal F. There is still room for disagreement about vaginal delivery of breech at term. *Br J Obstet Gynaecol* 2002;109:967–9.
41. Lilford RJ, Van Coeverden de Groot HA, Moore PJ, Bingham P. The relative risks of cesarean section (intrapartum and elective) and vaginal delivery: A detailed analysis to exclude the effects of medical disorders and other acute pre-existing physiological disturbances. *Br J Obstet Gynaecol* 1990;97:439–92.
42. Waites B. *Breech birth.* London: Free Association Books, 2003.
43. Queenan JT. Teaching infrequently used skills: Vaginal breech delivery (editorial). *Am J Obstet Gynecol* 2004;103:405–6.
44. Hogle KL, Kilburn L, Hewson S, Gafni A, Wall R, Hannah, ME. Impact of the International Term Breech Trial on clinical practice and concerns: A survey of centre collaborators. *J Obstet Gynaecol Can* 2003;25:14–26.
45. Kaushik V, Gudgeon C. Cesarean for breech: A paradigm shift? *Aust N Z J Obstet Gynaecol* 2004;43:298–301.
46. Leung WC, Pun TC, Wong WM. Undiagnosed breech revisited. *Br J Obstet Gynaecol* 1999;106:638–41.

182 Shoulder dystocia

F. Goffinet and D. Cabrol

Definition and mechanism

During normal labor and delivery, the fetal shoulder width (the bisacromial diameter) advances through one of the oblique diameters of the pelvic inlet: the posterior shoulder moves into the concavity of the sacrum or the sacrosciatic notch, while the anterior shoulder glides behind the symphysis. Then, as they descend, the shoulders turn into the anteroposterior diameter of the midpelvis. Shoulder width usually ranges between 12 and 13 cm; compressed, it passes easily through the pelvic inlet.

Shoulder dystocia (SD) can be categorized into three degrees of increasing severity:[1]

(1) Slight dystocia, in which the shoulders rotate normally, but the large size of the baby requires considerable compression of the shoulders in order to deliver.
(2) Unilateral dystocia, in which the posterior shoulder enters the pelvis, but the anterior shoulder remains above the symphysis.
(3) Bilateral dystocia, in which both shoulders remain above the pelvic inlet.

In the latter two types, downward traction on the fetal head when it has delivered serves only to aggravate the impaction of the shoulders in the pelvis. As the brachial plexus is already stretched once the head is delivered and one or both shoulders remains impacted, any further stretching through traction risks lacerations of the C5-T1 nerve roots. Prolonged forcible traction can lead to delivery only at the cost of injury to the mother and the child.

Because this anatomical classification is difficult to use in practice, more pragmatic definitions have been proposed and are sometimes used in the literature. These include: (1) a condition in which special maneuvers, in addition to downward traction and episiotomy, are required to deliver the shoulders; (2) the arrest of spontaneous delivery due to impaction of the anterior shoulder against the symphysis pubis; or (3) a time between the delivery of head and body longer than 60 s.[2]

Frequency

The variety of different definitions used in published series results in a great variability in the reported frequency of SD. If we consider only the third, most severe, stage, this accident occurs in 1 of every 4000 deliveries.[1] With more pragmatic definitions, the frequencies reported range from 0.2% to 2.1% of all vaginal deliveries.[3] The frequency also varies according to the population considered, and, in particular, according to the distribution of the principal risk factors, such as fetal macrosomia.

Maternal and neonatal consequences

Neonatal complications included mortality, asphyxial, neurologic, and orthopedic damage. Perinatal mortality may increase as much as ninefold among babies with SD,[4] although the perinatal mortality rate associated with it in a recent series was reported to be below 1%.[3] In a British study of 1,400,000 deliveries and 56 deaths directly associated with SD, the incidence of fatal SD was reported to be 0.04 per 1000 births and 0.025 per 1000 births when the definition of 'true SD' was used.[5] In this registry, the perinatal loss rate was 0.57 per 100 cases of SD, with a vaginal delivery rate of 70% and the SD incidence 1% of all vaginal deliveries. In their literature review, Rouse *et al.* reported two to four SD-associated deaths with SD per 100,000 births.[6]

Neonatal morbidity has been reported to complicate 24.9% of births with SD.[3] In addition to nerve injury and fractures, neonatal asphyxia, due to the long and difficult delivery, is a common causal mechanism. Hope *et al.* reported that in their series, the median interval between delivery of the head and the body for the 56 deaths caused by SD was only 5 min.[5] A 5-min Apgar score < 3 was found with a frequency 6–11 times greater in births with SD than in controls.[4]

The most common fractures are those of the clavicle and the humerus, associated with SD in 9.5% and 4.2% of cases, respectively.[3] The incidence of clavicle fractures in the general population is estimated as 2.7%;

among infants with a birth weight of 4000–4500 g it reaches 14%, and among those weighing more than 4500 g it reaches 38%.[1]

Gherman *et al.* reported brachial plexus injury (BPI) in 16.8% of SD cases and Rouse in 6–35%.[3,6] Most are temporary, persisting at 1 year among about 5–8% of babies.[3,6] The most common injury affects the C5 and C6 nerve roots and causes Duchenne–Erb paralysis. Paralysis of the C7 to T1 roots below the plexus (Klumpke paralysis) is quite rare, but has a worse prognosis, with a recovery rate of only 40% in 1 year.

Permanent brachial plexus palsy is not always associated with SD, or even with vaginal delivery: one study found that no perinatal risk factors could be identified in one-third of the cases of brachial plexus palsies identified in newborns.[7] Numerous other studies confirm that brachial palsies cannot be accurately predicted before delivery, either by risk factor scoring or by partographic analysis.[8,9] Finally, infants with transient brachial plexus neuropathies do not differ from those with permanent injuries with respect to most antepartum or intrapartum characteristics.[10] Birth weight is the only reproducibly identified risk factor; but a minority of large babies have brachial plexus injuries. In a series of 210,947 births, the overall incidence of BPI was 50 per 100,000.[11] This risk was 2.5-fold higher in neonates weighing 4000–4500 g and 10-fold higher in those > 4500 g.

Adverse maternal consequences of shoulder dysticia may include cervicovaginal injuries, third-stage hemorrhage, and infection.[3] The frequency of these complications is not well documented in the literature.

Table 182.1 Distribution of complications according to birth weight categories (from Gonen *et al.*[14])

	n (%)		
Birth weight	SD (*n*=92)	BPI (*n*=9)	Clavicle fracture (*n*=39)
< 4000	46 (50)	5 (56)	32 (82)
4000–4500	40 (43.5)	3 (33)	7 (18)
> 4500	6 (6.5)	1 (11)	0

Risk factors and predictability

Risk factors

Fetal macrosomia is the principal risk factor of SD. Two recent series found the risk of SD to be 11.4% for babies weighing 4200 g or more and 22% for babies weighing 4500 g or more.[12,13] Table 182.1 summarizes the distribution of birth weights in the series by Gonen *et al.*, according to the three most common traumatic injuries.[14] The clear relationship between birth weight and the risk of SD and BPI notwithstanding, predicting SD from the presence of estimated fetal weight (EFW) is associated with numerous false-positive and false-negative predictions. The vast majority of macrosomic babies delivered vaginally do not present with SD. Moreover, half the cases of SD and BPI occur in children with a birth weight less than 4000 g. A recent review reports that 26–58% of the cases of SD and 24–44% of the BPIs occur among babies weighing less than 4000 g, even though the risk of SD among infants with macrosomia is multiplied by nine [OR = 9.1, 95% CI (8.3–10.0)].[15]

Maternal diabetes mellitus is an important factor that, because of its common association with fetal macrosomia, increases the chance of delivery trauma. The incidence of SD among children of non-diabetic mothers varies by birth weight category as follows: 4000–4250 g, 5.2%; 4250–4500 g, 9.1%; 4500–4750 g, 14.6%; and 4750–5000 g, 21.1%; for those with mothers with diabetes, the frequencies in the same birth weight groups are 12.2%, 16.7%, 27.3%, and 34.8%, respectively.[16] In a large series of children with birth weights > 4000 g, Langer *et al.* found that the risk of SD was multiplied 3.6-fold when the mother had diabetes.[4]

Other risk factors that have been implicated include a history of SD in a prior pregnancy (risk multiplied by 17), high maternal weight gain during pregnancy, multiparity, long labor, and the need for forceps-assisted delivery.[17] Table 182.2 summarizes the principal risk factors of macrosomia and SD. Because so many of these criteria are cross-correlated, it is difficult to identify their independent contributions to risk. The use of these criteria for predicting macrosomia and SD is thus disappointing. While their sensitivity is good, their specificity is very mediocre, because most women with at least one of these risk factors give birth to a child weighing less than 4000 g and without SD.

Prediction of fetal macrosomia: Evaluation of the available diagnostic methods

Prenatal assessment of the risk of SD is often limited to an assessment of the risk of macrosomia. Unfortunately, prenatal diagnosis of macrosomia is also difficult. Screening during standard prenatal monitoring generally involves abdominal palpation and measurement of fundal height, but this technique is quite imprecise. One study found the precision of EFW by clinical examination to be ±500 g in 82.5% of all cases but in only 35.3% of those with a birth weight > 4500 g.[18]

With the introduction of ultrasound in the late 1970s, it was hoped that the problem of this imprecision would be solved. Numerous formulas and indices for predicting fetal macrosomia have been reported; they used various combinations of biparietal diameter, head circumference, transverse abdominal diameter, abdominal circumference, and femur length.[19–21] These

Table 182.2 Risk factors for fetal macrosomia and SD

History	Current pregnancy	Intrapartum events
High maternal birth weight SD Macrosomia Preexisting diabetes Gestational diabetes Obesity Multiparity Maternal age >35 years	Gestational diabetes Excessive weight gain Suspected fetal macrosomia Post-term	Abnormal labor, especially during second stage Instrumental delivery for failure to progress at mid pelvis

formulas for EFW differ little in precision, and none is clearly superior to any other. The mean error is significantly higher in cases of macrosomia, reaching approximately 15%,[21,22] while 50–70% of the estimates have a mean error less than 10%.[22–25] For example, McLaren *et al.* showed that for an EFW of 4000 g, there was a 95% chance that the birth weight would range between 3288 and 4798 g and for an EFW of 4500 g, between 3750 and 5269 g.[26] These data confirm the imprecision of the EFW calculated by ultrasound, which thus yields many false-positive and false-negative predictions.

Several studies have compared the relative utility of clinical and ultrasound estimates for predicting birth weight at term, and most have not found ultrasound to be clearly superior.[27,28] In an earlier study, predicted birth weight was similar for ultrasound, clinical examination, and the woman's own estimate at the onset of labor.[29] Similarly, Gonen *et al.* found diagnostic value to be better with clinical examination alone than with clinical examination and ultrasound for predicting newborns ≥4500 g.[14]

In view of the imprecision of ultrasound in predicting fetal macrosomia, most teams do not systematically use it to estimate birth weight at the end of pregnancy. Generally, screening involves standard prenatal monitoring with ultrasound then performed only if macrosomia is suspected.

Prediction of the risk of SD

Since the principal goal is to predict SD (or, better, BPI) and not fetal macrosomia, several authors have sought to identify criteria specifically predictive of SD. Some risk factors have been identified, but their extremely low sensitivity and specificity make them essentially useless for practical decision making. This applies as well to radiographic pelvimetry for which there exist no data to justify its use to predict SD.

Among the most predictive factors, we find the sequence dubbed 'DOPE' (diabetes, obesity, postdatism, excessive fetal weight or maternal weight gain). Although the concurrence of these factors does not justify systematic cesarean, it signals the need for extreme prudence during labor.

Shoulder width is thought to be greater in newborns with SD than in those who had uncomplicated deliveries [30]. The factors associated with increased shoulder width are the same as those linked to SD and are often interdependent, as Verspyck *et al.* showed in a prospective study.[17] In addition to greater shoulder width, newborns with SD have other biometric characteristics different from those with the same birth weight but without SD.[31] These findings have led some authors to seek antenatal ultrasound criteria to predict SD. Some data suggest that differences between ratios of measurements (e.g. thoracic diameter to biparietal diameter, as well as between abdominal diameter or thoracic circumference and the biparietal diameter)[19,32,33] can identify fetuses at increased risk of SD. Riska *et al.* found the ultrasound measurement of the distance between the humeral heads to be significantly correlated with the measurement of shoulder width.[34] Others showed that shoulder width can be measured by magnetic resonance imaging (MRI) and suggest that the comparison of its measurement by MRI and radiopelvimetry might be a decision criterion.[35] Their studies are generally preliminary and isolated: prospective confirmation of these results will require considerable supplementary data. Moreover, only one report assessed the predictive value of these different parameters for the risk of SD: Verspyck *et al.* measured shoulder width in 2222 consecutive births.[17] The prevalence of SD in that study was 1.2%, and the mean shoulder width was significantly higher in the cases of SD than among those without it (130.1±9.6 mm vs. 122.1±10.5 mm, $P < 0.001$). Table 182.3 summarizes the predictive values for SD of the various significant parameters, especially the shoulder width. Although the predictive values of some criteria appear interesting, specificity must be very high if they are to serve as a basis for decision making in a general population. The overall conclusion of these authors was that regardless of the criterion or shoulder width threshold chosen, predictive value is insufficient to justify the use of these indicators in daily practice. Thus, even if shoulder width could be measured perfectly, that is, with no false-positives or false-negatives before labor (the measurements in the study discussed were made at birth), its predictive value for SD would be inadequate.[17]

Table 182.3 Predictive value of maternal and neonatal criteria significantly associated with SD (from Verspyck *et al.*[17])

Predictive factors	Sen	Spe	PPV	NPV
Shoulder width (mm)				
≥130	68.2	69.3	2.7	99.4
≥140	27.3	91.8	4.0	99.0
≥145	9.1	98.5	7.1	98.9
Maternal weight gain (kg)				
≥15	72.1	64.3	2.5	99.5
≥20	31.8	92.6	5.2	92.6
Gestational age at delivery (weeks)				
≥41	36.4	85.7	3.1	99.1
≥42	9.1	96.7	3.4	98.8
Birth weight (g)				
≥4000	36.3	95.3	8.7	99.2
≥4250	22.7	98.8	19.2	99.0
≥4500	13.6	99.5	25.0	99.5
≥5000	4.5	99.9	50.0	98.8

Prevalence of SD = 1.2% (n = 22)
Sen, sensitivity; spe, specificity; PPV, positive predictive value; NPV, negative predictive value

Prevention of SD

Efforts proposed to prevent SD generally entail an attempt to identify cases of fetal macrosomia so that a cesarean delivery can be performed, or labor induced before the fetus gains even more weight. Two assumptions underlie this approach. The first is that the estimation of SD risk is clinically meaningful, and the second is that some effective preventive management would be possible once the risk is identified.

To be clinically useful, a method to predict SD would need to be associated with only a small percentage of false-positives and false-negatives. In practice, diagnostic resources are directed toward fetal macrosomia rather than its complications. Accordingly, even if the diagnosis of macrosomia were always correct, the number of false-positive diagnoses of complications would be very high (approximately 90% of cases of macrosomia are not accompanied by SD). Moreover, it is not clear that intervention to prevent SD could be rationalized. For example, cesareans for 10% of the total population based on estimated excess fetal weight would result in a rise in maternal morbidity (or even mortality), an increase in the number of uterine scars, and changes in the organization and cost of care. These changes must be assessed according to the number of complications avoided.

Cesarean in cases of suspected fetal macrosomia

Some physicians consider that an EFW > 4000 g or > 4500 g indicates the need for cesarean delivery, although no policy of that type has yet been subjected to systematic evaluation. We can, nevertheless, study the risks and benefits of such approaches using theoretical decision models, such as those employed by Rouse *et al.*[6] Table 182.4 summarizes the consequences of three intervention strategies on the rates of cesarean delivery, SD, and BPI per million pregnancies without diabetes after 39 weeks' gestation.

A policy of systematic cesarean for EFW > 4000 g would result in a cesarean rate of 27.6% for the total population, and 3695 cesareans would be performed to prevent one Erb palsy; systematic cesarean for EFW > 4500 g would reduce the cesareans required to prevent one BPI to 2345. The authors conclude that such a policy is indefensible, given the number of unnecessary cesareans that would be performed. This low 'yield' is due to the low frequency of SD (1%) and the low predictive value of EFW for macrosomia and SD. If the mother also has diabetes, 489 cesareans would be necessary to avoid one case of permanent BPI at a threshold of 4000 g and 443 cesareans at a threshold of 4500 g.

Weeks *et al.* reviewed their 6-year experience with 504 consecutive cases of infants born weighing more that 4200 g.[36] Macrosomia had been diagnosed prenatally for 102 of these. The principal findings of the study (Table 182.5) were a significant increase in the number of cesareans before labor, more inductions of labor, and more failed inductions in the group with 'diagnosed fetal macrosomia' compared with the 'undiagnosed fetal macrosomia' group. The two groups did not, however, differ in their rates of SD or

Table 182.4 Obstetrical results and cost according to three different management policies for 1 million pregnant women with diabetes after 39 weeks (USA) (from Rouse *et al.*[6])

Management policy	CS (%)	SD (%)	BPI (n)	n of CS to avoid one BPI	Cost ($)**
Classic management	19.1	1.00	157*		9.0
Systematic ultrasound and cesarean if EFW > 4500 g	27.6	0.84	134	3695	18.0
Systematic ultrasound and cesarean if EFW > 4000 g	30.6	0.64	108	2345	26.0

CS, overall rate of cesarean deliveries in the population; n, number
*Or 0.0157%. **Millions of US dollars

BPI. The authors concluded that ultrasonography and induction of labor for patients at risk of fetal macrosomia should be discouraged.[36] These results are similar to those found in a prospective study in 15 maternity hospitals in Paris and the Ile-de-France area.[37] Although these findings must be interpreted prudently (the most high-risk cases may have been screened and delivered by cesarean), they nonetheless show the limits of decisions based on EFW. In another retrospective study, similar results were found: the policy of elective cesarean section for diagnosed fetal macrosomia (EFW > 4500 g) did not have a significant effect on the incidence of brachial plexus palsy.[38]

The problem seems different, however, in cases in which macrosomia is associated with another important risk factor, such as maternal diabetes. In a historical study of 1200 pregnancies of mothers with diabetes, the authors compared a period during which fetal weight was not estimated and a second period where a cesarean was performed when the EFW was ≥4250 g.[39] They found a significant reduction of nearly 50% (2.8% vs. 1.5%) in the SD rate, with only a moderate increase in the number of cesareans (21.7% vs. 25.1%). Accordingly, most authors consider that when the mother has diabetes, an EFW of about 4250 or 4500 g requires cesarean delivery; there are, however, no data precisely on point, probably because of the difficulty of recruiting enough subjects to reach a conclusion.

Should labor be induced when fetal macrosomia is suspected?

Many obstetricians think it is reasonable to induce labor before the weight of the fetus becomes excessive and increases the risk of complications associated with macrosomia. A systematic review of observational studies found, however, that labor induction for suspected fetal macrosomia increased the cesarean delivery rate without improving perinatal outcome.[40] Table 182.6 reports the results of a meta-analysis based on the two published trials:[42,43] their combined results show that induction of labor does not reduce the risk of cesarean or instrumental delivery. Birth weight and gestational age were comparable in both groups. Neonatal morbidity was similar in both but their statistical power to demonstrate differences with this regard was weak. Based on what we now know, inducing labor for suspected macrosomia is not recommended.

Management at delivery

Our ability to predict SD is unfortunately very limited, as pointed out above. The audit by Hope *et al.* of 56 cases of fatal SD showed that its occurrence was most often unpredictable.[5] SD occurs and will continue to occur in numerous cases with no known predictive factors. In view of this unpredictability, the only real solution is to prevent its complications (nerve palsies, fractures) by appropriate management at delivery. Obstetricians and midwives must know the appropriate maneuvers thoroughly. Each department should have a written protocol, which lists the order in which the different maneuvers should be performed, and these should be regularly explained and reviewed.

General rules

In all cases of suspected macrosomia, the entire team must be informed at the woman's arrival in the delivery room. A case–control study in the Paris metropolitan area of 384 deliveries of babies with macrosomia found that the midwife was alone for 53.4% of the spontaneous vaginal deliveries with suspected macrosomia.[37] At delivery, an obstetrician, anesthetist, and pediatrician should be in the delivery room with the midwife. Prophylactic use of the McRoberts maneuver and suprapubic pressure is not recommended in a population of patients at increased risk of SD, since it appears to be ineffective. Delivery time did not differ in a randomized trial between the prophylactic and control patients (24 ± 18 s vs. 27 ± 20 s, $P = 0.38$).[44]

The first step in management is the rapid recognition of SD, so as to avoid inappropriate procedures with potentially irreversible adverse consequences. The accoucheur must remain calm and act rapidly, but neither precipitately nor impulsively. A large episiotomy should be performed. Analgesia must be

Table 182.5 Obstetrical results and risks of SD according to whether macrosomia was predicted before birth (from Weeks *et al.*[36])

	Macrosomia predicted (n D 102) (%)	Macrosomia not predicted (n D 402) (%)	*P*
Cesarean (rate)	52.0	30.0	< 0.01
Cesarean before labor	14.7	10.2	NS
Cesarean before 4 cm (among attempted vaginal deliveries)	49.0	16.5	< 0.01
Induction	42.5	26.6	< 0.01
Failure of induction	59.5	33.4	0.01
SD	11.8	11.7	NS

Table 182.6 Induction of labor in cases of suspected fetal macrosomia: meta-analysis of results of two clinical trials (from Irion and Boulvain[49])

	Induction of labor ($n=153$)	Expectant ($n-160$)	Relative risk (95% CI)
Cesarean	32	38	0.88 (0.59–1.34)
Instrumental interventions	17	18	0.98 (0.53–1.82)
SD	9	9	1.06 (0.44–2.56)
BPI	0	2	0.21 (0.01–4.28)
Birth weight (g)	4086	4149	NS

perfect; peridural anesthesia is often sufficient, but in case of agitation or pain, general anesthesia may be administered.

The '3 Ps' summarize what absolutely must not be done:[1] Panic-pulling, Pushing, or Pivoting.[45] That is, do not exert traction, which might rupture the brachial plexus of the anterior shoulder; do not exert fundal pressure; and do not pivot the head by twisting the neck.

Several maneuvers have been described that are potentially useful for the resolution of impacted shoulders. Operators must not only know them perfectly, at least in theory, but also must know the order in which they will employ them. The protocol in our department calls for beginning with McRoberts maneuver, because it is the least invasive and the least difficult, and then, if it fails, attempting a Jacquemier maneuver (delivery of the posterior arm). The advantage of having two principal preferred maneuvers is that they are explained regularly to the staff at the morning meetings when interns, midwives, and the senior obstetrician describe in detail to the rest of the team any maneuvers they performed during the night. If the Jacquemier maneuver fails, a careful Woods maneuver will be attempted. If these fail, we recommend beginning them over, in the same order.

The McRoberts maneuver[1,46]

This is a simple method with a high success rate and should be attempted first. In a retrospective study of 236 cases of SD, use of the McRoberts position alone successfully alleviated SD in 98 cases (42%).[47] The woman's feet should be removed from the stirrups and her legs hyperflexed at both the hip and the knee joints, so that her thighs rest on her abdomen, while her buttocks remain in complete contact with the delivery table. This maneuver elevates the pubic symphysis and thus brings the axis of descent closer to the umbilical–coccygeal axis of the pelvic inlet.

Oblique suprapubic pressure by an assistant on the median line above the symphysis is used in association with the thigh hyperflexion and is part of the maneuver. It pushes the posterior face of the anterior shoulder toward the ventral surface of the fetus, thereby reducing shoulder width. The operator applies downward traction in an attempt to accomplish delivery. Fundal pressure is expressly contraindicated.

The Jacquemier maneuver

This maneuver is designed to deliver the posterior arm of the fetus. The accoucheur, kneeling, introduces a lubricated hand into the vagina. The palm of the hand should face the fetal abdomen (left hand if the back is to the left, right hand if the back is to the right) and enter the uterus along the umbilical–coccygeal axis. The posterior shoulder is identified at the level of the sacral promontory; the arm is followed distally past the elbow and forearm (often flexed), and the hand grasped firmly. If the hand cannot be grasped initially, the humerus should be brought in front of the fetal thorax with the operator's fingers placed to support the humerus, to reduce the risk of its fracture.

Once the hand is grasped, the arm is withdrawn gently, by sweeping it across the front of the chest and face of the fetus. This maneuver transforms the bisacromial diameter (shoulder width) into an axillo–acromial diameter and may be sufficient to deliver the fetus. If delivery of the posterior arm is not sufficient, the body should be rotated 180° to transfer the anterior shoulder into the posterior shoulder and then repeat the Jacquemier maneuver.

Other maneuvers

The Woods maneuver

This approach involves transforming the posterior shoulder into the anterior shoulder. It is important to exert the rotational force on the shoulders, and not the head. To do this, the accoucheur places a palm behind the posterior shoulder and exerts pressure on it to force a 180° rotation of the shoulder axis. Exerting pressure in the opposite direction on the front of the anterior shoulder can facilitate rotation. This maneuver allows the engagement beneath the sacral promontory of the anterior shoulder, which becomes posterior at the end of the rotation.

The Zavanelli maneuver (replacement of the fetal head)

This method is used for dystocia considered intractable. It involves flexion of the fetal head, after tocolysis, in order to reintroduce it into the vagina, and then the uterus in order to perform a cesarean. In nearly 70 published cases, this maneuver has often been presented as easy to accomplish.[48] In a retrospective study, O'Leary *et al.* reported 59 women who underwent replacement of the fetal head after unsuccessful attempts at vaginal delivery.[49] All but six infants were successfully replaced and delivered by cesarean. Three neonates died and five had permanent brachial plexus palsy. Hysterectomy was required for two women. The authors conclude that cephalic replacement is a useful technique that need not be used as a last resort, but may be considered if any undue difficulty is encountered. It may have a place as an initial technique for those who are inexperienced with management of SD. It is difficult to interpret the results of this study because we know neither the severity of the cases of SD nor what maneuvers were attempted before the cesarean. The role of this maneuver must still be defined. We think that it is preferable to attempt the maneuvers described above rather than resort early to this technique. We have never had to use this extreme method in our hospital and have had no deaths associated with SD over the past 10 years.

Conclusion

The occurrence of SD in the delivery room, because it is so often unable to be predicted, cannot be attributed simply to poor medical practice. Even careful screening for macrosomia cannot eliminate this catastrophic complication. SD occurs and will continue to occur in numerous cases that have no known predictive factors. In view of this unpredictability, the only real solution is to prevent its complications (primarily BPI, fractures, and hypoxia) by optimizing management at delivery. Obstetricians and midwives must know the appropriate maneuvers thoroughly, and each department should have a written protocol, which lists the order in which they should be attempted. Moreover, these maneuvers must be regularly explained and their procedures repeated. It is also necessary that the entire obstetrical team – including the midwife, senior obstetrician, anesthetist, and pediatrician – be in the delivery room for cases of suspected fetal macrosomia.

REFERENCES

1. Langer B, Treisser A. Dystocie des épaules. In Cabrol D, Pons J, Goffinet F, eds. *Traité d'obstétrique*. Paris: Flammarion Médecine-Sciences, 2003:960–4.
2. Chang A, Lau T. Operative vaginal delivery. In Chamberlain G, Steer P, eds. *Turnbull's Obstetrics*, 3rd edn. London: Churchill Livingstone, 2001:581–600.
3. Gherman RB, Goodwin TM. Shoulder dystocia. *Curr Opin Obstet Gynecol* 1998;10:459–63.
4. Langer O, Berkus MD, Huff RW, Samueloff A. Shoulder dystocia: Should the fetus weighing greater than or equal to 4000 grams be delivered by cesarean section? *Am J Obstet Gynecol* 1991;165: 831–7.
5. Hope P, Breslin S, Lamont L, *et al.* Fatal shoulder dystocia: A review of 56 cases reported to the confidential enquiry into stillbirths and deaths in infancy. *Br J Obstet Gynaecol* 1998;105: 1256–61.
6. Rouse DJ, Owen J, Goldenberg RL, Cliver SP. The effectiveness and costs of elective cesarean delivery for fetal macrosomia diagnosed by ultrasound. *J Am Med Assoc* 1996;276:1480–6.
7. Peleg D, Hasnin J, Shalev E. Fractured clavicle and Erb's palsy unrelated to birth trauma. *Am J Obstet Gynecol* 1997;177:1038–40.
8. Donnelly V, Foran A, Murphy J, McParland P, Keane D, O'Herlihy C. Neonatal brachial plexus palsy: An unpredictable injury. *Am J Obstet Gynecol* 2002;187:1209–12.
9. Christoffersson M, Kannisto P, Rydhstroem H, Stale H, Walles B. Shoulder dystocia and brachial plexus injury: A case-control study. *Acta Obstet Gynecol Scand* 2003;82:147–51.
10. Gherman RB, Ouzounian JG, Satin AJ, Goodwin TM, Phelan JP. A comparison of shoulder dystocia-associated transient and permanent brachial plexus palsies. *Obstet Gynecol* 2003;102:544–8.
11. McFarland LV, Raskin M, Daling JR, Benedetti TJ. Erb/Duchenne's palsy: A consequence of fetal macrosomia and method of delivery. *Obstet Gynecol* 1986;68:784–8.
12. Berard J, Dufour P, Vinatier D, *et al.* Fetal macrosomia: Risk factors and outcome. A study of the outcome concerning 100 cases > 4500 g. *Eur J Obstet Gynecol Reprod Biol* 1998;77:51–9.
13. Blickstein I, Ben-Arie A, Hagay ZJ. Antepartum risks of shoulder dystocia and brachial plexus injury for infants weighing 4,200 g or more. *Gynecol Obstet Invest* 1998;45:77–80.
14. Gonen R, Spiegel D, Abend M. Is macrosomia predictable, and are shoulder dystocia and birth trauma preventable? *Obstet Gynecol* 1996;88:526–9.

15. Sacks DA, Chen W. Estimating fetal weight in the management of macrosomia. *Obstet Gynecol Surv* 2000;55:229–39.
16. Nesbitt TS, Gilbert WM, Herrchen B. Shoulder dystocia and associated risk factors with macrosomic infants born in California [see comments]. *Am J Obstet Gynecol* 1998;179:476–80.
17. Verspyck E, Goffinet F, Hellot M, Milliez J, Marpeau L. Newborn shoulder width: A prospective study of 2222 consecutive measurements. *Br J Obstet Gynecol* 1999;106:589–93.
18. Ong HC, Sen DK. Clinical estimation of fetal weight. *Am J Obstet Gynecol* 1972;112:877–80.
19. Elliott JP, Garite TJ, Freeman RK, McQuown DS, Patel JM. Ultrasonic prediction of fetal macrosomia in diabetic patients. *Obstet Gynecol* 1982;60:159–62.
20. Hirata GI, Medearis AL, Horenstein J, Bear MB, Platt LD. Ultrasonographic estimation of fetal weight in the clinically macrosomic fetus. *Am J Obstet Gynecol* 1990;162:238–42.
21. Hadlock FP. Sonographic estimation of fetal age and weight. *Radiol Clin North Am* 1990;28:39–50.
22. Alsulyman OM, Ouzounian JG, Kjos SL. The accuracy of intrapartum ultrasonographic fetal weight estimation in diabetic pregnancies [see comments]. *Am J Obstet Gynecol* 1997;177:503–6.
23. Benacerraf BR, Gelman R, Frigoletto FD Jr. Sonographically estimated fetal weights: Accuracy and limitation. *Am J Obstet Gynecol* 1988;159:1118–21.
24. Field NT, Piper JM, Langer O. The effect of maternal obesity on the accuracy of fetal weight estimation [see comments]. *Obstet Gynecol* 1995;86:102–7.
25. Hedriana HL, Moore TR. A comparison of single versus multiple growth ultrasonographic examinations in predicting birth weight. *Am J Obstet Gynecol* 1994;170:1600–6.
26. McLaren RA, Puckett JL, Chauhan SP. Estimators of birth weight in pregnant women requiring insulin: A comparison of seven sonographic models. *Obstet Gynecol* 1995;85:565–9.
27. Raman S, Urquhart R, Yusof M. Clinical versus ultrasound estimation of fetal weight. *Aust N Z J Obstet Gynaecol* 1992;32:196–9.
28. Watson WJ, Soisson AP, Harlass FE. Estimated weight of the term fetus. Accuracy of ultrasound vs. clinical examination. *J Reprod Med* 1988;33:369–71.
29. Chauhan SP, Lutton PM, Bailey KJ, Guerrieri JP, Morrison JC. Intrapartum clinical, sonographic, and parous patients' estimates of newborn birth weight. *Obstet Gynecol* 1992;79:956–8.
30. Bahar AM. Risk factors and fetal outcome in cases of shoulder dystocia compared with normal deliveries of a similar birthweight [see comments]. *Br J Obstet Gynaecol* 1996;103:868–72.
31. Hopwood HG Jr. Shoulder dystocia: Fifteen years' experience in a community hospital. *Am J Obstet Gynecol* 1982;144:162–6.
32. Cohen B, Penning S, Major C, Ansley D, Porto M, Garite T. Sonographic prediction of shoulder dystocia in infants of diabetic mothers. *Obstet Gynecol* 1996;88:10–3.
33. Winn HN, Holcomb W, Shumway JB, al-Malt A, Amon E, Hobbins JC. The neonatal bisacromial diameter: A prenatal sonographic evaluation. *J Perinat Med* 1997;25:484–7.
34. Riska A, Laine H, Voutilainen P, Kariniemi V. Estimation of fetal shoulder width by measurement of the humerospinous distance by ultrasound. *Ultrasound Obstet Gynecol* 1996;7:272–4.
35. Kastler B, Gangi A, Mathelin C, *et al.* Fetal shoulder measurements with MRI. *J Comput Assist Tomogr* 1993;17:777–80.
36. Weeks JW, Pitman T, Spinnato JA, II. Fetal macrosomia: Does antenatal prediction affect delivery route and birth outcome? *Am J Obstet Gynecol* 1995;173:1215–9.
37. Batallan A, Goffinet F, Paris-Llado J, *et al.* Fetal macrosomia: Management, obstetrical and neonatal results. Multicenter case-control study in 15 maternity hospitals in Paris and the Ile de France area. *Gynecol Obstet Fertil* 2002;30:483–91.
38. Gonen R, Bader D, Ajami M. Effects of a policy of elective cesarean delivery in cases of suspected fetal macrosomia on the incidence of brachial plexus injury and the rate of cesarean delivery. *Am J Obstet Gynecol* 2000;183:1296–300.
39. Conway DL, Langer O. Elective delivery of infants with macrosomia in diabetic women: Reduced shoulder dystocia versus increased cesarean deliveries [see comments]. *Am J Obstet Gynecol* 1998;178:922–5.
40. Sanchez-Ramos L, Bernstein S, Kaunitz AM. Expectant management versus labor induction for suspected fetal macrosomia: A systematic review. *Obstet Gynecol* 2002;100:997–1002.
41. Irion O, Boulvain M. Induction of labour for suspected fetal macrosomia. *Cochrane Database Syst Rev* 2000;2:CD000938.
42. Gonen O, Rosen DJ, Dolfin Z, Tepper R, Markov S, Fejgin MD. Induction of labor versus expectant management in macrosomia: A randomized study. *Obstet Gynecol* 1997;89:913–7.
43. Tey A, Eriksen N, Blanco J. A prospective randomized trial of induction versus expectant management in nondiabetic pregnancies with fetal macrosomia (abstract). *Am J Obstet Gynecol* 1995; 172:293.
44. Beall MH, Spong CY, Ross MG. A randomized controlled trial of prophylactic maneuvers to reduce head-to-body delivery time in patients at risk for shoulder dystocia. *Obstet Gynecol* 2003;102:31–5.
45. O'Leary JA, Leonetti HB. Shoulder dystocia: Prevention and treatment [see comments]. *Am J Obstet Gynecol* 1990;162:5–9.
46. Oury JF, Sibony O, Luton D, Feraud O, Volumenie JL, Blot P. Obstetrical strategies and emergency procedures for delivery of macrosomic fetuses. *J Gynecol Obstet Biol Reprod (Paris)* 2000; 29(Suppl 1):20–4.
47. Gherman RB, Goodwin TM, Souter I, Neumann K, Ouzounian JG, Paul RH. The McRoberts' maneuver for the alleviation of shoulder dystocia: How successful is it? *Am J Obstet Gynecol* 1997;176: 656–61.
48. Vollebergh JH, van Dongen PW. The Zavanelli manoeuvre in shoulder dystocia: Case report and review of published cases. *Eur J Obstet Gynecol Reprod Biol* 2000;89:81–4.
49. O'Leary JA. Cephalic replacement for shoulder dystocia: Present status and future role of the Zavanelli maneuver. *Obstet Gynecol* 1993;82:847–50.

183 The third stage of labor and the puerperium

G. Sylvestre and Y. S. Thornton

The third stage of labor is defined as the time between delivery of the infant (or infants) and that of the placenta. The puerperium, also referred to as the postpartum period, is broadly defined as the interval between placental delivery and 6–12 weeks after delivery. While a wealth of literature is available on prenatal care and on the first and second stages of labor, relatively little attention has been devoted to advance our understanding of the third stage of labor and the puerperium.

The puerperium is remarkable in that many of the physiologic changes that evolved gradually over the course of pregnancy in virtually every organ system revert to the non-pregnant state at an astonishing pace. These rapid changes are well tolerated by most women, but those with certain underlying pathologic conditions may not withstand them very well, and may suffer serious complications. For example, the sudden blood loss and fluctuations in the cardiovascular indices in the immediate postpartum period can cause acute decompensation in patients with cardiovascular conditions such as pulmonary hypertension or aortic stenosis. Not surprisingly, more women die from anomalies of the third stage of labor than during the two other stages combined.[1,2]

The third stage of labor

Normal third-stage physiology

The delivery of the infant at the end of the second stage causes a dramatic reduction in uterine volume. This rapid uterine involution leads to a proportional decrease in the decidual surface where the placenta is inserted, leading to the shearing of the placenta off its uterine attachment. Myometrial contractions then effectively compress the large blood vessels and venous sinuses lying in the placental bed, thereby minimizing excessive bleeding and assisting expulsion of the placenta and membranes. Uterine massage during that moment is uncomfortable for the mother, and is unlikely to hasten the process of placental expulsion. For most parturients, spontaneous placental separation occurs within two contractions after vaginal delivery of the neonate and placental expulsion is usually completed after a few more contractions. Although the length of the third stage does not vary significantly across gestational ages, with median durations of 8 and 5 min, at 26 and 40 weeks, respectively, many studies have noted an association between preterm delivery and prolonged third stage of labor.[3]

Minimizing blood loss in the third stage

Under normal circumstances, in the interval between delivery of the infant and effective compression of the placental bed vasculature by myometrial contractions, a substantial amount of blood loss normally takes place. Given the physiologic increase in blood volume associated with pregnancy, this blood loss is usually well tolerated and intervention to minimize it is probably unnecessary for most parturients. However, in some cases, such as patients with significant anemia or those with a history of postpartum hemorrhage, pharmacologic and non-pharmacologic interventions may be warranted to minimize puerperal blood loss. The association between prolonged third stage and postpartum hemorrhage is well documented, so most interventions are aimed at decreasing the duration of the third stage.

Controlled cord traction (Brandt–Andrews technique)

After delivery of the infant, many clinicians apply controlled cord traction (CCT) to the umbilical cord at the level of the introitus. At the same time, cephaloposterior pressure on the uterus or direct grasping of its fundus is used to prevent uterine inversion. The CCT method, widely used in Canada and elsewhere, is less popular in the United States, where expectant management and maternal pushing efforts are more commonly used to achieve placental delivery.

Khan *et al.* compared CCT to no intervention and found CCT was associated with significantly decreased incidences of postpartum hemorrhage, prolonged third stage, and the need for surgical intervention.[4] Another well-designed randomized controlled trial comparing CCT to expectant management failed to detect a difference in the need for surgical removal of the placenta, but confirmed reduced blood loss and shorter duration of the third stage[5] in the intervention group.

Oxytocin/oxytocin and ergotamine

The efficacy of oxytocin administered after delivery in reducing the risks of postpartum hemorrhage, the need for secondary uterotonic drugs, and postpartum anemia has been well established.[6,7] In theory, its administration prior to placental delivery could lead to contraction of the cervix and of the lower uterine segment, thus interfering with placental expulsion; but one study comparing administration of oxytocin pre- to postplacental delivery failed to show any difference in the incidence of placental retention and the need for surgical placental removal.[8]

Oxytocin is most commonly administered intravenously as a dilute solution after placental delivery, but can also be given intramuscularly and as a direct injection in the myometrium. Intravenous injection of an undiluted oxytocin bolus is best avoided, as sudden hypotension can occur with this route. The addition of the ergot derivative ergometrine to oxytocin substantially increases the rate of hypertensive episodes, nausea and vomiting after its administration and offers, at best, marginal superiority over oxytocin alone.[9,10]

Misoprostol

In the last decade, misoprostol, a prostaglandin E_1 analog, has been used more frequently in obstetrics and its use has been introduced for the prevention and treatment of postpartum hemorrhage. Oral, vaginal, and rectal routes of administration have been described, with varying degrees of success. Its greatest advantages over other drugs used to prevent postpartum hemorrhage are its low cost, ease of storage, and non-intravenous route of administration. One randomized controlled trial suggested superiority of rectal misoprostol over placebo,[11] so in countries where oxytocin is unavailable, misoprostol is a welcome alternative. Oxytocin is, however, superior to rectally or orally administered misoprostol, and is, therefore, the drug of choice for this purpose. The addition of oral misoprostol to intravenous oxytocin may be slightly superior to oxytocin alone in preventing postpartum hemorrhage.[12,13]

Retained placenta/abnormal placentation

Traditionally, a prolonged third stage is diagnosed when the placenta has been retained for more than 30 min. Irrespective of elapsed time, in the presence of heavy vaginal bleeding, manual removal of the retained placenta should be undertaken immediately. In a cohort study of third-stage duration, Dombrowski *et al.*[3] noted that 11.5%, 3.5%, and 2.1% of patients required surgical removal of the placenta at 26, 34, and 40 weeks' gestation, respectively. In addition to preterm birth, other factors that have been associated with a prolonged third stage include fetal anomalies, pre-eclampsia, nulliparity, and labor induction.[14]

Surgical removal of the placenta usually involves introducing a hand through the vagina, finding the plane between the uterus and placenta, and then separating the placenta from its uterine attachment. Regional or general anesthesia is usually appropriate for this procedure, although intravenous sedation can also be used. If cotyledons or pieces of membrane appear to be missing from the removed specimen, or if the specimen is extensively fragmented, the procedure should be completed with curettage of the uterine cavity, using a large curette. If difficulty is encountered in finding the plane between the uterus and placenta when attempting to extract the placenta, or if fragments are resistant to removal, or if bleeding becomes brisk, one should suspect placenta accreta. Excessive traction on the uterus or overaggressive curettage places the patient at risk of uterine inversion, perforation, and can contribute to severe hemorrhage. In such cases, it is usually wiser to proceed promptly to hysterectomy. The following factors place patients at particularly high risk for placenta accreta and percreta:

- Prior uterine incision (e.g. cesarean or myomectomy)
- Multiple previous curettages or intrauterine manipulations (such as hysteroscopic myomectomy or polypectomy)
- Abnormal placental location (e.g. placenta previa or low-lying placenta)
- Grand multiparity.

Before attempting manual removal of a placenta in a situation in which there is a high risk of placenta accreta, good intravenous access is important, and blood for transfusion should be available when possible.

Uterine inversion

This uncommon but serious complication occurs with an incidence of 1 in 3000–6000 deliveries. It is encountered more frequently with a fundal placenta, and may be more common with excessive traction on the umbilical cord between uterine contractions. Typically, partial delivery of the placenta is noted, and is followed rapidly by severe blood loss and hypotension. Uterine inversion is graded as incomplete, complete, or prolapsed. Incomplete inversion is limited to the fundus and does not reach the cervix. Complete uterine inversion refers to the delivery of the uterine fundus and corpus through the cervix. If the inverted uterus extends beyond the introitus, it is referred to as a prolapsed inversion. Uterine inversion is an obstetric emergency and, unless corrected rapidly, the cervix and lower uterine segment create a constricting band around the inverted fundus. The constriction causes edema of the uterus, reduction of its blood supply and, eventually, necrosis. The following sequence of steps should be followed to manage uterine inversion:

(1) If recognized early, before substantial edema is present, the uterus can be replaced without anesthesia through the constricting band, with transvaginal pressure over the inverted fundus.
(2) When the constricting band is too tight and the uterus too edematous, the maneuver described above should be tried using a combination of general anesthesia and uterine relaxants, which may assist in releasing the constriction.
(3) If still unsuccessful, laparotomy should be performed. A combination of traction on the round ligaments from above and upward pressure on the uterine fundus from below are applied.
(4) A posterior vertical incision can be made on the posterior wall of the uterus and is useful in many ways.[15,16] It allows the surgeon to visualize directly and to reverse the inversion; it makes upward traction easier; and it relieves the constricting band.

It is of utmost importance to replace the blood lost aggressively, as hemodynamic shock is a frequent complication. Intravenous access through two large-bore catheters is recommended. Unless it has already separated from the uterine wall, the placenta should not be detached during the above manipulation, as profuse bleeding may result. It should be removed only once the uterus is restored to its normal position and the patient is hemodynamically stable. Once the uterus is successfully repositioned, there is a great risk of atony. Therefore, all uterine relaxants should be discontinued and uterotonics administered.

The puerperium

Postpartum hospital stay

From the beginning of humanity until the 20th century, the vast majority of deliveries occurred at home, either unsupervised or monitored by lay attendants. In the early 1900s, a new trend began, and childbirth became a more 'medicalized' event in the industrialized world, taking place increasingly in hospitals (often referred to as 'lying-in hospitals') and supervised by medical personnel. There were many perceived advantages to hospital birth:

- Hospital births were safer. With more births taking place in hospital, a significant reduction in both perinatal and maternal morbidity was observed, attributable to some extent to hospital-based childbirth.
- Some interventions, such as analgesia, cesarean birth, antibiotics, and transfusions, were accessible only in a hospital setting.
- It allowed the opportunity for medical personnel to be trained in obstetrics.
- Women could rest more comfortably away from their home.

Until a few decades ago, hospital bed rest was recommended for the postpartum woman, often for an extended period of time. Since the 1980s, however, this trend changed, with more and more women wishing to return home as soon as possible after the delivery. The cause for this shift probably is a combination of the desire of women to 'demedicalize' childbirth and, in some countries, a desire to decrease the costs associated with childbirth and the puerperium.

In the United States, the law in most states requires hospitals to allow a minimum of 48 and 96 h postpartum stay after an uncomplicated vaginal birth and cesarean delivery, respectively. Discharge within 24–48 h after an uncomplicated birth, has proven safe in most contexts.[17] Prior to discharge, the following minimum conditions should be met:

- Common maternal and neonatal problems such as infection, bleeding, severe anemia, and hyperbilirubinemia have been ruled out.
- Neonatal screening has been completed, in accordance with local regulations. For example, neonatal screening for phenylketonuria is required by many states. This test must be performed after 24 h of life, and unless it has been arranged for testing as an outpatient, this precludes neonatal discharge before 24 h of life.
- The mother must be familiar with breast-feeding or, if applicable, other forms of infant nutrition. Frequently, optimal 'hands-on' education about breast-feeding cannot take place immediately postpartum, a period during which the breast milk cycle has not yet been established. This must be taken into consideration before discharge. Sometimes formal home visits during the days after early discharge are used for follow-up and patient education.
- The mother is properly educated about normal and abnormal postpartum and neonatal findings.
- Appropriate resources are available to ensure efficient and rapid assessment of the mother or newborn, should any acute problem occur at home, or should the parents have any questions or concerns.
- Potential social problems that could compromise care for the newborn have been addressed, such as financial difficulties or limited intellect.

In a Canadian study, Liu *et al.* reported a higher readmission rate in children discharged within 48 h, most commonly for neonatal hyperbilirubinemia, feeding problems, and suspected infection.[18] In another study, maternal readmission rates were found to have been similarly affected by early discharge. When compared to a 5-day postpartum stay after a cesarean delivery, women who were discharged at 2, 3, and 4 days postcesarean have a readmission rate increased by 21%, 18%, and 10%, respectively.[19] Ideally, preparation for short postpartum stays should take place early in prenatal care so that patients deemed suitable for early discharge, and, where it is optional, willing to participate, can be identified. Multiparas with proper home support are often good candidates.

Physiologic changes

From conception until delivery, many maternal organ systems have undergone some degree of physiologic or anatomic changes to adapt to the pregnant state. The return to prepregnant status is not immediate, and in some cases, the changes induced by the pregnancy are permanent (e.g. the cervix and the breast).

Postpartum weight loss

The rate of obesity in the Western hemisphere is increasing, particularly so in the United States, where over 50% of women have a body mass index of over 25 kg/m^2,[20] and where 18% of women are frankly obese, defined by a body mass index over 29 kg/m^2.[21] One event that most pregnant women look forward to is the dramatic weight loss that occurs during the puerperium. Although considerable weight is shed immediately through delivery of the fetus, amniotic fluid, and placenta, the remainder of the weight gained during pregnancy – increased fat stores and expanded intravascular and extracellular fluid – is lost more slowly. Rooney and Schauberger studied the postpartum weight pattern in a cohort of 795 women from Wisconsin.[22] At 2 weeks, 6 weeks, and 6 months postpartum, the average weight lost was 9.7, 10, and 11 kg, respectively. Twenty-two percent of patients had returned to their prepregnancy weight by 6 weeks and 37% by 6 months. Most women were still above their prepregnancy weight at 6 months postpartum, with an average net weight gain of 1.4 ± 4.8 kg. The persistence of net weight gain after pregnancy was confirmed by a large study from Smith *et al.* During a 5-year period, they studied the effects of pregnancy on weight in a racially diverse cohort of 2788 women. When compared to women who remain nulligravid throughout the study period, black and white women who experienced a first pregnancy gained an extra 4.3 and 2.3 kg, respectively. The findings did not differ significantly when corrected for behavioral factors such as baseline fitness, smoking status, and education.[23]

Although women who gain weight excessively during pregnancy lose more weight postpartum than those who gain more modestly, many authors have also noted that these women also retain more weight at 6 months postpartum and are at increased risk for long-term obesity.[24] Less weight is retained postpartum in smokers and in women who return to work promptly. In a large cohort of women studied during more than one pregnancy, Green *et al.* found that there was a direct correlation between weight gain during the first pregnancy and the weight at the onset of a subsequent pregnancy.[25] Cesarean delivery is also associated with delayed postpartum weight loss, but at 6 months that difference is no longer significant. Breast-feeding has not consistently been associated with more effective postpartum weight loss but, reassuringly, aggressive maternal weight loss through diet and exercise has no deleterious effect on the growth of breast-fed infants.[26]

It is important to note that although there are clear associations between pregnancy and postpartum weight patterns and long-term development of obesity, it has not been established whether or not interventions for weight control during pregnancy or the puerperium have any impact on enduring obesity.

Uterus

At term, the uterus weighs nearly 1 kg and its fundus reaches the level of the xyphoid process. Its cavity is large enough to accommodate one (or more) fetus(es). Immediately after delivery of its content, the uterus contracts and involutes down to the dimensions it had at 20 gestational weeks. The uterus then continues to decrease in size through a diminution in cell size and through dissolution of the connective tissue framework. Two weeks later, it usually has returned to its pelvic location. Uterine involution plateaus at 12 weeks postpartum and, for primiparas, the organ rarely returns to its original nulligravid size.

Endometrium

Within days following the delivery, the superficial decidual layer necroses and sloughs off in the form of lochia, a term used to describe the vaginal discharge during the puerperium. New endometrium is regenerated from the underlying basal layer and within 7–10 days after delivery, the endometrial surface has been completely regenerated with the exception of the area of placental implantation. The placental site is slowly resurfaced from the adjacent growth of new endometrium.

Lochial discharge is divided into three phases. Immediately postpartum, it consists of *lochia rubra*, a bloody discharge that lasts until the third or fourth day postpartum. It is then replaced by *lochia serosa*, a mucopurulent discharge with a more watery consistency that lasts up to a few weeks. Eventually, the blood and water content of the discharge decrease and its inflammatory cell content increases, forming the *lochia alba*, a yellowish-white discharge that lasts a few weeks further postpartum. Although it is often thought that lochial discharge stops after 2 weeks postpartum, more recent research suggests that many women experience a longer duration than previously thought. The duration of the lochia varies, and averages approximately 5 weeks, with a frequent waxing and waning amount of flow and color. In a cohort of 477 Filipina multiparous women, Visness *et al.* reported that postpartum vaginal discharge persisted beyond 6 weeks after delivery in nearly 10% of women.[27]

Cervix

Immediately after delivery of the uterine contents, the cervix retracts, looks edematous, loses much of its elasticity, and frequently bears minor lacerations, especially on its lateral edges. Although the cervix regresses back to its prepregnancy appearance and consistency after approximately 1 week, the external os never reachieves its pinpoint nulligravid appearance; it is wider, flat, or stellate in appearance.[28]

Perineum, perineal lacerations, and episiotomy

Some degree of perineal pain is almost universal during the immediate puerperal period, and is usually proportional to the severity of the lacerations or episiotomy. Ibuprofen is the analgesic of choice as it usually provides sufficient perineal analgesia, relieves the pain from postpartum uterine contractions, and, being present in very low levels in breast milk, is safe for the breast-fed newborn.[29] Further relief can be obtained by cold Sitz baths, where ice cubes are added to the water in which the perineum is immersed. The cold temperature provides immediate relief by decreased excitability of severed nerve endings.[30]

Perineal infections are surprisingly uncommon, given the high bacterial colonization of the lower genital tract and high frequency of perineal lacerations. This is probably explained, at least to some extent, by the dense vascularity of the perineal tissues. Perineal injury dehiscence usually presents within a few days or weeks postpartum, and is almost always associated with infection of the involved tissues.[31] For this reason, immediate reapproximation of episiotomy or laceration breakdown has been traditionally discouraged, with a period of 3 or 4 months usually allowed until secondary repair is contemplated. This period allows the tissue to revascularize, the infection to clear, and, in most cases, the injury to heal spontaneously by primary intent. Some authors advocate early repair of episiotomy or laceration breakdown, i.e. within a few days after the dehiscence.[32] If performed early, the repair must be preceded by meticulous debridement of necrotic tissue, diligent cleaning of the wound edges (using Sitz baths and local wound care) and clearance of infection, with systemic or local antibiotics. Once the wound edges are well granulated and show no evidence of necrosis or infection, usually after a few days, they are reapproximated using usual postpartum laceration repair techniques.

Bladder

There has recently been an extensive burst of new data concerning the effects of pregnancy and delivery on the urinary tract. Both hormonal and mechanical factors account for these changes. Vaginal delivery leads to marked distension of the lower genital tract and may cause some degree of trauma to the urethra, bladder, and pelvic floor. The most commonly observed postpartum urinary dysfunctions are urinary retention, usually a short-term, self-limited problem, and genuine urinary stress incontinence, which can be more of a chronic issue. Some authors have found increased rates of postpartum bladder dysfunction in the second stage complicated by macrosomia, use of forceps or vacuum, and perineal lacerations. Other authors suggest that vaginal delivery in itself is a risk factor for the subsequent onset of urinary dysfunction, such as genuine stress incontinence,[33,34] and go even further in suggesting that there may be, in selected cases, a role for elective cesarean delivery in preventing incontinence. Urinary incontinence is an underestimated and under-reported problem and some degree of urinary incontinence has been described in at least 12% of women following delivery. Factors associated with a more severe degree of incontinence include development of symptoms during pregnancy and anteceding pregnancy. It is unclear whether the use of Kegel exercises during pregnancy and the puerperium ameliorates the risk and course of urinary stress incontinence.[35]

Lactation and breast feeding

A full description of lactogenesis and breast feeding is beyond the scope of this chapter. Nevertheless, important considerations about breast-feeding are introduced here, and should be known by any clinician dealing with women in the puerperal period. After a period of relative unpopularity in the United States, breast feeding is regaining ground with over 60% women now having done some breast feeding by the time they leave the hospital. Breast feeding offers many advantages to both mother and newborn: transfer of immunoglobulins (IgA) to the newborn with consequent decrease in the incidence of gastroenteritis, colic, and other infections; decreased admission to the hospital during infancy; improved maternal–infant bonding; low cost; and reduced long-term development of diabetes and obesity. Maternal advantages include a reduced incidence of breast and ovarian cancer, a degree of contraception, and reduced anemia, from the delayed return of menses. Successful lactation relies on many factors: motivation of the mother; physicians and nurses who understand breast feeding and can provide assistance and advice; and a hospital or birthing center hospitable to breast feeding and able to provide adequate education on the topic.

Breast feeding relies on milk production (lactogenesis) and the ejection (let-down) reflex. Progesterone exerts an inhibitory effect on lactogenesis. The dramatic decrease in its concentration immediately after delivery allows lactogenesis to begin, a process that is mediated by prolactin. Milk production gradually increases from as little as 50 ml in the first 24 h to 750 ml/day by the eighth day.[36] Milk ejection is mediated through the release of oxytocin, which contracts the myoepithelial cells within the milk sinuses. Suckling of the infant stimulates both milk production from the lactotrophs and milk ejection from the milk sinuses and ducts, via the release of prolactin and oxytocin, respectively.

It is important that mothers (and their attendants) understand that the relatively limited production of milk in the first few days is a normal event, and that the infant can safely lose up to 5–10% of its body weight during that period. That weight is usually regained by days 7–10. The breast-fed infant should void and stool at least once, twice, and three times during the first, second, and third days of life, respectively. After this, at least six voids and three stools should be expected. Voids and stooling less than this or weight loss beyond 7% warrant reviewing breast feeding techniques with the mother. Breast feeding is not contraindicated in women who previously underwent breast surgery, such as reduction mammoplasty and breast augmentation, providing that the lactiferous ducts were not substantially disturbed. Patients who had mammoplasty via periareolar incisions, and those who had very little breast tissue prior to breast augmentation are more at risk for insufficient milk quantity.[37–39] Patients who had a breast cyst removal or a lumpectomy can usually breast feed without problems.[40] Adequate caloric intake in the newborn is confirmed by monitoring proper weight gain and frequency of voiding and stooling episodes as described above.

Table 183.1 Symptoms of major postpartum depression with postpartum onset (from American Psychiatric Association:[41] postpartum depression is defined in the DSM-IV as that which begins within 4 weeks after delivery)

Major depression is defined by the presence of five of the following symptoms, one of which must be either depressed mood or decreased interest or pleasure*
Depressed mood, often accompanied or overshadowed by severe anxiety
Markedly diminished interest or pleasure in activities
Appetite disturbance – usually loss of appetite with weight loss
Sleep disturbance – most often insomnia and fragmented sleep, even when the baby sleeps
Physical agitation (most commonly) or psychomotor slowing
Fatigue, decreased energy
Feelings of worthlessness or excessive or inappropriate guilt
Decreased concentration or ability to make decisions
Recurrent thoughts of death or suicidal ideation

*Symptoms must be present most of the day nearly every day for 2 weeks. A diagnosis of major depression also requires a decline from the woman's previous level of functioning and substantial impairment

Postpartum cognitive issues, postpartum depression (PPD), and postpartum psychosis

Even in the most uneventful pregnancy, significant physical, biochemical, and important psychosocial changes take place, at a relatively rapid pace. Consequently, pregnancy, delivery, and the puerperium bring about unique and complex stresses. The psychological changes noted during pregnancy are well documented but not fully understood and are probably the result of interactions among social, biological, and cultural factors. Forgetfulness, confusion, and inability to concentrate are often reported during the puerperal period. In addition, 'postpartum baby blues' are common, and manifested by anxiety, sadness, irritability, and some degree of confusion. Unlike PPD, the baby blues usually do not significantly interfere with daily functioning and resolve by the 10th postpartum day. These minor mood and cognitive changes are almost universal – and most likely benign in nature; but 10–15% of women suffer from more clinically concerning psychiatric disorders.

PPD is a well-recognized entity and has been reported in at least 10–12% of women in the postpartum period. The clinical findings associated with PPD are similar to non-puerperal depression, and its diagnostic criteria are identical,[41] except that they must be present within 4 weeks after birth (Table 183.1). The diagnosis is often delayed or the condition simply missed because mood changes, weight loss, or change in appetite – classical signs of depression – can easily be considered normal postpartum symptoms by the inexperienced clinician. As in non-puerperal depression, management usually consists of a combination of psychotherapy and pharmacotherapy. Although some antidepressants must be used cautiously in the breast feeding mother, most have little effect on the breast-fed infants. The agents of choice are the secondary amines and the selective serotonin reuptake inhibitors, which have gained increasing popularity in the last decade.

Risk factors for PPD include pregestational psychiatric conditions, antepartum pregnancy complications, especially those requiring hospitalization, complications during parturition, and poor social support. Women who experience PPD are at risk for a recurrence in a subsequent pregnancy as well as for non-puerperal depression.

Postpartum psychosis is a rarer, but serious condition. There is significant risk for both newborn and mother and it therefore should be considered a psychiatric emergency. Suicide or infanticide has been reported to occur in 5–10% of cases. Its onset is usually within the first 2 weeks postpartum and is characterized by marked disorganization, delusions, and hallucinations. Compared to non-puerperal psychotic episodes, postpartum psychosis is often more akin to psychosis caused by an organic syndrome. Neuroleptics, lithium carbonate, electro-convulsive therapy, and antidepressant drugs have all been used in the treatment of postpartum psychosis with some degree of success. However, the optimal management of PPD remains unclear, as there are limited numbers of comparative trials looking at the efficacy of the various pharmacologic agents. Given the lack of data at this point, the therapeutic approach is similar to the non-pregnant state. Compared to non-puerperal psychosis, recovery from postpartum psychosis is faster, and its overall long-term prognosis is better. The recurrence rate in subsequent pregnancies is 20%. Interestingly, some authors have described the use of sublingual estrogen, and reported significant efficacy, for the treatment of both postpartum psychosis[42] and PPD.[43]

Sexuality and the puerperium

Resumption of sexual activity

Physicians frequently recommend an arbitrary period of abstinence after delivery, usually between 2 and 6 weeks. There is little evidence that it is medically necessary but, obviously, there are many non-medical reasons that women choose to abstain from sexual activity during the postpartum period, including sleep deprivation, concerns about the newborn, sudden change in the family dynamics, lochia, perineal pain and tenderness, and fear of pregnancy. For many women who have had a vaginal birth and for all women who have had an abdominal delivery, intercourse shortly following delivery would be painful, as a certain period of time is needed for proper perineal and abdominal healing. Furthermore, the hypoestrogenism associated with breast feeding frequently contributes to vaginal dryness and consequent dyspareunia. After the vagina has healed properly, this problem is easily managed with a simple vaginal lubricant. If the problem is recalcitrant, local estrogen cream can also be used. Although a small amount of hormone is absorbed systemically with the local use of estrogen, breast feeding should not be affected.

Resumption of fertility and menstruation

The return of menstruation is highly variable during the postpartum period, and is significantly influenced by breast feeding. Campbell and Gray[44] and Gray *et al.*[45] extensively studied the relationships among lactation, ovulation, and menstruation. In their cohort of 22 non-lactating and 66 lactating mothers, first ovulation occurred on average 45 days after delivery among non-breast feeding mothers and 189 days among breast-feeding mothers. The initial menstruation is frequently anovulatory or its luteal phase is inadequate; but resumption of the normal ovulatory cycle is observed rapidly thereafter. All non-breast feeding mothers menstruated within the first 12 weeks postpartum, compared with just 20% of nursing mothers. Factors directly proportional to the risk of ovulation include duration of suckling per feed and the daily number of nursing episodes. Up to 6 months postpartum, exclusive breast feeding reduces the risk of pregnancy by 98–99% during amenorrhea and by 94–97% after anovulatory menstruation. Only amenorrheic women practicing exclusive breast feeding during the first 6 postpartum months can achieve a pregnancy rate below 2%, suggesting that contraceptive use is recommended among all other lactating women who resume menstruating before 6 postpartum months or who continue to breast feed beyond 6 months.

Birth control

The lactational amenorrhea associated with exclusive breast feeding provides effective contraception (98% effectiveness) for some time, but the failure rate is much higher if more than 10% of the caloric intake is not provided by breast milk. In a cohort study of 319 women who initiated breast feeding, Halderman and Nelson found that only 24% provided at least 90% of their child's caloric intake through breast feeding at 6 weeks postpartum.[46] This indicates that, as noted previously, effective contraception is frequently needed even among breast feeding women.

The most popular contraceptive methods used in the postpartum period are the barrier methods (condoms, diaphragm) and hormonal contraception. Because of their lack of influence on breast milk production, progestin-based contraceptive methods such as levonorgestrel pills and intramuscular medroxyprogesterone acetate are ideal choices. Compared to progestin-based oral contraception, estrogen–progestin combination oral contraception offers more effective contraception and more cycle regularity but has been discouraged in the breast feeding mother mainly because of its effect of decreasing milk production. This effect is less clinically significant when such contraceptives are initiated after 6 weeks postpartum. In women who have a well-established breast feeding pattern and who would be able to detect a clinically important decrease in milk supply, combination oral contraception can be considered after 6 weeks postpartum. Another reason to delay its use is the pregnancy-associated thrombogenic state, which could be worsened by estrogen. There are at this time insufficient data on the transdermal estrogen–progestin patch or on the transvaginal estrogen-releasing ring to consider their use in the breast feeding mother.

The timing of initiation of hormonal contraception in the postpartum period has been the object of much debate. Since ovulation rarely occurs prior to 45 days after delivery, and is even more delayed in the breast feeding mother, and since many couples wait a few weeks prior to resuming sexual activity, contraception can safely be withheld in most couples until 2–3 weeks postpartum. The United States Food and Drug Administration recommends waiting 6 weeks in the breast-feeding mother and 3 weeks in the non-breast feeding mother prior to initiation of progestin-based oral contraceptives, but practical reasons (e.g. questionable compliance with postpartum visit or medical insurance coverage issues) may call for earlier initiation of such contraception. This practice has not been shown to be deleterious to successful breast feeding or newborn growth. In many clinical settings, progestins are administered intramuscularly at 2–3 days postpartum, immediately before discharge from the hospital, and no adverse effects have been found.[47]

REFERENCES

1. Prendiville W. The prevention of post partum haemorrhage: Optimising routine management of the third stage of labour. *Eur J Obstet Gynecol Reprod Biol* 1996;69:19–24.
2. Royston E, Armstrong S. *Preventing Maternal Deaths.* Geneva: World Health Organization, 1989:30–42.
3. Khan GQ, John IS, Wani S, Doherty T, Sibai BM. Controlled cord traction versus minimal intervention techniques in delivery of the placenta: A randomized controlled trial. *Am J Obstet Gynecol* 1997;177:770–4.
4. Giacalone PL, Vignal J, Daures JP, Boulot P, Hedon B, Laffargue F. A randomised evaluation of two techniques of management of the third stage of labour in women at low risk of postpartum haemorrhage. *Br J Obstet Gynecol* 2000;107:396–400.
5. Nordstrom L, Fogelstam K, Fridman G, Larsson A, Rydhstroem H. Routine oxytocin in the third stage of labour: A placebo controlled randomised trial. *Br J Obstet Gynaecol* 1997;104:781–6.
6. Elbourne DR, Prendiville WJ, Carroli G, Wood J, McDonald S. Prophylactic use of oxytocin in the third stage of labour. *Cochrane Database Syst Rev* 2001:CD001808.
7. Jackson KW Jr, Allbert JR, Schemmer GK, Elliot M, Humphrey A, Taylor J. A randomized controlled trial comparing oxytocin administration before and after placental delivery in the prevention of postpartum hemorrhage. *Am J Obstet Gynecol* 2001; 185:873–7.
8. Soriano D, Dulitzki M, Schiff E, Barkai G, Mashiach S, Seidman DS. A prospective cohort study of oxytocin plus ergometrine compared with oxytocin alone for prevention of postpartum haemorrhage. *Br J Obstet Gynaecol* 1996;103:1068–73.
9. Carey M. Adverse cardiovascular sequelae of ergometrine. *Br J Obstet Gynaecol* 1993;100:865.
10. Bamigboye AA, Hofmeyr GJ, Merrell DA. Rectal misoprostol in the prevention of postpartum hemorrhage: A placebo-controlled trial. *Am J Obstet Gynecol* 1998;179:1043–6.
11. Villar J, Gulmezoglu AM, Hofmeyr GJ, Forna F. Systematic review of randomized controlled trials of misoprostol to prevent postpartum hemorrhage. *Obstet Gynecol* 2002;100:1301–12.
12. Gerstenfeld TS, Wing DA. Rectal misoprostol versus intravenous oxytocin for the prevention of postpartum hemorrhage after vaginal delivery. *Am J Obstet Gynecol* 200;185:878–82.
13. Dombrowski MP, Bottoms SF, Saleh AA, *et al.* Third stage of labor: Analysis of duration and clinical practice. *Am J Obstet Gynecol* 1995;172:1279–84.
14. Combs CA, Laros RK Jr. Prolonged third stage of labor: Morbidity and risk factors. *Obstet Gynecol* 1991;77:863–7.
15. Lee WK, Baggish MS, Lashgari M. Acute inversion of the uterus. *Obstet Gynecol* 1978;51:144–7.
16. Easterday CL, Reid DE. Inversion of the puerperal uterus managed by the Haultain technique. *Am J Obstet Gynecol* 1959;78:1224–6.
17. Mandl KD, Homer CJ, Harary O, Finkelstein JA. Effect of a reduced postpartum length of stay program on primary care services use by mothers and infants. *Pediatrics* 2000;106(Suppl 4):937–41.
18. Liu S, Wen SW, McMillan D, Trouton K, Fowler D, McCourt C. Increased neonatal readmission rate associated with decreased length of hospital stay at birth in Canada. *Can J Public Health* 2000;91:46–50.
19. Liu S, Heaman M, Kramer MS, Demissie K, Wen SW, Marcoux S, Maternal Health Study Group of the Canadian Perinatal Surveillance System. Length of hospital stay, obstetric conditions at childbirth, and maternal readmission: A population-based cohort study. *Am J Obstet Gynecol* 2002;187:681–7.
20. Flegal KM, Carroll MD, Kuczmarski RJ, Johnson CL. Overweight and obesity in the United States: Prevalence and trends, 1960–1994. *Int J Obes Relat Metab Disord* 1998;22:39–47.
21. Mokdad AH, Serdula MK, Dietz WH, Bowman BA, Marks JS, Koplan JP. The spread of the obesity epidemic in the United States, 1991–1998. *J Am Med Assoc* 1999;282:1519–22.
22. Rooney BL, Schauberger CW. Excess pregnancy weight gain and long-term obesity: One decade later. *Obstet Gynecol* 2002;100: 245–52.
23. Smith DE, Lewis CE, Caveny JL, Perkins LL, Burke GL, Bild DE. Longitudinal changes in adiposity associated with pregnancy. The CARDIA Study. Coronary Artery Risk Development in Young Adults Study. *J Am Med Assoc* 1994;271:1747–51.
24. Shauberger CW, Rooney BL, Brimer LM. Factors that influence weight loss in the puerperium. *Obstet Gynecol* 1992;79: 424–9.
25. Greene GW, Smiciklas-Wright H, Scholl TO, Karp RJ. Postpartum weight change: How much of the weight gained in pregnancy will be lost after delivery? *Obstet Gynecol* 1988;71:701–7.
26. Lovelady CA, Garner KE, Moreno KL, Williams JP. The effect of weight loss in overweight, lactating women on the growth of their infants. *N Engl J Med* 2000;342:449–53.
27. Visness CM, Kennedy KI, Ramos R. The duration and character of postpartum bleeding among breast-feeding women. *Obstet Gynecol* 1997;89:159–63.
28. Johnson LD, Sheps MC, Easterday CL. The cervix in pregnancy and the postpartum period. I. The correlation of certain clinical factors with the clinical appearance of the cervix. *Obstet Gynecol* 1959;14:452–60.
29. Windle ML, Booker LA, Rayburn WF. Postpartum pain after vaginal delivery. A review of comparative analgesic trials. *J Reprod Med* 1989;34:891–5.
30. Droegemuller W. Cold sitz baths for relief of postpartum perineal pain. *Clin Obstet Gynecol* 1980;23:1039–43.
31. Ramin SM, Ramus RM, Little BB, Gilstrap LC III. Early repair of episiotomy dehiscence associated with infection. *Am J Obstet Gynecol* 1992;167(4, Pt 1):1104–7.
32. Hankins GD, Hauth JC, Gilstrap LC III, Hammond TL, Yeomans ER, Snyder RR. Early repair of episiotomy dehiscence. *Obstet Gynecol* 1990;75:48–51.
33. Eason E, Labrecque M, Marcoux S, Mondor M. Effects of carrying a pregnancy and of method of delivery on urinary incontinence: A prospective cohort study. *BMC Pregnancy Childbirth* 2004;4:4.
34. Farrell SA, Allen VM, Baskett TF. Parturition and urinary incontinence in primiparas. *Obstet Gynecol* 2001;97:350–6.
35. Burgio KL, Zyczynski H, Locher JL, Richter HE, Redden DT, Wright KC. Urinary incontinence in the 12-month postpartum period. *Obstet Gynecol* 2003;102:1291–8.
36. Neville MC, Keller R, Seacat J, *et al.* Studies in human lactation: Milk volumes in lactating women during the onset of lactation and full lactation. *Am J Clin Nutr* 1988;48:1375–86.
37. Hurst NM. Breastfeeding after breast augmentation. *J Hum Lact* 2003;19:70–1.
38. Hurst NM. Lactation after augmentation mammoplasty. *Obstet Gynecol* 1996;87:30–4.
39. Cruz-Korchin N, Korchin L. *Plast Reconstr Surg* 2004;114:890–4.

40. Neifert M, DeMarzo S, Seacat J, Young D, Leff M, Orleans M. The influence of breast surgery, breast appearance, and pregnancy-induced breast changes on lactation sufficiency as measured by infant weight gain. *Birth* 1990;17:31–8.
41. American Psychiatric Association. *The Diagnostic and Statistical Manual of Mental Disorders*, DSM-IV, 4th edn. Washington, DC: American Psychiatric Association, 1994.
42. Ahokas A, Aito M, Rimon R. Positive treatment effect of estradiol in postpartum psychosis: A pilot study. *J Clin Psychiatry* 2000; 61:166–9.
43. Gregoire AJ, Kumar R, Everitt B, Henderson AF, Studd JW. Transdermal oestrogen for treatment of severe postnatal depression. *Lancet* 1996;347:930–3.
44. Campbell OM, Gray RH. Characteristics and determinants of postpartum ovarian function in women in the United States. *Am J Obstet Gynecol* 1993;169:55–60.
45. Gray RH, Campbell OM, Apelo R, *et al.* Risk of ovulation during lactation. *Lancet* 1990;335:25–9.
46. Halderman LD, Nelson AL. Impact of early postpartum administration of progestin-only hormonal contraceptives compared with nonhormonal contraceptives on short-term breast-feeding patterns. *Am J Obstet Gynecol* 2002;186:1250–6.
47. Halderman LD, Nelson AL. Impact of early postpartum administration of progestin-only hormonal contraceptives compared with nonhormonal contraceptives on short-term breast-feeding patterns. *Am J Obstet Gynecol* 2002;186:1250–6.

184 Postpartum hemorrhage

J. Herczeg

At the beginning of the 20th century, parturient mothers were fearful for their own lives during childbirth. Beginning some 40 years ago, an unprecedented and rapid development of the management of childbirth occurred, especially in the field of electronic surveillance and in the care of the critically ill obstetric patient.

Throughout recent decades in the developed world, fetal health has been the primary focus of prenatal and intrapartum care. Obstetrics in the 21st century will pose new challenges, many of which will be directed at the maintenance of maternal well-being. One contributor to this shift in emphasis relates to the change in maternal demographics that has occurred in many parts of the world. Some women are prepared to undertake high medical risks to their own lives by having a child close to or 'beyond' the extremes of their reproductive lives.

The peripartal period is one of the most dangerous times of life. Family expectations are very high, and the responsibilities of the obstetrician are expanding. It is very difficult to draw a line between good and substandard care, and practitioners of obstetrics are well aware of the fact that modern reproductive research does not eliminate all the risks and hazards associated with childbirth.

Direct causes of maternal mortality in modern obstetrics include:

(1) Postpartum hemorrhage (PPH)
(2) Infections during labor and delivery
(3) Puerperal sepsis
(4) Complications arising from the second stage of labor
(5) Pregnancy-induced hypertension
(6) Obstructed labor
(7) Abortion-related causes
(8) Uterine inversion.

Although modern medicine has made considerable progress in reducing the mortality from all these causes, PPH remains one of the most frequent causes of maternal mortality, arising most often from uterine hypotonia or atony. Ironically, with the availability of appropriate modern techniques of prevention and treatment, many of these deaths are avoidable.

Maternal death rates from infection and sepsis have shown a steady decrease over the last several decades, while hemorrhage-related maternal deaths have declined more slowly, pointing to the fact that they are more difficult to prevent.[1] PPH is still a leading cause of maternal mortality in some areas of the world. The incidence of PPH is 3–5% of all deliveries, and its incidence is doubled after induced labors.[2] It is the greatest single cause of maternal deaths in the majority of mortality surveys, and is directly responsible for 12–60% of maternal mortality in developing countries.

Postpartum hemorrhage can also be indirectly responsible, as an associated factor, for a further proportion of maternal deaths attributed directly to other causes, such as infection and obstructed labor. About one-third of all maternal mortality is related to obstetric hemorrhage. In sharp contrast to antepartum hemorrhages, which usually claim life after 10 h if left untreated, PPH kills swiftly, often in less than 2 h if not properly treated. In the overwhelming majority of cases, the PPH occurs unexpectedly, exploding into a drama in the labor room, where blood is seen everywhere. The mother's face and lips are pale and her skin is covered with a cold sweat. Her calm suggests that she thinks she is going to die. In such a severe clinical emergency, successful management requires immediate access to special expertise and facilities, and the outcome is dependent on instant availability of blood replacement facilities, and swift expert decisions on the steps necessary to bring the bleeding under control.

Clinical definitions

The widely accepted clinical definition of PPH is blood loss greater than 500 ml during the first 24 h after delivery. The excessive bleeding is usually evident within 5 min following birth. It should be pointed out that blood loss after spontaneous vaginal delivery may be up to 600 ml and can amount to 1000 ml or even as much as 1500 ml, following instrumental or operative delivery. Extensive obstetric experience is necessary to determine if bleeding is occurring too rapidly, and if it is responsive to conventional treatment. Excessive blood loss is especially dangerous in cases where the physiologic expansion of blood volume during pregnancy has not occurred, such as in cases with preeclampsia.

Bleeding during the third stage of labor occurring before delivery of the placenta (third stage of labor defined here as the period from delivery of the fetus to expulsion of the placenta and its membranes and establishment of satisfactory uterine tone) is also categorized not as intrapartum but as PPH.

Primary PPH

Primary PPH has been defined internationally as more than 500 ml of blood loss during the first 24 h following delivery. The main argument for this threshold rests on the fact that postpartum blood loss is notoriously and significantly underestimated. In addition, there are clinical cases in which the mother does not undergo the normal physiologic blood volume adaptation during pregnancy, or in which the mother is anemic (small stature women, pregnancy blood expansion not yet developed, or restricted, such as in preeclamptic patients). In such cases, a lower level of blood loss should prompt therapeutic measures.

Primary PPH is a frequent, unpredictable and potentially lethal complication of childbirth. In the vast majority of cases, primary PPH is caused by hypotonia or atony of the uterus. The most common causes of primary PPH are listed in Table 184.1.

Table 184.1 Common causes of primary postpartum hemorrhage

(1) Uterine hypotonia/atonia
(2) Retained placenta, placental fragments (succenturiate lobe or cotyledon)
(3) Subtle myometrial trophoblastic invasion (focal placenta accreta)
(4) Obvious myometrial trophoblastic invasion (placenta accreta, increta, percreta)
(5) Lacerations of the lower genital tract
(6) Intravascular coagulation
(7) Rupture of the uterus
(8) Uterine inversion

Secondary (late) PPH

Secondary PPH is defined as serious bleeding from the genital tract after the first 24 h and during the first 6 weeks of the postpartum period. Its most frequent causes are the subinvolution of the attachment site of the placenta, puerperal infection (endometritis), and retained placental fragments. Its prevention resides in awareness of the dangers and avoidance of mismanagement of the third stage of labor. Treatment includes oxytocic administration. In severe cases, administration of third-generation prostaglandin analogs may become necessary. In the author's experience these have proved to be extremely useful. It should also be noted that in rare cases a primary PPH (e.g. postcesarean hemorrhage) may be followed 10–15 days later by a secondary 'attack' necessitating the reintroduction of the original treatment. In late hemorrhage cases, gentle curettage and antibiotics are also in the mainstream of management.

Causes of PPH

Uterine atony

Uterine atony is defined as a loss of blood that is not arising from trauma to the birth canal or from placental tissue left in the uterine cavity. In modern obstetric practice, the increased use of labor induction carries an increased risk of postpartum atonic hemorrhage (PPAH).

The incidence of PPH due to uterine exhaustion or hypotonia (arrhythmia) is very high. Uterine atony is responsible for 90% of all PPHs (trauma is responsible for about 7% and coagulation failure for 3%).[3] Severe hemorrhage from uterine atony can be defined as a > 30 mmHg drop in blood pressure, a decrease of hemoglobin by 3g/dl or more, and an estimated blood loss > 1000 ml.

If routine oxytocics are not administered following delivery, the frequency of PPAH is between 10% and 20%.[4] Clinical investigations have proved that programmed routine use of oxytocics significantly reduces the incidence of PPH.[5]

Postpartum atonic hemorrhage is a dramatic clinical situation putting the life of the mother into immediate danger, because it may lead to circulatory collapse within a few minutes, and it is often accompanied by coagulation dysfunction, which can perpetuate severe bleeding. It is imperative to be aware of (1) predisposing factors, because postpartum uterine atony can sometimes be anticipated, and (2) the fact that PPAH often does not respond to conventional therapy.

Retained placental fragments

In the natural course of the third stage of labor, the placenta generally separates in about 10–15 min, then gradually descends to the lower part of the genital tract. In cases with a history of previous radical intrauterine instrumentation or infection, an unsuspected focal placenta accreta can develop, and part or all of the placenta remains in the uterine cavity. Retained placental fragments are the most common cause of delayed PPH.

Placenta accreta

The rising cesarean delivery rate has increased the incidence of placenta accreta. In these cases, the basal decidual layer is defective, and the trophoblast invades the myometrium. Manual removal of the placenta is difficult even in mild, focal cases, because there is no clear cleavage plane for placental separation. In most cases with significant placental invasion, manual removal of the placenta is impossible, and hysterectomy is usually required to control hemorrhage.

Bleeding from lacerations

Lower birth canal lacerations should be suspected if the uterus is firmly contracted but the bleeding is profuse. Adequate exploration with good exposure is necessary; lacerations must be repaired promptly and with careful attention to good hemostasis.

Uterine rupture

The most severe obstetric catastrophe is uterine rupture. Damage to this upper region of the genital tract is serious because this region is supplied by large vessels; therefore, any vascular tear in this region can result in immediate and catastrophic loss of blood. Its incidence is about 1 in 2000 deliveries (there is great variation among different places, ranging from 1:100 to 1:11,000). The dehiscence of a previous cesarean section scar is less dangerous than the rupture of an unscarred uterus, and in modern obstetrical institutions the use of the partogram has proved to be helpful in avoiding this serious complication.

Careful management of labor inductions, with close supervision of uterine stimulation with oxytocin infusion is an important preventive measure. The rate of the oxytocin infusion must be decreased when the partogram shows that the acceleration phase of labor has been reached. Preinduction ripening of the uterine cervix with a prostaglandin E_2 gel preparation should also be carefully supervised, because the prostaglandin might initiate strong contractility with the potential to rupture the uterus. Clinical management requires considerable surgical skills, because the uterus in most cases should be removed, and large hematomas may be present in the operative field.

Acute inversion of the uterus

Fortunately this problem is rare, if mismanagement of the third stage of labor is avoided. Its incomplete forms should also be recognized. Management sometimes requires uterine relaxation with betamimetics, manual repositioning, and administration of a prostaglandin analog to keep the uterus well contracted.

Coagulopathy

Bleeding from venous puncture sites or the sutured cesarean section wound suggests coagulopathy. A platelet count and D-dimer (a fibrin degradation product) level can be quickly obtained before any sophisticated tests; a low platelet count or the presence of elevated D-dimer concentrations raises the possibility of disseminated intravascular coagulation (DIC). DIC is often triggered by a sudden episode of blood loss, and the generated fibrin degradation products from the transient DIC episode further impair myometrial contractility.

To correct the coagulation disturbance, fresh whole blood (very difficult to obtain nowadays), fresh frozen plasma, and, if possible, thrombocyte preparations, should be administered.

Basic studies: exhaustion of cellular mechanisms of contractility

The human uterus has a highly sophisticated, multilayered bleeding control system. The first line of defense is the hemostatic contractions of the different myometrial layers, twisting and compressing the vessel tree. This myometrial contractile action is supplemented by constriction of the torn maternal vessels at the placental site.

The level of excitability and the condition of electrical coupling between myometrial cells determine the ability of the uterine muscle to contract. Hormonal, nervous and immune intrinsic factors, and many extrinsic pharmacologic factors, can modulate membrane potential, ionic exchange and electrical propagation. Between myometrial cells electrical coupling is possible via gap junctions; postdelivery disappearance of gap junctions is accompanied by a nearly total inability of the muscle to contract and respond to stimulation.[6] The exhaustion of cellular mechanisms (ionic exchange and electrical propagation) after delivery can be an explanation for uterine atony.[7] Exogenous prostaglandins in pharmacologic doses can sometimes restart the 'burned out' system.

Contractility of uterine muscle is regulated by calcium. Prostaglandins facilitate the entry of calcium into the cell through specific calcium channels or receptor-operated channels.[8]

The intracellular adenosine triphosphate-dependent Ca^{2+} transport pump is an important regulator of cytoplasmic calcium levels, and thus of the contractile state of the muscle.[8] Ca^{2+} is essential for myosin light-chain kinase activation, and is carried by the calmodulin–Ca^{2+} complex. An unknown calcium regulatory system may play a role, allowing uterine muscle to remain contracted at less than maximum levels of cellular calcium.[9] Subthreshold doses of prostaglandins potentiate the spasmogenic Ca^{2+}, even after removal of the prostaglandins.[10] Synergistic effects of Ca^{2+} and prostaglandins are utilized to enhance mid-trimester uterine activity.[11] Therefore Ca^{2+} entry blockers (nifedipine) should not be used close to delivery because of the high risk of postpartum atony, resistant to oxytocics.[12–14]

There is no anatomically demonstrable specific pacemaker and propagation system in the human uterus. There appears to be a physiologic pacemaker area. Contractions begin high in the lateral side of the fundus, and the speed of stimulus propagation downward is 2 cm/s. When the whole uterus is covered, the stimulus travels back.[15,16] Contractions are strongest near the pacemaker and have the longest duration there (high power area, HPA).[17] In the synchronous pattern, HPA is monofocal and is high in the fundus. The HPA propagates all over the uterus. HPA is of multifocal origin in false labor, proceeding in an asynchronous pattern leading to uterine arrhythmia.[17]

Disorders of HPA will be manifest as an inverted triple descending gradient, in terms of propagation, intensity, duration, and are called wandering HPA, resulting in impaired contractions. Asynchronous tocograms predict complicated labor, and may forecast uterine atonia.[17]

Table 184.2 Conditions predisposing to postpartum hemorrhage[4]

Case history	Prenatal factors	Labor factors
Primigravida	Placenta previa	Labor induction
Multigravida (5+)	Placental abruption	Prolonged/ obstructed labor
Myoma	Hydramnios	Short labor
Von Willebrand's disease	Multiple pregnancy	Cesarean section
Anemia	Intrauterine death	Epidural anesthesia
Purpura	Pre-eclampsia	Disseminated intravascular coagulation
Unknown	Placenta accreta	Chorioamnionitis

Risk factors for atonic PPH

Widely-known risk factors include previous PPH, manual removal of the placenta, abruptio placentae, placenta previa, prolonged labor with prolonged administration of oxytocin, precipitate labor, difficult vacuum extraction or forceps delivery, and breech extraction.

Following uterine inertia during labor, for which correction has been attempted by supportive administration of oxytocin, or following a short, precipitate labor, or following labor induction, the uterine muscle often fails to contract in the third stage. The failure of the normal hemostatic contraction and retraction of the myometrium is due to exhaustion of the cellular contractile system.

Postpartum uterine activity is also impaired under anesthesia. The resting tone remains unchanged, but contractility is inhibited, recovering with time.[18,19]

The predisposing conditions for uterine atony are listed in Table 184.2. However, the predictive values of antenatal factors is disturbingly low. Previous third-stage bleeding in the case history increases the likelihood of PPH twofold. Pregnant women with unfavorable characteristics, such as age over 35 years, infection, diabetes mellitus and cardiac disease, are not necessarily at increased risk for PPH, but these underlying conditions worsen the serious sequelae of PPH.

Maternal response to massive blood loss

Normal pregnant patients expand their original 5000 ml blood volume by at least 1500 ml, a hematologic adaptation that reduces the risk from hemorrhage at delivery. Some fraction of this extra volume can be lost without obvious signs of hypovolemic shock.

If an obstetric patient with a normally expanded blood volume bleeds profusely, symptoms of shock will usually appear following a loss of more than 1500 ml. Loss of 25% of intravascular volume may be fatal, but in the early stages of shock arterial blood pressure remains unaltered.[3]

Coagulation failure often accompanies severe postpartum bleeding.[20] Disseminated intravascular coagulopathy may be triggered by obstetric events such as release of thromboplastic substances during placental abruption, or may develop as a consequence of hypovolemic shock. When there has been massive blood replacement, an element of dilutional coagulopathy may also exist. Diagnosis may not await the results of sophisticated tests; observing the operative field and a tube of freshly drawn blood for the presence of clots and a thrombocyte count can aid prompt diagnosis.

Good myometrial contractions generally prevent fatal hemorrhage from the placental site, even when the maternal blood is incoagulable, but fatal bleeding can occur in the presence of uterine atony.

Prevention of PPAH

Nowadays, there are new aspects to the prevention of PPAH. Patients are concerned about receiving blood transfusions, because of the small HIV and hepatitis risk. Autologous blood can be taken and retransfused when needed, but this is not a simple method, and requires that excessive blood loss is anticipated.

Planning of labor inductions so that patients deliver during the daytime, when access to life-supporting facilities are optimal, can help, but induction itself is a predisposing factor to uterine exhaustion and atonic bleeding.[21] The introduction of active third-stage management, controlled cord traction, and use of oxytocics were major improvements, but these measures are not without risks. Oxytocin can cause a drop of blood pressure, and can lead to arrhythmias. Ergot derivatives can precipitate hypertension in one-third of cases and cause nausea or vomiting in a quarter of cases. Prostaglandins offer a better and more efficient choice to prevent and correct uterine hypotonia.

Prostaglandins in postpartum uterine hemostasis

Prostaglandins play a fundamental role in the maintenance of continued contractions, myometrial retraction, vasoconstriction and platelet activation. Prostaglandin metabolites rapidly increase in the peripheral circulation at the time of placental separation, pointing to a dramatic increase of myometrial prostaglandin synthesis, which is responsible for maintaining uterine tonicity and controlling postpartum hemostasis.[22,23]

Prostaglandins offer a logical choice to fight against uterine hypotonia, because endogenous prostaglandins are involved in maintaining postpartum resting uterine tone and stimulating myometrial contractions, which continue after delivery of the baby and the placenta.[24,25] Their usefulness has been demonstrated in many clinical studies during the last two decades.

When uterine activity and blood flow were studied, it was shown that intravenous sulprostone (16-phenoxy-prostaglandin E_2) infusion resulted in a uterine contracture (sustained contraction) response, which was obvious on photographs taken intraoperatively; a change of color of the uterine surface indicated reduction of perfusion.[26]

Early observations with prostaglandin $F_{2\alpha}$ in the third stage proved that intramyometrial injections cause myometrial ischemia and sustained contracture, with rapid spread over the uterine surface providing good hemostasis.[27] These early observations provided the basis for use of prostaglandins in atonic hemorrhage.

The pioneering clinical use of first-generation prostaglandins more than 15 years ago was not without problems. Takagi *et al.* injected prostaglandin $F_{2\alpha}$ intramyometrially.[28] Later, 15-methyl-prostaglandin $F_{2\alpha}$ was used,[29] but maternal arterial oxygen desaturation, secondary to increased intrapulmonary shunting, was reported after this prostaglandin was given for arresting postpartum atonic bleeding.[30] Continuing research has resulted in the development of second-generation prostaglandin analogs, with significant improvement in utero-selectivity and clinical acceptability.

A multisubstituted third-generation prostaglandin analog, the 16-phenoxy-E_2 molecule (sulprostone), has a highly selective effect on the uterus, since it does not influence the function of other smooth muscle tissues, as natural or first-generation prostaglandins do. From this observation, a significant clinical advantage originated: there is separation between the desirable, therapeutic effects and the unwanted, mainly gastrointestinal, side-effects.[31] The drug is available in Europe, but not in the United States.

Sulprostone has shown good tolerance in local and systemic routes of administration, focused action on the uterus, and an acceptably low incidence of side-effects. The use of relatively low doses is possible due to its marked biostability.[32] The main effect of the uterotopic sulprostone is induction of controllable uterine contractions, with simultaneous compression and constriction of the uterine blood vessels, especially at the placental site. Following intramuscular injection, sulprostone reaches maximal plasma levels within 5–15 min; its plasma level decreases by 50% in 1–2 h. The uterorelaxant effect and risk of atonic bleeding from tocolytics such as betamimetics, magnesium sulfate in toxemia, and prostaglandin synthetase inhibitors, can be quickly neutralized by postpartum administration of sulprostone infusion.[33–35]

Prevention and treatment of PPAH in the labor and delivery room

In cases of atonic bleeding quick action is necessary to save the life of the mother. The two simultaneous lines of treatment are: (1) control and stop the bleeding, and (2) correct hypovolemia (hematocrit is not reliable in sudden acute severe blood loss). The age-old observation should be kept in mind: 'An empty, well-contracted uterus with good myometrial contractile ability will not bleed'. The following management approach consists of 10 steps, assuming that the delivery takes place in a hospital and that active third-stage management was employed. The scheme is summarized in Table 184.3.

Step 1

React to excessive rates of bleeding even if the loss has not exceeded 500 ml. Reconsider the history and the clinical course for possible causes, remembering that more than one etiologic factor could be responsible.

Step 2

If the uterus is atonic by abdominal palpation, and the placenta has already been expelled, fundal massage should be started immediately, which helps to initiate good uterine contraction and expel accumulated clots from the uterine cavity. Do a bimanual examination and perform bimanual uterine massage and compression. Order oxytocin and intravenous ergometrine.

External fundal massage should be complemented by internal bimanual compression: with one hand in the lower birth canal the cervix and the paracervical region should be compressed, and with the other hand the uterus should be elevated. This forced anteflexion of the uterus should help to control the bleeding, and it also makes it possible to give a prostaglandin injection through the abdominal wall directly into the myometrium. For this purpose only the safest available prostaglandin analog should be used, such as sulprostone (described in step 5).

Step 3

If bleeding continues, and the uterus is still boggy and atonic, consider early intravenous administration of a

Table 184.3 Management of postpartum (atonic) hemorrhage

Step 1	React to excessive bleeding, even if it does not exceed 500 ml
Step 2	If the uterus is atonic, do fundal massage to expel clots; perform bimanual massage and compression; order oxytocin and intravenous ergometrine
Step 3	If bleeding continues with an atonic uterus, consider early intravenous prostaglandin analog; install a reliable intravenous line; ask for blood typing and cross-matching
Step 4	If the uterus is well contracted but the bleeding is continuing, prepare for manual exploration of the uterus
Step 5	Mild atonic hemorrhage will not exceed 1000 ml of lost blood; intravenous sulprostone 4.1 μg/min (40 drops/min) for 120 min, up to 16.7 μg/min
Step 6	For severe atonic bleeding exceeding 1000 ml of blood loss, immediately restore lost volume with fresh whole blood and estimate blood loss; sulprostone dose may be increased briefly up to 330 drops/min (33.3 μg/min)
Step 7	If bleeding is continuing, transfer patient to the operating room; intracervical prostaglandin analog injection might help
	Postcesarean atonic bleeding within 30 min is especially dangerous; transfer patient back to operating room; sulprostone intracervically on the operating table
	For intraoperative atonic bleeding during cesarean section give intraoperative, intramyometrial injection of sulprostone (100–300 μg)
Step 8	In cases of acute inversion of the uterus: after manual repositioning of the uterus give intravenous sulprostone infusion
Step 9	Ligation of the hypogastric artery or the uterine artery can control pelvic hemorrhage
Step 10	Hysterectomy is indicated when all attempts to control the bleeding have failed. Placenta previa with previous cesarean section and uteroplacental apoplexy are especially prone to uncontrollable bleeding, and are often hysterectomy indications

third-generation prostaglandin analog, as described in step 5. Install a reliable intravenous line, and ask for blood typing and cross-matching. Notify anesthesia and operating room personnel.

Step 4

If the uterus is well contracted and the bleeding is continuing, prepare for mandatory manual exploration of the uterus under general anesthesia, to remove possible placental fragments and rule out injury in the higher region of the genital tract. This exploration is extremely important, because it is the only defense against severe mistakes, such as overlooking cervical or high sulcus lacerations or, the most severe obstetric complication, rupture of the uterus. Lower genital tract lacerations are repaired under adequate exposure.

Step 5

Mild atonic hemorrhage will not exceed 1000 ml of lost blood. The patient is still in the labor and delivery room and the modern management list includes all of the above: massage and bimanual compression of the uterus, giving uterotonic drugs, exploring the uterus, placing an ice bag over the lower abdomen, and simultaneous establishment of an intravenous line for administering sulprostone, 500 μg in 250 ml of any isotonic crystalloid solution. The recommended dosage is 4.1 μg/min (40 drops/min) for 120 min, which can be increased up to 16.7 μg/min (120 drops/min) for 30 min as a maximum.

Step 6

For management of severe atonic bleeding exceeding 1000 ml of blood loss, immediately start restoring lost volume with an estimate of blood loss. Rapid volume replacement is crucial, even before deterioration in the patient's vital signs, because in the early stages of shock, arterial blood pressure can remain unaltered.[3]

Fresh whole blood is ideal for treatment of serious obstetric hemorrhage; but over the last 25 years, the availability of whole blood has decreased due to blood bank fractionation, and packed red blood cells are generally used, along with crystalloid solutions and fresh frozen plasma as required.

Prepare the operating room and inform the patient that surgery may become necessary. The sulprostone intravenous dose may be increased briefly to 330 drops/min (33.3 μg/min). Take a quick look at blood coagulation, looking for the presence of clots, because obstetric events often trigger a sudden, transitory episode of DIC.[20] Coagulation failure with decreased thrombocyte count suggests DIC, while fragile coagulums with normal thrombocyte count point to fibrinolysis as the main pathological event.

Rule out injury, and remove intrauterine clots. Chronic intravenous administration of sulprostone should be continued. The infused dose of sulprostone per hour should not exceed 500 μg (approximately 80 drops/min). The infusion should be continuously supervised, and the maximum total dose should be 1500 μg. With this therapy, atonic blood loss will be no more than 1000 ml, because the rapid, efficient and long-lasting myometrial contraction induced by the prostaglandin compresses the uterine vessels.

Step 7

The patient is transferred to the operating room if all the above measures fail to control the bleeding. Manual exploration has been done, and damage to the birth canal has already been ruled out in the labor and delivery room. On the operating table, while preparing for surgical intervention as a last resort, intracervical prostaglandin analog injection can be carried out under adequate exposure.

At the same time, accumulated intrauterine clots can be removed. At this stage a coagulation failure with DIC is usually present; therefore fresh frozen plasma should be administered. Even if the bleeding is decreasing, the patient is kept on the operating table, with full preparation for surgery. In such cases, usually 1–4 h are required to complete cessation of the bleeding. Intravenous prostaglandin analog treatment is continued as described above.

Postcesarean atonic bleeding is especially dangerous, and usually appears within 30 min following transfer to the recovery room. The patient should be immediately transferred back to the operating room and treatment should proceed as described in steps 5 and 6. Sulprostone can also be given intracervically under adequate exposure on the operating table. In high-risk atony-prone cases, postoperative prophylactic intravenous low-dose administration (2 μg/min) of sulprostone may be recommended.

Intraoperative atonic bleeding during cesarean section is quite common, especially if there was a preceding elective labor induction with oxytocin. In the author's experience, intraoperative, intramyometrial injection of sulprostone (100–300 mg) proves to be extremely helpful. Contraction is promptly initiated within seconds by the prostaglandin analog, given into the anterior wall of the uterus. Avoid direct intravascular injection of the prostaglandin.

Step 8

In case of acute inversion of the uterus, which is fortunately rare, a two-stage treatment is recommended: first, in some cases betamimetics are needed for relaxing the contraction ring; then, after manual repositioning of the uterus, intravenous infusion of sulprostone should be started immediately, while holding the repositioned uterus in its correct position by hand. This type of treatment has proved to be successful.

Step 9

Ligation of the hypogastric artery or the uterine artery is described in every standard textbook of obstetrics. The use of this method is advocated in cases of placenta previa, focal placenta accreta, and cervical pregnancy. However the author's experience has showed that in a real catastrophic obstetric scenario, the large uterus prevents adequate exposure of the vessels, especially if a hematoma is present. Such a case has been encountered when even a vascular surgeon was unable to locate the vessels for more than 30 min in the large pelvic hematoma. Although hypogastric artery ligation can control pelvic hemorrhage through eliminating uterine artery pulsation (the so-called 'trip-hammer effect'), it is a time-consuming approach with potential for serious operative field complications.[36]

Ligation of the ascending branch of the uterine artery on both sides requires the elevation of the uterus out of the abdominal cavity. The ureter is in close proximity, and there is a danger of ureteral ligation, because of the distorted anatomy of the postpartum uterus.

Step 10

Hysterectomy is indicated when all attempts to control the bleeding have failed. It is a striking observation that 26% of patients who require emergency hysterectomy cannot be identified before delivery by the existence of predisposing risk factors.[37]

The author's experience has shown that in cases in which severe PPH is combined with severe DIC and multiorgan failure, it is futile to try to preserve the uterus. In many such cases when the uterus was preserved, it became a focus of infection, and the patient, who already survived the bleeding and the DIC, died of sepsis.

The author had a case in which, after a placental abruption, the uterine bleeding and DIC were successfully controlled, but then multiorgan failure supervened. The patient became unconscious, and was transferred by helicopter in deep coma to a national center. There she underwent hysterectomy, and recovered after a long stay in a critical care unit.

Placenta previa with previous cesarean section is especially prone to uncontrollable bleeding and is often an indication for hysterectomy. Uteroplacental apoplexy (Couvelaire uterus) is very often accompanied by a total inability of the uterus to contract, due to intramural bleeding spots, and the fibrin degradation products (originating from the coagulopathy) further impair myometrial contractility; therefore hysterectomy is frequently needed.

In cases of uterine rupture and placenta accreta, removal of the uterus also serves the best interests of the patient. In a hemodynamically unstable patient, subtotal hysterectomy may be performed.

In the fortunately rare surgically unmanageable, case of diffuse posthysterectomy bleeding, a situation accompanied by DIC, a pelvic pressure pack can be used (Logothetopulos umbrella pack).[38]

Future clinical aspects

Obstetrics is a 'bloody arena', and in the new millennium practitioners of obstetrics are facing new challenges. The inability to predict PPH makes it necessary to be always prepared to deal with it. The main problem is the poor predictive power of screening, because low-risk women who have delivered normally previously, without complications, do sometimes develop serious postpartum bleeding.

Avoiding transfusion in obstetric management is increasingly demanded for various reasons, and at the same time the availability of fresh whole blood is also decreasing. Some have taken extraordinary measures in this regard. A placenta percreta case in a Jehovah's Witness, diagnosed by magnetic resonance imaging, has been posted previously on the Internet. The patient donated blood for herself and in week 37 she underwent laparotomy, the aorta was clamped, hysterotomy was performed, and then bilateral hypogastric artery ligation was carried out prior to hysterectomy.

The life-threatening association of massive hemorrhage and coagulation failure, which knocks out the stability of the hemostatic system, is the most feared cascade of events frequently seen in postpartum bleeding scenarios. Clotting factors are consumed (consumption type) or removed from the bloodstream (in case of placental abruption) and the fibrinolytic system is activated. Thromboplastic materials, cytokines, and interleukin-6 may enter the bloodstream; endothelial damage and intravascular hemolysis occur, with release of procoagulants. These factors explode into DIC, resulting in a critically ill obstetric patient with uncontrollable hemorrhage.

There are no 'evidence-based' markers or clear guidelines in this dark field: we have to wait many years until such knowledge will be available. In 2004, the author participated in the EUPHRATES expert meeting (**Eu**ropean **P**roject on Obstetric **H**emorrhage **R**eduction: **A**ttitudes, **T**rial, and **E**arly warning **S**ystem) in Paris, trying to reach a multinational minimum consensus on PPH management and raising the level of awareness of professionals, health care planners and governments of the magnitude and importance of this cornerstone of obstetrics. For the coming years our own clinical experience, professional judgment, clinical research data from the literature, and expert opinion are still the prime source of our management plans.

A large number of maternal deaths could be attributed to this deadly combination of PPH and coagulation disorder. The author's experience also showed that saving the life of these patients requires a concerted team effort, often including access to emergency air transport to a state-of-the art critical care facility, where there is experience in dealing with massive hemorrhage and its consequences. The availability of all modern blood-banking equipment, including plasmapheresis, can be life-saving.

Obstetricians are continuously trying to use novel approaches in such critical treatments, and also rediscover some old options, like uterine packing. Here are some examples of newly proposed approaches to PPH:

Compression sutures, B-Lynch suture[39]: This technique is designed to try to control uterine atony by compressing the uterus with large sutures. These may cause severe complications, and require a word of caution.[40] The use of prostaglandin analogs is the more logical treatment choice in uterine atony cases. In the author's experience over the last 30 years, since the availability of synthetic prostaglandins, there was not a single case of uterine atony that was not successfully managed by a prostaglandin analog.

The author was only forced to resort to hypogastric artery ligation in a case of cervical pregnancy, but never encountered a case in his large obstetric practice, when a uterine compression suture was thought to be needed.

In such a case of cervical pregnancy with profuse bleeding the author compressed the abdominal aorta transabdominally with his left hand, and opened the abdomen, without stopping to scrub, still compressing the abdominal aorta until the bleeding was controlled. The patient recovered smoothly and quickly without any fever. So, in the author's opinion, the 'best compression' is the age-old hand compression of the abdominal aorta, until the bleeding is brought under control.

Misoprostol,[41] a prostaglandin-E_1 analog that was developed for the management of peptic ulcer disease, has found some uses in obstetrics. Its use is plagued by legitimacy issues,[41] and in case of massive bleeding – when every passing second increases the risk, its rectal use is inadequate in the author's opinion.

Pelvic arterial selective embolization[42] requires a hemodynamically stable patient, when the bleeding is not immediately life-threatening, and a special unit with an interventional radiologist. The technique is not without serious complications, but has been used with success in selected situations.

Recombinant activated factor VII (rFVIIa)[43–45] is a new and promising option to fight intractable postpartum bleeding arising from the life-threatening combination of profuse bleeding and associated destabilization of the hemostatic system (DIC, hemolysis, elevated liver enzymes, low platelet count (HELLP syndrome)), especially the rampant variety, characterized by gross depletion of coagulation factors and very high levels of fibrin degradation products (D-dimer).[20] Its place in the management of PPH is still uncertain, and it suffers from the problems of a short half-life (about 2 h) and extremely high cost. Limited experience suggests that it may have a lifesaving role when DIC cannot be controlled by more conventional means.

Over the years the author has encountered many cases of horrendous postpartum bleeding, one in which the patient was operated on five times in 30 h, and got 25,000 ml of blood; another in our national critical care center received 100,000 ml of blood until stabilization. It is hoped that in the coming years rFVIIa will give us great help, and such heroic, extremely high-volume blood transfusions will be a relic of the past. The use of rFVIIa might prove to be a quantum leap in this murky field of obstetrics. The author recently had a case with acutely successful use of rFVIIa, which stopped the postcesarean, then posthysterectomy bleeding; however, due to its short half-life, the intra-abdominal bleeding restarted 6 h later, requiring another reoperation. The patient ultimately recovered smoothly.

Some adjunctive treatments like planned auto-transfusion, erythropoietin, synthetic blood also deserve research as potential tools in the management of patients during and after severe PPH.

Summarized conclusions from clinical experience

Strategy: Try to identify high-risk cases that are prone to PPH.

Tactics: Management should be carried out according to a logical plan, which should include the early or immediate use of third-generation prostaglandin analogs when atony is present.

Be alert: Always rule out damage to the higher and lower genital tract. In cases of a reluctantly atonic uterus with non-traumatic bleeding, use prostaglandin analogs as a first choice, especially in high-risk cases of atony.

Be aware: Labor induction or augmentation increases PPAH risk by uterine exhaustion.

Think prevention: By using intravenous third-generation prostaglandin analogs, prevention can be achieved. Accompanying coagulation disturbance is dynamic and self-limiting with time if the bleeding is controlled.

Keep in mind: The intravenous route for chronic administration of prostaglandin analog is especially good if atonic hemorrhage is persistent.

Count on: Prostaglandin analog treatment decreases bleeding within 2–4 min, and will stop non-traumatic bleeding within 5–15 min.

Remember: Atony following cesarean section is especially dangerous, and in cases at high risk for atony prophylactic intravenous administration of sulprostone is advisable, using a lower dose range (approximately 2 μg/min).

REFERENCES

1. Royston E, Armstrong S. *Preventing Maternal Deaths.* Geneva: World Health Organization, 1989:40–1.
2. Brinsden PRS, Clark AD. Postpartum hemorrhage after induced and spontaneous labour. *Br Med J* 1978;2:855–6.
3. Ratnam SS, Rauff M. Postpartum hemorrhage and abnormalities of the third stage of labour. In Turnbull AC, Chamberlain G, eds. *Obstetrics.* London: Churchill Livingstone, 1989:868–75.
4. World Health Organisation. The prevention and management of postpartum hemorrhage. In *WHO Technical Working Group Report,* Geneva, July, 1989, WHO/MCH/90.7.
5. Prendiville WJ, Elbourne D, Chalmers I. The effects of routine oxytocic administration in the management of the third stage of labour: An overview of the evidence from controlled trials. *Br J Obstet Gynaecol* 1988;95:3–16.
6. Garfield RE, Tabb T, Thilander G. Intercellular coupling and modulation of uterine contractility. In Garfield RE, ed. *Uterine Contractility.* Norwell, MA: Serono Symposia USA, 1990:21.
7. Pulkkinen M. Analysis of uterine contractility. In Garfield RE, ed. *Uterine Contractility,* Norwell, MA: Serono Symposium, USA, 1990:296.
8. Grover AK. Role of cellular membranes in calcium mobilization of uterine smooth muscle. In Huszar G, ed. *The Physiology and Biochemistry of the Uterus in Pregnancy and Labor.* Boca Raton, FL: CRC Press Inc., 1986:93–106.
9. Huszar G. Cellular regulation of myometrial contractility and essentials for tocolytic therapy. In Huszar G, ed. *The Physiology and Biochemistry of the Uterus in Pregnancy and Labor.* Boca Raton, FL: CRC Press Inc., 1986:107–26.
10. Clegg PC, Hopkinson P, Pickles VR. Some effects of calcium and magnesium ions on guinea pig uterine muscle. *J Physiol* 1963;167:1–17.
11. Weinstein L, Droegemueller W, Greer B. The synergistic effect of calcium and prostaglandin $F_{2\alpha}$ in second-trimester abortion. *Obstet Gynecol* 1976;48:469–71.
12. Janis RA, Triggle DJ. Effects of calcium channel antagonists on the myometrium. In Huszar G, ed. *The Physiology and Biochemistry of the Uterus in Pregnancy and Labor.* Boca Raton, FL: CRC Press Inc., 1986:201–5.
13. Thiery M, Amy JJ. Inhibition of labour. In Bygdeman M, Berger GS, Keith LG, eds. *Prostaglandins and their Inhibitors in Clinical Obstetrics and Gynaecology.* Lancaster, UK: MTP Press, 1986. 203–31.
14. Forman A, Gandrup P, Andersson KE, Ulmsten U. Effects of nifedipine on spontaneous and methyl-ergometrine-induced activity postpartum. *Am J Obstet Gynecol* 1982;144:442–5.
15. Caldeyro-Barcia R, Poseiro JJ. Physiology of the uterine contraction. *Clin Obstet Gynecol* 1960;3:386–9.
16. Csapo A, Takeda H. Electrical activity of the parturient human uterus. *Nature* 1963;200:680–1.
17. Takagi K, Matsuura M, Sakata H, Takagi S. A topographic investigation of the site of origin and subsequent propagation of uterine contractions in spontaneous labor and their clinical significance. *Asia Oceania J Obstet Gynaecol* 1986;12:371–83.
18. Zargham I, Leviss SR, Marx GF. Uterine pressure during fluoxene anesthesia. *Anesthesiology* 1974;53:568–72.
19. Marx GF, Kim YI, Lin CC, Halevy S, Schulman H. Post-partum uterine pressures under halothane or enflurane anesthesia. *Obstet Gynecol* 1978;51:695–8.
20. Letsky EA. Coagulation problems during pregnancy. *Curr Rev Obstet Gynecol* 1985;10:64–5.
21. Zahradnik HP, Kraft H, Quaas L, Prompeler J, Karck U, Neulen J. Postpartum uterine atonia. In Husslein P, Egarter C, eds. *Postpartum Uterine Atonia. Proceedings of a Special Satellite Symposium, 1st European Congress on Prostaglandins in Reproduction, Vienna.* Vienna: Facultats-Universitatsverlag, 1989:1–15.
22. Husslein P, Sinzinger H. Concentration of 13,14-dihydro-15-keto-$PGF_{2\alpha}$ in the maternal peripheral plasma during labor of spontaneous onset. *Br J Obstet Gynaecol* 1984;91:228–31.
23. Keirse MJNC. Treatment of postpartum uterine hypotonia with prostaglandins. In Husslein P, Egarter C, eds. *Postpartum Uterine Atonia. Proceedings of a Special Satellite Symposium, 1st European Congress on Prostaglandins in Reproduction, Vienna.* Vienna: Facultats-Universitatsverlag, 1989:25–32.
24. Hendricks CH, Eskes TKA, Saameli K. Uterine contractility at delivery and in the puerperium. *Am J Obstet Gynecol* 1962;83:890–8.
25. Toppozada MK. Postpartum hemorrhage. In Bygdeman M, Berger GS, Keith LG, eds. *Prostaglandins and their Inhibitors in Clinical Obstetrics and Gynaecology.* Lancaster, UK: MTP Press, 1986: 234–51.
26. Pulkkinen M. Uterine activity and blood flow in response to sulprostone during midtrimester pregnancy termination. *Arch Gynecol* 1981;581:10–12.
27. Kerekes L, Domokos N. The effect of $PGF_{2\alpha}$ on third-stage labor. *Prostaglandins* 1979;18:161–6.
28. Takagi S, Yoshida T, Togo Y, *et al.* The effects of intra-myometrial injection of $PGF_{2\alpha}$ on severe postpartum hemorrhage. *Prostaglandins* 1976;12:565–7.
29. Hayashi RK, Castillo MS, Noah ML. Management of severe postpartum hemorrhage with a $PGF_{2\alpha}$ analog. *Obstet Gynecol* 1984; 63:806–8.

30. Hankins GDV, Berryman GK, Scott RT, Hood D. Maternal arterial oxygen desaturation with 15-methyl-PGF$_{2\alpha}$ for uterine atony. *Obstet Gynecol* 1988;72:367–70.
31. Herczeg J. Pretreatment of the cervix prior to surgical evacuation of the uterus in the late first and early second trimester of pregnancy. In Bygdeman M, ed. *Clinical Obstetrics and Gynecology. International Practice and Research.* London: Bailliere Tindall, 1990;4(2):307–25.
32. Herczeg J, Gréen K, Bygdeman M. Physiological and biochemical implications of prostaglandins from the perspective of developing safer first- and second-trimester obstetrics. *Acta Physiol Hung* 1988;71:233–7.
33. Andersson KE, Forman A, Ulmsten U. Pharmacology of labor. *Clin Obstet Gynecol* 1983;26:56–77.
34. Török I, Herczeg J. Betamimetic effects on the electromechanical characteristics of the pregnant and postpartum myometrium *in vitro. Acta Physiol Hung* 1985;65:335–9.
35. Falkay G, Herczeg J, Kovács L. Effect of betamimetic isoxsuprine on prostaglandin biosynthesis in pregnant human myometrium *in vitro. Life Sci* 1978;23:2689–96.
36. O'Leary JL, O'Leary JA. Uterine artery ligation for control of post-Cesarean section hemorrhage. *Obstet Gynecol* 1974;43:849–53.
37. Clark SL, Yeh SY, Phelan JP, Bruce S, Paul RH. Emergency hysterectomy for obstetric hemorrhage. *Obstet Gynecol* 1984;64: 376–80.
38. Hallak M, Dildy GA, Hurley TJ, Moise KJ. Transvaginal pressure pack for life-threatening pelvic hemorrhage secondary to placenta accreta. *Obstet Gynecol* 1991;78:939–42.
39. Hayman RG, Arulkumaran S, Steer PJ. Uterine compression suture: Surgical management of postpartum hemorrhage. *Obstet Gynecol* 2002;99:502–6.
40. Ochoa M, Allaire AD, Stitely ML. Pyometra after hemostatic square suture technique. *Obstet Gynecol* 2002;99:506–9.
41. Chong YS, Su LL, Arulkumaran S. Misoprostol: A quarter century of use, abuse and creative misuse. *Obstet Gynecol Surv* 2004; 59:128–40.
42. Ornan D, White R, Pollak J, Tal M. Pelvic embolization for intractable postpartum hemorrhage: Long-term follow-up and implications for fertility. *Obstet Gynecol* 2003;102:904–10.
43. Branch WD, Rodgers GM. Recombinant activated factor VII: A new weapon in the fight against hemorrhage. *Obstet Gynecol* 2003;101:1155–6.
44. Bouwmeester FW, Jonkhoff AR, Verheijen RH, van Geijn HP. Successful treatment of life threatening postpartum hemorrhage with recombinant activated factor VII. *Obstet Gynecol* 2003;101: 1174–6.
45. Midathada MV, Mehta P, Waner M, Fink LM. Recombinant factor VIIa in the treatment of bleeding. *Am J Clin Pathol* 2004;121: 124–37.

185 Resuscitation and immediate care of the newborn

J. Babnik

There are few moments in life when humans are as vulnerable and as dependent on the help of others as at birth. In a few seconds the newborn must adapt from life in the warm, moist, sterile environment of the mother's womb to wholly different extrauterine surroundings. Every organ must adjust to this change over a few minutes or a few days; but the key to immediate survival of the newborn is a smooth cardiopulmonary transition. The neonate must successfully inflate his or her lungs and rearrange the fetal circulation. With modern obstetric care there are only a few newborns who do not succeed in this adaptation, primarily for reasons related to perinatal asphyxia. Immediately after delivery these infants are not vigorous, do not cry, and do not breathe regularly. Resuscitation, from the Latin *resuscitate*, 'to arouse again', implies those actions that restore life. Skillful resuscitation of the asphyxiated infant immediately after delivery can prevent brain damage and minimize subsequent neonatal disease.

Approximately 5–10% of all newborn infants require some form of resuscitation.[1] Jain and Vidyasagar[2] found that the percentage could be as high as 9.4% (excluding suctioning) and that 6% of newborn babies were intubated. Not all hospitals experience such high numbers of resuscitated infants. Our data from the Ljubljana Maternity Hospital for the 6-year period 1997–2002 include 33,357 live-born babies. Of these, 4.2% were born with a 1-min Apgar score < 7 and 0.6% with score < 3. The majority of babies (94.7%) accomplished their transition to extrauterine life without any help: 1.4% received only suctioning, 3.6% were ventilated with bag and mask, and an additional 0.4% required intubation, chest compression or medication.[3]

Causes of newborn depression

Intrapartum asphyxia cannot be easily differentiated clinically from neonatal depression caused by a variety of drugs during labor, congenital anomalies, prematurity and other diseases of the infant. Initial resuscitative measures are, nevertheless, similar in all situations and should be initiated without delay.[4] The major causes of neonatal depression at birth are shown in Table 185.1. The diagnosis of perinatal asphyxia should only be made when certain clinical criteria are met.

Table 185.1 Causes of delayed onset of regular respiration

Perinatal asphyxia
Excessive suctioning (vagal stimulation causes bradycardia and apnea)
Trauma, especially to central nervous system (tentorial tears) or cervical cord
Drugs that depress breathing (anesthetic, narcotic, alcohol, magnesium sulfate, tranquilizers)
Severe immaturity (surfactant-deficient lung, inadequate respiratory effort)
Perinatally acquired sepsis: group B streptococci, *Listeria monocytogenes*
Primary neuromuscular disease (Werdnig–Hoffmann disease, congenital myopathies, myotonic dystrophy, congenital muscular dystrophy)
Congenital malformation obstructing the airway or preventing lung expansion (choanal atresia, Pierre–Robin syndrome, laryngeal atresia, diaphragmatic hernia, pulmonary hypoplasia)

Definition of perinatal asphyxia

Perinatal asphyxia remains a concern of obstetricians, neonatologists and others involved in the care of women, infants, and children. Despite considerable advances in our knowledge of its epidemiology and pathophysiology, and despite the development of novel diagnostic tools and new treatments, a precise definition remains elusive. The American College of Obstetricians and Gynecologists' (ACOG) Committee on Maternal–Fetal Medicine and the American

Table 185.2 Essential characteristics of perinatal asphyxia[5]

Profound metabolic or mixed academia (pH < 7.00) in an umbilical cord arterial blood sample
Persistence of an Apgar score of 0–3 for > 5 min
Clinical neurological sequelae in the immediate neonatal period, including seizures, hypotonia, coma, or hypoxic–ischemic encephalopathy
Evidence of multiorgan system dysfunction in the immediate neonatal period

Academy of Pediatrics' (AAP) Committee on the Fetus and Newborn have defined certain criteria that must be met if neurologic deficits are to be attributed to perinatal asphyxia.[5] All of the characteristics listed in Table 185.2 must be present, including evidence of at least one organ dysfunction. If such evidence is lacking, it is difficult to conclude that perinatal asphyxia is the cause of later developmental disability.

Pathophysiology of asphyxia and resuscitation

In order to undertake the necessary and appropriate measures for resuscitation of the newborn, a firm understanding of pathophysiologic events that occur during asphyxia is vital. Asphyxia (which etymologically means 'without pulse') is defined as hypoxia combined with respiratory acidosis (organ gas exchange failure). When this occurs, the arterial carbon dioxide partial pressure ($PaCO_2$) rises, whereas the arterial oxygen partial pressure (PaO_2) and pH fall. During lack of oxygen the cell switches to anaerobic metabolism to meet energy requirements. Glycolysis is accelerated, but in anaerobic conditions 15 times more glucose is expended for the same amount of ATP production as occurs in aerobic conditions. Therefore, anaerobic glycolysis represents only a short-term compensation and leads to a large amount of lactic acid accumulation that is partially buffered by the bicarbonate in the blood.

The main causes of asphyxia are hypoxemia and ischemia, hence the term hypoxic–ischemic encephalopathy. Five principal mechanisms of asphyxia have been described in the human infant during labor, delivery, and the immediate postpartum period.[5] These are: (1) interruption of umbilical blood flow (cord compression, prolapse); (2) failure of gas exchange across the placenta (placental insufficiency, abruption, or previa); (3) inadequate perfusion of the maternal side of the placenta (severe maternal hypotension, hypertension from any cause, or excess uterine contractility); (4) impaired maternal oxygenation (cardiopulmonary disease, anemia); and (5) failure of adequate cardiopulmonary adaptation after birth (insufficient lung inflation and faulty rearrangement of the fetal circulation).

Classic changes of perinatal hypoxia were described in the rhesus monkey experimental model and probably imitate events in human fetuses.[6] Figure 185.1 illustrates the changes in heart rate, breathing movements, blood pressure and pH during 10 min of total asphyxia and after subsequent resuscitation. Immediately after delivery, the umbilical cord was tied, and the head of the monkey was covered with a bag of a warm saline. Within 30 s a short series of rhythmic respiratory efforts began, which was interrupted by a series of clonic movements accompanied by an abrupt and profound fall in heart rate to below 100 beats per minute (bpm), after which the animal lay inert with no muscular tone. The skin became cyanotic and during the next few minutes it gradually became pale as vasoconstriction appeared and produced asphyxia pallida. The initial period of apnea (primary apnea) lasted for 30–60 s. After primary apnea, the monkey made deep gasping efforts for 4–5 min. The gasping then weakened gradually until it ceased completely, with the last gasp about 8 min after the onset of total asphyxia. Secondary (terminal) apnea followed, during which the heart rate and blood pressure declined steadily. During the period of primary apnea, spontaneous respiration could be induced by tactile stimulation. Profound changes in pH, PCO_2, and PO_2 occurred during the 10 min of total asphyxia: pH decreased from 7.3 to 6.8; $PaCO_2$ increased from 45 to 200 mmHg; and PaO_2 decreased from the normal umbilical arterial level of 25 mmHg to nearly zero. During secondary apnea, tactile stimulation could not induce spontaneous respiration, and unless resuscitation with bag and mask ventilation began within a few minutes, death resulted. The longer is the delay in initiating resuscitation after the last gasp, the longer is the time to the beginning of spontaneous respiration (Figure 185.2).

Early in perinatal asphyxia, cardiac output is maintained, but its distribution changes radically. Blood flow to less vital organs such as gut, kidney, muscle and skin is reduced by selective regional vasoconstriction.[7] However, blood flow to brain and myocardium increases, and the delivery of oxygen to these organs is maintained despite reduced blood oxygen content.[8] If asphyxia progresses to the severe stage, oxygen delivery to the brain and heart decreases. At first, the myocardium uses its stored reserve of glycogen for energy; but when this has been consumed, the combined effect of hypoxia and acidosis impairs myocardial function.[9] The result is decreased blood flow to the brain, which can lead to brain damage.

The adaptive events described above probably reflect the responses of the human newborn to absolute asphyxia such as could occur during total placental abruption, rupture of the uterus or prolapse and compression of the umbilical cord. Such experimental knowledge is not always directly applicable to

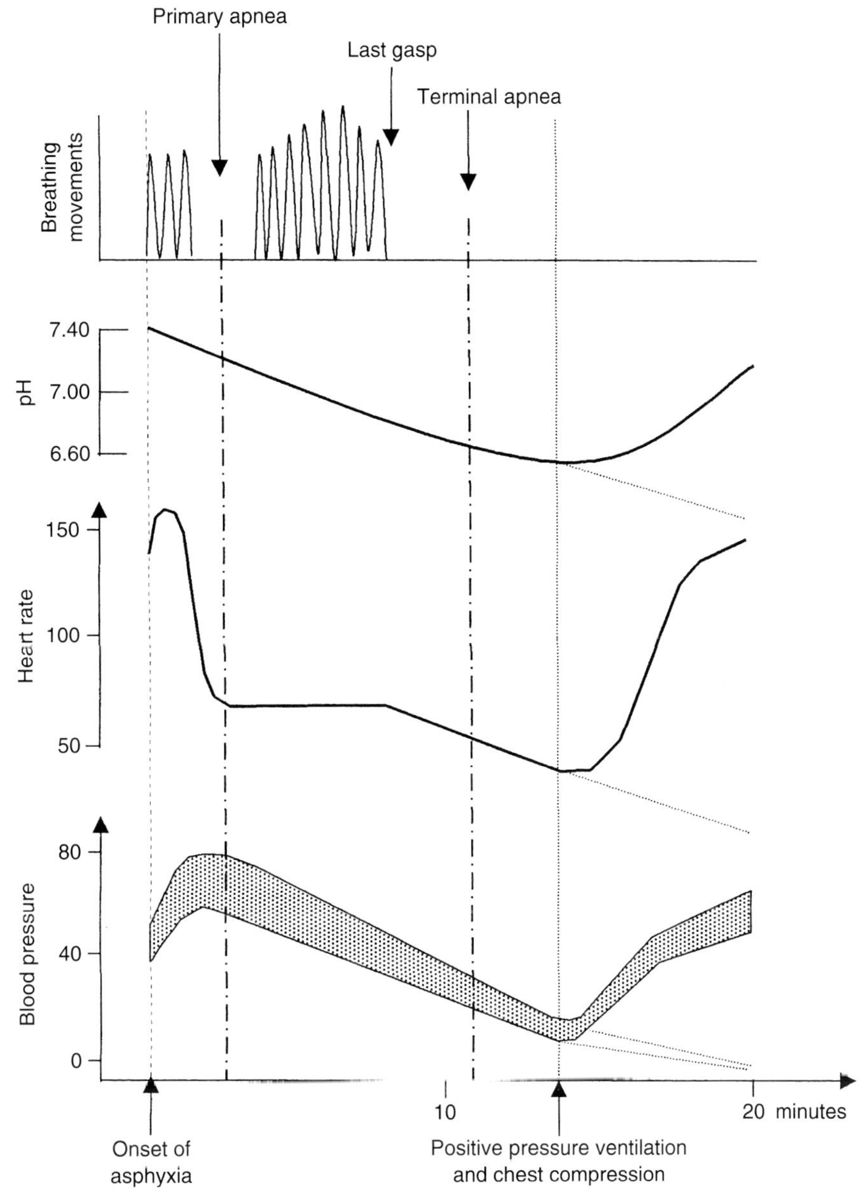

Figure 185.1 Physiological changes during asphyxia.[6]

the human fetus and newborn, because most clinically encountered asphyxia is intermittent, subacute or chronic. Nevertheless, the sequence of events in successful resuscitation is quantitatively similar in all species, including man.[10]

The apneic newborn who responds to tactile stimulation by gasping is in primary apnea. If the infant is till gasping, administration of air (oxygen) or gentle tactile stimulation is sufficient for recovery, unless the gasps are too feeble and arterial pressure too low.

If asphyxia is only moderate, the resuscitation begins when the infant is apneic but the myocardium has not yet failed. Effective ventilation with oxygen corrects acidosis by lowering PCO_2, while oxygenation of blood dilates the pulmonary vascular bed. During secondary apnea the human newborn is usually pale. The first sign of recovery once adequate ventilation is achieved is an acceleration of the heart rate. Following this, the blood pressure rises, the skin becomes pink, and gasping then reappears after an interval. The duration of this interval has some practical value in indicating the magnitude of the asphyxial insult that the infant has suffered. Rhythmic spontaneous respiratory efforts become established after a further interval and muscular tone reappears gradually over the course of the next hour or more.

If the asphyxia proceeds to myocardial failure, resuscitation must include the restoration of cardiac output as well as the establishment of effective ventilation and perfusion of the lung. Generally, myocardial failure does not occur until both pH and PaO_2 are extremely low, approximately 6.9 and 20 mmHg, respectively. Chest compression (external cardiac massage) should be performed until cardiac output is reestablished. As soon as the pH is raised to 7.1 and PaO_2 to 50 mmHg, the myocardium responds, and heart rate and aortic pressure rise, while the central venous pressure falls. Because vasoconstriction to non-vital organs is still present, the infant becomes hypertensive. With correction of acidosis and continuous oxygenation, vasoconstriction is relieved and pressure will fall toward normal. The skin becomes pink and well perfused. The improved perfusion to all organs means that lactic acid, sequestered in these tissues, enters the circulation and makes the metabolic acidosis even greater than before. Measuring lactic acid in the umbilical cord just after delivery does not always reflect the magnitude of the asphyxia, as lactate is also produced in the placenta, and an increased quantity may result from decreased uptake by the asphyxiated fetal liver.[11]

The blood volume of the asphyxiated infant may be abnormal. Usually there is no great shift of blood between the fetus and placenta and the infant is born with an adequate blood volume. In the clinical situation of external bleeding from the feto-placental unit, in feto-maternal or feto-fetal bleeding, the infant's blood volume is reduced. The other most common causes are cord compression (venous flow is compressed more than the arterial flow), and severe maternal hypotension and asphyxia occurring at the end of labor.[12]

Clinically it may be difficult to determine if the shock is hypoxic or hypovolemic, as both can cause bradycardia, metabolic acidosis, hypotension and poor peripheral perfusion. Only changes in the central venous pressure, which is low in hypovolemic shock, may be of discriminative value. The course of events during resuscitation usually determines the adequacy of blood volume. During asphyxia the systemic and pulmonary vasoconstriction maintain normal blood pressure, even with reduced blood volume. The administration of a blood volume expander at this point would only overload the circulation. The correction of asphyxia relieves vasoconstriction, and a small blood volume becomes inadequate to support circulation. Reperfusion of the ischemic tissues leads to intravascular water loss from the capillary bed and aggravates hypovolemia.

The signs of hypovolemic shock include low aortic pressure with narrow pulse pressure, falling hematocrit, persistent metabolic acidosis, low central venous PO_2 ($<$ 30 mmHg) after correction of arterial hypoxia, cold extremities, and delayed capillary refilling. Tachycardia is often absent, as the predominant regulator of cardiac output in the human fetus and newborn is the Frank–Starling mechanism and not the heart rate.[13] As in the adult, the fetal heart follows a Frank–Starling curve in such a manner that an increase in the filling pressure leads to an increase in stroke volume. However, the fetal heart operates, in its baseline state, high on its cardiac function curve. With increasing atrial pressure, there is diminished capacity to increase myocardial performance, as the length–tension relationship has already approached its maximal plateau.[14]

Hypovolemia should be treated promptly, lest prolonged under-perfusion of tissues leads to increased capillary permeability and pulmonary disease, which make resuscitation more difficult. Excessively rapid volume replacement can lead to myocardial failure; therefore, repeated small infusions of whole blood (5 ml/kg) or packed erythrocytes should be used.

Resuscitation

Based on extensive review of available information, neonatal resuscitation guidelines (basic and advanced life support) were revised extensively in 1999 by the International Liaison Committee on Resuscitation (ILCOR) Pediatric Working Group, with representatives from North America, Europe, Australia, New Zealand, Africa, and South America.[15] Consensus was reached on almost all aspects of neonatal resuscitation, was published,[16] and is widely accessible on the Internet (http://www.circulationaha.org, http://www.pediatrics.org/cgi/content/full/103/4/e56).

Although the guidelines focus on the newly born infant, most of the principles are applicable throughout the neonatal period (first 28 days of life) and early infancy. The term newly born refers specifically to the infant in the first minutes to hours after birth. The point at which neonatal resuscitation guidelines should be changed to a pediatrics resuscitation protocol varies for individual patients. The transition from fetal to extrauterine life involves dramatic changes in cardiopulmonary physiology (initial lung expansion, decrease in pulmonary vascular resistance, closure of intracardiac shunts), temperature regulation and metabolic adaptation. Although certain physiologic features are unique to the newly born, others pertain to infants, especially to premature infants, throughout the neonatal period. Therefore, until discharge from maternity hospital or from a neonatal intensive care unit newborn resuscitation guidelines should be followed; after readmission pediatric protocols should be used.

However useful the guidelines are it should be remembered that, much of what they proposed was based on opinions of experienced clinicians or on less than optimal studies.[17] Only two of the recommendations are Class I (based on the evidence from randomized, controlled trials that showed a large effect); therefore, areas of controversy and of high priority for additional research were delineated. Moreover, the guidelines made no distinction between the techniques used for term and very preterm infants and it is very likely that some of the proposed procedures may even hurt preterm infants instead of treating them. The current chapter includes the proposed guidelines, with special consideration devoted to areas of controversy.

Only basic resuscitation measures, discussed in this section, should be carried out in the labor ward. The aim should be to normalize the heart rate and to assure breathing, if necessary with the aid of intermittent positive-pressure ventilation and chest compression. To achieve these goals, the only medications, except for epinephrine and plasma expanders, which can be tried blindly, are naloxone, a single dose of bicarbonate, and an infusion of glucose. All other treatments are best postponed until the baby is in the neonatal intensive care unit.[4]

Anticipation of resuscitation and preparation for the delivery

A maternity hospital should be designed so that the delivery rooms and the neonatal unit are adjacent to each other. If this is not the case the labor ward should be prepared to carry out more prolonged resuscitation and for the care of the baby, until transport to the neonatal unit is accomplished.

Only about 5–10% of all newborn infants require some form of resuscitation[1] and this number increases exponentially for very low birth weight (VLBW) infants. The delivery of a baby requiring resuscitation may often be predicted, as more than 50% of such babies are born after some complications during pregnancy or labor. Whenever complications are expected, it is advisable, when possible, to transport the woman (transport *in utero*) to an institution where appropriate care can be offered and experienced personnel are available. Many of these high-risk categories, presented in Table 185.3, have been defined, and hospital practice is that such a delivery should be attended by the neonatologist/pediatrician. Optimally, the pediatrician should be present at more than 30% of all deliveries, although he or she will often not be needed. Cesarean section is the most common reason for calling the neonatologist, although an elective cesarean section is not necessarily a high-risk situation.[18,19] Usually the risk factors are combined (emergency cesarean section and fetal distress) but when considered alone, the most common reasons for skilled resuscitation are emergency cesarean section, forceps and vacuum delivery, newborn being covered with thick particulate meconium, breech delivery, prematurity, multiple birth, and fetal distress.[20,21]

Although the causes of asphyxia are numerous, review of the clinical situation and of the patient's history can help guide the physician's approach to the resuscitation. When time permits, the following information should be acquired: gestational age, fetal growth during pregnancy, findings of amniocentesis or ultrasound assessment (gastrointestinal anomaly, diaphragmatic hernia, bilateral renal anomaly), reasons for preterm delivery (chorioamnionitis), complications during pregnancy, course of labor, indications for operative intervention, drug administration, and maternal health during labor (evidence of infection).

Personnel

Although it has been suggested that around 60% of deliveries resulting in the need for neonatal

Table 185.3 Risk factors associated with the need for neonatal resuscitation (from Emergency Cardiac Care Committee and Subcommittees, American Heart Association[22] with permission)

Antepartum factors	Intrapartum factors
Maternal diabetes	Emergency cesarean section
Pregnancy-induced hypertension	Forceps- or vacuum-assisted delivery
Chronic hypertension	Breech or other abnormal presentation
Chronic maternal illness (cardiovascular, thyroid, neurological, pulmonary, renal)	Premature labor
Anemia or isoimmunization	Precipitate labor
Previous fetal or neonatal death	Long labor (>24 h)
Bleeding in second or third trimester	Prolonged second stage of labor (>2 h)
Maternal infection	Chorioamnionitis
Polyhydramnios	Fetal bradycardia
Oligohydramnios	Abnormal fetal heart rate patterns
Prelabor rupture of membranes	Use of general anesthesia
Post-term gestation	Narcotic administration to mother proximate to delivery
Multiple gestation	Meconium-stained amniotic fluid
Intrauterine growth restriction	Prolapsed cord
Drug therapy (lithium, magnesium, adrenergic blocking agents)	Abruptio placentae
Maternal drug abuse	Placenta previa
Fetal congenital anomalies	
Diminished fetal activity	
No prenatal care	
Age < 16 or > 35 years	

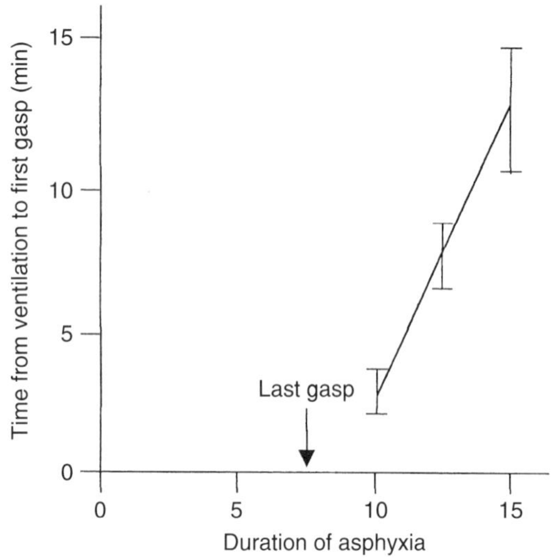

Figure 185.2 Mean time from the onset of asphyxia or anoxia to the last gasp, and mean time from the beginning of positive pressure ventilation to the first gasp in fetal monkeys asphyxiated for 10, 12.5 and 15 min.[6]

resuscitation can be anticipated,[2] many more are unpredictable events, and these usually require the most urgent and most aggressive resuscitation. The recommendation that someone who is trained in all aspects of neonatal resuscitation should be present at every delivery is impractical.[22] More reasonable is that such qualified person should be available in the hospital at all times and should attend only high-risk deliveries. Depending on the organization of the health service and the particular hospital policy, this person could be a pediatrician, an obstetrician, an anesthesiologist, an obstetric nurse or a respiratory care practitioner. It is imperative that he or she is well trained in neonatal resuscitation, which includes initial management, bag and mask ventilation, intubation, and umbilical catheter insertion. However, in cases of unpredictable events, resuscitation is given by the first person available who is skilled in basic procedures (prompt evaluation of the newborn's condition, clearing the airway, bag and mask ventilation). These goals must be achieved through carefully programmed training for all persons who could possibly be involved in resuscitation. It does not mean that every person knows all the steps; a nurse may not be expected to have the intubation skills, and a respiratory therapist may not be asked to provide medication.

Equipment

At every delivery the equipment and medication necessary for resuscitation should be prepared, and appropriate function should be checked before the anticipated need, and replenished after each use. It is recommended to have a list of the necessary equipment and medication, and every day the integrity should be guaranteed by the signature of a responsible person.

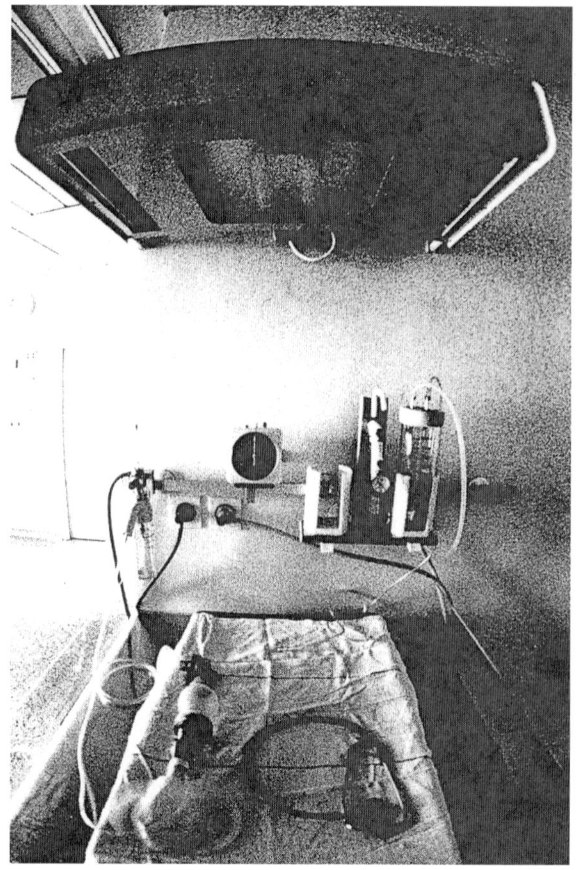

Figure 185.3 Place for resuscitation of newly born infants in the delivery room, with wall-mounted oxygen supply, suction device and radiant heater.

Most neonatal resuscitation is now carried out on resuscitation trolleys built for this purpose or in a special place in the delivery room (Figure 185.3), equipped with the essential components listed in Table 185.4 (radiant warmer, supply of oxygen, suction with manometer, large clock), and with good access from at least two sides. The shelf should be tiltable and at a comfortable height for the resuscitator. On arrival to the labor ward the resuscitator should check the equipment for resuscitation: radiant heater and room temperature, oxygen supply, adequate suctioning, functioning of self-inflating bag and laryngoscope, availability of the appropriate mask and endotracheal tubes, warm towels and linen.

Evaluation of the newborn's condition

Immediately after birth (and not after the umbilical cord is cut) the clock should be started and signs that show infant condition (meconium in the amniotic fluid or on the infant skin, cry or respiration, muscle tone, color, term or preterm gestation) should be evaluated simultaneously by visual inspection. Indications for further assessement and intervention under the radiant warmer include: meconium in the amniotic fluid

Table 185.4 Resuscitation equipment required in the delivery room[16,22]

Radiant warmer

Supply of oxygen with flowmeter (capable of delivering at least 10 l O_2/min) and tubing (including portable oxygen cylinders)

Suction with manometer: the suction should not exceed 200 mmHg, and for routine use should be set at 100 mmHg

Suction equipment
Bulb syringe
Suction catheters, 5F or 6F, 8F, and 10F or 12F
Meconium aspiration device

Bag-and-mask equipment
Face masks, newborn and preterm size (mask with cushioned rim preferred, should be easily detached from the bags and replaced with endotracheal tube connectors)
Resuscitation bags: self-inflating with pop-off valve opened at 30–35 cmH_2O or anesthesia bags

Intubation equipment
Tracheal tubes, size 2.0, 2.5, 3.0, 3.5 and 4.0 (internal diameter)
Laryngoscope with straight blades No. 0 (preterm) and 1 (term)
Endotracheal tube introducers (optional)
CO_2 detector (optional)
Magill forceps for nasotracheal intubation
Laringeal mask airway (optional)

Medication
Epinephrine ampule (1 mg/ml) (1:10,000 solution should be prepared)
Naloxone hydrochloride (1 or 0.4 mg/ml solution)
Sodium bicarbonate (0.5 mEq/ml solution)
Volume expander: normal saline (0.9% NaCl), Ringer's lactate

Umbilical vessel catheterization tray
Umbilical catheters (3.5F and 5.0F)
Three-way stopcocks

Miscellaneous
Nasogastric feeding tubes (6F and 8F) for gastric suction
A selection of syringes, needles, intravenous cannulas, specimen bottles
Scissors, adhesive tape of a type that will not damage very fragile preterm infant skin
Solution for skin disinfection, gloves
Stethoscope
Oropharyngeal airways, newborn and premature infant size
Cardiac monitor and pulse oximeter or fetal cardiac monitor are desirable

or on the infant's skin; absent or weak respiration; persistent cyanosis; and preterm birth.

In every labor ward, the Apgar score is traditionally used for the assessment of the newborn and to provide an overview of the degree of resuscitation likely to be necessary. Before and during resuscitation, however, it is enough to assess sequentially the respiratory effort, heart rate and color.

Respiratory efforts may be manifest as vigorous crying, regular breathing, gasping respiration or apnea. The assessment should be done by auscultation or inspection of breathing movements. If breathing is shallow or the infant is apneic, he or she needs physical stimulation and bag and mask ventilation. Regular respiration should be sufficient to maintain heart rate > 100 bpm.

The heart rate may be evaluated by auscultation with a stethoscope, with palpation of the pulse at the base of the umbilical cord, or with a fetal cardiac monitor (Doppler method). The palpation of femoral or brachial pulses is unreliable and even umbilical pulsation must not be relied upon if low or absent.[23] The Doppler method is most desirable, as all resuscitators can hear the heart beat and take appropriate steps in response to it. There is no need for exact counting of the pulse rate during resuscitation; a rapid estimation of whether the heart rate is above or below 100 bpm or whether it exists at all is most important. Therefore, all other resuscitation measures are discontinued for some seconds during auscultation.

Color can range from normal pink with acrocyanosis to central cyanosis or pallor. Color indirectly reflects the state of the circulation. Pallor is due to peripheral vasoconstriction and is a sign of shock (hypoxic or hypovolemic), acidosis or hypothermia, whereas cyanosis suggests normal circulation, with disturbed oxygenation. Preterm newborns are not infrequently covered with bruises, making evaluation of color difficult. A look at the lips usually suffices to evaluate cyanosis and the need for oxygenation.

Immediate newborn care: initial stabilization

Positioning

Just after delivery the face and nose should be wiped, and a healthy baby is placed on his or her side to aid drainage of the mucus from the nasopharynx and trachea. Usually, the healthy baby retains good muscle tone in the flexed position, and begins crying after initial drying. Most immediate care of the healthy newborn can be accomplished while the newborn is held on the mother's abdomen or under the radiant warmer, which may be placed near the parents so that they can see the baby. Because of reports of sudden unexpected neonatal death, the baby lying prone on the mother's abdomen should be constantly observed.[24]

The neonate requiring resuscitation should be placed supine or on his or her side with the neck in a neutral position. Overextension or flexion may produce airway obstruction and should be avoided.

Cord clamping

If time permits, umbilical cord should be clamped when pulsations cease, usually 30–60 s after birth; when resuscitation is required the umbilical cord should be clamped immediately. It is important that as much umbilical cord blood as possible is taken for further analysis: blood gas analysis, hematocrit, blood group studies, lactate, etc. For this purpose a section of cord is clamped between the newborn infant and the placenta. The results of blood gas analysis may be available within minutes and can be helpful in further management of the asphyxiated infant.

Maintaining warmth

The first priority is to provide and maintain warmth, because cold stress can increase oxygen consumption and impede effective resuscitation.[25] The newborn is, therefore, dried immediately and all wet linen is removed. Warmth can be maintained by covering the newborn with warm blankets or by placing it in skin-to-skin contact with the mother. There is no need for bathing and removing the vernix from the infant's skin. These procedures can be safely postponed until the end of the first day when the adaptation to extra-uterine life has been well accomplished.

When placing the infant under a radiant warmer, hyperthermia should be avoided because it is associated with respiratory depression.[26,27] Moreover, recent data suggest that even mild hyperthermia during or following a hypoxic–ischemic insult may exacerbate damage.[28] The mechanism of this adverse influence is unclear but may be related to a dramatic increase in the release of excitotoxins.[29]

Some animal studies revealed that hypothermia after hypoxic–ischemic injury reduced histologic evidence of brain damage,[30,31] delayed cerebral energy failure,[32] and improved behavioral outcome.[33] Cooling was achieved with the head and neck covered with ice bags and with peritoneal cold lavage performed when the spontaneous circulation was restored. The mechanism of therapeutic hypothermia is multifaceted and includes preserving energy, stabilizing membranes, decreasing oxygen demand, excitotoxicity, free radical reactions, and deleterious enzyme reactions.[34]

Under normal conditions the brain is metabolically highly active, and produces about 70% of total body heat in the newborn.[35] The heat produced is dissipated by conductive loss through the cerebral circulation and by radiant loss from the scalp. There is a normal core-to-skin gradient in the head of more than 1°C, which is lost when the external heating under a radiant warmer begins.[36] Considering that overhead heating prevents heat dissipation and even promotes cerebral hyperthermia, mild systemic hypothermia, with or without head cooling has been proposed as a therapeutic intervention in infants who suffer perinatal hypoxic–ischemic injury.[37,38] However, because of potential adverse effects, including metabolic, cardiovascular, pulmonary, coagulation, and immunologic complications, hypothermia cannot be recommended as a routine therapeutic intervention until appropriate controlled studies in human have been performed.[15]

Tactile stimulation

Most newborn infants begin to breathe and cry during wiping with a towel. However, rubbing the back and slapping or flicking the soles are two other safe methods of tactile stimulation. Tactile stimulation may initiate spontaneous respiration in a newborn with primary apnea. If no response occurs within 10–15 s, the infant should be placed under a radiant warmer on the resuscitation desk, and positive pressure ventilation should be initiated.

Type of resuscitation after initial stabilization

After initial evaluation and stabilization, one can classify the newborn as either healthy, with good tone, regular breathing and a loud cry, or as one with shallow breathing, apnea, pallor or cyanosis.

Healthy newborn crying loudly

Such a newborn needs no additional care. No pharyngeal or tracheal aspiration is needed unless the amniotic fluid is exceedingly bloody or meconium-stained. After clamping the umbilical cord, the infant should be thoroughly dried, and put into contact with the mother. The mother should be encouraged to put it against her breast because early suckling induces more efficient breastfeeding and quicker contraction of the uterus. When still in the delivery room, the infant must be identified and must receive 1 mg of vitamin K for protection against hemorrhagic disease of the newborn. Eye infection prophylaxis should be administered with topical 1% $AgNO_3$, 0.5% erythromycin or 1% tetracycline.

Newborn not breathing and cyanotic or pale

The umbilical cord should be clamped quickly, the infant put on the resuscitative trolley, and resuscitative measures started without delay. The promptness of the response to resuscitation efforts enables a retrospective diagnosis of primary or terminal apnea.

Most depressed newborns are in a state of primary apnea, and they start breathing after sensory stimulation (wiping or rubbing the soles or back) or after short bag and mask ventilation. Once they become pink, breathe regularly or cry, they may generally be admitted to the ward for healthy newborns, regardless of the 1-min Apgar score.

The newborn in terminal apnea experiences severe asphyxia and will not start breathing spontaneously without appropriate resuscitation measures. The longer the resuscitation is postponed, the more severe the metabolic and physiologic changes and the greater the possibility of brain damage. Resuscitation should be started immediately (Figure 185.4). Some newborns are born dead (with Apgar score of 0) but are still

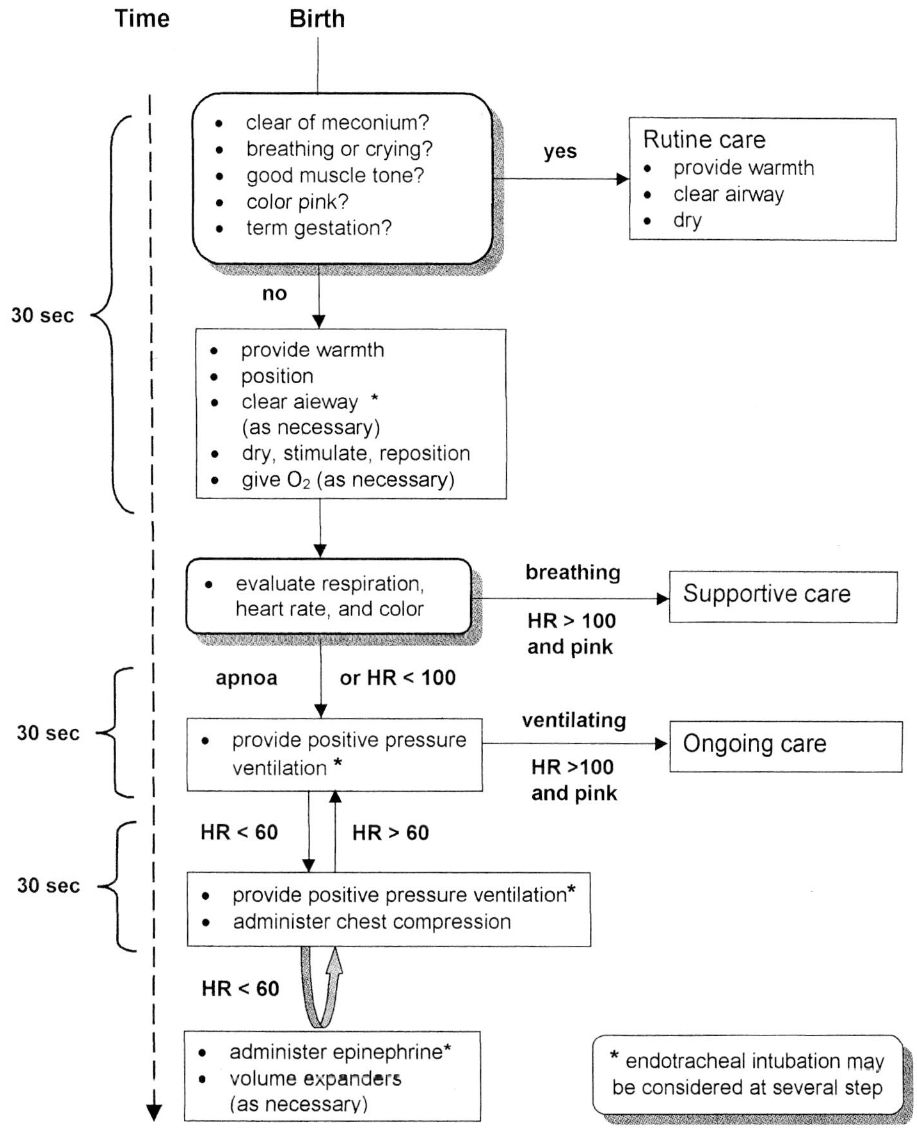

Figure 185.4 Algorithm for the resuscitation of the newly born infants.[16,22]

resuscitatable. In that situation, resuscitation is started unless the obstetrician is sure that the fetal heart ceased beating more than 10 min before delivery. If the heart rate does not appear within 10–15 min after birth, the resuscitation should be stopped.[39]

Techniques used during resuscitation

Suctioning

Guidelines for neonatal resuscitation[16] still recommend suctioning of the infant's nose and mouth with a bulb syringe after delivery of the shoulders, but before delivery of the chest. This task is often difficult to accomplish because, after delivery of the head, the rest of the body often delivers promptly. In addition, it has been shown that oropharyngeal suctioning at the perineum does not affect the rate of meconium aspiration syndrome (MAS).[40]

Immediately after the fetal head is delivered, whether vaginally or by cesarean, the newborn's face should be wiped with gauze or a towel, and, once delivered, a healthy baby should be put on its side or prone. At birth the baby has amniotic fluid and mucus in its mouth, nose and pharynx. We should remember that throughout its intrauterine life the fetus exercised respiratory movements and that the presence of amniotic fluid is indispensable for development of the fetal lungs. If the amniotic fluid is not meconium-stained and there is not much maternal blood in it, healthy, vigorous newly born infants generally do not require suctioning.[41] With the first few deep breaths the newborn expels the amniotic fluid, together with the rest of the fluid from the lungs, into the pharynx and swallows it. Some of the fluid is absorbed into the pulmonary interstitium and removed by blood or lymph. Aggressive suctioning of the pharynx may cause laryngeal spasm and vagal bradycardia.[42] Suctioning should be carried out only when the newborn is depressed and needs bag and mask ventilation or tracheal intubation, especially when amniotic fluid is meconium-stained or is exceedingly bloody.

Clearing the airway of meconium

Approximately 8–13% of infants are born with meconium in the amniotic fluid[43,44] and 3–7% of these develop MAS.[39,45] The meconium causes chemical pneumonitis, and at the same time inhibits surfactant activity and thus leads to severe respiratory distress. The first priority after delivery is, therefore, to clean the infant's airway. As noted, although guidelines and common practice counsel[15,16] suctioning of infant's mouth, pharynx and nose just after delivery of the head with a large-bore suction catheter (12F) or bulb syringe, it is not certain that oropharyngeal suctioning at the perineum reduces the risk of meconium aspiration.[39] To remove thick meconium a higher negative pressure is needed than provided by a De Lee oral aspirator or a bulb syringe. Efficient aspiration must be carried out as soon as possible on the resuscitation table with vacuum or air aspirators.

Results of several recent studies, summarized by the Cochrane database of systematic reviews[45–48] showed that intubation and suctioning of the apparently vigorous meconium-stained infant did not result in a decreased incidence of MAS or other respiratory disorders. Therefore, intubation and suctioning should be carried out only in depressed infants.

The initial aspiration of thick meconium may require negative pressures as high as 150 mmHg.[49] The 10F or 12F suction catheter is introduced under laryngoscope-guided control; the mouth and pharynx should be aspirated first, followed by the trachea. Should meconium be found in the trachea, aspiration is continued so that as much of the meconium as possible is aspirated in the shortest possible time before the first breath. During this time all actions which could induce breathing (drying, tactile stimulation) should be postponed, until the posterior pharynx is clean of meconium.[47–49]

If the meconium is extremely thick and infant is still depressed, the trachea should be intubated. Current recommendation is that aspiration and removal of the tube are carried out simultaneously. The procedure is repeated until the tracheal tube is almost cleared.[16] Between two aspirations, which must be brief, the newborn's condition is monitored. If the infant's heart rate or respiration is severely depressed, resuscitation with positive pressure ventilation should be initiated, despite the presence of the meconium in the airway. A large amount of meconium is usually present in the stomach and should be suctioned after cleaning the respiratory tree.

Ventilation

The indications for positive pressure ventilation after birth are: apnea or gasping respiration; heart rate less than 100 bpm; and persistent central cyanosis despite the delivery of 100% free-flow O_2.

Bilateral chest wall motion and audible breath sounds are adequate signs of successful ventilation. To establish effective ventilation after birth, the neonate must generate an opening negative pressure of 20–40 cmH_2O,[50] and even higher pressures may be required to inflate the fluid-filled lung of the baby who does not breathe spontaneously after birth. Inflation should be prolonged, lasting 3–5 s to establish a functional residual capacity (FRC).[51] Less pressure and shorter inflation times are required for succeeding breaths. The observation of chest wall movement is a more reliable sign of appropriate inflation pressure than any pressure read from the manometer. If the lungs cannot be inflated, attempt the following: (1) reposition the mask to ensure a tight seal between face and mask; (2) reposition the head in a case of overextension or flexion; (3) repeat suctioning if necessary; and (4) use increased inflation pressure. If these measures are inadequate, prompt intubation is necessary. Prolonged bag and mask ventilation may insufflate the stomach; therefore, after suctioning the mouth and nose a catheter left open to air should be inserted into the stomach. Ventilation should be at the rate of 40–60 breaths per minute, and after 15–30 s the infant's response should be checked.

Most infants respond to adequate ventilation within 10–15 s with increasing heart rate to more than 100 bpm, and with improvement in color. If spontaneous respiration is present, ventilation should be slowly discontinued. Gentle tactile stimulation, such as rubbing the skin, helps to commence and maintain spontaneous respiration.

If the infant is cyanotic or pale blue despite good chest wall movement, the heart rate should be re-evaluated, even before 15–30 s as recommended. If the heart rate is more than 60 bpm and rising, ventilation is continued. If the heart rate drops below 60 bpm, chest compressions are initiated and ventilation continued.[15,16]

Face masks

Most neonates requiring respiratory support can be adequately ventilated with a bag and mask at a rate of 40–60 breaths per minute. For proper ventilation, face masks fitting term or preterm infants should be available. Cushioned, soft rims are essential for achieving a tight seal between the mask and the face.

Ventilation bags. Two types of ventilation bags are available: self-inflating bags and anesthesia bags (Figure 185.5).

Self-inflating bags are independent of the gas flow. The elasticity of the bag permits its rapid refill through the intake valve that is open to air and to the O_2 reservoir. If there is sufficient O_2 flow, keeping the reservoir full, the bag can deliver nearly 100% O_2.

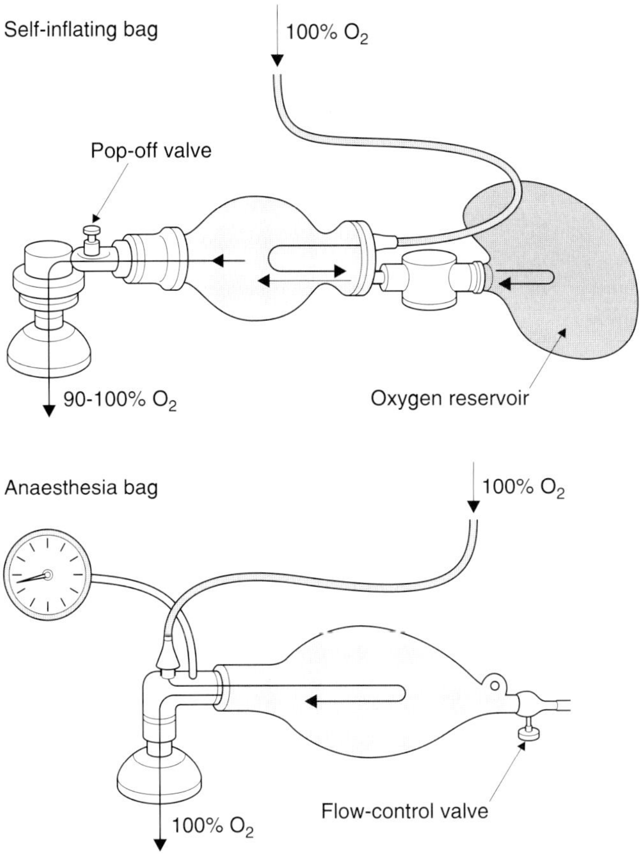

Figure 185.5 Self-inflating bag with reservoir and anesthesia bag.

Without the reservoir, O_2 is diluted with air. Many self-inflating bags are equipped with a pop-off valve that opens when the pressure exceeds 30–35 cmH_2O. If there is a leak around the face mask during bag and mask ventilation the pop-off valve can be closed to ensure a higher pressure. Bags without a pop-off valve should be used with caution, especially if the infant is intubated, because baro- or volutrauma from excessive peak inspiratory pressures is the most common complication during neonatal respiratory support. Many self-inflating resuscitators are commonly used with different characteristics in inspiratory or expiratory resistance, pressure relief valve, fraction of delivered O_2, and function at extreme temperature.[52] Bags that cannot be disassembled easily and are equipped with a reservoir to provide visual assurance of gas flow may have less margin for error and can be more easily used by resuscitators.[53]

The anesthesia bags require compressed air or O_2 flow for inflation. As they can deliver very high pressures, the pressure should be constantly monitored. Proper balance between the flow of gas and the flow control valve, and a tight seal around the face are required for effective use. Usually more training and experience is required for adequate use of anesthesia bags than for self-inflating bags.

Laryngeal mask airway

The laryngeal mask airway (LMA), developed in 1981 by Brain,[54] became available in 1988 for clinical use in anesthesiology. Initially, the LMA was designed for use in adults and has revolutionized routine airway treatment in the operating theater.[55] Later, many studies reported its successful use during newborn resuscitation,[56] and successful resuscitation of infants with Pierre–Robin syndrome when all the classical methods (bag and mask ventilation, oropharyngeal airway, tracheal intubation) failed.[57] It has been suggested that all pediatricians involved in neonatal resuscitation should become familiar with LMA use,[58] especially in the case of ineffective bag and mask ventilation and tracheal intubation. Neonatal guidelines do not recommend its routine use at this time, as the device cannot allow tracheal suctioning of thick meconium.

If the neonate requires positive pressure ventilation, the head is placed in the standard position for tracheal intubation, and a lubricated size 1 LMA, with the cuff fully deflated, is blindly inserted into the pharynx. The LMA is advanced, with the aperture facing anteriorly, until resistance is encountered. The cuff is then inflated with 2–4 ml of air to make a low pressure seal around the larynx.

The design of the LMA (Figure 185.6) prevents the distal end from entering the esophagus while it sits in the hypopharynx over the laryngeal inlet. When the cuff is inflated, a gas-tight seal exists between the larynx and the LMA which allows a peak inspiratory pressure of up to 30–40 cmH_2O; with some leaks this is around 20 cmH_2O.[59] In the hands of an experienced resuscitator it can be inserted within 8 s, nearly always at the first attempt, with successful ventilation within 20 s. The advantages over a facemask include better oxygenation, prevention of gastric distension, successful ventilation in cases of facial dysmorphism (e.g. Pierre–Robin syndrome, Treacher–Collins syndrome) and blind insertion, avoiding the need for laryngoscopy. The limiting features are that the airway is not protected from regurgitating gastric contents (not a serious problem in resuscitation of the newborn), and the low-pressure seal limiting inflation of a low-compliance lung. The size of the LMA-1 is appropriate for the newborn weighing more than 2.5 kg. Use of the LMA has not been sufficiently studied for patients who require chest compressions or who suffer from congenital anomalies (diaphragmatic hernia, abdominal wall anomalies). The LMA is not a substitute for tracheal intubation, which should be carried out when indicated.

Endotracheal intubation

Endotracheal intubation is indicated when: (1) bag and mask ventilation is ineffective; (2) tracheal suctioning of thick meconium or maternal blood is required; and (3) prolonged positive ventilation is anticipated. When chest compression is required,

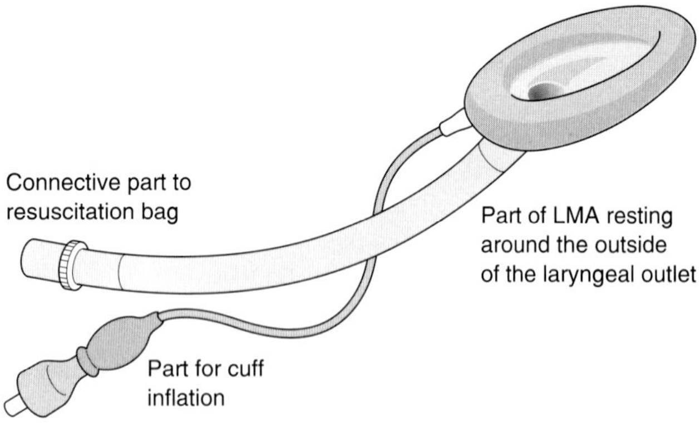

Figure 185.6 Laryngeal mask airway.

positive pressure ventilation is much more easily accomplished if the infant is intubated.

Successful intubation should be checked by observing for: (1) symmetric chest wall motion during inflation; (2) audible and equal breath sounds bilaterally, especially at the axillae; (3) improvement in heart rate and color; and (4) absent breath sounds over the stomach. When in doubt, the position of the tube should be visualized, and the infant reintubated if necessary. If the infant is to remain intubated, a chest radiograph should confirm the proper position of the tube before its fixation. When available, an exhaled-CO_2 monitor may be used to verify tracheal tube placement. Inadequate pulmonary expansion, decreased or absent pulmonary blood flow in cases with extreme bradycardia or asystole, and small tidal volume may limit its use in the delivery room.

The common ventilation rate is that of ventilation with bags: 40–60 breaths per minute. If chest compression is required, the ratio 3:1 should be applied (three chest compressions interposed with one breath at a common rate of 120/min).

The tracheal tube should be radio-opaque, without cuff, and with the same diameter throughout.[60] The Cole tube, with a small diameter at the distal end, is no longer recommended, as visualization of the larynx is more difficult, and the narrowed diameter prevents effective suctioning.[61] The Murphy tube is now preferred, with a uniform internal diameter, centimeter markers along the length, and a default marker 2 cm above the tip. The clinician can avoid deep insertion, leaving the default marker at the level of the glottis. Another guide to the proper depth of tracheal tube placement is a distance from the tube tip to the lip of the infant of 6 cm plus the infant's weight in kilograms (for infant weighing 3 kg, the 'tip-to-lip' distance would be 9 cm).[62] The guidelines for tracheal tube size are listed in Table 185.5.

Intubation can be performed orally or nasally. Oral intubation is generally easier, faster and less traumatic, and it is generally preferred in an emergency.

Table 185.5 Guidelines for endotracheal tube size

Tube internal diameter (mm)	Infant weight (g)	Suction catheter size
2.0	< 600	5F
2.5	600–1000	5F
3.0	1000–2000	6F
3.5	2000–3000	6F
3.5–4.0	> 3000	8F

Orotracheal intubation. The infant should be placed in the supine position and the chin extended slightly, but care should be taken not to hyperextend the neck. Hyperextension may impede venous return, increase intracranial pressure,[63] or kink the trachea.[64] A newborn glottis is in close proximity to the base of the tongue and visualization is easier if the neck is not extended. A laryngoscope with a Miller No. 0 or 1 straight blade, with the light close to the tip of the blade, is used to visualize the glottis. The blade No. 0 is usually sufficient for all newborns, except the largest ones. The laryngoscope is held between the thumb and the first finger of the left hand, the other fingers holding the chin. The blade is introduced from the right side between the tongue and palate and, while advancing, the tongue is pushed to the left. With the small finger of the left hand, pressure over the cricoid bone is applied to move the larynx posteriorly and visualize the glottis. The tip of the blade should advance into the vallecula epiglottis, and with a slight elevation the epiglottis is lifted anteriorly to expose the glottis (Figure 185.7). The tracheal tube, held in the right hand, is then introduced from the right corner of the mouth, along the side of the laryngoscope, through the glottis. When a properly sized tube does not pass easily into the trachea, the neck should be slightly flexed, and with rotating movement the tube should be slowly advanced. For difficult intubation in cases of dysmorphism of the upper airway a small bronchoscope should be available.[65] The bronchoscope should be inserted into the tracheal tube and then intubation can be endoscopically guided.

Nasotracheal intubation. Nasotracheal intubation is more time-consuming and technically more difficult for an inexperienced resuscitator. The tube should be lubricated with a water-base lubricant, inserted into one nostril, and with rotating movements advanced until the tip is seen in the posterior pharynx. In cases of difficult insertion a small suction catheter, pulled through the tube, should be a guide. After advancing through the nasal cavity the tube is easily passed and the catheter is then removed. The laryngoscope is placed into the mouth as described before, and the glottis visualized. With the aid of the Magill forceps

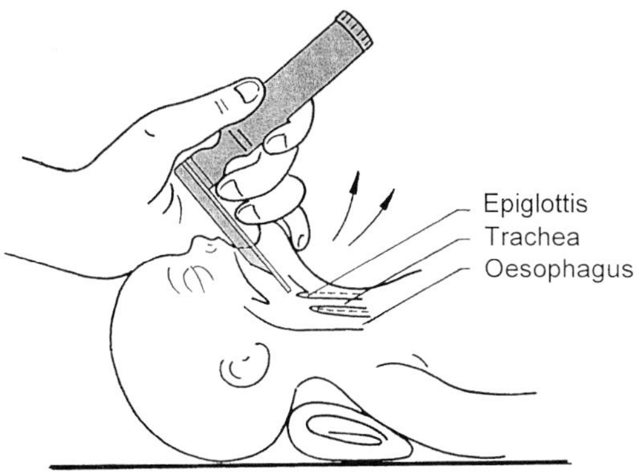

Figure 185.7 Placement of laryngoscope and landmark for intubation.

the nasotracheal tube is grasped short distance from its tip and advanced into the trachea.

Chest compression

Physiology

From the first report of cardiopulmonary resuscitation (CPR) by Kouwenhoven *et al.* in 1960,[66] it was believed that the blood flow caused by external chest compression was a result of direct squeezing of the heart between the sternum and the spinal column (cardiac pump mechanism). In 1976, Criley *et al.*[67] reported that by repeated coughing, several patients who developed ventricular fibrillation maintained a cardiac output adequate to maintain consciousness. These coughing spells were felt to increase the intrathoracic pressure, and the thoracic pump hypothesis soon followed. According to this hypothesis the external chest compression produces an increased intrathoracic pressure which translates to the lung and heart. Because of a competent venous valve at the thoracic inlet, the blood is squeezed out to the arterial system. According to this theory the heart plays no active role as a pump, but serves only as a passive conduit for the flow. It has been reported that simultaneous ventilation and external cardiac compression increase the intrathoracic vascular pressure to a greater extent than either measure alone, and enhance the cerebral and myocardial flow.[68]

Infants have a more pliable thorax, and during standard CPR a greater pressure in comparison with an adult model is generated. Secondly, a neonatal cardiac arrest differs from an adult cardiac arrest, which is usually of cardiac origin with an arrhythmia (ventricular fibrillation) as a terminal event. In infants and neonates there is generally a respiratory failure which leads to hypoxia and tissue acidosis with consequent bradycardia, decreased cardiac contractility and cardiac arrest. Therefore, establishing ventilation is of primary importance during CPR. This task is more easily accomplished with unobstructive ventilation coordinated with compression.

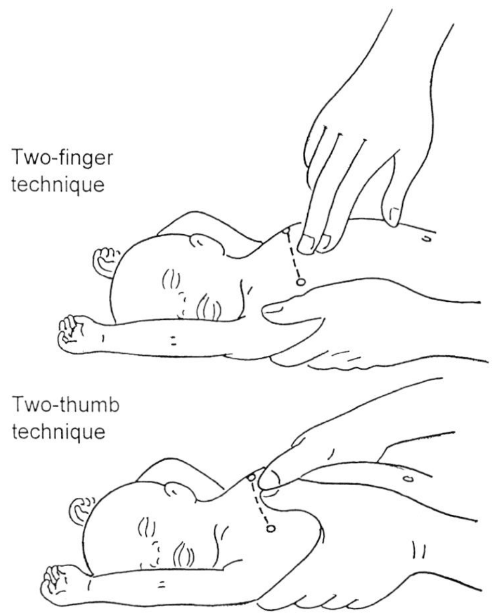

Figure 185.8 Methods of applying chest compression: two-finger technique and two-thumb technique. For a very small newborn the thumbs could overlap each other. Thumbs or fingers must be positioned on the sternum just below an imaginary line drawn between the nipples.

There are two recommended techniques for performing chest compression in the neonate (Figure 185.8).[69] In the two-thumb technique the hands are wrapped around the chest with thumbs placed on the lower third of the sternum, just below the line connecting the nipples. In the two-finger technique the index and middle fingers compress over the sternum, while the other hand supports the thorax. With the two-thumb technique the sternum is compressed and the thorax is simultaneously squeezed; therefore, cardiac and thoracic pump mechanisms are operating simultaneously. In animal studies it has been shown that with this technique higher arterial and coronary perfusion pressures are achieved.[70] For this reason, guidelines recommend two-thumb technique for chest compression in newborns whose size permits its use.[15,16]

Current recommendations

Chest compression should be started only after establishment of adequate ventilation, when a heart rate is below 60 bpm and not improving despite proper ventilation with 100% O_2 for 30 s. Both hands are placed around the thorax, with the thumb on the lower third of the sternum. Direct compression on the xiphoid or lower part of the sternum can damage abdominal organs and should be avoided. The sternum should be compressed firmly, approximately one-third of the anterior–posterior diameter of the chest, with a rate of 120 per minute (2 per second). Chest compressions should be interposed with intermittent ventilation (through bags or tracheal tube) in a 3:1 ratio.[71]

Table 185.6 Medications for neonatal resuscitation[73]

Drugs	Dose and route	Concentration	Total dose	Precautions
Epinephrine	0.01–0.03 mg/kg, IV or ET	Diluted to 1:10,000	0.1–0.3 ml/kg	Give rapidly
Volume expanders	10 ml/kg, IV			Infuse over 5 min
Sodium bicarbonate	1–2 mEq/kg, IV	0.5 mEq/ml	2–4 ml/kg	Give slowly over 2 min
Naloxone	0.1 mg/kg, IV, ET, IM or SC	0.4 or 1.0 mg/ml	0.25 or 0.1 ml/kg	Give rapidly, preferred IV or ET

IV, intravenously; ET, endotracheally; IM, intramuscularly; SC, subcutaneously

This means that the combined rate is 120 per minute: 90 chest compressions and 30 ventilations. It is recommended that the rescuer who performs chest compression counts loudly 'one-and-two-and-three-and-bag-and-one' so that synchrony is accomplished.[72] When the heart rate is greater than 60 bpm, chest compression should be discontinued.

Medications

Severe bradycardia that does not respond to adequate ventilation and chest compression is usually due to long-standing intrauterine hypoxia superimposed on acute deterioration during delivery. If after 30 s of chest compression and ventilation with 100% oxygen, bradycardia (heart rate < 60 bpm) persists, medications are indicated. This recommendation is restricted to delivery room resuscitation; therefore there is no place for medications other than epinephrine and volume expanders. Sodium bicarbonate is helpful only after prolonged resuscitation, and naloxone hydrochloride when respiratory depression secondary to maternal analgesia is suspected to exist. Medications, routes of administration, and currently recommended doses of commonly used drugs are provided in Table 185.6.[73]

Intravascular access

In the delivery room the umbilical vein can be rapidly identified and catheterized. A 3.5F or 5F single-hole radio-opaque catheter should be inserted, with the tip just below skin level, so that a free flow of blood returns on aspiration. When the catheter is inserted too deeply and without x-ray control, the tip of the catheter may be wedged in the liver, and the administration of vasoactive or hypertonic solutions may damage the liver parenchyma. A peripheral vein can be used, but can be difficult to cannulate in the presence of impaired circulation.

Tracheal access

Although this route of emergency drug administration has been widely accepted and frequently used, little scientific investigation on human subjects has been carried out. Epinephrine and naloxone can be administered by this route.[74]

Many issues concerning drug dose, route of instillation, and dilution have not been sufficiently clarified by current recommendations for resuscitation of the newborn infant. Several studies carried out on animals show that direct instillation of diluted drugs into the tube, followed by some inflation, produces the same concentration and lung distribution as other more cumbersome methods.[75] Direct instillation of epinephrine into the tube has also been found advantageous in a pediatric animal study.[76]

Drug dilution is very important for ensuring a good distribution over the largest possible surface area, providing a good pharmacological response. Redding *et al.*[77] found that 1 ml of endotracheal epinephrine was ineffective in adults unless diluted with 10 ml of water, and thereafter it has been generally accepted that endotracheal drugs should be diluted with 5–10 ml of distilled water or normal saline. Currently, there is no specific recommendation for diluting the drug in neonates, but for practical and theoretical reasons a common volume should be at least 0.5–1.0 ml.

Hypoxic neonates experience prolonged adaptation to extrauterine life. They are likely to have fluid-filled lungs and a right-to-left shunt at the level of the foramen ovale and ductus arteriosus.[78] No studies have been published on the pulmonary absorption of epinephrine in a neonatal animal model. In the first description of successful survival after the endotracheal administration of epinephrine to neonates, who did not respond to chest compression and ventilation, a standard dose (0.01 mg/kg) was used.[79]

The current recommendation states that, whether giving epinephrine intravenously or intratracheally, 0.01–0.03 mg/kg should be used. After giving the drug into the trachea, five quick insufflations are recommended before continuation of CPR.[15,16]

Intraosseous access

When a vascular line is difficult to achieve, intraosseous access can be useful for application of fluid and medication in children and adults. This is not the case in newborn infants, where the umbilical vein is easily accessible, small bones are fragile, and the intraosseous space is small, especially in premature infants.

Epinephrine. Administration of epinephrine is indicated when the heart rate is < 60 bpm after a minimum of 30 s of adequate ventilation and chest compression. The dose for neonates is 0.01–0.03 mg/kg (0.1–0.3 ml/kg of 1:10,000 solution), and the administration may be repeated every 3–5 min, if necessary. If there is no venous access, epinephrine may be administered intratracheally. Endotracheal epinephrine can be associated with low plasma levels,[80] and if there is no response the drug should be given intravenously without delay.

Epinephrine is an endogenous catecholamine with both alpha- and beta-adrenergic activity. It is released from the adrenal medulla during hypoxia and acidosis. Following intravenous administration of 0.01 mg/kg epinephrine, a further increase in plasma catecholamines is observed.[81,82] After saturation of the peripheral beta-receptors (which mediate vasodilatation) epinephrine, through the stimulation of alpha-1 receptors, decreases blood flow to the periphery (skin and skeletal muscles) and enhances myocardial and cerebral perfusion. This increase seems necessary to bring the myocardial blood flow to a sufficiently high level for restoration of spontaneous circulation (more than 20 ml/100 g/min).[83] Epinephrine also stimulates and enhances cardiac contractility, and increases heart rate.

During their early investigation, Redding and Pearson[84] found that 1 mg of epinephrine was effective in resuscitating dogs weighing approximately 10 kg, i.e. at a dose of 0.1 mg/kg. Nevertheless, the standard dose of epinephrine in adult and pediatric CPR has been for a long period considerably lower: 0.01 mg/kg. There have been reports in the pediatric and adult literature that a 10-times higher dose of epinephrine (0.1–0.2 mg/kg) is more effective than the standard dose regimen.[85,86] In the animal studies standard-dose epinephrine had a minimal effect on myocardial perfusion pressure and blood flow, whereas high-dose epinephrine (HDE) enhanced both, despite a significant reduction in cardiac output.[87] Later, randomized clinical studies revealed that HDE improved the return of spontaneous circulation, but no benefit in the discharge rates or neurological outcome was observed.[88,89]

Some of these clinical findings could be explained by a beta-1 agonist effect of epinephrine on increasing myocardial metabolism and oxygen demand, which offsets any increase in myocardial oxygen delivery during CPR. Moreover, many animal or human observational studies confirm that HDE has a detrimental effect on postresuscitation myocardial function, which includes prolonged hypertension, lactic acidemia, tachycardia, low cardiac index, low systemic oxygen delivery and consumption.[90–92] Besides, there is a substantial theoretical risk for the newly born, especially for premature infant, that rapid elevation of blood pressure may lead to intraventricular hemorrhage (IVH).[93]

Despite the existence of formal guidelines for the use of epinephrine in neonatal resuscitation, it should be emphasized that there have been no randomized controlled trials evaluating the administration of epinephrine to the apparently stillborn or extremely bradycardic newborn infant, the effect of high vs. standard doses, or the effect of intravenous vs. endotracheal administration of epinephrine.[94]

Volume expanders. Fetuses can suffer from significant blood loss into the placenta without any external evidence of acute hemorrhage. Therefore, hypovolemia should be suspected whenever a neonate is unresponsive to epinephrine, or when in spite of a normal heart rate the neonate remains pale, with a barely palpable pulse. Recommended volume expanders for such situations are normal saline (0.9% NaCl) and Ringer's lactate. Usually, a dose of 10 ml/kg is administered slowly over 5 min into the umbilical vein. Current recommendations do not support the use of albumin-containing solutions, because of risk of infectious disease and an observed association with increased mortality.[95] The use of albumin for resuscitation in acute hypovolemia in adults is still debated as well.[96,97]

A neonate in severe hypovolemic shock should receive plasma expanders at a dose of 20 ml/kg and an infusion of an inotropic agent such as dopamine at a rate of 5–20 μg/kg/min or epinephrine at a rate of 0.1–0.5 μg/kg/min. In cases of feto-fetal or feto-maternal hemorrhage, where acute blood loss is superimposed on more chronic blood loss, repeated small infusions of whole blood (5 ml/kg) or packed erythrocytes should be infused, or exchange transfusion should be carried out, if high central venous pressure already reflects myocardial failure.

Sodium bicarbonate. Perinatal hypoxia leads to lactic acidosis, which decreases myocardial contractility, lowers blood pressure, and decreases cardiac response to catecholamines. Theoretically, there are therefore many reasons for using sodium bicarbonate ($NaHCO_3$) during resuscitation.

The ability of $NaHCO_3$ to buffer an increase in H^+ depends upon the ability of the lung to exhale CO_2 produced by the buffering process: $H^+ + NaHCO_3 = Na^+ + H_2CO_3 = Na^+ + H_2O + CO_2$.

The ability of the lung to eliminate CO_2 depends on ventilation and pulmonary blood flow. At the beginning of resuscitation, in the state of low cardiac output, giving $NaHCO_3$ is counterproductive. Even with adequate ventilation, a low pulmonary blood flow does not allow CO_2 elimination, and metabolic acidosis is simply replaced by respiratory acidosis. As CO_2 easily crosses the cell membrane, it transiently lowers the intramyocardial pH and decreases myocardial contractility,[98] even if the pH in the arterial blood is normalized. After the restoration of pulmonary blood flow and ventilation, this effect can be quickly reversed. Furthermore, $NaHCO_3$ may even contribute to IVH[99] in preterm infants. IVH is thought to be secondary to hypernatremia and hypertonicity,[100] but any preterm infant requiring CPR is at increased risk for IVH.

Recently, the role of $NaHCO_3$ has been reevaluated. In an animal model it was found that during neonatal resuscitation, with hypoxia and compromised hemodynamics, metabolic acidemia significantly attenuated the hemodynamic responses to epinephrine and oxygen, suggesting that the correction of metabolic acidosis may be warranted.[101] However, a randomized controlled trial of $NaHCO_3$ in neonatal resuscitation did not provide evidence for improved survival or immediate neurologic outcome.[102] Even more, a thorough review of the physiologic evidence for use of bicarbonate in the neonatal intensive care unit showed that, should bicarbonate be introduced today as a new drug for the treatment of acidosis, its approval could not be supported on the basis of existing experimental data.[103]

During brief resuscitation the use of bicarbonate is discouraged. It should be administered only when CPR is prolonged, adequate ventilation has been established, and there is no response to epinephrine and volume expanders. The dose of 1–2 mEq/kg of 0.5 M solution is administered intravenously, at the slow rate of 1 mEq/kg/min, to minimize the acute effect of hypertonicity.[16,104]

Naloxone hydrochloride. Naloxone hydrochloride is a narcotic antagonist that reverses the respiratory depression induced by narcotics. It is indicated when there are no clinical signs of hypoxic–ischemic injury (adequate circulation is established) and with a history of maternal narcotic administration within 4 h prior to delivery. The dose is 0.1 mg/kg,[105] and should be given every 2–3 min, as the narcotic suppression of respiration exceeds the effect of the antagonist.

The preferred route of administration is intravenous or intratracheal, but the drug can also be given intramuscularly or subcutaneously. Continuous monitoring for at least 6 h after administration is indicated. In the neonate whose mother is suspected to be addicted to narcotics, the use of naloxone hydrochloride is contraindicated because narcotic withdrawal can induce severe seizures.[106]

Oxygen. Oxygen has been traditionally used for resuscitation of the newborn. Current guidelines[15,16] recommend using 100% oxygen in a breathing newborn during stabilization, whenever he or she is cyanotic, bradycardic, or has other signs of distress. Oxygen should be delivered close to the infant's face by oxygen mask, face mask or by flow-inflating bag. Many self-inflating bags do not deliver 100% oxygen if they are not squeezed simultaneously. Obviously, 100% oxygen should be provided during positive-pressure ventilation and, even more importantly, during chest compressions. If oxygen is not available, resuscitation should be initiated with positive-pressure ventilation and room air.

Oxygen paradox

The paradox of aerobic life is that higher eukaryotic aerobic organisms cannot exist without oxygen, yet oxygen is inherently dangerous to their existence through the formation of highly toxic free radical species. These molecules are highly reactive and are capable of damaging all biological macromolecules including proteins, DNA and lipids and have been implicated in inflammatory, toxic and metabolic insults, ischemia–reperfusion injury, carcinogenesis and atherosclerosis.[107] It has recently been proposed that many diseases affecting preterm infants are only different facets of the same oxygen radical disease.[108] Furthermore, it has become evident that hypoxic tissue injury is not caused only by lack of oxygen but occurs to a large extent from events in the posthypoxic reoxygenation period, which lasts long after the primary insult.[109]

In animal experiments it was found that room air was as effective as 100% oxygen for normalizing blood pressure, heart rate, base deficit, and plasma hypoxanthine after severe neonatal hypoxia, and that the extent of hypoxic brain damage was similar. There were also no differences in cerebral blood flow (CBF) or somatosensory-evoked potentials.[110,111]

Oxygen is not universally used in many situations during resuscitation outside hospitals, and in many developing countries supplementary oxygen is rarely available. The results of several clinical studies have also shown no differences between the groups of infants resuscitated with room air or 100% oxygen in heart rate response, acid–base status, or outcome at 28 days.[112,113] Furthermore, they found that infants resuscitated with air recovered more quickly as assessed by Apgar scores and time to first cry. The air-resuscitated babies achieved a sustained pattern of respiration more quickly, and required a shorter duration of positive-pressure ventilation. A trend toward lower mortality was noticed, although it was not statistically significant. It was also found that oxidative stress measured by the ratio of reduced to oxidized glutathione in whole blood and by superoxide dismutase activity in erythrocytes, was increased in newborns resuscitated with oxygen compared with room air.[114] Biochemical findings of prolonged oxygen stress were apparent even after 4 weeks of postnatal life.[115]

Despite these growing biochemical and clinical evidence of oxygen toxicity, Niermeyer and Vento[107] concluded that further research in the way of a prospective randomized clinical trial is needed before the use of room air instead of 100% of oxygen can be recommended. While waiting for the new recommendation, the goal of oxygen supplementation should be normoxemia. A recent international survey of a sample of academic centers disclosed that approximately

50% of neonatologists reported that they already had begun to modify the percentage of oxygen used during neonatal resuscitation in their institutions.[116] Obviously, adequate ventilation seems to be more important than oxygen supplementation during resuscitation. However, some newborns with severely impaired lungs may not be adequately oxygenated with room air and on such occasions monitoring with pulse oximetry is recommended.

Problems of resuscitation

Technical errors

In spite of apparently appropriate resuscitation, some newborns remain cyanotic and bradycardic or breathe irregularly. Sometimes the cause may be a congenital anomaly, but first one should consider the possibility of the following technical errors in resuscitation:

- not enough pressure delivered with the self-inflating bag (change bag for another),
- incorrectly sized face mask or loss of tight seal around the mask,
- collapsing upper airway because of neck hyperextension or flexion (change position of the head while observing chest movements),
- disconnection of the oxygen (anesthesia bag is not inflating, oxygen reservoir on self-inflating mask is empty),
- tube not in the trachea but inserted too deep in main bronchus, or tube slipped into the esophagus (observe chest movement, auscultate, reintubate if necessary),
- improperly sized tracheal tube, which is too small for the particular infant.

Pneumothorax

Pneumothorax should always be considered in the neonate responding poorly to resuscitation. The main clinical signs are a lateral shift of the heart sounds, sometimes with muffled tones, decreased movement of the thorax and difficult inflation, distended abdomen (especially in preterm infants), and sustained or secondary bradycardia.

As there is no time for an x-ray, cold-light examination can be of assistance. If the newborn's condition deteriorates rapidly, trial punctures on both sides of the thorax in the midclavicular line in the second intercostal space, must be carried out. If air comes out and the newborn's condition improves, a thoracic drainage is performed, or a venous cannula (18–20 gauge) is inserted at the side of the pneumothorax, the stylet removed, and the neonate prepared for transport.

Congenital malformations

Some newborns are vigorous and have a normal heart rate, but have increasingly severe respiratory distress and remain cyanotic in spite of oxygenation and bag and mask ventilation. In such cases the possibility of congenital malformation should be considered.

Some malformations of the upper respiratory tract (choanal atresia, Pierre–Robin syndrome) are disclosed clinically and during laryngoscopy. A prone position, insertion of an oropharyngeal tube or intubation will usually solve the problem. Laryngeal or tracheal atresia are found during an unsuccessful trial of intubation, and only emergency tracheotomy or puncturing of the trachea with a thicker vein cannula may help the baby to survive in the delivery room.

Neonates with lung malformations (pulmonary hypoplasia due to Potter syndrome or prolonged membrane rupture, congenital anomalies of the lung itself, pleural effusion) are usually intubated at birth because of respiratory deterioration; for diagnosis and management, transport to the neonatal intensive care unit is urgent.

There are many dysmorphic syndromes, such as some short-limb dwarfing syndromes, that are incompatible with life. Nevertheless, as the delivery room is not the proper place for a careful physical examination, and as the most experienced team is probably not present, it is more appropriate to stabilize and transport the baby to the intensive care unit where careful examination to identify the disorder can be done.

Very rarely, a newborn baby has a normal heart rate and good peripheral perfusion but is hypotonic and does not breathe by itself in spite of appropriate oxygenation, and correction of blood sugar and potential acidosis. If there is no history of maternal diseases or fetal distress during labor, a congenital neuromuscular disease (Werdnig–Hoffmann disease, transient neonatal myasthenia gravis, congenital myopathies, severe neonatal form of myotonic dystrophy, congenital muscular dystrophy) should be considered.

Anomalies of the abdominal wall

Diaphragmatic hernia, omphalocele and gastroschisis can be detected by ultrasound examination in pregnancy. Therefore, when labor begins there is enough time for the most experienced team to be prepared for delivery. Some hours after delivery, the intestines fill with air because of swallowing. This occurs even more rapidly if after birth ventilation with a mask is required. In cases of diaphragmatic hernia the air in the intestines disturbs breathing, while in cases of gastroschisis it interferes with vein return, which causes preoperative conditions to deteriorate. Therefore, it is recommended to intubate these newborns immediately after birth,[117] and to insert a wide catheter to decompress the stomach. The newborn with gastroschisis should be placed on its side to prevent venous stasis.

Fetuses with congenital diaphragmatic hernia (CDH) are at high risk for severe pulmonary hypoplasia. They should be ideally delivered in a perinatal center with a neonatal surgical department.[118] CDH presents with a deviation of the mediastinum to the right (shift of cardiac impulse), markedly reduced or absent breath sounds on the left (the most common side of the hernia), and a concave-appearing abdomen. Usually diagnosis has been established before delivery by ultrasound examination, but in any newborn with rapidly developing respiratory distress, urgent intubation without attempts at bag and mask ventilation is mandatory if there is any suspicion of CDH. In cases of clinically suspected or already diagnosed CDH, the resuscitation of the newborn includes tracheal intubation and positive pressure ventilation.

Hydrops fetalis

Clinically, hydrops is recognized at birth as anasarca, ascites and pleural effusion, and is generally classified as either immune or non-immune in nature. The introduction of Rh D immune globulin prophylaxis has so reduced the incidence of immune hydrops that more than 75% of neonatal hydrops cases show no evidence of associated hemolytic disease. Ultrasound examination in all pregnancies complicated by hypertension, preeclampsia, polyhydramnios or anemia could identify 80% of affected neonates before the 28th week of gestation.[119] The resuscitators should be experienced in tracheal intubation, chest compression, umbilical vessel catheterization, paracentesis, thoracentesis and pericardiocentesis.

Special considerations

Preterm neonates

Currently, VLBW infants account for more than 50% of perinatal mortality and more than 50% of neonatal deaths, and occupy more than two-thirds of the beds in neonatal intensive care units. As the survival of these infants depends more on experienced management than on the initial resuscitation,[120] every effort should be made to transfer the parturient to a perinatal center with experienced obstetricians and neonatologists, and neonatal intensive care facilities.

The incidence of perinatal depression, but not asphyxia, is increased among premature infants, because of their physiologic immaturity. Diminished lung compliance, weakness of respiratory musculature and reduced respiratory drive may increase necessity for assisted ventilation. Among 33,357 liveborn infants delivered at the Maternity Hospital of Ljubljana (1997–2002), 3.6% were bag and mask resuscitated (49% of them were preterm infants) and 0.4% were intubated and ventilated in the delivery room (65% of them were preterm; 35% had a gestational age of 27 weeks or less).[3] Very preterm infants have an increased risk of acute and chronic neonatal disorders (heat loss, IVH, periventricular leukomalacia, respiratory distress, necrotizing enterocolitis, chronic lung disease, retinopathy of prematurity). Current guidelines make no distinction between the techniques of resuscitation for term and very preterm infants with respect to ventilation and oxygen administration. Modifications of the basic approach may, nevertheless, be warranted for very immature infants.[121]

Volutrauma

It has been recognized that volutrauma (the adverse effects of a large tidal volume regardless of the pressure applied) plays an important role in lung injury.[122] The current practice, among other methods aimed at reducing lung injury, includes breathing on nasal continuous positive airway pressure (CPAP), low tidal volume ventilation (high-frequency ventilation), and gentle ventilation in the delivery room.[123] It has been demonstrated in a premature lamb model that a few large breaths applied manually at birth to a surfactant-deficient lung can produce lung injury, irrespective of whether artificial surfactant has been administered before or afterwards.[124,125] Self-inflating or flow-inflating bags either display no data on tidal volume or show only the pressure. It is known that positive end-expiratory pressure (PEEP) during ventilation increases lung surface area and compliance, preserves FRC, conserves surfactant, reduces hyaline membrane disease, and reduces expression of pro-inflammatory cytokines.[121] Adequate PEEP cannot be provided with self-inflating bags and is difficult to control with anesthesia bags. There are no formal recommendations regarding its use during resuscitation of the newborn.

CPAP is used ever more frequently in intensive care units and its early use together with surfactant administration reduces the need for intubation and subsequent mechanical ventilation of premature infants.[126] With the use of a T-piece or a Neopuff infant resuscitator (Fisher & Paykel, New Zealand), which is a modified T-piece, CPAP, variable PEEP and positive inspiratory pressure can be delivered, although they provide no data on tidal volume. The Neopuff is easy to use, even in the hands of inexperienced operators[127] and should be considered for resuscitation of preterm infants.

Oxygen toxicity

As noted above, clinical studies have shown that resuscitation can be carried out with room air without any adverse effect, and that there may in fact be some advantages of air over oxygen.[112,113] It was also found that oxidative stress is increased in newborn infants resuscitated with oxygen and is apparent even after 4 weeks of postnatal life.[114,115] Oxygen is even more toxic for preterm babies, as it has been shown that they have a lower capacity for induction of antioxidant enzymes than do term babies.[128] Recent results from several observational studies, summarized by Tin,[129] showed that keeping oxygen saturation levels below 90–95% in the first weeks postpartum, reduced the frequency of chronic lung disease and retinopathy (stage 3–4) in infants with birth weights < 1500 g.

Lower levels of saturation (< 94%) did not influence the mortality and neurodevelopmental outcome at 1 year.[130] Even if there is yet no definite answer to the question of what constitutes the lower safe limit of oxygen saturation, it is becoming clear that a more permissive approach to minor hypoxia may, like a permissive approach to hypercapnia, reduce the need for ventilatory support, the risk of chronic lung disease, and their associated health care costs.[131] It has also been shown that even short-term administration of 80% oxygen during initial stabilization at birth produces a persistent cerebral vasoconstriction with a lower CBF in preterm infants.[132] Oxidative stress influences apoptosis and cell growth, and may have long-term consequences on growth and development.[133] While we await the results of ongoing trials, it would seem wise to monitor oxygen saturation during resuscitation of preterm infants and use the lowest possible FiO_2 to reach normoxemia.

Limits of viability

Regionalization and new technology have increased the survival rate in preterm neonates. With survival of more and more of these tiny babies a lot of new questions have emerged: Are we using the new technology rationally and, more importantly, ethically? How small is too small and toward what goal should we aim: survival, or quality of life? Do we respect the ethical principles of beneficence and nonmaleficence; are we helping or hurting these tiny children? How do we determine what is in the best interests of the baby, and who is the most appropriate surrogate decision maker – parents or health care providers? Should we consider economic pressure to decrease expenses?[134] Every pediatrician working in the delivery room is sooner or later faced with these questions and is placed in the position of determining if resuscitation of a tiny baby is warranted. Characteristics of the individual physician, both personal and professional, and the presence of an ethics committee in the hospital influence this attitude.[135] With the decision to resuscitate comes the long-term commitment for the care of this child, and the emotional and financial investments are very high.[136] It is very difficult for the physician to be objective in the delivery room, where he or she may feel the pressure of the parents, obstetrician, and nurses, each of them with their own expectations.

Survival rates for extremely preterm infants have steadily increased in all weight or age groups during recent decades, whereas neurodevelopmental disability rates have, in general, remained unchanged.[137,138] Survival has increased from 20% to more than 50% between 23 and 24 weeks of gestation or, similarly, between 500 and 600 g of birth weight. Guidelines on life and death decisions in preterm infants have been formulated in different countries and varied from non-initiation of resuscitation at 22 weeks to provision of all reasonable care beyond 25 weeks.[139] In the gray zone between the opinions of the parents should be respected. Because in these tiny babies the risks of death and long-term morbidity are not negligible, it is important that, whenever possible, maternal interventions, mode of delivery, extent of resuscitative efforts, and discontinuance of therapy are discussed before the delivery begins.[140,141] The family should also be informed that resuscitation at delivery does not mandate continued support, that decision making continues beyond the first few critical hours, and that the child's future treatment will be based on almost continuous reassessment.

Does the preterm infant need prophylactic surfactant therapy?

Intratracheal surfactant administration at birth theoretically offers the advantage of optimal surfactant distribution within the alveoli. As the lung expands and fluid is reabsorbed, the surfactant is distributed to all parts of the lung. Even short-term ventilation of surfactant-deficient lungs results in areas of atelectasis and areas of hyperinflation, which causes uneven distribution of exogenous surfactant.[142] In several studies that compared prophylactic vs. rescue treatment, no great advantage of prophylaxis could be found, except in the smallest infants (26 weeks of gestation or less).[143] However, recent reports have shown that very preterm infants who received prophylactic surfactant developed less severe respiratory distress syndrome, needed lower peak inspiratory pressures, had a shorter duration of oxygen therapy, and less periventricular leukomalacia and IVH.[144,145]

When early surfactant administration is used it should be provided early, preferably in the delivery room or at least within 1 h of age.[146,147] Such treatment may interfere with initial resuscitation; nevertheless, preterm infants are intubated in the delivery room mostly for respiratory insufficiency and less often for severe asphyxia. Early surfactant administration improves ventilatory efficiency, which is of outmost importance for successful resuscitation.

Meconium-stained amniotic fluid

As noted above, morbidity and mortality from MAS seemed to improve after Gregory *et al.*[148] in 1974 recommended laryngoscopy and tracheal intubation with suctioning for all newborns delivered through thick particulate meconium. In 1976, Carson *et al.*[149] reported that additional obstetric suctioning of the oro- and hypopharynx before the shoulders were delivered further reduced the severity and frequency of MAS. The importance of tracheal intubation and suctioning for all newborns with meconium-stained amniotic fluid was, however, challenged by others who proposed selective tracheal suctioning only for severely depressed infants born through thick particulate meconium.[150,151] They believed that lung disease is primarily due to hypoxia, and that an unnecessary intubation of an infant with thin meconium or a vigorous infant with thick meconium-stained fluid can expose it to unnecessary risk.

The concept of unselected tracheal suctioning was based on the assumption that MAS is primarily a postnatal event, that oronasopharyngeal suctioning at the perineum and tracheal intubation just after delivery prevents the moving of meconium into the trachea, and that all deaths from MAS could be prevented by these measures. It was reported subsequently that the introduction of De Lee suctioning did not influence the presence of meconium below the vocal cords or the rate of MAS.[40] It is now believed that chronic fetal hypoxia can result in meconium passage, and, in the presence of oligohydramnios, the meconium becomes thick. Further hypoxia induces gasping respirations that move the meconium into the trachea. The compromised fetus with decreased lung fluid outflow fails to clear the meconium from the respiratory tree.[152]

In the Ljubljana Maternity Hospital, we perform selective tracheal suctioning under laryngoscopic control with a thick catheter. If meconium is found in the trachea and the infant is severely depressed, we intubate the baby and perform lung lavage with 1–2 ml of normal saline. When the condition of the infant allows, the procedure is repeated as long as meconium is achieved. During lavage the tracheal tube is not withdrawn, and suctioning is performed with the widest bore catheter possible. During a 6-year period, 4795 (15.9%) term infants were born through meconium-stained amniotic fluid; 2.5% were aspirated, an additional 3.4% were bag and mask ventilated, and only 0.3% were intubated in the delivery room. Altogether 14 infants had signs of MAS, seven were mechanically ventilated, and only one died of extreme hypoxia.

Care after resuscitation

After resuscitation blood should be taken for blood gas analysis and glucose determination. Special efforts to avoid hypo- and hyperthermia should be made. When the infant is stabilized he or she should be transported to the neonatal intensive care unit. Severe asphyxia could lead to multiorgan failure; therefore, appropriate control of respiration, circulation, blood gas and electrolyte balance is important. Complete documentation of all interventions and medications used during resuscitation should be recorded. The use of standard resuscitation records is desirable because it offers the further advantage of uniform data collection to facilitate study and comparison of resuscitation techniques and outcomes.

The Apgar score is traditionally used in the delivery room to evaluate the physical condition of the newborn at birth and the immediate need for resuscitation. Heart rate, breathing efforts, muscle tone, reflex irritability, and color are recorded at 1 and 5 min after birth and then sequentially every 5 min until vital signs have established. The score is designed to facilitate clinical assessment of the newborn and guide resuscitative interventions, which aid in accomplishing transition from the fetal to the neonatal environment. The Apgar score should not be used to define birth asphyxia, or to predict subsequent child development.[153]

Ethical considerations

Cardiopulmonary resuscitation in the delivery room is a therapeutic modality that initiates a cascade of events that usually results in admission to the neonatal intensive care unit with assisted ventilation, often painful and expensive therapy, and sometimes ends with an imperfect outcome. The decision either to resuscitate or not must be made instantaneously, always without the advice of the ethics committee, usually without full knowledge of the baby's condition and future outcome, and commonly without consultation with the parents.[154]

Competent practice of neonatal intensive care today requires more than the knowledge of the relevant medical science. At least some understanding of medical ethics and associated dilemmas that are nowadays the subject of wide public concern is required. In the search for practical guidelines for solving medical dilemmas, ethical theorists advocate four principles on which to ground ethical analysis.[155]

(1) Respect for autonomy (self determination) – everyone is free to choose what is best for him/her.
(2) Beneficence (doing good) – the practitioner has a moral obligation to act for the benefit of the patient.
(3) Nonmaleficence (avoiding harm) – the practitioner has an obligation not to harm intentionally.
(4) Justice (fair distribution) – the practitioner should distribute benefits and burdens fairly, to treat equals equally.

Many physicians believe that there is an ethical difference between stopping a treatment once it is started, and not starting it in the first place (withdrawing vs. withholding treatment). A survey of opinions of attending physicians, house-staff, and medical students indicated that all felt much more comfortable in withholding treatments than in withdrawing them.[156,157] This opinion is strikingly different from the prevailing views among ethicists and lawyers who consider the decision to withhold or withdraw as equivalent under the condition that in either case the patient receives an adequate trial of therapy.[158,159] While newborns share with children and adults the right to live, there will occasionally be some who by reason of severe malformation, asphyxial injury or extreme prematurity, have the right to die with dignity, without inappropriate or futile medical intervention. CPR should reasonably be withheld from such patients. The Royal College of Pediatrics and Child Health advised to withhold treatment in the following three situations: the no-chance situation, the no-purpose situation with massive physical or mental impairment, and the unbearable situation with progressive and irreversible illness.[160] Nevertheless, physicians should be aware that withholding CPR from critically ill newborns, based on assumptions of future mental and physical development or social adaptability, places decision makers on a slippery slope, the bottom of which holds that no person or value is sacred against social utility.[161]

The current guidelines recommend that non-initiation of resuscitation in the delivery room is appropriate for infants with confirmed gestation < 23 weeks or birth weight < 400 g, anencephaly or confirmed trisomy 13 or 18. In case of uncertainty, the resuscitation should be initiated and life preserved until enough information is gathered to provide counseling with the parents and to decide whether continuation or withdrawal of life support is in the best interests of the infant.

REFERENCES

1. Saugstad OD. Practical aspects of resuscitating asphyxiated newborn infants. *Eur J Pediatr* 1998;157(Suppl 1):S11–15.
2. Jain L, Vidyasagar D. Cardiopulmonary resuscitation of newborns. Its application to transport medicine. *Pediatr Clin N Am* 1993; 40:287–301.
3. Anonymous. National Perinatal Information System Republic Slovenia. *Yearly Report in Zdrav Vest,* 1996–2002;Suppl 5:36–41.
4. Roberton NRC. Resuscitation of the newborn. In Roberton NRC, ed. *Textbook of Neonatology,* 3rd edn. London: Churchill Livingstone, 1994:173–95.
5. American Academy of Pediatrics Committee on Fetus and Newborn, and Committee on Obstetric Practice, American College of Obstetricians and Gynecologists. Use and abuse of the Apgar score. *Pediatrics* 1996;98:141–2.
6. Dawes GS. Birth asphyxia, resuscitation and brain damage. In Dawes GS, ed. *Fetal and Neonatal Physiology.* Chicago, IL: Year Book Medical Publishers, 1968:141–59.
7. Cohn HE, Sack FJ, Heymann MA, Rudolph AM. Cardiovascular responses to hypoxemia and acidemia in fetal lambs. *Am J Obstet Gynecol* 1974;120:817–24.
8. Fisher DJ. Increased regional myocardial blood flows and oxygen deliveries during hypoxemia in lambs. *Pediatr Res* 1984;18:602–6.
9. Fisher DJ. Acidemia reduces cardiac output and left ventricular contractility in conscious lambs. *J Dev Physiol* 1986;8:23–31.
10. Cross KW. Resuscitation of the asphyxiated infant. *Br Med Bull* 1966;22:73–8.
11. Rudolph CD, Roman C, Rudolph AM. Effect of acute umbilical cord compression on hepatic carbohydrate metabolism in the fetal lamb. *Pediatr Res* 1989;25:228–33.
12. Linderkamp O, Versmold HT, Messow-Yahn K, Muller-Holve W, Riegel KP, Betke K. The effect of intrapartum and intrauterine asphyxia on placental transfusion in premature and full-term infants. *Eur J Pediatr* 1978;127:91–9.
13. Kenny J, Plappert T, Doubilet P. Effect of heart rate on ventricular size, stroke volume, and output in the normal human fetus: A prospective Doppler echocardiographic study. *Circulation* 1987;76:52–8.
14. Friedman AH, Fahey JT. The transition from fetal to neonatal circulation: Normal responses and implications for infants with heart disease. *Semin Perinatol* 1993;17:106–21.
15. Kattwinkel J, Niermeyer S, Nadkarni V, *et al.* An advisory statement from the Pediatric Working Group of the International Liaison Committee on Resuscitation. *Pediatrics* 1999;103:e56.
16. The American Heart Association in collaboration with the International Liaison Committee on Resuscitation. Guidelines 2000 for Cardiopulmonary Resuscitation and Emergency Cardiovascular Care. Part 11: Neonatal resuscitation. *Circulation* 2000; 102(Suppl):I343–57.
17. Wiswell TE. Neonatal resuscitation. *Respir Care* 2003;48:288–94.
18. Gordon A, McKechnie EJ, Jeffery H. Pediatric presence at cesarean section: justified or not? *Am J Obstet Gynecol* 2005;193: 599–605.
19. American Academy of Pediatrics, American College of Obstetrics and Gynecology. In Poland RL, Freeman RK, eds. *Guidelines for Perinatal Care,* 3rd edn. Elk Grove Village, IL: American Academy of Pediatrics; Washington DC: American College of Obstetrics and Gynecology, 1992.
20. Kroll L, Twohey L, Daubeney PE, Lynch D, Ducker DA. Risk factors at delivery and the need for skilled resuscitation. *Eur J Obstet Gynecol Reprod Biol* 1994;55:175–7.
21. Allwood ACL, Madar RJ, Baumer JH, Readdy L, Wright D. Changes in resuscitation practise at birth. *Arch Dis Child Fetal Neonatal Ed* 2003;88:F375–9.
22. Emergency Cardiac Care Committee and Subcommittees, American Heart Association. Guidelines for cardiopulmonary resuscitation and emergency cardiac care. *J Am Med Assoc* 1992; 268:2276–81.
23. Owen CJ, Wyllie JP. Determination of heart rate in the baby at birth. *Resuscitation* 2004;60:213–17.
24. Gatti H, Castel C, Andrini P, *et al.* Cardiorespiratory arrest in full term newborn infants: Six case reports. *Arch Pediatr* 2004;11: 432–5.
25. Dahm LS, James LS. Newborn temperature and calculated heat loss in the delivery room. *Pediatrics* 1972;49:504–13.
26. Perlman JM. Maternal fever and neonatal depression: Preliminary observation. *Clin Pediatr* 1999;38:287–91.
27. Lieberman E, Lang J, Richardson DK, Frigoletto FD, Heffner LJ, Cohen A. Intrapartum maternal fever and neonatal outcome. *Pediatrics* 2000;105:8–13.
28. Dietrich WD, Busto R, Valdes I, Loor Y. Effects of normothermic versus mild hypothermic forebrain ischemia in rats. *Stroke* 1990; 21:1318–25.
29. Takagi K, Ginsberg MD, Globus MY, Martinez E, Busto R. Effect of hyperthermia on glutamate release in ischemic penumbra after middle cerebral artery occlusion in rats. *Am J Physiol Heart Circ Phys* 1994;36:H1770–6.
30. Safar P, Xiao F, Radovsky A, *et al.* Improved cerebral resuscitation from cardiac arrest in dogs with mild hypothermia plus blood flow promotion. *Stroke* 1996;27:105–13.
31. Gunn AJ, Gunn TR, Gunning MI, Williams CE, Gluckman PD. Neuroprotection with prolonged head cooling started before postischemic seizures in fetal sheep. *Pediatrics* 1998;102:1098–106.
32. Thoresen M, Penrice J, Lorek A, *et al.* Mild hypothermia after severe transient hypoxia-ischemia ameliorates delayed cerebral energy failure in the newborn piglet. *Pediatr Res* 1995;37:667–70.
33. Bona E, Hagberg H, Loberg EM, Bagenholm R, Thoresen M. Protective effects of moderate hypothermia after neonatal hypoxia-ischemia: Short- and long-term outcome. *Pediatr Res* 1998;43:738–45.
34. Safar P. Cerebral resuscitation after cardiac arrest: Research initiatives and future directions. *Ann Emerg Med* 1993;22:324–9.
35. Stratton D. Aural temperature in the newborn infant. *Arch Dis Child* 1977;52:865–9.
36. Gunn AJ, Gunn TR. Effect of radiant heat on head temperature gradient in term infants. *Arch Dis Child* 1996;74:F200–3.
37. Battin MR, Penrice J, Gunn TR, Gunn AJ. Treatment of term infants with head cooling and mild systemic hypothermia (35.0°C and 34.5°C) after perinatal asphyxia. *Pediatrics* 2003;111:244–51.
38. Gunn AJ. Cerebral hypothermia for prevention of brain injury following perinatal asphyxia. *Curr Opin Pediatr* 2000;12:111–15.
39. Patel H, Beeby PJ. Resuscitation beyond 10 minutes of term babies born without signs of life. *J Paediatr Child Health* 2004;40: 136–8.

40. Falciglia HS, Henderschott C, Potter P, Helmchen R. Does DeLee suction at the perineum prevents meconium aspiration syndrome? *Am J Obstet Gynecol* 1992;167:1243–9.
41. Estol PC, Pariz H, Basalo S, Simini F, Grela C. Oro-naso-pharyngeal suction at birth: Effect on respiratory adaptation of normal term vaginally-born infants. *J Perinat Med* 1992;20:297–305.
42. Cordero LJ, Hon EH. Neonatal bradycardia following nasopharyngeal stimulation. *J Pediatr* 1971;78:441–7.
43. Liu WF, Harrington T. Delivery room risk factors for meconium aspiration syndrome. *Am J Perinatol* 2002;19:367–78.
44. Cleary GM, Wiswell TE. Meconium-stained amniotic fluid and the meconium aspiration syndrome. An update. *Pediatr Clin North Am* 1998;45:511–29.
45. Wiswell TE, Gannon CM, Jacob J, *et al.* Delivery room management of the apparently vigorous meconium-stained neonate: Results of the multicenter, international collaborative trial. *Pediatrics* 2000;105:1–7.
46. Chaturvedi P, Yadav B, Bharambe MS. Delivery room management of neonates born through meconium stained amniotic fluid. *Indian Pediatr* 2000;37:1251–5.
47. Linder N, Aranda JV, Tsur M, *et al.* Need for tracheal intubation and suction in the meconium-stained neonates. *J Pediatr* 1988;112:613–15.
48. Halliday HL, Sweet D. Endotracheal intubation at birth for preventing morbidity and mortality in vigorous, meconium-stained infants born at term. *The Cochrane Library* 2004;2.
49. Kattwinkel J. American Academy of Pediatrics, NRP Steering Committee. *Textbook of neonatal resuscitation.* American Academy of Pediatrics, Elk Grove Village 2000:1–40.
50. Milner AD, Vyas H. Lung expansion at birth. *J Pediatr* 1982;101: 879–86.
51. Vyas H, Milner AD, Hopkin IE, Boon AW. Physiologic responses to prolonged and slow-rise inflation in the resuscitation of the asphyxiated newborn infant. *J Pediatr* 1981;99:635–9.
52. Finer NN, Barrington KJ, Al-Fadley F, Paters KL. Limitation of self-inflating resuscitators. *Pediatrics* 1986;77:417–20.
53. Connors R, Kisson N, Tiffin N, Frewen TC. An evaluation of the physical and functional characteristics of infant resuscitators. *Pediatr Emerg Care* 1993;9:104–7.
54. Brain AIJ. The development of the laryngeal mask: A brief history of invention, early clinical studies and experimental work from which the laryngeal mask evolved. *Eur J Anaesthesiol* 1991;4: 5–17.
55. American Society of Anesthesiologists Task Force on Management of the Difficult Airway. Practice guidelines for management of the difficult airway. *Anesthesiology* 1993;78:597–602.
56. Paterson SJ, Byrne PJ, Molesky MG, Seal RF. Neonatal resuscitation using the laryngeal mask airway. *Anesthesiology* 1994;80: 1248–53.
57. Baraka A. Laryngeal mask airway for resuscitation of a newborn with Pierre–Robin syndrome. *Anesthesiology* 1995;83:645–6 [Letter].
58. Brimacombe J. The laryngeal mask airway for neonatal resuscitation. *Pediatrics* 1994;93:874 [Letter].
59. White DC. The laryngeal mask: A non-invasive airway. *Eur J Anaesthesiol* 1991;4(Suppl):1–4.
60. Colice GL. Technical standards of tracheal tubes. *Clin Chest Med* 1991;12:433–48.
61. Mitchell MD, Bailey CM. Dangers of neonatal intubation with the Cole tube. *Br Med J* 1990;301:602–3.
62. Tochen ML. Orotracheal intubation in the newborn infant: A method of determining depth of tube insertion. *J Pediatr* 1979;95:1050–1.
63. Gregory GA. Airway obstruction. In Pascoe D, Grossman M, eds. *Quick Reference to Pediatric Emergency*, 3rd edn. Philadelphia: J.B. Lippincott Co., 1984:15.
64. Fletcher MA. Tracheal intubation. In Fletcher MA, MacDonald MG, Avery G, eds. *Atlas of Procedures in Neonatology.* Philadelphia: J.B. Lippincott Co., 1983:213.
65. Finer NN, Muzyka D. Flexible endoscopic intubation of the neonate. *Pediatr Pulmonol* 1992;12:48–51.
66. Kouwenhoven WB, Jude JR, Knickerbocker GG. Closed-chest cardiac massage. *J Am Med Assoc* 1960;173:1064.
67. Criley JM, Blaufuss AH, Kissel GL. Cough-induced cardiac compression. *J Am Med Assoc* 1976;236:1246–8.
68. Koehler RC, Chandra N, Guerci AD, *et al.* Augmentation of cerebral perfusion by simultaneous chest compression and lung inflation with abdominal binding after cardiac arrest in dogs. *Circulation* 1983;67:266–75.
69. David R. Closed chest cardiac massage in the newborn infant. *Pediatrics* 1988;81:552–4.
70. Menegazzi JJ, Auble TE, Nicklas KA, Hosak GM, Rack L, Goode JS. Two-thumb versus two-finger chest compression during CPR in a swine infant model of cardiac arrest. *Ann Emerg Med* 1993;22:240–3.
71. Keenan WJ, Raye JR, Schell B. *NRP Instructor Update.* Elk Grove Village, IL: American Academy of Pediatrics, 1993:1.
72. Karlowitcz MG, Karotkin EH, Goldsmith JP. Resuscitation. In Goldsmith, JP, Karotkin EH, eds. *Assisted Ventilation of the Neonate*, 3rd edn. London: W.B. Saunders Company, 1996:83–99.
73. American Academy of Pediatrics/American Heart Association. *Textbook of Neonatal Resuscitation.* Dallas, TX: American Heart Association, 1994.
74. Hess D, Alagar R. Methods of emergency drug administration. *Resp Care* 1995;40:498–511.
75. Prengel AW, Lindner FH, Hahnel JH, Georgieff M. Pharmacokinetics and technique of endotracheal and deep endotracheal lidocain administration. *Anesth Analg* 1993;77:985–9.
76. Jasani MS, Nadkarni VM, Finkelstein MS, Mandell GA, Salzman SK, Norman ME. Effects of different techniques of endotracheal epinephrine administration in pediatric porcine hypoxic-hypercarbic cardiopulmonary arrest. *Crit Care Med* 1994;22:1174–80.
77. Redding JS, Asuncion JS, Pearson JW. Effective routes of drug administration during cardiac arrest. *Anesth Analg* 1967;l46: 253–8.
78. Burchfield DJ, Berkowitz ID, Berg RA, Goldberg RN. Medication in neonatal resuscitation. *Ann Emerg Med* 1993;22:435–9.
79. Lindemann R. Resuscitation of the newborn: Endotracheal administration of epinephrine. *Acta Paediatr Scand* 1984;73:210–12.
80. Orlowski JP, Gallagher JM, Porembka DT. Endotracheal epinephrine is unreliable. *Resuscitation* 1990;19:103–13.
81. Wortsman J, Frank S, Cryer PE. Adrenomedullary response to maximal stress in humans. *Am J Med* 1984;77:779–84.
82. Lindner KH, Ahnefeld FW, Bowdler IM, Prengel AW. Influence of epinephrine on systemic, myocardial and cerebral acid-base status during cardiopulmonary resuscitation. *Anesthesiology* 1991; 74:333–9.
83. Neimann IT. Differences in cerebral and myocardial perfusion during closed-chest resuscitation. *Ann Emerg Med* 1984;13: 849–53.
84. Redding IS, Pearson JW. Evaluation of drugs for cardiac resuscitation. *Anaesthesia* 1963;24:203–7.
85. Goetting MG, Paradis NA. High-dose epinephrine (HDE) improves outcome from pediatric cardiac arrest. *Ann Emerg Med* 1991;20:22–6.
86. Barton C, Callahan M. High-dose epinephrine improves the spontaneous circulation rates in human victims of cardiac arrest. *Ann Emerg Med* 1991;120:772–5.
87. Chase PB, Kern KB, Sanders AB, Otto CW, Ewy GA. Effect of a graded dose of epinephrine on both noninvasive and invasive measures of myocardial perfusion and blood flow during cardiopulmonary resuscitation. *Crit Care Med* 1993;21:413–19.
88. Callahan M, Madren CD, Barton CW, Saunders CE, Pointer J. A randomized clinical trial of high-dose epinephrine and norepinephrine vs. standard-dose epinephrine in prehospital cardiac arrest. *J Am Med Assoc* 1992;268:2667–72.
89. Brown CG, Martin DR, Pepe PE, *et al.* A comparison of standard-dose and high-dose epinephrine in cardiac arrest outside the hospital. The Multicenter High-Dose Epinephrine Study Group. *N Engl J Med* 1992;327:1051–5.
90. Tang W, Weil MH, Sun S, Noc M, Yang L, Gazmuri RJ. Epinephrine increases the severity of postresuscitative myocardial dysfunction. *Circulation* 1995;92:3089–93.
91. Neumar RW, Bircher NG, Sim KM, *et al.* Epinephrine and sodium bicarbonate during cardiopulmonary resuscitation following asphyxial cardiac arrest in rats. *Resuscitation* 1995;29:249–63.
92. Rivers EP, Wortsman J, Rady MY, Blake HC, McGeorge FT, Buderer NH. The effect of the total cumulative epinephrine dose administered during human CPR on hemodynamics, oxygen transport, and utilization variables in the postresuscitation period. *Chest* 1994;106:1499–507.
93. Berg RA, Otto CW, Kern KB, *et al.* A randomized, blinded trial of high-dose epinephrine versus standard-dose epinephrine in a swine model of pediatric asphyxial cardiac arrest. *Crit Care Med* 1996;24:1696–1700.
94. Ziino AJA, Davies MW, Davis PG. Epinephrine for the resuscitation of apparently stillborn or extremely bradycardic newborn infants. *The Cochrane Database of Systematic Reviews* 2002, Issue 3. Art No.: CD003849. DOI: 10.1002/14651858.CD003849.

95. Cochrane Injuries Group Albumin Reviewers. Human albumin administration in critically ill patients: Systematic review of randomised controlled trials. *BMJ* 1998;317:235–40.
96. Allison SP, Lobo DN. Debate: Albumin administration should not be avoided. *Crit Care* 2000;4:147–50.
97. Pulimood TB, Park GR. Debate: Albumin administration should be avoided in the critically ill. *Crit Care* 2000;4:151–5.
98. Graf H, Leach W, Arieff AI. Evidence for a detrimental effect of bicarbonate therapy in hypoxic lactic acidosis. *Science* 1985;227: 754–6.
99. Papile LA, Burnstein J, Burstein R, Koffler H, Koops B. Relationship of intravenous sodium bicarbonate infusions and cerebral intraventricular hemorrhage. *J Pediatr* 1978;93:834–6.
100. Simmons MA, Adcock EW, Berd H, Battaglia FC. Hypernatremia and intracranial hemorrhage in neonates. *N Engl J Med* 1974;291: 6–10.
101. Preziosi MP, Roig JC, Hargrove N, Burchfield DJ. Metabolic acidemia with hypoxia attenuates the hemodynamic responses to epinephrine during resuscitation in lambs. *Crit Care Med* 1993; 21:1901–7.
102. Lokesh L, Kumar P, Murki S, Narang A. A randomized controlled trial of sodium bicarbonate in neonatal resuscitation: Effect on immediate outcome. *Resuscitation* 2004;60:219–23.
103. Ammari AN, Schulze KF. Uses and abuses of sodium bicarbonate in the neonatal intensive care unit. *Curr Opin Pediatr* 2002;14: 151–6.
104. Leuthner SR, Jansen RD, Hageman JR. Cardiopulmonary resuscitation of the newborn: An update. *Pediatr Clin N Am* 1994;41: 893–907.
105. American Academy of Pediatrics Committee on Drugs. Emergency drug doses for infant and children and naloxone use in newborns: Clarification. *Pediatrics* 1989;83:803.
106. Gibbs J, Newson T, Williams J, Davidson DC. Naloxone hazard in an infant of an opioid abuser. *Lancet* 1989;2:159–60.
107. Niermeyer S, Vento M. Is 100% oxygen necessary for the resuscitation for the newborn infants? *J Matern Fetal Neonatal Med* 2004;15:75–84.
108. Saugstad OD. Oxygen toxicity in the neonatal period. Review article. *Acta Paediatr Scand* 1990;79:881–92.
109. Saugstad OD. Free radicals in neonatal intensive care. In Tibboel D, van der Vort E, eds. *Intensive Care in Childhood. A Challenge to the Future.* Berlin: Springer-Verlag, 1996:36–52.
110. Rootwelt T, Loeberg EM, Moen A, Oeyasaeter S, Saugstad OD. Hypoxemia and reoxygenation with 21% or 100% oxygen in newborn pigs: Changes in blood pressure, base deficit and hypoxanthine and brain morphology. *Pediatr Res* 1992;32:107–13.
111. Rootwelt T, Odden JP, Hall C, Ganes T, Saugstad OD. Cerebral blood flow and evoked potentials during reoxygenation with 21% or 100% O_2 in newborn pigs. *J Appl Physiol* 1995;75:2054–60.
112. Saugstad OD, Rootwelt T, Aalen O. Resuscitation of asphyxiated newborn infants with room air or oxygen: An international controlled trial: the Resair 2 study. *Pediatrics* 1998;102:e1.
113. Saugstad OD, Ramji S, Irani SF, *et al.* Resuscitation of newborn infants with 21% or 100% oxygen: Follow-up at 18 to 24 months. *Pediatrics* 2003;112:296–300.
114. Vento M, Asensi M, Sastre J, Lioret A, Garcia-Sala F, Viña J. Oxidative stress in asphyxiated term infants resuscitated with 100% oxygen. *J Pediatr* 2003;142:240–6.
115. Vento M, Asensi M, Sastre J, Garcia-Sala F, Pallardo FV, Vina J. Resuscitation with room air instead of 100% oxygen prevents oxidative stress in moderately asphyxiated term neonates. *Pediatrics* 2001;107:642–7.
116. Sinha S, Tin W. Oxygen therapy during neonatal resuscitation – too little or too much? *Indian Pediatr* 2003;40:507–9.
117. Engels M. Beeinflussende Faktoren des postpartalen Verlaufes von Kindern mit Gastroschisis. *Z Geburtsh Perinatol* 1994;194:131–3.
118. Morin L, Crombleholme TM, D'Alton ME. Prenatal diagnosis and management of fetal thoracic lesion. *Semin Perinatol* 1994;18: 228–53.
119. Hutchison AA, Drew JH, Yu VY, Williams ML, Fortune DW, Beischer NA. Nonimmunologic hydrops fetalis: A review of 61 cases. *Obstet Gynecol* 1982;59:347–52.
120. Babnik J, Kornhauser-Cerar L. Resuscitation of the newborn with 1-minute Apgar score <3: Population-based analysis. In *Abstracts of the 7th European Congress on Paediatric, Surgical and Neonatal Intensive Care*, Cambridge, 1995.
121. O'Donnell PF, Davis PG, Morley CJ. Resuscitation of premature infants: What are we doing wrong and can we do better? *Biol Neonate* 2003;84:76–82.
122. Jobe AH, Ikegami M. Mechanisms initiating lung injury in the preterm. *Early Hum Dev* 1998;53:81–94.
123. Burch K, Rhine W, Baker R, *et al.* Implementing potentially better practices to reduce lung injury in neonates. *Pediatrics* 2003;111: e432–6.
124. Ingimarsson J, Bjorklund LJ, Curstedt T, *et al.* Incomplete protection by prophylactic surfactant against the adverse effects of large lung inflations at birth in immature lambs. *Intensive Care Med* 2004;30:1446–53.
125. Bjorklund LJ, Ingimarsson J, Curstedt T, *et al.* Manual ventilation with a few large breaths at birth compromises the therapeutic effect of subsequent surfactant replacement in immature lambs. *Pediatr Res* 1997;42:348–55.
126. Verder H, Albertsen P, Ebbesen F, *et al.* Nasal continuous positive airway pressure and early surfactant therapy for respiratory distress syndrome in newborns of less than 30 weeks' gestation. *Pediatrics* 1999;103:E24.
127. Finer NN, Rich W, Craft A, Henderson C. Comparison of methods of bag and mask ventilation for neonatal resuscitation. *Resuscitation* 2001;49:299–305.
128. Frank L, Sosenko IRS. Failure of premature rabbits to increase antioxidant enzymes during hyperoxic exposure: Increased susceptibility to pulmonary oxygen toxicity compared with term rabbits. *Pediatr Res* 1991;129:292–6.
129. Tin W. Optimal oxygen saturation for preterm infants: Do we really know? *Biol Neonate* 2004;85:319–25.
130. Askie LM, Henderson-Smart DJ, Irwig L, Simpson JM. Oxygen saturation targets and outcomes in extremely preterm infants. *N Engl J Med* 2003;349:959–67.
131. Tin W, Milligan DW, Pennefather P, Hey E. Pulse oximetry, severe retinopathy, and outcome at one year in babies of less than 28 weeks gestation. *Arch Dis Child Fetal Neonatal Ed* 2001;84: F106–10.
132. Lundstroem KE, Pryds O, Griesen G. Oxygen at birth and prolonged cerebral vasoconstriction in preterm infants. *Arch Dis Child* 1995;73:F81–6.
133. Suzuki YJ, Forman HJ, Sevanian A. Oxidants as stimulators of signal transduction. *Free Radic Biol Med* 1997;22:269–85.
134. Peabody JL, Martin GI. From how small is too small to how much is too much. Ethical issues at the limits of neonatal viability. *Clin Perinatol* 1996;23:473–89.
135. De Leeuw R, Cuttini M, Nadai M, *et al*; EURONIC study group. Treatment choices for extremely preterm infants: An international perspective. *J Pediatr* 2000;137:608–16.
136. Babnik J. Ethical decisions in the delivery room. In Kurjak A ed. *Textbook of Perinatal Medicine.* London: The Parthenon Publishing Group Ltd, 1998:1880–5.
137. Boyle RJ, Kattwinkel J. Ethical issues surrounding resuscitation. *Clin Perinatol* 1999;26:779–92.
138. Hack M, Fanarrof AA. Outcome of extremely low birth-weight and gestational age in the 1990's. *Early Hum Dev* 1999;53: 193–218.
139. Van Reempts PJ, Van Acker KJ. Ethical aspects of cardiopulmonary resuscitation in premature neonates: Where do we stand? *Resuscitation* 2001;51:225–32.
140. American Academy of Pediatrics Committee on Fetus and Newborn. American College of Obstetricians and Gynecologists Committee on Obstetric Practise. Perinatal care at the threshold of viability. *Pediatrics* 1995;96;974–6.
141. Renie JM. Perinatal management at the lower margin of viability. *Arch Dis Child* 1996;74;F214–18.
142. Jobe AH, Ikegami M, Jacobs H, Jones S. Surfactant and pulmonary blood flow distributions following treatment of premature lambs with natural surfactant. *J Clin Invest* 1984;73:848–56.
143. Kendig JW, Notter RH, Cox C, *et al.* A comparison of surfactant as immediate prophylaxis and as rescue therapy in newborns of less than 30 weeks' gestation. *N Engl J Med* 1991;l324:865–71.
144. Bevilacqua G, Parmigiani S; OBSERVES Group. An observational study of surfactant treatment in infants of 23–30 weeks' gestation: Comparison of prophylaxis and early rescue. *J Matern Fetal Neonatal Med* 2003;14:197–204.
145. Walti H, Paris-Llado J, Egberts J, *et al.* Prophylactic administration of porcine-derived lung surfactant is a significant factor in reducing the odds for peri-intraventricular haemorrhage in premature infants. *Biol Neonate* 2002;81:182–7.
146. Stevens T, Blennow M, Soll R. Early surfactant administration with brief ventilation vs selective surfactant and continued mechanical ventilation for preterm infants with or at risk for respiratory distress syndrome. *Cochrane Database Syst Rev* 2004;3.

147. Horbar JD, Carpenter JH, Buzas J, *et al.* Vermont Oxford Network. Timing of initial surfactant treatment for infants 23 to 29 weeks' gestation: Is routine practice evidence based? *Pediatrics* 2004; 113:1593–602.
148. Gregory GA, Gooding CA, Phibbs RH, Tooley WH. Meconium aspiration in infants – A prospective study. *J Pediatr* 1974;85: 848–52.
149. Carson BS, Losey RW, Bowes WA, Simmons MA. Combined obstetrics and pediatrics approach to prevent meconium aspiration syndrome. *Am J Obstetr Gynecol* 1976;126:712–15.
150. Cunningham AS, Lowson EE, Martin RJ, Pildes RS. Tracheal suctioning and meconium: A proposed standard of care. *J Pediatr* 1990;116:153–4.
151. Yoder BA. Meconium-stained amniotic fluid and respiratory complications: Impact of selective tracheal suction. *Obstet Gynecol* 1994;83:77–84.
152. Berkus MD, Langer O, Samueloff A, Xenakis EMJ, Field NT, Ridgway LE. Meconium-stained amniotic fluid: Increased risk for adverse neonatal outcome. *Obstet Gynecol* 1994;84:115–20.
153. American Academy of Pediatrics Committee on Fetus and Newborn. Use and abuse of the Apgar score. *Pediatrics* 1986;78: 1148–9.
154. Goldsmith JP, Ginsberg HG, McGettigan MC. Ethical decision in the delivery room. *Clin Perinatol* 1996;23:529–50.
155. Beauchamp TL, Childress JF. *Principles of Biomedical Ethics*, 4th edn. New York: Oxford University Press, 1994.
156. Solomon MZ, O'Donnell L, Jennings B, *et al.* Decision near the end of life: Professional views on life-sustaining treatments. *Am J Public Health* 1993;83:14–23.
157. Caralis PV, Hammond JS. Attitudes of medical students, housestaff, and faculty phisicians toward euthanasia and termination of life-sustaining treatment. *Crit Care Med* 1992;20:683–90.
158. Annas GJ. Nancy Cruzan and the right to die. *N Engl J Med* 1990;323:670–3.
159. Annas GJ, Arnold B, Aroskar M, Battin D, Beauchamp T, *et al.* Bioethicists' statement on the U.S. Supreme Court's Cruzan decision. *N Engl J Med* 1990;323:686–7.
160. Van Reempts PJ, Van Acker KJ. Ethical aspects of cardiopulmonary resuscitation in premature neonates: Where do we stand? *Resuscitation* 2001;51:225–32.
161. Robertson JA, Fost N. Passive euthanasia of defective newborn infants: Legal consideration. *J Pediatr* 1976;88:883–9.

186 Childbirth and the pelvic floor

W. R. Cohen and R. Romero

A dramatic change in the distribution of delivery modes has occurred recently in many parts of the developed world. While the rise in cesarean rates that began in the 1970s had modulated by the 1990s, more recent changes have led cesarean rates to previously unimagined levels in many countries, and they continue to rise. Until recently, concerns about fetal and neonatal well-being drove most decisions for cesarean section; but now the need to protect maternal pelvic floor integrity has arisen as a justification for avoiding vaginal delivery. The medical profession and the lay public share the unease about the potential adverse effects of vaginal birth on the pelvic floor and the long-term consequences of such injury.

It is clear that damage to the musculofascial supports of the lower female genitourinary tract and anal continence mechanism can occur during vaginal birth, and there is evidence that such harm to pelvic floor structures and their innervation can cause or contribute to chronic genital, urinary, or defecatory pathology in later life (Table 186.1).[1–7] The magnitude of the contribution of parturitional trauma to the prevalence of pelvic organ prolapse and incontinence, which may not be manifest until many years after delivery, is not, however, known precisely. It is nevertheless increasingly cited to justify liberal use of cesarean delivery as well as to question the benefits of instrumental delivery and episiotomy.[8]

This nascent trend in obstetric thinking countervails the prevailing logic that has guided efforts to reduce the cesarean section rate during the last few decades and, if validated, would lead to a sea change in our concept of indications for cesarean delivery. The issue is of particular and increasing importance because pelvic floor disorders afflict primarily older women, and the aging of our population endows a practical urgency to develop a complete understanding of this complex area. Moreover, recent studies suggest that these disorders are considerably more prevalent than was recognized previously and that they contribute mightily to health care costs.[9–18] It is important that we determine what the etiology is of parturitional pelvic tissue injury, what the short- and long-term consequences of that injury are, and what obstetric or other factors make a patient vulnerable to serious adverse outcomes. Only with that information can we make informed medical judgments and rational obstetric care policies.

Table 186.1 Potential consequences of pelvic floor injury

Cystocele, rectocele, enterocele, urethrocele
Urinary incontinence
Fecal incontinence
Procidentia
Dyspareunia, other sexual dysfunction
Genital fistulas
Pelvic surgery

Prevalence and cost

The prevalence of the symptomatic consequences of obstetric pelvic floor disruption is difficult to determine. While many studies exist, the reported frequencies of incontinence and genital prolapse vary a great deal. This is probably the consequence of an inhomogeneity in survey methods of ascertainment, in definitions of incontinence, and in study population demographics.[9] Urinary incontinence probably exists in at least 5–10% of the female population; many estimate it is much more common. Using a questionnaire approach, Crist *et al.* found that 34% of women reported some degree of urinary incontinence, the frequency and severity of which was related directly to age and parity.[19]

In a population-based study, Samuelsson *et al.* identified some evidence of genital prolapse (cystocele, rectocele, uterine prolapse, or absence of the urethrovesical crease) in about 30% of the general female population in Sweden.[20] Among parous women aged 20–60 years 44% were affected; 5.8% of nulliparas had these signs of pelvic floor incompetence. While age and parity were strongly associated with prolapse, only a small minority of cases were symptomatic or of any functional significance. This observation emphasizes one of the important deficits in our knowledge of pelvic floor disorders in general. The rate at which minor degrees of anatomic prolapse, or subclinical abnormalities in the continence mechanism progress to a significantly symptomatic state is not discernible; neither do we understand how progression is influenced, or what therapeutic or lifestyle changes might hasten or slow its progress.

The prevalence of anal incontinence is also quite difficult to ascertain with certainty, but is doubtless more common than realized previously, and occurs predominantly in women.[4,10,11,13,21] A community survey in Wisconsin[10] showed that about 2–3% of women suffered from anal incontinence, with associated factors being advancing age, poor general health, and physical limitations. Anal incontinence often accompanies urinary incontinence and other pelvic floor disorders.[21,22] A population-based survey done in Australia in 1998[13] revealed that 35% of women had urinary incontinence and 3.5% had fecal incontinence. An additional 10.9% suffered from inability to control flatus. About one quarter of women had had previous surgery for incontinence or prolapse.

Kalantar *et al.*[23] found anal incontinence in 3.7% of a surveyed population of 65- to 93-year-olds in Australia, and Nelson *et al.*[10] reported an overall 2.2% incidence in the general population in a study done in the United States. Of the incontinent people, only 30% were older than 65 years, and 63% were women, findings consistent with those of other studies.[13] Some surveys suggest the problem of anal incontinence is even more widespread, and place the prevalence as high as 16%.[11] Several obstetric events and features have been identified as risk factors for anal incontinence. These include instrumental (especially forceps) delivery, episiotomy, and large birth weight.[1,4–6,24–27] All are factors known as well to be associated with risk of anal sphincter injury.

Pelvic floor dysfunction is more prevalent than previously realized. In addition to the inconvenience, risk, and emotional and physical disability that continence and genital prolapse disorders endow on individual women, the impact of these diseases on the public health and on health care costs is quite considerable. The lifetime risk of surgery for genital prolapse or urinary incontinence in an American female population was found to be about 11%;[28] a much larger number of affected women use non-surgical therapy or have no treatment. The number of women having surgery for urinary incontinence in the United States was 0.32 procedures per 1000 women per year in 1979; by 1997 the rate had increased to 0.60,[17] and in 1998 it was reported to have been 1.3.[15] It is likely higher today. This increase probably relates to several factors, including enhanced awareness of the problem among physicians and the lay public, the availability of new (and relatively simple) techniques for operative management, and the burgeoning size of the population at greatest risk.

The direct cost of care for urinary incontinence in women in the United States was estimated to be about $12.4 billion (in 1995 dollars),[29] and the cost of organ prolapse surgery more than $1 billion.[16] This amount is more than the cost of managing breast cancer, and in a league with that of many other chronic diseases. The need to understand and treat these problems has taken on a greater urgency recently because of the increasing longevity of the population and the transition of the post-World War II baby-boom generation into the age group in which pelvic floor problems become most prevalent. There is a need to develop our understanding of the causes of pelvic floor dysfunction if we are to make informed clinical judgments and fashion rational public heath policies to deal with them.

Mechanisms of obstetric injury

The mechanism of permanent parturitional injury to the birth canal and surrounding structures is the subject of controversy and uncertainty. We can predict *a priori* that possible mechanisms could include pudendal or autonomic nerve damage from excess direct pressure or traction, laceration and imperfect healing of pelvic tissues, stretching of muscle or connective tissue beyond its ability to recover strength and elasticity, and necrosis of pelvic soft tissues (from prolonged pressure by the fetus). One or more of these factors could cause or contribute to pelvic floor dysfunction in a particular case. Unfortunately, our inability to identify the mechanism of injury in many women and thereby to tailor treatment to address it confounds our efforts to help many patients.

Overt perineal trauma during vaginal delivery is not infrequent. Lacerations of the external anal sphincter (with or without accompanying tears of the anal–rectal wall) occur in about 1–4% of deliveries.[30–34] Risk factors include occiput posterior position, use of episiotomy, fetal macrosomia, and instrumental delivery. In addition to visible trauma, it is now clear that injuries to this area may be occult in a substantial number of cases.[26,35] Sultan *et al.*[26] showed that in a sample of primiparous women there was a 3% incidence of clinically diagnosed anal sphincter disruption; but anal sonography found sphincter defects in 35%. In another study, anal sonography done immediately after delivery revealed that 28% of patients had clinically undetectable anal sphincter disruptions.[36] These revelations raise many questions and concerns. While we have focused traditionally on the importance of repairing visible injuries, it is possible that most long-term damage is the consequence of invisible trauma that is perforce not repaired after delivery. Frudinger *et al.*[37] noted that some women with anal incontinence had intact sphincters. Thus, not only does occult sphincteric damage occur during delivery, but some women with anatomically intact sphincter mechanisms have postpartum incontinence, presumably the consequence of some functional (neurologic or traumatic) disruption of the continence mechanism.

In the lower pelvis the pudendal nerve lies relatively fixed in Alcock's Canal, where it is vulnerable to direct compression by the fetal head and to traction as the fetal presenting part distends the perineal structures and pushes them caudad late in the second stage of labor. The fact that pudendal nerve injury has not been observed after elective cesarean delivery but does occur after cesarean delivery in the first stage of labor suggests that compression injury can occur.[38,39] Therefore, prevention of pudendal nerve injury is not necessarily avoidable by cesarean section, unless it is done prior to labor. Even then, there is some evidence that pregnancy *per se* may have an effect on pelvic innervation.[39]

Pudendal nerve dysfunction probably underlies many cases of urinary and fecal incontinence.[2,40–42] The extent to which this denervation is the sole result of vaginal delivery is still unclear. In one study cohort, up to 80% of primiparous women had some evidence of denervation of the pelvic floor following vaginal delivery.[42] In the majority of cases, prolonged pudendal nerve terminal latencies recovered within 6 months of delivery. It does appear that women whose symptoms of incontinence persist for several months after delivery are highly likely to have these problems persist.[43]

In a 5-year follow-up of women who had evidence of pudendal neuropathy 2 months after vaginal delivery, Snooks *et al.*[7] showed evidence of persistent pudendal nerve damage in women who delivered vaginally, as determined by the observation of increased EMG-derived fiber density in the external anal sphincter, increased pudendal nerve terminal motor latency and reduced maximal anal canal pressure. Associated risk factors for nerve injury were multiparity, forceps delivery, third-degree perineal tear, long second stage, and high birth weight. This damage to the pelvic floor innervation is usually unrecognized after delivery, and is generally not associated with immediate symptoms of pelvic floor dysfunction. While such damage presumably predisposes to pelvic floor disability later in life, the frequency at which this occurs, and the degree to which such damage is repaired or compensated for over time are not known. Perhaps, the presence of cofactors is important or even necessary in order for most parturitional damage to become manifest as clinical incontinence or genital prolapse.

Some healing or compensatory mechanisms undoubtedly influence the degree to which overt or occult pelvic floor trauma contribute to long-term dysfunction. As noted, evidence of at least partial denervation of the pelvic floor can be demonstrated in 80% of primiparas.[42] If all such affected women developed incontinence or prolapse, observed prevalences later in life would be much higher than reported. In addition, the natural history of incontinence is understood incompletely. Some women have symptoms that subside spontaneously, or as a consequence of lifestyle changes (weight loss, smoking cessation, use of pelvic floor exercises, etc.). While the development of stress urinary incontinence shortly after delivery clearly places a woman at increased risk of such problems later in life, not all such individuals have persistent symptoms. It is likewise astounding that as many as one-third of women may sustain anal sphincter injuries during vaginal delivery that are not recognized.[5,26,35,44] This is an intriguing observation for two reasons. It is on the one hand sobering to realize that so normal a process as vaginal birth could cause significant injury so frequently; on the other, it is reassuring that the body is clearly able to heal or to compensate for many of these injuries. (Were it not competent in so doing, we would observe a much higher prevalence of anal incontinence than we do.)

The literature on pelvic floor injury is replete with references to pudendal nerve dysfunction and its effect on continence and the strength of the pelvic floor. While the pudendal nerve may indeed play an important role in this regard, its precise contribution to maintaining pelvic visceral support and urinary and fecal continence is not well understood. In fact, there is recent evidence from monkeys and humans that the levator ani muscles receive their innervation from sacral nerve roots (S4-5) and not from the pudendal nerve, as has been assumed.[45,46] This may explain why not all women, even with evidence of major pudendal nerve dysfunction, are incontinent. Such observations are of considerable importance for three reasons: they underscore our relative ignorance about the complex functional anatomy of this area; they require rethinking some traditional concepts of obstetric pelvic floor denervation; and they suggest potential avenues for diagnostic and therapeutic procedures.

The mechanisms that link childbirth to fecal incontinence are also not completely clear. There is no doubt that vaginal delivery may have a contributing role, and severe overt trauma to the pelvic floor and sphincter apparatus, especially if not properly repaired, can obviously lead to problems, as has been amply demonstrated in the developing world;[47] but other factors figure importantly in the risk of developing defecatory dysfunction. Among an Australian cohort of women who had vaginal instrumental delivery and/or delivered a baby weighing more than 4000 g, nearly 7% reported fecal incontinence 1 year after delivery.[13] In this group of high-risk women, fecal incontinence was significantly associated with maternal age above 35 years and with the presence of joint hypermobility. It often coexisted with urinary incontinence, but was not (contrary to other data) associated with multiparity.

Direct damage to the anal sphincters or pelvic floor muscular or connective tissue may also be etiologic in incontinence disorders and pelvic organ descent and is often persistent. Mechanical injury to the external anal sphincter does not always heal with restoration of competent function.[48,49] In one study, all women with symptoms of postpartum fecal urgency and anal incontinence had sonographically detectable mechanical disruption of the sphincter ani; these lesions persisted at 6 months.[50] The internal sphincter may be compressed, stretched, or lacerated during vaginal delivery. The integrity of this smooth muscle tissue and its autonomic innervation is also critically important in maintaining anal continence.[51] The thickness of the internal sphincter, as measured endosonographically, correlates well with anal luminal resting pressure and incontinence.[44] The importance of repairing a damaged internal anal sphincter during the repair of obstetric lacerations has not been sufficiently emphasized.[52,53]

In addition to its role in predisposing to incontinence, denervation of the muscles of the pelvic floor can also lead to genital prolapse.[2,22,41,54] By undergirding the female pelvic viscera, the levators and related musculature provide active support for the genital organs. When this support is lost, the levator hiatus widens and increased stress is placed upon the passive fascial supports of the pelvic viscera – the uterosacral and cardinal ligament complex and the endopelvic fascia – creating weaknesses or breaks in these supports and prolapse of the uterus, bladder or rectum. Often, several pelvic floor disorders occur concomitantly and require complex treatment strategies.

The role of parity and delivery mode

Implicit in the notion that vaginal delivery is a major risk factor for incontinence and prolapse is the assumption that parity has a direct relationship with risk, and that delivery by cesarean would eliminate risk. Not all studies support either assumption. Maclennan *et al.*[13] showed that pelvic floor problems were associated with pregnancy regardless of the mode of delivery, although other data[55] suggested that cesarean section reduced the risk of urinary incontinence regardless of the stage of labor in which it was performed.

In a cross-sectional population study, Rortveit *et al.*[56] administered a questionnaire to 27,900 women in Norway to analyze the relationships among age, parity and urinary incontinence. These data suggested that, while parity was directly related to the prevalence of urinary incontinence, so was age. Moreover, incontinence existed in a substantial proportion or nulliparous women, and the greatest effect of parity was in the youngest age groups, substantiating other data.[57] In other words, among women over 65 years old, the prevalence of urinary incontinence was not influenced by parity.

In a 15-year follow-up of a small cohort of women, Dolan *et al.*[40] found that increasing parity did not increase the risk of stress incontinence, suggesting that any pregnancy may expose a preexisting tendency to the disorder. Among women who had stress urinary incontinence either during or shortly after pregnancy, about two-thirds had symptoms 15 years later; one-third did not.

In an Australian study alluded to above[13] multivariate regression showed that in women advancing age, obesity, frequent coughing, and osteoporosis were significantly associated with pelvic floor disorders. Tobacco smoking may be a common denominator for many of the reported associations. Of interest is that while parity was a risk factor for pelvic floor dysfunction, the relationship was not linear, i.e. after the first child, increasing parity did not further enhance risk. Moreover, mode of delivery did not have a strong influence on risk. That is to say, women who had only cesareans were not significantly less likely to develop pelvic floor dysfunction than those who had delivered spontaneously; instrumental delivery did, however, have an adverse effect.

One may conclude from available data that, although vaginal delivery is clearly a contributor to, and sometimes a sole cause of, pelvic floor dysfunction, the degree to which increasing parity is an important risk factor is not clear. It is tempting to assume that if vaginal delivery causes or promotes pelvic floor pathology, then avoiding vaginal delivery would eliminate the risk of incontinence and prolapse; such is not the case. There is evidence that patients delivered late in the first stage of labor by cesarean section have documentable abnormalities in pudendal nerve function. This implies neurologic injury to the anal continence mechanism can occur, although in a series of such patients[27] no incontinence was noted 6 weeks after delivery. It is also clear that some injuries that occur during labor and delivery are self-repairable. For example, Arya *et al.*[58] studied urinary incontinence in patients after normal spontaneous delivery. Two weeks after delivery 13.3% of women had symptoms of urinary incontinence; only 2.9% did 1 year later.

It is presumed that most significant injuries to the pelvic floor structures occur during the second stage of labor. There is considerable substantiation for the idea that it is not appropriate to terminate the second stage of labor purely because an arbitrary amount of time has elapsed.[59–61] Rather, intervention by cesarean or instrumental vaginal delivery should be undertaken only when there is evidence of fetal compromise or an insurmountable labor dysfunction or cephalopelvic disproportion. None of the several studies that lend credence to that approach studied the effect of second-stage duration on the pelvic floor. Despite limited evidence linking the length of the second stage to birth canal injury, minimizing the duration of the second stage is viewed by some obstetricians as a strategy to help preserve pelvic floor integrity. This approach is not supported by all available evidence. Van Kessel *et al.*[62] demonstrated no relationship between second-stage length and the risk of stress urinary incontinence nearly 8 years after delivery; MacArthur *et al.*[63] and Arya *et al.*[58] reached the same conclusion regarding early onset of fecal and urinary incontinence, respectively. While other studies suggest long second-stage duration is a risk factor for pelvic floor dysfunction,[7,13] it is difficult to interpret this information. Studies generally lack information about whether the rate of descent was normal, and the intensity and duration of bearing-down efforts is not known; moreover, they do not always correct for cofactors that are associated with injury such as birth weight, malposition, or pelvic architecture.

It is during the second stage that the most extreme stretching and compression of the birth canal and its supporting tissues occurs. While data do not exist to guide evidence-based management for all aspects of late labor, some reasonable guidelines can be asserted based on experience and current knowledge. One should avoid long periods in the second stage during which there is no descent. Such situations can focus prolonged pressure on tissues in a limited area and provoke compression injury or even pressure necrosis. Similarly, as long as the fetus is well oxygenated, there is no reason to rush descent with extreme bearing-down efforts. It is probable that gradual steady distortion of tissues is less likely to result in overstretching or tearing than is very rapid deformation. Several lines of evidence have shown that delaying pushing until the head is well engaged, and using open-glottis pushing are reasonable alternatives to more active management of the second stage and yield equivalent outcomes.[64–66]

Some data show that pelvic floor problems were associated with pregnancy regardless of the mode of delivery,[13] although Farrell *et al.*[55] suggested that cesarean section reduced the risk of urinary incontinence regardless of the stage of labor in which it was performed. Nevertheless, even women who have delivered only by cesarean section still have a risk of pelvic floor disorders.[13,67] This suggests that pregnancy *per se* (as opposed to vaginal birth) may have an influence, or that in some women non-obstetric factors play a predominant or exclusive role in the development of incontinence and prolapse. Nulliparous women sometimes develop pelvic floor dysfunction, confirming that pregnancy and delivery are not pure prerequisites. This and the fact that, as noted, stress urinary incontinence occurs in those who have delivered only by cesarean and even in men indicates that factors other than vaginal delivery are involved.

Non-obstetric factors

The matrix of influences that determine the risks of parturitional trauma and the likelihood it will progress to permanent dysfunction is complex (Table 186.2). Factors in addition to obstetric characteristics that have been demonstrated or postulated to cause or function as cofactors in producing injury include age, obesity, smoking, posture, coexisting gastrointestinal pathology, estrogen deficiency, chronic pulmonary disease, peripheral neuropathy, and differences in collagen composition or metabolism.[68–80] Many of these are probably genetically determined; women or their health-care providers may influence others.

The evidence for a genetic predisposition to the development of pelvic floor weakness and its

Table 186.2 Pelvic floor dysfunction: non-obstetric causes and cofactors

Age
Obesity
Estrogen deficiency
Genetic factors
Posture
Gastrointestinal pathology
Chronic obstructive pulmonary disease
Peripheral neuropathy
Connective tissue disease

associated continence problems is supported by clinical and laboratory observations. Urinary incontinence has a familial tendency[21,71] and the prevalence of stress incontinence varies considerably by race.[68] Moreover, women who develop genital prolapse tend to have hyperextensible finger joints,[69,76,77] and may be more likely to have various forms of hernia. All of these observations suggest genetic influences are involved. A heritable mechanism would presumably derive from factors that affect connective tissue strength or integrity. Some data support the idea that connective tissue is somehow deficient in women who develop pelvic floor dysfunction. For example, Boreham *et al.*[78] found a disproportionate increase in caldesmon expression as compared to smooth muscle-myosin heavy-chain proteins in women with pelvic organ prolapse. This imbalance in contractile proteins, perhaps genetically determined, could contribute to reduction in pelvic support through altered collagen.

There has also been[79] demonstrated reduced collagen content and increased turnover in the vaginal tissue of premenopausal patients with prolapse compared with controls. Other data regarding changes in collagen enzymes support the notion that the connective tissue structure or metabolism in women who develop pelvic floor dysfunction somehow predisposes them to prolapse or incontinence; but the alternative explanation, i.e. that these biochemical and structural changes are the consequence of pelvic floor weakness rather than the cause remains to be explored.

Heavy smoking and obesity are associated with urinary incontinence and other forms of pelvic floor dysfunction.[72] So are a variety of medical problems, including chronic pulmonary disease, gastrointestinal pathology, diabetes, peripheral neuropathies, and connective tissue diseases.[80] Demographic factors, particularly age, make an important contribution to risk.[2,13,21,75]

Based on a great deal of epidemiologic and experimental data, it is possible to conclude that the development of pelvic floor dysfunction that leads to pelvic organ prolapse and to urinary or fecal incontinence is multifactorial (Figure 186.1). It is clear that obstetric injury plays a significant role in this kind of disability; but it is as certain that other factors contribute substantially, and sometimes exclusively, to these problems. Genetic factors are certainly important, and their involvement in the genesis of pelvic floor dysfunction

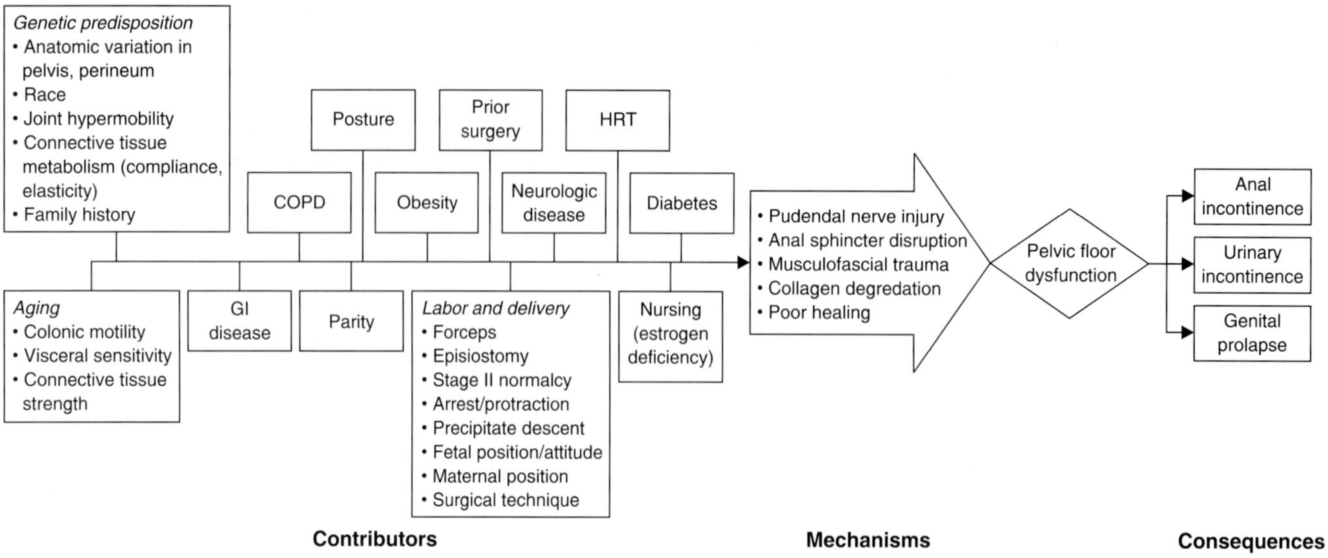

Figure 186.1 Factors that affect the risk of pelvic floor dysfunction.

is just beginning to be understood. Undoubtedly, host factors, both inherited and acquired, are important in determining whether an individual develops prolapse or incontinence, and when in life it will emerge.

While it is tempting to assume that delivering all babies by cesarean section would preclude the development of pelvic floor dysfunction in later life, this is clearly not the case.[27,38] This observation could indicate that pregnancy or labor *per se* are risk factors, irrespective of delivery mode, or that non-pregnancy-related factors cause pelvic floor problems. There is evidence to support both conclusions. Like all challenging health problems, those relating to female pelvic floor dysfunction are complex and will not yield to simple formulaic modes of treatment or prevention.

Episiotomy

Episiotomy was introduced to obstetrics in the mid-18th century in Europe. It came into use in America in the latter part of the next century, and became common as hospital birth, often by prophylactic forceps delivery, became widely practiced. Pomeroy[81] emphasized in 1918 that episiotomy could prevent pelvic tissue damage during delivery and suggested considering its routine use for nulliparas. DeLee,[82] a very influential obstetrician, advocated routine episiotomy along with elective forceps extraction, and by the 1940s these approaches were used commonly used in the United States. Over recent years, the benefits of routine episiotomy have been questioned, and its use has diminished considerably.[83,84] In the 1980s, episiotomy was performed in as many as 60–70% of vaginal deliveries in the United States; in 2000 the rate was about 20%.[85–87]

Although there is considerable polemic about the necessity for and the protective value of episiotomy, the procedure has been subjected to relatively little systematic investigation. This is unfortunate because the commonness of the procedure makes it a considerable contributor to discomfort and morbidity in the postpartum population. The study of episiotomy is challenging for several reasons, most prominent of which is that follow-up for a sufficient time to determine whether it prevents (or contributes to) pelvic floor dysfunction in late life is very difficult.

Gainey[88] examined 1000 consecutive women at their postpartum visits for evidence of pelvic floor damage. Among primiparas, the anovaginal portion of the urogenital trigone was spared trauma in those patients who had episiotomies. In another large series of women delivered by forceps, those who had routine episiotomy had less than half the incidence of clinically measured levator atrophy than those who had episiotomy done only when a laceration seemed imminent.[89] These and other data from that clinical era,[90] although neither controlled nor randomized, suggested a potential benefit from episiotomy. More recent data are less convincing in this regard, and make it difficult to support the use of routine episiotomy during vaginal delivery.[86,91–93] Some obstetricians use episiotomy selectively by resorting to it only when a spontaneous laceration seems about to occur; but there is evidence to suggest that this is not an effective approach to avoid major tears.[94]

While episiotomy is often used as a means to avoid serious perineal lacerations that would be anticipated otherwise to occur, this potential advantage of the procedure is not supported by the literature. In fact, almost all studies, including randomized trials, conclude that episiotomy increases the likelihood of anal sphincter and rectal wall lacerations. This is particularly true of median episiotomy, but applies as well to mediolateral incisions.[95–101]

There is no evidence that episiotomy preserves pelvic floor muscular function, at least in the short term. Röckner *et al.*[102] showed that pelvic floor muscle strength, studied 8 weeks postpartum, was weaker in women who had a mediolateral episiotomy than in those who delivered spontaneously or had a spontaneous laceration. Similar data exist for median incisions.[97]

Episiotomy and laceration repair

Two major approaches to obstetric perineotomy are used. The mediolateral technique (currently favored in most European obstetric services) involves an incision that extends laterally and posteriorly from the base of the introitus; the median approach (the most common technique in the United States) is directed posteriorly in the midline from the fourchette. Both techniques have passionate advocates, and reasonably well defined advantages and shortcomings. The median approach is easier to perform and repair, causes less immediate discomfort during the early puerperium, is less prone to hematoma formation, infection and dehiscence, and is associated with less long-term dyspareunia. These advantages accrue, however, at the considerable price of many more extensions through the anal sphincters and rectal wall.

Gustafson[103] made several suggestions in 1940 to help minimize the risk of cystocele formation after delivery that remain relevant. These included avoiding overdistension of the bladder, maternal bearing-down efforts prior to complete cervical dilatation, extremely rapid labors, and injudicious use of forceps. He also indicated, as have others subsequently, that in order to minimize trauma, early episiotomy should be accomplished before excessive stretching of the vaginal and surrounding fascial tissues has occurred.

It is logical that to the extent damage to the birth canal and pelvic floor may be avoided by episiotomy, the procedure should be accomplished prior to the considerable distention and elongation of the vaginal tube that occurs during crowning of the fetal head. Decisions about the potential benefits of episiotomy are fruitless if one awaits evidence of impending laceration; damage may have already occurred.

The pelvic architecture is an important (and too often overlooked) consideration. If the anterior segment of the pelvic outlet is narrow, delivery of the head will occur at the expense of the posterior portions of the perineum as the head is directed away from the constricted subpubic arch. Such a pelvis might benefit from episiotomy, or at least from very thorough ironing out of the perineal tissues during labor. With narrowing of the posterior segment of the outlet and an ample angle anteriorly, injury to perineal soft parts is less likely. However, anterior injury may occur. Obstetricians who eschew episiotomy commonly observe small periurethral or periclitoral lacerations as the head is directed anteriorly when it crosses an intact perineum. Whether there are long-term consequences from such (apparently) small injuries for urinary function is not known. In addition to pelvic architecture, fetal position, size, and attitude influence the risk of birth canal laceration, and these must all be considered in optimizing a delivery strategy.

One of the major difficulties in interpreting the effects of episiotomy is that its most important potential consequences may not be manifest until decades after the delivery. Although visible lacerations at delivery and evidence of pelvic tissue relaxation postpartum are important, the most significant parturitional damage may be invisible at that time. As noted, occult rectal sphincter injury is not uncommon; similarly, hidden damage to muscles and fascia may occur that contributes to pelvic visceral prolapse later in life.

Many questions remain unanswered about the virtues and risks of episiotomy, and will remain so for some time. For those who wish to avoid the procedure, gradual stretching of the perineal tissues during the second stage of labor may reduce the risk of lacerations. To this end, the use of some water-soluble lubricating gel can be beneficial. In addition, the use of a delivery position that tends to stretch the perineal tissues laterally should be avoided. Thus, the dorsal lithotomy position leads to episiotomy being done more often because the tension that flexion and abduction of the thighs places on the perineal tissues makes them less able to stretch further as the fetal head crosses them. The lateral position has benefits in this regard, as may squatting.

Repair technique

Whatever kind of episiotomy is done, it is wise to remember that the perineum is a complex structure, and failure to perform a proper surgical repair can result in considerable (and sometimes permanent) misery for the patient. A thorough knowledge of the functional anatomy of the pelvic floor and meticulous surgical technique are necessary to provide optimal results. Remember that episiotomy severs the supporting fascial structures of the lower vagina; the consequences of poor repair are considerable.

The repair of third- and fourth-degree lacerations is of particular importance, as these are obviously potential contributors to anal continence abnormalities. These should be repaired by an individual fluent in the anatomy of the perineal area. There should be a layered anatomic closure without any tension on the suture lines. It is very important, especially if there has been a complete perineal tear, to repair both the external and the internal sphincters. The latter is often ignored, but is of considerable importance in maintaining rectal tone. The internal and external anal sphincters both contribute importantly to anal continence.[50] Some data suggest that as much as 85% of the resting tone of the anal canal is contributed by the internal sphincter muscle.[104,105] Consequently, where there is a complete perineal laceration (extending from the vagina posteriorly into the anal canal) every effort should be made to do an anatomically faithful repair to reapproximate both sphincters independently. The external sphincter is usually identified easily, but sometimes may retract from the point of laceration.

Table 186.3 Episiotomy decision factors

Episiotomy decision factors
Fetal size
Fetal position and attitude
Pelvic architecture
Perineal length
Instrumental delivery
Prior pregnancy lacerations

The external sphincter muscle should be reapproximated, either end-to-end or overlapping; the important key is that it should not be under tension. The dense connective tissue sheath that surrounds the striated muscle of the sphincter should also be reapproximated. The internal sphincter can usually be identified during the repair. Good lighting is essential. It generally appears much paler and is considerably thinner than the robust muscle bundles of the external sphincter. Posterior to it is the anal canal's submucosa; anteriorly lies a thin condensation of connective tissue that separates it from the external sphincter and the vaginal submucosa. Remember that the internal sphincter extends cephalad at least 1 cm above the upper border of the external, and should be repaired to the full extent of its length using fine suture material.

Choosing whether or not to do an episiotomy should depend in part on the patient's anatomy (Table 186.3). Frudinger *et al.*[37] showed that more anal sphincter tears and anal incontinence were found in nulliparas with a narrow subpubic arch than in those with a wider arch. A narrow arch should prompt special attention to protection of the perineal and perianal structures. Women who have had third- or fourth-degree perineal lacerations in a previous pregnancy have a three- to fourfold increased risk of recurrence in a subsequent delivery.[106] This fact should also be considered when making decisions about management of the perineum.

Practical guidelines

Given the current state of our knowledge, what can be done by the clinician to minimize the risk of permanent pelvic floor injury that occurs during vaginal delivery? Several guidelines can be suggested, based on available evidence and the authors' experience:

(1) An organized and systematic approach to the management of labor is mandatory. Assess and judge the normality of labor by following progress in cervical dilatation and fetal descent and identifying dysfunctional labor with a consistent, reproducible and predictive system. That recommended by Friedman and coworkers[107,108] is the most widely used and best studied of such systems. It is important to recognize and treat labor abnormalities promptly. By so doing one can minimize the dangers to the birth canal when cephalopelvic disproportion is ultimately shown to be present.

(2) All decisions about allowing the labor to continue, or hastening its termination by oxytocin administration, or by cesarean or vaginal instrumentation should be made in the context of assessing the probability of a safe vaginal delivery. Safety in this case refers to the maternal pelvic floor as well as the fetus.

(3) Pay particular attention to marking progress in descent, fetal position, and the degree of cranial molding; all are useful clinical indicators of the probability of a vaginal delivery without maternal trauma. Occult and overt maternal injury is probably more likely in the presence of dysfunctional labor, especially if timely intervention is neglected.

(5) Use oxytocin judiciously. Creating unnecessarily rapid descent can lead to pelvic floor trauma.

(6) Minimize perineal tension as the head crosses the pelvic floor, i.e. do not fix the hips in extreme flexion when the patient is in the semi-sitting or lithotomy position. Extending the mother's legs somewhat during the terminal portion of expulsion may reduce injury risk. Consider other postures for delivery, such as squatting or lying in the lateral position.

(7) Consider lubrication of the lower vagina and outlet with water-soluble surgical lubricant as the head distends the perineum. This helps to aid the obstetric attendant to stretch the perineum manually and reduces shearing forces that contribute to the creation of lacerations.[61] There may be some benefit to antenatal perineal massage as well.[109,110]

(8) When instrumental injury is indicated, take into consideration that vacuum extraction is generally less likely to provoke major perineal laceration than forceps delivery.[58,111,112]

(9) Understand the pelvic architecture and its influence on the mechanism of labor and the risk of perineal trauma. More anal sphincter tears and anal incontinence occur in nulliparas with a narrow subpubic arch than in those with a wider arch.[37,113]

(10) Consider limiting strong maternal expulsive efforts to the time during the second stage when she feels a strong urge to bear down or (if she has sensory anesthetic blockade) until the head is well engaged in the pelvis.

(11) Perform a careful layered repair of episiotomies and perineal lacerations, using fine suture materials and meticulous surgical technique. Respect the imperative to restore anatomic integrity and to treat tissues gently.

(12) If a patient has had a third- or fourth-degree laceration in a previous pregnancy, is asymptomatic with regard to pelvic relaxation and symptoms of incontinence, and has an intact sphincter mechanism (determined clinically or by ultrasound), it is reasonable for her to have a vaginal delivery. But if these criteria are not met, cesarean delivery should be considered.

REFERENCES

1. Handa VL, Danielsen BH, Gilbert WM. Obstetric anal sphincter lacerations. *Obstet Gynecol* 2001;98:225–30.
2. Snooks SJ, Swash M, Henry MM, Setchell M. Risk factors in childbirth causing damage to the pelvic floor innervation. *Int J Colorectal Dis* 1986;1:20–4.
3. Okonkwo JEN, Obionu CO, Obiechina NJA. Factors contributing to urinary incontinence and pelvic prolapse in Nigeria. *Int J Gynecol Obstet* 2001;74:301–3.
4. Zetterstrom JP, Lopez A, Anzen B, Dolk A, Norman M, Mellgren A. Anal incontinence after vaginal delivery: A prospective study in primiparous women. *Br J Obstet Gynaecol* 1999; 106:324–30.
5. Sultan AH, Kamm MA, Hudson CN, Bartram CI. Third degree obstetric anal sphincter tears: Risk factors and outcome of primary repair. *BMJ* 1993;307:887–91.
6. Peschers UM, Schaer GN, DeLancey JOL, Schuessler B. Levator ani function before and after childbirth. *Br J Obstet Gynecol* 1997; 104:1004–8.
7. Snooks SJ, Swash M, Mathers SE, Henry MM. Effect of vaginal delivery on the pelvic floor: A 5-year follow-up. *Br J Surg* 1990; 77:1358–60.
8. Morrison J, MacKenzie IZ. Cesarean section on demand. *Semin Perinatol* 2003;27:20–33.
9. Hampel C, Weinhold D, Benken BN, Eggersmann C, Thüroff JW. Prevalence and natural history of female incontinence. *Eur Urol* 1997;32(Suppl 2):3–12.
10. Nelson R, Norton N, Cautley E, Furner S. Community-based prevalence of anal incontinence. *JAMA* 1995;274:559–61.
11. Johanson JF, Lafferty J. Epidemiology of fecal incontinence: The silent affliction. *Am J Gastroenterol* 1996;91:33–6.
12. Hendrix SL, Clark A, Nygaard I, Aragaki A, Barnabei V, McTiernan A. Pelvic organ prolapse in the Women's Health Initiative: Gravity and gravidity. *Am J Obstet Gynecol* 2002;186:1160–6.
13. MacLennan AH, Taylor AW, Wilson DH, Wilson D. The prevalence of pelvic floor disorders and their relationship to gender, age, parity and mode of delivery. *Br J Obstet Gynaecol* 2000;107: 1460–70.
14. Boyles SH, Weber AM, Meyn L. Procedures for pelvic organ prolapse in the United States, 1979–1997. *Am J Obstet Gynecol* 2003;188:108–15.
15. Waetjen LE, Subak LL, Shen H, *et al.* Stress urinary incontinence in the United States. *Obstet Gynecol* 2003;101:671–6.
16. Subak LL, Waetjen LE, van den Eeden S, Thom DH, Vittinghoff E, Brown JS. Cost of pelvic organ prolapse surgery in the United States. *Obstet Gynecol* 2001;98:646–51.
17. Boyles SH, Weber AM, Meyn L. Procedures for urinary incontinence in the United States 1979–1997. *Am J Obstet Gynecol* 2003;189:70–5.
18. Kamm MA. Obstetric damage and faecal incontinence. *Lancet* 1994;344:730–3.
19. Crist T, Shingelton HM, Koch GG. Stress incontinence and the nulliparous patient. *Obstet Gynecol* 1972;40:13–17.
20. Samuelsson EC, Victor FTA, Tibblin G, Svärdsudd KF. Signs of genital prolapse in a Swedish population of women 20 to 59 years of age and possible related factors. *Am J Obstet Gynecol* 1999; 180:299–305.
21. Fornell EU, Wingren G, Kjolhede P. Factors associated with pelvic floor dysfunction with emphasis on urinary and fecal incontinence and genital prolapse: An epidemiological study. *Acta Obstet Gynecol Scand* 2004;83:383–9.
22. Peters WA, Smith MR, Drescher CW. Rectal prolapse in women with other defects of pelvic support. *Am J Obstet Gynecol* 2001; 184:1488–95.
23. Kalantar JS, Howell S, Talley NJ. Prevalence of faecal incontinence and associated risk factors; an underdiagnosed problem in the Australian community? *Med J Aust* 2002;176:47–8.
24. Fitzpatrick M, Behan M, O'Connell PR. Randomized clinical trial to assess anal sphincter function following forceps or vacuum assisted vaginal delivery. *BJOG* 2003;110:424–9.
25. Signorello LB, Harlow BL, Chekos AK, Repke JT. Midline episiotomy and anal incontinence: Retrospective cohort study. *BMJ* 2000;320:86–90.
26. Sultan AH, Kamm MA, Hudson CN, Thomas JM, Bartram CI. Anal sphincter disruption during vaginal delivery. *N Engl J Med* 1993;329:1905–11.
27. Fynes M, Donnelly VS, O'Connell, O'Herlihy C. Cesarean delivery and anal sphincter injury. *Obstet Gynecol* 1998;92:496–500.
28. Olsen AL, Smith VJ, Bergstrom JO, Colling JC, Clark AL. Epidemiology of surgically managed pelvic organ prolapse and urinary incontinence. *Obstet Gynecol* 1997;89:501–6.
29. Wilson L, Brown JS, Shin GP, Luc K-O, Subak LL. Annual direct cost of urinary incontinence. *Obstet Gynecol* 2001;98:398–406.
30. Riskin-Mashiah S, Smith EO, Wilkins I. Risk factors for severe perineal tear: Can we do better? *Am J Perinatol* 2002;19:225–34.
31. Ingraham HA, Gardner MM, Heus EG. A report on 159 third degree lacerations. *Am J Obstet Gynecol* 1949;57:730–5.
32. de Leeuw JW, Struijk PC, Vierhout ME, Wallenburg HCS. Risk factors for third degree ruptures during delivery. *Br J Obstet Gynaecol* 2001;108:383–7.
33. Bodner-Adler B, Bodner K, Kaider A, *et al.* Risk factors for third-degree perineal tears in vaginal delivery, with an analysis of episiotomy types. *J Reprod Med* 2001;46:752–6.
34. Jones KD. Incidence and risk factors for third degree perineal tears. *Int J Gynecol Obstet* 2000;71:227–9.
35. Sandridge DA, Thorp JM Jr, Roddenberry P, Kuller J, Wild J. Vaginal delivery is associated with occult disruption of the anal sphincter mechanism. *Am J Perinatol* 1997;14:527–33.
36. Faltin DL, Boulvain M, Irion O, Bretones S, Stan C, Weil A. Diagnosis of anal sphincter tears by postpartum endosonography to predict fecal incontinence. *Obstet Gynecol* 2000;95:643–7.
37. Frudinger A, Halligan S, Spencer JAD, Bartram CI, Kamm MA, Winter R. Influence of the subpubic arch angle on anal sphincter trauma and anal incontinence following childbirth. *BJOG* 2002;109:1207–12.
38. Faúndes A, Guarisi T, Pinto-Neto AM. The risk of urinary incontinence of parous women who delivered only by cesarean section. *Int J Gynecol Obstet* 2001;72:41–6.
39. Lal M, Mann CH, Callender R, Radley S. Does cesarean delivery prevent anal incontinence? *Obstet Gynecol* 2003;101:305–12.
40. Dolan LM, Hosker GL, Mallett VT, Allen RE, Smith ARB. Stress incontinence and pelvic floor neurophysiology 15 years after the first delivery. *BJOG* 2003;110:1107–14.
41. Bartolo DCC, Jarratt JA, Read MG, Donnelly TC, Read NW. The role of partial denervation of the puborectalis in idiopathic faecal incontinence. *Br J Surg* 1983;70:664–7.
42. Allen RE, Hosker GL, Smith ARB, Warrell DW. Pelvic floor damage and childbirth: A neurophysiological study. *Br J Obstet Gynaecol* 1990;97:770–9.
43. Viktrup L, Lose G, Rolff M, Barfoed K. The symptom of stress incontinence caused by pregnancy or delivery in primiparas. *Obstet Gynaecol* 1992;79:945–9.
44. Law PJ, Kamm MA, Bartram CI. Anal endosonography in the investigation of faecal incontinence. *Br J Surg* 1991;78:312–14.
45. Barber MD, Bremer RE, Thor KB, Dolber PC, Kuehl TJ, Coates KW. Innervation of the female levator ani muscles. *Am J Obstet Gynecol* 2002;187:64–71.
46. Pierce LM, Reyes M, Thor KB, *et al.* Innervation of the levator ani muscles in the female squirrel monkey. *Am J Obstet Gynecol* 2003;188:1141–7.
47. Arrowsmith S, Hamlin EC, Wall LL. Obstructed labor injury complex: Obstetric fistula formation and the multifaceted morbidity of maternal birth trauma in the developing world. *Obstet Gynecol Surv* 1996;51:568–74.
48. Nygaard IE, Rao SSC, Dawson JD. Anal incontinence after anal sphincter disruption: A 30-year retrospective cohort study. *Obstet Gynecol* 1997;89:896–901.
49. Fenner DE, Genberg B, Brahma P, Marek L, DeLancey JOL. Fecal and urinary incontinence after vaginal delivery with anal sphincter disruption in an obstetrics unit in the United States. *Am J Obstet Gynecol* 2003;189:1543–50.
50. Lee S-J, Park J-W. Follow-up evaluation of the effect of vaginal delivery on the pelvic floor. *Dis Colon Rectum* 2000;43:1550–5.
51. Speakman CTM, Kamm MA. The internal anal sphincter-new insights into faecal incontinence. *Gut* 1991;32:345–6.
52. Donnelly V, Fynes M, Campbell D, Johnson H, O'Connell PR, O'Herlihy C. Obstetric events leading to anal sphincter damage. *Obstet Gynecol* 1998;92:955–61.
53. Nichols AM, Gill EJ, Nguyen T, Barber MD, Hurt WG. Anal sphincter injury in women with pelvic floor disorders. *Obstet Gynecol* 2004;104:690–6.
54. Smith ARB, Hosker GL, Warrell DW. The role of partial denervation of the pelvic floor in the aetiology of genitourinary prolapse and stress incontinence of urine. A neurophysiological study. *Br J Obstet Gynecol* 1989;96:24–8.

55. Farrell SA, Allen VM, Baskett TF. Parturition and urinary incontinence in primiparas. *Obstet Gynecol* 2001;97:350–6.
56. Rortveit G, Hannestad YS, Daltveit AK, Hunskaar S. Age- and type-dependent effects of parity on urinary incontinence: The Norwegian EPINCONT study. *Obstet Gynecol* 2001;98:1004–10.
57. Chiarelli P, Brown W, McElduff P. Leaking urine: Prevalence and associated factors in Australian women. *Neurourol Urodyn* 1999;18:567–77.
58. Arya LA, Jackson ND, Myers DL, Verma A. Risk of new-onset urinary incontinence after forceps and vacuum delivery in primiparous women. *Am J Obstet Gynecol* 2001;185:1318–23.
59. Menticoglou SM, Manning F, Harman C, Morrison I. Perinatal outcome in relation to second-stage duration. *Am J Obstet Gynecol* 1995;173:906–12.
60. Saunders NStG, Paterson CM, Wadsworth J. Neonatal and maternal morbidity in relation to the length of the second stage of labour. *Br J Obstet Gynaecol* 1992;99:381–5.
61. Cohen WR. Influence of the duration of second stage labor on perinatal outcome and puerperal morbidity. *Obstet Gynecol* 1977;49:266–9.
62. Van Kessel K, Reed S, Newton K, Meier A, Lentz G. The second stage of labor and stress urinary incontinence. *Am J Obstet Gynecol* 2001;184:1571–5.
63. MacArthur C, Glazener CMA, Wilson PD, *et al.* Obstetric practice and faecal incontinence three months after delivery. *Br J Obstet Gynecol* 2001;108:678–83.
64. Benyon CL. Normal second stage of labour. A plea for reform in its conduct. *J Obstet Gynaecol Br Commonw* 1957;64:815–20.
65. Parnell C, Langhoff-Roos J, Iverson R, Damgaard P. Pushing method in the expulsive phase of labor. *Acta Obstet Gynecol Scand* 1993;72:31–5.
66. Thomson AM. Pushing techniques in the second stage of labour. *J Adv Nurs* 1993;18:171–7.
67. Sze EHM, Sherard GB III, Dolezal JM. Pregnancy, labor, delivery, and pelvic organ prolapse. *Obstet Gynecol* 2002;100:981–6.
68. Graham CA, Mallett VT. Race as a predictor of urinary incontinence and pelvic organ prolapse. *Am J Obstet Gynecol* 2001;185: 116–20.
69. Bai SW, Choe BH, Kim JY, Park KH. Pelvic organ prolapse and connective tissue abnormalities in Korean women. *J Reprod Med* 2002;47:231–4.
70. Mattox TF, Lucente V, McIntyre P, Miklos JR, Tomezsko J. Abnormal spinal curvature and its relationship to pelvic organ prolapse. *Am J Obstet Gynecol* 2000;183:1381–4.
71. Elia G, Bergman J, Dye TD. Familial incidence of urinary incontinence. *Am J Obstet Gynecol* 2002;187:53–5.
72. Hannestas YS, Rortveit G, Daltveit AK, Hunskaar S. Are smoking and other lifestyle factors associated with female urinary incontinence? *BJOG* 2003;110:247–54.
73. Brown JS, Seeley DG, Fong J, Black DM, Ensrud KE, Grady D. Urinary incontinence in older women: Who is at risk? *Obstet Gynecol* 1996;87:715–21.
74. Moalli PA, Klingensmith WL, Meyn LA, Zyczynski HM. Regulation of matrix metalloproteinase expression by estrogen in fibroblasts that are derived from the pelvic floor. *Am J Obstet Gynecol* 2002;187:72–9.
75. Fornell E, Wingren G, Kjolhede P. Factors associated with pelvic floor dysfunction with emphasis on urinary and fecal incontinence and genital prolapse: An epidemiological study. *Acta Obstet Gynecol Scand* 2004;83:383–9.
76. Al-Rawi ZS, Al-Rawi ZT. Joint hypermobility in women with genital prolapse. *Lancet* 1982;1:1439–41.
77. Norton PA. Pelvic floor disorders: The role of fascia and ligaments. *Clin Obstet Gynecol* 1993;36:926–38.
78. Boreham MK, Miller RT, Schaffer JI, Word RA. Smooth muscle myosin heavy chain and caldesmon expression in the anterior vaginal wall of women with and without pelvic organ prolapse. *Am J Obstet Gynecol* 2001;185:944–52.
79. Jackson SR, Avery NC, Tarlton JF, Eckford SD, Abrams P, Bailey AJ. Changes in metabolism of collagen in genitourinary prolapse. *Lancet* 1996;347:1658–61.
80. Jameson JS, Scott AD. Medical causes of faecal incontinence. *Eur J Gastroenterol Hepatol* 1997;9:428–30.
81. Pomeroy RH. Shall we cut and reconstruct the perineum for every primipara? *Am J Obstet Gynecol* 1918;78:211–19.
82. DeLee JB. The prophylactic forceps operation. *Am J Obstet Gynecol* 1920;1:33–44.
83. Harrison RF, Brennan M, North PM, Reed JV, Wickham EA. Is routine episiotomy necessary? *Br Med J* 1984;288:1971–5.
84. Cogan R, Edmunds EP. The unkindest cut? *J Nurse-Midwifery* 1978;23:17–21.
85. Goldberg J, Holtz D, Hyslop, Tolosa JE. Has the use of routine episiotomy decreased? Examination of episiotomy rates from 1983 to 2000. *Obstet Gynecol* 2002;99:395–400.
86. Thacker SB, Banta HD. Benefits and risks of episiotomy: An interpretive review of the English language literature, 1860–1980. *Obstet Gynecol Surv* 1983;38:322–38.
87. Weber AM, Meyn L. Episiotomy use in the United States, 1979–1997. *Obstet Gynecol* 2002;100:1177–82.
88. Gainey HL. Postpartum observation of pelvic tissue damage. *Am J Obstet Gynecol* 1943;45:457–66.
89. Gainey HL. Postpartum observation of pelvic tissue damage. Further studies. *Am J Obstet Gynecol* 1955;70:800–7.
90. Nugent FB. The primiparous perineum after forceps delivery. *Am J Obstet Gynecol* 1935;30:249–55.
91. Cleary-Goldman J, Robinson JN. The role of episiotomy in current obstetric practice. *Semin Perinatol* 2003;27:3–12.
92. Sleep J, Grant A. West Berkshire perineal management trial: Three-year follow-up. *BMJ* 1998;295:749–51.
93. Carroli B, Belizan J, Stamp G. Episiotomy policies in vaginal birth. *The Cochrane Library* 1997;Issue 2:1–9.
94. Dannecker C, Hillemanns P, Strauss A, Hasbargen U, Hepp H, Anthuber C. Episiotomy and perineal tears presumed to be imminent: Randomized controlled trial. *Acta Obstet Gynecol Scand* 2004;83:364–8.
95. Borgotta L, Piening S, Cohen WR. Association of episiotomy and delivery position with deep perineal laceration during spontaneous delivery in nulliparous women. *Am J Obstet Gynecol* 1989; 160:294–8.
96. Nager CW, Helliwell JP. Episiotomy increases perineal laceration length in primiparous women. *Am J Obstet Gynecol* 2001;185: 444–50.
97. Klein MC, Gauthier RJ, Jorgensen SH, *et al.* Does episiotomy prevent perineal trauma and pelvic floor relaxation? *Online J Curr Clin Trials* 1992;July 1:Document No. 10.
98. Argentine Episiotomy Trial Collaborative Group. Routine vs. selective episiotomy: A randomized controlled trial. *Lancet* 1993;42: 517–18.
99. Sleep J, Grant A, Garcia J, Elbourne D, Spencer J, Chalmers I. West Berkshire perineal management trial. *BMJ* 1984;289:587–90.
100. Shiono P, Klebanoff MA, Carey JC. Midline episiotomies: More harm than good? *Obstet Gynecol* 1990;75:765–70.
101. Eason E, Labrecque M, Wells G, Feldman P. Preventing perineal trauma during childbirth: A systematic review. *Obstet Gynecol* 2000;95:464–71.
102. Röckner G, Jonasson A, Ölund A. The effect of mediolateral episiotomy at delivery on pelvic floor muscle strength evaluated with vaginal cones. *Acta Obstet Gynecol Scand* 1991;70:51–4.
103. Gustafson GW. The prevention and treatment of cystocele in the reproductive age. *Urol Cutan Rev* 1940;44:160.
104. Freckner B, Euler CV. Influence of pudendal block on the function of the anal sphincters. *Gut* 1975;16:482–9.
105. Schweiger M. Method for determining individual contributions of voluntary and involuntary anal sphincters to resting tone. *Dis Colon Rectum* 1979;175:13–27.
106. Payne TN, Carey JC, Rayburn WF. Prior third- or fourth-degree perineal tears and recurrence risks. *Int J Gynecol Obstet* 1999;64:55–7.
107. Friedman EA. *Labor: Clinical Evaluation and Management*, 2nd edn. New York: Appleton-Century-Crofts, 1978.
108. Cohen WR, Acker DA, Friedman EA. *Management of Labor*, 2nd edn. Rockville, MD: Aspen Publications, 1989.
109. Renfrew MJ, Hannah W, Albers L, Floyd E. Practices that minimize trauma to the genital tract in childbirth: A systematic review of the literature. *Birth* 1998;25:143–60.
110. Labrecque M, Eason E, Marcoux S, *et al.* Randomized controlled trial of prevention of perineal trauma by perineal massage during pregnancy. *Am J Obstet Gynecol* 1999;180:593–600.
111. Meyer S, Hohlfeld P, Achtari C, Russolo A, De Grandi P. Birth trauma: Short and long-term effects of forceps delivery compared with spontaneous delivery on various pelvic floor parameters. *Br J Obstet Gynecol* 2000;107:1360–5.
112. Sultan AH, Kamm MA, Bartram CI, Hudson CN. Anal sphincter trauma during instrumental delivery. *Int J Gynecol Obstet* 1993; 43:263–70.
113. Handa VL, Pannu HK, Siddique S, Gutman R, VanRooyen J, Cundiff G. Architectural differences in the bony pelvis of women with and without pelvic floor disorders. *Obstet Gynecol* 2003; 102:1283–90.

187 Effects of labor and delivery on the fetus

E. A. Friedman

There is little doubt that much of the untoward outcome encountered among fetuses and surviving infants is unrelated to events that occur during labor and delivery. Most often, bad results are either of unknown cause or due to identifiable problems afflicting the developing embryo and fetus during intrauterine life long before term. These latter include a wide range of influences from chromosomal defects, anatomic malformations, infections, metabolic disorders and toxins to the potentially devastating impact of preterm birth.[1–4] This observation that so many poor outcomes are unrelated to labor and delivery, however reassuring it may be, should not lull one into assuming that parturition is always a benign process for the fetus, lest obstetric practices and surveillance are not stressed in the interest of safeguarding fetal well-being during this crucial time *in utero*. Some have focused so much on the antepartum factors, essentially denying the impact of labor and delivery, as to imply that one can essentially ignore intrapartum risks.[5–8] Even such apologists, however, do reluctantly acknowledge that no fewer than 6% of bad results are attributable to problems encountered in labor or at delivery.[5] Others have demonstrated much higher frequencies of intrapartum causes, with rates as high as 34%.[9–12]

Regardless of the actual magnitude of the fetal risk from labor, it should be quite clear that the labor and delivery process is not always innocuous. Optimal clinical care requires (1) careful attention to the mother's labor progress to detect those abnormal labor patterns that place the fetus at risk; (2) close fetal surveillance to detect evidence of fetal compromise; and (3) gentle, cautious measures to ensure safe and atraumatic vaginal delivery. Recommendations for management have heretofore often been based largely on oracular pronouncements derived from accumulated clinical experience. In this era of evidence-based medicine with more confident decision making supported by objective information, it is essential to provide such documented evidence about which specific abnormalities of labor actually affect the fetus adversely and whether the deleterious effects of those disorders can be mitigated by appropriate clinical management.

Sources of injury

There are at least two major conditions that are recognized to expose the fetus to jeopardy in the course of labor and during the delivery process, namely, hypoxia and physical trauma. Intrauterine fetal hypoxia may develop in labor from the intermittent uterine contractions that compress uterine vessels traversing the myometrium to supply the intervillous space of the placenta with oxygen-rich maternal blood. While healthy, well-oxygenated fetuses usually withstand this stress well, the fetus that is already somewhat compromised by preexisting chronic hypoxia from some form of uteroplacental insufficiency may not. In such situations, the additional stress of uterine contractions may be sufficient to reduce marginally sustaining oxygenation to dangerous and damaging levels. Intrapartum hypoxia may also occur from umbilical cord compression. Fetal injury that results from oxygen deprivation may be mediated primarily by ischemia. When tissue hypoxia is severe, hemodynamic changes can occur that lead to selective or even global underperfusion of vital organs.

Physical trauma during labor and delivery may result from undue – that is, excessively prolonged and intense – mechanical forces exerted on the fetal head. These forces may cause extreme molding, which stretches or tears the supporting fasciae (specifically, falx cerebri and tentorium cerebelli) and the large venous sinuses coursing within them. The resulting intracranial hemorrhage can be devastating. Additionally, physical damage may be the consequence of excessive or inappropriately directed forces applied by instruments used to aid the delivery process, such as obstetric forceps and vacuum extractor.

There are no objective clinical means for determining when potentially deleterious extremes of molding are occurring. Fetal heart rate monitoring, which is so sensitive for detecting fetal hypoxia, is inadequate for disclosing impending physical trauma, although heart rate patterns may become abnormal after damage has occurred. Several specific major labor aberrations, the adverse impact of which is to be discussed in more detail here, are associated with cephalopelvic disproportion that is likely to be manifest by hazardous degrees of molding. Understanding which labor patterns put the fetus at risk and recognizing when they develop are thus important clinical considerations. The obstetric health care provider who is knowledgeable in this regard is appropriately equipped to be alert to recognize those relevant abnormalities in the course of labor as they arise. He or she will then be prepared to pursue evaluation of the case expeditiously and astutely and, if necessary, to intervene aggressively to avoid the expected adverse fetal outcome.

There has been an understandable paucity of recent studies in this area, given the fact that controlled investigations cannot be carried because of ethical, moral and legal constraints. The only data available, therefore, are from reports detailing collected experiential information on outcomes stratified according to labor and delivery events. The investigations upon which these reports are based were carried out mostly without cautionary measures having been taken to ensure against confounding by the many concurrent conditions that prevail among the population samples under study. The only publication in which some attempt was made to deal with this issue was the monograph emanating from the National Collaborative Perinatal Project (NCPP) under the aegis of the U.S. Public Health Service.[13] It provided extensive, sophisticated analyses of data gathered prospectively from a large population of some 60,000 gravidas and their offspring delivered at 14 university hospitals in the United States. The data, collected during the interval from 1958 to 1974, focused on a group of nearly 18,000 term infants who were free of anomalies incompatible with intact survival and whose mothers' records contained adequate documentation of the labor course to reconstruct a meaningful pattern of progression in dilatation and fetal descent. The large database thus compiled was subjected to a sequence of analytic techniques to ascertain the relative impact of more than 2400 different factors on the fetus and surviving infant, including maternal demographic attributes and antecedent illnesses, extensive observations during pregnancy, complicating antepartum conditions, exposures to infections and drugs, as well as the full range of labor variables, such as fetal presentation, position, mechanisms of labor, labor progress, membrane status, pain relief, uterotonic stimulation, and the gamut of delivery procedures. Outcome variables included not only perinatal morbidity, mortality and nursery course, but also periodic follow-up neurological evaluations for mental and motor disorders, speech, language and hearing problems, and intelligence quotient determinations through 7 years of age. The long and detailed follow-up of the study infants makes the NCPP database notable, perhaps unique, and unlikely to be replicated or improved upon in the foreseeable future.

This unequalled resource is of special interest because the analyses undertaken with it addressed the issues of potential confounding and interaction of factors other than the labor–delivery process (but also mindful of the interaction among labor–delivery factors) that might have been acting simultaneously to affect outcome. A singular shortcoming of these studies is that the deliveries all took place before widespread electronic fetal heart rate monitoring was available. This deficiency is counterbalanced somewhat by the frequent, careful, close auscultation of the fetal heart that was carried out on nearly all NCPP patients. Other practice patterns have also changed over the years, particularly with less use of narcotic analgesia, more peridural anesthesia, fewer operative vaginal deliveries, almost no difficult instrumental delivery procedures, and many more cesarean sections. Nonetheless, the sophisticated statistical techniques applied to the study – including univariate and multivariate regression, aggregative hierarchical cluster and logistic regression analyses – were able to assess the specific effects of each of these practices in regard to their individual contributions to outcome (regardless of the frequency of their use in clinical practice), isolating those effects from the impact of the labor process itself. Thus, the findings derived from this extensive study of the NCPP database with reference to the impact of specific labor disorders on outcome should still be considered relevant to current-day obstetric activities.

Prolonged latent phase

The common labor disorder of prolonged latent phase (defined and characterized in Chapter 174, p. 1822) appears to have a pervasively deleterious effect on the fetus and surviving infant. This adverse influence was not disclosed in several early studies that failed to take confounding factors into account.[14–17] Later and more critical investigations showed the labor abnormality to be considerably less innocuous than had been originally thought.[13,18]

The NCPP study data demonstrated a significantly worse perinatal outcome in association with labors complicated by prolonged latent phase than after a normal labor pattern [composite adverse results, relative risk (RR) 1.77, $P=0.024$], particularly in offspring of multiparas, when controlled for the concurrent effects of antepartum, intrapartum and delivery factors.[19] Simple univariate analysis, done without controlling for confounding factors, showed prolonged latent phase labors were associated with consistent increases in bad results across the range of outcomes that were studied from birth to 7 years of age: Stillbirths (RR 2.43 for multiparas and RR 3.0 for nulliparas, $P < 0.05$), neonatal deaths (RR 12.8 and 4.50, $P < 0.01$), depressed 5-min Apgar scores (RR 3.70 and 6.43, $P < 0.001$), and long-term sequelae reflected in Bayley mental (RR 1.99 and 1.90, $P < 0.05$), motor (RR 2.0, $P < 0.05$) and global scores at 8 months (RR 1.66, $P < 0.05$), abnormal neurological findings at 1 year (RR 1.71, $P < 0.05$), abnormal speech, language and hearing at 3 years (RR 1.28, $P < 0.05$) and low 4- and 7-year intelligent quotients (RR 1.18, 1.27 and 1.19, 1.34, $P < 0.05$).[20] These findings were further confirmed in logistic regression analyses, which showed significantly increased rates of perinatal mortality and birth asphyxia among infants born after prolonged latent phase (RR 1.55, $P < 0.05$). Increased frequencies of long-term effects were consistent with and paralleled those of the perinatal period. It was clear, however, that many babies who were born depressed, but survived, did well nevertheless, with no apparent ill effects from the stresses of labor and delivery.

Recently, confirmation and elaboration of these findings have been forthcoming in a report of an investigation by Chelmow *et al.*,[18] who studied 713 term gravidas with prolonged latent phase, excluding those with known antepartum risk factors for adverse outcome. These investigators also used logistic regression analysis to study the impact of labor on outcome, but limited their surveillance to the neonatal period only. Without the benefit of long-term follow-up, this otherwise good study could not provide the confirmation we seek of a truly persistent adverse impact. Poor perinatal results do tend to predict future bad outcomes among surviving infants, of course, but since the correlation is imperfect, they must be considered mere markers for that possibility. This limitation notwithstanding, Chelmow *et al.* found independent statistically significant associations with increased frequencies of neonatal depression [higher rates of low Apgar scores below 7 at 5 min of age, RR 1.97, confidence intervals (CI) 1.23–3.16] and the need for resuscitation (RR 1.37, CI 1.15–1.64). Cord blood pH determinations, however, were not found to be significantly decreased in this group. They also noted that prolonged latent phase labors were more likely to be associated with other labor aberrations: the total frequency of such disorders was 42.9% (vs. 16.3% among infants born after normal latent-phase durations, $P < 0.05$); subsequent active phase arrest and protraction abnormalities 30.3% (vs. 9.8%, $P < 0.05$); second-stage problems 20.5% (vs. 9.9%, $P < 0.05$); and a greater need for cesarean delivery (RR 1.65, CI 1.32–2.06). In addition, even after controlling for mode of delivery, there were more cases with thick meconium, maternal fever, intensive care nursery admission, prolonged maternal and neonatal hospital stay and maternal blood loss. Of interest, the criteria used by Chelmow *et al.* for the diagnosis of prolonged latent phase – namely, 12 h in nulliparas and 6 h in multiparas – were less stringent than those described by Friedman[21] and currently considered the standard for the definition (20 and 12 h, respectively).[22] That they demonstrated significantly adverse perinatal effects associated with these shorter 'prolonged' latent phases allows us to infer that a still greater impact could have been expected from their study if the longer cut-off durations had been used for diagnosis instead.

Having demonstrated with reasonable certainty that a prolonged latent phase exposes the fetus to harm, we should turn our attention to the more clinically pragmatic issue of whether that deleterious fetal impact can be mitigated by early diagnosis and timely intervention. Unfortunately, while this issue can be addressed inferentially, it cannot be satisfactorily resolved because no prospectively controlled investigation has as yet been carried out targeting the problem. Indeed, there has not even been a retrospective comparative study reported to date. There is information from the NCPP data bank, however, that shows the longer the latent phase is permitted to continue, the greater its potential harm to the fetus.[23] The frequency of neonatal depression (reflected in low Apgar scores at 5 min), for example, rose progressively with each passing hour in latent-phase duration in offspring of multiparas, from a low hovering at or below 3% up to 10 h, to a significantly increased 5.0% at 11 h, 7.7% at 12 h, 8.8% at 14 h (the cut-point for the diagnosis of prolonged latent phase in multiparas), 11.8% at 15 h, 12.8% at 16–19 h and 13.5% at 20 h or more. Similarly significant time trends were seen with a wide range of other outcomes among offspring of nulliparas when the latent-phase duration was stratified by its length, including the rates of stillbirths, neonatal deaths, mental and motor deficiencies at 8 months of age, neurologic defects at 1 year of age, and abnormal speech, language and hearing test results at 3 years of age; intelligence quotients were more often lower at 4 and 7 years of age as well, and the 7-year intelligence quotient data achieved statistical significance. It is clear from these data that the longer the latent phase is prolonged, the greater its adverse effect on the fetus.

To ensure that the effect shown in the foregoing univariate analysis of latent-phase prolongation did not reflect the confounding effects of other factors acting concurrently, logistic regression analyses were pursued.[24] Concern was appropriately generated over whether gravidas with prolongation of the latent phase might be those whose labors were augmented with oxytocin or whose subsequent labors were complicated by another labor disorders or some superimposed adverse influences to expose the fetus to potential harm. The analyses determined that some of the poor results associated with prolonged latent phase persisted even when the effect of many other variables were considered simultaneously. An RR of

1.77 ($P=0.024$), for example, was found for untoward perinatal outcomes in multiparas, but not in nulliparas. Other outcome variables either failed to show the same adverse effects or those effects were not so consistent or strong as they had been with the univariate analysis.[24]

This suggests that the impact documented previously was either subsumed by other factors acting on the fetus or somehow mitigated by subsequent interventions. Thus, whether efforts to shorten this labor aberration will improve outcome or not cannot be answered definitively. In the absence of such an answer, we are unable (and unwilling) to recommend an aggressive approach for the ostensible purpose of improving outcome. Our difficulty in this regard is compounded by the problem of clear prospective diagnosis of this condition. Too often, gravidas whose labors are not progressive for long periods may appear to have the labor aberration of prolonged latent phase, but they turn out in due course to have been in false labor instead, as diagnosed in hindsight when their contractions finally stop. To have intervened in those cases in which true labor had not yet actually begun would have exposed them and their fetuses to the recognized hazards of 'induction' of labor under suboptimal circumstances. Without the benefit of a well-conducted study to show the RRs and benefits of intervention in these cases – in which prolonged latent phase and false labor cannot be clinically distinguished prospectively – the conservative management regimen described earlier (see Chapter 174, pp. 1823–1825), therefore, seems more appropriate and logical for most cases.

Protracted labor patterns

The adverse impact of the two protraction disorders, protracted active-phase dilatation and protracted descent, as defined earlier (see Chapter 174, p. 1823), has been apparent from about the time these labor aberrations were first described.[15] All subsequent investigations of fetal and neonatal outcomes associated with these major labor aberrations, carried out in greater depth and sophistication, have only verified and strengthened the truth of this relationship.[15–17] From the beginning, perinatal mortality was found to be more than three times greater with these disorders than after normal labor, with recorded rates of 15.2 per 1000 and 4.9 per 1000, respectively, a statistically significant difference.[15] Long-term outcomes were similarly poor among surviving babies born after these types of labors, with more than twice the frequency of abnormalities found in tests of speech, language and hearing at 3 years of age (16.2% vs. 7.7%) and, in matched-pair analyses, significantly lower mean intelligence quotients at 4 and 7 years of age (reduced by 4.6 and 8.4 points, respectively).[16,17]

The ability to reduce or even eliminate confounding effects of other potentially deleterious influences acting simultaneously on the fetus, a capacity afforded by the large NCPP database, served to confirm the earlier findings and to make it clear that they were not spurious.[19] The composite perinatal risk increased, especially among those delivered of multiparas, more than twofold (RR 2.40, $P=0.05$).[19] Univariate analysis demonstrated that protracted labor patterns in nulliparas were associated with a trend toward increased risks of perinatal deaths (RR 1.57, not significant) and significantly more low Apgar scores at 5 min (RR 1.94, $P<0.05$).[25] Infants of multiparas showed even worse immediate effects, including perinatal mortality (RR 1.77, $P<0.05$), low 5-min Apgar scores (RR 1.97, $P<0.05$), as well as long-term adverse impact, such as abnormal neurological findings at 1 year of age (RR 1.41, $P<0.05$) and low mean intelligence quotient at 4 years (RR 1.22, $P<0.05$).[25]

When logistic regression analysis was applied to these data to diminish confounding and interactional effects, it became clear that protracted dilatation continued to yield bad outcomes. For nulliparas, for example, the RR for adverse composite results was 1.36 ($P=0.044$) and for perinatal morbidity and mortality 2.12 ($P=0.0052$). Step-up regression modeling, done to introduce variables seriatim, showed the composite risk to be still worse among babies born to nulliparas, at RR 2.38 ($P=0.021$); and for perinatal outcome, the results were even poorer, with RR of 3.75 ($P=0.00046$).[26] For offspring of multiparas, the results were comparable for perinatal outcome, producing an RR by step-up modeling of 3.04 ($P=0.0038$).[26]

As to protracted descent, outcome data for offspring resulting from such labors were just as impressive as those of protracted dilatation. For poor composite outcome in nulliparas, for example, there was an RR of 1.35 ($P=0.0037$) and in multiparas, 1.57 ($P=1.2\times10^{-6}$).[26,27] Logistic regression analysis showed this effect to be enhanced when confounding factors were taken into account (RR 2.55, $P=0.021$) for perinatal impact. Step-up modeling indicated this impact to be particularly resistant to the simultaneous effects of confounding factors, especially that of other labor disorders (RR 3.64, $P=0.3.5\times10^{-9}$).[26]

The question of whether these adverse effects can be mitigated by early diagnosis and expeditious management deserves to be answered, but cannot. No data are as yet available to help elucidate whether results are worse if the protraction disorder is allowed to continue for any length of time, as there was for prolonged latent phase (see above) and for arrest disorders, as will be shown below. The extensive NCPP analyses did not provide any insight into this matter because the duration of these disorders was neither recorded nor stratified. By contrast, we have already seen that logistic regression analysis verified that protraction disorders retained their adverse impact even when other factors were taken into account at the same time.

Inferentially, but without the kind of proof that ought to be forthcoming from a prospective controlled study, we can only surmise that intervention might succeed in diminishing those deleterious effects, but not entirely eliminate them. We are more confident that no measures used so far can eliminate them, but have to admit we have nothing objective to support the statement concerning the decrease in magnitude of effect. The latter is based on our conjecture that since so many of these cases are associated with cephalopelvic disproportion, some of the poor outcomes may reflect that factor rather than the labor disorder. Since the clinical diagnosis of cephalopelvic disproportion is not always made (or is sometimes made even though it may not exist), its presence may exert its ill effect without the health-care providers being aware of it. We have stressed the need to examine the cephalopelvic relations when confronted by either protraction or arrest disorders (see Chapter 174, pp. 1825–1828).

As stated, these investigations confirmed the bad effect that had been observed earlier and demonstrated that the impact seen was very likely the result of the labor disorder itself and not some other concurrently acting factor. It is regrettable, however, that there have been no more recent studies undertaken to verify these findings in an era when obstetrics is practiced with greater attention to continuous fetal surveillance and more expeditious intervention to effect delivery than was the case when the NCPP data were generated.

Arrest disorders

Arrest patterns of labor, which have been defined and characterized earlier (see Chapter 174, p. 1823), are recognized to be utilitarian clinical markers of cephalopelvic disproportion. When an arrest disorder is encountered in the course of labor, the probability of safe vaginal delivery is reduced to about half by virtue of the high likelihood that disproportion exists, ranging as high as 56%.[28–30] Accordingly, it is not unexpected that these abnormal labor patterns will perforce be associated with adverse outcomes among fetuses who are exposed to them in the course of labor and at delivery. This applies especially for those in whom vaginal delivery is attempted without the precaution of ensuring that the cephalopelvic relations are adequate and the prospects of such delivery are safe. Increased rates of perinatal deaths and morbidity in association with arrest disorders have been well documented.[31] The RR of perinatal deaths expected in association with arrest disorders of labor is 7.5, based on a rate of 36.6 per 1000 as contrasted with 4.9 per 1000 after normal labor progress.[31] Correcting for the type of delivery more than doubles the RR to 15.7, although the absolute mortality is reduced by this correction to 16.1 per 1000 as the perinatal mortality after normal labor is reduced even more to 1.5 per 1000.[32] A later study indicated higher perinatal losses of 40.2 per 1000 after arrest disorders compared with 11.8 per 1000 after normal labor patterns, showing a consistency of adverse effect.[33]

Even Nelson, who asserted that intrapartum events have little or no adverse effect on the fetus, has had to acknowledge that arrest disorders are clear exceptions (along with fetal heart rate and midforceps delivery).[1,34] She reported the results of a large case–control study examining many labor and delivery factors simultaneously in which there were nearly three times the frequency of arrest of progress among developmentally abnormal children, specifically 18.0% vs. 6.6%, a significant difference.[34] Not unexpectedly, significantly increased frequencies of midforceps procedures and cesarean delivery (RR 5.0), low Apgar scores (RR 1.6), requirement for intensive neonatal care (RR 1.4), and long-term neurologic handicap have also been reported following arrest of dilatation.[35] Of special interest in this last-cited report is that stratification by delivery method showed that vaginal delivery after an arrest disorder magnified the poor infant results, whereas cesarean delivery diminished the impact attributable to the labor disorder.

The NCPP investigation confirmed these outcome effects for arrest disorders.[36] Arrest of dilatation was associated with increased perinatal hazard, reaching statistical significance in multiparas (RR 1.68, $P=0.049$).[36] Infants delivered after arrest of descent fared just as poorly or worse, with deleterious perinatal outcomes much increased among them (RR 1.53 for nulliparas, $P=0.028$, and RR 4.02 for multiparas, $P=1\times10^{-6}$).[36] Prolonged deceleration, another variant of the arrested labor patterns, was also associated with marginally to significantly increased perinatal death rates in nulliparas (RR 1.43, $P=0.051$) and multiparas (RR 1.51, $P=0.019$).[36] However, there was no evidence that this adverse effect persisted into later life among surviving infants. Moreover, when logistic analytic methods were brought to bear to assess the impact of these disorders while other factors were taken into account simultaneously, the adverse perinatal effect disappeared from all the aforementioned arrest patterns, except arrest of descent in multiparas. Perinatal mortality remained significantly high among this latter group (RR 3.35, $P=1.4\times10^{-6}$).[26] The relationship was also upheld in the step-up logistic modeling assessment (RR 2.88, $P=0.0038$).[26]

Based on these findings, one could surmise that much of the impact of arrest disorders on the fetus is subsumed by other factors acting simultaneously. These other factors most probably include uterotonic stimulation, the presence or absence of cephalopelvic disproportion, and the timing and type of delivery intervention taken to address the labor problem. In addition, the duration of the arrest pattern may also play a role in this regard, as evidenced by the correlation between longer arrest periods and more intense and prolonged adverse effects.[37] For example, neonatal death rates increased progressively with duration of arrest of descent in nulliparas: the RR after a half hour of arrest in second stage was 1.45, which was increased, but not significantly different from those with normal second-stage progress; however, the RR of perinatal death was 3.97 after 1 h and 4.92 after 2 h of arrest ($P < 0.01$ for both).[37]

These findings clearly indicate that delayed diagnosis of an arrest disorder of labor is detrimental to the fetus. The benefit of early diagnosis can be assumed to have arisen because some form of evaluation may have been done to rule out cephalopelvic disproportion in those cases in which the labor was allowed to continue; alternatively, cephalopelvic disproportion was found – or presumed to exist – and cesarean delivery was then pursued. Operative delivery may thus have averted any adverse consequence from continuing the labor. If those cases in which the arrest pattern develops without concurrent cephalopelvic disproportion could have been specifically identified, as proposed earlier, labor might have been permitted to continue and an unnecessary abdominal delivery averted, presumably with no deleterious fetal effects. We have thus addressed the issue of possible mitigation of adverse effect of arrest disorders by early diagnosis and aggressive intervention, with somewhat clearer resolution. We do acknowledge, however, that we lack substantiation in the form of objective supportive data derived from a more reliable recent source, such as a well-designed clinical study.

Precipitate labor

It is generally accepted that fetuses may be damaged by labors that are very short in duration, or are characterized by excessively rapid cervical dilatation or fetal descent, or by quick delivery over an unsterile field without good control of the fetal head as it is expelled over the perineum. Because such rapid labors are often associated with tumultuous uterine contractions – that is, contractions that are powerful in strength, long in duration and quite frequently recurrent – such labors may thereby expose the fetus to the risks of both physical trauma and hypoxia. The mechanism by which precipitate labors cause fetal hypoxia is logically assumed to be one in which the intense and prolonged contractions obstruct the flow in the spiral arterioles that supply oxygenated maternal blood to the intervillous space of the placenta, thus depleting to hazardous levels the oxygen reserves from which the fetus can draw. Physical trauma may result from one of two different mechanisms, either from the rapid compression–decompression phenomenon of excessively rapid descent (causing tissue damage from the 'blast' effect) or from excessive molding of the fetal head resulting in damage to intracranial fasciae with ensuing hemorrhage.

This latter form of injury can be more easily understood by considering the tissue attribute of plasticity. This physical property permits tissues to be atraumatically stretched and reshaped when steady forces are applied to them over relatively long periods of time. An extreme example of tissue plasticity is orthodontic remodeling of teeth alignment; other examples include the changes the cervix and the perineum undergo in labor. If the same (or larger) forces are exerted instead at great speed, however, those tissues will fracture or lacerate instead. Thus, the normal fetal head molding process, which all fetuses in cephalic presentation experience in the course of vaginal delivery, is ordinarily harm-free. By contrast, the rapid deformation resulting from the excessive magnitude and speed of force to which that fetal head is exposed in many precipitate labors may not be so benign at all. The harm from this mechanism may also occur even without precipitate labor if the fetal head is unduly compressed and thereby remolded excessively over a relatively short time in the course of labor as the consequence of constraining cephalopelvic relations. This applies particularly if the uterine contractions are being simultaneously augmented by a uterotonic agent, such as oxytocin. The adverse fetal effects of cephalopelvic disproportion can thus be expected to compound those of uterine hypercontractility, if both occur concomitantly in a given labor, at minimum additively and perhaps synergistically as well.

We have addressed the clinical means for diagnosing precipitate labor patterns (see Chapter 174, p. 1829). What has not been well documented is the quantitation of the injurious impact of such labors on the fetus – that is, how bad the effect is and under what particular conditions in labor can it be expected to become manifest? There is a regrettable paucity of meaningful data available to probe these questions. One univariate clinical study dating back many years showed a statistically significant 45% relative increase in perinatal mortality among infants born after precipitate labor (15.5 per 1000 vs. 10.7 per 1000, $P < 0.05$).[38] Of those infants who died in this series, autopsies found 18.8% of the deaths were due to intracranial hemorrhage. Among surviving infants, neurological and developmental abnormalities were identified in significantly large numbers, including 20.0% with mental retardation (as opposed to 7.0% among those delivered after normal labor patterns, $P < 0.05$) and 20.0% with intelligent quotient scores of 70 or less (vs. 2.5% in the normal controls, $P < 0.01$).[39]

Some more recent studies have denied that precipitate labor is a risk factor for poor short- or long-term outcomes.[40–42] Others, however, have shown important adverse consequences, including increased perinatal mortality, need for neonatal intensive care and longer hospitalizations after birth, and neonatal complications.[43–45] The report by Bateman *et al.*, for example, demonstrated unattended births were associated with neonatal mortality of 20.3 per 1000 [vs. 7.3 per 1000, odds ratio (OR) 2.82, $P < 0.05$], hypothermia $< 35°$ (OR 20.8, $P < 0.01$), hypoglycemia < 40 mg/dl (OR 4.41, $P < 0.05$), and polycythemia with hematocrit $> 65\%$ (14% incidence).[43] These effects were felt to be attributable mostly to the high proportion of premature births in their series. Comparably increased mortality and morbidity rates were also encountered in two other studies of similar deliveries, even though the frequencies of prematurity were lower.[44,45] Certain characteristics, which may be considered to represent risk factors, were found to prevail among gravidas with precipitate labors and deliveries, all occurring with significantly increased frequencies: they included the aforementioned increased incidence of prematurity (OR 2.99), plus low educational level (OR 6.11), multiparity (OR 6.18), prior preterm delivery (OR 4.03), and no prenatal care.[46]

It is clear from these observations that several identified confounding factors do exist (and other confounders not yet identified may also exist). These have to be taken into account if we are to ascertain the real impact of precipitate labor on the offspring, devoid of the concomitant effect of such powerful hazards as prematurity, among others. To this end, we turn again to the NCPP data, which is unique in affording us the opportunity to assess simultaneously the effect of all the confounders as they impact upon perinatal and long-term results. Univariate analysis showed that precipitate dilatation – defined objectively by excessively rapid rate of cervical dilatation in the active phase of labor – was associated with increased perinatal mortality (RR 6.99, $P < 0.05$), low Apgar scores at 5 min (RR 4.28, $P < 0.05$), abnormal global neurological examination findings at age 8 months (RR 1.67, $P < 0.05$), abnormal speech, language and hearing at 3 years of age (RR 1.79, $P < 0.05$) and low intelligence quotients at 4 and 7 years (RR 1.98 and 1.62, respectively, $P < 0.05$ for both) in nulliparas; and comparable results were found among offspring of multiparas.[47] Precipitate descent – defined by very rapid slope of descent in second stage of labor – was also accompanied by high perinatal mortality (RR 2.49, $P < 0.05$), low 5-min Apgar scores, abnormal speech, language and hearing at 3 years of age (RR 1.27, $P < 0.05$) and low intelligence quotients at 4 and 7 years (RR 1.67 and 1.37, respectively, $P < 0.05$ for both) in infants of nulliparas, with parallel findings in those delivered of multiparas.[47] Precipitate delivery – that is, uncontrolled delivery over the perineum – was determined to carry even higher rates of adverse outcomes, including stillbirths (RR 6.14, $P < 0.00001$), neonatal deaths (RR 6.34, $P < 0.00001$), low Apgar scores at 5 min (RR 2.61, $P < 0.001$) in nulliparas; stillbirths (RR 3.34, $P < 0.00001$), neonatal deaths (RR 2.95, $P < 0.00001$), low 5-min Apgar scores (RR 2.77, $P < 0.00001$), abnormal mental and motor scores at 8 months (RR 2.15 and 2.62, $P < 0.05$ for both), and low intelligence quotients at 7 years (RR 1.34, $P < 0.05$) in multiparas. Other long-term outcome results were also poorer than among infants delivered with good control of the delivery of the fetal head over the perineum, but those rates did not reach statistical significance.[48]

Limiting analysis of the NCPP study population to those weighing between 2500 and 4000 g, to eliminate the acknowledged high-risk factor of prematurity, focused the analysis somewhat more closely on the impact of the labor disorder itself. While short active-phase duration was found to retain its adverse impact (perinatal composite outcome effect, including deaths and Apgar scores < 4, RR 1.40, $P = 0.034$), rapid maximum slope of dilatation paradoxically did not (perinatal composite RR 0.95, a slight, but not statistically significant protective effect). Precipitate descent, when reflected in a very short second-stage duration, was associated with poor perinatal composite results (RR 1.34, $P < 0.039$), but when defined by rapid maximum slope of descent, it was not.[36] All labor variables considered together in the logistic regression analysis demonstrated that precipitate dilatation retained its adverse perinatal impact (RR 1.92, $P = 0.0034$) in babies delivered of nulliparas (but not those of multiparas). Precipitate descent defined by second-stage duration had an adverse effect (RR 1.21, $P = 0.012$), but not when it was diagnosed by maximum slope of descent, which again had a marginally protective effect (RR 0.79, not significant).[26] In the step-up logistic sequence for perinatal outcome, these relationships continued to reflect the bad influence of precipitate dilatation (RR 1.83, $P = 0.0060$).[26] The aforementioned marginally protective effect of precipitate descent was subsumed by other factors in this last analysis, but reemerged as those other factors were identified and corrected for. When logistic regression analysis was finally brought to bear on the full panoply of variables in the NCPP study, encompassing demographic, preexisting illness, antepartum and intrapartum factors, and delivery variables, foreshortened active-phase duration was still holding its own as an adverse factor affecting both composite and perinatal outcomes (RR 1.29 and 1.67, $P < 0.05$ for both) in nulliparas, as did precipitate descent, which served as an apparently protective factor for composite outcomes only (RR 0.71, $P < 0.05$).[24]

These data are difficult to interpret because they seem inconsistent. Rapid cervical dilatation and short active-phase duration are two aspects of the same phenomenon and can both be expected to have the same influence of the fetus. The same applies to the two related factors of rapid descent and short second-stage duration. When examined separately, short active phase showed its expected adverse fetal effects, but rapid dilatation did not; and similarly, short second stage did, but rapid descent did not. When both members of a related pair of variables are examined at the same time by statistical testing, only one or the other is likely to demonstrate statistical significance, but not both because the information they share about outcome is subsumed by one of them. What cannot be explained so readily, however, are the paradoxical effects seen for the two related pairs of factors, rapid dilatation and short active phase, on the one hand, and rapid descent and short second-stage duration, on the other, given that the observed impact appeared to act in opposite directions. Confounding is the likeliest explanation, but there is probably another explanation: not all precipitate labors are comparable insofar as their potential for harm. Spontaneously occurring fast labors in multiparas may not be caused by tumultuous uterine contractions or uterotonic stimulation, but instead reflect the ready response of elastic maternal soft parts yielding atraumatically to normal (or even hypotonic) contractions. This latter form of facile, but rapid labor should not be anticipated to have the same bad effect on the fetus as the excessively forceful labor that is more likely to harm the fetus by means of physical trauma and hypoxia. While no study has been undertaken to elucidate the relative effects of these distinctive labor types, it is likely that their outcomes would be quite different. If the cases of precipitate labor in the NCPP data resource (which regrettably could not distinguish the two varieties), to which we have just alluded, were diluted with large numbers of such 'benign' labors, it would make it difficult to demonstrate the deleterious effects of the less benign form.

Conclusions

Labor abnormalities, as defined objectively on the basis of patterns of cervical dilatation and fetal descent, can, based on the evidence presented here, be associated with poor outcomes for the fetus and surviving infant. The adverse outcomes are apparently independent of the modality chosen for the delivery, although it should be clear that ill-advised attempts to effect delivery by traumatic instrumentation, such as difficult midforceps procedures, will probably diminish the potential for a good result. Contrastingly, timely intervention by cesarean delivery, when indicated, may have a beneficial impact by reducing the deleterious effect of the continuing abnormal labor progression pattern. This is not intended as license to proceed with cesarean delivery whenever such disorders are encountered during the course of labor, but rather to alert health-care providers to the need to recognize them early, to evaluate for potentially serious associated or etiological conditions that threaten the well-being and life of the fetus, and if such conditions are found, to proceed with the requisite intervention.

REFERENCES

1. Nelson KB, Ellenberg JH. Antecedents of cerebral palsy. Multivariate analysis of risk. *N Engl J Med* 1986;315:81–6.
2. Paneth N. Birth and the origins of cerebral palsy (Editorial). *N Engl J Med* 1986;315:124–5.
3. Paneth N, Stark RI. Cerebral palsy and mental retardation in relation to indicators of perinatal asphyxia. An epidemiologic overview. *Am J Obstet Gynecol* 1983;147:960–6.
4. Rosen MG, Debanne S, Thompson K, Lilenker RM. Long-term neurological morbidity in breech and vertex births. *Am J Obstet Gynecol* 1985;151:718–20.
5. Nelson KB. Can we prevent cerebral palsy? *N Engl J Med* 2004; 349:1765–9.
6. Richmond S, Niswander K, Snodgrass CD, Wagstaff I. The obstetric management of fetal distress and its association with cerebral palsy. *Obstet Gynecol* 1994;83:643–6.
7. *Fetal and Neonatal Neurological Injury*. Washington, DC: ACOG Technical Bulletin No. 163, 1992:1–5.
8. *Neonatal Encephalopathy and Cerebral Palsy: Defining the Pathogenesis and Pathophysiology*. Washington, DC: American College of Obstetricians and Gynecologists, 2003.
9. Krägeloh-Mann I, Hagberg G, Meisner C, *et al.* Bilateral spastic cerebral palsy. A collaborative study between Southwest Germany and Western Sweden. III. Aetiology. *Dev Med Child Neurol* 1995; 37:191–203.
10. Stanley F, Blair E, Hockey A, *et al.* Spastic quadriplegia in Western Australia: A genetic epidemiological study. I. Case population and perinatal risk factors. *Dev Med Child Neurol* 1993;35:191–201.
11. Badawi N, Kurinczuk JJ, Keogh JM, *et al.* Intrapartum risk factors for newborn encephalopathy. The Western Australia case–control study. *Br Med J* 1998;317:1554–8.
12. Hankins GDV, Koen S, Gei AF, *et al.* Neonatal organ system injury in acute birth asphyxia sufficient to result in neonatal encephalopathy. *Obstet Gynecol* 2002;99:688–91.
13. Friedman EA, Neff RK. *Labor and Delivery: Impact on Offspring*. Littleton, MA: PSG Publishing Co., 1987.
14. Friedman EA, Sachtleben MR. Dysfunctional labor. I. Prolonged latent phase in the nullipara. *Obstet Gynecol* 1961;17:135–48.
15. Friedman EA, Niswander KR, Sachtleben MR. Dysfunctional labor. XI. Neurological and developmental effects on surviving infants. *Obstet Gynecol* 1969;33:785–91.
16. Friedman EA, Sachtleben MR, Bresky PA. Dysfunctional labor. XII. Long-term effects on infant. *Am J Obstet Gynecol* 1977;127:779–83.
17. Friedman EA, Sachtleben-Murray MR, Dahrouge D, Neff RK. Long-term effects on offspring. A matched-pair analysis. *Am J Obstet Gynecol* 1984;150:941–5.
18. Chelmow D, Kilpatrick SJ, Laros RK Jr. Maternal and neonatal outcomes after prolonged latent phase. *Obstet Gynecol* 1993;81: 486–91.
19. Friedman EA, Neff RK. *Labor and Delivery: Impact on Offspring*. Littleton, MA: PSG Publishing Co., 1987:353–60.
20. Friedman EA, Neff RK. *Labor and Delivery: Impact on Offspring*. Littleton, MA: PSG Publishing Co., 1987:78–81.
21. Friedman EA. *Labor: Clinical Evaluation and Management*, 2nd edn. New York: Appleton-Century-Crofts, 1978:62–3, 73–5.
22. *Dystocia*. Washington, DC: ACOG Technical Bulletin No. 137, 1989:1–6.
23. Friedman EA, Neff RK. *Labor and Delivery: Impact on Offspring*. Littleton, MA: PSG Publishing Co., 1987:77–80.
24. Friedman EA, Neff RK. *Labor and Delivery: Impact on Offspring*. Littleton, MA: PSG Publishing Co., 1987:348–60.
25. Friedman EA, Neff RK. *Labor and Delivery: Impact on Offspring*. Littleton, MA: PSG Publishing Co., 1987:80–3.
26. Friedman EA, Neff RK. *Labor and Delivery: Impact on Offspring*. Littleton, MA: PSG Publishing Co., 1987:140–5.
27. Friedman EA, Neff RK. *Labor and Delivery: Impact on Offspring*. Littleton, MA: PSG Publishing Co., 1987:134–6.
28. Friedman EA. *Labor: Clinical Evaluation and Management*. New York: Appleton-Century-Crofts, 1978:102–23.
29. Friedman EA, Niswander KR, Sachtleben MR, Ashworth M. Dysfunctional labor. IX. Delivery outcome. *Am J Obstet Gynecol* 1970;106:219–26.
30. Friedman EA, Sachtleben MR. Dysfunctional labor. III. Secondary arrest of dilatation. *Obstet Gynecol* 1962;19:576–91.
31. Friedman EA, Niswander KR, Sachtleben MR, Naftaly N. Dysfunctional labor. X. Immediate result to infant. *Obstet Gynecol* 1969;33:776–83.
32. Friedman EA. Patterns of labor as indicators of risk. *Clin Obstet Gynecol* 1973;16:172–83.
33. Friedman EA. *Labor: Clinical Evaluation and Management*. New York: Appleton-Century-Crofts, 1978:105–6.

34. Nelson KB, Broman SH. Perinatal risk factors in children with serious motor and mental handicaps. *Ann Neurol* 1977;2:371–7.
35. Bottoms SF, Hirsch VJ, Sokol RJ. Medical management of arrest disorders of labor. A current overview. *Am J Obstet Gynecol* 1987;156:935–9.
36. Friedman EA, Neff RK. *Labor and Delivery: Impact on Offspring.* Littleton, MA: PSG Publishing Co., 1987:130–4.
37. Friedman EA, Neff RK. *Labor and Delivery: Impact on Offspring.* Littleton, MA: PSG Publishing Co., 1987:113–16.
38. Tucker BE, Benaron HB. The immediate effects of prolonged labor with forceps delivery, precipitate labor with spontaneous delivery, and natural labor with spontaneous delivery on the child. *Am J Obstet Gynecol* 1953;66:540–50.
39. Benaron HB, Brown M, Tucker BE, Wentz V, Yacorzynski GK. The remote effects of prolonged labor with forceps delivery, precipitate labor with spontaneous delivery, and natural labor with spontaneous delivery on the child. *Am J Obstet Gynecol* 1953;66: 551–68.
40. Nelson KB, Ellenberg JH. Antecedents of cerebral palsy. I. Univariate analysis of risks. *Am J Dis Child* 1985;139:1031–8.
41. Erkkola R, Nikkanen V. Precipitate labour. *Ann Chir Gynaecol* 1978;67:150–3.
42. Nkyekyer K. Arrival in the labour ward in second stage of labour. Any prognostic significance? *East Afr Med J* 1998;75:282–7.
43. Bateman DA, O'Bryan L, Nicholas SW, Heagarty MC. Outcome of unattended out-of-hospital births in Harlem. *Arch Pediatr Adolesc Med* 1994;148:147–52.
44. Sirimai K, Titapant V, Roongphornchai S. Morbidity and mortality from birth before arrival at Siriraj Hospital. *J Med Assoc Thai* 2002;85:1258–63.
45. Di Benedetti MR, Piazza JJ, Unfer V, *et al.* An obstetric and neonatal study on unplanned deliveries before arrival at hospital. *Clin Exp Obstet Gynecol* 1996;23:108–11.
46. Titapant V. Sirimai K, Roongphornchai S. Risk factors for birth before arrival at Siriraj Hospital. *J Med Assoc Thai* 2002;85: 1251–7.
47. Friedman EA, Neff RK. *Labor and Delivery: Impact on Offspring.* Littleton, MA: PSG Publishing Co., 1987:81–5.
48. Friedman EA, Neff RK. *Labor and Delivery: Impact on Offspring.* Littleton, MA: PSG Publishing Co., 1987:280–1.

188 Maternal stress and labor

K. M. Paarlberg, A. J. J. M. Vingerhoets and H. P. van Geijn

Labor and delivery are among the most intense events a woman faces in life. Maternal distress or maternal anxiety in reaction to stressors can probably trigger the onset of labor (at term or preterm), and can predispose to an abnormal course of labor.[1] These stressors may be related directly to pregnancy (e.g. a fetal or maternal complication, or bad experiences in an earlier pregnancy), or may arise from other circumstances (e.g. family, work, social life or personality characteristics). All these kinds of stressors may influence the onset and course of delivery.

Depending on her ability to cope with stressful circumstances and dramatic changes occurring in her body, the woman's experience of giving birth may range from an intense but satisfying occasion to a most traumatic event, resulting in extreme states of distress. The distress may be experienced before, during or after delivery.[2]

This chapter reviews our understanding of the interplay between maternal distress and the onset and course of labor. The effects of maternal stress on the onset and course of labor, its role in preterm labor and the relation to intrapartum complications are discussed. Attention is then given to the main causes of maternal distress during labor, and finally, interventions are suggested to decrease maternal stress during labor, with emphasis on the therapeutic implications of the relevant issues.

Maternal intrapartum stress

Onset of labor

The onset of parturition is the result of a complex interplay of fetal and maternal hormones, including cortisol, catecholamines, interleukins, prostaglandins, maternal and placental CRH,[3] vasopressin, oxytocin and the oxytocin receptors in the myometrium.[4] Because the considerable inter-species differences do not allow generalization to human beings, the precise role of these substances in human labor are not fully understood. It is clear, nevertheless, that in humans, secretion of many of the hormones that participate in the initiation of labor may be influenced by stressful stimuli.[5] For example, the uterus of a woman who delivers preterm appears to be more sensitive to oxytocin during pregnancy than that of a woman who delivers at term.[6] The effects of oxytocin during human labor result from an increased number of oxytocin receptors rather than from increased levels of the circulating hormone.[7–9] Small quantities of oxytocin can trigger uterine contractions at levels that are completely ineffective in the non-pregnant state.[9] The increase in receptors is not only confined to the myometrium, but is also found in the decidua. Oxytocin has an additional separate action of stimulating the release of prostaglandin $F_{2\alpha}$ ($PGF_{2\alpha}$), so that at the end of pregnancy there is a greatly increased secretion of $PGF_{2\alpha}$.[11] This represents a secondary effect of oxytocin on uterine contractility through prostaglandin release.[8] The transition from a relatively relaxed state to the onset of contractions can be seen as the result of stimulatory inputs or perhaps as a consequence of the loss or 'switching off' of mechanisms that promote relaxation. One such mechanism could be the activation of cyclic nucleotide (cAMP, cGMP) pathways. During the onset of labor, cAMP synthesis is decreased, and its catabolism is promoted, contributing to enhanced uterine contractility.[4]

Immunological activity is influenced via hormonal and neuronal pathways.[9,12–18] Increases in catecholamines or cortisol can suppress immune processes and may also rapidly alter numbers of immune cells via redistribution.[9,12–14] In addition, neuropeptides such as plasma β-endorphin, another hormone sensitive to stress exposure,[15,16] are known to mediate increases in natural killer (NK) cell activity. Exposure to chronic stressful situations (such as caregiving for Alzheimer patients and bereavement) has been shown to result in decreased NK cell activity.[14] Apart from hormonal factors, direct neural influences from the hypothalamus on the immune system have been described.[17,18]

A compromised immune system may have a negative effect on gestational length. Under circumstances of intrauterine infection (chorioamnionitis), decidual macrophages may be involved in premature labor through the premature release of prostaglandins and other inflammatory mediators in the decidua and fetal membranes, close to myometrial cells.[4] Given the established relationship between exposure to stressful conditions and increased risk of infectious diseases,[19–22] it may be postulated that adverse psychological conditions enhance the susceptibility to infections such as chorioamnionitis and in that way can induce preterm contractions and/or rupture of membranes.

Course of labor

In primates and sheep, stressful conditions during labor (e.g. presence of observers and unfamiliar sounds) reduce oxytocin release and can thus delay the birth process.[6,23] Naaktgeboren and Bontekoe[23] measured uterine activity during labor in ewes. In anxious ewes uterine activity sank to zero when human observers were present. Uterine activity was recorded and the lamb born only when no observers were present. In less anxious ewes, the presence of observers did not evoke any change in the contraction pattern. Assuming that biological stress reactions in primates and sheep are comparable to those in human beings, it is plausible to hypothesize that stressful stimulation can negatively influence the progress of labor. Which mechanisms are involved is as yet not completely clear.

Omer and Everly[9] and Omer[12] presented an arousal model based on the results of experimental studies with rodents and humans. Catecholamines and oxytocin are hypothesized to mediate the influence of psychosocial factors in preterm labor. It is theorized that the threshold for uterine contractility can be lowered by constitutional tendencies or by acutely intense or chronically repeated central nervous system (CNS) stimulation. This state of hypersensitivity might then be perpetuated in a vicious circle by high adrenergic activity, neuromuscular tension and cognitive excitation. Neurologic hyperreactivity manifests itself by a cascade of physiologic responses in all efferent components of the limbic circuitry. This multiple response chain might affect the uterus in different ways: through norepinephrine secretion; through prolonged epinephrine secretion, causing a rebound effect, characterized by initial inhibition of uterine contractility followed by stimulation of contractility; through oxytocin release; through skeletal-muscular activation, which in turn influences (through interneurons) sympathetic neurons responsible for uterine innervation; and indirectly, through immunosuppression and, consequently, heightened vulnerability to infectious diseases.

Preterm labor

The results of research on the effects of maternal exposure to stressful events on onset of labor are consistent and unambiguous. There is ample evidence that preterm deliveries have often been preceded by stressful situations. In a prospective study in 2593 pregnant women,[24] anxiety, stress, self-esteem, mastery and depression were assessed at 25–29 weeks of gestation. Stress was found to be a significant predictor of spontaneous preterm birth even after adjustment for adverse health behaviors (tobacco, alcohol and drug use).

In addition, the study by Pritchard and Teo[25] demonstrated that the influence of chronic stressor exposure on preterm birth should also not be overlooked. These authors found a strong association between experiencing high levels of perceived difficulty with the household at 20 weeks of gestation and preterm birth.

Studies from more recent date show less consistency in their results than those of previous decades have shown.[26] Levi *et al.*[27] found a negative association between trait-anxiety and the duration of pregnancy. However, preterm birth did not occur in this group. In a prospective study by Norbeck and Tilden,[28] state-anxiety appeared to be unrelated to gestational complications, including preterm labor. In contrast, a prospective study by Omer *et al.*[29] yielded evidence that state-anxiety was more prevalent in pregnant women with preterm contractions or delivery than in a comparable group with term labor. It is not clear to what extent these contradicting findings could be attributed to differences in research methodology. Omer *et al.*[29] focused on preterm labor, whereas the Norbeck and Tilden study[28] combined preterm labor, anemia and preeclampsia. The selection of study participants was also different. Norbeck and Tilden excluded all women with preexisting medical risk factors in the beginning of pregnancy, whereas Omer *et al.*[29] did not. Therefore, in the study of Omer *et al.*, in which anxiety was measured at 4–6 months, and there was no control for medical risk, it may be that anxiety reflected early indications of risk which, in turn, could have influenced outcome.

The majority of the studies that focused on the relationship between negative psychosocial factors and preterm labor reported a positive association.[24,25,27,29–36] A marginal or absent relation was found in three.[28,37,38] The most recent studies were carried out prospectively.[24,25,27–29,35–38]

Prospective[24,36,38] and retrospective studies[29,30,32–34,38] have reported that stressful life events are more common in pregnancies resulting in preterm delivery. A few researchers[35,37,38] observed no differences in reported life events between a preterm and full-term birth group, but life events may well play an important role in the onset of preterm labor.

In order to obtain a reliable picture of the influence of psychosocial factors on preterm labor, it is important to study specific psychosocial and background variables prospectively in a large group of women. Such a research project has been carried out by Hedegaard *et al.*,[36] who found a dose–response relationship between stressor exposure (i.e. stressful life events, physical job strain and psychological job strain) assessed in the 30th week of pregnancy and risk of preterm delivery. In contrast, the same factors measured in the 16th week of pregnancy were not related to preterm delivery.

Psychologic responses to stress are progressively attenuated throughout pregnancy. Glynn *et al.* examined the birth outcomes of women who had experienced an earthquake during pregnancy. The earthquake was rated as most stressful during the first trimester of pregnancy and as least stressful during the third trimester. Timing of the earthquake was inversely related to gestational age at birth: stress experienced early in pregnancy was associated with shorter gestation. Women who did not experience the earthquake during pregnancy had the longest mean gestational length.[39]

Given the results, it is tempting to hypothesize that stressful events can potentiate preterm contractions and may trigger preterm labor. However, the same kind of stressor may be perceived differently throughout pregnancy, depending on the phase of pregnancy, and therefore its effect may vary.

Intrapartum complications

Suppression of labor activity and prolonged deliveries due to anxiety, strong emotions, and stressful events has been reported in women since ancient times, and are known to occur in many other mammalian species.[23]

The literature shows a wide variety in severity and nature of the intrapartum complications that have been studied. Except for three studies,[40–42] the design was generally prospective. Most investigators found a positive relationship between psychosocial factors and the occurrence of intrapartum complications.[42–58] Reeb *et al.*[51] studied the occurrence of intrapartum complications in 140 urban black women. In the 8th month of pregnancy, demographic, biomedical and psychosocial factors (i.e. life events, maternal worries about adjusting to life with a new baby, emotional and instrumental support, depression and family size and functioning) were assessed. Intrapartum complications were defined as three or more significant problems occurring during labor and delivery. It was found that the four-factor equation: low family functioning, advanced maternal age, working during pregnancy and short stature, predicted intrapartum complications with a relative risk of 5.5 (95% confidence interval: 2.2–13.9). Clifford *et al.*[57] examined life events, social support and anxiety in the 16th, 28th and 36th week of pregnancy. Intrapartum complications were operationalized as 'noteworthy' medical events. Some serious outcomes were not included because their cause was either known or believed to be unrelated to psychosocial stress (e.g. cord around the neck, injury incurred at birth, malpresentation). It was found that the incidence of stressful life events and anxiety in the third trimester were significantly related to the risk of intrapartum complications.

A smaller number of publications reported no association.[27,40,41,59–67] In most investigations, trait-anxiety has been considered the main predictive variable of intrapartum complications. Retrospective[41,59] and prospective[27,46–49,64,67] studies have focused on the possible relationship between trait-anxiety and length of labor. Some investigators[46–49,67] found higher anxiety scores for women with prolonged labor compared with normally delivering women, while others[41,59,64] found no difference. One author[27] even reported shorter labor in women reporting high levels of trait-anxiety. These seemingly conflicting findings can be understood if one takes into account the course of the effects of epinephrine, which is the hormone most strongly associated with anxiety. The results of Lederman *et al.*,[47] who measured epinephrine plasma levels and self-reported anxiety of women during labor, showed a positive correlation between these two variables. High levels of anxiety and plasma epinephrine were associated with a pronounced decrease in uterine activity, particularly in the second stage of labor. However, after a while, uterine contractions returned to their initial level and a rebound effect often took place, leading to a pronounced increase in uterine contractility. The apparent contradiction between the stimulating and inhibiting effects of anxiety on duration of labor can be explained by taking into account the duration of receptor stimulation. Initially, epinephrine inhibits uterine contractility through stimulation of β_2-receptors in the uterine muscle, while norepinephrine stimulates contractility through α-receptors, which are also situated in the uterine muscle. As labor progresses, the amount of β_2-receptor stimulation decreases in favor of α-receptor stimulation. This phenomenon is probably due to upregulation or increased sensitivity of α-receptors caused by estrogen.[9,12] Epinephrine stimulation changes from an inhibiting to a stimulating effect on uterine activity, thereby reinforcing the effects of norepinephrine.

The clinical effects of epinephrine may be well illustrated by experiments in Guatamala and in the United States.[68–70] Sosa *et al.*[68] examined the effects of a supportive lay woman (doula) on the length of labor and intrapartum complications in healthy primigravid Guatemalan women. Hospital policies did not provide for any family member, friend, or continuous nurse caretaker to be present in the labor rooms, apparently as a consequence of the large number of deliveries, and limited space. It appeared that the length of time from admission to delivery was shorter in the supported groups than in the control groups. In addition, more mother–infant interactions were observed in the supported group. Klaus *et al.*[69] and Kennell *et al.*[70] further reported fewer perinatal complications and less medication (epidural analgesia and oxytocin stimulation) in the supported group than in the control group. Besides the possibility that the presence of a companion might account for the obstetrician making fewer interventions, a supportive companion may also reduce catecholamine levels by reducing maternal anxiety and facilitating uterine contractile activity and uterine blood flow.

Most studies used the dichotomous distinction of 'normal' and 'abnormal' in their outcome variables.[40,42–46,48,50,51,53–57,59–67,71,72] In these investigations abnormal outcome variables could be anything from umbilical cord around the neck to a cleft palate and stillbirth. It is therefore difficult to draw any definitive conclusions from them regarding the influence of maternal stress during labor. In the majority of studies focusing on the relationship between anxiety and complications, higher trait-anxiety in the 'abnormal' delivery group was observed than in the 'normal' delivery group.[43–46,48,50,54,55,57,71,72] A smaller number of publications reported no differences.[60,62,64–67]

In summary, trait-anxiety appears to be positively associated with 'abnormal' delivery, in particular prolonged labor, but the inadequate operationalization of intrapartum complications prevents us from drawing clear-cut conclusions.

Causes of maternal distress during labor

How a woman will experience and perceive her delivery depends on numerous factors. Fear of childbirth (FOC) can be so intense that it may qualify as a legitimate diagnosis, often described with terms like 'clinical FOC'. This is a disabling fear that interferes with occupational or academic functioning, with domestic and social activities, or with relationships.[73] Women who suffer the most from FOC during pregnancy are likely to have the most intense fear during the delivery, and also suffer the most from it afterwards, independent of the kind of delivery that occurs. Due to enormous methodological problems, sound research regarding FOC is uncommon. Areskog *et al.*[74] investigated background factors associated with FOC. Between 32 and 34 weeks of gestation, pregnant women ($n=153$) were categorized as 'suffering' ($n=92$) or 'not suffering' ($n=61$) from FOC. Nulliparous ($n=93$) and parous women ($n=60$) were analyzed separately. FOC was more prevalent in nulliparous than in parous women (33% vs. 26%). In nulliparous women, more background factors associated with FOC were identified than in parous women. The significant background factors are summarized in Table 188.1.

In an earlier investigation,[2] the same authors found that, among women with severe FOC, various attributions of fear were involved, such as shape and well-being of the unborn child, fear of physical damage to the woman herself (such as birth canal lacerations), fear of not being able to control herself during the delivery and fear of losing dignity. Fear of delivery in parous women was very often based on previous experiences of traumatic deliveries. In contrast to a woman with, for instance a pathologic fear of spiders, a pregnant woman who suffers from FOC cannot avoid the delivery she fears and is therefore captured in a situation in which she is (slowly) forced to approach delivery, which is regarded as an unknown, uncontrollable and unavoidable event. The only way out for her will be an abortion in early pregnancy or a cesarean section, in spite of the risks of this procedure. In Finland, Sweden, and the United Kingdom, FOC is the reason for about 7–22% of cesarean section births on maternal request.[75] A vivid debate about a woman's right to choose the mode of delivery is currently going on in the obstetric literature, but discussion and analysis of the reasons for women to request a cesarean section, or of ways to help them overcome the fear of vaginal birth is only scanty.[75] Anxious people have a bias to perceive information as threatening. It has been shown that, at the end of pregnancy, pregnant women with severe fear of labor had only heard negative stories about deliveries, while women with low or mild fear of delivery mostly had heard positive accounts. Thus, like certain individuals who develop a specific phobia by means of vicarious experience or informational transmission, anxious apprehension could ensure that mostly negative information is processed and women consequently become so alarmed, that in their view the approaching delivery already is a catastrophe before the event has taken place.[73]

Psychological trauma and post-traumatic stress disorder after birth

Childbirth can be so traumatic that the new mother fulfills the criteria for post-traumatic stress disorder (PTSD), with its well-known symptoms such as nightmares, intrusive memories, depression, anxiety, difficulty bonding with the infant, fear of sexual intimacy, and avoidance of future childbearing.[76–81] In addition, there is limited evidence that experiencing a psychologic trauma during childbirth may lead to difficulty in bonding between mother and child resulting in long-term attachment problems.[77]

According to the literature, the percentage of women experiencing a birth as traumatic ranges between 20% and 30%, and of developing PTSD, between 2% and 6%.[81] In contrast to what might be expected, the highest incidence of postpartum PTSD is found in the group with obstetrically normal deliveries.[73] Psychosocial factors before birth play an important role in these traumatic experiences. Psychosocial predictors include preexisting psychopathology,[77,78,82] expectations,[78,82] nulliparity,[78] high trait anxiety,[82] and history of sexual trauma.[81] Soet *et al.*[81] found that women who had experienced a past sexual trauma were 12 times more likely to experience the delivery as traumatic. Lack of confidence in the ability to control pain together with low coping skills may be related to women's negative perceptions of birth. Event characteristics predicting

Table 188.1 Personal life experiences significantly related to fear of delivery in nulliparous and parous women[74]

Type of life experience	Significant in nulliparous women	Significant in multiparous women
Present pregnancy		
Fetal movements perceived late (≥22 gestational weeks in nulliparous women; ≥20 weeks in parous women)		*
Less verbal communication with the fetus	*	
Sexuality		
Ignoring sexuality in parental home	*	
Non-permissive attitude toward sexuality in parental home	*	
Negative experience of first intercourse		*
Childhood		
Negative life experience of childhood	*	
Poor relationship with father	*	
Psychological well-being		
Significant anxiety during last 2 years		*
Significant other psychological problems during last 2 years	*	
Disturbed emotional balance during present pregnancy	*	*
Psychological tension during the interview	*	
Strong dissimulation tendency	*	
Medical treatment		
First gynecological examination experienced as a psychological trauma		*
Fear of gynecological examinations at present	*	
Fear of pain in general	*	*
Earlier traumatic experiences of pain (except deliveries)		*
Fear of attending hospital services	*	
Verbal tradition concerning delivery		
Negative aspects dominant in apprehension of verbal tradition about delivery	*	

childbirth as a traumatic experience are patient's feelings of powerlessness,[81] pain during childbirth,[77,81,83] delivery of an ill or stillborn infant,[77,83] hostile and uncaring treatment by medical personnel,[77,78,83] inadequate information given to the patient,[82,83] patient's lack of consent,[83] and increasing medical intervention.[81,84]

Pain in labor

The pain of childbirth is one of the most severe forms of pain.[85] Elevation of catecholamines in maternal blood during labor is associated with pain, anxiety and prolonged labor.[47,86] Pain relief by epidural block decreases catecholamines, cortisol and adrenocorticotropic hormone secretion during labor.[87] This suggests that the hypothalamo-pituitary-adrenal axis is involved in the maternal response to pain.

Whipple *et al.*[88] investigated pain thresholds in 10 women, five of whom had had childbirth preparation according to Lamaze. The pain thresholds were measured by applying a gradually increasing force to a finger. In the group of women with childbirth preparation the pain detection threshold during labor was higher than before labor (21%) and 24 h postpartum (33%), whereas in the group without childbirth preparation, the pain detection threshold significantly decreased during labor (19%) compared to predelivery values. There were no significant differences between the intrapartum and 24-h postpartum values in this group. The authors concluded that 'in the women with childbirth preparation, an analgesic process is activated during labor'. The differences in pain thresholds were attributed to differences in anxiety during labor. Charles *et al.*[89] and Melzack *et al.*[90,91] found that women who followed childbirth preparation courses reported less pain during the delivery than women without childbirth preparation, but there was still a lot of pain.

The phenomenon that pain detection thresholds may vary among women and even may vary over time in the same woman, may be explained by the 'gate-control' theory of Melzack.[92] The basis of this theory is that a neural mechanism (cells in the gelatinous substance) in the posterior horns of the spinal cord functions as a gate that can modulate the input of nerve impulses to the CNS. The extent to which the gate can increase or decrease the transfer is determined by the relative activity in thick (A-beta) and thin (A-delta and C) fibers and by descending influences from the brain. When the amount of information flowing through the gate exceeds a certain critical level, areas responsible for pain sensation and reaction to pain are activated. There is a central control system activating the special brain processes that keep nervous input under control. In addition, enforcing the 'gate-control' theory, a central inhibition mechanism has been localized in different areas in the brainstem.

Analgesia by overstimulation can be explained by high output of the transmission cells in the spinal cord. The output may exceed the critical level and cause pain, but could also activate the central system that inhibits the excitation level of the transmission cells. Psychologic processes, such as earlier experiences, attention and distraction, and positive and negative emotions, can influence pain experience by their effects on the gate system in the spinal cord. Some of these psychologic influences can open the gate and others can close it. The 'gate-control' theory elucidates the possibilities for pain relief by several different kinds of interventions including pharmacological means, acupuncture, massage, transcutaneous electrical nerve stimulation, application of heat and cold, as well as psychologic techniques.

Interventions to decrease maternal distress during labor

A limited number of efforts have been undertaken to prevent preterm labor and complications during labor by applying psychologic or social interventions. The kind of interventions can be roughly divided into two categories: (1) physical and mental relaxation techniques, and (2) social support. Physical and mental relaxation techniques have been used to prolong pregnancy in women at risk for preterm delivery.[9,93] Social support has been applied to prolong pregnancy duration[94] and to diminish perinatal complications.[68–70,94] Omer and Everly[9] referred to early Russian efforts to apply hypnosis in the prevention of preterm birth. They concluded that the results of these studies appeared promising. Relaxation techniques, in some cases combined with drug treatment, have contributed to clinically relevant prolongation of pregnancy.[93] In contrast, efforts to induced post-term delivery with the help of hypnosis failed.[9]

Earlier research showed that patients who had undergone a cholecystectomy used less pain medication and had more rapid recovery if they were in a room with a window so they could see natural surroundings than patients who only saw a blinded wall. It has been suggested, supported by biochemical measurements, that natural scenery has a powerful ability to promote relaxation.[95] Nowadays, experiments are carried out to mimic this effect by applying virtual reality as adjunct analgesic.[96] Whether this technique might be of help in obstetric patients still has to be investigated.

During prenatal care, a careful history, including relevant psychosocial factors, should always be taken.[97] The upcoming delivery should be discussed in a way that allows the woman as much control as possible. Joint decision making should be a pivotal part of counseling a women who is at risk for a traumatic experience during parturition. During the labor and delivery there should be ensured adequate communication and appropriate pain control. In contrast to earlier belief, PTSD cannot be prevented by psychologic debriefing.[98] It has, however, been suggested that by evaluation after birth a bridge may be provided for later screening and treatment, if required.[99]

As has been mentioned above, when supportive lay women (doulas) accompany laboring women, the length of time from admission to delivery in the supported women will be reduced, fewer perinatal complications will be seen, less intrapartum medication (epidural analgesia and oxytocin stimulation) will be necessary, and more mother–infant interaction will be expected.[68–70] These studies suggest that continuous human support during labor may be both beneficial for the labor course and perinatal outcome.

Conclusions

Maternal distress during labor can originate either from non-delivery-related background factors, such as negative life experiences in childhood, psychological problems, fear of pain in general, or from difficulties in coping with the intense experience of giving birth. The effects of exposure to psychosocial stressors may include initiating preterm labor, disrupting the normal labor course, experiencing labor as traumatic, and the development of PTSD.

Stressful events can promote the secretion of hormones that are involved in the onset of delivery, and that play a role in the regulation of the birth process. In addition, stress reactions may impair the immunologic defense against microorganisms that may colonize the uterus and initiate uterine contractions or weaken the chorion. Consequently, the membranes may become vulnerable and at risk for (preterm) premature rupture, resulting in preterm birth.

Once a woman is in labor, state-anxiety, due to loss of control and feelings of powerlessness, has been found to be positively related to 'abnormal' delivery, in particular prolonged labor, but the inadequate or inconsistent definitions of intrapartum complications used in the literature prevents the drawing of clear-cut conclusions in this regard. FOC is more frequent in nulliparous than in parous women. The most common causes of this FOC in nulliparous women are background factors, such as low psychologic well-being and negative life experiences in childhood, and in parous women previous experiences of traumatic deliveries. Pain experienced during parturition is mediated by psychological processes, such as earlier experiences, attention and emotions.[100] This can be understood by the 'gate-control' theory of Melzack, elucidating the possibilities for pain relief by, for instance, pharmacologic means, acupuncture and psychologic interventions. Several studies suggest that continuous human support during labor may be beneficial for the course of labor and perinatal outcome.

Therapeutic implications

Excessive maternal stress during delivery could be reduced by health-care providers in several ways. During pregnancy, a careful history should be taken, with particular attention to the patient's attitudes and feelings about pregnancy and delivery. During the delivery there should be ensured adequate communication and appropriate pain control. After the delivery it may be a good routine to evaluate the labor experience of the new mother. Postpartum depression should be acknowledged and treated when necessary. During subsequent pregnancies, a careful history should again be taken in order to be prepared for the upcoming delivery.[97] Joint decision making is a very important part of counseling women before and during labor.

Unfortunately, scientifically valid data about treatment of childbirth-related anxiety is almost nonexistent. The clinical practice of how to treat fear of pregnancy is based primarily on knowledge of treatment of similar problems in the non-pregnant state, clinical experience, and common sense. More basic knowledge of childbirth-related anxiety is crucial to develop adequate methods of treatment. There is ample evidence that many women experience great distress related to childbirth, which might have long-lasting consequences for their mental and emotional well-being.[73] In debates on women's right to choose elective caesarean section there should be more attention to the reasons why so many women apparently fear vaginal delivery. And a related question is how we can organize our labor ward in a way that it is more patient-friendly. In order to facilitate maternal–child bonding and future attachment, a new mother should welcome her baby in an atmosphere as peaceful as possible; health-care workers can, and have to, play a crucial role in this goal.

REFERENCES

1. Paarlberg KM, Vingerhoets AJJM, Passchier J, *et al.* Psychosocial factors and pregnancy outcome: A review with emphasis on methodological issues. *J Psychosom Res* 1995;39:563–96.
2. Areskog B, Uddenberg N, Kjessler B. Fear of childbirth in late pregnancy. *Gynecol Obstet Invest* 1981;12:262–6.
3. Kalantaridou SN, Makrigiannakis A, Zoumakis E, *et al.* Reproductive functions of corticotropin-releasing hormone. research and potential clinical utility ofantalarmins (CRH receptor type 1 antagonists). *Am J Reprod Immunol* 2004; 51:269–74.
4. Bernal AL. Mechanisms of labor-biochemical aspects. *BJOG* 2003;110(Suppl 20):39–45.
5. Istvan J. Stress, anxiety, and birth outcomes: A critical review of the evidence. *Psychol Bull* 1986;100:331–48.
6. Naaktgeboren C, Bontekoe EHM. Vergleichend-geburtskundliche Betrachtungen und experimentelle Untersuchungen über psychosomatische Störungen der Schwangerschaft und des Geburtsablaufes. *Z Tierzüchtg Züchtgsbiol* 1976;93:264–320.
7. Carsten ME, Miller JD. A new look at uterine muscle contraction. *Am J Obstet Gynecol* 1987;157:1303–15.
8. Fuchs AR, Fuchs F. Endocrinology of human parturition: A review. *Br J Obstet Gynaecol* 1984;91:948–67.
9. Omer H, Everly GS. Psychological factors in preterm labor: Critical review and theoretical synthesis. *Am J Psychiatry* 1988;145:1507–13.
10. Jenkins JS, Nussey SS. The role of oxytocin: Present concepts. *Clin Endocrinol* 1991;34:515–25.
11. Blanks AM, Thornton S. The role of oxytocin in parturition. *BJOG* 2003;110(Suppl 20):46–51.
12. Omer H. Possible psychophysiologic mechanisms in premature labour. *Psychosomatics* 1986;27:580–4.
13. Sterling P, Eyer J. Biological basis of stress-related mortality. *Soc Sci Med* 1981;15E:3–42.
14. Naliboff BD, Benton D, Solomon GF, *et al.* Immunological changes in young and old adults during brief laboratory stress. *Psychosom Med* 1991;53:121–32.
15. Meyerhoff JL, Olehansky MA, Mougey EH. Effects of psychological stress on pituitary hormones in man. In Chrousos GP, Loriaux DL, Gold W, eds. *Mechanisms of Physical and Emotional Stress.* New York: Plenum Press, 1988:465–78.
16. Fraioli F, Moretti C, Paolucci D, *et al.* Physical exercise stimulates marked concomitant release of β-endorphin and adrenocorticotropic hormone (ACTH) in peripheral blood in man. *Experientia* 1980;36:987–9.
17. Dantzer R, Kelley KW. Stress and immunity: An integrated view of relationships between the brain and the immune system. *Life Sci* 1989;44:1995–2008.
18. Ader R, Felten DL, Cohen N. Interactions between the brain and the immune system. *Annu Rev Pharmacol Toxicol* 1990;30:561–602.
19. Crary B, Hauser SL, Borysenko M, *et al.* Epinephrine-induced changes in the distribution of lymphocyte subsets in peripheral blood of humans. *J Immunol* 1983;131:1178–81.
20. Jemmott JB, Locke SE. Psychosocial factors, immunologic mediation, and human susceptibility to infectious diseases: How much do we know? *Psychol Bull* 1984;95:78–108.
21. Cohen S, Tyrrell DAJ, Smith AP. Psychological stress and susceptibility to the common cold. *N Engl J Med* 1991;325:606–12.
22. Jabaaij L, Grosheide PM, Heijtink RA, *et al.* Influence of perceived psychological stress and distress on antibody response to low dose rDNA Hepatitis B vaccine. *J Psychosom Res* 1993;37:361–9.
23. Naaktgeboren C, Bontekoe EHM. The uterus, a mirror of the soul. In Hirsch H, ed. *4th International Congress of Psychosomatic Obstetrics and Gynecology.* Tel Aviv, Basel: S Karger, 1974: 511–19.
24. Copper RL, Das A, Goldenberg RL, *et al.* The preterm prediction study: Maternal stress is associated with spontaneous preterm birth at less than thirty-five weeks' gestation. *Am J Obstet Gynecol* 1996;175:1286–92.
25. Pritchard CW, Teo PYK. Preterm birth, low birthweight and the stressfulness of the household role for pregnant women. *Soc Sci Med* 1994;38:89–96.

26. Johnson RC, Slade P. Obstetric complications and anxiety during pregnancy: Is there a relationship? *J Psychosom Obstet Gynaecol* 2003;24:1–14.
27. Levi R, Lundberg U, Hanson U, *et al.* Anxiety during pregnancy after the Chernobyl accident as related to obstetric outcome. *J Psychosom Obstet Gynaecol* 1989;10:221–30.
28. Norbeck JS, Tilden VP. Life stress, social support, and emotional disequilibrium in complications of pregnancy: A prospective multivariate study. *J Health Soc Behav* 1983;24:30–46.
29. Omer H, Elizur Y, Barnea T, *et al.* Psychological variables and premature labour: A possible solution for some methodological problems. *J Psychosom Res* 1986;30:559–65.
30. Gunter LM. Psychopathology and stress in the life experience of mothers of premature infants. *Am J Obstet Gynecol* 1963;86: 405–20.
31. Williams CC, Williams RA, Griswold MJ, *et al.* Pregnancy and life change. *J Psychosom Res* 1975;19:123–9.
32. Schwartz JL. A study of the relationship between maternal life-change events and premature delivery. In Schwartz JL, Schwartz LH, eds. *Vulnerable Infants: a Psychological Dilemma.* New York: McGraw-Hill, 1977:47–61.
33. Newton RW, Webster PAC, Binu PS, *et al.* Psychosocial stress in pregnancy and its relation to the onset of premature labour. *Br Med J* 1979;2:411–13.
34. Berkowitz GS, Kasl SV. The role of psychosocial factors in spontaneous preterm delivery. *J Psychosom Res* 1983;27:283–90.
35. Lobel M, Dunkel-Schetter C, Scrimshaw SCM. Prenatal maternal stress and prematurity: A prospective study of socioeconomically disadvantaged women. *Health Psychol* 1992;11:32–40.
36. Hedegaard M, Brink Henriksen T, Sabroe S, *et al.* Psychological distress in pregnancy and preterm delivery. *Br Med J* 1983;307:234–9.
37. Ching J, Newton N. A prospective study of psychological and social factors in pregnancy related to preterm and low-birthweight deliveries. In Prill HJ, Stauber M, eds. *Advances in Psychosomatic Obstetrics and Gynecology.* Berlin: Springer, 1982:384–5.
38. Omer H, Friedlander D, Palti Z, *et al.* Life stresses and premature labor: Real connection or artifactual findings? *Psychosom Med* 1986;48:362–9.
39. Glynn LM, Wadhwa PD, Dunkel-Schetter C, *et al.* When stress happens matters: Effects of earthquake timing on stress responsivity in pregnancy. *Am J Obstet Gynecol* 2001;184:637–42.
40. Smilkstein G, Helsper-Lucas A, Ashworth C, *et al.* Prediction of pregnancy complications: An application of the biopsychosocial model. *Soc Sci Med* 1984;18:315–21.
41. Cramond WA. Psychological aspects of uterine dysfunction. *Lancet* 1954;2:1241–5.
42. Kapp FT, Hornstein S, Graham VT. Some psychological factors in prolonged labor due to inefficient uterine action. *Compr Psychiatry* 1963;4:9–18.
43. Davids A, DeVault S, Talmadge M. Anxiety, pregnancy and childbirth abnormalities. *J Consult Psychol* 1961;25:74–7.
44. Davids A, DeVault S. Maternal anxiety during pregnancy and childbirth abnormalities. *Psychosom Med* 1962;24:464–70.
45. McDonald RL, Christakos AC. Relationship of emotional adjustment during pregnancy to obstetric complications. *Am J Obstet Gynecol* 1963;86:341–8.
46. McDonald RL, Gynther MD, Christakos AC. Relations between maternal anxiety and obstetric complications. *Psychosom Med* 1963;25:357–63.
47. Lederman RP, Lederman E, Work BA, *et al.* The relationship of maternal anxiety, plasma catecholamines, and plasma cortisol to progress in labor. *Am J Obstet Gynecol* 1978;132:495–500.
48. Crandon AJ. Maternal anxiety and obstetric complications. *J Psychosom Res* 1979;23:109–11.
49. Falorni ML, Fornasarig A, Stefanile C. Research about anxiety effects on the pregnant woman and her newborn child. In Carenza L, Zichella L, eds. *Emotion and Reproduction: Proceedings of the Serono Symposium,* Vol. 20B. London: Academic Press, 1979: 1147–53.
50. Molfese VJ, Bricker MC, Manion LG, *et al.* Anxiety, depression and stress in pregnancy: A multivariate model of intra-partum risks and pregnancy outcomes. *J Psychosom Obstet Gynaecol* 1987; 7:77–92.
51. Reeb KG, Graham AV, Zyzanski SJ, *et al.* Predicting low birth weight and complicated labor in urban black women: A biopsychological perspective. *Soc Sci Med* 1987;25:1321–7.
52. Vartiainen H. Effects of psychosocial factors, especially work-related stress, on fertility and pregnancy (abstract). *Acta Obstet Gynecol Scand* 1990;69:677–8.
53. Nuckolls KB, Cassel J, Kaplan BH. Psychosocial assets, life crisis and the prognosis of pregnancy. *Am J Epidemiol* 1972;95:431–41.
54. Gorsuch RL, Key MK. Abnormalities of pregnancy as a function of anxiety and life stress. *Psychosom Med* 1974;36:352–62.
55. Magni G, Rizzardo R, Andreoli C. Psychosocial stress and obstetrical complications. *Acta Obstet Gynecol Scand* 1986;65:273–6.
56. Obayuwana AO, Carter AL, Barnett RM. Psychosocial distress and pregnancy outcome: A three-year prospective study. *J Psychosom Obstet Gynaecol* 1984;3:173–83.
57. Clifford E, Weaver SM, Hay DM. Stress and pregnancy complications: A prospective study. In McGuigan FJ, Sime WE, MacDonald WJ, eds. *Stress and Tension Control 3. Stress Management.* New York: Plenum Press, 1989:47–61.
58. Da Costa D, Dritsa M, Larouche J, Brender W. Psychosocial predictors of labor/delivery complications and infant birth weight: A prospective multivariate study. *J Psychosom Obstet Gynaecol* 2000;21(3):137–48.
59. Grimm ER. Psychological tension in pregnancy. *Psychosom Med* 1961;23:520–7.
60. Edwards KR, Jones MR. Personality changes related to pregnancy and obstetric complications. In *Proceedings, 78th Annual Convention, American Psychiatric Association,* Miami, FL 1970:341–2.
61. Jones AC. Life change and psychological distress as predictors of pregnancy outcome. *Psychosom Med* 1978;40:402–12.
62. Morcos FH, Funke-Ferber J. Anxiety and depression in the mother and father and their relationship to physical complications of pregnancy and labor. In Carenza L, Zichella L, eds. *Emotion and Reproduction. Proceedings of the Serono Symposium,* Vol. 20B. London: Academic Press, 1979:757–65.
63. Boyce WT, Schaeffer C, Uitti C. Permanence and change: Psychosocial factors in the outcome of adolescent pregnancy. *Soc Sci Med* 1985;21:1279–87.
64. McDonald RL, Parham KJ. Relation of emotional changes during pregnancy to obstetric complications in unmarried primigravidas. *Am J Obstet Gynecol* 1964;90:195–201.
65. Grimm ER, Venet WR. The relationship of emotional adjustment and attitudes to the course and outcome of pregnancy. *Psychosom Med* 1966;28:34–49.
66. Burstein I, Kinch RA, Stern L. Anxiety, pregnancy, labor, and the neonate. *Am J Obstet Gynecol* 1974;118:195–9.
67. Beck NC, Siegel LJ, Davidson NP, *et al.* The prediction of pregnancy outcome: Maternal preparation, anxiety and additional sets. *J Psychosom Res* 1980;24:343–51.
68. Sosa R, Kennell JH, Klaus MH, *et al.* The effect of a supportive companion on perinatal problems, length of labor, and mother-infant interaction. *N Engl J Med* 1980;303:597–600.
69. Klaus MH, Kennel JH, Robertson SS, *et al.* Effects of social support during parturition on maternal and infant morbidity. *Br Med J* 1986;293:585–7.
70. Kennell JH, Klaus MH, McCrath S, *et al.* Continuous emotional support during labor in a US hospital. A randomized controlled trial. *J Am Med Assoc* 1991;265:2197–201.
71. Hansen KA, Opsahl MS, Nieman LK, *et al.* Natural killer cell activity from pregnant subjects is modulated by RU 486. *Am J Obstet Gynecol* 1992;166:87–90.
72. Crandon AJ. Maternal anxiety and neonatal wellbeing. *J Psychosom Res* 1979;23:113–15.
73. Wijma K. Why focus on 'fear of childbirth'? *J Psychosom Obstet Gynecol* 2003;24:141–3.
74. Areskog B, Uddenberg N, Kjessler B. Background factors in pregnant women with and without fear of childbirth. *J Psychosom Obstet Gynaecol* 1983;2:102–8.
75. Saisto T, Halmesmaki E. Fear of childbirth: A neglected dilemma. *Acta Obstet Gynecol Scand* 2003;82:201–8.
76. Ayers S, Pickering AD. Do women get posttraumatic stress disorder as a result of childbirth? A prospective study of incidence. *Birth* 2001;28:111–18.
77. Ballard CG, Stanley AK, Brockington IF. Post-traumatic stress disorder (PTSD) after childbirth. *Br J Psychiatry* 1995;166:525–8.
78. Wijma K, Soderquist J, Wijma B. Posttraumatic stress disorder after childbirth: A cross-sectional study. *J Anxiety Disord* 1997;11:587–97.
79. Creedy DK, Shochet IM, Horsfall J. Childbirth and the development of acute trauma symptoms: Incidence and contributing factors. *Birth* 2000;27:104–11.
80. Goldbeck-Wood S. Post-traumatic stress disorder may follow childbirth. *BMJ* 1996;313:774.
81. Soet JE, Brack GA, Dilorio C. Prevalence and predictors of women's experience of psychological trauma during childbirth. *Birth* 2003;30:36–46.

82. Czarnocka J, Slade P. Prevalence and predictors of post-traumatic stress symptoms following childbirth. *Br J Clin Psychol* 2000; 39(Pt 1):35–51.
83. Menage J. Post-traumatic stress disorder in women who have undergone obstetric and/or gynaecological procedures: A consecutive series of 30 cases of PTSD. *J Reprod Infant Psychol* 1993;11:221–8.
84. Ryding EL, Wijma B, Wijma K. Posttraumatic stress reactions after emergency cesarean section. *Acta Obstet Gynecol Scand* 1997; 76:856–61.
85. Melzack R. The myth of painless childbirth. *Pain* 1984;19: 321–37.
86. Lederman RP, Lederman E, Work BA, *et al.* Plasma epinephrine, norepinephrine, and cortisol of multigravidas in pregnancy and labor and in umbilical cord arteries after delivery. *J Psychosom Obstet Gynaecol* 1989;10:57–69.
87. Westgren M, Lindahl SGE, Nordén NE. Maternal and fetal endocrine stress response at vaginal delivery with and without epidural block. *J Perinat Med* 1986;14:235–41.
88. Whipple B, Josimovich JB, Komisaruk BR. Sensory thresholds during the antepartum, intrapartum and postpartum periods. *Int J Nurs Stud* 1990;27:213–21.
89. Charles AG, Norr KL, Block CR, *et al.* Obstetric and psychological effects of psychoprophylactic preparation for childbirth. *Am J Obstet Gynecol* 1978;31:44–52.
90. Melzack R, Taenzer P, Feldman P, *et al.* Labour is still painful after prepared childbirth training. *Can Med Assoc J* 1981;125:357–63.
91. Melzack R, Kinch RA, Dobkin P, *et al.* Severity of labour pain: Influences of physical as well as psychological variables. *Can Med Assoc J* 1984;130:579–84.
92. Melzack R. *The Puzzle of Pain.* Harmondsworth, Middlesex, UK: Penguin Books, 1973.
93. Derom H. Prevention of preterm labor through physiotherapy (abstract). *J Psychosom Obstet Gynaecol* 1983;2:171.
94. Villar J, Farnot U, Barros F, *et al.* A randomized trial of psychosocial support during high-risk pregnancies. *N Engl J Med* 1992;327: 1266–71.
95. Ulrich RS. View through a window may influence recovery from surgery. *Science* 1984;224:420–1.
96. Wissmeijer A, Vingerhoets AJJM. The use of virtual reality and audiovisual eyeglass systems as adjunct analgesic techniques: a review of the literature. *Ann Behav Med* 2005 Dec;30(3):268–78.
97. Reynolds, J. Post-traumatic stress disorder after childbirth: The phenomenon of traumatic birth. *Can Med Assoc J* 1997;156: 831–5.
98. Priest SR, Henderson J, Evans SF, *et al.* Stress debriefing after childbirth: a randomised controlled trial. *Med J Austral* 2003;178:542–5.
99. McFarlane AC. Debriefing: care and sympathy are not enough. Psychological first aid after traumatic events does not prevent later psychological disorders. *MJA* 2003;178:533–4.
100. Wuitchik M, Bakal D, Lipshitz J. Relationships between pain, cognitive activity and epidural analgesia during labor. *Pain* 1990; 41:125–32.

189 Intrapartum decision-making: a computational approach

J. E. Deaver

The medical literature provides clinicians with measures of effect that relate risks in patients exposed and unexposed to treatments and putative causative agents. Measures of effect include differences in risk between exposed and unexposed subjects and the ratio of these risks (relative risk), the latter being closely related to the odds ratio. Well-conducted trials in which exposures, usually treatments, are randomly assigned to patients are considered to provide the strongest evidence for effects. The high quality of evidence potentially generated by such trials is a function of the randomization process that produces equal proportions of potential confounders in exposed and unexposed groups. However, clinical decisions are made for individuals rather than groups. How should one extrapolate evidence obtained by the analysis of groups differing on a single exposure to the treatment of individual patients, each with his or her own multitude of traits? It has become popular to bridge the gap by attempting to make care uniform within groups. However, this approach only ignores the problem of within-group heterogeneity on a wide variety of factors including comorbid conditions and coexisting treatments for conditions other than the outcome addressed by a particular clinical guideline. Decision modeling is another approach to helping clinicians make the leap from clinical science to clinical practice. Decision modeling incorporates rather than ignores multiple factors that impact on outcomes and treatment decisions in individual patients. It is hoped that the reader will discover that decision modeling is helpful for difficult, not obvious, decisions.

As a practical example of decision modeling, this chapter examines the decision about whether to perform a cesarean section in order to prevent shoulder dystocia. This topic was selected because prevention of shoulder dystocia has been an intractable problem. It and its associated birth trauma (primarily brachial plexus injury) are largely regarded as complications that cannot usually be predicted or prevented. One approach to reducing risk would be to perform cesarean deliveries on all patients with antepartum or intrapartum risk factors associated with shoulder dystocia. However, current risk assessment is insufficiently specific for this approach; the number of unnecessary cesarean sections that would result have risks that are simply too large in relation to the number of shoulder dystocias that would be prevented.

Decision analysis utilizes many tools, including decision trees, Markov and Monte Carlo process modeling, regression analysis, neural networks, and Bayesian analysis. This chapter will focus on the techniques of multiple logistic regression and Bayesian analysis. It is intended that the reader develop a basic understanding of how a decision analysis is conducted using these two methods. An understanding of logistic regression and Bayesian analysis will provide the interested reader with a solid foundation from which to explore other methods of decision analysis.

There may be a temptation for readers of the medical literature to regard decision analysis as a 'black box', because all of the above methods are computationally intensive, and to focus on the results of decision analysis without an appreciation of the inherent limitations and assumptions. If the methods of decision analysis seem less daunting and the results more fallible after reading this chapter, then a useful purpose will have been served.

Basic probability concepts, definitions, and formulas

Two-by-two tables are used to illustrate many of the concepts to be presented. By convention, the left margin of a two-by-two table is labeled with the exposure, the top margin with the disease or outcome, the right margin with row totals, and the bottom margin with column totals as shown in the following:

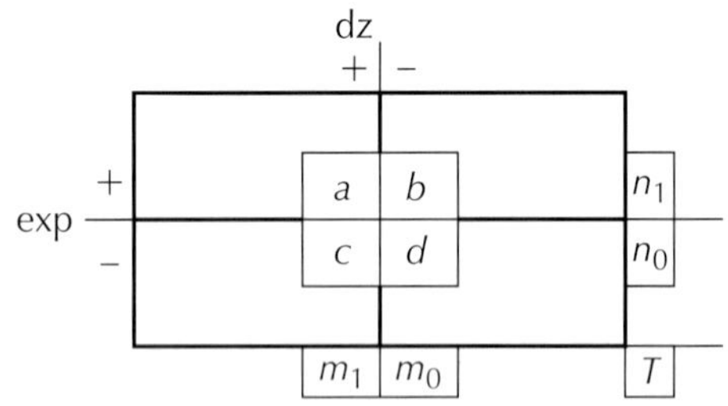

where 'exp' is the exposure including risk factors, tests, and treatments; 'dz' is the disease or outcome; '+' means positive (presence); and '–' means negative (absence). The cells 'a' through 'd', 'm_1', 'm_0', 'n_1', 'n_0', and 'T' have numbers (N) corresponding to the following:

$$
\begin{aligned}
&a=\text{exp}^{+}\text{dz}^{+}\ (N_{\text{(exposed diseased)}}),\\
&b=\text{exp}^{+}\text{dz}^{-}\ (N_{\text{(exposed disease-free)}}),\\
&c=\text{exp}^{-}\text{dz}^{+}\ (N_{\text{(non-exposed diseased)}}),\\
&d=\text{exp}^{-}\text{dz}^{-}\ (N_{\text{(non-exposed disease-free)}}),\\
&m_1=\text{dz}^{+}\ (N_{\text{(diseased)}}),\\
&m_0=\text{dz}^{-}\ (N_{\text{(disease-free)}}),\\
&n_1=\text{exp}^{+}\ (N_{\text{(exposed)}}),\\
&n_0=\text{exp}^{-}\ (N_{\text{(non-exposed)}}),\\
&T=a+b+c+d=n_1+n_0=m_1+m_0=(N_{\text{total}}).
\end{aligned}
$$

Probability notation can be understood in terms of a two-by-two table. The unconditional (baseline or prior) probabilities have the following notation:

$$P[\text{dz}^{+}]$$

read, 'the probability (or proportion) of diseased' prior to exposure, treatment or testing, and is equivalent to baseline disease prevalence. Prior probability of disease is derived from the two-by-two table *row* margin and is equal to m_1/T.

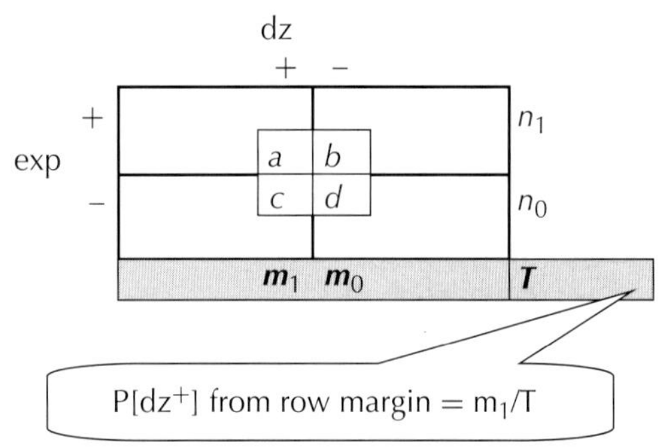

$$P[\text{exp}^{+}]$$

read, 'the probability (or proportion) of exposed (or treated or whose tests were positive)' without regard to disease, is equivalent to exposure prevalence. The prior probability of exposure is derived from the two-by-two table *column* margin and is equal to n_1/T.

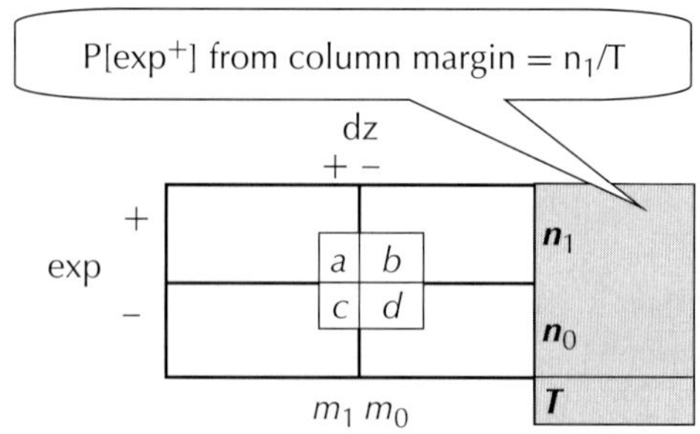

Conditional or posterior probabilities have the following notation:

$$P[\text{dz}^{+}\,|\,\text{exp}^{+}]$$

read, 'the probability of disease presence *given that* exposure is present', and is equivalent to risk in exposed or to positive predictive value when the exposure is a test (see below). The probability is conditioned on an exposure level, in this case on exposure being present. This conditional probability is determined from a *non-marginal row* of the two-by-two table and is equal to a/n_1.

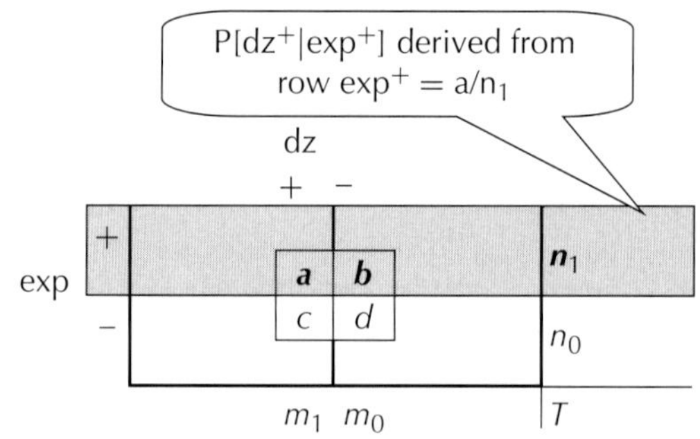

$$P[\text{exp}^{+}\,|\,\text{dz}^{+}]$$

read, 'the probability (or proportion) with positive test result *given that* disease is present', and is equivalent to sensitivity when exposure is a test (see below). The probability is conditioned on disease being present. This conditional probability is determined from a *non-marginal column* of the two-by-two table and is equal to a/m_1.

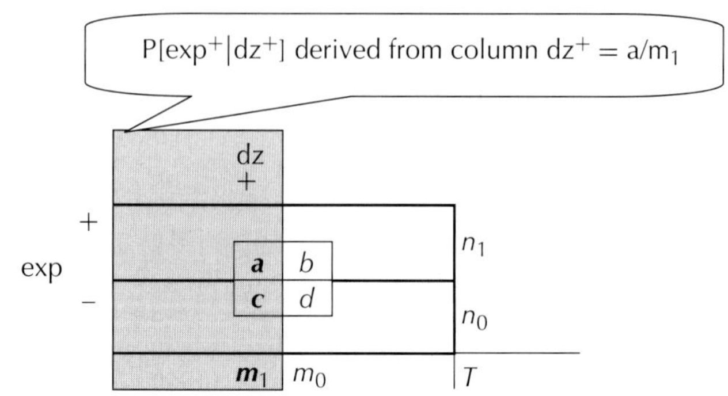

The following useful ratios, expressed in terms of a two-by-two table and in probability notation, are obtained from two-by-two table *columns*:

$a/(a+c) = a/m_1 = P[\text{exp}^+ \mid \text{dz}^+] =$ sensitivity (true-positive rate or detection rate), when exposure is a test;

$c/(a+c) = c/m_1 = P[\text{exp}^- \mid \text{dz}^+] =$ $1-$sensitivity (false-negative rate), when exposure is a test;

$d/(b+d) = d/m_0 = P[\text{exp}^- \mid \text{dz}^-] =$ specificity (true-negative rate), when exposure is a test;

$b/(b+d) = b/m_0 = P[\text{exp}^+ \mid \text{dz}^-] =$ $1-$specificity (false-positive rate), when exposure is a test.

The likelihood ratio of a positive test (LR^+) reflects how much greater are the odds of disease when a test result is positive and is found by the following:

Formula (1): Likelihood ratio (LR^+) = sensitivity/(1 − specificity) = true-positive rate/false-positive rate,

The probability (or proportion) of an attribute is the number with the attribute divided by the total of those with and without the attribute. After 100 tosses of a fair coin, one would expect 50 "heads" out of the total of 100 tosses. The probability (or proportion) of "heads" is 50/100 or 0.50.

The odds of an attribute are the number with the attribute divided by the remainder without the attribute. After 100 tosses of a fair coin, one would expect 50 "heads" and 50 "non heads" or "tails". The odds of "heads" are 50/50 or 1.

Exposure odds are the number exposed over the number unexposed.

Unconditional odds of exposure are the odds of exposure without consideration for whether disease is present or absent.

Unconditional or prior exposure odds, $\text{odds}[\text{exp}^+] = n_1/n_0$

Conditional exposure odds can be found for two strata, those with disease and those without disease.

$\text{odds}[\text{exp}^+ \mid \text{dz}^+] = a/c =$ exposure odds in diseased stratum

$\text{odds}[\text{exp}^+ \mid \text{dz}^-] = b/d =$ exposure odds in non-diseased stratum

Odds and probability (P) are interchangeable by using the following formulas:

Formula (2): $P = \text{odds}/(1+\text{odds})$

Formula (3): $\text{odds} = P/(1-P)$

Note that the exposure odds, $\text{odds}[\text{exp}^+|\text{dz}^+] = a/c$ and $\text{odds}[\text{exp}^+|\text{dz}^-] = b/d$ can converted to $P[\text{exp}^+|\text{dz}^+]$ (sensitivity; true-positive rate) and $P[\text{exp}^+|\text{dz}^-]$ (1 − specificity; false-positive rate), respectively.

The following useful ratios, expressed in terms of a two-by-two table and in probability notation, are obtained from two-by-two table *rows*:

$a/(a+b) = a/n_1 = P[\text{dz}^+ \mid \text{exp}^+]$

$b/(a+b) = b/n_1 = P[\text{dz}^- \mid \text{exp}^+]$

$c/(c+d) = c/n_0 = P[\text{dz}^+ \mid \text{exp}^-]$

$d/(c+d) = d/n_0 = P[\text{dz}^- \mid \text{exp}^-]$

Note that if exposure is a test, then $a/(a+b) = a/n_1 =$ positive predictive value (PPV). If the exposure is a risk factor, then $a/n_1 = \text{risk}_{(\text{exposed})}$ and $c/n_0 = \text{risk}_{(\text{unexposed})}$. Then

$(a/n_1)/(c/n_0) = \text{risk}_{(\text{exposed})}/\text{risk}_{(\text{unexposed})} =$ relative risk (RR).

Disease odds are the number with disease over the number without disease.

Unconditional odds of disease are the odds of disease without consideration for whether exposure is present or absent.

Unconditional odds or prior odds of disease, $\text{odds}[\text{dz}^+] = m_1/m_0$.

Conditional odds of disease can be found for two strata, those exposed and those unexposed.

$\text{odds}[\text{dz}^+ \mid \text{exp}^+] = a/b =$ disease odds in exposed stratum

$\text{odds}[\text{dz}^+ \mid \text{exp}^-] = c/d =$ disease odds in unexposed stratum

The odds of disease in exposed divided by odds of disease in unexposed, or

odds ratio (OR) = $\text{odds}[\text{dz}^+ \mid \text{exp}^+]/\text{odds}[\text{dz}^+ \mid \text{exp}^-] = (a/b)/(c/d) = (a \times d)/(b \times c)$,

i.e., the OR is the ratio of two-by-two table cross-products.

Note that when a disease is rare, i.e., when the numbers in cells 'a' and 'c' of the two-by-two table approach 0, then $a/(a+b)$ approaches a/b and $c/(c+d)$ approaches c/d. Relative risk (RR), $a/(a+b)/c/(c+d)$, then is approximately $(a/b)/(c/d)$, which is the odds ratio (OR). When disease prevalence is low, the OR becomes a reasonable approximation of RR.

Bayes' theorem can be expressed in the following useful form that relates prior or baseline disease odds ($\text{odds}[\text{dz}^+]$) to posterior odds or the conditional odds of disease given a positive test result ($\text{odds}[\text{dz}^+ \mid \text{exp}^+]$ where 'exp^+' is a positive test result) based on the likelihood ratio of a positive test (LR^+) which is the ratio of test characteristics (sensitivity/(1 – specificity)).

> *Formula (4):* Posterior odds =
> Likelihood ratio (LR^+) × Prior odds,
> i.e.,
> Conditional odds of disease given exposure =
> LR^+ × Unconditional odds of disease
> i.e.,
> $\text{odds}[dz^+|exp^+] = LR^+ \times \text{odds}[dz^+]$

Baseline prevalence (or prior probability) can be converted to prior odds using Formula (3); the posterior odds can be converted to post-test probability, or the positive predictive value of a test, using Formula (2).

As an example, suppose that we are given a baseline disease prevalence or prior probability, $P[dz^+]=0.25$, and test sensitivity, $P[exp^+|dz^+]=0.80$, and specificity, $P[exp^-|dz^-]=0.90$. Then,

$LR^+ = \text{sensitivity}/(1-\text{specificity}) = 0.80/(1-0.90) = 0.80/0.10 = 8.0$

$P[dz^+]$ = baseline disease prevalence = prior probability of disease = 0.25

Prior odds or $\text{odds}[dz^+]$, from $\text{odds} = P[dz^+]/(1-P[dz^+]) = 0.25/(1-0.25) = 0.25/0.75 = 0.333$

Posterior odds of disease given a positive test result or $\text{odds}[dz^+|exp^+] = LR^+ \times 0.33 = 8 \times 0.333 = 2.66$

Posterior probability $P[dz^+|exp^+]$, or positive predictive value (PPV) $= 2.66/(1+2.66) = 0.73$ (from $P = \text{odds}/(1+\text{odds})$).

A patient from a population with a baseline prevalence of disease 1-in-4 has a nearly 3-in-4 chance of disease given a positive test result. This result of Bayes' theorem can be confirmed by populating a two-by-two table to obtain PPV directly. Assume a population size (T) of 1000 patients.

	dz +	dz –	
exp +	a	b	n_1
exp –	c	d	n_0
	m_1	m_0	T **1000**

Then m_1 equals 250 given the baseline disease prevalence, $P[dz^+]$, that is $0.25 \times T$ and m_0, is the difference between T and $m_1=750$. This completes the row margin of the two-by-two table. Given that sensitivity, $P[exp^+|dz^+]=0.80$, the quantities 'a' and 'c' can be obtained where, $a=0.80 \times m_1 = 0.80 \times 250 = 200$; and $c = m_1 - a = 250 - 200 = 50$.

Given that specificity, $P[exp^-|dz^-]=0.90$, the quantities b and d can be obtained where,

$d = 0.90 \times m_0 = 675$; $b = m_0 - d = 750 - 675 = 75$.

The fully populated two-by-two table contains the following quantities:

$n_1 = a + b = 200 + 75 = 275$ and
$n_0 = c + d = 50 + 675 = 725$

	dz +	dz –	
exp +	200 (a)	75 (b)	n_1 275
exp –	50 (c)	675 (d)	n_0 725
	250 m_1	m_0 750	T 1000

The ratio a/n_1 is the positive predictive value (PPV) or the posterior probability of disease given a positive test result, $P[dz^+|exp^+] = 200/275 = 0.73$, confirming the earlier result obtained by using the likelihood ratio form of Bayes' theorem.

Given the same test, i.e., when test characteristics (sensitivity and specificity) are held constant, posterior probabilities vary directly in relation to baseline disease prevalence (prior probabilities). For instance, if our test with sensitivity 0.80 and specificity 0.90 were applied to a population with a baseline disease prevalence, $P[dz^+]$, of only 0.10 (rather than 0.25 as in the example above), then the following illustrates this point using Bayes theorem. Recall that the likelihood ratio of the given test, a constant, is 8. Prior probability of disease, $P[dz^+]=0.10$. Then our new prior odds is $0.10/(1-0.10) = 0.10/0.90 = 0.11$. The posterior odds = $LR^+ \times$ prior odds $= 8 \times 0.11 = 0.88$. Our new posterior probability, $P[dz^+|exp^+]$ or PPV, is equal to $0.88/(1+0.88) = 0.88/1.88 = 0.47$. The PPV associated with the same test is only 0.47 in contrast to the earlier result of 0.73. The difference is due to higher baseline prevalence in the first compared to the second example.

The general form of Bayes' theorem is written as

Formula (5):

$$P[A^+|X^+] = \frac{(P[X^+|A^+] \times P[A^+])}{(P[X^+|A^+] \times P[A^+]) + (P[X^+|A^-] \times P[A^-])}$$

If A = disease (dz) and X = exposure (exp), then:

$P[A^+|X^+] = P[dz^+|exp^+]$ = posterior probability of disease = positive predictive value,

> $P[X^+|A^+] = P[exp^+|dz^+]$ = true-positive rate = sensitivity, and
>
> $P[A^+] = P[dz^+]$ = prior probability of disease (baseline disease prevalence)

$P[X^+ | A^-] = P[\text{dz}^+ | \text{exp}^-]$ = false-positive rate = 1 − specificity

$P[A^-]$ = prior probability of non-disease = 1 − baseline prevalence of disease.

Therefore, if one is interested, as we have been, in deriving the probability of disease given an exposure level, in this case when exposure is present, and baseline disease prevalence and test characteristics are known, then Bayes theorem takes the following form [disease (dz) is substituted for *A* and the test exposure (exp) is substituted for *X*]:

Formula (6):

$$P[\text{dz}^+ | \text{exp}^+] = \frac{(P[\text{dz}^+ | \text{exp}^+] \times P[\text{dz}^+])}{(P[\text{dz}^+ | \text{exp}^+] \times P[\text{exp}^+]) + (P[\text{exp}+ | \text{dz}^-] \times P[\text{dz}^-])}$$

or, equivalently,

Formula (7):

$$\text{PPV} = \frac{(\text{Sens} \times \text{baseline dz prevalence})}{(\text{Sens} \times \text{baseline dz prevalence}) + [(1-\text{spec}) \times (1-\text{baseline dz prevalence})]}$$

To use our example of a test with sensitivity 0.80 and specificity 0.90 applied to a population with baseline disease prevalence 0.25, then the general form of Bayes theorem provides the same PPV of 0.73, as follows:

$$PPV = \frac{(0.80 \times 0.25)}{(0.80 \times 0.25) + (0.10 \times 0.75)} = \frac{(0.20)}{(0.275)} = 0.73$$

The utility of the general form of Bayes theorem, as given in Formula (5), can be seen by deriving sensitivity from baseline *exposure* prevalence and the relative risk of disease. Compared to the previous example, we reverse the substitution of exposure (exp) and disease (dz) for the terms '*A*' and '*X*' in Formula (5). Rather than *X* = exposure and *A* = disease, here we instead let *X* = disease and *A* = exposure, in which case:

$P[A^+ | X^+] = P[\text{exp}^+ | \text{dz}^+]$ = sensitivity,

$P[X^+ | A^+] = P[\text{dz}^+ | \text{exp}^+] = \text{risk}_{(\text{exposed})}$,

$P[X^+ | A^-] = P[\text{dz}^+ | \text{exp}^-] = \text{risk}_{(\text{unexposed})}$,

$P[A^+] = P[\text{exp}^+]$ = prior (baseline) exposure prevalence, and

$P[A^-] = P[\text{exp}^-]$ = prior non-exposure prevalence = (1 − prior exposure prevalence).

Then Bayes theorem takes the following form:

Formula (8):

$$P[\text{exp}^+ | \text{dz}^+] = \frac{(P[\text{dz}^+ | \text{exp}^+] \times P[\text{exp}^+])}{(P[\text{dz}^+ | \text{exp}^+] \times P[\text{exp}^+]) + (P[\text{dz}^+ | \text{exp}^-] \times P[\text{exp}^-])}$$

or, equivalently,

Formula (9):

$$\text{Sensitivity} = \frac{(\text{risk}_{(\text{exposed})} \times \text{baseline exp prevalence})}{((\text{risk}_{(\text{exposed})} \times \text{baseline exp prevalence}) + (\text{risk}_{(\text{unexposed})} \times (1-\text{baseline exp prevalence})))}$$

Assume that exposure is a risk factor with a baseline prevalence (prior probability of exposure) = 0.275. $\text{Risk}_{(\text{exposed})} = 0.73$. $\text{Risk}_{(\text{unexposed})} = 0.07$. Relative risk (RR) = 10.4. The 'sensitivity' of the risk factor for disease is $(0.73 \times 0.275)/((0.73 \times 0.275) + (0.07 \times (1-0.275))) = 0.80$. Sensitivity could be obtained alternatively by using the following forms of Bayes' theorem:

Formula (10): Posterior odds of exposure = RR × prior odds of exposure

or, when disease is rare, by,

Formula (11): Posterior odds of exposure = OR × prior odds of exposure

The prior odds of exposure = $0.275/(1-0.275) = 0.38$. Posterior odds of exposure given disease = $10.4 \times 0.38 = 3.95$. The posterior probability of exposure, $P[\text{exp}^+ | \text{dz}^+]$, or sensitivity = $3.95/(1+3.95) = 0.80$. From relative risk (RR) or odds ratio (OR) and baseline exposure prevalence, one can obtain sensitivity or the probability of exposure given disease, $P[\text{exp}^+ | \text{dz}^+]$.

Note that predictive value (the term used when exposure is a test) is synonymous with $\text{risk}_{(\text{exposed})}$ (the term used when exposure is a risk factor or treatment). Both are the posterior probability of disease given exposure, $P[\text{dz}^+ | \text{exp}^+]$.

One can determine $P[\text{dz}^+ | \text{exp}^+]$, the posterior probability of disease given exposure or positive predictive value or $\text{risk}_{(\text{exposed})}$, from $P[\text{exp}^+ | \text{dz}^+]/P[\text{exp}^+ | \text{dz}^-]$ (called the likelihood ratio if exposure is a test) and prior probability of disease.

One can determine $P[\text{exp}^+ | \text{dz}^+]$ (notice that 'exp' and 'dz' traded places), the posterior probability of exposure given disease or sensitivity, from $P[\text{dz}^+ | \text{exp}^+]/P[\text{dz}^+ | \text{exp}^-]$ (called the relative risk if exposure is a risk factor or treatment) and prior probability of exposure.

Creating a risk score for shoulder dystocia prevention

The above principles and formulas will be used to demonstrate the creation of a risk score for shoulder dystocia having a threshold (cutoff) value with sensitivity and specificity such that the number of additional cesarean sections needed to prevent a case of shoulder dystocia is acceptably small. The steps in creating such a risk scoring system are as follows:

(1) Use multiple logistic regression modeling to determine the adjusted regression coefficients for various risk factors that are associated with shoulder dystocia. For demonstration purposes, we will confine the analysis to three risk factors for shoulder dystocia (assisted vaginal delivery, i.e., vacuum extraction and forceps deliveries, diabetes, and fetal macrosomia).
(2) Use regression coefficients to determine, for various combinations of exposures, risk scores either as probabilities of shoulder dystocia or odds ratios of shoulder dystocia (where the denominator of the odds ratio is the odds in patients with none of these risk factors).
(3) Determine the probability distribution of risk scores.
(4) Determine the receiver-operator characteristics (sensitivity versus specificity) of various thresholds (cutoff values) of risk scores given the probability distribution of scores.
(5) Choose a score threshold that will result in the most cases of shoulder prevented at an acceptable cost in terms of the risks associated with additional cesarean sections.

Adjusted coefficients from multiple logistic regression modeling

Multiple logistic regression modeling is a technique for estimating the independent contribution of multiple exposures to outcomes measured as binary or dichotomous variables, such as shoulder dystocia that has the values 'present' or 'absent'. The regression coefficients can be used to determine the probabilities of the outcome for combinations of $i=1$ to j exposures, each having the value x_i,

Formula (12): $P[dz^+|\exp_{i=1,\ldots,j}$ having values $x_1,\ldots,x_j] = \dfrac{1}{1+e^{-(\beta_0+\Sigma_{i=1}^{j}\beta_i x_i)}}$

From a logistic regression analysis of binary predictors of coronary heart disease (CHD),[1] the coefficients given in Table 189.1 were obtained:

Notice that the values (x_is) of these binary variables are either 1 or 0.

A female patient with no risk factors ($x_{gender}=0$, $x_{smoking}=0$, $x_{age}=0$, $x_{hypertension}=0$, $x_{obesity}=0$) in the above study has the following estimated probability of developing CHD:

P[CHD$^+$|female, non-smoker, age <55, normotensive, non-obese] =

$$\frac{1}{1+e^{-[(\beta_0+(\beta_{gender}\times 0)+(\beta_{smoking}\times 0)+(\beta_{age}\times 0)+(\beta_{hypertension}\times 0)+(\beta_{obesity}\times 0)]}}$$

Formula (12), in this case, simplifies to

$$P[CHD^+|\exp_{i=1,\ldots,j}] = \frac{1}{1+e^{-\beta_0}}$$

so that the probability of CHD in a female with no risk factors is

P[CHD$^+$|female, non-smoker, age <55, normotensive, non-obese] =

$$\frac{1}{1+e^{-\beta_0}} = \frac{1}{1+e^{-(-4.567)}} = 0.0103,$$

i.e., there is only a 1% risk of CHD over the follow-up period defined by the study.

Therefore, only the coefficient for the intercept (β_0) is needed to estimate the probability of the outcome when the values of all predictors (x_is) are zero in which case all the $\beta_i x_i$s are also zero.

A male smoker who is young, hypertensive, and thin ($x_{gender}=1$, $x_{smoking}=1$, $x_{age}=0$, $x_{hypertension}=1$, $x_{obesity}=0$) has the following estimated probability for CHD:

P[CHD$^+$|male, smoker, age <55, hypertensive, non-obese] =

$$\frac{1}{1+e^{-[(\beta_0+(\beta_{gender}\times 1)+(\beta_{smoking}\times 1)+(\beta_{age}\times 0)+(\beta_{hypertension}\times 1)+(\beta_{obesity}\times 0)]}} =$$

$$\frac{1}{1+e^{-[(\beta_0+(\beta_{gender}\times 1)+(\beta_{smoking}\times 1)+(\beta_{hypertension}\times 1)]}} =$$

(since the x_is and $\beta_i x_i$s for age and obesity are zero). Therefore, the probability of CHD in this subject is

Table 189.1 CHD risk factors from the Atherosclerosis Risk in Communities (ARIC) study

Variables (i)/values (x_i)	β_i	Logistic regression coefficient	Odds ratio
Intercept	β_0	–4.567	
$i=1$, gender / male = 1, female = 0	β_1	1.311	3.71
$i=2$, smoking / yes = 1, no = 0	β_2	0.703	2.02
$i=3$, age > 54 years / yes = 1, no = 0	β_3	0.144	1.15
$i=4$, hypertension / yes = 1, no = 0	β_4	0.510	1.67
$i=5$, obesity / yes = 1, no = 0	β_5	0.192	1.21

P[CHD$^+$ | male, smoker, age < 55, hypertensive, non-obese] =

$$\frac{1}{1+e^{-(-4.567+1.311+0.703+0.510)}}=0.115,$$

i.e., there is a 11.5% risk of CHD over the same follow-up period.

Rather than using probability to quantify risk, the odds ratio can be used. Since odds $=P/(1-P)$, the odds of CHD is $0.115/(1-0.115)=0.13$ in young, hypertensive, thin male smokers; the odds of CHD is $0.0103/(1-0.0103)=0.0104$ when no risk factors are present. The ratio of odds in young, hypertensive, thin male smokers relative to odds in a referent group having no risk factors, or odds ratio (OR)=0.13/0.0104=12.5.

The odds ratio can also be calculated by obtaining, for each variable, the product term, β_i multiplied by the difference in x_is between the two groups, named 'a' and 'b' ($x_{ia}-x_{ib}$); the product terms are summed; this sum is exponentiated to obtain the odds for a combination of risk factors that are present (group a) contrasted to a group in which no risk factors are present (group b).

Formula (13):

$$\mathrm{OR}=\frac{\mathrm{Odds}[\mathrm{dz}^+|\exp_{i=1,\ldots,j}\text{ having value }x_{1a},\ldots,x_{ja}]}{\mathrm{Odds}[\mathrm{dz}^+|\exp_{i=1,\ldots,j}\text{ having value }x_{1b},\ldots,x_{jb}]}=e^{\Sigma_{i=1}^{i}\beta_i(x_{ia}-x_{ib})}$$

Young, hypertensive, thin, male smokers compared to young, normotensive, thin, female non-smokers have the following values (x_{ia} vs. x_{ib}) of these five variables: $x_1=x_{gender}=1$ vs. 0, respectively; $x_2=x_{smoking}=1$ vs. 0; $x_3=x_{age}=0$ vs. 0; $x_4=x_{hypertension}=1$ vs. 0; $x_5=x_{obesity}=0$ vs. 0. Each difference is multiplied by the respective coefficients and these values are summed, the result of which is exponentiated. The odds ratio (OR) is therefore:

$$\frac{\mathrm{Odds[CHD\,|\,young,\ hypertensive,\ thin,\ male\ smoker]}}{\mathrm{Odds[CHD\,|\,young\ normotensive\ thin,\ female\ non\text{-}smoker]}}=$$

$$e^{(\beta_{gender}\times(1-0))+(\beta_{smoking}\times(1-0))+(\beta_{age}\times(0-0))+(\beta_{hypertension}\times(1-0))+(\beta_{obesity}\times(0-0))}=$$
$$e^{(\beta_{gender}+\beta_{smoking}+\beta_{hypertension})}=$$
$$e^{(1.311+0.703+0.510)}=12.5$$

which is equivalent to the odds ratio we obtained by converting probabilities associated with the same two groups. Probabilities or relative probabilities (relative risks) or relative odds (odds ratios) can be used to construct risk scores. Odds ratios are commonly reported in the literature from which we will obtain our estimates of the effects of individual variables.

By using Formula (14), individual coefficients, β_is, can be obtained when odds ratios are reported in the literature.

Formula (14): $\beta_i=\ln(\mathrm{OR}_i)$,

presuming a difference of 1 between two exposure levels.

Conversely, Formula (15) can be used to convert a coefficient to an odds ratio.

Formula (15): $\mathrm{OR}_i=e^{\beta_i}$

Therefore, from the individual odds ratios reported in the literature, we can determine the individual coefficients by using Formula (14). Risk scores consisting of odds ratios for combinations of variables that differ from a referent group having no risk factors can be obtained using Formula (13). The advantage of this approach is that the coefficient for the intercept, which is usually not reported in the literature and which cannot be calculated by knowing odds ratios, is unnecessary for computing the score.

The literature was surveyed to identify, for a variety of exposures, their odds ratios for shoulder dystocia. The exposures surveyed included diabetes, fetal macrosomia, and assisted vaginal delivery by forceps or vacuum extractor.

The odds of shoulder dystocia are 1.7–6.0 times greater in diabetics compared to non-diabetics.[2–4] I assumed an odds ratio of 6 for the association of diabetes with shoulder dystocia.

The odds of shoulder dystocia are 3.5–20.4 times greater in neonates with birth weights more than 4000 g compared to smaller neonates.[2,4,5] I assumed an odds ratio of 20 for the association of macrosomia with shoulder dystocia.

The odds of shoulder dystocia are 1.9–3.5 times greater in assisted vaginal deliveries compared to spontaneous vaginal deliveries.[2,4] I assumed an odds ratio of 3.5 for the association of assisted vaginal deliveries with shoulder dystocia.

These selected odds ratios (OR_i) and their regression coefficients, calculated using Formula (14), are summarized in Table 189.2.

Table 189.2 Odds ratios for risk factors for shoulder dystocia (S)

Exposure (exp_i)	$OR_i = \frac{odds[S^+[exp_i^+]}{odds[S^+[exp_i^-]}$	Coefficients [ln(OR) $= \beta$]
i=A, assisted vaginal delivery*	3.5	$\beta_A = 1.25$
i=D, diabetes	6.0	$\beta_D = 1.79$
i=M, macrosomia	20	$\beta_M = 3.00$

*Vacuum extraction or forceps vaginal delivery

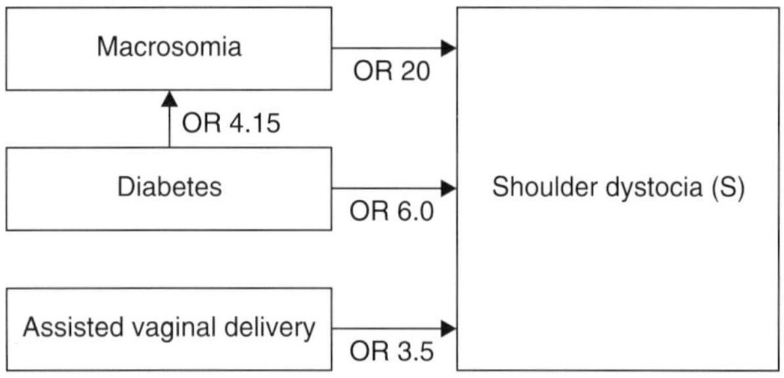

Figure 189.1 Associations between risk factors and shoulder dystocia.

Table 189.3 Selected prior probabilities based on literature review

Factor or outcome	Prevalence
Shoulder dystocia (S)	0.01
Macrosomia (M)	0.10
Diabetes (D)	0.05
Assisted delivery (A)	0.10

The direction and magnitudes of the effects of these risk factors on the outcome of shoulder dystocia are shown in Figure 189.1. Diabetes also influences the probability of macrosomia. The odds of macrosomia are 3–4.2 times greater in diabetic pregnancies.[6,7] I assumed an odds ratio of 4.2 for the association of diabetes with macrosomia.

One might expect for macrosomia and diabetes to negatively influence the probability of assisted vaginal delivery, although no data were available to support this hypothesis. One could also hypothesize that assisted vaginal deliveries, which are associated both with abnormal labor and with shoulder dystocia, merely confound an association between abnormal labor and shoulder dystocia. Shoulder dystocia might have occurred in these deliveries as a result of abnormal labor whether or not forceps had been applied. The prevalence of abnormal labor is likely to be increased with diabetes and macrosomia. Assisted delivery might also represent an intermediate (or intervening) variable in the effect of abnormal labor on shoulder dystocia, i.e., assisted vaginal delivery might be part of a causal pathway involving abnormal labor. Assisted vaginal delivery might also modify the effect of abnormal labor on shoulder dystocia. Since these causal pathways and interactions involving assisted vaginal delivery, abnormal labor, and either macrosomia or diabetes have not been studied, I assumed for purposes of this analysis that diabetes and macrosomia did not influence the probability of assisted vaginal delivery.

Whether macrosomia exists cannot be known prospectively. Our goal is a risk score based on prospectively available risk factors. Therefore, an ultrasound diagnosis of macrosomia should be substituted in our model for macrosomia. The odds ratios for the associations between an ultrasound finding of an EFW > 4 kg and both shoulder dystocia and diabetes are not available from the literature directly. We will determine these odds ratios using Bayesian methods and the reported associations between macrosomia and diabetes and between macrosomia and shoulder dystocia, and the reported sensitivities and specificities of an ultrasound diagnosis of macrosomia.

Prevalence data (prior probabilities) are necessary for what follows.

Langer *et al.* concluded from their review that shoulder dystocia complicates 0.1–1.7% of deliveries.[4] A prevalence of 1% will therefore be used for the prior probability of shoulder dystocia in our model.

Diabetes in some form complicates 2–8% of pregnancies.[3] The midpoint of this range, 5%, will be used for the prior probability of diabetes.

Vacuum extraction ands forceps deliveries account for 8–12% of all births.[8,9] The midpoint of this range, approximately 10%, will be used for the prior probability of assisted delivery.

Macrosomia, defined as birth weight more than 4000 g, occurs in 7.6–13.1% of pregnancies.[4,5] The midpoint of this range, approximately 10%, will be used for the prior probability of macrosomia.

The prior probabilities for purposes of this analysis are summarized in Table 189.3.

Based on their literature review, Rouse *et al.* concluded that typical sensitivities and specificities of ultrasound (USG > 4 kg) for fetal macrosomia (M) were 0.6 and 0.9, respectively.[10] The prior probability (baseline prevalence) of macrosomia, from Table 189.3,

Table 189.4 Association between ultrasound and macrosomia

USG >4 kg	M +		M −			
+	60 ($0.60 \times m_1$)	a	b	90	n_1	150
−	40	c	d	810 ($0.90 \times m_0$)	n_0	850
	100	m_1	m_0	900	T	1000

Table 189.5 Association between macrosomia and shoulder dystocia

M	S +		S −			
+	($0.69 \times 10 = 7$)	a	b	($n_1 - a = 93$)	$n_1 =$	100
−	($m_1 - a - 3$)	c	d	(m_0 $b = 897$)	$n_0 =$	900
	10	m_1	m_0	990	T	1000

is 0.10. These values allow us to populate a two-by-two table as shown (Table 189.4).

Note that the prevalence of an ultrasound EFW > 4 kg is 0.15, higher than the prevalence of macrosomia because false positives ($n = 90$) are in excess of false negatives ($n = 40$). Sensitivity = 60/100 = 0.6 and specificity = 810/900 = 0.9. The posterior probability of macrosomia given a positive ultrasound finding, $P[M^+|USG^+]$ or PPV = 60/150 = 0.4.

We can then find the posterior probability of shoulder dystocia given macrosomia, $P[S^+|M^+]$, and the posterior probability of shoulder dystocia given a normal birth weight neonate, $P[S^+|M^-]$, as follows.

Recall that the posterior odds, odds[exp$^+$|dz$^+$] (or in this case, odds[$M^+|S^+$]), are obtained by multiplying relative risk (RR) by the prior odds of exposure, odds[exp$^+$] (or in this case, odds[M^+]).

The requisite data are as follows: RR (of shoulder dystocia in macrosomia relative to non-macrosomia) = 20 (the odds ratio from Table 189.2 is used as a reasonable approximation of RR); From Table 189.3, $P[M^+]$ (baseline prevalence or prior probability of the macrosomia exposure) = 0.1.

Prior probability, $P[M^+] = 0.1$
Prior Odds$[M^+] = 0.1/(1 - 0.1) = 0.111$
Posterior Odds$[M^+|S^+] =$
RR $\times$ Prior Odds$[M^+] =$
$20 \times 0.111 = 2.22$
Posterior $P[M^+|S^+] = 2.22/(1 + 2.22) = 0.69$.

A two-by-two table of this association between the exposure (macrosomia) and the outcome (shoulder dystocia) can be populated (Table 189.5). The bottom margin is populated based on the prevalence of shoulder dystocia from Table 189.3 (0.01); the right margin is populated based on the prevalence of macrosomia from Table 189.3 (0.10). Cells 'a' and 'c' are populated based on the posterior probability $P[M^+|S^+] = 0.69$ (7/10). Cells 'b' and 'd' are populated when 'a' and 'c' are subtracted from 'n_1' and 'n_0', respectively.

Note that $P[S^+|M^+] = 7/100 = 0.07$ and that $P[S^+|M^-] = 3/900 = 0.0033$.

The 150 patients with a positive ultrasound finding of EFW > 4 kg (from Table 189.4), among whom 60 were macrosomic (n_1) and 90 were non-macrosomic (n_0), occupy the column margin of two-by-two (Table 189.6a).

The quantity 'a' $= P[S^+|M^+] \times 60 = 0.07 \times 60 = 4.2$. The quantity '$c$' $= P[S^+|M^-] \times 90 = 0.0033 \times 90 = 0.3$.

The 850 patients with a negative ultrasound finding of EFW > 4 kg, among whom 40 were macrosomic (n_1) and 810 were non-macrosomic (n_0), occupy the column margin of two-by-two (Table 189.6b).

The quantity 'a' $= P[S^+|M^+] \times 40 = 0.07 \times 40 = 2.8$. The quantity '$c$' $= P[S^+|M^-] \times 810 = 0.0033 \times 810 = 2.7$.

The marginal rows of Tables 189.6a and b are combined to show the association of ultrasound with shoulder dystocia (Table 189.7).

The original prior probabilities of positive ultrasounds (0.15) and shoulder dystocia (0.01) are preserved. Note that the odds ratio for the association of ultrasound findings of EFW > 4 kg and shoulder dystocia (Table 189.7),

$$\mathrm{OR} = \frac{(4.5 \times 844.5)}{(5.5 \times 145.5)} = 4.75$$

substantially lower than the OR for the association of macrosomia and shoulder dystocia because the positive ultrasound group has normal-weight neonates

Table 189.6a Association between macrosomia and shoulder dystocia given a positive ultrasound finding

USG+

		S +	S −			
M	(0.07 × 60 = 4.2)	a	b	($n_1 - a = 55.8$)	$n_1 =$	60 (given)
	(0.0033 × 90 = 0.3)	c	d	($n_0 - c = 89.7$)	$n_0 =$	90 (given)
	($a + c = 4.5$)	m_1	m_0	($b + d = 145.5$)	$T =$	150 (given)

Table 189.6b Association between macrosomia and shoulder dystocia given a negative ultrasound finding

USG−

			S +	S −			
M	+	(0.07 × 40 = 2.8)	a	b	($n_1 - a = 37.2$)	$n_1 =$	40 (given)
	−	(0.0033 × 810 = 2.7)	c	d	($n_0 - c = 807.3$)	$n_0 =$	810 (given)
		($a + c = 5.5$)	m_1	m_0	($b + d = 844.5$)		$T = 850$ (given)

Table 189.7 Association between ultrasound and shoulder dystocia

			S +	S −			
USG > 4kg	+	4.5	a	b	145.5	$n_1 =$	150
	−	5.5	c	d	844.5	$n_0 =$	850
		10	m_1	m_0	990	T	1000

and the negative ultrasound group has some macrosomic neonates.

The association between diabetes and an ultrasound EFW > 4 kg can be determined as follows: Prior probabilities (from Table 189.3) of diabetes, $P[D^+]$, and of macrosomia, $P[M^+]$, are 0.05 and 0.10, respectively, as shown in the two-by-two table margins (Tables 189.8a and b).

The prior probability of diabetes, $P[D^+]$, is converted to the prior odds of diabetes, odds$[D^+]$, using formula (3). Odds$[D^+]$ = $P[D^+]/(1 - P[D^+])$ = 0.05/(1 − 0.05) = 0.053.

An OR = 4.2 for macrosomia in diabetics relative to non-diabetics, as described previously, is used as a reasonable approximation of the RR.

Posterior Odds$[D^+|M^+]$ = OR × odds$[D^+]$ = 4.2 × 0.053 = 0.223

Posterior probability $P[D^+|M^+]$ = 1/(1 + 0.223) = 0.18

Then the quantity 'a' in Table 189.8b = $P[D^+|M^+] \times 100$ = 0.18 × 100 = 18. The values of 'b' and 'c' are determined by subtracting 'a' from 'n_1' and 'm_1', respectively. The value of 'd' is self-evident. Note that $P[D^+|M^-]$ = 32/900 = 0.036.

The 150 patients with a positive ultrasound finding of EFW > 4 kg (from Table 189.4), among whom 60 were macrosomic, occupy the following two-by-two table row margin (Table 189.9a). The quantity 'a' = $P[D^+|M^+] \times 60 = 0.18 \times 60 = 10.8$. The quantity '$b$' = $P[D^+|M^-] = 0.036 \times 90 = 3.2$.

The 850 patients with a negative ultrasound finding of EFW > 4 kg (from Table 189.4), among whom 40 were macrosomic, occupy the following two-by-two table row margin (Table 189.9b). The quantity 'a' = $P[D^+|M^+] \times 40 = 0.18 \times 40 = 7.2$. The quantity '$b$' = $P[D^+|M^-] = 0.036 \times 810 = 29.2$.

The column margins from these two tables are combined in Table 189.10, which shows the association between diabetes and ultrasound findings. Note that

Table 189.8a Prior probabilities of diabetes and macrosomia

D \ M	+	−		
+	a	b	n_1	50
−	c	d	n_0	950
	100 m_1	m_0 900	T	1000

Table 189.8b Association between diabetes and macrosomia

D \ M	+	−		
+	$(0.18 \times m_1 = 18)$ a	b $(n_1 - a = 32)$	n_1	50
−	$(m_1 - a = 82)$ c	d $(m_0 - b = 868)$	n_0	950
	100 m_1	m_0 900	T	1000

Table 189.9a Association between diabetes and macrosomia given a positive ultrasound

USG+

D \ M	+	−		
+	$(0.18 \times 60 = 10.8)$ a	b $(0.036 \times 90 = 3.2)$	n_1	14
−	$(m_1 - a = 49.2)$ c	d $(m_0 - b = 86.8)$	n_0	136
	60 (given) m_1	m_0 90 (given)	T	150

Table 189.9b Association between diabetes and macrosomia given a negative ultrasound

USG−

D \ M	+	−		
+	$(0.18 \times 40 = 7.2)$ a	b $(0.036 \times 810 = 29.2)$	n_1	36
−	$(m_1 - a = 32.8)$ c	d $(m_0 - b = 780.8)$	n_0	814
	40 (given) m_1	m_0 810 (given)	T	850

Table 189.10 Association between diabetes and ultrasound

D \ U	+	−		
+	14 a	b 36	n_1	50
−	136 c	d 814	n_0	950
	150 m_1	m_0 850	T	1000

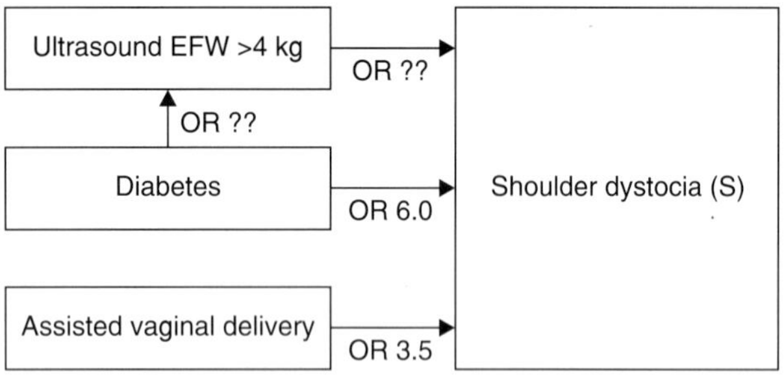

Figure 189.2 Unknown associations between prospective risk factors and shoulder dystocia.

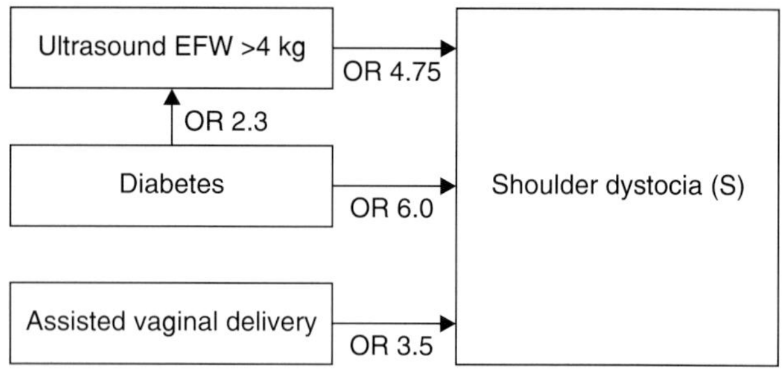

Figure 189.3 Results of Bayesian method to determine associations between prospective risk factors and shoulder dystocia.

Table 189.11 The effects of prospective risk factors (odds ratios)

Exposure (exp_i)	$OR_i = \dfrac{odds[S^+ \mid exp_i^+]}{odds[S^+ \mid exp_i^-]}$	**Coefficients ($\ln(OR) = \beta_i$)**
i=U, Ultrasound EFW >4 kg	4.75	$\beta_M = 1.56$
i=A, assisted vaginal delivery*	3.5	$\beta_A = 1.25$
i=D, diabetes	6.0	$\beta_D = 1.79$

*Vacuum extraction or forceps vaginal delivery

the prevalence of a positive ultrasound finding (0.15) and of diabetes (0.05) is preserved. The odds ratio for an ultrasound EFW >4 kg in diabetics relative to non-diabetics,

$$OR = ((a \times d)/(b \times c)) = ((14 \times 814)/(36 \times 136)) = 2.3,$$

is lower than the odds ratio describing the association of diabetes with macrosomia due to the misclassification of macrosomia by ultrasound as was described earlier.

The unknown effects in Figure 189.2 can now be replaced with these estimates determined using Bayesian methods (Figure 189.3).

Table 189.11 summarizes the selected odds ratios and their coefficients for these prospective risk factors. There are $2^3 = 8$ linear combinations of three exposures, each having two levels (present and absent). These combinations are as follows:

Assisted vaginal delivery (A^+)

	Ultrasound Present	EFW > 4 kg Absent
Diabetes Present	$U^+D^+A^+$	$U^-D^+A^+$
Absent	$U^+D^-A^+$	$U^-D^-A^+$

Spontaneous vaginal delivery (A^-)

	Ultrasound Present	EFW > 4 kg Absent
Diabetes Present	$U^+D^+A^-$	$U^-D^+A^-$
Absent	$U^+D^-A^-$	$U^-D^-A^-$

Scores are obtained by finding, for each combination, the odds ratio or the odds of shoulder dystocia in a given exposure combination divided by the odds of shoulder dystocia in a referent group. The referent group having no risk factors, i.e., where the values of all exposures (x_is) are zero, consists of patients with negative ultrasounds who are non-diabetic and have no indication for assisted vaginal delivery ($U^-D^-A^-$). These odds ratios for exposure combinations are obtained by exponentiating sums of the product terms, $\beta_i(x_{ia} - x_{ib})$, where β_is are the coefficients of individual exposures and $(x_{ia} - x_{ib})$ are the differences between values of individual exposures contrasting the combination of interest (group a) and the referent group (group b) as shown by Formula (13).

For instance, the odds ratio for shoulder dystocia (S) contrasting patients with an ultrasound EFW > 4000 g who are non-diabetic and have an indication for an assisted vaginal delivery, $U^+D^-A^+$, relative to the referent group having no risk factors, $U^-D^-A^-$, is determined based on the exposure differences, $(U^+ - U^- = 1 - 0 = 1)$, $(D^- - D^- = 0 - 0 = 0)$, and $(A^+ - A^- = 1 - 0 = 1)$ where U^+, D^+, and A^+ have the values 1, and U^-, D^-, and A^- have the values 0. The coefficient for each exposure is shown in Table 189.11.

$$OR = odds[S^+ \mid U^+D^-A^+]/odds[S^+ \mid U^-D^-A^-] =$$

$$e^{\beta_U(1-0) + \beta_D(0-0) + \beta_A(1-0)} = e^{\beta_U + \beta_A} = e^{1.56 + 1.26} = e^{2.81} = 16.6$$

The resulting odds ratios for all exposure combinations, which are the risk scores, are shown in Table 189.12.

Table 189.12 Odds ratios (risk scores) for exposure combinations

Exposure combination	OR	Formula	OR
$U^-D^-A^-$	$e^0=$	e^0	1
$U^-D^-A^+$	$e^{\beta_A}=$	$e^{1.25}$	3.5
$U^+D^-A^-$	$e^{\beta_U}=$	$e^{1.56}$	4.75
$U^-D^+A^-$	$e^{\beta_D}=$	$e^{1.79}$	6
$U^+D^-A^+$	$e^{\beta_U}+e^{\beta_A}=$	$e^{2.81}$	16.6
$U^-D^+A^+$	$e^{\beta_D}+e^{\beta_A}=$	$e^{3.04}$	21
$U^+D^+A^-$	$e^{\beta_U}+e^{\beta_D}=$	$e^{3.35}$	28.5
$U^+D^+A^+$	$e^{\beta_U+\beta_D+\beta_A}=$	$e^{4.60}$	99.75

Table 189.13 Final probability distribution of exposure combinations rank-ordered by risk score

Exposure combination	OR (risk score)	N
$U^-D^-A^-$	1	732.6
$U^-D^-A^+$	3.5	81.4
$U^+D^-A^-$	4.75	122.4
$U^-D^+A^-$	6	32.4
$U^+D^-A^+$	16.625	13.6
$U^-D^+A^+$	21	3.6
$U^+D^+A^-$	28.5	12.6
$U^+D^+A^+$	99.75	1.4
	Total	1000

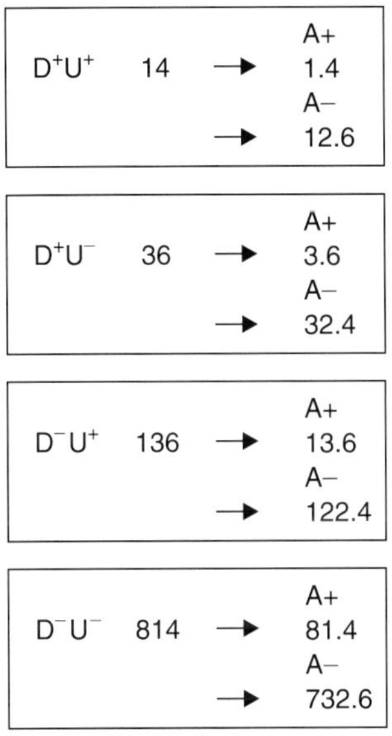

Figure 189.4 Combinations of diabetes and ultrasound stratified by assisted vaginal delivery.

Joint distribution of combinations of risk factors for shoulder dystocia

Given three risk factors for shoulder dystocia, namely ultrasound EFW > 4000 g (U), diabetes (D), and indication for assisted vaginal delivery (A), that have binary (dichotomous) values [either present (+) or absent (–)] we would like to know the joint probability distribution of the resulting combinations for which we now have risk scores.

From Table 189.10, we have the number with each combination of D and U. We assume for our purposes that the assisted vaginal deliveries (or the indications for operative vaginal delivery) are not conditioned on diabetes or ultrasound findings. Therefore, the prevalence of assisted vaginal delivery ($P[A^+]=0.10$) is presumed to be constant across all strata of diabetes and ultrasound findings (Figure 189.4).

Table 189.13 shows the final distribution of exposure combinations rank-ordered by risk scores. The receiver–operator characteristics for various score thresholds can then be determined. Any combination, e.g., $U^-D^-A^+$, relative to the referent group, $U^-D^-A^-$, can be shown in a two-by-two table. Assume that the probability of shoulder dystocia in the lowest risk group, $P[S^+ | U^-D^-A^-]=0.004$ (the reason for the choice of this probability will become clear). The two-by-two table quantity 'n_1' is N in Table 189.13 for the exposure $U^-D^-A^+$; the quantity 'n_0' is N for the exposure $U^-D^-A^-$. The quantity 'c' = $P[S^+ | U^-D^-A^-] \times n_0 = 0.004 \times 732.6 = 2.93$. This is the number of shoulder dystocia cases ($N_{(shoulder\ dystocia)}$) contributed by the $U^-D^-A^-$ exposure group (see Table 189.14)

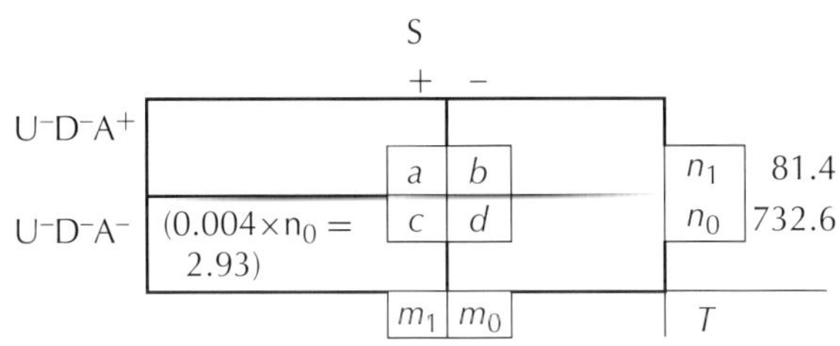

The prior odds of the exposure $U^-D^-A^+$ (where non-exposed $=U^-D^-A^-$) $=n_1/n_0=81.4/732.6 = 0.111$.

Recall that posterior odds of exposure given disease = OR × prior odds of exposure. The odds ratio from Table 189.12 is 3.5. Therefore,

$$\text{posterior odds, } P[U^-D^-A^+ | S^+] = 3.5 \times 0.111 = 0.39$$

This posterior odds of exposure given disease, in two-by-two table notation, is a/c = 0.39. By rearrangement, a = 0.39 × c. The quantity 'c', from above, is 2.93. Therefore, the quantity 'a' = 0.39 × 2.93 = 1.14. This is the number of shoulder dystocia cases ($N_{(shoulder\ dystocia)}$) contributed by the $U^-D^-A^+$ exposure group (see Table 189.14).

Table 189.14 shows the prior and posterior odds, calculated in a similar fashion, for the remaining exposure combinations and the resulting distribution of shoulder dystocia cases. Note that there are 10 shoulder dystocia cases across all exposure combinations that

	S +	S −	
Score ≥6	0.78 + 0.90 + 0.30 + 1.44 + 0.56 = **3.98** (a)	63.6 − 3.98 = **59.62** (b)	32.4 + 13.6 + 3.6 + 12.6 + 1.4 = **63.6** (n_1)
<6	2.93 + 1.14 + 2.33 = **6.40** (c)	936.4 − 6.4 = **930** (d)	732.6 + 81.4 + 122.4 = **936.4** (n_0)
	10.38 (m_1)	**989.62** (m_0)	1000 (T)

form the total population of 1000 subjects. In choosing a shoulder dystocia prevalence of 0.004 in the lowest-risk group ($U^-D^-A^-$), the original shoulder dystocia prevalence of 0.01 across all groups was preserved.

Table 189.13 and 189.14 were used to construct, for each score threshold, a table of sensitivities and specificities. Using a score threshold of 6 or higher, for example, the quantity 'n_1' in a two-by-two table, corresponding to the number of exposed (the number with a score ≥ 6) is found by summing the N's in Table 189.13 for OR's (risk scores) 6 and higher. The quantity 'n_0' is the sum of N's in table 189.13 for OR's < 6. The quantity 'a', corresponding to the number exposed and diseased (the number with a score ≥6 and shoulder dystocia) is found by summing the N's in Table 189.14

Table 189.14 Determination of probability distribution of shoulder dystocia by risk scores

Combination	OR (score)	N (total)	Prior odds of exposure	Posterior odds of exposure	*N* (shoulder dystocia)
$U^-D^-A^-$	1	732.6	1.00	1.00	2.93
$U^-D^-A^+$	3.5	81.4	0.11	0.39	1.14
$U^+D^-A^-$	4.75	122.4	0.17	0.79	2.33
$U^-D^+A^-$	6	32.4	0.04	0.27	0.78
$U^+D^-A^+$	16.6	13.6	0.02	0.31	0.90
$U^-D^+A^+$	21	3.6	0.00	0.10	0.30
$U^+D^+A^-$	28.5	12.6	0.02	0.49	1.44
$U^+D^+A^+$	99.75	1.4	0.00	0.19	0.56
		1000			10.38

Table 189.15 Sensitivities and specificities at score thresholds

	Shoulder dystocia (S)				
Score	Positive	Negative	Total		
≥3.5	7.44	259.96	267.40	sens	0.72
< 3.5	2.93	729.67	732.60	1 − spec	0.26
Total	10.38	989.63	1000.00		
≥4.75	6.31	179.70	186.00	sens	0.61
< 4.75	4.07	809.93	814.00	1 − spec	0.18
Total	10.38	989.63	1000.00		
≥6	3.98	59.62	63.60	sens	0.38
< 6	6.40	930.00	936.40	1 − spec	0.06
Total	10.38	989.63	1000.00		
≥16.6	3.20	28.00	31.20	sens	0.31
< 16.6	7.17	961.63	968.80	1 − spec	0.03
Total	10.38	989.63	1000.00		
≥21	2.30	15.30	17.60	sens	0.22
< 21	8.08	974.32	982.40	1 − spec	0.02
Total	10.38	989.63	1000.00		
≥28.5	2.00	12.01	14.00	sens	0.19
< 28.5	8.38	977.62	986.00	1 − spec	0.01
Total	10.38	989.63	1000.00		
≥99.75	0.56	0.84	1.40	sens	0.05
< 99.75	9.82	988.78	998.60	1 − spec	0.001
Total	10.38	989.63	1000.00		

Table 189.16 Receiver–operator characteristics of shoulder dystocia risk score

Score	1 – Specificity	Sensitivity
99.75	0.001	0.05
28.5	0.01	0.19
21	0.02	0.22
16.6	0.03	0.31
6	0.06	0.38
4.75	0.18	0.61
3.5	0.26	0.72

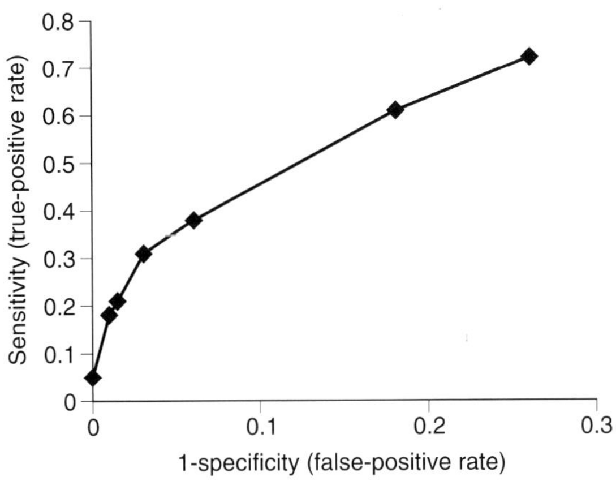

Figure 189.5 Receiver–operator characteristics of shoulder dystocia risk score.

for OR's 6 and higher. The quantity 'b' is the sum of N's in Table 189.14 for OR's <6. The remaining quantities are found by differences or sums. The quantity 'b' is n_1−a, 'd' is n_0−c, 'm_1' is a+c, and 'm_0' is b+d.

Sensitivity at this score threshold, $P[\text{Score} \geq 6 \mid S^+] = 3.98/10.38 = 0.38$. Specificity, $P[\text{Score} < 6 \mid S^-] = 930/989.62 = 0.94$. 1−specificity (the false-positive rate) = 0.06.

Similarly, the sensitivities and false-positive rates (1−specificity) for each score threshold were used to create Table 189.15.

The receiver–operator characteristics of the risk score are displayed in Table 189.16 and in Figure 189.5. We will explore the choice of a threshold value of the risk score at or above which cesarean section might be recommended to prevent shoulder dystocia. As noted, Langer *et al.*, based on literature review, reported that shoulder dystocia prevalence ranged from 0.001 to 0.17.[4] First, assume that baseline prevalence of shoulder dystocia in the population of interest is low (0.001). The baseline prevalence of shoulder dystocia affects the number needed to treat (NNT) or the number of cesarean sections required to prevent a single case of shoulder dystocia. The risk of shoulder dystocia in cesarean section, $\text{risk}_{(\text{cesarean})}$, is presumed to be zero. The risk of shoulder dystocia in vaginally delivered neonates, $\text{risk}_{(\text{vaginal})}$, is shown in Table 189.17. The absolute risk reduction (ARR) is the risk difference, $(\text{risk}_{(\text{vaginal})} - \text{risk}_{(\text{cesarean})})$. NNT = 1/ARR

Table 189.17 Number needed to treat (NNT) when shoulder dysocia risk is low ($P[S+]=0.001$)

Score	Shoulder dystocia Positive	 Negative	 Total	$\text{Risk}_{(\text{vaginal})}$	NNT
≥3.5	0.7	266.7	267.4	0.0028	359
<3.5	0.3	732.3	732.6		
	1.0	999.0	1000.0		
≥4.75	0.6	185.4	186.0	0.0034	295
<4.75	0.4	813.6	814.0		
	1.0	999.0	1000.0		
≥6	0.4	63.2	63.6	0.0063	160
<6	0.6	935.8	936.4		
	1.0	999.0	1000.0		
≥16.6	0.3	30.9	31.2	0.0103	97
<16.6	0.7	968.1	968.8		
	1.0	999.0	1000.0		
≥21	0.2	17.4	17.6	0.0131	77
<21	0.8	981.6	982.4		
	1.0	999.0	1000.0		
≥28.5	0.2	13.8	14.0	0.0143	70
<28.5	0.8	985.2	986.0		
	1.0	999.0	1000.0		
≥99.75	0.1	1.3	1.4	0.0399	25
<99.75	1.0	997.6	998.6		
	1.0	999.0	1000.0		

Table 189.18 Number needed to treat (NNT) when shoulder dysocia risk is high ($P[S+]=0.017$)

Score	Shoulder dystocia Positive	Negative	Total	$Risk_{(vaginal)}$	NNT
≥3.5	12.1	255.3	267.4	0.0452	22
<3.5	4.8	727.8	732.6		
	16.9	983.1	1000.0		
≥4.75	10.2	175.8	186.0	0.0551	18
<4.75	6.6	807.4	814.0		
	16.9	983.1	1000.0		
≥6	6.5	57.1	63.6	0.1017	10
<6	10.4	926.0	936.4		
	16.9	983.1	1000.0		
≥16.6	5.2	26.0	31.2	0.1668	6
<16.6	11.7	957.1	968.8		
	16.9	983.1	1000.0		
≥21	3.7	13.9	17.6	0.2121	5
<21	13.1	969.3	982.4		
	16.9	983.1	1000.0		
≥28.5	3.2	10.8	14.0	0.2316	4
<28.5	13.6	972.4	986.0		
	16.9	983.1	1000.0		
≥99.75	0.9	0.5	1.4	0.6484	2
<99.75	16.0	982.6	998.6		
	16.9	983.1	1000.0		

Table 189.19 Impact of risk scores on cesarean section rate (baseline=0.25)

Score threshold	Baseline number of cesareans	Number 'test positive'	New number of cesareans	N total	New cesarean section rate
≥3.5 vs. <3.5	333	267	600	1333	0.450
≥4.75 vs. <4.75	333	186	519	1333	0.389
≥6 vs. <6	333	64	397	1333	0.298
≥16.6 vs. <16.6	333	31	364	1333	0.273
≥21 vs. <21	333	18	351	1333	0.263
≥28.5 vs. <28.5	333	14	347	1333	0.260
≥99.75 vs. <99.75	333	1	334	1333	0.251

which, in this case where the risk in cesarean section is zero, equals $1/risk_{(vaginal)}$.

The risk scoring system in this low-prevalence scenario has no value. Even the highest risk score of 99.75 is an unacceptable threshold since 25 cesarean sections are required to prevent a single case of shoulder dystocia. Even then, only 10% of shoulder dystocia cases would be prevented.

When the baseline prevalence of shoulder dystocia in the population of interest is at the upper end of the range reported by Langer *et al.* ($P[S^+]=0.017$), $risk_{(vaginal)}$, is consequently higher and the NNT (number of cesarean sections to prevent a single case of shoulder dystocia) is lower, as shown in Table 189.18.

In this high-prevalence scenario, the risk scoring system performs quite well. A score threshold of 16.6 requires 6 cesarean sections to prevent a single case of shoulder dystocia and prevents nearly one-third of all shoulder dystocias.

We assume that our population, $T=1000$, consists only of vaginally delivered patients. Assume that the cesarean section rate is 25%. Let x = the baseline number of cesarean sections. Then,

$$0.25(x+1000)=x$$

$$0.25x+250=x$$

$$250=x-0.25x=0.75x$$

$x=250/0.75=333$ cesarean sections (at baseline).

The total number delivered is 1000 + 333 = 1333 by vaginal and abdominal routes. The number of additional cesarean sections (the number who are 'test positive') is added to the baseline number of 333 and the new cesarean section rate is calculated for each risk score, as shown in Table 189.19.

The risk score of 16.6 seems to be an acceptable threshold that would result in 31 additional cesarean sections, an increase in the cesarean section rate from 25% to 27%, and prevention of nearly one-third of 17 shoulder dystocia cases.

Practical issues

Prior probabilities of shoulder dystocia, macrosomia, diabetes, and assisted deliveries were selected from the literature, as were the effects of risk factors on shoulder dystocia and of diabetes on macrosomia, as well as the test characteristics (sensitivity and specificity) of ultrasound for diagnosis of macrosomia. While I used the midpoints of reported prevalence ranges, I used the highest reported estimates of effects. This suffices for illustration, but the reader is cautioned that a risk scoring system should ideally be examined across the full range of prior probabilities and effect estimates during a process of *sensitivity analysis*. The importance of sensitivity analysis is illustrated by the exploration of 'number needed to treat' across a range of shoulder dystocia prevalence. The risk scoring system had no value when the shoulder dystocia prevalence was at the lowest end of the range reported in the literature. Finally, I took the liberty of using unadjusted effect estimates since few adjusted estimates are available. Obviously, adjusted estimates are required before a model is suitable for further testing. Before a risk scoring system is put into practice, it should be tested against recent data from the actual population in which it will be used. Such data are often not available. However, as electronic patient records become increasingly available, there will emerge databases with a sufficient number of discretely coded variables to allow model testing. For that matter, such databases will provide more accurate prior probabilities and allow for logistic regression modeling to obtain adjusted effect estimates that are often not available from the literature. Regression modeling should be performed against a portion of the database; the remainder of the data are reserved for testing whether the resulting scoring system performs as expected against novel data.

REFERENCES

1. Chambless LC, Heiss G, Folsom AR. Association of coronary heart disease incidence with carotid arterial wall thickness and major risk factors: The Atherosclerosis Risk in Communities (ARIC) study. *Am J Epidemiol* 1997,146.483–94.
2. Nesbitt TS, Gilbert WM, Herrchen B. Shoulder dystocia and associated risk factors with macrosomic infants born in California. *Am J Obstet Gynecol* 1998;179:476–80.
3. Moore TR. Diabetes in Pregnancy. In Creasy RK, Resnik R, eds. *Maternal-Fetal Medicine: Principles and Practice*, 5th edn. Philadelphia, PA: Saunders, 2004:1023–61.
4. Langer O, Berkus MD, Huff RW, Samueloff A. Shoulder dystocia: Should the fetus weighing >4000 grams be delivered by cesarean section? *Am J Obstet Gynecol* 1991;165:831–7.
5. Perlow JH, Wigton T, Hart J, Strassner HT, Nageotte MP, Wolk BM. Birth trauma: A five-year review of incidence and associated perinatal factors. *J Reprod Med* 1996;41:754–60.
6. Combs CA, Gunderson E, Kitzmiller J. Relationship of macrosomia to maternal postprandial glucose control during pregnancy. *Diabetes Care* 1992;15:1251.
7. Hunter DJ, Burrows RF, Mohide PT. Influence of maternal insulin-dependent diabetes mellitus on neonatal morbidity. *Can Med Assoc J* 1993;149(1):47.
8. Martin JA, Hamilton BE, Sutton PD. Births: Final data for 2002. *Natl Vital Stat Rep* 2002;52:1.
9. Kozack LJ, Weeks JD. U.S. trends in obstetric procedures. *Birth* 2002;29:157.
10. Rouse DJ, Owen J, Goldenberg RL, Cliver SP. The effectiveness and costs of elective cesarean delivery for fetal macrosomia diagnosed by ultrasound. *J Am Med Assoc* 1996;276:1480–6.

SECTION XIX

Maternal disease

Section Editors: **A. Grunebaum and L. Voto**

190 Periconception care

A. Grunebaum

Introduction

Prenatal care is an important intervention in the early diagnosis and prevention of adverse pregnancy outcome. Since the introduction of prenatal care, early in the last century, women have been advised by their obstetricians to register for prenatal care only after they miss their period or when their pregnancy has been confirmed, and many obstetricians do not even give their patients an appointment for the first prenatal visit until late in the first trimester.

Periconception care, caring for couples before pregnancy, on the other hand is a relatively new approach to improve pregnancy outcome.

In its 'Healthy People 2010' report, the US Public Health Service has underscored the importance of preconception care by including several recommendations promoting the health of women before pregnancy (www.health.gov/healthypeople/). Benefits of periconception care, such as the early identification of potential problems and medical treatment before pregnancy, seem apparent, yet only recently evidence has emerged supporting improved outcomes in certain conditions (e.g. diabetes mellitus, phenylketonuria, and a previous pregnancy with a fetus with a neural tube defect).[1–3] De Weerd has shown that two of the major components of preconception care, smoking cessation and folic acid supplementation, can lead to a significant cost-saving balance.[4]

Periconception care begins prior to pregnancy at a time when preparations for pregnancy can be made. Periconception care usually involves one or more meetings prior to pregnancy between the couple trying to conceive and a doctor or another health care provider who is experienced in this area. Any doctor with interest in this area can provide many aspects of periconception care, but the obstetrician and gynecologist are best trained to handle most aspects of periconception care.

There is an evolving science showing that seeing a doctor prior to pregnancy, when the couple starts thinking about a family, can improve pregnancy outcomes for both the mother and the baby.

Since up to 50% of pregnancies are unintended,[5,6] promoting health and healthy lifestyles prior to pregnancy is crucial among all childbearing couples, especially as planned pregnancies have better outcomes than unplanned ones.[7] Thus, the overall goal of periconceptional care is to ensure that:

(1) Women and men are in their best health and practice healthy lifestyles before conception.
(2) Couples become aware that preconception, conception, pregnancy, birth, and childrearing are a continuum in which earlier events affect the present and the future.
(3) Physicians and care providers are able to identify prior to conception any issues and resolve them without being concerned about the ongoing pregnancy.

The best example of how periconception care can improve pregnancy outcome is supplementation with folic acid. An increase in the intake of folic acid among women planning a pregnancy was shown to prevent most neural tube defects.[8,9]

Freda *et al.*[10] summarized the thinking about preconception health into the following acronym: REFRAMED: Reproductive awareness; Environemental toxicants and teratogens; Folic acid supplementation; Review genetic history; Alcohol, tobacco, and other substance use; Medical conditions and medications; Evaluate immunizations and infectious diseases; Domestic violence and psychosocial issues.

The key elements of preconception care include the following.

(1) Obtaining a thorough personal, medical, and family history of the potential mother and father and an assessment of the health of both potential parents, although a greater emphasis is usually placed on that of the mother.
(2) Obtaining a genetic history about family members with genetic problems and congenital birth defects and conditions like hypertension, diabetes, mental retardation, blindness, and deafness and testing if indicated.
(3) Review of the reproductive and gynecologic history and prior pregnancies.

(4) Reviewing the couple's daily living habits and the environment, reviewing medications both prescription and over the counter and screening for exposure to potentially harmful substances both at home or at work; reviewing weight, diet, and food and providing specific nutritional and exercise counseling.
(5) Review and optimization of fertility.
(6) Medical and gynecologic examination, reviewing and screening for infectious diseases, and updating immunizations performing additional tests if indicated [e.g. blood samples and other tests of both parents if indicated, for example, human immunodeficiency virus (HIV), infectious diseases, and genetic predisposition].
(7) Male periconception counseling.

The key elements of periconception counseling include the following:

(1) Medical history and medication review

- Diabetes – identify prior to pregnancy and optimize control.
- Hypertension – avoid angiotensin-converting enzyme (ACE) inhibitors, angiotensin II receptor antagonists, and thiazide diuretics.
- Epilepsy – optimize control; folic acid, 1 mg/day.
- Deep venous thrombosis (DVT) – switch from warfarin (Coumadin) to heparin.
- Depression/anxiety – avoid benzodiazepines.

(2) Genetic history

- Review family history of genetic issues.
- Carrier screening (ethnic background): sickle cell anemia, thalassemia, Tay–Sachs disease.
- Carrier screening (family history): cystic fibrosis, non-syndromic hearing loss (connexin-26).

(3) Reproductive and gynecologic history

- Review prior pregnancy outcomes and counsel about recurrence.
- Review prior gynecologic history.
- Review history of pelvic inflammatory disease (PID) or other tubal issues.

(4) Living environment: diet, weight, food, and medications

- Folic acid supplement (400 μg routine, 1 mg diabetes/epilepsy, 4 mg previous neural tube defect).
- Assess weight, calculate body mass index (BMI), advise optimal BMI.
- Recommend regular exercise in moderation.
- Avoid hyperthermia (hot tubs, overheating).
- Assess risk of nutritional deficiencies (vegan, pica, milk intolerance, calcium or iron deficiency).
- Avoid overuse of vitamin A (limit to 3000 IU/day) and vitamin D (limit to 400 IU/day).
- Limit caffeine to two cups of coffee or six glasses of soda per day.
- Screen for domestic violence
- Household chemicals – avoid paint thinners and strippers, other solvents, and pesticides.
- Smoking cessation and avoidance of secondary smoking.
- Screen for alcoholism and use of illegal drugs.

(5) Fertility review and optimization

- Assess for regular ovulation, signs of polycystic ovarian syndrome (PCOS).
- Discuss fertility after birth control.
- Review frequency and timing of sexual intercourse.
- Refrain from using lubricants.

(6) Medical examination and testing; immunization

- Test for infectious diseases (e.g. HIV, syphilis).
- Hepatitis B immunization for at-risk patients.
- Preconception immunizations (rubella, varicella).
- Counsel about avoidance of infections [e.g. toxoplasmosis, cytomegalovirus (CMV), and parvovirus B19].
- Suggest a dental examination.

(7) Male periconception counseling and assessment

- Medical history and review.
- Review of potentially harmful exposure.
- Avoid exposure to heat.
- Avoid alcohol and smoking and other harmful substances.
- Suggest sperm analysis.

Medical history and health assessment

The first step

Because many medical problems place the mother and the fetus at risk,[11] the first step in identifying potential issues is to obtain a good medical and social history. Many doctors have their patients' first fill in a periconception questionnaire or health assessment form. This questionnaire can help in the counseling and care process and organizes the periconceptual approach.[12] Filling out this questionnaire is not only time-saving, but it also allows for a complete evaluation of the couple's medical and surgical history. In addition, it allows enough time to consider all answers and helps the provider to focus only on the significant issues.

Below is a sample questionnaire, which can be individualized for each special circumstance:

Sample periconception patient questionnaire

	Yes	No
Are you taking any prescription drugs?		
Are you using birth control pills or other hormonal contraceptives?		
Do you use over-the-counter (non-prescription) drugs?		
Do you take any vitamins, minerals, herbal supplements, or other food supplements?		
Do you take a multivitamin containing 0.4 mg of folic acid every day?		
Do you use any recreational or street drugs (e.g. marijuana, cocaine, crack, etc.)?		
Do you smoke cigarettes? If yes, how many per day?		
Do you breathe second-hand smoke?		
Do you drink beer, wine, or hard liquor?		
How many drinks does it take to make you feel high?		
Have people annoyed you by criticizing your drinking?		
Have you felt you ought to cut down on your drinking?		
Have you ever had a drink first thing in the morning to steady your nerves or get rid of a hangover?		
Have you recently seen a dentist?		
Are you over- or underweight?		
Personal information: Tell us about you and your partner		
Family and genetic history: Tell us about your family and your genetic history		
Your daily living and the environment: Tell us about your daily routines and your environment.		
Are you exposed to any harmful agents?		
Diet and food: Tell us about your diet and food		
Trying to conceive history: Tell us about your attempts trying to conceive		
Gynecologic history: Tell us about your gynecologic history		
Medical history: Tell us about your medical history		
Infections: Have you ever had an infection or a sexually transmitted disease?		
Immunizations: Are you immunized against common childhood diseases and hepatitis B?		
Prior pregnancies: Tell us about your prior pregnancies		
What is your ethnic background?		
Have you or the baby's father ever been screened for special diseases related to your ethnic background?		
Have you or your partner had a baby with a genetic (inherited) problem or have there been any birth defects or mental retardation in the family?		
Does anybody in the family have a history of a genetic disease, such as cystic fibrosis, Tay–Sachs disease, hemophilia?		
Do you have a close family member with a medical condition, such as diabetes or a history of seizures?		
Did your mother have toxemia or high blood pressure in any of her pregnancies?		
Do you or a close family member have a history of blood clots?		
Do you have a close family member with ovarian or breast cancer?		

Please enter here and explain for any question where you checked a 'YES'.

Diabetes mellitus

Women with poorly controlled diabetes have a significantly higher rate of spontaneous abortion and increased risk of severe fetal anomalies compared with women who have good control. Preconception diabetic management decreases the risk of abortions and congenital anomalies and lessens the complications of pregnancy. Preconception is the optimal time to identify, evaluate, and treat hypertension, nephropathy, retinopathy, and thyroid disease in these patients and provide counseling on risks of pregnancy, requirement for increased visits, and close monitoring. In addition, periconception provides the opportunity to evaluate patients for relative contraindications to pregnancy, such as those with blood urea nitrogen greater than 30 mg/dl (10.7 mmol/l), low creatinine clearance, and coronary artery disease.

Hypertension

Most patients with chronic hypertension can expect an uncomplicated pregnancy, but will require enhanced monitoring for the risks of pre-eclampsia, renal insufficiency, and fetal growth retardation. It is important that women with hypertension be evaluated before pregnancy to determine the severity of the hypertension and to recommend potential lifestyle modifications. Preconception is the best time to review and change medications for use during pregnancy. Methyldopa (Aldomet) and calcium channel blockers are commonly used during pregnancy. Drugs that should be avoided in the first and second trimesters of pregnancy are ACE inhibitors, angiotensin II receptor antagonists, and thiazide diuretics, which are associated with congenital defects.

Epilepsy

The incidence of malformations in infants of mothers with epilepsy who are treated with antiepileptic drugs is two to three times that of infants of mothers without epilepsy,[13] and they also have an increased risk of developing epilepsy. Preconception counseling should include optimizing seizure control, prescribing folic acid supplements, 1–4 mg/day, and offering referral to a genetic counselor. When possible, use of multiple anticonvulsants should be avoided. Using a single agent for the seizure type at the lowest protective level is preferable, and there is no single drug of choice. If a patient has been seizure-free for 2 years or longer, drug discontinuation with a long taper period (3 months) may be successful in individual cases, and tapering should begin 6 months prior to conception.[14]

Thromboembolism

Women with a history of a DVT have a 7–12% risk of recurrence during pregnancy, and those with a personal or family history of venous thromboembolism should be offered testing for thrombophilia before pregnancy. Those on warfarin (Coumadin) as maintenance therapy for DVT should be switched to heparin before conception, because warfarin is teratogenic. Heparin (in regular or low-molecular weight form) is indicated for prophylaxis and should be started as early in pregnancy as possible.

Depression and anxiety

About 10% of pregnant women have depression. Tricyclic antidepressants and selective serotonin reuptake inhibitors have not been shown to cause any teratogenic effects and may be used before conception. Rarely, maternal use of benzodiazepines has been associated with anomalies, such as cleft lip and palate, as well as a withdrawal syndrome in the newborn.

Asthma

Asthma is one of the most common medical illnesses likely to occur in women of childbearing age, with approximately 1% of pregnancies complicated by asthma. Optimizing preconceptional asthma control and reviewing use of the peak flow meter and personal best surveillance, and offering influenza vaccine ensures that the patient begins her pregnancy in optimal condition. The fewest medications needed to control symptoms of asthma should be recommended.

Cardiac diseases

Maternal morbidity from cardiac diseases is as high as 7% in combined New York Heart Association classes III and IV heart disease, compared to only 0.5% in combined classes I and II. Certain cardiac disorders, such as primary pulmonary hypertension, place women at very high risk during pregnancy (maternal mortality approaches 50%) and counseling prior to pregnancy may help couples decide on the best course. The preconception evaluation should therefore identify cardiac disease risk factors, determine the extent of disease, identify correctable problems, and provide the patient with detailed information about maternal and fetal risks. Close consultation before and during pregnancy with a cardiologist may help guide a patient though the pregnancy.

Autoimmune disorders

Autoimmune disorders, such as lupus, are not unusual among women of childbearing age. Patients should be counseled that the best time to attempt conception is during periods of inactive disease. Even women with quiescent disease or a distant history of disease should be carefully evaluated and counseled about maternal and fetal risks.

Obtaining a genetic history

Genetic issues

The woman's family history and ethnicity for genetic disorders (such as cystic fibrosis, sickle cell anemia, and Tay–Sachs disease) and malformations (such as neural tube defects) should be reviewed thoroughly during the periconception visit. The clinician should consider referring the patient to a genetic counselor or maternal–fetal specialist if there is a personal or family history of a child with a potential genetic disorder or if advanced maternal age is an issue.

Advanced maternal age

The periconception time period is the optimal time to educate patients about a woman's fertility 'biologic time clock' and the purposes and techniques of prenatal diagnosis during pregnancy.

Women becoming pregnant at more advanced ages are at increased risk of

- Infertility
- Having fetuses with chromosomal abnormalities
- An increased likelihood of chronic medical illness.

Advanced maternal age is becoming more common as women postpone pregnancy because of educational and career goals. Many women are postponing childbearing until after age 35 years, which poses a higher risk of medical problems during pregnancy and chromosomal abnormalities in the fetus. Older couples should be counseled about genetic risks and the availability of antenatal testing (amniocentesis and chorionic villus sampling), which may not be options if the first visit for prenatal care is delayed. The risk of infertility also increases with age, rising to 20% in couples older than 35 years.

Carrier screening

The ethnic background of either partner determines whether genetic screening should be recommended for sickle cell trait, thalassemias, and Tay–Sachs disease carrier state. A family history that is positive for certain diseases, such as cystic fibrosis and congenital hearing loss, indicates the need for additional screening. The American College of Obstetricians and Gynecologists recommends that screening for Tay–Sachs disease, Canavan disease, cystic fibrosis, and familial dysautonomia should be offered for couples of Ashkenazi Jewish ancestry.[15]

Carrier screening by ethnicity

Ethnic origin	Screening recommended	Test	Frequency(%)
Black	Sickle cell trait	Sickle cell smear	10
	β-thalassemia	MCV < 70	5
European Jewish	Tay–Sachs disease carrier; Canavan, cystic fibrosis, familial dysautonomia	Hexosaminidase A	4
French Canadian	Tay-Sachs disease carrier	Hexosaminidase A	> 5
Mediterranean	α-, β-thalassemia	MCV < 70	10–20
Southeast Asian (Laotian, Thai, Cambodian, Hmong)	α-, β-thalassemia	MCV < 70	20–40
Indian, Middle Eastern	Sickle cell trait	Sickle cell smear	Unknown
	α-, β-thalassemia	MCV < 70	Unknown

MCV, mean corpuscular volume
From Cowchock *et al.*[16]

Thromboembolic disease

A family history of thromboembolic disease may identify a woman at risk for pregnancy complications and requires a thorough workup prior to pregnancy.

A reproductive and gynecologic history and review of prior pregnancies

The time prior to pregnancy is the optimal time to review gynecologic and prior pregnancy issues and counsel couples about improving health and future pregnancy outcomes. A review of the gynecologic and obstetric history can identify possible signs of infertility or issues that may affect future pregnancies.

Are menstrual periods regular or irregular and are there signs of PCOS? Patients with irregular periods may have hormonal and ovulation problems or may have PCOS. Treating these problems will improve the patients' chances of getting pregnant. Patients with a history of recurrent miscarriages may benefit from a workup and baby aspirin prior to pregnancy.

Previous pregnancy complications, such as a history of a preterm delivery, a baby with intrauterine growth restriction, diabetes, hypertension, or pre-eclampsia, have an increased risk of repeating in future pregnancies and should be assessed prior to the next pregnancy.

If the patient has had a history of PID, then testing for fallopian tube patency may save many months of futile attempts attempting to get pregnant. Patients with a history of prior ectopic pregnancies have a 20-fold increased risk and should be counseled to see a doctor as soon as they believe that they are pregnant.

Living environment: diet, weight, and food

Exposure to harmful agents

In a retrospective, register-based cohort study[17] of 43,470 pregnant women, there were 20.4% of women who purchased at least one drug classified as potentially harmful during pregnancy, and 3.4% purchased at least one drug classified as clearly harmful. The authors concluded that their study places emphasis on the need for careful prepregnancy counseling. Preconception care should review exposure to any potentially harmful drugs, review the need to take them, and offer alternatives. Drug or chemical exposure causes 3–6% of anomalies and periconception care is ideal to prevent potential teratogenic effects on the developing fetus by stopping harmful influences or switching to safer medications. The Food and Drug Administration (FDA) has defined risk factor designations A, B, C, D, and X to classify drugs used during pregnancy. Category X drugs should never be used during pregnancy and while trying to conceive. Category X drugs include

- Folic acid antagonsist
- Warfarin
- Isotretinoin
- Valproic acid (should be avoided by all women likely to become pregnant).[5]

Periconception retinoic acid can lead to fetal embryopathy[18] and the American College of Obstetricians and Gynecologists recommends that pregnant and preconceptional women should avoid taking more than 5000 IU of vitamin A daily, though one study showed no association between periconceptional vitamin A exposures at doses of > 8000 IU/day or > 10,000 IU/day and malformations in general.[19]

Alcohol

Alcohol consumption during pregnancy can lead to adverse pregnancy outcome, such as fetal alcohol syndrome and lower birth weight babies,[20,21] and many women stop consuming alcohol once they know that they are pregnant. But there is also an adverse effect on alcohol on women who are trying to conceive as it decreases their fertility and increases their risk of having a miscarriage. Alcohol consumption prior to conception is a potential risk factor to fetal outcome and an important consideration for those females planning to have children. In a study involving mice,[22] long-term alcohol exposure prior to conception resulted in lower fetal body weights. The authors showed that fetal growth and development can be affected by alcohol consumption even prior to the time of conception. However, even modest amounts of alcohol consumption during pregnancy can cause a negative impact on the fetus.[21]

The Surgeon General in the USA has advised that 'the best way to improve pregnancy outcome is to not drink any alcohol when you are trying to conceive and during pregnancy'.

Smoking

Approximately 18% of pregnant women in the USA report smoking tobacco and their pregnancy is at increased risk for such complications as abruptio placenta, pre-eclampsia, and preterm labor.[23] Additionally, tobacco is associated with decreased fertility rates and increased oocyte depletion rates as well as ectopic pregnancy.[24] Periconception is thus the optimal time to inform women about the risks associated with smoking prior to and during pregnancy.

Environmental toxins and exposure

Women trying to conceive and pregnant women should minimize the use of common household products, such as paint and paint removal products, bleaches, lye, and oven cleaners. A detailed occupational history, including household and hobby activities, occupational exposure to organic solvents, anesthetic gases, and antineoplastic agents, can reveal potential teratogenic exposures. Women susceptible to toxoplasmosis should be advised to stay away from undercooked meat sources and have someone else change the cat litter.

Folic acid supplementation

A minimum of 400 μg folic acid supplementation with or without a multivitamin decreases the risk of fetal malformations, such as neural tube defects, miscarriages, and cardiac malformations.[25,26] This positive effect can only be achieved when the supplement is taken prior to conception, at least 1–2 months before conception. In the USA, the average woman receives about 100 μg of folic acid/day from fortified breads and grains. Women trying to conceive and beginning at least 1–2 months before conception and continuing through the first 3 months of pregnancy should take a daily vitamin supplement containing at least 400 μg of folic acid. Higher dosages are indicated for special-risk groups. A dosage of 1 mg/day is recommended for women with diabetes mellitus or epilepsy. Mothers who have given birth to children with neural tube defects should take 4 mg of folic acid/day for subsequent pregnancies. Studies have shown that addressing folic acid use even at a single periconception visit can significantly improve mean red cell folate levels.[27]

Diet

Women trying to conceive and pregnant women should have a diet rich in iron, calcium, vitamins B, and low in saturated fats.[28] There are even diets suggested for women to improve fertility.[29] Except for added calories during pregnancy, women trying to conceive should follow the same diet as if they were already pregnant. If a diet deficiency is identified, a visit with a dietician may help the woman understand the importance of a healthy diet.

Caffeine

A high caffeine intake delays conception[30] and increases the risk for a miscarriage.[31] Women therefore should be advised to have not more than 300 mg of caffeine/day, which is equal to two 5-oz. cups of coffee, three 5-oz. cups of tea, or two 12-oz. glasses of caffeinated soda.

Fish

Mercury can have a deleterious effect on the developing fetus and there is evidence that especially large fish can contain excessive amounts of mercury. To prevent potential mercury toxicity on the fetus, the American FDA recommends the following for fish consumption before, during, and after pregnancy:

- *Fish to be avoided*: shark, swordfish, king mackerel, tile fish.
- *Fish to be limited*: a total of no more than 12 oz. per week of shellfish, canned fish, canned tuna, or farm-raised fish.

Weight

Both extremes of a woman's weight can lead to decreased fertility and an increase in adverse pregnancy outcomes. Women who are underweight (BMI < 20) are less likely to ovulate, have amenorrhea, infertility, and a low birth weight baby.[32] Obesity also has a negative effect on fertility and increases the risks for gestational diabetes, hypertension, preeclampsia, and cesarean section.[33] The optimal time to lose weight and try to reach an ideal weight (BMI 20–25) is before conception.

Exercise and nutrition

Regular moderate exercise is generally beneficial and the current evidence continues to demonstrate marked benefit to both the mother and the fetus if women exercise during pregnancy. The current recommendation is for women to continue their prepregnancy activity level when they become pregnant. Hyperthermia in the first trimester has been associated with increases in congenital anomalies. Pregnant women should limit vigorous exercise to avoid an increase in core body temperature above 38°C (100.4°F). They should be adequately hydrated, wear loose clothing, and avoid extreme environmental temperatures and not spend too long time periods in saunas or hot tubs.

Social risk factors

Pregnancy can be adversely affected by a woman's mental and social health and there is an association between pregnancy and risk of domestic violence.[34] The physician can use a simple four-question screening tool modeled after the CAGE questionnaire for alcoholism:

(1) How often does your partner hurt you?
(2) How often does your partner insult or talk down to you?
(3) How often are you threatened with physical harm?
(4) How often does your partner scream or curse at you?

Responses of 'often' or 'frequent' to any of these questions place the women at risk of domestic violence. The patient should receive information about community resources for battered women and emergency shelters.

Illegal drugs

Using illegal drugs during pregnancy can have deleterious effects on pregnancy outcome. Advising patients to stop these drugs prior to pregnancy and referring patients to drug treatment can improve their pregnancy outcome. Women using illegal drugs, such as cocaine, marijuana, or heroin, should be encouraged to quit before pregnancy. Cocaine use in pregnancy is associated with miscarriage, prematurity, growth retardation, and congenital defects, while marijuana use can cause prematurity and jitteriness in the neonate. Use of heroin may lead to intrauterine growth restriction, hyperactivity, and severe neonatal withdrawal syndrome. Women who use illegal drugs may need a referral to a special withdrawal program to be completed before conception. A methadone maintenance program is an alternative if the patient is unable to complete the withdrawal.

Environmental toxins

Hazard	Types	Associated outcomes	Sources of exposure
Metals	Lead	Abnormal sperm, menstrual disorders, miscarriages, stillbirths, mental retardation	Solder, lead pipes, batteries, paints, ceramics, smelter emissions
	Mercury	Impaired fetal motor and mental development	Thermometers, mirror coating, dyes, inks, pesticides, dental fillings, fish from contaminated waters
Solvents	Trichloroethylene, chloroform, benzene, toluene	Birth defects	Dry cleaning fluids, degreasers, paint strippers, drug, and electronics industries
Plastics	Vinyl chloride	Decreased fertility, chromosomal aberrations, miscarriages, stillbirths, birth defects	Plastic manufacturing
Pollutants	Polychlorinated biphenyl, polybrominated biphenyl	Low birth weight, stillbirths	Pesticides; carbonless copy paper; rubber, chemicals, and electronics industries; fire retardants; food chain
Pesticides	2,4,5-T and 2,4-D organophosphates	Birth defects, miscarriages, low birth weight	Farm, home, and garden insect sprays, wood treatment
Gases	Carbon monoxide	Low birth weight, stillbirths	Auto exhaust, furnaces, kerosene heaters, cigarette smoke
	Anesthetic gases	Decreased fertility, miscarriages, birth defects	Dental offices, operating rooms, chemicals industries
Radiation	Radiographs, radioactive materials	Sterility, birth defects	Medical and dental offices, electronics industries

From Cefalo RC, Moos MK. Preconceptional health promotion. In Cefalo RC, Moos MK, eds. *Preconceptional Health Care: A Practical Guide*, 2nd edn. St. Louis: Mosby, 1995:41–2

Fertility review and optimization of fertility

Fertility review and testing

Women often assume that conception will happen quickly as soon as birth control has been stopped. However, only 50% of couples get pregnant after trying to get pregnant for 4–5 months, and 15% do not get pregnant even after trying for a year. Especially as women get older, they will encounter increased difficulties in getting pregnant. Any advice on how to improve fertility and maybe shorten the time period to get pregnant is important. Counseling couples about the basics of getting pregnant including timing and frequency of sexual intercourse and reviewing the mechanism of conception and the physiology of ovulation and the menstrual cycle is often crucial in helping them achieve a healthy pregnancy. Lubricants can decrease the chance of conceiving, and couples trying to conceive should be advised not to use any lubricants.

Unfortunately, many infertile couples are seen very late in their unsuccessful attempts to get pregnant. A quick review of fertility issues (e.g. regular ovulation and menstrual cycles, a history of PID, and a review of the mother's age) can assess whether an infertility evaluation may be indicated early on. For example, a sperm analysis is an easy test, which may be recommended before the attempt of trying to conceive. In about 50% of infertile couples there is a 'male' problem and if there is a problem it should be addressed before spending a long time trying to conceive in vain.

Conception after birth control

'When can I get pregnant after stopping the pill?' is among the first question women on the pill ask. There are several different ways this question can be answered: First, there is the safety of getting pregnant after stopping the pill. Women should be informed that there is no known fetal harm if conception happens right after the pill is stopped. So, there is no medical need to wait for fetal reasons. However, it may take some time for regular fertility to begin after stopping the pill. Ovulation may happen as soon as 2 weeks after the pill has been stopped, but can sometimes take longer. Women should be advised to seek consultation if ovulation and the menstrual period have not returned within 2–3 months after the pill was stopped.

Many physicians advise waiting for at least one cycle before getting pregnant after removal of the intrauterine device. But there is little scientific evidence in this suggestion.

Medical and gynecologic examination, reviewing and screening for infectious diseases, and updating immunizations

Examination

The periconception examination should include a full physical examination (e.g. lung, breast, heart, abdomen, skin, extremities) as well as a gynecologic history and examination including a Pap smear and a culture for chlamydia and gonorrhea. The examination should focus on possible problems that may affect the pregnancy. If a mammogram is indicated it is best done prior to conception.

Screening for infectious diseases

During the preconception evaluation, a history of high-risk behavior, including multiple sexual partners, sexually transmitted diseases, blood transfusions, or intravenous drug abuse, should be obtained from both the patient and her sexual partner. In addition, safe sex for prevention of sexually transmitted diseases and early medical care for vaginal discharge should be discussed.[35] Testing a women and her husband for infectious diseases prior to pregnancy allows for early interventions, before the developing fetus can be potentially affected. A history of sexually transmitted diseases and a history of a prior ectopic pregnancy increase the risk of ectopic pregnancy.[36] Patients with those histories should be counseled to see their doctor as soon as they believe that they are pregnant. Depending on individual circumstances, clinicians may perform the following infection tests prior to pregnancy:

(1) HIV (both in husband and in wife)
(2) Syphilis (both in husband and in wife)
(3) Hepatitis B antigen and antibody (both in husband and in wife)
(4) Gonorrhea
(5) Chlamydia
(6) Testing for prior exposure to parvovirus
(7) Testing for prior exposure to CMV
(8) Testing for prior exposure to toxoplasma
(9) Testing for prior exposure to herpes (both in husband and in wife)
(10) Testing for varicella immunity
(11) Testing for rubella immunity.

Women susceptible to any of these should be counseled about immunization and about prevention of infections.

Human immunodeficiency virus

All sexually active women should be offered HIV testing. Most women who might transmit the HIV infection to their fetus are asymptomatic. Preconception testing for HIV is important because the Pediatric AIDS Clinical Trials Study Group has shown that treatment with zidovudine (Retrovir) reduces the risk of transmission to the fetus from 25.5% to 8.3%. Earlier treatment of HIV and other sexually transmitted diseases decreases the risk of transmission to the fetus. Vertical transmission results in an approximately 30% chance of fetal infection from an untreated HIV-positive mother, a risk that can be reduced substantially with preconception or early pregnancy treatment. During the preconception period, women should be educated about high-risk behavior and given advice on contraception.

Syphilis

The time prior to pregnancy is optimal to identify and treat syphilis because at that time there is no fetus yet to be concerned about giving appropriate medications.

Gonorrhea, chlamydia

Both of these organisms can lead to adverse pregnancy outcomes and to infertility if not treated appropriately. Treatment of both partners prior to pregnancy is preferred as it prevents unnecessary exposure of the fetus.

Hepatitis B and other immunizations

All women should be screened for hepatitis B, and those at high risk should be tested for the presence of both hepatitis B surface antigen and hepatitis Be antigen. The preconception time period is optimal to provide immunization and women who have not received the hepatitis B vaccine should be considered for immunization if they are at risk of sexually transmitted diseases or blood exposure. The vaccine may be given during pregnancy. Hepatitis B is the most common type of hepatitis in the USA.

Influenza

Pregnancy is considered a high-risk condition for influenza. According to CDC guidelines, all women who expect to be pregnant during the influenza season (November to April) should be vaccinated against influenza. The specific guidelines for immunizations for adults can be found under 'Update on Adult Immunization Recommendations of the Immunization Practices Advisory Committee' at www.cdc.gov/mmwr/preview/mmwrhtml/00025228.htm.

Rubella and varicella

Preconception evaluation should include tests for immunity to rubella and varicella. Women who have no immunity to varicella are at risk of development of varicella pneumonia, which has a maternal mortality rate as high as 40%. Because immunization against these includes live-virus vaccines, women should be advised not to get pregnant for at least 1 month after immunization.

Toxoplasmosis

Toxoplasmosis may cause congenital infections if the mother becomes infected during pregnancy, and testing during pregnancy can sometimes yield confusing results. Preconception is the optimal time to test for past exposure to toxoplasma. Currently, no immunizations are available for these infections. Women who have not previously been exposed to toxoplasmosis should be counseled to avoid contact with cat feces in litter boxes, wear gloves while gardening, and avoid eating raw or undercooked meat.[37]

CMV and parvovirus B19 (fifth disease)

CMV and parvovirus exposure in susceptible women is especially risky for child care and health care workers.[23] Periconception testing for CMV or toxoplasmosis may be advantageous in counseling women about infection prevention during pregnancy. Women with negative titers prior to pregnancy should receive extensive counseling on how to avoid infections during pregnancy. Persons at risk should wash their hands frequently and use gloves to prevent transmission.[38]

Dental hygiene

There has recently been scientific evidence that gum disease increases the risk of preterm delivery.[39,40] Therefore, every woman should have dental care and treatment prior to pregnancy and during pregnancy to prevent adverse outcomes.

Male periconception care

There is expanding scientific evidence of an association between male-associated health issues and pregnancy outcomes. Optimally, a couple should attend the periconception visit together and the woman's partner should be encouraged to be included in periconception counseling and care. Seeing the couple together allows the clinician to also educate men about risks, review their family history for genetic disorders, and screen for sexually transmitted diseases and sexual dysfunction, or refer them to a specialist. Paternal smoking as well as alcohol consumption have been associated with decreased fertility and adverse neonatal outcomes, such as low birth weight and an increased incidence of fetal malformations. It takes on average 10–11 weeks for sperms to be produced. To optimize male fertility, men should abstain from alcohol and tobacco, and exposure to potentially damaging substances for at least 3 months prior to conception. Other substances and chemicals may adversely affect spermatogenesis and male fertility. In addition, smoking by the father and passive smoking by the prospective mother can equally have a potential negative effect on pregnancy. Sperm production in the testes requires a temperature that is lower than the core body temperature. To maximize sperm production, men should therefore refrain from staying too long in saunas or hot tubs and prevent overheating of testes (e.g. not wear too tight pants).

Summary

Every obstetrician and gynecologist should focus on periconception care during each annual visit of women of childbearing age. Patients should be asked about conception plans and early prenatal care when a pregnancy is confirmed should be encouraged. Clinicians should encourage all women of childbearing age to receive periconception care, and some may require a periconception consultation with a maternal–fetal medicine or other specialist. Encourage women to eat a healthy diet, try to reach their optimal weight, not drink any alcohol and stay away from smoking, limit consumption of certain fish, and supplement their diet with folic acid (0.4 mg/day). Encourage couples to enhance their probability of conception with regular midcycle coitus, ovulation monitoring, and avoidance of lubricants that can decrease fertility. Suggest early evaluation if infertility is an issue, especially in women older than 35 years.

REFERENCES

1. Cox M, Whittle MJ, Byrne A, *et al.* Prepregnancy counseling: Experience from 1,075 cases. *Br J Obstet Gynaecol* 1992; 99:873.
2. Kitzmiller JL, Gavin LA, Gin GD, *et al.* Preconception care of diabetes: Glycemic control prevents congenital anomalies. *J Am Med Assoc* 1991;265:731.
3. Waisbren SE, Hanley W, Levy HL, *et al.* Outcome at age 4 in the offspring of women with maternal phenylketonuria. *J Am Med Assoc* 2000;283:756.
4. De Weerd S, Polder JJ, Cohen-Overbeck TE, *et al.* Preconception care: Preliminary estimates of costs and effects of smoking cessation and folic acid supplementation. *J Reprod Med* 2004;49:338.
5. Adams MM, Bruce FC, Shulman HB, *et al.* Pregnancy planning and pre-conception counseling. *Obstet Gynecol* 1993;82:955.
6. Henshaw S. Unintended pregnancy in the United States. *Fam Plan Perspect* 1998;30:24.
7. Hellerstedt WL, Pirie PL, Lando HA, *et al.* Differences in preconceptional and prenatal behaviors in women with intended and unintended pregnancies. *Am J Public Health* 1998;88:663.
8. MRC Vitamin Study Research Group. Prevention of neural tube defects: Results of the MRC vitamin study. *Lancet* 1991;338:132–7.
9. Berry RJ, Li Z, Erickson JD, *et al.*, for China–U.S. Collaborative Project for Neural Tube Defect Prevention. Prevention of neural-tube defects with folic acid in China. *N Engl J Med* 1999;341: 1485–90.
10. Freda MC, Chazotte C, Bernstein P, *et al.* Interdisciplinary development of a preconception health curriculum for four medical specialities. *Obstet Gynecol* 2002;99:301.
11. Sablock U, Lindow SW, Arnott PI, Masson EA. Prepregnancy counseling for women with medical disorders. *J Obstet Gynecol* 2002;22:637.
12. De Weerd S, van der Bij AK, Cikot RJ, *et al.* Preconception care: A screening tool for health assessment and risk detection. *Prev Med* 2002;34(5):505:11.
13. Delgado-Escueta AV, Janz D. Consensus guideline: Preconception counseling, management, and care of the pregnant woman with epilepsy. *Neurology* 1992;42(4, Suppl 5):149.
14. Pennel PR. Pregnancy in women who have epilepsy. *Neurol Clin* 2004;22:799.
15. American College of Obstetricians and Gynecologists. *Committee Opinion: Prenatal and Preconceptional Carrier Screening for Genetic Diseases in Individuals of Easter European Jewish Descent,* August 2004, Number 298.
16. Cowchock FS, Johnson A, Jackson LG. Screening for genetic abnormalities. *Infertil Reprod Med Clin North Am* 1994;5: 177–95.
17. Malm H, Martikainen J, Klaukka T, *et al.* Prescription of hazardous drugs during pregnancy. *Druf Saf* 2004;27:899.
18. Lammer EJ, Chen DT, Hoar RM, *et al.* Retinoic acid embryopathy. *N Engl J Med* 1985;313:837.
19. Mills JL, Simpson JL, Cunningham GC, *et al.* Vitamin A and birth defects. *Am J Obstet Gynecol* 1997;177:1.
20. Marbury MC, Linn S, Monson R, *et al.* The association of alcohol consumption with outcome of pregnancy. *Am J Public Health* 1983;73:1165.
21. Lundsberg LS, Bracken MB, Saftlas AF. Low-to-moderate gestational alcohol use and intrauterine growth retardation, low birthweight, and preterm delivery. *Ann Epidemiol* 1997;7:498.
22. Livy DJ, Maier SE, West JR. Long-term alcohol exposure prior to conception results in lower fetal body weights. *Birth Defects Res B Dev Reprod Toxicol* 2004;71(3):135.
23. Brundage SC. Preconception health care. *Am Fam Physician* 2002;65:2507.
24. Saraiya M, Berg CJ, Kendrick JS, *et al.* Cigarette smoking as a risk factor for ectopic pregnancy. *Am J Obstet Gynaecol* 1998; 178:493.
25. Brent R, Oakley G, Mattis D. The unnecessary epidemic of folic acid-preventable spina bifida and anenecephaly. *Pediatrics* 2000;106:825.
26. Botto LD, Moore CA, Khoury MJ, *et al.* Neural tube defects. *N Engl J Med* 1999;341:1509.
27. De Weerd S, Thomas CMG, Cikot R, *et al.* Preconception counseling improves folate status of women planning pregnancy. *Obstet Gynecol* 2002;99:45.
28. Hindmarsh PC, Geary MP, Rodeck CH, *et al.* Effects of early maternal iron stores on placental weight and structure. *Lancet* 2000;356:719.
29. Wynn M, Wynn A. A fertility diet for planning pregnancy. *Nutr Health* 1995;10:219.
30. Stanton CK, Gray RH. Effects of caffeine consumption on delayed conception. *Am J Epidemiol* 1995;142:1322.
31. Cnattingius S, Signorello LB, Anneren G, *et al.* Caffeine intake and the risk of first trimester spontaneous abortion. *N Engl J Med* 2000;343:1839.
32. Grodstein F, Goldman MB, Cramer DW. Body mass index and ovulatory infertility. *Epidemiology* 1994;5:247.
33. Castro LC, Avina RL. Maternal obesity and pregnancy outcomes. *Curr Opin Obstet Gynecol* 2002;14:601.
34. Curry MA, Perrin N, Wall E. Effects of abuse on maternal complications and low birth weight in adult and adolescent women. *Obstet Gynecol* 1998;92:530.
35. Hanlin RB. Congenital infections and preconception counseling. *J SC Med Assoc* 2002;98:277.
36. Chow WH, Daling JR, Cates W, *et al.* Epidemiology of ectopic pregnancy. *Epidemiol Rev* 1987;9:70.
37. Lopez A, Dietz VJ, Wilson M, *et al.* Preventing congenital toxoplasmosis. *Morb Mortal Wkly Rep* 2000;49:59.
38. Allaire AD, Cefalo RC. Preconceptional health care model. *Eur J Obstet Gynecol Rep Biol* 1998;78:163.
39. Champagne CM, Madianos PN, Lieff S, *et al.* Periodontal medicine: Emerging concepts in pregnancy outcome. *J Intern Acad Periodontol* 2000;2:9.
40. Jeffcoat MK, Geurs NC, Reddy MS, *et al.* Periodontal infection and preterm birth: Results of a prospective study. *J Am Dent Assoc* 2001;132:875.

191 Maternal issues in thrombosis and thrombophilia

B. E. Grand and L. S. Voto

During normal pregnancy the hemostatic system changes to a hypercoagulable state. Pregnancy is associated with an increased risk of venous thrombosis, which is a leading cause of mortality at gestation.[1] Recently, acquired and inherited thrombophilia have been reported in women with early and late complications of pregnancy such as recurrent pregnancy loss, intrauterine growth restriction (IUGR), fetal loss and pre-eclampsia.[2,3]

Prevention and treatment of venous thromboembolism (VTE) and arterial thrombosis during pregnancy is an important issue. The relation of thrombophilia and fetal loss and the treatment of this complication are still controversial. This chapter focuses on recent advances in the management of thrombosis and thrombophilia in pregnancy with a special interest in the hematological aspects.

Hemostasis during normal pregnancy

Normal pregnancy is associated with an increase in clotting factors, a decrease of natural anticoagulants and an impairment of fibrinolytic activity. There is an increase in the concentration of fibrinogen, factors VIII, V, VII, IX, X, XII and von Willebrand factor. Protein C values remain within the normal non-pregnant range, while the protein S decreases during pregnancy. An acquired activated protein C (APC) resistance has also been described during pregnancy, and a reduction in the APC ratio has been associated with gestational vascular complications. There is an increase in the level of plasminogen activator inhibitor-2 (PAI-2) from the placenta, which leads to a reduction of fibrinolytic activity during the whole pregnancy, with a return to normal after delivery.[4] The D-dimer is elevated during pregnancy and may reflect increased coagulation activation and thrombin generation with increased secondary fibrinolysis. Finally, an increase in the level of platelet and endothelial microparticles is observed during pregnancy.[5] These microparticles have been associated with procoagulant complications.

In conclusion, these normal global hemostatic changes lead to an increase of the risk of thrombosis throughout pregnancy, which is particularly high after delivery.

Thrombosis, thrombophilia and pregnancy outcome

We can define thrombophilia as an acquired or hereditary hemostatic disorder that predisposes to thrombosis.

There is clear evidence in the literature that acquired and hereditary thrombophilias increase the risk of VTE and adverse pregnancy outcome. Recently, there has been a dramatic increase in the number of identifiable causes of thrombophilia.[6]

However, the heterogeneity in design and size of different studies makes it difficult to establish the real risk and to indicate adequate treatment if necessary. The presence of thrombophilia alone does not necessarily lead to a clinical event.

Maternal VTE

Epidemiology of VTE during pregnancy

There is an increased risk of VTE in pregnant women compared to non-pregnant women. VTE is one of the leading causes of maternal mortality and it could appear in any trimester with an increased risk during the puerperium. There is a striking predisposition for deep vein thrombosis to occur in the left leg (compressive effect by the right iliac artery on the left iliac vein).

Specific genetic defects that contribute to VTE include deficiencies of antithrombin, protein C, protein S, the G1691A mutation in the factor V gene (factor V Leiden), and the G20210A mutation in the prothrombin gene. These disorders underlie about 50% of episodes of VTE in pregnant and postpartum women.[7,8] The risk of VTE in women with thrombophilias is different when considering data obtained either from family studies or unselected women. The risk is higher in women with previous thrombosis and with symptomatic relatives. To date, there is no evidence to support routine screening of all pregnant

Table 191.1 Regimens of UFH and LMWH. ACCP Recommendations

- Minidose UFH: UFH 5000 U SC q12 h
- Moderate-dose UFH: UFH SC q12 h in doses adjusted to target an anti-Xa level of 0.1–0.3 U/ml
- Adjusted-dose UFH: UFH SC q12 h in doses adjusted to target a midinterval aPTT into the therapeutic range
- Prophylactic LMWH: e.g. dalteparin 5000 U SC q24 h, or enoxaparin 40 mg SC q24 h (although at extremes of body weight modification of dose may be required)
- Intermediate-dose LMWH: e.g. dalteparin 5000 U SC q12 h, or enoxaparin 40 mg SC q12 h
- Adjusted-dose LMWH: weight-adjusted, full-treatment doses of LMWH administered once or twice daily (e.g. dalteparin 200 U/kg, or tinzaparin 175 U/kg qd, or dalteparin 100 U/kg q12 h, or enoxaparin 1 mg/kg q12 h)
- Postpartum anticoagulants: warfarin for 4–6 weeks with a target international normalized ratio of 2.0–3.0

women for congenital thrombophilia. Thrombophilia screening is required in women with a personal or family history of VTE.[9]

Management of women with thrombophilia with or without VTE

Recently, information has been published on the management of women with VTE during pregnancy and primary and secondary thromboprophylaxis depending on quantification the risk of thrombosis or recurrence of thrombosis in women with a previous venous thrombosis. Risk factors are as follows: age above 35 years, unplanned cesarean section, bed rest, history of thrombosis, multiparity, gemellarity, severe ovarian hyperstimulation, antiphospholipid syndrome (APS) and hereditary thombophilia. Some women with prior VTE have an identifiable laboratory abnormality associated with thrombophilia; the significance of these abnormalities and the management of such individuals remain controversial. Despite the progress in risk stratification, in many cases without previous thrombosis, recommendations for prophylaxis are empirical.

The use of antithrombotic agents in pregnancy has been recently reviewed and is part of the *Seventh ACCP Conference on Antithrombotic and Thrombolytic Therapy: Evidence-Based Guidelines.*[10]

Antithrombotics in pregnancy

Recommendations about the use of anticoagulants during pregnancy are based on extrapolations of data from non-pregnant patients, from case reports and from case series of pregnant patients. The antithrombotic used in pregnancy include unfractionated heparin (UFH), low molecular weight heparin (LMWH), heparinoids (danaparoid), coumarin derivatives and aspirin. UFH has been the anticoagulant of choice in pregnancy. There is evidence that LMWH have potential advantages over UFH because they cause less heparin-induced thrombocytopenia (HIT), have a longer plasma half-life and a more predictable dose response. LMWH have a better bioavailability, a better safety profile with regard to osteoporosis and thrombocytopenia. A recent systematic review has addressed the safety of LMWH in pregnancy.[11] Heparins do not cross the placenta, so they are safe for the fetus. UFH doses should be adjusted to prolong a midinterval activate partial thromboplastin time (aPTT) into the therapeutic range [adjusted-dose subcutaneous (SC) heparin].

Coumarin derivatives cross the placenta and have the potential to cause both bleeding in the fetus and teratogenicity (nasal hypoplasia, stippled epiphyses) during the first trimester and central nervous system abnormalities after exposure during any trimester. Oral anticoagulants cause an anticoagulant effect in the fetus; we must be aware of this situation at the time of delivery. It is essential that some form of heparin therapy is instituted in the last 3–4 weeks of pregnancy. Optimally, there should be at least 1 week's washout of warfarin before delivery.

For women requiring long-term vitamin K anticoagulant therapy who are attempting conception, it is suggested to perform frequent pregnancy tests and substitute UFH or LMWH for warfarin when conception is achieved.

Heparin and LMWH are not secreted into breast milk and can be safely administered to nursing mothers. Suggested regimens of UFH and LMWH are given in Table 191.1.

Warfarin does not induce an anticoagulant effect in the breast-fed infant when the drug is given to a nursing mother. Therefore, the use of warfarin in women who require postpartum anticoagulant therapy is also safe, and women using this drug should be encouraged to breast feed.

Prevention of VTE in pregnancy

Although different recommendations have been published for the prevention of VTE,[12] levels of evidence are often low due to the lack of randomized trials in pregnancy and some studies have been done with small-sized samples. We must first examine if the women need VTE prophylaxis according to the risk factors. There is a consensus that the risk of VTE is higher in the postpartum period, and women with thrombophilia and/or history of VTE should receive prophylaxis during the postpartum for at least 6 weeks. In contrast, during the antepartum period recommendations are unclear. LMWH are commonly used, but the time to start and the doses are not well defined. A prophylaxis could be

Table 191.2 Prophilaxis of VTE in pregnancy. ACCP Recommendations

Prior VTE and pregnancy:

- In patients with a single episode of VTE associated with a transient risk factor that is no longer present, we recommend clinical surveillance and postpartum anticoagulants (**Grade 1C**). If the previous event is pregnancy or estrogen-related or there are additional risk factors (such as obesity), we suggest antenatal anticoagulant prophylaxis (**Grade 2C**).
- In patients with a single idiopathic episode of VTE who are not receiving long-term anticoagulants, we suggest prophylactic LMWH, or minidose UFH, or moderate-dose UFH, or clinical surveillance plus postpartum anticoagulants (**Grade 2C**).
- In patients with a single episode of VTE and thrombophilia (confirmed laboratory abnormality) or strong family history of thrombosis and not receiving long-term anticoagulants, we suggest prophylactic or intermediate-dose LMWH, or mini-dose or moderate dose UFH, plus postpartum anticoagulants (**Grade 2C**).
- In antithrombin-deficient women, compound heterozygotes for prothrombin G20210A and factor V Leiden and homozygotes for these conditions with a history of VTE, we suggest intermediate-dose LMWH prophylaxis or moderate-dose UFH (**Grade 2C**).
- In patients with multiple (two or more) episodes of VTE and/or women receiving long-term anticoagulants (e.g., single episode of VTE—either idiopathic or associated with thrombophilia) we suggest adjusted-dose UFH or adjusted-dose LMWH followed by resumption of longterm anticoagulants postpartum (**Grade 2C**).
- In all women with previous DVT, antenatally and postpartum, we suggest use of graduated elastic compression stockings (**Grade 2C**).

Thrombophilia and venous thromboembolism associated with pregnancy

- In antithrombin-deficient women, compound heterozygotes for prothrombin G20210A and factor V Leiden, and homozygotes for these conditions with no prior VTE, we suggest active prophylaxis (**Grade 2C**).
- In all other patients with no prior VTE and thrombophilia (confirmed laboratory abnormality), we suggest surveillance or prophylactic LMWH or minidose UFH, plus postpartum anticoagulants (**Grade 2C**).

administered throughout pregnancy in all women at risk of VTE. In other women the prophylaxis is often decided on a case-by-case basis. VTE has an equal distribution throughout gestation. The American College of Chest Physicians (ACCP) Guidelines[10] are given in Table 191.2.

Treatment of VTE in pregnancy

UFH has been the anticoagulant of choice during pregnancy. Actually, the results from randomized trials and meta-analyses comparing intravenous (IV) UFH and SC LMWH for the treatment of acute DVT and pulmonar thromboembolism (PE) in non-pregnant patients showed that LMWH is at least as safe and as effective as UFH. In pregnant women with acute VTE, two alternatives treatments are proposed: UFH followed by LMWH or adjusted SC dose of UFH. Some authors recommend that adjusted dose SC UFH or LMWH can be used for both initial and long-term treatments. Therapeutic LMWH must be discontinued 24 h prior to elective induction of labor or cesarean section.

In high-risk situations, we recommend the use of UFH, which can be initiated and discontinued a few hours prior to delivery. Postpartum anticoagulants should be administered for at least 6 weeks and in women with long-term indication of anticoagulation oral anticoagulants can be resumed.[11]

Prosthetic heart valves

Pregnant women with mechanical prosthetic heart valves represent a very high-risk group. There is consensus that these women need anticoagulation at the upper limit of the therapeutic range, but there is otherwise little agreement on the optimum management regimen. The role of LMWH during pregnancy in the treatment of women with mechanical heart valves is the subject of active debate. The publication quoted by Chan *et al.*[14] calculated the percentage risk of thromboembolic complications in women with mechanical valves and maternal death for three broad treatment strategies in pregnancy: only warfarin 3.9%; heparin in the first trimester, then switched to warfarin 9.2% and only heparin 33%. Some authors do not exclude the possibility of using LMWHs,[15] if administered in high enough doses and aggressively monitored. The publication of the *Seventh ACCP Conference Guidelines* on antithrombotic agents in pregnancy has specifically addressed this issue, so it is appropriate to review this controversial area. The authors of the recent consensus statement concluded that taking the current evidence into consideration there are still three treatment regimens that can be reasonably used in pregnant women with mechanical valves (Table 191.3).

Antiphospholipid syndrome

APS is defined by the combination of a clinical venous or arterial thrombotic event or an obstetric complication and the laboratory detection of antiphospholipid antibodies. The syndrome is primary when there is no evidence of an underlying disease and secondary mainly in the setting of systemic lupus erithematosus.[16]

Antiphospholipid antibodies are a heterogenous group of immunoglobulins IgG, IgM or, less frequently IgA. The association between antiphospholipid (aPL)

Table 191.3

- Adjusted-dose, twice-daily LMWH throughout pregnancy in doses adjusted either to keep a 4-h postinjection anti-Xa heparin level at approximately 1.0 to 1.2 U/mL or according to weight (**Grade 1C**), or
- Aggressive adjusted-dose UFH throughout pregnancy: *i.e.*, administered SC q12h in doses adjusted to keep the mid-interval aPTT at least twice control or to attain an anti-Xa heparin level of 0.35 to 0.70 U/mL (**Grade 1C**), or
- UFH or LMWH (as above) until the thirteenth week, change to warfarin (target INR: 3) until the middle of the third trimester, and then restart UFH or LMWH (**Grade 1C**).
- Long-term anticoagulants should be resumed postpartum with all regimens.
- In women with prosthetic heart valves at high risk,we suggest the addition of low-dose aspirin, 75 to 162 mg/d (**Grade 2C**).

Table 191.4 Revised classification criteria of the antiphospholipid syndrome[18]

Antiphospholipid antibody syndrome (APS) is present if at least one of the clinical criteria and one of the laboratory criteria that follow are met

Clinical criteria

1. Vascular thrombosis
   One or more clinical episodes of arterial, venous, or small vessel thrombosis, in any tissue or organ. Thrombosis must be confirrmed by objective validated criteria (i.e. unequivocal findings of appropriate imaging studies or histopathology). For histopathologic confirrmation, thrombosis should be present without significant evidence of inflammation in the vessel wall.
2. Pregnancy morbidity
   (a) One or more unexplained deaths of a morphologically normal fetus at or beyond the 10th week of gestation, with normal fetal morphology documented by ultrasound or by direct examination of the fetus, or
   (b) One or more premature births of a morphologically normal neonate before the 34th week of gestation because of: (i) eclampsia or severe preeclampsia defined according to SD, or (ii) recognized features of placental insufficiency, or
   (c) Three or more unexplained consecutive spontaneous abortions before the 10th week of gestation, with maternal anatomic or hormonal abnormalities and paternal and maternal chromosomal causes excluded.
   In studies of populations of patients who have more than one type of pregnancy morbidity, investigators are strongly encouraged to stratify groups of subjects according to a, b, or c above.

Laboratory criteria

1. Lupus anticoagulant (LA) present in plasma, on two or more occasions at least 12 weeks apart, detected according to the guidelines of the International Society on Thrombosis and Hemostasis (Scientific Subcommittee on LAs/phospholipid-dependent antibodies).
2. Anticardiolipin (aCL) antibody of IgG and/or IgM isotype in serum or plasma, present in medium or high titer (i.e. >40 GPL or MPL, or >the 99th percentile), on two or more occasions, at least 12 weeks apart, measured by a standardized ELISA
3. Anti-b2 glycoprotein-I antibody of IgG and/or IgM isotype in serum or plasma (in titer >the 99th percentile), present on two or more occasions, at least 12 weeks apart, measured by a standardized ELISA, according to recommended procedures.

antibodies and pregnancy loss was fist suggested more than 30 years ago, during the last meeting in Sapporo. Other pregnancy complications linked to placental insufficiency such as pre-eclampsia and fetal growth restriction are included in the definition of the APS. So the adverse obstetric outcomes included in the clinical criteria for the APS are recurrent early pregnancy loss, fetal death, pre-eclampsia and fetal growth restriction[17] (Table 191.4).

Antiphospholipid antibodies do not recognize anionic phospholipids, as has been believed for a long time.[18] These aPL antibodies recognize plasma proteins bound to suitable anionic surfaces; among them, b2-glycoprotein I and prothrombin are the most common and investigated antigenic targets.[18] b2-Glycoprotein I is required by the great majority of anticardiolipin antibodies to react with cardiolipin in immunoassays, whereas lupus anticoagulant activity in phospholipid-dependent coagulation tests is caused by subgroups of both antibodies. Other antigenic targets of the aPL are listed in Table 191.5. The interaction of aPL antibodies with their respective antigens at the phospholipid surface may lead to a prothrombotic condition. Most reactions that control the blood coagulation process occur at the phospholipid surface. The aPL antibodies used to define de APS in Sapporo Preliminary Criteria were: lupus anticoagulant (LAC) and anticardiolipin antibodies (17). Amendments to the Sapporo Criteria were proposed at a Workshop in Sydney before the Eleventh International Congress on antiphospholipid antibodies in 2004. Anti- b2-glycoprotein I Ig G and Ig M assays are added in the revised criteria (19). LAC assays should be done according to the International Society of Thrombosis and Haemostasis (ISTH) guidelines. In pregnancy we found that the most sensitive screening test to detect LAC was the diluted Russell viper venom time.[21]

Table 191.5 Antigenic targets for antiphospholipid antibodies

B2-Glicoprotein I
Activated protein C
Protein S
(human) prothrombin
Tissue type plasminogen activator
AnnexinV
Thrombomodulin
Oxidize low density lipoproteins
Factor XII , Factor VII/VIIa
Complement components H and C4b
High and low molecular weight kininogens
Endothelial protein C receptor (EPCR)

The mechanisms involved in the obstetric compromise are actually debated and the question about the possible causal role of the aPL is still an unanswered question. Multiple possible physiopathological mechanisms have been involved in the genesis of obstetric adverse complications. Whether there is a different mechanism when the obstetric complication comprises the early period of embryonic development and placentation or when placental insufficiency is the basis for late pregnancy complications is not known. Rand *et al.*[22] have proposed that the mechanism of recurrent pregnancy loss may be a consequence of aPL antibody-mediated disruption of annexin A5 binding to syncytiotrophoblasts. This finding would impact on the modulation of coagulation within the placenta, and predispose to intervillous clot formation and subsequent diminished capacity for nutrient and oxygen exchange. In a recent study antiannexin V antibodies were significantly increased in women with recurrent spontaneous miscarriage and recurrent implantation failures after *in vitro* fertilization.[23]

It has been suggested that the endothelial protein C receptor plays a relevant role in pregnancy maintenance, since EPCR knockout mice experience placental thrombosis and early embryonic mortality.[24] The EPCR is a potentially important target of aPL antibodies; it has been hypothesized that antibodies directed against endothelial protein C receptor (EPCR) may be involved in the development of the thrombotic and obstetric complications of the APS.[24]

Management of pregnant women with APS

The APS is an established and treatable cause of recurrent miscarriage.[25] The mechanism of aPL-associated pregnancy loss is related to the deleterious effect of these antibodies on embryonic implantation, trophoblast function and differentiation[26] and placental thrombosis.[27–29] Venous or arterial thrombosis can develop during the whole pregnancy and the postpartum period. Women with pregnancy loss and APS have a poor live birth rate in future untreated pregnancies. The treatment with a combination of aspirin and heparin significantly improves the live birth rate in these women. During the initial weeks of gestation, heparin can improve trophoblast invasion and differentiation, resulting in successful implantation. In later pregnancy, the anticoagulant effect can reduce placental thrombosis. The objectives of heparin treatment are prevention of maternal thrombosis and improvement of gestational outcome. In spite of the continued efforts in understanding the pathogenesis of obstetric complications of APS, there are few therapeutic trials. There is a recent excellent review of randomized therapeutic trials by Empson *et al.*[31] Low-dose aspirin and heparin are recommended for obstetric APS.[32] This recommendation lies in the results of a few trials with important differences in trial design.[33] In our experience, when we treated patients with prophylactic doses of enoxaparin 40 mg daily and 100 mg of aspirin, live birth occurred in 39 of the 49 treated pregnancies (79%).[34]

The major problem we actually face in the definition of the APS lies in the aPL assays. In spite of the international efforts to standardize laboratory testing for antiphospholipid antibodies, there is a considerable inter- and intralaboratory variation in their detection.

Assay problems contribute to the controversies in our understanding and definition of this syndrome. We hope that in the near future a better obstetric and laboratory definition of the APS, with different levels of risk, in well-designed therapeutic trials, will provide us better evidence regarding the management of obstetric APS.[35]

Inherited thrombophilias, pregnancy loss and gestational vascular complications

The increase in the number of identifiable causes of thrombophilia during the past 10 years introduces a new question: Are these thrombophilic abnormalities directly related to fetomaternal complications or can they increase thromboembolic risk and other obstetric complications?[36] Thromboembolism is a major cause of maternal death and thrombotic complications may also affect the uteroplacental circulation. Recent data have linked thrombophilia to other obstetric complications such as pregnancy loss, pre-eclampsia and IUGR. It has been hypothesized that recurrent pregnancy loss (RPL) represents an exaggerated hemostatic response to pregnancy leading to thrombosis of the uteroplacental vasculature and subsequent fetal loss.[37] Prevalence studies of inherited thrombophilic defects in women with pregnancy loss suggest an etiological role for inherited thrombophilias. Previous observations suggest an association between RPL and uncommon inherited thrombophilic states such as protein C, protein S, antithrombin and disfibrinogenemia. Actually, the association between the main thrombophilic polymorphisms factor V Leiden and prothrombin G20210 A mutation is well established. A large number of case–control studies found a high prevalence of factor V Leiden in women with RPL.[38,39] A systematic review noted an increased prevalence of the prothrombin G20210 mutation. Several other studies found no association with fetal loss. Rey *et al.*[40] reported an association between early and late loss. Various other thrombophilic defects may play a role in pregnancy loss: hypofibrinolysis, factor XII deficiency, high factor VIII levels and hyperhomocysteinemia.[41] A meta-analysis concluded that the C677T methylenetetrahydrofolate reductase (MTHFR) polymorphism was not associated with fetal loss. In spite of these results, maternal vascular disease of the placenta has been described, and these results highlight the importance of folic acid supplementation in patients with C677T homozygosity phenotypic expression. Inherited thrombophilias has been described in association with other pregnancy complications such as pre-eclampsia and IUGR.[42,43]

The prevalence of inherited thrombophilias is up to 20% in the normal population and the probability of a successful pregnancy outcome is high. Therefore, routine screening of all pregnant women is not warranted. Screening is recommended for women with the following previous complications: fetal loss including three or more in the first trimester, two or more in the second trimester, or any stillbirth, early, severe or recurrent pre-eclampsia or severe IUGR.[44]

Management of pregnant women with inherited thrombophilias, pregnancy loss and gestational vascular complications

The current evidence for antithrombotic therapy in women with inherited thrombophilia and recurrent pregnancy loss is limited to a few uncontrolled case series and a cohort study. A number of prospective studies have demonstrated the benefit of LMWH.[45–48]

A recent multicentric group coordinated by Brenner[49] published the results of the LIVE–ENOX study. The LMWH enoxaparin increases the rate of live births in comparison to what happened during previous pregnancies and decreases the incidence of complications in thrombophilic women with recurrent pregnancy loss. They also found that doses of 40 mg/day and 80 mg/day led to similar clinical results. The potential therapeutic benefits of LMWH for women with pregnancy complications and thrombophilia were presented in a recent debate.[50,51] Though preliminary data suggest that prophylactic anticoagulation may improve gestational outcome, confirmation in prospective randomized trials in thrombophilic women with unexplained recurrent fetal loss is needed.

Conclusions and comments

Pregnancy is an acquired hypercoagulable state and thromboembolism is a major cause of maternal death. There is growing evidence implicating congenital and acquired thrombophilias in the pathophysiological mechanism underlying miscarriage, fetal loss, pre-eclampsia and IUGR. The APS is an established and treatable cause of recurrent miscarriage. Maternal antithrombotic therapy is currently being evaluated in women with hereditary thrombophilia, fetal loss and gestational vascular complications.

Appropriate counseling should be offered to women with VTE and/or poor obstetric outcome associated with thrombophilia.

REFERENCES

1. Greer IA. Thrombosis in pregnancy: Maternal and fetal issues. *Lancet* 1999;353:1258–65.
2. Sibai BM. Thrombophilias and adverse outcomes of pregnancy – What should a clinician do? *N Engl J Med* 1999;340:50–2.
3. Kupferminc MJ, Eldor A, Steinman N, *et al.* Increased frequency of genetic thrombophilia in women with complications of pregnancy. *N Engl J Med* 1999;340:9–13.
4. Brenner B. Haemostatic changes in pregnancy. *Thromb Res* 2004;114:409–14.
5. Epiney M, Boehlen F, Boulvain M, De Moerloose P. D-dimer levels during delivery and the postpartum. *J Thromb Haemost* 2005;3:268–71.
6. Brenner B, Kupferminc M. Inherited thrombophilia and poor pregnancy outcome. *Best Pract Res Clin Obstet Gynecol* 2003;17:427–39.
7. Samama M, Rached R, Horellou M, *et al.* Pregnancy-associated venous thromboembolism (VTE) in combined heterozygous factor V Leiden (FVL) and prothrombin (FII) 20210 A mutation and in heterozygous FII single gene mutation alone. *Br J Haematol* 2003;123:327–34.
8. Meglic L, Stegnar M, Milanez T, *et al.* Factor V Leiden, prothrombin 20210G4A, methylenetetrahydrofolate reductase 677C4T and plasminogen activator inhibitor 4G/5G polymorphism in women with pregnancy related venous thromboembolism. *Eur J Obstet Gynaecol Reprod Biol* 2003;111:157–63.
9. Gerhardt A, Scharf R, Zotz R. Effect of hemostatic risk factors on the individual probability of thrombosis during pregnancy and the puerperium. *Thromb Haemost* 2003;90:77–85.
10. Bates S, Greer I, Hirsh J, Ginsberg J. Use of antithrombotic agents during pregnancy. The seventh ACCP conference on antithromboptic conference on antithrombotic and thrombolytc therapy. *Chest* 2004;126:179S–87S.
11. Sanson BJ, Lensing AW, Prins MH, *et al.* Safety of low-molecular-weight heparin in pregnancy: A systematic review. *Thromb Haemost* 1999;81(5):668–72.
12. Nelson-Piercy C, Letsky EA, de Swiet M. Low-molecular weight heparin for obstetric thromboprophylaxis: Experience of sixty-nine pregnancies in sixty-one women at high risk. *Am J Obstet Gynecol* 1997;176:1062–8.
13. Ginsberg J, Bates S. Management of venous thromboembolism during pregnancy. *J Thromb Haemost* 2003;1:1435–42.
14. Chan WS, Anand S, Ginsberg JS. Anticoagulation of pregnant women with mechanical heart valves: A systematic review of the literature. *Arch Intern Med* 2000;160(2):191–6.

15. Rowan JA, McCowan LM, Raudkivi PJ, North RA. Enoxaparin treatment in women with mechanical heart valves during pregnancy. *Am J Obstet Gynecol* 2001;185(3):633–7.
16. Galli M, Barbui T. Antiphospholipid syndrome: Definition and treatment. *Semin Thromb Haemost* 2003;29:195–203.
17. Wilson WA, Gharavi AE, Koike T, *et al.* International consensus statement on preliminary classification for definite antiphospholipid síndrome. *Arthritis Rheum* 1999;42:1309–11.
18. Miyakis S, Lockshin MD, Atsumi T, Branch DW, Brey RL, Cervera R, Derksen, RHWM, de Groot PG, Koike T, Meroni PL, Reber G, Shoenfeld Y, Tincani A, Vlachoyiannopoulos PG, Krilis SA. International consensus statement on an update of the classification criteria for definite antiphospholipid syndrome (APS). J Thromb Haemost 2005; DOI: 10.1111/j.1538-7836.2005.01753.x
19. Galli M, Comfurius P, Maassen C, *et al.* Anticardiolipin antibodies (ACA) directed not to cardiolipin but to a plasma protein cofactor. *Lancet* 1990;335:1544–7.
20. McNeil HP, Simpson RJ, Chesterman CN, Krilis SA. Antiphospholipid antibodies are directed against a complex antigen that include a lipid-binding inhibitor of coagulation: b2-glycoprotein I (apolipoprotein H). *Proc Natl Acad Sci USA* 1990;87:4120–7.
21. Grand B, Blanco A, Voto L, Lazzari M. Laboratory identification of the lupus anticoagulant in normal and pregnancy-induced hypertension. *Am J Obstet Gynecol* 1990;163:704–5.
22. Rand JH, Wu XX, Andree HA, *et al.* Pregnancy loss in the antiphospholipid-antibody syndrome – A possible thrombogenic mechanism. *N Engl J Med* 1997;337:154–60.
23. Matsubayashi H, Arai T, Izumi S, Sugi T, McIntyre JA, Makino T. Anti-annexin V antibodies in patients with early pregnancy loss or implantation failures. *Fertil Steril* 2001;76:694–9.
24. Hurtado V, Montes R, Gris JP, *et al.* Autoantibodies against EPCR are found in antiphospholipid syndrome and are a risk factor for fetal death. *Blood* 2004;104:1369–74.
25. Gu JM, Crawly JT, Ferrell G, *et al.* Disruption of the endothelial cell protein C receptor gene in mice causes placental thrombosis and early embryonic lethality. *J Biol Chem* 2002;277:43335–43.
26. Royal College of Obstetricians and Gynecologists. Immunological testing and interventions for reproductive failure. Scientific Advisory Committee Opinion Paper 5, 2003.
27. Sebire N, Fox H, Backos M, Rai R, Regan L. Defective endovascular trophoblast invasion in primary antiphospholipid antibody syndrome-associated early pregnancy failure. *Hum Reprod* 2002;17:1067–71.
28. Sebire N, Backos M, Rai R, Regan L. Placental pathology, antiphospholipid antibodies and pregnancy outcome in recurrent miscarriage patients. *Obstet Gynecol* 2003;101:258–63.
29. Pierangeli SS, Harris EN. In vivo models of thrombosis for the antiphospholipid syndrome. *Lupus* 1996;5:451–5.
30. Gharavi AE, Pierangeli SS, Levy RA, Harris EN. Mechanisms of pregnancy loss in antiphospholipid syndrome. *Clin Obstet Gynecol* 2001;44:11–9.
31. Empson M, Lassere M, Craig JC, *et al.* Recurrent pregnancy loss with antiphospholipid antibody: A systematic review of therapeutic trials. *Obstet Gynecol* 2002;99:135–44.
32. Rai R, Cohen H, Dave M, Regan L. Randomised controlled trial of aspirin and aspirin plus heparin in pregnant women with recurrent miscarriage associated with phospholipid antibodies. *Br Med J* 1997;314:253–7.
33. Lassere M, Empson M. Treatment of antiphospholipid syndrome in pregnancy – A systematic review of randomized therapeutic trials. *Thromb Res* 2004;114:419–26.
34. Grand B, Ventura A, Riveros D. Enoxaparin in pregnancy loss associated with antiphospholipid antibodies. *Thromb Res* 2004;114:653.
35. Branch DW. Antiphospholipid antibodies and fetal compromise. *Thromb Res* 2004;114:415–8.
36. Rai R. Is miscarriage a coagulopathy? *Curr Opin Obstet Gynaecol* 2003;15:265–8.
37. Martinelli I, Taioli E, Cetin I, *et al.* Mutations in coagulation factors in women with unexplained late fetal loss. *N Engl J Med* 2000;343:1015–8.
38. Dudding T, Attia J. The association between adverse pregnancy outcomes and maternal factor V Leiden genotype: A meta-analysis. *Thromb Haemost* 2004;91:700–11.
39. Kovalevsky G, Gracia C, Berlin J, *et al.* Evaluation of the association between hereditary thrombophilias and recurrent pregnancy loss: A meta-analysis. *Arch Intern Med* 2004;164:558–63.
40. Rey E, Kahn SR, David M, Shrier I. Thrombophilic disorders and fetal loss: A meta-analysis. *Lancet* 2003;361:901–8.
41. Hohlagschwandtner M, Unfried G, Heinze G, *et al.* Combined thrombophilic polymorphisms in women with idiopathic recurrent miscarriage. *Fertil Steril* 2003;79:1141–8.
42. Kosmas I, Tatsioni A, Ioannidis J. Association of Leiden mutation in factor V gene with hypertension in pregnancy and pre-eclampsia: A meta-analysis. *J Hypertens* 2003;21:1221–8.
43. Morrison ER, Miedzybrodzka ZH, Campbell DM, *et al.* Prothrombotic genotypes are not associated with pre-eclampsia and gestational hypertension: Results from a large population-based study and systematic review. *Thromb Haemost* 2002;87:779–85.
44. Brenner B, Grabowski E, Hellgran M, *et al.* Thrombophilia and pregnancy complications. *Thromb Haemost* 2004;92:678–81.
45. Gris J, Mercier E, Quere I, *et al.* Low-molecular-weight heparin versus low dose aspirin in women with one fetal loss and a constitutional thrombophilic disorder. *Blood* 2004;103:3695–9.
46. Brenner B, Homan R, Blumenfeld Z, Weiner Z, Younis JS. Gestational outcome in thrombophilic women with recurrent pregnancy loss treated by enoxaparin. *Thromb Haemost* 2000;83:693–7.
47. Carp H, Dolitzky M, Inbal A. Thromboprophylaxis improves the live birth rate in women with consecutive recurrent miscarriages and hereditary thrombophila. *J Thromb Haemost* 2003;1:433–8.
48. Grandone E, Brancaccio V, Colaizzo D, *et al.* Preventing adverse obstetric outcomes in women with genetic thrombophilia. *Fertil Steril* 2002;78:371–5.
49. Brenner B, Hoffman R, Carp H, Dulitsky M, Younis J. Efficacy and safety of two doses of enoxaparin in women with thrombophilia and recurrent pregnancy loss: The LIVE-ENOX study. *J Thromb Haemost* 2004;3:227–30.
50. Middeldorp S. Antithrombotic prophylaxis for women with thrombophilia and pregnancy complications – No. *J Thromb Haemost* 2003;1:2073–4.
51. Brenner B. Antithrombotic prophylaxis for women with thrombophilia and pregnancy complications – Yes. *J Thromb Haemost* 2003;1:2070–2.

192 Hypertension in pregnancy

L. S. Voto and J. Ortí

Introduction

Hypertension in pregnancy continues to be a major concern for perinatal health all over the world. When the cause of a disease is unknown, new theories are unavoidably generated and renewed hopes of progress emerge.

Hypertension is one of the main causes of prematurity, perinatal mortality, and maternal death in both industrialized and developing countries. According to the literature, its incidence worldwide ranges from 0.1% to 35%[1] as it is affected by a multiplicity of factors.

Edema in pregnancy is considered to be a controversial sign, as it may appear in pregnant women without necessarily being associated with any pathology. However, edema has been detected in the most severe cases of hypertension and has led to a diagnosis of eclampsia only in the presence of maternal seizures.

High levels of proteinuria are indeed good indicators of the severity of hypertension. Proteinuria appears late in the disease and has been found to be more significant with higher diastolic blood pressure.[2]

In any event, it is pre-eclampsia, i.e., hypertension plus proteinuria, pure or superimposed upon chronic (preexisting) hypertension, that will increase the risk of both maternal and perinatal morbilidy and mortality.

Physiopathology

Increased blood pressure in pregnancy results from a concatenation of polysemic events. Numerous clinical and experimental studies provide evidence that points to reduced trophoblastic perfusion, i.e., tissue ischemia, as the trigger of gestational hypertension.

In normal pregnant women, vasodilation of the spiral arteries can be up to four times their usual gauge, which reduces their peripheral resistance and favors intervillous space perfusion.[3] This is due to the trophoblastic invasion of the placental bed which ends at 20–21 weeks' gestation, and which destroys the vascular musculoelastic layer, thus preventing the action of vasopressor agents. In contrast, in preecalmpsia, the second trophoblastic migration does not take place; therefore, the musculoeslastic layer remains intact, reducing the gauge of blood vessels and giving rise to atheromatose plaques due to decreased blood flow. This paralysis of trophoblastic migration might be mediated by the maternal immune system.[4]

As stated by Gant in the early 1970s, pre-eclamptic pregnant women develop vascular sensitivity to angiotensin II. His studies demonstrated that in these patients the balance between the prostacyclin (vasasodilator) and thromboxane ring (the most powerful vasoconstrictor in the body) is lost in favor of the latter. As a result, blood pressure increases and the coagulation chain is activated.[5]

Gestational hypertension is a truly endothelial disorder, and among the multiple functions of the endothelium is the secretion of such substances as prostaglandins, endothelin, nitric oxide, and protein C. When a noxa causes endothelial damage, anticoagulant and vasodilator production decreases. Alterations in intercellular unions and in the water and protein transport expel these elements outside the cells.

Endothelin 1 levels have been shown to be more elevated in preeclamptic than in normal pregnant women, whereas prostacyclin and nitric oxide, the most important vasodilating and antiaggregating factors, are markedly reduced.[6]

We might then conclude that there is an inadequate expansion in plasma volume, an increased sensitivity to angiotensin II, a ruptured prostacyclin/thromboxane ring and an untimely activation of the coagulation mechanism, leading to decreased multiorgan perfusion. Therefore, pregnancy-induced hypertension is likely to be caused by an abnormal trophoblastic invasion, leading to decreased uteroplacental blood flow, placental ischemia, placental release of cytokines, endothelial dysfunction due to an increase in endothelin 1 and thromboxane A2 (two vasoconstricting substances), a reduction in prostacylin and nitric oxide levels (two powerful vasodilating substances), and a rise in vascular sensitivity to angiotensin II.

Epidemiologic studies agree that the immunological maladaptation of the fetal graft plays a major role in the defective placentation that gives rise to placental ischemia. This ischemia can be caused by several factors, the most important of which are:

a) immunological maladaptation
b) genetic predisposition
c) vascular mediators.

Endothelial dysfunction: all roads of the pathogenesis of hypertension in pregnancy lead to endothelial dysfunction.

The alterations found in the plasminogen activator and/or in the balance between the plasminogen activator and the inhibiting function of the prostacyclin/thromboxane balance seem to lead to increased platelet aggregation and vasoconstriction. These morphological and functional changes in endothelial cells would be responsible for triggering a clinical syndrome characterized by arterial vasospasm, and increased platelet aggregation and capillary permeability, manifested clinically as hypertension, edema, proteinuria and, sometimes, thrombocytopenia and organic hypoperfusion.

Epidemiologic findings seem to confirm the presence of a maladaptation syndrome:

- Pre-eclampsia is more frequent in primigravidas, but less frequent in subsequent gestations if pregnant by the same husband.
- Women with a history of abortion and blood transfusions are at a lower risk of pre-eclampsia.
- There is an inverse relationship between the length of cohabitation and the incidence of pre-eclampsia.
- Women who use barrier contraceptive methods are twice as likely to develop pre-eclampsia compared with those who do not.
- The incidence of pre-eclampsia is higher in women who have conceived with donor semen.

In spite of these epidemiologic facts, no alterations in IGM, IgA, IgG and IgD levels have been demonstrated yet in normal or pre-eclamptic pregnant women. HLA-G expressed on trophoblast would be responsible for immune tolerance. An alternative hypothesis suggests that maternal production of blocking antibodies plays a role in the survival of the fetal graft. The decrease in the production of these antibodies would result in a direct maternal reaction against both endovascular and intersticial trophoblastic invasion. Placental ischemia and the activation of polynuclear neutrophiles appear to be the most severe consequences of the altered maternal immune response, which in turn sets in motion a chain of events ending up in endothelial damage and dysfunction, and in typical pre-eclamptic symptomatology.

Genetic predisposition

It would be of great value in the prediction of pre-eclampsia to find the relationship between pre-eclampsia and a susceptible gene. Unfortunately, this gene – other than the one found in family relations – has not been discovered yet.

Vascular mediators

Pathologies such as chronic hypertension, diabetes, immune disorders, chronic renal failure, subclinical metabolic or hemostatic abnormalities facilitating thrombophilia (protein S deficiency, resistance to activated protein C, anticardiolipins, hyperhomocysteinemia), all of which have an impact on the vascular system, are associated with a higher risk of developing pre-eclampsia.

The unidentified point of union

The unidentified point of union between placental pathology and the chain of events leading to disorders in maternal circulation might be called the X factor. Genetic predisposition, the presence of a susceptible gene, and of vascular pathology are likely to be the modulating factors in the pre-eclamptic process.

The role of the placenta in the etiopathogenesis of pre-eclampsia

The presence of pre-eclampsia in women with trophoblastic disease or with an abdominal pregnancy points to the importance of the placental role and to the irrelevance of the decidua in the development of the pre-eclamptic syndrome.

As a result of trophoblastic invasion, the diameter of spiral arteries shows a four- to sixfold increase when compared to that in non-pregnant women; and disorders in that invasion can be demonstrated quite early in pregnancy, towards the end of the first trimester.

Some experimental findings suggest that, prior to trophoblastic invasion, there is reduced perfusion in the implantation site. Furthermore, pregnancy is associated with a 10-fold increase in uterine blood flow, 90% of which goes to the invervillous space. Towards the end of gestation, blood flow may reach 750 ml/min. The number of spiral arteries can be predicted early in pregnancy (about 120). In their adaptation to the increased blood flow, during the first trimester, the decidual segment of spiral arteries undergoes the degeneration of the internal elastic medial wall, as well as the disappearance of the smooth muscle and of elastin in the inner and outer medial tunic. A change is observed in the structure of vascular walls due to hyaline and fibrin. The second adaptation phase takes place during the second trimester and is characterized by intense trophoblastic invasion limited to the internal part of the medial tunic of spiral arteries.

Whereas blood pressure in the radial arteries is 70–80 mmHg, in the villous spaces it is about 10 mmHg, which shows a gradient that clearly benefits the fetus. Normal morphological changes in the placental bed prevent maternal spiral vessels from responding to vasopressor agents by reducing the number of smooth muscle cells capable of responding to them.

Cases with acute atherosclerosis show discontinuity of endothelial cells, focal interruption of the basal membrane, platelet deposits, mural thrombosis and fibrinoid necrosis. There are also disorderly proliferative changes in the vascular intima cells, resulting in hyperplasia of the myointimal and medial tunic smooth muscle cells, which could be caused by the mitogenic effects of platelet growth factors.

The marked reduction in fetal villous cell subendothelial fibronectin is a clear indicator of extensive endothelial damage in pre-eclampsia. An important characteristic of acute atherosis is the extensive lipoid necrosis of smooth muscle and myointimal cells, resulting from chronic hypoxia and/or from cytotoxin action. Acute atherosis is not only found in pre-eclamptic primigravidas, but also in the pre-eclamptic placentas of women with chronic hypertension, or with diabetes, renal failure and/or lupus, and it can lead to reduced intervillous blood flow, increased intrinsic vascular resistance and an elevated response to vasopressor substances.

The pathophysiology of pre-eclampsia

Normal pregnancy is associated with an increase in plasma renin activity and in the concentration of plasma renin, renin substrate, and angiotensin II. In contrast, pre-eclampsia is responsible for the suppression of the renin–angiotensin system. Regardless of the levels of renin present, aldosterone plays a role, either directly or indirectly, in the etiopathology of gestational hypertension.

In normal gestations, angiotensin stimulates prostacyclin production through the walls of uterine and systemic arterial blood vessels. Pre-eclampsia would therefore suggest a defective production of angiotensin II. In a recent study, Ito *et al.* demonstrated that angiotensin-converting enzyme (ACE) is present mainly in venous endothelial cells of placental villous stem cells, and that ACE activity, ACE protein expression, and ACE messenger RNA expression are higher in pre-eclamptic placentas than in normal pregnancy. Furthermore, they also found that, *in vitro*, hypoxia promotes the expression of ACE messenger RNA and its activity in endothelial vein cells. Consequently, venous endothelial cells both in the placenta and the umbilical vein would play a major role in the regulation of the fetoplacental renin–angiotensin system, and, in hypoxic conditions such as pre-eclampsia, the fetus can induce placental ACE activity.

The pathophysiological alterations characteristic of pre-eclampsia are manifested both at a local level (defective placentation and reduced placental perfusion) and at a systemic level (prostacyclin and nitric oxide deficiency in the vascular endothelium).

These changes raise endothelial sensitivity to vasopressor substances, platelet activity and thrombogenesis. Reduced placental perfusion enhances oxidative stress, and anomalous fetal and maternal vascular endothelium leads to prostacyclin deficiency. The increase of oxidative stress and prostacyclin and nitric oxide deficit result in vascular endothelium dysfunction, impairing other organs such as the placenta, kidneys, liver, pancreas, lungs, brain, and the hematopoietic system. The different clinical signs of pre-eclampsia stem from the dysfunction of all these organs.

To sum up, the pathophysiology of toxemia in pregnancy involves:

- Abnormal placentation leading to placental ischemia and oxidative stress.
- Prostacyclin and nitric oxide deficiency, which increases blood cell sensitivity to vasopressor agents, thrombin activity and platelet aggregation, and enhances the homeostatic system.
- Structural and functional disorders in endothelial cells.

Hypertension would therefore be the homeostatic response of the fetoplacental unit to these alterations, and should then be considered a consequence rather than a cause of the disease.

Diagnosis of gestational hypertension

The patient should be seated for a minimum of 5 min before blood pressure is measured. The sphygmomanometer cuff should be wrapped around the patient's upper arm at heart level. If the reading is abnormal, blood pressure should be measured three more times at 1-min intervals. In pregnant women, the first and the fifth Korotkoff sounds are recorded as systolic and diastolic blood pressure, respectively, as they are easily recognizable and better related to intra-arterial blood pressure.

Hermida *et al.* studied the effectiveness of the blood pressure load in the diagnosis of hypertension in pregnancy. They analyzed 2014 blood pressure series recorded by ambulatory monitoring for 48 h every 4 weeks, from the first antenatal visit until delivery in 205 normotensive pregnant women and 123 with gestational hypertension or pre-eclampsia. The blood pressure load test was defined as the 'percentage of values higher than 140/110/90 mmHg (systolic/mean arterial/diastolic blood pressure) during active hours or 120/95/80 mmHg during resting hours'. The blood pressure load was also obtained by comparing with the limits recorded while reducing the previous limits by 15 mmHg until a final threshold of 126/95/75 mmHg (day) and 105/80/65 mmHg (night) was reached.

The sensitivity for the blood pressure load was over 55% during all gestation when the highest limits used were considered. However, sensitivity was higher than 73% when day limits of 125/95/75 mmHg and night limits of 105/80/65 mmHg were used as references before 26 weeks' gestation, and when the tested limits of 130/100/80 and 110/35/70 (day and night, respectively) were used after week 26.

These findings show that the optimum reference limits to calculate blood pressure must take into account both gestational age and active and resting time values. In fact, the criteria for defining gestational hypertension according to blood pressure readings should be revised, as adverse outcomes have occurred with diastolic blood pressure equal to or higher than 85 and 95 mmHg before 36 weeks' gestation and at term, respectively.

A greater risk is also associated to the levels of proteinuria: fetal death rate is three times higher when proteinuria is ≥2+. When diastolic blood pressure is 95 mmHg or higher, there is also a threefold increase in fetal mortality rate (Perinatal Collaborative Study, USA).

However, fetal mortality can be nine times higher in the presence of both diastolic hypertension and proteinuria (95–105 mmHg with 2+ proteinuria), showing a synergic effect of diastolic blood pressure and proteinuria.

Risk factors for pre-eclampsia

- Primiparity: relative risk (RR) of 3
- Age: a J-shaped curve; women over 40 years of age show a RR of 3
- Multiple gestations: RR 5
- Chronic hypertension: RR 5
- Chronic renal disease: RR 20
- Antiphospholipid syndrome: RR 10
- Severe pre-eclampsia in previous gestation: RR 10
- Homozygous carriers of angiotensinogen T235 gene: RR 20
- Inverse correlation between gestational age when the disease is manifested and the risk for recurrence.

Proteinuria

Proteinuria is an excellent predictor of the extent of renal glomerular damage. Our experience shows that pre-eclampsia can be diagnosed when proteinuria is higher than 300 mg/l in 24-h urine samples. When renal dysfunction is already present, urinary levels of proteins, and mainly of albumin, will be elevated. However, as glomerular damage occurs late in the course of gestational hypertension, measurable proteinuria may not be useful for early detection of the disease. In any case, patients should be screened for proteinuria because its detection will affect both the prognosis and the treatment of this illness.[7]

Edema

The presence of edema has less predictive value than proteinuria in the diagnosis of pre-eclampsia. Edema is common in normal pregnancies and therefore lacks specificity. A ponderal sudden increase in weight gain (over 500 g in a week), especially if sustained through time, can be a clear indicator of edema in the absence of other complications.

Risk factors[8]

- Nulliparity
- Maternal age < 25 or > 35 years
- Multiple pregnancy
- Obesity
- Family history of pre-eclampsia–eclampsia
- History of pre-eclampsia in previous gestations
- Abnormal Doppler ultrasound scan of uterine arteries between 13 and 24 weeks' gestation
- Pregestational diabetes mellitus
- Thrombophilia.

Other diagnostic factors

If the first antenatal visit occurs after 20 weeks' gestation, the patient may not be aware of her blood pressure values, making diagnosis of either gestational or preexisting hypertension more difficult.

Cardiovascular function

Pregnancy-induced hypertension usually has little or no impact on cardiac function. Nevertheless, if the hypertensive condition is severe during the third trimester, the patient may present with reduced cardiac preload and minute volume, as well as increased postload. An electrocardiogram must be ordered in any event and, in cases where heart valve pathology is suspected, an echocardiogram is also recommended.[9]

Renal function

In the course of the disease, it is the kidneys that are most impaired, showing alterations in renal perfusion flow and depuration. Glomerular endotheliosis is a highly characteristic sign of pre-eclampsia and can be diagnosed after a careful study of renal function with urine cultures and screening tests for creatininemia, creatinine clearance, uricemia, and proteinuria in 24-h urine. Postpartum renal biopsy would be very useful to diagnose renal pathology, but due to its invasive nature, it should not be performed as a routine procedure.[10]

Ophthalmoscopy

Ophthalmoscopy can reveal vascular narrowing, edema, hemorrhage, exudates, and a cotton-like fundus If the patient complains of blurred vision, there is likely to be subretinal fluid coming from choroidal plexus exudation. In all cases, ocular changes usually resolve completely some time after delivery.

Hematologic follow-up

At present, coagulation disorders are known to be a consequence rather than the origin of this syndrome. Disorders in coagulation factors, thrombocytopenia and hemolysis, are the most common complications. Thrombocytopenia is secondary to endothelial damage and may be associated with the appearance of schistocytes (fragmented erythrocytes), spherocytes, reticulocytes and hemoglobinuria in peripheral blood, which are characteristic of the condition known as microangiopathic hemolysis.[11]

Liver function

Only in very severe cases is hepatic function altered. However, a hepatogram should be ordered in all cases, mainly after the patient is diagnosed with HELLP (hemolysis, elevated liver enzymes, low platelets).

Classification

The classification of hypertension in pregnancy continues to be a problem as the etiology of the disease is still unknown. None of the classifications attempted so far is broad enough to cover all the possible types. Recently, the US National Institutes of Health (NIH) and the Working Group on High Blood Pressure in Pregnancy have proposed a new classification, which has added the term *gestational hypertension* to describe patients presenting with hypertension in pregnancy but without proteinuria, leaving *pregnancy-induced* or *temporary hypertension* to be used for postpartum diagnosis.[12]

The classification proposed by both American institutions is as follows:

(1) Chronic hypertension
(2) Pre-eclampsia–eclampsia
(3) Chronic hypertension with superimposed pre-eclampsia
(4) Gestational hypertension: this comprises two subgroups:
  (a) Temporary hypertension in pregnancy without pre-eclampsia: where blood pressure values return to normal within 6 weeks postpartum
  (b) Chronic hypertension: this type is diagnosed during gestation and blood pressure values continue to be elevated after the sixth week postpartum.

In order to include all the pathologies of gestation in one classification, the International Society for the Study of Hypertension in Pregnancy (ISSHP) has classified the disease into four groups[13]:

Group A
A.1. Gestational hypertension
A.2. Gestational proteinuria
A.3. Gestational hypertension with proteinuria or pre-eclampsia

Group B
B.1. Chronic hypertension
B.2. Chronic renal disease
B.3. Chronic hypertension with superimposed pre-eclampsia

Group C
Unclassified hypertension and/or proteinuria

Group D
D.1. Hypertensive emergency
D.2. Eclampsia

Group A comprises all cases where proteinura or hypertension or a combination of both appears and resolves during pregnancy. Group B includes cases with preexisting hypertension or previous renal pathologies plus pre-eclampsia as an aggravating factor. All those cases where it is not possible to make an accurate diagnosis of the origin of hypertension, either because of a late prenatal visit or deficient follow-up in remote puerperium, are classified into Group C.

We recommend adopting this classification of hypertension in pregnancy because:

- It allows the classification of patients according to the characteristics of their own gestations.
- It enables physicians to reclassify the patient within each group according to the clinical evolution of the disease.
- It clearly distinguishes patients with pre-eclampsia (pure or superimposed) from those with preexisting hypertension.
- It includes a group for unclassifiable cases, which prevents inaccurate labeling.
- It allows the analysis of cases with nephropathy with or without hypertension.

Pathological anatomy of the placenta in pre-eclampsia

The extravillous trophoblast encompasses all the trophoblastic cells which are not in contact with the basal membrane of chorionic villi. It has two components: the interstitial trophoblast and the endovascular trophoblast. The giant multinuclear cells of the interstitial trophoblast infiltrate into the placental bed.

In 1967 Brosens described the trophoblastic permeation of decidual and myometrial spiral arteries by extravillous trophoblast, which penetrates the spiral arteries migrating through the distal end of decidual vessels at 9 weeks' gestations and reaching myometrial vessels at 14–15 weeks' gestation.

Trophoblastic invasion leads to the destruction of the muscular elastic tissue and of the nervous tissue, turning the uteroplacental vasculature into a low resistance, low pressure and high blood flow system without maternal vasomotor control.

Five years later, Brosens demonstrated the absence of a physiological transformation of uteroplacental arteries in pre-eclampsia. There are, however, other vascular lesions such as atherosis which was described by Hertig back in 1945. In 1985, Klurfel showed vascular endothelial infiltration by macrophages. In addition to atherosis, there is fibrinoid necrosis.

Over 60% of pre-eclamptic placentas show vascular atherosis mainly in decidual necrosis and infarcted areas. The endothelium is disrupted in 80% of the patients with pre-eclampsia, probably resulting from increased oxidative stress and production of vasoactive substances as well as from alterations in cytokine production. The vascular bed in pre-eclamptic patients is characterized by a higher number basal and spiral arteries with greater tortuosity and by a reduction in their luminal diameter. Medial disorganization and hyperplasia in myometrial arteries are also displayed, more frequently than atherosis, in pre-eclamptic patients.

In normal pregnancy, 40% of all decicual lymphocytes are CD56+ uterine natural killer cells, and 60%, CD3+ T-lymphocytes; about 30% of the latter are CD8+ T cells. In contrast, in pre-eclamptic pregnancies with intrauterine growth retardation (IUGR), there is a higher proportion of CD56+ uterine natural killer cells and CD8+ T lymphocytes in the decidua (70% of all CD3+ cells). In pregnancies without IUGR no increase in CD56+ uterine natural killer cells has been observed, while CD8+ T lymphocytes have been found to be significantly elevated compared with the normal level (50% of all CD3+ cells).[14]

Impact of pre-eclampsia on the placenta

Changes in the villous structure

Normally at 32 weeks' gestation placental membranes are vasculosyncytial and the syncytiotrophoblast forms clusters, knots or sprouts which are attached to the villi or remain loose in the intervillous lakes, comprising 30% of a term placenta villi.

In pre-eclampsia, the cytotrophoblast proliferates and the syncytiotrophoblast becomes thinner while the basal membrane grows thicker. These placentas show signs of reduced uteroplacental blood flow and are known as Tenney–Parker placentas. Macroscopically, they are little, fibrotic, and dark, which is due to the polyglobulia developed by fetuses with IUGR, placental color resulting from fetal blood circulating in villous capillaries. Besides, as a consequence of chronic hypoxia, fetal blood vessels in villous stem cells display fibromuscular hyperplasia and obliterant endarteritis,[15] often accompanied by thrombosis triggered by fetal blood hypercoagulability in the presence of prolonged hypoxia. Chronic hypoxia may also lead to syncytiotrophoblastic rugosity, which favors the thrombosis of circulating blood in the intervillous space.

Treatment of hypertension in pregnancy

The majority of treatments carried out at present are symptomatic and highly controversial; they do not cure the disease and are mainly aimed at preventing or reducing maternal and fetal risk.

Significantly lowering maternal blood pressure does not necessarily improve the pregnancy condition, as can be seen in cases of chronic hypertension where early reduction of blood pressure does not preclude the later development of superimposed pre-eclampsia.[16]

Ideally, an antihypertensive drug should be harmless for both mother and fetus, it should not have adverse side effects, and it should be effective, easy to dose, adequately presented and reasonably priced. It goes without saying that, unfortunately, no such drug is available on the market yet.

Rationale for treatment

The rationale for the treatment of hypertension in pregnancy is as follows:

- Pregnancy-induced hypertension should be defined according to changes in blood pressure values, but it is not a hypertensive disorder.
- Although its etiology is still unknown, it has been found to originate in alterations in the utero-placental unit.
- Elevated blood pressure might be triggered by the need for better fetoplacental perfusion
- Drug treatment of pre-eclamptic hypertension would reduce placental perfusion and affect normal fetal growth.
- Therefore, treatment is carried out in spite of its deleterious effect on the uteroplacental unit, and is aimed at protecting the mother. Treatment is indicated only when blood pressure values can lead to a cerebrovascular accident.[17]

Treatment principles

Our specialist team follows the principles below:

- Hypertension is considered moderate if blood pressure ranges from 140/90 to 159/99 mmHg, and severe if it is 160/100 mmHg or higher.
- Drug treatment is used when blood pressure is 160/100 mmHg or higher to avoid irreversible maternal cerebrovascular damage.
- The decision to start treatment is based on the highest blood pressure values recorded twice 24 h apart, with the patient at bedrest.[18]

The choice of treatment depends on the characteristics and severity of maternal hypertension, the age of pregnancy and fetal condition. At present, the following drugs are available.

Alpha-2 receptor agonists

Alpha-methyldopa
  Therapeutic action: central hypotensive action
  Reduced peripheral resistance
  Route of administration: oral
  Dose: 500–3000 mg/day.

Beta-blockers

Atenolol
  Therapeutic action: beta-receptor blockade. Atenolol antagonizes competitively endogenous and exogenous beta-sympathetic stimulation.
  Route of administration: oral
  Dose: 50–250 mg/day.

Calcium-channel blockers

Niphedipine
  Therapeutic action: calcium-channel blocker
  Route of administration: oral
  Dose: 20–40 mg/day.
Amlodipine
  Therapeutic action: selective calcium antagonist. Amlodipine reduces peripheral vascular resistance
  Route of administration: oral
  Dose: 10–40 mg/day.

Angiotensin converting enzyme inhibitors (ACE)

Enalapril
  Therapeutic action: enalapril curtails the conversion of angiotensin I to angiotensin II
  Route of administration: oral
  Dose: 5–30 mg/day
  Only used in cases of persistent postpartum hypertension.

Direct action vasodilators

Hydralazine
  Therapeutic action: arterial vasodilator which blocks calcium influx into the cell. It relaxes smooth muscle of arterioles
  Route of administration: IV or IM
  Dose: 5 mg/day as IV bolus, followed by 5–10 mg doses every 20 min (until a total dose of 40 mg is administered). Continue with the effective dose reached within 6 h.

Anticonvulsivants

Magnesium sulfate
  Therapeutic action: myoneural presynaptic inhibition; peripheral vasolidators; minimum hypotensive action
  Route of administration: IV
  Dose: (1) Slow IV bolus of 2 or 4 g; (2) 1 g infusion every hour, up to 3 g/h. Magnesemia is measured and possible reduction of patellar reflex, respiratory insufficiency and diuresis (oliguria) are strictly checked.
Diazepam
  Therapeutic action: anticonvulsant; myorelaxant
  Route of administration: IV
  Dose: (1) slow IV bolus of 40 mg; (2) 10 mg/h infusion

Management and treatment of moderate hypertension

(1) Weekly blood pressure measurement
(2) Reduced physical activity at home
(3) Laboratory tests
(4) Fetal vitality check-ups:
  (a) Ultrasound scan
  (b) Antepartum non-stress test
  (c) Vascular Doppler ultrasound scan
(5) No elective induction of labor unless for obstetric reasons.

Management and treatment of severe hypertension

(1) Hospitalization
(2) If blood pressure is not reduced with bed rest, one of the following drugs should be prescribed:
  (a) Atenolol: 50–250 mg/day
  (b) Alpha-methyldopa: 500–2000 mg/day
  (c) Amlodipine: 10–40 mg/day
(3) Laboratory tests (more frequent than in outpatients)
(4) Patients with chronic hypertension who respond to treatment can then be followed up as outpatients
(5) Patients with gestational hypertension should remain in hospital because the risk of seizures does not disappear with the use of hypotensive drugs.

Follow-up

If blood pressure continues to increase in spite of the therapeutic measures taken and/or if clinical symptoms appear (headache, visual problems, irritability), the protocol for the treatment of hypertensive emergencies must be followed (see below)

The guidelines for pregnancy interruption are as follows:

Before interruption. Assessment of fetal growth and vitality: The fetus will be affected by the disease, and will show alterations in both growth and vitality. Ultrasound scans should be used to follow fetal growth, and to study amniotic fluid volume and any changes that might occur in it. Any reduction in amniotic fluid volume will be an indication of compromised vitality and a sign of an adverse outcome.

Fetal vitality can be evaluated before the third trimester through the study of blood flow velocity waves: an increase in systolic peak and a reduction in end diastolic flow will be an indication of a higher resistance in the uteroplacental and umbilical beds, and therefore, of imminent compromise in fetal vitality. During the third trimester, evaluation of fetal vitality by means of antepartum non-stress tests is recommended since its effectiveness is not affected by the use of hypotensive drugs.[19]

Criteria for pregnancy interruption

- Moderated hypertensive condition with a mature fetus (over 37 weeks' gestation)
- Severe hypertensive condition with a fetus over 34 weeks gestational age
- Severe hypertensive condition with an immature fetus in the presence of damaged maternal health and/or treatment failure
- Eclampsia.

Route of delivery

The route of delivery will depend on the hypertensive condition and the degree of fetal distress and/or IUGR.

In the presence of mild or moderate hypertension, there is no contraindication to vaginal delivery, unless there is an obstetric indication for surgical delivery.

In cases with severe hypertension, the route of delivery will depend on the degree of fetal distress and of IUGR: if the fetus is highly compromised, surgical delivery through the abdominal wall is recommended. If the vaginal route is attempted, intrapartum fetal monitoring is mandatory. However, any complication in the progress of labor and/or any sign of intrapartum fetal distress must be taken as an indication for a cesarean section.

Anesthesia

General anesthesia is preferred in cases of severe hypertension and eclampsia. In mild or moderate hypertension, however, an epidural can be used if a sudden hypotension is avoided and if the dose is fractioned and administered through a catheter.[20]

Treatment of eclampsia

- Protect the patient:
  - Prevent tongue biting
  - Suction the pharynx
- Administer oxygen
- Do blood and urine tests
- Insert a Foley catheter to measure urine output
- Administer magnesium sulfate ($MgSO_4$).

(1) If the patient has seizures, start with a slow intravenous bolus (7–14 drops per minute) of 4–6 g of $MgSO_4$, diluted in 10 cm^3 of 5% dextrose solution. If seizures recur within 2 h, the same diluted bolus can be administered again.

(2) In the absence of seizures but with prodromic signs, we recommend administering an $MgSO_4$ infusion and avoiding a bolus.[21]

When a patient shows signs and/or symptoms of magnesium toxicity[22]:

- Interrupt magnesium administration immediately
- Maintain adequate oxygenation
- Perform an ECG (arrhythmias are likely)
- Administer diuretics
- IV calcium gluconate is an adequate antidote.

Treatment with $MgSO_4$ should be administered for at least 24 h after achieving its therapeutic effect or until the cause of its indication has ceased.

Alternative medications for the treatment of seizures

- Sodium thiopental: slow, diluted IV dose of 250 mg
- Diazepam: 100 mg in 500 cm^3 of 5% dextrose solution, 5–7 drops per minute. A slow IV bolus of 40 mg is also possible. (Diazepam is an important fetal and maternal respiratory depressant.)[23]

If the patient presents with high blood pressure concomitant with seizures, administer simultaneously parenteral hypotensive medication.

The patient's prognosis can be complicated by[24–26]:

Pulmonary edema
- Weak and fast pulse
- Pulmonary stertors
- Decrease in blood pressure

Prolonged coma
- Focus signs
- Cerebral hemorrhage

Renal failure
- Reduced urinary output.

Treatment of hypertensive emergencies

A hypertensive emergency is a condition in which a sudden increase in blood pressure is accompanied by clinical symptoms such as intense headaches, scotomas, blurred vision, photopsia, tinnitus, increased osteotendinous reflexes, and epigastralgia. It usually occurs in patients with preexisting hypertension, and can be treated with various drugs, but in all cases, a

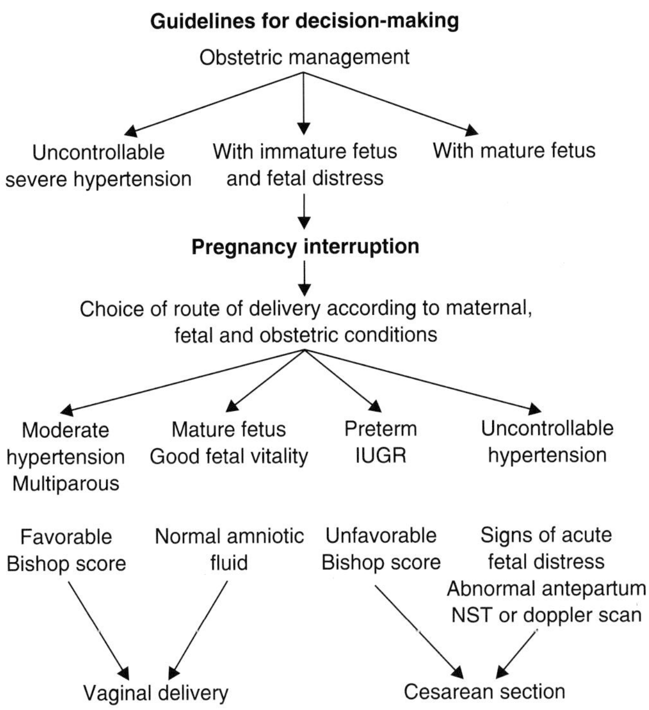

sudden decrease in blood pressure should be avoided as it can have a deleterious effect on the fetus.

Clonidine: Start with a slow 0.25 mg IV bolus and then continue with 0.75 mg diluted in 500 cm^3 of dextrose solution, at a rate of 7 drops per minute.[27]

Hydralazine: This drug is the most widely used all over the world in hypertensive emergencies in pregnant women with pre-eclampsia. It is less effective in patients with preexisting hypertension. Attack dose: slow 5 mg IV bolus (dilute the 20 mg ampoule in 10 cm^3 of dextrose solution). Wait for 15–20 min. If blood pressure does not go down, administer 5–10 mg at 20-min intervals until a 40 mg dose is given. Maintenance dose: this should be the same as the attack dose which resulted in a favorable response.

Sodium nitroprusiate has been shown to be effective in the treatment of non-pregnant patients, but its use can lead to cyanhydric poisoning. Diazoxide is no longer used at present. There are numerous articles in the literature reporting the effectiveness of the use of labetalol, which seems to have become the 'drug of choice' in the treatment of hypertensive emergencies. In contrast, hydralazine has not been on our market for long; therefore, our results with it can only be considered preliminary. Kean,[28] however, has published an interesting article about the use of hydralazine. Except in extreme cases and in the absence of other drugs, converting enzyme inhibitors such as intravenous enalapril are not recommended as they can result in acute fetal renal failure and even intrauterine fetal death. Enalapril has been found to be effective in cases of acute ventricular failure.[29] Our experience with the use of enalapril in the treatment of a hypertensive emergency during puerperium has been satisfactory.

Hypertensive emergencies and/or eclampsia are the most severe clinical conditions of the gestational hypertension syndrome. Appropriate diagnosis and timely therapeutic measures can help to prevent the worst outcome: maternal death.

Prevention of gestational hypertension

State of the art and future perspectives[30]

The efforts made to prevent a disease depend on its prevalence and on the consequences it has in both the individual and the community. Prevention is successful if it allows us to determine the cause of the disease, to detect an early and latent stage of the pathology and to establish effective and safe intervention measures.

The incidence of gestational hypertension without proteinuria ranges from 10% to 15% of pregnancies. Whereas pre-eclampsia occurs in 2–8% of pregnancies, eclampsia is observed in 5–8 out of 10,000 gestations.

Risk. The main risk entailed by pregnancy-induced hypertension is that it may develop into pre-eclampsia and therefore result in potentially severe complications in both the mother and the fetus/neonate.

Pre-eclampsia affects different systems and is characterized by:

- Vasoconstriction
- Blood flow disorders
- Endothelial cells dysfunction
- Hemostatic system alterations.

Maternal morbidity and mortality may occur due to:

- Renal failure
- Liver dysfunction
- Heart and lung failure
- Seizures (eclampsia)
- Cerebral hemorrhage
- Death.

These disorders are found to be more serious in countries with low-budget hospitals and where prenatal care is not easily accessible.

Perinatal morbidity and mortality may occur due to:

Abruptio placentae
Intrauterine fetal growth retardation
Acute and chronic fetal distress
Elective preterm delivery.

The epidemiologic studies detailed below are described in their corresponding articles as cited in the *References section.*

Risk factors for gestational hypertensive disorders

Maternal history
Nulliparity
Previous pre-eclampsia/eclampsia

Age: older than 40 years or younger than 20 years
Short intervals between gestations
Partner with whom the patient has had a pre-eclamptic pregnancy
New partner
Smoker
Mother or sister with a history of pre-eclampsia/eclampsia.

Maternal Disorders
Chronic hypertension and renal disease
Obesity, insulin resistance
Diabetes mellitus (gestational and type 1)
Factor V Leiden, protein S deficiency
Antiphospholipid antibodies
Lupic anticoagulant
Hyperhomocysteinemia

Fetal factors
Multiple gestation
Hydatidiform mole
Chromosomal abnormalities (trisomy 13, tryploidy)

Early markers with predictive value

These markers must be sensitive and specific and should detect the anomaly while prevention of the clinical development of the disease is still possible.

The test should be safe, simple, inexpensive, and appropriate for the patient. Unfortunately, in pre-eclampsia, none of the tests available leads to accurate diagnosis either in low- or high-risk patients; they do not comply with the all criteria mentioned above.

The predictive methods developed so far are the following:

Methods for the prediction of hypertensive disorders in pregnancy recommended between 1985 and 2003

Standard or modified methods of antinatal care
Elevated blood pressure (mean blood pressure)
Ambulatory automatized monitoring of blood pressure; chronobiological study of blood pressure
Tests for microproteinuria

Biophysical tests
Isometric exercise, roll-over test

Biochemical test and markers

- Sensitivity to angiotensin II
- Plasma volume, hemoglobin concentration, hematocrit
- Serum uric acid levels
- Different coagulation factors (activity of the antigen associated to factor VIII, antithrombin III, thrombin–antithrombin III, protein C)
- Platelet count, platelet volume, platelet volume and angiotensin 2 receptors
- Human chorionic gonadotrophin
- Endothelial activation markers (fibronectin, Von Willebrand factor, tissue plasminogen activator, plasminogen activator inhibitor, thrombomodulin, endothelin, laminin)
- Urinary calcium excretion
- Urinary excretion of prostacyclin metabolites
- Urinary kallikrein/creatinine ratio.

Doppler methods
Analysis of the velocity waveform in the uterine artery.

Given the multiple factors leading to pre-eclampsia, it is difficult to develop a sole test that is at the same time predictive, sensitive and specific. As a consequence, the decision to implement prophylactic measures in certain patients should be based on the presence of risk factors stemming from preexisting diseases, from their obstetric history or from their current gestation associated with an increased risk for pregnancy-induced hypertension.

Preventive approaches

The term *prevention* refers not only to primary prevention (stopping the disease from developing), but also to the act of reversing or slowing the process of the disease before it becomes clinically manifest (secondary prevention).

Primary prevention is achieved only if the cause of the disease is apprehended and then prevented or manipulated; therefore, it is not possible in gestational hypertension, where the etiology is unknown. We are still unable to determine why there is a faulty union between the trophoblast and maternal tissue leading to disorders in uteroplacental adaptation and trophoblastic invasion, and also to an exaggerated inflammatory response in the mother and to endothelial damage in pre-eclampsia.

Secondary prevention is the only prevention possible in pre-eclampsia, and can be summarized as follows:

Measures for secondary prevention of pre-eclampsia used between 1985 and 2003[31]

Intervention in lifestyle
Reduced physical activity: less stress

Intervention in diet
Low-sodium diet; energy, protein, magnesium, zinc, calcium, vitamin, linoleic acid, and fish oil supplementation

Pharmacologic intervention
Diuretics; antihypertensive drugs; anticoagulants and nitric oxide donors; acetyl salicylic acid.

Lifestyle

There is no evidence that changes in lifestyle have a preventive effect on the development of pregnancy-induced hypertension. Robilliard *et al.*, however, have found a strong correlation between gestational hypertension and the length of sexual cohabitation. The risk of developing this disease in primigravid and multiparous women is inversely proportional to the length of cohabitation.[32]

Diet

Observational studies indicate that a balanced diet with an adequate daily calorie intake benefits both the pregnant mother and the baby. This preventive measure is also taken into account in the prevention of cardiovascular diseases in general.

Below we will analyze some dietary components and their likely relation with hypertensive disorders of pregnancy.

Sodium restriction

In two clinical controlled trials of 603 women, no evidence was found of the prophylactic effect of sodium restriction in the patients' diets. Besides, clinical experimental studies indicate that strict sodium restriction in pregnancy may not be completely harmless as it interferes with the physiological increase in cardiac one-minute volume and the expansion of plasma volume, which are already markedly reduced in pre-eclamptic patients.

While there seems to be no reason to prescribe a low-sodium diet in healthy pregnant women, it should be recommended in patients sensitive to salt who suffer from chronic hypertension and are already on a sodium restricted diet.

Energy and proteins

A recent meta-analysis of 13 controlled studies of less than 25% of the total energy has shown a small but statistically significant reduction in low birth weight and fetal and neonatal death rates. The evidence, however, is not enough to evaluate other potential benefits. Although some studies show that a high-energy intake is associated with an increased risk for pre-eclampsia, in controlled studies there is no clear evidence that weight loss or reduced weight gain might lead to a decrease in the incidence of pregnancy-induced hypertension.

It is important to note that a severe limitation in weight gain reduces birth weight and, therefore, might be dangerous for the fetus.

Magnesium and zinc

Magnesium has been shown to relax vascular smooth muscle, by interfering with calcium entry, and to promote prostacyclin synthesis.

Recent controlled clinical trials have demonstrated the efficacy of magnesium sulfate in the prevention of eclampsia in pre-eclamptic women and in the management of eclampsia. However, prevention of hypertensive disorders of pregnancy with the use of magnesium supplements has so far been unsuccessful. The systematic review of seven controlled clinical trials involving 2689 women did not show any beneficial effect of the daily oral intake of a magnesium supplement during pregnancy.

Zinc is an essential oligo-element in many metabolic pathways. In a recent cohort study, no association was found between maternal plasma concentrations of zinc and any pregnancy outcome parameters in almost 3500 women from a low socioeconomic class.

Calcium

The hypothetical mechanism of action of calcium supplementation is the reduction in parathyroid hormone secretion,[33] which would in turn decrease the levels of free ionized calcium in the smooth muscle and lead to a reduced response of vasopressor agents and to vasodilation.

Bucher *et al.* undertook the meta-analysis of 14 controlled but heterogeneous clinical studies involving a total of 1218 pregnant women who received a daily 1.5–2 g calcium supplement. Results showed calcium supplementation to be associated with a significant reduction in systolic and diastolic blood pressure, with an odds ratio for pre-eclampsia of 0.38 (95% CI: 0.22–0.65), as compared with the placebo group. It also demonstrated that there is a tendency towards a lower incidence of preterm deliveries, IUGR, and perinatal death. Almost all these studies included populations with a low-calcium diet, which would explain why a randomized controlled study of the use of a daily 2 g calcium supplement in healthy nulliparous pregnant women from week 21 to delivery carried out in the United States did not have satisfactory results.

To conclude, currently available data seem to indicate that calcium supplement in pregnancy reduces the risk of pre-eclampsia in communities with a low calcium intake. Yet no beneficial effects on perinatal outcome have been demonstrated so far.

Linoleic acid and fish oil

The large chain omega-3 essential polysaturated fatty acid derivatives of linoleic acid, such as eicosapentaenoic acid or docosahexaenoic acid in sea fish oil, seem to protect against thromboembolic and hypertensive disorders.

Dietary polysaturated omega-3 fatty acids are the precursors of series 3 prostanoids, and combined with arachidonic acid, they produce changes in prostanoid synthesis leading to a reduction in the vasoconstriction and thrombotic effects of thromboxane A2.

The intake of omega-6 linoleic acid derivatives found in vegetable oils such as sunflower oil has been found to have similar effects.[34]

Controlled clinical studies carried out to assess their possible beneficial effects in gestational hypertension have demonstrated that the use of fish oil supplements helps to prolong the length of gestation. However, fish oil has not been found to prevent either the development of pre-eclampsia or its complications. The same conclusions apply to vegetable oils.

Vitamins

Oxidative stress is known to be a major pathophysiological mechanism leading to endothelial damage and malfunctioning in pre-eclampsia. Vitamins C and E are powerful inhibitors of reactive oxygen and lipid peroxidation. The levels of both these vitamins have been found to be rather low in pre-eclamptic patients.

In a randomized clinical study, a total of 283 women at high risk of developing pre-eclampsia, as determined by the anomalies in the uterine artery Doppler waveform or by a previous history of this disease, received a daily 1000 mg supplement of vitamin C and 400 IU of vitamin E from 16 to 22 weeks' gestation until delivery, and were compared with a placebo group. No difference was found in the incidence of pregnancy-induced hypertension in both groups, but the incidence of pre-eclampsia was 17% in the control group, and only 8% in the study group (OR 0.39, 95% CI: 0.17–0.90). Improvement in the biochemical indicators of endothelial and placental vascular function was also observed in the treated group.

As vitamins B6 (piridoxin), B12 (cobalamin) and folic acid, together with specific enzymes, are involved in metionin bioconversion to homocystein, their deficiency might result in hyperhomocysteinemia, which is associated with thromboembolic events and pregnancy complications including pre-eclampsia.

Pharmacologic interventions

Diuretics

Diuretics are known to reduce blood pressure and edema, which does not necessarily imply they have a beneficial effect on the pathophysiology of pre-eclampsia. Furthermore, all the articles in the literature reporting meta-analyses of controlled studies agree that there is not enough evidence to support a probable preventive effect of diuretics on the development of pre-eclampsia and its complications.

On the other hand, no deleterious effects on the fetus or gestation have been found with the use of diuretics. Therefore, treatment with diuretics may be continued in pregnant women who require it due to a preexisting pathology.

Antihypertensive drugs

If systolic and diastolic blood pressure is 160 and 110 mmHg or over, respectively, antihypertensive medication must be prescribed immediately given the high risk for such serious complications as abruptio placentae, cerebral hemorrhage, hepatic and renal failure. In patients with mild or moderate hypertension, the administration of antihypertensive drugs does not prevent the development of pre-eclampsia.

In a recent systematic review of 19 heterogeneous studies involving 2402 pregnant women who underwent antihypertensive treatment and were controlled with a placebo group, the risk of developing severe hypertension was found to be 50% lower in treated patients. However, no differences were found in the incidence of proteinuric pre-eclampsia, perinatal death, preterm delivery or low birth weight.

The use of beta-blockers, as compared with methyldopa, was analyzed in 11 studies involving 787 women. Beta-blockers were found to be more effective than and as safe as alpha-methyldopa. It is important to note that results which showed an association between atenolol and intrauterine growth retardation were not corroborated by other studies.

To conclude, there is no evidence in the controlled clinical studies available in the literature that the use of antihypertensive treatment in women with mild or moderate hypertension, whether chronic or gestational, might prevent the development of pre-eclampsia and eclampsia.

Angiotensin converting enzyme inhibitors and, therefore, angiotensin II receptor antagonists, seem to be the only contraindicated drugs during gestation as they have been found to be associated with fetal skull ossification defects, fetal growth restriction, oligohydramnios and neonatal renal failure.

Anticoagulants and nitric oxide donors

The high prevalence of genetic thrombophilia in patients with early and recurrent pre-eclampsia and intrauterine growth retardation might indicate that the hemostatic system is pathogenetically involved. As a consequence, many authors have proposed the use of aspirin and heparin as a preventive measure and to improve fetal outcome in patients with hereditary thrombofilia and also in patients at a high risk for renal disease.

In a randomized controlled study, Seki *et al.* administered ozagrel hydrochloride, a thromboxane A2 synthetase inhibitor, to 20 women at risk of developing pre-eclampsia from 20 weeks' gestation until delivery. These were compared with 20 women who received placebo. There was a significant decrease in the incidence of pre-eclampsia in the treatment group (RR 0.52) without affecting perinatal outcome.

Nitric oxide. In a controlled randomized study, transdermal nitric oxide (NO) donor glyceryl trinitrate patches and placebo patches were applied to 40 pregnant women at high risk of developing pre-eclampsia. The criterion for inclusion was the presence of abnormal Doppler waveforms in umbilical artery. No reduction in the incidence of pre-eclampsia and of intratuterine fetal growth restriction was observed in treated patients as compared with controls.

In conclusion there is still no evidence to support that heparin, thromboxane synthetase inhibitors and NO donors have a role in the prevention of pre-eclampsia.

Acetylsalicylic acid

Aspirin inhibits prostanoid synthesis through the acetylation and inhibition of cyclooxygenase, the key enzyme in the arachidonic acid cascade. The inhibition of prostanoid synthesis is selective and it depends on the aspirin dose: a low daily dose (0.5–1.5 mg/kg body weight) produces a dose-dependent inhibition in platelet TxA21 synthesis, reaching almost complete inhibition with a 1.5 mg/kg. As platelets do not have a nucleus, they are unable to resynthetize TxA21; consequently, their recovery depends on new platelet production by the bone marrow.

In contrast, the low concentration of aspirin in endothelial cells is not affected, and they continue producing PCI2, even when aspirin is no longer present in the patient's circulation.[35,36]

Several studies suggest that higher doses of aspirin may also affect the early interaction between the trophoblast and the decidua. In 1994, CLASP carried out a multicenter controlled clinical trial of a daily dose 60 mg of aspirin among 8021 women with mixed parity and at low to moderate risk for hypertensive disorders of pregnancy and/or fetal growth restriction. It is important to note that the reduction in the incidence of proteinuric pre-eclampsia (12%), fetal growth restriction (11%), and perinatal death (20%) observed in the group treated with aspirin, when compared with the placebo group, was not statistically significant. However, low-dose aspirin was found to reduce significantly the rate of preterm delivery (20%). Post hoc analysis of the data in the CLASP trial showed that the earlier the onset of treatment, the greater the reduction in the development of pre-eclampsia.

The results of this trial showed that aspirin had no therapeutic effect in 1343 women with pregnancy-induced hypertension or IUGR. The differences observed were not statistically significant either in women with moderate or low risk among a population of 28,000 women.

Through meta-analysis, it can be concluded that the results of the randomized controlled studies conducted in over 30,000 pregnant women at low, moderate, or high risk of developing pre-eclampsia indicate that prophylactic use of low-dose aspirin as from the 12th week of gestation will prevent the development of pre-eclampsia in about 15% of high-risk women. It will also lead to a similar reduction in the rate of low birth weight for gestational age and preterm deliveries. A lower and not statistically significant decrease in perinatal mortality will also be observed. The number of women at low or moderate risk who have to be treated in order to prevent one single case of pre-eclampsia is high (about 100), but it is much lower in high-risk patients.

It should be noted that neither in the CLASP trial nor in any other report has the prophylactic use of low-dose aspirin been associated with any deleterious effect on gestation, delivery or the newborn. Furthermore, follow-up of those babies from delivery to date has not revealed any aspirin-related complication.

Discrepancies among clinical studies

The decision to publish articles in the literature is usually biased towards those which report positive results even though the populations involved may be small. It is also a fact that in the large populations analyzed in multicenter studies high-risk patients may be overlooked and others may be wrongly classified as pre-eclamptic, thus underestimating the preventive effect of low-dose aspirin.

Sources of discrepancy among reported results:

- Gestational age at the time of inclusion in the trial (before or after 20 weeks' gestation)
- Time of the day when aspirin is administered: several controlled studies have demonstrated a more marked effect on blood pressure when aspirin is taken 8 h after waking up; even better results have been obtained if aspirin is taken at bedtime.
- Dose: early trials conducted in small populations report the use of daily doses of 100–150 mg, while later large multicenter studies have used much lower doses (50–75 mg daily). This dose will inhibit platelet thromboxane but may not be enough to affect placental thromboxane.
- We still do not know if a higher dose of aspirin might have other benefits without increasing side effects.
- Protocol adherence: in large multicenter studies it is not possible to corroborate whether the protocol has been followed correctly.
- Results reported in small randomized clinical studies should not be underestimated in favor of large multicenter trials as the former enable better control over eligibility criteria, objectives, time of treatment administration and protocol adherence by both researchers and patients.

Conclusions for obstetric practice

Preventive measures require the accurate identification of high-risk patients – about 2–8% of healthy nulliparous pregnant women. So far this selection can only be based on their obstetric and clinical histories and on the presence of known maternal and fetal risks. Unfortunately, no biophysical or biochemical markers are available yet which can predict the development of a hypertensive disorder during pregnancy.

Current studies do not support the prophylactic use of low-dose aspirin or calcium supplements in pregnant women at low or moderate risk for hypertension in pregnancy. This involves healthy nulliparous women, and those with a history of mild pregnancy-induced hypertension or with mild chronic hypertension.

A daily dose of 60–80 mg of aspirin from week 12 to delivery seems to be safe and effective when used in a definite group of high-risk patients in order to either prevent pre-eclampsia or delay its development and reduce its severity and complications.

In contrast, calcium supplement appears to be effective only in high-risk pregnant women with a low dietary calcium intake.

Recommended treatment protocol

(1) Daily administration of 60–80 mg of aspirin from week 12 to delivery in pregnant women with
   (a) a history of severe pre-eclampsia or elcampsia before 32 weeks' gestation
   (b) a history of severe fetal growth restriction, with or without pre-eclampsia, due to reduced uteroplacental blood flow
   (c) a family history of pre-eclampsia/eclampsia (in the mother or sister)
   (d) severe chronic hypertension and/or renal disease.

(2) Daily administration of 1.5–2 g elemental calcium supplement in high-risk women categorized as above and with a low dietary calcium intake, assessed according to their consumption of milk and other dairy products.

To conclude, given the multiplicity of clinical forms of this syndrome and the absence of early signs it is still not possible to predict its development. This, compounded by poor prenatal care, impedes the resolution of the disease.

We health care providers in Latin America should strive to reach the community *before* a gestation is conceived so that the antenatal visit does not constitute the first contact between the health center and the patient. The future is still uncertain; in the meantime, the medical community continues to provide new answers.[37]

REFERENCES

1. Saftlas AE, Olson DR, FrankAL, Atrash HK, Pokras R. Epidemiology in pre-eclampsia and eclampsia in the United States. *Am J Obstet Gynecol* 1990;163:460–5.
2. Voto LS, *et al.* Valor clínico de la proteinuria en los embarazos complicados con hipertensión arterial. I Congreso Argentino de Hipertensión en el Embarazo. Libro de resúmenes. Pag. 32. *Obstet Ginecol Lat Am* 1988;46(7–8):203–6.
3. Margulies M, Zin C, Margulies ND, Voto LS. Non-invasive ambulatory blood pressure control in normotensive pregnant women. *Am J Hypertens* 1989;2:924–6.
4. Brossens I, Robertson WB, Dixon HG. The role of the spiral arteries in the pathogenesis of pre-eclampsia. *Obstet Gynecol Ann* 1972;1:177–91.
5. Gant NF, Daley GI, Chand S, Whalley PJ, Mc Donald PC. A study of angiotensin II pressor response throughout primigravid pregnancy. *J Clin Invest* 1973;52:2682–9.
6. Florijn KW, Derkx FH, Visser W, *et al.* Plasma immunoreactive endothelin-1 in pregnant women with and without pre-eclampsia. *J Cardiovasc Pharmacol* 1991;17(Suppl 7):S446–8.
7. Gant NF, Worley RJ. *Hypertension in Pregnancy: Concepts and Management.* Appleton-Century Crofts, 1982.
8. Granger JP, Alexander BT, Bennet WA, Khalil RA. Pathophysiology of pregnancy-induced hypertension. *Am J Obstet Gynecol* 2001;14:178–85.
9. Visser W. Maternal hemodynamics, pathophysiology and implications for management in pre-eclamptic patients. The Rotterdam view. Erasmus University Rotterdam. The Netherlands. *VIII World Congress on Hypertension in Pregnancy,* 109, 1992.
10. Voto LS, *et al.* Seguimiento de la función renal en la embarazada normal e hipertensa. Ambiente Médico, Supl. 2, Sexta Sesión, 1984.
11. McKay DG. Discussion of Pritchard JA, Cunningham FG, Mason RA: Does coagulation have causative in eclampsia? In Lindheimer MD, Katz AI, Zuspan FP, eds. *Hypertension in Pregnancy.* New York: Wiley, 1976:102.
12. National High Blood Pressure Education Program. NIH Publication No. 00-3029 Originally printed 1990. Revised July 2000.
13. Davey DA, Mac Gillivray I. The classification and definition of the hypertensive disorders of pregnancy. *Clin Exp Hypertens B* 1986; 85:97–133.
14. Crocker IP, Tansindo DM, Baker PN. Altered cell kinetic in culture placental villous explants in pregnancies complicated by preeclapsia and intrauterine growth restriction. *J Pathol* 2004; 204(1):11–18.
15. Merviel P, Carbillon L, *et al.* Pathophysiology of pre-eclampsia: Links with implantations disorders. *Eur J Obstet Gynecol Reprod Biol* 2004;115(2):134–47.
16. Redman CWG, BelinLJ, Bonnar J. Fetal outcome in trial of antihypertensive treatment in pregnancy. *Lancet* 1976;2:753–6.
17. Redman CWG. Controlled trials of antihypertensive drugs in pregnancy. *Am J Kidney Dis* 1991;XVII(2):149–53.
18. Voto LS *et al.* Análisis comparativo del uso de las drogas hipotensoras en el tratamiento de la hipertensión en el embarazo. *Rev Argent Cardiol* 1987;55(4 Suppl):S44.
19. Barton JR, Stanziano GI, Sibai BM. Monitored outpatient management of mild gestational hypertension, remote from term. *Am J Obstet Gynaecol* 1994;170:765–9.
20. Ramanathan J. Pathophysiology and anesthesic implications in pre-eclampsia. *Clin Obstet Gynaecol* 1992;35(2):414–25.
21. Sibai BM. Magnesium sulfate is the ideal anticonvulsant in pre-eclampsia–eclampsia. *Am J Obstet Gynecol* 1990;162: 1141–5.
22. Dildy GA, ClarkSL. Managing eclampsia. *Contemp Obstet Gynecol* 1993;38(5):13–19.
23. Crowther C. Magnesium sulfate versus diazepam the management of eclampsia: A randomized controlled trial. *Br J Obstet Gynaecol* 1990;97:110–17.
24. López-Lera M. Complicated eclampsia. Fifteen years's experience in a referral medical center.
25. Sibai BM, Mabie BC, Harvey CJ, González AR. Pulmonary edema in severe pre-eclampsia–eclampsia: Analysis of thirty-seven consecutive cases. *Am J Obstet Gynecol* 1987;156:1174–9.
26. Clark SL, Gteenspoon JS, Aldahl D, Phelan JP. Severe pre-eclampsia with persistent oliguria: Management of hemodynamic subsets. *Am J Obstet Gynaecol* 1986;154:490–4.
27. Horvath JS, Phippard A, Korda A, Henderson-Smat DJ, Child A, Tiller DJ. Clonidine hydrochloride. A safe and effective antihypertensive agent in pregnancy. *Obstet Gynecol* 1985;66: 6348.
28. Kean L. Managing hypertension in pregnancy. *Curr Obstet Gynaecol* 2002;12:104–10.
29. Sibai BM, *et al.* Labetalol for intrapartum hypertension. *Contemp Obstet Gynecol* 1994;39(8):37–8.
30. *Desórdenes Hipertensivos durante la Gestación.* Clínicas Perinatológicas Argentinas. Vol 1, 2003. Ed. Panamericana.

31. Davies AM, Dunlop WW. Hypertension in pregnancy. In Barow SL, Thompson AM, eds. *Obstetrical Epidemiology*. London: Academic Press, 1983;Chap 6:167–208.
32. Roblliard, *et al.* Association of pregnancy-induced hypertension with duration of sexual cohabitation before conception. *Lancet* 1994;344:973–5.
33. Belizan JM, Villar J, Gozález L, Campodónico, Bergel E. Calcium supplementation to prevent hypertensive disorders in pregnancy. *N Engl J Med* 1991;325:1399–405.
34. Onwude JL, *et al.* A randomised double blink placebo controlled trial of fish oil high risk pregnancy. *Obstet Gynaecol* 1995;102: 95–100.
35. Sibai BM, Caritis SN, Thom E, *et al.* Prevention of pre-eclampsia with low-dose aspirin in healthy, nulliparous pregnant women. *N Engl J Med* 1993;329:1213–18.
36. Italian Study of Aspirin in Pregnancy. Low-dose aspirin in prevention of intrauterine growth retardation and pregnancy-induced hypertension. *Lancet* 1993;341:396–400.
37. Voto LS, Margulies M, *et al. Hipertensión en el Embarazo*. El Ateneo, 1997.
38. Consensus Report: National High Blood Pressure Education Program Working Group Report on High Blood Pressure in Pregancy. *Am J Obstet Gynecol* 1990;163:1689–712.
39. Paterson-Brown S, Robson SC, *et al.* Hydralazine boluses for the treatment of severe hypertension in pre-eclampsia.
40. Sibai B. Diagnosis and management of gestational hypertension and pregnancy. *Am Coll Obstet Gynecol* 2003;102(1).
41. Hermida RC, *et al.* Chronotherapy of hipertensión. *Curr Opin Nephrol Hyptentens* 2004;13(5):501–5.

193 Diabetes and pregnancy

F. A. Van Assche

Introduction

Although substantial progress has been made in the physiopathology and management of diabetes and pregnancy, major problems remain unsolved. Furthermore, diabetes in pregnancy remains an important medical complication, with implications for mother and child in the short and long term. Gestational diabetes does not significantly increase perinatal mortality; however, fetal hyperinsulinism and macrosomia are present. The case for the preexisting insulin-dependent pregnant diabetic has improved, but major complications, such as congenital malformations, sudden fetal death and the association with pre-eclampsia, need better understanding.

Screening for gestational diabetes

Gestational diabetes is defined as carbohydrate intolerance of variable severity with onset or first recognition during the current pregnancy.[1] Gestational diabetes occurs more frequently in older and overweight pregnant women. It is a heterogenous disorder and affects 2–3% of pregnancies in the Western world.[2,3] The metabolic adaptation that occurs during normal pregnancy involves apparent deterioration of glucose tolerance and hyperinsulinism, but only in a minority of women are the diagnostic criteria for gestational diabetes present.[4] Insulin secretions are increased during pregnancy and there is evidence that insulin resistance exists.[5,6] The morphological basis for this hyperinsulinism during pregnancy is marked B cell hypertrophy and hyperplasia, and hyperactivity of individual B cells.[7]

The diabetic ketoacidosis, hyperosmolar coma and vascular complications seen in type I diabetes are extremely rare in gestational diabetes. Cousins[8] found that the incidence of pre-eclampsia was increased in women with gestational diabetes. Perinatal mortality and morbidity are affected by this complication. Gestational diabetes is also a risk factor for the development of diabetes in later life. The first studies were those of O'Sullivan,[9] who reported a high incidence of diabetes mellitus many years after pregnancies complicated by gestational diabetes. Further studies have confirmed this original findings.[10–14]

In the past, gestational diabetes was reported to be associated with increased perinatal mortality.[15–17] More recently, it has been shown that perinatal mortality associated with gestational diabetes is not different from that of the general population. However, gestational diabetic women receive more obstetric attention and there is increased perinatal mortality in undiagnosed gestational diabetes.[18] Perinatal mortality therefore remains an indication to screen for gestational diabetes. Perinatal morbidity, in particular fetal macrosomia, is also increased in gestational diabetes. Fetal macrosomia is associated with an increased number of operative deliveries and with shoulder dystocia.[19,20] There is also evidence that infants born to mothers with gestational diabetes have an increased risk of becoming diabetic in later life.[21]

It therefore remains necessary to screen for gestational diabetes and if possible to perform general screening of all pregnant women.[22] However, there are a large number of glucose challenge procedures, with no agreement on the diagnostic criteria for gestational diabetes and there is not much hope of standardization in the near future.[22] Venous or capillary blood can be used and the glucose load can be oral or intravenous, with a glucose challenge of 50, 75 or 100 g. The original Somogyi–Nelson method of glucose measurement has been changed over the years to the glucose oxidase or hexokinase method. Furthermore, there are geographical, ethnic and racial differences in the deterioration of glucose metabolism.[23] Screening for glycosuria is not a strong index of gestational diabetes, since in pregnancy glucose in the urine does not reflect hyperglycemia. In the USA screening of the total pregnant population is advised using a 50-g 1-h challenge test; the American College of Obstetricians and Gynecologists advocate a glucose threshold of 140 mg/100 ml or 7.8 mmol/l (using venous plasma or serum and glucose oxidase or hexokinase techniques). Screening should be performed at 26–28 weeks, but retesting later in pregnancy might be reasonable for some patients such as obese and older women.[22] The use of the glucose reflectance meter may facilitate general screening in the future. However, lack of precision of the meters can be responsible for missing pregnant women who need further testing.[24,25] Other challenge tests and also random blood glucose testing have been

Table 193.1 Glucose challenge test criteria

	Glucose threshold mg/100 ml	mmol/l
Fasting	95	5.3
1 h	180	10.0
2 h	155	8.7
3 h	140	7.8

used but do not show any advantage over the 50-g challenge test.[22] The measurement of glycosylated hemoglobin and glycosylated proteins has inadequate sensitivity and specificity for screening.[26,27]

The standard method for the diagnosis of gestational diabetes still remains the 100-g oral glucose challenge, although the WHO has recommended a 75-g load (as in the non-pregnant population). The interpretation of the test goes back to the original study of O'Sullivan and Mahan.[28] Carpenter and Coustan,[29] using venous plasma and the glucose oxidase or hexokinase techniques, converted the O'Sullivan and Mahan[28] criteria as shown in Table 193.1. These criteria are close to the data of the European collaborative study where a glucose load of 75 g was used, but the blood sampling varied in the different centers.[30]

It must be stressed that international comparisons of the prevalence of diabetes during pregnancy are difficult because of the different methods and cutoff points for diagnosis. Furthermore, there are major ethnic variations.[31]

Gestational diabetes remains a risk factor for mother and child. It is therefore necessary to screen for this disorder during pregnancy. Universal screening with a 50-g 1-h glucose challenge is recommended. The final diagnosis is made with a 100-g oral glucose tolerance test. This clearly means that women with risk factors (severe obesity, a history of diabetes in the family, a personal birth weight of more than 4500 g, pre-eclampsia, polyhydramnios, fetal macrosomia, perinatal death and congenital anomalies) need a 100-g oral glucose tolerance test.

Prepregnancy care

There is growing evidence that tight control of diabetes before pregnancy improves fetal and maternal outcome. Education and management may prevent congenital malformations and early pregnancy loss and can also improve the maternal condition.[32] Many studies have shown that congenital malformations are more numerous in infants of type I diabetic mothers[33–38] and these are becoming the leading cause of perinatal morbidity and mortality in such infants. Kucera[39] reviewed the world literature between 1930 and 1964; the incidence of congenital malformations in diabetic pregnancies was 4.8% compared with 1.65% in normal pregnancies. Anomalies of the central nervous system, heart, skeleton, gastrointestinal tract and genitourinary tract are predominant. Poor metabolic control and the severity of diabetes is correlated with the high incidence of congenital anomalies.[34,40] An association is also found with a high level of glycosylated hemoglobin in the first trimester of pregnancy.[41] Furthermore, optimal treatment with insulin in the critical periods of organogenesis reduces the rate of fetal malformations in the rat.[42,43]

The first study in human pregnancy showing a reduction of congenital malformations by intensive diabetic management prior to conception was from Karlsburg, Germany.[44] The incidence of congenital malformations was 0.8% in the pregnancies of women given intensive treatment prior to conception and 7.8% in those pregnancies where intensive treatment started at 8 weeks. Studies in Europe and the USA confirmed these positive findings.[45–48] Strict metabolic control early in pregnancy reduces the number of congenital malformations at birth but does not prevent the excess frequency at conception, as is the case with tight glycemia control prior to conception.[38]

The relationship between poor diabetic control before conception or early in pregnancy and an increased rate of spontaneous abortion is not so clear. Miodovnik and colleagues[49] concluded that control of blood sugar is crucial around conception and in the early weeks of pregnancy to reduce the risk of an early abortion. Abortions after 10 weeks are probably due to congenital malformations. Studies in diabetic rats have shown delayed morphological development of blastocysts even in the preimplantation period and also more degenerate embryos.[50]

It therefore seems necessary for each diabetic woman planning a pregnancy to undergo preconception counseling. The presence of hypertension, vasculopathy, proliferative retinopathy and neuropathy must be investigated. Proliferative retinopathy should be treated by laser coagulation. The woman and her partner should be told that in the case of severe diabetes, certainly in association with hypertension, life-threatening complications for herself and the fetus do exist and exceptionally she should be advised not to become pregnant.

The most important goal of preconception care is to motivate intensive self-management in order to obtain normoglycemia. The woman must be instructed on self-monitoring her blood glucose and must learn about diet, physical activity and an efficient insulin regimen. Only when permanent normoglycemia is achieved can the future of the conceptus and maternal health be assured.

The key points of preconception counseling are clearly described by Steel,[51] who was one of the first to indicate the importance of this approach. After 20 years' experience in Scotland, it is still the case that all diabetic women should, at reproductive age, be visited by health-care providers, and that this should be regarded as a preconception visit.[51]

Medical approach of the pregnant diabetic woman

Normoglycemia from the preconception period until the time of delivery must be achieved in pregnant women with preexisting diabetes. In order to achieve this goal, intensive education of the diabetic woman is necessary. The skills, knowledge and experience of doctors and non-medical advisers are also important. During their reproductive years, diabetic women must be treated by a diabetologist with clinical and research interests in diabetic pregnancy. Of even more importance, a multidisciplinary approach is necessary, including general practitioner, nurse, dietician, physician, obstetrician and neonatologist. In most centers care is performed in a combined obstetric–diabetic antenatal clinic.

Self-monitoring of capillary blood glucose must be taught before conception and continued throughout pregnancy. There is no evidence that any special insulin regimen is better than others.[52] Frequent daily use of short- and medium-acting insulin and pen injectors or pumps delivering insulin subcutaneously are accepted alternatives. Optimal blood glucose levels are 4.0 mmol/l (80 mg/100 ml) preprandial and 6.0 mmol/l (120 mg/100 ml) postprandial. Since hypoglycemia can occur in the first trimester, it is advisable to use the same dose of insulin as that used before conception. With further progression of pregnancy the dose of insulin will increase. There is universal agreement that the measurement of glycosylated hemoglobin is the gold standard for the evaluation of good diabetic control. Levels below 7.5% should be achieved.[52] During labor and delivery, blood glucose is controlled by an intravenous infusion of dextrose and insulin.

Gestational diabetes can be treated by diet alone or by diet and insulin therapy. It is usual to start with dietary control. When blood sugar levels remain high or when fasting blood glucose is elevated, insulin should be given and adjusted in order to maintain normoglycemia. One insulin injection daily in the morning will control hyperglycemia. Weiss and associates[53] have suggested intensive management of the fetus in gestational diabetes by measuring insulin in the amniotic fluid. In the case of fetal hyperinsulinism, treatment with increasing doses of insulin is advised.

The intention of controlling fetal hyperinsulinism is to prevent macrosomia and neonatal complications. A review of current practice shows that only 15% of women with gestational diabetes require insulin.[54] However, intensive treatment with insulin has reduced the rate of macrosomia.[55] Moreover, experimental and epidemiological data indicate that long-term complications can be prevented by correct insulin therapy during gestational diabetes.[56]

There are no clear data available concerning the use of active agents in delaying digestion or absorption of nutrients. The use of oral hypoglycemic agents is a matter of controversy and is mostly regarded as contraindicated in Western medicine.

Obstetric approach of the pregnant diabetic woman

Perinatal mortality in the pregnancies of women with preexisting diabetes has been reduced over the last few decades. Congenital malformations and unexpected stillbirths remain the leading causes of death. Intrauterine deaths can still occur in type I diabetic pregnancies with poor control and in women with complications such as polyhydramnios, pre-eclampsia, macrosomia and intrauterine growth retardation.[57] The most important obstetric management therefore includes the detection of congenital anomalies, fetal surveillance and the prevention or early detection of complications of pregnancy. Congenital malformations can be detected by ultrasound examination between 16 and 20 weeks of pregnancy. Pedersen and Mølsted-Pedersen[58] have shown that fetuses with early growth retardation have a higher incidence of congenital malformations. Ultrasound is also the most suitable method for the evaluation of fetal growth. Increased thoracic diameter and increased abdominal circumference are markers for macrosomia.[59] However, the exact prediction of fetal weight remains difficult.[60] In diabetic vasculopathy, asymmetrical growth retardation can be detected during the second half of pregnancy.[61] Biophysical methods, such as fetal heart rate monitoring and the biophysical profile are superior to the older fetoplacental function tests for fetal surveillance, certainly during the third trimester. It is our experience that abnormalities of these tests are more ominous for the fetus of a diabetic woman than for the fetus of a woman with other complications of pregnancy.

Maternal complications are still frequently seen in pregnancy complicated by diabetes.[8] Hypertension during pregnancy and pre-eclampsia are increased in gestational diabetes and in the pregnant woman with preexisting diabetes. Garner and coworkers[62] found an incidence of preeclampsia of 9.9% in diabetic pregnancies compared with 4.3% in non-diabetic women. Van Assche and colleagues[63] found an increased production of thromboxane between 28 and 32 weeks of pregnancy in diabetic women without clinical vascular complications at the time of testing. The highest levels were found in those women who subsequently developed pre-eclampsia. It was concluded that increased thromboxane generation could be related to the occurrence of preeclampsia and the use of antiplatelet therapy to prevent pre-eclampsia warrants further investigation. However, preeclampsia will keep its secrets and prevention of the disease will be difficult. When polyhydramnios is found, fetal anomalies must be excluded and re-evaluation of strict diabetic control is advisable.[8] Polyhydramnios can be caused by excessive fetal urine production secondary to hyperglycemia. Premature rupture of the membranes, preterm labor, cord prolapse and abruptio placentae are known complications. Preterm labor can lead to the birth of a premature baby. On the other hand, the use of β-agonists and corticosteroids can result in maternal hyperglycemia, hyperinsulinemia, hypocalcemia, ketoacidosis, pulmonary edema and angina.[64] When these drugs are used, intensive diabetic monitoring is mandatory. Magnesium sulfate and calcium channel blockers may be worthwhile alternatives.[65] While the incidence of urinary tract infections is not increased in diabetic pregnancies, pyelonephritis increases the risk of perinatal morbidity.[66]

In older studies it was recommended that type I diabetic women were delivered between 35 and 36 weeks of pregnancy in order to avoid the high number of intrauterine deaths. In the last decade it has been suggested that diabetic pregnancies under tight control and without complications should be allowed to continue to term. Under these circumstances, an amniocentesis to determine fetal maturity seems unnecessary. For cervical ripening and induction of labor, local prostaglandin E_2 administration is of substantial benefit. Close supervision of the progress of labor and continuous electronic fetal monitoring are mandatory. The incidence of cesarean section varies between 17 and 83%.[60] Failed induction, macrosomia causing obstructed labor and fetal distress are the main reasons for abdominal delivery.[8] Coustan and associates[67] have shown that with close supervision the cesarean section rate can be reduced without increased perinatal risk. However, in the presence of a macrosomic fetus cesarean section is advisable in order to avoid shoulder dystocia. Indeed the physique of the infant with broad shoulders and a short neck may predispose to the dangerous complication of shoulder dystocia.

The obstetric management of the mother with gestational diabetes is mainly concentrated upon the detection of fetal macrosomia. Maresh and Beard[68] suggest that in the absence of any obstetric complication spontaneous labor can be awaited. However, in more severe gestational diabetes, certainly in the case of macrosomia, management similar to that of the pregestational diabetic is recommended.[69] Congenital malformations and early fetal loss are probably not increased in gestational diabetes.

The effect of maternal diabetes on the fetus and offspring

Alterations in the intrauterine environment affect fetal growth and development. In diabetic pregnancies not complicated by vasculopathy, fetal hyperinsulinism and macrosomia are mostly present. However, when vasculopathy and nephropathy are associated intrauterine growth restriction and hypoinsulinism are common findings. Both conditions may have long-term consequences. At present, human and experimental data in the rat are available. The advantage of research in the rat is that a better exploration of the working mechanisms is possible.

Offspring of rats that were hyperglycemic throughout the last week of gestation, at adulthood, appear as normal healthy animals with a normal body weight, normal basal glucose and insulin levels and a morphologically normal endocrine pancreas.[70,71] When stressed, however, glucose tolerance appears to be impaired, and the effect is divergent whether the youngster had passed its intrauterine life in a mildly or in a severely diabetic mother. When the maternal hyperglycemia was mild and resulted in fetal hyperinsulinemia, the induced increase in amino acid turnover is maintained in adulthood, and the β-cell response to glucose stimulation is deficient, while the insulin receptor system appears to be unaffected.[71–73] When the maternal hyperglycemia was severe and resulted in fetal hypoinsulinemia, the adult offspring not only displays a deregulation of the stimulated insulin output, but also insulin resistance in the liver and the peripheral tissues.[72,74] When the mothers were malnourished during pregnancy, whether in a qualitative (protein deficiency) or a quantitative (50% restriction) way, glucose tolerance is also impaired in the offspring.[75,76]

Pregnancy causes a considerable stress on the glucose and insulin metabolism of the mother and implies important adaptations of the endocrine pancreas at the structural and functional levels. The mass of islet tissue doubles and the activity of the β-cells is enhanced.[77] Normal pregnancy is associated with hyperinsulinemia and insulin resistance. When these youngsters of diabetic or malnourished mothers with impaired glucose tolerance become pregnant, they develop gestational diabetes.[71,78,79] This implies that their fetuses also will develop in an abnormal intrauterine milieu and have to adapt to it. Indeed, they display the typical features of fetuses from mildly diabetic mothers, and when they become adult they develop impaired glucose tolerance and gestational diabetes.[77,78] A diabetogenic tendency is thereby transmitted from one generation to another, without any genetic involvement, but as a result of the fact that the fetus developed in an abnormal intrauterine milieu. In the human a number of epidemiological studies also point to the importance of the intrauterine milieu for the development of the fetus. A higher incidence of non-insulin-dependent diabetes and of gestational diabetes is reported in children from diabetic mothers than from diabetic fathers,[80] and a higher incidence of diabetes is present in offspring from diabetic great-grandmothers via the maternal than via the paternal line.[81] Systematic treatments of diabetic mothers during pregnancy may result in a decreased incidence of diabetes in their children.[82] The most convincing data on the intrauterine transmission of the diabetogenic tendency in the human derive from studies of Pettitt and coworkers[83] on the Pima Indians, a population with a high incidence of diabetes. Glucose tolerance is much more frequent in children from mothers who had diabetes during pregnancy than in children from mothers who developed diabetes only after that pregnancy. The difference is convincing: 33% vs. 1%.[83] Recent epidemiological studies, relating birth files from 50 years ago with the health condition of these people now, also demonstrate a significant relationship between body weight at birth, whether or not related to a known metabolic pathology of the mother, and the incidence of impaired glucose tolerance and diabetes in adulthood.[84]

We can conclude that even a minor disturbance in maternal metabolism induces alterations in the fetal metabolism with lasting consequence for the offspring, even over several generations. The effect is situated at the level of insulin secretion (number, sensitivity, synthesis and secretion of β-cells) but also at the level of the insulin receptor system (number and sensitivity of receptor and postreceptor mechanisms).

Conclusion

At the beginning of the century a large number of diabetic women died before the age of reproduction or were too unwell to ovulate. When pregnancy occurred, maternal morbidity and mortality were high and only a few children were born alive. The discovery of insulin was beneficial for the mother but perinatal survival was still rare. With improvements in diabetic care, perinatal mortality improved but remained very high. Clinical and fundamental research brought the knowledge that for the treatment of the fetus of a diabetic mother, normoglycemia is obligatory. To protect the fetus during conception, tight control is necessary before conception. This implies commitment from physician, obstetrician, neonatologist and non-medical personnel. The diabetic woman herself and the environment take the major responsibility for care and management.

The most important goals for the future are the further reduction of congenital malformations, the early detection and prevention of pre-eclampsia, the prevention of diabetic complications during pregnancy and further investigation of the mechanisms of long-term effects.

REFERENCES

1. Freinkel N, Gable SG, Hadden DR, *et al.* Summary and recommendations of the second international workshop-conference on gestational diabetes mellitus. *Diabetes* 1985;34:123–6.
2. Sepe SJ, Connel FA, Geiss LS, *et al.* Gestational diabetes – incidence, maternal characteristics and perinatal outcome. *Diabetes* 1985;34:13–6.
3. Gabbe SG. Gestational diabetes mellitus. *N Engl J Med* 1986;315:1025–6.
4. Kühl C, Hornnes P, Andersen O. Aetiological factors in gestational diabetes. In Sutherland HW, Stowers KM, eds. *Carbohydrate Metabolism in Pregnancy and the Newborn.* Edinburgh: Churchill Livingstone, 1984:12–22.
5. Burt RL, Davidson IWF. Insulin half-life and utilization in normal pregnancy. *Obstet Gynecol* 1974;43:161–70.
6. Bellmann O, Hartmann E. Influence of pregnancy on the kinetics of insulin. *Am J Obstet Gynecol* 1975;122:829–33.
7. Van Assche FA, Aerts L, De Prins F. Morphological study of the endocrine pancreas in human pregnancy. *Br J Obstet Gynaecol* 1978,85:818–20.
8. Cousins L. Pregnancy complications among diabetic women. Review 1965–1985. *Obstet Gynecol Surv* 1987;42:140–9.
9. O'Sullivan JB. Long-term follow-up of gestational diabetics. In Camerini-Davalos RA, Cole HS, eds. *Early Diabetes in Early Life.* New York: Academic Press, 1975;503–10.
10. Stowers JM, Sutherland HW, Kerridge DF. Long-range implications for the mother: The Aberdeen experience. *Diabetes* 1985;34:106–10.
11. Grant PT, Oats JN, Beischer NA. The long-term follow-up of women with gestational diabetes. *Aust NZ J Obstet Gynaecol* 1986;26:17–22.
12. Mestman JH. Follow-up studies in women with gestational diabetes mellitus. The experience at Los Angeles County/University of Southern California Medical Center. In Weiss PAM, Coustan DR, eds. *Gestational Diabetes.* New York: Springer-Velag, 1988:191–8.
13. Oats JN, Beischer NA, Grant PT. The emergence of diabetes and impaired glucose tolesance in women who had gestational diabetes. In Weiss PAM, Coustan DR, eds. *Gestational Diabetes.* New York: Springer-Verlag, 1988:199–207.
14. Henry OA, Beischer NA. Long-term implications of gestational diabetes for the mother. In Oats JN, ed. *Diabetes in Pregnancy.* London: Baillière Tindall, 1991:461–83.
15. Jackson WPU, Woolf N. Maternal prediabetes as a cause of the unexplained stillbirth. *Diabetes* 1958;7:446–8.
16. Gabbe SG, Mestman JH, Freeman RK, *et al.* Management and the outcome of class A diabetes mellitus. *Am J Obstet Gynecol* 1977;127:465–9.
17. Merkatz IR, Duchon MA, Yamashita TS, *et al.* A pilot community based screening program for gestational diabetes. *Diabetes Care* 1980;3:453–7.
18. Pettitt DJ, Knowler WC, Baird HR, *et al.* Gestational diabetes: Infant and maternal complications of pregnancy in relation to third-trimester glucose tolerance in Pima Indians. *Diabetes Care* 1980,3:458–64.
19. Acker DB, Sachs BP, Friedmann EA. Risk factor for shoulder dystocia. *Obstet Gynecol* 1985;66:762–8.
20. Spellacy WN, Miller S, Winegar A, *et al.* Macrosomia – maternal characteristics and infant complications. *Obstet Gynecol* 1985;66:158–61.
21. Martin AO, Simpson JL, Ober C, *et al.* Frequency of diabetes mellitus in mothers of probands with gestational diabetes: Possible maternal influence on the predisposition to gestational diabetes. *Am J Obstet Gynecol* 1985;151:471–5.
22. Cousan DR. Screening and diagnosis of gestational diabetes. In Oats JN, ed. *Diabetes in Pregnancy.* London: Baillière Tindall, 1991:293–313.
23. Hadden DR. Geographic, ethnic, and racial variations in the incidence of gestational diabetes. *Diabetes* 1985;34:21–3.
24. Landon MB, Gabbe SG, Sachs L. Management of diabetes mellitus and pregnancy: A survey of obstetricians and maternal–fetal specialists. *Obstet Gynecol* 1990;75:635–40.
25. Weiner CP, Faustich MW, Burns J, *et al.* Diagnosis of gestational diabetes by capillary blood samples and a portable reflectant meter. Derivation of threshold values and prospective validation. *Am J Obstet Gynecol* 1987;156:1085–9.
26. Landon MB, Cembrowski GS, Gabbe SG. Capillary blood glucose screening for gestational diabetes: A preliminary investigation. *Am J Obstet Gynecol* 1986;155:717–21.

27. Cefalu WT, Prather KL, Chester DL, *et al.* Total serum glycosylated proteins in detection and monitoring of gestational diabetes. *Diabetes Care* 1990;13:872–5.
28. O'Sullivan JB, Mahan CM. Criteria for the oral glucose tolerance test in pregnancy. *Diabetes* 1964;13:278–85.
29. Carpenter MW, Coustan DR. Criteria for screening tests for gestational diabetes. *Am J Obstet Gynecol* 1982;144:768–73.
30. Lind T, Philips PR. A prospective multicentre study to determine the influence of pregnancy upon the 75-g oral glucose tolerance test (OGTT). In Sutherland HW, Stowers JM, Pearson DWM, eds. *Carbohydrate Metabolism in Pregnancy and the Newborn IV.* New York: Springer, 1989:209–26.
31. McCance DR. Classification and diagnosis of diabetes in pregnancy. In Dornhorst A, Hadden DR, eds. *Diabetes and Pregnancy: An International Approach to Diagnosis and Management.* New York: John Wiley and Sons, 1996:23–42.
32. Kitzmiller JL, Gavin LA, Gunderson E. Preconception counseling: Rationale for evaluation and management of diabetes prior to pregnancy. In Lee RV, Barron WM, Cotton DV, Coustan DR, eds. *Current Obstetric Medicine.* St Louis: Mosby Year Book, 1991:1–16.
33. Gabbe SG. Congenital malformations in infants of diabetic mothers. *Obstet Gynecol Surv* 1977;32:125–32.
34. Pedersen J. *The Pregnant Diabetic and Her Newborn,* 2nd edn. Baltimore: Williams and Wilkins, 1977.
35. Cousins L. Congenital anomalies among infants of diabetic mothers: Etiology, prevention, diagnosis. *Am J Obstet Gynecol* 1983;41:333–8.
36. Lowy C, Beard RW, Goldschmidt J. Congenital malformations in babies of diabetic mothers. *Diabet Med* 1986;3:458–62.
37. Reece EA, Hobbins JC. Diabetic embryopathy: Pathogenesis, prenatal diagnosis and prevention. *Obstet Gynecol Surv* 1986;41:325–35.
38. Mills JL, Knopp RH, Simpson JL, *et al.* Lack of relation of increased malformation rates in infants of diabetic mothers to glycemic control during organogenesis. *N Engl J Med* 1988;318:671–6.
39. Kucera J. Rate and type of congenital anomalies among offspring of diabetic women. *J Reprod Med* 1971;7:73.
40. Freinkel N, Cockroft DL, Lewis NJ, *et al.* Fuel-mediated teratogenesis during early organogenesis: The effects of increased concentrations of glucose, ketones, or somatomedin inhibitor during rat embryo culture. *Am J Clin Nutr* 1986;44:896–995.
41. Hanson U, Persson B, Thunell S. Relationship between haemoglobin A_{1c} in early type 1 (insulin dependent) diabetic pregnancy and the occurrence of spontaneous abortion and fetal malformation in Sweden. *Diabetologia* 1990;33:100–4.
42. Rashbass P, Ellington SKL. Development of rat embryos cultured in serum prepared from rats with streptozotocin-induced diabetes. *Teratology* 1988;37:51–61.
43. Eriksson RSM, Thunberg L, Eriksson UJ. Effects of interrupted insulin treatment on fetal outcome of pregnant diabetic rats. *Diabetes* 1989;38:764–72.
44. Fuhrmann K, Reiher H, Semmler K, *et al.* Prevention of congenital malformations in infants of insulin-dependent diabetic mothers. *Diabetes Care* 1983;6:219–23.
45. Damm P, Mølsted-Pedersen L. Significant decrease in congenital malformations in newborn infants of an unselected population of diabetic women. *Am J Obstet Gynecol* 1989;161:1163–7.
46. Goldman JA, Dickerd D, Feldberg D, *et al.* Pregnancy outcome in patients with insulin-dependent diabetes mellitus with preconceptual diabetic control: A comparative study. *Am J Obstet Gynecol* 1986;155:193–7.
47. Steel JM, Johnstone FD, Hepburn DA, *et al.* Can prepregnancy care of diabetic women reduce the risk of abnormal babies? *Br Med J* 1990;301:1070–4.
48. Kitzmiller JL, Gavin LA, Gin GD, *et al.* Pre-conception management of diabetes continued through early pregnancy prevents the excess of major congenital anomalies in infants of diabetic mothers. *J Am Med Assoc* 1991;265:731–6.
49. Miodovnik M, Mimouni F, Dignan PS, *et al.* Major malformations in infants of IDDM women: Vasculopathy and early first-trimester poor glycemic control. *Diabetes Care* 1988;11:713–8.
50. Pampfer S, De Hertogh R, Vanderheyden I, *et al.* Decreased inner cell mass proportion in blastocysts from diabetic rats. *Diabetes* 1990;39:471–6.
51. Steel JM. Pre-pregnancy care. In Dornhorst A, Hadden DR, eds. *Diabetes and Pregnancy: An International Approach to Diagnosis and Management.* 1996:101–19.
52. Hadden DR. Medical management of diabetes in pregnancy. In Oats JN, ed. *Diabetes in Pregnancy.* London: Baillière Tindall, 1991:369–94.
53. Weiss PAM, Winter R, Pürstner P, *et al.* Amniotic fluid glucose values in normal and abnormal pregnancies. *Obstet Gynecol* 1985;65:333.
54. Gabbe SG. Diabetes mellitus in pregnancy – how to manage. *Am J Obstet Gynecol* 1985;153:824.
55. Langer O. Prevention of macrosomia. In Oats JN, ed. *Diabetes in Pregnancy.* London: Baillière Tindall, 1991:333–47.
56. Aerts L, Van Assche FA. Islet transplantation in diabetic pregnant rats normalizes glucose homeostasis in their offspring. *J Dev Physiol* 1992;17:283–7.
57. Landon MB, Gabbe SG. Antepartum fetal surveillance and delivery timing in diabetic pregnancies. *Clin Diabetes* 1990;8:34–46.
58. Pedersen JF, Mølsted-Pedersen L. Early growth retardation in diabetic pregnancy. *Br Med J* 1979;1:18–9.
59. Landon MB, Mintz MC, Gabbe SG. Sonographic evaluation of fetal abdominal growth: Predictor of the large-for-gestational-age infant in pregnancies complicated by diabetes mellitus. *Am J Obstet Gynecol* 1989;160:115–21.
60. Coustan DR. Delivery timing mode and management. In Reece EA, Coustan DR, eds. *Diabetes Mellitus in Pregnancy: Principles and Practices.* New York: Churchill Livingstone, 1988:525–33.
61. Campbell S, Thomas A. Ultrasound measurement of the fetal head to abdomen circumference ratio in the assessment of growth retardation. *Br J Obstet Gynaecol* 1977;84:165–74.
62. Garner PR, D'Alton ME, Dudley DK, *et al.* Preeclampsia in diabetic pregnancies. *Am J Obstet Gynecol* 1990;163:505–8.
63. Van Assche FA, Spitz B, Hanssens M, *et al.* Increased thromboxane formation in diabetic pregnancy as a possible contributor to preeclampsia. *Am J Obstet Gynecol* 1993;168:84–7.
64. Kitzmiller JL, Gavin LA, Gin GD, *et al.* Managing diabetes and pregnancy *Curr Probl Obstet Gynecol Fertil* 1988;11:107–66.
65. Barss VA. Obstetrical complications. In Hare JW, ed. *Diabetes Complicating Pregnancy.* New York: Alan R Liss, 1989:125–34.
66. Diamond MP, Salyer SL, Vaughn WK, *et al.* Reassessment of White's classification and Pedersen's prognostically bad signs of diabetic pregnancies in insulin-dependent diabetic pregnancies. *Am J Obstet Gynecol* 1987;156:599–604.
67. Coustan D, Berkowitz R, Hobbins J. Tight metabolic control of overt diabetes in pregnancy. *Am J Med* 1980;68:845–52.
68. Maresh M, Beard RW. Screening and management of gestational diabetes mellitus. In Sutherland HW, Stowers JM, Pearson DWM, eds. *Carbohydrate Metabolism in Pregnancy and the Newborn IV.* London: Springer-Verlag, 1989:201–8.
69. Oats JN. Obstetrical management of patients with diabetes in pregnancy. In Oats JN, ed. *Diabetes in Pregnancy.* London: Balllière Tindall, 1991:395–411.
70. Aerts L, Van Assche FA. Endocrine pancreas in the offspring of rats with experimentally induced diabetes. *J Endocrinol* 1981;88:81–8.
71. Ktorza A, Gauguier D, Bihoreau MT, *et al.* Adult offspring from mildly hyperglycemic rats show impairment of glucose regulation and insulin secretion which is transmissible to the next generation. In Shafrir E, ed. *Frontiers of Diabetes Research. Lessons from Animal Diabetes III.* London: Smith-Gordon, 1990:555–60.
72. Aerts L, Sodoyez-Goffaux F, Sodoyez JC, *et al.* The diabetic intrauterine milieu has a long-lasting effect on insulin secretion by β-cells and on insulin uptake by target tissues. *Am J Obstet Gynecol* 1988;5:1287–92.
73. Susa JB, Boylan JM, Seghal P, *et al.* Persistence of impaired insulin secretion in infant rhesus markers that had been hyperinsulinemic *in utero. J Clin Endocrinol Metab* 1992;75:265–9.
74. Holemans K, Aerts L, Van Assche FA. Evidence for an insulin resistance in the adult offspring of pregnant steptozotocin-diabetic rats. *Diabetologia* 1991;34:81–5.
75. Dahri S, Snoeck A, Reusens-Billen B, *et al.* Islet function in offspring of mothers on low-protein diet during gestation. *Diabetes* 1991;40:115–20.
76. Holemans K, Verhaeghe J, Dequeker J, *et al.* Insulin sensitivity in adult female rats subjected to malnutrition during perinatal period. *J Soc Gynecol Invest* 1995;3:71–7.
77. Van Assche FA, Aerts L. Morphologic and ultrastructural modifications in the endocrine pancreas of pregnant rats. In Davlos C, ed. *Early Diabetes in Early Life.* New York: Academic Press, 1975: 333–41.
78. Aerts L, Holemans K, Van Assche FA. Maternal diabetes during pregnancy: Consequences for the offspring. *Diabetes Metab Rev* 1990;6:147–67.
79. Holemans K, Van Bree R, Verhaeghe J, *et al.* *In vivo* glucose utilization by individual tissues in virgin and pregnant offspring of severely diabetic rats. *Diabetes* 1993;42:530–6.

80. Martin AO, Simpson JL, Ober C, *et al.* Frequency of diabetes mellitus in probands with gestational diabetes: Possible maternal influence on the predisposition to diabetes. *Am J Obstet Gynecol* 1985;151:471–3.
81. Dorner G, Plagemann A, Reinagel H. Familial diabetes aggregation in type 2 diabetics: Gestational diabetes as apparent risk factor for increased diabetes susceptibility in the offspring. *Exp Clin Endocrinol* 1987;89:84–90.
82. Dörner G, Steindel E, Thoelke H, *et al.* Evidence for decreasing prevalence of diabetes mellitus in childhood apparently produced by prevention of hyperinsulinism in the foetus and newborn. *Exp Clin Endocrinol* 1984;84:134–42.
83. Pettitt DJ, Aleck KA, Baird HR, *et al.* Congenital susceptibility to NIDMM. Role of intrauterine environment. *Diabetes* 1988; 37:622–8.
84. Phipps K, Barker DJP, Hales CN, *et al.* Fetal growth and impaired glucose tolerance in men and women. *Diabetologia* 1993;36: 225–8.

194 Disorders of the respiratory system in pregnancy

C. Nelson-Piercy and J. Moore-Gillon

Introduction

Asthma is the commonest preexisting medical condition to complicate pregnancy, tuberculosis is becoming more common and pneumonia and cystic fibrosis are important causes of maternal mortality. This chapter discusses the physiological changes in the respiratory system during pregnancy, and the effect of asthma and other respiratory disease on pregnancy, as well as the effect of pregnancy on respiratory disease and the management of asthma, pneumonia, tuberculosis, sarcoidosis, cystic fibrosis and restrictive lung disease in pregnant women.

Physiological changes

There is a significant increase in oxygen demand in normal pregnancy due to the 15% increase in metabolic rate and the 20% increase in consumption of oxygen. There is a 40–50% increase in minute ventilation, mostly due to an increase in tidal volume, rather than in respiratory rate. This maternal hyperventilation leads to a reduction in partial pressure of arterial carbon dioxide, with a compensatory fall in serum bicarbonate and a mild respiratory alkalosis.

Later in pregnancy, the elevation of the diaphragm caused by the enlarging uterus leads to a decrease in functional residual capacity, but diaphragm excursion is unaffected so vital capacity is unchanged. A potential source of diagnostic confusion is awareness of the physiological hyperventilation of pregnancy, which leads to a subjective feeling of breathlessness in up to three-quarters of women at some time during pregnancy.

Patients with severe lung disease are less likely to deteriorate in pregnancy than those with severe cardiac disease. This is because there is a relatively greater reserve in respiratory function. Thus, although there is a comparative (about 40%) increase in both cardiac output and minute ventilation in pregnancy, for minute ventilation this represents a smaller fraction of the maximum increase possible by the body. If there is severe lung disease, however, right heart failure may be precipitated because of the increase in blood volume and cardiac output in pregnancy.

Asthma

Asthma is the commonest chronic illness of young adulthood, affecting at least 3% of women of childbearing age.[1] It is therefore often encountered in pregnancy, and this provides a valuable opportunity to diagnose asthma, and to optimize the treatment of women already known to have asthma.

Pregnancy and the severity of asthma

Pregnancy itself does not usually influence the severity of asthma. The course of asthma during pregnancy in individual patients is unpredictable. A review of more than 1000 pregnant asthmatics reported in nine studies found a worsening of asthma in 22%, improvement in 29% and no change in 49%.[2] Women with only mild disease are unlikely to experience problems, whereas severe asthmatics are at greater risk of deterioration, particularly late in pregnancy.[2,3] Those women whose symptoms improve during the last trimester of pregnancy may experience postnatal deterioration.[3,4]

Although in most individuals the severity of the disease process itself is probably unaffected by pregnancy, many asthmatics do experience a deterioration in symptoms. This may relate to increased awareness of the physiological hyperventilation of pregnancy. Of greater concern is the deterioration in disease control caused by reduction or even complete cessation of medication due to fears about its safety.

Asthma and the outcome of pregnancy

For the majority of women, asthma has no adverse effect on pregnancy outcome, and women should be reassured accordingly. Severe poorly controlled asthma, associated with chronic or intermittent maternal hypoxemia, may adversely affect the fetus and thus be associated with a significant decrease in mean birth weight, and an increase in the proportion of low birth weight neonates,[5,6] but recent studies have in general been very reassuring. Schatz and colleagues[7] compared nearly 500 pregnant asthmatics with non-asthmatic pregnant controls, and found the overall perinatal prognosis for women with actively managed asthma during pregnancy did not differ significantly from that of the non-asthmatic population. The incidence of pre-eclampsia, preterm births, low birth weight infants, intrauterine growth retardation, congenital malformations and perinatal mortality was similar in both groups.

Similarly, a retrospective study from India found no significant difference in antenatal complications, duration of pregnancy, mode of delivery, incidence of prematurity and low birth weight and perinatal mortality in asthmatic compared to non-asthmatic women.[6] A recent study looking specifically at the effects of acute attacks of asthma during pregnancy found no detrimental effect on birth weight, incidence of malformations, hypoglycemia or the need for phototherapy for jaundice during the neonatal period.[8] However, it is important to note that in this study the attacks were relatively mild and promptly treated.

There are other studies which do report a slight increase in the risk of premature labor[5,7,9–11] and low birth weight,[12–14] but some of the literature includes retrospective studies without adequate controls. Although a large prospective study did find a greater than twofold risk of preterm labor in asthmatics,[10] another prospective study[15] supports the findings of Schatz and coworkers[16] of no increase in either low birth weight or preterm delivery. A study from Quebec found that women with early and recurrent idiopathic preterm labor were significantly more likely to report asthma symptoms or physician diagnosed asthma than controls although there was no association with methacholine responsiveness, a measure of severity of asthma, suggesting that non-atopic noncholinergic mechanisms may link bronchial and uterine smooth muscle lability.[17] In summary, it would seem that any influence on birth weight and prematurity is small and related to the severity and control of the asthma.

Some studies have reported an increased incidence of pregnancy-induced hypertension/pre-eclampsia in asthmatic women.[5,8,18] Using a study population of over 24,000 women without essential hypertension, Lehrer and colleagues[18] found a significant association between pregnancy-induced hypertension and asthma. This is not a consistent finding[11,16] and caution is needed when interpreting these studies, since women with asthma are likely to be reviewed, and therefore to have their blood pressure measured more frequently than non-asthmatics during the antenatal period. It may be the detection rather than the incidence of raised blood pressure that is increased in asthmatics. A recent study from Finland demonstrated a significantly higher incidence of pre-eclampsia in asthmatics treated with theophylline (with more severe disease) but not in non-theophylline-treated asthmatics compared to non-asthmatic pregnant controls,[19] suggesting that the association with hypertensive disorders of pregnancy may be related to the severity of the asthma. Low-dose aspirin is gaining acceptance as prophylaxis for certain women at very high risk of early-onset pre-eclampsia,[20] but it is worth remembering that some asthmatics may develop severe bronchospasm with aspirin, and pregnant asthmatic women should be asked about a history of such sensitivity before being treated with low-dose aspirin.

Some studies suggest a possible increased incidence of transient tachypnea of the newborn,[21] neonatal hypoglycemia,[15] neonatal seizures[22] and admission to the neonatal intensive care unit,[11] in the babies of asthmatic women, but again these effects are small and are related to the degree of control of the asthma.

In summary, there is some evidence in asthmatic mothers for an increased incidence of small and preterm infants, but this risk appears to be small and may be minimized by maintaining good control of asthma throughout pregnancy. A relationship between asthma and hypertension or pre-eclampsia has also been suggested, but again any effect seems to be very small.

Management

Treatment of asthma in pregnancy differs little from the management in the non-pregnant patient. Effective control of the disease process and its accompanying symptoms is a priority. The focus should be on explanation and reassurance concerning the safety of the drugs used to treat asthma in pregnancy and during lactation. Education of asthmatic women prior to conception as well as during pregnancy are integral parts of management since decreasing or stopping inhaled anti-inflammatory therapy during pregnancy is a frequent cause of potentially dangerous deterioration in disease control. A team approach involving the obstetricians and midwives, the physician and the woman herself is the ideal. Emphasis on the safety of medication, including systemic steroids, helps ensure that women – and their doctors – do not discontinue, reduce or withhold vital drugs during pregnancy.

Two recent studies have shown that regular inhaled corticosteroids are beneficial in pregnant women with asthma. The first, a large prospective study from Finland, found that in women not initially treated with inhaled anti-inflammatory treatment during pregnancy the incidence of acute attacks of asthma was 17%, compared to only 4% in those on inhaled anti-inflammatory treatment from the start of pregnancy.[8] The second, smaller prospective study found the readmission rate for asthma exacerbations was decreased by 55% in women receiving inhaled beclomethasone at discharge following admission for asthma exacerbations compared to those not receiving this drug.[23]

Only minimal amounts of inhaled corticosteroid preparations are systemically absorbed.[24] Most of the information is for beclomethasone dipropionate (e.g. Becotide®, Becloforte®, Filair®, Beclazone® and other proprietary brands). Studies have shown no increased incidence of congenital malformations or adverse fetal effects attributable to the use of inhaled beclomethasone in pregnancy,[9,25,26] There is less information about budesonide (Pulmicort®), but it is widely used and appears to be safe. Fluticasone propionate (Flixotide®) is a newer inhaled corticosteroid and it too appears to be safe.

The addition of systemic corticosteroids to control exacerbations of asthma is safe, and these must not be withheld if current medications are inadequate. Prednisolone is metabolized by the placenta and very little (10%) active drug ever reaches the fetus. Sadly, media-fed concern about drugs falling within the broad category of 'steroids', combined with 'post-thalidomide' anxiety regarding the use of *any* drug in the first trimester, continue to hamper efforts to ensure that asthma remains optimally controlled throughout pregnancy. Findings from a single 40-year-old report of an increased incidence of cleft palate in the offspring of rabbits treated with massive doses of cortisone early in gestation[27] have been wrongly extrapolated to human pregnancy, where this has never been reproduced, despite the extensive use of steroids during pregnancy for a variety of conditions. There is no evidence of an increased risk of abortion, stillbirth, congenital malformations, adverse fetal effects or neonatal death attributable to maternal steroid therapy.[5,9,28] Although suppression of the fetal hypothalamic–pituitary–adrenal axis is a theoretical possibility with maternal systemic steroid therapy, there is no evidence from clinical practice to support this. The adrenocortical reserve of six newborns whose mothers had received long-term systemic steroids has been formally assessed and the response to exogenous adrenocorticotropic hormone was normal.[29]

Oral steroids will increase the risk of gestational diabetes, and cause a deterioration in blood glucose control in those women with established impairment of glucose tolerance in pregnancy. Blood glucose should be checked regularly, and the hyperglycemia is amenable to treatment with diet and, if required, insulin, and is reversible on cessation or reduction of steroid dose. The development of hyperglycemia is not an indication to discontinue or decrease the dose of oral steroids, the requirement for which must be determined by the asthma.

Transfer of β_2-agonists from the systemic circulation across the placenta is relatively rapid,[30] but very little of a given inhaled dose reaches the lungs, and only a minute fraction of this reaches the systemic circulation. A prospective study of 259 pregnant asthmatics treated with inhaled β_2-agonists showed no difference in perinatal mortality, congenital malformations, birth weight, Apgar scores or delivery complications when compared with asthmatics not using β-agonists and non-asthmatic controls.[31] Experience with the use of the inhaled long-acting β_2-agonist salmeterol (Serevent®) in pregnancy is growing. It appears free from fetal toxicity, it is not discontinued in pregnant asthmatics who require it for good asthma control, and may be introduced during pregnancy.

Inhaled disodium cromoglycate (Intal®), and the more recently introduced Nedocromil (Tilade®), appear to be safe for both mother and fetus, although there are, as yet, insufficient data to support routine use of the latter. Similarly, no adverse fetal affects have been reported with the use of anticholinergic drugs.

Both theophylline and aminophylline readily cross the placenta and fetal theophylline levels are similar to those of the mother.[32] Theophylline has been shown to be a cardiovascular teratogen in animals, and one report has suggested a possible link between theophylline and three cases of congenital cardiac anomalies in the human.[33] Stenius-Aarniala and colleagues[19] have recently published a series of 212 theophylline-treated asthmatics. The incidence of congenital malformations in the group receiving theophylline during the first trimester (2.5%) was not significantly higher than that in asthmatic or non-asthmatic controls, and only one of three abnormalities in the theophylline group was a case of congenital heart disease. There is no conclusive evidence of ill effect or malformation in the human fetus,[34] despite extensive use of theophylline in the past. Some have noted transient tachycardia or irritability in neonates of mothers receiving xanthines, but others have found that mean neonatal heart rate and Apgar scores were unaffected by maternal theophylline use.[19,32] The study of Stenius-Aarniala and colleagues[19] found a twofold increase in the frequency of jaundice in the neonates of theophylline-treated mothers, but this may relate to disease severity rather than the drug itself.

Acute severe attacks of asthma are treated as medical emergencies as in the non-pregnant[35] and, if needed, intravenous aminophylline or intravenous β_2-agonists should not be withheld.

The ionizing radiation from a chest x-ray is approximately 0.2 rad [less than 1/20th of the maximum recommended exposure in pregnancy (5 rad)], and abdominal shielding will minimize the exposure to the fetus. If a chest x-ray is clinically indicated, this investigation must not be withheld just because the patient is pregnant.

Asthmatic attacks in labor are rare. Women should not discontinue their prophylactic inhalers during labor, and there is no evidence to suggest that β-agonists given via the inhaled route impair uterine contraction or delay the onset of labor. Women receiving oral steroids (> 7.5 mg prednisolone daily for > 2 weeks prior to delivery) should receive parenteral hydrocortisone (100 mg three or four times a day) to cover the stress of labor, and until oral medication is restarted. Prostaglandin E_2, used to induce labor, to ripen the cervix or for early termination of pregnancy, is a bronchodilator and is safe. The use of prostaglandin F_{2a} to treat life-threatening postpartum hemorrhage may be unavoidable, but it can cause bronchospasm,[36,37] and should be used with caution in asthmatics. All forms of pain relief in labor, including epidural analgesia and Entonox, are appropriate for asthmatic women, although in the unlikely event of an acute severe asthmatic attack, opiates for pain relief should be avoided. Epidural rather than general anesthesia is preferable because of the increased risk of chest infection and atelectasis associated with the latter. Ergometrine has been reported to cause bronchospasm, but this does not seem to be a practical problem when syntometrine (oxytocin/ergometrine) is used for the prophylaxis of postpartum hemorrhage.

The risk of atopic disease developing in the child of an asthmatic woman is about 1 in 10, or one in three if both parents are atopic. There is some evidence that this risk may be reduced by breast feeding,[38,39] which provides another reason to encourage this practice.

All the drugs discussed above, including oral steroids, are safe to use in nursing mothers. Prednisolone is secreted in breast milk,[40,41] but there have been no reported clinical side effects in infants breast-fed by mothers receiving prednisolone and concerns regarding neonatal adrenal function are unwarranted with doses below 30 mg/day.

Pneumonia

Bacterial pneumonia is no more common in pregnancy than in non-pregnant women of the same age, matched for smoking status. However, viral pneumonia, for example, influenza pneumonia, is more severe in pregnancy[42] and pregnant women are particularly susceptible to varicella zoster (chicken pox) pneumonia and the maternal and fetal mortality is high.[43]

Patients with suggestive symptoms of cough (often dry at first), fever, rigors, breathlessness or pleuritic pain or signs of purulent sputum, coarse crackles or signs of consolidation on auscultation should have a chest x-ray.

Bacterial pneumonia

Bacterial pneumonia can kill previously fit young people, pregnant or not. Cases in pregnant women must always be regarded as potentially very serious, and always be managed in conjunction with a respiratory specialist. A respiratory rate of $\geq$30/min, a diastolic blood pressure of $\leq$60 mmHg and a serum urea of $\geq$7 mol/l are particularly poor prognostic signs.

Initial investigations should include an assessment of blood gases. Dangerous degrees of hypoxia may not be detectable clinically. Moreover, oximetry alone will only ensure adequate oxygenation, and a patient on oxygen supplementation may progress to the point of respiratory arrest from respiratory muscle fatigue without an oximeter giving any warning.

Initial antibiotic management must include drugs that will cover the likely pathogens (*Streptococcus pneumoniae, Hemophilus influenzae, Mycoplasma pneumoniae, Legionella*) and a regimen combining amoxycillin and clarithromycin or cefuroxime is usually used.[44] The precise microbial etiology may not be clear at the onset of treatment (and may never be established), and the possibility of non-bacterial causes (see below) should be kept in mind. Staphylococcal pneumonia is more common at times of influenza epidemics. It has a high mortality, and requires a different drug regimen.

Clearance of renally excreted drugs increases in pregnancy and therefore higher doses are required. Tetracyclines should be avoided after about 20 weeks' gestation since they can cause discoloration of the teeth. Iodine-containing cough medicines are also contraindicated because iodine is taken up by the fetal thyroid and may cause hypothyroidism and fetal goitre.

Remember that pleuritic chest pain, hemoptysis, breathlessness and cardiovascular collapse can be caused by the pneumococcus and not just by a pulmonary embolus.

Varicella

Chicken pox is more common and more severe in pregnancy than at other times and the maternal and fetal morbidity and mortality are high. Infection occurs in 0.05–0.07% of pregnancies[45] and about 10–20% of infected women develop varicella pneumonia associated with maternal mortality as high as 40%.[46,47] Later gestational age (perhaps due to increased immunosuppression) at the onset of varicella pneumonia is a significant risk factor for maternal mortality,[48] and the maternal disease appears to be worse in the latter half of pregnancy.[46] A history of previous infection, and therefore likely immunity, is usually reliable in the case of chicken pox since the clinical features are so unique. A live attenuated vaccine has recently become available in the USA and should be offered before conception to non-immune women.[45] Because of the substantial risk accompanying chicken pox infection in pregnancy, non-immune pregnant women exposed to varicella should be given zoster-immune globulin (ZIG).[47] Women should be asked about previous chicken pox infection before they are prescribed steroids in pregnancy, and those found not to be immune should be given ZIG. Those women who do develop clinical varicella should be treated with acyclovir.[49]

Anyone with varicella should be seen away from the antenatal clinic to minimize the risk to other pregnant women. Maternal and neonatal morbidity and mortality in cases of maternal varicella pneumonia may be improved by the use of intravenous acyclovir and mechanical ventilation.[50] This probably justifies the prophylactic use of intravenous acyclovir in those women who develop cutaneous varicella.[51] Smego and Asperilla[48] reviewed 21 cases of varicella pneumonia complicating pregnancy and found no adverse effects of acyclovir given in the second and third trimesters.

The fetus is at risk of congenital varicella with maternal infection in the first 12–16 weeks of pregnancy. The risk of teratogenicity is about 2%.[47] There is a risk of neonatal varicella if infection occurs within 10 days of, and especially 4 days before, delivery. ZIG administered at birth does not prevent all cases of neonatal infection, which has 30% mortality.[45]

Pneumocystis carinii pneumonia

The increasing number of women of child-bearing age who are seropositive for human immunodeficiency virus (HIV) has contributed to the increased incidence of pneumonia in pregnancy.[52] The most common opportunistic infection in patients progressing to AIDS is *Pneumocystis carinii* pneumonia (PCP). PCP is associated with adverse obstetric outcome, particularly if the diagnosis is not suspected.[53] PCP should be treated with high-dose cotrimoxazole (trimethoprim/sulfamethoxazole) with or without pentamidine. Despite the theoretical risks of neonatal kernicterus or hemolysis from sulfonamides given at term, there is increasing evidence that trimethoprim/sulfamethoxazole is safe in pregnancy.[53] Because PCP is an important cause of AIDS-related maternal mortality, HIV-infected pregnant women with a history of this opportunistic infection or with a $CD4^+$ cell count of < 200 cells/ml should receive prophylaxis with either cotrimoxazole or nebulized pentamidine.[54]

Tuberculosis

Rates of tuberculosis (TB) are increasing in Europe, the United States and developing countries. This recent resurgence is in part, but not wholly, due to the susceptibility of HIV-infected patients to TB infection. In Britain and the USA there are reports of increasing rates among the homeless and in inner city populations.

The onset is usually insidious with cough, hemoptysis, weight loss (or failure to gain weight) and night sweats. Diagnosis may be delayed in pregnancy because of inappropriate reluctance to carry out a chest x-ray. Less commonly, urinary tract, abdominal, lymph node or bone TB may present in pregnancy.

Tuberculosis is diagnosed by the typical appearances on a chest x-ray and sputum examination for acid-fast bacilli (Ziehl–Nielsen stain). Culture of the organism, *Mycobacterium tuberculosis* (MBTB) takes about 3 weeks, and if there is no sputum, washings from bronchoscopy must be obtained.

There is little evidence to suggest that tuberculosis has a detrimental effect on pregnancy or that pregnancy adversely affects disease progression and in neither HIV-positive nor HIV-negative women is recent pregnancy associated with an increased risk of developing active TB.[55]

Management

The principles of management are similar in pregnant and non-pregnant patients. The advice of a respiratory physician or infectious diseases specialist should always be sought. Active disease should be treated with a prolonged supervised course of more than one drug to which the organism is sensitive. Before sensitivities are available most patients are given triple/quadruple therapy with rifampicin, isoniazid and pyrazinamide and/or ethambutol. Liver function tests should be monitored regularly in patients taking rifampicin and all patients taking isoniazid should also be prescribed pyridoxine 10 mg/day to reduce the risk of peripheral neuropathy. The above drugs can all be safely given in pregnancy but streptomycin has been associated with a high (> 10%) incidence of eighth nerve damage[56] and should be avoided throughout pregnancy.

The risk of the neonate developing active tuberculosis is high and advice should be sought from the TB specialist supervising the mother's treatment as to the use of antituberculous chemoprophylaxis and BCG vaccination in the infant. HIV-negative infants born to HIV-positive mothers are at great risk of TB and should also routinely be given BCG.[57] The amounts of antituberculous drugs excreted in breast milk are not sufficient to dissuade women from breast-feeding.

Sarcoid

Sarcoid is uncommon in pregnancy, perhaps affecting 0.05% of all pregnancies in the UK. There may be chest symptoms, but the patient is often asymptomatic. Extrapulmonary manifestations include erythema nodosum (which may also occur as an isolated finding in pregnancy without evidence of an underlying associated cause), anterior uveitis, hypercalcemia, fever, or central nervous system (CNS) involvement.

Sarcoidosis is a multisystem granulomatous disorder of unknown etiology. It has pathological similarities to TB, but unlike tuberculosis, the granulomata are non-caseating. The commonest feature on chest x-ray is bilateral hilar lymphadenopathy but there may be extensive pulmonary infiltration progressing to fibrosis. Although there may be no obvious infiltration in the lung fields, the lung parenchyma is usually involved and diagnosis can be made by transbronchial biopsy. Serum levels of angiotensin converting enzyme may be altered in normal pregnancy and cannot therefore be used to help diagnosis or monitor disease activity as in the non-pregnant patient.

The course of sarcoidosis is largely unaffected by pregnancy, although those with active disease may have resolution of their x-ray changes during pregnancy,[58] and there is a tendency for sarcoidosis to relapse in the puerperium.[59] Any improvement that is seen antenatally may be due to the increased levels of endogenous cortisol present in pregnancy.[60]

Management

Sarcoidosis often resolves spontaneously, but indications for steroid treatment include extrapulmonary, especially CNS or eye disease, hypercalcemia or functional respiratory impairment. The safety of steroids in pregnancy has been discussed above, and they should be continued or started in pregnancy if clinically indicated. As with asthmatics on maintenance steroids, labor and delivery should be covered with parenteral hydrocortisone if women are taking more than 7.5 mg daily of prednisolone. Women should be advised not to take supplemental vitamin D, which may precipitate hypercalcemia in patients with sarcoidosis.

Cystic fibrosis

Advances in the care of children with cystic fibrosis (CF) have resulted in increasing numbers surviving into adulthood. The median age at death for CF patients is now over 30 years. This increase in longevity is due to several factors including increased emphasis on chest physiotherapy, early use of effective antipseudomonal antibiotics, improved fat absorption and nutrition using microsphere pancreatic enzyme supplements and the centralization of expertise in CF centers.[61]

Males with CF are usually sterile, but female fertility, especially in the well nourished, is normal. Women with CF who become pregnant are usually older at the time of diagnosis of CF, which probably reflects inherent differences in the severity of the disease itself. This may be due to different genetic errors or altered gene penetrance.[62] Pregnancy is well tolerated by many mothers with CF, but these women need expert joint care in a specialist obstetric unit and CF center.[63] CF is a multisystem disease, and during pregnancy, the obstetrician must work with the multidisciplinary team including physiotherapists, physicians and dieticians with particular expertise in the care of these patients.

Effect of pregnancy on CF

Most patients with CF die in early adult life, but with a few exceptions (see below) pregnancy does not increase this risk. Maternal mortality, although significantly increased compared with normal women, is not significantly greater than in non-pregnant age-matched women with cystic fibrosis.[62] But even if a CF woman survives pregnancy, she may deteriorate and die while the child is still young and it is important that such issues are discussed with the woman and her partner prior to pregnancy.

Factors adversely affecting maternal prognosis include maternal pulmonary hypertension, cyanosis and hypoxemia. Mortality is increased in women with moderate to severe lung disease [forced expiratory volume in 1 s (FEV_1) less than 60% of predicted normal values] at the onset of pregnancy,[62,64] and maternal survival is positively correlated with prepregnancy FEV_1%.[64]

Women with CF have difficulty gaining weight in pregnancy. Even those without pancreatic insufficiency are often underweight at the onset of pregnancy. The more underweight the mother prepregnancy, the greater the risk of cesarean section, and weight gain during pregnancy is positively correlated with prepregnancy FEV_1%. One year after delivery, however, there is no overall weight change.[64] Other problems encountered are deterioration in lung function with worsening dyspnea, exercise tolerance and oxygen saturation, pulmonary infective exacerbations and congestive cardiac failure. There is usually a loss of lung function during pregnancy, but this is regained following delivery. Edenborough and coworkers[64] described the outcome in lung function of 18 pregnancies in 17 women. They found a mean loss of FEV_1 of 13% and a loss of forced vital capacity of 11% by the end of pregnancy, but this was largely regained by 1 year postpartum. The patients showed a large variability in the pattern of lung function changes. The same authors found no change in microbiological status, and none of their women became colonized with *Pseudomonas* for the first time in pregnancy.

Effect of CF on pregnancy outcome

The rate of spontaneous abortion is not increased in CF pregnancies. Despite the frequent use of high doses of antibiotics in these women, the rate of congenital abnormalities in reported series is not increased.[62,64]

Factors predicting a poor obstetric outcome are the same as those adversely affecting maternal outcome and include pulmonary hypertension, cyanosis, arterial hypoxemia (oxygen saturation $< 90\%$), moderate to severe lung disease ($FEV_1 < 60\%$ predicted) and poor maternal nutrition. Perinatal mortality in the study of 129 pregnancies in 100 women in the USA[62] was 11.3% (all born to mothers with poor respiratory status), but a smaller, more recent study from the UK[64] of 22 pregnancies in 20 women had no perinatal losses. This may reflect advances in care, but also selection of lower-risk women with relatively preserved lung function. Those with very severe lung disease and deemed to be at high risk may be advised against pregnancy or are advised to have a termination of pregnancy.

The commonest complications during pregnancy are prematurity and intrauterine growth retardation. The preterm (< 37 weeks) delivery rate is increased in

CF pregnancies (26.8% in the series of Cohen and associates[62] and 33.3% in that of Edenborough and colleagues[64]). All mothers with moderate to severe lung disease in the study of Edenborough and coworkers[64] delivered preterm infants (all by cesarean section). The indication in all cases was deteriorating maternal pulmonary function. Chronic hypoxia (oxygen saturation < 90%) and cyanosis both increase the risk of small-for-gestational-age infants. Birth weight is positively correlated with prepregnancy lung function (probably related to longer gestations).[64] Women with preserved pancreatic function have an improved pregnancy outcome.[65] Poor maternal weight gains are predictive of both prematurity and stillbirth.[62]

Management

Prepregnancy counseling is desirable with determination of the carrier status of the partner. Since all women with CF are homozygous, all offspring will be carriers of the CF gene. The risk of a child being born with CF is 2–2.5% if the carrier status of the father is unknown (based on a carrier rate in the general UK population of about 1 in 25), and 50% if the father is heterozygous for the gene.

Pregnant women with CF should always be jointly managed in a CF center and an obstetric unit with experience in the management of such women. Medical management during pregnancy should include attention to adequate maternal nutrition, control of pulmonary infection, avoidance of prolonged hypoxia and regular assessment of fetal growth.

Over 90% of adult CF patients have pancreatic insufficiency and require enzyme supplements. High-calorie dietary supplements may be required in order to maintain maternal weight, since patients with CF (even without malabsorption) have high energy requirements, which will be further increased by pregnancy. Of adults with CF, 20% have diabetes and a further 15% have impaired glucose tolerance (IGT). Insulin requirements increase in pregnancy and those with IGT will be at risk of gestational diabetes.

Strict adherence to chest physiotherapy regimens must be encouraged. Some women decrease their physiotherapy due to fears concerning the fetus. These fears should be allayed. Most of the older, more established antibiotics used to treat pulmonary infective exacerbations in CF have a good safety record in pregnancy, and as stated above, the congenital abnormality rate in CF pregnancies is not increased. Appropriate caution is needed when considering the use of new drugs for which there is little information in pregnancy. The risks to the fetus from poor maternal health probably outweigh the risks to the fetus from transplacental passage of drugs.[63] Some patients may be taking prophylactic antibiotics either orally or via a nebulizer. Except in the case of tetracycline, which is contraindicated in pregnancy because of the effects on fetal teeth and skeleton, these should usually be continued throughout pregnancy. Infective exacerbations should be aggressively treated and this often requires admission to hospital and intravenous penicillins and aminoglycosides or cephalosporins in cases of resistant pseudomonas. Antibiotic therapy must be dictated by the results of sputum cultures. Caution is needed when using intravenous aminoglycosides, whether the patient is pregnant or not, and regular monitoring of drug levels is required. Some patients with CF respond to bronchodilators, and women should be reassured that inhaled and nebulized corticosteroids are safe in pregnancy.

Toward the middle and end of the third trimester, women with CF may become increasingly breathless often without any obvious infective exacerbation. If there is resting hypoxia, and especially if oxygen saturation is in the 80s or low 90s, admission for bed rest and oxygen therapy is advised. In some women, symptom deterioration warrants early delivery. Cesarean section is only necessary for obstetric indications and general anesthesia should be avoided if possible. Instrumental delivery may be indicated to avoid a prolonged second stage. Patients with CF are particularly prone to pneumothoraces, which may be precipitated by prolonged attempts at pushing and repeated Valsalva maneuvers in the second stage of labor.

In view of the risk of fetal growth retardation, the mother should be scanned regularly throughout pregnancy. If the growth rate slows down, it may sometimes be improved by admission of the mother for bed rest, nutritional supplements and oxygen.

In most cases, CF women deliver vaginally at term.[63] Breast feeding should usually be encouraged, although the mother may continue to require nutritional supplements in the puerperium especially if she is breast feeding. Most of the drugs used will be secreted into the breast milk, but this is rarely a contraindication to breast feeding.

Severe restrictive lung disease

Patients with restrictive lung disease, due to, for example, kyphoscoliosis, are less likely to deteriorate in pregnancy than those with severe cardiac disease for the reasons described above. It is difficult to predict with any accuracy the minimum vital capacity compatible with successful pregnancy outcome in patients with kyphoscoliosis and other causes of severe restrictive lung disease. Although figures such as 1 l[66] or 50% of predicted have been suggested, women with more severe impairment have had successful pregnancies.[67,68] Polycythemia gives an indirect assessment of the degree of hypoxia, and in itself is associated with an increased risk of thrombosis due to hyperviscosity.

Women with severe kyphoscoliosis are often delivered prematurely due to deterioration in respiratory function in the third trimester, and by cesarean section because of associated abnormalities of the bony pelvis and of abnormal presentations of the fetus.[69] Each case must be assessed individually, but, whatever the underlying cause of respiratory insufficiency, significant hypercapnia or hypoxia, and pulmonary hypertension and cor pulmonalae are associated with less favorable pregnancy outcome.

Conclusions

Respiratory diseases are common in the population generally and are thus common in pregnancy. They can cause much maternal morbidity – most of it preventable – even when the risk to the fetus is extremely small. Whilst severe respiratory disease may be apparent before pregnancy, and the woman already under specialist care, other cases may come to light for the first time during the antenatal period. All those involved in the care of pregnant women should have some knowledge of respiratory disease, and, in particular, how to recognize present or future problems and the need for specialist advice.

REFERENCES

1. Littlejohn PI, Ebrahim S, Anderson R. Prevalence and diagnosis of chronic respiratory symptoms in adults. *Br Med J* 1989;298:1556–60.
2. Gluck JC, Gluck P. The effects of pregnancy on asthma: A prospective study. *Ann Allergy* 1976;37:164–8.
3. White RJ, Coutts I, Gibbs CJ, *et al.* A prospective study of asthma during pregnancy and the puerperium. *Resp Med* 1989;83:103–6.
4. Juniper EF, Daniel EE, Roberts RS, *et al.* Improvement in airway responsiveness and asthma severity during pregnancy. A prospective study. *Am Rev Resp Dis* 1989;140:924–31.
5. Bahna SL, Bjerkedal T. The course and outcome of pregnancy in women with bronchial asthma. *Acta Allergologica* 1972;27:397–400.
6. Jana N, Vasishta K, Saha SC, *et al.* Effect of bronchial asthma on the course of pregnancy, labour and perinatal outcome. *J Obstet Gynaecol* 1995;21:227–32.
7. Schatz M, Patterson R, Zeitz S, *et al.* Corticosteroid therapy for the pregnant asthmatic patient. *J Am Med Assoc* 1975;233:804–7.
8. Stenius-Aarniala BSM, Hedman J, Teramo KA. Acute asthma during pregnancy. *Thorax* 1996;51:411–14.
9. Fitzsimons R, Greenberger PA, Patterson R. Outcome of pregnancy in women requiring corticosteroids for severe asthma. *J Allergy Clin Immunol* 1986;78:349–53.
10. Doucette JT, Bracken MB. Possible role of asthma in the risk of preterm labor and detivery. *Epidemiology* 1993;4:143–50.
11. Perlow JH, Montgomery D, Morgan MA, *et al.* Severity of asthma and perinatal outcome. *Am J Obstet Gynecol* 1992;167:963–7.
12. Sims CD, Chamberlain GVP, de Swiet M. Lung function tests in bronchial asthma during and after pregnancy. *Br J Obstet Gynaecol* 1976;83:434–7.
13. Greenberger PA, Patterson R. The outcome of pregnancy complicated by severe asthma. *Allergy Proc* 1988;9:539–43.
14. Schatz M, Zeiger RS, Hoffman CP. Intrauterine growth is related to gestational pulmonary function in pregnant asthmatic women. Kaiser–Permanente asthma and pregnancy study group. *Chest* 1990;98:389–92.
15. Stenius-Aarniala BSM, Piirila P, Teramo K. Asthma and pregnancy: A prospective study of 198 pregnancies. *Thorax* 1988;43:12–18.
16. Schatz M, Zeiger RS, Hoffman CP, *et al.* Perinatal outcomes in the pregnancies of asthmatic women: A prospective controlled analysis. *Am J Resp Crit Care Med* 1995;151:1170–4.
17. Kramer MS, Coates AL, Michoud MC, *et al.* Maternal asthma and idiopathic preterm labor. *Am J Epidemiol* 1995;142:1078–88.
18. Lehrer S, Stone J, Lapinski R, *et al.* Association between pregnancy-induced hypertension and asthma. *Am J Obstet Gynecol* 1993;168:1463–6.
19. Stenius-Aarniala B, Riikonen S, Teramo K. Slow-release theophylline in pregnant asthmatics. *Chest* 1995;107:642–7.
20. CLASP (Collaborative Low-Dose Aspirin Study in Pregnancy) Collaborative Group. CLASP: A randomised trial of low-dose aspirin for the prevention and treatment of pre-eclampsia among 9364 pregnant women. *Lancet* 1994;343:616–29.
21. Schatz M, Zeiger RS, Hoffman CP, *et al.* Increased transient tachypnoea of the newborn in infants of asthmatic mothers. *Am J Dis Child* 1991;145:156–8.
22. Patterson CA, Graves WL, Bugg G, *et al.* Antenatal and intrapartum factors associated with the occurrence of seizures in term infant. *Obstet Gynecol* 1989;74:361–5.
23. Wendel PJ, Ramin SM, Barnett-Hamm C, *et al.* Asthma treatment in pregnancy: A randomized controlled study. *Am J Obstet Gynecol* 1996;175:150–4.
24. Harris DM. Some properties of beclomethasone dipropionate and related steroids in man. *Postgrad Med J* 1975;51:20–5.
25. Marion-Brown H, Storey G. Beclomethasone dipropionate aerosol in long-term treatment of perennial and seasonal asthma in children and adults. A report of five and a half years experience in 600 asthmatic patients. *Br J Clin Pharmacol* 1977;4:529s–67s.
26. Greenberger P, Patterson R. Beclomethasone dipropionate for severe asthma during pregnancy. *Ann Intern Med* 1983;98:478–80.
27. Fainstat T. Cortisone-induced congenital cleft palate in rabbits. *Endocrinology* 1954;55:502.
28. Snyder RD, Snyder D. Corticosteroids for asthma during pregnancy. *Ann Allergy* 1978;41:340–1.
29. Arad I, Landau H. Adrenocortical reserve of neonates born of long-term, steroid-treated mothers. *Eur J Pediatr* 1984;142:279–80.
30. Morgan DJ. Clinical pharmacokinetics of beta-agonists. *Clin Pharmacokinet* 1990;18:270–94.
31. Schatz M, Zeiger RS, Harden KM, *et al.* The safety of inhaled beta-agonist bronchodilators during pregnancy. *J Allergy Clin Immunol* 1988;82:686–95.
32. Labovitz E, Spector S. Parental theophylline transfer in pregnant asthmatics. *J Am Med Assoc* 1982;247:786–8.
33. Park JM, Schmer V, Myers TL. Cardiovasacular anomalies associated with prenatal exposure to theophylline. *South Med J* 1990; 83:1487–8.
34. Greenberger P, Patterson R. Safety of therapy for allergic symptoms during pregnancy. *Ann Intern Med* 1978;89:234–7.
35. British Thoracic Society. The British Guidelines on asthma management: 1995 review and position statement. *Thorax* 1997; 52(Suppl 1):S1–21.
36. Fishburne JI Jr, Brenner WE, Braaksma JT, *et al.* Bronchospasm complicating intravenous prostaglandin F_{2a} for therapeutic abortion. *Obstet Gynecol* 1972;39:892–6.
37. Hyman AL, Spannhake EW, Kadowitz QJ. Prostaglandins and the lung: State of the art. *Am Rev Resp Dis* 1978;117:111–36.
38. Gruskay FL. Comparison of breast, cow, and soy feedings in the prevention of onset of allergic disease: A 15-year prospective study. *Clin Pediatr Phil* 1982;21:486–91.
39. Saarinen UM, Kajosaari M. Breast-feeding as prophylaxis against atopic disease: Prospective follow-up study until 17 years old. *Lancet* 1995;346:1065–9.
40. McKenzie SA, Selley JA, Agnew JE. Secretion of prednisolone into breast milk. *Arch Dis Child* 1975;50:894–6.
41. Katz FH, Duncan BR. Entry of prednisone into human milk. *N Engl J Med* 1975;293:1154.
42. Harris RE. Influenza during pregnancy. In Amstey MS, ed. *Virus Infection in Pregnancy.* Orlando, FL: Grune and Stratton, 1984:35–54.
43. Broussard RC, Payne DK, George RB. Treatment with acyclovir of varicella pneumonia during pregnancy. *Chest* 1991;99:1045–7.
44. Finch R, Mafarlane JT, Selkon JD, *et al.* Guidelines for the management of community-acquired pneumonia in adults admitted to hospital. *Br J Hosp Med* 1993;49:346–50.
45. Seidman DS, Stevenson DK, Arvin AM. Varicella vaccine in pregnancy. *Br Med J* 1996;313:701–2.

46. Katz VL, Kuller JA, McMahon MJ, *et al.* Varicella during pregnancy. Maternal and fetal effects. *West J Med* 1995;163:446–50.
47. Parayani SG, Arvin AM. Intrauterine infection with varicella-zoster virus after maternal varicella. *N Engl J Med* 1986;314: 1542–6.
48. Smego RA Jr, Asperilla MO. Use of acyclovir for varicella pneumonia during pregnancy. *Obstet Gynecol* 1991;78:1112–16.
49. Boyd K, Walker E. Use of acyclovir to treat chicken pox in pregnancy. *Br Med J* 1988;296:393–4.
50. Cox SM, Cunningham FG, Luby J. Management of varicella pneumonia complicating pregnancy. *Am J Perinatol* 1990;7:300–1.
51. Brown ZA, Baker DA. Acyclovir therapy during pregnancy. *Obstet Gynecol* 1989;73:526–31.
52. Berkowitz K, LaSala A. Risk factors associated with the increasing prevalence of pneumonia during pregnancy. *Am J Obstet Gynecol* 1990;163:981–5.
53. Schoenbaum EE, Davenny K, Holbrook K. The management of HIV disease in pregnancy. In Johnstone F, ed. *HIV Infection in Obstetrics and Gynaecology*. London: Bailliere Tindall, 1992:101.
54. Sperling RS, Stratton P. Treatment options for human immunodeficiency virus-infected pregnant women. Obstetric–Gynaecologic Working Goup of the AIDS Clinical Trials Group of the National Institute of Allergy and Infectious Diseases. *Obstet Gynecol* 1992;79:443–8.
55. Espinal MA, Reingold AL, Lavandera M. Effect of pregnancy on the risk of developing active tuberculosis. *J Infect Dis* 1996;173: 488–91.
56. Snider DE, Layde PM, Johnson MW, *et al.* Treatment of tuberculosis during pregnancy. *Am Rev Resp Dis* 1980;122:65–78.
57. Felten MK, Leichsenring M. Use of BCG in high prevalence areas for HIV. *Trop Med Parasitol* 1995;46:69–71.
58. Scadding JG. *Sarcoidosis*. London: Eyre and Spottiswoode, 1967.
59. Fried KH. Sarcoidosis and pregnancy. *Acta Med Scand* 1964; 176(Suppl 425):218–21.
60. Weinberger SE, Weiss ST. Pulmonary diseases. In Burrow GN, Ferris TF, eds. *Medical Complications during Pregnancy*, 4th edn. Philadelphia: W. B. Saunders, 1988:457–8.
61. Conway SP. Cystic fibrosis: Adult clinical aspects. *Br J Hosp Med* 1996;55:248–52.
62. Cohen LF, di Sant'Agnese PA, Friedlander J. Cystic fibrosis and pregnancy. *Lancet* 1980;18:842–4.
63. Geddes DM. Cystic fibrosis and pregnancy. *J R Soc Med* 1992; 85(Suppl 19):36–7.
64. Edenborough FP, Stableforth DE, Webb AK, *et al.* Outcome of pregnancy in women with cystic fibrosis. *Thorax* 1995;50:70–4.
65. Corkey CWB, Newth CJL, Corey M, *et al.* Pregnancy in cystic fibrosis: A better prognosis in patients with pancreatic function? *Am J Obstet Gynecol* 1981;140:737–42.
66. Novy MJ, Edwards MJ. Respiratory problems in pregnancy. *Am J Obstet Gynecol* 1967;99:1024.
67. de Swiet M. Respiratory diseases. In de Swiet M, ed. *Medical Disorders in Obstetric Practice*, 3rd edn. Oxford: Blackwell, 1995:20.
68. Hung CT, Pelosi M, Langer A, *et al.* Blood gas measurements in the kyphoscoliotic gravida and her fetus: Report of a case. *Am J Obstet Gynecol* 1975;121:287.
69. Lao TT, Yeung S, Leung BFH. Kyphoscoliosis and pregnancy. *J Obstet Gynaecol* 1986;7:11–15.

The reader is referred to the following British guideline [http://www.brit-thoracic.org.uk] on the management of asthma in pregnancy.

195 Cardiac disease in pregnancy

D. J. Williams and M. de Swiet

Introduction

Cardiac disease is after psychiatric causes, the second most common cause of maternal death in the UK.[1] Furthermore, symptoms such as breathlessness and signs such as an ejection systolic murmur reflect the physiological changes of healthy pregnancy and are present in up to 90% of the pregnant population.[2] Distinguishing between benign physiological change and significant pathology is an important part of good maternal and perinatal practice. In the developed world the pattern of maternal heart disease has changed radically over the last 50 years, but it has changed little in the developing world. As a prelude to a discussion of the assessment and management of heart disease during pregnancy, we describe the physiological changes of healthy pregnancy and how the pattern of heart disease in pregnancy has changed over a single generation.

Cardiovascular changes during healthy pregnancy

In normal pregnancy, cardiovascular changes are recognized as early as 5 weeks after the last menstrual period, i.e. 3 weeks after conception[3] (Table 195.1). At this time an increase in heart rate and ventricular function combine with a fall in total peripheral vascular resistance to significantly increase maternal cardiac output.[3,4] This trend persists until 24 weeks' gestation by which time cardiac output has increased by approximately 45%, from 4.8 to 7.2 l/min.[3] In the third trimester, cardiac output falls when the gravid uterus compresses the inferior vena cava.[6] Whether or not this fall is evident when measured in the left lateral position remains controversial.[3,7] During labor, cardiac output increases from a basal mean of 7.9 to

Table 195.1 Change in cardiovascular variables in pregnancy[3–5]

Variable	Non-pregnant	Pregnant	Change (%)
Aortic area (cm^2)	3.66	4.16	+13
Cardiac output (l/min)	4.9	7.2	+47
Heart rate (beats/min)	75	88	+17
Stroke volume (cm^3)	66	87	+32
Systolic blood pressure (mmHg)	115	111	−3
Diastolic blood pressure (mmHg)	72	55	−24
Peripheral vascular resistance (dynes/s/cm^5)	1326	875	−34
Pulmonary vascular resistance (arbitrary units)	2.85	2.17	−24
Blood volume (ml)	2600	3850	+48
Red cell mass (ml)	1400	1652	+18
Hemoglobin concentration (g/dl)	12.0	10.4	−15
LV end systolic diameter (cm)	2.90	3.04	+5
LV end diastolic diameter (cm)	4.49	4.79	+7
LA diameter (cm)	3.12	3.63	+16
LV wall thickness (cm)	1.48	1.89	+28
Left ventricular mass (g)	120	183	+53
Peak LV cavity d*D*/d*t** (cm/s)			
Systolic	7.8	10.7	+27
Diastolic	12.2	17.7	+45
Ejection fraction (%)	72.4	77.3	+7

Values for pregnancy are those at rest giving the maximum change from the non-pregnant state before labor, irrespective of gestational age; LV, left ventricle; LA, left atrium

*d*D*/d*t* is the rate of change of diameter

10.6 l/min during contractions,[8] returning to prelabor levels within 24 h. Within 2 weeks of delivery cardiac output almost returns to prepregnancy levels.[9]

Total extracellular fluid volume increases by 6–8 l, with a relatively greater increase in intravascular compared with interstitial fluid volume.[5] However, arterial and venous dilatation in the first and second trimesters creates a relatively underfilled state associated with a fall in blood pressure.[10,11] By 32 weeks' gestation, plasma volume has increased to a maximum of 40% above prepregnancy levels (approximately 1.2L).[12] Although the mechanism of vasodilatation in healthy pregnancy has not been fully elucidated, there is accumulating evidence that increased activity of nitric oxide synthase has an important role.[13,14]

Increased erythropoietin levels stimulate red cell production from early pregnancy,[15] but as the rise in plasma volume is relatively greater than the increase in red cell mass, there is an apparent anemia. Nevertheless, the hemoglobin concentration should not normally fall below 10 g/dl.[16] Plasma colloid oncotic pressure (COP) falls by about 15% in normal pregnancy secondary to a fall in plasma albumin concentration. Edema is usually prevented by a similar fall in interstitial COP.[17]

In anticipation of hemorrhage at childbirth, normal pregnancy is characterized by low-grade chronic intravascular coagulation within both the maternal and uteroplacental circulation.[18] There is evidence for increased levels of clotting factors, especially fibrinogen[19] and depression of fibrinolysis.[20]

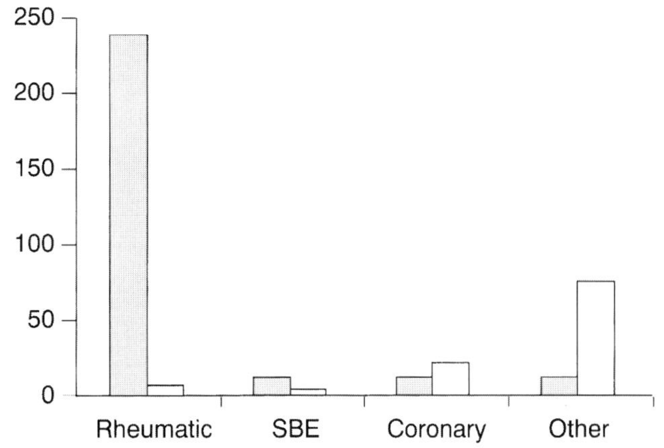

Figure 195.1 A comparison of the causes of death due to heart disease in pregnancy between 1952–1960 (shaded bars) and 1991–2002 (clear bars).[1]

Table 195.2 Deaths from rheumatic heart disease, 1952–1954

Disease	Deaths
Mitral valve disease (predominantly mitral stenosis)	96
Mitral and aortic valve disease	6
Mitral and tricuspid valve disease	1
Aortic valve disease	5
Total	108

Maternal mortality from heart disease

The best data regarding maternal mortality from heart disease in pregnancy come from the *Confidential Enquiries into Maternal Deaths in the UK*.[1] In the 9-year period following the beginning of the *Confidential Enquiries*, from 1952 to 1960, heart disease caused about one-quarter of all indirect (i.e. not 'direct' obstetric) maternal deaths. This amounted to 42 maternal deaths from heart disease per million maternities. During this period the picture was dominated by rheumatic heart disease, predominantly mitral stenosis, which caused 239 of the 277 cardiac deaths (Figure 195.1 and Table 195.2). There were also 12 deaths from endocarditis, 13 deaths from coronary artery disease and 13 deaths from other causes. This is probably a similar pattern to that seen at present in developing countries, though in Africa a considerable number of women die from dilated cardiomyopathy (not puerperal cardiomyopathy) associated with its high local prevalence, even in the non-pregnant population.

In the 12 years from 1991–2002, the death rate from heart disease represents about one-third of all indirect maternal deaths, but now this equates to 18 deaths per million maternities.[1] Furthermore, the pattern of death from heart disease in the UK is completely different from 1952 to 1960 (Figure 195.1). Between 1991–2002, there were 117 deaths from acquired heart disease (Table 195.3) and 38 deaths from congenital heart disease (Table 195.4). The majority of the 117 deaths from acquired heart disease were either ischemic (27) or due to rupture of aneurysm of the thoracic aorta or its branches (28). The women who died from ischemic heart disease were in general older than other women during pregnancy. It is not clear whether these data demonstrate an increased risk of dying from ischemic heart disease in pregnancy or merely reflect the older age at which women now become pregnant and the higher prevalence of smokers in this age group. Those dying from congenital heart disease included 22 with pulmonary vascular disease, who had either primary pulmonary hypertension or Eisenmenger's syndrome. Nearly all healthcare workers, with the exception of cardiologists, seem to be unaware of the seriousness of pulmonary hypertension in pregnancy.

Between 1991–2002, there were 28 deaths from dissecting aneurysm, a persistent observation in repeated maternal mortality reports, possibly related to increased shear stresses and thinner vessel walls in pregnancy. Indeed, rupture of other blood vessels in

Table 195.3 Deaths from heart disease in pregnancy, 1991–2002

Disease	Deaths
Cardiomyopathy and myocarditis	34
Aneurysm of thoracic aorta and its branches	28
Myocardial infarction	27
Pulmonary hypertension	22
Subacute bacterial endocarditis and valve disease	12
Other congenital heart disease	9
Other acquired heart disease	8
Sudden adult death syndrome	6
Myocardial fibrosis	4
Total	150

Table 195.4 Deaths from congenital heart disease in pregnancy, 1985–1993

Disease	Deaths
Primary pulmonary hypertension	8
Eisenmenger's syndrome	3
Atrial septal defect	4
Ventricular septal defect	4
Hypertrophic cardiomyopathy	2
Aortic valve disease	2
Mitral valve disease	1
Complex congenital cardiac lesion	3
Total	27

the brain or abdomen (splenic artery aneurysm, renal artery aneurysm) are more common in pregnancy. Again, an aging reproductive population may be part of the explanation, though women who died from aneurysm were not as old as those who died from ischemic heart disease.

With regard to the standard of care provided, deaths from ischemic heart disease (I.H.D.) were usually sudden and probably little more could have been done to prevent them. However, they all had risk factors, such as smoking and a family history of I.H.D. Patients with aneurysms had often been ill for several days before they finally died and usually the condition had not been considered a possibility.

Cardiovascular examination in pregnancy

History

As in all medical specialties, the history is of paramount importance in the assessment of patients with heart disease. In developed countries, women have frequent medical examinations throughout their lives and cardiac lesions are usually identified long before they attend an antenatal clinic. The family history is important for conditions such as hypertrophic cardiomyopathy and congenital heart disease.

The most frequent symptom of cardiac disease in pregnancy is dyspnea. However, this is difficult to assess as it is a variable feature of healthy pregnancy.[21] Furthermore, syncope is also common in normal pregnancy, but can be a symptom of severe aortic stenosis, hypertrophic cardiomyopathy (HCM), Fallot's tetralogy, Eisenmenger's syndrome or dysrrhythmias. Palpitations are often a symptom of dysrrhythmias. Chest pain is usually a symptom of ischemic heart disease, but is also associated with HCM or severe aortic stenosis. However, attempts to predict the outcome of heart disease in pregnancy by assessing the severity of symptoms in the first trimester have proved unreliable.[22] A precise anatomical diagnosis and knowledge of the outcome from previous pregnancies is more useful.[2]

Physical signs

The hyperdynamic circulation of pregnancy causes alterations in the cardiovascular system that mimic heart disease. The peripheral pulses are full, bounding and often collapsing suggesting aortic regurgitation to the untutored. Premature atrial and ventricular ectopic beats are common in normal pregnancy.[23] From midgestation onward, the jugular venous pressure becomes more obvious and may be raised due to increased intrathoracic pressure secondary to increased intra-abdominal pressure.[24] The apex beat is more forceful and because of the increase in cardiac output may suggest cardiomegaly in normal patients. However, if the apex beat is more than 2 cm outside the midclavicular line, this should be considered abnormal.[2] On auscultation, the first heart sound is loud and a third heart sound is audible in most pregnant women, reflecting rapid ventricular filling.[25] Rarely, during the last trimester, increased mammary blood flow can produce a bruit that varies with the pressure of the stethoscope.[2]

Investigations

Chest x-ray

The gestational increase in cardiac output and pulmonary blood flow causes an increase in cardiothoracic ratio and pulmonary vascular markings. A chest x-ray is indicated in a pregnant woman who has new onset of dyspnea. If the fetus is properly screened from x-rays the dose of radiation is less than 10 days of background radiation.

Electrocardiogram (ECG)

The heart rate increases gradually throughout normal pregnancy to reach a mean of 88 beats/min in the third trimester.[3] As the diaphragm becomes elevated, the heart gradually changes position and the QRS axis moves to the left.[26] Q waves and inverted T waves are frequently seen in lead III and aVR.

Echocardiography

Echocardiography is a safe and accurate method of discriminating significant heart disease from the physiological changes of healthy pregnancy. It is particularly useful when serially monitoring known valvular and myocardial lesions throughout pregnancy. A degree of regurgitant flow across the tricuspid, mitral and pulmonary valves was found in 41–90% of apparently normal pregnant women, depending on the valve and the stage of gestation.[27] Certain heart lesions are more accurately identified by transesophageal echocardiography. This involves passing a transducer mounted on the end of a flexible endoscope into the esophagus. Bacterial vegetations, intracavity thrombi and prosthetic valve dysfunction are all more accurately identified with transesophageal echocardiography.[2] Furthermore, non-invasive Doppler echocardiography can be used as effectively as Swan–Ganz catheterization for hemodynamic monitoring of the critically ill pregnant patient.[28]

Stress testing

The exercise ECG of healthy pregnant women reveals a shorter time to onset of maximum ST depression compared with non-pregnant women, but no difference in the time to resolve these changes.[29] In the absence of symptoms of ischemic heart disease these changes should be considered normal.[29] However, exercise testing prior to pregnancy, while monitoring the ECG and blood pressure, is useful for assessing cardiac reserve in women with ischemic heart disease, aortic stenosis or impaired ventricular function.[24]

Specific conditions occurring during pregnancy

Rheumatic heart disease

Although the incidence of rheumatic heart disease has fallen dramatically in the developed world, it used to be, and still is in the developing world, the most common cardiac cause of death during pregnancy. Acute rheumatic fever, following infection with a group A β-hemolytic streptococcus, is rare during pregnancy, even in developing countries.[30] However, the consequences of the acute disease, resulting in damage to heart valves, have major implications for the pregnant patient.

Mitral stenosis causes far more death and morbidity during pregnancy than any other rheumatic valve lesion (Table 195.2). Breathlessness is the most common presenting symptom of mitral stenosis, which becomes worse during pregnancy because affected women are unable to increase their cardiac output by the same degree as normal pregnant women.[31] This is due to the gestational increase in heart rate, which reduces diastolic filling time through the stenotic mitral valve. The consequent rise in left atrial pressure, and gestational increase in pulmonary blood volume, makes these women particularly vulnerable to pulmonary edema in the third trimester.[2] Furthermore, contraction of the uterus and relief of inferior vena cava compression immediately after delivery causes an increase in intravascular volume and a sharp rise in left atrial pressure, which can also result in acute pulmonary edema.[32,33] Conversely, peripartum hemorrhage can offset the increase in intravascular blood volume.[7] Patients who enter labor with a pulmonary artery wedge pressure of less than 14 mmHg are unlikely to develop pulmonary edema.[32]

The management of severe mitral stenosis should be aimed at improving left ventricular diastolic filling by slowing down the heart rate with β-blockers.[34] The dose should be titrated according to the patient's symptoms and heart rate.[30] Diuretics are necessary for the treatment of pulmonary edema and cardioversion may be needed to treat atrial fibrillation (see later). Pregnant women with mitral stenosis and atrial fibrillation should be anticoagulated with low molecular weight heparin e.g. dalteparin 5000 units daily (the risk of thromboembolism is not as high as with mechanical heart valves).[30] If the clinical condition deteriorates despite medical treatment, then balloon or surgical valvotomy during pregnancy gives good results.[35]

The cardiovascular adaptations to pregnancy allow women with mitral regurgitation to tolerate pregnancy well. Systemic vasodilatation off-loads the left ventricle and stretching of the left atrial wall keeps left atrial pressure down.[30] However, infective endocarditis remains a concern, so antibiotic prophylaxis is required for a complicated or surgical delivery.

Rheumatic aortic stenosis is less common in women than in men and is usually associated with mitral valve stenosis. Although the symptoms of coexistent mitral stenosis dominate, patients can present with chest pain, syncope or even sudden death. The severity of aortic stenosis can be estimated by calculating the pressure gradient across the valve with echocardiography. However, this gradient can be overestimated in pregnancy due to increased flow across the valve, while a fall in stroke volume, in patients with severe aortic stenosis, causes a reduction in gradient.[30] Medical treatment is aimed at improving function with coexistent mitral stenosis, but if the clinical condition deteriorates, then the fused commissures of the rheumatic aortic valve can be divided by balloon valvotomy, until valve replacement becomes necessary.[30] Epidural anesthesia causes peripheral vasodilatation and further increases the valvular gradient. Care should therefore be taken to avoid hypotension, while in those with a large pre-existing aortic valve gradient, epidural anesthesia should be avoided.

The gestational fall in peripheral vascular resistance improves cardiac output through a regurgitant aortic valve. Hence, aortic regurgitation is usually well tolerated during pregnancy, although pulmonary edema can occur with poor left ventricular function.[2]

Rheumatic tricuspid valve disease almost always coexists with mitral valve disease and the latter dominates the clinical picture.[36] Tricuspid regurgitation is more common than stenosis, but in healthy pregnancy there is also a functional regurgitation through the tricuspid valve.[37] Patients with tricuspid regurgitation have a raised right atrial pressure with 'v' waves in the jugular vein that become more obvious during pregnancy. Right heart failure presents with systemic edema and may require treatment with diuretics. Tricuspid stenosis in the presence of sinus rhythm is associated with an 'a' wave in the venous pulse and right atrial hypertrophy on an ECG. Echocardiography can recognize a rheumatic tricuspid valve, which if unsatisfactorily treated with diuretics requires definitive treatment with valvotomy.

Infective endocarditis

Infective endocarditis is a microbiological inflammation of the endothelial lining of the heart chambers, heart valves or great vessels.[38] It is characterized by fever, positive blood cultures, vegetations on heart valves or congenital defects, embolism and immunological phenomena.[39] Almost all patients with endocarditis have a heart murmur. However, increased blood flow during normal pregnancy intensifies murmurs from preexisting heart lesions and makes changes in auscultatory findings more difficult to interpret. The decline of rheumatic fever in the developed world has led to a reduction in the prevalence of abnormal heart valves and, consequently, a reduction in the incidence of infective endocarditis. Furthermore, puerperal sepsis related to criminal abortion remains a source of endocarditis only in the developing world.[39]

A group from Duke University have modified the criteria for a diagnosis of infective endocarditis to include echocardiographic evidence of a vegetation as well as fever and positive blood cultures with an organism that typically causes infective endocarditis.[40] Particularly virulent organisms, such as *Staphylococcus aureus*, can damage normal valves, but more usually, vegetations form at the site of known heart defects where there is damaged endothelium. The range of pathogenic organisms is similar to that of the non-pregnant state, although the urogenital tract is a source of enterococcal endocarditis following obstetric surgical intervention.[41] Previous antibiotics may suppress fever and cause negative blood cultures. Transesophageal echocardiography provides a better view of a vegetation or paravalvular abscess than transthoracic echocardiography. Once a clinical diagnosis has been made, three sets of blood cultures must be sent and then antibiotics initiated immediately. The most serious complications of infective endocarditis include valve destruction, embolism and immunological phenomena including a crescentic glomerulonephritis. As in the non-pregnant state, surgery is indicated for heart failure secondary to valve destruction.

In one series, there were no cases of infective endocarditis following a normal delivery in over 2000 cardiac patients.[42] Furthermore, although endocarditis was present in over 10% of cardiac deaths between 1985 and 1993,[1] very rarely was it acquired at the time of delivery. British microbiological[43] and cardiological[44] working parties have therefore been persuaded that, except for women with a history of previous infective endocarditis or prosthetic heart valves, this relatively high incidence of endocarditis is not a justification for routine antibiotic prophylaxis at the time of normal delivery. However, the *Confidential Enquiry* into maternal deaths during 2000–2002 included two women who died from bacterial endocarditis (one on a ventricular septal defect after a normal delivery), out of 44 deaths from cardiac disease.[1] This demonstrates that endocarditis can occur on heart lesions following normal delivery with catastrophic results. Since it is difficult to predict if a delivery will remain 'uncomplicated', it is the authors' personal recommendation to give antibiotic prophylaxis to all women with structural heart lesions at the time of normal delivery. We recommend a similar strategy to the UK recommendation for cardiac patients having an operative delivery.[43] This is to give 1 g amoxycillin intramuscularly and 120 mg of gentamicin intravenously at the time of induction of anesthesia (or onset of labor), and then 500 mg amoxycillin orally (we prefer intravenously) 6 h later (or every 6 h while the patient is still in labor). Drugs are variably absorbed during labor; therefore, we do not give 3 g oral amoxycillin to cover an anticipated normal delivery. Alternatives to amoxycillin include either vancomycin 1 g intravenously over 1 h or teicoplanin 400 mg intravenously.

Artificial heart valves and anticoagulation

Artificial heart valves are either mechanical or bioprosthetic (made of animal tissue). Women with diseased heart valves who are contemplating pregnancy should be advised to have children early, before a prosthetic valve becomes necessary.[45] When there is no alternative to heart valve replacement in a young woman, the risks of anticoagulation for a mechanical valve need to be weighed against the accelerated deterioration of a bioprosthetic valve during pregnancy.[46–48]

Warfarin crosses the placenta into the fetal circulation where it is a more potent anticoagulant. This is due to reduced production of vitamin K-dependent clotting factors by the fetal liver, rendering it at greater risk of hemorrhage throughout pregnancy and for up to 2 weeks after the mother stops warfarin.[45] The quoted risk of fetal embryopathy (chondrodysplasia punctata) from taking warfarin in the first trimester is 6%,[51] but this ignores the fact that warfarin-induced fetal embryopathy is dose-dependent.[45] In women taking less than 5 mg/day the risk of embryopathy is likely to be even less.[49]

Low molecular weight heparin does not cross the placenta, but it is less effective in preventing prosthetic valve thrombosis than warfarin.[47,48,50] Furthermore, heparin has a similar miscarriage rate to warfarin,[51] but otherwise has few maternal side effects.[52] There are small case-series of low molecular weight heparin successfully preventing mechanical valve thrombosis during pregnancy, but this mode of anti-coagulation to prevent valve thrombosis has yet to be evaluated.[53]

There is no optimal strategy for anticoagulation of women with metal heart valves during pregnancy. The author (D.W.) favours switching to LMW heparin at therapeutic doses aiming for a 3–4 hr. post dose anti Xa level of > 1.0 u/mL and a trough level of at least 0.5 u/mL. It might be possible to reduce the rate of valve thrombosis (currently estimated at approx. 10% on LMW heparin), by using higher doses, but this remains speculative. Low dose aspirin (75–150 mg) density is a safe and possibly effective adjunct to low molecular weight heparin in women with mechanical heart valves or an otherwise increased risk of intra cardiac thrombosis.[52]

Anticoagulation at the time of delivery is particularly difficult. Converting to i.v. infractionated heparin peripartum is very difficult to manage, due to variability in the APTT at term. Timing the dose of LMW heparin to minimise haemorrhage and restarting 4–6 hours post-partum may minimise the risk of valve thrombosis. Delaying reintroduction of warfarin for 3–5 days will reduce the risk of secondary postpartum haemorrhage.

A woman presenting with thrombosis of a heart valve will become acutely breathless. Sudden death is unusual, as the valves usually stick half open. This results in muffling of the prosthetic heart clicks and stenotic and regurgitant murmurs of the obstructed valve.[45] Echocardiography will confirm the diagnosis. Thrombolysis is the treatment of choice for thrombosis of right-sided heart valves,[45] but has also been successful for thrombosis of left-sided prosthetic heart valves.[54] However, emergency heart valve replacement is usually necessary.

The hemodynamic stress of pregnancy leads to accelerated damage of bioprosthetic valves, with all the attendant risks of subsequent valve replacement.[47,48,55] Consequently, these women should have serial echocardiography throughout pregnancy to assess valve integrity.[45]

Warfarin does not pass into breast milk, so is safe for the breast-fed infant.

Myocardial infarction

Coronary artery disease is an unusual occurrence in young women, but the incidence is increasing.[1] The reasons include more smokers, especially among young professional women, more obesity, more drug abuse, particularly with cocaine, and delay of pregnancy until a later age. Other rarer causes include vasculitis and congenital coronary anomalies.

Although early atheromatous disease of the coronary arteries is probably under-reported, myocardial infarction in pregnancy is often caused by coronary artery dissection.[56] Women therefore present suddenly, without prodromal angina and usually in the third trimester or postpartum.[57,58] The dissection usually begins within 2 cm of the ostium of the left anterior descending artery, causing an infarct of the anterior wall of the left ventricle.[59] The preponderance of arterial dissections associated with pregnancy may be related to increased hemodynamic shear stress on thin and dilated vessels.

Myocardial infarction is diagnosed in the usual way by noting typical ECG changes and enzyme rises. The MB isoenzyme of creatinine phosphokinase is released from the myometrium postpartum; therefore, cardiac troponin must be measured peripartum, to diagnose a myocardial infarction.[60] If possible, immediate coronary angiography is indicated to discover the cause of the infarct.[59] If an intracoronary artery thrombosis is identified, it can be lysed with a local injection of streptokinase, remembering that there is a risk of bleeding from the genital tract, if delivery has just occurred or is imminent. However, the first choice for treatment of acute coronary syndrome in pregnancy is percutaneous catheter intervention. Women with coronary artery dissection have survived thrombolysis with normal ejection fractions.[61] Major dissections threatening a large territory of anterior wall are best repaired with urgent coronary artery bypass grafting, preferably after delivery of a viable fetus.[59] However, both balloon angioplasty and coronary artery bypass grafting have been performed successfully during pregnancy.[59,62]

The size of the infarct can be reduced by β-blockers given as soon as possible after the diagnosis.[59] Although angiotensin converting enzyme inhibitors cause oligohydramnios and reduce renal blood flow in the fetus, the benefits to a mother, who has had a large infarct, probably outweigh the risks to the fetus. Cesarean section creates less physical demand on the impaired left ventricle and is therefore preferable to vaginal delivery. Epidural anesthesia is acceptable, especially in women who have had a small infarct, but some believe a general anesthetic causes less hemodynamic stress and is therefore preferable for patients with poor ventricular function.[59] Oxytocic drugs constrict coronary arteries as well as the uterus and should be avoided. Ergotamine, used to prevent postpartum hemorrhage, can also provoke coronary artery spasm and has caused fatal myocardial infarction in a previously healthy woman.[59]

Arrhythmias

As ischemic heart disease is rare in women of childbearing years, its clinical sequelae such as angina, heart failure and arrhythmias are also unusual. However, women with non-ischemic disease of cardiac conducting tissue, such as Wolff–Parkinson–White syndrome, have supraventricular tachycardias more frequently during pregnancy.[63] The precise reason for this observation must in some way relate to the cardiovascular and hormonal changes of healthy pregnancy.[64]

In general, antiarrhythmic drugs are safe in pregnancy and should be prescribed according to clinical need.[64] Most experience has been gained with digoxin, quinidine and β-adrenergic blocking drugs. Digoxin crosses the placenta to give similar drug levels in the fetus as in the mother,[65] hence its use as a first-line treatment of fetal supraventricular arrhythmias *in utero*.[66] Quinidine, procainamide and lignocaine are all well tolerated and relatively safe in pregnancy.[64] Similarly, β-blockers are also well tolerated, especially in later pregnancy, but atenolol can cause intrauterine growth retardation when taken during the first half of pregnancy.[64,67] Amiodarone can cause fetal thyroid dysfunction[68] and should be reserved for life-threatening arrhythmias.[64] Verapamil has been widely used for the treatment of maternal supraventricular arrhythmias, but adenosine is now gaining favor, especially in the second and third trimesters.[69]

Supraventricular arrhythmias

Almost all narrow complex tachycardias have a supraventricular origin. Chronic atrial fibrillation in women of childbearing age is usually associated with rheumatic mitral valve disease.[70] Under these circumstances, anticoagulation throughout pregnancy is essential, due to the increased risk of cardiac thrombus and embolization.[71] Fast atrial fibrillation can be treated with digoxin or combined with β-blockers if necessary.[72]

Atrial fibrillation in the absence of structural heart disease may be secondary to cardiomyopathy (particularly puerperal cardiomyopathy), thyroid disease, excessive alcohol, infection or sick sinus syndrome, but usually no cause is found.[73] In the presence of risk factors, anticoagulation is necessary and the choice between warfarin and low molecular weight heparin depends on the type of underlying heart disease (see sections on artificial valves and rheumatic fever).

The treatment of atrial fibrillation depends on the underlying cause, precipitating factors and duration of the episode. Direct current cardioversion is safe in pregnancy,[74] but there are only anecdotal data on the outcome of chemical cardioversion in pregnancy. Women who have had atrial fibrillation for longer than 2 days should be anticoagulated for 3 weeks prior to cardioversion. However, it may be possible to reduce this time and thereby improve the likelihood of successful cardioversion, by excluding atrial thrombi with transesophageal echo.[75] If no thrombus is detected, then patients can be fully anticoagulated at the time of cardioversion and for 4 weeks postcardioversion.[75] Type 1c antiarrhythmic drugs, such as flecanide, are most effective at maintaining sinus rhythm after cardioversion and treating paroxysmal atrial fibrillation. Flecanide is probably safe in pregnancy, as it is given to the mother for the treatment of fetal supraventricular tachycardia.[76] However, in the absence of controlled trials in pregnancy, β-blockers remain a sensible first choice, especially in relation to thyrotoxicosis, for the treatment of maternal paroxysmal atrial fibrillation.[73] Quinidine is useful and safe in pregnancy if a β-blocker fails. Digoxin is of no benefit in preventing paroxysms of atrial fibrillation.[77]

Ventricular tachycardia

It is important to make the diagnosis of a broad complex tachycardia, not only to avoid inappropriate treatment (that can be fatal in the case of verapamil given to a patient with ventricular tachycardia), but also to provide an accurate prognosis and plan for follow-up. Broad complex tachycardias can be either ventricular or supraventricular associated with bundle branch block or pre-excitation.[78] A wide complex tachycardia with atrioventricular dissociation is almost diagnostic of ventricular tachycardia.[78] The presence of fusion and capture beats and concordance of the QRS complex across the chest leads confirm the diagnosis. However, when the hemodynamic situation is stable, further clarification can be gained using echocardiography to identify dissociated atrial activity. If diagnostic difficulty persists, then atrioventricular block with either vagal stimulation or intravenous adenosine can terminate supraventricular tachycardia and a.v. nodal re-entry tachycardias.[79] In the same way, retrograde ventriculo- atrial conduction can be blocked to reveal the characteristic features of an underlying ventricular tachycardia.[78]

There is an increased awareness of ventricular arrhythmias in pregnancy.[64] If paroxysmal ventricular tachycardia is well tolerated, there is a place for conservative management.[80] The first-line treatment for idiopathic ventricular tachycardia during pregnancy should be β-blockade with metoprolol or failing that, sotalol.[64,81] Electrophysiological testing is usually not required for the treatment of most tachyarrhythmias and because of the high dose of radiation[82] associated with invasive electrophysiology, it has a limited role during pregnancy.

Bradyarrhythmias

Bradycardias are unusual in pregnancy. They may be secondary to vasovagal episodes, iatrogenic (b-blockade), or more rarely, sick sinus syndrome or complete heart block.[73] Congenital complete heart block can present for the first time during pregnancy with syncope. This is particularly true during the second stage of labor when the Valsalva maneuver can lead to further slowing of the heart rate.[83] It is therefore recommended that even asymptomatic women with complete heart block should have labor covered with a temporary pacing wire.[83] Physiological permanent pacemakers adapt to the physiological increase in heart rate during pregnancy. Women with fixed rate pacemakers also do well, presumably by increasing their stroke volume, but if symptoms related to an inappropriate bradycardia develop, then the pacemaker can be set at a faster rate.[2]

Cardiac arrest in pregnancy

In late pregnancy, resuscitation in the supine position may fail as venous return and cardiac output are compromised by aortocaval compression by the fetus.[5] Turning the patient to relieve the compression can overcome this problem.[84] If necessary, cardioversion can be used without apparent harm to the fetus.[74] If resuscitation is failing, emergency cesarean section in the accident and emergency department may help maternal cardiac output. If resuscitation has failed, but the fetus is still viable, an emergency cesarean section should be carried out within 15 min.[85]

Pericardial disease

Three main syndromes affect the pericardium: acute pericarditis, pericardial tamponade and constrictive pericarditis. Acute pericarditis is most commonly 'idiopathic' or related to a viral infection.[86] Rarer causes include tuberculosis, pyogenic infection, autoimmune disease, postinfarction, irradiation, neoplasia and trauma.[86] Chest pain and fever are the most common symptoms. Pericardial pain can be differentiated from the pain of myocardial ischemia by its accentuation on inspiration and movement of the thorax. There is a pericardial rub on auscultation and widespread, concave ST elevation on the ECG. Admission to hospital allows time to investigate an underlying etiology. Symptomatic relief with salicylates or non-steroidal anti-inflammatory drugs is acceptable, except close to term, when there is a risk of narrowing of the patent ductus arteriosus. Acute pericarditis may cause a pericardial effusion, which can be identified by echocardiography. If the effusion becomes too large, tamponade will develop, impeding ventricular filling and reducing cardiac output. This can present during pregnancy and is life-threatening unless aspiration or pericardiotomy is performed urgently.[87] Pregnant women with constrictive pericarditis are unable to accommodate the gestational increase in blood volume and may therefore present for the first time during pregnancy.[88] The ventricles cannot distend during diastole; therefore, the stroke volume is reduced and there is a compensatory tachycardia. Symptoms resemble those of right-sided cardiac failure, but with a normal-sized heart. There is an elevated venous pressure, systemic edema, which often includes hepatomegaly and ascites. Pulmonary edema is not a problem. There is frequently pericardial calcification on a chest x-ray, which together with a normal-sized heart and typical echocardiographic features, allows differentiation from a cardiomyopathy.[86] Without pericardectomy, maternal cardiovascular adaptation cannot take place and fetal outcome is compromised.[88]

Cardiomyopathies

Hypertrophic cardiomyopathy

Hypertrophic cardiomyopathy (HCM) is characterized by hypertrophy of the undilated left ventricle in the absence of an abnormal hemodynamic load, but in the presence of disorganized cardiac muscle.[89,90] It is an autosomal dominant condition with variable penetrance.[91] It can present as a chance finding, following investigations for an asymptomatic murmur, or as sudden death.[92] Other symptoms include syncope, palpitations, exertional chest pain and dyspnea.

On examination, there is a typical late systolic murmur, accentuated by standing and attenuated by squatting. Investigations include echocardiography, which will identify symmetrical or asymmetrical thickening of the left ventricular wall. An ECG will typically reveal left atrial P waves and left ventricular hypertrophy with strain. Once diagnosed, a 24-h ECG will identify arrhythmias and an exercise test will assess tolerance and changes in blood pressure. A failure of the blood pressure to rise may suggest an inability to increase stroke volume and an increased risk of syncope.

Asymptomatic pregnant women with HCM do well.[93] Although there are reports of women dying in pregnancy, sudden death in pregnancy is unusual.[94] It appears that the overall risk of sudden death from HCM is not increased by pregnancy.[90] However, a family history of sudden death or episodes of syncope or near syncope are poor prognostic signs. If there are symptoms of syncope then it must be deduced whether this is secondary to arrhythmias or hemodynamic instability. Short bursts of ventricular tachycardia can be treated with amiodarone, but there has been no controlled trial to test whether amiodarone is effective in preventing sudden death.[90] Indeed, asymptomatic bursts of ventricular tachycardia on ECG ambulatory monitoring are no longer thought to be a poor prognostic feature.[95] Similarly, the degree of outflow tract obstruction does not predict a poor outcome.[96] Arrhythmias should be treated appropriately, bearing in mind that the hypotensive action of verapamil may aggravate syncope in patients with HCM.[90] Symptoms of palpitations or chest pain might be improved with β-blockers, such as propranolol, as the bradycardia will improve coronary artery filling and left atrial emptying.[90]

Normal vaginal delivery is safe, but should take place in hospital with continuous ECG monitoring. Blood volume must be maintained throughout delivery, as a reduction in venous return will aggravate the gradient across the outflow obstruction. Therefore, peripartum blood loss must be replaced promptly and filling pressure kept up, if an epidural anesthesia is used. For similar reasons induction of labor with prostaglandins is best avoided.[90]

Peripartum cardiomyopathy

In the UK the incidence of peripartum cardiomyopathy is less than 1 in 5000.[2] There is no predisposing cause of the heart failure that develops peripartum (within 1 month of delivery and up to 6 months postpartum).[97] However, women with multiple pregnancies and gestational hypertension are more likely to develop peripartum cardiomyopathy.[98] Cases range from mild left ventricular dysfunction to sudden onset of gross heart failure and death within days of delivery. Symptoms include dyspnea, orthopnea and palpitations. Signs of heart failure include tachycardia, hypotension, elevated jugular venous pressure, basal crepitations, third heart sound and mitral regurgitation. Arrhythmias are common and thrombus within a dilated left heart can embolize systemically at presentation and before the clinical onset of heart failure.[99]

An ECG will show sinus tachycardia, possibly with runs of supraventricular or ventricular arrhythmias. A chest radiograph can reveal a grossly dilated heart and pulmonary edema.[99] Echocardiography usually reveals dilatation of all four chambers of the heart and hypokinesia of the left ventricule. Functional regurgitation through the mitral, tricuspid and pulmonary valves can be present in normal hearts during pregnancy, but will be more obvious in patients with a peripartum cardiomyopathy.[99]

The prognosis depends on the severity of the initial insult. While some women make a good recovery, others gradually decline to death or have a cardiac transplant.[100] Even women who have made an apparently full recovery are likely to have lost some cardiac reserve in the initial insult. Therefore, the hemodynamic challenge of a future pregnancy will always carry risks. Women who have made a good and sustained recovery will do best in a subsequent pregnancy, but serial echocardiography to assess left ventricular function is sensible as the possibility of relapse remains. Women with residual left ventricular dysfunction and an ejection fraction less than 50% should be discouraged from a further pregnancy.

Pulmonary vascular disease

Pulmonary hypertension may be either primary, when there is no demonstrable cause, or secondary to underlying cardiac or vascular disease. Whatever the etiology, pulmonary hypertension is life-threatening in pregnancy.[1]

Primary pulmonary hypertension

This is a rare disease characterized by increased pulmonary vascular resistance of unknown etiology. Diagnostic criteria used by the National Institutes of Health (NIH) include a mean pulmonary artery pressure of more than 25 mmHg at rest, without evidence of left-sided cardiac valvular disease, myocardial disease, congenital heart disease or clinically important respiratory, connective tissue or thromboembolic diseases.[101] However, clinical and pathological features of primary pulmonary hypertension (PPH) are seen in patients with human immunodeficiency virus (HIV), a history of cocaine abuse, portal hypertension and in those who take appetite suppressant drugs such as fenfluramine.[102] Women are affected twice as often as men.

Symptoms of PPH usually begin with dyspnea and easy fatigability.[102] However, the non-specific nature of these symptoms often means that the disease is not diagnosed until severe.[102] Consequently, women who become pregnant with recognized PPH have severe disease and a maternal mortality of about 40%.[103,104]

On examination, signs include a loud second heart sound, pulmonary ejection click and, occasionally, an early diastolic murmur of pulmonary regurgitation. An ECG may show right atrial P waves and evidence of right ventricular pressure overload.[103] An echocardiogram can exclude other cardiac disease, but also reveal elevated pulmonary artery systolic pressure and a dominant right ventricle.[103] A normal ventilation–perfusion scan will discriminate between PPH and the large perfusion defects typical of chronic major vessel thromboembolic pulmonary hypertension.[102]

Due to the 40% maternal mortality and possibility of disease progression during pregnancy, any patient with PPH should be advised to have a termination. If the patient insists on continuing the pregnancy, then maximum rest is advised due to the limited ability to increase cardiac output and the possibility of right ventricular failure.

Increased pulmonary vascular resistance is created by a combination of vasoconstriction, thrombosis *in situ* and medial hypertrophy of the vessel wall. Management of PPH is therefore aimed at correcting these abnormalities. Vasodilators such as calcium channel blockers produce a sustained improvement in 25–30% of patients.[105] Anticoagulation with LMW heparin will reduce the risk of thrombosis within the damaged pulmonary artery during the hypercoagulable state of pregnancy.[106] Oxygen and pulmonary vasodilator therapy can provide symptomatic relief for hypoxic patients and diuretics have a place when right heart failure causes gross hepatic congestion and ascites. However, a high right filling pressure is required for maintenance of cardiac output; therefore, any fall in intravascular volume due to blood loss must be replaced promptly. Postpartum management should take place in the intensive care unit with monitoring of the central venous pressure, systemic blood pressure and oxygen saturation.[103] Occasionally, right ventricular function recovers postpartum, but often, despite all precautions, symptomatic deterioration is relentless until death.[103] When death ensues, it is usually postpartum, precipitated by hypotension secondary to blood loss, arrhythmia, thromboembolism or right ventricular failure.[103]

Pulmonary embolism

When the hypercoagulable state of healthy pregnancy combines with a thrombophilia, immobilization, venous stasis, cesarean section or obesity, the incidence of thromboembolism increases markedly.[1] There were 25 maternal deaths from pulmonary embolus (PE) documented in the latest triennial *Confidential Enquiry into Maternal Deaths*.[1] Seventeen of these cases occurred postpartum (10 after cesarean section) and only 4 antepartum. A subclinical thrombophilia can manifest for the first time with thromboembolism during pregnancy. Thrombophilia may be secondary to deficiencies of antithrombin protein C and protein S as well as abnormalities of procoagulant factors, specifically factor V Leiden and prothrombin gene polymorphisms.[135]

Pulmonary embolism can be rapidly fatal or cause minor pleuritic pain. Although massive pulmonary embolism requires emergency treatment to save life, small PEs may herald a large fatal embolus and need to be fully investigated and anticoagulated.

A woman with massive PE may present with dyspnea and collapse. Examination may reveal an elevated venous pressure, a third heart sound and soft second sound. The cardiac monitor may show sinus tachycardia in the absence of a cardiac output, i.e. electromechanical dissociation. Emergency care should include elevation of the legs, turning the late pregnant patient onto her side, oxygen and colloid administration to improve right ventricular filling.[107] Inotropes are unnecessary due to maximal endogenous release of catecholamines.[107] When there is more time, as in a subacute PE, the ECG may show evidence of right atrial and ventricular dilatation with a typical S1 Q3 T3 pattern and T wave inversion in leads V1 to V4.[107] A chest X-ray may show dilatation of the pulmonary artery, then pulmonary oligemia. Echocardiography may reveal a dilated right ventricle that is hardly moving and a hypercontractile left ventricle. The patient should then be sent for immediate cardiac catheterization via the brachial artery, so as not to dislodge more clot from the inferior vena cava. The embolus can then be agitated and fragmented by the catheter itself.[107,108] The fragments of clot then pass into the peripheral pulmonary vasculature where they lyse rapidly and spontaneously.[108] If the facilities of a cardiac catheterization laboratory are not available, systemic thrombolysis should be used in acute massive pulmonary embolus. Subsequent treatment with intravenous heparin should start with 40,000 units/24 h, then adjusted to keep the partial thromboplastin time around two times control values.[109] Long-term prophylaxis could then continue with self-administered subcutaneous low molecular weight heparin. Twice daily injections of low molecular weight heparin (e.g. enoxaparin 1 mg/kg twice daily) are gaining popularity, and proving to be safe and effective.[112] About 1 week postpartum, women who find injections difficult can safely transfer to warfarin, as it does not pass into breast milk. Anticoagulation should continue for 3 months postpartum.

Small pulmonary emboli may present with mild pleuritic pain, hemoptysis or mild dyspnea. All preliminary investigations may be normal, but if suspicion persists, then there should be no hesitation in performing a perfusion scan (no need for a ventilation scan). The dose of radiation is not enough to be harmful to fetus. If available, magnetic resonance angiography is a sensitive and probably safe method for diagnosing pulmonary emboli in pregnancy.[113] Small PEs may become large and fatal; therefore, pregnant women should be anticoagulated in the same way as for larger PEs.

Around the time of delivery, sudden cardiovascular collapse with central cyanosis may be secondary to amniotic fluid embolus. This is almost invariably followed by disseminated intravascular coagulation and is often fatal.[114] The diagnosis can sometimes be confirmed by histological identification of fetal squames in maternal central venous blood,[115] although these have also been found in normal pregnancy. Treatment is aimed at supporting the circulation, contracting the uterus and correcting disseminated intravascular coagulation by monitored infusion of colloid and fresh frozen plasma.

Congenital heart disease

Improvements in cardiac surgery and pediatric care have meant that more women with congenital heart disease survive until a fertile age and become pregnant.

Acyanotic heart disease

Mitral valve prolapse

Mitral valve prolapse is a relatively common finding in young women of childbearing age. It is usually diagnosed when an asymptomatic systolic murmur leads to echocardiography. One or both of the mitral valve leaflets prolapse into the left atrium during systole, associated with or without mitral regurgitation.[116] Echocardiography recognizes some patients with a slight bowing of the mitral valve into the left atrium, but with an otherwise normal valve this is of no clinical consequence and should lead to reassurance of the patient.[116] Occasionally, patients present with palpitations caused by ectopic beats and even more rarely tachyarrhythmias.[116] However, generally mitral valve prolapse is a benign condition, which is well tolerated during pregnancy.

Mitral valve prolapse can be inherited as an autosomal dominant condition, usually associated with an asthenic habitus,[117] or secondary to acute rheumatic carditis, following mitral valvotomy and connective tissue disorders such as Marfan syndrome.[116] The typical auscultatory findings are of a late systolic click followed by a murmur with an accentuation at the end of systole. When regurgitation becomes more severe, the click and the murmur are heard earlier. However, the gestational increase in left ventricular volume during pregnancy causes a diminution of these auscultatory findings.[118]

Mitral valve prolapse is well tolerated in pregnancy. An increase in cardiac volume reduces valve prolapse and systemic vasodilatation diminishes mitral regurgitation.[116] However, infective endocarditis remains a significant concern.[119] Therefore, antibiotic prophylaxis is required for women who have more than trivial mitral regurgitation. Occasionally ulcerated areas on the mitral cusps attract non-bacterial platelet aggregates. These can separate and lead to cerebral embolism, but this possibility should not lead to prophylactic anticoagulation in all patients with mitral valve prolapse.[119]

Marfan syndrome

This is an autosomal dominant condition caused by a defect in the fibrillin gene that leads to abnormal collagen synthesis.[120] Characteristic clinical features affect the cardiovascular system, eyes and skeleton. The most important cardiac abnormalities are dissection of the aorta, aortic regurgitation and mitral valve prolapse. Advice to women with Marfan syndrome planning a pregnancy must be based on a cardiovascular assessment. If the aortic root is measured at less that 4 cm on echocardiography then the likelihood of aortic dissection is small.[121] Out of one series of 26 pregnant women with Marfan syndrome only one died, from endocarditis.[121] However, families 'breed true', as exemplified by two women who had a dissection of the aorta during pregnancy, despite an aortic root diameter less than 5 cm, but with a family history of aortic root dissection.[122] The risk of dissection persists for up to 6 months postpartum. During pregnancy hypertension must be aggressively treated with β-blockers to reduce hemodynamic stress on the aortic root. Identification of the putative gene is possible to make a prenatal and presymptomatic diagnosis.[123] Cesarean section is the safest form of delivery for women with an enlarged aortic root.

Atrial septal defects

An interatrial defect (ostium secundum type) allows blood to shunt from the left to the right atrium. Consequently, the right atrium and ventricle become dilated and pulmonary blood flow increases. This causes a pulmonary flow murmur and prominent venous pulsation, both of which become even more pronounced during pregnancy. However, an atrial septal defect is often not detected until adult life, when patients present with dyspnea or syncope from supraventricular arrhythmias. During pregnancy, acute blood loss must be avoided, as the consequent systemic vasoconstriction and reduced venous return leads to an increase in the left to right shunt, reduced left ventricular output and cardiac arrest.[124] More complicated atrioventricular defects (ostium primum defects) are associated with mitral regurgitation and direct shunts between the left ventricle and right atrium. Unlike secundum defects, which are not associated with endocarditis even in the non-pregnant state, these lesions require prophylactic antibiotics peripartum.[124]

Ventricular septal defect

Ventricular septal defects have usually been identified prior to pregnancy, but may be picked up by color flow Doppler, after referral for investigation of a pansystolic murmur. Patients are at risk of infective endocarditis and require antibiotic prophylaxis at the time of delivery. At delivery the shunt that is left to right in the acyanotic patient can reverse if there has been major blood loss on top of the gestational vasodilatation of pregnancy. If the ventricular septal defect is restrictive there is a loud pansystolic murmur, but with a large ventricular septal defect there is often pulmonary hypertension. Following closure of a ventricular septal defect in childhood there is no added risk due to pregnancy, except when there is residual pulmonary hypertension. This is of variable severity, so exercise tolerance and functional reserve of the right ventricle should be assessed before pregnancy.[124] Those with significant pulmonary hypertension should be treated in the same way as women with primary pulmonary hypertension (see above). One report suggests that nearly one-quarter of offspring will be born with ventricular septal defects.[125]

Persistent ductus arteriosus

During fetal life, blood flows from the pulmonary artery through the ductus arteriosus into the aorta. If the ductus does not close at the time of birth, then blood will flow in the opposite direction from the aorta into the pulmonary artery. This can be recognized with a collapsing pulse and a continuous murmur at the left second intercostal space. A large shunt leads to pulmonary artery hypertension and congestive cardiac failure and should be closed before pregnancy. Furthermore, widely patent persistent ductus arteriosus are at increased risk of dissection during pregnancy.[126] There is also a small risk of infective endocarditis.[124] Small persistent ductus arteriosus may be identified on auscultation and echocardiography, but if there is a normal pulmonary artery pressure then pregnancy does not present any added difficulty.

Coarctation of the aorta

Women who become pregnant with coarctation of the aorta are at increased risk of aortic dissection, rupture of an associated berry aneurysm, infective endocarditis and heart failure.[127] However, the overall mortality rate of a pregnant woman with coarctation of the aorta is currently less than 3%.[124] Hypertension should be aggressively treated, exercise curtailed and cesarean section performed (if labor is expected to be difficult or prolonged) to reduce the possibility of dissection. One-third of all patients with an aortic coarctation have an associated bicuspid valve, which is vulnerable to endocarditis. Surgical repair of the coarctation is usually performed in childhood with improvement of long-term outcome, but late local complications such as dissection or aneurysm are still possible.[124]

Ebstein's anomaly

Ebstein's anomaly consists of downward displacement of the tricuspid valve into the right ventricle, usually associated with an atrial septal defect. Cyanosis, arrhythmias and dyspnea are common problems, depending on the severity of the condition. Reduced systemic vascular resistance of pregnancy should aggravate cyanosis by increasing the right to left shunt. However, Ebstein's anomaly seems to be well tolerated during pregnancy.[128] There were no maternal deaths or serious complications following 111 pregnancies in 44 women (10 after surgical repair) with Ebstein's anomaly.[128] There were 85 live births, of which five had congenital heart disease. Women who were cyanosed had smaller babies than acyanotic women (2.53 kg vs. 3.14 kg, $P < 0.001$).[128]

Cyanotic heart disease

Women with cyanotic congenital heart disease even without Eisenmenger's complex (see below), carry a high risk of maternal cardiovascular complications 14/44 (32%).[129] These include heart failure (8), thromboses (2), bacterial endocarditis (2) and supraventricular tachycardia (2).[129] However, only 41 of 96 pregnancies resulted in a live birth, perhaps because of fetal hypoxemia secondary to maternal cyanosis.[129]

Eisenmenger's syndrome

The clinical picture of pulmonary hypertension and a right to left shunt through an atrial septal defect, ventricular septal defect or aortopulmonary shunt is known as the Eisenmenger complex. The patient is breathless and cyanosed. High pulmonary and low systemic vascular resistance aggravates the cyanosis. Consequently, gestational vasodilatation combined with even minor blood loss or a vasovagal episode can be fatal.[130] Women with Eisenmenger complex who continue with a pregnancy have at least a 30% maternal mortality rate.[131] Sadly, they should be advised against pregnancy and to terminate an ongoing pregnancy. If continuation of pregnancy is insisted upon, they should have as much bed rest as possible and complete bed rest in the lateral position, from the third trimester onward.[130] There is an increased risk of thromboembolism, which should be countered with prophylactic L.M.W. heparin e.g. enoxaparin 40 mg once daily. Overall experience in the management of delivery in this condition is limited and therefore no consensus regarding the mode of delivery has been reached. Vaginal delivery is recommended by some[130,131] while cesarean section under general anesthetic is favored by others[132] as it provides a controlled hemodynamic environment. Either way, there should be intensive cardiac and blood gas monitoring.[130] Hypotension must be avoided at all costs, whether induced by epidural anesthesia, blood loss or arrhythmias. Most maternal deaths occur peripartum; therefore, the mother must stay in hospital, near resuscitation facilities, for at least 7 days postpartum.[130]

Tetralogy of Fallot

The tetralogy of Fallot consists of pulmonary outflow obstruction, due to infundibular narrowing of the pulmonary outflow tract and pulmonary stenosis leading to right ventricular hypertrophy. There is a ventricular septal defect, over which lies the aorta. Due to the high resistance to flow through the pulmonary outflow obstruction, venous blood passes from right to left through the ventricular septal defect. Cyanosis worsens as the pulmonary stenosis progresses. During pregnancy, the fall in peripheral vascular resistance increases the right to left shunt and dyspnea gets worse. Any hypotension related to blood loss at the time of delivery will also increase the right to left shunt. Fetal outcome is poor in pregnant women with uncorrected tetralogy of Fallot and maternal cardiovascular complications are common.[130] After surgical correction of the anomaly there is a much improved maternal and fetal outcome.[133] Prepregnancy assessment with echocardiography and stress testing to assess cardiovascular reserve will help determine the likelihood of a successful outcome for the mother during pregnancy. There is an increased risk of a congenital heart defect in the offspring.

Transposition of the great vessels

Transposition of the great vessels occurs when the aorta arises from the right ventricle and the pulmonary artery from the left ventricle, associated with a communication between the two circulations. An operation to redirect oxygenated blood into the right ventricle and aorta and systemic venous blood into the left ventricle and pulmonary artery now allows women to survive until adulthood. One series of nine women who had 15 pregnancies, following this operation, resulted in 12 healthy live births.[134] There were two spontaneous abortions and one intrauterine death.[134] However, prepregnancy assessment of right ventricular function with echocardiography and exercise testing is essential before advising pregnancy.[130]

Tricuspid atresia and the Fontan procedure

In tricuspid atresia, blood is unable to pass through the tricuspid valve and therefore exits the right atrium through an atrial septal defect. Blood then passes through a ventricular septal defect back into the right ventricle and into the pulmonary circulation. The Fontan procedure creates a connection between the right atrium and pulmonary artery while closing off the atrial septal defect and ventricular septal defect. In general, maternal outcome depends on the state of health at the beginning of pregnancy and fetal outcome on the level of central cyanosis.[2]

Heart transplantation and pregnancy

A survey of international cardiac transplant centers identified 30 women who had had pregnancies following heart transplantation: 27 heart and 3 heart and lung recipients.[100] The cardiovascular changes of pregnancy were well tolerated. There were six episodes of mild to moderate rejection, requiring an increase in prednisolone. Different combinations of prednisolone, azathioprine and cyclosporin were used throughout all pregnancies. Of the women 48% had preexisting hypertension and 24% developed preeclampsia. There were no maternal deaths during pregnancy, but three women died within 30 months of delivery. Two died after stopping their immunosuppressive therapy and one developed cryptococcal meningitis 2 years postpartum. Four women had heart transplants following peripartum cardiomyopathy and all survived without any recurrence of their original heart disease. Preterm labor occurred in nine cases (36%). There were 27 live-born infants with two sets of twins. There were no fetal deaths or anomalies, but 20% had fetal growth retardation.[100] Overall, it is sensible to advise heart transplant patients who wish to conceive that although most pregnancies are successful, complications are common. Furthermore, those women with poor cardiac reserve may not survive to raise their children.

REFERENCES

1. RCOG Press, Confidential Enquiry into maternal and child health. Why mothers Die 2000–2002; CEMHCH, 2004.
2. De Swiet M. Heart disease in pregnancy. In de Swiet M, ed. *Medical Disorders in Obstetric Practice.* Oxford: Blackwell Science Ltd, 1995:143–81.
3. Robson SC, Hunter S, Boys RJ, *et al.* Serial study of factors influencing changes in cardiac output during human pregnancy. *Am J Physiol* 1989;256:H1060–5.
4. Robson SC, Hunter S, Boys RJ, *et al.* Serial changes in pulmonary haemodynamics during human pregnancy: A non-invasive study using Doppler echocardiography. *Clin Sci* 1991;80:113–7.
5. Brown MA, Gallery EDM. Volume homeostasis in normal pregnancy and pre-eclampsia: Physiology and clinical implications. *Baillieres Clin Obstet Gynaecol* 1994;8:287–310.
6. Kerr MG, Scott DB, Samuel E. Studies of the inferior vena cava in late pregnancy. *Br Med J* 1964;1:532–3.
7. Newman B, Derrington C, Dore C. Cardiac output and the recumbent position in late pregnancy. *Anaesthesia* 1983;38:322–35.
8. Robson SC, Dunlop W, Boys RJ, *et al.* Cardiac output during labour. *Br Med J* 1987;295:1169–72.
9. Robson SC, Dunlop W, Hunter S. Haemodynamic changes during the early puerperium. *Br Med J* 1987;294:1065.
10. MacGillivray I, Rose GA, Rowe B. Blood pressure survey in pregnancy. *Clin Sci* 1969;37:395–407.
11. Redman CWG. Hypertension in pregnancy. In de Swiet M, ed. *Medical Disorders in Obstetric Practice.* Oxford: Blackwell Science Ltd, 1995:182–225.
12. Gallery EDM, Hunyor SN, Gyory AZ. Plasma volume contraction: A significant factor in both pregnancy associated hypertension (pre-eclampsia) and chronic hypertension in pregnancy. *Q J Med* 1979;48:593–602.
13. Williams DJ, Vallance PJT, Neild GH, *et al.* Nitric oxide mediated vasdilatation in human pregnancy. *Am J Physiol* 1997;272: H748–52.
14. Sladek SM, Magness RR, Conrad KP. Nitric oxide and pregnancy. *Am J Physiol* 1997;272:R441–63.
15. Harstad TW, Madon RA, Cox SM. Serum erythropoietin quantitation in pregnancy using an enzyme linked immunoassay. *Am J Perinatol* 1992;9:233–5.
16. Leeuw NKM, de Lowenstein L, Hsieh YS. Iron deficiency and hydremia in normal pregnancy. *Med (Baltimore)* 1966;45: 291–315.
17. Sibai BM, Mabie WC. Hemodynamics of preeclampsia. *Clin Perinatol* 1991;18:727–47.
18. Letsky EA. Coagulation defects. In de Swiet M, ed. *Medical Disorders in Obstetric Practice,* 3rd edn. Oxford: Blackwell Science Ltd, 1995:71–115.
19. Bonnar J. Haemostasis and coagulation disorders in pregnancy. In Bloom AL, Thomas DP, eds. *Haemostasis and Thrombosis.* Edinburgh: Churchill Livingstone, 1987:570–84.
20. Kruithof EK, Tran-Thang C, Gudinchet A, *et al.* Fibrinolysis in pregnancy: A study of plasminogen activator inhibitors. *Blood* 1987;69:460–6.
21. Milne JA, Mowie AD, Pack AI. Dyspnoea during normal pregnancy. *Br J Obstet Gynaecol* 1978;85:260–3.
22. Szekely P, Turner R, Snaith L. Pregnancy and the changing pattern of rheumatic heart disease. *Br Heart J* 1973;35:1293–303.
23. Sugrue D, Blake S, MacDonald D. Pregnancy complicated by maternal heart disease at the National Maternity Hospital, Dublin, Ireland, 1969 to 1978. *Am J Obstet Gynecol* 1981;139:1–6.
24. Nihoyannopoulos P. Cardiovascular examination in pregnancy and the approach to diagnosis of cardiac disorder. In Oakley CM, ed. *Heart Disease in Pregnancy.* London: B.M.J. Publishing Group, 1997:52–62.
25. Cutforth R, MacDonald CB. Heart sounds and murmurs in pregnancy. *Am Heart J* 1966;71:741–7.
26. Carruth SE, Mirvis SB, Brogan DR, *et al.* The electrocardiogram in normal pregnancy. *Am Heart J* 1981;102:1075–8.

27. Robson SC, Richley D, Boys RJ, *et al.* Incidence of Doppler regurgitant flow velocities during normal pregnancy. *Eur Heart J* 1992;13:84–7.
28. Belfort MA, Rokey R, Saade GR, *et al.* Rapid echocardiographic assessment of left and right heart hemodynamics in critically ill obstetric patients. *Am J Obstet Gynecol* 1994;171:884–92.
29. Veille JC, Kitzman DW, Bacevice AE. Effects of pregnancy on the electrocardiogram in healthy subjects during strenuous exercise. *Am J Obstet Gynecol* 1996;175:1360–4.
30. Ribeiro P, Al Zaibag M. Rheumatic heart disease. In Oarkley CM, ed. *Heart Disease in Pregnancy.* London: B.M.J. Publishing Group, 1997:112–27.
31. Ueland K, Novy MJ, Metcalfe J. Hemodynamic responses of patients with heart disease to pregnancy and exercise. *Am J Obstet Gynecol* 1972;113:47–59.
32. Clark SL, Phelan JP, Greenspoon J, *et al.* Labour and delivery in the presence of mitral stenosis: Central hemodynamic observations. *Am J Obstet Gynecol* 1985;8:984–8.
33. Clark S, Phelan JP, Greenspoon J, *et al.* Labor and delivery in the presence of mitral stenosis: Central hemodynamic observation. *Am J Obstet Gynecol* 1985;152:984–8.
34. Al-Kasab S, Sabag T, Al-Zaibag M, *et al.* Beta adrenergic receptor blockade in the management of pregnant women with mitral stenosis. *Am J Obstet Gynecol* 1990;163:37–40.
35. Ribeiro PA, Fawzy ME, Awad M, *et al.* Balloon valvotomy for pregnant patients with severe pliable mitral stenosis using the Inoue technique with total abdominal and pelvic shielding. *Am Heart J* 1992;124:1558–62.
36. Hank AJ, Freeman DP, Ackerman DM, *et al.* Surgical pathology of the tricuspid valve: A study of 363 cases spanning 25 years. *Mayo Clin Proc* 1988;63:851–63.
37. Limacher MC, Ware JA, O'Meara ME, *et al.* Tricuspid regurgitation during pregnancy: Two-dimensional and pulsed Doppler echocardiographic observations. *Am J Cardiol* 1985;55:1059–62.
38. Gribbin B, Crook DWM. Infective endocarditis. In Weatherall DJ, Ledingham JGG, Warrell DA, eds. *Oxford Textbook of Medicine.* Oxford: Oxford Medical Publications, 1996:2436–51.
39. Oakley CM. Infective endocarditis. In Oakley CM, ed. *Heart Disease in Pregnancy.* London: B.M.J. Publishing Group, 1997:147–52.
40. Durack DT, Bright DK, Lukes AS. Duke Endocarditis Service: New criteria for diagnosis of infective endocarditis: Utilization of specific echocardiographic findings. *Am J Med* 1994;96:200–9.
41. Lein JN, Stander RW. Subacute bacterial endocarditis following obstetric and gynecologic procedures. *Obstet Gynecol* 1959;13: 568–73.
42. Sugrue D, Blake S, Troy P, *et al.* Antibiotic prophylaxis against infective endocarditis after normal delivery – Is it necessary? *Br Heart J* 1980;44:499–502.
43. Recommendations from Endocarditis Working Party of the British Society for Antimicrobial Chemotherapy. Antibiotic prophylaxis of infective endocarditis. *Lancet* 1990;335:88–9.
44. Working Party of the British Cardiac Society and the Research Unit of the Royal College of Physicians. Valvular heart disease: recommendations for investigation and management. Summary of guidelines. *J R Coll Physicians* 1996;30:309–15.
45. Oakley CM. Artificial heart valves. In Oakley CM, ed. *Heart Disease in Pregnancy.* London: B.M.J. Publishing Group, 1997:135–46.
46. Salazar E, Zajarias A, Gutiarraz N, *et al.* The problem of cardiac valve prostheses: anticoagulants and pregnancy. *Circulation* 1984;70:169–77.
47. Sbarouni E, Oakley CM. Outcome of pregnancy in women with valve prostheses. *Br Heart J* 1994;71:196–201.
48. Hanania G, Thomas D, Michel PL, *et al.* Pregnancy and prosthetic heart valves: A French cooperative retrospective study of 155 cases. *Eur Heart J* 1994;15:1651–8.
49. Cottrufo M, de Luca TSL, Calabro R, *et al.* Coumarin anticoagulation during pregnancy in patients with mechanical heart valve prostheses. *Eur J Cardiothorac Surg* 1991;5:300–5.
50. Iturbe-Alessio I, Delcarmen Fonesca M, Mutchinik D, *et al.* Risks of anticoagulant therapy in pregnancy: Women with articial heart valves. *N Engl J Med* 1986;27:1390–3.
51. Chan WS, Anand S, Ginsberg JS. Anticoagulation of pregnant women with mechanical heart valves: a systematic review of the literature. Arch Intern Med 2000;160:191–6.
52. Greer IA, Nelson-Piercy C. Low molecular weight heparins for thromboprophylaxis and treatment of venous thromboembolism in pregnancy: a systematic review of safety and efficacy. Blood 2005; 106:401–7.
53. Rowan JA, McCowan LM, Raudkivi PJ *et al.* Enoxaparin treatment in women with mechanical heart valves during pregnancy. *Am J Obstet Gynecol* 2001;185:633–7.
54. Birdi I, Angelini GD, Bryan AJ. Thrombolytic therapy for left sided prosthetic heart valve thromobosis. *J Heart Valve Dis* 1995;4: 154–9.
55. Taylor KM. *Report of the United Kingdom Heart Valve Registry 1993.* London: HMSO, 1995.
56. Kearney P, Singh H, Hutter J, *et al.* Spontaneous coronary artery dissection: A report of three cases and review of the literature. *Postgrad Med J* 1993;69:940–5.
57. Hankins GDV, Wendel GD, Leveno KL, *et al.* Myocardial infarction during pregnancy: A review. *Obstet Gynecol* 1985;65:139–46.
58. Bac DJ, Lotgering FK, Verkaaik APK, *et al.* Spontaneous coronary artery dissection during pregnancy and postpartum. *Eur Heart J* 12995;16:136–8.
59. Oakley CM. Coronary artery disease. In Oakley CM, ed. *Heart Disease in Pregnancy.* London: B.M.J. Publishing Group, 1997: 237–47.
60. Shade GH, Ross G, Bever FW, *et al.* Troponin I in the diagnosis of acute myocardial infarction in pregnancy, labour and post-partum. Am J Obstet Gynecol 2002;187:1719–20.
61. Zampieri P, Aggio S, Roncon L, *et al.* Follow up after spontaneous coronary artery dissection: A report of five cases. *Heart* 1996; 75:206–9.
62. Gonzalez JI, Hill JA, Conti CR. Spontaneous coronary artery dissection treated with percutaneous transluminal angioplasty. *Am J Cardiol* 1989;63:885–6.
63. Widerhorn J, Widerhorn AL, Rahimtoola SH, *et al.* WPW syndrome during pregnancy: Increased incidence of supraventricular arrhythmias. *Am Heart J* 1992;123:796–8.
64. Page RL. Treatment of arrythmias during pregnancy. *Am Heart J* 1995;130:871–6.
65. Saarikoski S. Placental transfer and fetal uptake of 3H-digoxin in humans. *Br J Obstet Gynaecol* 1976;83:879–84.
66. Azancot-Benisty A, Jacqz-Aigrain E, Guirgis NM, *et al.* Clinical and pharmacologic study of fetal supraventricular tachyarrhythmias. *J Pediatr* 1992;121:608–13.
67. Rubin PC, Butters L, Clark DM, *et al.* Placebo-controlled trial of atenolol in treatment of pregnancy-associated hypertension. *Lancet* 1983;1:431–4.
68. Magee LA, Downar E, Sermer M, *et al.* Pregnancy outcome after gestational exposure to amiodarone in Canada. *Am J Obstet Gynecol* 1995;172:1307–11.
69. Elkayam U, Goodwin TM. Adenosine therapy for supra ventricular tachycardia during pregnancy. *Am J Cardiol* 1995;75:521–3.
70. Mendelson CL. Disorders of the heart beat during pregnancy. *Am J Obstet Gynecol* 1956;72:1268–301.
71. Wolf PA, Dawber TR, Thomas HE, *et al.* Epidemiological assessment of chronic atrial fibrillation and risk of stroke: The Framingham study. *Neurology* 1978;28:973–7.
72. DiBianco R, Morganroth J, Freitag JA, *et al.* Effects of nadalol on the spontaneous and exercise-provoked heart rate of patients with chronic atrial fibrillation receiving stable doses of digoxin. *Am Heart J* 1984;108:1121–7.
73. Anderson MH. Rhythm disorders. In Oakley CM, ed. *Heart Disease in Pregnancy.* London: B.M.J. Publishing Group, 1997: 248–81.
74. Finlay AY, Edmunds V. DC cardioversion in pregnancy. *Br J Clin Pract* 1979;33:88–94.
75. Klein AL, Grimm RA, Black IW, *et al.* Cardioversion guided by transoesophageal echocardiography: the ACUTE Pilot Study. A randomized, controlled trial. Assessment of Cardioversion Using Transoesophageal Echocardiography. *Ann Intern Med* 1997;126: 200–9.
76. Frohn-Mulder IM, Stewart PA, Witsenburg M, *et al.* The efficacy of flecanide versus digoxin in the management of fetal supraventricular tachycardia. *Prenat Diagn* 1995;15:1209–13.
77. Rawles JM, Metcalfe MJ, Jennings K. Time of occurrence, duration and ventricular rate of paroxysmal atrial fibrillation: The effect of digoxin. *Br Heart J* 1990;63:225–7.
78. Cobbe SM, Rankin AC. Cardiac arrhythmias. In Weatherall DJ, Ledingham JGG, Warrell DA, eds. *Oxford Textbook of Medicine.* Oxford: Oxford University Press, 1996:2259–85.
79. Camm AJ, Garratt CJ. Adenosine and supraventricular tachycardia. *N Engl J Med* 1991;325:1621–9.
80. Chandra NC, Gates EA, Thamer M. Conservative treatment of paroxysmal ventricular tachycardia during pregnancy. *Clin Cardiol* 1991;14:347–50.

81. Brodsky M, Doria R, Allen B, *et al.* New onset ventricular tachycardia during pregnancy. *Am Heart J* 1992;123:933–41.
82. Calkins H, Nikalsson L, Sousa J, *et al.* Radiation exposure during radiofrequency catheter ablation of accessory atrioventricular connections. *Circulation* 1991;84:2376–82.
83. Dalvi BV, Chaudhuri A, Kulkarni HL, *et al.* Therapeutic guidelines for congenital complete heart block presenting in pregnancy. *Obstet Gynecol* 1992;79:802–4.
84. Goodwin APL, Pearce AJ. The human wedge. A manoeuvre to relieve aortocaval compression during resuscitation in late pregnancy. *Anaesthesia* 1992;47:433–4.
85. Lee RV, Rodgers BD, White LM, *et al.* Cardiopulmonary resuscitation of pregnant women. *Am J Med* 1986;81:311–18.
86. Oakley CM. Pericardial disease. In Oakley CM, ed. *Heart Disease in Pregnancy.* London: B.M.J. Publishing Group, 1997:226–36.
87. Hagley MT, Shaub TF. Acute pericarditis with a symptomatic pericardial effusion complicating pregnancy. A case report. *J Reprod Med* 1993;10:813–14.
88. Bakri YN, Martan A, Amri A, *et al.* Pregnancy complicating irradiation-induced constrictive pericarditis. *Acta Obstet Gynecol Scand* 1992;71:143–4.
89. Davies MJ. The current status of myocardial disarray in hypertrophic cardiomyopathy. *Br Heart J* 1984;51:361–3.
90. Oakley CM. Hypertrophic cardiomyopathy. In Oakley CM, ed. *Heart Disease in Pregnancy.* London: B.M.J. Publishing Group, 1997:201–9.
91. Ryan MP, French J, Al-Mahdawi S, *et al.* Genetic testing for familial hypertrophic cardiomyopathy in newborn infants. *Br Med J* 1995;310:856–7.
92. Maron BJ, Roberts WC, Epstein SE. Sudden death in hypertrophic cardiomyopathy: A profile of 78 patients. *Circulation* 1982;65: 1388–94.
93. Oakley GD, McGarry K, Limb DG, *et al.* Management of pregnancy in patients with hypertrophic cardiomyopathy. *Br Med J* 1979;1:1749–50.
94. Pelliccia F, Gainfrocca C, Gandio C, *et al.* Sudden death during pregnancy in hypertrophic cardiomyopathy. *Eur Heart J* 1992;13: 421–3.
95. Spirito P, Rapezzi C, Autore C, *et al.* Prognosis of asymptomatic patients with hypertrophic cardiomyopathy and non-sustained ventricular tachycardia. *Circulation* 1994;90:2743–7.
96. Fananapazir L, Chang AC, Epstein SE, *et al.* Prognostic determinants in hypertrophic cardiomyopathy. *Circulation* 1992;86: 730–40.
97. Homans DC. Peripartum cardiomyopathy. *N Engl J Med* 1985; 312:1432–7.
98. Demakis JG, Rahimtoola SH, Sutton GC, *et al.* Natural course of peripartum cardiomyopathy. *Circulation* 1971;44:1053–61.
99. Elkayam U, Akhter MW, Singh H *et al.* Pregnancy-associated cardiomyopathy: clinical characteristics and a comparison between early and late presentation. *Circulation* 2005;111:2050–5.
100. Scott JR, Wagoner LE, Olsen SL, *et al.* Pregnancy in heart transplant recipients: Management and outcome. *Obstet Gynecol* 1993; 82:324–7.
101. Rich S, Dantzker DR, Ayres SM, *et al.* Primary pulmonary hypertension: A national prospective study. *Ann Intern Med* 1987;107: 216–23.
102. Rubin LJ. Primary pulmonary hypertension. *N Engl J Med* 1997; 336:111–17.
103. Oakley CM. Pulmonary hypertension. In Oakley CM, ed. *Heart Disease in Pregnancy.* London: B.M.J. Publishing Group, 1997: 97–111.
104. Elkayam U, Gleicher N. Primary pulmonary hypertension in pregnancy. In Elkayam U, Gleicher N, eds. *Cardiac Problems in Pregnancy: Diagnosis and Management of Maternal and Fetal Disease.* New York: Alan R. Liss, 1982:153–60.
105. Rich S, Kaufmann E, Levy PS. The effect of high doses of calcium channel blockers on survival in primary pulmonary hypertension. *N Engl J Med* 1992;327:76–81.
106. Fuster V, Steele PM, Edwards WD, *et al.* Primary pulmonary hypertension: natural history and the importance of thrombosis. *Circulation* 1984;70:580–7.
107. Oakley CM. Pulmonary embolism. In Oakley CM, ed. *Heart Disease in Pregnancy.* London: B.M.J. Publishing Group, 1997: 282–92.
108. Brady AJB, Crake T, Oakley CM. Percutaneous catheter fragmentation and distal dispersion of proximal pulmonary embolus. *Lancet* 1991;338:1186–9.
109. de Swiet M. Thromboembolism. In de Swiet M, ed. *Medical Disorders in Obstetric Practice.* Oxford: Blackwell Science Ltd, 1995:116–42.
110. Brancazio LR, Roperti KA, Stierer R, *et al.* Pharmacokinetics and pharmacodynamics of subcutaneous heparin during the early third trimester of pregnancy. *Am J Obstet Gynecol* 1995;173: 1240–5.
111. Barbour LA, Smith JM, Marlar RA. Heparin levels to guide thromboembolism prophylaxis in pregnancy. *Am J Obstet Gynecol* 1995;173:1869–73.
112. Rowan JA, McLintock C, Taylor RS, *et al.* Prophylactic and therapeutic enoxaparin during pregnancy: indications, outcomes and monitoring. Aust NZJ Obstet Gynecol 2003;43:123–8.
113. Meaney JFM, Weg JG, Chenevert TL, *et al.* Diagnosis of pulmonary embolism with magnetic resonance angiography. *N Engl J Med* 1997;336:1422–7.
114. Herbert WNP. Complications of the immediate puerperium. *Clin Obstet Gynecol* 1982;25:219–32.
115. Masson RG. Amniotic fluid embolism. *Clin Chest Med* 1992;13: 657–65.
116. Oakley CM. Mitral valve prolapse. In Oakley CM, ed. *Heart Disease in Pregnancy.* London: B.M.J. Publishing Group, 1997: 128–34.
117. Beighton P. Mitral valve prolapse and a Marfanoid habitus. *Br Med J* 1982;284:920.
118. Haas JH. The effect of pregnancy on the mid-systolic click and murmur of the prolapsing posterior leaflet of the mitral valve. *Am Heart J* 1976;92:407–8.
119. Gibson DG. Valve disease. In Weatherall DJ, Ledingham JGG, Warrell DA, eds. *Oxford Textbook of Medicine.* Oxford: Oxford University Press, 1996:2451–72.
120. Smith R. The Marfan syndrome. In Weatherall DJ, Ledingham JGG, Warrell DA, eds. *Oxford Textbook of Medicine.* Oxford: Oxford Medical Publications, 1996:3083–4.
121. Pyeritz RE. Maternal and fetal complications of pregnancy in the Marfan syndrome. *Am J Med* 1981;71:784–90.
122. Child AH. Management of pregnancy in Marfan syndrome, Ehlers–Danlos syndrome, and other heritable connective tissue disorders. In Oakley CM, ed. *Heart Disease in Pregnancy.* London: B.M.J. Publishing Group, 1997:153–62.
123. Wang M, Mata J, Price CE, *et al.* Prenatal and presymptomatic diagnosis of the Marfan syndrome using fluorescence P.C.R. and an automated sequencer. *Prenat Diagn* 1995;15:499–507.
124. Oakley CM. Acyanotic congenital heart disease. In Oakley CM, ed. *Heart Disease in Pregnancy.* London: B.M.J. Publishing Group, 1997:63–82.
125. Wooley CF, Sparks EH. Congenital heart disease, inheritable cardiovascular disease and pregnancy. *Prog Cardiovasc Dis* 1992; 35:41–60.
126. Green NJ, Rollason TP. Pulmonary artery rupture in pregnancy complicating patent ductus arteriosus. *Br Heart J* 1992;68: 616–18.
127. Deal K, Wooley CF. Coarctation of the aorta and pregnancy. *Ann Intern Med* 1973;78:706–10.
128. Connolly HM, Warnes CA. Ebstein's anomaly: Outcome of pregnancy. *J Am Coll Cardiol* 1994;23:1194–8.
129. Presbitero P, Somerville J, Stone S, *et al.* Pregnancy in cyanotic congenital heart disease. Outcome of mother and fetus. *Circulation* 1994;89:2673–6.
130. Warnes CA. Cyanotic congenital heart disease. In Oakley CM, ed. *Heart Disease in Pregnancy.* London: B.M.J. Publishing Group, 1997:83–96.
131. Gleicher N, Midwall J, Hochberger D, *et al.* Eisenmenger's syndrome and pregnancy. *Obstet Gynecol Surv* 1975;34:721–41.
132. Avila WS, Grinberg M, Smitcowsky R, *et al.* Maternal and fetal outcome in pregnant women with Eisenmenger's syndrome. *Eur Heart J* 1995;16:460–4.
133. Singh H, Bolton PJ, Oakley CM. Pregnancy after surgical correction of tetralogy of Fallot. *Br Med J Clin Res Ed* 1982;285: 168–70.
134. Clarkson PM, Wilson NJ, Neutze JM, *et al.* Outcome of pregnancy after the Mustard operation for transposition of the great arteries with intact ventricular septum. *J Am Coll Cardiol* 1994; 24:190–3.
135. Robertson L., Wu O, Langhorne P, *et al.* Thrombophilia in pregnancy: a systematic review, Br J Haematol 2006;132:171–96.

196 Disorders of the musculoskeletal system in pregnancy

C. Gordon

Introduction

Musculoskeletal symptoms are common in pregnancy. Many women suffer mild non-specific arthralgia and myalgia, which require no specific intervention. Some pregnant women develop more clear-cut and distressing symptoms such as parasthesiae due to carpal tunnel syndrome, mechanical low-back or pelvic pain. Occasionally, transient osteoporosis of the hip or osteoporotic vertebral fractures occur. Most of these cases occur in women without underlying disease but about 3% of pregnant women will have a chronic musculoskeletal disorder. In addition to the effect of the pregnancy on the disease, the effect of the disease on the pregnancy needs to be considered.

Rheumatoid arthritis (RA) is the most common inflammatory arthropathy and the best studied, but other inflammatory rheumatic diseases will be mentioned in this review as well. Systemic lupus erythematosus (SLE) is the most common systemic connective tissue disease, usually develops in women of child-bearing age and may present for the first time in pregnancy or soon after delivery. Differentiation between a flare of lupus and pre-eclampsia and toxemia of pregnancy is important for appropriate management. Similarly, it is essential to detect and treat antiphospholipid syndrome, which may complicate SLE or present as a primary disorder often in pregnancy or the puerperium. Genetic disorders of collective tissue matrix proteins are a rare but important group of diseases to be aware of. These, like the inflammatory collective tissue disorders and vasculitides, can be life-threatening to the mother and fetus during pregnancy and delivery. These individual conditions will be considered in more detail below, but first a few general points will be discussed.

Management of musculoskeletal disorders during pregnancy must take into consideration the risk of investigations and drug therapy to the fetus. In general, radiological procedures should be kept to a minimum especially in early pregnancy but, with appropriate shielding, can be performed if the results will significantly affect management. Ultrasound is the safest way to look for synovial effusions and to guide needle aspiration, particularly in the hip. Isotope, computerized tomography (CT) and magnetic resonance imaging (MRI) scans can usually be deferred until after delivery.

Female patients of reproductive age with any rheumatic disease need to be aware of the implications of their disease and its treatment on their fertility, risk of fetal loss and ability to bring up children from the time of diagnosis. Close support from their partner, family and friends will be invaluable as pregnancy and parenthood can be very tiring and stressful for such women. It is often helpful for a family member or friend to come to clinics with them, to encourage the patient to ask relevant questions and to help remember what was said at the consultation. Close liaison is required between the obstetrician, rheumatologist and any other physicians involved in the care of the pregnant patient. Review by a physiotherapist and discussion with an anesthetist about pain relief and anesthesia should be arranged.

In some cases, difficult issues such as termination of pregnancy may have to be discussed if the patient has life-threatening systemic disease. However, in most patients therapy can be adjusted to control the disease without significant risk to the mother or fetus. In general, it is preferable to plan pregnancy in advance so that the disease is under good control and drug treatment is appropriate at the time of conception and throughout fetal development (Tables 196.1–196.3). Although it is often preferable to discontinue drugs in pregnancy, the likely consequences of this need to be considered as well as the risk of continuing therapy. There is little point in stopping all drugs if the disease will flare, putting the mother at risk of significant

Table 196.1 Analgesic and anti-inflammatory drug use in pregnancy

Drug	Main use in musculoskeletal disorders	Possible risks to fetus	Contraindicated in pregnancy	Contraindicated in breast feeding
Paracetamol	Analgesic (mild)	Unlikely	No	No
Codeine	Analgesic	Respiratory depression, withdrawal syndrome	No (caution)	Caution
Aspirin	NSAID, anti-thrombotic	Low with low doses, neonatal hemorrhage, pulmonary hypertension, renal anomalies?	No (low doses)	No (low doses)
Ibuprofen	Mild NSAID for RA	Renal anomalies?, premature closure ductus, pulmonary hypertension	Caution first and third trimester	No (low dose, and other arthritides short-acting)
Indometacin	Potent NSAID for AS	Congenital malformation, prolonged gestation, pulmonary hypertension	Yes	Yes

NSAID, non-steroidal anti-inflammatory drug; RA, rheumatoid arthritis; AS, ankylosing spondylitis

Table 196.2 Antirheumatic drug use in pregnancy

Drug	Main use in rheumatic disease	Possible risks to fetus	Contraindicated in pregnancy	Contraindicated in breast feeding
Hydroxychloroquine	SLE (RA)	Eye or ear abnormalities? (risks with chloroquine)	No (low dose)	No (low dose)
Sulfasalazine	RA	Congenital malformations?, possible kernicterus (none confirmed)	No (caution first and third trimesters)	No (avoid high dose)
Gold salts: Myocrisin	RA	None confirmed intramuscularly, Auranofin oral	No (low dose)	No (low dose)
D-Penicillamine	RA	Cutis laxa, connective tissue abnormalities	Yes	Yes

SLE, systemic lupus erythematosus; RA, rheumatoid arthritis

systemic disease and fetal loss. Combined clinics for patients with connective tissue diseases provide the most efficient service for these patients, as close monitoring of the pregnancy and the disease is required and this arrangement avoids the need for multiple clinic visits each month.[1,2]

Musculoskeletal disorders due to pregnancy

Carpal tunnel syndrome

Carpal tunnel syndrome is the most common entrapment neuropathy.[3] It is common in patients with synovitis of the wrist but also occurs frequently in healthy women in the third trimester of pregnancy (21% of women in one series), possibly due to fluid retention.[4] It causes sensations of burning, tingling and numbness in the distribution of the median nerve, usually on the palmar surface of the radial three and one-half digits and palm of the hand. More severe cases will have weakness of abductor pollicis brevis and the pain may radiate proximally in the forearm. Cases presenting in pregnancy without an associated arthropathy usually resolve after pregnancy and do not require surgery. Treatment consists of the provision of a wrist support splint, particularly for use at night when symptoms are often worst, and local steroid injection for more severe cases.

Transient osteoporosis of the hip

This is a rare but well-recognized condition, which presents in pregnancy as hip pain on movement or

Table 196.3 Immunosuppressive drugs used in pregnancy

Drug	Main uses in rheumatic disease	Possible risks to fetus	Contraindicated in pregnancy	Contraindicated in breast feeding
Methotrexate	RA, psoriatic arthritis	Facial and skeletal abnormalities	Yes	Yes
Cyclosporin A	RA, SLE, psoriatic arthritis	Spontaneous abortion? (not teratogenic in animals)	Caution (limited data)	Yes
Glucocorticoids	RA, AS, SLE, vasculitis	Cleft palate hypoadrenal, small for dates?, stillbirth?	No, caution high dose	No, caution high dose
Azathioprine	SLE, RA, vasculitis	None definite	No, caution high dose	Caution, conflicting
Cyclosphamide	SLE, vasculitis	Facial, skin, limb and visceral abnormalities	Yes	Yes

RA, rheumatoid arthritis; SLE, systemic lupus erythematosus; AS, ankylosing spondylitis

weight-bearing, more often on the left than the right, sometimes with radiation to the anterior thigh and knee.[5,6] It may be due to pregnancy-related hormonal changes and local compression of vessels or nerves resulting in a transient algodystrophy (reflex sympathetic dystrophy). However, it can occur early in pregnancy, in the non-pregnant state and in other joints, leaving the etiology unclear. It is important to distinguish other causes of pain in the hip region, which require different management. The pain may be due to a femoral or inguinal hernia or may be referred from the sacroiliac joints or lumbar spine. Obturator nerve compression at the pelvic brim due to engagement of the fetal head can cause pain in the upper anterior thigh. The hip pain may be part of a generalized preexisting arthropathy or may be an isolated joint flare in which case infective arthritis must be excluded (even if there is a history of previous hip involvement, for example in RA). Pregnancy-induced osteomalacia and osteonecrosis (aseptic necrosis, particularly in patients with sickle cell anemia or SLE) should also be considered.

X-rays, isotope and MRI scans should be avoided until after the delivery but can be used to confirm osteopenia with preservation of joint space and to exclude synovitis. Ultrasound can be used to look for an effusion and to guide aspiration in suspected infection. Treatment usually involves short-acting nonsteroidal anti-inflammatory drugs (NSAIDs) like ibuprofen, up to the third trimester and postpartum, with paracetamol and codeine if required in the third trimester (Table 196.1). Physiotherapy is advised as there is often significant muscle wasting. A walking stick or crutches may be necessary, but the prognosis is usually good with full clinical and radiological recovery within 6 months.

Vertebral osteoporosis

Severe osteoporosis may develop in pregnancy and cause vertebral fracture(s).[7,8] This presents with severe, localized back pain with loss of vertebral height, usually in the third trimester or puerperium of a first pregnancy. Sometimes there is evidence of generalized osteopenia, and occasionally fractures of the femur have occurred as well. Under 20% of reported cases have had a predisposing cause such as treatment with heparin or steroids, or previous anorexia nervosa, structural protein or metabolic bone disease. Bone biopsies suggest that there is a failure of osteoblast activity but the etiology remains obscure.[8] However, the prognosis is generally good with resolution of pain and no further vertebral collapse after delivery, and few patients suffer a recurrence in subsequent pregnancies.

Mechanical low-back and pelvic pain

Low-back and pelvic pain are very common in pregnancy, particularly in the last trimester. The pains probably result from postural changes (increased lordosis) due to the enlarging fetus, ligamentous laxity and increased mobility of the pelvic bones.[9] Relaxin, which enhances collagenase production and plasminogen activation, is present at increased levels in pregnant women with severe pain.[10] Pain settles after delivery and investigation is not indicated unless there are neurological signs suggesting nerve root or cord compression.

Inflammatory arthropathies

Rheumatoid arthritis

RA is the commonest inflammatory arthritis, which affects about 2% of the population and three times as many women as men. The peak age of onset is 40 years. RA presents as a symmetrical polyarthritis typically involving wrists, metacarpophalangeal and proximal interphalangeal joints. Active disease is usually associated with considerable fatigue, anemia of chronic disorders and a high erythrocyte sedimentation rate,

CRP (C–reactive protein) and viscosity. Rheumatoid factor positive patients may develop a more serious systemic disease with, for example, nodules, pleuropericarditis, lymphadenopathy, weight loss and vasculitis.

The effect of pregnancy on RA

Pregnancy is associated with a marked reduction in the symptoms of RA in about 70% of cases.[11] This improvement is most marked in the third trimester and often occurs despite patients stopping or reducing NSAIDs, and antirheumatic or immunosuppressive therapy (Tables 196.1–196.3). Unfortunately, the remaining 30% of patients have persistent symptoms and drug treatment needs to be given to prevent the mother from developing significant loss of function. RA rarely develops for the first time during pregnancy but there is an increased risk of RA appearing in the first year after a delivery. There is also considerable risk of a postpartum flare of existing arthritis within 3 months of delivery.[12]

Protection against the development and activity of RA in pregnancy may be due to neuroendocrine and sex hormone changes that suppress immunological and inflammatory processes.[9,11,13] Use of the oral contraceptive pill has also been reported to protect against the development of RA.[14] Natural immunosuppressive mechanisms that act in pregnancy to prevent rejection of the fetus and to reduce arthritis include changes in cytokines, such as increased interleukin (IL) 10 levels,[15] pregnancy-associated a_2-glycoprotein, induction of maternal antibodies or regulatory T cells in response to paternal HLA antigen exposure, or changes in the maternal T cell repertoire induced by fetal HLA peptides.[9,11]

The effect of RA on pregnancy

There is no evidence that RA patients have reduced fertility but they may take longer to conceive than healthy women.[11] RA in the mother is unlikely to affect the development of the fetus or increase the risk of maternal complications in pregnancy. Spontaneous abortion and stillbirth rates are slightly increased compared with healthy controls but successful pregnancy and uncomplicated delivery usually occur. Pre-eclampsia may be less common in RA patients than in the general population. Involvement of the hip joints, even if previously replaced, rarely interferes with delivery. If a general anesthetic is needed, temporomandibular and cricoarytenoid joint disease may make intubation difficult. The risk of atlantoaxial instability needs to be considered.[16] All RA patients should wear a cervical collar so that the staff takes greater care by being visibly reminded that the cervical spine, roots and cord are at risk of damage.

Other inflammatory arthropathies and spondyloarthropathies

There is an increased risk of systemic gonococcal disease with arthritis during pregnancy, especially in the third trimester, probably due to the state of relative immunosuppression. Reactive arthritis due to gut infections and *Chlamydia* may also present for the first time in pregnancy, although there are few data on this type of arthritis in pregnancy.[16,17] With appropriate and prompt antibiotic therapy for these infections, there is no evidence that the inflammatory processes in these arthropathies are associated with impaired fetal development or increased risk of maternal complications of pregnancy.

Lyme disease, a tick-borne inflammatory disease caused by the spirochete *Borrelia burgdorferi*, may present with erythema chronicum migrans or chronic inflammation in the joints, skin or nervous system during pregnancy. *B. burgdorferi* can cross the placenta and there have been a few cases of stillbirth and neonatal death ascribed to such transmission. However, it appears to be a rare event.[18,19] Nevertheless, a low threshold for aggressive antibiotic regimens for Lyme borreliosis in pregnancy has been recommended. There are no reports of congenital abnormalities or adverse maternal pregnancy complications in women with a history of Lyme disease.[19]

Acute gouty arthritis due to uric acid crystals is very rare in women before the menopause unless there is a specific enzyme defect that causes overproduction of purines (usually with a family history) or significant renal impairment. However, hyperuricemia (without arthritis) is common in preeclampsia and toxemia of pregnancy due to impaired renal clearance of urate.[18] High urate levels and raised diastolic blood pressure are associated with increased perinatal mortality. Transient hyperuricemia is seen during normal labor and for 1–2 days postpartum.[20]

Psoriatic arthritis, juvenile chronic arthritis and palindromic rheumatism behave similarly to RA, generally with improvement of symptoms during pregnancy and a high risk of postpartum flare. Adult Still's disease can flare or present in pregnancy and the postpartum period and may require treatment with prednisolone.[21] The spine disease associated with psoriasis and inflammatory bowel disease, which resembles ankylosing spondylitis, tends to improve in pregnancy. However, true ankylosing spondylitis is less likely to remit in pregnancy.[17,22] Spine and hip disease may make epidural anesthesia and vaginal delivery difficult. Postpartum flare is common in ankylosing spondylitis and the other inflammatory arthropathies.

Treatment of inflammatory arthropathies in pregnancy

Although most drugs used in the treatment of rheumatic disease do cross the placenta, few are definitely teratogenic in humans and many healthy babies have been born to mothers who were taking various antirheumatic drugs at the onset of pregnancy. Table 196.1 lists the analgesic and anti-inflammatory drugs. Advice on the use of antirheumatic drugs during pregnancy and lactation is given in Table 196.2. Immunosuppressive drugs are reviewed in Table 196.3.[11,23–26] Prednisolone, azathioprine and paracetamol are the safest drugs in pregnancy.[2,25,26] There has been considerable experience in their use during pregnancy for a variety of disorders. In inflammatory arthritis, which cannot easily be controlled by aspirin or low-dose NSAIDs, it is best to use intra-articular steroid injections or low-dose oral prednisolone. Gold (Myocrisin) injections may be continued in pregnancy at low doses (20 mg intramuscularly) monthly to prevent relapse but are usually avoided.[23,24] Ankylosing spondylitis can be difficult to treat, as patients are often very dependent on potent NSAIDs, such as indometacin, which have to be stopped in pregnancy. Steroid therapy is disappointing, but may be helpful if moderate doses (for example, 20 mg/day) are used with analgesics and physiotherapy to control the incapacitating pain and stiffness that may otherwise occur during periods of physical inactivity.

Connective tissue disorders

Systemic lupus erythematosus

This is the commonest systemic autoimmune disease, occurring in about 1 in 2000 women,[27] and is most prevalent in people from the Caribbean, the Indian subcontinent and the Far East. Almost any system in the body can be affected. The commonest manifestations include fatigue, non-erosive polyarthritis in rheumatoid distribution, photosensitive rashes, mouth ulcers, alopecia, Raynaud's phenomenon and pleurisy. More serious manifestations are endocarditis, lung fibrosis, pulmonary hypertension and various forms of renal and neurological disease.[28] SLE is associated with the production of autoantibodies directed against a variety of antigens, such as antinuclear antibodies and antibodies to double-stranded (ds) DNA, extractable nuclear antigens (e.g. Ro and La) and hematopoietic cells (resulting in hemolytic anemia, leukopenia or thrombocytopenia).

Effect of pregnancy on SLE

This has been a debatable issue for some time.[2,29] There is evidence that sex hormones may increase autoantibody formation. Estrogens, in particular, can predispose to the development of lupus in mouse models and human SLE.[10] Many patients do not tolerate the oral combined contraceptive pill due to exacerbation of lupus and, until recently, many physicians considered pregnancy relatively contraindicated, as pregnancy frequently caused SLE to deteriorate significantly. This impression may have developed because patients often reduced or stopped their drugs when pregnancy was diagnosed, an action that usually precipitates active disease.

There have been a number of retrospective and prospective studies assessing the risk of lupus flare in pregnancy.[2] These have suffered from a number of problems such as lack of controls, inappropriately matched controls, small numbers and failure to define flare. Overall, they have suggested that the frequency of flare is between 21% and 82%, and is similar or increased during pregnancy compared with non-pregnant patients. Only one study matched for disease activity at the beginning of the study. This showed that flare was reduced in patients with inactive disease at the time of conception, compared to those with active disease, and non-pregnant patients with inactive or active disease.[30] Two recent controlled prospective studies[31,32] using patients when not pregnant as their own controls as well as a separate non-pregnant group showed that lupus flared in about 65% of pregnancies. This was more common than in the controls (about 40% flared). The flares were usually mild, occurred after the first trimester or postpartum, were independent of therapy and were more likely in those with active disease at conception.

SLE in pregnancy with active renal involvement is the most worrying, as deterioration poses considerable risk to the mother and fetus.[2,16] Steroids should not be used prophylactically as they can aggravate pregnancy-induced hypertension and preeclampsia, and do not appear to reduce the risk of flare. However, prednisolone and azathioprine can be used in pregnancy (see Table 196.3) and should be continued at prepregnancy doses, and increased or started as clinically indicated to prevent serious clinical deterioration.

Identifying active lupus disease in pregnancy, particularly with renal involvement, can be difficult as it needs to be distinguished from preeclampsia, which may coexist. It is important to identify more specific features of active SLE such as malar rash, red cells in the urine and rising titers of anti-dsDNA antibodies (see Table 196.4). Proteinuria and hypertension due to pre-eclampsia can be associated with thrombocytopenia, pregnancy-induced musculoskeletal pain and palmar erythema.[29] Assessment of the complement proteins C3 and C4 is less helpful, as these levels usually rise in pregnancy and a fall in active SLE may not be detected unless frequently checked. Increased levels of complement degradation products (C3a, C3d, Ba and Bb) may be a more reliable measure of active lupus.[33]

Effect of SLE on the pregnancy

Retrospective and prospective studies have found that patients with SLE are at increased risk of fetal loss due to spontaneous abortion and stillbirth. Recent studies suggest that fetal loss occurs in about 20% of SLE pregnancies.[2,34] Different frequencies for fetal loss between studies are likely to reflect variable patient selection and disease activity, as well as differences in obstetric care and fetal monitoring between clinical centers. Factors that probably contribute to the increased risk of fetal loss include disease activity overall, type and severity of renal involvement and a hypercoagulable state due to the presence of antiphospholipid antibodies.

Table 196.4 Diagnosis of lupus flare in pregnancy

Unreliable features	Reliable features
Facial/palmar erythema	True lupus rash
Arthralgia	Synovitis
Anemia	Mucosal ulcers
Low platelets	Leukopenia
Hypertension	Red cells in urine
Proteinuria	Casts in urine
Low C4/high C4d	Anti-DNA antibodies
Classical pathway activation	Alternative pathway activation

Antiphospholipid antibodies have been associated with recurrent miscarriages and stillbirth. They are detected usually as a 'lupus anticoagulant' and/or anticardiolipin antibodies and are not necessarily associated with SLE (see 'the antiphospholipid syndrome' below).[2]

Preterm delivery is more common in SLE patients than in controls. In one study, 24% of pregnancies in diagnosed SLE patients ended in preterm labor compared with 6% of the pregnancies before SLE was diagnosed.[34] More recently, 43% of live births in a lupus cohort were preterm with a mean gestational age of 34 weeks.[35] In 76% of these cases fetal distress and/or intrauterine growth retardation had prompted induction of labor. This intervention appears to have improved outcome, with the live birth rate rising from 31% to 82% for these women compared with their own previous obstetric history.[35] In another study, premature rupture of membranes was found to be more common in SLE pregnancies than controls and accounted for 25% of preterm deliveries.[36] Active disease at conception, renal involvement, hypertension, Raynaud's phenomenon and antiphospholipid antibodies may indicate patients at risk of preterm delivery.[2]

Neonatal lupus syndrome

Fortunately, this is a rare manifestation of maternal autoantibody production, which may present with transient skin rashes, liver dysfunction, hematological abnormalities or congenital heart block in the newborn.[29,37] The condition is due to cellular damage by passively acquired maternal IgG autoantibodies. The skin rashes and cytopenias disappear after about 8 weeks as the maternal autoantibodies are cleared from the neonatal circulation and the tissues regenerate. As cardiac tissue cannot regenerate, heartblock is persistent but can be treated by the insertion of a pacemaker. This may be delayed until the child is about 10 years old but in severe cases, congenital heartblock may be associated with perinatal death due to myocarditis and cardiac failure. Maternal dexamethasone administration may reduce this inflammation and improve fetal outcome but the heartblock remains irreversible.[37]

The skin rashes and heartblock are associated with anti-Ro (SS-A) antibodies in the mother. There is some evidence that mothers with anti-La (SS-B) and anti-Ro antibodies are at increased risk of having a child with congenital heartblock. The mothers often have a history of photosensitive rashes and are usually known to have SLE. In some cases the birth of a child with neonatal lupus is the first and only manifestation of autoantibody formation in the mother. Over subsequent years, typical features of SLE develop in about 50% of these mothers. The remainder usually develops some lupus-like features such as photosensitivity and arthralgia. Only 5–10% of mothers with anti-Ro antibodies give birth to a child with neonatal lupus, but there is a one in three chance of a further child with congenital heartblock after the birth of a first child with this form of neonatal lupus.

Antiphospholipid syndrome

The antiphospholipid antibody syndrome is characterized by the development of recurrent venous and arterial thromboembolism, fetal loss due to placental thrombosis and infarction and thrombocytopenia associated with the production of high levels of IgG antiphospholipid antibodies.[2,38] Other clinical features include cardiac murmurs, pulmonary hypertension, hemolytic anemia, livedo reticularis and neurological disorders such as migraine, epilepsy, chorea and stroke. The antiphospholipid syndrome occurs in about 15% of SLE cases but can occur spontaneously (the primary antiphospholipid syndrome) or in association with other autoimmune conditions.[39] Antiphospholipid antibodies are present in about 10% of patients with recurrent miscarriage.[40]

Antiphospholipid antibodies can be identified by a variety of tests.[38] Antibodies to cardiolipin and other negatively charged phospholipids can be measured directly by ELISA techniques. Some antiphospholipid antibodies interfere with phospholipid-dependent coagulation tests. They can cause a prolonged activated partial thromboplastin time (APTT) by acting as an inhibitor of coagulation *in vitro*. The effect of this 'lupus anticoagulant' (LA) cannot be corrected by the addition of normal plasma. It is paradoxically associated with an increased risk of thrombosis, not bleeding, *in vivo*. The Russell viper venom test is a more sensitive and specific test for LA than the more commonly performed APTT screen.[2,40] As transiently positive results are found for both anticardiolipin antibodies and LA (e.g. in infection), it is important to obtain a confirmatory test at least 6 weeks later. Persistently high levels of IgG anticardiolipin antibodies and the Russel viper venom test appear to be the best predictors of fetal loss.[40,41]

The antiphospholipid syndrome may present for the first time during pregnancy, most commonly with deep vein thrombosis or recurrent second-trimester fetal loss. First- and third-trimester losses and intrauterine growth retardation (IUGR) may also occur. Hemolysis, elevated liver enzymes and low platelets (HELLP) syndrome and hepatic infarction have been reported in several patients with antiphospholipid antibodies. There is a risk of recurrence of all these complications in subsequent pregnancies.[42–44] The fetus should be assessed carefully for evidence of fetal distress and IUGR from 26 weeks onward, as premature delivery may reduce the risk of intrauterine death in a potentially viable fetus. Doppler blood flow waveforms can be used to assess utero-placental blood flow with conventional assessments of fetal growth, heart rate, movement, tone and maturity.[1,2]

Management of the antiphospholipid syndrome

This is a debatable issue as there are few randomized controlled studies. The evidence increasingly supports the use of low-dose aspirin (75 mg) in patients with anticardiolipin antibodies and/or LA and a history of recurrent miscarriages.[45] More recent work supports the addition of subcutaneous heparin.[46] Many doctors will prescribe low-dose aspirin, at least between weeks 10 and 34, to all patients with any serological evidence of antiphospholipid antibodies or SLE, to reduce the risk of fetal loss and IUGR as the risk of such aspirin therapy is minimal compared with the disease-associated risk.[47] For patients with antiphospholipid antibodies and a history of venous or arterial thrombosis, subcutaneous heparin (unfractionated or low molecular weight) is required. Low-dose aspirin is often given as well.[45,46] When not pregnant, they require high-dose warfarin therapy to keep the international normalized ratio greater than 3.0.[48]

There is no evidence that oral prednisolone therapy provides additional protection from the deleterious effects of antiphospholipid antibodies with the primary antiphospholipid syndrome. There is even some evidence to suggest that pregnant patients given steroids and low-dose aspirin do less well than those given aspirin alone (increased risk of hypertension and pre-eclampsia). For patients on heparin and prednisolone there is an increased (additive) risk of osteoporosis. However, patients with SLE who are taking prednisolone to control their overall disease should continue with this therapy, at the lowest dose possible to keep the disease suppressed. For the unfortunate patients with recurrent fetal loss despite heparin and aspirin therapy, uncontrolled studies suggest that treatment with intravenous γ-globulin or plasma exchange may be helpful monthly throughout pregnancy.[2,39,49–52]

Systemic sclerosis

Systemic sclerosis (scleroderma) is a multisystem disease of unknown etiology that is characterized by the overproduction and growth of connective tissue, especially collagen, with associated microvascular obliteration and vascular damage. Immune dysfunction, inflammation and endothelial damage involving growth factor and cytokine activation are probably involved in the pathogenesis. The prevalence is about 1 in 10,000 and it is three times more common in women than in men. The peak age of onset is 30–50 years. In the past, most women would have completed their families by this time but it is now becoming a more frequent problem in pregnancy. Typical features include thickened shiny skin (scleroderma), microstomia, telangiectasia, Raynaud's phenomenon, esophageal dysmotility, pulmonary fibrosis and hypertension. The most serious manifestations are cardiac failure, pulmonary hypertension, digital gangrene and renal failure.

There have been no prospective and very few case-controlled studies of pregnancy in systemic sclerosis. In contrast to previous reports, recent work suggests that infertility and fetal loss are not increased,[53] but prematurity and intrauterine growth retardation are more common than in controls.[54] The disease does not necessarily change during pregnancy. However, those with diffuse cutaneous disease and antitopoisomerase antibodies have a poorer prognosis than those with limited cutaneous disease and anticentromere antibodies. Patients with aggressive skin disease, especially those within 5 years of onset, are at most risk of deteriorating during pregnancy with life-threatening systemic complications, especially hypertensive renal crisis and pulmonary hypertension. Acid reflux, esophagitis, constipation, arthralgias and hypertension are common problems, which often deteriorate in pregnancy. Blood pressure should be checked several times a week in diffuse disease.

Nifedipine, paracetamol and ranitidine should be prescribed if needed. NSAIDs should not be given as they can precipitate hypertension and renal crisis in addition to fetal risks. Pre-eclampsia can be difficult to distinguish from renal involvement but this does not affect management. Angiotensin-converting enzyme (ACE) inhibitors are indicated in resistant systemic hypertension, particularly if there is proteinuria, elevation of serum creatinine or microangiopathic hemolytic anemia indicating life-threatening renal crisis.[53] The risks of ACE inhibitors causing fetal abnormalities, impaired placental perfusion and intrauterine death appear to be less than the risk of maternal and fetal death without such treatment. D-Penicillamine can cause fetal abnormalities and is usually stopped before pregnancy (Table 196.2). In patients with aggressive disease it has been continued in some cases without ill-effect.[53] Steroids increase the risk of renal crisis and should be avoided unless aggressive fibrosing alveolitis, pericarditis or inflammatory myopathy develop.[54] Anesthesia may be complicated if there is cardiac, respiratory or renal involvement, and if the skin and esophageal changes are severe. A Swan–Ganz catheter may be necessary for monitoring during and after delivery. Epidural anesthesia is often preferred, as it promotes peripheral vasodilatation and avoids problems with intubation and the risk of inhalation. Lower than normal doses of all agents are recommended as systemic sclerosis patients are often very sensitive. Systemic hypertension with renal impairment, acute pulmonary hypertension and cardiac failure may develop for the first time in the postnatal period.[55,56]

Vasculitis

Vasculitis is a term used to describe a heterogenous group of diseases characterized by an inflammatory cell infiltrate and necrosis of blood vessel walls. The size, site and number of blood vessels involved determine the clinical consequences of this vascular inflammation. Vasculitis may be primary, for example, Wegener's granulomatosis, or secondary to a systemic disease such as SLE. These conditions are all rare especially in pregnant women, as the onset is usually after the age of 40 years and cyclophosphamide therapy may induce premature menopause. However, as treatment of these previously lethal conditions improves, the association of vasculitis and pregnancy may be encountered more frequently. Polyarteritis nodosa and Wegener's granulomatosis may deteriorate or present for the first time in pregnancy with high risk of maternal morbidity and mortality.[56,57] The prognosis is best in patients who are in remission on low dose or no immunosuppression. Cessation of drugs may contribute to disease flare in pregnancy, so prednisolone and azathioprine should be continued or used as necessary but cyclophosphamide should be avoided (Table 196.3). Fetal outcome is usually good unless maternal disease is very severe in early pregnancy.

Genetic syndromes with musculoskeletal manifestations

Familial Mediterranean fever

This genetic disorder occurs predominantly in people of Mediterranean and Middle Eastern origin, especially Sephardi Jews and Armenians.[58] It is characterized by brief attacks of fever at irregular intervals, which may be associated with arthritis, pleurisy, peritonitis and erysipelas-like erythema. Untreated patients develop systemic amyloidosis, which causes proteinuria due to nephropathy and may result in death from renal failure before the age of 40. This can be prevented by continuous colchicine therapy,[59] which also prevents symptomatic attacks in about 65% and reduces the frequency and severity of attacks in a further 30%. Two cases each of trisomy 21 and Down's syndrome have been reported in 620 colchicine-treated pregnant women. It is not clear that the chromosomal aberrations were due to colchicine but amniocentesis is recommended for those who wish to assess this potential risk in pregnancy.[58]

Marfan's syndrome

This genetic disorder affecting the extracellular matrix protein fibrillin has an autosomal dominant inheritance, is relatively common in all racial groups and has a prevalence of about 1 in 20,000.[60,61] The characteristic clinical features include tall stature, disproportionately long limbs (and digits) relative to trunk length, chest wall deformities (e.g. pectus excavatum), scoliosis, high arched narrow palate and ligamentous laxity. The patients often have flat feet, which can increase the risk of mechanical back pain, and may have limited extension of some joints. Most are myopic and have non-progressive upward subluxation of the lens. The most serious problems are mitral valve prolapse and dilatation of the aorta due to cystic medial necrosis. Symmetrical aortic dilatation begins at the sinus of Valsalva and may cause aortic regurgitation as well as dissection or rupture. Timely surgical intervention when the aortic root is 55–60 mm may prevent such a catastrophic outcome. Pregnancy poses a very high risk of precipitating this in patients with moderate aortic dilatation.[60] Women should receive multidisciplinary advice both before and during pregnancy.

Ehlers–Danlos syndromes

This is a heterogenous group of genetic disorders affecting structural proteins, particularly type I and type III collagen, fibronectin, enzymes involved in connective tissue synthesis or copper metabolism.[60,61] Most show autosomal dominant inheritance but some are autosomal or X-linked recessive. It is the more severe, type IV Ehlers–Danlos syndrome (ecchymotic or arterial form) that is the most dangerous in pregnancy due to the additional risk of rupture of the uterus and preterm delivery at this time.[61,62]

These patients have characteristic faces with large eyes, thin nose and lips, easy bruising and thin skin with prominent venous pattern affecting the hands and feet Only the small joints of the hand are hypermobile and peripheral joint contractures may develop. Spontaneous pneumothorax and mitral valve prolapse occur frequently. Repeated gastrointestinal and arterial ruptures, usually involving the iliac, splenic or renal arteries or aorta, result in peritonitis, hematomas and eventually death. There is a defect in the synthesis or secretion of type III collagen, which is usually inherited in an autosomal dominant manner, but spontaneous mutations in one of the collagen type III alleles may occur.[61] Although pregnancy may be uneventful, the risk of uterine rupture and the tendency toward friable tissues means that delivery, anesthesia and surgery can be fraught with difficulties, so pregnancy should not be undertaken lightly.

Conclusion

In all cases, everyone involved in the care of the pregnant patient with a musculoskeletal disorder must be aware of the underlying disease and its potential effects on the mother and fetus. Full discussion of the likely advantages and disadvantages of any treatment plan must take place. Even with systemic rheumatic disease, providing that it is stable at the onset of pregnancy, the prognosis is usually good with careful monitoring of maternal disease and fetal development.

REFERENCES

1. Dudley DJ, Branch DW. Pregnancy in the patient with rheumatic disease: The obstetrician's perspective. *Bailliere's Clin Rheumatol* 1990;4:141–56.
2. Petri M. Systemic lupus erythematosus and pregnancy. *Rheumatic Dis Clin North Am* 1994;20:87–118.
3. Nashel DJ. Entrapment neuropathies. In Klippel JH, Dieppe PA, eds. *Rheumatology*. London: Mosby, 1994;5:19.1–12.
4. Gould JS, Wissinger A. Carpal tunnel syndrome in pregnancy. *South Med J* 1978;71:144–6.
5. George E. Hip pain during pregnancy. In Klippel JH, Dieppe PA, eds. *Rheumatology*. London: Mosby, 1994;5:15.6–7.
6. Schapira D. Transient osteoporosis of the hip. *Semin Arthritis Rheum* 1992;22:98–105.
7. Dunne F, Walters B, Marshall T, *et al.* Pregnancy associated osteoporosis. *Clin Endocrinol* 1993;39:487–90.
8. Smith R, Athanasou NA, Ostlere SJ, *et al.* Pregnancy-associated osteoporosis. *Q J Med* 1995;88:865–78.
9. Mcguire JL, Lambert RE. Arthropathies associated with endocrine disorders. In Kelley WN, Harris ED, Ruddy S, Sledge CB, eds. *Textbook of Rheumatology*. Philadelphia: W. B. Saunders Company, 1997:1499–513.
10. MacLennan AH, Nicholson R, Green RC, *et al.* Serum relaxin and pelvic pain of pregnancy. *Lancet* 1986;2:243–5.
11. Nelson JL, Ostensen M. Pregnancy and rehumatoid arthritis. *Rheumatic Dis Clin North Am* 1997;23:195–212.
12. Silman A, Kay A, Brennan P. Timing of pregnancy in relation to the onset of rheumatoid arthritis. *Arthritis Rheum* 1992;35:152–5.
13. Da Silva JAP, Hall GM. The effects of gender and sex hormones on outcome in rheumatoid arthritis. *Bailliere's Clin Rheumatol* 1992;6:193–219.
14. Spector TD, Roman E, Silman AJ. The pill, parity, and rheumatoid arthritis. *Arthritis Rheum* 1990;33:782–9.
15. Lin H, Mosmann TR, Guilbert L, *et al.* Synthesis of T helper 2-type cytokines at the maternal–fetal interface. *J Immunol* 1993;151: 1562 73.
16. Buchanan WW, Kean WF. Pregnancy and the rheumatic diseases. In Maddison PJ, Isenberg DA, Woo P, Glass DN, eds. *Oxford Textbook of Rheumatology*. Oxford: Oxford University Press, 1993:93–8.
17. Kean WF, Buchanan WW. Pregnancy and rheumatic disease. *Bailliere's Clin Rheumatol* 1990;4:125–40.
18. Liedholm H, Montan S, Aberg A. Risk grouping of 113 patients with hypertensive disorders during pregnancy, with respect to serum urate, proteinuria, and time of onset of hypertension. *Acta Obstet Gynecol Scand* 1984;118 (Suppl):43–8.
19. Rahn DW. Lyme disease. In Klippel JH, Dieppe PA, eds. *Rheumatology*. London: Mosby, 1994;4:4.1–12.
20. Kelley WN, Wortmann RL. Gout and hyperuricaemia. In Kelley WN, Harris ED, Ruddy S, Sledge CB, eds. *Textbook of Rheumatology*. Philadelphia: W. B. Saunders Company, 1997: 1313–51.
21. Pouchot J, Sampalis JS, Beaudet F, *et al.* Adult Still's disease: Manifestations, disease course, and outcome in 62 patients. *Med (Baltimore)* 1991;70:118–36.
22. Ostensen M, Husby G. A prospective clinical study of the effect of pregnancy on rheumatoid arhritis and ankylosing spondylitis. *Arthritis Rheum* 1983;26:1155–9.
23. Roubenoff R, Hoyt J, Petri M, *et al.* Effects of antiinflammatory and immunosuppressive drugs on pregnancy and fertility. *Semin Arthritis Rheum* 1988;18:88–110.
24. Needs C, Brooks P. Drugs, pregnancy and rheumatoid arthritis. In Klippel JH, Dieppe PA, eds. *Rheumatology*. London: Mosby, 1994,8.18.4–6.
25. Bermas BL, Hill JA. Effects of immunosuppressive drugs during pregnancy. *Arthritis Rheum* 1995;38:1722–32.
26. Ramsey-Goldman R, Schilling E. Immunosuppressive drug use during pregnancy. *Rheumatic Dis Clin North Am* 1997;23: 149–67.
27. Johnson AE, Gordon C, Palmer RG, *et al.* The prevalence and incidence of systemic lupus erythematosus in Birmingham, England – Relationship to ethnicity and country of birth. *Arthritis Rheum* 1995;38:551–8.
28. Isenberg DA, Horsfall AC. Systemic lupus erythematosus – Adult onset. In Maddison PJ, Isenberg DA, Woo P, Glass DN, eds. *Oxford Textbook of Rheumatology*. Oxford: Oxford Medical Publications, 1993:733–55.
29. Buyon JP. Systemic lupus erythematosus and the maternal–fetal dyad. *Bailliere's Clin Rheumatol* 1990;4:85–103.
30. Urowitz MB, Gladman DD, Farewell VT, *et al.* Lupus and pregnancy studies. *Arthritis Rheum* 1993;36:1392–7.
31. Petri M, Howard D, Repke J. Frequency of lupus flare in pregnancy: The Hopkins Lupus Pregnancy Center experience. *Arthritis Rheum* 1991;34:1538–45.
32. Ruiz-Irastorza G, Lima F, Alves J, *et al.* Increased rate of lupus flare during pregnancy and the puerperium: A prospective study of 78 pregnancies. *Br J Rheumatol* 1996;35:133–8.
33. Buyon JP, Tamerius J, Ordorica S, *et al.* Activation of alternative complement pathway accompanies disease flares in systemic lupus erythematosus during pregnancy. *Arthritis Rheum* 1992;35: 55–61.
34. Petri M, Allbritton J. Fetal outcome of lupus pregnancy: a retrospective case–control study of the Hopkins Lupus Cohort. *J Rheumatol* 1993;20:650–6.
35. Lima F, Buchanan NMM, Khamashta MA, *et al.* Obstetric outcome in systemic lupus-erythematosus. *Semin Arthritis Rheum* 1995;25: 184–92.
36. Johnson MJ, Petri M, Witter FR, *et al.* Evaluation of preterm delivery in a systemic lupus-erythematosus pregnancy clinic. *Obstet Gynecol* 1995;86:396–9.
37. Tseng CE, Buyon JP. Neonatal lupus syndromes. *Rheumatic Dis Clin North Am* 1997;23:31–54.
38. Petri M. Diagnosis of antiphospholipid antibodies. *Rheumatic Dis Clin North Am* 1994;20:443–69.
39. Ehrenfeld M, Schoenfeld Y. Haematology and oncology in rheumatology. In Maddison PJ, Isenberg DA, Woo P, Glass DN, eds. *Oxford Textbook of Rheumatology*. Oxford: Oxford University Press, 1993:154–62.
40. Rai RS, Regan L, Clifford K, *et al.* Antiphospholipid antibodies and beta-2-glycoprotein-i in 500 women with recurrent miscarriage – Results of a comprehensive screening approach. *Hum Reprod* 1995;10:2001–5.
41. Lynch A, Marlar R, Murphy J, *et al.* Antiphospholipid antibodies in predicting adverse pregnancy outcome: a prospective study. *Ann Intern Med* 1994;120:470–5.
42. Mor F, Beigel Y, Inbal A, *et al.* Hepatic infarction in a patient with lupus anticoagulant. *Arthritis Rheum* 1989;32:491–5.
43. Kilpatrick DC, Maclean C, Liston QA, *et al.* Antiphospholipid antibody syndrome and pre-eclampsia. *Lancet* 1989;2:987–8.
44. Kinoshita K. Hepatic infarction during pregnancy complicated by antiphospholipid syndrome. *Am J Obstet Gynecol* 1993;169: 199–202.
45. Lima F, Khamashta MA, Buchanan NMM, *et al.* A study of 60 pregnancies in patients with the antiphospholipid syndrome. *Clin Exp Rheumatol* 1996;14:131–6.
46. Rai R, Cohen H, Dave M, *et al.* Randomised controlled trial of aspirin and aspirin plus heparin in pregnant women with recurrent miscarriage associated with antiphospholipid antibodies (or antiphospholipid antibodies). *Br Med J* 1997;314:253–7.

47. Collaborative low dose aspirin study in pregnancy collaborative group CLASP. A randomised trial of low-dose aspirin for the prevention and treatment of pre-eclampsia among 9364 pregnant women. *Lancet* 1994;343:619–29.
48. Khamashta MA, Cuadrado MJ, Mujic F, *et al.* The management of thrombosis in the antiphospholipid syndrome-antibody syndrome. *N Engl J Med* 1995;332:993–7.
49. Lockshin MD. Which patients with antiphospholipid antibody should be treated and how? *Rheum Dis Clin North Am* 1993;19: 235–47.
50. Cowchock FS, Reece EA, Balaban D, *et al.* Repeated fetal losses associated with antiphospholipid antibodies: A collaborative randomized trial comparing prednisone with low-dose heparin treatment. *Am J Obstet Gynecol* 1992;166:1318–23.
51. Silver RK, MacGregor SN, Sholl JS, *et al.* Comparative trial of prednisolone plus aspirin versus aspirin alone in the treatment of anticardiolipin antibody-positive obstetric patients. *Am J Obstet Gynecol* 1993;169:1411–7.
52. Spinnato JA, Clark AL, Pierangeli SS, *et al.* Intravenous immunoglobulin therapy for the antiphospholipid syndrome in pregnancy. *Am J Obstet Gynecol* 1995;172:690–4.
53. Steen VD. Scleroderma and pregnancy. *Rheum Dis Clin North Am* 1997;23:133–47.
54. Kitridou RC. Pregnancy in systemic sclerosis. In Klippel JH, Dieppe PA, eds. *Rheumatology*. London: Mosby, 1994;6:11.11–3.
55. Black CM. Systemic sclerosis and pregnancy. *Bailliere's Clin Rheumatol* 1990;4:105–21.
56. Friedman SA, Bernstein MS, Kitzmiller JL. Pregnancy complicated by collagen vascular disease. *Obstet Gynecol Clin North Am* 1991;18:213–36.
57. Pauzner R, Mayan H, Hershko E, *et al.* Exacerbation of Wegener's granulomatosis during pregnancy: report of a case with tracheal stenosis and literature review. *J Rheumatol* 1991;21:1153–6.
58. Pras M, Sohar E, Familial Mediterranean fever. In Klippel JH, Dieppe PA, eds. *Rheumatology*. London: Mosby, 1994;6:30.1–4.
59. Zemer D, Pras M, Sohar E, *et al.* Colchicine in the prevention and treatment of the amyloidosis of familial Mediterranean fever. *N Engl J Med* 1986;314:1001–5.
60. Marini JC. Heritable collagen disorders. In Klippel JH, Dieppe PA, eds. *Rheumatology*. London: Mosby, 1994;7:44.1–8.
61. Rowe DW, Shapiro JR. Heritable disorders of structural proteins. In Kelley WN, Harris ED, Ruddy S, Sledge CB, eds. *Textbook of Rheumatology*. Philadelphia: W.B. Saunders Company, 1997;1535–62.
62. Peaceman AM, Cruikshank D. Ehlers–Danlos syndrome and pregnancy: Association of type IV disease with maternal death. *Obstet Gynecol* 1987;69:428–31.

197 Thyroid function in pregnancy

C. Paul

Introduction

Normal thyroid function in pregnancy is essential for the normal growth and maturation of the fetus. Any disturbance of thyroid function, either from disruption of the hypothalamic–pituitary–thyroid axis or from non-thyroid disease can have a profound effect on this process. The antibodies present in maternal serum in autoimmune thyroid disorders readily cross the placenta, as do many of the drugs used to treat maternal thyroid disease. These factors may also significantly influence fetal development. In this chapter, these processes in normal pregnancy and the ways in which they may be altered by disease will be discussed. The implications for both mother and fetus and the relevant treatments available will be considered.

Over recent years maternal and fetal thyroid physiology and the relationship between the two have been well studied. Improved understanding of these processes has opened up interesting possibilities in the field of fetal therapy. One such example is the use of thyroid hormones for the acceleration of fetal lung maturity in preterm labor. This is currently the subject of important research and will also be discussed later in this chapter.

Development of fetal thyroid

Embryology

The development of the thyroid gland commences during the fourth week of embryonic life. Initially, an endodermal thickening forms in the floor of the pharynx. This grows downward forming the thyroid diverticulum. This diverticulum branches into two and continues to migrate downward as the embryo grows. It passes in front of the developing hyoid bone and laryngeal cartilages during its descent. The developing gland is attached by a fine stalk, the thyroglossal duct, to its original site on the tongue – the foramen cecum.

By the seventh week the thyroid gland has usually reached its normal position in the neck. At this time it is composed of a right and a left lobe connected by the isthmus. The distal part of the thyroglossal duct forms the pyramidal lobe and the remainder usually disappears.

Placental transfer of thyroid hormones

The fetal hypothalamic–pituitary–thyroid axis and thyroid gland develop independently of maternal thyroid hormone status, and become functional toward the end of the first trimester. However, thyroxine (T4) has been isolated from celomic and amniotic fluid from as early as 6 weeks' gestation,[1] at concentrations that vary directly according to maternal serum concentrations. This T4 must therefore be derived from the maternal circulation.

After the first trimester, transfer of tri-iodothyronine (T3) and T4 across the placenta does occur, but it is slow and maternal levels remain higher than fetal levels.[2] Neither thyroid-stimulating hormone (TSH) nor thyroid-binding globulin (TBG) is able to cross the placenta. Maternal thyrotropin-releasing hormone (TRH) reaches the fetal circulation,[3] but is not required for the release of TSH from the fetal pituitary.[4]

Fetal thyroid function

By 12 weeks' gestation the fetal pituitary gland contains TSH. The thyroid gland is able to synthesize T3 and T4. TBG, T4 and TSH are all measurable in fetal serum.[5,6] The concentrations of TBG, TSH, free T3 and T4 and total T3 and T4 all increase with gestation.[7] Free and total T4 levels reach adult levels by 36 weeks, but T3 levels remain lower than adult levels throughout pregnancy. TSH levels in the fetus also continue to increase throughout gestation despite rising T4 concentration and remain higher than the maternal levels.

Hypothalamic maturation is an important part of thyroid system development. This process commences at between 4 and 5 weeks' gestation and continues until the third trimester. TRH has been detected in hypothalamic tissue by radioimmunoassay from 10 weeks' gestation.[6] The fetal pituitary is very sensitive to TRH.[8] A response is seen from around 20 weeks' gestation and negative feedback develops during the second trimester.[9]

Changes at delivery

Delivery results in stimulation of TSH release from the pituitary. This reaches a peak at 30 min of age. The level of TSH then falls rapidly during the first 24 h but more slowly over the next 2 days. T4 (both free and total) levels reach a peak at 24 h of age and then gradually decrease over the first few weeks of life.[6] There is a small peak in T3 production during the first hours after birth; this is followed by a more sustained rise commencing within 4 h and maintained for up to 36 h. These increased T3 levels are thought to arise from both increased secretion of T3 and increased conversion of T4 to T3. In preterm infants the pattern of TSH and T4 release are similar, but the magnitude of the changes is lower than in term infants.

Normal maternal thyroid function in pregnancy

During pregnancy, many of the normal maternal physiological changes that occur, such as increased heart rate, cardiac output and circulating blood volume, may complicate the assessment of maternal thyroid function. This difficulty is compounded by the fact that the size of the thyroid gland increases in pregnancy.[10] This has long been known to be so and, in fact, was a physical sign used in ancient times to diagnose the onset of pregnancy.[11] Despite this, most women in normal pregnancy are assumed to be euthyroid, and only the presence of an obvious goiter is considered pathological.[9]

The increased estrogen level in pregnancy stimulates the synthesis and reduces the hepatic clearance of TBG.[12] Serum TBG concentrations continue to rise from the beginning of the first trimester until around 24 weeks' gestation. The level then reaches a plateau, which is maintained until approximately 2 weeks after delivery.[13] There is a compensatory increase in the production of T4 and T3. The total serum levels of these hormones are significantly elevated in pregnancy; however, as in the non-pregnant state it is the unbound or free T3 and T4 that are responsible for thyroid activity.

Over the years there has been some disagreement regarding the exact nature of the changes in free thyroid hormone concentrations in pregnancy. This is probably due to difficulties in comparing different assay techniques. Now that measurements are more reliable and consistent it is accepted that there is a small increase in the free T4 concentration during the first trimester and a small decrease thereafter.[14].

Table 197.1 Summary of changes in thyroid function in normal pregnancy

	First trimester	Second and third trimesters
Thyroid volume	↑	↑
TBG	↓	↑
Total T3 and T4	↑	↑
Free T3 and T4	↑	↓
TSH	↓	↑
Iodine uptake	↑	↑
Iodine clearance	↑	↑

TBG, thyroid-binding globulin; T3, tri-iodothyronine; T4, thyroxine; TSH, thyroid-stimulating hormone

In most women these changes are within normal non-pregnant ranges.[15,16] There is a corresponding change in TSH levels, which fall in the first trimester and later rise as the T4 levels fall. Again, these levels remain within the normal limits in most women.[17]. The overall increase in thyroid function is thought to be primarily due to stimulation of the gland by substances released from the placenta. These are human chorionic gonadotropin (hCG),[17] chorionic TSH[18] and a placental TSH-releasing factor.[19] Chorionic TSH has only been found in one-third of pregnant women, and even in them the levels are so low that the hormone is unlikely to be of clinical significance in thyroid regulation. The effect of placental TRH on fetal and maternal thyroid function is, likewise, yet to be defined. There is, however, good evidence to suggest that hCG plays a significant role in maternal thyroid stimulation.[17] Throughout pregnancy there is a negative correlation between the levels of hCG and TSH. This supports the theory that it is hCG that stimulates the thyroid gland, leading to suppression of TSH in early pregnancy, and is thus responsible for the increase in maternal thyroid function.[6]

It has been suggested that the reduced serum concentration of iodine in late pregnancy may be another factor involved in the reduction of thyroid activity at this time.[13] The fall in serum iodine levels is due to the increased renal clearance of iodide and the increased requirements of the fetus. The increased demand for iodine is of little clinical significance in most developed countries where iodine intake is sufficient. A summary of the physiological changes occurring in pregnancy is given in Table 197.1.

Abnormalities of maternal thyroid function

Maternal hyperthyroidism

Incidence

The exact incidence of hyperthyroidism in pregnancy is unclear; however, it is generally estimated to occur in somewhere between 1 in 500 and 1 in 2000 pregnant women.[9,13]

Etiology

Autoimmune disorders. Autoimmune disorders, including the hypermetabolic phase of Hashimoto's thyroiditis, account for the majority of cases of maternal hyperthyroidism in pregnancy. The most common of these disorders is Graves' disease. In most women the onset of this disease precedes the pregnancy. Symptoms of thyrotoxicosis may be exacerbated in the first trimester of pregnancy due to the small increase in thyroid function at this time. As the pregnancy progresses, many women with Graves' and other autoimmune diseases experience some degree of remission, because of the mild immunosuppression occurring in normal pregnancy. The return of autoimmune activity in the postnatal period often results in relapse of the condition after delivery.[21]

Other thyroid causes. Acute thyroiditis is another relatively common thyroid disorder in pregnancy. This is commonly preceded by a viral illness, is usually self-limiting and seldom requires treatment. Solitary toxic adenomata and toxic multinodular goiter may also occur but are less common.

Non-thyroid conditions. As already discussed, hCG is known to have thyroid-stimulating properties. In trophoblastic disease the greatly increased levels of this hormone may result in biochemical or clinical evidence of hyperthyroidism.[22,23] In addition, there is production of acidic variants of hCG, which have even greater stimulatory properties.[24] Overt thyrotoxicosis is actually quite rare in these women, the hyperthyroidism resolves as the hCG levels fall following treatment for the trophoblastic disease, and antithyroid drug therapy is rarely indicated.

Although the cause of hyperemesis gravidarum is unknown, it is more common in pregnancies in which the levels of hCG are higher than normal. It is particularly common in multiple pregnancies and women with trophoblastic tumors. It is likely that in hyperemesis, as discussed above for trophoblastic disease, the elevated hCG levels are responsible for the increased thyroid stimulation. A recent study, demonstrating a direct correlation between the increased hCG levels in hyperemesis and thyroid stimulation *in vitro*, lends support to this theory.[25] In most cases the hyperthyroidism in this condition is mild and resolves spontaneously before the second trimester.[26]

Clinical features

Many women in pregnancy experience symptoms that in a non-pregnant woman would lead to a suspicion of hyperthyroidism. These symptoms include changes in appetite, weight and bowel function, tremor, palpitations, heat intolerance, mood changes, anxiety and tiredness.

The possibility of thyroid dysfunction should not be discounted in pregnancy, particularly in women with a past or family history of thyroid disease.

Diagnosis

This is confirmed biochemically by the detection of suppressed TSH and elevated T4 levels in maternal serum. In borderline cases it is sometimes useful to repeat the blood tests after 3–4 weeks in order to confirm or exclude the diagnosis. TSH is the single best indicator of thyroid function in pregnancy,[27,28] the diagnosis of hyperthyroidism being based on its low levels. T4 may be normal and T3 levels elevated in isolation.

Since Graves' disease is such a common cause of hyperthyroidism in pregnancy, the thyroid-stimulating antibodies should be measured in all cases in order to assess the risks to the fetus and neonate.

Effects of hyperthyroidism on pregnancy

Maternal. Although oligo- or amenorrhea and anovulation are associated with thyrotoxicosis,[29] mild hyperthyroidism has not been found to significantly affect fertility.[11] A rare but serious complication of thyrotoxicosis is congestive cardiac failure. Women with long-standing untreated disease and those remaining thyrotoxic despite treatment are most at risk of developing this problem.[30]

Fetal. Maternal thyrotoxicosis in pregnancy is associated with considerable risks to the fetus. The incidence of miscarriage, stillbirth, intrauterine growth retardation (IUGR), premature delivery and neonatal death are all greater than in normal pregnancy.[30–33] An increase in the number of babies with structural and chromosomal abnormalities, including Down's syndrome, has also been reported,[33–35] but the cause of this is not clear.

Antithyroid drugs have also been implicated, but recent evidence suggests that poor control of thyrotoxicosis is more likely to account for congenital defects.[34] Thyroid autoimmunity is thought to be a risk factor both for chromosomal abnormality[36] and for miscarriage.[37,38] Higher titers of TSH receptor antibody increase the fetal risks.[32]

Treatment

The maternal and fetal complications are significantly reduced if the disease is diagnosed and treated promptly.

Drug therapy. Thionamides are the most common agents used for the treatment of thyrotoxicosis in pregnancy. They include carbimazole, methimazole and propylthyrouracil (PTU). Carbimazole is rapidly metabolized to methimazole. These drugs have two actions. First, they inhibit thyroid hormone synthesis. This is achieved by the competitive blocking of the peroxidase enzyme, preventing the release of iodine from circulating iodides. The enzymes responsible for the iodination of tyrosine and the coupling of iodothyronine molecules are also inhibited. The second action is to cause a reduction in the levels of circulating thyroid autoantibodies. PTU has the additional effect of inhibiting the peripheral conversion of T4 to the more active T3. The release of thyroid hormones is not prevented, so it may be at least a week before a response is detectable and up to 6 weeks before a patient becomes euthyroid.

Although all the thionamide drugs cross the placenta, PTU does so more slowly than carbimazole and methimazole.[39] This has resulted in PTU becoming the treatment of first choice in pregnancy. There is ongoing concern that there may be a link between the use of methimazole and the development of a rare skin condition in the fetus, aplasia cutis congenita; although a direct causal relationship has not been confirmed, this has further decreased the popularity of this drug.[40] Despite its advantages, PTU is not without risks to the fetus. It is slowly metabolized by the fetus, and is present in higher concentrations in the fetal than the maternal circulation.[41] The resulting suppression of fetal thyroid function by this drug can lead to the development of fetal goiter,[42,43] or neonatal hypothyroidism.[44]

The treatment regimen commonly used in non-pregnant women with Graves' disease involves complete suppression of thyroid function with high doses of antithyroid drugs and T4 replacement. This treatment cannot be used in pregnancy because of the poor placental transfer of T4 compared to the thiourea drugs.

The aim of treatment should be to rapidly control the thyrotoxicosis and then to reduce the dose of drug to maintain the T4 level toward the upper limit of the normal range, or at mildly hyperthyroid levels.[40,45] Treatment should be monitored by measuring maternal free T4, which generally correlates well with fetal levels; TSH measurement is less useful in these patients.

Up to 5% of women experience mild side effects with thionamides. These include gastrointestinal upset, rashes, joint pains, pruritus, a metallic taste and nausea. More serious side effects such as bronchospasm, hepatitis and a lupus-like syndrome can also occur. Some patients will, however, be able to tolerate a different agent from the group. The most dangerous side effect, agranulo-cytosis, occurs in only 0.1% of patients. It tends to occur in women older than 40 years of age; it is dose related and reversible on stopping treatment.[46] It is a contraindication to further treatment with any thionamide agents.

Side effects are usually apparent within 2 months after commencing treatment. All women should have regular assessment of liver function and blood count, and be advised to report any problems.

β-Blockers may be used in the short term to control severe symptoms such as palpitations. They do not, however, treat the underlying condition. Prolonged use has been associated with a number of fetal side effects including IUGR, fetal bradycardia, hypoglycemia, a poor response to anoxic stress and respiratory depression at birth.[47,48]

Surgery. This is only indicated in pregnancy for those women who cannot tolerate antithyroid drugs, those in whom biochemical control is poor and in rare cases of suspected malignancy. It is best performed during the second trimester. The complications are the same as for non-pregnant patients and include hypothyroidism, recurrent hyperthyroidism, hypoparathyroidism and vocal cord paralysis.

Radioactive iodine therapy. This form of treatment is contraindicated in pregnancy and during breast feeding.[49] Termination of pregnancy should be offered to women inadvertently treated during early pregnancy, due to the risks of teratogenesis.

Maternal hypothyroidism

Incidence

Hypothyroidism is more common than hyperthyroidism, occurring in between 6 and 9 per 1000 women in pregnancy.[50]

Etiology

Autoimmune disorders. Most cases of hypothyroidism in women of child-bearing age have an autoimmune etiology. These conditions tend to reduce fertility and are unlikely to develop during pregnancy, thus most women will have been diagnosed, and treatment instituted, before the onset of pregnancy. The commonest cause in this group of women is Hashimoto's thyroiditis. Spontaneous atrophic hypothyroidism and treated Graves' disease with inadequate thyroxine replacement are other autoimmune conditions that should be considered.

Iatrogenic. Hypothyroidism may also be the consequence of thyroidectomy, radio-iodine ablation or excessive dosage with antithyroid drugs.

Iodine deficiency. During pregnancy the uptake of iodine is increased in order to maintain normal thyroid function. This is of little significance in developed countries, but in areas of the Third World where iodine deficiency is endemic it is a major health problem.

Clinical features. The symptoms of hypothyroidism including tiredness, poor concentration and weight gain with poor appetite, dry skin, hair loss and cold intolerance often occur only in severe cases. Physical signs including bradycardia, delayed relaxation of tendon reflexes and goiter are, likewise, not invariably present.[9]

Diagnosis

In hypothyroidism the serum concentration of TSH is significantly increased. Free T4 and T3 may be reduced; however, due to the increase in TBG found in pregnancy the total serum levels of these hormones may remain within the normal range, and are not useful in the diagnosis. Testing for maternal thyroid autoantibodies should be performed routinely.

Effects of hypothyroidism on pregnancy

Maternal. It is well recognized that the incidence of menstrual irregularity and anovulation are high in hypothyroid women. Pregnancy is uncommon in severe cases. Gestational hypertension is much more common in hypothyroid women than in the general obstetric population, even in those with subclinical disease.[51]

Fetal. In the past, hypothyroidism has been associated with high rates of miscarriage, stillbirth, neonatal death and congenital abnormality.[52–55] More recent evidence has been more reassuring, indicating that pregnancy outcome is usually good in these women.[56]

Treatment

Many women with hypothyroidism will already be taking T4 replacement therapy before becoming pregnant. Those in whom the diagnosis is made during pregnancy should be started immediately on T4. Adequate dosage should be confirmed by monitoring maternal TSH levels. It has been reported that the requirements for T4 are increased during pregnancy;[57] however, for women who are established on treatment, it is probably sufficient to check TSH and free T4 levels once in the first trimester, and to alter the dose at this point if necessary.[58] Subsequent adjustments can be made if the patient becomes symptomatic.

As with the treatment of hyperthyroidism, the serum free T4 levels should be kept in the upper normal or lower hyperthyroid range. This will allow adequate production of T3 via the peripheral conversion of T4. It is perfectly safe for mothers to breastfeed while taking thyroxine.

Abnormalities of fetal and neonatal thyroid function

Hyperthyroidism

Incidence

This is a rare condition affecting less than 1 in 4000 pregnancies.[59]

Etiology

Fetal and neonatal thyrotoxicosis generally occurs as a result of transplacental transfer of thyroid autoantibodies from the maternal circulation. All women with a history of autoimmune thyroid disorder (most commonly Graves' disease or Hashimoto's thyroiditis) may, even after successful treatment, pass antibodies to the fetus during pregnancy.

The risk to the fetus can be determined by measuring the maternal antibody levels. If the levels are low, the fetus is not at risk; if they are high, more careful monitoring is required.[60,61] However, it is only after 22–24 weeks' gestation that the fetus is at risk of developing thyrotoxicosis.[62] All women with a past or current history of thyroid disease should be monitored carefully during the second half of pregnancy. Increased thyroid activity has also been demonstrated in fetuses anemic as a result of rhesus isoimmunization.[63]

Clinical features

Fetal. The rates of preterm delivery and stillbirth are considerably higher for thyrotoxic fetuses.[64] Careful postmortem in cases of stillbirth may reveal features including thyromegaly, cardiomegaly, congestive visceromegaly, generalized adenopathy, reduction in subcutaneous fat and signs of pulmonary hypertension.[65]

Neonatal. A number of clinical signs may lead to a suspicion of thyrotoxicosis in the fetus at risk of this condition. These include poor feeding and failure to gain weight, irritability, tachypnea, tachycardia and sometimes the development of cardiac failure. Goiter may also be seen.[9]

Diagnosis

Fetal. Serial ultrasound scanning from 28 weeks' gestation is useful for the detection of IUGR, fetal tachycardia, hyperactivity and goiter. The characteristic findings of advanced bone age and craniosynostosis have also been described on ultrasound.[11] Polyhydramnios, which may be due to esophageal obstruction by fetal goiter and fetal hydrops from cardiac failure, can also be excluded.

Fetal thyroid function can be abnormal regardless of maternal thyroid status and occasionally a direct assessment of fetal thyroid function can be undertaken by performing fetal blood sampling. The results can be compared with established normal ranges.[7]

Neonatal. Cord blood should be taken at the time of delivery to check for thyroid autoantibodies, TSH, T4 and T3 in all at-risk cases. It is important to remember that autoantibodies will last longer in the neonatal circulation than antithyroid medication transferred from the maternal circulation. Therefore, if the mother has been taking antithyroid drugs the neonate may not present with features of thyrotoxicosis until 5–10 days of age. Untreated neonatal thyrotoxicosis has a mortality rate of up to 25%.[66] It is important to maintain a high index of suspicion, to make an early diagnosis and to institute treatment promptly.

Treatment

Fetal. If the diagnosis of fetal thyrotoxicosis is made, the mother should be treated with antithyroid medication in the same way as for maternal hyperthyroidism. PTU is the drug of choice, as already described.

The fetal condition can be closely monitored with cardiotocography (CTG) and ultrasound assessment. These should initially be performed weekly, but the frequency can be decreased as the condition stabilizes.

Neonatal. When the diagnosis is made in the neonate the thionamide agents are still the first-line choice of treatment. Other drugs such as propranolol for tachycardia, digoxin and diuretics for cardiac failure and sedatives can be used as appropriate.

Maternal autoantibodies will disappear from the neonatal circulation over the first 3–4 months, leading to spontaneous resolution of the hyperthyroidism, allowing gradual withdrawal of medication.

Hypothyroidism

Incidence

Screening programs performed in the USA have found the incidence of permanent abnormalities leading to hypothyroidism to be between 1 in 3500 and 4000 live births. Transient functional abnormalities occur in 1–2% of newborn babies, with premature infants being most commonly affected.[67–69]

Etiology

Thyroid dysgenesis. This term covers the spectrum of disorders from ectopic or hypoplastic thyroid gland tissue to complete agenesis. It is the most common cause of permanent hypothyroidism. Babies tend to be asymptomatic and are diagnosed by routine screening. The cause is unknown.

Dyshormonogenesis. Several defects in thyroid hormone synthesis and metabolism have been described. Most have an autosomal recessive inheritance. Goiter may be present at birth, but usually develops postnatally over a period of months or years.[6]

Secondary and tertiary hypothyroidism. Abnormal synthesis or metabolism of TSH and TRH are extremely rare. They may occur either as isolated abnormalities or in association with other hypothalamic or pituitary abnormality.[70] These conditions will not be detected by routine screening.

Transient primary hypothyroidism. This may result from passage across the placenta of antithyroid drugs or other drugs such as amiodarone or lithium.[71,72] It can also be caused by the transfer of maternal thyroid autoantibodies or high concentrations of iodine from excessive maternal intake.

Prematurity. Serum T4 concentration increases with gestational age, as the hypothalamic function matures.[6] All premature infants thus have low T4 levels at birth, which are physiological. TSH levels remain within the normal range. Sick premature infants may have lower levels of T4 than those who are well, and lower T3 levels due to reduced peripheral conversion of T4.[73] Thyroid function returns to normal as the babies recover.

Hypoxia and IUGR. Hypothyroidism has been found to be a feature of hypoxic growth retardation due to uteroplacental insufficiency. TSH is higher and T4 lower in these babies as compared to normally grown babies of the same gestation. The severity of the hypothyroidism reflects the severity of the hypoxia.[74] It is thought that this may be a result either of reduced supply of nutrients across the placenta due to impaired placental blood flow, or of hypoxia affecting the thyroid function itself.

Chromosomal abnormalities. More than 50% of adults with Down's syndrome suffer from hypothyroidism.[75] These patients have been found to have a greater degree of intellectual impairment than euthyroid Down's syndrome patients.[76]

It is only recently that the thyroid function of fetuses with chromosomal abnormalities has been investigated *in utero*.[77] It has been found that even though their thyroid hormones remain within the normal range, TSH levels are elevated. This may be an early sign of developing hypothyroidism. It has been suggested that this may contribute to the development of mental and neurological handicap in chromosomally abnormal patients.

Iodine deficiency. Around 800 million people live in areas of severe iodine deficiency and are thus at risk of developing related disorders.[78] This includes the development of cretinism, which is a major problem, commonly leading to irreversible mental deficiency, deaf-mutism and spastic diplegia.[9] In these countries the situation may be worsened by the high intake of foodstuffs such as cassava, which inhibit thyroid function. The condition can be prevented by the administration of iodine supplementation.

Clinical features

Fetal. IUGR, bradycardia, delayed skeletal development and goiter have all been identified in severely hypothyroid fetuses.[79] Goiter may cause polyhydramnios by mechanical obstruction of the esophagus, thus increasing the risk of preterm labor.

Neonatal. Often there are no obvious clinical features at birth in these babies. Depending on the cause and severity of the condition the classical features may take several weeks or months to become apparent. These features include poor feeding, constipation, respiratory problems, umbilical hernia, prolonged jaundice, dry skin, 'cretinoid facies' and an enlarged fontanelle.

Neurological development. Babies born with severe congenital hypothyroidism, even if treated promptly after birth, have been shown to have lower scores on intelligence testing than their normal siblings and moderately hypothyroid infants.[80] There seems to be a threshold level of T4 below which impaired brain development occurs.[81]

Screening

In the UK all babies are screened routinely for hypothyroidism at between 5 and 8 days of age. A blood sample is obtained from the baby by heel prick. Spots of blood are applied directly on to special filter papers and TSH measured. Similar programs are in operation in Europe, USA and Japan. These screening programs allow early diagnosis and treatment of affected babies, thus preventing the development of neurological and mental impairment.[82]

Babies born to mothers with a history of autoimmune disease or other babies thought to be particularly at risk can be investigated in more detail by obtaining cord blood at the time of delivery.

Diagnosis

Fetal. Fetal hypothyroidism may be suspected because of maternal history, or in the presence of the abnormal scan findings described earlier. Investigation of the mother is helpful to assess the thyroid hormone and autoantibody status. As mentioned previously, fetal thyroid function can only be measured directly by obtaining a fetal blood sample. A raised TSH will confirm the diagnosis.[83]

Neonatal. Screening programs will allow the detection of most cases in the first week of life. Further investigation, including measurement of autoantibodies and thyroglobulin or even radioisotope scanning, may be necessary in order to determine the cause. In the rare cases of secondary or tertiary hypothyroidism the TSH will not be increased, and thus these conditions will not be detected by normal screening.

Treatment

Careful assessment of maternal thyroid function and autoantibody levels is essential. In those women taking antithyroid medication or T4, the treatment dosage should be adjusted to keep the maternal thyroid function in the upper normal or low hyperthyroid range.

Unfortunately very little T4 crosses the placenta after the first trimester of pregnancy. If the fetus were to be adequately treated by maternal administration of T4, the doses required would result in the mother developing significant hyperthyroidism.[2] Treatment of the fetus by intra-amniotic administration of T4 at intervals of 7–10 days has been described by several authors.[83–85] Fetal blood sampling for assessment of thyroid function has been described in the management of thyrotoxicosis.[86] This technique is equally suitable for the management of hypothyroidism cases where the response to intra-amniotic treatment was poor.

There are many advantages of early treatment. These include the prevention of neurological sequelae of antenatal fetal hypothyroidism and also reduction of the polyhydramnios associated with fetal goiter, thereby decreasing the risk of preterm delivery and its complications.

Postpartum maternal thyroid dysfunction

Incidence

The reported incidence of postpartum thyroiditis varies widely between different studies, but is probably somewhere around 4.9%.[87]

Etiology

A mild state of immunosuppression exists in pregnancy, which results in the temporary remission of many autoimmune diseases. This is often followed by a relapse in the postnatal period as the autoimmune activity increases. Graves' disease is one condition that follows this pattern.[21]

Both Graves' disease and Hashimoto's thyroiditis may also present for the first time after pregnancy. There is another form of autoimmune thyroiditis that occurs specifically in postpartum women. This condition, known as postpartum thyroiditis, is characterized by its transient nature, and was first described by Amino and colleagues in 1976.[88] The classical picture of this disease comprises an initial hyperthyroid phase typically occurring 2–3 months after delivery. This is caused by a destructive process involving the thyroid gland and resulting in the release of thyroid hormones into the circulation. This phase is followed 2–6 months later by a hypothyroid phase. This phase generally resolves spontaneously within 3–5 months; however, it may be severe enough to require treatment and often results in goiter formation. It has also been associated with postnatal depression.[89]

The presentation of this condition may vary from the sequence of events described. Patients may experience transient hypothyroidism without the preceding hyperthyroid phase or an isolated transient hyperthyroidism. Interestingly, it has been found to occur more commonly in women giving birth to girls.[90]

Women developing postpartum thyroiditis are significantly more likely than those not affected to develop permanent hypothyroidism.[91]

Diagnosis

Levels of T4, T3 and TSH are different during the various phases of the disease. Thyroid antibodies, including microsomal antibodies, are present in high concentrations.[92] Measurement of microsomal antibodies during the first trimester may predict the development and degree of transient postpartum hypothyroidism.[93] If the mother is not breast-feeding, radioisotope scanning can be performed and will demonstrate decreased uptake, which is consistent with thyroiditis and the associated reduction in thyroid hormone synthesis.

Cytological examination of specimens obtained by fine-needle aspiration from the thyroid glands of women with this condition shows a lymphocytic infiltration consistent with an autoimmune diagnosis.[94]

Treatment

The hyperthyroid phase tends to be mild and of short duration, so that treatment is seldom indicated. If the symptoms are severe they should be treated with β-blockers or mild sedatives. Antithyroid medication is not indicated as the high levels of thyroid hormones result from destruction of the gland and release of stored hormone rather than increased production or secretion.

T4 therapy is, however, indicated for all women developing symptoms during the hypothyroid phase of the illness. This can be continued for up to 1 year. The thyroid function should be monitored carefully after stopping treatment to exclude the development of permanent hypothyroidism. The risk of recurrence in future pregnancies means that follow-up is particularly important at this time.

The effect of thyroid hormones on fetal lung maturation

Background

Thyroid hormones are among the many factors involved in the development and maturation of fetal lung function. This is important due to the high incidence of respiratory morbidity and mortality occurring in preterm infants. These complications of prematurity have been greatly reduced but not abolished by the introduction of maternal corticosteroid administration to women at risk of preterm labor.

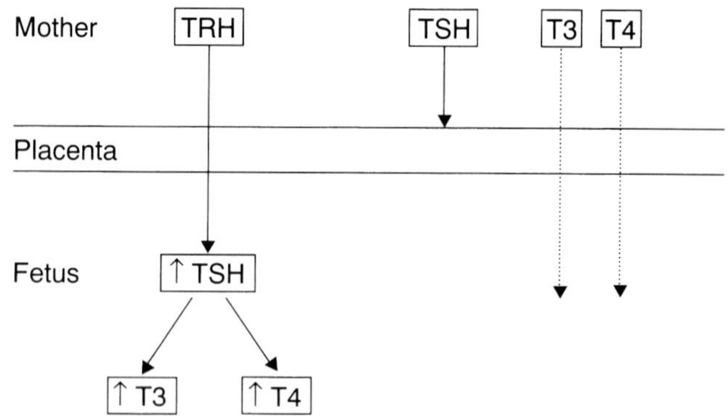

Figure 197.1 Placental transfer of thyroid-stimulating hormone (TSH), thyroid-releasing hormone (TRH), triiodothyronine (T3) and thyroxine (T4).

It has been known for some time that infants with respiratory distress syndrome (RDS) have lower levels of T3 and T4 than normal infants.[95] This has led to the investigation of the potential benefit of the antenatal use of thyroid hormones in an attempt to prevent the development of RDS.[96]

As already discussed TSH does not cross the placenta, and T3 and T4 cross only in small amounts. The maternal dose of T4 required to obtain satisfactory fetal levels is unacceptably high for the mother.[2] Both intra-amniotic and fetal intramuscular administration of T4 have therefore been attempted.[96,97] These routes are invasive and thus carry risks for the fetus. Another problem with the intra-amniotic route is that the volume of amniotic fluid, and hence the concentration of the hormones, is variable and fetal absorption may be different in different fetuses. These considerations have limited the adoption of this policy.

The safest and most effective way to stimulate fetal thyroid function is by the maternal administration of TRH. This small tripeptide molecule rapidly crosses the placenta and stimulates fetal production of TSH with the subsequent release of thyroid hormones (Figure 197.1).

Mechanism of action of TRH

There is no evidence to suggest that TRH alone, without corticosteroids, is of any benefit in promoting lung maturity. However, there is believed to be a synergistic effect when TRH and corticosteroids are used in combination.

Many mechanisms have been hypothesized. These include effects on increasing surfactant production;[98] effects on pulmonary fluid production and absorption;[99] stimulation of fetal breathing;[100] accelerated structural development, possibly mediated by prolactin secretion[101] and stimulation of the sympathetic nervous system via the neurotransmitter properties of TRH.[102] Despite these theories the exact mechanism has not yet been defined.[103]

Clinical trials

A number of randomized controlled trials comparing the outcome in women and their babies given TRH and corticosteroids antenatally to those given corticosteroids alone have now been conducted.[104–109] A meta-analysis of these trials has also been published.[110] These studies have used different dosages, dose intervals and number of doses of TRH. Various gestational ages have been used to qualify for entry into the trials.

Different subgroup analysis has also been performed, with a number of the trials reporting outcomes only for the 'optimally treated' infants, this being defined as those having received a complete course of treatment and then delivered within a certain time period. Even optimal treatment is defined differently in different papers. These discrepancies make direct comparison of the results of these trials quite difficult. So far, the combined results show few significant differences between the treatment and control groups. These differences are a reduction in the incidence of severe RDS and an increase in maternal side effects. There is no significant effect on the incidence of either chronic lung disease or perinatal mortality.

Further work is currently in progress to investigate the issue of antenatal TRH treatment. Long-term follow-up of the infants delivered after their mothers have received this therapy will also be necessary to address the question of pituitary–thyroid and neurodevelopmental effects.

Conclusion

Maternal thyroid disease in pregnancy may have important implications for both mother and fetus. Prompt diagnosis and treatment are therefore imperative. It is also important to remember that the babies of women with thyroid disease may be at risk despite normal maternal thyroid function throughout pregnancy. These pregnancies should thus be monitored carefully.

Antenatal TRH therapy is currently being investigated as a potentially useful addition to corticosteroids in reducing morbidity and mortality in preterm infants. The definitive results of this work are awaited.

REFERENCES

1. Contempre B, Jauniaux E, Calvo R, *et al.* Detection of thyroid hormones in human embryonic cavities during the first trimester of pregnancy. *J Clin Endocrinol Metab* 1993;77:1719–22.
2. Fisher DA, Lehman H, Lackey C. Placental transport of thyroxine. *J Clin Endocrinol Metab* 1964;24:393–400.
3. Azukizawa M, Murata Y, Ikenoue T, *et al.* Effect of thyrotropin-releasing hormone on secretion of thyrotropin, prolactin, thyroxine and tri-iodothyronine in pregnant and fetal rhesus monkeys. *J Clin Endocrinol Metab* 1976;43:1020–8.
4. Tonooka N, Greer MA. Evidence that control of fetal thyrotropin secretion is independent of both the fetal and maternal hypothalamus. *Endocrinology* 1978;102:852–8.
5. Burrow GN, Fisher DA, Larson PR. Mechanisms of disease: Maternal and fetal thyroid function. *N Engl J Med* 1997;331:1072–8.
6. Fisher DA, Klein AH. Thyroid development and disorders of thyroid function in the new-born. *N Engl J Med* 1981;304:702–12.
7. Thorpe-Beeston JG, Nicolaides KH, Felton CV, *et al.* Maturation of the secretion of thyroid hormone and thyroid stimulating hormone in the fetus. *N Engl J Med* 1991;324:532–6.
8. Ballabio M, Nicolini U, Jowett T, *et al.* Maturation of thyroid function in normal human fetuses. *Clin Endocrinol* 1989;31:565–71.
9. Kendall-Taylor P. Pregnancy and the thyroid. *Fetal Maternal Med Rev* 1993;5:89–103.
10. Rasmussen NG, Hornnes PJ, Hegedus L. Ultrasonically determined thyroid size in pregnancy and postpartum: The goitrogenic effect of pregnancy. *Am J Obstet Gynecol* 1989;160:1216–20.
11. Becks GP, Burrow G. Thyroid disease and pregnancy. *Med Clin N Am* 1991;75:121–36.
12. Ain KB, Mori Y, Refetoff S. Reduced clearance rate of thyroxine-binding globulin (TBG) with increased sialylation: A mechanism for oestrogen-induced elevation of serum TBG concentration. *J Clin Endocrinol Metab* 1987;65:689–96.
13. Kennedy RL, Darne FJ. Disorders of the thyroid gland during pregnancy and the postpartum period. In Studd J, ed. *Progress in Obstetrics and Gynaecology.* Edinburgh: Churchill Livingstone, 1994;11:125–40.
14. Guillaume J, Schussler GC, Goldman J. Components of the total serum thyroid hormone concentrations during pregnancy: high free thyroxine and blunted thyrotropin (TSH) response to TSH-releasing hormone in the first trimester. *J Clin Endocrinol Metab* 1985;60:678–84.
15. Glinoer D, de Nayer P, Bourdoux P, *et al.* Regulation of maternal thyroid during pregnancy. *J Clin Endocrinol Metab* 1990;71:276–87.
16. Weeke J, Dybkjaer L, Granlie K, *et al.* A longitudinal study of serum TSH and total and free iodothyronines during normal pregnancy. *Acta Endocrinol (Copenh)* 1982;101:531–7.
17. Ballabio M, Poshyachinda M, Ekins RP. Pregnancy induced changes in thyroid function: Role of human chorionic gonadotropin as putative regulator of maternal thyroid. *J Clin Endocrinol Metab* 1991;73:824–31.
18. Tojo S, Kanazawa S, Nakamura A, *et al.* Human chorionic TSH (hCTSH, HCT) during normal and molar pregnancy. *Endocrinol Jpn* 1973;20:505–15.
19. Gibbons JM, Mitnick M, Chieffo V. *In vitro* biosynthesis of TSH and LH releasing factors by the human placenta. *Am J Obstet Gynecol* 1975;121:127–31.
20. Harada A, Hershman JM, Reed AW, *et al.* Comparison of thyroid stimulators and thyroid hormone concentrations in the sera of pregnant women. *J Clin Endocrinol Metab* 1979;48:793–7.
21. Amino N, Tanizawa O, Mori H, *et al.* Aggravation of thyrotoxicosis in early pregnancy and after delivery in Grave's disease. *J Clin Endocrinol Metab* 1982;55:108–12.
22. Norman RJ, Green-Thompson RW, Jialal I, *et al.* Hyperthyroidism in gestational trophoblastic neoplasia. *Clin Endocrinol (Oxford)* 1981;15:395–401.
23. Desai RK, Norman RJ, Jialal I, *et al.* Spectrum of thyroid function abnormalities in gestational trophoblastic neoplasia. *Clin Endocrinol* 1988;29:583–92.
24. Mann K, Schneider N, Hoermann R. Thyrotropic activity of acidic isoelectric variants of human chorionic gonadotropin from trophoblastic tumors. *Endocrinology* 1986;118:1558–66.
25. Goodwin TM, Montoro M, Mestman JH, *et al.* The role of chorionic gonadotrophin in transient hyperthyroidism of hyperemesis gravidarum. *J Clin Endocrinol Metab* 1992;75:1333–7.
26. Bouillon R, Naesens M, Van Assche FA, *et al.* Thyroid function in patients with hyperemesis gravidarum. *Am J Obstet Gynecol* 1982;143:922–6.
27. Bassett F, Eastman CJ, Ma G, *et al.* Diagnostic value of thyrotropin concentrations in serum as measured by sensitive immunoradiometric assay. *Clin Chem* 1986;32:461–4.
28. De los Santos ET, Mazzaferri EL. Sensitive thyroid stimulating hormone assays: Clinical applications and limitations. *Compr Ther* 1988;14:26–33.

29. Thomas R, Reid RL. Thyroid disease and reproductive dysfunction. A review. *Obstet Gynecol* 1987;70:789–98.
30. Davis LE, Lucas MJ, Hankins GDV, *et al.* Thyrotoxicosis complicating pregnancy. *Am J Obstet Gynecol* 1989;160:63–70.
31. Mestman JH, Manning PR, Hodgman J. Hyperthyroidism and pregnancy. *Arch Int Med* 1974;134:434–9.
32. Mitsuda N, Tamaki H, Amino N, *et al.* Risk factors for developmental disorders in infants born to women with Graves' disease. *Obstet Gynecol* 1992;80:359–64.
33. Mujtaba Q, Burrow GN. Treatment of hyperthyroidism in pregnancy with propylthiouracil and methimazole. *Obstet Gynecol* 1975;46:282–6.
34. Momotami N, Ito K, Hamada N, *et al.* Maternal hyperthyroidism and congenital malformation in the offspring. *Clin Endocrinol* 1984;20:695–700.
35. Dinani S, Carpenter S. Down's syndrome and thyroid disorder. *J Ment Defic Res* 1990;34:187–93.
36. Kennedy RL, Jones TH, Cuckle HS. Down's syndrome and the thyroid. *Clin Endocrinol* 1992;37:471–6.
37. Stagnaro-Green A, Roman SH, Cobin RH, *et al.* Detection of at-risk pregnancy by means of highly sensitive assays for thyroid autoantibodies. *J Am Med Assoc* 1990;264:1422–5.
38. Glinoer D, Soto MF, Bourdoux P, *et al.* Pregnancy in patients with mild thyroid abnormalities: Maternal and neonatal repercussions. *J Clin Endocrinol Metab* 1991;73:421–7.
39. Marchant B, Brownlie BEW, Hart DM, *et al.* The placental transfer of propylthiouracil, methimazole and carbimazole. *J Clin Endocrinol Metab* 1977;45:1187–93.
40. Mandel SJ, Brent GA, Larsen PR. Review of antithyroid drug use during pregnancy and report of a case of aplasia cutis. *Thyroid* 1994;4:129–33.
41. Gardner DF, Cruikshank DP, Hays PM, *et al.* Pharmacology of propylthiouracil (PTU) in pregnant hyperthyroid women: Correlation of maternal PTU concentrations with cord serum thyroid function tests. *J Clin Endocrinol Metab* 1986;62:217–20.
42. Burrow GN. Neonatal goitre after maternal propylthiouracil therapy. *J Clin Endocrinol Metab* 1965;25:403–8.
43. Refetoff S, Ochi Y, Selenkow HA, *et al.* Neonatal hypothyroidism and goitre in one infant of each of two sets of twins due to maternal therapy with antithyroid drugs. *J Pediatr* 1974;85:240–4.
44. Werner SC. Hyperthyroidism in the pregnant woman and neonate. Two panel discussions on hyperthyroidism. *J Clin Endocrinol Metab* 1967;27:1637–54.
45. Momotani N, Noh J, Oyanagi H, *et al.* Antithyroid drug therapy optimal for Graves' disease during pregnancy: Optimal regimen for fetal thyroid status. *N Engl J Med* 1986;315:24–8.
46. Cooper DS, Goldminz D, Levin AA, *et al.* Agranulocytosis associated with antithyroid drugs: Effects of patient age and drug dose. *Ann Intern Med* 1983;98:26–9.
47. Gladstone GR, Hordof AJ, Gersony WM. Propranolol administration during pregnancy: Effects on the fetus. *J Pediatr* 1975;86:962–4.
48. Habib A, McCarthy JS. Effects on the neonate of propranolol administered during pregnancy. *J Pediatr* 1977;91:808–11.
49. Pekonen F, Lamberg B-A. Thyrotoxicosis during pregnancy. *Ann Chir Gynaecol* 1978;67:165–73.
50. Niswander KR, Gordon M, Berendes HW. The women and their pregnancies. In *The Collaborative Perinatal Study of the Institute of Neurological Disease and Stroke.* Philadelphia: W. B. Saunders, 1972:246–9.
51. Leung AS, Millar LK, Koonings PP, *et al.* Perinatal outcome in hypothyroid pregnancies. *Obstet Gynecol* 1993;81:349–53.
52. Hodges RE, Hamilton HE, Keettel WC. Pregnancy in myxedema. *Arch Int Med* 1952;90:863–8.
53. Greenman GW, Gabrielson MO, Howard-Flanders J, *et al.* Thyroid dysfunction in pregnancy: Fetal loss and follow-up evaluation of surviving infants. *N Engl J Med* 1962;267:426–31.
54. Jones WS, Man EB. Thyroid function in normal pregnancy. VI. Premature deliveries and reproductive failures of pregnant women with low serum butanol-extractable iodines. Maternal serum TBG and TBPA capacities. *Am J Obstet Gynecol* 1969;104:909–14.
55. Potter JD. Hypothyroidism and reproductive failure. *Surg Gynecol Obstet* 1980;150:251–5.
56. Montoro M, Collea JV, Frasier D, *et al.* Successful outcome of pregnancy in women with hypothyroidism. *Ann Int Med* 1981;94:31–4.
57. McDougall IR, Maclin N. Hypothyroid women need more thyroxine when pregnant. *J Fam Pract* 1995;41:238–40.
58. Girling JC, DeSwiet M. Thyroxine dosage during pregnancy in women with primary hypothyroidism. *Br J Obstet Gynaecol* 1992; 99:368–70.
59. Fisher DA. Neonatal thyroid disease in offspring of women with autoimmune thyroid disease. *Thyroid Today* 1986;9:1–7.
60. Zakarija M, McKenzie JM, Hoffman WH. Prediction and therapy of intrauterine and late onset neonatal hyperthyroidism. *J Clin Endocrinol Metab* 1986;62:368–71.
61. Tamaki H, Amino N, Aozasa M, *et al.* Universal predictive criteria for neonatal overt thyrotoxicosis requiring treatment. *Am J Perinatol* 1988;5:152–8.
62. Cove DH, Johnston P. Fetal hyperthyroidism: Experience of treatment in four siblings. *Lancet* 1985;1:430–2.
63. Thorpe-Beeston JG, Nicolaides KH, Snijders RJM, *et al.* Thyroid function in anaemic fetuses. *Fetal Ther* 1990;5:109–14.
64. Bruinse H, Vermeulen-Meiners C, Wit JM. Fetal treatment for thyrotoxicosis in non-thyrotoxic pregnant women. *Fetal Ther* 1988;3:152–7.
65. Page DV, Brady K, Mitchell J, *et al.* The pathology of intrauterine thyrotoxicosis: two case reports. *Obstet Gynecol* 1988;72:479–81.
66. Delange F. Effect of maternal thyroid function during pregnancy on fetal development. In Beckers C, Reinwein D, eds. *The Thyroid and Pregnancy.* New York: Wiley, 1992.
67. Fisher DA, Dussault JH, Foley TP, *et al.* Screening for congenital hypothyroidism: results of screening one million North American infants. *J Pediatr* 1979;94:700–5.
68. DeLange F. New-born Committee of the European Thyroid Association. Neonatal screening for congenital hypothyroidism in Europe. *Acta Endocrinol (Copenh)* 1979;90(Suppl):3–29.
69. Robertson EF, Oldfield R, Wilkins A, *et al.* Screening of new-born infants for hypothyroidism: Two years experience in South Australia. *Med J Aust* 1979;1:593–6.
70. Dussault JH, Letarte J, Guyda H, *et al.* Thyroid function in neonatal hypothyroidism. *J Pediatr* 1976;89:541–4.
71. Matsumara LK, Born D, Kunii IS, *et al.* Outcome of thyroid function in new-borns from mothers treated with amiodarone. *Thyroid* 1992;2:279–81.
72. DeCatte L, deWolfe D, Smitz J, *et al.* Fetal hypothyroidism as a complication of amiodarone treatment for persistent fetal supraventricular tachycardia. *Prenat Diagn* 1994;14:762–5.
73. Klein AH, Foley B, Kenny FM, *et al.* Thyroid hormone and thyrotropin responses to parturition in premature infants with and without the respiratory distress syndrome. *Pediatrics* 1979;63:380–5.
74. Thorpe-Beeston JG, Nicolaides KH, Snijders RJM, *et al.* Thyroid function in small for gestational age fetuses. *Obstet Gynecol* 1991;77:701–6.
75. Baxter RG, Martin FIR, Myles K, *et al.* Down syndrome and thyroid function in adults. *Lancet* 1975;2:794–6.
76. Pueschel SM, Pezzullo JC. Thyroid dysfunction in Down syndrome. *Am J Dis Child* 1985;139:636–9.
77. Thorpe-Beeston JG, Nicolaides KH, Gosden CM, *et al.* Thyroid function in fetuses with chromosomal abnormalities. *Br Med J* 1991;302:628.
78. Hetzel BS. Progression in the prevention and control of iodine deficiency disorders. *Lancet* 1987;2:266.
79. Utiger RD. Recognition of thyroid disease in the fetus. *N Engl J Med* 1991;324:559–61.
80. Glorieux J, Dussault JH, Morissette J, *et al.* Follow-up at ages 5 and 7 years on mental development in children with hypothyroidism detected by Quebec screening programme. *J Pediatr* 1985;107:913–15.
81. Tillotson SL, Fuggle PW, Smith I, *et al.* Relation between biochemical severity and intelligence in early treated congenital hypothyroidism: a threshold effect. *Br Med J* 1994;309:440–5.
82. New England Congenital Hypothyroidism Collaborative. Elementary school performance of children with congenital hypothyroidism. *J Pediatr* 1990;116:27–32.
83. Noia G, de Santis M, Tocci A, *et al.* Early prenatal diagnosis and therapy of fetal hypothyroid goitre. *Fetal Diagn Ther* 1992;7:138–43.
84. Johnson RL, Finberg HJ, Perlman AH, *et al.* Fetal goitrous hypothyroidism. *Fetal Ther* 1989;4:141–5.
85. Davidson KM, Richards DS, Schatz DA, *et al.* Successful *in utero* treatment of fetal goitre and hypothyroidism. *N Engl J Med* 1991;324:543–6.
86. Porreco RP, Bloch CA. Fetal blood sampling in the management of intrauterine thyrotoxicosis. *Obstet Gynecol* 1990;76:509–12.
87. Gerstein HC. How common is postpartum thyroiditis? A methodological overview of the literature. *Arch Int Med* 1990;150: 1397–400.
88. Amino N, Miyai K, Onishi T, *et al.* Transient hypothyroidism after delivery in autoimmune thyroiditis. *J Clin Endocrinol Metab* 1976; 42:296–301.

89. Pop VJM, de Rooy HAM, Vader HL, *et al.* Microsomal antibodies during gestation in relation to postpartum thyroid dysfunction and depression. *Acta Endocrinol* 1993;129:26–30.
90. Amino N, Mori H, Iwatani Y, *et al.* High prevalence of transient postpartum thyrotoxicosis and hypothyroidism *N Engl J Med* 1982;306:849–52.
91. Othman S, Phillips DIW, Parkes AB, *et al.* A long-term follow-up of postpartum thyroiditis. *Clin Endocrinol* 1990;32:559–64.
92. Amino N, Kuro R, Tanizawa O, *et al.* Changes of serum antithyroid antibodies during and after pregnancy in autoimmune thyroid diseases. *Clin Exp Immunol* 1978;31:30–7.
93. Jansson R, Bernander S, Karlsson A, *et al.* Autoimmune thyroid dysfunction in the postpartum period. *J Clin Endocrinol Metab* 1984;58:681–7.
94. Fein H, Goldman J, Weintraub B. Postpartum lymphocytic thyroiditis in American women: A spectrum of thyroid dysfunction. *Am J Obstet Gynecol* 1980;138:504–10.
95. Cuestas RA, Lindall A, Engel RR. Low thyroid hormones and RDS of the newborn: Studies on cord blood. *N Engl J Med* 1976;295: 297–302.
96. Mashiach S, Barkai J, Sack J, *et al.* The effect of intraamniotic thyroxine administration on fetal lung maturity in man. *J Perinat Med* 1979;7:161–70.
97. Romaguera J, Raminez M, Adamsons K. Intraamniotic thyroxine to accelerate fetal maturation. *Semin Perinatol* 1993;17:260–6.
98. Rooney S, Marino P, Gobran L, *et al.* Thyrotropin-releasing hormone increases the amount of surfactant in lung lavage from fetal rabbits. *Pediatr Res* 1979;13:623–5.
99. Ballard PL. Hormonal control of lung maturation. *Balliere's Clin Endocrinol Metab* 1989;3:723–53.
100. Umans JG, Umans HR, Szeto HH. Effects of thyrotropin releasing hormone in the fetal lamb. *Am J Obstet Gynecol* 1986;155:1266–71.
101. Ballard PL, Ballard RA, Creasy RK, *et al.* Plasma thyroid hormones and prolactin in premature infants and their mothers after prenatal treatment with thyrotropin releasing hormone. *Pediatr Res* 1992;32:673–8.
102. de Zegher F, Spitz B, Devlieger H. Prenatal treatment with thyrotropin releasing hormone to prevent neonatal respiratory distress. *Arch Dis Child* 1992;67:450–4.
103. Liggins GC. Thyrotropin releasing hormone (TRH) and lung maturation. *Reprod Fertil Dev* 1995;7:443–50.
104. ACTOBAT Study Group. Australian collaborative trial of antenatal thyrotropin-releasing hormone (ACTOBAT) for prevention of neonatal respiratory disease. *Lancet* 1995;345:877–82.
105. Knight DB, Liggins GC, Wealthall SR. A randomised controlled trial of antepartum thyrotropin releasing hormone and betamethasone in the prevention of respiratory disease in preterm infants. *Am J Obstet Gynecol* 1994;171:11–16.
106. Ballard RA, Ballard PL, Creasy RK, *et al.* Respiratory disease in very low birthweight infants after prenatal thyrotropin releasing hormone and glucocorticoid. *Lancet* 1992;339:510–15.
107. Jikihara H, Sawada Y, Imai S, *et al.* Maternal administration of thyrotropin releasing hormone for prevention of neonatal respiratory distress syndrome. *Proceedings of the Sixth Congress of the Federation of the Asia–Oceania Perinatal Societies*, Perth, Western Australia, May 1990:Abstr. 87.
108. Morales WJ, O'Brien WF, Angel JL, *et al.* Fetal lung maturation: the combined use of corticosteroids and thyrotropin releasing hormone. *Obstet Gynecol* 1989;73:111–16.
109. Ceriani JM, Fustinana C, Althabe F, *et al.* Controlled trial of prenatal betamethasone (B) plus TRH for prevention of respiratory distress syndrome (RDS) in preterm infants. *Pediatr Res* 1992; 32:738:A9.
110. Crowther CA, Grant AM. Antenatal thyrotropin-releasing hormone (TRH) prior to preterm delivery. *Cochrane Pregnancy and Childbirth Database*, 1995:Review 04749.

198 Management of severe pre-eclampsia and eclampsia

C. Sen

Introduction

Hypertension is a common problem occurring in around 12–15% of all pregnancies.[1] It remains one of the major causes of maternal mortality.[2] Because of the difficulty in deciding who has a problem and who does not, obstetricians often admit a patient to hospital for closer observation. This approach can cause much inconvenience to the patient and her family. In-patient management may vary between different hospitals but the cornerstone is hospitalization in order to maintain close monitoring.

The outcome of pre-eclampsia changes depends on severity. Maternal and perinatal mortality and morbidity in the hospitalized case with mild pre-eclampsia are extremely low and approach those of normotensive pregnancies. In contrast, in the case of severe pre-eclampsia, maternal and perinatal mortality is very high. Sibai and colleagues[3] reported that the corrected perinatal mortality rate in severe pre-eclampsia is 135 in 1000. In this study, the perinatal survival rate was zero in those cases up to 28 weeks' gestation, but rose to 100% after 36 weeks' gestation, especially in cases of pre-eclampsia with hemolysis, elevated liver enzymes and low platelet (HELLP) syndrome when the perinatal mortality ranged from 77 to 600 per 1000 and maternal mortality from 0% to 24%. Based on this experience, prompt delivery was recommended after stabilizing the maternal condition.[4,5]

Doppler studies on uterine artery and fibronectin measurements in maternal blood have been predictive methods for pre-eclampsia with 77% and 90% sensitivity, respectively.[6,7] In these high-risk patients low-dose aspirin can be given as a prophylaxis, but recent studies have shown that there is no apparent beneficial effect on clinical outcome.[8,9] At the present time there is no effective method that can prevent the complications of pre-eclampsia, and clinical management of severe cases is becoming an important issue.

The most important therapy for severe pre-eclampsia and eclampsia is delivery of the fetus and placenta and there is universal agreement that all such patients should be delivered at or after 32–34 weeks' gestation and, in cases of severe pre-eclampsia, delivery has to be taken into account between 28 and 32 weeks' gestation, depending on the situation. At this stage, the neonatal mortality rate is not very high depending on the ability and experience of the neonatal intensive care unit.[10] Timing the delivery in cases of severe pre-eclampsia at a gestational age of less than 28 weeks is a difficult decision for the mother and obstetrician to make. Aggressive management with immediate delivery will result in extremely high neonatal mortality and morbidity. In contrast, attempts to prolong pregnancy may result in fetal demise and high maternal morbidity and mortality. The perinatal survival rate is poor when the disease develops before 24 weeks' gestation (2%); however, after that stage the survival rate is good (50%).[11]

In a study with 252 cases of hypertension in pregnancy, the maternal mortality rate was 0.4% (eclamptic case with cesarean section). Overall perinatal mortality in those cases with hypertension in pregnancy was 182/1000, which is 2.5-fold higher compared to the perinatal mortality at this hospital.[12] In those cases of severe pre-eclampsia, the perinatal mortality was about 300/1000. Most of the cases had not received any antenatal care nor were referred patients who had received conservative management with antihypertensive therapy over a long period. In this study, the perinatal mortality was 116/1000 in those cases after 32 weeks' gestation and 686/1000 in those of less than 32 weeks' gestation. The rate of intrauterine growth retardation (IUGR) in patients with severe pre-eclampsia was 92.3% for those cases below 32 weeks' gestation and 40% in those cases above 32 weeks' gestation. The average rate of IUGR was 54.2% in the severe pre-eclamptic cases. For this reason maximum attention should be paid to the fetus [e.g. non-stress test (NST), Doppler assessment]. In addition, there was no beneficial effect of cesarean delivery on perinatal mortality in case of pre-eclampsia and eclampsia.

Maternal mortality in the case of eclampsia is usually associated with mismanaged or complicated cases. Maternal morbidity is greater in multigravidae than in primigravidae. This difference may be due to a higher incidence of chronic hypertension and underlying renal disease in multigravidae. The complication rate is also higher in patients who have had no antenatal care. The fetus of the eclamptic woman is particularly at risk from abruptio placentae, preterm delivery, IUGR and fetal distress during seizure. In a study from Turkey,[13] the rate of maternal mortality in cases of hypertension in pregnancy varied in the different regions, while the rate of maternal mortality was about 0.52–1.20% in urban areas; in the rural areas, where antenatal care is not satisfactory, the perinatal mortality was 2.90–5.20%.

The clinical course of patients with severe pre-eclampsia may be associated with progressive deterioration in maternal and fetal condition. In the case of severe pre-eclampsia, both the mother and the fetus are at risk for morbidity and mortality. Some clinical signs and symptoms, such as hypertension, proteinuria, edema or other parameters, might indicate the level of pathophysiology in relation to the severity of the disease and endothelial cell damage. With regard to endothelial cell damage and vascular pathology, the risk of vascular damage for the mother would appear to increase after the diastolic blood pressure had reached 110 mmHg, whereas an increased risk to the baby has been shown to correlate with a diastolic blood pressure above 95 mmHg.[14] There is universal agreement that all such patients should be delivered at or after 32–34 weeks' gestation or if there is any evidence of premature rupture of membranes, IUGR, oligohydramnios or fetal and/or maternal distress, at any gestational age. However, there is disagreement on the management of patients with severe pre-eclampsia before 32 weeks' gestation. Some authors consider delivery as a definitive therapy for all patients with severe pre-eclampsia regardless of gestational age; others recommend expectant management.[3,15] In the literature it is not always possible to compare the studies because their design differs in definition, clinical decision and follow-up and studies are retrospective. There is also no agreement on the classification of hypertension in pregnancy. The classifications of the American College of Obstetricians and Gynecologists and the International Society for the Study of Hypertension in Pregnancy are mostly used, but both are not clinically well applicable. The outcome of severe pre-eclamptic cases differs depending on definition and clinical management. If the pathology is severe enough in the case of severe pre-eclampsia, the maternal morbidity and mortality are very high. In some cases with severe pre-eclampsia where the blood pressure is high but the other clinical parameters are not severe, the pathophysiology may not be severe enough to put the mother at risk of severe morbidity or mortality. We need to differentiate therefore between which patient should have expectant management and induction of labor and which criteria we should apply to make a decision for delivery in the case of expectant management with severe pre-eclampsia.

Expectant management in severe pre-eclampsia

There is no controversy on the management of the cases with chronic hypertension, gestational hypertension and mild pre-eclampsia at any gestational age. These cases consist of a mild group and maternal–perinatal mortality and morbidity (mild pre-eclampsia has high perinatal morbidity) are not high and patients are delivered at term. In severe cases, because the maternal–perinatal morbidity and mortality are very high, delivery should be after 32 weeks' gestation, when fetal lung maturity is complete. However, there is controversy in the literature on management of cases with severe pre-eclampsia at a gestational age of less than 32 weeks because of high perinatal mortality. While delivery has long been felt to be the best therapeutic regimen for the mother with severe pre-eclampsia, in certain cases remote from term it may not be the best for the fetus. As methods for monitoring both maternal and fetal well-being have been improved, expectant management in an attempt to prolong gestation is an alternative option.

When the extent of the maternal antenatal management is compared with the costs of neonatal intensive care, it is obvious that intensive care for prolonged periods of time is more complicated and also therefore more costly. For developing countries with limited resources available for sophisticated treatment, expectant management is recommended providing that the level of care is adequate to detect any maternal complications early. The expectant management can be beneficial to the fetus without exposing the mother to severe risks.

In a study,[16] a randomized clinical trial was conducted in which patients with severe pre-eclampsia between 26 and 36 weeks' gestation were assigned to be treated with either nifedipine or hydralazine. The authors found better control of blood pressure and a lower incidence of fetal distress in the group managed with nifedipine. In addition, the group managed with nifedipine had a better perinatal outcome than those receiving hydralazine. They concluded that nifedipine is a safe and effective drug in the management of patients with severe pre-eclampsia remote from term.

Odendaal and colleagues[17] described the results of conservative management in 129 patients with severe pre-eclampsia before 34 weeks' gestation. The patients were managed with bed rest, antihypertensive therapy and frequent evaluation of maternal and fetal well-being. These pregnancies were prolonged for an average of 11 days. The overall perinatal mortality was 326/1000.

Moderate and severe pre-eclampsia

Some authors suggest that severe pre-eclampsia cases at a gestational age of between 26 and 32 weeks can be managed conservatively in a close follow-up at the hospital, but in the literature there is no clear definition of which case is suitable for expectant management.

In order to evaluate and properly manage the cases with hypertension in pregnancy we should identify which case is at high risk. In our practice we classify cases with hypertension in pregnancy as follows:

(1) Chronic hypertension;
(2) Gestational hypertension (hypertension in pregnancy without proteinuria);
(3) Mild pre-eclampsia (hypertension < 10 mmHg diastolic pressure and proteinuria > 0.5 g/l and < 5 g/l);
(4) Moderate pre-eclampsia (hypertension ≥ 10 mmHg diastolic pressure and proteinuria < 5 g/l, no other clinical/laboratory signs for severity);
(5) Severe pre-eclampsia (hypertension ≥110 mmHg and/or proteinuria > 5 g/l, and/or clinical/laboratory sign for severity such as oliguria, scotomata, headache, confusion, epigastric pain, retinal hemorrhage, pulmonary edema, HELLP syndrome) or a moderate pre-eclampsia that cannot be controlled by antihypertensive therapy;
(6) Superimposed pre-eclampsia and
(7) Eclampsia.

The cases with moderate pre-eclampsia, as classified above, can be managed with expectant management. At this stage of the pathophysiology the blood supply from mother to the placenta and hence to the fetus can be achieved by increased blood pressure. The pathophysiology is not generally systemic and the organ systems of the mother are not compromised. There is no increased risk for the mother but fetal morbidity and mortality are very high. The method of assessment for the fetus at risk will be discussed later (NST, Doppler and fetal blood sampling). Another important point is that the expectantly managed pregnant woman should be hospitalized and followed intensively for the probability of a severe form of pre-eclampsia that can cause severe maternal morbidity and mortality.

For this purpose the patients are hospitalized and given special care in the hospital. For moderate pre-eclampsia, proteinuria should not be higher than 5 g/l with no other clinical/laboratory sign for severity. After bed rest in the hospital, the diastolic blood pressure might be decreased to less than 110 mmHg without any medication. If not, an antihypertensive drug such as nifedipine can be given to keep the diastolic pressure level between 90 and 100 mmHg. If the patient is treated by antihypertensive therapy, it may cause relatively decreased blood flow in the uterine artery and fetal hypoxia. Also, fetal demise should be expected if the blood pressure is prominently decreased. We should remember that in both moderate and severe cases, perinatal morbidity such as IUGR (45.8%) is higher than in mild cases (10.2%).[12] The evidence of IUGR and oligohydramnios is an indication for induction of labor in the case of moderate pre-eclampsia.

If any of the following signs is becoming evident, the case should be categorized as severe pre-eclampsia and labor should be induced: diastolic pressure more than 110 mmHg in spite of antihypertensive therapy, increase in proteinuria to 5 g/l or more, any clinical/laboratory sign for severity during follow-up in the hospital. In that case, delivery should be the recommended approach to the patient because of high maternal morbidity and mortality as well as high perinatal mortality.

The aim of expectant management for cases with moderate pre-eclampsia is to gain more time for the fetus to mature. It is possible to prolong the pregnancy by approximately 7–10 days but usually no longer. It should be expected that the patient with expectant management may move to the severe category at any time. Daily NST and Doppler assessment should be carried out. Biochemical parameters for severe pre-eclampsia (uric acid, platelets, Hb, bilirubin, transaminases and fundoscopic evaluation) should be checked at least every other day. Close clinical follow-up and blood pressure monitoring at least four times a day are essential clinical workup. These moderate cases should be managed by a person who has experience of these cases, preferably at a tertiary center.

Fetal surveillance

The NST is a useful test, and has 88% specificity and 50% sensitivity for fetal well-being.[18,19] The oxytocin challenge test (OCT) has no extra value compared to the NST and also can be hazardous. Doppler study and NST are both more accurate in IUGR and oligohydramnios cases. In a study[20,21] of IUGR cases with oligohydramnios, 90% of the cases with abnormal Doppler findings were acidemic. In cases of oligohydramnios without IUGR with normal findings, both Doppler and NST were 20% acidemic. We should remember that in the case of IUGR, the risk for fetal hypoxemia is very high and delivery is mandatory. In the case of oligohydramnios there is a high risk of fetal hypoxemia, which remains at 20%. Fetal blood sampling may help to rule out the risk of fetal hypoxia or acidemia in a tertiary center. Fetal biophysical profile (FBP) may also help in high-risk cases but is time-consuming. Meanwhile the combination of NST and amniotic fluid volume measurement (AFV) is a reliable and time-saving method with similar sensitivity and specificity rates as FBP.[22] In any category of pre-eclampsia, any case with IUGR and oligohydramnios should be delivered. Some cases with moderate pre-eclampsia and borderline IUGR without oligohydramnios at a gestational age of less than 28 weeks, if NST and Doppler findings are normal, can be managed conservatively. Recently, it has been shown[23] that monitoring of the fetal venous circulation represents a more accurate method of determining the optimum time of delivery and also can predict fetal compromise earlier than antenatal cardiotocography. Another important factor to be taken into consideration in moderate pre-eclampsia managed expectantly is the risk of abruptio placentae and eclampsia.

Antihypertensive therapy in moderate/severe pre-eclampsia

In severe pre-eclampsia, a blood pressure more than 180/110 mmHg, mainly a diastolic pressure of more than 110 mmHg, is a risk factor for intracerebral bleeding, tissue hypoxia and abruptio placentae, which can cause maternal or fetal morbidity and mortality. In this situation, to control the blood pressure, antihypertensive medications should be given to the mother until delivery.

Pre-eclampsia might be better explained and defined as a platelet/endothelial cell disorder rather than a primary hypertensive disease. For that reason using antihypertensive drugs is not the best treatment for the disease. The clinical manifestations of moderate or severe pre-eclampsia are consistent with a systemic disorder in which severe hypertension is only one aspect of the pathophysiology. Patients presenting with such multiorgan disease are often both a diagnostic and a therapeutic challenge. For that reason treating the mother by antihypertensive medications should not be the main therapeutic approach. The control of hypertension may prevent some complications such as intracerebral hemorrhage and cardiac failure in which severe proteinuria and other compromised systemic organ functions are not evident. The aim of antihypertensive therapy in the case of moderate pre-eclampsia at less than 32 weeks' gestation is to gain more time and to reduce the risk of respiratory distress syndrome. If there is IUGR and oligohydramnios, the fetus is probably at risk as well as the mother. For that reason there is no indication for using antihypertensive therapy and in that situation the best option is delivery at any gestational age.

Different types of antihypertensive agents have been used for the long- or short-term treatment of hypertension in pregnancy.[24] Methyldopa is one of the antihypertensive agents whose long-term safety for both the mother and the fetus has been adequately assessed. It reduces systemic vascular resistance without significant physiological changes in heart or cardiac output, while renal blood flow is maintained. Plasma half-life and also peak plasma levels after oral administration are approximately 2 h. However, decrease in arterial pressure is maximal about 4–8 h after an oral dose of methyldopa. The usual dose is 1–2 g/day given in four divided doses although sometimes 4 g/day is needed.

Clonidine is a potent a_2 receptor to central stimulator and has some side effects such as sedation, dry mouth and rebound hypertension following an abrupt discontinuation. The usual oral dose is 0.1–0.3 mg/day given in two divided doses and up to a maximum of 1.2 mg/day as needed. Horvath and coworkers[25] studied this drug and concluded that clonidine was a safe and effective antihypertensive agent.

Sodium nitroprusside is a potent arterial and venous dilator, which is used extensively in the treatment of cases with malignant hypertension in non-pregnant patients. It has a rapid onset and a short duration of action. This agent should be used only in extreme emergencies in pregnancy because of the potential risks of fetal cyanide poisoning and metabolic acidosis.[26]

β-Blockers (propanolol, metropolol and atenolol) have different hemodynamic effects that depend on their receptor selectivity. The type of action of β-blockers is competitive inhibition of catecholamines at β_1 (heart) and β_2 (peripheral circulation, bronchi and uterus) adrenoreceptors. Side effects are bronchial spasm, hypoglycemia, cold extremities and a disturbance in lipid metabolism, neonatal bradycardia, neonatal hyperglycemia, fetal growth retardation and neonatal respiratory depression.[27] Because of the concern regarding side effects such as fetal growth retardation, the use of this drug should be limited.

Labetalol is a combined α- and β-adrenoreceptor blocker. The additional property of α-blockade induces vasodilatation improving the primary vasospasm in this disorder. The usual dose is 33 mg daily up to 2400 mg/day as required. It appears to be safe like methyldopa for short-term use in the third trimester, but it has an increased incidence of fetal growth retardation in the case of long-term use.[28]

Diuretics decrease the blood pressure by decreasing the intravascular volume and cardiac output. The most commonly used diuretics of the non-pregnant hypertensives are the thiazide diuretics. However, the use of diuretics in case of pre-eclampsia should be restricted to the patients whose pregnancy is complicated by pulmonary edema or excessive fluid retention or to certain patients with renal disease.

Hydralazine has a direct relaxation effect on arterial smooth muscle and is associated with stimulation of the sympathetic nervous system resulting in an increased heart rate and contractility. Maternal side effects are headache, flushing, palpitations, nausea and vomiting. Drug-induced lupus syndrome is generally observed only after long-term oral use. Uteroplacental blood flow may decrease following parenteral administration, which can cause fetal distress. Hydralazine may accumulate after continuous intravenous infusion resulting in hypertension and therefore it should be administered in small intravenous amounts of 5–10 g at intervals because the onset of the effect may be delayed for 15–20 min.

Comparative trials between hydralazine, nifedipine and labetalol have not shown one agent to be superior in the acute management of severe hypertension.[16,28,29] Calcium channel blockers (such as nifedipine, nicardipine, isradipine, nimodipine and verapamil) are potent antihypertensive agents that depress the myogenic tone of precapillary arterioles. The most frequent side effects associated with these drugs are secondary to the acute vasodilatation.

Nicardipine has been studied[30] and demonstrated to reduce maternal blood pressure without increasing neonatal morbidity. Additionally, Doppler flow studies of the umbilical artery were not significantly affected by nicardipine therapy. Long-term therapy was well tolerated by the mother with no adverse fetal/neonatal side effects.

Intravenous isradipine studied by Ingemarsson and associates[31] was found to normalize blood pressure 15–30 min after injection. There was no change in Doppler velocimetry of the umbilical arteries. Wide-Swensson and coworkers[32] performed a randomized placebo-controlled trial of a slow-release form of isradipine in women with gestational hypertension. Again, they demonstrated the effect of isradipine on decreasing maternal blood pressure without demonstrating an effect on vascular flow.

Belfort and colleagues[33] studied the hemodynamic effects of verapamil administration in nine women with proteinuric hypertension. These patients had an intravenous infusion of verapamil, after plasma volume expansion with dextran-70, until a 20% reduction in mean arterial pressure was obtained. They concluded that verapamil is a good antihypertensive agent to be used in hypertension in pregnancy but deemed that caution was indicated when it was used in combination with magnesium sulfate.

Nifedipine was found to be extremely effective in the acute treatment of severe hypertension in pregnancy. In patients treated with daily nifedipine and serially followed by maternal blood pressure and fetal Doppler studies, it was demonstrated that a significant decrease occurred in maternal blood pressure without any change in resistance index in the umbilical and uterine arteries or in the fetal aorta. The Apgar scores and arterial blood gases were not consistent with fetal compromise. In a retrospective study, Sibai and colleagues[34] studied the effect of nifedipine on 200 women between 26 and 36 weeks' gestation. Nifedipine was associated with significantly lower blood pressure and good perinatal outcome.

Many of the calcium channel blocker agents have been found to inhibit platelet aggregation, both *in vivo* and *in vitro*. Rubin and colleagues[35] studied 10 women with proteinuric gestational hypertension and noted a statistically significant increase in the mean platelet count, which they attributed to nifedipine. They concluded that nifedipine reversed thrombocytopenia and controlled blood pressure in patients with gestational hypertension.

In conclusion, calcium channel blockers such as nifedipine have been used for many years in pregnant women with good effect. In many cases, they are effective and safe for the mother and the fetus when used carefully and are inexpensive. Additional benefits may be derived from vasodilator and antiaggregational effects. In the acute situation, calcium channel blockers such as nifedipine can be given sublingually 10 mg two or three times at 15-min intervals. Blood pressure decreases slowly to an appropriate level and then is maintained with 10 mg three or four times a day at 6–8-h intervals. The onset of action occurs within 10 min of administration and the peak action occurs after 30 min, with the blood pressure control maintained for approximately 4 h. It should be remembered that the daily maximum dose should not exceed 120 mg/day because of maternal side effects. Mild side effects and a short half-life, plus a rapid but not very deep response, make this drug preferable to others. In moderate pre-eclampsia there is no need to add any alternative antihypertensive agent. In this situation the case should be classified as severe pre-eclampsia and be delivered after stabilization of the mother.

Maternal volume expansion

The clinical consequences of vasodilatation without volume expansion include precipitous falls in blood pressure as well as the onset of peripheral ischemia, most clearly evident as a fall in renal output and the development of fetal distress.[36] Preloading the patient prior to vasodilatation is known to prevent these complications and also facilitates subsequent vasodilatation.

Fluid therapy in pre-eclampsia has traditionally been monitored by the use of central venous pressure (CVP) lines, but CVP readings, while acting as a good index of overall intravascular volume, do not give any indication of the left ventricular response to acute volume expansion. Central monitoring, to be meaningful, requires right heart catheterization in order to measure pulmonary capillary wedge pressure. In practice, in these severe cases, patients should never be exposed to acute plasma volume expansion of more than 30 ml of fluid.

Eclampsia

Eclampsia is associated with multiple organ dysfunction. The question of whether or not eclampsia is a preventable complication is controversial. Campbell and coworkers[37] studied factors leading to the development of eclampsia in 66 women and concluded that convulsions were not preventable in 42% of the cases.

The first action should be to control convulsions. As a first line, 10 mg intravenous diazepam can be given as a bolus and then 3–4 mg of magnesium sulfate administered as a bolus. After convulsions have been abolished, the magnesium sulfate perfusion should be maintained at 1–1.5 g/h for at least 24 h. Arterial blood gas measurements, magnesium level in the blood and a chest radiograph should be obtained to ensure adequate maternal oxygenation and to avoid overperfusion of magnesium. Hypoxemia and acidemia should be corrected. Hydralazine or labetalol can be intravenously administered, or sublingual/oral calcium channel blockers can be used to control the blood pressure. Intensive care of the patient is necessary. Occasionally, it is not possible to control the convulsions. In that situation the woman should be cared for in the intensive care unit under the perfusion of sodium thiopental. The seizures can be prevented with this therapeutic approach.

In some cases, fetal bradycardia or signs of fetal distress can be seen during or just after seizures. In this situation, there is no hurry to perform immediate cesarean section. Because of maternal distress, the placental flow is not in the optimum condition and temporary fetoplacental insufficiency is present. After abolishing the seizures, maternal oxygenation and hemodynamic condition recover. At this stage, any sign of fetal distress disappears and fetal well-being returns. Immediate maternal oxygenation and control of seizures and blood pressure are significant steps for fetal well-being. Fetal heart rate usually returns to normal once convulsions cease. If the bradycardia persists or the uterus is hypertonic, placental abruption should be suspected. Following stabilization of maternal conditions, the next step should be delivery of the fetus. Induction of labor with oxytocin is often successful. The fetal heart rate and uterine activity must be closely monitored. Eclampsia is not an indication for cesarean section. Cesarean section solely for this indication should be avoided. In the case of seizure or just after convulsion, it can cause harmful effects on the maternal system and increase maternal morbidity and the heart rate.

Magnesium sulfate prophylaxis in severe pre-eclampsia

Considerable conflict exists regarding the need for seizure prophylaxis, the optimal anticonvulsant for this purpose and the type of hypertension in pregnancy that increases the patient's risk. The recommendations from the literature state that the essential management of pre-eclampsia includes preventing convulsions, which involves the use of parenteral magnesium sulfate.[38] Magnesium sulfate is the drug of choice in the United States, while it is less frequently used in other countries. Instead, standard anticonvulsants such as phenytoin, diazepam and phenobarbital are used frequently for the treatment of seizures. In Turkey, magnesium sulfate is the most preferred and used anticonvulsant for the treatment of convulsions and also for the prophylaxis of convulsions in the case of severe pre-eclampsia.[39]

Moodley and Moodley[40] addressed the necessity of anticonvulsant therapy in hypertension in pregnancy. They randomized 228 women with severe pre-eclampsia to receive magnesium sulfate with antihypertensive therapy vs. antihypertensive therapy alone. There was no significant difference in the number of convulsions, birth weight, Apgar score or maternal complications between these two groups. In 1993, Friedman and associates[41] performed a randomized clinical trial on the use of phenytoin vs. magnesium sulfate in 105 patients with severe pre-eclampsia or eclampsia. They found that patients receiving phenytoin had a more rapid cervical dilatation and a decreased incidence of postpartum anemia. There were no seizures in either group after initiation of therapy.

In 1995 the Eclampsia Trial Collaborative Group published data[42] on the anticonvulsant medication for the treatment of eclampsia and compared the efficacy of magnesium sulfate, phenytoin and diazepam with respect to reduction of seizures in women with eclampsia. They concluded that magnesium sulfate is a more effective agent than either of the other two medications in the prevention of further seizures, as well as being equally safe. The use of magnesium sulfate for the prevention of eclamptic seizures is not entirely without risk. Magnesium toxicity can culminate in cardio-respiratory arrest if it is not prevented or treated immediately. In addition, some studies have reported low Apgar scores, respiratory depression and hyperflexia in preterm neonates of mothers receiving magnesium sulfate.[43]

Recently, Odendaal and Hall[44] performed a study on maternal and perinatal outcomes by using prophylactic administration of magnesium sulfate to patients with early severe pre-eclampsia. They concluded that the prophylactic use of magnesium sulfate in patients with severe pre-eclampsia, especially when they are not in labor, is questionable, and that, although the use of magnesium sulfate did not cause severe morbidity, it is a potentially harmful drug that should be reserved for specific indications.

Cases with severe pre-eclampsia or eclampsia that present with cerebral or visual disturbances, right quadrant abdominal pain, severe headache, unconsciousness, acute exacerbation in blood pressure or uncontrolled blood pressure should have prophylatic therapy because of high seizure risk. Also, in the case of severe pre-eclampsia or eclampsia during labor or on the first day of the postpartum period, prophylactic therapy should be initiated. This prophylactic therapy can be administered as 3–4 g magnesium sulfate intravenously given as a bolus, with a caution about side effects, and then perfused 1.5 g/h for 24 h. Under these circumstances there is no evidence or reason for continuing prophylactic therapy for more than 24 h.

Intrapartum and postpartum management

Pre-eclampsia or eclampsia alone should not be an indication for cesarean section. All women with severe pre-eclampsia should receive anticonvulsant prophylaxis during labor or postpartum. In our institute, magnesium sulfate is administered by controlled intravenous infusion with a loading dose of 3 or 4 g over 20 min, followed by a maintenance dose of 1.5 g/h. The infusion is continued throughout labor and delivery, and at least 12 h postpartum. All patients should be monitored very closely, with special attention given to fluid intake and output. Patients with severe pre-eclampsia and eclampsia, particularly uncontrolled, or those remote from term and those with the HELLP syndrome are at increased risk for the development of pulmonary edema and acute renal failure.[4]

REFERENCES

1. Cunningham FG, Lindheimer MD. Hypertension in pregnancy. *N Engl Med J* 1992;326:927–32.
2. Redman CWG. Eclampsia still kills. *Br Med J* 1988;296:1209–10.
3. Sibai BM, Spinnato JA, Watson DL, *et al.* Pregnancy outcome in 303 cases with severe preeclampsia. *Obstet Gynecol* 1984;64: 319–23.
4. Sibai BM, Taslimi MM, el Nazer A, *et al.* Maternal–perinatal outcome associated with the syndrome of hemolysis, elevated liver enzymes, and low platelet in severe preeclampsia. *Am J Obstet Gynecol* 1986;155:501–4.
5. Lopez-Llera M, Linares GR, Horta JL. Maternal mortality rates in eclampsia. *Am J Obstet Gynecol* 1976;124:149–55.
6. Harrington K, Cooper D, Lees C, *et al.* Doppler ultrasound of the uterine arteries: The importance of bilateral notching in the prediction of preeclampsia, placental abruption or delivery of a small-for-gestational-age baby. *Ultrasound Obstet Gynecol* 1966;7:182–8.
7. Sen C, Madazli R, Kavuzlu C, *et al.* The value of antithrombin-III and fibronectin in hypertensive disorders of pregnancy. *J Perinat Med* 1994;22:29–38.
8. CLASP (Collaborate Low-Dose Aspirin Study in Pregnancy). A randomized trial of low dose aspirin for the prevention and treatment of preeclampsia among 9384 pregnant women. *Lancet* 1994; 343:619–29.
9. Italian study of aspirin in pregnancy. Low-dose aspirin in prevention and treatment of intrauterine growth retardation and pregnancy induced hypertension. *Lancet* 1993;341:753–4.
10. Pattinson RC, Odendaal HJ, Dutoit R. Conservative management of severe proteinuric hypertension before 28 weeks' gestation. *S Afr Med J* 1988;73:516–19.
11. Sibai BM, Akl S, Fairlie F, *et al.* A protocol for managing severe preeclampsia in the second trimester. *Am J Obstet Gynecol* 1990; 163:733–5.
12. Sen C, Karagozlu F, Ocak V. Clinical management of hypertension in pregnancy – Gebelik ve Hipertansiuonda klinik yonetim (in Turkish). *J Perinatol* 1993;1:37–44.
13. Erden AC, Yayla M. Maternal–fetal mortality and morbidity in preeclampsia and eclampsia (in Turkish). *J Perinatol* 1993;1:24–30.
14. Goldby FS, Beilin LJ. Relationship between arterial pressure and the permeability of arterioles to carbon particles in acute hypertension. *Cardiovasc Res* 1972;6:384–8.
15. Odendaal HJ, Pattinson RC, Bam R. Aggressive or expectant management for patients with severe preeclampsia between 28–34. weeks' gestation: A randomized controlled trial. *Obstet Gynecol* 1990;76:1070–3.
16. Fenakel K, Fenakel E, Appleman Z, *et al.* Nifedipine in the treatment of severe preeclampsia. *Obstet Gynecol* 1991;77:331–4.
17. Odendaal HJ, Pattinson RC, Dutoit RD. Fetal and neonatal outcome in patients with severe preeclampsia before 34 weeks. *S Afr Med J* 1987;71:555–8.
18. Ocak V, Sen C, Demirkiran F, *et al.* FHR monitoring and perinatal mortality in high-risk pregnancies. *Eur J Obstet Gynecol Reprod Biol* 1992;44:59–63.
19. Ocak V, Demirkiran F, Sen C, *et al.* The predictive value of fetal heart rate monitoring: retrospective analysis of 2165 high-risk pregnancies. *Eur J Obstet Gynecol Reprod Biol* 1992;44:53–8.
20. Sen C. Oligohydramnios and its management. Presented at the *XII International Congress – The Fetus as a Patient*, Grado, Italy, May 1996.
21. Sen C, Uludag S, Madazli R, *et al.* Doppler flow measurements, NST and fetal blood sampling in the prediction of fetal acidaemia. *Prenat Neonat Med* 1996;1(Suppl 1):9.
22. Ocak V, Sen C, Madazli R. Is fetal biophysical profile with all parameters needed? *Matern Fetal Invest* 1994;4:37–41.
23. Hecker K, Hackeloer BJ. Cardiotocogram compared to Doppler investigation of the fetal circulation in the premature growth-retarded fetus: Longitudinal observations. *Ultrasound Obstet Gynecol* 1997;9:152–61.
24. Cockburn J, Moar VA, Ounsted NM, *et al.* Final report of the study on hypertension during pregnancy: The effects of specific treatment on the growth and development of the children. *Lancet* 1982;1:647–9.
25. Horvath JS, Phippard A, Korda A, *et al.* Clonidine-hydrochloride: A safe and effective antihypertensive agent in pregnancy. *Obstet Gynecol* 1985;66:634–8.
26. Naulty JN, Cefalo RJ, Lewis PE. Fetal toxicity of nitroprusside in the pregnant ewe. *Am J Obstet Gynecol* 1981;139:708–11.
27. Van Zwieten PA, Timmermans PB. MVM: Differential pharmacological properties of beta adrenoreceptor blocking drugs. *J Cardiovasc Pharmacol* 1983;5(Suppl):55–7.
28. Blouin PF, Breart GL, Maillard F, *et al.* Comparison of antihypertensive efficacy and perinatal safety of labetalol and methyldopa in the treatment of hypertension in pregnancy: A randomised controlled trial. *Br J Obstet Gynaecol* 1988;95:868–76.
29. Mabie WC, Gonzales AR, Sibai BM, *et al.* A comparative trial of labetalol and hydralazine in the acute management of severe hypertension complicating pregnancy. *Obstet Gynecol* 1987;70: 328–33.
30. Carbonne B, Jannet D, Touboul C, *et al:* Nicardipine treatment of hypertension during pregnancy. *Obstet Gynecol* 1993;81:908–14.
31. Ingermarsson I, Wide-Swensson D, Andersson KR, *et al.* Maternal and fetal cardiovascular changes after intravenous injection of isradipine to pregnant women. *Drugs* 1990;40:58–9.
32. Wide-Swensson DH, Ingermarsson I, Lunell NO, *et al.* Calcium channel blockade (isradipine) in the treatment of hypertension in pregnancy: A randomized placebo-controlled study. *Am J Obstet Gynecol* 1995;173:872–8.
33. Belfort MA, Anthony J, Buccimazza A, *et al.* Hemodynamic changes associated with intravenous infusion of calcium antagonist verapamil in the treatment of severe gestational proteinuric hypertension. *Obstet Gynecol* 1990;75:970–4.
34. Sibai BM, Barton JR, Akl S, *et al.* A randomized prospective comparison of nifedipine and bed rest versus bed rest alone in the management of preeclampsia remote from term. *Am J Obstet Gynecol* 1992;167:879–84.
35. Rubin PC, Butters L, McCabe R. Nifedipine and platelets in preeclampsia. *Am J Hypertens* 1988;1:175–7.
36. Belfort MA, Anthony J, Kirshon B. Respiratory function in severe gestational proteinuric hypertension: the effects of rapid volume expansion and subsequent vasodilatation with verapamil. *Br J Obstet Gynaecol* 1991;98:964–72.
37. Campbell DM, Templeton AA. Is eclampsia preventable. In Bonnar J, MacGillivary I, Symonds EM, eds. *Pregnancy Hypertension.* Baltimore: University Park Press, 1980;483–9.
38. American College of Obstetricians and Gynecologists. *Management of preeclampsia.* Technical Bulletin 91. Washington, DC: American College of Obstetricians and Gynecologists, 1986.

39. Madazli R, Sen C, Ocak V. Clinical management of eclampsia (Eklampside klinik yonetim) (in Turkish). *J Perinatol* 1993;1:45–9.
40. Moodley J, Moodley VV. Prophylactic anticonvulsant therapy in hypertensive crises of pregnancy – The need for a large, randomized trial. *Hypertens Preg* 1994;13:245–52.
41. Friedman SA, Lim KH, Baker CA, *et al.* Phenytoin versus magnesium sulphate in preeclampsia: A pilot study. *Am J Obstet Perinatol* 1993;10:233–8.
42. Eclampsia Trial Collaborative Group. Which anticonvulsant for women with eclampsia? Evidence from the Collaborative Eclampsia Trial. *Lancet* 1995;345:1455–63.
43. McGuiness GA, Weinstein MM, Cruikshank DP, *et al.* Effects of magnesium sulphate treatment on perinatal clacium metabolism. II. Neonatal responses. *Obstet Gynecol* 1980;56:595–600.
44. Odendaal HJ, Hall DR. Is magnesium sulphate prophylaxis really necessary in patients with severe preeclampsia? *J Matern Fetal Invest* 1996;6:14–8.

SECTION XX

The challenge facing developing countries

Section Editors: **J. J. Sciarra and A. Adra**

199 Maternal mortality in developing countries

J. A. Fortney, J. B. Smith and P. E. Bailey

Levels of maternal mortality and the public health discrepancy

Overall mortality in developing countries has declined rapidly during the last half of the 20th century. Much of this decline is attributable to nearly universal immunization against childhood diseases, public health measures such as improved water and sanitation, and some economic development allowing higher living standards.[1] Differences between rich and poor countries in expectation of life at birth have narrowed, although discrepancies in various public health indices remain.[2]

Maternal mortality has failed to keep up with this progress in public health. Maternal mortality ratios (MMRs) in developing countries are about 20-fold greater than in the developed world.[3] By contrast, infant mortality is only ninefold greater, and life expectancy at birth is 20% lower in developing countries than in developed countries (24% lower if China is excluded).[4]

Maternal mortality is fundamentally different from other public health challenges in that curative services are more important than preventive services and in that a package of interventions is needed to address it. About 80% of maternal deaths are attributable to five direct obstetric complications, which can, for the most part, be neither predicted nor prevented. They are hemorrhage, sepsis, hypertensive disorders of pregnancy, prolonged or obstructed labor, and unsafe abortion.

While it is generally true that direct obstetric complications are not predictable or preventable, some complications can be prevented some of the time. Recent studies have now provided good evidence that active management of the third stage of labor has the potential to prevent a significant proportion of postpartum hemorrhage (PPH), perhaps in the range of 40% if well and widely implemented.[5–7] Evidence to date, however, requires that deliveries take place in the presence of an attendant trained and equipped to practice active management of the third stage. Research regarding the use of uterotonics (especially misoprostol) with less skilled attendants is under development.[8] It is important to note that even if active management of the third stage of labor is fully and perfectly implemented, some PPH will still occur and will require treatment by skilled attendants in a facility equipped to provide such care.

While prevention of sepsis in domiciliary deliveries attended by traditional birth attendants (TBAs) has been disappointing,[9] sepsis is preventable when deliveries are supervised by skilled attendants properly trained and equipped.[10] Preventing sepsis in cesarean deliveries is eminently possible.[11] Evidence for the ability to prevent hypertensive diseases of pregnancy is not compelling at the present time, but may be accumulating.[12–14]

Complications of abortion, either spontaneous or induced, typically include sepsis and/or blood loss. In places with good access to care for these complications, abortion mortality is extremely low. In places where access to care for abortion complications is poor (for either resource or policy reasons), abortion complications can account for as much as 20% of maternal mortality.[15] Of course, abortion complications can be prevented by making safe abortion available and accessible; and the need for abortion can be reduced (but not eliminated) by affordable, acceptable, and accessible family planning programs.

While the direct obstetric complications themselves may not usually be preventable, death resulting from them can usually be prevented if appropriate medical care is available. As we shall see, this is a big 'if'.

Developing countries today

The countries with the highest MMR today are in Africa. (The sole exception to this is Afghanistan.) Table 199.1 shows MMRs estimated by UN agencies.[16] While the developing world as a whole has MMRs 22 times greater than the developed world, the range among individual countries is vastly greater. Some developed countries may go for long periods (i.e. more than 1 year) without any maternal death and therefore

Table 199.1 UN estimates of maternal mortality in 2000* (adapted from AbouZahr and Wardlaw[16])

Region	MMR*	Number of maternal deaths	Lifetime risk of maternal death (1 in)
World total	400	529,000	74
Developed regions	20	2,500	2800
Developing regions	440	527,000	61
Northern Africa	130	4,600	210
Sub-Saharan Africa	920	247,000	16
Eastern Asia	55	11,000	840
South Central Asia	520	207,000	46
South Eastern Asia	210	25,000	140
Western Asia	190	9,800	120
Latin America and the Caribbean	190	22,000	160
Oceania	240	530	83

*Maternal deaths per 100,000 live births

Table 199.2 Maternal mortality ratios in 1920 in developed countries (adapted from Woodbury RM. *Maternal Mortality*. Washington, DC: Children's Bureau Publications, No. 15, 1926; quoted in Loudon[17])

Europe		Other developed countries	
Country	MMR	Country	MMR
Denmark	235	Uruguay	338
Netherlands	242	Japan	353
Sweden (1918)	258	South Africa*	410
Norway (1919)	297	Australia	501
Finland	360	New Zealand	648
Italy	367	Chile	748
England and Wales	433	United States	799
Spain	501		
Germany (1919)	515		
Ireland	553		
Belgium	609		
Scotland	615		
France	664		

*Probably (but not so specified) whites only

have an MMR of 0 for that year (e.g. Iceland). Other countries (e.g. Afghanistan, Sierra Leone) have MMRs in excess of 2000 deaths per 100,000 live births. In many countries, national estimates may mask wide subnational variations in MMRs – especially in remote or geographically challenging areas where MMRs may be considerably higher than the national ratio.

Considering the absolute number of deaths rather than the MMRs, the magnitude of the problem becomes even more apparent. The number of deaths in Asia (combined) is approximately equal to those in Africa. This is because the generally lower MMRs in Asia are applied to a larger population base. Certain countries account for large numbers of maternal deaths. India, alone, accounts for 136,000 – a staggering quarter of all the world's maternal deaths. Nigeria is a distant second with 37,000, and Pakistan is third with 26,000. China, on the other hand, has 'only' 11,000 in spite of having a population more or less the same as India's.

Developed countries historically

Historically, the countries currently labeled as developed had MMRs not very different from the developing world today.[17] Table 199.2 shows MMRs from the early 20th century for 21 of today's developed countries. Given the level of sophistication with regard to measurement at that time, these numbers should be interpreted with caution, and experience tells us that they are probably underestimates. It should also be noted that some of the countries at the high end had some remote (and therefore difficult to reach) populations, but so did Norway and Finland.

Table 199.3 Decline in MMRs from 1920 to 1960 in the United States, England and Wales, and the Netherlands (adapted from Loudon[17])

	1920	1940	1960
United States	799	376	37
England and Wales	433	261	39
The Netherlands	242	235	37

High as these 1920s numbers are, some had already declined substantially. Loudon graphs the decline in several of these countries showing in Scandinavia, the Netherlands, Belgium, and Paris a sharp decline from around 1880 to around 1910. He attributes this to acceptance of new aseptic techniques during this period and, to a lesser extent, the emergence of anesthesia. In other countries (England and Wales, Scotland, Australia, New Zealand, and the United States), there was no comparable decline in 1880–1920.

Table 199.3 shows how rapidly three disparate countries converged during the first half of the last century. Again, readers should view the numbers as indicative rather than completely accurate.

Maternal mortality in the developed world began its rapid decline to current levels in the 1930s (Table 199.3) following the widespread introduction of new drugs (sulfa drugs in the late 1930s, then antibiotics in the mid-1940s[18]) for management of infections,[19] blood transfusion technologies,[20,21] and improved surgical techniques developed during World War II. Cesarean sections, for example, carried a high risk of dying before the availability of antibiotics and blood transfusion. There was a further decline in the 1960s and 1970s, though far less spectacular, as many countries both legalized abortion and introduced safer techniques of pregnancy termination. Probably, the increasing proportion of deliveries taking place in medical facilities also contributed to the decline in many (but not all) countries.

Developed countries today

Developed countries today account for 2500 deaths or 0.005% of the world's total. Their combined MMR is 20. A score of countries have MMRs in the single digits, including some well-resourced Middle Eastern ones. The United States and the United Kingdom, both countries with pockets of poverty and/or substantial immigrant populations, are in the midteens. Developed countries with higher MMRs are most likely to be located in Eastern Europe where access to high-quality care may be limited in some areas.

Issues in measuring maternal mortality

Three measures of maternal mortality are used.*

(a) *Maternal mortality ratio*: The MMR is the most commonly used measure. It is defined as the number of maternal deaths per 100,000 live births. (Unfortunately, many people still refer to this by its old name – maternal mortality rate, which means something else.) There are issues related to both the numerator and the denominator.

(1) *Numerator*: Should only direct obstetric deaths be included? What about indirect obstetric deaths, and non-obstetric deaths? The trend is to be more inclusive. One reason for this is that it is increasingly recognized that it is not always simple to determine whether the death is related to pregnancy. The most glaring example of this is deaths related to domestic violence, homicide, suicide, and accidents.[23] One author reports that 40% of maternal deaths in New York City are due to injury, mostly homicide and suicide.[24] Furthermore, it seems likely that pregnancy contributes to the likelihood of violence.[25]

(2) What time frame should be used – 42 days, 3 months, 12 months?[26] Again, the trend is to be more inclusive for several reasons. In developed countries, where extreme measures are sometimes taken, women may survive well beyond the 42-day limit only to eventually succumb to a direct obstetric complication (for example, kidney failure due to eclampsia). Postpartum depression may lead to suicide more than 3 months after delivery. The advantage of 12 months is that maternal mortality would then be equivalent to infant death (deaths to infants under 12 months due to any cause per 1000 live births). The disadvantage, of course, is that the ratio would be inflated with deaths unrelated to pregnancy or childbirth.

(3) *Denominator*: Some writers prefer using 10,000 or even 1000. Smaller denominators turn the low levels of MMR in developed countries into an awkward statistic – the mean is 2 per 10,000 live births or 0.2 per 1000. Some writers have argued that the denominator should include all pregnancies, not just live births. This is a matter of convenience. National statistical offices report live births reasonably accurately; stillbirths are reported less completely, and data

*Calculations may be found in Fortney.[22]

on abortions (whether spontaneous or induced) are invariably underreported.

(b) *Maternal mortality rate*: This is defined as the number of maternal deaths per 100,000 women of reproductive age (15–45 years). It is a measure of both obstetric risk and the frequency with which women are exposed to the risk. If you wish to measure the impact of family planning on maternal mortality, this is the measure to use.[22]

(c) *Lifetime risk*: This is the risk of dying in childbirth for a woman in a specific country and is stated as a 1 in *X* risk. For example, it was recently reported that a girl in Sudan is more likely to die in childbirth than to finish primary school. The likelihood that she will finish primary school is 1 in 100, while her lifetime risk of death in childbirth is 1 in 9.[27] This, too, is a measure of the average number of births combined with the risk of dying at each birth.[22]

Why measure?

Maternal mortality is measured either to assess the magnitude of the problem or to evaluate the impact of improved services. However, all methods of measurement have significant shortcomings or are costly to implement. Furthermore, one commonly used method (sisterhood) refers to a period of time beginning 10 years (or so) before the measurement is taken, which has implications for its current usefulness for policy makers. Because of its cost and its lack of precision, it is recommended to undertake measurements of maternal mortality only rarely, i.e. not more than once every 10 years.[28] Whichever method is used, it is important to calculate 95% confidence limits as these are typically quite wide. This is especially important in making comparisons as confidence limits may overlap even though point estimates seem quite different.

Types of measurement

There are several ways of measuring maternal mortality. These are discussed below in approximate order of their appearance over time.

Hospital death rate: This is defined as the number of maternal deaths divided by the number of obstetric patients admitted. While most hospitals calculate this, it is of value only to that hospital and reflects the mix of patients and their condition on admission as well as the quality of care they receive. Conceivably, a hospital's death rate could increase as the quality of care improves and more patients come from ever greater distances. The case fatality rate (obstetric deaths per 100 obstetric complications admitted) is a better measure of quality of care, but this too is affected by the condition of patients at admission. The more inaccessible† the area served by the health facility the less informative the hospital death rate could be.

Vital statistics: Even in countries where reporting of death is complete, maternal deaths are underestimated in vital statistics.[29–31] There are several reasons for this, including the skills of the physician signing the death certificate and that of the person assigning the code for cause of death. Vital statistics should not be used as a measure of maternal death.

RAMOS: RAMOS stands for reproductive age mortality survey, and was developed in the late 1970s. It consists of determining (usually by verbal autopsy[32] through interviews with family members and health care workers) the cause of death in women of reproductive age (15–45 years). This generates a percentage that can be attributed to each of the major causes of death ('proportional mortality'). In developing countries, maternal deaths are typically between 20% and 25% of all deaths during the reproductive life span, but can be much higher for the prime child-bearing years.[33] RAMOS studies have fallen into some disfavor because of challenges in locating all deaths to women of reproductive age (usually in the absence of systematic death reports), but one was done in 2002 in four provinces of Afghanistan.[34]

Sisterhood: The limitations of the methods described above led to the development, in the 1980s of a method of estimating maternal mortality by asking people (both men and women) how many sisters they have ever had, how many are still living, the age at death of those who died, and their cause of death.[35] There is now very wide experience with this method; it is used in the demographic and health surveys that are implemented in many developing countries on a continuing basis. The sisterhood method tends to consistently underestimate maternal mortality by about one-third.[28] There are several reasons for this built-in bias.[36] In spite of its limitations, this method is currently the best there is and will continue to be used until newer methods are developed and refined. The IMMPACT program at the University of Aberdeen‡ is currently developing methods to assess the effectiveness and cost-effectiveness of maternal mortality reduction intervention strategies.[37]

Modeling: The continuing difficulty in arriving at good – and not too expensive – estimates of maternal mortality led WHO, in the 1990s, to collaborate with scholars at the Johns Hopkins University School of Public Health to develop estimates by using a computer model. This method has been used successfully to estimate infant mortality.[38] The maternal mortality estimates are updated regularly by the UN agencies

† Inaccessibility includes distance, lack of transport, cost, cultural avoidance of medical facilities, and beliefs in causes of complications that are at odds with medical science.

‡ Funded by the Bill and Melinda Gates Foundation, the European Union, DfID (UK's Department for International Development), and United States Agency for International Development.

Table 199.4 The UN process indicators (from United Nations[38])

Process indicator	Definition
Availability of EmOC	Number of facilities that provide EmOC per 500,000 population
Percentage of all births in EmOC facilities	Percentage of all births in EmOC facilities
Met need	Proportion of women estimated to have complications who are treated in EmOC facilities
Cesarean deliveries as a percentage of all births	Cesarean deliveries as a percentage of all births
Case fatality rate	Proportion of women with obstetric complications admitted to a facility who die

* Emergency obstetric care.

using this model.[16] This method has the advantage that it uses secondary data, the collection of which is less time-consuming and costs less than collecting new data in the field.

Monitoring progress

Progress in reducing maternal mortality can be assessed either through the use of a direct indicator (i.e. the MMR) or through changes in proxy indicators that are known (or strongly believed) to have a strong and *direct* association with maternal mortality. Indicators such as education or the status of women are strongly associated with maternal mortality, but the relationship is indirect – better educated women are more likely to seek care *if it is available*. Countries with a relatively high status of women are more likely to make maternity care available.

It is important to recognize that whether a woman survives an obstetric complication depends on many factors. A failure in one part of the health system can lead to death even when all the other parts are functioning correctly. If the MMR is used as the measure of success or failure, the measure will not identify which element is lacking or has failed to improve. The use of a package of proxy indicators can identify some of the elements in need of improvement.

UN indicators

The UN agencies with a mandate to address maternal mortality (WHO, UNICEF, and UNFPA) developed such a set of proxy indicators – described in the 'UN Guidelines' (Table 199.4).[39] The guidelines identify eight 'signal functions', which are deemed necessary to manage obstetric complications. Each should have been provided to at least one patient in the last 3 months for the facility to be considered able to provide it. The functions are provision of parenteral antibiotics, oxytocics, and antihypertensives; removal of retained products (preferably manual vacuum aspiration rather than D&C); manual removal of placenta; assisted vaginal delivery; cesarean section; and blood transfusion. If a medical facility can provide only the first six it is considered able to provide basic emergency obstetric care (EmOC). If it can provide all eight it is considered to provide comprehensive EmOC.

The UN Guidelines further note that there should be at least one comprehensive and at least four basic EmOC facilities per 500,000 population. Because approximately 15% of women will experience a potentially life-threatening complication during pregnancy or delivery, at least 15% of women should deliver in a medical facility able to provide EmOC, and 100% of women with complications should deliver in a medical facility. Cesarean section rates should be between 5% and 15%, and case fatality rates should not exceed 1% of women presenting with complications.

The UN indicators have now been used in many needs assessments in all regions of the world and have proven to be useful in national and regional planning.[40–45] It is probable they will be reviewed in the near future in the light of accumulated experience, and they may undergo minor modifications. The signal function that is least likely to be available is assisted vaginal delivery. Some countries no longer train midwives (or even doctors) to do this, preferring instead for women to proceed directly to cesarean section.[46] While most countries have an adequate number of comprehensive EmOC facilities (though not necessarily well located), most have far too few facilities providing basic EmOC. This means that women must travel further to seek care, causing them to be in poorer condition on arrival at the hospital. This may also cause an overload in the comprehensive EmOC facilities.

The theoretical framework

The three-delay model[47] describes the three points in time at which delay contributes to maternal death: the delay in deciding to seek care, the delay in reaching an adequate facility, and the delay in receiving adequate care once at the facility.

When a woman experiences an obstetric complication during a home delivery she and her family decide whether to seek help. First, they must decide whom they will ask to help – other family members, TBAs, staff at a health center nearby, or staff at a more distant hospital. Often all of these are consulted in roughly that order. Seeking care from the formal health system requires traveling there whether on foot, on human-powered devices, or on motorized transport of various types, public or private. This may or may not require the presence of roads and/or money.

When she arrives at the medical facility (sometimes after hours or even days of travel), her family may be required to provide a certain amount of money, which they may need time to get, or they may be asked to go outside the hospital to buy drugs. In addition, staff may not be there, drugs and equipment may not be available, or there may be no operating room or blood for transfusion. All may be present, but the staff may be unwilling or unable to do what is needed. It is obvious that many things need to be *simultaneously* in place and functioning before medical care of adequate quality is administered. Interventions may target any one or more of these opportunities in the pursuit of medical attention. Some of the more common interventions are described later.

Training TBAs

Training TBAs has long been a priority in many developing countries, but its effectiveness is being questioned. Typically, training lasts several weeks and covers the 'three cleans' (hands, delivery surface, cord care), management of a normal delivery, recognition of complications, and referral. Note the assumption that there is an appropriate place to which women can be referred if needed.

Evaluating the work of TBAs is not easy. Evaluations most often consist of the number of TBAs trained. Sometimes TBAs are given oral examinations asking about their knowledge, attitude, and practice. Rarely are they observed practicing their trade, and if they are, the presence of the observer may change the practice. Goodburn and colleagues[9] found that training in asepsis and antisepsis neither improved practice nor reduced infections. Smith and Fortney, comparing outcomes of pregnancy among women delivered by trained or untrained TBAs in Ghana, found a small improvement in management of the placenta and postpartum fever, but a tendency to wait longer before referral.[48] Bailey found that TBAs in Quetzaltenango, Guatemala, were actually less likely to detect women with complications after they were trained.[49] A recent meta-analysis of studies with quasi-experimental design[50] found small but significant benefits for neonatal morbidity and mortality, but no evidence of either cost-effectiveness or benefits for mothers.

There is anecdotal evidence that TBA effectiveness is enhanced when they are incorporated into the larger health system, accorded respect, and allowed to remain with their patients even when they are admitted to hospital. Payment is a crucial factor; if TBAs lose their fee when their patients are delivered elsewhere, then the motivation to refer is reduced. To address this issue, hospitals sometimes pay a small fee to TBAs for the referrals (anecdotal evidence only).

Antenatal care

The purpose of antenatal care is to improve women's health and nutrition during pregnancy, to detect the early signs of what could develop into a complication and potentially prevent it, to educate women to recognize symptoms of complications, and to help women make decisions about where to deliver (and 'birth preparedness'). Unfortunately, antenatal care in many resource-poor settings is little more than an injection of tetanus toxoid, and weighing and measuring the woman's height. Often, even when potential complications are detected (hypertension, for example), no further action is taken. In spite of their shortcomings, antenatal clinics are often overcrowded so that most women spend no more than 5 min with a physician during their entire pregnancy. Blood pressure machines often do not function and vitamins and iron supplements are inadequately supplied. Nonetheless, widespread use of tetanus toxoid has greatly reduced both neonatal and maternal mortality due to tetanus.

In fact, antenatal care has only a limited ability to reduce maternal mortality. Consider the five main causes of maternal death: complications of abortion, prolonged or obstructed labor, PPH, puerperal infection, and hypertensive disorder of pregnancy. Only the last can logically be affected by antenatal care. Some of its effectiveness depends on the availability of a not-too-distant referral hospital. A program in an area of Gambia provided high-quality antenatal care (and nutritional support) to pregnant women; nevertheless until the 24 h-a-day availability of a physician or qualified midwife, maternal mortality did not decline.[51]

The risk approach and risk assessment

Every obstetrician considers the risks to which each patient is subject. Some programs, however, calculate a score based on several factors. Many of these have been developed, some complex, others simple. Often the factors are demographic (age, parity), physical (height), and obstetric history (previous pregnancy loss, or previous complications).[52]

The paramount difficulty with any risk scoring system is that both sensitivity and specificity are low. In other words, many complications occur in 'low-risk' mothers, and most of the mothers defined as 'high risk' will deliver normally. As long as most women deliver in a medical facility, this presents little difficulty. However, it is when most women deliver at home, and only those 'at risk' deliver in medical facilities that difficulties arise. Being labeled as 'low risk' gives mothers and their families a false sense of security and reduces their 'birth preparedness'. The

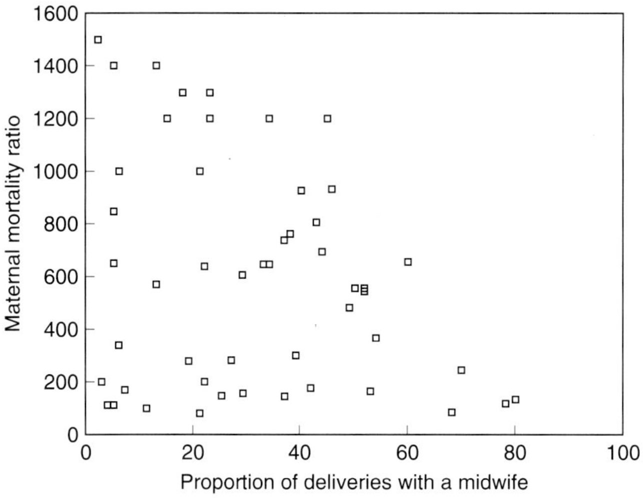

Figure 199.1 Proportion of deliveries with midwives and the maternal mortality ratio for 50 developing countries. Adapted from Graham *et al.*[57] with permission.

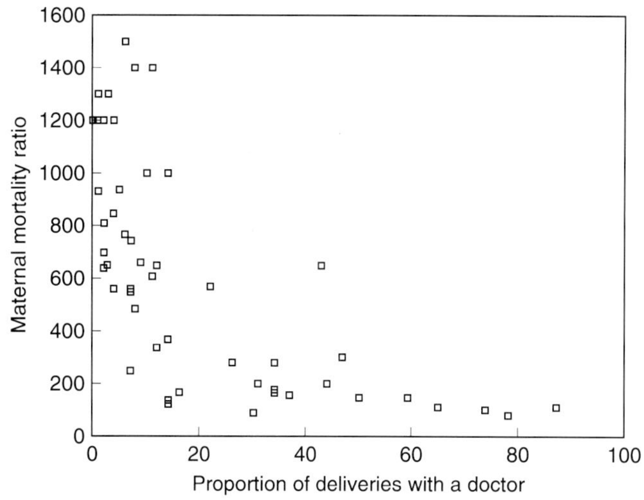

Figure 199.2 Proportion of deliveries with doctors and the maternal mortality ratio for 50 developing countries, 1990. Adapted from McCord *et al.*[56] with permission.

fact is that all women are at risk and should be prepared to seek medical help.[53]

Having said that, at least one country – Malaysia – used the risk approach to dramatically change its maternal health program.[54] Using a system of colored cards and careful follow-up with home visits if needed, 'high-risk' women were encouraged *and helped* to deliver in medical facilities. Definitions of risk were very broad and included geographic reasons – living a long way from the hospital. Furthermore, the number of risk factors was gradually expanded until a large proportion of women were included – acknowledging, tacitly, that indeed all women are at risk. Delivery in a medical facility increased from about 15% in 1950 to more than 80% in 1995, and maternal mortality plummeted from 534 to 19.[55] It is sometimes said that the disadvantage of a risk assessment approach is that medical facilities are 'flooded' with women who, although labeled as high risk, in fact have uncomplicated deliveries. The other side of this coin is that, as Malaysia found, increasing the proportion of deliveries in medical facilities is often desirable.

Note that even if accurate risk assessment were feasible, any program based on this approach would require the availability of high-quality maternity care, including EmOC, to manage those women who do develop complications – regardless of whether they were labeled high or low risk.

Institutional deliveries

We have said above that increasing the proportion of deliveries in medical facilities is often desirable. Institutional deliveries are more likely to be aseptic, to include active management of the third stage of labor, to use the partogram for early identification of obstructed labor, and to have rapid access to the drugs and equipment needed in case obstetric emergencies do arise. It is important to note, however, that not all medical facilities meet these standards.

An assessment of several hospitals in a country of medium development found clinical staff disregarded their training, ignored management protocols, and treated patients with little regard for their comfort and dignity.[55] Maternal and perinatal mortality were higher than might be expected despite the high rate of delivery by a skilled attendant. An analysis of the situation points to weak leadership and management, a lack of accountability in the health system, and women who are unaware of their rights to higher quality of care. Nevertheless, women defend their decisions to deliver in these facilities; they believe (probably correctly) this is where the highest quality of care is to be found.

In most developed countries virtually all deliveries take place in institutions, usually those able to provide a full range of life-saving services. The Netherlands is an exception to this rule (MMR=16) but hospitals are always in close proximity. Among developing countries, there is a very wide range of institutional deliveries. Often the problem is the inaccessibility of quality obstetric care when it is needed. McCord and his colleagues in southern India[56] have shown that, given confidence in the quality of medical services provided, women and their families do a good job of knowing when to seek care. Furthermore, they are willing to pay for it. Thus, we can see that, while increasing the proportion of births in institutions certainly facilitates a rapid decline in maternal mortality, it is neither necessary nor sufficient.

Figures 199.1 and 199.2 show scattergrams of MMRs with the percentage of births attended by midwives and doctors, respectively. Figure 199.1 (midwives) shows no clear pattern, while Figure 199.2 shows a clear relationship between physician-assisted delivery and lowered maternal mortality. While, in general, doctors practice in hospitals, midwives may practice in either communities or hospitals.

There is a building momentum within the donor community for increasing the availability of *skilled* (not merely trained) attendance at delivery. Skilled attendance is defined as a skilled attendant in an environment that enables referral to higher levels of skill as needed. While the rigorous evidence needed to support the claim that skilled attendance reduces maternal mortality is lacking, less rigorous evidence does support this claim.[56] Note that the effects of skilled attendance and those of institutional deliveries overlap to a considerable degree. Note also that the concept of skilled attendance includes access to EmOC and the two are highly complementary.

Community involvement

Community involvement, as a program, typically includes one or more of the following: community facilitation of transport to a medical institution, community-implemented insurance schemes, community education on the need for nurturing pregnant women, education on recognition of symptoms of complications,[58] community involvement in building a health center or maternity waiting home[59] and/or providing a welcoming environment for health workers in rural areas. A welcoming environment might include, for example, a cultural acceptance of single women (doctors, nurses, or midwives) living apart from their families, or the building of living quarters suitable for health professionals.

While community involvement often costs relatively little, sustainability is difficult and many programs fold when program support is withdrawn. Homegrown programs have greater viability. In the absence of accessible medical care, community involvement in maternity care is necessarily of limited effectiveness. At the end of the day, however, community involvement is an essential ingredient to enhance the utilization of obstetric services.

Emergency obstetric care

Accessible, acceptable, and affordable EmOC is the ingredient that is critical to the success of all other approaches. Implicit in almost all interventions designed to reduce maternal mortality is the intention to increase the proportion of women who are able to seek care when they need it. Surprisingly, this was not made explicit until relatively recently.[60] Nor were the components of EmOC defined until relatively recently. They include the following:

- availability of EmOC 24 h a day, 7 days a week (24/7)
- training of staff (at all levels) in the clinical and support skills needed for EmOC
- management protocols for each complication
- reliable and accessible supply of drugs and functioning equipment
- renovation of buildings to provide dedicated labor and delivery rooms and operating rooms that can be kept clean
- infection prevention measures
- laboratory support
- a functioning system of collecting and transfusing blood
- sensible management and logistics
- quality assurance including regular self-assessment (audits)[61]
- supportive supervision and mechanisms of quality improvement.

A recent program at Columbia University[§] has been elaborating the necessary components and implements programs through two UN agencies (UNICEF and UNFPA) and two non-governmental organizations (Care and Save the Children).[62] This program is now at the point where an assessment of impact can be made. The program met many challenges that had to be overcome – nonfunctioning equipment, drugs that remained in warehouses or on the docks, surgeons working in hospitals with no anesthetists or functioning operating room, staff untrained in obstetric procedures, low staff morale, no budgets for maintenance and repair, national policies against necessary practices, unwillingness to innovate, among others. The good news is that many of the problems could be solved with relatively little money simply by improving logistics and management practices.

Few of the interventions described above have been adequately evaluated. As we have stressed earlier, whether a woman survives an obstetric complication depends on many factors. If one element fails, others cannot function, as they should. Thus, no matter how well TBAs might recognize complications and understand the need for referral, if they cannot refer because there is nowhere to refer to, their training will have little impact on maternal mortality. A community may collaborate on developing means of transport, but if there is no medical facility to transport women to, their efforts are wasted.

There are well-established guidelines for evaluating individual interventions – such as active management of the third stage of labor.[5] But there is – as yet – no recognized hierarchy of evidence to support programs (which are, in essence, packages of interventions). While this is beginning to be developed for EmOC it remains at an early stage[63] and others would contest this.[64] It is important for researchers in this field to develop imaginative ways to provide evidence for the effectiveness of program interventions.

[§]Funded by the Bill and Melinda Gates Foundation.

Causes of maternal death

There are many causes of maternal death. In Fathalla's now famous 'Why did Mrs X die?' he describes the many off-ramps from the road to death.[65] In addition to PPH, Mrs X was high parity, without access to contraception, and the hospital to which she was taken had no blood available for transfusion. It is important to address the multiple causes of maternal death and this requires the attention of many in the government and the private sectors, not only those concerned with health.

Clinical causes

All obstetricians are familiar with the clinical causes of maternal death. In addition to the five main direct causes (abortion complications, hemorrhage, sepsis, obstructed/prolonged labor, hypertensive diseases of pregnancy) there are less frequent ones such as ectopic pregnancy, amniotic fluid embolism among others. Indirect and non-obstetric causes can be difficult to separate. In developing countries, malaria, tuberculosis, and AIDS all make a significant contribution. HIV/AIDS-associated disease is the leading cause of maternal death in some settings.[66] Anemia, while rarely a cause by itself, makes women less resistant to other complications. Violence is increasingly getting attention as a cause of maternal death, though it may not always come to the attention of maternal health workers.

Social causes

The low status of women contributes greatly to women's inability to obtain the medical care they need. It limits their access to money needed to pay for transport or for medical care, and it makes them less likely to demand high-quality care provided humanely and with dignity. Low levels of education and high rates of illiteracy in some developing countries make women less likely to know the symptoms of complications, less likely to understand the need for certain interventions, and less likely to be told the reason for treatment. Some widespread cultural beliefs (for example, obstructed labor is caused by adultery) mean that women and their families do not seek appropriate care for some complications. Many hospitals ignore women's preferences for such things as companions during labor, delivery position, or means of placenta disposal; this adds to women's reluctance to deliver in hospital. The social distance between women (especially, rural women) and medical staff means women may be reluctant to speak (and therefore to provide necessary information) to their doctors and midwives. Often they have no language in common, and even if they do, medical professionals often fail to state things in simple, non-medical terms.

Geographic and logistic causes

Many countries must contend with populations living in remote or difficult areas (curfews, mountains, deserts, rivers, floods). In developed countries, the solutions are often high-tech (such as telemedicine) or expensive – medical 'flying squads' that fly women to medical centers 2 or more weeks before the expected date of delivery. In low-resource countries, these solutions are usually out of the question. But there are maternity waiting homes in many countries that provide a convenient place to stay for a week or more prior to delivery. Because these populations are often quite small (and out of sight), and the solutions are difficult, they are seldom given high priority. Indeed, it is difficult to provide any kind of service to such populations and preventive health services are more easily given than curative ones. Lack of infrastructure – roads, transport, communication, security – presents further barriers to those seeking medical care.

Management and quality of obstetric services

Experience has shown us a multitude of ways in which poor management can jeopardize quality of care. All aspects of clinical care and support functions are compromised by poor management, from failure to replace light bulbs to assigning surgeons to hospitals with no operating room or anesthetist. It is difficult to overestimate the contribution made by poor management to maternal mortality, or indeed mortality from any cause. Poor management is the leading contributor to the 'third delay' (failure to receive prompt and appropriate care once in the medical facility).

Accountability for how professional staff perform and behave is likely to contribute to whether women receive the care they need.[67] Too often key staff are absent and sometimes for understandable reasons – public salaries are so low that medical professionals must maintain more than one job. Thus, management at the policy level must also be held accountable.

Quality of care is compromised by a very long list of factors including – but not limited to – lack of accountability, poor preservice training, lack of ongoing in-service training, lack of up-to-date skills, lack of clinical management protocols, lack of equipment and drugs, low morale of health workers, lack of concern for patients, poor condition of hospital buildings, and a policy environment that is not supportive of the needs of either health workers or their patients. Nevertheless, some hospitals are able to function well and provide high-quality care in spite of these many obstacles, which may help explain why some poor countries despite their limited financial resources have lower mortality than others with a similar level of poverty.

Prospects for the future

The Nairobi Conference on Safe Motherhood in 1987 set the goal of halving maternal mortality by 2000 and this goal was adopted by national governments and other international conferences including the International Conference on Population and Development in Cairo (1994) and the Fourth World Conference on Women in Beijing (1995). But the goal was not met. The international development community is currently using the Millennium Development Goals (MDGs) as a roadmap to reducing poverty. It includes only eight goals, one of which is to improve maternal health; its indicator target is to reduce maternal mortality by 3/4 by 2015 from the 1990 levels (whether the MMR or actual numbers is not specified). National governments and donor agencies are also adopting these goals. From a political perspective, keeping maternal mortality reduction at the center of long-term planning is critical.

While MMRs have declined, the population base has increased leading to an increase in the number of deaths. Several donors – multilateral agencies, national aid agencies, and private foundations – have provided several hundred million US dollars toward achievement of the goal. Much of the effort has, however, been directed to projects that were, and still are, small relative to the size of the target population. Few countries have embraced the challenge and moved beyond statements of goodwill and good intentions.

A significant barrier has been the perception that real progress would require a great deal of money and reform of health systems; the former was not forthcoming and the latter seemed too great a challenge. Many projects therefore remained small in scale and went around the health system rather than attempting wider reform.

Recently, it has been realized that revitalizing maternity services can lead to improvements in hospital services beyond obstetric departments. Functioning operating rooms and blood transfusion services benefit those needing surgery as well as obstetric emergencies. The same is true for training anesthetists and laboratory technicians, or renovating operating rooms. Improved drug logistics benefit far more patients than just those in the obstetric ward. Better infection prevention benefits medical staff, patients, and the community at large. Enabling people to do their jobs as they were trained to do them (through the components listed in 'Emergency Obstetric Care') improves morale, performance, and accountability. Thus, it appears that a focus on EmOC can lead to significant improvements in the way the broader health system functions.

As countries move from externally funded projects in limited geographic areas to nationwide programs, two questions dominate. First, how should a country 'scale up'? Second, how can we ensure sustainability when donors withdraw their technical and financial assistance?

Improvement in health services is incremental but successful expansion to a national level will undoubtedly require that the specific goal of reducing maternal mortality and the general goal of improving health systems be widely internalized. The increasing profile of the MDGs should reinforce these goals as countries must report to the UN their progress on the MDGs. Not only must all personnel in the health sector – from the Minister of Health down – understand what needs to be done, but so must counterparts in other sectors. Nevertheless, significant progress can be made with the involvement of only the health sector. And while improvement is facilitated by economic development, Sri Lanka and Malaysia have demonstrated that low mortality can be achieved even in low-resource countries.

The precise route to national expansion will vary with circumstances. Determining factors include whether the health sector (among others) is centralized, decentralized, or devolved; the geographic barriers that exist; the size of the population and whether the country (or regions of it) is densely or sparsely populated; whether services are free or fee-for-service; the mix of public and private services; and the commitment of the relevant professional organizations.

Similarly, there are many routes to expansion of health sector improvements that are sustainable when donors withdraw. The reader is referred to publications of the World Bank on this topic. Two important factors, though, are first, widespread commitment to health outside the health sector and second, widespread technical competence within the health sector. The latter includes competence in public health, management, awareness of international norms and standards of practice, and problem-solving skills. These skills are needed at the district level as well as at the central level, and the more so in devolved or decentralized systems.

REFERENCES

1. World Health Organization. Global Health: today's challenges. In *The World Health Report 2003 – Shaping the Future*. Geneva: World Health Organization, 2003:chap 1.
2. Starrs A. The safe motherhood action agenda: priorities for the next decade. Report on the safe motherhood technical consultation, October 18–23, 1997, Colombo, Sri Lanka. Family Care International, no date.
3. Population Reference Bureau. Women of the World data sheet 2002.
4. Population Reference Bureau, World Population data sheet 2003.
5. Prendiville W, Elbourne D, McDonald S. Active versus expectant management in the third stage of labour, issue 2. Oxford: The Cochrane Library, 2003.
6. Gülmezoglu M, Villar J, Ngoc N, *et al.* WHO multicentre randomized trial of misoprostol in the management of the third stage of labour. *Lancet* 2001;358:689–95.

7. McCormick M, Sanghvi H, Kinzie B, McIntosh N. Preventing postpartum hemorrhage in low-resource settings. *Int J Gynecol Obstet* 2002;77:267–75.
8. Tsu VD, Sutano O, Vaidya K, Coffey P, Widjaya A. Oxytocin in prefilled Uniject™ injection devices for managing third-stage labor in Indonesia. *Int J Gynencol Obstet* 2003;83: 103–11.
9. Goodburn E, Chowdhury M, Gazi R, Marshall T, Graham W. Training traditional birth attendants in clean delivery does not prevent postpartum infection. *Health Policy Plan* 2000;15:394–99.
10. Dare F, Bako A, Ezechi O. Puerperal sepsis: a preventable postpartum complication. *Trop Doct* 1998;28:92–5.
11. Smaill F, Hofmeyr GJ. Antibiotic prophylaxis for cesarean section (Cochrane Review). In *The Cochrane Library*, issue 2, Chichester, UK: John Wiley & Sons, 2004.
12. Hofmeyr G, Roodt A, Atallah A, Duley L. Calcium supplementation to prevent pre-eclampsia – a systematic review. *S Afr Med J* 2003;93:22–8.
13. McCaw-Binns A, Ashley D, Knight LP, McGillivray I, Golding J. Strategies to prevent eclampsia in a developing country: I. Reorganization of maternity services. *Int J Obstet Gynecol* 2004;87:286–94.
14. McGillivray I, McCaw-Binns A, Ashley D, Fedrick A, Golding J. Strategies to prevent eclampsia in a developing country: II. Use of a maternal pictorial card. *Int J Obstet Gynecol* 2004;87:295–300.
15. World Health Organization. The prevention and management of unsafe abortion: Report of a technical working group. Geneva: WHO/MSM 92.5, 2003.
16. AbouZahr C, Wardlaw T. Maternal mortality in 2000. Estimates developed by WHO, UNCEF and UNFPA. Geneva, 2003.
17. Loudon I. *Death in Childbirth: An International Study of Maternal Care and Maternal Mortality 1800–1950.* Oxford: Clarendon Press, 1992.
18. Welch H. Antibiotics 1943–1955: Their development and role in present-day society. In Gladstone I, ed. *The Impact of Antibiotics on Medicine and Society.* New York: International Universities Press, 1958:70–87.
19. Kerr J, Johnstone R, Phillips M. Puerperal infection 1800–1950. In *Historical Review of British Obstetrics and Gynaecology (1800–1950).* London: Livingstone, 1954:202–225.
20. Baskett TF, James B. The first transfusion of human blood. *Resuscitation* 2002;52:229–233.
21. Giangrande PL. Historical review: the history of blood transfusion. *Br J Haematol* 2000;110:758–67.
22. Fortney JA. The importance of family planning in reducing maternal mortality. *Stud Fam Plann* 1987;18(2):109–14.
23. Frautschi S, Cerulli A, Maine D. Suicide during pregnancy as a component of maternal mortality. *Int J Gynecol Obstet* 1994;47:275–84.
24. Dannenberg AL, Carter DM, Lawson HW, Ashton DM, Dorfman SF, Graham EH. Homicide and other injuries as causes of maternal death in New York City, 1987 through 1991. *Am J Obstet Gynecol* 1995;172(5):1557–64.
25. Gelles RJ. Violence and pregnancy: Are pregnant women at greater risk of abuse? *J Marriage Fam* 1988;50:841–7.
26. Anonymous. Editorial note. *Weekly Epidemiol Rec* 1991;46:341–2.
27. Moszynski P. Girls in southern Sudan are more likely to die in childbirth than complete primary school. *Br Med J* 2004;328:1514.
28. WHO, UNICEF. The sisterhood method for estimating maternal mortality: Guidance notes for potential users. Geneva: WHO/RHT/ 97.28, UNICEF/EPP/97.1, 1997.
29. Berg CJ, Antrash HK, Koonin LM, Tucker M. Pregnancy-related mortality in the United States. *Obstet Gynecol* 1996;88:161–7.
30. Bouvier-Colle MH, Varnoux N, Costes PH, Hatton F. Reasons for the underreporting of maternal mortality in France, as indicated by a survey of all deaths among women of childbearing age. *Int J Epidemiol* 1991;20:717–21.
31. Grubb GS, Fortney JA, Saleh S, *et al.* A comparison of two cause-of-death classification systems for deaths among women of reproductive age in Menoufia, Egypt, *Int J Epidemiol* 1988;17:201–7.
32. World Health Organization. Verbal autopsies for maternal deaths: Report of a technical working group. Geneva: WHO/FHE/MSM/ 95.15, 1995.
33. Kwast B, Rochat W, Kidane-Mariam W. Maternal mortality in Addis Ababa, Ethiopia. *Stud Fam Plann* 1986;17;6:288–301.
34. Bartlett LA, Mawji S, Whitehead S, *et al.* Afghan maternal mortality study team. Where giving birth is a forecast of death: maternal mortality in four districts of Afghanistan, 1999–2002. *Lancet* 2005;365(9462):864–70.
35. Graham W, Brass W, Snow R. Estimating maternal mortality: The sisterhood method. *Stud Fam Plann* 1989;20:125–35.
36. Smith JB, Fortney JA, Wong E, Amatya R, Coleman NA, de Graft-John J. Estimates of the maternal mortality ratio in two districts of Brong-Ahafo region of Ghana. *Bull World Health Organ* 2001;79(5):400–8.
37. www.abdn.ac.uk/immpact.
38. United Nations. Methods of estimating demographic measures from incomplete data. In *Manual IV. Manuals on Methods of Estimating Population*, Series A, Population Studies, No. 42, 1967.
39. WHO, UNICEF, UNFPA. *Guidelines for Monitoring the Availability and Use of Obstetric Services.* New York: UNICEF, 1997.
40. Bailey P, Paxton A. Program note. Using UN process indicators to assess needs in emergency obstetric services (Mozambique, Nepal and Senegal). *Int J Gynecol Obstet* 2002;76:299–305.
41. AMDD Working Group on Indicators. Program note. Using UN process indicators to assess needs in emergency obstetric services: Bhutan, Cameroon and Rajasthan, India. *Int J Gynecol Obstet* 2002;77:277–84.
42. AMDD Working Group on Indicators. Program note. Using UN process indicators to assess needs in emergency obstetric services: Pakistan, Peru and Vietnam. *Int J Gynecol Obstet* 2002;78: 275–82.
43. AMDD Working Group on Indicators. Program note. Using UN process indicators to assess needs in emergency obstetric services: Morocco, Nicaragua and Sri Lanka. *Int J Gynecol Obstet* 2003;80:222 30.
44. AMDD Working Group on Indicators. Program note. Using UN process indicators to assess needs in emergency obstetric services: Niger, Rwanda and Tanzania. *Int J Gynecol Obstet* 2003;83: 112–20.
45. AMDD Working Group on Indicators. Program note. Using the UN process indicators to assess needs in emergency obstetric services: Benin and Chad. *Int J Gynecol Obstet* 2004;86: 110–20.
46. Bailey P. The disappearing art of instrumental delivery: Time to reverse the trend. *Int J Obstet Gynecol* 2005;91:89–96.
47. Thaddeus S, Maine D. Too far to walk: Maternal mortality in context. *Soc Sci Med* 1994;38:1091–110.
48. Smith JB, Coleman NA, Fortney JA, de Graft-Johnson J, Blumhagen D, Grey T. The impact of traditional birth attendant training on the health of mothers and newborns in Brong-Ahafo, Ghana. *Health Policy and Plan* 2000;15:326–31.
49. Bailey P, Szászdi JA, Glover, L. Obstetric complications: Does training traditional birth attendants make a difference? *Pan Am J Public Health* 2002;11(1):15–22.
50. Sibley LM, Sipe TA. What can a meta-analysis tell us about traditional birth attendant training and pregnancy outcomes? *Midwifery* 2004;20:51–60.
51. Lamb WH, Foord FA, Lamb CM, Whitehead RG. Changes in maternal and child mortality rates in three isolated Gambian villages over ten years. *Lancet* 1984;2(8408):912–4.
52. Fortney JA. Antenatal risk screening and scoring: A new look. *Int J Gynecol Obstet* 1995;50:S53–S8.
53. Kaunitz AM, Spence C, Danielson TA, Rochat RW, Grimes DA. Perinatal and maternal mortality in a religious group avoiding obstetric care. *Am J Obstet Gynecol* 1984;150:826–31.
54. Pathmanathan I, Liljestrand J, Martins J, *et al. Investing in Maternal Health: Learning from Malaysia and Sri Lanka.* Washington, DC: World Bank, 2003.
55. Miller S, Cordero M, Coleman AL, *et al.*. Quality of care in institutionalized deliveries: The paradox of the Dominican Republic. *Int J Gynecol Obstet* 2003; 82:89–103.
56. McCord C, Premkumar R, Arole S, Arole R. Effective and efficient emergency obstetric care in a rural Indian community where most deliveries are at home. *Int J Gynecol Obstet* 2001;75:297–307.
57. Graham W, Bell JS, Bullough CH. Can skilled attendance at delivery reduce maternal mortality in developing countries? In De Brouwere V, Van Lerberghe W, eds. *Safe Motherhood Strategies: A Review of the Evidence.* Studies in Health Services Organisation and Policy, No. 17. Antwerp, Belguium: ITB Press, 2001:97–130.
58. Perreira K, Bailey P, Bocaletti E, Hurtado E, Recinos S, Matute J. Increasing awareness of danger signs in pregnancy through community- and clinic-based education in Guatemala. *Matern Child Health J* 2002;6(1):19–28.
59. Wilson JB, Collison AHK, Richardson D, Kwofie G, Senah KA, Tinkorang EK. The maternity waiting home concept: the Nsawam, Ghana experience. *Int J Gynecol Obstet* 1997;Suppl 2:S165–72.

60. Maine D, Rosenfield A. The Safe Motherhood Initiative: why has it failed? *Am J Public Health* 1999;89(4):480–2.
61. AMDD. *Reducing Maternal Mortality through the Criterion-Based Audit.* New York: Columbia University, 2002.
62. Maine D, Rosenfield A. The AMDD program: History, focus and structure. *Int J Gynecol Obstet* 2001;74:99–103.
63. Paxton A, Maine DP, Freedman L, Fry D, Lobis S. The evidence for emergency obstetric care. *Int J Gynecol Obstet* 2005;88:181–93.
64. Miller S, Sloan N, Winikoff B, Langer A, Fikree F. Where is the "E" in MCH? The need for an evidence-based approach in safe motherhood. *J Midwifery Womens Health* 2003;48(1):10–18.
65. Fathalla M. Why did Mrs X die? *People* 1987;14:8–9.
66. Kruger AM, Bhagwanjee S. HIV/AIDS: Impact on maternal mortality at the Johannesburg Hospital, South Africa, 1995–2001.
67. Van Lerberghe W, DeBrouwere V, JS, Bullough CH. Reducing maternal mortality in a context of poverty. In: De Brouwere V, Van Lerberghe W, eds. *Safe Motherhood Strategies: A Review of the Evidence.* Studies in Health Services Organisation and Policy, No. 17. Antwerp, Belgium: ITB Press, 2001:1–5.

200 Developing countries: the goals of safe motherhood

G. Benagiano and B. Thomas

Introduction

The 20th century witnessed a dramatic drop in maternal mortality throughout the western, industrialized world. For example, maternal death rates in England and Wales, between 1935 and 1978 dropped from 341 to 10 per 100,000[1] and in 1990 there were no deaths attributable to pregnancy and delivery in Iceland, Luxembourg and Malta.[2] Unfortunately, similar results were not achieved in the developing world and in most countries of the so-called 'south' deaths attributable to pregnancy, labor, delivery and the immediate postpartum continued to be unacceptably high throughout the second part of the 20th century.[2]

This means that most obstetricians practicing in developed countries end their professional careers without witnessing a single maternal death, whereas for obstetricians in the South of the world, "maternal deaths are real people, human faces seen in agony and distress: they have names, and continue to live in their memories. Indeed, for an obstetrician, there is no more tragic event than a maternal death".[3]

Because of the failure of the international community to effectively tackle the plight of so many young women and their children, it was not until the 1980s that the right to safe motherhood was recognized as an important health goal. The turning point in creating a global awareness about maternal mortality was achieved with the convening of the International Conference on Safe Motherhood, in Nairobi in 1987. The sponsors of the Conference then created an *Inter-Agency Group for Safe Motherhood*, whose members included the World Health Organization (WHO), the United Nation Population Fund (UNFPA), the World Bank, the United Nations Children Fund (UNICEF), the International Planned Parenthood Federation (IPPF) and The Population Council amongst others; the secretariat of Family Care International acted as secretariat.[4]

It must be pointed out that obstetricians were conspicuously absent in this initiative, because, at the time, their relevance was in doubt; there was a feeling that obstetricians were part of the problem, rather than a part of the solution. In fact, initially, there were many misconceptions about the role of obstetricians, with their professional privileges, their alleged obsession for high technology and inability to play the constructive role of team leaders.[3]

Fortunately, this attitude changed and – in the 1990s – the international community recognized that obstetricians in the South and North were very much concerned about this neglected tragedy, and that they had the know-how to alleviate this unnecessary suffering. Proof of this recognition was the invitation extended to the International Federation of Gynecology and Obstetrics (FIGO) to join the Inter-Agency Group.

The work to bring maternal morbidity and mortality to the forefront of the international agenda for development climaxed in the year 2000, when the largest-ever gathering of heads of state at the United Nations in New York, adopted the *UN Millennium Declaration*, made up of eight critical goals to fight poverty and accelerate development, named *Millennium Development Goals* (MDGs). Two of the eight MDGs deal with improving maternal health and reducing child mortality, thereby recognizing the importance of these health goals in promoting global development and in fighting poverty.[5] The target is to reduce by three-quarters, between 1990 and 2015, the maternal mortality ratio. As an indicator to measure progress toward the goal of reducing maternal and under-five mortalities, the MDGs selected the proportion of births attended by a skilled attendant. Targets were agreed for countries with high rates of both maternal mortality and under-five mortality. Thanks to the existence of these MDGs, today's policy-makers must, not only acknowledge that for the world's poor, pregnancy and delivery still carry an unacceptably high risk of morbidity and mortality, but also actively engage themselves to improve the situation.

Unfortunately, 5 years after the Declaration, the available data on reported proportion of births attended by a skilled attendant show poor progress in a number of countries, particularly in Asia and sub-Saharan Africa, the very places where maternal mortality is highest. At the same time, in spite of a slow start and of many obstacles, today, 25 years after the founding of the safe motherhood movement and many failed attempts, the international community seems ready to launch a unified struggle to reduce mortality related to pregnancy, including that due to unsafe abortion. Indeed, the beginning of a new era was marked in September of 2003, when all major organizations active in the field of maternal health, joined forces and launched, in Kuala Lumpur, the Partnership for Maternal and Neonatal Health.

Thanks to the new partnership, a global consensus has now been reached on what should be done to eliminate the menace of maternal deaths and disabilities hanging over so many women of the developing world.

Four major strategies have been identified to reach the MDGs of safer pregnancies and deliveries:

- Skilled attendance at all births,
- Basic emergency obstetric care (BEOC) in peripheral units,
- Comprehensive emergency obstetric care (CEOC) in referral hospitals, and
- Rapid transport of women in need of special care.

Ways to achieve these goals will be illustrated in this chapter.

Skilled attendance at birth

The first and most important strategy to reduce maternal mortality involves the presence – during childbirth – of a health professional who can manage a normal delivery as well as detect and manage complications such as hemorrhage, shock and infection. Skilled attendants should have access to a functioning emergency and transport system so that they can refer women to an appropriate health facility for higher level medical care (such as cesarean delivery or blood transfusion) when necessary.[6] Skilled attendants include doctors, nurses, midwives and other health workers with midwifery skills who can diagnose and manage complications during childbirth, as well as assist normal deliveries.

Already in 1999, a joint statement by several international organizations called on countries to 'ensure that all women and newborns have skilled care during pregnancy, childbirth and the immediate postnatal period'.[7]

According to a document jointly published by the WHO, FIGO and the International Confederation of Midwives (ICM),[8] 'Skilled care refers to the care provided to a woman (and her newborn) during pregnancy, childbirth or immediately after birth by an accredited and competent health care provider who has at her/his disposal the necessary equipment and the support of a functioning health system, including transport and referral facilities for emergency obstetric care'. Around the world skilled care can be provided by a range of health professionals, whose titles may vary according to specific countries. For this reason it has been agreed to refer to this health care provider as the 'skilled birth attendant' (SBA), so as to avoid confusion over titles.

Therefore, an SBA is 'an accredited health professional – such as a midwife, doctor or nurse – who has been educated and trained to proficiency in the skills needed to manage normal, uncomplicated pregnancies, childbirth and the immediate postnatal period, and in the identification, management or referral of complications in women and newborns'.[8]

The unique role of SBAs becomes clear when we realize that, at the community level, she/he will often be the only qualified and accredited health care worker who can take care of women during pregnancy, child birth and the immediate postpartum period. Unfortunately, communities in many developing countries often still lack sufficient numbers of skilled attendants and rely on unskilled personnel, such as the Traditional Birth Attendants (TBAs).

All skilled attendants must have the core midwifery skills. The additional skills required will vary from country to country, and possibly even within a country, to take account of local differences such as urban and rural settings. As detailed in the joint WHO, ICM, FIGO document,[8] the core functions must include:

- Communicate effectively cross-culturally in order to be able to provide holistic 'women-centered' care. To provide such care skilled attendants will need to cultivate effective interpersonal communication skills and an attitude of respect for the woman's right to be a full partner in the management of her pregnancy, childbirth and the postnatal period.
- In pregnancy care, take a detailed history by asking relevant questions, assess individual needs, give appropriate advice and guidance, calculate the expected date of delivery and perform specific screening tests as required, including voluntary counseling and testing for HIV.
- Assist pregnant women and their families in making a plan for birth (i.e. where the delivery will take place, who will be present and, in case of a complication, how timely referral will be arranged).
- Educate women (and their families and others supporting pregnant women) in self-care during pregnancy, childbirth and the postnatal period.
- Identify illnesses and conditions detrimental to health during pregnancy, perform first-line management (including performance of life-saving procedures when needed) and make arrangements for effective referral.
- Perform vaginal examination, ensuring the woman's and her/his own safety (by using gloves).
- Identify the onset of labor.
- Monitor maternal and fetal well-being during labor and provide supportive care.

- Record maternal and fetal well-being on a partograph and identify maternal and fetal distress and take appropriate action, including referral where required.
- Identify delayed progress in labor and take appropriate action, including referral where appropriate.
- Manage a normal vaginal delivery.
- Manage the third stage of labor actively, including using oxytocic drugs.
- Assess the newborn at birth and give immediate care.
- Identify any life-threatening conditions in the newborn and take essential life-saving measures, including, where necessary, active resuscitation as a component of the management of birth asphyxia, and referral where appropriate.
- Identify hemorrhage and hypertension in labor, provide first-line management (including life-saving skills where needed) and, if required, make an effective referral.
- Provide postnatal care to women and their newborn infants and post-abortion care where necessary.
- Assist women and their newborns in initiating and establishing exclusive breastfeeding, including educating women and their families and other helpers in maintaining successful breastfeeding.
- Identify illnesses and conditions detrimental to the health of women and/or their newborns in the postnatal period, apply first-line management (including the performance of life-saving procedures when needed) and, if required, make arrangements for effective referral.
- Supervise non-skilled attendants, including TBAs where they exist, in order to ensure that the care they provide during pregnancy, childbirth and early postpartum period is of sound quality and ensure continuous training of non-skilled attendants.
- Provide advice on postpartum family planning and birth spacing.
- Educate women (and their families) on how to prevent sexually transmitted infections including HIV.
- Collect and report relevant data and collaborate in data analysis and case audits.
- Promote an ethos of shared responsibility and partnership with individual women, their family members/supporters and the community for the care of women and newborns throughout pregnancy, childbirth and the postnatal period.

Obviously, depending on the setting and the availability of referral centers, additional and advanced skills should be identified and agreed upon by individual countries.

As part of the new, ongoing collaboration promoted and supported by the Partnership for Maternal and Newborn Health (and its predecessor, the Inter Agency Group for Safe Motherhood), WHO-UNICEF-UNFPA-the World Bank, with the endorsement of ICM, FIGO and the International Pediatric Association (IPA) have produced a Manual for the integrated management of pregnancy and child birth[9] that details essential practices for the management of pregnancy, childbirth and the postpartum and for proper neonatal care.

Emergency obstetric care

Contrary to common belief – most obstetric complications cannot be predicted or prevented,[10,11] but they can be treated and a woman's life saved in most cases. Therefore, the second pillar of safe motherhood is represented by the widespread availability of centers capable to provide BEOC. This involves the provision of antibiotics, oxytocics, anticonvulsants, the manual removal of placenta and – if necessary – of retained products and assisted vaginal delivery.[12]

The presence of skilled attendants at all home births should be sufficient to ensure an early identification of those complications requiring referral of the woman to a center where can BEOC be provided. It must be pointed out that, in a majority of developing countries, centers supposed to provide BEOC already exist, although – for a variety of reasons – the posts may not be equipped. It seems therefore that basic emergency care could be provided in most countries and that a modest financial input would be sufficient to enable skilled attendants to provide basic services to most women.

In the effort to provide BEOC, it is vital to ensure their proper distribution throughout a territory, taking care of studying the geography, the presence of roads, or the existence of natural barriers (rivers, mountains, etc.) that can make difficult the access to a health post. Under normal conditions, it should be sufficient to have one BEOC center for every 100,000 150,000 inhabitants.

Comprehensive obstetric care

A facility providing BEOC can perform a majority, but not all, emergency obstetric functions. There is therefore a need to ensure that, for each territory of 500,000 inhabitants or so (again, depending on the geography and overall easiness of access) a CEOC facility exists. Such a center must be able to provide all BEOC functions plus the possibility to perform cesarean sections and blood transfusions.[12]

All district hospitals are, in theory, capable of carrying out CEOC, although this is often not the case because existing equipment is not functioning, spare parts are not available, or the skills needed for repair do not exist. Given this situation, any attempt at ensuring CEOC for a given area must focus on upgrading existing facilities, not creating new ones. Monitoring the functioning of a facility providing comprehensive care is essential to ensure that lives will be saved. Experience has taught that efforts aimed at improving the situation in the developing world are often not sustainable, that once a project or a model intervention has been completed, because of lack of funding, personnel turnover or equipment break down, slowly but steadily the situation reverts to the *status quo ante*. This is probably the biggest danger that all safe motherhood programs run into; it is therefore fundamental that – when improving a CEOC facility – the self-sustainability of the effort be properly evaluated and measures to ensure it be undertaken.

Another major problem is that local physicians may not be adequately trained, or that they, as well as other auxiliary health personnel may not be available on a 24 h basis, or that drugs or blood supplies do not exist. In this respect, skills in surgery and anesthesiology are critical for the management of complications in pregnancy and childbirth. It is therefore essential that skilled attendants in the field or at primary health facilities who do not themselves have these skills, be able to refer women to centers where these skills are available. In such cases, skilled attendants must work closely with these professionals in order to ensure that speedy action is taken soon after the need for surgery has been established.

Countries that are facing a severe shortage of physicians trained in surgery and/or anesthesiology have successfully trained nurses, midwives and other cadres of health workers to perform or assist in cesarean sections. This however can pose problems, since if people with these skills are health care workers who are not skilled attendants, then the need to operate must be identified by the skilled attendant working in the field or at the BEOC unit; furthermore the skilled attendants must be able to provide ongoing and follow-up midwifery care.

Rapid transport

A safe pregnancy and a safe delivery require the provision of a continuum of care, which – in turn – necessitates, not only a functioning health care system, but also the necessary infrastructure, including transport between the primary level of health care and referral clinics and hospitals. It also needs effective, efficient and proactive collaboration between all those involved in the provision of care to pregnant women and newborns.

For this reason, improving facilities and ensuring their presence in a territory does not *per se* ensure that all women will reach a post in time for their lives to be saved. Often transportation, to be effective must be *rapid,* since conditions like intrapartum hemorrhage, must be dealt with within a very short time. Unfortunately, the rapid transport of patients in need involves complex interactions between the pregnant woman and the community in which she lives and this may be problematic.

In an effort to contribute to the solution of this problem, the Mailman School of Public Health at Columbia University in New York, has recommended a scheme focused on delays that could lead to maternal mortality, with the aim of identifying solutions to the causes of such delays[12,13] and to possible solutions.

The 'three delays' are defined as:

- Delay in deciding to seek care,
- Delay in reaching a treatment facility, and
- Delay in receiving adequate treatment at the facility.

It must be stressed that in many cases, a decision to seek care to resolve a labor complication occurring at the pregnant woman's home – where most deliveries still occur in the developing world – is often neither quick nor easy.

In societies where a long, painful labor is considered part of the process of giving birth, family members may not recognize a 'true' complication. Often, TBAs, who still assist a majority of home deliveries, may delay a decision to seek skilled care by days, because referral may be seen as a 'failure' on their part, especially if – once the woman has reached the facility – health center personnel will exclude the TBA from any further involvement. Furthermore, the lack of autonomy of women in many societies may necessitate a decision by the husband to seek help and the cost of transportation may negatively influence his decision.

Even when a decision has been made, a health post may be days away, especially if it can only be reached by foot. This is why the proper distribution of centers providing emergency obstetric care is so important in the fight for safe motherhood. For instance, if a woman has reached a BEOC facility and it is determined that she needs a cesarean section, the ability to immediately communicate with the referral CEOC center to request the ambulance needed for a speedy transport of the woman, may be the most important ring in the chain to save her life.

Finally, statistics show that many maternal deaths take place at a health post or hospital; this is why the delay in receiving care once reaching a center is still an important factor to be considered in attempting to achieve safe motherhood.

Implementing programs: the FIGO Save the Mothers Initiative

Over the last two decades many international, governmental or non-governmental organizations have created programs aimed at promoting safe motherhood, both in terms of decreasing mortality and morbidity. Only one program however, was promoted and implemented by obstetricians – gynecologists. For this reason, it was felt important – in providing an example of field activities – to single out the work carried out by the FIGO, the only organization capable of combining the experience of doctors in the industrialized world with the local knowledge of their colleagues in the developing world to combat the scourge of maternal mortality and morbidity. With this initiative, obstetricians–gynecologists all over the world provided clear proof that they are part of the solution, rather than being part of the problem.

FIGO's activities, named the FIGO Save the Mothers Initiative, have been ongoing since 1998 with funding from UNFPA, the World Bank and Pharmacia Corporation and FIGO's own resources and today span over several fields: prevention of maternal mortality, treatment of disabilities (vescico-vaginal fistulae) and prevention of hemorrhage during labor, delivery and the postpartum. These are the areas where obstetrician/gynecologists can contribute most and, at the same time, acknowledge the roots of the problem and the need for other interventions. The overall objective of the project was – and continues to be – to mobilize the obstetric/gynecological community in both the developed and developing world to work in partnership to reduce maternal mortality, and to show the feasibility and effectiveness of integrated essential and/or comprehensive obstetric services.

Reports of individual projects,[14–17] as well as a comprehensive summary[18] have already been published. The following is therefore an overview aimed at illustrating the uniqueness of FIGO's interventions.

The twinning system

From the outset, FIGO's initiative was confronted with an overwhelming demand for assistance that could not possibly be satisfied in full. For this reason, the number of partnerships to be created had to be limited to five, as follows:

- The Society of Obstetricians and Gynecologists of Canada (SOGC) was twinned with the Association of Obstetricians and Gynecologists of Uganda (AOGU).
- The American College of Obstetrics and Gynecology (ACOG) was twinned with the Central American Federation of Associations and Societies of Obstetrics and Gynecology (FECASOG).
- The Swedish Society of Obstetrics and Gynecology was twinned with the Ethiopian Society of Obstetricians & Gynecologists.
- The Royal College of Obstetricians and Gynaecologists was twinned with the Pakistani Society of Obstetricians and Gynaecologists.
- The Italian Society of Gynecology and Obstetrics was asked to work directly with the Government of Mozambique, since that country does not, as yet, have a dedicated society of obstetricians and gynecologists.

The countries in which activities took place were chosen on the basis of their high maternal mortality, the desire of the local society of obstetrics and gynecology to work with FIGO, the demonstration of government interest and commitment to improving women's health and an expression of interest from a FIGO member society of obstetricians and gynecologists in a developed country to work in the chosen region. Dedicated 'Country Teams' were established for each geographical area identified. Each team consisted of international experts and of local obstetricians–gynecologists, in a developing country together with representatives from both the 'developed' and the 'developing' country.

For each Country Team a Coordinator was selected to participate in the initial situational analysis and needs assessment visits to the developing country with a view to defining how maternity services can best be organized within the available and potentially available resources, and to work with the other members of the Country Team to evaluate the feasibility, impact and cost-effectiveness of the proposals made as a result of the assessment carried out.

Evaluating the situation

The first step in the implementation phase consisted of carrying out a situation analysis to assess the accessibility and efficiency of the existing health infrastructure for essential obstetric functions, the availability of facilities, equipment, supplies, training needs and personnel to provide easy access to obstetric functions. As part of the assessment, each Team evaluated the optimal allocation and redeployment of available resources, so that the ensuing demonstration project could be properly customized to meet the needs of the area selected in each country.

Particular attention was paid to ways to measure the success of the project. In the end, it was decided that only really measurable output would be the number of cases of life-threatening complications admitted to the health facilities and the outcome of their management.

In carrying out the needs assessment the Guidelines issued by the United Nations were used.[19] These Guidelines focus on process indicators of CEOC – in other words, the treatment of serious obstetric complications. Three key indicators are laid out in the Guidelines:

(1) *Coverage of services:* The Guidelines specify that for every 500,000 population there should be at least one facility providing CEOC and four facilities providing BEOC.
(2) *Unmet need for emergency obstetric care:* An estimated 15% of pregnant women will require medical treatment for obstetric complications. Unmet need is the proportion of these women who do not receive care in a medical facility.
(3) *Cesarean section rate:* At least 5% of women giving birth will require a cesarean section. (Note

that this is population-based rate and not a hospital-based rate.) By counting the number of cesarean sections performed in health facilities, the deficit in this life-saving service can be estimated (the recommended maximum for the cesarean section rate is 15% and care must be taken that all procedures are indicated).

When the teams conducted needs assessments, they found striking deficits. Not surprisingly, the greatest deficits were in the poorest countries. In the study areas of Ethiopia and Mozambique, for example, the unmet need for emergency obstetric care was over 98% and the cesarean section rate for the population was less than 1%. Even in Central America, serious shortages were discovered. While there were enough hospitals in the study areas of the four countries in this region, there were no lower level facilities (such as health centers) providing BEOC. The lack of basic care, often caused by shortages of trained staff, equipment and drugs, presents serious access problems for poor women in rural areas, where transportation is scarce and expensive.

The field projects

Each project carried out in partnership is different and therefore their characteristics have been unique, although they have all achieved the basic goal of helping to save mothers' lives. For this reason they represent useful examples of how, with limited resources, obstetricians–gynecologists can move out of their hospital natural setting and provide unique support to the fight for safe motherhood. For this reason, the main feature of all five projects will be briefly described here.

Central America

The Central America–USA demonstration projects took place in one rural province of El Salvador, Guatemala, Honduras, and Nicaragua. They focused on interventions aimed at implementing training courses in the management of BEOC and CEOC on the one hand and at improving relationships between the National Obstetric and Gynecology societies and the Ministries of Health, on the other.

The starting point was the realization that high maternal mortality rates were a common medical, social, as well as human problem and that no reliable information on maternal mortality was available in the four Central American countries. It was recognized that, notwithstanding the fact that properly trained obstetricians–gynecologists existed in all four countries, at rural level the capacity to render basic care for obstetric emergencies was virtually non-existent. Almost all of the institutions rendering total care were located in urban areas and were private facilities. As a result, the indigent population, which comprises the majority of the rural population, had very limited access to obstetric care during pregnancy and at delivery, since adequately trained health care personnel capable of managing obstetric emergencies at peripheral public hospitals and at health centers and offices were lacking and communication between health centers and regional hospitals was deficient.

Given this reality, activities centered around assessing and improving obstetric emergency care, establishing monitoring systems and committees at community and district hospital levels, properly carrying out audits of cases of maternal deaths and identifying strategies to effectively prevent these deaths.

A series of interventions were therefore planned and implemented, including:

- Training of field coordinators in the management of emergency obstetric care, including the development of *ad hoc* Instructors and Course Manuals with Updates in Obstetric Emergency Care.[20] These coordinators then trained the remainder of the staff in the entire province thereby ensuring that all health care personnel would be adequately trained.
- Introducing a routine protocol for the active management with oxytocin during the third period of labor in all the institutions providing childbirth services.
- Establishing a prospective and systematic data gathering system, including a detailed study of all maternal deaths with 'verbal autopsies' (interviews with family and community members), thereby determining a more realistic maternal mortality rate.
- Creating provincial maternal mortality committees to better understand causes and factors related to each death, with the aim of providing education to ensure better prevention.
- Training health providers in the manual endometrial vacuum aspiration for incomplete abortions.
- Installing radiotelephones at health centers and tertiary hospitals to ensure proper communication with tertiary hospitals.
- Establishing evaluation meetings to brief local and national health authorities and Obstetrics/Gynecology Society representatives.

In all areas, the *unmet need* for emergency obstetric care was in the order of 80%. When, after 3 years, results started to be evaluated, a slight decrease was observed to approximately 70%. However, one worrying feature emerged: no significant reduction in the number of maternal deaths was evident, contrary to the strong belief of everyone involved who had originally expected positive results within a 3-year time frame. However, looking more carefully at the situation, it became apparent that, as a result of the improved surveillance system, more maternal deaths were being identified. Indeed, the surveillance system developed by the project clearly demonstrated that the majority of maternal deaths were not being reported. This made any comparison with historical data impossible and forced the realization that the intervention would need to continue for a longer period in order to demonstrate a decrease in the real maternal mortality rate. An important finding, with very practical repercussions was that 74% of maternal deaths – approximately two-thirds of which due to postpartum hemorrhage – occur following delivery at home and only 22% occur in hospitals, pointing out to serious delays in transporting women to medical facilities.

The most important achievement of the activities in Central America was the training of almost all health care providers in the targeted provinces. Overall, 929 health care personnel received initial training and 502 follow-up training. Today, all health care facilities in each of the four provinces can provide BEOC.

Ethiopia

Maternal mortality in Ethiopia is one of the highest in the world, with a ratio of 1800 deaths per 100,000 live births and the prospect for a rapid decline in this rate is poor because of the limited availability of health services. In addition, in Ethiopia there is a substantial number of women who die because of complications caused by illegal abortions.

The FIGO project dealt with an area approximately 250 km from the capital, where a zonal hospital and two health centers are located. The area is among those with the lowest obstetric indicators for the entire country and emergency obstetric care services deemed below an acceptable standard and not provided around the clock, even at the zonal hospital. Coverage of emergency obstetric care in the targeted area was very low, at slightly more than 6% in 1999, raising to some 7.5% in 2001. This indicates an unmet need for emergency obstetric care of 91% and for Caesarean sections of 97%. In the area there was an acute shortage or absence of trained manpower at all levels; a poor administrative system and a lack of accountability by bureaucrats; non-conducive working environments for medical and paramedical personnel; shortages of essential drugs, supplies and medical equipment; absence of blood transfusion services and of an effective referral system.

Given this reality, the main aim of the intervention was to increase coverage in emergency obstetric care through training, accurate record keeping, securing adequate staff and creating cost-effective, community-based, integrated emergency obstetric care services. This was accomplished by upgrading existing facilities through the provision of equipment, supplies and materials.

The intervention included training physicians and other service providers from the Hospital and the health centers in emergency obstetric care; providing new equipment, materials and supplies; entering into agreements with the Ethiopian Red Cross Society for a regular supply of blood for transfusion in Ambo Hospital; securing a dependable supply of water and electricity to a new block for obstetric and gynecological services that had been built at the zonal hospital prior to the intervention, and had been standing idle for over 2 years. During the intervention period, all the obstetric and gynecological services – including the operating theatre were moved to the new block; encouraging community participation through a regular dialogue with community leaders and extending invitations to the local population to attend graduation ceremonies of trainees.

Specific care was given to training and motivating staff; this led to an improvement in record keeping already after the first round of training not only in the zonal hospital, but also in the two health centers. Midwives were assigned this responsibility in all facilities, and this activity has also been strengthened by regular supervision. Before the intervention, obstetric performance at the target Hospital was very poor, as documented by the number of referrals to Hospitals in the Capital. However, as soon as the implementation phase began, the total number of deliveries at the Hospital increased from a baseline of 709 in 1998 to 991 in 2001 (an increase of almost 40%). Particularly significant was the increase in cases with obstetric complications – from 128 in 1998 to 432 in 2001 (an increase of approximately 238%). The leading cause of hospitalization in the area is obstructed labor, accounting for 39% of all complications. Obstetric hemorrhage comes next, accounting for 24% of all admissions. Instrumental deliveries also increased from 6% in 1998 to 23% in 2001. Particularly noteworthy was the almost sixfold increase in the Caesarean section rate at the zonal hospital, from a base line level of 3.8% in 1998 to 17.3% in 2001. Case fatality rates, calculated taking into account direct maternal deaths, decreased from 7.2% in 1998 to 4.6% in 2001. The two health centers in the intervention area have been upgraded in terms of training of staff members, and provision of equipment and supplies. Regular supervision has been undertaken to ensure that the community in these areas has access to BEOC services.

The availability of high-quality emergency obstetric care in the hospital and in the sites involved in the project is shown by a significant decline in referrals to Addis Ababa. Annual deliveries at one of the health centers have increased from 38 in 1999 to 76 in 2001 and at the other from 206 in 1999 to 362 in 2001.

Mozambique

Mozambique is another African country where maternal mortality rates are very high, ranging – in 1997 – between 500 and 1500 per 100,000 live births. A recent analysis of 90 in-hospital maternal deaths in seven provinces during the period of January 1, 1997 and June 30, 1998 was conducted by the Ministry of Health in order to try to identify the principal determinants of maternal mortality; the results indicated that more than 80% of these deaths were attributed to direct obstetric causes.

One of the major determinants was obstructed labor: with a caesarean section rate of 2.7% and a range of 7.3% in urban areas and of 1.4% in rural areas, clearly the majority of cases of obstructed labor went untreated.

The FIGO project focused on six Rural Hospitals and two General Hospitals in the area around the capital, where a number of reasons were identified that accounted for a general inability to provide CEOC. These included: low number of trained personnel; scarcity of drugs and lack of surgical materials and equipment. When trying to design strategies to improve the situation, it soon was recognized that the major obstacle to improvement was the almost complete lack of trained medical practitioners qualified to provide obstetric care. Therefore, improving the country's ability to train physicians in general and obstetricians in particular, became a top long-term priority.

Although the floods that devastated Mozambique in 2000 affected the project areas and completely disturbed the normal activities at the country level, interventions went on aimed at upgrading three selected hospitals to allow them to become CEOC units. This was obtained through training of non-physicians (surgical technicians); supplementing the equipment of the BEOC and CEOC units in the selected Districts; improving the diagnosis and management of obstetric complications; improving the interpersonal communication and counseling skills of health providers; and improving data collection systems.

As a result of the interventions the number of centers offering BEOC in the project area doubled in 2 years and the number of units offering BEOC increased, during the same period from one to five. Within the first 3 years, emergency obstetric care had become available 24 h a day in one site, for part of the day in another and intermittently at the third site, with the aim of 24-h provision in all three centers by the end of the project activities. This resulted in an increase in the number of complications treated at the project hospitals where, globally, total deliveries decreased between 1998 and 2000, from 4289 to 3822, but concomitantly complications rose from 1816 to 2065 and the number of caesarean sections increased from 14 to 39.

An important result of the FIGO project was that the model of intervention used was adopted as a model for basic and comprehensive emergency care at the national level. As a result, a 5-year plan was developed for Mozambique, taking into account the difficulties, mistakes and problems that had arisen during the demonstration project. All the lessons learned have been incorporated into the national strategy for the reduction of maternal and perinatal mortality in the country, which essentially means the concepts utilized in the FIGO project have now been applied throughout the country. Work continues to ensure sustainability of the effort even in the difficult situation faced by Mozambique.

Pakistan

The FIGO-supported intervention took place in a rural district which was believed to be representative of the semi-urban and rural nature of many of the country's communities. Although the area would not rank as 'very poor' by Pakistani standards, it was considered representative of the country, as, prior to the commencement of activities, the provision of emergency obstetric care was virtually non-existent. Three Rural Health Centers (RHCs) – essentially 'cottage hospitals' with only modest inpatient facilities – each serving about six Basic Health Units (BHUs) – primary care facilities – were targeted. Once operational, the registers of all three RHCs were audited both for normal deliveries and for all interventions (including caesarean sections) carried out in the presence of complications, to evaluate which were potentially life-threatening if untreated. Specific attention was given to an evaluation of the impact that the new services might have throughout the area. Therefore, the village of origin of all women presenting themselves for delivery, or treatment of a pregnancy-related emergency, at hospitals in Lahore was also recorded. This ensured that, for the population of the study area, the total number of deliveries, treated complications and caesarean sections were recorded irrespective of whether they had taken place within and outside the area.

The interventions aimed at restoring structural facilities and upgrading the operating and delivery rooms within the RHCs, at ensuring that RHC ambulances were functional and that blood transfusion equipment became available. An important component of the project involved negotiating the filling of established health personnel positions, and offering in-service training in emergency obstetric care to existing medical and paramedical staff. Another specific feature dealt with the creation of a comprehensive educational program for local people, including males and civic dignitaries (customarily the decision makers) and 'dayas' (TBAs).

As a result of the intervention, the number of births in the project facilities increased in 1 year by almost 71%; caesarean sections increased in the same period by 48% and that of complications treated by almost 10%. By the middle of 2002, over 80% of all women living in the area of intervention who required a caesarean section, received it at the targeted centers. Good liaison and interaction with government authorities was established at all levels and the traditional cultural resistance shown by women to the idea of being examined or treated by male doctors has all but disappeared.

Uganda

Uganda is unquestionably one of the poorest countries in the world. Maternal mortality in Uganda is estimated at 510 per 100,000 live births. Only 38% of all births are attended by trained health personnel (skilled attendants), making the country perfectly eligible for a FIGO project.

The rural district selected for the intervention was of the appropriate size, with no other ongoing public health projects and one hospital with the capacity to become a referral hospital. Maternal mortality rates in the district had been estimated at 650 per 100,000 live births, even higher than the national average.

The main challenges to the provision of emergency obstetric care services identified in the district were: delays in transportation for women trying to reach a health center; lack of radio or telephone communication between the community dispensaries and the referral hospital; lack of trained midwives; lack of community health workers; and lack of basic equipment and supplies in some community dispensaries.

A number of interventions were planned to make emergency obstetric services available to the women of the District and reduce maternal morbidity and mortality. Among them prominent was increasing the skilled attendants' coverage and capabilities related to basic and CEOC. This was achieved by opening eight new Dispensary Maternity Units; recruiting 14 midwives to ensure 24-h coverage; recruiting a midwife-coordinator to coordinate the project's seminar series for midwives, collect the project data and organize the bimonthly visits of local or foreign volunteer obstetricians.

Another important task was upgrading health facilities by providing basic equipment, supplies and medication; identifying and addressing social and cultural barriers to maternal care by educating, through a partnership with the Department of Women and Gender Studies at Makerere University, women and their families on issues related to pregnancy, delivery and possible complications during birth; addressing the lack of emergency communication and transportation facilities in the district to ensure the timely transfer of women to health facilities.

Already after the first 18 months of continuing work, a number of improvements were noticed: one CEOC facility became fully functional, with two other facilities providing basic care; the number of births in the project's health facilities increased from 17% in 1998, to 23% in 1999, although it decreased slightly to 21% in 2000. The ability to treat all women with obstetric complications (the so-called 'met need'), in emergency obstetric care facilities increased from 8.5% in 1998, to 34% in 1999 and 38% in the year 2000.

Caesarean section rates increased from 1.3% in 1998 to 2.2% in 1999 and to 2.7% in the year 2000 and the number of antenatal cases seen and treated by midwives increased by more than 40%.

More work lies ahead: the number of births in all the BEOC centers and Dispensary Maternity Units has consistently remained less than 10% of women attending antenatal clinics, with the majority of deliveries taking place in the home. Overall 'unmet need' for general obstetrics services remains more than 60% and the cesarean section rate still needs to raise to the optimum calculated at around 12%.

Lessons from the FIGO Initiative

The Save the Mothers activities in all five areas have been quite different, although they have all achieved varying degrees of success. It must be stressed that FIGO set out to try to show that one of the direst medico-social problems affecting the lives of women in the developing world, could be addressed and resolved even under some of the worst logistic conditions and with very limited financial resources. It is fair to state that the results document that this approach is feasible and should be replicated.

A number of lessons can be drawn: first, although activities had been designed using the same basic parameters, as the work progressed, it became clear that each project was unique, reflecting the needs of the countries and regions concerned. Perhaps more importantly, it also became apparent that individual projects could easily be replicated wherever a set of similar circumstances prevailed, as it was the case in each of the countries where the Initiative was conducted. In many ways, whereas FIGO had expected to see one solution that could be applied across the board, it got five. All five projects developed findings that, whilst specific to their area, could also provide lessons for not just other similar interventions, but also for health care workers in developing nations worldwide.

In Central America, training of field coordinators who then trained the remainder of the staff of the entire province ensured better training for all health care personnel involved in delivering obstetric services. In Ethiopia, strengthening existing programs improved the availability of Emergency obstetric care services, and simple modification of routine practices produced startling results: adequate supplies of blood for transfusions at Ambo Hospital were obtained by simply discussing the matter with the local Red Cross. In Mozambique, the simple interventions advocated by the Initiative were adopted as a model for basic and comprehensive emergency care at the national level and a 5-year plan based on the project's template was developed. In Pakistan, the activities undertaken in a rural area, close to a large city, highlighted a number of interesting points that, whilst not anticipated, should be noted. For example, voluntary Lady Health Workers, who became major contributors particularly insofar as immunization and family planning aspects were concerned, facilitated the collection of data. Of particular note is the fact that a 300% increase over 5 years in the uptake of general (i.e. non-pregnancy-related) medical services was seen at the 'flagship' RHC, without any increase in costs or staffing. Finally, in Uganda, those working in the field noted that less than 20% of the relatively large number of women who attended antenatal classes returned to the same facility to deliver their baby, a fact which strongly suggested the existence of cultural barriers against delivery outside the home environment. In addition, although the number of women with obstetric complications referred to the hospital increased over the period of the interventions, between 40% and 60% of those who had been instructed to attend the hospital for treatment did not subsequently go. Up to 10% of the women referred to the hospital returned home to seek care from relatives or other community providers; unfortunately, some of these women died.

Conclusions

The work of the international community has begun to show that even an extremely difficult and logistically complex problem such as that of ensuring safe motherhood for all women of the planet can be attacked and eventually resolved: if there is a will, there is a way. What is needed today in a sustained effort capable of producing results over the long period in all the areas where women die unnecessarily.

Thanks to this work today we know that, not only progress is possible with modest resources, but improving emergency obstetric care is a cost-effective approach to reducing maternal mortality. At the same time, the effort must be global; in other words, success depends on strengthening the full range of existing reproductive health programs, of which availability of Emergency Obstetric Care services is a key component.

Success however, is also linked to modifications of existing routine practices; even minor modifications can result in startling improvements, as it is the case with the many solutions found across the developing world to the non-availability of adequate supplies of blood for transfusions. These are areas where the Community, if properly mobilized, can take a leading role.

More complex to resolve is the lack of trained professionals – particularly acute in some countries. This suggests that one of the top priorities in creating emergency obstetric centers is the need to develop human resources and to place trained personnel in areas where women are dying. A sustained 'cascading' of knowledge through training at the local level could allow replication of the results achieved in one area or country to another. All this means that success will not be achieved without the development of local capacity for support, supervision and monitoring. In this respect, the partnership of midwives, general practitioners and an obstetrician can have a significant impact on the availability of emergency obstetric care in rural districts.

The role of local communities, their sense of pride and 'ownership' in the fight to improve the health of women is also essential. In this respect, upgrading facilities can lead to a global better utilization of a health center for purposes that go well beyond safe motherhood. When a center 'belongs' to a community, even the age old and widespread reticence to deliver in medical facilities – a result of culture and tradition which requires an intensive effort to modify – may eventually be resolved. At a higher level, since Ministries of Health are the most important players in the struggle to resolve their countries' problems, involving Ministry officials becomes a primary objective.

In conclusion, there is one inescapable conclusion of all the efforts we have recently witnessed: with determination and a sustained effort, the lives of mothers and their babies can be saved with very little real financial outlay.

The real outlay is one, not of money, but of a will by doctors, nurses, midwives and all other arms of the medical profession to become a part of the solution rather than remain part of the problem, and by government to recognize that by diverting a comparatively modest part of their national budgets to providing, at a modest cost, CEOC, they will be helping to save countless thousands of lives.

Acknowledgments

The section of this chapter dealing with the FIGO Project is based on material originally supplied and written by the members of the country teams concerned, to whom due acknowledgment must be made.

REFERENCES

1. Macfarlane A, Mugford M, Henderson J, Furtado A, Stevens J, Dunn A. *Birth Counts: Statistics of Pregnancy and Childbirth*, Vol. 2, 2nd edn. London: The Stationery Office, 2000.
2. World Health Organization and United Nations Children Fund: *Revised 1990 Estimates of Maternal Mortality*. DOC WHO/FRH/MSM196.11. Geneva: World Health organization, 1996.
3. Benagiano G, Fathalla M, Lalonde A, Thomas B. The FIGO save the mothers initiative. *Int J Obstet Gynecol* 2004;86: 283–293.
4. Family Care International. *Safe Motherhood Fact Sheet: The Safe Motherhood Initiative*. New York: FCI, 1998.
5. United Nations Millennium Declaration UN A/RES.53.2 available from www.un.org/millennium/declaration/ares552e.pdf.
6. World Health Organization, International Federation of Gynecology and Obstetrics, International Confederation of Midwives. *Definition of the Midwife*. Geneva: World Health Organization, 1992.
7. World Health Organization, United Nations Population Fund, United Nations Children Fund and the World Bank. *Reducing Maternal Mortality. A Joint Statement by WHO–UNFPA–UNICEF–the World Bank*. Geneva: World Health Organization, 1999.
8. World Health Organization, International Confederation of Midwives, International Federation of Gynecology and Obstetrics. *Making Pregnancy Safer: The Critical Role of the Skilled Attendant. A Joint Statement by WHO-ICM-FIGO*. Geneva: World Health Organization, 2004.

9. World Health Organization, United Nations Population Fund, United Nations Children Program and the World Bank. *Pregnancy, Childbirth, Post-partum and Newborn Care: A Guide for Essential Practice.* Geneva: World Health Organization, 2003.
10. Rosenfield A, Maine D. Maternal mortality – a neglected tragedy: Where is the M in MCH? *Lancet* 1985;2(8446):83–5.
11. Rooney C. *Antenatal Care and Maternal Health: How Effective Is It?* Geneva: World Health Organization, 1991.
12. Maine D, Azakalin MD, Ward VM, Kamara A. *The Design and Evaluation of Maternal Mortality Programs.* New York: Center for Population and Family Health, School of Public Health, Columbia University, 1997.
13. Maine D. *Safe Motherhood programs: Options and Issues.* New York: Center for Population and Family Health, School of Public Health, Columbia University, 1991.
14. Curet LB, Foster-Rosales A, Hale R, *et al.* FIGO save the mothers initiative: the Central America and USA collaboration. *Int J Gynecol Obstet* 2003;80:213–21.
15. Lalonde AB, Okong P, Mugasa A, Perron L. FIGO save the mothers initiative: the Uganda—Canada collaboration. *Int J Gynecol Obstet* 2003;80:204–12.
16. Lodhi SK, Sohail R, Zaman F, *et al.* FIGO save the mothers initiative: the Pakistan—United Kingdom collaboration. *Int J Gynecol Obstet* 2004;87:79–87.
17. Mekbib TA, Kassaye E, Getachew A, Tadesse T, Debebe A. FIGO save the mothers initiative: the Ethiopia–Sweden collaboration. *Int J Gynecol Obstet* 2003;81:93–102.
18. Benagiano G, Thomas B. Safe motherhood: the FIGO initiative. *Int J Gynecol Obstet* (World Report on Women's Health) 2003;82:263–74.
19. United Nations Children Program. *Programming for Safe Motherhood – Guidelines for Maternal and Neonatal Survival.* New York: United Nations Children Program, 1999.
20. Baskett TF. *Essential Management of Obstetric Emergencies.* New York: John Wiley and Sons, 1985.

201 Vesico-vaginal fistulas in developing countries

P. Hilton

Introduction

Although it is likely that vesico-vaginal fistula (VVF) of obstetric etiology was known to the physicians of ancient Egypt, the association with difficult labor was not made until 1000 AD when it was described by the Perso-Arab physician Avicenna (Ibn Sinna) in his text 'Al Kanoun'.

Since then the literature on this subject has been extensive, although largely based on anecdote, small retrospective case series, and opinions rather than facts. As a result, much of our knowledge and practice in this area is based on the experience of a small number of individuals working in areas of high fistula prevalence, rather than firm scientific evidence.

Etiology and epidemiology

Urogenital fistulas may occur congenitally, but are most often acquired from obstetric, surgical, radiation, malignant, and miscellaneous causes. In much of the developing world over 90% of fistulae are of obstetric etiology,[1–4] whereas in the UK and USA over 70% follow pelvic surgery.[5]

Obstetric fistulas

The basic physical factors responsible for obstetric fistula include obstructed labor, accidental injury at the time of caesarean section, forceps delivery, craniotomy, symphysiotomy, traditional surgical practices including circumcision and gishiri, and complications of criminal abortion.

The overwhelming proportion of cases are complications of neglected obstructed labor. During normal labor the bladder is displaced upwards and the anterior vaginal wall, bladder base, and urethra are compressed between the fetal head and the posterior surface of the pubis. No harm results if compression lasts for a short time, but in prolonged obstructed labor the intervening tissues are devitalized by ischemia. Usually the anterior vaginal wall and underlying bladder neck are affected, although sometimes the area of necrosis is higher, in which case the anterior lip of the cervix and underlying trigone are involved. The devitalized area separates as a slough, usually between the third and 10th day of the puerperium, with resulting fistula formation and incontinence (see Figures 201.1 and 201.2).

In other instances accidental injury to the vaginal wall occurs during a difficult operative delivery and may involve damage to the underlying bladder wall, particularly if the tissues are devitalized by prolonged pressure. Forcible rotation of the head with Kielland's

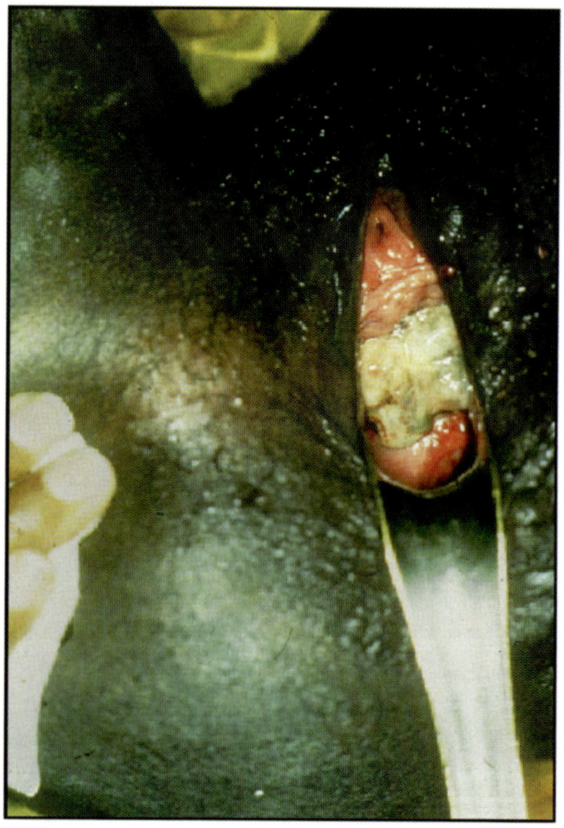

Figure 201.1 Area of slough on anterior vaginal wall 5 days following delivery.

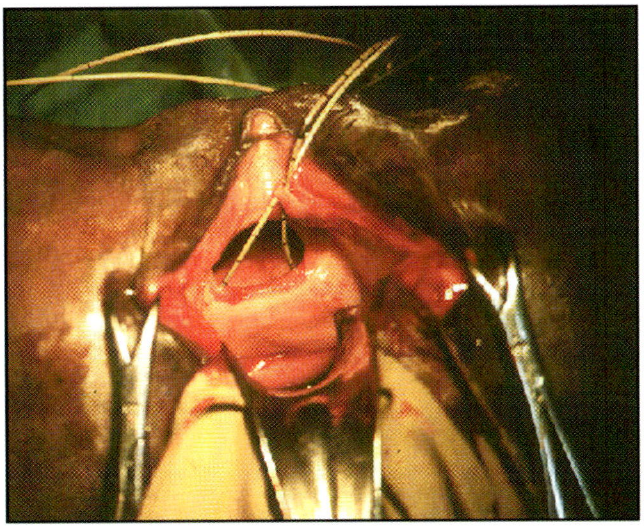

Figure 201.2 Large obstetric fistula involving the whole urethra and bladder base, up to the level of the ureteric orifices.

forceps is particularly liable to produce such an injury by shearing stresses. The bladder is exposed to injury following symphysiotomy if the pubic bones are too widely separated by forced abduction of the thighs. In these circumstances the unsupported bladder neck is very likely to be damaged especially if the head is rotated and extracted with forceps. The posterior wall of the bladder may be accidentally incised during lower segment cesarean section or repair of ruptured uterus, particularly if the bladder is not reflected sufficiently far downwards before the lower uterine segment is opened. Alternatively, sutures may be passed through the posterior bladder wall during repair of the uterine incision. The appearance of urinary incontinence in such cases is delayed until the intervening bladder tissue is caught up in the suture sloughs.

Traditional surgical practices play a significant role in the etiology of obstetric fistulas in several parts of Africa. The practice of yankan gishiri is still commonly employed among the Hausa, Fulani and Kanuri tribes of northern Nigeria. The traditional cut made with a razor blade or knife through the vaginal introitus is sometimes superficial, but still may result in fistula formation. Since the procedure is usually made by linear incision into healthy tissues, repair is often much easier than those fistulas which result from pressure necrosis (see Figure 201.3).

Female circumcision is practiced in various forms in much of North Africa, and is widespread in Sudan and other Moslem cultures. The most extreme form, pharaonic circumcision, involves removal of the labia minora, most of the labia majora, the mons veneris, and often the clitoris, the introitus being reduced to pinhole size. Coitus itself may result in perineal rupture and may be a primary cause of fistula formation. Delivery will often necessitate wide episiotomy, often with an anterior incision. Intuitively one might expect this to contribute to the development of both VVF, and recto-vaginal fistulas or third-degree tears, particularly where skilled obstetric care is not available; however, the exact relevance of female circumcision to obstetric VVF remains unclear. Tahzib reported on the epidemiological determinants of VVF in women and children in northern Nigeria.[6,7] In over 80% of cases obstructed labor was the major etiological factor; one-third of the total had undergone gishiri, and in 15% this was felt to be the main etiological factor.

In considering obstetric fistulas, however, it is equally relevant to consider the social, cultural and geographical influences of this condition. Obstructed labor is most often due to a contracted pelvis. This usually results from stunting of growth by malnutrition and untreated infections in childhood and adolescence. Where women retain a subservient role in society, and standards of education are limited, early marriage and the absence of family planning results in early childbearing. First pregnancies occur soon after menarche, before growth of the pelvis is complete, accentuating this risk. It is however important to recognize that whilst fistula are of high prevalence in areas where the educational and nutritional status of women is poor, where traditional surgical practices abound, and where early marriage, early childbearing and poor access to health care are the norm, these factors are not necessarily in themselves causative. In a case–control series from northern Nigeria it was found that whilst VVF patients had a lower educational and socioeconomic status than control women, age at marriage and first pregnancy, and uptake of antenatal care were not different.[8]

Surgical fistulas

Genital fistula may occur following a wide range of surgical procedures within the pelvis. The contribution of surgical fistulas to the total fistula prevalence in developing countries is small, however. It is often supposed that this complication results from direct injury to the lower urinary tract at the time of operation but this is certainly not always the result of careless, hurried, or rough surgical technique. Of the 165 urogenital fistulas referred to the author over the last 12 years, 117 have been associated with pelvic surgery, and 91 followed hysterectomies; of these only four (4%) presented with leakage of urine on the first day postoperatively. In the other cases it was presumed that tissue devascularization during dissection, inadvertent suture placement, or pelvic hematoma formation or infection developing postoperatively resulted in tissue necrosis with leakage usually developing 5–14 days later. Overdistension of the bladder postoperatively may be an additional factor in many of these latter cases.[9] It is likely that patients with a habit of infrequent voiding, or those with inefficient detrusor contractility, may be at increased risk of postoperative urinary retention; if this is not recognized early and managed appropriately, the risk of

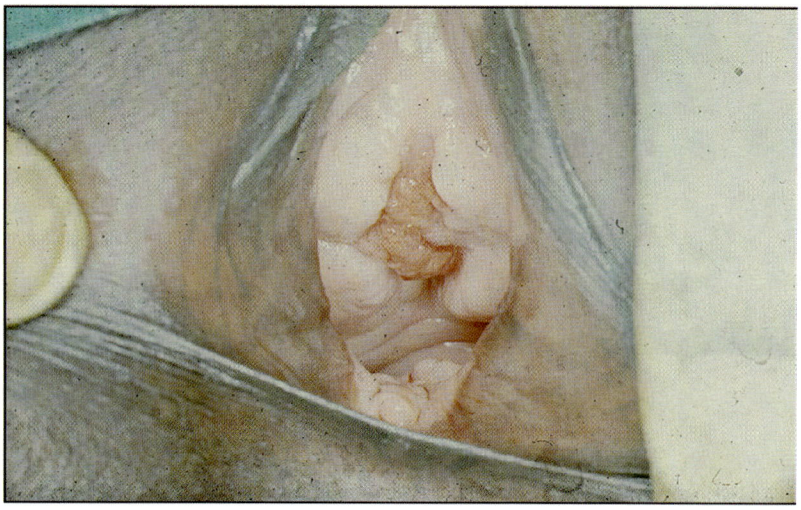

Figure 201.3 Urethro-vaginal fistula following 'gishiri cut'.

fistula formation may be increased. The use of prophylactic catheterization in the first 24–48 h might be expected to reduce the risk of postoperative fistula formation, but this has never been proven.

Radiation fistulas

The obliterative endarteritis associated with ionizing radiation in therapeutic dosage proceeds over many years and may result in a fistula long after the primary malignancy has been treated. Of the 19 radiation fistulas in the author's series, leakage developed at intervals between 1 and 30 years following radiotherapy. The associated devascularization in the adjacent tissues means that ordinary surgical repair has a high likelihood of failure,[10] and modified surgical techniques are required.

Malignant fistulas

Excluding the effects of treatment, malignant disease itself may result in genital tract fistula, particularly in areas where primary health care and screening programs are absent or ineffective. Carcinoma of cervix, vagina and rectum are the most common malignancies to present in this manner. It is relatively unusual for urothelial tumors to present with fistula formation, other than following surgery or radiotherapy. Although the development of a fistula may be a distressing aspect of the terminal phase of malignant disease, it is nevertheless deserving of a full consideration of the therapeutic or palliative possibilities rather than simply compassion.

Miscellaneous causes

Miscellaneous causes of fistulas in the genital tract include infection (lymphogranuloma venereum, schistosomiasis, tuberculosis, actinomycosis, measles, noma vaginae), trauma (penetrating trauma, coital injury, neglected pessary, or other foreign bodies), and catheter-related injuries.

Prevalence

The prevalence of genital fistulas varies from country to country and continent to continent, just as the main causative factors vary. In the developing world, many fistula cases never come to medical attention, as these women are separated from their husbands and ostracized from society. Although the true prevalence in the developing world is unknown, high prevalence rates have been reported from Sudan,[11] Ethiopia,[12] Chad,[13] Ghana,[3] and Nigeria.[6] An incidence of 1–2 per 1000 deliveries has been estimated worldwide, with an annual incidence of 50,000–100,000 and a prevalence of untreated fistulas of 500,000–2,000,000.[14] The incidence of fistulas clearly relates to the level of maternity care. Areas with high maternal mortality also tend to have high fistula rates. Danso *et al.* have suggested that a more realistic estimate of the incidence of fistulas in any community might be that it approaches the maternal mortality rate.[3] If this were true the annual incidence worldwide might approach 500,000.

The rate of fistula formation following hysterectomy has been calculated as between 1 per 642 (from the author's fistula cases) and 1 per 1330 operations in the UK (J. B. Lawson, 1990, personal communication). Figures of between 1% and 4% fistulas have been reported following radical hysterectomy,[15,16] with a similar incidence following radiation for gynecological malignancies.[17] The incidence of fistula formation following pelvic exenteration may be as high as 10%.[18]

Investigation

The four cardinal principles of investigation are simple: (1) confirm that the discharge is urinary; (2) confirm that leakage is extra-urethral; (3) identify site of leakage; and (4) identify or exclude multiple or complex fistulous tracks.

Investigation has traditionally been undertaken by dye testing, examination under anesthesia, cystourethroscopy, and intravenous urography. Phenazopyridine may be used orally or indigo carmine intravenously to stain the urine and hence confirm the presence of a fistula. The identification of the fistula site is best carried out by the instillation of colored dye (usually methylene blue) into the bladder with the patient in the lithotomy position. The traditional 'three swab test' has limitations and is not recommended; examination is best carried out with direct inspection. If leakage of clear fluid continues after dye instillation a ureteric fistula is likely, and this is most easily confirmed by a 'two dye test', using phenazopyridine to stain the renal urine, and methylene blue to stain bladder contents.[19]

Although intravenous urography is a particularly insensitive investigation for the diagnosis of VVF, assessment of upper urinary tract status may have a significant influence on treatment measures applied (see Figure 201.4). Where x-ray facilities are available, this test should be viewed as an essential part of the investigation. Some authorities would go so far as to advocate bilateral retrograde pyelography in the assessment of all VVFs. Compromise to ureteric function is a particularly common finding when a fistula occurs in relation to malignant disease or its treatment. Whilst this recommendation is not possible in much of the world, it remains underutilized where facilities are available.

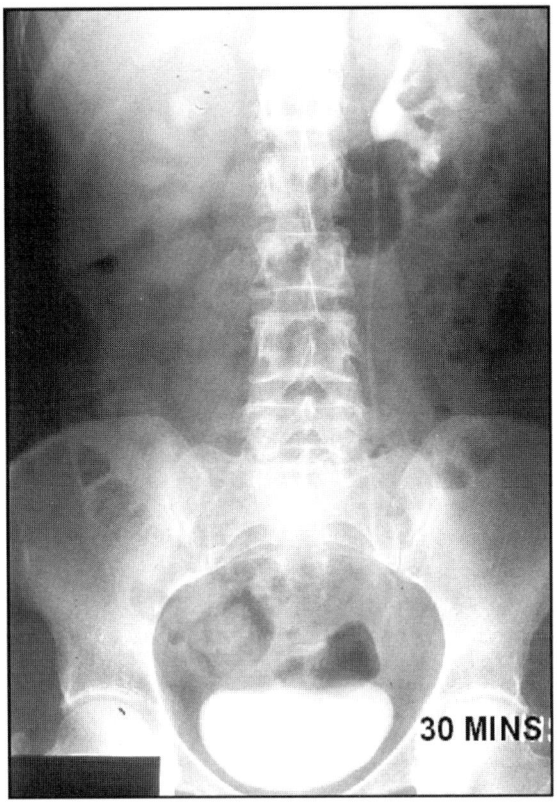

Figure 201.4 Intravenous urogram illustrating poorly functioning hydonephrosis right kidney in association with uretero-vaginal fistula.

Management

Immediate management by catheter drainage

An abnormal communication between viscera will tend to close spontaneously before epithelialization is complete, provided that the natural outflow is unobstructed. Bypassing the urethral sphincter mechanisms by catheterization may encourage early closure, especially in cases where the fistula is small. Obstetric fistulas developing after obstructed labor should be treated initially by continuous bladder drainage, combined with antibiotics to limit tissue damage from infection. Indeed, if a patient is known to have been in obstructed labor for any significant length of time, or is recognized to have areas of slough on the vaginal walls during the puerperium, prophylactic catheterization should be undertaken before the development of a fistula. This should be maintained for 6–8 weeks, since spontaneous closure in both surgical and obstetric cases may occur within this period.[14,20,21] Indeed, spontaneous closure of obstetric fistulas has been reported in up to 28% of cases where catheterization has been employed.[22]

Palliation and skin care

The vulvar skin is at considerable risk from ammoniacal dermatitis in fistula patients, and liberal use of barrier creams should be encouraged (see Figure 201.5). Steroid therapy was advocated in the past as a means of reducing tissue edema and fibrosis, although these benefits have been refuted more recently, and there may be a risk of compromise to subsequent healing. Local estrogen cream has been recommended by some authors, and whilst empirically one might expect benefit in postmenopausal women or those obstetric fistula patients with prolonged amenorrhea, the evidence for this is lacking.

Nutrition

Because of social ostracism and the effects of prolonged sepsis, patients with obstetric fistulas may also suffer from malnutrition and anemia. In order to maximize the prospects for postoperative healing, it is essential to optimize the general health of the patient. The admission of fistula patients to preoperative hostel facilities is encouraged by several of the larger third world fistula units. Where nursing staffs are

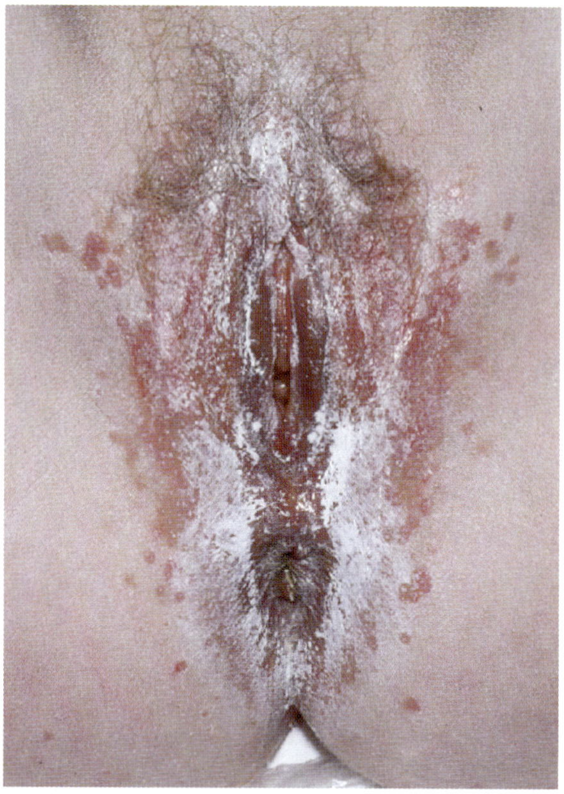

Figure 201.5 Ammoniacal dermatitis.

limited, family members may be required to help with cooking and general support.

Physiotherapy

Early involvement of the physiotherapist in preoperative management and rehabilitation of such patients is essential, as obstetric fistulas are commonly associated with lower limb weakness, foot drop and limb contracture. In a group of 479 patients studied prospectively, 27% had signs of peroneal nerve weakness at presentation, and a further 38% gave a history of relevant symptoms.

Antimicrobial therapy

Opinions differ on the desirability of prophylactic antibiotics at the time of surgery. Some authors avoid their use except for the treatment of specific infection; others advocate broad-spectrum treatment in all cases. One randomized trial of antibiotic prophylaxis in obstetric fistula patients from West Africa failed to show benefit.[23] The author's current practice is single-dose prophylaxis in urinary fistulas, and 5-day coverage for intestinal fistulas.

Counseling

Confident but realistic counseling by the surgeon is essential. Of equal importance is the involvement of nursing staff or counselors with experience of fistula patients. In addition, support from previously treated patients can be of immense value in maintaining patient morale, especially where a delay prior to definitive treatment is required.

General principles of surgical treatment

Timing of repair

The timing of surgical repair is perhaps the single most contentious aspect of fistula management. Whilst shortening the waiting period is of both social and psychological benefit, one must not compromise surgical success. The benefit of delay is to allow slough to separate and the inflammatory changes to resolve. Considerable sloughing of tissues occurs in both obstetric and radiation fistulas and it is imperative that this should have ceased before repair is undertaken. Most authorities suggest that a minimum of 3 months should be allowed to elapse in obstetric cases, although others advocate surgery as soon as the slough is separated.[14] It may be necessary to wait 12 months or more in radiation fistulas.

The same principles should apply with surgical fistulas. Here, although the extent of sloughing is limited, extravasation of urine into the pelvic tissues invariably sets up some inflammatory response. Although several authors advocate early repair most would agree that 10–12 weeks after the inciting event is the earliest appropriate time for repair.

Route of repair

Arguments continue as to whether the abdominal or vaginal route is most appropriate for fistula repair. Two recent small and uncontrolled studies suggested advantage from the abdominal transvesical[24] and transperitoneal[25] approaches. Recognizing that other authorities recommend the vaginal route,[2,26] these two series acknowledge the need for individualized management based upon anatomical relationships, extent of injury, and comorbidities. Larger series of obstetric[1,2] and surgical[5] fistulas indicate high success rates with the vaginal approach.

Regardless of personal preferences, surgeons involved in fistula management should be capable of all approaches, and must have the versatility to modify their techniques in order to select that most appropriate to the individual case. When access is good and vaginal tissues are sufficiently mobile, the vaginal route is usually most appropriate. If access is poor and the fistula cannot be brought down, on the contrary, the abdominal approach should be used. Overall more surgical than obstetric fistulas are likely to require an abdominal repair, although in the author's series of cases from the UK,[5] and those reviewed from Nigeria,[2] two-thirds of cases were satisfactorily treated by the vaginal route regardless of etiology.

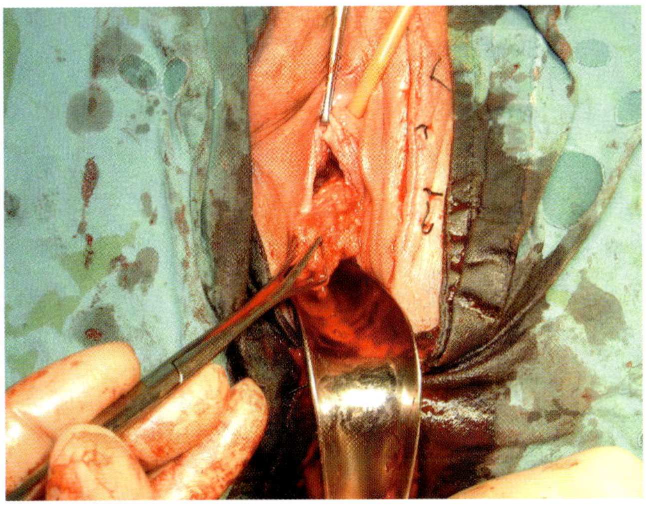

Figure 201.6 Martius bulbocavernous muscle/fat graft passed subcutaneously from left labium majus to overlie fistula repair.

Interposition grafts

Several techniques have been described to support fistula repair in different sites. In each instance, the interposed tissue serves to create an additional layer in the repair, to fill dead space, and to bring in new blood supply to the area. As such, interposition grafts have been most commonly in use in the repair of radiation fistulas, or to limit scarring and reduce postfistula repair stress incontinence in patients with urethral and bladder neck fistulas. The tissues used include: (a) labial fat and bulbocavernosus muscle passed subcutaneously to cover a vaginal repair (Martius graft)[27] (see Figure 201.6); (b) gracilis muscle, either passed via the obturator foramen[28] or subcutaneously[29] or rectus abdominis muscle[30] – both used in repairs by the vaginal route; (c) omental pedicle grafts[31,32] from the greater curve of the stomach and rotated into the pelvis on the right gastroepiploic artery (these may be used at any transperitoneal procedure, but have greatest advantage in postradiation fistulae); (d) peritoneal flap grafts[33] provide an additional layer for transperitoneal repair procedures by taking a flap of peritoneum from any available surface, most usually the paravesical area; (e) a pedicled flap of vaginal wall[34] (although the results were good in this case, concern exists over the risk of subvaginal cyst formation in the buried vaginal tissue); and (f) free bladder mucosal grafting.[35]

The role of interposition flaps in transabdominal repair procedures has recently reviewed by Evans *et al.*[36] These authors reported 37 patients with fistulas of largely surgical etiology. All of the 12 treated employing an omental or peritoneal interposition flap were cured, compared with 16 cures among 25 managed without interposition (64%). This finding was consistent for fistulas of both benign and malignant etiology. The authors acknowledge that their overall cure rate (75%) is lower than many series. Despite this, they recommend an interposition flap regardless of fistula etiology when a transabdominal repair is undertaken, particularly when the repair is performed by a surgeon without extensive prior experience.

Rangnekar *et al.* evaluated the role of the Martius graft in vaginal repair procedures in a series of mainly obstetric fistulas from Mumbai, India.[37] Forty-six cases were reviewed retrospectively, of which 12 were urethro-vaginal and 34 vesico-vaginal; a Martius graft was employed in 21 instances. Overall, 95% of those treated with a graft were cured, compared with 72% of those with simple anatomic repair. Despite small numbers, the authors of this series recommend the use of an interposition graft, particularly for urethro-vaginal fistulas and in patients with recurrent or multiple fistulas.

The difficulty with case series such as those cited here is that the use of grafting has not been randomized, and reflects the personal prejudices of the surgeon as to which patients are most likely to benefit form the procedure. In the author's practice, it has been standard for the last 15 years, to use a labial fat graft in all urethral and bladder neck fistulas, and an omental graft in VVFs treated by the transperitoneal approach, but not in those treated by either the vaginal or abdominal transvesical routes. With this approach, the cure rate at first operation has been 95% for those cases treated with a graft, and 97% for those where a graft has not been used. There were also no significant differences in cure rate between the urethral and bladder fistulas, or between primary and recurrent fistulas.

Urinary diversion

The acceptability of permanent urinary diversion in most developing countries is extremely limited, and the need is infrequent. In the series of cases from southeast Nigeria cited previously, only 0.6% of 2484 patients required diversion.[2] In a review of 55 cases from Denmark, Langkilde *et al.* report 90% success using either vaginal or transvesical approaches in postsurgical fistulas, but only 14% success in postradiation fistulas.[10] As a consequence, they advocate ileal conduit urinary diversion as the method of choice for the latter cases. Although currently 12% of patients with VVF undergo a diversionary procedure in the UK,[38] the requirement for urinary diversion in fistula patients should be very uncommon, and in series of both surgical[5] and obstetric[2] cases is less than 3%.

Specific repair techniques

Vaginal procedures

Dissection and repair in layers. Two main types of closure are applied to the vaginal repair of urinary fistulas, the classical saucerization technique described in 1852 by Sims (see below),[39] and the much more commonly used dissection and repair in layers. In this latter procedure sutures must be placed with meticulous accuracy in the bladder wall, care being taken not to penetrate the mucosa which should be inverted as far as possible. The repair should be started at either end, working toward the midline, so that the least accessible aspects are sutured first. Interrupted sutures are preferred and should be placed approximately 3 mm apart, taking as large a bite of tissue as feasible. Stitches that are too close together, or the use of continuous or purse-string sutures, tend to impair blood supply and interfere with healing. Knots must be secure with three hitches, so that they can be cut short, leaving the minimum amount of material within the body of the repair. With dissection and repair in layers the first layer of sutures in the bladder should invert the edges; the second adds bulk to the repair by taking a wide bite of bladder wall, but also closes off dead space by catching the back of the vaginal flaps. After testing the repair, a third layer of interrupted mattress sutures is used to evert and close the vaginal wall, consolidating the repair by picking up the underlying bladder wall.

Saucerization. The saucerization technique described by Sims involves converting the track into a shallow crater, which is closed without dissection of bladder from vagina using a single row of interrupted sutures. The method is only applicable to small fistulas and perhaps residual fistulas after closure of a larger defect; in other situations the technique does not allow secure closure without tension.

Vaginal repair procedures in specific circumstances

The conventional dissection and repair in layers described above is entirely appropriate for the majority of mid-vaginal fistulas, although modifications may be necessary in specific circumstances. In juxta-cervical fistulas in the anterior fornix vaginal repair may be feasible if the cervix can be drawn down to provide access. Dissection should include mobilization of the bladder from the cervix. The repair must be undertaken transversely to reconstruct the underlying trigone and prevent distortion of the ureteric orifices.

Vault fistulas, particularly those following hysterectomy, can again usually be managed vaginally. The vault is incised transversely and mobilization of the fistula is often aided by deliberate opening of the Pouch of Douglas.[40] The peritoneal opening does not require to be closed separately, but is incorporated into the vaginal closure.

Tissue loss may be extensive with subsymphyseal fistulas involving the bladder neck and proximal urethra as a consequence of obstructed labor, and fixity to underlying bone is a common problem. The lateral aspects of the fistula require careful mobilization to overcome disproportion between the defect in the bladder and the urethral stump. A racquet shape extension of the incision facilitates exposure of the proximal urethra. Although transverse repair is often necessary, longitudinal closure gives better prospects for urethral competence.

Where there is substantial urethral loss, reconstruction may be undertaken using the method described by Chassar Moir,[41] or Hamlin and Nicholson.[29] A strip of anterior vaginal wall is constructed into a tube over a catheter. Plication behind the bladder neck is probably important if continence is to be achieved. The interposition of a labial fat or muscle graft not only fills up the potential dead space, but provides additional bladder neck support and improves continence by reducing scarring between bladder neck and vagina.

The extensive dissection required with very large fistulas extending from the bladder neck to the vault may produce considerable bleeding. The main surgical difficulty is to avoid the ureters. They are usually situated close to the supero-lateral angles of the fistula, and if they can be identified they should be catheterized. Straight ureteric catheters passed transurethrally, or double pigtail catheters may both be useful in directing the intramural portion of the ureters internally.

Radiation fistulas present particular problems in that the area of devitalized tissue is usually considerably larger than the fistula itself. Mobilization is often impossible, and the flaps are likely to slough if repair in layers is attempted. Closure by colpocleisis is usually required. Some authors advocate total closure of the vagina although it is preferable to avoid dissection in the devitalized tissue entirely and to perform a lower partial colpocleisis converting the upper vagina into a diverticulum of the bladder. It is usually necessary to fill the dead space below this with an interposition graft.

Abdominal procedures

Transvesical repair. Repair by the abdominal route is indicated when high fistulas are fixed in the vault and are inaccessible *per vaginam*. Transvesical repair has the advantage of being entirely extraperitoneal. It is often helpful to elevate the fistula site by a vaginal pack, and the ureters should be catheterized under direct vision. The technique of closure is similar to that of the transvaginal flap-splitting repair except that for hemostasis the bladder mucosa is closed with a continuous suture.

Transperitoneal repair. It is often said that there is little place for a simple transperitoneal repair, although a combined transperitoneal and transvesical procedure is favored by urologists and is particularly useful for VVF following cesarean section. A midline split is made in the vault of the bladder; this is extended downward in a racquet shape around the fistula. The fistulous track is excised and the vaginal or cervical defect closed in a single layer. The bladder is then closed in two layers.

Results

It is difficult to compare the results of treatment in different series, since the lesions involved and the techniques of repair vary so greatly. Cure rates should be considered in terms of closure at first operation; these vary from 60% to 98%. Of the 165 patients in the author's series managed in the UK, 12 (7.2%) healed without operation, nine declined surgery, one (with coexistent detrusor instability) was asymptomatic on medical treatment, three underwent primary urinary diversion, and two patients with radiotherapy fistulae died without being operated upon (one from recurrent disease and one from cachexia without recurrence). Of the remaining 138 who underwent repair surgery, 133 (96%) were cured by the first operation. Of the 71 fistulas occurring after simple hysterectomy, 99% were cured at their first operation.

As in many other forms of surgery a law of diminishing returns is evident in fistula repair. Although repeat operations are certainly justified, the success rate decreases progressively with increasing numbers of previous unsuccessful procedures. Unfortunately, individual surgical series are rarely large enough for this fact to be evident. In one series of 2484 largely obstetric fistulas, the success rate fell from 81% for first procedures to 65% for those requiring two or more procedures.[2]

Postfistula stress incontinence

The occurrence of stress incontinence in patients following successful repair of obstetric VVF is well known, and estimated to range from 10% to 12%. Waaldijk documented the occurrence of postfistula stress incontinence in fistulas of varying type in a Nigerian population, describing 1% incidence where there was no sphincter involvement in the fistula, 13% incidence where there was sphincter involvement without tissue loss, and 16% incidence where there was both sphincter involvement and tissue loss.[1] Because of concern over the possible incidence of functional abnormalities of the lower urinary tract following fistula repair in the UK and the need to appropriately counsel patients prior to repair, Hilton undertook a series of urodynamic investigations in 30 patients with urogenital fistulas prior to repair.[9] Only one in six had normal findings, with 47% showing urodynamic stress incontinence, 40% detrusor instability, and 50% voiding dysfunction; those with urethral or bladder neck fistulas had the highest incidence of abnormality. Following repair of the fistulas in this small group of patients, stress incontinence persisted in 11%, and detrusor overactivity in 50% of those urethral fistula patients who had had these diagnoses prior to repair. In another series of urodynamic investigations in 30 women with persistent incontinence following anatomically successful repair of obstetric fistulas from Ethiopia, 31% had urodynamic stress incontinence, 4% detrusor overactivity, and 20% mixed incontinence.[42] In a long-term 'quality of life' follow-up of previously treated fistula patients in the UK, whilst seriously bothersome residual urinary symptoms were most uncommon, mildly bothersome symptoms were reported by 75% of patients.[43] Whilst the extrapolation of outcomes from patients with surgical fistulas in the UK to those with obstetric fistulas in the developing world might be questioned, it is unlikely that functional outcomes in the latter group would be better.

There have been a number of recent reports describing techniques for the management of post-fistula repair stress incontinence. These range from the relatively minimally invasive peri-urethral injection of autologous fat,[44] to a combined retropubic urethrolysis, fascial sling, and omental graft.[45] Most recently Browning has reported on the use of a sling procedure at the time of fistula for prophylaxis against postoperative stress incontinence, in women felt to be at particular risk for this complication.[46]

Subsequent pregnancy

Although many patients with obstetric VVF experience amenorrhea for 2 years or more after the causative pregnancy,[2] hypothalamic function often returns to normal immediately after successful repair if tissue loss is not great, and fertility may be relatively normal. The need for cesarean section in any subsequent pregnancy has been emphasized.[47] Kelly, however, reported 33 patients who became pregnant within 1 year of fistula repair, 12 of whom were delivered vaginally without damage to the repair.[48] The criteria he used for attempting vaginal delivery were that the fistula arose from a non-recurring cause (i.e. malpresentation as opposed to absolute pelvic contraction), that an interposition graft had been utilized in the repair, and that the labor is conducted under skilled supervision in hospital.

National and international strategies

The World Health Organization estimates that approximately 500,000 maternal deaths occur each year worldwide. It is clear that the prevalence of obstetric fistulas and maternal mortality rates are closely related. Indeed, one might consider the VVF patient as being the 'near miss' maternal death. In recognition of this fact, WHO established, through their 'Safe Motherhood Initiative', a technical working group to investigate the problems of prevention and management of obstetric fistulas. The recommendations from this working group included the extension of antenatal and intrapartum care, the transfer of women in prolonged labor for delivery by skilled personnel, the identification of areas where fistulas are still prevalent, so that resources could be mobilized to deal with fistulas more effectively, and the creation of specialized centers for management, training and research.[49]

Certainly obstetric fistulas would disappear if early intervention in obstructed labor were available and acceptable throughout the world. It has been pointed out, however, that this would require the establishment of some 75,000 obstetric units throughout Africa.[50] In addition to the provision of services for fistula management however, the achievement of the WHO's aims and recommendations is critically dependent on major social changes in areas where fistulas are most prevalent. These changes must include government recognition of fistulas as a major public health concern, improvement in the status of women in society, the extension of primary education for girls, deferment of marriage and childbearing, the abolition of female genital mutilation, improved nutritional status and contraceptive services, and affordable, accessible and acceptable services for all pregnant women.[51] These socio-political issues were the main concerns of an international workshop on fistula management and prevention in Abuja.[52]

REFERENCES

1. Waaldijk K. *The Surgical Management of Bladder Fistula in 775 Women in Northern Nigeria.* [MD thesis]: Amsterdam, 1989.
2. Hilton P, Ward A. Epidemiological and surgical aspects of urogenital fistulae: a review of 25 years experience in south-east Nigeria. *Int Urogynecol J Pelvic Floor Dysfunct* 1998;9:189–94.
3. Danso K, Martey J, Wall L, Elkins T. The epidemiology of genitourinary fistulae in Kumasi, Ghana, 1977–1992. *Int Urogynecol J Pelvic Floor Dysfunct* 1996;7(3):117–20.
4. Hilton P. Obstetric fistulae. In: Cardozo L, Staskin D, eds. *Textbook of Female Urology and Urogynaecology.* London: Isis Medical Media Ltd, 2001:711–19.
5. Hilton P. Surgical fistulae. In: Cardozo L, Staskin D, eds. *Textbook of Female Urology and Urogynaecology.* London: Isis Medical Media Ltd, 2001:691–709.
6. Tahzib F. Epidemiological determinants of vesicovaginal fistulas. *Br J Obstet Gynaecol* 1983;90:387–91.
7. Tahzib F. Vesicovaginal fistula in Nigerian children. *Lancet* 1985; 2:1291–3.
8. Onolemhemhen DO, Ekwempu CC. An investigation of sociomedical risk factors associated with vaginal fistula in northern Nigeria. *Women Health* 1999;28(3):103–16.
9. Hilton P. The urodynamic findings in patients with urogenital fistulae. *Br J Urol* 1998;81:539–42.
10. Langkilde NC, Pless TK, Lundbeck F, Nerstrom B. Surgical repair of vesicovaginal fistulae – a ten-year retrospective study. *Scand J Urol Nephrol* 1999;33(2):100–103.
11. Abbo A. New trends in the operative management of urinary fistulae. *Sudan Med J* 1975;13:126–32.
12. Hamlin R, Nicholson E. Experiences in the treatment of 600 vaginal fistulas and in the management of 80 labours which have followed the repair of these injuries. *Ethiop Med J* 1966;4:189–92.
13. Barnaud P, Veillard J, Richard J, *et al.* Les fistulas vesico-vaginales Africanes. *Med Trop* 1980;40:389–401.
14. Waaldijk K. The immediate surgical management of fresh obstetric fistulas with catheter and/or early closure. *Int J Gynaecol Obstet* 1994;45:11–16.
15. Averette HE, Nguyen HN, Donato DM, *et al.* Radical hysterectomy for invasive cervical cancer. A 25-year prospective experience with the Miami technique. *Cancer* 1993;71:1422–37.
16. Emmert C, Köhler U. Management of genital fistulas in patients with cervical cancer. *Arch Gynecol Obstet* 1996;259:19–24.
17. White A, Buchsbaum H, Blythe J, Lifshitz S. Use of the bulbocavernosus muscle (Martius procedure) for repair of radiation-induced rectovaginal fistulas. *Obstet Gynecol* 1982;60(1):114–18.
18. Bladou F, Houvenaeghel G, Delpero JR, Guerinel G. Incidence and management of major urinary complications after pelvic exenteration for gynecological malignancies. *J Surg Oncol* 1995;58:91–6.
19. Raghavaiah N. Double-dye test to diagnose various types of vaginal fistulas. *J Urol* 1974;112:811–12.
20. Gorrea A, Zuazu F, Sanchis MA, Jimenez-Cruz JF. Spontaneous healing of uretero-vesico-vaginal fistulas. *Eur Urol* 1985;11(5): 341–3.
21. Davits R, Miranda S. Conservative treatment of vesico-vaginal fistulas by bladder drainage alone. *Br J Urol* 1991;68:155–6.
22. Waaldijk K. Immediate indwelling bladder catheterisation at postpartum urine leakage – personal experience of 1200 patients. *Trop Doct* 1997;27:227–8.
23. Tomlinson AJ, Thornton JG. A randomised controlled trial of antibiotic prophylaxis for vesico-vaginal fistula repair. *Br J Obstet Gynaecol* 1998;105:397–9.
24. Leng WW, Amundsen CL, McGuire EJ. Management of female genitourinary fistulas: transvesical or transvaginal approach? *J Urol* 1998;160(6 Pt 1):1995–9.
25. Nesrallah LJ, Srougi M, Gittes RF. The O'Conor technique: the gold standard for supratrigonal vesicovaginal fistula repair. *J Urol* 1999;161(2):566–8.
26. Iselin CE, Aslan P, Webster GD. Transvaginal repair of vesicovaginal fistulas after hysterectomy by vaginal cuff excision. *J Urol* 1998;160:728–30.
27. Martius H. Die operative Wiederherstellung der vollkommen fehlenden Harnrohre und des Schiessmuskels derselben. *Zentralbl Gynakol* 1928;52:480.
28. Ingelman-Sundberg A. Surgical treatment of urinary fistulae. *Zentralbl Gynakol* 1978;100(20):1281–94.
29. Hamlin R, Nicholson E. Reconstruction of urethra totally destroyed in labour. *Br Med J* 1969;2:147–50.
30. Bruce RG, El-Galley RES, Galloway NTM. Use of rectus abdominis muscle flap for the treatment of complex and refractory urethrovaginal fistulas. *J Urol* 2000;163:1212–15.
31. Turner-Warwick R. The use of the omental pedicle graft in urinary tract reconstruction. *J Urol* 1976;116:341–7.
32. Kiricuta I, Goldstein A. The repair of extensive vesicovaginal fistulas with pedicled omentum: a review of 27 cases. *J Urol* 1972;108:724–7.
33. Jonas U, Petri E. Genitourinary fistulae. In: Stanton S, ed. *Clinical Gynecologic Urology.* St Louis, MO: CV Mosby, 1984:238–55.
34. Hurley LJ, Previte SR. Vaginal pedicled flap for closure of vesicovaginal fistula. *Urology* 2000;56(5):856.
35. Venema PL. Closing a vesico-vaginal fistula with a free bladder mucosal graft [Dutch]. Ned Tijdschr Urol 2001;9(3):68–9.
36. Evans DH, Madjar S, Politano VA, Bejany DE, Lynne CM, Gousse AE. Interposition flaps in transabdominal vesicovaginal fistula repairs: are they really necessary? *Urology* 2001;57(4):670–4.
37. Rangnekar NP, Imdad AN, Kaul SA, Pathak HR. Role of the Martius procedure in the management of urinary-vaginal fistulas. *J Am Coll Surg* 2000;191:259–63.
38. Hilton P. Debate: Post-operative urogenital fistulae are best managed by Gynaecologists in specialist centres. *Br J Urol* 1997;80(Suppl 1):35–42.
39. Sims J. On the treatment of vesico-vaginal fistula. *Am J Med Sci* 1852;XXIII:59–82.
40. Lawson J. Vesical fistulae into the vaginal vault. *Br J Urol* 1972;44:623–31.
41. Chassar Moir J. *The Vesico-vaginal Fistula*, 2nd edn. London: Bailliere, 1967.
42. Murray C, Goh JT, Fynes M, Carey MP. Urinary and faecal incontinence following delayed primary repair of obstetric genital fistula. *BJOG* 2002;109(7):828–32.
43. Dolan L, Dixon W, Hilton P. Quality of life and urodynamic abnormality in patients following urogenital fistula repair. *Int Urogynecol J Pelvic Floor Dysfunct* 2003;14(abstract):S42.
44. Hilton P, Ward A, Molloy M, Umana O. Periurethral injection of autologous fat for the treatment of post-fistula repair stress incontinence: a preliminary report. *Int Urogynecol J Pelvic Floor Dysfunct* 1998;9:118–21.

45. Carey MP, Goh JT, Fynes MM, Murray CJ. Stress urinary incontinence after delayed primary closure of genitourinary fistula: a technique for surgical management. *Am J Obstet Gynecol* 2002;186(5):948–53.
46. Browning A. Prevention of residual urinary incontinence following successful repair of obstetric vesico-vaginal fistula using a fibro-muscular sling. *BJOG Int J Obstet Gynaecol* 2004;111(4): 357–361.
47. Lawson J. The management of genito-urinary fistulae. *Clin Obstet Gynaecol* 1978;6:209–36.
48. Kelly J. Vesicovaginal fistulae. *Br J Urol* 1979;51:208–10.
49. World Health Organization. *The Prevention and Treatment of Obstetric Fistulae: A Report of a Technical Working Group.* Geneva: WHO, 1989.
50. Waaldijk K. *Evaluation Report XIV on VVF Projects in Northern Nigeria and Niger.* Katsina, Nigeria: Babbar Ruga Fistula Hospital, 1998.
51. Hilton P. Sims to SMIS – an historical perspective on vesico-vaginal fistulae. In: *The Yearbook of the RCOG,* 1994. London: RCOG, 1995:7–16.
52. Ejembi C. Communique on the International Workshop on Vesico-vaginal Fistula: A Persisting Threat to Womanhood. Kano: Nigerian National Taskforce of Vesico-vaginal Fistula, 1998.

202 Traditional birth attendant training

P. Buekens

Introduction

The training of traditional birth attendants (TBAs) was a priority strategy to reduce maternal and newborn mortality and morbidity in the late 1970s and throughout the 1980s, but its effectiveness is now questioned by many. Yet, little scientific evidence is available to support the enthusiasm of the past and the criticisms of today.[1] In many developing countries, the majority of the deliveries are not performed by health professionals.[2] Training TBAs seems thus a logical thing to do.

The term 'TBA' was coined by the international health development community and includes the vast array of birth attendants throughout the world who have not received formal Western medical training.[3] A shortcoming of the term is that it gives the impression that TBAs are one unified body of birth attendants and that health professionals have a choice of whether or not to collaborate with them. In fact, TBAs are quite heterogeneous and play such a central role in many societies that ignoring them does not seem realistic.

The role of TBAs varies across communities. In some cultures, TBAs only attend a few deliveries a year among family members, while in others they have a broader role.[1] On average, 24% of births were attended by TBAs in countries where data from 1995–2002 Demographic and Health Surveys were available, but the frequency varied from less than 1% to over 90%.[4] In most countries, TBAs do not provide prenatal care, with the exception of Guatemala, Honduras and Mexico.[5,6]

TBAs are an important source of social and cultural support to women, and the role of TBAs in providing support during childbirth is potentially important.[1] Support provided by TBAs could be compared with the support provided by 'doulas' or other accompanying persons during labor. A meta-analysis of 15 randomized trials concluded that continuous support for women during childbirth was associated with a reduction in the length of labor, better Apgar scores, increased women's satisfaction and increased breast feeding at 4–6 weeks.[7]

Clean delivery kits

The goal of TBA training is to improve each individual's skills and to strengthen links within the health care system.[1] Training programs put emphasis on infection prevention and include such approaches as the promotion of the 'three cleans' (Table 202.1) and the provision of clean delivery kits (CDKs).[8,9] CDKs generally include soap, a plastic sheet (1 × 1 m), a new razor blade and clean cord ties. A CDK that is packed in a sturdy plastic bag and includes pictorial instructions is available from UNFPA Procurement Services, and the kits can be produced locally as well (Figure 202.1).[8,9] In Nepal, the rate of cord infections found in deliveries that utilized CDKs was less than half of the infection rate among non-users who did not use a new or boiled razor blade and a clean cutting surface.[10] However, more than 90% of non-users did in fact use a new or boiled blade to cut the cord. Another study from Nepal suggests that CDKs have a limited influence on hygiene practices, as the majority of the respondents were not aware that the soap provided in the kit was intended for washing their hands during the delivery rather than for bathing the infant after delivery.[11] In rural Bangladesh, training TBAs in clean delivery did not prevent postpartum infection.[12] Furthermore, although a clean delivery should decrease the risk of maternal and neonatal tetanus, immunization with tetanus toxoid is overwhelmingly superior.[1]

Table 202.1 'Three cleans' and clean delivery kits[8,9]

'Three cleans'	clean delivery kit
1. Clean hands	Soap
2. Clean delivery surface	Plastic sheet
3. Clean cord cutting	New razor blade
	Clean cord ties

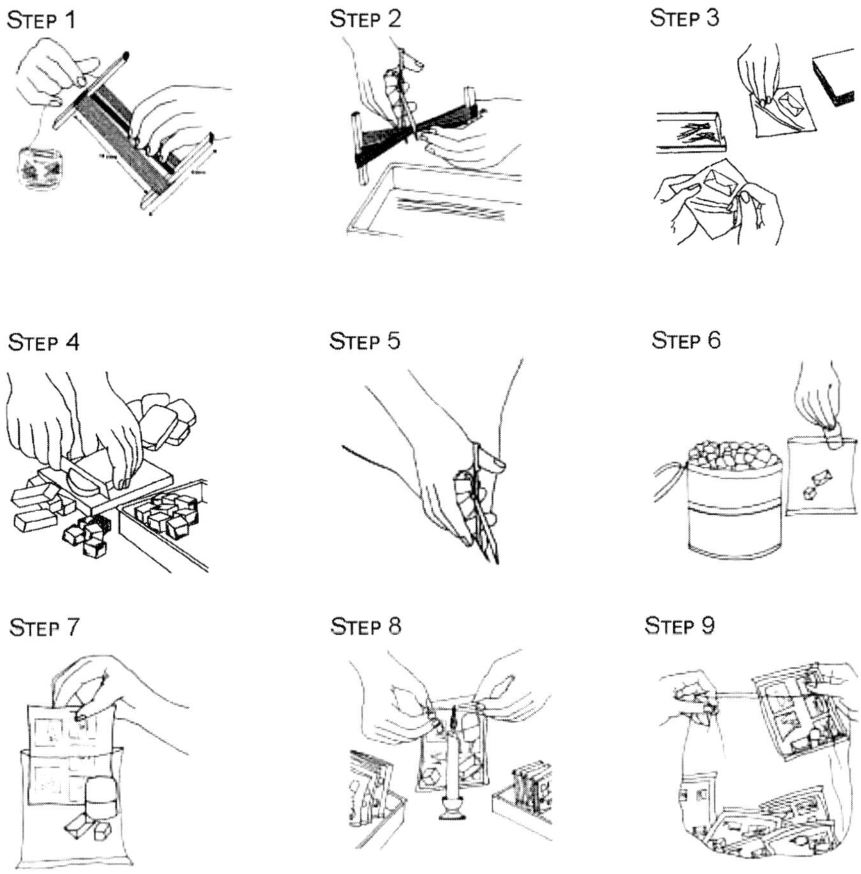

Figure 202.1 Assembly of clean delivery kit components. Figure courtesy of Program for Appropriate Technology in Health.[9] Step 1: Measuring string for cord ties; Step 2: Cutting string; Step 3: Wrapping cord ties and razor blade into paper packet; Step 4: Cutting soap pieces; Step 5: Cutting sheets of papers into squares; Step 6: Placing wrapped components into kit plastic bag; Step 7: Placing the pictorial instruction sheet into kit plastic bag; Step 8: Sealing kit plastic bag with candle flame; Step 9: Placing delivery kits in large plastic bags for storage.

Prevention and treatment of postpartum hemorrhage

Postpartum hemorrhage is a major cause of maternal mortality, and TBAs should refer bleeding women to an essential obstetric care facility.[1] Unfortunately, timely referrals are not always feasible, as transportation is difficult to obtain and essential obstetric care facilities are often unavailable. This is a major limitation in the role of TBAs. Early suckling and nipple stimulation have been proposed as simple alternatives to uterotonics, but a trial randomizing 23 TBAs to an early suckling intervention group and 26 TBAs to a control group did not show any difference in blood loss between the groups.[13] One alternative currently under study is the potential postpartum use of misoprostol.[14–16] A prostaglandin E_1 analog with strong uterotonic effects, misoprostol can be taken orally or administered rectally, does not require refrigeration and is not contraindicated for hypertensive patients.[16] However, for active management of the third stage of labor, oral misoprostol 600 μg has been shown to be less effective than injectable uterotonics, and trials comparing misoprostol vs. no uterotonics or a placebo were inconclusive.[17] Shivering, pyrexia, nausea and vomiting are common but not severe side-effects of misoprostol. Potential misuse of misoprostol during the first and second stage of labor is a concern.[18] However, a field demonstration project conducted in Indonesia suggests that self-administration of misoprostol is feasible.[15] Community health workers distributed misoprostol and counseling material to women for self-administration after delivery. Additionally, the use of misoprostol for managing postpartum hemorrhage rather than preventing it is promising and is under study.[15,16] A Tanzania study is examining the use of 1000 μg of misoprosotol administered rectally by TBAs when blood loss is greater than 500 ml.[15] It is too early to recommend making misoprostol widely available to TBAs until studies in the community show that it is both safe and effective.

Referral

A key element of TBA training should be the identification of obstetric complications and their referral. The author's experience in Burkina Faso suggests that TBAs can indeed detect complications and refer women.[19] However, a meta-analysis of 16 studies showed that the effect of TBA training on the referral of women with obstetric complications is relatively small.[4] Another meta-analysis suggested that TBAs may play a role in referring women to professional prenatal care during pregnancy.[20] The availability of an essential obstetric care unit to which the women can be referred is a necessary condition for TBAs to be effective.[1,21]

Impact on health outcomes

Evaluating the impact of TBA training on health outcomes is difficult. One of the challenges is that very large sample sizes are needed to study an impact on maternal mortality, which is a relatively rare event. Many evaluations have thus been focused on process rather than on outcome. A meta-analysis recently published by Sibley and Sipe summarized the results of 60 studies of the effectiveness of TBA training.[22,23] The data suggest that TBA training is associated with substantial improvement in TBA's 'knowledge, attitudes, behavior and advice'. There was also a small (8%) decrease in perinatal or neonatal mortality associated with training. Two studies included data on maternal mortality, and the meta-analysis concluded that there were 8% fewer deaths among women cared for or living in areas served by trained TBAs. However, the studies were not randomized controlled trials, and thus were not rigorous enough to firmly establish a causal relationship between TBA training and improved health outcomes. The results of this meta-analysis suggest that the impact of TBA training should not be expected to be large.

Conclusion

In addition to having a limited impact, TBA training programs are expensive and are difficult to sustain if not funded by international donors.[1] Thus, TBA training should not be given a high priority. While there is no single magic solution that will make pregnancy safer in developing countries, programs need to be multifaceted and improve every level of health care. As such, TBAs should not be ignored and should be trained and linked to the health system whenever possible.

Acknowledgments

The author thanks Jose Belizan, Richard Derman and Lynn Sibley for their comments and suggestions.

REFERENCES

1. Bergström S, Goodburn E. The role of traditional birth attendants in the reduction of maternal mortality. In De Brouwere V, Van Lerberghe W, eds. *Safe Motherhood Strategies: A Review of the Evidence.* Antwerp, Belgium: ITG Press, 2001:77–96.
2. Demographic and Health Surveys. http://www.measuredhs.com/. Accessed July 19, 2004.
3. Pigg SL. Acronyms and effacement: Traditional medical practitioners (TMP) in international health development. *Soc Sci Med* 1995;41:47–68.
4. Sibley L, Sipe TA, Koblinsky M. Does traditional birth attendant training improve referral of women with obstetric complications: A review of the evidence. *Soc Sci Med* 2004;59:1757–68.
5. Buekens P. Variations in provision and uptake of prenatal care. *Baillieres Clin Obstet Gynaecol* 1990;4(1):187–205.
6. Buekens P, Hernandez P, Infante C. La atención prenatal en América Latina. *Salud Publica Mex* 1990;32:673–84.
7. Hodnett ED. Caregiver support for women during childbirth. *Cochrane Database Syst Rev* 2002;1:CD000199.
8. UNICEF, WHO, UNFPA. *Maternal and Neonatal Tetanus Elimination by 2005. Strategies for Achieving and Maintaining Elimination.* Geneva, Switzerland: World Health Organization, 2000.
9. *Basic Delivery Kit Guide.* Seattle, WA: PATH, 2001.
10. Tsu V. *Nepal Clean Home Delivery Kit. Evaluation of the Health Impact.* Seattle, WA: PATH, 2000.
11. Beun M, Wood S. Acceptability and use of clean home delivery kits in Nepal: A qualitative study. *J Health Popul Nutr* 2003;21:367–73.
12. Goodburn EA, Chowdhury M, Gazi R, Marshall T, Graham W. Training traditional birth attendants in clean delivery does not prevent postpartum infection. *Health Policy Plan* 2000;15: 394–9.
13. Bullough CH, Msuku RS, Karonde L. Early suckling and postpartum hemorrhage: Controlled trial in deliveries by traditional birth attendants. *Lancet* 1989;2:522–5.
14. Derman R, Kodakany B. Misoprostol use for prevention of postpartum hemorrhage. Global Network for Women's and Children's Health Research. http://gn.rti.org. Accessed July 19, 2004.
15. Miller S, Lester F, Hensleigh P. Prevention and treatment of postpartum hemorrhage: New advances for low-resource setting. *J Midwifery Womens Health* 2004;49:283–92.
16. Tsu V, Langer A, Aldrich T. Postpartum hemorrhage in developing countries: Is the public health community using the right tools? *Int J Gynecol Obstet* 2004;85(Suppl 1):S42–51.
17. Gulmezoglu AM, Forna F, Villar J, Hofmeyr GJ. Prostaglandins for prevention of postpartum hemorrhage. *Cochrane Database Syst Rev* 2002;2:CD000494.
18. Hofmeyr GJ. Obstructed labor: Using better technologies to reduce mortality. *Int J Gynecol Obstet* 2004;85(Suppl 1):S62–72.
19. Wollast E, Renard F, Vandenbussche P, Buekens P. Detecting maternal morbidity and mortality by traditional birth attendants in Burkina Faso. *Health Policy Plan* 1993;8:161–8.
20. Sibley L, Sipe TA, Koblinsky M. Does traditional birth attendant training increase use of antenatal care? A review of the evidence. *J Midwifery Womens Health* 2004;49:298–305.
21. Maine D, Akalin MZ, Chakraborty J, de Francisco A, Strong M. Why did maternal mortality decline in Matlab? *Stud Fam Planning* 1996;27:179–87.
22. Sibley LM, Sipe TA. *Traditional Birth Attendant Training Effectiveness: A Meta-Analysis.* Washington, DC: Academy for Educational Development (SARA Project), 2002.
23. Sibley L, Sipe TA. What can a meta-analysis tell us about traditional birth attendant training and pregnancy outcomes? *Midwifery* 2004;20:51–60.

203 Collaborative perinatal neonatal networking in the Eastern Mediterranean Region

K. A. Yunis, G. Mumtaz, H. Tamim and A. Adra

Introduction

Maternal and perinatal health remain major contributors to the global burden of disease, on a par with HIV, tuberculosis, and malaria. The annual global burden of neonatal deaths is estimated at about four million, 98% of which occur in the developing countries.[1] In the Eastern Mediterranean Region (EMR) maternal and perinatal conditions rank second among the leading causes of death, as they account for 8.8% of all deaths.[2] About 99% of the half million women who die annually from pregnancy or childbirth complications occur in low- and middle-income countries.[3]

While developing countries suffer from the greatest load of the world's health burden, they have the least capacity to carry out quality research and to generate nation-specific data that will allow them the identification of their own health problems and priorities.[4] The first recommendation by the Commission on Macroeconomics and Health[5] is that 'Developing countries should begin to map out a path to universal access for essential health services based on epidemiological evidence and the health priorities of the poor', stressing the importance of scientific research in identifying national priorities.

Furthermore, most developing countries lack high-quality routine statistics that provide a consistent and continuous system of assessment that constitutes the first step in planning appropriate health strategies. Poverty, the lack of health care infrastructure and the limited resources are enormous barriers faced by governments trying to implement such systems. Statistics are mostly based on models or *ad hoc* surveys, with minimal training of personnel on interpretation of findings and few follow-up interventions. The sample sizes of *ad hoc* studies are often too small to allow decentralized problem identification and planning. In such settings with fragmented care and weak government regulation and capacity, research networks are likely to be one of the few successful approaches to building an infrastructure for evidence-based decision and policy making.

The multidimensional nature of the medical field makes networking in medicine very attractive and efficient. Practice, policy, education, and research are different facets of the domain. As a result, the relationships between these factors cannot be ignored and cannot be considered as separate items. The combination of resources from all dimensions and the collaboration of all persons within these dimensions are necessary to accomplish strength and productivity.

International experience has proven that building up regional networks among academic, research and health care institutions allows an accurate and continuous assessment of the population health status and is an efficient approach to respond to growing economic constraints faced by developing countries. Identification of common problems, pooling of resources and addressing solutions collectively increase the problem-solving potential of these countries. These South–South alliances contribute significantly to capacity building and are the basis for sustainable development. In this chapter, we present the experience of a perinatal neonatal network established in Lebanon as a model for a successful approach to research in the EMR.

Defining networks

A network is an infrastructure where individuals, institutions or organizations that have similar issues, aspirations or problems join their efforts to collaborate, share information and expertise, find solutions and as a result improve the quality of their services to reach higher standards in their quest for excellence. Flexibility and collaboration alongside with having a systematic structure and a long-term perspective are crucial concepts in insuring a network's scientific self-sufficiency and, most importantly, sustainablitiy.[6]

At the core of their activities, networks maintain databases. Collaborative databases provide a rich and functional resource for analysis and constitute a solid infrastructure to assess the impact of maternal and neonatal health care over time, carry out intervention programs aiming at improving perinatal health and health care, conduct multicenter randomized controlled research trials, efficiently practice continuous quality improvement, help member institutions reach national and international accreditation standards and most importantly, it helps in defining and implementing national health care policies based on accurate primary data.

Examples of existing networks in the world

Networking in research is not a novel approach. It has been applied in both developed and developing parts of the world and has proven successful. Examples of perinatal neonatal networks include the Vermont Oxford Neonatal Network (VON) which includes over 450 neonatal intensive care units across the world, the Latin American Center for Perinatology and Human development (CLAP) whose database covers information on more than one million births from hospitals in 19 Latin American and Caribbean countries and The National Institute of Child Health and Human Development (NICHD) Neonatal Research Network in the USA specialized in conducting clinical trials. The European Neonatal Network (Euro Neo Net) is a similar European-level initiative whose database was developed to meet the specific needs of the very-low-birthweight infants.

Introducing the National Collaborative Perinatal Neonatal Network

Lebanon, with relatively high fertility and perinatal mortality rates is in great need for vital and routine health statistics. Unfortunately similar to other developing countries, many obstacles, related mainly to the lack of a structured health care system and a restricted budget the government is allocating for scientific research, are impeding the way to generating accurate health statistics and to setting national priorities and programs. These problems are widespread in the region; the latest United Nations Development Programme (UNDP) Arab Human Development report identifies the region as suffering from a paucity of investment in research and information gathering.[7]

In such an environment, the National Collaborative Perinatal Neonatal Network (NCPNN) was created in 1998 by a group of investigators working in different private health care institutions in Beirut. Partially funded by grants from the World Health Organization (WHO), the Network is a voluntary collaborative effort of professionals from different disciplines including pediatrics, obstetrics, family medicine, nursing, epidemiology and public health. The primary objective of the NCPNN is to improve the health of the pregnant woman and her offspring through scientific research and the establishment of an integrated maternal and perinatal neonatal database.

Mission statement of the Network: The Network is a non-profit collaboration created to conduct scientific research, gather scientific and sociodemographic data, and maintain the database regarding the quality, utilization, costs, outcomes and effectiveness of medical treatments and health care practices as related to perinatal and neonatal elements.

Methodology of the NCPNN

Data covering all deliveries are collected prospectively at participating health care centers in the capital Beirut and its suburbs. With so far nine member hospitals in Beirut, the NCPNN has achieved a good coverage of the population of pregnant women and their newborns in the capital and its suburbs where 35% of the Lebanese population resides. The NCPNN is currently expanding to the rural more underprivileged areas of Lebanon where maternal and child health problems are of greater magnitude. Eight centers in different areas of Lebanon have joined the network so far and efforts are made in planning the regional expansion of the network to neighboring countries. The NCPNN database gathers data on over 60,000 newborns and their mothers.

Currently, the coordinating center of the NCPNN lies at the American University of Beirut Medical Center. It is composed of a project director (neonatologist), three co-investigators (a PhD epidemiologist and biostatistician and a family medicine professor and an obstetrician), one network coordinator, two data analysts (MSc Epidemiology and Biostatistics), five research assistants and several data entry persons. Obstetricians working in the different network centers are also close collaborators and key investigators in the network's integrated activities. A primary investigator (attending physician) is assigned in each member hospital to supervise the implementation of the system. Meetings are held on regular basis with the investigators for updates and discussions of current and future matters pertaining to the network. Data are collected daily at each participating hospital by a local nurse, midwife or research assistant. Data collectors undergo an extensive training on the questionnaire and on retrieval of the data from the medical charts of the mother and newborn. Training is done by the network coordinator in the locals of the participating hospital to insure applicability to the available medical charts. Two standardized instruments have been developed: one for the Normal Nursery and one more detailed version for the Neonatal Intensive Care Unit. These questionnaires are modified and updated as the need arises, depending on observations and experiences from current collection. The collected data is transported at the end of each month to the coordinating center where it is entered into the computerized database. Continuous auditing of data collection and entry is performed. The data are highly protected and access to the data is restricted to insure confidentiality of both patients and providers. One general annual report covering data on the entire network and individual reports for each center are generated and distributed to the member hospitals. Newsletters are issued and distributed periodically.

Projects by the NCPNN

In addition to the ongoing database, the NCPNN carried on several research projects that took advantage from the existing database for the identification of study objectives, data collection, access to medical records from hospitals, identification of cases and many other logistics. One example is the 'The study on morbidity and mortality among newborn babies, infants and under 5-year-old children in Greater Beirut' also known as the follow-up (FUP) study. This was the first cohort study of its kind in the region whereby 1320 newborns were recruited and followed up prospectively with the collaboration of over 117 pediatricians. The NCPNN has completed the first phase of the study, which is the first year of life follow-up.

The FUP study met its primary objective in identifying the causes of morbidity and mortality during the first year of life in our population. Among all morbidity outcomes, the overall infection rate till the age of 15 months was the highest. Of the entire cohort, 71.8% have had at least one infection episode during their first year of life. Upper respiratory tract infections were the most common type of infections (49.9%). High prevalence of otitis and bronchiolitis was also noted (26.5% and 20.1%, respectively). On the contrary, the cumulative hospital readmission rate during the first year of life was 15%, being highest at the age of 1–2 months. The high rate of antibiotic use identified in the analysis warrants further research into the reasons behind such a high rate and the extent of accompanying antibiotic resistance. The rate of antibiotic use during the first year was over 42%. Although not recommended during the first months of life, 4.3% of the infants received oral antibiotics at the age of 1–2 months.

In addition to morbidity patterns, the FUP study looked into behavioral and preventive practices such as breast feeding, vaccination patterns, car seat use and others. Low breast feeding rates at 4 months were noticed in our sample (24.7%) and a negative correlation was found between breast feeding and socioeconomic status. On the contrary, by the end of the first year of life, there was an almost complete coverage for the three doses of polio, diphtheria-tetanus-pertussis (DTP), and hemophilus influenza (Hib) vaccines, with a noticeable decrease in the third dose (87.7%) of Hib vaccination rate. The vast majority of the children received the cellular type of DTP. Although WHO recommends the exclusive use of oral poliovirus vaccine, the injectable form of polio was administered to more than 65.5% of the children.

The above-mentioned results have been published in the monograph summarizing results of the first year of life FUP[8] and that was distributed during the national dissemination workshop held in Beirut in February 2004. Results derived from the study carry several implications for further analysis, research and interventions.

Another project by the NCPNN is 'Group B streptococcal colonization of pregnant women and neonates in Beirut'. This is the first study conducted in Lebanon, whereby the prevalence of group B streptococcus (GBS) and its risk of infection are determined in attempt to assess the magnitude of the problem in our population. The study is still ongoing. However, preliminary results indicate relatively high rates of GBS colonization among pregnant women and among newborns. Predictors of GBS colonization are also looked at. The generated data would thus provide the guidelines for recommending and implementing appropriate policies regarding screening and prevention of neonatal GBS disease in the country.

Currently, the NCPNN is in the data collection phase of a study entitled 'Consanguinity and congenital malformations: a study of prevalence and association in the Lebanese population'. This projects looks into the health consequences of consanguinity. Consanguinity has been associated with increased morbidity and mortality in offsprings of consanguineous parents. Research by the NCPNN has already found significant association between consanguinity and congenital health disease,[9] apnea of prematurity[10] and intrauterine growth restriction (unpublished data, Mumtaz G, Tamim H, Khawaja M *et al.*)[11] in Beirut. Despite the adverse health consequences of consanguineous marriages, this practice is still common in the Lebanese community. The NCPNN data indicates a consanguinity rate of 12.8% in the Capital Beirut and its suburbs. Preliminary analyses on the data collected from the newly recruited hospitals in the rural areas shows significantly higher rates reaching up to 40% in some remote areas of Lebanon. The inclusion, in the sample, of hospitals located outside the capital Beirut, including the most underprivileged areas of the country, represents indeed a major feature of this study, as local research is usually confined to the capital Beirut. Results of this project will provide solid grounds for public health programs concerning the implications of consanguinity.

Achievements of the NCPNN

Research conducted by the NCPNN has identified health and health care problems and as such, has set the grounds for conducting intervention studies of public health significance. One of the most important observations is the high cesarean-section rate in most member centers of the NCPNN, reaching more than 30% in some hospitals. In addition to other adverse outcomes identified in the literature, a significant double-fold risk of hyaline membrane disease was found in babies delivered via cesarean route in the NCPNN newborn population.[12] Accordingly, the NCPNN is about to start a multicenter intervention study based on the implementation of practice guidelines and on auditing, in an attempt to reduce the cesarean-section rate.

Among the other major issues that pertain to the pregnant women, the indiscriminate use of oxytocin, the high rate of general anesthesia administered during cesarean delivery, postpartum depression and cigarette and/or hubble-bubble smoking during pregnancy were some of the major concerns identified. The NCPNN has also identified several problems that pertain to the care of the newborn, such as nosocomial infections, the abuse of antibiotics during the first months of life and the lack of long-term follow-up for premature infants.

In the absence of any published birthweight for gestational age growth charts for the Lebanese newborn population, a major achievement by the NCPNN was the development of its own fetal growth charts based on the NCPNN newborn population.[13] In Lebanon, the absence of a governmental entity responsible for the production and dissemination of perinatal health statistics has precluded data collection on a large scale and the generation of national standards for intrauterine growth. The availability of the NCPNN database allowed the development of our own population fetal growth charts based on 24,767 single live births delivered between 28 and 42 weeks of gestation. To our knowledge, this is the first attempt at devising intrauterine growth standards that are specific to a developing country in the EMR and thus they are useful tools for assessing the health of newborn infants delivered at sea level in the urban areas of Lebanon and other countries having a similar socioeconomic profile.

From our experience at the NCPNN, the establishment of research networks of collaborative nature has a considerable impact on the health care system. The NCPNN annual reports presented to each of the participating hospitals, and the NCPNN newsletters distributed to pediatricians, nurses, hospital administrators, and other health care providers have been instrumental in the ongoing self-evaluation and thus improvement of hospital services and pediatricians' practices. Furthermore, there has been a steady improvement in medical records documentation at the participating hospitals as per NCPNN recommendations. Some hospitals have even incorporated a questionnaire in their medical charts similar to that of the NCPNN. The NCPNN has also played a role in educating women about health issues related to the different stages of pregnancy such as breast feeding, postpartum follow-up, pap smear performance and newborn vaccination.

NCPNN, the future

So far, the main achievements of the NCPNN were in the capital Beirut where the network was created and maintained for the past few years. During the past two years, the NCPNN has initiated its local expansion in the different regions of Lebanon and new health centers have already joined the network successfully. The NCPNN near objectives are the consolidation of the perinatal care system in Lebanon, with more centers from the rural underprivileged areas joining the network, so as to insure a national coverage of the Lebanese population. However, the regional expansion of the network to neighboring countries remains the primary objective of the NCPNN. The NCPNN infrastructure provides a solid base for the network to be a model for a successful approach to medicine and public health research in these countries that share similar population characteristics, similar environmental and geographical features as well as similar challenges.

Consolidation and expansion of the network will not be feasible without lesson-learning from other multinational networks (e.g. CLAP) and links with governmental and international agencies, the network is anticipating to collaborate with. In that respect, the NCPNN is planning to initiate ties with professional/institutions having expertise in networking methodology such as the National Institute of Child Health neonatal network and Development and the Vermont-Oxford network. These North–South alliances will help strengthening the research capacity of the network member countries by providing expertise and knowledge. In addition, the NCPNN anticipates establishing links with regional groupings such as Pediatric and Obstetric Societies, with academic or research institutions that can be of help in issues of analysis and with professionals with expertise in the field of perinatal and neonatal network as well as in electronic data management and other technicalities.

Conclusion

The NCPNN has pioneered a unique system/model in Lebanon and the region. With over 88% of the deliveries in Lebanon occurring in hospitals,[14] hospital-based networks are effective and insure a good coverage of the population of pregnant women. However, financial constraints and the unavailability of adequate funding for planning and organizing have been the major limitation to the rapid expansion of the NCPNN in Lebanon and other neighboring countries. In developing countries with a low level of expenditure on health research, the input of the private sector (academic institutions, non-governmental agencies and private hospitals) is crucial. Inter- and intra-organizational arrangements, as well as partnership and collaboration among professionals can provide such settings with a productive, reliable and sustainable model/system where epidemiological evidence is gathered, the health priorities of the population under study are set and effective interventions are designed.

Funding remains the major challenge for the sustainability and evolution of such systems, but experience with this voluntary approach to date and projected estimates of the costs per patient entered in the database suggest that the anticipated cost is affordable in the settings concerned, making the proposed system appealing for governments to support and collaborate with.

REFERENCES

1. Troedsson H, Martines J. Introduction to the meeting "Perinatal and Neonatal Health Intervention Research". *J Perinatol* 2002; 22(Suppl 2):S5.
2. Mathers C, Stein C, Ma Fat D, *et al. Global Burden of Disease: Version 2, Methods and Results.* Geneva: World Health Organization, 2002.
3. Jha P, Mills A, Hanson K, *et al.* Improving the health of the Global Poor. *Science* 2002;295:2036–9.
4. Nchinda T. Research capacity strengthening in the South. *Soc Sci Med* 2002;54:1699–711.
5. World Health Organization. *Investing in Health: A Summary of the Findings of the Commission on Macroeconomics and Health.* Geneva: World Health Organization, 8.
6. Langthaler M for the Austrian Development Cooperation. *Networking and Capacity Development in Developing Countries: Reflections after the Annual Conferences of the European Association for International Education,* Austrian Development Corporation, Vienna, 2003.
7. UNDP. *Arab Human Development Report.* http://www.undp/rbas/ahdr/english2003.html UNDP, 2003.
8. National Collaborative Perinatal Neonatal Network. A Study on Morbidity and Mortality among Newborn Babies, Infants and under Five year old Children in Greater Beirut – Lebanon: The first year of life. National Collaborative Perinatal Neonatal Network, 2004.
9. Nabulsi MM, Tamim H, Sabbagh M, *et al.* Parental consanguinity and congenital heart malformations in a developing country. *Am J Med Genet* 2003;116A(4):342–7.
10. Tamim H, Khogali M, Beydoun H, *et al.* Consanguinity and apnea of prematurity. *Am J Epidemiol* 2003;158(10):942–6.
11. Mumtaz G, Tamim H, Khawaja M, *et al.* Consanguinity, a risk factor for small-for-gestational age in the affluent community of a low–middle income country. Submitted for publication, 2005.
12. Beydoun H, Yunis KA, Khogali M, *et al.* Caesarean route of delivery and hyaline membrane disease: A hospital-based case–control study in Greater Beirut. *Paediatr Perinat Epidemiol* 2003; 17(4):363–8.
13. Yunis K, Khawaja M, Beydoun H, *et al.* Intrauterine growth standards in a developing country: A study of single live births at 28 to 42 weeks' gestation. Provisional acceptance, Paediatric and Perinatal Epidemiology, 2006.
14. Ministry of Public Health. *Maternal and Child Health Survey.* Done as part of the Pan Arab Project for Child Development. Ministry of Public Health, Lebanon, 1998.

204 Perinatal genetics: preliminary experience from a developing country

P. Zalloua and A. Adra

Introduction

Being located in the Eastern Mediterranean Basin, Lebanon has been a crossroads between Europe, Asia and Africa, allowing the settlement and intermingling of successive different ethnic groups throughout history. Consequently, a melting pot of over three million people comprising 17 religious groups resides in Lebanon, contributing to its particular genetic heterogeneity. Intercommunity marriages are rare but consanguineous marriages exceed 25% in certain groups,[1] increasing the incidence of genetic diseases, particularly autosomal recessive diseases, such as hemoglobinopathies, cystic fibrosis (CF) and congenital sensorineural deafness.[2] For example, beta-thalassemia (β-thalassemia), an autosomal recessive disorder characterized by reduced (β^+) or absent (β^0) beta-globin chain synthesis, is the most predominant genetic defect and the most common hemoglobin disorder in Lebanon[3] and throughout the Middle East region. The challenges in diagnosis, treatment and prevention of this disease, as discussed in this chapter, are indicative of the difficulties in the management and prevention of genetic diseases in developing countries.

The early identification of genetic diseases could aid health care providers: obstetricians, neonatalogists and pediatricians, in treating the affected individuals and in providing support to their families. In addition, a comprehensive approach to early diagnosis as well as the creation of a centralized data bank concerning epidemiological characteristics could aid in planning and implementing the appropriate preventive measures.[4]

Furthermore, the comprehensive approach is never complete without the presence of genetic counselors who have a primordial role in discussing the medical aspects of the disorder, its mode of inheritance, the available diagnostic and treatment options as well as possible preventive measures.[5]

The role of genetic counseling in a developing country

Genetic counseling addresses the medical and psychosocial impact of a genetic disease on the individuals and their families who are either undergoing molecular genetic testing or who are afflicted with such a disease. Genetic counseling is an integral part of any genetic testing, screening or prevention programs and should be optimally offered before and after the genetic testing.[6]

In addition, it should be offered by medically trained clinical geneticists or trained genetic counselors.[6] These criteria are not always easy to implement in Lebanon. There are two genetic counseling programs available and they usually handle postdiagnostic counseling, often having difficulty in follow-up counseling. Education of the medical community and the population at large concerning the importance of the prediagnostic counseling is essential.

Furthermore, while one of the goals of prenatal genetic counseling and diagnosis is patient reassurance to foster reproduction in parents with genetic problems, the prenatal diagnosis of a genetic disorder may be followed by abortion of the affected fetus for many reasons, including the obvious monetary cost/benefit ratios in an economically struggling developing country.[5] A comprehensive genetic counseling program, in addition to counseling couples with a child afflicted with a genetic disease, should also support couples who have decided to abort their fetus, as these couples are at risk for depression or marital separation.[5]

The implementation of a good prevention program with one of its main axis based on prenatal diagnosis requires clear laws concerning abortion. This has to be kept in mind in any country where religion plays a major role in societal life.

Prenatal diagnosis and population screening in a developing country

Many prenatal diagnosis techniques have been incorporated into routine antenatal care in Lebanon. The request for prenatal diagnosis is most commonly made for aneuploidy testing and for disorders with onset in early childhood, associated with severe symptoms and/or with no treatment available. Individuals seeking prenatal diagnosis for a genetic disease are usually couples who already have an affected child, who have had a positive history of miscarriages or because of advanced maternal age.[5] In addition, there is a proportional relationship between the demand for genetic testing and the perceived individual and familial burden of a genetic disease.[7] The request for prenatal diagnosis may be made not only for the selective abortion of the affected fetus, but also for better preparation for an affected child.[6]

In Lebanon, prenatal diagnosis has rapidly been accepted in concordance with a changing cultural climate consisting of a reluctance to accept physical handicap and a struggle to balance the independent rights of the unborn fetus with limiting the perceived suffering of the unborn child. Prenatal diagnosis has an increasingly recognized role in confirming normality, optimizing antenatal management and providing the opportunity for intrauterine treatment.[8]

Furthermore, in order to decrease the incidence of genetic disease in Lebanon, carrier testing and prenatal diagnosis are very important.[5] Some limitations do occur and include the lack of social acceptability of genetic testing in some populations because of the fear of being labeled as 'abnormal', the lack of adequate genetic counseling and the cost-effectiveness in detecting heterozygous couples. More importantly, governmental support or subsidy for genetic testing is still limited and the cost/benefit ratio for public testing still needs to be adequately studied when considering funding carrier screening or prenatal diagnosis programs.

The new approach: preimplantation genetic diagnosis

Preimplantation genetic diagnosis (PGD) is used to detect many single gene disorders including β-thalassemia, CF and others.[9] It allows for the selection and transfers of unaffected embryos in high-risk couples[10] and thus may be used as an alternative to prenatal diagnosis in a country where abortion is not always preferred or even illegal. Furthermore, some patients undergoing *in vitro* fertilization (IVF) for male infertility factor may be CF male carriers having a congenital absence of their vas deferens. These patients could benefit from PDG.[9] Nevertheless today, because of the prohibitive cost of the test, PGD is mainly recommended for patients with a specific chromosomal abnormality.[11]

In order to perform PGD, couples need to undergo IVF.[11] To diagnose single gene defects, genetic testing centers need to biopsy one to two cells from an 8- to 10-cell embryo and use polymerase chain reaction (PCR) technology to detect the gene defect.[10] Embryo biopsy for PGD is usually performed on the morning of day 3 after egg collection. PGD only tests for one specific disease so it is important for IVF couples to consider prenatal diagnosis for other diseases.[9]

In Lebanon, efforts are being made to develop a comprehensive PGD program. The lack of advanced training in the field and the absence of adequate training in the procedure of embryo biopsy are hindering the rapid development of such a program.

Furthermore, in Lebanon and elsewhere, PGD is still considered an experimental procedure rather than a form of medical treatment or an extension of IVF, and health insurers do not have PGD as part of their coverage policy.[12] In Lebanon, patients would be required to cover the entire cost of PGD, without governmental subsidy or insurance coverage. Legislation is required to address and regulate genetic testing as well as PGD.

Thalassemia: a case study of perinatal genetics in a developing country

β-Thalassemia is an autosomal recessive disorder of hemoglobin metabolism in which there is a genetic defect in one of two or more genes which results in reduced synthesis of β-globin chains.[13] The disorder is manifested by a severe hemolytic anemia, requiring regular blood transfusions and iron chelating therapy. β-Thalassemia occurs with high frequency in areas endemic for malaria such as the Mediterranean countries, Africa and Southeast Asia, where carriers of the disease are genetically protected against malaria and therefore selectively advantaged.[14] It is the most common hemoglobin disorder in Lebanon and there is an estimated carrier frequency rate between 2% and 3%.[15] Based on the patients' registry of the 'Chronic Care Center (CCC)', a non-governmental, non-profit medico-social center that specializes in the treatment and care of patients with thalassemia and childhood diabetes, there are about 600 registered patients in Lebanon with hemoglobinopathies (86% β-thalassemia major and intermedia, 5% α-thalassemia, 4% sickle cell-thalassemia and 5% sickle cell disease).

Though non-curable, thalassemia is a preventable disease as learned from Cyprus and Sardinia, Italy. In a country like Lebanon, thalassemia prevention is desperately needed since treatment costs are a healthcare burden to a society where the health care system is private and medical expenses are very high. Prevention strategies have been implemented since

1994 and focus mainly on premarital testing, population screening and more recently prenatal diagnosis programs accompanied by public awareness and education campaigns. However, success has been limited due to a number of barriers including (1) limited individual education, (2) culture and religion obstacles mostly with regard to abortion issues, and (3) genetic test costs that are not included under any national health insurance coverage. All these factors limit the success of prevention and comprehensive screening programs.

Premarital testing

The law for premarital testing for β-thalassemia was implemented in 1994. This law helped tremendously in identifying couples at risk of having a child with this hemoglobinopathy, especially since around 25% of marriages in Lebanon are consanguineous, reaching 61% in some areas of Lebanon, as reported in a 1993 study done by the Lebanese Ministry of Public Health and UNICEF in underserved areas. Analysis of the percentage distribution of thalassemic patients from CCC by geographic area of origin (Figure 204.1), showed that the majority is from the North and South regions of Lebanon (49.7%) followed by the Bekaa region (17.7%). Since malaria was reported to have spread mostly in these marshy regions,[16,17] sparing Beirut, the central parts of the country and the mountains, these results might also explain the high prevalence of thalassemia among Muslims (Figure 204.2) who resided in these areas, corroborating the fact that malaria-infested regions exhibit the highest incidences of β-thalassemia with the Muslim Sunnis showing evidence of 16 different mutations (Figure 204.3). This high mutational heterogeneity may be partly explained by their interaction with neighboring Muslim countries for centuries, resulting in a genetic admixture.

Nevertheless, despite the goals of premarital screening, two major problems were encountered that hampered its success. On one hand, the primary laboratory screening test performed consists mainly of determining the mean corpuscular volume (MCV). Blood samples with an MCV value of $< 70\,\mu m^3$ were considered as having microcytosis and electrophoresis was then performed to determine the presence of a thalassemia trait. However, with a cut-off point of $70\,\mu m^3$ and the occurrence of errors in testing, some carriers of thalassemia are missed. On the other hand, couples identified at risk are offered very basic counseling by the laboratory technician or physician where the test was performed or by their referring physician. This type of genetic counseling seems insufficient because of the currently registered thalassemic patients at the CCC, 27.2% remain under the age of 10. The need for professional genetic counseling is evident.

Population screening

Screening patients' siblings is currently being conducted in order to identify those carrying the disease trait and thus make them or their parents aware of any future risk they might have in giving birth to a thalassemic child. Furthermore, a 'Thalassemia Youth Screening Project' was initiated in 2002 in schools, universities and other youth's clubs. This project was launched by a collaborative effort between the CCC and the Ministry of Social Affairs in Lebanon. Due to limited resources, the progress is unfortunately slow with no preliminary data available yet.

Genetic testing and prenatal diagnosis

β-Thalassemia mutations may be identified using the Amplification Refractory Mutation System (ARMS) PCR or direct gene sequencing. Haplotype analysis of a subset of the Lebanese population shows that the observed genetic diversity originates from both new mutational events and gene flow from population migration. Identification of both common and rare

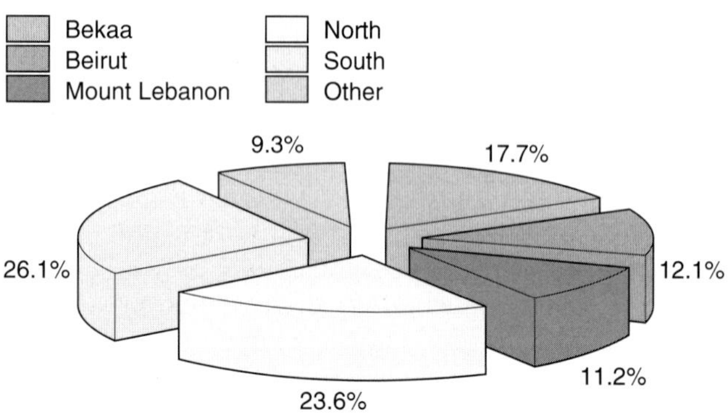

Figure 204.1 Geographic distribution of thalassemia patients.

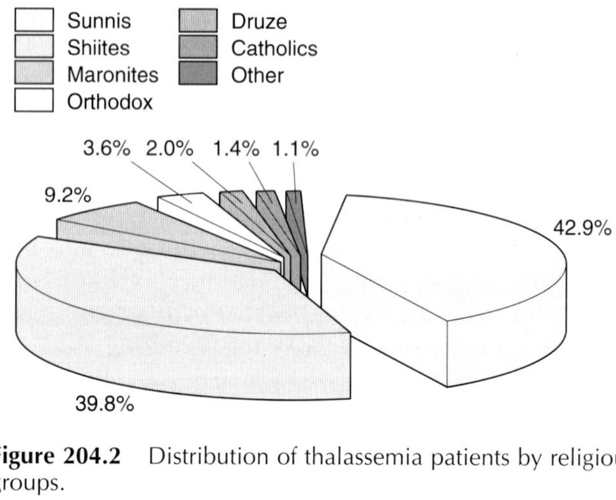

Figure 204.2 Distribution of thalassemia patients by religious groups.

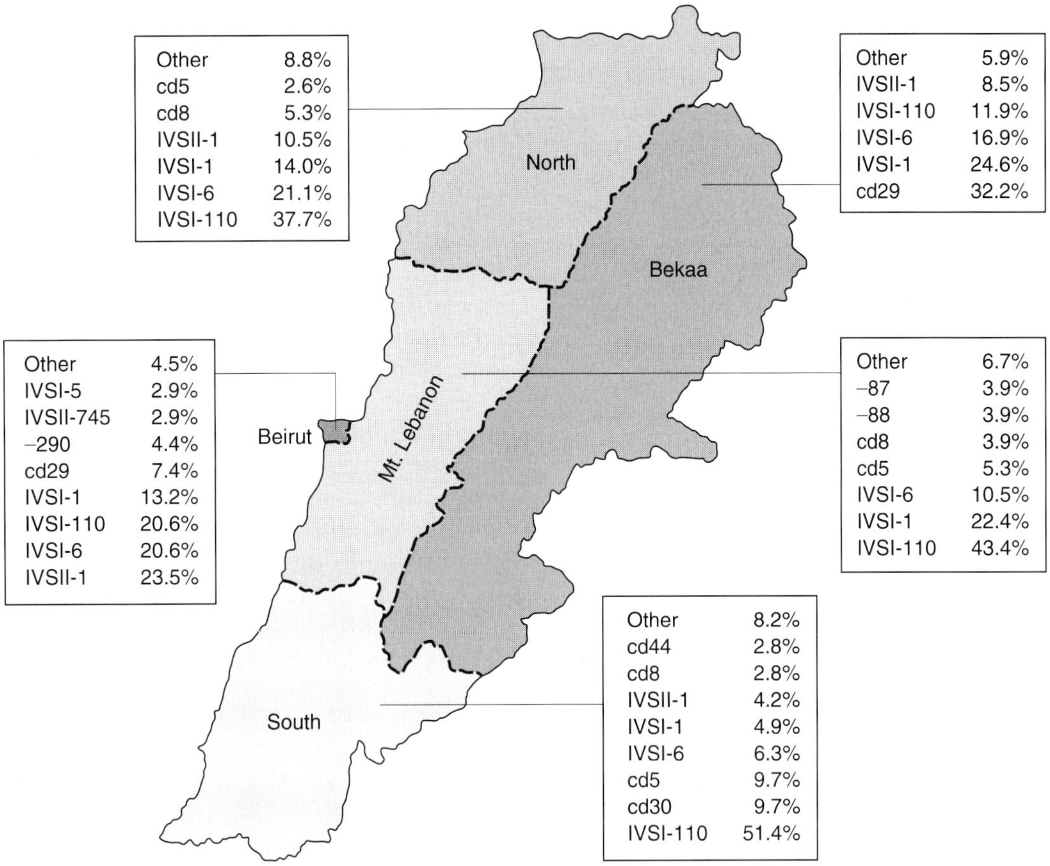

Figure 204.3 The relative frequencies and distribution of β-thalassemia mutations within five main geographic regions in Lebanon.

β-thalassemia mutations is essential for the implementation of screening and prenatal diagnosis programs.

In 1982, chorionic villous tissue was used for the first time to provide fetal DNA in order to diagnose fetal hemoglobinopathies. This procedure was not used in Lebanon for the detection of β-thalassemia until 1999 because of test costs, ignorance of the procedure, cultural and religious beliefs.[18] Furthermore, the required genetic testing procedure was exclusively performed abroad in Cyprus, the UK or the USA, which exacerbated the costs and made the actual testing more cumbersome and complicated. Local genetic prenatal diagnosis for thalassemia in Lebanon was started in 1999 at the Genetics Research Laboratory of the CCC. Diagnosis is based on mutation detection using ARMS PCR[19,20] and DNA sequencing on DNA from chorionic villi and in some cases fetal amniocytes. Most individuals (90%) who are referred for prenatal diagnosis in Lebanon already have an affected child or family member. Today, an increasing number of couples, suspected or confirmed to be β-thalassemia carriers, seek prenatal diagnosis, mostly encouraged by their obstetrician, family doctor or hematologist. The families are given limited genetic counseling at the CCC. Since most couples seeking prenatal diagnosis for thalassemia already have an affected child, they most often choose to terminate the pregnancy in the event of an affected fetus.

All these prevention strategies, though encouraging, seem insufficient. Recent data from the CCC shows that only 12% of thalassemia cases are being prevented each year! Several barriers need to be overcome in order to achieve a concrete success with existing and future prevention strategies.

Barriers: education

Education is the key ingredient to promoting awareness. Most families with thalassemia come from low socioeconomic backgrounds with limited schooling or university education. Many a times parents do not come to terms that their child is affected when there has never been any affected member of the family before. Furthermore, the mother is often blamed for the condition of her child. The notion that the genetic makeup of a child is determined by the genetic makeup of both the father and the mother is rarely accepted. To promote awareness and understanding of thalassemia as a genetic disease, parents of children afflicted with the disease are invited to attend seminars at the CCC given by nurses, doctors and/or members of thalassemic parents association. Educational material is distributed during these meetings and the language is simple and understandable to all.

Unfortunately, however, public awareness of the disease is limited. Some TV talk shows are presented each year on the International Thalassemia Day (May 8) but these remain insufficient since the focus is on patients, their families and how the disease is affecting them rather than on the different ways to prevent and treat thalassemia. Awareness campaigns at the national level involving the media, schools and universities are primordial.

Barriers: culture and religion

Sometimes, parents with an affected child, from both a legal and religious perspective, are found with no alternatives but to continue with the pregnancy. Despite these barriers, abortions are sometimes performed on affected fetuses.

Barriers: financial

The costs of amniocentesis and chorionic villous sampling procedures for genetic diagnosis as well the diagnostic laboratory testing itself are almost equivalent to the minimum monthly wage set by the government. These procedures and genetic tests are not covered by the National Social Security Foundation. Private health insurance companies still do not include genetic testing in their premium. In any public health policies, cost/benefit ratios need to be determined and funding provided if the problem is considered important.

Other barriers

Geographic and psychological factors also influence the success of prevention and awareness programs. Even though Lebanon is a small country, reaching remote villages and towns in order to promote knowledge on thalassemia and its prevention is very difficult. Residents of these villages are sometimes illiterate, they visit a doctor for emergencies only and may seek late or erratic prenatal care. Psychological fear from being labeled as 'outside the norms' is quite frequent and results in denial of the diagnosis or refusal to seek prenatal testing.

Steps toward improvement

In neighboring Cyprus, where the frequency of β-thalassemia carriers is highest (one in seven) among East Mediterranean countries, control programs have achieved close to 100% prevention of new thalassemia cases and specialized clinics and centers deliver the best treatment and management for affected individuals.[21] Successful screening programs were also implemented and encouraged by the Greek Orthodox Church who refused marriages unless the couple's carrier status for thalassemia was determined. Furthermore, although sanctioned by the church, abortion in Cyprus is legal for affected fetuses.[21,22]

In 1994, the WHO working group on hemoglobinopathies, in its publication 'Guidelines for the Control of Hemoglobin Disorders',[23] outlined the steps required for successful control programs implementation. In Lebanon, while management of thalassemia patients is optimized, the need for more extensive prevention programs is urgent. A collaborative effort between governmental, religious and legal sectors as well as healthcare institutions is necessary in order to create a national work task force for the prevention of hemoglobin disorders.

Obstetric and laboratory facilities are already available but not extensively exploited. Population screening programs and mutation detection are not very expensive when compared with the healthcare costs incurred during the treatment of thalassemia and thus they constitute the next step in the program. In addition, genetic counseling should be offered to families by trained genetic counselors and specialists who can properly explain the mode of inheritance, risk and treatment/diagnostic tools available to families. Of particular importance is the discussion, revision and resolution of important abortion laws, bioethical and religious issues.

The control program has to be carefully monitored by an expert program coordinator who would overlook the progress by continuous research. The establishment of a national birth registry, like in other Arab countries,[24] and a national reference center would allow the exact evaluation of the health and economic burden.[25]

Other genetic diseases

Congenital sensorineural hearing loss

Hearing loss in humans is not uncommon. In fact, one in 1000 children are hearing impaired and half of these cases appear to have a genetic cause.[2] The incidence of hearing loss in Lebanon is unknown, due to the lack of a national registry, but could be high because of the high rate of consanguineous marriages.

The congenital sensorineural hearing loss is a 'hearing impairment due to disorders of the cochlear division of the ninth cranial nerve (auditory nerve), the cochlea, or the retro cochlear nerve tracts'.[13] The major mode of inheritance is autosomal recessive.[26] As such, prelingual deafness is highly genetically heterogeneous.[26] Mutations in the Connexin 26 gene, producing a defunct gap junction protein, represent a major cause of the deafness.[26] In particular, the 30delG mutation is one of the most frequent mutations and was found to occur with a carrier frequency of 1/43 in one study of the Lebanese population, with no excess in any particular ethno-religious community.[2] This high prevalence is due to a 'hot spot' rather than from an ancestral mutation in the Lebanese population.[2,26]

In Lebanon and elsewhere, genetic counseling for patients with congenital sensorineural hearing loss and their families is limited because physicians are currently unable to distinguish between genetic non-syndromic and non-genetic deafness.[26] Based on recent findings of the prevalence of the Connexin 26 mutation, the possibility of developing a simple molecular test to distinguish between genetic and non-genetic deafness would greatly improve genetic counseling opportunities for affected families. Furthermore, early screening for the 30delG mutation would allow for the early detection of about one-third of non-syndromic autosomal recessive deafness cases in Lebanon.[2]

Cystic fibrosis

Cystic fibrosis is the most common lethal autosomal recessive disorder in Caucasians[27], yet its prevalence in Lebanon is unknown. It is an autosomal recessive congenital metabolic disorder characterized by chronic pulmonary disease, pancreatic exocrine insufficiency and increased sodium chloride composition of sweat.[13,28] Genetic allelic heterogeneity is associated with clinical heterogeneity.[28]

Cystic fibrosis results from a mutation in the gene encoding the cystic fibrosis transmembrane regulator (CFTR) involved in the transport of ions across the cell membrane.[28] It is imperative for the genetic counselor/genetic scientist to be aware of the relative frequency of the most common CFTR gene mutations among their respective patient population. Mutations of the CF gene are detected using ARMS PCR and Allele-Specific Oligonucleotide technology.[27] For at-risk families or consanguineous couples, linkage analysis based on the family's particular genetic markers may also be used to detect the mutation.[27,28] In addition, an amniocentesis may be performed for fetuses found to have a fetal meconium ileus with an unknown risk of CF.[28] To definitively diagnose a patient postnatally, a sweat and pancreatic sufficiency test is needed.[27]

Cystic fibrosis is thought to be rare among the Arab populations from the Middle East and little data have been reported so far. A recent study have been performed on several families living in Lebanon for several generations and who have at least one child with CF. The study found that there was a 50% rate of consanguineous marriage among these families, independent of the community of origin. Mutational analysis have been performed and a total of 10 different mutations accounting for 87.5% of 32 unrelated CF alleles were identified, including two novel putative mutations (E672del and IVS21-28G→A). Three mutations, delta F508 (37.5%), W1282X (15.6%), and N1303K (9.4%) accounted for 62.5% of CF alleles.

Treatment for CF requires long-term medical care, managing respiratory complications and replacing pancreatic enzymes. The disease is often fatal by the fourth decade.[28] Newborn CF screening in Lebanon could make a large difference in the quality of life of CF patients, allowing for early diagnosis or prophylactic treatment. Screening could prevent chronic malnutrition, allow for improved growth of patients, improved pulmonary function and reduce the number of hospital admissions.[29,30] In the future, genetic counseling could also allow parents to avoid having a second child with CF.[29]

Duchenne muscular dystrophy

Duchenne muscular dystrophy (DMD) is the most common childhood muscular dystrophy and is characterized by symmetrical weakness and muscle wasting.[13] It is an X-linked recessive disease with an incidence of 1/3000 male births in most parts of the world. It is caused by a mutation in the dystrophin gene resulting in grossly reduced or absent levels of dystrophin in muscles. Without dystrophin, muscle degeneration occurs. Fetuses with a positive family history for DMD may be tested using Southern Blotting or PCR analysis.[28]

Conclusion/future plans

In the future development of the field of genetics in Lebanon, it is imperative to develop an interconnected network of professionals consisting of genetic counselors, laboratory researchers, clinicians and nurses, in addition to establishing a comprehensive patient and family support system. In particular, fertility centers and clinical genetic scientists as well as neonatologists need to develop an interconnected perinatal network to provide more opportunities for couples with a positive family history for a genetic disease or who are themselves afflicted with a genetic disease. It is equally important to consider the development of graduate programs in the field of genetics and genetic counseling at universities within Lebanon and the Middle East.

Furthermore, the development of a national registry for genetic disorders is essential. In fact, in Lebanon, the National Collaborative Perinatal Neonatal Network is aiming at improving the lives of mothers and newborn infants. One of its goals is to establish a Lebanese National Birth Registry that would help in following the prevalence of certain diseases in the country and hopefully measure the success of future genetic counseling programs and PGD programs in Lebanon.

REFERENCES

1. Klat M, Khudr A. Religious endogamy and consanguinity in marriage patterns in Beirut, Lebanon. *Soc Biol* 1986;33:138–45.
2. Mustapha M, Salem N, Delague V, *et al.* Autosomal recessive non-syndromic hearing loss in the Lebanese population: prevalence of the 30delG mutation and report of two novel mutations in Connexin 26(GJB2) gene. *J Med Genet* 2001;38(10):E36.
3. Hamamy H, Alwan A. Hereditary disorders in the Eastern Mediterranean Region. *Bull World Health Organ* 1994;72:145–54.
4. Scarpelli E, Cosmi E. *Reviews in Perinatal Medicine*, Vol. 4. New York: Raven Press, 1981:192–214.
5. Bolognese R, Schwarz RH, Schneider J. *Perinatal Medicine: Management of the High Risk Fetus and Neonate.* Baltimore, MD: Williams and Wilkins, 1982:47–79.
6. Kersin-Storrar L. Genetic counseling and molecular testing. In Elles R, ed. *Molecular Diagnosis of Genetic Diseases.* Totowa, NJ: Humana Press, 1996:205–17.
7. Elles R. An overview of clinical molecular genetics. In Elles R, ed. *Molecular Diagnosis of Genetic Diseases.* Totowa, NJ: Humana Press, 1996:1–15.
8. Cockell A, Rodeck C. Prenatal diagnosis. In Harper J, Delhanty JDA, Handyside AH, eds. *Preimplantation Genetic Diagnosis.* Chichester, UK: John Wiley & Sons, Ltd, 2001:27–43.
9. Overton C, Serhal P, Davies M. Clinical aspects of preimplantation diagnosis. In Harper J, Delhanty JDA, Handyside AH, eds. *Preimplantation Genetic Diagnosis.* Chichester, UK: John Wiley & Sons, Ltd, 2001:123–40.
10. Ray P, Handyside AH. PCR from single cells for preimplantation diagnosis. In Elles R, ed. *Molecular Diagnosis of Genetic Diseases.* Totowa, NJ: Humana Press, 1996:245–58.
11. Harper J. Introduction. In Harper J, Delhanty JDA, Handyside AH, eds. *Preimplantation Genetic Diagnosis.* Chichester, UK: John Wiley & Sons, Ltd, 2001:3–12.
12. Viville S, Pergament D, Fiddler M. Ethical perspectives and regulation of preimplantation genetic diagnostic practice. In Harper J, Delhanty JDA, Handyside AH, eds. *Preimplantation Genetic Diagnosis.* Chichester, UK: John Wiley & Sons, Ltd, 2001:227–40.
13. Dirckx J. *Stedman's Concise Medical Dictionary for the Health Professions*, 4th edn. Baltimore, MD: Lippincott Williams & Wilkins, 2001.
14. Haldane JBS. The rate of mutations of human genes. *Hereditas* 1949;1049(Suppl 35):267–73.
15. Cabannes R, Taleb N, Ghorra F, Schmitt-Beurrier A. Studies of hemoglobin types in the population of Lebanon. *Nouv Rev Fr Hematol* 1969;5:851–6.
16. Rafie L, Rafie JJ (1984) *Thalassemia in Lebanon.* International Red Cross.
17. Taleb N, Loiselet J, Ghorra F, Sfeir A. Sur la deficience en glucose-6-phosphate dehydrogenase dans les populations autochtones du Liban. *Cr Acad Sci Paris* 1964;258:5749–51.
18. Zahed L, Bou-Dames J. Acceptance of first-trimester prenatal diagnosis for the haemoglobinopathies in Lebanon. *Prenat Diagn* 1997;17:423–8.
19. Newton CR, Graham A, Heptinstall LE, *et al.* Analysis of any point mutation in DNA. The amplification refractory mutation system (ARMS). *Nucleic Acids Res* 1989;17:2503–16.
20. Bravo M, Salazar R, Arends A, *et al.* Detection of beta thalassemia by the technique of refractory amplification of mutation systems (Arms-Pcr). *Invest Clin* 1999;40:203–13.
21. Angastiniotis M, Modell B. Global epidemiology of hemoglobin disorders. *Ann N Y Acad Sci* 1998;850:251–69.
22. Richards M. Families, kinship and genetics. In Marteau T, Richards M, eds. *The Troubled Helix: Social and Psychological Implications of the New Human Genetics.* Cambridge: Cambridge University Press, 1996:249–73.
23. WHO Working Group on Haemoglobinopathies. *Guidelines for the Control of Haemoglobin Disorders. VI Annual Meeting of the WHO Working Group on Haemoglobinopathies.* Sardinia: World Health Organization, 1994.
24. Rajab A, Patton MA. Major factors determining the frequencies of hemoglobinopathies in Oman. *Am J Med Genet* 1997;71: 240–2.
26. Denoyelle F, Weil D, Maw MA, *et al.* Prelingual deafness: high prevalence of a 30delG mutation in the Connexion 26 gene. *Hum Mol Genet* 1997;6:2173–7.
27. Schwarz M, Malone G. Methods for screening in cystic fibrosis. In Elles R, ed. *Molecular Diagnosis of Genetic Diseases.* Totowa, NJ: Humana Press, 1996:99–119.
28. Thompson M, McInnes R, Willard H. *Thompson & Thompson Genetics in Medicine*, 5th edn. Philadelphia: W.B. Saunders Company, 1991.
29. Young S, Kharrazi M, Pearly M, Cunnigham G. Cystic fibrosis screening in newborns: results from existing programs. *Curr Opin Pulm Med* 2001;7(6):427–33.
30. Grosse S, Gwinn M. Assisting states in assessing newborn screening options. *Public Health Rep* 2001;116(2):169–72.

205 Surgical management of postpartum hemorrhage: lessons learned

M. Seoud and A. Adra

Introduction

Postpartum hemorrhage (PPH) remains a leading cause of maternal morbidity and mortality in developing and developed countries. Maternal mortality varies from 1000 per 100,000 live births in countries like Mozambique to 11.8 per 100,000 live births in the USA.[1] PPH remains a leading cause of death accounting for around one-third of maternal deaths in USA and other developing countries.[1] The most frequent causes of death due to hemorrhage are abruptio placenta, uterine atony, uterine rupture and lacerations of the birth canal. The frequency of each of these causes varies depending on various risk factors including age, parity, place of delivery, presence and type of birth attendant, prior incidence of PPH, type of delivery, prior cesarean birth, as well as other maternal and fetal complications that are beyond the scope of discussion of this chapter.[2]

The definition of PPH is arbitrary. It is often defined as a blood loss of more than 500 cm^3 following a normal vaginal delivery and 1000 cm^3 following a cesarean delivery. In practical terms, however, it is very difficult to quantitate the amount of bleeding and it is left to the birth attendant to subjectively assess the amount of blood loss that is frequently underestimated. Blood loss estimate at cesarean section is even more difficult to assess since one cannot visualize the amount of blood loss until is has spilled over the table and onto the floor. Objectively, the American College of Obstetricians and Gynecologists (ACOG) defines PPH as a drop in hematocrit of more than 10% or a need for blood transfusion.[3]

The predictable increase in the red cell mass of 33% and blood volume of around 45% and the compensatory venous adaptation in pregnancy allows the pregnant women to tolerate moderate amount of blood loss with no significant hemodynamic compromise. However, with excessive blood loss, compensatory mechanisms fail and hypovolemic shock sets in resulting in hypoperfusion and its consequences on vital organs especially the kidneys. The birth attendant should be aware of the hemodynamics of the patient while trying to control PPH. He should call for the appropriate expert help to assist him both in the surgical and supportive management of the patient.

Practical approach to the initial evaluation and management of PPH

The management of PPH starts with steps taken before, during and after its occurrence. It is important to identify high-risk factors which increase the risk of a pregnant patient to develop PPH. This will ensure the right set up and support team to be available at delivery. In some situations, it may involve the early transfer of the patient to a better-equipped center. The presence of skilled and experienced obstetricians, anesthesiologists, intensive care unit, and blood bank are all necessary to ensure a good outcome.

It is beyond the scope of this chapter to discuss high-risk factors and their identification. It is also beyond our scope to discuss various medical and non-surgical means of management of PPH.

When all medical and supportive measures fail to control PPH, the obstetrician must intervene surgically to identify and control the source of bleeding. During surgery, the obstetrician must continue to assess the hemodynamic status of the patient and try to avoid hypovolemic shock with its deleterious effects on organ perfusion. In general, the patient should have two large-bore intravenous (i.v.) accesses. Dilute Pitocin should be infused continuously. A Foley catheter should be in place and continuous monitoring of urine output performed. An adequate urine output of more than 25–30 cm^3 per hour usually indicates an appropriate renal perfusion and avoids postpartum acute tubular necrosis. Although difficult, an estimate of the amount of blood loss should be promptly made in order to prepare the appropriate amount and type of blood products. Crystalloids are preferred solutions, however, in cases of sudden and excessive blood loss and while waiting for blood to be transfused, plasma expanders may be used with supervision of accurate input and output to avoid cardiac overload and pulmonary edema.

The most difficult decision to make is usually when to start packed red blood cells (RBCs) and blood component replacement. At the present time, blood is the best volume expander and ensures the best oxygenation and blood pressure support. Yet it has several potential disadvantages ranging from unavailability especially in unpredictable situations, possible untoward reactions, and blood born infections. Nonetheless, with massive hemorrhage, blood replacement is life-saving and should be available. Moreover, the use of clotting factors, especially fresh frozen plasma (FFP), is usually needed in cases of massive blood loss. A quick assessment of the bed-side-clotting time (wall clot) may indicate the need for FFP. However, the exact timing of the use of the FFP is often not clear and is arbitrary. The preparation of packed RBCs and FFP may take up to 30–60 min depending on their availability and the closeness of the blood bank. It is important for the obstetrician to anticipate the need for blood component replacement ahead of time and to ask for its preparation. The presence of a skilled anesthesiologist, familiar with the hemodynamics of pregnancy, may relieve the pressure on the obstetrician who subsequently can concentrate on the surgical management of PPH. Most of the time, placement of central monitoring (central venous line, arterial line, and pulmonary capillary pressure catheter) is left to the anesthesiologist, the maternal fetal medicine specialist, or intensive care specialist.

When medical management fails and surgery is contemplated, it is important for the obstetrician to formulate a differential diagnosis and proceed accordingly. Conditions requiring surgical intervention include: lacerations of maternal soft tissues, uterine atony, placental conditions (retained placenta, placenta accreta), uterine rupture, and uterine inversion.

Differential diagnosis and management of PPH

Faced with PPH, the birth attendant should immediately ask for additional help. This should include a senior experienced obstetrician, a skilled anesthesiologist and a high-risk nursing staff. An additional i.v. access should be inserted and continuous vital signs monitoring initiated including blood pressure, pulse, oxygen saturation, and urine output. The patient should be carefully inspected including assessment of the birth canal for lacerations, uterine tone for atony and the abdomen for blood collection.

Cervico-vaginal lacerations

With appropriate anesthesia (general is preferred to regional to avoid worsening of the hypotension), the birth canal should be carefully and gently inspected. Various risk factors may guide toward certain potential sites of bleeding. A vaginal birth after cesarean may necessitate a careful inspection of the prior uterine incision. A difficult vaginal delivery especially if associated with an operative delivery (vacuum or forceps) or if complicated by a macrosomic newborn or shoulder dystocia may result in a cervical or vaginal laceration. Inspection should start with the episiotomy especially the apex, even if it involves reopening the episiotomy. A rectal examination may also reveal the presence of a hematoma which should be evacuated, the bleeder identified if possible and ligated and, if one cannot be seen, a drain should be left in the episiotomy bed. The cervix should be examined and sutured if bleeding lacerations are noted, securing the base of the laceration. In referred cases of vaginal laceration, especially if previously inspected and manipulated, the vagina is often very edematous, eroded and individual bleeders are often difficult to identify. In these cases, careful packing of the vagina may be necessary. If bleeding from vaginal laceration continues despite these efforts, then one may resort to selective artery embolization as noted in the next section. Recently however, Hebisch and Huch described a method of vaginal uterine artery ligation which in their experience avoided other procedures.[4] If no cervico-vaginal lacerations are found, then one has to concentrate on the uterus as a source of bleeding. Sterile manual digital exploration of the uterine cavity is mandatory in order to identify uterine laceration, dehiscence/rupture of prior scar, or retained placental tissues. In case of dehiscence of a uterine scar or uterine laceration associated with brisk vaginal bleeding, an emergency exploratory laparotomy is usually needed as detailed in the following section.

If a vaginal pack is left in place for few hours, the patient should be frequently assessed for collection of blood behind the pack. A Foley catheter is left to asses the urine output and may be removed following removal of the pack if the patient vital signs are stable. Management of lacerations of the uterus and or uterine artery will be discussed later.

Placental conditions

Case 1

Mrs A.S. was undergoing a quaternary cesarean section at a small community hospital. Following the delivery of the newborn, the placenta was noted to be complete previa and attempt at its separation resulted in the avulsion of the lower uterine segment. This left a large crater with subsequent massive bleeding. Following a short attempt to control bleeding, the defect was packed and the abdomen closed. The patient was transferred immediately to our hospital and directly to the operating room (OR). In the OR, following dissection of the bladder from the remaining lower uterine segment, exposing the broad ligament, and identifying the uterine arteries and the ureters, an abdominal hysterectomy was performed. The patient was transfused with packed RBCs. The bleeding continued despite the hysterectomy and the whole surgical bed was oozing, with no specific major bleeder. Following careful revision of all pedicles, bilateral hypogastric artery ligation was performed with significant decrease in the bleeding. A drain was left in place and the abdomen closed. Post-op, the patient initially did well. However, 12 h later, she became hypotensive with progressive decrease in the hematocrit. Computerized tomographic scan of abdomen and pelvis revealed a pelvic hematoma. Uterine artery embolization was arranged, however the vital signs stabilized and the hematocrit as well. The patient was transfused with a total of 30 units of blood and FFP. She was discharged on the fifth post-op day, and remains well 1 year after the surgery.

Most cases of retained placenta can be managed conservatively. One can usually wait for the placenta to separate spontaneously. In the presence of heavy bleeding manual separation and removal are needed. Piece-meal removal of the placenta should be followed by curetting of the cavity. Inspection of the placenta may identify one or more missing cotyledons. In rare cases, careful uterine inspection may identify the presence of a succenturiate placental lobe. Inspection of the cavity with a large oval forceps and/or a gauze wrapped around the fingers, may be needed to remove large placental tissue followed by gentle curetting of the cavity with a blunt curette to avoid uterine synechiae in the future. In the majority of patients, this is enough to control the bleeding. In rare cases, it may reveal the presence of an adherent placenta or accreta.

The incidence of placenta accreta has increased 10 times in the last 50 years reaching an incidence of 1/2500 deliveries.[5] This increase is attributed to the increase in the cesarean section rate. Women who have two or more cesarean sections have a 40% risk of developing placenta accreta.[5,6] The use of ultrasonography, color Doppler and magnetic resonance imaging have improved our ability to diagnose abnormal placentation antenatally.[7] The ACOG advocates in cases where the diagnosis is strongly suspected to be prepared by properly counseling the patient, preparing blood products, timing and properly locating the delivery with the obstetric anesthesiologist on alert.[5] When attempts fail to control vaginal bleeding from a retained placenta the obstetrician usually resorts to a laparotomy to control the bleeding. Recently however, some have recommended the use of selective uterine artery embolization to control bleeding from a placenta accreta.[8,9] Others have left the placenta in place after ligating and cutting the umbilical cord, followed by the use of methotrexate. Others have combined this with the use of internal iliac balloon catheterization with limited success.[10] When a small segment of placenta is firmly adherent to the endometrium, segmental resection of the piece with the underlying myometrium can be attempted.[11] In case of profuse bleeding from a low lying or placenta previa/accreta, we and others have successfully sutured the lower uterine segment *en masse* or segmentaly.[11,12] When all conservative measures fail, a hysterectomy should be performed.

Uterine atony

Case 2

Mrs M.A. was a 28-year-old primigravida who failed tocolysis at 31 weeks and was undergoing a primary cesarean delivery for breech presentation. Following the delivery, the uterus was atonic with continued bleeding. All conservative measures, including ligation of the uterine and utero-ovarian ligaments, and hemostatic sutures failed. Bilateral hypogastric artery ligation also failed. News of the newborn not faring well only prolonged the attempt at preserving the uterus. Finally, an abdominal hysterectomy was performed. However, continuous oozing from the surgical bed was noted. In the end, multiple surgical pads were tied together, left in place and extruded through the vagina and slowly removed over the next 48 h. She was transfused with a total of 60 units of packed RBCs, FFPs, and platelets. She survived with bilateral moderate atrophy of her gluteal muscles.

Postpartum uterine atony is the most common cause of PPH. The birth attendant should be aware of the various risk factors in order to anticipate the occurrence of uterine atony. Various preventive measures have been found to be effective in significantly reducing the incidence and magnitude of PPH from atony. These include the prophylactic use of various uterotonic agents, in addition to the routine practice of manual uterine massage with gentle cord traction to assist in spontaneous placental separation.

When the medical management of uterine atony fails and the uterus remains hypotonic and continuously bleeding, one can resort to uterine packing while preparing the patient for the operating room. Traditionally, this involves packing the uterus with a long sterile pack while applying continuous pressure on the uterine fundus. Prior to surgical exploration the pack can be gently removed and the bleeding and uterine tone observed. In case the bleeding recurs, a ring forceps is placed on the anterior and posterior lips of the cervix to help identifying the cervix if an abdominal hysterectomy is later needed. This is especially useful when the patient is fully dilated and the cervico-vaginal junction cannot be easily palpated abdominally. Others have tried various devices to tamponade the uterus, such as using a 30–50 ml intrauterine Foley catheter balloon or a 75 ml ovoid fluted Foley catheter which will allow the drainage of blood as well as tamponading the uterus.[13]

If uterine atony is encountered during a cesarean section, uterine massage with a warm pack may be helpful. Compressing the anterior and posterior abdominal wall is important to decrease the amount of bleeding while preparing prostaglandin medications such as intra-myometrial 15-methyl-$F_{2\alpha}$.[14] Success of this preliminary maneuver may be also useful in identifying those patients who will benefit from placement of hemostatic sutures in the uterine wall. Various techniques have been tried in placing these compressing sutures, however, the most popular being the B-lynch using a 36 inch 0-vicryl through the uterine wall in the lower uterine segment, over the uterine fundus and across to the other side[14–16] Some authors have reported serious complications from such procedures such as the development of pyometra.[17]

If all these methods fail, one may resort to the ligation of the various blood supply to the uterus including the uterine vessels, the utero-ovarian vessels, and the internal iliac vessels. In cases of uterine atony, however, these may not be as useful as in cases of uterine laceration or accreta, and they are more difficult to perform by a general obstetrician (especially ligation of the internal iliac arteries). These may also take precious time that is best spent on proceeding with a hysterectomy. In our part of the world, we have witnessed on numerous occasions significant morbidity and mortality when time is wasted while attempting to safeguard the uterus especially if the patient is young, nulliparous, of low parity, and/or the newborn is not in a viable condition.

Uterine lacerations

Case 3

Mrs I.S. is a 31-year-old G3 P2 woman at 38 weeks who was undergoing a trial of labor following a vaginal delivery and a cesarean section for a non-reassuring fetal heart. The patient was expecting her third female newborn. She progressed smoothly to full dilatation and pushed for 2 h with arrest of dilatation. During the repeat cesarean section, and following the extraction, a lateral downward extension of the uterine scar was noted. Massive bleeding ensued. Careful dissection of the bladder off the cervix revealed a laceration of the descending branch of the uterine artery. The ureter on that site was carefully dissected and the uterine branch ligated effectively controlling the bleeding. The family was adamantly opposing a hysterectomy citing the need for a future male progeny. The patient subsequently had two more female children by repeat cesarean sections and still wants to continue conceiving.

Uterine laceration may be encountered during a vaginal delivery, such as during a trial of labor for a patient with a prior uterine scar, during operative vaginal delivery (much less these days), during an intrauterine rotation (much less common), or with extension of a cesarean incision.

Lacerations following a trial of labor with a prior cesarean section or during a primary or repeat cesarean section most often result from the extension of the incision toward the uterine vessels, at times leading to massive hemorrhage. Occasionally, the extension is toward the cervix and or vagina, where the bleeding is more difficult to see. The blood flow of the uterine artery at term may reach 500 cm^3/min, hence the urgency in rapidly controlling the bleeding. If the uterus has been exteriorized outside the abdomen, the vessels may retract and constrict, and hence be more difficult to identify. Replacing the uterus in the abdomen may reveal the source of bleeding. In controlling the bleeding from such extension, one should be aware of the path of the ureter and the position of the bladder, especially in patients with a prior cesarean section when the cervix is fully dilated and/or the bladder is adherent to the lower segment. In all cases, the bladder should be identified and sharply dissected as low as possible from the lower uterine segment. The broad ligament on the side of the laceration should be opened, and the ureter identified on its medial leaf. If suturing the edge of the uterus at the site of laceration does not control the bleeding, then one should ligate the uterine vessels at the site of the laceration. This suture, as originally described by O' Leary, is performed using number 1 or 0-vicryl suture placed above and below the laceration perpendicular to the uterine artery and in the uterine wall thus ligating the ascending branch of the uterine vessels.[18] In addition, occlusion of the utero-ovarian ligament on that side by a vascular clamp may further decrease the amount of bleeding. If bleeding decreases, the utero-ovarian vessels may be permanently ligated.

In cases where the bleeding results from more extensive lacerations in the lower uterine segment, such as in placenta previa/accreta, especially in repeat cesarean section, when the lower uterine segment cannot be identified, some advocate ligation of the hypogastric vessels. It is a rather easy procedure, but with which many obstetricians are not familiar. If not familiar with it, this is not the time to learn it and one should not waste precious time trying to perform it. If expertise is available, the dissection should start with opening the broad ligament at the level of the round ligament. The external iliac artery is easy to identify. The index finger is placed over it and used to dissect the tissues cephalad toward the bifurcation of common iliac arteries. The ureter passes over them and is followed caudally to identify the internal iliac vessels. The vessel is ligated using 2-0 silk sutures by passing a right-angle clamp starting laterally toward the midline below the artery and beyond the posterior division to avoid ligation of the superior gluteal artery. Occlusion of both hypogastric vessels may be needed to drop the pulse pressure enough to decrease the bleeding. The presence of extensive pelvic anastomosis is a mixed blessing. While it makes the uterus the best incubator for the fetus and makes it hard to control PPH, it also helps the uterus survive ligation of many of its blood supply with subsequent successful pregnancies.[7] Recently, however, identification and embolization of pelvic bleeders have been performed radiologically under fluoroscopy. In patients who are relatively more stable, this procedure in expert hands has helped avoid many surgeries.

When all measures fail to control PPH, hysterectomy is then indicated. Often, however, precious time is lost trying to preserve the uterus for future fertility. It is important to proceed with the hysterectomy before the onset of disseminated intravascular coagulopathy when all measures may fail to control the bleeding. It is the precise timing of the hysterectomy that helps avoiding many of the long-term complications. Hysterectomy on a pregnant uterus with a nondilated cervix is relatively simple and quick. When the cervix is fully dilated, it becomes more difficult to identify the cervico-vaginal junction. Placing ring forceps on the anterior and posterior cervical lips will make it easier. However, if the cervix is difficult to identify, one should not waste time looking for it, but rather proceed with a supracervical hysterectomy, unless the bleeding is from the cervix or upper vagina. In many cases, oozing is noted from the surgical bed. If it is minimal, and the patient is not hypotensive, one can leave a drain, exteriorize it from the vagina, and close the peritoneum over it.

In cases of a complete previa/accreta, especially after repeat cesarean sections, a large defect may be left in the lower uterine segment and pelvis. Bleeding in these cases may neither be controlled with ligation of the hypogastric arteries nor following hysterectomy. One should avoid the non-discriminate use of clamping as well the placement of blind sutures. This will not control bleeding and may injure vital organs such as ureters and veins. Applying pressure with pads exteriorized through the vagina or placed in a nylon bag and placed in the pelvis, exteriorized through vagina and placed under tension by attaching it to 1 l of an i.v. bag over the edge of the bed, may be life-saving. One may go back 24–48 h later to remove the pack, or slowly remove them from the vagina, when the patient is stable, and blood products made available.[19,20] The use of hemostatic powder over the area prior to the application of pressure may also be useful.

Selective embolization of the uterine artery

When medical management of PPH fails, and if the patient is clinically stable, selective embolization of the uterine artery, in the proper hands, may be attempted. It is becoming an increasingly popular alternative to hysterectomy or myomectomy for uterine fibroids.[21] It was originally used successfully to control intractable PPH.[22] A recent review indicated a high success rate (91%) when properly used by expert interventional radiologists.[23] Nevertheless, numerous complications have been reported, including uterine necrosis, labial necrosis, ovarian artery necrosis, and other serious complications.[24]

Conclusions

(1) The management of PPH starts with steps taken before (recognizing high-risk factors), during and after its occurrence.
(2) The obstetrician must continue to assess the hemodynamic status of the patient and try to avoid hypovolemic shock with its deleterious effects on organ perfusion.
(3) Faced with PPH, the birth attendant should immediately ask for additional help.
(4) In referred cases of vaginal laceration, because the vaginal mucosa is often very edematous, eroded and individual bleeders are often difficult to identify, careful packing of the vagina may be necessary.
(5) Most cases of retained placenta can be managed conservatively.
(6) Postpartum uterine atony is the most common cause of PPH. Various preventive measures including the use of pharmacologic agents have been found to be effective in significantly reducing the incidence and magnitude of PPH from atony.
(7) If hemorrhage secondary to uterine atony fails to respond to conventional methods and available pharmacologic agents, the obstetrician should proceed with surgical management starting with ligation of the uterine and ovarian arteries.
(8) When vascular ligation fails to control the bleeding, it is important to proceed with hysterectomy before the onset of disseminated intravascular coagulopathy. It is the precise timing of the hysterectomy that helps avoiding many of the long-term morbidity.
(9) Proceed with a supracervical hysterectomy to shorten operative time and reduce blood loss, unless the bleeding is from the cervix or upper vagina.
(10) Selective uterine artery embolization should be considered in women of low parity with persistent hemorrhage and stable vital signs, where preservation of the uterus is contemplated for future fertility.

REFERENCES

1. Benagiano G, Thomas B. Averting maternal death and disability. Saving mothers' lives: The FIGO Save the Mothers Initiative. *Internat J Obstet Gynecol* 2003;80:198–203.
2. Chikhakli L, Atrash H, Mackay A, Musani A, Berg C. Pregnancy-related mortality in the USA due to hemorrhage: 1979–1992. *Obstet Gynecol* 1999;94:721–5.
3. The American College of Obstetricians and Gynecologists. *Quality Assurance in Obstetrics and Gynecology*. Washington, DC: The American College of Obstetricians and Gynecologists, 1989.
4. Hebisch G, Huch A. Vaginal uterine artery ligation avoids high blood loss and puerperal hysterectomy in postpartum hemorrhage. *Obstet Gynecol* 2002;100:574–8.
5. American College of Obstetricians and Gynecologists. Placenta accreta. ACOG Committee Opinion No. 266. *Obstet Gynecol* 2002;99:169–70.
6. Gillima M, Rosenberg D, Davis D. The likelihood of placenta previa with greater number of cesarean deliveries and higher parity. *Obstet Gynecol* 2002;99:976–80.
7. American College of Obstetricians and Gynecologists. Uterine artery embolization. ACOG Committee Opinion No. 293. *Obstet Gynecol* 2004;103:403–4.
8. Tourne G, Collet F, Seffert P, Veyert C. Place of embolization of the uterine arteries in the management of post-partum hemorrhage: A study of 12 cases. *Eur J Obstet Gynecol Reprod Med* 2003;110: 29–34.
9. Butt K, Gagnon A, Delisle M-F. Failure of methotrexate and internal iliac balloon catheterization to manage placenta percreta. *Obstet Gynecol* 2002;99:981–2.
7. Kirkinen P, Helin-Martikainen HL, Vanninen, Partanen K. Placental accrete: Imaging by gray-scale and contrast enhanced color Doppler sonography and magnetic resonance imaging. *J Clin Ultrasound* 1998;26:90–4.
8. Cho JY, Kim SJ, Cha KY, Kay CW, Kim MI, Cha KS. Interrupted circular suture: Bleeding control during cesarean section delivery in placenta accreta. *Obstet Gynecol* 1991;78:876–9.
9. Abu-Musa A, Seoud M, Suidan F. A new technique for control of placental site bleeding. *Int J Obstet Gynecol* 1998;60:169–70.
10. Marcoviv I, Scoccia B. Postpartum hemorrhage and intrauterine balloon tamponade. A report of three cases. *J Reprod Med* 1999;44:122–6.
11. B-Lynch C, Coker A, Lawal AH, Abu J, Cowen MJ. The B-Lynch surgical technique for the control of massive postpartum hemorrhage: An alternative to hysterectomy? Five cases reported. *Br J Obstet Gynecol* 1997;104:372–5.
12. Ferguson JE II, Bourgeois FJ, Underwood PB. B-Lynch suture for postpartum hemorrhage. *Obstet Gynecol* 2000;95:1020–2.
13. Hayman RG, Arulkumaran S, Steer PJ. Uterine compressing sutures: Surgical management of postpartum hemorrhage. *Obstet Gynecol* 2002;99:502–6.
14. Ochoa M, Allaire AD, Stitely M. Pyometra after hemostatic square suture technique. *Obstet Gynecol* 2002;99:506–9.
15. O'Leary JL, O'Leary JA. Uterine artery ligation in control of intractable postpartum hemorrhage. *Am J Obstet Gynecol* 1966; 94:920–3.
16. Mengert WE, Burchell RC, Blumstein R, Daskal J. Pregnancy after bilateral ligation of the internal iliac and ovarian vessels. *Obstet Gynecol* 1969;34:664–6.
17. Hallack M, Dildy G, Hurley T, Moise K. Transvaginal pressure pack for life-threatening pelvic hemorrhage secondary to placenta accrete. *Obstet Gynecol* 1991;78:938–40.
18. Farag GEE, Susmita R, Ferguson A. Surgical packing as a means of controlling massive hemorrhage in association with advanced abdominal pregnancy. *Eur J Obstet Gynecol Reprod Biol* 2003; 109:106–7.
19. Heaston DK, Mineau DE, Brown BJ, Miller FJ Jr. Transcatheter arterial embolization for control of persistent massive puepural hemorrhage after bilateral hypogastric artery ligation. *AJR Am J Roentgenol* 1979;133:152–4.
20. Tourne G, Collet F, Seffert P, Veyret C. Place of embolization of the uterine arteries in the management of post-partum hemorrhage. *Eur J Obstet Gynecol Reprod Biol* 2003;110:29–34.
21. Cottier JP, Fignon A, Tranquart F, Herbreteau D. Uterine necrosis after arterial embolization for postpartum hemorrhage. *Obstet Gynecol* 2002;100:1074–7.
22. Yeagky TJ, Goldberg J, Klein TA, Bonn JB. Labial necrosis after uterine artery embolization for leimyomata. *Obstet Gynecol* 2002;100:881–2.
23. Payne JF, Staney JR, Haney AF. Embolic microspheres within ovarian arterial vasculature after uterine artery embolization. *Obstet Gynecol* 2002;100:883–6.
24. Spies JB, Spector A, Roth AR, Baker CM, Mauro L, Murphy-Skrynarz K. Complications after uterine artery embolization for leiomyomas. *Obstet Gynecol* 2002;100:873–80.

Index

Note – This is a comprehensive index for both Volume 1 and Volume 2